Access the BNF *your* way

The *British National Formulary* (*BNF*) and *BNF for Children* are updated monthly online via MedicinesComplete, ensuring healthcare professionals always have the latest prescribing advice.

ONLINE

 MedicinesComplete

BNF on MedicinesComplete
Access *BNF* and *BNF for Children* on MedicinesComplete and receive the very latest drug information through monthly online updates.

 FormularyComplete

FormularyComplete Create, edit and manage your own local formulary content built upon the trusted prescribing advice of the *BNF* and *BNF for Children*.

BNF on Evidence Search
Search the *BNF* and *BNF for Children* alongside other authoritative clinical and non-clinical evidence and best practice at www.evidence.nhs.uk from NICE.

PRINT

Eligible health professionals will now receive one print copy a year – the September issue – to supplement online access. If you are entitled to an NHS copy please refer to page ii for full details on distribution, call 01268 495 609 or email BNF@wilmingtonhealthcare.com.

Turn the page for more details...

BNF
76

September 2018
– March 2019

BMA

ROYAL
PHARMACEUTICAL
SOCIETY

Published jointly by
BMJ Group
Tavistock Square, London, WC1H 9JP, UK

and

Pharmaceutical Press
Pharmaceutical Press is the publishing division of the Royal
Pharmaceutical Society.
66-68 East Smithfield, London E1W 1AW, UK

Copyright © BMJ Group and the Royal Pharmaceutical
Society of Great Britain 2018.

ISBN: 978 0 85711 338 2

ISBN: 978 0 85711 340 5 (NHS Edition)

ISBN: 978 0 85711 339 9 (ePDF)

Printed by GGP Media GmbH, Pößneck, Germany

Typeset by Data Standards Ltd, UK

Text design by Peter Burgess

A catalogue record for this book is available from the British
Library.

Requesting copies of BNF publications

Paper copies may be obtained through any bookseller or
direct from:

Pharmaceutical Press
c/o Macmillan Distribution (MDL)
Hampshire International Business Park
Lime Tree Way
Basingstoke
Hampshire
RG24 8YJ
Tel: +44 (0) 1256 302 699
Fax: +44 (0) 1256 812 521
direct@macmillan.co.uk
or via our website www.pharmpress.com

For all bulk orders of more than 20 copies:
Tel: +44 (0) 207 572 2266
pharmpress-support@rpharms.com

The BNF is available as a mobile app, online (bnf.nice.org.uk/)
and also through MedicinesComplete; a PDA version is also
available. In addition, BNF content can be integrated into a
local formulary by using BNF on FormularyComplete; see
www.bnf.org for details.

Distribution of printed BNFs

In **England**, NICE purchases print editions of the BNF
(September editions only) for distribution within the
NHS. For details of who is eligible to receive a copy and
further contact details, please refer to the NICE website:
www.nice.org.uk/about/what-we-do/evidence-services/british-
national-formulary. If you are entitled to a shared copy of the
BNF, please call (0)1268 495 609 or email:
BNF@wilmingtonhealthcare.com.

In **Scotland**, email:
nss.psd-bnf@nhs.net

In **Wales**, contact NHS Wales Shared Services Partnership—
Contractor Services:
Tel: 01792 607420

In **Northern Ireland**, email:
ni.bnf@hscni.net

About BNF content

The BNF is designed as a digest for rapid reference and it
may not always include all the information necessary for
prescribing and dispensing. Also, less detail is given on areas
such as obstetrics, malignant disease, and anaesthesia since
it is expected that those undertaking treatment will have
specialist knowledge and access to specialist literature. *BNF
for Children* should be consulted for detailed information on
the use of medicines in children. The BNF should be
interpreted in the light of professional knowledge and
supplemented as necessary by specialised publications and
by reference to the product literature. Information is also
available from Medicines Information Services.

Please refer to digital versions of BNF for the most up-to-
date content. BNF is published in print but interim updates
are issued and published in the digital versions of BNF. The
publishers work to ensure that the information is as accurate
and up-to-date as possible at the date of publication, but
knowledge and best practice in this field change regularly.
BNF's accuracy and currency cannot be guaranteed and
neither the publishers nor the authors accept any
responsibility for errors or omissions. While considerable
efforts have been made to check the material in this
publication, it should be treated as a guide only. Prescribers,
pharmacists and other healthcare professionals are advised
to check www.bnf.org for information about key updates and
corrections.

Pharmaid

Numerous requests have been received from
developing countries for BNFs. The Pharmaid scheme
of the Commonwealth Pharmacists Association
will dispatch old BNFs to certain Commonwealth
countries. For more information on this scheme see
commonwealthpharmacy.org/what-we-do/pharmaid/. If you
would like to donate your copy email:
admin@commonwealthpharmacy.org

Preface

The BNF is a joint publication of the British Medical Association and the Royal Pharmaceutical Society. It is published under the authority of a Joint Formulary Committee which comprises representatives of the two professional bodies, the UK Health Departments, the Medicines and Healthcare products Regulatory Agency, and a national guideline producer. The Dental Advisory Group oversees the preparation of advice on the drug management of dental and oral conditions; the Group includes representatives of the British Dental Association and a representative from the UK Health Departments. The Nurse Prescribers' Advisory Group advises on the content relevant to nurses and includes representatives from different parts of the nursing community and from the UK Health Departments.

The BNF aims to provide prescribers, pharmacists, and other healthcare professionals with sound up-to-date information about the use of medicines.

The BNF includes key information on the selection, prescribing, dispensing and administration of medicines. Medicines generally prescribed in the UK are covered and those considered less suitable for prescribing are clearly identified. Little or no information is included on medicines promoted for purchase by the public.

Information on drugs is drawn from the manufacturers' product literature, medical and pharmaceutical literature, UK health departments, regulatory authorities, and professional bodies. Advice is constructed from clinical literature and reflects, as far as possible, an evaluation of the evidence from diverse sources. The BNF also takes account of authoritative national guidelines and emerging safety concerns. In addition, the editorial team receives advice on all therapeutic areas from expert clinicians; this ensures that the BNF's recommendations are relevant to practice.

The BNF is designed as a digest for rapid reference and it may not always include all the information necessary for prescribing and dispensing. Also, less detail is given on areas such as obstetrics, malignant disease, and anaesthesia since it is expected that those undertaking treatment will have specialist knowledge and access to specialist literature. Similarly, little or no information is included on medicines for very rare conditions. *BNF for Children* should be consulted for detailed information on the use of medicines in children. The BNF should be interpreted in the light of professional knowledge and supplemented as necessary by specialised publications and by reference to the product literature. Information is also available from medicines information services, see Medicines Information Services (see inside front cover).

It is **important** to use the most recent BNF information for making clinical decisions. The print edition of the BNF is updated in March and September each year. Monthly updates are provided online via Medicines Complete and the NHS Evidence portal. The more important changes are listed under Changes; changes listed online are cumulative (from one print edition to the next), and can be printed off each month to show the main changes since the last print edition as an aide memoire for those using print copies.

The BNF Publications website (www.bnf.org) includes additional information of relevance to healthcare professionals. Other digital formats of the BNF—including versions for mobile devices and integration into local formularies—are also available.

BNF Publications welcomes comments from healthcare professionals. Comments and constructive criticism should be sent to:

British National Formulary,
Royal Pharmaceutical Society,
66–68 East Smithfield
London
E1W 1AW
editor@bnf.org

The contact email for manufacturers or pharmaceutical companies wishing to contact BNF Publications is manufacturerinfo@bnf.org

Contents

Acknowledgements

The Joint Formulary Committee is grateful to individuals and organisations that have provided advice and information to the BNF.

The principal contributors for this update were:

K.W. Ah-See, M.N. Badminton, A.K. Bahl, P.R.J. Barnes, D. Bilton, S.L. Bloom, M.F. Bultitude, I.F. Burgess, D.J. Burn, C.E. Dearden, D.W. Denning, P.N. Durrington, D.A.C. Elliman, P. Emery, M.D. Feher, A. Freyer, B.G. Gazzard, A.M. Geretti, N.J.L. Gittoes, P.J. Goadsby, M. Gupta, T.L. Hawkins, B.G. Higgins, S.P. Higgins, S.H.D. Jackson, A. Jones, D.M. Keeling, J.R. Kirwan, P.G. Kopelman, T.H. Lee, A. Lekkas, D.N.J. Lockwood, A.M. Lovering, M.G. Lucas, L. Luzzatto, P.D. Mason, D.A. McArthur, K.E.L. McColl, L.M. Melvin, E. Miller, R.M. Mirakian, P. Morrison, S.M.S. Nasser, C. Nelson-Piercy, J.M. Neuberger, D.J. Nutt, R. Patel, W.J. Penny, A.B. Provan, A.S.C. Rice, D.J. Rowbotham, J.W. Sander, J.A.T. Sandoe, M. Schacter, S.E. Slater, J. Soar, S.C.E. Sporton, M.D. Stewart, S. Thomas, J.P. Thompson, A.D. Weeks, A. Wilcock, A.P.R. Wilson, M.M. Yaqoob.

Expert advice on neurological conditions was kindly provided by the Association of British Neurologists.

Expert advice on the management of oral and dental conditions was kindly provided by M. Addy, P. Coulthard, A. Crighton, M.A.O. Lewis, J.G. Meechan, N.D. Robb, C. Scully, R.A. Seymour, R. Welbury, and J.M. Zakrzewska. S. Kaur provided valuable advice on dental prescribing policy.

Members of the British Association of Dermatologists' Therapy & Guidelines Subcommittee, D.A. Buckley, N. Chiang, M. Cork, K. Gibbon, R.Y.P. Hunasehally, G.A. Johnston, T.A. Leslie, E.C. Mallon, P.M. McHenry, J. Natkunarajah, C. Saunders, S. Ungureanu, S. Wakelin, F.S. Worsnop, A.G. Brain (Secretariat), and M.F. Mohd Mustapa (Secretariat) have provided valuable advice.

Members of the Advisory Committee on Malaria Prevention, R.H. Behrens, D. Bell, P.L. Chiodini, V. Field, F. Genasi, L. Goodyer, A. Green, J. Jones, G. Kassianos, D.G. Lalloo, D. Patel, H. Patel, M. Powell, D.V. Shingadia, N.O. Subair, C.J.M. Whitty, M. Blaze (Secretariat), and V. Smith (Secretariat) have provided valuable advice.

The MHRA have provided valuable assistance.

Correspondents in the pharmaceutical industry have provided information on new products and commented on products in the BNF.

Numerous doctors, pharmacists, nurses, and others have sent comments and suggestions.

The BNF has valuable access to the Martindale data banks by courtesy of A. Brayfield and staff.

The BNF team are grateful for the support and access to in-house expertise at Pharmaceutical Press and acknowledge the assistance of A. Lourie, J. Macdonald, N. Potter, H. Sondh and their teams.

E. Hagos, A. Pryde, M. Smith, and K. Sproston provided considerable assistance during the production of this update of the BNF.

BNF Staff

Joint Formulary Committee

CHAIR
Derek G. Waller
BSc, MB BS, DM, FRCP

COMMITTEE MEMBERS
Gill Brown
MSc, Dip

Andy Burman
CMgr, FCMI, FRSA, FIAM

Jo Lyn Chooi
BMedSc, BM BS, FRCA

Carmel M. Darcy
BSc, MSc, IP, MPSNI, MRPharmS

Andrew Evans
BPharm, MPH, DipClinPharm, MRPharmS

Sue Faulding
BPharm, MSc, FRPharmS

Tracy Hall
BSc, MSc, Cert N, Dip N, RGN, DN

Simon Hurding
MB, ChB, MRCGP

W. Moira Kinnear
BSc, MSc, MRPharmS

Mark P. Lythgoe
MB BS, MRPharmS

Louise Picton
BSc, DipCommPharm, MSc, MRPharmS

Esther Wong
BSc, MPharm, MSc, DipEthics, DipPharmPract, IP, MRPharmS

Dental Advisory Group

CHAIR
Sarah Manton
BDS, FDSRCS Ed, FHEA, PhD

COMMITTEE MEMBERS
Andrew K. Brewer
BSc, BchD

Alexander Crighton

Kristina Fowlie
MPharm, CertPharmPract, MRPharmS

Michelle Moffat
BDS, MFDS RCS Ed, M Paed Dent RCPS, FDS (Paed Dent) RCS Ed

Kate Towers
BPharm (AU), GCClinPharm (AU)

SECRETARY
Arianne J. Matlin
MA, MSc, PhD

ADVICE ON DENTAL PRACTICE
The **British Dental Association** has contributed to the advice on medicines for dental practice through its representatives on the Dental Advisory Group.

Nurse Prescribers' Advisory Group

CHAIR
Molly Courtenay
PhD, MSc, Cert Ed, BSc, RGN

COMMITTEE MEMBERS
Kristina Fowlie
MPharm, CertPharmPract, MRPharmS

Penny M. Franklin
RN, RCN, RSCPHN(HV), MA, PGCE

Matt Griffiths
BA (Hons), FAETC, RGN, Cert A&E, NISP, PHECC

Tracy Hall
BSc, MSc, RGN, DN, Dip N, Cert N

Penny Harrison
BSc (Hons)

Julie MacAngus
BSc (Hons), RGN, RM, PGCE

Joan Myers
MSc, BSc, RGN, RSCN, Dip DN

Fiona Peniston-Bird
BSc (Hons), NIP, RHV, RGN

Kathy Radley
BSc, RGN

Kate Towers
BPharm (AU), GCClinPharm (AU)

How BNF Publications are constructed

Overview
The BNF is an independent professional publication that addresses the day-to-day prescribing information needs of healthcare professionals. Use of this resource throughout the health service helps to ensure that medicines are used safely, effectively, and appropriately.

Hundreds of changes are made between print editions, and are published monthly in a number of digital formats. The most clinically significant updates are listed under Changes p. xix.

The BNF is unique in bringing together authoritative, independent guidance on best practice with clinically validated drug information. Validation of information follows a standardised process, reviewing emerging evidence, best-practice guidelines, and advice from a network of clinical experts. Where the evidence base is weak, further validation is undertaken through a process of peer review. The process and its governance are outlined in greater detail in the sections that follow.

Joint Formulary Committee
The Joint Formulary Committee (JFC) is responsible for the content of the BNF. The JFC includes pharmacy, medical, nursing and lay representatives; there are also representatives from the Medicines and Healthcare products Regulatory Agency (MHRA), the UK Health Departments, and a national guideline producer. The JFC decides on matters of policy and reviews amendments to the BNF in the light of new evidence and expert advice.

Dental Advisory Group
The Dental Advisory Group oversees the preparation of advice on the drug management of dental and oral conditions; the group includes representatives from the British Dental Association and a representative from the UK Health Departments.

Nurse Prescribers' Advisory Group
The Nurse Prescribers' Advisory Group oversees the list of drugs approved for inclusion in the Nurse Prescribers' Formulary; the group includes representatives from a range of nursing disciplines and stakeholder organisations.

Expert advisers
The BNF uses about 60 expert clinical advisers (including doctors, pharmacists, nurses, and dentists) throughout the UK to help with clinical content. The role of these expert advisers is to review existing text and to comment on amendments drafted by the clinical writers. These clinical experts help to ensure that the BNF remains reliable by:

- commenting on the relevance of the text in the context of best clinical practice in the UK;
- checking draft amendments for appropriate interpretation of any new evidence;
- providing expert opinion in areas of controversy or when reliable evidence is lacking;
- providing independent advice on drug interactions, prescribing in hepatic impairment, renal impairment, pregnancy, breast-feeding, children, the elderly, palliative care, and the emergency treatment of poisoning.

In addition to consulting with regular advisers, the BNF calls on other clinical specialists for specific developments when particular expertise is required.

The BNF works closely with a number of expert bodies that produce clinical guidelines. Drafts or pre-publication copies of guidelines are often received for comment and assimilation into the BNF.

Editorial team
BNF clinical writers have all worked as pharmacists or possess a pharmacy degree and a further, relevant post-graduate qualification, and have a sound understanding of how drugs are used in clinical practice. As a team, the clinical writers are responsible for editing, maintaining, and updating BNF content. They follow a systematic prioritisation process in response to updates to the evidence base in order to ensure the most clinically important topics are reviewed as quickly as possible. In parallel the team of clinical writers undertakes a process of rolling revalidation, aiming to review all of the content in the BNF over a 3- to 4-year period.

Amendments to the text are drafted when the clinical writers are satisfied that any new information is reliable and relevant. A set of standard criteria define when content is referred to expert advisers, the Joint Formulary Committee or other advisory groups, or submitted for peer review.

Clinical writers prepare the text for publication and undertake a number of validation checks on the knowledge at various stages of the production process.

Sources of BNF information
The BNF uses a variety of sources for its information; the main ones are shown below.

Summaries of product characteristics
The BNF reviews summaries of product characteristics (SPCs) of all new products as well as revised SPCs for existing products. The SPCs are the principal source of product information and are carefully processed. Such processing involves:

- verifying the approved names of all relevant ingredients including 'non-active' ingredients (the BNF is committed to using approved names and descriptions as laid down by the Human Medicine Regulations 2012);
- comparing the indications, cautions, contra-indications, and side-effects with similar existing drugs. Where these are different from the expected pattern, justification is sought for their inclusion or exclusion;
- seeking independent data on the use of drugs in pregnancy and breast-feeding;
- incorporating the information into the BNF using established criteria for the presentation and inclusion of the data;
- checking interpretation of the information by a second clinical writer before submitting to a content manager; changes relating to doses receive a further check;
- identifying potential clinical problems or omissions and seeking further information from manufacturers or from expert advisers;
- constructing, with the help of expert advisers, a comment on the role of the drug in the context of similar drugs.

Much of this processing is applicable to the following sources as well.

Literature
Clinical writers monitor core medical and pharmaceutical journals. Research papers and reviews relating to drug therapy are carefully processed. When a difference between the advice in the BNF and the paper is noted, the new information is assessed for reliability (using tools based on SIGN methodology) and relevance to UK clinical practice. If necessary, new text is drafted and discussed with expert advisers and the Joint Formulary Committee. The BNF enjoys a close working relationship with a number of national information providers.

In addition to the routine process, which is used to identify 'triggers' for changing the content, systematic literature searches are used to identify the best quality evidence available to inform an update. Clinical writers receive training in critical appraisal, literature evaluation, and search strategies.

Consensus guidelines

The advice in the BNF is checked against consensus guidelines produced by expert bodies. The quality of the guidelines is assessed using adapted versions of the AGREE II tool. A number of bodies make drafts or pre-publication copies of the guidelines available to the BNF; it is therefore possible to ensure that a consistent message is disseminated. The BNF routinely processes guidelines from the National Institute for Health and Care Excellence (NICE), the All Wales Medicines Strategy Group (AWMSG), the Scottish Medicines Consortium (SMC), and the Scottish Intercollegiate Guidelines Network (SIGN).

Reference sources

Textbooks and reference sources are used to provide background information for the review of existing text or for the construction of new text. The BNF team works closely with the editorial team that produces *Martindale: The Complete Drug Reference*. The BNF has access to *Martindale* information resources and each team keeps the other informed of significant developments and shifts in the trends of drug usage.

Peer review

Although every effort is made to identify the most robust data available, inevitably there are areas where the evidence base is weak or contradictory. While the BNF has the valuable support of expert advisers and the Joint Formulary Committee, the recommendations made may be subject to a further level of scrutiny through peer review to ensure they reflect best practice.

Content for peer review is posted on bnf.org and interested parties are notified via a number of channels, including the BNF e-newsletter.

Statutory information

The BNF routinely processes relevant information from various Government bodies including Statutory Instruments and regulations affecting the Prescriptions only Medicines Order. Official compendia such as the British Pharmacopoeia and its addenda are processed routinely to ensure that the BNF complies with the relevant sections of the Human Medicines Regulations 2012.

The BNF maintains close links with the Home Office (in relation to controlled drug regulations) and the Medicines and Healthcare products Regulatory Agency (including the British Pharmacopoeia Commission). Safety warnings issued by the Commission on Human Medicines (CHM) and guidelines on drug are issued by the UK health departments are processed as a matter of routine.

Relevant professional statements issued by the Royal Pharmaceutical Society are included in the BNF as are guidelines from bodies such as the Royal College of General Practitioners.

Medicines and devices

NHS Prescription Services (from the NHS Business Services Authority) provides non-clinical, categorical information (including prices) on the medicines and devices included in the BNF.

Comments from readers

Readers of the BNF are invited to send in comments. Numerous letters and emails are received by the BNF team. Such feedback helps to ensure that the BNF provides practical and clinically relevant information. Many changes in the presentation and scope of the BNF have resulted from comments sent in by users.

Comments from industry

Close scrutiny of BNF by the manufacturers provides an additional check and allows them an opportunity to raise issues about BNF's presentation of the role of various drugs; this is yet another check on the balance of BNF's advice. All comments are looked at with care and, where necessary, additional information and expert advice are sought.

Market research

Market research is conducted at regular intervals to gather feedback on specific areas of development.

Assessing the evidence

From January 2016, recommendations made in BNF publications have been evidence graded to reflect the strength of the recommendation. The addition of evidence grading is to support clinical decision making based on the best available evidence.

The BNF aims to revalidate all content over a rolling 3- to 4-year period and evidence grading will be applied to recommendations as content goes through the revalidation process. Therefore, initially, only a small number of recommendations will have been graded.

Grading system

The BNF has adopted a five level grading system from A to E, based on the former SIGN grading system. This grade is displayed next to the recommendation within the text.

Evidence used to make a recommendation is assessed for validity using standardised methodology tools based on AGREE II and assigned a level of evidence. The recommendation is then given a grade that is extrapolated from the level of evidence, and an assessment of the body of evidence and its applicability.

Evidence assigned a level 1- or 2- score has an unacceptable level of bias or confounding and is not used to form recommendations.

Levels of evidence

- Level 1++
  High quality meta-analyses, systematic reviews of randomised controlled trials (RCTs), or RCTs with a very low risk of bias.

- Level 1+
  Well-conducted meta-analyses, systematic reviews, or RCTs with a low risk of bias.

- Level 1-
  Meta-analyses, systematic reviews, or RCTs with a high risk of bias.

- Level 2++
  High quality systematic reviews of case control or cohort studies; or high quality case control or cohort studies with a very low risk of confounding or bias and a high probability that the relationship is causal.

- Level 2+
  Well-conducted case control or cohort studies with a low risk of confounding or bias and a moderate probability that the relationship is causal.

- Level 2-
  Case control or cohort studies with a high risk of confounding or bias and a significant risk that the relationship is not causal.

- Level 3
  Non-analytic studies, e.g. case reports, case series.

- Level 4
  Expert advice or clinical experience from respected authorities.

Grades of recommendation

- Grade A: High strength
  NICE-accredited guidelines; or guidelines that pass AGREE II assessment; or at least one meta-analysis, systematic review, or RCT rated as 1++, and directly applicable to the target population; or a body of evidence consisting principally of studies rated as 1+, directly applicable to the target population, and demonstrating overall consistency of results.

- Grade B: Moderate strength
  A body of evidence including studies rated as 2++, directly applicable to the target population, and demonstrating

overall consistency of results; or extrapolated evidence from studies rated as 1++ or 1+.

- **Grade C: Low strength**
  A body of evidence including studies rated as 2+, directly applicable to the target population and demonstrating overall consistency of results; or extrapolated evidence from studies rated as 2++.

- **Grade D: Very low strength**
  Evidence level 3; or extrapolated evidence from studies rated as 2+; or tertiary reference source created by a transparent, defined methodology, where the basis for recommendation is clear.

- **Grade E: Practice point**
  Evidence level 4.

How to use BNF Publications in print

How to use the BNF

This edition of the BNF continues to display the fundamental change to the structure of the content that was first shown in BNF 70. The changes were made to bring consistency and clarity to BNF content, and to the way that the content is arranged within print and digital products, increasing the ease with which information can be found.

For reference, the most notable changes to the structure of the content include:

- Drug monographs – where possible, all information that relates to a single drug is contained within its drug monograph, moving information previously contained in the prescribing notes. Drug monographs have also changed structurally: additional sections have been added, ensuring greater regularity around where information is located within the publication.
- Drug class monographs – where substantial amounts of information are common to all drugs within a drug class (e.g. macrolides p. 528), a drug class monograph has been created to contain the common information.
- Medicinal forms – categorical information about marketed medicines, such as price and pack size, continues to be sourced directly from the Dictionary of Medicines and Devices provided by the NHS Business Services Authority. However, clinical information curated by the BNF team has been clearly separated from the categorical pricing and pack size information and is included in the relevant section of the drug monograph.
- Section numbering – the BNF section numbering has been removed. This section numbering tied the content to a rigid structure and enforced the retention of defunct classifications, such as mercurial diuretics, and hindered the relocation of drugs where therapeutic use had altered. It also caused constraints between the BNF and BNF *for Children*, where drugs had different therapeutic uses in children.
- Appendix 4 – the content has been moved to individual drug monographs. The introductory notes have been replaced with a new guidance section, Guidance on intravenous infusions p. 16.

Introduction

In order to achieve the safe, effective, and appropriate use of medicines, healthcare professionals must be able to use the BNF effectively, and keep up to date with significant changes in the BNF that are relevant to their clinical practice. This *How to Use the BNF* is key in reinforcing the details of the new structure of the BNF to all healthcare professionals involved with prescribing, monitoring, supplying, and administering medicines, as well as supporting the learning of students training to join these professions.

Structure of the BNF

This BNF edition continues to broadly follows the high-level structure of earlier editions of the BNF (i.e. those published before BNF 70):

Front matter, comprising information on how to use the BNF, the significant content changes in each edition, and guidance on various prescribing matters (e.g. prescription writing, the use of intravenous drugs, particular considerations for special patient populations).

Chapters, containing drug monographs describing the uses, doses, safety issues and other considerations involved in the use of drugs; drug class monographs; and treatment summaries, covering guidance on the selection of drugs. Monographs and treatment summaries are divided into chapters based on specific aspects of medical care, such as Chapter 5, Infections, or Chapter 16, Emergency treatment of poisoning; or drug use related to a particular system of the body, such as Chapter 2, Cardiovascular.

Within each chapter, content is organised alphabetically by therapeutic use (e.g. Airways disease, obstructive), with the treatment summaries first, (e.g. asthma), followed by the monographs of the drugs used to manage the conditions discussed in the treatment summary. Within each therapeutic use, the drugs are organised alphabetically by classification (e.g. Antimuscarinics, Beta $_2$-agonist bronchodilators) and then alphabetically within each classification (e.g. Aclidinium bromide, Glycopyrronium bromide, Ipratropium bromide).

Appendices, covering interactions, borderline substances, cautionary and advisory labels, and woundcare.

Back matter, covering the lists of medicines approved by the NHS for Dental and Nurse Practitioner prescribing, proprietary and specials manufacturers' contact details, and the index. Yellow cards are also included, to facilitate the reporting of adverse events, as well as quick reference guides for life support and key drug doses in medical emergencies, for ease of access.

Navigating the BNF

The contents page provides the high-level layout of information within the BNF; and in addition, each chapter begins with a small contents section, describing the therapeutic uses covered within that chapter. Once in a chapter, location is guided by the side of the page showing the chapter number (the *thumbnail*), alongside the chapter title. The top of the page includes the therapeutic use (the *running head*) alongside the page number.

Once on a page, visual cues aid navigation: treatment summary information is in black type, with therapeutic use titles similarly styled in black, whereas the use of colour indicates drug-related information, including drug classification titles, drug class monographs, and drug monographs.

Although navigation is possible by browsing, primarily access to the information is via the index, which covers the titles of drug class monographs, drug monographs, and treatment summaries. The index also includes the names of branded medicines and other topics of relevance, such as abbreviations, guidance sections, tables, and images.

Content types

Treatment summaries

Treatment summaries are of three main types;

- an overview of delivering a drug to a particular body system (e.g. Skin conditions, management p. 1185)
- a comparison between a group or groups of drugs (e.g. beta-adrenoceptor blockers (systemic) p. 146)
- an overview of the drug management or prophylaxis of common conditions intended to facilitate rapid appraisal of options (e.g. Hypertension p. 139, or Malaria, prophylaxis p. 596).

In order to select safe and effective medicines for individual patients, information in the treatment summaries must be used in conjunction with other prescribing details about the drugs and knowledge of the patient's medical and drug history.

Monographs

Overview

In earlier editions (i.e. before BNF 70), a systemically administered drug with indications for use in different body systems was split across the chapters relating to those body systems. So, for example, codeine phosphate p. 448 was found in chapter 1, for its antimotility effects and chapter 4 for its analgesic effects. However, the monograph in chapter

1 contained only the dose and some selected safety precautions.

Now, all of the information for the systemic use of a drug is contained within one monograph, so codeine phosphate p. 448 is now included in chapter 4. This carries the advantage of providing all of the information in one place, so the user does not need to flick back and forth across several pages to find all of the relevant information for that drug. Cross references are included in chapter 1, where the management of diarrhoea is discussed, to the drug monograph to assist navigation.

Where drugs have systemic and local uses, for example, chloramphenicol p. 558, 1139, 1161, and the considerations around drug use are markedly different according to the route of administration, the monograph is split, as with earlier editions, into the relevant chapters.

This means that the majority of drugs are still placed in the same chapters and sections as earlier editions, and although there may be some variation in order, all of the relevant information will be easier to locate.

One of the most significant changes to the monograph structure is the increased granularity, with a move from around 9 sections to over 20 sections; sections are only included when relevant information has been identified. The following information describes these sections and their uses in more detail.

Nomenclature
Monograph titles follow the convention of recommended international non-proprietary names (rINNs), or, in the absence of a rINN, British Approved Names. Relevant synonyms are included below the title and, in some instances a brief description of the drug action is included. Over future editions these drug action statements will be rolled out for all drugs.

In some monographs, immediately below the nomenclature or drug action, there are a number of cross references or flags used to signpost the user to any additional information they need to consider about a drug. This is most common for drugs formulated in combinations, where users will be signposted to the monographs for the individual ingredients (e.g. senna with ispaghula husk p. 63) or for drugs that are related to a drug class monograph (see Drug class monographs, below).

Indication and dose
User feedback has highlighted that one of the main uses of the BNF is identifying indications and doses of drugs. Therefore, indication and dose information has been promoted to the top of the monograph and highlighted by a coloured panel to aid quick reference.

The indication and dose section is more highly structured than in earlier editions, giving greater clarity around which doses should be used for which indications and by which route. In addition, if the dose varies with a specific preparation or formulation, that dosing information has been moved out of the preparations section and in to the indication and dose panel, under a heading of the preparation name.

Doses are either expressed in terms of a definite frequency (e.g. 1 g 4 times daily) or in the total daily dose format (e.g. 6 g daily in 3 divided doses); the total daily dose should be divided into individual doses (in the second example, the patient should receive 2 g 3 times daily).

Doses for specific patient groups (e.g. the elderly) may be included if they are different to the standard dose. Doses for children can be identified by the relevant age range and may vary according to their age or body-weight.

In earlier editions of the BNF, age ranges and weight ranges overlapped. For clarity and to aid selection of the correct dose, wherever possible these age and weight ranges now do not overlap. When interpreting age ranges it is important to understand that a patient is considered to be 64 up until the point of their 65th birthday, meaning that an age

range of adult 18 to 64 is applicable to a patient from the day of their 18th birthday until the day before their 65th birthday. All age ranges should be interpreted in this way. Similarly, when interpreting weight ranges, it should be understood that a weight of up to 30 kg is applicable to a patient up to, but not including, the point that they tip the scales at 30 kg and a weight range of 35 to 59 kg is applicable to a patient as soon as they tip the scales at 35 kg right up until, but not including, the point that they tip the scales at 60 kg. All weight ranges should be interpreted in this way.

In all circumstances, it is important to consider the patient in question and their physical condition, and select the dose most appropriate for the individual.

Other information relevant to Indication and dose
The dose panel also contains, where known, an indication of **pharmacokinetic considerations** that may affect the choice of dose, and **dose equivalence** information, which may aid the selection of dose when switching between drugs or preparations.

The BNF includes **unlicensed use** of medicines when the clinical need cannot be met by licensed medicines; such use should be supported by appropriate evidence and experience. When the BNF recommends an unlicensed medicine or the 'off-label' use of a licensed medicine, this is shown below the indication and dose panel in the unlicensed use section.

Minimising harm and drug safety
The drug chosen to treat a particular condition should minimise the patient's susceptibility to adverse effects and, where co-morbidities exist, have minimal detrimental effects on the patient's other diseases. To achieve this, the *Contra-indications*, *Cautions* and *Side-effects* of the relevant drug should be reviewed.

The information under Cautions can be used to assess the risks of using a drug in a patient who has co-morbidities that are also included in the Cautions for that drug—if a safer alternative cannot be found, the drug may be prescribed while monitoring the patient for adverse-effects or deterioration in the co-morbidity. Contra-indications are far more restrictive than Cautions and mean that the drug should be avoided in a patient with a condition that is contra-indicated.

The impact that potential side-effects may have on a patient's quality of life should also be assessed. For instance, in a patient who has difficulty sleeping, it may be preferable to avoid a drug that frequently causes insomnia.

Clinically relevant *Side-effects* for drugs are included in the monographs or class monographs. Side-effects are listed in order of frequency, where known, and arranged alphabetically. The frequency of side-effects follows the regulatory standard:

- Very common — occurs more frequently than 1 in 10 administrations of a drug
- Common — occurs between 1 in 10 and 1 in 100 administrations of a drug
- Uncommon — between 1 in 100 and 1 in 1,000 administrations of a drug
- Rare — between 1 in 1,000 and 1 in 10,000 administrations of a drug
- Very rare — occurs less than 1 in 10,000 administrations of a drug
- Frequency not known

An exhaustive list of side-effects is not included, particularly for drugs that are used by specialists (e.g. cytotoxic drugs and drugs used in anaesthesia). The BNF also omits effects that are likely to have little clinical consequence (e.g. transient increase in liver enzymes).

Recognising that hypersensitivity reactions can occur with virtually all medicines, this effect is generally not listed, unless the drug carries an increased risk of such reactions,

Typical layout of a monograph and associated medicinal forms

❶ Class Monographs and drug monographs

In most cases, all information that relates to an individual drug is contained in its drug monograph and there is no symbol. Class monographs have been created where substantial amounts of information are common to all drugs within a drug class, these are indicated by a flag symbol in a circle:

Drug monographs with a corresponding class monograph are indicated by a tab with a flag symbol:

The page number of the corresponding class monograph is indicated within the tab. For further information, see How to use BNF Publications

❷ Drug classifications

Used to inform users of the class of a drug and to assist in finding other drugs of the same class. May be based on pharmacological class (e.g. opioids) but can also be associated with the use of the drug (e.g. cough suppressants)

❸ Review date

The date of last review of the content

❹ Specific preparation name

If the dose varies with a specific preparation or formulation it appears under a heading of the preparation name

---

Class monograph ❶

CLASSIFICATION ❷

Drug monograph ❶   ❸ 01-Jun-2016

(Synonym) another name by which a drug may be known

● DRUG ACTION how a drug exerts its effect in the body

● **INDICATIONS AND DOSE**
  Indications are the clinical reasons a drug is used. The dose of a drug will often depend on the indications

  Indication
  ▶ ROUTE
  ▶ Age groups: [Child/Adult/Elderly]
    Dose and frequency of administration (max. dose)

  SPECIFIC PREPARATION NAME ❹

  Indication
  ▶ ROUTE
  ▶ Age groups: [Child/Adult/Elderly]
    Dose and frequency of administration (max. dose)

  DOSE ADJUSTMENTS DUE TO INTERACTIONS dosing information when used concurrently with other drugs

  DOSES AT EXTREMES OF BODY-WEIGHT dosing information for patients who are overweight or underweight

  DOSE EQUIVALENCE AND CONVERSION information around the bioequivalence between formulations of the same drug, or equivalent doses of drugs that are members of the same class

  PHARMACOKINETICS how the body affects a drug (absorption, distribution, metabolism, and excretion)

  POTENCY a measure of drug activity expressed in terms of the concentration required to produce an effect of given intensity

● UNLICENSED USE describes the use of medicines outside the terms of their UK licence (off-label use), or use of medicines that have no licence for use in the UK

  > IMPORTANT SAFETY INFORMATION
  > Information produced and disseminated by drug regulators often highlights serious risks associated with the use of a drug, and may include advice that is mandatory

● CONTRA-INDICATIONS circumstances when a drug should be avoided
● CAUTIONS details of precautions required
● INTERACTIONS when one drug changes the effects of another drug; the mechanisms underlying drug interactions are explained in Appendix 1
● SIDE-EFFECTS listed in order of frequency, where known, and arranged alphabetically
● ALLERGY AND CROSS-SENSITIVITY for drugs that carry an increased risk of hypersensitivity reactions
● CONCEPTION AND CONTRACEPTION potential for a drug to have harmful effects on an unborn child when prescribing for a woman of childbearing age or for a man trying to father a child; information on the effect of drugs on the efficacy of latex condoms or diaphragms

- PREGNANCY advice on the use of a drug during pregnancy
- BREAST FEEDING [EvGr] advice on the use of a drug during breast feeding Ⓐ Ⓔ
- HEPATIC IMPAIRMENT advice on the use of a drug in hepatic impairment
- RENAL IMPAIRMENT advice on the use of a drug in renal impairment
- PRE-TREATMENT SCREENING covers one off tests required to assess the suitability of a patient for a particular drug
- MONITORING REQUIREMENTS specifies any special monitoring requirements, including information on monitoring the plasma concentration of drugs with a narrow therapeutic index
- EFFECTS ON LABORATORY TESTS for drugs that can interfere with the accuracy of seemingly unrelated laboratory tests
- TREATMENT CESSATION specifies whether further monitoring or precautions are advised when the drug is withdrawn
- DIRECTIONS FOR ADMINISTRATION practical information on the preparation of intravenous drug infusions; general advice relevant to other routes of administration
- PRESCRIBING AND DISPENSING INFORMATION practical information around how a drug can be prescribed and dispensed including details of when brand prescribing is necessary
- HANDLING AND STORAGE includes information on drugs that can cause adverse effects to those who handle them before they are taken by, or administered to, a patient; advice on storage conditions
- PATIENT AND CARER ADVICE for drugs with a special need for counselling
- PROFESSION SPECIFIC INFORMATION provides details of the restrictions certain professions such as dental practitioners or nurse prescribers need to be aware of when prescribing on the NHS
- NATIONAL FUNDING/ACCESS DECISIONS details of NICE Technology Appraisals, SMC advice and AWMSG advice
- LESS SUITABLE FOR PRESCRIBING preparations that are considered by the Joint Formulary Committee to be less suitable for prescribing
- EXCEPTION TO LEGAL CATEGORY advice and information on drugs which may be sold without a prescription under specific conditions

---

- MEDICINAL FORMS
  Form
  CAUTIONARY AND ADVISORY LABELS if applicable
  EXCIPIENTS clinically important but not comprehensive [consult manufacturer information for full details]
  ELECTROLYTES if clinically significant quantities occur
  ▸ Preparation name (Manufacturer/Non-proprietary)
    Drug name and strength pack sizes [PoM] Ⓖ Prices

Combinations available this indicates a combination preparation is available and a cross reference page number is provided to locate this preparation

Ⓔ Evidence grading

Evidence grading to reflect the strengths of recommendations will be applied as content goes through the revalidation process. A five level evidence grading system based on the former SIGN grading system has been adopted. The grades Ⓐ Ⓑ Ⓒ Ⓓ Ⓔ are displayed next to the recommendations within the text, and are preceded by the symbol: [EvGr]

For further information, see How BNF Publications are constructed

Ⓖ Legal categories

[PoM] This symbol has been placed against those preparations that are available only on a prescription issued by an appropriate practitioner. For more detailed information see *Medicines, Ethics and Practice*, London, Pharmaceutical Press (always consult latest edition)

[CD1] [CD2] [CD3] [CD4-1] [CD4-2] [CD5] These symbols indicate that the preparations are subject to the prescription requirements of the Misuse of Drugs Act

For regulations governing prescriptions for such preparations, see Controlled Drugs and Drug Dependence

Not all monographs include all possible sections; sections are only included when relevant information has been identified

when the information is included under *Allergy and cross sensitivity*.

The *Important safety advice* section in the BNF, delineated by a coloured outline box, highlights important safety concerns, often those raised by regulatory authorities or guideline producers. Safety warnings issued by the Commission on Human Medicines (CHM) or Medicines and Healthcare products Regulatory Agency (MHRA) are found here.

Drug selection should aim to minimise drug interactions. If it is necessary to prescribe a potentially serious combination of drugs, patients should be monitored appropriately. The mechanisms underlying drug interactions are explained in Appendix 1, followed by details of drug interactions.

Use of drugs in specific patient populations
Drug selection should aim to minimise the potential for drug accumulation, adverse drug reactions, and exacerbation of pre-existing hepatic or renal disease. If it is necessary to prescribe drugs whose effect is altered by hepatic or renal disease, appropriate drug dose adjustments should be made, and patients should be monitored adequately. The general principles for prescribing are outlined under Prescribing in hepatic impairment p. 19, and Prescribing in renal impairment p. 19. Information about drugs that should be avoided or used with caution in hepatic disease or renal impairment can be found in drug monographs under *Hepatic impairment* and *Renal impairment* (e.g. fluconazole p. 584).

Similarly, drug selection should aim to minimise harm to the fetus, nursing infant, and mother. The infant should be monitored for potential side-effects of drugs used by the *mother during pregnancy or breast-feeding*. The general principles for prescribing are outlined under Prescribing in pregnancy p. 22 and Prescribing in breast-feeding p. 22. The Treatment Summaries provide guidance on the drug treatment of common conditions that can occur during pregnancy and breast-feeding (e.g. Asthma, acute p. 240). Information about the use of specific drugs during pregnancy and breast-feeding can be found in their drug monographs under *Pregnancy*, and *Breast-feeding* (e.g. fluconazole p. 584).

A section, *Conception and contraception*, containing information around considerations for females of childbearing potential or men who might father a child (e.g. isotretinoin p. 1234) has been included.

Administration and monitoring
When selecting the most appropriate drug, it may be necessary to screen the patient for certain genetic markers or metabolic states. This information is included within a section called *Pre-treatment screening* (e.g. abacavir p. 634). This section covers one-off tests required to assess the suitability of a patient for a particular drug.

Once the drug has been selected, it needs to be given in the most appropriate manner. A *Directions for administration* section contains the information about intravenous administration previously located in Appendix 4. This provides practical information on the preparation of intravenous drug infusions, including compatibility of drugs with standard intravenous infusion fluids, method of dilution or reconstitution, and administration rates. In addition, general advice relevant to other routes of administration is provided within this section (e.g. fentanyl p. 451).

After selecting and administering the most appropriate drug by the most appropriate route, patients should be monitored to ensure they are achieving the expected benefits from drug treatment without any unwanted side-effects. The *Monitoring* section specifies any special monitoring requirements, including information on monitoring the plasma concentration of drugs with a narrow therapeutic index (e.g. theophylline p. 273). Monitoring may, in certain cases, be affected by the impact of a drug on laboratory tests (e.g. hydroxocobalamin p. 994), and this information is included in *Effects on laboratory tests*.

In some cases, when a drug is withdrawn, further monitoring or precautions may be advised (e.g. clonidine hydrochloride p. 144): these are covered under *Treatment cessation*.

Choice and supply
The prescriber and the patient should agree on the health outcomes that the patient desires and on the strategy for achieving them (see *Taking Medicines to Best Effect*). Taking the time to explain to the patient (and carers) the rationale and the potential adverse effects of treatment may improve adherence. For some medicines there is a special need for counselling (e.g. appropriate posture during administration of doxycycline p. 555); this is shown in *Patient and carer advice*.

Other information contained in the latter half of the monograph also helps prescribers and those dispensing medicines choose medicinal forms by indicating information such as flavour or when branded products may not be interchangeable (e.g. diltiazem hydrochloride p. 157), assess the suitability of a drug for prescribing, understand the NHS funding status for a drug (e.g. sildenafil p. 794), or assess when a patient may be able to purchase a drug without prescription (e.g. loperamide hydrochloride p. 66).

Medicinal forms
In the BNF, preparations follow immediately after the monograph for the drug that is their main ingredient.

In earlier editions, when a particular preparation had safety information, dose advice or other clinical information specific to the product, it was contained within the preparations section. This information has been moved to the relevant section in the main body of the monograph under a heading of the name of the specific medicinal form (e.g. peppermint oil p. 47).

The medicinal forms (formerly preparations) section provides information on the type of formulation (e.g. tablet), the amount of active drug in a solid dosage form, and the concentration of active drug in a liquid dosage form. The legal status is shown for prescription-only medicines and controlled drugs, as well as pharmacy medicines and medicines on the general sales list. Practitioners are reminded, by a statement under the heading of "Medicinal Forms" that not all products containing a specific drug ingredient may be similarly licensed. To be clear on the precise licensing status of specific medicinal forms, practitioners should check the product literature for the particular product being prescribed or dispensed.

Details of all medicinal forms available on the dm+d for each drug in BNF Publications appears online on MedicinesComplete. In print editions, due to space constraints, only certain branded products are included in detail. Where medicinal forms are listed they should not be inferred as equivalent to the other brands listed under the same form heading. For example, all the products listed under a heading of "Modified release capsule" will be available as modified release capsules, however, the brands listed under that form heading may have different release profiles, the available strengths may vary and/or the products may have different licensing information. As with earlier editions of the BNF, practitioners must ensure that the particular product being prescribed or dispensed is appropriate.

As medicinal forms are derived from dm+d data, some drugs may appear under names derived from that data; this may vary slightly from those in previous BNF versions, e.g. sodium acid phosphate, is now sodium dihydrogen phosphate anhydrous.

Patients should be prescribed a preparation that complements their daily routine, and that provides the right dose of drug for the right indication and route of administration. When dispensing liquid preparations, a sugar-free preparation should always be used in preference to one containing sugar. Patients receiving medicines containing cariogenic sugars should be advised of appropriate dental hygiene measures to prevent caries.

In earlier editions, the BNF only included excipients and electrolyte information for proprietary medicines. This information is now covered at the level of the dose form (e.g. tablet). It is not possible to keep abreast of all of the generic products available on the UK market, and so this information serves as a reminder to the healthcare professional that, if the presence of a particular excipient is of concern, they should check the product literature for the particular product being prescribed or dispensed.

Cautionary and advisory labels that pharmacists are recommended to add when dispensing are included in the medicinal forms section. Details of these labels can be found in Appendix 3, Guidance for cautionary and advisory labels p. 1534. As these labels have now been applied at the level of the dose form, a full list of medicinal products with their relevant labels would be extensive. This list has therefore been removed, but the information is retained within the monograph.

In the case of compound preparations, the prescribing information for all constituents should be taken into account.

Prices in the BNF

Basic NHS **net prices** are given in the BNF to provide an indication of relative cost. Where there is a choice of suitable preparations for a particular disease or condition the relative cost may be used in making a selection. Cost-effective prescribing must, however, take into account other factors (such as dose frequency and duration of treatment) that affect the total cost. The use of more expensive drugs is justified if it will result in better treatment of the patient, or a reduction of the length of an illness, or the time spent in hospital.

Prices are regularly updated using the Drug Tariff and proprietary price information published by the NHS dictionary of medicines and devices (dm+d, www.dmd.nhs.uk). The weekly updated dm+d data (including prices) can be accessed using the dm+d browser of the NHS Business Services Authority (apps.nhsbsa.nhs.uk/DMDBrowser/DMDBrowser.do). Prices have been calculated from the net cost used in pricing NHS prescriptions and generally reflect whole dispensing packs. Prices for extemporaneously prepared preparations are not provided in the BNF as prices vary between different manufacturers. In Appendix 4, prices stated are per dressing or bandage.

BNF prices are not suitable for quoting to patients seeking private prescriptions or contemplating over-the-counter purchases because they do not take into account VAT, professional fees, and other overheads.

A fuller explanation of costs to the NHS may be obtained from the Drug Tariff. Separate drug tariffs are applicable to England and Wales (www.ppa.org.uk/ppa/edt_intro.htm), Scotland (www.isdscotland.org/Health-Topics/Prescribing-and-Medicines/Scottish-Drug-Tariff/), and Northern Ireland (www.hscbusiness.hscni.net/services/2034.htm); prices in the different tariffs may vary.

Drug class monographs

In earlier editions of the BNF, information relating to a class of drugs sharing the same properties (e.g. tetracyclines p. 554), was contained within the prescribing notes. In the updated structure, drug class monographs have been created to contain the common information; this ensures such information is easier to find, and has a more regularised structure.

For consistency and ease of use, the class monograph follows the same structure as a drug monograph. Class monographs are indicated by the presence of a flag ◉ (e.g. beta-adrenoceptor blockers (systemic) p. 146). If a drug monograph has a corresponding class monograph, that

needs to be considered in tandem, in order to understand the full information about a drug, the monograph is also indicated by a flag ◤ 1234 (e.g. metoprolol tartrate p. 154). Within this flag, the page number of the drug class monograph is provided (e.g. 1234), to help navigate the user to this information. This is particularly useful where occasionally, due to differences in therapeutic use, the drug monograph may not directly follow the drug class monograph (e.g. sotalol hydrochloride p. 108).

Evidence grading

The BNF has adopted a five level evidence grading system (see How BNF Publications are constructed p. ix). Recommendations that are evidence graded can be identified by a symbol appearing immediately before the recommendation. The evidence grade is displayed at the end of the recommendation.

Other content

Nutrition

Appendix 2, Borderline substances p. 1500, includes tables of ACBS-approved enteral feeds and nutritional supplements based on their energy and protein content. There are separate tables for specialised formulae for specific clinical conditions. Classified sections on foods for special diets and nutritional supplements for metabolic diseases are also included.

Wound dressings

A table on wound dressings in Appendix 4, Wound management products and elasticated garments p. 1537, allows an appropriate dressing to be selected based on the appearance and condition of the wound. Further information about the dressing can be found by following the cross-reference to the relevant classified section in the Appendix.

Advanced wound contact dressings have been classified in order of increasing absorbency.

Other useful information

Finding significant changes in the BNF

- *Changes*, provides a list of significant changes, dose changes, classification changes, new names, and new preparations that have been incorporated into the BNF, as well as a list of preparations that have been discontinued and removed from the BNF. Changes listed online are cumulative (from one print edition to the next), and can be printed off each month to show the main changes since the last print edition as an aide memoire for those using print copies. So many changes are made for each update of the BNF, that not all of them can be accommodated in the *Changes* section. We encourage healthcare professionals to regularly review the prescribing information on drugs that they encounter frequently;

- *Changes to the Dental Practitioners' Formulary*, are located at the end of the Dental List;

- *E-newsletter*, the BNF & BNFC e-newsletter service is available free of charge. It alerts healthcare professionals to details of significant changes in the clinical content of these publications and to the way that this information is delivered. Newsletters also review clinical case studies, provide tips on using these publications effectively, and highlight forthcoming changes to the publications. To sign up for e-newsletters go to www.bnf.org.

- An e-learning programme developed in collaboration with the Centre for Pharmacy Postgraduate Education (CPPE), enables pharmacists to identify and assess how significant changes in the BNF affect their clinical practice. The module can be found at www.cppe.ac.uk.

Using other sources for medicines information

The BNF is designed as a digest for rapid reference. Less detail is given on areas such as obstetrics, malignant disease, and anaesthesia since it is expected that those undertaking treatment will have specialist knowledge and access to specialist literature. *BNF for Children* should be consulted for detailed information on the use of medicines in children. The BNF should be interpreted in the light of professional knowledge and supplemented as necessary by specialised publications and by reference to the product literature. Information is also available from medicines information services.

Changes

Monthly updates are provided online via MedicinesComplete and the NHS Evidence portal. The changes listed below are cumulative (from one print edition to the next).

Significant changes

Significant changes that appear in the print edition of BNF 76 (September 2018–March 2019):

- Side-effects and their further information sections have been reviewed against the current product literature and terms used to define these have been standardised across all drug monographs in this edition of the BNF.
- Aflibercept p. 975 for treating choroidal neovascularisation [NICE guidance].
- Alendronic acid p. 710, ibandronic acid p. 711, risedronate sodium p. 713 and zoledronic acid p. 715 for treating osteoporosis [updated NICE guidance].
- Asthma, chronic p. 236: updated guidance on management.
- Atezolizumab p. 840 for treating locally advanced or metastatic non-small-cell lung cancer after chemotherapy [NICE guidance].
- Atezolizumab p. 840 for untreated locally advanced or metastatic urothelial cancer when cisplatin unsuitable [NICE guidance].
- Attention deficit hyperactivity disorder p. 343: updated guidance on management.
- Avelumab p. 841 for treating metastatic Merkel cell carcinoma [NICE guidance].
- *Braltus* ® (tiotropium p. 247): risk of inhalation of capsule if placed in the mouthpiece of the inhaler [MHRA/CHM advice].
- Brodalumab p. 1222 for treating moderate to severe plaque psoriasis [NICE guidance].
- Cabozantinib p. 943 for treating medullary thyroid cancer [NICE guidance].
- Ceritinib p. 945 for untreated ALK-positive non-small-cell lung cancer [NICE guidance].
- Cladribine p. 882 for leukaemia: reports of progressive multifocal encephalopathy (PML); stop treatment if PML suspected [MHRA/CHM advice].
- Cladribine p. 882 tablets for treating relapsing-remitting multiple sclerosis [NICE guidance].
- Corticosteroids [see Corticosteroids, general use p. 656]: rare risk of central serous chorioretinopathy with local and systemic administration [MHRA/CHM advice].
- Cystic fibrosis p. 291: updated guidance.
- Daclizumab (*Zinbryta* ®) and risk of severe liver injury: new restrictions to use and strengthened liver monitoring [MHRA/CHM advice].
- Daclizumab (*Zinbryta* ®) — marketing authorisation withdrawn for safety reasons.
- Daclizumab (*Zinbryta* ®) suspension and recall for safety reasons; review patients as soon as possible and start alternative therapy [MHRA/CHM advice].
- Daratumumab p. 846 monotherapy for treating relapsed and refractory multiple myeloma [NICE guidance].
- Dihydrocodeine with paracetamol p. 450 (co-dydramol): prescribe and dispense by strength to minimise risk of medication error (January 2018) [MHRA/CHM advice].
- Dihydrocodeine with paracetamol p. 450 [formerly co-dydramol].
- Drug name confusion: reminder to be vigilant for potential errors between clobazam and clonazepam, atenolol and amlodipine, propranolol and prednisolone, risperidone and ropinirole, sulfadiazine and sulfasalazine, amlodipine and nimodipine, mercaptamine and mercaptopurine, zuclopentixol acetate and zuclopentixol decanoate [MHRA/CHM advice].
- Eluxadoline p. 46 (*Truberzi* ®): risk of pancreatitis; do not use in patients who have undergone cholecystectomy or in those with biliary disorders [MHRA/CHM advice].
- Emergency contraception p. 775: updated guidance on management.
- Endometriosis p. 733: new guidance on management.
- Eribulin p. 909 for treating locally advanced or metastatic breast cancer after 1 chemotherapy regimen [NICE guidance].
- *Esmya* ® (ulipristal acetate p. 785) for uterine fibroids: do not initiate or re-start treatment; monitor liver function in current and recent users [MHRA/CHM advice].
- Fingolimod p. 834 (*Gilenya* ®): new contra-indications in relation to cardiac risk (December 2017) [MHRA/CHM advice].
- Fingolimod p. 834 (*Gilenya* ®): updated advice about risk of cancers and serious infections (December 2017) [MHRA/CHM advice].
- Fulvestrant p. 926 for untreated locally advanced or metastatic oestrogen-receptor positive breast cancer [NICE guidance].
- Glecaprevir with pibrentasvir p. 620 for treating chronic hepatitis C [NICE guidance].
- Golimumab p. 1080 for treating non-radiographic axial spondyloarthritis [NICE guidance].
- Ibrutinib p. 952 for treating relapsed or refractory mantle cell lymphoma [NICE guidance].
- Ibrutinib p. 952 for treating Waldenstrom's macroglobulinaemia [NICE guidance].
- Immunoglobulins p. 1252: updated guidance for Varicella-zoster immunoglobulin.
- Ixazomib p. 940 with lenalidomide p. 933 and dexamethasone for treating relapsed or refractory multiple myeloma [NICE guidance].
- Lenvatinib p. 957 with everolimus p. 950 for previously treated advanced renal cell carcinoma [NICE guidance].
- Mycophenolate mofetil p. 826, mycophenolic acid: updated contraception advice for male patients [MHRA/CHM advice].
- Malaria, prophylaxis p. 596: update to country recommendations and guidance.
- Naltrexone with bupropion p. 91 for managing overweight and obesity [NICE guidance].
- Nivolumab p. 850 for previously treated advanced renal cell carcinoma [updated NICE guidance].
- Nivolumab p. 850 for previously treated non-squamous non-small-cell lung cancer [NICE guidance].
- Nivolumab p. 850 for previously treated squamous non-small-cell lung cancer [NICE guidance].
- Nivolumab p. 850 for treating relapsed or refractory classical Hodgkin lymphoma [updated NICE guidance].
- Nivolumab p. 850 for treating squamous cell carcinoma of the head and neck after platinum-based chemotherapy [NICE guidance].
- Noradrenaline/norepinephrine 0.08 mg/mL (4 mg in 50 mL) solution for infusion p. 188 association with potential risk of medication errors.
- Obeticholic acid p. 88 (*Ocaliva* ®): risk of serious liver injury in patients with pre-existing moderate or severe hepatic impairment; reminder to adjust dosing according to liver function monitoring [MHRA/CHM advice].
- Obinutuzumab p. 852 for untreated advanced follicular lymphoma [NICE guidance].
- Osteoporosis p. 708: updated guidance.
- Palbociclib p. 961 with an aromatase inhibitor for previously untreated, hormone receptor-positive, HER-2 negative, locally advanced or metastatic breast cancer [NICE guidance].

- Pembrolizumab p. 856 for treating locally advanced or metastatic urothelial carcinoma after platinum-containing chemotherapy [NICE guidance].
- Pertuzumab p. 857 with trastuzumab p. 862 and docetaxel p. 900 for treating HER2-positive breast cancer [NICE guidance].
- Pirfenidone p. 296 for treating idiopathic pulmonary fibrosis [NICE guidance].
- Quinine p. 608: clarification of parenteral dose for the treatment of malaria [dose reduction necessary if parenteral treatment is required for more than 48 hours].
- Raloxifene hydrochloride p. 736 and teriparatide p. 716 for the secondary prevention of osteoporotic fragility fractures in postmenopausal women [updated NICE guidance].
- Raloxifene hydrochloride p. 736 for the primary prevention of osteoporotic fragility fractures in postmenopausal women [updated NICE guidance].
- Recombinant human erythropoietins (epoetin alfa p. 981, epoetin beta p. 982, epoetin zeta p. 983, darbepoetin alfa p. 979, methoxy polyethylene glycol-epoetin): very rare risk of severe cutaneous adverse reactions [MHRA/CHM advice].
- Regorafenib p. 964 for previously treated advanced hepatocellular carcinoma [NICE guidance].
- Regorafenib p. 964 for previously treated unresectable or metastatic gastrointestinal stomal tumours (November 2017) [NICE guidance].
- Ribociclib p. 965 with an aromatase inhibitor for previously untreated, hormone receptor-positive, HER2-negative, locally advanced or metastatic breast cancer [NICE guidance].
- Sarilumab p. 1065 for moderate to severe rheumatoid arthritis [NICE guidance].
- Sinusitis (acute) p. 1168: updated guidance.
- Skin infections p. 1193: head lice eradication products: risk of serious burns if treated hair is exposed to open flames or other sources of ignition [MHRA/CHM advice].
- Sofosbuvir with velpatasvir and voxilaprevir p. 619 for treating chronic hepatitis C [NICE guidance].
- Terbinafine p. 1200: clarification of hepatic monitoring advice.
- *Tivicay*® (dolutegravir p. 630), *Triumeq*® (dolutegravir, abacavir, lamivudine), *Juluca*® (dolutegravir, rilpivirine): neural tube defects reported in infants born to women exposed to dolutegravir at the time of conception [MHRA/CHM advice].
- Tivozanib p. 969 for treating advanced renal cell carcinoma [NICE guidance].
- Tocilizumab p. 1068 for treating giant cell arteritis [NICE guidance].
- Trastuzumab emtansine p. 863 for treating HER2-positive advanced breast cancer after trastuzumab and a taxane [updated NICE guidance].
- Vaccines p. 1259: updated guidance for Hepatitis A Vaccine.
- Vaccines for travel p. 1270: updated guidance on Hepatitis A.
- Valproic acid p. 351 and sodium valproate p. 325: valproate medicines contraindicated in women and girls of childbearing potential unless conditions of Pregnancy Prevention Programme are met [MHRA/CHM advice].
- Venetoclax p. 974 for treating chronic lymphocytic leukaemia (November 2017) [NICE guidance].
- Vismodegib p. 974 for treating basal cell carcinoma [NICE guidance].

Dose changes

Changes in dose statements that appear in the print edition of BNF 76 (September 2018–March 2019):
- Abatacept p. 1073 [update to dosing advice].
- Alprostadil p. 798 [Initial dose for erectile dysfunction and neurogenic erectile dysfunction for *Viridal*®*Duo*].

- Amitriptyline hydrochloride p. 369 [doses for depression, neuropathic pain and migraine prophylaxis].
- Bosutinib p. 942 [update to dose in renal impairment].
- Budesonide p. 43 [alternative dosing regimen for Crohn's disease updated for *Budenofalk*® capsules].
- Candesartan cilexetil p. 174 [clarification of maximum daily dose in heart failure]
- Chloroquine p. 604 [clarification of dose equivalence statement].
- Chloroquine p. 604 [clarification of dosing for rheumatoid arthritis, systemic and discoid lupus erythematosus].
- Clomifene citrate p. 750 [clarification of dosing].
- Daptomycin p. 558 [update to dosing advice].
- Dexibuprofen p. 1098.
- Ganciclovir p. 626.
- Gentamicin p. 510 [clarification of dosing for surgical prophylaxis, including joint replacement surgery].
- Haloperidol p. 382 [clarification of continuous subcutaneous dose for nausea and vomiting in palliative care].
- Hydroxycarbamide p. 910.
- Ivabradine p. 210.
- Lacosamide p. 315.
- Levonorgestrel p. 787 [update to effective duration for *Levosert*® intra-uterine device].
- Levonorgestrel p. 787 [update to timing for emergency contraception].
- Macrogol 3350 with potassium chloride, sodium bicarbonate and sodium chloride p. 56.
- Nilotinib p. 959 [update to dosing advice].
- Nivolumab p. 850 [doses for monotherapy].
- Olaparib p. 973 [dose in renal impairment].
- Sildenafil p. 794 Digital ulcers associated with systemic sclerosis [unlicensed].
- Sodium thiosulfate p. 1327.
- Tadalafil p. 796 [clarification of dosing for intermittent use in erectile dysfunction and dosing in hepatic and renal impairment].
- Temocillin p. 545.
- Tramadol with paracetamol p. 467 [clarification of dosing].
- Lisdexamfetamine mesilate p. 348 [dose for children updated].
- Lisdexamfetamine mesilate p. 348 [unlicensed use statement deleted].
- Papaveretum p. 462 [clarification of dosing].
- Raltegravir p. 631 [all doses updated].
- Vancomycin p. 525.

Classification changes
Classification changes that appear in the print edition of BNF 76 (September 2018–March 2019):

New names
Name changes that appear in the print edition of BNF 76 (September 2018–March 2019):

Deleted preparations
Preparations discontinued in the print edition of BNF 76 (September 2018–March 2019):

New preparations
New preparations that appear in the print edition of BNF 76 (September 2018–March 2019):
- *AirFluSal*® preparations [fluticasone with salmeterol p. 263].
- *Bavencio*® [avelumab p. 841].
- *Cetraxal*® [ciprofloxacin ear drops p. 1161].
- *Chenodeoxycholic acid* [chenodeoxycholic acid capsules p. 88].
- *Dupixent*® [dupilumab p. 1223].
- *Fasenra*® [benralizumab p. 266].
- *Fotivda*® [tivozanib p. 969].
- *Hemlibra*® [emicizumab p. 111].
- *Kyleena*® [levonorgestrel intrauterine device p. 787].
- *Mylotarg*® [gemtuzumab ozogamicin p. 847].

- *NACSYS*® [acetylcysteine effervescent tablets p. 290].
- *Ocrevus*® [ocrelizumab p. 838].
- *Penthrox*® [methoxyflurane p. 438].
- *Plenvu*® [macrogol 3350 with anhydrous sodium sulfate, ascorbic acid, potassium chloride, sodium ascorbate and sodium chloride p. 50].
- *RoActemra*® preparations [tocilizumab p. 1068].
- *Rydapt*® [midostaurin p. 958].
- *Skudexa*® [tramadol with dexketoprofen p. 466].
- *Symtuza*® [darunavir with cobicistat, emtricitabine and tenofovir alafenamide p. 644].
- *Synagis*® [palivizumab p. 651].
- *Testogel*® 16.2 mg/g [testosterone gel p. 751].
- *Trelegy Ellipta*® [fluticasone with umeclidinium and vilanterol p. 264].
- *Tremfya*® [guselkumab p. 1224].
- *Vemlidy*® [tenofovir alafenamide p. 611].
- *Xylonor*® [lidocaine with cetrimide p. 1314].
- *Zejula*® [niraparib p. 972].

Guidance on prescribing

General guidance

Medicines should be prescribed only when they are necessary, and in all cases the benefit of administering the medicine should be considered in relation to the risk involved. This is particularly important during pregnancy, when the risk to both mother and fetus must be considered. It is important to discuss treatment options carefully with the patient to ensure that the patient is content to take the medicine as prescribed. In particular, the patient should be helped to distinguish the adverse effects of prescribed drugs from the effects of the medical disorder. When the beneficial effects of the medicine are likely to be delayed, the patient should be advised of this.

Prescribing competency framework The Royal Pharmaceutical Society has published a Prescribing Competency Framework that includes a common set of competencies that form the basis for prescribing, regardless of professional background. The competencies have been developed to help healthcare professionals to be safe and effective prescribers, with the aim of supporting patients to get the best outcomes from their medicines. It is available at www.rpharms.com/resources/frameworks/prescribers-competency-framework.

Multimorbidity

The presence of two or more long-term health conditions in a patient (multimorbidity) is associated with reduced quality of life, higher mortality, higher rates of adverse drug reactions, greater use of the health service, and a higher treatment burden (due to polypharmacy or multiple appointments). EvGr Treatment decisions in these patients should involve consideration of the patient's needs, preferences for treatment, health priorities, and lifestyle with the aim of improving quality of life by reducing treatment burden, adverse events, and unplanned or uncoordinated care.

Prescribers should consider the risks and benefits of treatments recommended for patients with multimorbidity from guidance for single health conditions; evidence for these recommendations is commonly drawn from patients without multimorbidity or who are taking fewer prescribed regular medicines.

Treatments intended to relieve symptoms should be reviewed for effectiveness, including reducing or stopping the treatment and monitoring the effects. Alternatively, non-pharmacological treatments may be offered or treatments of limited benefit can be considered for discontinuation. ⒶThe management of risk factors for future disease can be a major treatment burden for patients with multimorbidity and is not always appropriate.

Deprescribing

Deprescribing is the process of discontinuing or reducing the dose of medicines, supervised by a healthcare professional, with the aim of managing polypharmacy and improving outcomes. Deprescribing requires careful counselling and shared decision-making with patients, and is considered part of routine clinical care.

Taking medicines to best effect

Difficulties in adherence to drug treatment occur regardless of age. Factors contributing to poor compliance with prescribed medicines include:

- prescription not collected or not dispensed;
- purpose of medicine not clear;
- perceived lack of efficacy;

- real or perceived adverse effects;
- patients' perception of the risk and severity of side-effects may differ from that of the prescriber;
- instructions for administration not clear;
- physical difficulty in taking medicines (e.g. swallowing the medicine, handling small tablets, or opening medicine containers);
- unattractive formulation (e.g. unpleasant taste);
- complicated regimen.

The prescriber and the patient should agree on the health outcomes that the patient desires and on the strategy for achieving them ('concordance'). The prescriber should be sensitive to religious, cultural, and personal beliefs that can affect a patient's acceptance of medicines.

Taking the time to explain to the patient (and relatives) the rationale and the potential adverse effects of treatment may improve adherence. Reinforcement and elaboration of the physician's instructions by the pharmacist and other members of the healthcare team also helps. Advising the patient of the possibility of alternative treatments may encourage the patient to seek advice rather than merely abandon unacceptable treatment.

Simplifying the drug regimen may help; the need for frequent administration may reduce adherence, although there appears to be little difference in adherence between once-daily and twice-daily administration. Combination products reduce the number of drugs taken but at the expense of the ability to titrate individual doses.

Biological medicines

Biological medicines are medicines that are made by or derived from a biological source using biotechnology processes, such as recombinant DNA technology. The size and complexity of biological medicines, as well as the way they are produced, may result in a degree of natural variability in molecules of the same active substance, particularly in different batches of the medicine. This variation is maintained within strict acceptable limits. Examples of biological medicines include insulins and monoclonal antibodies. EvGr Biological medicines must be prescribed by brand name and the brand name specified on the prescription should be dispensed in order to avoid inadvertent switching. Automatic substitution of brands at the point of dispensing is not appropriate for biological medicines. Ⓐ

Biosimilar medicines

A **biosimilar medicine** is a biological medicine that is highly similar and clinically equivalent (in terms of quality, safety, and efficacy) to an existing biological medicine that has already been authorised in the European Union (known as the reference biological medicine or originator medicine). The active substance of a biosimilar medicine is similar, but not identical, to the originator biological medicine. Once the patent for a biological medicine has expired, a biosimilar medicine may be authorised by the European Medicines Agency (EMA). A biosimilar medicine is not the same as a generic medicine, which contains a simpler molecular structure that is identical to the originator medicine.

Therapeutic equivalence EvGr Biosimilar medicines should be considered to be therapeutically equivalent to the originator biological medicine within their authorised indications. Ⓐ Biosimilar medicines are usually licensed for all the indications of the originator biological medicine, but this depends on the evidence submitted to the EMA for

Guidance on prescribing

authorisation and must be scientifically justified on the basis of demonstrated or extrapolated equivalence.

Prescribing and dispensing The choice of whether to prescribe a biosimilar medicine or the originator biological medicine rests with the clinician in consultation with the patient. EvGr Biological medicines (including biosimilar medicines) must be prescribed by brand name and the brand name specified on the prescription should be dispensed in order to avoid inadvertent switching. Automatic substitution of brands at the point of dispensing is not appropriate for biological medicines. A

Safety monitoring Biosimilar medicines are subject to a black triangle status (▼) at the time of initial authorisation. EvGr It is important to report suspected adverse reactions using the Yellow Card Scheme (see Adverse reactions to drugs p. 12). For all biological medicines, adverse reaction reports should clearly state the brand name and the batch number of the suspected medicine. A

UK Medicines Information centres have developed a validated tool to determine potential safety issues associated with all new medicines. These 'in-use product safety assessment reports' will be published for new biosimilar medicines as they become available, see www.sps.nhs.uk/home/medicines/.

National funding/access decisions The Department of Health has confirmed that, in England, NICE can decide to apply the same remit, and the resulting technology appraisal guidance, to relevant biosimilar medicines which appear on the market subsequent to their originator biological medicine. In other circumstances, where a review of the evidence for a particular biosimilar medicine is necessary, NICE will consider producing an evidence summary (see *Evidence summary: new medicines*, www.nice.org.uk/about/what-we-do/our-programmes/nice-advice/evidence-summaries-new-medicines).

National information In England, see www.nice.org.uk/Media/Default/About/what-we-do/NICE-guidance/NICE-technology-appraisals/biosimilars-statement.pdf.
In Northern Ireland, see niformulary.hscni.net/ManagedEntry/bios/Pages/default.aspx.
In Scotland, see www.scottishmedicines.org.uk/About_SMC/Policy_statements/Biosimilar_Medicines.
In Wales, see www.wales.nhs.uk/sites3/Documents/814/BIOSIMILARS-ABUHBpositionStatement%5BNov2015%5D.pdf.

Availability The following drugs are available as a biosimilar medicine:

- Adalimumab p. 1073
- Bevacizumab p. 841
- Enoxaparin sodium p. 131
- Epoetin alfa p. 981
- Epoetin zeta p. 983
- Etanercept p. 1078
- Filgrastim p. 997
- Follitropin alfa p. 728
- Infliximab p. 1082
- Insulin glargine p. 701
- Insulin lispro p. 698
- Rituximab p. 859
- Somatropin p. 731
- Teriparatide p. 716

Complementary and alternative medicine

An increasing amount of information on complementary and alternative medicine is becoming available. The scope of the BNF is restricted to the discussion of conventional medicines but reference is made to complementary treatments if they affect conventional therapy (e.g. interactions with St John's wort). Further information on herbal medicines is available at www.mhra.gov.uk.

Abbreviation of titles

In general, titles of drugs and preparations should be written in full. Unofficial abbreviations should not be used as they may be misinterpreted.

Non-proprietary titles

Where non-proprietary ('generic') titles are given, they should be used in prescribing. This will enable any suitable product to be dispensed, thereby saving delay to the patient and sometimes expense to the health service. The only exception is where there is a demonstrable difference in clinical effect between each manufacturer's version of the formulation, making it important that the patient should always receive the same brand; in such cases, the brand name or the manufacturer should be stated. Non-proprietary titles should not be invented for the purposes of prescribing generically since this can lead to confusion, particularly in the case of compound and modified-release preparations. Titles used as headings for monographs may be used freely in the United Kingdom but in other countries may be subject to restriction.

Many of the non-proprietary titles used in this book are titles of monographs in the European Pharmacopoeia, British Pharmacopoeia, or British Pharmaceutical Codex 1973. In such cases the preparations must comply with the standard (if any) in the appropriate publication, as required by the Human Medicines Regulations 2012.

Proprietary titles

Names followed by the symbol® are or have been used as proprietary names in the United Kingdom. These names may in general be applied only to products supplied by the owners of the trade marks.

Marketing authorisation and BNF advice

In general the *doses, indications, cautions, contra-indications,* and *side-effects* in the BNF reflect those in the manufacturers' data sheets or Summaries of Product Characteristics (SPCs) which, in turn, reflect those in the corresponding marketing authorisations (formerly known as Product Licences). The BNF does not generally include proprietary medicines that are not supported by a valid Summary of Product Characteristics or when the marketing authorisation holder has not been able to supply essential information. When a preparation is available from more than one manufacturer, the BNF reflects advice that is the most clinically relevant regardless of any variation in the marketing authorisations. Unlicensed products can be obtained from 'special-order' manufacturers or specialist importing companies.

Where an unlicensed drug is included in the BNF, this is indicated in square brackets after the entry. When the BNF suggests a use (or route) that is outside the licensed indication of a product ('off-label' use), this too is indicated. Unlicensed use of medicines becomes necessary if the clinical need cannot be met by licensed medicines; such use should be supported by appropriate evidence and experience.

The doses stated in the BNF are intended for general guidance and represent, unless otherwise stated, the usual range of doses that are generally regarded as being suitable for adults.

Prescribing unlicensed medicines

Prescribing medicines outside the recommendations of their marketing authorisation alters (and probably increases) the prescriber's professional responsibility and potential liability. The prescriber should be able to justify and feel competent in using such medicines, and also inform the patient or the patient's carer that the prescribed medicine is unlicensed.

Oral syringes

An **oral syringe** is supplied when oral liquid medicines are prescribed in doses other than multiples of 5 mL. The oral syringe is marked in 0.5 mL divisions from 1 to 5 mL to measure doses of less than 5 mL (other sizes of oral syringe may also be available). It is provided with an adaptor and an instruction leaflet. The 5–*mL spoon* is used for doses of 5 mL (or multiples thereof).

Important To avoid inadvertent intravenous administration of oral liquid medicines, only an appropriate oral or enteral syringe should be used to measure an oral liquid medicine (if a medicine spoon or graduated measure cannot be used); these syringes should not be compatible with intravenous or other parenteral devices. Oral or enteral syringes should be clearly labelled 'Oral' or 'Enteral' in a large font size; it is the healthcare practitioner's responsibility to label the syringe with this information if the manufacturer has not done so.

Excipients

Branded oral liquid preparations that do not contain *fructose, glucose,* or *sucrose* are described as 'sugar-free' in the BNF. Preparations containing hydrogenated glucose syrup, mannitol, maltitol, sorbitol, or xylitol are also marked 'sugar-free' since there is evidence that they do not cause dental caries. Patients receiving medicines containing cariogenic sugars should be advised of appropriate dental hygiene measures to prevent caries. Sugar-free preparations should be used whenever possible.

Where information on the presence of *aspartame, gluten, sulfites, tartrazine, arachis (peanut) oil* or *sesame oil* is available, this is indicated in the BNF against the relevant preparation.

Information is provided on selected excipients in skin preparations, in vaccines, and on *selected preservatives* and *excipients* in eye drops and injections.

The presence of *benzyl alcohol* and *polyoxyl castor oil* (polyethoxylated castor oil) in injections is indicated in the BNF. Benzyl alcohol has been associated with a fatal toxic syndrome in preterm neonates, and therefore, parenteral preparations containing the preservative should not be used in neonates. Polyoxyl castor oils, used as vehicles in intravenous injections, have been associated with severe anaphylactoid reactions.

The presence of *propylene glycol* in oral or parenteral medicines is indicated in the BNF; it can cause adverse effects if its elimination is impaired, e.g. in renal failure, in neonates and young children, and in slow metabolisers of the substance. It may interact with disulfiram p. 489 and metronidazole p. 533.

The *lactose* content in most medicines is too small to cause problems in most lactose-intolerant patients. However in severe lactose intolerance, the lactose content should be determined before prescribing. The amount of lactose varies according to manufacturer, product, formulation, and strength.

Important In the absence of information on excipients in the BNF and in the product literature (available at www.medicines.org.uk/emc), contact the manufacturer (see Index of Proprietary Manufacturers) if it is essential to check details.

Extemporaneous preparation

A product should be dispensed extemporaneously only when no product with a marketing authorisation is available.

The BP direction that a preparation must be *freshly prepared* indicates that it must be made not more than 24 hours before it is issued for use. The direction that a preparation should be *recently prepared* indicates that deterioration is likely if the preparation is stored for longer than about 4 weeks at 15–25° C.

The term **water** used without qualification means either potable water freshly drawn direct from the public supply and suitable for drinking or freshly boiled and cooled purified water. The latter should be used if the public supply is from a local storage tank or if the potable water is unsuitable for a particular preparation (Water for injections).

Drugs and driving

Prescribers and other healthcare professionals should advise patients if treatment is likely to affect their ability to perform skilled tasks (e.g. driving). This applies especially to drugs with sedative effects; patients should be warned that these effects are increased by alcohol. General information about a patient's fitness to drive is available from the Driver and Vehicle Licensing Agency at www.dvla.gov.uk.

A new offence of driving, attempting to drive, or being in charge of a vehicle, with certain specified controlled drugs in excess of specified limits, came into force on 2nd March 2015. This offence is an addition to the existing rules on drug impaired driving and fitness to drive, and applies to two groups of drugs—commonly abused drugs, including amfetamines, cannabis, cocaine, and ketamine p. 1305, and drugs used mainly for medical reasons, such as opioids and benzodiazepines. Anyone found to have any of the drugs (including related drugs, for example, apomorphine hydrochloride p. 413) above specified limits in their blood will be guilty of an offence, whether their driving was impaired or not. This also includes prescribed drugs which metabolise to those included in the offence, for example, selegiline hydrochloride p. 423. However, the legislation provides a statutory "medical defence" for patients taking drugs for medical reasons in accordance with instructions, *if their driving was not impaired*—it continues to be an offence to drive if actually impaired. Patients should therefore be advised to continue taking their medicines as prescribed, and when driving, to carry suitable evidence that the drug was prescribed, or sold, to treat a medical or dental problem, and that it was taken according to the instructions given by the prescriber, or information provided with the medicine (e.g. a repeat prescription form or the medicine's patient information leaflet). Further information is available from the Department for Transport at www.gov.uk/government/collections/drug-driving.

Patents

In the BNF, certain drugs have been included notwithstanding the existence of actual or potential patent rights. In so far as such substances are protected by Letters Patent, their inclusion in this Formulary neither conveys, nor implies, licence to manufacture.

Health and safety

When handling chemical or biological materials particular attention should be given to the possibility of allergy, fire, explosion, radiation, or poisoning. Substances such as corticosteroids, some antimicrobials, phenothiazines, and many cytotoxics, are irritant or very potent and should be handled with caution. Contact with the skin and inhalation of dust should be avoided.

Safety in the home

Patients must be warned to keep all medicines out of the reach of children. All solid dose and all oral and external liquid preparations must be dispensed in a reclosable *child-resistant container* unless:

- the medicine is in an original pack or patient pack such as to make this inadvisable;
- the patient will have difficulty in opening a child-resistant container;
- a specific request is made that the product shall not be dispensed in a child-resistant container;

- no suitable child-resistant container exists for a particular liquid preparation.

All patients should be advised to dispose of *unwanted medicines* by returning them to a supplier for destruction.

Labelling of prescribed medicines

There is a legal requirement for the following to appear on the label of any prescribed medicine:

- name of the patient;
- name and address of the supplying pharmacy;
- date of dispensing;
- name of the medicine;
- directions for use of the medicine;
- precautions relating to the use of the medicine.

The Royal Pharmaceutical Society recommends that the following also appears on the label:

- the words 'Keep out of the sight and reach of children';
- where applicable, the words 'Use this medicine only on your skin'.

A pharmacist can exercise professional skill and judgement to amend or include more appropriate wording for the name of the medicine, the directions for use, or the precautions relating to the use of the medicine.

Non-proprietary names of compound preparations

Non-proprietary names of **compound preparations** which appear in the BNF are those that have been compiled by the British Pharmacopoeia Commission or another recognised body; whenever possible they reflect the names of the active ingredients.

Prescribers should avoid creating their own compound names for the purposes of generic prescribing; such names do not have an approved definition and can be misinterpreted.

Special care should be taken to avoid errors when prescribing compound preparations; in particular the hyphen in the prefix 'co-' should be retained.

Special care should also be taken to avoid creating generic names for **modified-release** preparations where the use of these names could lead to confusion between formulations with different lengths of action.

EEA and Swiss prescriptions

Pharmacists can dispense prescriptions issued by doctors and dentists from the European Economic Area (EEA) or Switzerland (except prescriptions for controlled drugs in Schedules 1, 2, or 3, or for drugs without a UK marketing authorisation). Prescriptions should be written in ink or otherwise so as to be indelible, should be dated, should state the name of the patient, should state the address of the prescriber, should contain particulars indicating whether the prescriber is a doctor or dentist, and should be signed by the prescriber.

Security and validity of prescriptions

The Councils of the British Medical Association and the Royal Pharmaceutical Society have issued a joint statement on the security and validity of prescriptions.

In particular, prescription forms should:

- not be left unattended at reception desks;
- not be left in a car where they may be visible; and
- when not in use, be kept in a locked drawer within the surgery and at home.

Where there is any doubt about the authenticity of a prescription, the pharmacist should contact the prescriber. If this is done by telephone, the number should be obtained from the directory rather than relying on the information on the prescription form, which may be false.

Patient group direction (PGD)

In most cases, the most appropriate clinical care will be provided on an individual basis by a prescriber to a specific individual patient. However, a Patient Group Direction for supply and administration of medicines by other healthcare professionals can be used where it would benefit patient care without compromising safety.

A Patient Group Direction is a written direction relating to the supply and administration (or administration only) of a licensed prescription-only medicine (including some Controlled Drugs in specific circumstances) by certain classes of healthcare professionals; the Direction is signed by a doctor (or dentist) and by a pharmacist. Further information on Patient Group Directions is available in Health Service Circular HSC 2000/026 (England), HDL (2001) 7 (Scotland), and WHC (2000) 116 (Wales); see also the Human Medicines Regulations 2012.

NICE, Scottish Medicines Consortium and All Wales Medicines Strategy Group

Advice issued by the National Institute for Health and Care Excellence (NICE), the Scottish Medicines Consortium (SMC) and the All Wales Medicines Strategy Group (AWMSG) is included in the BNF when relevant. Details of the advice together with updates can be obtained from: www.nice.org.uk, www.scottishmedicines.org.uk and www.awmsg.org.

Prescription writing

Shared care

In its guidelines on responsibility for prescribing (circular EL (91) 127) between hospitals and general practitioners, the Department of Health has advised that legal responsibility for prescribing lies with the doctor who signs the prescription.

Requirements

Prescriptions should be written legibly in ink or otherwise so as to be indelible (it is permissible to issue carbon copies of NHS prescriptions as long as they are signed in ink), should be dated, should state the name and address of the patient, the address of the prescriber, an indication of the type of prescriber, and should be signed in ink by the prescriber (computer-generated facsimile signatures do not meet the legal requirement). The age and the date of birth of the patient should preferably be stated, and it is a legal requirement in the case of prescription-only medicines to state the age for children under 12 years. These recommendations are acceptable for **prescription-only medicines**. Prescriptions for controlled drugs have additional legal requirements.

Wherever appropriate the prescriber should state the current weight of the child to enable the dose prescribed to be checked. Consideration should also be given to including the dose per unit mass e.g. mg/kg or the dose per m^2 body-surface area e.g. mg/m^2 where this would reduce error. The following should be noted:

- The strength or quantity to be contained in capsules, lozenges, tablets etc. should be stated by the prescriber. In particular, strength of liquid preparations should be clearly stated (e.g. 125 mg/5 mL).
- The unnecessary use of decimal points should be avoided, e.g. 3 mg, not 3.0 mg. Quantities of 1 gram or more should be written as 1 g etc. Quantities less than 1 gram should be written in milligrams, e.g. 500 mg, not 0.5 g. Quantities less than 1 mg should be written in micrograms, e.g. 100 micrograms, not 0.1 mg. When decimals are unavoidable a zero should be written in front of the decimal point where there is no other figure, e.g. 0.5 mL, not .5 mL. Use of the decimal point is acceptable to express a range, e.g. 0.5 to 1 g.
- 'Micrograms' and 'nanograms' should **not** be abbreviated. Similarly 'units' should **not** be abbreviated.
- The term 'millilitre' (ml or mL) is used in medicine and pharmacy, and cubic centimetre, c.c., or cm^3 should not be used. (The use of capital 'L' in mL is a printing convention throughout the BNF; both 'mL' and 'ml' are recognised SI abbreviations).
- Dose and dose frequency should be stated; in the case of preparations to be taken 'as required' a **minimum dose interval** should be specified. Care should be taken to ensure children receive the correct dose of the active drug. Therefore, the dose should normally be stated in terms of the mass of the active drug (e.g. '125 mg 3 times daily'); terms such as '5 mL' or '1 tablet' should be avoided except for compound preparations. When doses other than multiples of 5 mL are prescribed for *oral liquid preparations* the dose-volume will be provided by means of an **oral syringe**, (except for preparations intended to be measured with a pipette). Suitable quantities:
  - Elixirs, Linctuses, and Paediatric Mixtures (5-mL dose), 50, 100, or 150 mL
  - Adult Mixtures (10 mL dose), 200 or 300 mL
  - Ear Drops, Eye drops, and Nasal Drops, 10 mL (or the manufacturer's pack)
  - Eye Lotions, Gargles, and Mouthwashes, 200 mL
- The names of drugs and preparations should be written clearly and **not** abbreviated, using approved titles **only**;

avoid creating generic titles for modified-release preparations.

- The quantity to be supplied may be stated by indicating the number of days of treatment required in the box provided on NHS forms. In most cases the exact amount will be supplied. This does not apply to items directed to be used as required—if the dose and frequency are not given then the quantity to be supplied needs to be stated. When several items are ordered on one form the box can be marked with the number of days of treatment provided the quantity is added for any item for which the amount cannot be calculated.
- Although directions should preferably be in **English without abbreviation**, it is recognised that some Latin abbreviations are used.

Sample prescription

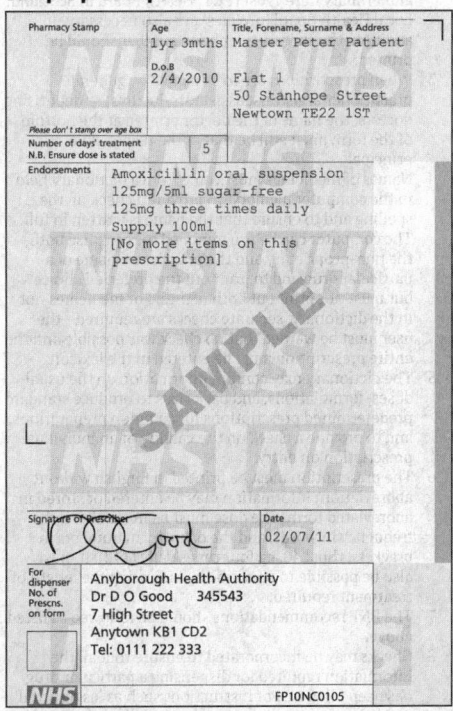

Prescribing by dentists

Until new prescribing arrangements are in place for NHS prescriptions, dentists should use form FP10D (GP14 in Scotland, WP10D in Wales) to prescribe only those items listed in the Dental Practitioners' Formulary. The Human Medicines Regulations 2012 does not set any limitations upon the number and variety of substances which the dentist may administer to patients in the surgery or may order by private prescription—provided the relevant legal requirements are observed the dentist may use or order whatever is required for the clinical situation. There is no statutory requirement for the dentist to communicate with a patient's medical practitioner when prescribing for dental use. There are, however, occasions when this would be in the patient's interest and such communication is to be encouraged. For legal requirements relating to prescriptions

Prescription writing

of Controlled Drugs, see Controlled drugs and drug dependence p. 8.

Computer-issued prescriptions

For computer-issued prescriptions the following advice, based on the recommendations of the Joint GP Information Technology Committee, should also be noted:

1 The computer must print out the date, the patient's surname, one forename, other initials, and address, and may also print out the patient's title and date of birth. The age of children under 12 years and of adults over 60 years must be printed in the box available; the age of children under 5 years should be printed in years and months. A facility may also exist to print out the age of patients between 12 and 60 years.

2 The doctor's name must be printed at the bottom of the prescription form; this will be the name of the doctor responsible for the prescription (who will normally sign it). The doctor's surgery address, reference number, and Primary Care Trust (PCT, Health Board in Scotland, Local Health Board in Wales) are also necessary. In addition, the surgery telephone number should be printed.

3 When prescriptions are to be signed by general practitioner registrars, assistants, locums, or deputising doctors, the name of the doctor printed at the bottom of the form must still be that of the responsible principal.

4 Names of medicines must come from a dictionary held in the computer memory, to provide a check on the spelling and to ensure that the name is written in full. The computer can be programmed to recognise both the non-proprietary and the proprietary name of a particular drug and to print out the preferred choice, but must not print out both names. For medicines not in the dictionary, separate checks are required—the user must be warned that no check was possible and the entire prescription must be entered in the lexicon.

5 The dictionary may contain information on the usual doses, formulations, and pack sizes to produce standard predetermined prescriptions for common preparations, and to provide a check on the validity of an individual prescription on entry.

6 The prescription must be printed in English without abbreviation; information may be entered or stored in abbreviated form. The dose must be in numbers, the frequency in words, and the quantity in numbers in brackets; thus: 40 mg four times daily (112). It must also be possible to prescribe by indicating the length of treatment required.

7 The BNF recommendations should be followed as listed above.

8 Checks may be incorporated to ensure that all the information required for dispensing a particular drug has been filled in. For instructions such as 'as directed' and 'when required', the maximum daily dose should normally be specified.

9 Numbers and codes used in the system for organising and retrieving data must never appear on the form.

10 Supplementary warnings or advice should be written in full, should not interfere with the clarity of the prescription itself, and should be in line with any warnings or advice in the BNF; numerical codes should not be used.

11 A mechanism (such as printing a series of nonspecific characters) should be incorporated to cancel out unused space, or wording such as 'no more items on this prescription' may be added after the last item. Otherwise the doctor should delete the space manually.

12 To avoid forgery the computer may print on the form the number of items to be dispensed (somewhere separate from the box for the pharmacist). The number of items per form need be limited only by the ability of the printer to produce clear and well-demarcated instructions with sufficient space for each item and a spacer line before each fresh item.

13 Handwritten alterations should only be made in exceptional circumstances—it is preferable to print out a new prescription. Any alterations must be made in the doctor's own handwriting and countersigned; computer records should be updated to fully reflect any alteration. Prescriptions for drugs used for contraceptive purposes (but which are not promoted as contraceptives) may need to be marked in handwriting with the symbol ♀, (or endorsed in another way to indicate that the item is prescribed for contraceptive purposes).

14 Prescriptions for controlled drugs can be printed from the computer, but the prescriber's signature must be handwritten (See Controlled Drugs and Drug Dependence; the prescriber may use a date stamp).

15 The strip of paper on the side of the FP10SS (GP10SS in Scotland, WP10SS in Wales) may be used for various purposes but care should be taken to avoid including confidential information. It may be advisable for the patient's name to appear at the top, but this should be preceded by 'confidential'.

16 In rural dispensing practices prescription requests (or details of medicines dispensed) will normally be entered in one surgery. The prescriptions (or dispensed medicines) may then need to be delivered to another surgery or location; if possible the computer should hold up to 10 alternatives.

17 Prescription forms that are reprinted or issued as a duplicate should be labelled clearly as such.

Emergency supply of medicines

Emergency supply requested by member of the public

Pharmacists are sometimes called upon by members of the public to make an emergency supply of medicines. The Human Medicines Regulations 2012 allows exemptions from the Prescription Only requirements for emergency supply to be made by a person lawfully conducting a retail pharmacy business provided:

a) that the pharmacist has interviewed the person requesting the prescription-only medicine and is satisfied:
   i) that there is immediate need for the prescription-only medicine and that it is impracticable in the circumstances to obtain a prescription without undue delay;
   ii) that treatment with the prescription-only medicine has on a previous occasion been prescribed for the person requesting it;
   iii) as to the dose that it would be appropriate for the person to take;

b) that no greater quantity shall be supplied than will provide 5 days' treatment of phenobarbital p. 331, *phenobarbital sodium*, or Controlled Drugs in Schedules 4 or 5 (doctors or dentists from the European Economic Area and Switzerland, or their patients, cannot request an emergency supply of Controlled Drugs in Schedules 1, 2, or 3, or drugs that do not have a UK marketing authorisation) or 30 days' treatment for other prescription-only medicines, except when the prescription-only medicine is:
   i) insulin, an ointment or cream, or a preparation for the relief of asthma in an aerosol dispenser when the smallest pack can be supplied;
   ii) an oral contraceptive when a full cycle may be supplied;
   iii) an antibiotic in liquid form for oral administration when the smallest quantity that will provide a full course of treatment can be supplied;

c) that an entry shall be made by the pharmacist in the prescription book stating:
   i) the date of supply;
   ii) the name, quantity and, where appropriate, the pharmaceutical form and strength;
   iii) the name and address of the patient;
   iv) the nature of the emergency;

d) that the container or package must be labelled to show:
   i) the date of supply;
   ii) the name, quantity and, where appropriate, the pharmaceutical form and strength;
   iii) the name of the patient;
   iv) the name and address of the pharmacy;
   v) the words 'Emergency supply';
   vi) the words 'Keep out of the reach of children' (or similar warning);

e) that the prescription-only medicine is not a substance specifically excluded from the emergency supply provision, and does not contain a Controlled Drug specified in Schedules 1, 2, or 3 to the Misuse of Drugs Regulations 2001 except for phenobarbital p. 331 or *phenobarbital sodium* for the treatment of epilepsy: for details see *Medicines, Ethics and Practice,* London, Pharmaceutical Press (always consult latest edition). Doctors or dentists from the European Economic Area and Switzerland, or their patients, cannot request an emergency supply of Controlled Drugs in Schedules 1, 2, or 3, or drugs that do not have a UK marketing authorisation.

Emergency supply requested by prescriber

Emergency supply of a prescription-only medicine may also be made at the request of a doctor, a dentist, a supplementary prescriber, a community practitioner nurse prescriber, a nurse, pharmacist, or optometrist independent prescriber, or a doctor or dentist from the European Economic Area or Switzerland, provided:

a) that the pharmacist is satisfied that the prescriber by reason of some emergency is unable to furnish a prescription immediately;
b) that the prescriber has undertaken to furnish a prescription within 72 hours;
c) that the medicine is supplied in accordance with the directions of the prescriber requesting it;
d) that the medicine is not a Controlled Drug specified in Schedules 1, 2, or 3 to the Misuse of Drugs Regulations 2001 except for phenobarbital p. 331 or *phenobarbital sodium* for the treatment of epilepsy: for details see *Medicines, Ethics and Practice,* London, Pharmaceutical Press (always consult latest edition); (Doctors or dentists from the European Economic Area and Switzerland, or their patients, cannot request an emergency supply of Controlled Drugs in Schedules 1, 2, or 3, or drugs that do not have a UK marketing authorisation).
e) that an entry shall be made in the prescription book stating:
   i) the date of supply;
   ii) the name, quantity and, where appropriate, the pharmaceutical form and strength;
   iii) the name and address of the practitioner requesting the emergency supply;
   iv) the name and address of the patient;
   v) the date on the prescription;
   vi) when the prescription is received the entry should be amended to include the date on which it is received.

Royal Pharmaceutical Society's guidelines

1. The pharmacist should consider the medical consequences of not supplying a medicine in an emergency.
2. If the pharmacist is unable to make an emergency supply of a medicine the pharmacist should advise the patient how to obtain essential medical care.

For conditions that apply to supplies made at the request of a patient see Medicines, Ethics and Practice, London Pharmaceutical Press, (always consult latest edition).

Controlled drugs and drug dependence

Regulations and classification

The Misuse of Drugs Act, 1971 as amended prohibits certain activities in relation to 'Controlled Drugs', in particular their manufacture, supply, and possession (except where permitted by the 2001 Regulations or under licence from the Secretary of State). The penalties applicable to offences involving the different drugs are graded broadly according to the *harmfulness attributable to a drug when it is misused* and for this purpose the drugs are defined in the following three classes:

- **Class A** includes: alfentanil p. 1304, cocaine, diamorphine hydrochloride (heroin) p. 449, dipipanone hydrochloride, fentanyl p. 451, lysergide (LSD), methadone hydrochloride p. 495, 3, 4-methylenedioxymethamfetamine (MDMA, 'ecstasy'), morphine p. 456, opium, oxycodone hydrochloride p. 459, pethidine hydrochloride p. 463, phencyclidine, remifentanil p. 1304, and class B substances when prepared for injection.
- **Class B** includes: oral amfetamines, barbiturates, cannabis, *Sativex* ®, codeine phosphate p. 448, dihydrocodeine tartrate p. 450, ethylmorphine, glutethimide, ketamine p. 1305, nabilone p. 425, pentazocine, phenmetrazine, and pholcodine p. 295.
- **Class C** includes: certain drugs related to the amfetamines such as benzfetamine and chlorphentermine, buprenorphine p. 442, mazindol, meprobamate, pemoline, pipradrol, most benzodiazepines, tramadol hydrochloride p. 464, zaleplon, zolpidem tartrate, zopiclone, androgenic and anabolic steroids, clenbuterol, chorionic gonadotrophin (HCG), non-human chorionic gonadotrophin, somatotropin, somatrem, and somatropin p. 731.

The Misuse of Drugs (Safe Custody) Regulations 1973 as amended details the storage and safe custody requirements for Controlled Drugs.

The Misuse of Drugs Regulations 2001 (and subsequent amendments) defines the classes of person who are authorised to supply and possess Controlled Drugs while acting in their professional capacities and lays down the conditions under which these activities may be carried out. In the 2001 regulations, drugs are divided into five Schedules, each specifying the requirements governing such activities as import, export, production, supply, possession, prescribing, and record keeping which apply to them.

- **Schedule 1** includes drugs not used medicinally such as hallucinogenic drugs (e.g. LSD), ecstasy-type substances, raw opium, and cannabis. A Home Office licence is generally required for their production, possession, or supply. A Controlled Drug register must be used to record details of any Schedule I Controlled Drugs received or supplied by a pharmacy.
- **Schedule 2** includes opiates (e.g. diamorphine hydrochloride (heroin) p. 449, morphine p. 456, methadone hydrochloride p. 495, oxycodone hydrochloride p. 459, pethidine hydrochloride p. 463), major stimulants (e.g. amfetamines), quinalbarbitone (secobarbital), cocaine and ketamine p. 1305. Schedule 2 Controlled Drugs are subject to the full Controlled Drug requirements relating to prescriptions, safe custody (except for quinalbarbitone (secobarbital) and some liquid preparations), and the need to keep a Controlled Drug register, (unless exempted in Schedule 5). Possession, supply and procurement is authorised for pharmacists and other classes of persons named in the 2001 Regulations.
- **Schedule 3** includes the barbiturates (except secobarbital, now Schedule 2), buprenorphine p. 442, mazindol, meprobamate, midazolam p. 336,

pentazocine, phentermine, temazepam p. 481, and tramadol hydrochloride p. 464. They are subject to the special prescription requirements. Safe custody requirements do apply, except for any 5,5 disubstituted barbituric acid (e.g. phenobarbital), mazindol, meprobamate, midazolam p. 336, pentazocine, phentermine, tramadol hydrochloride p. 464, or any stereoisomeric form or salts of the above. Records in registers do not need to be kept (although there are requirements for the retention of invoices for 2 years).

- **Schedule 4** includes in Part I drugs that are subject to minimal control, such as benzodiazepines (except temazepam p. 481 and midazolam p. 336, which are in Schedule 3), non-benzodiazepine hypnotics (zaleplon, zolpidem tartrate, and zopiclone) and *Sativex* ®. Part II includes androgenic and anabolic steroids, clenbuterol, chorionic gonadotrophin (HCG), non-human chorionic gonadotrophin, somatotropin, somatrem, and somatropin p. 731. Controlled drug prescription requirements do not apply and Schedule 4 Controlled Drugs are not subject to safe custody requirements. Records in registers do not need to be kept (except in the case of *Sativex* ®).
- **Schedule 5** includes preparations of certain Controlled Drugs (such as codeine, pholcodine p. 295 or morphine p. 456) which due to their low strength, are exempt from virtually all Controlled Drug requirements other than retention of invoices for two years.

Since the Responsible Pharmacist Regulations were published in 2008, standing operation procedures for the management of Controlled Drugs, are required in registered pharmacies.

The Health Act 2006 introduced the concept of the 'accountable officer' with responsibility for the management of Controlled Drugs and related governance issues in their organisation. Most recently, in 2013 The Controlled Drugs (Supervision of Management and Use) Regulations were published to ensure good governance concerning the safe management and use of Controlled Drugs in England and Scotland.

Prescriptions

Preparations in Schedules 1, 2, 3, 4 and 5 of the Misuse of Drugs Regulations 2001 (and subsequent amendments) are identified throughout the BNF and BNF *for children* using the following symbols:

CD1	for preparations in Schedule 1
CD2	for preparations in Schedule 2
CD3	for preparations in Schedule 3
CD4-1	for preparations in Schedule 4 (Part I)
CD4-2	for preparations in Schedule 4 (Part II)
CD5	for preparations in Schedule 5

The principal legal requirements relating to medical prescriptions are listed below (see also Department of Health Guidance at www.gov.uk/dh).

Prescription requirements Prescriptions for Controlled Drugs that are subject to prescription requirements (all preparations in Schedules 2 and 3) must be indelible, must be *signed* by the prescriber, include the *date* on which they were signed, and specify the prescriber's *address* (must be within the UK). A machine-written prescription is acceptable, but the prescriber's signature must be handwritten. Advanced electronic signatures can be accepted for Schedule 2 and 3 Controlled Drugs where the Electronic Prescribing Service (EPS) is used. All prescriptions for Controlled Drugs that are subject to the prescription requirements must always state:

- the name and address of the patient (use of a PO Box is not acceptable);
- in the case of a preparation, the form (the dosage form e.g. tablets must be included on a Controlled Drugs prescription irrespective of whether it is implicit in the proprietary name e.g. *MST Continus*, or whether only one form is available), and, where appropriate, the strength of the preparation (when more than one strength of a preparation exists the strength required must be specified); to avoid ambiguity, where a prescription requests multiple strengths of a medicine, each strength should be prescribed separately (i.e. separate dose, total quantity, etc);
- for liquids, the total volume in millilitres (in both words and figures) of the preparation to be supplied; for dosage units (tablets, capsules, ampoules), state the total number (in both words and figures) of dosage units to be supplied (e.g. 10 tablets [of 10 mg] rather than 100 mg total quantity);
- the dose, which must be clearly defined (i.e. the instruction 'one as directed' constitutes a dose but 'as directed' does not); it is not necessary that the dose is stated in both words and figures;
- the words 'for dental treatment only' if issued by a dentist.

A pharmacist is **not** allowed to dispense a Controlled Drug unless all the information required by law is given on the prescription. In the case of a prescription for a Controlled Drug in Schedule 2 or 3, a pharmacist can amend the prescription *if* it specifies the total quantity only in words or in figures or if it contains minor typographical errors, provided that such amendments are indelible and clearly attributable to the pharmacist (e.g. name, date, signature and GPhC registration number). The prescription should be marked with the date of supply at the time the Controlled Drug supply is made.

The Department of Health and the Scottish Government have issued a strong recommendation that the maximum quantity of Schedule 2, 3 or 4 Controlled Drugs prescribed should not exceed 30 days; exceptionally, to cover a justifiable clinical need and after consideration of any risk, a prescription can be issued for a longer period, but the reasons for the decision should be recorded on the patient's notes.

A prescription for a Controlled Drug in Schedules 2, 3, or 4 is valid for 28 days from the date stated thereon (the prescriber may forward-date the prescription; the start date may also be specified in the body of the prescription). Schedule 5 prescriptions are valid for 6 months from the appropriate date.

Medicines that are not Controlled Drugs should not be prescribed on the same form as a Schedule 2 or 3 Controlled Drug.

See sample prescription:

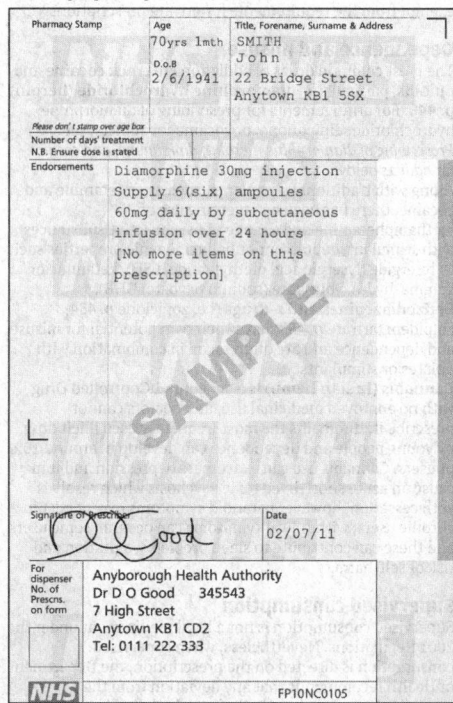

Instalments and repeatable prescriptions Prescriptions for Schedule 2 or 3 Controlled Drugs can be dispensed by instalments. An instalment prescription must have an instalment direction including both the dose and the instalment amount specified separately on the prescription, and it must also state the interval between each time the medicine can be supplied.

The first instalment must be dispensed within 28 days of the appropriate day (i.e. date of signing unless the prescriber indicates a date before which the Controlled Drug should not be dispensed) and the remainder should be dispensed in accordance with the instructions on the prescription. The prescription must be marked with the date of each supply. The instalment direction is a legal requirement and needs to be complied with, however, for certain situations (e.g. if a pharmacy is closed on the day an instalment is due) the Home Office has approved specific wording which provides pharmacists some flexibility for supply. For details, see Medicines, Ethics and Practice, London, Pharmaceutical Press (always consult latest edition) or see Home Office approved wording for instalment prescribing (Circular 027/2015), available at www.gov.uk/.

Repeatable prescriptions are prescriptions which contain a direction that they can be dispensed more than once (e.g. repeat × 3). Only Schedule 4 and 5 Controlled Drugs are permitted on repeatable prescriptions.

Private prescriptions Private prescriptions for Controlled Drugs in Schedules 2 and 3 must be written on specially designated forms which are provided by local NHS England area teams in England (form FP10PCD), local NHS Health Boards in Scotland (form PPCD) and Wales (form W10PCD); in addition, prescriptions must specify the *prescriber's identification number* (or a NHS prescriber code in Scotland).

Prescriptions to be supplied by a pharmacist in hospital are exempt from the requirements for private prescriptions.

Dependence and misuse

The most common drugs of addiction are **crack cocaine** and **opioids**, particularly **diamorphine hydrochloride (heroin) p. 449**. For arrangements for prescribing of diamorphine hydrochloride, dipipanone, or cocaine for addicts, see *Prescribing of diamorphine (heroin), dipipanone, and cocaine for addicts* below.

Along with traditional stimulants, such as amfetamine and cocaine, there has been an emerging use of methamphetamine and a range of psychoactive substances with stimulant, depressant or hallucinogenic properties such as lysergide (lysergic acid diethylamide, LSD), ketamine or gamma-hydroxybutyrate (sodium oxybate, GHB). **Benzodiazepines and z-drugs** (i.e. zopiclone p. 484, zolpidem tartrate p. 483) have their own potential for misuse and dependence and are often taken in combination with opiates or stimulants.

Cannabis (Indian hemp) is a Schedule 1 Controlled Drug with no approved medicinal use, and doctors cannot prescribe it. It remains the most frequently used illicit drug by young people and dependence can develop in around 10% of users. Cannabis use can exacerbate depression and it may cause an acute short-lived toxic psychosis which resolves with cessation, however paranoid symptoms may persist in chronic users; withdrawal symptoms can occur in some users and these can contribute to sleep problems, agitation and risk of self-harm.

Supervised consumption

Supervised consumption is not a legal requirement under the 2001 Regulations. Nevertheless, when supervised consumption is directed on the prescription, the Department of Health recommends that any deviation from the prescriber's intended method of supply should be documented and the justification for this recorded. Individuals prescribed opioid substitution therapy can take their daily dose under the supervision of a doctor, nurse, or pharmacist during the dose stabilisation phase (usually the first 3 months of treatment), after a relapse or period of instability, or if there is a significant increase in the dose of methadone. Supervised consumption should continue (in accordance with local protocols) until the prescriber is confident that the patient is compliant with their treatment. It is good practice for pharmacists to alert the prescriber when a patient has missed consecutive daily doses.

Prescribing drugs likely to cause dependence or misuse

The prescriber has three main responsibilities:

- To avoid creating dependence by introducing drugs to patients without sufficient reason. In this context, the proper use of the morphine-like drugs is well understood. The dangers of other Controlled Drugs are less clear because recognition of dependence is not easy and its effects, and those of withdrawal, are less obvious.
- To see that the patient does not gradually increase the dose of a drug, given for good medical reasons, to the point where dependence becomes more likely. This tendency is seen especially with hypnotics and anxiolytics. The prescriber should keep a close eye on the amount prescribed to prevent patients from accumulating stocks. A minimal amount should be prescribed in the first instance, or when seeing a patient for the first time.
- To avoid being used as an unwitting source of supply for addicts and being vigilant to methods for obtaining medicines. Methods include visiting more than one doctor, fabricating stories, and forging prescriptions.

Patients under temporary care should be given only small supplies of drugs unless they present an unequivocal letter from their own doctor. Doctors should also remember that their own patients may be attempting to collect prescriptions from other prescribers, especially in hospitals. It is sensible to reduce dosages steadily or to issue weekly or even daily prescriptions for small amounts if it is apparent that dependence is occurring.

Prescribers are responsible for the security of prescription forms once issued to them. The stealing and misuse of prescription forms could be minimised by the following precautions:

- records of serial numbers received and issued should be retained for at least three years;
- blank prescriptions should never be pre-signed;
- prescription forms should not be left unattended and should be locked in a secure drawer, cupboard, or carrying case when not in use;
- doctors', dentists' and surgery stamps should be kept in a secure location separate from the prescription forms;
- alterations are best avoided but if any are made and the prescription is to be used, best practice is for the prescriber to cross out the error, initial and date the error, then write the correct information;
- if an error made in a prescription cannot be corrected, best practice for the prescriber is to put a line through the script and write 'spoiled' on the form, or destroy the form and start writing a new prescription;
- prescribers and pharmacists dispensing drugs prone to abuse should ensure compliance with all relevant legal requirements specially when dealing with prescriptions for Controlled Drugs (see *Prescription requirements* and *Instalments* above);
- at the time of dispensing, prescriptions should be stamped with the pharmacy stamp and endorsed by the pharmacist or pharmacy technician with what has been supplied; where loss or theft is suspected, the police should be informed immediately.

Travelling abroad

Prescribed drugs listed in Schedule 4 Part II (CD Anab) for self-administration and Schedule 5 of the Misuse of Drugs Regulations 2001 (and subsequent amendments) are not subject to export or import licensing. A personal import/export licence is required for patients travelling abroad with Schedules 2, 3, or 4 Part I (CD Benz) and Part II (CD Anab) Controlled Drugs if, they are carrying more than 3 months' supply or are travelling for 3 calendar months or more. A Home Office licence is required for any amount of a Schedule 1 Controlled Drug imported into the UK for personal use regardless of the duration of travel. Further details can be obtained at www.gov.uk/guidance/controlled-drugs-licences-fees-and-returns or from the Home Office by contacting DFLU.ie@homeoffice.gsi.gov.uk. In cases of emergency, telephone (020) 7035 6330.

Applications for obtaining a licence must be supported by a cover letter signed by the prescribing doctor or drug worker, which must confirm:

- the patient's name and address;
- the travel itinerary;
- the names of the prescribed Controlled Drug(s), doses and total amounts to be carried.

Applications for licences should be sent to the Home Office, Drugs & Firearms Licensing Unit, Fry Building, 2 Marsham Street, London, SW1P 4DF.

Alternatively, completed application forms can be emailed to DFLU.ie@homeoffice.gsi.gov.uk. A minimum of 10 days should be allowed for processing the application.

Patients travelling for less than 3 months or carrying less than 3 months supply of Controlled Drugs do not require a personal export/import licence, but are advised to carry a cover letter signed by the prescribing doctor or drug worker.

Those travelling for more than 3 months are advised to make arrangements to have their medication prescribed by a practitioner in the country they are visiting.

Doctors who want to take Controlled Drugs abroad while accompanying patients may similarly be issued with licences. Licences are not normally issued to doctors who want to take Controlled Drugs abroad solely in case a family emergency should arise.

Personal export/import licences do not have any legal status outside the UK and are issued only to comply with the Misuse of Drugs Act 2001 and to facilitate passage through UK Customs and Excise control. For clearance in the country to be visited it is necessary to approach that country's consulate in the UK.

Notification of patients receiving structured drug treatment for substance dependence

In **England**, doctors should report cases where they are providing structured drug treatment for substance dependence to their local National Drug Treatment Monitoring System (NDTMS) Team. General information about NDTMS can be found at www.nta.nhs.uk/ndtms.aspx. Enquiries about NDTMS, and how to submit data, should initially be directed to:

- EvidenceApplicationteam@phe.gov.uk

In **Scotland**, doctors should report cases to the Substance Drug Misuse Database. General information about the Scottish Drug Misuse Database can be found in www.isdscotland.org/Health-Topics/Drugs-and-Alcohol-Misuse/Drugs-Misuse/Scottish-Drug-Misuse-Database/. Enquiries about reporting can be directed to:

- nss.isdsubstancemisuse@nhs.net

In **Northern Ireland**, the Misuse of Drugs (Notification of and Supply to Addicts) (Northern Ireland) Regulations 1973 require doctors to send particulars of persons whom they consider to be addicted to certain Controlled Drugs to the Chief Medical Officer of the Ministry of Health and Social Services. The Northern Ireland contact is:

Public Health Information & Research Branch
Department of Health,
Annexe 2,
Castle Buildings,
Stormont,
Belfast
BT4 3SQ
Tel: 028 9052 2340
phirb@health-ni.gov.uk

Public Health Information & Research Branch also maintains the Northern Ireland Drug Misuse Database (NIDMD) which collects detailed information on those presenting for treatment, on drugs misused and injecting behaviour; participation is not a statutory requirement.

In **Wales**, doctors should report cases where they are providing structured drug treatment for substance dependence on the Welsh National Database for Substance Misuse; enquiries should be directed to: substancemisuse-queries@wales.nhs.uk.

Prescribing of diamorphine (heroin), dipipanone, and cocaine for addicts

The Misuse of Drugs (Supply to Addicts) Regulations 1997 require that **only** medical practitioners who hold a special licence issued by the Home Secretary (or Scottish Government's Chief Medical Officer) may prescribe, administer, or supply diamorphine hydrochloride p. 449, dipipanone, or cocaine for *the treatment of drug addiction*. Medical prescribers, pharmacists independent prescribers, nurses independent prescribers and supplementary prescribers do not require a special licence for prescribing diamorphine hydrochloride p. 449, dipipanone, or cocaine for patients (including addicts) for relieving pain from organic disease or injury.

Adverse reactions to drugs

Yellow card scheme

Any drug may produce unwanted or unexpected adverse reactions. Rapid detection and recording of adverse drug reactions is of vital importance so that unrecognised hazards are identified promptly and appropriate regulatory action is taken to ensure that medicines are used safely. Healthcare professionals and coroners are urged to report suspected adverse drug reactions directly to the Medicines and Healthcare products Regulatory Agency (MHRA) through the Yellow Card Scheme using the electronic form at www.mhra. gov.uk/yellowcard. Alternatively, prepaid Yellow Cards for reporting are available from the address below and are also bound in the inside back cover of the *BNF*.

Send Yellow Cards to:

FREEPOST YELLOW CARD
(No other address details required).
Tel: 0800 731 6789

Suspected adverse drug reactions to any therapeutic agent should be reported, including drugs (*self-medication* as well as those *prescribed*), blood products, vaccines, radiographic contrast media, complementary and herbal products. For biosimilar medicines and vaccines, adverse reaction reports should clearly state the brand name and the batch number of the suspected medicine or vaccine.

Suspected adverse drug reactions should be reported through the Yellow Card Scheme at www.mhra.gov.uk/ yellowcard. Yellow Cards can be used for reporting suspected adverse drug reactions to medicines, vaccines, herbal or complementary products, whether self-medicated or prescribed. This includes suspected adverse drug reactions associated with misuse, overdose, medication errors or from use of unlicensed and off-label medicines. Yellow Cards can also be used to report medical device incidents, defective medicines, and suspected fake medicines.

Spontaneous reporting is particularly valuable for recognising possible new hazards rapidly. An adverse reaction should be reported even if it is not certain that the drug has caused it, or if the reaction is well recognised, or if other drugs have been given at the same time. Reports of overdoses (deliberate or accidental) can complicate the assessment of adverse drug reactions, but provide important information on the potential toxicity of drugs.

A freephone service is available to all parts of the UK for advice and information on suspected adverse drug reactions; contact the National Yellow Card Information Service at the MHRA on 0800 731 6789. Outside office hours a telephone-answering machine will take messages.

The following Yellow Card Centres can be contacted for further information:

Yellow Card Centre Northwest
2nd Floor, 70 Pembroke Place, Liverpool, L69 3GF
Tel: (0151) 794 8122

Yellow Card Centre Wales
All Wales Therapeutics and Toxicology Centre, Academic Building, University Hospital Llandough, Penlan Road, Penarth, Vale of Glamorgan, CF64 2XX
Tel: (029) 2074 5831

Yellow Card Centre Northern & Yorkshire
Regional Drug and Therapeutics Centre, 16/17 Framlington Place, Newcastle upon Tyne, NE2 4AB
Tel: (0191) 213 7855

Yellow Card Centre West Midlands
City Hospital, Dudley Road, Birmingham, B18 7QH
Tel: (0121) 507 5672

Yellow Card Centre Scotland
CARDS, Royal Infirmary of Edinburgh, 51 Little France Crescent, Old Dalkeith Road, Edinburgh, EH16 4SA
Tel: (0131) 242 2919
YCCScotland@luht.scot.nhs.uk

The MHRA's database facilitates the monitoring of adverse drug reactions. More detailed information on reporting and a list of products currently under additional monitoring can be found on the MHRA website: www.mhra.gov.uk.

MHRA Drug Safety Update *Drug Safety Update* is a monthly newsletter from the MHRA and the Commission on Human Medicines (CHM); it is available at www.gov.uk/drug-safety-update.

Self-reporting

Patients and their carers can also report suspected adverse drug reactions to the MHRA. Reports can be submitted directly to the MHRA through the Yellow Card Scheme using the electronic form at www.mhra.gov.uk/yellowcard, by telephone on 0808 100 3352, or by downloading the Yellow Card form from www.mhra.gov.uk. Alternatively, patient Yellow Cards are available from pharmacies and GP surgeries. Information for patients about the Yellow Card Scheme is available in other languages at www.mhra.gov.uk/ yellowcard.

Prescription-event monitoring

In addition to the MHRA's Yellow Card Scheme, an independent scheme monitors the safety of new medicines using a different approach. The Drug Safety Research Unit identifies patients who have been prescribed selected new medicines and collects data on clinical events in these patients. The data are submitted on a voluntary basis by general practitioners on green forms. More information about the scheme and the Unit's educational material is available from www.dsru.org.

Newer drugs and vaccines

Only limited information is available from clinical trials on the safety of new medicines. Further understanding about the safety of medicines depends on the availability of information from routine clinical practice.

The black triangle symbol identifies newly licensed medicines that require additional monitoring by the European Medicines Agency. Such medicines include new active substances, biosimilar medicines, and medicines that the European Medicines Agency consider require additional monitoring. The black triangle symbol also appears in the Patient Information Leaflets for relevant medicines, with a brief explanation of what it means. Products usually retain a black triangle for 5 years, but this can be extended if required.

Spontaneous reporting is particularly valuable for recognising possible new hazards rapidly. For medicines showing the black triangle symbol, the MHRA asks that **all** suspected reactions (including those considered not to be serious) are reported through the Yellow Card Scheme. An adverse reaction should be reported even if it is not certain that the drug has caused it, or if the reaction is well recognised, or if other drugs have been given at the same time.

Established drugs and vaccines

Healthcare professionals and coroners are asked to report all suspected reactions to established drugs (including over-the-counter, herbal, and unlicensed medicines and medicines used off-label) and vaccines that are **serious, medically significant, or result in harm**. Serious reactions include those that are fatal, life-threatening, disabling, incapacitating, or which result in or prolong hospitalisation, or a congenital abnormality; they should be reported even if the effect is well recognised. Examples include anaphylaxis, blood disorders, endocrine disturbances, effects on fertility, haemorrhage from any site, renal impairment, jaundice, ophthalmic disorders, severe CNS effects, severe skin reactions, reactions in pregnant women, and any drug interactions. Reports of serious adverse reactions are required to enable comparison with other drugs of a similar class. Reports of overdoses (deliberate or accidental) can complicate the assessment of adverse drug reactions, but provide important information on the potential toxicity of drugs.

For established drugs there is no need to report well-known, relatively minor side-effects, such as dry mouth with tricyclic antidepressants or constipation with opioids.

Medication errors

Adverse drug reactions where harm occurs as a result of a medication error are reportable as a Yellow Card or through the local risk management systems into the National Reporting and Learning System (NRLS). If reported to the NRLS, these will be shared with the MHRA. If the NRLS is not available and harm occurs, report using a Yellow Card.

Adverse reactions to medical devices

Suspected adverse reactions to medical devices including dental or surgical materials, intra-uterine devices, and contact lens fluids should be reported. Information on reporting these can be found at: www.mhra.gov.uk.

Side-effects in the BNF

The BNF includes clinically relevant side-effects for most drugs; an exhaustive list is not included for drugs that are used by specialists (e.g. cytotoxic drugs and drugs used in anaesthesia). Where causality has not been established, side-effects in the manufacturers' literature may be omitted from the BNF.

Recognising that hypersensitivity reactions (including anaphylactic and anaphylactoid reactions) can occur with virtually all drugs, this effect is not generally listed, unless the drug carries an increased risk of such reactions or specific management advice is provided by the manufacturer. Administration site reactions have been omitted from the BNF (e.g. pain at injection site). The BNF also omits effects that are likely to have little clinical consequence (e.g. transient increase in liver enzymes). Drugs that are applied locally or topically carry a theoretical or low risk of systemic absorption and therefore systemic side-effects for these drugs are not listed in the BNF unless they are associated with a high risk to patient safety. Infections are a known complication of treatment with drugs that affect the immune system (e.g. corticosteroids or immunosuppressants); this side-effect is listed in the BNF as 'increased risk of infection'. Symptoms of drug withdrawal reactions are not individually listed, but are collectively termed 'withdrawal syndrome'. Side-effects are generally listed alphabetically in order of frequency. In the product literature the frequency of side-effects is generally described as follows:

Description of the frequency of side-effects	
Very common	greater than 1 in 10
Common	1 in 100 to 1 in 10
Uncommon [formerly 'less commonly' in BNF publications]	1 in 1000 to 1 in 100
Rare	1 in 10 000 to 1 in 1000
Very rare	less than 1 in 10 000
Frequency not known	frequency is not defined by product literature or the side-effect has been reported from post-marketing surveillance data

For consistency, the terms used to describe side-effects are standardised using a defined vocabulary across all of the drug monographs in the BNF (e.g. postural hypotension is used for the term orthostatic hypotension).

Special problems

Delayed drug effects Some reactions (e.g. cancers, chloroquine retinopathy, and retroperitoneal fibrosis) may become manifest months or years after exposure. Any suspicion of such an association should be reported directly to the MHRA through the Yellow Card Scheme.

The elderly Particular vigilance is required to identify adverse reactions in the elderly.

Congenital abnormalities When an infant is born with a congenital abnormality or there is a malformed aborted fetus doctors are asked to consider whether this might be an adverse reaction to a drug and to report all drugs (including self-medication) taken during pregnancy.

Children Particular vigilance is required to identify and report adverse reactions in children, including those resulting from the unlicensed use of medicines; all suspected reactions should be reported directly to the MHRA through the Yellow Card Scheme (see also Adverse Drug Reactions in Children).

Prevention of adverse reactions

Adverse reactions may be prevented as follows:

- never use any drug unless there is a good indication. If the patient is pregnant do not use a drug unless the need for it is imperative;
- allergy and idiosyncrasy are important causes of adverse drug reactions. Ask if the patient had previous reactions to the drug or formulation;
- ask if the patient is already taking other drugs including self-medication drugs, health supplements, complementary and alternative therapies; interactions may occur;
- age and hepatic or renal disease may alter the metabolism or excretion of drugs, so that much smaller doses may be needed. Genetic factors may also be responsible for variations in metabolism, and therefore for the adverse effect of the drug; notably of isoniazid p. 576 and the tricyclic antidepressants;
- prescribe as few drugs as possible and give very clear instructions to the elderly or any patient likely to misunderstand complicated instructions;
- whenever possible use a familiar drug; with a new drug, be particularly alert for adverse reactions or unexpected events;
- consider if excipients (e.g. colouring agents) may be contributing to the adverse reaction. If the reaction is minor, a trial of an alternative formulation of the same drug may be considered before abandoning the drug;
- warn the patient if serious adverse reactions are liable to occur.

Adverse reactions to drugs

Drug allergy (suspected or confirmed)

Suspected drug allergy is any reaction caused by a drug with clinical features compatible with an immunological mechanism. All drugs have the potential to cause adverse drug reactions, but not all of these are allergic in nature. A reaction is more likely to be caused by drug allergy if:

- The reaction occurred while the patient was being treated with the drug, or
- The drug is known to cause this pattern of reaction, or
- The patient has had a similar reaction to the same drug or drug-class previously.

A suspected reaction is less likely to be caused by a drug allergy if there is a possible non-drug cause or if there are only gastro-intestinal symptoms present.

The following signs, allergic patterns and timing of onset can be used to help decide whether to suspect drug allergy:

Immediate, rapidly-evolving reactions (onset usually less than 1 hour after drug exposure)

- Anaphylaxis, with erythema, urticaria or angioedema, and hypotension and/or bronchospasm. See also Antihistamines, allergen immunotherapy and allergic emergencies p. 276
- Urticaria or angioedema without systemic features
- Exacerbation of asthma e.g. with non-steroidal anti-inflammatory drugs (NSAIDs)

*Non-immediate reactions, **without** systemic involvement* (onset usually 6–10 days after first drug exposure or 3 days after second exposure)

- Cutaneous reactions, e.g. widespread red macules and/or papules, or, fixed drug eruption (localised inflamed skin)

*Non-immediate reactions, **with** systemic involvement* (onset may be variable, usually 3 days to 6 weeks after first drug exposure, depending on features, or 3 days after second exposure)

- Cutaneous reactions with systemic features, e.g. drug reaction with eosinophilia and systemic signs (DRESS) or drug hypersensitivity syndrome (DHS), characterised by widespread red macules, papules or erythroderma, fever, lymphadenopathy, liver dysfunction or eosinophilia
- Toxic epidermal necrolysis or Stevens–Johnson syndrome
- Acute generalised exanthematous pustulosis (AGEP)

EvGr Suspected drug allergy information should be clearly and accurately documented in clinical notes and prescriptions, and shared among all healthcare professionals. Patients should be given information about which drugs and drug-classes to avoid and encouraged to share their drug allergy status.

If a drug allergy is suspected, consider stopping the suspected drug and advising the patient or carer to avoid this drug in future. Symptoms of the acute reaction should be treated, in hospital if severe. Patients presenting with a suspected anaphylactic reaction, or a severe or non-immediate cutaneous reaction, should be referred to a specialist drug allergy service. Patients presenting with a suspected drug allergic reaction or anaphylaxis to NSAIDs, and local and general anaesthetics may also need to be referred to a specialist drug allergy service, e.g. in cases of anaphylactoid reactions or to determine future treatment options. Patients presenting with a suspected drug allergic reaction or anaphylaxis associated with beta-lactam antibiotics should be referred to a specialist drug allergy service if their disease or condition can only be treated by a beta-lactam antibiotic or they are likely to need beta-lactam antibiotics frequently in the future (e.g. immunodeficient patients). Ⓐ For further information see Drug allergy: diagnosis and management. NICE Clinical Guideline 183 (September 2014) www.nice.org.uk/guidance/cg183.

Oral side-effects of drugs

Drug-induced disorders of the mouth may be due to a local action on the mouth or to a systemic effect manifested by oral changes. In the latter case urgent referral to the patient's medical practitioner may be necessary.

Oral mucosa Medicaments left in contact with or applied directly to the oral mucosa can lead to inflammation or ulceration; the possibility of allergy should also be borne in mind.

Aspirin tablets p. 121 allowed to dissolve in the sulcus for the treatment of toothache can lead to a white patch followed by ulceration.

Flavouring agents, particularly **essential oils**, may sensitise the skin, but mucosal swelling is not usually prominent.

The oral mucosa is particularly vulnerable to ulceration in patients treated with cytotoxic drugs, e.g. methotrexate p. 888. Other drugs capable of causing oral ulceration include **ACE inhibitors, gold, nicorandil p. 211, NSAIDs, pancreatin p. 96, penicillamine p. 1063, proguanil hydrochloride p. 607,** and **protease inhibitors.**

Erythema multiforme or Stevens-Johnson syndrome may follow the use of a wide range of drugs including **antibacterials, antiretrovirals, sulfonamide derivatives,** and **anticonvulsants;** the oral mucosa may be extensively ulcerated, with characteristic target lesions on the skin. Oral lesions of toxic epidermal necrolysis have been reported with a similar range of drugs.

Lichenoid eruptions are associated with **ACE inhibitors, NSAIDs,** methyldopa p. 144, chloroquine p. 604, **oral antidiabetics, thiazide diuretics,** and **gold.**

Candidiasis can complicate treatment with **antibacterials** and **immunosuppressants** and is an occasional side-effect of **corticosteroid inhalers.**

Teeth and jaw *Brown staining* of the teeth frequently follows the use of chlorhexidine mouthwash, spray or gel p. 1175, but can readily be removed by polishing. **Iron** salts in liquid form can stain the enamel black. Superficial staining has been reported rarely with co-amoxiclav suspension p. 542. *Intrinsic staining* of the teeth is most commonly caused by **tetracyclines.** They will affect the teeth if given at any time from about the fourth month *in utero* until the age of twelve years; they are contra-indicated during pregnancy, in breast-feeding women, and in children under 12 years. All tetracyclines can cause permanent, unsightly staining in children, the colour varying from yellow to grey.

Excessive ingestion of **fluoride** leads to *dental fluorosis* with mottling of the enamel and areas of hypoplasia or pitting; fluoride supplements occasionally cause mild mottling (white patches) if the dose is too large for the child's age (taking into account the fluoride content of the local drinking water and of toothpaste).

The risk of *osteonecrosis of the jaw* is substantially greater for patients receiving intravenous bisphosphonates in the treatment of cancer than for patients receiving oral bisphosphonates for osteoporosis or Paget's disease. All patients receiving bisphosphonates should have a dental check-up (and any necessary remedial work should be performed) before bisphosphonate treatment, or as soon as possible after starting treatment. Patients with cancer receiving bevacizumab p. 841 or sunitinib p. 967 may also be at risk of osteonecrosis of the jaw.

Periodontium *Gingival overgrowth* (gingival hyperplasia) is a side-effect of phenytoin p. 321 and sometimes of ciclosporin p. 818 or of nifedipine p. 162 (and some other calcium-channel blockers).

Thrombocytopenia may be drug related and may cause bleeding at the gingival margins, which may be spontaneous or may follow mild trauma (such as toothbrushing).

Salivary glands The most common effect that drugs have on the salivary glands is to *reduce flow* (xerostomia). Patients with a persistently dry mouth may have poor oral hygiene;

they are at an increased risk of dental caries and oral infections (particularly candidiasis). Many drugs have been implicated in xerostomia, particularly **antimuscarinics** (anticholinergics), **antidepressants** (including tricyclic antidepressants, and selective serotonin re-uptake inhibitors), **alpha-blockers, antihistamines, antipsychotics, baclofen p. 1092, bupropion hydrochloride p. 491, clonidine hydrochloride p. 144, 5HT$_1$ agonists, opioids**, and tizanidine p. 1094. Excessive use of **diuretics** can also result in xerostomia.

Some drugs (e.g. clozapine p. 392, neostigmine p. 1090) can *increase saliva production* but this is rarely a problem unless the patient has associated difficulty in swallowing.

Pain in the salivary glands has been reported with some **antihypertensives** (e.g. clonidine hydrochloride p. 144, methyldopa p. 144) and with **vinca alkaloids**.

Swelling of the salivary glands can occur with **iodides, antithyroid drugs, phenothiazines**, and **sulfonamides**.

Taste There can be *decreased* taste acuity or *alteration* in taste sensation. Many drugs are implicated, including amiodarone hydrochloride p. 105, **calcitonin, ACE inhibitors**, carbimazole p. 754, clarithromycin p. 529, **gold**, griseofulvin p. 590, **lithium salts**, metformin hydrochloride p. 678, metronidazole p. 533, penicillamine p. 1063, phenindione p. 139, propafenone hydrochloride p. 104, **protease inhibitors**, terbinafine p. 1200, and zopiclone p. 484.

Defective medicines

During the manufacture or distribution of a medicine an error or accident may occur whereby the finished product does not conform to its specification. While such a defect may impair the therapeutic effect of the product and could adversely affect the health of a patient, it should **not** be confused with an Adverse Drug Reaction where the product conforms to its specification.

The Defective Medicines Report Centre assists with the investigation of problems arising from licensed medicinal products thought to be defective and co-ordinates any necessary protective action. Reports on suspect defective medicinal products should include the brand or the non-proprietary name, the name of the manufacturer or supplier, the strength and dosage form of the product, the product licence number, the batch number or numbers of the product, the nature of the defect, and an account of any action already taken in consequence. The Centre can be contacted at:

The Defective Medicines Report Centre
Medicines and Healthcare products Regulatory Agency,
151 Buckingham Palace Road, London, SW1W 9SZ
Tel: (020) 3080 6574
dmrc@mhra.gsi.gov.uk

Guidance on intravenous infusions

Intravenous additives policies

A local policy on the addition of drugs to intravenous fluids should be drawn up by a multi-disciplinary team and issued as a document to the members of staff concerned. Centralised additive services are provided in a number of hospital pharmacy departments and should be used in preference to making additions on wards.

The information that follows should be read in conjunction with local policy documents.

Guidelines

- Drugs should only be added to infusion containers when constant plasma concentrations are needed or when the administration of a more concentrated solution would be harmful.
- In general, only one drug should be added to any infusion container and the components should be compatible. Ready-prepared solutions should be used whenever possible. Drugs should not normally be added to blood products, mannitol, or sodium bicarbonate. Only specially formulated additives should be used with fat emulsions or amino-acid solutions.
- Solutions should be thoroughly mixed by shaking and checked for absence of particulate matter before use.
- Strict asepsis should be maintained throughout and in general the giving set should not be used for more than 24 hours (for drug admixtures).
- The infusion container should be labelled with the patient's name, the name and quantity of additives, and the date and time of addition (and the new expiry date or time). Such additional labelling should not interfere with information on the manufacturer's label that is still valid. When possible, containers should be retained for a period after use in case they are needed for investigation.
- It is good practice to examine intravenous infusions from time to time while they are running. If cloudiness, crystallisation, change of colour, or any other sign of interaction or contamination is observed the infusion should be discontinued.

Problems

Microbial contamination The accidental entry and subsequent growth of micro-organisms converts the infusion fluid pathway into a potential vehicle for infection with micro-organisms, particularly species of *Candida*, *Enterobacter*, and *Klebsiella*. Ready-prepared infusions containing the additional drugs, or infusions prepared by an additive service (when available) should therefore be used in preference to making extemporaneous additions to infusion containers on wards etc. However, when this is necessary strict aseptic procedure should be followed.

Incompatibility Physical and chemical incompatibilities may occur with loss of potency, increase in toxicity, or other adverse effect. The solutions may become opalescent or precipitation may occur, but in many instances there is no visual indication of incompatibility. Interaction may take place at any point in the infusion fluid pathway, and the potential for incompatibility is increased when more than one substance is added to the infusion fluid.

Common incompatibilities Precipitation reactions are numerous and varied and may occur as a result of pH, concentration changes, 'salting-out' effects, complexation or other chemical changes. Precipitation or other particle formation must be avoided since, apart from lack of control of dosage on administration, it may initiate or exacerbate adverse effects. This is particularly important in the case of drugs which have been implicated in either thrombophlebitis (e.g. diazepam) or in skin sloughing or necrosis caused by extravasation (e.g. sodium bicarbonate and certain cytotoxic drugs). It is also especially important to effect solution of colloidal drugs and to prevent their subsequent precipitation in order to avoid a pyrogenic reaction (e.g. amphotericin). It is considered undesirable to mix beta-lactam antibiotics, such as semi-synthetic penicillins and cephalosporins, with proteinaceous materials on the grounds that immunogenic and allergenic conjugates could be formed.

A number of preparations undergo significant loss of potency when added singly or in combination to large volume infusions. Examples include ampicillin in infusions that contain glucose or lactates. The breakdown products of dacarbazine have been implicated in adverse effects.

Blood Because of the large number of incompatibilities, drugs should not normally be added to blood and blood products for infusion purposes. Examples of incompatibility with blood include hypertonic mannitol solutions (irreversible crenation of red cells), dextrans (rouleaux formation and interference with cross-matching), glucose (clumping of red cells), and oxytocin (inactivated). If the giving set is not changed after the administration of blood, but used for other infusion fluids, a fibrin clot may form which, apart from blocking the set, increases the likelihood of microbial growth.

Intravenous fat emulsions These may break down with coalescence of fat globules and separation of phases when additions such as antibacterials or electrolytes are made, thus increasing the possibility of embolism. Only specially formulated products such as *Vitlipid N*® may be added to appropriate intravenous fat emulsions.

Other infusions Infusions that frequently give rise to incompatibility include amino acids, mannitol, and sodium bicarbonate.

Bactericides Bactericides such as chlorocresol 0.1% or phenylmercuric nitrate 0.001% are present in some injection solutions. The total volume of such solutions added to a container for infusion on one occasion should not exceed 15 mL.

Method

Ready-prepared infusions should be used whenever available. **Potassium chloride** is usually available in concentrations of 20, 27, and 40 mmol/litre in sodium chloride intravenous infusion (0.9%), glucose intravenous infusion (5%) or sodium chloride and glucose intravenous infusion. **Lidocaine hydrochloride** is usually available in concentrations of 0.1 or 0.2% in glucose intravenous infusion (5%).

When addition is required to be made extemporaneously, any product reconstitution instructions such as those relating to concentration, vehicle, mixing, and handling precautions should be strictly followed using an aseptic technique throughout. Once the product has been reconstituted, addition to the infusion fluid should be made immediately in order to minimise microbial contamination and, with certain products, to prevent degradation or other formulation change which may occur; e.g. reconstituted ampicillin injection degrades rapidly on standing, and also may form polymers which could cause sensitivity reactions. It is also important in certain instances that an infusion fluid of specific pH be used (e.g. **furosemide** injection requires dilution in infusions of pH greater than 5.5).

When drug additions are made it is important to mix thoroughly; additions should not be made to an infusion container that has been connected to a giving set, as mixing is hampered. If the solutions are not thoroughly mixed a concentrated layer of the additive may form owing to differences in density. **Potassium chloride** is particularly prone to this 'layering' effect when added without adequate mixing to infusions packed in non-rigid infusion containers; if such a mixture is administered it may have a serious effect on the heart.

A time limit between addition and completion of administration must be imposed for certain admixtures to guarantee satisfactory drug potency and compatibility. For admixtures in which degradation occurs without the formation of toxic substances, an acceptable limit is the time taken for 10% decomposition of the drug. When toxic substances are produced stricter limits may be imposed. Because of the risk of microbial contamination a maximum time limit of 24 hours may be appropriate for additions made elsewhere than in hospital pharmacies offering central additive service.

Certain injections must be protected from light during continuous infusion to minimise oxidation, e.g. dacarbazine and sodium nitroprusside.

Dilution with a small volume of an appropriate vehicle and administration using a motorised infusion pump is advocated for preparations such as unfractionated heparin where strict control over administration is required. In this case the appropriate dose may be dissolved in a convenient volume (e.g. 24–48 mL) of sodium chloride intravenous infusion (0.9%).

Information provided in the *BNF*

The *BNF* gives information about preparations given by three methods:

- continuous infusion;
- intermittent infusion;
- addition via the drip tubing.

Drugs for **continuous infusion** must be diluted in a large volume infusion. Penicillins and cephalosporins are not usually given by continuous infusion because of stability problems and because adequate plasma and tissue concentrations are best obtained by intermittent infusion. Where it is necessary to administer them by continuous infusion, detailed literature should be consulted.

Drugs that are both compatible and clinically suitable may be given by **intermittent infusion** in a relatively small volume of infusion over a short period of time, e.g. 100 mL in 30 minutes. The method is used if the product is incompatible or unstable over the period necessary for continuous infusion; the limited stability of ampicillin or amoxicillin in large volume glucose or lactate infusions may be overcome in this way.

Intermittent infusion is also used if adequate plasma and tissue concentrations are not produced by continuous infusion as in the case of drugs such as dacarbazine, gentamicin, and ticarcillin.

An in-line burette may be used for intermittent infusion techniques in order to achieve strict control over the time and rate of administration, especially for infants and children and in intensive care units. Intermittent infusion may also make use of the 'piggy-back' technique provided that no additions are made to the primary infusion. In this method the drug is added to a small secondary container connected to a Y-type injection site on the primary infusion giving set; the secondary solution is usually infused within 30 minutes.

Addition *via* the drip tubing is indicated for a number of cytotoxic drugs in order to minimise extravasation. The preparation is added aseptically via the rubber septum of the injection site of a fast-running infusion. In general, drug preparations intended for a bolus effect should be given directly into a separate vein where possible. Failing this, administration may be made via the drip tubing provided that the preparation is compatible with the infusion fluid when given in this manner.

Drugs given by intravenous infusion The BNF includes information on addition to *Glucose intravenous infusion* 5 and 10%, and *Sodium chloride intravenous infusion* 0.9%. Compatibility with glucose 5% and with sodium chloride 0.9% indicates compatibility with *Sodium chloride and glucose intravenous infusion*. Infusion of a large volume of hypotonic solution should be avoided therefore care should be taken if water for injections is used. The information relates to the proprietary preparations indicated; for other preparations suitability should be checked with the manufacturer.

Prescribing in children

Overview

For detailed advice on medicines used for children, consult *BNF for Children*.

Children, and particularly neonates, differ from adults in their response to drugs. Special care is needed in the neonatal period (first 28 days of life) and doses should always be calculated with care. At this age, the risk of toxicity is increased by reduced drug clearance and differing target organ sensitivity.

Whenever possible, intramuscular injections should be **avoided** in children because they are painful.

Where possible, medicines for children should be prescribed within the terms of the marketing authorisation (product licence). However, many children may require medicines not specifically licensed for paediatric use.

Although medicines cannot be promoted outside the limits of the licence, the Human Medicines Regulations 2012 does not prohibit the use of unlicensed medicines. It is recognised that the informed use of unlicensed medicines or of licensed medicines for unlicensed applications ('off-label' use) is often necessary in paediatric practice.

Adverse drug reactions in children

Suspected adverse drug reactions in children and young adults under 18 years should be reported through the Yellow Card Scheme. Yellow cards can be used for reporting suspected adverse drug reactions to medicines, vaccines, herbal or complementary products, whether self-medicated or prescribed. This includes suspected adverse drug reactions associated with misuse, overdose, medication errors or from use of unlicensed and off-label medicines. Yellow Cards can also be used to report medical device incidents, defective medicines, and suspected fake medicines.

Report all suspected adverse drug reactions that are:

- **serious, medically significant or result in harm.** Serious events are fatal, life-threatening, a congenital abnormality, disabling or incapacitating, or resulting in hospitalisation;
- associated with **newer drugs and vaccines;** the most up to date list of black triangle medicines is available at: www.mhra.gov.uk/blacktriangle

If in doubt whether to report a suspected adverse drug reaction, please complete a Yellow Card.

The identification and reporting of adverse reactions to drugs in children and neonates is particularly important because:

- the action of the drug and its pharmacokinetics in children (especially in the very young) may be different from that in adults;
- drugs may not have been extensively tested in children;
- many drugs are not specifically licensed for use in children and are used either 'off-label' or as unlicensed products;
- drugs may affect the way a child grows and develops or may cause delayed adverse reactions which do not occur in adults;
- suitable formulations may not be available to allow precise dosing in children or they may contain excipients that should be used with caution in children;
- the nature and course of illnesses and adverse drug reactions may differ between adults and children.

Even if reported through the British Paediatric Surveillance Unit's Orange Card Scheme, any identified suspected adverse drug reactions should also be submitted to the Yellow Card Scheme.

Adverse drug reactions where harm occurs as a result of a medication error are reportable as a Yellow Card or through the local risk management systems into the National Reporting and Learning System (NRLS). If reported to the NRLS, these will be shared with the MHRA. If the NRLS is not available and harm occurs, report using a Yellow Card.

Prescription writing

Prescriptions should be written according to the guidelines in Prescription Writing. Inclusion of age is a legal requirement in the case of prescription-only medicines for children under 12 years of age, but it is preferable to state the age for **all** prescriptions for children.

It is particularly important to state the strengths of capsules or tablets. Although liquid preparations are particularly suitable for children, they may contain sugar which encourages dental decay. Sugar-free medicines are preferred for long-term treatment.

Many children are able to swallow tablets or capsules and may prefer a solid dose form; involving the child and parents in choosing the formulation is helpful.

When a prescription for a liquid oral preparation is written and the dose ordered is smaller than 5 mL an **oral syringe** will be supplied. Parents should be advised not to add any medicines to the infant's feed, since the drug may interact with the milk or other liquid in it; moreover the ingested dosage may be reduced if the child does not drink all the contents.

Parents must be warned to keep **all** medicines out of reach of children.

Rare paediatric conditions

Information on substances such as *biotin* and *sodium benzoate* used in rare metabolic conditions is included in *BNF for Children*; further information can be obtained from:

Alder Hey Children's Hospital
Drug Information Centre, Liverpool, L12 2AP
Tel: (0151) 252 5381

Great Ormond Street Hospital for Children
Pharmacy, Great Ormond St, London, WC1N 3JH
Tel: (020) 7405 9200

Dosage in children

Children's doses in the BNF are stated in the individual drug entries.

Doses are generally based on body-weight (in kilograms) or specific age ranges. In the BNF and BNF for *Children*, the term neonate is used to describe a newborn infant aged 0–28 days. The terms child or children are used generically to describe the entire range from infant to adolescent (1 month–17 years). An age range is specified when the dose information applies to a narrower age range than a child from 1 month–17 years.

Dose calculation

Many children's doses are standardised by **weight** (and therefore require multiplying by the body-weight in kilograms to determine the child's dose); occasionally, the doses have been standardised by **body surface area** (in m²). These methods should be used rather than attempting to calculate a child's dose on the basis of doses used in adults. For most drugs the adult maximum dose should not be exceeded. For example if the dose is stated as 8 mg/kg (max. 300 mg), a child weighing 10 kg should receive 80 mg but a child weighing 40 kg should receive 300 mg (rather than 320 mg).

Young children may require a higher dose per kilogram than adults because of their higher metabolic rates. Other problems need to be considered. For example, calculation by body-weight in the overweight child may result in much higher doses being administered than necessary; in such cases, dose should be calculated from an ideal weight, related to height and age.

Body surface area (BSA) estimates are sometimes preferable to body-weight for calculation of paediatric doses since many physiological phenomena correlate better with body surface area. Body surface area can be estimated from weight. For more information, refer to *BNF for Children*. Where the dose for children is not stated, prescribers should consult *BNF for Children* or seek advice from a medicines information centre.

Dose frequency

Antibacterials are generally given at regular intervals throughout the day. Some flexibility should be allowed in children to avoid waking them during the night. For example, the night-time dose may be given at the child's bedtime.

Where new or potentially toxic drugs are used, the manufacturers' recommended doses should be carefully followed.

Prescribing in hepatic impairment

Overview

Liver disease may alter the response to drugs in several ways as indicated below, and drug prescribing should be kept to a minimum in all patients with severe liver disease. The main problems occur in patients with jaundice, ascites, or evidence of encephalopathy.

Impaired drug metabolism

Metabolism by the liver is the main route of elimination for many drugs, but hepatic reserve is large and liver disease has to be severe before important changes in drug metabolism occur. Routine liver-function tests are a poor guide to the capacity of the liver to metabolise drugs, and in the individual patient it is not possible to predict the extent to which the metabolism of a particular drug may be impaired. A few drugs, e.g. rifampicin p. 571 and fusidic acid p. 561, are excreted in the bile unchanged and can accumulate in patients with intrahepatic or extrahepatic obstructive jaundice.

Hypoproteinaemia

The hypoalbuminaemia in severe liver disease is associated with reduced protein binding and increased toxicity of some highly protein-bound drugs such as phenytoin p. 321 and prednisolone p. 664.

Reduced clotting

Reduced hepatic synthesis of blood-clotting factors, indicated by a prolonged prothrombin time, increases the sensitivity to oral anticoagulants such as warfarin sodium p. 139 and phenindione p. 139.

Hepatic encephalopathy

In severe liver disease many drugs can further impair cerebral function and may precipitate hepatic encephalopathy. These include all sedative drugs, opioid analgesics, those diuretics that produce hypokalaemia, and drugs that cause constipation.

Fluid overload

Oedema and ascites in chronic liver disease can be exacerbated by drugs that give rise to fluid retention e.g. NSAIDs and corticosteroids.

Hepatotoxic drugs

Hepatotoxicity is either dose-related or unpredictable (idiosyncratic). Drugs that cause dose-related toxicity may do so at lower doses in the presence of hepatic impairment than in individuals with normal liver function, and some drugs that produce reactions of the idiosyncratic kind do so more frequently in patients with liver disease. These drugs should be avoided or used very carefully in patients with liver disease.

Where care is needed when prescribing in hepatic impairment, this is indicated under the relevant drug in the BNF.

Prescribing in renal impairment

Issues encountered in renal impairment

The use of drugs in patients with reduced renal function can give rise to problems for several reasons:

- reduced renal excretion of a drug or its metabolites may cause toxicity;
- sensitivity to some drugs is increased even if elimination is unimpaired;
- many side-effects are tolerated poorly by patients with renal impairment;
- some drugs are not effective when renal function is reduced.

Many of these problems can be avoided by reducing the dose or by using alternative drugs.

If even mild renal impairment is considered likely on clinical grounds, renal function should be checked before prescribing any drug which requires dose modification.

General guidance

Where care is needed when prescribing in renal impairment, this is indicated under the relevant drug monograph in the BNF.

When both efficacy and toxicity are closely related to plasma-drug concentration, recommended regimens should be regarded only as a guide to initial treatment; subsequent doses must be adjusted according to clinical response and plasma-drug concentration.

Dose recommendations are based on the severity of renal impairment. The total daily maintenance dose of a drug can be reduced either by reducing the size of the individual doses or by increasing the interval between doses.

For some drugs, although the size of the maintenance dose is reduced it is important to give a loading dose if an immediate effect is required. This is because it takes about five times the half-life of the drug to achieve steady-state plasma concentrations. Because the plasma half-life of drugs excreted by the kidney is prolonged in renal impairment it can take many doses for the reduced dosage to achieve a therapeutic plasma concentration.

Important: dosage adjustment advice in the BNF Clinical laboratories routinely report renal function in adults based on *estimated glomerular filtration rate* (eGFR) normalised to a body surface area of 1.73 m². This is derived from either the Chronic Kidney Disease Epidemiology Collaboration (CKD-EPI) formula or the Modification of Diet in Renal disease (MDRD) formula.

However, in product literature, the effects of renal impairment on drug elimination is usually stated in terms of *creatinine clearance* as a surrogate for GFR.

The information on dosage adjustment in the BNF is *usually* expressed in terms of eGFR. Exceptions to the use of eGFR include toxic drugs, in elderly patients and in patients at extremes of muscle mass (see *Estimating renal function in patients at extremes of muscle mass* and *Estimating renal function in elderly patients*, below) where calculation of CrCl is recommended. Although these two measures of renal function are not interchangeable, for most drugs and for most adult patients of average build and height, eGFR (rather than CrCl) can be used to determine dosage adjustments.

Nephrotoxic drugs Nephrotoxic drugs should, if possible, be avoided in patients with renal disease because the consequences of nephrotoxicity are likely to be more serious when renal reserve is already reduced. During intercurrent illness the risk of acute kidney injury is increased in patients with an eGFR of less than 60 mL/min/1.73 m²; potentially nephrotoxic or renally excreted drugs may require dose reduction or temporary discontinuation.

Renal replacement therapy and transplantation For prescribing in patients who have received a renal transplant or who are on renal replacement therapy (peritoneal dialysis or haemodialysis), consult specialist literature.

Estimating renal function

Direct measure of Glomerular filtration rate (GFR) using plasma or urinary clearance is considered the best overall index of renal function. However, this is difficult to do in practice.

As an alternative, the *estimated* Glomerular filtration rate (eGFR) based on serum creatinine is used to assess renal function. Creatinine clearance (CrCl) is also used as an estimate of GFR.

Various equations for estimating glomerular filtration rate exist, however there is no compelling evidence to support the superiority of any given method for drug dosing in *all* patient populations or clinical situations. There is also insufficient evidence to provide *definitive* guidance about dosage adjustment of all drugs in patients with reduced renal function. Therefore, an understanding of drug pharmacokinetics is necessary in order to make appropriate dosing decisions.

Using serum creatinine to derive eGFR has a number of limitations; serum creatinine levels are dependent on muscle mass and diet, therefore estimates should be interpreted with caution in certain individuals (such as the elderly, body builders, amputees, in muscle-wasting disorders and vegans)—estimates will be higher or lower than the true value. Creatinine-derived measurements are also **not** useful in periods of rapidly changing renal function or in patients with AKI.

Estimated glomerular filtration rate

Chronic Kidney Disease Epidemiology Collaboration (CKD-EPI) formula The CKD-EPI formula is the recommended method for estimating GFR and calculating drug doses in **most** patients with renal impairment.

CKD-EPI is adjusted for body surface area (BSA) and utilises serum creatinine, age, sex and race as variables. Clinical laboratories should use the CKD-EPI formula to routinely report eGFR.

CKD-EPI equation

$$\text{eGFR (ml/min/1.73 m}^2) = 141 \times \min(S_{Cr}/K, 1)^{\alpha} \times \max(S_{Cr}/K, 1)^{-1.209} \times 0.993^{Age}[\times 1.018 \text{ if female}] [\times 1.159 \text{ if black}]$$

Where:
- S_{Cr} = serum creatinine in mg/dL;
- K = 0.7 for females and 0.9 for males;
- α = -0.329 for females and -0.411 for males;
- $\min(S_{Cr}/K, 1)$ indicates the minimum of S_{Cr}/K or 1;
- $\max(S_{Cr}/K, 1)$ indicates the maximum of S_{Cr}/K or 1.

Modification of Diet in Renal disease (MDRD) The MDRD formula, like CKD-EPI, is expressed in terms of body surface area. It is less accurate than the CKD-EPI formula when eGFR is greater than 60 mL/min/1.73 m². It also overestimates GFR in elderly patients.

Estimated creatinine clearance

Cockcroft and Gault The Cockcroft and Gault formula is the preferred method for estimating renal function or calculating drug doses in patients with renal impairment who are elderly or at extremes of muscle mass (see below); it provides an estimate of CrCl (which is not equivalent to eGFR).

$$\text{Estimated Creatinine Clearance in mL/minute} = \frac{(140 - \text{Age}) \times \text{Weight} \times \text{Constant}}{\text{Serum creatinine}}$$

- Age in years
- Weight in kilograms (use ideal body weight where fat is likely to be the major contributor to body mass)
- Serum creatinine in micromol/litre
- Constant = 1.23 for men; 1.04 for women

Estimating renal function in patients at extremes of muscle mass In patients at both extremes of muscle mass, eGFR should be interpreted with caution. Reduced muscle mass will lead to overestimation of GFR and increased muscle mass will lead to underestimation of the GFR.

Creatinine clearance or *absolute glomerular filtration rate* should be used to adjust drug doses in patients with a BMI less than 18 kg/m² or greater than 40 kg/m².

Ideal body weight should be used to calculate the CrCl. Where the patient's actual body weight is less than their ideal body weight, actual body weight should be used instead.

The absolute glomerular filtration rate is determined by removing the normalisation for BSA from the eGFR using the following formula:

GFR (Absolute) = eGFR × (individual's body surface area / 1.73)

The ideal body weight is calculated as follows:

Ideal body weight (kilograms) = Constant + 0.91 (Height - 152.4)

Where:
- Constant = 50 for men; 45.5 for women
- Height in centimetres

Estimating renal function in elderly patients The Cockcroft and Gault formula is the preferred method for estimating renal function in elderly patients aged 75 years and over.

Chronic kidney disease

Classification of chronic kidney disease using GFR and ACR categories Chronic kidney disease is classified using a combination of GFR and albumin:creatinine ratio (ACR). A decreased GFR and an increased ACR is associated with an increased risk of adverse outcomes.

For example, a person with an eGFR of 25 ml/min/1.73 m² and an ACR of 15 mg/mmol has a CKD classification of G4A2.

GFR and ACR categories and risk of adverse outcomes		ACR categories (mg/mmol), description and range		
		<3 Normal to mild increase	3–30 Moderate increase	>30 Severe increase
		A1	A2	A3
GFR categories (ml/min/1.73m²), description and range	≥90 Normal or high	G1	No CKD in the absence of markers of kidney damage		
	60–89 Mild reduction relative to normal range for a young adult	G2			
	45–59 Mild-moderate reduction	G3a			
	30–44 Moderate-severe reduction	G3b			
	15–29 Severe reduction	G4			
	<15 Kidney failure	G5			

Increasing risk

Increasing risk

Abbreviations: ACR, albumin:creatinine ratio; CKD, chronic kidney disease; GFR, glomerular filtration rate

Adapted with the kind permission of the Kidney Disease: Improving Global Outcomes (KDIGO) CKD Work Group, 2013.

Prescribing in pregnancy

Prescribing in pregnancy

Overview

Drugs can have harmful effects on the embryo or fetus at any
time during pregnancy. It is important to bear this in mind
when prescribing for a woman of *childbearing age* or for men
trying to *father* a child.

During the *first trimester* drugs can produce congenital
malformations (teratogenesis), and the period of greatest
risk is from the third to the eleventh week of pregnancy.
During the *second* and *third trimesters* drugs can affect the
growth or functional development of the fetus, or they can
have toxic effects on fetal tissues.

Drugs given shortly before term or during labour can have
adverse effects on labour or on the neonate after delivery.
Not all the damaging effects of intra-uterine exposure to
drugs are obvious at birth, some may only manifest later in
life. Such late-onset effects include malignancy, e.g.
adenocarcinoma of the vagina after puberty in females
exposed to diethylstilbestrol in the womb, and adverse
effects on intellectual, social, and functional development.
The *BNF* and *BNF for Children* identifies drugs which:

- may have harmful effects in pregnancy and indicates the
  trimester of risk
- are not known to be harmful in pregnancy

The information is based on human data, but information
from *animal* studies has been included for some drugs when
its omission might be misleading. Maternal drug doses may
require adjustment during pregnancy due to changes in
maternal physiology but this is beyond the scope of the *BNF*
and *BNF for Children*.

Where care is needed when prescribing in pregnancy, this is
indicated under the relevant drug in the *BNF* and *BNF for
Children*.

Important

Drugs should be prescribed in pregnancy only if the expected
benefit to the mother is thought to be greater than the risk to
the fetus, and all drugs should be avoided if possible during
the first trimester. Drugs which have been extensively used
in pregnancy and appear to be usually safe should be
prescribed in preference to new or untried drugs; and the
smallest effective dose should be used. Few drugs have been
shown conclusively to be teratogenic in humans, but no drug
is safe beyond all doubt in early pregnancy. Screening
procedures are available when there is a known risk of
certain defects.

Absence of information does not imply safety. It should
be noted that the *BNF* and *BNF for Children* provide
independent advice and may not always agree with the
product literature.

Information on drugs and pregnancy is also available from
the UK Teratology Information Service. www.uktis.org.
Tel: 0344 892 0909 (09.00–17:00 Monday to Friday; urgent
enquiries only outside these hours).

Prescribing in breast-feeding

Overview

Breast-feeding is beneficial; the immunological and
nutritional value of breast milk to the infant is greater than
that of formula feeds.

Although there is concern that drugs taken by the mother
might affect the infant, there is very little information on
this. In the absence of evidence of an effect, the potential for
harm to the infant can be inferred from:

- the amount of drug or active metabolite of the drug
  delivered to the infant (dependent on the
  pharmacokinetic characteristics of the drug in the
  mother);
- the efficiency of absorption, distribution, and
  elimination of the drug by the infant (infant
  pharmacokinetics);
- the nature of the effect of the drug on the infant
  (pharmacodynamic properties of the drug in the infant).

The amount of drug transferred in breast milk is rarely
sufficient to produce a discernible effect on the infant. This
applies particularly to drugs that are poorly absorbed and
need to be given parenterally. However, there is a theoretical
possibility that a small amount of drug present in breast milk
can induce a hypersensitivity reaction.

A clinical effect can occur in the infant if a pharmacologically
significant quantity of the drug is present in milk. For some
drugs (e.g. fluvastatin p. 201), the ratio between the
concentration in milk and that in maternal plasma may be
high enough to expose the infant to adverse effects. Some
infants, such as those born prematurely or who have
jaundice, are at a slightly higher risk of toxicity.

Some drugs inhibit the infant's sucking reflex (e.g.
phenobarbital p. 331) while others can affect lactation (e.g.
bromocriptine p. 414).

The *BNF* identifies drugs:

- that should be used with caution or are contra-indicated
  in breast-feeding;
- that can be given to the mother during breast-feeding
  because they are present in milk in amounts which are
  too small to be harmful to the infant;
- that might be present in milk in significant amount but
  are not known to be harmful.

Where care is needed when prescribing in breast-feeding,
this is indicated under the relevant drug in the *BNF*.

Important

For many drugs insufficient evidence is available to provide
guidance and it is advisable to administer only essential
drugs to a mother during breast-feeding. Because of the
inadequacy of information on drugs in breast-feeding,
absence of information does not imply safety.

Prescribing in palliative care

Overview

Palliative care is an approach that improves the quality of life of patients and their families facing life-threatening illness, through the prevention and relief of suffering by means of early identification and impeccable assessment and treatment of pain and other problems, physical, psychosocial, and spiritual. Careful assessment of symptoms and needs of the patient should be undertaken by a multidisciplinary team.

Specialist palliative care is available in most areas as day hospice care, home-care teams (often known as Macmillan teams), in-patient hospice care, and hospital teams. Many acute hospitals and teaching centres now have consultative, hospital-based teams.

Hospice care of terminally ill patients has shown the importance of symptom control and psychosocial support of the patient and family. Families should be included in the care of the patient if they wish.

Many patients wish to remain at home with their families. Although some families may at first be afraid of caring for the patient at home, support can be provided by community nursing services, social services, voluntary agencies and hospices together with the general practitioner. The family may be reassured by the knowledge that the patient will be admitted to a hospital or hospice if the family cannot cope.

Drug treatment The number of drugs should be as few as possible, for even the taking of medicine may be an effort. Oral medication is usually satisfactory unless there is severe nausea and vomiting, dysphagia, weakness, or coma, when parenteral medication may be necessary.

Pain

Pain management in palliative care is focused on achieving control of pain by administering the right drug in the right dose at the right time. Analgesics can be divided into three broad classes: non-opioid (paracetamol p. 438, NSAID), opioid (e.g. codeine phosphate p. 448 'weak', morphine p. 456 'strong') and adjuvant (e.g. antidepressants, antiepileptics). Drugs from the different classes are used alone or in combination according to the type of pain and response to treatment. Analgesics are more effective in preventing pain than in the relief of established pain; it is important that they are given regularly.

Paracetamol p. 438 or a **NSAID** given regularly will often be sufficient to manage mild pain. If non-opioid analgesics alone are not sufficient, then an opioid analgesic alone or in combination with a non-opioid analgesic at an adequate dosage, may be helpful in the control of moderate pain. Codeine phosphate p. 448 or tramadol hydrochloride p. 464 can be considered for moderate pain. If these preparations do not control the pain then morphine p. 456 is the most useful opioid analgesic. Alternatives to morphine, including transdermal buprenorphine p. 442, transdermal fentanyl p. 451, hydromorphone hydrochloride p. 456, methadone hydrochloride p. 495, or oxycodone hydrochloride p. 459, should be initiated by those with experience in palliative care. Initiation of an opioid analgesic should not be delayed by concern over a theoretical likelihood of psychological dependence (addiction).

Bone metastases In addition to the above approach, radiotherapy, **bisphosphonates**, and radioactive isotopes of strontium chloride (*Metastron*® available from GE Healthcare) may be useful for pain due to bone metastases.

Neuropathic pain Patients with **neuropathic pain** may benefit from a trial of a tricyclic antidepressant. An antiepileptic may be added or substituted if pain persists; gabapentin p. 314 and pregabalin p. 322 are licensed for neuropathic pain. Ketamine p. 1305 is sometimes used under

specialist supervision for neuropathic pain that responds poorly to opioid analgesics. Pain due to nerve compression may be reduced by a corticosteroid such as dexamethasone p. 660, which reduces oedema around the tumour, thus reducing compression. Nerve blocks or regional anaesthesia techniques (including the use of epidural and intrathecal catheters) can be considered when pain is localised to a specific area.

Pain management with opioids

Oral route Treatment with morphine p. 456 is given by mouth as immediate-release or modified-release preparations. During the titration phase the initial dose is based on the previous medication used, the severity of the pain, and other factors such as presence of renal impairment, increasing age, or frailty. The dose is given either as an immediate-release preparation 4-hourly or as a modified-release preparation 12-hourly, in addition to rescue doses. If pain occurs between regular doses of morphine ('breakthrough pain'), an additional dose ('rescue dose') of immediate-release morphine should be given. An additional dose should also be given 30 minutes before an activity that causes pain, such as wound dressing. The standard dose of a strong opioid for breakthrough pain is usually one-tenth to one-sixth of the regular 24-hour dose, repeated every 2–4 hours as required (up to hourly may be needed if pain is severe or in the last days of life). Review pain management if rescue analgesic is required frequently (twice daily or more). Each patient should be assessed on an individual basis. Formulations of fentanyl p. 451 that are administered nasally, buccally or sublingually are also licensed for breakthrough pain.

When adjusting the dose of morphine p. 456, the number of rescue doses required and the response to them should be taken into account; increments of morphine should not exceed one-third to one-half of the total daily dose every 24 hours. Thereafter, the dose should be adjusted with careful assessment of the pain, and the use of adjuvant analgesics should also be considered. Upward titration of the dose of morphine stops when either the pain is relieved or unacceptable adverse effects occur, after which it is necessary to consider alternative measures.

Morphine immediate-release 30mg 4-hourly (or modified-release 100 mg 12-hourly) is usually adequate for most patients; some patients require morphine immediate-release up to 200mg 4-hourly (or modified-release 600 mg 12-hourly), occasionally more is needed.

Once their pain is controlled, patients started on 4-hourly immediate-release morphine can be transferred to the same total 24-hour dose of morphine given as the modified-release preparation for 12-hourly or 24-hourly administration. The first dose of the modified-release preparation is given with, or within 4 hours of, the last dose of the immediate-release preparation. For preparations suitable for 12-hourly or 24-hourly administration see modified-release preparations under morphine. Increments should be made to the dose, not to the frequency of administration. The patient must be monitored closely for efficacy and side-effects, particularly constipation, and nausea and vomiting. A suitable laxative should be prescribed routinely.

Oxycodone hydrochloride p. 459 can be used in patients who require an opioid but cannot tolerate morphine. If the patient is already receiving an opioid, oxycodone hydrochloride should be started at a dose equivalent to the current analgesic (see below). Oxycodone hydrochloride immediate-release preparations can be given for breakthrough pain.

Equivalent doses of opioid analgesics.

This table is only an **approximate** guide (doses may not correspond with those given in clinical practice); patients should be carefully monitored after any change in medication and dose titration may be required.

Analgesic/Route	Dose
Codeine: PO	100 mg
Diamorphine: IM, IV, SC	3 mg
Dihydrocodeine: PO	100 mg
Hydromorphone: PO	2 mg
Morphine: PO	10 mg
Morphine: IM, IV, SC	5 mg
Oxycodone: PO	6.6 mg
Tramadol: PO	100 mg

PO = by mouth; IM = intramuscular; IV = intravenous; SC = subcutaneous

Parenteral route The equivalent parenteral dose of morphine p. 456 (subcutaneous, intramuscular, or intravenous) is about half of the oral dose. If the patient becomes unable to swallow, generally morphine is administered as a continuous subcutaneous infusion (for details, see Continuous Subcutaneous Infusions below). Diamorphine hydrochloride p. 449 is sometimes preferred, because being more soluble, it can be given in a smaller volume. The equivalent subcutaneous dose of diamorphine hydrochloride is about one-third of the oral dose of morphine.
If the patient can resume taking medicines by mouth, then oral morphine may be substituted for subcutaneous infusion of morphine or diamorphine hydrochloride, see table above of approximate equivalent doses of morphine and diamorphine hydrochloride. The infusion is discontinued when the first oral dose of morphine is given.

Rectal route Morphine p. 456 is also available for rectal administration as suppositories; alternatively oxycodone hydrochloride suppositories p. 459 can be obtained on special order.

Transdermal route Transdermal preparations of fentanyl p. 451 and buprenorphine p. 442 are available, they are not suitable for acute pain or in patients whose analgesic requirements are changing rapidly because the long time to steady state prevents rapid titration of the dose. Prescribers should ensure that they are familiar with the correct use of transdermal preparations, see under buprenorphine p. 442 and fentanyl p. 451 (inappropriate use has caused fatalities). Immediate-release morphine p. 456 can be given for breakthrough pain.
The following 24-hour oral doses of morphine are considered to be *approximately* equivalent to the buprenorphine and fentanyl patches shown, however when switching due to possible opioid-induced hyperalgesia, reduce the calculated equivalent dose of the new opioid by one-quarter to one-half.

Buprenorphine patches are *approximately* equivalent to the following 24-hour doses of oral morphine

morphine salt 12 mg daily	≡ buprenorphine '5' patch
morphine salt 24 mg daily	≡ buprenorphine '10' patch
morphine salt 36 mg daily	≡ buprenorphine '15' patch
morphine salt 48 mg daily	≡ buprenorphine '20' patch
morphine salt 84 mg daily	≡ buprenorphine '35' patch
morphine salt 126 mg daily	≡ buprenorphine '52.5' patch
morphine salt 168 mg daily	≡ buprenorphine '70' patch

Formulations of transdermal patches are available as 72-hourly, 96-hourly and 7-day patches, for further information see buprenorphine p. 442. Conversion ratios vary and these figures are a guide only. Morphine equivalences for transdermal opioid preparations have been approximated to allow comparison with available preparations of oral morphine.

72-hour Fentanyl patches are *approximately* equivalent to the following 24-hour doses of oral morphine

morphine salt 30 mg daily	≡ fentanyl '12' patch
morphine salt 60 mg daily	≡ fentanyl '25' patch
morphine salt 120 mg daily	≡ fentanyl '50' patch
morphine salt 180 mg daily	≡ fentanyl '75' patch
morphine salt 240 mg daily	≡ fentanyl '100' patch

Fentanyl equivalences in this table are for patients on well-tolerated opioid therapy for long periods; for patients who are opioid naive or who have been stable on oral morphine or other immediate release opioid for only several weeks, see Transdermal Route. Conversion ratios vary and these figures are a guide only. Morphine equivalences for transdermal opioid preparations have been approximated to allow comparison with available preparations of oral morphine.

Symptom control

Several recommendations in this section involve unlicensed indications or routes.

Anorexia Anorexia may be helped by prednisolone p. 664 or dexamethasone p. 660.

Bowel colic and excessive respiratory secretions Bowel colic and excessive respiratory secretions may be reduced by a subcutaneous injection of hyoscine hydrobromide p. 433, hyoscine butylbromide p. 85, or glycopyrronium bromide p. 246. These antimuscarinics are generally given every 4 hours when required, but hourly use is occasionally necessary, particularly in excessive respiratory secretions. If symptoms persist, they can be given regularly via a continuous infusion device. Care is required to avoid the discomfort of dry mouth.

Capillary bleeding Capillary bleeding can be treated with tranexamic acid p. 110 by mouth; treatment is usually discontinued one week after the bleeding has stopped, or, if necessary, it can be continued at a reduced dose. Alternatively, gauze soaked in tranexamic acid 100 mg/mL p. 110 or adrenaline/epinephrine solution 1 mg/mL (1 in 1000) p. 221 can be applied to the affected area.
Vitamin K may be useful for the treatment and prevention of bleeding associated with prolonged clotting in liver disease. In severe chronic cholestasis, absorption of vitamin K may be impaired; either parenteral or water-soluble oral vitamin K (see phytomenadione p. 1056 and menadiol sodium phosphate p. 1056) should be considered.

Constipation Constipation is a common cause of distress and is almost invariable after administration of an opioid analgesic. It should be prevented if possible by the regular administration of laxatives; a faecal softener with a peristaltic stimulant (e.g. co-danthramer p. 61) or lactulose solution p. 56 with a senna preparation p. 63 should be used. Methylnaltrexone bromide p. 64 is licensed for the treatment of opioid-induced constipation.

Convulsions Patients with cerebral tumours or uraemia may be susceptible to convulsions. Prophylactic treatment with phenytoin p. 321 or carbamazepine p. 309 should be considered. When oral medication is no longer possible, diazepam p. 340 given rectally, or phenobarbital p. 331 by injection is continued as prophylaxis. For the use of midazolam p. 336 by subcutaneous infusion using a continuous infusion device see below.

Dry mouth Dry mouth may be relieved by good mouth care and measures such as chewing sugar-free gum, sucking ice or pineapple chunks, or the use of artificial saliva,dry mouth associated with candidiasis can be treated by oral preparations of nystatin p. 1184 or miconazole p. 811, alternatively, fluconazole p. 584 can be given by mouth. Dry mouth may be caused by certain medications including opioids, antimuscarinic drugs (e.g. hyoscine), antidepressants and some antiemetics; if possible, an alternative preparation should be considered.

Dysphagia A corticosteroid such as dexamethasone p. 660 may help, temporarily, if there is an obstruction due to tumour. See also *Dry mouth*, above.

Dyspnoea Breathlessness at rest may be relieved by regular oral morphine p. 456 in carefully titrated doses. Diazepam p. 340 may be helpful for dyspnoea associated with anxiety. A corticosteroid, such as dexamethasone p. 660, may also be helpful if there is bronchospasm or partial obstruction.

Fungating tumours Fungating tumours can be treated by regular dressing and antibacterial drugs; systemic treatment with metronidazole p. 533 is often required to reduce malodour but topical metronidazole p. 533 is also used.

Gastro-intestinal pain The pain of bowel colic may be reduced by loperamide hydrochloride p. 66. Hyoscine hydrobromide p. 433 may also be helpful, given sublingually as *Kwells* ® tablets. Subcutaneous injections of hyoscine butylbromide p. 85, hyoscine hydrobromide p. 433, and glycopyrronium bromide p. 246 can also be used to treat bowel colic.
Gastric distension pain due to pressure on the stomach may be helped by a preparation incorporating an antacid with an antiflatulent and a prokinetic such as domperidone p. 426 before meals.

Hiccup Hiccup due to gastric distension may be helped by a preparation incorporating an antacid with an antiflatulent. If this fails, metoclopramide hydrochloride p. 426 by mouth or by subcutaneous or intramuscular injection can be added; if this also fails, baclofen p. 1092, or nifedipine p. 162, or chlorpromazine hydrochloride p. 381 can be tried.

Insomnia Patients with advanced cancer may not sleep because of discomfort, cramps, night sweats, joint stiffness, or fear. There should be appropriate treatment of these problems before hypnotics are used. Benzodiazepines, such as temazepam p. 481, may be useful.

Intractable cough Intractable cough may be relieved by moist inhalations or by regular administration of oral morphine p. 456. Methadone hydrochloride linctus p. 495 should be avoided because it has a long duration of action and tends to accumulate.

Muscle spasm The pain of muscle spasm can be helped by a muscle relaxant such as diazepam p. 340 or baclofen p. 1092.

Nausea and vomiting Nausea and vomiting are common in patients with advanced cancer. Ideally, the cause should be determined before treatment with an antiemetic is started.

A prokinetic antiemetic may be a preferred choice for first-line therapy.
Nausea and vomiting may occur with opioid therapy particularly in the initial stages but can be prevented by giving an antiemetic such as haloperidol p. 382 or metoclopramide hydrochloride p. 426. An antiemetic is usually necessary only for the first 4 or 5 days and therefore combined preparations containing an opioid with an antiemetic are not recommended because they lead to unnecessary antiemetic therapy (and associated side-effects when used long-term).
Metoclopramide hydrochloride p. 426 has a prokinetic action and is used by mouth for nausea and vomiting associated with gastritis, gastric stasis, and functional bowel obstruction. Drugs with antimuscarinic effects antagonise prokinetic drugs and, if possible, should not be used concurrently.
Haloperidol p. 382 is used by mouth for most metabolic causes of vomiting (e.g. hypercalcaemia, renal failure).
Cyclizine p. 424 is given by mouth. It is used for nausea and vomiting due to mechanical bowel obstruction, raised intracranial pressure, and motion sickness.
Levomepromazine p. 435 is used as an antiemetic; it is given by mouth or by subcutaneous injection at bedtime. For the dose by subcutaneous infusion see below. Dexamethasone p. 660 by mouth can be used as an adjunct.
Antiemetic therapy should be reviewed every 24 hours; it may be necessary to substitute the antiemetic or to add another one.
For the administration of antiemetics by subcutaneous infusion using a continuous infusion device, see below.
For the treatment of nausea and vomiting associated with cancer chemotherapy see Cytotoxic drugs p. 865.

Pruritus Pruritus, even when associated with obstructive jaundice, often responds to simple measures such as application of emollients. In the case of obstructive jaundice, further measures include administration of colestyramine p. 196.

Raised intracranial pressure Headache due to raised intracranial pressure often responds to a high dose of a corticosteroid, such as dexamethasone p. 660 and should be given before 6 p.m. to reduce the risk of insomnia.

Restlessness and confusion Restlessness and confusion may require treatment with an antipsychotic, e.g. haloperidol p. 382 or levomepromazine p. 435, by mouth or by subcutaneous injection, both repeated every 2 hours if required. The dose and frequency is adjusted according to the level of patient distress and the response. A regular maintenance dose should also be considered, given twice daily either by mouth or by subcutaneous injection; alternatively use a continuous infusion device.
Levomepromazine p. 435 is licensed to treat pain in palliative care—this use is reserved for distressed patients with severe pain unresponsive to other measures (seek specialist advice).

Continuous subcutaneous infusions

Although drugs can usually be administered *by mouth* to control the symptoms of advanced cancer, the parenteral route may sometimes be necessary. Repeated administration of *intramuscular injections* can be difficult in a cachectic patient. This has led to the use of portable continuous infusion devices, such as syringe drivers, to give a *continuous subcutaneous infusion*, which can provide good control of symptoms with little discomfort or inconvenience to the patient.
Indications for the **parenteral route** are:

• the patient is unable to take medicines by mouth owing to *nausea and vomiting, dysphagia, severe weakness,* or *coma*

- there is *malignant bowel obstruction* in patients for whom further surgery is inappropriate (avoiding the need for an intravenous infusion or for insertion of a nasogastric tube)
- occasionally when the patient *does not wish* to take regular medication by mouth.

Syringe driver rate settings Staff using syringe drivers should be **adequately trained** and different rate settings should be **clearly identified** and **differentiated**; incorrect use of syringe drivers is a common cause of medication errors.

Bowel colic and excessive respiratory secretions Hyoscine hydrobromide p. 433 effectively reduces respiratory secretions and bowel colic and is sedative (but occasionally causes paradoxical agitation).
Hyoscine butylbromide p. 85 is used for bowel colic and for excessive respiratory secretions, and is less sedative than hyoscine hydrobromide.
Glycopyrronium bromide p. 246 may also be used to treat bowel colic or excessive respiratory secretions.

Confusion and restlessness Haloperidol p. 382 has little sedative effect.
Levomepromazine p. 435 has a sedative effect.
Midazolam p. 336 is a sedative and an antiepileptic that may be used in addition to an antipsychotic drug in a very restless patient. Midazolam is also used for myoclonus.

Convulsions If a patient has previously been receiving an antiepileptic drug *or* has a primary or secondary cerebral tumour *or* is at risk of convulsion (e.g. owing to uraemia) antiepileptic medication should not be stopped. Midazolam p. 336 is the benzodiazepine antiepileptic of choice for *continuous subcutaneous infusion*.

Nausea and vomiting Haloperidol p. 382 and levomepromazine p. 435 can both be given as a *subcutaneous infusion* but sedation can limit the dose of levomepromazine. Cyclizine is particularly likely to precipitate if mixed with diamorphine or other drugs (see under Mixing and Compatibility, below)
Metoclopramide hydrochloride p. 426 can cause skin reactions.
Octreotide p. 924, which stimulates water and electrolyte absorption and inhibits water secretion in the small bowel, can be used by subcutaneous infusion to reduce intestinal secretions and to reduce vomiting due to bowel obstruction.

Pain control Diamorphine hydrochloride p. 449 is the preferred opioid since its high solubility permits a large dose to be given in a small volume (see under Mixing and Compatibility, below). The table shows approximate equivalent doses of morphine p. 456 and diamorphine hydrochloride p. 449.

Mixing and compatibility The general principle that injections should be given into separate sites (and should not be mixed) does not apply to the use of syringe drivers in palliative care. Provided that there is evidence of compatibility, selected injections can be mixed in syringe drivers. Not all types of medication can be used in a subcutaneous infusion. In particular, chlorpromazine hydrochloride p. 381, prochlorperazine p. 385, and diazepam p. 340 are **contra-indicated** as they cause skin reactions at the injection site; to a lesser extent cyclizine p. 424 and levomepromazine p. 435 also sometimes cause local irritation.
In theory injections dissolved in water for injections are more likely to be associated with pain (possibly owing to their hypotonicity). The use of physiological saline (sodium chloride 0.9% p. 1008) however increases the likelihood of precipitation when more than one drug is used; moreover subcutaneous infusion rates are so slow (0.1– 0.3 mL/hour) that pain is not usually a problem when water is used as a diluent.

Compatibility with diamorphine Diamorphine can be given by *subcutaneous infusion* in a strength of up to 250 mg/mL; up to a strength of 40 mg/mL either *water for injections* or *physiological saline* (sodium chloride 0.9%) is a suitable diluent—above that strength only *water for injections* is used (to avoid precipitation).
The following can be mixed with *diamorphine*:

- **Cyclizine**, may precipitate at concentrations above 10 mg/mL *or* in the presence of sodium chloride 0.9% *or* as the concentration of diamorphine relative to cyclizine increases; mixtures of diamorphine and cyclizine are also likely to precipitate after 24 hours.
- **Dexamethasone**, special care is needed to avoid precipitation of dexamethasone when preparing it.
- **Haloperidol**, mixtures of haloperidol and diamorphine are likely to precipitate after 24 hours if haloperidol concentration is above 2 mg/mL.
- **Hyoscine butylbromide**
- **Hyoscine hydrobromide**
- **Levomepromazine**
- **Metoclopramide**, under some conditions infusions containing metoclopramide become discoloured; such solutions should be discarded.
- **Midazolam**

Subcutaneous infusion solution should be monitored regularly both to check for precipitation (and discolouration) and to ensure that the infusion is running at the correct rate.

Problems encountered with syringe drivers The following are problems that may be encountered with syringe drivers and the action that should be taken:

- if the subcutaneous infusion runs *too quickly* check the rate setting and the calculation;
- if the subcutaneous infusion runs *too slowly* check the start button, the battery, the syringe driver, the cannula, and make sure that the injection site is not inflamed;
- if there is an *injection site reaction* make sure that the site does not need to be changed—firmness or swelling at the site of injection is not in itself an indication for change, but pain or obvious inflammation is.

Equivalent doses of morphine sulfate and diamorphine hydrochloride given over 24 hours

These equivalences are *approximate only* and should be adjusted according to response

ORAL MORPHINE	PARENTERAL MORPHINE	PARENTERAL DIAMORPHINE
Oral morphine sulfate over 24 hours	Subcutaneous infusion of morphine sulfate over 24 hours	Subcutaneous infusion of diamorphine hydrochloride over 24 hours
30 mg	15 mg	10 mg
60 mg	30 mg	20 mg
90 mg	45 mg	30 mg
120 mg	60 mg	40 mg
180 mg	90 mg	60 mg
240 mg	120 mg	80 mg
360 mg	180 mg	120 mg
480 mg	240 mg	160 mg
600 mg	300 mg	200 mg
780 mg	390 mg	260 mg
960 mg	480 mg	320 mg
1200 mg	600 mg	400 mg

If breakthrough pain occurs give a subcutaneous (preferable) or intramuscular injection equivalent to one-tenth to one-sixth of the total 24-hour subcutaneous infusion dose. It is kinder to give an intermittent bolus injection *subcutaneously*—absorption is smoother so that the risk of adverse effects at peak absorption is avoided (an even better method is to use a subcutaneous butterfly needle). To minimise the risk of infection no individual subcutaneous infusion solution should be used for longer than 24 hours.

Prescribing in the elderly

Overview
Old people, especially the very old, require special care and consideration from prescribers. *Medicines for Older People*, a component document of the National Service Framework for Older People (Department of Health. National Service Framework for Older People. London: Department of Health, March 2001), describes how to maximise the benefits of medicines and how to avoid excessive, inappropriate, or inadequate consumption of medicines by older people.

Appropriate prescribing
Elderly patients often receive multiple drugs for their multiple diseases. This greatly increases the risk of drug interactions as well as adverse reactions, and may affect compliance. The balance of benefit and harm of some medicines may be altered in the elderly. Therefore, elderly patients' medicines should be reviewed regularly and medicines which are not of benefit should be stopped. Non-pharmacological measures may be more appropriate for symptoms such as headache, sleeplessness, and light-headedness when associated with social stress as in widowhood, loneliness, and family dispersal.

In some cases prophylactic drugs are inappropriate if they are likely to complicate existing treatment or introduce unnecessary side-effects, especially in elderly patients with poor prognosis or with poor overall health. However, elderly patients should not be denied medicines which may help them, such as anticoagulants or antiplatelet drugs for atrial fibrillation, antihypertensives, statins, and drugs for osteoporosis.

Form of medicine
Frail elderly patients may have difficulty swallowing tablets; if left in the mouth, ulceration may develop. They should always be encouraged to take their tablets or capsules with enough fluid, and whilst in an upright position to avoid the possibility of oesophageal ulceration. It can be helpful to discuss with the patient the possibility of taking the drug as a liquid if available.

Manifestations of ageing
In the very old, manifestations of normal ageing may be mistaken for disease and lead to inappropriate prescribing. In addition, age-related muscle weakness and difficulty in maintaining balance should not be confused with neurological disease. Disorders such as light-headedness not associated with postural or postprandial hypotension are unlikely to be helped by drugs.

Sensitivity
The nervous system of elderly patients is more sensitive to many commonly used drugs, such as opioid analgesics, benzodiazepines, antipsychotics, and antiparkinsonian drugs, all of which must be used with caution. Similarly, other organs may also be more susceptible to the effects of drugs such as anti-hypertensives and NSAIDs.

Pharmacokinetics
Pharmacokinetic changes can markedly increase the tissue concentration of a drug in the elderly, especially in debilitated patients.

The most important effect of age is reduced renal clearance. Many aged patients thus *excrete drugs slowly*, and are *highly susceptible to nephrotoxic drugs*. Acute illness can lead to rapid reduction in renal clearance, especially if accompanied by dehydration. Hence, a patient stabilised on a drug with a narrow margin between the therapeutic and the toxic dose (e.g. digoxin p. 109) can rapidly develop adverse effects in the aftermath of a myocardial infarction or a respiratory-tract infection. The hepatic metabolism of lipid soluble drugs is reduced in elderly patients because there is a reduction in liver volume. This is important for drugs with a narrow therapeutic window.

Adverse reactions
Adverse reactions often present in the elderly in a vague and non-specific fashion. *Confusion* is often the presenting symptom (caused by almost any of the commonly used drugs). Other common manifestations are *constipation* (with antimuscarinics and many tranquillisers) and postural *hypotension* and *falls* (with diuretics and many psychotropics).

Hypnotics
Many hypnotics with long half-lives have serious hangover effects, including drowsiness, unsteady gait, slurred speech, and confusion. Hypnotics with short half-lives should be used but they too can present problems. Short courses of hypnotics are occasionally useful for helping a patient through an acute illness or some other crisis but every effort must be made to avoid dependence. Benzodiazepines impair balance, which can result in falls.

Diuretics
Diuretics are overprescribed in old age and should **not** be used on a long-term basis to treat simple gravitational oedema which will usually respond to increased movement, raising the legs, and support stockings. A few days of diuretic treatment may speed the clearing of the oedema but it should rarely need continued drug therapy.

NSAIDs
Bleeding associated with aspirin and other NSAIDs is more common in the elderly who are more likely to have a fatal or serious outcome. NSAIDs are also a special hazard in patients with cardiac disease or renal impairment which may again place older patients at particular risk.

Owing to the *increased susceptibility of the elderly* to the *side-effects of NSAIDs* the following recommendations are made:
- for *osteoarthritis, soft-tissue lesions,* and *back pain*, first try measures such as weight reduction (if obese), warmth, exercise, and use of a walking stick;
- for *osteoarthritis, soft-tissue lesions, back pain,* and *pain in rheumatoid arthritis*, paracetamol p. 438 should be used first and can often provide adequate pain relief;
- alternatively, a low-dose NSAID (e.g. ibuprofen p. 1106 up to 1.2 g daily) may be given;
- for pain relief when either drug is inadequate, paracetamol in a full dose plus a low-dose NSAID may be given;
- if necessary, the NSAID dose can be increased or an opioid analgesic given with paracetamol p. 438;
- do not give two NSAIDs at the same time.

Prophylaxis of NSAID-induced peptic ulcers may be required if continued NSAID treatment is necessary see, *NSAID-associated ulcers* under Peptic ulceration p. 71.

Other drugs
Other drugs which commonly cause adverse reactions are *antiparkinsonian drugs, antihypertensives, psychotropics*, and digoxin p. 109. The usual maintenance dose of digoxin in very old patients is 125 micrograms daily (62.5 micrograms in those with renal disease); lower doses are often inadequate but toxicity is common in those given 250 micrograms daily. Drug-induced blood disorders are much more common in the elderly. Therefore drugs with a tendency to cause bone marrow depression (e.g. co-trimoxazole p. 552, mianserin

hydrochloride p. 367) should be avoided unless there is no acceptable alternative.

The elderly generally require a lower maintenance dose of warfarin sodium p. 139 than younger adults; once again, the outcome of bleeding tends to be more serious.

Guidelines

Always consider whether a drug is indicated at all.

Limit range It is a sensible policy to prescribe from a limited range of drugs and to be thoroughly familiar with their effects in the elderly.

Reduce dose Dosage should generally be substantially lower than for younger patients and it is common to start with about 50% of the adult dose. Some drugs (e.g. long-acting antidiabetic drugs such as glibenclamide p. 692) should be avoided altogether.

Review regularly Review repeat prescriptions regularly. In many patients it may be possible to stop some drugs, provided that clinical progress is monitored. It may be necessary to reduce the dose of some drugs as renal function declines.

Simplify regimens Elderly patients benefit from simple treatment regimens. Only drugs with a clear indication should be prescribed and whenever possible given once or twice daily. In particular, regimens which call for a confusing array of dosage intervals should be avoided.

Explain clearly Write full instructions on every prescription (*including* repeat prescriptions) so that containers can be properly labelled with full directions. Avoid imprecisions like 'as directed'. Child-resistant containers may be unsuitable.

Repeats and disposal Instruct patients what to do when drugs run out, and also how to dispose of any that are no longer necessary. Try to prescribe matching quantities.

If these guidelines are followed most elderly people will cope adequately with their own medicines. If not then it is essential to enrol the help of a third party, usually a relative or a friend.

Drugs and sport

Anti-doping

UK Anti-Doping, the national body responsible for the UK's anti-doping policy, advises that athletes are personally responsible should a prohibited substance be detected in their body. Information regarding the use of medicines in sport is available from:

UK Anti-doping
Fleetbank House
2-6 Salisbury Square
London
EC4Y 8AE
(020) 7842 3450
ukad@ukad.org.uk
www.ukad.org.uk

Information about the prohibited status of specific medications based on the current World Anti-Doping Agency Prohibited List is available from Global Drug Reference Online: www.globaldro.com/UK/search

General Medical Council's advice

Doctors who prescribe or collude in the provision of drugs or treatment with the intention of improperly enhancing an individual's performance in sport contravene the GMC's guidance, and such actions would usually raise a question of a doctor's continued registration. This does not preclude the provision of any care or treatment where the doctor's intention is to protect or improve the patient's health.

Prescribing in dental practice

General guidance

Advice on the drug management of dental and oral conditions has been integrated into the main text. For ease of access, guidance on such conditions is usually identified by means of a relevant heading (e.g. Dental and Orofacial Pain) in the appropriate sections of the BNF.
The following is a list of topics of particular relevance to dentists.

> Prescribing by dentists, see Prescription writing p. 5
> Oral side-effects of drugs, see Adverse reactions to drugs p. 12
> Medical emergencies in dental practice, see below
> Medical problems in dental practice, see below

Drug management of dental and oral conditions
Dental and orofacial pain

> Neuropathic pain p. 475
> Non-opioid analgesics and compound analgesic preparations, see Analgesics p. 436
> Opioid analgesics, see Analgesics p. 436
> Non-steroidal anti-inflammatory drugs p. 1094

Oral infections

> Bacterial infections, see Antibacterials, principles of therapy p. 498
>> Phenoxymethylpenicillin p. 538
>> Broad-spectrum penicillins (amoxicillin p. 539 and ampicillin p. 540)
>> Cephalosporins (cefalexin p. 516 and cefradine p. 516)
>> Tetracyclines p. 554
>> Macrolides (clarithromycin p. 529, erythromycin p. 530 and azithromycin p. 528)
>> Clindamycin p. 526
>> Metronidazole p. 533
>> Fusidic acid p. 561

> Fungal infections, see Antifungals, systemic use p. 580
>> Local treatment, see Oropharyngeal fungal infections p. 1182
>> Systemic treatment, see Antifungals, systemic use p. 580

> Viral infections
>> Herpetic gingivostomatitis, local treatment, see Oropharyngeal viral infections p. 1184
>> Herpetic gingivostomatitis, systemic treatment, see Oropharyngeal viral infections p. 1184 and Herpesvirus infections p. 621
>> Herpes labialis, see Skin infections p. 1193

Anaesthetics, anxiolytics and hypnotics

> Sedation, anaesthesia, and resuscitation in dental practice p. 1290
> Hypnotics, see Hypnotics and anxiolytics p. 477
> Sedation for dental procedures, see Hypnotics and anxiolytics p. 477
> Anaesthesia (local) p. 1307

Minerals

> Fluoride p. 1177

Oral ulceration and inflammation p. 1178
Mouthwashes, gargles and dentifrices, see Mouthwashes and other preparations for oropharyngeal use p. 1175
Dry mouth, see Treatment of dry mouth p. 1173
Aromatic inhalations, see Aromatic inhalations, cough preparations and systemic nasal decongestants p. 294
Nasal decongestants, see Aromatic inhalations, cough preparations and systemic nasal decongestants p. 294

Dental Practitioners' Formulary p. 1562

Medical emergencies in dental practice

This section provides guidelines on the management of the more common medical emergencies which may arise in dental practice. Dentists and their staff should be familiar with standard resuscitation procedures, but in all circumstances it is advisable to summon medical assistance as soon as possible. See also **algorithm** of the procedure for Cardiopulmonary resuscitation p. 221.

The drugs referred to in this section include:

> Adrenaline/epinephrine Injection, adrenaline 1 in 1000, (adrenaline 1 mg/mL as acid tartrate), 1 mL amps p. 221
> Aspirin Dispersible Tablets 300 mg p. 121
> Glucagon Injection p. 707, glucagon (as hydrochloride), 1- unit vial (with solvent) p. 707
> Glucose (for administration by mouth) p. 1009
> Glyceryl trinitrate Spray p. 217
> Midazolam Oromucosal Solution p. 336
> Oxygen
> Salbutamol Aerosol Inhalation, salbutamol 100 micrograms/metered inhalation p. 252

Adrenal insufficiency

Adrenal insufficiency may follow prolonged therapy with corticosteroids and can persist for years after stopping. A patient with adrenal insufficiency may become hypotensive under the stress of a dental visit (important: see individual monographs for details of corticosteroid cover before dental surgical procedures under general anaesthesia).

Management
- Lay the patient flat
- Give **oxygen**
- Transfer patient urgently to hospital

Anaphylaxis

A severe allergic reaction may follow oral or parenteral administration of a drug. Anaphylactic reactions in dentistry may follow the administration of a drug or contact with substances such as latex in surgical gloves. In general, the more rapid the onset of the reaction the more profound it tends to be. Symptoms may develop within minutes and rapid treatment is essential.

Anaphylactic reactions may also be associated with *additives* and *excipients* in foods and medicines. Refined arachis (peanut) oil, which may be present in some medicinal products, is unlikely to cause an allergic reaction—nevertheless it is wise to check the full formula of preparations which may contain allergens (including those for topical application, particularly if they are intended for use in the mouth or for application to the nasal mucosa).

Symptoms and signs
- Paraesthesia, flushing, and swelling of face
- Generalised itching, especially of hands and feet
- Bronchospasm and laryngospasm (with wheezing and difficulty in breathing)
- Rapid weak pulse together with fall in blood pressure and pallor; finally cardiac arrest

Management

First-line treatment includes securing the airway, restoration of blood pressure (laying the patient flat and raising the feet, or in the recovery position if unconscious or nauseous and at risk of vomiting), and administration of adrenaline/epinephrine injection p. 221. This is given **intramuscularly** in a dose of 500 micrograms (0.5 mL adrenaline injection 1 in 1000); a dose of 300 micrograms (0.3 mL adrenaline injection 1 in 1000) may be appropriate for immediate self-administration. The dose is repeated if necessary at 5-minute intervals according to blood pressure, pulse, and respiratory function. **Oxygen** administration is also of primary importance. Arrangements should be made to transfer the patient to hospital urgently.

Asthma

Patients with asthma may have an attack while at the dental surgery. Most attacks will respond to 2 puffs of the patient's short-acting beta$_2$ agonist inhaler such as salbutamol 100 micrograms/puff p. 252; further puffs are required if the patient does not respond rapidly. If the patient is unable to use the inhaler effectively, further puffs should be given through a large-volume spacer device (or, if not available, through a plastic or paper cup with a hole in the bottom for the inhaler mouthpiece). If the response remains unsatisfactory, or if further deterioration occurs, then the patient should be transferred urgently to hospital. Whilst awaiting transfer, **oxygen** should be given with salbutamol 5 mg p. 252 or terbutaline sulfate 10 mg by nebuliser p. 254; if a nebuliser is unavailable, then 2–10 puffs of salbutamol 100 micrograms/metered inhalation p. 252 should be given (preferably by a large-volume spacer), and repeated every 10–20 minutes if necessary. If asthma is part of a more generalised anaphylactic reaction, an intramuscular injection of adrenaline/epinephrine p. 221 (as detailed under Anaphylaxis) should be given.

Patients with severe chronic asthma or whose asthma has deteriorated previously during a dental procedure may require an increase in their prophylactic medication before a dental procedure. This should be discussed with the patient's medical practitioner and may include increasing the dose of inhaled or oral corticosteroid.

Cardiac emergencies

If there is a history of *angina* the patient will probably carry glyceryl trinitrate spray or tablets p. 217 (or isosorbide dinitrate tablets p. 219) and should be allowed to use them. Hospital admission is not necessary if symptoms are mild and resolve rapidly with the patient's own medication. See also Coronary Artery Disease below.

Arrhythmias may lead to a sudden reduction in cardiac output with loss of consciousness. Medical assistance should be summoned. For advice on pacemaker interference, see also Pacemakers below.

The pain of *myocardial infarction* is similar to that of angina but generally more severe and more prolonged. For general advice see also Coronary Artery Disease below.

Symptoms and signs of myocardial infarction:

- Progressive onset of severe, crushing pain across front of chest; pain may radiate towards the shoulder and down arm, or into neck and jaw
- Skin becomes pale and clammy
- Nausea and vomiting are common
- Pulse may be weak and blood pressure may fall
- Breathlessness

Initial management of myocardial infarction:

Call immediately for medical assistance and an ambulance, as appropriate.

Allow the patient to rest in the position that feels most comfortable; in the presence of breathlessness this is likely to be sitting position, whereas the syncopal patient should be laid flat; often an intermediate position (dictated by the patient) will be most appropriate. **Oxygen** may be administered.

Sublingual glyceryl trinitrate p. 217 may relieve pain. Intramuscular injection of drugs should be avoided because absorption may be too slow (particularly when cardiac output is reduced) and pain relief is inadequate. Intramuscular injection also increases the risk of local bleeding into the muscle if the patient is given a thrombolytic drug.

Reassure the patient as much as possible to relieve further anxiety. If available, aspirin p. 121 in a single dose of 300 mg should be given. A note (to say that aspirin has been given) should be sent with the patient to the hospital. For further details on the initial management of myocardial infarction, see Management of ST-Segment Elevation Myocardial Infarction.

If the patient collapses and loses consciousness attempt standard resuscitation measures. See also **algorithm** of the procedure for Cardiopulmonary resuscitation p. 221.

Epileptic seizures

Patients with epilepsy must continue with their normal dosage of anticonvulsant drugs when attending for dental treatment. It is not uncommon for epileptic patients not to volunteer the information that they are epileptic but there should be little difficulty in recognising a tonic-clonic (grand mal) seizure.

Symptoms and signs

- There may be a brief warning (but variable)
- Sudden loss of consciousness, the patient becomes rigid, falls, may give a cry, and becomes cyanotic (tonic phase)
- After 30 seconds, there are jerking movements of the limbs; the tongue may be bitten (clonic phase)
- There may be frothing from mouth and urinary incontinence
- The seizure typically lasts a few minutes; the patient may then become flaccid but remain unconscious. After a variable time the patient regains consciousness but may remain confused for a while

Management

During a convulsion try to ensure that the patient is not at risk from injury but make no attempt to put anything in the mouth or between the teeth (in mistaken belief that this will protect the tongue). Give **oxygen** to support respiration if necessary.

Do not attempt to restrain convulsive movements.

After convulsive movements have subsided place the patient in the coma (recovery) position and check the airway.

After the convulsion the patient may be confused ('post-ictal confusion') and may need reassurance and sympathy. The patient should not be sent home until fully recovered. Seek medical attention or transfer the patient to hospital if it was the first episode of epilepsy, or if the convulsion was atypical, prolonged (or repeated), or if injury occurred. Medication should only be given if convulsive seizures are prolonged (convulsive movements lasting 5 minutes or longer) or repeated rapidly.

Midazolam oromucosal solution p. 336 can be given by the buccal route in adults as a single dose of 10 mg [unlicensed]. For further details on the management of status epilepticus, including details of paediatric doses of midazolam p. 336, see Drugs used in status epilepticus (Epilepsy p. 304).

Focal seizures similarly need very little active management (in an automatism only a minimum amount of restraint should be applied to prevent injury). Again, the patient should be observed until post-ictal confusion has completely resolved.

Hypoglycaemia

Insulin-treated diabetic patients attending for dental treatment under local anaesthesia should inject insulin and eat meals as normal. If food is omitted the blood glucose will fall to an abnormally low level (hypoglycaemia). Patients can often recognise the symptoms themselves and this state responds to sugar in water or a few lumps of sugar. Children may not have such prominent changes but may appear unduly lethargic.

Symptoms and signs

- Shaking and trembling
- Sweating
- 'Pins and needles' in lips and tongue
- Hunger
- Palpitation
- Headache (occasionally)
- Double vision
- Difficulty in concentration
- Slurring of speech
- Confusion
- Change of behaviour; truculence
- Convulsions
- Unconsciousness

Management

Initially glucose 10–20 g is given by mouth either in liquid form or as granulated sugar or sugar lumps. Approximately 10 g of glucose is available from non-diet versions of *Lucozade*® *Energy Original* 110 mL, *Coca- Cola*® 100 mL, *Ribena*® *Blackcurrant* 19 mL (to be diluted), 2 teaspoons sugar, and also from 3 sugar lumps. (Proprietary products of quick-acting carbohydrate (e.g. *GlucoGel*®, *Dextrogel*®, *GSF-Syrup*®, *Rapilose*® gel) are available on prescription for the patient to keep to hand in case of hypoglycaemia.) If necessary this may be repeated in 10–15 minutes. **Note: the carbohydrate content of some commercially available glucose-containing drinks is currently subject to change—individual product labels should be checked.** Patients should be aware that for a time, both old and new bottles and cans may be available—individual product labels should be checked.

If glucose cannot be given by mouth, if it is ineffective, or if the hypoglycaemia causes unconsciousness, **glucagon** 1 mg (1 unit) should be given by intramuscular (or subcutaneous) injection; a child under 8 years or of body-weight under 25 kg should be given 500 micrograms. Once the patient regains consciousness oral glucose should be administered as above. If glucagon is ineffective or contra-indicated, the patient should be transferred urgently to hospital. The patient must also be admitted to hospital if hypoglycaemia is caused by an oral antidiabetic drug.

Syncope

Insufficient blood supply to the brain results in loss of consciousness. The commonest cause is a vasovagal attack or simple faint (syncope) due to emotional stress.

Symptoms and signs

- Patient feels faint
- Low blood pressure
- Pallor and sweating
- Yawning and slow pulse
- Nausea and vomiting
- Dilated pupils
- Muscular twitching

Management

- Lay the patient as flat as is reasonably comfortable and, in the absence of associated breathlessness, raise the legs to improve cerebral circulation
- Loosen any tight clothing around the neck
- Once consciousness is regained, give sugar in water or a cup of sweet tea

Other possible causes Postural hypotension can be a consequence of rising abruptly or of standing upright for too long; antihypertensive drugs predispose to this. When rising, susceptible patients should take their time. Management is as for a vasovagal attack.

Under stressful circumstances, some patients hyperventilate. This gives rise to feelings of faintness but does not usually result in syncope. In most cases reassurance is all that is

necessary; rebreathing from cupped hands or a bag may be helpful but calls for careful supervision.

Adrenal insufficiency or arrhythmias are other possible causes of syncope.

Medical problems in dental practice

Individuals presenting at the dental surgery may also suffer from an unrelated medical condition; this may require modification to the management of their dental condition. If the patient has systemic disease or is taking other medication, the matter may need to be discussed with the patient's general practitioner or hospital consultant.

Allergy

Patients should be asked about any history of allergy; those with a history of atopic allergy (asthma, eczema, hay fever, etc.) are at special risk. Those with a history of a severe allergy or of anaphylactic reactions are at high risk—it is essential to confirm that they are not allergic to any medication, or to any dental materials or equipment (including latex gloves). See also Anaphylaxis above.

Arrhythmias

Patients, especially those who suffer from heart failure or who have sustained a myocardial infarction, may have irregular cardiac rhythm. Atrial fibrillation is a common arrhythmia even in patients with normal hearts and is of little concern except that dentists should be aware that such patients may be receiving anticoagulant therapy. The patient's medical practitioner should be asked whether any special precautions are necessary. Premedication (e.g. with temazepam p. 481) may be useful in some instances for very anxious patients.

See also Cardiac emergencies above, and Dental Anaesthesia (Anaesthesia (local) p. 1307).

Cardiac prostheses

For an account of the risk of infective endocarditis in patients with prosthetic heart valves, see Infective Endocarditis below. For advice on patients receiving anticoagulants, see Thromboembolic disease below.

Coronary artery disease

Patients are vulnerable for at least 4 weeks following a myocardial infarction or following any sudden increase in the symptoms of angina. It would be advisable to check with the patient's medical practitioner before commencing treatment. See also Cardiac Emergencies above.

Treatment with low-dose aspirin (75 mg daily), clopidogrel p. 122, or dipyridamole p. 123 should not be stopped routinely nor should the dose be altered before dental procedures.

A Working Party of the British Society for Antimicrobial Chemotherapy has not recommended antibiotic prophylaxis for patients following coronary artery bypass surgery.

Cyanotic heart disease

Patients with cyanotic heart disease are at risk in the dental chair, particularly if they have pulmonary hypertension. In such patients a syncopal reaction increases the shunt away from the lungs, causing more hypoxia which worsens the syncopal reaction—a vicious circle that may prove fatal. The advice of the cardiologist should be sought on any patient with congenital cyanotic heart disease. Treatment in hospital is more appropriate for some patients with this condition.

Hypertension

Patients with hypertension are likely to be receiving antihypertensive drugs. Their blood pressure may fall dangerously low under general anaesthesia, see also under Dental Anaesthesia (Anaesthesia (local) p. 1307).

Immunosuppression and indwelling intraperitoneal catheters

Advice of a Working Party of the British Society for Antimicrobial Chemotherapy is that patients who are immunosuppressed (including transplant patients) and patients with indwelling intraperitoneal catheters do not require antibiotic prophylaxis for dental treatment provided there is no other indication for prophylaxis.

The Working Party has commented that there is little evidence that dental treatment is followed by infection in immunosuppressed and immunodeficient patients nor is there evidence that dental treatment is followed by infection in patients with indwelling intraperitoneal catheters.

Infective endocarditis

While almost any dental procedure can cause bacteraemia, there is no clear association with the development of infective endocarditis. Routine daily activities such as tooth brushing also produce a bacteraemia and may present a greater risk of infective endocarditis than a single dental procedure.

Antibacterial prophylaxis and chlorhexidine mouthwash p. 1175 are **not** recommended for the prevention of endocarditis in patients undergoing dental procedures. Such prophylaxis may expose patients to the adverse effects of antimicrobials when the evidence of benefit has not been proven.

Reduction of oral bacteraemia Patients at risk of endocarditis including those with valve replacement, acquired valvular heart disease with stenosis or regurgitation, structural congenital heart disease (including surgically corrected or palliated structural conditions, but excluding isolated atrial septal defect, fully repaired ventricular septal defect, fully repaired patent ductus arteriosus, and closure devices considered to be endothelialised), hypertrophic cardiomyopathy, or a previous episode of infective endocarditis, should be advised to maintain the highest possible standards of oral hygiene in order to reduce the:

- need for dental extractions or other surgery;
- chances of severe bacteraemia if dental surgery is needed;
- possibility of 'spontaneous' bacteraemia.

Postoperative care Patients at risk of endocarditis including those with valve replacement, acquired valvular heart disease with stenosis or regurgitation, structural congenital heart disease (including surgically corrected or palliated structural conditions, but excluding isolated atrial septal defect, fully repaired ventricular septal defect, fully repaired patent ductus arteriosus, and closure devices considered to be endothelialised), hypertrophic cardiomyopathy, or a previous episode of infective endocarditis, should be warned to report to the doctor or dentist any unexplained illness that develops after dental treatment.

Any infection in patients at risk of endocarditis should be investigated promptly and treated appropriately to reduce the risk of endocarditis.

Patients on anticoagulant therapy

For general advice on dental surgery in patients receiving oral anticoagulant therapy see Thromboembolic Disease below.

Joint prostheses

Advice of a Working Party of the British Society for Antimicrobial Chemotherapy is that patients with prosthetic joint implants (including total hip replacements) do not require antibiotic prophylaxis for dental treatment. The Working Party considers that it is unacceptable to expose patients to the adverse effects of antibiotics when there is no evidence that such prophylaxis is of any benefit, but that those who develop any intercurrent infection require prompt treatment with antibiotics to which the infecting organisms are sensitive.

The Working Party has commented that joint infections have rarely been shown to follow dental procedures and are even more rarely caused by oral streptococci.

Pacemakers

Pacemakers prevent asystole or severe bradycardia. Some ultrasonic scalers, electronic apex locators, electro-analgesic devices, and electrocautery devices interfere with the normal function of pacemakers (including shielded pacemakers) and should not be used. The manufacturer's literature should be consulted whenever possible. If severe bradycardia occurs in a patient fitted with a pacemaker, electrical equipment should be switched off and the patient placed supine with the legs elevated. If the patient loses consciousness and the pulse remains slow or is absent, cardiopulmonary resuscitation may be needed. Call immediately for medical assistance and an ambulance, as appropriate.

A Working Party of the British Society for Antimicrobial Chemotherapy does not recommend antibacterial prophylaxis for patients with pacemakers.

Thromboembolic disease

Patients receiving a **heparin** or an oral anticoagulant such as warfarin sodium p. 139, acenocoumarol (nicoumalone) p. 138, phenindione p. 139, apixaban p. 124, dabigatran etexilate p. 135 or rivaroxaban p. 127 may be liable to excessive bleeding after extraction of teeth or other dental surgery. Often dental surgery can be delayed until the anticoagulant therapy has been completed.

For a patient requiring long-term therapy with warfarin sodium, the patient's medical practitioner should be consulted and the International Normalised Ratio (INR) should be assessed 72 hours before the dental procedure. This allows sufficient time for dose modification if necessary. In those with an unstable INR (including those who require weekly monitoring of their INR, or those who have had some INR measurements greater than 4.0 in the last 2 months), the INR should be assessed within 24 hours of the dental procedure. Patients requiring minor dental procedures (including extractions) who have an INR below 4.0 may continue warfarin sodium without dose adjustment. There is no need to check the INR for a patient requiring a non-invasive dental procedure.

If it is necessary to remove several teeth, a single extraction should be done first; if this goes well further teeth may be extracted at subsequent visits (two or three at a time). Measures should be taken to minimise bleeding during and after the procedure. This includes the use of sutures and a haemostatic such as oxidised cellulose, collagen sponge or resorbable gelatin sponge. Scaling and root planing should initially be restricted to a limited area to assess the potential for bleeding.

For a patient on long-term warfarin sodium, the advice of the clinician responsible for the patient's anticoagulation should be sought if:

- the INR is unstable, or if the INR is greater than 4.0;
- the patient has thrombocytopenia, haemophilia, or other disorders of haemostasis, or suffers from liver impairment, alcoholism, or renal failure;
- the patient is receiving antiplatelet drugs, cytotoxic drugs or radiotherapy.

Intramuscular injections are *contra-indicated* in patients taking anticoagulants with an INR above the therapeutic range, and in those with any disorder of haemostasis. In patients taking anticoagulants who have a stable INR within the therapeutic range, intramuscular injections should be avoided if possible; if an intramuscular injection is necessary, the patient should be informed of the increased risk of localised bleeding and monitored carefully.

A local anaesthetic containing a vasoconstrictor should be given by infiltration, or by intraligamentary or mental nerve injection if possible. If regional nerve blocks cannot be avoided the local anaesthetic should be given cautiously using an aspirating syringe.

Drugs which have potentially serious interactions with anticoagulants include aspirin and other NSAIDs, carbamazepine p. 309, imidazole and triazole antifungals (including miconazole p. 811), erythromycin p. 530, clarithromycin p. 529, and metronidazole p. 533; for details of these and other interactions with anticoagulants, see Appendix 1 (dabigatran etexilate, heparins, phenindione, rivaroxaban, and coumarins).

Although studies have failed to demonstrate an interaction, common experience in anticoagulant clinics is that the INR can be altered following a course of an oral broad-spectrum antibiotic, such as ampicillin p. 540 or amoxicillin p. 539. Information on the treatment of patients who take anticoagulants is available at www.npsa.nhs.uk/patientsafety/alerts-and-directives/alerts/anticoagulant.

Liver disease

Liver disease may alter the response to drugs and drug prescribing should be kept to a minimum in patients with severe liver disease. Problems are likely mainly in patients with *jaundice, ascites,* or evidence of *encephalopathy.* For guidance on prescribing for patients with hepatic impairment, see Prescribing in hepatic impairment p. 19. Where care is needed when prescribing in hepatic impairment, this is indicated under the relevant drug in the BNF.

Renal impairment

The use of drugs in patients with reduced renal function can give rise to many problems. Many of these problems can be avoided by reducing the dose or by using alternative drugs. Special care is required in renal transplantation and immunosuppressed patients; if necessary such patients should be referred to specialists.

For guidance on prescribing in patients with renal impairment, see Prescribing in renal impairment p. 19. Where care is needed when prescribing in renal impairment, this is indicated under the relevant drug in the BNF.

Pregnancy

Drugs taken during pregnancy can be harmful to the fetus and should be prescribed only if the expected benefit to the mother is thought to be greater than the risk to the fetus; all drugs should be avoided if possible during the first trimester. For guidance on prescribing in pregnancy, see Prescribing in pregnancy p. 22. Where care is needed when prescribing in pregnancy, this is indicated under the relevant drug in the BNF.

Breast-feeding

Some drugs taken by the mother whilst breast-feeding can be transferred to the breast milk, and may affect the infant. For guidance on prescribing in breast-feeding, see Prescribing in breast-feeding p. 22. Where care is needed when prescribing in breast-feeding, this is indicated under the relevant drug in the BNF.

Chapter 1
Gastro-intestinal system

CONTENTS

1 Chronic bowel disorders
1.1 Coeliac disease

Coeliac disease
25-Jul-2016

Description of condition
Coeliac disease is an autoimmune condition which is associated with chronic inflammation of the small intestine. Dietary proteins known as gluten, which are present in wheat, barley and rye, activate an abnormal immune response in the intestinal mucosa, which can lead to malabsorption of nutrients.

Aims of treatment
The management of coeliac disease is aimed at eliminating symptoms (such as diarrhoea, bloating and abdominal pain) and reducing the risk of complications, including those resulting from malabsorption.

Non-drug treatment
EvGr The only effective treatment for coeliac disease is a strict, life-long, gluten-free diet. A range of gluten-free products is available for prescription (see *Borderline substances*). ⟨A⟩

Drug treatment
EvGr Patients who have coeliac disease are at an increased risk of malabsorption of key nutrients (such as calcium and vitamin D). Their risk of osteoporosis and the need for active treatment of bone disease should form part of the ongoing management of coeliac disease. Supplementation of key nutrients may be required if dietary intake is insufficient.

Patients who have coeliac disease should be advised **not** to self-medicate with over-the-counter vitamins or mineral supplements. Initiation of supplementation should involve a discussion with a member of the patient's healthcare team in order to identify the individual needs of the patient and to allow for appropriate ongoing monitoring.

Confirmed cases of refractory coeliac disease should be referred to a specialist centre. Treatment with prednisolone

p. 664 can be considered for initial management while awaiting specialist advice. ⟨A⟩

Useful Resources
Coeliac disease: recognition, assessment and management. National Institute for Health and Care Excellence. Clinical guideline 20. September 2015.
www.nice.org.uk/guidance/ng20

1.2 Diverticular disease and diverticulitis

Diverticular disease and diverticulitis
24-Feb-2016

Description of condition
Diverticular disease is a condition where diverticula (sac-like protrusions of mucosa through the muscular colonic wall) cause intermittent lower abdominal pain in the absence of inflammation or infection. The prevalence of diverticula increases with age, with the majority of patients older than 50 years.

Diverticulitis occurs when the diverticula become inflamed and infected, causing marked lower abdominal pain usually accompanied by fever and general malaise, and occasionally, with large rectal bleeds. Complicated diverticulitis includes episodes associated with an abscess, free perforation, fistula, obstruction, or stricture.

To ensure that an accurate diagnosis of diverticular disease and diverticulitis is made, consider and exclude all other causes of lower abdominal pain prior to treatment.

Aims of treatment
The aim of treatment is to relieve symptoms of diverticular disease, cure episodes of diverticulitis, and reduce the risk of recurrences and complications.

Drug treatment

EvGr A high-fibre diet is recommended for the treatment of symptomatic diverticular disease, although evidence supporting this is inconsistent and of low quality. Bulk-forming drugs have also been used, but evidence of their effectiveness is lacking.

Treatment of uncomplicated diverticulitis includes a low residue diet and bowel rest. Antibacterials are recommended only when the patient presents with signs of infection or is immunocompromised, as there is no evidence to support routine administration.

Patients with complicated diverticulitis or with severe presentation, require hospital admission, treatment with intravenous antibacterials (covering Gram-negative organisms and anaerobes), and bowel rest.

There is insufficient evidence to justify the role of fibre, rifaximin p. 565, antispasmodics, mesalazine p. 39, and probiotics in the prevention or treatment of diverticulitis.

Elective surgery to provide symptomatic relief or prevent recurrence, should be considered for patients following recovery from an episode of complicated diverticulitis. This includes episodes associated with free perforation, abscess, fistula, obstruction, or stricture. Urgent sigmoid colectomy is required for patients with diffuse peritonitis or for those in whom non-operative management of acute diverticulitis fails. Ⓐ

1.3 Inflammatory bowel disease

Inflammatory bowel disease

Chronic inflammatory bowel diseases include Crohn's disease below and Ulcerative colitis p. 37.

Drugs used in chronic bowel disorders

Aminosalicylates

Sulfasalazine p. 42 is a combination of 5-aminosalicylic acid ('5-ASA') and sulfapyridine; sulfapyridine acts only as a carrier to the colonic site of action but still causes side-effects. In the newer aminosalicylates, mesalazine (5-aminosalicylic acid) p. 39, balsalazide sodium p. 39 (a pro-drug of 5-aminosalicylic acid) and olsalazine sodium p. 42 (a dimer of 5-aminosalicylic acid which cleaves in the lower bowel), the sulfonamide-related side-effects of sulfasalazine are avoided, but 5-aminosalicylic acid alone can still cause side-effects including blood disorders and lupus-like syndrome also seen with sulfasalazine.

Drugs affecting the immune response

Folic acid p. 993 should be given to reduce the possibility of methotrexate toxicity [unlicensed indication]. Folic acid is usually given once weekly on a different day to the methotrexate; alternative regimens may be used in some settings.

Cytokine modulators

Infliximab p. 1082, adalimumab p. 1073, and golimumab p. 1080 are monoclonal antibodies which inhibit the pro-inflammatory cytokine, tumour necrosis factor alpha. They should be used under specialist supervision.

Crohn's disease

20-Dec-2016

Description of condition

Crohn's disease is a chronic, inflammatory bowel disease that mainly affects the gastro-intestinal tract. It is characterised by thickened areas of the gastro-intestinal wall with inflammation extending through all layers, deep ulceration and fissuring of the mucosa, and the presence of granulomas; affected areas may occur in any part of the gastro-intestinal tract, interspersed with areas of relatively normal tissue. Crohn's disease may present as recurrent attacks, with acute exacerbations combined with periods of remission or less active disease. Symptoms depend on the site of disease but may include abdominal pain, diarrhoea, fever, weight loss and rectal bleeding.

Complications of Crohn's disease include intestinal strictures, abscesses in the wall of the intestine or adjacent structures, fistulae, anaemia, malnutrition, colorectal and small bowel cancers, and growth failure and delayed puberty in children. Crohn's disease may also be associated with extra-intestinal manifestation: the most common are arthritis and abnormalities of the joints, eyes, liver and skin. Crohn's disease is also a cause of secondary osteoporosis and those at greatest risk should be monitored for osteopenia and assessed for the risk of fractures.

Fistulating Crohn's disease

Fistulating Crohn's disease is a complication that involves the formation of a fistula between the intestine and adjacent structures, such as perianal skin, bladder, and vagina. It occurs in about one quarter of patients, mostly when the disease involves the ileocolonic area.

Aims of treatment

Treatment is largely directed at the induction and maintenance of remission and the relief of symptoms. Active treatment of acute Crohn's disease should be distinguished from preventing relapse. The aims of drug treatment are to reduce symptoms and maintain or improve quality of life, while minimising toxicity related to drugs over both the short and long term.

In fistulating Crohn's disease, surgery and medical treatment aim to close and maintain closure of the fistula.

Non-drug treatment

EvGr In addition to drug treatment, management options for Crohn's disease include smoking cessation and attention to nutrition, which plays an important role in supportive care. Surgery may be considered in certain patients with early disease limited to the distal ileum and in severe or chronic active disease. Ⓐ

Drug treatment

Treatment of acute disease

Monotherapy

EvGr A corticosteroid (either prednisolone p. 664 or methylprednisolone p. 663 or intravenous hydrocortisone p. 662), is used to induce remission in patients with a first presentation or a single inflammatory exacerbation of Crohn's disease in a 12-month period.

In patients with distal ileal, ileocaecal or right-sided colonic disease, in whom a conventional corticosteroid is unsuitable or contra-indicated, budesonide p. 43 may be considered. Budesonide is less effective but may cause fewer side-effects than other corticosteroids, as systemic exposure is limited. Aminosalicylates (such as sulfasalazine p. 42 and mesalazine p. 39) are an alternative option in these patients. They are less effective than a corticosteroid or budesonide, but may be preferred because they have fewer side-effects. Aminosalicylates and budesonide are not appropriate for severe presentations or exacerbations. Ⓐ

Add-on treatment

EvGr Add on treatment is prescribed if there are two or more inflammatory exacerbations in a 12-month period, or the corticosteroid dose cannot be reduced.

Azathioprine p. 816 or mercaptopurine p. 887 [unlicensed indications] can be added to a corticosteroid or budesonide to induce remission. In patients who cannot tolerate azathioprine or mercaptopurine or in whom thiopurine methyltransferase (TPMT) activity is deficient, methotrexate p. 888 can be added to a corticosteroid.

Under specialist supervision, monoclonal antibody therapies, adalimumab p. 1073 and infliximab p. 1082, are options for the treatment of severe, active Crohn's disease, following inadequate response to conventional therapies or in those who are intolerant of or have contra-indications to conventional therapy. Vedolizumab p. 44 is recommended as a treatment option for moderate to severely active Crohn's disease when therapy with adalimumab or infliximab is unsuccessful, is contra-indicated or not tolerated. See also *National funding/access decisions* for adalimumab, infliximab and vedolizumab.

Adalimumab and infliximab can be used as monotherapy or combined with an immunosuppressant although there is uncertainty about the comparative effectiveness and long-term side-effects of therapy. Ⓐ

Maintenance of remission
EvGr Patients who choose not to receive maintenance treatment during remission should be made aware of the symptoms that may suggest a relapse (most frequently unintended weight loss, abdominal pain, diarrhoea and general ill-health). For those who choose not to receive maintenance treatment during remission, a suitable follow up plan should be agreed upon and information provided on how to access healthcare if a relapse should occur.

Azathioprine or mercaptopurine [unlicensed indications] as monotherapy can be used to maintain remission when previously used with a corticosteroid to induce remission. They may also be used in patients who have not previously received these drugs (particularly those with adverse prognostic factors such as early age of onset, perianal disease, corticosteroid use at presentation, and severe presentations). Methotrexate can be used to maintain remission only in patients who required methotrexate to induce remission, or who are intolerant of or are not suitable for azathioprine or mercaptopurine for maintenance. Corticosteroids or budesonide should not be used. Ⓐ

Maintaining remission following surgery
EvGr Azathioprine or mercaptopurine [unlicensed indications] can be considered to maintain remission after surgery in patients with adverse prognostic factors such as more than one resection, or previously complicated or debilitating disease (for example abscess, involvement of adjacent structures, fistulating or penetrating disease). Aminosalicylates can also be considered as an option, however budesonide or enteral nutrition should not be used. Ⓐ

Other treatments
EvGr Loperamide hydrochloride p. 66 or codeine phosphate p. 448 can be used to manage diarrhoea associated with Crohn's disease in those who do not have colitis. Ⓐ Colestyramine p. 196 is licensed for the relief of diarrhoea associated with Crohn's disease. See also Diarrhoea (acute) p. 65.

Fistulating Crohn's disease
Perianal fistulae are the most common occurrence in patients with fistulating Crohn's disease. EvGr Treatment may not be necessary for simple, asymptomatic perianal fistulae. When fistulae are symptomatic, local drainage and surgery may be required in conjunction with the medical therapy.

Metronidazole p. 533 or ciprofloxacin p. 548 [unlicensed indications], alone or in combination, can improve symptoms of fistulating Crohn's disease but complete healing occurs rarely. Metronidazole is usually given for 1 month, but no longer than 3 months because of concerns about peripheral neuropathy. Other antibacterials should be given if specifically indicated (e.g. in sepsis associated with fistulae and perianal disease) and for managing bacterial overgrowth in the small bowel.

Either azathioprine or mercaptopurine [unlicensed indications] is used to control the inflammation in fistulating Crohn's disease and they are continued for maintenance.

Infliximab p. 1082 is recommended for patients with active fistulating Crohn's disease who have not responded to conventional therapy (including antibacterials, drainage and immunosuppressive treatments), or who are intolerant of or have contra-indications to conventional therapy. Infliximab should be used after ensuring that all sepsis is actively draining.

Abscess drainage, fistulotomy, and seton insertion may be appropriate, particularly before infliximab treatment.

Azathioprine, mercaptopurine, or infliximab should be continued as maintenance treatment for at least one year.

For the management of non-perianal fistulating Crohn's disease (including entero-gynaecological and enterovesical fistulae) surgery is the only recommended approach. Ⓐ

Useful Resources
Crohn's disease: management in adults, children and young people. Clinical guideline 152. October 2012 (updated May 2016).
www.nice.org.uk/guidance/cg152

Ulcerative colitis   20-Feb-2017
Description of condition
Ulcerative colitis is a chronic inflammatory condition, characterised by diffuse mucosal inflammation—it has a relapsing-remitting pattern. It is a life-long disease that is associated with significant morbidity. It most commonly presents between the ages of 15 and 25 years, although diagnosis can be made at any age.

The pattern of inflammation is continuous, extending from the rectum upwards to a varying degree. Inflammation of the rectum is referred to as **proctitis**, and inflammation of the rectum and sigmoid colon as **proctosigmoiditis**. **Left-sided colitis** refers to disease involving the colon distal to the splenic flexure. **Extensive colitis** affects the colon proximal to the splenic flexure, and includes pan-colitis, where the whole colon is involved. Common symptoms of active disease or relapse include bloody diarrhoea, an urgent need to defaecate, and abdominal pain.

Ulcerative colitis is classified as **subacute** if it is moderate-to-severely active disease which can be managed in an outpatient setting, and does not require hospitalisation or consideration of urgent surgical intervention.

Complications associated with ulcerative colitis include an increased risk of colorectal cancer, secondary osteoporosis, venous thromboembolism and toxic megacolon.

Aims of treatment
Treatment is focussed on treating active disease to manage symptoms and to induce and maintain remission.

Drug treatment
Overview
EvGr Management of ulcerative colitis is dependent on factors such as clinical severity, extent of disease, and patient preference. Clinical and laboratory investigations are used to determine the extent and severity of disease and to guide treatment. Severity is classified as mild, moderate or severe by using the Truelove and Witts' Severity Index to assess bowel movements, heart rate, erythrocyte sedimentation rate and the presence of pyrexia, melaena or anaemia—see the NICE guideline for Ulcerative Colitis for further information (*Useful resources* below). Ⓐ
EvGr The extent of disease should be considered when choosing the route of administration for aminosalicylates and corticosteroids; whether oral treatment, topical treatment or both are to be used. If the inflammation is

distal, a rectal preparation is adequate but if the inflammation is extended, systemic medication is required. Either suppositories or enemas can be offered, taking into account the patient's preferences. Ⓐ

EvGr Rectal foam preparations and suppositories can be used when patients have difficulty retaining liquid enemas.

Diarrhoea associated with ulcerative colitis is sometimes treated with anti-diarrhoeal drugs (such as loperamide hydrochloride p. 66 or codeine phosphate p. 448) on the advice of a specialist; however their use is contra-indicated in acute ulcerative colitis as they can increase the risk of toxic megacolon.

A macrogol-containing osmotic laxative (such as macrogol 3350 with potassium chloride, sodium bicarbonate and sodium chloride p. 56) may be useful for proximal faecal loading in proctitis. Ⓔ

Oral aminosalicylates for the treatment of ulcerative colitis are available in different preparations and release forms. EvGr The preparation and dosing schedule should be chosen taking into account the delivery characteristics and suitability for the patient. When used to maintain remission, single daily doses of oral aminosalicylates can be more effective than multiple daily dosing, but may result in more side-effects. Ⓐ

Treatment of acute mild-to-moderate ulcerative colitis

EvGr Acute treatment to induce remission generally consists of an aminosalicylate with or without a corticosteroid. Ⓐ

EvGr Oral and rectal aminosalicylate in combination can be used as first line treatment in patients with acute, mild-to-moderate extensive ulcerative colitis; as this is associated with higher rates of improvement in disease activity. Ⓔ

Proctitis and proctosigmoiditis

EvGr **Aminosalicylates** are recommended as first-line treatment for patients with a mild-to-moderate initial presentation or inflammatory exacerbation. Using a rectal aminosalicylate (mesalazine p. 39 or sulfasalazine p. 42) alone is likely to be more effective for patients with **proctitis** and **proctosigmoiditis**. Monotherapy with an oral aminosalicylate (balsalazide sodium p. 39, mesalazine, olsalazine sodium p. 42, sulfasalazine) can be considered for patients who prefer not to use enemas or suppositories, although this may not be as effective.

A rectal **corticosteroid** (budesonide p. 43, hydrocortisone p. 662 or prednisolone p. 664) or oral prednisolone can be considered in patients who are intolerant to, decline, or have a contra-indication to aminosalicylates.

Oral prednisolone should be considered for the treatment of patients with subacute proctitis or proctosigmoiditis. Ⓐ

Left-sided or extensive ulcerative colitis

EvGr First-line treatment in patients with **left-sided** or **extensive** ulcerative colitis is a high induction dose of an oral aminosalicylate, with addition of a rectal aminosalicylate or oral beclometasone dipropionate if necessary. Oral prednisolone alone is recommended for patients who cannot tolerate or who decline aminosalicylates, in whom aminosalicylates are contra-indicated or in patients with subacute left-sided or extensive ulcerative colitis. Ⓐ

Initial treatment failure in all extents of mild-to-moderate disease

EvGr In all patients who are treated with an aminosalicylate, if there are no improvements within four weeks of initial treatment or if symptoms worsen, addition of oral prednisolone to aminosalicylate therapy can be considered (discontinue beclometasone dipropionate p. 43 if adding oral prednisolone). If there is still no response after 2–4 weeks of prednisolone, consider adding oral tacrolimus p. 821 [unlicensed indication] to induce remission. Ⓐ Budesonide multimatrix (a corticosteroid that is taken orally but exerts its action topically in the colon) is licensed for inducing remission in mild-to-moderate active ulcerative colitis in

adults for whom aminosalicylate treatment is not sufficient and can be considered as an additional therapeutic option.

EvGr Moderate disease may require treatment with a monoclonal antibody due to inadequate response to conventional treatment or if conventional treatment is not tolerated or contra-indicated (see *Monoclonal antibodies for ulcerative colitis* below). Ⓐ

Treatment of acute severe ulcerative colitis

Acute severe ulcerative colitis of any extent can be life-threatening and is regarded as a medical emergency. EvGr Immediate hospital admission is required for treatment.

Intravenous corticosteroids (such as hydrocortisone or methylprednisolone p. 663) should be given to induce remission in patients with acute severe ulcerative colitis (at first presentation or an exacerbation) while assessing the need for surgery. If intravenous corticosteroids are contra-indicated, declined or cannot be tolerated, then intravenous ciclosporin p. 818 [unlicensed indication] or surgery should be considered. A combination of intravenous ciclosporin with intravenous corticosteroids, or surgery is second line therapy for patients who have little or no improvement within 72 hours of starting intravenous corticosteroids or whose symptoms worsen despite treatment. Ⓐ

EvGr Research has shown that infliximab p. 1082 is as effective as ciclosporin and, in practice, it is commonly used in these patients instead of ciclosporin—see also *Monoclonal antibodies for acute ulcerative colitis*, below.

In patients who experience an initial response to steroids followed by deterioration, stool cultures should be taken to exclude the presence of pathogens; cytomegalovirus activation should be considered. Ⓔ

Monoclonal antibodies for acute ulcerative colitis

EvGr Adalimumab p. 1073, golimumab p. 1080, infliximab p. 1082 and vedolizumab p. 44 can be used to treat moderate-to-severe active ulcerative colitis following an inadequate response to conventional treatment options, or if conventional treatment options are not tolerated or contra-indicated. Treatment with these agents is continued into the maintenance phase, if effective and tolerated. See also *National funding/access decisions* for adalimumab, golimumab, infliximab and vedolizumab.

Infliximab can be used to treat acute exacerbations of severely active ulcerative colitis if ciclosporin is contra-indicated or clinically inappropriate. Ⓐ

Maintaining remission in mild, moderate or severe ulcerative colitis

EvGr To reduce the chances of relapse occurring, maintenance therapy with an aminosalicylate is recommended in most patients. Corticosteroids are **not** suitable for maintenance treatment because of their side-effects.

After a mild-to-moderate inflammatory exacerbation of *proctitis* or *proctosigmoiditis*, a rectal aminosalicylate can be started alone or in combination with an oral aminosalicylate, administered daily or as part of an intermittent regimen (such as twice to three times weekly or the first seven days of each month). An oral aminosalicylate can be used alone in patients who prefer not to use enemas or suppositories, although, this may not be as effective.

A low-dose of oral aminosalicylate is given to maintain remission in patients after a mild-to-moderate inflammatory exacerbation of left-sided or extensive ulcerative colitis.

When used to maintain remission, single daily doses of oral aminosalicylates can be more effective than multiple daily dosing, but may result in more side-effects.

Oral azathioprine p. 816 or mercaptopurine p. 887 [unlicensed indications] can be considered to maintain remission, if there has been two or more inflammatory exacerbations in a 12-month period that required treatment with systemic corticosteroids, or if remission is not maintained by aminosalicylates, or following a single acute severe episode. ⟨A⟩

There is no evidence to support the use of methotrexate p. 888 to induce or maintain remission in ulcerative colitis, though its use is common in clinical practice.

Monoclonal antibodies for maintaining remission of ulcerative colitis

Treatment with these agents is continued into the maintenance phase, if effective and tolerated in acute disease. See also *National funding/access decisions* for adalimumab, golimumab, infliximab and vedolizumab.

Non-drug treatment

EvGr Surgery may be necessary as emergency treatment for severe ulcerative colitis that does not respond to drug treatment. Patients can also choose to have elective surgery for unresponsive or frequently relapsing disease that is affecting their quality of life. ⟨A⟩

Useful Resources

NICE. Ulcerative colitis: management in adults, children and young people. Clinical guideline 166. June 2013.
www.nice.org.uk/guidance/CG166/

> **Other drugs used for Inflammatory bowel disease**
> Ustekinumab, p. 1069

AMINOSALICYLATES

Aminosalicylates

- SIDE-EFFECTS
- **Common or very common** Arthralgia · cough · diarrhoea · dizziness · fever · gastrointestinal discomfort · headache · leucopenia · nausea · skin reactions · vomiting
- **Uncommon** Alopecia · depression · dyspnoea · myalgia · photosensitivity reaction · thrombocytopenia
- **Rare or very rare** Agranulocytosis · bone marrow disorders · cardiac inflammation · hepatitis · neutropenia · pancreatitis · peripheral neuropathy · renal impairment · respiratory disorders
- **Frequency not known** Angioedema · eosinophilia · haemolytic anaemia · nephritis tubulointerstitial · oligozoospermia (reversible) · ulcerative colitis aggravated

  SIDE-EFFECTS, FURTHER INFORMATION A blood count should be performed and the drug stopped immediately if there is suspicion of a blood dyscrasia.
- ALLERGY AND CROSS-SENSITIVITY Contra-indicated in salicylate hypersensitivity.
- RENAL IMPAIRMENT
  Monitoring Renal function should be monitored more frequently in renal impairment.
- MONITORING REQUIREMENTS Renal function should be monitored before starting an oral aminosalicylate, at 3 months of treatment, and then annually during treatment.
- PATIENT AND CARER ADVICE
  Blood disorders Patients receiving aminosalicylates, and their carers, should be advised to report any unexplained bleeding, bruising, purpura, sore throat, fever or malaise that occurs during treatment.

📕 above

Balsalazide sodium

- INDICATIONS AND DOSE

Treatment of mild to moderate ulcerative colitis, acute attack
- BY MOUTH
- Adult: 2.25 g 3 times a day until remission occurs or for up to maximum of 12 weeks

Maintenance of remission of ulcerative colitis
- BY MOUTH
- Adult: 1.5 g twice daily (max. per dose 3 g), adjusted according to response; maximum 6 g per day

- CAUTIONS History of asthma
- INTERACTIONS → Appendix 1: balsalazide
- SIDE-EFFECTS Acute kidney injury · blood disorder · cholelithiasis · lupus-like syndrome
- PREGNANCY Manufacturer advises avoid.
- BREAST FEEDING Diarrhoea may develop in the infant.
  Monitoring Monitor breast-fed infants for diarrhoea.
- HEPATIC IMPAIRMENT Avoid in severe impairment.
- RENAL IMPAIRMENT Manufacturer advises avoid in moderate to severe impairment.

- MEDICINAL FORMS
  There can be variation in the licensing of different medicines containing the same drug.
  Capsule
  CAUTIONARY AND ADVISORY LABELS 21, 25
  - Colazide (Almirall Ltd)
    Balsalazide disodium 750 mg Colazide 750mg capsules |
    130 capsule PoM £30.42 DT = £30.42

📕 above

Mesalazine

- INDICATIONS AND DOSE

DOSE EQUIVALENCE AND CONVERSION
There is no evidence to show that any one oral preparation of mesalazine is more effective than another; however, the delivery characteristics of oral mesalazine preparations may vary.

ASACOL ® MR 400MG TABLETS

Treatment of mild to moderate ulcerative colitis, acute attack
- BY MOUTH
- Child 12–17 years: 800 mg 3 times a day
- Adult: 2.4 g daily in divided doses

Maintenance of remission of ulcerative colitis and Crohn's ileo-colitis
- BY MOUTH
- Child 12–17 years: 400–800 mg 2–3 times a day
- Adult: 1.2–2.4 g daily in divided doses

ASACOL ® MR 800MG TABLETS

Treatment of mild to moderate ulcerative colitis, acute attack
- BY MOUTH
- Adult: 2.4–4.8 g daily in divided doses

Maintenance of remission of ulcerative colitis
- BY MOUTH
- Adult: Up to 2.4 g once daily, alternatively up to 2.4 g daily in divided doses

Maintenance of remission of Crohn's ileo-colitis
- BY MOUTH
- Adult: Up to 2.4 g daily in divided doses   continued →

ASACOL® FOAM ENEMA

Treatment of acute attack of mild to moderate ulcerative colitis affecting the rectosigmoid region
▸ BY RECTUM
▸ Adult: 1 g daily for 4–6 weeks, to be administered into the rectum

Treatment of acute attack of mild to moderate ulcerative colitis, affecting the descending colon
▸ BY RECTUM
▸ Adult: 2 g once daily for 4–6 weeks, to be administered into the rectum

ASACOL® SUPPOSITORIES

Treatment of acute attack of mild to moderate ulcerative colitis and maintenance of remission
▸ BY RECTUM
▸ Adult: 0.75–1.5 g daily in divided doses, last dose to be administered at bedtime

MEZAVANT® XL

Treatment of mild to moderate ulcerative colitis, acute attack
▸ BY MOUTH
▸ Adult: 2.4 g once daily, increased if necessary to 4.8 g once daily, review treatment at 8 weeks

Maintenance of remission of ulcerative colitis
▸ BY MOUTH
▸ Adult: 2.4 g once daily

OCTASA®

Treatment of mild to moderate ulcerative colitis, acute attack
▸ BY MOUTH
▸ Adult: 2.4–4.8 g once daily, alternatively 2.4–4.8 g daily in divided doses, dose over 2.4 g daily in divided doses only

Maintenance of remission of ulcerative colitis and Crohn's ileo-colitis
▸ BY MOUTH
▸ Adult: 1.2–2.4 g once daily, alternatively daily in divided doses

PENTASA® GRANULES

Treatment of mild to moderate ulcerative colitis, acute attack
▸ BY MOUTH
▸ Child 5–17 years (body-weight up to 40 kg): 10–20 mg/kg 3 times a day
▸ Child 5–17 years (body-weight 40 kg and above): 1–2 g twice daily, total daily dose may alternatively be given in 3–4 divided doses
▸ Adult: Up to 4 g once daily, alternatively up to 4 g daily in 2–4 divided doses

Maintenance of remission of ulcerative colitis
▸ BY MOUTH
▸ Child 5–17 years (body-weight up to 40 kg): 7.5–15 mg/kg twice daily, total daily dose may alternatively be given in 3 divided doses
▸ Child 5–17 years (body-weight 40 kg and above): 2 g once daily
▸ Adult: 2 g once daily

PENTASA® RETENTION ENEMA

Treatment of acute attack of mild to moderate ulcerative colitis or maintenance of remission
▸ BY RECTUM
▸ Adult: 1 g once daily, dose to be administered at bedtime

Treatment of acute attack of mild to moderate ulcerative colitis affecting the rectosigmoid region
▸ BY RECTUM
▸ Child 12–17 years: 1 g once daily, dose to be administered at bedtime

PENTASA® SUPPOSITORIES

Treatment of acute attack, ulcerative proctitis
▸ BY RECTUM
▸ Adult: 1 g daily for 2–4 weeks

Maintenance, ulcerative proctitis
▸ BY RECTUM
▸ Adult: 1 g daily

PENTASA® TABLETS

Treatment of mild to moderate ulcerative colitis, acute attack
▸ BY MOUTH
▸ Adult: Up to 4 g once daily, alternatively up to 4 g daily in 2–3 divided doses

Maintenance of remission of ulcerative colitis
▸ BY MOUTH
▸ Adult: 2 g once daily

SALOFALK® ENEMA

Treatment of acute attack of mild to moderate ulcerative colitis or maintenance of remission
▸ BY RECTUM
▸ Adult: 2 g once daily, dose to be administered at bedtime

SALOFALK® GRANULES

Treatment of mild to moderate ulcerative colitis, acute attack
▸ BY MOUTH
▸ Child 5–17 years (body-weight up to 40 kg): 30–50 mg/kg once daily, dose preferably given in the morning, alternatively 10–20 mg/kg 3 times a day
▸ Child 5–17 years (body-weight 40 kg and above): 1.5–3 g once daily, dose preferably given in the morning, alternatively 0.5–1 g 3 times a day
▸ Adult: 1.5–3 g once daily, dose preferably taken in the morning, alternatively 0.5–1 g 3 times a day

Maintenance of remission of ulcerative colitis
▸ BY MOUTH
▸ Child 5–17 years (body-weight up to 40 kg): 7.5–15 mg/kg twice daily, total daily dose may alternatively be given in 3 divided doses
▸ Child 5–17 years (body-weight 40 kg and above): 500 mg 3 times a day
▸ Adult: 500 mg 3 times a day

SALOFALK® RECTAL FOAM

Treatment of mild ulcerative colitis affecting sigmoid colon and rectum
▸ BY RECTUM
▸ Child 12–17 years: 2 g once daily, dose to be administered into the rectum at bedtime, alternatively 2 g daily in 2 divided doses
▸ Adult: 2 g once daily, dose to be administered into the rectum at bedtime, alternatively 2 g daily in 2 divided doses

SALOFALK® SUPPOSITORIES

Treatment of acute attack of mild to moderate ulcerative colitis affecting the rectum, sigmoid colon and descending colon
▸ BY RECTUM
▸ Adult: 0.5–1 g 2–3 times a day, adjusted according to response, dose to be given using 500 mg suppositories

Treatment of acute attack of mild to moderate ulcerative colitis affecting the rectum
▸ BY RECTUM
▸ Adult: 1 g daily, preferably at bedtime, dose to be given using 1 g suppositories

SALOFALK® TABLETS

Treatment of mild to moderate ulcerative colitis, acute attack
▶ BY MOUTH
▶ Child 5–17 years (body-weight up to 40 kg): 10–20 mg/kg 3 times a day
▶ Child 5–17 years (body-weight 40 kg and above): 0.5–1 g 3 times a day
▶ Adult: 0.5–1 g 3 times a day

Maintenance of remission of ulcerative colitis
▶ BY MOUTH
▶ Child 5–17 years (body-weight up to 40 kg): 7.5–15 mg/kg twice daily, total daily dose may alternatively be given in 3 divided doses
▶ Child 5–17 years (body-weight 40 kg and above): 500 mg 3 times a day
▶ Adult: 500 mg 3 times a day

● UNLICENSED USE
▶ With oral use in children *Asacol*® (all preparations) not licensed for use in children under 18 years. *Pentasa*® granules and *Salofalk*® tablets and granules not licensed for use in children under 6 years.
▶ With rectal use in children *Salofalk*® rectal foam no dose recommendations for children (age range not specified by manufacturer).

● CONTRA-INDICATIONS Blood clotting abnormalities (in children)
● CAUTIONS Elderly · pulmonary disease
● INTERACTIONS → Appendix 1: mesalazine
● SIDE-EFFECTS
GENERAL SIDE-EFFECTS
▶ Rare or very rare Flatulence · hepatic disorders · nephritis
SPECIFIC SIDE-EFFECTS
▶ Rare or very rare
▶ With rectal use Constipation

● PREGNANCY Negligible quantities cross placenta.
● BREAST FEEDING Diarrhoea reported in breast-fed infants, but negligible amounts of mesalazine detected in breast milk.
Monitoring Monitor breast-fed infant for diarrhoea.
● HEPATIC IMPAIRMENT Avoid in severe impairment.
● RENAL IMPAIRMENT
▶ In adults Use with caution. Avoid if eGFR less than 20 mL/minute/1.73 m².
▶ In children Use with caution. Avoid if estimated glomerular filtration rate less than 20 mL/minute/1.73 m².

● DIRECTIONS FOR ADMINISTRATION
PENTASA® TABLETS Tablets may be halved, quartered, or dispersed in water, but should not be chewed.
PENTASA® GRANULES Granules should be placed on tongue and washed down with water or orange juice without chewing.
▶ In children Contents of one sachet should be weighed and divided immediately before use; discard any remaining granules.
SALOFALK® GRANULES Granules should be placed on tongue and washed down with water without chewing.

● PRESCRIBING AND DISPENSING INFORMATION There is no evidence to show that any one oral preparation of mesalazine is more effective than another; however, the delivery characteristics of oral mesalazine preparations may vary.
Flavours of granule formulations of *Salofalk*® may include vanilla.

● PATIENT AND CARER ADVICE If it is necessary to switch a patient to a different brand of mesalazine, the patient should be advised to report any changes in symptoms.

Some products may require special administration advice; patients and carers should be informed.
Medicines for Children leaflet: Mesalazine (oral) for inflammatory bowel disease www.medicinesforchildren.org.uk/mesalazine-oral-for-inflammatory-bowel-disease
Medicines for Children leaflet: Mesalazine foam enema for inflammatory bowel disease www.medicinesforchildren.org.uk/mesalazine-foam-enema-for-inflammatory-bowel-disease
Medicines for Children leaflet: Mesalazine liquid enema for inflammatory bowel disease www.medicinesforchildren.org.uk/mesalazine-liquid-enema-for-inflammatory-bowel-disease

● MEDICINAL FORMS
There can be variation in the licensing of different medicines containing the same drug.

Modified-release tablet
CAUTIONARY AND ADVISORY LABELS 21(does not apply to Pentasa® tablets), 25 (does not apply to Pentasa® tablets)
▶ Mezavant XL (Shire Pharmaceuticals Ltd)
Mesalazine 1.2 gram Mezavant XL 1200mg tablets | 60 tablet [PoM] £42.95 DT = £42.95
▶ Pentasa (Ferring Pharmaceuticals Ltd)
Mesalazine 500 mg Pentasa 500mg modified-release tablets | 100 tablet [PoM] £30.74 DT = £30.74
Mesalazine 1 gram Pentasa 1g modified-release tablets | 60 tablet [PoM] £36.89 DT = £36.89

Foam
EXCIPIENTS: May contain Cetostearyl alcohol (including cetyl and stearyl alcohol), disodium edetate, hydroxybenzoates (parabens), polysorbates, propylene glycol, sodium metabisulfite
▶ Salofalk (Dr. Falk Pharma UK Ltd)
Mesalazine 1 gram per 1 application Salofalk 1g/application foam enema | 14 dose [PoM] £30.17 DT = £30.17

Gastro-resistant tablet
CAUTIONARY AND ADVISORY LABELS 5(does not apply to Octasa®), 25
▶ Asacol MR (Allergan Ltd)
Mesalazine 400 mg Asacol 400mg MR gastro-resistant tablets | 84 tablet [PoM] £27.45 DT = £27.45 | 168 tablet [PoM] £54.90
Mesalazine 800 mg Asacol 800mg MR gastro-resistant tablets | 84 tablet [PoM] £54.90 DT = £54.90
▶ Octasa MR (Tillotts Pharma Ltd)
Mesalazine 400 mg Octasa 400mg MR gastro-resistant tablets | 90 tablet [PoM] £16.58 DT = £16.58 | 120 tablet [PoM] £22.10
Mesalazine 800 mg Octasa 800mg MR gastro-resistant tablets | 90 tablet [PoM] £40.38 | 180 tablet [PoM] £80.75 DT = £80.75
▶ Salofalk (Dr. Falk Pharma UK Ltd)
Mesalazine 250 mg Salofalk 250mg gastro-resistant tablets | 100 tablet [PoM] £16.19 DT = £16.19
Mesalazine 500 mg Salofalk 500mg gastro-resistant tablets | 100 tablet [PoM] £32.38 DT = £32.38

Suppository
▶ Asacol (Allergan Ltd)
Mesalazine 250 mg Asacol 250mg suppositories | 20 suppository [PoM] £4.82 DT = £4.82
Mesalazine 500 mg Asacol 500mg suppositories | 10 suppository [PoM] £4.82 DT = £4.82
▶ Pentasa (Ferring Pharmaceuticals Ltd)
Mesalazine 1 gram Pentasa 1g suppositories | 28 suppository [PoM] £40.01 DT = £40.01
▶ Salofalk (Dr. Falk Pharma UK Ltd)
Mesalazine 500 mg Salofalk 500mg suppositories | 30 suppository [PoM] £14.81
Mesalazine 1 gram Salofalk 1g suppositories | 30 suppository [PoM] £29.62

Modified-release granules
CAUTIONARY AND ADVISORY LABELS 25 (does not apply to Pentasa® granules)
EXCIPIENTS: May contain Aspartame
▶ Pentasa (Ferring Pharmaceuticals Ltd)
Mesalazine 1 gram Pentasa 1g modified-release granules sachets sugar-free | 50 sachet [PoM] £30.74 DT = £30.74
Mesalazine 2 gram Pentasa 2g modified-release granules sachets sugar-free | 60 sachet [PoM] £73.78 DT = £73.78
▶ Salofalk (Dr. Falk Pharma UK Ltd)
Mesalazine 1 gram Salofalk 1g gastro-resistant modified-release granules sachets sugar-free | 50 sachet [PoM] £28.74 DT = £28.74

Mesalazine 1.5 gram Salofalk 1.5g gastro-resistant modified-release granules sachets sugar-free | 60 sachet [PoM] £48.85 DT = £48.85
Mesalazine 3 gram Salofalk 3g gastro-resistant modified-release granules sachets sugar-free | 60 sachet [PoM] £97.70 DT = £97.70

Enema
▸ Pentasa (Ferring Pharmaceuticals Ltd)
Mesalazine 10 mg per 1 ml Pentasa Mesalazine 1g/100ml enema | 7 enema [PoM] £17.73 DT = £17.73
▸ Salofalk (Dr. Falk Pharma UK Ltd)
Mesalazine 33.9 mg per 1 ml Salofalk 2g/59ml enema | 7 enema [PoM] £29.92 DT = £29.92

Olsalazine sodium

● INDICATIONS AND DOSE
Treatment of acute attack of mild ulcerative colitis
▸ BY MOUTH
▸ Adult: 1 g daily in divided doses, doses to be taken after meals, then increased if necessary up to 3 g daily in divided doses (max. per dose 1 g), dose to be increased over 1 week

Maintenance of remission of mild ulcerative colitis
▸ BY MOUTH
▸ Adult: Maintenance 500 mg twice daily, dose to be taken after food

● INTERACTIONS → Appendix 1: olsalazine
● SIDE-EFFECTS
▸ Uncommon Paraesthesia · tachycardia
▸ Frequency not known Palpitations · vision blurred
● PREGNANCY Manufacturer advises avoid unless potential benefit outweighs risk.
● BREAST FEEDING
Monitoring Monitor breast-fed infants for diarrhoea.
● RENAL IMPAIRMENT Use with caution; manufacturer advises avoid in significant impairment.
● DIRECTIONS FOR ADMINISTRATION Capsules can be opened and contents sprinkled on food.

● MEDICINAL FORMS
There can be variation in the licensing of different medicines containing the same drug. Forms available from special-order manufacturers include: oral suspension, oral solution
Tablet
CAUTIONARY AND ADVISORY LABELS 21
▸ Olsalazine sodium (Non-proprietary)
Olsalazine sodium 500 mg Olsalazine 500mg tablets | 60 tablet [PoM] £161.00 DT = £161.00
Capsule
CAUTIONARY AND ADVISORY LABELS 21
▸ Olsalazine sodium (Non-proprietary)
Olsalazine sodium 250 mg Olsalazine 250mg capsules | 112 capsule [PoM] £144.00 DT = £144.00

Sulfasalazine
07-Feb-2018
(Sulphasalazine)

● INDICATIONS AND DOSE
Treatment of acute attack of mild to moderate and severe ulcerative colitis | Active Crohn's disease
▸ BY MOUTH
▸ Adult: 1–2 g 4 times a day until remission occurs, corticosteroids may also be given, if necessary
▸ BY RECTUM
▸ Adult: 0.5–1 g twice daily, administered alone or in conjunction with oral therapy, morning and night after a bowel movement

Maintenance of remission of mild to moderate and severe ulcerative colitis
▸ BY MOUTH
▸ Adult: 500 mg 4 times a day
▸ BY RECTUM
▸ Adult: 0.5–1 g twice daily, administered alone or in conjunction with oral therapy, morning and night after a bowel movement

Active rheumatoid arthritis (administered on expert advice)
▸ BY MOUTH
▸ Adult: Initially 500 mg daily, increased in steps of 500 mg every week, increased to 2–3 g daily in divided doses, enteric coated tablets to be administered

IMPORTANT SAFETY INFORMATION
SAFE PRACTICE
Sulfasalazine has been confused with sulfadiazine; care must be taken to ensure the correct drug is prescribed and dispensed.

● CAUTIONS Acute porphyrias p. 1025 · G6PD deficiency · history of allergy · history of asthma · maintain adequate fluid intake · risk of haematological toxicity · risk of hepatic toxicity · slow acetylator status
● INTERACTIONS → Appendix 1: sulfasalazine
● SIDE-EFFECTS
▸ Common or very common Insomnia · stomatitis · taste altered · tinnitus · urine abnormalities
▸ Uncommon Face oedema · seizure · vasculitis · vertigo
▸ Frequency not known Anaemia · appetite decreased · ataxia · cyanosis · encephalopathy · haematuria · hallucination · hepatic disorders · hypoprothrombinaemia · idiopathic pulmonary fibrosis · lymphadenopathy · macrocytosis · meningitis aseptic · methaemoglobinaemia · myocarditis allergic · nephrotic syndrome · parotitis · periorbital oedema · pseudomembranous enterocolitis · serum sickness · severe cutaneous adverse reactions (SCARs) · smell disorders · systemic lupus erythematosus (SLE) · yellow discolouration of body fluids
SIDE-EFFECTS, FURTHER INFORMATION Incidence of side-effects increases with higher doses.
Blood disorders Haematological abnormalities occur usually in the first 3 to 6 months of treatment—discontinue if these occur.
● PREGNANCY Theoretical risk of neonatal haemolysis in third trimester; adequate folate supplements should be given to mother.
● BREAST FEEDING Small amounts in milk (1 report of bloody diarrhoea); theoretical risk of neonatal haemolysis especially in G6PD-deficient infants.
● HEPATIC IMPAIRMENT Use with caution.
● RENAL IMPAIRMENT Risk of toxicity, including crystalluria, in moderate impairment—ensure high fluid intake. Avoid in severe impairment.
● MONITORING REQUIREMENTS
▸ Blood disorders Close monitoring of full blood counts (including differential white cell count and platelet count) is necessary initially, and at monthly intervals during the first 3 months.
▸ Renal function Although the manufacturer recommends renal function tests in rheumatic diseases, evidence of practical value is unsatisfactory.
▸ Liver function Liver function tests should be performed at monthly intervals for first 3 months.
● PATIENT AND CARER ADVICE
Contact lenses Some soft contact lenses may be stained.

● MEDICINAL FORMS
There can be variation in the licensing of different medicines containing the same drug. Forms available from special-order manufacturers include: oral suspension

Oral suspension
CAUTIONARY AND ADVISORY LABELS 14
EXCIPIENTS: May contain Alcohol
▸ Sulfasalazine (Non-proprietary)
Sulfasalazine 50 mg per 1 ml Sulfasalazine 250mg/5ml oral suspension sugar free sugar-free | 500 ml PoM £42.76 DT = £42.76

Gastro-resistant tablet
CAUTIONARY AND ADVISORY LABELS 5, 14, 25
▸ Sulfasalazine (Non-proprietary)
Sulfasalazine 500 mg Sulfasalazine 500mg gastro-resistant tablets | 112 tablet PoM £8.43 DT = £8.43
▸ Salazopyrin EN(Pfizer Ltd)
Sulfasalazine 500 mg Salazopyrin EN-Tabs 500mg | 112 tablet PoM £8.43 DT = £8.43
▸ Sulazine EC(Genesis Pharmaceuticals Ltd)
Sulfasalazine 500 mg Sulazine EC 500mg tablets | 112 tablet PoM £6.74 DT = £8.43

Tablet
CAUTIONARY AND ADVISORY LABELS 14
▸ Sulfasalazine (Non-proprietary)
Sulfasalazine 500 mg Sulfasalazine 500mg tablets | 112 tablet PoM £9.00 DT = £7.83
▸ Salazopyrin(Pfizer Ltd)
Sulfasalazine 500 mg Salazopyrin 500mg tablets | 112 tablet PoM £6.97 DT = £7.83

Suppository
CAUTIONARY AND ADVISORY LABELS 14
▸ Salazopyrin(Pfizer Ltd)
Sulfasalazine 500 mg Salazopyrin 500mg suppositories | 10 suppository PoM £3.30

CORTICOSTEROIDS

F 658

Beclometasone dipropionate

04-Jan-2016

(Beclomethasone dipropionate)

● INDICATIONS AND DOSE

Adjunct to aminosalicylates in acute mild to moderate ulcerative colitis
▸ BY MOUTH
▸ Adult: 5 mg daily maximum duration of treatment of 4 weeks, dose to be taken in the morning

● INTERACTIONS → Appendix 1: corticosteroids

● SIDE-EFFECTS
▸ **Uncommon** Abdominal pain · constipation · idiopathic intracranial hypertension · menorrhagia · muscle cramps · throat candidiasis

● HEPATIC IMPAIRMENT Manufacturer advises avoid in severe impairment—no information available.

● MEDICINAL FORMS
There can be variation in the licensing of different medicines containing the same drug.
Modified-release tablet
CAUTIONARY AND ADVISORY LABELS 25
▸ Clipper(Chiesi Ltd)
Beclometasone dipropionate 5 mg Clipper 5mg gastro-resistant modified-release tablets | 30 tablet PoM £56.56

F 658

Budesonide

21-Dec-2017

● DRUG ACTION Budesonide is a glucocorticoid, which exerts significant local anti-inflammatory effects.

● INDICATIONS AND DOSE

BUDENOFALK ® CAPSULES

Mild to moderate Crohn's disease affecting the ileum or ascending colon
▸ BY MOUTH
▸ Adult: 9 mg once daily for 8 weeks, to be taken in the morning, alternatively 3 mg 3 times a day for 8 weeks, reduce dose gradually over two weeks following treatment

Collagenous colitis
▸ BY MOUTH
▸ Adult: 9 mg once daily for 8 weeks, to be taken in the morning, reduce dose gradually over two weeks following treatment

Autoimmune hepatitis, induction of remission
▸ BY MOUTH
▸ Adult: 3 mg 3 times a day

Autoimmune hepatitis, maintenance
▸ BY MOUTH
▸ Adult: 3 mg twice daily

BUDENOFALK ® GRANULES

Mild to moderate Crohn's disease affecting the ileum or ascending colon | Collagenous colitis
▸ BY MOUTH
▸ Adult: 9 mg once daily for 8 weeks, to be taken in the morning about 30 minutes before breakfast, reduce dose gradually over two weeks following treatment

BUDENOFALK ® RECTAL FOAM

Ulcerative colitis affecting sigmoid colon and rectum
▸ BY RECTUM
▸ Adult: 1 metered application once daily for up to 8 weeks

DOSE EQUIVALENCE AND CONVERSION
▸ For *Budenofalk*® rectal foam: 1 metered application is equivalent to budesonide 2 mg.

CORTIMENT ®

Induction of remission of mild-to-moderate active ulcerative colitis
▸ BY MOUTH
▸ Adult: 9 mg once daily for up to 8 weeks, dose to be taken in the morning

ENTOCORT ® CAPSULES

Active microscopic colitis
▸ BY MOUTH
▸ Adult: 9 mg once daily, to be taken in the morning

Mild to moderate Crohn's disease affecting the ileum or ascending colon
▸ BY MOUTH
▸ Adult: 9 mg once daily for up to 8 weeks; reduce dose for the last 2–4 weeks of treatment, to be taken in the morning

ENTOCORT ® ENEMA

Ulcerative colitis involving rectal and recto-sigmoid disease
▸ BY RECTUM
▸ Adult: 1 enema daily for 4 weeks, to be administered at bedtime

● CAUTIONS
▸ With systemic use Autoimmune hepatitis
● INTERACTIONS → Appendix 1: corticosteroids

1

Gastro-intestinal system

- SIDE-EFFECTS
  ▸ **Common or very common**
    ▸ With oral use Muscle twitching · oedema
    ▸ With rectal use Diarrhoea · gastrointestinal disorders
  ▸ **Rare or very rare**
    ▸ With oral use Fatigue · malaise
- HEPATIC IMPAIRMENT
  Monitoring When used in autoimmune hepatitis liver function tests should be monitored every 2 weeks for 1 month, then at least every 3 months.
- DIRECTIONS FOR ADMINISTRATION Granules should be placed on tongue and washed down with water without chewing.
- PRESCRIBING AND DISPENSING INFORMATION Flavours of granule formulations may include lemon.
  ENTOCORT® CAPSULES Dispense modified-release capsules in original container (contains desiccant).
- PATIENT AND CARER ADVICE Patients or carers should be given advice on how to administer budesonide granules.
- NATIONAL FUNDING/ACCESS DECISIONS
  CORTIMENT®

  Scottish Medicines Consortium (SMC) Decisions
  The *Scottish Medicines Consortium* has advised (October 2016) that budesonide (*Cortiment*®) is accepted for restricted use within NHS Scotland for induction of remission of mild-to-moderate active ulcerative colitis where aminosalicylate treatment is not sufficient, and only if patients present with active left-sided disease and/or proctosigmoiditis who are not suitable for oral prednisolone, as an alternative to budesonide rectal formulations or off-label oral budesonide.

  BUDENOFALK® CAPSULES

  Scottish Medicines Consortium (SMC) Decisions
  ▸ With oral use The *Scottish Medicines Consortium* has advised (April 2015) that *Budenofalk*® gastro-resistant capsules are accepted for restricted use within NHS Scotland for the treatment of autoimmune hepatitis in non-cirrhotic patients who are intolerant of conventional oral corticosteroids (prednisolone) with severe corticosteroid-related side effects (actual or anticipated) such as psychosis, poorly controlled diabetes or osteoporosis.

- MEDICINAL FORMS
  There can be variation in the licensing of different medicines containing the same drug.
  Modified-release tablet
  CAUTIONARY AND ADVISORY LABELS 25
  ▸ Cortiment (Ferring Pharmaceuticals)
    Budesonide 9 mg Cortiment 9mg modified-release tablets | 30 tablet PoM £75.00 DT = £75.00
  Gastro-resistant capsule
  CAUTIONARY AND ADVISORY LABELS 5, 10, 22, 25
  ▸ Budenofalk (Dr. Falk Pharma UK Ltd)
    Budesonide 3 mg Budenofalk 3mg gastro-resistant capsules | 100 capsule PoM £75.05 DT = £75.05
  Foam
  EXCIPIENTS: May contain Cetostearyl alcohol (including cetyl and stearyl alcohol), disodium edetate, propylene glycol, sorbic acid
  ▸ Budenofalk (Dr. Falk Pharma UK Ltd)
    Budesonide 2 mg per 1 actuation Budenofalk 2mg foam enema | 14 dose PoM £57.11
  Modified-release capsule
  CAUTIONARY AND ADVISORY LABELS 5, 10, 25
  ▸ Entocort CR (Tillotts Pharma Ltd)
    Budesonide 3 mg Entocort CR 3mg capsules | 100 capsule PoM £84.15 DT = £84.15
  Gastro-resistant granules
  CAUTIONARY AND ADVISORY LABELS 5, 10, 22, 25
  ▸ Budenofalk (Dr. Falk Pharma UK Ltd)
    Budesonide 9 mg Budenofalk 9mg gastro-resistant granules sachets | 60 sachet PoM £135.00 DT = £135.00

Enema
- Entocort (Tillotts Pharma Ltd)
  Budesonide 20 microgram per 1 ml Entocort 2mg/100ml enema | 7 enema PoM £33.66

IMMUNOSUPPRESSANTS › MONOCLONAL ANTIBODIES, ANTI-LYMPHOCYTE

Vedolizumab

04-Apr-2016

- DRUG ACTION Vedolizumab is a monoclonal antibody that binds specifically to the $\alpha_4\beta_7$ integrin, which is expressed on gut homing T helper lymphocytes and causes a reduction in gastrointestinal inflammation.

- INDICATIONS AND DOSE

  Moderate to severe active ulcerative colitis in patients who have had an inadequate response with, lost response to, or are intolerant to either conventional therapy or a tumour necrosis factor alpha inhibitor (under expert supervision)
  ▸ BY INTRAVENOUS INFUSION
    ▸ Adult: Initially 300 mg, then 300 mg after 2 weeks, followed by 300 mg after 4 weeks, followed by 300 mg every 8 weeks, dose to be given over 30 minutes, if treatment is interrupted or response decreases, dosing frequency may be increased—consult product literature; review treatment if no response within 10 weeks of initial dose

  Moderate to severe active Crohn's disease in patients who have had an inadequate response with, lost response to, or are intolerant to either conventional therapy or a tumour necrosis factor alpha inhibitor (under expert supervision)
  ▸ BY INTRAVENOUS INFUSION
    ▸ Adult: Initially 300 mg, then 300 mg after 2 weeks, followed by 300 mg after 4 weeks, followed by 300 mg every 8 weeks, dose to be given over 30 minutes, if no response is observed, an additional dose of 300 mg may be given 10 weeks after initial dose; if treatment is interrupted or response decreases, dosing frequency may be increased—consult product literature; review treatment if no response within 14 weeks of initial dose

- CONTRA-INDICATIONS Severe active infection
- CAUTIONS Controlled chronic severe infection · history of recurring severe infection · previous treatment with natalizumab (wait at least 12 weeks between natalizumab use and initiation of vedolizumab unless potential benefit outweighs risk) · previous treatment with rituximab
  CAUTIONS, FURTHER INFORMATION
  ▸ Risk of infection Patients must be screened for tuberculosis before starting treatment; if latent tuberculosis is diagnosed, appropriate treatment must be initiated prior to vedolizumab treatment; if tuberculosis is diagnosed during treatment, discontinue vedolizumab until infection is resolved.
    Patients should be brought up to date with current immunisation schedule before initiating treatment.
- INTERACTIONS → Appendix 1: monoclonal antibodies
- SIDE-EFFECTS
  ▸ **Common or very common** Arthralgia · constipation · cough · fatigue · fever · gastrointestinal discomfort · gastrointestinal disorders · headache · hypertension · increased risk of infection · muscle spasms · muscle weakness · nasal congestion · nausea · night sweats · oropharyngeal pain · pain · paraesthesia · skin reactions
  ▸ **Uncommon** Chills · feeling cold
  ▸ **Frequency not known** Hypersensitivity
  SIDE-EFFECTS, FURTHER INFORMATION Infusion-related and hypersensitivity reactions have been reported. Patients should be observed continuously during each

infusion for signs and symptoms of acute hypersensitivity reactions; they should also be observed for 2 hours after the initial two infusions, and for 1 hour after subsequent infusions. Discontinue treatment if a severe infusion-related or other severe reaction occurs and initiate appropriate treatment (e.g. adrenaline and antihistamines); if a mild to moderate infusion-related reaction occurs, interrupt infusion or reduce infusion rate and initiate appropriate treatment (if reaction subsides the infusion may be continued)—consider pretreatment with an antihistamine, hydrocortisone, and/or paracetamol prior to subsequent infusions in patients who experience mild to moderate infusion-related reactions.

- CONCEPTION AND CONTRACEPTION Manufacturer advises effective contraception required during and for at least 18 weeks after treatment.
- PREGNANCY Manufacturer advises use only if potential benefit outweighs risk.
- BREAST FEEDING Manufacturer advises avoid—present in milk in *animal* studies.
- MONITORING REQUIREMENTS
  ▸ Manufacturer advises monitor closely for infection before, during and after treatment—potential increased risk of opportunistic infection.
  ▸ Manufacturer advises monitor for new onset or worsening neurological signs and symptoms (withhold treatment if progressive multifocal leukoencephalopathy (PML) is suspected.
- DIRECTIONS FOR ADMINISTRATION For *intravenous infusion* (*Entyvio*®), give intermittently *in* Sodium chloride 0.9%; allow vial to reach room temperature then reconstitute with 4.8 mL of water for injection (using a syringe with a 21–25 gauge needle); gently swirl vial for at least 15 seconds, do not shake vigorously or invert; allow to stand for up to 20 minutes (gently swirl vial if needed), leave for an additional 10 minutes if not dissolved; gently invert vial three times, withdraw 5 mL of reconstituted solution (using a syringe with a 21–25 gauge needle), and add to 250 mL of infusion fluid; gently mix and give over 30 minutes.
- PATIENT AND CARER ADVICE Patients should be provided with a patient alert card.
- NATIONAL FUNDING/ACCESS DECISIONS

  NICE decisions
  ▸ **Vedolizumab for treating moderately to severely active Crohn's disease after prior therapy (August 2015)** NICE TA352
  Vedolizumab is recommended as an option for the treatment of moderate to severe active Crohn's disease in adults if:
  - a tumour necrosis factor-alpha inhibitor has failed (that is, the disease has responded inadequately or has lost response to treatment) **or**
  - a tumour necrosis factor-alpha inhibitor cannot be tolerated or is contra-indicated,
  - **and** the manufacturer provides vedolizumab with the discount agreed in the patient access scheme.

  Vedolizumab should be given as a planned course of treatment until treatment fails, or surgery is needed, or until 12 months after starting treatment, whichever is the shorter. Treatment should be continued only if there is clear evidence of a response. Patients who continue treatment should be reassessed at least every 12 months to determine whether ongoing treatment is still clinically appropriate.

  Patients currently receiving vedolizumab whose disease does not meet the above criteria should be able to continue treatment until they and their clinician consider it appropriate to stop.
  www.nice.org.uk/TA352

Scottish Medicines Consortium (SMC) Decisions
The *Scottish Medicines Consortium* has advised (July 2015) that vedolizumab (*Entyvio*®) is accepted for restricted use within NHS Scotland for the treatment of adult patients with moderately to severely active Crohn's disease who have had an inadequate response with, lost response to, or were intolerant to a TNFα antagonist; it is also accepted for use in NHS Scotland for the treatment of adult patients with moderately to severely active ulcerative colitis who have had an inadequate response with, lost response to, or were intolerant to either conventional therapy or a TNFα antagonist.

- MEDICINAL FORMS
  There can be variation in the licensing of different medicines containing the same drug.

  Powder for solution for infusion
  ▸ Entyvio (Takeda UK Ltd) ▼
    Vedolizumab 300 mg Entyvio 300mg powder for concentrate for solution for infusion vials | 1 vial [PoM] £2,050.00

1.4 Irritable bowel syndrome

Irritable bowel syndrome   24-Feb-2016

Description of condition

Irritable bowel syndrome (IBS) is a common, chronic, relapsing, and often life-long condition, mainly affecting people aged between 20 and 30 years. It is more common in women. Symptoms include abdominal pain or discomfort, disordered defaecation (either diarrhoea, or constipation with straining, urgency, and incomplete evacuation), passage of mucus, and bloating. Symptoms are usually relieved by defaecation. Obtaining an accurate clinical diagnosis of IBS prior to treatment is crucial.

Aims of treatment

The treatment of IBS is focused on symptom control, in order to improve quality of life.

Non-drug treatment

[EvGr] Diet and lifestyle changes are important for effective self-management of IBS. Patients should be encouraged to increase physical activity, and advised to eat regularly, without missing meals or leaving long gaps between meals. Dietary advice should also include, limiting fresh fruit consumption to no more than 3 portions per day. The fibre intake of patients with IBS should be reviewed. If an increase in dietary fibre is required, soluble fibre such as ispaghula husk p. 54, or foods high in soluble fibre such as oats, are recommended. Intake of insoluble fibre (e.g. bran) and 'resistant starch' should be reduced or discouraged as they may exacerbate symptoms. Fluid intake (mostly water) should be increased to at least 8 cups each day and the intake of caffeine, alcohol and fizzy drinks reduced. The artificial sweetener sorbitol should be avoided in patients with diarrhoea. Where probiotics are being used, continue for at least 4 weeks while monitoring the effect.

If a patient's symptoms persist following lifestyle and dietary advice, single food avoidance and exclusion diets may be an option under the supervision of a dietitian or medical specialist. Ⓐ

Drug treatment

[EvGr] The choice of drug treatment depends on the nature and severity of the symptoms. Many drug treatment options for IBS are available over-the-counter.

Antispasmodic drugs (such as alverine citrate p. 86, mebeverine hydrochloride p. 86 and peppermint oil p. 47) can be taken in addition to dietary and lifestyle changes. A laxative (excluding lactulose p. 56 as it may cause bloating) can be used to treat constipation. Patients who have not responded to laxatives from the different classes and who have had constipation for at least 12 months, can be treated with linaclotide p. 47. Loperamide hydrochloride p. 66 is the first-line choice of anti-motility drug for relief of diarrhoea. Patients with IBS should be advised how on to adjust their dose of laxative or anti-motility drug according to stool consistency, with the aim of achieving a soft, well-formed stool. Ⓐ See Constipation p. 52, for information on other drugs used for chronic constipation.

EvGr A low-dose tricyclic antidepressant, such as amitriptyline hydrochloride p. 369 [unlicensed indication], can be used for abdominal pain or discomfort as a second-line option in patients who have not responded to antispasmodics, anti-motility drugs, or laxatives. A selective serotonin reuptake inhibitor may be considered in those who do not respond to a tricyclic antidepressant [unlicensed indication].

Psychological intervention can be offered to patients who have no relief of IBS symptoms after 12 months of drug treatment. Ⓐ

Useful Resources

Irritable bowel syndrome in adults: diagnosis and management. Clinical guideline 61. February 2015
www.nice.org.uk/guidance/cg61

ANTIDIARRHOEALS ⟩ ANTIPROPULSIVES

Eluxadoline
03-Jan-2018

- **DRUG ACTION** Eluxadoline acts locally on opioid receptors in the gut to reduce gastro-intestinal contractility and fluid secretion.

- **INDICATIONS AND DOSE**

Irritable bowel syndrome with diarrhoea (specialist use only)

▶ BY MOUTH
▶ Adult: 100 mg twice daily; reduced if not tolerated to 75 mg twice daily, dose should be administered in the morning and evening, the reduced dose may be more appropriate for elderly patients

IMPORTANT SAFETY INFORMATION

MHRA/CHM ADVICE: ELUXADOLINE (*TRUBERZI*®): RISK OF PANCREATITIS; DO NOT USE IN PATIENTS WHO HAVE UNDERGONE CHOLECYSTECTOMY OR IN THOSE WITH BILIARY DISORDERS (DECEMBER 2017)

Cases of pancreatitis, with or without sphincter of Oddi spasm, have been reported in patients taking eluxadoline. Some cases have resulted in hospitalisation and death, primarily in patients who have undergone cholecystectomy—see Contra-indications and Patient and carer advice for further information. Eluxadoline should be initiated and supervised by a specialist physician experienced in diagnosis and management of gastrointestinal disorders.

- **CONTRA-INDICATIONS** Alcoholism · cholecystectomy · diseases of the biliary tract · diseases of the pancreas · excessive alcohol use · gall bladder agenesis · gastro-intestinal obstruction · history of chronic constipation · history of hepatic impairment · history of pancreatitis · history of severe constipation · known or suspected biliary tree or pancreatic duct obstruction · sphincter of Oddi disease or dysfunction

- **CAUTIONS** Genetic predisposition for poor function of OATP1B1 transporter (increased risk of adverse events)

- **INTERACTIONS** → Appendix 1: eluxadoline

- **SIDE-EFFECTS**
▶ **Common or very common** Constipation · dizziness · drowsiness · gastrointestinal discomfort · gastrointestinal disorders · nausea · skin reactions · vomiting
▶ **Uncommon** Sphincter of Oddi spasm (discontinue)

- **PREGNANCY** Manufacturer advises avoid—limited information available.

- **BREAST FEEDING** Manufacturer advises avoid—present in milk in *animal* studies.

- **HEPATIC IMPAIRMENT** Manufacturer advises avoid—risk of significantly increased plasma-drug concentration.

- **MONITORING REQUIREMENTS** Manufacturer advises monitor for symptoms suggestive of sphincter of Oddi spasm and pancreatitis.

- **PATIENT AND CARER ADVICE** Manufacturer advises that patients should be told to avoid alcohol during treatment; patients should also be advised to stop treatment and seek medical attention if they experience symptoms suggestive of pancreatitis or sphincter of Oddi spasm, (such as acute worsening of abdominal pain that may radiate to the back or shoulder, with or without nausea and vomiting), or if they develop severe constipation lasting for more than 4 days.

- **NATIONAL FUNDING/ACCESS DECISIONS**

NICE decisions
▶ **Eluxadoline for treating irritable bowel syndrome with diarrhoea (August 2017)** NICE TA471
Eluxadoline is recommended as an option for treating irritable bowel syndrome with diarrhoea in patients, only if:
- the condition has not responded to other pharmacological treatments (for example, antimotility agents, antispasmodics, tricyclic antidepressants), **or**
- pharmacological treatments are contra-indicated or not tolerated, **and**
- it is started in secondary care.
Stop eluxadoline at four weeks if there is inadequate relief of the symptoms of irritable bowel syndrome with diarrhoea.

Patients whose treatment was started within the NHS before this guidance was published should have the option to continue treatment, without change to their funding arrangements, until they and their clinician consider it appropriate to stop.
www.nice.org.uk/guidance/ta471

Scottish Medicines Consortium (SMC) Decisions
The *Scottish Medicines Consortium* has advised (January 2018) that eluxadoline (*Truberzi*®) is **not** recommended for use within NHS Scotland in adults for the treatment of irritable bowel syndrome with diarrhoea as the economic case was not demonstrated.

- **MEDICINAL FORMS**
There can be variation in the licensing of different medicines containing the same drug.

Tablet
CAUTIONARY AND ADVISORY LABELS 3, 21
▶ Truberzi (Allergan Ltd) ▼
Eluxadoline 75 mg Truberzi 75mg tablets | 56 tablet [PoM] £88.20
Eluxadoline 100 mg Truberzi 100mg tablets | 56 tablet [PoM] £88.20

ANTISPASMODICS

Alverine with simeticone

27-Jul-2017

The properties listed below are those particular to the combination only. For the properties of the components please consider, alverine citrate p. 86.

- ● INDICATIONS AND DOSE
  Abdominal pain in irritable bowel syndrome
  ▸ BY MOUTH
  ▸ Adult: 60/300 mg 2–3 times a day, to be taken at the beginning of meals
  DOSE EQUIVALENCE AND CONVERSION
  ▸ Dose expressed as x/y mg alverine/simeticone.

- ● MEDICINAL FORMS
  There can be variation in the licensing of different medicines containing the same drug.
  Capsule
  ▸ SimAlvia (HFA Healthcare Products Ltd)
    Alverine citrate 60 mg, Simeticone 300 mg SimAlvia 60mg/300mg capsules | 90 capsule [PoM] £11.00

Mebeverine with ispaghula husk

04-Feb-2016

The properties listed below are those particular to the combination only. For the properties of the components please consider, mebeverine hydrochloride p. 86, ispaghula husk p. 54.

- ● INDICATIONS AND DOSE
  Irritable bowel syndrome
  ▸ BY MOUTH
  ▸ Child 12–17 years: 1 sachet twice daily, in water, morning and evening, 30 minutes before food and 1 sachet daily if required, taken 30 minutes before midday meal
  ▸ Adult: 1 sachet twice daily, in water, morning and evening, 30 minutes before food and 1 sachet daily if required, taken 30 minutes before midday meal

- ● DIRECTIONS FOR ADMINISTRATION Contents of one sachet should be stirred into a glass (approx. 150 mL) of cold water and drunk immediately.

- ● PATIENT AND CARER ADVICE Patients or carers should be given advice on how to administer ispaghula husk with mebeverine granules.

- ● MEDICINAL FORMS
  There can be variation in the licensing of different medicines containing the same drug.
  Effervescent granules
  CAUTIONARY AND ADVISORY LABELS 13, 22
  EXCIPIENTS: May contain Aspartame
  ELECTROLYTES: May contain Potassium
  ▸ Fybogel Mebeverine (Reckitt Benckiser Healthcare (UK) Ltd)
    Mebeverine hydrochloride 135 mg, Ispaghula husk 3.5 gram Fybogel Mebeverine effervescent granules sachets orange sugar-free | 10 sachet [P] £4.64 DT = £4.64

Peppermint oil

- ● INDICATIONS AND DOSE
  COLPERMIN ®
  Relief of abdominal colic and distension, particularly in irritable bowel syndrome
  ▸ BY MOUTH
  ▸ Child 15–17 years: 1–2 capsules 3 times a day for up to 3 months if necessary, capsule to be swallowed whole with water
  ▸ Adult: 1–2 capsules 3 times a day for up to 3 months if necessary, capsule to be swallowed whole with water
  MINTEC ®
  Relief of abdominal colic and distension, particularly in irritable bowel syndrome
  ▸ BY MOUTH
  ▸ Adult: 1–2 capsules 3 times a day for up to 2–3 months if necessary, dose to be taken before meals, swallowed whole with water

- ● CAUTIONS Sensitivity to menthol

- ● INTERACTIONS → Appendix 1: peppermint oil

- ● SIDE-EFFECTS Ataxia · bradycardia · gastrointestinal discomfort · gastrooesophageal reflux disease · headache · nausea · paraesthesia · rash erythematous · tremor · vomiting

- ● PREGNANCY Not known to be harmful.

- ● BREAST FEEDING Significant levels of menthol in breast milk unlikely.

- ● DIRECTIONS FOR ADMINISTRATION Capsules should not be broken or chewed because peppermint oil may irritate mouth or oesophagus.

- ● MEDICINAL FORMS
  There can be variation in the licensing of different medicines containing the same drug.
  Gastro-resistant capsule
  CAUTIONARY AND ADVISORY LABELS 5, 22, 25
  ▸ Mintec (Almirall Ltd)
    Peppermint oil 200 microlitre Mintec 0.2ml gastro-resistant capsules | 84 capsule [GSL] £7.04 DT = £7.04
  Modified-release capsule
  CAUTIONARY AND ADVISORY LABELS 5, 22, 25
  EXCIPIENTS: May contain Arachis (peanut) oil
  ▸ Colpermin (McNeil Products Ltd)
    Peppermint oil 200 microlitre Colpermin gastro-resistant modified-release capsules | 20 capsule [GSL] £3.77 | 100 capsule [GSL] £14.33 DT = £13.09

LAXATIVES 〉 GUANYLATE CYCLASE-C RECEPTOR AGONISTS

Linaclotide

24-Feb-2016

- ● INDICATIONS AND DOSE
  Moderate to severe irritable bowel syndrome with constipation
  ▸ BY MOUTH
  ▸ Adult: 290 micrograms once daily, dose to be taken at least 30 minutes before meals, review treatment if no response after 4 weeks

- ● CONTRA-INDICATIONS Gastro-intestinal obstruction · inflammatory bowel disease

- ● CAUTIONS Predisposition to fluid and electrolyte disturbances

- ● SIDE-EFFECTS
  ▸ Common or very common Diarrhoea · dizziness · gastrointestinal discomfort · gastrointestinal disorders

Gastro-intestinal system

1

▸ **Uncommon** Appetite decreased · dehydration · haemorrhage · hypokalaemia · nausea · postural hypotension · vomiting
▸ **Frequency not known** Rash

SIDE-EFFECTS, FURTHER INFORMATION Manufacturer advises if diarrhoea severe or prolonged, consider suspending treatment.

● PREGNANCY Manufacturer advises avoid.

● BREAST FEEDING Unlikely to be present in milk in significant amounts, but manufacturer advises avoid.

● PRESCRIBING AND DISPENSING INFORMATION Dispense capsules in original container (contains desiccant); discard any capsules remaining 18 weeks after opening.

● NATIONAL FUNDING/ACCESS DECISIONS
Scottish Medicines Consortium (SMC) Decisions
The *Scottish Medicines Consortium* has advised (May 2013) that linaclotide (*Constella*®) is accepted for restricted use within NHS Scotland for moderate to severe irritable bowel syndrome in patients whose condition has not responded adequately to all other treatments, or who are intolerant of them.

● MEDICINAL FORMS
There can be variation in the licensing of different medicines containing the same drug.
Capsule
CAUTIONARY AND ADVISORY LABELS 22
▸ Linaclotide (Non-proprietary)
Linaclotide 290 microgram Linaclotide 290microgram capsules | 28 capsule PoM ⓢ DT = £37.56
▸ Constella (Allergan Ltd)
Linaclotide 290 microgram Constella 290microgram capsules | 28 capsule PoM £37.56 DT = £37.56

1.5 Short bowel syndrome

Short bowel syndrome
31-Aug-2016

Description of condition
Patients with a shortened bowel due to large surgical resection (with or without stoma formation) may require medical management to ensure adequate absorption of nutrients and fluid. Absorption of oral medication is also often impaired.

Aims of treatment
The management of short bowel syndrome focuses on ensuring adequate nutrition and drug absorption, thereby reducing the risk of complications resulting from these effects.

Drug treatment
Nutritional deficiencies
EvGr Patients with a short bowel may require replacement of vitamins and minerals depending on the extent and position of the bowel resection. Deficiencies in vitamins A, B$_{12}$, D, E, and K, essential fatty acids, zinc, and selenium can occur.

Hypomagnesaemia is common and is treated with oral or intravenous magnesium supplementation (see under *Magnesium*, p. 1017), though administration of oral magnesium may cause diarrhoea. Occasionally the use of oral alfacalcidol p. 1050 and correction of sodium depletion may be useful. Nutritional support can range from oral supplements to parenteral nutrition, depending on the severity of intestinal failure. Ⓐ

Diarrhoea and high output stomas
Diarrhoea is common in short bowel syndrome and can be due to multiple factors. EvGr The use of oral rehydration salts can be considered in order to promote adequate

hydration. Oral intake influences the volume of stool passed, so reducing food intake will lessen diarrhoea, but will also exacerbate the problems of undernutrition. A patient may require parenteral nutrition to allow them to eat less, if the extent of diarrhoea is unacceptable.

Pharmacological treatment may be necessary, with the choice of drug depending on the potential for side-effects and the degree of resection. Ⓐ

Antimotility drugs
EvGr Loperamide hydrochloride p. 66 and codeine phosphate p. 448 reduce intestinal motility and thus exert antidiarrhoeal actions. Loperamide hydrochloride is preferred as it is not sedative and does not cause dependence or fat malabsorption. High doses of loperamide hydrochloride [unlicensed] may be required in patients with a short bowel due to disrupted enterohepatic circulation and rapid gastrointestinal transit time. If the desired response is not obtained with loperamide hydrochloride, codeine phosphate may be added to therapy.

Co-phenotrope p. 66 has traditionally been used alone or in combination with other medications to help decrease faecal output. Co-phenotrope crosses the blood–brain barrier and can produce central nervous system side-effects, which may limit its use; the potential for dependence and anticholinergic effects may also restrict its use. Ⓐ

Colestyramine
EvGr In patients with an intact colon and less than 100 cm of ileum resected, colestyramine p. 196 can be used to bind the unabsorbed bile salts and reduce diarrhoea. When colestyramine is given to these patients, it is important to monitor for evidence of fat malabsorption (steatorrhoea) or fat-soluble vitamin deficiencies. Ⓐ

Antisecretory drugs
EvGr Drugs that reduce gastric acid secretion reduce jejunostomy output. Omeprazole p. 80 is readily absorbed in the duodenum and upper small bowel, but if less than 50 cm of jejunum remains, it may need to be given intravenously. Use of a proton pump inhibitor alone does not eliminate the need for further intervention for fluid control (such as antimotility agents, intravenous fluids, or oral rehydration salts).

Octreotide [unlicensed indication] reduces ileostomy diarrhoea and large volume jejunostomy output by inhibiting multiple pro-secretory substances. There is insufficient evidence to establish its role in the management of short bowel syndrome. Ⓐ

Growth factors
Growth factors can be used to facilitate intestinal adaptation after surgery in patients with short bowel syndrome, thus enhancing fluid, electrolyte, and micronutrient absorption.

Teduglutide p. 49 is an analogue of endogenous human glucagon-like peptide 2 (GLP-2) which is licensed for use in the management of short bowel syndrome. It may be considered after a period of stabilisation following surgery, during which intravenous fluids and nutritional support should have been optimised.

Drug absorption
For *Prescribing in patients with stoma*, see Stoma care p. 97.

EvGr Many drugs are incompletely absorbed by patients with a short bowel and may need to be prescribed in much higher doses than usual (such as levothyroxine, warfarin, oral contraceptives, and digoxin) or may need to be given intravenously. Ⓐ

Several factors can alter the absorption of drugs taken by mouth in patients with a compromised gastrointestinal system. The most important factors are the length of intestine available for drug absorption, and which section has been removed. The small intestine, with its large surface area and high blood flow, is the most important site of drug absorption. The larger amount of the small intestine that has been removed, the higher the possibility that drug absorption will be affected. Other factors, such as gastric emptying and gastric transit time, also affect drug handling.

EvGr Enteric-coated and modified-release preparations are unsuitable for use in patients with short bowel syndrome, particularly in patients with an ileostomy, as there may not be sufficient release of the active ingredient.

Dosage forms with quick dissolution (soluble tablets) should be used. Uncoated tablets and liquid formulations may also be suitable. A EvGr Before prescribing liquid formulations, prescribers should consider the osmolarity, excipient content and volume required. Hyperosmolar liquids and some excipients (such as sorbitol) can result in fluid loss. The calorie density of oral supplements should also be considered, as it will influence the volume to be taken. E

> **Other drugs used for Short bowel syndrome** Cimetidine, p. 74

AMINO ACIDS AND DERIVATIVES

▌Teduglutide

15-May-2018

● DRUG ACTION Teduglutide is an analogue of human glucagon-like peptide-2 (GLP-2), which preserves mucosal integrity by promoting growth and repair of the intestine.

● **INDICATIONS AND DOSE**

Short bowel syndrome (initiated under specialist supervision)
▶ BY SUBCUTANEOUS INJECTION
▶ Adult: 0.05 mg/kg once daily, dose to be administered to alternating quadrants of the abdomen; alternatively the thigh can be used, for optimal injection volume per body weight, consult product literature. Review treatment after 6 months

● CONTRA-INDICATIONS Active or suspected malignancy · history of gastro-intestinal malignancy (in previous 5 years)

● CAUTIONS Abrupt withdrawal of parenteral support (reduce gradually with concomitant monitoring of fluid status) · cardiac insufficiency · cardiovascular disease · colo-rectal polyps · hypertension

● SIDE-EFFECTS
▶ **Common or very common** Anxiety · appetite decreased · congestive heart failure · cough · dyspnoea · fluid imbalance · gallbladder disorders · gastrointestinal discomfort · gastrointestinal disorders · headache · influenza like illness · insomnia · nausea · pancreatitis · peripheral oedema · respiratory tract infection · vomiting
▶ **Uncommon** Syncope

● ALLERGY AND CROSS-SENSITIVITY Manufacturer advises caution in patients with tetracycline hypersensitivity.

● PREGNANCY EvGr Specialist sources indicate use if necessary—no human data available. D

● BREAST FEEDING Manufacturer advises avoid—toxicity in *animal* studies.

● RENAL IMPAIRMENT
Dose adjustments Manufacturer advises use half the daily dose in moderate or severe impairment and end-stage renal disease.

● MONITORING REQUIREMENTS Manufacturer advises monitoring of small bowel function, gall bladder, bile ducts and pancreas during treatment.

● TREATMENT CESSATION Caution when discontinuing treatment—risk of dehydration.

● PATIENT AND CARER ADVICE Patients with cardiovascular disease should seek medical attention if they notice

sudden weight gain, swollen ankles or dyspnoea—may indicate increased fluid absorption.

● MEDICINAL FORMS
There can be variation in the licensing of different medicines containing the same drug.
Powder and solvent for solution for injection
▶ Revestive (Shire Pharmaceuticals Ltd) ▼
  Teduglutide 1.25 mg Revestive 1.25mg powder and solvent for solution for injection vials | 28 vial PoM £7,307.70
  Teduglutide 5 mg Revestive 5mg powder and solvent for solution for injection vials | 28 vial PoM £14,615.39

2 Constipation and bowel cleansing

2.1 Bowel cleansing

> **Other drugs used for Bowel cleansing** Bisacodyl, p. 61 · Docusate sodium, p. 60 · Magnesium sulfate, p. 1019

LAXATIVES > OSMOTIC LAXATIVES

▌Citric acid with magnesium carbonate
(Formulated as a bowel cleansing preparation)

● **INDICATIONS AND DOSE**

Bowel evacuation for surgery, colonoscopy or radiological examination
▶ BY MOUTH
▶ Child 5-9 years: One-third of a sachet to be given at 8 a.m. the day before the procedure and, one-third of a sachet to be given between 2 and 4 p.m. the day before the procedure
▶ Child 10-17 years: 0.5-1 sachet, given at 8 a.m. the day before the procedure and 0.5-1 sachet, given between 2 and 4 p.m. the day before the procedure
▶ Adult: 1 sachet, given 8 a.m. the day before the procedure and 1 sachet, given between 2 and 4 p.m. the day before the procedure, use half the dose in frail elderly patients

● CONTRA-INDICATIONS Acute severe colitis · gastric retention · gastro-intestinal obstruction · gastro-intestinal perforation · toxic megacolon

● CAUTIONS Children · colitis (avoid if acute severe colitis) · debilitated · elderly · hypovolaemia (should be corrected before administration of bowel cleansing preparations) · impaired gag reflex or possibility of regurgitation or aspiration · patients with fluid and electrolyte disturbances
CAUTIONS, FURTHER INFORMATION Adequate hydration should be maintained during treatment.

● INTERACTIONS → Appendix 1: bowel cleansing preparations

● SIDE-EFFECTS
▶ **Common or very common** Gastrointestinal discomfort · nausea · vomiting
▶ **Uncommon** Dehydration · dizziness · electrolyte imbalance · headache
SIDE-EFFECTS, FURTHER INFORMATION Abdominal pain is usually transient and can be reduced by taking preparation more slowly.

● PREGNANCY Use with caution.

● BREAST FEEDING Use with caution.

● HEPATIC IMPAIRMENT Avoid in hepatic coma if risk of renal failure.

- RENAL IMPAIRMENT
- In adults Avoid if eGFR less than 30 mL/minute/1.73 m²—risk of hypermagnesaemia.
- In children Avoid if estimated glomerular filtration rate less than 30 mL/minute/1.73 m²—risk of hypermagnesaemia.
- MONITORING REQUIREMENTS Renal function should be measured before starting treatment in patients at risk of fluid and electrolyte disturbances.
- DIRECTIONS FOR ADMINISTRATION One sachet should be reconstituted with 200 mL of hot water; the solution should be allowed to cool for approx. 30 minutes before drinking.
- PRESCRIBING AND DISPENSING INFORMATION Reconstitution of one sachet containing 11.57 g magnesium carbonate and 17.79 g anhydrous citric acid produces a solution containing magnesium citrate with 118 mmol Mg²⁺.

  Flavours of oral powders may include lemon and lime.
- PATIENT AND CARER ADVICE Low residue or fluid only diet (e.g. water, fruit squash, clear soup, black tea or coffee) recommended before procedure (according to prescriber's advice) and copious intake of clear fluids recommended until procedure. Patient or carers should be given advice on how to administer oral powder.

- MEDICINAL FORMS
  There can be variation in the licensing of different medicines containing the same drug.

  Effervescent powder
  CAUTIONARY AND ADVISORY LABELS 13, 10
  ELECTROLYTES: May contain Magnesium
  - Citramag (Sanochemia Diagnostics UK Ltd)
    Magnesium carbonate heavy 11.57 gram, Citric acid anhydrous 17.79 gram Citramag effervescent powder sachets sugar-free | 10 sachet [P] £18.92

Macrogol 3350 with anhydrous sodium sulfate, ascorbic acid, potassium chloride, sodium ascorbate and sodium chloride

01-Mar-2018

(Polyethylene glycols)

- INDICATIONS AND DOSE

MOVIPREP ®

Bowel cleansing [before any procedure requiring a clean bowel]
- BY MOUTH
- Adult: 1 litre daily for 2 doses; first dose of reconstituted solution taken on the evening before procedure and the second dose on the morning of procedure, alternatively 2 litres daily for 1 dose; reconstituted solution to be taken on the evening before the procedure, or on the morning of the procedure, treatment should be completed at least 1 hour before clinical procedures conducted without general anaesthesia, and at least 2 hours before clinical procedures conducted under general anaesthesia

PLENVU ®

Bowel cleansing [before any procedure requiring a clean bowel]
- BY MOUTH
- Adult: 500 mL daily for 2 doses; first dose of reconstituted solution taken on the evening before procedure and the second dose on the morning of procedure, alternatively 1 litre daily in 2 divided doses, reconstituted solution to be taken either on the evening before the procedure, or in the morning of the procedure—separate doses by at least 1 hour,

treatment should be completed at least 1 hour before clinical procedures conducted without general anaesthesia, and at least 2 hours before clinical procedures conducted under general anaesthesia

- CONTRA-INDICATIONS Disorders of gastric emptying · G6PD deficiency · gastro-intestinal obstruction · gastro-intestinal perforation · ileus · toxic megacolon
- CAUTIONS Debilitated patients · dehydration (correct before administration) · impaired consciousness · impaired gag reflex or possibility of regurgitation or aspiration · moderate-to-severe cardiac impairment · patients at risk of arrhythmia (including those with thyroid disease or electrolyte imbalance) · severe acute inflammatory bowel disease
- INTERACTIONS → Appendix 1: bowel cleansing preparations
- SIDE-EFFECTS
- **Common or very common** Dehydration · nausea
- **Uncommon** Asthenia · chills · drowsiness · dry mouth · dry throat · electrolyte imbalance · gastrointestinal discomfort · headaches · hot flush · pain · palpitations · sinus tachycardia · temperature sensation altered · thirst · vomiting

  SIDE-EFFECTS, FURTHER INFORMATION Abdominal pain is usually transient and can be reduced by taking preparation more slowly.
- PREGNANCY Manufacturer advises use only if essential—no or limited information available.
- BREAST FEEDING Manufacturer advises use only if essential—no information available.
- RENAL IMPAIRMENT Manufacturer advises caution if eGFR less than 30 mL/minute/1.73 m².
- MONITORING REQUIREMENTS Manufacturer advises consider monitoring baseline and post-treatment electrolytes, renal function and ECG as appropriate, in debilitated patients, those with significant renal impairment, arrhythmia, or at risk of electrolyte imbalance.
- DIRECTIONS FOR ADMINISTRATION
  PLENVU ® Manufacturer advises the contents of the single sachet for Dose 1 should be made up to 500 mL with water and taken over 30 minutes; the contents of the 2 sachets (A and B) for Dose 2 should be made up to 500 mL with water and taken over 30 minutes. Each dose should be followed by 500 mL of clear fluid taken over 30 minutes.
  MOVIPREP ® Manufacturer advises one pair of sachets (A and B) should be made up to 1 litre with water and taken over 1–2 hours; 1 litre of other clear fluid should also be taken during treatment.
- PRESCRIBING AND DISPENSING INFORMATION
  PLENVU ® Dose 1 (single sachet) when reconstituted up to 500 mL with water provides Na⁺ 160.9 mmol, K⁺ 13.3 mmol, Cl⁻ 47.6 mmol; Dose 2 (sachets A and B) when reconstituted up to 500 mL with water provides Na⁺ 297.6 mmol, K⁺ 16.1 mmol, Cl⁻ 70.9 mmol.
  MOVIPREP ® 1 pair of sachets (A+B) when reconstituted up to 1 litre with water provides Na⁺ 181.6 mmol (Na⁺ 56.2 mmol absorbable), K⁺ 14.2 mmol, Cl⁻ 59.8 mmol.
- PATIENT AND CARER ADVICE Manufacturer advises solid food should not be taken during treatment until procedure completed.

● MEDICINAL FORMS
There can be variation in the licensing of different medicines
containing the same drug.

Oral powder
CAUTIONARY AND ADVISORY LABELS 10, 13
EXCIPIENTS: May contain Aspartame
ELECTROLYTES: May contain Chloride, potassium, sodium
▸ Moviprep (Norgine Pharmaceuticals Ltd)
Moviprep oral powder sachets sugar-free | 4 sachet P £10.36
▸ Plenvu (Norgine Pharmaceuticals Ltd)
Plenvu oral powder sachets sugar-free | 3 sachet P £12.43

Macrogol 3350 with anhydrous sodium sulfate, potassium chloride, sodium bicarbonate and sodium chloride

(Formulated as a bowel cleansing preparation)

● INDICATIONS AND DOSE
Bowel cleansing before radiological examination, colonoscopy, or surgery
▸ INITIALLY BY MOUTH
▸ Adult: Initially 2 litres daily for 2 doses: first dose of
reconstituted solution taken on the evening before
procedure and the second dose on the morning of
procedure, alternatively (by mouth) initially 250 mL
every 10–15 minutes, reconstituted solution to be
administered, alternatively (by nasogastric tube)
initially 20–30 mL/minute, starting on the day before
procedure until 4 litres have been consumed

● CONTRA-INDICATIONS Acute severe colitis · gastric
retention · gastro-intestinal obstruction · gastro-intestinal
perforation · toxic megacolon
● CAUTIONS Colitis (avoid if acute severe colitis) · debilitated
patients · elderly · fluid and electrolyte disturbances · heart
failure · hypovolaemia (should be corrected before
administration of bowel cleansing preparations) · impaired
gag reflex or possibility of regurgitation or aspiration
● INTERACTIONS → Appendix 1: bowel cleansing
preparations
● SIDE-EFFECTS Angioedema · arrhythmia · chills · confusion
· dehydration · dizziness · dyspnoea · electrolyte imbalance
· fever · flatulence · gastrointestinal discomfort · headache ·
malaise · nausea · palpitations · seizure · skin reactions ·
thirst · vomiting
SIDE-EFFECTS, FURTHER INFORMATION Abdominal pain is
usually transient and can be reduced by taking preparation
more slowly.
● PREGNANCY Manufacturers advise use only if essential—
no information available.
● BREAST FEEDING Manufacturers advise use only if
essential—no information available.
● MONITORING REQUIREMENTS Renal function should be
measured before starting treatment in patients at risk of
fluid and electrolyte disturbances.
● DIRECTIONS FOR ADMINISTRATION 1 sachet should be
reconstituted with 1 litre of water. Flavouring such as clear
fruit cordials may be added if required. After
reconstitution the solution should be kept in a refrigerator
and discarded if unused after 24 hours.
● PRESCRIBING AND DISPENSING INFORMATION Each *Klean-
Prep*® sachet provides Na+ 125 mmol, K+ 10 mmol, Cl-
35 mmol and HCO3 - 20mmol when reconstituted with
1 litre of water.
● PATIENT AND CARER ADVICE Solid food should not be
taken for 2 hours before starting treatment. Adequate
hydration should be maintained during treatment.

Treatment can be stopped if bowel motions become watery
and clear.

● MEDICINAL FORMS
There can be variation in the licensing of different medicines
containing the same drug.

Oral powder
CAUTIONARY AND ADVISORY LABELS 10, 13
EXCIPIENTS: May contain Aspartame
ELECTROLYTES: May contain Bicarbonate, chloride, potassium, sodium
▸ Klean-Prep (Norgine Pharmaceuticals Ltd)
**Potassium chloride 742.5 mg, Sodium chloride 1.465 gram,
Sodium bicarbonate 1.685 gram, Sodium sulfate anhydrous
5.685 gram, Polyethylene glycol 3350 59 gram** Klean-Prep oral
powder 69g sachets sugar-free | 4 sachet P £10.48

LAXATIVES > STIMULANT LAXATIVES

Magnesium citrate with sodium picosulfate

(Formulated as a bowel cleansing preparation)

● INDICATIONS AND DOSE
CITRAFLEET® SACHETS
Bowel evacuation on day before radiological examination, endoscopy, or surgery
▸ BY MOUTH
▸ Adult: 1 sachet taken before 8 a.m, then 1 sachet after
6–8 hours
PHARMACOKINETICS
▸ For *CitraFleet*®: acts within 3 hours of first dose.
PICOLAX® SACHETS
Bowel evacuation on day before radiological procedure, endoscopy, or surgery
▸ BY MOUTH
▸ Child 1 year: 0.25 sachet taken before 8 a.m, then
0.25 sachet after 6–8 hours
▸ Child 2-3 years: 0.5 sachet taken before 8 a.m, then
0.5 sachet after 6–8 hours
▸ Child 4-8 years: 1 sachet taken before 8 a.m, then
0.5 sachet after 6–8 hours
▸ Child 9-17 years: 1 sachet taken before 8 a.m, then
1 sachet after 6–8 hours
▸ Adult: 1 sachet taken before 8 a.m, then 1 sachet after
6–8 hours
PHARMACOKINETICS
▸ For *Picolax*®: acts within 3 hours of first dose.

● CONTRA-INDICATIONS Acute severe colitis · ascites ·
congestive cardiac failure · gastric retention · gastrointestinal obstruction · gastro-intestinal perforation ·
gastro-intestinal ulceration · toxic megacolon
● CAUTIONS Cardiac disease (avoid in congestive cardiac
failure) · children · colitis (avoid if acute severe colitis) ·
debilitated patients · elderly · fluid and electrolyte
disturbances · hypovolaemia (should be corrected before
administration) · impaired gag reflex or possibility of
regurgitation or aspiration · recent gastro-intestinal
surgery
● SIDE-EFFECTS
▸ Common or very common Gastrointestinal discomfort ·
headache · nausea
▸ Uncommon Confusion · electrolyte imbalance ·
gastrointestinal disorders · seizures · skin reactions ·
vomiting
● PREGNANCY Caution.
● BREAST FEEDING Caution.
● HEPATIC IMPAIRMENT Avoid in hepatic coma if risk of
renal failure.

• RENAL IMPAIRMENT
▶ In adults Avoid if eGFR less than 30 mL/minute/1.73 m^2—risk of hypermagnesaemia.
▶ In children Avoid if estimated glomerular filtration rate less than 30 mL/minute/1.73 m^2—risk of hypermagnesaemia.
• DIRECTIONS FOR ADMINISTRATION One sachet of sodium picosulfate with magnesium citrate powder should be reconstituted with 150 mL (approx. half a glass) of cold water; patients should be warned that heat is generated during reconstitution and that the solution should be allowed to cool before drinking.
PICOLAX ® SACHETS, CITRAFLEET ® SACHETS One sachet should be reconstituted with 150 mL (approx. half a glass) of cold water.
• PRESCRIBING AND DISPENSING INFORMATION Flavours of oral powder formulations may include lemon.
PICOLAX ® SACHETS One reconstituted sachet contains K$^+$ 5 mmol and Mg^{2+} 87 mmol.
CITRAFLEET ® SACHETS One reconstituted sachet contains K$^+$ 5 mmol and Mg^{2+} 86 mmol.
• PATIENT AND CARER ADVICE Low residue diet recommended on the day before procedure and copious intake of water or other clear fluids recommended during treatment. Patients or carers should be given advice on how to administer sodium picosulfate with magnesium citrate oral powder.
PICOLAX ® SACHETS, CITRAFLEET ® SACHETS Low residue diet recommended on the day before procedure and copious intake of water or other clear fluids recommended during treatment.
Patients and carers should be given advice on how to administer oral powder; they should be warned that heat is generated during reconstitution and that the solution should be allowed to cool before drinking.

• MEDICINAL FORMS
There can be variation in the licensing of different medicines containing the same drug.
Powder
CAUTIONARY AND ADVISORY LABELS 10, 13
ELECTROLYTES: May contain Magnesium, potassium
▶ CitraFleet (Casen Recordati S.L.)
Sodium picosulfate 10 mg, Magnesium oxide light 3.5 gram, Citric acid anhydrous 10.97 gram CitraFleet oral powder 15.08g sachets sugar-free | 2 sachet Ⓟ £3.25
▶ Picolax (Ferring Pharmaceuticals Ltd)
Sodium picosulfate 10 mg, Magnesium oxide 3.5 gram, Citric acid anhydrous 12 gram Picolax oral powder 16.1g sachets sugar-free | 2 sachet Ⓟ £3.39

2.2 Constipation

Constipation

06-Jun-2017

Description of condition

Constipation is defaecation that is unsatisfactory because of infrequent stools, difficult stool passage, or seemingly incomplete defaecation. It can occur at any age and is commonly seen in women, the elderly, and during pregnancy.
It is important for those who complain of constipation to understand that bowel habit can vary considerably in frequency without doing harm. Some people erroneously consider themselves constipated if they do not have a bowel movement each day.
New onset constipation, especially in patients over 50 years of age, or accompanying symptoms such as anaemia, abdominal pain, weight loss, or overt or occult blood in the stool should provoke urgent investigation because of the risk of malignancy or other serious bowel

disorder. In those patients with secondary constipation caused by a drug, the drug should be reviewed.

Overview

EvGr In all patients with constipation, an increase in dietary fibre, adequate fluid intake and exercise is advised. Diet should be balanced and contain whole grains, fruits and vegetables. Fibre intake should be increased gradually (to minimise flatulence and bloating). The effects of a high-fibre diet may be seen in a few days although it can take as long as 4 weeks. Adequate fluid intake is important (particularly with a high-fibre diet or fibre supplements), but can be difficult for some people (for example, the frail or elderly). Fruits high in fibre and sorbitol, and fruit juices high in sorbitol, can help prevent and treat constipation. Ⓐ
Misconceptions about bowel habits have led to excessive laxative use. Laxative abuse may lead to hypokalaemia. Before prescribing laxatives it is important to be sure that the patient is constipated and that the constipation is not secondary to an underlying undiagnosed complaint.

Laxatives
Bulk-forming laxatives
Bulk-forming laxatives include bran, ispaghula husk p. 54, methylcellulose p. 54 and sterculia p. 54. They are of particular value in adults with small hard stools if fibre cannot be increased in the diet. Onset of action is up to 72 hours. Symptoms of flatulence, bloating, and cramping may be exacerbated. Adequate fluid intake must be maintained to avoid intestinal obstruction.
Methylcellulose, ispaghula husk and sterculia may be used in patients who cannot tolerate bran. Methylcellulose also acts as a faecal softener.
Stimulant laxatives
Stimulant laxatives include bisacodyl p. 61, sodium picosulfate p. 63, and members of the anthraquinone group (senna p. 63, co-danthramer p. 61 and co-danthrusate p. 62). Stimulant laxatives increase intestinal motility and often cause abdominal cramp; manufacturer advises they should be avoided in intestinal obstruction.
The use of co-danthramer and co-danthrusate is limited to constipation in terminally ill patients because of potential carcinogenicity (based on animal studies) and evidence of genotoxicity.
Docusate sodium p. 60 is believed to act as both a stimulant laxative and as a faecal softener (below). Glycerol suppositories act as a lubricant and as a rectal stimulant by virtue of the mildly irritant action of glycerol.
Faecal softeners
Faecal softeners are claimed to act by decreasing surface tension and increasing penetration of intestinal fluid into the faecal mass. Docusate sodium and glycerol suppositories p. 59 have softening properties. Enemas containing arachis oil p. 60 (ground-nut oil, peanut oil) lubricate and soften impacted faeces and promote a bowel movement. Liquid paraffin p. 61 has also been used as a lubricant for the passage of stools but manufacturer advises that it should be used with caution because of its adverse effects, which include anal seepage and the risks of granulomatous disease of the gastro-intestinal tract or of lipoid pneumonia on aspiration.
Osmotic laxatives
Osmotic laxatives increase the amount of water in the large bowel, either by drawing fluid from the body into the bowel or by retaining the fluid they were administered with. Lactulose p. 56 is a semi-synthetic disaccharide which is not absorbed from the gastro-intestinal tract. It produces an osmotic diarrhoea of low faecal pH, and discourages the proliferation of ammonia-producing organisms. It is therefore useful in the treatment of hepatic encephalopathy. Macrogols (such as macrogol 3350 with potassium chloride, sodium bicarbonate and sodium chloride p. 56) are inert

polymers of ethylene glycol which sequester fluid in the bowel; giving fluid with macrogols may reduce the dehydrating effect sometimes seen with osmotic laxatives.

Other drugs used in constipation

Linaclotide p. 47 is a guanylate cyclase-C receptor agonist that is licensed for the treatment of moderate to severe irritable bowel syndrome associated with constipation. It increases intestinal fluid secretion and transit, and decreases visceral pain.

Lubiprostone p. 55 is a chloride-channel activator that is licensed for the treatment of chronic idiopathic constipation in adults whose condition has not responded adequately to lifestyle changes (including dietary changes).

Prucalopride p. 59 is a selective serotonin 5HT$_4$-receptor agonist with prokinetic properties. It is licensed for the treatment of chronic constipation in adults, when other laxatives have failed to provide an adequate response.

Bowel cleansing preparations

Bowel cleansing preparations are used before colonic surgery, colonoscopy or radiological examination to ensure the bowel is free of solid contents; examples include macrogol 3350 with anhydrous sodium sulfate, potassium chloride, sodium bicarbonate and sodium chloride p. 51, citric acid with magnesium carbonate p. 49, magnesium citrate with sodium picosulfate p. 51 and sodium acid phosphate with sodium phosphate p. 58. Bowel cleansing treatments are not treatments for constipation.

Management

Short-duration constipation

ᴇᴠɢʳ In the management of short-duration constipation (where dietary measures are ineffective) treatment should be started with a bulk-forming laxative, ensuring adequate fluid intake. If stools remain hard, add or switch to an osmotic laxative. If stools are soft but difficult to pass or the person complains of inadequate emptying, a stimulant laxative should be added. ⒶⒶ

Opioid-induced constipation

See also *Constipation* under Prescribing in palliative care p. 23. ᴇᴠɢʳ In patients with opioid-induced constipation, an osmotic laxative (or docusate sodium to soften the stools) and a stimulant laxative is recommended. Bulk-forming laxatives should be avoided.

Naloxegol p. 64 is recommended for the treatment of opioid-induced constipation when response to other laxatives is inadequate. ⒶⒶ

Methylnaltrexone bromide p. 64 is licensed for the treatment of opioid-induced constipation when response to other laxatives is inadequate. Manufacturer advises that in patients receiving palliative care, methylnaltrexone bromide should be used as an adjunct to existing laxative therapy.

Faecal impaction

The treatment of faecal impaction depends on the stool consistency. ᴇᴠɢʳ In patients with hard stools, a high dose of an oral macrogol (such as macrogol 3350 with potassium chloride, sodium bicarbonate and sodium chloride) may be considered. In those with soft stools, or with hard stools after a few days treatment with a macrogol, an oral stimulant laxative should be started or added to the previous treatment. If the response to oral laxatives is inadequate, for soft stools consider rectal administration of bisacodyl, and for hard stools rectal administration of glycerol alone, or glycerol plus bisacodyl. Alternatively, a docusate sodium p. 60 or sodium citrate enema p. 770 may be tried. ⒶⒶ

ᴇᴠɢʳ If the response is still insufficient, a sodium acid phosphate with sodium phosphate p. 58 or arachis oil p. 60 retention enema may be necessary. For hard faeces it can be helpful to give the arachis oil enema overnight before giving a sodium acid phosphate with sodium phosphate or sodium citrate enema the following day. Enemas may need to be repeated several times to clear hard impacted faeces. ⒶⒶ

Chronic constipation

ᴇᴠɢʳ In the management of chronic constipation, treatment should be started with a bulk-forming laxative, whilst ensuring good hydration. If stools remain hard, add or change to an osmotic laxative such as a macrogol. Lactulose p. 56 is an alternative if macrogols are not effective, or not tolerated. If the response is inadequate, a stimulant laxative can be added. The dose of laxative should be adjusted gradually to produce one or two soft, formed stools per day.

If at least two laxatives (from different classes) have been tried at the highest tolerated recommended doses for at least 6 months, the use of prucalopride p. 59 (in women only) or lubiprostone p. 55 should be considered. If treatment with prucalopride is not effective after 4 weeks, or lubiprostone is not effective after 2 weeks, the patient should be re-examined and the benefit of continuing treatment reconsidered.

Laxatives can be slowly withdrawn when regular bowel movements occur without difficulty, according to the frequency and consistency of the stools. If a combination of laxatives has been used, reduce and stop one laxative at a time; if possible, the stimulant laxative should be reduced first. However, it may be necessary to also adjust the dose of the osmotic laxative to compensate. ⒶⒶ

Constipation in pregnancy and breast-feeding

ᴇᴠɢʳ If dietary and lifestyle changes fail to control constipation in pregnancy, fibre supplements in the form of bran or wheat are likely to help women experiencing constipation in pregnancy, and raise no serious concerns about side-effects to the mother or fetus.

A bulk-forming laxative is the first choice during pregnancy if fibre supplements fail. An osmotic laxative, such as lactulose, can also be used. Bisacodyl p. 61 or senna p. 63 may be suitable if a stimulant effect is necessary but use of senna should be avoided near term or if there is a history of unstable pregnancy. Stimulant laxatives are more effective than bulk-forming laxatives but are more likely to cause side-effects (diarrhoea and abdominal discomfort), reducing their acceptability to patients. Docusate sodium and glycerol suppositories p. 62 can also be used.

A bulk-forming laxative is the first choice during breast-feeding, if dietary measures fail. Lactulose or a macrogol may be used if stools remain hard. As an alternative, a short course of a stimulant laxative such as bisacodyl or senna can be considered. ⒶⒶ

Constipation in children

Early identification of constipation and effective treatment can improve outcomes for children. Without early diagnosis and treatment, an acute episode of constipation can lead to anal fissure and become chronic.

ᴇᴠɢʳ The first-line treatment for children with constipation requires the use of a laxative in combination with dietary modification or with behavioural interventions. Diet modification alone is not recommended as first-line treatment.

In children an increase in dietary fibre, adequate fluid intake, and exercise is advised. Diet should be balanced and contain fruits, and vegetables, high-fibre bread, baked beans, and wholegrain breakfast cereals. Unprocessed bran (which may cause bloating and flatulence and reduces the absorption of micronutrients) is **not** recommended.

If faecal impaction is not present (or has been treated), the child should be treated promptly with a laxative. A macrogol (such as macrogol 3350 with potassium chloride, sodium bicarbonate and sodium chloride p. 56) is preferred as first-line management. If the response is inadequate, add a stimulant laxative or change to a stimulant laxative if the first-line therapy is not tolerated. If stools remain hard, lactulose or another laxative with softening effects, such as docusate sodium can be added.

In children with chronic constipation, laxatives should be continued for several weeks after a regular pattern of bowel movements or toilet training is established. The dose of laxatives should then be tapered gradually, over a period of months, according to response. Some children may require laxative therapy for several years.

A shorter duration of laxative treatment may be possible in some children with a short history of constipation.

Laxatives should be administered at a time that produces an effect that is likely to fit in with the child's toilet routine. Ⓐ

Faecal impaction in children

EvGr Treatment of faecal impaction may initially increase symptoms of soiling and abdominal pain. In children over 1 year of age with faecal impaction, an oral preparation containing a macrogol (such as macrogol 3350 with potassium chloride, sodium bicarbonate and sodium chloride) is used to clear faecal mass and to establish and maintain soft well-formed stools, using an escalating dose regimen depending on symptoms and response. If disimpaction does not occur after 2 weeks, a stimulant laxative can be added or if stools are hard, used in combination with an osmotic laxative such as lactulose. Long-term regular use of laxatives is essential to maintain well-formed stools and prevent recurrence of faecal impaction; intermittent use may provoke relapses. Ⓐ

LAXATIVES > BULK-FORMING LAXATIVES

Ispaghula husk

24-Feb-2016

- **DRUG ACTION** Bulk-forming laxatives relieve constipation by increasing faecal mass which stimulates peristalsis.

- **INDICATIONS AND DOSE**

Constipation
▸ BY MOUTH
▸ Child 1 month-5 years: 2.5–5 mL twice daily, dose to be taken only when prescribed by a doctor, as half or whole level spoonful in water, preferably after meals, morning and evening
▸ Child 6-11 years: 2.5–5 mL twice daily, dose to be given as a half or whole level spoonful in water, preferably after meals, morning and evening
▸ Child 12-17 years: 1 sachet twice daily, dose to be given in water preferably after meals, morning and evening
▸ Adult: 1 sachet twice daily, dose to be given in water preferably taken after food, morning and evening
DOSE EQUIVALENCE AND CONVERSION
▸ 1 sachet equivalent to 2 level 5 ml spoonful.

- **CONTRA-INDICATIONS** Colonic atony · faecal impaction · intestinal obstruction · reduced gut motility
- **CAUTIONS** Adequate fluid intake should be maintained to avoid intestinal obstruction
- **SIDE-EFFECTS** Abdominal distension · bronchospasm · conjunctivitis · gastrointestinal disorders · hypersensitivity · rhinitis · skin reactions
- **DIRECTIONS FOR ADMINISTRATION** Dose to be taken with at least 150 mL liquid.
- **PRESCRIBING AND DISPENSING INFORMATION** Flavours of soluble granules formulations may include plain, lemon, or orange.
- **HANDLING AND STORAGE** Ispaghula husk contains potent allergens. Individuals exposed to the product (including those handling the product) can develop hypersensitivity reactions such as rhinitis, conjunctivitis, bronchospasm and in some cases, anaphylaxis.
- **PATIENT AND CARER ADVICE** Manufacturer advises that preparations that swell in contact with liquid should always be carefully swallowed with water and should not

be taken immediately before going to bed. Patients and their carers should be advised that the full effect may take some days to develop and should be given advice on how to administer ispaghula husk.

- **MEDICINAL FORMS** There can be variation in the licensing of different medicines containing the same drug.
Effervescent granules
CAUTIONARY AND ADVISORY LABELS 13
EXCIPIENTS: May contain Aspartame
▸ Ispaghula husk (Non-proprietary)
  Ispaghula husk 3.5 gram Ispaghula husk 3.5g effervescent granules sachets gluten free sugar free sugar-free | 30 sachet Ⓟ Ⓢ DT = £2.72
Granules
CAUTIONARY AND ADVISORY LABELS 13
EXCIPIENTS: May contain Aspartame
▸ Ispaghula husk (Non-proprietary)
  Ispaghula husk 3.5 gram Ispaghula husk 3.5g granules sachets gluten free | 30 sachet GSL £2.72

Combinations available: *Senna with ispaghula husk,* p. 63

Methylcellulose

- **DRUG ACTION** Bulk-forming laxatives relieve constipation by increasing faecal mass which stimulates peristalsis.

- **INDICATIONS AND DOSE**

Constipation | Diarrhoea
▸ BY MOUTH USING TABLETS
▸ Adult: 3–6 tablets twice daily

- **CONTRA-INDICATIONS** Colonic atony · difficulty in swallowing · faecal impaction · infective bowel disease · intestinal obstruction
- **CAUTIONS** Adequate fluid intake should be maintained to avoid intestinal obstruction
  CAUTIONS, FURTHER INFORMATION It may be necessary to supervise elderly or debilitated patients or those with intestinal narrowing or decreased motility to ensure adequate fluid intake.
- **SIDE-EFFECTS** Abdominal distension · gastrointestinal disorders
- **DIRECTIONS FOR ADMINISTRATION** In constipation the dose should be taken with at least 300 mL liquid. In diarrhoea, ileostomy, and colostomy control, avoid liquid intake for 30 minutes before and after dose.
- **PATIENT AND CARER ADVICE** Patients and their carers should be advised that the full effect may take some days to develop. Preparations that swell in contact with liquid should always be carefully swallowed with water and should not be taken immediately before going to bed.

- **MEDICINAL FORMS** There can be variation in the licensing of different medicines containing the same drug.
Tablet
▸ Celevac (AMCo)
  Methylcellulose "450" 500 mg Celevac 500mg tablets | 112 tablet GSL £5.31 DT = £5.31

Sterculia

19-Feb-2016

- **DRUG ACTION** Sterculia is a bulk-forming laxative. It relieves constipation by increasing faecal mass which stimulates peristalsis.

- **INDICATIONS AND DOSE**

Constipation
▸ BY MOUTH
▸ Child 6-11 years: 0.5–1 sachet 1–2 times a day, alternatively, half to one heaped 5-mL spoonful once

or twice a day; washed down without chewing with plenty of liquid after meals
‣ Child 12-17 years: 1–2 sachets 1–2 times a day, alternatively, one to two heaped 5-mL spoonfuls once or twice a day; washed down without chewing with plenty of liquid after meals
‣ Adult: 1–2 sachets 1–2 times a day, alternatively, one to two heaped 5-mL spoonfuls once or twice a day; washed down without chewing with plenty of liquid after meals

● CONTRA-INDICATIONS Colonic atony · difficulty in swallowing · faecal impaction · intestinal obstruction
● CAUTIONS Adequate fluid intake should be maintained to avoid intestinal obstruction
CAUTIONS, FURTHER INFORMATION
‣ In adults It may be necessary to supervise elderly or debilitated patients or those with intestinal narrowing or decreased motility to ensure adequate fluid intake.
● SIDE-EFFECTS Diarrhoea · gastrointestinal discomfort · gastrointestinal disorders · nausea
● DIRECTIONS FOR ADMINISTRATION May be mixed with soft food (e.g. yoghurt) before swallowing, followed by plenty of liquid.
● PATIENT AND CARER ADVICE Patients and their carers should be advised that the full effect may take some days to develop. Preparations that swell in contact with liquid should always be carefully swallowed with water and should not be taken immediately before going to bed.

● MEDICINAL FORMS
There can be variation in the licensing of different medicines containing the same drug.
Granules
CAUTIONARY AND ADVISORY LABELS 25, 27
‣ Normacol (Norgine Pharmaceuticals Ltd)
Sterculia 620 mg per 1 gram Normacol granules 7g sachets | 60 sachet GSL £6.67 DT = £6.67
Normacol granules | 500 gram GSL £7.92 DT = £7.92

Sterculia with frangula

The properties listed below are those particular to the combination only. For the properties of the components please consider, sterculia p. 54.

● INDICATIONS AND DOSE
After haemorrhoidectomy
‣ BY MOUTH
‣ Adult: 1–2 sachets 1–2 times a day, alternatively, 1–2 heaped 5 mL spoonfuls once or twice a day; washed down without chewing with plenty of liquid after meals
Constipation
‣ BY MOUTH
‣ Adult: 1–2 sachets 1–2 times a day, alternatively, 1–2 heaped 5 mL spoonfuls once or twice a day; washed down without chewing with plenty of liquid after meals

● PREGNANCY Manufacturer advises avoid.
● BREAST FEEDING Manufacturer advises avoid.
● PATIENT AND CARER ADVICE Patients and their carers should be advised that the full effect may take some days to develop. Preparations that swell in contact with liquid should always be carefully swallowed with water and should not be taken immediately before going to bed.

● MEDICINAL FORMS
There can be variation in the licensing of different medicines containing the same drug.
Granules
‣ Normacol Plus (Norgine Pharmaceuticals Ltd)
Frangula 80 mg per 1 gram, Sterculia 620 mg per 1 gram Normacol Plus granules 7g sachets | 60 sachet GSL £7.12 DT = £7.12
Normacol Plus granules | 500 gram GSL £8.45 DT = £8.45

LAXATIVES > CHLORIDE-CHANNEL AGONISTS

Lubiprostone
23-Mar-2016

● DRUG ACTION Lubiprostone is a chloride-channel activator that acts locally in the gut to increase intestinal fluid secretion and intestinal motility, resulting in a laxative effect.

● INDICATIONS AND DOSE
Chronic idiopathic constipation when response to lifestyle changes (including diet) inadequate
‣ BY MOUTH
‣ Adult: 24 micrograms twice daily for 2–4 weeks, discontinue if no response after initial 2 weeks

● CONTRA-INDICATIONS Gastro-intestinal obstruction
● SIDE-EFFECTS
‣ **Common or very common** Chest discomfort · diarrhoea · dizziness · dyspnoea · gastrointestinal discomfort · gastrointestinal disorders · headache · hot flush · hyperhidrosis · nausea · oedema · palpitations
‣ **Uncommon** Muscle spasms · syncope · vomiting
‣ **Frequency not known** Hypotension · influenza like illness · skin reactions · tachycardia · throat tightness
● PREGNANCY Manufacturer advises avoid—toxicity in *animal* studies.
● BREAST FEEDING Unknown if excreted in milk. EvGr If benefits of use outweigh the risk, monitor infant for side effects (e.g. diarrhoea). Ⓔ
● HEPATIC IMPAIRMENT
Dose adjustments In moderate to severe impairment initially 24 micrograms once daily; if tolerated, and if necessary, increased to 24 micrograms twice daily.
● PRESCRIBING AND DISPENSING INFORMATION Dispense capsules in original container; discard any capsules remaining 4 weeks after opening.
● NATIONAL FUNDING/ACCESS DECISIONS
NICE decisions
‣ **Lubiprostone for treating chronic idiopathic constipation (July 2014)** NICE TA318
Lubiprostone is recommended as an option for treating chronic idiopathic constipation for adults in whom treatment with at least 2 laxatives from different classes, at the highest tolerated recommended doses for at least 6 months, has failed to provide adequate relief and for whom invasive treatment for constipation is being considered. If treatment with lubiprostone is not effective after 2 weeks, the patient should be re-examined and the benefit of continuing treatment reconsidered.
  Lubiprostone should only be prescribed by a clinician with experience of treating chronic idiopathic constipation, after careful review of the patient's previous courses of laxative treatments.
www.nice.org.uk/TA318
Scottish Medicines Consortium (SMC) Decisions
The *Scottish Medicines Consortium* has advised (July 2014) that lubiprostone (*Amitiza*) ® is **not** recommended for use within NHS Scotland.

- MEDICINAL FORMS
There can be variation in the licensing of different medicines containing the same drug.

Capsule

CAUTIONARY AND ADVISORY LABELS 21

▸ Amitiza (Sucampo Pharma Europe Ltd) ▼
Lubiprostone 24 microgram Amitiza 24microgram capsules | 28 capsule PoM £29.68 | 56 capsule PoM £53.48

LAXATIVES > OSMOTIC LAXATIVES

Lactulose

- INDICATIONS AND DOSE

Constipation

▸ BY MOUTH

▸ Child 1–11 months: 2.5 mL twice daily, adjusted according to response

▸ Child 1–4 years: 2.5–10 mL twice daily, adjusted according to response

▸ Child 5–17 years: 5–20 mL twice daily, adjusted according to response

▸ Adult: Initially 15 mL twice daily, adjusted according to response

Hepatic encephalopathy (portal systemic encephalopathy)

▸ BY MOUTH

▸ Adult: Adjusted according to response to 30–50 mL 3 times a day, subsequently adjusted to produce 2–3 soft stools per day

PHARMACOKINETICS

▸ Lactulose may take up to 48 hours to act.

- UNLICENSED USE
▸ In adults Lactulose doses in the BNF may differ from those in product literature.

- CONTRA-INDICATIONS Galactosaemia · intestinal obstruction

- CAUTIONS Lactose intolerance

- SIDE-EFFECTS

▸ **Common or very common** Abdominal pain · diarrhoea · flatulence · nausea · vomiting

▸ **Uncommon** Electrolyte imbalance

- PREGNANCY Not known to be harmful.

- PATIENT AND CARER ADVICE
Medicines for Children leaflet: Lactulose for constipation www.medicinesforchildren.org.uk/lactulose-for-constipation

- MEDICINAL FORMS
There can be variation in the licensing of different medicines containing the same drug.

Oral solution

▸ Lactulose (Non-proprietary)
Lactulose 666.667 mg per 1 ml Lactulose 10g/15ml oral solution 15ml sachets sugar free sugar-free | 10 sachet P £2.51 DT = £2.51
Lactulose 680 mg per 1 ml Lactulose 3.1-3.7g/5ml oral solution | 300 ml P £1.39–£2.73 | 500 ml P £4.55 DT = £2.32

▸ Duphalac (Mylan)
Lactulose 680 mg per 1 ml Duphalac 3.35g/5ml syrup | 200 ml P £1.92

▸ Lactugal (Intrapharm Laboratories Ltd)
Lactulose 680 mg per 1 ml Lactugal 3.1-3.7g/5ml oral solution | 500 ml P £4.56 DT = £2.32 | 2000 ml P £16.42

Macrogol 3350

21-Aug-2017

- INDICATIONS AND DOSE

Chronic constipation

▸ BY MOUTH

▸ Adult: 2 sachets once daily usually for up to 2 weeks, dose to be taken preferably in the morning

PHARMACOKINETICS

▸ Onset of action 24–48 hours.

- CONTRA-INDICATIONS Ileus · intestinal obstruction · intestinal perforation · risk of intestinal perforation · severe inflammatory bowel disease · toxic megacolon

- SIDE-EFFECTS

▸ **Common or very common** Flatulence · gastrointestinal discomfort · nausea · vomiting

▸ **Uncommon** Anaemia · angioedema · appetite disorder · dehydration · dizziness · fatigue · hiccups · hypertension · hypoglycaemia · hypothyroidism · increased risk of infection · local swelling · migraine · muscle twitching · neuritis · oedema · pain · pelvic pain · sinus congestion · skin reactions · tachycardia · taste altered

- PREGNANCY Limited data, but manufacturer advises no effects anticipated as systemic exposure is negligible.

- DIRECTIONS FOR ADMINISTRATION Manufacturer advises contents of each sachet to be dissolved in half a glass (approx. 100 mL) of water just before administration.

- MEDICINAL FORMS
There can be variation in the licensing of different medicines containing the same drug.

Powder

CAUTIONARY AND ADVISORY LABELS 13

▸ TransiSoft (HFA Healthcare Products Ltd)
Macrogol '3350' 85 gram per 1 litre TransiSoft oral powder 8.5g sachets sugar-free | 28 sachet P £3.89 DT = £3.89

Macrogol 3350 with potassium chloride, sodium bicarbonate and sodium chloride

18-Apr-2018

- INDICATIONS AND DOSE

Chronic constipation (dose for 'paediatric' sachets) | Prevention of faecal impaction (dose for 'paediatric' sachets)

▸ BY MOUTH

▸ Child 2–5 years: 1 sachet daily, adjust dose to produce regular soft stools; maximum 4 sachets per day

▸ Child 6–11 years: 2 sachets daily, adjust dose to produce regular soft stools; maximum 4 sachets per day

Faecal impaction (dose for 'paediatric' sachets)

▸ BY MOUTH

▸ Child 5–11 years: 4 sachets on first day, then increased in steps of 2 sachets daily, total daily dose to be taken over a 12-hour period, after disimpaction, switch to maintenance laxative therapy; maximum 12 sachets per day

Chronic constipation (dose for 'half-strength' sachets)

▸ BY MOUTH

▸ Child 12–17 years: 2–6 sachets daily in divided doses usually for up to 2 weeks; maintenance 2–4 sachets daily

▸ Adult: 2–6 sachets daily in divided doses usually for up to 2 weeks; maintenance 2–4 sachets daily

Faecal impaction (dose for 'half-strength' sachets)

▸ BY MOUTH

▸ Child 12–17 years: 8 sachets on first day, then increased in steps of 4 sachets daily, total daily dose to be drunk within a 6 hour period, after disimpaction, switch to maintenance laxative therapy if required; maximum 16 sachets per day

▸ Adult: 8 sachets on first day, then increased in steps of 4 sachets daily, total daily dose to be drunk within a 6 hour period, after disimpaction, switch to maintenance laxative therapy if required; maximum 16 sachets per day

Chronic constipation (dose for 'full-strength' sachets)
▸ BY MOUTH
▸ Child 12-17 years: 1–3 sachets daily in divided doses usually for up to 2 weeks; maintenance 1–2 sachets daily
▸ Adult: 1–3 sachets daily in divided doses usually for up to 2 weeks; maintenance 1–2 sachets daily

Faecal impaction (dose for 'full-strength' sachets)
▸ BY MOUTH
▸ Child 12-17 years: 4 sachets on first day, then increased in steps of 2 sachets daily, total daily dose to be drunk within a 6 hour period, after disimpaction, switch to maintenance laxative therapy if required; maximum 8 sachets per day
▸ Adult: 4 sachets on first day, then increased in steps of 2 sachets daily, total daily dose to be drunk within a 6 hour period, after disimpaction, switch to maintenance laxative therapy if required; maximum 8 sachets per day

DOSE EQUIVALENCE AND CONVERSION
▸ Each 'paediatric' sachet contains 6.563 g of macrogol 3350; each 'half-strength' sachet contains 6.563 g of macrogol 3350; each 'full-strength' sachet contains 13.125 g of macrogol 3350.

MOVICOL ® READY TO TAKE SACHETS

Chronic constipation
▸ BY MOUTH
▸ Child 12-17 years: 1–3 sachets daily in divided doses usually for up to 2 weeks; maintenance 1–2 sachets daily
▸ Adult: 1–3 sachets daily in divided doses usually for up to 2 weeks; maintenance 1–2 sachets daily

Faecal impaction
▸ BY MOUTH
▸ Child 12-17 years: 4 sachets on first day, then increased in steps of 2 sachets daily, total daily dose to be drunk within a 6 hour period; patients should also take an additional 1 litre of fluid daily, after disimpaction, switch to maintenance laxative therapy if required; maximum 8 sachets per day
▸ Adult: 4 sachets on first day, then increased in steps of 2 sachets daily, total daily dose to be drunk within a 6 hour period; patients should also take an additional 1 litre of fluid daily, after disimpaction, switch to maintenance laxative therapy if required; maximum 8 sachets per day

MOVICOL ® LIQUID

Chronic constipation
▸ BY MOUTH
▸ Child 12-17 years: 25 mL 1–3 times a day usually for up to 2 weeks; maintenance 25 mL 1–2 times a day
▸ Adult: 25 mL 1–3 times a day usually for up to 2 weeks; maintenance 25 mL 1–2 times a day

VISTAPREP ® ORAL POWDER

Bowel cleansing before colonoscopy
▸ BY MOUTH
▸ Adult: 3–4 litres, reconstituted solution taken over 4 hours, generally on the day of procedure; alternatively, it can be taken on the evening before procedure *or* started on the evening before procedure and completed on the morning of procedure

● UNLICENSED USE
▸ In children Macrogol 3350 with potassium chloride, sodium bicarbonate and sodium chloride may be used as detailed below, although these situations are considered outside the scope of its licence:
  ● EvGr dose for chronic constipation/prevention of faecal impaction in children aged 6 years;

● dose titration schedule for faecal impaction in children aged 12–17 years Ⓐ.
▸ In adults Macrogol 3350 with potassium chloride, sodium bicarbonate and sodium chloride may be used as detailed below, although this is considered outside the scope of its licence: EvGr dose titration schedule for faecal impaction Ⓔ

● CONTRA-INDICATIONS Intestinal obstruction · intestinal perforation · paralytic ileus · severe inflammatory conditions of the intestinal tract (including Crohn's disease, ulcerative colitis and toxic megacolon) · use of 'paediatric' sachets for faecal impaction in impaired cardiovascular function (no information available) (in children)

VISTAPREP ® ORAL POWDER Impaired consciousness · impaired swallowing reflex · moderate-to-severe heart failure—limited safety information available · risk of regurgitation or aspiration · severe dehydration—limited safety information available

● CAUTIONS Cardiovascular impairment (should not take more than 2 'full-strength' sachets or 4 'half-strength' sachets in any one hour) · impaired consciousness (with high doses) · impaired gag reflex (with high doses) · reflux oesophagitis (with high doses)

VISTAPREP ® ORAL POWDER Chronic inflammatory bowel disease · elderly · heart rhythm abnormalities · reflux oesophagitis

● SIDE-EFFECTS Flatulence · gastrointestinal discomfort · nausea

● PREGNANCY Manufacturers advise may be used—limited data available.

● HEPATIC IMPAIRMENT
VISTAPREP ® ORAL POWDER Manufacturer advises avoid—limited safety information available.

● RENAL IMPAIRMENT
▸ In children Manufacturers advise avoid use of 'paediatric' sachets for faecal impaction—no information available.
VISTAPREP ® ORAL POWDER Manufacturer advises avoid—limited safety information available.

● DIRECTIONS FOR ADMINISTRATION Manufacturers advise dissolve contents of each 'half-strength' sachet of oral powder in 62.5 mL of water, and each 'full-strength' sachet of oral powder in 125 mL of water; after reconstitution the solution should be kept in a refrigerator—for further information consult product literature.
▸ In children Manufacturers advise dissolve contents of each 'paediatric' sachet of oral powder in 62.5 mL of water; after reconstitution the solution should be kept in a refrigerator—for further information consult product literature.
MOVICOL ® LIQUID Manufacturer advises dilute 25 mL of oral concentrate with 100 mL of water; after dilution the solution should be discarded if unused after 24 hours.
VISTAPREP ® ORAL POWDER Manufacturer advises dissolve the contents of each sachet in 1 L water; if not consumed immediately, the reconstituted solution should be kept in a refrigerator and discarded if unused after 48 hours.

● PATIENT AND CARER ADVICE Patients or carers should be counselled on how to take the oral powder and oral solution.
Medicines for Children leaflet: Movicol for constipation
www.medicinesforchildren.org.uk/movicol-for-constipation
VISTAPREP ® ORAL POWDER Manufacturer advises treatment can be stopped if bowel motions become watery and clear.

• MEDICINAL FORMS
There can be variation in the licensing of different medicines containing the same drug.

Oral solution
CAUTIONARY AND ADVISORY LABELS 13
ELECTROLYTES: May contain Bicarbonate, chloride, potassium, sodium
▸ Movicol (Norgine Pharmaceuticals Ltd)
Macrogol '3350' 105 gram per 1 litre, Potassium 5.4 mmol per 1 litre, Bicarbonate 17 mmol per 1 litre, Chloride 53 mmol per 1 litre, Sodium 65 mmol per 1 litre Movicol Liquid sugar-free | 500 ml P £5.41 DT = £5.41
Macrogol '3350' 13.125 gram, Potassium 27 mmol per 1 litre, Bicarbonate 85 mmol per 1 litre, Chloride 267 mmol per 1 litre, Sodium 325 mmol per 1 litre Movicol Ready to Take oral solution 25ml sachets sugar-free | 30 sachet P £7.72

Powder
CAUTIONARY AND ADVISORY LABELS 10, 13
ELECTROLYTES: May contain Bicarbonate, chloride, potassium, sodium
▸ Macrogol 3350 with potassium chloride, sodium bicarbonate and sodium chloride (Non-proprietary)
Macrogol '3350' 52.5 gram per 1 litre, Potassium 5.4 mmol per 1 litre, Bicarbonate 17 mmol per 1 litre, Chloride 53 mmol per 1 litre, Sodium 65 mmol per 1 litre Macrogol compound half-strength oral powder sachets NPF sugar free sugar-free | 30 sachet PoM ⓢ DT = £4.38
Macrogol '3350' 105 gram per 1 litre, Potassium 5.4 mmol per 1 litre, Bicarbonate 17 mmol per 1 litre, Chloride 53 mmol per 1 litre, Sodium 65 mmol per 1 litre Macrogol compound oral powder sachets sugar free sugar-free | 20 sachet P £2.63–£4.45 sugar-free | 30 sachet P £6.68 DT = £3.95
Macrogol compound oral powder sachets sugar free plain sugar-free | 20 sachet P £2.63 sugar-free | 30 sachet P £3.95 DT = £3.95
▸ CosmoCol (Stirling Anglian Pharmaceuticals Ltd)
Macrogol '3350' 52.5 gram per 1 litre, Potassium 5.4 mmol per 1 litre, Bicarbonate 17 mmol per 1 litre, Chloride 53 mmol per 1 litre, Sodium 65 mmol per 1 litre CosmoCol Half oral powder 6.9g sachets sugar-free | 30 sachet P £2.99 DT = £4.38
CosmoCol Paediatric oral powder 6.9g sachets sugar-free | 30 sachet PoM £2.99 DT = £4.38
Macrogol '3350' 105 gram per 1 litre, Potassium 5.4 mmol per 1 litre, Bicarbonate 17 mmol per 1 litre, Chloride 53 mmol per 1 litre, Sodium 65 mmol per 1 litre CosmoCol Orange Lemon and Lime oral powder sachets sugar-free | 30 sachet P £3.95 DT = £3.95
CosmoCol Plain oral powder sachets sugar-free | 30 sachet P £3.95 DT = £3.95
CosmoCol Orange Flavour oral powder sachets sugar-free | 20 sachet P £2.75 sugar-free | 30 sachet P £3.95 DT = £3.95
CosmoCol Lemon and Lime Flavour oral powder sachets sugar-free | 20 sachet P £2.75 sugar-free | 30 sachet P £3.95 DT = £3.95
▸ Laxido (Galen Ltd)
Macrogol '3350' 52.5 gram per 1 litre, Potassium 5.4 mmol per 1 litre, Bicarbonate 17 mmol per 1 litre, Chloride 53 mmol per 1 litre, Sodium 65 mmol per 1 litre Laxido Paediatric Plain oral powder 6.9g sachets sugar-free | 30 sachet PoM £2.99 DT = £4.38
Macrogol '3350' 105 gram per 1 litre, Potassium 5.4 mmol per 1 litre, Bicarbonate 17 mmol per 1 litre, Chloride 53 mmol per 1 litre, Sodium 65 mmol per 1 litre Laxido Orange oral powder sachets sugar free sugar-free | 20 sachet P £2.75 sugar-free | 30 sachet P £3.95 DT = £3.95
▸ Molative (Mylan)
Macrogol '3350' 52.5 gram per 1 litre, Potassium 5.4 mmol per 1 litre, Bicarbonate 17 mmol per 1 litre, Chloride 53 mmol per 1 litre, Sodium 65 mmol per 1 litre Molative Paediatric oral powder 6.9g sachets sugar-free | 30 sachet PoM £4.30 DT = £4.38
Macrogol '3350' 105 gram per 1 litre, Potassium 5.4 mmol per 1 litre, Bicarbonate 17 mmol per 1 litre, Chloride 53 mmol per 1 litre, Sodium 65 mmol per 1 litre Molative oral powder 13.8g sachets sugar-free | 20 sachet P £2.85 sugar-free | 30 sachet P £4.27 DT = £3.95 sugar-free | 50 sachet P £7.17
▸ Molaxole (Meda Pharmaceuticals Ltd)
Macrogol '3350' 105 gram per 1 litre, Potassium 5.4 mmol per 1 litre, Bicarbonate 17 mmol per 1 litre, Chloride 53 mmol per 1 litre, Sodium 65 mmol per 1 litre Molaxole oral powder sachets sugar-free | 20 sachet P £3.78 sugar-free | 30 sachet P £5.68 DT = £3.95
▸ Movicol (Norgine Pharmaceuticals Ltd)
Macrogol '3350' 52.5 gram per 1 litre, Potassium 5.4 mmol per 1 litre, Bicarbonate 17 mmol per 1 litre, Chloride 53 mmol per

1 litre, Sodium 65 mmol per 1 litre Movicol Paediatric Plain oral powder 6.9g sachets sugar-free | 30 sachet PoM £4.38 DT = £4.38
Movicol Paediatric Chocolate oral powder 6.9g sachets sugar-free | 30 sachet PoM £4.38 DT = £4.38
Macrogol '3350' 105 gram per 1 litre, Potassium 5.4 mmol per 1 litre, Bicarbonate 17 mmol per 1 litre, Chloride 53 mmol per 1 litre, Sodium 65 mmol per 1 litre Movicol Plain oral powder 13.7g sachets sugar-free | 30 sachet P £8.11 DT = £3.95 sugar-free | 50 sachet P £13.49
Movicol Chocolate oral powder 13.9g sachets sugar-free | 30 sachet P £8.11 DT = £3.95
Movicol oral powder 13.8g sachets lemon & lime sugar-free | 20 sachet P £5.41 sugar-free | 30 sachet P £8.11 DT = £3.95 sugar-free | 50 sachet P £13.49
▸ VistaPrep (Tillotts Pharma Ltd)
Macrogol '3350' 105 gram per 1 litre, Potassium 5.4 mmol per 1 litre, Bicarbonate 17 mmol per 1 litre, Chloride 53 mmol per 1 litre, Sodium 65 mmol per 1 litre VistaPrep oral powder 110g sachets sugar-free | 4 sachet P £7.92

Magnesium hydroxide

• INDICATIONS AND DOSE

Constipation
▸ BY MOUTH
▸ Adult: 30–45 mL as required, dose to be given mixed with water at bedtime

• CONTRA-INDICATIONS Acute gastro-intestinal conditions
• CAUTIONS Debilitated patients · elderly
• INTERACTIONS → Appendix 1: magnesium
• HEPATIC IMPAIRMENT Avoid in hepatic coma if risk of renal failure.
• RENAL IMPAIRMENT Increased risk of toxicity in renal impairment.
Dose adjustments Avoid or reduce dose.
• PRESCRIBING AND DISPENSING INFORMATION When prepared extemporaneously, the BP states Magnesium Hydroxide Mixture, BP consists of an aqueous suspension containing about 8% hydrated magnesium oxide.

• MEDICINAL FORMS
There can be variation in the licensing of different medicines containing the same drug.
Oral suspension
▸ Magnesium hydroxide (Non-proprietary)
Magnesium hydroxide 79 mg per 1 ml Magnesium hydroxide 7.45-8.35% oral suspension BP | 500 ml GSL £5.15-£5.31
Magnesium hydroxide 80 mg per 1 ml Magnesium hydroxide 8% oral suspension | 200 ml GSL £3.22 DT = £3.22 | 500 ml GSL £7.99-£8.05
▸ Brands may include Phillips' Milk of Magnesia

Sodium acid phosphate with sodium phosphate

• INDICATIONS AND DOSE

Constipation (using Phosphates Enema BP Formula B) | Bowel evacuation before abdominal radiological procedures, endoscopy, and surgery (using Phosphates Enema BP Formula B)
▸ BY RECTUM
▸ Child 3-6 years: 45–65 mL once daily
▸ Child 7-11 years: 65–100 mL once daily
▸ Child 12-17 years: 100–128 mL once daily
▸ Adult: 128 mL daily

FLEET ® READY-TO-USE ENEMA

Constipation | Bowel evacuation before abdominal radiological procedures | Bowel evacuation before endoscopy | Bowel evacuation before surgery
▸ BY RECTUM
▸ Adult: 118 mL

FLEET ® PHOSPHO-SODA

Bowel evacuation before colonic surgery | Bowel evacuation before colonoscopy | Bowel evacuation before radiological examination
▸ BY MOUTH
▸ Adult: 45 mL twice daily, each dose must be diluted with half a glass (120 mL) of cold water, followed by one full glass (240 mL) of cold water, timing of doses is dependent on the time of the procedure, for morning procedure, the first dose should be taken at 7 a.m. and second at 7 p.m. on day before the procedure.; for afternoon procedure, first dose should be taken at 7 p.m. on day before and second dose at 7 a.m. on day of the procedure

PHARMACOKINETICS
▸ For *Fleet® phospho-soda*: onset of action is within half to 6 hours of first dose.

● CONTRA-INDICATIONS
▸ With oral use Acute severe colitis · ascites · congestive cardiac failure · gastric retention · gastro-intestinal obstruction · gastro-intestinal perforation · toxic megacolon
▸ With rectal use conditions associated with increased colonic absorption · gastro-intestinal obstruction · inflammatory bowel disease
● CAUTIONS
▸ With oral use cardiac disease (avoid in congestive cardiac failure) · colitis (avoid if acute severe colitis) · elderly and debilitated patients · fluid and electrolyte disturbances · hypovolaemia (should be corrected before administration) · impaired gag reflex or possibility of regurgitation or aspiration
▸ With rectal use Ascites · congestive heart failure · elderly and debilitated patients · electrolyte disturbances · uncontrolled hypertension
● INTERACTIONS → Appendix 1: bowel cleansing preparations
● SIDE-EFFECTS
GENERAL SIDE-EFFECTS
▸ **Common or very common** Chills · gastrointestinal discomfort · nausea · vomiting
▸ **Uncommon** Dehydration
▸ **Rare or very rare** Electrolyte imbalance · metabolic acidosis
SPECIFIC SIDE-EFFECTS
▸ **Common or very common**
▸ With oral use Asthenia · chest pain · dizziness · headache
▸ **Rare or very rare**
▸ With oral use Allergic dermatitis · arrhythmia · hypotension · loss of consciousness · muscle cramps · myocardial infarction · nephrocalcinosis · paraesthesia · renal impairment · tetany
▸ With rectal use Pain
● PREGNANCY
▸ With oral use Caution.
● BREAST FEEDING
▸ With oral use Caution.
● HEPATIC IMPAIRMENT Use with caution in cirrhosis.
● RENAL IMPAIRMENT
▸ With oral use Avoid if eGFR less than 60 mL/minute/1.73 m^2.
▸ With rectal use Use with caution.

● MONITORING REQUIREMENTS
▸ With oral use Renal function should be measured before starting treatment in patients at risk of fluid and electrolyte disturbances.
● DIRECTIONS FOR ADMINISTRATION
FLEET ® PHOSPHO-SODA Copious intake of water or other clear fluids (e.g. clear soup, strained fruit juice without pulp, black tea or coffee) recommended until midnight before morning procedure and until 8 a.m. before afternoon procedure. At least one glass (approx 240 mL) of water or other clear fluid should also be taken immediately before each dose.
● PRESCRIBING AND DISPENSING INFORMATION When prepared extemporaneously, the BP states Phosphates Enema BP Formula B consists of sodium dihydrogen phosphate dihydrate 12.8 g, disodium phosphate dodecahydrate 10.24 g, purified water, freshly boiled and cooled, to 128 mL.
● PATIENT AND CARER ADVICE
FLEET ® PHOSPHO-SODA Intake of solid food should be stopped for at least 6 hours before starting treatment and until procedure completed.
Patients or carers should be advised that adequate hydration should be maintained during treatment.
Patients or carers should be given advice on administration of *Fleet ® Phospho-soda* oral solution.

● MEDICINAL FORMS
There can be variation in the licensing of different medicines containing the same drug.
Oral solution
CAUTIONARY AND ADVISORY LABELS 10
ELECTROLYTES: May contain Phosphate, sodium
▸ Fleet Phospho-soda (Casen Recordati S.L.)
   Disodium hydrogen phosphate dodecahydrate 240 mg per 1 ml, Sodium dihydrogen phosphate dihydrate 562 mg per 1 ml Phospho-soda 24.4g/10.8g oral solution sugar-free | 90 ml Ⓟ £4.79
Enema
▸ Sodium acid phosphate with sodium phosphate (Non-proprietary)
   Disodium hydrogen phosphate dodecahydrate 80 mg per 1 ml, Sodium dihydrogen phosphate dihydrate 100 mg per 1 ml Phosphates enema (Formula B) 128ml long tube | 1 enema Ⓟ £27.93 DT = £27.93
   Phosphates enema (Formula B) 128ml standard tube | 1 enema Ⓟ £3.98 DT = £3.98
▸ Fleet Ready-to-use (Casen Recordati S.L.)
   Disodium hydrogen phosphate dodecahydrate 80 mg per 1 ml, Sodium dihydrogen phosphate dihydrate 181 mg per 1 ml Cleen Ready-to-use 133ml enema | 1 enema Ⓟ £0.68

LAXATIVES ⟩ SELECTIVE 5-HT$_4$ RECEPTOR AGONISTS

Prucalopride
24-Feb-2016

● DRUG ACTION A selective serotonin 5HT$_4$-receptor agonist with prokinetic properties.

● INDICATIONS AND DOSE
Chronic constipation when other laxatives fail to provide an adequate response
▸ BY MOUTH
▸ Adult: 2 mg once daily, review treatment if no response after 4 weeks
▸ Elderly: Initially 1 mg once daily, increased if necessary to 2 mg once daily, review treatment if no response after 4 weeks

● CONTRA-INDICATIONS Crohn's disease · intestinal obstruction · intestinal perforation · toxic megacolon · ulcerative colitis

Gastro-intestinal system

- CAUTIONS History of arrhythmias · history of ischaemic heart disease
- SIDE-EFFECTS
  ▸ **Common or very common** Appetite decreased · diarrhoea · dizziness · fatigue · gastrointestinal discomfort · gastrointestinal disorders · headache · nausea · vomiting
  ▸ **Uncommon** Anorectal haemorrhage · fever · malaise · palpitations · tremor · urinary frequency increased
  SIDE-EFFECTS, FURTHER INFORMATION Side-effects generally occur at the start of treatment and are usually transient.
- CONCEPTION AND CONTRACEPTION Manufacturer recommends effective contraception during treatment.
- PREGNANCY Manufacturer advises avoid—limited data available.
- BREAST FEEDING Manufacturer advises avoid—present in milk.
- HEPATIC IMPAIRMENT
  Dose adjustments In severe impairment, manufacturer advises reduced dose of 1 mg once daily; increased if necessary to 2 mg once daily.
- RENAL IMPAIRMENT
  Dose adjustments Manufacturer recommends a reduced dose of 1 mg daily if eGFR less than 30 mL/minute/1.73 m^2.
- PATIENT AND CARER ADVICE
  Driving and skilled tasks Manufacturer advises that dizziness and fatigue may initially affect ability to drive or operate machinery.
- NATIONAL FUNDING/ACCESS DECISIONS
  NICE decisions
  ▸ **Prucalopride for the treatment of chronic constipation in women (December 2010) NICE TA211**
  Prucalopride is recommended as an option for the treatment of chronic constipation in women for whom treatment with at least 2 laxatives from different classes, at the highest tolerated recommended doses for at least 6 months, has failed to provide adequate relief and invasive treatment for constipation is being considered. If treatment with prucalopride is not effective after 4 weeks, the patient should be re-examined and the benefit of continuing treatment reconsidered.
  Prucalopride should only be prescribed by a clinician with experience of treating chronic constipation, after careful review of the patient's previous courses of laxative treatments.
  www.nice.org.uk/TA211
  Scottish Medicines Consortium (SMC) Decisions
  The *Scottish Medicines Consortium* has advised (June 2011) that prucalopride (*Resolor*®) is not recommended for use within NHS Scotland for the symptomatic treatment of chronic constipation of women in whom laxatives fail to provide adequate relief.
- MEDICINAL FORMS
  There can be variation in the licensing of different medicines containing the same drug.
  Tablet
  ▸ Resolor (Shire Pharmaceuticals Ltd)
  Prucalopride (as Prucalopride succinate) **1 mg** Resolor 1mg tablets | 28 tablet PoM £38.69 DT = £38.69
  Prucalopride (as Prucalopride succinate) **2 mg** Resolor 2mg tablets | 28 tablet PoM £59.52 DT = £59.52

LAXATIVES ⟩ SOFTENING LAXATIVES

Arachis oil

- INDICATIONS AND DOSE
  To soften impacted faeces
  ▸ BY RECTUM
  ▸ Adult: 130 mL as required

- CAUTIONS Hypersensitivity to soya · intestinal obstruction
- ALLERGY AND CROSS-SENSITIVITY Contra-indicated if history of hypersensitivity to arachis oil or peanuts.
- DIRECTIONS FOR ADMINISTRATION Warm enema in warm water before use.

- MEDICINAL FORMS
  There can be variation in the licensing of different medicines containing the same drug.
  Enema
  ▸ Arachis oil (Non-proprietary)
  Arachis oil **1 ml per 1 ml** Arachis oil 130ml enema | 1 enema P £47.50 DT = £47.50

Docusate sodium

20-Apr-2016

(Dioctyl sodium sulphosuccinate)

- INDICATIONS AND DOSE
  Chronic constipation
  ▸ BY MOUTH
  ▸ Child 6 months–1 year: 12.5 mg 3 times a day, adjusted according to response, use paediatric oral solution
  ▸ Child 2–11 years: 12.5–25 mg 3 times a day, adjusted according to response, use paediatric oral solution
  ▸ Child 12–17 years: Up to 500 mg daily in divided doses, adjusted according to response
  ▸ Adult: Up to 500 mg daily in divided doses, adjusted according to response
  ▸ BY RECTUM
  ▸ Adult: 120 mg for 1 dose
  Adjunct in abdominal radiological procedures
  ▸ BY MOUTH
  ▸ Adult: 400 mg, to be administered with barium meal
  ▸ BY RECTUM
  ▸ Adult: 120 mg for 1 dose
  PHARMACOKINETICS
  ▸ Oral preparations act within 1–2 days; response to rectal administration usually occurs within 20 minutes.

- UNLICENSED USE *Adult oral solution and capsules* not licensed for use in children under 12 years.
- CONTRA-INDICATIONS Avoid in intestinal obstruction
- CAUTIONS Do not give with liquid paraffin · excessive use of stimulant laxatives can cause diarrhoea and related effects such as hypokalaemia · rectal preparations not indicated if haemorrhoids or anal fissure
- SIDE-EFFECTS
  ▸ **Rare or very rare**
  ▸ With oral use Abdominal cramps · nausea · rash
- PREGNANCY Not known to be harmful—manufacturer advises caution.
- BREAST FEEDING Present in milk following oral administration— manufacturer advises caution.
  Rectal administration not known to be harmful.
- DIRECTIONS FOR ADMINISTRATION
  ▸ With oral use in children For administration *by mouth*, solution may be mixed with milk or squash.

● MEDICINAL FORMS
There can be variation in the licensing of different medicines containing the same drug.

Oral solution
▸ Docusate sodium (Non-proprietary)
Docusate sodium 2.5 mg per 1 ml Docusate 12.5mg/5ml oral solution sugar free sugar-free | 300 ml P £7.79 DT = £7.79
Docusate sodium 10 mg per 1 ml Docusate 50mg/5ml oral solution sugar free sugar-free | 300 ml P £7.99-£8.01 DT = £8.01
▸ Docusol (Typharm Ltd)
Docusate sodium 2.5 mg per 1 ml Docusol Paediatric 12.5mg/5ml oral solution sugar-free | 125 ml P £4.46

Enema
▸ Norgalax (Essential Pharma Ltd)
Docusate sodium 12 mg per 1 gram Norgalax 120mg/10g enema | 6 enema P £28.00

Capsule
▸ Dioctyl (UCB Pharma Ltd)
Docusate sodium 100 mg Dioctyl 100mg capsules | 30 capsule P £2.09 DT = £2.09 | 100 capsule P £6.98
▸ DulcoEase (Sanofi)
Docusate sodium 100 mg DulcoEase 100mg capsules | 30 capsule GSL £3.20 DT = £2.09

Combinations available: *Co-danthrusate*, p. 62

Liquid paraffin

12-Apr-2016

● INDICATIONS AND DOSE

Constipation
▸ BY MOUTH
▸ Adult: 10–30 mL daily if required, to be administered at night

● CONTRA-INDICATIONS Children under 3 years
● CAUTIONS Avoid prolonged use
● SIDE-EFFECTS Anal irritation · contact dermatitis · granuloma · pneumonia lipoid · rectal discharge of drug
● PRESCRIBING AND DISPENSING INFORMATION When prepared extemporaneously, the BP states Liquid Paraffin Oral Emulsion, BP consists of liquid paraffin 5 mL, vanillin 5 mg, chloroform 0.025 mL, benzoic acid solution 0.2 mL, methylcellulose-20 200 mg, saccharin sodium 500 micrograms, water to 10 mL.
● PATIENT AND CARER ADVICE Oral emulsion should not be taken immediately before going to bed.
● LESS SUITABLE FOR PRESCRIBING Liquid Paraffin Oral Emulsion BP is less suitable for prescribing.
● MEDICINAL FORMS
There can be variation in the licensing of different medicines containing the same drug.

Liquid
▸ Liquid paraffin (Non-proprietary)
Liquid paraffin 1 ml per 1 ml Liquid paraffin liquid | 150 ml P £1.37-£1.49 | 2000 ml GSL £10.24 | 5000 ml GSL £20.57

LAXATIVES ❭ STIMULANT LAXATIVES

Bisacodyl

● INDICATIONS AND DOSE

Constipation
▸ BY MOUTH
▸ Child 4-17 years: 5–20 mg once daily, adjusted according to response, dose to be taken at night
▸ Adult: 5–10 mg once dailyIncreased if necessary up to 20 mg once daily, dose to be taken at night
▸ BY RECTUM
▸ Child 2-17 years: 5–10 mg once daily, adjusted according to response
▸ Adult: 10 mg once daily, dose to be taken in the morning

Bowel clearance before radiological procedures and surgery
▸ INITIALLY BY MOUTH
▸ Adult: 10 mg twice daily, does to be taken in the morning and evening on the day before procedure and (by rectum) 10 mg, to be administered 1–2 hours before procedure the following day

PHARMACOKINETICS
▸ Tablets act in 10–12 hours; suppositories act in 20–60 minutes.

● CONTRA-INDICATIONS Acute abdominal conditions (in children) · acute inflammatory bowel disease · acute surgical abdominal conditions (in adults) · intestinal obstruction · severe dehydration
● CAUTIONS Excessive use of stimulant laxatives can cause diarrhoea and related effects such as hypokalaemia · risk of electrolyte imbalance with prolonged use (in children)
● SIDE-EFFECTS

GENERAL SIDE-EFFECTS
▸ **Common or very common** Gastrointestinal discomfort · nausea
▸ **Uncommon** Vomiting
▸ **Rare or very rare** Angioedema · colitis · dehydration
SPECIFIC SIDE-EFFECTS
▸ **Uncommon**
▸ With oral use Haemorrhage
▸ With rectal use Haematochezia
● PREGNANCY May be suitable for constipation in pregnancy, if a stimulant effect is necessary.

● MEDICINAL FORMS
There can be variation in the licensing of different medicines containing the same drug. Forms available from special-order manufacturers include: oral suspension, suppository, enema

Gastro-resistant tablet
CAUTIONARY AND ADVISORY LABELS 5, 25
▸ Bisacodyl (Non-proprietary)
Bisacodyl 5 mg Bisacodyl 5mg gastro-resistant tablets | 60 tablet P £5.13 DT = £5.13 | 100 tablet P £5.40 | 500 tablet P £25.73-£50.00 | 1000 tablet P £51.45-£100.00
▸ Dulco-Lax (bisacodyl) (Sanofi)
Bisacodyl 5 mg Dulcolax 5mg gastro-resistant tablets | 40 tablet P £2.44 | 100 tablet P £3.60

Enema
▸ Bisacodyl (Non-proprietary)
Bisacodyl 333.333 microgram per 1 ml Fleet Bisacodyl 10mg/30ml enema | 1 enema PoM ⚠ DT = £30.38

Suppository
▸ Bisacodyl (Non-proprietary)
Bisacodyl 10 mg Bisacodyl 10mg suppositories | 12 suppository P £3.53 DT = £3.53
▸ Dulco-Lax (bisacodyl) (Sanofi)
Bisacodyl 5 mg Dulcolax 5mg suppositories for children | 5 suppository P £1.04 DT = £1.04
Bisacodyl 10 mg Dulcolax 10mg suppositories | 12 suppository P £2.35 DT = £3.53

Co-danthramer

● INDICATIONS AND DOSE

Constipation in terminally ill patients (standard strength capsules)
▸ BY MOUTH USING CAPSULES
▸ Child 6-11 years: 1 capsule once daily, dose should be taken at night
▸ Child 12-17 years: 1–2 capsules once daily, dose should be taken at night
▸ Adult: 1–2 capsules once daily, dose should be taken at night

continued →

Gastro-intestinal system

1

Constipation in terminally ill patients (strong capsules)
▶ BY MOUTH USING CAPSULES
▸ Child 12–17 years: 1–2 capsules once daily, dose should be given at night
▸ Adult: 1–2 capsules once daily, dose should be given at night

Constipation in terminally ill patients (standard strength suspension)
▶ BY MOUTH USING ORAL SUSPENSION
▸ Child 2–11 years: 2.5–5 mL once daily, dose should be taken at night
▸ Child 12–17 years: 5–10 mL once daily, dose should be taken at night
▸ Adult: 5–10 mL once daily, dose should be taken at night

Constipation in terminally ill patients (strong suspension)
▶ BY MOUTH USING ORAL SUSPENSION
▸ Child 12–17 years: 5 mL once daily, dose should be taken at night
▸ Adult: 5 mL once daily, dose should be taken at night

DOSE EQUIVALENCE AND CONVERSION
▸ Co-danthramer (standard strength) capsules contain dantron 25 mg with poloxamer '188' 200 mg per capsule.
▸ Co-danthramer (standard strength) oral suspension contains dantron 25 mg with poloxamer '188' 200 mg per 5 mL.
▸ Co-danthramer **strong** capsules contain dantron 37.5 mg with poloxamer '188' 500 mg.
▸ Co-danthramer **strong** oral suspension contains dantron 75 mg with poloxamer '188' 1 g per 5 mL.
▸ Co-danthramer suspension 5 mL = one co-danthramer capsule, **but** strong co-danthramer suspension 5 mL = two strong co-danthramer capsules.

● CONTRA-INDICATIONS Acute abdominal conditions (in children) · acute inflammatory bowel disease · acute surgical abdominal conditions (in adults) · intestinal obstruction · severe dehydration
● CAUTIONS Excessive use of stimulant laxatives can cause diarrhoea and related effects such as hypokalaemia · may cause local irritation · *rodent* studies indicate potential carcinogenic risk
CAUTIONS, FURTHER INFORMATION
▸ Local irritation Avoid prolonged contact with skin (as in incontinent patients or infants wearing nappies—risk of irritation and excoriation).
● SIDE-EFFECTS Abdominal cramps · asthenia · gastrointestinal disorders · hypermagnesaemia · skin reactions · urine red
● PREGNANCY Manufacturers advise avoid—limited information available.
● BREAST FEEDING Manufacturers advise avoid—no information available.

● MEDICINAL FORMS
There can be variation in the licensing of different medicines containing the same drug.
Oral suspension
CAUTIONARY AND ADVISORY LABELS 14 (urine red)
▸ Co-danthramer (Non-proprietary)
  Dantron 5 mg per 1 ml, Poloxamer 188 40 mg per 1 ml Co-danthramer 25mg/200mg/5ml oral suspension sugar free sugar-free | 300 ml PoM £169.28 DT = £168.93
  Dantron 15 mg per 1 ml, Poloxamer 188 200 mg per 1 ml Co-danthramer 75mg/1000mg/5ml oral suspension sugar free sugar-free | 300 ml PoM £337.73 DT = £337.05

Co-danthrusate
20-Apr-2016

● INDICATIONS AND DOSE
Constipation in terminally ill patients
▶ BY MOUTH USING CAPSULES
▸ Child 6–11 years: 1 capsule once daily, to be taken at night
▸ Child 12–17 years: 1–3 capsules once daily, to be taken at night
▸ Adult: 1–3 capsules once daily, to be taken at night
▶ BY MOUTH USING ORAL SUSPENSION
▸ Child 6–11 years: 5 mL once daily, to be taken at night
▸ Child 12–17 years: 5–15 mL once daily, to be taken at night
▸ Adult: 5–15 mL once daily, to be taken at night

DOSE EQUIVALENCE AND CONVERSION
▸ Co-danthrusate suspension contains dantron 50 mg and docusate 60 mg per 5 mL.
▸ Co-danthrusate capsules contain dantron 50 mg and docusate 60 mg per capsule.

● CONTRA-INDICATIONS Acute abdominal conditions (in children) · acute inflammatory bowel disease · acute surgical abdominal conditions (in adults) · intestinal obstruction · severe dehydration
● CAUTIONS Excessive use of stimulant laxatives can cause diarrhoea and related effects such as hypokalaemia · may cause local irritation · *rodent* studies indicate potential carcinogenic risk
CAUTIONS, FURTHER INFORMATION
▸ Local irritation Avoid prolonged contact with skin (as in incontinent patients—risk of irritation and excoriation).
● SIDE-EFFECTS Gastrointestinal disorders · skin reactions · urine orange
● PREGNANCY Manufacturers advise avoid—limited information available.
● BREAST FEEDING Manufacturers advise avoid—no information available.

● MEDICINAL FORMS
There can be variation in the licensing of different medicines containing the same drug.
Oral suspension
CAUTIONARY AND ADVISORY LABELS 14 (urine orange)
▸ Co-danthrusate (Non-proprietary)
  Dantron 10 mg per 1 ml, Docusate sodium 12 mg per 1 ml Co-danthrusate 50mg/60mg/5ml oral suspension sugar free sugar-free | 200 ml PoM £154.40 DT = £154.40
Capsule
CAUTIONARY AND ADVISORY LABELS 14 (urine orange)
▸ Co-danthrusate (Non-proprietary)
  Dantron 50 mg, Docusate sodium 60 mg Co-danthrusate 50mg/60mg capsules | 63 capsule PoM ⓧ

Glycerol
(Glycerin)

● INDICATIONS AND DOSE
Constipation
▶ BY RECTUM
▸ Child 1–11 months: 1 g as required
▸ Child 1–11 years: 2 g as required
▸ Child 12–17 years: 4 g as required
▸ Adult: 4 g as required

● SIDE-EFFECTS Gastrointestinal discomfort
● DIRECTIONS FOR ADMINISTRATION Moisten suppositories with water before insertion.
● PRESCRIBING AND DISPENSING INFORMATION When prepared extemporaneously, the BP states Glycerol

Suppositories, BP consists of gelatin 140 mg, glycerol 700 mg, purified water to 1 g.

● PATIENT AND CARER ADVICE
Medicines for Children leaflet: Glycerin (glycerol) suppositories for constipation www.medicinesforchildren.org.uk/glycerin-glycerol-suppositories-for-constipation

● MEDICINAL FORMS
There can be variation in the licensing of different medicines containing the same drug. Forms available from special-order manufacturers include: suppository
Suppository
▸ Glycerol (Non-proprietary)
Glycerol 700 mg Glycerol 1g suppositories | 12 suppository GSL
£1.75 DT = £1.04
Glycerol 1400 mg Glycerol 2g suppositories | 12 suppository GSL
£1.78 DT = £1.70
Glycerol 2800 mg Glycerol 4g suppositories | 12 suppository GSL
£1.31 DT = £1.16

Senna
20-Jul-2017

● DRUG ACTION Senna is a stimulant laxative. After metabolism of sennosides in the gut the anthrone component stimulates peristalsis thereby increasing the motility of the large intestine.

● INDICATIONS AND DOSE
Constipation
▸ BY MOUTH USING TABLETS
▹ Child 6–17 years: 7.5–30 mg once daily, adjusted according to response
▹ Adult: 7.5–15 mg daily (max. per dose 30 mg daily), dose usually taken at bedtime; initial dose should be low then gradually increased, higher doses may be prescribed under medical supervision
▸ BY MOUTH USING SYRUP
▹ Child 1 month–3 years: 3.75–15 mg once daily, adjusted according to response
▹ Child 4–17 years: 3.75–30 mg once daily, adjusted according to response
▹ Adult: 7.5–15 mg once daily (max. per dose 30 mg daily), dose usually taken at bedtime, higher doses may be prescribed under medical supervision
PHARMACOKINETICS
▸ Onset of action 8–12 hours.

● UNLICENSED USE *Tablets* not licensed for use in children under 6 years. *Syrup* not licensed for use in children under 2 years.
    Doses in BNF adhere to national guidelines and may differ from those in product literature.

● CONTRA-INDICATIONS Intestinal obstruction · undiagnosed abdominal pain

● SIDE-EFFECTS Albuminuria · diarrhoea · electrolyte imbalance · fluid imbalance · gastrointestinal discomfort · haematuria · pseudomelanosis coli · skin reactions · urine discolouration
SIDE-EFFECTS, FURTHER INFORMATION Prolonged or excessive use can cause hypokalaemia.

● PREGNANCY EvGr Specialist sources indicate suitable for use in pregnancy. ◇

● BREAST FEEDING EvGr Specialist sources indicate suitable for use in breast-feeding in infants over 1 month. ◇

● PATIENT AND CARER ADVICE
Medicines for Children leaflet: Senna for constipation
www.medicinesforchildren.org.uk/senna-for-constipation

● NATIONAL FUNDING/ACCESS DECISIONS
NHS restrictions *Senokot*® tablets are not prescribable in NHS primary care.

● EXCEPTIONS TO LEGAL CATEGORY Senna is on sale to the public for use in children over 12 years; doses on packs may vary from those in BNF Publications.

● MEDICINAL FORMS
There can be variation in the licensing of different medicines containing the same drug.
Oral solution
▸ Senokot (Forum Health Products Ltd, Reckitt Benckiser Healthcare (UK) Ltd)
Sennoside B (as Sennosides) 1.5 mg per 1 ml Senokot 7.5mg/5ml Syrup Pharmacy sugar free sugar-free | 500 ml P £4.76 DT = £4.76
Tablet
▸ Senna (Non-proprietary)
Sennoside B (as Sennosides) 7.5 mg Senna 7.5mg tablets | 20 tablet P £1.00 | 60 tablet P £1.78 DT = £1.61 | 100 tablet P £2.15
▸ Senokot (Reckitt Benckiser Healthcare (UK) Ltd, Forum Health Products Ltd)
Sennoside B (as Sennosides) 15 mg Senokot Max Strength 15mg tablets | 24 tablet GSL £3.23 | 48 tablet GSL £5.69 DT = £5.69

Senna with ispaghula husk
24-Feb-2016

The properties listed below are those particular to the combination only. For the properties of the components please consider, senna above, ispaghula husk p. 54.

● INDICATIONS AND DOSE
Constipation
▸ BY MOUTH
▹ Child 12–17 years: 5–10 g once daily, to be taken at night, 5 g equivalent to one level spoonful of granules
▹ Adult: 5–10 g once daily, to be taken at night, 5 g equivalent to one level spoonful of granules

● PREGNANCY Manufacturer advises avoid during first trimester. To be used only intermittently and only if dietary and lifestyle changes fail.

● DIRECTIONS FOR ADMINISTRATION Take at night with at least 150 mL liquid.

● MEDICINAL FORMS
There can be variation in the licensing of different medicines containing the same drug.
Granules
CAUTIONARY AND ADVISORY LABELS 25
EXCIPIENTS: May contain Sucrose
▸ Manevac (Meda Pharmaceuticals Ltd)
Senna fruit 124 mg per 1 gram, Ispaghula 542 mg per 1 gram Manevac granules | 400 gram P £9.50 DT = £9.50

Sodium picosulfate
06-May-2016

(Sodium picosulphate)

● DRUG ACTION Sodium picosulfate is a stimulant laxative. After metabolism in the colon it stimulates the mucosa thereby increasing the motility of the large intestine.

● INDICATIONS AND DOSE
Constipation
▸ BY MOUTH
▹ Child 1 month–3 years: 2.5–10 mg once daily, adjusted according to response
▹ Child 4–17 years: 2.5–20 mg once daily, adjusted according to response
▹ Adult: 5–10 mg once daily, dose to be taken at bedtime
PHARMACOKINETICS
▸ Onset of action 6–12 hours.

● UNLICENSED USE Sodium picosulfate doses in BNF Publications adhere to national guidelines and may differ from those in product literature.

- CONTRA-INDICATIONS Intestinal obstruction ·
  undiagnosed abdominal pain
- INTERACTIONS → Appendix 1: sodium picosulfate
- SIDE-EFFECTS
  ▸ **Common or very common** Diarrhoea · gastrointestinal
  discomfort
  ▸ **Uncommon** Dizziness · nausea · vomiting
  ▸ **Frequency not known** Angioedema · skin reactions ·
  syncope
  SIDE-EFFECTS, FURTHER INFORMATION Prolonged or
  excessive use can cause diarrhoea and related effects such
  as hypokalaemia.
- PREGNANCY Manufacturer states evidence limited but not
  known to be harmful.
- BREAST FEEDING [EvGr] Specialist sources indicate suitable
  for use in breast-feeding in infants over 1 month—not
  known to be present in milk. Ⓓ
- PATIENT AND CARER ADVICE
  Medicines for Children leaflet: Sodium picosulfate for
  constipation www.medicinesforchildren.org.uk/sodium-
  picosulfate-for-constipation

- MEDICINAL FORMS
  There can be variation in the licensing of different medicines
  containing the same drug.
  Oral solution
  EXCIPIENTS: May contain Alcohol
  ▸ Sodium picosulfate (Non-proprietary)
  Sodium picosulfate 1 mg per 1 ml Sodium picosulfate 5mg/5ml oral
  solution sugar free sugar-free | 100 ml [P] £2.37 sugar-free |
  300 ml [P] £7.10 DT = £7.10
  ▸ Laxoberal (Sanofi)
  Sodium picosulfate 1 mg per 1 ml Dulcolax Pico 5mg/5ml liquid
  sugar-free | 100 ml [P] £1.94 sugar-free | 300 ml [P] £4.62 DT =
  £7.10

OPIOID RECEPTOR ANTAGONISTS

Methylnaltrexone bromide   12-Dec-2016

- DRUG ACTION Methylnaltrexone bromide is a peripherally
  acting opioid-receptor antagonist. It therefore blocks the
  gastro-intestinal (constipating) effects of opioids without
  altering their central analgesic effects.

- INDICATIONS AND DOSE
  **Opioid-induced constipation in patients with chronic pain
  (except palliative care patients with advanced illness)**
  ▸ BY SUBCUTANEOUS INJECTION
  ▸ Adult: 12 mg once daily if required, to be given as
  4–7 doses weekly
  **Adjunct to other laxatives in opioid-induced constipation
  in advanced illness (palliative care patients)**
  ▸ BY SUBCUTANEOUS INJECTION
  ▸ Adult (body-weight up to 38 kg): 150 micrograms/kg once
  daily on alternate days for maximum duration of
  treatment 4 months, two consecutive doses may be
  given 24 hours apart if no response to treatment on the
  preceding day
  ▸ Adult (body-weight 38–61 kg): 8 mg once daily on
  alternate days for maximum duration of treatment
  4 months, two consecutive doses may be given
  24 hours apart if no response to treatment on the
  preceding day
  ▸ Adult (body-weight 62–114 kg): 12 mg once daily on
  alternate days for maximum duration of treatment
  4 months, two consecutive doses may be given
  24 hours apart if no response to treatment on the
  preceding day
  ▸ Adult (body-weight 115 kg and above): 150 micrograms/kg
  once daily on alternate days for maximum duration of
  treatment 4 months, two consecutive doses may be

given 24 hours apart if no response to treatment on the
preceding day
PHARMACOKINETICS
▸ May act within 30–60 minutes.

- CONTRA-INDICATIONS Acute surgical abdominal
  conditions · gastro-intestinal obstruction
- CAUTIONS Diverticular disease (when active) · faecal
  impaction · gastro-intestinal tract lesions (known or
  suspected) · patients with colostomy · patients with
  peritoneal catheter
- SIDE-EFFECTS
  ▸ **Common or very common** Abdominal pain · diarrhoea ·
  dizziness · gastrointestinal disorders · nausea · opioid
  withdrawal-like syndrome · vomiting
  Overdose Symptoms of overdosage include orthostatic
  hypotension.
- PREGNANCY Manufacturer advises avoid unless
  essential—toxicity at high doses in *animal* studies.
- BREAST FEEDING Manufacturer advises use only if
  potential benefit outweighs risk—present in milk in *animal*
  studies.
- HEPATIC IMPAIRMENT Manufacturer advises avoid in
  severe impairment—no information available.
- RENAL IMPAIRMENT
  Dose adjustments If eGFR less than 30 mL/minute/1.73 m^2,
  reduce dose as follows: body-weight under 62 kg,
  75 micrograms/kg on alternate days; body-weight
  62–114 kg, 8 mg on alternate days; body-weight over
  114 kg, 75 micrograms/kg on alternate days.
- DIRECTIONS FOR ADMINISTRATION Rotate injection site.
- PRESCRIBING AND DISPENSING INFORMATION
  Palliative care For further information on the use of
  methylnaltrexone in palliative care, see
  www.palliativedrugs.com/formulary/en/opioid-antagonists.
  html.
- HANDLING AND STORAGE Protect from light.

- MEDICINAL FORMS
  There can be variation in the licensing of different medicines
  containing the same drug.
  Solution for injection
  ▸ Relistor (Swedish Orphan Biovitrum Ltd)
  Methylnaltrexone bromide 20 mg per 1 ml Relistor 12mg/0.6ml
  solution for injection vials | 1 vial [PoM] £21.05 | 7 vial [PoM] £147.35

Naloxegol   20-Jun-2016

- DRUG ACTION Naloxegol is a peripherally acting opioid
  receptor antagonist. It therefore decreases the
  constipating effects of opioids without altering their
  central analgesic effects.

- INDICATIONS AND DOSE
  **Opioid-induced constipation when response to laxatives
  inadequate**
  ▸ BY MOUTH
  ▸ Adult: 25 mg once daily, to be taken in the morning
  DOSE ADJUSTMENTS DUE TO INTERACTIONS
  ▸ Manufacturer advises reduce initial dose to 12.5 mg
  daily with concurrent use of moderate inhibitors of
  CYP3A4, increasing to 25 mg daily if well tolerated.

- CONTRA-INDICATIONS Gastro-intestinal or peritoneum
  malignancy (risk of gastro-intestinal perforation) · known
  or suspected gastro-intestinal obstruction · patients at risk
  of recurrent gastro-intestinal obstruction · recurrent or
  advanced ovarian cancer (risk of gastro-intestinal
  perforation) · vascular endothelial growth factor (VEGF)
  inhibitor treatment (risk of gastro-intestinal perforation)

- CAUTIONS Alzheimer's disease (advanced) · cardiovascular disease · CNS metastases · congestive heart failure (symptomatic) · Crohn's disease · diverticulitis (active or recurrent) · multiple sclerosis (active) · peptic ulcer disease (severe) · primary brain malignancies · QT interval over 500 milliseconds · recent history of myocardial infarction (within 6 months)

  CAUTIONS, FURTHER INFORMATION
  ‣ Disruptions to blood-brain barrier Manufacturer advises caution in patients with clinically important disruptions to the blood-brain barrier (e.g. advanced Alzheimer's disease, active multiple sclerosis, primary brain malignancies)—risk of uptake into the CNS.
  ‣ Cardiovascular disorders Safety and efficacy has not been established in patients with these conditions.
- INTERACTIONS → Appendix 1: naloxegol
- SIDE-EFFECTS
  ‣ **Common or very common** Abdominal pain · diarrhoea · flatulence · headache · hyperhidrosis · nasopharyngitis · nausea · vomiting
  ‣ **Uncommon** Withdrawal syndrome

  SIDE-EFFECTS, FURTHER INFORMATION Manufacturer advises that gastrointestinal side-effects typically occur shortly after initiation of treatment—consider reducing the dose.
- PREGNANCY Manufacturer advises avoid—limited data available but toxicity at high doses in *animal* studies; theoretical risk of opioid withdrawal in fetus.
- BREAST FEEDING Manufacturer advises avoid—present in milk in *animal* studies and theoretical risk of opioid withdrawal in breast-fed infants.
- HEPATIC IMPAIRMENT Manufacturer advises avoid in severe impairment—safety and efficacy not established.
- RENAL IMPAIRMENT
  Dose adjustments Manufacturer advises lower initial dose in moderate to severe impairment—initially 12.5 mg daily, increase to 25 mg if well tolerated.
- DIRECTIONS FOR ADMINISTRATION Manufacturer advises tablets can be crushed, mixed with 120 mL of water and taken immediately if patients are unable to swallow tablets whole. The mixture may be administered via a nasogastric tube, if required.
- PATIENT AND CARER ADVICE Manufacturer advises patients report severe, persistent or worsening gastro-intestinal effects (such as abdominal pain) to their prescriber.
- NATIONAL FUNDING/ACCESS DECISIONS
  NICE decisions
  ‣ **Naloxegol for treating opioid induced constipation (July 2015)** NICE TA345
  Naloxegol is recommended as a possible treatment for opioid induced constipation in patients whose response to laxatives is inadequate.
  www.nice.org.uk/TA345

- MEDICINAL FORMS
  There can be variation in the licensing of different medicines containing the same drug.
  Tablet
  CAUTIONARY AND ADVISORY LABELS 23
  ‣ Moventig (Kyowa Kirin Ltd) ▼
    Naloxegol (as Naloxegol oxalate) 12.5 mg Moventig 12.5mg tablets | 30 tablet PoM £55.20 DT = £55.20
    Naloxegol (as Naloxegol oxalate) 25 mg Moventig 25mg tablets | 30 tablet PoM £55.20 DT = £55.20

3 Diarrhoea

Diarrhoea (acute)
01-Aug-2017

Description of condition
Diarrhoea is the abnormal passing of loose or liquid stools, with increased frequency, increased volume, or both. Acute diarrhoea is that which lasts less than 14 days, but symptoms usually improve within 2–4 days. It can result from infection, as a side-effect of a drug, or as an acute symptom of a chronic gastro-intestinal disorder (such as Inflammatory bowel disease p. 36 or Irritable bowel syndrome p. 45). It may also result from the accumulation of non-absorbed osmotically active solutes in the gastro-intestinal lumen (e.g. in lactase deficiency) or from the gastro-intestinal effects of secretory stimuli (other than the enterotoxins from an infection). It may also occur when intestinal motility or morphology is altered.

Prompt investigation is required to identify or exclude any serious underlying cause if the patient has any red flag symptoms such as unexplained weight loss, rectal bleeding, persistent diarrhoea, a systemic illness, has received recent hospital treatment or antibiotic treatment, or following foreign travel (other than to Western Europe, North America, Australia or New Zealand).

Aims of treatment
The priority of acute diarrhoea treatment, as in gastro-enteritis, is the prevention or reversal of fluid and electrolyte depletion and the management of dehydration when it is present. This is particularly important in infants, frail and elderly patients, when excessive water and electrolyte loss and dehydration can be life-threatening.

Treatment
Most episodes of acute diarrhoea will settle spontaneously without the need for any medical treatment. EvGr Oral rehydration therapy (ORT, such as disodium hydrogen citrate with glucose, potassium chloride and sodium chloride p. 1010; potassium chloride with sodium chloride p. 1008; potassium chloride with rice powder, sodium chloride and sodium citrate p. 1011) is the mainstay of treatment for acute diarrhoea to prevent or correct diarrhoea dehydration and to maintain the appropriate fluid intake once rehydration is achieved—see Fluids and electrolytes p. 1003.

However, in patients with severe dehydration and in those unable to drink, immediate admission to hospital and urgent replacement treatment with an intravenous rehydration fluid is recommended—see Fluids and electrolytes p. 1003.

The antimotility drug loperamide hydrochloride p. 66 is usually considered to be the standard treatment when rapid control of symptoms is required. It can also be used for mild-to-moderate travellers' diarrhoea (e.g. where toilet amenities are limited or unavailable) but should be avoided in bloody or suspected inflammatory diarrhoea (febrile patients) and in cases of significant abdominal pain (which also suggests inflammatory diarrhoea).

Loperamide hydrochloride is also the first-line treatment for patients with faecal incontinence [unlicensed indication] after the underlying cause of incontinence has been addressed. Ⓐ

Racecadotril p. 67 is licensed as an adjunct to rehydration for the symptomatic treatment of uncomplicated acute diarrhoea in adults and children over 3 months.

There is insufficient evidence to recommend adsorbent preparations (such as kaolin p. 68) in acute diarrhoea.

Antibacterial drugs for acute diarrhoea
EvGr Ciprofloxacin p. 548 is occasionally used for prophylaxis against travellers' diarrhoea, but routine use is

not recommended. Ⓐ See also Gastro-intestinal system infections, antibacterial therapy p. 505.

Related drugs

Other drugs used for diarrhoea: codeine phosphate p. 448, colestyramine, p. 196, methylcellulose p. 54, rifaximin p. 565.

ANTIDIARRHOEALS › ANTIPROPULSIVES

⌖ 441

Co-phenotrope

- **INDICATIONS AND DOSE**

Adjunct to rehydration in acute diarrhoea

▸ BY MOUTH
- ‣ Child 4–8 years: 1 tablet 3 times a day
- ‣ Child 9–11 years: 1 tablet 4 times a day
- ‣ Child 12–15 years: 2 tablets 3 times a day
- ‣ Child 16–17 years: Initially 4 tablets, followed by 2 tablets every 6 hours until diarrhoea controlled
- ‣ Adult: Initially 4 tablets, followed by 2 tablets every 6 hours until diarrhoea controlled

Control of faecal consistency after colostomy or ileostomy

▸ BY MOUTH
- ‣ Child 4–8 years: 1 tablet 3 times a day
- ‣ Child 9–11 years: 1 tablet 4 times a day
- ‣ Child 12–15 years: 2 tablets 3 times a day
- ‣ Child 16–17 years: Initially 4 tablets, then 2 tablets 4 times a day
- ‣ Adult: Initially 4 tablets, then 2 tablets 4 times a day

- **UNLICENSED USE** Not licensed for use in children under 4 years.
- **CONTRA-INDICATIONS** Gastro-intestinal obstruction · intestinal atony · myasthenia gravis (but some antimuscarinics may be used to decrease muscarinic side-effects of anticholinesterases) · paralytic ileus · prostatic enlargement (in adults) · pyloric stenosis · severe ulcerative colitis · significant bladder outflow obstruction · toxic megacolon · urinary retention
- **CAUTIONS** Presence of subclinical doses of atropine may give rise to atropine side-effects in susceptible individuals or in overdosage · young children are particularly susceptible to **overdosage**; symptoms may be delayed and observation is needed for at least 48 hours after ingestion
- **INTERACTIONS** → Appendix 1: atropine · opioids
- **SIDE-EFFECTS** Abdominal discomfort · angioedema · angle closure glaucoma · appetite decreased · arrhythmia · cardiac disorder · depression · dry skin · dysuria · fever · gastrointestinal disorders · lethargy · malaise · mucosal dryness · mydriasis · restlessness · vision disorders
- **PREGNANCY** Manufacturer advises caution.
- **BREAST FEEDING** May be present in milk.
- **HEPATIC IMPAIRMENT** Avoid in jaundice.
- **DIRECTIONS FOR ADMINISTRATION** For administration *by mouth* tablets may be crushed.
- **PRESCRIBING AND DISPENSING INFORMATION** A mixture of diphenoxylate hydrochloride and atropine sulfate in the mass proportions 100 parts to 1 part respectively.
- **EXCEPTIONS TO LEGAL CATEGORY** Co-phenotrope 2.5/0.025 can be sold to the public for adults and children over 16 years (provided packs do not contain more than 20 tablets) as an adjunct to rehydration in acute diarrhoea (max. daily dose 10 tablets).

- **MEDICINAL FORMS**
There can be variation in the licensing of different medicines containing the same drug.

Tablet
- ‣ Co-phenotrope (Non-proprietary)
Atropine sulfate 25 microgram, Diphenoxylate hydrochloride 2.5 mg Lomotil 2.5mg/25microgram tablets | 100 tablet [PoM] Ⓢ [CD5]
Lofenoxal 2.5mg/25microgram tablets | 20 tablet [PoM] Ⓢ [CD5]

⌖ 441

Kaolin with morphine

- **INDICATIONS AND DOSE**

Acute diarrhoea

▸ BY MOUTH
- ‣ Adult: 10 mL every 6 hours, dose to be given in water

- **CONTRA-INDICATIONS** Acute abdomen · delayed gastric emptying · heart failure secondary to chronic lung disease · phaeochromocytoma
- **CAUTIONS** Cardiac arrhythmias · pancreatitis · severe cor pulmonale
- **INTERACTIONS** → Appendix 1: kaolin · opioids
- **SIDE-EFFECTS** Constipation · drowsiness · dry mouth · flushing · hyperhidrosis · miosis · nausea · vomiting
- **BREAST FEEDING** Therapeutic doses unlikely to affect infant.
- **RENAL IMPAIRMENT** Avoid use or reduce dose; opioid effects increased and prolonged, and increased cerebral sensitivity occurs.
- **PRESCRIBING AND DISPENSING INFORMATION** When prepared extemporaneously, the BP states Kaolin and Morphine Mixture, BP consists of light kaolin or light kaolin (natural) 20%, sodium bicarbonate 5%, and chloroform and morphine tincture 4% in a suitable vehicle. Contains anhydrous morphine 550–800 micrograms/10 mL.
- **LESS SUITABLE FOR PRESCRIBING** Kaolin and Morphine Mixture, BP (Kaolin and Morphine Oral Suspension) is less suitable for prescribing.

- **MEDICINAL FORMS**
There can be variation in the licensing of different medicines containing the same drug.

Oral suspension
- ‣ Kaolin with morphine (Non-proprietary)
Morphine hydrochloride 91.6 mg per 1 litre, Sodium bicarbonate 50 gram per 1 litre, Kaolin light 200 gram per 1 litre, Chloroform 5 ml per 1 litre Kaolin and Morphine mixture | 200 ml Ⓟ £1.71 DT = £1.71 [CD5]

Loperamide hydrochloride

11-Oct-2017

- **INDICATIONS AND DOSE**

Symptomatic treatment of acute diarrhoea

▸ BY MOUTH
- ‣ Child 4–7 years: 1 mg 3–4 times a day for up to 3 days only
- ‣ Child 8–11 years: 2 mg 4 times a day for up to 5 days
- ‣ Child 12–17 years: Initially 4 mg, followed by 2 mg for up to 5 days, dose to be taken after each loose stool; usual dose 6–8 mg daily; maximum 16 mg per day
- ‣ Adult: Initially 4 mg, followed by 2 mg for up to 5 days, dose to be taken after each loose stool; usual dose 6–8 mg daily; maximum 16 mg per day

Chronic diarrhoea
▶ BY MOUTH
▶ Adult: Initially 4–8 mg daily in divided doses, adjusted according to response; maintenance up to 16 mg daily in 2 divided doses

Faecal incontinence
▶ BY MOUTH
▶ Adult: Initially 500 micrograms daily, adjusted according to response, maximum daily dose to be given in divided doses; maximum 16 mg per day

Pain of bowel colic in palliative care
▶ BY MOUTH
▶ Adult: 2–4 mg 4 times a day

● UNLICENSED USE *Capsules* not licensed for use in children under 8 years.
▶ In adults Use for faecal incontinence is an unlicensed indication.

IMPORTANT SAFETY INFORMATION
MHRA/CHM ADVICE: REPORTS OF SERIOUS CARDIAC ADVERSE REACTIONS WITH HIGH DOSES OF LOPERAMIDE ASSOCIATED WITH ABUSE OR MISUSE (SEPTEMBER 2017)
Serious cardiovascular events (such as QT prolongation, torsades de pointes, and cardiac arrest), including fatalities, have been reported in association with large overdoses of loperamide.
  Healthcare professionals are reminded that if symptoms of overdose occur, naloxone can be given as an antidote. The duration of action of loperamide is longer than that of naloxone (1–3 hours), so repeated treatment with naloxone might be indicated; patients should be monitored closely for at least 48 hours to detect possible CNS depression.
  Pharmacists should remind patients not to take more than the recommended dose on the label.

● CONTRA-INDICATIONS Active ulcerative colitis · antibiotic-associated colitis · conditions where abdominal distension develops · conditions where inhibition of peristalsis should be avoided
● CAUTIONS Not recommended for children under 12 years
● INTERACTIONS → Appendix 1: loperamide
● SIDE-EFFECTS
▶ Common or very common Gastrointestinal disorders · headache · nausea
▶ Uncommon Dizziness · drowsiness · dry mouth · gastrointestinal discomfort · skin reactions · vomiting
▶ Rare or very rare Angioedema · consciousness impaired · coordination abnormal · fatigue · miosis · muscle tone increased · severe cutaneous adverse reactions (SCARs) · urinary retention
● PREGNANCY Manufacturers advise avoid—no information available.
● BREAST FEEDING Amount probably too small to be harmful.
● HEPATIC IMPAIRMENT Risk of accumulation—manufacturer advises caution.
● PRESCRIBING AND DISPENSING INFORMATION
Palliative care For further information on the use of loperamide in palliative care, see www.palliativedrugs.com/formulary/en/loperamide.html.
● PATIENT AND CARER ADVICE
Medicines for Children leaflet: Loperamide for diarrhoea www.medicinesforchildren.org.uk/loperamide-for-diarrhoea
● EXCEPTIONS TO LEGAL CATEGORY Loperamide can be sold to the public, for use in adults and children over 12 years, provided it is licensed and labelled for the treatment of acute diarrhoea.

▶ In adults Loperamide can be sold to the public, provided it is licensed and labelled for the treatment of acute diarrhoea associated with irritable bowel syndrome (after initial diagnosis by a doctor) in adults over 18 years of age.

● MEDICINAL FORMS
There can be variation in the licensing of different medicines containing the same drug. Forms available from special-order manufacturers include: oral suspension, oral solution

Tablet
▶ Loperamide hydrochloride (Non-proprietary)
  Loperamide hydrochloride 2 mg Loperamide 2mg tablets | 30 tablet [PoM] £2.93 DT = £2.93
▶ Norimode (Tillomed Laboratories Ltd)
  Loperamide hydrochloride 2 mg Norimode 2mg tablets | 30 tablet [PoM] £2.15 DT = £2.93

Oral solution
▶ Imodium (Janssen-Cilag Ltd)
  Loperamide hydrochloride 200 microgram per 1 ml Imodium 1mg/5ml oral solution sugar-free | 100 ml [PoM] £1.17 DT = £1.17

Capsule
▶ Loperamide hydrochloride (Non-proprietary)
  Loperamide hydrochloride 2 mg Loperamide 2mg capsules | 30 capsule [PoM] £2.99 DT = £0.68

Orodispersible tablet
▶ Imodium (McNeil Products Ltd)
  Loperamide hydrochloride 2 mg Imodium Instant Melts 2mg orodispersible tablets sugar-free | 12 tablet [P] £4.38 sugar-free | 18 tablet [P] £5.85 DT = £5.39

Loperamide with simeticone

The properties listed below are those particular to the combination only. For the properties of the components please consider, loperamide hydrochloride p. 66, simeticone p. 71.

● INDICATIONS AND DOSE

Acute diarrhoea with abdominal colic
▶ BY MOUTH
▶ Child 12-17 years: Initially 1 tablet, then 1 tablet, after each loose stool, for up to 2 days; maximum 4 tablets per day
▶ Adult: Initially 2 tablets, then 1 tablet, after each loose stool, for up to 2 days; maximum 4 tablets per day

● INTERACTIONS → Appendix 1: loperamide

● MEDICINAL FORMS
There can be variation in the licensing of different medicines containing the same drug.

Tablet
▶ Imodium Plus (McNeil Products Ltd)
  Loperamide hydrochloride 2 mg, Dimeticone (as Simeticone) 125 mg Imodium Plus caplets | 12 tablet [P] £4.21

ANTIDIARRHOEALS > ENKEPHALINASE INHIBITORS

Racecadotril
11-Feb-2016

● INDICATIONS AND DOSE

Adjunct to rehydration, for the symptomatic treatment of uncomplicated acute diarrhoea
▶ BY MOUTH USING CAPSULES
▶ Adult: Initially 100 mg, then 100 mg 3 times a day until diarrhoea stops; maximum duration of treatment 7 days, dose to be taken preferably before food
▶ BY MOUTH USING GRANULES
▶ Child 3 months-17 years (body-weight up to 9 kg): 10 mg 3 times a day until diarrhoea stops; maximum duration of treatment 7 days

continued →

▸ Child 3 months-17 years (body-weight 9-12 kg): 20 mg
3 times a day until diarrhoea stops; maximum duration
of treatment 7 days
▸ Child 3 months-17 years (body-weight 13-27 kg): 30 mg
3 times a day until diarrhoea stops; maximum duration
of treatment 7 days
▸ Child 3 months-17 years (body-weight 28 kg and
above): 60 mg 3 times a day until diarrhoea stops;
maximum duration of treatment 7 days

● CONTRA-INDICATIONS Antibiotic-associated diarrhoea
● SIDE-EFFECTS
▸ **Uncommon** Skin reactions · tonsillitis
▸ **Frequency not known** Angioedema · erythema nodosum ·
eyelid oedema · face oedema · oral disorders
  SIDE-EFFECTS, FURTHER INFORMATION Severe skin
  reactions have been reported—discontinue treatment
  immediately.
● PREGNANCY Manufacturer advises avoid—no information
available.
● BREAST FEEDING Manufacturer advises avoid—no
information available.
● HEPATIC IMPAIRMENT
▸ In adults Manufacturer advises caution.
▸ In children Manufacturer advises avoid.
● RENAL IMPAIRMENT
▸ In adults Manufacturer advises caution.
▸ In children Manufacturer advises avoid.
● DIRECTIONS FOR ADMINISTRATION Granules may be added
to food or mixed with water or bottle feeds and then taken
immediately.
● PATIENT AND CARER ADVICE Patients and carers should be
given advice on how to administer racecadotril granules.
● NATIONAL FUNDING/ACCESS DECISIONS
  Scottish Medicines Consortium (SMC) Decisions
  The *Scottish Medicines Consortium*, has advised (July 2014)
  that racecadotril (*Hidrasec* ®) is **not** recommended for use
  within NHS Scotland for the treatment of acute diarrhoea
  in children because there is insufficient evidence that it
  improves the recovery rate.

● MEDICINAL FORMS
  There can be variation in the licensing of different medicines
  containing the same drug.
  Granules
  EXCIPIENTS: May contain Sucrose
▸ Hidrasec (Lincoln Medical Ltd)
  Racecadotril 10 mg Hidrasec Infants 10mg granules sachets |
  20 sachet PoM £8.42
  Racecadotril 30 mg Hidrasec Children 30mg granules sachets |
  20 sachet PoM £8.42

ANTIDIARRHOEALS > INTESTINAL ADSORBENTS

Kaolin

● INDICATIONS AND DOSE
Diarrhoea (not recommended for acute diarrhoea)
▸ BY MOUTH
▸ Adult: 10–20 mL every 4 hours

● INTERACTIONS → Appendix 1: kaolin
● DIRECTIONS FOR ADMINISTRATION Warm and apply
poultice directly or between layers of muslin; avoid
application of overheated poultice.
● PRESCRIBING AND DISPENSING INFORMATION Flavours of
oral liquid formulations may include peppermint.
  When prepared extemporaneously, the BP states Kaolin
  Mixture, BP consists of light kaolin or light kaolin (natural)
  20%, light magnesium carbonate 5%, sodium bicarbonate
  5% in a suitable vehicle with a peppermint flavour.

● LESS SUITABLE FOR PRESCRIBING Kaolin Mixture BP is less
suitable for prescribing.

● MEDICINAL FORMS
  No licensed medicines listed.

  Combinations available: *Kaolin with morphine,* p. 66

4 Disorders of gastric acid and ulceration

4.1 Dyspepsia

Dyspepsia

Overview

Dyspepsia covers upper abdominal pain, fullness, early
satiety, bloating, and nausea. It can occur with gastric and
duodenal ulceration and, gastric cancer, but most commonly
it is of uncertain origin.

Urgent endoscopic investigation is required if dyspepsia is
accompanied by 'alarm features' (e.g. bleeding, dysphagia,
recurrent vomiting, or weight loss). Urgent investigation
should also be considered for patients over 55 years with
unexplained, recent-onset dyspepsia that has not responded
to treatment.

Patients with dyspepsia should be advised about lifestyle
changes (avoidance of excess alcohol and of aggravating
foods such as fats); other measures include weight reduction,
smoking cessation, and raising the head of the bed. Some
medications may cause dyspepsia—these should be stopped,
if possible.

Antacids may provide some symptomatic relief, however if
symptoms persist in *uninvestigated dyspepsia*, treatment
involves a **proton pump inhibitor** for up to 4 weeks. A
proton pump inhibitor can be used intermittently to control
symptoms long term. Patients with uninvestigated
dyspepsia, who do not respond to an initial trial with a
proton pump inhibitor, should be tested for *Helicobacter
pylori* and given eradication therapy if *H. pylori* is present.
Alternatively, particularly in populations where *H. pylori*
infection is more likely, the 'test and treat' strategy for *H.
pylori* can be used before a trial with a proton pump
inhibitor.

If *H. pylori* is present in patients with *functional
(investigated, non-ulcer) dyspepsia*, eradication therapy
should be provided. If symptoms persist, treatment with
either a **proton pump inhibitor** or a **histamine H$_2$-
receptor antagonist** can be given for 4 weeks. These
antisecretory drugs can be used intermittently to control
symptoms long term. However, most patients with
functional dyspepsia do not benefit symptomatically from *H.
pylori* eradication therapy or antisecretory drugs.

ANTACIDS

Antacids

Overview

Antacids (usually containing aluminium or magnesium
compounds) can often relieve symptoms in *ulcer dyspepsia*
and in *non-erosive gastro-oesophageal reflux* ; they are also
sometimes used in functional (non-ulcer) dyspepsia but the
evidence of benefit is uncertain. Antacids are best given
when symptoms occur or are expected, usually between
meals and at bedtime, although additional doses may be
required. Conventional doses of liquid magnesium–
aluminium antacids promote ulcer healing, but less well
than antisecretory drugs; proof of a relationship between

healing and neutralising capacity is lacking. Liquid preparations are more effective than tablet preparations.

Aluminium- and **magnesium-containing** antacids (e.g. aluminium hydroxide p. 1020, magnesium carbonate p. 70, co-magaldrox p. 70 and magnesium trisilicate p. 71), being relatively insoluble in water, are long-acting if retained in the stomach. They are suitable for most antacid purposes. Magnesium-containing antacids tend to be laxative whereas aluminium-containing antacids may be constipating; antacids containing both magnesium and aluminium may reduce these colonic side-effects. Aluminium accumulation does not appear to be a risk if renal function is normal.

The acid-neutralising capacity of preparations that contain more than one antacid may be the same as simpler preparations. Complexes such as **hydrotalcite** confer no special advantage.

Sodium bicarbonate p. 1006 should no longer be prescribed alone for the relief of dyspepsia but it is present as an ingredient in many indigestion remedies. However, it retains a place in the management of urinary-tract disorders and acidosis.

Bismuth-containing antacids (unless chelates) are not recommended because absorbed bismuth can be neurotoxic, causing encephalopathy; they tend to be constipating. **Calcium-containing** antacids can induce rebound acid secretion: with modest doses the clinical significance is doubtful, but prolonged high doses also cause hypercalcaemia and alkalosis, and can precipitate the milk-alkali syndrome.

Simeticone

Simeticone (activated dimeticone) p. 71 is added to an antacid as an antifoaming agent to relieve flatulence. These preparations may be useful for the relief of hiccup in palliative care.

Alginates

Alginates taken in combination with an antacid increases the viscosity of stomach contents and can protect the oesophageal mucosa from acid reflux. Some alginate-containing preparations form a viscous gel ('raft') that floats on the surface of the stomach contents, thereby reducing symptoms of reflux.

The amount of additional ingredient or antacid in individual preparations varies widely, as does their sodium content, so that preparations may not be freely interchangeable.

ANTACIDS > ALGINATE

Alginic acid

● **INDICATIONS AND DOSE**

GAVISCON INFANT ® POWDER SACHETS

Management of gastro-oesophageal reflux disease
▸ BY MOUTH
▸ Child 1–23 months (body-weight up to 4.5 kg): 1 dose as required, to be mixed with feeds (or water, for breast-fed infants); maximum 6 doses per day
▸ Child 1–23 months (body-weight 4.5 kg and above): 2 doses as required, to be mixed with feeds (or water, for breast-fed infants); maximum 12 doses per day

● **CONTRA-INDICATIONS** Intestinal obstruction · preterm neonates · where excessive water loss likely (e.g. fever, diarrhoea, vomiting, high room temperature)
GAVISCON INFANT ® POWDER SACHETS Concurrent use of preparations containing thickening agents

● **HEPATIC IMPAIRMENT** In patients with fluid retention, avoid antacids containing large amounts of sodium. Avoid

antacids containing magnesium salts in hepatic coma if there is a risk of renal failure.

● **RENAL IMPAIRMENT** In patients with fluid retention, avoid antacids containing large amounts of sodium.

● **PRESCRIBING AND DISPENSING INFORMATION** Each half of the dual-sachet is identified as 'one dose'.
To avoid errors prescribe with directions in terms of 'dose'.

● **MEDICINAL FORMS**
There can be variation in the licensing of different medicines containing the same drug.
Powder
ELECTROLYTES: May contain Sodium
▸ Gaviscon Infant (Forum Health Products Ltd)
Magnesium alginate 87.5 mg, Sodium alginate 225 mg Gaviscon Infant oral powder sachets sugar-free | 15 dual dose sachet ℗ £4.82 DT = £4.82

Sodium alginate with potassium bicarbonate

The properties listed below are those particular to the combination only. For the properties of the components please consider, alginic acid above.

● **INDICATIONS AND DOSE**

Management of mild symptoms of dyspepsia and gastro-oesophageal reflux disease
▸ BY MOUTH USING CHEWABLE TABLETS
▸ Child 6–11 years (under medical advice only): 1 tablet, to be chewed after meals and at bedtime
▸ Child 12–17 years: 1–2 tablets, to be chewed after meals and at bedtime
▸ Adult: 1–2 tablets, to be chewed after meals and at bedtime
▸ BY MOUTH USING ORAL SUSPENSION
▸ Child 2–11 years (under medical advice only): 2.5–5 mL, to be taken after meals and at bedtime
▸ Child 12–17 years: 5–10 mL, to be taken after meals and at bedtime
▸ Adult: 5–10 mL, to be taken after meals and at bedtime

● **PRESCRIBING AND DISPENSING INFORMATION** Flavours of oral liquid formulations may include aniseed or peppermint.

● **MEDICINAL FORMS**
There can be variation in the licensing of different medicines containing the same drug.
Oral suspension
ELECTROLYTES: May contain Potassium, sodium
▸ Acidex Advance (Pinewood Healthcare)
Potassium bicarbonate 20 mg per 1 ml, Sodium alginate 100 mg per 1 ml Acidex Advance oral suspension peppermint sugar-free | 250 ml ℗ £2.05 sugar-free | 500 ml ℗ £4.10 DT = £5.12
Acidex Advance oral suspension aniseed sugar-free | 250 ml ℗ £2.05 sugar-free | 500 ml ℗ £4.10 DT = £5.12
▸ Gaviscon Advance (Reckitt Benckiser Healthcare (UK) Ltd)
Potassium bicarbonate 20 mg per 1 ml, Sodium alginate 100 mg per 1 ml Gaviscon Advance oral suspension aniseed sugar-free | 150 ml ℗ £3.23 sugar-free | 250 ml ℗ £2.56 sugar-free | 300 ml ℗ £5.82 sugar-free | 500 ml ℗ £5.12 DT = £5.12
Gaviscon Advance oral suspension peppermint sugar-free | 250 ml ℗ £2.56 sugar-free | 300 ml ℗ £5.82 sugar-free | 500 ml ℗ £5.12 DT = £5.12
Chewable tablet
EXCIPIENTS: May contain Aspartame
ELECTROLYTES: May contain Potassium, sodium
▸ Sodium alginate with potassium bicarbonate (Non-proprietary)
Potassium bicarbonate 100 mg, Sodium alginate 500 mg Sodium alginate 500mg / Potassium bicarbonate 100mg chewable tablets sugar free sugar-free | 60 tablet GSL ⊠ DT = £3.07
▸ Brands may include Gaviscon Advance

Gastro-intestinal system

1

ANTACIDS > ALUMINIUM AND MAGNESIUM

Co-magaldrox

The properties listed below are those particular to the combination only. For the properties of the components please consider, aluminium hydroxide p. 1020, magnesium hydroxide p. 58.

● **INDICATIONS AND DOSE**

MAALOX ®

Dyspepsia
▶ BY MOUTH
▶ Child 14-17 years: 10–20 mL, to be taken 20–60 minutes after meals, and at bedtime or when required
▶ Adult: 10–20 mL, to be taken 20–60 minutes after meals, and at bedtime or when required

MUCOGEL ®

Dyspepsia
▶ BY MOUTH
▶ Child 12-17 years: 10–20 mL 3 times a day, to be taken 20–60 minutes after meals, and at bedtime, or when required
▶ Adult: 10–20 mL 3 times a day, to be taken 20–60 minutes after meals, and at bedtime, or when required

● INTERACTIONS → Appendix 1: antacids · magnesium
● PRESCRIBING AND DISPENSING INFORMATION Co-magaldrox is a mixture of aluminium hydroxide and magnesium hydroxide; the proportions are expressed in the form x/y where x and y are the strengths in milligrams per unit dose of magnesium hydroxide and aluminium hydroxide respectively.

MAALOX ® Maalox ® suspension is low in sodium.
MUCOGEL ® Mucogel ® suspension is low in sodium.

● MEDICINAL FORMS
There can be variation in the licensing of different medicines containing the same drug.
Oral suspension
▶ Maalox (Sanofi)
Aluminium hydroxide 35 mg per 1 ml, Magnesium hydroxide 40 mg per 1 ml Maalox 175mg/200mg/5ml oral suspension sugar-free | 250 ml GSL £2.33 DT = £2.33
▶ Mucogel (Chemidex Pharma Ltd)
Magnesium hydroxide 39 mg per 1 ml, Aluminium hydroxide gel dried 44 mg per 1 ml Mucogel oral suspension sugar-free | 500 ml GSL £2.99 DT = £2.99

Co-simalcite

● **INDICATIONS AND DOSE**
Dyspepsia
▶ BY MOUTH
▶ Child 8-11 years: 5 mL 4 times a day as required, to be taken between meals and at bedtime
▶ Child 12-17 years: 10 mL 4 times a day as required, to be taken between meals and at bedtime
▶ Adult: 10 mL 4 times a day as required, to be taken between meals and at bedtime

● CONTRA-INDICATIONS Hypophosphataemia · infants · neonates
CONTRA-INDICATIONS, FURTHER INFORMATION
▶ Aluminium-containing antacids Aluminium-containing antacids should not be used in neonates and infants because accumulation may lead to increased plasma-aluminium concentrations.

● HEPATIC IMPAIRMENT Avoid; can cause constipation which can precipitate coma. Avoid in hepatic coma; risk of renal failure.
● RENAL IMPAIRMENT
Dose adjustments Antacids containing magnesium salts should be avoided or used at a reduced dose because there is an increased risk of toxicity.
▶ In adults There is a risk of accumulation and aluminium toxicity with antacids containing aluminium salts. Absorption of aluminium from aluminium salts is increased by citrates, which are contained in many effervescent preparations (such as effervescent analgesics).
▶ In children Aluminium-containing antacids should not be used in children with renal impairment, because accumulation may lead to increased plasma-aluminium concentrations.
● PRESCRIBING AND DISPENSING INFORMATION Altacite Plus ® is low in Na+.

● MEDICINAL FORMS
There can be variation in the licensing of different medicines containing the same drug.
Oral suspension
▶ Altacite Plus (Peckforton Pharmaceuticals Ltd)
Simeticone 25 mg per 1 ml, Hydrotalcite 100 mg per 1 ml Altacite Plus oral suspension sugar-free | 100 ml P £4.00 sugar-free | 500 ml P £5.20 DT = £5.20

Simeticone with aluminium hydroxide and magnesium hydroxide

The properties listed below are those particular to the combination only. For the properties of the components please consider, simeticone p. 71, aluminium hydroxide p. 1020.

● **INDICATIONS AND DOSE**
Dyspepsia
▶ BY MOUTH
▶ Child 12-17 years: 5–10 mL 4 times a day, to be taken after meals and at bedtime, or when required
▶ Adult: 5–10 mL 4 times a day, to be taken after meals and at bedtime, or when required

● INTERACTIONS → Appendix 1: antacids

● MEDICINAL FORMS
There can be variation in the licensing of different medicines containing the same drug.
Oral suspension
▶ Maalox Plus (Sanofi)
Simeticone 5 mg per 1 ml, Magnesium hydroxide 39 mg per 1 ml, Aluminium hydroxide gel dried 44 mg per 1 ml Maalox Plus oral suspension sugar-free | 250 ml GSL £2.91

ANTACIDS > MAGNESIUM

Magnesium carbonate

● **INDICATIONS AND DOSE**
Dyspepsia
▶ BY MOUTH USING ORAL SUSPENSION
▶ Adult: 10 mL 3 times a day, dose to be taken in water

● CONTRA-INDICATIONS Hypophosphataemia
● INTERACTIONS → Appendix 1: antacids
● SIDE-EFFECTS Diarrhoea
● HEPATIC IMPAIRMENT In patients with fluid retention, avoid antacids containing large amounts of sodium. Avoid antacids containing magnesium salts in hepatic coma if there is a risk of renal failure.

- RENAL IMPAIRMENT Magnesium carbonate mixture has a high sodium content; avoid in patients with fluid retention.
  Dose adjustments Avoid or use at a reduced dose; increased risk of toxicity.
- PRESCRIBING AND DISPENSING INFORMATION When prepared extemporaneously, the BP states Aromatic Magnesium Carbonate Mixture, BP consists of light magnesium carbonate 3%, sodium bicarbonate 5%, in a suitable vehicle containing aromatic cardamom tincture.
- MEDICINAL FORMS
  No licensed medicines listed.

Magnesium trisilicate

- INDICATIONS AND DOSE
Dyspepsia
- BY MOUTH USING CHEWABLE TABLETS
- Adult: 1–2 tablets as required

- CONTRA-INDICATIONS Hypophosphataemia
- INTERACTIONS → Appendix 1: antacids
- SIDE-EFFECTS Diarrhoea · nephrolithiasis (long term use)
- HEPATIC IMPAIRMENT Avoid in hepatic coma; risk of renal failure.
- RENAL IMPAIRMENT
  Dose adjustments Avoid or used at a reduced dose (increased risk of toxicity).
- MEDICINAL FORMS
  No licensed medicines listed.

Magnesium trisilicate with magnesium carbonate and sodium bicarbonate

The properties listed below are those particular to the combination only. For the properties of the components please consider, magnesium trisilicate above, magnesium carbonate p. 70, sodium bicarbonate p. 1006.

- INDICATIONS AND DOSE
Dyspepsia
- BY MOUTH
- Child 5–11 years: 5–10 mL 3 times a day, alternatively as required, dose to be made up with water
- Child 12–17 years: 10–20 mL 3 times a day, alternatively as required, dose to be made up with water
- Adult: 10–20 mL 3 times a day, alternatively as required, dose to be made up with water

- CONTRA-INDICATIONS Hypophosphataemia · Severe renal failure
- CAUTIONS Heart failure · hypermagnesaemia · hypertension · metabolic alkalosis · respiratory alkalosis
- INTERACTIONS → Appendix 1: antacids · sodium bicarbonate
- HEPATIC IMPAIRMENT In patients with fluid retention avoid antacids containing large amounts of sodium. Avoid antacids containing magnesium salts in hepatic coma if there is a risk of renal failure.
- RENAL IMPAIRMENT Magnesium trisilicate and magnesium carbonate mixtures have high sodium content; avoid in patients with fluid retention.
- PRESCRIBING AND DISPENSING INFORMATION When prepared extemporaneously, the BP states Magnesium Trisilicate Mixture, BP consists of 5% each of magnesium trisilicate, light magnesium carbonate, and sodium bicarbonate in a suitable vehicle with a peppermint flavour.

- MEDICINAL FORMS
  There can be variation in the licensing of different medicines containing the same drug.
  Oral suspension
  - Magnesium trisilicate with magnesium carbonate and sodium bicarbonate (Non-proprietary)
    Magnesium carbonate light 50 mg per 1 ml, Magnesium trisilicate 50 mg per 1 ml, Sodium bicarbonate 50 mg per 1 ml Magnesium trisilicate oral suspension | 200 ml GSL £1.65 DT = £1.65

ANTIFOAMING DRUGS

Simeticone

(Activated dimeticone)

- DRUG ACTION Simeticone (activated dimeticone) is an antifoaming agent.

- INDICATIONS AND DOSE
DENTINOX ®
Colic | Wind pains
- BY MOUTH
- Child 1 month–1 year: 2.5 mL, to be taken with or after each feed; may be added to bottle feed; maximum 6 doses per day
INFACOL ®
Colic | Wind pains
- BY MOUTH
- Child 1 month–1 year: 0.5–1 mL, to be taken before feeds

- PRESCRIBING AND DISPENSING INFORMATION
  DENTINOX ® The brand name *Dentinox*® is also used for other preparations including teething gel.
- PATIENT AND CARER ADVICE
  INFACOL ® Patients or carers should be given advice on use of the *Infacol*® dropper.
- LESS SUITABLE FOR PRESCRIBING
  INFACOL ® *Infacol*® is less suitable for prescribing (evidence of benefit in infantile colic uncertain).
  DENTINOX ® *Dentinox*® colic drops are less suitable for prescribing (evidence of benefit in infantile colic uncertain).

- MEDICINAL FORMS
  There can be variation in the licensing of different medicines containing the same drug.
  Oral suspension
  - Infacol (Teva UK Ltd)
    Simeticone 40 mg per 1 ml Infacol 40mg/ml oral suspension sugar-free | 50 ml GSL £2.71 DT = £2.71
  Oral drops
  - Dentinox Infant (Dendron Ltd)
    Simeticone 8.4 mg per 1 ml Dentinox Infant colic drops | 100 ml GSL £1.80 DT = £1.80

Combinations available: *Co-simalcite,* p. 70 · *Simeticone with aluminium hydroxide and magnesium hydroxide,* p. 70

4.2 Gastric and duodenal ulceration

Peptic ulceration

Overview

Peptic ulceration commonly involves the stomach, duodenum, and lower oesophagus; after gastric surgery it involves the gastro-enterostomy stoma. Healing can be promoted by general measures, stopping smoking and taking antacids and by antisecretory drug treatment, but relapse is

Recommended regimens for *Helicobacter pylori* eradication in adults

Acid suppressant	Antibacterial			Price for 7-day course
	Amoxicillin	Clarithromycin	Metronidazole	
Esomeprazole 20 mg twice daily	1 g twice daily	500 mg twice daily	–	£6.63
	–	250 mg twice daily	400 mg twice daily	£4.30
Lansoprazole 30 mg twice daily	1 g twice daily	500 mg twice daily	–	£5.52
	1 g twice daily	–	400 mg twice daily	£3.70
	–	250 mg twice daily	400 mg twice daily	£3.19
Omeprazole 20 mg twice daily	1 g twice daily	500 mg twice daily	–	£5.36
	500 mg 3 times a day	–	400 mg 3 times a day	£3.40
	–	250 mg twice daily	400 mg twice daily	£3.03
Pantoprazole 40 mg twice daily	1 g twice daily	500 mg twice daily	–	£5.48
	–	250 mg twice daily	400 mg twice daily	£3.15
Rabeprazole sodium 20 mg twice daily	1 g twice daily	500 mg twice daily	–	£6.04
	–	250 mg twice daily	400 mg twice daily	£3.71

common when treatment ceases. Nearly all duodenal ulcers and most gastric ulcers not associated with NSAIDs are caused by *Helicobacter pylori*.

Helicobacter pylori infection

Eradication of *Helicobacter pylori* reduces recurrence of gastric and duodenal ulcers and the risk of rebleeding. It also causes regression of most localised gastric mucosa associated lymphoid-tissue (MALT) lymphomas. The presence of *H. pylori* should be confirmed before starting eradication treatment. Acid inhibition combined with antibacterial treatment is highly effective in the eradication of *H. pylori*; reinfection is rare. Antibiotic associated colitis is an uncommon risk.

For initial treatment, a one-week triple-therapy regimen that comprises a proton pump inhibitor, clarithromycin p. 529, and *either* amoxicillin p. 539 *or* metronidazole p. 533 can be used. However, if a patient has been treated with metronidazole for other infections, a regimen containing a proton pump inhibitor, amoxicillin and clarithromycin is preferred for initial therapy. If a patient has been treated with a macrolide for other infections, a regimen containing a proton pump inhibitor, amoxicillin and metronidazole is preferred for initial therapy. These regimens eradicate *H. pylori* in about 85% of cases. There is usually no need to continue antisecretory treatment (with a proton pump inhibitor or H_2-receptor antagonist), however, if the ulcer is large, or complicated by haemorrhage or perforation, then antisecretory treatment is continued for a further 3 weeks. Treatment failure usually indicates antibacterial resistance or poor compliance. Resistance to amoxicillin is rare. However, resistance to clarithromycin and metronidazole is common and can develop during treatment.

Two-week triple-therapy regimens offer the possibility of higher eradication rates compared to one-week regimens, but adverse effects are common and poor compliance is likely to offset any possible gain.

Two-week dual-therapy regimens using a proton pump inhibitor and a single antibacterial are licensed, but produce low rates of *H. pylori* eradication and are **not** recommended.

Tinidazole p. 534 is also used occasionally for *H. pylori* eradication as an alternative to metronidazole; tinidazole should be combined with antisecretory drugs and other antibacterials.

Routine retesting, to confirm eradication, is not necessary unless the patient has gastric MALT lymphoma or complicated *H. pylori* associated peptic ulcer.

A two-week regimen comprising a proton pump inhibitor *plus* tripotassium dicitratobismuthate, *plus* tetracycline p. 557, *plus* metronidazole can be used for eradication failure. Alternatively, the patient can be referred for endoscopy and treatment based on the results of culture and sensitivity testing.

See under *NSAID-associated ulcers* for the role of *H. pylori* eradication therapy in patients starting or taking a NSAID. Also see Dyspepsia p. 68 for *H. pylori* eradication in patients with dyspepsia.

Test for *Helicobacter pylori*

^{13}C-Urea breath test kits are available for the diagnosis of gastro-duodenal infection with *Helicobacter pylori*. The test involves collection of breath samples before and after ingestion of an oral solution of ^{13}C-urea; the samples are sent for analysis by an appropriate laboratory. The test should not be performed within 4 weeks of treatment with an antibacterial or within 2 weeks of treatment with an antisecretory drug. A specific ^{13}C-urea breath test kit for children is available (*Helicobacter Test INFAI for children of the age* 3–11 ®). However, the appropriateness of testing for *H. pylori* infection in children has not been established.

NSAID-associated ulcers

Gastro-intestinal bleeding and ulceration can occur with NSAID use. The risk of serious upper gastro-intestinal side-effects varies between individual NSAIDs. Whenever possible, the NSAID should be **withdrawn** if an ulcer occurs.

Patients at high risk of developing gastro-intestinal complications with a NSAID include those aged over 65 years, those with a history of peptic ulcer disease or serious gastro-intestinal complication, those taking other medicines that increase the risk of gastro-intestinal side-effects, or those with serious co-morbidity (e.g. cardiovascular disease, diabetes, renal or hepatic impairment). In those at risk of ulceration, a proton pump inhibitor can be considered for protection against gastric and duodenal ulcers associated with non-selective NSAIDs; a H_2-receptor antagonist such as ranitidine p. 75 given at twice the usual dose or misoprostol p. 77 are alternatives. Colic and diarrhoea may limit the dose of misoprostol. Its use is most appropriate for the frail or very elderly from whom NSAIDs cannot be withdrawn. A combination of a cyclo-oxygenase-2 selective inhibitor with a proton pump inhibitor may be more appropriate for those with a history of upper gastro-intestinal bleeding or 3 or more risk factors for gastro-intestinal ulceration, but see NSAIDs and Cardiovascular Events.

NSAID use and *H. pylori* infection are independent risk factors for gastro-intestinal bleeding and ulceration. In patients already taking a NSAID, eradication of *H. pylori* is unlikely to reduce the risk of NSAID-induced bleeding or ulceration. However, in patients with dyspepsia or a history of gastric or duodenal ulcer, who are *H. pylori* positive, and who are about to start long-term treatment with a non-selective NSAID, eradication of *H. pylori* may reduce the overall risk of ulceration.

In a patient who has developed an ulcer, if the *NSAID can be discontinued*, a proton pump inhibitor usually produces the most rapid healing; alternatively, the ulcer can be treated with a H$_2$-receptor antagonist or misoprostol. On healing, patients should be tested for *H. pylori* and given eradication therapy if *H. pylori* is present (see also Test for *Helicobacter pylori*).

If *treatment with a non-selective NSAID needs to continue*, the following options are suitable:

- Treat ulcer with a proton pump inhibitor and on healing continue the proton pump inhibitor (dose does not normally reduced because asymptomatic ulcer recurrence may occur);
- Treat ulcer with a proton pump inhibitor and on healing switch to misoprostol for maintenance therapy (colic and diarrhoea may limit the dose of misoprostol);
- Treat ulcer with a proton pump inhibitor and switch non-selective NSAID to a cyclo-oxygenase-2 selective inhibitor, but see NSAIDs and Cardiovascular Events; on healing, continuation of the proton pump inhibitor in patients with a history of upper gastro-intestinal bleeding may provide further protection against recurrence.

If *treatment with a cyclo-oxygenase-2 selective inhibitor needs to continue,* treat ulcer with a proton pump inhibitor; on healing continuation of the proton pump inhibitor in patients with a history of upper gastro-intestinal bleeding may provide further protection against recurrence.

GASTROPROTECTIVE COMPLEXES AND CHELATORS

Chelates and complexes

Overview

Sucralfate below may act by protecting the mucosa from acid-pepsin attack in gastric and duodenal ulcers. It is a complex of aluminium hydroxide and sulfated sucrose but has minimal antacid properties.

Sucralfate

- **INDICATIONS AND DOSE**

Benign gastric ulceration | Benign duodenal ulceration
▸ BY MOUTH
▸ Child 15–17 years: 2 g twice daily, dose to be taken on rising and at bedtime, alternatively 1 g 4 times a day for 4–6 weeks, or in resistant cases up to 12 weeks, dose to be taken 1 hour before meals and at bedtime; maximum 8 g per day
▸ Adult: 2 g twice daily, dose to be taken on rising and at bedtime, alternatively 1 g 4 times a day for 4–6 weeks, or in resistant cases up to 12 weeks, dose to be taken 1 hour before meals and at bedtime; maximum 8 g per day

Chronic gastritis
▸ BY MOUTH
▸ Adult: 2 g twice daily, dose to be taken on rising and at bedtime, alternatively 1 g 4 times a day for 4–6 weeks, or in resistant cases up to 12 weeks, dose to be taken 1 hour before meals and at bedtime; maximum 8 g per day

Prophylaxis of stress ulceration in child under intensive care
▸ BY MOUTH
▸ Child 15–17 years: 1 g 6 times a day; maximum 8 g per day

Prophylaxis of stress ulceration
▸ BY MOUTH
▸ Adult: 1 g 6 times a day; maximum 8 g per day

- **CAUTIONS** Patients under intensive care (**Important:** reports of bezoar formation)

CAUTIONS, FURTHER INFORMATION
▸ Bezoar formation Following reports of bezoar formation associated with sucralfate, caution is advised in seriously ill patients, especially those receiving concomitant enteral feeds or those with predisposing conditions such as delayed gastric emptying.

- **INTERACTIONS** → Appendix 1: sucralfate

- **SIDE-EFFECTS**
▸ **Common or very common** Constipation
▸ **Uncommon** Dry mouth · nausea
▸ **Rare or very rare** Bezoar · rash
▸ **Frequency not known** Back pain · bone disorders · diarrhoea · dizziness · drowsiness · encephalopathy · flatulence · headache · vertigo

- **PREGNANCY** No evidence of harm; absorption from gastro-intestinal tract negligible.

- **BREAST FEEDING** Amount probably too small to be harmful.

- **RENAL IMPAIRMENT** Use with caution; aluminium is absorbed and may accumulate.

- **DIRECTIONS FOR ADMINISTRATION** Administration of sucralfate and enteral feeds should be separated by 1 hour and for administration by *mouth*, sucralfate should be given 1 hour before meals. *Oral suspension* blocks fine-bore feeding tubes. Crushed *tablets* may be dispersed in water.

- **PRESCRIBING AND DISPENSING INFORMATION** Flavours of oral liquid formulations may include aniseed and caramel.

- **MEDICINAL FORMS**
There can be variation in the licensing of different medicines containing the same drug. Forms available from special-order manufacturers include: tablet, oral suspension
Tablet
CAUTIONARY AND ADVISORY LABELS 5
▸ Sucralfate (Non-proprietary)
Sucralfate 1 gram Sulcrate 1g tablets | 100 tablet [ⓧ]
Carafate 1g tablets | 100 tablet [ⓧ]

H$_2$-RECEPTOR ANTAGONISTS

H$_2$-receptor antagonists

Overview

Histamine H$_2$-receptor antagonists heal *gastric and duodenal ulcers* by reducing gastric acid output as a result of histamine H$_2$-receptor blockade; they are also used to relieve symptoms of *gastro-oesophageal reflux disease*. H$_2$-receptor antagonists should not normally be used for *Zollinger-Ellison syndrome* because proton pump inhibitors are more effective.

Maintenance treatment with low doses for the prevention of peptic ulcer disease has largely been replaced in *Helicobacter pylori* positive patients by eradication regimens.

In adults, H$_2$-receptor antagonists are used for the treatment of *functional dyspepsia* and may be used for the treatment of *uninvestigated dyspepsia* without alarm features.

H$_2$-receptor antagonist therapy can promote healing of NSAID-associated ulcers (particularly duodenal).

Treatment with a H$_2$-receptor antagonist has not been shown to be beneficial in haematemesis and melaena, but prophylactic use reduces the frequency of bleeding from *gastroduodenal erosions in hepatic coma*, and possibly in other conditions requiring intensive care. H$_2$- receptor antagonists also reduce the risk of *acid aspiration* in obstetric patients at delivery (Mendelson's syndrome).

H₂-receptor antagonists

- CAUTIONS Signs and symptoms of gastric cancer (in adults)

  CAUTIONS, FURTHER INFORMATION
  ‣ Gastric cancer
  ‣ In adults H₂-receptor antagonists might mask symptoms of gastric cancer; particular care is required in patients presenting with 'alarm features' in such cases gastric malignancy should be ruled out before treatment.

- SIDE-EFFECTS
  ‣ **Common or very common** Constipation · diarrhoea · dizziness · fatigue · headache · myalgia · skin reactions
  ‣ **Uncommon** Confusion · depression · erectile dysfunction · gynaecomastia · hallucination · hepatic disorders · leucopenia · nausea · tachycardia
  ‣ **Rare or very rare** Agranulocytosis · alopecia · arthralgia · atrioventricular block · fever · galactorrhoea · pancytopenia · thrombocytopenia · vasculitis

  ◀ above

Cimetidine

- INDICATIONS AND DOSE

Benign duodenal ulceration
‣ BY MOUTH
  ‣ Adult: 400 mg twice daily for at least 4 weeks, to be taken with breakfast and at night, alternatively 800 mg once daily for at least 4 weeks, to be taken at night; increased if necessary up to 400 mg 4 times a day; maintenance 400 mg once daily, to be taken at night, alternatively maintenance 400 mg twice daily, to be taken in the morning and at night

Benign gastric ulceration
‣ BY MOUTH
  ‣ Adult: 400 mg twice daily for 6 weeks, to be taken with breakfast and at night, alternatively 800 mg daily for 6 weeks, to be taken at night; increased if necessary up to 400 mg 4 times a day; maintenance 400 mg once daily, to be taken at night, alternatively maintenance 400 mg twice daily, to be taken in the morning and at night

NSAID-associated ulceration
‣ BY MOUTH
  ‣ Adult: 400 mg twice daily for 8 weeks, to be taken with breakfast and at night, alternatively 800 mg daily for 8 weeks, to be taken at night; increased if necessary up to 400 mg 4 times a day; maintenance 400 mg daily, to be taken at night, alternatively maintenance 400 mg twice daily, to be taken in the morning and at night

Reflux oesophagitis
‣ BY MOUTH
  ‣ Adult: 400 mg 4 times a day for 4–8 weeks

Prophylaxis of stress ulceration
‣ BY MOUTH
  ‣ Adult: 200–400 mg every 4–6 hours

Gastric acid reduction in obstetrics
‣ BY MOUTH
  ‣ Adult: Initially 400 mg, to be administered at start of labour, then increased if necessary up to 400 mg every 4 hours, do not use syrup in prophylaxis of acid aspiration; maximum 2.4 g per day

Gastric acid reduction during surgical procedures
‣ BY MOUTH
  ‣ Adult: 400 mg, to be given 90–120 minutes before induction of general anaesthesia

Short-bowel syndrome
‣ BY MOUTH
  ‣ Adult: 400 mg twice daily, adjusted according to response, to be taken with breakfast and at bedtime

To reduce degradation of pancreatic enzyme supplements
‣ BY MOUTH
  ‣ Adult: 0.8–1.6 g daily in 4 divided doses, dose to be taken 1–1½ hours before meals

- INTERACTIONS → Appendix 1: H2 receptor antagonists
- SIDE-EFFECTS
  ‣ **Rare or very rare** Anaphylactic reaction · aplastic anaemia · hypersensitivity vasculitis · nephritis tubulointerstitial · pancreatitis · sinus bradycardia
- PREGNANCY Manufacturer advises avoid unless essential.
- BREAST FEEDING Significant amount present in milk—not known to be harmful but manufacturer advises avoid.
- HEPATIC IMPAIRMENT Increased risk of confusion. **Dose adjustments** Reduce dose.
- RENAL IMPAIRMENT Occasional risk of confusion. **Dose adjustments** Reduce dose to 200 mg 4 times daily if eGFR 30–50 mL/minute/1.73 m². Reduce dose to 200 mg 3 times daily if eGFR 15–30 mL/minute/1.73 m². Reduce dose to 200 mg twice daily if eGFR less than 15 mL/minute/1.73 m².
- EXCEPTIONS TO LEGAL CATEGORY Cimetidine can be sold to the public for adults and children over 16 years (provided packs do not contain more than 2 weeks' supply) for the short-term symptomatic relief of heartburn, dyspepsia, and hyperacidity (max. single dose 200 mg, max. daily dose 800 mg), and for the prophylactic management of nocturnal heartburn (single night-time dose 100 mg).

- MEDICINAL FORMS
  There can be variation in the licensing of different medicines containing the same drug. Forms available from special-order manufacturers include: oral suspension

Oral solution
EXCIPIENTS: May contain Propylene glycol
  ‣ Cimetidine (Non-proprietary)
    Cimetidine 40 mg per 1 ml Cimetidine 200mg/5ml oral solution sugar free sugar-free | 300 ml [PoM] £14.24–£14.25 DT = £14.25
  ‣ Tagamet (Essential Pharma Ltd)
    Cimetidine 40 mg per 1 ml Tagamet 200mg/5ml syrup | 600 ml [PoM] £28.49 DT = £28.49

Tablet
  ‣ Cimetidine (Non-proprietary)
    Cimetidine 200 mg Cimetidine 200mg tablets | 60 tablet £9.98–£45.59 | 120 tablet [PoM] £120.00
    Cimetidine 400 mg Cimetidine 400mg tablets | 60 tablet £120.00 DT = £16.37
    Cimetidine 800 mg Cimetidine 800mg tablets | 30 tablet [PoM] £15.31 DT = £15.31
  ‣ Tagamet (Chemidex Pharma Ltd)
    Cimetidine 400 mg Tagamet 400mg tablets | 60 tablet [PoM] £22.62 DT = £16.37
    Cimetidine 800 mg Tagamet 800mg tablets | 30 tablet [PoM] £22.62 DT = £15.31

  ◀ above

Famotidine

- INDICATIONS AND DOSE

Treatment of benign gastric and duodenal ulceration
‣ BY MOUTH
  ‣ Adult: 40 mg once daily for 4–8 weeks, dose to be taken at night

Maintenance treatment of duodenal ulceration
‣ BY MOUTH
  ‣ Adult: 20 mg once daily, dose to be taken at night

Reflux oesophagitis
‣ BY MOUTH
  ‣ Adult: 20–40 mg twice daily for 6–12 weeks; maintenance 20 mg twice daily

the most rapid healing; alternatively, the ulcer can be treated with a H$_2$-receptor antagonist or misoprostol. On healing, patients should be tested for *H. pylori* and given eradication therapy if *H. pylori* is present (see also Test for *Helicobacter pylori*).

If *treatment with a non-selective NSAID needs to continue*, the following options are suitable:

- Treat ulcer with a proton pump inhibitor and on healing continue the proton pump inhibitor (dose does not normally reduced because asymptomatic ulcer recurrence may occur);
- Treat ulcer with a proton pump inhibitor and on healing switch to misoprostol for maintenance therapy (colic and diarrhoea may limit the dose of misoprostol);
- Treat ulcer with a proton pump inhibitor and switch non-selective NSAID to a cyclo-oxygenase-2 selective inhibitor, but see NSAIDs and Cardiovascular Events; on healing, continuation of the proton pump inhibitor in patients with a history of upper gastro-intestinal bleeding may provide further protection against recurrence.

If *treatment with a cyclo-oxygenase-2 selective inhibitor needs to continue,* treat ulcer with a proton pump inhibitor; on healing continuation of the proton pump inhibitor in patients with a history of upper gastro-intestinal bleeding may provide further protection against recurrence.

GASTROPROTECTIVE COMPLEXES AND CHELATORS

Chelates and complexes

Overview
Sucralfate below may act by protecting the mucosa from acid-pepsin attack in gastric and duodenal ulcers. It is a complex of aluminium hydroxide and sulfated sucrose but has minimal antacid properties.

Sucralfate

- **INDICATIONS AND DOSE**

Benign gastric ulceration | Benign duodenal ulceration
▸ BY MOUTH
▸ Child 15–17 years: 2 g twice daily, dose to be taken on rising and at bedtime, alternatively 1 g 4 times a day for 4–6 weeks, or in resistant cases up to 12 weeks, dose to be taken 1 hour before meals and at bedtime; maximum 8 g per day
▸ Adult: 2 g twice daily, dose to be taken on rising and at bedtime, alternatively 1 g 4 times a day for 4–6 weeks, or in resistant cases up to 12 weeks, dose to be taken 1 hour before meals and at bedtime; maximum 8 g per day

Chronic gastritis
▸ BY MOUTH
▸ Adult: 2 g twice daily, dose to be taken on rising and at bedtime, alternatively 1 g 4 times a day for 4–6 weeks or in resistant cases up to 12 weeks, dose to be taken 1 hour before meals and at bedtime; maximum 8 g per day

Prophylaxis of stress ulceration in child under intensive care
▸ BY MOUTH
▸ Child 15–17 years: 1 g 6 times a day; maximum 8 g per day

Prophylaxis of stress ulceration
▸ BY MOUTH
▸ Adult: 1 g 6 times a day; maximum 8 g per day

- **CAUTIONS** Patients under intensive care (**Important:** reports of bezoar formation)
  CAUTIONS, FURTHER INFORMATION
▸ Bezoar formation Following reports of bezoar formation associated with sucralfate, caution is advised in seriously ill patients, especially those receiving concomitant enteral feeds or those with predisposing conditions such as delayed gastric emptying.
- **INTERACTIONS** → Appendix 1: sucralfate
- **SIDE-EFFECTS**
▸ **Common or very common** Constipation
▸ **Uncommon** Dry mouth · nausea
▸ **Rare or very rare** Bezoar · rash
▸ **Frequency not known** Back pain · bone disorders · diarrhoea · dizziness · drowsiness · encephalopathy · flatulence · headache · vertigo
- **PREGNANCY** No evidence of harm; absorption from gastro-intestinal tract negligible.
- **BREAST FEEDING** Amount probably too small to be harmful.
- **RENAL IMPAIRMENT** Use with caution; aluminium is absorbed and may accumulate.
- **DIRECTIONS FOR ADMINISTRATION** Administration of sucralfate and enteral feeds should be separated by 1 hour and for administration by *mouth*, sucralfate should be given 1 hour before meals. *Oral suspension* blocks fine-bore feeding tubes. Crushed *tablets* may be dispersed in water.
- **PRESCRIBING AND DISPENSING INFORMATION** Flavours of oral liquid formulations may include aniseed and caramel.
- **MEDICINAL FORMS**
  There can be variation in the licensing of different medicines containing the same drug. Forms available from special-order manufacturers include: tablet, oral suspension
  Tablet
  CAUTIONARY AND ADVISORY LABELS 5
  ▸ Sucralfate (Non-proprietary)
    Sucralfate 1 gram Sulcrate 1g tablets | 100 tablet ⓢ
    Carafate 1g tablets | 100 tablet ⓢ

H$_2$-RECEPTOR ANTAGONISTS

H$_2$-receptor antagonists

Overview
Histamine H$_2$-receptor antagonists heal *gastric and duodenal ulcers* by reducing gastric acid output as a result of histamine H$_2$-receptor blockade; they are also used to relieve symptoms of *gastro-oesophageal reflux disease*. H$_2$-receptor antagonists should not normally be used for *Zollinger-Ellison syndrome* because proton pump inhibitors are more effective.

Maintenance treatment with low doses for the prevention of peptic ulcer disease has largely been replaced in *Helicobacter pylori* positive patients by eradication regimens.

In adults, H$_2$-receptor antagonists are used for the treatment of *functional dyspepsia* and may be used for the treatment of *uninvestigated dyspepsia* without alarm features.

H$_2$-receptor antagonist therapy can promote healing of NSAID-associated ulcers (particularly duodenal).

Treatment with a H$_2$-receptor antagonist has not been shown to be beneficial in haematemesis and melaena, but prophylactic use reduces the frequency of bleeding from *gastroduodenal erosions in hepatic coma*, and possibly in other conditions requiring intensive care. H$_2$- receptor antagonists also reduce the risk of *acid aspiration* in obstetric patients at delivery (Mendelson's syndrome).

Gastro-intestinal system

1

H₂-receptor antagonists

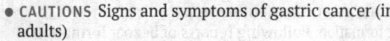

- CAUTIONS Signs and symptoms of gastric cancer (in adults)

  CAUTIONS, FURTHER INFORMATION
  ▸ Gastric cancer
  ▸ In adults H₂-receptor antagonists might mask symptoms of gastric cancer; particular care is required in patients presenting with 'alarm features' in such cases gastric malignancy should be ruled out before treatment.
- SIDE-EFFECTS
  ▸ **Common or very common** Constipation · diarrhoea · dizziness · fatigue · headache · myalgia · skin reactions
  ▸ **Uncommon** Confusion · depression · erectile dysfunction · gynaecomastia · hallucination · hepatic disorders · leucopenia · nausea · tachycardia
  ▸ **Rare or very rare** Agranulocytosis · alopecia · arthralgia · atrioventricular block · fever · galactorrhoea · pancytopenia · thrombocytopenia · vasculitis

⌐ above

Cimetidine

- **INDICATIONS AND DOSE**
  Benign duodenal ulceration
  ▸ BY MOUTH
  ▸ Adult: 400 mg twice daily for at least 4 weeks, to be taken with breakfast and at night, alternatively 800 mg once daily for at least 4 weeks, to be taken at night; increased if necessary up to 400 mg 4 times a day; maintenance 400 mg once daily, to be taken at night, alternatively maintenance 400 mg twice daily, to be taken in the morning and at night

  Benign gastric ulceration
  ▸ BY MOUTH
  ▸ Adult: 400 mg twice daily for 6 weeks, to be taken with breakfast and at night, alternatively 800 mg daily for 6 weeks, to be taken at night; increased if necessary up to 400 mg 4 times a day; maintenance 400 mg once daily, to be taken at night, alternatively maintenance 400 mg twice daily, to be taken in the morning and at night

  NSAID-associated ulceration
  ▸ BY MOUTH
  ▸ Adult: 400 mg twice daily for 8 weeks, to be taken with breakfast and at night, alternatively 800 mg daily for 8 weeks, to be taken at night; increased if necessary up to 400 mg 4 times a day; maintenance 400 mg daily, to be taken at night, alternatively maintenance 400 mg twice daily, to be taken in the morning and at night

  Reflux oesophagitis
  ▸ BY MOUTH
  ▸ Adult: 400 mg 4 times a day for 4–8 weeks

  Prophylaxis of stress ulceration
  ▸ BY MOUTH
  ▸ Adult: 200–400 mg every 4–6 hours

  Gastric acid reduction in obstetrics
  ▸ BY MOUTH
  ▸ Adult: Initially 400 mg, to be administered at start of labour, then increased if necessary up to 400 mg every 4 hours, do not use syrup in prophylaxis of acid aspiration; maximum 2.4 g per day

  Gastric acid reduction during surgical procedures
  ▸ BY MOUTH
  ▸ Adult: 400 mg, to be given 90–120 minutes before induction of general anaesthesia

  Short-bowel syndrome
  ▸ BY MOUTH
  ▸ Adult: 400 mg twice daily, adjusted according to response, to be taken with breakfast and at bedtime

To reduce degradation of pancreatic enzyme supplements
▸ BY MOUTH
▸ Adult: 0.8–1.6 g daily in 4 divided doses, dose to be taken 1–1½ hours before meals

- INTERACTIONS → Appendix 1: H2 receptor antagonists
- SIDE-EFFECTS
  ▸ **Rare or very rare** Anaphylactic reaction · aplastic anaemia · hypersensitivity vasculitis · nephritis tubulointerstitial · pancreatitis · sinus bradycardia
- PREGNANCY Manufacturer advises avoid unless essential.
- BREAST FEEDING Significant amount present in milk—not known to be harmful but manufacturer advises avoid.
- HEPATIC IMPAIRMENT Increased risk of confusion.
  Dose adjustments Reduce dose.
- RENAL IMPAIRMENT Occasional risk of confusion.
  Dose adjustments Reduce dose to 200 mg 4 times daily if eGFR 30–50 mL/minute/1.73 m².
  Reduce dose to 200 mg 3 times daily if eGFR 15–30 mL/minute/1.73 m².
  Reduce dose to 200 mg twice daily if eGFR less than 15 mL/minute/1.73 m².
- EXCEPTIONS TO LEGAL CATEGORY Cimetidine can be sold to the public for adults and children over 16 years (provided packs do not contain more than 2 weeks' supply) for the short-term symptomatic relief of heartburn, dyspepsia, and hyperacidity (max. single dose 200 mg, max. daily dose 800 mg), and for the prophylactic management of nocturnal heartburn (single night-time dose 100 mg).
- MEDICINAL FORMS
  There can be variation in the licensing of different medicines containing the same drug. Forms available from special-order manufacturers include: oral suspension

  Oral solution
  EXCIPIENTS: May contain Propylene glycol
  ▸ Cimetidine (Non-proprietary)
    Cimetidine **40 mg per 1 ml** Cimetidine 200mg/5ml oral solution sugar free | 300 ml PoM £14.24-£14.25 DT = £14.25
  ▸ Tagamet (Essential Pharma Ltd)
    Cimetidine **40 mg per 1 ml** Tagamet 200mg/5ml syrup | 600 ml PoM £28.49 DT = £28.49

  Tablet
  ▸ Cimetidine (Non-proprietary)
    Cimetidine **200 mg** Cimetidine 200mg tablets | 60 tablet PoM £9.98-£45.59 | 120 tablet PoM £120.00
    Cimetidine **400 mg** Cimetidine 400mg tablets | 60 tablet PoM £120.00 DT = £16.37
    Cimetidine **800 mg** Cimetidine 800mg tablets | 30 tablet PoM £15.31 DT = £15.31
  ▸ Tagamet (Chemidex Pharma Ltd)
    Cimetidine **400 mg** Tagamet 400mg tablets | 60 tablet PoM £22.62 DT = £16.37
    Cimetidine **800 mg** Tagamet 800mg tablets | 30 tablet PoM £22.62 DT = £15.31

⌐ above

Famotidine

- **INDICATIONS AND DOSE**
  Treatment of benign gastric and duodenal ulceration
  ▸ BY MOUTH
  ▸ Adult: 40 mg once daily for 4–8 weeks, dose to be taken at night

  Maintenance treatment of duodenal ulceration
  ▸ BY MOUTH
  ▸ Adult: 20 mg once daily, dose to be taken at night

  Reflux oesophagitis
  ▸ BY MOUTH
  ▸ Adult: 20–40 mg twice daily for 6–12 weeks; maintenance 20 mg twice daily

● INTERACTIONS → Appendix 1: H2 receptor antagonists
● SIDE-EFFECTS
▶ **Uncommon** Appetite decreased · dry mouth · pruritus · taste altered · vomiting
▶ **Rare or very rare** Anxiety · chest tightness · disorientation · drowsiness · insomnia · interstitial pneumonia · jaundice cholestatic · libido decreased · muscle cramps · neutropenia · paraesthesia · psychiatric disorder · seizures · severe cutaneous adverse reactions (SCARs)
● PREGNANCY Manufacturer advises avoid unless potential benefit outweighs risk.
● BREAST FEEDING Present in milk—not known to be harmful but manufacturer advises avoid.
● RENAL IMPAIRMENT Seizures reported very rarely.
Dose adjustments Use normal dose every 36–48 hours or use half normal dose if eGFR less than 50 mL/minute/1.73 m^2.
● EXCEPTIONS TO LEGAL CATEGORY Famotidine can be sold to the public for adults and children over 16 years (provided packs do not contain more than 2 weeks' supply) for the short-term symptomatic relief of heartburn, dyspepsia, and hyperacidity, and for the prevention of these symptoms when associated with consumption of food or drink including when they cause sleep disturbance (max. single dose 10 mg, max. daily dose 20 mg).

● MEDICINAL FORMS
There can be variation in the licensing of different medicines containing the same drug.
Tablet
▶ Famotidine (Non-proprietary)
Famotidine 20 mg Famotidine 20mg tablets | 28 tablet PoM £22.00 DT = £21.97
Famotidine 40 mg Famotidine 40mg tablets | 28 tablet PoM £39.00 DT = £38.98

F 74

Nizatidine

● INDICATIONS AND DOSE
Benign gastric, duodenal or NSAID-associated ulceration
▶ BY MOUTH
▶ Adult: 300 mg once daily for 4–8 weeks, dose to be taken in the evening, alternatively 150 mg twice daily for 4–8 weeks; maintenance 150 mg once daily, dose to be taken at night
Gastro-oesophageal reflux disease
▶ BY MOUTH
▶ Adult: 150–300 mg twice daily for up to 12 weeks

● INTERACTIONS → Appendix 1: H2 receptor antagonists
● SIDE-EFFECTS
▶ **Rare or very rare** Anaemia · cholestatic liver injury · exfoliative dermatitis · hyperuricaemia · serum sickness · thrombocytopenic purpura
▶ **Frequency not known** Hyperhidrosis
● PREGNANCY Manufacturer advises avoid unless essential.
● BREAST FEEDING Amount too small to be harmful.
● HEPATIC IMPAIRMENT Manufacturer advises caution.
● RENAL IMPAIRMENT
Dose adjustments Use half normal dose if eGFR 20–50 mL/minute/1.73 m^2.
Use one-quarter normal dose if eGFR less than 20 mL/minute/1.73 m^2.
● EXCEPTIONS TO LEGAL CATEGORY Nizatidine can be sold to the public for the prevention and treatment of symptoms of food-related heartburn and meal-induced indigestion in adults and children over 16 years; max. single dose 75 mg, max. daily dose 150 mg for max. 14 days.

● MEDICINAL FORMS
There can be variation in the licensing of different medicines containing the same drug. Forms available from special-order manufacturers include: oral suspension, oral solution
Capsule
▶ Nizatidine (Non-proprietary)
Nizatidine 150 mg Nizatidine 150mg capsules | 30 capsule PoM £12.20 DT = £3.73
Nizatidine 300 mg Nizatidine 300mg capsules | 30 capsule PoM £15.43 DT = £15.43

F 74

Ranitidine

● INDICATIONS AND DOSE
Benign gastric ulceration | Duodenal ulceration
▶ BY MOUTH
▶ Child 1-5 months: 1 mg/kg 3 times a day (max. per dose 3 mg/kg 3 times a day)
▶ Child 6 months-2 years: 2–4 mg/kg twice daily
▶ Child 3-11 years: 2–4 mg/kg twice daily (max. per dose 150 mg)
▶ Child 12-17 years: 150 mg twice daily, alternatively 300 mg once daily, dose to be taken at night
▶ Adult: 150 mg twice daily for 4–8 weeks, alternatively 300 mg once daily for 4–8 weeks, dose to be taken at night
Chronic episodic dyspepsia
▶ BY MOUTH
▶ Adult: 150 mg twice daily for 6 weeks, alternatively 300 mg once daily for 6 weeks, dose to be taken at night
NSAID-associated gastric ulceration
▶ BY MOUTH
▶ Adult: 150 mg twice daily for up to 8 weeks, alternatively 300 mg once daily for up to 8 weeks, dose to be taken at night
NSAID-associated duodenal ulcer
▶ BY MOUTH
▶ Adult: 300 mg twice daily for 4 weeks, to achieve a higher healing rate
Prophylaxis of NSAID-associated gastric ulcer | Prophylaxis of NSAID-associated duodenal ulcer
▶ BY MOUTH
▶ Adult: 300 mg twice daily
Gastro-oesophageal reflux disease
▶ BY MOUTH
▶ Adult: 150 mg twice daily for up to 8 weeks or if necessary 12 weeks, alternatively 300 mg once daily for up to 8 weeks or if necessary 12 weeks, dose to be taken at night
Moderate to severe gastro-oesophageal reflux disease
▶ BY MOUTH
▶ Adult: 600 mg daily in 2–4 divided doses for up to 12 weeks
Long-term treatment of healed gastro-oesophageal reflux disease
▶ BY MOUTH
▶ Adult: 150 mg twice daily
Gastric acid reduction (prophylaxis of acid aspiration) in obstetrics
▶ BY MOUTH
▶ Adult: 150 mg, dose to be given at onset of labour, then 150 mg every 6 hours
Gastric acid reduction (prophylaxis of acid aspiration) in surgical procedures
▶ INITIALLY BY INTRAMUSCULAR INJECTION, OR BY SLOW INTRAVENOUS INJECTION
▶ Adult: 50 mg, to be given 45–60 minutes before induction of anaesthesia, intravenous injection diluted to 20 mL and given over at least 2 minutes, continued →

alternatively (by mouth) 150 mg, to be given 2 hours before induction of anaesthesia and also when possible on the preceding evening

Prophylaxis of stress ulceration
▸ INITIALLY BY SLOW INTRAVENOUS INJECTION
▸ Adult: 50 mg every 8 hours, dose to be diluted to 20 mL and given over at least 2 minutes, then (by mouth) 150 mg twice daily, may be given when oral feeding commences

Reflux oesophagitis and other conditions where gastric acid reduction is beneficial
▸ BY MOUTH
▸ Child 1–5 months: 1 mg/kg 3 times a day (max. per dose 3 mg/kg 3 times a day)
▸ Child 6 months–2 years: 2–4 mg/kg twice daily
▸ Child 3–11 years: 2–4 mg/kg twice daily (max. per dose 150 mg); increased to up to 5 mg/kg twice daily (max. per dose 300 mg), dose increase for severe gastro-oesophageal disease
▸ Child 12–17 years: 150 mg twice daily, alternatively 300 mg once daily, dose to be taken at night, then increased if necessary to 300 mg twice daily for up to 12 weeks in moderate to severe gastro-oesophageal reflux disease, alternatively increased if necessary to 150 mg 4 times a day for up to 12 weeks in moderate to severe gastro-oesophageal reflux disease

Conditions where reduction of gastric acidity is beneficial and oral route not available
▸ BY INTRAMUSCULAR INJECTION
▸ Adult: 50 mg every 6–8 hours
▸ BY SLOW INTRAVENOUS INJECTION
▸ Adult: 50 mg, dose to be diluted to 20 mL and given over at least 2 minutes; may be repeated every 6–8 hours

● UNLICENSED USE
▸ In children *Oral* preparations not licensed for use in children under 3 years.
▸ In adults Doses given for prophylaxis of NSAID-associated gastric or duodenal ulcer, and prophylaxis of stress ulceration, are not licensed.
● INTERACTIONS → Appendix 1: H2 receptor antagonists
● SIDE-EFFECTS
GENERAL SIDE-EFFECTS
▸ **Rare or very rare** Bone marrow depression · bradycardia · breast conditions · dyskinesia · erythema multiforme · hepatitis cholestatic · nephritis acute interstitial · pancreatitis acute · vision blurred
▸ **Frequency not known** Dyspnoea
SPECIFIC SIDE-EFFECTS
▸ **Rare or very rare**
▸ With parenteral use Anaphylactic shock · cardiac arrest
● PREGNANCY Manufacturer advises avoid unless essential, but not known to be harmful.
● BREAST FEEDING Significant amount present in milk, but not known to be harmful.
● RENAL IMPAIRMENT
Dose adjustments ▸ In adults Use half normal dose if eGFR less than 50 mL/minute/1.73 m^2.
▸ In children Use half normal dose if estimated glomerular filtration rate less than 50 mL/minute/1.73 m^2.
● DIRECTIONS FOR ADMINISTRATION For *intravenous infusion* (*Zantac*®), give intermittently in Glucose 5% or Sodium Chloride 0.9%.
● PATIENT AND CARER ADVICE In fat malabsorption syndrome, give oral doses 1–2 hours before food to enhance effects of pancreatic enzyme replacement.
Medicines for Children leaflet: Ranitidine for acid reflux
www.medicinesforchildren.org.uk/ranitidine-for-acid-reflux

● EXCEPTIONS TO LEGAL CATEGORY Ranitidine can be sold to the public for adults and children over 16 years (provided packs do not contain more than 2 weeks' supply) for the short-term symptomatic relief of heartburn, dyspepsia, and hyperacidity, and for the prevention of these symptoms when associated with consumption of food or drink (max. single dose 75 mg, max. daily dose 300 mg).

● MEDICINAL FORMS
There can be variation in the licensing of different medicines containing the same drug. Forms available from special-order manufacturers include: oral suspension, oral solution, infusion

Tablet
▸ Ranitidine (Non-proprietary)
Ranitidine (as Ranitidine hydrochloride) 150 mg Ranitidine 150mg tablets | 60 tablet [PoM] £1.27 DT = £0.76
Ranitidine (as Ranitidine hydrochloride) 300 mg Ranitidine 300mg tablets | 30 tablet [PoM] £1.27 DT = £0.75
▸ Ranitil (Tillomed Laboratories Ltd)
Ranitidine (as Ranitidine hydrochloride) 150 mg Ranitil 150mg tablets | 60 tablet [PoM] £18.13 DT = £0.76
Ranitidine (as Ranitidine hydrochloride) 300 mg Ranitil 300mg tablets | 30 tablet [PoM] £17.64 DT = £0.75
▸ Zantac (Omega Pharma Ltd, GlaxoSmithKline UK Ltd)
Ranitidine (as Ranitidine hydrochloride) 75 mg 24 tablet [P] £5.16 | 48 tablet [P] £7.75 **DT = £7.75**
Ranitidine (as Ranitidine hydrochloride) 150 mg Zantac 150mg tablets | 60 tablet [PoM] £1.30 DT = £0.76
Ranitidine (as Ranitidine hydrochloride) 300 mg Zantac 300mg tablets | 30 tablet [PoM] £1.30 DT = £0.75

Solution for injection
▸ Ranitidine (Non-proprietary)
Ranitidine (as Ranitidine hydrochloride) 25 mg per 1 ml Ranitidine 50mg/2ml solution for injection ampoules | 5 ampoule [PoM] £2.69–£5.00 DT = £2.69
▸ Zantac (GlaxoSmithKline UK Ltd)
Ranitidine (as Ranitidine hydrochloride) 25 mg per 1 ml Zantac 50mg/2ml solution for injection ampoules | 5 ampoule [PoM] £2.82 DT = £2.69

Effervescent tablet
CAUTIONARY AND ADVISORY LABELS 13
ELECTROLYTES: May contain Sodium
▸ Ranitidine (Non-proprietary)
Ranitidine (as Ranitidine hydrochloride) 150 mg Ranitidine 150mg effervescent tablets | 60 tablet [PoM] £36.50 DT = £34.98
Ranitidine (as Ranitidine hydrochloride) 300 mg Ranitidine 300mg effervescent tablets | 30 tablet [PoM] £36.50 DT = £34.98

Oral solution
EXCIPIENTS: May contain Alcohol
▸ Ranitidine (Non-proprietary)
Ranitidine (as Ranitidine hydrochloride) 15 mg per 1 ml Ranitidine 75mg/5ml oral solution sugar free sugar-free | 100 ml [PoM] £2.07–£2.43 sugar-free | 300 ml [PoM] £21.55 DT = £6.24
Ranitidine (as Ranitidine hydrochloride) 30 mg per 1 ml Ranitidine 150mg/5ml oral solution sugar free sugar-free | 150 ml [PoM] £5.50 DT = £5.50
▸ Zantac (GlaxoSmithKline UK Ltd)
Ranitidine (as Ranitidine hydrochloride) 15 mg per 1 ml Zantac 150mg/10ml syrup sugar-free | 300 ml [PoM] £20.76 DT = £6.24

PROSTAGLANDIN ANALOGUES AND PROSTAMIDES > PROSTAGLANDINS, GASTROPROTECTIVE

Misoprostol
21-Feb-2018

- **DRUG ACTION** Misoprostol is a synthetic prostaglandin analogue that has antisecretory and protective properties, promoting healing of gastric and duodenal ulcers.

- **INDICATIONS AND DOSE**

Benign gastric ulcer | Benign duodenal ulcer | NSAID-induced peptic ulcer
▸ BY MOUTH
  ▸ Adult: 400 micrograms twice daily, alternatively 200 micrograms 4 times a day continued for at least 4 weeks or may be continued for up to 8 weeks if required, dose to be taken with breakfast (or main meals) and at bedtime

Prophylaxis of NSAID-induced peptic ulcer
▸ BY MOUTH
  ▸ Adult: 200 micrograms 2–4 times a day

- **CAUTIONS** Conditions where hypotension might precipitate severe complications (e.g. cerebrovascular disease, cardiovascular disease) · conditions which predispose to diarrhoea (e.g. inflammatory bowel disease)
- **SIDE-EFFECTS**
▸ **Common or very common** Constipation · diarrhoea · dizziness · flatulence · gastrointestinal discomfort · headache · nausea · rash · vomiting
▸ **Uncommon** Fever · haemorrhage · menstrual cycle irregularities · postmenopausal haemorrhage · uterine cramps
▸ **Frequency not known** Chills · uterine rupture
  SIDE-EFFECTS, FURTHER INFORMATION Diarrhoea may occasionally be severe and require withdrawal, reduced by giving single doses not exceeding 200 micrograms and by avoiding magnesium-containing antacids.
- **CONCEPTION AND CONTRACEPTION** Manufacturer advises do not use in women of childbearing potential unless pregnancy has been excluded; patients must use effective contraception during treatment, and be informed of the risks of taking misoprostol if pregnant.
- **PREGNANCY** Manufacturer advises avoid—induces uterine contractions, and associated with abortion and birth defects; teratogenic in first trimester.
- **BREAST FEEDING** Manufacturer advises avoid—present in milk, and may cause diarrhoea in nursing infants. EvGr Tertiary sources state present in milk but amount probably too small to be harmful; to further reduce risk following termination of pregnancy, consider interrupting breastfeeding for 5 hours after a dose. ⟨D⟩
- **PATIENT AND CARER ADVICE**
Driving and skilled tasks Manufacturer advises patients should be cautioned on the effects on driving and performance of skilled tasks—increased risk of dizziness.

- **MEDICINAL FORMS**
  There can be variation in the licensing of different medicines containing the same drug.
  Tablet
  CAUTIONARY AND ADVISORY LABELS 21
  ▸ Cytotec (Pfizer Ltd)
    Misoprostol 200 microgram Cytotec 200microgram tablets | 60 tablet PoM £10.03 DT = £10.03

PROTON PUMP INHIBITORS

Proton pump inhibitors

Overview

Proton pump inhibitors are effective short-term treatments for *gastric* and *duodenal ulcers*; they are also used in combination with antibacterials for the eradication of *Helicobacter pylori* (see specific regimens). Following endoscopic treatment of severe peptic ulcer bleeding, an intravenous, high-dose proton pump inhibitor reduces the risk of rebleeding and the need for surgery. Proton pump inhibitors can be used for the treatment of *dyspepsia* and *gastro-oesophageal reflux disease*.

Proton pump inhibitors are also used for the prevention and treatment of NSAID-associated ulcers. In patients who need to continue NSAID treatment after an ulcer has healed, the dose of proton pump inhibitor should normally not be reduced because asymptomatic ulcer deterioration may occur.

A proton pump inhibitor can be used to reduce the degradation of pancreatic enzyme supplements in patients with cystic fibrosis. They can also be used to control excessive secretion of gastric acid in *Zollinger–Ellison syndrome*; high doses are often required.

Proton pump inhibitors

- **DRUG ACTION** Proton pump inhibitors inhibit gastric acid secretion by blocking the hydrogen-potassium adenosine triphosphatase enzyme system (the 'proton pump') of the gastric parietal cell.

> **IMPORTANT SAFETY INFORMATION**
> MHRA ADVICE: PROTON PUMP INHIBITORS (PPIs): VERY LOW RISK OF SUBACUTE CUTANEOUS LUPUS ERYTHEMATOSUS (SEPTEMBER 2015)
> Very infrequent cases of subacute cutaneous lupus erythematosus (SCLE) have been reported in patients taking PPIs. Drug-induced SCLE can occur weeks, months or even years after exposure to the drug.
> If a patient treated with a PPI develops lesions—especially in sun-exposed areas of the skin—and it is accompanied by arthralgia:
> - advise them to avoid exposing the skin to sunlight;
> - consider SCLE as a possible diagnosis;
> - consider discontinuing PPI treatment unless it is imperative for a serious acid-related condition; a patient who develops SCLE with a particular PPI may be at risk of the same reaction with another;
> - in most cases, symptoms resolve on PPI withdrawal; topical or systemic steroids might be necessary for treatment of SCLE only if there are no signs of remission after a few weeks or months.

- **CAUTIONS** Can increase the risk of fractures (particularly when used at high doses for over a year in the elderly) · may increase the risk of gastro-intestinal infections (including *Clostridium difficile* infection) · may mask the symptoms of gastric cancer (in adults) · patients at risk of osteoporosis
  CAUTIONS, FURTHER INFORMATION
  ▸ Risk of osteoporosis Patients at risk of osteoporosis should maintain an adequate intake of calcium and vitamin D, and if necessary, receive other preventative therapy.
  ▸ Gastric cancer
  ▸ In adults Particular care is required in those presenting with 'alarm features', in such cases gastric malignancy should be ruled out before treatment.

Gastro-intestinal system

1

- SIDE-EFFECTS
▶ **Common or very common** Abdominal pain · constipation · diarrhoea · dizziness · dry mouth · gastrointestinal disorders · headache · insomnia · nausea · skin reactions · vomiting
▶ **Uncommon** Arthralgia · bone fractures · confusion · depression · drowsiness · leucopenia · malaise · myalgia · paraesthesia · peripheral oedema · thrombocytopenia · vertigo · vision disorders
▶ **Rare or very rare** Agranulocytosis · alopecia · gynaecomastia · hallucination · hepatic disorders · hyperhidrosis · hyponatraemia · nephritis tubulointerstitial · pancytopenia · photosensitivity reaction · severe cutaneous adverse reactions (SCARs) · stomatitis · taste altered
▶ **Frequency not known** Hypomagnesaemia (more common after 1 year of treatment, but sometimes after 3 months of treatment) · subacute cutaneous lupus erythematosus

- MONITORING REQUIREMENTS Measurement of serum-magnesium concentrations should be considered before and during prolonged treatment with a proton pump inhibitor, especially when used with other drugs that cause hypomagnesaemia or with digoxin.

- PRESCRIBING AND DISPENSING INFORMATION A proton pump inhibitor should be prescribed for appropriate indications at the lowest effective dose for the shortest period; the need for long-term treatment should be reviewed periodically.

F 77

Esomeprazole

- INDICATIONS AND DOSE

NSAID-associated gastric ulcer
▶ BY MOUTH
  ▸ Adult: 20 mg once daily for 4–8 weeks
▶ BY INTRAVENOUS INJECTION, OR BY INTRAVENOUS INFUSION
  ▸ Adult: 20 mg daily continue until oral administration possible, injection to be given over at least 3 minutes

Prophylaxis of NSAID-associated gastric ulcer in patients with an increased risk of gastroduodenal complications who require continued NSAID treatment
▶ BY MOUTH
  ▸ Adult: 20 mg daily

Prophylaxis of NSAID-associated gastric or duodenal ulcer
▶ BY INTRAVENOUS INJECTION, OR BY INTRAVENOUS INFUSION
  ▸ Adult: 20 mg daily continue until oral administration possible, injection to be given over at least 3 minutes

Gastro-oesophageal reflux disease (in the presence of erosive reflux oesophagitis)
▶ BY MOUTH
  ▸ Child 1-11 years (body-weight 10-19 kg): 10 mg once daily for 8 weeks
  ▸ Child 1-11 years (body-weight 20 kg and above): 10–20 mg once daily for 8 weeks
  ▸ Child 12-17 years: Initially 40 mg once daily for 4 weeks, continued for further 4 weeks if not fully healed or symptoms persist; maintenance 20 mg daily
  ▸ Adult: Initially 40 mg once daily for 4 weeks, continued for further 4 weeks if not fully healed or symptoms persist; maintenance 20 mg daily
▶ BY INTRAVENOUS INJECTION, OR BY INTRAVENOUS INFUSION
  ▸ Adult: 40 mg daily continue until oral administration possible, injection to be given over at least 3 minutes

Symptomatic treatment of gastro-oesophageal reflux disease (in the absence of oesophagitis)
▶ BY MOUTH
  ▸ Child 1-11 years (body-weight 10 kg and above): 10 mg once daily for up to 8 weeks
  ▸ Child 12-17 years: 20 mg once daily for up to 4 weeks

  ▸ Adult: 20 mg once daily for up to 4 weeks, then 20 mg daily if required
▶ BY INTRAVENOUS INJECTION, OR BY INTRAVENOUS INFUSION
  ▸ Adult: 20 mg once daily continue until oral administration is possible, injection to be given over at least 3 minutes

Zollinger–Ellison syndrome
▶ BY MOUTH
  ▸ Adult: Initially 40 mg twice daily, adjusted according to response; usual dose 80–160 mg daily, daily doses above 80 mg should be given in 2 divided doses

Severe peptic ulcer bleeding (following endoscopic treatment)
▶ INITIALLY BY INTRAVENOUS INFUSION
  ▸ Adult: Initially 80 mg, to be given over 30 minutes, then (by continuous intravenous infusion) 8 mg/hour for 72 hours, then (by mouth) 40 mg once daily for 4 weeks

***Helicobacter pylori* eradication in combination with clarithromycin and amoxicillin or metronidazole**
▶ BY MOUTH
  ▸ Adult: 20 mg twice daily

- UNLICENSED USE Tablets and capsules not licensed for use in children 1–11 years.

- INTERACTIONS → Appendix 1: proton pump inhibitors

- SIDE-EFFECTS
  GENERAL SIDE-EFFECTS
▶ **Uncommon** Encephalopathy
▶ **Rare or very rare** Aggression · agitation · bronchospasm · increased risk of infection · muscle weakness
▶ **Frequency not known** Colitis microscopic
  SPECIFIC SIDE-EFFECTS
▶ **Rare or very rare**
▶ With parenteral use Renal failure
▶ **Frequency not known**
▶ With parenteral use Electrolyte imbalance · vitamin B12 deficiency

- PREGNANCY Manufacturer advises caution—no information available.

- BREAST FEEDING Manufacturer advises avoid—no information available.

- HEPATIC IMPAIRMENT
  Dose adjustments ▸ In adults In severe hepatic impairment max. 20 mg daily. Severe peptic ulcer bleeding in severe hepatic impairment, initial intravenous infusion of 80 mg, then by continuous intravenous infusion, 4 mg/hour for 72 hours.
  ▸ In children 1–11 years max. 10 mg daily in severe impairment. 12–17 years max. 20 mg daily in severe impairment.

- RENAL IMPAIRMENT Manufacturer advises caution in severe renal insufficiency.

- DIRECTIONS FOR ADMINISTRATION
▶ With intravenous use in adults For *intravenous infusion* (*Nexium®*), give continuously or intermittently in Sodium Chloride 0.9%; reconstitute 40–80 mg with up to 100 ml infusion fluid; for intermittent infusion, give requisite dose over 10–30 minutes; stable for 12 hours in Sodium Chloride 0.9%.
▶ With oral use Do not chew or crush capsules; swallow whole or mix capsule contents in water and drink within 30 minutes. Do not crush or chew tablets; swallow whole or disperse in water and drink within 30 minutes. Disperse the contents of each sachet of gastro-resistant granules in approx. 15 mL water. Stir and leave to thicken for a few minutes; stir again before administration and use within 30 minutes; rinse container with 15 mL water to obtain full dose. For administration through a gastric tube, consult product literature.

● PATIENT AND CARER ADVICE
▸ **With oral use** Counselling on administration of gastro-resistant capsules, tablets, and granules advised.

● MEDICINAL FORMS
There can be variation in the licensing of different medicines containing the same drug. Forms available from special-order manufacturers include: oral suspension

Gastro-resistant capsule
▸ Esomeprazole (Non-proprietary)
Esomeprazole (as Esomeprazole magnesium dihydrate)
20 mg Esomeprazole 20mg gastro-resistant capsules |
28 capsule [PoM] £12.95 DT = £2.64
Esomeprazole (as Esomeprazole magnesium dihydrate)
40 mg Esomeprazole 40mg gastro-resistant capsules |
28 capsule [PoM] £17.63 DT = £3.30
▸ Emozul (Consilient Health Ltd)
Esomeprazole (as Esomeprazole magnesium dihydrate)
20 mg Emozul 20mg gastro-resistant capsules | 28 capsule [PoM]
£2.64 DT = £2.64
Esomeprazole (as Esomeprazole magnesium dihydrate)
40 mg Emozul 40mg gastro-resistant capsules | 28 capsule [PoM]
£3.30 DT = £3.30
▸ Ventra (Ethypharm UK Ltd)
Esomeprazole (as Esomeprazole magnesium dihydrate)
20 mg Ventra 20mg gastro-resistant capsules | 28 capsule [PoM]
£2.55 DT = £2.64
Esomeprazole (as Esomeprazole magnesium dihydrate)
40 mg Ventra 40mg gastro-resistant capsules | 28 capsule [PoM]
£2.97 DT = £3.30

Gastro-resistant tablet
▸ Esomeprazole (Non-proprietary)
Esomeprazole (as Esomeprazole magnesium trihydrate)
20 mg Esomeprazole 20mg gastro-resistant tablets | 28 tablet [PoM]
£18.50 DT = £2.32
Esomeprazole (as Esomeprazole magnesium trihydrate)
40 mg Esomeprazole 40mg gastro-resistant tablets | 28 tablet [PoM]
£25.19 DT = £2.91
▸ Nexium (AstraZeneca UK Ltd, Pfizer Consumer Healthcare Ltd)
Esomeprazole (as Esomeprazole magnesium trihydrate)
20 mg Nexium 20mg gastro-resistant tablets | 28 tablet [PoM]
£18.50 DT = £2.32
Nexium Control 20mg gastro-resistant tablets | 7 tablet [GSL] £4.37
| 14 tablet [GSL] £7.49
Esomeprazole (as Esomeprazole magnesium trihydrate)
40 mg Nexium 40mg gastro-resistant tablets | 28 tablet [PoM]
£25.19 DT = £2.91

Powder for solution for injection
▸ Esomeprazole (Non-proprietary)
Esomeprazole (as Esomeprazole sodium) 40 mg Esomeprazole
40mg powder for solution for injection vials | 1 vial [PoM] £3.13
(Hospital only) | 1 vial [PoM] £3.07
▸ Nexium (AstraZeneca UK Ltd)
Esomeprazole (as Esomeprazole sodium) 40 mg Nexium I.V 40mg
powder for solution for injection vials | 1 vial [PoM] £4.25 (Hospital
only)

Gastro-resistant granules
CAUTIONARY AND ADVISORY LABELS 25
▸ Nexium (AstraZeneca UK Ltd)
Esomeprazole (as Esomeprazole magnesium trihydrate)
10 mg Nexium 10mg gastro-resistant granules sachets |
28 sachet [PoM] £25.19 DT = £25.19

F 77

Lansoprazole

07-Jun-2017

● INDICATIONS AND DOSE

**Helicobacter pylori eradication in combination with
amoxicillin and clarithromycin; or in combination with
amoxicillin and metronidazole; or in combination with
clarithromycin and metronidazole**
▸ BY MOUTH
▸ Adult: 30 mg twice daily

Benign gastric ulcer
▸ BY MOUTH
▸ Adult: 30 mg once daily for 8 weeks, dose to be taken in
the morning

Duodenal ulcer
▸ BY MOUTH
▸ Adult: 30 mg once daily for 4 weeks, dose to be taken in
the morning; maintenance 15 mg once daily

**NSAID-associated duodenal ulcer | NSAID-associated
gastric ulcer**
▸ BY MOUTH
▸ Adult: 30 mg once daily for 4 weeks, continued for
further 4 weeks if not fully healed

**Prophylaxis of NSAID-associated duodenal ulcer |
Prophylaxis of NSAID-associated gastric ulcer**
▸ BY MOUTH
▸ Adult: 15–30 mg once daily

**Zollinger–Ellison syndrome (and other hypersecretory
conditions)**
▸ BY MOUTH
▸ Adult: Initially 60 mg once daily, adjusted according to
response, daily doses of 120 mg or more given in two
divided doses

Gastro-oesophageal reflux disease
▸ BY MOUTH
▸ Adult: 30 mg once daily for 4 weeks, continued for
further 4 weeks if not fully healed; maintenance
15–30 mg once daily, doses to be taken in the morning

Severe oesophagitis
▸ BY MOUTH
▸ Adult: 30 mg once daily for 8 weeks, continue as
maintenance treatment if appropriate

Severe oesophagitis, refractory to initial treatment
▸ BY MOUTH
▸ Adult: 30 mg twice daily

Acid-related dyspepsia
▸ BY MOUTH
▸ Adult: 15–30 mg once daily for 2-4 weeks, doses to be
taken in the morning

● UNLICENSED USE Lansoprazole doses in BNF may differ
from those in product literature. [EvGr] Not licensed at
30 mg twice daily for severe oesophagitis refractory to
initial treatment. ◁

● INTERACTIONS → Appendix 1: proton pump inhibitors

● SIDE-EFFECTS
▸ **Common or very common** Dry throat · fatigue
▸ **Uncommon** Eosinophilia · oedema
▸ **Rare or very rare** Anaemia · angioedema · appetite
decreased · colitis · erectile dysfunction · fever · glossitis ·
oesophageal candidiasis · pancreatitis · restlessness ·
tremor

● PREGNANCY Manufacturer advises avoid.

● BREAST FEEDING Avoid—present in milk in *animal* studies.

● HEPATIC IMPAIRMENT
Dose adjustments Use half normal dose in moderate to
severe liver disease.

● DIRECTIONS FOR ADMINISTRATION Orodispersible tablets
should be placed on the tongue, allowed to disperse and
swallowed, or may be swallowed whole with a glass of
water. Alternatively, tablets can be dispersed in a small
amount of water and administered by an oral syringe or
nasogastric tube.

● PATIENT AND CARER ADVICE Counselling on
administration of orodispersible tablet advised.

● PROFESSION SPECIFIC INFORMATION

Dental practitioners' formulary
Lansoprazole capsules may be prescribed.

1

Gastro-intestinal system

● MEDICINAL FORMS
There can be variation in the licensing of different medicines containing the same drug. Forms available from special-order manufacturers include: oral suspension, oral solution

Gastro-resistant capsule

CAUTIONARY AND ADVISORY LABELS 5, 22, 25

▸ Lansoprazole (Non-proprietary)
Lansoprazole 15 mg Lansoprazole 15mg gastro-resistant capsules | 28 capsule [PoM] £12.92 DT = £0.57
Lansoprazole 30 mg Lansoprazole 30mg gastro-resistant capsules | 28 capsule [PoM] £23.63 DT = £0.89

Orodispersible tablet

CAUTIONARY AND ADVISORY LABELS 5, 22
EXCIPIENTS: May contain Aspartame

▸ Lansoprazole (Non-proprietary)
Lansoprazole 15 mg Lansoprazole 15mg orodispersible tablets | 28 tablet [PoM] £3.99 DT = £2.55
Lansoprazole 30 mg Lansoprazole 30mg orodispersible tablets | 28 tablet [PoM] £6.99 DT = £4.26

▸ Zoton FasTab (Pfizer Ltd)
Lansoprazole 15 mg Zoton FasTab 15mg | 28 tablet [PoM] £2.99 DT = £2.55
Lansoprazole 30 mg Zoton FasTab 30mg | 28 tablet [PoM] £5.50 DT = £4.26

�F 77

Omeprazole

21-Mar-2018

● INDICATIONS AND DOSE

Helicobacter pylori eradication in combination with amoxicillin and clarithromycin; or in combination with amoxicillin and metronidazole; or in combination with clarithromycin and metronidazole

▸ BY MOUTH
▸ Adult: 20 mg twice daily

Benign gastric ulceration

▸ BY MOUTH
▸ Adult: 20 mg once daily for 8 weeks, increased if necessary to 40 mg once daily, in severe or recurrent cases

Duodenal ulceration

▸ BY MOUTH
▸ Adult: 20 mg once daily for 4 weeks, increased if necessary to 40 mg once daily, in severe or recurrent cases

Prevention of relapse in gastric ulcer

▸ BY MOUTH
▸ Adult: 20 mg once daily, increased if necessary to 40 mg once daily

Prevention of relapse in duodenal ulcer

▸ BY MOUTH
▸ Adult: 20 mg once daily, dose may range between 10–40 mg daily

NSAID-associated duodenal ulcer | NSAID-associated gastric ulcer | NSAID-associated gastroduodenal erosions

▸ BY MOUTH
▸ Adult: 20 mg once daily for 4 weeks, continued for a further 4 weeks if not fully healed

Prophylaxis in patients with a history of NSAID-associated duodenal ulcer who require continued NSAID treatment | Prophylaxis in patients with a history of NSAID-associated gastric ulcer who require continued NSAID treatment | Prophylaxis in patients with a history of NSAID-associated gastroduodenal lesions who require continued NSAID treatment | Prophylaxis in patients with a history of NSAID-associated dyspeptic symptoms who require continued NSAID treatment

▸ BY MOUTH
▸ Adult: 20 mg once daily

Zollinger–Ellison syndrome

▸ BY MOUTH
▸ Adult: Initially 60 mg once daily; usual dose 20–120 mg daily, total daily doses greater than 80 mg should be given in 2 divided doses
▸ BY INTRAVENOUS INJECTION, OR BY INTRAVENOUS INFUSION
▸ Adult: Initially 60 mg once daily, adjusted according to response, total daily doses greater than 60 mg should be given in 2 divided doses, injection to be given over 5 minutes, infusion to be given over 20–30 minutes

Gastro-oesophageal reflux disease

▸ BY MOUTH
▸ Adult: 20 mg once daily for 4 weeks, continued for a further 4–8 weeks if not fully healed; maintenance 20 mg once daily

Gastro-oesophageal reflux disease refractory to other treatment

▸ BY MOUTH
▸ Adult: 40 mg once daily for 8 weeks; maintenance 20 mg once daily

Acid reflux disease (long-term management)

▸ BY MOUTH
▸ Adult: 10 mg once daily, increased to 20 mg once daily, dose only increased if symptoms return

Acid-related dyspepsia

▸ BY MOUTH
▸ Adult: 10–20 mg once daily for 2–4 weeks according to response

Treatment and prevention of benign gastric ulcers | Treatment and prevention of duodenal ulcers | Treatment and prevention of NSAID-associated ulcers | Treatment and prevention of gastro-oesophageal reflux disease

▸ BY INTRAVENOUS INJECTION, OR BY INTRAVENOUS INFUSION
▸ Adult: 40 mg once daily until oral administration possible, injection to be given over 5 minutes, infusion to be given over 20–30 minutes

Major peptic ulcer bleeding (following endoscopic treatment)

▸ INITIALLY BY INTRAVENOUS INFUSION
▸ Adult: Initially 80 mg, to be given over 40–60 minutes, then (by continuous intravenous infusion) 8 mg/hour for 72 hours, subsequent dose then changed to oral therapy

● UNLICENSED USE Treatment of major peptic ulcer bleeding (following endoscopic treatment) is an unlicensed indication.

● INTERACTIONS → Appendix 1: proton pump inhibitors

● SIDE-EFFECTS
▸ **Rare or very rare** Aggression · agitation · bronchospasm · colitis microscopic · encephalopathy · gastrointestinal candidiasis · muscle weakness

● PREGNANCY Not known to be harmful.

● BREAST FEEDING Present in milk but not known to be harmful.

● HEPATIC IMPAIRMENT
Dose adjustments Not more than 20 mg daily should be needed.

● DIRECTIONS FOR ADMINISTRATION For administration by *mouth*, swallow whole, or disperse *Losec MUPS®* tablets in water, *or* mix capsule contents or *Losec MUPS®* tablets with fruit juice or yoghurt. Preparations consisting of an e/c tablet within a capsule should **not** be opened.

▸ With intravenous use For *intravenous infusion* (*Losec®*), give intermittently or continuously in Glucose 5% or Sodium chloride 0.9%; reconstitute each 40 mg vial with infusion fluid and dilute to 100 mL; for intermittent infusion give 40 mg over 20–30 minutes; stable for 3 hours in glucose 5% or 12 hours in sodium chloride 0.9%.

- **PATIENT AND CARER ADVICE**
- ▶ With oral use Counselling on administration advised.
- **PROFESSION SPECIFIC INFORMATION**

  Dental practitioners' formulary
  Gastro-resistant omeprazole capsules may be prescribed.
- **EXCEPTIONS TO LEGAL CATEGORY** Omeprazole 10 mg tablets can be sold to the public for the short-term relief of reflux-like symptoms (e.g. heartburn) in adults over 18 years, max. daily dose 20 mg for max. 4 weeks, and a pack size of 28 tablets.

- **MEDICINAL FORMS**
  There can be variation in the licensing of different medicines containing the same drug. Forms available from special-order manufacturers include: oral suspension, oral solution

Gastro-resistant capsule

- ▶ Omeprazole (Non-proprietary)
  Omeprazole 10 mg Omeprazole 10mg gastro-resistant capsules | 28 capsule PoM £9.30 DT = £0.59
  Omeprazole 20 mg Omeprazole 20mg gastro-resistant capsules | 28 capsule PoM £13.50 DT = £0.60
  Omeprazole 40 mg Omeprazole 40mg gastro-resistant capsules | 7 capsule PoM £6.96 DT = £0.36 | 28 capsule PoM £1.44–£19.72
- ▶ Losec (AstraZeneca UK Ltd)
  Omeprazole 10 mg Losec 10mg gastro-resistant capsules | 28 capsule PoM £11.16 DT = £0.59
  Omeprazole 20 mg Losec 20mg gastro-resistant capsules | 28 capsule PoM £16.70 DT = £0.60
  Omeprazole 40 mg Losec 40mg gastro-resistant capsules | 7 capsule PoM £8.35 DT = £0.36
- ▶ Mepradec (Discovery Pharmaceuticals)
  Omeprazole 10 mg Mepradec 10mg gastro-resistant capsules | 28 capsule PoM £0.58 DT = £0.59
  Omeprazole 20 mg Mepradec 20mg gastro-resistant capsules | 28 capsule PoM £0.59 DT = £0.60

Gastro-resistant tablet
CAUTIONARY AND ADVISORY LABELS 25

- ▶ Omeprazole (Non-proprietary)
  Omeprazole 10 mg Omeprazole 10mg gastro-resistant tablets | 28 tablet PoM £18.91 DT = £7.90
  Omeprazole (as Omeprazole magnesium) 10 mg Omeprazole 10mg dispersible gastro-resistant tablets | 28 tablet PoM £9.30 DT = £9.30
  Omeprazole 20 mg Omeprazole 20mg gastro-resistant tablets | 28 tablet PoM £28.56 DT = £6.39
  Omeprazole (as Omeprazole magnesium) 20 mg Omeprazole 20mg dispersible gastro-resistant tablets | 28 tablet PoM £13.92 DT = £13.92
  Omeprazole 40 mg Omeprazole 40mg gastro-resistant tablets | 7 tablet PoM £14.28 DT = £6.42
  Omeprazole (as Omeprazole magnesium) 40 mg Omeprazole 40mg dispersible gastro-resistant tablets | 7 tablet PoM £6.96 DT = £6.96
- ▶ Losec MUPS (AstraZeneca UK Ltd)
  Omeprazole (as Omeprazole magnesium) 10 mg Losec MUPS 10mg gastro-resistant tablets | 28 tablet PoM £9.30 DT = £9.30
  Omeprazole (as Omeprazole magnesium) 20 mg Losec MUPS 20mg gastro-resistant tablets | 28 tablet PoM £13.92 DT = £13.92
  Omeprazole (as Omeprazole magnesium) 40 mg Losec MUPS 40mg gastro-resistant tablets | 7 tablet PoM £6.96 DT = £6.96
- ▶ Mezzopram (Sandoz Ltd)
  Omeprazole (as Omeprazole magnesium) 10 mg Mezzopram 10mg dispersible gastro-resistant tablets | 28 tablet PoM £6.58 DT = £9.30
  Omeprazole (as Omeprazole magnesium) 20 mg Mezzopram 20mg dispersible gastro-resistant tablets | 28 tablet PoM £9.86 DT = £13.92
  Omeprazole (as Omeprazole magnesium) 40 mg Mezzopram 40mg dispersible gastro-resistant tablets | 7 tablet PoM £4.93 DT = £6.96

Powder for solution for infusion

- ▶ Omeprazole (Non-proprietary)
  Omeprazole (as Omeprazole sodium) 40 mg Omeprazole 40mg powder for solution for infusion vials | 5 vial PoM £32.45 (Hospital only) | 5 vial PoM £26.00

Pantoprazole

▶ 77

- **INDICATIONS AND DOSE**

  Helicobacter pylori eradication in combination with amoxicillin and clarithromycin; or in combination with clarithromycin and metronidazole
  - ▶ BY MOUTH
  - ▶ Adult: 40 mg twice daily

  Benign gastric ulcer
  - ▶ BY MOUTH
  - ▶ Adult: 40 mg daily for 8 weeks; increased if necessary up to 80 mg daily, dose increased in severe cases

  Gastric ulcer
  - ▶ BY INTRAVENOUS INJECTION, OR BY INTRAVENOUS INFUSION
  - ▶ Adult: 40 mg daily until oral administration can be resumed, injection to be given over at least 2 minutes

  Duodenal ulcer
  - ▶ BY MOUTH
  - ▶ Adult: 40 mg daily for 4 weeks; increased if necessary up to 80 mg daily, dose increased in severe cases
  - ▶ BY INTRAVENOUS INJECTION, OR BY INTRAVENOUS INFUSION
  - ▶ Adult: 40 mg daily until oral administration can be resumed, injection to be given over at least 2 minutes

  Prophylaxis of NSAID-associated gastric ulcer in patients with an increased risk of gastroduodenal complications who require continued NSAID treatment | Prophylaxis of NSAID-associated duodenal ulcer in patients with an increased risk of gastroduodenal complications who require continued NSAID treatment
  - ▶ BY MOUTH
  - ▶ Adult: 20 mg daily

  Gastro-oesophageal reflux disease
  - ▶ BY MOUTH
  - ▶ Adult: 20–80 mg daily for 4 weeks, continued for further 4 weeks if not fully healed, dose to be taken in the morning; maintenance 20 mg daily and increased to 40 mg daily, increased only if symptoms return
  - ▶ BY INTRAVENOUS INJECTION, OR BY INTRAVENOUS INFUSION
  - ▶ Adult: 40 mg daily until oral administration can be resumed, injection to be given over at least 2 minutes

  Zollinger–Ellison syndrome (and other hypersecretory conditions)
  - ▶ BY MOUTH
  - ▶ Adult: Initially 80 mg daily (max. per dose 80 mg), adjusted according to response
  - ▶ Elderly: 40 mg daily
  - ▶ BY INTRAVENOUS INJECTION, OR BY INTRAVENOUS INFUSION
  - ▶ Adult: Initially 80 mg, alternatively 160 mg in 2 divided doses, if rapid acid control required, then 80 mg once daily (max. per dose 80 mg), adjusted according to response

- **INTERACTIONS** → Appendix 1: proton pump inhibitors
- **SIDE-EFFECTS**
  GENERAL SIDE-EFFECTS
  - ▶ **Uncommon** Asthenia · gastrointestinal discomfort · sleep disorder
  - ▶ **Rare or very rare** Angioedema · depression exacerbated · disorientation · hyperlipidaemia · weight change
  - ▶ **Frequency not known** Hepatocellular injury
  SPECIFIC SIDE-EFFECTS
  - ▶ **Frequency not known**
  - ▶ With intravenous use Electrolyte imbalance · muscle spasms
- **PREGNANCY** Manufacturer advises avoid unless potential benefit outweighs risk—fetotoxic in _animals_.
- **BREAST FEEDING** Manufacturer advises avoid unless potential benefit outweighs risk—small amount present in milk.

Gastro-intestinal system

1

- **HEPATIC IMPAIRMENT**
  Dose adjustments Max. 20 mg daily in severe impairment and cirrhosis.
  Monitoring Monitor liver function in hepatic impairment (discontinue if deterioration).
- **RENAL IMPAIRMENT**
  Dose adjustments Max. oral dose 40 mg daily.
- **DIRECTIONS FOR ADMINISTRATION** For *intravenous infusion* (*Protium* ®), give intermittently in Glucose 5% or Sodium chloride 0.9%; reconstitute 40 mg with 10 mL sodium chloride 0.9% and dilute with 100 mL of infusion fluid; give 40 mg over 15 minutes.
- **EXCEPTIONS TO LEGAL CATEGORY** Pantoprazole 20 mg tablets can be sold to the public for the short-term treatment of reflux symptoms (e.g. heartburn) in adults over 18 years, max. daily dose 20 mg for max. 4 weeks.

- **MEDICINAL FORMS**
  There can be variation in the licensing of different medicines containing the same drug. Forms available from special-order manufacturers include: oral suspension

Gastro-resistant tablet
CAUTIONARY AND ADVISORY LABELS 25
- Pantoprazole (Non-proprietary)
  Pantoprazole (as Pantoprazole sodium sesquihydrate)
  20 mg Pantoprazole 20mg gastro-resistant tablets | 28 tablet PoM £11.83 DT = £0.62
  Pantoprazole (as Pantoprazole sodium sesquihydrate)
  40 mg Pantoprazole 40mg gastro-resistant tablets | 28 tablet PoM £20.57 DT = £0.77

Powder for solution for injection
- Pantoprazole (Non-proprietary)
  Pantoprazole (as Pantoprazole sodium sesquihydrate)
  40 mg Pantoprazole 40mg powder for solution for injection vials | 1 vial PoM £5.00 | 5 vial PoM £22.50–£23.25
- Protium (Takeda UK Ltd)
  Pantoprazole (as Pantoprazole sodium sesquihydrate)
  40 mg Protium I.V. 40mg powder for solution for injection vials | 5 vial PoM £25.53

Rabeprazole sodium

F 77

07-Jun-2017

- **INDICATIONS AND DOSE**

Benign gastric ulcer
- BY MOUTH
- Adult: 20 mg daily for 8 weeks, dose to be taken in the morning

Duodenal ulcer
- BY MOUTH
- Adult: 20 mg daily for 4 weeks, dose to be taken in the morning

Gastro-oesophageal reflux disease
- BY MOUTH
- Adult: 20 mg once daily for 4-8 weeks; maintenance 10–20 mg daily

Gastro-oesophageal reflux disease (symptomatic treatment in the absence of oesophagitis)
- BY MOUTH
- Adult: 10 mg daily for up to 4 weeks, then 10 mg daily if required

Severe oesophagitis
- BY MOUTH
- Adult: 20 mg once daily for 8 weeks, continue as maintenance treatment if appropriate

Severe oesophagitis, refractory to initial treatment
- BY MOUTH
- Adult: 20 mg twice daily

Zollinger–Ellison syndrome
- BY MOUTH
- Adult: Initially 60 mg once daily, adjusted according to response, doses above 100 mg daily given in 2 divided doses; maximum 120 mg per day

Helicobacter pylori **eradication in combination with amoxicillin or metronidazole and clarithromycin**
- BY MOUTH
- Adult: 20 mg twice daily

- **UNLICENSED USE** EvGr Not licensed at 20 mg twice daily for severe oesophagitis refractory to initial treatment. Ⓐ
- **INTERACTIONS** → Appendix 1: proton pump inhibitors
- **SIDE-EFFECTS**
- **Common or very common** Asthenia · cough · increased risk of infection · influenza like illness · pain
- **Uncommon** Burping · dyspepsia · leg cramps · nervousness
- **Rare or very rare** Appetite decreased · gastritis · hepatic encephalopathy · leucocytosis · neutropenia · weight increased
- **Frequency not known** Chest pain · chills · fever
- **PREGNANCY** Manufacturer advises avoid—no information available.
- **BREAST FEEDING** Manufacturer advises avoid—no information available.
- **HEPATIC IMPAIRMENT** Manufacturer advises caution in severe hepatic dysfunction.

- **MEDICINAL FORMS**
  There can be variation in the licensing of different medicines containing the same drug.

Gastro-resistant tablet
CAUTIONARY AND ADVISORY LABELS 25
- Rabeprazole sodium (Non-proprietary)
  Rabeprazole sodium 10 mg Rabeprazole 10mg gastro-resistant tablets | 28 tablet PoM £11.56 DT = £0.99
  Rabeprazole sodium 20 mg Rabeprazole 20mg gastro-resistant tablets | 28 tablet PoM £19.55 DT = £1.34
- Pariet (Eisai Ltd)
  Rabeprazole sodium 10 mg Pariet 10mg gastro-resistant tablets | 28 tablet PoM £5.78 DT = £0.99
  Rabeprazole sodium 20 mg Pariet 20mg gastro-resistant tablets | 28 tablet PoM £11.34 DT = £1.34

4.3 Gastro-oesophageal reflux disease

Gastro-oesophageal reflux disease

Management

Gastro-oesophageal reflux disease (including non-erosive gastro-oesophageal reflux and erosive oesophagitis) is associated with heartburn, acid regurgitation, and sometimes, difficulty in swallowing (dysphagia); oesophageal inflammation (oesophagitis), ulceration, and stricture formation may occur and there is an association with asthma.

The management of gastro-oesophageal reflux disease includes drug treatment, lifestyle changes and, in some cases, surgery. Initial treatment is guided by the severity of symptoms and treatment is then adjusted according to response. The extent of healing depends on the severity of the disease, the treatment chosen, and the duration of therapy.

Patients with gastro-oesophageal reflux disease should be advised about lifestyle changes (avoidance of excess alcohol and of aggravating foods such as fats); other measures include weight reduction, smoking cessation, and raising the head of the bed.

For *mild symptoms* of gastro-oesophageal reflux disease, initial management may include the use of **antacids** and **alginates**. Alginate-containing antacids can form a 'raft' that floats on the surface of the stomach contents to reduce reflux and protect the oesophageal mucosa. **Histamine H₂-receptor antagonists** may relieve symptoms and permit reduction in antacid consumption. However, **proton pump inhibitors** provide more effective relief of symptoms than H₂-receptor antagonists. When symptoms abate, treatment is titrated down to a level which maintains remission (e.g. by giving treatment intermittently).

For *severe symptoms* of gastro-oesophageal reflux disease or for patients with a proven or severe pathology (e.g. *oesophagitis, oesophageal ulceration, oesophagopharyngeal reflux, Barrett's oesophagus*), initial management involves the use of a **proton pump inhibitor**; patients need to be reassessed if symptoms persist despite treatment for 4–6 weeks with a proton pump inhibitor. When symptoms abate, treatment is titrated down to a level which maintains remission (e.g. by reducing the dose of the proton pump inhibitor or by giving it intermittently, or by substituting treatment with a histamine H₂-receptor antagonist). However, for endoscopically confirmed *erosive, ulcerative*, or *stricturing* disease, or *Barrett's oesophagus*, treatment with a proton pump inhibitor usually needs to be maintained at the minimum effective dose.

Pregnancy

If dietary and lifestyle changes fail to control gastro-oesophageal reflux disease in pregnancy, an antacid or an alginate can be used. If this is ineffective, ranitidine p. 75 can be tried. Omeprazole p. 80 is reserved for women with severe or complicated reflux disease.

Gastro-oesophageal reflux disease in children

Gastro-oesophageal reflux disease is common in infancy but most symptoms resolve without treatment between 12 and 18 months of age. In infants, mild or moderate reflux without complications can be managed initially by changing the frequency and volume of feed; a feed thickener or thickened formula feed can be used (with advice of a dietitian). If necessary, a suitable alginate-containing preparation can be used instead of thickened feeds. For older children, life-style changes similar to those for adults may be helpful followed if necessary by treatment with an alginate-containing preparation.

Children who do not respond to these measures or who have problems such as respiratory disorders or suspected oesophagitis need to be referred to hospital; an H₂-receptor antagonist may be needed to reduce acid secretion. If the oesophagitis is resistant to H₂-receptor blockade, the proton pump inhibitor omeprazole can be tried.

ANTACIDS > ALGINATE

Sodium alginate with calcium carbonate and sodium bicarbonate

The properties listed below are those particular to the combination only. For the properties of the components please consider, alginic acid p. 69, sodium bicarbonate p. 1006, calcium carbonate p. 1013.

- ● **INDICATIONS AND DOSE**

Mild symptoms of gastro-oesophageal reflux disease
▶ BY MOUTH
  ▸ Child 6–11 years: 5–10 mL, to be taken after meals and at bedtime
  ▸ Child 12–17 years: 10–20 mL, to be taken after meals and at bedtime
  ▸ Adult: 10–20 mL, to be taken after meals and at bedtime

- ● INTERACTIONS → Appendix 1: calcium salts · sodium bicarbonate
- ● PRESCRIBING AND DISPENSING INFORMATION Flavours of oral liquid formulations may include aniseed or peppermint.
- ● PATIENT AND CARER ADVICE
  Medicines for Children leaflet: Gaviscon for gastro-oesophageal reflux disease www.medicinesforchildren.org.uk/gaviscon-gastro-oesophageal-reflux-disease
- ● MEDICINAL FORMS
  There can be variation in the licensing of different medicines containing the same drug.
  Oral suspension
  ELECTROLYTES: May contain Sodium
  ▸ Sodium alginate with calcium carbonate and sodium bicarbonate (Non-proprietary)
    Calcium carbonate 16 mg per 1 ml, Sodium bicarbonate 26.7 mg per 1 ml, Sodium alginate 50 mg per 1 ml Alginate raft-forming oral suspension sugar free aniseed sugar-free | 500 ml GSL 🅺 DT = £1.95
    Alginate raft-forming oral suspension sugar free sugar-free | 500 ml GSL 🅺 DT = £1.95
    Alginate raft-forming oral suspension sugar free peppermint sugar-free | 500 ml GSL 🅺 DT = £1.95
  ▸ Brands may include Acidex, Entrocalm Heartburn and Indigestion Relief, Gaviscon, Gaviscon Cool, Gaviscon Liquid Relief, Peptac

4.4 *Helicobacter pylori* diagnosis

DIAGNOSTIC AGENTS

Urea (13C)

- ● INDICATIONS AND DOSE
  Diagnosis of gastro-duodenal *Helicobacter pylori* infection
  ▶ BY MOUTH
    ▸ Adult: (consult product literature)

- ● MEDICINAL FORMS
  There can be variation in the licensing of different medicines containing the same drug.
  Soluble tablet
  ▸ Pylobactell (Torbet Laboratories Ltd)
    Urea [13-C] 100 mg Pylobactell breath test kit | 1 kit PoM £20.75
  Powder
  ▸ Helicobacter Test INFAI (INFAI UK Ltd)
    Urea [13-C] 45 mg Helicobacter Test INFAI for children breath test kit sugar-free | 1 kit PoM £19.10
    Urea [13-C] 75 mg Helicobacter Test INFAI breath test kit sugar-free | 1 kit PoM £21.70
  Tablet
  ▸ Diabact UBT (HFA Healthcare Products Ltd)
    Urea [13-C] 50 mg diabact UBT 50mg tablets | 1 tablet PoM £21.25

5 Food allergy

Food allergy

15-Dec-2016

Description of condition

Food allergy is an adverse immune response to a food, commonly associated with cutaneous and gastro-intestinal reactions, and less frequently associated with respiratory reactions and anaphylaxis. It is distinct from food intolerance which is non-immunological. Cow's milk, hen's eggs, soy, wheat, peanuts, tree nuts, fish, and shellfish are the most common allergens. Cross-reactivity between similar foods can occur (e.g. allergy to other mammalian milk in patients with cow's milk allergy).

1

Gastro-intestinal system

Management of food allergy

EvGr Allergy caused by specific foods should be managed by strict avoidance of the causal food. Sodium cromoglicate p. 270 is licensed as an adjunct to dietary avoidance in patients with food allergy. Educating patients about appropriate nutrition, food preparation, and the risks of accidental exposure is recommended, such as food and drinks to avoid, ensuring adequate nutritional intake, and interpreting food labels. Ⓐ

Drug treatment

EvGr There is low quality evidence to support the use of antihistamines to treat acute, **non-life-threatening** symptoms (such as flushing and urticaria) if accidental ingestion of allergenic food has occurred (see *Antihistamines*, under Antihistamines, allergen immunotherapy and allergic emergencies p. 276). Chlorphenamine maleate p. 283 is licensed for the symptomatic control of food allergy. In case of food-induced anaphylaxis, adrenaline/epinephrine p. 221 is the first-line immediate treatment (see also *Allergic emergencies*, under Antihistamines, allergen immunotherapy and allergic emergencies p. 276). Patients who are at risk of anaphylaxis should be trained to use self-injectable adrenaline/epinephrine. Ⓐ

6   Gastro-intestinal smooth muscle spasm

Antispasmodics

Antimuscarinics

The intestinal smooth muscle relaxant properties of antimuscarinic and other antispasmodic drugs may be useful in *irritable bowel syndrome*.

Antimuscarinics (formerly termed 'anticholinergics') reduce intestinal motility. They can be used for the management of *irritable bowel syndrome*.

Antimuscarinics that are used for gastro-intestinal smooth muscle spasm include the tertiary amines atropine sulfate p. 1295 and dicycloverine hydrochloride below and the quaternary ammonium compounds propantheline bromide p. 85 and hyoscine butylbromide p. 85. The quaternary ammonium compounds are less lipid soluble than atropine sulfate and are less likely to cross the blood–brain barrier; they are also less well absorbed from the gastro-intestinal tract.

Dicycloverine hydrochloride has a much less marked antimuscarinic action than atropine sulfate and may also have some direct action on smooth muscle. Hyoscine butylbromide is advocated as a gastro-intestinal antispasmodic, but it is poorly absorbed; the injection is useful in endoscopy and radiology. Atropine sulfate and the belladonna alkaloids are outmoded treatments, any clinical virtues being outweighed by atropinic side-effects.

Other indications for antimuscarinic drugs include arrhythmias, asthma and airways disease, motion sickness, parkinsonism, urinary incontinence, mydriasis and cycloplegia, premedication, and as an antidote to organophosphorus poisoning.

Other antispasmodics

Alverine citrate p. 86, mebeverine hydrochloride p. 86, and peppermint oil p. 47 are believed to be direct relaxants of intestinal smooth muscle and may relieve pain in *irritable bowel syndrome*. They have no serious adverse effects but, like all antispasmodics, should be avoided in paralytic ileus.

⟋ 759

Dicycloverine hydrochloride

(Dicyclomine hydrochloride)

● **INDICATIONS AND DOSE**

Symptomatic relief of gastro-intestinal disorders characterised by smooth muscle spasm

▸ BY MOUTH
▸ Child 6–23 months: 5–10 mg 3–4 times a day, dose to be taken 15 minutes before feeds
▸ Child 2–11 years: 10 mg 3 times a day
▸ Child 12–17 years: 10–20 mg 3 times a day
▸ Adult: 10–20 mg 3 times a day

● CONTRA-INDICATIONS Child under 6 months
● INTERACTIONS → Appendix 1: dicycloverine
● SIDE-EFFECTS Appetite decreased · fatigue · sedation · thirst
● PREGNANCY Not known to be harmful; manufacturer advises use only if essential.
● BREAST FEEDING Avoid—present in milk; apnoea reported in infant.
● EXCEPTIONS TO LEGAL CATEGORY Dicycloverine hydrochloride can be sold to the public provided that max. single dose is 10 mg and max. daily dose is 60 mg.
● MEDICINAL FORMS
There can be variation in the licensing of different medicines containing the same drug.

Oral solution
▸ Dicycloverine hydrochloride (Non-proprietary)
   Dicycloverine hydrochloride 2 mg per 1 ml Dicycloverine 10mg/5ml oral solution | 120 ml PoM £196.36 DT = £179.73
Tablet
▸ Dicycloverine hydrochloride (Non-proprietary)
   Dicycloverine hydrochloride 10 mg Dicycloverine 10mg tablets | 100 tablet PoM £201.22 DT = £184.25
   Dicycloverine hydrochloride 20 mg Dicycloverine 20mg tablets | 84 tablet PoM £203.42 DT = £196.69

Dicycloverine hydrochloride with aluminium hydroxide, magnesium oxide and simeticone

The properties listed below are those particular to the combination only. For the properties of the components please consider, dicycloverine hydrochloride above, aluminium hydroxide p. 1020, simeticone p. 71.

● **INDICATIONS AND DOSE**

Symptomatic relief of gastro-intestinal disorders characterised by smooth muscle spasm

▸ BY MOUTH
▸ Child 12-17 years: 10–20 mL every 4 hours as required
▸ Adult: 10–20 mL every 4 hours as required

● INTERACTIONS → Appendix 1: antacids · dicycloverine
● MEDICINAL FORMS
There can be variation in the licensing of different medicines containing the same drug.

Oral suspension
▸ Kolanticon (Peckforton Pharmaceuticals Ltd)
   Dicycloverine hydrochloride 500 microgram per 1 ml, Simeticone 4 mg per 1 ml, Magnesium oxide light 20 mg per 1 ml, Aluminium hydroxide dried 40 mg per 1 ml Kolanticon gel sugar-free | 200 ml Ⓟ £4.00 sugar-free | 500 ml Ⓟ £6.00

Hyoscine butylbromide

⚑ 759
13-Mar-2017

- **INDICATIONS AND DOSE**

Symptomatic relief of gastro-intestinal or genito-urinary disorders characterised by smooth muscle spasm

▸ BY MOUTH

- ‣ Child 6–11 years: 10 mg 3 times a day
- ‣ Child 12–17 years: 20 mg 4 times a day
- ‣ Adult: 20 mg 4 times a day

Irritable bowel syndrome

▸ BY MOUTH

- ‣ Adult: 10 mg 3 times a day; increased if necessary up to 20 mg 4 times a day

Acute spasm | Spasm in diagnostic procedures

▸ INITIALLY BY INTRAMUSCULAR INJECTION, OR BY SLOW INTRAVENOUS INJECTION

- ‣ Adult: 20 mg, then (by intramuscular injection or by slow intravenous injection) 20 mg after 30 minutes if required, dose may be repeated more frequently in endoscopy; maximum 100 mg per day

Excessive respiratory secretions in palliative care

▸ BY MOUTH

- ‣ Child 1 month–1 year: 300–500 micrograms/kg 3–4 times a day (max. per dose 5 mg)
- ‣ Child 2–4 years: 5 mg 3–4 times a day
- ‣ Child 5–11 years: 10 mg 3–4 times a day
- ‣ Child 12–17 years: 10–20 mg 3–4 times a day

▸ BY INTRAMUSCULAR INJECTION, OR BY INTRAVENOUS INJECTION

- ‣ Child 1 month–4 years: 300–500 micrograms/kg 3–4 times a day (max. per dose 5 mg)
- ‣ Child 5–11 years: 5–10 mg 3–4 times a day
- ‣ Child 12–17 years: 10–20 mg 3–4 times a day

▸ BY SUBCUTANEOUS INJECTION

- ‣ Adult: 20 mg every 4 hours if required, adjusted according to response to up to 20 mg every 1 hour

▸ BY SUBCUTANEOUS INFUSION

- ‣ Adult: 20–120 mg/24 hours

Bowel colic (in palliative care)

▸ BY MOUTH

- ‣ Child 1 month–1 year: 300–500 micrograms/kg 3–4 times a day (max. per dose 5 mg)
- ‣ Child 2–4 years: 5 mg 3–4 times a day
- ‣ Child 5–11 years: 10 mg 3–4 times a day
- ‣ Child 12–17 years: 10–20 mg 3–4 times a day

▸ BY INTRAMUSCULAR INJECTION, OR BY INTRAVENOUS INJECTION

- ‣ Child 1 month–4 years: 300–500 micrograms/kg 3–4 times a day (max. per dose 5 mg)
- ‣ Child 5–11 years: 5–10 mg 3–4 times a day
- ‣ Child 12–17 years: 10–20 mg 3–4 times a day

▸ BY SUBCUTANEOUS INJECTION

- ‣ Adult: 20 mg every 4 hours if required, adjusted according to response to up to 20 mg every 1 hour

▸ BY SUBCUTANEOUS INFUSION

- ‣ Adult: 60–300 mg/24 hours

PHARMACOKINETICS

- ‣ Administration by mouth is associated with poor absorption.

- **UNLICENSED USE** *Tablets* not licensed for use in children under 6 years. *Injection* not licensed for use in children (age range not specified by manufacturer).

IMPORTANT SAFETY INFORMATION

MHRA/CHM ADVICE: HYOSCINE BUTYLBROMIDE (*BUSCOPAN*®) INJECTION: RISK OF SERIOUS ADVERSE EFFECTS IN PATIENTS WITH UNDERLYING CARDIAC DISEASE (FEBRUARY 2017)

The MHRA advises that hyoscine butylbromide injection can cause serious adverse effects including tachycardia, hypotension, and anaphylaxis; several reports have noted that anaphylaxis is more likely to be fatal in patients with underlying coronary heart disease. Hyoscine butylbromide injection is contra-indicated in patients with tachycardia and should be used with caution in patients with cardiac disease; the MHRA recommends that these patients are monitored and that resuscitation equipment and trained personnel are readily available.

- **CONTRA-INDICATIONS**
- ‣ With intramuscular use or intravenous use or subcutaneous use Tachycardia
- **INTERACTIONS** → Appendix 1: hyoscine
- **SIDE-EFFECTS**

GENERAL SIDE-EFFECTS

- ‣ **Uncommon** Skin reactions
- ‣ **Frequency not known** Dyspnoea

SPECIFIC SIDE-EFFECTS

- ‣ With parenteral use Mydriasis
- **PREGNANCY** Manufacturer advises avoid.
- **BREAST FEEDING** Amount too small to be harmful.
- **DIRECTIONS FOR ADMINISTRATION**
- ‣ With oral use in children For administration by *mouth*, injection solution may be used; content of ampoule may be stored in a refrigerator for up to 24 hours after opening.
- ‣ With intravenous use in children For *intravenous injection*, may be diluted with Glucose 5% or Sodium Chloride 0.9%; give over at least 1 minute.
- **PRESCRIBING AND DISPENSING INFORMATION**

Palliative care For further information on the use of hyoscine butylbromide in palliative care, see www.palliativedrugs.com/formulary/en/hyoscine-butylbromide. html .

- **EXCEPTIONS TO LEGAL CATEGORY** Hyoscine butylbromide tablets can be sold to the public for medically confirmed irritable bowel syndrome, provided single dose does not exceed 20 mg, daily dose does not exceed 80 mg, and pack does not contain a total of more than 240 mg.

- **MEDICINAL FORMS**

There can be variation in the licensing of different medicines containing the same drug. Forms available from special-order manufacturers include: oral suspension, oral solution

Solution for injection

- ‣ Buscopan (Sanofi)

Hyoscine butylbromide 20 mg per 1 ml Buscopan 20mg/1ml solution for injection ampoules | 10 ampoule PoM £2.92 DT = £2.92

Tablet

- ‣ Buscopan (Sanofi)

Hyoscine butylbromide 10 mg Buscopan Cramps 10mg tablets | 20 tablet P £2.77
Buscopan 10mg tablets | 56 tablet PoM £3.00 DT = £3.00
Buscopan IBS Relief 10mg tablets | 20 tablet GSL £2.77 |
40 tablet GSL £4.64

Propantheline bromide

⚑ 759

- **INDICATIONS AND DOSE**

Symptomatic relief of gastro-intestinal disorders characterised by smooth muscle spasm

▸ BY MOUTH

- ‣ Child 12–17 years: 15 mg 3 times a day, dose to be taken at least one hour before food and 30 mg, dose to be taken at night; maximum 120 mg per day
- ‣ Adult: 15 mg 3 times a day, dose to be taken at least one hour before food and 30 mg, dose to be taken at night; maximum 120 mg per day

continued →

Adult enuresis
► BY MOUTH
► Adult: Initially 15 mg 3 times a day, dose to be taken at least one hour before food and 30 mg, dose to be taken at bedtime, subsequently adjusted according to response; maximum 120 mg per day

● INTERACTIONS → Appendix 1: propantheline
● SIDE-EFFECTS Arrhythmias · bronchial secretion decreased · mydriasis · photophobia · urinary hesitation
● PREGNANCY Manufacturer advises avoid unless essential—no information available.
● BREAST FEEDING May suppress lactation.
● HEPATIC IMPAIRMENT Manufacturer advises caution.
● RENAL IMPAIRMENT Manufacturer advises caution.

● MEDICINAL FORMS
There can be variation in the licensing of different medicines containing the same drug. Forms available from special-order manufacturers include: oral suspension, oral solution

Tablet
CAUTIONARY AND ADVISORY LABELS 23
► Pro-Banthine(Kyowa Kirin Ltd)
Propantheline bromide 15 mg Pro-Banthine 15mg tablets | 112 tablet [PoM] £20.74 DT = £20.74

ANTISPASMODICS

Alverine citrate

24-Feb-2016

● INDICATIONS AND DOSE
Symptomatic relief of gastro-intestinal disorders characterised by smooth muscle spasm | Dysmenorrhoea
► BY MOUTH
► Child 12-17 years: 60–120 mg 1–3 times a day
► Adult: 60–120 mg 1–3 times a day

● CONTRA-INDICATIONS Intestinal obstruction · paralytic ileus
● SIDE-EFFECTS Dizziness · dyspnoea · headache · jaundice (reversible on discontinuation) · nausea · skin reactions · wheezing
● PREGNANCY Manufacturer advises avoid—limited information available.
● BREAST FEEDING Manufacturer advises avoid—limited information available.
● PATIENT AND CARER ADVICE
Driving and skilled tasks Dizziness may affect performance of skilled tasks (e.g. driving).

● MEDICINAL FORMS
There can be variation in the licensing of different medicines containing the same drug.

Capsule
► Alverine citrate (Non-proprietary)
Alverine citrate 60 mg Alverine 60mg capsules | 100 capsule [P] £19.49 DT = £4.78
Alverine citrate 120 mg Alverine 120mg capsules | 60 capsule [P] £23.28 DT = £23.28
► Audmonal(Teva UK Ltd)
Alverine citrate 60 mg Audmonal 60mg capsules | 100 capsule [P] £14.80 DT = £4.78
Alverine citrate 120 mg Audmonal Forte 120mg capsules | 60 capsule [P] £17.75 DT = £23.28
► Gielism(HFA Healthcare Products Ltd)
Alverine citrate 60 mg Gielism 60mg capsules | 100 capsule [P] £19.48 DT = £4.78
► Spasmonal(Meda Pharmaceuticals Ltd)
Alverine citrate 60 mg Spasmonal 60mg capsules | 100 capsule [P] £16.45 DT = £4.78
Alverine citrate 120 mg Spasmonal Forte 120mg capsules | 60 capsule [P] £19.42 DT = £23.28

Mebeverine hydrochloride

● INDICATIONS AND DOSE
Adjunct in gastro-intestinal disorders characterised by smooth muscle spasm
► BY MOUTH USING IMMEDIATE-RELEASE MEDICINES
► Child 10-17 years: 135–150 mg 3 times a day, dose preferably taken 20 minutes before meals
► Adult: 135–150 mg 3 times a day, dose preferably taken 20 minutes before meals

Irritable bowel syndrome
► BY MOUTH USING MODIFIED-RELEASE MEDICINES
► Child 12-17 years: 200 mg twice daily
► Adult: 200 mg twice daily

● UNLICENSED USE *Granules* not licensed for use in children under 12 years. *Modified-release capsules* not licensed for use in children under 18 years.
● CONTRA-INDICATIONS Paralytic ileus
● SIDE-EFFECTS Angioedema · face oedema · skin reactions
● PREGNANCY Not known to be harmful—manufacturers advise avoid.
● BREAST FEEDING Manufacturers advise avoid—no information available.
● PATIENT AND CARER ADVICE Patients or carers should be given advice on the timing of administration of mebeverine hydrochloride tablets and oral suspension. Medicines for Children leaflet: Mebeverine for intestinal spasm www.medicinesforchildren.org.uk/mebeverine-for-intestinal-spasms
● EXCEPTIONS TO LEGAL CATEGORY
► In adults Mebeverine hydrochloride can be sold to the public for symptomatic relief of irritable bowel syndrome provided that max. single dose is 135 mg and max. daily dose is 405 mg; for uses other than symptomatic relief of irritable bowel syndrome provided that max. single dose is 100 mg and max. daily dose is 300 mg.

● MEDICINAL FORMS
There can be variation in the licensing of different medicines containing the same drug.
Oral suspension
► Mebeverine hydrochloride (Non-proprietary)
Mebeverine hydrochloride (as Mebeverine pamoate) 10 mg per 1 ml Mebeverine 50mg/5ml oral suspension sugar free sugar-free | 300 ml [PoM] £187.00 DT = £187.00
Modified-release capsule
CAUTIONARY AND ADVISORY LABELS 25
► Mebeverine hydrochloride (Non-proprietary)
Mebeverine hydrochloride 200 mg Mebeverine 200mg modified-release capsules | 60 capsule [PoM] £6.92 DT = £6.92
► Aurobeverine MR(Milpharm Ltd)
Mebeverine hydrochloride 200 mg Aurobeverine MR 200mg capsules | 60 capsule [PoM] £6.92 DT = £6.92
► Colofac MR(Mylan)
Mebeverine hydrochloride 200 mg Colofac MR 200mg capsules | 60 capsule [PoM] £6.92 DT = £6.92
Tablet
► Mebeverine hydrochloride (Non-proprietary)
Mebeverine hydrochloride 135 mg Mebeverine 135mg tablets | 100 tablet [PoM] £20.00 DT = £4.35
► Colofac(Mylan)
Mebeverine hydrochloride 135 mg Colofac 135mg tablets | 100 tablet [PoM] £9.02 DT = £4.35
Colofac IBS 135mg tablets | 15 tablet [P] £2.83

7 Liver disorders and related conditions

7.1 Biliary disorders

Cholestasis

01-May-2017

Description of condition

Cholestasis is an impairment of bile formation and/or bile flow, which may clinically present with fatigue, pruritus, dark urine, pale stools and, in its most overt form, jaundice and signs of fat soluble vitamin deficiencies.

Treatment of cholestatic pruritus

Several drugs are used to relieve cholestatic pruritus, even if evidence to support their use is limited.

EvGr Colestyramine p. 196 is the drug of choice for treating cholestatic pruritus. It is an anion-exchange resin that is not absorbed from the gastro-intestinal tract. It relieves pruritus by forming an insoluble complex in the intestine with bile acids and other compounds—the reduction of serum bile acid levels reduces excess deposition in the dermal tissue with a resultant decrease in pruritus. Ⓐ

EvGr Ursodeoxycholic acid p. 89 has a small and variable impact on cholestatic pruritus. Ⓔ

EvGr Rifampicin p. 571 [unlicensed indication] can be used as an alternative treatment for pruritus, but should be used with caution in patients with pre-existing liver disease because of possible hepatotoxicity. Ⓐ

EvGr Where previous therapy has proved ineffective or was not tolerated, other drugs including sertraline p. 364 [unlicensed indication] and naltrexone hydrochloride p. 491 [unlicensed indication], may be used to treat cholestatic pruritus. However, their use is limited due to significant side-effects. Ⓔ

Intrahepatic cholestasis in pregnancy

EvGr Ursodeoxycholic acid is effective for the treatment of pruritus associated with intrahepatic cholestasis in pregnancy. Ⓔ

Intrahepatic cholestasis usually occurs in late pregnancy and is associated with adverse fetal outcomes. EvGr There is no evidence that ursodeoxycholic acid used in late pregnancy affects birth weight in the infant or the risk of preterm delivery. There is limited data about the effect of fetal exposure during the first trimester. Ⓓ

Gallstones

01-May-2017

Description of condition

Gallstones (cholelithiases) occur when hard mineral or fatty deposits form in the gallbladder. Gallstone disease is a general term that describes the presence of one or more stones in the gallbladder or in the bile duct, and the symptoms and complications that they may cause.

The majority of patients with gallstones remain asymptomatic. When the stones irritate the gallbladder or block part of the biliary system, the patient can experience symptoms such as pain, or infection and inflammation that if left untreated, can lead to severe complications such as biliary colic, acute cholecystitis, cholangitis, pancreatitis, and obstructive jaundice.

Non-drug treatment

EvGr Asymptomatic gallbladder stones do not need to be treated unless symptoms develop.

The definitive treatment of symptomatic gallstones (and all bile duct stones) is surgical removal by laparoscopic cholecystectomy. Ⓐ

Drug treatment

EvGr Analgesia should be offered to control pain symptoms. Paracetamol p. 438 or a nonsteroidal anti-inflammatory drug (see Non-steroidal anti-inflammatory drugs p. 1094) is recommended for intermittent mild-to-moderate pain. Intramuscular diclofenac sodium p. 1101 can be given for severe pain or, if not suitable, an intramuscular opioid (such as morphine p. 456 or pethidine hydrochloride p. 463). Ⓐ

Although ursodeoxycholic acid p. 89 has been used for the management of gallstone disease, there is no evidence to support its use.

Useful Resources

Gallstone disease: diagnosis and management. National Institute for Health and Care Excellence. Clinical guideline 188. October 2014.
www.nice.org.uk/guidance/cg188

Inborn errors of primary bile acid synthesis

27-Apr-2018

Description of condition

Inborn errors of primary bile acid synthesis are a group of diseases in which the liver does not produce enough primary bile acids due to enzyme deficiencies. These acids are the main components of the bile, and include cholic acid and chenodeoxycholic acid.

Treatment

Cholic acid p. 88 is licensed for the treatment of inborn errors in primary bile acid synthesis due to an inborn deficiency of two specific liver enzymes. It acts by replacing some of the missing bile acids, therefore relieving the symptoms of the disease.

Chenodeoxycholic acid p. 88 is licensed for the treatment of inborn errors of primary bile acid synthesis due to a deficiency of one specific enzyme in the bile acid synthesis pathway when presenting as cerebrotendinous xanthomatosis.

Ursodeoxycholic acid p. 89 [unlicensed indication] has been used to treat inborn errors of primary bile acid synthesis, but there is an absence of evidence to recommend its use.

Primary biliary cholangitis

30-May-2017

Description of condition

Primary biliary cholangitis (or primary biliary cirrhosis) is a chronic cholestatic disease which develops due to progressive destruction of small and intermediate bile ducts within the liver, subsequently evolving to fibrosis and cirrhosis.

Treatment

EvGr Ursodeoxycholic acid p. 89 is recommended for the management of primary biliary cholangitis, including those with asymptomatic disease. It slows disease progression, but the effect on overall survival is uncertain. Liver transplantation can be considered in patients with advanced primary biliary cholangitis. Ⓐ

Gastro-intestinal system

1

Gastro-intestinal system

1

BILE ACIDS

Chenodeoxycholic acid

05-Apr-2018

- INDICATIONS AND DOSE

Cerebrotendinous xanthomatosis (specialist use only)
▶ BY MOUTH
▸ Adult: Initially 750 mg daily in 3 divided doses, increased if necessary up to 1000 mg daily in divided doses

- CONTRA-INDICATIONS Non-functioning gall bladder · radio-opaque stones
- INTERACTIONS → Appendix 1: chenodeoxycholic acid
- SIDE-EFFECTS Constipation
- PREGNANCY Manufacturer advises avoid—fetotoxicity reported in *animal* studies.
- HEPATIC IMPAIRMENT Manufacturer advises monitor—no information available.
- RENAL IMPAIRMENT Manufacturer advises monitor—no information available.
- MONITORING REQUIREMENTS Manufacturer advises to monitor serum cholestanol levels and/or urine bile alcohols every 3 months during the initiation of therapy and dose adjustment, and then at least annually; liver function should also be monitored during initiation of therapy and then at least annually; additional or more frequent investigations may need to be undertaken to monitor therapy during periods of fast growth or concomitant disease.
- DIRECTIONS FOR ADMINISTRATION For administration *by mouth* in patients who are unable to swallow capsules and/or need to take a dose below 250 mg, manufacturer advises to add capsule contents to sodium bicarbonate solution 8.4%—for further information, consult product literature.
- MEDICINAL FORMS
There can be variation in the licensing of different medicines containing the same drug.
Capsule
▸ Chenodeoxycholic acid (non-proprietary) ▼
Chenodeoxycholic acid 250 mg Chenodeoxycholic acid 250mg capsules | 100 capsule [PoM] £14,000.00

Cholic acid

21-Mar-2016

- DRUG ACTION Cholic acid is the predominant primary bile acid in humans, which can be used to provide a source of bile acid in patients with inborn deficiencies in bile acid synthesis.

- INDICATIONS AND DOSE

Inborn errors of primary bile acid synthesis (initiated by a specialist)
▶ BY MOUTH
▸ Adult: Usual dose 5–15 mg/kg daily; increased in steps of 50 mg daily in divided doses if required, dose to be given with food at the same time each day; Usual maximum 500 mg/24 hours

- INTERACTIONS → Appendix 1: cholic acid
- SIDE-EFFECTS Cholelithiasis (long term use) · diarrhoea · pruritus
SIDE-EFFECTS, FURTHER INFORMATION Patients presenting with pruritus and/or persistent diarrhoea should be investigated for potential overdose by a serum and/or urine bile acid assay.
- PREGNANCY Limited data available—not known to be harmful, manufacturer advises continue treatment.

Monitoring Manufacturer advises monitor patient parameters more frequently in pregnancy.
- BREAST FEEDING Present in milk but not known to be harmful.
- HEPATIC IMPAIRMENT
Monitoring Manufacturer advises monitor closely.
- MONITORING REQUIREMENTS Manufacturer advises monitor serum and/or urine bile-acid concentrations every 3 months for the first year, then every 6 months for three years, then annually; monitor liver function tests at the same or greater frequency.
- DIRECTIONS FOR ADMINISTRATION Manufacturer advises capsules may be opened and the content added to infant formula, juice, fruit compote, or yoghurt for administration.
- PATIENT AND CARER ADVICE Counselling advised on administration.
- MEDICINAL FORMS
There can be variation in the licensing of different medicines containing the same drug.
Capsule
CAUTIONARY AND ADVISORY LABELS 25
▸ Orphacol (Laboratoires CTRS) ▼
Cholic acid 50 mg Orphacol 50mg capsules | 30 capsule £1,860.00 | 60 capsule [PoM] £3,720.00
Cholic acid 250 mg Orphacol 250mg capsules | 30 capsule [PoM] £6,630.00

Obeticholic acid

15-May-2018

- DRUG ACTION Obeticholic acid is a selective farnesoid X receptor agonist, which decreases circulating bile acid.

- INDICATIONS AND DOSE

Primary biliary cholangitis in combination with ursodeoxycholic acid when response to ursodeoxycholic acid has been inadequate, or as monotherapy in patients intolerant of ursodeoxycholic acid
▶ BY MOUTH
▸ Adult: Initially 5 mg once daily for 6 months, then increased if tolerated to 10 mg once daily, for dose adjustments due to severe pruritus, consult product literature

> **IMPORTANT SAFETY INFORMATION**
> MHRA/CHM ADVICE: OBETICHOLIC ACID (*OCALIVA*®): RISK OF SERIOUS LIVER INJURY IN PATIENTS WITH PRE-EXISTING MODERATE OR SEVERE HEPATIC IMPAIRMENT; REMINDER TO ADJUST DOSING ACCORDING TO LIVER FUNCTION MONITORING (APRIL 2018)
> The MHRA is aware of reports of serious liver injuries and deaths in patients with primary biliary cholangitis with pre-existing moderate or severe liver impairment who were not adequately dose-adjusted. Follow dose reduction and monitoring advice in these patients to reduce the risk of serious liver injury; for further information, see *Hepatic impairment* and *Monitoring*.

- CONTRA-INDICATIONS Complete biliary obstruction
- INTERACTIONS → Appendix 1: obeticholic acid
- SIDE-EFFECTS
▶ Common or very common Arthralgia · constipation · dizziness · fatigue · fever · gastrointestinal discomfort · oropharyngeal pain · palpitations · peripheral oedema · skin reactions
▶ Frequency not known Hepatic failure
- PREGNANCY
Dose adjustments No evidence of harm but manufacturer advises avoid.

- BREAST FEEDING Not known to be harmful but manufacturer advises avoid.
- HEPATIC IMPAIRMENT
  Dose adjustments Manufacturer advises reduce initial dose to 5 mg once weekly in moderate-to-severe impairment; dose may be increased if necessary according to level of alkaline phosphatase and/or total bilirubin—consult product literature.
- MONITORING REQUIREMENTS Manufacturer advises assess hepatic status before treatment initiation and then monitor for progression of primary biliary cholangitis with laboratory and clinical assessment to evaluate the need for dose reduction; patients at an increased risk of hepatic decompensation, including those with laboratory evidence of worsening liver function and/or progression to cirrhosis, should be monitored more closely.
- NATIONAL FUNDING/ACCESS DECISIONS

  NICE decisions
  ▶ **Obeticholic acid for treating primary biliary cholangitis (April 2017)** NICE TA443
  Obeticholic acid (*Ocaliva®*) is recommended as an option for treating primary biliary cholangitis, in combination with ursodeoxycholic acid when response to ursodeoxycholic acid is inadequate, or as monotherapy when ursodeoxycholic acid is not tolerated and only if the manufacturer provides obeticholic acid with the discount agreed in the patient access scheme. Response to obeticholic acid should be assessed after 12 months and treatment continued only if there is evidence of clinical benefit.
  www.nice.org.uk/guidance/ta443

  Scottish Medicines Consortium (SMC) Decisions
  The *Scottish Medicines Consortium* has advised (June 2017) that obeticholic acid (*Ocaliva®*) is accepted for use within NHS Scotland for the treatment of primary biliary cholangitis in combination with ursodeoxycholic acid when response to ursodeoxycholic acid is inadequate, or as monotherapy when ursodeoxycholic acid is not tolerated. This advice is contingent upon the continuing availability of the patient access scheme in NHS Scotland or a list price that is equivalent or lower.

- MEDICINAL FORMS
  There can be variation in the licensing of different medicines containing the same drug.
  Tablet
  ▶ Ocaliva (Intercept Pharma UK & Ireland Ltd) ▼
  Obeticholic acid 5 mg Ocaliva 5mg tablets | 30 tablet [PoM] £2,384.04 (Hospital only)
  Obeticholic acid 10 mg Ocaliva 10mg tablets | 30 tablet [PoM] £2,384.04 (Hospital only)

Ursodeoxycholic acid

- INDICATIONS AND DOSE
  Dissolution of gallstones
  ▶ BY MOUTH
  ▶ Adult: 8–12 mg/kg once daily, dose to be taken at bedtime, alternatively 8–12 mg/kg daily in 2 divided doses for up to 2 years; treatment is continued for 3–4 months after stones dissolve

  Primary biliary cirrhosis
  ▶ BY MOUTH
  ▶ Adult: 12–16 mg/kg daily in 3 divided doses for 3 months, then 12–16 mg/kg once daily, dose to be taken at bedtime

- CONTRA-INDICATIONS Acute inflammation of the gall bladder · frequent episodes of biliary colic · inflammatory diseases and other conditions of the colon, liver or small intestine which interfere with enterohepatic circulation of

bile salts · non-functioning gall bladder · radio-opaque stones
- CAUTIONS Liver disease
- INTERACTIONS → Appendix 1: ursodeoxycholic acid
- SIDE-EFFECTS
  ▶ **Common or very common** Diarrhoea · pale faeces
  ▶ **Rare or very rare** Cholelithiasis calcification · skin reactions
  ▶ **Frequency not known** Nausea · vomiting
- PREGNANCY No evidence of harm but manufacturer advises avoid.
- BREAST FEEDING Not known to be harmful but manufacturer advises avoid.
- HEPATIC IMPAIRMENT Avoid in chronic liver disease (but used in primary biliary cirrhosis).
- MONITORING REQUIREMENTS In primary biliary cirrhosis, monitor liver function every 4 weeks for 3 months, then every 3 months.
- PATIENT AND CARER ADVICE Patients should be given dietary advice (including avoidance of excessive cholesterol and calories).

- MEDICINAL FORMS
  There can be variation in the licensing of different medicines containing the same drug. Forms available from special-order manufacturers include: oral suspension, oral solution
  Oral suspension
  CAUTIONARY AND ADVISORY LABELS 21
  ▶ Ursofalk (Dr. Falk Pharma UK Ltd)
  Ursodeoxycholic acid 50 mg per 1 ml Ursofalk 250mg/5ml oral suspension sugar-free | 250 ml [PoM] £26.98 DT = £26.98
  Tablet
  CAUTIONARY AND ADVISORY LABELS 21
  ▶ Ursodeoxycholic acid (Non-proprietary)
  Ursodeoxycholic acid 150 mg Ursodeoxycholic acid 150mg tablets | 60 tablet [PoM] £19.02 DT = £19.02
  Ursodeoxycholic acid 300 mg Ursodeoxycholic acid 300mg tablets | 60 tablet [PoM] £47.63 DT = £47.63
  ▶ Cholurso (HFA Healthcare Products Ltd)
  Ursodeoxycholic acid 250 mg Cholurso 250mg tablets | 60 tablet [PoM] £15.49 DT = £15.49
  Ursodeoxycholic acid 500 mg Cholurso 500mg tablets | 60 tablet [PoM] £45.00
  ▶ Destolit (Norgine Pharmaceuticals Ltd)
  Ursodeoxycholic acid 150 mg Destolit 150mg tablets | 60 tablet [PoM] £18.39 DT = £19.02
  ▶ Ursofalk (Dr. Falk Pharma UK Ltd)
  Ursodeoxycholic acid 500 mg Ursofalk 500mg tablets | 100 tablet [PoM] £80.00 DT = £80.00
  Capsule
  CAUTIONARY AND ADVISORY LABELS 21
  ▶ Ursodeoxycholic acid (Non-proprietary)
  Ursodeoxycholic acid 250 mg Ursodeoxycholic acid 250mg capsules | 60 capsule [PoM] £31.50 DT = £15.75 | 100 capsule [PoM] £26.25
  ▶ Ursofalk (Dr. Falk Pharma UK Ltd)
  Ursodeoxycholic acid 250 mg Ursofalk 250mg capsules | 60 capsule [PoM] £30.17 DT = £15.75 | 100 capsule [PoM] £31.88

TERPENES

Borneol with camphene, cineole, menthol, menthone and pinene

- INDICATIONS AND DOSE
  Biliary disorders
  ▶ BY MOUTH
  ▶ Adult: 1–2 capsules 3 times a day, to be taken before food

- LESS SUITABLE FOR PRESCRIBING *Rowachol®* is less suitable for prescribing.

7.2   Oesophageal varices

Other drugs used for Oesophageal varices Vasopressin,
p. 655

PITUITARY AND HYPOTHALAMIC HORMONES
AND ANALOGUES ⟩ VASOPRESSIN AND
ANALOGUES

Terlipressin acetate

● **INDICATIONS AND DOSE**

GLYPRESSIN ® INJECTION

Bleeding from oesophageal varices
▸ BY INTRAVENOUS INJECTION
▸ Adult (body-weight up to 50 kg): Initially 2 mg every
  4 hours until bleeding controlled, then reduced to 1 mg
  every 4 hours if required, maximum duration 48 hours
▸ Adult (body-weight 50 kg and above): Initially 2 mg every
  4 hours until bleeding controlled, reduced if not
  tolerated to 1 mg every 4 hours, maximum duration
  48 hours

VARIQUEL ® INJECTION

Bleeding from oesophageal varices
▸ BY INTRAVENOUS INJECTION
▸ Adult (body-weight up to 50 kg): Initially 1 mg, then 1 mg
  every 4–6 hours for up to 72 hours, to be administered
  over 1 minute
▸ Adult (body-weight 50-69 kg): Initially 1.5 mg, then 1 mg
  every 4–6 hours for up to 72 hours, to be administered
  over 1 minute
▸ Adult (body-weight 70 kg and above): Initially 2 mg, then
  1 mg every 4–6 hours for up to 72 hours, to be
  administered over 1 minute

● CAUTIONS Arrhythmia · elderly · electrolyte and fluid
  disturbances · heart disease · history of QT-interval
  prolongation · respiratory disease · septic shock ·
  uncontrolled hypertension · vascular disease
● SIDE-EFFECTS
▸ **Common or very common** Abdominal cramps · arrhythmias
  · diarrhoea · headache · hypertension · hypotension · pallor
  · peripheral ischaemia · vasoconstriction
▸ **Uncommon** Chest pain · cyanosis · fluid overload · heart
  failure · hot flush · hyponatraemia · intestinal ischaemia ·
  ischaemic heart disease · lymphangitis · myocardial
  infarction · nausea · pulmonary oedema · respiratory
  disorders · seizure · skin necrosis · uterine disorders ·
  vomiting
▸ **Rare or very rare** Dyspnoea · hyperglycaemia · stroke
● PREGNANCY Avoid unless benefits outweigh risk—uterine
  contractions and increased intra-uterine pressure in early
  pregnancy, and decreased uterine blood flow reported.
● BREAST FEEDING Avoid unless benefits outweigh risk—no
  information available.
● RENAL IMPAIRMENT Use with caution in chronic renal
  failure.

8   Obesity

Obesity

01-Jun-2016

Description of condition

Obesity is directly linked to many health problems including
cardiovascular disease, type 2 diabetes, fatty liver disease,
gallstones, and gastro-oesophageal reflux disease. It is also
linked to psychological and psychiatric morbidities.
   In adults, obesity is generally classified as a body mass
index (BMI) of $\geq 30\ \mathrm{kg/m^2}$, though BMI should be interpreted
with caution as it is not a direct measure of adiposity,
particularly in patients who are very muscular or have
muscle weakness or atrophy.
   Waist circumference should also be considered as it may
provide an indication of total body fat and a risk of obesity-
related health problems. Men with a waist circumference
$\geq 94\ \mathrm{cm}$ ($\geq 90\ \mathrm{cm}$ for Asian men), and women with a waist
circumference of $\geq 80\ \mathrm{cm}$ are at increased risk of obesity-
related health problems. A waist circumference of $\geq 102\ \mathrm{cm}$
in men and $\geq 88\ \mathrm{cm}$ in women indicates a very high risk of
obesity-related health problems.

Aims of treatment

Management should be aimed at modest, sustainable weight
loss and maintenance of a healthy weight, to reduce the risk
factors associated with obesity.

Overview

EvGr Obesity should be managed in an appropriate setting
by staff who have been trained in the management of
obesity. Patients should be monitored for changes in weight,
as well as changes in blood pressure and blood lipids, and for
other associated conditions.
   An initial assessment should consider potential
underlying causes (e.g. hypothyroidism) and a review of the
appropriateness of current medications which are known to
cause weight gain, e.g. atypical antipsychotics, beta-
adrenoceptor blocking drugs, insulin (when used in the
treatment of type 2 diabetes), lithium carbonate, lithium
citrate, sodium valproate, sulphonylureas,
thiazolidinediones, and tricyclic antidepressants. Ⓐ

Lifestyle changes

EvGr Patients should be encouraged to engage in a
sustainable weight management programme which includes
strategies to change behaviour, increase physical activity,
and improve diet and eating behaviour. Ⓐ

Drug treatment

EvGr Drug treatment should **never** be used as the sole
element of treatment and should be used as part of an
overall weight management plan. An anti-obesity drug
should be considered only for those with a BMI of
$\geq 30\ \mathrm{kg/m^2}$, in whom diet, exercise and behaviour changes
fail to achieve a realistic reduction in weight. In the presence
of associated risk factors, it may be appropriate to prescribe
an anti-obesity drug to individuals with a BMI of $\geq 28\ \mathrm{kg/m^2}$.
A vitamin and mineral supplement may also be considered if

there is concern about inadequate micronutrient intake, particularly for vulnerable groups such as in the elderly and younger patients.

The effect of management should be monitored on a regular basis with reinforcement of supporting lifestyle advice. Rates of weight loss may be slower in patients with type 2 diabetes, so less strict goals than in those without diabetes may be appropriate.

Orlistat below, is the only drug currently available in the UK that is recommended specifically for the management of obesity; it acts by reducing the absorption of dietary fat.

Orlistat is licensed for use as an adjunct in the management of obesity in patients with a BMI of $\geq 30 \text{ kg/m}^2$, or, in individuals with a BMI of $\geq 28 \text{ kg/m}^2$ in the presence of other risk factors. Treatment with orlistat may also be used to maintain weight loss rather than to continue to lose weight. Discontinuation of treatment with orlistat should be considered after 12 weeks if weight loss has not exceeded 5% since the start of treatment. Ⓐ

Drugs which produce a feeling of satiety (such as methylcellulose p. 54 and sterculia p. 54 [unlicensed indications]) have been used in an attempt to control appetite, but there is little evidence for their efficacy. Various centrally acting appetite suppressants, including stimulants and serotonergic drugs (such as dexfenfluramine, fenfluramine, sibutramine, and rimonabant), have been used in the management of obesity but have been withdrawn or are no longer recommended due to serious safety concerns or their addictive potential.

Surgery

ᴇᵥᴳʳ Bariatric surgery may be considered for patients who have a BMI of $\geq 40 \text{ kg/m}^2$ (Obesity III, morbid obesity), or between 35–39.9 kg/m^2 (Obesity II) and a significant disease (such as type 2 diabetes or high blood pressure) which could be improved with weight loss, and if all appropriate non-surgical measures have been tried but clinically beneficial weight loss has not been achieved or maintained. Ⓐ

Useful Resources

Obesity: identification, assessment and management. Clinical Guideline 189. National Institute for Health and Care Excellence. November 2014.
www.nice.org.uk/guidance/cg189

> **Other drugs used for Obesity** Liraglutide, p. 685

ANTIDEPRESSANTS > SEROTONIN AND NORADRENALINE RE-UPTAKE INHIBITORS

Naltrexone with bupropion   30-Jan-2018

The properties listed below are those particular to the combination only. For the properties of the components please consider, bupropion hydrochloride p. 491, naltrexone hydrochloride p. 491.

- ● **INDICATIONS AND DOSE**

  Adjunct in obesity (in conjunction with dietary measures and increased physical activity in individuals with a body mass index (BMI) of 30 kg/m^2 or more or in individuals with a BMI of 27 kg/m^2 or more in the presence of one or more weight related co-morbidity)
  - ▸ BY MOUTH
  - ▸ Adult 18-75 years: Initially 1 tablet daily for 7 days, then increased to 1 tablet twice daily for 7 days, then increased to 3 tablets daily in divided doses for 7 days, two tablets to be taken in the morning, and one tablet to be taken in the evening, then maintenance 2 tablets twice daily, review treatment after 16 weeks and then annually

- ▸ Each tablet contains 8 mg naltrexone with 90 mg bupropion.

- ● **CONTRA-INDICATIONS** Uncontrolled hypertension
- ● **CAUTIONS** History of mania · hypertension
- ● **INTERACTIONS** → Appendix 1: bupropion · naltrexone
- ● **HEPATIC IMPAIRMENT** Manufacturer advises avoid—no information available.
- ● **RENAL IMPAIRMENT** Manufacturer advises avoid in moderate-to-severe impairment—limited information available.
- ● **PRESCRIBING AND DISPENSING INFORMATION** Prescribers should consult the *Mysimba® Physician Prescribing Checklist* provided by the manufacturer, before initiation of treatment.
- ● **NATIONAL FUNDING/ACCESS DECISIONS**

  NICE decisions
  - ▸ **Naltrexone–bupropion for managing overweight and obesity (December 2017)** NICE TA494

  Naltrexone–bupropion is not recommended within its marketing authorisation for managing overweight and obesity in adults alongside a reduced-calorie diet and increased physical activity.

  Patients whose treatment was started within the NHS before this guidance was published should have the option to continue treatment, without change to their funding arrangements, until they and their NHS clinician consider it appropriate to stop.
  www.nice.org.uk/guidance/ta494

- ● **MEDICINAL FORMS** There can be variation in the licensing of different medicines containing the same drug.

  Modified-release tablet
  CAUTIONARY AND ADVISORY LABELS 21, 25
  - ▸ Mysimba (Consilient Health Ltd) ▼

    Naltrexone hydrochloride 8 mg, Bupropion hydrochloride 90 mg Mysimba 8mg/90mg modified-release tablets | 112 tablet ᴘᴏᴍ £73.00

PERIPHERALLY ACTING ANTIOBESITY PRODUCTS > LIPASE INHIBITORS

Orlistat

- ● **DRUG ACTION** Orlistat, a lipase inhibitor, reduces the absorption of dietary fat.

- ● **INDICATIONS AND DOSE**

  Adjunct in obesity (in conjunction with a mildly hypocaloric diet in individuals with a body mass index (BMI) of 30 kg/m^2 or more or in individuals with a BMI of 28 kg/m^2 or more in the presence of other risk factors such as type 2 diabetes, hypertension, or hypercholesterolaemia)
  - ▸ BY MOUTH
  - ▸ Adult: 120 mg up to 3 times a day, dose to be taken immediately before, during, or up to 1 hour after each main meal, continue treatment beyond 12 weeks only if weight loss since start of treatment exceeds 5% (target for initial weight loss may be lower in patients with type 2 diabetes), if a meal is missed or contains no fat, the dose of orlistat should be omitted

- ● **CONTRA-INDICATIONS** Cholestasis · chronic malabsorption syndrome
- ● **CAUTIONS** Chronic kidney disease · may impair absorption of fat-soluble vitamins · volume depletion
  CAUTIONS, FURTHER INFORMATION Vitamin supplementation (especially of vitamin D) may be

1

Gastro-intestinal system

considered if there is concern about deficiency of fat-soluble vitamins.

● INTERACTIONS → Appendix 1: orlistat

● SIDE-EFFECTS

▸ **Common or very common** Abdominal pain (may be minimised by reduced fat intake) · anxiety · diarrhoea · gastrointestinal disorders

▸ **Frequency not known** Anorectal haemorrhage · bullous dermatitis · cholelithiasis · diverticulitis · hepatitis · oxalate nephropathy · pancreatitis · renal failure

● PREGNANCY Use with caution.

● BREAST FEEDING Avoid—no information available.

● MEDICINAL FORMS
There can be variation in the licensing of different medicines containing the same drug.

Capsule

▸ Orlistat (Non-proprietary)
Orlistat 120 mg Orlistat 120mg capsules | 84 capsule PoM £35.43 DT = £15.90

▸ Alli (GlaxoSmithKline Consumer Healthcare)
Orlistat 60 mg Alli 60mg capsules | 84 capsule P £30.70

▸ Beacita (Actavis UK Ltd)
Orlistat 120 mg Beacita 120mg capsules | 84 capsule PoM £31.63 DT = £15.90

▸ Orlos (Crescent Pharma Ltd)
Orlistat 60 mg Orlos 60mg capsules | 84 capsule P £9.89

▸ Xenical (Cheplapharm Arzneimittel GmbH)
Orlistat 120 mg Xenical 120mg capsules | 84 capsule PoM £31.63 DT = £15.90

9 Rectal and anal disorders

9.1 Anal fissures

Anal fissure

31-Aug-2016

Description of condition

An anal fissure is a tear or ulcer in the lining of the anal canal, immediately within the anal margin. Clinical features of anal fissure include bleeding and persistent pain on defecation, and a linear split in the anal mucosa.

Aims of treatment

The aim of treatment is to relieve pain and promote healing of the fissure.

Drug treatment

Acute anal fissure

EvGr Initial management of acute anal fissures (present for less than 6 weeks) should focus on ensuring that stools are soft and easily passed. Bulk-forming laxatives (such as ispaghula husk p. 54) are recommended and an osmotic laxative (such as lactulose p. 56) can be considered as an alternative—see also Constipation p. 52, for further information about these laxatives. Short-term use of a topical preparation containing a local anaesthetic (such as lidocaine hydrochloride p. 1312) or a simple analgesic (such as paracetamol p. 438 or ibuprofen p. 1106) may be offered for prolonged burning pain following defecation. If these measures are inadequate, the patient should be referred for specialist treatment in hospital. Ⓐ

Chronic anal fissure

EvGr Chronic anal fissures (present for 6 weeks or longer), and associated pain, may be treated with glyceryl trinitrate rectal ointment 0.4% or 0.2% p. 217 [unlicensed] (available from Special-order manufacturers p. 1573 or specialist importing companies). Limited evidence suggests that the strength used does not influence the effectiveness, but that the higher strength potentially increases the incidence of

side-effects. Healing rates with topical glyceryl trinitrate are marginally superior to placebo, but the incidence of headache as an adverse effect is quite high (about 20-30% of patients). Recurrence of the fissure after treatment is common.

As an alternative to glyceryl trinitrate rectal ointment, chronic anal fissure may also be treated with topical diltiazem hydrochloride 2% [unlicensed] or nifedipine 0.2-0.5% [unlicensed] (available from Special-order manufacturers or specialist importing companies), which have a lower incidence of adverse effects than topical glyceryl trinitrate. Oral nifedipine p. 162 [unlicensed indication] and oral diltiazem hydrochloride p. 157 [unlicensed indication] may be as effective as topical treatment, but the incidence of adverse effects are likely to be higher and topical preparations are preferred.

Patients who do not respond to first-line treatment may be referred to a specialist for local injection of botulinum toxin type A [unlicensed indication]. Ⓐ

Non-drug treatment

EvGr Surgery is an effective option for the management of chronic anal fissure in adults but is generally reserved for those who do not respond to drug treatment. Ⓐ

9.2 Haemorrhoids

Haemorrhoids

01-Dec-2016

Description of condition

Haemorrhoids, or piles, are abnormal swellings of the vascular mucosal anal cushions around the anus. Internal haemorrhoids arise above the dentate line and are usually painless unless they become strangulated. External haemorrhoids originate below the dentate line and can be itchy or painful. Women are predisposed to developing haemorrhoids during pregnancy.

Aims of treatment

The aims of treatment are to reduce the symptoms (pain, bleeding and swelling), promote healing, and prevent recurrence.

Non-drug treatment

EvGr Stools should be kept soft and easy to pass (to minimise straining) by increasing dietary fibre and fluid intake. Advice about perianal hygiene is helpful to aid healing and reduce irritation and itching. Ⓐ

Drug treatment

EvGr If constipation is reported, it should be treated. A bulk-forming laxative can be prescribed (see Constipation p. 52)

A simple analgesic such as paracetamol p. 438 can be used for pain relief. Opioid analgesics should be avoided as they can cause constipation, and NSAIDs should be avoided if rectal bleeding is present. Ⓐ

Topical preparations that contain a combination of local anaesthetics, corticosteroids, astringents, lubricants, and antiseptics are available—see *Related drugs* below. EvGr They can offer symptomatic relief of local pain and itching but evidence does not suggest that any preparation is more effective than any other.

Topical preparations containing local anaesthetics (lidocaine, benzocaine, cinchocaine and pramocaine) should only be used for a few days as they may cause sensitisation of the anal skin. Local anaesthetics can be absorbed through the rectal mucosa (with a theoretical risk of systemic side effects) and very rarely may cause increased irritation; therefore excessive application should be **avoided**. Ⓐ

Topical preparations combining corticosteroids with local anaesthetics and soothing agents are available for the management of haemorrhoids. They may ameliorate local perianal inflammation, but no data suggest that they actually reduce haemorrhoidal swelling, bleeding, or protrusion.

EvGr Topical corticosteroids are suitable for occasional short-term use (no more than 7 days) after exclusion of infections (such as perianal streptococcal infection, *herpes simplex* or perianal thrush). Long-term use of corticosteroid creams can cause ulceration or permanent damage due to thinning of the perianal skin and should be avoided. Ⓐ Continuous or excessive use carries a risk of adrenal suppression and systemic corticosteroid effects.

EvGr Recurrent symptoms, should be referred to secondary care for further investigation and management.

Treatments available from *specialists* include rubber band ligation, injection sclerotherapy (using phenol in oil p. 95), infrared coagulation/photocoagulation, bipolar diathermy and direct-current electrotherapy, haemorrhoidectomy, stapled haemorrhoidectomy, and haemorrhoidal artery ligation. Ⓐ

Pregnancy
EvGr Bulk forming laxatives are not absorbed, and are therefore safe for use in pregnant women (see Pregnancy, under Constipation p. 52). Ⓐ No topical haemorrhoidal preparations are licensed for use during pregnancy.

EvGr If treatment with a topical haemorrhoidal preparation is required, a soothing preparation containing simple, soothing products (**not** local anaesthetics or corticosteroids) can be considered. Ⓐ

Related drugs
Topical preparations used for haemorrhoids: lidocaine hydrochloride p. 1312, benzyl benzoate with bismuth oxide, bismuth subgallate, hydrocortisone acetate, peru balsam and zinc oxide below, cinchocaine hydrochloride with fluocortolone caproate and fluocortolone pivalate below, cinchocaine with hydrocortisone p. 94, cinchocaine with prednisolone p. 94.

CORTICOSTEROIDS

Benzyl benzoate with bismuth oxide, bismuth subgallate, hydrocortisone acetate, peru balsam and zinc oxide
21-Dec-2017

● INDICATIONS AND DOSE
Haemorrhoids | Pruritus ani
▶ BY RECTUM USING OINTMENT
▶ Adult: Apply twice daily for no longer than 7 days, to be applied morning and night, an additional dose should be applied after a bowel movement
▶ BY RECTUM USING SUPPOSITORIES
▶ Adult: 1 suppository twice daily for no longer than 7 days, to be inserted night and morning, additional dose after a bowel movement

IMPORTANT SAFETY INFORMATION
MHRA/CHM ADVICE: CORTICOSTEROIDS: RARE RISK OF CENTRAL SEROUS CHORIORETINOPATHY WITH LOCAL AS WELL AS SYSTEMIC ADMINISTRATION (AUGUST 2017)
See *Corticosteroids, general use* p. 656.

● CAUTIONS Local anaesthetic component can be absorbed through the rectal mucosa (avoid excessive application, particularly in children and infants) · local anaesthetic component may cause sensitisation (use for short periods only—no longer than a few days)

● PRESCRIBING AND DISPENSING INFORMATION A proprietary brand *Anusol Plus HC®* (ointment and suppositories) is on sale to the public.

● MEDICINAL FORMS
There can be variation in the licensing of different medicines containing the same drug.
Ointment
▶ Anusol-Hc (Church & Dwight UK Ltd)
Hydrocortisone acetate 2.5 mg per 1 gram, Bismuth oxide 8.75 mg per 1 gram, Benzyl benzoate 12.5 mg per 1 gram, Peru Balsam 18.75 mg per 1 gram, Bismuth subgallate 22.5 mg per 1 gram, Zinc oxide 107.5 mg per 1 gram Anusol HC ointment | 30 gram PoM £2.49
Suppository
▶ Anusol-Hc (Church & Dwight UK Ltd)
Hydrocortisone acetate 10 mg, Bismuth oxide 24 mg, Benzyl benzoate 33 mg, Peru Balsam 49 mg, Bismuth subgallate 59 mg, Zinc oxide 296 mg Anusol HC suppositories | 12 suppository PoM £1.74

Cinchocaine hydrochloride with fluocortolone caproate and fluocortolone pivalate
21-Dec-2017

● INDICATIONS AND DOSE
Haemorrhoids | Pruritus ani
▶ BY RECTUM USING OINTMENT
▶ Adult: Apply twice daily for 5–7 days, apply 3–4 times a day if required, on the first day of treatment, then apply once daily for a few days after symptoms have cleared
▶ BY RECTUM USING SUPPOSITORIES
▶ Adult: Initially 1 suppository daily for 5–7 days, to be inserted after a bowel movement, then 1 suppository once daily on alternate days for 1 week
Haemorrhoids (severe cases) | Pruritus ani (severe cases)
▶ BY RECTUM USING SUPPOSITORIES
▶ Adult: Initially 1 suppository 2–3 times a day for 5–7 days, then 1 suppository once daily on alternate days for 1 week

IMPORTANT SAFETY INFORMATION
MHRA/CHM ADVICE: CORTICOSTEROIDS: RARE RISK OF CENTRAL SEROUS CHORIORETINOPATHY WITH LOCAL AS WELL AS SYSTEMIC ADMINISTRATION (AUGUST 2017)
See *Corticosteroids, general use* p. 656.

● CAUTIONS Local anaesthetic component can be absorbed through the rectal mucosa (avoid excessive application) · local anaesthetic component may cause sensitisation (use for short periods only—no longer than a few days)

● MEDICINAL FORMS
There can be variation in the licensing of different medicines containing the same drug.
Ointment
▶ Ultraproct (Meadow Laboratories Ltd)
Fluocortolone pivalate 920 microgram per 1 gram, Fluocortolone caproate 950 microgram per 1 gram, Cinchocaine hydrochloride 5 mg per 1 gram Ultraproct ointment | 30 gram PoM £8.27
Suppository
▶ Ultraproct (Meadow Laboratories Ltd)
Fluocortolone pivalate 610 microgram, Fluocortolone caproate 630 microgram, Cinchocaine hydrochloride 1 mg Ultraproct suppositories | 12 suppository PoM £4.06

Cinchocaine with hydrocortisone

21-Dec-2017

● **INDICATIONS AND DOSE**

PROCTOSEDYL ® OINTMENT

Haemorrhoids | Pruritus ani
▶ TO THE SKIN, OR BY RECTUM
▶ Child: Apply twice daily, to be administered morning and night and after a bowel movement. Apply externally or by rectum. Do not use for longer than 7 days
▶ Adult: Apply twice daily, to be administered morning and night and after a bowel movement. Apply externally or by rectum. Do not use for longer than 7 days

PROCTOSEDYL ® SUPPOSITORIES

Haemorrhoids | Pruritus ani
▶ BY RECTUM
▶ Child 12-17 years: 1 suppository, insert suppository night and morning and after a bowel movement. Do not use for longer than 7 days
▶ Adult: 1 suppository, insert suppository night and morning and after a bowel movement. Do not use for longer than 7 days

UNIROID-HC ® OINTMENT

Haemorrhoids | Pruritus ani
▶ TO THE SKIN, OR BY RECTUM
▶ Child 12-17 years: Apply twice daily, and apply after a bowel movement, apply externally or by rectum, do not use for longer than 7 days
▶ Adult: Apply twice daily, and apply after a bowel movement, apply externally or by rectum, do not use for longer than 7 days

UNIROID-HC ® SUPPOSITORIES

Haemorrhoids | Pruritus ani
▶ BY RECTUM
▶ Child 12-17 years: 1 suppository, insert twice daily and after a bowel movement. Do not use for longer than 7 days
▶ Adult: 1 suppository, insert twice daily and after a bowel movement. Do not use for longer than 7 days

---

IMPORTANT SAFETY INFORMATION
MHRA/CHM ADVICE: CORTICOSTEROIDS: RARE RISK OF CENTRAL SEROUS CHORIORETINOPATHY WITH LOCAL AS WELL AS SYSTEMIC ADMINISTRATION (AUGUST 2017)
See *Corticosteroids, general use* p. 656.

● CAUTIONS Local anaesthetic component can be absorbed through the rectal mucosa (avoid excessive application, particularly in children and infants) · local anaesthetic component may cause sensitisation (use for short periods only—no longer than a few days)

● MEDICINAL FORMS
There can be variation in the licensing of different medicines containing the same drug.
Ointment
▶ Proctosedyl (Sanofi)
   Cinchocaine hydrochloride 5 mg per 1 gram, Hydrocortisone 5 mg per 1 gram Proctosedyl ointment | 30 gram [PoM] £10.34 DT = £10.34
▶ Uniroid HC (Chemidex Pharma Ltd)
   Cinchocaine hydrochloride 5 mg per 1 gram, Hydrocortisone 5 mg per 1 gram Uniroid HC ointment | 30 gram [PoM] £4.23 DT = £10.34

Suppository
▶ Proctosedyl (Sanofi)
   Cinchocaine hydrochloride 5 mg, Hydrocortisone 5 mg Proctosedyl suppositories | 12 suppository [PoM] £5.08 DT = £5.08
▶ Uniroid HC (Chemidex Pharma Ltd)
   Cinchocaine hydrochloride 5 mg, Hydrocortisone 5 mg Uniroid HC suppositories | 12 suppository [PoM] £1.91 DT = £5.08

Cinchocaine with prednisolone
21-Dec-2017

● **INDICATIONS AND DOSE**

Haemorrhoids | Pruritus ani
▶ BY RECTUM USING OINTMENT
▶ Adult: Apply twice daily for 5–7 days, apply 3–4 times a day on the first day if necessary, then apply once daily for a few days after symptoms have cleared
▶ BY RECTUM USING SUPPOSITORIES
▶ Adult: 1 suppository daily for 5–7 days, to be inserted after a bowel movement

Haemorrhoids (severe cases) | Pruritus ani (severe cases)
▶ BY RECTUM USING SUPPOSITORIES
▶ Adult: Initially 1 suppository 2–3 times a day, then 1 suppository daily for a total of 5–7 days, to be inserted after a bowel movement

---

IMPORTANT SAFETY INFORMATION
MHRA/CHM ADVICE: CORTICOSTEROIDS: RARE RISK OF CENTRAL SEROUS CHORIORETINOPATHY WITH LOCAL AS WELL AS SYSTEMIC ADMINISTRATION (AUGUST 2017)
See *Corticosteroids, general use* p. 656.

● CAUTIONS Local anaesthetic component can be absorbed through the rectal mucosa (avoid excessive application) · local anaesthetic component may cause sensitisation (use for short periods only—no longer than a few days)

● MEDICINAL FORMS
There can be variation in the licensing of different medicines containing the same drug.
Ointment
▶ Scheriproct (Bayer Plc)
   Prednisolone hexanoate 1.9 mg per 1 gram, Cinchocaine hydrochloride 5 mg per 1 gram Scheriproct ointment | 30 gram [PoM] £3.23 DT = £3.23
Suppository
▶ Scheriproct (Bayer Plc)
   Cinchocaine hydrochloride 1 mg, Prednisolone hexanoate 1.3 mg Scheriproct suppositories | 12 suppository [PoM] £1.52 DT = £1.52

Hydrocortisone with lidocaine
21-Dec-2017

● **INDICATIONS AND DOSE**

Haemorrhoids | Pruritus ani
▶ BY RECTUM USING AEROSOL SPRAY
▶ Adult: 1 spray up to 3 times a day for no longer than 7 days without medical advice, spray once over the affected area
▶ BY RECTUM USING OINTMENT
▶ Adult: Apply several times daily, for short term use only

IMPORTANT SAFETY INFORMATION
MHRA/CHM ADVICE: CORTICOSTEROIDS: RARE RISK OF CENTRAL SEROUS CHORIORETINOPATHY WITH LOCAL AS WELL AS SYSTEMIC ADMINISTRATION (AUGUST 2017)
See *Corticosteroids, general use* p. 656.

● CAUTIONS Local anaesthetic component can be absorbed through the rectal mucosa (avoid excessive application) ·

local anaesthetic component may cause sensitisation (use for short periods only—no longer than a few days)

● MEDICINAL FORMS
There can be variation in the licensing of different medicines containing the same drug.

Ointment
▸ Hydrocortisone with lidocaine (Non-proprietary)
Hydrocortisone acetate 2.75 mg per 1 gram, Lidocaine 50 mg per 1 gram Lidocaine 5% / Hydrocortisone acetate 0.275% ointment | 20 gram [PoM] [Ⓢ] DT = £4.19
▸ Xyloproct (Aspen Pharma Trading Ltd)
Hydrocortisone acetate 2.75 mg per 1 gram, Lidocaine 50 mg per 1 gram Xyloproct 5%/0.275% ointment | 20 gram [PoM] £4.19 DT = £4.19

Spray
▸ Perinal (Dermal Laboratories Ltd)
Hydrocortisone 2 mg per 1 gram, Lidocaine hydrochloride 10 mg per 1 gram Perinal spray | 30 ml [P] £6.11

Hydrocortisone with pramocaine

21-Dec-2017

● INDICATIONS AND DOSE

Haemorrhoids | Proctitis
▸ BY RECTUM
▸ Adult: 1 applicatorful 2–3 times a day and 1 applicatorful, after a bowel movement, do not use for longer than 7 days; maximum 4 applicatorfuls per day

---

IMPORTANT SAFETY INFORMATION

MHRA/CHM ADVICE: CORTICOSTEROIDS: RARE RISK OF CENTRAL SEROUS CHORIORETINOPATHY WITH LOCAL AS WELL AS SYSTEMIC ADMINISTRATION (AUGUST 2017)

See *Corticosteroids, general use* p. 656.

● CAUTIONS Local anaesthetic component can be absorbed through the rectal mucosa (avoid excessive application) · local anaesthetic component may cause sensitisation (use for short periods only—no longer than a few days)

● MEDICINAL FORMS
There can be variation in the licensing of different medicines containing the same drug.

Foam
▸ Proctofoam HC (Meda Pharmaceuticals Ltd)
Hydrocortisone acetate 10 mg per 1 gram, Pramocaine hydrochloride 10 mg per 1 gram Proctofoam HC foam enema | 40 dose [PoM] £6.07 DT = £6.07

SCLEROSANTS

Phenol

● INDICATIONS AND DOSE

Haemorrhoids (particularly when unprolapsed)
▸ BY SUBMUCOSAL INJECTION
▸ Adult: 2–3 mL, dose (using phenol 5%) to be injected into the submucosal layer at the base of the pile; several injections may be given at different sites, max. total injected 10 mL at any one time

● SIDE-EFFECTS Abdominal sepsis · abscess · dizziness · erectile dysfunction · fever · hepatitis · increased risk of infection · ulcer · urinary disorders

● PRESCRIBING AND DISPENSING INFORMATION When prepared extemporaneously, the BP states Oily Phenol Injection, BP consists of phenol 5% in a suitable fixed oil.

● MEDICINAL FORMS
There can be variation in the licensing of different medicines containing the same drug. Forms available from special-order manufacturers include: solution for injection

Solution for injection
▸ Phenol (Non-proprietary)
Phenol 50 mg per 1 ml Oily phenol 5% solution for injection 5ml ampoules | 10 ampoule [PoM] £63.92 DT = £63.92

10   Reduced exocrine secretions

Exocrine pancreatic insufficiency

14-Dec-2016

Description of condition

Exocrine pancreatic insufficiency is characterised by reduced secretion of pancreatic enzymes into the duodenum.

The main clinical manifestations are maldigestion and malnutrition, associated with low circulating levels of micronutrients, fat-soluble vitamins and lipoproteins. Patients also present with gastro-intestinal symptoms such as diarrhoea, abdominal cramps and steatorrhoea.

Exocrine pancreatic insufficiency can result from chronic pancreatitis, cystic fibrosis, obstructive pancreatic tumours, coeliac disease, Zollinger-Ellison syndrome, and gastro-intestinal or pancreatic surgical resection.

Aims of treatment

The aim of treatment is to relieve gastro-intestinal symptoms and to achieve a normal nutritional status.

Drug treatment

Pancreatic enzyme replacement therapy with pancreatin p. 96 is the mainstay of treatment for exocrine pancreatic insufficiency.

Pancreatin contains the three main groups of digestive enzymes: lipase, amylase and protease. These enzymes respectively digest fats, carbohydrates and proteins into their basic components so that they can be absorbed and utilised by the body. [EvGr] Pancreatin should be administered with meals and snacks. The dose should be adjusted, as necessary, to the lowest effective dose according to the symptoms of maldigestion and malabsorption. [Ⓐ]

Fibrosing colonopathy has been reported in patients with cystic fibrosis taking high dose pancreatic enzyme replacement therapy (in excess of 10 000 units/kg/day of lipase). Possible risk factors are gender (in children, boys are at greater risk than girls), more severe cystic fibrosis, and concomitant use of laxatives. The peak age for developing fibrosing colonopathy is between 2 and 8 years. Manufacturers of *Pancrease HL*® and *Nutrizym* 22® recommend that the total dose of pancreatin used in patients with cystic fibrosis should not usually exceed 10 000 units/kg/day of lipase. Manufacturers of pancreatin recommend that if a patient taking pancreatin develops new abdominal symptoms (or any change in existing abdominal symptoms) the patient should be reviewed to exclude the possibility of colonic damage.

There is limited evidence that acid suppression may improve the effectiveness of pancreatin. [EvGr] Acid-suppressing drugs (proton pump inhibitors or H_2-receptor antagonists) may be trialled in patients who continue to experience symptoms despite high doses of pancreatin.

Levels of fat-soluble vitamins and micronutrients (such as zinc and selenium) should be routinely assessed and supplementation advised whenever necessary. [Ⓐ]

Gastro-intestinal system

Gastro-intestinal system

1

Pancreatin preparations

Preparation	Protease units	Amylase units	Lipase units
Creon® 10 000 capsule, e/c granules	600	8000	10 000
Creon® Micro e/c granules (per 100 mg)	200	3600	5000
Pancrex® granules (per gram)	300	4000	5000
Pancrex V® capsule, powder	430	9000	8000
Pancrex V '125'® capsule, powder	160	3300	2950
Pancrex V® e/c tablet	110	1700	1900
Pancrex V® Forte e/c tablet	330	5000	5600
Pancrex V® powder (per gram)	1400	30 000	25 000

Higher-strength pancreatin preparations

Preparation	Protease units	Amylase units	Lipase units
Creon® 25 000 capsule, e/c pellets	1000	18 000	25 000
Creon® 40000 capsule, e/c granules	1600	25 000	40 000
Nutrizym 22® capsule, e/c minitablets	1100	19 800	22 000
Pancrease HL® capsule, e/c minitablets	1250	22 500	25 000

Non-drug treatment

[EvGr] Dietary advice should be provided. Food intake should be distributed between three main meals per day, and two or three snacks. Food that is difficult to digest should be avoided, such as legumes (peas, beans, lentils) and high-fibre foods. Alcohol should be avoided completely. Reduced fat diets are not recommended. ◁

Medium-chain triglycerides (see MCT oil, in *Borderline substances*), which are directly absorbed by the intestinal mucosa, were thought to be useful in some patients. However evidence has shown that MCT-enriched preparations offer no advantage over a normal balanced diet.

PANCREATIC ENZYMES

| Pancreatin

08-Mar-2017

● DRUG ACTION Supplements of pancreatin are given to compensate for reduced or absent exocrine secretion. They assist the digestion of starch, fat, and protein.

● **INDICATIONS AND DOSE**

CREON® 10000

Pancreatic insufficiency

▶ BY MOUTH
▶ Child: Initially 1–2 capsules, dose to be taken with each meal either taken whole or contents mixed with acidic fluid or soft food (then swallowed immediately without chewing)
▶ Adult: Initially 1–2 capsules, dose to be taken with each meal either taken whole or contents mixed with acidic fluid or soft food (then swallowed immediately without chewing)

CREON® 25000

Pancreatic insufficiency

▶ BY MOUTH
▶ Child 2-17 years: Initially 1–2 capsules, dose to be taken with each meal either taken whole or contents mixed with acidic fluid or soft food (then swallowed immediately without chewing)
▶ Adult: Initially 1–2 capsules, dose to be taken with each meal either taken whole or contents mixed with acidic fluid or soft food (then swallowed immediately without chewing)

CREON® 40000

Pancreatic insufficiency

▶ BY MOUTH
▶ Child 2-17 years: Initially 1–2 capsules, dose to be taken with each meal either taken whole or contents mixed with acidic fluid or soft food (then swallowed immediately without chewing)
▶ Adult: Initially 1–2 capsules, dose to be taken with each meal either taken whole or contents mixed with acidic fluid or soft food (then swallowed immediately without chewing)

CREON® MICRO

Pancreatic insufficiency

▶ BY MOUTH
▶ Child: Initially 100 mg, for administration advice, see *Directions for administration*
▶ Adult: Initially 100 mg, for administration advice, see *Directions for administration*

DOSE EQUIVALENCE AND CONVERSION

▶ For *Creon® Micro*: 100 mg granules = one measured scoopful (scoop supplied with product).

NUTRIZYM 22® GASTRO-RESISTANT CAPSULES

Pancreatic insufficiency

▶ BY MOUTH
▶ Adult: Initially 1–2 capsules, dose to be taken with meals and 1 capsule as required, dose to be taken with snacks, doses should be swallowed whole or contents taken with water, or mixed with acidic fluid or soft food (then swallowed immediately without chewing)

PANCREASE HL®

Pancreatic insufficiency

▶ BY MOUTH
▶ Child 15-17 years: Initially 1–2 capsules, dose to be taken during each meal and 1 capsule, to be taken with snacks, all doses either taken whole or contents mixed with slightly acidic liquid or soft food (then swallowed immediately without chewing)
▶ Adult: Initially 1–2 capsules, dose to be taken during each meal and 1 capsule, to be taken with snacks, all doses either taken whole or contents mixed with slightly acidic liquid or soft food (then swallowed immediately without chewing)

PANCREX®

Pancreatic insufficiency

▶ BY MOUTH
▶ Child 2-17 years: 5–10 g, to be taken just before meals, washed down or mixed with milk or water
▶ Adult: 5–10 g, to be taken just before meals; washed down or mixed with milk or water

PANCREX® V

Pancreatic insufficiency

▶ BY MOUTH

▶ Child 1-11 months: 1–2 capsules, contents of capsule to be mixed with feeds

▶ Child 1-17 years: 2–6 capsules, dose to be taken with each meal either swallowed whole or sprinkled on food

▶ Adult: 2–6 capsules, dose to be taken with each meal either swallowed whole or sprinkled on food

PANCREX® V POWDER

Pancreatic insufficiency

▶ BY MOUTH

▶ Child: 0.5–2 g, to be taken before or with meals, washed down or mixed with milk or water

▶ Adult: 0.5–2 g, to be taken before or with meals, washed down or mixed with milk or water

PANCREX® V TABLETS

Pancreatic insufficiency

▶ BY MOUTH

▶ Child 2-17 years: 5–15 tablets, to be taken before meals

▶ Adult: 5–15 tablets, to be taken before meals

PANCREX® V TABLETS FORTE

Pancreatic insufficiency

▶ BY MOUTH

▶ Child 2-17 years: 6–10 tablets, to be taken before meals

▶ Adult: 6–10 tablets, to be taken before meals

● CONTRA-INDICATIONS

PANCREASE HL® Should not be used in children aged 15 years or less with cystic fibrosis

NUTRIZYM 22® GASTRO-RESISTANT CAPSULES Should not be used in children aged 15 years or less with cystic fibrosis

● CAUTIONS Can irritate the perioral skin and buccal mucosa if retained in the mouth · excessive doses can cause perianal irritation

● INTERACTIONS → Appendix 1: pancreatin

● SIDE-EFFECTS

▶ **Common or very common** Abdominal distension · constipation · nausea · vomiting

▶ **Uncommon** Skin reactions

▶ **Frequency not known** Fibrosing colonopathy

● PREGNANCY Not known to be harmful.

● DIRECTIONS FOR ADMINISTRATION Pancreatin is inactivated by gastric acid therefore manufacturer advises pancreatin preparations are best taken with food (or immediately before or after food). Since pancreatin is inactivated by heat, excessive heat should be avoided if preparations are mixed with liquids or food; manufacturer advises the resulting mixtures should not be kept for more than one hour and any left-over food or liquid containing pancreatin should be discarded. Enteric-coated preparations deliver a higher enzyme concentration in the duodenum (provided the capsule contents are swallowed whole without chewing). Manufacturer advises gastro-resistant granules should be mixed with slightly acidic soft food or liquid such as apple juice, and then swallowed immediately without chewing. Capsules containing enteric-coated granules can be opened and the granules administered in the same way. For infants, *Creon Micro*® granules can be mixed with a small amount of milk on a spoon and administered immediately—granules should not be added to the baby's bottle. Manufacturer advises *Pancrex*® V powder may be administered via nasogastric tube or gastrostomy tube—consult local and national official guidelines.

● PRESCRIBING AND DISPENSING INFORMATION Preparations may contain pork pancreatin—consult product literature.

● HANDLING AND STORAGE Hypersensitivity reactions occur occasionally and may affect those handling the powder.

● PATIENT AND CARER ADVICE Patients or carers should be given advice on administration. It is important to ensure adequate hydration at all times in patients receiving higher-strength pancreatin preparations.
Medicines for Children leaflet: Pancreatin for pancreatic insufficiency www.medicinesforchildren.org.uk/pancreatin-for-pancreatic-insufficiency

● MEDICINAL FORMS
There can be variation in the licensing of different medicines containing the same drug.

Gastro-resistant capsule

▶ Creon (Mylan)
Protease 600 unit, Amylase 8000 unit, Lipase 10000 unit Creon 10000 gastro-resistant capsules | 100 capsule ℗ £12.93
Protease 1000 unit, Amylase 18000 unit, Lipase 25000 unit Creon 25000 gastro-resistant capsules | 100 capsule PoM £28.25
Protease 1600 unit, Amylase 25000 unit, Lipase 40000 unit Creon 40000 gastro-resistant capsules | 100 capsule PoM £47.55

▶ Nutrizym (Merck Serono Ltd)
Protease 1100 unit, Amylase 19800 unit, Lipase 22000 unit Nutrizym 22 gastro-resistant capsules | 100 capsule PoM £33.33

▶ Pancrease (Janssen-Cilag Ltd)
Protease 1250 unit, Amylase 22500 unit, Lipase 25000 unit Pancrease HL gastro-resistant capsules | 100 capsule PoM £40.38

Gastro-resistant tablet

CAUTIONARY AND ADVISORY LABELS 5, 25

▶ Pancrex (Essential Pharmaceuticals Ltd)
Protease 110 unit, Amylase 1700 unit, Lipase 1900 unit Pancrex V gastro-resistant tablets | 300 tablet ℗ £38.79
Protease 330 unit, Amylase 5000 unit, Lipase 5600 unit Pancrex V Forte gastro-resistant tablets | 300 tablet ℗ £48.11

Gastro-resistant granules

CAUTIONARY AND ADVISORY LABELS 25

▶ Creon (Mylan)
Protease 200 unit, Amylase 3600 unit, Lipase 5000 unit Creon Micro Pancreatin 60.12mg gastro-resistant granules | 20 gram ℗ £31.50

▶ Pancrex (Essential Pharmaceuticals Ltd)
Protease 300 unit, Amylase 4000 unit, Lipase 5000 unit Pancrex gastro-resistant granules | 300 gram ℗ £57.00

Powder

▶ Pancrex (Essential Pharmaceuticals Ltd)
Protease 1400 unit, Lipase 25000 unit, Amylase 30000 unit Pancrex V oral powder sugar-free | 300 gram ℗ £58.88

Capsule

▶ Pancrex (Essential Pharmaceuticals Ltd)
Protease 430 unit, Lipase 8000 unit, Amylase 9000 unit Pancrex V capsules | 300 capsule ℗ £53.20

11   Stoma care

Stoma care

24-Feb-2016

Description of condition

A stoma is an artificial opening on the abdomen to divert flow of faeces or urine into an external pouch located outside of the body. This procedure may be temporary or permanent. Colostomy and ileostomy are the most common forms of stoma but a gastrostomy, jejunostomy, duodenostomy or caecostomy may also be performed. Understanding the type and extent of surgical intervention in each patient is crucial in managing the patient's pharmaceutical needs correctly.

Overview

Prescribing for patients with stoma calls for special care due to modifications in drug delivery, resulting in a higher risk of sub-optimal absorption. The following is a brief account of some of the main points to be borne in mind.

Enteric-coated and modified-release medicines are **unsuitable**, particularly in patients with an ileostomy, as there may not be sufficient release of active ingredient. Soluble tablets, liquids, capsules or uncoated tablets are more suitable due to their quicker dissolution. When a solid-dose form such as a capsule or a tablet is given, the contents of the ostomy bag should be checked for any remnants.

Preparations containing sorbitol as an excipient should be avoided, due to its laxative side effects.

Analgesics

Opioid analgesics may cause troublesome constipation in colostomy patients. When a non-opioid analgesic is required, paracetamol is usually suitable. Anti-inflammatory analgesics may cause gastric irritation and bleeding; faecal output should be monitored for traces of blood.

Antacids

The tendency to diarrhoea from magnesium salts or constipation from aluminium or calcium salts may be increased in patients with stoma.

Antisecretory drugs

The gastric acid secretion often increases stoma output. Proton pump inhibitors and somatostatin analogues (octreotide p. 924 and lanreotide p. 923) are often used to reduce this risk.

Antidiarrhoeal drugs

Loperamide hydrochloride p. 66 and codeine phosphate p. 448 reduce intestinal motility and decrease water and sodium output from an ileostomy. Loperamide hydrochloride circulates through the enterohepatic circulation, which is disrupted in patients with a short bowel; high doses of loperamide hydrochloride may be required. Codeine phosphate can be added if response with loperamide hydrochloride alone is inadequate.

Digoxin

Patients with a stoma are particularly susceptible to hypokalaemia if taking digoxin p. 109, due to fluid and sodium depletion. Potassium supplements or a potassium-sparing diuretic may be advisable with monitoring for early signs of toxicity.

Diuretics

Diuretics should be used with caution in patients with an ileostomy or with urostomy as they may become excessively dehydrated and potassium depletion may easily occur. It is usually advisable to use a potassium-sparing diuretic.

Iron preparations

Iron preparations may cause loose stools and sore skin in these patients. If this is troublesome and if iron is definitely indicated, an intramuscular iron preparation should be used. Modified-release preparations should be avoided for the reasons given above.

Laxatives

Laxatives should not be used in patients with an ileostomy where possible as they may cause rapid and severe loss of water and electrolytes.

Colostomy patients may suffer from constipation and whenever possible should be treated by increasing fluid intake or dietary fibre. Bulk-forming drugs can be tried. If they are insufficient, as small a dose as possible of a stimulant laxative such as senna p. 63 can be used with caution.

Potassium supplements

Liquid formulations are preferred to modified-release formulations. The daily dose should be split to avoid osmotic diarrhoea.

Care of stoma

Patients and their carers are usually given advice about the use of cleansing agents, protective creams, lotions, deodorants, or sealants whilst in hospital, either by the surgeon or by stoma care nurses. Voluntary organisations offer help and support to patients with stoma.

Chapter 2
Cardiovascular system

CONTENTS

1   Arrhythmias

Arrhythmias

Overview

Management of an arrhythmia requires precise diagnosis of the type of arrhythmia, and electrocardiography is essential; underlying causes such as heart failure require appropriate treatment.

Ectopic beats

If ectopic beats are spontaneous and the patient has a normal heart, treatment is rarely required and reassurance to the patient will often suffice. If they are particularly troublesome, beta-blockers are sometimes effective and may be safer than other suppressant drugs.

Atrial fibrillation

Treatment of patients with atrial fibrillation aims to reduce symptoms and prevent complications, especially stroke. All patients with atrial fibrillation should be assessed for their risk of stroke and thromboembolism. Atrial fibrillation can be managed by either controlling the ventricular rate ('rate control') or by attempting to restore and maintain sinus rhythm ('rhythm control'). At any stage if treatment fails to control symptoms, or, if symptoms reoccur after cardioversion and specialised management is required, referral should be made within 4 weeks. If drug treatment fails to control the symptoms of atrial fibrillation or is unsuitable, ablation strategies can be considered. Review anticoagulation, stroke, and bleeding risk at least annually in all patients with atrial fibrillation.

Acute presentation

All patients with life-threatening haemodynamic instability caused by new-onset atrial fibrillation should undergo emergency electrical cardioversion without delaying to achieve anticoagulation. In patients presenting acutely but without life-threatening haemodynamic instability, rate or rhythm control can be offered if the onset of arrhythmia is less than 48 hours; rate control is preferred if onset is more than 48 hours or uncertain. Consideration of pharmacological or electrical cardioversion should be based on clinical circumstances. If pharmacological cardioversion

has been agreed, intravenous amiodarone hydrochloride p. 105, or alternatively flecainide acetate p. 103, can be used (amiodarone hydrochloride is preferred if there is structural heart disease). If urgent rate control is required, a beta-blocker or verapamil hydrochloride p. 163 can be given intravenously.

Cardioversion

Sinus rhythm can be restored by electrical cardioversion, or pharmacological cardioversion with an oral or intravenous antiarrhythmic drug e.g. flecainide acetate or amiodarone hydrochloride. If atrial fibrillation has been present for more than 48 hours, electrical cardioversion is preferred and should not be attempted until the patient has been fully anticoagulated for at least 3 weeks; if this is not possible, parenteral anticoagulation should be commenced, and a left atrial thrombus ruled out immediately before cardioversion; oral anticoagulation should be given after cardioversion and continued for at least 4 weeks; prior to cardioversion, offer rate control as appropriate.

Drug treatment

Rate control is the preferred first-line drug treatment strategy for atrial fibrillation except in patients with new-onset atrial fibrillation, heart failure secondary to atrial fibrillation, atrial flutter suitable for an ablation strategy, atrial fibrillation with a reversible cause, or if rhythm control is more suitable based on clinical judgement. Ventricular rate can be controlled with a standard beta-blocker (not sotalol hydrochloride p. 108) or a rate-limiting calcium channel blocker such as diltiazem hydrochloride p. 157 [unlicensed indication], or verapamil hydrochloride as monotherapy. Choice of drug should be based on individual symptoms, heart rate, comorbidities, and patient preference. Digoxin p. 109 is usually only effective for controlling the ventricular rate at rest, and should therefore only be used as monotherapy in predominantly sedentary patients with non-paroxysmal atrial fibrillation. When a single drug fails to adequately control the ventricular rate, a combination of two drugs including a beta-blocker, digoxin, or diltiazem hydrochloride can be used. If symptoms are not controlled with a combination of two drugs, a rhythm-control strategy should be considered. If ventricular function is diminished, the combination of a beta-blocker (that is licensed for use in heart failure) and digoxin is preferred. Digoxin is also used when atrial fibrillation is accompanied by congestive heart failure.

Cardiovascular system

2

If drug treatment is required to maintain sinus rhythm ('rhythm control') post-cardioversion, a standard beta-blocker is used. If a standard beta-blocker is not appropriate or is ineffective, consider an oral anti-arrhythmic drug such as sotalol hydrochloride, flecainide acetate, propafenone hydrochloride p. 104, or amiodarone hydrochloride; dronedarone p. 106 may be considered in paroxysmal or persistent atrial fibrillation (see NICE guidance). If necessary, amiodarone hydrochloride can be started 4 weeks before and continuing for up to 12 months after electrical cardioversion to increase success of the procedure, and to maintain sinus rhythm. Flecainide acetate or propafenone hydrochlorideshould not be given when there is known ischaemic or structural heart disease. Consider amiodarone hydrochloride in patients with left ventricular impairment or heart failure.

Paroxysmal atrial fibrillation

In symptomatic paroxysmal atrial fibrillation, ventricular rhythm is controlled with a standard beta-blocker. Alternatively, if symptoms persist or a standard beta-blocker is not appropriate, an oral anti-arrhythmic drug such as dronedarone (see NICE guidance), sotalol hydrochloride, flecainide acetate, propafenone hydrochloride, or amiodarone hydrochloride can be given (see also Paroxysmal supraventricular tachycardia and Supraventricular arrhythmias). In selected patients with infrequent episodes of symptomatic paroxysmal atrial fibrillation, sinus rhythm can be restored using the 'pill-in-the-pocket' approach; this involves the patient taking oral flecainide acetate or propafenone hydrochloride to self-treat an episode of atrial fibrillation when it occurs.

Stroke prevention

All patients with atrial fibrillation should be assessed for their risk of stroke and the need for thromboprophylaxis; this needs to be balanced with the patient's risk of bleeding; a NICE guideline (NICE clinical guideline 180 (June 2014). Atrial fibrillation: The management of atrial fibrillation) recommends using the $CHA_2 DS_2$-VASc assessment tool for stroke risk and the HAS-BLED tool for bleeding risk prior to and during anticoagulation. Risk factors for stroke taken into account by $CHA_2 DS_2$-VASc include prior ischaemic stroke, transient ischaemic attacks, or thromboembolic events, heart failure, left ventricular systolic dysfunction, vascular disease, diabetes, hypertension, females, and patients over 65 years. Patients with a very low risk of stroke ($CHA_2 DS_2$-VASc score of 0 for men or 1 for women) do not require an antithrombotic for stroke prevention. Parenteral anticoagulation should be offered to patients with new-onset atrial fibrillation who are receiving subtherapeutic or no anticoagulation therapy until assessment is made, and appropriate anticoagulation is started. Oral anticoagulation should be offered to patients with confirmed diagnosis of atrial fibrillation in whom sinus rhythm has not been successfully restored within 48 hours of onset, patients who have had, or are at high risk of recurrence of atrial fibrillation such as those with structural heart disease, prolonged history of atrial fibrillation (more than 12 months), a history of failed attempts at cardioversion, and patients whom the risk of stroke outweighs the risk of bleeding. Anticoagulation treatment should not be withheld solely because of the risk of falls, and choice of treatment should be based on clinical features and patient preferences. Oral anticoagulation may be with a vitamin K antagonist (e.g warfarin sodium p. 139, or in non-valvular atrial fibrillation with apixaban p. 124, dabigatran etexilate p. 135, edoxaban p. 125, or rivaroxaban p. 127. Anticoagulants are also indicated during cardioversion procedures. Aspirin p. 121 is less effective than warfarin sodium at preventing emboli; the modest benefit is offset by the risk of bleeding, and aspirin should not be offered as monotherapy solely for stroke prevention in atrial fibrillation. If anticoagulant treatment is contra-indicated or

not tolerated, left atrial appendage occlusion can be considered.

Atrial flutter

Like atrial fibrillation, treatment options for atrial flutter involve either controlling the ventricular rate or attempting to restore and maintain sinus rhythm. However, atrial flutter generally responds less well to drug treatment than atrial fibrillation.

Control of the ventricular rate is usually an interim measure pending restoration of sinus rhythm. Ventricular rate can be controlled by administration of a beta-blocker, diltiazem hydrochloride p. 157 [unlicensed indication], or verapamil hydrochloride p. 163; an intravenous beta-blocker or verapamil hydrochloride is preferred for rapid control. Digoxin p. 109 can be added if rate control remains inadequate, and may be particularly useful in those with heart failure.

Conversion to sinus rhythm can be achieved by electrical cardioversion (by cardiac pacing or direct current), pharmacological cardioversion, or catheter ablation. If the duration of atrial flutter is unknown, or it has lasted for over 48 hours, cardioversion should not be attempted until the patient has been fully anticoagulated for at least 3 weeks; if this is not possible, parenteral anticoagulation should be commenced and a left atrial thrombus ruled out immediately before cardioversion; oral anticoagulation should be given after cardioversion and continued for at least 4 weeks.

Direct current cardioversion is usually the treatment of choice when rapid conversion to sinus rhythm is necessary (e.g. when atrial flutter is associated with haemodynamic compromise); catheter ablation is preferred for the treatment of recurrent atrial flutter. There is a limited role for anti-arrhythmic drugs as their use is not always successful. Flecainide acetate p. 103 or propafenone hydrochloride p. 104 can slow atrial flutter, resulting in 1:1 conduction to the ventricles, and should therefore be prescribed in conjunction with a ventricular rate controlling drug such as a beta-blocker, diltiazem hydrochloride [unlicensed indication], or verapamil hydrochloride. Amiodarone hydrochloride p. 105 can be used when other drug treatments are contra-indicated or ineffective.

All patients should be assessed for their risk of stroke and the need for thromboprophylaxis; the choice of anticoagulant is based on the same criteria as for atrial fibrillation.

Paroxysmal supraventricular tachycardia

This will often terminate spontaneously or with reflex vagal stimulation such as a Valsalva manoeuvre, immersing the face in ice-cold water, or carotid sinus massage; such manoeuvres should be performed with ECG monitoring.

If the effects of reflex vagal stimulation are transient or ineffective, or if the arrhythmia is causing severe symptoms, intravenous adenosine p. 107 should be given. If adenosine is ineffective or contra-indicated, intravenous verapamil hydrochloride is an alternative, but it should be avoided in patients recently treated with beta-blockers.

Failure to terminate paroxysmal supraventricular tachycardia with reflex vagal stimulation or drug treatment may suggest an arrhythmia of atrial origin, such as focal atrial tachycardia or atrial flutter.

Treatment with direct current cardioversion is needed in haemodynamically unstable patients or when the above measures have failed to restore sinus rhythm (and an alternative diagnosis has not been found).

Recurrent episodes of paroxysmal supraventricular tachycardia can be treated by catheter ablation, or prevented with drugs such as diltiazem hydrochloride, verapamil hydrochloride, beta-blockers including sotalol hydrochloride p. 108, flecainide acetate or propafenone hydrochloride.

Arrhythmias after myocardial infarction

In patients with a paroxysmal tachycardia or rapid irregularity of the pulse it is best not to administer an anti-arrhythmic until an ECG record has been obtained. Bradycardia, particularly if complicated by hypotension, should be treated with an intravenous dose of atropine sulfate p. 1295 the dose may be repeated if necessary. If there is a risk of asystole, or if the patient is unstable and has failed to respond to atropine sulfate, adrenaline/epinephrine p. 221 should be given by intravenous infusion, and the dose adjusted according to response.

For further advice, refer to the most recent recommendations of the Resuscitation Council (UK) available at www.resus.org.uk.

Ventricular tachycardia

Pulseless ventricular tachycardia or ventricular fibrillation should be treated with immediate defibrillation (see Cardiopulmonary resuscitation).

Patients with unstable sustained ventricular tachycardia, who continue to deteriorate with signs of hypotension or reduced cardiac output, should receive direct current cardioversion to restore sinus rhythm. If this fails, intravenous amiodarone hydrochloride should be administered and direct current cardioversion repeated.

Patients with sustained ventricular tachycardia who are haemodynamically stable can be treated with intravenous anti-arrhythmic drugs. Amiodarone hydrochloride is the preferred drug. Flecainide acetate, propafenone hydrochloride, and, although less effective, lidocaine hydrochloride p. 103 have all been used. If sinus rhythm is not restored, direct current cardioversion or pacing should be considered. Catheter ablation is an alternative if cessation of the arrhythmia is not urgent. Non-sustained ventricular tachycardia can be treated with a beta-blocker.

All patients presenting with ventricular tachycardia should be referred to a specialist. Following restoration of sinus rhythm, patients who remain at high risk of cardiac arrest will require maintenance therapy. Most patients will be treated with an implantable cardioverter defibrillator. Beta-blockers or sotalol hydrochloride (in place of a standard beta-blocker), or amiodarone hydrochloride (in combination with a standard beta-blocker), can be used in addition to the device in some patients; alternatively, they can be used alone when use of an implantable cardioverter defibrillator is not appropriate.

Torsade de pointes

Torsade de pointes is a form of ventricular tachycardia associated with a long QT syndrome (usually drug-induced, but other factors including hypokalaemia, severe bradycardia, and genetic predisposition are also implicated). Episodes are usually self-limiting, but are frequently recurrent and can cause impairment or loss of consciousness. If not controlled, the arrhythmia can progress to ventricular fibrillation and sometimes death. Intravenous infusion of magnesium sulfate p. 1019 is usually effective. A beta-blocker (but not sotalol hydrochloride) and atrial (or ventricular) pacing can be considered. Anti-arrhythmics can further prolong the QT interval, thus worsening the condition.

Anti-arrhythmic drugs

Anti-arrhythmic drugs can be classified clinically into those that act on supraventricular arrhythmias (e.g. verapamil hydrochloride), those that act on both supraventricular and ventricular arrhythmias (e.g. amiodarone hydrochloride), and those that act on ventricular arrhythmias (e.g. lidocaine hydrochloride).

Anti-arrhythmic drugs can also be classified according to their effects on the electrical behaviour of myocardial cells

during activity (the Vaughan Williams classification) although this classification is of less clinical significance:

- Class I: membrane stabilising drugs (e.g. lidocaine, flecainide)
- Class II: beta-blockers
- Class III: amiodarone; sotalol (also Class II)
- Class IV: calcium-channel blockers (includes verapamil but not dihydropyridines)

The negative inotropic effects of anti-arrhythmic drugs tend to be additive. Therefore special care should be taken if two or more are used, especially if myocardial function is impaired. Most drugs that are effective in countering arrhythmias can also provoke them in some circumstances; moreover, hypokalaemia enhances the arrhythmogenic (pro-arrhythmic) effect of many drugs.

Supraventricular arrhythmias

Adenosine p. 107 is usually the treatment of choice for terminating paroxysmal supraventricular tachycardia. As it has a very short duration of action (half-life only about 8 to 10 seconds, but prolonged in those taking dipyridamole p. 123), most side-effects are short lived. Unlike verapamil hydrochloride p. 163, adenosine can be used after a beta-blocker. Verapamil hydrochloride may be preferable to adenosine in asthma.

Oral administration of a **cardiac glycoside** (such as digoxin p. 109) slows the ventricular response in cases of atrial fibrillation and atrial flutter. However, intravenous infusion of digoxin is rarely effective for rapid control of ventricular rate. Cardiac glycosides are contra-indicated in supraventricular arrhythmias associated with accessory conducting pathways (e.g. Wolff- Parkinson-White syndrome).

Verapamil hydrochloride is usually effective for supraventricular tachycardias. An initial intravenous dose (**important:** serious beta-blocker interaction hazard) may be followed by oral treatment; hypotension may occur with large doses. It should not be used for tachyarrhythmias where the QRS complex is wide (i.e. broad complex) unless a supraventricular origin has been established beyond reasonable doubt. It is also contra-indicated in atrial fibrillation or atrial flutter associated with accessory conducting pathways (e.g. Wolff-Parkinson-White syndrome). It should not be used in children with arrhythmias without specialist advice; some supraventricular arrhythmias in childhood can be accelerated by verapamil hydrochloride with dangerous consequences.

Intravenous administration of a **beta-blocker** such as esmolol hydrochloride p. 153 or propranolol hydrochloride p. 149, can achieve rapid control of the ventricular rate.

Drugs for both supraventricular and ventricular arrhythmias include amiodarone hydrochloride p. 105, **beta-blockers**, disopyramide p. 102, flecainide acetate p. 103, **procainamide** (available from 'special-order' manufacturers or specialist importing companies), and propafenone hydrochloride p. 104.

Supraventricular and ventricular arrhythmias

Amiodarone hydrochloride is used in the treatment of arrhythmias, particularly when other drugs are ineffective or contra-indicated. It can be used for paroxysmal supraventricular, nodal and ventricular tachycardias, atrial fibrillation and flutter, and ventricular fibrillation. It can also be used for tachyarrhythmias associated with Wolff-Parkinson- White syndrome. It should be initiated only under hospital or specialist supervision. Amiodarone hydrochloride may be given by intravenous infusion as well as by mouth, and has the advantage of causing little or no myocardial depression. Unlike oral amiodarone hydrochloride, intravenous amiodarone hydrochloride acts relatively rapidly.

Intravenous injection of amiodarone hydrochloride can be used in cardiopulmonary resuscitation for ventricular

Cardiovascular system

2

fibrillation or pulseless tachycardia unresponsive to other interventions.

Amiodarone hydrochloride has a very long half-life (extending to several weeks) and only needs to be given once daily (but high doses can cause nausea unless divided). Many weeks or months may be required to achieve steady-state plasma-amiodarone concentration; this is particularly important when drug interactions are likely.

Beta-blockers act as anti-arrhythmic drugs principally by attenuating the effects of the sympathetic system on automaticity and conductivity within the heart. Sotalol hydrochloride p. 108 has a role in the management of ventricular arrhythmias.

Disopyramide can be given by intravenous injection to control arrhythmias after myocardial infarction (including those not responding to lidocaine hydrochloride), but it impairs cardiac contractility. Oral administration of disopyramide is useful, but it has an antimuscarinic effect which limits its use in patients susceptible to angle-closure glaucoma or with prostatic hyperplasia.

Flecainide acetate belongs to the same general class as lidocaine hydrochloride and may be of value for serious symptomatic ventricular arrhythmias. It may also be indicated for junctional re-entry tachycardias and for paroxysmal atrial fibrillation. However, it can precipitate serious arrhythmias in a small minority of patients (including those with otherwise normal hearts).

Propafenone hydrochloride is used for the prophylaxis and treatment of ventricular arrhythmias and also for some supraventricular arrhythmias. It has complex mechanisms of action, including weak beta-blocking activity (therefore caution is needed in obstructive airways disease—contra-indicated if severe).

Drugs for supraventricular arrhythmias include adenosine, **cardiac glycosides**, and verapamil hydrochloride. Drugs for ventricular arrhythmias include lidocaine hydrochloride.

Mexiletine and procainamide are both available from 'special-order' manufacturers or specialist importing companies. Mexiletine can be used for life-threatening ventricular arrhythmias; procainamide is given by intravenous injection to control ventricular arrhythmias.

Ventricular arrhythmias
Intravenous lidocaine hydrochloride can be used for the treatment of ventricular tachycardia in haemodynamically stable patients, and ventricular fibrillation and pulseless ventricular tachycardia in cardiac arrest refractory to defibrillation, however it is no longer the anti-arrhythmic drug of first choice.

Drugs for both supraventricular and ventricular arrhythmias include amiodarone hydrochloride, **beta-blockers**, disopyramide, flecainide acetate, **procainamide** (available from 'special- order' manufacturers or specialist importing companies), and propafenone hydrochloride.

Mexiletine is available from 'special-order' manufacturers or specialist importing companies for treatment of life-threatening ventricular arrhythmias.

Other drugs used for Arrhythmias Acebutolol, p. 151 · Atenolol, p. 151 · Metoprolol tartrate, p. 154 · Nadolol, p. 148 · Oxprenolol hydrochloride, p. 149

ANTIARRHYTHMICS 〉 CLASS IA

Disopyramide

● **INDICATIONS AND DOSE**

Prevention and treatment of ventricular and supraventricular arrhythmias, including after myocardial infarction | Maintenance of sinus rhythm after cardioversion

▸ BY MOUTH USING IMMEDIATE-RELEASE MEDICINES
▸ **Adult:** 300–800 mg daily in divided doses
▸ BY MOUTH USING MODIFIED-RELEASE MEDICINES
▸ **Adult:** 250–375 mg every 12 hours

● **CONTRA-INDICATIONS** Bundle-branch block associated with first-degree AV block · second- and third-degree AV block or bifascicular block (unless pacemaker fitted) · severe heart failure (unless secondary to arrhythmia) · severe sinus node dysfunction

● **CAUTIONS** Atrial flutter or atrial tachycardia with partial block · avoid in Acute porphyrias p. 1025 · elderly · heart failure (avoid if severe) · myasthenia gravis · prostatic enlargement · structural heart disease · susceptibility to angle-closure glaucoma

● **INTERACTIONS** → Appendix 1: antiarrhythmics

● **SIDE-EFFECTS** Abdominal pain · appetite decreased · arrhythmias · cardiac conduction disorders · cardiogenic shock · cognitive disorder · constipation · diarrhoea · dizziness · dry mouth · erectile dysfunction · headache · heart failure · hyperhidrosis · hypoglycaemia · hypotension · jaundice cholestatic · nausea · neutropenia · psychotic disorder · QT interval prolongation · rash · urinary disorders · vision disorders · vomiting

● **PREGNANCY** Manufacturer advises use only if potential benefit outweighs risk; may induce labour if used in third trimester.

● **BREAST FEEDING** Present in milk—use only if essential. **Monitoring** Monitor infant for antimuscarinic effects.

● **HEPATIC IMPAIRMENT** Avoid modified-release preparation. **Dose adjustments** Half-life prolonged—may need dose reduction.

● **RENAL IMPAIRMENT** Avoid modified-release preparation. **Dose adjustments** Reduce dose by increasing dose interval; adjust according to response.

● **MONITORING REQUIREMENTS**
▸ Monitor for hypotension, hypoglycaemia, ventricular tachycardia, ventricular fibrillation or torsade de pointes (discontinue if occur).
▸ Monitor serum potassium.

● **MEDICINAL FORMS**
There can be variation in the licensing of different medicines containing the same drug. Forms available from special-order manufacturers include: capsule, oral suspension, oral solution

Modified-release tablet
CAUTIONARY AND ADVISORY LABELS 25
▸ Rythmodan Retard(Sanofi)
 Disopyramide (as Disopyramide phosphate) 250 mg Rythmodan Retard 250mg tablets | 60 tablet [PoM] £32.08 DT = £32.08

Capsule
▸ Disopyramide (Non-proprietary)
 Disopyramide 100 mg Disopyramide 100mg capsules | 84 capsule [PoM] £25.00 DT = £22.09
 Disopyramide 150 mg Disopyramide 150mg capsules | 84 capsule [PoM] £33.40 DT = £27.58
▸ Rythmodan(Sanofi)
 Disopyramide 100 mg Rythmodan 100mg capsules | 84 capsule [PoM] £14.14 DT = £22.09

ANTIARRHYTHMICS > CLASS IB

Lidocaine hydrochloride

(Lignocaine hydrochloride)

- ● INDICATIONS AND DOSE

Cardiopulmonary resuscitation (as an alternative if amiodarone is not available)
- ▸ BY INTRAVENOUS INJECTION
- ▸ Adult: 1 mg/kg, do not exceed 3 mg/kg over the first hour

Ventricular arrhythmias, especially after myocardial infarction in patients without gross circulatory impairment
- ▸ INITIALLY BY INTRAVENOUS INJECTION
- ▸ Adult: 100 mg, to be given as a bolus dose over a few minutes, followed immediately by (by intravenous infusion) 4 mg/minute for 30 minutes, then (by intravenous infusion) 2 mg/minute for 2 hours, then (by intravenous infusion) 1 mg/minute, reduce concentration further if infusion continued beyond 24 hours (ECG monitoring and specialist advice for infusion), following intravenous injection lidocaine has a short duration of action (lasting for 15–20 minutes). If an intravenous infusion is not immediately available the initial intravenous injection of 100 mg can be repeated if necessary once or twice at intervals of not less than 10 minutes

Ventricular arrhythmias, especially after myocardial infarction in lighter patients or those whose circulation is severely impaired
- ▸ INITIALLY BY INTRAVENOUS INJECTION
- ▸ Adult: Initially 50 mg, to be given as a bolus dose over a few minutes, followed immediately by (by intravenous infusion) 4 mg/minute for 30 minutes, then (by intravenous infusion) 2 mg/minute for 2 hours, then (by intravenous infusion) 1 mg/minute, reduce concentration further if infusion continued beyond 24 hours (ECG monitoring and specialist advice for infusion), following intravenous injection lidocaine has a short duration of action (lasting for 15–20 minutes). If an intravenous infusion is not immediately available the initial intravenous injection of 50 mg can be repeated if necessary once or twice at intervals of not less than 10 minutes

- ● CONTRA-INDICATIONS All grades of atrioventricular block · severe myocardial depression · sino-atrial disorders
- ● CAUTIONS Acute porphyrias p. 1025 (consider infusion with glucose for its anti-porphyrinogenic effects) · congestive cardiac failure (consider lower dose) · post cardiac surgery (consider lower dose)
- ● INTERACTIONS → Appendix 1: antiarrhythmics
- ● SIDE-EFFECTS Anxiety · arrhythmias · atrioventricular block · cardiac arrest · circulatory collapse · confusion · dizziness · drowsiness · euphoric mood · headache · hypotension (may lead to cardiac arrest) · loss of consciousness · methaemoglobinaemia · muscle twitching · myocardial contractility decreased · nausea · neurological effects · nystagmus · pain · psychosis · respiratory disorders · seizure · sensation abnormal · temperature sensation altered · tinnitus · tremor · vision blurred · vomiting
- ● PREGNANCY Crosses the placenta but not known to be harmful in *animal* studies—use if benefit outweighs risk.
- ● BREAST FEEDING Present in milk but amount too small to be harmful.
- ● HEPATIC IMPAIRMENT Caution—increased risk of side-effects.
- ● RENAL IMPAIRMENT Possible accumulation of lidocaine and active metabolite; caution in severe impairment.

- ● MONITORING REQUIREMENTS Monitor ECG and have resuscitation facilities available.
- ● MEDICINAL FORMS There can be variation in the licensing of different medicines containing the same drug. Forms available from special-order manufacturers include: solution for injection

Solution for injection
- ▸ Lidocaine hydrochloride (Non-proprietary)
  - **Lidocaine hydrochloride 5 mg per 1 ml** Lidocaine 50mg/10ml (0.5%) solution for injection ampoules | 10 ampoule ⯀PoM⯀ £7.00
  - **Lidocaine hydrochloride 10 mg per 1 ml** Lidocaine 100mg/10ml (1%) solution for injection Mini-Plasco ampoules | 20 ampoule ⯀PoM⯀ £11.21
  - Lidocaine 100mg/10ml (1%) solution for injection ampoules | 10 ampoule ⯀PoM⯀ £4.40 DT = £4.40
  - Lidocaine 100mg/10ml (1%) solution for injection Sure-Amp ampoules | 20 ampoule ⯀PoM⯀ £8.80
  - Lidocaine 200mg/20ml (1%) solution for injection vials | 10 vial ⯀PoM⯀ £19.00
  - Lidocaine 200mg/20ml (1%) solution for injection ampoules | 10 ampoule ⯀PoM⯀ £7.00–£9.63 DT = £9.63
  - Lidocaine 50mg/5ml (1%) solution for injection ampoules | 10 ampoule ⯀PoM⯀ £2.59–£3.10 DT = £2.59
  - Lidocaine 20mg/2ml (1%) solution for injection ampoules | 10 ampoule ⯀PoM⯀ £3.50 DT = £2.20
  - Lidocaine 50mg/5ml (1%) solution for injection Sure-Amp ampoules | 20 ampoule ⯀PoM⯀ £6.00
  - **Lidocaine hydrochloride 20 mg per 1 ml** Lidocaine 100mg/5ml (2%) solution for injection ampoules | 10 ampoule ⯀PoM⯀ £2.70–£3.80 DT = £2.70
  - Lidocaine 400mg/20ml (2%) solution for injection vials | 10 vial ⯀PoM⯀ £19.50
  - Lidocaine 200mg/10ml (2%) solution for injection Mini-Plasco ampoules | 20 ampoule ⯀PoM⯀ £14.95
  - Lidocaine 40mg/2ml (2%) solution for injection ampoules | 10 ampoule ⯀PoM⯀ £4.00 DT = £2.37
  - Lidocaine 100mg/5ml (2%) solution for injection Sure-Amp ampoules | 20 ampoule ⯀PoM⯀ £6.00
  - Lidocaine 400mg/20ml (2%) solution for injection ampoules | 10 ampoule ⯀PoM⯀ £8.00–£9.90 DT = £9.90

ANTIARRHYTHMICS > CLASS IC

Flecainide acetate

- ● INDICATIONS AND DOSE

AV nodal reciprocating tachycardia, arrhythmias associated with accessory conducting pathways (e.g. Wolff-Parkinson-White syndrome), disabling symptoms of paroxysmal atrial fibrillation in patients without left ventricular dysfunction (arrhythmias of recent onset will respond more readily) (specialist supervision in hospital) | Ventricular tachyarrhythmias resistant to other treatment (specialist supervision in hospital)
- ▸ INITIALLY BY SLOW INTRAVENOUS INJECTION
- ▸ Adult: Initially 2 mg/kg (max. per dose 150 mg), to be given over 10–30 minutes with ECG monitoring, followed by (by intravenous infusion) 1.5 mg/kg/hour if required for 1 hour, then (by intravenous infusion) reduced to 100–250 micrograms/kg/hour for up to 24 hours, maximum cumulative dose of 600 mg in first 24 hours, then transfer to oral treatment

Supraventricular arrhythmias
- ▸ BY MOUTH USING IMMEDIATE-RELEASE MEDICINES
- ▸ Adult: Initially 50 mg twice daily, increased if necessary up to 300 mg daily
- ▸ BY MOUTH USING MODIFIED-RELEASE MEDICINES
- ▸ Adult: 200 mg daily

Ventricular arrhythmias (initiated under direction of hospital consultant)
- ▸ BY MOUTH USING IMMEDIATE-RELEASE MEDICINES
- ▸ Adult: Initially 100 mg twice daily for 3–5 days, maximum 400 mg daily reserved for rapid control or in heavily built patients; for maintenance, reduce to the lowest dose that controls the arrhythmia continued →

Cardiovascular system

2

DOSE ADJUSTMENTS DUE TO INTERACTIONS
▶ Manufacturer advises reduce dose by half with concurrent use of amiodarone.

DOSE EQUIVALENCE AND CONVERSION
▶ Patients stabilised on 200 mg daily immediate-release flecainide may be transferred to modified-release medicines.

● UNLICENSED USE Capsules, tablets and injection: licensed for AV nodal reciprocating tachycardia, arrhythmias associated with accessory conducting pathways (e.g. Wolff-Parkinson-White syndrome), disabling symptoms of paroxysmal atrial fibrillation in patients without left ventricular dysfunction (arrhythmias of recent onset will respond more readily). Immediate-release tablets only: licensed for symptomatic sustained ventricular tachycardia, disabling symptoms of premature ventricular contractions and/or non-sustained ventricular tachycardia in patients resistant to or intolerant of other therapy. Injection only: licensed for ventricular tachyarrhythmias resistant to other treatment.

● CONTRA-INDICATIONS Abnormal left ventricular function · atrial conduction defects (unless pacing rescue available) · bundle branch block (unless pacing rescue available) · control of arrhythmias in acute situations (for modified-release forms only) · distal block (unless pacing rescue available) · haemodynamically significant valvular heart disease · heart failure · history of myocardial infarction and either asymptomatic ventricular ectopics or asymptomatic non-sustained ventricular tachycardia · long-standing atrial fibrillation where conversion to sinus rhythm not attempted · second-degree or greater AV block (unless pacing rescue available) · sinus node dysfunction (unless pacing rescue available)

● CAUTIONS Atrial fibrillation following heart surgery · elderly (accumulation may occur) · patients with pacemakers (especially those who may be pacemaker dependent because stimulation threshold may rise appreciably)

● INTERACTIONS → Appendix 1: antiarrhythmics

● SIDE-EFFECTS
▶ **Common or very common** Arrhythmias · asthenia · dizziness · dyspnoea · fever · oedema · vision disorders
▶ **Uncommon** Alopecia · appetite decreased · constipation · diarrhoea · flatulence · gastrointestinal discomfort · nausea · skin reactions · vomiting
▶ **Rare or very rare** Anxiety · confusion · corneal deposits · depression · drowsiness · flushing · hallucination · headache · hepatic disorders · hyperhidrosis · insomnia · memory loss · movement disorders · peripheral neuropathy · photosensitivity reaction · respiratory disorders · seizure · sensation abnormal · syncope · tinnitus · tremor · vertigo
▶ **Frequency not known** Altered pacing threshold · atrioventricular block · cardiac arrest · chest pain · heart failure · hypotension · myocardial infarction · palpitations · QT interval prolongation

● PREGNANCY Used in pregnancy to treat maternal and fetal arrhythmias in specialist centres; toxicity reported in *animal* studies; infant hyperbilirubinaemia also reported.

● BREAST FEEDING Significant amount present in milk but not known to be harmful.

● HEPATIC IMPAIRMENT
Dose adjustments Avoid or reduce dose in severe impairment.

● RENAL IMPAIRMENT
Dose adjustments Reduce initial oral dose to max. 100 mg daily or reduce intravenous dose by 50%, if eGFR less than 35 mL/minute/1.73 m^2.

● MONITORING REQUIREMENTS
▶ With intravenous use ECG monitoring and resuscitation facilities must be available.

● DIRECTIONS FOR ADMINISTRATION For *intravenous infusion* (*Tambocor*®), give continuously or intermittently in Glucose 5% or Sodium Chloride 0.9%. Minimum volume in infusion fluids containing chlorides 500 mL.

● MEDICINAL FORMS
There can be variation in the licensing of different medicines containing the same drug. Forms available from special-order manufacturers include: oral suspension, oral solution

Tablet
▶ Flecainide acetate (Non-proprietary)
Flecainide acetate 50 mg Flecainide 50mg tablets | 60 tablet PoM £7.68 DT = £7.46
Flecainide acetate 100 mg Flecainide 100mg tablets | 60 tablet PoM £8.06 DT = £7.68
▶ Tambocor (Teva UK Ltd)
Flecainide acetate 50 mg Tambocor 50mg tablets | 60 tablet PoM £11.57 DT = £7.46
Flecainide acetate 100 mg Tambocor 100mg tablets | 60 tablet PoM £16.53 DT = £7.68

Solution for injection
▶ Tambocor (Teva UK Ltd)
Flecainide acetate 10 mg per 1 ml Tambocor 150mg/15ml solution for injection ampoules | 5 ampoule PoM £21.99

Modified-release capsule
CAUTIONARY AND ADVISORY LABELS 25
▶ Tambocor XL (Teva UK Ltd)
Flecainide acetate 200 mg Tambocor XL 200mg capsules | 30 capsule PoM £14.77

Propafenone hydrochloride

● INDICATIONS AND DOSE

Ventricular arrhythmias (specialist supervision in hospital) | Paroxysmal supraventricular tachyarrhythmias which include paroxysmal atrial flutter or fibrillation and paroxysmal re-entrant tachycardias involving the AV node or accessory pathway, where standard therapy ineffective or contra-indicated (specialist supervision in hospital)
▶ BY MOUTH
▶ **Adult:** Initially 150 mg 3 times a day, dose to be taken after food, monitor ECG and blood pressure, if QRS interval prolonged by more than 20%, reduce dose or discontinue until ECG returns to normal limits; increased if necessary to 300 mg twice daily (max. per dose 300 mg 3 times a day), dose to be increased at intervals of at least 3 days, reduce total daily dose for patients under 70 kg
▶ **Elderly:** Initially 150 mg 3 times a day, dose to be taken after food, monitor ECG and blood pressure, if QRS interval prolonged by more than 20%, reduce dose or discontinue until ECG returns to normal limits; increased if necessary to 300 mg twice daily (max. per dose 300 mg 3 times a day), dose to be increased at intervals of at least 5 days, reduce total daily dose for patients under 70 kg

● CONTRA-INDICATIONS Atrial conduction defects (unless adequately paced) · Brugada syndrome · bundle branch block (unless adequately paced) · cardiogenic shock (except arrhythmia induced) · distal block (unless adequately paced) · electrolyte disturbances · marked hypotension · myasthenia gravis · myocardial infarction within last 3 months · second degree or greater AV block (unless adequately paced) · severe bradycardia · severe obstructive pulmonary disease (due to weak beta-blocking activity) · sinus node dysfunction (unless adequately paced) · uncontrolled congestive heart failure with left ventricular ejection fraction less than 35%

- **CAUTIONS** Elderly · great caution in mild to moderate obstructive airways disease owing to beta-blocking activity · heart failure · pacemaker patients · potential for conversion of paroxysmal atrial fibrillation to atrial flutter with 2:1 or 1:1 conduction block
- **INTERACTIONS** → Appendix 1: antiarrhythmics
- **SIDE-EFFECTS**
- ▸ **Common or very common** Anxiety · arrhythmias · asthenia · cardiac conduction disorder · chest pain · constipation · diarrhoea · dizziness · dry mouth · dyspnoea · fever · gastrointestinal discomfort · headache · hepatic disorders · nausea · palpitations · sleep disorders · taste altered · vision blurred · vomiting
- ▸ **Uncommon** Appetite decreased · erectile dysfunction · gastrointestinal disorders · hypotension · movement disorders · paraesthesia · skin reactions · syncope · thrombocytopenia · vertigo
- ▸ **Frequency not known** Agranulocytosis · confusion · granulocytopenia · heart failure · leucopenia · lupus-like syndrome · seizure
- **PREGNANCY** Use only if potential benefit outweighs risk.
- **BREAST FEEDING** Use with caution—present in milk.
- **PATIENT AND CARER ADVICE**
  Driving and skilled tasks May affect performance of skilled tasks e.g. driving.

- **MEDICINAL FORMS**
  There can be variation in the licensing of different medicines containing the same drug. Forms available from special-order manufacturers include: oral suspension, oral solution
  Tablet
  CAUTIONARY AND ADVISORY LABELS 21, 25
  ▸ Propafenone hydrochloride (Non-proprietary)
    Propafenone hydrochloride 150 mg Propafenone 150mg tablets | 90 tablet [PoM] £7.37 DT = £7.37
    Propafenone hydrochloride 300 mg Propafenone 300mg tablets | 60 tablet [PoM] £9.34 DT = £9.34
  ▸ Arythmol (Mylan)
    Propafenone hydrochloride 150 mg Arythmol 150mg tablets | 90 tablet [PoM] £7.37 DT = £7.37
    Propafenone hydrochloride 300 mg Arythmol 300mg tablets | 60 tablet [PoM] £9.34 DT = £9.34

ANTIARRHYTHMICS > CLASS III

Amiodarone hydrochloride

- **INDICATIONS AND DOSE**

Treatment of arrhythmias, particularly when other drugs are ineffective or contra-indicated (including paroxysmal supraventricular, nodal and ventricular tachycardias, atrial fibrillation and flutter, ventricular fibrillation, and tachyarrhythmias associated with Wolff-Parkinson-White syndrome) (initiated in hospital or under specialist supervision)

- ▸ BY MOUTH
- ▸ Adult: 200 mg 3 times a day for 1 week, then reduced to 200 mg twice daily for a further week, followed by maintenance dose, usually 200 mg daily or the minimum dose required to control arrhythmia
- ▸ BY INTRAVENOUS INFUSION
- ▸ Adult: Initially 5 mg/kg, to be given over 20–120 minutes with ECG monitoring, subsequent infusions given if necessary according to response; maximum 1.2 g per day

Ventricular fibrillation or pulseless ventricular tachycardia refractory to defibrillation (for cardiopulmonary resuscitation)

- ▸ INITIALLY BY INTRAVENOUS INJECTION
- ▸ Adult: Initially 300 mg, dose to be considered after administration of adrenaline, dose should be given from a pre-filled syringe or diluted in 20 mL Glucose

5%, then (by intravenous injection) 150 mg if required, followed by (by intravenous infusion) 900 mg/24 hours

> **IMPORTANT SAFETY INFORMATION**
> MHRA/CHM ADVICE: SOFOSBUVIR WITH DACLATASVIR; SOFOSBUVIR AND LEDIPASVIR (MAY 2015); SIMEPREVIR WITH SOFOSBUVIR (AUGUST 2015): RISK OF SEVERE BRADYCARDIA AND HEART BLOCK WHEN TAKEN WITH AMIODARONE
> Avoid concomitant use unless other antiarrhythmics cannot be given.

- **CONTRA-INDICATIONS**
  GENERAL CONTRA-INDICATIONS
  Avoid in severe conduction disturbances (unless pacemaker fitted) · avoid in sinus node disease (unless pacemaker fitted) · iodine sensitivity · sino-atrial heart block (except in cardiac arrest) · sinus bradycardia (except in cardiac arrest) · thyroid dysfunction
  SPECIFIC CONTRA-INDICATIONS
  ▸ With intravenous use Avoid bolus injection in cardiomyopathy · avoid bolus injection in congestive heart failure · avoid in circulatory collapse · avoid in severe arterial hypotension · avoid in severe respiratory failure

- **CAUTIONS**
  GENERAL CAUTIONS Acute porphyrias p. 1025 · conduction disturbances (in excessive dosage) · elderly · heart failure · hypokalaemia · severe bradycardia (in excessive dosage)
  SPECIFIC CAUTIONS
  ▸ With intravenous use moderate and transient fall in blood pressure (circulatory collapse precipitated by rapid administration or overdosage) · severe hepatocellular toxicity

- **INTERACTIONS** → Appendix 1: antiarrhythmics
- **SIDE-EFFECTS**
  GENERAL SIDE-EFFECTS
  ▸ **Common or very common** Arrhythmias · hepatic disorders · hyperthyroidism · nausea · respiratory disorders · skin reactions
  ▸ **Rare or very rare** Bronchospasm (in patients with severe respiratory failure) · headache · idiopathic intracranial hypertension · nerve disorders · SIADH
  ▸ **Frequency not known** Angioedema · confusion · delirium · pancreatitis · severe cutaneous adverse reactions (SCARs)
  SPECIFIC SIDE-EFFECTS
  ▸ **Common or very common**
  ▸ With oral use Constipation · corneal deposits · hypothyroidism · movement disorders · photosensitivity reaction · sleep disorders · taste altered · vomiting
  ▸ With parenteral use Hypotension (following rapid injection)
  ▸ **Uncommon**
  ▸ With oral use Cardiac conduction disorders · dry mouth · myopathy (usually reversible on discontinuation) · peripheral neuropathy (usually reversible on discontinuation)
  ▸ **Rare or very rare**
  ▸ With oral use Alopecia · aplastic anaemia · epididymo-orchitis · erectile dysfunction · haemolytic anaemia · pulmonary haemorrhage · thrombocytopenia · vertigo
  ▸ With parenteral use Hot flush · hyperhidrosis
  ▸ **Frequency not known**
  ▸ With oral use Altered smell sensation · appetite decreased · parkinsonism · vasculitis
  ▸ With parenteral use Agranulocytosis · libido decreased · neutropenia
  SIDE-EFFECTS, FURTHER INFORMATION
  Corneal microdeposits Patients taking amiodarone may develop corneal microdeposits (reversible on withdrawal of treatment). However, if vision is impaired or if optic neuritis or optic neuropathy occur, amiodarone must be stopped to prevent blindness and expert advice sought.

Thyroid function Amiodarone contains iodine and can cause disorders of thyroid function; both hypothyroidism and hyperthyroidism can occur. Hypothyroidism can be treated with replacement therapy without withdrawing amiodarone if it is essential; careful supervision is required.

Hepatotoxicity Amiodarone is also associated with hepatotoxicity and treatment should be discontinued if severe liver function abnormalities or clinical signs of liver disease develop.

Pulmonary toxicity Pneumonitis should always be suspected if new or progressive shortness of breath or cough develops in a patient taking amiodarone.

● PREGNANCY Possible risk of neonatal goitre; use only if no alternative.

● BREAST FEEDING Avoid; present in milk in significant amounts; theoretical risk of neonatal hypothyroidism from release of iodine.

● MONITORING REQUIREMENTS

▸ Thyroid function tests should be performed before treatment and then every 6 months. Clinical assessment of thyroid function alone is unreliable. Thyroxine (T4) may be raised in the absence of hyperthyroidism; therefore tri-iodothyronine (T3), T4, and thyroid-stimulating hormone (thyrotrophin, TSH) should all be measured. A raised T3 and T4 with a very low or undetectable TSH concentration suggests the development of thyrotoxicosis.

▸ Liver function tests required before treatment and then every 6 months.

▸ Serum potassium concentration should be measured before treatment.

▸ Chest x-ray required before treatment.

▸ If concomitant use of amiodarone with sofosbuvir and daclatasvir, simeprevir and sofosbuvir, or sofosbuvir and ledipasvir cannot be avoided because other anti-arrhythmics are not tolerated or contra-indicated, patients should be closely monitored, particularly during the first weeks of treatment. Patients at high risk of bradycardia should be monitored continuously for 48 hours in an appropriate clinical setting after starting concomitant treatment. Patients who have stopped amiodarone within the last few months and need to start sofosbuvir and daclatasvir, simeprevir and sofosbuvir, or sofosbuvir and ledipasvir should be monitored.

▸ With intravenous use ECG monitoring and resuscitation facilities must be available. Monitor liver transaminases closely.

● DIRECTIONS FOR ADMINISTRATION

▸ With intravenous use For *intravenous infusion* (*Cordarone X*®), give continuously or intermittently in Glucose 5%. Suggested initial infusion volume 250 mL given over 20–120 minutes; for repeat infusions up to 1.2 g in max. 500 mL; should not be diluted to less than 600 micrograms/mL. See cardio-pulmonary resuscitation for details of infusion in extreme emergency. Incompatible with Sodium Chloride infusion fluids; avoid equipment containing the plasticizer di-2-ethylhexphthalate (DEHP).

▸ With oral use For administration *by mouth*, tablets may be crushed and dispersed in water; injection solution should **not** be given orally (irritant).

● PATIENT AND CARER ADVICE Because of the possibility of phototoxic reactions, patients should be advised to shield the skin from light during treatment and for several months after discontinuing amiodarone; a wide-spectrum sunscreen to protect against both long-wave ultraviolet and visible light should be used.

If taking amiodarone with concomitant sofosbuvir and daclatasvir, simeprevir and sofosbuvir, or sofosbuvir and ledipasvir, patients and their carers should be told how to recognise signs and symptoms of bradycardia and heart block and advised to seek immediate medical attention if

symptoms such as shortness of breath, light-headedness, palpitations, fainting, unusual tiredness or chest pain develop.

● MEDICINAL FORMS
There can be variation in the licensing of different medicines containing the same drug. Forms available from special-order manufacturers include: oral suspension, oral solution

Tablet

CAUTIONARY AND ADVISORY LABELS 11

▸ Amiodarone hydrochloride (Non-proprietary)
Amiodarone hydrochloride 100 mg Amiodarone 100mg tablets | 28 tablet [PoM] £4.25 DT = £1.63
Amiodarone hydrochloride 200 mg Amiodarone 200mg tablets | 28 tablet [PoM] £7.80 DT = £2.02

▸ Cordarone X (Sanofi)
Amiodarone hydrochloride 100 mg Cordarone X 100 tablets | 28 tablet [PoM] £4.28 DT = £1.63
Amiodarone hydrochloride 200 mg Cordarone X 200 tablets | 28 tablet [PoM] £6.99 DT = £2.02

Solution for injection

EXCIPIENTS: May contain Benzyl alcohol

▸ Amiodarone hydrochloride (Non-proprietary)
Amiodarone hydrochloride 30 mg per 1 ml Amiodarone 300mg/10ml solution for injection pre-filled syringes | 1 pre-filled disposable injection [PoM] £13.80 DT = £13.80
Amiodarone hydrochloride 50 mg per 1 ml Amiodarone 150mg/3ml concentrate for solution for injection ampoules | 5 ampoule [PoM] £7.75 | 10 ampoule [PoM] £15.00

▸ Cordarone X (Sanofi)
Amiodarone hydrochloride 50 mg per 1 ml Cordarone X 150mg/3ml solution for injection ampoules | 6 ampoule [PoM] £9.60

Dronedarone

● DRUG ACTION Dronedarone is a multi-channel blocking anti-arrhythmic drug.

● INDICATIONS AND DOSE

Maintenance of sinus rhythm after cardioversion in clinically stable patients with paroxysmal or persistent atrial fibrillation, when alternative treatments are unsuitable (initiated under specialist supervision)
▸ BY MOUTH
▸ Adult: 400 mg twice daily

● CONTRA-INDICATIONS Atrial conduction defects · bradycardia · complete bundle branch block · distal block · existing or previous heart failure or left ventricular systolic dysfunction · haemodynamically unstable patients · liver toxicity associated with previous amiodarone use · lung toxicity associated with previous amiodarone use · permanent atrial fibrillation · prolonged QT interval · second- or third- degree AV block · sick sinus syndrome (unless pacemaker fitted) · sinus node dysfunction

● CAUTIONS Coronary artery disease · correct hypokalaemia and hypomagnesaemia before starting and during treatment

● INTERACTIONS → Appendix 1: antiarrhythmics

● SIDE-EFFECTS

▸ **Common or very common** Asthenia · bradycardia · congestive heart failure · diarrhoea · gastrointestinal discomfort · nausea · QT interval prolongation · skin reactions · vomiting

▸ **Uncommon** Photosensitivity reaction · respiratory disorders · taste altered

▸ **Rare or very rare** Hepatic disorders · vasculitis

SIDE-EFFECTS, FURTHER INFORMATION

Liver injury Liver injury including life-threatening acute liver failure reported rarely; discontinue treatment if 2 consecutive alanine aminotransferase concentrations exceed 3 times upper limit of normal.

Heart failure New onset or worsening heart failure reported. If heart failure or left ventricular systolic dysfunction develops, discontinue treatment.
Pulmonary toxicity Interstitial lung disease, pneumonitis and pulmonary fibrosis reported. Investigate if symptoms such as dyspnoea or dry cough develop and discontinue if confirmed.

● PREGNANCY Manufacturer advises avoid—toxicity in *animal* studies.

● BREAST FEEDING Manufacturer advises avoid—present in milk in *animal* studies.

● HEPATIC IMPAIRMENT Avoid in severe impairment.

● RENAL IMPAIRMENT Avoid if eGFR less than 30 mL/minute/1.73 m².

● MONITORING REQUIREMENTS
▸ Ongoing monitoring should occur under specialist supervision.
▸ Monitor for heart failure.
▸ Perform ECG at least every 6 months—consider discontinuation if atrial fibrillation reoccurs.
▸ Measure serum creatinine before treatment and 7 days after initiation—if raised, measure again after a further 7 days and consider discontinuation if creatinine continues to rise.
▸ Monitor liver function before treatment, 1 week and 1 month after initiation of treatment, then monthly for 6 months, then every 3 months for 6 months and periodically thereafter.

● PATIENT AND CARER ADVICE
Heart failure Patients or their carers should be told how to recognise signs of heart failure and advised to seek prompt medical attention if symptoms such as weight gain, dependent oedema, or dyspnoea develop or worsen.
Hepatic disorders Patients or their carers should be told how to recognise signs of liver disorder and advised to seek prompt medical attention if symptoms such as abdominal pain, anorexia, nausea, vomiting, fever, malaise, itching, dark urine, or jaundice develop.

● NATIONAL FUNDING/ACCESS DECISIONS
NICE decisions
▸ **Dronedarone for the treatment of non-permanent atrial fibrillation (December 2012) NICE TA197**
Dronedarone is an option for the maintenance of sinus rhythm after successful cardioversion in paroxysmal or persistent atrial fibrillation which is not controlled by first-line therapy (usually including beta-blockers), **and** after alternative options have been considered in patients:
  ● who have at least 1 of the following cardiovascular risk factors: hypertension requiring drugs of at least 2 different classes, diabetes mellitus, previous transient ischaemic attack, stroke or systemic embolism, left atrial diameter of 50 mm or greater, or age 70 years or older **and**
  ● who do not have left ventricular systolic dysfunction nor a history of, or current, heart failure
Patients who do not meet the above criteria who are currently receiving dronedarone should have the option to continue treatment until they and their clinicians consider it appropriate to stop.
www.nice.org.uk/TA197

● MEDICINAL FORMS
There can be variation in the licensing of different medicines containing the same drug.
Tablet
CAUTIONARY AND ADVISORY LABELS 21
▸ Multaq (Sanofi)
  Dronedarone (as Dronedarone hydrochloride) 400 mg Multaq 400mg tablets | 20 tablet [PoM] £22.50 DT = £22.50 | 60 tablet [PoM] £67.50

ANTIARRHYTHMICS ⟩ OTHER

Adenosine

● INDICATIONS AND DOSE
Rapid reversion to sinus rhythm of paroxysmal supraventricular tachycardias, including those associated with accessory conducting pathways (e.g. Wolff-Parkinson-White syndrome) | Used to aid in diagnosis of broad or narrow complex supraventricular tachycardias
▸ BY RAPID INTRAVENOUS INJECTION
▸ Adult: Initially 6 mg, administer into central or large peripheral vein and give over 2 seconds, cardiac monitoring required, followed by 12 mg after 1–2 minutes if required, then 12 mg after 1–2 minutes if required, increments should not be given if high level AV block develops at any particular dose

Rapid reversion to sinus rhythm of paroxysmal supraventricular tachycardias, including those associated with accessory conducting pathways (e.g. Wolff-Parkinson-White syndrome) in patients with a heart transplant | Aid to diagnosis of broad or narrow complex supraventricular tachycardias in patients with a heart transplant
▸ BY RAPID INTRAVENOUS INJECTION
▸ Adult: Initially 3 mg, administer into a central or large peripheral vein and give over 2 seconds, followed by 6 mg after 1–2 minutes if required, then 12 mg after 1–2 minutes if required, patients with a heart transplant are very sensitive to the effects of adenosine

Used in conjunction with radionuclide myocardial perfusion imaging in patients who cannot exercise adequately or for whom exercise is inappropriate
▸ BY INTRAVENOUS INFUSION
▸ Adult: (consult product literature)

● UNLICENSED USE Adenosine doses in the BNF may differ from those in the product literature.

● CONTRA-INDICATIONS Asthma · chronic obstructive lung disease · decompensated heart failure · long QT syndrome · second- or third-degree AV block and sick sinus syndrome (unless pacemaker fitted) · severe hypotension

● CAUTIONS Atrial fibrillation with accessory pathway (conduction down anomalous pathway may increase) · atrial flutter with accessory pathway (conduction down anomalous pathway may increase) · autonomic dysfunction · bundle branch block · first-degree AV block · heart transplant · left main coronary artery stenosis · left to right shunt · pericardial effusion · pericarditis · QT-interval prolongation · recent myocardial infarction · severe heart failure · stenotic carotid artery disease with cerebrovascular insufficiency · stenotic valvular heart disease · uncorrected hypovolaemia

● INTERACTIONS → Appendix 1: antiarrhythmics

● SIDE-EFFECTS
▸ **Common or very common** Abdominal discomfort · arrhythmias · atrioventricular block · chest discomfort · chest pain (discontinue) · dizziness · dry mouth · dyspnoea · flushing · headache · hypotension (discontinue if severe) · pain · paraesthesia · throat discomfort
▸ **Uncommon** Asthenia · back discomfort · bradycardia (discontinue if asystole or severe bradycardia occur) · hyperhidrosis · limb discomfort · nervousness · taste metallic
▸ **Rare or very rare** Drowsiness · nasal congestion · nipple tenderness · respiratory disorders · respiratory failure (discontinue) · tinnitus · tremor · urinary urgency · vision blurred
▸ **Frequency not known** Apnoea · cardiac arrest · loss of consciousness · nausea · seizure · syncope · vomiting

2

Cardiovascular system

- **PREGNANCY** Large doses may produce fetal toxicity; manufacturer advises use only if potential benefit outweighs risk.
- **BREAST FEEDING** No information available—unlikely to be present in milk owing to short half-life.
- **MONITORING REQUIREMENTS** Monitor ECG and have resuscitation facilities available.
- **DIRECTIONS FOR ADMINISTRATION** For *rapid intravenous injection* give over 2 seconds into central or large peripheral vein followed by rapid Sodium Chloride 0.9% flush; injection solution may be diluted with Sodium Chloride 0.9% if required.

- **MEDICINAL FORMS**
  There can be variation in the licensing of different medicines containing the same drug. Forms available from special-order manufacturers include: solution for injection, infusion, solution for infusion

  Solution for injection
  ELECTROLYTES: May contain Sodium
  ▸ Adenosine (Non-proprietary)
  Adenosine 3 mg per 1 ml Adenosine 6mg/2ml solution for injection vials | 5 vial PoM £7.00 (Hospital only) | 6 vial PoM £26.70–£29.24 (Hospital only)
  ▸ Adenocor (Sanofi)
  Adenosine 3 mg per 1 ml Adenocor 6mg/2ml solution for injection vials | 6 vial PoM £6.45 (Hospital only)

  Solution for infusion
  ELECTROLYTES: May contain Sodium
  ▸ Adenosine (Non-proprietary)
  Adenosine 3 mg per 1 ml Adenosine 30mg/10ml solution for infusion vials | 5 vial PoM £12.00 (Hospital only) | 6 vial PoM £70.00–£85.57 (Hospital only)
  ▸ Adenoscan (Sanofi)
  Adenosine 3 mg per 1 ml Adenoscan 30mg/10ml solution for infusion vials | 6 vial PoM £16.05

BETA-ADRENOCEPTOR BLOCKERS ›
NON-SELECTIVE

F 146

Sotalol hydrochloride

- **INDICATIONS AND DOSE**

Symptomatic non-sustained ventricular tachyarrhythmias | Prophylaxis of paroxysmal atrial tachycardia or fibrillation, paroxysmal AV re-entrant tachycardias (both nodal and involving accessory pathways), and paroxysmal supraventricular tachycardia after cardiac surgery | Maintenance of sinus rhythm following cardioversion of atrial fibrillation or flutter
▸ BY MOUTH
▸ Adult: Initially 80 mg daily in 1–2 divided doses, then increased to 160–320 mg daily in 2 divided doses, dose to be increased gradually at intervals of 2–3 days

Life-threatening arrhythmias including ventricular tachyarrhythmias
▸ BY MOUTH
▸ Adult: Initially 80 mg daily in 1–2 divided doses, then increased to 160–320 mg daily in 2 divided doses, dose to be increased gradually at intervals of 2–3 days, higher doses of 480–640 mg daily may be required for life-threatening ventricular arrhythmias (under specialist supervision)

IMPORTANT SAFETY INFORMATION

Sotalol may prolong the QT interval, and it occasionally causes life threatening ventricular arrhythmias (**important**: particular care is required to avoid hypokalaemia in patients taking sotalol—electrolyte disturbances, particularly hypokalaemia and hypomagnesaemia should be corrected before sotalol started and during use).

- **CONTRA-INDICATIONS** Long QT syndrome (congenital or acquired) · torsade de pointes
- **CAUTIONS** Diarrhoea (severe or prolonged)
- **INTERACTIONS** → Appendix 1: beta blockers, non-selective
- **SIDE-EFFECTS**
  ▸ **Common or very common** Anxiety · arrhythmia · chest pain · dyspepsia · fever · flatulence · hearing impairment · mood altered · muscle spasms · oedema · palpitations · presyncope · sexual dysfunction · taste altered · torsade de pointes (increased risk in females)
- **BREAST FEEDING** Water soluble beta-blockers such as sotalol are present in breast milk in greater amounts than other beta blockers.
- **RENAL IMPAIRMENT** Avoid if eGFR less than 10 mL/minute/1.73 m².
  Dose adjustments Use half normal dose if eGFR 30–60 mL/minute/1.73 m²; use one-quarter normal dose if eGFR 10–30 mL/minute/1.73 m².
- **MONITORING REQUIREMENTS** Measurement of corrected QT interval, and monitoring of ECG and electrolytes required; correct hypokalaemia, hypomagnesaemia, or other electrolyte disturbances.

- **MEDICINAL FORMS**
  There can be variation in the licensing of different medicines containing the same drug. Forms available from special-order manufacturers include: oral suspension, oral solution

  Tablet
  CAUTIONARY AND ADVISORY LABELS 8
  ▸ Sotalol hydrochloride (Non-proprietary)
  Sotalol hydrochloride 40 mg Sotalol 40mg tablets | 28 tablet PoM £1.53 DT = £1.53
  Sotalol hydrochloride 80 mg Sotalol 80mg tablets | 28 tablet PoM £3.75 DT = £1.08 | 56 tablet PoM £1.81
  Sotalol hydrochloride 160 mg Sotalol 160mg tablets | 28 tablet PoM £6.25 DT = £5.25
  ▸ Beta-Cardone (Focus Pharmaceuticals Ltd)
  Sotalol hydrochloride 200 mg Beta-Cardone 200mg tablets | 28 tablet PoM £2.40 DT = £2.40
  ▸ Sotacor (Bristol-Myers Squibb Pharmaceuticals Ltd)
  Sotalol hydrochloride 80 mg Sotacor 80mg tablets | 30 tablet PoM £3.28

CARDIAC GLYCOSIDES

Cardiac glycosides

Digoxin-specific antibody

Serious cases of digoxin toxicity should be discussed with the National Poisons Information Service (see further information, under Poisoning, emergency treatment p. 1319). Digoxin-specific antibody p. 1328 fragments are indicated for the treatment of known or strongly suspected life-threatening digoxin toxicity associated with ventricular arrhythmias or bradyarrhythmias unresponsive to atropine sulfate p. 1295 and when measures beyond the withdrawal of digoxin p. 109 and correction of any electrolyte abnormalities are considered necessary.

Digoxin

Digoxin is most useful for controlling ventricular response in persistent and permanent atrial fibrillation and atrial flutter. Digoxin also has a role in heart failure.

For management of atrial fibrillation the maintenance dose of digoxin can usually be determined by the ventricular rate at rest, which should not usually be allowed to fall persistently below 60 beats per minute.

Digoxin is now rarely used for rapid control of heart rate (see management of supraventricular arrhythmias). Even with intravenous administration, response may take many hours; persistence of tachycardia is therefore not an indication for exceeding the recommended dose. The intramuscular route is **not** recommended.

In patients with heart failure who are in sinus rhythm a loading dose is not required, and a satisfactory plasma-digoxin concentration can be achieved over a period of about a week.

Digoxin has a long half-life and maintenance doses need to be given only once daily (although higher doses may be divided to avoid nausea); renal function is the most important determinant of digoxin dosage.

Unwanted effects depend both on the concentration of digoxin in the plasma and on the sensitivity of the conducting system or of the myocardium, which is often increased in heart disease. It can sometimes be difficult to distinguish between toxic effects and clinical deterioration because symptoms of both are similar. The plasma concentration alone cannot indicate toxicity reliably, but the likelihood of toxicity increases progressively through the range 1.5 to 3 micrograms/litre for digoxin. Digoxin should be used with special care in the elderly, who may be particularly susceptible to digitalis toxicity.

Regular monitoring of plasma-digoxin concentration during maintenance treatment is not necessary unless problems are suspected. Hypokalaemia predisposes the patient to digitalis toxicity; it is managed by giving a potassium-sparing diuretic or, if necessary, potassium supplementation.

If toxicity occurs, digoxin should be withdrawn; serious manifestations require urgent specialist management. Digoxin-specific antibody fragments are available for reversal of life-threatening overdosage.

Digoxin

16-Jun-2017

● **DRUG ACTION** Digoxin is a cardiac glycoside that increases the force of myocardial contraction and reduces conductivity within the atrioventricular (AV) node.

● **INDICATIONS AND DOSE**

Rapid digitalisation, for atrial fibrillation or flutter
▶ BY MOUTH
▶ Adult: 0.75–1.5 mg in divided doses, dose to be given over 24 hours, reduce dose in the elderly

Maintenance, for atrial fibrillation or flutter
▶ BY MOUTH
▶ Adult: Maintenance 125–250 micrograms daily, dose according to renal function and initial loading dose, reduce dose in the elderly

Heart failure (for patients in sinus rhythm)
▶ BY MOUTH
▶ Adult: 62.5–125 micrograms once daily, reduce dose in the elderly

Emergency loading dose, for atrial fibrillation or flutter
▶ INITIALLY BY INTRAVENOUS INFUSION
▶ Adult: Loading dose 0.75–1 mg, to be given over at least 2 hours, then (by mouth) maintenance, loading dose is rarely necessary, maintenance dose to be started on the day following the loading dose, reduce dose in the elderly

DOSE ADJUSTMENTS DUE TO INTERACTIONS
▶ Manufacturer advises reduce dose by half with concurrent use of amiodarone, dronedarone and quinine.

DOSE EQUIVALENCE AND CONVERSION
▶ Dose may need to be reduced if digoxin (or another cardiac glycoside) has been given in the preceding 2 weeks.
▶ When switching from intravenous to oral route may need to increase dose by 20–33% to maintain the same plasma-digoxin concentration.

● **UNLICENSED USE** Digoxin doses in the BNF may differ from those in product literature.

● **CONTRA-INDICATIONS** Constrictive pericarditis (unless to control atrial fibrillation or improve systolic dysfunction—but use with caution) · hypertrophic cardiomyopathy (unless concomitant atrial fibrillation and heart failure—but use with caution) · intermittent complete heart block · myocarditis · second degree AV block · supraventricular arrhythmias associated with accessory conducting pathways e.g. Wolff-Parkinson-White syndrome (although can be used in infancy) · ventricular tachycardia or fibrillation

● **CAUTIONS** Hypercalcaemia (risk of digitalis toxicity) · hypokalaemia (risk of digitalis toxicity) · hypomagnesaemia (risk of digitalis toxicity) · hypoxia (risk of digitalis toxicity) · recent myocardial infarction · severe respiratory disease · sick sinus syndrome · thyroid disease

● **INTERACTIONS** → Appendix 1: digoxin

● **SIDE-EFFECTS**
▶ **Common or very common** Arrhythmias · cardiac conduction disorder · cerebral impairment · diarrhoea · dizziness · eosinophilia · nausea · skin reactions · vision disorders · vomiting
▶ **Uncommon** Depression
▶ **Rare or very rare** Appetite decreased · asthenia · confusion · gastrointestinal disorders · gynaecomastia · headache · malaise · psychosis · thrombocytopenia

Overdose If toxicity occurs, digoxin should be withdrawn; serious manifestations require urgent specialist management.

● **PREGNANCY**
Dose adjustments May need dosage adjustment.

● **BREAST FEEDING** Amount too small to be harmful.

● **RENAL IMPAIRMENT**
Dose adjustments Reduce dose.
Monitoring Monitor plasma-digoxin concentration in renal impairment.

● **MONITORING REQUIREMENTS**
▶ For plasma-digoxin concentration assay, blood should be taken at least 6 hours after a dose.
▶ Monitor serum electrolytes and renal function. Toxicity increased by electrolyte disturbances.

● **DIRECTIONS FOR ADMINISTRATION**
▶ With intravenous use Avoid rapid intravenous administration (risk of hypertension and reduced coronary flow). For *intravenous infusion* (*Lanoxin*®), give intermittently in Glucose 5% or Sodium chloride 0.9%; dilute to a concentration of not more than 62.5 micrograms/mL. To be given over at least 2 hours.
▶ With oral use For *oral* administration, oral solution must **not** be diluted.

● **PATIENT AND CARER ADVICE** Patient counselling is advised for digoxin elixir (use pipette).

● **MEDICINAL FORMS**
There can be variation in the licensing of different medicines containing the same drug. Forms available from special-order manufacturers include: oral suspension, oral solution, solution for injection

Tablet
▶ Digoxin (Non-proprietary)
Digoxin 62.5 microgram Digoxin 62.5microgram tablets | 28 tablet PoM £9.99 DT = £1.23
Digoxin 125 microgram Digoxin 125microgram tablets | 28 tablet PoM £4.99 DT = £1.22
Digoxin 250 microgram Digoxin 250microgram tablets | 28 tablet PoM £4.99 DT = £1.22
▶ Lanoxin (Aspen Pharma Trading Ltd)
Digoxin 62.5 microgram Lanoxin PG 62.5microgram tablets | 500 tablet PoM £8.09
Digoxin 125 microgram Lanoxin 125 tablets | 500 tablet PoM £8.09

Cardiovascular system

2

Digoxin 250 microgram Lanoxin 250microgram tablets |
500 tablet PoM £8.09

Solution for infusion
▸ Digoxin (Non-proprietary)
  Digoxin 250 microgram per 1 ml Digoxin 500micrograms/2ml
  solution for infusion ampoules | 10 ampoule PoM £7.00
▸ Lanoxin (Aspen Pharma Trading Ltd)
  Digoxin 250 microgram per 1 ml Lanoxin 500micrograms/2ml
  solution for infusion ampoules | 5 ampoule PoM £3.30

Oral solution
▸ Lanoxin (Aspen Pharma Trading Ltd)
  Digoxin 50 microgram per 1 ml Lanoxin PG 50micrograms/ml elixir
  | 60 ml PoM £5.35 DT = £5.35

2   Bleeding disorders

Antifibrinolytic drugs and haemostatics

Overview

Fibrin dissolution can be impaired by the administration of
tranexamic acid below, which inhibits fibrinolysis. It can be
used to prevent bleeding or to treat bleeding associated with
excessive fibrinolysis (e.g. in surgery, dental extraction,
obstetric disorders, and traumatic hyphaema) and in the
management of menorrhagia. Tranexamic acid may also be
used in hereditary angioedema, epistaxis, and in
thrombolytic overdose.

Desmopressin p. 653 is used in the management of mild to
moderate haemophilia and von Willebrand's disease. It is
also used for fibrinolytic response testing.

Etamsylate p. 111 reduces capillary bleeding in the
presence of a normal number of platelets; it does not act by
fibrin stabilisation, but probably by correcting abnormal
adhesion. Etamsylate is less effective than other treatments
in the management of heavy menstrual bleeding and its use
is no longer recommended.

ANTIHAEMORRHAGICS > ANTIFIBRINOLYTICS

| Tranexamic acid

26-Apr-2017

● **INDICATIONS AND DOSE**

Local fibrinolysis
▸ BY MOUTH
▸ Adult: 1–1.5 g 2–3 times a day, alternatively
  15–25 mg/kg 2–3 times a day
▸ INITIALLY BY SLOW INTRAVENOUS INJECTION
▸ Adult: 0.5–1 g 2–3 times a day, to be administered at a
  rate not exceeding 100 mg/minute, followed by (by
  continuous intravenous infusion) 25–50 mg/kg if
  required, dose to be given over 24 hours

Menorrhagia
▸ BY MOUTH
▸ Adult: 1 g 3 times a day for up to 4 days, to be initiated
  when menstruation has started; maximum 4 g per day

Hereditary angioedema
▸ BY MOUTH
▸ Adult: 1–1.5 g 2–3 times a day, for short-term
  prophylaxis of hereditary angioedema, tranexamic acid
  is started several days before planned procedures
  which may trigger an acute attack of hereditary
  angioedema (e.g. dental work) and continued for
  2–5 days afterwards

Epistaxis
▸ BY MOUTH
▸ Adult: 1 g 3 times a day for 7 days

General fibrinolysis
▸ BY SLOW INTRAVENOUS INJECTION
▸ Adult: 1 g every 6–8 hours, alternatively 15 mg/kg
  every 6–8 hours, dose to be given at a rate not
  exceeding 100 mg/minute

**Prevention and treatment of significant haemorrhage
following trauma**
▸ INITIALLY BY SLOW INTRAVENOUS INJECTION
▸ Adult: Loading dose 1 g to be given over 10 minutes,
  treatment should commence within 8 hours of injury,
  followed by (by intravenous infusion) 1 g to be given
  over 8 hours

● UNLICENSED USE Use of tranexamic acid by continuous
  intravenous infusion for treatment of local fibrinolysis is
  an unlicensed route of administration.
  EvGr Not licensed for prevention and treatment of
  significant haemorrhage following trauma. ◈

● CONTRA-INDICATIONS Fibrinolytic conditions following
  disseminated intravascular coagulation (unless
  predominant activation of fibrinolytic system with severe
  bleeding) · history of convulsions · thromboembolic
  disease

● CAUTIONS Irregular menstrual bleeding (establish cause
  before initiating therapy) · massive haematuria (avoid if
  risk of ureteric obstruction) · patients receiving oral
  contraceptives (increased risk of thrombosis)

  CAUTIONS, FURTHER INFORMATION
▸ Menorrhagia Before initiating treatment for menorrhagia,
  exclude structural or histological causes or fibroids causing
  distortion of uterine cavity.

● INTERACTIONS → Appendix 1: tranexamic acid

● SIDE-EFFECTS
  GENERAL SIDE-EFFECTS
▸ **Common or very common** Diarrhoea (reduce dose) · nausea ·
  vomiting
▸ **Uncommon** Allergic dermatitis
▸ **Rare or very rare** Colour vision change (discontinue) ·
  embolism and thrombosis
▸ **Frequency not known** Seizure (more common at high
  doses) · visual impairment (discontinue)
  SPECIFIC SIDE-EFFECTS
▸ With intravenous use Hypotension · malaise (on rapid
  intravenous injection)

● PREGNANCY No evidence of teratogenicity in *animal*
  studies; manufacturer advises use only if potential benefit
  outweighs risk—crosses the placenta.

● BREAST FEEDING Small amount present in milk—
  antifibrinolytic effect in infant unlikely.

● RENAL IMPAIRMENT
  Dose adjustments Reduce dose—consult product literature
  for details.

● MONITORING REQUIREMENTS Regular liver function tests
  in long-term treatment of hereditary angioedema.

● DIRECTIONS FOR ADMINISTRATION For *intravenous infusion*
  (Cyklokapron®), give continuously in Glucose 5% or
  Sodium chloride 0.9%.

● MEDICINAL FORMS
  There can be variation in the licensing of different medicines
  containing the same drug. Forms available from special-order
  manufacturers include: oral suspension, oral solution
  Tablet
▸ Tranexamic acid (Non-proprietary)
  Tranexamic acid 500 mg Tranexamic acid 500mg tablets |
  60 tablet PoM £32.10 DT = £12.85
▸ Cyklokapron (Meda Pharmaceuticals Ltd)
  Tranexamic acid 500 mg Cyklokapron 500mg tablets |
  60 tablet PoM £14.30 DT = £12.85

Solution for injection

▸ Tranexamic acid (Non-proprietary)

Tranexamic acid 100 mg per 1 ml Tranexamic acid 500mg/5ml solution for injection ampoules | 5 ampoule PoM £7.50 (Hospital only) | 5 ampoule PoM £7.50 | 10 ampoule PoM £13.99–£15.47 (Hospital only)

▸ Cyklokapron (Pfizer Ltd)

Tranexamic acid 100 mg per 1 ml Cyklokapron 500mg/5ml solution for injection ampoules | 10 ampoule PoM £15.47

ANTIHAEMORRHAGICS > HAEMOSTATICS

Emicizumab

09-May-2018

- **DRUG ACTION** Emicizumab is a monoclonal antibody that bridges activated factor IX and factor X to restore function of missing activated factor VIII, which is needed for haemostasis.

- **INDICATIONS AND DOSE**

Prophylaxis of haemorrhage in patients with haemophilia A (initiated by a specialist)

▸ BY SUBCUTANEOUS INJECTION

▸ Adult: Initially 3 mg/kg once weekly for 4 weeks, then maintenance 1.5 mg/kg once weekly, administer into the thigh, abdomen or upper arm

- **CAUTIONS** Concomitant bypassing agent · risk factors for thrombotic microangiopathy

CAUTIONS, FURTHER INFORMATION

▸ Concomitant bypassing agent Manufacturer advises discontinue bypassing agents the day before starting emicizumab; if a bypassing agent is required—consult product literature.

- **SIDE-EFFECTS**

▸ **Common or very common** Arthralgia · diarrhoea · fever · headache · myalgia · thrombotic microangiopathy

▸ **Uncommon** Cavernous sinus thrombosis · skin necrosis · thrombophlebitis

- **CONCEPTION AND CONTRACEPTION** Manufacturer advises effective contraception during and for 6 months after treatment in women of childbearing potential.

- **PREGNANCY** Manufacturer advises use only if potential benefit outweighs risk—no information available.

- **BREAST FEEDING** Manufacturer advises avoid—no information available.

- **EFFECT ON LABORATORY TESTS** Manufacturer advises to avoid intrinsic pathway clotting-based laboratory tests or use with caution as results may be misinterpreted—consult product literature.

- **DIRECTIONS FOR ADMINISTRATION** Manufacturer advises max. 2 mL per injection site; rotate injection site and avoid skin that is tender, damaged or scarred. Patients or their caregivers may self-administer *Hemlibra*® after appropriate training.

- **PRESCRIBING AND DISPENSING INFORMATION** Emicizumab is a biological medicine. Biological medicines must be prescribed and dispensed by brand name, see *Biological medicines* and *Biosimilar medicines*, under Guidance on prescribing p. 1; manufacturer advises to record the brand name and batch number after each administration.

- **PATIENT AND CARER ADVICE**

Missed doses Manufacturer advises if a dose is missed by more than 5 days, the missed dose should not be taken and the next dose administered at the normal time.

- **MEDICINAL FORMS**
There can be variation in the licensing of different medicines containing the same drug.

Solution for injection

▸ Hemlibra (Roche Products Ltd) ▼

Emicizumab 30 mg per 1 ml Hemlibra 30mg/1ml solution for injection vials | 1 vial PoM £2,415.30

Emicizumab 150 mg per 1 ml Hemlibra 150mg/1ml solution for injection vials | 1 vial PoM £12,076.50

Hemlibra 105mg/0.7ml solution for injection vials | 1 vial PoM £8,453.55

Hemlibra 60mg/0.4ml solution for injection vials | 1 vial PoM £4,830.60

Etamsylate

(Ethamsylate)

- **INDICATIONS AND DOSE**

Short-term blood loss in menorrhagia

▸ BY MOUTH

▸ Adult: 500 mg 4 times a day during menstruation

- **CONTRA-INDICATIONS** Acute porphyrias p. 1025

- **CAUTIONS** Exclude structural or histological causes of menorrhagia, or fibroids causing distortion of the uterine cavity, before initiating treatment

- **SIDE-EFFECTS** Diarrhoea · fever (discontinue) · headache · nausea · rash · vomiting

- **BREAST FEEDING** Present in milk—manufacturer advises avoid.

- **LESS SUITABLE FOR PRESCRIBING** Less suitable for prescribing.

- **MEDICINAL FORMS**
Forms available from special-order manufacturers include: oral solution

2.1 Coagulation factor deficiencies

BLOOD AND RELATED PRODUCTS >
COAGULATION PROTEINS

Dried prothrombin complex

(Human prothrombin complex)

- **INDICATIONS AND DOSE**

Treatment and peri-operative prophylaxis of haemorrhage in patients with congenital deficiency of factors II, VII, IX, or X if purified specific coagulation factors not available | Treatment and peri-operative prophylaxis of haemorrhage in patients with acquired deficiency of factors II, VII, IX, or X (e.g. during warfarin treatment)

▸ BY INTRAVENOUS INFUSION

▸ Adult: (consult haematologist)

Major bleeding in patients on warfarin following phytomenadione (initiated under specialist supervision)

▸ BY INTRAVENOUS INFUSION

▸ Adult: 25–50 units/kg

- **CONTRA-INDICATIONS** Angina · history of heparin induced thrombocytopenia · recent myocardial infarction (except in life-threatening haemorrhage following overdosage of oral anticoagulants, and before induction of fibrinolytic therapy)

Cardiovascular system

- CAUTIONS Disseminated intravascular coagulation · history of myocardial infarction or coronary heart disease · postoperative use · risk of thrombosis
- SIDE-EFFECTS
- ▶ Rare or very rare Fever · headache · hypersensitivity
- ▶ Frequency not known Disseminated intravascular coagulation · nephrotic syndrome · thromboembolism
- HEPATIC IMPAIRMENT
  Monitoring Monitor closely in hepatic impairment (risk of thromboembolic complications).
- PRESCRIBING AND DISPENSING INFORMATION Dried prothrombin complex is prepared from human plasma by a suitable fractionation technique, and contains factor IX, together with variable amounts of factors II, VII, and X.
  Available from CSL Behring (*Beriplex ® P/N*), Octapharma (*Octaplex ®*).
- MEDICINAL FORMS
  No licensed medicines listed.

Factor VIIa (recombinant)

(Eptacog alfa (activated))

- INDICATIONS AND DOSE

Treatment and prophylaxis of haemorrhage in patients with haemophilia A or B with inhibitors to factors VIII or IX, acquired haemophilia, factor VII deficiency, or Glanzmann's thrombasthenia
- ▶ BY INTRAVENOUS INJECTION
- ▶ Adult: (consult haematologist)

- CAUTIONS Disseminated intravascular coagulation · risk of thrombosis
- SIDE-EFFECTS
- ▶ Uncommon Embolism and thrombosis · fever · hepatic disorders · intestinal ischaemia · skin reactions
- ▶ Rare or very rare Angina pectoris · cerebrovascular insufficiency · coagulation disorders · headache · myocardial infarction · nausea · peripheral ischaemia
- ▶ Frequency not known Angioedema · flushing

- MEDICINAL FORMS
  There can be variation in the licensing of different medicines containing the same drug.
  Powder and solvent for solution for injection
- ▶ NovoSeven (Novo Nordisk Ltd)
  Eptacog alfa activated 50000 unit NovoSeven 1mg (50,000units) powder and solvent for solution for injection pre-filled syringes | 1 pre-filled disposable injection [PoM] £525.20 (Hospital only)
  NovoSeven 1mg (50,000units) powder and solvent for solution for injection vials | 1 vial [PoM] £525.20 (Hospital only)
  Eptacog alfa activated 100000 unit NovoSeven 2mg (100,000units) powder and solvent for solution for injection vials | 1 vial [PoM] £1,050.40 (Hospital only)
  NovoSeven 2mg (100,000units) powder and solvent for solution for injection pre-filled syringes | 1 pre-filled disposable injection [PoM] £1,050.40 (Hospital only)
  Eptacog alfa activated 250000 unit NovoSeven 5mg (250,000units) powder and solvent for solution for injection pre-filled syringes | 1 pre-filled disposable injection [PoM] £2,626.00 (Hospital only)
  NovoSeven 5mg (250,000units) powder and solvent for solution for injection vials | 1 vial [PoM] £2,626.00 (Hospital only)
  Eptacog alfa activated 400000 unit NovoSeven 8mg (400,000units) powder and solvent for solution for injection vials | 1 vial [PoM] £4,201.60 (Hospital only)
  NovoSeven 8mg (400,000units) powder and solvent for solution for injection pre-filled syringes | 1 pre-filled disposable injection [PoM] £4,201.60 (Hospital only)

Factor VIII fraction, dried

(Human coagulation factor VIII, dried)

- INDICATIONS AND DOSE

Treatment and prophylaxis of haemorrhage in congenital factor VIII deficiency (haemophilia A), acquired factor VIII deficiency | Von Willebrand's disease
- ▶ BY INTRAVENOUS INJECTION, OR BY INTRAVENOUS INFUSION, OR BY CONTINUOUS INTRAVENOUS INFUSION
- ▶ Adult: (consult haematologist)

- CAUTIONS Intravascular haemolysis after large or frequently repeated doses in patients with blood groups A, B, or AB—less likely with high potency concentrates
- SIDE-EFFECTS
- ▶ Uncommon Angioedema · cardiac discomfort · chills · flushing · headache · hypersensitivity · hypotension · lethargy · nausea · paraesthesia · restlessness · skin reactions · tachycardia · vomiting · wheezing
- ▶ Rare or very rare Fever
- MONITORING REQUIREMENTS Monitor for development of factor VIII inhibitors.
- PRESCRIBING AND DISPENSING INFORMATION Dried factor VIII fraction is prepared from human plasma by a suitable fractionation technique; it may also contain varying amounts of von Willebrand factor. *Optivate ®*, *Fanhdi ®*, and *Octanate ®* are not indicated for use in von Willebrand's disease.
  Recombinant human coagulation factor VIII including octocog alfa, moroctocog alfa, and simoctocog alfa are not indicated for use in von Willebrand's disease.

- MEDICINAL FORMS
  There can be variation in the licensing of different medicines containing the same drug.
  Powder and solvent for solution for injection
- ▶ Advate (Baxalta UK Ltd)
  Octocog alfa 250 unit Advate 250unit powder and solvent for solution for injection vials | 1 vial [PoM] £177.50
  Octocog alfa 500 unit Advate 500unit powder and solvent for solution for injection vials | 1 vial [PoM] £355.00
  Octocog alfa 1000 unit Advate 1,000unit powder and solvent for solution for injection vials | 1 vial [PoM] £710.00
  Octocog alfa 2000 unit Advate 2,000unit powder and solvent for solution for injection vials | 1 vial [PoM] £1,420.00
- ▶ Elocta (Swedish Orphan Biovitrum Ltd) ▼
  Efmoroctocog alfa 250 unit Elocta 250unit powder and solvent for solution for injection vials | 1 vial [PoM] 🛇 (Hospital only)
  Efmoroctocog alfa 500 unit Elocta 500unit powder and solvent for solution for injection vials | 1 vial [PoM] 🛇 (Hospital only)
  Efmoroctocog alfa 1000 unit Elocta 1,000unit powder and solvent for solution for injection vials | 1 vial [PoM] 🛇 (Hospital only)
  Efmoroctocog alfa 1500 unit Elocta 1,500unit powder and solvent for solution for injection vials | 1 vial [PoM] 🛇 (Hospital only)
  Efmoroctocog alfa 2000 unit Elocta 2,000unit powder and solvent for solution for injection vials | 1 vial [PoM] 🛇 (Hospital only)
  Efmoroctocog alfa 3000 unit Elocta 3,000unit powder and solvent for solution for injection vials | 1 vial [PoM] 🛇 (Hospital only)
- ▶ Fanhdi (Grifols UK Ltd)
  Factor VIII high purity 500 unit Fanhdi 500unit powder and solvent for solution for injection vials | 1 vial [PoM] £165.00 (Hospital only)
  Factor VIII high purity 1000 unit Fanhdi 1,000unit powder and solvent for solution for injection vials | 1 vial [PoM] £330.00 (Hospital only)
  Factor VIII high purity 1500 unit Fanhdi 1,500unit powder and solvent for solution for injection vials | 1 vial [PoM] £495.00
- ▶ Haemoctin (Biotest Ltd)
  Factor VIII high purity 250 unit Haemoctin 250unit powder and solvent for solution for injection vials | 1 vial [PoM] £150.00 (Hospital only)
  Factor VIII high purity 500 unit Haemoctin 500unit powder and solvent for solution for injection vials | 1 vial [PoM] £300.00 (Hospital only)

Factor VIII high purity 1000 unit Haemoctin 1,000unit powder and solvent for solution for injection vials | 1 vial [PoM] £600.00 (Hospital only)

▸ Helixate NexGen (CSL Behring UK Ltd)
Octocog alfa 250 unit Helixate NexGen 250unit powder and solvent for solution for injection vials | 1 vial [PoM] £139.50
Octocog alfa 500 unit Helixate NexGen 500unit powder and solvent for solution for injection vials | 1 vial [PoM] £279.00
Octocog alfa 1000 unit Helixate NexGen 1,000unit powder and solvent for solution for injection vials | 1 vial [PoM] £558.00
Octocog alfa 2000 unit Helixate NexGen 2,000unit powder and solvent for solution for injection vials | 1 vial [PoM] £1,116.00
▸ Kogenate (Bayer Plc)
Octocog alfa 250 unit Kogenate Bayer 250unit powder and solvent for solution for injection vials | 1 vial [PoM] £157.50
Octocog alfa 500 unit Kogenate Bayer 500unit powder and solvent for solution for injection vials | 1 vial [PoM] £315.00
Octocog alfa 1000 unit Kogenate Bayer 1,000unit powder and solvent for solution for injection vials | 1 vial [PoM] £630.00
Octocog alfa 2000 unit Kogenate Bayer 2,000unit powder and solvent for solution for injection vials | 1 vial [PoM] £1,260.00
▸ Nuwiq (Octapharma Ltd) ▼
Simoctocog alfa 250 unit Nuwiq 250unit powder and solvent for solution for injection vials | 1 vial [PoM] £190.00 (Hospital only)
Simoctocog alfa 500 unit Nuwiq 500unit powder and solvent for solution for injection vials | 1 vial [PoM] £380.00 (Hospital only)
Simoctocog alfa 1000 unit Nuwiq 1,000unit powder and solvent for solution for injection vials | 1 vial [PoM] £760.00 (Hospital only)
Simoctocog alfa 2000 unit Nuwiq 2,000unit powder and solvent for solution for injection vials | 1 vial [PoM] £1,520.00 (Hospital only)
▸ Octanate LV (Octapharma Ltd)
Factor VIII high purity 500 unit Octanate LV 500unit powder and solvent for solution for injection vials | 1 vial [PoM] £300.00 (Hospital only)
Factor VIII high purity 1000 unit Octanate LV 1,000unit powder and solvent for solution for injection vials | 1 vial [PoM] £600.00 (Hospital only)
▸ Optivate (Bio Products Laboratories Ltd)
Factor VIII 500 unit Optivate 500unit powder and solvent for solution for infusion vials | 1 vial [PoM] £180.00
Factor VIII 1000 unit Optivate 1,000unit powder and solvent for solution for infusion vials | 1 vial [PoM] £360.00

Powder and solvent for solution for infusion
▸ Advate (Baxalta UK Ltd)
Octocog alfa 1500 unit Advate 1,500unit powder and solvent for solution for infusion vials | 1 vial [PoM] £1,065.00
Octocog alfa 3000 unit Advate 3,000unit powder and solvent for solution for infusion vials | 1 vial [PoM] £2,130.00
▸ Kogenate (Bayer Plc)
Octocog alfa 3000 unit Kogenate Bayer 3,000unit powder and solvent for solution for injection vials | 1 vial [PoM] £1,890.00

Factor IX fraction, dried

● **INDICATIONS AND DOSE**

Treatment and prophylaxis of haemorrhage in congenital factor IX deficiency (haemophilia B)
▸ BY INTRAVENOUS INJECTION, OR BY CONTINUOUS INTRAVENOUS INFUSION
▸ Adult: (consult haematologist)

● CONTRA-INDICATIONS Disseminated intravascular coagulation
● CAUTIONS Risk of thrombosis—principally with former low purity products
● SIDE-EFFECTS
▸ **Common or very common** Anxiety · back pain · dyspnoea · hypersensitivity · nausea · sensation abnormal · skin reactions · vasodilation
▸ **Rare or very rare** Angioedema · cardiac discomfort · chills · disseminated intravascular coagulation · embolism · thrombosis · headache · hypotension · lethargy · myocardial infarction · tachycardia · vomiting · wheezing
▸ **Frequency not known** Nephrotic syndrome
● PRESCRIBING AND DISPENSING INFORMATION Dried factor IX fraction is prepared from human plasma by a suitable

fractionation technique; it may also contain clotting factors II, VII, and X.

● MEDICINAL FORMS
There can be variation in the licensing of different medicines containing the same drug.
Powder and solvent for solution for injection
▸ AlphaNine (Grifols UK Ltd)
Factor IX high purity 1000 unit AlphaNine 1,000unit powder and solvent for solution for injection vials | 1 vial [PoM] £390.00
Factor IX high purity 1500 unit AlphaNine 1,500unit powder and solvent for solution for injection vials | 1 vial [PoM] [Ⓢ]
▸ Haemonine (Biotest (UK) Ltd)
Factor IX high purity 500 unit Haemonine 500unit powder and solvent for solution for injection vials | 1 vial [PoM] £300.00 (Hospital only)
Factor IX high purity 1000 unit Haemonine 1,000unit powder and solvent for solution for injection vials | 1 vial [PoM] £600.00 (Hospital only)
▸ Replenine-VF (Bio Products Laboratory Ltd)
Factor IX high purity 500 unit Replenine-VF 500unit powder and solvent for solution for injection vials | 1 vial [PoM] £180.00
Factor IX high purity 1000 unit Replenine-VF 1,000unit powder and solvent for solution for injection vials | 1 vial [PoM] £360.00
Powder and solvent for solution for infusion
▸ BeneFIX (Pfizer Ltd)
Nonacog alfa 250 unit BeneFIX 250unit powder and solvent for solution for infusion vials | 1 vial [PoM] £151.80 (Hospital only)
Nonacog alfa 500 unit BeneFIX 500unit powder and solvent for solution for infusion vials | 1 vial [PoM] £303.60 (Hospital only)
Nonacog alfa 1000 unit BeneFIX 1,000unit powder and solvent for solution for infusion vials | 1 vial [PoM] £607.20 (Hospital only)
Nonacog alfa 2000 unit BeneFIX 2,000unit powder and solvent for solution for infusion vials | 1 vial [PoM] £1,214.40 (Hospital only)
Nonacog alfa 3000 unit BeneFIX 3,000unit powder and solvent for solution for infusion vials | 1 vial [PoM] £1,821.60 (Hospital only)

Factor XIII fraction, dried

(Human fibrin-stabilising factor, dried)

● **INDICATIONS AND DOSE**

Congenital factor XIII deficiency
▸ BY INTRAVENOUS INJECTION, OR BY INTRAVENOUS INFUSION
▸ Adult: (consult haematologist)

● SIDE-EFFECTS
▸ **Rare or very rare** Anaphylactoid reaction · dyspnoea · skin reactions

● MEDICINAL FORMS
There can be variation in the licensing of different medicines containing the same drug.
Powder and solvent for solution for injection
▸ Fibrogammin P (CSL Behring UK Ltd)
Factor XIII 250 unit Fibrogammin 250unit powder and solvent for solution for injection vials | 1 vial [PoM] £106.58
Factor XIII 1250 unit Fibrogammin 1,250unit powder and solvent for solution for injection vials | 1 vial [PoM] £532.90

Fibrinogen, dried

(Human fibrinogen)

● **INDICATIONS AND DOSE**

Treatment of haemorrhage in congenital hypofibrinogenaemia or afibrinogenaemia
▸ BY INTRAVENOUS INJECTION, OR BY INTRAVENOUS INFUSION
▸ Adult: (consult haematologist)

● CAUTIONS Risk of thrombosis
● SIDE-EFFECTS
▸ **Common or very common** Fever · thromboembolism
▸ **Frequency not known** Chest pain · chills · cough · dyspnoea · nausea · skin reactions · tachycardia · vomiting

2

Cardiovascular system

- PREGNANCY Manufacturer advises not known to be harmful—no information available.
- BREAST FEEDING Manufacturer advises avoid—no information available.
- PRESCRIBING AND DISPENSING INFORMATION Fibrinogen is prepared from human plasma.

- MEDICINAL FORMS
There can be variation in the licensing of different medicines containing the same drug.
Powder for solution for infusion
  ▸ Riastap (CSL Behring UK Ltd)
  Fibrinogen 1 gram Riastap 1g powder for solution for infusion vials | 1 vial [PoM] £400.00

Protein C concentrate

- **INDICATIONS AND DOSE**
Congenital protein C deficiency
  ▸ BY INTRAVENOUS INJECTION
  ▸ Adult: (consult haematologist)

- CAUTIONS Hypersensitivity to heparins
- SIDE-EFFECTS
  ▸ **Rare or very rare** Dizziness · fever · skin reactions
  ▸ **Frequency not known** Haemothorax · hyperhidrosis · restlessness
- PRESCRIBING AND DISPENSING INFORMATION Protein C is prepared from human plasma.

- MEDICINAL FORMS
There can be variation in the licensing of different medicines containing the same drug.
Powder and solvent for solution for injection
  ▸ Ceprotin (Baxalta UK Ltd)
  Protein C 500 unit Ceprotin 500unit powder and solvent for solution for injection vials | 1 vial [PoM] £2,000.00
  Protein C 1000 unit Ceprotin 1000unit powder and solvent for solution for injection vials | 1 vial [PoM] £1,000.00

BLOOD AND RELATED PRODUCTS ›
HAEMOSTATIC PRODUCTS

Factor VIII inhibitor bypassing fraction

- **INDICATIONS AND DOSE**
Treatment and prophylaxis of haemorrhage in patients with congenital factor VIII deficiency (haemophilia A) and factor VIII inhibitors | Treatment of haemorrhage in non-haemophiliac patients with acquired factor VIII inhibitors
  ▸ BY INTRAVENOUS INFUSION, OR BY INTRAVENOUS INJECTION
  ▸ Adult: (consult haematologist)

- CONTRA-INDICATIONS Disseminated intravascular coagulation
- SIDE-EFFECTS
  ▸ **Common or very common** Dizziness · headache · hypersensitivity · hypotension · skin reactions
  ▸ **Frequency not known** Abdominal discomfort · anamnestic reaction · angioedema · chest discomfort · chills · cough · diarrhoea · disseminated intravascular coagulation · drowsiness · dyspnoea · embolism and thrombosis · fever · flushing · hypertension · ischaemic stroke · malaise · myocardial infarction · nausea · paraesthesia · respiratory disorders · restlessness · tachycardia · taste altered · vomiting
- PRESCRIBING AND DISPENSING INFORMATION
Preparations with factor VIII inhibitor bypassing activity are prepared from human plasma.

- MEDICINAL FORMS
There can be variation in the licensing of different medicines containing the same drug.
Powder and solvent for solution for injection
  ▸ FEIBA Imuno (Baxalta UK Ltd)
  Factor VIII inhibitor bypassing fraction 500 unit FEIBA 500unit powder and solvent for solution for injection vials | 1 vial [PoM] £390.00
Powder and solvent for solution for infusion
  ▸ FEIBA Imuno (Baxalta UK Ltd)
  Factor VIII inhibitor bypassing fraction 1000 unit FEIBA 1,000unit powder and solvent for solution for infusion vials | 1 vial [PoM] £780.00

BLOOD AND RELATED PRODUCTS › PLASMA PRODUCTS

Fresh frozen plasma

- **INDICATIONS AND DOSE**
Replacement of coagulation factors or other plasma proteins where their concentration or functional activity is critically reduced
  ▸ BY INTRAVENOUS INFUSION
  ▸ Adult: (consult haematologist)
Major bleeding in patients on warfarin following phytomenadione (if dried prothrombin complex is unavailable)
  ▸ Adult: 15 mL/kilogram

- CONTRA-INDICATIONS Avoid use as a volume expander · IgA deficiency with confirmed antibodies to IgA
- CAUTIONS Cardiac decompensation · need for compatibility · pulmonary oedema · severe protein S deficiency (avoid products with low protein S activity e.g. *OctaplasLG*®)
- SIDE-EFFECTS
  ▸ **Common or very common** Nausea · skin reactions
  ▸ **Uncommon** Oedema · vomiting
  ▸ **Rare or very rare** Agitation · arrhythmias · bronchospasm · cardio-respiratory distress · chills · fever · hypersensitivity · hypertension · thromboembolism
- PRESCRIBING AND DISPENSING INFORMATION Fresh frozen plasma is prepared from the supernatant liquid obtained by centrifugation of one donation of whole blood.
A preparation of solvent/detergent treated human plasma (frozen) from pooled donors is available from Octapharma (*OctaplasLG*®).

- MEDICINAL FORMS
There can be variation in the licensing of different medicines containing the same drug.
Infusion
  ▸ OctaplasLG (Octap;harma Ltd)
  Human plasma proteins 57.5 mg per 1 ml OctaplasLG Blood Group A Infusion 200 ml bags | 1 bag [PoM] no price available | 10 bag [PoM] no price available
  Human plasma proteins 57.5 mg per 1 ml OctaplasLG Blood Group AB Infusion 200 ml bags | 1 bag [PoM] no price available | 10 bag [PoM] no price available
  Human plasma proteins 57.5 mg per 1 ml OctaplasLG Blood Group B Infusion 200 ml bags | 1 bag [PoM] no price available | 10 bag [PoM] no price available
  Human plasma proteins 57.5 mg per 1 ml OctaplasLG Blood Group O Infusion 200 ml bags | 1 bag [PoM] no price available | 10 bag [PoM] no price available

2.2 Subarachnoid haemorrhage

CALCIUM-CHANNEL BLOCKERS

☛ 155

Nimodipine

07-Feb-2018

- DRUG ACTION Nimodipine is a dihydropyridine calcium-channel blocker.

- ● INDICATIONS AND DOSE

Prevention of ischaemic neurological defects following aneurysmal subarachnoid haemorrhage
▸ BY MOUTH
▸ Adult: 60 mg every 4 hours, to be started within 4 days of aneurysmal subarachnoid haemorrhage and continued for 21 days

Treatment of ischaemic neurological defects following aneurysmal subarachnoid haemorrhage
▸ BY INTRAVENOUS INFUSION
▸ Adult (body-weight up to 70 kg): Initially up to 0.5 mg/hour, increased after 2 hours if no severe fall in blood pressure; increased to 2 mg/hour and continue for at least 5 days (max. 14 days); if surgical intervention during treatment, continue for at least 5 days after surgery; max. total duration of nimodipine use 21 days, to be given via central catheter
▸ Adult (body-weight 70 kg and above): Initially 1 mg/hour, increased after 2 hours if no severe fall in blood pressure; increased to 2 mg/hour and continue for at least 5 days (max. 14 days); if surgical intervention during treatment, continue for at least 5 days after surgery; max. total duration of nimodipine use 21 days, to be given via central catheter

Treatment of ischaemic neurological defects following aneurysmal subarachnoid haemorrhage in patients with unstable blood pressure
▸ BY INTRAVENOUS INFUSION
▸ Adult: Initially up to 0.5 mg/hour, increased after 2 hours if no severe fall in blood pressure; increased to 2 mg/hour and continue for at least 5 days (max. 14 days); if surgical intervention during treatment, continue for at least 5 days after surgery; max. total duration of nimodipine use 21 days, to be given via central catheter

- IMPORTANT SAFETY INFORMATION
SAFE PRACTICE
Nimodipine has been confused with amlodipine; care must be taken to ensure the correct drug is prescribed and dispensed.

- ● CONTRA-INDICATIONS Unstable angina · within 1 month of myocardial infarction
- ● CAUTIONS Cerebral oedema · hypotension · severely raised intracranial pressure
- ● INTERACTIONS → Appendix 1: calcium channel blockers
- ● SIDE-EFFECTS
▸ **Uncommon** Thrombocytopenia · vasodilation
▸ **Rare or very rare** Bradycardia · ileus
- ● PREGNANCY Manufacturer advises use only if potential benefit outweighs risk.
- ● BREAST FEEDING Manufacturer advises avoid—present in milk.
- ● HEPATIC IMPAIRMENT
Monitoring Elimination reduced in cirrhosis—monitor blood pressure.

- ● RENAL IMPAIRMENT
Monitoring ▸ With intravenous use Manufacturer advises monitor renal function closely in renal impairment.
- ● DIRECTIONS FOR ADMINISTRATION Avoid concomitant administration of nimodipine infusion and tablets.
▸ With oral use For administration *by mouth*, tablets may be crushed or halved but are light sensitive—administer immediately.
▸ With intravenous use For *intravenous infusion*, give via drip tubing in Glucose 5% or Sodium chloride 0.9%. Not to be added to infusion container; administer via an infusion pump through a Y-piece into a central catheter; incompatible with polyvinyl chloride giving sets or containers; protect infusion from light. Polyethylene, polypropylene, or glass apparatus should be used. PVC should be avoided.

- ● MEDICINAL FORMS
There can be variation in the licensing of different medicines containing the same drug. Forms available from special-order manufacturers include: oral suspension
Solution for infusion
▸ Nimotop (Bayer Plc)
Nimodipine 200 microgram per 1 ml Nimotop 0.02% solution for infusion 50ml vials | 5 vial [PoM] £68.00 (Hospital only)
Tablet
▸ Nimotop (Bayer Plc)
Nimodipine 30 mg Nimotop 30mg tablets | 100 tablet [PoM] £40.00

3 Blood clots
3.1 Blocked catheters and lines

Other drugs used for Blocked catheters and lines Heparin (unfractionated), p. 132 · Urokinase, p. 137

ANTITHROMBOTIC DRUGS > PROSTAGLANDINS, CARDIOVASCULAR

Epoprostenol

(Prostacyclin)

- DRUG ACTION Epoprostenol is a prostaglandin and a potent vasodilator. It is also a powerful inhibitor of platelet aggregation.

- ● INDICATIONS AND DOSE

Inhibition of platelet aggregation during renal dialysis when heparins are unsuitable or contra-indicated | Treatment of primary pulmonary hypertension resistant to other treatments, usually with oral anti-coagulation (initiated by a specialist)
▸ BY CONTINUOUS INTRAVENOUS INFUSION
▸ Adult: (consult product literature)
PHARMACOKINETICS
▸ Short half-life of approximately 3 minutes, therefore it must be administered by continuous intravenous infusion.

- ● CONTRA-INDICATIONS Severe left ventricular dysfunction
- ● CAUTIONS Avoid abrupt withdrawal when used for primary pulmonary hypertension (risk of rebound pulmonary hypertension) · extreme caution in coronary artery disease · haemorrhagic diathesis · pulmonary veno-occlusive disease · reconstituted solution highly alkaline—avoid extravasation (irritant to tissues) · risk of pulmonary oedema (dose titration for pulmonary hypertension should be in hospital)
- ● INTERACTIONS → Appendix 1: epoprostenol

- SIDE-EFFECTS
▸ **Common or very common** Abdominal pain · anxiety · arrhythmias · arthralgia · chest discomfort · diarrhoea · flushing · haemorrhage · headache · intracranial haemorrhage · nausea · pain · rash · sepsis · vomiting
▸ **Uncommon** Dry mouth · hyperhidrosis
▸ **Rare or very rare** Fatigue · hyperthyroidism · local infection · pallor
▸ **Frequency not known** Ascites · pulmonary oedema (avoid chronic use if occurs during dose titration) · spleen abnormalities
- PREGNANCY Use if potential benefit outweighs risk.
- BREAST FEEDING Manufacturer advises avoid—no information available.
- MONITORING REQUIREMENTS Anticoagulant monitoring required when given with anticoagulants.
- TREATMENT CESSATION Avoid abrupt withdrawal when used for primary pulmonary hypertension (risk of rebound pulmonary hypertension).
- DIRECTIONS FOR ADMINISTRATION For *intravenous infusion* (*Flolan*®), give continuously in Sodium chloride 0.9%; reconstitute using the filter and solvent (glycine buffer diluent) provided to make a concentrate; may be diluted further (consult product literature); for *pulmonary hypertension* dilute further with glycine buffer diluent only and administer via a central venous catheter (can give via peripheral vein until central venous access established); for *renal dialysis* may be diluted further with sodium chloride 0.9%; protect infusion from light. For *intravenous infusion* (*Veletri*®), give continuously in Sodium chloride 0.9%; reconstitute each vial with 5 mL sodium chloride 0.9% then dilute to required concentration with sodium chloride 0.9% (consult product literature); administer through an in-line 0.22 micron filter; for *pulmonary hypertension*, administer via a central venous catheter (can give via peripheral vein until central venous access established); protect infusion from direct sunlight.

- MEDICINAL FORMS
There can be variation in the licensing of different medicines containing the same drug.
Powder for solution for infusion
▸ Veletri (Actelion Pharmaceuticals UK Ltd)
Epoprostenol (as Epoprostenol sodium) 500 microgram Veletri 500microgram powder for solution for infusion vials | 1 vial [PoM] £24.44
Epoprostenol (as Epoprostenol sodium) 1.5 mg Veletri 1.5mg powder for solution for infusion vials | 1 vial [PoM] £49.24
Powder and solvent for solution for infusion
▸ Flolan (GlaxoSmithKline UK Ltd)
Epoprostenol (as Epoprostenol sodium) 500 microgram Flolan 500microgram powder and solvent (pH12) for solution for infusion vials | 1 vial [PoM] £22.22
Epoprostenol (as Epoprostenol sodium) 1.5 mg Flolan 1.5mg powder and solvent (pH12) for solution for infusion vials | 1 vial [PoM] £44.76

3.2 Thromboembolism

Venous thromboembolism

Overview

Venous thromboembolism includes deep-vein thrombosis and pulmonary embolism, and occurs as a result of thrombus formation in a vein.

Venous thromboembolism prophylaxis

All patients admitted to hospital should undergo a risk assessment for venous thromboembolism on admission. Patients considered to be at high risk include those

anticipated to have a substantial reduction in mobility, those with obesity, malignant disease, history of venous thromboembolism, thrombophilic disorder, or patients over 60 years. Patients with risk factors for bleeding (e.g. acute stroke, thrombocytopenia, acquired or untreated inherited bleeding disorders) should only receive pharmacological prophylaxis when the risk of bleeding does not outweigh the risk of venous thromboembolism. NICE clinical guideline 92 (January 2010) provides a full list of risk factors, and gives recommendations for prophylaxis. A venous thromboembolism risk assessment checklist is also available from the Department of Health (www.gov.uk/dh).

Patients scheduled for surgery should be offered mechanical prophylaxis (e.g. anti-embolism stockings) on admission if appropriate; prophylaxis should continue until the patient is sufficiently mobile. Choice of mechanical prophylaxis will depend on factors such as the type of surgery, suitability for the patient, and their condition.

Patients undergoing general or orthopaedic surgery, who are considered to be at high risk of venous thromboembolism, should be offered pharmacological prophylaxis. Choice of prophylaxis will depend on the type of surgery, suitability for the patient, and local policy. A low molecular weight heparin is suitable in all types of general and orthopaedic surgery; heparin (unfractionated) p. 132 is preferred for patients in renal failure. Fondaparinux sodium p. 126 is an option for patients undergoing hip or knee replacement surgery, hip fracture surgery, gastro-intestinal, bariatric, or day surgery procedures. The oral anticoagulants apixaban p. 124, dabigatran etexilate p. 135, and rivaroxaban p. 127 are indicated for thromboprophylaxis following hip or knee replacement surgery.

Pharmacological prophylaxis in general surgery should usually continue for 5–7 days, or until sufficient mobility has been re-established. Pharmacological prophylaxis should be extended to 28 days after major cancer surgery in the abdomen or pelvis. Hip or knee replacement surgery, and hip fracture surgery, require an extended duration of pharmacological prophylaxis, depending on the preparation used (consult product literature).

General medical patients who are considered to be at high risk of venous thromboembolism should be offered pharmacological prophylaxis on admission. Choice of prophylaxis will depend on the medical condition, suitability for the patient, and local policy. Patients should receive either a low molecular weight heparin, heparin (unfractionated) (if patient in renal failure), or fondaparinux sodium. Prophylaxis should continue until the patient is no longer considered to be at significant risk of venous thromboembolism. Mechanical prophylaxis (e.g. anti-embolism stockings) can be offered to medical patients in whom pharmacological prophylaxis is contra-indicated, and continued until the patient is sufficiently mobile.

Edoxaban

Edoxaban p. 125, an inhibitor of factor Xa, is given orally for the treatment and prophylaxis of venous thromboembolism, although, it should not be used as an alternative to unfractionated heparin in pulmonary embolism in patients with haemodynamic instability, or who may receive thrombolysis or pulmonary embolectomy. Duration of therapy should be determined by balancing the benefit of treatment with the bleeding risk; shorter duration of treatment (at least 3 months) should be based on transient risk factors i.e. recent surgery, trauma, immobilisation, and longer durations should be based on permanent risk factors or idiopathic deep-vein thrombosis or pulmonary embolism. Edoxaban is also licensed for the prophylaxis of stroke and systemic embolism in patients with non-valvular atrial fibrillation and at least one other risk factor.

Treatment of venous thromboembolism

For the initial treatment of deep-vein thrombosis and pulmonary embolism a low molecular weight heparin is used; alternatively, heparin (unfractionated) is given as an intravenous loading dose, followed by continuous intravenous infusion (using an infusion pump) or (for deep-vein thrombosis only) by intermittent subcutaneous injection. Intermittent intravenous injection of heparin (unfractionated) is no longer recommended. An oral anticoagulant (usually warfarin sodium p. 139 is started at the same time as unfractionated or low molecular weight heparin (the heparin needs to be continued for at least 5 days and until the INR is $\geq$2 for at least 24 hours). Laboratory monitoring for heparin (unfractionated), preferably on a daily basis, is essential; determination of the activated partial thromboplastin time (APTT) is the most widely used measure (for heparin (unfractionated). A low molecular weight heparin or, in some circumstances, heparin (unfractionated) is also used in regimens for the management of myocardial infarction and unstable angina.

Venous thromboembolism in pregnancy

Heparins are used for the management of venous thromboembolism in pregnancy because they do not cross the placenta. Low molecular weight heparins are preferred because they have a lower risk of osteoporosis and of heparin-induced thrombocytopenia. Low molecular weight heparins are eliminated more rapidly in pregnancy, requiring alteration of the dosage regimen for drugs such as dalteparin sodium p. 130, enoxaparin sodium p. 131, and tinzaparin sodium p. 133. Treatment should be stopped at the onset of labour and advice sought from a specialist on continuing therapy after birth.

Extracorporeal circuits

Heparin (unfractionated) is also used in the maintenance of extracorporeal circuits in cardiopulmonary bypass and haemodialysis.

Haemorrhage

If haemorrhage occurs it is usually sufficient to withdraw unfractionated or low molecular weight heparin, but if rapid reversal of the effects of the heparin is required, protamine sulfate p. 1328 is a specific antidote (but only partially reverses the effects of low molecular weight heparins).

Management of stroke
16-May-2017

Overview

Stroke is associated with a significant risk of morbidity and mortality. Patients presenting with acute symptoms should be immediately transferred to hospital for accurate diagnosis of stroke type, and urgent initiation of appropriate treatment; patients should be managed by a specialist multidisciplinary stroke team.

The following notes give an overview of the initial and long-term management of transient ischaemic attack, ischaemic stroke, and intracerebral haemorrhage.

Transient ischaemic attack

Patients suspected of having a transient ischaemic attack should immediately receive aspirin p. 121 (patients with aspirin hypersensitivity, or those intolerant of aspirin despite the addition of a proton pump inhibitor, should receive clopidogrel p. 122 [unlicensed use] as an alternative). Following a confirmed diagnosis, patients should receive treatment for secondary prevention (see Long-term Management, under Ischaemic Stroke).

Ischaemic stroke

Initial management

Alteplase p. 215 is recommended in the treatment of acute ischaemic stroke if it can be administered within 4.5 hours of symptom onset; it should be given by medical staff experienced in the administration of thrombolytics and the treatment of acute stroke, preferably within a specialist stroke centre. Treatment with aspirin should be initiated 24 hours after thrombolysis (or as soon as possible within 48 hours of symptom onset in patients not receiving thrombolysis); patients with aspirin hypersensitivity, or those intolerant of aspirin despite the addition of a proton pump inhibitor, should receive clopidogrel [unlicensed use] as an alternative.

Anticoagulants are not recommended as an alternative to antiplatelet drugs in acute ischaemic stroke in patients who are in sinus rhythm. However, parenteral anticoagulants may be indicated in patients who are symptomatic of, or at high risk of developing, deep vein thrombosis or pulmonary embolism; warfarin sodium p. 139 should not be commenced in the acute phase of ischaemic stroke.

Anticoagulants should be considered after cardio-embolic ischaemic stroke in patients with atrial fibrillation, however patients presenting with atrial fibrillation following a disabling ischaemic stroke should receive aspirin before being considered for anticoagulant treatment. Patients already receiving anticoagulation for a prosthetic heart valve who experience a disabling ischaemic stroke and are at significant risk of haemorrhagic transformation, should have their anticoagulant treatment stopped for 7 days and substituted with aspirin.

Treatment of hypertension in the acute phase of ischaemic stroke can result in reduced cerebral perfusion, and should therefore only be instituted in the event of a hypertensive emergency, or in those patients considered for thrombolysis.

Long-term management

Patients should receive long-term treatment following a transient ischaemic attack or an ischaemic stroke to reduce the risk of further cardiovascular events.

Following a *transient ischaemic attack* or an *ischaemic stroke* (not associated with atrial fibrillation), long-term treatment with clopidogrel [unlicensed in transient ischaemic attack] is recommended. If clopidogrel is contra-indicated or not tolerated, patients can receive modified-release dipyridamole p. 123 in combination with aspirin; if both aspirin and clopidogrel are contra-indicated or not tolerated, then modified-release dipyridamole alone is recommended; if both modified-release dipyridamole and clopidogrel are contra-indicated or not tolerated, then aspirin alone is recommended.

Patients with stroke associated with atrial fibrillation should be reviewed for long-term treatment with warfarin sodium or an alternative anticoagulant (see Initial Management under Ischaemic Stroke).

Anticoagulants are not routinely recommended in the long-term prevention of recurrent stroke, except in patients with atrial fibrillation.

A statin should be initiated 48 hours after stroke symptom onset, irrespective of the patient's serum-cholesterol concentration.

Following the acute phase of ischaemic stroke, blood pressure should be measured and treatment initiated to achieve a target blood pressure of <130/80 mmHg. Beta-blockers should not be used in the management of hypertension following a stroke, unless they are indicated for a co-existing condition.

All patients should be advised to make lifestyle modifications that include beneficial changes to diet, exercise, weight, alcohol intake, and smoking.

Intracerebral haemorrhage

Initial Management

Surgical intervention may be required following intracerebral haemorrhage to remove the haematoma and relieve intracranial pressure. Patients taking anticoagulants should have this treatment stopped and reversed; anticoagulant therapy has, however, been used in patients with intracerebral haemorrhage who are symptomatic of deep vein thrombosis or pulmonary embolism; placement of a caval filter is an alternative in this situation.

Long-term management

Aspirin therapy should only be given to patients at a high risk of a cardiac ischaemic event. Anticoagulant therapy is not recommended following an intracerebral haemorrhage, even in those with atrial fibrillation, unless the patient is at very high risk of an ischaemic stroke or cardiac ischaemic events; advice from a specialist should be sought in this situation. Blood pressure should be measured and treatment initiated where appropriate, taking care to avoid hypoperfusion. Statins should be avoided following intracerebral haemorrhage, however they can be used with caution when the risk of a vascular event outweighs the risk of further haemorrhage.

Oral anticoagulants

Overview

The main use of anticoagulants is to prevent thrombus formation or extension of an existing thrombus in the slower-moving venous side of the circulation, where the thrombus consists of a fibrin web enmeshed with platelets and red cells.

Anticoagulants are of less use in preventing thrombus formation in arteries, for in faster-flowing vessels thrombi are composed mainly of platelets with little fibrin.

Coumarins and phenindione

The oral anticoagulants warfarin sodium p. 139, acenocoumarol p. 138 and phenindione p. 139, antagonise the effects of vitamin K, and take at least 48 to 72 hours for the anticoagulant effect to develop fully; warfarin sodium is the drug of choice. If an immediate effect is required, unfractionated or low molecular weight heparin must be given concomitantly.

These oral anticoagulants should not be used in cerebral artery thrombosis or peripheral artery occlusion as first-line therapy; aspirin p. 121 is more appropriate for reduction of risk in transient ischaemic attacks. Unfractionated or a low molecular weight heparin (see under Parenteral anticoagulants p. 119) is usually preferred for the prophylaxis of venous thromboembolism in patients undergoing surgery; alternatively, warfarin sodium can be continued in selected patients currently taking long-term warfarin sodium and who are at high risk of thromboembolism (seek expert advice).

Dose

The base-line prothrombin time should be determined but the initial dose should not be delayed whilst awaiting the result.

Target INR

The following indications and target INRs for adults for warfarin take into account recommendations of the British Society for Haematology guidelines on oral anticoagulation with warfarin—fourth edition. *Br J Haematol* 2011; **154**: 311–324:

An INR which is within 0.5 units of the target value is generally satisfactory; larger deviations require dosage adjustment. Target values (rather than ranges) are now recommended.

INR 2.5 for:

- treatment of deep-vein thrombosis or pulmonary embolism (including those associated with antiphospholipid syndrome or for recurrence in patients no longer receiving warfarin sodium)
- atrial fibrillation
- cardioversion—target INR should be achieved at least 3 weeks before cardioversion and anticoagulation should continue for at least 4 weeks after the procedure (higher target values, such as an INR of 3, can be used for up to 4 weeks before the procedure to avoid cancellations due to low INR)
- dilated cardiomyopathy
- mitral stenosis or regurgitation in patients with either atrial fibrillation, a history of systemic embolism, a left atrial thrombus, or an enlarged left atrium
- bioprosthetic heart valves in the mitral position (treat for 3 months), or in patients with a history of systemic embolism (treat for at least 3 months), or with a left atrial thrombus at surgery (treat until clot resolves), or with other risk factors (e.g. atrial fibrillation or a low ventricular ejection fraction)
- acute arterial embolism requiring embolectomy (consider long-term treatment)
- myocardial infarction

INR 3.5 for:

- recurrent deep-vein thrombosis or pulmonary embolism in patients currently receiving anticoagulation and with an INR above 2;

Mechanical prosthetic heart valves:

- the recommended target INR depends on the type and location of the valve, and patient-related risk factors
- consider increasing the INR target or adding an antiplatelet drug, if an embolic event occurs whilst anticoagulated at the target INR.

Duration

The risks of thromboembolism recurrence and anticoagulant-related bleeding should be considered when deciding the duration of anticoagulation.

The following durations of warfarin sodium for the treatment of deep-vein thrombosis and pulmonary embolism reflect the recommendations of the British Society for Haematology (Guidelines on Oral Anticoagulation with Warfarin—fourth edition. *Br J Haematol* 2011; **154**: 311–324):

- 6 weeks for isolated calf-vein deep-vein thrombosis
- 3 months for venous thromboembolism provoked by surgery or other transient risk factor (e.g. combined oral contraceptive use, pregnancy, plaster cast)
- *at least* 3 months for unprovoked proximal deep-vein thrombosis or pulmonary embolism; long-term anticoagulation may be required.

Haemorrhage

The main adverse effect of all oral anticoagulants is haemorrhage. Checking the INR and omitting doses when appropriate is essential; if the anticoagulant is stopped but not reversed, the INR should be measured 2–3 days later to ensure that it is falling. The cause of an elevated INR should be investigated. The following recommendations (which take into account the recommendations of the British Society for Haematology Guidelines on Oral Anticoagulation with Warfarin—fourth edition. *Br J Haematol* 2011; **154**: 311–324) are based on the result of the INR and whether there is major or minor bleeding; the recommendations apply to adults taking warfarin:

- Major bleeding—stop warfarin sodium; give phytomenadione p. 1056 (vitamin K₁) by slow intravenous injection; give dried prothrombin complex p. 111 (factors II, VII, IX, and X); if dried prothrombin complex unavailable, fresh frozen plasma can be given but is less effective; recombinant factor VIIa is not recommended for emergency anticoagulation reversal

- INR >8.0, minor bleeding—stop warfarin sodium; give phytomenadione (vitamin K$_1$) by slow intravenous injection; repeat dose of phytomenadione if INR still too high after 24 hours; restart warfarin sodium when INR <5.0
- INR >8.0, no bleeding—stop warfarin sodium; give phytomenadione (vitamin K$_1$) by mouth using the intravenous preparation orally [unlicensed use]; repeat dose of phytomenadione if INR still too high after 24 hours; restart warfarin when INR <5.0
- INR 5.0–8.0, minor bleeding—stop warfarin sodium; give phytomenadione (vitamin K$_1$) by slow intravenous injection; restart warfarin sodium when INR <5.0
- INR 5.0–8.0, no bleeding—withhold 1 or 2 doses of warfarin sodium and reduce subsequent maintenance dose
- Unexpected bleeding at therapeutic levels—always investigate possibility of underlying cause e.g. unsuspected renal or gastro-intestinal tract pathology

Peri-operative anticoagulation

Warfarin sodium should usually be stopped 5 days before elective surgery; phytomenadione (vitamin K$_1$) by mouth (using the intravenous preparation orally [unlicensed use]) should be given the day before surgery if the INR is ≥1.5. If haemostasis is adequate, warfarin sodium can be resumed at the normal maintenance dose on the evening of surgery or the next day.

Patients stopping warfarin sodium prior to surgery who are considered to be at high risk of thromboembolism (e.g. those with a venous thromboembolic event within the last 3 months, atrial fibrillation with previous stroke or transient ischaemic attack, or mitral mechanical heart valve) may require interim therapy ('bridging') with a low molecular weight heparin (using treatment dose). The low molecular weight heparin should be stopped at least 24 hours before surgery; if the surgery carries a high risk of bleeding, the low molecular weight heparin should not be restarted until at least 48 hours after surgery.

Patients on warfarin sodium p. 139 who require emergency surgery that can be delayed for 6–12 hours can be given intravenous phytomenadione p. 1056 (vitamin K$_1$) to reverse the anticoagulant effect. If surgery cannot be delayed, dried prothrombin complex p. 111 can be given in addition to intravenous phytomenadione (vitamin K$_1$) and the INR checked before surgery.

Combined anticoagulant and antiplatelet therapy

Existing antiplatelet therapy following an acute coronary syndrome or percutaneous coronary intervention should be continued for the necessary duration according to the indication being treated. The addition of warfarin sodium, when indicated (e.g. for venous thromboembolism or atrial fibrillation) should be considered following an assessment of the patient's risk of bleeding and discussion with a cardiologist. The duration of treatment with dual therapy (e.g. aspirin p. 121 and warfarin sodium) or triple therapy (e.g. aspirin with clopidogrel p. 122 and warfarin sodium) should be kept to a minimum where possible. The risk of bleeding with aspirin and warfarin sodium dual therapy is lower than with clopidogrel and warfarin sodium Depending on the indications being treated and the patient's risk of thromboembolism, it may be possible to withhold antiplatelet therapy until warfarin sodium therapy is complete, or vice versa (on specialist advice) in order to reduce the length of time on dual or triple therapy.

Parenteral anticoagulants

Overview

The main use of anticoagulants is to prevent thrombus formation or extension of an existing thrombus in the slower-moving venous side of the circulation, where the thrombus consists of a fibrin web enmeshed with platelets and red cells.

Anticoagulants are of less use in preventing thrombus formation in arteries, for in faster-flowing vessels thrombi are composed mainly of platelets with little fibrin.

Heparin

Heparin initiates anticoagulation rapidly but has a short duration of action. It is often referred to as **'standard'** or heparin (unfractionated) p. 132 to distinguish it from the **low molecular weight heparins**, which have a longer duration of action. Although a low molecular weight heparin is generally preferred for routine use, heparin (unfractionated) can be used in those at high risk of bleeding because its effect can be terminated rapidly by stopping the infusion.

Low molecular weight heparins

Low molecular weight heparins (dalteparin sodium p. 130, enoxaparin sodium p. 131, and tinzaparin sodium p. 133) are usually preferred over heparin (unfractionated) in the *prevention* of Venous thromboembolism p. 116 because they are as effective and they have a lower risk of heparin-induced thrombocytopenia. The standard prophylactic regimen does not require anticoagulant monitoring. The duration of action of low molecular weight heparins is longer than that of heparin (unfractionated) and *once-daily subcutaneous* administration is possible for some indications, making them convenient to use.

Low molecular weight heparins are generally preferred over heparin (unfractionated) in the *treatment* of deep vein thrombosis and pulmonary embolism, and are also used in the treatment of myocardial infarction, unstable coronary artery disease (see under Acute coronary syndromes p. 212) and for the prevention of clotting in extracorporeal circuits.

Dalteparin sodium and tinzaparin sodium (only 20 000 unit/mL syringe) are also licensed for the extended treatment and prophylaxis of venous thromboembolism in patients with solid tumours; treatment is recommended for a duration of 6 months. Treatment should be initiated by healthcare professionals experienced in the treatment of venous thromboembolism.

Heparinoids

Danaparoid sodium p. 129 is a heparinoid used for prophylaxis of deep-vein thrombosis in patients undergoing general or orthopaedic surgery. Providing there is no evidence of cross-reactivity, it also has a role in patients who develop heparin-induced thrombocytopenia.

Argatroban

An oral anticoagulant can be given with argatroban monohydrate p. 134, but it should only be started once thrombocytopenia has substantially resolved.

Hirudins

Bivalirudin, a hirudin analogue, is a thrombin inhibitor which is licensed for unstable angina or non-ST-segment elevation myocardial infarction in patients planned for urgent or early intervention, and as an anticoagulant for patients undergoing percutaneous coronary intervention (including patients with ST-segment elevation myocardial infarction undergoing primary percutaneous coronary intervention—see also Management of ST-segment elevation myocardial infarction (STEMI) in Acute coronary syndromes p. 212).

Heparin flushes

The use of heparin flushes should be kept to a minimum. For maintaining patency of peripheral venous catheters, sodium chloride injection 0.9% is as effective as heparin flushes. The role of heparin flushes in maintaining patency of arterial and central venous catheters is unclear.

Epoprostenol

Epoprostenol (prostacyclin) can be given to inhibit platelet aggregation during renal dialysis when heparins are unsuitable or contra-indicated. It is also licensed for the treatment of primary pulmonary hypertension resistant to other treatment, usually with oral anticoagulation; it should be initiated by specialists in pulmonary hypertension. Epoprostenol is a potent vasodilator. It has a short half-life of approximately 3 minutes and therefore it must be administered by continuous intravenous infusion.

Fondaparinux

Fondaparinux sodium is a synthetic pentasaccharide that inhibits activated factor X.

> **Other drugs used for Thromboembolism** Streptokinase, p. 216

ANTIDOTES AND CHELATORS

Idarucizumab
17-Mar-2017

- **DRUG ACTION** Idarucizumab is a humanised monoclonal antibody fragment that binds specifically to dabigatran and its metabolites, thereby reversing the anticoagulant effect.

- **INDICATIONS AND DOSE**

  Rapid reversal of dabigatran for emergency procedures, or in life-threatening or uncontrolled bleeding (specialist supervision in hospital)
  ▸ BY INTRAVENOUS INJECTION, OR BY INTRAVENOUS INFUSION
  ▸ Adult: 5 g, followed by 5 g if required

- **CAUTIONS** Risk of thrombosis
  CAUTIONS, FURTHER INFORMATION Manufacturer advises to consider re-starting anticoagulant therapy as soon as medically appropriate to reduce the risk of thrombosis. Dabigatran can be re-started 24 hours after administration of idarucizumab; other anticoagulant therapy can be started at any time.

- **PREGNANCY** Manufacturer advises use only if potential benefit outweighs risk—no information available.

- **DIRECTIONS FOR ADMINISTRATION** Manufacturer advises that one dose of *Praxbind®* is administered as either two consecutive intravenous infusions, each given over 5–10 minutes, *or* as a bolus injection.

- **HANDLING AND STORAGE** Manufacturer advises store in a refrigerator at 2–8°C.

- **NATIONAL FUNDING/ACCESS DECISIONS**
  Scottish Medicines Consortium (SMC) Decisions
  The *Scottish Medicines Consortium* has advised (September 2016) that idarucizumab (*Praxbind®*) is accepted for use within NHS Scotland for adult patients treated with dabigatran etexilate when rapid reversal of its anticoagulant effects is required for emergency surgery/urgent procedures or in life-threatening or uncontrolled bleeding.

- **MEDICINAL FORMS**
  There can be variation in the licensing of different medicines containing the same drug.
  Solution for infusion
  EXCIPIENTS: May contain Polysorbates, sorbitol
  ELECTROLYTES: May contain Sodium
  ▸ Praxbind (Boehringer Ingelheim Ltd) ▼
  Idarucizumab 50 mg per 1 ml Praxbind 2.5g/50ml solution for infusion vials | 2 vial [PoM] £2,400.00 (Hospital only)

ANTITHROMBOTIC DRUGS > ANTIPLATELET DRUGS

Antiplatelet drugs

Overview

Antiplatelet drugs decrease platelet aggregation and inhibit thrombus formation in the arterial circulation, because in faster-flowing vessels, thrombi are composed mainly of platelets with little fibrin.

Use of aspirin p. 121 in primary prevention of cardiovascular events, in patients with or without diabetes, is of unproven benefit. Long-term use of aspirin is of benefit in established cardiovascular disease (secondary prevention); unduly high blood pressure must be controlled before aspirin is given. If the patient is at a high risk of gastro-intestinal bleeding, a proton pump inhibitor can be added.

Aspirin is given following coronary bypass surgery. It is also used in atrial fibrillation, for intermittent claudication, for stable angina and acute coronary syndromes, for use following placement of coronary stents and for use in stroke.

Clopidogrel p. 122 is licensed for the prevention of atherothrombotic events in patients with a history of symptomatic ischaemic disease. Clopidogrel, in combination with low-dose aspirin, is also licensed for acute coronary syndrome without ST-segment elevation; in these circumstances the combination is given for up to 12 months (most benefit occurs during the first 3 months; there is no evidence of benefit beyond 12 months). Clopidogrel, in combination with low-dose aspirin, is also licensed for acute myocardial infarction with ST-segment elevation; the combination is licensed for at least 4 weeks, but the optimum treatment duration has not been established. In patients undergoing percutaneous coronary intervention, clopidogrel is used as an adjunct with aspirin. Patients who are not already taking clopidogrel should receive a loading dose prior to procedure.

Clopidogrel is also licensed, in combination with low-dose aspirin, for the prevention of atherothrombotic and thromboembolic events in patients with atrial fibrillation (and at least one risk factor for a vascular event), and for whom warfarin sodium p. 139 is unsuitable.

Use of clopidogrel with aspirin increases the risk of bleeding. Clopidogrel monotherapy may be an alternative when aspirin is contra-indicated, for example in those with aspirin hypersensitivity, or when aspirin is not tolerated despite the addition of a proton pump inhibitor (see also NICE guidance).

Clopidogrel also has uses in stroke.

Dipyridamole p. 123 is used by mouth as an adjunct to oral anticoagulation for prophylaxis of thromboembolism associated with prosthetic heart valves. Modified-release preparations are licensed for secondary prevention of ischaemic stroke and transient ischaemic attacks.

Prasugrel p. 213, in combination with aspirin, is licensed for the prevention of atherothrombotic events in patients with acute coronary syndrome undergoing percutaneous coronary intervention; the combination is usually given for up to 12 months.

Ticagrelor p. 214, in combination with aspirin, is licensed for the prevention of atherothrombotic events in patients with acute coronary syndrome; the combination is usually given for up to 12 months.

Cangrelor p. 208, in combination with aspirin, is licensed for the reduction of thrombotic cardiovascular events in patients with coronary artery disease undergoing percutaneous coronary intervention (PCI) who have not received treatment with oral clopidogrel, prasugrel or ticagrelor prior to the procedure and in whom oral therapy with these drugs is not suitable. Cangrelor is to be used under expert supervision only.

Antiplatelet drugs and coronary stents
Patients selected for percutaneous coronary intervention, with the placement of a coronary stent, will require dual antiplatelet therapy with aspirin and either cangrelor, clopidogrel, prasugrel, or ticagrelor. Aspirin therapy should continue indefinitely. Clopidogrel is recommended for 1 month following elective percutaneous coronary intervention with placement of a bare-metal stent, and for 12 months if percutaneous coronary intervention with placement of a bare-metal stent was for an acute coronary syndrome; clopidogrel should be given for 12 months following placement of a drug-eluting stent. Clopidogrel should not be discontinued prematurely in patients with a drug-eluting stent—there is an increased risk of stent thrombosis as a result of the eluted drug slowing the re-endothelialisation process. Patients considered to be at high risk of developing late stent thrombosis with a drug-eluting stent may require a longer duration of treatment with clopidogrel. Prasugrel or ticagrelor are alternatives to clopidogrel in certain patients undergoing percutaneous coronary intervention.

Glycoprotein IIb/IIIa inhibitors
Glycoprotein IIb/IIIa inhibitors prevent platelet aggregation by blocking the binding of fibrinogen to receptors on platelets. Abciximab p. 208 is a monoclonal antibody which binds to glycoprotein IIb/IIIa receptors and to other related sites; it is licensed as an adjunct to heparin (unfractionated) p. 132 and aspirin for the prevention of ischaemic complications in high-risk patients undergoing percutaneous transluminal coronary intervention. Abciximab should be used once only (to avoid additional risk of thrombocytopenia). Eptifibatide p. 209 (in combination with heparin (unfractionated) and aspirin) and tirofiban p. 209 (in combination with heparin (unfractionated), aspirin, and clopidogrel) also inhibit glycoprotein IIb/IIIa receptors; they are licensed for use to prevent early myocardial infarction in patients with unstable angina or non-ST-segment-elevation myocardial infarction. Tirofiban is also licensed for use in combination with heparin (unfractionated), aspirin, and clopidogrel, for the reduction of major cardiovascular events in patients with ST-segment elevation myocardial infarction intended for primary percutaneous coronary intervention. Abciximab, eptifibatide and tirofiban should be used by specialists only.

Epoprostenol p. 115 is also used to inhibit platelet aggregation during renal dialysis when heparins are unsuitable or contra-indicated.

Aspirin
(Acetylsalicylic Acid)

● INDICATIONS AND DOSE
Cardiovascular disease (secondary prevention)
▶ BY MOUTH
▶ Adult: 75 mg daily

Management of unstable angina and non-ST-segment elevation myocardial infarction (NSTEMI) | Management of ST-segment elevation myocardial infarction (STEMI)
▶ BY MOUTH
▶ Adult: 300 mg, chewed or dispersed in water

Suspected transient ischaemic attack
▶ BY MOUTH
▶ Adult: 300 mg once daily until diagnosis established

Transient ischaemic attack (long-term treatment in combination with dipyridamole) | Ischaemic stroke not associated with atrial fibrillation (in combination with dipyridamole if clopidogrel contra-indicated or not tolerated) | Ischaemic stroke not associated with atrial fibrillation (used alone if clopidogrel and dipyridamole contra-indicated or not tolerated)
▶ BY MOUTH
▶ Adult: 75 mg once daily

Acute ischaemic stroke
▶ BY MOUTH
▶ Adult: 300 mg once daily for 14 days, to be initiated 24 hours after thrombolysis or as soon as possible within 48 hours of symptom onset in patients not receiving thrombolysis

Atrial fibrillation following a disabling ischaemic stroke (before being considered for anticoagulant treatment)
▶ BY MOUTH
▶ Adult: 300 mg once daily for 14 days

Following disabling ischaemic stroke in patients receiving anticoagulation for a prosthetic heart valve and who are at significant risk of haemorrhagic transformation
▶ BY MOUTH
▶ Adult: 300 mg once daily, anticoagulant treatment stopped for 7 days and to be substituted with aspirin

Following coronary by-pass surgery
▶ BY MOUTH
▶ Adult: 75–300 mg daily

Mild to moderate pain | Pyrexia
▶ BY MOUTH
▶ Adult: 300–900 mg every 4–6 hours as required; maximum 4 g per day
▶ BY RECTUM
▶ Adult: 450–900 mg every 4 hours; maximum 3.6 g per day

● CONTRA-INDICATIONS Active peptic ulceration · bleeding disorders (antiplatelet dose) · children under 16 years (risk of Reye's syndrome) · haemophilia · previous peptic ulceration (analgesic dose) · severe cardiac failure (analgesic dose)

CONTRA-INDICATIONS, FURTHER INFORMATION
▶ Reye's syndrome Owing to an association with Reye's syndrome, aspirin-containing preparations should not be given to children under 16 years, unless specifically indicated, e.g. for Kawasaki disease.

● CAUTIONS Allergic disease · anaemia · asthma · dehydration · elderly · G6PD deficiency · preferably avoid during fever or viral infection in children (risk of Reye's syndrome) · previous peptic ulceration (but manufacturers may advise avoidance of low-dose aspirin in history of peptic ulceration) · thyrotoxicosis · uncontrolled hypertension

● INTERACTIONS → Appendix 1: aspirin
● SIDE-EFFECTS
▶ Common or very common Dyspepsia · haemorrhage
▶ Uncommon Dyspnoea · rhinitis · severe cutaneous adverse reactions (SCARs) · skin reactions
▶ Rare or very rare Aplastic anaemia · asthmatic attack · bronchospasm · erythema nodosum · gastrointestinal haemorrhage (severe) · granulocytosis · haemorrhagic vasculitis · intracranial haemorrhage · menorrhagia · nausea · thrombocytopenia · vomiting
▶ Frequency not known Fluid retention · gastrointestinal disorders · headache · hearing impairment · hepatic failure · hyperuricaemia · iron deficiency anaemia · renal impairment · sodium retention · vertigo

Overdose The main features of salicylate poisoning are hyperventilation, tinnitus, deafness, vasodilatation, and sweating. Coma is uncommon but indicates very severe poisoning.

For specific details on the management of poisoning, see Aspirin, under Emergency treatment of poisoning p. 1319.

- ALLERGY AND CROSS-SENSITIVITY Aspirin is **contra-indicated** in history of hypersensitivity to aspirin or any other NSAID—which includes those in whom attacks of asthma, angioedema, urticaria, or rhinitis have been precipitated by aspirin or any other NSAID.

- PREGNANCY Use antiplatelet doses with caution during third trimester; impaired platelet function and risk of haemorrhage; delayed onset and increased duration of labour with increased blood loss; avoid analgesic doses if possible in last few weeks (low doses probably not harmful); high doses may be related to intra-uterine growth restriction, teratogenic effects, closure of fetal ductus arteriosus in utero and possibly persistent pulmonary hypertension of newborn; kernicterus may occur in jaundiced neonates.

- BREAST FEEDING Avoid—possible risk of Reye's syndrome; regular use of high doses could impair platelet function and produce hypoprothrombinaemia in infant if neonatal vitamin K stores low.

- HEPATIC IMPAIRMENT Avoid in severe impairment—increased risk of gastro-intestinal bleeding.

- RENAL IMPAIRMENT Use with caution; avoid in severe impairment; sodium and water retention; deterioration in renal function; increased risk of gastro-intestinal bleeding.

- PRESCRIBING AND DISPENSING INFORMATION BP directs that when no strength is stated the 300 mg strength should be dispensed, and that when soluble aspirin tablets are prescribed, dispersible aspirin tablets shall be dispensed.

- PROFESSION SPECIFIC INFORMATION

  Dental practitioners' formulary
  Aspirin Dispersible Tablets 300 mg may be prescribed.

- EXCEPTIONS TO LEGAL CATEGORY Can be sold to the public provided packs contain no more than 32 capsules or tablets; pharmacists can sell multiple packs up to a total quantity of 100 capsules or tablets in justifiable circumstances.

- MEDICINAL FORMS
  There can be variation in the licensing of different medicines containing the same drug. Forms available from special-order manufacturers include: capsule, oral suspension, oral solution

  Gastro-resistant tablet
  CAUTIONARY AND ADVISORY LABELS 5, 25, 32
  ▶ Aspirin (Non-proprietary)
  Aspirin 75 mg Aspirin 75mg gastro-resistant tablets | 28 tablet P £0.52 DT = £0.52
  Aspirin 300 mg Aspirin 300mg gastro-resistant tablets | 100 tablet PoM £20.34 DT = £20.34
  ▶ Micropirin (Dexcel-Pharma Ltd)
  Aspirin 75 mg Micropirin 75mg gastro-resistant tablets | 28 tablet P £1.45 DT = £0.52 | 56 tablet P £2.87
  ▶ Nu-Seals (Alliance Pharmaceuticals Ltd)
  Aspirin 75 mg Nu-Seals 75 gastro-resistant tablets | 56 tablet P £3.12

  Tablet
  CAUTIONARY AND ADVISORY LABELS 21, 32
  ▶ Aspirin (Non-proprietary)
  Aspirin 75 mg Aspirin 75mg tablets | 28 tablet PoM £1.13 DT = £1.12
  Aspirin 300 mg Aspirin 300mg tablets | 100 tablet PoM £1.12-£10.47

Suppository
CAUTIONARY AND ADVISORY LABELS 32
▶ Aspirin (Non-proprietary)
Aspirin 150 mg Aspirin 150mg suppositories | 10 suppository P £18.67 DT = £18.67
Aspirin 300 mg Aspirin 300mg suppositories | 10 suppository P £35.89 DT = £35.89

Dispersible tablet
CAUTIONARY AND ADVISORY LABELS 13, 21, 32
▶ Aspirin (Non-proprietary)
Aspirin 75 mg Aspirin 75mg dispersible tablets | 1000 tablet PoM £11.79-£18.57
Aspirin 300 mg Aspirin 300mg dispersible tablets | 32 tablet PoM Ⓢ DT = £0.66 | 100 tablet PoM £2.06 DT = £2.06
▶ Danamep (Ecogen Europe Ltd)
Aspirin 75 mg Danamep 75mg dispersible tablets | 28 tablet PoM £0.50 DT = £0.33

Clopidogrel

- INDICATIONS AND DOSE

Prevention of atherothrombotic events in percutaneous coronary intervention (adjunct with aspirin) in patients not already on clopidogrel
▶ BY MOUTH
▶ Adult: Loading dose 300 mg, to be taken prior to the procedure, alternatively loading dose 600 mg, higher dose may produce a greater and more rapid inhibition of platelet aggregation

Transient ischaemic attack for patients with aspirin hypersensitivity, or those intolerant of aspirin despite the addition of a proton pump inhibitor | Acute ischaemic stroke for patients with aspirin hypersensitivity, or those intolerant of aspirin despite the addition of a proton pump inhibitor
▶ BY MOUTH
▶ Adult: 75 mg once daily

Prevention of atherothrombotic events in peripheral arterial disease or within 35 days of myocardial infarction, or within 6 months of ischaemic stroke
▶ BY MOUTH
▶ Adult: 75 mg once daily

Prevention of atherothrombotic events in acute coronary syndrome without ST-segment elevation (given with aspirin)
▶ BY MOUTH
▶ Adult: Initially 300 mg, then 75 mg daily for up to 12 months

Prevention of atherothrombotic events in acute myocardial infarction with ST-segment elevation (given with aspirin)
▶ BY MOUTH
▶ Adult 18-75 years: Initially 300 mg, then 75 mg for at least 4 weeks
▶ Adult 76 years and over: 75 mg daily for at least 4 weeks

Prevention of atherothrombotic and thromboembolic events in patients with atrial fibrillation and at least one risk factor for a vascular event (with aspirin) and for whom warfarin is unsuitable
▶ BY MOUTH
▶ Adult: 75 mg once daily

- UNLICENSED USE 600 mg loading dose prior to percutaneous coronary intervention is an unlicensed dose. Use in transient ischaemic attack or acute ischaemic stroke, in patients with aspirin hypersensitivity or intolerant of aspirin, is unlicensed.

- CONTRA-INDICATIONS Active bleeding

- CAUTIONS Discontinue 7 days before elective surgery if antiplatelet effect not desirable · patients at risk of increased bleeding from trauma, surgery, or other pathological conditions

- **INTERACTIONS** → Appendix 1: clopidogrel
- **SIDE-EFFECTS**
▶ **Common or very common** Diarrhoea · gastrointestinal discomfort · haemorrhage · skin reactions
▶ **Uncommon** Constipation · dizziness · eosinophilia · gastrointestinal disorders · headache · intracranial haemorrhage · leucopenia · nausea · paraesthesia · thrombocytopenia · vomiting
▶ **Rare or very rare** Acquired haemophilia · agranulocytosis · anaemia · angioedema · arthralgia · arthritis · bone marrow disorders · confusion · fever · glomerulonephritis · gynaecomastia · hallucination · hepatic disorders · hypersensitivity · hypotension · myalgia · neutropenia · pancreatitis · respiratory disorders · severe cutaneous adverse reactions (SCARs) · stomatitis · taste altered · ulcerative colitis · vasculitis · vertigo
▶ **Frequency not known** Kounis syndrome
- **ALLERGY AND CROSS-SENSITIVITY** Caution with history of hypersensitivity reactions to thienopyridines (e.g. prasugrel).
- **PREGNANCY** Manufacturer advises avoid—no information available.
- **BREAST FEEDING** Manufacturer advises avoid.
- **HEPATIC IMPAIRMENT** Manufacturer advises caution (risk of bleeding). Avoid in severe impairment.
- **RENAL IMPAIRMENT** Manufacturer advises caution.
- **NATIONAL FUNDING/ACCESS DECISIONS**
  NICE decisions
▶ Clopidogrel and modified-release dipyridamole in the prevention of occlusive vascular events (December 2010) NICE TA210
The guidance applies to patients who have had an occlusive vascular event, or who have established peripheral arterial disease. The guidance does not apply to patients who have had, or are at risk of, stroke associated with atrial fibrillation, or who need prophylaxis for occlusive events following coronary revascularisation or carotid artery procedures.

Clopidogrel monotherapy is recommended as an option to prevent occlusive vascular events in patients who have had:
- an ischaemic stroke, or who have peripheral arterial disease or multivascular disease, **or**
- a myocardial infarction, only if aspirin is contra-indicated or not tolerated.
www.nice.org.uk/TA210

Scottish Medicines Consortium (SMC) Decisions
The *Scottish Medicines Consortium* has advised (February 2004) that clopidogrel be accepted for restricted use for the treatment of confirmed acute coronary syndrome (without ST-segment elevation), in combination with aspirin. Clopidogrel should be initiated in hospital inpatients **only**.

The *Scottish Medicines Consortium* has also advised (July 2007) that clopidogrel be accepted for restricted use for patients with ST-segment elevation acute myocardial infarction in combination with aspirin; treatment with clopidogrel is restricted to 4 weeks only.

- **MEDICINAL FORMS**
There can be variation in the licensing of different medicines containing the same drug. Forms available from special-order manufacturers include: oral suspension, oral solution

Tablet
▶ Clopidogrel (Non-proprietary)
Clopidogrel 75 mg Clopidogrel 75mg tablets | 28 tablet [PoM]
£30.53 DT = £1.30 | 30 tablet [PoM] £1.39–£32.71
▶ Grepid (Kent Pharmaceuticals Ltd)
Clopidogrel 75 mg Grepid 75mg tablets | 28 tablet [PoM] £33.93 DT
= £1.30 | 30 tablet [PoM] £32.28

▶ Plavix (Sanofi)
Clopidogrel 75 mg Plavix 75mg tablets | 30 tablet [PoM] £35.64
Clopidogrel (as Clopidogrel hydrogen sulfate) 300 mg Plavix
300mg tablets | 30 tablet [PoM] £142.54 DT = £142.54

Dipyridamole

- **INDICATIONS AND DOSE**
Secondary prevention of ischaemic stroke (not associated with atrial fibrillation) and transient ischaemic attacks (used alone or with aspirin) | Adjunct to oral anticoagulation for prophylaxis of thromboembolism associated with prosthetic heart valves
▶ BY MOUTH USING MODIFIED-RELEASE MEDICINES
▶ Adult: 200 mg twice daily, to be taken preferably with food

Adjunct to oral anticoagulation for prophylaxis of thromboembolism associated with prosthetic heart valves
▶ BY MOUTH USING IMMEDIATE-RELEASE MEDICINES
▶ Adult: 300–600 mg daily in 3–4 divided doses

Myocardial imaging—diagnostic use only
▶ BY INTRAVENOUS INJECTION
▶ Adult: (consult product literature)

- **CAUTIONS** Aortic stenosis · coagulation disorders · heart failure · hypotension · left ventricular outflow obstruction · may exacerbate migraine · myasthenia gravis (risk of exacerbation) · rapidly worsening angina · recent myocardial infarction
- **INTERACTIONS** → Appendix 1: dipyridamole
- **SIDE-EFFECTS**
▶ **Common or very common** Angina pectoris · diarrhoea · dizziness · headache · myalgia · nausea · skin reactions · vomiting
▶ **Frequency not known** Angioedema · bronchospasm · haemorrhage · hot flush · hypotension · tachycardia · thrombocytopenia
- **PREGNANCY** Not known to be harmful.
- **BREAST FEEDING** Manufacturers advise use only if essential—small amount present in milk.
- **PRESCRIBING AND DISPENSING INFORMATION** Modified-release capsules should be dispensed in original container (pack contains a desiccant) and any capsules remaining should be discarded 6 weeks after opening.
- **NATIONAL FUNDING/ACCESS DECISIONS**
  NICE decisions
▶ Clopidogrel and modified-release dipyridamole in the prevention of occlusive vascular events (December 2010) NICE TA210
The guidance applies to patients who have had an occlusive vascular event, or who have established peripheral arterial disease. The guidance does not apply to patients who have had, or are at risk of, stroke associated with atrial fibrillation, or who need prophylaxis for occlusive events following coronary revascularisation or carotid artery procedures.

Modified-release dipyridamole, in combination with aspirin, is recommended as an option to prevent occlusive vascular events in patients who have had:
- a transient ischaemic attack, **or**
- an ischaemic stroke, only if clopidogrel is contra-indicated or not tolerated.
Modified-release dipyridamole monotherapy is recommended as an option to prevent occlusive vascular events in patients who have had:
- an ischaemic stroke, only if aspirin and clopidogrel are contra-indicated or not tolerated, **or**
- a transient ischaemic attack, only if aspirin is contra-indicated or not tolerated.
www.nice.org.uk/TA210

● MEDICINAL FORMS
There can be variation in the licensing of different medicines containing the same drug. Forms available from special-order manufacturers include: oral suspension, oral solution

Oral suspension

▸ Dipyridamole (Non-proprietary)
Dipyridamole 10 mg per 1 ml Dipyridamole 50mg/5ml oral suspension sugar free sugar-free | 150 ml [PoM] £39.40 DT = £39.40
Dipyridamole 40 mg per 1 ml Dipyridamole 200mg/5ml oral suspension sugar free sugar-free | 150 ml [PoM] £133.53 DT = £133.53

Modified-release capsule

CAUTIONARY AND ADVISORY LABELS 21, 25

▸ Dipyridamole (Non-proprietary)
Dipyridamole 200 mg Dipyridamole 200mg modified-release capsules | 60 capsule [PoM] [Ⓢ] DT = £10.06

▸ Attia (Dr Reddy's Laboratories (UK) Ltd)
Dipyridamole 200 mg Attia 200mg modified-release capsules | 60 capsule [PoM] £9.56 DT = £10.06

▸ Ofcram PR (Focus Pharmaceuticals Ltd)
Dipyridamole 200 mg Ofcram PR 200mg capsules | 60 capsule [PoM] £10.06 DT = £10.06

▸ Persantin Retard (Boehringer Ingelheim Ltd, Consilient Health Ltd)
Dipyridamole 200 mg Persantin Retard 200mg capsules | 60 capsule [PoM] £8.55–£10.06 DT = £10.06

▸ Trolactin (Actavis UK Ltd)
Dipyridamole 200 mg Trolactin 200mg modified-release capsules | 60 capsule [PoM] £10.05 DT = £10.06

Tablet

CAUTIONARY AND ADVISORY LABELS 22

▸ Dipyridamole (Non-proprietary)
Dipyridamole 25 mg Dipyridamole 25mg tablets | 84 tablet [PoM] £9.40 DT = £9.40
Dipyridamole 100 mg Dipyridamole 100mg tablets | 84 tablet [PoM] £12.50 DT = £3.88

▸ Persantin (Boehringer Ingelheim Ltd)
Dipyridamole 100 mg Persantin 100mg tablets | 84 tablet [PoM] £6.30 DT = £3.88

Dipyridamole with aspirin

The properties listed below are those particular to the combination only. For the properties of the components please consider, dipyridamole p. 123, aspirin p. 121.

● INDICATIONS AND DOSE

Secondary prevention of ischaemic stroke and transient ischaemic attacks

▸ BY MOUTH USING MODIFIED-RELEASE MEDICINES
▸ Adult: 25/200 mg twice daily

● INTERACTIONS → Appendix 1: aspirin · dipyridamole

● PRESCRIBING AND DISPENSING INFORMATION Dispense in original container (pack contains a desiccant) and discard any capsules remaining 6 weeks after opening.

● MEDICINAL FORMS
There can be variation in the licensing of different medicines containing the same drug.

Modified-release capsule

CAUTIONARY AND ADVISORY LABELS 21, 25, 32

▸ Dipyridamole with aspirin (Non-proprietary)
Aspirin 25 mg, Dipyridamole 200 mg Dipyridamole 200mg modified-release / Aspirin 25mg capsules | 100 capsule [PoM] [Ⓢ] DT = £9.35

▸ Atransipar (Par Laboratories Europe Ltd)
Aspirin 25 mg, Dipyridamole 200 mg Atransipar 200mg/25mg modified-release capsules | 60 capsule [PoM] £9.84

▸ Molita (Dr Reddy's Laboratories (UK) Ltd)
Aspirin 25 mg, Dipyridamole 200 mg Molita 200mg/25mg modified-release capsules | 100 capsule [PoM] £9.35 DT = £9.35

ANTITHROMBOTIC DRUGS ❭ FACTOR XA INHIBITORS

Apixaban
20-Apr-2017

● DRUG ACTION Apixaban is a direct inhibitor of activated factor X (factor Xa).

● INDICATIONS AND DOSE

Prophylaxis of venous thromboembolism following knee replacement surgery

▸ BY MOUTH
▸ Adult: 2.5 mg twice daily for 10–14 days, to be started 12–24 hours after surgery

Prophylaxis of venous thromboembolism following hip replacement surgery

▸ BY MOUTH
▸ Adult: 2.5 mg twice daily for 32–38 days, to be started 12–24 hours after surgery

Treatment of deep-vein thrombosis | Treatment of pulmonary embolism

▸ BY MOUTH
▸ Adult: Initially 10 mg twice daily for 7 days, then maintenance 5 mg twice daily

Prophylaxis of recurrent deep-vein thrombosis | Prophylaxis of recurrent pulmonary embolism

▸ BY MOUTH
▸ Adult: 2.5 mg twice daily, following completion of 6 months anticoagulant treatment

Prophylaxis of stroke and systemic embolism in non-valvular atrial fibrillation and at least one risk factor (such as previous stroke or transient ischaemic attack, symptomatic heart failure, diabetes mellitus, hypertension, or age 75 years and over)

▸ BY MOUTH
▸ Adult: 5 mg twice daily, reduce dose to 2.5 mg twice daily in patients with at least two of the following characteristics: age 80 years and over, body-weight less than 61 kg, or serum creatinine 133 micromol/litre and over

DOSE EQUIVALENCE AND CONVERSION

▸ For information on changing from, or to, other anticoagulants, consult product literature.

● CONTRA-INDICATIONS Active, clinically significant bleeding · risk factors for major bleeding

CONTRA-INDICATIONS, FURTHER INFORMATION

▸ Risk factors for major bleeding Manufacturer advises avoid in conditions with significant risk factors for major bleeding, including current or recent gastrointestinal ulceration, malignant neoplasms at high risk of bleeding, recent brain, spinal or ophthalmic surgery, recent intracranial haemorrhage, known or suspected oesophageal varices, arteriovenous malformations, vascular aneurysms or major intraspinal or intracerebral vascular abnormalities.

● CAUTIONS Anaesthesia with postoperative indwelling epidural catheter (risk of paralysis—monitor neurological signs and wait 20–30 hours after apixaban dose before removing catheter and do not give next dose until at least 5 hours after catheter removal) · prosthetic heart valve (efficacy not established) · risk of bleeding

● INTERACTIONS → Appendix 1: apixaban

● SIDE-EFFECTS
▸ **Common or very common** Anaemia · haemorrhage · nausea · skin reactions
▸ **Uncommon** CNS haemorrhage · hypotension · thrombocytopenia

● PREGNANCY Manufacturer advises avoid—no information available.

- BREAST FEEDING Manufacturer advises avoid—present in milk in *animal* studies.
- HEPATIC IMPAIRMENT Manufacturer advises use with caution in mild-to-moderate impairment; avoid in severe impairment and in hepatic disease associated with coagulopathy and clinically relevant bleeding risk.
- RENAL IMPAIRMENT Manufacturer advises avoid if creatinine clearance less than 15 mL/minute—no information available. When used for *prophylaxis of venous thromboembolism following knee or hip replacement surgery, prophylaxis of recurrent deep-vein thrombosis or pulmonary embolism, and treatment of deep-vein thrombosis or pulmonary embolism*, use with caution if creatinine clearance 15–29 mL/minute.

  Dose adjustments When used for *prophylaxis of stroke and systemic embolism in non-valvular atrial fibrillation*, reduce dose to 2.5 mg twice daily if serum-creatinine 133 micromol/litre and over is associated with age 80 years and over or body-weight less than 61 kg; reduce dose to 2.5 mg twice daily if creatinine clearance 15–29 mL/minute.
- MONITORING REQUIREMENTS
- ▶ Patients should be monitored for signs of bleeding or anaemia; treatment should be stopped if severe bleeding occurs.
- ▶ No routine anticoagulant monitoring required (INR tests are unreliable).
- PRESCRIBING AND DISPENSING INFORMATION Duration of treatment should be determined by balancing the benefit of treatment with the bleeding risk; shorter duration of treatment (at least 3 months) should be based on transient risk factors i.e recent surgery, trauma, immobilisation.

  Apixaban should not be used as an alternative to unfractionated heparin in pulmonary embolism in patients with haemodynamic instability, or who may receive thrombolysis or pulmonary embolectomy.
- NATIONAL FUNDING/ACCESS DECISIONS

  NICE decisions
- ▶ **Apixaban for the prevention of venous thromboembolism after total hip or knee replacement in adults (January 2012)** NICE TA245
  Apixaban is an option for the prevention of venous thromboembolism in adults after elective hip or knee replacement surgery.
  www.nice.org.uk/TA245
- ▶ **Apixaban for the prevention of stroke and systemic embolism in non-valvular atrial fibrillation (February 2013)** NICE TA275
  Apixaban is an option for the prevention of stroke and systemic embolism in non-valvular atrial fibrillation in accordance with its licensed indication; with one or more of the following risk factors:
  - previous stroke or transient ischaemic attack
  - symptomatic heart failure
  - age ≥75 years
  - diabetes mellitus
  - hypertension
  The risks and benefits of apixaban compared to warfarin, dabigatran etexilate, and rivaroxaban should be discussed with the patient.
  www.nice.org.uk/TA275
- ▶ **Apixaban for the treatment and secondary prevention of deep vein thrombosis and/or pulmonary embolism (June 2015)** NICE TA341
  Apixaban is an option for the treatment and prevention of recurrent deep vein thrombosis and pulmonary embolism in adults.
  www.nice.org.uk/TA341

- MEDICINAL FORMS
  There can be variation in the licensing of different medicines containing the same drug.

  Tablet
- ▶ Eliquis (Bristol-Myers Squibb Pharmaceuticals Ltd)
  Apixaban 2.5 mg Eliquis 2.5mg tablets | 10 tablet [PoM] £9.50 | 20 tablet [PoM] £19.00 | 60 tablet [PoM] £57.00 DT = £57.00
  Apixaban 5 mg Eliquis 5mg tablets | 28 tablet [PoM] £26.60 | 56 tablet [PoM] £53.20 DT = £53.20

Edoxaban

25-Apr-2016

- DRUG ACTION Edoxaban is a direct and reversible inhibitor of activated factor X (factor Xa), which prevents conversion of prothrombin to thrombin and prolongs clotting time, thereby reducing the risk of thrombus formation.

- INDICATIONS AND DOSE

  Prophylaxis of stroke and systemic embolism in non-valvular atrial fibrillation, in patients with at least one risk factor (such as congestive heart failure, hypertension, aged 75 years and over, diabetes mellitus, previous stroke or transient ischaemic attack)
  - ▶ BY MOUTH
  - ▶ Adult (body-weight up to 61 kg): 30 mg once daily
  - ▶ Adult (body-weight 61 kg and above): 60 mg once daily

  Treatment of deep-vein thrombosis | Prophylaxis of recurrent deep-vein thrombosis | Treatment of pulmonary embolism | Prophylaxis of recurrent pulmonary embolism
  - ▶ BY MOUTH
  - ▶ Adult (body-weight up to 61 kg): 30 mg once daily, duration of treatment adjusted according to risk factors—consult product literature, treatment should follow initial use of parenteral anticoagulant for at least 5 days
  - ▶ Adult (body-weight 61 kg and above): 60 mg once daily, duration of treatment adjusted according to risk factors—consult product literature, treatment should follow initial use of parenteral anticoagulant for at least 5 days

  DOSE ADJUSTMENTS DUE TO INTERACTIONS
  - ▶ Manufacturer advises max. dose of 30 mg once daily with concurrent ciclosporin, dronedarone, erythromycin, or ketoconazole.

  DOSE EQUIVALENCE AND CONVERSION
  - ▶ For information on changing from, or to, other anticoagulants, consult product literature.

- CONTRA-INDICATIONS Active bleeding · arteriovenous malformations · current or recent gastro-intestinal ulceration · hepatic disease (associated with coagulopathy and clinically relevant bleeding risk) · known or suspected oesophageal varices · major intraspinal or intracerebral vascular abnormalities · presence of malignant neoplasms at high risk of bleeding · recent brain or spinal injury · recent brain, spinal or ophthalmic surgery · recent intracranial haemorrhage · uncontrolled severe hypertension · vascular aneurysms

  CONTRA-INDICATIONS, FURTHER INFORMATION
  - ▶ Risk for major bleeding Edoxaban treatment is contra-indicated in patients with significant risk factors for major bleeding, these include those listed above.

- CAUTIONS Moderate to severe mitral stenosis (safety and efficacy not established) · prosthetic heart valve (safety and efficacy not established) · risk of bleeding · surgery

  CAUTIONS, FURTHER INFORMATION
  - ▶ Surgery Manufacturer recommends to discontinue treatment at least 24 hours before a surgical procedure;

the risk of bleeding should be weighed against the urgency of the intervention—consult product literature.

- INTERACTIONS → Appendix 1: edoxaban
- SIDE-EFFECTS
▶ **Common or very common** Anaemia · haemorrhage · nausea · skin reactions
▶ **Uncommon** CNS haemorrhage
 SIDE-EFFECTS, FURTHER INFORMATION Should a bleeding complication arise in a patient receiving edoxaban, the manufacturer recommends to delay the next dose or treatment should be discontinued as appropriate.
- PREGNANCY Manufacturer advises avoid—toxicity in *animal* studies.
- BREAST FEEDING Manufacturer advises avoid—present in milk in *animal* studies.
- HEPATIC IMPAIRMENT Manufacturer advises avoid in severe impairment; use with caution in mild to moderate impairment.
- RENAL IMPAIRMENT Manufacturer advises avoid if creatinine clearance less than 15 mL/minute.
 Dose adjustments Manufacturer advises use a dose of 30 mg once daily if creatinine clearance 15–50 mL/minute.
- MONITORING REQUIREMENTS
▶ Manufacturer advises monitor renal function before treatment and when clinically indicated during treatment; monitor hepatic function before treatment and repeat periodically if treatment duration longer than 1 year.
▶ Manufacturer advises monitor for signs of mucosal bleeding and anaemia in patients at increased risk; treatment should be stopped if severe bleeding occurs.
▶ No routine anticoagulant monitoring required (INR tests are unreliable).
- PATIENT AND CARER ADVICE Patients should be provided with an alert card and advised to keep it with them at all times.
- NATIONAL FUNDING/ACCESS DECISIONS
 NICE decisions
▶ **Edoxaban for treating and preventing deep vein thrombosis and pulmonary embolism (August 2015)** NICE TA354
 Edoxaban (*Lixiana* ®) is recommended as an option for treating and preventing recurrent deep vein thrombosis and pulmonary embolism.
 www.nice.org.uk/guidance/TA354
▶ **Edoxaban for preventing stroke and systemic embolism in non-valvular atrial fibrillation (September 2015)** NICE TA355
 Edoxaban (*Lixiana* ®) is an option for the prevention of stroke and systemic embolism in non-valvular atrial fibrillation, with one or more of the following risk factors:
 - previous stroke or transient ischaemic attack
 - congestive heart failure
 - age ≥75 years
 - diabetes mellitus
 - hypertension
 The risks and benefits of edoxaban treatment compared to warfarin, apixaban, dabigatran etexilate, and rivaroxaban should be discussed with the patient.
 www.nice.org.uk/TA355

- MEDICINAL FORMS
 There can be variation in the licensing of different medicines containing the same drug.
 Tablet
▶ Lixiana (Daiichi Sankyo UK Ltd) ▼
 Edoxaban (as Edoxaban tosilate) 15 mg Lixiana 15mg tablets | 10 tablet PoM £17.50 DT = £17.50
 Edoxaban (as Edoxaban tosilate) 30 mg Lixiana 30mg tablets | 28 tablet PoM £49.00 DT = £49.00
 Edoxaban (as Edoxaban tosilate) 60 mg Lixiana 60mg tablets | 28 tablet PoM £49.00 DT = £49.00

Fondaparinux sodium

21-May-2018

- DRUG ACTION Fondaparinux sodium is a synthetic pentasaccharide that inhibits activated factor X.

- INDICATIONS AND DOSE

Prophylaxis of venous thromboembolism in patients after undergoing major orthopaedic surgery of the hip or leg, or abdominal surgery
▶ BY SUBCUTANEOUS INJECTION
▹ Adult: Initially 2.5 mg, dose to be given 6 hours after surgery, then 2.5 mg once daily

Prophylaxis of venous thromboembolism in medical patients immobilised because of acute illness
▶ BY SUBCUTANEOUS INJECTION
▹ Adult: 2.5 mg once daily

Treatment of superficial-vein thrombosis
▶ BY SUBCUTANEOUS INJECTION
▹ Adult (body-weight 50 kg and above): 2.5 mg once daily for at least 30 days (max. 45 days if high risk of thromboembolic complications), treatment should be stopped 24 hours before surgery and restarted at least 6 hours post operatively

Treatment of unstable angina and non-ST-segment elevation myocardial infarction
▶ BY SUBCUTANEOUS INJECTION
▹ Adult: 2.5 mg once daily for up to 8 days (or until hospital discharge if sooner), treatment should be stopped 24 hours before coronary artery bypass graft surgery (where possible) and restarted 48 hours post operatively

Treatment of ST-segment elevation myocardial infarction
▶ INITIALLY BY INTRAVENOUS INJECTION, OR BY INTRAVENOUS INFUSION
▹ Adult: Initially 2.5 mg daily for the first day, then (by subcutaneous injection) 2.5 mg once daily for up to 8 days (or until hospital discharge if sooner), treatment should be stopped 24 hours before coronary artery bypass graft surgery (where possible) and restarted 48 hours post operatively

Treatment of deep-vein thrombosis and pulmonary embolism
▶ BY SUBCUTANEOUS INJECTION
▹ Adult (body-weight up to 50 kg): 5 mg every 24 hours, an oral anticoagulant (usually warfarin) is started at the same time as fondaparinux (fondaparinux should be continued for at least 5 days and until INR ≥ 2 for at least 24 hours)
▹ Adult (body-weight 50–100 kg): 7.5 mg every 24 hours, an oral anticoagulant (usually warfarin) is started at the same time as fondaparinux (fondaparinux should be continued for at least 5 days and until INR ≥ 2 for at least 24 hours)
▹ Adult (body-weight 101 kg and above): 10 mg every 24 hours, an oral anticoagulant (usually warfarin) is started at the same time as fondaparinux (fondaparinux should be continued for at least 5 days and until INR ≥ 2 for at least 24 hours)

- CONTRA-INDICATIONS Active bleeding · bacterial endocarditis
- CAUTIONS Active gastro-intestinal ulcer disease · bleeding disorders · brain surgery · elderly patients · low body-weight · ophthalmic surgery · recent intracranial haemorrhage · risk of catheter thrombus during percutaneous coronary intervention · spinal or epidural anaesthesia (risk of spinal haematoma—avoid if using treatment doses) · spinal surgery
- INTERACTIONS → Appendix 1: fondaparinux
- SIDE-EFFECTS
▶ **Common or very common** Anaemia · haemorrhage

- ▸ **Uncommon** Chest pain · coagulation disorder · dyspnoea · fever · hepatic function abnormal · nausea · oedema · platelet abnormalities · skin reactions · thrombocytopenia · vomiting · wound secretion
- ▸ **Rare or very rare** Anxiety · confusion · constipation · cough · diarrhoea · dizziness · drowsiness · fatigue · gastritis · gastrointestinal discomfort · genital oedema · headache · hyperbilirubinaemia · hypersensitivity · hypokalaemia · hypotension · leg pain · syncope · vasodilation · vertigo
- ● **PREGNANCY** Manufacturer advises avoid unless potential benefit outweighs possible risk—no information available.
- ● **BREAST FEEDING** Present in milk in *animal* studies—manufacturer advises avoid.
- ● **HEPATIC IMPAIRMENT** Caution in severe impairment (increased risk of bleeding).
- ● **RENAL IMPAIRMENT** Increased risk of bleeding in renal impairment.
- ▸ When used for treatment of acute coronary syndromes or prophylaxis of venous thromboembolism and treatment of superficial-vein thrombosis Avoid if eGFR less than 20 mL/minute/1.73 m².
- ▸ When used for treatment of venous thromboembolism Use with caution if eGFR 30–50 mL/minute/1.73 m², avoid if eGFR less than 30 mL/minute/1.73 m².

  Dose adjustments
- ▸ When used for prophylaxis of venous thromboembolism and treatment of superficial-vein thrombosis Reduce dose to 1.5 mg daily if eGFR 20–50 mL/minute/1.73 m².
- ● **DIRECTIONS FOR ADMINISTRATION** For *intravenous infusion* (*Arixtra*®), give intermittently in Sodium chloride 0.9%. For ST-segment elevation myocardial infarction, add requisite dose to 25-50 mL infusion fluid and give over 1-2 minutes.

- ● **MEDICINAL FORMS**
  There can be variation in the licensing of different medicines containing the same drug.

  Solution for injection
  - ▸ Fondaparinux sodium (Non-proprietary)
    Fondaparinux sodium 5 mg per 1 ml Fondaparinux sodium 2.5mg/0.5ml solution for injection pre-filled syringes | 10 pre-filled disposable injection PoM £59.65
    Fondaparinux sodium 12.5 mg per 1 ml Fondaparinux sodium 5mg/0.4ml solution for injection pre-filled syringes | 10 pre-filled disposable injection PoM £110.70
    Fondaparinux sodium 10mg/0.8ml solution for injection pre-filled syringes | 10 pre-filled disposable injection PoM £110.70
    Fondaparinux sodium 7.5mg/0.6ml solution for injection pre-filled syringes | 10 pre-filled disposable injection PoM £110.70-£116.53
  - ▸ Arixtra (Aspen Pharma Trading Ltd)
    Fondaparinux sodium 5 mg per 1 ml Arixtra 2.5mg/0.5ml solution for injection pre-filled syringes | 10 pre-filled disposable injection PoM £62.79
    Arixtra 1.5mg/0.3ml solution for injection pre-filled syringes | 10 pre-filled disposable injection PoM £62.79 (Hospital only)
    Fondaparinux sodium 12.5 mg per 1 ml Arixtra 7.5mg/0.6ml solution for injection pre-filled syringes | 10 pre-filled disposable injection PoM £116.53
    Arixtra 5mg/0.4ml solution for injection pre-filled syringes | 10 pre-filled disposable injection PoM £116.53
    Arixtra 10mg/0.8ml solution for injection pre-filled syringes | 10 pre-filled disposable injection PoM £116.53

Rivaroxaban

- ● **DRUG ACTION** Rivaroxaban is a direct inhibitor of activated factor X (factor Xa).

- ● **INDICATIONS AND DOSE**

  Prophylaxis of venous thromboembolism following knee replacement surgery
  - ▸ BY MOUTH
  - ▸ Adult: 10 mg once daily for 2 weeks, to be started 6–10 hours after surgery

  Prophylaxis of venous thromboembolism following hip replacement surgery
  - ▸ BY MOUTH
  - ▸ Adult: 10 mg once daily for 5 weeks, to be started 6–10 hours after surgery

  Initial treatment of deep-vein thrombosis | Initial treatment of pulmonary embolism
  - ▸ BY MOUTH
  - ▸ Adult: Initially 15 mg twice daily for 21 days, to be taken with food

  Continued treatment of deep-vein thrombosis (following initial treatment) | Continued treatment of pulmonary embolism (following initial treatment) | Prophylaxis of recurrent deep-vein thrombosis | Prophylaxis of recurrent pulmonary embolism
  - ▸ BY MOUTH
  - ▸ Adult: 20 mg once daily, to be taken with food, consult product literature for duration of treatment; also consult product literature for adjustment of dose for prophylaxis of recurrent deep-vein thrombosis or pulmonary embolism

  Prophylaxis of stroke and systemic embolism in patients with non-valvular atrial fibrillation and with at least one of the following risk factors: congestive heart failure, hypertension, previous stroke or transient ischaemic attack, age ≥ 75 years, or diabetes mellitus
  - ▸ BY MOUTH
  - ▸ Adult: 20 mg once daily, to be taken with food

  Prophylaxis of atherothrombotic events following an acute coronary syndrome with elevated cardiac biomarkers (in combination with aspirin alone or aspirin and clopidogrel)
  - ▸ BY MOUTH
  - ▸ Adult: 2.5 mg twice daily usual duration 12 months

  DOSE EQUIVALENCE AND CONVERSION
  - ▸ For information on changing from, or to, other anticoagulants—consult product literature.

- ● **CONTRA-INDICATIONS** Active bleeding · in *acute coronary syndrome*—previous stroke · in *acute coronary syndrome*—transient ischaemic attack · malignant neoplasms · oesophageal varices · recent brain surgery · recent gastro-intestinal ulcer · recent intracranial haemorrhage · recent ophthalmic surgery · recent spine surgery · significant risk of major bleeding · vascular aneurysm
- ● **CAUTIONS** Anaesthesia with postoperative indwelling epidural catheter (risk of paralysis—monitor neurological signs and wait at least 18 hours after rivaroxaban dose before removing catheter and do not give next dose until at least 6 hours after catheter removal) · bronchiectasis · prosthetic heart valve (efficacy not established) · risk of bleeding · rivaroxaban should not be used as an alternative to unfractionated heparin in pulmonary embolism in patients with haemodynamic instability, or who may receive thrombolysis or pulmonary embolectomy · severe hypertension · vascular retinopathy
- ● INTERACTIONS → Appendix 1: rivaroxaban
- ● SIDE-EFFECTS
  - ▸ **Common or very common** Anaemia · asthenia · constipation · diarrhoea · dizziness · fever · gastrointestinal discomfort ·

haemorrhage · headache · hypotension · menorrhagia · nausea · oedema · pain in extremity · renal impairment · skin reactions · vomiting
▶ **Uncommon** Allergic oedema · angioedema · dry mouth · hepatic disorders · intracranial haemorrhage · malaise · syncope · tachycardia · thrombocytopenia · thrombocytosis
▶ **Rare or very rare** Vascular pseudoaneurysm
● PREGNANCY Manufacturer advises avoid—toxicity in *animal* studies.
● BREAST FEEDING Manufacturer advises avoid—present in milk in *animal* studies.
● HEPATIC IMPAIRMENT Avoid in liver disease with coagulopathy.
● RENAL IMPAIRMENT Use with caution if concomitant use of drugs that increase plasma-rivaroxaban concentration (consult product literature). Avoid if creatinine clearance less than 15 mL/minute; manufacturer recommends Cockroft and Gault formula to calculate creatinine clearance. When used for *prophylaxis of venous thromboembolism following knee or hip replacement surgery and prophylaxis of atherothrombotic events in acute coronary syndrome*, use with caution if creatinine clearance 15–29 mL/minute.
Dose adjustments When used for *treatment of deep-vein thrombosis or pulmonary embolism and prophylaxis of recurrent deep-vein thrombosis and pulmonary embolism*, initially 15 mg twice daily for 21 days, then 20 mg once daily (but consider reducing to 15 mg once daily if risk of bleeding outweighs risk of recurrent deep-vein thrombosis or pulmonary embolism) if creatinine clearance 15–49 mL/minute.
For *prophylaxis of stroke and systemic embolism in atrial fibrillation,* reduce dose to 15 mg once daily if creatinine clearance 15–49 mL/minute.
● MONITORING REQUIREMENTS
▶ Patients should be monitored for signs of bleeding or anaemia; treatment should be stopped if severe bleeding occurs.
▶ No routine anticoagulant monitoring required (INR tests are unreliable).
● DIRECTIONS FOR ADMINISTRATION Tablets may be crushed and mixed with water or apple puree just before administration.
● PRESCRIBING AND DISPENSING INFORMATION Low-dose rivaroxaban, in combination with aspirin alone *or* aspirin and clopidogrel, is licensed for the prevention of atherothrombotic events following an acute coronary syndrome with elevated cardiac biomarkers. Treatment should be started as soon as possible after the patient has been stabilised following the acute coronary event, at the earliest 24 hours after admission to hospital, and at the time when parenteral anticoagulation therapy would normally be discontinued; the usual duration of treatment is 12 months.
● NATIONAL FUNDING/ACCESS DECISIONS
NICE decisions
▶ **Rivaroxaban for the prevention of venous thromboembolism after total hip or total knee replacement in adults (April 2009)** NICE TA170
Rivaroxaban is an option for the prophylaxis of venous thromboembolism in adults after total hip replacement or total knee replacement surgery.
www.nice.org.uk/TA170
▶ **Rivaroxaban for the prevention of stroke and systemic embolism in atrial fibrillation (May 2012)** NICE TA256
Rivaroxaban is an option for the prevention of stroke and systemic embolism (in accordance with its licensed indication) in patients with non-valvular atrial fibrillation and with at least one of the following risk factors:
● previous stroke or transient ischaemic attack
● congestive heart failure

● age ≥75 years
● diabetes mellitus
● hypertension
The risks and benefits of rivaroxaban compared with warfarin should be discussed with the patient.
www.nice.org.uk/TA256
▶ **Rivaroxaban for the treatment of deep-vein thrombosis and prevention of recurrent deep-vein thrombosis and pulmonary embolism (July 2012)** NICE TA261
Rivaroxaban is an option for the treatment of deep-vein thrombosis and prevention of recurrent deep-vein thrombosis and pulmonary embolism in adults after diagnosis of acute deep-vein thrombosis.
www.nice.org.uk/TA261
▶ **Rivaroxaban for treating pulmonary embolism and preventing recurrent venous thromboembolism (June 2013)** NICE TA287
Rivaroxaban is an option for treating pulmonary embolism and preventing recurrent deep-vein thrombosis and pulmonary embolism in adults.
www.nice.org.uk/TA287
▶ **Rivaroxaban for preventing adverse outcomes after acute management of acute coronary syndrome (March 2015)** NICE TA335
Rivaroxaban is an option within its marketing authorisation, in combination with aspirin plus clopidogrel or aspirin alone, for preventing atherothrombotic events in patients who have had an acute coronary syndrome with elevated cardiac biomarkers.
The patient's risk of bleeding should be carefully assessed before treatment is initiated and the risks and benefits of rivaroxaban in combination with aspirin plus clopidogrel or with aspirin alone, compared with aspirin plus clopidogrel or aspirin alone should be discussed with the patient.
A decision on continuation of treatment should be taken no later than 12 months after starting treatment.
www.nice.org.uk/TA335
Scottish Medicines Consortium (SMC) Decisions
The *Scottish Medicines Consortium* has advised (January 2012) that rivaroxaban (*Xarelto*®) is accepted for restricted use within NHS Scotland for the prevention of stroke and systemic embolism in accordance with the licensed indication; use is restricted to patients with poor INR control despite compliance with coumarin anticoagulant therapy, or to patients who are allergic to, or unable to tolerate, a coumarin anticoagulant.

● MEDICINAL FORMS
There can be variation in the licensing of different medicines containing the same drug.
Tablet
▶ Xarelto (Bayer Plc) ▼
Rivaroxaban 2.5 mg Xarelto 2.5mg tablets | 56 tablet [PoM] £50.40 DT = £50.40
Rivaroxaban 10 mg Xarelto 10mg tablets | 10 tablet [PoM] £18.00 | 30 tablet [PoM] £54.00 DT = £54.00 | 100 tablet [PoM] £180.00
Rivaroxaban 15 mg Xarelto 15mg tablets | 14 tablet [PoM] £25.20 | 28 tablet [PoM] £50.40 DT = £50.40 | 42 tablet [PoM] £75.60 | 100 tablet [PoM] £180.00
Rivaroxaban 20 mg Xarelto 20mg tablets | 28 tablet [PoM] £50.40 DT = £50.40 | 100 tablet [PoM] £180.00

ANTITHROMBOTIC DRUGS > HEPARINOIDS

Danaparoid sodium

- **INDICATIONS AND DOSE**

Prevention of deep-vein thrombosis in general or orthopaedic surgery
- ▸ BY SUBCUTANEOUS INJECTION
- ▸ Adult: 750 units twice daily for 7–10 days, initiate treatment before operation, with last pre-operative dose 1–4 hours before surgery

Thromboembolic disease in patients with history of heparin-induced thrombocytopenia
- ▸ INITIALLY BY INTRAVENOUS INJECTION
- ▸ Adult (body-weight up to 55 kg): Initially 1250 units, then (by continuous intravenous infusion) 400 units/hour for 2 hours, then (by continuous intravenous infusion) 300 units/hour for 2 hours, then (by continuous intravenous infusion) 200 units/hour for 5 days
- ▸ Adult (body-weight 55–89 kg): Initially 2500 units, then (by continuous intravenous infusion) 400 units/hour for 2 hours, then (by continuous intravenous infusion) 300 units/hour for 2 hours, then (by continuous intravenous infusion) 200 units/hour for 5 days
- ▸ Adult (body-weight 90 kg and above): Initially 3750 units, then (by continuous intravenous infusion) 400 units/hour for 2 hours, then (by continuous intravenous infusion) 300 units/hour for 2 hours, then (by continuous intravenous infusion) 200 units/hour for 5 days

- **CONTRA-INDICATIONS** Active peptic ulcer (unless this is the reason for operation) · acute bacterial endocarditis · diabetic retinopathy · epidural anaesthesia (with treatment doses) · haemophilia and other haemorrhagic disorders · recent cerebral haemorrhage · severe hypertension · spinal anaesthesia (with treatment doses) · thrombocytopenia (unless patient has heparin-induced thrombocytopenia)

- **CAUTIONS** Antibodies to heparins (risk of antibody-induced thrombocytopenia) · body-weight over 90 kg · recent bleeding · risk of bleeding

- **INTERACTIONS** → Appendix 1: danaparoid

- **SIDE-EFFECTS**
- ▸ **Common or very common** Haemorrhage · heparin-induced thrombocytopenia · skin reactions · thrombocytopenia

- **PREGNANCY** Manufacturer advises avoid—limited information available but not known to be harmful.

- **BREAST FEEDING** Amount probably too small to be harmful but manufacturer advises avoid.

- **HEPATIC IMPAIRMENT** Caution in moderate impairment (increased risk of bleeding). Avoid in severe impairment unless patient has heparin-induced thrombocytopenia and no alternative available.

- **RENAL IMPAIRMENT** Use with caution in moderate impairment. Avoid in severe impairment unless patient has heparin-induced thrombocytopenia and no alternative available.
  Monitoring Increased risk of bleeding in renal impairment, monitor anti-Factor Xa activity.

- **MONITORING REQUIREMENTS** Monitor anti factor Xa activity in patients with body-weight over 90 kg.

- **MEDICINAL FORMS**
  There can be variation in the licensing of different medicines containing the same drug.
  Solution for injection
- ▸ Danaparoid sodium (Non-proprietary)
  Danaparoid sodium 1250 unit per 1 ml Danaparoid sodium 750units/0.6ml solution for injection ampoules | 10 ampoule PoM £599.99

ANTITHROMBOTIC DRUGS > HEPARINS

Heparins

- **CONTRA-INDICATIONS** Acute bacterial endocarditis · after major trauma · epidural anaesthesia with treatment doses · haemophilia and other haemorrhagic disorders · peptic ulcer · recent cerebral haemorrhage · recent surgery to eye · recent surgery to nervous system · severe hypertension · spinal anaesthesia with treatment doses · thrombocytopenia (including history of heparin-induced thrombocytopenia)

- **CAUTIONS** Elderly

- **SIDE-EFFECTS**
- ▸ **Common or very common** Haemorrhage · heparin-induced thrombocytopenia · skin reactions · thrombocytopenia · thrombocytosis
- ▸ **Uncommon** CNS haemorrhage
- ▸ **Rare or very rare** Alopecia · hyperkalaemia · osteoporosis · priapism
- ▸ **Frequency not known** Hypoaldosteronism

  SIDE-EFFECTS, FURTHER INFORMATION
  Haemorrhage If haemorrhage occurs it is usually sufficient to withdraw unfractionated or low molecular weight heparin, but if rapid reversal of the effects of the heparin is required, protamine sulfate is a specific antidote (but only partially reverses the effects of low molecular weight heparins).
  Heparin-induced thrombocytopenia Clinically important heparin-induced thrombocytopenia is immune-mediated and can be complicated by thrombosis. Signs of heparin-induced thrombocytopenia include a 30% reduction of platelet count, thrombosis, or skin allergy. If heparin-induced thrombocytopenia is strongly suspected or confirmed, the heparin should be stopped and an alternative anticoagulant, such as danaparoid, should be given. Ensure platelet counts return to normal range in those who require warfarin.
  Hyperkalaemia Inhibition of aldosterone secretion by unfractionated or low molecular weight heparin can result in hyperkalaemia; patients with diabetes mellitus, chronic renal failure, acidosis, raised plasma potassium or those taking potassium-sparing drugs seem to be more susceptible. The risk appears to increase with duration of therapy.

- **ALLERGY AND CROSS-SENSITIVITY** Hypersensitivity to unfractionated or low molecular weight heparin.

- **MONITORING REQUIREMENTS**
- ▸ Heparin-induced thrombocytopenia Platelet counts should be measured just before treatment with unfractionated or low molecular weight heparin, and regular monitoring of platelet counts may be required if given for longer than 4 days. See the British Society for Haematology's Guidelines on the diagnosis and management of heparin-induced thrombocytopenia: second edition. *Br J Haematol* 2012; **159**: 528–540.
- ▸ Hyperkalaemia Plasma-potassium concentration should be measured in patients at risk of hyperkalaemia before starting the heparin and monitored regularly thereafter, particularly if treatment is to be continued for longer than 7 days.

▶ 129

Dalteparin sodium

● **INDICATIONS AND DOSE**

FRAGMIN ®

Treatment of deep-vein thrombosis | Treatment of pulmonary embolism
▶ BY SUBCUTANEOUS INJECTION
▸ Adult: 200 units/kg daily (max. per dose 18 000 units) until adequate oral anticoagulation with vitamin K antagonist established (at least 5 days of combined treatment is usually required)

Treatment of deep-vein thrombosis (in patients at increased risk of haemorrhage) | Treatment of pulmonary embolism (in patients at increase risk of haemorrhage)
▶ BY SUBCUTANEOUS INJECTION
▸ Adult: 100 units/kg twice daily until adequate oral anticoagulation with vitamin K antagonist established (at least 5 days of combined treatment is usually required)

Unstable coronary artery disease
▶ BY SUBCUTANEOUS INJECTION
▸ Adult: 120 units/kg every 12 hours (max. per dose 10 000 units twice daily) for 5–8 days

Prevention of clotting in extracorporeal circuits
▶ TO THE DEVICE AS A FLUSH
▸ Adult: (consult product literature)

FRAGMIN ® GRADUATED SYRINGES

Unstable coronary artery disease (including non-ST-segment-elevation myocardial infarction)
▶ BY SUBCUTANEOUS INJECTION
▸ Adult: 120 units/kg every 12 hours (max. per dose 10 000 units twice daily) for up to 8 days

Patients with unstable coronary artery disease (including non-ST-segment-elevation myocardial infarction) awaiting angiography or revascularisation and having already had 8 days treatment with dalteparin
▶ BY SUBCUTANEOUS INJECTION
▸ Adult (body-weight up to 70 kg and male): 5000 units every 12 hours until the day of the procedure (max. 45 days).
▸ Adult (body-weight up to 80 kg and female): 5000 units every 12 hours until the day of the procedure (max. 45 days).
▸ Adult (body-weight 70 kg and above and male): 7500 units every 12 hours until the day of the procedure (max. 45 days).
▸ Adult (body-weight 80 kg and above and female): 7500 units every 12 hours until the day of the procedure (max. 45 days).

FRAGMIN ® SINGLE-DOSE SYRINGES

Prophylaxis of deep-vein thrombosis in surgical patients—moderate risk
▶ BY SUBCUTANEOUS INJECTION
▸ Adult: Initially 2500 units for 1 dose, dose to be given 1–2 hours before surgery, then 2500 units every 24 hours

Prophylaxis of deep-vein thrombosis in surgical patients—high risk
▶ BY SUBCUTANEOUS INJECTION
▸ Adult: Initially 2500 units for 1 dose, to be administered 1–2 hours before surgery, followed by 2500 units after 8–12 hours, then 5000 units every 24 hours, alternatively initially 5000 units for 1 dose, dose to be given on the evening before surgery, followed by 5000 units after 24 hours, then 5000 units every 24 hours

Prophylaxis of deep-vein thrombosis in medical patients
▶ BY SUBCUTANEOUS INJECTION
▸ Adult: 5000 units every 24 hours

Treatment of deep-vein thrombosis | Treatment of pulmonary embolism
▶ BY SUBCUTANEOUS INJECTION
▸ Adult (body-weight up to 46 kg): 7500 units once daily until adequate oral anticoagulation with vitamin K antagonist established (at least 5 days of combined treatment is usually required)
▸ Adult (body-weight 46–56 kg): 10 000 units once daily until adequate oral anticoagulation with vitamin K antagonist established (at least 5 days of combined treatment is usually required)
▸ Adult (body-weight 57–68 kg): 12 500 units once daily until adequate oral anticoagulation with vitamin K antagonist established (at least 5 days of combined treatment is usually required)
▸ Adult (body-weight 69–82 kg): 15 000 units once daily until adequate oral anticoagulation with vitamin K antagonist established (at least 5 days of combined treatment is usually required)
▸ Adult (body-weight 83 kg and above): 18 000 units once daily until adequate oral anticoagulation with vitamin K antagonist established (at least 5 days of combined treatment is usually required)

Extended treatment of venous thromboembolism and prevention of recurrence in patients with solid tumours
▶ BY SUBCUTANEOUS INJECTION
▸ Adult (body-weight 40–45 kg): 7500 units once daily for 30 days, then 7500 units once daily for a further 5 months, interrupt treatment or reduce dose in chemotherapy-induced thrombocytopenia—consult product literature
▸ Adult (body-weight 46–56 kg): 10 000 units once daily for 30 days, then 7500 units once daily for a further 5 months, interrupt treatment or reduce dose in chemotherapy-induced thrombocytopenia—consult product literature
▸ Adult (body-weight 57–68 kg): 12 500 units once daily for 30 days, then 10 000 units once daily for a further 5 months, interrupt treatment or reduce dose in chemotherapy-induced thrombocytopenia—consult product literature
▸ Adult (body-weight 69–82 kg): 15 000 units once daily for 30 days, then 12 500 units once daily for a further 5 months, interrupt treatment or reduce dose in chemotherapy-induced thrombocytopenia—consult product literature
▸ Adult (body-weight 83–98 kg): 18 000 units once daily for 30 days, then 15 000 units once daily for a further 5 months, interrupt treatment or reduce dose in chemotherapy-induced thrombocytopenia—consult product literature
▸ Adult (body-weight 99 kg and above): 18 000 units once daily for 30 days, then 18 000 units once daily for a further 5 months, interrupt treatment or reduce dose in chemotherapy-induced thrombocytopenia—consult product literature

Treatment of venous thromboembolism in pregnancy
▶ BY SUBCUTANEOUS INJECTION
▸ Adult (body-weight up to 50 kg): 5000 units twice daily, use body-weight in early pregnancy to calculate the dose
▸ Adult (body-weight 50–69 kg): 6000 units twice daily, use body-weight in early pregnancy to calculate the dose
▸ Adult (body-weight 70–89 kg): 8000 units twice daily, use body-weight in early pregnancy to calculate the dose
▸ Adult (body-weight 90 kg and above): 10 000 units twice daily, use body-weight in early pregnancy to calculate the dose

- UNLICENSED USE Not licensed for treatment of venous thromboembolism in pregnancy.
- INTERACTIONS → Appendix 1: low molecular-weight heparins
- PREGNANCY Not known to be harmful, low molecular weight heparins do not cross the placenta. Multidose vial contains benzyl alcohol—manufacturer advises avoid.
- BREAST FEEDING Due to the relatively high molecular weight and inactivation in the gastro-intestinal tract, passage into breast-milk and absorption by the nursing infant are likely to be negligible, however manufacturers advise avoid.
- HEPATIC IMPAIRMENT
Dose adjustments Dose reduction may be required in severe impairment—risk of bleeding may be increased.
- RENAL IMPAIRMENT Use of unfractionated heparin may be preferable.
Dose adjustments Risk of bleeding may be increased—dose reduction may be required.
- MONITORING REQUIREMENTS
- For monitoring during treatment of deep-vein thrombosis and of pulmonary embolism, blood should be taken 3–4 hours after a dose (recommended plasma concentration of anti-Factor Xa 0.5–1 unit/mL); monitoring not required for once-daily treatment regimen and not generally necessary for twice-daily regimen.
- Routine monitoring of anti-Factor Xa activity is not usually required during treatment with dalteparin, but may be necessary in patients at increased risk of bleeding (e.g. in renal impairment and those who are underweight or overweight).
- NATIONAL FUNDING/ACCESS DECISIONS
Scottish Medicines Consortium (SMC) Decisions
The *Scottish Medicines Consortium* has advised (February 2011) that dalteparin (*Fragmin®*) is accepted for restricted use within NHS Scotland as extended treatment of symptomatic venous thromboembolism and prevention of its recurrence in patients with solid tumours.
- MEDICINAL FORMS
There can be variation in the licensing of different medicines containing the same drug.
Solution for injection
EXCIPIENTS: May contain Benzyl alcohol
- Fragmin (Pfizer Ltd)
Dalteparin sodium 2500 unit per 1 ml Fragmin 10,000units/4ml solution for injection ampoules | 10 ampoule [PoM] £51.22
Dalteparin sodium 10000 unit per 1 ml Fragmin 10,000units/1ml solution for injection pre-filled syringes | 5 pre-filled disposable injection [PoM] £28.23 DT = £28.23
Fragmin 10,000units/1ml solution for injection ampoules | 10 ampoule [PoM] £51.22
Dalteparin sodium 12500 unit per 1 ml Fragmin 2,500units/0.2ml solution for injection pre-filled syringes | 10 pre-filled disposable injection [PoM] £18.58 DT = £18.58
Dalteparin sodium 25000 unit per 1 ml Fragmin 18,000units/0.72ml solution for injection pre-filled syringes | 5 pre-filled disposable injection [PoM] £50.82 DT = £50.82
Fragmin 15,000units/0.6ml solution for injection pre-filled syringes | 5 pre-filled disposable injection [PoM] £42.34 DT = £42.34
Fragmin 5,000units/0.2ml solution for injection pre-filled syringes | 10 pre-filled disposable injection [PoM] £28.23 DT = £28.23
Fragmin 12,500units/0.5ml solution for injection pre-filled syringes | 5 pre-filled disposable injection [PoM] £35.29 DT = £35.29
Fragmin 7,500units/0.3ml solution for injection pre-filled syringes | 10 pre-filled disposable injection [PoM] £42.34 DT = £42.34
Fragmin 100,000units/4ml solution for injection vials | 1 vial [PoM] £48.66
Fragmin 10,000units/0.4ml solution for injection pre-filled syringes | 5 pre-filled disposable injection [PoM] £28.23 DT = £28.23

F 129

Enoxaparin sodium

F 129

- INDICATIONS AND DOSE
Treatment of venous thromboembolism in pregnancy
- BY SUBCUTANEOUS INJECTION
- Adult (body-weight up to 50 kg): 40 mg twice daily, dose based on early pregnancy body-weight
- Adult (body-weight 50–69 kg): 60 mg twice daily, dose based on early pregnancy body-weight
- Adult (body-weight 70–89 kg): 80 mg twice daily, dose based on early pregnancy body-weight
- Adult (body-weight 90 kg and above): 100 mg twice daily, dose based on early pregnancy body-weight

Prophylaxis of deep-vein thrombosis, especially in surgical patients—moderate risk
- BY SUBCUTANEOUS INJECTION
- Adult: 20 mg for 1 dose, dose to be given approximately 2 hours before surgery, then 20 mg every 24 hours

Prophylaxis of deep-vein thrombosis, especially surgical patients—high risk (e.g. orthopaedic surgery)
- BY SUBCUTANEOUS INJECTION
- Adult: 40 mg for 1 dose, dose to be given 12 hours before surgery, then 40 mg every 24 hours

Prophylaxis of deep-vein thrombosis in medical patients
- BY SUBCUTANEOUS INJECTION
- Adult: 40 mg every 24 hours

Treatment of deep-vein thrombosis in uncomplicated patients with low risk of recurrence | Treatment of pulmonary embolism in uncomplicated patients with low risk of recurrence
- BY SUBCUTANEOUS INJECTION
- Adult: 1.5 mg/kg every 24 hours until adequate oral anticoagulation established

Treatment of deep-vein thrombosis in patients with risk factors such as obesity, cancer, recurrent VTE, or proximal thrombosis | Treatment of pulmonary embolism in patients with risk factors such as obesity, symptomatic pulmonary embolism, cancer, or recurrent VTE
- BY SUBCUTANEOUS INJECTION
- Adult: 1 mg/kg every 12 hours until adequate oral anticoagulation established

Treatment of acute ST-segment elevation myocardial infarction (patients not undergoing percutaneous coronary intervention)
- INITIALLY BY INTRAVENOUS INJECTION
- Adult 18–74 years: Initially 30 mg, followed by (by subcutaneous injection) 1 mg/kg for 1 dose, then (by subcutaneous injection) 1 mg/kg every 12 hours (max. per dose 100 mg) for up to 8 days, maximum dose applies for the first two subcutaneous doses only
- BY SUBCUTANEOUS INJECTION
- Adult 75 years and over: 750 micrograms/kg every 12 hours (max. per dose 75 mg), maximum dose applies for the first two doses only

Treatment of acute ST-segment elevation myocardial infarction (patients undergoing percutaneous coronary intervention)
- INITIALLY BY INTRAVENOUS INJECTION
- Adult 18–74 years: Initially 30 mg, followed by (by subcutaneous injection) 1 mg/kg every 12 hours (max. per dose 100 mg) for up to 8 days, maximum dose applies for the first two subcutaneous doses only, then (by intravenous injection) 300 micrograms/kg for 1 dose, dose to be given at the time of procedure if the last subcutaneous dose was given more than 8 hours previously

continued →

2

Cardiovascular system

‣ INITIALLY BY SUBCUTANEOUS INJECTION
‣ Adult 75 years and over: 750 micrograms/kg every 12 hours (max. per dose 75 mg), maximum dose applies for the first two doses only, then (by intravenous injection) 300 micrograms/kg for 1 dose, dose to be given at the time of procedure if the last subcutaneous dose was given more than 8 hours previously

Unstable angina | Non-ST-segment-elevation myocardial infarction
‣ BY SUBCUTANEOUS INJECTION
‣ Adult: 1 mg/kg every 12 hours usually for 2–8 days (minimum 2 days)

Prevention of clotting in extracorporeal circuits
‣ TO THE DEVICE AS A FLUSH
‣ Adult: (consult product literature)

DOSE EQUIVALENCE AND CONVERSION
‣ 1 mg equivalent to 100 units.

● UNLICENSED USE Not licensed for treatment of venous thromboembolism in pregnancy.
● CAUTIONS Low body-weight (increased risk of bleeding)
● INTERACTIONS → Appendix 1: low molecular-weight heparins
● SIDE-EFFECTS
‣ **Common or very common** Hypersensitivity
‣ **Frequency not known** Cutaneous vasculitis · eosinophilia · haemorrhagic anaemia · headache · hepatic disorders
● PREGNANCY Not known to be harmful, low molecular weight heparins do not cross the placenta. Multidose vial contains benzyl alcohol—avoid.
● BREAST FEEDING Due to the relatively high molecular weight of enoxaparin and inactivation in the gastro-intestinal tract, passage into breast-milk and absorption by the nursing infant are likely to be negligible; however manufacturers advise avoid.
● HEPATIC IMPAIRMENT Manufacturer advises caution—no information available.
● RENAL IMPAIRMENT Risk of bleeding increased; use of unfractionated heparin may be preferable. Manufacturer advises avoid if creatinine clearance less than 15 mL/minute.
Dose adjustments Manufacturer advises reduce dose if creatinine clearance 15–30 mL/minute—consult product literature for details.
● MONITORING REQUIREMENTS Routine monitoring of anti-Factor Xa activity is not usually required during treatment with enoxaparin, but may be necessary in patients at increased risk of bleeding (e.g. in renal impairment and those who are underweight or overweight).
● DIRECTIONS FOR ADMINISTRATION When administered in conjunction with a thrombolytic, enoxaparin should be given between 15 minutes before and 30 minutes after the start of thrombolytic therapy.
● PRESCRIBING AND DISPENSING INFORMATION Enoxaparin sodium is a biological medicine. Biological medicines must be prescribed and dispensed by brand name, see *Biological medicines* and *Biosimilar medicines*, under Guidance on prescribing p. 1.

● MEDICINAL FORMS
There can be variation in the licensing of different medicines containing the same drug.
Solution for injection
EXCIPIENTS: May contain Benzyl alcohol
‣ Enoxaparin sodium (non-proprietary) ▼
Enoxaparin sodium 100 mg per 1 ml Enoxaparin Becat 40mg/0.4ml solution for injection pre-filled syringes | 10 pre-filled disposable injection [PoM] £30.27 DT = £30.27
Enoxaparin Becat 60mg/0.6ml solution for injection pre-filled syringes | 10 pre-filled disposable injection [PoM] £39.26 DT = £39.26

Enoxaparin Becat 100mg/1ml solution for injection pre-filled syringes | 10 pre-filled disposable injection [PoM] £72.30 DT = £72.30
Enoxaparin Becat 20mg/0.2ml solution for injection pre-filled syringes | 10 pre-filled disposable injection [PoM] £20.86 DT = £20.86
Enoxaparin Becat 80mg/0.8ml solution for injection pre-filled syringes | 10 pre-filled disposable injection [PoM] £55.13 DT = £55.13
‣ Clexane (Sanofi)
Enoxaparin sodium 100 mg per 1 ml Clexane 60mg/0.6ml solution for injection pre-filled syringes | 10 pre-filled disposable injection [PoM] £39.26 DT = £39.26
Clexane 300mg/3ml solution for injection multidose vials | 1 vial [PoM] £21.33 DT = £21.33
Clexane 80mg/0.8ml solution for injection pre-filled syringes | 10 pre-filled disposable injection [PoM] £55.13 DT = £55.13
Clexane 40mg/0.4ml solution for injection pre-filled syringes | 10 pre-filled disposable injection [PoM] £30.27 DT = £30.27
Clexane 100mg/1ml solution for injection pre-filled syringes | 10 pre-filled disposable injection [PoM] £72.30 DT = £72.30
Clexane 20mg/0.2ml solution for injection pre-filled syringes | 10 pre-filled disposable injection [PoM] £20.86 DT = £20.86
Enoxaparin sodium 150 mg per 1 ml Clexane Forte 120mg/0.8ml solution for injection pre-filled syringes | 10 pre-filled disposable injection [PoM] £87.93 DT = £87.93
Clexane Forte 150mg/1ml solution for injection pre-filled syringes | 10 pre-filled disposable injection [PoM] £99.91 DT = £99.91
‣ Inhixa (Techdow Pharma England Ltd) ▼
Enoxaparin sodium 100 mg per 1 ml Inhixa 40mg/0.4ml solution for injection pre-filled syringes | 10 pre-filled disposable injection [PoM] £24.22 DT = £30.27
Inhixa 80mg/0.8ml solution for injection pre-filled syringes | 10 pre-filled disposable injection [PoM] £44.10 DT = £55.13
Inhixa 60mg/0.6ml solution for injection pre-filled syringes | 10 pre-filled disposable injection [PoM] £31.41 DT = £39.26
Inhixa 100mg/1ml solution for injection pre-filled syringes | 10 pre-filled disposable injection [PoM] £57.84 DT = £72.30
Inhixa 20mg/0.2ml solution for injection pre-filled syringes | 10 pre-filled disposable injection [PoM] £16.69 DT = £20.86

◀ 129

Heparin (unfractionated)

● INDICATIONS AND DOSE

Treatment of mild to moderate pulmonary embolism | Treatment of unstable angina | Treatment of acute peripheral arterial occlusion
‣ INITIALLY BY INTRAVENOUS INJECTION
‣ Adult: Loading dose 5000 units, alternatively (by intravenous injection) loading dose 75 units/kg, followed by (by continuous intravenous infusion) 18 units/kg/hour, laboratory monitoring essential—preferably on a daily basis, and dose adjusted accordingly

Treatment of severe pulmonary embolism
‣ INITIALLY BY INTRAVENOUS INJECTION
‣ Adult: Loading dose 10 000 units, followed by (by continuous intravenous infusion) 18 units/kg/hour, laboratory monitoring essential—preferably on a daily basis, and dose adjusted accordingly

Treatment of deep-vein thrombosis
‣ INITIALLY BY INTRAVENOUS INJECTION
‣ Adult: Loading dose 5000 units, alternatively (by intravenous injection) loading dose 75 units/kg, followed by (by continuous intravenous infusion) 18 units/kg/hour, alternatively (by subcutaneous injection) 15 000 units every 12 hours, laboratory monitoring essential—preferably on a daily basis, and dose adjusted accordingly

Thromboprophylaxis in medical patients
‣ BY SUBCUTANEOUS INJECTION
‣ Adult: 5000 units every 8–12 hours

Thrombophylaxis in surgical patients
‣ BY SUBCUTANEOUS INJECTION
‣ Adult: 5000 units for 1 dose, to be taken 2 hours before surgery, then 5000 units every 8–12 hours

Thromboprophylaxis during pregnancy
▸ BY SUBCUTANEOUS INJECTION
▸ Adult: 5000–10 000 units every 12 hours, to be administered with monitoring, **Important:** prevention of prosthetic heart-valve thrombosis in pregnancy calls for **specialist management**

Haemodialysis
▸ INITIALLY BY INTRAVENOUS INJECTION
▸ Adult: Initially 1000–5000 units, followed by (by continuous intravenous infusion) 250–1000 units/hour

Prevention of clotting in extracorporeal circuits
▸ TO THE DEVICE AS A FLUSH
▸ Adult: (consult product literature)

To maintain patency of catheters, cannulas, other indwelling intravenous infusion devices
▸ TO THE DEVICE AS A FLUSH
▸ Adult: 10–200 units, to be flushed through every 4–8 hours, not for therapeutic use

● INTERACTIONS → Appendix 1: heparin (unfractionated)
● SIDE-EFFECTS Adrenal insufficiency · hypokalaemia · rebound hyperlipidaemia
● PREGNANCY Does not cross the placenta; maternal osteoporosis reported after prolonged use; multidose vials may contain benzyl alcohol—some manufacturers advise avoid.
● BREAST FEEDING Not excreted into milk due to high molecular weight.
● HEPATIC IMPAIRMENT
  Dose adjustments Risk of bleeding increased—reduce dose or avoid in severe impairment (including oesophageal varices).
● RENAL IMPAIRMENT
  Dose adjustments Risk of bleeding increased in severe impairment—dose may need to be reduced.
● DIRECTIONS FOR ADMINISTRATION For *intravenous infusion*, give continuously in Glucose 5% or Sodium chloride 0.9%; administration with a motorised pump is advisable.
● PRESCRIBING AND DISPENSING INFORMATION Doses listed take into account the guidelines of the British Society for Haematology.

● MEDICINAL FORMS
  There can be variation in the licensing of different medicines containing the same drug. Forms available from special-order manufacturers include: solution for injection, solution for infusion

  Solution for injection
  EXCIPIENTS: May contain Benzyl alcohol
  ▸ Heparin (unfractionated) (Non-proprietary)
  Heparin sodium 1000 unit per 1 ml Heparin sodium 1,000units/1ml solution for injection ampoules | 10 ampoule [PoM] £14.85
  Heparin sodium 5,000units/5ml solution for injection vials | 10 vial [PoM] £16.50–£37.41
  Heparin sodium 20,000units/20ml solution for injection ampoules | 10 ampoule [PoM] £70.80–£70.88
  Heparin sodium 5,000units/5ml solution for injection ampoules | 10 ampoule [PoM] £37.45–£37.47
  Heparin sodium 10,000units/10ml solution for injection ampoules | 10 ampoule [PoM] £64.50–£64.59
  Heparin sodium 5000 unit per 1 ml Heparin sodium 5,000units/1ml solution for injection ampoules | 10 ampoule [PoM] £29.04
  Heparin sodium 25,000units/5ml solution for injection vials | 10 vial [PoM] £45.00–£84.60
  Heparin sodium 25,000units/5ml solution for injection ampoules | 10 ampoule [PoM] £75.78
  Heparin calcium 25000 unit per 1 ml Heparin calcium 5,000units/0.2ml solution for injection ampoules | 10 ampoule [PoM] £44.70
  Heparin sodium 25000 unit per 1 ml Heparin sodium 25,000units/1ml solution for injection ampoules | 10 ampoule [PoM] £76.95
  Heparin sodium 5,000units/0.2ml solution for injection ampoules | 10 ampoule [PoM] £37.35

  Intravenous flush
  EXCIPIENTS: May contain Benzyl alcohol
  ▸ Heparin (unfractionated) (Non-proprietary)
  Heparin sodium 10 unit per 1 ml Heparin sodium 50units/5ml patency solution ampoules | 10 ampoule [PoM] £14.96 DT = £14.96
  Heparin sodium 50units/5ml I.V. flush solution ampoules | 10 ampoule [PoM] £14.96 DT = £14.96
  Heparin sodium 100 unit per 1 ml Heparin sodium 200units/2ml I.V. flush solution ampoules | 10 ampoule [PoM] £15.68 DT = £15.68
  Heparin sodium 200units/2ml patency solution ampoules | 10 ampoule [PoM] £15.68 DT = £15.68

  Infusion
  ▸ Heparin (unfractionated) (Non-proprietary)
  Heparin sodium 2 unit per 1 ml Heparin sodium 1,000units/500ml infusion Viaflex bags | 1 bag [PoM] [℞]
  Heparin sodium 2,000units/1litre infusion Viaflex bags | 1 bag [PoM] [℞]
  Heparin sodium 5 unit per 1 ml Heparin sodium 5,000units/1litre infusion Viaflex bags | 1 bag [PoM] [℞]

▶ 129

| Tinzaparin sodium

● INDICATIONS AND DOSE
INNOHEP® 10,000 UNITS/ML

Prophylaxis of deep-vein thrombosis (general surgery)
▸ BY SUBCUTANEOUS INJECTION
▸ Adult: 3500 units for 1 dose, dose to be given 2 hours before surgery, then 3500 units every 24 hours

Prophylaxis of deep-vein thrombosis (orthopaedic surgery)
▸ BY SUBCUTANEOUS INJECTION
▸ Adult: Initially 50 units/kg for 1 dose, dose to be given 2 hours before surgery, then 50 units/kg every 24 hours, alternatively initially 4500 units for 1 dose, dose to be given 12 hours before surgery, then 4500 units every 24 hours

Prevention of clotting in extracorporeal circuits
▸ TO THE DEVICE AS A FLUSH
▸ Adult: (consult product literature)

INNOHEP® 20,000 UNITS/ML

Extended treatment of venous thromboembolism and prevention of recurrence in patients with active cancer
▸ BY SUBCUTANEOUS INJECTION
▸ Adult: 175 units/kg once daily for 6 months; the benefit of continued treatment beyond 6 months should be evaluated

Treatment of deep-vein thrombosis | Treatment of pulmonary embolism
▸ BY SUBCUTANEOUS INJECTION
▸ Adult: 175 units/kg once daily until adequate oral anticoagulation established, treatment regimens do not require anticoagulation monitoring

Treatment of venous thromboembolism in pregnancy
▸ BY SUBCUTANEOUS INJECTION
▸ Adult: 175 units/kg once daily, dose based on early pregnancy body-weight, treatment regimens do not require anticoagulation monitoring

● UNLICENSED USE Not licensed for the treatment of venous thromboembolism in pregnancy.
● INTERACTIONS → Appendix 1: low molecular-weight heparins
● SIDE-EFFECTS
▸ **Common or very common** Anaemia
▸ **Rare or very rare** Angioedema · Stevens-Johnson syndrome
● PREGNANCY Not known to be harmful, low molecular weight heparins do not cross the placenta. Vials contain benzyl alcohol—manufacturer advises avoid.
● BREAST FEEDING Due to the relatively high molecular weight of tinzaparin and inactivation in the gastro-intestinal tract, passage into breast-milk and absorption

by the nursing infant are likely to be negligible; however manufacturer advise avoid.

- RENAL IMPAIRMENT Risk of bleeding may be increased. Unfractionated heparin may be preferable. Manufacturer advises caution if eGFR less than 30 mL/minute/1.73 m². **Monitoring** In renal impairment monitoring of anti-Factor Xa may be required if eGFR less than 30 mL/minute/1.73 m².

- MONITORING REQUIREMENTS Routine monitoring of anti-Factor Xa activity is not usually required during treatment with tinzaparin, but may be necessary in patients at increased risk of bleeding (e.g. in renal impairment and those who are underweight or overweight).

- MEDICINAL FORMS
  There can be variation in the licensing of different medicines containing the same drug.
  Solution for injection
  EXCIPIENTS: May contain Benzyl alcohol, sulfites
  ▸ Innohep (LEO Pharma)
  Tinzaparin sodium 10000 unit per 1 ml Innohep 20,000units/2ml solution for injection vials | 10 vial [PoM] £105.66 DT = £105.66
  Tinzaparin sodium 20000 unit per 1 ml Innohep 18,000units/0.9ml solution for injection pre-filled syringes | 6 pre-filled disposable injection [PoM] £64.25 | 10 pre-filled disposable injection [PoM] £107.08 DT = £107.08
  Innohep 40,000units/2ml solution for injection vials | 1 vial [PoM] £34.20 DT = £34.20
  Innohep 14,000units/0.7ml solution for injection pre-filled syringes | 6 pre-filled disposable injection [PoM] £49.98 | 10 pre-filled disposable injection [PoM] £83.30 DT = £83.30
  Innohep 10,000units/0.5ml solution for injection pre-filled syringes | 6 pre-filled disposable injection [PoM] £35.70 | 10 pre-filled disposable injection [PoM] £59.50 DT = £59.50

ANTITHROMBOTIC DRUGS ⟩ THROMBIN INHIBITORS, DIRECT

Argatroban monohydrate

- **INDICATIONS AND DOSE**

Anticoagulation in patients with heparin-induced thrombocytopenia type II who require parenteral antithrombotic treatment
▸ INITIALLY BY CONTINUOUS INTRAVENOUS INFUSION
▸ Adult: Initially 2 micrograms/kg/minute, dose to be adjusted according to activated partial thromboplastin time, (by intravenous infusion) increased to up to 10 micrograms/kg/minute maximum duration of treatment 14 days

Anticoagulation in patients with heparin-induced thrombocytopenia type II who require parenteral antithrombotic treatment (for dose in cardiac surgery, percutaneous coronary intervention, or critically ill patients)
▸ BY CONTINUOUS INTRAVENOUS INFUSION
▸ Adult: (consult product literature)

Anticoagulation in patients with heparin-induced thrombocytopenia type II who require parenteral antithrombotic treatment (when initiating concomitant warfarin treatment)
▸ BY CONTINUOUS INTRAVENOUS INFUSION
▸ Adult: Reduced to 2 micrograms/kg/minute, dose should be temporarily reduced and INR measured after 4–6 hours; warfarin should be initiated at intended maintenance dose (do not give loading dose of warfarin); consult product literature for further details

- CAUTIONS Bleeding disorders · diabetic retinopathy · gastro-intestinal ulceration · immediately after lumbar puncture · major surgery (especially of brain, spinal cord, or eye) · risk of bleeding · severe hypertension · spinal anaesthesia

- INTERACTIONS → Appendix 1: argatroban
- SIDE-EFFECTS
  ▸ **Common or very common** Anaemia · haemorrhage · nausea · skin reactions
  ▸ **Uncommon** Alopecia · appetite decreased · arrhythmias · cardiac arrest · confusion · constipation · deafness · diarrhoea · dizziness · dysphagia · dyspnoea · fatigue · fever · gastritis · headache · hepatic disorders · hiccups · hyperbilirubinaemia · hyperhidrosis · hypertension · hypoglycaemia · hyponatraemia · hypotension · hypoxia · increased risk of infection · leucopenia · muscle tone decreased · muscle weakness · myalgia · myocardial infarction · pericardial effusion · peripheral ischaemia · peripheral oedema · pleural effusion · renal failure · shock · speech disorder · stroke · syncope · thrombocytopenia · tongue disorder · visual impairment · vomiting

- PREGNANCY Manufacturer advises avoid unless essential—limited information available.

- BREAST FEEDING Avoid—no information available.

- HEPATIC IMPAIRMENT Avoid in severe impairment *or* in patients with hepatic impairment undergoing percutaneous coronary intervention.
  Dose adjustments Reduce initial dose to 500 nanograms/kg/minute in moderate impairment.

- MONITORING REQUIREMENTS Determine activated partial thromboplastin time 2 hours after start of treatment, then 2 or 4 hours after infusion rate altered (consult product literature), and at least once daily thereafter.

- DIRECTIONS FOR ADMINISTRATION For *intravenous infusion* (*Exembol®*) give continuously in Glucose 5% or Sodium chloride 0.9%. Dilute each 2.5-mL vial with 250 mL infusion fluid.

- MEDICINAL FORMS
  There can be variation in the licensing of different medicines containing the same drug.
  Solution for infusion
  EXCIPIENTS: May contain Ethanol
  ▸ Exembol (Mitsubishi Tanabe Pharma Europe Ltd)
  Argatroban monohydrate 1 mg per 1 ml Exembol 50mg/50ml solution for infusion vials | 4 vial £198.80
  Argatroban monohydrate 100 mg per 1 ml Exembol 250mg/2.5ml concentrate for solution for infusion vials | 4 vial 🔣

Bivalirudin

- DRUG ACTION Bivalirudin, a hirudin analogue, is a thrombin inhibitor.

- **INDICATIONS AND DOSE**

Unstable angina or non-ST-segment elevation myocardial infarction in patients planned for urgent or early intervention (in addition to aspirin and clopidogrel)
▸ INITIALLY BY INTRAVENOUS INJECTION
▸ Adult: Initially 100 micrograms/kg, then (by intravenous infusion) 250 micrograms/kg/hour (for up to 72 hours in medically managed patients)

Unstable angina or non-ST-segment elevation myocardial infarction (in addition to aspirin and clopidogrel) in patients proceeding to percutaneous coronary intervention or coronary artery bypass surgery without cardiopulmonary bypass
▸ INITIALLY BY INTRAVENOUS INJECTION
▸ Adult: Initially 100 micrograms/kg for 1 dose, then (by intravenous injection) 500 micrograms/kg for 1 dose, then (by intravenous infusion) 1.75 mg/kg/hour for duration of procedure; (by intravenous infusion) reduced to 250 micrograms/kg/hour for 4–12 hours as necessary following percutaneous coronary intervention, for patients proceeding to coronary artery bypass surgery with cardiopulmonary bypass,

discontinue intravenous infusion 1 hour before procedure and treat with unfractionated heparin

Anticoagulation in patients undergoing percutaneous coronary intervention including patients with ST-segment elevation myocardial infarction undergoing primary percutaneous coronary intervention (in addition to aspirin and clopidogrel)

▶ INITIALLY BY INTRAVENOUS INJECTION
▶ Adult: Initially 750 micrograms/kg, followed immediately by (by intravenous infusion) 1.75 mg/kg/hour during procedure and for up to 4 hours after procedure, then (by intravenous infusion) reduced to 250 micrograms/kg/hour for a further 4–12 hours if necessary

● CONTRA-INDICATIONS Active bleeding · bleeding disorders · severe hypertension · subacute bacterial endocarditis
● CAUTIONS Brachytherapy procedures · previous exposure to lepirudin (theoretical risk from lepirudin antibodies)
● INTERACTIONS → Appendix 1: bivalirudin
● SIDE-EFFECTS
▶ Common or very common Skin reactions
▶ Uncommon Anaemia · headache · hypersensitivity · hypotension · nausea · shock · thrombocytopenia
▶ Rare or very rare Arrhythmias · cardiac tamponade · chest pain · compartment syndrome · dyspnoea · embolism and thrombosis · intracranial haemorrhage · pain · vascular disorders · vomiting
● PREGNANCY Manufacturer advises avoid unless potential benefit outweighs risk—no information available.
● BREAST FEEDING Manufacturer advises caution—no information available.
● RENAL IMPAIRMENT Avoid if eGFR less than 30 mL/minute/1.73 m^2.
Dose adjustments
▶ When used for percutaneous coronary intervention Reduce rate of infusion to 1.4 mg/kg/hour if eGFR 30–60 mL/minute/1.73 m^2 and monitor blood clotting parameters.
● DIRECTIONS FOR ADMINISTRATION For *intravenous infusion* (*Angiox*®), give continuously in Glucose 5% or Sodium chloride 0.9%. Reconstitute each 250-mg vial with 5 mL water for injections then withdraw 5 mL and dilute to 50 mL with infusion fluid.
● NATIONAL FUNDING/ACCESS DECISIONS
NICE decisions
▶ Bivalirudin for the treatment of ST-segment elevation myocardial infarction (July 2011) NICE TA230
Bivalirudin in combination with aspirin and clopidogrel is recommended for the treatment of adults with ST-segment elevation myocardial infarction undergoing primary percutaneous coronary intervention.
www.nice.org.uk/TA230

Scottish Medicines Consortium (SMC) Decisions
The *Scottish Medicines Consortium* has advised (November 2008) that bivalirudin (*Angiox*®) is accepted for restricted use within NHS Scotland for patients with acute coronary syndromes planned for urgent or early intervention who would have been considered for treatment with unfractionated heparin in combination with a glycoprotein IIb/IIIa inhibitor; it should not be used as an alternative to heparin alone.
The *Scottish Medicines Consortium* has advised (August 2010) that bivalirudin (*Angiox*®) is accepted for restricted use within NHS Scotland as an anticoagulant in patients undergoing percutaneous coronary intervention who would have been considered for treatment with unfractionated heparin in combination with a glycoprotein IIb/IIIa inhibitor; it should not be used as an alternative to heparin alone.

● MEDICINAL FORMS
There can be variation in the licensing of different medicines containing the same drug.
Powder for solution for infusion
▶ Bivalirudin (Non-proprietary)
Bivalirudin 250 mg Bivalirudin 250mg powder for concentrate for solution for infusion vials | 1 vial PoM £175.00
▶ Angiox (The Medicines Company UK Ltd)
Bivalirudin 250 mg Angiox 250mg powder for concentrate for solution for infusion vials | 10 vial PoM ⓢ

Dabigatran etexilate

● DRUG ACTION Dabigatran etexilate is a direct thrombin inhibitor with a rapid onset of action.

● INDICATIONS AND DOSE
Prophylaxis of venous thromboembolism following total knee replacement surgery
▶ BY MOUTH
▶ Adult 18–74 years: 110 mg, to be taken 1–4 hours after surgery, followed by 220 mg once daily for 9 days, to be taken 12–24 hours after initial dose
▶ Adult 75 years and over: 75 mg, to be taken 1–4 hours after surgery, followed by 150 mg once daily for 9 days, to be taken 12–24 hours after initial dose

Prophylaxis of venous thromboembolism following total knee replacement surgery in patients receiving concomitant treatment with amiodarone or verapamil
▶ BY MOUTH
▶ Adult 18–74 years: 110 mg, to be taken 1–4 hours after surgery, followed by 150 mg once daily for 9 days, to be taken 12–24 hours after initial dose
▶ Adult 75 years and over: 75 mg, to be taken 1–4 hours after surgery, followed by 150 mg once daily for 9 days, to be taken 12–24 hours after initial dose

Prophylaxis of venous thromboembolism following total hip replacement surgery
▶ BY MOUTH
▶ Adult 18–74 years: 110 mg, to be taken 1–4 hours after surgery, followed by 220 mg once daily for 27–34 days, to be taken 12–24 hours after initial dose
▶ Adult 75 years and over: 75 mg, to be taken 1–4 hours after surgery, followed by 150 mg once daily for 27–34 days, to be taken 12–24 hours after initial dose

Prophylaxis of venous thromboembolism following total hip replacement surgery in patients receiving concomitant treatment with amiodarone or verapamil
▶ BY MOUTH
▶ Adult 18–74 years: 110 mg, to be taken 1–4 hours after surgery, followed by 150 mg daily for 27–34 days, to be taken 12–24 hours after initial dose
▶ Adult 75 years and over: 75 mg, to be taken 1–4 hours after surgery, followed by 150 mg once daily for 27–34 days, to be taken 12–24 hours after initial dose

Treatment of deep-vein thrombosis | Treatment of pulmonary embolism | Prophylaxis of recurrent deep-vein thrombosis | Prophylaxis of recurrent pulmonary embolism
▶ BY MOUTH
▶ Adult 18–74 years: 150 mg twice daily, following at least 5 days treatment with a parenteral anticoagulant
▶ Adult 75–79 years: 110–150 mg twice daily, following at least 5 days treatment with a parenteral anticoagulant
▶ Adult 80 years and over: 110 mg twice daily, following at least 5 days treatment with a parenteral anticoagulant

continued →

Treatment of deep-vein thrombosis in patients with moderate renal impairment | Treatment of deep-vein thrombosis in patients at increased risk of bleeding | Treatment of pulmonary embolism in patients with moderate renal impairment | Treatment of pulmonary embolism in patients at increased risk of bleeding | Prophylaxis of recurrent deep-vein thrombosis in patients with moderate renal impairment | Prophylaxis of recurrent deep-vein thrombosis in patients at increased risk of bleeding | Prophylaxis of recurrent pulmonary embolism in patients with moderate renal impairment | Prophylaxis of recurrent pulmonary embolism in patients at increased risk of bleeding

▸ BY MOUTH
▸ Adult: 110–150 mg twice daily, following at least 5 days treatment with a parenteral anticoagulant

Treatment of deep-vein thrombosis in patients receiving concomitant treatment with verapamil | Treatment of pulmonary embolism in patients receiving concomitant treatment with verapamil | Prophylaxis of recurrent deep-vein thrombosis in patients receiving concomitant treatment with verapamil | Prophylaxis of recurrent pulmonary embolism in patients receiving concomitant treatment with verapamil

▸ BY MOUTH
▸ Adult: 110 mg twice daily, following at least 5 days treatment with a parenteral anticoagulant

Prophylaxis of stroke and systemic embolism in non-valvular atrial fibrillation and with one or more risk factors such as previous stroke or transient ischaemic attack, symptomatic heart failure, age ≥ 75 years, diabetes mellitus, or hypertension

▸ BY MOUTH
▸ Adult 18-74 years: 150 mg twice daily
▸ Adult 75-79 years: 110–150 mg twice daily
▸ Adult 80 years and over: 110 mg twice daily

Prophylaxis of stroke and systemic embolism in non-valvular atrial fibrillation and with one or more risk factors such as previous stroke or transient ischaemic attack, symptomatic heart failure, age ≥ 75 years, diabetes mellitus, or hypertension in patients receiving concomitant treatment with verapamil

▸ BY MOUTH
▸ Adult: 110 mg twice daily

Prophylaxis of stroke and systemic embolism in non-valvular atrial fibrillation and with one or more risk factors such as previous stroke or transient ischaemic attack, symptomatic heart failure, age ≥ 75 years, diabetes mellitus, or hypertension, in patients at increased risk of bleeding | Prophylaxis of stroke and systemic embolism in non-valvular atrial fibrillation and with one or more risk factors such as previous stroke or transient ischaemic attack, symptomatic heart failure, age ≥ 75 years, diabetes mellitus, or hypertension, in patients with moderate renal impairment

▸ BY MOUTH
▸ Adult: 110–150 mg twice daily

DOSE EQUIVALENCE AND CONVERSION
▸ For information on changing from, or to, other anticoagulants, consult product literature.

● CONTRA-INDICATIONS Active bleeding · do not use as anticoagulant for prosthetic heart valve · malignant neoplasms · oesophageal varices · recent brain surgery · recent gastro-intestinal ulcer · recent intracranial haemorrhage · recent ophthalmic surgery · recent spine surgery · significant risk of major bleeding · vascular aneurysm

● CAUTIONS Anaesthesia with postoperative indwelling epidural catheter (risk of paralysis—give initial dose at least 2 hours after catheter removal and monitor

neurological signs) · bacterial endocarditis · bleeding disorders · body-weight less than 50 kg · elderly · gastritis · gastro-oesophageal reflux · oesophagitis · recent biopsy · recent major trauma · thrombocytopenia

● INTERACTIONS → Appendix 1: dabigatran

● SIDE-EFFECTS
▸ **Common or very common** Hepatic function abnormal
▸ **Uncommon** Anaemia · diarrhoea · haemorrhage · hyperbilirubinaemia · nausea · vomiting
▸ **Rare or very rare** Angioedema · dysphagia · gastrointestinal discomfort · gastrointestinal disorders · intracranial haemorrhage · skin reactions · thrombocytopenia
▸ **Frequency not known** Bronchospasm

● PREGNANCY Manufacturer advises avoid unless essential—toxicity in *animal* studies.

● BREAST FEEDING Manufacturer advises avoid—no information available.

● HEPATIC IMPAIRMENT Avoid in severe liver disease, especially if prothrombin time already prolonged.

● RENAL IMPAIRMENT Avoid if creatinine clearance less than 30 mL/minute.
Dose adjustments When used for *prophylaxis of venous thromboembolism following knee or hip replacement surgery*, reduce initial dose to 75 mg and subsequent doses to 150 mg once daily if creatinine clearance 30–50 mL/minute; reduce dose to 75 mg once daily if creatinine clearance 30–50 mL/minute and patient receiving concomitant treatment with verapamil.
When used for *treatment of deep-vein thrombosis and pulmonary embolism, prophylaxis of recurrent deep-vein thrombosis and pulmonary embolism, prophylaxis of stroke and systemic embolism in non-valvular atrial fibrillation*, consider reduced dose of 110 mg twice daily if creatinine clearance 30–50 mL/minute, based on individual assessment of thromboembolic risk and risk of bleeding.
Monitoring In renal impairment monitor renal function at least annually (manufacturer recommends Cockroft and Gault formula to calculate creatinine clearance).

● MONITORING REQUIREMENTS
▸ Patients should be monitored for signs of bleeding or anaemia; treatment should be stopped if severe bleeding occurs.
▸ No routine anticoagulant monitoring required (INR tests are unreliable).
▸ Assess renal function (manufacturer recommends Cockroft and Gault formula to calculate creatinine clearance) before treatment in all patients and at least annually in elderly.

● DIRECTIONS FOR ADMINISTRATION When given concomitantly with amiodarone or verapamil, doses should be taken at the same time.

● PRESCRIBING AND DISPENSING INFORMATION Dabigatran etexilate, is given orally for prophylaxis of venous thromboembolism in adults after total hip replacement or total knee replacement surgery; it is also licensed for the treatment of deep-vein thrombosis and pulmonary embolism, and prophylaxis of recurrent deep-vein thrombosis and pulmonary embolism in adults. Duration of treatment should be determined by balancing the benefit of treatment with the bleeding risk; shorter duration of treatment (at least 3 months) should be based on transient risk factors i.e recent surgery, trauma, immobilisation, and longer duration of treatment should be based on permanent risk factors, or idiopathic deep-vein thrombosis or pulmonary embolism.

● NATIONAL FUNDING/ACCESS DECISIONS

NICE decisions

▶ **Dabigatran etexilate for the prevention of venous thromboembolism after hip or knee replacement surgery in adults (September 2008)** NICE TA157

Dabigatran etexilate is an option for the prophylaxis of venous thromboembolism in adults after total hip replacement or total knee replacement surgery.

www.nice.org.uk/TA157

▶ **Dabigatran etexilate for the prevention of stroke and systemic embolism in atrial fibrillation (March 2012)** NICE TA249

Dabigatran etexilate is an option for the prevention of stroke and systemic embolism in patients with non-valvular atrial fibrillation and with one or more of the following risk factors:

- previous stroke, transient ischaemic attack, or systemic embolism
- left ventricular ejection fraction <40%
- symptomatic heart failure
- age ≥75 years
- age ≥65 years in patients with diabetes mellitus, coronary artery disease, or hypertension

The risks and benefits of dabigatran compared to warfarin should be discussed with the patient.

www.nice.org.uk/TA249

▶ **Dabigatran etexilate for the treatment and secondary prevention of deep vein thrombosis and /or pulmonary embolism (December 2014)** NICE TA327

Dabigatran etexilate is recommended, within its marketing authorisation, as an option for treating and for preventing recurrent deep vein thrombosis and pulmonary embolism in adults.

www.nice.org.uk/TA327

● MEDICINAL FORMS

There can be variation in the licensing of different medicines containing the same drug.

Capsule

CAUTIONARY AND ADVISORY LABELS 25

▶ Pradaxa (Boehringer Ingelheim Ltd)

Dabigatran etexilate (as Dabigatran etexilate mesilate) 75 mg Pradaxa 75mg capsules | 10 capsule PoM £8.50 | 60 capsule PoM £51.00 DT = £51.00

Dabigatran etexilate (as Dabigatran etexilate mesilate) 110 mg Pradaxa 110mg capsules | 10 capsule PoM £8.50 | 60 capsule PoM £51.00 DT = £51.00

Dabigatran etexilate (as Dabigatran etexilate mesilate) 150 mg Pradaxa 150mg capsules | 60 capsule PoM £51.00 DT = £51.00

ANTITHROMBOTIC DRUGS › TISSUE PLASMINOGEN ACTIVATORS

⊩ 215

Urokinase

● INDICATIONS AND DOSE

Deep-vein thrombosis (thromboembolic occlusive vascular disease)

▶ BY INTRAVENOUS INFUSION

▸ Adult: Initially 4400 units/kg, to be given over 10–20 minutes, followed by 100 000 units/hour for 2–3 days

Pulmonary embolism (thromboembolic occlusive vascular disease)

▶ BY INTRAVENOUS INFUSION

▸ Adult: Initially 4400 units/kg, to be given over 10–20 minutes, followed by 4400 units/kg/hour for 12 hours

Occlusive peripheral arterial disease (thromboembolic occlusive vascular disease)

▶ BY INTRA-ARTERIAL INFUSION

▸ Adult: (consult product literature)

Occluded central venous catheters (blocked by fibrin clots)

▶ BY INTRAVENOUS INJECTION

▸ Adult: Inject directly into occluded catheter, to be dissolved in sodium chloride 0.9% to a concentration of 5000 units/mL; use a volume sufficient to fill the catheter lumen; leave for 20–60 minutes then aspirate the lysate; repeat if necessary

Occluded arteriovenous haemodialysis shunts (blocked by fibrin clots)

▶ BY INTRAVENOUS INFUSION, OR BY INTRA-ARTERIAL INFUSION

▸ Adult: (consult product literature)

SYNER-KINASE®

Deep-vein thrombosis (thromboembolic occlusive vascular disease)

▶ BY INTRAVENOUS INFUSION

▸ Adult: Initially 4400 units/kg, to be given over 10 minutes, dose to be made up in 15 mL sodium chloride 0.9%, followed by 4400 units/kg/hour for 12–24 hours

Pulmonary embolism (thromboembolic occlusive vascular disease)

▶ INITIALLY BY INTRAVENOUS INFUSION

▸ Adult: Initially 4400 units/kg, to be given over 10 minutes, dose to be made up in 15 mL sodium chloride 0.9%, followed by (by intravenous infusion) 4400 micrograms/kg/hour for 12 hours, alternatively (by intra-arterial injection) 15 000 units/kg, to be injected into pulmonary artery, subsequent doses adjusted according to response; maximum 3 doses per day

Occlusive peripheral arterial disease

▶ BY INTRA-ARTERIAL INFUSION

▸ Adult: (consult product literature)

Occluded intravenous catheters and cannulas (blocked by fibrin clots)

▶ BY INTRA-ARTERIAL INJECTION, OR BY INTRAVENOUS INJECTION

▸ Adult: 5000–25 000 units, to be injected directly into catheter or cannula, dose dissolved in suitable volume of sodium chloride 0.9% to fill the catheter or cannula lumen; leave for 20–60 minutes then aspirate the lysate; repeat if necessary

● INTERACTIONS → Appendix 1: urokinase

● SIDE-EFFECTS

▶ **Common or very common** Artery dissection · stroke

▶ **Uncommon** Renal failure

● BREAST FEEDING Manufacturer advises avoid—no information available.

● HEPATIC IMPAIRMENT

Dose adjustments Dose reduction may be required.

● RENAL IMPAIRMENT

Dose adjustments Dose reduction may be required.

● DIRECTIONS FOR ADMINISTRATION For *intravenous infusion* (*Syner-KINASE*®), give continuously or intermittently in Sodium chloride 0.9%.

● MEDICINAL FORMS

There can be variation in the licensing of different medicines containing the same drug.

Powder for solution for injection

▶ Urokinase (Non-proprietary)

Urokinase 10000 unit Urokinase 10,000unit powder for solution for injection vials | 1 vial PoM £33.79

Urokinase 50000 unit Urokinase 50,000unit powder for solution for injection vials | 1 vial PoM £69.70

Urokinase 100000 unit Urokinase 100,000unit powder for solution for injection vials | 1 vial PoM £106.17

Urokinase 250000 unit Urokinase 250,000unit powder for solution for injection vials | 1 vial PoM £185.65

Urokinase 500000 unit Urokinase 500,000unit powder for solution for injection vials | 1 vial [PoM] £365.00
▸ Syner-KINASE (Syner-Med (Pharmaceutical Products) Ltd)
Urokinase 10000 unit Syner-KINASE 10,000unit powder for solution for injection vials | 1 vial [PoM] £35.95 (Hospital only)
Urokinase 25000 unit Syner-KINASE 25,000unit powder for solution for injection vials | 1 vial [PoM] £45.95 (Hospital only)
Urokinase 100000 unit Syner-KINASE 100,000unit powder for solution for injection vials | 1 vial [PoM] £112.95 (Hospital only)
Urokinase 250000 unit Syner-KINASE 250,000unit powder for solution for injection vials | 1 vial [PoM] [S] (Hospital only)
Urokinase 500000 unit Syner-KINASE 500,000unit powder for solution for injection vials | 1 vial [PoM] [S] (Hospital only)

ANTITHROMBOTIC DRUGS › VITAMIN K ANTAGONISTS

Vitamin K antagonists

IMPORTANT SAFETY INFORMATION
MHRA/CHM ADVICE: DIRECT-ACTING ANTIVIRALS TO TREAT CHRONIC HEPATITIS C: RISK OF INTERACTION WITH VITAMIN K ANTAGONISTS AND CHANGES IN INR (JANUARY 2017)
A EU-wide review has identified that changes in liver function, secondary to hepatitis C treatment with direct-acting antivirals, may affect the efficacy of vitamin K antagonists; the MHRA has advised that INR should be monitored closely in patients receiving concomitant treatment.

● CONTRA-INDICATIONS Avoid use within 48 hours postpartum · haemorrhagic stroke · significant bleeding
● CAUTIONS Bacterial endocarditis (use only if warfarin otherwise indicated) · conditions in which risk of bleeding is increased · history of gastrointestinal bleeding · hyperthyroidism · hypothyroidism · peptic ulcer · postpartum (delay warfarin until risk of haemorrhage is low—usually 5–7 days after delivery) · recent ischaemic stroke · recent surgery · uncontrolled hypertension
● SIDE-EFFECTS
▸ Common or very common Haemorrhage
▸ Rare or very rare Alopecia · appetite decreased · hepatic disorders · nausea · skin necrosis haemorrhagic (increased risk in patients with protein C or protein S deficiency) · vasculitis · vomiting
▸ Frequency not known Agranulocytosis · albuminuria · blue toe syndrome · calciphylaxis · CNS haemorrhage · diarrhoea · eosinophilia · fever · haemothorax · increased leucocytes · kidney injury · leucopenia · lymphadenopathy · pancreatitis · pancytopenia · renal tubular necrosis · skin necrosis (increased risk in patients with protein C or protein S deficiency) · skin reactions · taste altered
● CONCEPTION AND CONTRACEPTION Women of child-bearing age should be warned of the danger of teratogenicity.
● PREGNANCY Should not be given in the first trimester of pregnancy. Warfarin, acenocoumarol, and phenindione cross the placenta with risk of congenital malformations, and placental, fetal, or neonatal haemorrhage, especially during the last few weeks of pregnancy and at delivery. Therefore, if at all possible, they should be avoided in pregnancy, especially in the first and third trimesters (difficult decisions have to be made, particularly in women with prosthetic heart valves, atrial fibrillation, or with a history of recurrent venous thrombosis or pulmonary embolism). Stopping these drugs before the sixth week of gestation may largely avoid the risk of fetal abnormality.
● MONITORING REQUIREMENTS
▸ The base-line prothrombin time should be determined but the initial dose should not be delayed whilst awaiting the result.

▸ It is essential that the INR be determined daily or on alternate days in early days of treatment, *then* at longer intervals (depending on response), *then* up to every 12 weeks.
▸ Change in patient's clinical condition, particularly associated with liver disease, intercurrent illness, or drug administration, necessitates more frequent testing.
● PATIENT AND CARER ADVICE Anticoagulant treatment booklets should be issued to all patients or their carers; these booklets include advice for patients on anticoagulant treatment, an alert card to be carried by the patient at all times, and a section for recording of INR results and dosage information. In **England**, **Wales**, and **Northern Ireland**, they are available for purchase from:
3M Security Print and Systems Limited
Gorse Street, Chadderton
Oldham
OL9 9QH
Tel: 0845 610 1112
   GP practices can obtain supplies through their Local Area Team stores. NHS Trusts can order supplies from www.nhsforms.co.uk or by emailing nhsforms@spsl.uk.com.
   In **Scotland**, treatment booklets and starter information packs can be obtained by emailing stockorders.DPPAS@apsgroup.co.uk or by fax on (0131) 6299 967.
   Electronic copies of the booklets and further advice are also available at www.npsa.nhs.uk/nrls/alerts-and-directives/alerts/anticoagulant.

▸ above

Acenocoumarol
(Nicoumalone)

● INDICATIONS AND DOSE
Prophylaxis of embolisation in rheumatic heart disease and atrial fibrillation | Prophylaxis after insertion of prosthetic heart valve | Prophylaxis and treatment of venous thrombosis and pulmonary embolism | Transient ischaemic attacks
▸ BY MOUTH
▸ Adult: Initially 2–4 mg once daily for 2 days, alternatively initially 6 mg on day 1, then 4 mg on day 2; maintenance 1–8 mg daily, adjusted according to response, dose to be taken at the same time each day, lower doses may be required in patients over 65 years, liver disease, severe heart failure with hepatic congestion, and malnutrition

● CAUTIONS Patients over 65 years
● INTERACTIONS → Appendix 1: coumarins
● BREAST FEEDING Risk of haemorrhage; increased by vitamin K deficiency—manufacturer recommends prophylactic vitamin K for the infant (consult product literature).
● HEPATIC IMPAIRMENT Use with caution in mild to moderate impairment. Avoid in severe impairment, especially if prothrombin time is already prolonged.
● RENAL IMPAIRMENT Caution in mild to moderate impairment. Avoid in severe impairment.
● PATIENT AND CARER ADVICE Anticoagulant card to be provided.

- **MEDICINAL FORMS**
There can be variation in the licensing of different medicines containing the same drug.
Tablet
CAUTIONARY AND ADVISORY LABELS 10
‣ Acenocoumarol (Non-proprietary)
Acenocoumarol 1 mg Acenocoumarol 1mg tablets | 100 tablet [PoM] [x̄] DT = £4.62
‣ Sinthrome (Merus Labs Luxco S.a R.L.)
Acenocoumarol 1 mg Sinthrome 1mg tablets | 100 tablet [PoM] £4.62 DT = £4.62

⟟ 138

Phenindione

- **INDICATIONS AND DOSE**

Prophylaxis of embolisation in rheumatic heart disease and atrial fibrillation | Prophylaxis after insertion of prosthetic heart valve | Prophylaxis and treatment of venous thrombosis and pulmonary embolism
‣ BY MOUTH
‣ Adult: Initially 200 mg on day 1, then 100 mg on day 2, then, adjusted according to response; maintenance 50–150 mg daily

- **INTERACTIONS** → Appendix 1: phenindione
- **BREAST FEEDING** Avoid. Risk of haemorrhage; increased by vitamin K deficiency.
- **HEPATIC IMPAIRMENT** Avoid in severe impairment, especially if prothrombin time is already prolonged.
- **RENAL IMPAIRMENT** Caution in mild to moderate impairment. Avoid in severe impairment.
- **PATIENT AND CARER ADVICE** Patient counselling is advised for phenindione tablets (may turn urine pink or orange). Anticoagulant card to be provided.

- **MEDICINAL FORMS**
There can be variation in the licensing of different medicines containing the same drug.
Tablet
CAUTIONARY AND ADVISORY LABELS 10, 14
‣ Phenindione (Non-proprietary)
Phenindione 10 mg Phenindione 10mg tablets | 28 tablet [PoM] £538.18 DT = £538.18
Phenindione 25 mg Phenindione 25mg tablets | 28 tablet [PoM] £538.18 DT = £538.18
Phenindione 50 mg Phenindione 50mg tablets | 28 tablet [PoM] £51.84

⟟ 138

Warfarin sodium

10-Oct-2016

- **INDICATIONS AND DOSE**

Prophylaxis of embolisation in rheumatic heart disease and atrial fibrillation | Prophylaxis after insertion of prosthetic heart valve | Prophylaxis and treatment of venous thrombosis and pulmonary embolism | Transient ischaemic attacks
‣ BY MOUTH
‣ Adult: Initially 5–10 mg, to be taken on day 1; subsequent doses dependent on the prothrombin time, reported as INR (international normalised ratio), a lower induction dose can be given over 3–4 weeks in patients who do not require rapid anticoagulation, elderly patients to be given a lower induction dose; maintenance 3–9 mg daily, to be taken at the same time each day

IMPORTANT SAFETY INFORMATION
MHRA/CHM ADVICE: WARFARIN: REPORTS OF CALCIPHYLAXIS (JULY 2016)
An EU-wide review has concluded that on rare occasions, warfarin use may lead to calciphylaxis—patients should

be advised to consult their doctor if they develop a painful skin rash; if calciphylaxis is diagnosed, appropriate treatment should be started and consideration should be given to stopping treatment with warfarin. The MHRA has advised that calciphylaxis is most commonly observed in patients with known risk factors such as end-stage renal disease, however cases have also been reported in patients with normal renal function.

- **INTERACTIONS** → Appendix 1: coumarins
- **PREGNANCY** Babies of mothers taking warfarin at the time of delivery need to be offered immediate prophylaxis with intramuscular phytomenadione (vitamin K₁).
- **BREAST FEEDING** Not present in milk in significant amounts and appears safe. Risk of haemorrhage which is increased by vitamin K deficiency.
- **HEPATIC IMPAIRMENT** Avoid in severe impairment, especially if prothrombin time is already prolonged.
- **RENAL IMPAIRMENT** Use with caution in mild to moderate impairment.
Monitoring In severe renal impairment, monitor INR more frequently.
- **PATIENT AND CARER ADVICE** Anticoagulant card to be provided.

- **MEDICINAL FORMS**
There can be variation in the licensing of different medicines containing the same drug. Forms available from special-order manufacturers include: oral suspension, oral solution
Oral suspension
CAUTIONARY AND ADVISORY LABELS 10
‣ Warfarin sodium (Non-proprietary)
Warfarin sodium 1 mg per 1 ml Warfarin 1mg/ml oral suspension sugar free sugar-free | 150 ml [PoM] £108.00 DT = £108.00
Tablet
CAUTIONARY AND ADVISORY LABELS 10
‣ Warfarin sodium (Non-proprietary)
Warfarin sodium 500 microgram Warfarin 500microgram tablets | 28 tablet [PoM] £1.70 DT = £1.27
Warfarin sodium 1 mg Warfarin 1mg tablets | 28 tablet [PoM] £1.16 DT = £0.33 | 500 tablet [PoM] £5.89
Warfarin sodium 3 mg Warfarin 3mg tablets | 28 tablet [PoM] £1.20 DT = £0.37 | 500 tablet [PoM] £6.61
Warfarin sodium 5 mg Warfarin 5mg tablets | 28 tablet [PoM] £1.29 DT = £0.42 | 500 tablet [PoM] £7.50

4   Blood pressure conditions

4.1   Hypertension

Hypertension

Overview

Lowering raised blood pressure decreases the risk of stroke, coronary events, heart failure, and renal impairment. Advice on antihypertensive therapy in this section takes into account the recommendations of NICE clinical guidance 127 (August 2011), Hypertension—Clinical management of primary hypertension in adults.

Possible causes of hypertension (e.g. renal disease, endocrine causes), contributory factors, risk factors, and the presence of any complications of hypertension, such as left ventricular hypertrophy, should be established. Patients should be given advice on lifestyle changes to reduce blood pressure or cardiovascular risk; these include smoking cessation, weight reduction, reduction of excessive intake of alcohol and caffeine, reduction of dietary salt, reduction of total and saturated fat, increasing exercise, and increasing fruit and vegetable intake.

Hypertension thresholds and targets for treatment

Patients presenting with a blood pressure of 140/90 mmHg or higher when measured in a clinic setting, should be offered ambulatory blood pressure monitoring (or home blood pressure monitoring if ambulatory blood pressure monitoring is unsuitable) to confirm the diagnosis and stage of hypertension.

Stage 1 hypertension:

- Clinic blood pressure 140/90 mmHg or higher, *and* ambulatory daytime average or home blood pressure average 135/85 mmHg or higher
- Treat patients under 80 years who have stage 1 hypertension and target-organ damage (e.g. left ventricular hypertrophy, chronic kidney disease, hypertensive retinopathy), cardiovascular disease, renal disease, diabetes, or a 10 year cardiovascular risk ≥20%; in the absence of these conditions, advise lifestyle changes and review annually. For patients under 40 years with stage 1 hypertension but **no** overt target-organ damage, cardiovascular disease, renal disease, or diabetes, consider seeking specialist advice for evaluation of secondary causes of hypertension

Stage 2 hypertension:

- Clinic blood pressure 160/100 mmHg or higher, *and* ambulatory daytime average or home blood pressure average 150/95 mmHg or higher
- Treat all patients who have stage 2 hypertension, regardless of age

Severe hypertension:

- Clinic systolic blood pressure ≥180 mmHg or clinic diastolic blood pressure ≥110 mmHg; treat promptly—see Hypertensive Crises, below.

A target clinic blood pressure below 140/90 mmHg is suggested for patients under 80 years; a target ambulatory or home blood pressure average (during the patient's waking hours) of below 135/85 mmHg is suggested for patients under 80 years; see also Hypertension in the Elderly, below. A target clinic blood pressure below 130/80 mmHg should be considered for those with established atherosclerotic cardiovascular disease, or diabetes in the presence of kidney, eye, or cerebrovascular disease. In some individuals it may not be possible to reduce blood pressure below the suggested targets despite the use of appropriate therapy.

Drugs for hypertension

A single antihypertensive drug is often inadequate in the management of hypertension, and additional antihypertensive drugs are usually added in a step-wise manner until control is achieved. Unless it is necessary to lower the blood pressure urgently (see Hypertensive Crises), an interval of at least 4 weeks should be allowed to determine response; clinicians should ensure antihypertensive drugs are titrated to the optimum or maximum tolerated dose at each step of treatment. Response to drug treatment may be affected by age and ethnicity.

Patients under 55 years:

Step 1

- **ACE inhibitor**; if not tolerated, offer an **angiotensin-II receptor antagonist**. If both ACE inhibitors and angiotensin-II receptor antagonists are contra-indicated or not tolerated, consider a **beta-blocker**; beta-blockers, especially when combined with a thiazide diuretic, should be avoided for the routine treatment of uncomplicated hypertension in patients with diabetes or at high risk of developing diabetes

Step 2

- ACE inhibitor or angiotensin-II receptor antagonist in combination with a **calcium-channel blocker**. If a calcium-channel blocker is not tolerated or if there is

evidence of, or a high risk of, heart failure, give a **thiazide-related diuretic** (e.g. chlortalidone or indapamide). If a beta-blocker was given at Step 1, add a calcium channel blocker in preference to a thiazide-related diuretic (see Step 1)

Step 3

- ACE inhibitor or angiotensin-II receptor antagonist in combination with a calcium-channel blocker *and* a thiazide-related diuretic

Step 4 (resistant hypertension)

- Consider seeking specialist advice
- Add low-dose **spironolactone** [unlicensed indication], *or* use high-dose thiazide related diuretic if plasma-potassium concentration above 4.5 mmol/litre
- Monitor renal function and electrolytes
- If additional diuretic therapy is contra-indicated, ineffective, or not tolerated, consider an **alpha-blocker** *or* a beta-blocker

Patients over 55 years, and patients of any age who are of African or Caribbean family origin:

Step 1

- Calcium-channel blocker; if not tolerated or if there is evidence of, or a high risk of, heart failure, give a thiazide-related diuretic (e.g. chlortalidone or indapamide)

Step 2

- Calcium-channel blocker *or* thiazide-related diuretic in combination with an ACE inhibitor or angiotensin-II receptor antagonist (an angiotensin-II receptor antagonist in combination with a calcium-channel blocker is preferred in patients of African or Caribbean family origin)

Steps 3 and 4

- Treat as for patients under 55 years

Cardiovascular risk reduction

Aspirin p. 121 reduces the risk of cardiovascular events and myocardial infarction. Unduly high blood pressure must be controlled before aspirin is given. Unless contra-indicated, aspirin is recommended for all patients with established cardiovascular disease. Use of aspirin in primary prevention, in those with or without diabetes, is of unproven benefit. For the role of aspirin in the prevention of stroke in patients with atrial fibrillation, see Arrhythmias p. 99.

Statins are also of benefit in cardiovascular disease or in those who are at high risk of developing cardiovascular disease.

Hypertension in the elderly

Benefit from antihypertensive therapy is evident up to at least 80 years of age, but it is probably inappropriate to apply a strict age limit when deciding on drug therapy. Patients who reach 80 years of age while taking antihypertensive drugs should continue treatment, provided that it continues to be of benefit and does not cause significant side-effects. If patients are aged over 80 years when diagnosed with stage 1 hypertension, the decision to treat should be based on the presence of other comorbidities; patients with stage 2 hypertension should be treated as for patients over 55 years. A target clinic blood pressure below 150/90 mmHg is suggested for patients over 80 years; the suggested target ambulatory or home blood pressure average (during the patient's waking hours) is below 145/85 mmHg.

Isolated systolic hypertension

Isolated systolic hypertension (systolic pressure ≥160 mmHg, diastolic pressure < 90 mmHg) is common in patients over 60 years, and is associated with an increased cardiovascular disease risk; it should be treated as for patients with both a raised systolic and diastolic blood pressure. Patients with severe postural hypotension should be referred to a specialist.

Hypertension in diabetes

For patients with diabetes, a target clinic blood pressure below 140/80 mmHg is suggested (below 130/80 mmHg is advised if kidney, eye, or cerebrovascular disease are also present). However, in some individuals, it may not be possible to achieve this level of control despite appropriate therapy. Most patients require a combination of antihypertensive drugs.

Hypertension is common in type 2 diabetes, and antihypertensive treatment prevents macrovascular and microvascular complications. In type 1 diabetes, hypertension usually indicates the presence of diabetic nephropathy. An ACE inhibitor (or an angiotensin-II receptor antagonist) may have a specific role in the management of diabetic nephropathy; in patients with type 2 diabetes, an ACE inhibitor (or an angiotensin-II receptor antagonist) can delay progression of microalbuminuria to nephropathy.

Hypertension in renal disease

A target clinic blood pressure below 140/90 mmHg is suggested (below 130/80 mmHg is advised in patients with chronic kidney disease and diabetes, or if proteinuria exceeds 1 g in 24 hours). An ACE inhibitor (or an angiotensin-II receptor antagonist) should be considered for patients with proteinuria; however, ACE inhibitors should be used with caution in renal impairment. Thiazide diuretics may be ineffective and high doses of loop diuretics may be required.

Hypertension in pregnancy

Hypertensive complications in pregnancy can be hazardous for both the mother and the fetus, and are associated with a significant risk of morbidity and mortality; complications can occur in pregnant women with pre-existing chronic hypertension, or in those who develop hypertension in the latter half of pregnancy.

Labetalol hydrochloride p. 147 is widely used for treating hypertension in pregnancy. Methyldopa p. 144 is considered safe for use in pregnancy. Modified-release preparations of nifedipine p. 162 [unlicensed] are also used.

The following advice takes into account the recommendations of NICE Clinical Guideline 107 (August 2010), Hypertension in Pregnancy.

Pregnant women with chronic hypertension who are already receiving antihypertensive treatment should have their drug therapy reviewed. In uncomplicated chronic hypertension, a target blood pressure of <150/100 mmHg is recommended; women with target-organ damage as a result of chronic hypertension, and in women with chronic hypertension who have given birth, a target blood pressure of <140/90 mmHg is advised. Long-term antihypertensive treatment should be reviewed 2 weeks following the birth. Women managed with methyldopa during pregnancy should discontinue treatment and restart their original antihypertensive medication within 2 days of the birth.

Pregnant women are at high risk of developing pre-eclampsia if they have chronic kidney disease, diabetes mellitus, autoimmune disease, chronic hypertension, or if they have had hypertension during a previous pregnancy; these women are advised to take aspirin p. 121 once daily [unlicensed indication] from week 12 of pregnancy until the baby is born. Women with more than one moderate risk factor (first pregnancy, aged ≥40 years, pregnancy interval >10 years, BMI ≥ 35 kg/m² at first visit, multiple pregnancy, or family history of pre-eclampsia) for developing pre-eclampsia are also advised to take aspirin once daily [unlicensed indication] from week 12 of pregnancy until the baby is born.

Women with pre-eclampsia or gestational hypertension who present with a blood pressure over 150/100 mmHg, should receive initial treatment with oral labetalol hydrochloride to achieve a target blood pressure of <150 mmHg systolic, and diastolic 80–100 mmHg. If labetalol hydrochloride is unsuitable, methyldopa or modified-release nifedipine may be considered. Women with gestational hypertension or pre-eclampsia who have been managed with methyldopa during pregnancy should discontinue treatment within 2 days of the birth. Women with a blood pressure of ≥160/110 mmHg who require critical care during pregnancy or after birth should receive immediate treatment with either oral or intravenous labetalol hydrochloride, intravenous hydralazine hydrochloride p. 180, or oral modified-release nifedipine to achieve a target blood pressure of <150 mmHg systolic, and diastolic 80–100 mmHg.

Also see use of magnesium sulfate p. 1019 in pre-eclampsia and eclampsia. [EvGr] In women with pre-eclampsia where birth is considered likely within 7 days, intramuscular betamethasone p. 660 [unlicensed indication] is recommended for fetal lung maturation. Ⓐ

Hypertensive crises

If blood pressure is reduced too quickly in the management of hypertensive crises, there is a risk of reduced organ perfusion leading to cerebral infarction, blindness, deterioration in renal function, and myocardial ischaemia.

A *hypertensive emergency* is defined as severe hypertension with acute damage to the target organs (e.g. signs of papilloedema or retinal haemorrhage, or the presence of clinical conditions such as acute coronary syndromes, acute aortic dissection, acute pulmonary oedema, hypertensive encephalopathy, acute cerebral infarction, intracerebral or subarachnoid haemorrhage, eclampsia, or rapidly progressing renal failure); prompt treatment with intravenous antihypertensive therapy is generally required. Over the first few minutes or within 2 hours, blood pressure should be reduced by 20–25%. When intravenous therapy is indicated, treatment options include sodium nitroprusside p. 182 [unlicensed], nicardipine hydrochloride p. 161, labetalol hydrochloride, glyceryl trinitrate p. 217, phentolamine mesilate p. 181, hydralazine hydrochloride, or esmolol hydrochloride p. 153; choice of drug is dependent on concomitant conditions and clinical status of the patient.

Severe hypertension (blood pressure ≥ 180/110 mmHg) without acute target-organ damage is defined as a *hypertensive urgency*; blood pressure should be reduced gradually over 24–48 hours with oral antihypertensive therapy, such as labetalol hydrochloride, or the calcium-channel blockers amlodipine p. 155 or felodipine p. 159. Use of sublingual nifedipine is not recommended.

Also see advice on short-term management of hypertensive episodes in phaeochromocytoma.

Phaeochromocytoma

Long-term management of phaeochromocytoma involves surgery. However, surgery should not take place until there is adequate blockade of both alpha- and beta-adrenoceptors; the optimal choice of drug therapy remains unclear. Alpha-blockers are used in the short-term management of hypertensive episodes in phaeochromocytoma. Once alpha blockade is established, tachycardia can be controlled by the cautious addition of a beta-blocker; a cardioselective beta-blocker is preferred.

Phenoxybenzamine hydrochloride p. 181, a powerful alpha-blocker, is effective in the management of phaeochromocytoma but it has many side-effects. Phentolamine mesilate is a short-acting alpha-blocker used mainly during surgery of phaeochromocytoma; its use for the diagnosis of phaeochromocytoma has been superseded by measurement of catecholamines in blood and urine.

Metirosine (available from 'special-order' manufacturers or specialist importing companies) inhibits the enzyme tyrosine hydroxylase, and hence the synthesis of catecholamines. It is rarely used in the pre-operative management of phaeochromocytoma, and long term in patients unsuitable for surgery; an alpha-adrenoceptor blocking drug may also be required. Metirosine should **not** be used to treat essential hypertension.

Antihypertensive drugs

Vasodilator antihypertensive drugs

Vasodilators have a potent hypotensive effect, especially when used in combination with a beta-blocker and a thiazide. **Important:** see Hypertension (hypertensive crises) for a warning on the hazards of a very rapid fall in blood pressure.

Hydralazine hydrochloride p. 180 is given by mouth as an adjunct to other antihypertensives for the treatment of resistant hypertension but is rarely used; when used alone it causes tachycardia and fluid retention.

Sodium nitroprusside p. 182 [unlicensed] is given by intravenous infusion to control severe hypertensive emergencies when parenteral treatment is necessary.

Minoxidil p. 181 should be reserved for the treatment of severe hypertension resistant to other drugs. Vasodilatation is accompanied by increased cardiac output and tachycardia and the patients develop fluid retention. For this reason the addition of a beta-blocker and a diuretic (usually furosemide p. 226, in high dosage) are mandatory. Hypertrichosis is troublesome and renders this drug unsuitable for females.

Prazosin p. 766, doxazosin p. 765, and terazosin p. 768 have alpha-blocking and vasodilator properties.

Ambrisentan p. 184, bosentan p. 184, iloprost p. 183, macitentan p. 185, sildenafil p. 794, and tadalafil p. 796 are licensed for the treatment of pulmonary arterial hypertension and should be used under specialist supervision. Epoprostenol p. 115 can be used in patients with primary pulmonary hypertension resistant to other treatments. Bosentan is also licensed to reduce the number of new digital ulcers in patients with systemic sclerosis and ongoing digital ulcer disease. Riociguat p. 185 is licensed for the treatment of pulmonary arterial hypertension and chronic thromboembolic pulmonary hypertension; it should be used under specialist supervision.

Sitaxentan has been withdrawn from the market because the benefit of treatment does not outweigh the risk of severe hepatotoxicity.

Centrally acting antihypertensive drugs

Methyldopa p. 144 is a centrally acting antihypertensive; it may be used for the management of hypertension in pregnancy.

Clonidine hydrochloride p. 144 has the disadvantage that sudden withdrawal of treatment may cause severe rebound hypertension.

Moxonidine p. 145, a centrally acting drug, is licensed for mild to moderate essential hypertension. It may have a role when thiazides, calcium-channel blockers, ACE inhibitors, and beta-blockers are not appropriate or have failed to control blood pressure.

Adrenergic neurone blocking drugs

Adrenergic neurone blocking drugs prevent the release of noradrenaline from postganglionic adrenergic neurones. These drugs do not control supine blood pressure and may cause postural hypotension. For this reason they have largely fallen from use, but may be necessary with other therapy in resistant hypertension.

Guanethidine monosulfate p. 182, which also depletes the nerve endings of noradrenaline, is licensed for rapid control of blood pressure, however alternative treatments are preferred.

Alpha-adrenoceptor blocking drugs

Prazosin has post-synaptic alpha-blocking and vasodilator properties and rarely causes tachycardia. It may, however, reduce blood pressure rapidly after the first dose and should be introduced with caution. Doxazosin, indoramin p. 766, and terazosin have properties similar to those of prazosin.

Alpha-blockers can be used with other antihypertensive drugs in the treatment of resistant hypertension.

Prostatic hyperplasia

Alfuzosin hydrochloride p. 764, doxazosin, indoramin, prazosin, tamsulosin hydrochloride p. 767, and terazosin are indicated for benign prostatic hyperplasia.

Drugs affecting the renin-angiotensin system

Angiotensin-converting enzyme inhibitors

Angiotensin-converting enzyme inhibitors (ACE inhibitors) inhibit the conversion of angiotensin I to angiotensin II. They have many uses and are generally well tolerated. The main indications of ACE inhibitors are shown below.

Heart failure

ACE inhibitors are used in all grades of heart failure, usually combined with a beta-blocker. Potassium supplements and potassium-sparing diuretics should be discontinued before introducing an ACE inhibitor because of the risk of hyperkalaemia. However, a low dose of spironolactone p. 190 may be beneficial in severe heart failure and can be used with an ACE inhibitor provided serum potassium is monitored carefully. Profound first-dose hypotension may occur when ACE inhibitors are introduced to patients with heart failure who are already taking a high dose of a loop diuretic (e.g. furosemide p. 226 80 mg daily or more). Temporary withdrawal of the loop diuretic reduces the risk, but may cause severe rebound pulmonary oedema. Therefore, for patients on high doses of loop diuretics, the ACE inhibitor may need to be initiated under specialist supervision. An ACE inhibitor can be initiated in the community in patients who are receiving a low dose of a diuretic or who are not otherwise at risk of serious hypotension; nevertheless, care is required and a very low dose of the ACE inhibitor is given initially.

Hypertension

An ACE inhibitor may be the most appropriate initial drug for hypertension in younger Caucasian patients; Afro-Caribbean patients, those aged over 55 years, and those with primary aldosteronism respond less well. ACE inhibitors are particularly indicated for hypertension in patients with type 1 diabetes with nephropathy. They may reduce blood pressure very rapidly in some patients particularly in those receiving diuretic therapy.

Diabetic nephropathy

ACE inhibitors have a role in the management of diabetic nephropathy.

Prophylaxis of cardiovascular events

ACE inhibitors are used in the early and long-term management of patients who have had a myocardial infarction. ACE inhibitors may also have a role in preventing cardiovascular events.

Initiation under specialist supervision

ACE inhibitors should be initiated under specialist supervision and with careful clinical monitoring in those with severe heart failure or in those:

- receiving multiple or high-dose diuretic therapy (e.g. more than 80 mg of furosemide daily or its equivalent);
- receiving concomitant angiotensin-II receptor antagonist or aliskiren;

- with hypovolaemia;
- with hyponatraemia (plasma-sodium concentration below 130 mmol/litre);
- with hypotension (systolic blood pressure below 90 mmHg);
- with unstable heart failure;
- receiving high-dose vasodilator therapy;
- known renovascular disease.

Renal effects

Renal function and electrolytes should be checked before starting ACE inhibitors (or increasing the dose) and monitored during treatment (more frequently if features mentioned below present); hyperkalaemia and other side-effects of ACE inhibitors are more common in those with impaired renal function and the dose may need to be reduced. Although ACE inhibitors now have a specialised role in some forms of renal disease, including chronic kidney disease, they also occasionally cause impairment of renal function which may progress and become severe in other circumstances (at particular risk are the elderly). A specialist should be involved if renal function is significantly reduced as a result of treatment with an ACE inhibitor.

Concomitant treatment with NSAIDs increases the risk of renal damage, and potassium-sparing diuretics (or potassium-containing salt substitutes) increase the risk of hyperkalaemia.

In patients with severe bilateral renal artery stenosis (or severe stenosis of the artery supplying a single functioning kidney), ACE inhibitors reduce or abolish glomerular filtration and are likely to cause severe and progressive renal failure. They are therefore not recommended in patients known to have these forms of critical renovascular disease.

ACE inhibitor treatment is unlikely to have an adverse effect on overall renal function in patients with severe unilateral renal artery stenosis and a normal contralateral kidney, but glomerular filtration is likely to be reduced (or even abolished) in the affected kidney and the long-term consequences are unknown.

ACE inhibitors are therefore best avoided in patients with known or suspected renovascular disease, unless the blood pressure cannot be controlled by other drugs. If ACE inhibitors are used, they should be initiated only under specialist supervision and renal function should be monitored regularly.

ACE inhibitors should also be used with particular caution in patients who may have undiagnosed and clinically silent renovascular disease. This includes patients with peripheral vascular disease or those with severe generalised atherosclerosis.

ACE inhibitors in combination with other drugs

See also, *Concomitant use of drugs affecting the renin-angiotensin system*, below.

Concomitant diuretics

ACE inhibitors can cause a very rapid fall in blood pressure in volume-depleted patients; treatment should therefore be initiated with very low doses. If the dose of diuretic is greater than 80 mg furosemide or equivalent, the ACE inhibitor should be initiated under close supervision and in some patients the diuretic dose may need to be reduced or the diuretic discontinued at least 24 hours beforehand (may not be possible in heart failure—risk of pulmonary oedema). If high-dose diuretic therapy cannot be stopped, close observation is recommended after administration of the first dose of ACE inhibitor, for at least 2 hours or until the blood pressure has stabilised.

Combination products

Products incorporating an ACE inhibitor with a thiazide diuretic or a calcium-channel blocker are available for the management of hypertension. Use of these combination products should be reserved for patients whose blood pressure has not responded adequately to a single antihypertensive drug and who have been stabilised on the individual components of the combination in the same proportions.

Angiotensin-II receptor antagonists

Azilsartan medoxomil p. 174, candesartan cilexetil p. 174, eprosartan p. 175, irbesartan p. 175, losartan potassium p. 176, olmesartan medoxomil p. 177, telmisartan p. 178, and valsartan p. 178 are angiotensin-II receptor antagonists with many properties similar to those of the ACE inhibitors. However, unlike ACE inhibitors, they do not inhibit the breakdown of bradykinin and other kinins, and thus are less likely to cause the persistent dry cough which can complicate ACE inhibitor therapy. They are therefore a useful alternative for patients who have to discontinue an ACE inhibitor because of persistent cough.

An angiotensin-II receptor antagonist may be used as an alternative to an ACE inhibitor in the management of heart failure or diabetic nephropathy. Candesartan cilexetil and valsartan are also licensed as adjuncts to ACE inhibitors under specialist supervision, in the management of heart failure when other treatments are unsuitable.

Renal effects

Angiotensin-II receptor antagonists should be used with caution in renal artery stenosis (see also Renal effects under Angiotensin-converting enzyme inhibitors, above).

Renin inhibitor

Aliskiren is a renin inhibitor that is licensed for the treatment of hypertension.

Concomitant use of drugs affecting the renin-angiotensin system

Combination therapy with two drugs affecting the renin-angiotensin system (ACE inhibitors, angiotensin-II receptor antagonists, and aliskiren p. 179 is not recommended due to an increased risk of hyperkalaemia, hypotension, and renal impairment, compared to use of a single drug. Patients with diabetic nephropathy are particularly susceptible to developing hyperkalaemia and should not be given an ACE inhibitor with an angiotensin-II receptor antagonist. There is some evidence that the benefits of combination use of an ACE inhibitor with candesartan or valsartan may outweigh the risks in selected patients with heart failure for whom other treatments are unsuitable, however, the concomitant use of this combination, together with an aldosterone antagonist or a potassium-sparing diuretic is not recommended.

For patients currently taking combination therapy, the need for continued combined therapy should be reviewed. If combination therapy is considered essential, it should be carried out under specialist supervision, with close monitoring of blood pressure, renal function, and electrolytes (particularly potassium); monitoring should be considered at the start of treatment, then monthly, and also after any change in dose or during intercurrent illness.

Other drugs used for Hypertension Amiloride hydrochloride, p. 228 · Chlortalidone, p. 229 · Co-triamterzide, p. 230 · Cyclopenthiazide, p. 230 · Metolazone, p. 230 · Torasemide, p. 227 · Triamterene with chlortalidone, p. 229 · Xipamide, p. 231

2

Cardiovascular system

ANTIHYPERTENSIVES, CENTRALLY ACTING

Clonidine hydrochloride   01-Jun-2017

- **INDICATIONS AND DOSE**

Hypertension
▸ BY MOUTH
▸ Adult: Initially 50–100 micrograms 3 times a day, increase dose every second or third day, usual maximum dose 1.2 mg daily

Prevention of recurrent migraine | Prevention of vascular headache | Menopausal symptoms, particularly flushing and vasomotor conditions
▸ BY MOUTH
▸ Adult: Initially 50 micrograms twice daily for 2 weeks, then increased if necessary to 75 micrograms twice daily

- **UNLICENSED USE** Clonidine may also be used for Tourette syndrome and sedation—unlicensed indications.
- **CONTRA-INDICATIONS** Severe bradyarrhythmia secondary to second- or third-degree AV block or sick sinus syndrome
- **CAUTIONS** Cerebrovascular disease · constipation · heart failure · history of depression · mild to moderate bradyarrhythmia · polyneuropathy · Raynaud's syndrome or other occlusive peripheral vascular disease
- **INTERACTIONS** → Appendix 1: clonidine
- **SIDE-EFFECTS**
  ▸ **Common or very common** Constipation · depression · dizziness · dry mouth · fatigue · headache · nausea · postural hypotension · salivary gland pain · sedation · sexual dysfunction · sleep disorders · vomiting
  ▸ **Uncommon** Delusions · hallucination · malaise · paraesthesia · Raynaud's phenomenon · skin reactions
  ▸ **Rare or very rare** Alopecia · atrioventricular block · dry eye · gynaecomastia · intestinal pseudo-obstruction · nasal dryness
  ▸ **Frequency not known** Accommodation disorder · arrhythmias · confusion
- **PREGNANCY** May lower fetal heart rate. Avoid oral use unless potential benefit outweighs risk. Avoid using injection.
- **BREAST FEEDING** Avoid—present in milk.
- **RENAL IMPAIRMENT**
  Dose adjustments Use with caution in severe impairment—reduce initial dose and increase gradually.
- **TREATMENT CESSATION** In hypertension, must be withdrawn gradually to avoid severe rebound hypertension.
- **PATIENT AND CARER ADVICE**
  Driving and skilled tasks Drowsiness may affect performance of skilled tasks (e.g. driving); effects of alcohol may be enhanced.
- **LESS SUITABLE FOR PRESCRIBING** Clonidine is less suitable for prescribing.
- **MEDICINAL FORMS**
  There can be variation in the licensing of different medicines containing the same drug. Forms available from special-order manufacturers include: oral suspension, oral solution
  Tablet
  CAUTIONARY AND ADVISORY LABELS 3, 8
  ▸ Clonidine hydrochloride (Non-proprietary)
  Clonidine hydrochloride 25 microgram Clonidine 25microgram tablets | 112 tablet PoM £9.15 DT = £4.18
  ▸ Catapres (Boehringer Ingelheim Ltd)
  Clonidine hydrochloride 100 microgram Catapres 100microgram tablets | 100 tablet PoM £8.04 DT = £8.04

Methyldopa

- **INDICATIONS AND DOSE**

Hypertension
▸ BY MOUTH
▸ Adult: Initially 250 mg 2–3 times a day, dose should be increased gradually at intervals of at least 2 days; maximum 3 g per day
▸ Elderly: Initially 125 mg twice daily, dose should be increased gradually; maximum 2 g per day

- **CONTRA-INDICATIONS** Acute porphyrias p. 1025 · depression · phaeochromocytoma
- **CAUTIONS** History of depression
- **INTERACTIONS** → Appendix 1: methyldopa
- **SIDE-EFFECTS** Abdominal distension · amenorrhoea · angina pectoris · angioedema · arthralgia · asthenia · atrioventricular block · bone marrow failure · bradycardia · breast enlargement · cardiac inflammation · carotid sinus syndrome · cerebrovascular insufficiency · choreoathetosis · cognitive impairment · constipation · depression · diarrhoea · dizziness · dry mouth · eosinophilia · facial paralysis · fever · gastrointestinal disorders · granulocytopenia · gynaecomastia · haemolytic anaemia · headache · hepatic disorders · hyperprolactinaemia · lactation disorder · leucopenia · lupus-like syndrome · myalgia · nasal congestion · nausea · nightmare · oedema · oral disorders · pancreatitis · paraesthesia · parkinsonism · postural hypotension · psychiatric disorder · psychosis · sedation · sexual dysfunction · sialadenitis · skin reactions · thrombocytopenia · toxic epidermal necrolysis · vomiting
  SIDE-EFFECTS, FURTHER INFORMATION Side-effects are minimised if the daily dose is kept below 1g.
- **PREGNANCY** Not known to be harmful.
- **BREAST FEEDING** Amount too small to be harmful.
- **HEPATIC IMPAIRMENT** Manufacturer advises caution in history of liver disease. Avoid in active liver disease.
- **RENAL IMPAIRMENT** Increased sensitivity to hypotensive and sedative effect.
  Dose adjustments Start with small dose.
- **MONITORING REQUIREMENTS** Monitor blood counts and liver-function before treatment and at intervals during first 6–12 weeks or if unexplained fever occurs.
- **EFFECT ON LABORATORY TESTS** Interference with laboratory tests. Positive direct Coombs' test in up to 20% of patients (may affect blood cross-matching).
- **PATIENT AND CARER ADVICE**
  Driving and skilled tasks Drowsiness may affect performance of skilled tasks (e.g. driving); effects of alcohol may be enhanced.
- **MEDICINAL FORMS**
  There can be variation in the licensing of different medicines containing the same drug. Forms available from special-order manufacturers include: oral suspension, oral solution
  Tablet
  CAUTIONARY AND ADVISORY LABELS 3, 8
  ▸ Methyldopa (Non-proprietary)
  Methyldopa anhydrous 125 mg Methyldopa 125mg tablets | 56 tablet PoM £103.56 DT = £103.56
  Methyldopa anhydrous 250 mg Methyldopa 250mg tablets | 56 tablet PoM £16.26 DT = £5.37
  Methyldopa anhydrous 500 mg Methyldopa 500mg tablets | 56 tablet PoM £25.18 DT = £9.88
  ▸ Aldomet (Aspen Pharma Trading Ltd)
  Methyldopa anhydrous 250 mg Aldomet 250mg tablets | 60 tablet PoM £6.15
  Methyldopa anhydrous 500 mg Aldomet 500mg tablets | 30 tablet PoM £4.55

Moxonidine

- **INDICATIONS AND DOSE**

Mild to moderate essential hypertension

▶ BY MOUTH

▶ Adult: 200 micrograms once daily for 3 weeks, dose to be taken in the morning, then increased if necessary to 400 micrograms daily in 1–2 divided doses (max. per dose 400 micrograms), maximum daily dose to be given in 2 divided doses; maximum 600 micrograms per day

- **CONTRA-INDICATIONS** Bradycardia · conduction disorders · second- or third-degree AV block · severe heart failure · sick sinus syndrome · sino-atrial block
- **CAUTIONS** First-degree AV block · moderate heart failure · severe coronary artery disease · unstable angina
- **INTERACTIONS** → Appendix 1: moxonidine
- **SIDE-EFFECTS**
▶ **Common or very common** Asthenia · diarrhoea · dizziness · drowsiness · dry mouth · dyspepsia · headache · insomnia · nausea · pain · skin reactions · vertigo · vomiting
▶ **Uncommon** Angioedema · bradycardia · nervousness · oedema · syncope · tinnitus
- **PREGNANCY** Manufacturer advises avoid—no information available.
- **BREAST FEEDING** Present in milk—manufacturer advises avoid.
- **RENAL IMPAIRMENT** Avoid if eGFR less than 30 mL/minute/1.73 m^2.
Dose adjustments Max. single dose 200 micrograms and max. daily dose 400 micrograms if eGFR 30–60 mL/minute/1.73 m^2.
- **TREATMENT CESSATION** Avoid abrupt withdrawal (if concomitant treatment with beta-blocker has to be stopped, discontinue beta-blocker first, then moxonidine after a few days).

- **MEDICINAL FORMS**
There can be variation in the licensing of different medicines containing the same drug.

Tablet
CAUTIONARY AND ADVISORY LABELS 3
▶ Moxonidine (Non-proprietary)
Moxonidine 200 microgram Moxonidine 200microgram tablets | 28 tablet [PoM] £10.40 DT = £0.97
Moxonidine 300 microgram Moxonidine 300microgram tablets | 28 tablet [PoM] £12.30 DT = £1.09
Moxonidine 400 microgram Moxonidine 400microgram tablets | 28 tablet [PoM] £14.24 DT = £1.07
▶ Physiotens (Mylan)
Moxonidine 200 microgram Physiotens 200microgram tablets | 28 tablet [PoM] £9.72 DT = £0.97
Moxonidine 300 microgram Physiotens 300microgram tablets | 28 tablet [PoM] £11.49 DT = £1.09
Moxonidine 400 microgram Physiotens 400microgram tablets | 28 tablet [PoM] £13.26 DT = £1.07

BETA-ADRENOCEPTOR BLOCKERS

Beta-adrenoceptor blocking drugs

Overview

Beta-adrenoceptor blocking drugs (beta-blockers) block the beta-adrenoceptors in the heart, peripheral vasculature, bronchi, pancreas, and liver.

Many beta-blockers are now available and in general they are all equally effective. There are, however, differences between them, which may affect choice in treating particular diseases or individual patients.

Intrinsic sympathomimetic activity (ISA, partial agonist activity) represents the capacity of beta-blockers to stimulate as well as to block adrenergic receptors.

Oxprenolol hydrochloride p. 149, pindolol p. 149, acebutolol p. 151, and celiprolol hydrochloride p. 153 have intrinsic sympathomimetic activity; they tend to cause less bradycardia than the other beta-blockers and may also cause less coldness of the extremities.

Some beta-blockers are lipid soluble and some are water soluble. Atenolol p. 151, celiprolol hydrochloride, nadolol p. 148, and sotalol hydrochloride p. 108 are the most water-soluble; they are less likely to enter the brain, and may therefore cause less sleep disturbance and nightmares. Water-soluble beta-blockers are excreted by the kidneys and dosage reduction is often necessary in renal impairment.

Beta-blockers with a relatively short duration of action have to be given two or three times daily. Many of these are, however, available in modified-release formulations so that administration once daily is adequate for hypertension. For angina twice-daily treatment may sometimes be needed even with a modified-release formulation. Some beta-blockers, such as atenolol, bisoprolol fumarate p. 152, celiprolol hydrochloride, and nadolol, have an intrinsically longer duration of action and need to be given only once daily.

Beta-blockers slow the heart and can depress the myocardium; they are contra-indicated in patients with second- or third-degree heart block. Beta-blockers should also be avoided in patients with worsening unstable heart failure; care is required when initiating a beta-blocker in those with stable heart failure.

Labetalol hydrochloride p. 147, celiprolol hydrochloride, carvedilol p. 147, and nebivolol p. 154 are beta-blockers that have, in addition, an arteriolar vasodilating action, by diverse mechanisms, and thus lower peripheral resistance. There is no evidence that these drugs have important advantages over other beta-blockers in the treatment of hypertension.

Beta-blockers can precipitate bronchospasm and should therefore usually be avoided in patients with a history of asthma. When there is no suitable alternative, it may be necessary for a patient with well-controlled asthma, or chronic obstructive pulmonary disease (without significant reversible airways obstruction), to receive treatment with a beta-blocker for a co-existing condition (e.g. heart failure or following myocardial infarction). In this situation, a cardioselective beta-blocker should be selected and initiated at a low dose by a specialist; the patient should be closely monitored for adverse effects. Atenolol, bisoprolol fumarate, metoprolol tartrate p. 154, nebivolol, and (to a lesser extent) acebutolol, have less effect on the beta$_2$(bronchial) receptors and are, therefore, relatively *cardioselective*, but they are not *cardiospecific*. They have a lesser effect on airways resistance but are not free of this side-effect.

Beta-blockers are also associated with fatigue, coldness of the extremities (may be less common with those with ISA), and sleep disturbances with nightmares (may be less common with the water-soluble beta-blockers).

Beta-blockers can affect carbohydrate metabolism, causing hypoglycaemia or hyperglycaemia in patients with or without diabetes; they can also interfere with metabolic and autonomic responses to hypoglycaemia, thereby masking symptoms such as tachycardia. However, beta-blockers are not contra-indicated in diabetes, although the cardioselective beta-blockers may be preferred. Beta-blockers should be avoided altogether in those with frequent episodes of hypoglycaemia. Beta-blockers, especially when combined with a thiazide diuretic, should be avoided for the routine treatment of uncomplicated hypertension in patients with diabetes or in those at high risk of developing diabetes.

Hypertension

The mode of action of beta-blockers in hypertension is not understood, but they reduce cardiac output, alter baroceptor

2

Cardiovascular system

reflex sensitivity, and block peripheral adrenoceptors. Some beta-blockers depress plasma renin secretion. It is possible that a central effect may also partly explain their mode of action.

Beta-blockers are effective for reducing blood pressure but other antihypertensives are usually more effective for reducing the incidence of stroke, myocardial infarction, and cardiovascular mortality, especially in the elderly. Other antihypertensives are therefore preferred for routine initial treatment of uncomplicated hypertension.

In general, the dose of a beta-blocker does not have to be high.

Beta-blockers can be used to control the pulse rate in patients with *phaeochromocytoma*. However, they should never be used alone as beta-blockade without concurrent alpha-blockade may lead to a hypertensive crisis. For this reason phenoxybenzamine hydrochloride p. 181 should always be used together with the beta-blocker.

Angina

By reducing cardiac work beta-blockers improve exercise tolerance and relieve symptoms in patients with *angina* (see management of stable angina and acute coronary syndromes for further details). As with hypertension there is no good evidence of the superiority of any one drug, although occasionally a patient will respond better to one beta-blocker than to another. There is some evidence that sudden withdrawal may cause an exacerbation of angina and therefore gradual reduction of dose is preferable when beta-blockers are to be stopped. There is a risk of precipitating heart failure when beta-blockers and verapamil are used together in established ischaemic heart disease.

Myocardial infarction

For specific comments see management of ST-segment elevation myocardial infarction and non-ST-segment elevation myocardial infarction.

Several studies have shown that some beta-blockers can reduce the recurrence rate of *myocardial infarction*. However, uncontrolled heart failure, hypotension, bradyarrhythmias, and obstructive airways disease render beta-blockers unsuitable in some patients following a myocardial infarction. Atenolol and metoprolol tartrate may reduce early mortality after intravenous and subsequent oral administration in the acute phase, while acebutolol, metoprolol tartrate, propranolol hydrochloride p. 149, and timolol maleate p. 150 have protective value when started in the early convalescent phase. The evidence relating to other beta-blockers is less convincing; some have not been tested in trials of secondary prevention.

Arrhythmias

Beta-blockers act as *anti-arrhythmic drugs* principally by attenuating the effects of the sympathetic system on automaticity and conductivity within the heart. They can be used in conjunction with digoxin to control the ventricular response in atrial fibrillation, especially in patients with thyrotoxicosis. Beta-blockers are also useful in the management of supraventricular tachycardias, and are used to control those following myocardial infarction.

Esmolol hydrochloride p. 153 is a relatively cardioselective beta-blocker with a very short duration of action, used intravenously for the short-term treatment of supraventricular arrhythmias, sinus tachycardia, or hypertension, particularly in the peri-operative period. It may also be used in other situations, such as acute myocardial infarction, when sustained beta-blockade might be hazardous.

Sotalol hydrochloride p. 108, a non-cardioselective beta-blocker with additional class III anti-arrhythmic activity, is used for prophylaxis in paroxysmal supraventricular arrhythmias. It also suppresses ventricular ectopic beats and

non-sustained ventricular tachycardia. It has been shown to be more effective than lidocaine in the termination of spontaneous sustained ventricular tachycardia due to coronary disease or cardiomyopathy. However, it may induce torsade de pointes in susceptible patients.

Heart failure

Beta-blockers may produce benefit in heart failure by blocking sympathetic activity. Bisoprolol fumarate p. 152 and carvedilol p. 147 reduce mortality in any grade of stable heart failure; nebivolol p. 154 is licensed for stable mild to moderate heart failure in patients over 70 years. Treatment should be initiated by those experienced in the management of heart failure.

Thyrotoxicosis

Beta-blockers are used in pre-operative preparation for thyroidectomy. Administration of propranolol hydrochloride p. 149 can reverse clinical symptoms of *thyrotoxicosis* within 4 days. Routine tests of increased thyroid function remain unaltered. The thyroid gland is rendered less vascular thus making surgery easier.

Other uses

Beta-blockers have been used to alleviate some symptoms of *anxiety*; probably patients with palpitation, tremor, and tachycardia respond best. Beta-blockers are also used in the *prophylaxis of migraine*. Betaxolol p. 1145, levobunolol hydrochloride p. 1146, and timolol maleate p. 150 are used topically in *glaucoma*.

Beta-adrenoceptor blockers (systemic)

- **CONTRA-INDICATIONS** Asthma · cardiogenic shock · hypotension · marked bradycardia · metabolic acidosis · phaeochromocytoma (apart from specific use with alpha-blockers) · Prinzmetal's angina · second-degree AV block · severe peripheral arterial disease · sick sinus syndrome · third-degree AV block · uncontrolled heart failure
  CONTRA-INDICATIONS, FURTHER INFORMATION
- ▶ Bronchospasm Beta-blockers, including those considered to be cardioselective, should usually be avoided in patients with a history of asthma, bronchospasm or a history of obstructive airways disease. However, when there is no alternative, a cardioselective beta-blocker can be given to these patients with caution and under specialist supervision. In such cases the risk of inducing bronchospasm should be appreciated and appropriate precautions taken.
- **CAUTIONS** Diabetes · first-degree AV block · history of obstructive airways disease (introduce cautiously) · myasthenia gravis · portal hypertension (risk of deterioration in liver function) · psoriasis · symptoms of hypoglycaemia may be masked · symptoms of thyrotoxicosis may be masked
- **SIDE-EFFECTS**
- ▶ Common or very common Abdominal discomfort · bradycardia · bronchospasm · confusion · constipation · depression · diarrhoea · dizziness · dry eye (rare in children, reversible on discontinuation) · dry mouth · dyspnoea · erectile dysfunction · fatigue · headache · heart failure · hyperglycaemia · hyperhidrosis · hypoglycaemia · hypoglycaemia masked · nausea · paraesthesia · peripheral coldness · peripheral vascular disease · postural hypotension · rash (reversible on discontinuation) · sleep disorders · syncope · visual impairment · vomiting
- ▶ Uncommon Alopecia · atrioventricular block · skin reactions · urinary disorders

▶ **Rare or very rare** Hallucination · psoriasis exacerbated · thrombocytopenia

SIDE-EFFECTS, FURTHER INFORMATION
Bradycardia With administration by intravenous injection, excessive bradycardia can occur and may be countered with **intravenous injection** of atropine sulfate.
Overdose Therapeutic overdosages with beta-blockers may cause lightheadedness, dizziness, and possibly syncope as a result of bradycardia and hypotension; heart failure may be precipitated or exacerbated. For details on the management of poisoning, see Beta-blockers, under Emergency treatment of poisoning p. 1319.

● ALLERGY AND CROSS-SENSITIVITY Caution is advised in patients with a history of hypersensitivity—may increase sensitivity to allergens and result in more serious hypersensitivity response. Furthermore beta-adrenoceptor blockers may reduce response to adrenaline (epinephrine).

● PREGNANCY Beta-blockers may cause intra-uterine growth restriction, neonatal hypoglycaemia, and bradycardia; the risk is greater in severe hypertension.

● BREAST FEEDING With systemic use in the mother, infants should be monitored as there is a risk of possible toxicity due to beta-blockade. However, the amount of most beta-blockers present in milk is too small to affect infants.

● MONITORING REQUIREMENTS Monitor lung function (in patients with a history of obstructive airway disease).

● TREATMENT CESSATION Avoid abrupt withdrawal especially in ischaemic heart disease. Sudden cessation of a beta-blocker can cause a rebound worsening of myocardial ischaemia and therefore gradual reduction of dose is preferable when beta-blockers are to be stopped.

BETA-ADRENOCEPTOR BLOCKERS ›
ALPHA- AND BETA-ADRENOCEPTOR
BLOCKERS

⚑ 146

Carvedilol

● INDICATIONS AND DOSE

Hypertension
▶ BY MOUTH
▶ Adult: Initially 12.5 mg once daily for 2 days, then increased to 25 mg once daily; increased if necessary up to 50 mg daily, dose to be increased at intervals of at least 2 weeks and can be given as a single dose or in divided doses
▶ Elderly: Initially 12.5 mg daily, initial dose may provide satisfactory control

Angina
▶ BY MOUTH
▶ Adult: Initially 12.5 mg twice daily for 2 days, then increased to 25 mg twice daily

Adjunct to diuretics, digoxin, or ACE inhibitors in symptomatic chronic heart failure
▶ BY MOUTH
▶ Adult: Initially 3.125 mg twice daily, dose to be taken with food, then increased to 6.25 mg twice daily, then increased to 12.5 mg twice daily, then increased to 25 mg twice daily, dose should be increased at intervals of at least 2 weeks up to the highest tolerated dose, max. 25 mg twice daily in patients with severe heart failure or body-weight less than 85 kg; max. 50 mg twice daily in patients over 85 kg

● CONTRA-INDICATIONS Acute or decompensated heart failure requiring intravenous inotropes

● INTERACTIONS → Appendix 1: beta blockers, non-selective

● SIDE-EFFECTS
▶ **Common or very common** Anaemia · asthma · eye irritation · fluid imbalance · genital oedema · hypercholesterolaemia ·

increased risk of infection · oedema · pulmonary oedema · renal impairment · weight increased
▶ **Rare or very rare** Hypersensitivity · leucopenia · nasal congestion · severe cutaneous adverse reactions (SCARs)

● PREGNANCY Information on the safety of carvedilol during pregnancy is lacking. If carvedilol is used close to delivery, infants should be monitored for signs of alpha-blockade (as well as beta-blockade).

● BREAST FEEDING Infants should be monitored as there is a risk of possible toxicity due to alpha-blockade (in addition to beta-blockade).

● HEPATIC IMPAIRMENT Avoid in hepatic impairment.

● MONITORING REQUIREMENTS Monitor renal function during dose titration in patients with heart failure who also have renal impairment, low blood pressure, ischaemic heart disease, or diffuse vascular disease.

● MEDICINAL FORMS
There can be variation in the licensing of different medicines containing the same drug. Forms available from special-order manufacturers include: oral suspension

Tablet
CAUTIONARY AND ADVISORY LABELS 8
▶ Carvedilol (Non-proprietary)
  Carvedilol 3.125 mg Carvedilol 3.125mg tablets | 28 tablet PoM £8.00 DT = £0.55
  Carvedilol 6.25 mg Carvedilol 6.25mg tablets | 28 tablet PoM £8.99 DT = £0.77
  Carvedilol 12.5 mg Carvedilol 12.5mg tablets | 28 tablet PoM £9.99 DT = £0.57
  Carvedilol 25 mg Carvedilol 25mg tablets | 28 tablet PoM £12.50 DT = £1.01

⚑ 146

Labetalol hydrochloride

● INDICATIONS AND DOSE

Controlled hypotension in anaesthesia
▶ BY INTRAVENOUS INFUSION, OR BY INTRAVENOUS INJECTION
▶ Adult: (consult product literature or local protocols)

Hypertension of pregnancy
▶ BY INTRAVENOUS INFUSION
▶ Adult: Initially 20 mg/hour, then increased if necessary to 40 mg/hour after 30 minutes, then increased if necessary to 80 mg/hour after 30 minutes, then increased if necessary to 160 mg/hour after 30 minutes, adjusted according to response; Usual maximum 160 mg/hour
▶ BY MOUTH
▶ Adult: Use dose for hypertension

Hypertension following myocardial infarction
▶ BY INTRAVENOUS INFUSION
▶ Adult: 15 mg/hour, then increased to up to 120 mg/hour, dose to be increased gradually

Hypertensive emergencies
▶ BY INTRAVENOUS INJECTION
▶ Adult: 50 mg, to be given over at least 1 minute, then 50 mg every 5 minutes if required until a satisfactory response occurs; maximum 200 mg per course
▶ BY INTRAVENOUS INFUSION
▶ Adult: Initially 2 mg/minute until a satisfactory response is achieved, then discontinue; usual dose 50–200 mg

Hypertension
▶ BY MOUTH
▶ Adult: Initially 100 mg twice daily, dose to be increased at intervals of 14 days; usual dose 200 mg twice daily, increased if necessary up to 800 mg daily in 2 divided doses, to be taken with food, higher doses to be given in 3–4 divided doses; maximum 2.4 g per day

continued →

2

Cardiovascular system

▸ **Elderly:** Initially 50 mg twice daily, dose to be increased at intervals of 14 days; usual dose 200 mg twice daily, increased if necessary up to 800 mg daily in 2 divided doses, to be taken with food, higher doses to be given in 3–4 divided doses; maximum 2.4 g per day

▸ **BY INTRAVENOUS INJECTION**

▸ **Adult:** 50 mg, dose to be given over at least 1 minute, then 50 mg after 5 minutes if required; maximum 200 mg per course

▸ **BY INTRAVENOUS INFUSION**

▸ **Adult:** Initially 2 mg/minute until a satisfactory response is achieved, then discontinue; usual dose 50–200 mg

● **CAUTIONS** Liver damage

● **INTERACTIONS** → Appendix 1: beta blockers, non-selective

● **SIDE-EFFECTS**

▸ **Common or very common** Drug fever · hypersensitivity

▸ **Rare or very rare** Hepatic disorders · systemic lupus erythematosus (SLE) · toxic myopathy · tremor

▸ **Frequency not known** Cyanosis · hyperkalaemia · interstitial lung disease · lethargy · lichenoid keratosis · muscle cramps · nasal congestion · peripheral oedema · photosensitivity reaction · psychosis

● **PREGNANCY** The use of labetalol in maternal hypertension is not known to be harmful, except possibly in the first trimester. If labetalol is used close to delivery, infants should be monitored for signs of alpha-blockade (as well as beta blockade).

● **BREAST FEEDING** Infants should be monitored as there is a risk of possible toxicity due to alpha-blockade (in addition to beta-blockade).

● **HEPATIC IMPAIRMENT** Avoid—severe hepatocellular injury reported.

● **RENAL IMPAIRMENT**
Dose adjustments Dose reduction may be required.

● **MONITORING REQUIREMENTS**

▸ **Liver damage** Severe hepatocellular damage reported after both short-term and long-term treatment. Appropriate laboratory testing needed at first symptom of liver dysfunction and if laboratory evidence of damage (or if jaundice) labetalol should be stopped and not restarted.

● **EFFECT ON LABORATORY TESTS** Interferes with laboratory tests for catecholamines.

● **DIRECTIONS FOR ADMINISTRATION** For *intravenous infusion*, give intermittently *in* Glucose 5% *or* Sodium chloride and glucose. Dilute to a concentration of 1 mg/mL; suggested volume 200 mL; adjust rate with in-line burette. Avoid upright position during and for 3 hours after intravenous administration.

● **MEDICINAL FORMS**
There can be variation in the licensing of different medicines containing the same drug. Forms available from special-order manufacturers include: oral suspension, oral solution
Solution for injection

▸ Labetalol hydrochloride (Non-proprietary)
Labetalol hydrochloride 5 mg per 1 ml Labetalol 100mg/20ml solution for injection ampoules | 5 ampoule [PoM] £61.34 DT = £57.06

Tablet
CAUTIONARY AND ADVISORY LABELS 8, 21

▸ Labetalol hydrochloride (Non-proprietary)
Labetalol hydrochloride 100 mg Labetalol 100mg tablets | 56 tablet [PoM] £7.21 DT = £5.73
Labetalol hydrochloride 200 mg Labetalol 200mg tablets | 56 tablet [PoM] £9.97 DT = £9.48
Labetalol hydrochloride 400 mg Labetalol 400mg tablets | 56 tablet [PoM] £21.12 DT = £15.41

▸ Trandate (RPH Pharmaceuticals AB)
Labetalol hydrochloride 50 mg Trandate 50mg tablets | 56 tablet [PoM] £3.79 DT = £3.79
Labetalol hydrochloride 100 mg Trandate 100mg tablets | 56 tablet [PoM] £4.64 DT = £5.73 | 250 tablet [PoM] £15.62

Labetalol hydrochloride 200 mg Trandate 200mg tablets | 56 tablet [PoM] £7.41 DT = £9.48 | 250 tablet [PoM] £24.76
Labetalol hydrochloride 400 mg Trandate 400mg tablets | 56 tablet [PoM] £10.15 DT = £15.41

BETA-ADRENOCEPTOR BLOCKERS ❯
NON-SELECTIVE

F 146

Nadolol

● **INDICATIONS AND DOSE**

Hypertension

▸ **BY MOUTH**

▸ **Adult:** Initially 80 mg once daily, then increased in steps of up to 80 mg every week if required, doses higher than the maximum are rarely necessary; maximum 240 mg per day

Angina

▸ **BY MOUTH**

▸ **Adult:** Initially 40 mg once daily, then increased if necessary up to 160 mg daily, doses should be increased at weekly intervals, maximum dose rarely is used; maximum 240 mg per day

Arrhythmias

▸ **BY MOUTH**

▸ **Adult:** Initially 40 mg once daily, then increased if necessary up to 160 mg once daily, doses should be increased at weekly intervals; reduced to 40 mg daily if bradycardia occurs

Migraine prophylaxis

▸ **BY MOUTH**

▸ **Adult:** Initially 40 mg once daily, then increased in steps of 40 mg every week, adjusted according to response; maintenance 80–160 mg once daily

Thyrotoxicosis (adjunct)

▸ **BY MOUTH**

▸ **Adult:** 80–160 mg once daily

● **INTERACTIONS** → Appendix 1: beta blockers, non-selective

● **SIDE-EFFECTS**

▸ **Uncommon** Appetite decreased · behaviour abnormal · cough · dyspepsia · facial swelling · flatulence · nasal congestion · sedation · speech slurred · tinnitus · vision blurred · weight increased

● **BREAST FEEDING** Water soluble beta-blockers such as nadolol are present in breast milk in greater amounts than other beta blockers.

● **HEPATIC IMPAIRMENT** Manufacturer advises caution.

● **RENAL IMPAIRMENT**
Dose adjustments Increase dosage interval if eGFR less than 50 mL/minute/1.73 m^2.

● **MEDICINAL FORMS**
There can be variation in the licensing of different medicines containing the same drug. Forms available from special-order manufacturers include: tablet, oral suspension, oral solution
Tablet
CAUTIONARY AND ADVISORY LABELS 8

▸ Corgard (Sanofi)
Nadolol 80 mg Corgard 80mg tablets | 28 tablet [PoM] £6.00 DT = £6.00

F 146

Oxprenolol hydrochloride

● **INDICATIONS AND DOSE**

Hypertension | Angina

▶ BY MOUTH USING IMMEDIATE-RELEASE MEDICINES
▶ Adult: 80–160 mg daily in 2–3 divided doses, then increased if necessary up to 320 mg daily
▶ BY MOUTH USING MODIFIED-RELEASE MEDICINES
▶ Adult: Initially 160 mg once daily, then increased if necessary up to 320 mg daily

Arrhythmias

▶ BY MOUTH USING IMMEDIATE-RELEASE MEDICINES
▶ Adult: 40–240 mg daily in 2–3 divided doses; maximum 240 mg per day

Anxiety symptoms (short-term use)

▶ BY MOUTH USING IMMEDIATE-RELEASE MEDICINES
▶ Adult: 40–80 mg daily in 1–2 divided doses

● INTERACTIONS → Appendix 1: beta blockers, non-selective

● SIDE-EFFECTS
▶ **Uncommon** Vision blurred
▶ **Frequency not known** Agranulocytosis · arthralgia · cutaneous lupus erythematosus · dyspepsia · muscle complaints · myasthenia gravis · psychosis · toxic epidermal necrolysis · vasculitis necrotising

● HEPATIC IMPAIRMENT
Dose adjustments Reduce dose.

● MEDICINAL FORMS
There can be variation in the licensing of different medicines containing the same drug. Forms available from special-order manufacturers include: oral solution

Tablet
CAUTIONARY AND ADVISORY LABELS 8
▶ Oxprenolol hydrochloride (Non-proprietary)
Oxprenolol hydrochloride 20 mg Oxprenolol 20mg tablets | 56 tablet [PoM] £5.37 DT = £5.37
Oxprenolol hydrochloride 40 mg Oxprenolol 40mg tablets | 56 tablet [PoM] £7.22 DT = £7.22

F 146

Pindolol

● **INDICATIONS AND DOSE**

Hypertension

▶ BY MOUTH
▶ Adult: Initially 5 mg 2–3 times a day, alternatively 15 mg once daily, doses to be increased as required at weekly intervals; maintenance 15–30 mg daily; maximum 45 mg per day

Angina

▶ BY MOUTH
▶ Adult: 2.5–5 mg up to 3 times a day

● INTERACTIONS → Appendix 1: beta blockers, non-selective
● SIDE-EFFECTS Agranulocytosis · arthralgia · cutaneous lupus erythematosus · gastrointestinal disorders · muscle complaints · myasthenia gravis · psychosis · thyrotoxicosis masked · toxic epidermal necrolysis · tremor · vasculitis necrotising · vision blurred
● RENAL IMPAIRMENT May adversely affect renal function in severe impairment—manufacturer advises avoid.

● MEDICINAL FORMS
There can be variation in the licensing of different medicines containing the same drug.

Tablet
CAUTIONARY AND ADVISORY LABELS 8
▶ Pindolol (Non-proprietary)
Pindolol 5 mg Pindolol 5mg tablets | 100 tablet [PoM] £15.00 DT = £8.22

▶ Visken (AMCo)
Pindolol 5 mg Visken 5mg tablets | 56 tablet [PoM] £5.85
Pindolol 15 mg Visken 15mg tablets | 28 tablet [PoM] £10.55

Pindolol with clopamide

The properties listed below are those particular to the combination only. For the properties of the components please consider, pindolol above.

● **INDICATIONS AND DOSE**

Hypertension

▶ BY MOUTH
▶ Adult: Initially 1 tablet daily for 2–3 weeks, increased if necessary to 2 tablets once daily, dose to be taken in the morning; maximum 3 tablets per day

● INTERACTIONS → Appendix 1: beta blockers, non-selective · thiazide diuretics

● MEDICINAL FORMS
There can be variation in the licensing of different medicines containing the same drug.

Tablet
CAUTIONARY AND ADVISORY LABELS 8
▶ Viskaldix (AMCo)
Clopamide 5 mg, Pindolol 10 mg Viskaldix tablets | 28 tablet [PoM] £6.70 DT = £6.70

F 146

Propranolol hydrochloride

07-Feb-2018

● **INDICATIONS AND DOSE**

Thyrotoxicosis (adjunct)

▶ BY MOUTH
▶ Adult: 10–40 mg 3–4 times a day

Thyrotoxic crisis

▶ BY INTRAVENOUS INJECTION
▶ Adult: 1 mg, to be given over 1 minute, dose may be repeated if necessary at intervals of 2 minutes, maximum total dose is 5 mg in anaesthesia; maximum 10 mg per course

Hypertension

▶ BY MOUTH
▶ Adult: Initially 80 mg twice daily, dose should be increased at weekly intervals as required; maintenance 160–320 mg daily

Prophylaxis of variceal bleeding in portal hypertension

▶ BY MOUTH
▶ Adult: Initially 40 mg twice daily, then increased to 80 mg twice daily (max. per dose 160 mg twice daily), dose to be adjusted according to heart rate

Phaeochromocytoma (only with an alpha-blocker) in preparation for surgery

▶ BY MOUTH
▶ Adult: 60 mg daily for 3 days before surgery

Phaeochromocytoma (only with an alpha-blocker) in patients unsuitable for surgery

▶ BY MOUTH
▶ Adult: 30 mg daily

Angina

▶ BY MOUTH
▶ Adult: Initially 40 mg 2–3 times a day; maintenance 120–240 mg daily

Hypertrophic cardiomyopathy | Anxiety tachycardia

▶ BY MOUTH
▶ Adult: 10–40 mg 3–4 times a day

continued →

Anxiety with symptoms such as palpitation, sweating and tremor

▸ BY MOUTH

▸ Adult: 40 mg once daily, then increased if necessary to 40 mg 3 times a day

Prophylaxis after myocardial infarction

▸ BY MOUTH

▸ Adult: Initially 40 mg 4 times a day for 2–3 days, then 80 mg twice daily, start treatment 5 to 21 days after infarction

Essential tremor

▸ BY MOUTH

▸ Adult: Initially 40 mg 2–3 times a day; maintenance 80–160 mg daily

Migraine prophylaxis

▸ BY MOUTH

▸ Adult: 80–240 mg daily in divided doses

Arrhythmias

▸ BY MOUTH

▸ Adult: 10–40 mg 3–4 times a day

▸ BY INTRAVENOUS INJECTION

▸ Adult: 1 mg, to be given over 1 minute, dose may be repeated if necessary at intervals of 2 minutes, maximum 10 mg per course (5 mg in anaesthesia)

IMPORTANT SAFETY INFORMATION

SAFE PRACTICE

Propranolol has been confused with prednisolone; care must be taken to ensure the correct drug is prescribed and dispensed.

● INTERACTIONS → Appendix 1: beta blockers, non-selective

● SIDE-EFFECTS

▸ Rare or very rare Memory loss · mood altered · neuromuscular dysfunction · psychosis

● HEPATIC IMPAIRMENT

Dose adjustments Reduce oral dose.

● RENAL IMPAIRMENT

Dose adjustments Manufacturer advises caution; dose reduction may be required.

● PRESCRIBING AND DISPENSING INFORMATION Modified-release preparations can be used for once daily administration.

● MEDICINAL FORMS

There can be variation in the licensing of different medicines containing the same drug. Forms available from special-order manufacturers include: oral suspension, oral solution

Oral solution

CAUTIONARY AND ADVISORY LABELS 8

▸ Propranolol hydrochloride (Non-proprietary)

Propranolol hydrochloride 1 mg per 1 ml Propranolol 5mg/5ml oral solution sugar free sugar-free | 150 ml PoM £21.67 DT = £21.59

Propranolol hydrochloride 2 mg per 1 ml Propranolol 10mg/5ml oral solution sugar free sugar-free | 150 ml PoM £26.66 DT = £26.56

Propranolol hydrochloride 8 mg per 1 ml Propranolol 40mg/5ml oral solution sugar free sugar-free | 150 ml PoM £34.77 DT = £34.64

Propranolol hydrochloride 10 mg per 1 ml Propranolol 50mg/5ml oral solution sugar free sugar-free | 150 ml PoM £35.26 DT = £35.12

Modified-release capsule

CAUTIONARY AND ADVISORY LABELS 8, 25

▸ Propranolol hydrochloride (Non-proprietary)

Propranolol hydrochloride 80 mg Propranolol 80mg modified-release capsules | 28 capsule PoM £4.95 DT = £4.95

Propranolol hydrochloride 160 mg Propranolol 160mg modified-release capsules | 28 capsule PoM £4.88 DT = £4.88

▸ Bedranol SR (Sandoz Ltd, Almus Pharmaceuticals Ltd)

Propranolol hydrochloride 80 mg Bedranol SR 80mg capsules | 28 capsule PoM £4.16 DT = £4.95

Propranolol hydrochloride 160 mg Bedranol SR 160mg capsules | 28 capsule PoM £4.59–£5.09 DT = £4.88

▸ Beta-Prograne (Tillomed Laboratories Ltd, Actavis UK Ltd, Teva UK Ltd)

Propranolol hydrochloride 160 mg Beta-Prograne 160mg modified-release capsules | 28 capsule PoM £6.11 DT = £4.88

▸ Half Beta-Prograne (Teva UK Ltd, Tillomed Laboratories Ltd, Actavis UK Ltd)

Propranolol hydrochloride 80 mg Half Beta-Prograne 80mg modified-release capsules | 28 capsule PoM £4.95 DT = £4.95

Tablet

CAUTIONARY AND ADVISORY LABELS 8

▸ Propranolol hydrochloride (Non-proprietary)

Propranolol hydrochloride 10 mg Propranolol 10mg tablets | 28 tablet PoM £1.47 DT = £0.89

Propranolol hydrochloride 40 mg Propranolol 40mg tablets | 28 tablet PoM £1.85 DT = £0.89

Propranolol hydrochloride 80 mg Propranolol 80mg tablets | 56 tablet PoM £9.33 DT = £1.19

Propranolol hydrochloride 160 mg Propranolol 160mg tablets | 56 tablet PoM £5.87 DT = £5.87

⚑ 146

Timolol maleate

● INDICATIONS AND DOSE

Hypertension

▸ BY MOUTH

▸ Adult: Initially 10 mg daily in 1–2 divided doses, then increased if necessary up to 60 mg daily, doses to be increased gradually. Doses above 30 mg daily given in divided doses, usual maintenance 10–30 mg daily; maximum 60 mg per day

Angina

▸ BY MOUTH

▸ Adult: Initially 5 mg twice daily, then increased in steps of 10 mg daily (max. per dose 30 mg twice daily), to be increased every 3–4 days

Prophylaxis after myocardial infarction

▸ BY MOUTH

▸ Adult: Initially 5 mg twice daily for 2 days, then increased if tolerated to 10 mg twice daily

Migraine prophylaxis

▸ BY MOUTH

▸ Adult: 10–20 mg daily in 1–2 divided doses

● INTERACTIONS → Appendix 1: beta blockers, non-selective

● SIDE-EFFECTS

▸ Rare or very rare Arthralgia · retroperitoneal fibrosis

▸ Frequency not known Cyanosis · disorientation · drowsiness · dyspepsia · psychosis · vertigo

● BREAST FEEDING Manufacturer advises avoidance.

● HEPATIC IMPAIRMENT

Dose adjustments Dose reduction may be necessary.

● RENAL IMPAIRMENT

Dose adjustments Manufacturer advises caution—dose reduction may be required.

● MEDICINAL FORMS

There can be variation in the licensing of different medicines containing the same drug.

Tablet

CAUTIONARY AND ADVISORY LABELS 8

▸ Timolol maleate (Non-proprietary)

Timolol maleate 10 mg Timolol 10mg tablets | 30 tablet PoM £39.93 DT = £39.75

Timolol with amiloride and hydrochlorothiazide

The properties listed below are those particular to the combination only. For the properties of the components please consider, timolol maleate p. 150, amiloride hydrochloride p. 228, hydrochlorothiazide p. 166.

● **INDICATIONS AND DOSE**

Hypertension

▶ BY MOUTH

▶ Adult: 1–2 tablets daily

● INTERACTIONS → Appendix 1: beta blockers, non-selective · potassium-sparing diuretics · thiazide diuretics

● MEDICINAL FORMS
There can be variation in the licensing of different medicines containing the same drug.

Tablet
CAUTIONARY AND ADVISORY LABELS 8
▶ Timolol with amiloride and hydrochlorothiazide (Non-proprietary)
  Amiloride hydrochloride 2.5 mg, Timolol maleate 10 mg, Hydrochlorothiazide 25 mg Timolol 10mg / Amiloride 2.5mg / Hydrochlorothiazide 25mg tablets | 28 tablet [PoM] £29.87

Timolol with bendroflumethiazide

The properties listed below are those particular to the combination only. For the properties of the components please consider, timolol maleate p. 150, bendroflumethiazide p. 165.

● **INDICATIONS AND DOSE**

Hypertension

▶ BY MOUTH

▶ Adult: 1–2 tablets daily; maximum 4 tablets per day

● INTERACTIONS → Appendix 1: beta blockers, non-selective · thiazide diuretics

● MEDICINAL FORMS
There can be variation in the licensing of different medicines containing the same drug.

Tablet
CAUTIONARY AND ADVISORY LABELS 8
▶ Timolol with bendroflumethiazide (Non-proprietary)
  Bendroflumethiazide 2.5 mg, Timolol maleate 10 mg Timolol 10mg / Bendroflumethiazide 2.5mg tablets | 30 tablet [PoM] £23.75–£63.14 DT = £62.83

BETA-ADRENOCEPTOR BLOCKERS ⟩ SELECTIVE

F 146

Acebutolol

● **INDICATIONS AND DOSE**

Hypertension

▶ BY MOUTH

▶ Adult: Initially 400 mg daily for 2 weeks, alternatively initially 200 mg twice daily for 2 weeks, then increased if necessary to 400 mg twice daily; maximum 1.2 g per day

Angina

▶ BY MOUTH

▶ Adult: Initially 400 mg daily, alternatively initially 200 mg twice daily; maximum 1.2 g per day

Arrhythmias

▶ BY MOUTH

▶ Adult: 0.4–1.2 g daily in 2–3 divided doses

Severe angina

▶ BY MOUTH

▶ Adult: Initially 300 mg 3 times a day; maximum 1.2 g per day

● INTERACTIONS → Appendix 1: beta blockers, selective

● SIDE-EFFECTS

▶ **Common or very common** Gastrointestinal disorder

▶ **Frequency not known** Cyanosis · hepatic disorders · lupus-like syndrome · nervous system disorder · psychosis · respiratory disorders

● BREAST FEEDING Acebutolol and water soluble beta-blockers are present in breast milk in greater amounts than other beta-blockers.

● RENAL IMPAIRMENT
Dose adjustments Halve dose if eGFR 25–50 mL/minute/1.73 m^2; use quarter dose if eGFR less than 25 mL/minute/1.73 m^2; do not administer more than once daily.

● MEDICINAL FORMS
There can be variation in the licensing of different medicines containing the same drug.

Tablet
CAUTIONARY AND ADVISORY LABELS 8
▶ Acebutolol (Non-proprietary)
  Acebutolol (as Acebutolol hydrochloride) 400 mg Acebutolol 400mg tablets | 28 tablet [PoM] DT = £18.62
▶ Sectral (Sanofi)
  Acebutolol (as Acebutolol hydrochloride) 400 mg Sectral 400mg tablets | 28 tablet [PoM] £18.62 DT = £18.62

Capsule
CAUTIONARY AND ADVISORY LABELS 8
▶ Acebutolol (Non-proprietary)
  Acebutolol (as Acebutolol hydrochloride) 100 mg Acebutolol 100mg capsules | 84 capsule [PoM] [℥] DT = £14.97
  Acebutolol (as Acebutolol hydrochloride) 200 mg Acebutolol 200mg capsules | 56 capsule [PoM] [℥] DT = £19.18
▶ Sectral (Sanofi)
  Acebutolol (as Acebutolol hydrochloride) 100 mg Sectral 100mg capsules | 84 capsule [PoM] £14.97 DT = £14.97
  Acebutolol (as Acebutolol hydrochloride) 200 mg Sectral 200mg capsules | 56 capsule [PoM] £19.18 DT = £19.18

F 146

Atenolol

07-Feb-2018

● **INDICATIONS AND DOSE**

Hypertension

▶ BY MOUTH

▶ Adult: 25–50 mg daily, higher doses are rarely necessary

Angina

▶ BY MOUTH

▶ Adult: 100 mg daily in 1–2 divided doses

Arrhythmias

▶ BY MOUTH

▶ Adult: 50–100 mg daily

▶ BY INTRAVENOUS INJECTION

▶ Adult: 2.5 mg every 5 minutes if required, to be given at a rate of 1 mg/minute, treatment course may be repeated every 12 hours if required; maximum 10 mg per course

▶ BY INTRAVENOUS INFUSION

▶ Adult: 150 micrograms/kg every 12 hours if required, to be given over 20 minutes

Migraine prophylaxis

▶ BY MOUTH

▶ Adult: 50–200 mg daily in divided doses

continued →

Early intervention within 12 hours of myocardial infarction
▸ INITIALLY BY INTRAVENOUS INJECTION
▸ Adult: 5–10 mg, to be given at a rate of 1 mg/minute, followed by (by mouth) 50 mg after 15 minutes, then (by mouth) 50 mg after 12 hours, then (by mouth) 100 mg after 12 hours, then (by mouth) 100 mg once daily

● UNLICENSED USE Use of atenolol for migraine prophylaxis is an unlicensed indication.

> IMPORTANT SAFETY INFORMATION
> SAFE PRACTICE
> Atenolol has been confused with amlodipine; care must be taken to ensure the correct drug is prescribed and dispensed.

● INTERACTIONS → Appendix 1: beta blockers, selective

● SIDE-EFFECTS
GENERAL SIDE-EFFECTS
▸ **Common or very common** Gastrointestinal disorder
▸ **Rare or very rare** Mood altered · psychosis
▸ **Frequency not known** Hypersensitivity · lupus-like syndrome
SPECIFIC SIDE-EFFECTS
▸ **Rare or very rare** Hepatic disorders

● BREAST FEEDING Water soluble beta-blockers such as atenolol are present in breast milk in greater amounts than other beta blockers.

● RENAL IMPAIRMENT
Dose adjustments
▸ With oral use Max. 50 mg daily if eGFR 15–35 mL/minute/1.73 m^2; max. 25 mg daily or 50 mg on alternate days if eGFR less than 15 mL/minute/1.73 m^2.
▸ With intravenous use Max. 10 mg on alternate days if eGFR 15–35 mL/minute/1.73 m^2; max.10 mg every 4 days if eGFR less than 15 mL/minute/1.73 m^2.

● DIRECTIONS FOR ADMINISTRATION For *intravenous infusion* (*Tenormin*®), give intermittently in Glucose 5% or Sodium chloride 0.9%. Suggested infusion time 20 minutes.

● MEDICINAL FORMS
There can be variation in the licensing of different medicines containing the same drug. Forms available from special-order manufacturers include: oral suspension, oral solution
Solution for injection
▸ Tenormin (AstraZeneca UK Ltd)
Atenolol 500 microgram per 1 ml Tenormin 5mg/10ml solution for injection ampoules | 10 ampoule [PoM] £34.45 (Hospital only)
Oral solution
▸ Atenolol (Non-proprietary)
Atenolol 5 mg per 1 ml Atenolol 25mg/5ml oral solution sugar free sugar-free | 300 ml [PoM] £6.72 DT = £5.59
Tablet
CAUTIONARY AND ADVISORY LABELS 8
▸ Atenolol (Non-proprietary)
Atenolol 25 mg Atenolol 25mg tablets | 28 tablet [PoM] £1.39 DT = £0.38
Atenolol 50 mg Atenolol 50mg tablets | 28 tablet [PoM] £4.09 DT = £0.43
Atenolol 100 mg Atenolol 100mg tablets | 28 tablet [PoM] £5.19 DT = £0.47
▸ Tenormin (AstraZeneca UK Ltd)
Atenolol 50 mg Tenormin LS 50mg tablets | 28 tablet [PoM] £10.22 DT = £0.43
Atenolol 100 mg Tenormin 100mg tablets | 28 tablet [PoM] £12.98 DT = £0.47

Atenolol with nifedipine

The properties listed below are those particular to the combination only. For the properties of the components please consider, atenolol p. 151, nifedipine p. 162.

● INDICATIONS AND DOSE
Hypertension
▸ BY MOUTH
▸ Adult: 1 capsule daily, increased if necessary to 1 capsule twice daily
▸ Elderly: 1 capsule daily
Angina
▸ BY MOUTH
▸ Adult: 1 capsule twice daily

● INTERACTIONS → Appendix 1: beta blockers, selective · calcium channel blockers

● PRESCRIBING AND DISPENSING INFORMATION Only indicated when calcium-channel blocker or beta-blocker alone proves inadequate.

● MEDICINAL FORMS
There can be variation in the licensing of different medicines containing the same drug.
Modified-release capsule
CAUTIONARY AND ADVISORY LABELS 8, 25
▸ Tenif (AstraZeneca UK Ltd)
Nifedipine 20 mg, Atenolol 50 mg Tenif 50mg/20mg modified-release capsules | 28 capsule [PoM] £15.30 DT = £15.30

☞ 146

Bisoprolol fumarate

● INDICATIONS AND DOSE
Hypertension | Angina
▸ BY MOUTH
▸ Adult: 5–10 mg once daily; maximum 20 mg per day
Adjunct in heart failure
▸ BY MOUTH
▸ Adult: Initially 1.25 mg once daily for 1 week, dose to be taken in the morning, then increased if tolerated to 2.5 mg once daily for 1 week, then increased if tolerated to 3.75 mg once daily for 1 week, then increased if tolerated to 5 mg once daily for 4 weeks, then increased if tolerated to 7.5 mg once daily for 4 weeks, then increased if tolerated to 10 mg once daily; maximum 10 mg per day

● CONTRA-INDICATIONS Acute or decompensated heart failure requiring intravenous inotropes · sino–atrial block

● CAUTIONS Ensure heart failure not worsening before increasing dose

● INTERACTIONS → Appendix 1: beta blockers, selective

● SIDE-EFFECTS
▸ **Uncommon** Muscle cramps · muscle weakness
▸ **Rare or very rare** Allergic rhinitis · auditory disorder · conjunctivitis · flushing · hepatitis · hypersensitivity · pruritus

● HEPATIC IMPAIRMENT
Dose adjustments Max. 10 mg daily in severe impairment.

● RENAL IMPAIRMENT
Dose adjustments Reduce dose if eGFR less than 20 mL/minute/1.73 m^2 (max. 10 mg daily).

- **MEDICINAL FORMS**
  There can be variation in the licensing of different medicines containing the same drug. Forms available from special-order manufacturers include: oral suspension, oral solution

Tablet
CAUTIONARY AND ADVISORY LABELS 8
- ▸ Bisoprolol fumarate (Non-proprietary)
  Bisoprolol fumarate 1.25 mg Bisoprolol 1.25mg tablets | 28 tablet [PoM] £7.43 DT = £0.48
  Bisoprolol fumarate 2.5 mg Bisoprolol 2.5mg tablets | 28 tablet [PoM] £4.39 DT = £0.43
  Bisoprolol fumarate 3.75 mg Bisoprolol 3.75mg tablets | 28 tablet [PoM] £6.50 DT = £0.64
  Bisoprolol fumarate 5 mg Bisoprolol 5mg tablets | 28 tablet [PoM] £5.89 DT = £0.38
  Bisoprolol fumarate 7.5 mg Bisoprolol 7.5mg tablets | 28 tablet [PoM] £5.90 DT = £0.68
  Bisoprolol fumarate 10 mg Bisoprolol 10mg tablets | 28 tablet [PoM] £5.89 DT = £0.45
- ▸ Cardicor (Merck Serono Ltd)
  Bisoprolol fumarate 1.25 mg Cardicor 1.25mg tablets | 28 tablet [PoM] £2.35 DT = £0.48
  Bisoprolol fumarate 2.5 mg Cardicor 2.5mg tablets | 28 tablet [PoM] £2.35 DT = £0.43
  Bisoprolol fumarate 3.75 mg Cardicor 3.75mg tablets | 28 tablet [PoM] £4.90 DT = £0.64
  Bisoprolol fumarate 5 mg Cardicor 5mg tablets | 28 tablet [PoM] £5.90 DT = £0.38
  Bisoprolol fumarate 7.5 mg Cardicor 7.5mg tablets | 28 tablet [PoM] £5.90 DT = £0.68
  Bisoprolol fumarate 10 mg Cardicor 10mg tablets | 28 tablet [PoM] £5.90 DT = £0.45
- ▸ Congescor (Tillomed Laboratories Ltd)
  Bisoprolol fumarate 1.25 mg Congescor 1.25mg tablets | 28 tablet [PoM] £5.90 DT = £0.48
  Bisoprolol fumarate 2.5 mg Congescor 2.5mg tablets | 28 tablet [PoM] £3.90 DT = £0.43

F 146

Celiprolol hydrochloride

- **INDICATIONS AND DOSE**

Mild to moderate hypertension
- ▸ BY MOUTH
- ▸ Adult: 200 mg once daily, dose to be taken in the morning, then increased if necessary to 400 mg once daily

- **INTERACTIONS** → Appendix 1: beta blockers, selective
- **SIDE-EFFECTS** Alveolitis allergic · drowsiness · palpitations · thyrotoxicosis masked · tremor
- **BREAST FEEDING** Manufacturers advise avoidance.
- **HEPATIC IMPAIRMENT**
  Dose adjustments Consider dose reduction.
- **RENAL IMPAIRMENT** Avoid if eGFR less than 15 mL/minute/1.73 m^2.
  Dose adjustments Reduce dose by half if eGFR 15–40 mL/minute/1.73 m^2.

- **MEDICINAL FORMS**
  There can be variation in the licensing of different medicines containing the same drug. Forms available from special-order manufacturers include: oral suspension

Tablet
CAUTIONARY AND ADVISORY LABELS 8, 22
- ▸ Celiprolol hydrochloride (Non-proprietary)
  Celiprolol hydrochloride 200 mg Celiprolol 200mg tablets | 28 tablet [PoM] £15.00 DT = £13.27
  Celiprolol hydrochloride 400 mg Celiprolol 400mg tablets | 28 tablet [PoM] £23.10 DT = £23.10
- ▸ Celectol (Zentiva)
  Celiprolol hydrochloride 200 mg Celectol 200mg tablets | 28 tablet [PoM] £19.83 DT = £13.27
  Celiprolol hydrochloride 400 mg Celectol 400mg tablets | 28 tablet [PoM] £39.65 DT = £23.10

F 146

Co-tenidone

- **INDICATIONS AND DOSE**

Hypertension
- ▸ BY MOUTH
- ▸ Adult: 50/12.5 mg daily, alternatively increased if necessary to 100/25 mg daily, doses higher than 50 mg atenolol rarely necessary

DOSE EQUIVALENCE AND CONVERSION
- ▸ A mixture of atenolol and chlortalidone in mass proportions corresponding to 4 parts of atenolol and 1 part chlortalidone.

- **INTERACTIONS** → Appendix 1: beta blockers, selective · thiazide diuretics
- **SIDE-EFFECTS**
- ▸ **Common or very common** Gastrointestinal disorder · hyperuricaemia
- ▸ **Rare or very rare** Hepatic disorders · mood altered · neutropenia · pancreatitis · psychosis
- ▸ **Frequency not known** Hypomagnesaemia · lupus-like syndrome
- **PREGNANCY** Avoid. Diuretics not used to treat hypertension in pregnancy.
- **BREAST FEEDING** Atenolol present in milk in greater amounts than some other beta-blockers. Possible toxicity due to beta-blockade—monitor infant. Large doses of chlortalidone may suppress lactation.
- **RENAL IMPAIRMENT** Avoid if eGFR less than 30 mL/minute/1.73 m^2—consider alternative treatment.

- **MEDICINAL FORMS**
  There can be variation in the licensing of different medicines containing the same drug. Forms available from special-order manufacturers include: oral suspension, oral solution

Tablet
CAUTIONARY AND ADVISORY LABELS 8
- ▸ Co-tenidone (Non-proprietary)
  Chlortalidone 12.5 mg, Atenolol 50 mg Co-tenidone 50mg/12.5mg tablets | 28 tablet [PoM] £4.85 DT = £1.50
  Chlortalidone 25 mg, Atenolol 100 mg Co-tenidone 100mg/25mg tablets | 28 tablet [PoM] £4.85 DT = £1.66
- ▸ Tenoret (AstraZeneca UK Ltd)
  Chlortalidone 12.5 mg, Atenolol 50 mg Tenoret 50mg/12.5mg tablets | 28 tablet [PoM] £10.36 DT = £1.50
- ▸ Tenoretic (AstraZeneca UK Ltd)
  Chlortalidone 25 mg, Atenolol 100 mg Tenoretic 100mg/25mg tablets | 28 tablet [PoM] £10.36 DT = £1.66

F 146

Esmolol hydrochloride

- **INDICATIONS AND DOSE**

Short-term treatment of supraventricular arrhythmias (including atrial fibrillation, atrial flutter, sinus tachycardia) | Tachycardia and hypertension in peri-operative period
- ▸ BY INTRAVENOUS INFUSION
- ▸ Adult: 50–200 micrograms/kg/minute, consult product literature for details of dose titration and doses during peri-operative period

- **INTERACTIONS** → Appendix 1: beta blockers, selective
- **SIDE-EFFECTS**
- ▸ **Common or very common** Anxiety · appetite decreased · concentration impaired · drowsiness
- ▸ **Uncommon** Chills · costochondritis · dyspepsia · fever · flushing · nasal congestion · oedema · pallor · pulmonary oedema · respiratory disorders · seizure · speech disorder · taste altered · thinking abnormal
- ▸ **Rare or very rare** Cardiac arrest

2 Cardiovascular system

▶ **Frequency not known** Angioedema · coronary vasospasm · hyperkalaemia · metabolic acidosis

● BREAST FEEDING Manufacturer advises avoidance.

● RENAL IMPAIRMENT Manufacturer advises caution.

● MEDICINAL FORMS
There can be variation in the licensing of different medicines containing the same drug.
Solution for injection
▶ Esmolol hydrochloride (Non-proprietary)
Esmolol hydrochloride 10 mg per 1 ml Esmolol hydrochloride 100mg/10ml solution for injection vials | 5 vial [PoM] £38.95 (Hospital only)
▶ Brevibloc (Baxter Healthcare Ltd)
Esmolol hydrochloride 10 mg per 1 ml Brevibloc Premixed 100mg/10ml solution for injection vials | 5 vial [PoM] [Ⓢ]
Solution for infusion
▶ Brevibloc (Baxter Healthcare Ltd)
Esmolol hydrochloride 10 mg per 1 ml Brevibloc Premixed 2.5g/250ml infusion bags | 1 bag [PoM] £89.69

⬛ 146

Metoprolol tartrate

● INDICATIONS AND DOSE
Hypertension
▶ BY MOUTH USING IMMEDIATE-RELEASE MEDICINES
▶ Adult: Initially 100 mg daily, increased if necessary to 200 mg daily in 1–2 divided doses, high doses are rarely required; maximum 400 mg per day
▶ BY MOUTH USING MODIFIED-RELEASE MEDICINES
▶ Adult: 200 mg once daily
Angina
▶ BY MOUTH USING IMMEDIATE-RELEASE MEDICINES
▶ Adult: 50–100 mg 2–3 times a day
▶ BY MOUTH USING MODIFIED-RELEASE MEDICINES
▶ Adult: 200–400 mg daily
Arrhythmias
▶ BY MOUTH USING IMMEDIATE-RELEASE MEDICINES
▶ Adult: Usual dose 50 mg 2–3 times a day, then increased if necessary up to 300 mg daily in divided doses
▶ BY INTRAVENOUS INJECTION
▶ Adult: Up to 5 mg, dose to be given at a rate of 1–2 mg/minute, then up to 5 mg after 5 minutes if required, total dose of 10–15 mg
Migraine prophylaxis
▶ BY MOUTH USING IMMEDIATE-RELEASE MEDICINES
▶ Adult: 100–200 mg daily in divided doses
▶ BY MOUTH USING MODIFIED-RELEASE MEDICINES
▶ Adult: 200 mg daily
Hyperthyroidism (adjunct)
▶ BY MOUTH USING IMMEDIATE-RELEASE MEDICINES
▶ Adult: 50 mg 4 times a day
In surgery
▶ BY SLOW INTRAVENOUS INJECTION
▶ Adult: Initially 2–4 mg, given at induction or to control arrhythmias developing during anaesthesia, then 2 mg, repeated if necessary; maximum 10 mg per course
Early intervention within 12 hours of infarction
▶ INITIALLY BY INTRAVENOUS INJECTION
▶ Adult: Initially 5 mg every 2 minutes, to a max. of 15 mg, followed by (by mouth) 50 mg every 6 hours for 48 hours, to be taken 15 minutes after intravenous injection; (by mouth) maintenance 200 mg daily in divided doses

● INTERACTIONS → Appendix 1: beta blockers, selective
● SIDE-EFFECTS
GENERAL SIDE-EFFECTS
▶ **Common or very common** Palpitations

▶ **Uncommon** Chest pain · drowsiness · dystrophic skin lesion · insomnia · muscle cramps · oedema · weight increased
▶ **Rare or very rare** Conjunctivitis · eye irritation · gangrene · hepatitis · rhinitis
SPECIFIC SIDE-EFFECTS
▶ **Uncommon**
▶ With intravenous use Cardiogenic shock · concentration impaired
▶ **Rare or very rare**
▶ With intravenous use Anxiety · arthralgia · memory loss · photosensitivity reaction · taste altered · tinnitus
▶ With oral use Alertness decreased · arthritis · auditory disorder · personality disorder
▶ **Frequency not known**
▶ With oral use Peyronie's disease · retroperitoneal fibrosis
● HEPATIC IMPAIRMENT
Dose adjustments Reduce dose in severe impairment.

● MEDICINAL FORMS
There can be variation in the licensing of different medicines containing the same drug. Forms available from special-order manufacturers include: capsule, oral suspension, oral solution
Tablet
CAUTIONARY AND ADVISORY LABELS 8
▶ Metoprolol tartrate (Non-proprietary)
Metoprolol tartrate 50 mg Metoprolol 50mg tablets | 28 tablet [PoM] £3.00 DT = £0.69 | 56 tablet [PoM] £1.38–£1.80
Metoprolol tartrate 100 mg Metoprolol 100mg tablets | 28 tablet [PoM] £3.00 DT = £0.76 | 56 tablet [PoM] £1.52–£1.78
Solution for injection
▶ Betaloc (AstraZeneca UK Ltd)
Metoprolol tartrate 1 mg per 1 ml Betaloc I.V. 5mg/5ml solution for injection ampoules | 5 ampoule [PoM] £5.02 (Hospital only)

⬛ 146

Nebivolol

● INDICATIONS AND DOSE
Essential hypertension
▶ BY MOUTH
▶ Adult: 5 mg daily
▶ Elderly: Initially 2.5 mg daily, then increased if necessary to 5 mg daily
Hypertension in patient with renal impairment
▶ BY MOUTH
▶ Adult: Initially 2.5 mg once daily, then increased if necessary to 5 mg once daily
Adjunct in stable mild to moderate heart failure
▶ BY MOUTH
▶ Adult 70 years and over: Initially 1.25 mg once daily for 1–2 weeks, then increased if tolerated to 2.5 mg once daily for 1–2 weeks, then increased if tolerated to 5 mg once daily for 1–2 weeks, then increased if tolerated to 10 mg once daily

● CONTRA-INDICATIONS Acute or decompensated heart failure requiring intravenous inotropes
● INTERACTIONS → Appendix 1: beta blockers, selective
● SIDE-EFFECTS
▶ **Common or very common** Oedema
▶ **Uncommon** Dyspepsia · flatulence
● BREAST FEEDING Manufacturers advise avoidance.
● HEPATIC IMPAIRMENT No information available— manufacturer advises avoid.
● RENAL IMPAIRMENT Manufacturer advises avoid in heart failure if serum creatinine greater than 250 micromol/litre.

● MEDICINAL FORMS
There can be variation in the licensing of different medicines containing the same drug.

Tablet
CAUTIONARY AND ADVISORY LABELS 8
▸ Nebivolol (Non-proprietary)
Nebivolol (as Nebivolol hydrochloride) 2.5 mg Nebivolol 2.5mg tablets | 28 tablet [PoM] £69.84 DT = £18.38
Nebivolol (as Nebivolol hydrochloride) 5 mg Nebivolol 5mg tablets | 28 tablet [PoM] £6.39 DT = £0.89
Nebivolol (as Nebivolol hydrochloride) 10 mg Nebivolol 10mg tablets | 28 tablet [PoM] £22.50 DT = £14.41
▸ Nebilet (A. Menarini Farmaceutica Internazionale SRL)
Nebivolol (as Nebivolol hydrochloride) 5 mg Nebilet 5mg tablets | 28 tablet [PoM] £9.23 DT = £0.89

CALCIUM-CHANNEL BLOCKERS

Calcium-channel blockers

Overview

Calcium-channel blockers differ in their predilection for the various possible sites of action and, therefore, their therapeutic effects are disparate, with much greater variation than those of beta-blockers. There are important differences between verapamil hydrochloride p. 163, diltiazem hydrochloride p. 157, and the dihydropyridine calcium-channel blockers (amlodipine below, felodipine p. 159, lacidipine p. 160, lercanidipine hydrochloride p. 160, nicardipine hydrochloride p. 161, nifedipine p. 162, and nimodipine p. 115). Verapamil hydrochloride and diltiazem hydrochloride should usually be **avoided** in heart failure because they may further depress cardiac function and cause clinically significant deterioration.

Verapamil hydrochloride is used for the treatment of angina, hypertension, and arrhythmias. It is a highly negatively inotropic calcium channel-blocker and it reduces cardiac output, slows the heart rate, and may impair atrioventricular conduction. It may precipitate heart failure, exacerbate conduction disorders, and cause hypotension at high doses and should **not** be used with beta-blockers. Constipation is the most common side-effect.

Nifedipine relaxes vascular smooth muscle and dilates coronary and peripheral arteries. It has more influence on vessels and less on the myocardium than does verapamil hydrochloride, and unlike verapamil hydrochloride has no anti-arrhythmic activity. It rarely precipitates heart failure because any negative inotropic effect is offset by a reduction in left ventricular work.

Nicardipine hydrochloride has similar effects to those of nifedipine and may produce less reduction of myocardial contractility. Amlodipine and felodipine also resemble nifedipine and nicardipine hydrochloride in their effects and do not reduce myocardial contractility and they do not produce clinical deterioration in heart failure. They have a longer duration of action and can be given once daily. Nifedipine, nicardipine hydrochloride, amlodipine, and felodipine are used for the treatment of angina or hypertension. All are valuable in forms of angina associated with coronary vasospasm. Side-effects associated with vasodilatation such as flushing and headache (which become less obtrusive after a few days), and ankle swelling (which may respond only partially to diuretics) are common.

Intravenous nicardipine hydrochloride is licensed for the treatment of acute life-threatening hypertension, for example in the event of malignant arterial hypertension or hypertensive encephalopathy; aortic dissection, when a short-acting beta-blocker is not suitable, or in combination with a beta-blocker when beta-blockade alone is not effective; severe pre-eclampsia, when other intravenous anti-hypertensives are not recommended or are contra-indicated; and for treatment of postoperative hypertension.

Lacidipine and lercanidipine hydrochloride have similar effects to those of nifedipine and nicardipine hydrochloride; they are indicated for hypertension only.

Nimodipine is related to nifedipine but the smooth muscle relaxant effect preferentially acts on cerebral arteries. Its use is confined to prevention and treatment of vascular spasm following aneurysmal subarachnoid haemorrhage.

Diltiazem hydrochloride is effective in most forms of angina; the longer-acting formulation is also used for hypertension. It may be used in patients for whom beta-blockers are contra-indicated or ineffective. It has a less negative inotropic effect than verapamil hydrochloride and significant myocardial depression occurs rarely. Nevertheless because of the risk of bradycardia it should be used with caution in association with beta-blockers.

Unstable angina

Calcium-channel blockers do not reduce the risk of myocardial infarction in unstable angina. The use of diltiazem hydrochloride or verapamil hydrochloride should be reserved for patients resistant to treatment with beta-blockers.

Calcium-channel blockers

● DRUG ACTION Calcium-channel blockers (less correctly called 'calcium-antagonists') interfere with the inward displacement of calcium ions through the slow channels of active cell membranes. They influence the myocardial cells, the cells within the specialised conducting system of the heart, and the cells of vascular smooth muscle. Thus, myocardial contractility may be reduced, the formation and propagation of electrical impulses within the heart may be depressed, and coronary or systemic vascular tone may be diminished.

● SIDE-EFFECTS
▸ **Common or very common** Dizziness · flushing · gastrointestinal disorders · headache · nausea · palpitations · peripheral oedema · sexual dysfunction · skin reactions · tachycardia · vomiting
▸ **Uncommon** Gingival hyperplasia
Overdose Features of calcium-channel blocker poisoning include nausea, vomiting, dizziness, agitation, confusion, and coma in severe poisoning. Metabolic acidosis and hyperglycaemia may occur.

In overdose, the dihydropyridine calcium-channel blockers cause severe hypotension secondary to profound peripheral vasodilatation.

For details on the management of poisoning, see Calcium-channel blockers, under Emergency treatment of poisoning p. 1319.

● TREATMENT CESSATION There is some evidence that sudden withdrawal of calcium-channel blockers may be associated with an exacerbation of myocardial ischaemia.

⌐ **above**

| Amlodipine
07-Feb-2018

● DRUG ACTION Amlodipine is a dihydropyridine calcium-channel blocker.

● INDICATIONS AND DOSE
Prophylaxis of angina
▸ BY MOUTH
▸ Adult: Initially 5 mg once daily; maximum 10 mg per day
Hypertension
▸ BY MOUTH
▸ Adult: Initially 5 mg once daily; maximum 10 mg per day
continued →

2 Cardiovascular system

DOSE EQUIVALENCE AND CONVERSION
▸ Tablets from various suppliers may contain different salts (e.g. amlodipine besilate, amlodipine maleate, and amlodipine mesilate) but the strength is expressed in terms of amlodipine (base); tablets containing different salts are considered interchangeable.

IMPORTANT SAFETY INFORMATION
SAFE PRACTICE
Amlodipine has been confused with nimodipine and atenolol; care must be taken to ensure the correct drug is prescribed and dispensed.

● CONTRA-INDICATIONS Cardiogenic shock · significant aortic stenosis · unstable angina
● INTERACTIONS → Appendix 1: calcium channel blockers
● SIDE-EFFECTS
▸ **Common or very common** Asthenia · constipation · diarrhoea · drowsiness · dyspnoea · gastrointestinal discomfort · joint disorders · muscle complaints · oedema · vision disorders
▸ **Uncommon** Alopecia · anxiety · arrhythmias · chest pain · cough · depression · dry mouth · gynaecomastia · hyperhidrosis · hypotension · insomnia · malaise · mood altered · pain · rhinitis · sensation abnormal · syncope · taste altered · tinnitus · tremor · urinary disorders · weight changes
▸ **Rare or very rare** Angioedema · confusion · hepatic disorders · hyperglycaemia · hypersensitivity · leucopenia · muscle tone increased · pancreatitis · peripheral neuropathy · photosensitivity reaction · Stevens-Johnson syndrome · thrombocytopenia · vasculitis
▸ **Frequency not known** Extrapyramidal symptoms · pulmonary oedema
● PREGNANCY No information available—manufacturer advises avoid, but risk to fetus should be balanced against risk of uncontrolled maternal hypertension.
● BREAST FEEDING Manufacturer advises avoid—no information available.
● HEPATIC IMPAIRMENT
Dose adjustments May need dose reduction—half-life prolonged.
● DIRECTIONS FOR ADMINISTRATION Tablets may be dispersed in water.

● MEDICINAL FORMS
There can be variation in the licensing of different medicines containing the same drug. Forms available from special-order manufacturers include: oral suspension, oral solution
Oral solution
▸ Amlodipine (Non-proprietary)
Amlodipine 1 mg per 1 ml Amlodipine 5mg/5ml oral solution sugar free sugar-free | 150 ml [PoM] £75.76 DT = £75.76
Amlodipine 2 mg per 1 ml Amlodipine 10mg/5ml oral solution sugar free sugar-free | 150 ml [PoM] £115.73 DT = £115.73
Tablet
▸ Amlodipine (Non-proprietary)
Amlodipine 5 mg Amlodipine 5mg tablets | 28 tablet [PoM] £9.99 DT = £1.43
Amlodipine 10 mg Amlodipine 10mg tablets | 28 tablet [PoM] £14.07 DT = £1.58
▸ Istin (Pfizer Ltd)
Amlodipine 5 mg Istin 5mg tablets | 28 tablet [PoM] £11.08 DT = £1.43
Amlodipine 10 mg Istin 10mg tablets | 28 tablet [PoM] £16.55 DT = £1.58

Combinations available: *Olmesartan with amlodipine,* p. 177 · *Olmesartan with amlodipine and hydrochlorothiazide,* p. 177

Amlodipine with valsartan

The properties listed below are those particular to the combination only. For the properties of the components please consider, amlodipine p. 155, valsartan p. 178.

● INDICATIONS AND DOSE
Hypertension in patients stabilised on the individual components in the same proportions
▸ BY MOUTH
▸ Adult: (consult product literature)
● INTERACTIONS → Appendix 1: angiotensin-II receptor antagonists · calcium channel blockers
● MEDICINAL FORMS
There can be variation in the licensing of different medicines containing the same drug.
Tablet
▸ Exforge (Novartis Pharmaceuticals UK Ltd)
Amlodipine (as Amlodipine besilate) 5 mg, Valsartan 80 mg Exforge 5mg/80mg tablets | 28 tablet [PoM] £20.11 DT = £20.11
Amlodipine (as Amlodipine besilate) 10 mg, Valsartan 160 mg Exforge 10mg/160mg tablets | 28 tablet [PoM] £26.51 DT = £26.51
Amlodipine (as Amlodipine besilate) 5 mg, Valsartan 160 mg Exforge 5mg/160mg tablets | 28 tablet [PoM] £26.51 DT = £26.51

▸ 155

Clevidipine
01-Feb-2017

● INDICATIONS AND DOSE
Hypertension in the peri-operative setting (specialist use only)
▸ BY INTRAVENOUS INFUSION
▸ Adult: Initially 2 mg/hour, dose may be doubled every 90 seconds as necessary; usual dose 4–6 mg/hour (max. per dose 32 mg/hour); maximum 500 mg per day
● CONTRA-INDICATIONS Defective lipid metabolism · uncorrected critical aortic stenosis
● CAUTIONS Hypertrophic obstructive cardiomyopathy (risk of reduced oxygen delivery) · lipid load restrictions (injection has a high lipid content) · mitral stenosis (risk of reduced oxygen delivery) · patients who are unable to increase their heart rate adequately to compensate for reduced blood pressure
● INTERACTIONS → Appendix 1: calcium channel blockers
● SIDE-EFFECTS
▸ **Common or very common** Acute kidney injury · arrhythmias · chest pain · feeling hot · hypotension · polyuria
▸ **Uncommon** Cardiac conduction disorders · congestive heart failure · constipation · hypoxia · pulmonary congestion
▸ **Rare or very rare** Ileus
SIDE-EFFECTS, FURTHER INFORMATION Manufacturer advises that systemic hypotension and reflex tachycardia have been reported - consider decreasing the dose by half or stopping the infusion.
● ALLERGY AND CROSS-SENSITIVITY Contra-indicated in patients with hypersensitivity to peanut, soy products, or egg products.
● PREGNANCY Manufacturer advises avoid unless essential—toxicity in *animal* studies (recommendation also supported by specialist sources).
● BREAST FEEDING Manufacturer advises avoid—no information available.
● MONITORING REQUIREMENTS Manufacturer advises monitor heart rate and blood pressure continuously during infusion, until vital signs are stable; continue to monitor patients who receive prolonged infusions and are not

transitioned to other antihypertensive therapies for at least 8 hours after the infusion is stopped.

- HANDLING AND STORAGE Manufacturer advises store in a refrigerator at 2–8°C.

- MEDICINAL FORMS
There can be variation in the licensing of different medicines containing the same drug.

Emulsion for infusion
EXCIPIENTS: May contain Disodium edetate
▸ Cleviprex (Chiesi Ltd)
   Clevidipine 500 microgram per 1 ml Cleviprex 25mg/50ml emulsion for infusion vials | 10 vial PoM £1,200.00 (Hospital only)

F 155

Diltiazem hydrochloride

- INDICATIONS AND DOSE

Prophylaxis and treatment of angina
▸ BY MOUTH
▸ Adult: Initially 60 mg 3 times a day, adjusted according to response; maximum 360 mg per day
▸ Elderly: Initially 60 mg twice daily, adjusted according to response; maximum 360 mg per day

ADIZEM-SR® CAPSULES
Mild to moderate hypertension
▸ BY MOUTH
▸ Adult: 120 mg twice daily, dose form not appropriate for initial dose titration

Angina
▸ BY MOUTH
▸ Adult: Initially 90 mg twice daily; increased if necessary to 180 mg twice daily, dose form not appropriate for initial dose titration in the elderly

ADIZEM-XL®
Angina | Mild to moderate hypertension
▸ BY MOUTH
▸ Adult: Initially 240 mg once daily, increased if necessary to 300 mg once daily
▸ Elderly: Initially 120 mg once daily, increased if necessary up to 300 mg once daily

ANGITIL® SR
Angina | Mild to moderate hypertension
▸ BY MOUTH
▸ Adult: Initially 90 mg twice daily; increased if necessary to 120–180 mg twice daily

ANGITIL® XL
Angina | Mild to moderate hypertension
▸ BY MOUTH
▸ Adult: Initially 240 mg once daily; increased if necessary to 300 mg once daily, dose form not appropriate for initial dose titration in the elderly

DILCARDIA® SR
Angina | Mild to moderate hypertension
▸ BY MOUTH
▸ Adult: Initially 90 mg twice daily; increased if necessary to 180 mg twice daily
▸ Elderly: Initially 60 mg twice daily; increased if necessary to 90 mg twice daily

DILZEM® SR
Angina | Mild to moderate hypertension
▸ BY MOUTH
▸ Adult: Initially 90 mg twice daily; increased if necessary up to 180 mg twice daily
▸ Elderly: Initially 60 mg twice daily; increased if necessary up to 180 mg twice daily

DILZEM® XL
Angina | Mild to moderate hypertension
▸ BY MOUTH
▸ Adult: Initially 180 mg once daily; increased if necessary to 360 mg once daily
▸ Elderly: Initially 120 mg once daily; increased if necessary to 360 mg once daily

SLOZEM®
Angina | Mild to moderate hypertension
▸ BY MOUTH
▸ Adult: Initially 240 mg once daily; increased if necessary to 360 mg once daily
▸ Elderly: Initially 120 mg once daily; increased if necessary to 360 mg once daily

TILDIEM RETARD®
Mild to moderate hypertension
▸ BY MOUTH
▸ Adult: Initially 90–120 mg twice daily; increased if necessary to 360 mg daily in divided doses
▸ Elderly: Initially 120 mg once daily; increased if necessary to 120 mg twice daily

Angina
▸ BY MOUTH
▸ Adult: Initially 90–120 mg twice daily; increased if necessary to 480 mg daily in divided doses
▸ Elderly: Up to 120 mg twice daily, dose form not appropriate for initial dose titration

TILDIEM® LA
Angina | Mild to moderate hypertension
▸ BY MOUTH
▸ Adult: Initially 200 mg once daily, to be taken with or before food, increased if necessary to 300–400 mg once daily; maximum 500 mg per day
▸ Elderly: Initially 200 mg once daily, increased if necessary to 300 mg once daily

VIAZEM® XL
Angina | Mild to moderate hypertension
▸ BY MOUTH
▸ Adult: Initially 180 mg once daily, adjusted according to response to 240 mg once daily; maximum 360 mg per day
▸ Elderly: Initially 120 mg once daily, adjusted according to response

ZEMTARD®
Angina
▸ BY MOUTH
▸ Adult: 180–300 mg once daily, increased if necessary to 480 mg once daily
▸ Elderly: Initially 120 mg once daily, increased if necessary to 480 mg once daily

Mild to moderate hypertension
▸ BY MOUTH
▸ Adult: 180–300 mg once daily, increased if necessary to 360 mg once daily
▸ Elderly: Initially 120 mg once daily, increased if necessary to 360 mg once daily

- CONTRA-INDICATIONS Acute porphyrias p. 1025 · left ventricular failure with pulmonary congestion · second- or third-degree AV block (unless pacemaker fitted) · severe bradycardia · sick sinus syndrome

- CAUTIONS Bradycardia (avoid if severe) · first degree AV block · heart failure · prolonged PR interval · significantly impaired left ventricular function

- INTERACTIONS → Appendix 1: calcium channel blockers

- SIDE-EFFECTS
▸ **Common or very common** Cardiac conduction disorders · constipation · gastrointestinal discomfort · malaise

▸ **Uncommon** Arrhythmias · diarrhoea · insomnia · nervousness · postural hypotension
▸ **Rare or very rare** Dry mouth
▸ **Frequency not known** Angioedema · cardiac arrest · congestive heart failure · depression · extrapyramidal symptoms · fever · gynaecomastia · hepatitis · hyperglycaemia · hyperhidrosis · mood altered · photosensitivity reaction · severe cutaneous adverse reactions (SCARs) · thrombocytopenia · vasculitis

Overdose In overdose, diltiazem has a profound cardiac depressant effect causing hypotension and arrhythmias, including complete heart block and asystole.

● PREGNANCY Avoid.
● BREAST FEEDING Significant amount present in milk—no evidence of harm but avoid unless no safer alternative.
● HEPATIC IMPAIRMENT
Dose adjustments Reduce dose.

TILDIEM RETARD ® Dose for mild to moderate hypertension—initially 120 mg once a day; increased if necessary to 120 mg twice a day.
    For treatment of angina, dose form not appropriate for initial titration; up to 120 mg twice a day may be required.

ADIZEM-XL ® Dose for angina and mild to moderate hypertension—initially 120 mg once daily.

DILZEM ® XL Dose for angina and mild to moderate hypertension—initially 120 mg once daily.

ZEMTARD ® Dose for angina and mild to moderate hypertension—initially 120 mg once daily.

DILCARDIA ® SR Dose for angina and mild to moderate hypertension—initially 60 mg twice a day; maximum 90 mg twice a day.

ANGITIL ® XL Dose form not appropriate for initial dose titration.

SLOZEM ® Dose for angina and mild to moderate hypertension—initially 120 mg once daily.

TILDIEM ® LA Dose for angina and mild to moderate hypertension—initially 200 mg daily; increased if necessary to 300 mg daily.

VIAZEM ® XL Dose for angina and mild to moderate hypertension—initially 120 mg once daily, adjusted according to response.

● RENAL IMPAIRMENT
Start with smaller dose.

TILDIEM RETARD ® Dose for mild to moderate hypertension—initially 120 mg once a day; increased if necessary to 120 mg twice a day.
    For treatment of angina, dose form not appropriate for initial titration; up to 120 mg twice a day may be required.

ADIZEM-XL ® Dose for angina and mild to moderate hypertension—initially 120 mg once daily.

DILZEM ® XL Dose for angina and mild to moderate hypertension—initially 120 mg once daily.

ZEMTARD ® Dose for angina and mild to moderate hypertension—initially 120 mg once daily.

DILCARDIA ® SR Dose for angina and mild to moderate hypertension—initially 60 mg twice a day; maximum 90 mg twice a day.

ANGITIL ® XL Dose form not appropriate for initial dose titration.

SLOZEM ® Dose for angina and mild to moderate hypertension—initially 120 mg once daily.

TILDIEM ® LA Dose for angina and mild to moderate hypertension—initially 200 mg daily; increased if necessary to 300 mg daily.

VIAZEM ® XL Dose for angina and mild to moderate hypertension—initially 120 mg once daily, adjusted according to response.

● PRESCRIBING AND DISPENSING INFORMATION The standard formulations containing 60 mg diltiazem hydrochloride are licensed as generics and there is no requirement for brand name dispensing. Although their means of formulation has called for the strict designation 'modified-release', their duration of action corresponds to that of tablets requiring administration more frequently.
    Different versions of modified-release preparations containing more than 60 mg diltiazem hydrochloride may not have the same clinical effect. To avoid confusion between these different formulations of diltiazem, prescribers should specify the brand to be dispensed.

● PATIENT AND CARER ADVICE
TILDIEM RETARD ® Tablet membrane may pass through gastro-intestinal tract unchanged, but being porous has no effect on efficacy.

● MEDICINAL FORMS
There can be variation in the licensing of different medicines containing the same drug. Forms available from special-order manufacturers include: oral suspension, oral solution

Modified-release tablet
CAUTIONARY AND ADVISORY LABELS 25
▸ Diltiazem hydrochloride (Non-proprietary)
   Diltiazem hydrochloride 60 mg Diltiazem 60mg modified-release tablets | 84 tablet [PoM] £41.59 DT = £41.59 | 100 tablet [PoM] £49.51
   Diltiazem hydrochloride 90 mg Diltiazem 90mg modified-release tablets | 56 tablet [PoM] [Ṡ] DT = £7.27
   Diltiazem hydrochloride 120 mg Diltiazem 120mg modified-release tablets | 56 tablet [PoM] [Ṡ] DT = £7.15
▸ Retalzem (Kent Pharmaceuticals Ltd)
   Diltiazem hydrochloride 60 mg Retalzem 60 modified-release tablets | 84 tablet [PoM] £7.43 DT = £41.59
▸ Tildiem (Sanofi)
   Diltiazem hydrochloride 60 mg Tildiem 60mg modified-release tablets | 90 tablet [PoM] £7.96
▸ Tildiem Retard (Sanofi)
   Diltiazem hydrochloride 90 mg Tildiem Retard 90mg tablets | 56 tablet [PoM] £7.27 DT = £7.27
   Diltiazem hydrochloride 120 mg Tildiem Retard 120mg tablets | 56 tablet [PoM] £7.15 DT = £7.15

Modified-release capsule
CAUTIONARY AND ADVISORY LABELS 25
▸ Diltiazem hydrochloride (Non-proprietary)
   Diltiazem hydrochloride 60 mg Diltiazem 60mg modified-release capsules | 56 capsule [PoM] £6.04 DT = £6.04
   Diltiazem hydrochloride 90 mg Diltiazem 90mg modified-release capsules | 56 capsule [PoM] £8.50 DT = £8.50
   Diltiazem hydrochloride 120 mg Diltiazem 120mg modified-release capsules | 28 capsule [PoM] £48.40 DT = £9.14 | 56 capsule [PoM] [Ṡ] DT = £9.45
   Diltiazem hydrochloride 180 mg Diltiazem 180mg modified-release capsules | 28 capsule [PoM] £54.20 DT = £10.37 | 56 capsule [PoM] [Ṡ] DT = £14.15
   Diltiazem hydrochloride 240 mg Diltiazem 240mg modified-release capsules | 28 capsule [PoM] £11.52 DT = £11.52
   Diltiazem hydrochloride 300 mg Diltiazem 300mg modified-release capsules | 28 capsule [PoM] £9.01 DT = £9.01
   Diltiazem hydrochloride 360 mg Diltiazem 360mg modified-release capsules | 28 capsule [PoM] [Ṡ] DT = £13.85
▸ Adizem-SR (Napp Pharmaceuticals Ltd)
   Diltiazem hydrochloride 90 mg Adizem-SR 90mg capsules | 56 capsule [PoM] £8.50 DT = £8.50
   Diltiazem hydrochloride 120 mg Adizem-SR 120mg capsules | 56 capsule [PoM] £9.45 DT = £9.45
   Diltiazem hydrochloride 180 mg Adizem-SR 180mg capsules | 56 capsule [PoM] £14.15 DT = £14.15
▸ Adizem-XL (Napp Pharmaceuticals Ltd)
   Diltiazem hydrochloride 120 mg Adizem-XL 120mg capsules | 28 capsule [PoM] £9.14 DT = £9.14
   Diltiazem hydrochloride 180 mg Adizem-XL 180mg capsules | 28 capsule [PoM] £10.37 DT = £10.37
   Diltiazem hydrochloride 200 mg Adizem-XL 200mg capsules | 28 capsule [PoM] £6.30 DT = £6.29
   Diltiazem hydrochloride 240 mg Adizem-XL 240mg capsules | 28 capsule [PoM] £11.52 DT = £11.52

Diltiazem hydrochloride 300 mg Adizem-XL 300mg capsules |
28 capsule [PoM] £9.14 DT = £9.01

▸ **Angitil SR** (Ethypharm UK Ltd)
Diltiazem hydrochloride 90 mg Angitil SR 90 capsules |
56 capsule [PoM] £7.03 DT = £8.50
Diltiazem hydrochloride 120 mg Angitil SR 120 capsules |
56 capsule [PoM] £6.91 DT = £9.45
Diltiazem hydrochloride 180 mg Angitil SR 180 capsules |
56 capsule [PoM] £13.27 DT = £14.15

▸ **Angitil XL** (Ethypharm UK Ltd)
Diltiazem hydrochloride 240 mg Angitil XL 240 capsules |
28 capsule [PoM] £7.94 DT = £11.52
Diltiazem hydrochloride 300 mg Angitil XL 300 capsules |
28 capsule [PoM] £6.98 DT = £9.01

▸ **Bi-Carzem SR** (Tillomed Laboratories Ltd)
Diltiazem hydrochloride 90 mg Bi-Carzem SR 90mg capsules |
56 capsule [PoM] £10.23 DT = £8.50
Diltiazem hydrochloride 120 mg Bi-Carzem SR 120mg capsules |
56 capsule [PoM] £11.16 DT = £9.45

▸ **Bi-Carzem XL** (Tillomed Laboratories Ltd)
Diltiazem hydrochloride 240 mg Bi-Carzem XL 240mg capsules |
28 capsule [PoM] £12.55 DT = £11.52
Diltiazem hydrochloride 300 mg Bi-Carzem XL 300mg capsules |
28 capsule [PoM] £10.70 DT = £9.01

▸ **Dilcardia SR** (Mylan)
Diltiazem hydrochloride 60 mg Dilcardia SR 60mg capsules |
56 capsule [PoM] £6.03 DT = £6.04
Diltiazem hydrochloride 90 mg Dilcardia SR 90mg capsules |
56 capsule [PoM] £9.61 DT = £8.50
Diltiazem hydrochloride 120 mg Dilcardia SR 120mg capsules |
56 capsule [PoM] £10.69 DT = £9.45

▸ **Dilzem XL** (Teva UK Ltd)
Diltiazem hydrochloride 120 mg Dilzem XL 120 capsules |
28 capsule [PoM] £7.78 DT = £9.14
Diltiazem hydrochloride 180 mg Dilzem XL 180 capsules |
28 capsule [PoM] £11.55 DT = £10.37
Diltiazem hydrochloride 240 mg Dilzem XL 240 capsules |
28 capsule [PoM] £11.03 DT = £11.52

▸ **Kenzem SR** (Kent Pharmaceuticals Ltd)
Diltiazem hydrochloride 60 mg Kenzem SR 60mg capsules |
56 capsule [PoM] £10.00 DT = £6.04
Diltiazem hydrochloride 90 mg Kenzem SR 90mg capsules |
56 capsule [PoM] £11.35 DT = £8.50
Diltiazem hydrochloride 120 mg Kenzem SR 120mg capsules |
56 capsule [PoM] £14.00 DT = £9.45

▸ **Slozem** (Merck Serono Ltd)
Diltiazem hydrochloride 120 mg Slozem 120mg capsules |
28 capsule [PoM] £7.00 DT = £9.14
Diltiazem hydrochloride 180 mg Slozem 180mg capsules |
28 capsule [PoM] £7.80 DT = £10.37
Diltiazem hydrochloride 240 mg Slozem 240mg capsules |
28 capsule [PoM] £8.20 DT = £11.52
Diltiazem hydrochloride 300 mg Slozem 300mg capsules |
28 capsule [PoM] £8.50 DT = £9.01

▸ **Tildiem LA** (Sanofi)
Diltiazem hydrochloride 200 mg Tildiem LA 200 capsules |
28 capsule [PoM] £6.29 DT = £6.29
Diltiazem hydrochloride 300 mg Tildiem LA 300 capsules |
28 capsule [PoM] £9.01 DT = £9.01

▸ **Uard XL** (Ennogen Healthcare Ltd)
Diltiazem hydrochloride 120 mg Uard 120XL capsules |
28 capsule [PoM] £7.31 DT = £9.14
Diltiazem hydrochloride 180 mg Uard 180XL capsules |
28 capsule [PoM] £8.30 DT = £10.37
Diltiazem hydrochloride 240 mg Uard 240XL capsules |
28 capsule [PoM] £9.22 DT = £11.52
Diltiazem hydrochloride 300 mg Uard 300XL capsules |
28 capsule [PoM] £7.21 DT = £9.01

▸ **Viazem XL** (Thornton & Ross Ltd)
Diltiazem hydrochloride 120 mg Viazem XL 120mg capsules |
28 capsule [PoM] £6.60 DT = £9.14
Diltiazem hydrochloride 180 mg Viazem XL 180mg capsules |
28 capsule [PoM] £7.36 DT = £10.37
Diltiazem hydrochloride 240 mg Viazem XL 240mg capsules |
28 capsule [PoM] £7.74 DT = £11.52
Diltiazem hydrochloride 300 mg Viazem XL 300mg capsules |
28 capsule [PoM] £8.03 DT = £9.01
Diltiazem hydrochloride 360 mg Viazem XL 360mg capsules |
28 capsule [PoM] £13.85 DT = £13.85

▸ **Zemret XL** (Tillomed Laboratories Ltd)
Diltiazem hydrochloride 180 mg Zemret 180 XL capsules |
28 capsule [PoM] £7.00 DT = £10.37
Diltiazem hydrochloride 240 mg Zemret 240 XL capsules |
28 capsule [PoM] £7.00 DT = £11.52
Diltiazem hydrochloride 300 mg Zemret 300 XL capsules |
28 capsule [PoM] £7.00 DT = £9.01

▸ **Zemtard XL** (Galen Ltd)
Diltiazem hydrochloride 120 mg Zemtard 120 XL capsules |
28 capsule [PoM] £6.10 DT = £9.14
Diltiazem hydrochloride 180 mg Zemtard 180 XL capsules |
28 capsule [PoM] £6.20 DT = £10.37
Diltiazem hydrochloride 240 mg Zemtard 240 XL capsules |
28 capsule [PoM] £6.30 DT = £11.52
Diltiazem hydrochloride 300 mg Zemtard 300 XL capsules |
28 capsule [PoM] £6.70 DT = £9.01

☞ 155

Felodipine

● **DRUG ACTION** Felodipine is a dihydropyridine calcium-channel blocker.

● **INDICATIONS AND DOSE**

Prophylaxis of angina
▸ BY MOUTH
▸ **Adult:** Initially 5 mg once daily; increased if necessary to 10 mg once daily, to be taken in the morning
▸ **Elderly:** Initially 2.5 mg once daily; increased if necessary to 10 mg once daily, to be taken in the morning

Hypertension
▸ BY MOUTH
▸ **Adult:** Initially 5 mg once daily; usual maintenance 5–10 mg once daily, to be taken in the morning, doses above 20 mg daily rarely needed
▸ **Elderly:** Initially 2.5 mg daily; usual maintenance 5–10 mg once daily, to be taken in the morning, doses above 20 mg daily rarely needed

● **CONTRA-INDICATIONS** Cardiac outflow obstruction · significant cardiac valvular obstruction (e.g. aortic stenosis) · uncontrolled heart failure · unstable angina · within 1 month of myocardial infarction

● **CAUTIONS** Predisposition to tachycardia · severe left ventricular dysfunction · withdraw if cardiogenic shock develops · withdraw if existing pain worsens shortly after initiating treatment · withdraw if ischaemic pain occurs shortly after initiating treatment

● **INTERACTIONS** → Appendix 1: calcium channel blockers

● **SIDE-EFFECTS**
▸ **Uncommon** Abdominal pain · fatigue · paraesthesia
▸ **Rare or very rare** Arthralgia · hypersensitivity vasculitis · myalgia · photosensitivity reaction · syncope · urinary frequency increased

● **PREGNANCY** Avoid; toxicity in *animal* studies; may inhibit labour.

● **BREAST FEEDING** Present in milk but amount probably too small to be harmful.

● **HEPATIC IMPAIRMENT**
Dose adjustments Dose reduction may be required.

● **MEDICINAL FORMS**
There can be variation in the licensing of different medicines containing the same drug. Forms available from special-order manufacturers include: oral solution

Modified-release tablet
CAUTIONARY AND ADVISORY LABELS 25
▸ **Felodipine** (Non-proprietary)
Felodipine 2.5 mg Felodipine 2.5mg modified-release tablets |
28 tablet [PoM] [Ⓢ] DT = £22.08
Felodipine 5 mg Felodipine 5mg modified-release tablets |
28 tablet [PoM] [Ⓢ] DT = £4.21

2 Cardiovascular system

Felodipine 10 mg Felodipine 10mg modified-release tablets | 28 tablet [PoM] [▼] DT = £5.66

▸ Cardioplen XL (Chiesi Ltd)
Felodipine 2.5 mg Cardioplen XL 2.5mg tablets | 28 tablet [PoM] £5.68 DT = £22.08
Felodipine 5 mg Cardioplen XL 5mg tablets | 28 tablet [PoM] £3.87 DT = £4.21
Felodipine 10 mg Cardioplen XL 10mg tablets | 28 tablet [PoM] £4.81 DT = £5.66

▸ Felendil XL (Teva UK Ltd)
Felodipine 2.5 mg Folpik XL 2.5mg tablets | 28 tablet [PoM] £6.31 DT = £22.08
Felodipine 5 mg Folpik XL 5mg tablets | 28 tablet [PoM] £4.21 DT = £4.21
Felodipine 10 mg Folpik XL 10mg tablets | 28 tablet [PoM] £7.21 DT = £5.66

▸ Neofel XL (Kent Pharmaceuticals Ltd, Actavis UK Ltd)
Felodipine 2.5 mg Neofel XL 2.5mg tablets | 28 tablet [PoM] £6.31 DT = £22.08
Felodipine 5 mg Neofel XL 5mg tablets | 28 tablet [PoM] £4.21 DT = £4.21
Felodipine 10 mg Neofel XL 10mg tablets | 28 tablet [PoM] £5.66 DT = £5.66

▸ Parmid XL (Sandoz Ltd)
Felodipine 2.5 mg Parmid XL 2.5mg tablets | 28 tablet [PoM] £5.36 DT = £22.08

▸ Pinefeld XL (Tillomed Laboratories Ltd)
Felodipine 10 mg Pinefeld XL 10mg tablets | 28 tablet [PoM] £11.98 DT = £5.66

▸ Plendil (AstraZeneca UK Ltd)
Felodipine 2.5 mg Plendil 2.5mg modified-release tablets | 98 tablet [PoM] £22.08
Felodipine 5 mg Plendil 5mg modified-release tablets | 28 tablet [PoM] £4.21 DT = £4.21
Felodipine 10 mg Plendil 10mg modified-release tablets | 28 tablet [PoM] £5.66 DT = £5.66

▸ Vascalpha (Actavis UK Ltd)
Felodipine 5 mg Vascalpha 5mg modified-release tablets | 28 tablet [PoM] £7.16 DT = £4.21
Felodipine 10 mg Vascalpha 10mg modified-release tablets | 28 tablet [PoM] £9.63 DT = £5.66

Combinations available: *Ramipril with felodipine,* p. 173

▸ 155

Lacidipine

● DRUG ACTION Lacidipine is a dihydropyridine calcium-channel blocker.

● INDICATIONS AND DOSE

Hypertension
▸ BY MOUTH
▸ Adult: Initially 2 mg daily; increased if necessary to 4 mg daily, then increased if necessary to 6 mg daily, dose increases should occur at intervals of 3–4 weeks, to be taken preferably in the morning

● CONTRA-INDICATIONS Acute porphyrias p. 1025 · aortic stenosis · avoid within 1 month of myocardial infarction · cardiogenic shock · unstable angina

● CAUTIONS Cardiac conduction abnormalities · poor cardiac reserve

● INTERACTIONS → Appendix 1: calcium channel blockers

● SIDE-EFFECTS
▸ **Common or very common** Abdominal discomfort · asthenia · polyuria
▸ **Uncommon** Ischaemic heart disease · syncope
▸ **Rare or very rare** Angioedema · depression · muscle cramps · tremor

● PREGNANCY Manufacturer advises avoid; may inhibit labour.

● BREAST FEEDING Manufacturer advises avoid—no information available.

● HEPATIC IMPAIRMENT Antihypertensive effect possibly increased.

● MEDICINAL FORMS
There can be variation in the licensing of different medicines containing the same drug.

Tablet
▸ Lacidipine (Non-proprietary)
Lacidipine 2 mg Lacidipine 2mg tablets | 28 tablet [PoM] £6.85 DT = £2.71
Lacidipine 4 mg Lacidipine 4mg tablets | 28 tablet [PoM] £6.85 DT = £3.57
▸ Molap (Rivopharm (UK) Ltd)
Lacidipine 4 mg Molap 4mg tablets | 28 tablet [PoM] £2.90 DT = £3.57
▸ Motens (GlaxoSmithKline UK Ltd)
Lacidipine 2 mg Motens 2mg tablets | 28 tablet [PoM] £2.95 DT = £2.71
Lacidipine 4 mg Motens 4mg tablets | 28 tablet [PoM] £3.10 DT = £3.57

▸ 155

Lercanidipine hydrochloride

● DRUG ACTION Lercanidipine is a dihydropyridine calcium-channel blocker.

● INDICATIONS AND DOSE

Mild to moderate hypertension
▸ BY MOUTH
▸ Adult: Initially 10 mg once daily; increased if necessary to 20 mg daily, dose can be adjusted after 2 weeks

● CONTRA-INDICATIONS Aortic stenosis · uncontrolled heart failure · unstable angina · within 1 month of myocardial infarction

● CAUTIONS Left ventricular dysfunction · sick sinus syndrome (if pacemaker not fitted)

● INTERACTIONS → Appendix 1: calcium channel blockers

● SIDE-EFFECTS
▸ **Rare or very rare** Angina pectoris · asthenia · chest pain · diarrhoea · drowsiness · gastrointestinal discomfort · myalgia · syncope · urinary disorders

● PREGNANCY Manufacturer advises avoid—no information available.

● BREAST FEEDING Manufacturer advises avoid.

● HEPATIC IMPAIRMENT Avoid in severe disease.

● RENAL IMPAIRMENT Avoid if eGFR less than 30 mL/minute/1.73 m^2.

● MEDICINAL FORMS
There can be variation in the licensing of different medicines containing the same drug.

Tablet
CAUTIONARY AND ADVISORY LABELS 22
▸ Lercanidipine hydrochloride (Non-proprietary)
Lercanidipine hydrochloride 10 mg Lercanidipine 10mg tablets | 28 tablet [PoM] £12.99 DT = £3.28
Lercanidipine hydrochloride 20 mg Lercanidipine 20mg tablets | 28 tablet [PoM] £15.99 DT = £3.91
▸ Zanidip (Recordati Pharmaceuticals Ltd)
Lercanidipine hydrochloride 10 mg Zanidip 10mg tablets | 28 tablet [PoM] £5.70 DT = £3.28
Lercanidipine hydrochloride 20 mg Zanidip 20mg tablets | 28 tablet [PoM] £10.82 DT = £3.91

⚑ 155

Nicardipine hydrochloride

- **DRUG ACTION** Nicardipine is a dihydropyridine calcium-channel blocker.

- **INDICATIONS AND DOSE**

Prophylaxis of angina
- ▸ BY MOUTH USING IMMEDIATE-RELEASE MEDICINES
- ▸ Adult: Initially 20 mg 3 times a day, then increased to 30 mg 3 times a day, dose increased after at least 3 days; usual dose 60–120 mg daily

Mild to moderate hypertension
- ▸ BY MOUTH USING IMMEDIATE-RELEASE MEDICINES
- ▸ Adult: Initially 20 mg 3 times a day, then increased to 30 mg 3 times a day, dose increased after at least 3 days; usual dose 60–120 mg daily
- ▸ BY MOUTH USING MODIFIED-RELEASE MEDICINES
- ▸ Adult: Initially 30 mg twice daily; increased if necessary up to 45 mg twice daily. usual dose 30–60 mg twice daily

Life-threatening hypertension (specialist use only) | Post-operative hypertension (specialist use only)
- ▸ BY CONTINUOUS INTRAVENOUS INFUSION
- ▸ Adult: Initially 3–5 mg/hour for 15 minutes, increased in steps of 0.5–1 mg every 15 minutes, adjusted according to response, maximum rate 15 mg/hour, reduce dose gradually when target blood pressure achieved; maintenance 2–4 mg/hour
- ▸ Elderly: Initially 1–5 mg/hour, then adjusted in steps of 500 micrograms/hour after 30 minutes, adjusted according to response, maximum rate 15 mg/hour

Life-threatening hypertension in patients with hepatic or renal impairment (specialist use only) | Postoperative hypertension in patients with hepatic or renal impairment (specialist use only)
- ▸ BY CONTINUOUS INTRAVENOUS INFUSION
- ▸ Adult: Initially 1–5 mg/hour, then adjusted in steps of 500 micrograms/hour after 30 minutes, adjusted according to response, maximum rate 15 mg/hour

Acute life-threatening hypertension in pregnancy (specialist use only)
- ▸ BY CONTINUOUS INTRAVENOUS INFUSION
- ▸ Adult: Initially 1–5 mg/hour, then adjusted in steps of 500 micrograms/hour after 30 minutes, adjusted according to response, usual maximum rate 4 mg/hour in treatment of pre-eclampsia (maximum rate 15 mg/hour)

- **CONTRA-INDICATIONS**

GENERAL CONTRA-INDICATIONS Acute porphyrias p. 1025 · cardiogenic shock · significant or advanced aortic stenosis · unstable or acute attacks of angina

SPECIFIC CONTRA-INDICATIONS
- ▸ With intravenous use avoid within 8 days of myocardial infarction · compensatory hypertension
- ▸ With oral use avoid within 1 month of myocardial infarction
- **CAUTIONS**

GENERAL CAUTIONS Congestive heart failure · elderly · pulmonary oedema · significantly impaired left ventricular function · stroke · withdraw if ischaemic pain occurs or existing pain worsens within 30 minutes of initiating treatment or increasing dose

SPECIFIC CAUTIONS
- ▸ With intravenous use Elevated intracranial pressure · portal hypertension
- **INTERACTIONS** → Appendix 1: calcium channel blockers
- **SIDE-EFFECTS**

GENERAL SIDE-EFFECTS
- **Common or very common** Hypotension

- ▸ **Frequency not known** Hepatic disorders · Pulmonary oedema · thrombocytopenia

SPECIFIC SIDE-EFFECTS
- ▸ With intravenous use Atrioventricular block · erythema · ischaemic heart disease · paralytic ileus
- ▸ With oral use Asthenia · depression · drowsiness · dyspnoea · feeling hot · insomnia · nervous system disorder · paraesthesia · renal impairment · tinnitus · urinary frequency increased

SIDE-EFFECTS, FURTHER INFORMATION Systemic hypotension and reflex tachycardia with rapid reduction of blood pressure may occur—during intravenous use consider stopping infusion or decreasing dose by half.

- **PREGNANCY** May inhibit labour. Not to be used in multiple pregnancy (twins or more) unless there is no other acceptable alternative. Toxicity in *animal* studies. Risk of severe maternal hypotension and fatal fetal hypoxia—avoid excessive decrease in blood pressure. For treatment of acute life-threatening hypertension only.

- **BREAST FEEDING** Manufacturer advises avoid—present in breast milk.

- **HEPATIC IMPAIRMENT**

Dose adjustments ▸ With oral use Use with caution—consider using lowest initial dose and extending dosing interval according to individual response.
- ▸ With intravenous use Use with caution—use lower initial dose.

- **RENAL IMPAIRMENT**

Dose adjustments ▸ With oral use Consider using lowest initial dose and extending dosing interval according to individual response.
- ▸ With intravenous use Use with caution—use lower initial dose.

- **MONITORING REQUIREMENTS** Monitor blood pressure and heart rate at least every 5 minutes during intravenous infusion, and then until stable, and continue monitoring for at least 12 hours after end of infusion.

- **DIRECTIONS FOR ADMINISTRATION** Intravenous nicardipine should only be administered under the supervision of a specialist and in a hospital or intensive care setting in which patients can be closely monitored.

  For *intravenous infusion* give continuously in Glucose 5%; dilute dose in infusion fluid to a final concentration of 100–200 micrograms/mL (undiluted solution *via* central venous line only) and give *via* volumetric infusion pump or syringe driver; protect from light; to minimise peripheral venous irritation, change site of infusion every 12 hours; risk of adsorption on to plastic of infusion set in the presence of saline solutions; incompatible with bicarbonate or alkaline solutions—consult product literature.

- **MEDICINAL FORMS**
There can be variation in the licensing of different medicines containing the same drug. Forms available from special-order manufacturers include: oral suspension, oral solution

Modified-release capsule
CAUTIONARY AND ADVISORY LABELS 25
- ▸ Cardene SR (Astellas Pharma Ltd)
  Nicardipine hydrochloride 30 mg Cardene SR 30mg capsules | 56 capsule PoM £7.15 DT = £7.15
  Nicardipine hydrochloride 45 mg Cardene SR 45mg capsules | 56 capsule PoM £10.40 DT = £10.40

Solution for infusion
- ▸ Nicardipine hydrochloride (Non-proprietary)
  Nicardipine hydrochloride 1 mg per 1 ml Nicardipine 10mg/10ml solution for injection ampoules | 5 ampoule PoM £50.00
  Nicardipine hydrochloride 2.5 mg per 1 ml Cardene I.V. 25mg/10ml solution for infusion ampoules | 10 ampoule PoM Ⓢ

Cardiovascular system

2

Capsule

▶ Nicardipine hydrochloride (Non-proprietary)
Nicardipine hydrochloride 20 mg Nicardipine 20mg capsules |
56 capsule PoM £8.38 DT = £6.00
Nicardipine hydrochloride 30 mg Nicardipine 30mg capsules |
56 capsule PoM £9.73 DT = £6.96

▶ Cardene (Astellas Pharma Ltd)
Nicardipine hydrochloride 20 mg Cardene 20mg capsules |
56 capsule PoM £6.00 DT = £6.00
Nicardipine hydrochloride 30 mg Cardene 30mg capsules |
56 capsule PoM £6.96 DT = £6.96

⚑ 155

Nifedipine

21-Nov-2016

● **DRUG ACTION** Nifedipine is a dihydropyridine calcium-channel blocker.

● **INDICATIONS AND DOSE**

Raynaud's syndrome
▶ BY MOUTH USING IMMEDIATE-RELEASE MEDICINES
▶ Adult: Initially 5 mg 3 times a day, then adjusted according to response to 20 mg 3 times a day

Angina prophylaxis (not recommended)
▶ BY MOUTH USING IMMEDIATE-RELEASE MEDICINES
▶ Adult: Initially 5 mg 3 times a day, then adjusted according to response to 20 mg 3 times a day

Postponement of premature labour
▶ BY MOUTH USING IMMEDIATE-RELEASE MEDICINES
▶ Adult: Initially 20 mg, followed by 10–20 mg 3–4 times a day, adjusted according to uterine activity

Hiccup in palliative care
▶ BY MOUTH USING IMMEDIATE-RELEASE MEDICINES
▶ Adult: 10 mg 3 times a day

ADALAT RETARD ®
Hypertension | Angina prophylaxis
▶ BY MOUTH
▶ Adult: 10 mg twice daily, adjusted according to response to 40 mg twice daily

ADALAT ®
Angina prophylaxis (not recommended) | Raynaud's phenomenon
▶ BY MOUTH USING IMMEDIATE-RELEASE MEDICINES
▶ Adult: Initially 5 mg 3 times a day, then adjusted according to response to 20 mg 3 times a day

DOSE EQUIVALENCE AND CONVERSION
▶ *Adalat*® liquid gel capsules contain 5 mg nifedipine in 0.17 mL and 10 mg nifedipine in 0.34 mL.

ADALAT ® LA
Hypertension
▶ BY MOUTH
▶ Adult: 20–30 mg once daily, increased if necessary up to 90 mg once daily

Angina prophylaxis
▶ BY MOUTH
▶ Adult: 30 mg once daily, increased if necessary up to 90 mg once daily

ADIPINE ® MR
Hypertension | Angina prophylaxis
▶ BY MOUTH
▶ Adult: 10 mg twice daily, adjusted according to response to 40 mg twice daily

ADIPINE ® XL
Hypertension | Angina prophylaxis
▶ BY MOUTH
▶ Adult: 30 mg daily, increased if necessary up to 90 mg daily

CORACTEN ® SR
Hypertension | Angina prophylaxis
▶ BY MOUTH
▶ Adult: Initially 10 mg twice daily, increased if necessary up to 40 mg twice daily

CORACTEN ® XL
Hypertension | Angina prophylaxis
▶ BY MOUTH
▶ Adult: Initially 30 mg daily, increased if necessary up to 90 mg daily

FORTIPINE ® LA 40
Hypertension | Angina prophylaxis
▶ BY MOUTH
▶ Adult: Initially 40 mg once daily, increased if necessary to 80 mg daily in 1–2 divided doses

NIFEDIPRESS ® MR
Hypertension | Angina prophylaxis
▶ BY MOUTH
▶ Adult: 10 mg twice daily, adjusted according to response to 40 mg twice daily

TENSIPINE ® MR
Hypertension | Angina prophylaxis
▶ BY MOUTH
▶ Adult: Initially 10 mg twice daily, adjusted according to response to 40 mg twice daily

VALNI ® XL
Severe hypertension | Prophylaxis of angina
▶ BY MOUTH
▶ Adult: 30 mg once daily, increased if necessary up to 90 mg once daily

● **UNLICENSED USE** Not licensed for use in postponing premature labour.

● **CONTRA-INDICATIONS** Acute attacks of angina · cardiogenic shock · significant aortic stenosis · unstable angina · within 1 month of myocardial infarction

● **CAUTIONS** Diabetes mellitus · elderly · heart failure · poor cardiac reserve · severe hypotension · short-acting formulations are not recommended for angina or long-term management of hypertension; their use may be associated with large variations in blood pressure and reflex tachycardia · significantly impaired left ventricular function (heart failure deterioration observed) · withdraw if ischaemic pain occurs or existing pain worsens shortly after initiating treatment

ADALAT® LA Crohn's disease · decreased lumen diameter of the gastro-intestinal tract · history of gastro-intestinal obstruction · history of oesophageal obstruction · inflammatory bowel disease

CAUTIONS, FURTHER INFORMATION Dose form not appropriate for use where there is a history of oesophageal or gastro-intestinal obstruction, decreased lumen diameter of the gastro-intestinal tract, or inflammatory bowel disease (including Crohn's disease).

VALNI® XL Decreased lumen diameter of gastro-intestinal tract · history of gastro-intestinal obstruction · history of oesophageal obstruction · ileostomy after proctocolectomy · inflammatory bowel disease

CAUTIONS, FURTHER INFORMATION Dose form not appropriate for use where there is a history of oesophageal or gastro-intestinal obstruction, decreased lumen diameter of the gastro-intestinal tract, inflammatory bowel disease, or ileostomy after proctocolectomy.

● **INTERACTIONS** → Appendix 1: calcium channel blockers

● **SIDE-EFFECTS**
▶ **Common or very common** Constipation · malaise · oedema · vasodilation

▸ **Uncommon** Allergic oedema · angioedema · anxiety · chills · dry mouth · epistaxis · gastrointestinal discomfort · hypotension · joint disorders · laryngeal oedema · migraine · muscle complaints · nasal congestion · pain · sleep disorder · syncope · tremor · urinary disorders · vertigo · visual impairment

▸ **Rare or very rare** Sensation abnormal

▸ **Frequency not known** Agranulocytosis · angina pectoris · chest pain · drowsiness · dyspnoea · eye pain · hyperglycaemia · jaundice · leucopenia · photoallergic reaction · pulmonary oedema · toxic epidermal necrolysis

● PREGNANCY May inhibit labour; manufacturer advises avoid before week 20, but risk to fetus should be balanced against risk of uncontrolled maternal hypertension. Use only if other treatment options are not indicated or have failed.

● BREAST FEEDING Amount too small to be harmful but manufacturers advise avoid.

● HEPATIC IMPAIRMENT
Dose adjustments Dose reduction may be required in severe liver disease.
Some modified-release formulations may not be suitable for dose titration in hepatic disease—consult product literature.
ADALAT ® LA Dose form not appropriate.
VALNI ® XL Dose form not appropriate.

● DIRECTIONS FOR ADMINISTRATION
FORTIPINE ® LA 40 Take with or just after food, or a meal.

● PRESCRIBING AND DISPENSING INFORMATION Different versions of modified-release preparations may not have the same clinical effect. To avoid confusion between these different formulations of nifedipine, prescribers should specify the brand to be dispensed.
Palliative care For further information on the use of nifedipine in palliative care, see www.palliativedrugs.com/formulary/en/nifedipine.html.

● PATIENT AND CARER ADVICE
ADALAT ® LA Tablet membrane may pass through gastrointestinal tract unchanged, but being porous has no effect on efficacy.

● MEDICINAL FORMS
There can be variation in the licensing of different medicines containing the same drug. Forms available from special-order manufacturers include: oral suspension, oral drops, ointment

Modified-release tablet
CAUTIONARY AND ADVISORY LABELS 25
▸ Adalat LA (Bayer Plc)
Nifedipine 20 mg Adalat LA 20mg tablets | 28 tablet [PoM] £5.27 DT = £5.27
Nifedipine 30 mg Adalat LA 30mg tablets | 28 tablet [PoM] £6.85 DT = £6.85
Nifedipine 60 mg Adalat LA 60mg tablets | 28 tablet [PoM] £9.03 DT = £9.03
▸ Adalat retard (Bayer Plc)
Nifedipine 10 mg Adalat retard 10mg tablets | 56 tablet [PoM] £7.34 DT = £7.34
Nifedipine 20 mg Adalat retard 20mg tablets | 56 tablet [PoM] £8.81 DT = £8.81
▸ Adipine MR (Chiesi Ltd)
Nifedipine 10 mg Adipine MR 10 tablets | 56 tablet [PoM] £3.73 DT = £7.34
Nifedipine 20 mg Adipine MR 20 tablets | 56 tablet [PoM] £5.21 DT = £8.81
▸ Adipine XL (Chiesi Ltd)
Nifedipine 30 mg Adipine XL 30mg tablets | 28 tablet [PoM] £4.70 DT = £6.85
Nifedipine 60 mg Adipine XL 60mg tablets | 28 tablet [PoM] £7.10 DT = £9.03
▸ Fortipine LA (AMCo)
Nifedipine 40 mg Fortipine LA 40 tablets | 30 tablet [PoM] £17.28 DT = £17.28

▸ Nifedipress MR (Dexcel-Pharma Ltd)
Nifedipine 10 mg Nifedipress MR 10 tablets | 56 tablet [PoM] £9.23 DT = £7.34
Nifedipine 20 mg Nifedipress MR 20 tablets | 56 tablet [PoM] £10.06 DT = £8.81
▸ Tensipine MR (Thornton & Ross Ltd)
Nifedipine 10 mg Tensipine MR 10 tablets | 56 tablet [PoM] £4.30 DT = £7.34
Nifedipine 20 mg Tensipine MR 20 tablets | 56 tablet [PoM] £5.49 DT = £8.81
▸ Valni Retard (Tillomed Laboratories Ltd)
Nifedipine 20 mg Valni 20 Retard tablets | 56 tablet [PoM] £10.06 DT = £8.81
▸ Valni XL (Zentiva)
Nifedipine 30 mg Valni XL 30mg tablets | 28 tablet [PoM] £9.14 DT = £6.85
Nifedipine 60 mg Valni XL 60mg tablets | 28 tablet [PoM] £21.85 DT = £9.03

Modified-release capsule
CAUTIONARY AND ADVISORY LABELS 25
▸ Coracten SR (UCB Pharma Ltd)
Nifedipine 10 mg Coracten SR 10mg capsules | 60 capsule [PoM] £3.90 DT = £3.90
Nifedipine 20 mg Coracten SR 20mg capsules | 60 capsule [PoM] £5.41 DT = £5.41
▸ Coracten XL (UCB Pharma Ltd)
Nifedipine 30 mg Coracten XL 30mg capsules | 28 capsule [PoM] £4.89 DT = £4.89
Nifedipine 60 mg Coracten XL 60mg capsules | 28 capsule [PoM] £7.34 DT = £7.34

Oral drops
▸ Nifedipine (Non-proprietary)
Nifedipine 20 mg per 1 ml Nifedipin-ratiopharm 20mg/ml oral drops | 30 ml [PoM] [℞]

Capsule
▸ Nifedipine (Non-proprietary)
Nifedipine 5 mg Nifedipine 5mg capsules | 84 capsule [PoM] £2.97-£19.99
Nifedipine 10 mg Nifedipine 10mg capsules | 84 capsule [PoM] £4.00-£21.00
▸ Adalat (Bayer Plc)
Nifedipine 5 mg Adalat 5mg capsules | 90 capsule [PoM] £5.73 DT = £5.73
Nifedipine 10 mg Adalat 10mg capsules | 90 capsule [PoM] £7.30 DT = £7.30

Combinations available: *Atenolol with nifedipine,* p. 152

F 155

Verapamil hydrochloride

● INDICATIONS AND DOSE
Treatment of supraventricular arrhythmias
▸ BY MOUTH USING IMMEDIATE-RELEASE MEDICINES
▸ Adult: 40–120 mg 3 times a day
▸ BY SLOW INTRAVENOUS INJECTION
▸ Adult: 5–10 mg, to be given over 2 minutes, preferably with ECG monitoring
▸ Elderly: 5–10 mg, to be given over 3 minutes, preferably with ECG monitoring

Paroxysmal tachyarrhythmias
▸ BY SLOW INTRAVENOUS INJECTION
▸ Adult: Initially 5–10 mg, followed by 5 mg after 5–10 minutes if required, to be given over 2 minutes, preferably with ECG monitoring
▸ Elderly: Initially 5–10 mg, followed by 5 mg after 5–10 minutes if required, to be given over 3 minutes, preferably with ECG monitoring

Angina
▸ BY MOUTH USING IMMEDIATE-RELEASE MEDICINES
▸ Adult: 80–120 mg 3 times a day

Hypertension
▸ BY MOUTH USING IMMEDIATE-RELEASE MEDICINES
▸ Adult: 240–480 mg daily in 2–3 divided doses

continued →

Prophylaxis of cluster headache (initiated under specialist supervision)
▸ BY MOUTH USING IMMEDIATE-RELEASE MEDICINES
▸ Adult: 240–960 mg daily in 3–4 divided doses

HALF SECURON ® SR

Hypertension (in patients new to verapamil)
▸ BY MOUTH
▸ Adult: Initially 120 mg daily, increased if necessary up to 480 mg daily, doses above 240 mg daily as 2 divided doses

Hypertension
▸ BY MOUTH
▸ Adult: 240 mg daily, increased if necessary up to 480 mg daily, doses above 240 mg daily as 2 divided doses

Angina
▸ BY MOUTH
▸ Adult: 240 mg twice daily, may sometimes be reduced to once daily

Prophylaxis after myocardial infarction where beta-blockers not appropriate
▸ BY MOUTH
▸ Adult: 360 mg daily in divided doses, started at least 1 week after infarction, given as either 240 mg in the morning and 120 mg in the evening *or* 120 mg 3 times daily

SECURON ® SR

Hypertension (in patients new to verapamil)
▸ BY MOUTH
▸ Adult: Initially 120 mg daily, increased if necessary up to 480 mg daily, doses above 240 mg daily as 2 divided doses

Hypertension
▸ BY MOUTH
▸ Adult: 240 mg daily, increased if necessary up to 480 mg daily, doses above 240 mg daily as 2 divided doses

Angina
▸ BY MOUTH
▸ Adult: 240 mg twice daily, may sometimes be reduced to once daily

Prophylaxis after myocardial infarction where beta-blockers not appropriate
▸ BY MOUTH
▸ Adult: 360 mg daily in divided doses, started at least 1 week after infarction, given as either 240 mg in the morning and 120 mg in the evening *or* 120 mg 3 times daily

VERAPRESS ® MR

Hypertension
▸ BY MOUTH
▸ Adult: 240 mg daily, increased if necessary to 240 mg twice daily

Angina
▸ BY MOUTH
▸ Adult: 240 mg twice daily, may sometimes be reduced to once daily

VERTAB ® SR 240

Mild to moderate hypertension
▸ BY MOUTH
▸ Adult: 240 mg daily, increased if necessary to 240 mg twice daily

Angina
▸ BY MOUTH
▸ Adult: 240 mg twice daily, may sometimes be reduced to once daily

● UNLICENSED USE
▸ With oral use Prophylaxis of cluster headaches is an unlicensed indication.

● CONTRA-INDICATIONS Acute porphyrias p. 1025 · atrial flutter or fibrillation associated with accessory conducting pathways (e.g. Wolff-Parkinson-White-syndrome) · bradycardia · cardiogenic shock · history of heart failure (even if controlled by therapy) · history of significantly impaired left ventricular function (even if controlled by therapy) · hypotension · second- and third-degree AV block · sick sinus syndrome · sino-atrial block

● CAUTIONS Acute phase of myocardial infarction (avoid if bradycardia, hypotension, left ventricular failure) · first-degree AV block

● INTERACTIONS → Appendix 1: calcium channel blockers

● SIDE-EFFECTS
GENERAL SIDE-EFFECTS
▸ **Common or very common** Hypotension
▸ **Frequency not known** Atrioventricular block · extrapyramidal symptoms · gynaecomastia · Stevens-Johnson syndrome · vertigo
SPECIFIC SIDE-EFFECTS
▸ **Common or very common**
▸ With intravenous use Bradycardia
▸ **Frequency not known**
▸ With intravenous use Cardiac arrest · drowsiness · hepatic impairment · hyperhidrosis · myocardial contractility decreased · nervousness · seizure
▸ With oral use Alopecia · angioedema · arthralgia · constipation · fatigue · galactorrhoea · gastrointestinal discomfort · heart failure · ileus · muscle weakness · myalgia · paraesthesia · tinnitus · tremor

Overdose In overdose, verapamil has a profound cardiac depressant effect causing hypotension and arrhythmias, including complete heart block and asystole.

● PREGNANCY May reduce uterine blood flow with fetal hypoxia. Manufacturer advises avoid in first trimester unless absolutely necessary. May inhibit labour.

● BREAST FEEDING Amount too small to be harmful.

● HEPATIC IMPAIRMENT
Dose adjustments Oral dose may need to be reduced.

● MEDICINAL FORMS
There can be variation in the licensing of different medicines containing the same drug. Forms available from special-order manufacturers include: oral suspension, oral solution
Modified-release tablet
CAUTIONARY AND ADVISORY LABELS 25
▸ Half Securon (Mylan)
Verapamil hydrochloride 120 mg Half Securon SR 120mg tablets | 28 tablet [PoM] £7.71 DT = £7.71
▸ Securon SR (Mylan)
Verapamil hydrochloride 240 mg Securon SR 240mg tablets | 28 tablet [PoM] £5.55 DT = £5.55
▸ Verapress MR (Dexcel-Pharma Ltd)
Verapamil hydrochloride 240 mg Verapress MR 240mg tablets | 28 tablet [PoM] £9.90 DT = £5.55
▸ Vertab SR (Chiesi Ltd)
Verapamil hydrochloride 240 mg Vertab SR 240 tablets | 28 tablet [PoM] £5.45 DT = £5.55
Tablet
▸ Verapamil hydrochloride (Non-proprietary)
Verapamil hydrochloride 40 mg Verapamil 40mg tablets | 84 tablet [PoM] £2.07 DT = £1.40
Verapamil hydrochloride 80 mg Verapamil 80mg tablets | 84 tablet [PoM] £2.33 DT = £1.74
Verapamil hydrochloride 120 mg Verapamil 120mg tablets | 28 tablet [PoM] £2.43 DT = £1.18
Verapamil hydrochloride 160 mg Verapamil 160mg tablets | 56 tablet [PoM] £28.20 DT = £28.20

Solution for injection
▶ Securon (Mylan)
Verapamil hydrochloride 2.5 mg per 1 ml Securon IV 5mg/2ml
solution for injection ampoules | 5 ampoule PoM £5.41

Oral solution
▶ Verapamil hydrochloride (Non-proprietary)
Verapamil hydrochloride 8 mg per 1 ml Verapamil 40mg/5ml oral
solution sugar free sugar-free | 150 ml PoM £39.00 DT = £39.00

DIURETICS > POTASSIUM-SPARING DIURETICS

Amiloride with cyclopenthiazide

The properties listed below are those particular to the
combination only. For the properties of the components
please consider, amiloride hydrochloride p. 228,
cyclopenthiazide p. 230.

- **INDICATIONS AND DOSE**
Hypertension
▶ BY MOUTH
▶ Adult: 1–2 tablets daily, dose to be taken in the
  morning

- **INTERACTIONS** → Appendix 1: potassium-sparing diuretics
  · thiazide diuretics

- **MEDICINAL FORMS**
  There can be variation in the licensing of different medicines
  containing the same drug.
  Tablet
  EXCIPIENTS: May contain Gluten
  ▶ Navispare (AMCo)
  **Cyclopenthiazide 250 microgram, Amiloride hydrochloride
  2.5 mg** Navispare 2.5mg/250microgram tablets | 28 tablet PoM
  £3.24 DT = £3.24

DIURETICS > THIAZIDES AND RELATED DIURETICS

Thiazides and related diuretics 🔓

- **CONTRA-INDICATIONS** Addison's disease · hypercalcaemia ·
  hyponatraemia · refractory hypokalaemia · symptomatic
  hyperuricaemia

- **CAUTIONS** Diabetes · gout · hyperaldosteronism ·
  malnourishment · nephrotic syndrome · systemic lupus
  erythematosus

  CAUTIONS, FURTHER INFORMATION
▶ **Potassium loss** Hypokalaemia can occur with both thiazide
  and loop diuretics. The risk of hypokalaemia depends on
  the duration of action as well as the potency and is thus
  greater with thiazides than with an equipotent dose of a
  loop diuretic.
    Hypokalaemia is dangerous in severe cardiovascular
  disease and in patients also being treated with cardiac
  glycosides. Often the use of potassium-sparing diuretics
  avoids the need to take potassium supplements.
    Potassium supplements or potassium-sparing diuretics
  are seldom necessary when thiazides are used in the
  routine treatment of hypertension.
    In hepatic failure, hypokalaemia caused by diuretics can
  precipitate encephalopathy, particularly in alcoholic
  cirrhosis.
▶ **Elderly** Lower initial doses of diuretics should be used in
  the elderly because they are particularly susceptible to the
  side-effects. The dose should then be adjusted according
  to renal function. Diuretics should not be used
  continuously on a long-term basis to treat simple
  gravitational oedema (which will usually respond to
  increased movement, raising the legs, and support
  stockings).
▶ **Existing conditions** Thiazides and related diuretics can
  exacerbate diabetes, gout, and systemic lupus
  erythematosus.

- **SIDE-EFFECTS**
▶ **Common or very common** Constipation · electrolyte
  imbalance · headache · postural hypotension · severe
  cutaneous adverse reactions (SCARs) · skin reactions
▶ **Rare or very rare** Leucopenia · thrombocytopenia

- **PREGNANCY** Thiazides and related diuretics should not be
  used to treat gestational hypertension. They may cause
  neonatal thrombocytopenia, bone marrow suppression,
  jaundice, electrolyte disturbances, and hypoglycaemia;
  placental perfusion may also be reduced. Stimulation of
  labour, uterine inertia, and meconium staining have also
  been reported.

- **HEPATIC IMPAIRMENT** Caution in mild to moderate
  impairment. Avoid in severe liver disease. Hypokalaemia
  may precipitate coma in hepatic impairment, although
  hypokalaemia can be prevented by using a potassium-
  sparing diuretic. There is an increased risk of
  hypomagnesaemia in alcoholic cirrhosis.

- **RENAL IMPAIRMENT** Thiazides and related diuretics are
  ineffective if eGFR is less than 30 mL/minute/1.73 m^2 and
  should be avoided. Metolazone remains effective if eGFR is
  less than 30 mL/minute/1.73 m^2 but is associated with a
  risk of excessive diuresis.
  Monitoring Electrolytes should be monitored in renal
  impairment.

- **MONITORING REQUIREMENTS** Electrolytes should be
  monitored, particularly with high doses and long-term
  use.

⬛ above

Bendroflumethiazide

(Bendrofluazide)

- **INDICATIONS AND DOSE**
Oedema
▶ BY MOUTH
▶ Adult: Initially 5–10 mg once daily or on alternate
  days, dose to be taken in the morning, then
  maintenance 5–10 mg 1–3 times a week
Hypertension
▶ BY MOUTH
▶ Adult: 2.5 mg daily, dose to be taken in the morning,
  higher doses are rarely necessary

- **INTERACTIONS** → Appendix 1: thiazide diuretics

- **SIDE-EFFECTS** Agranulocytosis · alkalosis hypochloraemic
  · aplastic anaemia · blood disorder · cholestasis · diarrhoea ·
  electrolyte imbalance · erectile dysfunction ·
  gastrointestinal disorder · gout · hyperglycaemia ·
  hyperuricaemia · neutropenia · pancreatitis ·
  photosensitivity reaction · pneumonitis · pulmonary
  oedema

- **BREAST FEEDING** The amount present in milk is too small
  to be harmful. Large doses may suppress lactation.

- **MEDICINAL FORMS**
  There can be variation in the licensing of different medicines
  containing the same drug. Forms available from special-order
  manufacturers include: oral suspension, oral solution
  Tablet
  ▶ Bendroflumethiazide (Non-proprietary)
    Bendroflumethiazide 2.5 mg Bendroflumethiazide 2.5mg tablets |
    28 tablet PoM £3.68 DT = £0.28 | 500 tablet PoM £5.00–£21.85
    Bendroflumethiazide 5 mg Bendroflumethiazide 5mg tablets |
    28 tablet PoM £9.80 DT = £0.34
  ▶ Aprinox (AMCo)
    Bendroflumethiazide 2.5 mg Aprinox 2.5mg tablets |
    500 tablet PoM £27.31
  ▶ Neo-Naclex (AMCo)
    Bendroflumethiazide 2.5 mg Neo-Naclex 2.5mg tablets |
    28 tablet PoM £0.33 DT = £0.28

  Combinations available: *Timolol with bendroflumethiazide*,
  p. 151

2 Cardiovascular system

☞ 165

Co-amilozide

- **INDICATIONS AND DOSE**

Hypertension
▸ BY MOUTH
- Adult: Initially 2.5/25 mg daily, increased if necessary up to 5/50 mg daily

Congestive heart failure
▸ BY MOUTH
- Adult: Initially 2.5/25 mg daily; increased if necessary up to 10/100 mg daily, reduce dose for maintenance if possible

Oedema and ascites in cirrhosis of the liver
▸ BY MOUTH
- Adult: Initially 5/50 mg daily; increased if necessary up to 10/100 mg daily, reduce dose for maintenance if possible

DOSE EQUIVALENCE AND CONVERSION
- A mixture of amiloride hydrochloride and hydrochlorothiazide in the mass proportions of 1 part amiloride hydrochloride to 10 parts hydrochlorothiazide.

- **CONTRA-INDICATIONS** Anuria · hyperkalaemia
- **CAUTIONS** Diabetes mellitus · elderly
- **INTERACTIONS** → Appendix 1: potassium-sparing diuretics · thiazide diuretics
- **SIDE-EFFECTS** Angina pectoris · appetite abnormal · arrhythmias · arthralgia · asthenia · chest pain · confusion · depression · diarrhoea · dizziness · drowsiness · dyspnoea · electrolyte imbalance · erectile dysfunction · flatulence · flushing · gastrointestinal discomfort · gastrointestinal haemorrhage · gout · hiccups · hyperhidrosis · insomnia · malaise · muscle cramps · nasal congestion · nausea · nervousness · pain · paraesthesia · renal impairment · stupor · syncope · taste unpleasant · urinary disorders · vertigo · visual impairment · vomiting
- **BREAST FEEDING** Avoid—no information regarding amiloride component available. Amount of hydrochlorothiazide in milk probably too small to be harmful. Large doses of hydrochlorothiazide may suppress lactation.
- **RENAL IMPAIRMENT** Manufacturers advise avoid in severe impairment.
  Monitoring Monitor plasma-potassium concentration (high risk of hyperkalaemia in renal impairment).
- **MONITORING REQUIREMENTS** Monitor electrolytes.

- **MEDICINAL FORMS**
There can be variation in the licensing of different medicines containing the same drug. Forms available from special-order manufacturers include: oral solution
Tablet
  ▸ Co-amilozide (Non-proprietary)
    Amiloride hydrochloride 2.5 mg, Hydrochlorothiazide 25 mg Co-amilozide 2.5mg/25mg tablets | 28 tablet [PoM] £7.56 DT = £6.05
    Amiloride hydrochloride 5 mg, Hydrochlorothiazide 50 mg Co-amilozide 5mg/50mg tablets | 28 tablet [PoM] £1.68 DT = £1.24
  ▸ Moduret (Merck Sharp & Dohme Ltd)
    Amiloride hydrochloride 2.5 mg, Hydrochlorothiazide 25 mg Moduret 25 tablets | 28 tablet [PoM] £0.86 DT = £6.05
  ▸ Moduretic (Merck Sharp & Dohme Ltd)
    Amiloride hydrochloride 5 mg, Hydrochlorothiazide 50 mg Moduretic 5mg/50mg tablets | 28 tablet [PoM] £1.29 DT = £1.24

☞ 165

Hydrochlorothiazide

- **INDICATIONS AND DOSE**

Indications listed in combination monographs (available in the UK only in combination with other drugs)
▸ BY MOUTH
- Adult: Doses listed in combination monographs

- **INTERACTIONS** → Appendix 1: thiazide diuretics

- **MEDICINAL FORMS**
No licensed medicines listed.

  Combinations available: Co-zidocapt, p. 168 ·
  Enalapril with hydrochlorothiazide, p. 169 ·
  Irbesartan with hydrochlorothiazide, p. 175 ·
  Lisinopril with hydrochlorothiazide, p. 170 ·
  Losartan with hydrochlorothiazide, p. 176 ·
  Olmesartan with amlodipine and hydrochlorothiazide, p. 177 ·
  Olmesartan with hydrochlorothiazide, p. 177 ·
  Quinapril with hydrochlorothiazide, p. 172 ·
  Telmisartan with hydrochlorothiazide, p. 178 ·
  Timolol with amiloride and hydrochlorothiazide, p. 151 ·
  Valsartan with hydrochlorothiazide, p. 179

☞ 165

Indapamide

- **DRUG ACTION** Indapamide is a thiazide-like diuretic with antihypertensive effects. At lower doses, vasodilatation is more prominent than diuresis; the diuretic effect becomes more apparent with higher doses.

- **INDICATIONS AND DOSE**

Essential hypertension
▸ BY MOUTH USING IMMEDIATE-RELEASE MEDICINES
- Adult: 2.5 mg daily, dose to be taken in the morning
▸ BY MOUTH USING MODIFIED-RELEASE MEDICINES
- Adult: 1.5 mg daily, dose to be taken preferably in the morning

- **CAUTIONS** Acute porphyrias p. 1025
- **INTERACTIONS** → Appendix 1: thiazide diuretics
- **SIDE-EFFECTS**
▸ **Common or very common** Hypersensitivity
▸ **Uncommon** Vomiting
▸ **Rare or very rare** Agranulocytosis · angioedema · aplastic anaemia · arrhythmias · dry mouth · fatigue · haemolytic anaemia · hepatic disorders · hypercalcaemia · nausea · pancreatitis · paraesthesia · renal failure · vertigo
▸ **Frequency not known** Hepatic encephalopathy · photosensitivity reaction · QT interval prolongation · syncope · systemic lupus erythematosus exacerbated · vision disorders

- **ALLERGY AND CROSS-SENSITIVITY** Contra-indicated if history of hypersensitivity to sulfonamides.
- **BREAST FEEDING** Present in milk—manufacturer advises avoid.

- **MEDICINAL FORMS**
There can be variation in the licensing of different medicines containing the same drug. Forms available from special-order manufacturers include: oral suspension
Modified-release tablet
CAUTIONARY AND ADVISORY LABELS 25
  ▸ Indapamide (Non-proprietary)
    Indapamide 1.5 mg Indapamide 1.5mg modified-release tablets | 30 tablet [PoM] £3.40 DT = £3.40
  ▸ Alkapamid XL (HBS Healthcare Ltd)
    Indapamide 1.5 mg Alkapamid XL 1.5mg tablets | 30 tablet [PoM] £2.20 DT = £3.40
  ▸ Cardide SR (Teva UK Ltd)
    Indapamide 1.5 mg Cardide SR 1.5mg tablets | 30 tablet [PoM] £4.32 DT = £3.40

▸ Indipam XL (Actavis UK Ltd)
Indapamide 1.5 mg Indipam XL 1.5mg tablets | 30 tablet PoM
£4.32 DT = £3.40

▸ Natrilix SR (Servier Laboratories Ltd)
Indapamide 1.5 mg Natrilix SR 1.5mg tablets | 30 tablet PoM £3.40
DT = £3.40

▸ Rawel XL (Consilient Health Ltd)
Indapamide 1.5 mg Rawel XL 1.5mg tablets | 30 tablet PoM £2.89
DT = £3.40

▸ Tensaid XL (Mylan)
Indapamide 1.5 mg Tensaid XL 1.5mg tablets | 30 tablet PoM
£3.40 DT = £3.40

Tablet

▸ Indapamide (Non-proprietary)
Indapamide hemihydrate 2.5 mg Indapamide 2.5mg tablets |
28 tablet PoM £29.00 DT = £0.70 | 56 tablet PoM £1.40–£12.68

▸ Natrilix (Servier Laboratories Ltd)
Indapamide hemihydrate 2.5 mg Natrilix 2.5mg tablets |
30 tablet PoM £3.40 | 60 tablet PoM £6.80

Combinations available: *Perindopril arginine with*
indapamide, p. 171

DRUGS ACTING ON THE RENIN-ANGIOTENSIN SYSTEM > ACE INHIBITORS

Angiotensin-converting enzyme inhibitors

- CONTRA-INDICATIONS The combination of an ACE
  inhibitor with aliskiren is contra-indicated in patients with
  an eGFR less than 60 mL/minute/1.73 m^2 · the combination
  of an ACE inhibitor with aliskiren is contra-indicated in
  patients with diabetes mellitus

- CAUTIONS Afro-Caribbean patients (may respond less well
  to ACE inhibitors) · concomitant diuretics · diabetes (may
  lower blood glucose) · first dose hypotension (especially in
  patients taking high doses of diuretics, on a low-sodium
  diet, on dialysis, dehydrated, or with heart failure) ·
  peripheral vascular disease or generalised atherosclerosis
  (risk of clinically silent renovascular disease) · primary
  aldosteronism (patients may respond less well to ACE
  inhibitors) · the risk of agranulocytosis is possibly
  increased in collagen vascular disease (blood counts
  recommended) · use with care (or avoid) in those with a
  history of idiopathic or hereditary angioedema · use with
  care in patients with hypertrophic cardiomyopathy · use
  with care in patients with severe or symptomatic aortic
  stenosis (risk of hypotension)

  CAUTIONS, FURTHER INFORMATION
▸ Anaphylactoid reactions To prevent anaphylactoid reactions,
  ACE inhibitors should be avoided during dialysis with
  high-flux polyacrylonitrile membranes and during low-
  density lipoprotein apheresis with dextran sulfate; they
  should also be withheld before desensitisation with wasp
  or bee venom.

- SIDE-EFFECTS
▸ **Common or very common** Alopecia · angina pectoris ·
  angioedema (may be delayed; more common in Afro-
  Caribbean patients · arrhythmias · asthenia · chest pain ·
  constipation · cough · diarrhoea · dizziness · drowsiness ·
  dry mouth · dyspnoea · electrolyte imbalance ·
  gastrointestinal discomfort · headache · hypotension ·
  myalgia · nausea · palpitations · paraesthesia · renal
  impairment · rhinitis · skin reactions (uncommon in
  children) · sleep disorder · syncope · taste altered · tinnitus ·
  vertigo · vomiting
▸ **Uncommon** Arthralgia · confusion · eosinophilia · erectile
  dysfunction · fever · haemolytic anaemia · hyperhidrosis ·
  myocardial infarction · pancreatitis · peripheral oedema ·
  photosensitivity reaction · respiratory disorders · stroke

▸ **Rare or very rare** Agranulocytosis · hepatic disorders ·
  leucopenia · neutropenia · pancytopenia · Stevens-Johnson
  syndrome · thrombocytopenia

  SIDE-EFFECTS, FURTHER INFORMATION In light of reports
  of cholestatic jaundice, hepatitis, fulminant hepatic
  necrosis, and hepatic failure, ACE inhibitors should be
  discontinued if marked elevation of hepatic enzymes or
  jaundice occur.

- ALLERGY AND CROSS-SENSITIVITY ACE inhibitors are
  contra-indicated in patients with hypersensitivity to ACE
  inhibitors (including angioedema).

- PREGNANCY ACE inhibitors should be avoided in
  pregnancy unless essential. They may adversely affect fetal
  and neonatal blood pressure control and renal function;
  skull defects and oligohydramnios have also been
  reported.

- BREAST FEEDING Information on the use of ACE inhibitors
  in breast-feeding is limited.

- RENAL IMPAIRMENT
  Dose adjustments Use with caution, starting with low dose,
  and adjust according to response. Hyperkalaemia and
  other side-effects of ACE inhibitors are more common in
  those with impaired renal function and the dose may need
  to be reduced.

- MONITORING REQUIREMENTS Renal function and
  electrolytes should be checked before starting ACE
  inhibitors (or increasing the dose) and monitored during
  treatment (more frequently if side effects mentioned are
  present).

- DIRECTIONS FOR ADMINISTRATION For hypertension the
  first dose should preferably be given at bedtime.

▸ above

Captopril

- **INDICATIONS AND DOSE**

Hypertension
▸ BY MOUTH
▸ Adult: Initially 12.5–25 mg twice daily, then increased
  if necessary up to 150 mg daily in 2 divided doses,
  doses to be increased at intervals of at least 2 weeks,
  once-daily dosing may be appropriate if other
  concomitant antihypertensive drugs taken
▸ Elderly: Initially 6.25 mg twice daily, then increased if
  necessary up to 150 mg daily in 2 divided doses, doses
  to be increased at intervals of at least 2 weeks, once-
  daily dosing may be appropriate if other concomitant
  antihypertensive drugs taken

**Essential hypertension if used in volume depletion,
cardiac decompensation, or renovascular hypertension**
▸ BY MOUTH
▸ Adult: Initially 6.25–12.5 mg for 1 dose (under close
  medical supervision), then 6.25–12.5 mg twice daily;
  increased if necessary up to 100 mg daily in 1–2 divided
  doses, doses to be increased at intervals of at least
  2 weeks, once-daily dosing may be appropriate if other
  concomitant antihypertensive drugs taken

Heart failure
▸ BY MOUTH
▸ Adult (under close medical supervision): Initially
  6.25–12.5 mg 2–3 times a day, then increased if
  tolerated to up to 150 mg daily in divided doses, dose
  to be increased gradually at intervals of at least 2 weeks

**Short-term treatment within 24 hours of onset of
myocardial infarction in clinically stable patients**
▸ BY MOUTH
▸ Adult: Initially 6.25 mg, then increased to 12.5 mg after
  2 hours, followed by 25 mg after 12 hours; increased if
  tolerated to 50 mg twice daily for 4 weeks continued →

Prophylaxis of symptomatic heart failure after myocardial infarction in clinically stable patients with asymptomatic left ventricular dysfunction (starting 3–16 days after infarction) (under close medical supervision)
▸ BY MOUTH
▸ Adult: Initially 6.25 mg daily, then increased to 12.5 mg 3 times a day for 2 days, then increased if tolerated to 25 mg 3 times a day, then increased if tolerated to 75–150 mg daily in 2–3 divided doses, doses exceeding 75 mg per day to be increased gradually

Diabetic nephropathy in type 1 diabetes mellitus
▸ BY MOUTH
▸ Adult: 75–100 mg daily in divided doses

● CAUTIONS Children (efficacy and safety not fully established)

● INTERACTIONS → Appendix 1: ACE inhibitors

● SIDE-EFFECTS
▸ **Common or very common** Epigastric discomfort · peptic ulcer
▸ **Uncommon** Appetite decreased · flushing · malaise · pallor · postural hypotension · Raynaud's phenomenon
▸ **Rare or very rare** Alveolitis allergic · anaemia · aplastic anaemia · autoimmune disorder · cardiac arrest · cardiogenic shock · cerebrovascular insufficiency · depression · gynaecomastia · hypoglycaemia · lymphadenopathy · nephrotic syndrome · oliguria · oral disorders · proteinuria · urinary disorders · vision blurred

● BREAST FEEDING Avoid in first few weeks after delivery, particularly in preterm infants—risk of profound neonatal hypotension; can be used in mothers breast-feeding older infants if essential but monitor infant's blood pressure.

● RENAL IMPAIRMENT
Dose adjustments Reduce dose; max. initial dose 50 mg if eGFR above 40 mL/minute/1.73 m^2; max. initial dose 25 mg daily (do not exceed 100 mg daily) if eGFR 20–40 mL/minute/1.73 m^2; max. initial dose 12.5 mg daily (do not exceed 75 mg daily) if eGFR 10–20 mL/minute/1.73 m^2; max. initial dose 6.25 mg daily (do not exceed 37.5 mg daily) if eGFR less than 10 mL/minute/1.73 m^2.

● MEDICINAL FORMS
There can be variation in the licensing of different medicines containing the same drug. Forms available from special-order manufacturers include: tablet, capsule, oral suspension, oral solution
Tablet
▸ Captopril (Non-proprietary)
   Captopril 12.5 mg Captopril 12.5mg tablets | 56 tablet [PoM] £2.80 DT = £2.06 | 100 tablet [PoM] £5.00
   Captopril 25 mg Captopril 25mg tablets | 56 tablet [PoM] £4.52 DT = £0.56 | 100 tablet [PoM] £8.07
   Captopril 50 mg Captopril 50mg tablets | 56 tablet [PoM] £5.83 DT = £2.15 | 100 tablet [PoM] £10.41
▸ Ecopace (AMCo)
   Captopril 12.5 mg Ecopace 12.5mg tablets | 56 tablet [PoM] £0.48 DT = £2.06
   Captopril 25 mg Ecopace 25mg tablets | 56 tablet [PoM] £0.60 DT = £0.56
   Captopril 50 mg Ecopace 50mg tablets | 56 tablet [PoM] £0.72 DT = £2.15
Oral solution
ELECTROLYTES: May contain Sodium
▸ Noyada (Martindale Pharmaceuticals Ltd)
   Captopril 1 mg per 1 ml Noyada 5mg/5ml oral solution sugar-free | 100 ml [PoM] £98.21 DT = £98.21
   Captopril 5 mg per 1 ml Noyada 25mg/5ml oral solution sugar-free | 100 ml [PoM] £108.94 DT = £108.94

Co-zidocapt

The properties listed below are those particular to the combination only. For the properties of the components please consider, captopril p. 167, hydrochlorothiazide p. 166.

● INDICATIONS AND DOSE

Mild to moderate hypertension in patients stabilised on the individual components in the same proportions
▸ BY MOUTH
▸ Adult: (consult product literature)

● INTERACTIONS → Appendix 1: ACE inhibitors · thiazide diuretics

● MEDICINAL FORMS
There can be variation in the licensing of different medicines containing the same drug.
Tablet
▸ Co-zidocapt (Non-proprietary)
   Hydrochlorothiazide 12.5 mg, Captopril 25 mg Co-zidocapt 12.5mg/25mg tablets | 28 tablet [PoM] £11.00
   Hydrochlorothiazide 25 mg, Captopril 50 mg Co-zidocapt 25mg/50mg tablets | 28 tablet [PoM] £14.00

☞ 167

Enalapril maleate

● INDICATIONS AND DOSE

Hypertension
▸ BY MOUTH
▸ Adult: Initially 5 mg once daily, lower initial doses may be required when used in addition to diuretic or in renal impairment; maintenance 20 mg once daily; maximum 40 mg per day

Heart failure
▸ BY MOUTH
▸ Adult (under close medical supervision): Initially 2.5 mg once daily, increased if tolerated to 10–20 mg twice daily, dose to be increased gradually over 2–4 weeks

Prevention of symptomatic heart failure in patients with asymptomatic left ventricular dysfunction
▸ BY MOUTH
▸ Adult (under close medical supervision): Initially 2.5 mg once daily, increased if tolerated to 10–20 mg twice daily, dose to be increased gradually over 2–4 weeks

● INTERACTIONS → Appendix 1: ACE inhibitors

● SIDE-EFFECTS
▸ **Common or very common** Depression · hypersensitivity · postural hypotension · vision blurred
▸ **Uncommon** Anaemia · appetite decreased · asthma · bone marrow disorders · epigastric discomfort · flushing · gastrointestinal disorders · hoarseness · hypoglycaemia · malaise · muscle cramps · nervousness · proteinuria · rhinorrhoea · throat pain
▸ **Rare or very rare** Autoimmune disorder · gynaecomastia · lymphadenopathy · oliguria · oral disorders · Raynaud's phenomenon · toxic epidermal necrolysis
▸ **Frequency not known** Arthritis · leucocytosis · myositis · serositis · SIADH · vasculitis

● BREAST FEEDING Avoid in first few weeks after delivery, particularly in preterm infants—risk of profound neonatal hypotension; can be used in mothers breast-feeding older infants if essential but monitor infant's blood pressure.

● HEPATIC IMPAIRMENT
Monitoring Enalapril is a prodrug and requires close monitoring in patients with hepatic impairment.

● RENAL IMPAIRMENT
Dose adjustments Max. initial dose 2.5 mg daily if eGFR less than 30 mL/minute/1.73 m^2.

● DIRECTIONS FOR ADMINISTRATION Tablets may be crushed and suspended in water immediately before use.

● MEDICINAL FORMS
There can be variation in the licensing of different medicines containing the same drug. Forms available from special-order manufacturers include: oral suspension, oral solution

Tablet
▸ Enalapril maleate (Non-proprietary)
Enalapril maleate 2.5 mg Enalapril 2.5mg tablets | 28 tablet PoM
£5.63 DT = £4.84
Enalapril maleate 5 mg Enalapril 5mg tablets | 28 tablet PoM
£4.13 DT = £2.28
Enalapril maleate 10 mg Enalapril 10mg tablets | 28 tablet PoM
£5.64 DT = £2.14
Enalapril maleate 20 mg Enalapril 20mg tablets | 28 tablet PoM
£6.63 DT = £1.94
▸ Innovace (Merck Sharp & Dohme Ltd)
Enalapril maleate 2.5 mg Innovace 2.5mg tablets | 28 tablet PoM
£5.35 DT = £4.84
Enalapril maleate 5 mg Innovace 5mg tablets | 28 tablet PoM
£7.51 DT = £2.28
Enalapril maleate 10 mg Innovace 10mg tablets | 28 tablet PoM
£10.53 DT = £2.14
Enalapril maleate 20 mg Innovace 20mg tablets | 28 tablet PoM
£12.51 DT = £1.94

Enalapril with hydrochlorothiazide

The properties listed below are those particular to the combination only. For the properties of the components please consider, enalapril maleate p. 168, hydrochlorothiazide p. 166.

● INDICATIONS AND DOSE
Mild to moderate hypertension in patients stabilised on the individual components in the same proportions
▸ BY MOUTH
▸ Adult: (consult product literature)

● INTERACTIONS → Appendix 1: ACE inhibitors · thiazide diuretics

● MEDICINAL FORMS
There can be variation in the licensing of different medicines containing the same drug.
Tablet
▸ Enalapril with hydrochlorothiazide (Non-proprietary)
Hydrochlorothiazide 12.5 mg, Enalapril maleate 20 mg Enalapril 20mg / Hydrochlorothiazide 12.5mg tablets | 28 tablet PoM £20.00
DT = £19.98
▸ Innozide (Merck Sharp & Dohme Ltd)
Hydrochlorothiazide 12.5 mg, Enalapril maleate 20 mg Innozide 20mg/12.5mg tablets | 28 tablet PoM £13.90 DT = £19.98

F 167

Fosinopril sodium

● INDICATIONS AND DOSE
Hypertension
▸ BY MOUTH
▸ Adult: Initially 10 mg daily for 4 weeks, then increased if necessary up to 40 mg daily, doses over 40 mg not shown to increase efficacy
Congestive heart failure (adjunct) (under close medical supervision)
▸ BY MOUTH
▸ Adult: Initially 10 mg once daily, then increased if tolerated to 40 mg once daily, doses to be increased gradually

● INTERACTIONS → Appendix 1: ACE inhibitors
● SIDE-EFFECTS
▸ **Common or very common** Eye disorder · increased risk of infection · mood altered · oedema · pain · postural hypotension · urinary disorder · visual impairment
▸ **Frequency not known** Abdominal distension · appetite abnormal · arthritis · balance impaired · behaviour abnormal · cardiac arrest · cardiac conduction disorder ·

cerebrovascular insufficiency · depression · dysphagia · dysphonia · ear pain · flatulence · flushing · gout · haemorrhage · hypertensive crisis · lymphadenopathy · memory loss · muscle weakness · oral disorders · prostatic disorder · tremor · weight changes
● BREAST FEEDING Not recommended; alternative treatment options, with better established safety information during breast-feeding, are available.
● HEPATIC IMPAIRMENT
Monitoring Fosinopril is a prodrug and requires close monitoring in patients with hepatic impairment.

● MEDICINAL FORMS
There can be variation in the licensing of different medicines containing the same drug. Forms available from special-order manufacturers include: oral suspension, oral solution
Tablet
▸ Fosinopril sodium (Non-proprietary)
Fosinopril sodium 10 mg Fosinopril 10mg tablets | 28 tablet PoM
£28.50 DT = £5.36
Fosinopril sodium 20 mg Fosinopril 20mg tablets | 28 tablet PoM
£38.98 DT = £4.86

F 167

Imidapril hydrochloride

● INDICATIONS AND DOSE
Essential hypertension
▸ BY MOUTH
▸ Adult: Initially 5 mg daily, increased if necessary to 10 mg daily, dose to be taken before food, doses to be increased at intervals of at least 3 weeks; maximum 20 mg per day
▸ Elderly: Initially 2.5 mg daily, increased if necessary to 10 mg daily, dose to be taken before food, doses to be increased at intervals of at least 3 weeks
Essential hypertension in patients with heart failure, angina or cerebrovascular disease, or in renal or hepatic impairment
▸ BY MOUTH
▸ Adult: Initially 2.5 mg daily, increased if necessary to 10 mg daily, dose to be taken before food, dose to be increased at intervals of at least 3 weeks; maximum 20 mg per day

● INTERACTIONS → Appendix 1: ACE inhibitors
● SIDE-EFFECTS
▸ **Uncommon** Cerebrovascular disorder · epigastric pain · increased risk of infection · joint swelling · limb pain · oedema
▸ **Rare or very rare** Anaemia
● BREAST FEEDING Not recommended; alternative treatment options, with better established safety information during breast-feeding, are available.
● HEPATIC IMPAIRMENT
Monitoring Imidapril is a prodrug and requires close monitoring in patients with hepatic impairment.
● RENAL IMPAIRMENT Avoid if eGFR less than 30 mL/minute/1.73 m^2.
Dose adjustments Initial dose 2.5 mg daily if eGFR 30–80 mL/minute/1.73 m^2.

● MEDICINAL FORMS
There can be variation in the licensing of different medicines containing the same drug.
Tablet
▸ Tanatril (Mitsubishi Tanabe Pharma Europe Ltd)
Imidapril hydrochloride 5 mg Tanatril 5mg tablets |
28 tablet PoM £6.40 DT = £6.40
Imidapril hydrochloride 10 mg Tanatril 10mg tablets |
28 tablet PoM £7.22 DT = £7.22
Imidapril hydrochloride 20 mg Tanatril 20mg tablets |
28 tablet PoM £8.67 DT = £8.67

Cardiovascular system 2

Lisinopril
F 167
19-Mar-2018

● INDICATIONS AND DOSE

Hypertension
▸ BY MOUTH
▸ Adult: Initially 10 mg once daily; usual maintenance 20 mg once daily; maximum 80 mg per day

Hypertension, when used in addition to diuretic, in cardiac decompensation or in volume depletion
▸ BY MOUTH
▸ Adult: Initially 2.5–5 mg once daily; usual maintenance 20 mg once daily; maximum 80 mg per day

Short-term treatment following myocardial infarction in haemodynamically stable patients—systolic blood pressure over 120 mmHg
▸ BY MOUTH
▸ Adult: Initially 5 mg, taken within 24 hours of myocardial infarction, followed by 5 mg, to be taken 24 hours after initial dose, then 10 mg, to be taken 24 hours after second dose, then 10 mg once daily for 6 weeks (or continued if heart failure), temporarily reduce maintenance dose to 5 mg and if necessary 2.5 mg daily if systolic blood pressure 100 mmHg or less during treatment; withdraw if prolonged hypotension occurs during treatment (systolic blood pressure less than 90 mmHg for more than 1 hour)

Short-term treatment following myocardial infarction in haemodynamically stable patients—systolic blood pressure 100–120 mmHg
▸ BY MOUTH
▸ Adult: Initially 2.5 mg once daily, maintenance 5 mg once daily, increase to maintenance dose only after at least 3 days of the initial dose, should not be started after myocardial infarction if systolic blood pressure less than 100 mmHg, temporarily reduce maintenance dose to 2.5 mg daily if systolic blood pressure 100 mmHg or less during treatment; withdraw if prolonged hypotension occurs (systolic blood pressure less than 90 mmHg for more than 1 hour)

Renal complications of diabetes mellitus
▸ BY MOUTH
▸ Adult: Initially 2.5–5 mg once daily, adjusted according to response; usual dose 10–20 mg once daily

Heart failure (adjunct) (under close medical supervision)
▸ BY MOUTH
▸ Adult: Initially 2.5 mg once daily; increased in steps of up to 10 mg at least every 2 weeks; maximum 35 mg per day

● INTERACTIONS → Appendix 1: ACE inhibitors

● SIDE-EFFECTS
▸ **Common or very common** Postural disorders
▸ **Uncommon** Hallucination · mood altered · Raynaud's phenomenon
▸ **Rare or very rare** Alveolitis allergic · anaemia · autoimmune disorder · azotaemia · bone marrow depression · gynaecomastia · hypersensitivity · hypoglycaemia · lymphadenopathy · olfactory nerve disorder · SIADH · sinusitis · toxic epidermal necrolysis
▸ **Frequency not known** Leucocytosis · vasculitis

● BREAST FEEDING Not recommended; alternative treatment options, with better established safety information during breast-feeding, are available.

● RENAL IMPAIRMENT
Dose adjustments Max. initial doses 5–10 mg daily if eGFR 30–80 mL/minute/1.73 m^2 (max. 40 mg daily); 2.5–5 mg daily if eGFR 10–30 mL/minute/1.73 m^2 (max. 40 mg daily); 2.5 mg daily if eGFR less than 10 mL/minute/1.73 m^2.

● MEDICINAL FORMS
There can be variation in the licensing of different medicines containing the same drug. Forms available from special-order manufacturers include: oral suspension, oral solution

Oral solution
▸ Lisinopril (Non-proprietary)
Lisinopril 1 mg per 1 ml Lisinopril 5mg/5ml oral solution sugar free sugar-free | 150 ml [PoM] £154.11 DT = £154.11

Tablet
▸ Lisinopril (Non-proprietary)
Lisinopril 2.5 mg Lisinopril 2.5mg tablets | 28 tablet [PoM] £4.81 DT = £0.48
Lisinopril 5 mg Lisinopril 5mg tablets | 28 tablet [PoM] £7.80 DT = £0.46
Lisinopril 10 mg Lisinopril 10mg tablets | 28 tablet [PoM] £11.81 DT = £0.61
Lisinopril 20 mg Lisinopril 20mg tablets | 28 tablet [PoM] £10.90 DT = £0.58
▸ Zestril (AstraZeneca UK Ltd)
Lisinopril 5 mg Zestril 5mg tablets | 28 tablet [PoM] £9.42 DT = £0.46
Lisinopril 10 mg Zestril 10mg tablets | 28 tablet [PoM] £14.76 DT = £0.61
Lisinopril 20 mg Zestril 20mg tablets | 28 tablet [PoM] £13.02 DT = £0.58

Lisinopril with hydrochlorothiazide

The properties listed below are those particular to the combination only. For the properties of the components please consider, lisinopril above, hydrochlorothiazide p. 166.

● INDICATIONS AND DOSE

Mild to moderate hypertension in patients stabilised on the individual components in the same proportions
▸ BY MOUTH
▸ Adult: (consult product literature)

● INTERACTIONS → Appendix 1: ACE inhibitors · thiazide diuretics

● MEDICINAL FORMS
There can be variation in the licensing of different medicines containing the same drug.
Tablet
▸ Lisinopril with hydrochlorothiazide (Non-proprietary)
Lisinopril 10 mg, Hydrochlorothiazide 12.5 mg Lisinopril 10mg / Hydrochlorothiazide 12.5mg tablets | 28 tablet [PoM] £3.15 DT = £3.06
Hydrochlorothiazide 12.5 mg, Lisinopril 20 mg Lisinopril 20mg / Hydrochlorothiazide 12.5mg tablets | 28 tablet [PoM] £2.25 DT = £1.83
▸ Zestoretic (AstraZeneca UK Ltd)
Lisinopril 10 mg, Hydrochlorothiazide 12.5 mg Zestoretic 10 tablets | 28 tablet [PoM] £13.62 DT = £3.06
Hydrochlorothiazide 12.5 mg, Lisinopril 20 mg Zestoretic 20 tablets | 28 tablet [PoM] £13.82 DT = £1.83

Perindopril arginine
F 167

● INDICATIONS AND DOSE

Hypertension
▸ BY MOUTH
▸ Adult: Initially 5 mg once daily for 1 month, dose to be taken in the morning, then, adjusted according to response; maximum 10 mg per day
▸ Elderly: Initially 2.5 mg once daily for 1 month, dose to be taken in the morning, then, adjusted according to response; maximum 10 mg per day

Hypertension, if used in addition to diuretic, or in cardiac decompensation or volume depletion
▸ BY MOUTH
▸ Adult: Initially 2.5 mg once daily for 1 month, dose to be taken in the morning, then, adjusted according to response; maximum 10 mg per day

Symptomatic heart failure (adjunct) (under close medical supervision)
▶ BY MOUTH
▶ Adult: Initially 2.5 mg once daily for 2 weeks, then increased if tolerated to 5 mg once daily, dose to be taken in the morning

Prophylaxis of cardiac events following myocardial infarction or revascularisation in stable coronary artery disease
▶ BY MOUTH
▶ Adult: Initially 5 mg once daily for 2 weeks, then increased if tolerated to 10 mg once daily, dose to be taken in the morning
▶ Elderly: Initially 2.5 mg once daily for 1 week, then increased if tolerated to 5 mg once daily for 1 week, then increased if tolerated to 10 mg once daily, dose to be taken in the morning

● INTERACTIONS → Appendix 1: ACE inhibitors
● SIDE-EFFECTS
▶ **Common or very common** Muscle cramps · visual impairment
▶ **Uncommon** Fall · hypoglycaemia · malaise · mood altered · vasculitis
● HEPATIC IMPAIRMENT
Monitoring Perindopril is a prodrug and requires close monitoring in patients with hepatic impairment.
● RENAL IMPAIRMENT
Dose adjustments Max. initial dose 2.5 mg once daily if eGFR 30–60 mL/minute/1.73 m^2; 2.5 mg once daily on alternate days if eGFR 15–30 mL/minute/1.73 m^2.

● MEDICINAL FORMS
There can be variation in the licensing of different medicines containing the same drug.
Tablet
CAUTIONARY AND ADVISORY LABELS 22
▶ Coversyl Arginine (Servier Laboratories Ltd)
   Perindopril arginine 2.5 mg Coversyl Arginine 2.5mg tablets | 30 tablet [PoM] £4.43 DT = £4.43
   Perindopril arginine 5 mg Coversyl Arginine 5mg tablets | 30 tablet [PoM] £6.28 DT = £6.28
   Perindopril arginine 10 mg Coversyl Arginine 10mg tablets | 30 tablet [PoM] £10.65 DT = £10.65

Perindopril arginine with indapamide

The properties listed below are those particular to the combination only. For the properties of the components please consider, perindopril arginine p. 170, indapamide p. 166.

● INDICATIONS AND DOSE
Hypertension not adequately controlled by perindopril alone
▶ BY MOUTH
▶ Adult: (consult product literature)

● INTERACTIONS → Appendix 1: ACE inhibitors · thiazide diuretics

● MEDICINAL FORMS
There can be variation in the licensing of different medicines containing the same drug.
Tablet
CAUTIONARY AND ADVISORY LABELS 22
▶ Coversyl Arginine Plus (Servier Laboratories Ltd)
   Indapamide 1.25 mg, Perindopril arginine 5 mg Coversyl Arginine Plus 5mg/1.25mg tablets | 30 tablet [PoM] £9.51 DT = £9.51

📖 167

Perindopril erbumine

● INDICATIONS AND DOSE
Hypertension
▶ BY MOUTH
▶ Adult: Initially 4 mg once daily for 1 month, dose to be taken in the morning, then, adjusted according to response; maximum 8 mg per day
▶ BY MOUTH
▶ Elderly: Initially 2 mg once daily for 1 month, dose to be taken in the morning, then, adjusted according to response; maximum 8 mg per day

Hypertension, if used in addition to diuretic, or in cardiac decompensation or volume depletion
▶ BY MOUTH
▶ Adult: Initially 2 mg once daily for 1 month, dose to be taken in the morning, then, adjusted according to response; maximum 8 mg per day

Heart failure (adjunct) (under close medical supervision)
▶ BY MOUTH
▶ Adult: Initially 2 mg once daily for at least 2 weeks, dose to be taken in the morning, then increased if tolerated to 4 mg once daily

Prophylaxis of cardiac events following myocardial infarction or revascularisation in stable coronary artery disease
▶ BY MOUTH
▶ Adult: Initially 4 mg once daily for 2 weeks, dose to be taken in the morning, then increased if tolerated to 8 mg once daily
▶ Elderly: Initially 2 mg once daily for 1 week, then increased if tolerated to 4 mg once daily for 1 week, then increased if tolerated to 8 mg once daily

● INTERACTIONS → Appendix 1: ACE inhibitors
● SIDE-EFFECTS
▶ **Common or very common** Muscle cramps · visual impairment
▶ **Uncommon** Fall · hypoglycaemia · malaise · mood altered · vasculitis
● BREAST FEEDING Not recommended; alternative treatment options, with better established safety information during breast-feeding, are available.
● HEPATIC IMPAIRMENT
Monitoring Perindopril is a prodrug and requires close monitoring in patients with hepatic impairment.
● RENAL IMPAIRMENT
Dose adjustments Max. initial dose 2 mg once daily if eGFR 30–60 mL/minute/1.73 m^2; 2 mg once daily on alternate days if eGFR 15–30 mL/minute/1.73 m^2.

● MEDICINAL FORMS
There can be variation in the licensing of different medicines containing the same drug. Forms available from special-order manufacturers include: oral suspension, oral solution
Tablet
CAUTIONARY AND ADVISORY LABELS 22
▶ Perindopril erbumine (Non-proprietary)
   Perindopril erbumine 2 mg Perindopril erbumine 2mg tablets | 30 tablet [PoM] £12.99 DT = £3.08 | 56 tablet [PoM] £3.34 | 60 tablet [PoM] £13.90
   Perindopril erbumine 4 mg Perindopril erbumine 4mg tablets | 30 tablet [PoM] £12.99 DT = £1.91 | 56 tablet [PoM] £3.38 | 60 tablet [PoM] £27.80
   Perindopril erbumine 8 mg Perindopril erbumine 8mg tablets | 30 tablet [PoM] £12.99 DT = £3.82 | 56 tablet [PoM] £3.88 | 60 tablet [PoM] £40.00

2

Cardiovascular system

Quinapril
⚑ 167

● **INDICATIONS AND DOSE**

Essential hypertension
▸ BY MOUTH
▸ Adult: Initially 10 mg once daily; maintenance 20–40 mg daily in up to 2 divided doses; maximum 80 mg per day
▸ Elderly: Initially 2.5 mg once daily; maintenance 20–40 mg daily in up to 2 divided doses; maximum 80 mg per day

Essential hypertension if used in addition to diuretic
▸ BY MOUTH
▸ Adult: Initially 2.5 mg once daily; maintenance 20–40 mg daily in up to 2 divided doses; maximum 80 mg per day

Heart failure (adjunct) (under close medical supervision)
▸ BY MOUTH
▸ Adult: Initially 2.5 mg daily, increased if tolerated to 10–20 mg daily in 1–2 divided doses, doses to be increased gradually; maximum 40 mg per day

● **INTERACTIONS** → Appendix 1: ACE inhibitors
● **SIDE-EFFECTS**
▸ **Common or very common** Back pain · increased risk of infection
▸ **Uncommon** Depression · dry throat · gastrointestinal disorders · generalised oedema · nervousness · proteinuria · vasodilation · vision disorders
▸ **Rare or very rare** Balance impaired · glossitis
▸ **Frequency not known** Arthritis · hypersensitivity · jaundice cholestatic · leucocytosis · postural hypotension · pulmonary oedema · serositis · toxic epidermal necrolysis · vasculitis necrotising

● **BREAST FEEDING** Avoid in the first few weeks after delivery, particularly in preterm infants, due to the risk of profound neonatal hypotension; if essential, may be used in mothers breast-feeding older infants—the infant's blood pressure should be monitored.

● **HEPATIC IMPAIRMENT**
Monitoring Quinapril is a prodrug and requires close monitoring in patients with hepatic impairment.

● **RENAL IMPAIRMENT**
Dose adjustments Max. initial dose 2.5 mg once daily if eGFR less than 40 mL/minute/1.73 m^2.

● **MEDICINAL FORMS**
There can be variation in the licensing of different medicines containing the same drug.
Tablet
▸ Quinapril (Non-proprietary)
Quinapril (as Quinapril hydrochloride) 5 mg Quinapril 5mg tablets | 28 tablet [PoM] £8.59 DT = £8.60
Quinapril (as Quinapril hydrochloride) 10 mg Quinapril 10mg tablets | 28 tablet [PoM] £8.59 DT = £8.60
Quinapril (as Quinapril hydrochloride) 20 mg Quinapril 20mg tablets | 28 tablet [PoM] £3.05 DT = £3.52
Quinapril (as Quinapril hydrochloride) 40 mg Quinapril 40mg tablets | 28 tablet [PoM] £3.51 DT = £4.00
▸ Accupro (Pfizer Ltd)
Quinapril (as Quinapril hydrochloride) 5 mg Accupro 5mg tablets | 28 tablet [PoM] £8.60 DT = £8.60
Quinapril (as Quinapril hydrochloride) 10 mg Accupro 10mg tablets | 28 tablet [PoM] £8.60 DT = £8.60
Quinapril (as Quinapril hydrochloride) 20 mg Accupro 20mg tablets | 28 tablet [PoM] £10.79 DT = £3.52
Quinapril (as Quinapril hydrochloride) 40 mg Accupro 40mg tablets | 28 tablet [PoM] £9.75 DT = £4.00

Quinapril with hydrochlorothiazide
The properties listed below are those particular to the combination only. For the properties of the components please consider, quinapril above, hydrochlorothiazide p. 166.

● **INDICATIONS AND DOSE**

Hypertension in patients stabilised on the individual components in the same proportions
▸ BY MOUTH
▸ Adult: (consult product literature)

● **INTERACTIONS** → Appendix 1: ACE inhibitors · thiazide diuretics

● **MEDICINAL FORMS**
There can be variation in the licensing of different medicines containing the same drug.
Tablet
▸ Quinapril with hydrochlorothiazide (Non-proprietary)
Quinapril (as Quinapril hydrochloride) 10 mg, Hydrochlorothiazide 12.5 mg Quinapril 10mg / Hydrochlorothiazide 12.5mg tablets | 28 tablet [PoM] £11.75 DT = £11.75
▸ Accuretic (Pfizer Ltd)
Quinapril (as Quinapril hydrochloride) 10 mg, Hydrochlorothiazide 12.5 mg Accuretic 12.5mg/10mg tablets | 28 tablet [PoM] £11.75 DT = £11.75

Ramipril
⚑ 167

● **INDICATIONS AND DOSE**

Hypertension
▸ BY MOUTH
▸ Adult: Initially 1.25–2.5 mg once daily, increased if necessary up to 10 mg once daily, dose to be increased at intervals of 2–4 weeks

Symptomatic heart failure (adjunct) (under close medical supervision)
▸ BY MOUTH
▸ Adult: Initially 1.25 mg once daily, increased if tolerated to 10 mg daily, preferably taken in 2 divided doses, increase dose gradually at intervals of 1–2 weeks

Prophylaxis after myocardial infarction in patients with clinical evidence of heart failure (started at least 48 hours after infarction)
▸ BY MOUTH
▸ Adult: Initially 2.5 mg twice daily for 3 days, then increased to 5 mg twice daily

Prophylaxis after myocardial infarction in patients with clinical evidence of heart failure (started at least 48 hours after infarction) when initial dose not tolerated
▸ BY MOUTH
▸ Adult: 1.25 mg twice daily for 2 days, then increased to 2.5 mg twice daily, then increased to 5 mg twice daily, withdraw treatment if dose cannot be increased to 2.5 mg twice daily

Prevention of cardiovascular events in patients with atherosclerotic cardiovascular disease or with diabetes mellitus and at least one additional risk factor for cardiovascular disease
▸ BY MOUTH
▸ Adult: Initially 2.5 mg once daily for 1–2 weeks, then increased to 5 mg once daily for a further 2–3 weeks, then increased to 10 mg once daily

Nephropathy (consult product literature)
▸ BY MOUTH
▸ Adult: Initially 1.25 mg once daily for 2 weeks, then increased to 2.5 mg once daily for a further 2 weeks, then increased if tolerated to 5 mg once daily

● **INTERACTIONS** → Appendix 1: ACE inhibitors

- SIDE-EFFECTS
▶ **Common or very common** Gastrointestinal discomfort · gastrointestinal disorders · increased risk of infection · muscle spasms
▶ **Uncommon** Anxiety · appetite decreased · asthma exacerbated · depressed mood · flushing · libido decreased · myocardial ischaemia · nasal congestion · proteinuria aggravated · vision disorders
▶ **Rare or very rare** Conjunctivitis · hearing impairment · hypoperfusion · movement disorders · onycholysis · oral disorders · tremor · vascular stenosis · vasculitis
▶ **Frequency not known** Altered smell sensation · bone marrow failure · cerebrovascular insufficiency · concentration impaired · gynaecomastia · hypersensitivity · Raynaud's phenomenon · SIADH · toxic epidermal necrolysis

- BREAST FEEDING Not recommended; alternative treatment options, with better established safety information during breast-feeding, are available.

- HEPATIC IMPAIRMENT
Dose adjustments Max. daily dose 2.5 mg.
Monitoring Ramipril is a prodrug and requires close monitoring in patients with hepatic impairment.

- RENAL IMPAIRMENT
Dose adjustments Max. daily dose 5 mg if eGFR 30–60 mL/minute/1.73 m^2; max. initial dose 1.25 mg once daily (do not exceed 5 mg daily) if eGFR less than 30 mL/minute/1.73 m^2.

- MEDICINAL FORMS
There can be variation in the licensing of different medicines containing the same drug. Forms available from special-order manufacturers include: oral suspension, oral solution

Oral solution
▶ Ramipril (Non-proprietary)
Ramipril 500 microgram per 1 ml Ramipril 2.5mg/5ml oral solution sugar free sugar-free | 150 ml PoM £96.00 DT = £96.00

Tablet
▶ Ramipril (Non-proprietary)
Ramipril 1.25 mg Ramipril 1.25mg tablets | 28 tablet PoM £5.25 DT = £1.20
Ramipril 2.5 mg Ramipril 2.5mg tablets | 28 tablet PoM £7.49 DT = £0.60
Ramipril 5 mg Ramipril 5mg tablets | 28 tablet PoM £10.40 DT = £0.63
Ramipril 10 mg Ramipril 10mg tablets | 28 tablet PoM £14.20 DT = £0.78
▶ Tritace (Sanofi)
Ramipril 1.25 mg Tritace 1.25mg tablets | 28 tablet PoM £5.09 DT = £1.20
Ramipril 2.5 mg Tritace 2.5mg tablets | 28 tablet PoM £7.22 DT = £0.60
Ramipril 5 mg Tritace 5mg tablets | 28 tablet PoM £10.05 DT = £0.63
Ramipril 10 mg Tritace 10mg tablets | 28 tablet PoM £13.68 DT = £0.78

Capsule
▶ Ramipril (Non-proprietary)
Ramipril 1.25 mg Ramipril 1.25mg capsules | 28 capsule PoM £2.00 DT = £1.27
Ramipril 2.5 mg Ramipril 2.5mg capsules | 28 capsule PoM £1.99 DT = £1.22
Ramipril 5 mg Ramipril 5mg capsules | 28 capsule PoM £2.05 DT = £0.78
Ramipril 10 mg Ramipril 10mg capsules | 28 capsule PoM £2.20 DT = £0.94

Ramipril with felodipine

The properties listed below are those particular to the combination only. For the properties of the components please consider, ramipril p. 172, felodipine p. 159.

- INDICATIONS AND DOSE
Hypertension in patients stabilised on the individual components in the same proportions
▶ BY MOUTH
▶ Adult: (consult product literature)

- INTERACTIONS → Appendix 1: ACE inhibitors · calcium channel blockers

- MEDICINAL FORMS
There can be variation in the licensing of different medicines containing the same drug.
Modified-release tablet
CAUTIONARY AND ADVISORY LABELS 25
▶ Triapin (Sanofi)
Felodipine 2.5 mg, Ramipril 2.5 mg Triapin 2.5mg/2.5mg modified-release tablets | 28 tablet PoM £24.55
Felodipine 5 mg, Ramipril 5 mg Triapin 5mg/5mg modified-release tablets | 28 tablet PoM £16.13 DT = £16.13

☞ 167

Trandolapril

- INDICATIONS AND DOSE
Mild to moderate hypertension
▶ BY MOUTH
▶ Adult: Initially 500 micrograms once daily; increased to 1–2 mg once daily, dose to be increased at intervals of 2–4 weeks; maximum 4 mg per day

Prophylaxis after myocardial infarction in patients with left ventricular dysfunction (starting as early as 3 days after infarction)
▶ BY MOUTH
▶ Adult: Initially 500 micrograms once daily, then increased to up to 4 mg once daily, doses to be increased gradually

- INTERACTIONS → Appendix 1: ACE inhibitors
- SIDE-EFFECTS
▶ **Uncommon** Feeling abnormal · gastrointestinal disorders · hot flush · increased risk of infection · libido decreased · malaise · muscle spasms · pain · rhinorrhoea
▶ **Rare or very rare** Anaemia · anxiety · appetite abnormal · arrhythmias · azotaemia · cerebrovascular insufficiency · depression · enzyme abnormality · eye disorder · eye inflammation · gout · haemorrhage · hallucination · hyperbilirubinaemia · hyperglycaemia · hypersensitivity · hyperuricaemia · migraine · movement disorders · myocardial ischaemia · oedema · osteoarthritis · platelet disorder · postural hypotension · throat irritation · urinary disorders · vascular disorders · visual impairment · white blood cell disorder
▶ **Frequency not known** Atrioventricular block · cardiac arrest · jaundice · proteinuria · toxic epidermal necrolysis
SIDE-EFFECTS, FURTHER INFORMATION If symptomatic hypotension develops during titration, do not increase dose further; if possible, reduce dose of any adjunctive treatment and if this is not effective or feasible, reduce dose of trandolapril.

- BREAST FEEDING Not recommended; alternative treatment options, with better established safety information during breast-feeding, are available.

- HEPATIC IMPAIRMENT
Monitoring Trandolapril is a prodrug and requires close monitoring in patients with hepatic impairment.

Cardiovascular system

2

- RENAL IMPAIRMENT
  Dose adjustments Max. 2 mg daily if eGFR less than 10 mL/minute/1.73 m^2.

- MEDICINAL FORMS
  There can be variation in the licensing of different medicines containing the same drug. Forms available from special-order manufacturers include: oral suspension
  Capsule
  ▸ Trandolapril (Non-proprietary)
    Trandolapril 500 microgram Trandolapril 500microgram capsules | 14 capsule [PoM] £1.66 DT = £1.66
    Trandolapril 1 mg Trandolapril 1mg capsules | 28 capsule [PoM] £19.99 DT = £19.99
    Trandolapril 2 mg Trandolapril 2mg capsules | 28 capsule [PoM] £3.08 DT = £3.08
    Trandolapril 4 mg Trandolapril 4mg capsules | 28 capsule [PoM] £13.24 DT = £13.24

DRUGS ACTING ON THE RENIN-ANGIOTENSIN SYSTEM ⟩ ANGIOTENSIN II RECEPTOR ANTAGONISTS

Angiotensin II receptor antagonists

- CONTRA-INDICATIONS The combination of an angiotensin-II receptor antagonist with aliskiren is contra-indicated in patients with an eGFR less than 60 mL/minute/1.73 m^2 · the combination of an angiotensin-II receptor antagonist with aliskiren is contra-indictated in patients with diabetes mellitus
- CAUTIONS Afro-Caribbean patients—particularly those with left ventricular hypertrophy (may not benefit from an angiotensin-II receptor antagonist) · aortic or mitral valve stenosis · elderly (lower initial doses may be appropriate) · hypertrophic cardiomyopathy · patients with a history of angioedema · patients with primary aldosteronism (may not benefit from an angiotensin-II receptor antagonist) · renal artery stenosis
- SIDE-EFFECTS
  ▸ **Common or very common** Abdominal pain · asthenia · back pain · cough · diarrhoea · dizziness · headache · hyperkalaemia (uncommon in children) · hypotension · nausea · postural hypotension (more common in patients with intravascular volume depletion, e.g. those taking high-dose diuretics) · renal impairment · vertigo · vomiting
  ▸ **Uncommon** Angioedema · myalgia · skin reactions (very common in children) · thrombocytopenia
  ▸ **Rare or very rare** Arthralgia · hepatic function abnormal (uncommon in children)
- PREGNANCY Angiotensin-II receptor antagonists should be avoided in pregnancy unless essential. They may adversely affect fetal and neonatal blood pressure control and renal function; neonatal skull defects and oligohydramnios have also been reported.
- BREAST FEEDING Information on the use of angiotensin-II receptor antagonists in breast-feeding is limited. They are not recommended in breast-feeding and alternative treatment options, with better established safety information during breast-feeding, are available.
- RENAL IMPAIRMENT
  Dose adjustments Use with caution, starting with low dose, and adjust according to response.
- MONITORING REQUIREMENTS Monitor plasma-potassium concentration, particularly in the elderly and in patients with renal impairment.

Azilsartan medoxomil

- INDICATIONS AND DOSE
  Hypertension
  ▸ BY MOUTH
  ▸ Adult 18-74 years: Initially 40 mg once daily, increased if necessary to 80 mg once daily
  ▸ Adult 75 years and over: Initially 20–40 mg once daily, increased if necessary to 80 mg once daily
  Hypertension with intravascular volume depletion
  ▸ BY MOUTH
  ▸ Adult: Initially 20–40 mg daily, increased if necessary to 80 mg daily

- CAUTIONS Heart failure
- INTERACTIONS → Appendix 1: angiotensin-II receptor antagonists
- SIDE-EFFECTS
  ▸ **Uncommon** Hyperuricaemia · muscle spasms · peripheral oedema
- HEPATIC IMPAIRMENT Manufacturer advises avoid in severe impairment (no information available).
  Dose adjustments Manufacturer advises to consider initial dose of 20 mg in mild to moderate impairment (limited information available).
  Monitoring Manufacturer advises monitor closely in mild to moderate hepatic impairment (limited information available).
- RENAL IMPAIRMENT Manufacturer advises caution in severe impairment—no information available.

- MEDICINAL FORMS
  There can be variation in the licensing of different medicines containing the same drug.
  Tablet
  ▸ Edarbi (Takeda UK Ltd)
    Azilsartan medoxomil 20 mg Edarbi 20mg tablets | 28 tablet [PoM] £16.80 DT = £16.80
    Azilsartan medoxomil 40 mg Edarbi 40mg tablets | 28 tablet [PoM] £16.80 DT = £16.80
    Azilsartan medoxomil 80 mg Edarbi 80mg tablets | 28 tablet [PoM] £19.95 DT = £19.95

Candesartan cilexetil

- INDICATIONS AND DOSE
  Hypertension
  ▸ BY MOUTH
  ▸ Adult: Initially 8 mg once daily, increased if necessary up to 32 mg once daily, doses to be increased at intervals of 4 weeks; usual dose 8 mg once daily
  Hypertension with intravascular volume depletion
  ▸ BY MOUTH
  ▸ Adult: Initially 4 mg once daily, increased if necessary up to 32 mg daily, doses to be increased at intervals of 4 weeks; usual dose 8 mg once daily
  Heart failure with impaired left ventricular systolic function when ACE inhibitors are not tolerated | Heart failure with impaired left ventricular systolic function in conjunction with an ACE inhibitor (under expert supervision)
  ▸ BY MOUTH
  ▸ Adult: Initially 4 mg once daily, increased at intervals of at least 2 weeks to 'target' dose of 32 mg once daily or to maximum tolerated dose; maximum 32 mg per day

- CONTRA-INDICATIONS Cholestasis
- INTERACTIONS → Appendix 1: angiotensin-II receptor antagonists

- SIDE-EFFECTS
- ► **Common or very common** Increased risk of infection
- ► **Rare or very rare** Agranulocytosis · hepatitis · hyponatraemia · leucopenia · neutropenia
- HEPATIC IMPAIRMENT Avoid in severe hepatic impairment.
  Dose adjustments Initially 4 mg once daily in mild or moderate impairment.
- RENAL IMPAIRMENT Use with caution if eGFR less than 15 mL/minute/1.73 m² —limited experience.
  Dose adjustments Initially 4 mg daily.

- MEDICINAL FORMS
  There can be variation in the licensing of different medicines containing the same drug. Forms available from special-order manufacturers include: oral suspension, oral solution

  Tablet
  ► Candesartan cilexetil (Non-proprietary)
    Candesartan cilexetil 2 mg Candesartan 2mg tablets | 7 tablet [PoM] £2.86 DT = £1.90
    Candesartan cilexetil 4 mg Candesartan 4mg tablets | 7 tablet [PoM] £3.88 DT = £0.30 | 28 tablet [PoM] £0.49–£9.78
    Candesartan cilexetil 8 mg Candesartan 8mg tablets | 28 tablet [PoM] £9.89 DT = £0.84
    Candesartan cilexetil 16 mg Candesartan 16mg tablets | 28 tablet [PoM] £12.72 DT = £1.14
    Candesartan cilexetil 32 mg Candesartan 32mg tablets | 28 tablet [PoM] £16.13 DT = £1.75
  ► Amias (Takeda UK Ltd)
    Candesartan cilexetil 2 mg Amias 2mg tablets | 7 tablet [PoM] £3.58 DT = £1.90
    Candesartan cilexetil 4 mg Amias 4mg tablets | 7 tablet [PoM] £3.88 DT = £0.30 | 28 tablet [PoM] £9.78
    Candesartan cilexetil 8 mg Amias 8mg tablets | 28 tablet [PoM] £9.89 DT = £0.84
    Candesartan cilexetil 16 mg Amias 16mg tablets | 28 tablet [PoM] £12.72 DT = £1.14
    Candesartan cilexetil 32 mg Amias 32mg tablets | 28 tablet [PoM] £16.13 DT = £1.75

Eprosartan

- INDICATIONS AND DOSE
  Hypertension
  ► BY MOUTH
  ► Adult: 600 mg once daily

- INTERACTIONS → Appendix 1: angiotensin-II receptor antagonists
- SIDE-EFFECTS
- ► **Common or very common** Gastrointestinal disorder · rhinitis
- HEPATIC IMPAIRMENT Caution in mild or moderate liver disease. Avoid in severe impairment.
- RENAL IMPAIRMENT
  Dose adjustments Caution if eGFR less than 30 mL/minute/1.73 m².

- MEDICINAL FORMS
  There can be variation in the licensing of different medicines containing the same drug. Forms available from special-order manufacturers include: oral suspension, oral solution

  Tablet
  CAUTIONARY AND ADVISORY LABELS 21
  ► Eprosartan (Non-proprietary)
    Eprosartan (as Eprosartan mesilate) 300 mg Eprosartan 300mg tablets | 28 tablet [PoM] £7.31 DT = £6.20
    Eprosartan (as Eprosartan mesilate) 400 mg Eprosartan 400mg tablets | 56 tablet [PoM] £25.85 DT = £15.58
    Eprosartan (as Eprosartan mesilate) 600 mg Eprosartan 600mg tablets | 28 tablet [PoM] £14.31 DT = £12.05
  ► Teveten (Mylan)
    Eprosartan (as Eprosartan mesilate) 300 mg Teveten 300mg tablets | 28 tablet [PoM] £7.31 DT = £6.20
    Eprosartan (as Eprosartan mesilate) 600 mg Teveten 600mg tablets | 28 tablet [PoM] £14.31 DT = £12.05

Irbesartan

- INDICATIONS AND DOSE
  Hypertension
  ► BY MOUTH
  ► Adult 18-74 years: Initially 150 mg once daily, increased if necessary to 300 mg once daily
  ► Adult 75 years and over: Initially 75–150 mg once daily, increased if necessary to 300 mg once daily

  Hypertension in patients receiving haemodialysis
  ► BY MOUTH
  ► Adult: Initially 75–150 mg once daily, increased if necessary to 300 mg once daily

  Renal disease in hypertensive type 2 diabetes mellitus
  ► BY MOUTH
  ► Adult 18-74 years: Initially 150 mg once daily, increased if tolerated to 300 mg once daily
  ► Adult 75 years and over: Initially 75–150 mg once daily, increased if tolerated to 300 mg once daily

  Renal disease in hypertensive type 2 diabetes mellitus in patients receiving haemodialysis
  ► BY MOUTH
  ► Adult: Initially 75–150 mg once daily, increased if tolerated to 300 mg once daily

- INTERACTIONS → Appendix 1: angiotensin-II receptor antagonists
- SIDE-EFFECTS
- ► **Common or very common** Musculoskeletal pain
- ► **Uncommon** Chest pain · dyspepsia · flushing · hepatic disorders · sexual dysfunction · tachycardia
- ► **Frequency not known** Hypersensitivity vasculitis · muscle cramps · taste altered · tinnitus

- MEDICINAL FORMS
  There can be variation in the licensing of different medicines containing the same drug. Forms available from special-order manufacturers include: oral suspension

  Tablet
  ► Irbesartan (Non-proprietary)
    Irbesartan 75 mg Irbesartan 75mg tablets | 28 tablet [PoM] £8.24 DT = £0.80
    Irbesartan 150 mg Irbesartan 150mg tablets | 28 tablet [PoM] £10.06 DT = £1.08
    Irbesartan 300 mg Irbesartan 300mg tablets | 28 tablet [PoM] £13.54 DT = £1.77
  ► Aprovel (Sanofi)
    Irbesartan 75 mg Aprovel 75mg tablets | 28 tablet [PoM] £9.69 DT = £0.80
    Irbesartan 150 mg Aprovel 150mg tablets | 28 tablet [PoM] £11.84 DT = £1.08
    Irbesartan 300 mg Aprovel 300mg tablets | 28 tablet [PoM] £15.93 DT = £1.77
  ► Ifirmasta (Consilient Health Ltd)
    Irbesartan 75 mg Ifirmasta 75mg tablets | 28 tablet [PoM] £8.23 DT = £0.80
    Irbesartan 150 mg Ifirmasta 150mg tablets | 28 tablet [PoM] £10.06 DT = £1.08
    Irbesartan 300 mg Ifirmasta 300mg tablets | 28 tablet [PoM] £13.54 DT = £1.77

Irbesartan with hydrochlorothiazide

The properties listed below are those particular to the combination only. For the properties of the components please consider, irbesartan above, hydrochlorothiazide p. 166.

- INDICATIONS AND DOSE
  Hypertension not adequately controlled with irbesartan alone
  ► BY MOUTH
  ► Adult: (consult product literature)

Cardiovascular system

2

- INTERACTIONS → Appendix 1: angiotensin-II receptor antagonists · thiazide diuretics

- MEDICINAL FORMS
There can be variation in the licensing of different medicines containing the same drug.

Tablet

▸ Irbesartan with hydrochlorothiazide (Non-proprietary)
Hydrochlorothiazide 12.5 mg, Irbesartan 150 mg Irbesartan 150mg / Hydrochlorothiazide 12.5mg tablets | 28 tablet PoM £10.06 DT = £4.65
Hydrochlorothiazide 25 mg, Irbesartan 300 mg Irbesartan 300mg / Hydrochlorothiazide 25mg tablets | 28 tablet PoM £13.54 DT = £6.46
Hydrochlorothiazide 12.5 mg, Irbesartan 300 mg Irbesartan 300mg / Hydrochlorothiazide 12.5mg tablets | 28 tablet PoM £13.54 DT = £1.73

▸ CoAprovel (Sanofi)
Hydrochlorothiazide 12.5 mg, Irbesartan 150 mg CoAprovel 150mg/12.5mg tablets | 28 tablet PoM £11.84 DT = £4.65
Hydrochlorothiazide 25 mg, Irbesartan 300 mg CoAprovel 300mg/25mg tablets | 28 tablet PoM £15.93 DT = £6.46
Hydrochlorothiazide 12.5 mg, Irbesartan 300 mg CoAprovel 300mg/12.5mg tablets | 28 tablet PoM £15.93 DT = £1.73

🏳 174

Losartan potassium

- **INDICATIONS AND DOSE**

Diabetic nephropathy in type 2 diabetes mellitus
▸ BY MOUTH
▸ Adult 18-75 years: Initially 50 mg once daily for several weeks, then increased if necessary to 100 mg once daily
▸ Adult 76 years and over: Initially 25 mg once daily for several weeks, then increased if necessary to 100 mg once daily

Chronic heart failure when ACE inhibitors are unsuitable or contra-indicated
▸ BY MOUTH
▸ Adult: Initially 12.5 mg once daily, increased if tolerated to up to 150 mg once daily, doses to be increased at weekly intervals

Hypertension (including reduction of stroke risk in hypertension with left ventricular hypertrophy)
▸ BY MOUTH
▸ Adult 18-75 years: Initially 50 mg once daily for several weeks, then increased if necessary to 100 mg once daily
▸ Adult 76 years and over: Initially 25 mg once daily for several weeks, then increased if necessary to 100 mg once daily

Hypertension with intravascular volume depletion
▸ BY MOUTH
▸ Adult 18-75 years: Initially 25 mg once daily for several weeks, then increased if necessary up to 100 mg once daily

- CAUTIONS Severe heart failure

- INTERACTIONS → Appendix 1: angiotensin-II receptor antagonists

- SIDE-EFFECTS
▸ **Common or very common** Anaemia · hypoglycaemia
▸ **Uncommon** Angina pectoris · constipation · drowsiness · dyspnoea · oedema · palpitations · sleep disorder
▸ **Rare or very rare** Angioedema · atrial fibrillation · hepatitis · hypersensitivity · paraesthesia · stroke · syncope · vasculitis
▸ **Frequency not known** Depression · erectile dysfunction · hyponatraemia · increased risk of infection · influenza like illness · malaise · migraine · pancreatitis · photosensitivity reaction · rhabdomyolysis · taste altered · tinnitus

- HEPATIC IMPAIRMENT Manufacturer advises avoid in severe impairment—no information available.

Dose adjustments Consider dose reduction in mild to moderate impairment.

- PRESCRIBING AND DISPENSING INFORMATION Flavours of oral liquid formulations may include berry-citrus.

- MEDICINAL FORMS
There can be variation in the licensing of different medicines containing the same drug. Forms available from special-order manufacturers include: oral suspension, oral solution

Oral suspension

▸ Cozaar (Merck Sharp & Dohme Ltd)
Losartan potassium 2.5 mg per 1 ml Cozaar 2.5mg/ml oral suspension sugar-free | 200 ml PoM £53.68 DT = £53.68

Tablet

▸ Losartan potassium (Non-proprietary)
Losartan potassium 12.5 mg Losartan 12.5mg tablets | 28 tablet PoM £30.00 DT = £4.50
Losartan potassium 25 mg Losartan 25mg tablets | 28 tablet PoM £16.18 DT = £0.55
Losartan potassium 50 mg Losartan 50mg tablets | 28 tablet PoM £12.80 DT = £0.57
Losartan potassium 100 mg Losartan 100mg tablets | 28 tablet PoM £16.18 DT = £1.16

▸ Cozaar (Merck Sharp & Dohme Ltd)
Losartan potassium 12.5 mg Cozaar 12.5mg tablets | 28 tablet PoM £9.70 DT = £4.50
Losartan potassium 25 mg Cozaar 25mg tablets | 28 tablet PoM £16.18 DT = £0.55
Losartan potassium 50 mg Cozaar 50mg tablets | 28 tablet PoM £12.80 DT = £0.57
Losartan potassium 100 mg Cozaar 100mg tablets | 28 tablet PoM £16.18 DT = £1.16

Losartan with hydrochlorothiazide

The properties listed below are those particular to the combination only. For the properties of the components please consider, losartan potassium above, hydrochlorothiazide p. 166.

- **INDICATIONS AND DOSE**

Hypertension not adequately controlled with losartan alone
▸ BY MOUTH
▸ Adult: (consult product literature)

- INTERACTIONS → Appendix 1: angiotensin-II receptor antagonists · thiazide diuretics

- MEDICINAL FORMS
There can be variation in the licensing of different medicines containing the same drug.

Tablet

▸ Losartan with hydrochlorothiazide (Non-proprietary)
Hydrochlorothiazide 12.5 mg, Losartan potassium 50 mg Losartan 50mg / Hydrochlorothiazide 12.5mg tablets | 28 tablet PoM £12.80 DT = £1.13
Hydrochlorothiazide 25 mg, Losartan potassium 100 mg Losartan 100mg / Hydrochlorothiazide 25mg tablets | 28 tablet PoM £16.18 DT = £1.48
Hydrochlorothiazide 12.5 mg, Losartan potassium 100 mg Losartan 100mg / Hydrochlorothiazide 12.5mg tablets | 28 tablet PoM £16.18 DT = £9.83

▸ Cozaar-Comp (Merck Sharp & Dohme Ltd)
Hydrochlorothiazide 12.5 mg, Losartan potassium 50 mg Cozaar-Comp 50mg/12.5mg tablets | 28 tablet PoM £12.80 DT = £1.13
Hydrochlorothiazide 25 mg, Losartan potassium 100 mg Cozaar-Comp 100mg/25mg tablets | 28 tablet PoM £16.18 DT = £1.48
Hydrochlorothiazide 12.5 mg, Losartan potassium 100 mg Cozaar-Comp 100mg/12.5mg tablets | 28 tablet PoM £16.18 DT = £9.83

F 174

Olmesartan medoxomil

● **INDICATIONS AND DOSE**

Hypertension

▶ BY MOUTH

▶ Adult: Initially 10 mg daily, increased if necessary to 20 mg daily; maximum 40 mg per day

● CONTRA-INDICATIONS Biliary obstruction

● INTERACTIONS → Appendix 1: angiotensin-II receptor antagonists

● SIDE-EFFECTS

▶ **Common or very common** Arthritis · chest pain · dyspepsia · haemorrhage · hypertriglyceridaemia · hyperuricaemia · increased risk of infection · influenza like illness · oedema

▶ **Uncommon** Angina pectoris · malaise · skin reactions

▶ **Rare or very rare** Lethargy · muscle spasms · sprue-like enteropathy

● HEPATIC IMPAIRMENT Manufacturer advises avoid in severe impairment—no information available.

Dose adjustments Dose should not exceed 20 mg daily in moderate impairment.

● RENAL IMPAIRMENT Avoid if eGFR less than 20 mL/minute/1.73 m^2.

Dose adjustments Max. 20 mg daily if eGFR 20–60 mL/minute/1.73 m^2.

● MEDICINAL FORMS

There can be variation in the licensing of different medicines containing the same drug. Forms available from special-order manufacturers include: oral suspension, oral solution

Tablet

▶ Olmesartan medoxomil (Non-proprietary)

Olmesartan medoxomil 10 mg Olmesartan medoxomil 10mg tablets | 28 tablet [PoM] £1.24–£10.40 DT = £1.24

Olmesartan medoxomil 20 mg Olmesartan medoxomil 20mg tablets | 28 tablet [PoM] £1.51–£12.30 DT = £1.51

Olmesartan medoxomil 40 mg Olmesartan medoxomil 40mg tablets | 28 tablet [PoM] £2.18–£16.63 DT = £2.26

▶ Olmetec (Daiichi Sankyo UK Ltd)

Olmesartan medoxomil 10 mg Olmetec 10mg tablets | 28 tablet [PoM] £10.95 DT = £1.24

Olmesartan medoxomil 20 mg Olmetec 20mg tablets | 28 tablet [PoM] £12.95 DT = £1.51

Olmesartan medoxomil 40 mg Olmetec 40mg tablets | 28 tablet [PoM] £17.50 DT = £2.26

Olmesartan with amlodipine

The properties listed below are those particular to the combination only. For the properties of the components please consider, olmesartan medoxomil above, amlodipine p. 155.

● **INDICATIONS AND DOSE**

Hypertension in patients stabilised on the individual components in the same proportions

▶ BY MOUTH

▶ Adult: (consult product literature)

● INTERACTIONS → Appendix 1: angiotensin-II receptor antagonists · calcium channel blockers

● MEDICINAL FORMS

There can be variation in the licensing of different medicines containing the same drug.

Tablet

▶ Sevikar (Daiichi Sankyo UK Ltd)

Amlodipine (as Amlodipine besilate) 5 mg, Olmesartan medoxomil 20 mg Sevikar 20mg/5mg tablets | 28 tablet [PoM] £16.95 DT = £16.95

Amlodipine (as Amlodipine besilate) 10 mg, Olmesartan medoxomil 40 mg Sevikar 40mg/10mg tablets | 28 tablet [PoM] £16.95 DT = £16.95

Amlodipine (as Amlodipine besilate) 5 mg, Olmesartan medoxomil 40 mg Sevikar 40mg/5mg tablets | 28 tablet [PoM] £16.95 DT = £16.95

Olmesartan with amlodipine and hydrochlorothiazide

The properties listed below are those particular to the combination only. For the properties of the components please consider, olmesartan medoxomil above, amlodipine p. 155, hydrochlorothiazide p. 166.

● **INDICATIONS AND DOSE**

Hypertension in patients stabilised on the individual components in the same proportions, or for hypertension not adequately controlled with olmesartan and amlodipine

▶ BY MOUTH

▶ Adult: (consult product literature)

● INTERACTIONS → Appendix 1: angiotensin-II receptor antagonists · calcium channel blockers · thiazide diuretics

● MEDICINAL FORMS

There can be variation in the licensing of different medicines containing the same drug.

Tablet

▶ Sevikar HCT (Daiichi Sankyo UK Ltd)

Amlodipine besilate 5 mg, Hydrochlorothiazide 12.5 mg, Olmesartan medoxomil 20 mg Sevikar HCT 20mg/5mg/12.5mg tablets | 28 tablet [PoM] £16.95

Amlodipine besilate 5 mg, Hydrochlorothiazide 25 mg, Olmesartan medoxomil 40 mg Sevikar HCT 40mg/5mg/25mg tablets | 28 tablet [PoM] £16.95

Amlodipine besilate 10 mg, Hydrochlorothiazide 25 mg, Olmesartan medoxomil 40 mg Sevikar HCT 40mg/10mg/25mg tablets | 28 tablet [PoM] £16.95

Amlodipine besilate 5 mg, Hydrochlorothiazide 12.5 mg, Olmesartan medoxomil 40 mg Sevikar HCT 40mg/5mg/12.5mg tablets | 28 tablet [PoM] £16.95

Amlodipine besilate 10 mg, Hydrochlorothiazide 12.5 mg, Olmesartan medoxomil 40 mg Sevikar HCT 40mg/10mg/12.5mg tablets | 28 tablet [PoM] £16.95

Olmesartan with hydrochlorothiazide

The properties listed below are those particular to the combination only. For the properties of the components please consider, olmesartan medoxomil above, hydrochlorothiazide p. 166.

● **INDICATIONS AND DOSE**

Hypertension not adequately controlled with olmesartan alone

▶ BY MOUTH

▶ Adult: (consult product literature)

● INTERACTIONS → Appendix 1: angiotensin-II receptor antagonists · thiazide diuretics

● MEDICINAL FORMS
There can be variation in the licensing of different medicines
containing the same drug.

Tablet

▶ Olmetec Plus (Daiichi Sankyo UK Ltd)
**Hydrochlorothiazide 12.5 mg, Olmesartan medoxomil
20 mg** Olmetec Plus 20mg/12.5mg tablets | 28 tablet [PoM] £12.95
DT = £12.95
**Olmesartan medoxomil 20 mg, Hydrochlorothiazide
25 mg** Olmetec Plus 20mg/25mg tablets | 28 tablet [PoM] £12.95 DT
= £12.95
**Hydrochlorothiazide 12.5 mg, Olmesartan medoxomil
40 mg** Olmetec Plus 40mg/12.5mg tablets | 28 tablet [PoM] £17.50
DT = £17.50

⚑ 174

Telmisartan

● INDICATIONS AND DOSE

Hypertension
▶ BY MOUTH
▶ Adult: Initially 20–40 mg once daily for at least
4 weeks, increased if necessary up to 80 mg once daily

**Prevention of cardiovascular events in patients with
established atherosclerotic cardiovascular disease, or
type 2 diabetes mellitus with target-organ damage**
▶ BY MOUTH
▶ Adult: 80 mg once daily

● INTERACTIONS → Appendix 1: angiotensin-II receptor
antagonists

● SIDE-EFFECTS
▶ **Uncommon** Anaemia · arrhythmias · chest pain · cystitis ·
depression · dyspnoea · flatulence · gastrointestinal
discomfort · hyperhidrosis · increased risk of infection ·
insomnia · muscle spasms · sciatica · syncope
▶ **Rare or very rare** Anxiety · drowsiness · dry mouth ·
eosinophilia · hypoglycaemia · influenza like illness ·
interstitial lung disease · liver disorder · pain in extremity ·
sepsis · taste altered · tendon pain · visual impairment

● HEPATIC IMPAIRMENT Avoid in severe impairment or
biliary obstruction.
Dose adjustments 20–40 mg once daily in mild or moderate
impairment.

● RENAL IMPAIRMENT
Dose adjustments Manufacturer advises initial dose of
20 mg once daily in severe impairment.

● MEDICINAL FORMS
There can be variation in the licensing of different medicines
containing the same drug.

Tablet

▶ Telmisartan (Non-proprietary)
Telmisartan 20 mg Telmisartan 20mg tablets | 28 tablet [PoM]
£1.05–£10.55 DT = £0.63
Telmisartan 40 mg Telmisartan 40mg tablets | 28 tablet [PoM]
£1.05–£12.93 DT = £1.05
Telmisartan 80 mg Telmisartan 80mg tablets | 28 tablet [PoM]
£1.36–£16.15 DT = £1.36
▶ Micardis (Boehringer Ingelheim Ltd)
Telmisartan 20 mg Micardis 20mg tablets | 28 tablet [PoM] £11.10
DT = £0.63
Telmisartan 40 mg Micardis 40mg tablets | 28 tablet [PoM] £13.61
DT = £1.05
Telmisartan 80 mg Micardis 80mg tablets | 28 tablet [PoM] £17.00
DT = £1.36
▶ Tolura (Consilient Health Ltd)
Telmisartan 20 mg Tolura 20mg tablets | 28 tablet [PoM] £11.10 DT
= £0.63
Telmisartan 40 mg Tolura 40mg tablets | 28 tablet [PoM] £13.61 DT
= £1.05
Telmisartan 80 mg Tolura 80mg tablets | 28 tablet [PoM] £17.00 DT
= £1.36

Telmisartan with hydrochlorothiazide

The properties listed below are those particular to the
combination only. For the properties of the components
please consider, telmisartan above, hydrochlorothiazide
p. 166.

● INDICATIONS AND DOSE

**Hypertension not adequately controlled by telmisartan
alone**
▶ BY MOUTH
▶ Adult: (consult product literature)

● INTERACTIONS → Appendix 1: angiotensin-II receptor
antagonists · thiazide diuretics

● MEDICINAL FORMS
There can be variation in the licensing of different medicines
containing the same drug.

Tablet

▶ Telmisartan with hydrochlorothiazide (Non-proprietary)
Hydrochlorothiazide 12.5 mg, Telmisartan 40 mg Telmisartan
40mg / Hydrochlorothiazide 12.5mg tablets | 28 tablet [PoM] £13.61
DT = £13.61
Hydrochlorothiazide 25 mg, Telmisartan 80 mg Telmisartan 80mg
/ Hydrochlorothiazide 25mg tablets | 28 tablet [PoM] £9.99–£17.00 DT
= £17.00
Hydrochlorothiazide 12.5 mg, Telmisartan 80 mg Telmisartan
80mg / Hydrochlorothiazide 12.5mg tablets | 28 tablet [PoM] £8.99–
£17.00 DT = £17.00
▶ Actelsar HCT (Actavis UK Ltd)
Hydrochlorothiazide 12.5 mg, Telmisartan 40 mg Actelsar HCT
40mg/12.5mg tablets | 28 tablet [PoM] £13.61 DT = £13.61
Hydrochlorothiazide 25 mg, Telmisartan 80 mg Actelsar HCT
80mg/25mg tablets | 28 tablet [PoM] £17.00 DT = £17.00
Hydrochlorothiazide 12.5 mg, Telmisartan 80 mg Actelsar HCT
80mg/12.5mg tablets | 28 tablet [PoM] £17.00 DT = £17.00
▶ MicardisPlus (Boehringer Ingelheim Ltd)
Hydrochlorothiazide 12.5 mg, Telmisartan 40 mg MicardisPlus
40mg/12.5mg tablets | 28 tablet [PoM] £13.61 DT = £13.61
Hydrochlorothiazide 12.5 mg, Telmisartan 80 mg MicardisPlus
80mg/12.5mg tablets | 28 tablet [PoM] £17.00 DT = £17.00
▶ MicardisPlus 80/25 (Boehringer Ingelheim Ltd)
Hydrochlorothiazide 25 mg, Telmisartan 80 mg MicardisPlus
80mg/25mg tablets | 28 tablet [PoM] £17.00 DT = £17.00
▶ Tolucombi (Consilient Health Ltd)
Hydrochlorothiazide 12.5 mg, Telmisartan 40 mg Tolucombi
40mg/12.5mg tablets | 28 tablet [PoM] £13.61 DT = £13.61
Hydrochlorothiazide 25 mg, Telmisartan 80 mg Tolucombi
80mg/25mg tablets | 28 tablet [PoM] £17.00 DT = £17.00
Hydrochlorothiazide 12.5 mg, Telmisartan 80 mg Tolucombi
80mg/12.5mg tablets | 28 tablet [PoM] £17.00 DT = £17.00

⚑ 174

Valsartan

● INDICATIONS AND DOSE

Hypertension
▶ BY MOUTH
▶ Adult: Initially 80 mg once daily, increased if necessary
up to 320 mg daily, doses to be increased at intervals of
4 weeks

Hypertension with intravascular volume depletion
▶ BY MOUTH
▶ Adult: Initially 40 mg once daily, increased if necessary
up to 320 mg daily, doses to be increased at intervals of
4 weeks

Heart failure when ACE inhibitors cannot be used, or in conjunction with an ACE inhibitor when a beta-blocker cannot be used | Heart failure, in conjunction with an ACE inhibitor when a beta-blocker cannot be used (under expert supervision)
▸ BY MOUTH
▸ Adult: Initially 40 mg twice daily, increased to up to 160 mg twice daily, doses to be increased at intervals of at least 2 weeks

Myocardial infarction with left ventricular failure or left ventricular systolic dysfunction (adjunct)
▸ BY MOUTH
▸ Adult: Initially 20 mg twice daily, increased if necessary up to 160 mg twice daily, doses to be increased over several weeks if tolerated

● CONTRA-INDICATIONS Biliary cirrhosis · cholestasis
● INTERACTIONS → Appendix 1: angiotensin-II receptor antagonists
● SIDE-EFFECTS
▸ **Uncommon** Heart failure · syncope
▸ **Frequency not known** Neutropenia · serum sickness · vasculitis
● HEPATIC IMPAIRMENT Avoid in severe hepatic impairment. **Dose adjustments** Max. dose 80 mg daily in mild to moderate impairment.
● RENAL IMPAIRMENT Use with caution if eGFR less than $10 \text{ mL/minute}/1.73 \text{ m}^2$—no information available.

● MEDICINAL FORMS
There can be variation in the licensing of different medicines containing the same drug. Forms available from special-order manufacturers include: oral suspension, oral solution
Oral solution
▸ Diovan (Novartis Pharmaceuticals UK Ltd)
Valsartan 3 mg per 1 ml Diovan 3mg/1ml oral solution | 160 ml [PoM] £7.20 DT = £7.20
Tablet
▸ Valsartan (Non-proprietary)
Valsartan 40 mg Valsartan 40mg tablets | 7 tablet [PoM] £5.00 DT = £4.29
Valsartan 80 mg Valsartan 80mg tablets | 28 tablet [PoM] £13.69 DT = £13.69
Valsartan 160 mg Valsartan 160mg tablets | 28 tablet [PoM] £14.69 DT = £14.69
Valsartan 320 mg Valsartan 320mg tablets | 28 tablet [PoM] £20.23 DT = £18.69
Capsule
▸ Valsartan (Non-proprietary)
Valsartan 40 mg Valsartan 40mg capsules | 28 capsule [PoM] £13.97 DT = £3.66
Valsartan 80 mg Valsartan 80mg capsules | 28 capsule [PoM] £13.97 DT = £4.76
Valsartan 160 mg Valsartan 160mg capsules | 28 capsule [PoM] £18.41 DT = £4.83

Combinations available: *Amlodipine with valsartan*, p. 156

Valsartan with hydrochlorothiazide

The properties listed below are those particular to the combination only. For the properties of the components please consider, valsartan p. 178, hydrochlorothiazide p. 166.

● INDICATIONS AND DOSE
Hypertension not adequately controlled by valsartan alone
▸ BY MOUTH
▸ Adult: (consult product literature)

● INTERACTIONS → Appendix 1: angiotensin-II receptor antagonists · thiazide diuretics

● MEDICINAL FORMS
There can be variation in the licensing of different medicines containing the same drug.
Tablet
▸ Valsartan with hydrochlorothiazide (Non-proprietary)
Hydrochlorothiazide 12.5 mg, Valsartan 80 mg Valsartan 80mg / Hydrochlorothiazide 12.5mg tablets | 28 tablet [PoM] £13.97 DT = £12.25
Hydrochlorothiazide 25 mg, Valsartan 160 mg Valsartan 160mg / Hydrochlorothiazide 25mg tablets | 28 tablet [PoM] £18.41 DT = £10.31
Hydrochlorothiazide 12.5 mg, Valsartan 160 mg Valsartan 160mg / Hydrochlorothiazide 12.5mg tablets | 28 tablet [PoM] £18.41 DT = £1.85
▸ Co-Diovan (Novartis Pharmaceuticals UK Ltd)
Hydrochlorothiazide 12.5 mg, Valsartan 80 mg Co-Diovan 80mg/12.5mg tablets | 28 tablet [PoM] £16.76 DT = £12.25
Hydrochlorothiazide 25 mg, Valsartan 160 mg Co-Diovan 160mg/25mg tablets | 28 tablet [PoM] £22.09 DT = £10.31
Hydrochlorothiazide 12.5 mg, Valsartan 160 mg Co-Diovan 160mg/12.5mg tablets | 28 tablet [PoM] £22.09 DT = £1.85

DRUGS ACTING ON THE RENIN-ANGIOTENSIN SYSTEM > RENIN INHIBITORS

Aliskiren

● DRUG ACTION Renin inhibitors inhibit renin directly; renin converts angiotensinogen to angiotensin I.

● INDICATIONS AND DOSE
Essential hypertension either alone or in combination with other antihypertensives
▸ BY MOUTH
▸ Adult: 150 mg once daily, increased if necessary to 300 mg once daily

● CONTRA-INDICATIONS Concomitant treatment with an ACE inhibitor or an angiotensin-II receptor antagonist in patients with an eGFR less than $60 \text{ mL/minute}/1.73 \text{ m}^2$ · concomitant treatment with an ACE inhibitor or an angiotensin-II receptor antagonist in patients with diabetes mellitus · hereditary angioedema · idiopathic angioedema
● CAUTIONS Combination treatment with an ACE inhibitor · combination treatment with an angiotensin-II receptor antagonist · concomitant use of diuretics (first doses may cause hypotension—initiate with care) · history of angioedema · moderate to severe congestive heart failure · patients at risk of renal impairment · salt depletion (first doses may cause hypotension—initiate with care) · volume depletion (first doses may cause hypotension—initiate with care)
CAUTIONS, FURTHER INFORMATION
▸ Concomitant use of drugs affecting the renin-angiotensin system Combination therapy with two drugs affecting the renin-angiotensin system (ACE inhibitors, angiotensin-II receptor antagonists, and aliskiren) is not recommended due to an increased risk of hyperkalaemia, hypotension, and renal impairment, compared to use of a single drug. Patients with diabetic nephropathy are particularly susceptible to developing hyperkalaemia and should not be given an ACE inhibitor with an angiotensin-II receptor antagonist. There is some evidence that the benefits of combination use of an ACE inhibitor with candesartan or valsartan may outweigh the risks in selected patients with heart failure for whom other treatments are unsuitable, however, the concomitant use of this combination, together with an aldosterone antagonist or a potassium-sparing diuretic is not recommended. For patients currently taking combination therapy, the need for continued combined therapy should be reviewed. If combination therapy is considered essential, it should be carried out under specialist supervision, with close

2

Cardiovascular system

monitoring of blood pressure, renal function, and electrolytes (particularly potassium); monitoring should be considered at the start of treatment, then monthly, and also after any change in dose or during intercurrent illness.

● INTERACTIONS → Appendix 1: aliskiren

● SIDE-EFFECTS

▶ **Common or very common** Arthralgia · diarrhoea · dizziness · electrolyte imbalance

▶ **Uncommon** Cough · oral disorder · palpitations · peripheral oedema · renal impairment · severe cutaneous adverse reactions (SCARs) · skin reactions

▶ **Rare or very rare** Angioedema · hypersensitivity

▶ **Frequency not known** Dyspnoea · hepatic disorders · nausea · vertigo · vomiting

SIDE-EFFECTS, FURTHER INFORMATION If diarrhoea is severe or persistent discontinue treatment.

● PREGNANCY Manufacturer advises avoid—no information available; other drugs acting on the renin-angiotensin system have been associated with fetal malformations and neonatal death.

● BREAST FEEDING Present in milk in *animal* studies—manufacturer advises avoid.

● RENAL IMPAIRMENT Avoid if eGFR is less than 30 mL/minute/1.73 m^2—no information available. Use with caution in renal artery stenosis—no information available.

Monitoring Monitor plasma-potassium concentration in renal impairment.

● MONITORING REQUIREMENTS Monitor patients with a history of angioedema closely during treatment.

● NATIONAL FUNDING/ACCESS DECISIONS

Scottish Medicines Consortium (SMC) Decisions
The *Scottish Medicines Consortium* has advised (January 2010) that aliskiren (*Rasilez*®) is **not** recommended for use within NHS Scotland.

● MEDICINAL FORMS
There can be variation in the licensing of different medicines containing the same drug.

Tablet
CAUTIONARY AND ADVISORY LABELS 21
▶ Rasilez (Noden Pharma DAC)
Aliskiren (as Aliskiren hemifumarate) 150 mg Rasilez 150mg tablets | 28 tablet PoM £28.51 DT = £28.51
Aliskiren (as Aliskiren hemifumarate) 300 mg Rasilez 300mg tablets | 28 tablet PoM £34.27 DT = £34.27

VASODILATORS ⟩ VASODILATOR
ANTIHYPERTENSIVES

Hydralazine hydrochloride

● INDICATIONS AND DOSE
Moderate to severe hypertension (adjunct)
▶ BY MOUTH
▶ Adult: Initially 25 mg twice daily, increased if necessary up to 50 mg twice daily

Heart failure (with long acting nitrate) (initiated in hospital or under specialist supervision)
▶ BY MOUTH
▶ Adult: Initially 25 mg 3–4 times a day, subsequent doses to be increased every 2 days if necessary; usual maintenance 50–75 mg 4 times a day

Hypertensive emergencies (including during pregnancy) | Hypertension with renal complications
▶ BY INTRAVENOUS INFUSION
▶ Adult: Initially 200–300 micrograms/minute; usual maintenance 50–150 micrograms/minute

▶ BY SLOW INTRAVENOUS INJECTION
▶ Adult: 5–10 mg, to be diluted with 10 mL sodium chloride 0.9%; dose may be repeated after 20–30 minutes

● CONTRA-INDICATIONS Acute porphyrias p. 1025 · cor pulmonale · dissecting aortic aneurysm · high output heart failure · idiopathic systemic lupus erythematosus · myocardial insufficiency due to mechanical obstruction · severe tachycardia

● CAUTIONS Cerebrovascular disease · coronary artery disease (may provoke angina, avoid after myocardial infarction until stabilised) · occasionally blood pressure reduction too rapid even with low parenteral doses

● INTERACTIONS → Appendix 1: hydralazine

● SIDE-EFFECTS

▶ **Common or very common** Angina pectoris · diarrhoea · dizziness · flushing · gastrointestinal disorders · headache · hypotension · joint disorders · lupus-like syndrome after long-term therapy with over 100 mg daily (or less in women and in slow acetylator individuals) · myalgia · nasal congestion · nausea · palpitations · tachycardia · vomiting

▶ **Rare or very rare** Acute kidney injury · agranulocytosis · anaemia · anxiety · appetite decreased · conjunctivitis · depression · dyspnoea · eosinophilia · eye disorders · fever · glomerulonephritis · haematuria · haemolytic anaemia · hallucination · heart failure · hepatic disorders · leucocytosis · leucopenia · lymphadenopathy · malaise · nerve disorders · neutropenia · oedema · pancytopenia · paradoxical pressor response · paraesthesia · pleuritic pain · proteinuria · skin reactions · splenomegaly · thrombocytopenia · urinary retention · vasculitis · weight decreased

SIDE-EFFECTS, FURTHER INFORMATION The incidence of side-effects is lower if the dose is kept below 100mg daily, but systemic lupus erythematosus should be suspected if there is unexplained weight loss, arthritis, or any other unexplained ill health.

● PREGNANCY Neonatal thrombocytopenia reported, but risk should be balanced against risk of uncontrolled maternal hypertension. Manufacturer advises avoid before third trimester.

● BREAST FEEDING Present in milk but not known to be harmful.

Monitoring Monitor infant in breast-feeding.

● HEPATIC IMPAIRMENT
Dose adjustments Reduce dose.

● RENAL IMPAIRMENT
Dose adjustments Reduce dose if eGFR less than 30 mL/minute/1.73 m^2.

● MONITORING REQUIREMENTS Manufacturer advises test for antinuclear factor and for proteinuria every 6 months and check acetylator status before increasing dose above 100 mg daily, but evidence of clinical value unsatisfactory.

● DIRECTIONS FOR ADMINISTRATION For *intravenous infusion* (*Apresoline*®) give continuously in Sodium chloride 0.9%. Suggested infusion volume 500 mL.

● MEDICINAL FORMS
There can be variation in the licensing of different medicines containing the same drug. Forms available from special-order manufacturers include: oral suspension, oral solution

Tablet
EXCIPIENTS: May contain Gluten, propylene glycol
▶ Hydralazine hydrochloride (Non-proprietary)
Hydralazine hydrochloride 25 mg Hydralazine 25mg tablets | 56 tablet PoM £7.37 DT = £5.82 | 84 tablet PoM £14.00
Hydralazine hydrochloride 50 mg Hydralazine 50mg tablets | 56 tablet PoM £15.46 DT = £9.63
▶ Apresoline (AMCo)
Hydralazine hydrochloride 25 mg Apresoline 25mg tablets | 84 tablet PoM £3.38

Powder for solution for injection
▸ Hydralazine hydrochloride (Non-proprietary)
Hydralazine hydrochloride 20 mg Hydralazine 20mg powder for concentrate for solution for injection ampoules | 5 ampoule [PoM] £64.50

Minoxidil

● **INDICATIONS AND DOSE**

Severe hypertension, in addition to a diuretic and a beta-blocker
▸ BY MOUTH
▸ Adult: Initially 5 mg daily in 1–2 divided doses, then increased in steps of 5–10 mg, increased at intervals of at least 3 days, seldom necessary to exceed 50 mg daily; maximum 100 mg per day
▸ Elderly: Initially 2.5 mg daily in 1–2 divided doses, then increased in steps of 5–10 mg, increased at intervals of at least 3 days, seldom necessary to exceed 50 mg daily; maximum 100 mg per day

● CONTRA-INDICATIONS Phaeochromocytoma
● CAUTIONS Acute porphyrias p. 1025 · after myocardial infarction (until stabilised) · angina
● INTERACTIONS → Appendix 1: minoxidil
● SIDE-EFFECTS
▸ **Common or very common** Fluid retention · hair changes · oedema · pericardial disorders · tachycardia
▸ **Rare or very rare** Leucopenia · skin reactions · Stevens-Johnson syndrome · thrombocytopenia
▸ **Frequency not known** Angina pectoris · breast tenderness · gastrointestinal disorder · pleural effusion · sodium retention · weight increased
● PREGNANCY Avoid—possible toxicity including reduced placental perfusion. Neonatal hirsutism reported.
● BREAST FEEDING Present in milk but not known to be harmful.
● RENAL IMPAIRMENT Use with caution in significant impairment.

● MEDICINAL FORMS
There can be variation in the licensing of different medicines containing the same drug.
Tablet
▸ Loniten (Pfizer Ltd)
Minoxidil 2.5 mg Loniten 2.5mg tablets | 60 tablet [PoM] £8.88 DT = £8.88
Minoxidil 5 mg Loniten 5mg tablets | 60 tablet [PoM] £15.83 DT = £15.83
Minoxidil 10 mg Loniten 10mg tablets | 60 tablet [PoM] £30.68 DT = £30.68

4.1a Hypertension associated with phaeochromocytoma

Other drugs used for Hypertension associated with phaeochromocytoma Propranolol hydrochloride, p. 149

VASODILATORS 〉 PERIPHERAL VASODILATORS

Phenoxybenzamine hydrochloride

● **INDICATIONS AND DOSE**

Hypertension in phaeochromocytoma
▸ BY MOUTH
▸ Adult: Initially 10 mg daily, increased in steps of 10 mg daily until hypertension controlled or treatment not tolerated; maintenance 1–2 mg/kg daily in 2 divided doses

● CONTRA-INDICATIONS During recovery period after myocardial infarction (usually 3–4 weeks) · history of cerebrovascular accident
● CAUTIONS Avoid contact with skin (risk of contact sensitisation) · avoid in Acute porphyrias p. 1025 · carcinogenic in *animals* · cerebrovascular disease · congestive heart failure · elderly · severe ischaemic heart disease
● SIDE-EFFECTS Abdominal distress · dizziness · ejaculation failure · fatigue · miosis · nasal congestion · postural hypotension · reflex tachycardia
● PREGNANCY Hypotension may occur in newborn.
● BREAST FEEDING May be present in milk.
● RENAL IMPAIRMENT Use with caution.
● HANDLING AND STORAGE Owing to risk of contact sensitisation healthcare professionals should avoid contamination of hands.

● MEDICINAL FORMS
There can be variation in the licensing of different medicines containing the same drug. Forms available from special-order manufacturers include: oral suspension, oral solution
Capsule
▸ Phenoxybenzamine hydrochloride (Non-proprietary)
Phenoxybenzamine hydrochloride 10 mg Phenoxybenzamine 10mg capsules | 30 capsule [PoM] £106.61 DT = £106.61

Phentolamine mesilate

● **INDICATIONS AND DOSE**

Hypertensive episodes due to phaeochromocytoma e.g. during surgery
▸ BY INTRAVENOUS INJECTION
▸ Adult: 2–5 mg, repeated if necessary
Diagnosis of phaeochromocytoma
▸ BY INTRAVENOUS INJECTION, OR BY INTRAMUSCULAR INJECTION
▸ Adult: (consult product literature)

● CONTRA-INDICATIONS Angina · coronary insufficiency · evidence of coronary artery disease · history of myocardial infarction · hypotension
● CAUTIONS Elderly · gastritis · peptic ulcer
● SIDE-EFFECTS
▸ **Common or very common** Arrhythmias · headache · hypertension · oral pain
▸ **Uncommon** Abdominal pain upper · diarrhoea · facial swelling · pain · paraesthesia · pruritus · vomiting
● PREGNANCY Use with caution—may cause marked decrease in maternal blood pressure with resulting fetal anoxia.
● BREAST FEEDING Manufacturer advises avoid—no information available.
● RENAL IMPAIRMENT Manufacturer advises caution—no information available.
● MONITORING REQUIREMENTS Monitor blood pressure and heart rate.

● MEDICINAL FORMS
Forms available from special-order manufacturers include: solution for injection

2

Cardiovascular system

4.1b Hypertensive crises

Other drugs used for Hypertensive crises Hydralazine hydrochloride, p. 180 · Labetalol hydrochloride, p. 147

ANTIADRENERGIC AGENTS, PERIPHERALLY ACTING

Guanethidine monosulfate

● **INDICATIONS AND DOSE**
Hypertensive crisis (but no longer recommended)
▶ BY INTRAMUSCULAR INJECTION
▶ Adult: 10–20 mg, dose may be repeated after 3 hours if necessary

● CONTRA-INDICATIONS Heart failure · phaeochromocytoma
● CAUTIONS Asthma · cerebral arteriosclerosis · coronary arteriosclerosis · history of peptic ulceration
● INTERACTIONS → Appendix 1: guanethidine
● SIDE-EFFECTS
▶ **Uncommon** Depression · dermatitis · dry mouth · heart failure · nausea · vision blurred · vomiting
▶ **Rare or very rare** Alopecia · asthma · ischaemic heart disease · myalgia · parotid gland enlargement · tremor
▶ **Frequency not known** Abdominal distension gaseous · anaemia · arrhythmias · azotaemia · cerebral ischaemia · diarrhoea · dizziness · ejaculation disorder · fatigue · headache · intermittent claudication exacerbated · lethargy · leucopenia · nasal congestion · oedema · paraesthesia · postural hypotension · thrombocytopenia
● PREGNANCY Postural hypotension and reduced uteroplacental perfusion. Should not be used to treat hypertension in pregnancy.
● RENAL IMPAIRMENT Avoid if eGFR less than 40 mL/minute/1.73 m^2.
  Dose adjustments Reduce dose if eGFR 40–65 mL/minute/1.73 m^2.
● LESS SUITABLE FOR PRESCRIBING Guanethidine monosulfate is less suitable for prescribing.

● MEDICINAL FORMS
There can be variation in the licensing of different medicines containing the same drug.
Solution for injection
▶ Guanethidine monosulfate (Non-proprietary)
  Guanethidine monosulfate 10 mg per 1 ml Guanethidine 10mg/1ml solution for injection ampoules | 5 ampoule [PoM] £224.15

VASODILATORS ⟩ VASODILATOR ANTIHYPERTENSIVES

Sodium nitroprusside

● **INDICATIONS AND DOSE**
Hypertensive emergencies
▶ BY INTRAVENOUS INFUSION
▶ Adult: Initially 0.5–1.5 micrograms/kg/minute, adjusted in steps of 500 nanograms/kg/minute every 5 minutes, usual dose 0.5–8 micrograms/kg/minute, use lower doses if already receiving other antihypertensives, stop if response unsatisfactory with max. dose in 10 minutes, lower initial dose of 300 nanograms/kg/minute has been used

Maintenance of blood pressure at 30–40% lower than pretreatment diastolic blood pressure
▶ BY INTRAVENOUS INFUSION
▶ Adult: 20–400 micrograms/minute, use lower doses for patients being treated with other antihypertensives
Controlled hypotension in anaesthesia during surgery
▶ BY INTRAVENOUS INFUSION
▶ Adult: Up to 1.5 micrograms/kg/minute
Acute or chronic heart failure
▶ BY INTRAVENOUS INFUSION
▶ Adult: Initially 10–15 micrograms/minute, increased every 5–10 minutes as necessary; usual dose 10–200 micrograms/minute normally for max. 3 days

● UNLICENSED USE Not licensed for use in the UK.
● CONTRA-INDICATIONS Compensatory hypertension · Leber's optic atrophy · severe vitamin B$_{12}$ deficiency
● CAUTIONS Elderly · hyponatraemia · hypothermia · hypothyroidism · impaired cerebral circulation · ischaemic heart disease
● INTERACTIONS → Appendix 1: sodium nitroprusside
● SIDE-EFFECTS Abdominal pain · anxiety · chest discomfort · dizziness · headache · hyperhidrosis · nausea · palpitations · phlebitis (transient) · vomiting
  SIDE-EFFECTS, FURTHER INFORMATION Side-effects associated with over rapid reduction in blood pressure: Headache, dizziness, nausea, retching, abdominal pain, perspiration, palpitation, anxiety, retrosternal discomfort—reduce infusion rate if any of these side-effects occur.
  Overdose Side-effects caused by excessive plasma concentration of the cyanide metabolite include tachycardia, sweating, hyperventilation, arrhythmias, marked metabolic acidosis (discontinue and give antidote, see Cyanide in Emergency treatment of poisoning p. 1319).
● PREGNANCY Avoid prolonged use—potential for accumulation of cyanide in fetus.
● BREAST FEEDING No information available. Caution advised due to thiocyanate metabolite.
● HEPATIC IMPAIRMENT Use with caution. Avoid in hepatic failure—cyanide or thiocyanate metabolites may accumulate.
● RENAL IMPAIRMENT Avoid prolonged use—cyanide or thiocyanate metabolites may accumulate.
● MONITORING REQUIREMENTS Monitor blood pressure (including intra-arterial blood pressure) and blood-cyanide concentration, and if treatment exceeds 3 days, also blood thiocyanate concentration.
● TREATMENT CESSATION Avoid sudden withdrawal—terminate infusion over 15–30 minutes.
● DIRECTIONS FOR ADMINISTRATION For *continuous intravenous infusion* in Glucose 5%, infuse *via* infusion device to allow precise control. For further details, consult product literature. Protect infusion from light.

● MEDICINAL FORMS
There can be variation in the licensing of different medicines containing the same drug.
Powder and solvent for solution for infusion
▶ Sodium nitroprusside (Non-proprietary)
  Sodium nitroprusside dihydrate 50 mg Sodium nitroprusside 50mg powder and solvent for solution for infusion vials | 1 vial [PoM] ▣

4.1c Pulmonary hypertension

Other drugs used for Pulmonary hypertension
Epoprostenol, p. 115 · Sildenafil, p. 794 · Tadalafil, p. 796

ANTITHROMBOTIC DRUGS > ANTIPLATELET DRUGS

Selexipag

23-May-2018

- **DRUG ACTION** Selexipag is a selective prostacyclin (IP) receptor agonist.

- **INDICATIONS AND DOSE**

Pulmonary arterial hypertension either as combination therapy (if insufficiently controlled with an endothelin receptor antagonist and/or a phosphodiesterase type-5 inhibitor), or as monotherapy (initiated under specialist supervision)
  ▸ BY MOUTH
  ▸ Adult: Initially 200 micrograms twice daily, increased in steps of 200 micrograms twice daily at weekly intervals up to the highest tolerated dose, usual maintenance 200–1600 micrograms twice daily, initial dose and first dose after each dose increase should be taken in the evening; maximum 3200 micrograms per day

- **CONTRA-INDICATIONS** Cerebrovascular event (within the last 3 months) · congenital or acquired valvular defects with myocardial function disorders (not related to pulmonary hypertension) · decompensated cardiac failure (unless under close medical supervision) · myocardial infarction (within last 6 months) · severe arrhythmias · severe coronary heart disease · unstable angina

- **CAUTIONS** Elderly (limited information available)

- **INTERACTIONS** → Appendix 1: selexipag

- **SIDE-EFFECTS**
- **Common or very common** Abdominal pain · anaemia · appetite decreased · arthralgia · diarrhoea · flushing · headache · hyperthyroidism · hypotension · myalgia · nasal congestion · nasopharyngitis · nausea · pain · skin reactions · vomiting · weight decreased
- **Uncommon** Sinus tachycardia

- **PREGNANCY** Manufacturer advises avoid—no information available.

- **BREAST FEEDING** Manufacturer advises avoid—present in milk in *animal* studies.

- **HEPATIC IMPAIRMENT** Manufacturer advises avoid in severe impairment.
  Dose adjustments Manufacturer advises reduce initial dose to 200 micrograms once daily in moderate impairment and increase in steps of 200 micrograms once daily at weekly intervals, as tolerated.

- **RENAL IMPAIRMENT** Manufacturer advises caution with dose titration in severe impairment.

- **PATIENT AND CARER ADVICE**
  Missed doses Manufacturer advises if a dose is more than 6 hours late, the missed dose should not be taken and the next dose should be taken at the normal time; if a dose is missed for 3 days or more, treatment should be restarted at a lower dose and then increased—consult product literature.

- **NATIONAL FUNDING/ACCESS DECISIONS**
  Scottish Medicines Consortium (SMC) Decisions
  SMC No. 1235/17
  The *Scottish Medicines Consortium* has advised (updated May 2018) that selexipag (*Uptravi*®) is accepted for

restricted use within NHS Scotland for the long-term treatment of pulmonary arterial hypertension in adults with WHO functional class III, as combination therapy in patients insufficiently controlled with an endothelin receptor antagonist and a phosphodiesterase type-5 inhibitor, and who would be considered for treatment with inhaled iloprost. This advice is contingent upon the continuing availability of the patient access scheme in NHS Scotland or a list price that is equivalent or lower.

- **MEDICINAL FORMS**
  There can be variation in the licensing of different medicines containing the same drug.

Tablet
CAUTIONARY AND ADVISORY LABELS 21, 25
  ▸ Uptravi (Actelion Pharmaceuticals UK Ltd) ▼
  Selexipag 200 microgram Uptravi 200microgram tablets | 60 tablet [PoM] £3,000.00 | 140 tablet [PoM] £7,000.00
  Selexipag 400 microgram Uptravi 400microgram tablets | 60 tablet [PoM] £3,000.00
  Selexipag 600 microgram Uptravi 600microgram tablets | 60 tablet [PoM] £3,000.00
  Selexipag 800 microgram Uptravi 800microgram tablets | 60 tablet [PoM] £3,000.00
  Selexipag 1 mg Uptravi 1,000microgram tablets | 60 tablet [PoM] £3,000.00
  Selexipag 1.2 mg Uptravi 1,200microgram tablets | 60 tablet [PoM] £3,000.00
  Selexipag 1.4 mg Uptravi 1,400microgram tablets | 60 tablet [PoM] £3,000.00
  Selexipag 1.6 mg Uptravi 1,600microgram tablets | 60 tablet [PoM] £3,000.00

ANTITHROMBOTIC DRUGS > PROSTAGLANDINS, CARDIOVASCULAR

Iloprost

- **INDICATIONS AND DOSE**

Idiopathic or familial pulmonary arterial hypertension (initiated under specialist supervision)
  ▸ BY INHALATION OF NEBULISED SOLUTION
  ▸ Adult: Initially 2.5 micrograms for 1 dose, increased to 5 micrograms for 1 dose, increased if tolerated to 5 micrograms 6–9 times a day, adjusted according to response; reduced if not tolerated to 2.5 micrograms 6–9 times a day, reduce to lower maintenance dose if high dose not tolerated

- **CONTRA-INDICATIONS** Conditions which increase risk of haemorrhage · congenital or acquired valvular defects of the myocardium · decompensated cardiac failure (unless under close medical supervision) · pulmonary veno-occlusive disease · severe arrhythmias · unstable angina · within 3 months of cerebrovascular events · within 6 months of myocardial infarction

- **CAUTIONS** Acute pulmonary infection · chronic obstructive pulmonary disease · hypotension (do not initiate if systolic blood pressure below 85 mmHg) · severe asthma · unstable pulmonary hypertension with advanced right heart failure

- **INTERACTIONS** → Appendix 1: iloprost

- **SIDE-EFFECTS**
- **Common or very common** Chest discomfort · cough · diarrhoea · dizziness · dyspnoea · haemorrhage · headache · hypotension · nausea · oral disorders · pain · palpitations · rash · syncope · tachycardia · throat complaints · vasodilation · vomiting
- **Frequency not known** Respiratory disorders · taste altered · thrombocytopenia

- **PREGNANCY** Use if potential benefit outweighs risk.

- **BREAST FEEDING** Manufacturer advises avoid—no information available.

- **HEPATIC IMPAIRMENT** Elimination reduced.

Dose adjustments Initially 2.5 micrograms at intervals of 3–4 hours (max. 6 times daily), adjusted according to response (consult product literature).

● DIRECTIONS FOR ADMINISTRATION For *inhaled treatment*, to minimise accidental exposure use only with nebulisers listed in *Ventavis* ® product literature in a well ventilated room.

● PRESCRIBING AND DISPENSING INFORMATION Delivery characteristics of nebuliser devices may vary—only switch devices under medical supervision.

● NATIONAL FUNDING/ACCESS DECISIONS

Scottish Medicines Consortium (SMC) Decisions
The *Scottish Medicines Consortium* has advised (November 2005) that iloprost (*Ventavis* ®) is accepted for restricted use within NHS Scotland in patients in whom bosentan is ineffective or not tolerated, and should only be prescribed by specialists in the Scottish Pulmonary Vascular Unit.

● MEDICINAL FORMS
There can be variation in the licensing of different medicines containing the same drug.
Nebuliser liquid
▸ Ventavis (Bayer Plc)
Iloprost (as Iloprost trometamol) 10 microgram per 1 ml Ventavis 10micrograms/ml nebuliser solution 1ml ampoules | 30 ampoule PoM £400.19 | 168 ampoule PoM £2,241.08
Iloprost (as Iloprost trometamol) 20 microgram per 1 ml Ventavis 20micrograms/ml nebuliser solution 1ml ampoules | 30 ampoule PoM £400.19 | 168 ampoule PoM £2,241.08

ENDOTHELIN RECEPTOR ANTAGONISTS

Ambrisentan

● INDICATIONS AND DOSE

Pulmonary arterial hypertension (initiated under specialist supervision)
▸ BY MOUTH
▸ Adult: 5 mg once daily, increased if necessary to 10 mg once daily

DOSE ADJUSTMENTS DUE TO INTERACTIONS
▸ Manufacturer advises max. dose 5 mg daily and close monitoring with concurrent use of ciclosporin.

● CONTRA-INDICATIONS Idiopathic pulmonary fibrosis
● CAUTIONS Not to be initiated in significant anaemia
● INTERACTIONS → Appendix 1: ambrisentan
● SIDE-EFFECTS
▸ **Common or very common** Abdominal pain · anaemia · asthenia · constipation · diarrhoea · dizziness · epistaxis · flushing · headaches · hearing impairment · hypersensitivity · increased risk of infection · nasal congestion · nausea · palpitations · skin reactions · syncope · vision disorders · vomiting
▸ **Uncommon** Hepatic disorders
● CONCEPTION AND CONTRACEPTION Exclude pregnancy before treatment and ensure effective contraception during treatment. Monthly pregnancy tests advised.
● PREGNANCY Avoid (teratogenic in *animal studies*).
● BREAST FEEDING Manufacturer advises avoid—no information available.
● HEPATIC IMPAIRMENT Avoid in severe impairment.
● RENAL IMPAIRMENT Use with caution if eGFR less than 30 mL/minute/1.73 m².
● MONITORING REQUIREMENTS
▸ Monitor haemoglobin concentration or haematocrit after 1 month and 3 months of starting treatment, and periodically thereafter (reduce dose or discontinue treatment if significant decrease in haemoglobin concentration or haematocrit observed).

▸ Monitor liver function before treatment, and monthly thereafter—discontinue if liver enzymes raised significantly or if symptoms of liver impairment develop.

● NATIONAL FUNDING/ACCESS DECISIONS

Scottish Medicines Consortium (SMC) Decisions
The *Scottish Medicines Consortium* has advised (October 2008) that ambrisentan (*Volibris* ®) should be prescribed only by specialists in the Scottish Pulmonary Vascular Unit or other similar specialists.

● MEDICINAL FORMS
There can be variation in the licensing of different medicines containing the same drug.
Tablet
▸ Volibris (GlaxoSmithKline UK Ltd)
Ambrisentan 5 mg Volibris 5mg tablets | 30 tablet PoM £1,618.08
Ambrisentan 10 mg Volibris 10mg tablets | 30 tablet PoM £1,618.08

Bosentan

● INDICATIONS AND DOSE

Pulmonary arterial hypertension (initiated under specialist supervision)
▸ BY MOUTH
▸ Adult: Initially 62.5 mg twice daily for 4 weeks, then increased to 125 mg twice daily (max. per dose 250 mg); maximum 500 mg per day

Systemic sclerosis with ongoing digital ulcer disease (to reduce number of new digital ulcers)
▸ BY MOUTH
▸ Adult: Initially 62.5 mg twice daily for 4 weeks, then increased to 125 mg twice daily

● CONTRA-INDICATIONS Acute porphyrias p. 1025
● CAUTIONS Not to be initiated if systemic systolic blood pressure is below 85 mmHg
● INTERACTIONS → Appendix 1: bosentan
● SIDE-EFFECTS
▸ **Common or very common** Anaemia · diarrhoea · flushing · gastrooesophageal reflux disease · headache · nasal congestion · palpitations · skin reactions · syncope
▸ **Uncommon** Hepatic disorders · leucopenia · neutropenia · thrombocytopenia
▸ **Rare or very rare** Angioedema
▸ **Frequency not known** Vision blurred
● CONCEPTION AND CONTRACEPTION Effective contraception required during administration (hormonal contraception not considered effective). Monthly pregnancy tests advised.
● PREGNANCY Avoid (teratogenic in *animal* studies).
● BREAST FEEDING Manufacturer advises avoid—no information available.
● HEPATIC IMPAIRMENT Avoid in moderate and severe impairment.
● MONITORING REQUIREMENTS
▸ Monitor haemoglobin before and during treatment (monthly for first 4 months, then 3-monthly).
▸ Monitor liver function before treatment, at monthly intervals during treatment, and 2 weeks after dose increase (reduce dose or suspend treatment if liver enzymes raised significantly)—discontinue if symptoms of liver impairment.
● TREATMENT CESSATION Avoid abrupt withdrawal—withdraw treatment gradually.

- **MEDICINAL FORMS**
  There can be variation in the licensing of different medicines containing the same drug.

  Tablet
  - ▸ Bosentan (Non-proprietary)
    Bosentan (as Bosentan monohydrate) 62.5 mg Bosentan 62.5mg tablets | 56 tablet [PoM] £1,359.19–£1,510.21
    Bosentan (as Bosentan monohydrate) 125 mg Bosentan 125mg tablets | 56 tablet [PoM] £1,359.19–£1,510.21
  - ▸ Stayveer (AMCo)
    Bosentan (as Bosentan monohydrate) 62.5 mg Stayveer 62.5mg tablets | 56 tablet [PoM] £1,510.21
    Bosentan (as Bosentan monohydrate) 125 mg Stayveer 125mg tablets | 56 tablet [PoM] £1,510.21
  - ▸ Tracleer (Actelion Pharmaceuticals UK Ltd)
    Bosentan (as Bosentan monohydrate) 62.5 mg Tracleer 62.5mg tablets | 56 tablet [PoM] £1,510.21
    Bosentan (as Bosentan monohydrate) 125 mg Tracleer 125mg tablets | 56 tablet [PoM] £1,510.21

Macitentan

- **INDICATIONS AND DOSE**

  Pulmonary arterial hypertension (initiated under specialist supervision)
  - ▸ BY MOUTH
  - ▸ Adult: 10 mg daily

- **CONTRA-INDICATIONS** Severe anaemia
- **CAUTIONS** Patients over 75 years · pulmonary veno-occlusive disease
- **INTERACTIONS** → Appendix 1: macitentan
- **SIDE-EFFECTS**
- ▸ **Common or very common** Anaemia · headache · increased risk of infection · nasal congestion
- **CONCEPTION AND CONTRACEPTION** Manufacturer advises exclude pregnancy before treatment and ensure effective contraception during and for one month after stopping treatment. Monthly pregnancy tests advised.
- **PREGNANCY** Toxicity in *animal* studies.
- **BREAST FEEDING** Manufacturer advises avoid—present in milk in *animal* studies.
- **HEPATIC IMPAIRMENT** Do not initiate if serum transaminases exceed 3 times upper limit of normal. Avoid in moderate and severe impairment.
- **RENAL IMPAIRMENT** Manufacturer advises caution in severe impairment and avoid in patients undergoing dialysis (no information available).
  Monitoring In renal impairment consider monitoring blood pressure (risk of hypotension).
- **MONITORING REQUIREMENTS**
- ▸ Monitor liver function before treatment, then monthly thereafter (discontinue if unexplained persistent raised serum transaminases or signs of hepatic injury—can restart on advice on hepatologist if liver function tests return to normal and no hepatic injury).
- ▸ Monitor haemoglobin concentration before treatment and then as indicated.
- **PATIENT AND CARER ADVICE** Patients should be told how to recognise signs of liver disorder and advised to seek immediate medical attention if symptoms such as dark urine, nausea, vomiting, fatigue, abdominal pain, or pruritus develop.
  Patient card should be provided.
- **NATIONAL FUNDING/ACCESS DECISIONS**

  Scottish Medicines Consortium (SMC) Decisions
  The *Scottish Medicines Consortium* has advised (March 2014) that macitentan (*Opsumit*®) should be initiated and prescribed only by specialists in the Scottish Pulmonary Vascular Unit or other similar specialists.

- **MEDICINAL FORMS**
  There can be variation in the licensing of different medicines containing the same drug.

  Tablet
  - ▸ Opsumit (Actelion Pharmaceuticals UK Ltd) ▼
    Macitentan 10 mg Opsumit 10mg tablets | 30 tablet [PoM] £2,306.00

GUANYLATE CYCLASE STIMULATORS

Riociguat

19-Oct-2016

- **INDICATIONS AND DOSE**

  Chronic thromboembolic pulmonary hypertension that is recurrent or persistent following surgery, or is inoperable (initiated under specialist supervision) | Monotherapy or in combination with an endothelin receptor antagonist for idiopathic or hereditary pulmonary arterial hypertension, or pulmonary arterial hypertension associated with connective tissue disease (initiated under specialist supervision)
  - ▸ BY MOUTH
  - ▸ Adult: Initially 1 mg 3 times a day for 2 weeks, increased in steps of 0.5 mg 3 times a day, dose to be increased every 2 weeks, increased to up to 2.5 mg 3 times a day (max. per dose 2.5 mg 3 times a day), increase up to maximum dose only if systolic blood pressure $\geq$ 95 mmHg and no signs of hypotension, if treatment interrupted for 3 or more days, restart at 1 mg three times daily for 2 weeks and titrate as before, during titration, reduce dose by 0.5 mg three times daily if systolic blood pressure falls below 95 mmHg and patient shows signs of hypotension

  IMPORTANT SAFETY INFORMATION
  MHRA/CHM ADVICE: PULMONARY HYPERTENSION ASSOCIATED WITH IDIOPATHIC INTERSTITIAL PNEUMONIAS (PH-IIP) (AUGUST 2016)
  Interim results from a terminated study to investigate the efficacy and safety of riociguat in patients with symptomatic PH-IIP, showed increased mortality and increased risk of serious adverse events in the riociguat group compared with the placebo group. The MHRA has advised that use of riociguat is contra-indicated in these patients and that existing treatment for this unauthorised indication should be discontinued.

- **CONTRA-INDICATIONS** History of serious haemoptysis · previous bronchial artery embolisation · pulmonary hypertension associated with idiopathic interstitial pneumonias · pulmonary veno-occlusive disease
- **CAUTIONS** Autonomic dysfunction · elderly (risk of hypotension) · hypotension (do not initiate if systolic blood pressure below 95 mmHg) · hypovolaemia · severe left ventricular outflow obstruction
  CAUTIONS, FURTHER INFORMATION
  - ▸ Smoking Smoking cessation advised (response possibly reduced); dose adjustment may be necessary if smoking started or stopped during treatment.
- **INTERACTIONS** → Appendix 1: riociguat
- **SIDE-EFFECTS**
- ▸ **Common or very common** Anaemia · constipation · diarrhoea · dizziness · dysphagia · gastroenteritis · gastrointestinal discomfort · gastrointestinal disorders · haemorrhage · headache · hypotension · nasal congestion · nausea · palpitations · peripheral oedema · vomiting
- **CONCEPTION AND CONTRACEPTION** Effective contraception required during treatment. Monthly pregnancy tests advised.
- **PREGNANCY** Avoid—toxicity in *animal* studies.

- **BREAST FEEDING** Manufacturer advises avoid—present in milk in *animal* studies.
- **HEPATIC IMPAIRMENT** Manufacturer advises avoid in severe impairment—no information available.
  Dose adjustments Titrate dose cautiously in moderate impairment.
- **RENAL IMPAIRMENT** Manufacturer advises avoid if eGFR less than 30 mL/minute/1.73 m^2—limited information available.
  Dose adjustments Titrate dose cautiously—risk of hypotension.
- **DIRECTIONS FOR ADMINISTRATION** Tablets may be crushed and mixed with water or soft foods and swallowed immediately.
- **PATIENT AND CARER ADVICE** Smoking cessation advised (response possibly reduced). Patients should inform prescriber if smoking started or stopped during treatment; dose adjustment may be necessary.
- **NATIONAL FUNDING/ACCESS DECISIONS**
  Scottish Medicines Consortium (SMC) Decisions
  The *Scottish Medicines Consortium* has advised (November 2014) that riociguat (*Adempas*®) is accepted for restricted use within NHS Scotland for the treatment of chronic thromboembolic pulmonary hypertension in patients for whom a phosphodiesterase type-5 inhibitor is inappropriate, not tolerated, or ineffective, and should only be prescribed by specialists in the Scottish Pulmonary Vascular Unit.

- **MEDICINAL FORMS**
  There can be variation in the licensing of different medicines containing the same drug.
  Tablet
  CAUTIONARY AND ADVISORY LABELS 5
  ▸ Adempas (Merck Sharp & Dohme Ltd) ▼
  Riociguat 500 microgram Adempas 0.5mg tablets | 42 tablet [PoM] £997.36
  Riociguat 1 mg Adempas 1mg tablets | 42 tablet [PoM] £997.36
  Riociguat 1.5 mg Adempas 1.5mg tablets | 42 tablet [PoM] £997.36
  Riociguat 2 mg Adempas 2mg tablets | 42 tablet [PoM] £997.36 | 84 tablet [PoM] £1,994.72
  Riociguat 2.5 mg Adempas 2.5mg tablets | 42 tablet [PoM] £997.36 | 84 tablet [PoM] £1,994.72

4.2 Hypotension and shock

Sympathomimetics

Inotropic sympathomimetics
Shock
Shock is a medical emergency associated with a high mortality. The underlying causes of shock such as haemorrhage, sepsis, or myocardial insufficiency should be corrected. The profound hypotension of shock must be treated promptly to prevent tissue hypoxia and organ failure. Volume replacement is essential to correct the hypovolaemia associated with haemorrhage and sepsis but may be detrimental in cardiogenic shock. Depending on haemodynamic status, cardiac output may be improved by the use of sympathomimetic inotropes such as adrenaline/epinephrine p. 221, dobutamine p. 220 or dopamine hydrochloride below. In septic shock, when fluid replacement and inotropic support fail to maintain blood pressure, the vasoconstrictor noradrenaline/norepinephrine p. 188 may be considered. In cardiogenic shock peripheral resistance is frequently high and to raise it further may worsen myocardial performance and exacerbate tissue ischaemia.

The use of sympathomimetic inotropes and vasoconstrictors should preferably be confined to the intensive care setting and undertaken with invasive haemodynamic monitoring.

See also advice on the management of anaphylactic shock in Antihistamines, allergen immunotherapy and allergic emergencies p. 276.

Vasoconstrictor sympathomimetics
Vasoconstrictor sympathomimetics raise blood pressure transiently by acting on alpha-adrenergic receptors to constrict peripheral vessels. They are sometimes used as an emergency method of elevating blood pressure where other measures have failed.

The danger of vasoconstrictors is that although they raise blood pressure they also reduce perfusion of vital organs such as the kidney.

Spinal and epidural anaesthesia may result in sympathetic block with resultant hypotension. Management may include intravenous fluids (which are usually given prophylactically), oxygen, elevation of the legs, and injection of a pressor drug such as ephedrine hydrochloride p. 271. As well as constricting peripheral vessels ephedrine hydrochloride also accelerates the heart rate (by acting on beta receptors). Use is made of this dual action of ephedrine hydrochloride to manage associated bradycardia (although intravenous injection of atropine sulfate p. 1295 may also be required if bradycardia persists).

SYMPATHOMIMETICS › INOTROPIC

Dopamine hydrochloride

- **DRUG ACTION** Dopamine is a cardiac stimulant which acts on beta$_1$ receptors in cardiac muscle, and increases contractility with little effect on rate.

- **INDICATIONS AND DOSE**
  Cardiogenic shock in infarction or cardiac surgery
  ▸ BY INTRAVENOUS INFUSION
  ▸ **Adult:** Initially 2–5 micrograms/kg/minute

- **CONTRA-INDICATIONS** Phaeochromocytoma · tachyarrhythmia
- **CAUTIONS** Correct hypovolaemia · hypertension (may raise blood pressure) · hyperthyroidism · low dose in shock due to acute myocardial infarction
- **INTERACTIONS** → Appendix 1: sympathomimetics, inotropic
- **SIDE-EFFECTS** Angina pectoris · anxiety · arrhythmias · azotaemia · cardiac conduction disorder · dyspnoea · gangrene · headache · hypertension · mydriasis · nausea · palpitations · piloerection · polyuria · tremor · vasoconstriction · vomiting
- **PREGNANCY** No evidence of harm in *animal* studies—manufacturer advises use only if potential benefit outweighs risk.
- **BREAST FEEDING** May suppress lactation—not known to be harmful.
- **DIRECTIONS FOR ADMINISTRATION** Dopamine concentrate for intravenous infusion to be diluted before use.
  For *intravenous infusion* give continuously in Glucose 5% or Sodium chloride 0.9%. Dilute to max. concentration of 3.2 mg/mL; incompatible with bicarbonate.

● MEDICINAL FORMS
There can be variation in the licensing of different medicines containing the same drug. Forms available from special-order manufacturers include: solution for infusion

Solution for infusion

▸ Dopamine hydrochloride (Non-proprietary)
Dopamine hydrochloride 40 mg per 1 ml Dopamine 200mg/5ml solution for infusion ampoules | 5 ampoule [PoM] £20.00 (Hospital only) | 5 ampoule [PoM] £20.00 | 10 ampoule [PoM] £9.04
Dopamine 200mg/5ml concentrate for solution for infusion ampoules | 10 ampoule [PoM] [⬛]
Dopamine hydrochloride 160 mg per 1 ml Dopamine 800mg/5ml solution for infusion ampoules | 10 ampoule [PoM] £34.00

SYMPATHOMIMETICS ⟩ VASOCONSTRICTOR

Metaraminol

● INDICATIONS AND DOSE

Acute hypotension
▸ BY INTRAVENOUS INFUSION
▸ Adult: 15–100 mg, adjusted according to response
Emergency treatment of acute hypotension
▸ INITIALLY BY INTRAVENOUS INJECTION
▸ Adult: Initially 0.5–5 mg, then (by intravenous infusion) 15–100 mg, adjusted according to response

● CONTRA-INDICATIONS Hypertension

● CAUTIONS Cirrhosis · coronary vascular thrombosis · diabetes mellitus · elderly · extravasation at injection site may cause necrosis · following myocardial infarction · hypercapnia · hyperthyroidism · hypoxia · mesenteric vascular thrombosis · peripheral vascular thrombosis · Prinzmetal's variant angina · uncorrected hypovolaemia

CAUTIONS, FURTHER INFORMATION
▸ Hypertensive response Metaraminol has a longer duration of action than noradrenaline, and an excessive vasopressor response may cause a prolonged rise in blood pressure.

● INTERACTIONS → Appendix 1: sympathomimetics, vasoconstrictor

● SIDE-EFFECTS
▸ **Common or very common** Headache · hypertension
▸ **Rare or very rare** Skin exfoliation · soft tissue necrosis
▸ **Frequency not known** Abscess · arrhythmias · nausea · palpitations · peripheral ischaemia

● PREGNANCY May reduce placental perfusion—manufacturer advises use only if potential benefit outweighs risk.

● BREAST FEEDING Manufacturer advises caution—no information available.

● MONITORING REQUIREMENTS Monitor blood pressure and rate of flow frequently.

● MEDICINAL FORMS
There can be variation in the licensing of different medicines containing the same drug. Forms available from special-order manufacturers include: solution for injection

Solution for injection

▸ Metaraminol (Non-proprietary)
Metaraminol (as Metaraminol tartrate) 10 mg per 1 ml Metaraminol 10mg/1ml solution for injection ampoules | 10 ampoule [PoM] £39.40

Midodrine hydrochloride   01-Apr-2016

● DRUG ACTION Midodrine hydrochloride is a pro-drug of desglymidodrine. Desglymidodrine is a sympathomimetic agent, which acts on peripheral alpha-adrenergic receptors to increase arterial resistance, resulting in an increase in blood pressure.

● INDICATIONS AND DOSE

Severe orthostatic hypotension due to autonomic dysfunction when corrective factors have been ruled out and other forms of treatment are inadequate
▸ BY MOUTH
▸ Adult: Initially 2.5 mg 3 times a day, increased if necessary up to 10 mg 3 times a day, dose to be increased at weekly intervals, according to blood pressure measurements; usual maintenance 10 mg 3 times a day, avoid administration at night; the last daily dose should be taken at least 4 hours before bedtime

● CONTRA-INDICATIONS Aortic aneurysm · blood vessel spasm · bradycardia · cardiac conduction disturbances · cerebrovascular occlusion · congestive heart failure · hypertension · hyperthyroidism · myocardial infarction · narrow-angle glaucoma · phaeochromocytoma · proliferative diabetic retinopathy · serious obliterative blood vessel disease · serious prostate disorder · urinary retention

● CAUTIONS Atherosclerotic cardiovascular disease (especially with symptoms of intestinal angina or claudication of the legs) · autonomic dysfunction · elderly (manufacturer recommends cautious dose titration) · prostate disorders

● INTERACTIONS → Appendix 1: sympathomimetics, vasoconstrictor

● SIDE-EFFECTS
▸ **Common or very common** Chills · flushing · gastrointestinal discomfort · headache · nausea · paraesthesia · piloerection · supine hypertension (dose-dependent) · scalp pruritus · skin reactions · stomatitis · urinary disorders
▸ **Uncommon** Anxiety · arrhythmias · irritability · sleep disorders
▸ **Rare or very rare** Hepatic function abnormal · palpitations
▸ **Frequency not known** Confusion · diarrhoea · vomiting
SIDE-EFFECTS, FURTHER INFORMATION Manufacturer advises that treatment must be stopped if supine hypertension is not controlled by reducing the dose.

● CONCEPTION AND CONTRACEPTION Manufacturer recommends effective contraception during treatment in women of childbearing potential.

● PREGNANCY Manufacturer advises avoid—toxicity in *animal* studies.

● BREAST FEEDING Manufacturer advises avoid—no information available.

● RENAL IMPAIRMENT Manufacturer advises avoid in severe or acute impairment.

● MONITORING REQUIREMENTS
▸ Manufacturer advises measure hepatic and renal function before treatment and at regular intervals during treatment.
▸ Manufacturer advises regular monitoring of supine and standing blood pressure due to the risk of hypertension in the supine position.

● PATIENT AND CARER ADVICE Manufacturer advises that patients report symptoms of supine hypertension (such as chest pain, palpitations, shortness of breath, headache and blurred vision) immediately. The risk of supine hypertension at night can be reduced by raising the head of the bed.

- MEDICINAL FORMS
There can be variation in the licensing of different medicines containing the same drug.
Tablet
▸ Midodrine hydrochloride (Non-proprietary)
Midodrine hydrochloride 2.5 mg Midodrine 2.5mg tablets | 100 tablet [PoM] £55.05 DT = £55.05
Midodrine hydrochloride 5 mg Midodrine 5mg tablets | 100 tablet [PoM] £75.05 DT = £75.05
▸ Bramox (Brancaster Pharma Ltd)
Midodrine hydrochloride 2.5 mg Bramox 2.5mg tablets | 100 tablet [PoM] £55.05 DT = £55.05
Midodrine hydrochloride 5 mg Bramox 5mg tablets | 100 tablet [PoM] £75.05 DT = £75.05
▸ Midotense (Transdermal Ltd)
Midodrine hydrochloride 2.5 mg Midotense 2.5mg tablets | 30 tablet [PoM] £15.69

Noradrenaline/norepinephrine   03-Apr-2018

- **INDICATIONS AND DOSE**

Acute hypotension [initial and on-going treatment]
▸ BY INTRAVENOUS INFUSION
▸ Adult: Initially 0.16–0.33 mL/minute, adjusted according to response, dose applies to a solution containing noradrenaline 40 micrograms(base)/mL only; dilute the 1 mg/mL concentrate for infusion for this solution—consult product literature

On-going treatment of acute hypotension [with escalating dose requirements]
▸ BY INTRAVENOUS INFUSION
▸ Adult (body-weight 50 kg and above): Use the 0.08 mg/mL solution for infusion (consult product literature)

DOSE EQUIVALENCE AND CONVERSION
▸ 1 mg of noradrenaline base is equivalent to 2 mg of noradrenaline acid tartrate. **Doses expressed as the base.**

IMPORTANT SAFETY INFORMATION

ASSOCIATION OF NORADRENALINE/NOREPINEPHRINE 0.08 MG/ML (4 MG IN 50 ML) SOLUTION FOR INFUSION WITH POTENTIAL RISK OF MEDICATION ERRORS
Healthcare professionals should be aware of the differences in strength and presentation between noradrenaline/norepinephrine products—manufacturer advises noradrenaline 0.08 mg/mL solution for infusion must **not** be diluted before use and should only be used for the on-going treatment of patients already established on noradrenaline therapy, whose dose requirements are clinically confirmed to be escalating.

- CONTRA-INDICATIONS Hypertension
- CAUTIONS Coronary vascular thrombosis · diabetes mellitus · elderly · extravasation at injection site may cause necrosis · following myocardial infarction · hypercapnia · hyperthyroidism · hypoxia · mesenteric vascular thrombosis · peripheral vascular thrombosis · Prinzmetal's variant angina · uncorrected hypovolaemia
- INTERACTIONS → Appendix 1: sympathomimetics, vasoconstrictor
- SIDE-EFFECTS Anxiety · arrhythmias · dyspnoea · extravasation necrosis · headache · hypertension · hypovolaemia · peripheral ischaemia
- PREGNANCY Manufacturer advises use if potential benefit outweighs risk—may reduce placental perfusion and induce fetal bradycardia.
- MONITORING REQUIREMENTS Monitor blood pressure and rate of flow frequently.
- DIRECTIONS FOR ADMINISTRATION For *intravenous infusion* using a solution containing noradrenaline 40 micrograms (base)/mL, manufacturer advises give continuously in

Glucose 5% or Sodium Chloride and Glucose via a controlled infusion device. For administration via syringe pump, dilute 2 mg (2 mL of 1 mg/mL concentrate for infusion) noradrenaline base with 48 mL infusion fluid. For administration via drip counter dilute 20 mg (20 mL of 1 mg/mL concentrate for infusion) noradrenaline base with 480 mL infusion fluid; give through a central venous catheter; incompatible with alkalis.

- PRESCRIBING AND DISPENSING INFORMATION For a period of time, preparations on the UK market may be described as either noradrenaline base or noradrenaline acid tartrate; doses in the BNF are expressed as the base.

- MEDICINAL FORMS
There can be variation in the licensing of different medicines containing the same drug. Forms available from special-order manufacturers include: infusion, solution for infusion
Solution for infusion
▸ Noradrenaline/norepinephrine (Non-proprietary)
Noradrenaline (as Noradrenaline acid tartrate) 80 microgram per 1 ml Noradrenaline (base) 4mg/50ml solution for infusion vials | 10 vial [PoM] [℞]
Noradrenaline (as Noradrenaline acid tartrate) 1 mg per 1 ml Noradrenaline (Norepinephrine) 4mg/4ml concentrate for solution for infusion ampoules | 10 ampoule [PoM] £44.00
Noradrenaline (base) 8mg/8ml concentrate for solution for infusion ampoules | 10 ampoule [PoM] £116.00
Noradrenaline (base) 2mg/2ml solution for infusion ampoules | 5 ampoule [PoM] £12.00 (Hospital only)
Noradrenaline (base) 4mg/4ml solution for infusion ampoules | 5 ampoule [PoM] £22.00 (Hospital only)
Noradrenaline (base) 4mg/4ml concentrate for solution for infusion ampoules | 10 ampoule [PoM] £58.00
Noradrenaline (Norepinephrine) 2mg/2ml concentrate for solution for Infusion ampoules | 5 ampoule [PoM] £11.00

Phenylephrine hydrochloride

- **INDICATIONS AND DOSE**

Acute hypotension
▸ BY SUBCUTANEOUS INJECTION, OR BY INTRAMUSCULAR INJECTION
▸ Adult: Initially 2–5 mg, followed by 1–10 mg, after at least 15 minutes if required
▸ BY SLOW INTRAVENOUS INJECTION
▸ Adult: 100–500 micrograms, repeated as necessary after at least 15 minutes
▸ BY INTRAVENOUS INFUSION
▸ Adult: Initially up to 180 micrograms/minute, reduced to 30–60 micrograms/minute, adjusted according to response

- CONTRA-INDICATIONS Hypertension · severe hyperthyroidism
- CAUTIONS
Coronary disease · coronary vascular thrombosis · diabetes · elderly · extravasation at injection site may cause necrosis · following myocardial infarction · hypercapnia · hyperthyroidism · hypoxia · mesenteric vascular thrombosis · peripheral vascular thrombosis · Prinzmetal's variant angina · susceptibility to angle-closure glaucoma · uncorrected hypovolaemia

CAUTIONS, FURTHER INFORMATION
▸ Hypertensive response Phenylephrine has a longer duration of action than noradrenaline (norepinephrine), and an excessive vasopressor response may cause a prolonged rise in blood pressure.

- INTERACTIONS → Appendix 1: sympathomimetics, vasoconstrictor
- SIDE-EFFECTS Angina pectoris · arrhythmias · cardiac arrest · dizziness · dyspnoea · flushing · glucose tolerance impaired · headache · hyperhidrosis · hypersalivation · hypotension · intracranial haemorrhage · metabolic change

· mydriasis · palpitations · paraesthesia · peripheral coldness · pulmonary oedema · soft tissue necrosis · syncope · urinary disorders · vomiting

● PREGNANCY Avoid if possible; malformations reported following use in first trimester; fetal hypoxia and bradycardia reported in late pregnancy and labour.

● MONITORING REQUIREMENTS Contra-indicated in hypertension—monitor blood pressure and rate of flow frequently.

● DIRECTIONS FOR ADMINISTRATION For *intravenous infusion* give intermittently in Glucose 5% or Sodium chloride 0.9%. Dilute 10 mg in 500 mL infusion fluid.

● MEDICINAL FORMS
There can be variation in the licensing of different medicines containing the same drug. Forms available from special-order manufacturers include: solution for injection, eye drops

Solution for injection

▸ Phenylephrine hydrochloride (Non-proprietary)

Phenylephrine (as Phenylephrine hydrochloride) 50 microgram per 1 ml Phenylephrine 500micrograms/10ml solution for injection pre-filled syringes | 1 pre-filled disposable injection PoM £15.00 | 10 pre-filled disposable injection PoM £150.00

Phenylephrine hydrochloride 100 microgram per 1 ml Phenylephrine 1mg/10ml solution for injection ampoules | 10 ampoule PoM £40.00

Phenylephrine hydrochloride 10 mg per 1 ml Phenylephrine 10mg/1ml solution for injection ampoules | 10 ampoule PoM £99.12

5   Heart failure

Heart failure

Drug treatment

Drug treatment of **heart failure** associated with a reduced left ventricular ejection fraction (left ventricular systolic dysfunction) is covered below; optimal management of heart failure with a preserved left ventricular ejection fraction has not been established.

The treatment of chronic heart failure aims to relieve symptoms, improve exercise tolerance, reduce the incidence of acute exacerbations, and reduce mortality. An **ACE inhibitor**, titrated to a 'target dose' (or the maximum tolerated dose if lower), together with a **beta-blocker**, form the basis of treatment for all patients with heart failure due to left ventricular systolic dysfunction.

An ACE inhibitor is generally advised for patients with asymptomatic left ventricular systolic dysfunction or symptomatic heart failure. An **angiotensin-II receptor antagonist** may be a useful alternative for patients who, because of side-effects such as cough, cannot tolerate ACE inhibitors; a relatively high dose of the angiotensin-II receptor antagonist may be required to produce benefit. Candesartan cilexetil p. 174 or valsartan p. 178 may be given under specialist supervision as adjuncts to an ACE inhibitor in the treatment of heart failure when other treatments are unsuitable; the concomitant use of this combination, together with an aldosterone antagonist or a potassium-sparing diuretic is not recommended. The combination of sacubitril with valsartan p. 191, an angiotensin-II receptor antagonist with a neprilysin inhibitor, may be a suitable alternative for those patients already stabilised on an ACE inhibitor or angiotensin-II receptor antagonist.

The beta-blockers bisoprolol fumarate p. 152 and carvedilol p. 147 are of value in any grade of stable heart failure due to left ventricular systolic dysfunction; nebivolol p. 154 is licensed for stable mild to moderate heart failure in patients over 70 years. Beta-blocker treatment should be started by those experienced in the management of heart failure, at a very low dose and titrated very slowly over a

period of weeks or months. Symptoms may deteriorate initially, calling for adjustment of concomitant therapy.

The aldosterone antagonist spironolactone p. 190 can be added to an ACE inhibitor and a beta-blocker in patients who continue to remain symptomatic (particularly in those with moderate to severe heart failure); low doses of spironolactone reduce symptoms and mortality in these patients. If spironolactone cannot be used, eplerenone p. 190 may be considered for the management of heart failure after an acute myocardial infarction with evidence of left ventricular systolic dysfunction, or for chronic mild heart failure with left ventricular systolic dysfunction. Close monitoring of serum creatinine, eGFR, and potassium is necessary, particularly following any change in treatment or any change in the patient's clinical condition.

Patients who cannot tolerate an ACE inhibitor or an angiotensin-II receptor antagonist, or in whom they are contra-indicated, may be given isosorbide dinitrate p. 219 with hydralazine hydrochloride p. 180 but this combination may be poorly tolerated. The combination of isosorbide dinitrate and hydralazine hydrochloride may be considered in addition to standard therapy with an ACE inhibitor and a beta-blocker in patients who continue to remain symptomatic (particularly in patients of African or Caribbean origin who have moderate to severe heart failure).

Digoxin p. 109 improves symptoms of heart failure and exercise tolerance and reduces hospitalisation due to acute exacerbations but it does not reduce mortality. Digoxin is reserved for patients with worsening or severe heart failure due to left ventricular systolic dysfunction who remain symptomatic despite treatment with an ACE inhibitor and a beta-blocker in combination with either an aldosterone antagonist, candesartan cilexetil, or isosorbide dinitrate with hydralazine hydrochloride.

Patients with fluid overload should also receive either a loop or a thiazide diuretic (with salt or fluid restriction where appropriate). A **thiazide diuretic** may be of benefit in patients with mild heart failure and good renal function; however, thiazide diuretics are ineffective in patients with poor renal function (eGFR less than 30 mL/minute/1.73 m²) and a **loop diuretic** is preferred. If diuresis with a single diuretic is insufficient, a combination of a loop diuretic and a thiazide diuretic may be tried; addition of metolazone p. 230 may also be considered but the resulting diuresis may be profound and care is needed to avoid potentially dangerous electrolyte disturbances.

Other drugs used for Heart failure Bendroflumethiazide, p. 165 · Captopril, p. 167 · Chlortalidone, p. 229 · Co-amilozide, p. 166 · Cyclopenthiazide, p. 230 · Enalapril maleate, p. 168 · Fosinopril sodium, p. 169 · Glyceryl trinitrate, p. 217 · Isosorbide mononitrate, p. 219 · Ivabradine, p. 210 · Lisinopril, p. 170 · Losartan potassium, p. 176 · Metoprolol tartrate, p. 154 · Perindopril arginine, p. 170 · Perindopril erbumine, p. 171 · Prazosin, p. 766 · Quinapril, p. 172 · Ramipril, p. 172 · Sodium nitroprusside, p. 182

DIURETICS > POTASSIUM-SPARING DIURETICS > ALDOSTERONE ANTAGONISTS

Co-flumactone

The properties listed below are those particular to the combination only. For the properties of the components please consider, spironolactone below.

● **INDICATIONS AND DOSE**

Congestive heart failure
▶ BY MOUTH
▶ Adult: Initially 100/100 mg daily; maintenance 25/25–200/200 mg daily, maintenance dose not recommended because spironolactone generally given in lower dose

● INTERACTIONS → Appendix 1: aldosterone antagonists · thiazide diuretics

● LESS SUITABLE FOR PRESCRIBING Co-flumactone tablets are less suitable for prescribing.

● **MEDICINAL FORMS**
There can be variation in the licensing of different medicines containing the same drug.
Tablet
▶ Aldactide (Pfizer Ltd)
  Hydroflumethiazide 25 mg, Spironolactone 25 mg Aldactide 25 tablets | 100 tablet PoM £20.23 DT = £20.23
  Hydroflumethiazide 50 mg, Spironolactone 50 mg Aldactide 50 tablets | 28 tablet PoM £10.70 | 100 tablet PoM £38.23 DT = £38.23

Eplerenone

● **INDICATIONS AND DOSE**

Adjunct in stable patients with left ventricular ejection fraction ≤40% with evidence of heart failure, following myocardial infarction (start therapy within 3–14 days of event) | Adjunct in chronic mild heart failure with left ventricular ejection fraction ≤30%
▶ BY MOUTH
▶ Adult: Initially 25 mg daily, then increased to 50 mg daily, increased within 4 weeks of initial treatment

DOSE ADJUSTMENTS DUE TO INTERACTIONS
▶ Manufacturer advises max. dose 25 mg daily with concurrent use of amiodarone or moderate inhibitors of CYP3A4.

● CONTRA-INDICATIONS Hyperkalaemia
● CAUTIONS Elderly
● INTERACTIONS → Appendix 1: aldosterone antagonists
● SIDE-EFFECTS
▶ **Common or very common** Arrhythmias · asthenia · constipation · cough · diarrhoea · dizziness · dyslipidaemia · electrolyte imbalance · headache · insomnia · muscle spasms · nausea · pain · renal impairment · skin reactions · syncope · vomiting
▶ **Uncommon** Angioedema · arterial thrombosis · cholecystitis · eosinophilia · flatulence · gynaecomastia · hyperhidrosis · hypothyroidism · increased risk of infection · malaise · numbness · postural hypotension

● PREGNANCY Manufacturer advises caution—no information available.
● BREAST FEEDING Manufacturer advises use only if potential benefit outweighs risk.
● HEPATIC IMPAIRMENT Avoid in severe impairment.
● RENAL IMPAIRMENT Avoid if eGFR less than 30 mL/minute/1.73 m².
  Dose adjustments Initially 25 mg on alternate days if eGFR 30–60 mL/minute/1.73 m², adjust dose according to

serum-potassium concentration—consult product literature.
  Monitoring Increased risk of hyperkalaemia in renal impairment—close monitoring required.
● MONITORING REQUIREMENTS Monitor plasma-potassium concentration before treatment, during initiation, and when dose changed.

● **MEDICINAL FORMS**
There can be variation in the licensing of different medicines containing the same drug.
Tablet
▶ Eplerenone (Non-proprietary)
  Eplerenone 25 mg Eplerenone 25mg tablets | 28 tablet PoM £42.72 DT = £14.52
  Eplerenone 50 mg Eplerenone 50mg tablets | 28 tablet PoM £42.72 DT = £11.52
▶ Inspra (Pfizer Ltd)
  Eplerenone 25 mg Inspra 25mg tablets | 28 tablet PoM £42.72 DT = £14.52
  Eplerenone 50 mg Inspra 50mg tablets | 28 tablet PoM £42.72 DT = £11.52

Spironolactone

19-Mar-2018

● **INDICATIONS AND DOSE**

Oedema | Ascites in cirrhosis of the liver
▶ BY MOUTH
▶ Adult: 100–400 mg daily, adjusted according to response

Malignant ascites
▶ BY MOUTH
▶ Adult: Initially 100–200 mg daily, then increased if necessary to 400 mg daily, maintenance dose adjusted according to response

Nephrotic syndrome
▶ BY MOUTH
▶ Adult: 100–200 mg daily

Oedema in congestive heart failure
▶ BY MOUTH
▶ Adult: Initially 100 mg daily, alternatively initially 25–200 mg daily, dose may be taken as a single dose or divided doses, maintenance dose adjusted according to response

Moderate to severe heart failure (adjunct)
▶ BY MOUTH
▶ Adult: Initially 25 mg once daily, then adjusted according to response to 50 mg once daily

Resistant hypertension (adjunct)
▶ BY MOUTH
▶ Adult: 25 mg once daily

Primary hyperaldosteronism in patients awaiting surgery
▶ BY MOUTH
▶ Adult: 100–400 mg daily, may be used for long-term maintenance if surgery inappropriate, use lowest effective dose

● UNLICENSED USE Resistant hypertension (adjunct) unlicensed indication.
● CONTRA-INDICATIONS Addison's disease · anuria · hyperkalaemia
● CAUTIONS Acute porphyrias p. 1025 · elderly · potential metabolic products carcinogenic in *rodents*
● INTERACTIONS → Appendix 1: aldosterone antagonists
● SIDE-EFFECTS Acidosis hyperchloraemic · acute kidney injury · agranulocytosis · alopecia · breast neoplasm benign · breast pain · confusion · dizziness · electrolyte imbalance · gastrointestinal disorder · gynaecomastia · hepatic function abnormal · hyperkalaemia (discontinue) · hypertrichosis · leg cramps · leucopenia · libido disorder · malaise · menstrual disorder · nausea · severe cutaneous

adverse reactions (SCARs) · skin reactions · thrombocytopenia

● PREGNANCY Use only if potential benefit outweighs risk—feminisation of male fetus in *animal* studies.

● BREAST FEEDING Metabolites present in milk, but amount probably too small to be harmful.

● RENAL IMPAIRMENT Avoid in acute renal insufficiency or severe impairment.
Monitoring Monitor plasma-potassium concentration (high risk of hyperkalaemia in renal impairment).

● MONITORING REQUIREMENTS Monitor electrolytes—discontinue if hyperkalaemia occurs (in *severe heart failure* monitor potassium and creatinine 1 week after initiation and after any dose increase, monthly for first 3 months, then every 3 months for 1 year, and then every 6 months).

● MEDICINAL FORMS
There can be variation in the licensing of different medicines containing the same drug. Forms available from special-order manufacturers include: oral suspension, oral solution
Tablet
CAUTIONARY AND ADVISORY LABELS 21
▶ Spironolactone (Non-proprietary)
Spironolactone 25 mg Spironolactone 25mg tablets |
28 tablet PoM £1.95 DT = £0.99
Spironolactone 50 mg Spironolactone 50mg tablets |
28 tablet PoM £9.99 DT = £4.74
Spironolactone 100 mg Spironolactone 100mg tablets |
28 tablet PoM £2.96 DT = £1.76
▶ Aldactone (Pfizer Ltd)
Spironolactone 25 mg Aldactone 25mg tablets | 100 tablet PoM
£8.89
Spironolactone 50 mg Aldactone 50mg tablets | 100 tablet PoM
£17.78
Spironolactone 100 mg Aldactone 100mg tablets | 28 tablet PoM
£9.96 DT = £1.76 | 100 tablet PoM £35.56

DRUGS ACTING ON THE RENIN-ANGIOTENSIN SYSTEM > ANGIOTENSIN II RECEPTOR ANTAGONISTS

| Sacubitril with valsartan
11-Sep-2017

The properties listed below are those particular to the combination only. For the properties of the components please consider, valsartan p. 178.

● DRUG ACTION Sacubitril (a prodrug) inhibits the breakdown of natriuretic peptides resulting in varied effects including increased diuresis, natriuresis, and vasodilation.

● INDICATIONS AND DOSE

Symptomatic chronic heart failure with reduced ejection fraction (in patients not currently taking an ACE inhibitor or angiotensin II receptor antagonist, or stabilised on low doses of either of these agents)
▶ BY MOUTH
▶ Adult: Initially 24/26 mg twice daily for 3–4 weeks, increased if tolerated to 49/51 mg twice daily for 3–4 weeks, then increased if tolerated to 97/103 mg twice daily

Symptomatic chronic heart failure with reduced ejection fraction (in patients currently stabilised on an ACE inhibitor or angiotensin II receptor antagonist)
▶ BY MOUTH
▶ Adult: Initially 49/51 mg twice daily for 2–4 weeks, increased if tolerated to 97/103 mg twice daily, consider a starting dose of 24/26 mg if systolic blood pressure less than 110 mmHg

DOSE EQUIVALENCE AND CONVERSION
▶ *Entresto*® tablets contain sacubitril and valsartan; the proportions are expressed in the form x/y where x and y

are the strength in milligrams of sacubitril and valsartan respectively. Valsartan, in this formulation, is more bioavailable than other tablet formulations—26 mg, 51 mg, and 103 mg valsartan is equivalent to 40 mg, 80 mg and 160 mg, respectively. Furthermore, note that the 24/26 mg, 49/51 mg and 97/103 mg strengths are sometimes referred to as a total of both drug strengths, that is, 50 mg, 100 mg and 200 mg, respectively.

● CONTRA-INDICATIONS Systolic blood pressure less than 100 mmHg

● INTERACTIONS → Appendix 1: angiotensin-II receptor antagonists · sacubitril

● SIDE-EFFECTS
▶ **Common or very common** Anaemia · asthenia · cough · diarrhoea · dizziness · electrolyte imbalance · gastritis · headache · hypoglycaemia · hypotension · nausea · renal impairment · syncope · vertigo
▶ **Uncommon** Angioedema · skin reactions

● PREGNANCY Manufacturer advises avoid—toxicity with sacubitril in *animal* studies.

● BREAST FEEDING Manufacturer advises avoid—present in milk in *animal* studies.

● HEPATIC IMPAIRMENT Contra-indicated in severe impairment.
Dose adjustments Manufacturer advises starting dose of 26/24 mg twice daily in moderate impairment.

● RENAL IMPAIRMENT
Dose adjustments Manufacturer recommends a starting dose of 26/24 mg twice daily if eGFR less than 30 mL/minute/1.73m^2. Also consider this starting dose if eGFR 30 to 60 mL/minute/1.73m^2.

● NATIONAL FUNDING/ACCESS DECISIONS
NICE decisions
▶ **Sacubitril valsartan for treating symptomatic chronic heart failure with reduced ejection fraction (April 2016)** NICE TA388
Sacubitril valsartan is recommended as an option for treating symptomatic chronic heart failure with reduced ejection fraction, only in adults:
● with New York Heart Association class II to IV symptoms **and**
● a left ventricular ejection fraction of 35% or less **and**
● who are already taking a stable dose of an ACE inhibitor or angiotensin II receptor antagonist.
www.nice.org.uk/ta388

● MEDICINAL FORMS
There can be variation in the licensing of different medicines containing the same drug.
Tablet
▶ Entresto (Novartis Pharmaceuticals UK Ltd) ▼
Sacubitril 24 mg, Valsartan 26 mg Entresto 24mg/26mg tablets |
28 tablet PoM £45.78 DT = £45.78
Sacubitril 49 mg, Valsartan 51 mg Entresto 49mg/51mg tablets |
28 tablet PoM £45.78 | 56 tablet PoM £91.56 DT = £91.56
Sacubitril 97 mg, Valsartan 103 mg Entresto 97mg/103mg tablets
| 56 tablet PoM £91.56 DT = £91.56

PHOSPHODIESTERASE TYPE-3 INHIBITORS

Enoximone

- **DRUG ACTION** Enoximone is a phosphodiesterase type-3 inhibitor that exerts most effect on the myocardium; it has positive inotropic properties and vasodilator activity.

- **INDICATIONS AND DOSE**

Congestive heart failure where cardiac output reduced and filling pressures increased
  - ► BY SLOW INTRAVENOUS INJECTION
  - ► Adult: Initially 0.5–1 mg/kg, rate not exceeding 12.5 mg/minute, then 500 micrograms/kg every 30 minutes until satisfactory response or total of 3 mg/kg given; maintenance, initial dose of up to 3 mg/kg may be repeated every 3–6 hours as required
  - ► BY INTRAVENOUS INFUSION
  - ► Adult: Initially 90 micrograms/kg/minute, dose to be given over 10–30 minutes, followed by 5–20 micrograms/kg/minute, dose to be given as either a continuous or intermittent infusion; maximum 24 mg/kg per day

- **CAUTIONS** Heart failure associated with hypertrophic cardiomyopathy, stenotic or obstructive valvular disease or other outlet obstruction

- **SIDE-EFFECTS**
  - ► **Common or very common** Headache · hypotension · insomnia
  - ► **Uncommon** Arrhythmias · diarrhoea · dizziness · nausea · vomiting
  - ► **Rare or very rare** Chills · fever · fluid retention · myalgia · oliguria · urinary retention

- **PREGNANCY** Manufacturer advises use only if potential benefit outweighs risk.

- **BREAST FEEDING** Manufacturer advises caution—no information available.

- **HEPATIC IMPAIRMENT**
Dose adjustments Dose reduction may be required.

- **RENAL IMPAIRMENT**
Dose adjustments Consider dose reduction.

- **MONITORING REQUIREMENTS** Monitor blood pressure, heart rate, ECG, central venous pressure, fluid and electrolyte status, renal function, platelet count and hepatic enzymes.

- **DIRECTIONS FOR ADMINISTRATION** Incompatible with glucose solutions. Use only plastic containers or syringes; crystal formation if glass used. Avoid extravasation.
  For *intravenous infusion (Perfan®)*, give continuously or intermittently in Sodium chloride 0.9% or Water for injections; dilute to a concentration of 2.5 mg/mL.

- **PRESCRIBING AND DISPENSING INFORMATION** Sustained haemodynamic benefit has been observed after administration of phosphodiesterase type-3 inhibitors, but there is no evidence of any beneficial effect on survival.

- **MEDICINAL FORMS**
There can be variation in the licensing of different medicines containing the same drug.
Solution for injection
EXCIPIENTS: May contain Alcohol, propylene glycol
  - ► Perfan (Myogen GmbH)
    Enoximone 5 mg per 1 ml Perfan 100mg/20ml solution for injection ampoules | 10 ampoule [PoM] [⚠] (Hospital only)

Milrinone

- **DRUG ACTION** Milrinone is a phosphodiesterase type-3 inhibitor that exerts most effect on the myocardium; it has positive inotropic properties and vasodilator activity.

- **INDICATIONS AND DOSE**

Short-term treatment of severe congestive heart failure unresponsive to conventional maintenance therapy (not immediately after myocardial infarction) | Acute heart failure, including low output states following heart surgery
  - ► INITIALLY BY INTRAVENOUS INJECTION
  - ► Adult: Initially 50 micrograms/kg, given over 10 minutes, followed by (by intravenous infusion) 375–750 nanograms/kg/minute usually given following surgery for up to 12 hours or in congestive heart failure for 48-72 hours; maximum 1.13 mg/kg per day

- **CONTRA-INDICATIONS** Severe hypovolaemia

- **CAUTIONS** Correct hypokalaemia · heart failure associated with hypertrophic cardiomyopathy, stenotic or obstructive valvular disease or other outlet obstruction

- **SIDE-EFFECTS**
  - ► **Common or very common** Arrhythmia supraventricular (increased risk in patients with pre-existing arrhythmias) · headache · hypotension
  - ► **Uncommon** Angina pectoris · chest pain · hypokalaemia · thrombocytopenia · tremor
  - ► **Rare or very rare** Anaphylactic shock · bronchospasm · skin eruption
  - ► **Frequency not known** Renal failure

- **PREGNANCY** Manufacturer advises use only if potential benefit outweighs risk.

- **BREAST FEEDING** Manufacturer advises avoid—no information available.

- **RENAL IMPAIRMENT**
Dose adjustments Reduce dose and monitor response if eGFR less than 50 mL/minute/1.73 m² —consult product literature for details.

- **MONITORING REQUIREMENTS** Monitor blood pressure, heart rate, ECG, central venous pressure, fluid and electrolyte status, renal function, platelet count and hepatic enzymes.

- **DIRECTIONS FOR ADMINISTRATION** Avoid extravasation.
  For *intravenous injection*, may be given either undiluted or diluted before use.
  For *intravenous infusion (Primacor®)* give continuously in Glucose 5% or Sodium chloride 0.9%; dilute to a suggested concentration of 200 micrograms/mL.

- **PRESCRIBING AND DISPENSING INFORMATION** Sustained haemodynamic benefit has been observed after administration of phosphodiesterase type-3 inhibitors, but there is no evidence of any beneficial effect on survival.

- **MEDICINAL FORMS**
There can be variation in the licensing of different medicines containing the same drug. Forms available from special-order manufacturers include: solution for infusion
Solution for injection
  - ► Milrinone (Non-proprietary)
    Milrinone 1 mg per 1 ml Milrinone 10mg/10ml solution for injection ampoules | 5 ampoule [PoM] £35.00 | 10 ampoule [PoM] £199.06
  - ► Primacor (Sanofi)
    Milrinone 1 mg per 1 ml Primacor 10mg/10ml solution for injection ampoules | 10 ampoule [PoM] £199.06

6   Hyperlipidaemia

Lipid-regulating drugs

Cardiovascular disease, primary and secondary prevention

Preventative measures should be taken in individuals with a high risk of developing cardiovascular disease (primary prevention) and to prevent recurrence of events in those with established cardiovascular disease (secondary prevention).

Cardiovascular disease, primary prevention

Individuals at high risk of developing cardiovascular disease include those who have diabetes mellitus, chronic kidney disease (eGFR < 60 mL/minute/1.73 m^2) and/or albuminuria, and those with familial hypercholesterolaemia. The risk also increases with age; those aged 85 years and over are at particularly high risk, especially if they smoke or have hypertension. Preventative measures are also required for other individuals who are considered to be at high risk of developing atherosclerotic cardiovascular disease based on risk estimated using risk calculators (see Risk calculators); those with a 10-year risk of cardiovascular disease of 10% or more stand to benefit most from drug treatment. Patients with a 10-year cardiovascular risk of less than 10% may benefit from an assessment of their lifetime risk (using the JBS3 tool—see Risk calculators for more detail), discussion on the impact of lifestyle interventions and, if necessary, drug therapy.

Cardiovascular disease risk calculators

Risk assessment calculators are recommended by both NICE (clinical guideline 181 (July 2014). Lipid Modification— Cardiovascular risk assessment and the modification of blood lipids for the primary and secondary prevention of cardiovascular disease) and JBS3 (Joint British Societies' consensus recommendations for the prevention of cardiovascular disease 2014). They should not be used in patients at high cardiovascular risk. Both calculators are unsuitable for assessing risk in those aged 85 years and over, and NICE advises against using a risk assessment tool in those with type 1 diabetes mellitus.

The QRISK® 2 risk calculator www.qrisk.org/ is recommended by NICE clinical guideline 181, and the JBS3 risk calculator www.jbs3risk.com/pages/risk_calculator.htm is endorsed by JBS3. Both tools assess cardiovascular risk— coronary heart disease (angina and myocardial infarction), stroke, and transient ischaemic attack, on the basis of lipid profile, systolic blood pressure, gender, age, ethnicity, smoking status, BMI, chronic kidney disease, diabetes mellitus, atrial fibrillation, treated hypertension, rheumatoid arthritis, or a family history of premature cardiovascular disease. Risk assessment tools underestimate risk in patients with additional risk due to existing conditions or medication, such as:

- serious mental disorder
- autoimmune disorders such as systemic lupus erythematosus and other systemic inflammatory disorders
- antiretroviral treatment
- medication causing dyslipidaemia as a side-effect e.g. antipsychotics, corticosteroids, or immunosuppressants
- triglyceride concentration > 4.5 mmol/litre

Cardiovascular disease risk is also underestimated in those who are already taking antihypertensive or lipid-regulating drugs, and in those who have recently stopped smoking. Severe obesity (BMI > 40 kg/m^2) also increases cardiovascular risk; the need for further treatment of risk factors in patients below the cardiovascular risk threshold for treatment should be based on clinical judgement.

Cardiovascular disease, measures for primary prevention

All patients at high risk of cardiovascular disease should be advised to make lifestyle modifications that include beneficial changes to diet, exercise, weight management, alcohol consumption, and smoking cessation.

Offer a statin as first-line drug treatment if lifestyle modifications are inappropriate or ineffective (see also Statins for the prevention of cardiovascular disease). Lipid-regulating drug treatment must be combined with advice on diet and lifestyle measures, and where appropriate, treatment of comorbidities and secondary causes of dyslipidaemia.

Cardiovascular disease, secondary prevention

Statins should be offered to all patients, including the elderly, with cardiovascular disease such as those with coronary heart disease (including history of angina or acute myocardial infarction), occlusive arterial disease (including peripheral vascular disease, non-haemorrhagic stroke, or transient ischaemic attacks).

Cardiovascular disease, measures for secondary prevention

Patients should be advised to make lifestyle modifications that include beneficial changes to diet, exercise, weight management, alcohol consumption, and smoking cessation, however, initiation of lipid-regulating drug treatment should not be delayed to manage modifiable risk factors, and must be combined with advice on diet and lifestyle measures, and where appropriate, treatment of co-morbidities and secondary causes of dyslipidaemia.

Statins for the prevention of cardiovascular disease

A statin reduces the risk of cardiovascular disease events, and is the drug of first choice for primary and secondary prevention of cardiovascular disease. Before starting treatment with statins, secondary causes of dyslipidaemia should be addressed; these include uncontrolled diabetes mellitus, hepatic disease, nephrotic syndrome, and excessive alcohol consumption. Patients with hypothyroidism should receive adequate thyroid replacement therapy (before assessing the requirement for lipid-regulating treatment if for primary prevention) because correcting hypothyroidism itself may resolve the lipid abnormality. Untreated hypothyroidism increases the risk of myositis with lipid-regulating drugs.

For the purpose of reducing cardiovascular risk, NICE Clinical Guideline 181 (NICE clinical guideline 181 (July 2014). Lipid Modification—Cardiovascular risk assessment and the modification of blood lipids for the primary and secondary prevention of cardiovascular disease) defines statins by the percentage reduction in LDL-cholesterol they achieve:

For *primary prevention*, NICE Clinical Guideline 181 recommends that atorvastatin p. 200 a high-intensity statin (when prescribed at a dose of at least 20 mg/day [unlicensed dose]), should be offered to those with a 10-year risk of cardiovascular disease of 10% or more; patients aged 85 years and over may benefit from atorvastatin to reduce the risk of non-fatal myocardial infarction. For *secondary prevention*, atorvastatin is also recommended [unlicensed indication]. Patients taking a low- or medium-intensity statin should discuss the benefits and risks of switching to a high intensity statin at their next medication review.

A statin should be considered for *all* adults with type 1 diabetes mellitus, particularly those aged 40 years and over, or who have had diabetes for more than 10 years, or who have established nephropathy, or other risk factors for

2

Cardiovascular system

cardiovascular disease. JBS3 recommendations (Joint British Societies' consensus recommendations for the prevention of cardiovascular disease (JBS3) 2014) in diabetes mellitus differ in certain respects from NICE Clinical Guideline 181 (NICE clinical guideline 181 (July 2014). Lipid Modification—Cardiovascular risk assessment and the modification of blood lipids for the primary and secondary prevention of cardiovascular disease)—see JBS3 recommendations for further details. In type 2 diabetes, assess level of risk using the risk calculator and treat for primary prevention if necessary.

Total cholesterol, HDL-cholesterol, and non-HDL cholesterol concentrations should be checked 3 months after starting treatment with a high intensity statin. NICE Clinical Guideline 181 recommends aiming for a reduction in non-HDL cholesterol concentration greater than 40%; JBS3 recommends a target non-HDL cholesterol concentration below 2.5 mmol/litre. If these are not achieved, ensure lifestyle modifications are optimised and consider increasing the dose of the statin if started on less than atorvastatin 80 mg and the patient is judged to be at higher risk because of comorbidities, risk score or, using clinical judgement.

Specialist advice should be sought about treatment options for patients at high risk of cardiovascular disease or those with existing cardiovascular disease, who are intolerant of three different statins.

Fibrates should not be routinely used for primary or secondary prevention. Nicotinic acid p. 199, **bile acid sequestrants**, and **omega-3 fatty acid compounds** are not recommended for primary or secondary prevention.

Hypercholesterolaemia, hypertriglyceridaemia, and familial hypercholesterolaemia

A statin is also the drug of first choice for treating hypercholesterolaemia and moderate hypertriglyceridaemia. Severe hyperlipidaemia not adequately controlled with a maximal dose of a statin may require the use of an additional lipid-regulating drug such as ezetimibe p. 196; such treatment should generally be supervised by a specialist.

A number of conditions, some familial, are characterised by very high LDL-cholesterol concentration, high triglyceride concentration, or both. Fenofibrate p. 198 may be added to statin therapy if triglycerides remain high even after the LDL-cholesterol concentration has been reduced adequately; nicotinic acid may also be used to further lower triglyceride or LDL-cholesterol concentration.

Combination of a statin with a fibrate or with nicotinic acid carries an increased risk of side-effects (including rhabdomyolysis) and should be used under specialist supervision; monitoring of liver function and creatine kinase should also be considered. The concomitant administration of gemfibrozil with a statin increases the risk of rhabdomyolysis considerably—this combination should **not** be used.

A statin is recommended for all patients with familial hypercholesterolaemia. A 'high-intensity' statin (as defined in NICE Clinical Guideline 71, August 2008. Identification and management of familial hypercholesterolaemia) e.g. rosuvastatin p. 202 (initiated by a specialist) or atorvastatin p. 200 should be considered in order to achieve the recommended reduction in LDL-cholesterol concentration of greater than 50% from baseline; a 'high-intensity' statin is one that produces a greater LDL-cholesterol reduction than simvastatin 40 mg. Patients with heterozygous familial hypercholesterolaemia who have contra-indications to, or are intolerant of, statins should receive ezetimibe. The combination of a statin and ezetimibe can be considered if a statin alone fails to provide adequate control (or if intolerance limits dose titration), and when a switch to an alternative statin is being considered. Patients for whom statins and ezetimibe are inappropriate, should be referred to a specialist for the consideration of treatment with a bile acid sequestrant, nicotinic acid, or a fibrate.

The prescribing of drug therapy in homozygous familial hypercholesterolaemia should be undertaken in a specialist centre.

Reduction in low-density lipoprotein cholesterol		
Therapy intensity	**Drug**	**Daily dose (reduction in LDL cholesterol)**
High-intensity	Atorvastatin	20 mg (43%)
		40 mg (49%)
		80 mg (55%)
	Rosuvastatin	10 mg (43%)
		20 mg (48%)
		40 mg (53%)
	Simvastatin	80 mg (42%)
Medium-intensity	Atorvastatin	10 mg (37%)
	Fluvastatin	80 mg (33%)
	Rosuvastatin	5 mg (38%)
	Simvastatin	20 mg (32%)
		40 mg (37%)
Low-intensity	Fluvastatin	20 mg (21%)
		40 mg (27%)
	Pravastatin	10 mg (20%)
		20 mg (24%)
		40 mg (29%)
	Simvastatin	10 mg (27%)

Advice from the MHRA: there is an increased risk of myopathy associated with high-dose (80 mg) simvastatin. The 80 mg dose should be considered only in patients with severe hypercholesterolaemia and high risk of cardiovascular complications who have not achieved their treatment goals on lower doses, when the benefits are expected to outweigh the potential risks.

Statins

Statins are more effective than other lipid-regulating drugs at lowering LDL-cholesterol concentration but they are less effective than the fibrates in reducing triglyceride concentration. However, statins reduce cardiovascular disease events and total mortality irrespective of the initial cholesterol concentration.

Alirocumab and evolocumab

Alirocumab p. 204 and evolocumab p. 205 are licensed for the treatment of primary hypercholesterolaemia (heterozygous familial and non-familial) or mixed dyslipidaemia as an adjunct to dietary measures. They can be used in combination with a statin, or with a statin and other lipid-regulating therapies, in patients unable to achieve their LDL-cholesterol treatment goals with the maximum tolerated dose of a statin. They can be used alone or in combination with other lipid-regulating therapies if a statin is contra-indicated or not tolerated. Evolocumab is also licensed for the treatment of homozygous familial hypercholesterolaemia in combination with other lipid-lowering therapies.

Bile acid sequestrants

Bile acid sequestrants effectively reduce LDL-cholesterol but can aggravate hypertriglyceridaemia. Treatment with bile acid sequestrants may be appropriate under specialist supervision if statins and ezetimibe are inappropriate, and when LDL-cholesterol is severely raised, for example in familial hypercholesterolaemia.

Fibrates

Fibrates are mainly used in those whose serum-triglyceride concentration is greater than 10 mmol/litre or in those who cannot tolerate a statin (specialist use).

Lomitapide

Lomitapide p. 206 is licensed as an adjunct to dietary measures and other lipid-regulating drugs for the treatment of homozygous familial hypercholesterolaemia.

Nicotinic acid group

The value of nicotinic acid is limited by its side-effects, especially vasodilatation.

Nicotinic acid is used by specialists in combination with a statin if the statin alone cannot adequately control dyslipidaemia (raised LDL-cholesterol, triglyceridaemia, and low HDL-cholesterol).

Acipimox p. 199 seems to have fewer side-effects than nicotinic acid but may be less effective in its lipid-regulating capabilities.

Omega-3 fatty acid compounds

There is no evidence that omega-3 fatty acid compounds reduce the risk of cardiovascular disease.

> **Other drugs used for Hyperlipidaemia** Inositol nicotinate, p. 232

LIPID MODIFYING DRUGS > BILE ACID SEQUESTRANTS

Bile acid sequestrants ▣

- **DRUG ACTION** Bile acid sequestrants act by binding bile acids, preventing their reabsorption; this promotes hepatic conversion of cholesterol into bile acids; the resultant increased LDL-receptor activity of liver cells increases the clearance of LDL-cholesterol from the plasma.
- **CAUTIONS** Interference with the absorption of fat-soluble vitamins (supplements of vitamins A, D, K, and folic acid may be required when treatment is prolonged).
- **SIDE-EFFECTS**
- ► **Common or very common** Constipation · gastrointestinal discomfort · gastrointestinal disorders · headaches · nausea · vomiting
- ► **Uncommon** Appetite decreased · diarrhoea · dysphagia · haemorrhage · hypoprothrombinaemia · myalgia · night blindness · osteoporosis · skin reactions · tongue irritation · vitamin deficiencies
- ► **Rare or very rare** Pancreatitis
- ► **Frequency not known** Angina pectoris · arthralgia · arthritis · asthenia · burping · chest pain · dizziness · dyspnoea · gallbladder disorders · inflammation · insomnia · pain · tachycardia
- **PREGNANCY** Bile acid sequestrants should be used with caution as although the drugs are not absorbed, they may cause fat-soluble vitamin deficiency on prolonged use.
- **BREAST FEEDING** Bile acid sequestrants should be used with caution as although the drugs are not absorbed, they may cause fat-soluble vitamin deficiency on prolonged use.

▶ above

Colesevelam hydrochloride

- **INDICATIONS AND DOSE**

Primary hypercholesterolaemia as an adjunct to dietary measures (monotherapy)
- ► BY MOUTH
- ► Adult: 3.75 g daily in 1–2 divided doses; maximum 4.375 g per day

Primary hypercholesterolaemia as an adjunct to dietary measures, in combination with a statin | Primary and familial hypercholesterolaemia, in combination with ezetimibe, either with or without a statin
- ► BY MOUTH
- ► Adult: 2.5–3.75 g daily in 1–2 divided doses, may be taken at the same time as the statin and ezetimibe

- **CONTRA-INDICATIONS** Biliary obstruction · bowel obstruction
- **CAUTIONS** Gastro-intestinal motility disorders · inflammatory bowel disease · major gastro-intestinal surgery
- **INTERACTIONS** → Appendix 1: colesevelam
- **HEPATIC IMPAIRMENT** Manufacturer advises caution.
- **MONITORING REQUIREMENTS** Patients receiving ciclosporin should have their blood-ciclosporin concentration monitored before, during, and after treatment with colesevelam.
- **PATIENT AND CARER ADVICE** Patient counselling on administration is advised for colesevelam hydrochloride tablets (avoid other drugs at same time).

- **MEDICINAL FORMS**
There can be variation in the licensing of different medicines containing the same drug.
Tablet
CAUTIONARY AND ADVISORY LABELS 21
► Cholestagel (Sanofi)
Colesevelam hydrochloride 625 mg Cholestagel 625mg tablets | 180 tablet [PoM] £115.32 DT = £115.32

▶ above

Colestipol hydrochloride

- **INDICATIONS AND DOSE**

Hyperlipidaemias, particularly type IIa, in patients who have not responded adequately to diet and other appropriate measures
- ► BY MOUTH
- ► Adult: Initially 5 g 1–2 times a day, increased in steps of 5 g every month if required, total daily dose may be given in 1–2 divided doses; maximum 30 g per day

- **INTERACTIONS** → Appendix 1: colestipol
- **DIRECTIONS FOR ADMINISTRATION** The contents of each sachet should be mixed with at least 100 mL of water or other suitable liquid such as fruit juice or skimmed milk; alternatively it can be mixed with thin soups, cereals, yoghurt, or pulpy fruits ensuring at least 100 mL of liquid is provided.
- **PATIENT AND CARER ADVICE** Patient counselling on administration is advised for colestipol hydrochloride granules (avoid other drugs at same time).

- **MEDICINAL FORMS**
There can be variation in the licensing of different medicines containing the same drug.
Granules
CAUTIONARY AND ADVISORY LABELS 13
► Colestid (Pfizer Ltd)
Colestipol hydrochloride 5 gram Colestid 5g granules sachets plain sugar-free | 30 sachet [PoM] £15.05

Cardiovascular system

2

Colestid Orange 5g granules sachets sugar-free | 30 sachet PoM
£15.05

Tablet
▸ Colestid (Imported (Canada))
 Colestipol hydrochloride 1 gram Colestid 1g tablets |
 120 tablet PoM ⑤

◀ 195

Colestyramine

(Cholestyramine)

● **INDICATIONS AND DOSE**

**Hyperlipidaemias, particularly type IIa, in patients who
have not responded adequately to diet and other
appropriate measures | Primary prevention of coronary
heart disease in men aged 35–59 years with primary
hypercholesterolaemia who have not responded to diet
and other appropriate measures**
▸ BY MOUTH
▸ Adult: Initially 4 g daily, increased in steps of 4 g every
 week; increased to 12–24 g daily in 1–4 divided doses,
 adjusted according to response; maximum 36 g per day

**Pruritus associated with partial biliary obstruction and
primary biliary cirrhosis**
▸ BY MOUTH
▸ Adult: 4–8 g once daily

**Diarrhoea associated with Crohn's disease, ileal resection,
vagotomy, diabetic vagal neuropathy, and radiation**
▸ BY MOUTH
▸ Adult: Initially 4 g daily, increased in steps of 4 g every
 week; increased to 12–24 g daily in 1–4 divided doses,
 adjusted according to response, if no response within
 3 days an alternative therapy should be initiated;
 maximum 36 g per day

Accelerated elimination of teriflunomide
▸ BY MOUTH
▸ Adult: 8 g 3 times a day for 11 days; reduced to 4 g
 3 times a day, dose should only be reduced if not
 tolerated

**Accelerated elimination of leflunomide (washout
procedure)**
▸ BY MOUTH
▸ Adult: 8 g 3 times a day for 11 days

● CONTRA-INDICATIONS Complete biliary obstruction (not
likely to be effective)

● INTERACTIONS → Appendix 1: colestyramine

● DIRECTIONS FOR ADMINISTRATION The contents of each
sachet should be mixed with at least 150 mL of water or
other suitable liquid such as fruit juice, skimmed milk, thin
soups, and pulpy fruits with a high moisture content.

● PATIENT AND CARER ADVICE Patient counselling on
administration is advised for colestyramine powder (avoid
other drugs at same time).

● MEDICINAL FORMS
There can be variation in the licensing of different medicines
containing the same drug. Forms available from special-order
manufacturers include: oral suspension, oral solution

Powder
CAUTIONARY AND ADVISORY LABELS 13
EXCIPIENTS: May contain Aspartame, sucrose
▸ Colestyramine (Non-proprietary)
 Colestyramine anhydrous 4 gram Colestyramine 4g oral powder
 sachets | 50 sachet PoM ⑤ DT = £10.76
 Colestyramine 4g oral powder sachets sugar free sugar-free |
 50 sachet PoM £30.00 DT = £16.15
▸ Questran (Bristol-Myers Squibb Pharmaceuticals Ltd)
 Colestyramine anhydrous 4 gram Questran 4g oral powder sachets
 | 50 sachet PoM £10.76 DT = £10.76
▸ Questran Light (Bristol-Myers Squibb Pharmaceuticals Ltd)
 Colestyramine anhydrous 4 gram Questran Light 4g oral powder
 sachets sugar-free | 50 sachet PoM £16.15 DT = £16.15

Ezetimibe

19-May-2016

● DRUG ACTION Ezetimibe inhibits the intestinal absorption
of cholesterol.
 If used alone, it has a modest effect on lowering LDL-
cholesterol, with little effect on other lipoproteins.

● **INDICATIONS AND DOSE**

**Adjunct to dietary measures and statin treatment in
primary hypercholesterolaemia | Adjunct to dietary
measures and statin in homozygous familial
hypercholesterolaemia | Primary hypercholesterolaemia
(if statin inappropriate or not tolerated) | Adjunct to
dietary measures in homozygous sitosterolaemia**
▸ BY MOUTH
▸ Adult: 10 mg daily

● INTERACTIONS → Appendix 1: ezetimibe

● SIDE-EFFECTS
▸ **Common or very common** Asthenia · diarrhoea ·
 gastrointestinal disorders
▸ **Uncommon** Appetite decreased · arthralgia · chest pain ·
 cough · hot flush · hypertension · muscle complaints ·
 nausea · pain
▸ **Frequency not known** Constipation · depression · dizziness ·
 dyspnoea · hepatitis · myopathy · pancreatitis ·
 paraesthesia · skin reactions · thrombocytopenia

● PREGNANCY Manufacturer advises use only if potential
benefit outweighs risk—no information available.

● BREAST FEEDING Manufacturer advises avoid—present in
milk in *animal* studies.

● HEPATIC IMPAIRMENT Avoid in moderate and severe
impairment—may accumulate.

● NATIONAL FUNDING/ACCESS DECISIONS

NICE decisions
▸ **Ezetimibe for treating primary heterozygous-familial and non-
 familial hypercholesterolaemia (February 2016)** NICE TA385
 This guidance should be used with NICE's guidelines on
 cardiovascular disease: risk assessment and reduction,
 including lipid modification and familial
 hypercholesterolaemia: identification and management
 (see Lipid-regulating drugs p. 193).
 Ezetimibe, alone, is recommended as an option for the
 treatment of primary (heterozygous-familial or
 non-familial) hypercholesterolaemia in adult patients in
 whom initial statin therapy is contra-indicated, or who are
 intolerant of initial statin therapy.
 Ezetimibe, in combination with initial statin therapy, is
 also recommended as an option for the treatment of
 primary (heterozygous-familial or non-familial)
 hypercholesterolaemia in adult patients when:
 ● serum total or low-density lipoprotein (LDL) cholesterol
  concentration is not appropriately controlled either
  after appropriate dose titration of initial statin therapy
  or because dose titration is limited by intolerance to the
  initial statin therapy **and**
 ● a change from initial statin therapy to an alternative
  statin is being considered.
 When prescribing ezetimibe in combination with statin,
 ezetimibe should be prescribed on the basis of lowest
 acquisition cost.
 www.nice.org.uk/TA385

- **MEDICINAL FORMS**
There can be variation in the licensing of different medicines containing the same drug.
Tablet
▸ Ezetimibe (Non-proprietary)
Ezetimibe 10 mg Ezetimibe 10mg tablets | 28 tablet P₀M £22.36-£26.31 DT = £26.31
▸ Ezetrol (Merck Sharp & Dohme Ltd)
Ezetimibe 10 mg Ezetrol 10mg tablets | 28 tablet P₀M £26.31 DT = £26.31

Combinations available: *Simvastatin with ezetimibe,* p. 204

LIPID MODIFYING DRUGS ⟩ FIBRATES

Bezafibrate

- **DRUG ACTION** Fibrates act by decreasing serum triglycerides; they have variable effect on LDL-cholestrol.

- **INDICATIONS AND DOSE**
Adjunct to diet and other appropriate measures in mixed hyperlipidaemia if statin contra-indicated or not tolerated | Adjunct to diet and other appropriate measures in severe hypertriglyceridaemia
▸ BY MOUTH USING IMMEDIATE-RELEASE MEDICINES
▸ Adult: 200 mg 3 times a day
▸ BY MOUTH USING MODIFIED-RELEASE MEDICINES
▸ Adult: 400 mg once daily, modified-release dose form is not appropriate in patients with renal impairment

- **CONTRA-INDICATIONS** Gall bladder disease · hypoalbuminaemia · nephrotic syndrome · photosensitivity to fibrates
- **CAUTIONS** Correct hypothyroidism before initiating treatment
- **INTERACTIONS** → Appendix 1: fibrates
- **SIDE-EFFECTS**
▸ **Common or very common** Appetite decreased · gastrointestinal disorder
▸ **Uncommon** Acute kidney injury · alopecia · cholestasis · constipation · diarrhoea · dizziness · erectile dysfunction · gastrointestinal discomfort · headache · muscle complaints · muscle weakness · nausea · photosensitivity reaction · skin reactions
▸ **Rare or very rare** Cholelithiasis · depression · insomnia · interstitial lung disease · pancreatitis · pancytopenia · paraesthesia · peripheral neuropathy · rhabdomyolysis (increased risk in renal impairment) · severe cutaneous adverse reactions (SCARs) · thrombocytopenic purpura
- **PREGNANCY** Manufacturers advise avoid—no information available.
- **BREAST FEEDING** Manufacturer advises avoid—no information available.
- **HEPATIC IMPAIRMENT** Avoid in severe liver disease.
- **RENAL IMPAIRMENT** Avoid *immediate-release* preparations if eGFR less than 15 mL/minute/1.73 m².
  Avoid *modified-release* preparations if eGFR less than 60 mL/minute/1.73 m².
  Dose adjustments Reduce dose to 400 mg daily if eGFR 40–60 mL/minute/1.73 m².
  Reduce dose to 200 mg every 1–2 days if eGFR 15–40 mL/minute/1.73 m².
  Myotoxicity Special care needed in patients with renal disease, as progressive increases in serum creatinine concentration or failure to follow dosage guidelines may result in myotoxicity (rhabdomyolysis); discontinue if myotoxicity suspected or creatine kinase concentration increases significantly.
- **MONITORING REQUIREMENTS** Consider monitoring of liver function and creatine kinase when fibrates used in combination with a statin.

- **PRESCRIBING AND DISPENSING INFORMATION** Fibrates are mainly used in those whose serum-triglyceride concentration is greater than 10 mmol/litre or in those who cannot tolerate a statin (specialist use).

- **MEDICINAL FORMS**
There can be variation in the licensing of different medicines containing the same drug. Forms available from special-order manufacturers include: oral suspension
Modified-release tablet
CAUTIONARY AND ADVISORY LABELS 21, 25
▸ Bezafibrate (Non-proprietary)
Bezafibrate 400 mg Bezafibrate 400mg modified-release tablets | 30 tablet P₀M ⒮ DT = £7.63
▸ Bezalip Mono (Teva UK Ltd)
Bezafibrate 400 mg Bezalip Mono 400mg modified-release tablets | 30 tablet P₀M £7.63 DT = £7.63
▸ Fibrazate XL (Sandoz Ltd)
Bezafibrate 400 mg Fibrazate XL 400mg tablets | 30 tablet P₀M £6.87 DT = £7.63
Tablet
CAUTIONARY AND ADVISORY LABELS 21
▸ Bezafibrate (Non-proprietary)
Bezafibrate 200 mg Bezafibrate 200mg tablets | 100 tablet P₀M £8.50 DT = £4.69
▸ Bezalip (Teva UK Ltd)
Bezafibrate 200 mg Bezalip 200mg tablets | 100 tablet P₀M £8.63 DT = £4.69

Ciprofibrate

- **DRUG ACTION** Fibrates act by decreasing serum triglycerides; they have variable effect on LDL-cholestrol.

- **INDICATIONS AND DOSE**
Adjunct to diet and other appropriate measures in mixed hyperlipidaemia if statin contra-indicated or not tolerated | Adjunct to diet and other appropriate measures in severe hypertriglyceridaemia
▸ BY MOUTH
▸ Adult: 100 mg daily

- **CONTRA-INDICATIONS** Gall bladder disease · hypoalbuminaemia · nephrotic syndrome · photosensitivity to fibrates
- **CAUTIONS** Correct hypothyroidism before initiating treatment
- **INTERACTIONS** → Appendix 1: fibrates
- **SIDE-EFFECTS**
▸ **Common or very common** Alopecia · diarrhoea · dizziness · drowsiness · fatigue · gastrointestinal discomfort · headache · myalgia · nausea · skin reactions · vertigo · vomiting
▸ **Frequency not known** Cholelithiasis · erectile dysfunction · hepatic disorders · leucopenia · myopathy · photosensitivity reaction · respiratory disorders · rhabdomyolysis (increased risk in renal impairment) · thrombocytopenia
- **PREGNANCY** Manufacturers advise avoid—toxicity in *animal* studies.
- **BREAST FEEDING** Manufacturer advises avoid—present in milk in *animal* studies.
- **HEPATIC IMPAIRMENT** Use with caution in mild to moderate impairment. Avoid in severe impairment.
- **RENAL IMPAIRMENT** Avoid in severe impairment.
  Dose adjustments Reduce dose to 100 mg on alternate days in moderate impairment.
  Myotoxicity Special care needed in patients with renal disease, as progressive increases in serum creatinine concentration or failure to follow dosage guidelines may result in myotoxicity (rhabdomyolysis); discontinue if myotoxicity suspected or creatine kinase concentration increases significantly.

- MONITORING REQUIREMENTS
- ▶ Liver function tests recommended every 3 months for first year (discontinue treatment if significantly raised).
- ▶ Consider monitoring liver function and creatine kinase when fibrates used in combination with a statin.
- PRESCRIBING AND DISPENSING INFORMATION Fibrates are mainly used in those whose serum-triglyceride concentration is greater than 10 mmol/litre or in those who cannot tolerate a statin (specialist use).

- MEDICINAL FORMS
There can be variation in the licensing of different medicines containing the same drug.

Tablet

- ▶ Ciprofibrate (Non-proprietary)
  Ciprofibrate 100 mg Ciprofibrate 100mg tablets | 28 tablet [PoM]
  £134.21 DT = £112.06

Fenofibrate

14-Jun-2017

- DRUG ACTION Fibrates act by decreasing serum triglycerides; they have variable effect on LDL-cholesterol.

- INDICATIONS AND DOSE

Adjunct to diet and other appropriate measures in mixed hyperlipidaemia if statin contra-indicated or not tolerated | Adjunct to diet and other appropriate measures in severe hypertriglyceridaemia | Adjunct to statin in mixed hyperlipidaemia if triglycerides and HDL-cholesterol inadequately controlled in patients at high cardiovascular risk

- ▶ BY MOUTH USING CAPSULES
- ▶ Adult: Initially 200 mg daily, then increased if necessary to 267 mg daily, maximum 200 mg daily with concomitant statin, 267 mg capsules not appropriate for initial dose titration
- ▶ BY MOUTH USING TABLETS
- ▶ Adult: 160 mg daily

DOSE ADJUSTMENTS DUE TO INTERACTIONS
- ▶ Manufacturer advises max. dose 200 mg daily with concurrent use of a statin.

- CONTRA-INDICATIONS Gall bladder disease · pancreatitis (unless due to severe hypertriglyceridaemia) · photosensitivity to ketoprofen
- CAUTIONS Correct hypothyroidism before initiating treatment
- INTERACTIONS → Appendix 1: fibrates
- SIDE-EFFECTS
- ▶ **Common or very common** Abdominal pain · diarrhoea · flatulence · nausea · vomiting
- ▶ **Uncommon** Cholelithiasis · embolism and thrombosis · headache · muscle complaints · myopathy · pancreatitis · sexual dysfunction · skin reactions
- ▶ **Rare or very rare** Alopecia · hepatic disorders · photosensitivity reaction
- ▶ **Frequency not known** Fatigue · interstitial lung disease · rhabdomyolysis (increased risk in renal impairment) · severe cutaneous adverse reactions (SCARs)
- PREGNANCY Avoid—embryotoxicity in *animal* studies.
- BREAST FEEDING Manufacturers advise avoid—no information available.
- HEPATIC IMPAIRMENT Avoid.
- RENAL IMPAIRMENT Manufacturer advises use with caution in mild-to-moderate impairment; avoid if eGFR less than 30 mL/minute/1.73 m^2.
  Dose adjustments Manufacturer advises max. 67 mg daily if eGFR 30–59 mL/minute/1.73 m^2.
  Myotoxicity Special care needed in patients with renal disease, as progressive increases in serum creatinine concentration or failure to follow dosage guidelines may

result in myotoxicity (rhabdomyolysis); discontinue if myotoxicity suspected or creatine kinase concentration increases significantly.

- MONITORING REQUIREMENTS Manufacturer advises monitor hepatic transaminases every 3 months during the first 12 months of treatment and periodically thereafter—discontinue treatment if levels increase to more than 3 times the upper limit of normal; monitor serum creatinine levels during the first 3 months of treatment and periodically thereafter—interrupt treatment if creatinine level is 50% above the upper limit of normal.
- PRESCRIBING AND DISPENSING INFORMATION Fibrates are mainly used in those whose serum-triglyceride concentration is greater than 10 mmol/litre or in those who cannot tolerate a statin (specialist use).

- MEDICINAL FORMS
There can be variation in the licensing of different medicines containing the same drug.

Tablet

CAUTIONARY AND ADVISORY LABELS 21
- ▶ Fenofibrate (Non-proprietary)
  Fenofibrate micronised 160 mg Fenofibrate micronised 160mg tablets | 28 tablet [PoM] £6.69 DT = £4.20
- ▶ Supralip (Mylan)
  Fenofibrate micronised 160 mg Supralip 160mg tablets | 28 tablet [PoM] £6.69 DT = £4.20

Capsule

CAUTIONARY AND ADVISORY LABELS 21
- ▶ Fenofibrate (Non-proprietary)
  Fenofibrate micronised 67 mg Fenofibrate micronised 67mg capsules | 90 capsule [PoM] £23.30 DT = £22.64
  Fenofibrate micronised 200 mg Fenofibrate micronised 200mg capsules | 28 capsule [PoM] £21.75 DT = £3.65
  Fenofibrate micronised 267 mg Fenofibrate micronised 267mg capsules | 28 capsule [PoM] £21.75 DT = £5.32
- ▶ Lipantil Micro (Mylan)
  Fenofibrate micronised 67 mg Lipantil Micro 67 capsules | 90 capsule [PoM] £23.30 DT = £22.64
  Fenofibrate micronised 200 mg Lipantil Micro 200 capsules | 28 capsule [PoM] £14.23 DT = £3.65
  Fenofibrate micronised 267 mg Lipantil Micro 267 capsules | 28 capsule [PoM] £21.75 DT = £5.32

Combinations available: *Simvastatin with fenofibrate*, p. 204

Gemfibrozil

- DRUG ACTION Fibrates act by decreasing serum triglycerides; they have variable effect on LDL-cholesterol.

- INDICATIONS AND DOSE

Adjunct to diet and other appropriate measures in mixed hyperlipidaemia if statin contra-indicated or not tolerated | Adjunct to diet and other appropriate measures in primary hypercholesterolaemia if statin contra-indicated or not tolerated | Adjunct to diet and other appropriate measures in severe hypertriglyceridaemia | Adjunct to diet and other appropriate measures in primary prevention of cardiovascular disease in men with hyperlipidaemias if statin contra-indicated or not tolerated

- ▶ BY MOUTH
- ▶ Adult: 1.2 g daily in 2 divided doses, maintenance 0.9–1.2 g daily

- CONTRA-INDICATIONS History of gall-bladder or biliary tract disease including gallstones · photosensitivity to fibrates
- CAUTIONS Correct hypothyroidism before initiating treatment · elderly
- INTERACTIONS → Appendix 1: fibrates

- SIDE-EFFECTS
▸ **Common or very common** Constipation · diarrhoea · fatigue · flatulence · gastrointestinal discomfort · headache · nausea · skin reactions · vertigo · vomiting
▸ **Uncommon** Atrial fibrillation
▸ **Rare or very rare** Alopecia · anaemia · angioedema · appendicitis · bone marrow failure · depression · dizziness · drowsiness · eosinophilia · gallbladder disorders · hepatic disorders · joint disorders · laryngeal oedema · leucopenia · muscle weakness · myopathy · pain in extremity · pancreatitis · paraesthesia · peripheral neuropathy · photosensitivity reaction · sexual dysfunction · thrombocytopenia · vision blurred
- PREGNANCY Manufacturers advise avoid unless essential— toxicity in *animal* studies.
- BREAST FEEDING Manufacturer advises avoid—no information available.
- HEPATIC IMPAIRMENT Avoid.
- RENAL IMPAIRMENT Avoid if eGFR less than 30 mL/minute/1.73 m^2.
  Dose adjustments Initially 900 mg daily if eGFR 30–80 mL/minute/1.73 m^2.
  Myotoxicity Special care needed in patients with renal disease, as progressive increases in serum creatinine concentration or failure to follow dosage guidelines may result in myotoxicity (rhabdomyolysis); discontinue if myotoxicity suspected or creatine kinase concentration increases significantly.
- MONITORING REQUIREMENTS
▸ Monitor blood counts for first year.
▸ Monitor liver-function (discontinue treatment if abnormalities persist).
▸ Consider monitoring creatine kinase if used in combination with a statin.
- PRESCRIBING AND DISPENSING INFORMATION Fibrates are mainly used in those whose serum-triglyceride concentration is greater than 10 mmol/litre or in those who cannot tolerate a statin (specialist use).
- MEDICINAL FORMS
  There can be variation in the licensing of different medicines containing the same drug.
  Tablet
  CAUTIONARY AND ADVISORY LABELS 22
  ▸ Gemfibrozil (Non-proprietary)
    Gemfibrozil 600 mg Gemfibrozil 600mg tablets | 30 tablet [PoM] £15.00 DT = £15.00 | 56 tablet [PoM] £35.57 DT = £35.57
  ▸ Lopid (Pfizer Ltd)
    Gemfibrozil 600 mg Lopid 600mg tablets | 56 tablet [PoM] £35.57 DT = £35.57
  Capsule
  CAUTIONARY AND ADVISORY LABELS 22
  ▸ Lopid (Pfizer Ltd)
    Gemfibrozil 300 mg Lopid 300mg capsules | 100 capsule [PoM] £31.76 DT = £31.76

LIPID MODIFYING DRUGS > NICOTINIC ACID DERIVATIVES

Acipimox

- INDICATIONS AND DOSE

Adjunct or alternative treatment in hyperlipidaemias of types IIb and IV in patients who have not responded adequately to other lipid-regulating drugs such as a statin or fibrate, and lifestyle changes (including diet, exercise, and weight reduction)
▸ BY MOUTH
▸ Adult: 250 mg 2–3 times a day

- CONTRA-INDICATIONS Peptic ulcer

- SIDE-EFFECTS
▸ **Common or very common** Asthenia · gastrointestinal discomfort · headache · skin reactions · vasodilation
▸ **Uncommon** Angioedema · arthralgia · feeling hot · malaise · myalgia · myositis · nausea
▸ **Frequency not known** Bronchospasm · diarrhoea · dry eye · eye disorder
- PREGNANCY Manufacturer advises avoid—no information available.
- BREAST FEEDING Manufacturer advises avoid—no information available.
- RENAL IMPAIRMENT Avoid if eGFR less than 30 mL/minute/1.73 m^2.
  Dose adjustments Reduce dose to 250 mg 1–2 times daily if eGFR 30–60 mL/minute/1.73 m^2.
- MONITORING REQUIREMENTS Monitor hepatic and renal function.

- MEDICINAL FORMS
  There can be variation in the licensing of different medicines containing the same drug.
  Capsule
  CAUTIONARY AND ADVISORY LABELS 21
  ▸ Olbetam (Pfizer Ltd)
    Acipimox 250 mg Olbetam 250mg capsules | 90 capsule [PoM] £46.33 DT = £46.33

Nicotinic acid

- DRUG ACTION In doses of 1.5 to 3 g daily, it lowers both cholesterol and triglyceride concentrations by inhibiting synthesis; it also increases HDL-cholesterol.

- INDICATIONS AND DOSE

Adjunct to statin in dyslipidaemia or used alone if statin not tolerated
▸ BY MOUTH
▸ Adult: (consult product literature)

- CONTRA-INDICATIONS Active peptic ulcer disease · arterial bleeding
- CAUTIONS Acute myocardial infarction · diabetes mellitus · gout · history of peptic ulceration · unstable angina
- INTERACTIONS → Appendix 1: nicotinic acid
- SIDE-EFFECTS
▸ **Common or very common** Diarrhoea · flushing · gastrointestinal discomfort · nausea · skin reactions · vomiting
▸ **Uncommon** Dizziness · dyspnoea · headache · hypophosphataemia · palpitations · peripheral oedema · tachycardia
▸ **Rare or very rare** Appetite decreased · hypotension · insomnia · myalgia · myopathy · rhinitis · syncope · visual impairment
▸ **Frequency not known** Jaundice

SIDE-EFFECTS, FURTHER INFORMATION Prostaglandin-mediated flushing is common, typically within an hour of dosing and lasting for 15–30 minutes (particularly with the initial doses). Taking after a meal or taking aspirin before dosing minimises flushing.

- PREGNANCY No information available—manufacturer advises avoid unless potential benefit outweighs risk.
- BREAST FEEDING Present in milk—avoid.
- HEPATIC IMPAIRMENT Avoid in severe impairment. Discontinue if severe abnormalities in liver function tests.
  Monitoring Manufacturer advises monitor liver function in mild to moderate hepatic impairment.
- RENAL IMPAIRMENT Manufacturer advises use with caution—no information available.

2

Cardiovascular system

- MEDICINAL FORMS
There can be variation in the licensing of different medicines containing the same drug. Forms available from special-order manufacturers include: tablet, modified-release tablet, capsule

Capsule
▸ Nicotinic acid (Non-proprietary)
Nicotinic acid 500 mg Solgar Niacin 500mg capsules | 100 capsule ⬚

LIPID MODIFYING DRUGS ⟩ STATINS

Statins

- DRUG ACTION Statins competitively inhibit 3-hydroxy-3-methylglutaryl coenzyme A (HMG CoA) reductase, an enzyme involved in cholesterol synthesis, especially in the liver.
- CAUTIONS Elderly · high alcohol intake · history of liver disease · hypothyroidism · patients at increased risk of muscle toxicity, including myopathy or rhabdomyolysis (e.g. those with a personal or family history of muscular disorders, previous history of muscular toxicity and a high alcohol intake)

CAUTIONS, FURTHER INFORMATION
▸ Muscle effects Muscle toxicity can occur with all statins, however the likelihood increases with higher doses and in certain patients (see below). Statins should be used with caution in patients at increased risk of muscle toxicity, including those with a personal or family history of muscular disorders, previous history of muscular toxicity, a high alcohol intake, renal impairment or hypothyroidism.
In patients at increased risk of muscle effects, a statin should not usually be started if the baseline creatine kinase concentration is more than 5 times the upper limit of normal (some patients may present with an extremely elevated baseline creatine kinase concentration, for example because of a physical occupation or rigorous exercise—specialist advice should be sought regarding consideration of statin therapy in these patients).
▸ Hypothyroidism Hypothyroidism should be managed adequately before starting treatment with a statin.

- SIDE-EFFECTS
▸ **Common or very common** Asthenia · constipation · diarrhoea · dizziness · flatulence · gastrointestinal discomfort · headache · myalgia · nausea · sleep disorders · thrombocytopenia
▸ **Uncommon** Alopecia · hepatic disorders · memory loss · pancreatitis · paraesthesia · sexual dysfunction · skin reactions · vomiting
▸ **Rare or very rare** Myopathy · peripheral neuropathy · tendinopathy
▸ **Frequency not known** Depression · diabetes mellitus (in those at risk) · interstitial lung disease

SIDE-EFFECTS, FURTHER INFORMATION
Muscle effects The risk of myopathy, myositis, and rhabdomyolysis associated with statin use is rare. Although myalgia has been reported commonly in patients receiving statins, muscle toxicity truly attributable to statin use is rare. When a statin is suspected to be the cause of myopathy, and creatine kinase concentration is markedly elevated or if muscular symptoms are severe, treatment should be discontinued. If symptoms resolve and creatine kinase concentrations return to normal, the statin should be reintroduced at a lower dose and the patient monitored closely. Statins should not be discontinued if there is an increase in the blood-glucose concentration as the benefits continue to outweigh the risks
Interstitial lung disease If patients develop symptoms such as dyspnoea, cough, and weight loss, they should seek medical attention.

- CONCEPTION AND CONTRACEPTION Adequate contraception is required during treatment and for 1 month afterwards.
- PREGNANCY Statins should be avoided in pregnancy (discontinue 3 months before attempting to conceive) as congenital anomalies have been reported and the decreased synthesis of cholesterol possibly affects fetal development.
- HEPATIC IMPAIRMENT Statins should be used with caution in those with a history of liver disease. Avoid in active liver disease or when there are unexplained persistent elevations in serum transaminases.
- MONITORING REQUIREMENTS
▸ Before starting treatment with statins, at least one full lipid profile (non-fasting) should be measured, including total cholesterol, HDL-cholesterol, non-HDL-cholesterol (calculated as total cholesterol minus HDL-cholesterol), and triglyceride concentrations, thyroid-stimulating hormone, and renal function should also be assessed.
▸ Liver function There is little information available on a rational approach to liver-function monitoring; however, NICE suggests that liver enzymes should be measured before treatment, and repeated within 3 months and at 12 months of starting treatment, unless indicated at other times by signs or symptoms suggestive of hepatotoxicity (NICE clinical guideline 181 (July 2014). Lipid Modification—Cardiovascular risk assessment and the modification of blood lipids for the primary and secondary prevention of cardiovascular disease).
Those with serum transaminases that are raised, but less than 3 times the upper limit of the reference range, should **not** be routinely excluded from statin therapy. Those with serum transaminases of more than 3 times the upper limit of the reference range should discontinue statin therapy.
▸ Creatine kinase Before initiation of statin treatment, creatine kinase concentration should be measured in patients who have had persistent, generalised, unexplained muscle pain (whether associated or not with previous lipid-regulating drugs); if the concentration is more than 5 times the upper limit of normal, a repeat measurement should be taken after 7 days. If the repeat concentration remains above 5 times the upper limit, statin treatment should not be started; if concentrations are still raised but less than 5 times the upper limit, the statin should be started at a lower dose.
▸ Diabetes Patients at high risk of diabetes mellitus should have fasting blood-glucose concentration or HbA_{1c} checked before starting statin treatment, and then repeated after 3 months.
- PATIENT AND CARER ADVICE Advise patients to report promptly unexplained muscle pain, tenderness, or weakness.

⬛ ▸ above

Atorvastatin

07-Jun-2017

- INDICATIONS AND DOSE

Primary hypercholesterolaemia in patients who have not responded adequately to diet and other appropriate measures | Combined (mixed) hyperlipidaemia in patients who have not responded adequately to diet and other appropriate measures
▸ BY MOUTH
▸ Adult: Usual dose 10 mg once daily; increased if necessary up to 80 mg once daily, dose to be increased at intervals of at least 4 weeks

Heterozygous familial hypercholesterolaemia in patients who have not responded adequately to diet and other appropriate measures | Homozygous familial hypercholestrolaemia in patients who have not responded adequately to diet and other appropriate measures

▶ BY MOUTH
▶ Adult: Initially 10 mg once daily, then increased to 40 mg once daily, dose to be increased at intervals of at least 4 weeks; maximum 80 mg per day

Primary prevention of cardiovascular events in patients at high risk of a first cardiovascular event

▶ BY MOUTH
▶ Adult: 20 mg once daily, dose can be increased if necessary

Secondary prevention of cardiovascular events

▶ BY MOUTH
▶ Adult: 80 mg once daily

DOSE ADJUSTMENTS DUE TO INTERACTIONS
▶ Manufacturer advises if concurrent use of ciclosporin is unavoidable, max. dose cannot exceed 10 mg daily.
▶ Manufacturer advises max. dose 40 mg daily when combined with anion-exchange resin for heterozygous familial hypercholesterolaemia.
▶ Manufacturer advises max. dose 20 mg daily with concurrent use of elbasvir with grazoprevir.

● UNLICENSED USE [EvGr] Not licensed for secondary prevention of cardiovascular events. Starting dose of 20 mg once daily is not licensed for the primary prevention of cardiovascular events. ◇

● CAUTIONS Haemorrhagic stroke

● INTERACTIONS → Appendix 1: statins

● SIDE-EFFECTS
▶ **Common or very common** Epistaxis · hyperglycaemia · hypersensitivity · joint disorders · laryngeal pain · pain
▶ **Uncommon** Appetite decreased · burping · chest pain · fatigue · fever · hearing impairment · hypoglycaemia · malaise · numbness · peripheral oedema · taste altered · vision disorders · weight increased
▶ **Rare or very rare** Angioedema · gynaecomastia · severe cutaneous adverse reactions (SCARs)

● BREAST FEEDING Manufacturer advises avoid—no information available.

● RENAL IMPAIRMENT
Dose adjustments In chronic kidney disease, for primary and secondary prevention of cardiovascular events [unlicensed starting dose in *primary* prevention; unlicensed in *secondary* prevention], initially 20 mg once daily, increased if necessary (on specialist advice if eGFR < 30 mL/minute/1.73 m^2); max. 80 mg once daily.

● PATIENT AND CARER ADVICE Patient counselling is advised for atorvastatin tablets (muscle effects).

● MEDICINAL FORMS
There can be variation in the licensing of different medicines containing the same drug. Forms available from special-order manufacturers include: oral suspension, oral solution

Tablet
▶ Atorvastatin (Non-proprietary)
Atorvastatin (as Atorvastatin calcium trihydrate)
10 mg Atorvastatin 10mg tablets | 28 tablet [PoM] £13.00 DT = £0.57 | 90 tablet [PoM] £41.78
Atorvastatin (as Atorvastatin calcium trihydrate)
20 mg Atorvastatin 20mg tablets | 28 tablet [PoM] £24.64 DT = £0.70 | 90 tablet [PoM] £79.20
Atorvastatin (as Atorvastatin calcium trihydrate)
30 mg Atorvastatin 30mg tablets | 28 tablet [PoM] £24.76 DT = £24.63
Atorvastatin (as Atorvastatin calcium trihydrate)
40 mg Atorvastatin 40mg tablets | 28 tablet [PoM] £24.64 DT = £0.98 | 90 tablet [PoM] £79.20

Atorvastatin (as Atorvastatin calcium trihydrate)
60 mg Atorvastatin 60mg tablets | 28 tablet [PoM] £28.39 DT = £28.20
Atorvastatin (as Atorvastatin calcium trihydrate)
80 mg Atorvastatin 80mg tablets | 28 tablet [PoM] £28.21 DT = £2.06 | 90 tablet [PoM] £90.67
▶ Lipitor (Pfizer Ltd)
Atorvastatin (as Atorvastatin calcium trihydrate) 10 mg Lipitor 10mg tablets | 28 tablet [PoM] £13.00 DT = £0.57
Atorvastatin (as Atorvastatin calcium trihydrate) 20 mg Lipitor 20mg tablets | 28 tablet [PoM] £24.64 DT = £0.70
Atorvastatin (as Atorvastatin calcium trihydrate) 40 mg Lipitor 40mg tablets | 28 tablet [PoM] £24.64 DT = £0.98
Atorvastatin (as Atorvastatin calcium trihydrate) 80 mg Lipitor 80mg tablets | 28 tablet [PoM] £28.21 DT = £2.06

Chewable tablet
CAUTIONARY AND ADVISORY LABELS 24
▶ Lipitor (Pfizer Ltd)
Atorvastatin (as Atorvastatin calcium trihydrate) 10 mg Lipitor 10mg chewable tablets sugar-free | 30 tablet [PoM] £13.80 DT = £13.80
Atorvastatin (as Atorvastatin calcium trihydrate) 20 mg Lipitor 20mg chewable tablets sugar-free | 30 tablet [PoM] £26.40 DT = £26.40

▣ 200

Fluvastatin

12-Apr-2017

● INDICATIONS AND DOSE

Adjunct to diet in primary hypercholesterolaemia or combined (mixed) hyperlipidaemia (types IIa and IIb)

▶ BY MOUTH USING IMMEDIATE-RELEASE MEDICINES
▶ Adult: Initially 20–40 mg daily, dose to be taken in the evening, increased if necessary up to 80 mg daily in 2 divided doses, dose to be adjusted at intervals of at least 4 weeks
▶ BY MOUTH USING MODIFIED-RELEASE MEDICINES
▶ Adult: 80 mg daily, dose form is not appropriate for initial dose titration

Prevention of coronary events after percutaneous coronary intervention

▶ BY MOUTH USING IMMEDIATE-RELEASE MEDICINES
▶ Adult: 80 mg daily
▶ BY MOUTH USING MODIFIED-RELEASE MEDICINES
▶ Adult: 80 mg daily, dose form is not appropriate for initial dose titration

DOSE ADJUSTMENTS DUE TO INTERACTIONS
▶ Max. dose 20 mg daily with concomitant elbasvir with grazoprevir.

● INTERACTIONS → Appendix 1: statins

● SIDE-EFFECTS
▶ **Rare or very rare** Angioedema · face oedema · lupus-like syndrome · sensation abnormal · vasculitis

● BREAST FEEDING Manufacturer advises avoid—no information available.

● RENAL IMPAIRMENT
Dose adjustments Manufacturer advises doses above 40 mg daily should be initiated with caution if eGFR less than 30 mL/minute/1.73 m^2.

● PATIENT AND CARER ADVICE Patient counselling is advised for fluvastatin tablets/capsules (muscle effects).

● NATIONAL FUNDING/ACCESS DECISIONS

Scottish Medicines Consortium (SMC) Decisions
The *Scottish Medicines Consortium* has advised (February 2004) that fluvastatin is accepted for restricted use for the secondary prevention of coronary events after percutaneous coronary angioplasty; if the patient has previously been receiving another statin, then there is no need to change the statin.

2

Cardiovascular system

● MEDICINAL FORMS
There can be variation in the licensing of different medicines containing the same drug.

Modified-release tablet
CAUTIONARY AND ADVISORY LABELS 25
▸ Fluvastatin (Non-proprietary)
  Fluvastatin (as Fluvastatin sodium) 80 mg Fluvastatin 80mg modified-release tablets | 28 tablet [PoM] ⅀ DT = £19.20
▸ Dorisin XL (Aspire Pharma Ltd)
  Fluvastatin (as Fluvastatin sodium) 80 mg Dorisin XL 80mg tablets | 28 tablet [PoM] £19.20 DT = £19.20
▸ Lescol XL (Novartis Pharmaceuticals UK Ltd)
  Fluvastatin (as Fluvastatin sodium) 80 mg Lescol XL 80mg tablets | 28 tablet [PoM] £19.20 DT = £19.20
▸ Nandovar XL (Sandoz Ltd)
  Fluvastatin (as Fluvastatin sodium) 80 mg Nandovar XL 80mg tablets | 28 tablet [PoM] £16.32 DT = £19.20

Capsule
▸ Fluvastatin (Non-proprietary)
  Fluvastatin (as Fluvastatin sodium) 20 mg Fluvastatin 20mg capsules | 28 capsule [PoM] £6.96 DT = £2.01
  Fluvastatin (as Fluvastatin sodium) 40 mg Fluvastatin 40mg capsules | 28 capsule [PoM] £7.42 DT = £2.22

⅏ 200

Pravastatin sodium
04-Jun-2017

● INDICATIONS AND DOSE

Adjunct to diet for primary hypercholesterolaemia or combined (mixed) hyperlipidaemias in patients who have not responded adequately to dietary control
▸ BY MOUTH
▸ Adult: 10–40 mg daily, dose to be taken at night, dose to be adjusted at intervals of at least 4 weeks

Prevention of cardiovascular events in patients with previous myocardial infarction or unstable angina | Adjunct to diet to prevent cardiovascular events in patients with hypercholesterolaemia
▸ BY MOUTH
▸ Adult: 40 mg daily, dose to be taken at night

Reduction of hyperlipidaemia in patients receiving immunosuppressive therapy following solid-organ transplantation
▸ BY MOUTH
▸ Adult: Initially 20 mg daily, then increased if necessary up to 40 mg daily, dose to be taken at night, close medical supervision is required if dose is increased to maximum dose

DOSE ADJUSTMENTS DUE TO INTERACTIONS
▸ Manufacturer advises reduce dose by half with concurrent use of ombitasvir with paritaprevir and ritonavir.
▸ Manufacturer advises max. 20 mg daily with concurrent use of glecaprevir with pibrentasvir.
▸ Manufacturer advises max. 40 mg daily with concurrent use of sofosbuvir with velpatasvir and voxaleprevir.

● INTERACTIONS → Appendix 1: statins
● SIDE-EFFECTS
▸ **Uncommon** Fatigue · hair abnormal · scalp abnormal · urinary disorders · vision disorders
▸ **Rare or very rare** Fulminant hepatic necrosis · polymyositis
● BREAST FEEDING Manufacturer advises avoid—small amount of drug present in breast milk.
● RENAL IMPAIRMENT
  Dose adjustments Manufacturer advises initial dose of 10 mg once daily in moderate to severe impairment.
● PATIENT AND CARER ADVICE Patient counselling is advised for pravastatin tablets (muscle effects).

● MEDICINAL FORMS
There can be variation in the licensing of different medicines containing the same drug. Forms available from special-order manufacturers include: oral suspension, oral solution

Tablet
▸ Pravastatin sodium (Non-proprietary)
  Pravastatin sodium 10 mg Pravastatin 10mg tablets | 28 tablet [PoM] £16.10 DT = £0.55
  Pravastatin sodium 20 mg Pravastatin 20mg tablets | 28 tablet [PoM] £29.60 DT = £0.87
  Pravastatin sodium 40 mg Pravastatin 40mg tablets | 28 tablet [PoM] £29.60 DT = £1.10

⅏ 200

Rosuvastatin
05-Feb-2018

● INDICATIONS AND DOSE

Primary hypercholesterolaemia (type IIa including heterozygous familial hypercholesterolaemia), mixed dyslipidaemia (type IIb), or homozygous familial hypercholesterolaemia in patients who have not responded adequately to diet and other appropriate measures
▸ BY MOUTH
▸ Adult 18–69 years: Initially 5–10 mg once daily, then increased if necessary up to 20 mg once daily, dose to be increased gradually at intervals of at least 4 weeks
▸ Adult (patients of Asian origin): Initially 5 mg once daily, then increased if necessary up to 20 mg once daily, dose to be increased gradually at intervals of at least 4 weeks.
▸ Adult 70 years and over: Initially 5 mg once daily, then increased if necessary up to 20 mg once daily, dose to be increased gradually at intervals of at least 4 weeks

Primary hypercholesterolaemia (type IIa including heterozygous familial hypercholesterolaemia), mixed dyslipidaemia (type IIb), or homozygous familial hypercholesterolaemia in patients who have not responded adequately to diet and other appropriate measures and who have risk factors for myopathy or rhabdomyolysis
▸ BY MOUTH
▸ Adult: Initially 5 mg once daily, then increased if necessary up to 20 mg once daily, dose to be increased gradually at intervals of at least 4 weeks

Severe primary hypercholesterolaemia (type IIa including heterozygous familial hypercholesterolaemia), mixed dyslipidaemia (type IIb), or homozygous familial hypercholesterolaemia in patients with high cardiovascular risk who have not responded adequately to diet and other appropriate measures (specialist use only)
▸ BY MOUTH
▸ Adult 18–69 years: Initially 5–10 mg once daily, then increased if necessary up to 40 mg once daily, dose to be increased gradually at intervals of at least 4 weeks
▸ Adult (patients of Asian origin): Initially 5 mg once daily, then increased if necessary up to 20 mg once daily, dose to be increased gradually at intervals of at least 4 weeks.
▸ Adult 70 years and over: Initially 5 mg once daily, then increased if necessary up to 40 mg once daily, dose to be increased gradually at intervals of at least 4 weeks

Severe primary hypercholesterolaemia (type IIa including heterozygous familial hypercholesterolaemia), mixed dyslipidaemia (type IIb), or homozygous familial hypercholesterolaemia in patients with high cardiovascular risk who have not responded adequately to diet and other appropriate measures, and who have risk factors for myopathy or rhabdomyolysis (specialist use only)

▸ BY MOUTH

▸ Adult: Initially 5 mg once daily, then increased if necessary up to 20 mg once daily, dose to be increased gradually at intervals of at least 4 weeks

Prevention of cardiovascular events in patients at high risk of a first cardiovascular event

▸ BY MOUTH

▸ Adult 18–69 years: 20 mg once daily

▸ Adult (patients of Asian origin): Initially 5 mg once daily, then increased if tolerated to 20 mg once daily, dose to be increased gradually at intervals of at least 4 weeks.

▸ Adult 70 years and over: Initially 5 mg once daily, then increased if tolerated to 20 mg once daily, dose to be increased gradually at intervals of at least 4 weeks

Prevention of cardiovascular events in patients at high risk of a first cardiovascular event and with risk factors for myopathy or rhabdomyolysis

▸ BY MOUTH

▸ Adult: Initially 5 mg once daily, then increased if tolerated to 20 mg once daily, dose to be increased gradually at intervals of at least 4 weeks

DOSE ADJUSTMENTS DUE TO INTERACTIONS

▸ Manufacturer advises initially 5 mg daily with concurrent use of bezafibrate, ciprofibrate, and fenofibrate—40 mg dose is contra-indicated.

▸ Manufacturer advises initially 5 mg daily with concurrent use of clopidogrel—max. dose 20 mg daily.

▸ Manufacturer advises initially 5 mg daily with concurrent use of simeprevir—max. dose 10 mg daily.

▸ Manufacturer advises max. dose 5 mg daily with concurrent ombitasvir, paritaprevir, and ritonavir given with dasabuvir, but max. 10 mg daily with concurrent ombitasvir, paritaprevir, and ritonavir given without dasabuvir.

▸ Manufacturer advises max. dose 10 mg daily with concurrent use of sofosbuvir with velpatasvir, or elbasvir with grazoprevir.

▸ Manufacturer advises reduce dose by half with concurrent use of teriflunomide.

▸ Manufacturer advises max. 5 mg daily with concurrent use of glecaprevir with pibrentasvir.

● CAUTIONS Known genetic polymorphisms—consult product literature · patients of Asian origin

● INTERACTIONS → Appendix 1: statins

● SIDE-EFFECTS

▸ **Rare or very rare** Arthralgia · gynaecomastia · haematuria · polyneuropathy

▸ **Frequency not known** Cough · dyspnoea · oedema · proteinuria · Stevens-Johnson syndrome · tendon disorders

● BREAST FEEDING Manufacturer advises avoid—no information available.

● RENAL IMPAIRMENT Avoid if eGFR less than 30 mL/minute/1.73 m^2.
Dose adjustments Initially 5 mg once daily (do not exceed 20 mg daily) if eGFR 30–60 mL/minute/1.73 m^2.

● MONITORING REQUIREMENTS Manufacturer advises consider routine monitoring of renal function when using 40 mg daily dose.

● PATIENT AND CARER ADVICE Patient counselling is advised for rosuvastatin tablets (muscle effects).

● MEDICINAL FORMS
There can be variation in the licensing of different medicines containing the same drug. Forms available from special-order manufacturers include: oral suspension

Tablet
▸ Rosuvastatin (Non-proprietary)
Rosuvastatin (as Rosuvastatin calcium) 5 mg Rosuvastatin 5mg tablets | 28 tablet [PoM] £18.03 DT = £2.92
Rosuvastatin (as Rosuvastatin calcium) 10 mg Rosuvastatin 10mg tablets | 28 tablet [PoM] £18.03 DT = £2.92
Rosuvastatin (as Rosuvastatin calcium) 20 mg Rosuvastatin 20mg tablets | 28 tablet [PoM] £26.02 DT = £4.48
Rosuvastatin (as Rosuvastatin calcium) 40 mg Rosuvastatin 40mg tablets | 28 tablet [PoM] £29.69 DT = £5.97
▸ Crestor (AstraZeneca UK Ltd)
Rosuvastatin (as Rosuvastatin calcium) 5 mg Crestor 5mg tablets | 28 tablet [PoM] £18.03 DT = £2.92
Rosuvastatin (as Rosuvastatin calcium) 10 mg Crestor 10mg tablets | 28 tablet [PoM] £18.03 DT = £2.92
Rosuvastatin (as Rosuvastatin calcium) 20 mg Crestor 20mg tablets | 28 tablet [PoM] £26.02 DT = £4.48
Rosuvastatin (as Rosuvastatin calcium) 40 mg Crestor 40mg tablets | 28 tablet [PoM] £29.69 DT = £5.97

F 200

Simvastatin

● INDICATIONS AND DOSE

Primary hypercholesterolaemia, or combined (mixed) hyperlipidaemia in patients who have not responded adequately to diet and other appropriate measures

▸ BY MOUTH

▸ Adult: 10–20 mg once daily, then increased if necessary up to 80 mg once daily, adjusted at intervals of at least 4 weeks, dose to be taken at night; 80 mg dose only for those with severe hypercholesterolaemia and at high risk of cardiovascular complications

Homozygous familial hypercholesterolaemia in patients who have not responded adequately to diet and other appropriate measures

▸ BY MOUTH

▸ Adult: Initially 40 mg once daily, then increased if necessary up to 80 mg once daily, adjusted at intervals of at least 4 weeks, dose to be taken at night; 80 mg dose only for those with severe hypercholesterolaemia and at high risk of cardiovascular complications

Prevention of cardiovascular events in patients with atherosclerotic cardiovascular disease or diabetes mellitus

▸ BY MOUTH

▸ Adult: Initially 20–40 mg once daily, increased if necessary up to 80 mg once daily, adjusted at intervals of at least 4 weeks, dose to be taken at night; 80 mg dose only for those with severe hypercholesterolaemia and at high risk of cardiovascular complications

DOSE ADJUSTMENTS DUE TO INTERACTIONS

▸ Manufacturer advises max. 10 mg daily with concurrent use of bezafibrate or ciprofibrate.

▸ Manufacturer advises max. 20 mg daily with concurrent use of amiodarone, amlodipine, or ranolazine.

▸ Manufacturer advises reduce dose with concurrent use of some moderate inhibitors of CYP3A4 (max. 20 mg daily with verapamil and diltiazem).

▸ Manufacturer advises max. 40 mg daily with concurrent use of lomitapide or ticagrelor.

▸ Manufacturer advises max. 20 mg daily with concurrent use of elbasvir with grazoprevir.

● INTERACTIONS → Appendix 1: statins

● SIDE-EFFECTS

▸ **Rare or very rare** Acute kidney injury · anaemia · muscle cramps

▸ **Frequency not known** Cognitive impairment

- **BREAST FEEDING** Manufacturer advises avoid—no information available.
- **RENAL IMPAIRMENT** Doses above 10 mg daily should be used with caution if eGFR less than 30 mL/minute/1.73 m^2.
- **PATIENT AND CARER ADVICE** Patient counselling is advised for simvastatin tablets/oral suspension (muscle effects).
- **EXCEPTIONS TO LEGAL CATEGORY** Simvastatin 10 mg tablets can be sold to the public to reduce risk of first coronary event in individuals at moderate risk of coronary heart disease (approx. 10–15 % risk of major event in 10 years), max. daily dose 10 mg and pack size of 28 tablets; treatment should form part of a programme to reduce risk of coronary heart disease.

- **MEDICINAL FORMS** There can be variation in the licensing of different medicines containing the same drug. Forms available from special-order manufacturers include: oral suspension, oral solution

Oral suspension
EXCIPIENTS: May contain Propylene glycol
▸ Simvastatin (Non-proprietary)
Simvastatin 4 mg per 1 ml Simvastatin 20mg/5ml oral suspension sugar free sugar-free | 150 ml [PoM] £126.87 DT = £126.87
Simvastatin 8 mg per 1 ml Simvastatin 40mg/5ml oral suspension sugar free sugar-free | 150 ml [PoM] £193.80 DT = £193.80

Tablet
▸ Simvastatin (Non-proprietary)
Simvastatin 10 mg Simvastatin 10mg tablets | 28 tablet [PoM] £18.00 DT = £0.35
Simvastatin 20 mg Simvastatin 20mg tablets | 28 tablet [PoM] £29.60 DT = £0.45
Simvastatin 40 mg Simvastatin 40mg tablets | 28 tablet [PoM] £29.60 DT = £0.65
Simvastatin 80 mg Simvastatin 80mg tablets | 28 tablet [PoM] £29.61 DT = £1.28
▸ Simvador (Discovery Pharmaceuticals)
Simvastatin 10 mg Simvador 10mg tablets | 28 tablet [PoM] £0.34 DT = £0.35
Simvastatin 20 mg Simvador 20mg tablets | 28 tablet [PoM] £0.44 DT = £0.45
Simvastatin 40 mg Simvador 40mg tablets | 28 tablet [PoM] £0.64 DT = £0.65
Simvastatin 80 mg Simvador 80mg tablets | 28 tablet [PoM] £1.27 DT = £1.28
▸ Zocor (Merck Sharp & Dohme Ltd)
Simvastatin 10 mg Zocor 10mg tablets | 28 tablet [PoM] £18.03 DT = £0.35
Simvastatin 20 mg Zocor 20mg tablets | 28 tablet [PoM] £29.69 DT = £0.45
Simvastatin 40 mg Zocor 40mg tablets | 28 tablet [PoM] £29.69 DT = £0.65
Simvastatin 80 mg Zocor 80mg tablets | 28 tablet [PoM] £29.69 DT = £1.28

Simvastatin with ezetimibe

The properties listed below are those particular to the combination only. For the properties of the components please consider, simvastatin p. 203, ezetimibe p. 196.

- **INDICATIONS AND DOSE**

Homozygous familial hypercholesterolaemia, primary hypercholesterolaemia, and mixed hyperlipidaemia in patients over 10 years stabilised on the individual components in the same proportions, or for patients not adequately controlled by statin alone
▸ BY MOUTH
▸ Adult: (consult product literature)

- **INTERACTIONS** → Appendix 1: ezetimibe · statins

- **MEDICINAL FORMS** There can be variation in the licensing of different medicines containing the same drug.
Tablet
▸ Inegy (Merck Sharp & Dohme Ltd)
Ezetimibe 10 mg, Simvastatin 20 mg Inegy 10mg/20mg tablets | 28 tablet [PoM] £33.42 DT = £33.42
Ezetimibe 10 mg, Simvastatin 40 mg Inegy 10mg/40mg tablets | 28 tablet [PoM] £38.98 DT = £38.98
Ezetimibe 10 mg, Simvastatin 80 mg Inegy 10mg/80mg tablets | 28 tablet [PoM] £41.21 DT = £41.21

Simvastatin with fenofibrate   19-Apr-2016

The properties listed below are those particular to the combination only. For the properties of the components please consider, simvastatin p. 203, fenofibrate p. 198.

- **INDICATIONS AND DOSE**

Adjunct to diet and exercise in mixed dyslipidaemia, when LDL-cholesterol levels are adequately controlled with the corresponding dose of simvastatin monotherapy (in patients at high cardiovascular risk)
▸ BY MOUTH
▸ Adult: 20/145 mg once daily, alternatively 40/145 mg once daily, dose should be based on previous simvastatin monotherapy dose

- **CAUTIONS** History of pulmonary embolism
- **INTERACTIONS** → Appendix 1: fibrates · statins
- **RENAL IMPAIRMENT** Manufacturer advises avoid if eGFR less than 60 mL/minute/1.73 m^2; use with caution if eGFR 60–89 mL/minute/1.73 m^2.

- **MEDICINAL FORMS** There can be variation in the licensing of different medicines containing the same drug.
Tablet
CAUTIONARY AND ADVISORY LABELS 25
EXCIPIENTS: May contain Butylated hydroxyanisole, lecithin
▸ Cholib (Mylan)
Simvastatin 20 mg, Fenofibrate 145 mg Cholib 145mg/20mg tablets | 30 tablet [PoM] £7.71 DT = £7.71
Simvastatin 40 mg, Fenofibrate 145 mg Cholib 145mg/40mg tablets | 30 tablet [PoM] £8.33 DT = £8.33

LIPID MODIFYING DRUGS 〉 OTHER

Alirocumab   24-Oct-2016

- **DRUG ACTION** Alirocumab binds to a pro-protein involved in the regulation of LDL receptors on liver cells; receptor numbers are increased, which results in increased uptake of LDL-cholesterol from the blood.

- **INDICATIONS AND DOSE**

Primary hypercholesterolaemia or mixed dyslipidaemia in patients who have not responded adequately to other appropriate measures (in combination with a statin, or with a statin and other lipid-lowering therapies, or with other lipid-lowering therapies or alone if a statin contra-indicated or not tolerated)
▸ BY SUBCUTANEOUS INJECTION
▸ Adult: 75–150 mg every 2 weeks, adjusted according to response, to be administered into the thigh, abdomen or upper arm, dose adjustments should be made at 4-weekly intervals

- **SIDE-EFFECTS**
▸ **Common or very common** Nasal complaints · oropharyngeal pain · pulmonary reaction · skin reactions
▸ **Rare or very rare** Hypersensitivity vasculitis

- PREGNANCY Manufacturer advises avoid unless clinical condition requires treatment—maternal toxicity in *animal* studies.
- BREAST FEEDING Manufacturer advises avoid—no information available.
- HEPATIC IMPAIRMENT Manufacturer advises use with caution in severe impairment—no information available.
- RENAL IMPAIRMENT Manufacturer advises use with caution in severe impairment—no information available.
- HANDLING AND STORAGE Manufacturer advises store in a refrigerator (2–8 °C)—consult product literature for further information regarding storage outside refrigerator.
- NATIONAL FUNDING/ACCESS DECISIONS

NICE decisions
▸ Alirocumab for treating primary hypercholesterolaemia and mixed dyslipidaemia (June 2016) NICE TA393
Alirocumab is recommended as an option for treating primary hypercholesterolaemia or mixed dyslipidaemia, only if :
- low-density lipoprotein cholesterol (LDL-C) concentrations are persistently above the thresholds specified in the NICE documentation **and**
- the manufacturer provides alirocumab with the discount agreed in the patient access scheme.

Patients whose treatment was started before this guidance was published should continue treatment until they and their clinician consider it appropriate to stop.
www.nice.org.uk/TA393

Scottish Medicines Consortium (SMC) Decisions
The *Scottish Medicines Consortium* has advised (Aug 2016) that alirocumab (*Praluent*®) is accepted for restricted use within NHS Scotland for treatment of primary hypercholesterolaemia or mixed dyslipidaemia (alone or in combination with other lipid lowering therapies, as specified within it's license), for specialist use only and only in patients at high cardiovascular risk as follows:
- patients with heterozygous familial hypercholesterolaemia (HeFH) and LDL-C $\geq$5.0mmol/L, for primary prevention of cardiovascular events, or
- patients with HeFH and LDL-C $\geq$3.5mmol/L, for secondary prevention of cardiovascular events, or
- patients at high risk due to previous cardiovascular events and LDL-C $\geq$4.0mmol/L, or
- patients with recurrent/polyvascular disease and LDL-C $\geq$3.5mmol/L

This advice is contingent upon the continuing availability of the Patient Access Scheme (PAS) in NHS Scotland or a list price that is equivalent or lower.

- MEDICINAL FORMS
There can be variation in the licensing of different medicines containing the same drug.
Solution for injection
EXCIPIENTS: May contain Polysorbates
▸ Praluent (Sanofi) ▼
Alirocumab 75 mg per 1 ml Praluent 75mg/1ml solution for injection pre-filled pen | 1 pre-filled disposable injection PoM £168.00 | 2 pre-filled disposable injection PoM £336.00
Alirocumab 150 mg per 1 ml Praluent 150mg/1ml solution for injection pre-filled pen | 1 pre-filled disposable injection PoM £168.00 | 2 pre-filled disposable injection PoM £336.00

Evolocumab

24-Apr-2017

- DRUG ACTION Evolocumab binds to a pro-protein involved in the regulation of LDL receptors on liver cells; receptor numbers are increased, which results in increased uptake of LDL-cholesterol from the blood.

- INDICATIONS AND DOSE

Primary hypercholesterolaemia or mixed dyslipidaemia in patients who have not responded adequately to other appropriate measures (in combination with a statin, or with a statin and other lipid-lowering therapies, or with other lipid-lowering therapies or alone if a statin contra-indicated or not tolerated)
▸ BY SUBCUTANEOUS INJECTION
▹ Adult: 140 mg every 2 weeks, alternatively 420 mg every month, to be administered into the thigh, abdomen or upper arm

Homozygous familial hypercholesterolaemia (in combination with other lipid-lowering therapies)
▸ BY SUBCUTANEOUS INJECTION
▹ Adult: Initially 420 mg every month; increased if necessary to 420 mg every 2 weeks, if inadequate response after 12 weeks of treatment, to be administered into the thigh, abdomen or upper arm

Homozygous familial hypercholesterolaemia in patients on apheresis (in combination with other lipid-lowering therapies)
▸ BY SUBCUTANEOUS INJECTION
▹ Adult: 420 mg every 2 weeks, to correspond with apheresis schedule, to be administered into the thigh, abdomen or upper arm

- SIDE-EFFECTS
▸ Common or very common Arthralgia · back pain · increased risk of infection · nausea · skin reactions
- PREGNANCY Manufacturer advises avoid unless essential—limited information available.
- BREAST FEEDING Manufacturer advises avoid—no information available.
- HEPATIC IMPAIRMENT Manufacturer advises monitor in moderate impairment—possible reduced efficacy; use with caution in severe impairment—no information available.
- RENAL IMPAIRMENT Manufacturer advises caution if eGFR less than 30 mL/minute/1.73 m^2—no information available.
- HANDLING AND STORAGE Manufacturer advises store in a refrigerator (2–8°C)—consult product literature for further information regarding storage outside refrigerator.
- PATIENT AND CARER ADVICE Patients and their carers should be given training in subcutaneous injection technique.
- NATIONAL FUNDING/ACCESS DECISIONS

NICE decisions
▸ Evolocumab for treating primary hypercholesterolaemia and mixed dyslipidaemia (June 2016) NICE TA394
Evolocumab is recommended as an option for treating primary hypercholesterolaemia or mixed dyslipidaemia, only if:
- it is given at a dose of 140 mg every 2 weeks; **and**
- low-density lipoprotein cholesterol (LDL-C) concentrations are persistently above the thresholds specified in the NICE documentation; **and**
- the manufacturer provides evolocumab with the discount agreed in the patient access scheme.

Patients whose treatment was started within the NHS before this guidance was published should have the option to continue treatment, without change to their funding arrangements, until they and their clinician consider it appropriate to stop.
www.nice.org.uk/TA394

2

Cardiovascular system

Scottish Medicines Consortium (SMC) Decisions
The *Scottish Medicines Consortium* has advised (February 2017) that evolocumab (*Repatha®*) is accepted for restricted use within NHS Scotland for the treatment of primary hypercholesterolaemia (heterozygous familial hypercholesterolaemia and non-familial) *or* mixed dyslipidaemia (alone or in combination with other lipid lowering therapies, as specified within it's license), for specialist use only when administered at a dose of 140 mg every 2 weeks and only in patients at high cardiovascular risk as follows:

- patients with heterozygous familial hypercholesterolaemia (HeFH) and LDL-C 5 mmol/L or greater for primary prevention of cardiovascular events, or
- patients with HeFH and LDL-C 3.5 mmol/L or greater for secondary prevention of cardiovascular disease, or
- patients with high risk due to previous cardiovascular events and LDL-C 4 mmol/L or greater, or
- patients with recurrent/polyvascular disease and LDL-C 3.5 mmol/L or greater
  This advice is contingent upon the continuing availability of the Patient Access Scheme in NHS Scotland or a list price that is equivalent or lower.

- MEDICINAL FORMS
There can be variation in the licensing of different medicines containing the same drug.
Solution for injection
▸ Repatha (Amgen Ltd) ▼
  Evolocumab 140 mg per 1 ml Repatha 140mg/1ml solution for injection pre-filled syringes | 1 pre-filled disposable injection PoM £170.10
▸ Repatha SureClick (Amgen Ltd) ▼
  Evolocumab 140 mg per 1 ml Repatha SureClick 140mg/1ml solution for injection pre-filled disposable devices | 2 pre-filled disposable injection PoM £340.20

Lomitapide

- DRUG ACTION Lomitapide, an inhibitor of microsomal triglyceride transfer protein (MTP), reduces lipoprotein secretion and circulating concentrations of lipoprotein-borne lipids such as cholesterol and triglycerides.

- INDICATIONS AND DOSE
Adjunct to dietary measures and other lipid-regulating drugs with or without low-density lipoprotein apheresis in homozygous familial hypercholesterolaemia (under expert supervision)
▸ BY MOUTH
▸ Adult: Initially 5 mg daily for 2 weeks, dose to be taken at least 2 hours after evening meal, then increased if necessary to 10 mg daily, for at least 4 weeks, then increased to 20 mg daily for at least 4 weeks, then increased in steps of 20 mg daily, adjusted at intervals of at least 4 weeks; maximum 60 mg per day

- CONTRA-INDICATIONS Significant or chronic bowel disease
- CAUTIONS Concomitant use of hepatotoxic drugs · lomitapide can interfere with the absorption of fat-soluble nutrients and supplementation of vitamin E and fatty acids is required · patients over 65 years
- INTERACTIONS → Appendix 1: lomitapide
- SIDE-EFFECTS
▸ Common or very common Aerophagia · appetite abnormal · asthenia · burping · constipation · diarrhoea · dizziness · gastrointestinal discomfort · gastrointestinal disorders · haemorrhage · headaches · hepatic disorders · increased risk of infection · muscle complaints · nausea · skin reactions · vomiting · weight decreased
▸ Uncommon Anaemia · chest pain · chills · dehydration · drowsiness · dry mouth · eye swelling · fever · gait abnormal

· hyperhidrosis · joint disorders · malaise · pain in extremity · paraesthesia · throat lesion · upper-airway cough syndrome · vertigo
▸ Frequency not known Alopecia

SIDE-EFFECTS, FURTHER INFORMATION Reduce dose if serum transaminases raised during treatment (consult product literature).

- CONCEPTION AND CONTRACEPTION Manufacturer advises exclude pregnancy before treatment and ensure effective contraception used.
- PREGNANCY Avoid—teratogenicity and embryotoxicity in *animal* studies.
- BREAST FEEDING Manufacturer advises avoid—no information available.
- HEPATIC IMPAIRMENT Avoid in moderate to severe impairment, or if unexplained persistent abnormal liver function tests.
  Dose adjustments Reduce dose if serum transaminases raised during treatment (consult product literature). Max. 40 mg daily in mild impairment.
- RENAL IMPAIRMENT
  Dose adjustments Max. 40 mg daily in end-stage renal disease.
- MONITORING REQUIREMENTS
▸ Monitor liver function tests before treatment, then at least monthly and before each dose increase for first year, then at least every 3 months and before each dose increase thereafter.
▸ Screen for hepatic steatosis and fibrosis before treatment, then annually thereafter.

- MEDICINAL FORMS
There can be variation in the licensing of different medicines containing the same drug.
Capsule
▸ Lojuxta (Amryt Pharma) ▼
  Lomitapide 5 mg Lojuxta 5mg capsules | 28 capsule PoM £17,765.00
  Lomitapide 10 mg Lojuxta 10mg capsules | 28 capsule PoM £17,765.00
  Lomitapide 20 mg Lojuxta 20mg capsules | 28 capsule PoM £17,765.00

Omega-3-acid ethyl esters

- INDICATIONS AND DOSE
Adjunct to diet and statin in type IIb or III hypertriglyceridaemia | Adjunct to diet in type IV hypertriglyceridaemia
▸ BY MOUTH
▸ Adult: Initially 2 capsules daily, dose to be taken with food, increased if necessary to 4 capsules daily

Adjunct in secondary prevention in those who have had a myocardial infarction in the preceding 3 months
▸ BY MOUTH
▸ Adult: 1 capsule daily, dose to be taken with food

- CAUTIONS Anticoagulant treatment (bleeding time increased) · haemorrhagic disorders
- INTERACTIONS → Appendix 1: omega-3-acid ethyl esters
- SIDE-EFFECTS
▸ Common or very common Burping · constipation · diarrhoea · gastrointestinal discomfort · gastrointestinal disorders · nausea · vomiting
▸ Uncommon Dizziness · gout · haemorrhage · headache · hyperglycaemia · hypotension · skin reactions · taste altered
▸ Rare or very rare Liver disorder
- PREGNANCY Manufacturers advise use only if potential benefit outweighs risk—no information available.

- BREAST FEEDING Manufacturers advise avoid—no information available.
- HEPATIC IMPAIRMENT
Monitoring Monitor liver function in hepatic impairment.
- NATIONAL FUNDING/ACCESS DECISIONS

Scottish Medicines Consortium (SMC) Decisions
The *Scottish Medicines Consortium* has advised (November 2002) that omega-3-acid ethyl esters are **not** recommended for use within NHS Scotland for the treatment of hypertriglyceridaemia.

- MEDICINAL FORMS
There can be variation in the licensing of different medicines containing the same drug.

Capsule
CAUTIONARY AND ADVISORY LABELS 21
▸ Omega-3-acid ethyl esters (Non-proprietary)
Eicosapentaenoic acid 60 mg, Docosahexaenoic acid 300 mg Omega-3 600mg capsules | 28 capsule 🔀
Docosahexaenoic acid 380 mg, Eicosapentaenoic acid 460 mg Eicosapentaenoic acid 460mg / Docosahexaenoic acid 380mg capsules | 28 capsule £14.24 DT = £14.24 | 100 capsule PoM £50.86
▸ Dualtis (Mylan)
Docosahexaenoic acid 380 mg, Eicosapentaenoic acid 460 mg Dualtis 1000mg capsules | 28 capsule P £11.37 DT = £14.24
▸ Omacor (Mylan)
Docosahexaenoic acid 380 mg, Eicosapentaenoic acid 460 mg Omacor capsules | 28 capsule P £14.24 DT = £14.24 | 100 capsule P £50.84
▸ Omega 3 (Glenmark Pharmaceuticals Europe Ltd)
Docosahexaenoic acid 380 mg, Eicosapentaenoic acid 460 mg Omega 3-acid-ethyl esters 1000mg capsules | 28 capsule PoM £6.00 DT = £14.24 | 100 capsule PoM £21.00
▸ Prestylon (Teva UK Ltd)
Docosahexaenoic acid 380 mg, Eicosapentaenoic acid 460 mg Prestylon 1g capsules | 28 capsule PoM £10.68 DT = £14.24 | 100 capsule PoM £38.13
▸ Teromeg (AMCo)
Docosahexaenoic acid 380 mg, Eicosapentaenoic acid 460 mg Teromeg 1000mg capsules | 28 capsule PoM £11.39 DT = £14.24 | 100 capsule PoM £40.67

7　Myocardial ischaemia

Stable angina

Overview
It is important to distinguish stable angina from unstable angina. *Stable angina* usually results from atherosclerotic plaques in the coronary arteries that restrict blood flow and oxygen supply to the heart; it is often precipitated by exertion and relieved by rest. Treatment involves management of acute anginal pain, and long term management to prevent angina attacks and to reduce the risk of cardiovascular events.

Management
Acute attacks of stable angina should be managed with sublingual glyceryl trinitrate p. 217 which can be taken immediately before performing activities that are known to bring on an attack. If attacks occur more than twice a week, regular drug therapy is required and should be introduced in a step-wise manner according to response.

Patients with stable angina should be given a **beta-blocker** or a **calcium-channel blocker**. In those with left-ventricular dysfunction, beta-blocker treatment should be started at a very low dose and titrated very slowly over a period of weeks or months. If a beta-blocker or a calcium-channel blocker alone fails to control symptoms adequately,

a combination of a beta-blocker and a dihydropyridine calcium-channel blocker (e.g. amlodipine p. 155, felodipine p. 159, modified-release nifedipine p. 162) should be used; if this combination is not appropriate due to intolerance of, or contra-indication to, *either* beta-blockers *or* calcium-channel blockers, addition of a long-acting **nitrate**, ivabradine p. 210, nicorandil p. 211, or ranolazine p. 210 can be considered.

For those patients in whom both beta-blockers *and* calcium-channel blockers are not tolerated or are contra-indicated, monotherapy with a long-acting nitrate, ivabradine, nicorandil, or ranolazine should be considered.

Response to treatment should be assessed every 2–4 weeks after initiating or changing drug therapy; the drug should be titrated (according to symptom control) to the maximum tolerated dose. Consider referring the patient to a specialist if a combination of two drugs fails to control symptoms. Addition of a third antianginal drug should only be considered if symptom control is not achieved with two drugs and the patient is either due to undergo a revascularisation procedure, or a revascularisation procedure is considered inappropriate. See the use of antiplatelet drugs in patients undergoing coronary stenting.

For long-term prevention of cardiovascular events, see Prevention of cardiovascular events.

Antianginal drugs
Nitrates, calcium-channel blockers, and potassium channel activators (use in adults only) have a vasodilating and, consequently, blood pressure lowering effect. Vasodilators can act in heart failure by arteriolar dilatation which reduces both peripheral vascular resistance and left ventricular pressure during systole resulting in improved cardiac output. They can also cause venous dilatation which results in dilatation of capacitance vessels, increase of venous pooling, and diminution of venous return to the heart (decreasing left ventricular end-diastolic pressure).

Nicorandil, a potassium-channel activator with a nitrate component, has both arterial and venous vasodilating properties and is licensed for the prevention and long-term treatment of angina. Nicorandil has similar efficacy to other antianginal drugs in controlling symptoms; it may produce additional symptomatic benefit in combination with other antianginal drugs [unlicensed indication].

Ivabradine lowers the heart rate by its action on the sinus node. It is licensed for the treatment of angina in patients who are in normal sinus rhythm in combination with a beta-blocker, or when beta-blockers are contra-indicated or not tolerated. Ivabradine, in combination with standard therapy including a beta-blocker (unless contra-indicated or not tolerated), is also licensed for mild to severe stable chronic heart failure in patients who are in sinus rhythm.

Ranolazine is licensed as adjunctive therapy in patients who are inadequately controlled or intolerant of first-line antianginal drugs.

Other drugs used for Myocardial ischaemia Acebutolol, p. 151 · Aspirin, p. 121 · Atenolol, p. 151 · Bisoprolol fumarate, p. 152 · Bivalirudin, p. 134 · Carvedilol, p. 147 · Diltiazem hydrochloride, p. 157 · Fondaparinux sodium, p. 126 · Metoprolol tartrate, p. 154 · Nadolol, p. 148 · Nicardipine hydrochloride, p. 161 · Oxprenolol hydrochloride, p. 149 · Pindolol, p. 149 · Propranolol hydrochloride, p. 149 · Timolol maleate, p. 150 · Verapamil hydrochloride, p. 163

Cardiovascular system

2

ANTITHROMBOTIC DRUGS > ANTIPLATELET DRUGS

Cangrelor   16-Feb-2016

- **DRUG ACTION** Cangrelor is a direct $P2Y_{12}$ platelet receptor antagonist that blocks adenosine diphosphate induced platelet activation and aggregation.

- **INDICATIONS AND DOSE**

In combination with aspirin for the reduction of thrombotic cardiovascular events in patients with coronary artery disease undergoing percutaneous coronary intervention (PCI) who have not received an oral $P2Y_{12}$ inhibitor (e.g. clopidogrel, prasugrel, ticagrelor) prior to the PCI procedure and in whom oral therapy with a $P2Y_{12}$ inhibitor is not suitable (under expert supervision)
  - ► INITIALLY BY INTRAVENOUS INJECTION
  - ► Adult: Initially 30 micrograms/kg, to be given as a bolus dose, followed immediately by (by intravenous infusion) 4 micrograms/kg/minute, start treatment before percutaneous coronary intervention and continue infusion for at least 2 hours or for the duration of intervention if longer; maximum duration of infusion 4 hours

- **CONTRA-INDICATIONS** Active bleeding · history of stroke · history of transient ischaemic attack · patients at increased risk of bleeding (e.g. impaired haemostasis, irreversible coagulation disorders, major surgery or trauma, uncontrolled severe hypertension)

- **CAUTIONS** Disease states associated with increased bleeding risk

- **INTERACTIONS** → Appendix 1: cangrelor

- **SIDE-EFFECTS**
  - ► **Common or very common** Dyspnoea · haemorrhage · skin reactions
  - ► **Uncommon** Cardiac tamponade · haemodynamic instability · renal impairment · retroperitoneal haemorrhage (including fatal cases)
  - ► **Rare or very rare** Anaemia · intracranial haemorrhage · menorrhagia · stroke · thrombocytopenia

- **PREGNANCY** Manufacturer advises avoid—toxicity in *animal* studies.

- **BREAST FEEDING** Manufacturer advises potential risk to infant —no information available.

- **RENAL IMPAIRMENT** Manufacturer advises caution in severe renal impairment—increased risk of bleeding.

- **DIRECTIONS FOR ADMINISTRATION** For *intravenous bolus injection* and *intravenous infusion*, reconstitute each 50 mg vial with 5 mL of water for injection and gently swirl, do not shake vigorously. Withdraw 5 mL of reconstituted solution, add to 250 mL of either Sodium Chloride 0.9% *or* Glucose 5% and mix thoroughly. The bolus injection and infusion should be administered from the infusion solution.

- **MEDICINAL FORMS**
  There can be variation in the licensing of different medicines containing the same drug.
  Powder for solution for injection
  - ► Kengrexal (Chiesi Ltd) ▼
    Cangrelor (as Cangrelor tetrasodium) 50 mg Kengrexal 50mg powder for concentrate for solution for injection / infusion vials | 10 vial [PoM] ⑤ (Hospital only)

ANTITHROMBOTIC DRUGS > GLYCOPROTEIN IIB/IIIA INHIBITORS

Abciximab

- **INDICATIONS AND DOSE**

Prevention of ischaemic cardiac complications in patients undergoing percutaneous coronary intervention (specialist use only)
  - ► INITIALLY BY INTRAVENOUS INJECTION
  - ► Adult: Initially 250 micrograms/kg, to be given over 1 minute, then (by intravenous infusion) 125 nanograms/kg/minute (max. per dose 10 micrograms/minute), to be started 10–60 minutes before percutaneous coronary intervention and continue for 12 hours

Short-term prevention of myocardial infarction in patients with unstable angina not responding to conventional treatment and who are scheduled for percutaneous coronary intervention (specialist use only)
  - ► INITIALLY BY INTRAVENOUS INJECTION
  - ► Adult: Initially 250 micrograms/kg, to be given over 1 minute, then (by intravenous infusion) 125 nanograms/kg/minute (max. per dose 10 micrograms/minute), to be started up to 24 hours before possible percutaneous coronary intervention and continue infusion for 12 hours after intervention

- **CONTRA-INDICATIONS** Active internal bleeding · arteriovenous malformation or aneurysm · haemorrhagic diathesis · hypertensive retinopathy · intracranial neoplasm · intracranial or intraspinal surgery or trauma within last 2 months · major surgery within last 2 months · severe hypertension · stroke within last 2 years · thrombocytopenia · vasculitis

- **CAUTIONS** Discontinue if uncontrollable serious bleeding occurs or emergency cardiac surgery needed (consult product literature for details of procedures to minimise bleeding) · elderly

- **INTERACTIONS** → Appendix 1: abciximab

- **SIDE-EFFECTS**
  - ► **Common or very common** Abdominal pain · back pain · bradycardia · chest pain · fever · haemorrhage · headache · hypotension · nausea · peripheral oedema · thrombocytopenia · vomiting
  - ► **Uncommon** Intracranial haemorrhage
  - ► **Rare or very rare** Acute respiratory distress syndrome (ARDS) · cardiac tamponade · hypersensitivity

- **PREGNANCY** Manufacturer advises use only if potential benefit outweighs risk—no information available.

- **BREAST FEEDING** Manufacturer advises avoid—no information available.

- **HEPATIC IMPAIRMENT** Avoid in severe liver disease—increased risk of bleeding.

- **RENAL IMPAIRMENT** Caution in severe impairment—increased risk of bleeding.

- **MONITORING REQUIREMENTS**
  - ► Measure baseline prothrombin time, activated clotting time, activated partial thromboplastin time, platelet count, haemoglobin and haematocrit.
  - ► Monitor haemoglobin and haematocrit 12 hours and 24 hours after start of treatment and platelet count 2–4 hours and 24 hours after start of treatment.

- **DIRECTIONS FOR ADMINISTRATION** For *intravenous infusion* (*ReoPro®*), give continuously in Glucose 5% or Sodium Chloride 0.9%. Dilute requisite dose in infusion fluid and give via infusion pump; filter upon dilution through a non-pyrogenic low proteinbinding 0.2, 0.22, or 5 micron filter or upon administration through an in-line non-progenic low protein-binding 0.2 or 0.22 micron filter.

● MEDICINAL FORMS
No licensed medicines listed.

Eptifibatide

● INDICATIONS AND DOSE

In combination with aspirin and unfractionated heparin for the prevention of early myocardial infarction in patients with unstable angina or non-ST-segment-elevation myocardial infarction and with last episode of chest pain within 24 hours (specialist use only)
▸ INITIALLY BY INTRAVENOUS INJECTION
▸ Adult: Initially 180 micrograms/kg, then (by intravenous infusion) 2 micrograms/kg/minute for up to 72 hours (up to 96 hours if percutaneous coronary intervention during treatment)

● CONTRA-INDICATIONS Abnormal bleeding within 30 days · aneurysm · arteriovenous malformation · haemorrhagic diathesis · history of haemorrhagic stroke · increased INR · increased prothrombin time · intracranial disease · major surgery or severe trauma within 6 weeks · neoplasm · severe hypertension · stroke within last 30 days · thrombocytopenia

● CAUTIONS Discontinue if emergency cardiac surgery necessary · discontinue if intra-aortic balloon pump necessary · discontinue if thrombolytic therapy necessary · risk of bleeding—discontinue immediately if uncontrolled serious bleeding

● INTERACTIONS → Appendix 1: eptifibatide

● SIDE-EFFECTS
▸ **Common or very common** Arrhythmias · atrioventricular block · cardiac arrest · congestive heart failure · haemorrhage · hypotension · intracranial haemorrhage · shock
▸ **Uncommon** Cerebral ischaemia · thrombocytopenia
▸ **Rare or very rare** Rash

● PREGNANCY Manufacturer advises use only if potential benefit outweighs risk—no information available.

● BREAST FEEDING Manufacturer advises avoid—no information available.

● HEPATIC IMPAIRMENT Avoid in severe liver disease—increased risk of bleeding.

● RENAL IMPAIRMENT Avoid if eGFR less than 30 mL/minute/1.73 m².
Dose adjustments Reduce infusion to 1 microgram/kg/minute if eGFR 30–50 mL/minute/1.73 m².

● MONITORING REQUIREMENTS
▸ Measure baseline prothrombin time, activated partial thromboplastin time, platelet count, haemoglobin, haematocrit and serum creatinine.
▸ Monitor haemoglobin, haematocrit and platelets within 6 hours after start of treatment, then at least once daily.

● MEDICINAL FORMS
There can be variation in the licensing of different medicines containing the same drug.
Solution for injection
▸ Eptifibatide (Non-proprietary)
  Eptifibatide 2 mg per 1 ml Eptifibatide 20mg/10ml solution for injection vials | 1 vial [PoM] £5.14 (Hospital only)
▸ Integrilin (GlaxoSmithKline UK Ltd)
  Eptifibatide 2 mg per 1 ml Integrilin 20mg/10ml solution for injection vials | 1 vial [PoM] £13.61 (Hospital only)
Solution for infusion
▸ Eptifibatide (Non-proprietary)
  Eptifibatide 750 microgram per 1 ml Eptifibatide 75mg/100ml solution for infusion vials | 1 vial [PoM] £17.14 (Hospital only)

▸ Integrilin (GlaxoSmithKline UK Ltd)
  Eptifibatide 750 microgram per 1 ml Integrilin 75mg/100ml solution for infusion vials | 1 vial [PoM] £42.79 (Hospital only)

Tirofiban

● INDICATIONS AND DOSE

In combination with unfractionated heparin, aspirin, and clopidogrel for prevention of early myocardial infarction in patients with unstable angina or non-ST-segment-elevation myocardial infarction (NSTEMI) and with last episode of chest pain within 12 hours (with angiography planned for 4–48 hours after diagnosis) (initiated under specialist supervision)
▸ BY INTRAVENOUS INFUSION
▸ Adult: Initially 400 nanograms/kg/minute for 30 minutes, then 100 nanograms/kg/minute for at least 48 hours (continue during and for 12–24 hours after percutaneous coronary intervention), maximum duration of treatment 108 hours

In combination with unfractionated heparin, aspirin, and clopidogrel for prevention of early myocardial infarction in patients with unstable angina or non-ST-segment-elevation myocardial infarction (NSTEMI) and with last episode of chest pain within 12 hours (with angiography within 4 hours of diagnosis) (initiated under specialist supervision)
▸ INITIALLY BY INTRAVENOUS INJECTION
▸ Adult: 25 micrograms/kg, to be given over 3 minutes at start of percutaneous coronary intervention, then (by intravenous infusion) 150 nanograms/kg/minute for 12–24 hours, maximum duration of treatment 48 hours

In combination with unfractionated heparin, aspirin, and clopidogrel for reduction of major cardiovascular events in patients with ST-segment elevation myocardial infarction (STEMI) intended for primary percutaneous coronary intervention (PCI) (initiated under specialist supervision)
▸ INITIALLY BY INTRAVENOUS INJECTION
▸ Adult: 25 micrograms/kg, to be given over 3 minutes at start of percutaneous coronary intervention, then (by intravenous infusion) 150 nanograms/kg/minute for 12–24 hours, maximum duration of treatment 48 hours

● CONTRA-INDICATIONS Abnormal bleeding within 30 days · history of aneurysm · history of arteriovenous malformation · history of haemorrhagic stroke · history of intracranial disease · history of neoplasm · increased INR · increased prothrombin time · severe hypertension · stroke within 30 days · thrombocytopenia

● CAUTIONS Active peptic ulcer (within 3 months) · acute pericarditis · anaemia · aortic dissection · cardiogenic shock · discontinue if intra-aortic balloon pump necessary · discontinue if thrombolytic therapy necessary · discontinue immediately if serious or uncontrollable bleeding occurs · discontiue if emergency cardiac surgery necessary · elderly · faecal occult blood · haematuria · haemorrhagic retinopathy · low body-weight · major surgery within 3 months (avoid if within 6 weeks) · organ biopsy or lithotripsy within last 2 weeks · puncture of non-compressible vessel within 24 hours · risk of bleeding (within 3 months) · severe heart failure · severe trauma within 3 months (avoid if within 6 weeks) · traumatic or protracted cardiopulmonary resuscitation within last 2 weeks · uncontrolled severe hypertension · vasculitis

● INTERACTIONS → Appendix 1: tirofiban

● SIDE-EFFECTS
▸ **Common or very common** Ecchymosis · fever · haemorrhage · headache · nausea · thrombocytopenia
▸ **Frequency not known** Intracranial haemorrhage

- **PREGNANCY** Manufacturer advises use only if potential benefit outweighs risk—no information available.
- **BREAST FEEDING** Manufacturer advises avoid—no information available.
- **HEPATIC IMPAIRMENT** Caution in mild to moderate liver disease. Avoid in severe liver disease—increased risk of bleeding.
- **RENAL IMPAIRMENT** Increased risk of bleeding.
  Dose adjustments Use half normal dose if eGFR less than 30 mL/minute/1.73 m².
  Monitoring Monitor carefully if eGFR less than 60 mL/minute/1.73 m².
- **MONITORING REQUIREMENTS** Monitor platelet count, haemoglobin and haematocrit before treatment, 2–6 hours after start of treatment and then at least once daily.
- **DIRECTIONS FOR ADMINISTRATION** For *intravenous infusion* (*Aggrastat*®), give continuously in Glucose 5% or Sodium chloride 0.9%. Withdraw 50 mL infusion fluid from 250 mL bag and replace with 50 mL tirofiban concentrate (250 micrograms/mL) to give a final concentration of 50 micrograms/mL.

- **MEDICINAL FORMS**
  There can be variation in the licensing of different medicines containing the same drug.
  Solution for infusion
  ELECTROLYTES: May contain Sodium
  ▸ Aggrastat (Correvio GmbH)
    Tirofiban 250 microgram per 1 ml Aggrastat 12.5mg/50ml concentrate for solution for infusion vials | 1 vial [PoM] 🛇 (Hospital only)
  Infusion
  ELECTROLYTES: May contain Sodium
  ▸ Tirofiban (Non-proprietary)
    Tirofiban 50 microgram per 1 ml Tirofiban 12.5mg/250ml infusion bags | 1 bag [PoM] £159.00–£160.72 (Hospital only)
  ▸ Aggrastat (Correvio GmbH)
    Tirofiban 50 microgram per 1 ml Aggrastat 12.5mg/250ml infusion bags | 1 bag [PoM] 🛇 (Hospital only)

PIPERAZINE DERIVATIVES

Ranolazine

- **INDICATIONS AND DOSE**
  As adjunctive therapy in the treatment of stable angina in patients inadequately controlled or intolerant of first-line antianginal therapies
  ▸ BY MOUTH
  ▸ Adult: Initially 375 mg twice daily for 2–4 weeks, then increased to 500 mg twice daily, then adjusted according to response to 750 mg twice daily; reduced if not tolerated to 375–500 mg twice daily

- **CAUTIONS** Body-weight less than 60 kg · elderly · moderate to severe congestive heart failure · QT interval prolongation
- **INTERACTIONS** → Appendix 1: ranolazine
- **SIDE-EFFECTS**
  ▸ **Common or very common** Asthenia · constipation · headache · vomiting
  ▸ **Uncommon** Anxiety · appetite decreased · confusion · cough · dehydration · dizziness postural · drowsiness · dry mouth · gastrointestinal discomfort · gastrointestinal disorders · haemorrhage · hallucination · hearing impairment · hot flush · hypotension · insomnia · joint swelling · muscle cramps · muscle weakness · pain in extremity · peripheral oedema · QT interval prolongation · sensation abnormal · skin reactions · syncope · tremor · urinary disorders · urine discolouration · vertigo · vision disorders · weight decreased

- ▸ **Rare or very rare** Acute kidney injury · altered smell sensation · angioedema · consciousness impaired · coordination abnormal · erectile dysfunction · gait abnormal · hyponatraemia · memory loss · oral hypoaesthesia · pancreatitis · peripheral coldness
- **PREGNANCY** Manufacturer advises avoid unless essential—no information available.
- **BREAST FEEDING** Manufacturer advises avoid—no information available.
- **HEPATIC IMPAIRMENT** Use with caution in mild impairment; avoid in moderate and severe impairment.
- **RENAL IMPAIRMENT** Use with caution if eGFR 30–80 mL/minute/1.73 m²; avoid if eGFR less than 30 mL/minute/1.73 m².
- **PATIENT AND CARER ADVICE** Patient alert card to be provided.
- **NATIONAL FUNDING/ACCESS DECISIONS**
  Scottish Medicines Consortium (SMC) Decisions
  The *Scottish Medicines Consortium* has advised (October 2012) that ranolazine (*Ranexa*®) is **not** recommended for use within NHS Scotland.

- **MEDICINAL FORMS**
  There can be variation in the licensing of different medicines containing the same drug.
  Modified-release tablet
  CAUTIONARY AND ADVISORY LABELS 25
  ▸ Ranexa (A. Menarini Farmaceutica Internazionale SRL)
    Ranolazine 375 mg Ranexa 375mg modified-release tablets | 60 tablet [PoM] £48.98 DT = £48.98
    Ranolazine 500 mg Ranexa 500mg modified-release tablets | 60 tablet [PoM] £48.98 DT = £48.98
    Ranolazine 750 mg Ranexa 750mg modified-release tablets | 60 tablet [PoM] £48.98 DT = £48.98

SELECTIVE SINUS NODE I$_F$ INHIBITORS

Ivabradine   10-May-2018

- **INDICATIONS AND DOSE**
  Treatment of angina in patients in normal sinus rhythm
  ▸ BY MOUTH
  ▸ Adult 18–74 years: Initially 2.5–5 mg twice daily for 3–4 weeks, then increased if necessary up to 7.5 mg twice daily, dose to be increased gradually; reduced if not tolerated to 2.5–5 mg twice daily, heart rate at rest should not be allowed to fall below 50 beats per minute, discontinue treatment if no improvement in symptoms within 3 months
  ▸ Adult 75 years and over: Initially 2.5 mg twice daily for 3–4 weeks, then increased if necessary up to 7.5 mg twice daily, dose to be increased gradually; reduced if not tolerated to 2.5–5 mg twice daily, heart rate at rest should not be allowed to fall below 50 beats per minute, discontinue treatment if no improvement in symptoms within 3 months
  Mild to severe chronic heart failure
  ▸ BY MOUTH
  ▸ Adult 18–74 years: Initially 5 mg twice daily for 2 weeks, then increased if necessary to 7.5 mg twice daily; reduced if not tolerated to 2.5–5 mg twice daily, heart rate at rest should not be allowed to fall below 50 beats per minute
  ▸ Adult 75 years and over: Initially 2.5 mg twice daily for 2 weeks, then increased if necessary up to 7.5 mg twice daily, dose to be increased gradually; reduced if not tolerated to 2.5–5 mg twice daily, heart rate at rest should not be allowed to fall below 50 beats per minute

DOSE ADJUSTMENTS DUE TO INTERACTIONS
▶ Manufacturer advises reduce initial dose to 2.5 mg twice daily with concurrent use of moderate CYP3A4 inhibitors (except diltiazem, erythromycin and verapamil where concurrent use is contra-indicated).

● CONTRA-INDICATIONS Acute myocardial infarction · cardiogenic shock · congenital QT syndrome · do not initiate for angina if heart rate below 70 beats per minute · do not initiate for chronic heart failure if heart rate below 75 beats per minute · immediately after cerebrovascular accident · patients dependent on pacemaker · second- and third-degree heart block · severe hypotension · sick-sinus syndrome · sino-atrial block · unstable angina · unstable or acute heart failure

● CAUTIONS Atrial fibrillation or other arrhythmias (treatment ineffective) · elderly · in angina, consider stopping if there is no or limited symptom improvement after 3 months · intraventricular conduction defects · mild to moderate hypotension (avoid if severe) · retinitis pigmentosa

● INTERACTIONS → Appendix 1: ivabradine

● SIDE-EFFECTS
▶ **Common or very common** Arrhythmias · atrioventricular block · dizziness · headache · hypertension · vision disorders
▶ **Uncommon** Abdominal pain · angioedema · constipation · diarrhoea · eosinophilia · hyperuricaemia · hypotension · muscle cramps · nausea · QT interval prolongation · skin reactions · syncope · vertigo

● PREGNANCY Manufacturer advises avoid— *toxicity* in animal studies.

● BREAST FEEDING Present in milk in *animal* studies— manufacturer advises avoid.

● HEPATIC IMPAIRMENT Manufacturer advises caution in moderate impairment. Avoid in severe impairment.

● RENAL IMPAIRMENT Manufacturer advises use with caution if eGFR less than 15 mL/minute/1.73 m^2—no information available.

● MONITORING REQUIREMENTS
▶ Monitor regularly for atrial fibrillation (consider benefits and risks of continued treatment if atrial fibrillation occurs).
▶ Monitor for bradycardia, especially after any dose increase, and discontinue if resting heart rate persistently below 50 beats per minute or continued symptoms of bradycardia despite dose reduction.

● NATIONAL FUNDING/ACCESS DECISIONS

NICE decisions
▶ **Ivabradine for the treatment of chronic heart failure (November 2012) NICE TA267**
Ivabradine, in combination with standard therapy including a beta-blocker (unless contra-indicated or not tolerated), an ACE inhibitor, and an aldosterone antagonist, is an option for treating mild to severe stable chronic heart failure in patients who:
● have a left ventricular ejection fraction of ≤ 35%, *and*
● are in sinus rhythm with a heart rate of ≥75 beats per minute

Ivabradine should be initiated only by a heart failure specialist after 4 weeks of stable optimal standard therapy; monitoring and dose titration should be carried out by a heart failure specialist, or a GP with special interest in heart failure, or by a heart failure specialist nurse.
www.nice.org.uk/TA267

Scottish Medicines Consortium (SMC) Decisions
The *Scottish Medicines Consortium* has advised (September 2012) that ivabradine (*Procoralan*®) is accepted for restricted use within NHS Scotland in accordance with its licensed indication for heart failure only if resting heart rate remains ≥75 beats per minute despite optimal standard therapy.

● MEDICINAL FORMS
There can be variation in the licensing of different medicines containing the same drug.

Tablet
▶ Ivabradine (non-proprietary) ▼
　Ivabradine (as Ivabradine hydrochloride) 2.5 mg Ivabradine 2.5mg tablets | 56 tablet [PoM] £40.17
　Ivabradine (as Ivabradine hydrochloride) 5 mg Ivabradine 5mg tablets | 56 tablet [PoM] £8.99–£40.17 DT = £40.17
　Ivabradine (as Ivabradine hydrochloride) 7.5 mg Ivabradine 7.5mg tablets | 56 tablet [PoM] £8.99–£40.17 DT = £40.17
▶ Procoralan (Servier Laboratories Ltd) ▼
　Ivabradine (as Ivabradine hydrochloride) 5 mg Procoralan 5mg tablets | 56 tablet [PoM] £40.17 DT = £40.17
　Ivabradine (as Ivabradine hydrochloride) 7.5 mg Procoralan 7.5mg tablets | 56 tablet [PoM] £40.17 DT = £40.17

VASODILATORS > POTASSIUM-CHANNEL OPENERS

Nicorandil
　　　　　　　　　　　　　　　　　　　　　　　24-Feb-2016

● INDICATIONS AND DOSE
Prophylaxis and treatment of stable angina (second-line)
▶ BY MOUTH
▶ Adult: Initially 5–10 mg twice daily, then increased if tolerated to 40 mg twice daily; usual dose 10–20 mg twice daily, use lower initial dose regimen if patient susceptible to headache

● CONTRA-INDICATIONS Acute pulmonary oedema · cardiogenic shock · hypovolaemia · left ventricular failure with low filling pressures · severe hypotension

● CAUTIONS Acute myocardial infarction with acute left ventricular failure and low filling pressures · diverticular disease (risk of fistula formation or bowel perforation) · G6PD deficiency · heart failure (class III–IV) · hyperkalaemia · low systolic blood pressure

● INTERACTIONS → Appendix 1: nicorandil

● SIDE-EFFECTS
▶ **Common or very common** Asthenia · dizziness · haemorrhage · headache (more common on initiation, usually transitory) · nausea · vasodilation · vomiting
▶ **Rare or very rare** Abdominal pain · angioedema · conjunctivitis · eye disorders · gastrointestinal disorders · genital ulceration · hepatic disorders · hyperkalaemia · mucosal ulceration · myalgia · oral disorders · skin reactions
▶ **Frequency not known** Diplopia

SIDE-EFFECTS, FURTHER INFORMATION Nicorandil can cause serious skin, mucosal, and eye ulceration; including gastrointestinal ulcers, which may progress to perforation, haemorrhage, fistula or abscess. Stop treatment if ulceration occurs and consider an alternative.

● PREGNANCY Manufacturer advises use only if potential benefit outweighs risk—no information available.

● BREAST FEEDING No information available—manufacturer advises avoid.

● PATIENT AND CARER ADVICE
Driving and skilled tasks Patients should be warned not to drive or operate machinery until it is established that their performance is unimpaired.

2

Cardiovascular system

● MEDICINAL FORMS
There can be variation in the licensing of different medicines containing the same drug.

Tablet

▸ Nicorandil (Non-proprietary)

Nicorandil 10 mg Nicorandil 10mg tablets | 60 tablet PoM £7.71 DT = £1.60

Nicorandil 20 mg Nicorandil 20mg tablets | 60 tablet PoM £14.64 DT = £3.88

▸ Ikorel (Zentiva)

Nicorandil 10 mg Ikorel 10mg tablets | 60 tablet PoM £7.71 DT = £1.60

Nicorandil 20 mg Ikorel 20mg tablets | 60 tablet PoM £14.64 DT = £3.88

7.1 Acute coronary syndromes

Acute coronary syndromes

Overview

Acute coronary syndromes encompass a spectrum of conditions which include unstable angina, and myocardial infarction with or without ST-segment elevation. Patients with different acute coronary syndromes may present similarly; definitive diagnosis is made on the basis of clinical presentation, ECG changes, and measurement of biochemical cardiac markers.

Unstable angina and non-ST-segment elevation myocardial infarction (NSTEMI)

These are related acute coronary syndromes that fall between the classifications of stable angina and ST-segment elevation myocardial infarction (STEMI). They usually occur as a result of atheromatous plaque rupture, and are often characterised by stable angina that suddenly worsens, recurring or prolonged angina at rest, or new onset of severe angina. Patients with unstable angina have no evidence of myocardial necrosis, whereas in NSTEMI, myocardial necrosis (less significant than with STEMI) will be evident. There is a risk of progression to STEMI or sudden death, particularly in patients who experience pain at rest.

Management of unstable angina and non-ST-segment elevation myocardial infarction (NSTEMI)

These conditions are managed similarly; the aims of management are to provide supportive care and pain relief during the acute attack and to prevent further cardiac events and death. For advice on the management of patients with acute ST-segment elevation myocardial infarction (STEMI), see below.

Initial management

Oxygen should be administered if there is evidence of hypoxia, pulmonary oedema, or continuing myocardial ischaemia; hyperoxia should be avoided and particular care is required in patients with chronic obstructive airways disease.

Nitrates are used to relieve ischaemic pain. If sublingual glyceryl trinitrate p. 217 is not effective, intravenous or buccal glyceryl trinitrate p. 219 or intravenous isosorbide dinitrate p. 219 is given. If pain continues, diamorphine hydrochloride p. 449 or morphine p. 456 can be given by slow intravenous injection; an antiemetic such as metoclopramide hydrochloride p. 426 should also be given.

Aspirin p. 121 (chewed or dispersed in water) is given for its antiplatelet effect. If aspirin is given before arrival at hospital, a note saying that it has been given should be sent with the patient. Clopidogrel p. 122 should also be given. Prasugrel p. 213 is an alternative to clopidogrel in certain patients undergoing percutaneous coronary intervention (see NICE guidance). Ticagrelor p. 214 is also an alternative to clopidogrel (see NICE guidance). Patients should also

receive either heparin (unfractionated) p. 132, a **low molecular weight heparin**, or fondaparinux sodium p. 126.

Patients without contra-indications should receive **beta-blockers** which should be continued indefinitely. In patients without left ventricular dysfunction and in whom beta-blockers are inappropriate, diltiazem hydrochloride p. 157 or verapamil hydrochloride p. 163 can be given.

The glycoprotein IIb/IIIa inhibitors eptifibatide p. 209 (in combination with heparin (unfractionated) and aspirin) and tirofiban p. 209 (in combination with heparin (unfractionated), aspirin, and clopidogrel) can be used for unstable angina or for NSTEMI in patients at a high risk of either myocardial infarction or death.

In intermediate- and high-risk patients, abciximab p. 208 or eptifibatide (in combination with heparin (unfractionated) and aspirin), or tirofiban (in combination with heparin (unfractionated), aspirin, and clopidogrel) can also be used in patients undergoing percutaneous coronary intervention, to reduce the immediate risk of vascular occlusion. In intermediate- and high-risk patients in whom early intervention is planned, bivalirudin p. 134 can be considered as an alternative to the combination of a glyocprotein IIb/IIIa inhibitor plus a heparin.

Revascularisation procedures are often appropriate for patients with unstable angina or NSTEMI; see Antiplatelet drugs p. 120 for the use of antiplatelet drugs in patients undergoing coronary stenting.

Long-term management

The need for long-term angina treatment or for coronary angiography should be assessed. Most patients will require standard angina treatment to prevent recurrence of symptoms.

ST-segment elevation myocardial infarction (STEMI)

This is an acute coronary syndrome where atheromatous plaque rupture leads to thrombosis and myocardial ischaemia, with irreversible necrosis of the heart muscle, often leading to long-term complications. STEMI can also occasionally occur as a result of coronary spasm or embolism, arteritis, spontaneous thrombosis, or sudden severe elevation in blood pressure.

Management of ST-segment elevation myocardial infarction (STEMI)

These notes give an overview of the initial and long-term management of myocardial infarction with ST segment elevation (STEMI). For advice on the management of non-ST-segment elevation myocardial infarction (NSTEMI) and unstable angina, see above. The aims of management of STEMI are to provide supportive care and pain relief, to promote reperfusion and to reduce mortality. Oxygen, nitrates, and diamorphine hydrochloride or morphine can provide initial support and pain relief; aspirin and percutaneous coronary intervention or thrombolytics promote reperfusion; anticoagulants help to reduce re-occlusion and systemic embolisation; long-term use of aspirin, beta-blockers, ACE inhibitors, and statins help to reduce mortality further.

Local guidelines for the management of myocardial infarction should be followed where they exist.

Initial management

Oxygen should be administered if there is evidence of hypoxia, pulmonary oedema, or continuing myocardial ischaemia; hyperoxia should be avoided and particular care is required in patients with chronic obstructive airways disease.

The pain (and anxiety) of myocardial infarction is managed with slow intravenous injection of diamorphine hydrochloride or morphine; an antiemetic such as metoclopramide hydrochloride (or, if left ventricular function is not compromised, cyclizine p. 424) by intravenous injection should also be given.

Aspirin (chewed or dispersed in water) is given for its antiplatelet effect. If aspirin is given before arrival at hospital, a note saying that it has been given should be sent with the patient. Clopidogrel, should also be given. Prasugrel, is an alternative to clopidogrel in certain patients undergoing percutaneous coronary intervention (see NICE guidance). Ticagrelor, is also an alternative to clopidogrel (see NICE guidance).

Patency of the occluded artery can be restored by percutaneous coronary intervention or by giving a **thrombolytic drug**, unless contra-indicated. Percutaneous coronary intervention is the preferred method; a **glycoprotein IIb/IIIa inhibitor** can be used to reduce the risk of immediate vascular occlusion in intermediate- and high-risk patients. Patients undergoing percutaneous coronary intervention should also receive either heparin (unfractionated) or a low molecular weight heparin (e.g. enoxaparin sodium p. 131); bivalirudin is an alternative to the combination of a glycoprotein IIb/IIIa inhibitor plus a heparin (see also NICE guidance). In patients who cannot be offered percutaneous coronary intervention within 90 minutes of diagnosis, a thrombolytic drug should be administered along with either heparin (unfractionated) (for maximum 2 days), a low molecular weight heparin (e.g. enoxaparin sodium), or fondaparinux sodium. See use of antiplatelet drugs in patients undergoing coronary stenting in Antiplatelet drugs p. 120.

Patients who do not receive reperfusion therapy (with percutaneous coronary intervention or a thrombolytic) should be treated with either fondaparinux sodium, enoxaparin sodium, or heparin (unfractionated). Prescribers should consult product literature and local protocols (where they exist) for details of anticoagulant dose and duration.

Nitrates are used to relieve ischaemic pain. If sublingual glyceryl trinitrate p. 217 is not effective, intravenous glyceryl trinitrate or isosorbide dinitrate p. 219 is given.

Early administration of some **beta-blockers** has been shown to be of benefit and should be given to patients without contra-indications.

ACE inhibitors, and angiotensin-II receptor antagonists if an ACE inhibitor cannot be used, are also of benefit to patients who have no contra-indications; in hypertensive and normotensive patients treatment with an ACE inhibitor, or an angiotensin-II receptor antagonist, can be started within 24 hours of the myocardial infarction and continued for at least 5–6 weeks (see below for long-term treatment).

All patients should be closely monitored for hyperglycaemia; those with diabetes or raised blood-glucose concentration should receive insulin p. 696.

Long-term management

Long-term management following STEMI involves the use of several drugs which should ideally be started before the patient is discharged from hospital.

Aspirin p. 121 should be given to all patients, unless contra-indicated. The addition of clopidogrel p. 122 has been shown to reduce morbidity and mortality. Prasugrel below or ticagrelor p. 214 are alternatives to clopidogrel in certain patients. For those intolerant of clopidogrel, and who are at low risk of bleeding, the combination of warfarin sodium p. 139 and aspirin should be considered. In those intolerant of both aspirin and clopidogrel, warfarin sodium alone can be used. Warfarin sodium should be continued for those who are already being treated for another indication, such as atrial fibrillation, with the addition of aspirin if there is a low risk of bleeding. The combination of aspirin with clopidogrel or warfarin sodium increases the risk of bleeding. Low-dose rivaroxaban p. 127, in combination with aspirin alone *or* aspirin and clopidogrel, is licensed for the prevention of atherothrombotic events following STEMI—see Prevention of cardiovascular events. For details of antiplatelet drug duration following coronary stenting—see also Antiplatelet drugs and coronary stents in Antiplatelet drugs p. 120.

Beta-blockers should be given to all patients in whom they are not contra-indicated. Acebutolol p. 151, metoprolol tartrate p. 154, propranolol hydrochloride p. 149 and timolol maleate p. 150 are suitable; for patients with left ventricular dysfunction, carvedilol p. 147, bisoprolol fumarate p. 152, or long-acting metoprolol tartrate may be appropriate

Diltiazem hydrochloride p. 157 [unlicensed] or verapamil hydrochloride p. 163 can be considered if a beta-blocker cannot be used; however, they are contra-indicated in those with left ventricular dysfunction. Other calcium-channel blockers have no place in routine long-term management after a myocardial infarction.

An **ACE inhibitor** should be considered for all patients, especially those with evidence of left ventricular dysfunction. If an ACE inhibitor cannot be used, an angiotensin-II receptor antagonist may be used for patients with heart failure. A relatively high dose of either the ACE inhibitor or angiotensin-II receptor antagonist may be required to produce benefit.

Nitrates are used for patients with angina.

Eplerenone p. 190 is licensed for use following a myocardial infarction in those with left ventricular dysfunction and evidence of heart failure.

See also the role of **statins** in preventing recurrent cardiovascular events in Lipid-regulating drugs p. 193.

Prevention of cardiovascular events

Patients with stable angina, unstable angina, or NSTEMI should be given advice and treatments to reduce their cardiovascular risk. The importance of life-style changes, especially stopping smoking, should be emphasised. Aspirin should be given indefinitely. Antihypertensive treatment should be initiated if appropriate, and a **statin** should also be given.

In patients with stable angina, addition of an **ACE inhibitor** should be considered for patients with diabetes (and should be continued if indicated for a co-morbidity).

In patients with unstable angina or NSTEMI, clopidogrel is given, in combination with aspirin, for up to 12 months—most benefit occurs during the first 3 months. Prasugrel or ticagrelor are alternatives to clopidogrel in certain patients. An ACE inhibitor should also be given.

Low-dose rivaroxaban, in combination with aspirin alone *or* aspirin and clopidogrel, is licensed for the prevention of atherothrombotic events following an acute coronary syndrome with elevated cardiac biomarkers.

> **Other drugs used for Acute coronary syndromes**
> Captopril, p. 167 · Dalteparin sodium, p. 130 · Lisinopril,
> p. 170 · Perindopril arginine, p. 170 · Perindopril erbumine,
> p. 171 · Ramipril, p. 172 · Trandolapril, p. 173 · Valsartan,
> p. 178

ANTITHROMBOTIC DRUGS › ANTIPLATELET DRUGS

Prasugrel

● **INDICATIONS AND DOSE**

In combination with aspirin for the prevention of atherothrombotic events in patients with acute coronary syndrome undergoing percutaneous coronary intervention

▸ BY MOUTH

▸ Adult 18–74 years (body-weight up to 60 kg): Initially 60 mg for 1 dose, then 5 mg once daily usually for up to 12 months

▸ Adult 18–74 years (body-weight 60 kg and above): Initially 60 mg for 1 dose, then 10 mg once daily usually for up to 12 months

▸ Adult 75 years and over: Initially 60 mg for 1 dose, then 5 mg once daily usually for up to 12 months   continued →

Patients undergoing coronary angiography within 48 hours of admission for unstable angina or NSTEMI
▸ BY MOUTH
▸ Adult: Loading dose 60 mg, not to be administered until the time of percutaneous coronary intervention in order to minimise the risk of bleeding, maintenance dose of 10 mg or 5 mg daily should then be selected as appropriate based on age and weight

Alternative to clopidogrel in certain patients undergoing percutaneous coronary intervention
▸ BY MOUTH
▸ Adult: 60 mg, as a single dose

● CONTRA-INDICATIONS Active bleeding · history of stroke or transient ischaemic attack
● CAUTIONS Body-weight less than 60 kg · discontinue at least 7 days before elective surgery if antiplatelet effect not desirable · elderly · patients at increased risk of bleeding (e.g. from recent trauma, surgery, gastro-intestinal bleeding, or active peptic ulcer disease)
● INTERACTIONS → Appendix 1: prasugrel
● SIDE-EFFECTS
▸ **Common or very common** Anaemia · haemorrhage · skin reactions
▸ **Uncommon** Angioedema
▸ **Rare or very rare** Thrombocytopenia
● ALLERGY AND CROSS-SENSITIVITY Caution in patients with history of hypersensitivity reactions to thienopyridines (e.g. clopidogrel).
● PREGNANCY Manufacturer advises use only if potential benefit outweighs risk.
● BREAST FEEDING Manufacturer advises avoid—no information available.
● HEPATIC IMPAIRMENT Use with caution in moderate impairment—increased risk of bleeding. Avoid in severe impairment.
● RENAL IMPAIRMENT Use with caution—increased risk of bleeding.
● NATIONAL FUNDING/ACCESS DECISIONS
NICE decisions
▸ **Prasugrel with percutaneous coronary intervention for treating acute coronary syndromes (July 2014)** NICE TA317
Prasugrel 10 mg in combination with aspirin is recommended as an option, within its marketing authorisation, for preventing atherothrombotic events in adults with acute coronary syndrome (unstable angina (UA), non-ST segment elevation myocardial infarction (NSTEMI) or ST segment elevation myocardial infarction (STEMI)) having primary or delayed percutaneous coronary intervention.
www.nice.org.uk/TA317

Scottish Medicines Consortium (SMC) Decisions
The *Scottish Medicines Consortium* has advised (August 2009) that prasugrel (*Efient*®), in combination with aspirin, be accepted for restricted use within NHS Scotland for the prevention of atherothrombotic events in patients with acute coronary syndrome undergoing percutaneous coronary intervention who are eligible to receive the 10 mg dose of prasugrel.

● MEDICINAL FORMS
There can be variation in the licensing of different medicines containing the same drug.
Tablet
▸ Efient (Eli Lilly and Company Ltd)
Prasugrel (as Prasugrel hydrochloride) 5 mg Efient 5mg tablets | 28 tablet [PoM] £47.56 DT = £47.56
Prasugrel (as Prasugrel hydrochloride) 10 mg Efient 10mg tablets | 28 tablet [PoM] £47.56 DT = £47.56

Ticagrelor

● INDICATIONS AND DOSE
In combination with aspirin for the prevention of atherothrombotic events in patients with acute coronary syndrome
▸ BY MOUTH
▸ Adult: Initially 180 mg for 1 dose, then 90 mg twice daily usually for up to 12 months

Alternative to clopidogrel in patients undergoing percutaneous coronary intervention
▸ BY MOUTH
▸ Adult: 180 mg, as a single dose

● CONTRA-INDICATIONS Active bleeding · history of intracranial haemorrhage
● CAUTIONS Asthma · bradycardia (unless pacemaker fitted) · chronic obstructive pulmonary disease · discontinue 7 days before elective surgery if antiplatelet effect not desirable · history of hyperuricaemia · patients at increased risk of bleeding (e.g. from recent trauma, surgery, gastro-intestinal bleeding, or coagulation disorders) · second- or third-degree AV block (unless pacemaker fitted) · sick sinus syndrome (unless pacemaker fitted)
● INTERACTIONS → Appendix 1: ticagrelor
● SIDE-EFFECTS
▸ **Common or very common** Constipation · diarrhoea · dizziness · dyspepsia · dyspnoea · gout · gouty arthritis · haemorrhage · headache · hyperuricaemia · hypotension · nausea · skin reactions · syncope · vertigo
▸ **Uncommon** Angioedema · confusion · intracranial haemorrhage
● PREGNANCY Manufacturer advises avoid—toxicity in *animal* studies.
● BREAST FEEDING Manufacturer advises avoid—present in milk in *animal* studies.
● HEPATIC IMPAIRMENT Avoid in moderate or severe impairment—no information available.
● MONITORING REQUIREMENTS Monitor renal function 1 month after initiation.
● NATIONAL FUNDING/ACCESS DECISIONS
NICE decisions
▸ **Ticagrelor for the treatment of acute coronary syndromes (October 2011)** NICE TA236
Ticagrelor, in combination with low-dose aspirin, is recommended for up to 12 months as a treatment option in adults with acute coronary syndromes, that is, people:
● with ST-segment elevation myocardial infarction— defined as ST elevation or new left bundle branch block on electrocardiogram—that cardiologists intend to treat with primary percutaneous coronary intervention, **or**
● with non-ST-segment elevation myocardial infarction (NSTEMI), **or**
● admitted to hospital with unstable angina—defined as ST or T wave changes on electrocardiogram suggestive of ischaemia plus one of the characteristics defined below. Before ticagrelor is continued beyond the initial treatment, the diagnosis of unstable angina should first be confirmed, ideally by a cardiologist. Characteristics to be used in defining treatment with ticagrelor for unstable angina are:
● age 60 years or older;
● previous myocardial infarction or previous coronary artery bypass grafting;
● coronary artery disease with stenosis of 50% or more in at least two vessels;
● previous ischaemic stroke;
● previous transient ischaemic attack, carotid stenosis of at least 50%, or cerebral revascularisation;
● diabetes mellitus;

- peripheral arterial disease, **or**
- chronic renal dysfunction (creatinine clearance less than 60 mL/minute/1.73 m^2).
www.nice.org.uk/TA236

▸ **Ticagrelor for preventing atherothrombotic events after myocardial infarction (December 2016)** NICE TA420
Ticagrelor, in combination with aspirin, is recommended within its marketing authorisation as an option for preventing atherothrombotic events in adults who had a myocardial infarction and who are at high risk of a further event. Treatment should be stopped when clinically indicated or at a maximum of 3 years.
www.nice.org.uk/TA420

● MEDICINAL FORMS
There can be variation in the licensing of different medicines containing the same drug.

Tablet

▸ Brilique (AstraZeneca UK Ltd)
Ticagrelor 60 mg Brilique 60mg tablets | 56 tablet [PoM] £54.60 DT = £54.60
Ticagrelor 90 mg Brilique 90mg tablets | 56 tablet [PoM] £54.60 DT = £54.60

ANTITHROMBOTIC DRUGS ＞TISSUE PLASMINOGEN ACTIVATORS

Fibrinolytic drugs

Overview

The value of thrombolytic drugs for the treatment of *myocardial infarction* has been established. Streptokinase p. 216 and alteplase below have been shown to reduce mortality. Reteplase and tenecteplase p. 216 are also licensed for acute myocardial infarction. Thrombolytic drugs are indicated for any patient with acute myocardial infarction for whom the benefit is likely to outweigh the risk of treatment. Trials have shown that the benefit is greatest in those with ECG changes that include ST segment elevation (especially in those with anterior infarction) and in patients with bundle branch block. Patients should not be denied thrombolytic treatment on account of age alone because mortality in the elderly is high and the reduction in mortality is the same as in younger patients. Alteplase should be given within 6–12 hours of symptom onset, reteplase and streptokinase within 12 hours of symptom onset, but ideally all should be given within 1 hour; use after 12 hours requires specialist advice. Tenecteplase should be given as early as possible and usually within 6 hours of symptom onset.

Alteplase, streptokinase and urokinase p. 137 can be used for other thromboembolic disorders such as deep-vein thrombosis and pulmonary embolism. Alteplase is also used for acute ischaemic stroke.

Urokinase is also licensed to restore the patency of occluded intravenous catheters and cannulas blocked with fibrin clots.

Fibrinolytics

- DRUG ACTION Fibrinolytic drugs act as thrombolytics by activating plasminogen to form plasmin, which degrades fibrin and so breaks up thrombi.
- CONTRA-INDICATIONS Active pulmonary disease with cavitation · acute pancreatitis · aneurysm · aortic dissection · bacterial endocarditis · bleeding diatheses · coagulation defects · coma · heavy vaginal bleeding · history of cerebrovascular disease (especially recent events or with any residual disability) · oesophageal varices · pericarditis · recent haemorrhage · recent surgery (including dental extraction) · recent symptoms of possible peptic ulceration · recent trauma · severe hypertension

- CAUTIONS Conditions in which thrombolysis might give rise to embolic complications such as enlarged left atrium with atrial fibrillation (risk of dissolution of clot and subsequent embolisation) · elderly · external chest compression · hypertension · risk of bleeding (including that from venepuncture or invasive procedures)
- SIDE-EFFECTS
▸ **Common or very common** Anaphylactic reaction · angina pectoris · cardiac arrest · cardiogenic shock · chills · CNS haemorrhage · ecchymosis · fever · haemorrhage · haemorrhagic stroke · heart failure · hypotension · ischaemia recurrent (when used in myocardial infarction) · nausea · pericarditis · pulmonary oedema · vomiting
▸ **Uncommon** Aphasia · mitral valve incompetence · myocardial rupture · pericardial disorders · reperfusion arrhythmia (when used in myocardial infarction) · seizure
SIDE-EFFECTS, FURTHER INFORMATION Serious bleeding calls for discontinuation of the thrombolytic and may require administration of coagulation factors and antifibrinolytic drugs.
- PREGNANCY Thrombolytic drugs can possibly lead to premature separation of the placenta in the first 18 weeks of pregnancy. There is also a risk of maternal haemorrhage throughout pregnancy and post-partum, and also a theoretical risk of fetal haemorrhage throughout pregnancy.
- HEPATIC IMPAIRMENT Avoid in severe hepatic impairment as there is an increased risk of bleeding.

☞ above

Alteplase

(rt-PA; Tissue-type plasminogen activator)

● INDICATIONS AND DOSE
Acute myocardial infarction, accelerated regimen
▸ INITIALLY BY INTRAVENOUS INJECTION
▸ Adult (body-weight up to 65 kg): Initially 15 mg, to be initiated within 6 hours of symptom onset, followed by (by intravenous infusion) 0.75 mg/kg, to be given over 30 minutes, then (by intravenous infusion) 0.5 mg/kg, to be given over 60 minutes, maximum total dose of 100 mg administered over 90 minutes
▸ Adult (body-weight 65 kg and above): Initially 15 mg, to be initiated within 6 hours of symptom onset, followed by (by intravenous infusion) 50 mg, to be given over 30 minutes, then (by intravenous infusion) 35 mg, to be given over 60 minutes, maximum total dose of 100 mg administered over 90 minutes

Acute myocardial infarction
▸ INITIALLY BY INTRAVENOUS INJECTION
▸ Adult: Initially 10 mg, to be initiated within 6–12 hours of symptom onset, followed by (by intravenous infusion) 50 mg, to be given over 60 minutes, then (by intravenous infusion) 10 mg for 4 infusions, each 10 mg infusion dose to be given over 30 minutes, total dose of 100 mg over 3 hours; maximum 1.5 mg/kg in patients less than 65 kg

Pulmonary embolism
▸ INITIALLY BY INTRAVENOUS INJECTION
▸ Adult: Initially 10 mg, to be given over 1–2 minutes, followed by (by intravenous infusion) 90 mg, to be given over 2 hours, maximum 1.5 mg/kg in patients less than 65 kg

Acute ischaemic stroke (under specialist neurology physician only)
▸ BY INTRAVENOUS INFUSION
▸ Adult 18-79 years: Initially 900 micrograms/kg (max. per dose 90 mg), treatment **must** begin within 4.5 hours of symptom onset, to be given over 60 minutes, the initial 10% of dose is to be   continued →

administered by intravenous injection and the remainder by intravenous infusion

ACTILYSE CATHFLO ®

Thrombolytic treatment of occluded central venous access devices (including those used for haemodialysis)
▸ BY INTRAVENOUS INJECTION
▸ Adult: (consult product literature)

● CONTRA-INDICATIONS
▸ When used for acute ischaemic stroke Convulsion accompanying stroke · history of stroke in patients with diabetes · hyperglycaemia · hypoglycaemia · severe stroke · stroke in last 3 months
● INTERACTIONS → Appendix 1: alteplase
● SIDE-EFFECTS
▸ Uncommon Cerebral embolism · haemothorax
▸ Rare or very rare Agitation · confusion · delirium · depression · epilepsy · psychosis · speech disorder
▸ Frequency not known Brain oedema (caused by reperfusion)
● ALLERGY AND CROSS-SENSITIVITY Contra-indicated if history of hypersensitivity to gentamicin (residue from manufacturing process).
● MONITORING REQUIREMENTS
▸ When used for acute ischaemic stroke Monitor for intracranial haemorrhage, and monitor blood pressure (antihypertensive recommended if systolic above 180 mmHg or diastolic above 105 mmHg).
● DIRECTIONS FOR ADMINISTRATION For *intravenous infusion* (*Actilyse* ®), give intermittently or continuously in Sodium chloride 0.9%; dissolve in water for injections to a concentration of 1 mg/mL or 2 mg/mL and infuse intravenously; alternatively dilute the solution further in the infusion fluid to a concentration of not less than 200 micrograms/mL; not to be infused in glucose solution.
● NATIONAL FUNDING/ACCESS DECISIONS

NICE decisions
▸ Alteplase for the treatment of acute ischaemic stroke (September 2012) NICE TA264
Alteplase is recommended for the treatment of acute ischaemic stroke in adults in accordance with its licensed indication if:
  ● treatment is started as early as possible within 4.5 hours of onset of stroke symptoms, *and*
  ● intracranial haemorrhage has been excluded by appropriate imaging techniques.
www.nice.org.uk/TA264

● MEDICINAL FORMS
There can be variation in the licensing of different medicines containing the same drug. Forms available from special-order manufacturers include: solution for injection
Powder and solvent for solution for injection
▸ Actilyse (Boehringer Ingelheim Ltd)
  Alteplase 10 mg Actilyse 10mg powder and solvent for solution for injection vials | 1 vial PoM £172.80
  Alteplase 20 mg Actilyse 20mg powder and solvent for solution for injection vials | 1 vial PoM £259.20
Powder and solvent for solution for infusion
▸ Actilyse (Boehringer Ingelheim Ltd)
  Alteplase 50 mg Actilyse 50mg powder and solvent for solution for infusion vials | 1 vial PoM £432.00

F 215

Streptokinase

● INDICATIONS AND DOSE

Acute myocardial infarction
▸ BY INTRAVENOUS INFUSION
▸ Adult: 1 500 000 units, to be initiated within 12 hours of symptom onset, dose to be given over 60 minutes

Deep-vein thrombosis | Pulmonary embolism | Acute arterial thromboembolism | Central retinal venous or arterial thrombosis
▸ BY INTRAVENOUS INFUSION
▸ Adult: 250 000 units, dose to be given over 30 minutes, then 100 000 units every 1 hour for up to 12–72 hours, duration is adjusted according to condition with monitoring of clotting parameters (consult product literature)

● INTERACTIONS → Appendix 1: streptokinase
● SIDE-EFFECTS
▸ Common or very common Arrhythmias · asthenia · diarrhoea · epigastric pain · headache · malaise · pain
▸ Uncommon Respiratory arrest · splenic rupture
▸ Rare or very rare Arthritis · eye inflammation · nephritis · nerve disorders · neurological effects · pulmonary oedema non-cardiogenic (caused by reperfusion) · shock · vasculitis
● ALLERGY AND CROSS-SENSITIVITY Contra-indicated if previous allergic reaction to either streptokinase or anistreplase (no longer available). Prolonged persistence of antibodies to streptokinase and anistreplase can reduce the effectiveness of subsequent treatment; therefore, streptokinase should not be used again beyond 4 days of first administration of either streptokinase or anistreplase.
● DIRECTIONS FOR ADMINISTRATION For *intravenous infusion* (*Streptase* ®), give continuously or intermittently; reconstitute with sodium chloride 0.9%, then dilute further with Glucose 5% or Sodium Chloride 0.9% after reconstitution.

● MEDICINAL FORMS
No licensed medicines listed.

F 215

Tenecteplase

● INDICATIONS AND DOSE

Acute myocardial infarction
▸ BY INTRAVENOUS INJECTION
▸ Adult: 30–50 mg (max. per dose 50 mg), dose to be given over 10 seconds and Initiated within 6 hours of symptom onset, dose varies according to body weight—consult product literature

● INTERACTIONS → Appendix 1: tenecteplase
● SIDE-EFFECTS
▸ Uncommon Drowsiness · hemiparesis
● BREAST FEEDING Manufacturer advises avoid breast-feeding for 24 hours after dose (express and discard milk during this time).

● MEDICINAL FORMS
There can be variation in the licensing of different medicines containing the same drug.
Powder and solvent for solution for injection
▸ Metalyse (Boehringer Ingelheim Ltd)
  Tenecteplase 8000 unit Metalyse 8,000unit powder and solvent for solution for injection vials | 1 vial PoM £602.70
  Tenecteplase 10000 unit Metalyse 10,000unit powder and solvent for solution for injection vials | 1 vial PoM £602.70

NITRATES

Nitrates

Overview

Nitrates have a useful role in *angina*. Although they are potent coronary vasodilators, their principal benefit follows from a reduction in venous return which reduces left ventricular work. Unwanted effects such as flushing, headache, and postural hypotension may limit therapy, especially when angina is severe or when patients are unusually sensitive to the effects of nitrates.

Sublingual glyceryl trinitrate below is one of the most effective drugs for providing rapid symptomatic relief of angina, but its effect lasts only for 20 to 30 minutes; the 300-microgram tablet is often appropriate when glyceryl trinitrate is first used. The *aerosol* spray provides an alternative method of rapid relief of symptoms for those who find difficulty in dissolving sublingual preparations. Duration of action may be prolonged by *transdermal* preparations (but tolerance may develop).

Isosorbide dinitrate p. 219 is active *sublingually* and is a more stable preparation for those who only require nitrates infrequently. It is also effective by mouth for prophylaxis; although the effect is slower in onset, it may persist for several hours. Duration of action of up to 12 hours is claimed for *modified-release* preparations. The activity of isosorbide dinitrate may depend on the production of active metabolites, the most important of which is isosorbide mononitrate p. 219. Isosorbide mononitrate itself is also licensed for angina prophylaxis; modified-release formulations (for once daily administration) are available.

Glyceryl trinitrate or isosorbide dinitrate may be tried by *intravenous injection* when the sublingual form is ineffective in patients with chest pain due to myocardial infarction or severe ischaemia. Intravenous injections are also useful in the treatment of congestive heart failure.

Nitrates

- CONTRA-INDICATIONS Aortic stenosis · cardiac tamponade · constrictive pericarditis · hypertrophic cardiomyopathy · hypotensive conditions · hypovolaemia · marked anaemia · mitral stenosis · raised intracranial pressure due to cerebral haemorrhage · raised intracranial pressure due to head trauma · toxic pulmonary oedema
- CAUTIONS Heart failure due to obstruction · hypothermia · hypothyroidism · hypoxaemia · malnutrition · metal-containing transdermal systems should be removed before magnetic resonance imaging procedures, cardioversion, or diathermy · recent history of myocardial infarction · susceptibility to angle-closure glaucoma · tolerance · ventilation and perfusion abnormalities

CAUTIONS, FURTHER INFORMATION
- Tolerance Many patients on long-acting or transdermal nitrates rapidly develop tolerance (with reduced therapeutic effects). Reduction of blood-nitrate concentrations to low levels for 4 to 12 hours each day usually maintains effectiveness in such patients. If tolerance is suspected during the use of transdermal patches they should be left off for 8–12 hours (usually overnight) in each 24 hours; in the case of modified-release tablets of isosorbide dinitrate (and conventional formulations of isosorbide mononitrate), the second of the two daily doses should be given after about 8 hours rather than after 12 hours. Conventional formulations of isosorbide mononitrate should not usually be given more than twice daily unless small doses are used; modified-release formulations of isosorbide mononitrate should only be given once daily, and used in this way do not produce tolerance.

- SIDE-EFFECTS
- Common or very common Arrhythmias · asthenia · cerebral ischaemia · dizziness · drowsiness · flushing · headache · hypotension · nausea · peripheral oedema · vomiting
- Uncommon Anorectal disorder · cardiac disorder · circulatory collapse · cyanosis · diarrhoea · gastrointestinal discomfort · haemorrhage · skin reactions · syncope
- Rare or very rare Angioedema · angle closure glaucoma · hypoxia · methaemoglobinaemia · myalgia · respiratory disorders · restlessness · Stevens-Johnson syndrome

- Frequency not known Drug tolerance · hyperhidrosis · palpitations · tongue blistering · vertigo
- ALLERGY AND CROSS-SENSITIVITY Contra-indicated in nitrate hypersensitivity.
- BREAST FEEDING No information available—manufacturers advise use only if potential benefit outweighs risk.
- HEPATIC IMPAIRMENT Caution in severe impairment.
- RENAL IMPAIRMENT Manufacturers advise use with caution in severe impairment.
- MONITORING REQUIREMENTS Monitor blood pressure and heart rate during intravenous infusion.
- TREATMENT CESSATION Avoid abrupt withdrawal.

Glyceryl trinitrate   09-Mar-2018

- INDICATIONS AND DOSE
Prophylaxis of angina
- BY SUBLINGUAL ADMINISTRATION USING SUBLINGUAL TABLETS
- Adult: 1 tablet, to be administered prior to activity likely to cause angina

Treatment of angina
- BY SUBLINGUAL ADMINISTRATION USING SUBLINGUAL TABLETS
- Adult: 1 tablet, dose may be repeated at 5 minute intervals if required; if symptoms have not resolved after 3 doses, medical attention should be sought

Prophylaxis of angina
- BY SUBLINGUAL ADMINISTRATION USING AEROSOL SPRAY
- Adult: 400–800 micrograms, to be administered under the tongue and then close mouth prior to activity likely to cause angina

Treatment of angina
- BY SUBLINGUAL ADMINISTRATION USING AEROSOL SPRAY
- Adult: 400–800 micrograms, to be administered under the tongue and then close mouth, dose may be repeated at 5 minute intervals if required; if symptoms have not resolved after 3 doses, medical attention should be sought

Control of hypertension and myocardial ischaemia during and after cardiac surgery | Induction of controlled hypotension during surgery | Congestive heart failure | Unstable angina
- BY INTRAVENOUS INFUSION
- Adult: 10–200 micrograms/minute (max. per dose 400 micrograms/minute), adjusted according to response, consult product literature for recommended starting doses specific to indication

Anal fissure
- BY RECTUM USING OINTMENT
- Adult: Apply 2.5 centimetres every 12 hours until pain stops. Max. duration of use 8 weeks, apply to anal canal, 2.5 cm of ointment contains 1.5 mg of glyceryl trinitrate

DEPONIT ®
Prophylaxis of angina
- BY TRANSDERMAL APPLICATION
- Adult: One '5' or one '10' patch to be applied to lateral chest wall, upper arm, thigh, abdomen, or shoulder; increase to two '10' patches every 24 hours if necessary, to be replaced every 24 hours, siting replacement patch on different area

MINITRAN ®
Prophylaxis of angina
- BY TRANSDERMAL APPLICATION
- Adult: One '5' patch to be applied to chest or upper arm; replace every 24 hours, siting replacement patch on different area, dose to be adjusted according to response   continued →

Maintenance of venous patency ('5' patch only)
▶ BY TRANSDERMAL APPLICATION
▸ Adult: (consult product literature)

NITRO-DUR ®

Prophylaxis of angina
▶ BY TRANSDERMAL APPLICATION
▸ Adult: One '0.2mg/h' patch to be applied to chest or outer upper arm and replaced every 24 hours, siting replacement patch on different area, dose adjusted according to response; maximum 15 mg per day

PERCUTOL ®

Prophylaxis of angina
▶ TO THE SKIN
▸ Adult: Usual dose 1–2 inches every 3–4 hours as required, to be measured on to *Applirule*® and applied (usually to chest, arm, or thigh) without rubbing in and secured with surgical tape, approx. 800 micrograms/hour absorbed from 1 inch of ointment.

Prophylaxis of angina (to determine dose)
▶ TO THE SKIN
▸ Adult: ½ inch to be administered on first day then increased by ½ inch/day until headache occurs, then reduced by ½ inch, to be measured on to *Applirule*® and applied (usually to chest, arm, or thigh) without rubbing in and secured with surgical tape, approx. 800 micrograms/hour absorbed from 1 inch of ointment.

TRANSIDERM-NITRO ®

Prophylaxis of angina
▶ BY TRANSDERMAL APPLICATION
▸ Adult: One '5' or one '10' patch to be applied to lateral chest wall and replaced every 24 hours, siting replacement patch on different area, max. two '10' patches daily

Prophylaxis of phlebitis and extravasation ('5' patch only)
▶ BY TRANSDERMAL APPLICATION
▸ Adult: (consult product literature)

● INTERACTIONS → Appendix 1: nitrates
● PREGNANCY Not known to be harmful.
● DIRECTIONS FOR ADMINISTRATION
▸ With intravenous use For *intravenous infusion* (*Nitrocine*®, *Nitronal*®), give continuously in Glucose 5% or Sodium Chloride 0.9%. For *Nitrocine*®, suggested infusion concentration 100 micrograms/mL; incompatible with polyvinyl chloride infusion containers such as *Viaflex*® or *Steriflex*®; use glass or polyethylene containers or give via a syringe pump.
   Glass or polyethylene apparatus is preferable; loss of potency will occur if PVC is used. Glyceryl trinitrate 1 mg/ml to be diluted before use or given undiluted with syringe pump. Glyceryl trinitrate 5 mg/ml to be diluted before use.

● PRESCRIBING AND DISPENSING INFORMATION
▸ With sublingual use Glyceryl trinitrate tablets are available in strengths of 300-, 500- and 600-micrograms—manufacturer advises tablets should be supplied in glass containers of not more than 100 tablets, closed with a foil-lined cap, and containing no cotton wool wadding; they should be discarded after 8 weeks in use.

● PATIENT AND CARER ADVICE Rectal ointment should be discarded 8 weeks after first opening.

PERCUTOL ® Patients or carers should be given advice on how to administer glyceryl trinitrate ointment.

● NATIONAL FUNDING/ACCESS DECISIONS
Scottish Medicines Consortium (SMC) Decisions
The *Scottish Medicines Consortium* has advised (January 2008) that glyceryl trinitrate 0.4% ointment (*Rectogesic*®)

is **not** recommended for use within NHS Scotland for the relief of pain associated with chronic anal fissure.

● MEDICINAL FORMS
There can be variation in the licensing of different medicines containing the same drug. Forms available from special-order manufacturers include: ointment

Solution for infusion
EXCIPIENTS: May contain Ethanol, propylene glycol
▸ Glyceryl trinitrate (Non-proprietary)
   Glyceryl trinitrate 1 mg per 1 ml Glyceryl trinitrate 50mg/50ml solution for infusion vials | 1 vial PoM £15.90
   Glyceryl trinitrate 5 mg per 1 ml Glyceryl trinitrate 50mg/10ml solution for infusion ampoules | 5 ampoule PoM £64.90 (Hospital only)
   Glyceryl trinitrate 25mg/5ml solution for infusion ampoules | 5 ampoule PoM £32.45 (Hospital only)
▸ Nitrocine (Aspire Pharma Ltd)
   Glyceryl trinitrate 1 mg per 1 ml Nitrocine 10mg/10ml solution for infusion ampoules | 10 ampoule PoM £58.75 (Hospital only)
▸ Nitronal (Intrapharm Laboratories Ltd)
   Glyceryl trinitrate 1 mg per 1 ml Nitronal 5mg/5ml solution for infusion ampoules | 10 ampoule PoM £18.04
   Nitronal 50mg/50ml solution for infusion vials | 1 vial PoM £14.76

Sublingual tablet
CAUTIONARY AND ADVISORY LABELS 16
▸ Glyceryl trinitrate (Non-proprietary)
   Glyceryl trinitrate 300 microgram GTN 300microgram sublingual tablets | 100 tablet P £2.71 DT = £2.71
   Glyceryl trinitrate 300microgram sublingual tablets | 100 tablet P ⊠ DT = £2.71
   Glyceryl trinitrate 500 microgram Glyceryl trinitrate 500microgram sublingual tablets | 100 tablet P £3.90 DT = £1.86
   Glyceryl trinitrate 600 microgram Glyceryl trinitrate 600microgram sublingual tablets | 100 tablet P ⊠

Transdermal patch
▸ Deponit (Aspire Pharma Ltd)
   Glyceryl trinitrate 5 mg per 24 hour Deponit 5 transdermal patches | 28 patch P £12.77
   Glyceryl trinitrate 10 mg per 24 hour Deponit 10 transdermal patches | 28 patch P £14.06
▸ Minitran (Meda Pharmaceuticals Ltd)
   Glyceryl trinitrate 5 mg per 24 hour Minitran 5 transdermal patches | 30 patch P £11.62
   Glyceryl trinitrate 10 mg per 24 hour Minitran 10 transdermal patches | 30 patch P £12.87
   Glyceryl trinitrate 15 mg per 24 hour Minitran 15 transdermal patches | 30 patch P £14.19
▸ Transiderm-Nitro (Novartis Pharmaceuticals UK Ltd)
   Glyceryl trinitrate 5 mg per 24 hour Transiderm-Nitro 5 transdermal patches | 28 patch P £20.46
   Glyceryl trinitrate 10 mg per 24 hour Transiderm-Nitro 10 transdermal patches | 28 patch P £22.49

Rectal ointment
EXCIPIENTS: May contain Propylene glycol, woolfat and related substances (including lanolin)
▸ Rectogesic (Kyowa Kirin Ltd)
   Glyceryl trinitrate 4 mg per 1 gram Rectogesic 0.4% rectal ointment | 30 gram PoM £39.30 DT = £39.30

Ointment
EXCIPIENTS: May contain Woolfat and related substances (including lanolin)
▸ Percutol (Aspire Pharma Ltd)
   Glyceryl trinitrate 20 mg per 1 gram Percutol 2% ointment | 60 gram P £79.00 DT = £79.00

Sublingual spray
CAUTIONARY AND ADVISORY LABELS 15
▸ Glyceryl trinitrate (Non-proprietary)
   Glyceryl trinitrate 400 microgram per 1 dose Glyceryl trinitrate 400micrograms/dose pump sublingual spray | 180 dose P £2.63 DT = £1.46 | 200 dose P £2.71 DT = £1.49
   Glyceryl trinitrate 400micrograms/dose aerosol sublingual spray | 180 dose P £3.20 DT = £3.01 | 200 dose P £3.50 DT = £3.50
▸ Coro-Nitro (J M Loveridge Ltd)
   Glyceryl trinitrate 400 microgram per 1 dose Coro-Nitro 400micrograms/dose pump sublingual spray | 200 dose GSL £3.44 DT = £1.49

▸ Glytrin (Aspire Pharma Ltd)
Glyceryl trinitrate 400 microgram per 1 dose Glytrin
400micrograms/dose aerosol sublingual spray | 200 dose P £3.44
DT = £3.50
▸ Nitrolingual (Intrapharm Laboratories Ltd)
Glyceryl trinitrate 400 microgram per 1 dose Nitrolingual
400micrograms/dose pump sublingual spray | 180 dose P £3.10 DT
= £1.46 | 200 dose P £3.44 DT = £1.49
▸ Nitromin (Teva UK Ltd)
Glyceryl trinitrate 400 microgram per 1 dose Nitromin
400micrograms/dose pump sublingual spray | 180 dose P £2.63 DT
= £1.46 | 200 dose P £2.71 DT = £1.49

F 217

Isosorbide dinitrate

● **INDICATIONS AND DOSE**

Prophylaxis and treatment of angina
▸ BY MOUTH USING IMMEDIATE-RELEASE MEDICINES
▸ Adult: 30–120 mg daily in divided doses
▸ BY INTRAVENOUS INFUSION
▸ Adult: 2–10 mg/hour, increased if necessary up to
20 mg/hour
▸ BY SUBLINGUAL ADMINISTRATION USING AEROSOL SPRAY
▸ Adult: 1–3 sprays, to be administered under tongue
whilst holding breath, allow a 30 second interval
between each dose

Left ventricular failure
▸ BY MOUTH USING IMMEDIATE-RELEASE MEDICINES
▸ Adult: 40–160 mg daily in divided doses, increased if
necessary up to 240 mg daily in divided doses
▸ BY INTRAVENOUS INFUSION
▸ Adult: Initially 2–10 mg/hour, increased if necessary up
to 20 mg/hour

Prophylaxis of angina
▸ BY MOUTH USING MODIFIED-RELEASE MEDICINES
▸ Adult: 40 mg daily in 1–2 divided doses, increased if
necessary to 60–80 mg daily in 2–3 divided doses

● INTERACTIONS → Appendix 1: nitrates

● PREGNANCY May cross placenta—manufacturers advise
avoid unless potential benefit outweighs risk.

● DIRECTIONS FOR ADMINISTRATION For *intravenous infusion*
(*Isoket* 0.05% ®, *Isoket* 0.1% ®), give continuously in
Glucose 5% or Sodium chloride 0.9%. Adsorbed to some
extent by polyvinyl chloride infusion containers;
preferably use glass or polyethylene containers or give via
a syringe pump; *Isoket* 0.05% ® can alternatively be
administered undiluted using a syringe pump with a glass
or rigid plastic syringe. Glass or polyethylene infusion
apparatus is preferable; loss of potency if PVC used.

● MEDICINAL FORMS
There can be variation in the licensing of different medicines
containing the same drug. Forms available from special-order
manufacturers include: oral suspension, oral solution

Modified-release tablet
CAUTIONARY AND ADVISORY LABELS 25
▸ Isosorbide dinitrate (Non-proprietary)
Isosorbide dinitrate 20 mg Isosorbide dinitrate 20mg modified-
release tablets | 56 tablet P S DT = £2.58
Isosorbide dinitrate 40 mg Isosorbide dinitrate 40mg modified-
release tablets | 56 tablet P S DT = £6.36
▸ Isoket Retard (Aspire Pharma Ltd)
Isosorbide dinitrate 20 mg Isoket Retard 20 tablets | 56 tablet P
£2.58 DT = £2.58
Isosorbide dinitrate 40 mg Isoket Retard 40 tablets | 56 tablet P
£6.36 DT = £6.36

Tablet
▸ Isosorbide dinitrate (Non-proprietary)
Isosorbide dinitrate 10 mg Isosorbide dinitrate 10mg tablets |
56 tablet P £34.00 DT = £13.41
Isosorbide dinitrate 20 mg Isosorbide dinitrate 20mg tablets |
56 tablet PoM S DT = £14.38 | 56 tablet P £70.00 DT = £14.38

Solution for injection
▸ Isosorbide dinitrate (Non-proprietary)
Isosorbide dinitrate 1 mg per 1 ml Isosorbide dinitrate 10mg/10ml
concentrate for solution for injection ampoules | 10 ampoule PoM
£23.40
▸ Isoket (Aspire Pharma Ltd)
Isosorbide dinitrate 1 mg per 1 ml Isoket 0.1% solution for injection
10ml ampoules | 10 ampoule PoM £26.93 (Hospital only)

Solution for infusion
▸ Isosorbide dinitrate (Non-proprietary)
Isosorbide dinitrate 500 microgram per 1 ml Isosorbide dinitrate
25mg/50ml solution for infusion vials | 10 vial PoM £55.00
Isosorbide dinitrate 1 mg per 1 ml Isosorbide dinitrate 50mg/50ml
concentrate for solution for infusion vials | 10 vial PoM £71.20

F 217

Isosorbide mononitrate

● **INDICATIONS AND DOSE**

Prophylaxis of angina | Adjunct in congestive heart failure
▸ BY MOUTH USING IMMEDIATE-RELEASE MEDICINES
▸ Adult: Initially 20 mg 2–3 times a day, alternatively
initially 40 mg twice daily, increased if necessary up to
120 mg daily in divided doses

**Prophylaxis of angina (for patients who have not
previously had a nitrate) | Adjunct in congestive heart
failure (for patients who have not previously had a
nitrate)**
▸ BY MOUTH USING IMMEDIATE-RELEASE MEDICINES
▸ Adult: Initially 10 mg twice daily, increased if necessary
up to 120 mg daily in divided doses

CHEMYDUR ® 60XL
Prophylaxis of angina
▸ BY MOUTH
▸ Adult: Initially 0.5 tablet daily for 2–4 days, to
minimise possibility of headache, then 1 tablet daily,
increased if necessary to 2 tablets daily, dose to be
taken in the morning

ELANTAN ® LA
Prophylaxis of angina
▸ BY MOUTH
▸ Adult: 25–50 mg once daily, then increased if necessary
to 50–100 mg once daily, dose to be taken in the
morning, the lowest effective dose should be used

IMDUR ®
Prophylaxis of angina
▸ BY MOUTH
▸ Adult: Initially 0.5 tablet once daily, to minimise the
occurrence of headache, then 1 tablet once daily, then
increased if necessary to 2 tablets once daily, dose to be
taken in the morning

ISIB ® 60XL
Prophylaxis of angina
▸ BY MOUTH
▸ Adult: Initially 0.5 tablet once daily for 2–4 days, to
minimise the occurrence of headache, then 1 tablet
once daily, increased if necessary to 2 tablets once
daily, dose to be taken in the morning

ISMO RETARD ®
Prophylaxis of angina
▸ BY MOUTH
▸ Adult: 1 tablet once daily, dose to be taken in the
morning

ISODUR ®
Prophylaxis of angina
▸ BY MOUTH
▸ Adult: 25–50 mg once daily, then increased if necessary
to 50–100 mg once daily, dose to be taken in the
morning continued →

2

Cardiovascular system

ISOTARD®

Prophylaxis of angina

▶ BY MOUTH

▶ Adult: 25–60 mg once daily, if headaches occur with 60 mg tablet, half a 60 mg tablet may be given for 2–4 days, then increased if necessary to 50–120 mg once daily, dose to be taken in the morning

MODISAL® XL

Prophylaxis of angina

▶ BY MOUTH

▶ Adult: Initially 0.5 tablet once daily for 2–4 days, to minimise the occurrence of headache, then 1 tablet once daily, increased if necessary to 2 tablets once daily, dose to be taken in the morning

MONOMAX® SR

Prophylaxis of angina

▶ BY MOUTH

▶ Adult: 40–60 mg daily, increased if necessary to 120 mg daily, dose to be taken in the morning

MONOMAX® XL

Prophylaxis of angina

▶ BY MOUTH

▶ Adult: Initially 0.5 tablet once daily for 2–4 days, to minimise occurrence of headache, then 1 tablet once daily, increased if necessary to 2 tablets once daily, dose to be taken in the morning

MONOMIL® XL

Prophylaxis of angina

▶ BY MOUTH

▶ Adult: Initially 0.5 tablet daily for 2–4 days, to minimise possibility of headache, then 1 tablet daily, increased if necessary to 2 tablets once daily, to be taken in the morning

MONOSORB® XL60

Prophylaxis of angina

▶ BY MOUTH

▶ Adult: Initially 0.5 tablet once daily for the first 2–4 days, to minimise the occurrence of headache, then 1 tablet once daily, increased if necessary to 2 tablets once daily, dose to be taken in the morning

ZEMON®

Prophylaxis of angina

▶ BY MOUTH

▶ Adult: Initially 30 mg once daily for 2–4 days, to minimise the occurrence of headache, then 40–60 mg once daily, increased if necessary to 80–120 mg once daily, dose to be taken in the morning

● INTERACTIONS → Appendix 1: nitrates

● PREGNANCY Manufacturers advise avoid unless potential benefit outweighs risk.

● MEDICINAL FORMS
There can be variation in the licensing of different medicines containing the same drug. Forms available from special-order manufacturers include: oral suspension, oral solution

Modified-release tablet

CAUTIONARY AND ADVISORY LABELS 25

▶ Chemydur 60XL(AMCo)
Isosorbide mononitrate 60 mg Chemydur 60XL tablets | 28 tablet PoM £3.49 DT = £10.50

▶ Imdur (AstraZeneca UK Ltd)
Isosorbide mononitrate 60 mg Imdur 60mg modified-release tablets | 28 tablet P £10.50 DT = £10.50

▶ Isib XL (Alliance Pharmaceuticals Ltd)
Isosorbide mononitrate 60 mg Isib 60XL tablets | 28 tablet P £8.15 DT = £10.50

▶ Ismo Retard (Intrapharm Laboratories Ltd)
Isosorbide mononitrate 40 mg Ismo Retard 40mg tablets | 30 tablet P £10.71

▶ Isotard XL (Kyowa Kirin Ltd)
Isosorbide mononitrate 25 mg Isotard 25XL tablets | 28 tablet P £6.75 DT = £6.75
Isosorbide mononitrate 40 mg Isotard 40XL tablets | 28 tablet P £6.75 DT = £6.75
Isosorbide mononitrate 50 mg Isotard 50XL tablets | 28 tablet P £6.75 DT = £6.75
Isosorbide mononitrate 60 mg Isotard 60XL tablets | 28 tablet P £5.75 DT = £10.50

▶ Modisal XL (Ennogen Pharma Ltd)
Isosorbide mononitrate 40 mg Modisal XL 40mg tablets | 28 tablet PoM £50.64 DT = £6.75

▶ Monomax XL (Chiesi Ltd)
Isosorbide mononitrate 60 mg Monomax XL 60mg tablets | 28 tablet P £5.25 DT = £10.50

▶ Monomil XL (Teva UK Ltd)
Isosorbide mononitrate 60 mg Monomil XL 60mg tablets | 28 tablet PoM £3.49 DT = £10.50

▶ Monosorb XL (Dexcel-Pharma Ltd)
Isosorbide mononitrate 60 mg Monosorb XL 60 tablets | 28 tablet P £15.53 DT = £10.50

▶ Zemon XL (Kent Pharmaceuticals Ltd)
Isosorbide mononitrate 40 mg Zemon 40 XL tablets | 28 tablet PoM £14.25 DT = £6.75

Tablet

CAUTIONARY AND ADVISORY LABELS 25

▶ Isosorbide mononitrate (Non-proprietary)
Isosorbide mononitrate 10 mg Isosorbide mononitrate 10mg tablets | 56 tablet P £25.00 DT = £0.97
Isosorbide mononitrate 20 mg Isosorbide mononitrate 20mg tablets | 56 tablet P £22.00 DT = £0.95 | 56 tablet PoM £1.14 DT = £0.95
Isosorbide mononitrate 40 mg Isosorbide mononitrate 40mg tablets | 56 tablet PoM £2.19 DT = £1.28 | 56 tablet P £35.00 DT = £1.28

▶ Ismo (Intrapharm Laboratories Ltd)
Isosorbide mononitrate 10 mg Ismo 10 tablets | 60 tablet P £2.98
Isosorbide mononitrate 20 mg Ismo 20 tablets | 60 tablet P £4.12

Modified-release capsule

CAUTIONARY AND ADVISORY LABELS 25

▶ Elantan LA (Aspire Pharma Ltd)
Isosorbide mononitrate 25 mg Elantan LA25 capsules | 28 capsule P £3.40 DT = £3.40
Isosorbide mononitrate 50 mg Elantan LA50 capsules | 28 capsule P £3.69 DT = £3.69

▶ Isodur XL (Galen Ltd)
Isosorbide mononitrate 25 mg Isodur 25XL capsules | 28 capsule P £4.63 DT = £3.40
Isosorbide mononitrate 50 mg Isodur 50XL capsules | 28 capsule P £6.45 DT = £3.69

▶ Monomax SR (Ethypharm UK Ltd)
Isosorbide mononitrate 40 mg Nyzamac SR 40mg capsules | 28 capsule P £6.52 DT = £6.52
Isosorbide mononitrate 60 mg Nyzamac SR 60mg capsules | 28 capsule P £8.86 DT = £8.86

SYMPATHOMIMETICS > SYMPATHOMIMETICS, INOTROPIC

Dobutamine

● DRUG ACTION Dobutamine is a cardiac stimulant which acts on beta$_1$ receptors in cardiac muscle, and increases contractility.

● INDICATIONS AND DOSE

Inotropic support in infarction, cardiac surgery, cardiomyopathies, septic shock, cardiogenic shock, and during positive end expiratory pressure ventilation

▶ BY INTRAVENOUS INFUSION

▶ Adult: Usual dose 2.5–10 micrograms/kg/minute, adjusted according to response, alternatively 0.5–40 micrograms/kg/minute

Cardiovascular system

Cardiac stress testing
▶ BY INTRAVENOUS INFUSION
▶ Adult: (consult product literature)

● CONTRA-INDICATIONS Phaeochromocytoma
● CAUTIONS Acute heart failure · acute myocardial infarction · arrhythmias · correct hypercapnia before starting and during treatment · correct hypovolaemia before starting and during treatment · correct hypoxia before starting and during treatment · correct metabolic acidosis before starting and during treatment · diabetes mellitus · elderly · extravasation may cause tissue necrosis · extreme caution or avoid in marked obstruction of cardiac ejection (such as idiopathic hypertrophic subaortic stenosis) · hyperthyroidism · ischaemic heart disease · occlusive vascular disease · severe hypotension · susceptibility to angle-closure glaucoma · tachycardia · tolerance may develop with continuous infusions longer than 72 hours
● INTERACTIONS → Appendix 1: sympathomimetics, inotropic
● SIDE-EFFECTS
▶ Common or very common Arrhythmias · bronchospasm · chest pain · dyspnoea · eosinophilia · fever · headache · inflammation localised · ischaemic heart disease · nausea · palpitations · platelet aggregation inhibition (on prolonged administration) · skin reactions · urinary urgency · vasoconstriction
▶ Uncommon Myocardial infarction
▶ Rare or very rare Atrioventricular block · cardiac arrest · coronary vasospasm · hypertension · hypokalaemia · hypotension
▶ Frequency not known Anxiety · cardiomyopathy · feeling hot · myoclonus · paraesthesia · tremor
● PREGNANCY No evidence of harm in *animal* studies—manufacturers advise use only if potential benefit outweighs risk.
● BREAST FEEDING Manufacturers advise avoid—no information available.
● MONITORING REQUIREMENTS Monitor serum-potassium concentration.
● DIRECTIONS FOR ADMINISTRATION Dobutamine injection should be diluted before use or given undiluted with syringe pump. Dobutamine concentrate for intravenous infusion should be diluted before use.
   For *intravenous infusion*, give continuously in Glucose 5% or Sodium chloride 0.9%. Dilute to a concentration of 0.5–1 mg/mL and give via an infusion pump; give higher concentration (max. 5 mg/mL) through central venous catheter; incompatible with bicarbonate and other strong alkaline solutions.

● MEDICINAL FORMS
There can be variation in the licensing of different medicines containing the same drug. Forms available from special-order manufacturers include: solution for infusion
Solution for infusion
EXCIPIENTS: May contain Sulfites
▶ Dobutamine (Non-proprietary)
   Dobutamine (as Dobutamine hydrochloride) 5 mg per 1 ml Dobutamine 250mg/50ml solution for infusion vials | 1 vial PoM £7.50
   Dobutamine (as Dobutamine hydrochloride) 12.5 mg per 1 ml Dobutamine 250mg/20ml concentrate for solution for infusion ampoules | 5 ampoule PoM £10.00-£26.25

7.1a Cardiac arrest

Cardiopulmonary resuscitation

Overview
The algorithm for cardiopulmonary resuscitation (Life support algorithm (image) p. 1618) reflects the most recent recommendations of the Resuscitation Council (UK). These guidelines are available at www.resus.org.uk.
   Cardiac arrest can be associated with ventricular fibrillation, pulseless ventricular tachycardia, asystole, and pulseless electrical activity (electromechanical dissociation). Adrenaline/epinephrine below 1 in 10000 (100 micrograms/mL) is recommended by intravenous injection repeated every 3–5 minutes if necessary. Administration through a central line results in a faster response than peripheral administration, however placement of a central line must not interfere with chest compressions; drugs administered peripherally must be followed by a flush of at least 20 mL Sodium Chloride 0.9% injection to aid entry into the central circulation. Intravenous injection of amiodarone hydrochloride p. 105 should be considered after adrenaline/epinephrine to treat ventricular fibrillation or pulseless ventricular tachycardia in cardiac arrest refractory to defibrillation. An additional dose of amiodarone hydrochloride can be given if necessary, followed by an intravenous infusion of amiodarone hydrochloride. Lidocaine hydrochloride p. 103, is an alternative if amiodarone hydrochloride is not available. Atropine sulfate p. 1295 is no longer recommended in the treatment of asystole or pulseless electrical activity.
   During cardiopulmonary arrest if intravenous access cannot be obtained, the intraosseous route can be used instead. Drug administration via the endotracheal route is no longer recommended.
   For the management of acute anaphylaxis, see allergic emergencies under Antihistamines, allergen immunotherapy and allergic emergencies p. 276.

SYMPATHOMIMETICS ⟩ VASOCONSTRICTOR

Ⅰ Adrenaline/epinephrine   27-Sep-2017

● DRUG ACTION Acts on both alpha and beta receptors and increases both heart rate and contractility (beta$_1$ effects); it can cause peripheral vasodilation (a beta$_2$ effect) or vasoconstriction (an alpha effect).

● INDICATIONS AND DOSE
Cardiopulmonary resuscitation
▶ BY INTRAVENOUS INJECTION
▶ Adult: 1 mg every 3–5 minutes as required, a 1 in 10 000 (100 micrograms/mL) solution is recommended
Acute hypotension
▶ BY CONTINUOUS INTRAVENOUS INFUSION
▶ Neonate: Initially 100 nanograms/kg/minute, adjusted according to response, higher doses up to 1.5 micrograms/kg/minute have been used in acute hypotension
▶ Child: Initially 100 nanograms/kg/minute, adjusted according to response, higher doses up to 1.5 micrograms/kg/minute have been used in acute hypotension
continued →

Emergency treatment of acute anaphylaxis (under expert supervision) | Angioedema (if laryngeal oedema is present) (under expert supervision)
▶ BY INTRAMUSCULAR INJECTION
▸ Child 1 month-5 years: 150 micrograms, doses may be repeated several times if necessary at 5 minute intervals according to blood pressure, pulse, and respiratory function, suitable syringe to be used for measuring small volume; injected preferably into the anterolateral aspect of the middle third of the thigh
▸ Child 6-11 years: 300 micrograms, doses may be repeated several times if necessary at 5 minute intervals according to blood pressure, pulse, and respiratory function, to be injected preferably into the anterolateral aspect of the middle third of the thigh
▸ Child 12-17 years: 500 micrograms, to be injected preferably into the anterolateral aspect of the middle third of the thigh, doses may be repeated several times if necessary at 5 minute intervals according to blood pressure, pulse, and respiratory function, 300 micrograms (0.3 mL) to be administered if child small or prepubertal
▸ Adult: 500 micrograms, to be injected preferably into the anterolateral aspect of the middle third of the thigh, doses may be repeated several times if necessary at 5 minute intervals according to blood pressure, pulse, and respiratory function

Acute anaphylaxis when there is doubt as to the adequacy of the circulation (specialist use only) | Angioedema (if laryngeal oedema is present) (specialist use only)
▶ BY SLOW INTRAVENOUS INJECTION
▸ Adult: 50 micrograms, using 0.5 mL of the dilute 1 in 10 000 adrenaline injection, dose to be repeated according to response, if multiple doses required, adrenaline should be given as a slow intravenous infusion stopping when a response has been obtained

Control of bradycardia in patients with arrhythmias after myocardial infarction, if there is a risk of asystole, or if the patient is unstable and has failed to respond to atropine
▶ BY INTRAVENOUS INFUSION
▸ Adult: 2–10 micrograms/minute, adjusted according to response

EMERADE ® 150 MICROGRAMS
Acute anaphylaxis (for self-administration)
▶ BY INTRAMUSCULAR INJECTION
▸ Child (body-weight up to 15 kg): 150 micrograms, then 150 micrograms after 5–15 minutes as required
▸ Child (body-weight 15-30 kg): 150 micrograms, then 150 micrograms after 5–15 minutes as required, on the basis of a dose of 10 micrograms/kg, 300 micrograms may be more appropriate for some children

EMERADE ® 300 MICROGRAMS
Acute anaphylaxis (for self-administration)
▶ BY INTRAMUSCULAR INJECTION
▸ Child (body-weight 30 kg and above): 300 micrograms, then 300 micrograms after 5–15 minutes as required
▸ Adult (body-weight 30 kg and above): 300 micrograms, then 300 micrograms after 5–15 minutes as required

EMERADE ® 500 MICROGRAMS
Acute anaphylaxis (for self-administration for patients at risk of severe anaphylaxis)
▶ BY INTRAMUSCULAR INJECTION
▸ Child 12-17 years: 500 micrograms, then 500 micrograms after 5–15 minutes as required
▸ Adult: 500 micrograms, then 500 micrograms after 5–15 minutes as required

EPIPEN ® AUTO-INJECTOR 0.3MG
Acute anaphylaxis (for self-administration)
▶ BY INTRAMUSCULAR INJECTION
▸ Child (body-weight 30 kg and above): 300 micrograms, then 300 micrograms after 5–15 minutes as required
▸ Adult (body-weight 30 kg and above): 300 micrograms, then 300 micrograms after 5–15 minutes as required

EPIPEN ® JR AUTO-INJECTOR 0.15MG
Acute anaphylaxis (for self-administration)
▶ BY INTRAMUSCULAR INJECTION
▸ Child (body-weight up to 15 kg): 150 micrograms, then 150 micrograms after 5–15 minutes as required
▸ Child (body-weight 15-30 kg): 150 micrograms, then 150 micrograms after 5–15 minutes as required, on the basis of a dose of 10 micrograms/kg, 300 micrograms may be more appropriate for some children

JEXT ® 150 MICROGRAMS
Acute anaphylaxis (for self-administration)
▶ BY INTRAMUSCULAR INJECTION
▸ Child (body-weight up to 15 kg): 150 micrograms, then 150 micrograms after 5–15 minutes as required
▸ Child (body-weight 15-30 kg): 150 micrograms, then 150 micrograms after 5–15 minutes as required, on the basis of a dose of 10 micrograms/kg, 300 micrograms may be more appropriate for some children

JEXT ® 300 MICROGRAMS
Acute anaphylaxis (for self-administration)
▶ BY INTRAMUSCULAR INJECTION
▸ Child (body-weight 30 kg and above): 300 micrograms, then 300 micrograms after 5–15 minutes as required
▸ Adult (body-weight 30 kg and above): 300 micrograms, then 300 micrograms after 5–15 minutes as required

● UNLICENSED USE
▸ With intramuscular use for acute anaphylaxis in children Auto-injectors delivering 150-microgram dose of adrenaline may not be licensed for use in children with body-weight under 15 kg.
▸ With intravenous use for acute hypotension in children Adrenaline 1 in 1000 (1 mg/mL) solution is not licensed for intravenous administration.

IMPORTANT SAFETY INFORMATION
SAFE PRACTICE
Intravenous route should be used with **extreme care** by specialists only.

MHRA/CHM ADVICE: ADRENALINE AUTO-INJECTORS: UPDATED ADVICE AFTER EUROPEAN REVIEW (AUGUST 2017)
Following a European review of all adrenaline auto-injectors approved in the EU, the MHRA recommend that 2 adrenaline auto-injectors are prescribed, which patients should carry at all times. This is particularly important for patients with allergic asthma, who are at increased risk of a severe anaphylactic reaction. Patients with allergies and their carers should be trained to use the particular auto-injector they have been prescribed and encouraged to practise using a trainer device. Patients are advised to check the expiry date of the adrenaline auto-injectors and obtain replacements before they expire.

● CAUTIONS Arteriosclerosis (in adults) · arrhythmias · cerebrovascular disease · cor pulmonale · diabetes mellitus · elderly · hypercalcaemia · hyperreflexia · hypertension · hyperthyroidism · hypokalaemia · ischaemic heart disease · obstructive cardiomyopathy · occlusive vascular disease · organic brain damage · phaeochromocytoma · prostate disorders · psychoneurosis · severe angina · susceptibility to angle-closure glaucoma

CAUTIONS, FURTHER INFORMATION Cautions listed are only for non-life-threatening situations.

● INTERACTIONS → Appendix 1: sympathomimetics, vasoconstrictor

● SIDE-EFFECTS

GENERAL SIDE-EFFECTS

Angina pectoris · angle closure glaucoma · anxiety · appetite decreased · arrhythmias · asthenia · cardiomyopathy · CNS haemorrhage · confusion · dizziness · dry mouth · dyspnoea · headache · hepatic necrosis · hyperglycaemia · hyperhidrosis · hypersalivation · hypertension (increased risk of cerebral haemorrhage) · hypokalaemia · insomnia · intestinal necrosis · metabolic acidosis · mydriasis · myocardial infarction · nausea · pallor · palpitations · peripheral coldness · psychosis · pulmonary oedema (on excessive dosage or extreme sensitivity) · renal necrosis · soft tissue necrosis · tremor · urinary disorders · vomiting

SPECIFIC SIDE-EFFECTS

▸ **Frequency not known**

▸ With intramuscular use Muscle necrosis · necrotising fasciitis · peripheral ischaemia

▸ With intravenous use Hemiplegia · muscle rigidity

● PREGNANCY May reduce placental perfusion and cause tachycardia, cardiac irregularities, and extrasystoles in fetus. Can delay second stage of labour. Manufacturers advise use only if benefit outweighs risk.

● BREAST FEEDING Present in milk but unlikely to be harmful as poor oral bioavailability.

● RENAL IMPAIRMENT Manufacturers advise use with caution in severe impairment.

● MONITORING REQUIREMENTS Monitor blood pressure and ECG.

● DIRECTIONS FOR ADMINISTRATION

Acute hypotension

▸ With intravenous use in children For *continuous intravenous infusion*, dilute with Glucose 5% or Sodium Chloride 0.9% and give through a central venous catheter. Incompatible with bicarbonate and alkaline solutions. *Neonatal intensive care*, dilute 3 mg/kg body-weight to a final volume of 50 mL with infusion fluid; an intravenous infusion rate of 0.1 mL/hour provides a dose of 100 nanograms/kg/minute; infuse through a central venous catheter. Incompatible with bicarbonate and alkaline solutions. These infusions are usually made up with adrenaline 1 in 1000 (1 mg/mL) solution.

Cardiopulmonary resuscitation

▸ With intravenous use in adults Administration through a central line results in a faster response than peripheral administration, however placement of a central line must not interfere with chest compressions; drugs administered peripherally must be followed by a flush of at least 20 mL Sodium Chloride 0.9% injection to aid entry into the central circulation.

● PRESCRIBING AND DISPENSING INFORMATION It is important, in acute anaphylaxis where intramuscular injection might still succeed, time should not be wasted seeking intravenous access.

Great vigilance is needed to ensure that the *correct strength* of adrenaline injection is used; anaphylactic shock kits need to make a *very clear distinction* between the 1 in 10 000 strength and the 1 in 1000 strength.

Patients with severe allergy should be instructed in the self-administration of adrenaline by intramuscular injection.

Packs for self-administration need to be **clearly labelled with instructions** on how to administer adrenaline (intramuscularly, preferably at the midpoint of the outer thigh, through light clothing if necessary) so that in the case of rapid collapse someone else is able to give it. It is important to ensure individuals at risk and their carers understand that:

● two injection devices should be carried at all times to treat symptoms until medical assistance is available; if, after the first injection, the individual does not start to feel better, the second injection should be given 5 to 15 minutes after the first;

● an ambulance should be called after every administration, even if symptoms improve;

● the individual should lie down with their legs raised (unless they have breathing difficulties, in which case they should sit up) and should not be left alone.

Adrenaline for administration by intramuscular injection is available in 'auto-injectors' (e.g. *Emerade®*, *EpiPen®*, or *Jext®*), pre-assembled syringes fitted with a needle suitable for very rapid administration (if necessary by a bystander or a healthcare provider if it is the only preparation available); injection technique is device specific.

To ensure patients receive the auto-injector device that they have been trained to use, prescribers should specify the brand to be dispensed.

● PATIENT AND CARER ADVICE

Medicines for Children leaflet: Adrenaline auto-injector for anaphylaxis www.medicinesforchildren.org.uk/adrenaline-for-anaplyaxis

▸ With intramuscular use Individuals at considerable risk of anaphylaxis need to carry (or have available) adrenaline at all times and the patient, or their carers, need to be *instructed in advance* when and how to inject it.

The MHRA has produced an advice sheet on the use of adrenaline auto-injectors, which should be provided to patients and their carers.

JEXT® 300 MICROGRAMS 1.1 mL of the solution remains in the auto-injector device after use.

JEXT® 150 MICROGRAMS 1.25 mL of the solution remains in the auto-injector device after use.

EPIPEN® JR AUTO-INJECTOR 0.15MG 1.7 mL of the solution remains in the auto-injector device after use.

EMERADE® 150 MICROGRAMS 0.35 mL of the solution remains in the auto-injector device after use.

EMERADE® 500 MICROGRAMS No solution remains in the auto-injector device after use.

EMERADE® 300 MICROGRAMS 0.2 mL of the solution remains in the auto-injector device after use.

EPIPEN® AUTO-INJECTOR 0.3MG 1.7 mL of the solution remains in the auto-injector device after use.

● EXCEPTIONS TO LEGAL CATEGORY POM restriction does not apply to the intramuscular administration of up to 1 mg of adrenaline injection 1 in 1000 (1 mg/mL) for the emergency treatment of anaphylaxis.

● MEDICINAL FORMS
There can be variation in the licensing of different medicines containing the same drug. Forms available from special-order manufacturers include: solution for injection

Solution for injection

EXCIPIENTS: May contain Sulfites

▸ Adrenaline/epinephrine (Non-proprietary)

Adrenaline 100 microgram per 1 ml Adrenaline (base) 100micrograms/1ml (1 in 10,000) dilute solution for injection ampoules | 10 ampoule [PoM] £69.40

Adrenaline (base) 1mg/10ml (1 in 10,000) dilute solution for injection pre-filled syringes | 1 pre-filled disposable injection [PoM] £6.87 | 1 pre-filled disposable injection [PoM] £18.00 (Hospital only) | 10 pre-filled disposable injection [PoM] £180.00 (Hospital only)

Adrenaline (as Adrenaline acid tartrate) 100 microgram per 1 ml Adrenaline (base) 1mg/10ml (1 in 10,000) dilute solution for injection ampoules | 1 ampoule [PoM] £43.53 | 10 ampoule [PoM] £80.44

Adrenaline (base) 500micrograms/5ml (1 in 10,000) dilute solution for injection ampoules | 10 ampoule [PoM] £73.94

2

Adrenaline 1 mg per 1 ml Adrenaline (base) 10mg/10ml (1 in 1,000) solution for injection ampoules | 10 ampoule PoM £87.62
Adrenaline (base) for anaphylaxis 1mg/1ml (1 in 1,000) solution for injection pre-filled syringes | 1 pre-filled disposable injection PoM £10.40
Adrenaline (base) 1mg/1ml (1 in 1,000) solution for injection pre-filled syringes | 1 pre-filled disposable injection PoM £10.40
Adrenaline (as Adrenaline acid tartrate) 1 mg per 1 ml Adrenaline (base) 5mg/5ml (1 in 1,000) solution for injection ampoules | 10 ampoule PoM £85.07
Adrenaline (base) 500micrograms/0.5ml (1 in 1,000) solution for injection ampoules | 10 ampoule PoM £67.72 DT = £67.72
Adrenaline (base) 1mg/1ml (1 in 1,000) solution for injection ampoules | 10 ampoule PoM £6.01 DT = £6.01

▸ Emerade (Bausch & Lomb UK Ltd)
Adrenaline 1 mg per 1 ml Emerade 300micrograms/0.3ml (1 in 1,000) solution for injection auto-injectors | 1 pre-filled disposable injection PoM £25.99 DT = £26.45
Adrenaline (as Adrenaline acid tartrate) 1 mg per 1 ml Emerade 150micrograms/0.15ml (1 in 1,000) solution for injection auto-injectors | 1 pre-filled disposable injection PoM £25.99 DT = £23.99
Emerade 500micrograms/0.5ml (1 in 1,000) solution for injection auto-injectors | 1 pre-filled disposable injection PoM £26.99

▸ EpiPen (Meda Pharmaceuticals Ltd)
Adrenaline 500 microgram per 1 ml EpiPen Jr. 150micrograms/0.3ml (1 in 2,000) solution for injection auto-injectors | 1 pre-filled disposable injection PoM £26.45 DT = £26.45 | 2 pre-filled disposable injection PoM £52.90 DT = £52.90
Adrenaline 1 mg per 1 ml EpiPen 300micrograms/0.3ml (1 in 1,000) solution for injection auto-injectors | 1 pre-filled disposable injection PoM £26.45 DT = £26.45 | 2 pre-filled disposable injection PoM £52.90

▸ Jext (ALK-Abello Ltd)
Adrenaline 1 mg per 1 ml Jext 300micrograms/0.3ml (1 in 1,000) solution for injection auto-injectors | 1 pre-filled disposable injection PoM £23.99 DT = £26.45
Adrenaline (as Adrenaline acid tartrate) 1 mg per 1 ml Jext 150micrograms/0.15ml (1 in 1,000) solution for injection auto-injectors | 1 pre-filled disposable injection PoM £23.99 DT = £23.99

8 Oedema

Diuretics

Overview

Thiazides are used to relieve oedema due to chronic heart failure and, in lower doses, to reduce blood pressure.

Loop diuretics are used in pulmonary oedema due to left ventricular failure and in patients with chronic heart failure.

Combination diuretic therapy may be effective in patients with oedema resistant to treatment with one diuretic. Vigorous diuresis, particularly with loop diuretics, may induce acute hypotension; rapid reduction of plasma volume should be avoided.

Thiazides and related diuretics

Thiazides and related compounds are moderately potent diuretics; they inhibit sodium reabsorption at the beginning of the distal convoluted tubule. They act within 1 to 2 hours of oral administration and most have a duration of action of 12 to 24 hours; they are usually administered early in the day so that the diuresis does not interfere with sleep.

In the management of *hypertension* a low dose of a thiazide produces a maximal or near-maximal blood pressure lowering effect, with very little biochemical disturbance. Higher doses cause more marked changes in plasma potassium, sodium, uric acid, glucose, and lipids, with little advantage in blood pressure control. Chlortalidone p. 229 and indapamide p. 166 are the preferred diuretics in the management of hypertension. Thiazides also have a role in chronic heart failure.

Bendroflumethiazide p. 165 can be used for mild or moderate heart failure; it is licensed for the treatment of hypertension but is no longer considered the first-line

diuretic for this indication, although patients with stable and controlled blood pressure currently taking bendroflumethiazide can continue treatment.

Chlortalidone, a thiazide-related compound, has a longer duration of action than the thiazides and may be given on alternate days to control oedema. It is also useful if acute retention is liable to be precipitated by a more rapid diuresis or if patients dislike the altered pattern of micturition caused by other diuretics. Chlortalidone can also be used under close supervision for the treatment of ascites due to cirrhosis in stable patients.

Xipamide p. 231 and indapamide are chemically related to chlortalidone. Indapamide is claimed to lower blood pressure with less metabolic disturbance, particularly less aggravation of diabetes mellitus.

Metolazone p. 230 is particularly effective when combined with a loop diuretic (even in renal failure); profound diuresis can occur and the patient should therefore be monitored carefully.

The thiazide diuretics benzthiazide, clopamide, cyclopenthiazide p. 230, hydrochlorothiazide, and hydroflumethiazide do not offer any significant advantage over other thiazides and related diuretics.

Loop diuretics

Loop diuretics are used in pulmonary oedema due to left ventricular failure; intravenous administration produces relief of breathlessness and reduces pre-load sooner than would be expected from the time of onset of diuresis. Loop diuretics are also used in patients with chronic heart failure. Diuretic-resistant oedema (except lymphoedema and oedema due to peripheral venous stasis or calcium-channel blockers) can be treated with a loop diuretic combined with a thiazide or related diuretic (e.g. bendroflumethiazide or metolazone).

If necessary, a loop diuretic can be added to antihypertensive treatment to achieve better control of blood pressure in those with resistant hypertension, or in patients with impaired renal function or heart failure.

Loop diuretics can exacerbate diabetes (but hyperglycaemia is less likely than with thiazides) and gout. If there is an enlarged prostate, urinary retention can occur, although this is less likely if small doses and less potent diuretics are used initially.

Furosemide p. 226 and bumetanide p. 225 are similar in activity; both act within 1 hour of oral administration and diuresis is complete within 6 hours so that, if necessary, they can be given twice in one day without interfering with sleep. Following intravenous administration furosemide has a peak effect within 30 minutes. The diuresis associated with these drugs is dose related.

Torasemide p. 227 has properties similar to those of furosemide and bumetanide, and is indicated for oedema and for hypertension.

Potassium-sparing diuretics and aldosterone antagonists

Amiloride hydrochloride p. 228 and triamterene p. 229 on their own are weak diuretics. They cause retention of potassium and are therefore given with thiazide or loop diuretics as a more effective alternative to potassium supplements. See compound preparations with thiazides or loop diuretics.

Potassium supplements must **not** be given with potassium-sparing diuretics. Administration of a potassium sparing diuretic to a patient receiving an ACE inhibitor or an angiotensin-II receptor antagonist can also cause severe hyperkalaemia.

Aldosterone antagonists

Spironolactone p. 190 potentiates thiazide or loop diuretics by antagonising aldosterone; it is a potassium-sparing diuretic. Spironolactone is of value in the treatment of oedema and ascites caused by cirrhosis of the liver; furosemide can be used as an adjunct. Low doses of spironolactone are beneficial in moderate to severe heart failure and when used in resistant hypertension [unlicensed indication].

Spironolactone is also used in primary hyperaldosteronism (Conn's syndrome). It is given before surgery or if surgery is not appropriate, in the lowest effective dose for maintenance.

Eplerenone p. 190 is licensed for use as an adjunct in left ventricular dysfunction with evidence of heart failure after a myocardial infarction; it is also licensed as an adjunct in chronic mild heart failure with left ventricular systolic dysfunction.

Potassium supplements must **not** be given with aldosterone antagonists

Potassium-sparing diuretics with other diuretics

Although it is preferable to prescribe thiazides and potassium-sparing diuretics separately, the use of fixed combinations may be justified if compliance is a problem. Potassium-sparing diuretics are not usually necessary in the routine treatment of hypertension, unless hypokalaemia develops.

Other diuretics

Mannitol p. 228 is an osmotic diuretic that can be used to treat cerebral oedema and raised intra-ocular pressure.

Mercurial diuretics are effective but are now almost never used because of their nephrotoxicity.

The carbonic anhydrase inhibitor acetazolamide p. 1147 is a weak diuretic and is little used for its diuretic effect. It is used for prophylaxis against mountain sickness [unlicensed indication] but is not a substitute for acclimatisation.

Eye drops of dorzolamide p. 1148 and brinzolamide p. 1147 inhibit the formation of aqueous humour and are used in glaucoma.

Diuretics with potassium

Many patients on diuretics do not need potassium supplements. For many of those who do, the amount of potassium in combined preparations may not be enough, and for this reason their use is to be discouraged.

Diuretics with potassium and potassium-sparing diuretics should **not** usually be given together. Diuretics and potassium supplements should be prescribed separately for children.

> **Other drugs used for Oedema** Diamorphine hydrochloride, p. 449

DIURETICS > LOOP DIURETICS

Loop diuretics

- DRUG ACTION Loop diuretics inhibit reabsorption from the ascending limb of the loop of Henlé in the renal tubule and are powerful diuretics.

- CONTRA-INDICATIONS Anuria · comatose and precomatose states associated with liver cirrhosis · renal failure due to nephrotoxic or hepatotoxic drugs · severe hypokalaemia · severe hyponatraemia

- CAUTIONS Can exacerbate diabetes (but hyperglycaemia less likely than with thiazides) · can exacerbate gout · hypotension should be corrected before initiation of treatment · hypovolaemia should be corrected before initiation of treatment · urinary retention can occur in prostatic hyperplasia

CAUTIONS, FURTHER INFORMATION
▸ Elderly Lower initial doses of diuretics should be used in the elderly because they are particularly susceptible to the

side-effects. The dose should then be adjusted according to renal function. Diuretics should not be used continuously on a long-term basis to treat simple gravitational oedema (which will usually respond to increased movement, raising the legs, and support stockings).

▸ Potassium loss Hypokalaemia can occur with both thiazide and loop diuretics. The risk of hypokalaemia depends on the duration of action as well as the potency and is thus greater with thiazides than with an equipotent dose of a loop diuretic.

Hypokalaemia is dangerous in severe cardiovascular disease and in patients also being treated with cardiac glycosides. Often the use of potassium-sparing diuretics avoids the need to take potassium supplements.

In hepatic failure, hypokalaemia caused by diuretics can precipitate encephalopathy, particularly in alcoholic cirrhosis.

▸ Urinary retention If there is an enlarged prostate, urinary retention is less likely, although this is less likely if small doses and less potent diuretics are used initially; an adequate urinary output should be established before initiating treatment.

- SIDE-EFFECTS
▸ **Common or very common** Asthenia · dehydration · dizziness · electrolyte imbalance · gastrointestinal disorder · headache · hypotension · metabolic alkalosis · muscle complaints · nausea · skin reactions
▸ **Uncommon** Bladder dilation · breast pain · chest discomfort · diarrhoea · ear pain · urinary disorders · vertigo
▸ **Rare or very rare** Bone marrow disorders · hearing impairment · photosensitivity reaction
▸ **Frequency not known** Acute kidney injury · agranulocytosis · anaemia · arthralgia · auditory disorder (more common with rapid intravenous administration, and in renal impairment) · cerebral ischaemia · confusion · deafness (more common in renal impairment) · diabetes mellitus · dry mouth · embolism · encephalopathy · eosinophilia · fever · gastrointestinal discomfort · gout · gynaecomastia · haemolytic anaemia · hepatic disorders · hyperglycaemia · hyperuricaemia · ischaemic heart disease · leucopenia · malaise · metabolic acidosis · mucosal reaction · musculoskeletal pain (with high doses in renal failure) · myocardial infarction · nephritis tubulointerstitial · pancreatitis · paraesthesia · psychiatric disorder · severe cutaneous adverse reactions (SCARs) · shock · syncope · tetany · thrombocytopenia · tinnitus (more common with rapid intravenous administration, and in renal impairment) · vasculitis · visual impairment · vomiting

- HEPATIC IMPAIRMENT Hypokalaemia induced by loop diuretics may precipitate hepatic encephalopathy and coma—potassium-sparing diuretics can be used to prevent this. Diuretics can increase the risk of hypomagnesaemia in alcoholic cirrhosis, leading to arrhythmias.

- RENAL IMPAIRMENT High doses or rapid intravenous administration can cause tinnitus and deafness.
Dose adjustments High doses of loop diuretics may occasionally be needed in renal impairment.

- MONITORING REQUIREMENTS Monitor electrolytes during treatment.

◤ above

Bumetanide

- INDICATIONS AND DOSE
Oedema
▸ BY MOUTH
▸ Adult: 1 mg, dose to be taken in the morning, then 1 mg after 6–8 hours if required
▸ Elderly: 500 micrograms daily, this lower dose may be sufficient in elderly patients continued →

2

Cardiovascular system

Oedema, severe cases
▶ BY MOUTH
▶ Adult: Initially 5 mg daily, increased in steps of 5 mg every 12–24 hours, adjusted according to response

● INTERACTIONS → Appendix 1: loop diuretics

● PREGNANCY Bumetanide should not be used to treat gestational hypertension because of the maternal hypovolaemia associated with this condition.

● BREAST FEEDING No information available. May inhibit lactation.

● MEDICINAL FORMS
There can be variation in the licensing of different medicines containing the same drug. Forms available from special-order manufacturers include: oral suspension

Oral solution
▶ Bumetanide (Non-proprietary)
Bumetanide 200 microgram per 1 ml Bumetanide 1mg/5ml oral solution sugar free sugar-free | 150 ml [PoM] £198.00 DT = £198.00

Tablet
▶ Bumetanide (Non-proprietary)
Bumetanide 1 mg Bumetanide 1mg tablets | 28 tablet [PoM] £7.35 DT = £1.20
Bumetanide 5 mg Bumetanide 5mg tablets | 28 tablet [PoM] £7.00 DT = £6.98

Combinations available: *Amiloride with bumetanide*, p. 229

Co-amilofruse

● INDICATIONS AND DOSE
Oedema
▶ BY MOUTH
▶ Adult: 2.5/20–10/80 mg daily, dose to be taken in the morning

DOSE EQUIVALENCE AND CONVERSION
▶ A mixture of amiloride hydrochloride and furosemide (frusemide) in the mass proportions of 1 part amiloride hydrochloride to 8 parts furosemide (frusemide).

● CONTRA-INDICATIONS Addison's disease · anuria · comatose or precomatose states associated with liver cirrhosis · dehydration · hyperkalaemia · hypovolaemia · renal failure · severe hypokalaemia · severe hyponatraemia

● CAUTIONS Correct hypovolaemia before using in oliguria · diabetes mellitus · elderly · gout · hepatorenal syndrome · hypoproteinaemia · hypotension · impaired micturition · prostatic enlargement

● INTERACTIONS → Appendix 1: loop diuretics · potassium-sparing diuretics

● PREGNANCY Not used to treat hypertension in pregnancy.

● BREAST FEEDING Manufacturers advise avoid—no information regarding amiloride component available. Amount of furosemide in milk too small to be harmful. Furosemide may inhibit lactation.

● HEPATIC IMPAIRMENT Increased risk of hypomagnesaemia in alcoholic cirrhosis.

● RENAL IMPAIRMENT Risk of hyperkalaemia in renal impairment but may need higher doses. Avoid if eGFR less than 30 mL/minute/1.73 m².
Monitoring Monitor plasma-potassium concentration.

● MONITORING REQUIREMENTS Monitor electrolytes.

● MEDICINAL FORMS
There can be variation in the licensing of different medicines containing the same drug. Forms available from special-order manufacturers include: oral suspension, oral solution

Tablet
▶ Co-amilofruse (Non-proprietary)
Amiloride hydrochloride 2.5 mg, Furosemide 20 mg Co-amilofruse 2.5mg/20mg tablets | 28 tablet [PoM] £6.00 DT = £5.20 | 56 tablet [PoM] £4.01–£10.40
Amiloride hydrochloride 5 mg, Furosemide 40 mg Co-amilofruse 5mg/40mg tablets | 28 tablet [PoM] £7.50 DT = £6.67 | 56 tablet [PoM] £4.01–£13.34
Amiloride hydrochloride 10 mg, Furosemide 80 mg Co-amilofruse 10mg/80mg tablets | 28 tablet [PoM] £15.52 DT = £15.52
▶ Frumil (Sanofi)
Amiloride hydrochloride 2.5 mg, Furosemide 20 mg Frumil LS 20mg/2.5mg tablets | 28 tablet [PoM] £4.32 DT = £5.20
Amiloride hydrochloride 5 mg, Furosemide 40 mg Frumil 40mg/5mg tablets | 28 tablet [PoM] £5.29 DT = £6.67

☞ 225

Furosemide

(Frusemide)

● INDICATIONS AND DOSE
Oedema
▶ BY MOUTH
▶ Adult: Initially 40 mg daily, dose to be taken in the morning, then maintenance 20–40 mg daily
▶ INITIALLY BY INTRAMUSCULAR INJECTION, OR BY SLOW INTRAVENOUS INJECTION, OR BY INTRAVENOUS INFUSION
▶ Adult: Initially 20–50 mg, then (by intramuscular injection or by intravenous injection or by intravenous infusion) increased in steps of 20 mg every 2 hours if required, doses greater than 50 mg given by intravenous infusion only; maximum 1.5 g per day

Resistant oedema
▶ BY MOUTH
▶ Adult: 80–120 mg daily
▶ INITIALLY BY INTRAMUSCULAR INJECTION, OR BY SLOW INTRAVENOUS INJECTION, OR BY INTRAVENOUS INFUSION
▶ Adult: Initially 20–50 mg, then (by intramuscular injection or by intravenous injection or by intravenous infusion) increased in steps of 20 mg every 2 hours if required, doses greater than 50 mg given by intravenous infusion only; maximum 1.5 g per day

Resistant hypertension
▶ BY MOUTH
▶ Adult: 40–80 mg daily
▶ INITIALLY BY INTRAMUSCULAR INJECTION, OR BY SLOW INTRAVENOUS INJECTION, OR BY INTRAVENOUS INFUSION
▶ Adult: Initially 20–50 mg, then (by intramuscular injection or by intravenous injection or by intravenous infusion) increased in steps of 20 mg every 2 hours if required, doses greater than 50 mg given by intravenous infusion only; maximum 1.5 g per day

● CAUTIONS Hepatorenal syndrome · hypoproteinaemia may reduce diuretic effect and increase risk of side-effects

● INTERACTIONS → Appendix 1: loop diuretics

● PREGNANCY Furosemide should not be used to treat gestational hypertension because of the maternal hypovolaemia associated with this condition.

● BREAST FEEDING Amount too small to be harmful. May inhibit lactation.

● DIRECTIONS FOR ADMINISTRATION Intravenous administration rate should not usually exceed 4 mg/minute however single doses of up to 80 mg may be administered more rapidly; a lower rate of infusion may be necessary in renal impairment.

● MEDICINAL FORMS
There can be variation in the licensing of different medicines containing the same drug. Forms available from special-order manufacturers include: oral suspension, oral solution

Tablet
▸ Furosemide (Non-proprietary)
   Furosemide 20 mg Furosemide 20mg tablets | 28 tablet [PoM]
   £1.02 DT = £0.37
   Furosemide 40 mg Furosemide 40mg tablets | 28 tablet [PoM]
   £1.03 DT = £0.33 | 1000 tablet [PoM] £11.79–£28.21
   Furosemide 500 mg Furosemide 500mg tablets | 28 tablet [PoM]
   £70.00 DT = £38.58
▸ Diuresal (Ennogen Pharma Ltd)
   Furosemide 500 mg Diuresal 500mg tablets | 28 tablet [PoM] [℥] DT
   = £38.58

Solution for injection
▸ Furosemide (Non-proprietary)
   Furosemide 10 mg per 1 ml Furosemide 250mg/25ml solution for
   injection ampoules | 10 ampoule [PoM] £25.00–£40.00
   Furosemide 50mg/5ml solution for injection ampoules |
   10 ampoule £2.38–£7.60
   Furosemide 20mg/2ml solution for injection ampoules |
   10 ampoule [PoM] £4.58 DT = £3.28

Oral solution
EXCIPIENTS: May contain Alcohol
▸ Furosemide (Non-proprietary)
   Furosemide 4 mg per 1 ml Furosemide 20mg/5ml oral solution
   sugar free sugar-free | 150 ml [PoM] £14.81 DT = £14.81
   Furosemide 8 mg per 1 ml Furosemide 40mg/5ml oral solution
   sugar free sugar-free | 150 ml [PoM] £19.57 DT = £19.57
   Furosemide 10 mg per 1 ml Furosemide 50mg/5ml oral solution
   sugar free sugar-free | 150 ml [PoM] £20.21 DT = £20.21
▸ Frusol (Rosemont Pharmaceuticals Ltd)
   Furosemide 4 mg per 1 ml Frusol 20mg/5ml oral solution sugar-free
   | 150 ml [PoM] £12.07 DT = £14.81
   Furosemide 8 mg per 1 ml Frusol 40mg/5ml oral solution sugar-free
   | 150 ml [PoM] £15.58 DT = £19.57
   Furosemide 10 mg per 1 ml Frusol 50mg/5ml oral solution sugar-
   free | 150 ml [PoM] £16.84 DT = £20.21

Combinations available: *Spironolactone with furosemide,*
p. 228

Furosemide with potassium chloride

The properties listed below are those particular to the combination only. For the properties of the components please consider, furosemide p. 226, potassium chloride p. 1025.

● INDICATIONS AND DOSE
Oedema
▸ BY MOUTH
▸ Adult: (consult product literature)

● INTERACTIONS → Appendix 1: loop diuretics · potassium chloride
● DIRECTIONS FOR ADMINISTRATION Furosemide with modified-release potassium chloride tablets should be swallowed whole with plenty of fluid during meals while sitting or standing.
● PATIENT AND CARER ADVICE Patients or carers should be given advice on how to administer furosemide with potassium chloride tablets.
● LESS SUITABLE FOR PRESCRIBING Furosemide with potassium chloride tablets are less suitable for prescribing.

● MEDICINAL FORMS
There can be variation in the licensing of different medicines containing the same drug.
Modified-release tablet
CAUTIONARY AND ADVISORY LABELS 25, 27
▸ Diumide-K Continus (Teofarma)
   Furosemide 40 mg, Potassium chloride 600 mg Diumide-K
   Continus tablets | 30 tablet [PoM] £3.00

Furosemide with triamterene

The properties listed below are those particular to the combination only. For the properties of the components please consider, furosemide p. 226, triamterene p. 229.

● INDICATIONS AND DOSE
Oedema
▸ BY MOUTH
▸ Adult: 0.5–2 tablets daily, dose to be taken in the morning

● CONTRA-INDICATIONS Anuria · comatose or precomatose states associated with liver cirrhosis · dehydration · hyperkalaemia · hypovolaemia · renal failure · severe hypokalaemia · severe hyponatraemia
● CAUTIONS Diabetes mellitus · elderly · gout · hepatorenal syndrome · hypotension · impaired micturition · may cause blue fluorescence of urine · prostatic enlargement
● INTERACTIONS → Appendix 1: loop diuretics · potassium-sparing diuretics
● BREAST FEEDING Triamterene present in milk—manufacturer advises avoid. Furosemide may inhibit lactation.
● HEPATIC IMPAIRMENT Increased risk of hypomagnesaemia in alcoholic cirrhosis. Hypokalaemia may precipitate coma.
● RENAL IMPAIRMENT Avoid in severe impairment.
   Dose adjustments May need high doses.
   Monitoring Monitor plasma-potassium concentration in renal impairment (high risk of hyperkalaemia).
● MONITORING REQUIREMENTS Monitor electrolytes.
● PATIENT AND CARER ADVICE Urine may look slightly blue in some lights.

● MEDICINAL FORMS
There can be variation in the licensing of different medicines containing the same drug.
Tablet
CAUTIONARY AND ADVISORY LABELS 14
▸ Frusene (Orion Pharma (UK) Ltd)
   Furosemide 40 mg, Triamterene 50 mg Frusene 50mg/40mg
   tablets | 56 tablet [PoM] £4.34 DT = £4.34

⯈ 225

Torasemide

● INDICATIONS AND DOSE
Oedema
▸ BY MOUTH
▸ Adult: 5 mg once daily, to be taken preferably in the morning, then increased if necessary to 20 mg once daily; maximum 40 mg per day

Hypertension
▸ BY MOUTH
▸ Adult: 2.5 mg daily, then increased if necessary to 5 mg once daily

● INTERACTIONS → Appendix 1: loop diuretics
● PREGNANCY Manufacturer advises avoid—toxicity in *animal* studies.
● BREAST FEEDING Manufacturer advises avoid—no information available.

● MEDICINAL FORMS
There can be variation in the licensing of different medicines containing the same drug.
Tablet
▸ Torasemide (Non-proprietary)
   Torasemide 5 mg Torasemide 5mg tablets | 28 tablet [PoM] £14.50
   DT = £5.53
   Torasemide 10 mg Torasemide 10mg tablets | 28 tablet [PoM]
   £18.50 DT = £8.14

Cardiovascular system

2

▸ Torem (Meda Pharmaceuticals Ltd)
Torasemide 2.5 mg Torem 2.5mg tablets | 28 tablet [PoM] £3.78 DT
= £3.78
Torasemide 5 mg Torem 5mg tablets | 28 tablet [PoM] £5.53 DT =
£5.53
Torasemide 10 mg Torem 10mg tablets | 28 tablet [PoM] £8.14 DT =
£8.14

DIURETICS > OSMOTIC DIURETICS

Mannitol

● **INDICATIONS AND DOSE**

Cerebral oedema
▸ **BY INTRAVENOUS INFUSION**
▸ Adult: 0.25–2 g/kg, repeated if necessary, to be
administered over 30–60 minutes, dose may be
repeated 1–2 times after 4–8 hours

Raised intra-ocular pressure
▸ **BY INTRAVENOUS INFUSION**
▸ Adult: 0.25–2 g/kg, repeated if necessary, to be
administered over 30–60 minutes, dose may be
repeated 1–2 times after 4–8 hours

● **CONTRA-INDICATIONS** Anuria · intracranial bleeding
(except during craniotomy) · severe cardiac failure · severe
dehydration · severe pulmonary oedema

● **CAUTIONS** Extravasation causes inflammation and
thrombophlebitis

● **SIDE-EFFECTS**
▸ **Common or very common** Cough · headache · vomiting
▸ **Uncommon** Dizziness · fever · malaise · nausea · pain · skin
reactions
▸ **Frequency not known** Arrhythmia · asthenia · azotaemia ·
chest pain · chills · coma · compartment syndrome ·
confusion · congestive heart failure · dry mouth ·
electrolyte imbalance · fluid imbalance · hyperhidrosis ·
hypersensitivity · hypertension · lethargy · metabolic
acidosis · muscle complaints · musculoskeletal stiffness ·
nephrotic syndrome · neurotoxicity · peripheral oedema ·
pulmonary oedema · rebound intracranial pressure
increase · renal impairment · rhinitis · seizure · thirst ·
urinary disorders · vision blurred

● **PREGNANCY** Manufacturer advises avoid unless
essential— no information available.

● **BREAST FEEDING** Manufacturer advises avoid unless
essential—no information available.

● **RENAL IMPAIRMENT** Use with caution in severe
impairment.

● **PRE-TREATMENT SCREENING** Assess cardiac function
before treatment.

● **MONITORING REQUIREMENTS** Monitor fluid and electrolyte
balance, serum osmolality, and cardiac, pulmonary and
renal function.

● **DIRECTIONS FOR ADMINISTRATION** For mannitol 20%, an
in-line filter is recommended (15-micron filters have been
used).

● **MEDICINAL FORMS**
There can be variation in the licensing of different medicines
containing the same drug. Forms available from special-order
manufacturers include: infusion, solution for infusion

Infusion
▸ Mannitol (Non-proprietary)
Mannitol 100 mg per 1 ml Mannitol 50g/500ml (10%) infusion Viaflo
bags | 1 bag [PoM] [℞]
Mannitol 50g/500ml (10%) infusion Viaflex bags | 1 bag [PoM] [℞]
Polyfusor K mannitol 10% infusion 500ml bottles | 1 bottle [PoM]
£4.92
Mannitol 150 mg per 1 ml Mannitol 75g/500ml (15%) infusion Viaflo
bags | 20 bag [PoM] [℞]

Mannitol 200 mg per 1 ml Polyfusor M mannitol 20% infusion
500ml bottles | 1 bottle [PoM] £6.46
Mannitol 100g/500ml (20%) infusion Viaflex bags | 1 bag [PoM] [℞]
Mannitol 50g/250ml (20%) infusion Viaflex bags | 1 bag [PoM] [℞]
Mannitol 100g/500ml (20%) infusion Viaflo bags | 1 bag [PoM] [℞]

DIURETICS > POTASSIUM-SPARING DIURETICS > ALDOSTERONE ANTAGONISTS

Spironolactone with furosemide

The properties listed below are those particular to the
combination only. For the properties of the components
please consider, spironolactone p. 190, furosemide p. 226.

● **INDICATIONS AND DOSE**

Resistant oedema
▸ **BY MOUTH**
▸ Adult: 20/50–80/200 mg daily

● **INTERACTIONS** → Appendix 1: aldosterone antagonists ·
loop diuretics

● **MEDICINAL FORMS**
There can be variation in the licensing of different medicines
containing the same drug.
Capsule
▸ Lasilactone (Sanofi)
Furosemide 20 mg, Spironolactone 50 mg Lasilactone 20mg/50mg
capsules | 28 capsule [PoM] £7.97

DIURETICS > POTASSIUM-SPARING DIURETICS > OTHER

Amiloride hydrochloride

● **INDICATIONS AND DOSE**

Oedema (monotherapy)
▸ **BY MOUTH**
▸ Adult: Initially 10 mg daily, alternatively initially 5 mg
twice daily, adjusted according to response; maximum
20 mg per day

**Potassium conservation when used as an adjunct to
thiazide or loop diuretics for hypertension or congestive
heart failure**
▸ **BY MOUTH**
▸ Adult: Initially 5–10 mg daily

**Potassium conservation when used as an adjunct to
thiazide or loop diuretics for hepatic cirrhosis with
ascites**
▸ **BY MOUTH**
▸ Adult: Initially 5 mg daily

● **CONTRA-INDICATIONS** Addison's disease · anuria ·
hyperkalaemia

● **CAUTIONS** Diabetes mellitus · elderly

● **INTERACTIONS** → Appendix 1: potassium-sparing diuretics

● **SIDE-EFFECTS** Alopecia · angina pectoris · aplastic anaemia
· appetite decreased · arrhythmia · arthralgia · asthenia ·
atrioventricular block exacerbated · bladder spasm · chest
pain · confusion · constipation · cough · depression ·
diarrhoea · dizziness · drowsiness · dry mouth · dyspnoea ·
dysuria · electrolyte imbalance · encephalopathy ·
gastrointestinal discomfort · gastrointestinal disorders ·
gastrointestinal haemorrhage · gout · headache · insomnia ·
jaundice · muscle cramps · nasal congestion · nausea ·
nervousness · neutropenia · pain · palpitations ·
paraesthesia · postural hypotension · sexual dysfunction ·
skin reactions · tinnitus · tremor · vertigo · visual
impairment · vomiting

● **PREGNANCY** Not to be used to treat gestational
hypertension.

- BREAST FEEDING Manufacturer advises avoid—no information available.
- RENAL IMPAIRMENT Manufacturers advise avoid in severe impairment.
  Monitoring Monitor plasma-potassium concentration (high risk of hyperkalaemia in renal impairment).
- MONITORING REQUIREMENTS Monitor electrolytes.

- MEDICINAL FORMS
  There can be variation in the licensing of different medicines containing the same drug. Forms available from special-order manufacturers include: oral suspension, oral solution
  Oral solution
  EXCIPIENTS: May contain Propylene glycol
  ▸ Amiloride hydrochloride (Non-proprietary)
  Amiloride hydrochloride 1 mg per 1 ml Amiloride 5mg/5ml oral solution sugar free sugar-free | 150 ml [PoM] £37.35 DT = £37.35
  Tablet
  ▸ Amiloride hydrochloride (Non-proprietary)
  Amiloride hydrochloride 5 mg Amiloride 5mg tablets | 28 tablet [PoM] £13.99 DT = £3.24

  Combinations available: *Co-amilofruse*, p. 226

Amiloride with bumetanide

The properties listed below are those particular to the combination only. For the properties of the components please consider, amiloride hydrochloride p. 228, bumetanide p. 225.

- INDICATIONS AND DOSE
  Oedema
  ▸ BY MOUTH
  ▸ Adult: 1–2 tablets daily

- INTERACTIONS → Appendix 1: loop diuretics · potassium-sparing diuretics

- MEDICINAL FORMS
  There can be variation in the licensing of different medicines containing the same drug.
  Tablet
  ▸ Amiloride with bumetanide (Non-proprietary)
  Bumetanide 1 mg, Amiloride hydrochloride 5 mg Amiloride 5mg / Bumetanide 1mg tablets | 28 tablet [PoM] £56.00 DT = £56.00

Triamterene

- INDICATIONS AND DOSE
  Oedema | Potassium conservation with thiazide and loop diuretics
  ▸ BY MOUTH
  ▸ Adult: Initially 150–250 mg daily for 1 week, lower initial dose when given with other diuretics, then reduced to 150–250 mg daily on alternate days, to be taken in divided doses after breakfast and lunch

- CONTRA-INDICATIONS Addison's disease · anuria · hyperkalaemia
- CAUTIONS Diabetes mellitus · elderly · gout · may cause blue fluorescence of urine
- INTERACTIONS → Appendix 1: potassium-sparing diuretics
- SIDE-EFFECTS
  ▸ **Common or very common** Diarrhoea · hyperkalaemia · nausea · vomiting
  ▸ **Uncommon** Dry mouth · headache · hyperuricaemia · renal failure (reversible on discontinuation) · skin reactions
  ▸ **Rare or very rare** Megaloblastic anaemia · nephritis tubulointerstitial · pancytopenia · photosensitivity reaction · serum sickness · urolithiasis
  ▸ **Frequency not known** Asthenia · jaundice · metabolic acidosis

- PREGNANCY Not used to treat gestational hypertension. Avoid unless essential.
- BREAST FEEDING Present in milk—manufacturer advises avoid.
- HEPATIC IMPAIRMENT Use with caution. Avoid in progressive impairment.
- RENAL IMPAIRMENT Avoid in progressive impairment.
  Monitoring Monitor plasma-potassium concentration (high risk of hyperkalaemia in renal impairment).
- MONITORING REQUIREMENTS Monitor electrolytes.
- PATIENT AND CARER ADVICE Urine may look slightly blue in some lights.

- MEDICINAL FORMS
  There can be variation in the licensing of different medicines containing the same drug.
  Capsule
  CAUTIONARY AND ADVISORY LABELS 14, 21
  ▸ Triamterene (Non-proprietary)
  Triamterene 50 mg Triamterene 50mg capsules | 30 capsule [PoM] £41.90 DT = £41.90

  Combinations available: *Co-triamterzide*, p. 230 · *Furosemide with triamterene*, p. 227

Triamterene with chlortalidone

The properties listed below are those particular to the combination only. For the properties of the components please consider, triamterene above, chlortalidone below.

- INDICATIONS AND DOSE
  Hypertension | Oedema
  ▸ BY MOUTH
  ▸ Adult: 50/50–100/100 mg once daily, dose to be taken in the morning
  DOSE EQUIVALENCE AND CONVERSION
  ▸ Dose expressed as x/y mg of triamterene/chlortalidone.

- INTERACTIONS → Appendix 1: potassium-sparing diuretics · thiazide diuretics

- MEDICINAL FORMS
  There can be variation in the licensing of different medicines containing the same drug.
  Tablet
  CAUTIONARY AND ADVISORY LABELS 14, 21
  ▸ Kalspare (DHP Healthcare Ltd)
  Chlortalidone 50 mg, Triamterene 50 mg Kalspare tablets | 28 tablet [PoM] £9.90

DIURETICS ❭ THIAZIDES AND RELATED DIURETICS

⌐ 165

Chlortalidone

(Chlorthalidone)

- INDICATIONS AND DOSE
  Ascites due to cirrhosis in stable patients (under close supervision) | Oedema due to nephrotic syndrome
  ▸ BY MOUTH
  ▸ Adult: Up to 50 mg daily
  Hypertension
  ▸ BY MOUTH
  ▸ Adult: 25 mg daily, dose to be taken in the morning, then increased if necessary to 50 mg daily
  Mild to moderate chronic heart failure
  ▸ BY MOUTH
  ▸ Adult: 25–50 mg daily, dose to be taken in the morning, then increased if necessary to 100–200 mg daily, reduce to lowest effective dose for maintenance
  continued →

Nephrogenic diabetes insipidus | Partial pituitary diabetes insipidus

▸ BY MOUTH
▸ Adult: Initially 100 mg twice daily, then reduced to 50 mg daily

● INTERACTIONS → Appendix 1: thiazide diuretics
● SIDE-EFFECTS
▸ **Common or very common** Appetite decreased · dizziness · electrolyte imbalance · erectile dysfunction · gastrointestinal discomfort · hyperglycaemia · hyperuricaemia · skin reactions
▸ **Uncommon** Gout
▸ **Rare or very rare** Agranulocytosis · alkalosis hypochloraemic · arrhythmia · diabetes mellitus exacerbated · diarrhoea · eosinophilia · glycosuria · hepatic disorders · nausea · nephritis tubulointerstitial · pancreatitis · paraesthesia · photosensitivity reaction · pulmonary oedema · respiratory disorder · vomiting
● BREAST FEEDING The amount present in milk is too small to be harmful. Large doses may suppress lactation.

● MEDICINAL FORMS
There can be variation in the licensing of different medicines containing the same drug. Forms available from special-order manufacturers include: oral suspension
Tablet
▸ Chlortalidone (Non-proprietary)
  Chlortalidone 25 mg Chlortalidone 25mg tablets | 100 tablet [PoM] [S]
  Chlortalidone 50 mg Chlortalidone 50mg tablets | 30 tablet [PoM] £90.55 DT = £88.04

Combinations available: *Triamterene with chlortalidone*, p. 229

Co-triamterzide

The properties listed below are those particular to the combination only. For the properties of the components please consider, triamterene p. 229, hydrochlorothiazide p. 166.

● INDICATIONS AND DOSE
Hypertension
▸ BY MOUTH
▸ Adult: 50/25 mg daily, increased if necessary up to 200/100 mg daily, dose to be taken after breakfast
Oedema
▸ BY MOUTH
▸ Adult: 50/25 mg twice daily, to be taken after breakfast and after midday meal, increased if necessary to 150/75 mg daily, to be taken as 100/50 mg after breakfast and 50/25 mg after midday meal; maintenance 50/25 mg daily, alternatively maintenance 100/50 mg once daily on alternate days; maximum 200/100 mg per day
DOSE EQUIVALENCE AND CONVERSION
▸ Dose expressed as x/y mg of triamterene/hydrochlorothiazide.

● INTERACTIONS → Appendix 1: potassium-sparing diuretics · thiazide diuretics
● PATIENT AND CARER ADVICE Urine may look slightly blue in some lights.

● MEDICINAL FORMS
There can be variation in the licensing of different medicines containing the same drug.
Tablet
CAUTIONARY AND ADVISORY LABELS 14, 21
▸ Dyazide (AMCo)
  Hydrochlorothiazide 25 mg, Triamterene 50 mg Dyazide 50mg/25mg tablets | 30 tablet [PoM] £0.95 DT = £0.95

Cyclopenthiazide

🏴 165

● INDICATIONS AND DOSE
Heart failure
▸ BY MOUTH
▸ Adult: 250–500 micrograms daily, take in the morning, then increased if necessary to 1 mg daily, reduce to lowest effective dose for maintenance
Hypertension
▸ BY MOUTH
▸ Adult: Initially 250 micrograms daily, take in the morning, then increased if necessary to 500 micrograms daily
Oedema
▸ BY MOUTH
▸ Adult: Up to 500 micrograms daily for a short period

● INTERACTIONS → Appendix 1: thiazide diuretics
● SIDE-EFFECTS Agranulocytosis · alkalosis hypochloraemic · appetite decreased · arrhythmia · bone marrow depression · cholestasis · consciousness impaired · cutaneous lupus erythematosus · depression · diabetes mellitus exacerbated · diarrhoea · dizziness · electrolyte imbalance · erectile dysfunction · gastrointestinal discomfort · glycosuria · gout · haemolytic anaemia · hyperglycaemia · hyperuricaemia · nausea · pancreatitis · paraesthesia · photosensitivity reaction · pulmonary oedema · respiratory disorders · skin reactions · sleep disorder · thrombocytopenic purpura · toxic epidermal necrolysis · vasculitis necrotising · visual impairment · vomiting
● BREAST FEEDING The amount present in milk is too small to be harmful. Large doses may suppress lactation.

● MEDICINAL FORMS
No licensed medicines listed.

Metolazone

🏴 165

● INDICATIONS AND DOSE
Oedema
▸ BY MOUTH
▸ Adult: 5–10 mg daily, dose to be taken in the morning; increased if necessary to 20 mg daily, dose increased in resistant oedema; maximum 80 mg per day
Hypertension
▸ BY MOUTH
▸ Adult: Initially 5 mg daily, dose to be taken in the morning; maintenance 5 mg once daily on alternate days

● CAUTIONS Acute porphyrias p. 1025
● INTERACTIONS → Appendix 1: thiazide diuretics
● SIDE-EFFECTS Chest pain · chills
● BREAST FEEDING The amount present in milk is too small to be harmful. Large doses may suppress lactation.
● DIRECTIONS FOR ADMINISTRATION Tablets may be crushed and mixed with water immediately before use.

● MEDICINAL FORMS
There can be variation in the licensing of different medicines containing the same drug. Forms available from special-order manufacturers include: tablet, oral suspension, oral solution
Tablet
▸ Zaroxolyn (Imported (Canada))
  Metolazone 2.5 mg Zaroxolyn 2.5mg tablets | 100 tablet [PoM] [S]
  Metolazone 5 mg Zaroxolyn 5mg tablets | 50 tablet [PoM] [S]

⚑ 165

Xipamide

● **INDICATIONS AND DOSE**

Oedema

▶ BY MOUTH

▸ Adult: Initially 40 mg daily, dose to be taken in the morning, increased if necessary to 80 mg daily, higher dose to be used in resistant cases; maintenance 20 mg daily, dose to be taken in the morning

Hypertension

▶ BY MOUTH

▸ Adult: 20 mg daily, dose to be taken in the morning

● CAUTIONS Acute porphyrias p. 1025

● INTERACTIONS → Appendix 1: thiazide diuretics

● SIDE-EFFECTS

▶ **Common or very common** Alkalosis hypochloraemic · anxiety · diarrhoea · dizziness · dry mouth · fatigue · gastrointestinal discomfort · gouty arthritis · hyperhidrosis · hypomagnesaemia · lethargy · muscle complaints · palpitations

▶ **Uncommon** Photosensitivity reaction

▶ **Rare or very rare** Agranulocytosis · aplastic anaemia · cholecystitis acute · hyperlipidaemia · jaundice · nephritis acute interstitial · pancreatitis haemorrhagic · skin reactions · vision disorders

● BREAST FEEDING No information available.

● MEDICINAL FORMS
There can be variation in the licensing of different medicines containing the same drug.

Tablet

▸ Diurexan (Meda Pharmaceuticals Ltd)
Xipamide 20 mg Diurexan 20mg tablets | 140 tablet PoM £19.46
DT = £19.46

9   Vascular disease

Peripheral vascular disease

Classification and management

Peripheral vascular disease can be either occlusive (e.g. *intermittent claudication*) in which occlusion of the peripheral arteries is caused by atherosclerosis, or vasospastic (e.g. *Raynaud's syndrome*). Peripheral arterial occlusive disease is associated with an increased risk of cardiovascular events; this risk is reduced by measures such as smoking cessation, effective control of blood pressure, regulating blood lipids, optimising glycaemic control in diabetes, taking aspirin p. 121 in a dose of 75 mg daily, and possibly weight reduction in obesity. Exercise training can improve symptoms of intermittent claudication; revascularisation procedures may be appropriate.

Naftidrofuryl oxalate p. 233 can alleviate symptoms of intermittent claudication and improve pain-free walking distance in moderate disease. Patients taking naftidrofuryl oxalate should be assessed for improvement after 3–6 months.

Cilostazol below is licensed for use in intermittent claudication to improve walking distance in patients without peripheral tissue necrosis who do not have pain at rest; use is restricted to second-line treatment where lifestyle modifications and other appropriate interventions have failed to improve symptoms. Cilostazol should be initiated by those experienced in the management of intermittent claudication. Patients receiving cilostazol should be assessed for improvement after 3 months; consider discontinuation of

treatment if there is no clinically relevant improvement in walking distance.

Inositol nicotinate p. 232 and pentoxifylline p. 233 are not established as being effective for the treatment of intermittent claudication.

Intravenous iloprost p. 183 [unlicensed] is a treatment option for critical limb ischaemia in patients unsuitable for surgery.

Management of *Raynaud's syndrome* includes avoidance of exposure to cold and stopping smoking. More severe symptoms may require vasodilator treatment, which is most often successful in primary Raynaud's syndrome. Nifedipine p. 162 is useful for reducing the frequency and severity of vasospastic attacks. Alternatively, naftidrofuryl oxalate may produce symptomatic improvement; inositol nicotinate (a nicotinic acid derivative) may also be considered. Pentoxifylline, prazosin p. 766, and moxisylyte p. 232 are not established as being effective for the treatment of Raynaud's syndrome.

Vasodilator therapy is not established as being effective for *chilblains*.

ANTITHROMBOTIC DRUGS 〉 ANTIPLATELET DRUGS

Cilostazol

● **INDICATIONS AND DOSE**

Intermittent claudication in patients without rest pain and no peripheral tissue necrosis

▶ BY MOUTH

▸ Adult: 100 mg twice daily, to be taken 30 minutes before food, cilostazol should be initiated by those experienced in the management of intermittent claudication, patients receiving cilostazol should be assessed for improvement after 3 months; consider discontinuation of treatment if there is no clinically relevant improvement in walking distance

DOSE ADJUSTMENTS DUE TO INTERACTIONS

▸ Manufacturer advises reduce dose to 50 mg twice daily with concurrent use of potent inhibitors of CYP3A4, potent inhibitors of CYP2C19, omeprazole and erythromycin.

● CONTRA-INDICATIONS Active peptic ulcer · congestive heart failure · coronary intervention in previous 6 months · haemorrhagic stroke in previous 6 months · history of severe tachyarrhythmia · myocardial infarction in previous 6 months · poorly controlled hypertension · predisposition to bleeding · proliferative diabetic retinopathy · prolongation of QT interval · severe atrial flutter · unstable angina

● CAUTIONS Atrial fibrillation · atrial or ventricular ectopy · diabetes mellitus (higher risk of intraocular bleeding) · mild to moderate atrial flutter · stable coronary disease · surgery

● INTERACTIONS → Appendix 1: cilostazol

● SIDE-EFFECTS

▶ **Common or very common** Appetite decreased · arrhythmias · diarrhoea · dizziness · gastrointestinal discomfort · gastrointestinal disorders · headache · increased risk of infection · nausea · oedema · palpitations · skin reactions · vomiting

▶ **Uncommon** Anaemia · anxiety · congestive heart failure · cough · dyspnoea · haemorrhage · hyperglycaemia · hypotension · sleep disorders · syncope

▶ **Rare or very rare** Renal impairment · thrombocytosis

▶ **Frequency not known** Agranulocytosis · bone marrow disorders · conjunctivitis · fever · granulocytopenia · hepatic disorders · hot flush · hypertension · intracranial haemorrhage · leucopenia · paresis · severe cutaneous adverse reactions (SCARs) · thrombocytopenia · tinnitus · urinary frequency increased

- **PREGNANCY** Avoid—toxicity in *animal* studies.
- **BREAST FEEDING** Present in milk in *animal* studies—manufacturer advises avoid.
- **HEPATIC IMPAIRMENT** Avoid in moderate or severe liver disease.
- **RENAL IMPAIRMENT** Avoid if eGFR less than 25 mL/minute/1.73 m².
- **PATIENT AND CARER ADVICE**
Blood disorders Patients should be advised to report any unexplained bleeding, bruising, sore throat, or fever.
- **NATIONAL FUNDING/ACCESS DECISIONS**
NICE decisions
  ▸ Cilostazol, naftidrofuryl oxalate, pentoxifylline and inositol nicotinate for the treatment of intermittent claudication in people with peripheral arterial disease (May 2011) NICE TA223
Cilostazol is not recommended for the treatment of intermittent claudication in patients with peripheral arterial disease; patients currently receiving this treatment should have the option to continue until they and their clinician consider it appropriate to stop.
www.nice.org.uk/TA223

Scottish Medicines Consortium (SMC) Decisions
The *Scottish Medicines Consortium* has advised (October 2005) that cilostazol is not recommended for the treatment of intermittent claudication within NHS Scotland.

- **MEDICINAL FORMS**
There can be variation in the licensing of different medicines containing the same drug.
Tablet
  ▸ Cilostazol (Non-proprietary)
Cilostazol 50 mg Cilostazol 50mg tablets | 56 tablet PoM £40.05 DT = £40.05
Cilostazol 100 mg Cilostazol 100mg tablets | 56 tablet PoM £31.70 DT = £5.03
  ▸ Pletal (Otsuka Pharmaceuticals (U.K.) Ltd) ▼
Cilostazol 50 mg Pletal 50mg tablets | 56 tablet PoM £35.31 DT = £40.05
Cilostazol 100 mg Pletal 100mg tablets | 56 tablet PoM £33.37 DT = £5.03

LIPID MODIFYING DRUGS › NICOTINIC ACID DERIVATIVES

Inositol nicotinate

- **INDICATIONS AND DOSE**
Peripheral vascular disease
  ▸ BY MOUTH
  ▸ Adult: 3 g daily in 2–3 divided doses; maximum 4 g per day

- **CONTRA-INDICATIONS** Acute phase of a cerebrovascular accident · recent myocardial infarction
- **CAUTIONS** Cerebrovascular insufficiency · unstable angina
- **SIDE-EFFECTS**
  ▸ **Uncommon** Dizziness · flushing · headache · nausea · oedema · paraesthesia · postural hypotension · rash · syncope · vomiting
  ▸ **Frequency not known** Myalgia
- **PREGNANCY** No information available—manufacturer advises avoid unless potential benefit outweighs risk.

- **NATIONAL FUNDING/ACCESS DECISIONS**
NICE decisions
  ▸ Cilostazol, naftidrofuryl oxalate, pentoxifylline and inositol nicotinate for the treatment of intermittent claudication in people with peripheral arterial disease (May 2011) NICE TA223
Inositol nicotinate is not recommended for the treatment of intermittent claudication in patients with peripheral arterial disease; patients currently receiving treatment should have the option to continue until they and their clinician consider it appropriate to stop.
www.nice.org.uk/TA223
- **LESS SUITABLE FOR PRESCRIBING** Less suitable for prescribing.
- **MEDICINAL FORMS**
There can be variation in the licensing of different medicines containing the same drug. Forms available from special-order manufacturers include: oral suspension
Capsule
  ▸ Inositol nicotinate (Non-proprietary)
Inositol nicotinate 500 mg Solgar No-Flush Niacin 500mg capsules | 50 capsule ⓢ

VASODILATORS › FLAVONOIDS

Oxerutins

- **INDICATIONS AND DOSE**
Relief of symptoms of oedema associated with chronic venous insufficiency
  ▸ BY MOUTH
  ▸ Adult: 500 mg twice daily

- **SIDE-EFFECTS**
  ▸ **Rare or very rare** Alopecia · arthralgia · diarrhoea · dizziness · fatigue · flushing · gastrointestinal discomfort · gastrointestinal disorders · headache · photosensitivity reaction · skin reactions
- **LESS SUITABLE FOR PRESCRIBING** Oxerutins (rutosides) are not vasodilators and are not generally regarded as effective preparations as capillary sealants or for the treatment of cramps; they are less suitable for prescribing.
- **MEDICINAL FORMS**
There can be variation in the licensing of different medicines containing the same drug.
Capsule
  ▸ Paroven (GlaxoSmithKline Consumer Healthcare)
Oxerutins 250 mg Paroven 250mg capsules | 120 capsule Ⓟ £24.61 DT = £24.61

VASODILATORS › PERIPHERAL VASODILATORS

Moxisylyte
(Thymoxamine)

- **INDICATIONS AND DOSE**
Primary Raynaud's syndrome (short-term treatment)
  ▸ BY MOUTH
  ▸ Adult: Initially 40 mg 4 times a day, increased if necessary to 80 mg 4 times a day, increase dose if poor initial response, discontinue after 2 weeks if no response

- **CONTRA-INDICATIONS** Active liver disease
- **CAUTIONS** Diabetes mellitus
- **INTERACTIONS** → Appendix 1: moxisylyte
- **SIDE-EFFECTS**
  ▸ **Rare or very rare** Hepatic disorders · rash
  ▸ **Frequency not known** Diarrhoea · flushing · headache · nausea · vertigo
- **PREGNANCY** Manufacturer advises avoid.

- LESS SUITABLE FOR PRESCRIBING Less suitable for prescribing.
- MEDICINAL FORMS
There can be variation in the licensing of different medicines containing the same drug.
Tablet
CAUTIONARY AND ADVISORY LABELS 21
▸ Opilon (Kyowa Kirin Ltd)
  Moxisylyte (as Moxisylyte hydrochloride) 40 mg Opilon 40mg tablets | 112 tablet [PoM] £90.22 DT = £90.22

Naftidrofuryl oxalate

- INDICATIONS AND DOSE
Peripheral vascular disease
▸ BY MOUTH
▸ Adult: 100–200 mg 3 times a day, patients taking naftidrofuryl should be assessed for improvement after 3–6 months
Cerebral vascular disease
▸ BY MOUTH
▸ Adult: 100 mg 3 times a day, patients taking naftidrofuryl should be assessed for improvement after 3–6 months

- SIDE-EFFECTS
▸ **Uncommon** Diarrhoea · epigastric pain · nausea · rash · vomiting
▸ **Rare or very rare** Liver injury · oxalate nephrolithiasis
▸ **Frequency not known** Oesophagitis
- NATIONAL FUNDING/ACCESS DECISIONS
NICE decisions
▸ Cilostazol, naftidrofuryl oxalate, pentoxifylline and inositol nicotinate for the treatment of intermittent claudication in people with peripheral arterial disease (May 2011) NICE TA223
Naftidrofuryl oxalate is an option for the treatment of intermittent claudication in patients with peripheral arterial disease in whom vasodilator therapy is considered appropriate.
www.nice.org.uk/TA223
- MEDICINAL FORMS
There can be variation in the licensing of different medicines containing the same drug. Forms available from special-order manufacturers include: oral solution
Capsule
CAUTIONARY AND ADVISORY LABELS 25, 27
▸ Naftidrofuryl oxalate (Non-proprietary)
  Naftidrofuryl oxalate 100 mg Naftidrofuryl 100mg capsules | 84 capsule [PoM] £8.10 DT = £6.17
▸ Praxilene (Merck Serono Ltd)
  Naftidrofuryl oxalate 100 mg Praxilene 100mg capsules | 84 capsule [PoM] £8.10 DT = £6.17

Pentoxifylline
(Oxpentifylline)

- INDICATIONS AND DOSE
Peripheral vascular disease | Venous leg ulcer (adjunct)
▸ BY MOUTH
▸ Adult: 400 mg 2–3 times a day

- UNLICENSED USE Use of pentoxifylline as adjunct therapy for venous leg ulcers is an unlicensed indication.
- CONTRA-INDICATIONS Acute myocardial infarction · cerebral haemorrhage · extensive retinal haemorrhage · severe cardiac arrhythmias
- CAUTIONS Avoid in Acute porphyrias p. 1025 · coronary artery disease · diabetes (may lower blood glucose) · hypotension

- INTERACTIONS → Appendix 1: pentoxifylline
- SIDE-EFFECTS Agitation · angina pectoris · angioedema · arrhythmias · bronchospasm · cholestasis · constipation · diarrhoea · dizziness · gastrointestinal discomfort · gastrointestinal disorder · haemorrhage · headache · hot flush · hypersalivation · hypotension · leucopenia · meningitis aseptic · nausea · neutropenia · skin reactions · sleep disorder · thrombocytopenia · vomiting
- PREGNANCY Manufacturer advises avoid—no information available.
- BREAST FEEDING Present in milk—manufacturer advises use only if potential benefit outweighs risk.
- HEPATIC IMPAIRMENT
Dose adjustments Manufacturer advises reduce dose in severe impairment.
- RENAL IMPAIRMENT
Dose adjustments Reduce dose by 30–50% if eGFR less than 30 mL/minute/1.73 m^2.
- NATIONAL FUNDING/ACCESS DECISIONS
NICE decisions
▸ Cilostazol, naftidrofuryl oxalate, pentoxifylline and inositol nicotinate for the treatment of intermittent claudication in people with peripheral arterial disease (May 2011) NICE TA223
Pentoxifylline is not recommended for the treatment of intermittent claudication in patients with peripheral arterial disease; patients currently receiving this treatment should have the option to continue until they and their clinician consider it appropriate to stop.
www.nice.org.uk/TA223
- LESS SUITABLE FOR PRESCRIBING Less suitable for prescribing.
- MEDICINAL FORMS
There can be variation in the licensing of different medicines containing the same drug. Forms available from special-order manufacturers include: oral solution
Modified-release tablet
CAUTIONARY AND ADVISORY LABELS 21, 25
▸ Trental (Sanofi)
  Pentoxifylline 400 mg Trental 400 modified-release tablets | 90 tablet [PoM] £19.39 DT = £19.39

9.1 Vein malformations

SCLEROSANTS

Sodium tetradecyl sulfate

- INDICATIONS AND DOSE
Sclerotherapy of reticular veins and spider veins in legs and varicose veins
▸ BY INTRAVENOUS INJECTION
▸ Adult: Test dose recommended before each treatment (consult product literature)

- CONTRA-INDICATIONS Acute infection · asthma · blood disorders · deep vein thrombosis · high risk of thromboembolism · hyperthyroidism · inability to walk · neoplasm · occlusive arterial disease · phlebitis · pulmonary embolism · recent acute superficial thrombophlebitis · recent surgery · respiratory disease · significant valvular incompetence in deep veins · skin disease · symptomatic patent foramen ovale (if administered as foam) · uncontrolled diabetes mellitus · varicose veins caused by tumours (unless tumour removed)
- CAUTIONS Arterial disease · asymptomatic patent foramen ovale (use smaller volumes and avoid Valsalva manoeuvre immediately after administration) · extravasation may cause necrosis of tissues · history of migraine (use smaller volumes) · resuscitation facilities must be available ·

venous insufficiency with lymphoedema (pain and inflammation may worsen)

● SIDE-EFFECTS
▸ **Common or very common** Embolism and thrombosis · pain · paraesthesia
▸ **Uncommon** Skin reactions · telangiectasia
▸ **Rare or very rare** Arterial spasm · asthenia · asthma · cerebrovascular insufficiency · chest pressure · circulatory collapse · confusion · cough · diarrhoea · dry mouth · dyspnoea · fever · headaches · hot flush · hypersensitivity · local exfoliation · nausea · nerve damage · palpitations · presyncope · soft tissue necrosis · tongue swelling · vasculitis · vision disorders · vomiting

● PREGNANCY Avoid unless benefits outweigh risks—no information available.

● BREAST FEEDING Use with caution—no information available.

● MEDICINAL FORMS
There can be variation in the licensing of different medicines containing the same drug.
Solution for injection
EXCIPIENTS: May contain Benzyl alcohol
▸ Fibro-Vein (STD Pharmaceutical Products Ltd)
Sodium tetradecyl sulfate 2 mg per 1 ml Fibrovein 0.2% solution for injection 5ml vials | 10 vial PoM £73.61
Sodium tetradecyl sulfate 5 mg per 1 ml Fibrovein 0.5% solution for injection 2ml ampoules | 5 ampoule PoM £18.93
Sodium tetradecyl sulfate 10 mg per 1 ml Fibrovein 1% solution for injection 2ml ampoules | 5 ampoule PoM £22.61
Sodium tetradecyl sulfate 30 mg per 1 ml Fibrovein 3% solution for injection 2ml ampoules | 5 ampoule PoM £33.65
Fibrovein 3% solution for injection 5ml vials | 10 vial PoM £166.66

Chapter 3
Respiratory system

CONTENTS

Respiratory system, drug delivery

Inhalation

This route delivers the drug directly to the airways; the dose required is smaller than when given by mouth and side-effects are reduced.

Inhaler devices

These include *pressurised metered-dose inhalers*, *breath-actuated inhalers*, and *dry powder inhalers*. Many patients can be taught to use a pressurised metered-dose inhaler effectively but some patients, particularly the elderly and children, find them difficult to use. *Spacer devices* can help such patients because they remove the need to co-ordinate actuation with inhalation. Dry powder inhalers may be useful in adults and children over 5 years who are unwilling or unable to use a pressurised metered-dose inhaler. Alternatively, breath-actuated inhalers are suitable for adults and older children provided they can use the device effectively.

Pressurised metered-dose inhalers are an effective and convenient method of drug administration in mild to moderate asthma.

On changing from a pressurised metered-dose inhaler to a dry powder inhaler, patients may notice a lack of sensation in the mouth and throat previously associated with each actuation. Coughing may also occur.

The patient should be instructed carefully on the use of the inhaler and it is important to check that the inhaler continues to be used correctly because inadequate inhalation technique may be mistaken for a lack of response to the drug.

Spacer devices

Spacer devices remove the need for coordination between actuation of a pressurised metered-dose inhaler and inhalation. The spacer device reduces the velocity of the aerosol and subsequent impaction on the oropharynx and allows more time for evaporation of the propellant so that a larger proportion of the particles can be inhaled and deposited in the lungs. Spacer devices are particularly useful for patients with poor inhalation technique, for children, for patients requiring high doses of inhaled corticosteroids, for nocturnal asthma, and for patients prone to candidiasis with inhaled corticosteroids. The size of the spacer is important, the larger spacers with a one-way valve (*Volumatic®*) being most effective. It is important to prescribe a spacer device that is compatible with the metered-dose inhaler, see devices below. Spacer devices should not be regarded as interchangeable; patients should be advised not to switch between spacer devices.

Use and care of spacer devices

Patients should inhale from the spacer device as soon as possible after actuation because the drug aerosol is very short-lived; single-dose actuation is recommended. Tidal breathing is as effective as single breaths. The device should be cleaned once a month by washing in mild detergent and then allowed to dry in air without rinsing; the mouthpiece should be wiped clean of detergent before use. Some manufacturers recommend more frequent cleaning, but this should be avoided since any electrostatic charge may affect drug delivery. Spacer devices should be replaced every 6–12 months.

Respiratory drug delivery, nebulisers

Solutions for nebulisation are available for use in severe acute asthma. They are administered over 5–10 minutes from a nebuliser usually driven by oxygen in hospital.

Patients with a severe attack of asthma should preferably have oxygen during nebulisation since beta$_2$ agonists can increase arterial hypoxaemia.

A nebuliser converts a solution of a drug into an aerosol for inhalation. It is used to deliver higher doses of drug to the airways than is usual with standard inhalers. The main indications for use of a nebuliser are to deliver:

- a beta$_2$ agonist or ipratropium bromide p. 246 to a patient with an *acute exacerbation* of asthma or of chronic obstructive pulmonary disease;
- a beta$_2$ agonist, corticosteroid, or ipratropium bromide on a *regular basis* to a patient with severe asthma or reversible airways obstruction when the patient is unable to use other inhalational devices;
- an antibiotic (such as colistimethate sodium p. 546) or a mucolytic to a patient with cystic fibrosis;
- Budesonide p. 259 or adrenaline/epinephrine p. 221 to a child with severe croup;
- Pentamidine isetionate p. 591 for the prophylaxis and treatment of pneumocystis pneumonia.

The use of nebulisers in chronic persistent asthma and chronic obstructive pulmonary disease should be considered only:

- after a review of the diagnosis;
- after review of therapy (see also Chronic Obstructive Pulmonary Disease) and the patient's ability to use hand-held devices;
- after increased doses of inhaled therapy from hand-held inhalers (with a spacer if necessary) have been tried for 2 weeks;
- if the patient remains breathless, despite correctly using optimal therapy.

Before prescribing a nebuliser, a home trial should preferably be undertaken to monitor response for up to 2 weeks on standard treatment and up to 2 weeks on nebulised treatment. If prescribed, patients must:

- have clear instructions from a doctor, specialist nurse, physiotherapist, or pharmacist on the use of the nebuliser (including maintenance and cleaning) and on peak-flow monitoring;
- be instructed not to treat acute attacks at home without also seeking help;
- have regular follow up by a doctor, specialist nurse or physiotherapist after about 1 month and annually thereafter.

The proportion of a nebuliser solution that reaches the lungs depends on the type of nebuliser and although it can be as high as 30%, it is more frequently close to 10% and sometimes below 10%. The remaining solution is left in the nebuliser as residual volume or is deposited in the mouthpiece and tubing. The extent to which the nebulised solution is deposited in the airways or alveoli depends on the droplet size, pattern of breath inhalation, and condition of the lung. Droplets with a mass median diameter of 1–5 microns are deposited in the airways and are therefore appropriate for asthma, whereas a particle size of 1–2 microns is needed for alveolar deposition of pentamidine isetionate to combat pneumocystis infection. The type of nebuliser is therefore chosen according to the deposition required and according to the viscosity of the solution.

Jet nebulisers

Jet nebulisers are more widely used than ultrasonic nebulisers. Most jet nebulisers require an optimum gas flow rate of 6–8 litres/minute and in hospital can be driven by piped air or oxygen; in acute asthma the nebuliser should be driven by oxygen. Domiciliary oxygen cylinders do not provide an adequate flow rate therefore an electrical compressor is required for domiciliary use.

For patients at risk of hypercapnia, such as those with chronic obstructive pulmonary disease, oxygen can be dangerous and the nebuliser should be driven by air. If oxygen is required, it should be given simultaneously by nasal cannula.

Tubing

The Department of Health has reminded users of the need to use the correct grade of tubing when connecting a nebuliser to a medical gas supply or compressor.

Ultrasonic nebulisers

Ultrasonic nebulisers produce an aerosol by ultrasonic vibration of the drug solution and therefore do not require a gas flow; they are not suitable for the nebulisation of some drugs, such as dornase alfa p. 292 and nebulised suspensions.

Nebuliser diluent

Nebulisation may be carried out using an undiluted nebuliser solution or it may require dilution beforehand. The usual diluent is sterile sodium chloride 0.9% (physiological saline).

In England and Wales nebulisers and compressors are not available on the NHS (but they are free of VAT); some nebulisers (but not compressors) are available on form GP10A in Scotland (for details consult Scottish Drug Tariff).

Oral

The oral route is used when administration by inhalation is not possible. Systemic side-effects occur more frequently when a drug is given orally rather than by inhalation. Drugs given by mouth for the treatment of asthma include beta$_2$ agonists, corticosteroids, theophylline p. 273, and leukotriene receptor antagonists.

Parenteral

Drugs such as beta$_2$ agonists, corticosteroids, and aminophylline p. 272 can be given by injection in acute severe asthma when administration by nebulisation is inadequate or inappropriate. If the patient is being treated in the community, urgent transfer to hospital should be arranged.

Peak flow meters

When used in addition to symptom-based monitoring, peak flow monitoring has not been proven to improve asthma control in either adults or children, however measurement of peak flow may be of benefit in adult patients who are 'poor perceivers' and hence slow to detect deterioration in their asthma, and for those with more severe asthma.

When peak flow meters are used, patients must be given clear guidelines as to the action they should take if their peak flow falls below a certain level. Patients can be encouraged to adjust some of their own treatment (within specified limits) according to changes in peak flow rate.

Peak flow charts should be issued to patients where appropriate, and are available to purchase from:

3M Security Print and Systems Limited. Gorse Street, Chadderton, Oldham, OL9 9QH. Tel: 0845 610 1112

GP practices can obtain supplies through their Area Team stores.

NHS Hospitals can order supplies from www.nhsforms.co.uk/ or by emailing nhsforms@mmm.com.

In Scotland, peak flow charts can be obtained by emailing stockorders.dppas@apsgroup.co.uk.

NICE decisions
Inhaler devices for children under 5 years with chronic asthma (August 2000) NICE TA10

When selecting inhaler devices for children under 5 years with chronic asthma, a child's needs and likelihood of good compliance should govern the choice of inhaler and spacer device; only then should cost be considered.

- corticosteroid and bronchodilator therapy should be delivered by pressurised metered-dose inhaler and spacer device, with a facemask if necessary;
- if this is not effective, and depending on the child's condition, nebulised therapy may be considered and, in children over 3 years, a dry powder inhaler may also be considered.

www.nice.org.uk/TA10

Inhaler devices for children 5–15 years with chronic asthma (March 2002) NICE TA38

When selecting inhaler devices for children between 5–15 years with chronic asthma, a child's needs, ability to develop and maintain effective technique, and likelihood of good compliance should govern the choice of inhaler and spacer device; only then should cost be considered.

- corticosteroid therapy should be routinely delivered by a pressurised metered-dose inhaler and spacer device;
- for other inhaled drugs, particularly bronchodilators, a wider range of devices should be considered;
- children and their carers should be trained in the use of the chosen device; suitability of the device should be reviewed at least annually. Inhaler technique and compliance should be monitored.

www.nice.org.uk/TA38

1   Airways disease, obstructive

Asthma, chronic

05-Apr-2018

Description of condition

Asthma is a common chronic inflammatory condition of the airways, associated with airway hyperresponsiveness and variable airflow obstruction. The most frequent symptoms of asthma are cough, wheeze, chest tightness, and breathlessness. Asthma symptoms vary over time and in intensity and can gradually or suddenly worsen, provoking an acute asthma attack that, if severe, may require hospitalisation.

Aims of treatment

The aim of treatment is to achieve control of asthma. Complete control of asthma is defined as no daytime symptoms, no night-time awakening due to asthma, no asthma attacks, no need for rescue medication, no limitations on activity including exercise, normal lung function (in practical terms forced expiratory volume in 1 second (FEV$_1$) and/or peak expiratory flow (PEF) > 80% predicted or best), and minimal side-effects from treatment. In clinical practice, patients may choose to balance the aims of asthma management against the potential side-effects or inconvenience of taking medication necessary to achieve perfect control.

Lifestyle changes

[EvGr] Weight loss in overweight patients may lead to an improvement in asthma symptoms. Parents with asthma should be advised about the danger of smoking, to themselves and to their children with asthma, and be offered appropriate support to stop smoking. Breathing exercise programmes (including physiotherapist-taught methods) can be offered as an adjuvant to drug treatment to improve quality of life and reduce symptoms. [A]

Management

[EvGr] A stepwise approach aims to stop symptoms quickly and to improve peak flow. Treatment should be started at the level most appropriate to initial severity of asthma. The aim is to achieve early control and to maintain it by stepping up treatment as necessary and decreasing treatment when control is good. Before initiating a new drug or adjusting treatment consider whether diagnosis is correct, check adherence and inhaler technique, and eliminate trigger factors for acute attacks.

A self-management programme comprising of a written personalised action plan and education should be offered to all patients with asthma (and/or their family or carers). [A]

Recommendations on the management of chronic asthma from the *National Institute for Health and Care Excellence (NICE)—Asthma: diagnosis, monitoring and chronic asthma management guidelines (NG80, November 2017)*, and *British Thoracic Society (BTS) and Scottish Intercollegiate Guidelines Network (SIGN)—British guideline on the management of asthma (SIGN 153, September 2016)* differ significantly. Recommendations in BNF publications are based on NICE guidelines, and differences with BTS/SIGN (2016) have been highlighted.

Adult

NICE (2017) treatment recommendations for adults apply to patients aged 17 years and over. BTS/SIGN (2016) treatment recommendations for adults apply to patients over 12 years.

Intermittent reliever therapy

[EvGr] Start an inhaled short-acting beta$_2$ agonist (such as salbutamol p. 252 or terbutaline sulfate p. 254), to be used as required, in all patients with asthma. For those with infrequent short-lived wheeze, occasional use of reliever therapy may be the only treatment required. Patients using more than one short-acting beta$_2$ agonist inhaler device a month should have their asthma urgently assessed and action taken to improve poorly controlled asthma. [A]

Regular preventer (maintenance) therapy

NICE (2017) define inhaled corticosteroid doses for adults as low, moderate, or high. BTS/SIGN (2016) instead define inhaled corticosteroid doses for adults as low, medium or high (refer to individual guidelines for inhaled corticosteroid dosing information).

[EvGr] A low dose of inhaled corticosteroid should be started as maintenance therapy in patients who present with any one of the following features: using an inhaled short-acting beta$_2$ agonist three times a week or more, symptomatic three times a week or more, or waking at night due to asthma symptoms at least once a week. BTS/SIGN (2016) also recommend initiation in patients who have had an asthma attack in the last 2 years, and starting inhaled corticosteroids at a dose appropriate to the severity of asthma.

BTS/SIGN (2016) recommend that inhaled corticosteroids (except ciclesonide p. 262) should be initially taken twice daily, however, the same total daily dose, taken once a day, can be considered in patients with milder disease if good or complete control of asthma is established. The dose of inhaled corticosteroid should be adjusted over time to the lowest effective dose at which control of asthma is maintained.

BTS/SIGN (2016) recommend the prescribing of inhalers by brand. [A]

Initial add-on therapy

[EvGr] If asthma is uncontrolled on a low dose of inhaled corticosteroid as maintenance therapy, a leukotriene receptor antagonist (such as montelukast p. 268 or zafirlukast p. 269) should be offered in addition to the inhaled corticosteroid, and the response to treatment reviewed in 4 to 8 weeks.

BTS/SIGN (2016) instead recommend a long-acting beta$_2$ agonist (LABA—such as salmeterol p. 251 or formoterol fumarate p. 250) as initial add-on therapy to inhaled corticosteroids if asthma is uncontrolled. [A]

Additional add-on therapy

[EvGr] If asthma is uncontrolled on a low dose of inhaled corticosteroid and a leukotriene receptor antagonist as maintenance therapy, a LABA in combination with the inhaled corticosteroid should be offered with or without continued leukotriene receptor antagonist treatment, depending on the response achieved from the leukotriene receptor antagonist.

If asthma remains uncontrolled, offer to change the inhaled corticosteroid and LABA maintenance therapy to a MART regimen (Maintenance And Reliever Therapy—a combination of an inhaled corticosteroid and a fast-acting LABA such as formoterol in a single inhaler), with a low dose of inhaled corticosteroid as maintenance. See beclometasone with formoterol p. 258 and budesonide with formoterol p. 260.

If asthma remains uncontrolled on a MART regimen with a low dose of inhaled corticosteroid as maintenance with or without a leukotriene antagonist, consider increasing to a moderate dose of inhaled corticosteroid (either continuing a MART regimen or changing to a fixed-dose regimen of an inhaled corticosteroid and a LABA, with a short-acting beta$_2$ agonist as reliever therapy).

If asthma is still uncontrolled in patients on a moderate dose of inhaled corticosteroid as maintenance with a LABA (either as MART or a fixed-dose regimen), with or without a leukotriene receptor antagonist, consider the following options:

- increasing the inhaled corticosteroid dose to a high-dose as maintenance (this should only be offered as part of a fixed-dose regimen, with a short-acting beta$_2$ agonist used as a reliever therapy), or
- a trial of an additional drug, for example, a long-acting muscarinic receptor antagonist (such as tiotropium p. 247) or modified-release theophylline p. 273, or
- seek advice from an asthma specialist.

BTS/SIGN (2016) instead recommend that if the patient is gaining some benefit from addition of a LABA but control remains inadequate, that the LABA be continued and the dose of inhaled corticosteroid be increased to a medium-dose, if not already on this dose. If increasing the dose of inhaled corticosteroid is ineffective, consider continuing on a low dose of inhaled corticosteroid and a LABA and try adding a leukotriene receptor antagonist, or a long-acting muscarinic receptor antagonist, or modified-release theophylline p. 273.

If there is no response to the LABA, discontinue it and increase the dose of the inhaled corticosteroid to a medium-dose, if not already on this dose. If increasing the dose of inhaled corticosteroid is ineffective, consider continuing on a low dose of inhaled corticosteroid and try adding a leukotriene receptor antagonist or a long-acting muscarinic receptor antagonist. Ⓐ

High-dose inhaled corticosteroids and further add-on treatment
ᴇᵛᴳʳ BTS/SIGN (2016) recommend that if control remains inadequate on a combination of short-acting beta₂ agonist as required, a medium dose of inhaled corticosteroid, plus an additional drug, usually a LABA, to consider the following interventions:

• increase the inhaled corticosteroid to a high-dose—with high doses of inhaled corticosteroid via a pressurised metered dose inhaler (pMDI), a spacer should be used, or
• add a leukotriene receptor antagonist, or
• add modified-release theophylline p. 273, or
• add tiotropium p. 247.

If a trial of a further add-on treatment is ineffective, stop the drug (or in the case of increased dose of inhaled corticosteroid, reduce to the original dose) and refer to specialist care. Ⓐ

Continuous or frequent use of oral corticosteroids
ᴇᵛᴳʳ BTS/SIGN (2016) recommend adding a regular oral corticosteroid (prednisolone p. 664) at the lowest dose to provide adequate control (under specialist care) in patients with very severe asthma uncontrolled on high-dose inhaled corticosteroids, and who have also tried (or are still receiving) a LABA, a leukotriene receptor antagonist, or modified-release theophylline p. 273. Ⓐ

Monoclonal antibodies and immunosuppressants
ᴇᵛᴳʳ BTS/SIGN (2016) recommend, that under specialist initiation, immunosuppressants such as methotrexate p. 888 [unlicensed], and monoclonal antibodies such as omalizumab (for severe persistent allergic asthma), and mepolizumab and reslizumab (in adults for severe eosinophilic asthma), may be considered in patients with severe asthma to achieve control and reduce the use of oral corticosteroids. Ⓐ See mepolizumab p. 266, omalizumab p. 267, reslizumab p. 267 National funding/access decisions.

Child over 5 years
For children over 5 years, NICE (2017) treatment recommendations for children apply to children aged 5–16 years and adult treatment recommendations apply to those aged 17 years and over. Whereas, for children over 5 years, BTS/SIGN (2016) treatment recommendations for children apply to children aged 5–12 years and adult treatment recommendations apply to those aged over 12 years.

Intermittent reliever therapy
ᴇᵛᴳʳ Start an inhaled short-acting beta₂ agonist (such as salbutamol p. 252 or terbutaline sulfate p. 254), to be used as required, in all children with asthma. For those with infrequent short-lived wheeze, occasional use of reliever therapy may be the only treatment required. Children using more than one short-acting beta₂ agonist inhaler device a month should have their asthma urgently assessed and action taken to improve poorly controlled asthma. Ⓐ

Regular preventer (maintenance) therapy
NICE (2017) define inhaled corticosteroid doses for children (5–16 years) as paediatric low, moderate, or high. BTS/SIGN (2016) instead define inhaled corticosteroid doses for children (5–12 years) as very low, low, or medium, and for children over 12 years as low, medium or high (refer to individual guidelines for inhaled corticosteroid dosing information).

ᴇᵛᴳʳ A paediatric low dose of inhaled corticosteroid should be started as maintenance therapy in children who present with any one of the following features: using an inhaled short-acting beta₂ agonist three times a week or more, symptomatic three times a week or more, or waking at night due to asthma symptoms at least once a week.

BTS/SIGN (2016) instead recommend starting a very low dose (child 5–12 years) or a low dose (child over 12 years) of inhaled corticosteroid in children presenting with any one of the following features: using an inhaled short-acting beta₂ agonist three times a week or more, symptomatic three times a week or more, or waking at night due to asthma symptoms at least once a week, or have had an asthma attack in the last 2 years, and starting inhaled corticosteroids at a dose appropriate to the severity of asthma.

BTS/SIGN (2016) recommend that inhaled corticosteroids (except ciclesonide p. 262) should be initially taken twice daily, however, the same total daily dose, taken once a day, can be considered in patients with milder disease if good or complete control of asthma is established. The dose of inhaled corticosteroid should be adjusted over time, to the lowest effective dose at which control of asthma is maintained.

BTS/SIGN (2016) recommend the prescribing of inhalers by brand. Ⓐ

Initial add-on therapy
ᴇᵛᴳʳ If asthma is uncontrolled on a paediatric low dose of inhaled corticosteroid as maintenance therapy, consider a leukotriene receptor antagonist (such as montelukast p. 268 or zafirlukast p. 269 [unlicensed in under 12 years]) in addition to the inhaled corticosteroid, and review the response to treatment in 4 to 8 weeks.

BTS/SIGN (2016) instead recommend a long-acting beta₂ agonist (LABA—such as salmeterol p. 251 or formoterol fumarate p. 250) in children over 12 years, or a LABA or a leukotriene receptor antagonist in children 5–12 years, as initial add-on therapy to inhaled corticosteroids if asthma is uncontrolled. Ⓐ

Additional add-on therapy
ᴇᵛᴳʳ If asthma is uncontrolled on a paediatric low dose of inhaled corticosteroid and a leukotriene receptor antagonist as maintenance therapy, consider discontinuation of the leukotriene receptor antagonist and initiation of a LABA in combination with the inhaled corticosteroid.

If asthma remains uncontrolled on a paediatric low dose of inhaled corticosteroid and a LABA as maintenance therapy, consider changing to a MART regimen (Maintenance And Reliever Therapy—a combination of an inhaled corticosteroid and fast-acting beta₂ agonist such as formoterol in a single inhaler) with a paediatric low dose of inhaled corticosteroid as maintenance. See budesonide with formoterol p. 260 [not licensed in all age groups].

If asthma remains uncontrolled on a MART regimen with a paediatric low dose of inhaled corticosteroid as maintenance, consider increasing to a paediatric moderate dose of inhaled corticosteroid (either continuing a MART regimen or changing to a fixed-dose regimen of an inhaled corticosteroid and a LABA, with a short-acting beta₂ agonist as reliever therapy).

If asthma is still uncontrolled on a paediatric moderate dose of inhaled corticosteroid as maintenance with a LABA (either as MART or a fixed-dose regimen), consider seeking advice from an asthma specialist and the following options:

- increasing the inhaled corticosteroid dose to a paediatric high dose as maintenance (this should only be offered as part of a fixed-dose regimen, with a short-acting beta$_2$ agonist as reliever therapy), or

- a trial of an additional drug, such as modified-release theophylline p. 273.

BTS/SIGN (2016) instead recommend that if the child is gaining some benefit from addition of a LABA but control remains inadequate, continue the LABA and increase the dose of the inhaled corticosteroid to a low-dose (child 5–12 years) or medium-dose (child over 12 years), if not already on this dose. If increasing the dose of inhaled corticosteroid is ineffective, consider continuing a very low dose (child 5–12 years) or low dose (child over 12 years) of inhaled corticosteroid and a LABA and try adding a leukotriene receptor antagonist, or modified-release theophylline p. 273, or long-acting muscarinic receptor antagonist (in children over 12 years).

If there is no response to the LABA, discontinue it and increase the dose of inhaled corticosteroid to a low-dose (child 5–12 years) or medium-dose (child over 12 years), if not already on this dose. If increasing the dose of inhaled corticosteroid is ineffective, consider continuing on a very low dose (child 5–12 years) or low dose (child over 12 years) of inhaled corticosteroid and try adding a leukotriene receptor antagonist or long-acting muscarinic receptor antagonist (in children over 12 years). Ⓐ

High-dose inhaled corticosteroids and further add-on treatment
EvGr BTS/SIGN (2016) recommend that if control remains inadequate on a combination of a short-acting beta$_2$ agonist as required, a low dose (child 5–12 years) or medium dose (child over 12 years) of inhaled corticosteroid, plus an additional drug, usually a LABA, to consider the following interventions:

- increase the inhaled corticosteroid to a medium-dose (child 5–12 years) or high-dose (child over 12 years)—with high doses of inhaled corticosteroid via a pressurised metered dose inhaler (pMDI), a spacer should be used, or
- add a leukotriene receptor antagonist, or
- add modified-release theophylline p. 273, or
- add tiotropium p. 247 (in children over 12 years).

If a trial of a further add-on treatment is ineffective, stop the drug (or in the case of increased dose of inhaled corticosteroid, reduce to the original dose) and refer to specialist care. Ⓐ

Continuous or frequent use of oral corticosteroids
EvGr BTS/SIGN (2016) recommend adding a regular oral corticosteroid (prednisolone p. 664) at the lowest dose to provide adequate control (under specialist care) in children with very severe asthma uncontrolled on a medium dose (child 5–12 years) or high dose (child over 12 years) of inhaled corticosteroid, and who have also tried (or are still receiving) a LABA, a leukotriene receptor antagonist, or modified-release theophylline p. 273. Ⓐ

Monoclonal antibodies and immunosuppressants
EvGr BTS/SIGN (2016) recommend, that under specialist initiation, immunosuppressants such as methotrexate p. 888 [unlicensed], and monoclonal antibodies such as omalizumab (child over 6 years for severe persistent allergic asthma) can be considered in children with severe asthma to achieve control and reduce the use of oral corticosteroids. Ⓐ See omalizumab p. 267 National funding/access decisions.

Child under 5 years
Intermittent reliever therapy
EvGr A short-acting beta$_2$ agonist (such as salbutamol p. 252) as reliever therapy should be offered to children under 5 years with suspected asthma. A short-acting beta$_2$ agonist should be used for symptom relief alongside maintenance treatment.

Children using more than one short-acting beta$_2$ agonist inhaler device a month should have their asthma urgently assessed and action taken to improve poorly controlled asthma. Ⓐ

Regular preventer (maintenance) therapy
NICE (2017) define inhaled corticosteroid doses for children under 5 years as paediatric low or moderate. BTS/SIGN (2016) instead define inhaled corticosteroid doses for children under 5 years as very low (refer to individual guidelines for inhaled corticosteroid dosing information).

EvGr Consider an 8-week trial of a paediatric moderate dose of inhaled corticosteroid in children presenting with any of the following features: asthma-related symptoms three times a week or more, experiencing night-time awakening at least once a week, or suspected asthma that is uncontrolled with a short-acting beta$_2$ agonist alone.

BTS/SIGN (2016) recommend the prescribing of inhalers by brand.

After 8 weeks, stop inhaled corticosteroid treatment and continue to monitor the child's symptoms:

- if symptoms did not resolve during the trial period, review whether an alternative diagnosis is likely;
- if symptoms resolved then reoccurred within 4 weeks of stopping inhaled corticosteroid treatment, restart the inhaled corticosteroid at a paediatric low-dose as first-line maintenance therapy;
- if symptoms resolved but reoccurred beyond 4 weeks after stopping inhaled corticosteroid treatment, repeat the 8-week trial of a paediatric moderate dose of inhaled corticosteroid.

BTS/SIGN (2016) instead recommend starting a very low dose of inhaled corticosteroid as initial regular preventer therapy in children presenting with any one of the following features: using an inhaled short-acting beta$_2$ agonist three times a week or more, symptomatic three times a week or more, or waking at night due to asthma symptoms at least once a week. In children unable to take an inhaled corticosteroid, a leukotriene receptor antagonist (such as montelukast p. 268) may be used an alternative. Ⓐ

Initial add-on therapy
EvGr If suspected asthma is uncontrolled in children under 5 years on a paediatric low dose of inhaled corticosteroid as maintenance therapy, consider a leukotriene receptor antagonist (such as montelukast p. 268) in addition to the inhaled corticosteroid.

If suspected asthma is uncontrolled in children under 5 years on a paediatric low dose of inhaled corticosteroid and a leukotriene receptor antagonist as maintenance therapy, stop the leukotriene receptor antagonist and refer the child to an asthma specialist. Ⓐ

Decreasing treatment
EvGr Consider decreasing maintenance therapy when a patient's asthma has been controlled with their current maintenance therapy for at least three months. When deciding which drug to decrease first and at what rate, the severity of asthma, the side-effects of treatment, duration on current dose, the beneficial effect achieved, and the patient's preference, should be considered. Patients should be regularly reviewed when decreasing treatment.

Patients should be maintained at the lowest possible dose of inhaled corticosteroid. Reductions should be considered every three months, decreasing the dose by approximately 25–50% each time. Reduce the dose slowly as patients deteriorate at different rates. Only consider stopping inhaled corticosteroid treatment completely for people who are using a paediatric or adult low dose inhaled corticosteroid alone as maintenance therapy and are symptom-free. Ⓐ

3

Respiratory system

Exercise-induced asthma

EvGr For most patients, exercise-induced asthma is an illustration of poorly controlled asthma and regular treatment including inhaled corticosteroids should therefore be reviewed. If exercise is a specific problem in patients already taking inhaled corticosteroids who are otherwise well controlled, consider adding either a leukotriene receptor antagonist, a long-acting beta₂ agonist, an oral beta₂ agonist, sodium cromoglicate p. 270 or nedocromil sodium p. 270, or theophylline p. 273. An inhaled short-acting beta₂ agonists used immediately before exercise is the drug of choice. ⚠A

Pregnancy

EvGr Women with asthma should be closely monitored during pregnancy. It is particularly important that asthma be well controlled during pregnancy; when this is achieved there is little or no increased risk of adverse maternal or fetal complications.

Women should be counselled about the importance and safety of taking their asthma medication during pregnancy to maintain good control. Women who smoke should be advised about the dangers to themselves and to their baby and be offered appropriate support to stop smoking.

Short-acting beta₂ agonists, LABAs, oral and inhaled corticosteroids, sodium cromoglicate p. 270 and nedocromil sodium p. 270, and oral and intravenous theophylline p. 273 (with appropriate monitoring) can be used as normal during pregnancy. There is limited information on use of a leukotriene receptor antagonist during pregnancy, however, where indicated to achieve adequate control, they should not be withheld. ⚠A

Useful Resources

Asthma: diagnosis, monitoring and chronic asthma management. National Institute for Health and Care Excellence. NICE guideline 80. November 2017. www.nice.org.uk/guidance/ng80

British guideline on the management of asthma. British Thoracic Society and Scottish Intercollegiate Guidelines Network. Full guidance - A national clinical guideline 153. September 2016. www.sign.ac.uk/assets/sign153.pdf

Asthma, acute

30-Nov-2016

Adults

Levels of severity

The nature of treatment required for the management of acute asthma depends on the level of severity, described as follows:

Moderate acute asthma

- Increasing symptoms
- Peak flow > 50-75% best or predicted
- No features of acute severe asthma

Severe acute asthma

Any one of the following:

- Peak flow 33-50% best or predicted
- Respiratory rate ≥ 25/min
- Heart rate ≥ 110/min
- Inability to complete sentences in one breath

Life-threatening acute asthma

Any one of the following, in a patient with severe asthma:

- Peak flow < 33% best or predicted
- Arterial oxygen saturation (SpO₂) < 92%
- Partial arterial pressure of oxygen (PaO₂) < 8 kPa
- Normal partial arterial pressure of carbon dioxide (PaCO₂) (4.6–6.0 kPa)
- Silent chest
- Cyanosis

- Poor respiratory effort
- Arrhythmia
- Exhaustion
- Altered conscious level
- Hypotension

Near-fatal acute asthma

- Raised PaCO₂, requiring mechanical ventilation with raised inflation pressures, or both

Management

EvGr Patients with moderate asthma should be treated at home or in primary care according to response to treatment, while patients with severe or life-threatening acute asthma should start treatment as soon as possible and be admitted to hospital immediately following initial assessment.

Supplementary oxygen should be given to all hypoxaemic patients with acute severe asthma to maintain a SpO₂ level between 94–98%.

First-line treatment for acute asthma is a high-dose inhaled short-acting beta₂ agonist (salbutamol p. 252 or terbutaline sulfate p. 254) given as soon as possible. A pressurised metered dose inhaler with spacer device is preferred in patients with non-life-threatening acute asthma. Whereas, in patients with life-threatening acute asthma, a beta₂ agonist administered by an oxygen-driven nebuliser is recommended. If the response to an initial dose of short-acting beta₂ agonist is poor, consider continuous nebulisation with an appropriate nebuliser. Intravenous beta₂ agonists are reserved for those patients in whom inhaled therapy cannot be used reliably.

In all cases of acute asthma, patients should be prescribed an adequate dose of oral prednisolone p. 664 once daily for at least 5 days or until recovery. Parenteral hydrocortisone p. 662 or intramuscular methylprednisolone p. 663 are alternatives in patients who are unable to take oral prednisolone.

Nebulised ipratropium bromide p. 246 may be combined with a nebulised beta₂ agonist in patients with acute severe or life-threatening asthma or in those with a poor initial response to beta₂ agonist therapy to provide greater bronchodilation.

There is some evidence that magnesium sulfate p. 1019 has bronchodilator effects. A single intravenous dose of magnesium sulfate may be considered in patients with severe acute asthma (peak flow < 50% best or predicted) who have not had a good initial response to inhaled bronchodilator therapy [unlicensed use]. In an acute asthma attack, intravenous aminophylline p. 272 is not likely to produce any additional bronchodilation compared to standard therapy with inhaled bronchodilators and corticosteroids. However, in some patients with near-fatal or life-threatening acute asthma with a poor response to initial therapy, intravenous aminophylline may provide some benefit. Magnesium sulfate by intravenous infusion or aminophylline should only be used after consultation with, or on the recommendation of, senior medical staff. ⚠A

Child over 2 years

Levels of severity

The nature of treatment required for the management of acute asthma depends on the level of severity, described as follows:

Moderate acute asthma

- Able to talk in sentences
- Arterial oxygen saturation (SpO₂) ≥ 92%
- Peak flow ≥ 50% best or predicted
- Heart rate ≤ 140/minute in children aged 2–5 years; heart rate ≤ 125/minute in children over 5 years
- Respiratory rate ≤ 40/minute in children aged 2–5 years; respiratory rate ≤ 30/minute in children over 5 years

Severe acute asthma

- Can't complete sentences in one breath or too breathless to talk or feed
- $SpO_2 < 92\%$
- Peak flow 33–50% best or predicted
- Heart rate > 140/minute in children aged 2–5 years; heart rate > 125/minute in children aged over 5 years
- Respiratory rate > 40/minute in children aged 2–5 years; respiratory rate > 30/minute in children aged over 5 years

Life-threatening acute asthma

Any one of the following in a child with severe asthma:

- $SpO_2 < 92\%$
- Peak flow < 33% best or predicted
- Silent chest
- Cyanosis
- Poor respiratory effort
- Hypotension
- Exhaustion
- Confusion

Management

EvGr Following initial assessment, supplementary high flow oxygen should be given to all children with life-threatening acute asthma or $SpO_2 < 94\%$ to achieve normal saturations of 94–98%.

First-line treatment for acute asthma is an inhaled short-acting beta₂ agonist (salbutamol or terbutaline sulfate) given as soon as possible, ideally via a metered dose inhaler and spacer device in mild to moderate acute asthma. Children with severe or life-threatening acute asthma should be transferred to hospital urgently.

In all cases of acute asthma, children should be prescribed an adequate once daily dose of oral prednisolone. Treatment for up to 3 days is usually sufficient, but the length of course should be tailored to the number of days necessary to bring about recovery. Intravenous hydrocortisone should be reserved for severely affected children who are unable to retain oral medication.

Nebulised ipratropium bromide can be combined with beta₂ agonist treatment for children with severe or life-threatening acute asthma or in those with a poor initial response to beta₂ agonist therapy to provide greater bronchodilation. Consider adding magnesium sulfate to nebulised salbutamol and ipratropium bromide in the first hour in children with a short duration of acute severe asthma symptoms presenting with an oxygen saturation less than 92%.

Children with continuing severe asthma despite frequent nebulised beta₂ agonists and ipratropium bromide plus oral corticosteroids, and those with life-threatening features, need urgent review by a specialist with a view to transfer to a high dependency unit or paediatric intensive care unit (PICU) to receive second-line intravenous therapies.

In a severe asthma attack where the child has not responded to initial inhaled therapy, early addition of a single bolus dose of intravenous salbutamol may be an option. Continuous intravenous infusion of salbutamol, administered under specialist supervision with continuous ECG and electrolyte monitoring, should be considered in children with unreliable inhalation or severe refractory asthma. Aminophylline may be considered in children with severe or life-threatening acute asthma unresponsive to maximal doses of bronchodilators and corticosteroids. Aminophylline is not recommended in children with mild to moderate acute asthma. Intravenous magnesium sulfate p. 1019 has been used for acute asthma [unlicensed use] although its place in management is not yet established. ⒶⒼ

Child under 2 years

EvGr Inhaled short-acting beta₂ agonists are the initial treatment of choice for acute asthma in children under 2 years. For mild to moderate acute asthma attacks, a metered-dose inhaler with a spacer and mask is the optimal drug delivery device. In a hospital setting, consider oral prednisolone daily for up to 3 days, early in the management of severe asthma attacks. For more severe symptoms, inhaled ipratropium bromide p. 246 in combination with an inhaled beta₂ agonist is also an option. ⒶⒼ

Follow up in all cases

EvGr Episodes of acute asthma may be a failure of preventative therapy, review is required to prevent further episodes. A careful history should be taken to establish the reason for the asthma attack. Inhaler technique should be checked and regular treatment should be reviewed. Patients should be given a written asthma action plan aimed at preventing relapse, optimising treatment, and preventing delay in seeking assistance in future attacks. It is essential that the patient's GP practice is informed within 24 hours of discharge from the emergency department or hospital following an asthma attack. Patients who have had a near-fatal asthma attack should be kept under specialist supervision indefinitely. A respiratory specialist should follow up all patients admitted with a severe asthma attack for at least one year after the admission. ⒶⒼ

Bronchodilators

29-Nov-2017

Adrenoceptor agonists (sympathomimetics)

Selective beta₂ agonists produce bronchodilation. A short-acting beta₂ agonist (such as salbutamol p. 252 and terbutaline sulfate p. 254) is used for immediate relief of asthma symptoms while some long-acting beta₂ agonists are added to an inhaled corticosteroid in patients requiring prophylactic treatment.

Adrenaline/epinephrine p. 221 (which has both alpha-and beta-adrenoceptor agonist properties) is used in the emergency management of acute allergic and anaphylactic reactions, in angioedema, in cardiopulmonary resuscitation, and in the management of severe croup.

Long-acting beta₂ agonists

Formoterol fumarate p. 250 and salmeterol p. 251 are longer-acting beta₂ agonists which are administered by inhalation. They should be used for asthma only in patients who regularly use an inhaled corticosteroid.

Combination inhalers that contain a long-acting beta₂ agonist and a corticosteroid ensure that long-acting beta₂ agonists are not used without concomitant corticosteroids.

Indacaterol p. 251 and olodaterol p. 251 are long-acting beta₂ agonists licensed for chronic obstructive pulmonary disease in adults; they are not indicated for the relief of acute bronchospasm.

Vilanterol is a long-acting beta₂ agonist available only in a combination inhaler with fluticasone furoate *or/and* with umeclidinium p. 248.

Oral

Oral preparations of beta₂ agonists may be used by patients who cannot manage the inhaled route. They are sometimes used for children and the elderly, but inhaled beta₂ agonists are more effective and have fewer side-effects. The longer-acting oral preparations, including bambuterol hydrochloride p. 249, may be of value in nocturnal asthma but they have a limited role and inhaled long-acting beta₂ agonists are usually preferred.

Parenteral

Salbutamol or terbutaline sulfate can be given intravenously for severe or life-threatening acute asthma; patients should be carefully monitored and the dose adjusted according to response and heart rate. The regular use of beta$_2$ agonists by the subcutaneous route is not recommended since the evidence of benefit is uncertain and it may be difficult to withdraw such treatment once started. In adults, beta$_2$ agonists may also be given by intramuscular injection.

Children

A pressurised metered-dose inhaler should be used with a spacer device in children under 5 years. A beta$_2$ agonist may also be given by mouth but administration by inhalation is preferred; a long-acting inhaled beta$_2$ agonist may be used where appropriate. In severe attacks nebulisation using a selective beta$_2$ agonist or ipratropium bromide p. 246 is advisable.

Antimuscarinic bronchodilators

Ipratropium bromide can provide short-term relief in chronic asthma, but short-acting beta$_2$ agonists act more quickly and are preferred. Ipratropium bromide by nebulisation can be added to other standard treatment in life-threatening asthma or if acute asthma fails to improve with standard therapy.

The aerosol inhalation of ipratropium bromide can be used for short-term relief in mild chronic obstructive pulmonary disease in patients who are not using a long-acting antimuscarinic drug. Its maximal effect occurs 30–60 minutes after use; its duration of action is 3 to 6 hours and bronchodilation can usually be maintained with treatment 3 times a day.

Aclidinium bromide p. 245, glycopyrronium bromide p. 246, tiotropium p. 247, and umeclidinium p. 248 are licensed for the maintenance treatment of adults with chronic obstructive pulmonary disease. They are not suitable for the relief of acute bronchospasm.

Theophylline

Theophylline p. 273 is a xanthine used as a bronchodilator in *asthma* and stable *chronic obstructive pulmonary disease*; it is not generally effective in exacerbations of chronic obstructive pulmonary disease. Theophylline may have an additive effect when used in conjunction with small doses of beta$_2$ agonists; the combination may increase the risk of side-effects, including hypokalaemia.

Theophylline is given by injection as aminophylline p. 272, a mixture of theophylline with ethylenediamine, which is 20 times more soluble than theophylline alone. Aminophylline injection is needed rarely for severe acute asthma.

Compound bronchodilator preparations

In general, patients are best treated with single-ingredient preparations, such as a selective beta$_2$ agonist or ipratropium bromide, so that the dose of each drug can be adjusted. However, a combination product may be appropriate for patients stabilised on individual components in the same proportion.

Chronic obstructive pulmonary disease

Management

Smoking cessation reduces the progressive decline in lung function in chronic obstructive pulmonary disease (COPD, chronic bronchitis, or emphysema). Infection can complicate chronic obstructive pulmonary disease and may be prevented by vaccination (pneumococcal polysaccharide conjugate vaccine (adsorbed) p. 1277 and influenza vaccine p. 1282).

A trial of a high-dose inhaled corticosteroid *or* an oral corticosteroid is recommended for patients with moderate or severe airflow obstruction if the diagnosis is in doubt.

Symptoms of chronic obstructive pulmonary disease may be alleviated by an inhaled **short-acting beta$_2$ agonist** or a **short-acting antimuscarinic bronchodilator** used as required.

When the airways obstruction is more severe, regular inhaled therapy should be used. It is important to check compliance and inhaler technique before initiating a new drug.

If the Forced Expiratory Volume in 1 second (FEV$_1$), is 50% of predicted or more, *either* a long-acting antimuscarinic bronchodilator *or* a long-acting beta$_2$ agonist should be used. Short-acting antimuscarinic bronchodilators should be discontinued when a long-acting antimuscarinic bronchodilator is started. A long-acting beta$_2$ agonist with a corticosteroid in a combination inhaler can be used for patients who remain symptomatic despite regular treatment with a long-acting beta$_2$ agonist.

If FEV$_1$ is less than 50% of predicted, *either* a long-acting antimuscarinic bronchodilator *or* a long-acting beta$_2$ agonist with a corticosteroid in a combination inhaler should be used.

In any patient who remains breathless or continues to have exacerbations, triple therapy with a long-acting beta$_2$ agonist and a corticosteroid in a combination inhaler *plus* a long-acting antimuscarinic bronchodilator should be used.

If an inhaled corticosteroid is not appropriate, a long-acting antimuscarinic bronchodilator can be used with a long-acting beta$_2$ agonist, (see Use of inhaled therapies in chronic obstructive pulmonary disease algorithm, below).

If symptoms persist or if the patient is unable to use an inhaler, oral modified-release aminophylline p. 272 or theophylline p. 273 can be used.

Indacaterol p. 251 is a long-acting beta$_2$ agonist licensed for the maintenance treatment of chronic obstructive pulmonary disease.

In patients with severe chronic obstructive pulmonary disease associated with chronic bronchitis and a history of frequent exacerbations, roflumilast p. 271 is licensed as an adjunct to existing bronchodilator treatment.

A **mucolytic** drug may be considered for a patient with a chronic productive cough.

Long-term **oxygen** therapy prolongs survival in patients with severe chronic obstructive pulmonary disease and hypoxaemia.

During an exacerbation of chronic obstructive pulmonary disease, bronchodilator therapy can be administered through a nebuliser if necessary and oxygen given if appropriate. Aminophylline can be given intravenously if response to nebulised bronchodilators is poor. A short course of **oral corticosteroid**, such as prednisolone for 7–14 days, should be given if increased breathlessness interferes with daily activities. **Antibacterial** treatment is required if sputum becomes more purulent than usual, or if there are other signs of infection.

Patients who have had an episode of hypercapnic respiratory failure should be given a 24% or 28% Venturi mask and an *oxygen alert card* endorsed with the oxygen saturations required during previous exacerbations. Patients and their carers should be instructed to show the card to emergency healthcare providers in the event of an exacerbation.

Oxygen alert card based on British Thoracic Society guideline for emergency oxygen use in adult patients (October 2008)

Oxygen alert card

Name: _____

I am at risk of type II respiratory failure with a raised CO_2 level.

Please use my _____% Venturi mask to achieve an oxygen saturation of _____% to _____% during exacerbations.

Use compressed air to drive nebulisers (with nasal oxygen at 2 litres/minute). If compressed air not available, limit oxygen-driven nebulisers to 6 minutes.

Oxygen alert card is available at www.brit-thoracic.org.uk.

Oxygen

Overview

Oxygen should be regarded as a drug. It is prescribed for hypoxaemic patients to increase alveolar oxygen tension and decrease the work of breathing. The concentration of oxygen required depends on the condition being treated; the administration of an inappropriate concentration of oxygen can have serious or even fatal consequences.

Oxygen is probably the most common drug used in medical emergencies. It should be prescribed initially to achieve a normal or near–normal oxygen saturation; in most acutely ill patients with a normal or low arterial carbon dioxide ($P_a CO_2$), oxygen saturation should be 94–98% oxygen saturation. However, in some clinical situations such as cardiac arrest and carbon monoxide poisoning it is more appropriate to aim for the highest possible oxygen saturation until the patient is stable. A lower target of 88–92% oxygen saturation is indicated for patients at risk of hypercapnic respiratory failure.

High concentration oxygen therapy is safe in uncomplicated cases of conditions such as pneumonia, pulmonary thromboembolism, pulmonary fibrosis, shock, severe trauma, sepsis, or anaphylaxis. In such conditions low arterial oxygen ($P_a O_2$) is usually associated with low or normal arterial carbon dioxide ($P_a CO_2$), and therefore there is little risk of hypoventilation and carbon dioxide retention.

In acute severe asthma, the arterial carbon dioxide ($P_a CO_2$) is usually subnormal but as asthma deteriorates it may rise steeply (particularly in children). These patients usually require high concentrations of oxygen and if the arterial carbon dioxide ($P_a CO_2$) remains high despite other treatment, intermittent positive-pressure ventilation needs to be considered urgently.

Low concentration oxygen therapy (controlled oxygen therapy) is reserved for patients at risk of hypercapnic respiratory failure, which is more likely in those with:

- chronic obstructive pulmonary disease;
- advanced cystic fibrosis;
- severe non-cystic fibrosis bronchiectasis;
- severe kyphoscoliosis or severe ankylosing spondylitis;
- severe lung scarring caused by tuberculosis;
- musculoskeletal disorders with respiratory weakness, especially if on home ventilation;
- an overdose of opioids, benzodiazepines, or other drugs causing respiratory depression.

Until blood gases can be measured, initial oxygen should be given using a controlled concentration of 28% or less,

titrated towards a target oxygen saturation of 88–92%. The aim is to provide the patient with enough oxygen to achieve an acceptable arterial oxygen tension without worsening carbon dioxide retention and respiratory acidosis. Patients may carry an *oxygen alert card*.

Domiciliary oxygen
Oxygen should only be prescribed for use in the home after careful evaluation in hospital by respiratory experts. Patients should be advised of the risks of continuing to smoke when receiving oxygen therapy, including the risk of fire. Smoking cessation therapy should be recommended before home oxygen prescription.

Air travel
Some patients with arterial hypoxaemia require supplementary oxygen for air travel. The patient's requirement should be discussed with the airline before travel.

Long-term oxygen therapy

Long-term administration of oxygen (usually at least 15 hours daily) prolongs survival in some patients with chronic obstructive pulmonary disease.

Assessment for long-term oxygen therapy requires measurement of arterial blood gas tensions. Measurements should be taken on 2 occasions at least 3 weeks apart to demonstrate clinical stability, and not sooner than 4 weeks after an acute exacerbation of the disease. Long-term oxygen therapy should be considered for patients with:

- chronic obstructive pulmonary disease with $P_a O_2 < 7.3$ kPa when breathing air during a period of clinical stability;
- chronic obstructive pulmonary disease with $P_a O_2$ 7.3–8 kPa in the presence of secondary polycythaemia, nocturnal hypoxaemia, peripheral oedema, or evidence of pulmonary hypertension;
- severe chronic asthma with $P_a O_2 < 7.3$ kPa or persistent disabling breathlessness;
- interstitial lung disease with $P_a O_2 < 8$ kPa and in patients with $P_a O_2 > 8$ kPa with disabling dyspnoea;
- cystic fibrosis when $P_a O_2 < 7.3$ kPa or if $P_a O_2$ 7.3–8 kPa in the presence of secondary polycythaemia, nocturnal hypoxaemia, pulmonary hypertension, or peripheral oedema;
- pulmonary hypertension, without parenchymal lung involvement when $P_a O_2 < 8$ kPa;
- neuromuscular or skeletal disorders, after specialist assessment;
- obstructive sleep apnoea despite continuous positive airways pressure therapy, after specialist assessment;
- pulmonary malignancy or other terminal disease with disabling dyspnoea;
- heart failure with daytime $P_a O_2 < 7.3$ kPa when breathing air or with nocturnal hypoxaemia;
- paediatric respiratory disease, after specialist assessment.

Increased respiratory depression is seldom a problem in patients with stable respiratory failure treated with low concentrations of oxygen although it may occur during exacerbations; patients and relatives should be warned to call for medical help if drowsiness or confusion occur.

Short-burst oxygen therapy

Oxygen is occasionally prescribed for short-burst (intermittent) use for episodes of breathlessness not relieved by other treatment in patients with severe chronic obstructive pulmonary disease, interstitial lung disease, heart failure, and in palliative care. It is important, however, that the patient does not rely on oxygen instead of obtaining medical help or taking more specific treatment. Short-burst oxygen therapy can be used to improve exercise capacity and recovery; it should only be continued if there is proven improvement in breathlessness or exercise tolerance.

3

Respiratory system

3

Respiratory system

Use of inhaled therapies in chronic obstructive pulmonary disease

Advice on the use of inhaled therapies in chronic obstructive pulmonary disease is based on the recommendations of the National Institute for Health and Care Excellence (2010). Management of chronic obstructive pulmonary disease in adults in primary and secondary care. London: NICE.
Available from www.nice.org.uk/CG101 Reproduced with permission

Ambulatory oxygen therapy

Ambulatory oxygen is prescribed for patients on long-term oxygen therapy who need to be away from home on a regular basis. Patients who are not on long-term oxygen therapy can be considered for ambulatory oxygen therapy if there is evidence of exercise-induced oxygen desaturation and of improvement in blood oxygen saturation and exercise capacity with oxygen. Ambulatory oxygen therapy is not recommended for patients with heart failure or those who smoke.

Oxygen therapy equipment

Under the NHS oxygen may be supplied as **oxygen cylinders**. Oxygen flow can be adjusted as the cylinders are equipped with an oxygen flow meter with 'medium' (2 litres/minute) and 'high' (4 litres/minute) settings. Oxygen delivered from a cylinder should be passed through a humidifier if used for long periods.

Oxygen concentrators are more economical for patients who require oxygen for long periods, and in England and Wales can be ordered on the NHS on a regional tendering basis. A concentrator is recommended for a patient who

requires oxygen for more than 8 hours a day (or 21 cylinders per month). Exceptionally, if a higher concentration of oxygen is required the output of 2 oxygen concentrators can be combined using a 'Y' connection.

A nasal cannula is usually preferred for long-term oxygen therapy from an oxygen concentrator. It can, however, produce dermatitis and mucosal drying in sensitive individuals.

Giving oxygen by nasal cannula allows the patient to talk, eat, and drink, but the concentration of oxygen is not controlled; this may not be appropriate for acute respiratory failure. When oxygen is given through a nasal cannula at a rate of 1–2 litres/minute the inspiratory oxygen concentration is usually low, but it varies with ventilation and can be high if the patient is underventilating.

Arrangements for supplying oxygen

The following oxygen services may be ordered in England and Wales:

- emergency oxygen;
- short-burst (intermittent) oxygen therapy;
- long-term oxygen therapy;
- ambulatory oxygen.

The type of oxygen service (or combination of services) should be ordered on a Home Oxygen Order Form (HOOF); the amount of oxygen required (hours per day) and flow rate should be specified. The clinician will determine the appropriate equipment to be provided. Special needs or preferences should be specified on the HOOF.

The clinician should obtain the patient or carers consent, to pass on the patient's details to the supplier, the fire brigade, and other relevant organisations. The supplier will contact the patient to make arrangements for delivery, installation, and maintenance of the equipment. The supplier will also train the patient or carer to use the equipment.

The clinician should send the HOOF to the supplier who will continue to provide the service until a revised HOOF is received, or until notified that the patient no longer requires the home oxygen service.

- East of England, North East: BOC Medical: Tel: 0800 136 603 Fax: 0800 169 9989
- South West: Air Liquide: Tel: 0808 202 2229 Fax: 0191 497 4340
- London, East Midlands, North West: Air Liquide: Tel: 0500 823 773 Fax: 0800 781 4610
- Yorkshire and Humberside, West Midlands, Wales: Air Products: Tel: 0800 373 580 Fax: 0800 214 709
- South East Coast, South Central: Dolby Vivisol: Tel: 08443 814 402 Fax: 0800 781 4610

In **Scotland** refer the patient for assessment by a respiratory consultant. If the need for a concentrator is confirmed the consultant will arrange for the provision of a concentrator through the Common Services Agency. Prescribers should complete a Scottish Home Oxygen Order Form (SHOOF) and email it to Health Facilities Scotland. Health Facilities Scotland will then liaise with their contractor to arrange the supply of oxygen. Further information can be obtained at: www.dolbyvivisol.com/our-services/healthcare-professionals/home-oxygen-services-sco.aspx.

In **Northern Ireland** oxygen concentrators and cylinders should be prescribed on form HS21; oxygen concentrators are supplied by a local contractor. Prescriptions for oxygen cylinders and accessories can be dispensed by pharmacists contracted to provide domiciliary oxygen services.

Croup

Management

Mild croup is largely self-limiting, but treatment with a single dose of a corticosteroid (e.g. dexamethasone p. 660) by mouth may be of benefit.

More severe croup (or mild croup that might cause complications) calls for hospital admission; a single dose of a corticosteroid (e.g. dexamethasone or prednisolone p. 664 by mouth) should be administered before transfer to hospital. In hospital, dexamethasone (by mouth or by injection) or budesonide p. 259 (by nebulisation) will often reduce symptoms; the dose may need to be repeated after 12 hours if necessary.

For severe croup not effectively controlled with corticosteroid treatment, nebulised adrenaline/epinephrine solution 1 in 1000 (1 mg/mL) p. 221 should be given with close clinical monitoring; the effects of nebulised adrenaline/epinephrine last 2–3 hours and the child needs to be monitored carefully for recurrence of the obstruction.

ANTIMUSCARINICS

Antimuscarinics (inhaled)

09-Feb-2016

- CAUTIONS Bladder outflow obstruction · paradoxical bronchospasm · prostatic hyperplasia · susceptibility to angle-closure glaucoma
- SIDE-EFFECTS
- ► **Common or very common** Arrhythmias · cough · dizziness · dry mouth · epistaxis · headache · nausea
- ► **Uncommon** Constipation · dysphonia · glaucoma · palpitations · skin reactions · stomatitis · urinary disorders · vision blurred

⏎ **above**

Aclidinium bromide

15-Feb-2016

- ● INDICATIONS AND DOSE

Maintenance treatment of chronic obstructive pulmonary disease
- ► BY INHALATION OF POWDER
- ► Adult: 375 micrograms twice daily

DOSE EQUIVALENCE AND CONVERSION
- ► Each 375 microgram inhalation of aclidinium bromide delivers 322 micrograms of aclidinium.

- ● CAUTIONS Arrhythmia (when newly diagnosed within last 3 months) · heart failure (hospitalisation with moderate or severe heart failure within last 12 months) · myocardial infarction within last 6 months · unstable angina
- ● INTERACTIONS → Appendix 1: aclidinium
- ● SIDE-EFFECTS
- ► **Common or very common** Diarrhoea · nasopharyngitis
- ► **Uncommon** Angioedema
- ► **Rare or very rare** Hypersensitivity
- ● PREGNANCY Manufacturer advises use only if potential benefit outweighs risk.
- ● BREAST FEEDING Manufacturer advises only use if potential benefits outweigh risks.
- ● PATIENT AND CARER ADVICE Patients or carers should be given advice on appropriate inhaler technique.

- ● MEDICINAL FORMS
There can be variation in the licensing of different medicines containing the same drug.
Inhalation powder
- ► Aclidinium bromide (non-proprietary) ▼
 Aclidinium bromide 375 microgram per 1 dose Aclidinium bromide 375micrograms/dose dry powder inhaler | 60 dose PoM Ⓢ DT = £28.60
- ► Eklira (AstraZeneca UK Ltd) ▼
 Aclidinium bromide 375 microgram per 1 dose Eklira 322micrograms/dose Genuair | 60 dose PoM £28.60 DT = £28.60

Aclidinium bromide with formoterol

19-Feb-2016

The properties listed below are those particular to the combination only. For the properties of the components please consider, aclidinium bromide above, formoterol fumarate p. 250.

- ● INDICATIONS AND DOSE

Maintenance treatment of chronic obstructive pulmonary disease
- ► BY INHALATION OF POWDER
- ► Adult: 1 inhalation twice daily

- ● CAUTIONS Convulsive disorders · phaeochromocytoma
- ● INTERACTIONS → Appendix 1: aclidinium · beta₂ agonists

Respiratory system
3

- PATIENT AND CARER ADVICE Patients or carers should be given advice on appropriate inhaler technique.

- MEDICINAL FORMS
There can be variation in the licensing of different medicines containing the same drug.
Inhalation powder
▸ Duaklir (AstraZeneca UK Ltd) ▼
Formoterol fumarate dihydrate 11.8 microgram per 1 dose, Aclidinium bromide 396 microgram per 1 dose Duaklir 340micrograms/dose / 12micrograms/dose Genuair | 60 dose PoM
£32.50 DT = £32.50

F 245

Glycopyrronium bromide
13-Sep-2017

(Glycopyrrolate)

- INDICATIONS AND DOSE
Maintenance treatment of chronic obstructive pulmonary disease
▸ BY INHALATION OF POWDER
▸ Adult: 1 capsule once daily
DOSE EQUIVALENCE AND CONVERSION
▸ Each capsule delivers 55 micrograms of glycopyrronium bromide (equivalent to 44 micrograms of glycopyrronium).

- CAUTIONS Arrhythmia (excluding chronic stable atrial fibrillation) · history of myocardial infarction · history of QT-interval prolongation · left ventricular failure · unstable ischaemic heart disease
- INTERACTIONS → Appendix 1: glycopyrronium
- SIDE-EFFECTS
▸ Common or very common Increased risk of infection · insomnia · pain
▸ Uncommon Asthenia · cystitis · dental caries · hyperglycaemia · hypersensitivity · numbness · productive cough · respiratory disorders · throat irritation
SIDE-EFFECTS, FURTHER INFORMATION The possibility of systemic side-effects should be considered; however, glycopyrronium is poorly absorbed and systemic effects are unlikely with topical use.
- PREGNANCY Manufacturer advises use only if potential benefit outweighs risk.
- BREAST FEEDING Manufacturer advises use only if potential benefit outweighs risk.
- RENAL IMPAIRMENT Manufacturer advises use only if potential benefit outweighs risk if eGFR less than 30 mL/minute/1.73 m².
- PATIENT AND CARER ADVICE Patients or carers should be given advice on appropriate inhaler technique.

- MEDICINAL FORMS
There can be variation in the licensing of different medicines containing the same drug.
Inhalation powder
▸ Glycopyrronium bromide (non-proprietary) ▼
Glycopyrronium bromide 55 microgram Glycopyrronium bromide 55microgram inhalation powder capsules with device | 30 capsule PoM ⓢ DT = £27.50
▸ Seebri Breezhaler (Novartis Pharmaceuticals UK Ltd) ▼
Glycopyrronium bromide 55 microgram Seebri Breezhaler 44microgram inhalation powder capsules with device | 10 capsule PoM £9.17 | 30 capsule PoM £27.50 DT = £27.50

Combinations available: *Beclometasone with formoterol and glycopyrronium*, p. 259

Glycopyrronium with indacaterol
17-Feb-2016

The properties listed below are those particular to the combination only. For the properties of the components please consider, glycopyrronium bromide above, indacaterol p. 251.

- INDICATIONS AND DOSE
Maintenance treatment of chronic obstructive pulmonary disease
▸ BY INHALATION OF POWDER
▸ Adult: 1 inhalation daily

- CAUTIONS Convulsive disorders
- INTERACTIONS → Appendix 1: beta₂ agonists · glycopyrronium
- PATIENT AND CARER ADVICE Patients or carers should be given advice on appropriate inhaler technique and reminded that the capsules are not for oral administration.

- MEDICINAL FORMS
There can be variation in the licensing of different medicines containing the same drug.
Inhalation powder
▸ Ultibro Breezhaler (Novartis Pharmaceuticals UK Ltd) ▼
Glycopyrronium bromide 54 microgram per 1 dose, Indacaterol (as Indacaterol maleate) 85 microgram per 1 dose Ultibro Breezhaler 85microgram/43microgram inhalation powder capsules with device | 10 capsule PoM £10.83 DT = £10.83 | 30 capsule PoM £32.50 DT = £32.50

F 245

Ipratropium bromide
22-Jan-2018

- INDICATIONS AND DOSE
Reversible airways obstruction
▸ BY INHALATION OF AEROSOL
▸ Child 1 month–5 years: 20 micrograms 3 times a day
▸ Child 6–11 years: 20–40 micrograms 3 times a day
▸ Child 12–17 years: 20–40 micrograms 3–4 times a day
Reversible airways obstruction, particularly in chronic obstructive pulmonary disease
▸ BY INHALATION OF AEROSOL
▸ Adult: 20–40 micrograms 3–4 times a day
▸ BY INHALATION OF NEBULISED SOLUTION
▸ Adult: 250–500 micrograms 3–4 times a day
Acute bronchospasm
▸ BY INHALATION OF NEBULISED SOLUTION
▸ Child 1 month–5 years: 125–250 micrograms as required; maximum 1 mg per day
▸ Child 6–11 years: 250 micrograms as required; maximum 1 mg per day
▸ Child 12–17 years: 500 micrograms as required, doses higher than max. can be given under medical supervision; maximum 2 mg per day
▸ Adult: 500 micrograms as required, doses higher than max. can be given under medical supervision; maximum 2 mg per day
Severe or life-threatening acute asthma
▸ BY INHALATION OF NEBULISED SOLUTION
▸ Child 1 month–11 years: 250 micrograms every 20–30 minutes for the first 2 hours, then 250 micrograms every 4–6 hours as required
▸ Child 12–17 years: 500 micrograms every 4–6 hours as required
▸ Adult: 500 micrograms every 4–6 hours as required
PHARMACOKINETICS
▸ The maximal effect of inhaled ipratropium occurs 30–60 minutes after use; its duration of action is 3 to 6 hours and bronchodilation can usually be maintained with treatment 3 times a day.

- UNLICENSED USE EvGr The dose of ipratropium for severe or life-threatening acute asthma is unlicensed. ⒶInhalvent® not licensed for use in children under 6 years.
- CAUTIONS Avoid spraying near eyes · cystic fibrosis

CAUTIONS, FURTHER INFORMATION

▸ Glaucoma *Acute angle-closure glaucoma* has been reported with nebulised ipratropium, particularly when given with nebulised salbutamol (and possibly other beta₂ agonists); care needed to protect the patient's eyes from nebulised drug or from drug powder.

- INTERACTIONS → Appendix 1: ipratropium
- SIDE-EFFECTS
▸ **Common or very common** Gastrointestinal motility disorder · throat complaints
▸ **Uncommon** Corneal oedema · diarrhoea · eye disorders · eye pain · respiratory disorders · vision disorders · vomiting
- ALLERGY AND CROSS-SENSITIVITY Contra-indicated in patients with hypersensitivity to atropine or its derivatives.
- PREGNANCY Manufacturer advises only use if potential benefit outweighs the risk.
- BREAST FEEDING No information available—manufacturer advises only use if potential benefit outweighs risk.
- DIRECTIONS FOR ADMINISTRATION If dilution of ipratropium bromide nebuliser solution is necessary use only sterile sodium chloride 0.9%.
- PATIENT AND CARER ADVICE Patients or carers should be counselled on appropriate administration technique and warned against accidental contact with the eye (due to risk of ocular complications).
Driving and skilled tasks Manufacturer advises patients and carers should be counselled on the effects on driving and performance of skilled tasks—increased risk of dizziness and vision disorders.

- MEDICINAL FORMS
There can be variation in the licensing of different medicines containing the same drug.
Nebuliser liquid
▸ Ipratropium bromide (Non-proprietary)
Ipratropium bromide 250 microgram per 1 ml Ipratropium bromide 500micrograms/2ml nebuliser liquid unit dose vials | 20 unit dose PoM £5.60 DT = £3.36
Ipratropium bromide 250micrograms/1ml nebuliser liquid unit dose vials | 20 unit dose PoM £4.83 DT = £4.65
▸ Atrovent UDV (Boehringer Ingelheim Ltd)
Ipratropium bromide 250 microgram per 1 ml Atrovent 500micrograms/2ml nebuliser liquid UDVs | 20 unit dose PoM £4.87 DT = £3.36 | 60 unit dose PoM £14.59
Atrovent 250micrograms/1ml nebuliser liquid UDVs | 20 unit dose PoM £4.14 DT = £4.65 | 60 unit dose PoM £12.44
Pressurised inhalation
▸ Atrovent (Boehringer Ingelheim Ltd)
Ipratropium bromide 20 microgram per 1 dose Atrovent 20micrograms/dose inhaler CFC free | 200 dose PoM £5.56 DT = £5.56
▸ Inhalvent (Alissa Healthcare Research Ltd)
Ipratropium bromide 20 microgram per 1 dose Inhalvent 20micrograms/dose inhaler | 200 dose PoM £5.56 DT = £5.56

Ipratropium with salbutamol   17-Feb-2016

The properties listed below are those particular to the combination only. For the properties of the components please consider, ipratropium bromide p. 246, salbutamol p. 252.

- INDICATIONS AND DOSE
Bronchospasm in chronic obstructive pulmonary disease
▸ BY INHALATION OF NEBULISED SOLUTION
▸ Adult: 0.5/2.5 mg 3–4 times a day

- INTERACTIONS → Appendix 1: beta₂ agonists · ipratropium

- PRESCRIBING AND DISPENSING INFORMATION A mixture of ipratropium bromide and salbutamol (as sulphate); the proportions are expressed in the form x/y where x and y are the strengths in milligrams of ipratropium and salbutamol respectively.

- MEDICINAL FORMS
There can be variation in the licensing of different medicines containing the same drug.
Nebuliser liquid
▸ Ipratropium with salbutamol (Non-proprietary)
Ipratropium bromide 200 microgram per 1 ml, Salbutamol (as Salbutamol sulfate) 1 mg per 1 ml Salbutamol 2.5mg/2.5ml / Ipratropium bromide 500micrograms/2.5ml nebuliser liquid unit dose vials | 60 unit dose PoM ⚠ DT = £24.10
▸ Combivent (Boehringer Ingelheim Ltd)
Ipratropium bromide 200 microgram per 1 ml, Salbutamol (as Salbutamol sulfate) 1 mg per 1 ml Combivent nebuliser liquid 2.5ml UDVs | 60 unit dose PoM £24.10 DT = £24.10
▸ Ipramol (Teva UK Ltd)
Ipratropium bromide 200 microgram per 1 ml, Salbutamol (as Salbutamol sulfate) 1 mg per 1 ml Ipramol nebuliser solution 2.5ml Steri-Neb unit dose vials | 60 unit dose PoM £23.83 DT = £24.10
▸ Salipraneb (Actavis UK Ltd)
Ipratropium bromide 200 microgram per 1 ml, Salbutamol (as Salbutamol sulfate) 1 mg per 1 ml Salipraneb 0.5mg/2.5mg nebuliser solution 2.5ml ampoules | 60 ampoule PoM £17.50 DT = £17.50

📕 245

Tiotropium   12-Jun-2018

- INDICATIONS AND DOSE
Maintenance treatment of chronic obstructive pulmonary disease
▸ BY INHALATION OF POWDER
▸ Adult: 1 capsule once daily

DOSE EQUIVALENCE AND CONVERSION

▸ For *Spiriva*® inhalation powder, 1 capsule contains a metered dose of 18 micrograms tiotropium; for *Braltus*® inhalation powder, 1 capsule contains a metered dose of 13 micrograms tiotropium.
▸ The delivered dose of *Spiriva*® and *Braltus*® inhalation powder products are the same (10 micrograms); no dose adjustment is necessary when switching between brands.

SPIRIVA RESPIMAT®

Maintenance treatment of chronic obstructive pulmonary disease | Severe asthma [add-on to inhaled corticosteroid (at least 800 micrograms budesonide daily or equivalent) and at least 1 controller in patients who have suffered one or more severe exacerbations in the last year]
▸ BY INHALATION OF AEROSOL
▸ Adult: 5 micrograms once daily

Severe asthma [add-on to inhaled corticosteroid (over 400 micrograms budesonide daily or equivalent) and 1 controller, or inhaled corticosteroid (200–400 micrograms budesonide daily or equivalent) and 2 controllers, in patients who have suffered one or more severe exacerbations in the last year]
▸ BY INHALATION OF AEROSOL
▸ Child 6-11 years: 5 micrograms once daily

Severe asthma [add-on to inhaled corticosteroid (over 800 micrograms budesonide daily or equivalent) and 1 controller, or inhaled corticosteroid (400–800 micrograms budesonide daily or equivalent) and 2 controllers, in patients who have suffered one or more severe exacerbations in the last year]
▸ BY INHALATION OF AEROSOL
▸ Child 12-17 years: 5 micrograms once daily   continued →

DOSE EQUIVALENCE AND CONVERSION
▶ For *Spiriva Respimat*® 2 puffs is equivalent to 5 micrograms tiotropium.

IMPORTANT SAFETY INFORMATION

MHRA/CHM ADVICE: *BRALTUS*® (TIOTROPIUM): RISK OF INHALATION OF CAPSULE IF PLACED IN THE MOUTHPIECE OF THE INHALER (MAY 2018)

The MHRA have received reports of patients who have inhaled a *Braltus*® capsule from the mouthpiece into the back of the throat, resulting in coughing and risking aspiration or airway obstruction. Patients should be trained in the correct use of their inhaler and told to store capsules in the screw-top bottle provided (never in the inhaler) and to always check the mouthpiece is clear before inhaling.

Pharmacists dispensing *Braltus*® capsules should remind patients always to read the instructions for use in the package leaflet and that they must never place a capsule directly into the mouthpiece.

● CAUTIONS Arrhythmia (unstable, life-threatening or requiring intervention in the previous 12 months) · heart failure (hospitalisation for moderate to severe heart failure in the previous 12 months) · myocardial infarction in the previous 6 months
● INTERACTIONS → Appendix 1: tiotropium
● SIDE-EFFECTS
▶ **Uncommon** Gastrointestinal disorders · increased risk of infection · taste altered
▶ **Rare or very rare** Bronchospasm · dysphagia · insomnia · oral disorders
▶ **Frequency not known** Dehydration · dry skin · joint swelling · skin ulcer
● PREGNANCY Manufacturer advises avoid—limited data available.
● BREAST FEEDING Manufacturer advises avoid—no information available.
● RENAL IMPAIRMENT Manufacturer advises use only if potential benefit outweighs risk if creatinine clearance less than or equal to 50 mL/minute—plasma-tiotropium concentration raised.
● PATIENT AND CARER ADVICE Patients or carers should be given advice on appropriate inhaler technique and reminded that the powder inhalation capsules are not for oral administration; for *Braltus*®, see also *Important safety Information*.
● NATIONAL FUNDING/ACCESS DECISIONS
SPIRIVA RESPIMAT®

Scottish Medicines Consortium (SMC) Decisions
▶ In adults The *Scottish Medicines Consortium* has advised (August 2015) that tiotropium (*Spiriva Respimat*®) is accepted for use within NHS Scotland as add-on maintenance bronchodilator treatment in adults with asthma who are currently treated with the maintenance combination of inhaled corticosteroids (≥800 micrograms budesonide/day or equivalent) and long-acting beta₂-agonists and who experienced one or more severe exacerbations in the previous year.
▶ In adults The *Scottish Medicines Consortium* has advised (December 2017) that tiotropium (*Spiriva Respimat*®) is accepted for use within NHS Scotland as a maintenance bronchodilator treatment to relieve symptoms of patients with chronic obstructive pulmonary disease.

All Wales Medicines Strategy Group (AWMSG) Decisions
▶ In adults The *All Wales Medicines Strategy Group* has advised (October 2017) that tiotropium (*Spiriva Respimat*®) is recommended as an option for use within NHS Wales as an add-on maintenance bronchodilator treatment in adults with asthma who are currently treated

with the maintenance combination of inhaled corticosteroids (≥800 micrograms budesonide daily or equivalent) and long-acting beta₂-agonists and who experienced one or more severe exacerbations in the previous year.

● MEDICINAL FORMS
There can be variation in the licensing of different medicines containing the same drug.
Inhalation powder
▶ Braltus (Teva UK Ltd)
Tiotropium (as Tiotropium bromide) 10 microgram Braltus 10microgram inhalation powder capsules with Zonda inhaler | 30 capsule [PoM] £25.80 DT = £25.80
▶ Spiriva (Boehringer Ingelheim Ltd)
Tiotropium (as Tiotropium bromide) 18 microgram Spiriva 18microgram inhalation powder capsules | 30 capsule [PoM] £33.50 DT = £33.50 | 60 capsule [PoM] £67.00
Spiriva 18microgram inhalation powder capsules with HandiHaler | 30 capsule [PoM] £34.87 DT = £34.87
Pressurised inhalation
▶ Spiriva Respimat (Boehringer Ingelheim Ltd)
Tiotropium (as Tiotropium bromide) 2.5 microgram per 1 dose Spiriva Respimat 2.5micrograms/dose solution for inhalation cartridge with device | 60 dose [PoM] £23.00 DT = £23.00

Tiotropium with olodaterol   15-Feb-2016

The properties listed below are those particular to the combination only. For the properties of the components please consider, tiotropium p. 247, olodaterol p. 251.

● INDICATIONS AND DOSE

Maintenance treatment of chronic obstructive pulmonary disease
▶ BY INHALATION OF AEROSOL
▶ **Adult:** 2 puffs once daily

● INTERACTIONS → Appendix 1: beta₂ agonists · tiotropium
● PATIENT AND CARER ADVICE Patient or carers should be given advice on appropriate inhaler technique.

● MEDICINAL FORMS
There can be variation in the licensing of different medicines containing the same drug.
Pressurised inhalation
▶ Spiolto Respimat (Boehringer Ingelheim Ltd) ▼
Olodaterol (as Olodaterol hydrochloride) 2.5 microgram per 1 dose, Tiotropium (as Tiotropium bromide) 2.5 microgram per 1 dose Spiolto Respimat 2.5micrograms/dose / 2.5micrograms/dose solution for inhalation cartridge with device | 60 dose [PoM] £32.50 DT = £32.50

⏴ 245

Umeclidinium   19-Feb-2016

● INDICATIONS AND DOSE

Maintenance treatment of chronic obstructive pulmonary disease
▶ BY INHALATION OF POWDER
▶ **Adult:** 55 micrograms once daily
DOSE EQUIVALENCE AND CONVERSION
▶ Each 65 microgram inhalation of umeclidinium bromide delivers 55 micrograms of umeclidinium.

● CAUTIONS Cardiac disorders (particularly cardiac rhythm disorders)
● INTERACTIONS → Appendix 1: umeclidinium
● SIDE-EFFECTS
▶ **Uncommon** Taste altered
▶ **Rare or very rare** Eye pain
● PREGNANCY Manufacturer advises use only if potential benefit outweighs risk.

- BREAST FEEDING Manufacturer advises avoid—no information available.
- HEPATIC IMPAIRMENT Manufacturer advises to use with caution in severe impairment—no information available.
- PATIENT AND CARER ADVICE Patient or carers should be given advice on appropriate inhaler technique.

- MEDICINAL FORMS
  There can be variation in the licensing of different medicines containing the same drug.
  Inhalation powder
  ▸ Incruse Ellipta (GlaxoSmithKline UK Ltd) ▼
    Umeclidinium bromide 65 microgram per 1 dose Incruse Ellipta 55micrograms/dose dry powder inhaler | 30 dose PoM £27.50 DT = £27.50

  Combinations available: *Fluticasone with umeclidinium and vilanterol*, p. 264

Umeclidinium with vilanterol 19-Feb-2016

The properties listed below are those particular to the combination only. For the properties of the components please consider, umeclidinium p. 248.

- INDICATIONS AND DOSE
  Maintenance treatment of chronic obstructive pulmonary disease
  ▸ BY INHALATION OF POWDER
  ▸ Adult: 1 inhalation once daily

- CONTRA-INDICATIONS Severe pre-eclampsia
- CAUTIONS Arrhythmias · cardiovascular disease · diabetes (risk of hyperglycaemia and ketoacidosis) · hypertension · hyperthyroidism · hypokalaemia · susceptibility to QT-interval prolongation
  CAUTIONS, FURTHER INFORMATION
  ▸ Hypokalaemia Potentially serious hypokalaemia may result from beta$_2$ agonist therapy. Particular caution is required in severe asthma, because this effect may be potentiated by concomitant treatment with theophylline and its derivatives, corticosteroids, diuretics, and by hypoxia.
- INTERACTIONS → Appendix 1: beta$_2$ agonists · umeclidinium
- SIDE-EFFECTS
  ▸ **Common or very common** Constipation · dry mouth · headache · oropharyngeal pain · sinusitis
  ▸ **Uncommon** Dysphonia · palpitations · taste altered · tremor
  ▸ **Rare or very rare** Bronchospasm paradoxical · glaucoma · urinary disorders
- MONITORING REQUIREMENTS
  ▸ In severe asthma, plasma-potassium concentration should be monitored (risk of hypokalaemia).
  ▸ In patients with diabetes, monitor blood glucose (risk of hyperglycaemia and ketoacidosis, especially when beta$_2$ agonist given intravenously).
- PATIENT AND CARER ADVICE Patient or carers should be given advice on appropriate inhaler technique.

- MEDICINAL FORMS
  There can be variation in the licensing of different medicines containing the same drug.
  Inhalation powder
  ▸ Umeclidinium with vilanterol (non-proprietary) ▼
    Vilanterol (as Vilanterol trifenatate) 22 microgram per 1 dose, Umeclidinium bromide 65 microgram per 1 dose Umeclidinium bromide 65micrograms/dose / Vilanterol 22micrograms/dose dry powder inhaler | 30 dose Ⓢ DT = £32.50
  ▸ Anoro Ellipta (GlaxoSmithKline UK Ltd) ▼
    Vilanterol (as Vilanterol trifenatate) 22 microgram per 1 dose, Umeclidinium bromide 65 microgram per 1 dose Anoro Ellipta 55micrograms/dose / 22micrograms/dose dry powder inhaler | 30 dose PoM £32.50 DT = £32.50

BETA$_2$-ADRENOCEPTOR AGONISTS, SELECTIVE

Beta$_2$-adrenoceptor agonists, selective 12-Feb-2016

- CONTRA-INDICATIONS Severe pre-eclampsia
- CAUTIONS Arrhythmias · cardiovascular disease · diabetes (risk of hyperglycaemia and ketoacidosis, especially with intravenous use) · hypertension · hyperthyroidism · hypokalaemia · susceptibility to QT-interval prolongation
  CAUTIONS, FURTHER INFORMATION
  ▸ Hypokalaemia Potentially serious hypokalaemia may result from beta$_2$ agonist therapy. Particular caution is required in severe asthma, because this effect may be potentiated by concomitant treatment with theophylline and its derivatives, corticosteroids, diuretics, and by hypoxia.
- SIDE-EFFECTS
  ▸ **Common or very common** Arrhythmias · dizziness · headache · hypokalaemia (with high doses) · nausea · palpitations · tremor
  ▸ **Uncommon** Hyperglycaemia · myocardial ischaemia
  ▸ **Rare or very rare** Bronchospasm paradoxical (sometimes severe)
- PREGNANCY Women planning to become pregnant should be counselled about the importance of taking their asthma medication regularly to maintain good control.
- MONITORING REQUIREMENTS
  ▸ In severe asthma, plasma-potassium concentration should be monitored (risk of hypokalaemia).
  ▸ In patients with diabetes, monitor blood glucose (risk of hyperglycaemia and ketoacidosis, especially when beta$_2$ agonist given intravenously).
- PATIENT AND CARER ADVICE
  ▸ When used by inhalation The **dose**, the frequency, and the maximum number of inhalations in 24 hours of the beta$_2$ agonist should be **stated explicitly** to the patient or their carer. The patient or their carer should be advised to seek medical advice when the prescribed dose of beta$_2$ agonist fails to provide the usual degree of symptomatic relief because this usually indicates a worsening of the asthma and the patient may require a prophylactic drug. Patients or their carers should be advised to follow manufacturers' instructions on the care and cleansing of inhaler devices.

BETA$_2$-ADRENOCEPTOR AGONISTS, SELECTIVE ⟩ LONG-ACTING

Bambuterol hydrochloride

- DRUG ACTION Bambuterol is a pro-drug of terbutaline.

- INDICATIONS AND DOSE
  Asthma (patients who have previously tolerated beta$_2$-agonists) | Other conditions associated with reversible airways obstruction (patients who have previously tolerated beta$_2$-agonists)
  ▸ BY MOUTH
  ▸ Adult: 20 mg once daily, dose to be taken at bedtime

  Asthma (patients who have not previously tolerated beta$_2$-agonists) | Other conditions associated with reversible airways obstruction (patients who have not previously tolerated beta$_2$-agonists)
  ▸ BY MOUTH
  ▸ Adult: Initially 10 mg once daily for 1–2 weeks, then increased if necessary to 20 mg once daily, dose to be taken at bedtime

- INTERACTIONS → Appendix 1: beta$_2$ agonists

- SIDE-EFFECTS
- ▶ **Common or very common** Anxiety · behaviour abnormal · muscle cramps · sleep disorder
- ▶ **Frequency not known** Akathisia · angioedema · circulatory collapse · hypersensitivity · hypotension · skin reactions
- PREGNANCY Manufacturer advises avoid—no information available.
- BREAST FEEDING Manufacturer advises avoid—no information available.
- HEPATIC IMPAIRMENT Avoid in severe impairment.
- RENAL IMPAIRMENT
  Dose adjustments Reduce initial dose by half if eGFR less than 50 mL/minute/1.73 m^2.

- MEDICINAL FORMS
  There can be variation in the licensing of different medicines containing the same drug.

  Tablet
  - ▶ Bambec (AstraZeneca UK Ltd)
    Bambuterol hydrochloride 10 mg Bambec 10mg tablets | 28 tablet [PoM] £28.92 DT = £28.92
    Bambuterol hydrochloride 20 mg Bambec 20mg tablets | 28 tablet [PoM] £15.77 DT = £15.77

F 249

Formoterol fumarate

(Eformoterol fumarate)

- INDICATIONS AND DOSE
  Reversible airways obstruction in patients requiring long-term regular bronchodilator therapy | Nocturnal asthma in patients requiring long-term regular bronchodilator therapy | Prophylaxis of exercise-induced bronchospasm in patients requiring long-term regular bronchodilator therapy | Chronic asthma in patients who regularly use an inhaled corticosteroid
  - ▶ BY INHALATION OF POWDER
  - ▶ Child 6–11 years: 12 micrograms twice daily, a daily dose of 24 micrograms of formoterol should be sufficient for the majority of children, particularly for younger age-groups; higher doses should be used rarely, and only when control is not maintained on the lower dose
  - ▶ Child 12–17 years: 12 micrograms twice daily, dose may be increased in more severe airway obstruction; increased to 24 micrograms twice daily, a daily dose of 24 micrograms of formoterol should be sufficient for the majority of children, particularly for younger age-groups; higher doses should be used rarely, and only when control is not maintained on the lower dose
  - ▶ Adult: 12 micrograms twice daily, dose may be increased in more severe airway obstruction; increased to 24 micrograms twice daily
  - ▶ BY INHALATION OF AEROSOL
  - ▶ Child 12–17 years: 12 micrograms twice daily, dose may be increased in more severe airway obstruction; increased to 24 micrograms twice daily, a daily dose of 24 micrograms of formoterol should be sufficient for the majority of children, particularly for younger age-groups; higher doses should be used rarely, and only when control is not maintained on the lower dose
  - ▶ Adult: 12 micrograms twice daily, dose may be increased in more severe airway obstruction; increased to 24 micrograms twice daily

Chronic obstructive pulmonary disease
  - ▶ BY INHALATION OF POWDER
  - ▶ Adult: 12 micrograms twice daily
  - ▶ BY INHALATION OF AEROSOL
  - ▶ Adult: 12 micrograms twice daily (max. per dose 24 micrograms), for symptom relief additional doses may be taken to maximum daily dose; maximum 48 micrograms per day

OXIS ®

Chronic asthma
  - ▶ BY INHALATION OF POWDER
  - ▶ Child 6–17 years: 6–12 micrograms 1–2 times a day (max. per dose 12 micrograms), occasionally doses up to the maximum daily may be needed, reassess treatment if additional doses required on more than 2 days a week; maximum 48 micrograms per day
  - ▶ Adult: 6–12 micrograms 1–2 times a day, increased if necessary up to 24 micrograms twice daily (max. per dose 36 micrograms), occasionally doses up to the maximum daily may be needed, reassess treatment if additional doses required on more than 2 days a week; maximum 72 micrograms per day

Relief of bronchospasm
  - ▶ BY INHALATION OF POWDER
  - ▶ Child 6–17 years: 6–12 micrograms
  - ▶ Adult: 6–12 micrograms

Prophylaxis of exercise-induced bronchospasm
  - ▶ BY INHALATION OF POWDER
  - ▶ Child 6–17 years: 6–12 micrograms, dose to be taken before exercise
  - ▶ Adult: 12 micrograms, dose to be taken before exercise

Chronic obstructive pulmonary disease
  - ▶ BY INHALATION OF POWDER
  - ▶ Adult: 12 micrograms 1–2 times a day (max. per dose 24 micrograms), for symptom relief additional doses up to maximum daily dose can be taken; maximum 48 micrograms per day

PHARMACOKINETICS
  - ▶ At recommended inhaled doses, the duration of action of formoterol is about 12 hours.

IMPORTANT SAFETY INFORMATION

CHM ADVICE

To ensure safe use, the CHM has advised that for the management of chronic asthma, long-acting beta$_2$ agonist (formoterol) should:
- be added only if regular use of standard-dose inhaled corticosteroids has failed to control asthma adequately;
- not be initiated in patients with rapidly deteriorating asthma;
- be introduced at a low dose and the effect properly monitored before considering dose increase;
- be discontinued in the absence of benefit;
- not be used for the relief of exercise-induced asthma symptoms unless regular inhaled corticosteroids are also used;
- be reviewed as clinically appropriate: stepping down therapy should be considered when good long-term asthma control has been achieved.

- CAUTIONS High doses of beta$_2$ agonists can be dangerous in some children
- INTERACTIONS → Appendix 1: beta$_2$ agonists
- SIDE-EFFECTS
- ▶ **Common or very common** Muscle cramps
- ▶ **Uncommon** Angina pectoris · bronchospasm · skin reactions · sleep disorder · taste altered
- ▶ **Rare or very rare** Anxiety · QT interval prolongation
- PREGNANCY Inhaled drugs for asthma can be taken as normal during pregnancy.
- BREAST FEEDING Inhaled drugs for asthma can be taken as normal during breast-feeding.
- PATIENT AND CARER ADVICE Advise patients not to exceed prescribed dose, and to follow manufacturer's directions; if a previously effective dose of inhaled formoterol fails to provide adequate relief, a doctor's advice should be obtained as soon as possible. Patients should be advised to

report any deterioration in symptoms following initiation of treatment with a long-acting beta$_2$ agonist. Patient or carer should be given advice on how to administer formoterol fumarate inhalers.

● MEDICINAL FORMS
There can be variation in the licensing of different medicines containing the same drug.
Inhalation powder
‣ Easyhaler (formoterol) (Orion Pharma (UK) Ltd)
Formoterol fumarate dihydrate 12 microgram per 1 dose Formoterol Easyhaler 12micrograms/dose dry powder inhaler | 120 dose PoM £23.75 DT = £23.75
‣ Foradil (Novartis Pharmaceuticals UK Ltd)
Formoterol fumarate dihydrate 12 microgram Foradil 12microgram inhalation powder capsules with device | 60 capsule PoM £28.06 DT = £28.06
‣ Oxis Turbohaler (AstraZeneca UK Ltd)
Formoterol fumarate dihydrate 6 microgram per 1 dose Oxis 6 Turbohaler | 60 dose PoM £24.80 DT = £24.80
Formoterol fumarate dihydrate 12 microgram per 1 dose Oxis 12 Turbohaler | 60 dose PoM £24.80 DT = £24.80
Pressurised inhalation
‣ Atimos Modulite (Chiesi Ltd)
Formoterol fumarate dihydrate 12 microgram per 1 dose Atimos Modulite 12micrograms/dose inhaler | 100 dose PoM £30.06 DT = £30.06

Combinations available: *Aclidinium bromide with formoterol,* p. 245 · *Beclometasone with formoterol,* p. 258 · *Beclometasone with formoterol and glycopyrronium,* p. 259 · *Budesonide with formoterol,* p. 260 · *Fluticasone with formoterol,* p. 262

Indacaterol

● INDICATIONS AND DOSE
Maintenance treatment of chronic obstructive pulmonary disease
▸ BY INHALATION OF POWDER
‣ Adult: 150 micrograms once daily, then increased to 300 micrograms once daily

● CAUTIONS Convulsive disorders
● INTERACTIONS → Appendix 1: beta$_2$ agonists
● SIDE-EFFECTS
▸ Common or very common Chest pain · cough · increased risk of infection · muscle complaints · oropharyngeal pain · peripheral oedema · rhinorrhoea · throat irritation
▸ Uncommon Diabetes mellitus · hypersensitivity · musculoskeletal pain · paraesthesia · skin reactions
● PREGNANCY Manufacturer advises use only if potential benefit outweighs risk.
● BREAST FEEDING Manufacturer advises avoid—present in milk in *animal* studies.
● HEPATIC IMPAIRMENT Use with caution in severe impairment—no information available.
● PATIENT AND CARER ADVICE Patients or carers should be given advice on how to administer indacaterol inhalation powder.

● MEDICINAL FORMS
There can be variation in the licensing of different medicines containing the same drug.
Inhalation powder
‣ Onbrez Breezhaler (Novartis Pharmaceuticals UK Ltd)
Indacaterol (as Indacaterol maleate) 150 microgram Onbrez Breezhaler 150microgram inhalation powder capsules with device | 30 capsule PoM £32.19 DT = £32.19
Indacaterol (as Indacaterol maleate) 300 microgram Onbrez Breezhaler 300microgram inhalation powder capsules with device | 30 capsule PoM £32.19 DT = £32.19

Combinations available: *Glycopyrronium with indacaterol,* p. 246

Olodaterol

● INDICATIONS AND DOSE
Maintenance treatment of chronic obstructive pulmonary disease
▸ BY INHALATION
‣ Adult: 5 micrograms once daily
DOSE EQUIVALENCE AND CONVERSION
‣ 2 puffs is equivalent to 5 micrograms.

● CAUTIONS Aneurysm · convulsive disorders
● INTERACTIONS → Appendix 1: beta$_2$ agonists
● SIDE-EFFECTS
▸ Uncommon Nasopharyngitis · rash
▸ Rare or very rare Arthralgia · hypertension
▸ Frequency not known Angina pectoris · dry mouth · fatigue · hypotension · insomnia · malaise · metabolic acidosis · muscle spasms · nervousness
● PREGNANCY Manufacturer advises avoid—no information available.
● BREAST FEEDING Manufacturer advises avoid— present in milk in *animal* studies.
● HEPATIC IMPAIRMENT Use with caution in severe hepatic impairment—no information available.
● PATIENT AND CARER ADVICE Patients or carers should be given advice on how to administer olodaterol solution for inhalation.

● MEDICINAL FORMS
There can be variation in the licensing of different medicines containing the same drug.
Pressurised inhalation
‣ Striverdi Respimat (Boehringer Ingelheim Ltd) ▼
Olodaterol (as Olodaterol hydrochloride) 2.5 microgram per 1 dose Striverdi Respimat 2.5micrograms/dose solution for inhalation cartridge with device | 60 dose PoM £26.35 DT = £26.35

Combinations available: *Tiotropium with olodaterol,* p. 248

Salmeterol

● INDICATIONS AND DOSE
Reversible airways obstruction in patients requiring long-term regular bronchodilator therapy | Nocturnal asthma in patients requiring long-term regular bronchodilator therapy | Prevention of exercise-induced bronchospasm in patients requiring long-term regular bronchodilator therapy | Chronic asthma only in patients who regularly use an inhaled corticosteroid (not for immediate relief of acute asthma)
▸ BY INHALATION OF AEROSOL, OR BY INHALATION OF POWDER
‣ Child 5–11 years: 50 micrograms twice daily
‣ Child 12–17 years: 50 micrograms twice daily, dose may be increased in more severe airway obstruction; increased to 100 micrograms twice daily
‣ Adult: 50 micrograms twice daily, dose may be increased in more severe airway obstruction; increased to 100 micrograms twice daily

Chronic obstructive pulmonary disease
▸ BY INHALATION OF AEROSOL, OR BY INHALATION OF POWDER
‣ Adult: 50 micrograms twice daily
PHARMACOKINETICS
▸ At recommended inhaled doses, the duration of action of salmeterol is about 12 hours.

3

Respiratory system

- UNLICENSED USE *Neovent*® not licensed for use in children under 12 years.

> IMPORTANT SAFETY INFORMATION
> CHM ADVICE
> To ensure safe use, the CHM has advised that for the management of chronic asthma, long-acting beta₂ agonist (salmeterol) should:
> - be added only if regular use of standard-dose inhaled corticosteroids has failed to control asthma adequately;
> - not be initiated in patients with rapidly deteriorating asthma;
> - be introduced at a low dose and the effect properly monitored before considering dose increase;
> - be discontinued in the absence of benefit;
> - not be used for the relief of exercise-induced asthma symptoms unless regular inhaled corticosteroids are also used;
> - be reviewed as clinically appropriate: stepping down therapy should be considered when good long-term asthma control has been achieved.

- CAUTIONS High doses of beta₂ agonists can be dangerous in some children
- INTERACTIONS → Appendix 1: beta₂ agonists
- SIDE-EFFECTS
- **Common or very common** Muscle cramps
- **Uncommon** Nervousness · skin reactions
- **Rare or very rare** Arthralgia · bronchospasm · chest pain · insomnia · oedema · oropharyngeal irritation
- PREGNANCY Inhaled drugs for asthma can be taken as normal during pregnancy.
- BREAST FEEDING Inhaled drugs for asthma can be taken as normal during breast-feeding.
- PATIENT AND CARER ADVICE Advise patients that salmeterol should **not** be used for relief of acute attacks, not to exceed prescribed dose, and to follow manufacturer's directions; if a previously effective dose of inhaled salmeterol fails to provide adequate relief, a doctor's advice should be obtained as soon as possible. Patients should be advised to report any deterioration in symptoms following initiation of treatment with a long-acting beta₂ agonist.
  Medicines for Children leaflet: Salmeterol inhaler for asthma prevention (prophylaxis) www.medicinesforchildren.org.uk/salmeterol-inhaler-for-asthma-prevention

- MEDICINAL FORMS
  There can be variation in the licensing of different medicines containing the same drug.
  Inhalation powder
  - Serevent Accuhaler (GlaxoSmithKline UK Ltd)
    Salmeterol (as Salmeterol xinafoate) 50 microgram per 1 dose Serevent 50micrograms/dose Accuhaler | 60 dose PoM
    £35.11 DT = £35.11
  Pressurised inhalation
  - Salmeterol (Non-proprietary)
    Salmeterol (as Salmeterol xinafoate) 25 microgram per 1 dose Salmeterol 25micrograms/dose inhaler CFC free | 120 dose PoM £29.26 DT = £29.26
  - Neovent (Kent Pharmaceuticals Ltd)
    Salmeterol (as Salmeterol xinafoate) 25 microgram per 1 dose Neovent 25micrograms/dose inhaler CFC free | 120 dose PoM £29.26 DT = £29.26
  - Serevent Evohaler (GlaxoSmithKline UK Ltd)
    Salmeterol (as Salmeterol xinafoate) 25 microgram per 1 dose Serevent 25micrograms/dose Evohaler | 120 dose £29.26 DT = £29.26
  - Soltel (Kent Pharmaceuticals Ltd)
    Salmeterol (as Salmeterol xinafoate) 25 microgram per 1 dose Soltel 25micrograms/dose inhaler CFC free | 120 dose PoM £19.95 DT = £29.26

- Vertine (Teva UK Ltd)
  Salmeterol (as Salmeterol xinafoate) 25 microgram per 1 dose Vertine 25micrograms/dose inhaler CFC free | 120 dose PoM £23.40 DT = £29.26

Combinations available: *Fluticasone with salmeterol,* p. 263

BETA₂-ADRENOCEPTOR AGONISTS, SELECTIVE › SHORT-ACTING

☞ 249

Salbutamol
(Albuterol)

- INDICATIONS AND DOSE

Asthma | Other conditions associated with reversible airways obstruction
- BY MOUTH USING IMMEDIATE-RELEASE MEDICINES
- Adult: 4 mg 3–4 times a day, maximum single dose 8 mg (but unlikely to provide much extra benefit or to be tolerated), inhalation route preferred over oral route, use elderly dose for sensitive patients
- Elderly: Initially 2 mg 3–4 times a day, maximum single dose 8 mg (but unlikely to provide much extra benefit or to be tolerated), inhalation route preferred over oral route
- BY SUBCUTANEOUS INJECTION, OR BY INTRAMUSCULAR INJECTION
- Adult: 500 micrograms every 4 hours if required
- BY SLOW INTRAVENOUS INJECTION
- Adult: 250 micrograms, repeated if necessary, injection to be diluted to a concentration of 50 micrograms/mL, reserve intravenous beta₂ agonists for those in whom inhaled therapy cannot be used reliably
- BY INTRAVENOUS INFUSION
- Adult: Initially 5 micrograms/minute, adjusted according to response and heart rate, usual dose 3–20 micrograms/minute, higher doses may be required, reserve intravenous beta₂ agonists for those in whom inhaled therapy cannot be used reliably
- BY INHALATION OF AEROSOL
- Adult: 100–200 micrograms, up to 4 times a day for persistent symptoms
- BY INHALATION OF NEBULISED SOLUTION
- Adult: 2.5–5 mg, repeated up to 4 times daily or more frequently in severe cases

Prophylaxis of allergen- or exercise-induced bronchospasm
- BY INHALATION OF AEROSOL
- Adult: 200 micrograms

Acute asthma
- BY INTRAVENOUS INJECTION
- Child 1–23 months: 5 micrograms/kg for 1 dose, dose to be administered over 5 minutes, reserve intravenous beta₂ agonists for those in whom inhaled therapy cannot be used reliably or there is no current effect
- Child 2–17 years: 15 micrograms/kg (max. per dose 250 micrograms) for 1 dose, dose to be administered over 5 minutes, reserve intravenous beta₂ agonists for those in whom inhaled therapy cannot be used reliably or there is no current effect

Moderate, severe, or life-threatening acute asthma
- BY INHALATION OF NEBULISED SOLUTION
- Child 1 month–4 years: 2.5 mg, repeat every 20–30 minutes or when required, give via oxygen-driven nebuliser if available
- Child 5–11 years: 2.5–5 mg, repeat every 20–30 minutes or when required, give via oxygen-driven nebuliser if available
- Child 12–17 years: 5 mg, repeat every 20–30 minutes or when required, give via oxygen-driven nebuliser if available

‣ Adult: 5 mg, repeat every 20–30 minutes or when required, give via oxygen-driven nebuliser if available

Moderate and severe acute asthma

▸ BY INHALATION OF AEROSOL

‣ Child: 2–10 puffs, each puff is to be inhaled separately, repeat every 10–20 minutes or when required, give via large volume spacer (and a close-fitting face mask in children under 3 years), each puff is equivalent to 100 micrograms

‣ Adult: 2–10 puffs, each puff is to be inhaled separately, repeat every 10–20 minutes or when required, give via large volume spacer, each puff is equivalent to 100 micrograms

Exacerbation of reversible airways obstruction (including nocturnal asthma) | Prophylaxis of allergen- or exercise-induced bronchospasm

▸ BY INHALATION OF AEROSOL

‣ Child: 100–200 micrograms, up to 4 times a day for persistent symptoms

▸ BY MOUTH USING IMMEDIATE-RELEASE MEDICINES

‣ Child 1 month–1 year: 100 micrograms/kg 3–4 times a day (max. per dose 2 mg), inhalation route preferred over oral route

‣ Child 2–5 years: 1–2 mg 3–4 times a day, inhalation route preferred over oral route

‣ Child 6–11 years: 2 mg 3–4 times a day, inhalation route preferred over oral route

‣ Child 12–17 years: 2–4 mg 3–4 times a day, inhalation route preferred over oral route

Chronic asthma

▸ BY MOUTH USING MODIFIED-RELEASE MEDICINES

‣ Child 3–11 years: 4 mg twice daily

‣ Child 12–17 years: 8 mg twice daily

‣ Adult: 8 mg twice daily

Uncomplicated premature labour (between 22 and 37 weeks of gestation) (specialist supervision in hospital)

▸ BY INTRAVENOUS INFUSION

‣ Adult: Initially 10 micrograms/minute, rate increased gradually according to response at 10-minute intervals until contractions diminish then increase rate slowly until contractions cease (maximum rate 45 micrograms/minute), maintain rate for 1 hour after contractions have stopped, then gradually reduce by 50% every 6 hours, maximum duration 48 hours

EASYHALER ® SALBUTAMOL

Acute bronchospasm

▸ BY INHALATION OF POWDER

‣ Adult: Initially 100–200 micrograms, increased if necessary to 400 micrograms; maximum 800 micrograms per day

Prophylaxis of allergen- or exercise-induced bronchospasm

▸ BY INHALATION OF POWDER

‣ Adult: 200 micrograms

PULVINAL ® SALBUTAMOL

Acute bronchospasm

▸ BY INHALATION OF POWDER

‣ Child 5–17 years: Initially 200 micrograms, up to 800 micrograms daily for persistent symptoms

‣ Adult: Initially 200 micrograms, up to 800 micrograms daily for persistent symptoms

Prophylaxis of allergen- or exercise-induced bronchospasm

▸ BY INHALATION OF POWDER

‣ Child 5–17 years: 200 micrograms

‣ Adult: 200 micrograms

SALBULIN NOVOLIZER ®

Acute bronchospasm

▸ BY INHALATION OF POWDER

‣ Adult: Initially 100–200 micrograms, up to 800 micrograms daily for persistent symptoms

Prophylaxis of allergen- or exercise-induced bronchospasm

▸ BY INHALATION OF POWDER

‣ Adult: 200 micrograms

VENTOLIN ACCUHALER ®

Acute bronchospasm

▸ BY INHALATION OF POWDER

‣ Adult: Initially 200 micrograms, up to 4 times daily for persistent symptoms

Prophylaxis of allergen- or exercise-induced bronchospasm

▸ BY INHALATION OF POWDER

‣ Adult: 200 micrograms

PHARMACOKINETICS

‣ At recommended inhaled doses, the duration of action of salbutamol is about 3 to 5 hours.

● UNLICENSED USE Syrup and tablets not licensed for use in children under 2 years. Modified-release tablets not licensed for use in children under 3 years. Injection and solution for intravenous infusion not licensed for use in children under 12 years.

‣ With intravenous use in children Administration of undiluted salbutamol injection through a central venous catheter is not licensed.

● CONTRA-INDICATIONS

‣ When used for uncomplicated premature labour under specialist supervision Abruptio placenta · antepartum haemorrhage · cord compression · eclampsia · history of cardiac disease · intra-uterine fetal death · intra-uterine infection · placenta praevia · pulmonary hypertension · severe pre-eclampsia · significant risk factors for myocardial ischaemia · threatened miscarriage

● CAUTIONS

GENERAL CAUTIONS High doses of beta$_2$ agonists can be dangerous in some children

SPECIFIC CAUTIONS

‣ With intravenous use Mild to moderate pre-eclampsia (when used for uncomplicated premature labour) · suspected cardiovascular disease (should be assessed by a cardiologist before initiating therapy for uncomplicated premature labour)

● INTERACTIONS → Appendix 1: beta$_2$ agonists

● SIDE-EFFECTS

GENERAL SIDE-EFFECTS

▸ Rare or very rare Akathisia · vasodilation

▸ Frequency not known Metabolic change

SPECIFIC SIDE-EFFECTS

▸ Common or very common Muscle complaints

▸ Uncommon

▸ When used by inhalation Oral and throat irritation

▸ With parenteral use Pulmonary oedema

▸ Frequency not known

▸ With parenteral use Lactic acidosis (with high doses) · vomiting

● BREAST FEEDING Inhaled drugs for asthma can be taken as normal during breast-feeding.

● MONITORING REQUIREMENTS In uncomplicated premature labour it is important to monitor blood pressure, pulse rate (should not exceed 120 beats per minute), ECG (discontinue treatment if signs of myocardial ischaemia develop), blood glucose and lactate concentrations, and the patient's fluid and electrolyte status (avoid over-

3

Respiratory system

Respiratory system

3

hydration—discontinue drug immediately and initiate diuretic therapy if pulmonary oedema occurs).

* DIRECTIONS FOR ADMINISTRATION
▸ With intravenous use in children For *continuous intravenous infusion*, dilute to a concentration of 200 micrograms/mL with Glucose 5% *or* Sodium Chloride 0.9%. If fluid-restricted, can be given undiluted through central venous catheter [unlicensed]. For *intravenous injection*, dilute to a concentration of 50 micrograms/mL with Glucose 5%, Sodium Chloride 0.9%, *or* Water for injections.
▸ When used by inhalation For *nebulisation*, dilute nebuliser solution with a suitable volume of sterile Sodium Chloride 0.9% solution according to nebuliser type and duration of administration; salbutamol and ipratropium bromide solutions are compatible and can be mixed for nebulisation.
▸ With intravenous use in adults For *bronchodilation* by *continuous intravenous infusion*, dilute to a concentration of 200 micrograms/mL with glucose 5% or sodium chloride 0.9%. For *premature labour* by *continuous intravenous infusion*, dilute with glucose 5% to a concentration of 200 micrograms/mL for use in a syringe pump *or* for other infusion methods (preferably *via* controlled infusion device), dilute to a concentration of 20 micrograms/mL; close attention to patient's fluid and electrolyte status essential.

* PATIENT AND CARER ADVICE For *inhalation by aerosol or dry powder*, advise patients and carers not to exceed prescribed dose and to follow manufacturer's directions; if a previously effective dose of inhaled salbutamol fails to provide at least 3 hours relief, a doctor's advice should be obtained as soon as possible. *For inhalation by nebuliser*, the dose given by nebuliser is substantially higher than that given by inhaler. Patients should therefore be warned that it is dangerous to exceed the prescribed dose and they should seek medical advice if they fail to respond to the usual dose of the respirator solution.
Medicines for Children leaflet: Salbutamol inhaler for asthma and wheeze www.medicinesforchildren.org.uk/salbutamol-inhaler-for-asthma-and-wheeze

* MEDICINAL FORMS
There can be variation in the licensing of different medicines containing the same drug.

Tablet
▸ Salbutamol (Non-proprietary)
Salbutamol (as Salbutamol sulfate) 2 mg Salbutamol 2mg tablets | 28 tablet [PoM] £106.43 DT = £100.52
Salbutamol (as Salbutamol sulfate) 4 mg Salbutamol 4mg tablets | 28 tablet [PoM] £108.95 DT = £102.90

Inhalation powder
▸ Easyhaler (salbutamol) (Orion Pharma (UK) Ltd)
Salbutamol 100 microgram per 1 dose Easyhaler Salbutamol sulfate 100micrograms/dose dry powder inhaler | 200 dose [PoM] £3.31 DT = £3.31
Salbutamol 200 microgram per 1 dose Easyhaler Salbutamol sulfate 200micrograms/dose dry powder inhaler | 200 dose [PoM] £6.63 DT = £6.63
▸ Salbulin Novolizer (Meda Pharmaceuticals Ltd)
Salbutamol (as Salbutamol sulfate) 100 microgram per 1 dose Salbulin Novolizer 100micrograms/dose inhalation powder | 200 dose [PoM] £4.95
Salbulin Novolizer 100micrograms/dose inhalation powder refill | 200 dose [PoM] £2.75
▸ Ventolin Accuhaler (GlaxoSmithKline UK Ltd)
Salbutamol 200 microgram per 1 dose Ventolin 200micrograms/dose Accuhaler | 60 dose [PoM] £3.60 DT = £3.60

Solution for injection
▸ Ventolin (GlaxoSmithKline UK Ltd)
Salbutamol (as Salbutamol sulfate) 500 microgram per 1 ml Ventolin 500micrograms/1ml solution for injection ampoules | 5 ampoule [PoM] £1.91

Solution for infusion
▸ Ventolin (GlaxoSmithKline UK Ltd)
Salbutamol (as Salbutamol sulfate) 1 mg per 1 ml Ventolin 5mg/5ml solution for infusion ampoules | 10 ampoule [PoM] £24.81

Oral solution
▸ Salbutamol (Non-proprietary)
Salbutamol (as Salbutamol sulfate) 400 microgram per 1 ml Salbutamol 2mg/5ml oral solution sugar free sugar-free | 150 ml [PoM] [℞] DT = £1.15
▸ Ventolin (GlaxoSmithKline UK Ltd)
Salbutamol (as Salbutamol sulfate) 400 microgram per 1 ml Ventolin 2mg/5ml syrup sugar-free | 150 ml [PoM] £1.15 DT = £1.15

Pressurised inhalation
▸ Salbutamol (Non-proprietary)
Salbutamol (as Salbutamol sulfate) 100 microgram per 1 dose Salbutamol 100micrograms/dose inhaler CFC free | 200 dose [PoM] £1.50 DT = £1.50
▸ Airomir (Teva UK Ltd)
Salbutamol (as Salbutamol sulfate) 100 microgram per 1 dose Airomir 100micrograms/dose inhaler | 200 dose [PoM] £1.97 DT = £1.50
▸ Airomir Autohaler (Teva UK Ltd)
Salbutamol (as Salbutamol sulfate) 100 microgram per 1 dose Airomir 100micrograms/dose Autohaler | 200 dose [PoM] £6.02 DT = £6.30
▸ Salamol (Teva UK Ltd)
Salbutamol (as Salbutamol sulfate) 100 microgram per 1 dose Salamol 100micrograms/dose inhaler CFC free | 200 dose [PoM] £1.46 DT = £1.50
▸ Salamol Easi-Breathe (Teva UK Ltd)
Salbutamol (as Salbutamol sulfate) 100 microgram per 1 dose Salamol 100micrograms/dose Easi-Breathe inhaler | 200 dose [PoM] £6.30 DT = £6.30
▸ Ventolin Evohaler (GlaxoSmithKline UK Ltd)
Salbutamol (as Salbutamol sulfate) 100 microgram per 1 dose Ventolin 100micrograms/dose Evohaler | 200 dose [PoM] £1.50 DT = £1.50

Nebuliser liquid
▸ Salbutamol (Non-proprietary)
Salbutamol (as Salbutamol sulfate) 1 mg per 1 ml Salbutamol 2.5mg/2.5ml nebuliser liquid unit dose vials | 20 unit dose [PoM] £1.91 DT = £1.91
Salbutamol (as Salbutamol sulfate) 2 mg per 1 ml Salbutamol 5mg/2.5ml nebuliser liquid unit dose vials | 20 unit dose [PoM] £3.82 DT = £3.82
▸ Salamol Steri-Neb (Teva UK Ltd)
Salbutamol (as Salbutamol sulfate) 1 mg per 1 ml Salamol 2.5mg/2.5ml nebuliser liquid Steri-Neb unit dose vials | 20 unit dose [PoM] £1.91 DT = £1.91
Salbutamol (as Salbutamol sulfate) 2 mg per 1 ml Salamol 5mg/2.5ml nebuliser liquid Steri-Neb unit dose vials | 20 unit dose [PoM] £3.82 DT = £3.82
▸ Ventolin (GlaxoSmithKline UK Ltd)
Salbutamol (as Salbutamol sulfate) 5 mg per 1 ml Ventolin 5mg/ml respirator solution | 20 ml [PoM] £2.18 DT = £2.18
▸ Ventolin Nebules (GlaxoSmithKline UK Ltd)
Salbutamol (as Salbutamol sulfate) 1 mg per 1 ml Ventolin 2.5mg Nebules | 20 unit dose [PoM] £1.65 DT = £1.91
Salbutamol (as Salbutamol sulfate) 2 mg per 1 ml Ventolin 5mg Nebules | 20 unit dose [PoM] £2.78 DT = £3.82

Combinations available: *Ipratropium with salbutamol*, p. 247

◤ 249

Terbutaline sulfate

* INDICATIONS AND DOSE

Asthma | Other conditions associated with reversible airways obstruction
▸ BY MOUTH
▸ Adult: Initially 2.5 mg 3 times a day for 1–2 weeks, then increased to up to 5 mg 3 times a day, use by inhalation preferred over by mouth

▸ BY SUBCUTANEOUS INJECTION, OR BY SLOW INTRAVENOUS INJECTION
▸ Adult: 250–500 micrograms up to 4 times a day, reserve intravenous beta$_2$ agonists for those in whom inhaled therapy cannot be used reliably or there is no current effect
▸ BY CONTINUOUS INTRAVENOUS INFUSION
▸ Adult: 90–300 micrograms/hour for 8-10 hours, to be administered as a solution containing 3–5 micrograms/mL, high doses require close monitoring, reserve intravenous beta$_2$ agonists for those in whom inhaled therapy cannot be used reliably or there is no current effect
▸ BY INHALATION OF POWDER
▸ Adult: 500 micrograms up to 4 times a day, for persistent symptoms
▸ BY INHALATION OF NEBULISED SOLUTION
▸ Adult: 5–10 mg 2–4 times a day, additional doses may be necessary in severe acute asthma

Acute asthma
▸ BY SUBCUTANEOUS INJECTION, OR BY SLOW INTRAVENOUS INJECTION
▸ Child 2-14 years: 10 micrograms/kg up to 4 times a day (max. per dose 300 micrograms), reserve intravenous beta$_2$ agonists for those in whom inhaled therapy cannot be used reliably or there is no current effect
▸ Child 15-17 years: 250–500 micrograms up to 4 times a day, reserve intravenous beta$_2$ agonists for those in whom inhaled therapy cannot be used reliably or there is no current effect
▸ BY CONTINUOUS INTRAVENOUS INFUSION
▸ Child: Loading dose 2–4 micrograms/kg, then 1–10 micrograms/kg/hour, dose to be adjusted according to response and heart rate, close monitoring is required for doses above 10 micrograms/kg/hour, reserve intravenous beta$_2$ agonists for those in whom inhaled therapy cannot be used reliably or there is no current effect

Moderate, severe, or life-threatening acute asthma
▸ BY INHALATION OF NEBULISED SOLUTION
▸ Child 1 month-4 years: 5 mg, repeat every 20–30 minutes or when required, give via oxygen-driven nebuliser if available
▸ Child 5-11 years: 5–10 mg, repeat every 20–30 minutes or when required, give via oxygen-driven nebuliser if available
▸ Child 12-17 years: 10 mg, repeat every 20–30 minutes or when required, give via oxygen-driven nebuliser if available
▸ Adult: 10 mg, repeat every 20–30 minutes or when required, give via oxygen-driven nebuliser if available

Exacerbation of reversible airways obstruction (including nocturnal asthma) | Prevention of exercise-induced bronchospasm
▸ BY INHALATION OF POWDER
▸ Child 5-17 years: 500 micrograms up to 4 times a day, for occasional use only
▸ BY MOUTH
▸ Child 1 month-6 years: 75 micrograms/kg 3 times a day (max. per dose 2.5 mg), administration by mouth is not recommended
▸ Child 7-14 years: 2.5 mg 2–3 times a day, administration by mouth is not recommended
▸ Child 15-17 years: Initially 2.5 mg 3 times a day, then increased if necessary to 5 mg 3 times a day, administration by mouth is not recommended

Uncomplicated premature labour (between 22 and 37 weeks of gestation) (specialist supervision in hospital)
▸ BY INTRAVENOUS INFUSION
▸ Adult: Initially 5 micrograms/minute for 20 minutes, then increased in steps of 2.5 micrograms/minute every 20 minutes until contractions have ceased (more than 10 micrograms/minute should **seldom** be given—20 micrograms/minute should **not** be exceeded), continue for 1 hour, then reduced in steps of 2.5 micrograms/minute every 20 minutes to lowest dose that maintains suppression (maximum total duration 48 hours)

PHARMACOKINETICS
▸ At recommended inhaled doses, the duration of action of terbutaline is about 3 to 5 hours.

● UNLICENSED USE Tablets not licensed for use in children under 7 years. Injection not licensed for use in children under 2 years.
● CONTRA-INDICATIONS
▸ When used for uncomplicated premature labour Abruptio placenta · antepartum haemorrhage · cord compression · eclampsia · history of cardiac disease · intra-uterine fetal death · intra-uterine infection · placenta praevia · pulmonary hypertension · severe pre-eclampsia · significant risk factors for myocardial ischaemia · threatened miscarriage
● CAUTIONS High doses of beta$_2$ agonists can be dangerous in some children · mild to moderate pre-eclampsia (when used for uncomplicated premature labour) · suspected cardiovascular disease (should be assessed by a cardiologist before initiating therapy for uncomplicated premature labour)
● INTERACTIONS → Appendix 1: beta$_2$ agonists
● SIDE-EFFECTS
GENERAL SIDE-EFFECTS
▸ **Common or very common** Hypotension · muscle spasms
▸ **Rare or very rare** Vasodilation
▸ **Frequency not known** Angioedema · anxiety · behaviour abnormal · bronchospasm · circulatory collapse · oral irritation · skin reactions · sleep disorder · throat irritation
SPECIFIC SIDE-EFFECTS
▸ **Uncommon**
▸ With parenteral use Pulmonary oedema
▸ **Rare or very rare**
▸ With parenteral use Lactic acidosis
▸ **Frequency not known**
▸ With parenteral use Akathisia · bleeding tendency
● PREGNANCY Inhaled drugs for asthma can be taken as normal during pregnancy.
● BREAST FEEDING Inhaled drugs for asthma can be taken as normal during breast-feeding.
● MONITORING REQUIREMENTS In uncomplicated premature labour it is important to monitor blood pressure, pulse rate (should not exceed 120 beats per minute), ECG (discontinue treatment if signs of myocardial ischaemia develop), blood glucose and lactate concentrations, and the patient's fluid and electrolyte status (avoid over-hydration—discontinue drug immediately and initiate diuretic therapy if pulmonary oedema occurs).
● DIRECTIONS FOR ADMINISTRATION
▸ With intravenous use in children For *continuous intravenous infusion*, dilute to a concentration of 5 micrograms/mL with Glucose 5% or Sodium Chloride 0.9%; if fluid-restricted, dilute to a concentration of 100 micrograms/mL.
▸ When used by inhalation For *nebulisation*, dilute nebuliser solution with sterile Sodium Chloride 0.9% solution according to nebuliser type and duration of

administration; terbutaline and ipratropium bromide solutions are compatible and may be mixed for nebulisation.

▶ With intravenous use in adults For *bronchodilation* by *continuous intravenous infusion*, dilute 1.5–2.5 mg with 500 mL glucose 5% or sodium chloride 0.9% and give over 8–10 hours. For *premature labour* by *continuous intravenous infusion*, dilute in glucose 5% and give *via* controlled infusion device preferably a syringe pump; if syringe pump available dilute to a concentration of 100 micrograms/mL; if syringe pump not available dilute to a concentration of 10 micrograms/mL; close attention to patient's fluid and electrolyte status essential.

● PATIENT AND CARER ADVICE *For inhalation by dry powder*, advise patients and carers not to exceed prescribed dose and to follow manufacturer's directions; if a previously effective dose of inhaled terbutaline fails to provide at least 3 hours relief, a doctor's advice should be obtained as soon as possible. *For inhalation by nebuliser*, the dose given by nebuliser is substantially higher than that given by inhaler. Patients should therefore be warned that it is dangerous to exceed the prescribed dose and they should seek medical advice if they fail to respond to the usual dose of the respirator solution.

● MEDICINAL FORMS
There can be variation in the licensing of different medicines containing the same drug. Forms available from special-order manufacturers include: solution for injection

Solution for injection
▶ Bricanyl (AstraZeneca UK Ltd)
Terbutaline sulfate 500 microgram per 1 ml Bricanyl 2.5mg/5ml solution for injection ampoules | 10 ampoule [PoM] £20.09 DT = £20.09
Bricanyl 500micrograms/1ml solution for injection ampoules | 5 ampoule [PoM] £6.48 DT = £6.48

Inhalation powder
▶ Bricanyl Turbohaler (AstraZeneca UK Ltd)
Terbutaline sulfate 500 microgram per 1 dose Bricanyl 500micrograms/dose Turbohaler | 100 dose [PoM] £8.30 DT = £8.30

Nebuliser liquid
▶ Terbutaline sulfate (Non-proprietary)
Terbutaline sulfate 2.5 mg per 1 ml Terbutaline 5mg/2ml nebuliser liquid unit dose vials | 20 unit dose [PoM] £4.04 DT = £4.04
▶ Bricanyl Respules (AstraZeneca UK Ltd)
Terbutaline sulfate 2.5 mg per 1 ml Bricanyl 5mg/2ml Respules | 20 unit dose [PoM] £11.64 DT = £4.04

Tablet
▶ Bricanyl (AstraZeneca UK Ltd)
Terbutaline sulfate 5 mg Bricanyl 5mg tablets | 100 tablet [PoM] £14.73 DT = £14.73

CORTICOSTEROIDS

Airways disease, use of corticosteroids

30-Nov-2017

Asthma, use of corticosteroids

Inhaled corticosteroids
Corticosteroids are effective in *asthma*; they reduce airway inflammation (and hence reduce oedema and secretion of mucus into the airway).

An inhaled corticosteroid is used regularly for prophylaxis of asthma. *Regular use* of inhaled corticosteroids reduces the risk of exacerbation of asthma.

Current and previous smoking reduces the effectiveness of inhaled corticosteroids and higher doses may be necessary.

Corticosteroid inhalers must be used regularly for maximum benefit. Beclometasone dipropionate p. 257, budesonide p. 259, fluticasone p. 262, and mometasone furoate p. 265 appear to be equally effective.

In adults using an inhaled corticosteroid and a long-acting beta₂ agonist for the prophylaxis of asthma, but who are poorly controlled, *Symbicort®* or *DuoResp Spiromax®* (both containing budesonide with formoterol p. 260) or *Fostair®* beclometasone with formoterol p. 258 can be used as relievers (instead of a short-acting beta₂ agonist), in addition to their regular use for the prophylaxis of asthma.

Oral corticosteroids
Systemic corticosteroid therapy may be necessary during episodes of stress, such as severe infection, or when airway obstruction or mucus prevent drug access to smaller airways.

An acute attack of asthma should be treated with a short course of an oral corticosteroid starting with a high dose. Patients whose asthma has deteriorated rapidly usually respond quickly to corticosteroids. The dose can usually be stopped abruptly; tapering is not needed provided that the patient receives an inhaled corticosteroid in an adequate dose (apart from those on maintenance oral corticosteroid treatment or where oral corticosteroids are required for 3 or more weeks). In patients who have needed several courses of oral corticosteroids and in whom the possibility of a period on maintenance corticosteroids is being considered, it may be useful to taper the corticosteroid dose gradually to identify a threshold dose for asthma control. This should only be done after other standard options for controlling asthma have been tried.

An oral corticosteroid should normally be taken as a single dose in the morning to reduce the disturbance to circadian cortisol secretion. Dosage should always be titrated to the lowest dose that controls symptoms. Regular peak-flow measurements help to optimise the dose.

Parenteral corticosteroids
Hydrocortisone injection p. 662 has a role in the emergency treatment of acute severe asthma.

Chronic obstructive pulmonary disease, use of corticosteroids

Inhaled corticosteroids
In *chronic obstructive pulmonary disease* inhaled corticosteroid therapy may reduce exacerbations when given in combination with an inhaled long-acting beta₂ agonist.

Oral corticosteroids
During an acute exacerbation of chronic obstructive pulmonary disease, prednisolone p. 664 should be given; treatment can be stopped abruptly. Prolonged treatment with oral prednisolone is of no benefit and maintenance treatment is not normally recommended.

Corticosteroids (inhaled)

IMPORTANT SAFETY INFORMATION
MHRA/CHM ADVICE: CORTICOSTEROIDS: RARE RISK OF CENTRAL SEROUS CHORIORETINOPATHY WITH LOCAL AS WELL AS SYSTEMIC ADMINISTRATION (AUGUST 2017)
Central serous chorioretinopathy is a retinal disorder that has been linked to the systemic use of corticosteroids. Recently, it has also been reported after local administration of corticosteroids via inhaled and intranasal, epidural, intra-articular, topical dermal, and periocular routes. The MHRA recommends that patients should be advised to report any blurred vision or other visual disturbances with corticosteroid treatment given by any route; consider referral to an ophthalmologist for evaluation of possible causes if a patient presents with vision problems.

● SIDE-EFFECTS
▶ Common or very common Altered smell sensation · Cushing's syndrome · epistaxis · headache · nasal complaints · oral candidiasis · skin reactions · taste altered · throat irritation · voice alteration

▸ **Uncommon** Adrenal suppression · anxiety · bronchospasm paradoxical · cataract · glaucoma · vision blurred
▸ **Rare or very rare** Behaviour abnormal · growth retardation (in children) · hypertrichosis · sleep disorder
▸ **Frequency not known** Pneumonia (in patients with COPD)

SIDE-EFFECTS, FURTHER INFORMATION Systemic absorption may follow inhaled administration particularly if high doses are used or if treatment is prolonged. Therefore also consider the side-effects of systemic corticosteroids.

Candidiasis The risk of oral candidiasis can be reduced by using a spacer device with the corticosteroid inhaler; rinsing the mouth with water after inhalation of a dose may also be helpful. An anti-fungal oral suspension or oral gel can be used to treat oral candidiasis without discontinuing corticosteroid therapy.

Paradoxical bronchospasm The potential for paradoxical bronchospasm (calling for discontinuation and alternative therapy) should be borne in mind. Mild bronchospasm may be prevented by inhalation of a short-acting beta₂ agonist beforehand (or by transfer from an aerosol inhalation to a dry powder inhalation).

● PREGNANCY Inhaled drugs for asthma can be taken as normal during pregnancy.

● BREAST FEEDING Inhaled corticosteroids for asthma can be taken as normal during breast-feeding.

● MONITORING REQUIREMENTS The height and weight of children receiving prolonged treatment with inhaled corticosteroids should be monitored annually; if growth is slowed, referral to a paediatrician should be considered.

● NATIONAL FUNDING/ACCESS DECISIONS

NICE decisions

▸ **Inhaled corticosteroids for the treatment of chronic asthma in children under 12 years (November 2007)** NICE TA131
For children under 12 years with chronic asthma in whom treatment with an inhaled corticosteroid is considered appropriate, the least costly product that is suitable for an individual child (taking into consideration NICE TAs 38 and 10), within its marketing authorisation, is recommended. For children under 12 years with chronic asthma in whom treatment with an inhaled corticosteroid and a long-acting beta₂ agonist is considered appropriate, the following apply:
● the use of a combination inhaler within its marketing authorisation is recommended as an option;
● the decision to use a combination inhaler or two agents in separate inhalers should be made on an individual basis, taking into consideration therapeutic need and the likelihood of treatment adherence;
● if a combination inhaler is chosen, then the least costly inhaler that is suitable for the individual child is recommended.
www.nice.org.uk/TA131

▸ **Inhaled corticosteroids for the treatment of chronic asthma in adults and children over 12 years (March 2008)** NICE TA138
For adults and children over 12 years with chronic asthma in whom treatment with an inhaled corticosteroid is considered appropriate, the least costly product that is suitable for an individual (taking into consideration NICE TAs 38 and 10), within its marketing authorisation is recommended.
For adults and children over 12 years with chronic asthma in whom treatment with an inhaled corticosteroid and a long-acting beta₂ agonist is considered appropriate, the following apply:
● the use of a combination inhaler within its marketing authorisation is recommended as an option;
● the decision to use a combination inhaler or two agents in separate inhalers should be made on an individual basis, taking into consideration therapeutic need, and the likelihood of treatment adherence;

● if a combination inhaler is chosen, then the least costly inhaler that is suitable for the individual is recommended.
www.nice.org.uk/TA138

F 256

Beclometasone dipropionate   04-Jan-2016

(Beclomethasone dipropionate)

● INDICATIONS AND DOSE

Prophylaxis of asthma
▸ BY INHALATION OF POWDER
▸ Child 5–11 years: 100–200 micrograms twice daily, dose to be adjusted as necessary
▸ Child 12–17 years: 200–400 micrograms twice daily; increased if necessary up to 800 micrograms twice daily, dose to be adjusted as necessary
▸ Adult: 200–400 micrograms twice daily; increased if necessary up to 800 micrograms twice daily, dose to be adjusted as necessary

DOSE EQUIVALENCE AND CONVERSION
▸ Dose adjustments may be required for some inhaler devices, see under individual preparations.

CLENIL MODULITE ®

Prophylaxis of asthma
▸ BY INHALATION OF AEROSOL
▸ Child 2–11 years: 100–200 micrograms twice daily
▸ Child 12–17 years: 200–400 micrograms twice daily, adjusted according to response; increased if necessary up to 1 mg twice daily
▸ Adult: 200–400 micrograms twice daily, adjusted according to response; increased if necessary up to 1 mg twice daily

QVAR ® PREPARATIONS

Prophylaxis of asthma
▸ BY INHALATION OF AEROSOL
▸ Child 12–17 years: 50–200 micrograms twice daily; increased if necessary up to 400 micrograms twice daily
▸ Adult: 50–200 micrograms twice daily; increased if necessary up to 400 micrograms twice daily

POTENCY
▸ *Qvar* ® has extra-fine particles, is more potent than traditional beclometasone dipropionate CFC-containing inhalers and is approximately twice as potent as *Clenil Modulite* ®.

● UNLICENSED USE *Easyhaler* ® *Beclometasone Dipropionate* is not licensed for use in children under 18 years. *Clenil Modulite* ®-200 and -250 are not licensed for use in children under 12 years.

> **IMPORTANT SAFETY INFORMATION**
> MHRA/CHM ADVICE (JULY 2008)
> Beclometasone dipropionate CFC-free pressurised metered-dose inhalers (*Qvar* ® and *Clenil Modulite* ®) are **not** interchangeable and should be prescribed by brand name; *Qvar* ® has extra-fine particles, is more potent than traditional beclometasone dipropionate CFC-containing inhalers, and is approximately twice as potent as *Clenil Modulite* ®.

● INTERACTIONS → Appendix 1: corticosteroids

● PRESCRIBING AND DISPENSING INFORMATION The MHRA has advised (July 2008) that beclometasone dipropionate CFC-free inhalers should be prescribed by brand name.
QVAR ® PREPARATIONS When switching a patient with well-controlled asthma from another corticosteroid inhaler, initially a 100-microgram metered dose of *Qvar* ® should be prescribed for 200–250 micrograms of beclometasone dipropionate or budesonide and for

100 micrograms of fluticasone propionate. When switching a patient with poorly controlled asthma from another corticosteroid inhaler, initially a 100-microgram metered dose of *Qvar*® should be prescribed for 100 micrograms of beclometasone dipropionate, budesonide, or fluticasone propionate; the dose of *Qvar*® should be adjusted according to response.

CLENIL MODULITE ® *Clenil Modulite*® is not interchangeable with other CFC-free beclometasone dipropionate inhalers.

- PATIENT AND CARER ADVICE Steroid card should be issued with high doses of inhaled beclometasone dipropionate. Medicines for Children leaflet: Beclometasone for asthma prevention (prophylaxis) www.medicinesforchildren.org.uk/beclometasone-inhaler-asthma-prevention-prophylaxis-0

- PROFESSION SPECIFIC INFORMATION

Dental practitioners' formulary
Clenil Modulite® 50 micrograms/metered inhalation may be prescribed.

- MEDICINAL FORMS
There can be variation in the licensing of different medicines containing the same drug.

Inhalation powder
CAUTIONARY AND ADVISORY LABELS 8, 10
- Easyhaler (beclometasone) (Orion Pharma (UK) Ltd)
Beclometasone dipropionate 200 microgram per 1 dose Easyhaler Beclometasone 200micrograms/dose dry powder inhaler | 200 dose PoM £14.93 DT = £14.93

Pressurised inhalation
CAUTIONARY AND ADVISORY LABELS 8, 10
- Clenil Modulite (Chiesi Ltd)
Beclometasone dipropionate 50 microgram per 1 dose Clenil Modulite 50micrograms/dose inhaler | 200 dose PoM £3.70 DT = £3.70
Beclometasone dipropionate 100 microgram per 1 dose Clenil Modulite 100micrograms/dose inhaler | 200 dose PoM £7.42 DT = £7.42
Beclometasone dipropionate 200 microgram per 1 dose Clenil Modulite 200micrograms/dose inhaler | 200 dose PoM £16.17 DT = £16.17
Beclometasone dipropionate 250 microgram per 1 dose Clenil Modulite 250micrograms/dose inhaler | 200 dose PoM £16.29 DT = £16.29
- Qvar (Teva UK Ltd)
Beclometasone dipropionate 50 microgram per 1 dose Qvar 50 inhaler | 200 dose PoM £7.87 DT = £3.70
Beclometasone dipropionate 100 microgram per 1 dose Qvar 100 inhaler | 200 dose PoM £17.21 DT = £7.42
- Qvar Autohaler (Teva UK Ltd)
Beclometasone dipropionate 50 microgram per 1 dose Qvar 50 Autohaler | 200 dose PoM £7.87 DT = £7.87
Beclometasone dipropionate 100 microgram per 1 dose Qvar 100 Autohaler | 200 dose PoM £17.21 DT = £17.21
- Qvar Easi-Breathe (Teva UK Ltd)
Beclometasone dipropionate 50 microgram per 1 dose Qvar 50micrograms/dose Easi-Breathe inhaler | 200 dose PoM £7.74 DT = £7.87
Beclometasone dipropionate 100 microgram per 1 dose Qvar 100micrograms/dose Easi-Breathe inhaler | 200 dose PoM £16.95 DT = £17.21

Beclometasone with formoterol
09-Jun-2017

The properties listed below are those particular to the combination only. For the properties of the components please consider, beclometasone dipropionate p. 257, formoterol fumarate p. 250.

- INDICATIONS AND DOSE

FOSTAIR NEXTHALER ® 100/6
Asthma maintenance therapy
- BY INHALATION OF POWDER
- Adult: 1–2 inhalations twice daily; maximum 4 inhalations per day

Chronic obstructive pulmonary disease with forced expiratory volume in 1 second < 50% of predicted
- BY INHALATION OF POWDER
- Adult: 2 inhalations twice daily

DOSE EQUIVALENCE AND CONVERSION
- For inhalation of powder, when switching patients from other beclometasone dipropionate formulations with non-extrafine particle size distribution to *Fostair NEXThaler*®, the dose should be adjusted according to response.
- 1 inhalation is equivalent to 100 micrograms beclometasone dipropionate and 6 micrograms formoterol fumarate.

FOSTAIR NEXTHALER ® 200/6
Asthma maintenance therapy
- BY INHALATION OF POWDER
- Adult: 2 inhalations twice daily; maximum 4 inhalations per day

DOSE EQUIVALENCE AND CONVERSION
- For inhalation of powder, when switching patients from other beclometasone dipropionate formulations with non-extrafine particle size distribution to *Fostair NEXThaler*®, the dose should be adjusted according to response.
- 1 inhalation is equivalent to 200 micrograms beclometasone dipropionate and 6 micrograms formoterol fumarate.

FOSTAIR ® 100/6
Asthma maintenance therapy
- BY INHALATION OF AEROSOL
- Adult: 1–2 inhalations twice daily; maximum 4 inhalations per day

Asthma, maintenance and reliever therapy
- BY INHALATION OF AEROSOL
- Adult: Maintenance 1 inhalation twice daily; 1 inhalation as required, for relief of symptoms; maximum 8 inhalations per day

Chronic obstructive pulmonary disease with forced expiratory volume in 1 second < 50% of predicted
- BY INHALATION OF AEROSOL
- Adult: 2 inhalations twice daily

DOSE EQUIVALENCE AND CONVERSION
- For inhalation of aerosol, when switching patients from other beclometasone dipropionate and formoterol fumarate inhalers, dose should be adjusted according to response—100 micrograms of beclometasone dipropionate extrafine in *Fostair*® is equivalent to 250 micrograms of beclometasone dipropionate in a non-extrafine formulation.
- 1 inhalation is equivalent to 100 micrograms beclometasone dipropionate and 6 micrograms formoterol fumarate.

FOSTAIR® 200/6

Asthma maintenance therapy
▶ BY INHALATION OF AEROSOL
▶ Adult: 2 inhalations twice daily; maximum 4 inhalations per day

DOSE EQUIVALENCE AND CONVERSION
▶ For inhalation of aerosol, when switching patients from other beclometasone dipropionate and formoterol fumarate inhalers, dose should be adjusted according to response—100 micrograms of beclometasone dipropionate extrafine in *Fostair*® is equivalent to 250 micrograms of beclometasone dipropionate in a non-extrafine formulation.
▶ 1 inhalation is equivalent to 200 micrograms beclometasone dipropionate and 6 micrograms formoterol fumarate.

IMPORTANT SAFETY INFORMATION
MHRA/CHM ADVICE (JULY 2008)
Fostair® contains extra-fine particles of beclometasone dipropionate and is more potent than traditional beclometasone dipropionate CFC-free inhalers. The dose of beclometasone dipropionate in *Fostair*® should be lower than non-extra-fine formulations of beclometasone dipropionate and will need to be adjusted to the individual needs of the patient.

● INTERACTIONS → Appendix 1: beta₂ agonists · corticosteroids
● PATIENT AND CARER ADVICE Patients or carers should be given advice on how to administer beclometasone with formoterol aerosol for inhalation.
   With high doses, a steroid card should be supplied.

● MEDICINAL FORMS
There can be variation in the licensing of different medicines containing the same drug.
Inhalation powder
CAUTIONARY AND ADVISORY LABELS 8, 10
▶ Fostair NEXThaler (Chiesi Ltd)
   Formoterol fumarate dihydrate 6 microgram per 1 dose, Beclometasone dipropionate 100 microgram per 1 dose Fostair NEXThaler 100micrograms/dose / 6micrograms/dose dry powder inhaler | 120 dose [PoM] £29.32 DT = £29.32
   Formoterol fumarate dihydrate 6 microgram per 1 dose, Beclometasone dipropionate 200 microgram per 1 dose Fostair NEXThaler 200micrograms/dose / 6micrograms/dose dry powder inhaler | 120 dose [PoM] £29.32 DT = £29.32
Pressurised inhalation
CAUTIONARY AND ADVISORY LABELS 8, 10
▶ Fostair (Chiesi Ltd)
   Formoterol fumarate dihydrate 6 microgram, Beclometasone dipropionate 200 microgram Fostair 200micrograms/dose / 6micrograms/dose inhaler | 120 dose [PoM] £29.32 DT = £29.32
   Formoterol fumarate dihydrate 6 microgram per 1 dose, Beclometasone dipropionate 100 microgram per 1 dose Fostair 100micrograms/dose / 6micrograms/dose inhaler | 120 dose [PoM] £29.32 DT = £29.32

Beclometasone with formoterol and glycopyrronium
18-Oct-2017

The properties listed below are those particular to the combination only. For the properties of the components please consider, beclometasone dipropionate p. 257, formoterol fumarate p. 250, glycopyrronium bromide p. 246.

● INDICATIONS AND DOSE
Moderate-to-severe chronic obstructive pulmonary disease
▶ BY INHALATION OF AEROSOL
▶ Adult: 2 inhalations twice daily

● INTERACTIONS → Appendix 1: beta₂ agonists · corticosteroids · glycopyrronium
● BREAST FEEDING Manufacturer advises avoid—no information available.
● HEPATIC IMPAIRMENT Manufacturer advises caution in severe impairment—no information available.
● NATIONAL FUNDING/ACCESS DECISIONS
Scottish Medicines Consortium (SMC) Decisions
The *Scottish Medicines Consortium* has advised (October 2017) that beclometasone with formoterol and glycopyrronium (*Trimbow*®) is accepted for restricted use within NHS Scotland for the maintenance treatment of adults with severe chronic obstructive pulmonary disease.

● MEDICINAL FORMS
There can be variation in the licensing of different medicines containing the same drug.
Pressurised inhalation
CAUTIONARY AND ADVISORY LABELS 8, 10
▶ Trimbow (Chiesi Ltd)
   Formoterol fumarate dihydrate 5 microgram per 1 dose, Glycopyrronium (as Glycopyrronium bromide) 9 microgram per 1 dose, Beclometasone dipropionate 87 microgram per 1 dose Trimbow 87micrograms/dose / 5micrograms/dose / 9micrograms/dose inhaler | 120 dose [PoM] £44.50

◄ 256

Budesonide
21-Dec-2017

● DRUG ACTION Budesonide is a glucocorticoid, which exerts significant local anti-inflammatory effects.

● INDICATIONS AND DOSE
Prophylaxis of mild to moderate asthma (in patients stabilised on twice daily dose)
▶ BY INHALATION OF POWDER
▶ Child 6-11 years: 200–400 micrograms once daily, dose to be given in the evening
▶ Child 12-17 years: 200–400 micrograms once daily (max. per dose 800 micrograms), dose to be given in the evening
▶ Adult: 200–400 micrograms once daily (max. per dose 800 micrograms), dose to be given in the evening
Prophylaxis of asthma
▶ BY INHALATION OF POWDER
▶ Child 6-11 years: 100–400 micrograms twice daily, dose to be adjusted as necessary
▶ Child 12-17 years: 100–800 micrograms twice daily, dose to be adjusted as necessary
▶ Adult: 100–800 micrograms twice daily, dose to be adjusted as necessary
▶ BY INHALATION OF NEBULISED SUSPENSION
▶ Child 6 months-11 years: 125–500 micrograms twice daily, adjusted according to response; maximum 2 mg per day
▶ Child 12-17 years: Initially 0.25–1 mg twice daily, adjusted according to response, doses higher than recommended max. may be used in severe disease; maximum 2 mg per day
▶ Adult: Initially 0.25–1 mg twice daily, adjusted according to response, doses higher than recommended max. may be used in severe disease; maximum 2 mg per day
POTENCY
▶ Dose adjustments may be required for some inhaler devices, see under individual preparations.

BUDELIN NOVOLIZER®
Prophylaxis of asthma
▶ BY INHALATION OF POWDER
▶ Adult: 200–800 micrograms twice daily, dose is adjusted as necessary   continued →

Alternative in mild to moderate asthma, for patients previously stabilised on a twice daily dose
▶ BY INHALATION OF POWDER
▶ Adult: 200–400 micrograms once daily (max. per dose 800 micrograms), to be taken in the evening

PULMICORT® RESPULES

Prophylaxis of asthma
▶ BY INHALATION OF NEBULISED SUSPENSION
▶ Child 3 months–11 years: Initially 0.5–1 mg twice daily, reduced to 250–500 micrograms twice daily
▶ Child 12–17 years: Initially 1–2 mg twice daily, reduced to 0.5–1 mg twice daily
▶ Adult: Initially 1–2 mg twice daily, reduced to 0.5–1 mg twice daily

PULMICORT® TURBOHALER

Prophylaxis of asthma
▶ BY INHALATION OF POWDER
▶ Adult: 100–800 micrograms twice daily, dose to be adjusted as necessary

Alternative in mild to moderate asthma, for patients previously stabilised on a twice daily dose
▶ BY INHALATION OF POWDER
▶ Adult: 200–400 micrograms once daily (max. per dose 800 micrograms), to be taken in the evening

● INTERACTIONS → Appendix 1: corticosteroids

● DIRECTIONS FOR ADMINISTRATION Budesonide nebuliser suspension is not suitable for use in ultrasonic nebulisers.

● PATIENT AND CARER ADVICE With high doses, a steroid card should be supplied. Patients or carers should be given advice on how to administer budesonide dry powder inhaler and nebuliser suspension.
Medicines for Children leaflet: Budesonide inhaler for asthma prevention (prophylaxis) www.medicinesforchildren.org.uk/budesonide-inhaler-asthma-prevention-prophylaxis

BUDELIN NOVOLIZER® Patients or carers should be given advice on adminstration of *Budelin NovolizerA®*.

● MEDICINAL FORMS
There can be variation in the licensing of different medicines containing the same drug.
Inhalation powder
CAUTIONARY AND ADVISORY LABELS 8, 10
▶ Budelin Novolizer (Meda Pharmaceuticals Ltd)
Budesonide 200 microgram per 1 dose Budelin Novolizer 200micrograms/dose inhalation powder | 100 dose PoM £14.86
Budelin Novolizer 200micrograms/dose inhalation powder refill | 100 dose PoM £9.59
▶ Easyhaler (budesonide) (Orion Pharma (UK) Ltd)
Budesonide 100 microgram per 1 dose Easyhaler Budesonide 100micrograms/dose dry powder inhaler | 200 dose PoM £8.86 DT = £14.25
Budesonide 200 microgram per 1 dose Easyhaler Budesonide 200micrograms/dose dry powder inhaler | 200 dose PoM £17.71
Budesonide 400 microgram per 1 dose Easyhaler Budesonide 400micrograms/dose dry powder inhaler | 100 dose PoM £17.71
▶ Pulmicort Turbohaler (AstraZeneca UK Ltd)
Budesonide 100 microgram per 1 dose Pulmicort 100 Turbohaler | 200 dose PoM £14.25 DT = £14.25
Budesonide 200 microgram per 1 dose Pulmicort 200 Turbohaler | 100 dose PoM £14.25 DT = £14.25
Budesonide 400 microgram per 1 dose Pulmicort 400 Turbohaler | 50 dose PoM £14.25 DT = £14.25
Nebuliser liquid
CAUTIONARY AND ADVISORY LABELS 8, 10
▶ Budesonide (Non-proprietary)
Budesonide 250 microgram per 1 ml Budesonide 500micrograms/2ml nebuliser liquid unit dose vials | 20 unit dose PoM £30.40 DT = £24.86
Budesonide 500 microgram per 1 ml Budesonide 1mg/2ml nebuliser liquid unit dose vials | 20 unit dose PoM £42.41 DT = £39.00

▶ Pulmicort Respules (AstraZeneca UK Ltd)
Budesonide 250 microgram per 1 ml Pulmicort 0.5mg Respules | 20 unit dose PoM £31.70 DT = £24.86
Budesonide 500 microgram per 1 ml Pulmicort 1mg Respules | 20 unit dose PoM £48.00 DT = £39.00

Budesonide with formoterol
08-Feb-2018

The properties listed below are those particular to the combination only. For the properties of the components please consider, budesonide p. 259, formoterol fumarate p. 250.

● INDICATIONS AND DOSE
DUORESP SPIROMAX® 160MICROGRAMS/4.5MICROGRAMS

Asthma, maintenance therapy
▶ BY INHALATION OF POWDER
▶ Adult: 1–2 inhalations twice daily, increased if necessary up to 4 inhalations twice daily

Asthma, maintenance and reliever therapy
▶ BY INHALATION OF POWDER
▶ Adult: Maintenance 2 inhalations daily in 1–2 divided doses, increased if necessary to 2 inhalations twice daily. 1 inhalation as required, for relief of symptoms, increased if necessary up to 6 inhalations as required, max. 8 inhalations per day; up to 12 inhalations daily can be used for a limited time but medical assessment is recommended

Chronic obstructive pulmonary disease with forced expiratory volume in 1 second <70% of predicted
▶ BY INHALATION OF POWDER
▶ Adult: 2 inhalations twice daily

DUORESP SPIROMAX® 320MICROGRAMS/9MICROGRAMS

Asthma, maintenance therapy
▶ BY INHALATION OF POWDER
▶ Adult: 1 inhalation twice daily, increased if necessary up to 2 inhalations twice daily

Chronic obstructive pulmonary disease with forced expiratory volume in 1 second < 70% of predicted
▶ BY INHALATION OF POWDER
▶ Adult: 1 inhalation twice daily

FOBUMIX® 160/4.5 EASYHALER

Asthma, maintenance therapy
▶ BY INHALATION OF POWDER
▶ Adult: 1–2 inhalations twice daily, increased if necessary up to 4 inhalations twice daily

Asthma, maintenance and reliever therapy
▶ BY INHALATION OF POWDER
▶ Adult: Maintenance 2 inhalations daily in 1–2 divided doses, increased if necessary to 2 inhalations twice daily. 1 inhalation as required for relief of symptoms, increased if necessary up to 6 inhalations as required, max. 8 inhalations per day; up to 12 inhalations daily can be used for a limited time but medical assessment is recommended

Chronic obstructive pulmonary disease with forced expiratory volume in 1 second < 70% of predicted (post-bronchodilator)
▶ BY INHALATION OF POWDER
▶ Adult: 2 inhalations twice daily

FOBUMIX® 320/9 EASYHALER

Asthma, maintenance therapy
▶ BY INHALATION OF POWDER
▶ Adult: 1 inhalation twice daily; increased if necessary up to 2 inhalations twice daily

Chronic obstructive pulmonary disease with forced expiratory volume in 1 second < 70% of predicted (post-bronchodilator)
▸ BY INHALATION OF POWDER
▸ Adult: 1 inhalation twice daily

FOBUMIX ® 80/4.5 EASYHALER

Asthma, maintenance therapy
▸ BY INHALATION OF POWDER
▸ Adult: 1–2 inhalations twice daily, increased if necessary up to 4 inhalations twice daily

Asthma, maintenance and reliever therapy
▸ BY INHALATION OF POWDER
▸ Adult: Maintenance 2 inhalations daily in 1–2 divided doses. 1 inhalation as required for relief of symptoms, increased if necessary up to 6 inhalations as required, max. 8 inhalations per day; up to 12 inhalations daily can be used for a limited time but medical assessment is recommended

SYMBICORT 100/6 TURBOHALER ®

Asthma, maintenance therapy
▸ BY INHALATION OF POWDER
▸ Child 6–17 years: Initially 1–2 puffs twice daily; reduced to 1 puff daily, dose reduced only if control is maintained
▸ Adult: Initially 1–2 puffs twice daily, increased if necessary up to 4 puffs twice daily; reduced to 1 puff daily, dose reduced only if control is maintained

Asthma, maintenance and reliever therapy
▸ BY INHALATION OF POWDER
▸ Child 12–17 years: Maintenance 2 puffs daily in 1–2 divided doses; 1 puff as required for relief of symptoms, increased if necessary up to 6 puffs as required, max. 8 puffs per day; up to 12 puffs daily can be used for a limited time but medical assessment is recommended
▸ Adult: Maintenance 2 puffs daily in 1–2 divided doses; 1 puff as required for relief of symptoms, increased if necessary up to 6 puffs as required, max. 8 puffs per day; up to 12 puffs daily can be used for a limited time but medical assessment is recommended

SYMBICORT 200/6 TURBOHALER ®

Asthma, maintenance therapy
▸ BY INHALATION OF POWDER
▸ Child 12–17 years: Initially 1–2 puffs twice daily; reduced to 1 puff daily, dose reduced only if control is maintained
▸ Adult: Initially 1–2 puffs twice daily, increased if necessary up to 4 puffs twice daily; reduced to 1 puff daily, dose reduced only if control is maintained

Asthma, maintenance and reliever therapy
▸ BY INHALATION OF POWDER
▸ Child 12–17 years: Maintenance 2 puffs daily in 1–2 divided doses, increased if necessary to 2 puffs twice daily; 1 puff as required for relief of symptoms, increased if necessary up to 6 puffs as required, max. 8 puffs per day; up to 12 puffs daily can be used for a limited time but medical assessment is recommended
▸ Adult: Maintenance 2 puffs daily in 1–2 divided doses, increased if necessary to 2 puffs twice daily; 1 puff as required for relief of symptoms, increased if necessary up to 6 puffs as required, max. 8 puffs per day; up to 12 puffs daily can be used for a limited time but medical assessment is recommended

Chronic obstructive pulmonary disease with forced expiratory volume in 1 second < 70% of predicted (post bronchodilator)
▸ BY INHALATION OF POWDER
▸ Adult: 2 puffs twice daily

SYMBICORT 400/12 TURBOHALER ®

Asthma, maintenance therapy
▸ BY INHALATION OF POWDER
▸ Child 12–17 years: Initially 1 puff twice daily; reduced to 1 puff daily, dose reduced only if control is maintained
▸ Adult: Initially 1 puff twice daily, increased if necessary up to 2 puffs twice daily; reduced to 1 puff daily, dose reduced only if control is maintained

Chronic obstructive pulmonary disease with forced expiratory volume in 1 second < 70% of predicted (post bronchodilator)
▸ BY INHALATION OF POWDER
▸ Adult: 1 puff twice daily

SYMBICORT ® 200/6 PRESSURISED INHALER

Chronic obstructive pulmonary disease with forced expiratory volume in 1 second <70% of predicted (post bronchodilator)
▸ BY INHALATION OF AEROSOL
▸ Adult: 2 inhalations twice daily

● INTERACTIONS → Appendix 1: beta$_2$ agonists · corticosteroids

● PATIENT AND CARER ADVICE Patient counselling is advised for budesonide with formoterol inhalation (administration).
     With high doses, a steroid card should be supplied.

● NATIONAL FUNDING/ACCESS DECISIONS

Scottish Medicines Consortium (SMC) Decisions
▸ In adults The *Scottish Medicines Consortium* has advised (June 2007) that budesonide/formoterol 100 micrograms/6 micrograms and 200 micrograms/6 micrograms (*Symbicort* ® SMART ®) is accepted for use within NHS Scotland, in adults, for regular treatment of asthma where use of a combination (inhaled corticosteroid and a long-acting β_2 agonist) is appropriate; *Symbicort* is taken as regular maintenance treatment and as needed in response to symptoms.
▸ In children The *Scottish Medicines Consortium* has advised (June 2017) that budesonide/formoterol 100 micrograms/6 micrograms and 200 micrograms/6 micrograms (*Symbicort* ® SMART ®) is accepted for use within NHS Scotland for regular treatment of asthma where use of a combination (inhaled corticosteroid and a long-acting β_2 adrenoceptor agonist) is appropriate: patients already adequately controlled on both or patients not adequately controlled with inhaled corticosteroids and "as needed" short-acting β_2 adrenoceptor agonists. This advice relates to the extension of the license for *Symbicort* maintenance and reliever therapy (SMART ®) to adolescents aged 12 years and over.

● MEDICINAL FORMS
There can be variation in the licensing of different medicines containing the same drug.

Inhalation powder
CAUTIONARY AND ADVISORY LABELS 8, 10 (high doses)
▸ DuoResp Spiromax (Teva UK Ltd)
    Formoterol fumarate dihydrate 6 microgram per 1 dose, Budesonide 200 microgram per 1 dose DuoResp Spiromax 160micrograms/dose / 4.5micrograms/dose dry powder inhaler | 120 dose [PoM] £27.97 DT = £28.00
    Formoterol fumarate dihydrate 12 microgram per 1 dose, Budesonide 400 microgram per 1 dose DuoResp Spiromax 320micrograms/dose / 9micrograms/dose dry powder inhaler | 60 dose [PoM] £27.97 DT = £28.00
▸ Fobumix Easyhaler (Orion Pharma (UK) Ltd)
    Formoterol fumarate dihydrate 6 microgram per 1 dose, Budesonide 100 microgram per 1 dose Fobumix Easyhaler 80micrograms/dose / 4.5micrograms/dose dry powder inhaler | 120 dose [PoM] £26.99 DT = £28.00
    Formoterol fumarate dihydrate 6 microgram per 1 dose, Budesonide 200 microgram per 1 dose Fobumix Easyhaler

3

Respiratory system

160micrograms/dose / 4.5micrograms/dose dry powder inhaler | 60 dose [PoM] £16.99 | 120 dose [PoM] £26.99 DT = £28.00
Formoterol fumarate dihydrate 12 microgram per 1 dose, Budesonide 400 microgram per 1 dose Fobumix Easyhaler 320micrograms/dose / 9micrograms/dose dry powder inhaler | 60 dose [PoM] £26.99 DT = £28.00
▸ Symbicort Turbohaler (AstraZeneca UK Ltd)
Formoterol fumarate dihydrate 6 microgram per 1 dose, Budesonide 100 microgram per 1 dose Symbicort 100/6 Turbohaler | 120 dose [PoM] £28.00 DT = £28.00
Formoterol fumarate dihydrate 6 microgram per 1 dose, Budesonide 200 microgram per 1 dose Symbicort 200/6 Turbohaler | 120 dose [PoM] £28.00 DT = £28.00
Formoterol fumarate dihydrate 12 microgram per 1 dose, Budesonide 400 microgram per 1 dose Symbicort 400/12 Turbohaler | 60 dose [PoM] £28.00 DT = £28.00
Pressurised inhalation
CAUTIONARY AND ADVISORY LABELS 8, 10 (high doses)
▸ Symbicort (AstraZeneca UK Ltd)
Formoterol fumarate dihydrate 6 microgram per 1 dose, Budesonide 200 microgram per 1 dose Symbicort 200micrograms/dose / 6micrograms/dose pressurised inhaler | 120 dose [PoM] £28.00 DT = £28.00

�, 256

Ciclesonide

21-Dec-2017

● **INDICATIONS AND DOSE**
Prophylaxis of asthma
▸ BY INHALATION OF AEROSOL
▸ Child 12-17 years: 160 micrograms once daily; reduced to 80 micrograms daily, if control maintained
▸ Adult: Initially 160 micrograms once daily; reduced to 80 micrograms once daily, if control maintained; increased if necessary up to 320 micrograms twice daily, in severe asthma

● **UNLICENSED USE**
▸ In adults High dose recommended in severe asthma is unlicensed.
● **INTERACTIONS** → Appendix 1: corticosteroids
● **PATIENT AND CARER ADVICE** Patients or carers should be given advice on how to administer ciclesonide aerosol inhaler.
● **MEDICINAL FORMS**
There can be variation in the licensing of different medicines containing the same drug.
Pressurised inhalation
CAUTIONARY AND ADVISORY LABELS 8
▸ Alvesco (AstraZeneca UK Ltd)
Ciclesonide 80 microgram per 1 dose Alvesco 80 inhaler | 120 dose [PoM] £32.83 DT = £32.83
Ciclesonide 160 microgram per 1 dose Alvesco 160 inhaler | 60 dose [PoM] £19.31 DT = £19.31 | 120 dose [PoM] £38.62 DT = £38.62

▸, 256

Fluticasone

21-Dec-2017

● **INDICATIONS AND DOSE**
Prophylaxis of asthma
▸ BY INHALATION OF POWDER
▸ Child 5-15 years: Initially 50-100 micrograms twice daily (max. per dose 200 micrograms twice daily), dose to be adjusted as necessary
▸ Child 16-17 years: Initially 100-500 micrograms twice daily (max. per dose 1 mg twice daily), dose may be increased according to severity of asthma. Doses above 500 micrograms twice daily initiated by a specialist
▸ Adult: Initially 100-500 micrograms twice daily (max. per dose 1 mg twice daily), dose may be increased according to severity of asthma. Doses above 500 micrograms twice daily initiated by a specialist

▸ BY INHALATION OF AEROSOL
▸ Child 4-15 years: Initially 50-100 micrograms twice daily (max. per dose 200 micrograms twice daily), dose to be adjusted as necessary
▸ Child 16-17 years: Initially 100-500 micrograms twice daily (max. per dose 1 mg twice daily), dose may be increased according to severity of asthma. Doses above 500 micrograms twice daily initiated by a specialist
▸ Adult: Initially 100-500 micrograms twice daily (max. per dose 1 mg twice daily), dose may be increased according to severity of asthma. Doses above 500 micrograms twice daily initiated by a specialist
▸ BY INHALATION OF NEBULISED SUSPENSION
▸ Child 4-15 years: 1 mg twice daily
▸ Child 16-17 years: 0.5-2 mg twice daily
▸ Adult: 0.5-2 mg twice daily

● **INTERACTIONS** → Appendix 1: corticosteroids
● **DIRECTIONS FOR ADMINISTRATION** Fluticasone nebuliser liquid may be diluted with sterile sodium chloride 0.9%. It is not suitable for use in ultrasonic nebulisers.
● **PATIENT AND CARER ADVICE** Patients or carers should be given advice on how to administer all fluticasone inhalations preparations.
    With high doses, a steroid card should be supplied.
Medicines for Children leaflet: Fluticasone inhaler for asthma prevention (prophylaxis) www.medicinesforchildren.org.uk/fluticasone-inhaler-for-asthma-prevention

● **MEDICINAL FORMS**
There can be variation in the licensing of different medicines containing the same drug.
Inhalation powder
CAUTIONARY AND ADVISORY LABELS 8, 10
▸ Flixotide Accuhaler (GlaxoSmithKline UK Ltd)
Fluticasone propionate 50 microgram per 1 dose Flixotide 50micrograms/dose Accuhaler | 60 dose [PoM] £4.00 DT = £4.00
Fluticasone propionate 100 microgram per 1 dose Flixotide 100micrograms/dose Accuhaler | 60 dose [PoM] £8.00 DT = £8.00
Fluticasone propionate 250 microgram per 1 dose Flixotide 250micrograms/dose Accuhaler | 60 dose [PoM] £25.51 DT = £25.51
Fluticasone propionate 500 microgram per 1 dose Flixotide 500micrograms/dose Accuhaler | 60 dose [PoM] £43.37 DT = £43.37
Pressurised inhalation
CAUTIONARY AND ADVISORY LABELS 8, 10
▸ Flixotide Evohaler (GlaxoSmithKline UK Ltd)
Fluticasone propionate 50 microgram per 1 dose Flixotide 50micrograms/dose Evohaler | 120 dose [PoM] £5.44 DT = £5.44
Fluticasone propionate 125 microgram per 1 dose Flixotide 125micrograms/dose Evohaler | 120 dose [PoM] £12.50 DT = £12.50
Fluticasone propionate 250 microgram per 1 dose Flixotide 250micrograms/dose Evohaler | 120 dose [PoM] £20.00 DT = £20.00
Nebuliser liquid
CAUTIONARY AND ADVISORY LABELS 8, 10
▸ Flixotide Nebules (GlaxoSmithKline UK Ltd)
Fluticasone propionate 250 microgram per 1 ml Flixotide 0.5mg/2ml Nebules | 10 unit dose [PoM] £9.34
Fluticasone propionate 1 mg per 1 ml Flixotide 2mg/2ml Nebules | 10 unit dose [PoM] £37.35

Fluticasone with formoterol

The properties listed below are those particular to the combination only. For the properties of the components please consider, fluticasone above, formoterol fumarate p. 250.

● **INDICATIONS AND DOSE**
FLUTIFORM® 125
Prophylaxis of asthma
▸ BY INHALATION OF AEROSOL
▸ Child 12-17 years: 2 puffs twice daily
▸ Adult: 2 puffs twice daily

FLUTIFORM® 250

Prophylaxis of asthma
▸ BY INHALATION OF AEROSOL
▸ Adult: 2 puffs twice daily

FLUTIFORM® 50

Prophylaxis of asthma
▸ BY INHALATION OF AEROSOL
▸ Child 12-17 years: 2 puffs twice daily
▸ Adult: 2 puffs twice daily

● INTERACTIONS → Appendix 1: beta₂ agonists ·
corticosteroids

● PATIENT AND CARER ADVICE Patients or carers should be
given advice on how to administer fluticasone with
formoterol aerosol inhalation.
    With high doses, a steroid card should be provided.

● MEDICINAL FORMS
There can be variation in the licensing of different medicines
containing the same drug.
Pressurised inhalation
CAUTIONARY AND ADVISORY LABELS 8, 10 (high doses)
▸ Flutiform (Napp Pharmaceuticals Ltd)
    Formoterol fumarate dihydrate 5 microgram per 1 dose,
    Fluticasone propionate 50 microgram per 1 dose Flutiform
    50micrograms/dose / 5micrograms/dose inhaler | 120 dose PoM
    £14.40 DT = £14.40
    Formoterol fumarate dihydrate 5 microgram per 1 dose,
    Fluticasone propionate 125 microgram per 1 dose Flutiform
    125micrograms/dose / 5micrograms/dose inhaler | 120 dose PoM
    £28.00 DT = £28.00
    Formoterol fumarate dihydrate 10 microgram per 1 dose,
    Fluticasone propionate 250 microgram per 1 dose Flutiform
    250micrograms/dose / 10micrograms/dose inhaler | 120 dose PoM
    £45.56 DT = £45.56

Fluticasone with salmeterol   26-Apr-2018

The properties listed below are those particular to the
combination only. For the properties of the components
please consider, fluticasone p. 262, salmeterol p. 251.

● INDICATIONS AND DOSE

AIRFLUSAL FORSPIRO®

Chronic obstructive pulmonary disease with forced
expiratory volume in 1 second <60% of predicted |
Prophylaxis of asthma
▸ BY INHALATION OF POWDER
▸ Adult: 1 inhalation twice daily

AIRFLUSAL® 125

Prophylaxis of moderate-to-severe asthma
▸ BY INHALATION OF AEROSOL
▸ Adult: 2 inhalations twice daily

AIRFLUSAL® 250

Prophylaxis of moderate-to-severe asthma
▸ BY INHALATION OF AEROSOL
▸ Adult: 2 inhalations twice daily

SEREFLO® 125

Moderate-to-severe asthma
▸ BY INHALATION OF AEROSOL
▸ Adult: 2 inhalations twice daily

SEREFLO® 250

Moderate-to-severe asthma
▸ BY INHALATION OF AEROSOL
▸ Adult: 2 inhalations twice daily

SERETIDE 100 ACCUHALER®

Prophylaxis of asthma
▸ BY INHALATION OF POWDER
▸ Child 5-17 years: 1 inhalation twice daily, reduced to
1 inhalation daily, use reduced dose only if control
maintained
▸ Adult: 1 inhalation twice daily, reduced to 1 inhalation
daily, use reduced dose only if control maintained

SERETIDE 125 EVOHALER®

Prophylaxis of asthma
▸ BY INHALATION OF AEROSOL
▸ Child 12-17 years: 2 puffs twice daily
▸ Adult: 2 puffs twice daily

SERETIDE 250 ACCUHALER®

Prophylaxis of asthma
▸ BY INHALATION OF POWDER
▸ Child 12-17 years: 1 inhalation twice daily
▸ Adult: 1 inhalation twice daily

SERETIDE 250 EVOHALER®

Prophylaxis of asthma
▸ BY INHALATION OF AEROSOL
▸ Child 12-17 years: 2 puffs twice daily
▸ Adult: 2 puffs twice daily

SERETIDE 50 EVOHALER®

Prophylaxis of asthma
▸ INITIALLY BY INHALATION OF AEROSOL
▸ Child 5-17 years: 2 puffs twice daily, (by inhalation)
reduced to 2 puffs once daily, use reduced dose only if
control maintained
▸ Adult: 2 puffs twice daily, (by inhalation) reduced to
2 puffs once daily, use reduced dose only if control
maintained

SERETIDE 500 ACCUHALER®

Prophylaxis of asthma
▸ BY INHALATION OF POWDER
▸ Child 12-17 years: 1 inhalation twice daily
▸ Adult: 1 inhalation twice daily

Chronic obstructive pulmonary disease with forced
expiratory volume in 1 second <60% of predicted
▸ BY INHALATION OF POWDER
▸ Adult: 1 inhalation twice daily

● INTERACTIONS → Appendix 1: beta₂ agonists ·
corticosteroids

● PRESCRIBING AND DISPENSING INFORMATION
SEREFLO® 125 Manufacturer advises spacer devices are
not compatible—if spacer device required, switch to
alternative fixed-dose combination preparation.

● PATIENT AND CARER ADVICE Patients or carers should be
given advice on how to administer fluticasone with
salmeterol dry powder inhalation and aerosol inhalation.
    With preparations containing greater than
100 micrograms fluticasone, a steroid card should be
provided.

● NATIONAL FUNDING/ACCESS DECISIONS
Scottish Medicines Consortium (SMC) Decisions
▸ In adults The *Scottish Medicines Consortium* has advised
(December 2008) that *Seretide* 500 *Accuhaler*® is **not**
recommended for use within NHS Scotland for chronic
obstructive pulmonary disease in patients with a forced
expiratory volume in 1 second (FEV₁) less than 60% and
greater than 50% of the predicted normal value, with
significant symptoms despite regular bronchodilator
therapy, and a history of repeated exacerbations.

Respiratory system

3

- MEDICINAL FORMS
  There can be variation in the licensing of different medicines containing the same drug.
  Inhalation powder
  CAUTIONARY AND ADVISORY LABELS 8, 10 (excluding Seretide 100 Accuhaler ®)

  ▶ AirFluSal Forspiro (Sandoz Ltd)
    Salmeterol (as Salmeterol xinafoate) 50 microgram per 1 dose, Fluticasone propionate 500 microgram per 1 dose AirFluSal Forspiro 50micrograms/dose / 500micrograms/dose dry powder inhaler | 60 dose [PoM] £29.97 DT = £40.92

  ▶ Seretide Accuhaler (GlaxoSmithKline UK Ltd)
    Salmeterol (as Salmeterol xinafoate) 50 microgram per 1 dose, Fluticasone propionate 100 microgram per 1 dose Seretide 100 Accuhaler | 60 dose [PoM] £18.00 DT = £18.00
    Salmeterol (as Salmeterol xinafoate) 50 microgram per 1 dose, Fluticasone propionate 250 microgram per 1 dose Seretide 250 Accuhaler | 60 dose [PoM] £35.00 DT = £35.00
    Salmeterol (as Salmeterol xinafoate) 50 microgram per 1 dose, Fluticasone propionate 500 microgram per 1 dose Seretide 500 Accuhaler | 60 dose [PoM] £40.92 DT = £40.92

  Pressurised inhalation
  CAUTIONARY AND ADVISORY LABELS 8, 10 (excluding Seretide 50 Evohaler ®)

  ▶ AirFluSal (Sandoz Ltd)
    Salmeterol (as Salmeterol xinafoate) 25 microgram per 1 dose, Fluticasone propionate 125 microgram per 1 dose AirFluSal 25micrograms/dose / 125micrograms/dose inhaler | 120 dose [PoM] £18.50 DT = £35.00
    Salmeterol (as Salmeterol xinafoate) 25 microgram per 1 dose, Fluticasone propionate 250 microgram per 1 dose AirFluSal 25micrograms/dose / 250micrograms/dose inhaler | 120 dose [PoM] £29.95 DT = £59.48

  ▶ Sereflo (Kent Pharmaceuticals Ltd)
    Salmeterol (as Salmeterol xinafoate) 25 microgram per 1 dose, Fluticasone propionate 125 microgram per 1 dose Sereflo 25micrograms/dose / 125micrograms/dose inhaler | 120 dose [PoM] £18.50 DT = £35.00
    Salmeterol (as Salmeterol xinafoate) 25 microgram per 1 dose, Fluticasone propionate 250 microgram per 1 dose Sereflo 25micrograms/dose / 250micrograms/dose inhaler | 120 dose [PoM] £29.95 DT = £59.48

  ▶ Seretide Evohaler (GlaxoSmithKline UK Ltd)
    Salmeterol (as Salmeterol xinafoate) 25 microgram per 1 dose, Fluticasone propionate 50 microgram per 1 dose Seretide 50 Evohaler | 120 dose [PoM] £18.00 DT = £18.00
    Salmeterol (as Salmeterol xinafoate) 25 microgram per 1 dose, Fluticasone propionate 125 microgram per 1 dose Seretide 125 Evohaler | 120 dose [PoM] £35.00 DT = £35.00
    Salmeterol (as Salmeterol xinafoate) 25 microgram per 1 dose, Fluticasone propionate 250 microgram per 1 dose Seretide 250 Evohaler | 120 dose [PoM] £59.48 DT = £59.48

Fluticasone with umeclidinium and vilanterol

16-Mar-2018

The properties listed below are those particular to the combination only. For the properties of the components please consider, fluticasone p. 262, umeclidinium p. 248.

- INDICATIONS AND DOSE
  Maintenance of moderate-to-severe chronic obstructive pulmonary disease
  ▶ BY INHALATION OF POWDER
  ▶ Adult: 1 inhalation once daily, dose should be taken at the same time each day

- CAUTIONS Convulsive disorders · pulmonary tuberculosis · thyrotoxicosis
- INTERACTIONS → Appendix 1: beta$_2$ agonists · corticosteroids · umeclidinium
- SIDE-EFFECTS
  ▶ **Common or very common** Back pain
  ▶ **Uncommon** Oropharyngeal pain

- HEPATIC IMPAIRMENT Manufacturer advises use with caution in moderate-to-severe impairment.
- PATIENT AND CARER ADVICE Patients or carers should be given advice on appropriate inhaler technique.
- NATIONAL FUNDING/ACCESS DECISIONS
  Scottish Medicines Consortium (SMC) Decisions
  The *Scottish Medicines Consortium* has advised (February 2018) that fluticasone furoate with umeclidinium and vilanterol (as trifenatate) (*Trelegy® Ellipta®*) is accepted for restricted use within NHS Scotland for the maintenance treatment in adults with severe chronic obstructive pulmonary disease (forced expiratory volume in one second [FEV1] <50% predicted normal).

- MEDICINAL FORMS
  There can be variation in the licensing of different medicines containing the same drug.
  Inhalation powder
  ▶ Trelegy Ellipta (GlaxoSmithKline UK Ltd) ▼
    Vilanterol (as Vilanterol trifenatate) 22 microgram per 1 dose, Umeclidinium bromide 65 microgram per 1 dose, Fluticasone furoate 92 microgram per 1 dose Trelegy Ellipta 92micrograms/dose / 55micrograms/dose / 22micrograms/dose dry powder inhaler | 30 dose [PoM] £44.50

Fluticasone with vilanterol

01-Nov-2017

The properties listed below are those particular to the combination only. For the properties of the components please consider, fluticasone p. 262.

- INDICATIONS AND DOSE
  RELVAR ELLIPTA ® 184 MICROGRAMS/22 MICROGRAMS
  Prophylaxis of asthma
  ▶ BY INHALATION OF POWDER
  ▶ Child 12–17 years: 1 inhalation once daily
  ▶ Adult: 1 inhalation once daily

  RELVAR ELLIPTA ® 92 MICROGRAMS/22 MICROGRAMS
  Prophylaxis of asthma
  ▶ BY INHALATION OF POWDER
  ▶ Child 12–17 years: 1 inhalation once daily
  ▶ Adult: 1 inhalation once daily

  Chronic obstructive pulmonary disease with forced expiratory volume in 1 second < 70% of predicted
  ▶ BY INHALATION OF POWDER
  ▶ Adult: 1 inhalation once daily

- INTERACTIONS → Appendix 1: beta$_2$ agonists · corticosteroids
- SIDE-EFFECTS
  ▶ **Common or very common** Abdominal pain · arthralgia · back pain · bone fracture · cough · dysphonia · fever · muscle spasms · oropharyngeal pain
  ▶ **Uncommon** Vision blurred
  ▶ **Rare or very rare** Angioedema · anxiety
- PREGNANCY Manufacturer advises use only if potential benefit outweighs risk.
- BREAST FEEDING Manufacturer advises avoid—no information available.
- HEPATIC IMPAIRMENT Manufacturer advises use with caution.
  RELVAR ELLIPTA ®
  184 MICROGRAMS/22 MICROGRAMS Avoid in moderate to severe impairment.
- PATIENT AND CARER ADVICE Patients or carers should be given advice on how to administer fluticasone with vilanterol powder for inhalation.
  A steroid card should be provided.

- NATIONAL FUNDING/ACCESS DECISIONS

Scottish Medicines Consortium (SMC) Decisions

▶ In adults The *Scottish Medicines Consortium* has advised (March 2014) that fluticasone furoate/vilanterol (*Relvar Ellipta*®) is accepted for restricted use within NHS Scotland in patients with severe chronic obstructive pulmonary disease with a forced expiratory volume in 1 second (FEV$_1$) less than 50% of the predicted normal value.

- MEDICINAL FORMS
There can be variation in the licensing of different medicines containing the same drug.

Inhalation powder

CAUTIONARY AND ADVISORY LABELS 8, 10

▶ Relvar Ellipta (GlaxoSmithKline UK Ltd) ▼
Vilanterol 22 microgram per 1 dose, Fluticasone furoate 92 microgram per 1 dose Relvar Ellipta 92micrograms/dose / 22micrograms/dose dry powder inhaler | 30 dose [PoM] £22.00 DT = £22.00
Vilanterol 22 microgram per 1 dose, Fluticasone furoate 184 microgram per 1 dose Relvar Ellipta 184micrograms/dose / 22micrograms/dose dry powder inhaler | 30 dose [PoM] £29.50 DT = £29.50

F 256

Mometasone furoate
21-Dec-2017

- INDICATIONS AND DOSE

Prophylaxis of asthma

▶ BY INHALATION OF POWDER
▶ Child 12-17 years: Initially 400 micrograms daily in 1–2 divided doses, single dose to be inhaled in the evening, reduced to 200 micrograms once daily, if control maintained
▶ Adult: Initially 400 micrograms daily in 1–2 divided doses, single dose to be inhaled in the evening, reduced to 200 micrograms once daily, if control maintained

Prophylaxis of severe asthma

▶ BY INHALATION OF POWDER
▶ Child 12-17 years: Increased if necessary up to 400 micrograms twice daily
▶ Adult: Increased if necessary up to 400 micrograms twice daily

- INTERACTIONS → Appendix 1: corticosteroids
- PATIENT AND CARER ADVICE Patients or carers should be given advice on how to administer mometasone by inhaler. With high doses, a steroid card should be supplied.
Medicines for Children leaflet: Mometasone furoate inhaler for asthma prevention (prophylaxis) www.medicinesforchildren.org.uk/mometasone-furoate-inhaler-for-asthma-prevention-prophylaxis

- NATIONAL FUNDING/ACCESS DECISIONS

Scottish Medicines Consortium (SMC) Decisions

The *Scottish Medicines Consortium* has advised (November 2003) that *Asmanex*® is restricted for use following failure of first-line inhaled corticosteroids.

- MEDICINAL FORMS
There can be variation in the licensing of different medicines containing the same drug.

Inhalation powder

CAUTIONARY AND ADVISORY LABELS 8, 10

▶ Asmanex Twisthaler (Merck Sharp & Dohme Ltd)
Mometasone furoate 200 microgram per 1 dose Asmanex 200micrograms/dose Twisthaler | 30 dose [PoM] £15.70 DT = £15.70 | 60 dose [PoM] £23.54 DT = £23.54
Mometasone furoate 400 microgram per 1 dose Asmanex 400micrograms/dose Twisthaler | 30 dose [PoM] £21.78 DT = £21.78 | 60 dose [PoM] £36.05 DT = £36.05

ENZYME INHIBITORS

Human alpha$_1$-proteinase inhibitor
17-Aug-2017

- DRUG ACTION Human alpha$_1$-proteinase inhibitor is a normal plasma constituent; it inhibits neutrophil elastase (an enzyme released in response to inflammation) in the lungs.

- INDICATIONS AND DOSE

Progression of emphysema in patients with severe alpha$_1$-proteinase inhibitor deficiency, despite optimal treatment with other standard therapies (specialist use only)

▶ BY INTRAVENOUS INFUSION
▶ Adult: 60 mg/kg once weekly

- CONTRA-INDICATIONS IgA deficiency with confirmed antibodies against IgA—increased risk of severe hypersensitivity reactions
- CAUTIONS Consider vaccination against hepatitis A and hepatitis B · hypersensitivity reactions · IgA deficiency (without known antibodies to IgA)—increased risk of hypersensitivity reactions

CAUTIONS, FURTHER INFORMATION

▶ Hypersensitivity reactions Hypersensitivity reactions may occur, even in patients who have previously tolerated treatment. Manufacturer advises close monitoring, including vital signs, during the first infusions. If a reaction occurs, manufacturer advises to decrease the rate of infusion or discontinue treatment; if symptoms improve promptly after stopping, the infusion may be resumed at a slower infusion rate.

- SIDE-EFFECTS
▶ **Common or very common** Dizziness · headache · nausea
▶ **Uncommon** Asthenia · confusion · flushing · hypersensitivity · hypotension · sensation abnormal · skin reactions · syncope · tachycardia · throat oedema
▶ **Rare or very rare** Chest pain · chills · fever · hyperhidrosis
▶ **Frequency not known** Eye swelling · facial swelling · lip swelling · lymph node pain

- PREGNANCY Manufacturer advises caution—no information available.

- BREAST FEEDING Manufacturer advises avoid—no information available.

- PRESCRIBING AND DISPENSING INFORMATION Manufacturer advises to record the brand name and batch number after each administration (in case of transmission of infective agents).

- PATIENT AND CARER ADVICE Manufacturer advises patients receiving treatment at home should receive appropriate training regarding self-administration, and be informed of the signs of hypersensitivity reactions.
Driving and skilled tasks Manufacturer advises patients and carers should be counselled on the effects on driving and performance of skilled tasks—increased risk of dizziness.

- NATIONAL FUNDING/ACCESS DECISIONS

Scottish Medicines Consortium (SMC) Decisions

The *Scottish Medicines Consortium* has advised (August 2016) that human alpha-$_1$ proteinase inhibitor (*Respreeza*®) is **not** recommended for use within NHS Scotland for maintenance treatment, to slow the progression of emphysema in adults with documented severe alpha$_1$-proteinase inhibitor deficiency. The manufacturer did not present a sufficiently robust clinical or economic analysis.

All Wales Medicines Strategy Group (AWMSG) Decisions

The *All Wales Medicines Strategy Group* has advised (March 2017) that human alpha-$_1$ proteinase inhibitor

(*Respreeza*®) is **not** recommended for use within NHS Wales for maintenance treatment, to slow the progression of emphysema in adults with documented severe alpha₁-proteinase inhibitor deficiency. The case for clinical and cost-effectiveness has not been proven.

- MEDICINAL FORMS
There can be variation in the licensing of different medicines containing the same drug.
Powder and solvent for solution for infusion
ELECTROLYTES: May contain Sodium
‣ Respreeza (CSL Behring UK Ltd) ▼
Human alpha1-proteinase inhibitor 1 gram Respreeza 1000mg powder and solvent for solution for infusion vials | 1 vial [PoM] £220.00

IMMUNOSUPPRESSANTS › MONOCLONAL ANTIBODIES

Benralizumab

02-May-2018

- DRUG ACTION Benralizumab is a humanised monoclonal antibody that interferes with interleukin-5 receptor binding, thereby reducing the survival of eosinophils and basophils.

- INDICATIONS AND DOSE
Severe eosinophilic asthma (specialist use only)
‣ BY SUBCUTANEOUS INJECTION
‣ Adult: Initially 30 mg every 4 weeks for the first 3 doses, then maintenance 30 mg every 8 weeks, to be administered into the thigh, abdomen or upper arm
PHARMACOKINETICS
‣ The half-life of benralizumab is approx. 15 days.

- CAUTIONS Pre-existing helminth infection
CAUTIONS, FURTHER INFORMATION
‣ Helminth infection Manufacturer advises to treat pre-existing helminth infections before starting benralizumab—if patient becomes infected during therapy and does not respond to anti-helminth treatment, discontinue benralizumab until infection is resolved.

- INTERACTIONS → Appendix 1: monoclonal antibodies

- SIDE-EFFECTS
‣ Common or very common Fever · headache · hypersensitivity (may be delayed) · pharyngitis

- PREGNANCY Manufacturer advises avoid unless potential benefit outweighs risk—limited data available.

- BREAST FEEDING Manufacturer advises avoid—no information available.

- DIRECTIONS FOR ADMINISTRATION Manufacturer advises to take the syringe out of the refrigerator at least 30 minutes before administration, and to avoid injecting into areas of the skin that are tender, bruised, erythematous, or hardened—consult product literature for further information.

- HANDLING AND STORAGE Manufacturer advises store in a refrigerator (2–8°C) and protect from light.

- PATIENT AND CARER ADVICE Manufacturer advises patients and their carers should be instructed to seek medical advice if their asthma remains uncontrolled or if symptoms worsen after initiation of treatment.

- MEDICINAL FORMS
There can be variation in the licensing of different medicines containing the same drug.
Solution for injection
‣ Fasenra (AstraZeneca UK Ltd) ▼
Benralizumab 30 mg per 1 ml Fasenra 30mg/1ml solution for injection pre-filled syringes | 1 pre-filled disposable injection [PoM] £1,955.00 (Hospital only)

Mepolizumab

09-Feb-2017

- DRUG ACTION Mepolizumab is a humanised anti-interleukin-5 (anti-IL-5) monoclonal antibody; it reduces the production and survival of eosinophils

- INDICATIONS AND DOSE
Add on treatment for severe refractory eosinophilic asthma (under expert supervision)
‣ BY SUBCUTANEOUS INJECTION
‣ Adult: 100 mg every 4 weeks

- CAUTIONS Helminth infection
CAUTIONS, FURTHER INFORMATION
‣ Helminth infections Manufacturer advises pre-existing helminth infections should be treated before initiation of therapy; if patients become infected during treatment and do not respond to anti-helminth treatment, consider treatment interruption.

- SIDE-EFFECTS
‣ Common or very common Abdominal pain upper · back pain · eczema · fever · headache · hypersensitivity · increased risk of infection · nasal congestion

- PREGNANCY Manufacturer advises avoid unless potential benefit outweighs risk—limited data available.

- BREAST FEEDING Manufacturer advises avoid—present in milk in *animal* studies.

- PATIENT AND CARER ADVICE
Asthma Patients and their carers should be advised to seek medical advice if their asthma remains uncontrolled or worsens after initiation of treatment.

- NATIONAL FUNDING/ACCESS DECISIONS
NICE decisions
‣ **Mepolizumab for treating severe refractory eosinophilic asthma (January 2017)** NICE TA431
Mepolizumab, as an add-on to optimised standard therapy, is recommended as an option for treating severe refractory eosinophilic asthma in adults, only if:
  • the blood eosinophil count is 300 cells/microlitre or more in the previous 12 months **and**
  • the person has agreed to and followed the optimised standard treatment plan **and** has had 4 or more asthma exacerbations requiring systemic corticosteroids in the previous 12 months **or** had continuous oral corticosteroids over the previous 6 months **and**
  • the manufacturer provides mepolizumab with the discount agreed in the patient access scheme
www.nice.org.uk/TA431

Scottish Medicines Consortium (SMC) Decisions
The *Scottish Medicines Consortium* has advised (June 2016) that mepolizumab (*Nucala*®) is accepted for restricted use within NHS Scotland as an add-on treatment for severe refractory eosinophilic asthma in adult patients who have eosinophils of at least 150 cells/microlitre (0.15×10^9/L) at initiation of treatment and have had at least four asthma exacerbations in the preceding year or are receiving maintenance treatment with oral corticosteroids.

- MEDICINAL FORMS
There can be variation in the licensing of different medicines containing the same drug.
Powder for solution for injection
‣ Nucala (GlaxoSmithKline UK Ltd) ▼
Mepolizumab 100 mg Nucala 100mg powder for solution for injection vials | 1 vial [PoM] £840.00 (Hospital only)

Omalizumab

- **INDICATIONS AND DOSE**

Prophylaxis of severe persistent allergic asthma
▸ BY SUBCUTANEOUS INJECTION
▸ Adult: Dose according to immunoglobulin E concentration and body-weight (consult product literature)

Add-on therapy for chronic spontaneous urticaria in patients who have had an inadequate response to H₁ antihistamine treatment
▸ BY SUBCUTANEOUS INJECTION
▸ Adult: 300 mg every 4 weeks

- CAUTIONS Autoimmune disease · susceptibility to helminth infection—discontinue if infection does not respond to anthelmintic

- SIDE-EFFECTS
▸ **Common or very common** Headache · skin reactions
▸ **Uncommon** Cough · diarrhoea · dizziness · drowsiness · fatigue · flushing · gastrointestinal discomfort (very common in children) · increased risk of infection · influenza like illness · limb swelling · nausea · paraesthesia · photosensitivity reaction · postural hypotension · respiratory disorders · syncope · weight increased
▸ **Rare or very rare** Angioedema · hypersensitivity · systemic lupus erythematosus (SLE)
▸ **Frequency not known** Alopecia · eosinophilic granulomatosis with polyangiitis · immune thrombocytopenic purpura · joint disorders · lymphadenopathy · myalgia

SIDE-EFFECTS, FURTHER INFORMATION

Eosinophilic granulomatosis with polyangiitis (Churg-Strauss syndrome) Churg-Strauss syndrome has occurred rarely in patients given omalizumab; the reaction is usually associated with the reduction of oral corticosteroid therapy. Churg-Strauss syndrome can present as eosinophilia, vasculitic rash, cardiac complications, worsening pulmonary symptoms, or peripheral neuropathy.

Hypersensitivity reactions Hypersensitivity reactions can also occur immediately following treatment with omalizumab or sometimes more than 24 hours after the first injection.

- PREGNANCY Manufacturer advises avoid unless essential—crosses the placenta.

- BREAST FEEDING Manufacturer advises avoid—present in milk in *animal* studies.

- HEPATIC IMPAIRMENT Manufacturer advises caution—no information available.

- RENAL IMPAIRMENT Manufacturer advises caution—no information available.

- NATIONAL FUNDING/ACCESS DECISIONS
NICE decisions
▸ Omalizumab for severe persistent allergic asthma (April 2013) NICE TA278
Omalizumab is recommended as an option for treating severe persistent confirmed allergic IgE-mediated asthma as an add-on to optimised standard therapy in patients aged 6 years and over:
- who need continuous or frequent treatment with oral corticosteroids (defined as 4 or more courses in the previous year), **and**
- only if the manufacturer makes omalizumab available with the discount agreed in the patient access scheme.
Optimised standard therapy is defined as a full trial of and, if tolerated, documented compliance with inhaled high-dose corticosteroids, long-acting beta₂ agonists, leukotriene receptor antagonists, theophyllines, oral corticosteroids, and smoking cessation if clinically appropriate.

Patients currently receiving omalizumab whose disease does not meet the criteria should be able to continue treatment until they and their clinician consider it appropriate to stop.
www.nice.org.uk/TA278
▸ Omalizumab for previously treated chronic spontaneous urticaria (June 2015) NICE TA339
Omalizumab is an option as add-on therapy for the treatment of severe chronic spontaneous urticaria in patients 12 years and over, only if:
- the severity of the condition is assessed objectively, for example, using a weekly urticaria activity score of 28 or more,
- the patient's condition has not responded to standard treatment with H₁-antihistamines and leukotriene receptor antagonists,
- omalizumab is stopped at or before the fourth dose if the condition has not responded,
- omalizumab is stopped at the end of a course of treatment (6 doses) if the condition has responded and is restarted only if the condition relapses,
- omalizumab is administered under the management of a secondary care specialist in dermatology, immunology or allergy,
- the manufacturer provides omalizumab with the discount agreed in the patient access scheme.
Patients currently receiving omalizumab whose disease does not meet the above criteria should have the option to continue treatment until they and their clinician consider it appropriate to stop.
www.nice.org.uk/TA339
Scottish Medicines Consortium (SMC) Decisions
The *Scottish Medicines Consortium* has advised (December 2014) that omalizumab (*Xolair®*) is accepted for restricted use within NHS Scotland for the treatment of chronic spontaneous urticaria in patients aged 12 years and over, who have had an inadequate response to combination therapy with H₁-antihistamines, leukotriene receptor antagonists and H₂-antihistamines, used according to current treatment guidelines.

- MEDICINAL FORMS
There can be variation in the licensing of different medicines containing the same drug.
Solution for injection
▸ Xolair (Novartis Pharmaceuticals UK Ltd)
Omalizumab 150 mg per 1 ml Xolair 150mg/1ml solution for injection pre-filled syringes | 1 pre-filled disposable injection PoM £256.15
Xolair 75mg/0.5ml solution for injection pre-filled syringes | 1 pre-filled disposable injection PoM £128.07

Reslizumab
01-Nov-2017

- DRUG ACTION Reslizumab is a humanised monoclonal antibody that interferes with interleukin-5 receptor binding, thereby reducing the survival and activity of eosinophils.

- **INDICATIONS AND DOSE**

Severe eosinophilic asthma (adjunctive therapy when inadequately controlled by high-dose corticosteroids plus another standard treatment) (specialist use only)
▸ BY INTRAVENOUS INFUSION
▸ Adult: (consult product literature)
PHARMACOKINETICS
▸ The half-life of reslizumab is approx. 24 days.

- CAUTIONS Hypersensitivity reactions · pre-existing helminth infection
CAUTIONS, FURTHER INFORMATION
▸ Helminth infection Manufacturer advises to treat pre-existing helminth infections before starting reslizumab—

consider temporarily discontinuing reslizumab if patient becomes infected during therapy and does not respond to anti-helminth treatment.

▸ **Hypersensitivity reactions** Serious hypersensitivity reactions, including life-threatening anaphylaxis, can occur and manufacturer advises to monitor closely during treatment and for at least 20 minutes after completion of infusion; in the event of a hypersensitivity reaction, treatment should be permanently discontinued.

● **SIDE-EFFECTS**
▸ **Uncommon** Anaphylactic reaction · myalgia
▸ **Frequency not known** Secondary malignancy

● **PREGNANCY** Manufacturer advises avoid—limited information available.

● **BREAST FEEDING** Manufacturer advises avoid during first few days after birth—risk of transfer of antibodies to infant cannot be excluded; present in milk in *animal* studies.

● **DIRECTIONS FOR ADMINISTRATION** For *intravenous infusion*, manufacturer advises give intermittently in Sodium chloride 0.9%; administer over 20–50 minutes through an in-line 0.2 micron filter.

● **HANDLING AND STORAGE** Manufacturer advises store in a refrigerator (2–8°C); consult product literature for storage conditions after preparation of infusion.

● **PATIENT AND CARER ADVICE** Manufacturer advises patients and their carers should be instructed to seek medical advice if their asthma remains uncontrolled or if symptoms worsen after initiation of treatment.

● **NATIONAL FUNDING/ACCESS DECISIONS**

NICE decisions
▸ **Reslizumab for treating severe eosinophilic asthma (October 2017) NICE TA479**
Reslizumab, as an add-on therapy, is recommended as an option for the treatment of severe eosinophilic asthma that is inadequately controlled in adults despite maintenance therapy with high-dose inhaled corticosteroids plus another drug, only if:
● the blood eosinophil count has been recorded as 400 cells per microlitre or more, **and**
● the person has had 3 or more severe asthma exacerbations needing systemic corticosteroids in the past 12 months, **and**
● the manufacturer provides reslizumab with the discount agreed in the patient access scheme.
At 12 months, stop reslizumab if the asthma has not responded adequately or continue reslizumab if the asthma has responded adequately and assess response each year.

Patients whose treatment was started within the NHS before this guidance was published should have the option to continue treatment, without change to their funding arrangements, until they and their NHS clinician consider it appropriate to stop.
www.nice.org.uk/guidance/ta479

Scottish Medicines Consortium (SMC) Decisions
The *Scottish Medicines Consortium* has advised (December 2017) that reslizumab (*Cinqaero®*) is **not** recommended for use within NHS Scotland as add-on therapy in adults with severe eosinophilic asthma inadequately controlled with high-dose inhaled corticosteroids plus another medicinal product for maintenance treatment, as the economic case was not demonstrated.

● **MEDICINAL FORMS**
There can be variation in the licensing of different medicines containing the same drug.
Solution for infusion
EXCIPIENTS: May contain Sucrose
▸ Cinqaero (Teva UK Ltd) ▼
Reslizumab 10 mg per 1 ml Cinqaero 100mg/10ml concentrate for solution for infusion vials | 1 vial P̲o̲M̲ £499.99
Cinqaero 25mg/2.5ml concentrate for solution for infusion vials | 1 vial P̲o̲M̲ £124.99

LEUKOTRIENE RECEPTOR ANTAGONISTS

Leukotriene receptor antagonists
29-Nov-2017

Overview
The leukotriene receptor antagonists, montelukast below and zafirlukast p. 269, block the effects of cysteinyl leukotrienes in the airways.

Montelukast has not been shown to be more effective than a standard dose of inhaled corticosteroid, but the two drugs appear to have an additive effect. The leukotriene receptor antagonists may be of benefit in exercise-induced asthma and in those with concomitant rhinitis, but they are less effective in those with severe asthma who are also receiving high doses of other drugs.

Montelukast

● **INDICATIONS AND DOSE**

Prophylaxis of asthma
▸ BY MOUTH
▸ **Child 6 months–5 years:** 4 mg once daily, dose to be taken in the evening
▸ **Child 6–14 years:** 5 mg once daily, dose to be taken in the evening
▸ **Child 15–17 years:** 10 mg once daily, dose to be taken in the evening
▸ **Adult:** 10 mg once daily, dose to be taken in the evening

Symptomatic relief of seasonal allergic rhinitis in patients with asthma.
▸ BY MOUTH
▸ **Child 15–17 years:** 10 mg once daily, dose to be taken in the evening
▸ **Adult:** 10 mg once daily, dose to be taken in the evening

● **INTERACTIONS** → Appendix 1: montelukast

● **SIDE-EFFECTS**
▸ **Common or very common** Diarrhoea · fever · gastrointestinal discomfort · headache · nausea · skin reactions · upper respiratory tract infection · vomiting
▸ **Uncommon** Akathisia · anxiety · arthralgia · asthenia · behaviour abnormal · depression · dizziness · drowsiness · dry mouth · haemorrhage · irritability · malaise · muscle complaints · oedema · seizure · sensation abnormal · sleep disorders
▸ **Rare or very rare** Angioedema · concentration impaired · disorientation · eosinophilic granulomatosis with polyangiitis · erythema nodosum · hallucination · hepatic disorders · memory loss · palpitations · pulmonary eosinophilia · suicidal tendencies · tremor

SIDE-EFFECTS, FURTHER INFORMATION Eosinophilic granulomatosis with polyangiitis (Churg-Strauss syndrome) has occurred very rarely in association with the use of montelukast; in many of the reported cases the reaction followed the reduction or withdrawal of oral corticosteroid therapy. Prescribers should be alert to the development of eosinophilia, vasculitic rash, worsening pulmonary symptoms, cardiac complications, or peripheral neuropathy.

- **PREGNANCY** Manufacturer advises avoid unless essential. There is limited evidence for the safe use of montelukast during pregnancy; however, it can be taken as normal in women who have shown a significant improvement in asthma not achievable with other drugs before becoming pregnant.
- **BREAST FEEDING** Manufacturer advises avoid unless essential.
- **DIRECTIONS FOR ADMINISTRATION** Granules may be swallowed or mixed with cold, soft food (not liquid) and taken immediately.
- **PRESCRIBING AND DISPENSING INFORMATION** Flavours of chewable tablet formulations may include cherry.
- **PATIENT AND CARER ADVICE** Patients or carers should be given advice on how to administer montelukast granules. Medicines for Children leaflet: Montelukast for asthma www.medicinesforchildren.org.uk/montelukast-for-asthma
- **NATIONAL FUNDING/ACCESS DECISIONS**
  SINGULAIR ® GRANULES
  Scottish Medicines Consortium (SMC) Decisions
  The *Scottish Medicines Consortium* has advised (June 2007) that *Singulair* ® granules are restricted for use as an alternative to low-dose inhaled corticosteroids for children 2–14 years with mild persistent asthma who have not recently had serious asthma attacks that required oral corticosteroid use and who are not capable of using inhaled corticosteroids; *Singulair* ® granules should be initiated by a specialist in paediatric asthma.
  SINGULAIR ® CHEWABLE TABLETS
  Scottish Medicines Consortium (SMC) Decisions
  The *Scottish Medicines Consortium* has advised (June 2007) that *Singulair* ® chewable tablets are restricted for use as an alternative to low-dose inhaled corticosteroids for children 2–14 years with mild persistent asthma who have not recently had serious asthma attacks that required oral corticosteroid use and who are not capable of using inhaled corticosteroids; *Singulair* ® chewable tablets should be initiated by a specialist in paediatric asthma.

- **MEDICINAL FORMS**
  There can be variation in the licensing of different medicines containing the same drug.
  Granules
  - Montelukast (Non-proprietary)
    Montelukast (as Montelukast sodium) 4 mg Montelukast 4mg granules sachets sugar free sugar-free | 28 sachet PoM £4.85–£19.99 DT = £4.85
  - Singulair (Merck Sharp & Dohme Ltd)
    Montelukast (as Montelukast sodium) 4 mg Singulair Paediatric 4mg granules sachets sugar-free | 28 sachet PoM £25.69 DT = £4.85
  Tablet
  - Montelukast (Non-proprietary)
    Montelukast (as Montelukast sodium) 10 mg Montelukast 10mg tablets | 28 tablet PoM £26.97 DT = £1.10
  - Singulair (Merck Sharp & Dohme Ltd)
    Montelukast (as Montelukast sodium) 10 mg Singulair 10mg tablets | 28 tablet PoM £26.97 DT = £1.10
  Chewable tablet
  CAUTIONARY AND ADVISORY LABELS 23, 24
  EXCIPIENTS: May contain Aspartame
  - Montelukast (Non-proprietary)
    Montelukast (as Montelukast sodium) 4 mg Montelukast 4mg chewable tablets sugar free sugar-free | 28 tablet PoM £25.69 DT = £0.89
    Montelukast (as Montelukast sodium) 5 mg Montelukast 5mg chewable tablets sugar free sugar-free | 28 tablet PoM £25.69 DT = £1.06
  - Singulair (Merck Sharp & Dohme Ltd)
    Montelukast (as Montelukast sodium) 4 mg Singulair Paediatric 4mg chewable tablets sugar-free | 28 tablet PoM £25.69 DT = £0.89
    Montelukast (as Montelukast sodium) 5 mg Singulair Paediatric 5mg chewable tablets sugar-free | 28 tablet PoM £25.69 DT = £1.06

Zafirlukast

- **INDICATIONS AND DOSE**
  Prophylaxis of asthma
  ▸ BY MOUTH
  ▸ Child 12–17 years: 20 mg twice daily
  ▸ Adult: 20 mg twice daily

- **CAUTIONS** Elderly
- **SIDE-EFFECTS**
  ▸ **Common or very common** Abdominal pain · headache · infection · myalgia · nausea · skin reactions · vomiting
  ▸ **Uncommon** Angioedema · arthralgia · hyperbilirubinaemia · malaise · oedema · sleep disorders
  ▸ **Rare or very rare** Haemorrhagic disorder · hepatic disorders · menorrhagia · thrombocytopenia
  ▸ **Frequency not known** Agranulocytosis · dizziness · sensation abnormal
  SIDE-EFFECTS, FURTHER INFORMATION
  Eosinophilic granulomatosis with polyangiitis (Churg-Strauss syndrome) Churg-Strauss syndrome has occurred rarely in association with the use of zafirlukast; in many of the reported cases the reaction followed the reduction or withdrawal of oral corticosteroid therapy. Prescribers should be alert to the development of eosinophilia, vasculitic rash, worsening pulmonary symptoms, cardiac complications, or neuropathy.
  Hepatic disorder Symptoms such as persistent nausea, vomiting, malaise, or jaundice may develop, and indicate the development of a liver disorder.
- **PREGNANCY** Manufacturer advises use only if potential benefit outweighs risk. There is limited evidence for the safe use of zafirlukast during pregnancy; however, it can be taken as normal in women who have shown a significant improvement in asthma not achievable with other drugs before becoming pregnant.
- **BREAST FEEDING** Present in milk—manufacturer advises avoid.
- **HEPATIC IMPAIRMENT** Manufacturer advises avoid.
- **RENAL IMPAIRMENT**
  ▸ In adults Manufacturer advises caution in moderate to severe impairment.
  ▸ In children Manufacturer advises caution.
- **PATIENT AND CARER ADVICE**
  Medicines for Children leaflet: Zafirlukast for asthma prevention (prophylaxis) www.medicinesforchildren.org.uk/zafirlukast-for-asthma-prevention

- **MEDICINAL FORMS**
  No licensed medicines listed.

MAST-CELL STABILISERS

Cromoglicate and related therapy

Overview

The mode of action of sodium cromoglicate p. 270 and nedocromil sodium p. 270 is not completely understood. They may be of value in asthma with an allergic basis, but, in practice, it is difficult to predict who will benefit; they could probably be given for 4 to 6 weeks to assess response. Dose frequency is adjusted according to response but is usually 3 to 4 times a day initially; this may subsequently be reduced.

In general, *prophylaxis* with sodium cromoglicate is less effective than prophylaxis with corticosteroid inhalations. There is evidence of efficacy of nedocromil sodium in children aged 5–12 years. Sodium cromoglicate and nedocromil sodium are of no value in the treatment of acute attacks of asthma.

3

Respiratory system

3

Respiratory system

Sodium cromoglicate can prevent exercise-induced asthma. However, exercise-induced asthma may reflect poor overall control and the patient should be reassessed.

Sodium cromoglicate and nedocromil sodium may also have a role in allergic conjunctivitis; sodium cromoglicate is used also in allergic rhinitis and allergy-related diarrhoea.

Nedocromil sodium

● **INDICATIONS AND DOSE**

Prophylaxis of asthma
▸ BY INHALATION OF AEROSOL
▸ Child 5–17 years: Initially 4 mg 4 times a day, when control achieved may be possible to reduce to twice daily
▸ Adult: Initially 4 mg 4 times a day, when control achieved may be possible to reduce to twice daily
DOSE EQUIVALENCE AND CONVERSION
▸ 2 puffs = 4 mg.

● **UNLICENSED USE** Not licensed for use in children under 6 years.
● **SIDE-EFFECTS**
▸ **Common or very common** Bronchospasm · cough · gastrointestinal discomfort · headache · nausea · taste altered · vomiting
▸ **Frequency not known** Pharyngitis · throat irritation
SIDE-EFFECTS, FURTHER INFORMATION If paradoxical bronchospasm occurs, fast-acting inhaled bronchodilator such as salbutamol or terbutaline should be used to control symptoms; treatment with nedocromil should be discontinued.
● **PREGNANCY** Inhaled drugs can be taken as normal during pregnancy.
● **BREAST FEEDING** Inhaled drugs can be taken as normal during breast-feeding.
● **TREATMENT CESSATION** Withdrawal should be done gradually over a period of one week—symptoms of asthma may recur.
● **PRESCRIBING AND DISPENSING INFORMATION** Flavours of inhalers may include mint.
● **PATIENT AND CARER ADVICE** Regular use is necessary. Patient counselling is advised for Nedocromil aerosol for inhalation (administration).

● **MEDICINAL FORMS**
There can be variation in the licensing of different medicines containing the same drug.
Pressurised inhalation
CAUTIONARY AND ADVISORY LABELS 8
▸ Tilade (Sanofi)
  Nedocromil sodium 2 mg per 1 dose Tilade 2mg/dose inhaler CFC free | 112 dose [PoM] £39.94

Sodium cromoglicate

(Sodium cromoglycate)

● **INDICATIONS AND DOSE**

Prophylaxis of asthma
▸ BY INHALATION OF AEROSOL
▸ Child 5–17 years: Initially 10 mg 4 times a day, additional dose may also be taken before exercise, increased if necessary to 10 mg 6–8 times a day; maintenance 5 mg 4 times a day, 5 mg is equivalent to 1 puff
▸ Adult: Initially 10 mg 4 times a day, additional dose may also be taken before exercise, increased if necessary to 10 mg 6–8 times a day; maintenance 5 mg 4 times a day, 5 mg is equivalent to 1 puff

Food allergy (in conjunction with dietary restriction)
▸ BY MOUTH
▸ Child 2–13 years: Initially 100 mg 4 times a day for 2–3 weeks, then increased if necessary up to 40 mg/kg daily, then reduced according to response, to be taken before meals
▸ Child 14–17 years: Initially 200 mg 4 times a day for 2–3 weeks, then increased if necessary up to 40 mg/kg daily, then reduced according to response, to be taken before meals
▸ Adult: Initially 200 mg 4 times a day for 2–3 weeks, then increased if necessary up to 40 mg/kg daily, then reduced according to response, to be taken before meals

● **CAUTIONS**
▸ When used by inhalation Discontinue if eosinophilic pneumonia occurs
● **SIDE-EFFECTS**
▸ When used by inhalation Cough · headache · pneumonia eosinophilic · rhinitis · throat irritation
▸ With oral use Arthralgia · nausea · rash
SIDE-EFFECTS, FURTHER INFORMATION When used by inhalation, if paradoxical bronchospasm occurs, a short-acting beta$_2$ agonist should be used to control symptoms; treatment with sodium cromoglicate should be discontinued.
● **PREGNANCY** Not known to be harmful.
▸ When used by inhalation Can be taken as normal during pregnancy.
● **BREAST FEEDING** Unlikely to be present in milk.
▸ When used by inhalation Can be taken as normal during breast-feeding.
● **TREATMENT CESSATION**
▸ When used by inhalation Withdrawal of sodium cromoglicate should be done gradually over a period of one week—symptoms of asthma may recur.
● **DIRECTIONS FOR ADMINISTRATION** Capsules may be swallowed whole or the contents dissolved in hot water and diluted with cold water before taking.
● **PATIENT AND CARER ADVICE**
▸ With oral use Patient counselling is advised for sodium cromoglicate capsules (administration).
▸ When used by inhalation Patient counselling is advised for sodium cromoglicate pressurised inhalation (administration).

● **MEDICINAL FORMS**
There can be variation in the licensing of different medicines containing the same drug. Forms available from special-order manufacturers include: oral solution
Capsule
CAUTIONARY AND ADVISORY LABELS 22
▸ Nalcrom (Sanofi)
  Sodium cromoglicate 100 mg Nalcrom 100mg capsules | 100 capsule [PoM] £41.14 DT = £41.14
Pressurised inhalation
CAUTIONARY AND ADVISORY LABELS 8
▸ Intal (Sanofi)
  Sodium cromoglicate 5 mg per 1 dose Intal 5mg/dose inhaler CFC free | 112 dose [PoM] £18.33 DT = £18.33

PHOSPHODIESTERASE TYPE-4 INHIBITORS

Roflumilast

30-Jun-2017

- DRUG ACTION Roflumilast is a phosphodiesterase type-4 inhibitor with anti-inflammatory properties.

- INDICATIONS AND DOSE

Adjunct to bronchodilators for the maintenance treatment of patients with severe chronic obstructive pulmonary disease associated with chronic bronchitis and a history of frequent exacerbations
▶ BY MOUTH
▸ Adult: 500 micrograms once daily

- CONTRA-INDICATIONS Cancer (except basal cell carcinoma) · concomitant treatment with immunosuppressive drugs (except short-term systemic corticosteroids) · history of depression associated with suicidal ideation or behaviour · moderate to severe cardiac failure · severe acute infectious disease · severe immunological disease

- CAUTIONS History of psychiatric illness (discontinue if new or worsening psychiatric symptoms occur) · latent infection (such as tuberculosis, viral hepatitis, herpes infection)

- INTERACTIONS → Appendix 1: roflumilast

- SIDE-EFFECTS
▶ **Common or very common** Appetite decreased · diarrhoea · gastrointestinal discomfort · headache · insomnia · nausea · weight decreased
▶ **Uncommon** Anxiety · asthenia · back pain · dizziness · gastrointestinal disorders · malaise · muscle complaints · muscle weakness · palpitations · skin reactions · tremor · vertigo · vomiting
▶ **Rare or very rare** Angioedema · constipation · depression · gynaecomastia · haematochezia · respiratory tract infection · suicidal tendencies · taste altered

- CONCEPTION AND CONTRACEPTION Women of child-bearing age should use effective contraception.

- PREGNANCY Manufacturer advises avoid—toxicity in *animal* studies.

- BREAST FEEDING Manufacturer advises avoid—present in milk in *animal* studies.

- HEPATIC IMPAIRMENT Caution in mild impairment. Avoid in moderate to severe impairment.

- MONITORING REQUIREMENTS Monitor body-weight.

- PATIENT AND CARER ADVICE Patients should be given a patient card before starting treatment and advised to record body-weight at regular intervals.

- NATIONAL FUNDING/ACCESS DECISIONS

NICE decisions
▶ **Roflumilast for treating chronic obstructive pulmonary disease (July 2017)** NICE TA461
Roflumilast, as an add-on to bronchodilator therapy, is recommended as an option for treating severe chronic obstructive pulmonary disease in patients with chronic bronchitis, only if:
  ● the disease is severe, defined as a forced expiratory volume in one second (FEV_1) after a bronchodilator of less than 50% of predicted normal, **and**
  ● the person has had two or more exacerbations in the previous 12 months despite triple inhaled therapy with a long-acting muscarinic antagonist, a long-acting beta-2 agonist and an inhaled corticosteroid.
Treatment with roflumilast should be started by a specialist in respiratory medicine.
  Patients currently receiving roflumilast whose disease does not meet the above criteria should be able to continue treatment until they and their clinician consider it appropriate to stop.
www.nice.org.uk/guidance/TA461

Scottish Medicines Consortium (SMC) Decisions
The *Scottish Medicines Consortium* has advised (September 2017) that roflumilast (*Daxas*®) is not recommended for use within NHS Scotland for maintenance treatment of severe chronic obstructive pulmonary disease (forced expiratory volume in one second [FEV_1] after a bronchodilator of less than 50% predicted) associated with chronic bronchitis in adults with a history of frequent exacerbations as add on to bronchodilator treatment as there was insufficient evidence submitted and the economic case was not demonstrated.

- MEDICINAL FORMS
There can be variation in the licensing of different medicines containing the same drug.

Tablet
▸ Daxas (AstraZeneca UK Ltd) ▼
  Roflumilast 500 microgram Daxas 500microgram tablets |
  30 tablet [PoM] £37.71 DT = £37.71

SYMPATHOMIMETICS ⟩ VASOCONSTRICTOR

Ephedrine hydrochloride

- INDICATIONS AND DOSE

Reversal of hypotension from spinal or epidural anaesthesia
▶ BY SLOW INTRAVENOUS INJECTION
▸ Adult: 3–6 mg every 3–4 minutes (max. per dose 9 mg), adjusted according to response, injection solution to contain ephedrine hydrochloride 3 mg/ml; maximum 30 mg per course

Reversible airways obstruction
▶ BY MOUTH
▸ Adult: 15–60 mg 3 times a day

Neuropathic oedema
▶ BY MOUTH
▸ Adult: 30–60 mg 3 times a day

- UNLICENSED USE Not licensed for neuropathic oedema.

- CAUTIONS
GENERAL CAUTIONS Diabetes mellitus · elderly · hypertension · hyperthyroidism · ischaemic heart disease · prostatic hypertrophy (risk of acute urinary retention)
SPECIFIC CAUTIONS
▶ With intravenous use Susceptibility to angle-closure glaucoma

- INTERACTIONS → Appendix 1: sympathomimetics, vasoconstrictor

- SIDE-EFFECTS
GENERAL SIDE-EFFECTS
▶ **Common or very common** Anxiety · headache · insomnia · nausea
▶ **Frequency not known** Tremor
SPECIFIC SIDE-EFFECTS
▶ **Common or very common**
▶ With intravenous use Arrhythmias · asthenia · confusion · depression · dyspnoea · hyperhidrosis · irritability · palpitations · vomiting
▶ **Rare or very rare**
▶ With intravenous use Acute urinary retention
▶ With oral use Myocardial infarction
▶ **Frequency not known**
▶ With intravenous use Acute angle closure glaucoma · angina pectoris · appetite decreased · cardiac arrest · dizziness · hypokalaemia · intracranial haemorrhage · psychotic disorder · pulmonary oedema

- With oral use Arrhythmias · circulation impaired · drug tolerance · dry mouth · enuresis · hypertension · sedation
- **PREGNANCY**
- With oral use Manufacturer advises avoid.
- With intravenous use Increased fetal heart rate reported with parenteral ephedrine.
- **BREAST FEEDING** Present in milk; manufacturer advises avoid—irritability and disturbed sleep reported.
- **RENAL IMPAIRMENT** Use with caution.
- **LESS SUITABLE FOR PRESCRIBING** Ephedrine tablets are less suitable and less safe for use as a bronchodilator than the selective beta₂ agonists.
- **EXCEPTIONS TO LEGAL CATEGORY** For exceptions relating to ephedrine tablets see *Medicines, Ethics and Practice*, London, Pharmaceutical Press (always consult latest edition).

- **MEDICINAL FORMS**
There can be variation in the licensing of different medicines containing the same drug. Forms available from special-order manufacturers include: oral suspension, oral solution, solution for injection

Tablet
- Ephedrine hydrochloride (Non-proprietary)
  Ephedrine hydrochloride 15 mg Ephedrine hydrochloride 15mg tablets | 28 tablet [PoM] £55.28 DT = £44.45
  Ephedrine hydrochloride 30 mg Ephedrine hydrochloride 30mg tablets | 28 tablet [PoM] £83.73 DT = £67.35

Solution for injection
- Ephedrine hydrochloride (Non-proprietary)
  Ephedrine hydrochloride 3 mg per 1 ml Ephedrine 30mg/10ml solution for injection ampoules | 10 ampoule [PoM] £84.56
  Ephedrine 30mg/10ml solution for injection pre-filled syringes | 1 pre-filled disposable injection [PoM] £7.59–£9.50 | 12 pre-filled disposable injection [PoM] £114.00
  Ephedrine hydrochloride 30 mg per 1 ml Ephedrine 30mg/1ml solution for injection ampoules | 10 ampoule [PoM] £5.48–£54.80

XANTHINES

Aminophylline

- **INDICATIONS AND DOSE**

Severe acute asthma in patients not previously treated with theophylline
▶ BY SLOW INTRAVENOUS INJECTION
- Child: 5 mg/kg (max. per dose 500 mg), to be followed by intravenous infusion
- Adult: 250–500 mg (max. per dose 5 mg/kg), to be followed by intravenous infusion

Severe acute asthma
▶ BY INTRAVENOUS INFUSION
- Child 1 month–11 years: 1 mg/kg/hour, adjusted according to plasma-theophylline concentration
- Child 12–17 years: 500–700 micrograms/kg/hour, adjusted according to plasma-theophylline concentration
- Adult: 500–700 micrograms/kg/hour, adjusted according to plasma-theophylline concentration
- Elderly: 300 micrograms/kg/hour, adjusted according to plasma-theophylline concentration

Severe acute exacerbation of chronic obstructive pulmonary disease in patients not previously treated with theophylline
▶ BY SLOW INTRAVENOUS INJECTION
- Adult: 250–500 mg (max. per dose 5 mg/kg), to be followed by intravenous infusion

Severe acute exacerbation of chronic obstructive pulmonary disease
▶ BY INTRAVENOUS INFUSION
- Adult: 500–700 micrograms/kg/hour, adjusted according to plasma-theophylline concentration

- Elderly: 300 micrograms/kg/hour, adjusted according to plasma-theophylline concentration

Chronic asthma
▶ BY MOUTH USING MODIFIED-RELEASE MEDICINES
- Child (body-weight 40 kg and above): Initially 225 mg twice daily for 1 week, then increased if necessary to 450 mg twice daily, adjusted according to plasma-theophylline concentration

Reversible airway obstruction
▶ BY MOUTH USING MODIFIED-RELEASE MEDICINES
- Adult (body-weight 40 kg and above): Initially 225 mg twice daily for 1 week, then increased if necessary to 450 mg twice daily, adjusted according to plasma-theophylline concentration

PHYLLOCONTIN CONTINUS ® FORTE

Reversible airways obstruction
▶ BY MOUTH USING MODIFIED-RELEASE MEDICINES
- Adult: Initially 350 mg twice daily for 1 week, then increased if necessary to 700 mg twice daily, increase dose according to plasma-theophylline concentration

DOSE ADJUSTMENTS DUE TO INTERACTIONS
- Dose adjustment may be necessary if smoking started or stopped during treatment.

DOSES AT EXTREMES OF BODY-WEIGHT
- To avoid excessive dosage in obese patients, dose should be calculated on the basis of ideal weight for height.

PHARMACOKINETICS
- Aminophylline is a stable mixture or combination of theophylline and ethylenediamine; the ethylenediamine confers greater solubility in water.
- Theophylline is metabolised in the liver. The plasma-theophylline concentration is increased in heart failure, hepatic impairment, and in viral infections. The plasma-theophylline concentration is decreased in smokers, and by alcohol consumption. Differences in the half-life of aminophylline are important because the toxic dose is close to the therapeutic dose.

- **UNLICENSED USE** Aminophylline injection not licensed for use in children under 6 months.
- **CAUTIONS** Arrhythmias following rapid intravenous injection · cardiac arrhythmias or other cardiac disease · elderly (increased plasma-theophylline concentration) · epilepsy · fever · hypertension · hyperthyroidism · peptic ulcer · risk of hypokalaemia
- **INTERACTIONS** → Appendix 1: aminophylline
- **SIDE-EFFECTS**

GENERAL SIDE-EFFECTS Arrhythmia (more common when given too rapidly by intravenous injection) · headache · nausea · palpitations · seizure (more common when given too rapidly by intravenous injection)

SPECIFIC SIDE-EFFECTS
- With intravenous use Abdominal pain · anxiety · confusion · delirium · diarrhoea · dizziness · electrolyte imbalance · gastrointestinal haemorrhage · gastrooesophageal reflux disease · hyperthermia · hyperventilation · hypotension (more common when given too rapidly by intravenous injection) · insomnia · mania · metabolic disorder · pain · skin reactions · tachycardia (more common when given too rapidly by intravenous injection) · thirst · tremor · vertigo · visual impairment · vomiting
- With oral use Central nervous system stimulation · epigastric discomfort

SIDE-EFFECTS, FURTHER INFORMATION Potentially serious hypokalaemia may result from beta 2 agonist therapy. Particular caution is required in severe asthma, because this effect may be potentiated by concomitant treatment with theophylline and its derivatives, corticosteroids, and diuretics, and by hypoxia. Plasma-potassium concentration should therefore be monitored in severe asthma.

Overdose Theophylline and related drugs are often prescribed as modified-release formulations and toxicity can therefore be delayed. They cause vomiting (which may be severe and intractable), agitation, restlessness, dilated pupils, sinus tachycardia, and hyperglycaemia. More serious effects are haematemesis, convulsions, and supraventricular and ventricular arrhythmias. Severe hypokalaemia may develop rapidly.

For specific details on the management of poisoning, see *Theophylline*, under Emergency treatment of poisoning p. 1319 .

- ● ALLERGY AND CROSS-SENSITIVITY Allergy to ethylenediamine can cause urticaria, erythema, and exfoliative dermatitis.

- ● PREGNANCY Neonatal irritability and apnoea have been reported. Theophylline can be taken as normal during pregnancy as it is particularly important that asthma should be well controlled during pregnancy.

- ● BREAST FEEDING Present in milk—irritability in infant reported; modified-release preparations preferable. Theophylline can be taken as normal during breast-feeding.

- ● HEPATIC IMPAIRMENT **Dose adjustments** Reduce dose.

- ● MONITORING REQUIREMENTS
  - ▸ Aminophylline is monitored therapeutically in terms of plasma-theophylline concentrations.
  - ▸ Measurement of plasma-theophylline concentration may be helpful and is **essential** if a loading dose of intravenous aminophylline is to be given to patients who are already taking theophylline, because serious side-effects such as convulsions and arrhythmias can occasionally precede other symptoms of toxicity.
  - ▸ In most individuals, a plasma-theophylline concentration of 10–20 mg/litre (55–110 micromol/litre) is required for satisfactory bronchodilation, although a lower plasma-theophylline concentration of 5–15 mg/litre may be effective. Adverse effects can occur within the range 10–20 mg/litre and both the frequency and severity increase at concentrations above 20 mg/litre.
  - ▸ If aminophylline is given intravenously, a blood sample should be taken 4–6 hours after starting treatment.
  - ▸ With oral use Plasma-theophylline concentration is measured 5 days after starting oral treatment and at least 3 days after any dose adjustment. A blood sample should usually be taken 4–6 hours after an oral dose of a modified-release preparation (sampling times may vary—consult local guidelines).

- ● DIRECTIONS FOR ADMINISTRATION
  - ▸ With intravenous use For *intravenous injection*, give **very slowly** over at least 20 minutes (with close monitoring).
  - ▸ With intravenous use in children For *intravenous infusion*, dilute to a concentration of 1 mg/mL with Glucose 5% *or* Sodium Chloride 0.9%.
  - ▸ With intravenous use in adults For *intravenous infusion*, give continuously in Glucose 5% *or* Sodium Chloride 0.9%.
  - ▸ With intramuscular use Aminophylline is too irritant for intramuscular use.

- ● PRESCRIBING AND DISPENSING INFORMATION Patients taking oral theophylline or aminophylline should not normally receive a loading dose of intravenous aminophylline.

  Consider intravenous aminophylline for treatment of severe and life-threatening acute asthma only after consultation with senior medical staff.

  Modified release The rate of absorption from modified-release preparations can vary between brands. If a prescription for a modified-release oral aminophylline preparation does not specify a brand name, the pharmacist should contact the prescriber and agree the brand to be dispensed. Additionally, it is essential that a patient discharged from hospital should be maintained on the brand on which that patient was stabilised as an in-patient.

PHYLLOCONTIN CONTINUS ® FORTE *Phyllocontin Continus*® Forte tablets are for smokers and other patients where theophylline half-life is shorter.

- ● MEDICINAL FORMS
  There can be variation in the licensing of different medicines containing the same drug. Forms available from special-order manufacturers include: solution for infusion

  Solution for injection
  - ▸ Aminophylline (Non-proprietary)
    Aminophylline 25 mg per 1 ml Aminophylline 250mg/10ml solution for injection ampoules | 10 ampoule [PoM] £6.50 DT = £6.50

  Modified-release tablet
  CAUTIONARY AND ADVISORY LABELS 25
  - ▸ Phyllocontin Continus (Napp Pharmaceuticals Ltd)
    Aminophylline hydrate 225 mg Phyllocontin Continus 225mg tablets | 56 tablet [P] £2.40 DT = £2.40
    Aminophylline hydrate 350 mg Phyllocontin Forte Continus 350mg tablets | 56 tablet [P] £4.22 DT = £4.22

Theophylline

- ● INDICATIONS AND DOSE

NUELIN SA ® 175MG TABLETS

Reversible airways obstruction | Severe acute asthma | Chronic asthma
- ▸ BY MOUTH USING MODIFIED-RELEASE MEDICINES
- ▸ Adult: 175–350 mg every 12 hours

Chronic asthma
- ▸ BY MOUTH USING MODIFIED-RELEASE MEDICINES
- ▸ Child 6–11 years: 175 mg every 12 hours
- ▸ Child 12–17 years: 175–350 mg every 12 hours

NUELIN SA ® 250 TABLETS

Reversible airways obstruction | Severe acute asthma | Chronic asthma
- ▸ BY MOUTH USING MODIFIED-RELEASE MEDICINES
- ▸ Adult: 250–500 mg every 12 hours

Chronic asthma
- ▸ BY MOUTH USING MODIFIED-RELEASE MEDICINES
- ▸ Child 6–11 years: 125–250 mg every 12 hours
- ▸ Child 12–17 years: 250–500 mg every 12 hours

SLO-PHYLLIN ®

Chronic asthma
- ▸ BY MOUTH USING MODIFIED-RELEASE MEDICINES
- ▸ Child 2–5 years: 60–120 mg every 12 hours
- ▸ Child 6–11 years: 125–250 mg every 12 hours
- ▸ Child 12–17 years: 250–500 mg every 12 hours

Reversible airways obstruction | Severe acute asthma | Chronic asthma
- ▸ BY MOUTH USING MODIFIED-RELEASE MEDICINES
- ▸ Adult: 250–500 mg every 12 hours

UNIPHYLLIN CONTINUS ®

Chronic asthma
- ▸ BY MOUTH USING MODIFIED-RELEASE MEDICINES
- ▸ Child 2–11 years: 9 mg/kg every 12 hours (max. per dose 200 mg), dose may be increased in some children with chronic asthma; increased to 10–16 mg/kg every 12 hours (max. per dose 400 mg), may be appropriate to give larger evening or morning dose to achieve optimum therapeutic effect when symptoms most severe; in patients whose night or daytime symptoms persist despite other therapy, who are not currently receiving theophylline, total daily requirement may be added as single evening or morning dose continued →

> Child 12–17 years: 200 mg every 12 hours, adjusted according to response to 400 mg every 12 hours, may be appropriate to give larger evening or morning dose to achieve optimum therapeutic effect when symptoms most severe; in patients whose night or daytime symptoms persist despite other therapy, who are not currently receiving theophylline, total daily requirement may be added as single evening or morning dose

Reversible airways obstruction | Severe acute asthma | Chronic asthma

▶ BY MOUTH USING MODIFIED-RELEASE MEDICINES

▶ Adult: 200 mg every 12 hours, adjusted according to response to 400 mg every 12 hours, may be appropriate to give larger evening or morning dose to achieve optimum therapeutic effect when symptoms most severe; in patients whose night or daytime symptoms persist despite other therapy, who are not currently receiving theophylline, total daily requirement may be added as single evening or morning dose

DOSE ADJUSTMENTS DUE TO INTERACTIONS

▶ Dose adjustment may be necessary if smoking started or stopped during treatment.

PHARMACOKINETICS

▶ Theophylline is metabolised in the liver. The plasma-theophylline concentration is increased in heart failure, hepatic impairment, and in viral infections. The plasma-theophylline concentration is decreased in smokers, and by alcohol consumption. Differences in the half-life of theophylline are important because the toxic dose is close to the therapeutic dose.

● CAUTIONS Cardiac arrhythmias or other cardiac disease · elderly (increased plasma-theophylline concentration) · epilepsy · fever · hypertension · hyperthyroidism · peptic ulcer · risk of hypokalaemia

● INTERACTIONS → Appendix 1: theophylline

● SIDE-EFFECTS Anxiety · arrhythmias · diarrhoea · dizziness · gastrointestinal discomfort · gastrooesophageal reflux disease · headache · hyperuricaemia · nausea · palpitations · seizure · skin reactions · sleep disorders · tremor · urinary disorders · vomiting

SIDE-EFFECTS, FURTHER INFORMATION Potentially serious hypokalaemia may result from beta$_2$ agonist therapy. Particular caution is required in severe asthma, because this effect may be potentiated by concomitant treatment with theophylline and its derivatives, corticosteroids, and diuretics, and by hypoxia. Plasma-potassium concentration should therefore be monitored in severe asthma.

Overdose Theophylline in overdose can cause vomiting (which may be severe and intractable), agitation, restlessness, dilated pupils, sinus tachycardia, and hyperglycaemia. More serious effects are haematemesis, convulsions, and supraventricular and ventricular arrhythmias. Severe hypokalaemia may develop rapidly.
　For details on the management of poisoning, see *Theophylline*, under Emergency treatment of poisoning p. 1319.

● PREGNANCY Neonatal irritability and apnoea have been reported. Theophylline can be taken as normal during pregnancy as it is particularly important that asthma should be well controlled during pregnancy.

● BREAST FEEDING Present in milk—irritability in infant reported; modified-release preparations preferable. Theophylline can be taken as normal during breast-feeding.

● HEPATIC IMPAIRMENT **Dose adjustments** Reduce dose.

● MONITORING REQUIREMENTS

▶ In most individuals, a plasma-theophylline concentration of 10–20 mg/litre (55–110 micromol/litre) is required for satisfactory bronchodilation, although a lower plasma-theophylline concentration of 5–15 mg/litre may be effective. Adverse effects can occur within the range 10–20 mg/litre and both the frequency and severity increase at concentrations above 20 mg/litre.

▶ Plasma-theophylline concentration is measured 5 days after starting oral treatment and at least 3 days after any dose adjustment. A blood sample should usually be taken 4–6 hours after an oral dose of a modified-release preparation (sampling times may vary—consult local guidelines).

● DIRECTIONS FOR ADMINISTRATION

SLO-PHYLLIN ®

▶ In adults Swallow whole with fluid or swallow enclosed granules with soft food (e.g. yoghurt).

▶ In children Contents of the capsule (enteric-coated granules) may be sprinkled on to a spoonful of soft food (e.g. yoghurt) and swallowed without chewing.

● PRESCRIBING AND DISPENSING INFORMATION The rate of absorption from modified-release preparations can vary between brands. If a prescription for a modified-release oral theophylline preparation does not specify a brand name, the pharmacist should contact the prescriber and agree the brand to be dispensed. Additionally, it is essential that a patient discharged from hospital should be maintained on the brand on which that patient was stabilised as an in-patient.

● PATIENT AND CARER ADVICE

SLO-PHYLLIN ® Patient or carer should be given advice on how to administer theophylline modified release capsules.

● MEDICINAL FORMS
There can be variation in the licensing of different medicines containing the same drug.

Modified-release tablet

CAUTIONARY AND ADVISORY LABELS 21, 25

▶ Nuelin SA (Meda Pharmaceuticals Ltd)
　Theophylline 175 mg Nuelin SA 175mg tablets | 60 tablet Ⓟ £6.38 DT = £6.38
　Theophylline 250 mg Nuelin SA 250 tablets | 60 tablet Ⓟ £8.92 DT = £8.92

▶ Uniphyllin Continus (Napp Pharmaceuticals Ltd)
　Theophylline 200 mg Uniphyllin Continus 200mg tablets | 56 tablet Ⓟ £2.96 DT = £2.96
　Theophylline 300 mg Uniphyllin Continus 300mg tablets | 56 tablet Ⓟ £4.77 DT = £4.77
　Theophylline 400 mg Uniphyllin Continus 400mg tablets | 56 tablet Ⓟ £5.65 DT = £5.65

Modified-release capsule

CAUTIONARY AND ADVISORY LABELS 25

▶ Slo-Phyllin (Merck Serono Ltd)
　Theophylline 60 mg Slo-Phyllin 60mg capsules | 56 capsule Ⓟ £2.76 DT = £2.76
　Theophylline 125 mg Slo-Phyllin 125mg capsules | 56 capsule Ⓟ £3.48 DT = £3.48
　Theophylline 250 mg Slo-Phyllin 250mg capsules | 56 capsule Ⓟ £4.34 DT = £4.34

Nebuliser solutions

● HYPERTONIC SODIUM CHLORIDE SOLUTIONS

● INDICATIONS AND DOSE

MUCOCLEAR ® 3%

Mobilise lower respiratory tract secretions in mucous consolidation (e.g. cystic fibrosis) | Mild to moderate acute viral bronchiolitis in infants

▶ BY INHALATION OF NEBULISED SOLUTION

▶ Adult: 4 mL 2–4 times a day, temporary irritation, such as coughing, hoarseness, or reversible bronchoconstriction may occur; an inhaled bronchodilator can be used before treatment with hypertonic sodium chloride to reduce the risk of these adverse effects

MucoClear 3% inhalation solution 4ml ampoules (Pari Medical Ltd) **Sodium chloride 30 mg per 1 ml** | 20 ampoule · NHS indicative price = £12.98 · Drug Tariff (Part IXa) | 60 ampoule · NHS indicative price = £27.00 · Drug Tariff (Part IXa)

● **INDICATIONS AND DOSE**
MUCOCLEAR ® 6%

Mobilise lower respiratory tract secretions in mucous consolidation (e.g. cystic fibrosis)
▸ BY INHALATION OF NEBULISED SOLUTION
▸ Adult: 4 mL twice daily, temporary irritation, such as coughing, hoarseness, or reversible bronchoconstriction may occur; an inhaled bronchodilator can be used before treatment with hypertonic sodium chloride to reduce the risk of these adverse effects

MucoClear 6% inhalation solution 4ml ampoules (Pari Medical Ltd) **Sodium chloride 60 mg per 1 ml** | 20 ampoule · NHS indicative price = £12.98 · Drug Tariff (Part IXa) | 60 ampoule · NHS indicative price = £27.00 · Drug Tariff (Part IXa)

● **INDICATIONS AND DOSE**
NEBUSAL ®

Mobilise lower respiratory tract secretions in mucous consolidation (e.g. cystic fibrosis)
▸ BY INHALATION OF NEBULISED SOLUTION
▸ Adult: 4 mL up to twice daily, temporary irritation, such as coughing, hoarseness, or reversible bronchoconstriction may occur; an inhaled bronchodilator can be used before treatment with hypertonic sodium chloride to reduce the risk of these adverse effects

Nebusal 7% inhalation solution 4ml vials (Forest Laboratories UK Ltd) **Sodium chloride 70 mg per 1 ml** | 60 vial · NHS indicative price = £27.00 · Drug Tariff (Part IXa)

Peak flow meters: low range

● LOW RANGE PEAK FLOW METERS
MEDI ® LOW RANGE

Range 40–420 litres/minute.
Compliant to standard EN ISO 23747:2007 except for scale range.

Medi peak flow meter low range (Medicareplus International Ltd)
1 device · NHS indicative price = £6.50 · Drug Tariff (Part IXa) price = £6.50

MINI-WRIGHT ® LOW RANGE
Range 30–400 litres/minute.
Compliant to standard EN ISO 23747:2007 except for scale range.

Mini-Wright peak flow meter low range (Clement Clarke International Ltd)
1 device · NHS indicative price = £7.14 · Drug Tariff (Part IXa) price = £6.50
POCKETPEAK ® LOW RANGE
Range 50–400 litres/minute.
Compliant to standard EN ISO 23747:2007 except for scale range.

nSpire Pocket Peak peak flow meter low range (nSpire Health Ltd)
1 device · NHS indicative price = £6.53 · Drug Tariff (Part IXa) price = £6.50

Peak flow meters: standard range

● STANDARD RANGE PEAK FLOW METERS
AIRZONE ®

Range 60–720 litres/minute.
Conforms to standard EN ISO 23747:2007.

AirZone peak flow meter standard range (Clement Clarke International Ltd)
1 device · NHS indicative price = £4.69 · Drug Tariff (Part IXa) price = £4.50
MEDI ® STANDARD RANGE
Range 60–800 litres/minute.
Conforms to standard EN ISO 23747:2007.

Medi peak flow meter standard range (Medicareplus International Ltd)
1 device · NHS indicative price = £4.50 · Drug Tariff (Part IXa) price = £4.50
MICROPEAK ®
Range 60–900 litres/minute.
Conforms to standard EN ISO 23747:2007.

MicroPeak peak flow meter standard range (Micro Medical Ltd)
1 device · NHS indicative price = £6.50 · Drug Tariff (Part IXa) price = £4.50
MINI-WRIGHT ® STANDARD RANGE
Range 60–800 litres/minute.
Conforms to standard EN ISO 23747:2007.

Mini-Wright peak flow meter standard range (Clement Clarke International Ltd)
1 device · NHS indicative price = £7.08 · Drug Tariff (Part IXa) price = £4.50
PIKO-1 ®
Range 15–999 litres/minute.
Conforms to standard EN ISO 23747:2007.

nSpire PiKo-1 peak flow meter standard range (nSpire Health Ltd)
1 device · NHS indicative price = £9.50 · Drug Tariff (Part IXa) price = £4.50
PINNACLE ®
Range 60–900 litres/minute.
Conforms to standard EN ISO 23747:2007.

Fyne Dynamics Pinnacle peak flow meter standard range (Fyne Dynamics Ltd)
1 device · NHS indicative price = £6.50 · Drug Tariff (Part IXa) price = £4.50
POCKETPEAK ® STANDARD RANGE
Range 60–800 litres/minute.
Conforms to standard EN ISO 23747:2007.

nSpire Pocket Peak peak flow meter standard range (nSpire Health Ltd)
1 device · NHS indicative price = £6.53 · Drug Tariff (Part IXa) price = £4.50
VITALOGRAPH ®
Range 50–800 litres/minute.
Conforms to standard EN ISO 23747:2007.

Vitalograph peak flow meter standard range (Vitalograph Ltd)
1 device · NHS indicative price = £4.83 · Drug Tariff (Part IXa) price = £4.50

Spacers

● SPACERS
A2A SPACER ®

For use with all pressurised (aerosol) inhalers.

A2A Spacer (Clement Clarke International Ltd)
1 device · NHS indicative price = £4.15 · Drug Tariff (Part IXa)

A2A Spacer with medium mask (Clement Clarke International Ltd)
1 device · NHS indicative price = £6.68 · Drug Tariff (Part IXa)

A2A Spacer with small mask (Clement Clarke International Ltd)
1 device · NHS indicative price = £6.68 · Drug Tariff (Part IXa)
ABLE SPACER ®
Small-volume device. For use with all pressurised (aerosol) inhalers.

Able Spacer (Clement Clarke International Ltd)
1 device · NHS indicative price = £4.39 · Drug Tariff (Part IXa)

3

Respiratory system

Able Spacer with medium mask (Clement Clarke International Ltd)
1 device · NHS indicative price = £7.16 · Drug Tariff (Part IXa)

Able Spacer with small mask (Clement Clarke International Ltd)
1 device · NHS indicative price = £7.16 · Drug Tariff (Part IXa)

AEROCHAMBER PLUS ®
Medium-volume device. For use with all pressurised (aerosol) inhalers.

AeroChamber Plus (Trudell Medical UK Ltd)
1 device · NHS indicative price = £4.90 · Drug Tariff (Part IXa)

AeroChamber Plus with adult mask (Trudell Medical UK Ltd)
1 device · NHS indicative price = £8.17 · Drug Tariff (Part IXa)

AeroChamber Plus with child mask (Trudell Medical UK Ltd)
1 device · NHS indicative price = £8.17 · Drug Tariff (Part IXa)

AeroChamber Plus with infant mask (Trudell Medical UK Ltd)
1 device · NHS indicative price = £8.17 · Drug Tariff (Part IXa)

BABYHALER ®
For paediatric use with *Flixotide*®, and *Ventolin*® inhalers.

● PRESCRIBING AND DISPENSING INFORMATION
Not available for NHS prescription.

Babyhaler (GlaxoSmithKline UK Ltd)
1 device · No NHS indicative price available · Drug Tariff (Part IXa)

HALERAID ®
Device to place over pressurised (aerosol) inhalers to aid when strength in hands is impaired (e.g. in arthritis). For use with *Flixotide*®, *Seretide*®, *Serevent*®, and *Ventolin*® inhalers.

● PRESCRIBING AND DISPENSING INFORMATION
Not available for NHS prescription.

Haleraid-120 (GlaxoSmithKline UK Ltd)
1 device · No NHS indicative price available · Drug Tariff (Part IXa)

Haleraid-200 (GlaxoSmithKline UK Ltd)
1 device · No NHS indicative price available · Drug Tariff (Part IXa)

OPTICHAMBER ®
For use with all pressurised (aerosol) inhalers.

OptiChamber (Respironics (UK) Ltd)
1 device · NHS indicative price = £4.28 · Drug Tariff (Part IXa)

OPTICHAMBER ® DIAMOND
For use with all pressurised (aerosol) inhalers.

OptiChamber Diamond (Respironics (UK) Ltd)
1 device · NHS indicative price = £4.49 · Drug Tariff (Part IXa)

OptiChamber Diamond with large LiteTouch mask 5 years-adult (Respironics (UK) Ltd)
1 device · NHS indicative price = £7.49 · Drug Tariff (Part IXa)

OptiChamber Diamond with medium LiteTouch mask 1-5 years (Respironics (UK) Ltd)
1 device · NHS indicative price = £7.49 · Drug Tariff (Part IXa)

OptiChamber Diamond with small LiteTouch mask 0-18 months (Respironics (UK) Ltd)
1 device · NHS indicative price = £7.49 · Drug Tariff (Part IXa)

POCKET CHAMBER ®
Small volume device. For use with all pressurised (aerosol) inhalers.

Pocket Chamber (nSpire Health Ltd)
1 device · NHS indicative price = £4.18 · Drug Tariff (Part IXa)

Pocket Chamber with adult mask (nSpire Health Ltd)
1 device · NHS indicative price = £9.75 · Drug Tariff (Part IXa)

Pocket Chamber with child mask (nSpire Health Ltd)
1 device · NHS indicative price = £9.75 · Drug Tariff (Part IXa)

Pocket Chamber with infant mask (nSpire Health Ltd)
1 device · NHS indicative price = £9.75 · Drug Tariff (Part IXa)

Pocket Chamber with teenager mask (nSpire Health Ltd)
1 device · NHS indicative price = £9.75 · Drug Tariff (Part IXa)

SPACE CHAMBER PLUS ®
For use with all pressurised (aerosol) inhalers.

Space Chamber Plus (Medical Developments International Ltd)
1 device · NHS indicative price = £4.26 · Drug Tariff (Part IXa)

Space Chamber Plus with large mask (Medical Developments International Ltd)
1 device · NHS indicative price = £6.98 · Drug Tariff (Part IXa)

Space Chamber Plus with medium mask (Medical Developments International Ltd)
1 device · NHS indicative price = £6.98 · Drug Tariff (Part IXa)

Space Chamber Plus with small mask (Medical Developments International Ltd)
1 device · NHS indicative price = £6.98 · Drug Tariff (Part IXa)

VOLUMATIC ®
Large-volume device. For use with *Clenil Modulite*®, *Flixotide*®, *Seretide*®, *Serevent*®, and *Ventolin*® inhalers.

Volumatic (GlaxoSmithKline UK Ltd)
1 device · NHS indicative price = £3.88 · Drug Tariff (Part IXa)

Volumatic with paediatric mask (GlaxoSmithKline UK Ltd)
1 device · NHS indicative price = £6.83 · Drug Tariff (Part IXa)

VORTEX ®
Medium-volume device. For use with all pressurised (aerosol) inhalers.

Vortex Spacer (Pari Medical Ltd)
1 device · NHS indicative price = £6.28 · Drug Tariff (Part IXa)

Vortex with baby mask 0-2 years (Pari Medical Ltd)
1 device · NHS indicative price = £7.99 · Drug Tariff (Part IXa)

Vortex with child mask 2 years+ (Pari Medical Ltd)
1 device · NHS indicative price = £7.99 · Drug Tariff (Part IXa)

2   Allergic conditions

Antihistamines, allergen immunotherapy and allergic emergencies

Antihistamines

All antihistamines are of potential value in the treatment of nasal allergies, particularly seasonal allergic rhinitis (hayfever), and they may be of some value in vasomotor rhinitis. They reduce rhinorrhoea and sneezing but are usually less effective for nasal congestion. Antihistamines are used topically in the eye, in the nose, and on the skin.

Oral antihistamines are also of some value in preventing urticaria and are used to treat urticarial rashes, pruritus, and insect bites and stings; they are also used in drug allergies. Injections of chlorphenamine maleate p. 283 or promethazine hydrochloride p. 286 are used as an adjunct to adrenaline/epinephrine p. 221 in the emergency treatment of anaphylaxis and angioedema. Antihistamines (including cinnarizine p. 432, cyclizine p. 424, and promethazine teoclate p. 432) may also have a role in nausea and vomiting. Buclizine is included as an anti-emetic in a preparation for migraine. Antihistamines may also have a role in occasional insomnia.

All older antihistamines cause sedation but alimemazine tartrate p. 282 and **promethazine** may be more sedating whereas chlorphenamine maleate and cyclizine may be less so. This sedating activity is sometimes used to manage the pruritus associated with some allergies. There is little evidence that any one of the older, 'sedating' antihistamines is superior to another and patients vary widely in their response.

Non-sedating antihistamines such as acrivastine p. 278, bilastine p. 278, cetirizine hydrochloride p. 279, desloratadine p. 279 (an active metabolite of loratadine p. 281), fexofenadine hydrochloride p. 280 (an active metabolite of terfenadine), levocetirizine hydrochloride p. 280 (an isomer of cetirizine hydrochloride), loratadine and mizolastine p. 281 cause less sedation and psychomotor impairment than the older antihistamines because they penetrate the blood brain barrier only to a slight extent.

3

Respiratory system

Allergen immunotherapy

Immunotherapy using allergen vaccines containing house dust mite, animal dander (cat or dog), or extracts of grass and tree pollen can reduce symptoms of asthma and allergic rhinoconjunctivitis. A vaccine containing extracts of wasp and bee venom is used to reduce the risk of severe anaphylaxis and systemic reactions in individuals with hypersensitivity to wasp and bee stings. An oral preparation of grass pollen extract (*Grazax*®) is also licensed for disease-modifying treatment of grass pollen-induced rhinitis and conjunctivitis. Those requiring immunotherapy must be referred to a hospital specialist for accurate diagnosis, assessment, and treatment.

Omalizumab p. 267 is a monoclonal antibody that binds to immunoglobulin E (IgE). It is used as additional therapy in individuals with proven IgE-mediated sensitivity to inhaled allergens, whose severe persistent allergic asthma cannot be controlled adequately with high dose inhaled corticosteroid together with a long-acting beta$_2$ agonist. Omalizumab should be initiated by physicians in specialist centres experienced in the treatment of severe persistent asthma. Omalizumab is also indicated as add-on therapy for the treatment of chronic spontaneous urticaria in patients who have had an inadequate response to H$_1$ antihistamine treatment.

Anaphylaxis and allergic emergencies

Anaphylaxis

Anaphylaxis is a severe, life-threatening, generalised or systemic hypersensitivity reaction. It is characterised by the rapid onset of respiratory and/or circulatory problems and is usually associated with skin and mucosal changes; prompt treatment is required. Patients with pre-existing asthma, especially poorly controlled asthma, are at particular risk of life-threatening reactions. Insect stings are a recognised risk (in particular wasp and bee stings). Latex and certain foods, including eggs, fish, cow's milk protein, peanuts, sesame, shellfish, soy, and tree nuts may also precipitate anaphylaxis (see Food allergy p. 83). Medicinal products particularly associated with anaphylaxis include blood products, vaccines, hyposensitising (allergen) preparations, antibacterials, aspirin and other NSAIDs, and neuromuscular blocking drugs. In the case of drugs, anaphylaxis is more likely after parenteral administration; resuscitation facilities must always be available for injections associated with special risk. Anaphylactic reactions may also be associated with *additives and excipients* in foods and medicines. Refined arachis (peanut) oil, which may be present in some medicinal products, is unlikely to cause an allergic reaction—nevertheless it is wise to check the full formula of preparations which may contain allergens.

Treatment of anaphylaxis

Adrenaline/epinephrine provides physiological reversal of the immediate symptoms associated with hypersensitivity reactions such as *anaphylaxis* and *angioedema*.

First-line treatment includes:

- securing the airway, restoration of blood pressure (laying the patient flat and raising the legs, or in the recovery position if unconscious or nauseous or at risk of vomiting);
- administering adrenaline/epinephrine (by **intramuscular** injection in a dose of 500 micrograms (a dose of 300 micrograms may be appropriate for *immediate self-administration*); the dose should be repeated if necessary at 5-minute intervals according to blood pressure, pulse, and respiratory function. Patients receiving beta-blockers require special consideration;
- administering high-flow **oxygen** and **intravenous fluids** is also of primary importance;
- administering an antihistamine, such as chlorphenamine maleate, by slow intravenous injection or intramuscular

injection is a useful adjunctive treatment, given after adrenaline.

- Administering an intravenous corticosteroid such as hydrocortisone p. 662 (preferably as sodium succinate) is of secondary value in the initial management of anaphylaxis because the onset of action is delayed for several hours, but should be given to prevent further deterioration in severely affected patients.

Continuing respiratory deterioration requires further treatment with **bronchodilators** including inhaled or intravenous salbutamol p. 252, inhaled ipratropium bromide p. 246, intravenous aminophylline p. 272, or intravenous magnesium sulfate p. 1019 [unlicensed indication] (as for acute severe asthma); in addition to oxygen, assisted respiration and possibly emergency tracheotomy may be necessary.

When a patient is so ill that there is doubt about the adequacy of the circulation, the initial injection of adrenaline/epinephrine may need to be given as a *dilute solution by the intravenous route.*

Cardiopulmonary arrest may follow an anaphylactic reaction; resuscitation should be started immediately.

On discharge, patients should be considered for further treatment with an oral antihistamine and an oral corticosteroid for up to 3 days to reduce the risk of further reaction. Patients should be instructed to return to hospital if symptoms recur and to contact their general practitioner for follow-up.

Patients who are suspected of having had an anaphylactic reaction should be referred to a specialist for specific allergy diagnosis. Avoidance of the allergen is the principal treatment; if appropriate, an adrenaline/epinephrine auto-injector should be given for self-administration or a replacement supplied.

Intramuscular adrenaline (epinephrine)

The *intramuscular route* is the *first choice route* for the administration of adrenaline/epinephrine in the management of anaphylaxis. Adrenaline/epinephrine is best given as an intramuscular injection into the anterolateral aspect of the middle third of the thigh; it has a rapid onset of action after intramuscular administration and in the shocked patient its absorption from the intramuscular site is faster and more reliable than from the subcutaneous site.

Patients with severe allergy should be instructed in the self-administration of adrenaline/epinephrine p. 221 by intramuscular injection.

Prompt injection of adrenaline/epinephrine is of paramount importance. The adrenaline/epinephrine doses recommended for the emergency treatment of anaphylaxis by appropriately trained healthcare professionals are based on the revised recommendations of the Working Group of the Resuscitation Council (UK).

Dose of intramuscular injection of adrenaline (epinephrine) for the emergency treatment of anaphylaxis by healthcare professionals

Age	Dose	Volume of adrenaline
▶ Child 1 month–5 years	150 micrograms	0.15 mL 1 in 1000 (1 mg/mL) adrenaline[1]
▶ Child 6–11 years	300 micrograms	0.3 mL 1 in 1000 (1 mg/mL) adrenaline
▶ Child 12–17 years	500 micrograms	0.5 mL 1 in 1000 (1 mg/mL) adrenaline[2]
▶ Adult	500 micrograms	0.5 mL 1 in 1000 (1 mg/mL) adrenaline

These doses may be repeated several times if necessary at 5-minute intervals according to blood pressure, pulse and respiratory function.

1. Use suitable syringe for measuring small volume
2. 300 micrograms (0.3 mL) if child is small or prepubertal

Intravenous adrenaline (epinephrine)

Intravenous adrenaline/epinephrine should be given only by those experienced in its use, in a setting where patients can be carefully monitored.

When the patient is severely ill and there is real doubt about the adequacy of the circulation and absorption after intramuscular injection, adrenaline/epinephrine can be given by **slow** *intravenous injection* repeated according to response; if multiple doses are required, adrenaline/epinephrine should be given as a **slow** intravenous infusion *stopping when a response has been obtained.*

It is important that, where intramuscular injection might still succeed, time should not be wasted seeking intravenous access.

The intravenous route is also used for *cardiac resuscitation.*

Angioedema

Angioedema is dangerous if *laryngeal oedema* is present. In this circumstance adrenaline/epinephrine injection and **oxygen** should be given as described under **Anaphylaxis**; antihistamines and corticosteroids should also be given. Tracheal intubation may be necessary.

Hereditary angioedema

The treatment of hereditary angioedema should be under specialist supervision. Unlike allergic angioedema, adrenaline/epinephrine, corticosteroids, and antihistamines should not be used for the treatment of acute attacks, including attacks involving laryngeal oedema, as they are ineffective and may delay appropriate treatment—intubation may be necessary. The administration of C1-esterase inhibitor p. 289, an endogenous complement blocker derived from human plasma, (in fresh frozen plasma or in partially purified form) can terminate acute attacks of *hereditary angioedema*; it can also be used for short-term prophylaxis before dental, medical or surgical procedures. Conestat alfa p. 289 and icatibant p. 290 are licensed for the treatment of acute attacks of hereditary angioedema in adults with C1-esterase inhibitor deficiency.

Tranexamic acid p. 110 and danazol p. 725 [unlicensed indication] are used for short-term and long-term prophylaxis of hereditary angioedema. Short-term prophylaxis with tranexamic acid or danazol is started several days before planned procedures (e.g. dental work) and continued for 2–5 days afterwards. Danazol should be avoided in children because of its androgenic effects

ANTIHISTAMINES > NON-SEDATING

Acrivastine

19-May-2017

● **INDICATIONS AND DOSE**

Symptomatic relief of allergy such as hayfever, chronic idiopathic urticaria
▸ BY MOUTH
▸ Child 12–17 years: 8 mg 3 times a day
▸ Adult: 8 mg 3 times a day

● CONTRA-INDICATIONS Avoid in Acute porphyrias p. 1025 · elderly

● INTERACTIONS → Appendix 1: antihistamines, non-sedating

● SIDE-EFFECTS
▸ **Common or very common** Drowsiness · dry mouth
▸ **Frequency not known** Dizziness · rash

SIDE-EFFECTS, FURTHER INFORMATION Non-sedating antihistamines such as acrivastine cause less sedation and psychomotor impairment than the older antihistamines, but can still occur; sedation is generally minimal. This is because non-sedating antihistamines penetrate the blood brain barrier to a much lesser extent.

● ALLERGY AND CROSS-SENSITIVITY Contra-indicated if history of hypersensitivity to triprolidine.

● PREGNANCY Most manufacturers of antihistamines advise avoiding their use during pregnancy; however, there is no evidence of teratogenicity.

● BREAST FEEDING Most antihistamines are present in breast milk in varying amounts; although not known to be harmful, most manufacturers advise avoiding their use in mothers who are breast-feeding.

● RENAL IMPAIRMENT Avoid in severe impairment.

● PATIENT AND CARER ADVICE
Driving and skilled tasks Although drowsiness is rare, nevertheless patients should be advised that it can occur and may affect performance of skilled tasks (e.g. cycling or driving); alcohol should be avoided.

● MEDICINAL FORMS
There can be variation in the licensing of different medicines containing the same drug.
Capsule
▸ Benadryl Allergy Relief (McNeil Products Ltd)
 Acrivastine 8 mg Benadryl Allergy Relief 8mg capsules | 24 capsule ℗ £5.45

Bilastine

22-May-2017

● **INDICATIONS AND DOSE**

Symptomatic relief of allergic rhinoconjunctivitis and urticaria
▸ BY MOUTH
▸ Child 12–17 years: 20 mg once daily
▸ Adult: 20 mg once daily

● CONTRA-INDICATIONS Avoid in Acute porphyrias p. 1025

● INTERACTIONS → Appendix 1: antihistamines, non-sedating

● SIDE-EFFECTS
▸ **Common or very common** Drowsiness · headache
▸ **Uncommon** Anxiety · appetite increased · asthenia · bundle branch block · diarrhoea · dry mouth · dyspnoea · fever · gastritis · gastrointestinal discomfort · insomnia · nasal complaints · nausea · oral herpes · pre-existing condition improved · pruritus · QT interval prolongation · sinus arrhythmia · thirst · tinnitus · vertigo · weight increased

SIDE-EFFECTS, FURTHER INFORMATION Non-sedating antihistamines such as bilastine cause less sedation and psychomotor impairment than the older antihistamines, but can still occur; sedation is generally minimal. This is because non-sedating antihistamines penetrate the blood brain barrier to a much lesser extent.

● PREGNANCY Avoid—limited information available. Most manufacturers of antihistamines advise avoiding their use during pregnancy; however, there is no evidence of teratogenicity.

● BREAST FEEDING Avoid—no information available. Most antihistamines are present in breast milk in varying amounts; although not known to be harmful, most manufacturers advise avoiding their use in mothers who are breast-feeding.

● DIRECTIONS FOR ADMINISTRATION Take tablet 1 hour before or 2 hours after food or fruit juice.

● PATIENT AND CARER ADVICE Patients or carers should be given advice on how to administer bilastine tablets.
Driving and skilled tasks Although drowsiness is rare, nevertheless patients should be advised that it can occur and may affect performance of skilled tasks (e.g. cycling or driving); alcohol should be avoided.

- **MEDICINAL FORMS**
There can be variation in the licensing of different medicines containing the same drug.
Tablet
CAUTIONARY AND ADVISORY LABELS 23
▸ Ilaxten (A. Menarini Farmaceutica Internazionale SRL)
Bilastine 20 mg Ilaxten 20mg tablets | 30 tablet PoM £15.09

Cetirizine hydrochloride

- **INDICATIONS AND DOSE**

Symptomatic relief of allergy such as hay fever, chronic idiopathic urticaria, atopic dermatitis
▸ BY MOUTH
- Child 2–5 years: 2.5 mg twice daily
- Child 6–11 years: 5 mg twice daily
- Child 12–17 years: 10 mg once daily
- Adult: 10 mg once daily

- **CAUTIONS** Epilepsy
- **INTERACTIONS** → Appendix 1: antihistamines, non-sedating
- **SIDE-EFFECTS**
▸ **Uncommon** Agitation · asthenia · diarrhoea · malaise · paraesthesia · skin reactions
▸ **Rare or very rare** Aggression · angioedema · confusion · depression · hallucination · hepatic function abnormal · insomnia · movement disorders · oculogyration · oedema · seizure · syncope · tachycardia · taste altered · thrombocytopenia · tic · tremor · urinary disorders · vision disorders · weight increased
▸ **Frequency not known** Abdominal pain · appetite increased · dizziness · drowsiness · dry mouth · headache · memory loss · nausea · pharyngitis · suicidal ideation · vertigo
SIDE-EFFECTS, FURTHER INFORMATION Non-sedating antihistamines such as certirizine cause less sedation and psychomotor impairment than the older antihistamines, but can still occur; sedation is generally minimal. This is because non-sedating antihistamines penetrate the blood brain barrier to a much lesser extent.
- **PREGNANCY** Most manufacturers of antihistamines advise avoiding their use during pregnancy; however, there is no evidence of teratogenicity.
- **BREAST FEEDING** Most antihistamines are present in breast milk in varying amounts; although not known to be harmful, most manufacturers advise avoiding their use in mothers who are breast-feeding.
- **RENAL IMPAIRMENT**
▸ In adults Avoid if eGFR less than 10 mL/minute/1.73 m^2.
▸ In children Avoid if estimated glomerular filtration rate less than 10 mL/minute/1.73 m^2.
Dose adjustments ▸ In adults Use half normal dose if eGFR 30–50 mL/minute/1.73 m^2. Use half normal dose and reduce dose frequency to alternate days if eGFR 10–30 mL/minute/1.73 m^2.
▸ In children Use half normal dose if estimated glomerular filtration rate 30–50 mL/minute/1.73 m^2. Use half normal dose and reduce dose frequency to alternate days if estimated glomerular filtration rate 10–30 mL/minute/1.73 m^2.
- **PATIENT AND CARER ADVICE**
Medicines for Children leaflet: Cetirizine hydrochloride for hay fever www.medicinesforchildren.org.uk/cetirizine-hay-fever-0
Driving and skilled tasks Although drowsiness is rare, nevertheless patients should be advised that it can occur and may affect performance of skilled tasks (e.g. cycling or driving); alcohol should be avoided.

- **PROFESSION SPECIFIC INFORMATION**
Dental practitioners' formulary
Cetirizine Tablets 10 mg may be prescribed.
Cetirizine Oral Solution 5 mg/5 mL may be prescribed.
- **MEDICINAL FORMS**
There can be variation in the licensing of different medicines containing the same drug.
Oral solution
EXCIPIENTS: May contain Propylene glycol
▸ Cetirizine hydrochloride (Non-proprietary)
Cetirizine hydrochloride 1 mg per 1 ml Cetirizine 1mg/ml oral solution sugar free sugar-free | 200 ml PoM £1.02 DT = £1.02
▸ Benadryl Allergy (McNeil Products Ltd)
Cetirizine hydrochloride 1 mg per 1 ml Benadryl Allergy Children's 1mg/ml oral solution sugar-free | 100 ml P £3.49
▸ Zirtek (UCB Pharma Ltd)
Cetirizine hydrochloride 1 mg per 1 ml Zirtek Allergy 1mg/ml oral solution sugar-free | 150 ml P £3.70 sugar-free | 200 ml P £9.77 DT = £1.02
Tablet
▸ Cetirizine hydrochloride (Non-proprietary)
Cetirizine hydrochloride 10 mg Cetirizine 10mg tablets | 30 tablet PoM £3.89 DT = £0.70
Capsule
▸ Benadryl Allergy (McNeil Products Ltd)
Cetirizine hydrochloride 10 mg Benadryl Allergy Liquid Release 10mg capsules | 7 capsule GSL £3.09 DT = £3.09

Desloratadine

23-May-2017

- **INDICATIONS AND DOSE**

Symptomatic relief of allergy such as allergic rhinitis, urticaria, chronic idiopathic urticaria
▸ BY MOUTH
- Child 1–5 years: 1.25 mg once daily
- Child 6–11 years: 2.5 mg once daily
- Child 12–17 years: 5 mg once daily
- Adult: 5 mg once daily
PHARMACOKINETICS
▸ Desloratadine is a metabolite of loratadine.

- **INTERACTIONS** → Appendix 1: antihistamines, non-sedating
- **SIDE-EFFECTS**
▸ **Common or very common** Asthenia · dry mouth · headache
▸ **Rare or very rare** Akathisia · arrhythmias · diarrhoea · dizziness · drowsiness · gastrointestinal discomfort · hallucination · hepatic disorders · insomnia · myalgia · nausea · palpitations · seizure · vomiting
▸ **Frequency not known** Behaviour abnormal · photosensitivity reaction · QT interval prolongation
SIDE-EFFECTS, FURTHER INFORMATION Non-sedating antihistamines such as desloratadine cause less sedation and psychomotor impairment than the older antihistamines, but can still occur; sedation is generally minimal. This is because non-sedating antihistamines penetrate the blood brain barrier to a much lesser extent.
- **ALLERGY AND CROSS-SENSITIVITY** Contra-indicated if history of hypersensitivity to loratadine.
- **PREGNANCY** Most manufacturers of antihistamines advise avoiding their use during pregnancy; however, there is no evidence of teratogenicity.
- **BREAST FEEDING** Most antihistamines are present in breast milk in varying amounts; although not known to be harmful, most manufacturers advise avoiding their use in mothers who are breast-feeding.
- **RENAL IMPAIRMENT** Use with caution in severe impairment.
- **PRESCRIBING AND DISPENSING INFORMATION** Flavours of oral liquid formulations may include bubblegum.

- PATIENT AND CARER ADVICE

  Driving and skilled tasks Although drowsiness is rare, nevertheless patients should be advised that it can occur and may affect performance of skilled tasks (e.g. cycling or driving); excess alcohol should be avoided.

- MEDICINAL FORMS

  There can be variation in the licensing of different medicines containing the same drug.

  Oral solution

  EXCIPIENTS: May contain Propylene glycol, sorbitol

  ▸ Desloratadine (Non-proprietary)

  Desloratadine 500 microgram per 1 ml Desloratadine 2.5mg/5ml oral solution sugar free sugar-free | 100 ml [PoM] £6.43–£6.77 sugar-free | 150 ml [PoM] £8.00–£10.15 DT = £10.15

  ▸ Neoclarityn (Merck Sharp & Dohme Ltd)

  Desloratadine 500 microgram per 1 ml Neoclarityn 2.5mg/5ml oral solution sugar-free | 100 ml [PoM] £6.77 sugar-free | 150 ml [PoM] £10.15 DT = £10.15

  Tablet

  ▸ Desloratadine (Non-proprietary)

  Desloratadine 5 mg Desloratadine 5mg tablets | 30 tablet [PoM] £6.77 DT = £0.86

  ▸ Neoclarityn (Merck Sharp & Dohme Ltd)

  Desloratadine 5 mg Neoclarityn 5mg tablets | 30 tablet [PoM] £6.77 DT = £0.86

Fexofenadine hydrochloride

22-May-2017

- INDICATIONS AND DOSE

  Symptomatic relief of seasonal allergic rhinitis

  ▸ BY MOUTH

  ▸ Child 6–11 years: 30 mg twice daily

  ▸ Child 12–17 years: 120 mg once daily

  ▸ Adult: 120 mg once daily

  Symptomatic relief of chronic idiopathic urticaria

  ▸ BY MOUTH

  ▸ Child 12–17 years: 180 mg once daily

  ▸ Adult: 180 mg once daily

  PHARMACOKINETICS

  ▸ Fexofenadine is a metabolite of terfenadine.

- INTERACTIONS → Appendix 1: antihistamines, non-sedating

- SIDE-EFFECTS

- **Common or very common** Dizziness · drowsiness · headache · nausea

- **Uncommon** Fatigue

- **Frequency not known** Diarrhoea · nervousness · palpitations · skin reactions · sleep disorders · tachycardia

  SIDE-EFFECTS, FURTHER INFORMATION Non-sedating antihistamines such as fexofenadine cause less sedation and psychomotor impairment than the older antihistamines, but can still occur; sedation is generally minimal. This is because non-sedating antihistamines penetrate the blood brain barrier to a much lesser extent.

- PREGNANCY Most manufacturers of antihistamines advise avoiding their use during pregnancy; however, there is no evidence of teratogenicity.

- BREAST FEEDING Most antihistamines are present in breast milk in varying amounts; although not known to be harmful, most manufacturers advise avoiding their use in mothers who are breast-feeding.

- PATIENT AND CARER ADVICE

  Driving and skilled tasks Although drowsiness is rare, nevertheless patients should be advised that it can occur and may affect performance of skilled tasks (e.g. cycling or driving); alcohol should be avoided.

- MEDICINAL FORMS

  There can be variation in the licensing of different medicines containing the same drug. Forms available from special-order manufacturers include: oral suspension, oral solution

  Tablet

  CAUTIONARY AND ADVISORY LABELS 5

  ▸ Fexofenadine hydrochloride (Non-proprietary)

  Fexofenadine hydrochloride 120 mg Fexofenadine 120mg tablets | 30 tablet [PoM] £6.23 DT = £1.76

  Fexofenadine hydrochloride 180 mg Fexofenadine 180mg tablets | 30 tablet [PoM] £7.89 DT = £2.84

  ▸ Telfast (Sanofi)

  Fexofenadine hydrochloride 30 mg Telfast 30mg tablets | 60 tablet [PoM] £5.46 DT = £5.46

  Fexofenadine hydrochloride 120 mg Telfast 120mg tablets | 30 tablet [PoM] £5.99 DT = £1.76

  Fexofenadine hydrochloride 180 mg Telfast 180mg tablets | 30 tablet [PoM] £7.58 DT = £2.84

Levocetirizine hydrochloride

24-May-2017

- INDICATIONS AND DOSE

  Symptomatic relief of allergy such as hay fever, urticaria

  ▸ BY MOUTH

  ▸ Child 6–17 years: 5 mg once daily

  ▸ Adult: 5 mg once daily

  PHARMACOKINETICS

  ▸ Levocetirizine is an isomer of cetirizine.

- CONTRA-INDICATIONS Avoid in Acute porphyrias p. 1025

- INTERACTIONS → Appendix 1: antihistamines, non-sedating

- SIDE-EFFECTS

- **Common or very common** Asthenia · constipation (in children) · drowsiness · dry mouth

- **Uncommon** Abdominal pain

- **Frequency not known** Aggression · agitation · angioedema · appetite increased · arthralgia · depression · diarrhoea (very common in children) · dizziness · dyspnoea · hallucination · hepatitis · myalgia · nausea · oedema · palpitations · paraesthesia · seizure · skin reactions · sleep disorders (very common in children) · suicidal ideation · syncope · tachycardia · taste altered · tremor · urinary disorders · vertigo · vision disorders · vomiting · weight increased

  SIDE-EFFECTS, FURTHER INFORMATION Non-sedating antihistamines such as levocetirizine cause less sedation and psychomotor impairment than the older antihistamines, but can still occur; sedation is generally minimal. This is because non-sedating antihistamines penetrate the blood brain barrier to a much lesser extent.

- PREGNANCY Most manufacturers of antihistamines advise avoiding their use during pregnancy; however, there is no evidence of teratogenicity.

- BREAST FEEDING Most antihistamines are present in breast milk in varying amounts; although not known to be harmful, most manufacturers advise avoiding their use in mothers who are breast-feeding.

- RENAL IMPAIRMENT

  ▸ In adults Avoid if eGFR less than 10 mL/minute/1.73 m^2.

  ▸ In children Avoid if estimated glomerular filtration rate less than 10 mL/minute/1.73 m^2.

  Dose adjustments ▸ In adults 5 mg on alternate days if eGFR 30–50 mL/minute/1.73 m^2. 5 mg every 3 days if eGFR 10–30 mL/minute/1.73 m^2.

  ▸ In children Reduce dose frequency to alternate days if estimated glomerular filtration rate 30–50 mL/minute/1.73 m^2. Reduce dose frequency to every 3 days if estimated glomerular filtration rate 10–30 mL/minute/1.73 m^2.

- PATIENT AND CARER ADVICE
Driving and skilled tasks Although drowsiness is rare, nevertheless patients should be advised that it can occur and may affect performance of skilled tasks (e.g. cycling or driving); alcohol should be avoided.

- MEDICINAL FORMS
There can be variation in the licensing of different medicines containing the same drug.
Oral solution
▸ Xyzal (UCB Pharma Ltd)
Levocetirizine dihydrochloride 500 microgram per 1 ml Xyzal 0.5mg/ml oral solution sugar-free | 200 ml PoM £6.00 DT = £6.00
Tablet
▸ Levocetirizine hydrochloride (Non-proprietary)
Levocetirizine dihydrochloride 5 mg Levocetirizine 5mg tablets | 30 tablet PoM £4.45 DT = £4.37
▸ Xyzal (UCB Pharma Ltd)
Levocetirizine dihydrochloride 5 mg Xyzal 5mg tablets | 30 tablet PoM £4.39 DT = £4.37

Loratadine
22-May-2017

- INDICATIONS AND DOSE
Symptomatic relief of allergy such as hay fever, chronic idiopathic urticaria
▸ BY MOUTH
▸ Child 2-11 years (body-weight up to 31 kg): 5 mg once daily
▸ Child 2-11 years (body-weight 31 kg and above): 10 mg once daily
▸ Child 12-17 years: 10 mg once daily
▸ Adult: 10 mg once daily

- INTERACTIONS → Appendix 1: antihistamines, non-sedating
- SIDE-EFFECTS
▸ **Common or very common** Drowsiness · nervousness (in children)
▸ **Uncommon** Appetite increased · headache (very common in children) · insomnia
▸ **Rare or very rare** Alopecia · angioedema · dizziness · dry mouth · fatigue (very common in children) · gastritis · hepatic function abnormal · nausea · palpitations · rash · seizure · tachycardia
SIDE-EFFECTS, FURTHER INFORMATION Non-sedating antihistamines such as loratadine cause less sedation and psychomotor impairment than the older antihistamines, but can still occur; sedation is generally minimal. This is because non-sedating antihistamines penetrate the blood brain barrier to a much lesser extent.
- PREGNANCY Most manufacturers of antihistamines advise avoiding their use during pregnancy; however, there is no evidence of teratogenicity.
- BREAST FEEDING Most antihistamines are present in breast milk in varying amounts; although not known to be harmful, most manufacturers advise avoiding their use in mothers who are breast-feeding.
- HEPATIC IMPAIRMENT **Dose adjustments** Reduce dose frequency to alternate days in severe impairment.
- PATIENT AND CARER ADVICE
Driving and skilled tasks Although drowsiness is rare, nevertheless patients and their carers should be advised that it can occur and may affect performance of skilled tasks (e.g. cycling or driving); alcohol should be avoided.
- PROFESSION SPECIFIC INFORMATION
Dental practitioners' formulary
Loratadine 10 mg tablets may be prescribed.
Loratadine syrup 5 mg/5 mL may be prescribed.

- MEDICINAL FORMS
There can be variation in the licensing of different medicines containing the same drug.
Oral solution
EXCIPIENTS: May contain Propylene glycol
▸ Loratadine (Non-proprietary)
Loratadine 1 mg per 1 ml Loratadine 5mg/5ml oral solution | 100 ml PoM £2.24 DT = £1.33
Tablet
▸ Loratadine (Non-proprietary)
Loratadine 10 mg Loratadine 10mg tablets | 30 tablet P £1.44 DT = £0.45
▸ Clarityn (Loratadine) (Bayer Plc)
Loratadine 10 mg Clarityn Allergy 10mg tablets | 60 tablet P £8.85
Oral lyophilisate
▸ Clarityn (Loratadine) (Bayer Plc)
Loratadine 10 mg Clarityn Rapide Allergy 10mg tablets sugar-free | 10 tablet GSL £3.24 DT = £3.24

Mizolastine
22-May-2017

- INDICATIONS AND DOSE
Symptomatic relief of allergy such as hay fever, urticaria
▸ BY MOUTH
▸ Child 12-17 years: 10 mg once daily
▸ Adult: 10 mg once daily

- CONTRA-INDICATIONS Cardiac disease · hypokalaemia · susceptibility to QT-interval prolongation
- INTERACTIONS → Appendix 1: antihistamines, non-sedating
- SIDE-EFFECTS
▸ **Common or very common** Appetite increased · asthenia · diarrhoea · dizziness · drowsiness · dry mouth · gastrointestinal discomfort · headache · nausea · weight increased
▸ **Uncommon** Anxiety · arrhythmias · arthralgia · depression · myalgia · palpitations
▸ **Rare or very rare** Hypersensitivity
▸ **Frequency not known** Asthma exacerbated · bronchospasm · QT interval prolongation
SIDE-EFFECTS, FURTHER INFORMATION Non-sedating antihistamines such as mizolastine cause less sedation and psychomotor impairment than the older antihistamines, but can still occur; sedation is generally minimal. This is because non-sedating antihistamines penetrate the blood brain barrier to a much lesser extent.
- PREGNANCY Most manufacturers of antihistamines advise avoiding their use during pregnancy; however, there is no evidence of teratogenicity.
- BREAST FEEDING Most antihistamines are present in breast milk in varying amounts; although not known to be harmful, most manufacturers advise avoiding their use in mothers who are breast-feeding.
- HEPATIC IMPAIRMENT Manufacturer advises avoid in significant impairment.
- PATIENT AND CARER ADVICE
Driving and skilled tasks Although drowsiness is rare, nevertheless patients and their carers should be advised that it can occur and may affect performance of skilled tasks (e.g. cycling or driving); alcohol should be avoided.

- MEDICINAL FORMS
There can be variation in the licensing of different medicines containing the same drug.
Modified-release tablet
CAUTIONARY AND ADVISORY LABELS 25
▸ Mizollen (Sanofi)
Mizolastine 10 mg Mizollen 10mg modified-release tablets | 30 tablet PoM £6.92 DT = £6.92

Rupatadine

14-Aug-2017

- **DRUG ACTION** Rupatadine is a second generation non-sedating antihistamine.

- **INDICATIONS AND DOSE**

Symptomatic relief of allergic rhinitis and urticaria
  - ▸ BY MOUTH
  - ▸ Child 12–17 years: 10 mg once daily
  - ▸ Adult: 10 mg once daily

- **CAUTIONS** Elderly—limited information available · history of QT-interval prolongation · predisposition to arrhythmia · uncorrected hypokalaemia

- **INTERACTIONS** → Appendix 1: antihistamines, non-sedating

- **SIDE-EFFECTS**
  - ▸ **Common or very common** Asthenia · dizziness · drowsiness · dry mouth · headache
  - ▸ **Uncommon** Appetite increased · arthralgia · back pain · concentration impaired · constipation · cough · diarrhoea · dry throat · epistaxis · fever · gastrointestinal discomfort · increased risk of infection · irritability · malaise · myalgia · nasal dryness · nausea · oropharyngeal pain · rash · thirst · vomiting · weight increased
  - ▸ **Rare or very rare** Palpitations · tachycardia

  SIDE-EFFECTS, FURTHER INFORMATION Non-sedating antihistamines such as rupatadine cause less sedation and psychomotor impairment than the older antihistamines, but can still occur; sedation is generally minimal. This is because non-sedating antihistamines penetrate the blood brain barrier to a much lesser extent.

- **PREGNANCY** Most manufacturers of antihistamines advise avoiding their use during pregnancy; however, there is no evidence of teratogenicity.

- **BREAST FEEDING** Most antihistamines are present in breast milk in varying amounts; although not known to be harmful, most manufacturers advise avoiding their use in mothers who are breast-feeding.

- **HEPATIC IMPAIRMENT** Manufacturer advises avoid—no information available.

- **RENAL IMPAIRMENT** Manufacturer advises avoid—no information available.

- **MEDICINAL FORMS**
  There can be variation in the licensing of different medicines containing the same drug.
  Tablet
  - ▸ Rupatadine (Non-proprietary)
    Rupatadine (as Rupatadine fumarate) 10 mg Rupatadine 10mg tablets | 30 tablet PoM £30.00 DT = £30.00

ANTIHISTAMINES > SEDATING

Alimemazine tartrate

(Trimeprazine tartrate)

- **INDICATIONS AND DOSE**

Urticaria | Pruritus
  - ▸ BY MOUTH
  - ▸ Child 2–4 years: 2.5 mg 3–4 times a day
  - ▸ Child 5–11 years: 5 mg 3–4 times a day
  - ▸ Child 12–17 years: 10 mg 2–3 times a day, in severe cases up to maximum daily dose has been used; maximum 100 mg per day
  - ▸ Adult: 10 mg 2–3 times a day, in severe cases up to maximum daily dose has been used; maximum 100 mg per day
  - ▸ Elderly: 10 mg 1–2 times a day

- **CONTRA-INDICATIONS** Children under 2 years except on specialist advice (safety of such use has not been established) · epilepsy · hepatic dysfunction · history of narrow angle glaucoma · hypothyroidism · myasthenia gravis · Parkinson's disease · phaeochromocytoma · prostatic hypertrophy (in adults) · renal dysfunction

- **CAUTIONS** Cardiovascular diseases (due to tachycardia-inducing and hypotensive effects of phenothiazines) · elderly · exposure to sunlight should be avoided during treatment with high doses · pyloroduodenal obstruction · urinary retention · volume depleted patients who are more susceptible to orthostatic hypotension

- **INTERACTIONS** → Appendix 1: antihistamines, sedating

- **SIDE-EFFECTS** Agitation · agranulocytosis · amenorrhoea · atrioventricular block · autonomic dysfunction · bile thrombus · consciousness impaired · drug fever · dry mouth · eosinophilia · erectile dysfunction · eye disorder · galactorrhoea · gynaecomastia · hepatic disorders · hyperprolactinaemia · hyperthermia · hypotension · insomnia · leucopenia (on prolonged high dose) · movement disorders · muscle rigidity · nasal congestion · neuroleptic malignant syndrome · pallor · parkinsonism · photosensitivity reaction · postural hypotension (more common in the elderly or in volume depletion) · QT interval prolongation · respiratory depression · seizure · skin reactions · tardive dyskinesia (more common after long term high doses) · tremor · ventricular fibrillation (increased risk with hypokalamia and cardiac disease) · ventricular tachycardia (increased risk with hypokalamia and cardiac disease)

  SIDE-EFFECTS, FURTHER INFORMATION Drowsiness may diminish after a few days. Patients on high dosage may develop photosensitivity and should avoid exposure to direct sunlight.
  Children and elderly patients are more susceptible to side-effects.

- **PREGNANCY** Most manufacturers of antihistamines advise avoiding their use during pregnancy; however, there is no evidence of teratogenicity. Use in the latter part of the third trimester may cause adverse effects in neonates such as irritability, paradoxical excitability, and tremor.

- **BREAST FEEDING** Most antihistamines are present in breast milk in varying amounts; although not known to be harmful, most manufacturers advise avoiding their use in mothers who are breast-feeding.

- **HEPATIC IMPAIRMENT** Avoid in severe liver disease—increased risk of coma.

- **RENAL IMPAIRMENT** Avoid.

- **PATIENT AND CARER ADVICE**
  Driving and skilled tasks Drowsiness may affect performance of skilled tasks (e.g. cycling or driving); sedating effects enhanced by alcohol.

- **MEDICINAL FORMS**
  There can be variation in the licensing of different medicines containing the same drug. Forms available from special-order manufacturers include: oral solution
  Oral solution
  CAUTIONARY AND ADVISORY LABELS 2
  - ▸ Alimemazine tartrate (Non-proprietary)
    Alimemazine tartrate 1.5 mg per 1 ml Alimemazine 7.5mg/5ml oral solution | 100 ml PoM £179.55 DT = £179.55
    Alimemazine tartrate 6 mg per 1 ml Alimemazine 30mg/5ml oral solution | 100 ml PoM £243.51 DT = £243.51
  Tablet
  CAUTIONARY AND ADVISORY LABELS 2
  - ▸ Alimemazine tartrate (Non-proprietary)
    Alimemazine tartrate 10 mg Alimemazine 10mg tablets | 28 tablet PoM £112.85 DT = £112.85

Chlorphenamine maleate

(Chlorpheniramine maleate)

- **INDICATIONS AND DOSE**

Symptomatic relief of allergy such as hay fever, urticaria, food allergy, drug reactions | Relief of itch associated with chickenpox

▸ BY MOUTH
- Child 1-23 months: 1 mg twice daily
- Child 2-5 years: 1 mg every 4-6 hours; maximum 6 mg per day
- Child 6-11 years: 2 mg every 4-6 hours; maximum 12 mg per day
- Child 12-17 years: 4 mg every 4-6 hours; maximum 24 mg per day
- Adult: 4 mg every 4-6 hours; maximum 24 mg per day
- Elderly: 4 mg every 4-6 hours; maximum 12 mg per day
▸ BY INTRAMUSCULAR INJECTION, OR BY INTRAVENOUS INJECTION
- Child 1-5 months: 250 micrograms/kg (max. per dose 2.5 mg), repeated if necessary; maximum 4 doses per day
- Child 6 months-5 years: 2.5 mg, repeated if necessary; maximum 4 doses per day
- Child 6-11 years: 5 mg, repeated if necessary; maximum 4 doses per day
- Child 12-17 years: 10 mg, repeated if necessary; maximum 4 doses per day
- Adult: 10 mg, repeated if necessary; maximum 4 doses per day

Emergency treatment of anaphylactic reactions

▸ BY INTRAMUSCULAR INJECTION, OR BY INTRAVENOUS INJECTION
- Child 1-5 months: 250 micrograms/kg (max. per dose 2.5 mg), repeated if necessary; maximum 4 doses per day
- Child 6 months-5 years: 2.5 mg, repeated if necessary; maximum 4 doses per day
- Child 6-11 years: 5 mg, repeated if necessary; maximum 4 doses per day
- Child 12-17 years: 10 mg, repeated if necessary; maximum 4 doses per day
- Adult: 10 mg, repeated if necessary; maximum 4 doses per day

- **UNLICENSED USE** *Tablets* not licensed for use in children under 6 years. *Syrup* not licensed for use in children under 1 year.

IMPORTANT SAFETY INFORMATION

MHRA/CHM ADVICE (MARCH 2008 AND FEBRUARY 2009) OVER-THE-COUNTER COUGH AND COLD MEDICINES FOR CHILDREN

Children under 6 years should not be given over-the-counter cough and cold medicines containing chlorphenamine.

- **CAUTIONS** Epilepsy · prostatic hypertrophy (in adults) · pyloroduodenal obstruction · susceptibility to angle-closure glaucoma · urinary retention
- **INTERACTIONS** → Appendix 1: antihistamines, sedating
- **SIDE-EFFECTS**

GENERAL SIDE-EFFECTS

▸ **Common or very common** Concentration impaired · coordination abnormal · dizziness · dry mouth · fatigue · headache · nausea · vision blurred
▸ **Frequency not known** Agitation · appetite decreased · blood disorder · bronchial secretion viscosity increased · depression · diarrhoea · gastrointestinal disorder · haemolytic anaemia · hypotension · irritability · muscle twitching · muscle weakness · nightmare · palpitations ·

photosensitivity reaction · skin reactions · tinnitus · urinary retention · vomiting

SPECIFIC SIDE-EFFECTS
▸ **Common or very common**
▸ With oral use Drowsiness
▸ **Frequency not known**
▸ With oral use Angioedema · arrhythmias · chest tightness · confusion · hepatic disorders
▸ With parenteral use Central nervous system stimulation · confusional psychosis (in adults) · dyspepsia · hepatitis · sedation

SIDE-EFFECTS, FURTHER INFORMATION Children and elderly patients are more susceptible to side-effects.

- **PREGNANCY** Most manufacturers of antihistamines advise avoiding their use during pregnancy; however, there is no evidence of teratogenicity. Use in the latter part of the third trimester may cause adverse effects in neonates such as irritability, paradoxical excitability, and tremor.
- **BREAST FEEDING** Most antihistamines are present in breast milk in varying amounts; although not known to be harmful, most manufacturers advise avoiding their use in mothers who are breast-feeding.
- **HEPATIC IMPAIRMENT** Avoid in severe liver disease—increased risk of coma.
- **DIRECTIONS FOR ADMINISTRATION** For *intravenous injection*, give over 1 minute; if small dose required, dilute with Sodium Chloride 0.9%.
- **PATIENT AND CARER ADVICE**

Medicines for Children leaflet: Chlorphenamine maleate for allergy symptoms www.medicinesforchildren.org.uk/chlorphenamine-maleate-allergy-symptoms-0

Driving and skilled tasks Drowsiness may affect performance of skilled tasks (e.g. cycling or driving); sedating effects enhanced by alcohol.

- **PROFESSION SPECIFIC INFORMATION**

Dental practitioners' formulary
Chlorphenamine tablets may be prescribed.
Chlorphenamine oral solution may be prescribed.

- **EXCEPTIONS TO LEGAL CATEGORY**
▸ With intramuscular use or intravenous use Prescription only medicine restriction does not apply to chlorphenamine injection where administration is for saving life in emergency.

- MEDICINAL FORMS
There can be variation in the licensing of different medicines containing the same drug. Forms available from special-order manufacturers include: oral solution

Solution for injection

▸ Chlorphenamine maleate (Non-proprietary)
Chlorphenamine maleate 10 mg per 1 ml Chlorphenamine 10mg/1ml solution for injection ampoules | 5 ampoule PoM £22.48-£22.50 DT = £22.50

Oral solution

CAUTIONARY AND ADVISORY LABELS 2

▸ Chlorphenamine maleate (Non-proprietary)
Chlorphenamine maleate 400 microgram per 1 ml Chlorphenamine maleate 2mg/5ml oral solution sugar free sugar-free | 150 ml P £2.78 DT = £2.62
▸ Allerief (Crescent Pharma Ltd)
Chlorphenamine maleate 400 microgram per 1 ml Allerief 2mg/5ml oral solution sugar-free | 150 ml P £2.21 DT = £2.62
▸ Piriton (GlaxoSmithKline Consumer Healthcare)
Chlorphenamine maleate 400 microgram per 1 ml Piriton 2mg/5ml syrup | 150 ml P £2.78 DT = £2.78

Tablet

CAUTIONARY AND ADVISORY LABELS 2

▸ Chlorphenamine maleate (Non-proprietary)
Chlorphenamine maleate 4 mg Chlorphenamine 4mg tablets | 28 tablet P £1.00 DT = £0.76
▸ Hayleve (Genesis Pharmaceuticals Ltd)
Chlorphenamine maleate 4 mg Hayleve 4mg tablets | 28 tablet P £0.76 DT = £0.76

▶ Piriton (GlaxoSmithKline Consumer Healthcare)
Chlorphenamine maleate 4 mg Piriton 4mg tablets | 500 tablet P £6.96
Piriton Allergy 4mg tablets | 30 tablet P £2.06 | 60 tablet P £3.73
▶ Pollenase (chlorphenamine) (E M Pharma)
Chlorphenamine maleate 4 mg Pollenase Antihistamine 4mg tablets | 30 tablet P £1.00

Clemastine

● **INDICATIONS AND DOSE**

Symptomatic relief of allergy such as hay fever, urticaria
▶ BY MOUTH
  ▶ Adult: 1 mg twice daily, increased if necessary up to 6 mg daily

● CONTRA-INDICATIONS Avoid in Acute porphyrias p. 1025
● CAUTIONS Epilepsy · prostatic hypertrophy · pyloroduodenal obstruction · susceptibility to angle-closure glaucoma · urinary retention
● INTERACTIONS → Appendix 1: antihistamines, sedating
● SIDE-EFFECTS
  ▶ **Common or very common** Asthenia · sedation
  ▶ **Uncommon** Dizziness
  ▶ **Rare or very rare** Abdominal pain · agitation · constipation · dry mouth · dyspnoea · headache · nausea · palpitations · rash · tachycardia
● PREGNANCY Most manufacturers of antihistamines advise avoiding their use during pregnancy; however, there is no evidence of teratogenicity. Use in the latter part of the third trimester may cause adverse effects in neonates such as irritability, paradoxical excitability, and tremor.
● BREAST FEEDING Most antihistamines are present in breast milk in varying amounts; although not known to be harmful, most manufacturers advise avoiding their use in mothers who are breast-feeding.
● HEPATIC IMPAIRMENT Avoid in severe liver disease—increased risk of coma.
● PATIENT AND CARER ADVICE
  Driving and skilled tasks Drowsiness may affect performance of skilled tasks (e.g. driving); sedating effects enhanced by alcohol.
● MEDICINAL FORMS
  There can be variation in the licensing of different medicines containing the same drug.
  Tablet
  CAUTIONARY AND ADVISORY LABELS 2
  ▶ Tavegil (GlaxoSmithKline Consumer Healthcare)
  Clemastine (as Clemastine hydrogen fumarate) 1 mg Tavegil 1mg tablets | 60 tablet P £6.66 DT = £6.66

Cyproheptadine hydrochloride

● **INDICATIONS AND DOSE**

Symptomatic relief of allergy such as hay fever, urticaria | Pruritus
▶ BY MOUTH
  ▶ Adult: 4 mg 3 times a day, usual dose 4–20 mg daily; maximum 32 mg per day

● CONTRA-INDICATIONS Avoid in Acute porphyrias p. 1025
● CAUTIONS Epilepsy · prostatic hypertrophy · pyloroduodenal obstruction · susceptibility to angle-closure glaucoma · urinary retention
● INTERACTIONS → Appendix 1: antihistamines, sedating
● SIDE-EFFECTS Aggression · agranulocytosis · anxiety · appetite abnormal · arrhythmias · bronchial secretion viscosity increased · chest tightness · chills · confusion · constipation · coordination abnormal · diarrhoea ·

dizziness · drowsiness · dry mouth · dry throat · epigastric distress · epistaxis · fatigue · haemolytic anaemia · hallucination · headache · hepatic disorders · hyperhidrosis · hypotension · insomnia · labyrinthitis · leucopenia · menstruation irregular · mood altered · nasal complaints · nausea · neuritis · oedema · palpitations · paraesthesia · photosensitivity reaction · seizure · skin reactions · thrombocytopenia · tinnitus · tremor · urinary disorders · vertigo · vision disorders · vomiting · weight increased · wheezing
● PREGNANCY Most manufacturers of antihistamines advise avoiding their use during pregnancy; however, there is no evidence of teratogenicity. Use in the latter part of the third trimester may cause adverse effects in neonates such as irritability, paradoxical excitability, and tremor.
● BREAST FEEDING Most antihistamines are present in breast milk in varying amounts; although not known to be harmful, most manufacturers advise avoiding their use in mothers who are breast-feeding.
● HEPATIC IMPAIRMENT Avoid in severe liver disease—increased risk of coma.
● PATIENT AND CARER ADVICE
  Driving and skilled tasks Drowsiness may affect performance of skilled tasks (e.g. driving); sedating effects enhanced by alcohol.

● MEDICINAL FORMS
  There can be variation in the licensing of different medicines containing the same drug. Forms available from special-order manufacturers include: oral suspension, oral solution
  Tablet
  CAUTIONARY AND ADVISORY LABELS 2
  ▶ Periactin (Teva UK Ltd)
  Cyproheptadine hydrochloride 4 mg Periactin 4mg tablets | 30 tablet P £5.99 DT = £5.99

Hydroxyzine hydrochloride

22-Feb-2016

● DRUG ACTION Hydroxyzine is a sedating antihistamine which exerts its actions by antagonising the effects of histamine.

● **INDICATIONS AND DOSE**

Pruritus
▶ BY MOUTH
  ▶ Child 6 months–5 years: 5–15 mg daily in divided doses, dose adjusted according to weight; maximum 2 mg/kg per day
  ▶ Child 6–17 years (body-weight up to 40 kg): Initially 15–25 mg daily in divided doses, dose increased as necessary, adjusted according to weight; maximum 2 mg/kg per day
  ▶ Child 6–17 years (body-weight 40 kg and above): Initially 15–25 mg daily in divided doses, increased if necessary to 50–100 mg daily in divided doses, dose adjusted according to weight
  ▶ Adult: Initially 25 mg daily, dose to be taken at night; increased if necessary to 25 mg 3–4 times a day
  ▶ Elderly: Initially 25 mg daily, dose to be taken at night; increased if necessary to 25 mg twice daily

IMPORTANT SAFETY INFORMATION

MHRA/CHM ADVICE: RISK OF QT-INTERVAL PROLONGATION AND TORSADE DE POINTES (APRIL 2015)

Following concerns of heart rhythm abnormalities, the safety and efficacy of hydroxyzine has been reviewed by the European Medicines Agency. The review concludes that hydroxyzine is associated with a small risk of QT-interval prolongation and torsade de pointes; these events are most likely to occur in patients who have risk factors for QT prolongation, e.g. concomitant use of drugs that prolong the QT-interval, cardiovascular disease, family history of sudden cardiac death, significant electrolyte imbalance (low plasma-potassium or plasma-magnesium concentrations), or significant bradycardia. To minimise the risk of such adverse effects, the following dose restrictions have been made and new cautions and contra-indications added:

- Hydroxyzine is contra-indicated in patients with prolonged QT-interval or who have risk factors for QT-interval prolongation;
- Avoid use in the elderly due to increased susceptibility to the side-effects of hydroxyzine;
- Consider the risks of QT-interval prolongation and torsade de pointes before prescribing to patients taking drugs that lower heart rate or plasma-potassium concentration;
- In children with body-weight up to 40 kg, the maximum daily dose is 2 mg/kg;
- In adults, the maximum daily dose is 100 mg;
- In the elderly, the maximum daily dose is 50 mg (if use of hydroxyzine cannot be avoided);
- The lowest effective dose for the shortest period of time should be prescribed.

● CONTRA-INDICATIONS Acquired or congenital QT interval prolongation · predisposition to QT interval prolongation

CONTRA-INDICATIONS, FURTHER INFORMATION

▸ QT interval prolongation Risk factors for QT interval prolongation include significant electrolyte imbalance, bradycardia, cardiovascular disease, and family history of sudden cardiac death.

● CAUTIONS Bladder outflow obstruction · breathing problems · cardiovascular disease · children · decreased gastrointestinal motility · dementia · elderly · epilepsy · hypertension · hyperthyroidism · myasthenia gravis · prostatic hypertrophy (in adults) · pyloroduodenal obstruction · stenosing peptic ulcer · susceptibility to angle-closure glaucoma · urinary retention

CAUTIONS, FURTHER INFORMATION Elderly patients are particularly susceptible to side-effects; manufacturers advise avoid or reduce dose.

Children have an increased susceptibility to side-effects, particularly CNS effects.

● INTERACTIONS → Appendix 1: antihistamines, sedating

● SIDE-EFFECTS

▸ **Rare or very rare** Severe cutaneous adverse reactions (SCARs) · skin reactions

▸ **Frequency not known** Agranulocytosis · alopecia · anticholinergic syndrome · anxiety · appetite decreased · arrhythmias · asthenia · blood disorder · bronchial secretion viscosity increased · chest tightness · chills · coma · concentration impaired · confusion · constipation · depression · diarrhoea · dizziness · drowsiness · dry mouth · dry throat · dyskinesia (on discontinuation) · epigastric pain · fever · flushing · gastrointestinal disorders · haemolytic anaemia · hallucination · headache · hepatic function abnormal · hyperhidrosis · hypotension · irritability · labyrinthitis · leucopenia · malaise · menstruation irregular · movement disorders · myalgia · nasal congestion · nausea · palpitations · paraesthesia · QT interval prolongation · respiratory disorders · respiratory tract dryness · seizure (with high doses) · sexual dysfunction · sleep disorders · speech slurred · taste bitter · thrombocytopenia · tinnitus · tremor (with high doses) · urinary disorders · vertigo · vision disorders · vomiting

SIDE-EFFECTS, FURTHER INFORMATION Paradoxical stimulation may occur rarely, especially with high doses or in the elderly. Drowsiness may diminish after a few days of treatment.

● ALLERGY AND CROSS-SENSITIVITY Manufacturer advises hydroxyzine should be avoided in patients with previous

hypersensitivity to cetirizine or other piperazine derivatives, and aminophylline.

● PREGNANCY Manufacturers advise avoid—toxicity in *animal* studies with higher doses. Use in the latter part of the third trimester may cause irritability, paradoxical excitability, and tremor in the neonate.

● BREAST FEEDING Manufacturer advises avoid—expected to be present in milk but effect unknown.

● HEPATIC IMPAIRMENT Manufacturer advises avoid in severe liver disease—increased risk of coma.
Dose adjustments Manufacturer advises reduce daily dose by one-third.

● RENAL IMPAIRMENT
Dose adjustments Manufacturers advise reduce daily dose by half in moderate to severe renal impairment.

● EFFECT ON LABORATORY TESTS May interfere with methacholine test—manufacturer advises stop treatment 96 hours prior to test. May interfere with skin testing for allergy—manufacturer advises stop treatment one week prior to test.

● PATIENT AND CARER ADVICE
Driving and skilled tasks Drowsiness may affect performance of skilled tasks (e.g. cycling or driving); sedating effects enhanced by alcohol.

● MEDICINAL FORMS
There can be variation in the licensing of different medicines containing the same drug. Forms available from special-order manufacturers include: oral suspension, oral solution
Tablet
CAUTIONARY AND ADVISORY LABELS 2
▸ Hydroxyzine hydrochloride (Non-proprietary)
Hydroxyzine hydrochloride 10 mg Hydroxyzine 10mg tablets |
84 tablet [PoM] £1.20–£1.53 DT = £1.37
Hydroxyzine hydrochloride 25 mg Hydroxyzine 25mg tablets |
28 tablet [PoM] £0.62–£0.80 DT = £0.71
▸ Atarax (Alliance Pharmaceuticals Ltd)
Hydroxyzine hydrochloride 10 mg Atarax 10mg tablets |
84 tablet [PoM] £1.20 DT = £1.37
Hydroxyzine hydrochloride 25 mg Atarax 25mg tablets |
28 tablet [PoM] £0.62 DT = £0.71

Ketotifen

● INDICATIONS AND DOSE
Allergic rhinitis
▸ BY MOUTH
▸ Child 3–17 years: 1 mg twice daily
▸ Adult: 1 mg twice daily, increased if necessary to 2 mg twice daily, to be taken with food
Allergic rhinitis in readily sedated patients
▸ BY MOUTH
▸ Adult: Initially 0.5–1 mg once daily, dose to be taken at night

● CONTRA-INDICATIONS Avoid in Acute porphyrias p. 1025

● CAUTIONS Epilepsy · prostatic hypertrophy (in adults) · pyloroduodenal obstruction · susceptibility to angle-closure glaucoma · urinary retention

● INTERACTIONS → Appendix 1: antihistamines, sedating

● SIDE-EFFECTS

▸ **Common or very common** Anxiety · insomnia · irritability

▸ **Uncommon** Cystitis · dizziness · dry mouth · skin reactions

▸ **Rare or very rare** Hepatitis · sedation · seizure · Stevens-Johnson syndrome · weight increased

SIDE-EFFECTS, FURTHER INFORMATION Drowsiness is a significant side-effect with most of the older antihistamines although paradoxical stimulation may occur rarely, especially with high doses or in children and the elderly. Drowsiness may diminish after a few days of treatment and is considerably less of a problem with the newer antihistamines.

- **PREGNANCY** Most manufacturers of antihistamines advise avoiding their use during pregnancy; however, there is no evidence of teratogenicity. Use in the latter part of the third trimester may cause adverse effects in neonates such as irritability, paradoxical excitability, and tremor.
- **BREAST FEEDING** Most antihistamines are present in breast milk in varying amounts; although not known to be harmful, most manufacturers advise avoiding their use in mothers who are breast-feeding.
- **HEPATIC IMPAIRMENT** Avoid in severe liver disease— increased risk of coma.
- **PATIENT AND CARER ADVICE**
Driving and skilled tasks Drowsiness may affect performance of skilled tasks (e.g. driving or cycling); sedating effects enhanced by alcohol.

- **MEDICINAL FORMS**
There can be variation in the licensing of different medicines containing the same drug.
Oral solution
CAUTIONARY AND ADVISORY LABELS 2, 21
▸ Zaditen (CD Pharma AB)
Ketotifen (as Ketotifen fumarate) 200 microgram per 1 ml Zaditen 1mg/5ml elixir sugar-free | 300 ml [PoM] £8.91 DT = £8.91
Tablet
CAUTIONARY AND ADVISORY LABELS 2, 21
▸ Zaditen (CD Pharma AB)
Ketotifen (as Ketotifen fumarate) 1 mg Zaditen 1mg tablets | 60 tablet [PoM] £7.53

Promethazine hydrochloride

- **INDICATIONS AND DOSE**
Symptomatic relief of allergy such as hay fever and urticaria | Insomnia associated with urticaria and pruritus
▸ BY MOUTH
▸ Child 2-4 years: 5 mg twice daily, alternatively 5–15 mg once daily, dose to be taken at night
▸ Child 5-9 years: 5–10 mg twice daily, alternatively 10–25 mg once daily, dose to be taken at night
▸ Child 10-17 years: 10–20 mg 2–3 times a day, alternatively 25 mg once daily, dose to be taken at night, increased if necessary to 25 mg twice daily
▸ Adult: 10–20 mg 2–3 times a day
▸ BY DEEP INTRAMUSCULAR INJECTION
▸ Adult: 25–50 mg (max. per dose 100 mg)
Emergency treatment of anaphylactic reactions
▸ BY SLOW INTRAVENOUS INJECTION
▸ Adult: 25–50 mg, to be administered as a solution containing 2.5 mg/mL in water for injections; maximum 100 mg per course
Sedation (short-term use)
▸ BY MOUTH
▸ Child 2-4 years: 15–20 mg
▸ Child 5-9 years: 20–25 mg
▸ Child 10-17 years: 25–50 mg
▸ Adult: 25–50 mg
▸ BY DEEP INTRAMUSCULAR INJECTION
▸ Adult: 25–50 mg
Nausea | Vomiting | Vertigo | Labyrinthine disorders | Motion sickness
▸ BY MOUTH
▸ Child 2-4 years: 5 mg, to be taken at bedtime on night before travel, repeat following morning if necessary
▸ Child 5-9 years: 10 mg, to be taken at bedtime on night before travel, repeat following morning if necessary

▸ Child 10-17 years: 20–25 mg, to be taken at bedtime on night before travel, repeat following morning if necessary
▸ Adult: 20–25 mg, to be taken at bedtime on night before travel, repeat following morning if necessary

> **IMPORTANT SAFETY INFORMATION**
> MHRA/CHM ADVICE (MARCH 2008 AND FEBRUARY 2009) OVER-THE-COUNTER COUGH AND COLD MEDICINES FOR CHILDREN
> Children under 6 years should not be given over-the-counter cough and cold medicines containing promethazine.

- **CONTRA-INDICATIONS** Should not be given to children under 2 years, except on specialist advice, because the safety of such use has not been established
- **CAUTIONS**
GENERAL CAUTIONS Epilepsy · prostatic hypertrophy (in adults) · pyloroduodenal obstruction · severe coronary artery disease · susceptibility to angle-closure glaucoma · urinary retention
SPECIFIC CAUTIONS
▸ With intravenous use Avoid extravasation with intravenous injection
- **INTERACTIONS** → Appendix 1: antihistamines, sedating
- **SIDE-EFFECTS**
GENERAL SIDE-EFFECTS
Arrhythmia · blood disorder · confusion · dizziness · drowsiness · dry mouth · headache · hypotension · jaundice · movement disorders · palpitations · photosensitivity reaction · urinary retention · vision blurred
SPECIFIC SIDE-EFFECTS
▸ With oral use Agranulocytosis · angle closure glaucoma · anticholinergic syndrome · anxiety · insomnia · leucopenia · nasal congestion · nausea · rash · seizure · thrombocytopenia · tinnitus · tremor · vomiting
▸ With parenteral use Appetite decreased · epigastric discomfort · fatigue · haemolytic anaemia · hypersensitivity · muscle spasms · nightmare · restlessness · skin reactions
SIDE-EFFECTS, FURTHER INFORMATION Elderly patients are more susceptible to anticholinergic side-effects.
- **PREGNANCY** Most manufacturers of antihistamines advise avoiding their use during pregnancy; however, there is no evidence of teratogenicity. Use in the latter part of the third trimester may cause adverse effects in neonates such as irritability, paradoxical excitability, and tremor.
- **BREAST FEEDING** Most antihistamines are present in breast milk in varying amounts; although not known to be harmful, most manufacturers advise avoiding their use in mothers who are breast-feeding.
- **HEPATIC IMPAIRMENT** Avoid in severe liver disease— increased risk of coma.
- **RENAL IMPAIRMENT** Use with caution.
- **PATIENT AND CARER ADVICE**
Driving and skilled tasks Drowsiness may affect the performance of skilled tasks (e.g. cycling or driving); sedating effects enhanced by alcohol.
- **PROFESSION SPECIFIC INFORMATION**
Dental practitioners' formulary
Promethazine Hydrochloride Tablets 10 mg or 25 mg may be prescribed.
    Promethazine Hydrochloride Oral Solution (elixir) 5 mg/5 mL may be prescribed.
- **LESS SUITABLE FOR PRESCRIBING** Promethazine is less suitable for prescribing for sedation.
- **EXCEPTIONS TO LEGAL CATEGORY** Prescription only medicine restriction does not apply to promethazine

hydrochloride injection where administration is for saving life in emergency.

● MEDICINAL FORMS
There can be variation in the licensing of different medicines containing the same drug. Forms available from special-order manufacturers include: oral suspension, oral solution

Solution for injection
EXCIPIENTS: May contain Sulfites
▶ Phenergan (Sanofi)
   Promethazine hydrochloride 25 mg per 1 ml Phenergan 25mg/1ml solution for injection ampoules | 10 ampoule [PoM] £6.74

Oral solution
CAUTIONARY AND ADVISORY LABELS 2
EXCIPIENTS: May contain Sulfites
ELECTROLYTES: May contain Sodium
▶ Phenergan (Sanofi)
   Promethazine hydrochloride 1 mg per 1 ml Phenergan 5mg/5ml elixir sugar-free | 100 ml [P] £2.85 DT = £2.85

Tablet
CAUTIONARY AND ADVISORY LABELS 2
▶ Promethazine hydrochloride (Non-proprietary)
   Promethazine hydrochloride 10 mg Promethazine hydrochloride 10mg tablets | 56 tablet [PoM] £2.96 DT = £2.96
   Promethazine hydrochloride 25 mg Promethazine hydrochloride 25mg tablets | 56 tablet [P] £4.00 DT = £4.65
▶ Phenergan (Sanofi)
   Promethazine hydrochloride 25 mg Phenergan 25mg tablets | 56 tablet [P] £4.65 DT = £4.65
▶ Sominex (Teva UK Ltd)
   Promethazine hydrochloride 20 mg Sominex 20mg tablets | 8 tablet [P] £1.89 | 16 tablet [P] £2.69

VACCINES > ALLERGEN-TYPE VACCINES

Bee venom extract

● INDICATIONS AND DOSE

Hypersensitivity to bee venom
▶ BY SUBCUTANEOUS INJECTION
▶ Adult: (consult product literature)

IMPORTANT SAFETY INFORMATION
DESENSITISING VACCINES
In view of concerns about the safety of desensitising vaccines, it is recommended that they are used by specialists and only for the following indications:
● seasonal allergic hay fever (caused by pollen) that has not responded to anti-allergic drugs;
● hypersensitivity to wasp and bee venoms.
Desensitising vaccines should generally be avoided or used with particular care in patients with asthma.

● CONTRA-INDICATIONS Consult product literature
● CAUTIONS Consult product literature
● INTERACTIONS → Appendix 1: bee venom extract
● SIDE-EFFECTS
   SIDE-EFFECTS, FURTHER INFORMATION Life-threatening hypersensitivity reactions can occur. Cardiopulmonary resuscitation must be immediately available. Manufacturer advises monitoring for at least 1 hour after injection.
● PREGNANCY Avoid.
● PRESCRIBING AND DISPENSING INFORMATION Each set of allergen extracts usually contains vials for the administration of graded amounts of allergen to patients undergoing hyposensitisation. Maintenance sets containing vials at the highest strength are also available. Product literature must be consulted for details of allergens, vial strengths, and administration.

● NATIONAL FUNDING/ACCESS DECISIONS
NICE decisions
▶ *Pharmalgen®* for bee and wasp venom allergy (February 2012) NICE TA246
Pharmalgen® is an option for the treatment of IgE-mediated bee and wasp venom allergy in those who have had:
● a severe systemic reaction to bee or wasp venom;
● a moderate systemic reaction to bee or wasp venom and who have a raised baseline serum-tryptase concentration, a high risk of future stings, or anxiety about future stings.
Treatment with *Pharmalgen®* should be initiated and monitored in a specialist centre experienced in venom immunotherapy.
www.nice.org.uk/TA246

● MEDICINAL FORMS
There can be variation in the licensing of different medicines containing the same drug.
Powder and solvent for solution for injection
▶ Bee Venom (ALK-Abello Ltd)
   Bee venom 120 nanogram Pharmalgen Bee Venom 120nanogram powder and solvent for solution for injection vials | 1 vial [PoM] [✸]
   Bee venom 1.2 microgram Pharmalgen Bee Venom 1.2microgram powder and solvent for solution for injection vials | 1 vial [PoM] [✸]
   Bee venom 12 microgram Pharmalgen Bee Venom 12microgram powder and solvent for solution for injection vials | 1 vial [PoM] [✸]
   Bee venom 120 microgram Pharmalgen Bee Venom maintenance set 120microgram powder and solvent for solution for injection vials | 4 vial [PoM] £150.00

Grass pollen extract

● INDICATIONS AND DOSE

Treatment of seasonal allergic hay fever due to grass pollen in patients who have failed to respond to anti-allergy drugs
▶ BY SUBCUTANEOUS INJECTION
▶ Adult: (consult product literature)

Treatment of seasonal allergic hay fever due to grass pollen in patients who have failed to respond to anti-allergy drugs (initiated under specialist supervision)
▶ BY MOUTH
▶ Adult: 1 tablet daily, treatment to be started at least 4 months before start of pollen season and continue for up to 3 years

---

IMPORTANT SAFETY INFORMATION
DESENSITISING VACCINES
In view of concerns about the safety of desensitising vaccines, it is recommended that they are used by specialists and only for the following indications:
● seasonal allergic hay fever (caused by pollen) that has not responded to anti-allergic drugs;
● hypersensitivity to wasp and bee venoms.
Desensitising vaccines should generally be avoided or used with particular care in patients with asthma.

● CONTRA-INDICATIONS Consult product literature
● CAUTIONS Consult product literature
● INTERACTIONS → Appendix 1: grass pollen extract
● SIDE-EFFECTS
   SIDE-EFFECTS, FURTHER INFORMATION Hypersensitivity reactions to immunotherapy can be life-threatening; bronchospasm usually develops within 1 hour and anaphylaxis within 30 minutes of injection. Therefore, cardiopulmonary resuscitation must be immediately available and patients need to be monitored for at least 1 hour after injection. If symptoms or signs of hypersensitivity develop (e.g. rash, urticaria,

3

Respiratory system

bronchospasm, faintness), **even when mild**, the patient should be observed until these have resolved completely.

- PREGNANCY Should be avoided in pregnant women—consult product literature.
- MONITORING REQUIREMENTS The first dose of grass pollen extract should be (*Grazax*®) should be taken under medical supervision and the patient should be monitored for 20–30 minutes.
- DIRECTIONS FOR ADMINISTRATION Oral lyophilisates should be placed under the tongue and allowed to disperse. Advise patient not to swallow for 1 minute, or eat or drink for 5 minutes after taking the tablet. The first should be taken under medical supervision and the patient should be monitored for 20–30 minutes.
- PRESCRIBING AND DISPENSING INFORMATION Each set of allergen extracts usually contains vials for the administration of graded amounts of allergen to patients undergoing hyposensitisation. Maintenance sets containing vials at the highest strength are also available. Product literature must be consulted for details of allergens, vial strengths, and administration.
- PATIENT AND CARER ADVICE Patients or carers should be given advice on how to administer oral lyophilisates.
- MEDICINAL FORMS
There can be variation in the licensing of different medicines containing the same drug.
Suspension for injection
▸ Pollinex Grasses + Rye (Allergy Therapeutics (UK) Ltd)
Pollinex Grasses + Rye suspension for injection treatment and extension course vials | 4 vial [PoM] £450.00
Oral lyophilisate
▸ Grazax (ALK-Abello Ltd)
Phleum pratense 75000 SQ-T Grazax 75,000 SQ-T oral lyophilisates sugar-free | 30 tablet [PoM] £80.12

Tree pollen extract

- INDICATIONS AND DOSE

Treatment of seasonal allergic hay fever due to tree pollen in patients who have failed to respond to anti-allergy drugs
▸ BY SUBCUTANEOUS INJECTION
▸ Adult: (consult product literature)

IMPORTANT SAFETY INFORMATION
DESENSITISING VACCINES
In view of concerns about the safety of desensitising vaccines, it is recommended that they are used by specialists and only for the following indications:
- seasonal allergic hay fever (caused by pollen) that has not responded to anti-allergic drugs;
- hypersensitivity to wasp and bee venoms.
Desensitising vaccines should generally be avoided or used with particular care in patients with asthma.

- CONTRA-INDICATIONS Consult product literature
- CAUTIONS Consult product literature
- INTERACTIONS → Appendix 1: tree pollen extract
- SIDE-EFFECTS
SIDE-EFFECTS, FURTHER INFORMATION Hypersensitivity reactions to immunotherapy can be life-threatening. Cardiopulmonary resuscitation must be immediately available and patients need to be monitored for at least 1 hour after injection. If symptoms or signs of hypersensitivity develop (e.g. rash, urticaria, bronchospasm, faintness), **even when mild**, the patient should be observed until these have resolved completely.
- PREGNANCY Should be avoided in pregnant women—consult product literature.

- PRESCRIBING AND DISPENSING INFORMATION Each set of allergen extracts usually contains vials for the administration of graded amounts of allergen to patients undergoing hyposensitisation. Maintenance sets containing vials at the highest strength are also available. Product literature must be consulted for details of allergens, vial strengths, and administration.

- MEDICINAL FORMS
There can be variation in the licensing of different medicines containing the same drug.
Suspension for injection
▸ Pollinex Trees (Allergy Therapeutics (UK) Ltd)
Pollinex Trees No 3 suspension for injection 1ml vials | 1 vial [PoM] [S]
Pollinex Trees No 2 suspension for injection 1ml vials | 1 vial [PoM] [S]
Pollinex Trees No 1 suspension for injection 1ml vials | 1 vial [PoM] [S]
Pollinex Trees suspension for injection treatment and extension course vials | 4 vial [PoM] £450.00

Wasp venom extract

- INDICATIONS AND DOSE

Hypersensitivity to wasp venom
▸ BY SUBCUTANEOUS INJECTION
▸ Adult: (consult product literature)

IMPORTANT SAFETY INFORMATION
DESENSITISING VACCINES
In view of concerns about the safety of desensitising vaccines, it is recommended that they are used by specialists and only for the following indications:
- seasonal allergic hay fever (caused by pollen) that has not responded to anti-allergic drugs;
- hypersensitivity to wasp and bee venoms.
Desensitising vaccines should generally be avoided or used with particular care in patients with asthma.

- CONTRA-INDICATIONS Consult product literature
- CAUTIONS Consult product literature
- INTERACTIONS → Appendix 1: wasp venom extract
- SIDE-EFFECTS
SIDE-EFFECTS, FURTHER INFORMATION Hypersensitivity reactions to wasp venom extracts can be life-threatening; cardiopulmonary resuscitation must be immediately available and patients need to be monitored for at least 1 hour after injection. If symptoms or signs of hypersensitivity develop (e.g. rash, urticaria, bronchospasm, faintness, **even when mild**, the patient should be observed until these have resolved completely.
- PREGNANCY Avoid.
- PRESCRIBING AND DISPENSING INFORMATION Each set of allergen extracts usually contains vials for the administration of graded amounts of allergen to patients undergoing hyposensitisation. Maintenance sets containing vials at the highest strength are also available. Product literature must be consulted for details of allergens, vial strengths, and administration.
- NATIONAL FUNDING/ACCESS DECISIONS
NICE decisions
▸ *Pharmalgen*® for bee and wasp venom allergy (February 2012) NICE TA246
Pharmalgen® is an option for the treatment of IgE-mediated bee and wasp venom allergy in those who have had:
- a severe systemic reaction to bee or wasp venom;
- a moderate systemic reaction to bee or wasp venom and who have a raised baseline serum-tryptase concentration, a high risk of future stings, or anxiety about future stings.

Treatment with *Pharmalgen®* should be initiated and monitored in a specialist centre experienced in venom immunotherapy.
www.nice.org.uk/TA246

● MEDICINAL FORMS
There can be variation in the licensing of different medicines containing the same drug.

Powder and solvent for solution for injection
▸ Wasp Venom (ALK-Abello Ltd)
Wasp venom 120 nanogram Pharmalgen Wasp Venom 120nanogram powder and solvent for solution for injection vials | 1 vial PoM Ⓢ
Wasp venom 1.2 microgram Pharmalgen Wasp Venom 1.2microgram powder and solvent for solution for injection vials | 1 vial PoM Ⓢ
Wasp venom 12 microgram Pharmalgen Wasp Venom 12microgram powder and solvent for solution for injection vials | 1 vial PoM Ⓢ
Wasp venom 120 microgram Pharmalgen Wasp Venom maintenance set 120microgram vaccine powder and solvent for solution for injection vials | 4 vial PoM £150.00

2.1 Angioedema

Other drugs used for Angioedema Adrenaline/epinephrine, p. 221

DRUGS USED IN HEREDITARY ANGIOEDEMA ›
COMPLEMENT REGULATORY PROTEINS

C1-esterase inhibitor

05-Dec-2017

● INDICATIONS AND DOSE

BERINERT®

Acute attacks of hereditary angioedema (under expert supervision)
▸ BY SLOW INTRAVENOUS INJECTION, OR BY INTRAVENOUS INFUSION
▸ Adult: 20 units/kg

Short-term prophylaxis of hereditary angioedema before dental, medical, or surgical procedures (under expert supervision)
▸ BY SLOW INTRAVENOUS INJECTION, OR BY INTRAVENOUS INFUSION
▸ Adult: 1000 units for 1 dose, to be administered less than 6 hours before procedure

CINRYZE®

Acute attacks of hereditary angioedema (under expert supervision)
▸ BY SLOW INTRAVENOUS INJECTION
▸ Adult: 1000 units, repeated if necessary for 1 dose, dose may be repeated if necessary after 60 minutes (or sooner for patients experiencing laryngeal attacks or if treatment initiation is delayed)

Short-term prophylaxis of hereditary angioedema before dental, medical, or surgical procedures (under expert supervision)
▸ BY SLOW INTRAVENOUS INJECTION
▸ Adult: 1000 units for 1 dose, to be administered up to 24 hours before procedure

Long-term prophylaxis of severe, recurrent attacks of hereditary angioedema where acute treatment is inadequate, or when oral prophylaxis is inadequate or not tolerated (under expert supervision)
▸ BY SLOW INTRAVENOUS INJECTION
▸ Adult: 1000 units every 3–4 days, interval between doses to be adjusted according to response

● CAUTIONS Vaccination against hepatitis A and hepatitis B may be required

● SIDE-EFFECTS
▸ **Rare or very rare** Dizziness · dyspnoea · flushing · headache · hypersensitivity · hypertension · hypotension · nausea · tachycardia · thrombosis (with high doses) · urticaria

● PREGNANCY Manufacturer advises avoid unless essential.

● PRESCRIBING AND DISPENSING INFORMATION C1-esterase inhibitor is prepared from human plasma.

● NATIONAL FUNDING/ACCESS DECISIONS

CINRYZE®

All Wales Medicines Strategy Group (AWMSG) Decisions
The *All Wales Medicines Strategy Group* has advised (October 2017) that C1-esterase inhibitor (*Cinryze®*) is recommended as an option for use within NHS Wales for the treatment and pre-procedure prevention of angioedema attacks in adults with hereditary angioedema (HAE); routine prevention of angioedema attacks in adults with severe and recurrent attacks of HAE, who are intolerant to or insufficiently protected by oral prevention treatments, or patients who are inadequately managed with repeated acute treatment.

● MEDICINAL FORMS
There can be variation in the licensing of different medicines containing the same drug.

Powder and solvent for solution for injection
ELECTROLYTES: May contain Sodium
▸ Berinert P (CSL Behring UK Ltd)
C1-esterase inhibitor 500 unit Berinert 500unit powder and solvent for solution for injection vials | 1 vial PoM £550.00
C1-esterase inhibitor 1500 unit Berinert 1,500unit powder and solvent for solution for injection vials | 1 vial PoM £1,650.00
▸ Cinryze (Shire Pharmaceuticals Ltd) ▼
C1-esterase inhibitor 500 unit Cinryze 500unit powder and solvent for solution for injection vials | 2 vial PoM £1,336.00

Conestat alfa

● INDICATIONS AND DOSE

Acute attacks of hereditary angioedema in patients with C1-esterase inhibitor deficiency
▸ BY SLOW INTRAVENOUS INJECTION
▸ Adult (body-weight up to 84 kg): 50 units/kg for 1 dose, to be administered over 5 minutes, dose may be repeated if necessary; maximum 2 doses per day
▸ Adult (body-weight 84 kg and above): 4200 units for 1 dose, to be administered over 5 minutes, dose may be repeated if necessary; maximum 2 doses per day

● CONTRA-INDICATIONS Rabbit allergy

● SIDE-EFFECTS
▸ **Common or very common** Headache
▸ **Uncommon** Abdominal discomfort · diarrhoea · nausea · oral paraesthesia · paraesthesia · throat irritation · urticaria · vertigo

● PREGNANCY Use only if potential benefit outweighs risk—toxicity in *animal* studies.

● BREAST FEEDING Use only if potential benefit outweighs risk—no information available.

● PRE-TREATMENT SCREENING Test for immunoglobulin E (IgE) antibodies against rabbit allergens before starting treatment.

● MONITORING REQUIREMENTS Repeat immunoglobulin E (IgE) antibody testing annually or after 10 treatments—consult product literature.

Respiratory system

3

- MEDICINAL FORMS
There can be variation in the licensing of different medicines containing the same drug.
Powder for solution for injection
  - Ruconest (Pharming Group N.V.)
  Conestat alfa 2100 unit Ruconest 2,100unit powder for solution for injection vials | 1 vial PoM £750.00

DRUGS USED IN HEREDITARY ANGIOEDEMA >
SELECTIVE BRADYKININ B₂ ANTAGONISTS

Icatibant

- INDICATIONS AND DOSE
Acute attacks of hereditary angioedema in patients with C1-esterase inhibitor deficiency
  - BY SUBCUTANEOUS INJECTION
  - Adult: 30 mg for 1 dose, then 30 mg after 6 hours if required, then 30 mg after 6 hours if required; maximum 3 doses per day

- CAUTIONS Ischaemic heart disease · stroke
- INTERACTIONS → Appendix 1: icatibant
- SIDE-EFFECTS
  - Common or very common Dizziness · fever · headache · nausea · skin reactions
- PREGNANCY Manufacturer advises use only if potential benefit outweighs risk—toxicity in *animal* studies.
- BREAST FEEDING Manufacturer advises avoid for 12 hours after administration.

- MEDICINAL FORMS
There can be variation in the licensing of different medicines containing the same drug.
Solution for injection
  - Firazyr (Shire Pharmaceuticals Ltd)
  Icatibant (as Icatibant acetate) 10 mg per 1 ml Firazyr 30mg/3ml solution for injection pre-filled syringes | 1 pre-filled disposable injection PoM £1,395.00

3   Conditions affecting sputum viscosity

MUCOLYTICS

Acetylcysteine
03-Apr-2018

- INDICATIONS AND DOSE
NACSYS ® EFFERVESCENT TABLETS
Reduction of sputum viscosity
  - BY MOUTH
  - Adult: 600 mg once daily

- CAUTIONS History of peptic ulceration
- SIDE-EFFECTS
  - Uncommon Diarrhoea · fever · gastrointestinal discomfort · headache · hypotension · nausea · stomatitis · tinnitus · vomiting
  - Rare or very rare Haemorrhage
  - Frequency not known Face oedema

- MEDICINAL FORMS
There can be variation in the licensing of different medicines containing the same drug.
Effervescent tablet
CAUTIONARY AND ADVISORY LABELS 13
ELECTROLYTES: May contain Sodium
  - NACSYS (Atlantic Pharma Ltd)
  Acetylcysteine 600 mg NACSYS 600mg effervescent tablets sugar-free | 30 tablet PoM £5.50 DT = £89.50

Carbocisteine

- INDICATIONS AND DOSE
Reduction of sputum viscosity
  - BY MOUTH
  - Adult: Initially 2.25 g daily in divided doses, then reduced to 1.5 g daily in divided doses, as condition improves

- CONTRA-INDICATIONS Active peptic ulceration
- CAUTIONS History of peptic ulceration (may disrupt the gastric mucosal barrier)
- SIDE-EFFECTS Gastrointestinal haemorrhage · skin reactions · Stevens-Johnson syndrome · vomiting
- PREGNANCY Manufacturer advises avoid in first trimester.
- BREAST FEEDING No information available.
- PRESCRIBING AND DISPENSING INFORMATION Flavours of oral liquid formulations may include cherry, raspberry, cinnamon, or rum.

- MEDICINAL FORMS
There can be variation in the licensing of different medicines containing the same drug.
Oral solution
  - Carbocisteine (Non-proprietary)
  Carbocisteine 50 mg per 1 ml Carbocisteine 250mg/5ml oral solution | 300 ml PoM £8.55 DT = £8.39
  Carbocisteine 75 mg per 1 ml Carbocisteine 750mg/10ml oral solution 10ml sachets sugar free sugar-free | 15 sachet PoM £3.85 DT = £3.85
  - Mucodyne (Sanofi)
  Carbocisteine 50 mg per 1 ml Mucodyne Paediatric 250mg/5ml syrup | 125 ml PoM £12.60
  Mucodyne 250mg/5ml syrup | 300 ml PoM £8.39 DT = £8.39
Capsule
  - Carbocisteine (Non-proprietary)
  Carbocisteine 375 mg Carbocisteine 375mg capsules | 120 capsule PoM £18.98 DT = £4.84
  - Mucodyne (Sanofi)
  Carbocisteine 375 mg Mucodyne 375mg capsules | 120 capsule PoM £18.98 DT = £4.84

Erdosteine

- INDICATIONS AND DOSE
Symptomatic treatment of acute exacerbations of chronic bronchitis
  - BY MOUTH
  - Adult: 300 mg twice daily for up to 10 days

- CAUTIONS History of peptic ulceration (may disrupt the gastric mucosal barrier)
- SIDE-EFFECTS
  - Common or very common Epigastric pain · taste altered
  - Uncommon Allergic dermatitis · angioedema · common cold · diarrhoea · dyspnoea · headache · nausea · vomiting
- PREGNANCY Manufacturer advises avoid—no information available.
- BREAST FEEDING Manufacturer advises avoid—no information available.
- HEPATIC IMPAIRMENT Avoid in severe impairment.
Dose adjustments Manufacturer advises max. 300 mg daily in mild to moderate impairment.
- RENAL IMPAIRMENT Avoid if eGFR less than 25 mL/minute/1.73 m² —no information available.
- NATIONAL FUNDING/ACCESS DECISIONS
Scottish Medicines Consortium (SMC) Decisions
The *The Scottish Medicines Consortium* (October 2007) has advised that erdosteine (*Erdotin* ®) is not recommended for the symptomatic treatment of acute exacerbations of chronic bronchitis.

3

- MEDICINAL FORMS
There can be variation in the licensing of different medicines containing the same drug.

Capsule
▸ Erdotin (Galen Ltd)
Erdosteine 300 mg Erdotin 300mg capsules | 20 capsule [PoM]
£5.00 DT = £5.00

3.1 Cystic fibrosis

Cystic fibrosis

10-Nov-2017

Description of condition

Cystic fibrosis is a genetic disorder affecting the lungs, pancreas, liver, intestine, and reproductive organs. The main clinical signs are pulmonary disease, with recurrent infections and the production of copious viscous sputum, and malabsorption due to pancreatic insufficiency. Other complications include hepatobiliary disease, osteoporosis, cystic fibrosis-related diabetes, and distal intestinal obstruction syndrome.

Aims of treatment

The aim of treatment includes preventing and managing lung infections, loosening and removing thick, sticky mucus from the lungs, preventing or treating intestinal obstruction, and providing sufficient nutrition and hydration.

Lung function is a key predictor of life expectancy in people with cystic fibrosis and optimising lung function is a major aim of care.

Non-drug treatment

Specialist physiotherapists should assess patients with cystic fibrosis and provide advice on airway clearance, nebuliser use, musculoskeletal disorders, physical activity, and urinary incontinence. The importance of airway clearance techniques should be discussed with patients and their parents or carers and appropriate training provided. Patients should be advised that regular exercise improves both lung function and overall fitness.

Drug treatment

Treatment for cystic fibrosis lung disease is based on the prevention of lung infection and the maintenance of lung function. [EvGr] In patients with cystic fibrosis, who have clinical evidence of lung disease, the frequency of routine review should be based on their clinical condition, but adults should be reviewed at least every 3 months. More frequent review is required immediately after diagnosis. ⟨A⟩

Mucolytics

[EvGr] Patients with cystic fibrosis who have evidence of lung disease should be offered a mucolytic. Dornase alfa p. 292 is the first choice mucolytic. If there is an inadequate response, dornase alfa and hypertonic sodium chloride p. 274, or hypertonic sodium chloride alone should be considered.

Mannitol dry powder for inhalation is recommended as an option when dornase alfa is unsuitable (because of ineligibility, intolerance, or inadequate response), when lung function is rapidly declining, and if other osmotic drugs are not considered appropriate (see Mannitol p. 294 National funding/access decisions). ⟨A⟩

Lumacaftor with ivacaftor is not recommended for treating cystic fibrosis within its marketing authorisation (see Lumacaftor with ivacaftor p. 293 National funding/access decisions).

Pulmonary infection

Staphylococcus aureus

[EvGr] Patients who are not taking prophylaxis and have a new *Staphylococcus aureus* infection can be given an oral anti-

Staph. aureus antibacterial, if they are clinically well. If they are clinically unwell and have pulmonary disease, oral or intravenous (depending on infection severity) broad-spectrum antibacterials with activity against *Staph. aureus* should be given (consult local protocol).

A long-term antibacterial should be considered to suppress **chronic** *Staph. aureus* respiratory infections in patients whose pulmonary disease is stable. In patients with chronic *Staph. aureus* respiratory infections who become clinically unwell with pulmonary disease, oral or intravenous (depending on infection severity) broad-spectrum antibacterials with activity against *Staph. aureus* should be given. In those patients with new evidence of **meticillin-resistant *Staphylococcus aureus* (MRSA)** respiratory infection (with or without pulmonary exacerbation), specialist microbiological advice should be sought.

Antibacterials should not be routinely used to suppress chronic MRSA in patients with stable pulmonary disease.

If a patient with cystic fibrosis and chronic MRSA respiratory infection becomes unwell with a pulmonary exacerbation or shows a decline in pulmonary function, specialist microbiological advice should be sought. ⟨A⟩

Pseudomonas aeruginosa

[EvGr] If a patient with cystic fibrosis develops a new *Pseudomonas aeruginosa* infection, eradication therapy with a course of oral antibacterial should be started (by intravenous injection, if they are clinically unwell), in combination with an inhaled antibacterial. An extended course of oral and inhaled antibacterial should follow (consult local protocol).

If eradication therapy is not successful, sustained treatment with an inhaled antibacterial should be offered. Nebulised colistimethate sodium p. 546 should be considered as first-line treatment (but see also colistimethate sodium by dry powder inhalation p. 546 National funding/access decisions).

In patients with **chronic** *Ps. aeruginosa* infection (when treatment has not eradicated the infection) who become clinically unwell with pulmonary exacerbations, an oral antibacterial or a combination of two intravenous antibacterial drugs of different classes (depending on infection severity) should be used. Changing antibacterial regimens should be considered to treat exacerbations (consult local protocol).

Nebulised aztreonam p. 532, nebulised tobramycin, or tobramycin dry powder for inhalation (see Tobramycin p. 512 National funding/access decisions) should be considered for those who are deteriorating despite regular inhaled colistimethate sodium p. 546. ⟨A⟩

Burkholderia cepacia **complex**

[EvGr] Patients who develop a new *Burkholderia cepacia* complex infection, should be given eradication therapy with a combination of intravenous antibacterial drugs (specialist microbiological advice should be sought on the choice of antibacterials). ⟨A⟩ There is no evidence to support using antibacterials to suppress **chronic** *Burkholderia cepacia* complex infection in patients with cystic fibrosis who have stable pulmonary status.

[EvGr] Specialist microbiological advice should be sought for patients with chronic *Burkholderia cepacia* complex infection (when treatment has not eradicated the infection) and who become clinically unwell with a pulmonary disease exacerbation.

An inhaled antibacterial should be considered for those who have chronic *Burkholderia cepacia* complex infection and declining pulmonary status; treatment should be stopped if there is no observed benefit. ⟨A⟩

Haemophilus influenzae

[EvGr] *Haemophilus influenzae* infection in the absence of clinical evidence of pulmonary infection should be treated with an appropriate oral antibacterial drug. In those who are unwell with clinical evidence of pulmonary infection, an

3

Respiratory system

appropriate antibacterial should be given by mouth or intravenously depending on the severity of the illness (consult local protocol). ⒶEvGr

Non-tuberculous mycobacteria

EvGr Non-tuberculous mycobacterial eradication therapy should be considered for patients with cystic fibrosis who are clinically unwell and whose pulmonary disease has not responded to other recommended treatments. Specialist microbiological advice should be sought on the choice of antibacterial and on the duration of treatment. Ⓐ

Aspergillus fumigatus complex

EvGr Treatment with an antifungal drug should only be considered to suppress **chronic** Aspergillus fumigatus complex respiratory infection in patients with declining pulmonary status. Specialist microbiological advice should be sought on the choice of antifungal drug. Ⓐ

Unidentified infections

EvGr An oral or intravenous (depending on the exacerbation severity) broad-spectrum antibacterial should be used for patients who have a pulmonary disease exacerbation and no clear cause. If a causative pathogen is identified, an appropriate treatment should be selected (consult local protocol). Ⓐ

Immunomodulatory drugs

EvGr Long-term treatment with azithromycin p. 528 [unlicensed indication], at an immunomodulatory dose, should be offered to patients with deteriorating lung function or repeated pulmonary exacerbations. In those patients with continued deterioration in lung function or continuing pulmonary exacerbations, long-term azithromycin should be discontinued and the use of an oral corticosteroid considered. Ⓐ

Nutrition and exocrine pancreatic insufficiency

EvGr The cystic fibrosis specialist dietitian should offer advice on optimal nutrition.

Pancreatin p. 96 should be offered to patients with exocrine pancreatic insufficiency. Dose should be adjusted as needed to minimise any symptoms or signs of malabsorption (see Exocrine pancreatic insufficiency p. 95). An acid-suppressing drug, such as an H₂ receptor antagonist or a proton pump inhibitor [unlicensed indications] can be considered for patients who have persistent symptoms or signs of malabsorption.

A short-term trial of an appetite stimulant (for example up to 3 months) [unlicensed indication] can be considered in adult patients if attempts to increase calorie intake are not effective. Ⓐ

Distal intestinal obstruction syndrome

EvGr Oral or intravenous fluids should be offered to ensure adequate hydration for patients with distal intestinal obstruction syndrome. Meglumine amidotrizoate with sodium amidotrizoate solution (orally or via an enteral tube) should be considered as first-line treatment for distal intestinal obstruction syndrome. An iso-osmotic polyethylene glycol and electrolyte solution (macrogols) (orally or via an enteral tube) can be considered as a second-line treatment. Surgery is a last resort, if prolonged treatment with a polyethylene glycol solution is not effective. Suspected distal intestinal obstruction syndrome should be managed in a specialist cystic fibrosis centre. Ⓐ

Liver disease

EvGr If liver function blood tests are abnormal in patients with cystic fibrosis, ursodeoxycholic acid p. 89 [unlicensed indication] can be given until liver function is restored. Ⓐ

Bone mineral density

EvGr Patients should be monitored for cystic fibrosis-related low bone mineral density. Ⓐ

Cystic fibrosis-related diabetes

EvGr Patients should be monitored for cystic fibrosis-related diabetes. Ⓐ

Useful Resources

Cystic fibrosis: diagnosis and management. National Institute for Health and Care Excellence. NICE guideline 78. October 2017

www.nice.org.uk/guidance/NG78

MUCOLYTICS

Dornase alfa

(Phosphorylated glycosylated recombinant human deoxyribonuclease 1 (rhDNase))

- **DRUG ACTION** Dornase alfa is a genetically engineered version of a naturally occurring human enzyme which cleaves extracellular deoxyribonucleic acid (DNA).

- **INDICATIONS AND DOSE**

Management of cystic fibrosis patients with a forced vital capacity (FVC) of greater than 40% of predicted to improve pulmonary function
  ▸ BY INHALATION OF NEBULISED SOLUTION
  ▸ Adult: 2500 units once daily, administered by jet nebuliser, patients over 21 years may benefit from twice daily dosage

DOSE EQUIVALENCE AND CONVERSION
  ▸ Dornase alfa 1000 units is equivalent to 1 mg

- **SIDE-EFFECTS** Chest pain · conjunctivitis · dyspepsia · dysphonia · dyspnoea · fever · increased risk of infection · skin reactions

- **PREGNANCY** No evidence of teratogenicity; manufacturer advises use only if potential benefit outweighs risk.

- **BREAST FEEDING** Amount probably too small to be harmful—manufacturer advises caution.

- **DIRECTIONS FOR ADMINISTRATION** Dornase alfa is administered by inhalation using a jet nebuliser, usually once daily at least 1 hour before physiotherapy; however, alternate-day therapy may be as effective as daily treatment.

  For use undiluted with jet nebulisers only; ultrasonic nebulisers are unsuitable.

- **MEDICINAL FORMS**
There can be variation in the licensing of different medicines containing the same drug.
Nebuliser liquid
  ▸ Pulmozyme (Roche Products Ltd)
  Dornase alfa 1 mg per 1 ml Pulmozyme 2.5mg nebuliser liquid 2.5ml ampoules | 30 ampoule PoM £496.43 DT = £496.43

Ivacaftor

22-Mar-2017

- **INDICATIONS AND DOSE**

Cystic fibrosis (specialist use only)
  ▸ BY MOUTH
  ▸ Adult: 150 mg every 12 hours

DOSE ADJUSTMENTS DUE TO INTERACTIONS
  ▸ Manufacturer advises reduce dose to 150 mg twice a week with concurrent use of potent inhibitors of CYP3A4.
  ▸ Manufacturer advises reduce dose to 150 mg once daily with concurrent use of moderate inhibitors of CYP3A4.

- **CONTRA-INDICATIONS** Organ transplantation (no information available)
- **INTERACTIONS** → Appendix 1: ivacaftor

- SIDE-EFFECTS
  - **Common or very common** Breast abnormalities · diarrhoea · dizziness · ear discomfort · headache · hearing impairment · rash · tympanic membrane hyperaemia
  - **Uncommon** Gynaecomastia
- PREGNANCY Manufacturer advises use only if potential benefit outweighs risk—no information available.
- BREAST FEEDING Manufacturer advises use only if potential benefit outweighs risk—no information available.
- HEPATIC IMPAIRMENT
  Dose adjustments Max. 150 mg once daily in moderate impairment; in severe impairment, manufacturer recommends use only if potential benefit outweighs risk— starting dose 150 mg on alternate days, dosing interval adjusted according to clinical response and tolerability.
- RENAL IMPAIRMENT Caution in severe impairment.
- MONITORING REQUIREMENTS Manufacturer advises monitor liver function before treatment, every 3 months during the first year of treatment, then annually thereafter (more frequent monitoring should be considered in patients with a history of transaminase elevations).
- DIRECTIONS FOR ADMINISTRATION Tablets should be taken with fat-containing food.
- PRESCRIBING AND DISPENSING INFORMATION Ivacaftor should be prescribed by a physician experienced in the treatment of cystic fibrosis.
- PATIENT AND CARER ADVICE Patients or carers should be given advice on how to administer ivacaftor tablets.
  Driving and skilled tasks Manufacturer advises that patients and their carers should be counselled on the effects on driving and skilled tasks—increased risk of dizziness.
- NATIONAL FUNDING/ACCESS DECISIONS
  Scottish Medicines Consortium (SMC) Decisions
  The *Scottish Medicines Consortium* has advised (December 2016) that ivacaftor (*Kalydeco®*) is **not** recommended for use within NHS Scotland for the treatment of patients with cystic fibrosis aged 18 years and above who have an R117H mutation in the cystic fibrosis transmembrane conductance regulator (CFTR) gene, as insufficient clinical and economic evidence was submitted.

  All Wales Medicines Strategy Group (AWMSG) Decisions
  The *All Wales Medicines Strategy Group* has advised (October 2017) that ivacaftor (*Kalydeco®*) is recommended for restricted use within NHS Wales for the treatment of adults with cystic fibrosis (CF) who have an R117H mutation in the CF transmembrane conductance regulator (CFTR) gene. This recommendation will apply only when people are treated in line with the relevant Welsh clinical access policy **and** only in circumstances where the approved Wales Patient Access Scheme (WPAS) is utilised or where the list/contract price is equivalent or lower.

- MEDICINAL FORMS
  There can be variation in the licensing of different medicines containing the same drug.
  Tablet
  CAUTIONARY AND ADVISORY LABELS 25
  - Kalydeco (Vertex Pharmaceuticals (UK) Ltd) ▼
    Ivacaftor 150 mg Kalydeco 150mg tablets | 56 tablet [PoM]
    £14,000.00

Lumacaftor with ivacaftor

22-Nov-2016

The properties listed below are those particular to the combination only. For the properties of the components please consider, ivacaftor p. 292.

- INDICATIONS AND DOSE
  Treatment of cystic fibrosis in patients who are homozygous for the F508del mutation in the cystic fibrosis transmembrane conductance regulator (CFTR) gene (under expert supervision)
  - BY MOUTH
  - Adult: 400/250 mg every 12 hours
  DOSE ADJUSTMENTS DUE TO INTERACTIONS
  - Manufacturer advises reduce initial dose to 200/125 mg daily for the first week in those also taking a potent inhibitor of CYP3A4.
  DOSE EQUIVALENCE AND CONVERSION
  - Dose expressed as x/y mg of lumacaftor/ivacaftor.

- CAUTIONS Forced expiratory volume in 1 second (FEV_1) less than 40% of the predicted normal value—additional monitoring required at initiation of treatment · pulmonary exacerbation—no information available
- INTERACTIONS → Appendix 1: ivacaftor · lumacaftor
- SIDE-EFFECTS
  - **Common or very common** Breast abnormalities · diarrhoea · dizziness · ear discomfort · flatulence · headache · hearing impairment · menstrual cycle irregularities · nausea · rash · tympanic membrane hyperaemia · vomiting
  - **Uncommon** Gynaecomastia · hepatic encephalopathy · hepatitis cholestatic · hypertension
  - **Frequency not known** Cataract · chest pain
- BREAST FEEDING Manufacturer advises avoid—present in milk in *animal* studies.
- HEPATIC IMPAIRMENT Manufacturer advises use with caution in severe impairment.
  Dose adjustments Manufacturer advises reduce dose to 400/250 mg in the morning and 200/125 mg in the evening (600/375 mg total daily dose) in moderate impairment; reduce dose to 200/125 mg every 12 hours (400/250 mg total daily dose) in severe impairment.
- PRE-TREATMENT SCREENING If the patient's genotype is unknown, a validated genotyping method should be performed to confirm the presence of the F508del mutation on both alleles of the CFTR gene before starting treatment.
- MONITORING REQUIREMENTS Manufacturer advises monitor blood pressure periodically during treatment.
- DIRECTIONS FOR ADMINISTRATION Tablets should be taken with fat-containing food.
- PATIENT AND CARER ADVICE Patients or carers should be given advice on how to administer tablets.
  Missed doses Manufacturer advises if a dose is more than 6 hours late, the missed dose should not be taken and the next dose should be taken at the normal time.
- NATIONAL FUNDING/ACCESS DECISIONS
  NICE decisions
  - **Lumacaftor with ivacaftor for treating cystic fibrosis homozygous for the F508del mutation (July 2016)** NICE TA398
    Lumacaftor with ivacaftor is **not** recommended, within its marketing authorisation, for treating cystic fibrosis in patients who are homozygous for the F508del mutation in the cystic fibrosis transmembrane conductance regulator (CFTR) gene.
    Patients whose treatment was started before this guidance was published may continue treatment until they (or their carers) and their clinician consider it appropriate to stop.
    www.nice.org.uk/TA398

Respiratory system

3

Scottish Medicines Consortium (SMC) Decisions
The *Scottish Medicines Consortium* has advised (May 2016) that lumacaftor with ivacaftor (*Orkambi*®) is **not** recommended within NHS Scotland for the treatment of cystic fibrosis in patients who are homozygous for the F508del mutation in the cystic fibrosis transmembrane conductance regulator (CFTR) gene.

● MEDICINAL FORMS
There can be variation in the licensing of different medicines containing the same drug.
Tablet
CAUTIONARY AND ADVISORY LABELS 25
EXCIPIENTS: May contain Propylene glycol
▸ Orkambi (Vertex Pharmaceuticals (UK) Ltd) ▼
  Ivacaftor 125 mg, Lumacaftor 200 mg Orkambi 200mg/125mg tablets | 112 tablet [PoM] £8,000.00

Mannitol

● INDICATIONS AND DOSE

Treatment of cystic fibrosis as an add-on therapy to standard care
▸ BY INHALATION OF POWDER
▸ Adult: Maintenance 400 mg twice daily, an initiation dose assessment must be carried out under medical supervision, for details of the initiation dose regimen, consult product literature

● CONTRA-INDICATIONS Bronchial hyperresponsiveness to inhaled mannitol · impaired lung function (forced expiratory volume in 1 second < 30% of predicted) · non-CF bronchiectasis
● CAUTIONS Asthma · haemoptysis
● SIDE-EFFECTS
▸ **Common or very common** Chest discomfort · condition aggravated · cough · haemoptysis · headache · respiratory disorders · throat complaints · vomiting
▸ **Uncommon** Abdominal pain upper · appetite decreased · asthma · burping · cold sweat · cystic fibrosis related diabetes · dehydration · diarrhoea · dizziness · dysphonia · dyspnoea · ear pain · fatigue · fever · gastrointestinal disorders · hypoxia · increased risk of infection · influenza like illness · insomnia · joint disorders · malaise · morbid thoughts · nausea · odynophagia · oral disorders · pain · rhinorrhoea · skin reactions · sputum discolouration · urinary incontinence
● PREGNANCY Manufacturer advises avoid.
● BREAST FEEDING Manufacturer advises avoid.
● PRE-TREATMENT SCREENING Patients must be assessed for bronchial hyperresponsiveness to inhaled mannitol before starting the therapeutic dose regimen; an initiation dose assessment must be carried out under medical supervision—for details of the initiation dose regimen, consult product literature.
● DIRECTIONS FOR ADMINISTRATION The dose should be administered 5–15 minutes after a bronchodilator and before physiotherapy; the second daily dose should be taken 2–3 hours before bedtime.
● PATIENT AND CARER ADVICE Patients or carers should be given advice on how to administer mannitol inhalation powder.
● NATIONAL FUNDING/ACCESS DECISIONS
NICE decisions
▸ **Mannitol dry powder for inhalation for treating cystic fibrosis** (November 2012) NICE TA266
Mannitol dry powder for inhalation is recommended as an option for treating cystic fibrosis in adults:
  ● who cannot use dornase alfa (rhDNase) because of ineligibility, intolerance or inadequate response to dornase alfa (rhDNase), **and**

  ● whose lung function is rapidly declining (forced expiratory volume in 1 second decline greater than 2% annually), **and**
  ● for whom other osmotic agents are not considered appropriate.
  www.nice.org.uk/TA266

Scottish Medicines Consortium (SMC) Decisions
The *Scottish Medicines Consortium*, has advised (November 2013) that mannitol (*Bronchitol*®) is accepted for restricted use within NHS Scotland for the treatment of cystic fibrosis in adults aged 18 years and over as an add-on therapy to best standard of care. Mannitol is restricted to patients who are not currently using dornase alfa due to lack of response, intolerance, or ineligibility and have rapidly declining lung function and in whom other osmotic agents are considered unsuitable.

● MEDICINAL FORMS
There can be variation in the licensing of different medicines containing the same drug.
Inhalation powder
▸ Osmohale (Mawdsley-Brooks & Company Ltd)
  Mannitol 5 mg Osmohale 5mg inhalation powder capsules | 1 capsule [PoM] 🅢
  Mannitol 10 mg Osmohale 10mg inhalation powder capsules | 1 capsule [PoM] 🅢
  Mannitol 20 mg Osmohale 20mg inhalation powder capsules | 1 capsule [PoM] 🅢
  Mannitol 40 mg Osmohale 40mg inhalation powder capsules | 15 capsule [PoM] 🅢
▸ Bronchitol (Chiesi Ltd)
  Mannitol 40 mg Bronchitol 40mg inhalation powder capsules with two devices | 280 capsule [PoM] £231.66
  Bronchitol 40mg inhalation powder capsules with device | 10 capsule [PoM] 🅢

4 Cough and congestion

Aromatic inhalations, cough preparations and systemic nasal decongestants

Aromatic inhalations in adults

Inhalations containing volatile substances such as eucalyptus oil are traditionally used and although the vapour may contain little of the additive it encourages deliberate inspiration of warm moist air which is often comforting in bronchitis; boiling water should not be used owing to the risk of scalding. In practice, inhalations are also used for the relief of nasal obstruction in acute rhinitis or sinusitis.

Cough preparations in adults

Cough suppressants
Cough may be a symptom of an underlying disorder, such as asthma, gastro-oesophageal reflux disease, or rhinitis, which should be addressed before prescribing cough suppressants. Cough may be a side-effect of another drug, such as an ACE inhibitor, or it can be associated with smoking or environmental pollutants. Cough can also have a significant habit component. When there is no identifiable cause, cough suppressants may be useful, for example if sleep is disturbed. They may cause sputum retention and this may be harmful in patients with chronic bronchitis and bronchiectasis.

Codeine phosphate p. 448 may be effective but it is constipating and can cause dependence;
dextromethorphan and pholcodine p. 295 have fewer side-effects.

Sedating antihistamines are used as the cough suppressant component of many compound cough preparations on sale to the public; all tend to cause drowsiness which may reflect their main mode of action.

Palliative care
Diamorphine hydrochloride p. 449 and methadone hydrochloride p. 495 have been used to control distressing cough in terminal lung cancer although morphine p. 456 is now preferred. In other circumstances they are contra-indicated because they induce sputum retention and ventilatory failure as well as causing opioid dependence. Methadone hydrochloride linctus should be avoided because it has a long duration of action and tends to accumulate.

Demulcent and expectorant cough preparations
Demulcent cough preparations contain soothing substances such as syrup or glycerol and some patients believe that such preparations relieve a dry irritating cough. Preparations such as **simple linctus** have the advantage of being harmless and inexpensive; **paediatric simple linctus** is particularly useful in children.

Expectorants are claimed to promote expulsion of bronchial secretions, but there is no evidence that any drug can specifically facilitate expectoration.

Compound preparations are on sale to the public for the treatment of cough and colds but should not be used in children under 6 years; the rationale for some is dubious. Care should be taken to give the correct dose and to not use more than one preparation at a time.

Nasal decongestants, systemic
Nasal decongestants for administration by mouth may not be as effective as preparations for local application but they do not give rise to rebound nasal congestion on withdrawal. Pseudoephedrine hydrochloride p. 1167 is available over the counter; it has few sympathomimetic effects.

Aromatic inhalations in children
The use of strong aromatic decongestants (applied as rubs or to pillows) is not advised for infants under the age of 3 months. Carers of young infants in whom nasal obstruction with mucus is a problem can readily be taught appropriate techniques of suction aspiration but sodium chloride 0.9% p. 1008 given as nasal drops is preferred; administration before feeds may ease feeding difficulties caused by nasal congestion.

Cough preparations in children
The use of over-the-counter cough suppressants containing codeine phosphate should be avoided in children under 12 years and in children of any age known to be CYP2D6 ultra-rapid metabolisers. Cough suppressants containing similar opioid analgesics such as dextromethorphan and pholcodine are not generally recommended in children and should be avoided in children under 6 years.

MHRA/CHM advice (March 2008 and February 2009)
Children under 6 years should not be given over-the-counter cough and cold medicines containing the following ingredients:
- brompheniramine, chlorphenamine maleate p. 283, diphenhydramine, doxylamine, promethazine, or triprolidine (antihistamines);
- dextromethorphan or pholcodine (cough suppressants);
- guaifenesin or ipecacuanha (expectorants);
- Phenylephrine hydrochloride p. 188, pseudoephedrine hydrochloride, ephedrine hydrochloride p. 271, oxymetazoline, or xylometazoline hydrochloride p. 1167 (decongestants).

Over-the-counter cough and cold medicines can be considered for children aged 6–12 years after basic principles of best care have been tried, but treatment should be restricted to five days or less. Children should not be given more than 1 cough or cold preparation at a time because

different brands may contain the same active ingredient; care should be taken to give the correct dose.

COUGH AND COLD PREPARATIONS > COUGH SUPPRESSANTS

Pholcodine

- **INDICATIONS AND DOSE**

Dry cough
▶ BY MOUTH USING LINCTUS
  ▶ Child 6–11 years: 2–5 mg 3–4 times a day
  ▶ Child 12–17 years: 5–10 mg 3–4 times a day
  ▶ Adult: 5–10 mg 3–4 times a day

IMPORTANT SAFETY INFORMATION
MHRA/CHM ADVICE (MARCH 2008 AND FEBRUARY 2009) OVER-THE-COUNTER COUGH AND COLD MEDICINES FOR CHILDREN
Children under 6 years should not be given over-the-counter cough and cold medicines containing pholcodine (cough suppressant).

Over-the-counter cough and cold medicines can be considered for children aged 6–12 years after basic principles of best care have been tried, but treatment should be restricted to 5 days or less. Children should not be given more than 1 cough or cold preparation at a time because different brands may contain the same active ingredient; care should be taken to give the correct dose.

- CONTRA-INDICATIONS Bronchiectasis · bronchiolitis (in children) · chronic bronchitis · chronic obstructive pulmonary disease (in adults) · patients at risk of respiratory failure
- CAUTIONS Asthma · chronic cough · persistent cough · productive cough
- INTERACTIONS → Appendix 1: pholcodine
- SIDE-EFFECTS Agitation · confusion · constipation · dizziness · drowsiness · gastrointestinal disorder · nausea · skin reactions · sputum retention · vomiting
- PREGNANCY Manufacturer advises avoid unless potential benefit outweighs risk.
- BREAST FEEDING Manufacturer advises avoid unless potential benefit outweighs risk—no information available.
- HEPATIC IMPAIRMENT Avoid in hepatic impairment.
- RENAL IMPAIRMENT Use with caution in renal impairment. Avoid in severe renal impairment.
- PRESCRIBING AND DISPENSING INFORMATION Pholcodine is not generally recommended for children.
  Flavours of oral liquid formulations may include orange.
  When prepared extemporaneously, the BP states Pholcodine Linctus, BP consists of pholcodine 5 mg/5 mL in a suitable flavoured vehicle, containing citric acid monohydrate 1% and Pholcodine Linctus, Strong, BP consists of pholcodine 10 mg/5 mL in a suitable flavoured vehicle, containing citric acid monohydrate 2%

- MEDICINAL FORMS
There can be variation in the licensing of different medicines containing the same drug.
Oral solution
▶ Pholcodine (Non-proprietary)
  Pholcodine 1 mg per 1 ml Pholcodine 5mg/5ml linctus | 200 ml [P] £1.23-£1.32 DT = £1.32 [CD5]
  Pholcodine 5mg/5ml linctus sugar free sugar-free | 200 ml [P] £1.34 DT = £1.34 [CD5] sugar-free | 2000 ml [P] £13.40 [CD5]
  Pholcodine 2 mg per 1 ml Pholcodine 10mg/5ml linctus strong sugar free sugar-free | 2000 ml [P] £9.88 DT = £9.88 [CD5]
  Pholcodine 10mg/5ml linctus strong | 200 ml [P] £1.67 [CD5]

- Covonia Dry Cough (Thornton & Ross Ltd)
  Pholcodine 1 mg per 1 ml Covonia Dry Cough Sugar Free Formula 5mg/5ml oral solution sugar-free | 150 ml ℗ £3.30 [CD5]
- Galenphol (Thornton & Ross Ltd)
  Pholcodine 1 mg per 1 ml Galenphol 5mg/5ml linctus sugar-free | 2000 ml ℗ £8.50 [CD5]
  Pholcodine 2 mg per 1 ml Galenphol Strong 10mg/5ml linctus sugar-free | 2000 ml ℗ £9.88 DT = £9.88 [CD5]
- Pavacol-D (Alliance Pharmaceuticals Ltd)
  Pholcodine 1 mg per 1 ml Pavacol-D 5mg/5ml mixture sugar-free | 150 ml ℗ £1.69 [CD5] sugar-free | 300 ml ℗ £2.55 [CD5]

COUGH AND COLD PREPARATIONS > OTHER

Citric acid

(Formulated as Simple Linctus)

- **INDICATIONS AND DOSE**

Cough
▶ BY MOUTH
- Adult: 5 mL 3–4 times a day, this dose is for Simple Linctus, BP (2.5%)

- **PRESCRIBING AND DISPENSING INFORMATION** Flavours of oral liquid formulations may include anise.
  When prepared extemporaneously, the BP states Simple Linctus, BP consists of citric acid monohydrate 2.5%, in a suitable vehicle with an anise flavour.

- **MEDICINAL FORMS**
There can be variation in the licensing of different medicines containing the same drug.
Oral solution
- Citric acid (Non-proprietary)
  Citric acid monohydrate 25 mg per 1 ml Simple linctus sugar free sugar-free | 200 ml [GSL] £1.25 DT = £0.92 sugar-free | 2000 ml [GSL] £9.20
  Simple linctus | 200 ml [GSL] £0.96 DT = £0.93

MENTHOL AND DERIVATIVES

Eucalyptus with menthol

- **INDICATIONS AND DOSE**

Aromatic inhalation for relief of nasal congestion
▶ BY INHALATION
- Adult: Add one teaspoonful to a pint of hot, **not** boiling, water and inhale the vapour

- **PRESCRIBING AND DISPENSING INFORMATION** When prepared extemporaneously, the BP states Menthol and Eucalyptus Inhalation, BP 1980 consists of racementhol or levomenthol 2 g, eucalyptus oil 10 mL, light magnesium carbonate 7 g, water to 100 mL.
- **PROFESSION SPECIFIC INFORMATION**

Dental practitioners' formulary
Menthol and Eucalyptus Inhalation BP, 1980 may be prescribed.

- **MEDICINAL FORMS**
There can be variation in the licensing of different medicines containing the same drug.
Inhalation vapour
- Eucalyptus with menthol (Non-proprietary)
  Menthol 20 mg per 1 ml, Magnesium carbonate light 70 mg per 1 ml, Eucalyptus oil 100 microlitre per 1 ml Menthol and Eucalyptus inhalation | 100 ml [GSL] £1.38–£1.39 DT = £1.38

RESINS

Benzoin tincture

(Friars' Balsam)

- **INDICATIONS AND DOSE**

Aromatic inhalation for relief of nasal congestion
▶ BY INHALATION
- Child: Add 5 mL to a pint of hot, **not** boiling, water and inhale the vapour; repeat after 4 hours if necessary
- Adult: Add 5 mL to a pint of hot, **not** boiling, water and inhale the vapour; repeat after 4 hours if necessary

- **SIDE-EFFECTS** Skin sensitisation
- **PRESCRIBING AND DISPENSING INFORMATION** Not recommended (applied as a rub or to pillows) for infants under 3 months.
  When prepared extemporaneously, the BP states Benzoin Tincture, Compound, BP consists of balsamic acids approx. 4.5%.

- **MEDICINAL FORMS**
There can be variation in the licensing of different medicines containing the same drug.
Liquid
CAUTIONARY AND ADVISORY LABELS 15
- Benzoin tincture (Non-proprietary)
  Balsamic acids 16.5 mg per 1 ml Benzoin tincture | 500 ml [GSL] £9.95 DT = £9.95

5 Idiopathic pulmonary fibrosis

Other drugs used for Idiopathic pulmonary fibrosis
Nintedanib, p. 960

ANTIFIBROTICS

Pirfenidone

06-Jul-2017

- **DRUG ACTION** The exact mechanism of action of pirfenidone is not yet understood, but it is believed to slow down the progression of idiopathic pulmonary fibrosis by exerting both antifibrotic and anti-inflammatory properties.

- **INDICATIONS AND DOSE**

Treatment of mild to moderate idiopathic pulmonary fibrosis (initiated under specialist supervision)
▶ BY MOUTH
- Adult: Initially 267 mg 3 times a day for 7 days, then increased to 534 mg 3 times a day for 7 days, then increased to 801 mg 3 times a day
DOSE ADJUSTMENTS DUE TO INTERACTIONS
- Caution with concomitant use with ciprofloxacin—reduce dose of pirfenidone to 534 mg three times daily with high-dose ciprofloxacin (750 mg twice daily).

- **CONTRA-INDICATIONS** Cigarette smoking
- **CAUTIONS**
CAUTIONS, FURTHER INFORMATION
- Photosensitivity Avoid exposure to direct sunlight—if photosensitivity reaction or rash occurs, dose adjustment or treatment interruption may be required (consult product literature).
- Treatment interruption If treatment is interrupted for 14 consecutive days or more, the initial 2 week titration regimen should be repeated; if treatment is interrupted for

less than 14 consecutive days, the dose can be resumed at the previous daily dose without titration.

● INTERACTIONS → Appendix 1: pirfenidone

● SIDE-EFFECTS

▶ **Common or very common** Appetite decreased · arthralgia · asthenia · constipation · cough · diarrhoea · dizziness · drowsiness · dyspnoea · gastrointestinal discomfort · gastrointestinal disorders · headache · hot flush · increased risk of infection · insomnia · musculoskeletal chest pain · myalgia · nausea · photosensitivity reaction · skin reactions · sunburn · taste altered · vomiting · weight decreased

▶ **Uncommon** Angioedema

▶ **Rare or very rare** Agranulocytosis

SIDE-EFFECTS, FURTHER INFORMATION Gastrointestinal side-effects may require dose reduction or treatment interruption—consult product literature.

● PREGNANCY Manufacturer advises avoid—no information available.

● BREAST FEEDING Manufacturer advises avoid—no information available.

● HEPATIC IMPAIRMENT Use with caution in mild to moderate hepatic impairment, particularly if concomitant use of CYP1A2 inhibitors. Avoid use in severe hepatic impairment.

● RENAL IMPAIRMENT Avoid use if eGFR less than 30 mL/minute/1.73 m^2.

● MONITORING REQUIREMENTS

▶ Monitor for weight loss.

▶ Test liver function before treatment, then at monthly intervals for the next 6 months, and then every 3 months thereafter; review if abnormal liver function tests—dose reduction, treatment interruption or discontinuation may be required (consult product literature).

● PATIENT AND CARER ADVICE

Driving and skilled tasks Dizziness or malaise may affect performance of skilled tasks (e.g. driving).

● NATIONAL FUNDING/ACCESS DECISIONS

NICE decisions

▶ **Pirfenidone for treating idiopathic pulmonary fibrosis (February 2018) NICE TA504**

Pirfenidone is recommended as an option for treating idiopathic pulmonary fibrosis in adults only if:

● the patient has a forced vital capacity (FVC) between 50% and 80% predicted, **and**

● the manufacturer provides pirfenidone with the discount agreed in the patient access scheme, **and**

● treatment is stopped if there is evidence of disease progression (an absolute decline of 10% or more in predicted FVC within any 12-month period).

Patients whose treatment was started within the NHS before this guidance was published should have the option to continue treatment, without change to their funding arrangements, until they and their NHS clinician consider it appropriate to stop.

www.nice.org.uk/guidance/ta504

Scottish Medicines Consortium (SMC) Decisions

The *Scottish Medicines Consortium* has advised (August 2013) that pirfenidone is accepted for restricted use within NHS Scotland for the treatment of mild to moderate idiopathic pulmonary fibrosis. Pirfenidone is restricted for use in patients with a predicted forced vital capacity less than or equal to 80%, and only whilst pirfenidone is available at the price agreed in the patient access scheme.

● MEDICINAL FORMS
There can be variation in the licensing of different medicines containing the same drug.

Tablet

▶ Esbriet (Roche Products Ltd) ▼
    Pirfenidone 267 mg Esbriet 267mg tablets | 63 tablet [PoM]
£501.92 | 252 tablet [PoM] £2,007.70
    Pirfenidone 801 mg Esbriet 801mg tablets | 84 tablet [PoM]
£2,007.70

Capsule

CAUTIONARY AND ADVISORY LABELS 21, 25, 11

▶ Esbriet (Roche Products Ltd) ▼
    Pirfenidone 267 mg Esbriet 267mg capsules | 63 capsule [PoM]
£501.92 | 252 capsule [PoM] £2,007.70 | 270 capsule [PoM]
£2,151.10

6   Respiratory depression, respiratory distress syndrome and apnoea

Respiratory stimulants

Overview

Respiratory stimulants (analeptic drugs) have a limited place in the treatment of ventilatory failure in patients with chronic obstructive pulmonary disease. They are effective only when given by intravenous injection or infusion and have a short duration of action. Their use has largely been replaced by ventilatory support including nasal intermittent positive pressure ventilation. However, occasionally when ventilatory support is contra-indicated and in patients with hypercapnic respiratory failure who are becoming drowsy or comatose, respiratory stimulants in the short term may arouse patients sufficiently to co-operate and clear their secretions.

Respiratory stimulants can also be harmful in respiratory failure since they stimulate non-respiratory as well as respiratory muscles. They should only be given under **expert supervision** in hospital and must be combined with active physiotherapy. There is at present no oral respiratory stimulant available for long-term use in chronic respiratory failure.

RESPIRATORY STIMULANTS

Doxapram hydrochloride

● INDICATIONS AND DOSE

Postoperative respiratory depression

▶ INITIALLY BY INTRAVENOUS INJECTION

▶ Adult: Initially 1–1.5 mg/kg, to be administered over at least 30 seconds, repeated if necessary after intervals of one hour, alternatively (by intravenous infusion) 2–3 mg/minute, adjusted according to response

Acute respiratory failure

▶ BY INTRAVENOUS INFUSION

▶ Adult: 1.5–4 mg/minute, adjusted according to response, to be given concurrently with oxygen and whenever possible monitor with frequent measurement of blood gas tensions

● CONTRA-INDICATIONS Cerebral oedema · cerebrovascular accident · coronary artery disease · epilepsy and other convulsive disorders · hyperthyroidism · physical obstruction of respiratory tract · severe hypertension · status asthmaticus

● CAUTIONS Give with beta$_2$ agonist in bronchoconstriction · give with oxygen in severe irreversible airways obstruction or severely decreased lung compliance (because of increased work load of breathing) · hypertension · impaired cardiac reserve · phaeochromocytoma

● INTERACTIONS → Appendix 1: doxapram

● SIDE-EFFECTS Arrhythmias · chest discomfort · confusion · cough · dizziness · dyspnoea · fever · flushing · hallucination · headache · hyperhidrosis · movement disorders · nausea · neuromuscular dysfunction · oral disorders · perineal warmth · reflexes abnormal · respiratory disorders · seizure · urinary disorders · vomiting

● PREGNANCY No evidence of harm, but manufacturer advises avoid unless benefit outweighs risk.

● HEPATIC IMPAIRMENT Use with caution.

● MONITORING REQUIREMENTS Frequent arterial blood gas and pH measurements are necessary during treatment to ensure correct dosage.

● MEDICINAL FORMS
There can be variation in the licensing of different medicines containing the same drug.

Solution for injection
▶ Doxapram hydrochloride (Non-proprietary)
  Doxapram hydrochloride 20 mg per 1 ml Doxapram 100mg/5ml solution for injection ampoules | 5 ampoule [PoM] £110.00

Infusion
▶ Doxapram hydrochloride (Non-proprietary)
  Doxapram hydrochloride 2 mg per 1 ml Doxapram 1g/500ml infusion bags | 1 bag [PoM] [Ⓢ]

Chapter 4
Nervous system

CONTENTS

1 Dementia

Dementia
27-Sep-2016

Description of condition

Dementia is a progressive and largely irreversible clinical syndrome that is characterised by a widespread impairment of mental function. There are a number of conditions that cause the symptoms of dementia. Alzheimer's disease accounts for most cases; other common causes include vascular dementia (due to cerebrovascular disease) and dementia with Lewy bodies. The symptoms of dementia include cognitive dysfunction (such as problems with memory, concentration and problem-solving), non-cognitive symptoms (such as psychiatric and behavioural problems) and difficulties with activities of daily living.

Aims of treatment

The aims of treatment are to promote independence, maintain function and treat symptoms.

Non-drug treatment

EvGr Patients with all types of *mild-to-moderate* dementia presenting with **cognitive symptoms** should be given the opportunity to participate in a structured group cognitive stimulation programme. Ⓐ

Drug treatment

Management of cognitive symptoms

EvGr When pharmacological treatments are used, they should be initiated and supervised by a specialist experienced in the management of dementia. Ⓐ The manufacturers of donepezil hydrochloride p. 300, galantamine p. 301, rivastigmine p. 302 and memantine hydrochloride p. 303 recommend that treatment should be reassessed on a regular basis.

EvGr Treatment should be continued only when it is considered to be having a worthwhile effect on symptoms.

Donepezil hydrochloride, galantamine and rivastigmine (acetylcholinesterase inhibitors) are recommended for the treatment of cognitive symptoms of *mild-to-moderate* dementia due to Alzheimer's disease. Memantine hydrochloride is a suitable alternative for patients with *moderate* Alzheimer's disease when acetylcholinesterase inhibitors are contra-indicated or are not tolerated. Memantine hydrochloride is the drug of choice for patients with *severe* Alzheimer's disease.

Pharmacological treatments are **not** recommended for the treatment of cognitive symptoms in cases of vascular dementia. Ⓐ

Management of non-cognitive symptoms

EvGr Patients with dementia who develop non-cognitive symptoms (such as delusions or anxiety) or 'behaviour that challenges' (such as aggression or agitation) should only be offered a pharmacological intervention if they are severely distressed or if there is an immediate risk of harm to the patient or others. Less severe non-cognitive symptoms are treated with non-pharmacological interventions, such as multisensory stimulation or aromatherapy. Ⓐ

Antipsychotic drugs

EvGr Patients with *mild-to-moderate* non-cognitive symptoms due to Alzheimer's disease, vascular dementia, mixed dementias or dementia with Lewy bodies should **not** be prescribed antipsychotic drugs.

Patients with *severe* non-cognitive symptoms due to Alzheimer's disease, vascular dementia, mixed dementias or dementia with Lewy bodies which are causing significant distress can be offered treatment with an antipsychotic drug (see *Antipsychotic drugs* under Psychoses and related disorders p. 377). Careful consideration should be given to the patient's co-morbid conditions and the benefits and risks of treatment. Ⓐ The MHRA has reported (2009) a clear increased risk of stroke and a small increased risk of death when antipsychotic drugs are used in elderly patients with dementia. The balance of risks and benefits should be carefully assessed, including any previous history of stroke or transient ischaemic attack and any risk factors for cerebrovascular disease including hypertension, diabetes, smoking and atrial fibrillation.

EvGr Treatment with antipsychotic drugs should be started with a low dose and titrated upwards, with regular review. In patients who have dementia with Lewy bodies, careful monitoring for severe untoward reactions, such as neuroleptic sensitivity reactions, is recommended. Ⓐ

Acetylcholinesterase inhibitors and memantine

[EvGr] An acetylcholinesterase inhibitor may be used to manage non-cognitive symptoms in patients with *mild-to-moderate* dementia due to Alzheimer's disease, if a non-pharmacological approach or an antipsychotic drug is inappropriate or ineffective.

Memantine hydrochloride may be considered in patients with *severe* symptoms, if a non-pharmacological approach or an antipsychotic drug is inappropriate or ineffective. Memantine hydrochloride may also be used in patients with *moderate* symptoms in whom acetylcholinesterase inhibitors are contra-indicated.

Patients who have dementia with Lewy bodies should be offered an acetylcholinesterase inhibitor for the treatment of non-cognitive symptoms. Acetylcholinesterase inhibitors are **not** recommended in patients with vascular dementia. Ⓐ

Management of violence, aggression, and extreme agitation

[EvGr] In cases of dementia associated with *severe* behavioural disturbance that requires urgent treatment (if violence, aggression and extreme agitation threaten the safety of the patient or others), an antipsychotic drug or a benzodiazepine may be given (see *Antipsychotic drugs* under Psychoses and related disorders p. 377; see *Benzodiazepines* under Hypnotics and anxiolytics p. 477). High doses or combinations of drugs should be avoided, and the lowest effective dose should be used. Oral treatment should be offered before parenteral administration. If intramuscular administration is needed for behavioural control, lorazepam p. 335, haloperidol p. 382 or olanzapine p. 394 should be used. Diazepam and chlorpromazine hydrochloride are **not** recommended. Intravenous administration should be used only in exceptional circumstances. Ⓐ

Useful Resources

Dementia: supporting people with dementia and their carers in health and social care. National Institute for Health and Care Excellence. Clinical guideline 42. November 2006 (updated May 2016).
www.nice.org.uk/guidance/CG42/

Other drugs used for Dementia Risperidone, p. 398

ANTICHOLINESTERASES › CENTRALLY ACTING

Donepezil hydrochloride
26-Sep-2016

● **DRUG ACTION** Donepezil is a reversible inhibitor of acetylcholinesterase.

● **INDICATIONS AND DOSE**

Mild to moderate dementia in Alzheimer's disease

▸ BY MOUTH
▸ Adult: Initially 5 mg once daily for one month, then increased if necessary up to 10 mg daily, doses to be given at bedtime

● **CAUTIONS** Asthma · chronic obstructive pulmonary disease · sick sinus syndrome · supraventricular conduction abnormalities · susceptibility to peptic ulcers

● **INTERACTIONS** → Appendix 1: anticholinesterases, centrally acting

● **SIDE-EFFECTS**
▸ **Common or very common** Aggression · agitation · appetite decreased · common cold · diarrhoea · dizziness · fatigue · gastrointestinal disorders · hallucination · headache · injury · muscle cramps · nausea · pain · skin reactions · sleep disorders · syncope · urinary incontinence · vomiting
▸ **Uncommon** Bradycardia · gastrointestinal haemorrhage · hypersalivation · seizure

▸ **Rare or very rare** Cardiac conduction disorders · extrapyramidal symptoms · hepatic disorders · neuroleptic malignant syndrome · rhabdomyolysis

SIDE-EFFECTS, FURTHER INFORMATION Dose should be started low and increased if tolerated and necessary.

● **HEPATIC IMPAIRMENT** Caution in mild to moderate impairment. No information available for severe impairment.

● **DIRECTIONS FOR ADMINISTRATION** Donepezil orodispersible tablet should be placed on the tongue, allowed to disperse, and swallowed.

● **PATIENT AND CARER ADVICE** Patient or carers should be given advice on how to administer donepezil hydrochloride orodispersible tablets.

● **NATIONAL FUNDING/ACCESS DECISIONS**

NICE decisions
▸ **Donepezil, galantamine, rivastigmine, and memantine for the treatment of Alzheimer's disease—updated May 2016**
NICE TA217
Donepezil can be used for the treatment of mild to moderate Alzheimer's disease. Treatment should only be prescribed under the following conditions:
● treatment should be initiated on the advice of a specialist
● ensure that local arrangements for prescribing, supply and treatment review follow the NICE guideline on medicines optimisation
● treatment should continue only if it is considered to have a worthwhile effect on cognitive, global, functional, or behavioural symptoms.
Healthcare professionals should not rely solely on assessment scales to determine the severity of Alzheimer's disease when the patient has learning or other disabilities, or other communication difficulties.
www.nice.org.uk/TA217

● MEDICINAL FORMS
There can be variation in the licensing of different medicines containing the same drug. Forms available from special-order manufacturers include: oral suspension

Oral solution
▸ Donepezil hydrochloride (Non-proprietary)
Donepezil hydrochloride 1 mg per 1 ml Donepezil 1mg/ml oral solution sugar free sugar-free | 150 ml [PoM] £48.00 DT = £48.00

Orodispersible tablet
▸ Donepezil hydrochloride (Non-proprietary)
Donepezil hydrochloride 5 mg Donepezil 5mg orodispersible tablets | 28 tablet [PoM] £59.85
Donepezil 5mg orodispersible tablets sugar free sugar-free | 28 tablet [PoM] £6.27–£50.87 DT = £7.12
Donepezil hydrochloride 10 mg Donepezil 10mg orodispersible tablets sugar free sugar-free | 28 tablet [PoM] £7.95–£71.31 DT = £8.44
Donepezil 10mg orodispersible tablets | 28 tablet [PoM] £83.89
▸ Aricept Evess (Eisai Ltd)
Donepezil hydrochloride 5 mg Aricept Evess 5mg orodispersible tablets sugar-free | 28 tablet [PoM] £59.85 DT = £7.12
Donepezil hydrochloride 10 mg Aricept Evess 10mg orodispersible tablets sugar-free | 28 tablet [PoM] £83.89 DT = £8.44

Tablet
▸ Donepezil hydrochloride (Non-proprietary)
Donepezil hydrochloride 5 mg Donepezil 5mg tablets | 28 tablet [PoM] £59.85 DT = £0.52
Donepezil hydrochloride 10 mg Donepezil 10mg tablets | 28 tablet [PoM] £83.89 DT = £0.76
▸ Aricept (Eisai Ltd)
Donepezil hydrochloride 5 mg Aricept 5mg tablets | 28 tablet [PoM] £59.85 DT = £0.52
Donepezil hydrochloride 10 mg Aricept 10mg tablets | 28 tablet [PoM] £83.89 DT = £0.76

Galantamine

26-Sep-2016

- **DRUG ACTION** Galantamine is a reversible inhibitor of acetylcholinesterase and it also has nicotinic receptor agonist properties.

- ### INDICATIONS AND DOSE

Mild to moderately severe dementia in Alzheimer's disease

▸ BY MOUTH USING IMMEDIATE-RELEASE MEDICINES
▹ Adult: Initially 4 mg twice daily for 4 weeks, increased to 8 mg twice daily for at least 4 weeks; maintenance 8–12 mg twice daily

▸ BY MOUTH USING MODIFIED-RELEASE CAPSULES
▹ Adult: Initially 8 mg once daily for 4 weeks, increased to 16 mg once daily for at least 4 weeks; maintenance 16–24 mg daily

- **CAUTIONS** Avoid in gastro-intestinal obstruction · avoid in urinary outflow obstruction · avoid whilst recovering from bladder surgery · avoid whilst recovering from gastro-intestinal surgery · cardiac disease · chronic obstructive pulmonary disease · congestive heart failure · electrolyte disturbances · history of seizures · history of severe asthma · pulmonary infection · sick sinus syndrome · supraventricular conduction abnormalities · susceptibility to peptic ulcers · unstable angina

- **INTERACTIONS** → Appendix 1: anticholinesterases, centrally acting

- **SIDE-EFFECTS**

▸ **Common or very common** Appetite decreased · arrhythmias · asthenia · depression · diarrhoea · dizziness · drowsiness · fall · gastrointestinal discomfort · hallucinations · headache · hypertension · malaise · muscle spasms · nausea · skin reactions · syncope · tremor · vomiting · weight decreased

▸ **Uncommon** Atrioventricular block · dehydration · flushing · hyperhidrosis · hypersomnia · hypotension · muscle weakness · palpitations · paraesthesia · seizure · taste altered · tinnitus · vision blurred

▸ **Rare or very rare** Hepatitis · severe cutaneous adverse reactions (SCARs)

SIDE-EFFECTS, FURTHER INFORMATION Manufacturer advises increasing dose according to response and tolerability.
Serious skin reactions Serious skin reactions (including Stevens-Johnson syndrome and acute generalized exanthematous pustulosis) have been reported—manufacturer advises discontinue at the first appearance of skin rash.

- **PREGNANCY** Use with caution—toxicity in *animal* studies.

- **BREAST FEEDING** Avoid—no information available.

- **HEPATIC IMPAIRMENT**
Dose adjustments For *immediate-release* preparations in moderate impairment, initially 4 mg once daily (preferably in the morning) for at least 7 days, then 4 mg twice daily for at least 4 weeks; max. 8 mg twice daily; avoid in severe impairment.
For *modified-release* preparations in moderate impairment, initially 8 mg on alternate days (preferably in the morning) for 7 days, then 8 mg once daily for 4 weeks; max. 16 mg daily; avoid in severe impairment.

- **RENAL IMPAIRMENT** Avoid if eGFR less than 9 mL/minute/1.73 m².

- **PATIENT AND CARER ADVICE** Manufacturer recommends that patients are warned of the signs of serious skin reactions; they should be advised to stop taking galantamine immediately and seek medical advice if symptoms occur.

- **NATIONAL FUNDING/ACCESS DECISIONS**

NICE decisions

▸ **Donepezil, galantamine, rivastigmine, and memantine for the treatment of Alzheimer's disease—updated May 2016**
NICE TA217
Galantamine can be used for the treatment of mild to moderate Alzheimer's disease. Treatment should only be prescribed under the following conditions:
- treatment should be initiated on the advice of a specialist
- ensure that local arrangements for prescribing, supply and treatment review follow the NICE guideline on medicines optimisation
- treatment should continue only if it is considered to have a worthwhile effect on cognitive, global, functional, or behavioural symptoms.
Healthcare professionals should not rely solely on assessment scales to determine the severity of Alzheimer's disease when the patient has learning or other disabilities, or other communication difficulties.
www.nice.org.uk/TA217

- **MEDICINAL FORMS**
There can be variation in the licensing of different medicines containing the same drug. Forms available from special-order manufacturers include: tablet

Oral solution
CAUTIONARY AND ADVISORY LABELS 3, 21
▹ Galantamine (Non-proprietary)
Galantamine (as Galantamine hydrobromide) 4 mg per 1 ml Galantamine 20mg/5ml oral solution sugar free sugar-free | 100 ml PoM £120.00 DT = £120.00
▹ Galzemic (Creo Pharma Ltd)
Galantamine (as Galantamine hydrobromide) 4 mg per 1 ml Galzemic 4mg/ml oral solution sugar-free | 100 ml PoM £90.00 DT = £120.00
▹ Reminyl (Shire Pharmaceuticals Ltd)
Galantamine (as Galantamine hydrobromide) 4 mg per 1 ml Reminyl 4mg/ml oral solution sugar-free | 100 ml PoM £120.00 DT = £120.00

Modified-release capsule
CAUTIONARY AND ADVISORY LABELS 3, 21, 25
▹ Acumor XL (Mylan)
Galantamine (as Galantamine hydrobromide) 8 mg Acumor XL 8mg capsules | 28 capsule PoM £49.26 DT = £51.88
Galantamine (as Galantamine hydrobromide) 16 mg Acumor XL 16mg capsules | 28 capsule PoM £61.65 DT = £64.90
Galantamine (as Galantamine hydrobromide) 24 mg Acumor XL 24mg capsules | 28 capsule PoM £75.81 DT = £79.80
▹ Consion XL (Dr. Reddy's Laboratories (UK) Ltd)
Galantamine (as Galantamine hydrobromide) 8 mg Consion XL 8mg capsules | 28 capsule PoM £25.94 DT = £51.88
Galantamine (as Galantamine hydrobromide) 16 mg Consion XL 16mg capsules | 28 capsule PoM £32.45 DT = £64.90
Galantamine (as Galantamine hydrobromide) 24 mg Consion XL 24mg capsules | 28 capsule PoM £39.90 DT = £79.80
▹ Elmino (Zentiva)
Galantamine (as Galantamine hydrobromide) 8 mg Elmino XL 8mg capsules | 28 capsule PoM £51.88 DT = £51.88
Galantamine (as Galantamine hydrobromide) 16 mg Elmino XL 16mg capsules | 28 capsule PoM £64.90 DT = £64.90
Galantamine (as Galantamine hydrobromide) 24 mg Elmino XL 24mg capsules | 28 capsule PoM £79.80 DT = £79.80
▹ Galantex XL (Creo Pharma Ltd)
Galantamine (as Galantamine hydrobromide) 8 mg Galzemic XL 8mg capsules | 28 capsule PoM £19.05 DT = £51.88
Galantamine (as Galantamine hydrobromide) 16 mg Galzemic XL 16mg capsules | 28 capsule PoM £23.84 DT = £64.90
Galantamine (as Galantamine hydrobromide) 24 mg Galzemic XL 24mg capsules | 28 capsule PoM £29.32 DT = £79.80
▹ Galsya XL (Consilient Health Ltd)
Galantamine (as Galantamine hydrobromide) 8 mg Galsya XL 8mg capsules | 28 capsule PoM £44.09 DT = £51.88
Galantamine (as Galantamine hydrobromide) 16 mg Galsya XL 16mg capsules | 28 capsule PoM £55.16 DT = £64.90
Galantamine (as Galantamine hydrobromide) 24 mg Galsya XL 24mg capsules | 28 capsule PoM £67.83 DT = £79.80

▶ Gatalin XL (Aspire Pharma Ltd)
Galantamine (as Galantamine hydrobromide) 8 mg Gatalin XL
8mg capsules | 28 capsule [PoM] £25.94 DT = £51.88
Galantamine (as Galantamine hydrobromide) 16 mg Gatalin XL
16mg capsules | 28 capsule [PoM] £32.45 DT = £64.90
Galantamine (as Galantamine hydrobromide) 24 mg Gatalin XL
24mg capsules | 28 capsule [PoM] £39.90 DT = £79.80

▶ Gazylan XL (Teva UK Ltd)
Galantamine (as Galantamine hydrobromide) 8 mg Gazylan XL
8mg capsules | 28 capsule [PoM] £19.04 DT = £51.88
Galantamine (as Galantamine hydrobromide) 16 mg Gazylan XL
16mg capsules | 28 capsule [PoM] £23.83 DT = £64.90
Galantamine (as Galantamine hydrobromide) 24 mg Gazylan XL
24mg capsules | 28 capsule [PoM] £29.31 DT = £79.80

▶ Lotprosin XL (Actavis UK Ltd)
Galantamine (as Galantamine hydrobromide) 8 mg Lotprosin XL
8mg capsules | 28 capsule [PoM] £51.88 DT = £51.88
Galantamine (as Galantamine hydrobromide) 16 mg Lotprosin XL
16mg capsules | 28 capsule [PoM] £64.90 DT = £64.90
Galantamine (as Galantamine hydrobromide) 24 mg Lotprosin XL
24mg capsules | 28 capsule [PoM] £79.80 DT = £79.80

▶ Luventa XL (Fontus Health Ltd)
Galantamine (as Galantamine hydrobromide) 8 mg Luventa XL
8mg capsules | 28 capsule [PoM] £25.42 DT = £51.88
Galantamine (as Galantamine hydrobromide) 16 mg Luventa XL
16mg capsules | 28 capsule [PoM] £31.80 DT = £64.90
Galantamine (as Galantamine hydrobromide) 24 mg Luventa XL
24mg capsules | 28 capsule [PoM] £39.10 DT = £79.80

▶ Reminyl XL (Shire Pharmaceuticals Ltd)
Galantamine (as Galantamine hydrobromide) 8 mg Reminyl XL
8mg capsules | 28 capsule [PoM] £51.88 DT = £51.88
Galantamine (as Galantamine hydrobromide) 16 mg Reminyl XL
16mg capsules | 28 capsule [PoM] £64.90 DT = £64.90
Galantamine (as Galantamine hydrobromide) 24 mg Reminyl XL
24mg capsules | 28 capsule [PoM] £79.80 DT = £79.80

Tablet
CAUTIONARY AND ADVISORY LABELS 3, 21
▶ Galantamine (Non-proprietary)
Galantamine (as Galantamine hydrobromide) 8 mg Galantamine
8mg tablets | 56 tablet [PoM] £59.25–£64.90 DT = £61.13
Galantamine (as Galantamine hydrobromide) 12 mg Galantamine
12mg tablets | 56 tablet [PoM] £71.25–£79.80 DT = £74.10
▶ Reminyl (Shire Pharmaceuticals Ltd)
Galantamine (as Galantamine hydrobromide) 8 mg Reminyl 8mg
tablets | 56 tablet [PoM] £68.32 DT = £61.13
Galantamine (as Galantamine hydrobromide) 12 mg Reminyl
12mg tablets | 56 tablet [PoM] £84.00 DT = £74.10

Rivastigmine

26-Sep-2016

● DRUG ACTION Rivastigmine is a reversible non-competitive inhibitor of acetylcholinesterases.

● INDICATIONS AND DOSE
Mild to moderate dementia in Alzheimer's disease
▶ BY MOUTH
▶ Adult: Initially 1.5 mg twice daily, increased in steps of 1.5 mg twice daily, dose to be increased at intervals of at least 2 weeks according to response and tolerance; usual dose 3–6 mg twice daily (max. per dose 6 mg twice daily), if treatment interrupted for more than several days, retitrate from 1.5 mg twice daily
▶ BY TRANSDERMAL APPLICATION USING PATCHES
▶ Adult: Apply 4.6 mg/24 hours daily for at least 4 weeks, increased if tolerated to 9.5 mg/24 hours daily for a further 6 months, then increased if necessary to 13.3 mg/24 hours daily, increase to 13.3 mg/24 hours patch if well tolerated and cognitive deterioration or functional decline demonstrated; use caution in patients with body-weight less than 50 kg, if treatment interrupted for more than 3 days, retitrate from 4.6 mg/24 hours patch

Mild to moderate dementia in Parkinson's disease
▶ BY MOUTH
▶ Adult: Initially 1.5 mg twice daily, increased in steps of 1.5 mg twice daily, dose to be increased at intervals of at least 2 weeks according to response and tolerance; usual dose 3–6 mg twice daily (max. per dose 6 mg twice daily), if treatment interrupted for more than several days, retitrate from 1.5 mg twice daily
DOSE EQUIVALENCE AND CONVERSION
▶ When switching from oral to transdermal therapy, patients taking 3–6 mg by mouth daily should initially switch to 4.6 mg/24 hours patch, then titrate as above. Patients taking 9 mg by mouth daily should switch to 9.5 mg/24 hours patch if oral dose stable and well tolerated; if oral dose not stable or well tolerated, patients should switch to 4.6 mg/24 hours patch, then titrate as above. Patients taking 12 mg by mouth daily should switch to 9.5 mg/24 hours patch. The first patch should be applied on the day following the last oral dose

● CAUTIONS Bladder outflow obstruction · conduction abnormalities · duodenal ulcers · gastric ulcers · history of asthma · history of chronic obstructive pulmonary disease · history of seizures · risk of fatal overdose with patch administration errors · sick sinus syndrome · susceptibility to ulcers

● INTERACTIONS → Appendix 1: anticholinesterases, centrally acting

● SIDE-EFFECTS
GENERAL SIDE-EFFECTS
▶ **Common or very common** Anxiety · appetite decreased · arrhythmias · asthenia · dehydration · depression · diarrhoea · dizziness · drowsiness · fall · gastrointestinal discomfort · headache · hyperhidrosis · hypersalivation · hypertension · movement disorders · nausea · skin reactions · syncope · tremor · urinary incontinence · urinary tract infection · vomiting · weight decreased
▶ **Uncommon** Aggression · atrioventricular block
▶ **Rare or very rare** Pancreatitis · seizure
▶ **Frequency not known** Hepatitis
SPECIFIC SIDE-EFFECTS
▶ **Common or very common**
▶ With oral use Confusion · gait abnormal · hallucinations · malaise · parkinsonism · sleep disorders
▶ **Uncommon**
▶ With oral use Hypotension
▶ With transdermal use Gastric ulcer
▶ **Rare or very rare**
▶ With oral use Angina pectoris · gastrointestinal disorders · gastrointestinal haemorrhage
▶ **Frequency not known**
▶ With transdermal use Hallucination · nightmare
SIDE-EFFECTS, FURTHER INFORMATION Dose should be started low and increased according to response if tolerated.
  Treatment should be interrupted if dehydration resulting from prolonged vomiting or diarrhoea occurs and withheld until resolution—retitrate dose if necessary.
  Transdermal administration less likely to cause side-effects.

● HEPATIC IMPAIRMENT Use with caution in severe impairment—no information available.
Dose adjustments Titrate according to individual tolerability in mild to moderate impairment.
● RENAL IMPAIRMENT
Dose adjustments Titrate according to individual tolerability.
● MONITORING REQUIREMENTS Monitor body-weight.

- DIRECTIONS FOR ADMINISTRATION
▶ With transdermal use Apply patches to clean, dry, non-hairy, non-irritated skin on back, upper arm, or chest, removing after 24 hours and siting a replacement patch on a different area (avoid using the same area for 14 days).

- PATIENT AND CARER ADVICE
EXELON ® PATCHES Advise patients and carers of patch administration instructions, particularly to remove the previous day's patch before applying the new patch—consult product literature.

- NATIONAL FUNDING/ACCESS DECISIONS
NICE decisions
▶ **Donepezil, galantamine, rivastigmine, and memantine for the treatment of Alzheimer's disease—updated May 2016**
NICE TA217
Rivastigmine can be used for the treatment of mild to moderate Alzheimer's disease. Treatment should only be prescribed under the following conditions:
- treatment should be initiated on the advice of a specialist
- ensure that local arrangements for prescribing, supply and treatment review follow the NICE guideline on medicines optimisation
- treatment should continue only if it is considered to have a worthwhile effect on cognitive, global, functional, or behavioural symptoms.
Healthcare professionals should not rely solely on assessment scales to determine the severity of Alzheimer's disease when the patient has learning or other disabilities, or other communication difficulties.
www.nice.org.uk/TA217

EXELON ® PATCHES
Scottish Medicines Consortium (SMC) Decisions
The *Scottish Medicines Consortium* has advised (October 2007) that *Exelon* ® patches should be restricted for use in patients with moderately severe Alzheimer's disease under the conditions of the NICE guidance (September 2007) and when a transdermal patch is an appropriate choice of formulation.

- MEDICINAL FORMS
There can be variation in the licensing of different medicines containing the same drug.
Oral solution
CAUTIONARY AND ADVISORY LABELS 21
▶ Rivastigmine (Non-proprietary)
Rivastigmine (as Rivastigmine hydrogen tartrate) 2 mg per 1 ml Rivastigmine 2mg/ml oral solution sugar free sugar-free | 120 ml PoM £96.82 DT = £96.82
Capsule
CAUTIONARY AND ADVISORY LABELS 21, 25
▶ Rivastigmine (Non-proprietary)
Rivastigmine (as Rivastigmine hydrogen tartrate) 1.5 mg Rivastigmine 1.5mg capsules | 28 capsule PoM £33.25 DT = £1.89 | 56 capsule PoM £3.78–£66.51
Rivastigmine (as Rivastigmine hydrogen tartrate) 3 mg Rivastigmine 3mg capsules | 28 capsule PoM £33.25 DT = £2.60 | 56 capsule PoM £5.20–£6.12
Rivastigmine (as Rivastigmine hydrogen tartrate) 4.5 mg Rivastigmine 4.5mg capsules | 28 capsule PoM £33.25 DT = £23.52 | 56 capsule PoM £28.66–£47.06
Rivastigmine (as Rivastigmine hydrogen tartrate) 6 mg Rivastigmine 6mg capsules | 28 capsule PoM £33.25 DT = £28.78 | 56 capsule PoM £31.78–£58.56
▶ Nimvastid (Consilient Health Ltd)
Rivastigmine (as Rivastigmine hydrogen tartrate) 1.5 mg Nimvastid 1.5mg capsules | 28 capsule PoM £28.26 DT = £1.89
Rivastigmine (as Rivastigmine hydrogen tartrate) 3 mg Nimvastid 3mg capsules | 28 capsule PoM £28.26 DT = £2.60
Rivastigmine (as Rivastigmine hydrogen tartrate) 4.5 mg Nimvastid 4.5mg capsules | 28 capsule PoM £28.26 DT = £23.52

Rivastigmine (as Rivastigmine hydrogen tartrate) 6 mg Nimvastid 6mg capsules | 28 capsule PoM £28.26 DT = £28.78
Transdermal patch
▶ Rivastigmine (Non-proprietary)
Rivastigmine 4.6 mg per 24 hour Rivastigmine 4.6mg/24hours transdermal patches | 30 patch PoM £77.97 DT = £77.97
Rivastigmine 9.5 mg per 24 hour Rivastigmine 9.5mg/24hours transdermal patches | 30 patch PoM £30.02 DT = £30.02
▶ Almuriva (Sandoz Ltd)
Rivastigmine 4.6 mg per 24 hour Almuriva 4.6mg/24hours transdermal patches | 30 patch PoM £77.97 DT = £77.97
Rivastigmine 9.5 mg per 24 hour Almuriva 9.5mg/24hours transdermal patches | 30 patch PoM £77.97 DT = £30.02
▶ Alzest (Dr Reddy's Laboratories (UK) Ltd)
Rivastigmine 4.6 mg per 24 hour Alzest 4.6mg/24hours transdermal patches | 30 patch PoM £35.10 DT = £77.97
Rivastigmine 9.5 mg per 24 hour Alzest 9.5mg/24hours transdermal patches | 30 patch PoM £19.97 DT = £30.02
▶ Exelon (Novartis Pharmaceuticals UK Ltd)
Rivastigmine 4.6 mg per 24 hour Exelon 4.6mg/24hours transdermal patches | 30 patch PoM £77.97 DT = £77.97
Rivastigmine 9.5 mg per 24 hour Exelon 9.5mg/24hours transdermal patches | 30 patch PoM £77.97 DT = £30.02
Rivastigmine 13.3 mg per 24 hour Exelon 13.3mg/24hours transdermal patches | 30 patch PoM £77.97 DT = £77.97
▶ Rivatev (Teva UK Ltd)
Rivastigmine 13.3 mg per 24 hour Erastig 13.3mg/24hours transdermal patches | 30 patch PoM £73.90 DT = £77.97
▶ Voleze (Focus Pharmaceuticals Ltd)
Rivastigmine 4.6 mg per 24 hour Voleze 4.6mg/24hours transdermal patches | 30 patch PoM £77.97 DT = £77.97
Rivastigmine 9.5 mg per 24 hour Voleze 9.5mg/24hours transdermal patches | 30 patch PoM £77.97 DT = £30.02
Rivastigmine 13.3 mg per 24 hour Voleze 13.3mg/24hours transdermal patches | 30 patch PoM £77.97 DT = £77.97

DOPAMINERGIC DRUGS > NMDA RECEPTOR ANTAGONISTS

Memantine hydrochloride   22-Nov-2016

- DRUG ACTION Memantine is a glutamate receptor antagonist.

- INDICATIONS AND DOSE
Moderate to severe dementia in Alzheimer's disease
▶ BY MOUTH
▶ Adult: Initially 5 mg once daily, then increased in steps of 5 mg every week; usual maintenance 20 mg daily; maximum 20 mg per day

- CAUTIONS Epilepsy · history of convulsions · risk factors for epilepsy

- INTERACTIONS → Appendix 1: memantine

- SIDE-EFFECTS
▶ **Common or very common** Balance impaired · constipation · dizziness · drowsiness · dyspnoea · headache · hypersensitivity · hypertension
▶ **Uncommon** Confusion · embolism and thrombosis · fatigue · fungal infection · hallucination · heart failure · vomiting
▶ **Rare or very rare** Seizure
▶ **Frequency not known** Hepatitis · pancreatitis · psychotic disorder

- PREGNANCY Manufacturer advises avoid unless essential—no information available.

- BREAST FEEDING Manufacturer advises avoid—no information available.

- HEPATIC IMPAIRMENT Avoid in severe impairment—no information available.

- RENAL IMPAIRMENT Avoid if eGFR less than 5 mL/minute/1.73 m^2.
Dose adjustments Reduce dose to 10 mg daily if eGFR 30–49 mL/minute/1.73 m^2, if well tolerated after at least 7 days dose can be increased in steps to 20 mg daily;

Nervous system

4

reduce dose to 10 mg daily if eGFR
5–29 mL/minute/1.73 m².

● DIRECTIONS FOR ADMINISTRATION For *oral solution*,
manufacturer advises solution should be dosed onto a
spoon or into a glass of water. For *soluble tablets*,
manufacturer advises drink resulting solution immediately
when dissolved in water.

● NATIONAL FUNDING/ACCESS DECISIONS
NICE decisions
▶ **Donepezil, galantamine, rivastigmine, and memantine for the
treatment of Alzheimer's disease—updated May 2016**
NICE TA217
Memantine is recommended as an option for managing
moderate Alzheimer's disease in patients who are unable
to take acetylcholinesterase inhibitors, and for patients
with severe disease; combination treatment with
memantine and an acetylcholinesterase inhibitor is not
recommended. Treatment should only be prescribed under
the following conditions:
● treatment should be initiated on the advice of a
specialist
● ensure that local arrangements for prescribing, supply
and treatment review follow the NICE guideline on
medicines optimisation
● treatment should continue only if it is considered to
have a worthwhile effect on cognitive, global,
functional, or behavioural symptoms.
Healthcare professionals should not rely solely on
assessment scales to determine the severity of Alzheimer's
disease when the patient has learning or other disabilities,
or other communication difficulties.
www.nice.org.uk/TA217

● MEDICINAL FORMS
There can be variation in the licensing of different medicines
containing the same drug.
Soluble tablet
CAUTIONARY AND ADVISORY LABELS 13
▶ Alzhok (Glenmark Pharmaceuticals Europe Ltd)
Memantine hydrochloride 5 mg Alzhok 5mg soluble tablets sugar-
free | 7 tablet [PoM] [℀]
Memantine hydrochloride 10 mg Alzhok 10mg soluble tablets
sugar-free | 28 tablet [PoM] £29.09
Memantine hydrochloride 15 mg Alzhok 15mg soluble tablets
sugar-free | 7 tablet [PoM] [℀]
Memantine hydrochloride 20 mg Alzhok 20mg soluble tablets
sugar-free | 28 tablet [PoM] £58.18
Alzhok soluble tablets treatment initiation pack sugar-free |
28 tablet [PoM] £40.97
Tablet
▶ Memantine hydrochloride (Non-proprietary)
Memantine hydrochloride 5 mg Memantine 5mg tablets |
7 tablet [PoM] [℀]
Memantine hydrochloride 10 mg Memantine 10mg tablets |
28 tablet [PoM] £34.50 DT = £1.37 | 56 tablet [PoM] £2.36–£69.01
Memantine hydrochloride 15 mg Memantine 15mg tablets |
7 tablet [PoM] [℀]
Memantine hydrochloride 20 mg Memantine 20mg tablets |
28 tablet [PoM] £69.01 DT = £1.60
Memantine 5mg/10mg/15mg/20mg tablets treatment initiation pack
| 28 tablet [PoM] £43.13
▶ Ebixa (Lundbeck Ltd)
Memantine hydrochloride 5 mg Ebixa 5mg tablets |
7 tablet [PoM] [℀]
Memantine hydrochloride 10 mg Ebixa 10mg tablets |
28 tablet [PoM] £34.50 DT = £1.37
Memantine hydrochloride 15 mg Ebixa 15mg tablets |
7 tablet [PoM] [℀]
Memantine hydrochloride 20 mg Ebixa 20mg tablets |
28 tablet [PoM] £69.01 DT = £1.60
Ebixa tablets treatment initiation pack | 28 tablet [PoM] £43.13
▶ Maruxa (Consilient Health Ltd)
Memantine hydrochloride 10 mg Marixino 10mg tablets |
28 tablet [PoM] £29.32 DT = £1.37
Memantine hydrochloride 20 mg Marixino 20mg tablets |
28 tablet [PoM] £58.65 DT = £1.60

▶ Nemdatine (Actavis UK Ltd)
Memantine hydrochloride 5 mg Nemdatine 5mg tablets |
7 tablet [PoM] [℀]
Memantine hydrochloride 10 mg Nemdatine 10mg tablets |
28 tablet [PoM] £34.50 DT = £1.37 | 56 tablet [PoM] £69.01
Memantine hydrochloride 15 mg Nemdatine 15mg tablets |
7 tablet [PoM] [℀]
Memantine hydrochloride 20 mg Nemdatine 20mg tablets |
28 tablet [PoM] £69.01 DT = £1.60
Nemdatine tablets treatment initiation pack | 28 tablet [PoM] £43.12
Oral solution
▶ Memantine hydrochloride (Non-proprietary)
Memantine hydrochloride 10 mg per 1 ml Memantine 10mg/ml
oral solution sugar free sugar-free | 50 ml [PoM] £61.61 DT = £53.85
sugar-free | 100 ml [PoM] £93.76–£123.23
▶ Ebixa (Lundbeck Ltd)
Memantine hydrochloride 10 mg per 1 ml Ebixa 5mg/0.5ml pump
actuation oral solution sugar free | 50 ml [PoM] £61.61 DT = £53.85
sugar-free | 100 ml [PoM] £123.23
Orodispersible tablet
EXCIPIENTS: May contain Aspartame
▶ Valios (Dr Reddy's Laboratories (UK) Ltd)
Memantine hydrochloride 5 mg Valios 5mg orodispersible tablets
sugar free sugar-free | 7 tablet [PoM] [℀]
Memantine hydrochloride 10 mg Valios 10mg orodispersible
tablets sugar free sugar-free | 28 tablet [PoM] £24.99 DT = £24.99
Memantine hydrochloride 15 mg Valios 15mg orodispersible tablets
sugar free sugar-free | 7 tablet [PoM] [℀]
Memantine hydrochloride 20 mg Valios 20mg orodispersible
tablets sugar free sugar-free | 28 tablet [PoM] £49.98 DT = £49.98
Valios 5mg/10mg/15mg/20mg orodispersible tablets initiation pack
sugar-free | 28 tablet [PoM] £31.24

2   Epilepsy and other seizure disorders

Epilepsy

26-May-2017

Epilepsy control

The object of treatment is to prevent the occurrence of
seizures by maintaining an effective dose of one or more
antiepileptic drugs. Careful adjustment of doses is necessary,
starting with low doses and increasing gradually until
seizures are controlled or there are significant adverse
effects.

When choosing an antiepileptic drug, the presenting
epilepsy syndrome should first be considered. If the
syndrome is not clear, the seizure type should determine the
choice of treatment. Concomitant medication, co-morbidity,
age, and sex should also be taken into account.

The dosage frequency is often determined by the plasma-
drug half-life, and should be kept as low as possible to
encourage adherence with the prescribed regimen. Most
antiepileptics, when used in the usual dosage, can be given
twice daily. Lamotrigine p. 316, perampanel p. 320,
phenobarbital p. 331, and phenytoin p. 321, which have long
half-lives, can be given once daily at bedtime. However, with
large doses, some antiepileptics may need to be given more
frequently to avoid adverse effects associated with high peak
plasma-drug concentration.

Management

When monotherapy with a first-line antiepileptic drug has
failed, monotherapy with a second drug should be tried; the
diagnosis should be checked before starting an alternative
drug if the first drug showed lack of efficacy. The change
from one antiepileptic drug to another should be cautious,
slowly withdrawing the first drug only when the new regimen
has been established. Combination therapy with two or more
antiepileptic drugs may be necessary, but the concurrent use
of antiepileptic drugs increases the risk of adverse effects
and drug interactions. If combination therapy does not bring

about worthwhile benefits, revert to the regimen (monotherapy or combination therapy) that provided the best balance between tolerability and efficacy. A single antiepileptic drug should be prescribed wherever possible.

MHRA/CHM advice: Antiepileptic drugs: new advice on switching between different manufacturers' products for a particular drug (November 2013)
The CHM has reviewed spontaneous adverse reactions received by the MHRA and publications that reported potential harm arising from switching of antiepileptic drugs in patients previously stabilised on a branded product to a generic. The CHM concluded that reports of loss of seizure control and/or worsening of side-effects around the time of switching between products could be explained as chance associations, but that a causal role of switching could not be ruled out in all cases. The following guidance has been issued to help minimise risk:

- Different antiepileptic drugs vary considerably in their characteristics, which influences the risk of whether switching between different manufacturers' products of a particular drug may cause adverse effects or loss of seizure control;
- Antiepileptic drugs have been divided into three risk-based categories to help healthcare professionals decide whether it is necessary to maintain continuity of supply of a specific manufacturer's product. These categories are listed below;
- If it is felt desirable for a patient to be maintained on a specific manufacturer's product this should be prescribed either by specifying a brand name, or by using the generic drug name and name of the manufacturer (otherwise known as the Marketing Authorisation Holder);
- This advice relates only to antiepileptic drug use for treatment of epilepsy; it does not apply to their use in other indications (e.g. mood stabilisation, neuropathic pain);
- Please report on a Yellow Card any suspected adverse reactions to antiepileptic drugs;
- Dispensing pharmacists should ensure the continuity of supply of a particular product when the prescription specifies it. If the prescribed product is unavailable, it may be necessary to dispense a product from a different manufacturer to maintain continuity of treatment of that antiepileptic drug. Such cases should be discussed and agreed with both the prescriber and patient (or carer);
- Usual dispensing practice can be followed when a specific product is not stated.

Category 1
Phenytoin, carbamazepine p. 309, phenobarbital, primidone p. 332. For these drugs, doctors are advised to ensure that their patient is maintained on a specific manufacturer's product.

Category 2
Valproate, lamotrigine, perampanel, rufinamide p. 324, clobazam p. 333, clonazepam p. 334, oxcarbazepine p. 319, eslicarbazepine acetate p. 312, zonisamide p. 330, topiramate p. 328. For these drugs, the need for continued supply of a particular manufacturer's product should be based on clinical judgement and consultation with the patient and/or carer taking into account factors such as seizure frequency and treatment history.

Category 3
Levetiracetam p. 318, lacosamide p. 315, tiagabine p. 327, gabapentin p. 314, pregabalin p. 322, ethosuximide p. 312, vigabatrin p. 329. For these drugs, it is usually unnecessary to ensure that patients are maintained on a specific manufacturer's product unless there are specific concerns such as patient anxiety, and risk of confusion or dosing errors.

Antiepileptic hypersensitivity syndrome
Antiepileptic hypersensitivity syndrome is a rare but potentially fatal syndrome associated with some antiepileptic drugs (**carbamazepine, lacosamide, lamotrigine, oxcarbazepine, phenobarbital, phenytoin, primidone**, and **rufinamide**); rarely cross-sensitivity occurs between some of these antiepileptic drugs. Some other antiepileptics (**eslicarbazepine, stiripentol**, and **zonisamide**) have a theoretical risk. The symptoms usually start between 1 and 8 weeks of exposure; fever, rash, and lymphadenopathy are most commonly seen. Other systemic signs include liver dysfunction, haematological, renal, and pulmonary abnormalities, vasculitis, and multi-organ failure. If signs or symptoms of hypersensitivity syndrome occur, the drug should be withdrawn immediately, and expert advice should be sought.

Risk of suicidal thoughts and behaviour
The MHRA has advised (August 2008) that all antiepileptic drugs are associated with a small increased risk of suicidal thoughts and behaviour. Symptoms may occur as early as one week after starting treatment. Patients should be advised to seek medical advice if they develop any mood changes, distressing thoughts, or feelings about suicide or harming themselves, and should be referred for appropriate treatment if necessary.

Interactions
Interactions between antiepileptics are complex and may increase toxicity without a corresponding increase in antiepileptic effect. Interactions are usually caused by hepatic enzyme induction or inhibition; displacement from protein binding sites is not usually a problem. These interactions are highly variable and unpredictable.

Withdrawal
Antiepileptic drugs should be withdrawn under specialist supervision. Avoid abrupt withdrawal, particularly of barbiturates and benzodiazepines, because this can precipitate severe rebound seizures. Reduction in dosage should be gradual and, in the case of barbiturates, withdrawal of the drug may take months.

The decision to withdraw antiepileptic drugs from a seizure-free patient, and its timing, is often difficult and depends on individual circumstances. Even in patients who have been seizure-free for several years, there is a significant risk of seizure recurrence on drug withdrawal. In patients receiving several antiepileptic drugs, only one drug should be withdrawn at a time.

Driving
If a driver has a seizure (of any type) they must stop driving immediately and inform the Driver and Vehicle Licensing Agency (DVLA)

Patients who have had a first unprovoked epileptic seizure or a single isolated seizure must not drive for 6 months; driving may then be resumed, provided the patient has been assessed by a specialist as fit to drive and investigations do not suggest a risk of further seizures.

Patients with established epilepsy may drive a motor vehicle provided they are not a danger to the public and are compliant with treatment and follow up. To continue driving, these patients must be seizure-free for at least one year (or have a pattern of seizures established for one year where there is no influence on their level of consciousness or the ability to act); also, they must not have a history of unprovoked seizures.

Note: additional criteria apply for drivers of large goods or passenger carrying vehicles—consult DVLA guidance.

Patients who have had a *seizure while asleep* are not permitted to drive for one year from the date of each seizure, unless:

- a history or pattern of sleep seizures occurring **only** ever while asleep has been established over the course of at least one year from the date of the first sleep seizure; or
- an established pattern of purely asleep seizures can be demonstrated over the course of three years if the patient has previously had seizures whilst awake (or awake and asleep).

The DVLA recommends that patients should not drive during medication changes or withdrawal of antiepileptic drugs, and for 6 months after their last dose. If a seizure occurs due to a prescribed change or withdrawal of epilepsy treatment, the patient will have their driving license revoked for 1 year; relicensing may be considered earlier if treatment has been reinstated for 6 months and no further seizures have occurred.

Pregnancy

Women of child-bearing potential should discuss with a specialist the impact of both epilepsy, and its treatment, on the outcome of pregnancy.

There is an increased risk of teratogenicity associated with the use of antiepileptic drugs (especially if used during the first trimester and particularly if the patient takes two or more antiepileptic drugs). Valproate is associated with the highest risk of serious developmental disorders (up to 30–40% risk) and congenital malformations (approx. 10% risk). Valproate must **not** be used in females of childbearing potential unless the conditions of the Pregnancy Prevention Programme are met and alternative treatments are ineffective or not tolerated; during pregnancy, it must not be used for epilepsy, unless it is the only possible treatment. There is also an increased risk of teratogenicity with phenytoin, primidone, phenobarbital, lamotrigine, and carbamazepine. Topiramate carries an increased risk of congenital malformations (including cleft palate, hypospadias, and anomalies involving various body systems) if taken in the first trimester of pregnancy. There is not enough evidence to establish the risk of teratogenicity with other antiepileptic drugs.

Prescribers should also consider carefully the choice of antiepileptic therapy in pre-pubescent girls who may later become pregnant. Women of child-bearing potential who take antiepileptic drugs should be given advice about the need for an effective contraception method to avoid unplanned pregnancy—for further information, see *Conception and contraception* in the individual drug monographs. Some antiepileptic drugs can reduce the efficacy of hormonal contraceptives, and the efficacy of some antiepileptics may be affected by hormonal contraceptives.

Women who want to become pregnant should be referred to a specialist for advice in advance of conception. For some women, the severity of seizure or the seizure type may not pose a serious threat, and drug withdrawal may be considered; therapy may be resumed after the first trimester. If treatment with antiepileptic drugs must continue throughout pregnancy, then monotherapy is preferable at the lowest effective dose.

Once an unplanned pregnancy is discovered it is usually too late for changes to be made to the treatment regimen; the risk of harm to the mother and fetus from convulsive seizures outweighs the risk of continued therapy. The likelihood of a woman who is taking antiepileptic drugs having a baby with no malformations is at least 90%, and it is important that women do not stop taking essential treatment because of concern over harm to the fetus. To reduce the risk of neural tube defects, folate supplementation is advised before conception and throughout the first trimester. In the case of sodium valproate p. 325 and valproic acid p. 351 an urgent consultation is required to reconsider the benefits and risks of valproate therapy.

The concentration of antiepileptic drugs in the plasma can change during pregnancy. Doses of phenytoin, carbamazepine, and lamotrigine should be adjusted on the basis of plasma-drug concentration monitoring; the dose of other antiepileptic drugs should be monitored carefully during pregnancy and after birth, and adjustments made on a clinical basis. Plasma-drug concentration monitoring during pregnancy is also useful to check compliance. Additionally, in patients taking topiramate or levetiracetam, it is recommended that fetal growth should be monitored. Women who have seizures in the second half of pregnancy should be assessed for eclampsia before any change is made to antiepileptic treatment. Status epilepticus should be treated according to the standard protocol.

Routine injection of vitamin K at birth minimises the risk of neonatal haemorrhage associated with antiepileptics. Withdrawal effects in the newborn may occur with some antiepileptic drugs, in particular benzodiazepines and phenobarbital.

Epilepsy and Pregnancy Register

All pregnant women with epilepsy, whether taking medication or not, should be encouraged to notify the UK Epilepsy and Pregnancy Register (Tel: 0800 389 1248).

Breast-feeding

Women taking antiepileptic monotherapy should generally be encouraged to breast-feed; if a woman is on combination therapy or if there are other risk factors, such as premature birth, specialist advice should be sought.

All infants should be monitored for sedation, feeding difficulties, adequate weight gain, and developmental milestones. Infants should also be monitored for adverse effects associated with the antiepileptic drug particularly with newer antiepileptics, if the antiepileptic is readily transferred into breast-milk causing high infant serum-drug concentrations (e.g. ethosuximide, lamotrigine, primidone, and zonisamide), or if slower metabolism in the infant causes drugs to accumulate (e.g. phenobarbital and lamotrigine). Serum-drug concentration monitoring should be undertaken in breast-fed infants if suspected adverse reactions develop; if toxicity develops it may be necessary to introduce formula feeds to limit the infant's drug exposure, or to wean the infant off breast-milk altogether.

Primidone, phenobarbital, and the benzodiazepines are associated with an established risk of drowsiness in breast-fed babies and caution is required.

Withdrawal effects may occur in infants if a mother suddenly stops breast-feeding, particularly if she is taking phenobarbital, primidone, or lamotrigine.

Focal seizures with or without secondary generalisation

Carbamazepine p. 309 and lamotrigine p. 316 are first-line options for treating newly diagnosed focal seizures; oxcarbazepine p. 319, sodium valproate p. 325 and levetiracetam p. 318 may be used if carbamazepine or lamotrigine are unsuitable or not tolerated. If monotherapy is unsuccessful with two of these first-line antiepileptic drugs, adjunctive treatment may be considered. Options for adjunctive treatment include carbamazepine, clobazam p. 333, gabapentin p. 314, lamotrigine, levetiracetam, oxcarbazepine, sodium valproate, or topiramate p. 328. If adjunctive treatment is ineffective or not tolerated, a tertiary epilepsy specialist should be consulted who may consider eslicarbazepine acetate p. 312, lacosamide p. 315, phenobarbital p. 331, phenytoin p. 321, pregabalin p. 322, tiagabine p. 327, vigabatrin p. 329 and zonisamide p. 330.

Generalised seizures

Tonic-clonic seizures

Sodium valproate is the first-line treatment for newly diagnosed generalised tonic-clonic seizures (except in female patients who are premenopausal, see *Valproate* below). Lamotrigine is the alternative choice if sodium valproate is not suitable, but may exacerbate myoclonic seizures. In those with established epilepsy with generalised tonic-clonic seizures only, lamotrigine or sodium valproate may be prescribed as the first-line treatment. Carbamazepine and oxcarbazepine may also be considered in newly diagnosed and established tonic-clonic seizures, but may exacerbate myoclonic and absence seizures. Clobazam, lamotrigine, levetiracetam, sodium valproate or topiramate may be used as adjunctive treatment if monotherapy is ineffective or not tolerated.

Absence seizures
Ethosuximide p. 312, or sodium valproate (except in female patients who are premenopausal, see *Valproate* below), are the drugs of choice in absence seizures and syndromes; lamotrigine is a suitable alternative when ethosuximide and sodium valproate are unsuitable, ineffective or not tolerated. Sodium valproate should be used as the first choice if there is a high risk of generalised tonic-clonic seizures. A combination of any two of these drugs may be used if monotherapy is ineffective. Clobazam, clonazepam p. 334, levetiracetam, topiramate or zonisamide may be considered by a tertiary epilepsy specialist if adjunctive treatment fails. Carbamazepine, gabapentin, oxcarbazepine, phenytoin, pregabalin, tiagabine and vigabatrin are not recommended in absence seizures or syndromes.

Myoclonic seizures
Myoclonic seizures (myoclonic jerks) occur in a variety of syndromes, and response to treatment varies considerably. Sodium valproate is the drug of choice in newly diagnosed myoclonic seizures (except in female patients who are premenopausal, see *Valproate* below); topiramate and levetiracetam are alternative options if sodium valproate is unsuitable but consideration should be given to the less favourable side-effect profile of topiramate. A combination of two of these drugs may be used if monotherapy is ineffective or not tolerated. If adjunctive treatment fails, a tertiary epilepsy specialist should be consulted and may consider clobazam, clonazepam, zonisamide or piracetam p. 402. Carbamazepine, gabapentin, oxcarbazepine, phenytoin, pregabalin, tiagabine and vigabatrin are not recommended for the treatment of myoclonic seizures.

Sodium valproate and levetiracetam are effective in treating the generalised tonic-clonic seizures that coexist with myoclonic seizures in idiopathic generalised epilepsy.

Atonic and tonic seizures
Atonic and tonic seizures are usually seen in childhood, in specific epilepsy syndromes, or associated with cerebral damage or mental retardation. They may respond poorly to the traditional drugs. Sodium valproate is the drug of choice (except in female patients who are premenopausal, see *Valproate* below); lamotrigine can be added as adjunctive treatment. If adjunctive treatment is ineffective or not tolerated, a tertiary epilepsy specialist should be consulted, and may consider rufinamide p. 324 or topiramate. Carbamazepine, gabapentin, oxcarbazepine, pregabalin, tiagabine or vigabatrin are not recommended in atonic and tonic seizures.

Epilepsy syndromes
Some drugs are licensed for use in particular epilepsy syndromes, such as lamotrigine and rufinamide in Lennox-Gastaut syndrome. The epilepsy syndromes are specific types of epilepsy that are characterised according to a number of features including seizure type, age of onset, and EEG characteristics.

Antiepileptic drugs
Carbamazepine and related antiepileptics
Carbamazepine is a drug of choice for simple and complex focal seizures and is a first-line treatment option for generalised tonic-clonic seizures. It can be used as adjunctive treatment for focal seizures when monotherapy has been ineffective. It is essential to initiate carbamazepine therapy at a low dose and build this up slowly. Carbamazepine may exacerbate tonic, atonic, myoclonic and absence seizures and is therefore not recommended if these seizures are present.

Oxcarbazepine is licensed as monotherapy or adjunctive therapy for the treatment of focal seizures with or without secondary generalised tonic-clonic seizures. It can also be considered for the treatment of primary generalised tonic-clonic seizures [unlicensed]. Oxcarbazepine is not recommended in tonic, atonic, absence or myoclonic seizures due to the risk of seizure exacerbation.

Eslicarbazepine acetate is licensed for adjunctive treatment in adults with focal seizures with or without secondary generalisation.

Ethosuximide
Ethosuximide is a first-line treatment option for absence seizures. It may also be prescribed as adjunctive treatment for absence seizures when monotherapy is ineffective. Ethosuximide is also licensed for myoclonic seizures.

Gabapentin and pregabalin
Gabapentin and pregabalin are used for the treatment of focal seizures with or without secondary generalisation. They are not recommended if tonic, atonic, absence or myoclonic seizures are present. Both are also licensed for the treatment of neuropathic pain. Pregabalin is licensed for the treatment of generalised anxiety disorder. Gabapentin is an effective treatment for migraine prophylaxis [unlicensed].

Lamotrigine
Lamotrigine is an antiepileptic drug recommended as a first-line treatment for focal seizures and primary and secondary generalised tonic-clonic seizures. It is also licensed for typical absence seizures in children (but efficacy may not be maintained in all children) and is an unlicensed treatment option in adults if first-line treatments have been unsuccessful. Lamotrigine can also be used as adjunctive treatment in atonic or tonic seizures if first-line treatment has failed [unlicensed]. Myoclonic seizures may be exacerbated by lamotrigine and it can cause serious rashes especially in children; dose recommendations should be adhered to closely.

Lamotrigine is used either as sole treatment or as an adjunct to treatment with other antiepileptic drugs. Valproate increases plasma-lamotrigine concentration, whereas the enzyme-inducing antiepileptics reduce it; care is therefore required in choosing the appropriate initial dose and subsequent titration. When the potential for interaction is not known, treatment should be initiated with lower doses, such as those used with valproate.

Levetiracetam and brivaracetam
Levetiracetam p. 318 is used for monotherapy and adjunctive treatment of focal seizures with or without secondary generalisation, and for adjunctive treatment of myoclonic seizures in patients with juvenile myoclonic epilepsy and primary generalised tonic-clonic seizures. Levetiracetam may be prescribed alone and in combination for the treatment of myoclonic seizures, and under specialist supervision for absence seizures [both unlicensed].

Brivaracetam p. 309 is used as adjunctive therapy in the treatment of partial-onset seizures with or without secondary generalisation.

Phenobarbital and primidone
Phenobarbital p. 331 is effective for tonic-clonic and focal seizures but may be sedative in adults. It may be tried for atypical absence, atonic, and tonic seizures. Rebound seizures may be a problem on withdrawal.

Primidone p. 332 is largely converted to phenobarbital and this is probably responsible for its antiepileptic action. A low initial dose of primidone is essential.

Phenytoin

Phenytoin p. 321 is licensed for tonic-clonic and focal seizures but may exacerbate absence or myoclonic seizures and should be avoided if these seizures are present. It has a narrow therapeutic index and the relationship between dose and plasma-drug concentration is non-linear; small dosage increases in some patients may produce large increases in plasma concentration with acute toxic side-effects. Similarly, a few missed doses or a small change in drug absorption may result in a marked change in plasma-drug concentration. Monitoring of plasma-drug concentration improves dosage adjustment.

When only parenteral administration is possible, fosphenytoin sodium p. 313, a pro-drug of phenytoin, may be convenient to give. Unlike phenytoin (which should only be given intravenously), fosphenytoin sodium may also be given by intramuscular injection.

Rufinamide

Rufinamide p. 324 is licensed for the adjunctive treatment of seizures in Lennox-Gastaut syndrome. It may be considered by a tertiary specialist for the treatment of refractory tonic or atonic seizures [unlicensed].

Topiramate

Topiramate p. 328 can be given alone or as adjunctive treatment in generalised tonic-clonic seizures or focal seizures with or without secondary generalisation. It can be used as adjunctive treatment for seizures associated with Lennox-Gastaut syndrome and for absence, tonic and atonic seizures under specialist supervision [unlicensed]. It can also be considered as an option in myoclonic seizures [unlicensed]. Female patients should be fully informed of the risks related to the use of topiramate during pregnancy and the need to use effective contraception—for further information, see *Conception and contraception* and *Pregnancy* in the topiramate drug monograph.

Valproate

Sodium valproate p. 325 is effective in controlling tonic-clonic seizures, particularly in primary generalised epilepsy. It is a drug of choice in primary generalised tonic-clonic seizures, focal seizures, generalised absences and myoclonic seizures, and can be tried in atypical absence seizures. It is recommended as a first-line option in atonic and tonic seizures. Sodium valproate has widespread metabolic effects and monitoring of liver function tests and full blood count is essential. Because of its high teratogenic potential, valproate must not be used in females of childbearing potential unless the conditions of the Pregnancy Prevention Programme are met and alternative treatments are ineffective or not tolerated. During pregnancy, it must not be used for epilepsy unless it is the only possible treatment. For further information see *Important safety information, Conception and contraception*, and *Pregnancy* in the sodium valproate and valproic acid p. 351 drug monographs.

Valproic acid (as semisodium valproate) is licensed for acute mania associated with bipolar disorder.

Zonisamide

Zonisamide p. 330 can be used alone for the treatment of focal seizures with or without secondary generalisation in adults with newly diagnosed epilepsy, and as adjunctive treatment for refractory focal seizures with or without secondary generalisation in adults and children aged 6 years and above. It can also be used under the supervision of a specialist for refractory absence and myoclonic seizures [unlicensed indications].

Benzodiazepines

Clobazam p. 333 may be used as adjunctive therapy in the treatment of generalised tonic-clonic and refractory focal seizures. It may be prescribed under the care of a specialist for refractory absence and myoclonic seizures. Clonazepam p. 334 may be prescribed by a specialist for refractory

absence and myoclonic seizures, but its sedative side-effects may be prominent.

Other drugs

Acetazolamide p. 1147, a carbonic anhydrase inhibitor, has a specific role in treating epilepsy associated with menstruation. Piracetam p. 402 is used as adjunctive treatment for cortical myoclonus.

Status epilepticus

Convulsive status epilepticus

Immediate measures to manage status epilepticus include positioning the patient to avoid injury, supporting respiration including the provision of oxygen, maintaining blood pressure, and the correction of any hypoglycaemia. Parenteral thiamine p. 1048 should be considered if alcohol abuse is suspected; pyridoxine hydrochloride p. 1047 should be given if the status epilepticus is caused by pyridoxine hydrochloride deficiency.

Seizures lasting longer than 5 minutes should be treated urgently with intravenous lorazepam p. 335 (repeated once after 10 minutes if seizures recur or fail to respond). Intravenous diazepam p. 340 is effective but it carries a high risk of thrombophlebitis (reduced by using an emulsion formulation). Absorption of diazepam from intramuscular injection or from suppositories is too slow for treatment of status epilepticus. Patients should be monitored for respiratory depression and hypotension.

Where facilities for resuscitation are not immediately available, diazepam can be administered as a rectal solution or midazolam p. 336 oromucosal solution can be given into the buccal cavity.

Important

If, after initial treatment with benzodiazepines, seizures recur or fail to respond 25 minutes after onset, phenytoin sodium, fosphenytoin sodium, or phenobarbital sodium should be used; contact intensive care unit if seizures continue. If these measures fail to control seizures 45 minutes after onset, anaesthesia with thiopental sodium p. 335, midazolam, or a non-barbiturate anaesthetic such as propofol p. 1291 [unlicensed indication], should be instituted with full intensive care support.

Phenytoin sodium can be given by slow intravenous injection, followed by the maintenance dosage if appropriate.

Alternatively, fosphenytoin sodium (a pro-drug of phenytoin), can be given more rapidly and when given intravenously causes fewer injection-site reactions than phenytoin sodium. Although it can also be given intramuscularly, absorption is too slow by this route for treatment of status epilepticus. Doses of fosphenytoin sodium should be expressed in terms of phenytoin sodium.

Non-convulsive status epilepticus

The urgency to treat non-convulsive status epilepticus depends on the severity of the patient's condition. If there is incomplete loss of awareness, usual oral antiepileptic therapy should be continued or restarted. Patients who fail to respond to oral antiepileptic therapy or have complete lack of awareness can be treated in the same way as for convulsive status epilepticus, although anaesthesia is rarely needed.

Febrile convulsions

Brief febrile convulsions need no specific treatment; antipyretic medication (e.g. paracetamol p. 438), is commonly used to reduce fever and prevent further convulsions but evidence to support this practice is lacking. *Prolonged febrile convulsions* (those lasting 5 minutes or longer), or *recurrent febrile convulsions* without recovery must be treated actively (as for convulsive status epilepticus). Long-term anticonvulsant prophylaxis for febrile convulsions is rarely indicated.

Other drugs used for Epilepsy and other seizure disorders Magnesium sulfate, p. 1019

ANTIEPILEPTICS

Brivaracetam

13-Feb-2017

- **INDICATIONS AND DOSE**

Adjunctive therapy of partial-onset seizures with or without secondary generalisation
  - BY MOUTH, OR BY INTRAVENOUS INJECTION, OR BY INTRAVENOUS INFUSION
  - Child 16–17 years: Initially 25–50 mg twice daily, adjusted according to response; usual maintenance 25–100 mg twice daily
  - Adult: Initially 25–50 mg twice daily, adjusted according to response; usual maintenance 25–100 mg twice daily

- **INTERACTIONS** → Appendix 1: antiepileptics

- **SIDE-EFFECTS**
  - **Common or very common** Anxiety · appetite decreased · constipation · cough · depression · dizziness · drowsiness · fatigue · increased risk of infection · insomnia · irritability · nausea · vertigo · vomiting
  - **Uncommon** Aggression · psychotic disorder

- **PREGNANCY** Manufacturer advises avoid unless potential benefit outweighs risk—limited information available.

- **BREAST FEEDING** Manufacturer advises avoid—present in milk in *animal* studies.

- **HEPATIC IMPAIRMENT**
  Dose adjustments Manufacturer advises consider a starting dose of 25 mg twice daily in chronic liver disease; max. maintenance dose 75 mg twice daily in all stages of impairment.

- **TREATMENT CESSATION** Manufacturer advises avoid abrupt withdrawal—reduce daily dose in steps of 50 mg at weekly intervals, then reduce to 20 mg daily for a final week.

- **DIRECTIONS FOR ADMINISTRATION**
  - With intravenous use For intermittent *intravenous infusion*, manufacturer advises dilute in Glucose 5% *or* Sodium Chloride 0.9% *or* Lactated Ringer's solution; give over 15 minutes.
  - With oral use Manufacturer advises oral solution can be diluted in water or juice shortly before swallowing.

- **PRESCRIBING AND DISPENSING INFORMATION**
  Manufacturer advises if switching between oral therapy and intravenous therapy (for those temporarily unable to take oral medication), the total daily dose and the frequency of administration should be maintained.

- **PATIENT AND CARER ADVICE**
  Missed doses Manufacturer advises if one or more doses are missed, a single dose should be taken as soon as possible and the next dose should be taken at the usual time.
  Driving and skilled tasks Manufacturer advises patients and carers should be cautioned on the effects on driving and performance of skilled tasks—increased risk of dizziness.

- **NATIONAL FUNDING/ACCESS DECISIONS**
  Scottish Medicines Consortium (SMC) Decisions
  The *Scottish Medicines Consortium* has advised (July 2016) that brivaracetam (*Briviact ®*) is accepted for restricted use within NHS Scotland as adjunctive therapy in the treatment of partial-onset seizures with or without secondary generalisation in patients with refractory epilepsy. Treatment should be initiated by physicians who have appropriate experience in the treatment of epilepsy.

All Wales Medicines Strategy Group (AWMSG) Decisions
The *All Wales Medicines Strategy Group* has advised (October 2016) that Brivaracetam (*Briviact ®*) is recommended as an option for restricted use within NHS Wales. Brivaracetam (*Briviact ®*) should be restricted to use in the treatment of patients with refractory epilepsy, who remain uncontrolled with, or are intolerant to, other adjunctive anti-epileptic medicines, within its licensed indication as adjunctive therapy in the treatment of partial-onset seizures (POS) with or without secondary generalisation in adult and adolescent patients from 16 years of age with epilepsy. Brivaracetam (*Briviact ®*) is not recommended for use within NHS Wales outside of this subpopulation.

- **MEDICINAL FORMS**
  There can be variation in the licensing of different medicines containing the same drug.
  Solution for injection
  CAUTIONARY AND ADVISORY LABELS 2
  ELECTROLYTES: May contain Sodium
  - Briviat (UCB Pharma Ltd) ▼
    Brivaracetam 10 mg per 1 ml Briviat 50mg/5ml solution for injection vials | 10 vial [PoM] £222.75
  Oral solution
  CAUTIONARY AND ADVISORY LABELS 2, 8
  EXCIPIENTS: May contain Sorbitol
  ELECTROLYTES: May contain Sodium
  - Briviat (UCB Pharma Ltd) ▼
    Brivaracetam 10 mg per 1 ml Briviat 10mg/ml oral solution sugar-free | 300 ml [PoM] £115.83 DT = £115.83
  Tablet
  CAUTIONARY AND ADVISORY LABELS 2, 8, 25
  - Briviat (UCB Pharma Ltd) ▼
    Brivaracetam 10 mg Briviat 10mg tablets | 14 tablet [PoM] £34.64
    Brivaracetam 25 mg Briviat 25mg tablets | 56 tablet [PoM] £129.64
    Brivaracetam 50 mg Briviat 50mg tablets | 56 tablet [PoM] £129.64
    Brivaracetam 75 mg Briviat 75mg tablets | 56 tablet [PoM] £129.64
    Brivaracetam 100 mg Briviat 100mg tablets | 56 tablet [PoM] £129.64

Carbamazepine

- **INDICATIONS AND DOSE**

Focal and secondary generalised tonic-clonic seizures | Primary generalised tonic-clonic seizures
  - BY MOUTH USING IMMEDIATE-RELEASE MEDICINES
  - Adult: Initially 100–200 mg 1–2 times a day, increased in steps of 100–200 mg every 2 weeks; usual dose 0.8–1.2 g daily in divided doses; increased if necessary up to 1.6–2 g daily in divided doses
  - Elderly: Reduce initial dose
  - BY RECTUM
  - Adult: Up to 1 g daily in 4 divided doses for up to 7 days, for short-term use when oral therapy temporarily not possible

Trigeminal neuralgia
  - BY MOUTH USING IMMEDIATE-RELEASE MEDICINES
  - Adult: Initially 100 mg 1–2 times a day, some patients may require higher initial dose, increase gradually according to response; usual dose 200 mg 3–4 times a day, increased if necessary up to 1.6 g daily

Prophylaxis of bipolar disorder unresponsive to lithium
  - BY MOUTH USING IMMEDIATE-RELEASE MEDICINES
  - Adult: Initially 400 mg daily in divided doses, increased until symptoms controlled; usual dose 400–600 mg daily; maximum 1.6 g per day

continued →

Adjunct in acute alcohol withdrawal
▶ BY MOUTH USING IMMEDIATE-RELEASE MEDICINES
▶ Adult: Initially 800 mg daily in divided doses, then reduced to 200 mg daily for usual treatment duration of 7–10 days, dose to be reduced gradually over 5 days

Diabetic neuropathy
▶ BY MOUTH USING IMMEDIATE-RELEASE MEDICINES
▶ Adult: Initially 100 mg 1–2 times a day, increased gradually according to response; usual dose 200 mg 3–4 times a day, increased if necessary up to 1.6 g daily

Focal and generalised tonic-clonic seizures
▶ BY MOUTH USING IMMEDIATE-RELEASE MEDICINES
▶ Child 1 month-11 years: Initially 5 mg/kg once daily, dose to be taken at night, alternatively initially 2.5 mg/kg twice daily, then increased in steps of 2.5–5 mg/kg every 3–7 days as required; maintenance 5 mg/kg 2–3 times a day, increased if necessary up to 20 mg/kg daily
▶ Child 12-17 years: Initially 100–200 mg 1–2 times a day, then increased to 200–400 mg 2–3 times a day, increased if necessary up to 1.8 g daily, dose should be increased slowly

DOSE EQUIVALENCE AND CONVERSION
▶ Suppositories of 125 mg may be considered to be approximately equivalent in therapeutic effect to tablets of 100 mg but final adjustment should always depend on clinical response (plasma concentration monitoring recommended).

CARBAGEN ® SR

Focal and secondary generalised tonic-clonic seizures | Primary generalised tonic-clonic seizures
▶ BY MOUTH
▶ Adult: Initially 100–400 mg daily in 1–2 divided doses, increased in steps of 100–200 mg every 2 weeks, dose should be increased slowly; usual dose 0.8–1.2 g daily in 1–2 divided doses, increased if necessary up to 1.6–2 g daily in 1–2 divided doses
▶ Elderly: Reduce initial dose

Trigeminal neuralgia
▶ BY MOUTH
▶ Adult: Initially 100–200 mg daily in 1–2 divided doses, some patients may require higher initial dose, increase gradually according to response; usual dose 600–800 mg daily in 1–2 divided doses, increased if necessary up to 1.6 g daily in 1–2 divided doses

Prophylaxis of bipolar disorder unresponsive to lithium
▶ BY MOUTH
▶ Adult: Initially 400 mg daily in 1–2 divided doses, increased until symptoms controlled; usual dose 400–600 mg daily in 1–2 divided doses; maximum 1.6 g per day

Focal and generalised tonic-clonic seizures | Prophylaxis of bipolar disorder
▶ BY MOUTH
▶ Child 5-11 years: Initially 5 mg/kg daily in 1–2 divided doses, then increased in steps of 2.5–5 mg/kg every 3–7 days as required, dose should be increased slowly; maintenance 10–15 mg/kg daily in 1–2 divided doses, increased if necessary up to 20 mg/kg daily in 1–2 divided doses
▶ Child 12-17 years: Initially 100–400 mg daily in 1–2 divided doses, then increased to 400–1200 mg daily in 1–2 divided doses, increased if necessary up to 1.8 g daily in 1–2 divided doses, dose should be increased slowly

TEGRETOL ® PROLONGED RELEASE

Focal and secondary generalised tonic-clonic seizures | Primary generalised tonic-clonic seizures
▶ BY MOUTH
▶ Adult: Initially 100–400 mg daily in 2 divided doses, increased in steps of 100–200 mg every 2 weeks, dose should be increased slowly; usual dose 0.8–1.2 g daily in 2 divided doses, increased if necessary up to 1.6–2 g daily in 2 divided doses
▶ Elderly: Reduce initial dose

Focal and generalised tonic-clonic seizures | Prophylaxis of bipolar disorder
▶ BY MOUTH
▶ Child 5-11 years: Initially 5 mg/kg daily in 2 divided doses, then increased in steps of 2.5–5 mg/kg every 3–7 days as required; maintenance 10–15 mg/kg daily in 2 divided doses, increased if necessary up to 20 mg/kg daily in 2 divided doses
▶ Child 12-17 years: Initially 100–400 mg daily in 2 divided doses, dose should be increased slowly; maintenance 400–1200 mg daily in 2 divided doses, increased if necessary up to 1.8 g daily in 2 divided doses

Trigeminal neuralgia
▶ BY MOUTH
▶ Adult: Initially 100–200 mg daily in 2 divided doses, some patients may require higher initial dose. After initial dose, increase according to response; usual dose 600–800 mg daily in 2 divided doses, increased if necessary up to 1.6 g daily in 2 divided doses, dose should be increased slowly

Prophylaxis of bipolar disorder unresponsive to lithium
▶ BY MOUTH
▶ Adult: Initially 400 mg daily in 2 divided doses, increased until symptoms controlled; usual dose 400–600 mg daily in 2 divided doses; maximum 1.6 g per day

● UNLICENSED USE Not licensed for use in acute alcohol withdrawal. Use in diabetic neuropathy is an unlicensed indication.

● CONTRA-INDICATIONS Acute porphyrias p. 1025 · AV conduction abnormalities (unless paced) · history of bone-marrow depression

● CAUTIONS Cardiac disease · history of haematological reactions to other drugs · may exacerbate absence and myoclonic seizures · skin reactions · susceptibility to angle-closure glaucoma

CAUTIONS, FURTHER INFORMATION Consider vitamin D supplementation in patients who are immobilised for long periods or who have inadequate sun exposure or dietary intake of calcium.
▶ Blood, hepatic, or skin disorders Carbamazepine should be withdrawn immediately in cases of aggravated liver dysfunction or acute liver disease. Leucopenia that is severe, progressive, or associated with clinical symptoms requires withdrawal (if necessary under cover of a suitable alternative).

● INTERACTIONS → Appendix 1: antiepileptics

● SIDE-EFFECTS

GENERAL SIDE-EFFECTS
▶ **Common or very common** Dizziness · drowsiness · dry mouth · eosinophilia · fatigue · fluid imbalance · headache · hyponatraemia · leucopenia · movement disorders · nausea · oedema · skin reactions · thrombocytopenia · vision disorders · vomiting · weight increased
▶ **Uncommon** Constipation · diarrhoea · eye disorders · tic · tremor
▶ **Rare or very rare** Aggression · agranulocytosis · albuminuria · alopecia · anaemia · angioedema · anxiety · appetite decreased · arrhythmias · arthralgia · azotaemia ·

bone disorders · bone marrow disorders · cardiac conduction disorders · circulatory collapse · confusion · congestive heart failure · conjunctivitis · coronary artery disease aggravated · depression · dyspnoea · embolism and thrombosis · erythema nodosum · fever · folate deficiency · galactorrhoea · gynaecomastia · haematuria · haemolytic anaemia · hallucinations · hearing impairment · hepatic disorders · hirsutism · hyperacusia · hyperhidrosis · hypersensitivity · hypertension · hypogammaglobulinaemia · hypotension · lens opacity · leucocytosis · lymphadenopathy · meningitis aseptic · muscle complaints · muscle weakness · nephritis tubulointerstitial · nervous system disorder · neuroleptic malignant syndrome · oral disorders · pancreatitis · paraesthesia · paresis · peripheral neuropathy · photosensitivity reaction · pneumonia · pneumonitis · pseudolymphoma · psychosis · red blood cell abnormalities · renal impairment · severe cutaneous adverse reactions (SCARs) · sexual dysfunction · speech impairment · spermatogenesis abnormal · syncope · systemic lupus erythematosus (SLE) · taste altered · urinary disorders · vanishing bile duct syndrome · vasculitis

▸ **Frequency not known** Bone fracture · colitis · human herpesvirus 6 infection reactivation · memory loss · nail loss

SPECIFIC SIDE-EFFECTS

▸ **Common or very common**
▸ With oral or rectal use Gastrointestinal discomfort

SIDE-EFFECTS, FURTHER INFORMATION Some side-effects (such as headache, ataxia, drowsiness, nausea, vomiting, blurring of vision, dizziness and allergic skin reactions) are dose-related, and may be dose-limiting. These side-effects are more common at the start of treatment and in the elderly.

Overdose For details on the management of poisoning, see Active elimination techniques, under Emergency treatment of poisoning p. 1319 .

● ALLERGY AND CROSS-SENSITIVITY Antiepileptic hypersensitivity syndrome associated with carbamazepine. See under Epilepsy p. 304 for more information. Caution—cross-sensitivity reported with oxcarbazepine and with phenytoin.

● PREGNANCY
Monitoring Doses should be adjusted on the basis of plasma-drug concentration monitoring.

● BREAST FEEDING Amount probably too small to be harmful.
Monitoring Monitor infant for possible adverse reactions.

● HEPATIC IMPAIRMENT Metabolism impaired in advanced liver disease.

● RENAL IMPAIRMENT Use with caution.

● PRE-TREATMENT SCREENING Test for HLA-B*1502 allele in individuals of Han Chinese or Thai origin (avoid unless no alternative—risk of Stevens-Johnson syndrome in presence of HLA-B*1502 allele).

● MONITORING REQUIREMENTS
▸ Plasma concentration for optimum response 4–12 mg/litre (20–50 micromol/litre) measured after 1–2 weeks.
▸ Manufacturer recommends blood counts and hepatic and renal function tests (but evidence of practical value uncertain).

● TREATMENT CESSATION When stopping treatment with carbamazepine for bipolar disorder, reduce the dose gradually over a period of at least 4 weeks.

● DIRECTIONS FOR ADMINISTRATION
▸ In children Oral liquid has been used rectally—should be retained for at least 2 hours (but may have laxative effect).

TEGRETOL ® PROLONGED RELEASE *Tegretol® Prolonged Release* tablets can be halved but should not be chewed.

● PRESCRIBING AND DISPENSING INFORMATION
Switching between formulations Different formulations of oral preparations may vary in bioavailability. Patients being treated for epilepsy should be maintained on a specific manufacturer's product.

● PATIENT AND CARER ADVICE
Medicines for Children leaflet: Carbamazepine (oral) for preventing seizures www.medicinesforchildren.org.uk/carbamazepine-oral-preventing-seizures-0

Blood, hepatic, or skin disorders Patients or their carers should be told how to recognise signs of blood, liver, or skin disorders, and advised to seek immediate medical attention if symptoms such as fever, rash, mouth ulcers, bruising, or bleeding develop.

● PROFESSION SPECIFIC INFORMATION
Dental practitioners' formulary
Carbamazepine Tablets may be prescribed.

● MEDICINAL FORMS
There can be variation in the licensing of different medicines containing the same drug. Forms available from special-order manufacturers include: oral suspension, oral solution

Modified-release tablet
CAUTIONARY AND ADVISORY LABELS 3, 8, 25
▸ Carbagen SR (Mylan)
Carbamazepine 200 mg Carbagen SR 200mg tablets | 56 tablet [PoM] £4.16 DT = £5.20
Carbamazepine 400 mg Carbagen SR 400mg tablets | 56 tablet [PoM] £8.20 DT = £10.24
▸ Tegretol Retard (Novartis Pharmaceuticals UK Ltd)
Carbamazepine 200 mg Tegretol Prolonged Release 200mg tablets | 56 tablet [PoM] £5.20 DT = £5.20
Carbamazepine 400 mg Tegretol Prolonged Release 400mg tablets | 56 tablet [PoM] £10.24 DT = £10.24

Tablet
CAUTIONARY AND ADVISORY LABELS 3, 8
▸ Carbamazepine (Non-proprietary)
Carbamazepine 100 mg Carbamazepine 100mg tablets | 84 tablet [PoM] ▤ DT = £2.07
Carbamazepine 200 mg Carbamazepine 200mg tablets | 84 tablet [PoM] ▤ DT = £3.83
Carbamazepine 400 mg Carbamazepine 400mg tablets | 56 tablet [PoM] ▤ DT = £5.02
▸ Carbagen (Mylan)
Carbamazepine 100 mg Carbagen 100mg tablets | 28 tablet [PoM] £5.74 | 84 tablet [PoM] ▤ DT = £2.07 (Hospital only)
Carbamazepine 200 mg Carbagen 200mg tablets | 28 tablet [PoM] £4.99 | 84 tablet [PoM] ▤ DT = £3.83 (Hospital only)
Carbamazepine 400 mg Carbagen 400mg tablets | 28 tablet [PoM] £4.27 | 56 tablet [PoM] ▤ DT = £5.02 (Hospital only)
▸ Tegretol (Novartis Pharmaceuticals UK Ltd)
Carbamazepine 100 mg Tegretol 100mg tablets | 84 tablet [PoM] £2.07 DT = £2.07
Carbamazepine 200 mg Tegretol 200mg tablets | 84 tablet [PoM] £3.83 DT = £3.83
Carbamazepine 400 mg Tegretol 400mg tablets | 56 tablet [PoM] £5.02 DT = £5.02

Suppository
CAUTIONARY AND ADVISORY LABELS 3, 8
▸ Carbamazepine (Non-proprietary)
Carbamazepine 125 mg Carbamazepine 125mg suppositories | 5 suppository [PoM] £120.00 DT = £120.00
Carbamazepine 250 mg Carbamazepine 250mg suppositories | 5 suppository [PoM] £140.00 DT = £140.00

Oral suspension
CAUTIONARY AND ADVISORY LABELS 3, 8
▸ Carbamazepine (Non-proprietary)
Carbamazepine 20 mg per 1 ml Carbamazepine 100mg/5ml oral suspension sugar free sugar-free | 300 ml [PoM] £7.35 DT = £6.94
▸ Tegretol (Novartis Pharmaceuticals UK Ltd)
Carbamazepine 20 mg per 1 ml Tegretol 100mg/5ml liquid sugar-free | 300 ml [PoM] £6.12 DT = £6.94

Nervous system

4

Eslicarbazepine acetate

● **INDICATIONS AND DOSE**

Adjunctive treatment in adults with focal seizures with or without secondary generalisation
▸ BY MOUTH
▸ Adult: Initially 400 mg once daily for 1–2 weeks, then increased to 800 mg once daily (max. per dose 1.2 g)

● CONTRA-INDICATIONS Second- or third-degree AV block
● CAUTIONS Elderly · hyponatraemia · PR-interval prolongation
● INTERACTIONS → Appendix 1: antiepileptics
● SIDE-EFFECTS
▸ **Common or very common** Appetite decreased · asthenia · concentration impaired · diarrhoea · dizziness · drowsiness · electrolyte imbalance · gait abnormal · headaches · movement disorders · nausea · skin reactions · sleep disorders · vertigo · vision disorders · vomiting
▸ **Uncommon** Alopecia · anaemia · anxiety · bradycardia · chest pain · chills · confusion · constipation · depression · dry mouth · eye disorders · flushing · gastritis · gastrointestinal discomfort · haemorrhage · hearing impairment · hyperhidrosis · hypertension · hypotension · hypothyroidism · increased risk of infection · liver disorder · malaise · mood altered · muscle weakness · myalgia · pain in extremity · palpitations · peripheral coldness · peripheral neuropathy · peripheral oedema · psychomotor retardation · psychotic disorder · sensation abnormal · speech impairment · toothache · weight decreased
▸ **Frequency not known** Leucopenia · pancreatitis · thrombocytopenia
● ALLERGY AND CROSS-SENSITIVITY Antiepileptic hypersensitivity syndrome theoretically associated with eslicarbazepine. See under Epilepsy p. 304 for more information.
● PREGNANCY
Monitoring The dose should be monitored carefully during pregnancy and after birth, and adjustments made on a clinical basis.
● HEPATIC IMPAIRMENT Avoid in severe impairment—no information available.
● RENAL IMPAIRMENT Avoid if eGFR less than 30 mL/minute/1.73 m^2.
Dose adjustments Reduce initial dose to 400 mg every other day for 2 weeks then 400 mg once daily if eGFR 30–60 mL/minute/1.73 m^2, adjusted according to response.
● PRE-TREATMENT SCREENING Test for HLA-B*1502 allele in individuals of Han Chinese or Thai origin (avoid unless no alternative— risk of Stevens-Johnson syndrome in presence of HLA-B*1502 allele).
● MONITORING REQUIREMENTS Monitor plasma-sodium concentration in patients at risk of hyponatraemia and discontinue treatment if hyponatraemia occurs.
● PRESCRIBING AND DISPENSING INFORMATION
Switching between formulations Care should be taken when switching between oral formulations. The need for continued supply of a particular manufacturer's product should be based on clinical judgement and consultation with the patient or their carer, taking into account factors such as seizure frequency and treatment history.
● NATIONAL FUNDING/ACCESS DECISIONS
Scottish Medicines Consortium (SMC) Decisions
The *Scottish Medicines Consortium* has advised (October 2010) that eslicarbazepine (*Zebinix*®) is accepted for restricted use within NHS Scotland as adjunctive therapy in adults with focal seizures with or without secondary generalisation. It is restricted for use in refractory epilepsy.

● MEDICINAL FORMS
There can be variation in the licensing of different medicines containing the same drug.
Tablet
CAUTIONARY AND ADVISORY LABELS 8
▸ Zebinix (Eisai Ltd)
 Eslicarbazepine acetate 200 mg Zebinix 200mg tablets | 60 tablet [PoM] £68.00 DT = £68.00
 Eslicarbazepine acetate 800 mg Zebinix 800mg tablets | 30 tablet [PoM] £136.00 DT = £136.00

Ethosuximide

● **INDICATIONS AND DOSE**

Absence seizures | Atypical absence seizures (adjunct) | Myoclonic seizures
▸ BY MOUTH
▸ Child 1 month-5 years: Initially 5 mg/kg twice daily (max. per dose 125 mg), dose to be increased every 5–7 days; maintenance 10–20 mg/kg twice daily (max. per dose 500 mg), total daily dose may rarely be given in 3 divided doses
▸ Child 6-17 years: Initially 250 mg twice daily, then increased in steps of 250 mg every 5–7 days; usual dose 500–750 mg twice daily, increased if necessary up to 1 g twice daily
▸ Adult: Initially 500 mg daily in 2 divided doses, then increased in steps of 250 mg every 5–7 days; usual dose 1–1.5 g daily in 2 divided doses, increased if necessary up to 2 g daily

● CAUTIONS Avoid in Acute porphyrias p. 1025
● INTERACTIONS → Appendix 1: antiepileptics
● SIDE-EFFECTS Aggression · agranulocytosis · appetite decreased · blood disorder · bone marrow disorders · concentration impaired · depression · diarrhoea · dizziness · drowsiness · erythema nodosum · fatigue · gastrointestinal discomfort · generalised tonic-clonic seizure · headache · hiccups · leucopenia · libido increased · lupus-like syndrome · mood altered · movement disorders · nausea · nephrotic syndrome · oral disorders · psychosis · rash · sleep disorders · Stevens-Johnson syndrome · vaginal haemorrhage · vision disorders · vomiting · weight decreased
SIDE-EFFECTS, FURTHER INFORMATION Blood counts required if features of fever, sore throat, mouth ulcers, bruising or bleeding.
● PREGNANCY
Monitoring The dose should be monitored carefully during pregnancy and after birth, and adjustments made on a clinical basis.
● BREAST FEEDING Present in milk. Hyperexcitability and sedation reported.
● HEPATIC IMPAIRMENT Use with caution.
● RENAL IMPAIRMENT Use with caution.
● PATIENT AND CARER ADVICE
Medicines for Children leaflet: Ethosuximide for preventing seizures www.medicinesforchildren.org.uk/ethosuximide-for-preventing-seizures
Blood disorders Patients or their carers should be told how to recognise signs of blood disorders, and advised to seek immediate medical attention if symptoms such as fever, mouth ulcers, bruising, or bleeding develop.

● MEDICINAL FORMS
There can be variation in the licensing of different medicines containing the same drug.

Oral solution
CAUTIONARY AND ADVISORY LABELS 8
▶ Ethosuximide (Non-proprietary)
  Ethosuximide 50 mg per 1 ml Ethosuximide 250mg/5ml syrup | 200 ml [PoM] £173.00 DT = £173.00

Capsule
CAUTIONARY AND ADVISORY LABELS 8
▶ Ethosuximide (Non-proprietary)
  Ethosuximide 250 mg Ethosuximide 250mg capsules | 56 capsule [PoM] £173.00 DT = £173.00

Fosphenytoin sodium

● DRUG ACTION Fosphenytoin is a pro-drug of phenytoin.

● INDICATIONS AND DOSE

Status epilepticus
▶ BY INTRAVENOUS INFUSION
▶ Adult: Initially 20 mg(PE)/kg, dose to be administered at a rate of 100–150 mg(PE)/minute, then 4–5 mg (PE)/kg daily in 1–2 divided doses, dose to be administered at a rate of 50–100 mg(PE)/minute, dose to be adjusted according to response and trough plasma-phenytoin concentration
▶ Elderly: Consider 10–25% reduction in dose or infusion rate

Prophylaxis or treatment of seizures associated with neurosurgery or head injury
▶ BY INTRAMUSCULAR INJECTION, OR BY INTRAVENOUS INFUSION
▶ Adult: Initially 10–15 mg(PE)/kg, intravenous infusion to be administered at a rate of 50–100 mg(PE)/minute, then 4–5 mg(PE)/kg daily in 1–2 divided doses, intravenous infusion to be administered at a rate of 50–100 mg(PE)/minute, dose to be adjusted according to response and trough plasma-phenytoin concentration
▶ Elderly: Consider 10–25% reduction in dose or infusion rate

Temporary substitution for oral phenytoin
▶ BY INTRAMUSCULAR INJECTION, OR BY INTRAVENOUS INFUSION
▶ Adult: Same dose and same dosing frequency as oral phenytoin therapy, intravenous infusion to be administered at a rate of 50–100 mg(PE)/minute
▶ Elderly: Consider 10–25% reduction in dose or infusion rate

DOSE EQUIVALENCE AND CONVERSION
▶ Doses are expressed as phenytoin sodium equivalent (PE); fosphenytoin sodium 1.5 mg ≡ phenytoin sodium 1 mg.

● UNLICENSED USE Fosphenytoin sodium doses in BNF may differ from those in product literature.

● CONTRA-INDICATIONS Acute porphyrias p. 1025 · second-degree heart block · sino-atrial block · sinus bradycardia · Stokes-Adams syndrome · third-degree heart block

● CAUTIONS Heart failure · hypotension · injection solutions alkaline (irritant to tissues) · respiratory depression · resuscitation facilities must be available

● INTERACTIONS → Appendix 1: antiepileptics

● SIDE-EFFECTS
▶ **Common or very common** Asthenia · chills · dizziness · drowsiness · dry mouth · dysarthria · euphoric mood · headache · hearing impairment · hypotension · movement disorders · nausea · nystagmus · sensation abnormal · skin reactions · stupor · taste altered · tremor · vasodilation · vertigo · vision disorders · vomiting
▶ **Uncommon** Cardiac arrest · confusion · muscle complaints · muscle weakness · nervousness · oral disorders · reflexes

abnormal · severe cutaneous adverse reactions (SCARs) · systemic lupus erythematosus (SLE) · thinking abnormal
▶ **Frequency not known** Acute psychosis · agranulocytosis · appetite disorder · atrial conduction depression (more common if injection too rapid) · atrioventricular block · bone disorders · bone fracture · bone marrow disorders · bradycardia · cardiotoxicity · cerebrovascular insufficiency · circulatory collapse (more common if injection too rapid) · coarsening of the facial features · constipation · delirium · Dupuytren's contracture · encephalopathy · granulocytopenia · groin tingling · hair changes · hepatic disorders · hyperglycaemia · hypersensitivity · insomnia · leucopenia · lymphadenopathy · nephritis tubulointerstitial · Peyronie's disease · polyarteritis nodosa · polyarthritis · purple glove syndrome · respiratory disorders · sensory peripheral polyneuropathy · thrombocytopenia · tonic seizure · ventricular conduction depression (more common if injection too rapid) · ventricular fibrillation (more common if injection too rapid)

SIDE-EFFECTS, FURTHER INFORMATION Fosphenytoin has been associated with severe cardiovascular reactions including asystole, ventricular fibrillation, and cardiac arrest. Hypotension, bradycardia, and heart block have also been reported. The following are recommended: monitor heart rate, blood pressure, and respiratory function for duration of infusion; observe patient for at least 30 minutes after infusion; if hypotension occurs, reduce infusion rate or discontinue; reduce dose or infusion rate in elderly, and in renal or hepatic impairment.

● ALLERGY AND CROSS-SENSITIVITY Cross-sensitivity reported with carbamazepine.

● PREGNANCY
Monitoring Changes in plasma-protein binding make interpretation of plasma-phenytoin concentrations difficult—monitor unbound fraction.
　The dose should be monitored carefully during pregnancy and after birth, and adjustments made on a clinical basis.

● BREAST FEEDING Small amounts present in milk, but not known to be harmful.

● HEPATIC IMPAIRMENT
Dose adjustments Consider 10–25% reduction in dose or infusion rate (except initial dose for status epilepticus).

● RENAL IMPAIRMENT
Dose adjustments Consider 10–25% reduction in dose or infusion rate (except initial dose for status epilepticus).

● PRE-TREATMENT SCREENING HLA-B* 1502 allele in individuals of Han Chinese or Thai origin—avoid unless essential (increased risk of Stevens-Johnson syndrome).

● MONITORING REQUIREMENTS
▶ Manufacturer recommends blood counts (but evidence of practical value uncertain).
▶ With intravenous use Monitor heart rate, blood pressure, ECG, and respiratory function for during infusion.

● DIRECTIONS FOR ADMINISTRATION For *intermittent intravenous infusion (Pro-Epanutin®)*, give in Glucose 5% or Sodium chloride 0.9%; dilute to a concentration of 1.5–25 mg (phenytoin sodium equivalent (PE))/mL.

● PRESCRIBING AND DISPENSING INFORMATION
Prescriptions for fosphenytoin sodium should state the dose in terms of phenytoin sodium equivalent (PE); fosphenytoin sodium 1.5 mg ≡ phenytoin sodium 1 mg.

● MEDICINAL FORMS
There can be variation in the licensing of different medicines containing the same drug.

Solution for injection

ELECTROLYTES: May contain Phosphate

▸ Pro-Epanutin (Pfizer Ltd)
Fosphenytoin sodium 75 mg per 1 ml Pro-Epanutin 750mg/10ml concentrate for solution for injection vials | 10 vial [PoM] £400.00 (Hospital only)

Gabapentin

19-Jul-2017

● INDICATIONS AND DOSE

Adjunctive treatment of focal seizures with or without secondary generalisation

▸ BY MOUTH

▸ Child 6–11 years: 10 mg/kg once daily (max. per dose 300 mg) on day 1, then 10 mg/kg twice daily (max. per dose 300 mg) on day 2, then 10 mg/kg 3 times a day (max. per dose 300 mg) on day 3; usual dose 25–35 mg/kg daily in 3 divided doses, some children may not tolerate daily increments; longer intervals (up to weekly) may be more appropriate, daily dose maximum to be given in 3 divided doses; maximum 70 mg/kg per day

▸ Child 12–17 years: Initially 300 mg once daily on day 1, then 300 mg twice daily on day 2, then 300 mg 3 times a day on day 3, alternatively initially 300 mg 3 times a day on day 1, then increased in steps of 300 mg every 2–3 days in 3 divided doses, adjusted according to response; usual dose 0.9–3.6 g daily in 3 divided doses (max. per dose 1.6 g 3 times a day), some children may not tolerate daily increments; longer intervals (up to weekly) may be more appropriate

▸ Adult: Initially 300 mg once daily on day 1, then 300 mg twice daily on day 2, then 300 mg 3 times a day on day 3, alternatively initially 300 mg 3 times a day on day 1, then increased in steps of 300 mg every 2–3 days in 3 divided doses, adjusted according to response; usual dose 0.9–3.6 g daily in 3 divided doses (max. per dose 1.6 g 3 times a day)

Monotherapy for focal seizures with or without secondary generalisation

▸ BY MOUTH

▸ Child 12–17 years: Initially 300 mg once daily on day 1, then 300 mg twice daily on day 2, then 300 mg 3 times a day on day 3, alternatively initially 300 mg 3 times a day on day 1, then increased in steps of 300 mg every 2–3 days in 3 divided doses, adjusted according to response; usual dose 0.9–3.6 g daily in 3 divided doses (max. per dose 1.6 g 3 times a day), some children may not tolerate daily increments; longer intervals (up to weekly) may be more appropriate

▸ Adult: Initially 300 mg once daily on day 1, then 300 mg twice daily on day 2, then 300 mg 3 times a day on day 3, alternatively initially 300 mg 3 times a day on day 1, then increased in steps of 300 mg every 2–3 days in 3 divided doses, adjusted according to response; usual dose 0.9–3.6 g daily in 3 divided doses (max. per dose 1.6 g 3 times a day)

Peripheral neuropathic pain

▸ BY MOUTH

▸ Adult: Initially 300 mg once daily on day 1, then 300 mg twice daily on day 2, then 300 mg 3 times a day on day 3, alternatively initially 300 mg 3 times a day on day 1, then increased in steps of 300 mg every 2–3 days in 3 divided doses, adjusted according to response; maximum 3.6 g per day

Migraine prophylaxis

▸ BY MOUTH

▸ Adult: Initially 300 mg daily, then increased to up to 2.4 g daily in divided doses, adjusted according to response

Menopausal symptoms, particularly hot flushes, in women with breast cancer

▸ BY MOUTH

▸ Adult: 300 mg 3 times a day, initial dose should be lower and titrated up over three days

● UNLICENSED USE Not licensed at doses over 50 mg/kg daily in children under 12 years. Not licensed for migraine prophylaxis. [EvGr] Not licensed for menopausal symptoms. Ⓐ

> IMPORTANT SAFETY INFORMATION
>
> The levels of propylene glycol, acesulfame K and saccharin sodium may exceed the recommended WHO daily intake limits if high doses of gabapentin oral solution (Rosemont brand) are given to adolescents or adults with low body-weight (39–50 kg)—consult product literature.
>
> MHRA/CHM ADVICE: GABAPENTIN (*NEURONTIN*®): RISK OF SEVERE RESPIRATORY DEPRESSION (OCTOBER 2017)
> Gabapentin has been associated with a rare risk of severe respiratory depression even without concomitant opioid medicines. Patients with compromised respiratory function, respiratory or neurological disease, renal impairment, concomitant use of central nervous system (CNS) depressants, and elderly people might be at higher risk of experiencing severe respiratory depression and dose adjustments may be necessary in these patients.

● CAUTIONS Diabetes mellitus · elderly · high doses of oral solution in adolescents and adults with low body-weight · history of psychotic illness · mixed seizures (including absences)

● INTERACTIONS → Appendix 1: antiepileptics

● SIDE-EFFECTS

▸ **Common or very common** Anxiety · appetite abnormal · arthralgia · asthenia · behaviour abnormal (frequency not known in children) · confusion · constipation · cough · depression · diarrhoea · dizziness · drowsiness · dry mouth · dysarthria · dyspnoea · emotional lability · flatulence · gait abnormal · gastrointestinal discomfort · headache · hypertension · increased risk of infection · insomnia · leucopenia · malaise · movement disorders · muscle complaints · nausea · nystagmus · oedema · pain · reflexes abnormal · seizure (in children) · sensation abnormal · sexual dysfunction · skin reactions · thinking abnormal · tooth disorder · tremor · vasodilation · vertigo · visual impairment · vomiting

▸ **Uncommon** Cognitive impairment · palpitations

▸ **Frequency not known** Acute kidney injury · alopecia · angioedema · breast enlargement · gynaecomastia · hallucination · hepatic disorders · hyponatraemia · pancreatitis · rhabdomyolysis · severe cutaneous adverse reactions (SCARs) · thrombocytopenia · tinnitus · urinary incontinence

● PREGNANCY
Monitoring The dose should be monitored carefully during pregnancy and after birth, and adjustments made on a clinical basis.

● BREAST FEEDING Present in milk—manufacturer advises use only if potential benefit outweighs risk.

● RENAL IMPAIRMENT
Dose adjustments ▸ In adults Reduce dose to 0.6–1.8 g daily in 3 divided doses if eGFR 50–80 mL/minute/1.73 m². Reduce dose to 300–900 mg daily in 3 divided doses if eGFR 30–50 mL/minute/1.73 m². Reduce dose to 300 mg

on alternate days (up to max. 600 mg daily) in 3 divided doses if eGFR 15–30 mL/minute/1.73 m². Reduce dose to 300 mg on alternate days (up to max. 300 mg daily) in 3 divided doses if eGFR less than 15 mL/minute/1.73 m²—consult product literature.

▸ In children Reduce dose if estimated glomerular filtration rate less than 80 mL/minute/1.73 m²; consult product literature.

● EFFECT ON LABORATORY TESTS False positive readings with some urinary protein tests.

● DIRECTIONS FOR ADMINISTRATION Capsules can be opened but the bitter taste is difficult to mask.

● PATIENT AND CARER ADVICE
Medicines for Children leaflet: Gabapentin for preventing seizures www.medicinesforchildren.org.uk/gabapentin-for-preventing-seizures

● MEDICINAL FORMS
There can be variation in the licensing of different medicines containing the same drug. Forms available from special-order manufacturers include: oral suspension, oral solution

Tablet
CAUTIONARY AND ADVISORY LABELS 3, 5, 8, 25
▸ Gabapentin (Non-proprietary)
  Gabapentin 600 mg Gabapentin 600mg tablets | 100 tablet [PoM] £106.00 DT = £6.45
  Gabapentin 800 mg Gabapentin 800mg tablets | 100 tablet [PoM] £98.13 DT = £29.85
▸ Neurontin (Pfizer Ltd)
  Gabapentin 600 mg Neurontin 600mg tablets | 100 tablet [PoM] £84.80 DT = £6.45
  Gabapentin 800 mg Neurontin 800mg tablets | 100 tablet [PoM] £98.13 DT = £29.85

Oral solution
CAUTIONARY AND ADVISORY LABELS 3, 5, 8
EXCIPIENTS: May contain Propylene glycol
ELECTROLYTES: May contain Potassium, sodium
▸ Gabapentin (Non-proprietary)
  Gabapentin 50 mg per 1 ml Gabapentin 50mg/ml oral solution sugar-free | 150 ml [PoM] £69.00 DT = £69.00

Capsule
CAUTIONARY AND ADVISORY LABELS 3, 5, 8, 25
▸ Gabapentin (Non-proprietary)
  Gabapentin 100 mg Gabapentin 100mg capsules | 100 capsule [PoM] £18.29 DT = £2.41
  Gabapentin 300 mg Gabapentin 300mg capsules | 100 capsule [PoM] £42.40 DT = £8.09
  Gabapentin 400 mg Gabapentin 400mg capsules | 100 capsule [PoM] £49.06 DT = £5.94
▸ Neurontin (Pfizer Ltd)
  Gabapentin 100 mg Neurontin 100mg capsules | 100 capsule [PoM] £18.29 DT = £2.41
  Gabapentin 300 mg Neurontin 300mg capsules | 100 capsule [PoM] £42.40 DT = £8.09
  Gabapentin 400 mg Neurontin 400mg capsules | 100 capsule [PoM] £49.06 DT = £5.94

Lacosamide

22-Feb-2018

● INDICATIONS AND DOSE

Monotherapy of focal seizures with or without secondary generalisation
▸ BY MOUTH, OR BY INTRAVENOUS INFUSION
▸ Child (body-weight 50 kg and above): Initially 50 mg twice daily, then increased to 100 mg twice daily, after one week, alternatively initially 100 mg twice daily; increased in steps of 50 mg twice daily (max. per dose 300 mg twice daily) if necessary and if tolerated, dose to be increased at weekly intervals
▸ Child 4-17 years (body-weight up to 50 kg): (consult product literature)
▸ Adult: Initially 50 mg twice daily, then increased to 100 mg twice daily, after one week, alternatively initially 100 mg twice daily; increased in steps of 50 mg

twice daily (max. per dose 300 mg twice daily) if necessary and if tolerated, dose to be increased at weekly intervals

Monotherapy of focal seizures with or without secondary generalisation (alternative loading dose regimen when it is necessary to rapidly attain therapeutic plasma concentrations) (under close medical supervision)
▸ BY MOUTH, OR BY INTRAVENOUS INFUSION
▸ Child (body-weight 50 kg and above): Loading dose 200 mg, followed by 100 mg twice daily, to be given 12 hours after initial dose; increased in steps of 50 mg twice daily (max. per dose 300 mg twice daily) if necessary and if tolerated, dose to be increased at weekly intervals
▸ Adult: Loading dose 200 mg, followed by 100 mg twice daily, to be given 12 hours after initial dose; increased in steps of 50 mg twice daily (max. per dose 300 mg twice daily) if necessary and if tolerated, dose to be increased at weekly intervals

Adjunctive treatment of focal seizures with or without secondary generalisation
▸ BY MOUTH, OR BY INTRAVENOUS INFUSION
▸ Child (body-weight 50 kg and above): Initially 50 mg twice daily, then increased to 100 mg twice daily, after one week; increased in steps of 50 mg twice daily (max. per dose 200 mg twice daily) if necessary and if tolerated, dose to be increased at weekly intervals
▸ Child 4-17 years (body-weight up to 50 kg): (consult product literature)
▸ Adult: Initially 50 mg twice daily, then increased to 100 mg twice daily, after one week; increased in steps of 50 mg twice daily (max. per dose 200 mg twice daily) if necessary and if tolerated, dose to be increased at weekly intervals

Adjunctive treatment of focal seizures with or without secondary generalisation (alternative loading dose regimen when it is necessary to rapidly attain therapeutic plasma concentrations) (under close medical supervision)
▸ BY MOUTH, OR BY INTRAVENOUS INFUSION
▸ Child (body-weight 50 kg and above): Loading dose 200 mg, followed by 100 mg twice daily, to be given 12 hours after initial dose; increased in steps of 50 mg twice daily (max. per dose 200 mg twice daily) if necessary and if tolerated, dose to be increased at weekly intervals
▸ Adult: Loading dose 200 mg, followed by 100 mg twice daily, to be given 12 hours after initial dose; increased in steps of 50 mg twice daily (max. per dose 200 mg twice daily) if necessary and if tolerated, dose to be increased at weekly intervals

● CONTRA-INDICATIONS Second- or third-degree AV block
● CAUTIONS Conduction problems · elderly · risk of PR-interval prolongation · severe cardiac disease
● INTERACTIONS → Appendix 1: antiepileptics
● SIDE-EFFECTS
▸ Common or very common Asthenia · concentration impaired · confusion · constipation · depression · diarrhoea · dizziness · drowsiness · dry mouth · dysarthria · dyspepsia · flatulence · gait abnormal · headache · insomnia · mood altered · movement disorders · muscle spasms · nausea · nystagmus · sensation abnormal · skin reactions · tinnitus · vertigo · vision disorders · vomiting
▸ Uncommon Aggression · agitation · angioedema · arrhythmias · atrioventricular block · hallucination · psychotic disorder · suicidal tendencies · syncope
▸ Frequency not known Agranulocytosis
● ALLERGY AND CROSS-SENSITIVITY Antiepileptic hypersensitivity syndrome associated with lacosamide. See under Epilepsy p. 304 for more information.

4

Nervous system

- PREGNANCY
  Monitoring The dose should be monitored carefully during pregnancy and after birth, and adjustments made on a clinical basis.
- BREAST FEEDING Manufacturer advises avoid—present in milk in *animal* studies.
- HEPATIC IMPAIRMENT
  Dose adjustments Consult product literature.
- RENAL IMPAIRMENT Consult product literature.
- DIRECTIONS FOR ADMINISTRATION For *intermittent intravenous infusion*, manufacturer advises give undiluted or dilute with Glucose 5% *or* Sodium Chloride 0.9% *or* Lactated Ringer's Solution; give over 15–60 minutes—give doses greater than 200 mg over at least 30 minutes.
- PRESCRIBING AND DISPENSING INFORMATION Flavours of syrup may include strawberry.
- PATIENT AND CARER ADVICE
  Medicines for Children leaflet: Lacosamide for preventing seizures www.medicinesforchildren.org.uk/lacosamide-for-preventing-seizures
- NATIONAL FUNDING/ACCESS DECISIONS

Scottish Medicines Consortium (SMC) Decisions
SMC No. 532/09
The *Scottish Medicines Consortium* has advised (February 2009) that lacosamide (*Vimpat*®) is accepted for restricted use within NHS Scotland as adjunctive treatment for focal seizures with or without secondary generalisation in patients from 16 years. It is restricted for specialist use in refractory epilepsy.
SMC No. 1301/18
The *Scottish Medicines Consortium* has advised (February 2018) that lacosamide (*Vimpat*®) is accepted for restricted use within NHS Scotland as adjunctive treatment for focal seizures with or without secondary generalisation in adolescents and children from 4 years of age with epilepsy. It is restricted for specialist use in refractory epilepsy.

All Wales Medicines Strategy Group (AWMSG) Decisions
AWMSG No. 3343
The *All Wales Medicines Strategy Group* has advised (March 2018) that lacosamide (*Vimpat*®) is recommended as an option for use within NHS Wales as adjunctive therapy in the treatment of focal seizures with or without secondary generalisation in children from 4 years of age up to 15 years of age with epilepsy.

- MEDICINAL FORMS
  There can be variation in the licensing of different medicines containing the same drug.
  Solution for infusion
  ELECTROLYTES: May contain Sodium
  ▸ Vimpat (UCB Pharma Ltd)
  Lacosamide 10 mg per 1 ml Vimpat 200mg/20ml solution for infusion vials | 1 vial PoM £29.70
  Oral solution
  CAUTIONARY AND ADVISORY LABELS 8
  EXCIPIENTS: May contain Aspartame, propylene glycol
  ELECTROLYTES: May contain Sodium
  ▸ Vimpat (UCB Pharma Ltd)
  Lacosamide 10 mg per 1 ml Vimpat 10mg/ml syrup sugar-free | 200 ml PoM £25.74 DT = £25.74
  Tablet
  CAUTIONARY AND ADVISORY LABELS 8
  ▸ Vimpat (UCB Pharma Ltd)
  Lacosamide 50 mg Vimpat 50mg tablets | 14 tablet PoM £10.81 DT = £10.81
  Lacosamide 100 mg Vimpat 100mg tablets | 14 tablet PoM £21.62 | 56 tablet PoM £86.50 DT = £86.50
  Lacosamide 150 mg Vimpat 150mg tablets | 14 tablet PoM £32.44 | 56 tablet PoM £129.74 DT = £129.74
  Lacosamide 200 mg Vimpat 200mg tablets | 56 tablet PoM £144.16 DT = £144.16

Lamotrigine

- INDICATIONS AND DOSE

Monotherapy of focal seizures | Monotherapy of primary and secondary generalised tonic-clonic seizures | Monotherapy of seizures associated with Lennox-Gastaut syndrome
▸ BY MOUTH
▸ Child 12–17 years: Initially 25 mg once daily for 14 days, then increased to 50 mg once daily for further 14 days, then increased in steps of up to 100 mg every 7–14 days; maintenance 100–200 mg daily in 1–2 divided doses; increased if necessary up to 500 mg daily, dose titration should be repeated if restarting after interval of more than 5 days
▸ Adult: Initially 25 mg once daily for 14 days, then increased to 50 mg once daily for further 14 days, then increased in steps of up to 100 mg every 7–14 days; maintenance 100–200 mg daily in 1–2 divided doses; increased if necessary up to 500 mg daily, dose titration should be repeated if restarting after interval of more than 5 days

Adjunctive therapy of focal seizures with valproate | Adjunctive therapy of primary and secondary generalised tonic-clonic seizures with valproate | Adjunctive therapy of seizures associated with Lennox-Gastaut syndrome with valproate
▸ BY MOUTH
▸ Child 2–11 years (body-weight up to 13 kg): Initially 2 mg once daily on alternate days for first 14 days, then 300 micrograms/kg once daily for further 14 days, then increased in steps of up to 300 micrograms/kg every 7–14 days; maintenance 1–5 mg/kg daily in 1–2 divided doses, dose titration should be repeated if restarting after interval of more than 5 days; maximum 200 mg per day
▸ Child 2–11 years (body-weight 13 kg and above): Initially 150 micrograms/kg once daily for 14 days, then 300 micrograms/kg once daily for further 14 days, then increased in steps of up to 300 micrograms/kg every 7–14 days; maintenance 1–5 mg/kg daily in 1–2 divided doses, dose titration should be repeated if restarting after interval of more than 5 days; maximum 200 mg per day
▸ Child 12–17 years: Initially 25 mg once daily on alternate days for 14 days, then 25 mg once daily for further 14 days, then increased in steps of up to 50 mg every 7–14 days; maintenance 100–200 mg daily in 1–2 divided doses, dose titration should be repeated if restarting after interval of more than 5 days
▸ Adult: Initially 25 mg once daily on alternate days for 14 days, then 25 mg once daily for further 14 days, then increased in steps of up to 50 mg every 7–14 days; maintenance 100–200 mg daily in 1–2 divided doses, dose titration should be repeated if restarting after interval of more than 5 days

Adjunctive therapy of focal seizures (with enzyme inducing drugs) without valproate | Adjunctive therapy of primary and secondary generalised tonic-clonic seizures (with enzyme inducing drugs) without valproate | Adjunctive therapy of seizures associated with Lennox-Gastaut syndromes (with enzyme inducing drugs) without valproate
▸ BY MOUTH
▸ Child 2–11 years: Initially 300 micrograms/kg twice daily for 14 days, then 600 micrograms/kg twice daily for further 14 days, then increased in steps of up to 1.2 mg/kg every 7–14 days; maintenance 5–15 mg/kg daily in 1–2 divided doses, dose titration should be repeated if restarting after interval of more than 5 days; maximum 400 mg per day

- Child 12–17 years: Initially 50 mg once daily for 14 days, then 50 mg twice daily for further 14 days, then increased in steps of up to 100 mg every 7–14 days; maintenance 200–400 mg daily in 2 divided doses, increased if necessary up to 700 mg daily, dose titration should be repeated if restarting after interval of more than 5 days
- Adult: Initially 50 mg once daily for 14 days, then 50 mg twice daily for further 14 days, then increased in steps of up to 100 mg every 7–14 days; maintenance 200–400 mg daily in 2 divided doses, increased if necessary up to 700 mg daily, dose titration should be repeated if restarting after interval of more than 5 days

Adjunctive therapy of focal seizures (without enzyme inducing drugs) without valproate | Adjunctive therapy of primary and secondary generalised tonic-clonic seizures (without enzyme inducing drugs) without valproate | Adjunctive therapy of seizures associated with Lennox-Gastaut syndromes (without enzyme inducing drugs) without valproate
- BY MOUTH
- Child 2–11 years: Initially 300 micrograms/kg daily in 1–2 divided doses for 14 days, then 600 micrograms/kg daily in 1–2 divided doses for further 14 days, then increased in steps of up to 600 micrograms/kg every 7–14 days; maintenance 1–10 mg/kg daily in 1–2 divided doses, dose titration should be repeated if restarting after interval of more than 5 days; maximum 200 mg per day
- Child 12–17 years: Initially 25 mg once daily for 14 days, then increased to 50 mg once daily for further 14 days, then increased in steps of up to 100 mg every 7–14 days; maintenance 100–200 mg daily in 1–2 divided doses, dose titration should be repeated if restarting after interval of more than 5 days
- Adult: Initially 25 mg once daily for 14 days, then increased to 50 mg once daily for further 14 days, then increased in steps of up to 100 mg every 7–14 days; maintenance 100–200 mg daily in 1–2 divided doses, dose titration should be repeated if restarting after interval of more than 5 days

Monotherapy or adjunctive therapy of bipolar disorder (without enzyme inducing drugs) without valproate
- BY MOUTH
- Adult: Initially 25 mg once daily for 14 days, then 50 mg daily in 1–2 divided doses for further 14 days, then 100 mg daily in 1–2 divided doses for further 7 days; maintenance 200 mg daily in 1–2 divided doses, patients stabilised on lamotrigine for bipolar disorder may require dose adjustments if other drugs are added to or withdrawn from their treatment regimens—consult product literature, dose titration should be repeated if restarting after interval of more than 5 days; maximum 400 mg per day

Adjunctive therapy of bipolar disorder with valproate
- BY MOUTH
- Adult: Initially 25 mg once daily on alternate days for 14 days, then 25 mg once daily for further 14 days, then 50 mg daily in 1–2 divided doses for further 7 days; maintenance 100 mg daily in 1–2 divided doses, patients stabilised on lamotrigine for bipolar disorder may require dose adjustments if other drugs are added to or withdrawn from their treatment regimens—consult product literature, dose titration should be repeated if restarting after interval of more than 5 days; maximum 200 mg per day

Adjunctive therapy of bipolar disorder (with enzyme inducing drugs) without valproate
- BY MOUTH
- Adult: Initially 50 mg once daily for 14 days, then 50 mg twice daily for further 14 days, then increased to

100 mg twice daily for further 7 days, then increased to 150 mg twice daily for further 7 days; maintenance 200 mg twice daily, patients stabilised on lamotrigine for bipolar disorder may require dose adjustments if other drugs are added to or withdrawn from their treatment regimens—consult product literature, dose titration should be repeated if restarting after interval of more than 5 days

> **IMPORTANT SAFETY INFORMATION**
> SAFE PRACTICE
> Do not confuse the different combinations or indications.

- CAUTIONS Myoclonic seizures (may be exacerbated) · Parkinson's disease (may be exacerbated)
- INTERACTIONS → Appendix 1: antiepileptics
- SIDE-EFFECTS
- Common or very common Aggression · agitation · arthralgia · diarrhoea · dizziness · drowsiness · dry mouth · fatigue · headache · irritability · nausea · pain · rash · sleep disorders · tremor · vomiting
- Uncommon Alopecia · movement disorders · vision disorders
- Rare or very rare Confusion · conjunctivitis · disseminated intravascular coagulation · face oedema · fever · hallucination · hepatic disorders · lupus-like syndrome · lymphadenopathy · meningitis aseptic · multi organ failure · nystagmus · seizure · severe cutaneous adverse reactions (SCARs) · tic

SIDE-EFFECTS, FURTHER INFORMATION Serious skin reactions including Stevens-Johnson syndrome and toxic epidermal necrolysis have developed (especially in children); most rashes occur in the first 8 weeks. Rash is sometimes associated with hypersensitivity syndrome and is more common in patients with history of allergy or rash from other antiepileptic drugs. Consider withdrawal if rash or signs of hypersensitivity syndrome develop. Factors associated with increased risk of serious skin reactions include concomitant use of valproate, initial lamotrigine dosing higher than recommended, and more rapid dose escalation than recommended.

- ALLERGY AND CROSS-SENSITIVITY Antiepileptic hypersensitivity syndrome associated with lamotrigine. See under Epilepsy p. 304 for more information.
- PREGNANCY
  Monitoring Doses should be adjusted on the basis of plasma-drug concentration monitoring.
- BREAST FEEDING Present in milk, but limited data suggest no harmful effect on infant.
- HEPATIC IMPAIRMENT
  Dose adjustments Halve dose in moderate impairment. Quarter dose in severe impairment.
- RENAL IMPAIRMENT Caution in renal failure; metabolite may accumulate.
  Dose adjustments Consider reducing maintenance dose in significant impairment.
- TREATMENT CESSATION Avoid abrupt withdrawal (taper off over 2 weeks or longer) unless serious skin reaction occurs.
- PRESCRIBING AND DISPENSING INFORMATION Patients being treated for epilepsy may need to be maintained on a specific manufacturer's branded or generic lamotrigine product.
  Switching between formulations Care should be taken when switching between oral formulations in the treatment of epilepsy. The need for continued supply of a particular manufacturer's product should be based on clinical judgement and consultation with the patient or their carer, taking into account factors such as seizure frequency and treatment history.

● PATIENT AND CARER ADVICE

Medicines for Children leaflet: Lamotrigine for preventing seizures www.medicinesforchildren.org.uk/lamotrigine-for-preventing-seizures

Skin reactions Warn patients and carers to see their doctor immediately if rash or signs or symptoms of hypersensitivity syndrome develop.

Blood disorders Patients and their carers should be alert for symptoms and signs suggestive of bone-marrow failure, such as anaemia, bruising, or infection. Aplastic anaemia, bone-marrow depression, and pancytopenia have been associated rarely with lamotrigine.

● MEDICINAL FORMS

There can be variation in the licensing of different medicines containing the same drug. Forms available from special-order manufacturers include: oral suspension, oral solution

Dispersible tablet

CAUTIONARY AND ADVISORY LABELS 8, 13

▸ Lamotrigine (Non-proprietary)

Lamotrigine 5 mg Lamotrigine 5mg dispersible tablets sugar free sugar-free | 28 tablet PoM £15.00 DT = £7.09

Lamotrigine 25 mg Lamotrigine 25mg dispersible tablets sugar free sugar-free | 56 tablet PoM £20.41 DT = £1.86

Lamotrigine 100 mg Lamotrigine 100mg dispersible tablets sugar free sugar-free | 56 tablet PoM £58.68 DT = £3.93

▸ Lamictal (GlaxoSmithKline UK Ltd)

Lamotrigine 2 mg Lamictal 2mg dispersible tablets sugar-free | 30 tablet PoM £18.81 DT = £18.81

Lamotrigine 5 mg Lamictal 5mg dispersible tablets sugar-free | 28 tablet PoM £9.38 DT = £7.09

Lamotrigine 25 mg Lamictal 25mg dispersible tablets sugar-free | 56 tablet PoM £23.53 DT = £1.86

Lamotrigine 100 mg Lamictal 100mg dispersible tablets sugar-free | 56 tablet PoM £69.04 DT = £3.93

Tablet

CAUTIONARY AND ADVISORY LABELS 8

▸ Lamotrigine (Non-proprietary)

Lamotrigine 25 mg Lamotrigine 25mg tablets | 56 tablet PoM £20.41 DT = £1.08

Lamotrigine 50 mg Lamotrigine 50mg tablets | 56 tablet PoM £8.00 DT = £1.22

Lamotrigine 100 mg Lamotrigine 100mg tablets | 56 tablet PoM £62.14 DT = £1.76

Lamotrigine 200 mg Lamotrigine 200mg tablets | 56 tablet PoM £105.62 DT = £2.55

▸ Lamictal (GlaxoSmithKline UK Ltd)

Lamotrigine 25 mg Lamictal 25mg tablets | 56 tablet PoM £23.53 DT = £1.08

Lamotrigine 50 mg Lamictal 50mg tablets | 56 tablet PoM £40.02 DT = £1.22

Lamotrigine 100 mg Lamictal 100mg tablets | 56 tablet PoM £69.04 DT = £1.76

Lamotrigine 200 mg Lamictal 200mg tablets | 56 tablet PoM £117.35 DT = £2.55

Levetiracetam

03-Apr-2018

● INDICATIONS AND DOSE

Monotherapy of focal seizures with or without secondary generalisation

▸ BY MOUTH, OR BY INTRAVENOUS INFUSION

▸ **Child 16-17 years:** Initially 250 mg once daily for 1 week, then increased to 250 mg twice daily, then increased in steps of 250 mg twice daily (max. per dose 1.5 g twice daily), adjusted according to response, dose to be increased every 2 weeks

▸ **Adult:** Initially 250 mg once daily for 1-2 weeks, then increased to 250 mg twice daily, then increased in steps of 250 mg twice daily (max. per dose 1.5 g twice daily), adjusted according to response, dose to be increased every 2 weeks

Adjunctive therapy of focal seizures with or without secondary generalisation

▸ BY MOUTH

▸ **Child 1-5 months:** Initially 7 mg/kg once daily, then increased in steps of up to 7 mg/kg twice daily (max. per dose 21 mg/kg twice daily), dose to be increased every 2 weeks

▸ **Child 6 months-17 years (body-weight up to 50 kg):** Initially 10 mg/kg once daily, then increased in steps of up to 10 mg/kg twice daily (max. per dose 30 mg/kg twice daily), dose to be increased every 2 weeks

▸ **Child 12-17 years (body-weight 50 kg and above):** Initially 250 mg twice daily, then increased in steps of 500 mg twice daily (max. per dose 1.5 g twice daily), dose to be increased every 2-4 weeks

▸ **Adult:** Initially 250 mg twice daily, then increased in steps of 500 mg twice daily (max. per dose 1.5 g twice daily), dose to be increased every 2-4 weeks

▸ BY INTRAVENOUS INFUSION

▸ **Child 4-17 years (body-weight up to 50 kg):** Initially 10 mg/kg once daily, then increased in steps of up to 10 mg/kg twice daily (max. per dose 30 mg/kg twice daily), dose to be increased every 2 weeks

▸ **Child 12-17 years (body-weight 50 kg and above):** Initially 250 mg twice daily, then increased in steps of 500 mg twice daily (max. per dose 1.5 g twice daily), dose to be increased every 2 weeks

▸ **Adult:** Initially 250 mg twice daily, then increased in steps of 500 mg twice daily (max. per dose 1.5 g twice daily), dose to be increased every 2-4 weeks

Adjunctive therapy of myoclonic seizures and tonic-clonic seizures

▸ BY MOUTH, OR BY INTRAVENOUS INFUSION

▸ **Child 12-17 years (body-weight up to 50 kg):** Initially 10 mg/kg once daily, then increased in steps of up to 10 mg/kg twice daily (max. per dose 30 mg/kg twice daily), dose to be increased every 2 weeks

▸ **Child 12-17 years (body-weight 50 kg and above):** Initially 250 mg twice daily, then increased in steps of 500 mg twice daily (max. per dose 1.5 g twice daily), dose to be increased every 2 weeks

▸ **Adult:** Initially 250 mg twice daily, then increased in steps of 500 mg twice daily (max. per dose 1.5 g twice daily), dose to be increased every 2-4 weeks

● UNLICENSED USE EvGr Initial dosing recommendations for levetiracetam ⓔ in BNF Publications differ from product licence.

Manufacturer advises granules not licensed for use in children under 6 years, for initial treatment in children with body-weight less than 25 kg, or for the administration of doses below 250 mg—oral solution should be used.

● INTERACTIONS → Appendix 1: antiepileptics

● SIDE-EFFECTS

▸ **Common or very common** Anxiety · appetite decreased · asthenia · behaviour abnormal · cough · depression · diarrhoea · dizziness · drowsiness · gastrointestinal discomfort · headache · increased risk of infection · insomnia · mood altered · movement disorders · nausea · skin reactions · vertigo · vomiting

▸ **Uncommon** Alopecia · concentration impaired · confusion · hallucination · leucopenia · muscle weakness · myalgia · paraesthesia · psychotic disorder · suicidal tendencies · thrombocytopenia · vision disorders · weight changes

▸ **Rare or very rare** Acute kidney injury · agranulocytosis · hepatic disorders · hyponatraemia · neutropenia · pancreatitis · pancytopenia · personality disorder · rhabdomyolysis · severe cutaneous adverse reactions (SCARs) · thinking abnormal

- PREGNANCY
Monitoring The dose should be monitored carefully during pregnancy and after birth, and adjustments made on a clinical basis.

It is recommended that the fetal growth should be monitored.

- BREAST FEEDING Present in milk—manufacturer advises avoid.

- HEPATIC IMPAIRMENT
Dose adjustments ▶ In adults Halve dose in severe hepatic impairment if eGFR less than 60 mL/minute/1.73 m².
▶ In children Halve dose in severe hepatic impairment if estimated glomerular filtration rate less than 60 mL/minute/1.73 m².

- RENAL IMPAIRMENT
Dose adjustments ▶ In children Reduce dose if estimated glomerular filtration rate less than 80 mL/minute/1.73 m² (consult product literature).
▶ In adults Maximum 2 g daily if eGFR 50–80 mL/minute/1.73 m². Maximum 1.5 g daily if eGFR 30–50 mL/minute/1.73 m². Maximum 1 g daily if eGFR less than 30 mL/minute/1.73 m².

- DIRECTIONS FOR ADMINISTRATION
▶ With intravenous use For *intravenous infusion (Keppra®)*, dilute requisite dose with at least 100 mL Glucose 5% or Sodium Chloride 0.9%; give over 15 minutes.
▶ With oral use For administration of *oral solution*, requisite dose may be diluted in a glass of water.

- PRESCRIBING AND DISPENSING INFORMATION If switching between oral therapy and intravenous therapy (for those temporarily unable to take oral medication), the intravenous dose should be the same as the established oral dose.

- PATIENT AND CARER ADVICE
Medicines for Children leaflet: Levetiracetam for preventing seizures www.medicinesforchildren.org.uk/levetiracetam-for-preventing-seizures

- MEDICINAL FORMS
There can be variation in the licensing of different medicines containing the same drug. Forms available from special-order manufacturers include: oral suspension, oral solution

Granules
CAUTIONARY AND ADVISORY LABELS 8
▶ Desitrend (Desitin Pharma Ltd)
Levetiracetam 250 mg Desitrend 250mg granules sachets sugar-free | 60 sachet [PoM] £22.41 DT = £22.41
Levetiracetam 500 mg Desitrend 500mg granules sachets sugar-free | 60 sachet [PoM] £39.46 DT = £39.46
Levetiracetam 1 gram Desitrend 1000mg granules sachets sugar-free | 60 sachet [PoM] £76.27 DT = £76.27

Tablet
CAUTIONARY AND ADVISORY LABELS 8
▶ Levetiracetam (Non-proprietary)
Levetiracetam 250 mg Levetiracetam 250mg tablets | 60 tablet [PoM] £26.86 DT = £19.31
Levetiracetam 500 mg Levetiracetam 500mg tablets | 60 tablet [PoM] £47.31 DT = £30.73
Levetiracetam 750 mg Levetiracetam 750mg tablets | 60 tablet [PoM] £84.02 DT = £43.15
Levetiracetam 1 gram Levetiracetam 1g tablets | 60 tablet [PoM] £93.09 DT = £54.76
▶ Keppra (UCB Pharma Ltd)
Levetiracetam 250 mg Keppra 250mg tablets | 60 tablet [PoM] £28.01 DT = £19.31
Levetiracetam 500 mg Keppra 500mg tablets | 60 tablet [PoM] £49.32 DT = £30.73
Levetiracetam 750 mg Keppra 750mg tablets | 60 tablet [PoM] £84.02 DT = £43.15
Levetiracetam 1 gram Keppra 1g tablets | 60 tablet [PoM] £95.34 DT = £54.76

Solution for infusion
ELECTROLYTES: May contain Sodium
▶ Levetiracetam (Non-proprietary)
Levetiracetam 100 mg per 1 ml Levetiracetam 500mg/5ml concentrate for solution for infusion vials | 10 vial [PoM] £125.00-£127.31 | 10 vial [PoM] £114.57 (Hospital only)
▶ Desitrend (Desitin Pharma Ltd)
Levetiracetam 100 mg per 1 ml Desitrend 500mg/5ml concentrate for solution for infusion ampoules | 10 ampoule [PoM] £127.31 DT = £127.31
▶ Keppra (UCB Pharma Ltd)
Levetiracetam 100 mg per 1 ml Keppra 500mg/5ml concentrate for solution for infusion vials | 10 vial [PoM] £127.31

Oral solution
CAUTIONARY AND ADVISORY LABELS 8
▶ Levetiracetam (Non-proprietary)
Levetiracetam 100 mg per 1 ml Levetiracetam 100mg/ml oral solution sugar-free | 150 ml [PoM] £27.00 sugar-free | 300 ml [PoM] £63.60 DT = £6.76
▶ Desitrend (Desitin Pharma Ltd)
Levetiracetam 100 mg per 1 ml Desitrend 100mg/ml oral solution sugar-free | 300 ml [PoM] £15.90 DT = £6.76
▶ Keppra (UCB Pharma Ltd)
Levetiracetam 100 mg per 1 ml Keppra 100mg/ml oral solution sugar-free | 150 ml [PoM] £33.48 sugar-free | 300 ml [PoM] £66.95 DT = £6.76

Oxcarbazepine

- INDICATIONS AND DOSE

Monotherapy for the treatment of focal seizures with or without secondary generalised tonic-clonic seizures
▶ BY MOUTH
▶ Child 6–17 years: Initially 4–5 mg/kg twice daily (max. per dose 300 mg), then increased in steps of up to 5 mg/kg twice daily, adjusted according to response, dose to be adjusted at weekly intervals; maximum 46 mg/kg per day
▶ Adult: Initially 300 mg twice daily, then increased in steps of up to 600 mg daily, adjusted according to response, dose to be adjusted at weekly intervals; usual dose 0.6–2.4 g daily in divided doses

Adjunctive therapy for the treatment of focal seizures with or without secondary generalised tonic-clonic seizures
▶ BY MOUTH
▶ Child 6–17 years: Initially 4–5 mg/kg twice daily (max. per dose 300 mg), then increased in steps of up to 5 mg/kg twice daily, adjusted according to response, dose to be adjusted at weekly intervals; maintenance 15 mg/kg twice daily; maximum 46 mg/kg per day
▶ Adult: Initially 300 mg twice daily, then increased in steps of up to 600 mg daily, adjusted according to response, dose to be adjusted at weekly intervals; usual dose 0.6–2.4 g daily in divided doses

Treatment of primary generalised tonic-clonic seizures
▶ BY MOUTH
▶ Adult: Initially 300 mg twice daily, then increased in steps of up to 600 mg daily, adjusted according to response, dose to be increased at weekly intervals; usual dose 0.6–2.4 g daily in divided doses

DOSE ADJUSTMENTS DUE TO INTERACTIONS
▶ In adjunctive therapy, the dose of concomitant antiepileptics may need to be reduced when using high doses of oxcarbazepine.

- UNLICENSED USE Not licensed for the treatment of primary generalised tonic-clonic seizures.

- CAUTIONS Avoid in Acute porphyrias p. 1025 · cardiac conduction disorders · heart failure · hyponatraemia

- INTERACTIONS → Appendix 1: antiepileptics

4

Nervous system

- SIDE-EFFECTS
▸ **Common or very common** Abdominal pain · agitation · alopecia · asthenia · ataxia · concentration impaired · constipation · depression · diarrhoea · dizziness · drowsiness · emotional lability · headache · hyponatraemia · nausea · nystagmus · skin reactions · vertigo · vision disorders · vomiting
▸ **Uncommon** Leucopenia
▸ **Rare or very rare** Angioedema · arrhythmia · atrioventricular block · hepatitis · hypothyroidism · pancreatitis · severe cutaneous adverse reactions (SCARs) · systemic lupus erythematosus (SLE) · thrombocytopenia
▸ **Frequency not known** Agranulocytosis · bone disorders · bone marrow disorders · hypertension · inappropriate antidiuretic hormone secretion like-syndrome · neutropenia · speech impairment

- ALLERGY AND CROSS-SENSITIVITY Caution in patients with hypersensitivity to carbamazepine. Antiepileptic hypersensitivity syndrome associated with oxcarbazepine. See under Epilepsy p. 304 for more information.

- PREGNANCY
Monitoring The dose should be monitored carefully during pregnancy and after birth, and adjustments made on a clinical basis.

- BREAST FEEDING Amount probably too small to be harmful but manufacturer advises avoid.

- HEPATIC IMPAIRMENT Caution in severe impairment—no information available.

- RENAL IMPAIRMENT
Dose adjustments ▸ In adults Halve initial dose if eGFR less than 30 mL/minute/1.73 m²; increase according to response at intervals of at least 1 week.
▸ In children Halve initial dose if estimated glomerular filtration rate less than 30 mL/minute/1.73 m², increase according to response at intervals of at least 1 week.

- PRE-TREATMENT SCREENING Test for HLA-B*1502 allele in individuals of Han Chinese or Thai origin (avoid unless no alternative—risk of Stevens-Johnson syndrome in presence of HLA-B*1502 allele).

- MONITORING REQUIREMENTS
▸ Monitor plasma-sodium concentration in patients at risk of hyponatraemia.
▸ Monitor body-weight in patients with heart failure.

- PRESCRIBING AND DISPENSING INFORMATION Patients may need to be maintained on a specific manufacturer's branded or generic oxcarbazepine product.
Switching between formulations Care should be taken when switching between oral formulations. The need for continued supply of a particular manufacturer's product should be based on clinical judgement and consultation with the patient or their carer, taking into account factors such as seizure frequency and treatment history.

- PATIENT AND CARER ADVICE
Medicines for Children: Oxcarbazepine for preventing seizures www.medicinesforchildren.org.uk/oxcarbazepine-for-preventing-seizures
Blood, hepatic, or skin disorders Patients or their carers should be told how to recognise signs of blood, liver, or skin disorders, and advised to seek immediate medical attention if symptoms such as lethargy, confusion, muscular twitching, fever, rash, blistering, mouth ulcers, bruising, or bleeding develop.

- MEDICINAL FORMS
There can be variation in the licensing of different medicines containing the same drug. Forms available from special-order manufacturers include: oral suspension

Oral suspension
CAUTIONARY AND ADVISORY LABELS 3, 8
EXCIPIENTS: May contain Propylene glycol
▸ Trileptal (Novartis Pharmaceuticals UK Ltd)
Oxcarbazepine 60 mg per 1 ml Trileptal 60mg/ml oral suspension sugar-free | 250 ml PoM £48.96 DT = £48.96

Tablet
CAUTIONARY AND ADVISORY LABELS 3, 8
▸ Oxcarbazepine (Non-proprietary)
Oxcarbazepine 150 mg Oxcarbazepine 150mg tablets | 50 tablet PoM £11.14 DT = £8.37
Oxcarbazepine 300 mg Oxcarbazepine 300mg tablets | 50 tablet PoM £22.61 DT = £6.43
Oxcarbazepine 600 mg Oxcarbazepine 600mg tablets | 50 tablet PoM £45.19 DT = £38.71
▸ Trileptal (Novartis Pharmaceuticals UK Ltd)
Oxcarbazepine 150 mg Trileptal 150mg tablets | 50 tablet PoM £12.24 DT = £8.37
Oxcarbazepine 300 mg Trileptal 300mg tablets | 50 tablet PoM £24.48 DT = £6.43
Oxcarbazepine 600 mg Trileptal 600mg tablets | 50 tablet PoM £48.96 DT = £38.71

Perampanel

- INDICATIONS AND DOSE
Adjunctive treatment of focal seizures with or without secondary generalised seizures
▸ BY MOUTH
▸ Child 12–17 years: Initially 2 mg once daily, dose to be taken before bedtime, then increased, if tolerated, in steps of 2 mg at intervals of at least every 2 weeks, adjusted according to response; maintenance 4–8 mg once daily; maximum 12 mg per day
▸ Adult: Initially 2 mg once daily, dose to be taken before bedtime, then increased, if tolerated, in steps of 2 mg at intervals of at least every 2 weeks, adjusted according to response; maintenance 4–8 mg once daily; maximum 12 mg per day

DOSE ADJUSTMENTS DUE TO INTERACTIONS
▸ Titrate at intervals of at least 1 week with concomitant carbamazepine, fosphenytoin, oxcarbazepine, or phenytoin.

- INTERACTIONS → Appendix 1: antiepileptics

- SIDE-EFFECTS
▸ **Common or very common** Anxiety · appetite abnormal · back pain · behaviour abnormal · confusion · dizziness · drowsiness · dysarthria · fatigue · gait abnormal · irritability · movement disorders · nausea · vertigo · vision disorders · weight increased

- PREGNANCY Manufacturer advises avoid.
Monitoring The dose should be monitored carefully during pregnancy and after birth, and adjustments made on a clinical basis.

- BREAST FEEDING Avoid—present in milk in *animal* studies.

- HEPATIC IMPAIRMENT Avoid in severe impairment.
Dose adjustments Increase at intervals of at least 2 weeks, up to max. 8 mg daily in mild or moderate impairment.

- RENAL IMPAIRMENT Avoid in moderate or severe impairment.

- PRESCRIBING AND DISPENSING INFORMATION
Switching between formulations Care should be taken when switching between oral formulations. The need for continued supply of a particular manufacturer's product should be based on clinical judgement and consultation with the patient or their carer, taking into account factors such as seizure frequency and treatment history.

Patients may need to be maintained on a specific manufacturer's branded or generic perampanel product.

● MEDICINAL FORMS
There can be variation in the licensing of different medicines containing the same drug.

Tablet
CAUTIONARY AND ADVISORY LABELS 3, 8, 25
▸ Fycompa (Eisai Ltd)

Perampanel 2 mg Fycompa 2mg tablets | 7 tablet PoM £35.00 = £35.00 | 28 tablet PoM £140.00 DT = £140.00

Perampanel 4 mg Fycompa 4mg tablets | 28 tablet PoM £140.00 DT = £140.00

Perampanel 6 mg Fycompa 6mg tablets | 28 tablet PoM £140.00 DT = £140.00

Perampanel 8 mg Fycompa 8mg tablets | 28 tablet PoM £140.00 DT = £140.00

Perampanel 10 mg Fycompa 10mg tablets | 28 tablet PoM £140.00 DT = £140.00

Perampanel 12 mg Fycompa 12mg tablets | 28 tablet PoM £140.00 DT = £140.00

Phenytoin

19-Apr-2017

● INDICATIONS AND DOSE

Tonic-clonic seizures | Focal seizures
▸ BY MOUTH
▸ Child 1 month–11 years: Initially 1.5–2.5 mg/kg twice daily, then adjusted according to response to 2.5–5 mg/kg twice daily (max. per dose 7.5 mg/kg twice daily), dose also adjusted according to plasma-phenytoin concentration; maximum 300 mg per day
▸ Child 12–17 years: Initially 75–150 mg twice daily, then adjusted according to response to 150–200 mg twice daily (max. per dose 300 mg twice daily), dose also adjusted according to plasma-phenytoin concentration

Tonic-clonic seizures | Focal seizures | Prevention and treatment of seizures during or following neurosurgery or severe head injury
▸ BY MOUTH
▸ Adult: Initially 3–4 mg/kg daily, alternatively 150–300 mg once daily, alternatively 150–300 mg daily in 2 divided doses; usual maintenance 200–500 mg daily, to be taken preferably with or after food, dose to be increased gradually as necessary (with plasma-phenytoin concentration monitoring), exceptionally, higher doses may be used

Prevention and treatment of seizures during or following neurosurgery or severe head injury
▸ BY MOUTH
▸ Child: Initially 2.5 mg/kg twice daily, then adjusted according to response to 4–8 mg/kg daily, dose also adjusted according to plasma-phenytoin concentration; maximum 300 mg per day

Status epilepticus | Acute symptomatic seizures associated with head trauma or neurosurgery
▸ INITIALLY BY SLOW INTRAVENOUS INJECTION, OR BY INTRAVENOUS INFUSION
▸ Child 1 month–11 years: Loading dose 20 mg/kg, then (by slow intravenous injection or by intravenous infusion) 2.5–5 mg/kg twice daily
▸ Child 12–17 years: Loading dose 20 mg/kg, then (by intravenous infusion or by slow intravenous injection) up to 100 mg 3–4 times a day
▸ Adult: Loading dose 20 mg/kg (max. per dose 2 g), then (by intravenous infusion or by slow intravenous injection or by mouth) maintenance 100 mg every 6–8 hours adjusted according to plasma-concentration monitoring

DOSE EQUIVALENCE AND CONVERSION
▸ Preparations containing phenytoin sodium are **not** bioequivalent to those containing phenytoin base

(such as *Epanutin Infatabs* ® and *Epanutin* ® suspension); 100 mg of phenytoin sodium is approximately equivalent in therapeutic effect to 92 mg phenytoin base. The dose is the same for all phenytoin products when initiating therapy. However, if switching between these products the difference in phenytoin content may be clinically significant. Care is needed when making changes between formulations and plasma-phenytoin concentration monitoring is recommended.

● UNLICENSED USE Licensed for use in children (age range not specified by manufacturer).
▸ With intravenous use Phenytoin doses in BNF publications may differ from those in product literature.

> IMPORTANT SAFETY INFORMATION
> NHS IMPROVEMENT PATIENT SAFETY ALERT: RISK OF DEATH AND SEVERE HARM FROM ERROR WITH INJECTABLE PHENYTOIN (NOVEMBER 2016)
> Use of injectable phenytoin is error-prone throughout the prescribing, preparation, administration and monitoring processes; all relevant staff should be made aware of appropriate guidance on the safe use of injectable phenytoin to reduce the risk of error.

● CONTRA-INDICATIONS
GENERAL CONTRA-INDICATIONS Acute porphyrias p. 1025
SPECIFIC CONTRA-INDICATIONS
▸ With intravenous use Second- and third-degree heart block · sino-atrial block · sinus bradycardia · Stokes-Adams syndrome

● CAUTIONS
GENERAL CAUTIONS Enteral feeding (interrupt feeding for 2 hours before and after dose; more frequent monitoring may be necessary)
SPECIFIC CAUTIONS
▸ With intravenous use Heart failure · hypotension · injection solutions alkaline (irritant to tissues) · respiratory depression · resuscitation facilities must be available
CAUTIONS, FURTHER INFORMATION Consider vitamin D supplementation in patients who are immobilised for long periods or who have inadequate sun exposure or dietary intake of calcium.
Intramuscular phenytoin should not be used (absorption is slow and erratic).

● INTERACTIONS → Appendix 1: antiepileptics

● SIDE-EFFECTS
GENERAL SIDE-EFFECTS Agranulocytosis · bone disorders · bone fracture · bone marrow disorders · cerebrovascular insufficiency · coarsening of the facial features · confusion · constipation · dizziness · drowsiness · Dupuytren's contracture · dysarthria · eosinophilia · fever · gingival hyperplasia (maintain good oral hygiene) · granulocytopenia · hair changes · headache · hepatic disorders · hypersensitivity · insomnia · joint disorders · leucopenia · lip swelling · lymphatic abnormalities · macrocytosis · megaloblastic anaemia · movement disorders · muscle twitching · nausea · neoplasms · nephritis tubulointerstitial · nervousness · nystagmus · paraesthesia · Peyronie's disease · polyarteritis nodosa · pseudolymphoma · sensory peripheral polyneuropathy · severe cutaneous adverse reactions (SCARs) · skin reactions · systemic lupus erythematosus (SLE) · taste altered · thrombocytopenia · tremor · vertigo · vomiting
SPECIFIC SIDE-EFFECTS
▸ With oral use Electrolyte imbalance · pneumonitis · vitamin D deficiency
▸ With parenteral use Arrhythmias · atrial conduction depression (more common if injection too rapid) · cardiac arrest · hypotension · purple glove syndrome · respiratory

4

Nervous system

arrest (more common if injection too rapid) · respiratory disorders · tonic seizure (more common if injection too rapid) · ventricular conduction depression (more common if injection too rapid) · ventricular fibrillation (more common if injection too rapid)

SIDE-EFFECTS, FURTHER INFORMATION

Rash Discontinue; if mild re-introduce cautiously but discontinue immediately if recurrence.

Bradycardia and hypotension With intravenous use; reduce rate of administration if bradycardia or hypotension occurs.

Overdose Symptoms of phenytoin toxicity include nystagmus, diplopia, slurred speech, ataxia, confusion, and hyperglycaemia.

● ALLERGY AND CROSS-SENSITIVITY Cross-sensitivity reported with carbamazepine. Antiepileptic hypersensitivity syndrome associated with phenytoin. See under Epilepsy p. 304 for more information.

● PREGNANCY

Monitoring Changes in plasma-protein binding make interpretation of plasma-phenytoin concentrations difficult—monitor unbound fraction.

Doses should be adjusted on the basis of plasma-drug concentration monitoring.

● BREAST FEEDING Small amounts present in milk, but not known to be harmful.

● HEPATIC IMPAIRMENT

Dose adjustments Reduce dose to avoid toxicity.

● PRE-TREATMENT SCREENING HLAB* 1502 allele in individuals of Han Chinese or Thai origin—avoid unless essential (increased risk of Stevens- Johnson syndrome).

● MONITORING REQUIREMENTS

▸ Manufacturer recommends blood counts (but evidence of practical value uncertain).

▸ In adults The usual total plasma-phenytoin concentration for optimum response is 10–20 mg/litre (or 40–80 micromol/litre). In pregnancy, the elderly, and certain disease states where protein binding may be reduced, careful interpretation of total plasma-phenytoin concentration is necessary; it may be more appropriate to measure free plasma-phenytoin concentration.

▸ In children Therapeutic plasma-phenytoin concentrations reduced in first 3 months of life because of reduced protein binding. Trough plasma concentration for optimum response: neonate–3 months, 6–15 mg/litre (25–60 micromol/litre); child 3 months–18 years, 10–20 mg/litre (40–80 micromol/litre).

▸ With intravenous use Monitor ECG and blood pressure.

● DIRECTIONS FOR ADMINISTRATION Manufacturer advises each injection or infusion should be preceded and followed by an injection of Sodium Chloride 0.9% through the same needle or catheter to avoid local venous irritation.

▸ With intravenous use in children [EvGr] For *intravenous injection*, give into a large vein at a rate not exceeding 1 mg/kg/minute (max. 50 mg/minute). ⓓ Manufacturer advises for *intravenous infusion*, dilute to a concentration not exceeding 10 mg/mL with Sodium Chloride 0.9% and give into a large vein through an in-line filter (0.22–0.50 micron). [EvGr] Give at a rate not exceeding 1 mg/kg/minute (max. 50 mg/minute). ⓓ Complete administration within 1 hour of preparation.

▸ With intravenous use in adults Manufacturer advises for *intravenous injection*, give into a large vein at a rate not exceeding 50 mg/minute; rate of 25 mg/minute or lower may be more appropriate in some patients (including the elderly and those with heart disease). Manufacturer advises for *intravenous infusion*, dilute in 50–100 mL Sodium Chloride 0.9% (final concentration not to exceed 10 mg/mL) and give into a large vein through an in-line filter (0.22–0.50 micron) at a rate not exceeding 50 mg/minute; rate of 25 mg/minute or lower may be more

appropriate in some patients (including the elderly and those with heart disease). Complete administration within 1 hour of preparation.

● PRESCRIBING AND DISPENSING INFORMATION Switching between formulations Different formulations of oral preparations may vary in bioavailability. Patients being treated for epilepsy should be maintained on a specific manufacturer's product.

● PATIENT AND CARER ADVICE

Medicines for Children leaflet: Phenytoin for preventing seizures www.medicinesforchildren.org.uk/phenytoin-for-preventing-seizures

Blood or skin disorders Patients or their carers should be told how to recognise signs of blood or skin disorders, and advised to seek immediate medical attention if symptoms such as fever, rash, mouth ulcers, bruising, or bleeding develop. Leucopenia that is severe, progressive, or associated with clinical symptoms requires withdrawal (if necessary under cover of a suitable alternative).

● MEDICINAL FORMS

There can be variation in the licensing of different medicines containing the same drug. Forms available from special-order manufacturers include: oral suspension, oral solution

Tablet

CAUTIONARY AND ADVISORY LABELS 8

▸ Phenytoin (Non-proprietary)

Phenytoin sodium 100 mg Phenytoin sodium 100mg tablets | 28 tablet [PoM] £30.00 DT = £13.89

Solution for injection

EXCIPIENTS: May contain Alcohol, propylene glycol
ELECTROLYTES: May contain Sodium

▸ Phenytoin (Non-proprietary)

Phenytoin sodium 50 mg per 1 ml Phenytoin sodium 250mg/5ml solution for injection ampoules | 5 ampoule [PoM] £24.40 (Hospital only)

▸ Epanutin (Pfizer Ltd)

Phenytoin sodium 50 mg per 1 ml Epanutin Ready-Mixed Parenteral 250mg/5ml solution for injection ampoules | 10 ampoule [PoM] £48.79 (Hospital only)

Oral suspension

CAUTIONARY AND ADVISORY LABELS 8

▸ Epanutin (Pfizer Ltd)

Phenytoin 6 mg per 1 ml Epanutin 30mg/5ml oral suspension | 500 ml [PoM] £4.27 DT = £4.27

Chewable tablet

CAUTIONARY AND ADVISORY LABELS 8, 24

▸ Epanutin (Pfizer Ltd)

Phenytoin 50 mg Epanutin Infatabs 50mg chewable tablets | 200 tablet [PoM] £13.18

Capsule

CAUTIONARY AND ADVISORY LABELS 8

▸ Phenytoin (Non-proprietary)

Phenytoin sodium 25 mg Phenytoin sodium 25mg capsules | 28 capsule [PoM] £7.24 DT = £7.24

Phenytoin sodium 50 mg Phenytoin sodium 50mg capsules | 28 capsule [PoM] £7.07 DT = £7.07

Phenytoin sodium 100 mg Phenytoin sodium 100mg capsules | 84 capsule [PoM] £67.50 DT = £9.14

Phenytoin sodium 300 mg Phenytoin sodium 300mg capsules | 28 capsule [PoM] £9.11 DT = £9.11

Pregabalin

● INDICATIONS AND DOSE

Peripheral and central neuropathic pain

▸ BY MOUTH

▸ Adult: Initially 150 mg daily in 2–3 divided doses, then increased if necessary to 300 mg daily in 2–3 divided doses, dose to be increased after 3–7 days, then increased if necessary up to 600 mg daily in 2–3 divided doses, dose to be increased after 7 days

Adjunctive therapy for focal seizures with or without secondary generalisation

▸ BY MOUTH

▸ Adult: Initially 25 mg twice daily, then increased in steps of 50 mg daily, dose to be increased at 7 day intervals, increased to 300 mg daily in 2–3 divided doses for 7 days, then increased if necessary up to 600 mg daily in 2–3 divided doses

Generalised anxiety disorder

▸ BY MOUTH

▸ Adult: Initially 150 mg daily in 2–3 divided doses, then increased in steps of 150 mg daily if required, dose to be increased at 7 day intervals, increased if necessary up to 600 mg daily in 2–3 divided doses

● UNLICENSED USE Pregabalin doses in BNF may differ from those in product literature.

● CAUTIONS Conditions that may precipitate encephalopathy · severe congestive heart failure

● INTERACTIONS → Appendix 1: antiepileptics

● SIDE-EFFECTS

▸ **Common or very common** Abdominal distension · appetite abnormal · asthenia · cervical spasm · concentration impaired · confusion · constipation · diarrhoea · dizziness · drowsiness · dry mouth · feeling abnormal · gait abnormal · gastrointestinal disorders · headache · increased risk of infection · joint disorders · memory loss · mood altered · movement disorders · muscle complaints · nausea · oedema · pain · sensation abnormal · sexual dysfunction · sleep disorders · speech impairment · vertigo · vision disorders · vomiting · weight changes

▸ **Uncommon** Aggression · anxiety · arrhythmias · atrioventricular block · breast abnormalities · chest tightness · chills · consciousness impaired · cough · depression · dry eye · dyspnoea · epistaxis · eye discomfort · eye disorders · eye inflammation · fever · hallucination · hyperacusia · hypertension · hypoglycaemia · hypotension · malaise · menstrual cycle irregularities · nasal complaints · neutropenia · oral disorders · peripheral coldness · psychiatric disorders · reflexes decreased · skin reactions · snoring · sweat changes · syncope · taste loss · thirst · urinary disorders · vasodilation

▸ **Rare or very rare** Altered smell sensation · ascites · dysgraphia · dysphagia · gynaecomastia · hepatic disorders · pancreatitis · QT interval prolongation · renal impairment · rhabdomyolysis · Stevens-Johnson syndrome · throat tightness

● RENAL IMPAIRMENT

Dose adjustments Initially 75 mg daily and maximum 300 mg daily if eGFR 30–60 mL/minute/1.73 m².

Initially 25–50 mg daily and maximum 150 mg daily in 1–2 divided doses if eGFR 15–30 mL/minute/1.73 m².

Initially 25 mg once daily and maximum 75 mg once daily if eGFR less than 15 mL/minute/1.73 m².

● TREATMENT CESSATION Avoid abrupt withdrawal (taper over at least 1 week).

● PRESCRIBING AND DISPENSING INFORMATION Flavours of oral liquid formulations may include strawberry.

● NATIONAL FUNDING/ACCESS DECISIONS

Scottish Medicines Consortium (SMC) Decisions

The *Scottish Medicines Consortium* has advised (July 2007) that pregabalin (*Lyrica*®) is not recommended for the treatment of central neuropathic pain.

The *Scottish Medicines Consortium* has advised (April 2009) that pregabalin (*Lyrica*®) is accepted for restricted use within NHS Scotland for the treatment of peripheral neuropathic pain in adults who have not achieved adequate pain relief with, or have not tolerated, first- or second-line treatments; discontinue treatment if sufficient

benefit is not achieved within 8 weeks of reaching the maximum tolerated dose.

● MEDICINAL FORMS
There can be variation in the licensing of different medicines containing the same drug. Forms available from special-order manufacturers include: oral suspension, oral solution

Oral solution

CAUTIONARY AND ADVISORY LABELS 3, 8

▸ Pregabalin (Non-proprietary)

Pregabalin 20 mg per 1 ml Pregabalin 20mg/ml oral solution sugar free sugar-free | 473 ml [PoM] £99.48 DT = £99.48 sugar-free | 500 ml [PoM] £75.00–£105.16

▸ Lyrica (Pfizer Ltd)

Pregabalin 20 mg per 1 ml Lyrica 20mg/ml oral solution sugar-free | 473 ml [PoM] £99.48 DT = £99.48

Capsule

CAUTIONARY AND ADVISORY LABELS 3, 8

▸ Pregabalin (Non-proprietary)

Pregabalin 25 mg Pregabalin 25mg capsules | 56 capsule [PoM] £64.40 DT = £5.84 | 84 capsule [PoM] £6.25–£96.60

Pregabalin 50 mg Pregabalin 50mg capsules | 84 capsule [PoM] £96.60 DT = £8.72

Pregabalin 75 mg Pregabalin 75mg capsules | 56 capsule [PoM] £64.40 DT = £5.42

Pregabalin 100 mg Pregabalin 100mg capsules | 84 capsule [PoM] £96.60 DT = £7.75

Pregabalin 150 mg Pregabalin 150mg capsules | 56 capsule [PoM] £64.40 DT = £5.88

Pregabalin 200 mg Pregabalin 200mg capsules | 84 capsule [PoM] £96.60 DT = £7.89

Pregabalin 225 mg Pregabalin 225mg capsules | 56 capsule [PoM] £64.40 DT = £5.26

Pregabalin 300 mg Pregabalin 300mg capsules | 56 capsule [PoM] £64.40 DT = £5.50

▸ Alzain (Dr Reddy's Laboratories (UK) Ltd)

Pregabalin 25 mg Alzain 25mg capsules | 56 capsule [PoM] £9.95 DT = £5.84

Pregabalin 50 mg Alzain 50mg capsules | 56 capsule [PoM] £9.95 | 84 capsule [PoM] £13.95 DT = £8.72

Pregabalin 75 mg Alzain 75mg capsules | 56 capsule [PoM] £9.95 DT = £5.42

Pregabalin 100 mg Alzain 100mg capsules | 84 capsule [PoM] £13.95 DT = £7.75

Pregabalin 150 mg Alzain 150mg capsules | 56 capsule [PoM] £9.95 DT = £5.88

Pregabalin 200 mg Alzain 200mg capsules | 84 capsule [PoM] £13.95 DT = £7.89

Pregabalin 225 mg Alzain 225mg capsules | 56 capsule [PoM] £9.95 DT = £5.26

Pregabalin 300 mg Alzain 300mg capsules | 56 capsule [PoM] £9.95 DT = £5.50

▸ Axalid (Kent Pharmaceuticals Ltd)

Pregabalin 25 mg Axalid 25mg capsules | 56 capsule [PoM] £19.95 DT = £5.84

Pregabalin 50 mg Axalid 50mg capsules | 56 capsule [PoM] £19.95

Pregabalin 75 mg Axalid 75mg capsules | 56 capsule [PoM] £19.95 DT = £5.42

Pregabalin 100 mg Axalid 100mg capsules | 56 capsule [PoM] £19.95

Pregabalin 150 mg Axalid 150mg capsules | 56 capsule [PoM] £19.95 DT = £5.88

Pregabalin 200 mg Axalid 200mg capsules | 56 capsule [PoM] £19.95

Pregabalin 225 mg Axalid 225mg capsules | 56 capsule [PoM] £19.95 DT = £5.26

Pregabalin 300 mg Axalid 300mg capsules | 56 capsule [PoM] £19.95 DT = £5.50

▸ Lecaent (Actavis UK Ltd)

Pregabalin 25 mg Lecaent 25mg capsules | 56 capsule [PoM] £64.39 DT = £5.84 | 84 capsule [PoM] £96.59

Pregabalin 50 mg Lecaent 50mg capsules | 84 capsule [PoM] £96.59 DT = £8.72

Pregabalin 75 mg Lecaent 75mg capsules | 56 capsule [PoM] £64.39 DT = £5.42

Pregabalin 100 mg Lecaent 100mg capsules | 84 capsule [PoM] £96.59 DT = £7.75

Pregabalin 150 mg Lecaent 150mg capsules | 56 capsule [PoM] £64.39 DT = £5.88

Pregabalin 200 mg Lecaent 200mg capsules | 84 capsule [PoM]
£96.59 DT = £7.89
Pregabalin 225 mg Lecaent 225mg capsules | 56 capsule [PoM]
£64.39 DT = £5.26
Pregabalin 300 mg Lecaent 300mg capsules | 56 capsule [PoM]
£64.39 DT = £5.50
▸ Lyrica (Pfizer Ltd)
Pregabalin 25 mg Lyrica 25mg capsules | 56 capsule [PoM] £64.40
DT = £5.84 | 84 capsule [PoM] £96.60
Pregabalin 50 mg Lyrica 50mg capsules | 84 capsule [PoM] £96.60
DT = £8.72
Pregabalin 75 mg Lyrica 75mg capsules | 56 capsule [PoM] £64.40
DT = £5.42
Pregabalin 100 mg Lyrica 100mg capsules | 84 capsule [PoM]
£96.60 DT = £7.75
Pregabalin 150 mg Lyrica 150mg capsules | 56 capsule [PoM]
£64.40 DT = £5.88
Pregabalin 200 mg Lyrica 200mg capsules | 84 capsule [PoM]
£96.60 DT = £7.89
Pregabalin 225 mg Lyrica 225mg capsules | 56 capsule [PoM]
£64.40 DT = £5.26
Pregabalin 300 mg Lyrica 300mg capsules | 56 capsule [PoM]
£64.40 DT = £5.50

Rufinamide

● **INDICATIONS AND DOSE**

**Adjunctive treatment of seizures in Lennox-Gastaut
syndrome**
▸ BY MOUTH
▸ Child 4-17 years (body-weight up to 30 kg): Initially
100 mg twice daily, then increased in steps of 100 mg
twice daily (max. per dose 500 mg twice daily), adjusted
according to response, dose to be increased at intervals
of not less than 2 days
▸ Child 4-17 years (body-weight 30-49 kg): Initially 200 mg
twice daily, then increased in steps of 200 mg twice
daily (max. per dose 900 mg twice daily), adjusted
according to response, dose to be increased at intervals
of not less than 2 days
▸ Child 4-17 years (body-weight 50-69 kg): Initially 200 mg
twice daily, then increased in steps of 200 mg twice
daily (max. per dose 1.2 g twice daily), adjusted
according to response, dose to be increased at intervals
of not less than 2 days
▸ Child 4-17 years (body-weight 70 kg and above): Initially
200 mg twice daily, then increased in steps of 200 mg
twice daily (max. per dose 1.6 g twice daily), adjusted
according to response, dose to be increased at intervals
of not less than 2 days
▸ Adult (body-weight 30-49 kg): Initially 200 mg twice
daily, then increased in steps of 200 mg twice daily
(max. per dose 900 mg twice daily), adjusted according
to response, dose to be increased at intervals of not less
than 2 days
▸ Adult (body-weight 50-69 kg): Initially 200 mg twice
daily, then increased in steps of 200 mg twice daily
(max. per dose 1.2 g twice daily), adjusted according to
response, dose to be increased at intervals of not less
than 2 days
▸ Adult (body-weight 70 kg and above): Initially 200 mg
twice daily, then increased in steps of 200 mg twice
daily (max. per dose 1.6 g twice daily), adjusted
according to response, dose to be increased at intervals
of not less than 2 days

**Adjunctive treatment of seizures in Lennox-Gastaut
syndrome with valproate**
▸ BY MOUTH
▸ Child 4-17 years (body-weight up to 30 kg): Initially
100 mg twice daily, then increased in steps of 100 mg
twice daily (max. per dose 300 mg twice daily), adjusted
according to response, dose to be increased at intervals
of not less than 2 days

● **INTERACTIONS** → Appendix 1: antiepileptics

● **SIDE-EFFECTS**

▸ **Common or very common** Anxiety · appetite decreased ·
back pain · constipation · diarrhoea · dizziness · drowsiness
· eating disorder · epistaxis · fatigue · gait abnormal ·
gastrointestinal discomfort · headache · increased risk of
infection · insomnia · movement disorders · nausea ·
nystagmus · oligomenorrhoea · seizures · skin reactions ·
tremor · vertigo · vision disorders · vomiting · weight
decreased

▸ **Uncommon** Hypersensitivity

● **ALLERGY AND CROSS-SENSITIVITY** Antiepileptic
hypersensitivity syndrome associated with rufinamide. See
under Epilepsy p. 304 for more information.

● **PREGNANCY**
Monitoring The dose should be monitored carefully during
pregnancy and after birth, and adjustments made on a
clinical basis.

● **BREAST FEEDING** Manufacturer advises avoid—no
information available.

● **HEPATIC IMPAIRMENT** Avoid in severe impairment.
Dose adjustments Caution and careful dose titration in
mild to moderate impairment.

● **DIRECTIONS FOR ADMINISTRATION** Tablets may be crushed
and given in half a glass of water.

● **PRESCRIBING AND DISPENSING INFORMATION**
Switching between formulations Care should be taken when
switching between oral formulations. The need for
continued supply of a particular manufacturer's product
should be based on clinical judgement and consultation
with the patient or their carer, taking into account factors
such as seizure frequency and treatment history.
  Patients may need to be maintained on a specific
manufacturer's branded or generic rufinamide product.

● **PATIENT AND CARER ADVICE** Counselling on antiepileptic
hypersensitivity syndrome is advised.
Medicines for Children leaflet: Rufinamide for preventing
seizures www.medicinesforchildren.org.uk/rufinamide-for-
preventing-seizures

● **NATIONAL FUNDING/ACCESS DECISIONS**

Scottish Medicines Consortium (SMC) Decisions
The *Scottish Medicines Consortium* has advised (October
2008) that rufinamide (*Inovelon*®) is accepted for restricted
use within NHS Scotland as adjunctive therapy in the
treatment of seizures associated with Lennox-Gastaut
syndrome in patients 4 years and above. It is restricted for
use when alternative traditional antiepileptic drugs are
unsatisfactory.

● **MEDICINAL FORMS**
There can be variation in the licensing of different medicines
containing the same drug.
Oral suspension
CAUTIONARY AND ADVISORY LABELS 8, 21
EXCIPIENTS: May contain Propylene glycol
▸ Inovelon (Eisai Ltd)
  Rufinamide 40 mg per 1 ml Inovelon 40mg/ml oral suspension
  sugar-free | 460 ml [PoM] £94.71 DT = £94.71
Tablet
CAUTIONARY AND ADVISORY LABELS 8, 21
▸ Inovelon (Eisai Ltd)
  Rufinamide 100 mg Inovelon 100mg tablets | 10 tablet [PoM] £5.15
  Rufinamide 200 mg Inovelon 200mg tablets | 60 tablet [PoM]
  £61.77
  Rufinamide 400 mg Inovelon 400mg tablets | 60 tablet [PoM]
  £102.96

Sodium valproate
<small>24-Apr-2018</small>

● INDICATIONS AND DOSE

All forms of epilepsy
▸ BY MOUTH USING IMMEDIATE-RELEASE MEDICINES
▸ Child 1 month–11 years: Initially 10–15 mg/kg daily in 1–2 divided doses (max. per dose 600 mg); maintenance 25–30 mg/kg daily in 2 divided doses, doses up to 60 mg/kg daily in 2 divided doses may be used in infantile spasms; monitor clinical chemistry and haematological parameters if dose exceeds 40 mg/kg daily
▸ Child 12–17 years: Initially 600 mg daily in 1–2 divided doses, increased in steps of 150–300 mg every 3 days; maintenance 1–2 g daily in 2 divided doses; maximum 2.5 g per day
▸ Adult: Initially 600 mg daily in 1–2 divided doses, then increased in steps of 150–300 mg every 3 days; maintenance 1–2 g daily, alternatively maintenance 20–30 mg/kg daily; maximum 2.5 g per day

Initiation of valproate treatment
▸ INITIALLY BY INTRAVENOUS INJECTION
▸ Adult: Initially 10 mg/kg, (usually 400–800 mg), followed by (by intravenous infusion or by intravenous injection) up to 2.5 g daily in 2–4 divided doses, alternatively (by continuous intravenous infusion) up to 2.5 g daily; (by intravenous injection or by intravenous infusion or by continuous intravenous infusion) usual dose 1–2 g daily, alternatively (by intravenous injection or by intravenous infusion or by continuous intravenous infusion) usual dose 20–30 mg/kg daily, intravenous injection to be administered over 3–5 minutes

Continuation of valproate treatment
▸ BY INTRAVENOUS INJECTION, OR BY INTRAVENOUS INFUSION, OR BY CONTINUOUS INTRAVENOUS INFUSION
▸ Adult: If switching from oral therapy to intravenous therapy give the same dose as current oral daily dose, give over 3–5 minutes by intravenous injection *or* in 2–4 divided doses by intravenous infusion

Migraine prophylaxis
▸ BY MOUTH USING IMMEDIATE-RELEASE MEDICINES
▸ Adult: Initially 200 mg twice daily, then increased if necessary to 1.2–1.5 g daily in divided doses

EPILIM CHRONOSPHERE ®

All forms of epilepsy
▸ BY MOUTH
▸ Adult: Total daily dose to be given in 1–2 divided doses (consult product literature)

EPILIM CHRONO ®

All forms of epilepsy
▸ BY MOUTH
▸ Adult: Total daily dose to be given in 1–2 divided doses (consult product literature)

EPISENTA ® CAPSULES

All forms of epilepsy
▸ BY MOUTH
▸ Adult: Total daily dose to be given in 1–2 divided doses (consult product literature)

Mania
▸ BY MOUTH
▸ Adult: Initially 750 mg daily in 1–2 divided doses, adjusted according to response, usual dose 1–2 g daily in 1–2 divided doses, doses greater than 45 mg/kg daily require careful monitoring

EPISENTA ® GRANULES

All forms of epilepsy
▸ BY MOUTH
▸ Adult: Total daily dose to be given in 1–2 divided doses (consult product literature)

Mania
▸ BY MOUTH
▸ Adult: Initially 750 mg daily in 1–2 divided doses, adjusted according to response, usual dose 1–2 g daily in 1–2 divided doses, doses greater than 45 mg/kg daily require careful monitoring

EPIVAL ®

All forms of epilepsy
▸ BY MOUTH
▸ Adult: Total daily dose to be given in 1–2 divided doses (consult product literature)

● UNLICENSED USE Not licensed for migraine prophylaxis.

IMPORTANT SAFETY INFORMATION

MHRA/CHM ADVICE: VALPROATE MEDICINES: CONTRA-INDICATED IN WOMEN AND GIRLS OF CHILDBEARING POTENTIAL UNLESS CONDITIONS OF PREGNANCY PREVENTION PROGRAMME ARE MET (APRIL 2018)

Valproate is highly teratogenic and evidence supports that use in pregnancy leads to neurodevelopmental disorders (approx. 30–40% risk) and congenital malformations (approx. 10% risk).

Valproate must not be used in women and girls of childbearing potential unless the conditions of the Pregnancy Prevention Programme are met (see *Conception and contraception*) and only if other treatments are ineffective or not tolerated, as judged by an experienced specialist.

Use of valproate in pregnancy is contra-indicated for migraine prophylaxis [unlicensed] and bipolar disorder; it must only be considered for epilepsy if there is no suitable alternative treatment (see *Pregnancy*).

Women and girls (and their carers) must be fully informed of the risks and the need to avoid exposure to valproate medicines in pregnancy; supporting materials have been provided to use in the implementation of the Pregnancy Prevention Programme (see *Prescribing and dispensing Information*). The MHRA advises that:
- GPs must recall all women and girls who may be of childbearing potential, provide the Patient Guide, check they have been reviewed by a specialist in the last year and are on highly effective contraception;
- Specialists must book in review appointments at least annually with women and girls under the Pregnancy Prevention Programme, re-evaluate treatment as necessary, explain clearly the conditions as outlined in the supporting materials and complete and sign the Risk Acknowledgement Form—copies of the form must be given to the patient or carer and sent to their GP;
- Pharmacists must ensure valproate medicines are dispensed in whole packs whenever possible—all packs dispensed to women and girls of childbearing potential should have a warning label either on the carton or via a sticker. They must also discuss risks in pregnancy with female patients each time valproate medicines are dispensed, ensure they have the Patient Guide and have seen their GP or specialist to discuss their treatment and the need for contraception.

● CONTRA-INDICATIONS Acute porphyrias p. 1025 · known or suspected mitochondrial disorders (higher rate of acute liver failure and liver-related deaths) · personal or family history of severe hepatic dysfunction

● CAUTIONS Systemic lupus erythematosus
CAUTIONS, FURTHER INFORMATION Consider vitamin D supplementation in patients that are immobilised for long

periods or who have inadequate sun exposure or dietary intake of calcium.

▶ Liver toxicity Liver dysfunction (including fatal hepatic failure) has occurred in association with valproate (especially in children under 3 years and in those with metabolic or degenerative disorders, organic brain disease or severe seizure disorders associated with mental retardation) usually in first 6 months and usually involving multiple antiepileptic therapy. Raised liver enzymes during valproate treatment are usually transient but patients should be reassessed clinically and liver function (including prothrombin time) monitored until return to normal—discontinue if abnormally prolonged prothrombin time (particularly in association with other relevant abnormalities).

● INTERACTIONS → Appendix 1: antiepileptics

● SIDE-EFFECTS

GENERAL SIDE-EFFECTS

▶ **Common or very common** Abdominal pain · agitation · alopecia (regrowth may be curly) · anaemia · behaviour abnormal · concentration impaired · confusion · deafness · diarrhoea · dizziness · drowsiness · haemorrhage · headache · hepatic disorders · hypersensitivity · hyponatraemia · memory loss · menstrual cycle irregularities · movement disorders · nausea · nystagmus · seizures · stupor · thrombocytopenia · tremor · weight increased

▶ **Uncommon** Angioedema · bone disorders · bone fracture · bone marrow disorders · coma · encephalopathy · leucopenia · pancreatitis · paraesthesia · parkinsonism · peripheral oedema · pleural effusion · SIADH · skin reactions · vasculitis

▶ **Rare or very rare** Agranulocytosis · cerebral atrophy · cognitive disorder · dementia · enuresis · gynaecomastia · hirsutism · hyperammonaemia · hypothyroidism · infertility male · learning disability · myelodysplastic syndrome · polycystic ovaries · red blood cell abnormalities · severe cutaneous adverse reactions (SCARs) · systemic lupus erythematosus (SLE) · urine abnormalities

▶ **Frequency not known** Alertness increased · hallucination

SIDE-EFFECTS, FURTHER INFORMATION

Hepatic dysfunction Withdraw treatment immediately if persistent vomiting and abdominal pain, anorexia, jaundice, oedema, malaise, drowsiness, or loss of seizure control.

Pancreatitis Discontinue treatment if symptoms of pancreatitis develop.

● CONCEPTION AND CONTRACEPTION The MHRA advises that all women and girls of childbearing potential being treated with valproate medicines must be supported on a Pregnancy Prevention Programme—pregnancy should be excluded before treatment initiation and highly effective contraception must be used during treatment.

● PREGNANCY For *migraine prophylaxis* [unlicensed] and *bipolar disorder*, the MHRA advises that valproate must not be used. For *epilepsy*, the MHRA advises valproate must not be used unless there is no suitable alternative treatment; in such cases, access to counselling about the risks should be provided (see Healthcare Professional Guide for more information) and a Risk Acknowledgement Form signed by both specialist and patient. If valproate is to be used during pregnancy, the lowest effective dose should be prescribed in divided doses or as modified-release tablets to avoid peaks in plasma-valproate concentrations; doses greater than 1 g daily are associated with an increased risk of teratogenicity. Neonatal bleeding (related to hypofibrinaemia) reported. Neonatal hepatotoxicity also reported.

Monitoring Specialist prenatal monitoring should be instigated when valproate has been taken in pregnancy.

The dose should be monitored carefully during pregnancy and after birth, and adjustments made on a clinical basis.

● BREAST FEEDING Present in milk—risk of haematological disorders in breast-fed newborns and infants.

● HEPATIC IMPAIRMENT Avoid if possible—hepatotoxicity and hepatic failure may occasionally occur (usually in first 6 months). Avoid in active liver disease.

● RENAL IMPAIRMENT

Dose adjustments Reduce dose.

● MONITORING REQUIREMENTS

▶ Plasma-valproate concentrations are not a useful index of efficacy, therefore routine monitoring is unhelpful.

▶ Monitor liver function before therapy and during first 6 months especially in patients most at risk.

▶ Measure full blood count and ensure no undue potential for bleeding before starting and before surgery.

● EFFECT ON LABORATORY TESTS False-positive urine tests for ketones.

● TREATMENT CESSATION [EvGr] Avoid abrupt withdrawal; if treatment with valproate is stopped, reduce the dose gradually over at least 4 weeks. ⟨A⟩

● DIRECTIONS FOR ADMINISTRATION

▶ With intravenous use in children For *intravenous injection*, may be diluted in Glucose 5% *or* Sodium Chloride 0.9% and given over 3–5 minutes. For *intravenous infusion*, dilute injection solution with Glucose 5% *or* Sodium Chloride 0.9%.

▶ With intravenous use in adults For *intravenous infusion* (*Epilim*®, *Episenta*®), give continuously *or* intermittently *in* Glucose 5% *or* Sodium Chloride 0.9%. Reconstitute *Epilim*® with solvent provided then dilute with infusion fluid.

▶ With rectal use in children For *rectal administration*, sodium valproate oral solution may be given rectally and retained for 15 minutes (may require dilution with water to prevent rapid expulsion).

EPIVAL® Tablets may be halved but not crushed or chewed.

EPISENTA® CAPSULES Contents of capsule may be mixed with cold soft food or drink and swallowed immediately without chewing.

EPILIM® SYRUP May be diluted, preferably in Syrup BP; use within 14 days.

EPISENTA® GRANULES Granules may be mixed with cold soft food or drink and swallowed immediately without chewing.

EPILIM CHRONOSPHERE® Granules may be mixed with soft food or drink that is cold or at room temperature, and swallowed immediately without chewing.

● PRESCRIBING AND DISPENSING INFORMATION The Pregnancy Prevention Programme is supported by the following materials provided by the manufacturer: *Patient Guide, Guide for Healthcare Professionals, Risk Acknowledgement Form*, and for pharmacists, *Patient Cards* and *Stickers with warning symbols*; the MHRA has also produced a patient information sheet providing advice for women and girls taking valproate medicines.

Switching between formulations Care should be taken when switching between oral formulations in the treatment of epilepsy. The need for continued supply of a particular manufacturer's product should be based on clinical judgement and consultation with the patient or their carer, taking into account factors such as seizure frequency and treatment history.

Patients being treated for epilepsy may need to be maintained on a specific manufacturer's branded or generic oral sodium valproate product.

EPILIM CHRONOSPHERE® Prescribe dose to the nearest whole 50-mg sachet.

● PATIENT AND CARER ADVICE

Medicines for Children leaflet: Sodium valproate for preventing seizures www.medicinesforchildren.org.uk/sodium-valproate-for-preventing-seizures

Valproate use by women and girls The MHRA advises women and girls should **not** stop taking valproate without first discussing it with their doctor.

Blood or hepatic disorders Patients or their carers should be told how to recognise signs and symptoms of blood or liver disorders and advised to seek immediate medical attention if symptoms develop.

Pancreatitis Patients or their carers should be told how to recognise signs and symptoms of pancreatitis and advised to seek immediate medical attention if symptoms such as abdominal pain, nausea, or vomiting develop.

Pregnancy Prevention Programme Pharmacists must ensure that female patients have a patient card—see also *Important safety information*.

EPISENTA ® CAPSULES Patients and carers should be counselled on the administration of capsules.

EPISENTA ® GRANULES Patients and carers should be counselled on the administration of granules.

EPILIM CHRONOSPHERE ® Patients and carers should be counselled on the administration of granules.

● MEDICINAL FORMS

There can be variation in the licensing of different medicines containing the same drug. Forms available from special-order manufacturers include: oral suspension, oral solution, suppository

Modified-release tablet

CAUTIONARY AND ADVISORY LABELS 8, 10, 21, 25

▸ Epilim Chrono (Sanofi) ▼
  Sodium valproate 200 mg Epilim Chrono 200 tablets | 100 tablet [PoM] £11.65 DT = £11.65
  Sodium valproate 300 mg Epilim Chrono 300 tablets | 100 tablet [PoM] £17.47 DT = £17.47
  Sodium valproate 500 mg Epilim Chrono 500 tablets | 100 tablet [PoM] £29.10 DT = £29.10

▸ Epival CR (Chanelle Medical UK Ltd) ▼
  Sodium valproate 300 mg Epival CR 300mg tablets | 100 tablet [PoM] £17.47 DT = £17.47
  Sodium valproate 500 mg Epival CR 500mg tablets | 100 tablet [PoM] £29.10 DT = £29.10

Gastro-resistant tablet

CAUTIONARY AND ADVISORY LABELS 5, 8, 10, 25

▸ Sodium valproate (non-proprietary) ▼
  Sodium valproate 200 mg Sodium valproate 200mg gastro-resistant tablets | 100 tablet [PoM] £7.70 DT = £4.04
  Sodium valproate 500 mg Sodium valproate 500mg gastro-resistant tablets | 100 tablet [PoM] £19.25 DT = £7.50

▸ Epilim (Sanofi) ▼
  Sodium valproate 200 mg Epilim 200 gastro-resistant tablets | 100 tablet [PoM] £7.70 DT = £4.04
  Sodium valproate 500 mg Epilim 500 gastro-resistant tablets | 100 tablet [PoM] £19.25 DT = £7.50

Tablet

CAUTIONARY AND ADVISORY LABELS 8, 10, 21

▸ Epilim (Sanofi) ▼
  Sodium valproate 100 mg Epilim 100mg crushable tablets | 100 tablet [PoM] £5.60 DT = £5.60

Powder and solvent for solution for injection

▸ Sodium valproate (non-proprietary) ▼
  Sodium valproate 400 mg Sodium valproate 400mg powder and solvent for solution for injection vials | 4 vial [PoM] £49.00

Solution for injection

▸ Sodium valproate (non-proprietary) ▼
  Sodium valproate 100 mg per 1 ml Sodium valproate 400mg/4ml solution for injection ampoules | 5 ampoule [PoM] £57.90

Modified-release capsule

CAUTIONARY AND ADVISORY LABELS 8, 10, 21, 25

▸ Episenta (Desitin Pharma Ltd) ▼
  Sodium valproate 150 mg Episenta 150mg modified-release capsules | 100 capsule [PoM] £7.00
  Sodium valproate 300 mg Episenta 300mg modified-release capsules | 100 capsule [PoM] £13.00 DT = £13.00

Oral solution

CAUTIONARY AND ADVISORY LABELS 8, 10, 21

▸ Sodium valproate (non-proprietary) ▼
  Sodium valproate 40 mg per 1 ml Sodium valproate 200mg/5ml oral solution sugar free sugar-free | 300 ml [PoM] £4.46-£7.78 DT = £4.46

▸ Epilim (Sanofi) ▼
  Sodium valproate 40 mg per 1 ml Epilim 200mg/5ml liquid sugar-free | 300 ml [PoM] £7.78 DT = £4.46
  Epilim 200mg/5ml syrup | 300 ml [PoM] £9.33 DT = £9.33

Modified-release granules

CAUTIONARY AND ADVISORY LABELS 8, 10, 21, 25

▸ Epilim Chronosphere MR (Sanofi) ▼
  Sodium valproate 50 mg Epilim Chronosphere MR 50mg granules sachets sugar-free | 30 sachet [PoM] £30.00
  Sodium valproate 100 mg Epilim Chronosphere MR 100mg granules sachets sugar-free | 30 sachet [PoM] £30.00 DT = £30.00
  Sodium valproate 250 mg Epilim Chronosphere MR 250mg granules sachets sugar-free | 30 sachet [PoM] £30.00 DT = £30.00
  Sodium valproate 500 mg Epilim Chronosphere MR 500mg granules sachets sugar-free | 30 sachet [PoM] £30.00 DT = £30.00
  Sodium valproate 750 mg Epilim Chronosphere MR 750mg granules sachets sugar-free | 30 sachet [PoM] £30.00 DT = £30.00
  Sodium valproate 1 gram Epilim Chronosphere MR 1000mg granules sachets sugar-free | 30 sachet [PoM] £30.00 DT = £30.00

▸ Episenta (Desitin Pharma Ltd) ▼
  Sodium valproate 500 mg Episenta 500mg modified-release granules sachets sugar-free | 100 sachet [PoM] £21.00 DT = £21.00
  Sodium valproate 1 gram Episenta 1000mg modified-release granules sachets sugar-free | 100 sachet [PoM] £41.00 DT = £41.00

Tiagabine

● INDICATIONS AND DOSE

Adjunctive treatment for focal seizures with or without secondary generalisation that are not satisfactorily controlled by other antiepileptics (with enzyme-inducing drugs)

▸ BY MOUTH

▸ Child 12-17 years: Initially 5–10 mg daily in 1–2 divided doses, then increased in steps of 5–10 mg/24 hours every week; maintenance 30–45 mg daily in 2–3 divided doses

▸ Adult: Initially 5–10 mg daily in 1–2 divided doses, then increased in steps of 5–10 mg/24 hours every week; maintenance 30–45 mg daily in 2–3 divided doses

Adjunctive treatment for focal seizures with or without secondary generalisation that are not satisfactorily controlled by other antiepileptics (without enzyme-inducing drugs)

▸ BY MOUTH

▸ Child 12-17 years: Initially 5–10 mg daily in 1–2 divided doses, then increased in steps of 5–10 mg/24 hours every week; maintenance 15–30 mg daily in 2–3 divided doses

▸ Adult: Initially 5–10 mg daily in 1–2 divided doses, then increased in steps of 5–10 mg/24 hours every week; maintenance 15–30 mg daily in 2–3 divided doses

● CAUTIONS Avoid in Acute porphyrias p. 1025

CAUTIONS, FURTHER INFORMATION Tiagabine should be avoided in absence, myoclonic, tonic and atonic seizures due to risk of seizure exacerbation.

● INTERACTIONS → Appendix 1: antiepileptics

● SIDE-EFFECTS

▸ **Common or very common** Abdominal pain · behaviour abnormal · concentration impaired · depression · diarrhoea · dizziness · emotional lability · fatigue · gait abnormal · insomnia · nausea · nervousness · speech disorder · tremor · vision disorders · vomiting

▸ **Uncommon** Drowsiness · psychosis · skin reactions

▸ **Rare or very rare** Delusions · hallucination

- PREGNANCY
Monitoring The dose should be monitored carefully during pregnancy and after birth, and adjustments made on a clinical basis.

- HEPATIC IMPAIRMENT Avoid in severe impairment.
Dose adjustments In mild to moderate impairment reduce dose, prolong the dose interval, or both.

- PATIENT AND CARER ADVICE
Medicines for Children leaflet: Tiagabine for preventing seizures www.medicinesforchildren.org.uk/tiagabine-for-preventing-seizures
Driving and skilled tasks May impair performance of skilled tasks (e.g. driving).

- MEDICINAL FORMS
There can be variation in the licensing of different medicines containing the same drug. Forms available from special-order manufacturers include: oral suspension
Tablet
CAUTIONARY AND ADVISORY LABELS 21
▸ Gabitril (Teva UK Ltd)
Tiagabine (as Tiagabine hydrochloride monohydrate)
5 mg Gabitril 5mg tablets | 100 tablet [PoM] £52.04
Tiagabine (as Tiagabine hydrochloride monohydrate)
10 mg Gabitril 10mg tablets | 100 tablet [PoM] £104.09
Tiagabine (as Tiagabine hydrochloride monohydrate)
15 mg Gabitril 15mg tablets | 100 tablet [PoM] £156.13

Topiramate

25-Jan-2018

- INDICATIONS AND DOSE

Monotherapy of generalised tonic-clonic seizures or focal seizures with or without secondary generalisation
▸ BY MOUTH
▸ **Child 6-17 years:** Initially 0.5–1 mg/kg once daily (max. per dose 25 mg) for 1 week, dose to be taken at night, then increased in steps of 250–500 micrograms/kg twice daily, dose to be increased by a maximum of 25 mg twice daily at intervals of 1–2 weeks; usual dose 50 mg twice daily (max. per dose 7.5 mg/kg twice daily), if child cannot tolerate titration regimens recommended above then smaller steps or longer interval between steps may be used; maximum 500 mg per day
▸ **Adult:** Initially 25 mg once daily for 1 week, dose to be taken at night, then increased in steps of 25–50 mg every 1–2 weeks, dose to be taken in 2 divided doses; usual dose 100–200 mg daily in 2 divided doses, adjusted according to response, doses of 1 g daily have been used in refractory epilepsy; maximum 500 mg per day

Adjunctive treatment of generalised tonic-clonic seizures or focal seizures with or without secondary generalisation | Adjunctive treatment for seizures associated with Lennox-Gastaut syndrome
▸ BY MOUTH
▸ **Child 2-17 years:** Initially 1–3 mg/kg once daily (max. per dose 25 mg) for 1 week, dose to be taken at night, then increased in steps of 0.5–1.5 mg/kg twice daily, dose to be increased by a maximum of 25 mg twice daily at intervals of 1–2 weeks; usual dose 2.5–4.5 mg/kg twice daily (max. per dose 7.5 mg/kg twice daily), if child cannot tolerate recommended titration regimen then smaller steps or longer interval between steps may be used; maximum 400 mg per day
▸ **Adult:** Initially 25–50 mg once daily for 1 week, dose to be taken at night, then increased in steps of 25–50 mg every 1–2 weeks, dose to be taken in 2 divided doses; usual dose 200–400 mg daily in 2 divided doses; maximum 400 mg per day

Migraine prophylaxis
▸ BY MOUTH
▸ **Adult:** Initially 25 mg once daily for 1 week, dose to be taken at night, then increased in steps of 25 mg every week; usual dose 50–100 mg daily in 2 divided doses; maximum 200 mg per day

- CAUTIONS Avoid in Acute porphyrias p. 1025 · risk of metabolic acidosis · risk of nephrolithiasis—ensure adequate hydration (especially in strenuous activity or warm environment)

- INTERACTIONS → Appendix 1: antiepileptics

- SIDE-EFFECTS
▸ **Common or very common** Alopecia · anaemia · anxiety · appetite abnormal · asthenia · behaviour abnormal · cognitive impairment · concentration impaired · confusion · constipation · cough · depression · diarrhoea · dizziness · drowsiness · dry mouth · dyspnoea · ear discomfort · eye disorders · feeling abnormal · fever (in children) · gait abnormal · gastrointestinal discomfort · gastrointestinal disorders · haemorrhage · hearing impairment · hypersensitivity · joint disorders · malaise · memory loss · mood altered · movement disorders (uncommon in children) · muscle complaints · muscle weakness · nasal complaints · nasopharyngitis · nausea · oral disorders · pain · seizures · sensation abnormal · skin reactions · sleep disorders · speech impairment · taste altered · tremor · urinary disorders · urolithiases · vertigo (in children) · vision disorders · vomiting (in children) · weight changes
▸ **Uncommon** Abnormal sensation in eye · anhidrosis · arrhythmias · aura · cerebellar syndrome · consciousness impaired · crying · drooling · dry eye · dysgraphia · dysphonia · eosinophilia (in children) · facial swelling · hallucinations · hyperthermia (in children) · hypokalaemia · hypotension · influenza like illness · learning disability (in children) · leucopenia · lymphadenopathy · metabolic acidosis · musculoskeletal stiffness · palpitations · pancreatitis · paranasal sinus hypersecretion · peripheral coldness · peripheral neuropathy · polydipsia · psychotic disorder · renal pain · sexual dysfunction · smell altered · suicidal tendencies · syncope · thinking abnormal · thirst · thrombocytopenia · vasodilation
▸ **Rare or very rare** Eye inflammation · face oedema · glaucoma · hepatic disorders · limb discomfort · neutropenia · Raynaud's phenomenon · renal tubular acidosis · severe cutaneous adverse reactions (SCARs) · unresponsive to stimuli

SIDE-EFFECTS, FURTHER INFORMATION Topiramate has been associated with acute myopia with secondary angle-closure glaucoma, typically occurring within 1 month of starting treatment. Choroidal effusions resulting in anterior displacement of the lens and iris have also been reported. If raised intra-ocular pressure occurs: seek specialist ophthalmological advice; use appropriate measures to reduce intra-ocular pressure and stop topiramate as rapidly as feasible.

- CONCEPTION AND CONTRACEPTION Manufacturer advises perform pregnancy test before the initiation of treatment—a highly effective contraceptive method is advised in women of child-bearing potential; patients should be fully informed of the risks related to the use of topiramate during pregnancy.

- PREGNANCY Increased risk of major congenital malformations following exposure during the first trimester. *For migraine prophylaxis* manufacturer advises avoid. *For epilepsy* manufacturer advises consider alternative treatment options.
Monitoring Manufacturer advises in case of administration during first trimester, careful prenatal monitoring should be performed.

It is recommended that the fetal growth should be monitored.

The dose should be monitored carefully during pregnancy and after birth, and adjustments made on a clinical basis.

● BREAST FEEDING Manufacturer advises avoid—present in milk.

● HEPATIC IMPAIRMENT Use with caution in moderate to severe impairment—clearance may be reduced.

● RENAL IMPAIRMENT Use with caution.

Dose adjustments ▸ In adults Half usual starting and maintenance dose if eGFR less than 70 mL/minute/1.73 m^2—reduced clearance and longer time to steady-state plasma concentration.

▸ In children Half usual starting and maintenance dose if estimated glomerular filtration less than 70 mL/minute/1.73 m^2—reduced clearance and longer time to steady-state plasma concentration.

● DIRECTIONS FOR ADMINISTRATION *Topamax*® *Sprinkle* capsules can either be swallowed whole or the contents of the capsule can be sprinkled on soft food and swallowed immediately without chewing.

● PRESCRIBING AND DISPENSING INFORMATION
Switching between formulations Care should be taken when switching between oral formulations in the treatment of epilepsy. The need for continued supply of a particular manufacturer's product should be based on clinical judgement and consultation with the patient or their carer, taking into account factors such as seizure frequency and treatment history.

Patients being treated for epilepsy may need to be maintained on a specific manufacturer's branded or generic topiramate product.

● PATIENT AND CARER ADVICE
Patients or carers should be given advice on how to administer *Topamax*® *Sprinkle* capsules.
Medicines for Children leaflet: Topiramate for preventing seizures www.medicinesforchildren.org.uk/topiramate-for-preventing-seizures

● MEDICINAL FORMS
There can be variation in the licensing of different medicines containing the same drug. Forms available from special-order manufacturers include: oral suspension, oral solution

Tablet
CAUTIONARY AND ADVISORY LABELS 3, 8
▸ Topiramate (Non-proprietary)
  Topiramate 25 mg Topiramate 25mg tablets | 60 tablet PoM
  £10.00 DT = £1.01
  Topiramate 50 mg Topiramate 50mg tablets | 60 tablet PoM
  £19.00 DT = £1.40
  Topiramate 100 mg Topiramate 100mg tablets | 60 tablet PoM
  £28.38 DT = £2.29
  Topiramate 200 mg Topiramate 200mg tablets | 60 tablet PoM
  £55.12 DT = £33.35
▸ Topamax (Janssen-Cilag Ltd)
  Topiramate 25 mg Topamax 25mg tablets | 60 tablet PoM £19.29
  DT = £1.01
  Topiramate 50 mg Topamax 50mg tablets | 60 tablet PoM £31.69
  DT = £1.40
  Topiramate 100 mg Topamax 100mg tablets | 60 tablet PoM
  £56.76 DT = £2.29
  Topiramate 200 mg Topamax 200mg tablets | 60 tablet PoM
  £110.23 DT = £33.35

Capsule
CAUTIONARY AND ADVISORY LABELS 3, 8
▸ Topiramate (Non-proprietary)
  Topiramate 15 mg Topiramate 15mg capsules | 60 capsule PoM
  £30.00 DT = £27.82
  Topiramate 25 mg Topiramate 25mg capsules | 60 capsule PoM
  £25.95 DT = £17.02
  Topiramate 50 mg Topiramate 50mg capsules | 60 capsule PoM
  £60.00 DT = £56.35

▸ Topamax (Janssen-Cilag Ltd)
  Topiramate 15 mg Topamax 15mg sprinkle capsules |
  60 capsule PoM £14.79 DT = £27.82
  Topiramate 25 mg Topamax 25mg sprinkle capsules |
  60 capsule PoM £22.18 DT = £17.02
  Topiramate 50 mg Topamax 50mg sprinkle capsules |
  60 capsule PoM £36.45 DT = £56.35

Vigabatrin

● INDICATIONS AND DOSE

Adjunctive treatment of focal seizures with or without secondary generalisation not satisfactorily controlled with other antiepileptics (under expert supervision)
▸ BY MOUTH
▸ Child 1–23 months: Initially 15–20 mg/kg twice daily (max. per dose 250 mg), to be increased over 2–3 weeks to usual maintenance dose, usual maintenance 30–40 mg/kg twice daily (max. per dose 75 mg/kg)
▸ Child 2–11 years: Initially 15–20 mg/kg twice daily (max. per dose 250 mg), to be increased over 2–3 weeks to usual maintenance dose, usual maintenance 30–40 mg/kg twice daily (max. per dose 1.5 g)
▸ Child 12–17 years: Initially 250 mg twice daily, to be increased over 2–3 weeks to usual maintenance dose, usual maintenance 1–1.5 g twice daily
▸ Adult: Initially 1 g once daily, alternatively initially 1 g daily in 2 divided doses, then increased in steps of 500 mg every week, adjusted according to response; usual dose 2–3 g daily; maximum 3 g per day
▸ BY RECTUM
▸ Child 1–23 months: Initially 15–20 mg/kg twice daily (max. per dose 250 mg), to be increased over 2–3 weeks to usual maintenance dose, usual maintenance 30–40 mg/kg twice daily (max. per dose 75 mg/kg)
▸ Child 2–11 years: Initially 15–20 mg/kg twice daily (max. per dose 250 mg), to be increased over 2–3 weeks to usual maintenance dose, usual maintenance 30–40 mg/kg twice daily (max. per dose 1.5 g)
▸ Child 12–17 years: Initially 250 mg twice daily, to be increased over 2–3 weeks to usual maintenance dose, usual maintenance 1–1.5 g twice daily

● UNLICENSED USE Granules not licensed for rectal use. Tablets not licensed to be crushed and dispersed in liquid. Vigabatrin doses in BNF publications may differ from those in product literature.

● CONTRA-INDICATIONS Visual field defects

● CAUTIONS Elderly · history of behavioural problems · history of depression · history of psychosis

CAUTIONS, FURTHER INFORMATION Vigabatrin may worsen absence, myoclonic, tonic and atonic seizures.
▸ Visual field defects Vigabatrin is associated with visual field defects. The onset of symptoms varies from 1 month to several years after starting. In most cases, visual field defects have persisted despite discontinuation, and further deterioration after discontinuation cannot be excluded. Product literature advises visual field testing before treatment and at 6-month intervals. Patients and their carers should be warned to report any new visual symptoms that develop and those with symptoms should be referred for an urgent ophthalmological opinion. Gradual withdrawal of vigabatrin should be considered.

● INTERACTIONS → Appendix 1: antiepileptics

● SIDE-EFFECTS
▸ **Common or very common** Abdominal pain · anaemia · anxiety · arthralgia · behaviour abnormal · concentration impaired · depression · dizziness · drowsiness · eye disorders · fatigue · headache · memory loss · mood altered · nausea · oedema · paraesthesia · speech disorder ·

thinking abnormal · tremor · vision disorders · vomiting · weight increased
▶ **Uncommon** Movement disorders · psychotic disorder · seizure (patients with myoclonic seizures at greater risk) · skin reactions
▶ **Rare or very rare** Angioedema · encephalopathy · hallucination · hepatitis · optic neuritis · suicide attempt
▶ **Frequency not known** Muscle tone increased

SIDE-EFFECTS, FURTHER INFORMATION
Encephalopathic symptoms Encephalopathic symptoms including marked sedation, stupor, and confusion with non-specific slow wave EEG can occur rarely—reduce dose or withdraw.
Visual field defects About one-third of patients treated with vigabatrin have suffered visual field defects; counselling and careful monitoring for this side-effect are required.

● PREGNANCY
Monitoring The dose should be monitored carefully during pregnancy and after birth, and adjustments made on a clinical basis.

● BREAST FEEDING Present in milk—manufacturer advises avoid.

● RENAL IMPAIRMENT
Dose adjustments ▶ In adults Consider reduced dose or increased dose interval if eGFR less than 60 mL/minute/1.73 m^2.
▶ In children Consider reduced dose or increased dose interval if estimated glomerular filtration rate less than 60 mL/minute/1.73 m^2.

● MONITORING REQUIREMENTS Closely monitor neurological function.

● DIRECTIONS FOR ADMINISTRATION
▶ With oral use The contents of a sachet should be dissolved in water or a soft drink immediately before taking. Tablets may be crushed and dispersed in liquid.
▶ With rectal use Dissolve contents of sachet in small amount of water and administer rectally [unlicensed use].

● PATIENT AND CARER ADVICE Patients and their carers should be warned to report any new visual symptoms that develop.
Medicines for Children leaflet: Vigabatrin for preventing seizures www.medicinesforchildren.org.uk/vigabatrin-for-preventing-seizures

● MEDICINAL FORMS
There can be variation in the licensing of different medicines containing the same drug. Forms available from special-order manufacturers include: oral solution

Powder
CAUTIONARY AND ADVISORY LABELS 3, 8, 13
▶ Sabril (Sanofi)
Vigabatrin 500 mg Sabril 500mg oral powder sachets sugar-free | 50 sachet [PoM] £24.60 DT = £24.60

Tablet
CAUTIONARY AND ADVISORY LABELS 3, 8
▶ Sabril (Sanofi)
Vigabatrin 500 mg Sabril 500mg tablets | 100 tablet [PoM] £44.41 DT = £44.41

Zonisamide

14-Mar-2018

● INDICATIONS AND DOSE
Monotherapy for treatment of focal seizures with or without secondary generalisation in adults with newly diagnosed epilepsy
▶ BY MOUTH
▶ Adult: Initially 100 mg once daily for 2 weeks, then increased in steps of 100 mg every 2 weeks, usual maintenance dose 300 mg once daily; maximum 500 mg per day

Adjunctive treatment for refractory focal seizures with or without secondary generalisation
▶ BY MOUTH
▶ Child 6-17 years (body-weight 20-54 kg): Initially 1 mg/kg once daily for 7 days, then increased in steps of 1 mg/kg every 7 days, usual maintenance 6–8 mg/kg once daily (max. per dose 500 mg once daily), dose to be increased at 2-week intervals in patients who are **not** receiving concomitant carbamazepine, phenytoin, phenobarbital or other potent inducers of cytochrome P450 enzyme CYP3A4
▶ Child 6-17 years (body-weight 55 kg and above): Initially 1 mg/kg once daily for 7 days, then increased in steps of 1 mg/kg every 7 days, usual maintenance 300–500 mg once daily, dose to be increased at 2-week intervals in patients who are **not** receiving concomitant carbamazepine, phenytoin, phenobarbital or other potent inducers of cytochrome P450 enzyme CYP3A4
▶ Adult: Initially 50 mg daily in 2 divided doses for 7 days, then increased to 100 mg daily in 2 divided doses, then increased in steps of 100 mg every 7 days, usual maintenance 300–500 mg daily in 1–2 divided doses, dose to be increased at 2-week intervals in patients who are **not** receiving concomitant carbamazepine, phenytoin, phenobarbital or other potent inducers of cytochrome P450 enzyme CYP3A4

● CAUTIONS Elderly · low body-weight or poor appetite—monitor weight throughout treatment (fatal cases of weight loss reported in children) · metabolic acidosis—monitor serum bicarbonate concentration in children and those with other risk factors (consider dose reduction or discontinuation if metabolic acidosis develops) · risk factors for renal stone formation (particularly predisposition to nephrolithiasis)

CAUTIONS, FURTHER INFORMATION Avoid overheating and ensure adequate hydration especially in children, during strenuous activity or if in warm environment (fatal cases of heat stroke reported in children).

● INTERACTIONS → Appendix 1: antiepileptics

● SIDE-EFFECTS
▶ **Common or very common** Alopecia · anxiety · appetite decreased · ataxia · bradyphrenia · concentration impaired · confusion · constipation · depression · diarrhoea · dizziness · drowsiness · fatigue · fever · gastrointestinal discomfort · hypersensitivity · influenza like illness · insomnia · memory loss · mood altered · nausea · nystagmus · paraesthesia · peripheral oedema · psychosis · rash (consider discontinuation) · skin reactions · speech disorder · tremor · urolithiases · vision disorders · vomiting · weight decreased
▶ **Uncommon** Behaviour abnormal · gallbladder disorders · hallucination · hypokalaemia · increased risk of infection · leucopenia · respiratory disorders · seizures · suicidal tendencies · thrombocytopenia
▶ **Rare or very rare** Agranulocytosis · angle closure glaucoma · anhidrosis · bone marrow disorders · coma · dyspnoea · eye pain · heat stroke · hepatocellular injury · hydronephrosis · leucocytosis · lymphadenopathy · metabolic acidosis · myasthenic syndrome · neuroleptic malignant syndrome · pancreatitis · renal failure · renal tubular acidosis · rhabdomyolysis · severe cutaneous adverse reactions (SCARs) · urine abnormal
▶ **Frequency not known** Sudden unexplained death in epilepsy

● ALLERGY AND CROSS-SENSITIVITY Contra-indicated in sulfonamide hypersensitivity.
Antiepileptic hypersensitivity syndrome theoretically associated with zonisamide. See under Epilepsy p. 304 for more information.

- CONCEPTION AND CONTRACEPTION Manufacturer advises women of childbearing potential should use effective contraception during treatment and for one month after last dose—avoid in women of childbearing potential not using effective contraception unless clearly necessary and the potential benefit outweighs risk; patients should be fully informed of the risks related to the use of zonisamide during pregnancy.
- PREGNANCY Manufacturer advises use only if clearly necessary and the potential benefit outweighs risk— toxicity in *animal* studies; patients should be fully informed of the risks related to the use of zonisamide during pregnancy.
  Monitoring The dose should be monitored carefully during pregnancy and after birth, and adjustments made on a clinical basis.
- BREAST FEEDING Manufacturer advises avoid for 4 weeks after last dose.
- HEPATIC IMPAIRMENT Avoid in severe impairment.
  Dose adjustments Initially increase dose at 2-week intervals if mild or moderate impairment.
- RENAL IMPAIRMENT
  Dose adjustments Initially increase dose at 2-week intervals; discontinue if renal function deteriorates.
- TREATMENT CESSATION Avoid abrupt withdrawal (consult product literature for recommended withdrawal regimens in children).
- PRESCRIBING AND DISPENSING INFORMATION
  Switching between formulations Care should be taken when switching between oral formulations. The need for continued supply of a particular manufacturer's product should be based on clinical judgement and consultation with the patient or their carer, taking into account factors such as seizure frequency and treatment history.
  Patients may need to be maintained on a specific manufacturer's branded or generic zonisamide product.
- PATIENT AND CARER ADVICE Children and their carers should be made aware of how to prevent and recognise overheating and dehydration.
  Medicines for Children leaflet: Zonisamide for preventing seizures www.medicinesforchildren.org.uk/zonisamide-for-preventing-seizures
- NATIONAL FUNDING/ACCESS DECISIONS
  Scottish Medicines Consortium (SMC) Decisions
  The *Scottish Medicines Consortium* has advised (February 2014) that zonisamide (*Zonegran®*) is accepted for restricted use within NHS Scotland as adjunctive treatment of focal seizures, with or without secondary generalisation, in adolescents and children aged 6 years and above. It is restricted to use on advice from specialists in paediatric neurology or epilepsy.

- MEDICINAL FORMS
  There can be variation in the licensing of different medicines containing the same drug. Forms available from special-order manufacturers include: oral suspension, oral solution

  Capsule
  CAUTIONARY AND ADVISORY LABELS 3, 8, 10
  ▹ Zonisamide (Non-proprietary)
  Zonisamide 25 mg Zonisamide 25mg capsules | 14 capsule [PoM] £4.49–£8.82 DT = £6.66
  Zonisamide 50 mg Zonisamide 50mg capsules | 56 capsule [PoM] £21.50–£47.04 DT = £34.51
  Zonisamide 100 mg Zonisamide 100mg capsules | 56 capsule [PoM] £11.04–£62.72 DT = £11.04
  ▹ Zonegran (Eisai Ltd)
  Zonisamide 25 mg Zonegran 25mg capsules | 14 capsule [PoM] £8.82 DT = £6.66
  Zonisamide 50 mg Zonegran 50mg capsules | 56 capsule [PoM] £47.04 DT = £34.51
  Zonisamide 100 mg Zonegran 100mg capsules | 56 capsule [PoM] £62.72 DT = £11.04

ANTIEPILEPTICS > BARBITURATES

Phenobarbital

(Phenobarbitone)

- INDICATIONS AND DOSE
  All forms of epilepsy except typical absence seizures
  ▸ BY MOUTH
  ▹ Child 1 month–11 years: Initially 1–1.5 mg/kg twice daily, then increased in steps of 2 mg/kg daily as required; maintenance 2.5–4 mg/kg 1–2 times a day
  ▹ Child 12–17 years: 60–180 mg once daily
  ▹ Adult: 60–180 mg once daily, dose to be taken at night

  Status epilepticus
  ▸ BY INTRAVENOUS INJECTION
  ▹ Adult: 10 mg/kg (max. per dose 1 g), dose to be administered at a rate not more than 100 mg/minute, injection to be diluted 1 in 10 with water for injections
  ▸ BY SLOW INTRAVENOUS INJECTION
  ▹ Neonate: Initially 20 mg/kg, dose to be administered at a rate no faster than 1 mg/kg/minute, then 2.5–5 mg/kg 1–2 times a day.
  ▹ Child 1 month–11 years: Initially 20 mg/kg, dose to be administered at a rate no faster than 1 mg/kg/minute, then 2.5–5 mg/kg 1–2 times a day
  ▹ Child 12–17 years: Initially 20 mg/kg (max. per dose 1 g), dose to be administered at a rate no faster than 1 mg/kg/minute, then 300 mg twice daily

  DOSE EQUIVALENCE AND CONVERSION
  ▹ For therapeutic purposes phenobarbital and phenobarbital sodium may be considered equivalent in effect.

- CAUTIONS Avoid in Acute porphyrias p. 1025 · children · debilitated · elderly · history of alcohol abuse · history of drug abuse · respiratory depression (avoid if severe)
  CAUTIONS, FURTHER INFORMATION Consider vitamin D supplementation in patients who are immobilised for long periods or who have inadequate sun exposure or dietary intake of calcium.
- INTERACTIONS → Appendix 1: antiepileptics
- SIDE-EFFECTS
  GENERAL SIDE-EFFECTS
  Agranulocytosis · anticonvulsant hypersensitivity syndrome · behaviour abnormal · bone disorders · bone fracture · cognitive impairment · confusion · depression · drowsiness · folate deficiency · hepatic disorders · memory loss · movement disorders · nystagmus · respiratory depression · skin reactions
  SPECIFIC SIDE-EFFECTS
  ▸ With oral use Anxiety · hallucination · hypotension · megaloblastic anaemia · severe cutaneous adverse reactions (SCARs) · thrombocytopenia
  ▸ With parenteral use Agitation · anaemia · aplastic anaemia · Dupuytren's contracture · hypocalcaemia · irritability · toxic epidermal necrolysis
  Overdose For details on the management of poisoning, see Active elimination techniques, under Emergency treatment of poisoning p. 1319.
- ALLERGY AND CROSS-SENSITIVITY Antiepileptic hypersensitivity syndrome associated with phenobarbital. See under Epilepsy p. 304 for more information.
- PREGNANCY
  Monitoring The dose should be monitored carefully during pregnancy and after birth, and adjustments made on a clinical basis.
- BREAST FEEDING Avoid if possible; drowsiness may occur.

Nervous system

4

- HEPATIC IMPAIRMENT May precipitate coma. Avoid in severe impairment.
- RENAL IMPAIRMENT Use with caution.
- MONITORING REQUIREMENTS
▶ Plasma-phenobarbital concentration for optimum response is 15–40 mg/litre (60–180 micromol/litre); however, monitoring the plasma-drug concentration is less useful than with other drugs because tolerance occurs.
- TREATMENT CESSATION Avoid abrupt withdrawal (dependence with prolonged use).
- DIRECTIONS FOR ADMINISTRATION
▶ With oral use For administration by *mouth*, tablets may be crushed.
▶ With intravenous use in adults Solution for injection must be diluted before intravenous administration.
▶ With intravenous use in children For *intravenous injection*, dilute to a concentration of 20 mg/mL with Water for Injections; give over 20 minutes (no faster than 1 mg/kg/minute).
- PRESCRIBING AND DISPENSING INFORMATION Some hospitals supply **alcohol-free** formulations of varying phenobarbital strengths.
  The RCPCH and NPPG recommend that, when a liquid special of phenobarbital is required, the following strength is used: 50 mg/5 mL.
  Switching between formulations Different formulations of oral preparations may vary in bioavailability. Patients should be maintained on a specific manufacturer's product.
- PATIENT AND CARER ADVICE
Medicines for Children leaflet: Phenobarbital for preventing seizures www.medicinesforchildren.org.uk/phenobarbital-for-preventing-seizures
- MEDICINAL FORMS
There can be variation in the licensing of different medicines containing the same drug. Forms available from special-order manufacturers include: tablet, capsule, oral suspension, oral solution

Tablet
CAUTIONARY AND ADVISORY LABELS 2, 8
▶ Phenobarbital (Non-proprietary)
Phenobarbital 15 mg Phenobarbital 15mg tablets | 28 tablet [PoM] £24.95 DT = £16.72 [CD3]
Phenobarbital 30 mg Phenobarbital 30mg tablets | 28 tablet [PoM] £5.99 DT = £0.44 [CD3]
Phenobarbital 60 mg Phenobarbital 60mg tablets | 28 tablet [PoM] £7.99 DT = £6.03 [CD3]

Solution for injection
EXCIPIENTS: May contain Propylene glycol
▶ Phenobarbital (Non-proprietary)
Phenobarbital sodium 30 mg per 1 ml Phenobarbital 30mg/1ml solution for injection ampoules | 10 ampoule [PoM] £89.47 DT = £89.47 [CD3]
Phenobarbital sodium 60 mg per 1 ml Phenobarbital 60mg/1ml solution for injection ampoules | 10 ampoule [PoM] £94.40 [CD3]
Phenobarbital sodium 200 mg per 1 ml Phenobarbital 200mg/1ml solution for injection ampoules | 10 ampoule [PoM] £76.96 DT = £76.96 [CD3]

Oral solution
CAUTIONARY AND ADVISORY LABELS 2, 8
EXCIPIENTS: May contain Alcohol
▶ Phenobarbital (Non-proprietary)
Phenobarbital 3 mg per 1 ml Phenobarbital 15mg/5ml elixir | 500 ml [PoM] £83.00–£83.16 DT = £83.08 [CD3]

Primidone

- INDICATIONS AND DOSE
All forms of epilepsy except typical absence seizures
▶ BY MOUTH
▶ Child 1 month-1 year: Initially 125 mg daily, dose to be taken at bedtime, then increased in steps of 125 mg every 3 days, adjusted according to response; maintenance 125–250 mg twice daily
▶ Child 2-4 years: Initially 125 mg once daily, dose to be taken at bedtime, then increased in steps of 125 mg every 3 days, adjusted according to response; maintenance 250–375 mg twice daily
▶ Child 5-8 years: Initially 125 mg once daily, dose to be taken at bedtime, then increased in steps of 125 mg every 3 days, adjusted according to response; maintenance 375–500 mg twice daily
▶ Child 9-17 years: Initially 125 mg once daily, dose to be taken at bedtime, then increased in steps of 125 mg every 3 days, increased to 250 mg twice daily, then increased in steps of 250 mg every 3 days (max. per dose 750 mg twice daily), adjusted according to response
▶ Adult: Initially 125 mg once daily, dose to be taken at bedtime, then increased in steps of 125 mg every 3 days, increased to 500 mg daily in 2 divided doses, then increased in steps of 250 mg every 3 days, adjusted according to response; maintenance 0.75–1.5 g daily in 2 divided doses

Essential tremor
▶ BY MOUTH
▶ Adult: Initially 50 mg daily, then adjusted according to response to up to 750 mg daily, dose to be increased over 2–3 weeks

- CAUTIONS Avoid in Acute porphyrias p. 1025 · children · debilitated · elderly · history of alcohol abuse · history of drug abuse · respiratory depression (avoid if severe)
CAUTIONS, FURTHER INFORMATION Consider vitamin D supplementation in patients who are immobilised for long periods or who have inadequate sun exposure or dietary intake of calcium.
- INTERACTIONS → Appendix 1: antiepileptics
- SIDE-EFFECTS
▶ Common or very common Apathy · ataxia · drowsiness · nausea · nystagmus · visual impairment
▶ Uncommon Dizziness · headache · hypersensitivity · skin reactions · vomiting
▶ Rare or very rare Arthralgia · blood disorder · bone disorders · Dupuytren's contracture · megaloblastic anaemia (may be treated with folic acid) · personality change · psychotic disorder · severe cutaneous adverse reactions (SCARs) · systemic lupus erythematosus (SLE)
▶ Frequency not known Bone fracture
- ALLERGY AND CROSS-SENSITIVITY Antiepileptic hypersensitivity syndrome associated with primidone. See under Epilepsy p. 304 for more information.
- PREGNANCY
Monitoring The dose should be monitored carefully during pregnancy and after birth, and adjustments made on a clinical basis.
- HEPATIC IMPAIRMENT May precipitate coma.
Dose adjustments Reduce dose.
- RENAL IMPAIRMENT Use with caution.
- MONITORING REQUIREMENTS
▶ Monitor plasma concentrations of derived phenobarbital; plasma concentration for optimum response is 15–40 mg/litre (60–180 micromol/litre).
- TREATMENT CESSATION Avoid abrupt withdrawal (dependence with prolonged use).

- PRESCRIBING AND DISPENSING INFORMATION
Switching between formulations Different formulations of oral preparations may vary in bioavailability. Patients being treated for epilepsy should be maintained on a specific manufacturer's product.

- MEDICINAL FORMS
There can be variation in the licensing of different medicines containing the same drug. Forms available from special-order manufacturers include: capsule, oral suspension

Tablet
CAUTIONARY AND ADVISORY LABELS 2, 8
▸ Primidone (Non-proprietary)
Primidone 50 mg Primidone 50mg tablets | 100 tablet PoM £110.00–£112.37 DT = £111.58
Primidone 250 mg Primidone 250mg tablets | 100 tablet PoM £99.65–£121.94 DT = £114.51

HYPNOTICS, SEDATIVES AND ANXIOLYTICS › BENZODIAZEPINES

F 339

Clobazam
07-Feb-2018

- INDICATIONS AND DOSE
Adjunct in epilepsy
▸ BY MOUTH
▸ Child 6–17 years: Initially 5 mg daily, dose to be increased if necessary at intervals of 5 days, maintenance 0.3–1 mg/kg daily, daily doses of up to 30 mg may be given as a single dose at bedtime, higher doses should be divided; maximum 60 mg per day
▸ Adult: 20–30 mg daily, then increased if necessary up to 60 mg daily

Anxiety (short-term use)
▸ BY MOUTH
▸ Adult: 20–30 mg daily in divided doses, alternatively 20–30 mg once daily, dose to be taken at bedtime; increased if necessary up to 60 mg daily in divided doses, dose only increased in severe anxiety (in hospital patients), for debilitated patients, use elderly dose
▸ Elderly: 10–20 mg daily

- UNLICENSED USE
▸ In children Not licensed as monotherapy.

IMPORTANT SAFETY INFORMATION
SAFE PRACTICE
Clobazam has been confused with clonazepam; care must be taken to ensure the correct drug is prescribed and dispensed.

- CONTRA-INDICATIONS Chronic psychosis (in adults) · hyperkinesis · not for use alone to treat anxiety associated with depression (in adults) · obsessional states · phobic states · respiratory depression

- CAUTIONS Muscle weakness · organic brain changes
CAUTIONS, FURTHER INFORMATION The effectiveness of clobazam may decrease significantly after weeks or months of continuous therapy.

- INTERACTIONS → Appendix 1: clobazam

- SIDE-EFFECTS Appetite decreased · consciousness impaired · constipation · drug abuse · dry mouth · fall · fine tremor · gait unsteady · libido loss · movement disorders · muscle spasms · nystagmus · psychotic disorder · respiratory disorder · severe cutaneous adverse reactions (SCARs) · skin reactions · speech impairment · vision disorder · weight increased

- BREAST FEEDING Benzodiazepines are present in milk, and should be avoided if possible during breast-feeding.

Monitoring All infants should be monitored for sedation, feeding difficulties, adequate weight gain, and developmental milestones.

- HEPATIC IMPAIRMENT Can precipitate coma. Avoid in severe impairment.
Dose adjustments Start with smaller initial doses or reduce dose.

- RENAL IMPAIRMENT
Dose adjustments Start with small doses in severe impairment.

- MONITORING REQUIREMENTS Routine measurement of plasma concentrations of antiepileptic drugs is not usually justified, because the target concentration ranges are arbitrary and often vary between individuals. However, plasma drug concentrations may be measured in children with worsening seizures, status epilepticus, suspected noncompliance, or suspected toxicity. Similarly, haematological and biochemical monitoring should not be undertaken unless clinically indicated.

- PRESCRIBING AND DISPENSING INFORMATION
Switching between formulations Care should be taken when switching between oral formulations in the treatment of epilepsy. The need for continued supply of a particular manufacturer's product should be based on clinical judgement and consultation with the patient or their carer, taking into account factors such as seizure frequency and treatment history.
Patients being treated for epilepsy may need to be maintained on a specific manufacturer's branded or generic clobazam product.

- PATIENT AND CARER ADVICE
Medicines for Children leaflet: Clobazam for preventing seizures www.medicinesforchildren.org.uk/clobazam-preventing-seizures-0

- NATIONAL FUNDING/ACCESS DECISIONS
NHS restrictions Clobazam is not prescribable in NHS primary care except for epilepsy and endorsed 'SLS'.

- MEDICINAL FORMS
There can be variation in the licensing of different medicines containing the same drug. Forms available from special-order manufacturers include: capsule, oral suspension

Oral suspension
CAUTIONARY AND ADVISORY LABELS 2, 8, 19
▸ Clobazam (Non-proprietary)
Clobazam 1 mg per 1 ml Clobazam 5mg/5ml oral suspension sugar free sugar-free | 150 ml PoM £90.00 DT = £90.00 CD4-1 sugar-free | 250 ml PoM £150.00 CD4-1
Clobazam 2 mg per 1 ml Clobazam 10mg/5ml oral suspension sugar free sugar-free | 150 ml PoM £95.00 DT = £95.00 CD4-1 sugar-free | 250 ml PoM £158.33 CD4-1
▸ Perizam (Rosemont Pharmaceuticals Ltd)
Clobazam 1 mg per 1 ml Perizam 1mg/ml oral suspension sugar-free | 150 ml PoM £90.00 = £90.00 CD4-1
Clobazam 2 mg per 1 ml Perizam 2mg/ml oral suspension sugar-free | 150 ml PoM £95.00 = £95.00 CD4-1
▸ Tapclob (Martindale Pharmaceuticals Ltd)
Clobazam 1 mg per 1 ml Tapclob 5mg/5ml oral suspension sugar-free | 150 ml PoM £90.00 DT = £90.00 CD4-1 sugar-free | 250 ml PoM £150.00 CD4-1
Clobazam 2 mg per 1 ml Tapclob 10mg/5ml oral suspension sugar-free | 150 ml PoM £95.00 DT = £95.00 CD4-1 sugar-free | 250 ml PoM £158.34 CD4-1
▸ Zacco (Thame Laboratories Ltd)
Clobazam 1 mg per 1 ml Zacco 5mg/5ml oral suspension sugar-free | 150 ml PoM £82.00 DT = £90.00 CD4-1
Clobazam 2 mg per 1 ml Zacco 10mg/5ml oral suspension sugar-free | 150 ml PoM £87.00 DT = £95.00 CD4-1

Nervous system

4

Tablet

CAUTIONARY AND ADVISORY LABELS 2, 8, 19
▸ Clobazam (Non-proprietary)
  Clobazam 10 mg Clobazam 10mg tablets | 30 tablet PoM £3.65 DT = £3.58 CD4–1
▸ Frisium (Sanofi)
  Clobazam 10 mg Frisium 10mg tablets | 30 tablet PoM £2.51 DT = £3.58 CD4–1

⚑ 339

Clonazepam

07-Feb-2018

● **INDICATIONS AND DOSE**

All forms of epilepsy
▸ BY MOUTH
  ▸ Child 1–11 months: Initially 250 micrograms once daily for 4 nights, dose to be increased over 2–4 weeks, usual dose 0.5–1 mg daily, dose to be taken at night; may be given in 3 divided doses if necessary
  ▸ Child 1–4 years: Initially 250 micrograms once daily for 4 nights, dose to be increased over 2–4 weeks, usual dose 1–3 mg daily, dose to be taken at night; may be given in 3 divided doses if necessary
  ▸ Child 5–11 years: Initially 500 micrograms once daily for 4 nights, dose to be increased over 2–4 weeks, usual dose 3–6 mg daily, dose to be taken at night; may be given in 3 divided doses if necessary
  ▸ Child 12–17 years: Initially 1 mg once daily for 4 nights, dose to be increased over 2–4 weeks, usual dose 4–8 mg daily, dose usually taken at night; may be given in 3–4 divided doses if necessary

All forms of epilepsy | Myoclonus
▸ BY MOUTH
  ▸ Adult: Initially 1 mg once daily for 4 nights, dose to be increased over 2–4 weeks, usual dose 4–8 mg daily, adjusted according to response, dose usually taken at night; may be given in 3–4 divided doses if necessary
  ▸ Elderly: Initially 500 micrograms once daily for 4 nights, dose to be increased over 2–4 weeks, usual dose 4–8 mg daily, adjusted according to response, dose usually taken at night; may be given in 3–4 divided doses if necessary

Panic disorders (with or without agoraphobia) resistant to antidepressant therapy
▸ BY MOUTH
  ▸ Adult: 1–2 mg daily

● UNLICENSED USE Clonazepam doses in BNF may differ from those in product literature. Use for panic disorders (with or without agoraphobia) resistant to antidepressant therapy is an unlicensed indication.

┌───┐
│ IMPORTANT SAFETY INFORMATION   │
│ SAFE PRACTICE   │
│ Clonazepam has been confused with   │
│ clobazam; care must be taken to ensure   │
│ the correct drug is prescribed and   │
│ dispensed.   │
└───┘

● CONTRA-INDICATIONS Coma · current alcohol abuse · current drug abuse · respiratory depression

● CAUTIONS Acute porphyrias p. 1025 · airways obstruction · brain damage · cerebellar ataxia · depression · spinal ataxia · suicidal ideation

  CAUTIONS, FURTHER INFORMATION The effectiveness of clonazepam may decrease significantly after weeks or months of continuous therapy.

● INTERACTIONS → Appendix 1: clonazepam

● SIDE-EFFECTS Abnormal dreams · alopecia · bronchial secretion increased (in children) · concentration impaired · coordination abnormal · disorientation · drooling (in children) · hostility · hypersalivation (in children) · incomplete precocious puberty · increased risk of fall (in adults) · increased risk of fracture (in adults) · muscle tone decreased · nervousness · nystagmus · psychotic disorder · seizures · sexual dysfunction · skin reactions · speech impairment · vision disorder

● BREAST FEEDING Present in milk, and should be avoided if possible during breast-feeding.
  Monitoring All infants should be monitored for sedation, feeding difficulties, adequate weight gain, and developmental milestones.

● HEPATIC IMPAIRMENT Can precipitate coma. Avoid in severe impairment.
  Dose adjustments Start with smaller initial doses or reduce dose.

● RENAL IMPAIRMENT
  Dose adjustments Start with small doses in severe impairment.

● MONITORING REQUIREMENTS Routine measurement of plasma concentrations of antiepileptic drugs is not usually justified, because the target concentration ranges are arbitrary and often vary between individuals. However, plasma drug concentrations may be measured in children with worsening seizures, status epilepticus, suspected noncompliance, or suspected toxicity. Similarly, haematological and biochemical monitoring should not be undertaken unless clinically indicated.

● PRESCRIBING AND DISPENSING INFORMATION The RCPCH and NPPG recommend that, when a liquid special of clonazepam is required, the following strength is used: 2 mg/5 mL.
  Switching between formulations Care should be taken when switching between oral formulations in the treatment of epilepsy. The need for continued supply of a particular manufacturer's product should be based on clinical judgement and consultation with the patient or their carer, taking into account factors such as seizure frequency and treatment history.

  Patients being treated for epilepsy may need to be maintained on a specific manufacturer's branded or generic oral clonazepam product.

● PATIENT AND CARER ADVICE Medicines for Children leaflet: Clonazepam for preventing seizures www.medicinesforchildren.org.uk/clonazepam-preventing-seizures-0

● MEDICINAL FORMS There can be variation in the licensing of different medicines containing the same drug. Forms available from special-order manufacturers include: orodispersible tablet, oral suspension, oral solution, oral drops

Tablet

CAUTIONARY AND ADVISORY LABELS 2, 8
▸ Clonazepam (Non-proprietary)
  Clonazepam 500 microgram Clonazepam 500microgram tablets | 100 tablet PoM £27.70 DT = £27.70 CD4–1
  Clonazepam 2 mg Clonazepam 2mg tablets | 100 tablet PoM £30.75 DT = £29.79 CD4–1

Oral solution

CAUTIONARY AND ADVISORY LABELS 2, 8
EXCIPIENTS: May contain Ethanol
▸ Clonazepam (Non-proprietary)
  Clonazepam 100 microgram per 1 ml Clonazepam 500micrograms/5ml oral solution sugar free | 150 ml PoM £69.50 DT = £69.50 CD4–1
  Clonazepam 400 microgram per 1 ml Clonazepam 2mg/5ml oral solution sugar free | 150 ml PoM £108.36 DT = £108.36 CD4–1

2.1 Status epilepticus

> **Other drugs used for Status epilepticus** Diazepam, p. 340 ·
> Fosphenytoin sodium, p. 313 · Phenobarbital, p. 331 ·
> Phenytoin, p. 321

ANTIEPILEPTICS > BARBITURATES

Thiopental sodium

(Thiopentone sodium)

● **INDICATIONS AND DOSE**

Status epilepticus (only if other measures fail)
▶ BY SLOW INTRAVENOUS INJECTION
▶ Adult: 75–125 mg for 1 dose, to be administered as a
  2.5% (25 mg/mL) solution

Induction of anaesthesia
▶ BY SLOW INTRAVENOUS INJECTION
▶ Adult: Initially 100–150 mg, to be administered over
  10–15 seconds usually as a 2.5% (25 mg/mL) solution,
  followed by 100–150 mg after 0.5–1 minute if required,
  dose to be given in fit and premedicated adults;
  debilitated patients or adults over 65 years may require
  a lower dose or increased administration time,
  alternatively initially up to 4 mg/kg (max. per dose
  500 mg)

Anaesthesia of short duration
▶ BY SLOW INTRAVENOUS INJECTION
▶ Adult: Initially 100–150 mg, to be administered over
  10–15 seconds usually as a 2.5% (25 mg/mL) solution,
  followed by 100–150 mg after 0.5–1 minute if required,
  dose to be given in fit and premedicated adults;
  debilitated patients or adults over 65 years may require
  a lower dose or increased administration time,
  alternatively initially up to 4 mg/kg (max. per dose
  500 mg)

**Reduction of raised intracranial pressure if ventilation
controlled**
▶ BY SLOW INTRAVENOUS INJECTION
▶ Adult: 1.5–3 mg/kg, repeated if necessary

> **IMPORTANT SAFETY INFORMATION**
> Thiopental sodium should only be administered by, or
> under the direct supervision of, personnel experienced
> in its use, with adequate training in anaesthesia and
> airway management, and when resuscitation equipment
> is available.

● CONTRA-INDICATIONS Acute porphyrias p. 1025 ·
  myotonic dystrophy
● CAUTIONS Acute circulatory failure (shock) · avoid intra-
  arterial injection · cardiovascular disease · elderly · fixed
  cardiac output · hypovolaemia · reconstituted solution is
  highly alkaline (extravasation causes tissue necrosis and
  severe pain)
● INTERACTIONS → Appendix 1: thiopental
● SIDE-EFFECTS
▶ **Common or very common** Arrhythmia · myocardial
  contractility decreased
▶ **Frequency not known** Appetite decreased · circulatory
  collapse · cough · electrolyte imbalance · extravasation ·
  hypotension · respiratory disorders · skin eruption ·
  sneezing
● PREGNANCY May depress neonatal respiration when used
  during delivery.
● BREAST FEEDING Breast-feeding can be resumed as soon
  as mother has recovered sufficiently from anaesthesia.

● HEPATIC IMPAIRMENT
  Dose adjustments Use with caution—reduce dose.
● RENAL IMPAIRMENT Caution in severe impairment.
● PATIENT AND CARER ADVICE
  Driving and skilled tasks Patients given sedatives and
  analgesics during minor outpatient procedures should be
  very carefully warned about the risk of driving or
  undertaking skilled tasks afterwards. For a short general
  anaesthetic the risk extends to **at least 24 hours** after
  administration. Responsible persons should be available to
  take patients home. The dangers of taking **alcohol** should
  also be emphasised.

● MEDICINAL FORMS
  There can be variation in the licensing of different medicines
  containing the same drug. Forms available from special-order
  manufacturers include: solution for injection
  Powder for solution for injection
  ▶ Thiopental sodium (Non-proprietary)
    Thiopental sodium 500 mg Thiopental 500mg powder for solution
    for injection vials | 10 vial PoM £69.00 | 25 vial PoM £172.50

HYPNOTICS, SEDATIVES AND
ANXIOLYTICS > BENZODIAZEPINES

F 339

Lorazepam

● **INDICATIONS AND DOSE**

Short-term use in anxiety
▶ BY MOUTH
▶ Adult: 1–4 mg daily in divided doses, for debilitated
  patients, use elderly dose
▶ Elderly: 0.5–2 mg daily in divided doses

Short-term use in insomnia associated with anxiety
▶ BY MOUTH
▶ Adult: 1–2 mg daily, to be taken at bedtime

Acute panic attacks
▶ BY INTRAMUSCULAR INJECTION, OR BY SLOW INTRAVENOUS
  INJECTION
▶ Adult: 25–30 micrograms/kg every 6 hours if required;
  usual dose 1.5–2.5 mg every 6 hours if required,
  intravenous injection to be administered into a large
  vein, only use intramuscular route when oral and
  intravenous routes not possible

Conscious sedation for procedures
▶ BY MOUTH
▶ Adult: 2–3 mg, to be taken the night before operation;
  2–4 mg, to be taken 1–2 hours before operation
▶ BY SLOW INTRAVENOUS INJECTION
▶ Adult: 50 micrograms/kg, to be administered
  30–45 minutes before operation
▶ BY INTRAMUSCULAR INJECTION
▶ Adult: 50 micrograms/kg, to be administered
  60–90 minutes before operation

Premedication
▶ BY MOUTH
▶ Adult: 2–3 mg, to be taken the night before operation;
  2–4 mg, to be taken 1–2 hours before operation
▶ BY SLOW INTRAVENOUS INJECTION
▶ Adult: 50 micrograms/kg, to be administered
  30–45 minutes before operation
▶ BY INTRAMUSCULAR INJECTION
▶ Adult: 50 micrograms/kg, to be administered
  60–90 minutes before operation

**Status epilepticus | Febrile convulsions | Convulsions
caused by poisoning**
▶ BY SLOW INTRAVENOUS INJECTION
▶ Child 1 month–11 years: 100 micrograms/kg (max. per
  dose 4 mg) for 1 dose, then 100 micrograms/kg after
  10 minutes (max. per dose 4 mg) if required for 1 dose,
  to be administered into a large vein continued →

> Child 12-17 years: 4 mg for 1 dose, then 4 mg after 10 minutes if required for 1 dose, to be administered into a large vein
> Adult: 4 mg for 1 dose, then 4 mg after 10 minutes if required for 1 dose, to be administered into a large vein

● UNLICENSED USE
> In children Not licensed for use in febrile convulsions. Not licensed for use in convulsions caused by poisoning.

┌───┐
IMPORTANT SAFETY INFORMATION
ANAESTHESIA
Benzodiazepines should only be administered for anaesthesia by, or under the direct supervision of, personnel experienced in their use, with adequate training in anaesthesia and airway management.
└───┘

● CONTRA-INDICATIONS Avoid injections containing benzyl alcohol in neonates · chronic psychosis (in adults) · CNS depression · compromised airway · hyperkinesis · not for use alone to treat depression (or anxiety associated with depression) (in adults) · obsessional states · phobic states · respiratory depression

● CAUTIONS Muscle weakness · organic brain changes · parenteral administration
CAUTIONS, FURTHER INFORMATION
> Paradoxical effects A paradoxical increase in hostility and aggression may be reported by patients taking benzodiazepines. The effects range from talkativeness and excitement to aggressive and antisocial acts. Adjustment of the dose (up or down) sometimes attenuates the impulses. Increased anxiety and perceptual disorders are other paradoxical effects.
> Special precautions for parenteral administration When given parenterally, facilities for managing respiratory depression with mechanical ventilation must be available. Close observation required until full recovery from sedation.

● INTERACTIONS → Appendix 1: lorazepam
● SIDE-EFFECTS
GENERAL SIDE-EFFECTS
> **Common or very common** Apnoea · asthenia · coma · disinhibition · euphoric mood · extrapyramidal symptoms · hypothermia · memory loss · speech slurred · suicide attempt · vision blurred
> **Uncommon** Allergic dermatitis · constipation · sexual dysfunction
> **Rare or very rare** Agranulocytosis · hyponatraemia · pancytopenia · SIADH · thrombocytopenia
SPECIFIC SIDE-EFFECTS
> **Rare or very rare**
> With oral use Saliva altered
> **Frequency not known**
> With parenteral use Leucopenia
● BREAST FEEDING Benzodiazepines are present in milk, and should be avoided if possible during breast-feeding.
● HEPATIC IMPAIRMENT Can precipitate coma. Avoid in severe impairment.
Dose adjustments Start with smaller initial doses or reduce dose.
> In adults If treatment is necessary, benzodiazepines with shorter half-lives are safer.
● RENAL IMPAIRMENT
Dose adjustments Start with small doses in severe impairment.
● DIRECTIONS FOR ADMINISTRATION
> With intravenous use in children For *intravenous injection*, dilute with an equal volume of Sodium Chloride 0.9% (for neonates, dilute injection solution to a concentration of 100 micrograms/mL). Give over 3–5 minutes; max. rate 50 micrograms/kg over 3 minutes.

> With intramuscular use in adults For intramuscular injection, solution for injection should be diluted with an equal volume of water for injections or sodium chloride 0.9% (but only use when oral and intravenous routes not possible).
> With intravenous use in adults For slow intravenous injection, solution for injection should preferably be diluted with an equal volume of water for injections or sodium chloride 0.9%.
● PATIENT AND CARER ADVICE
Driving and skilled tasks May impair judgement and increase reaction time, and so affect ability to drive or operate machinery; they increase the effects of alcohol. Moreover the hangover effects of a night dose may impair driving on the following day.

Patients given sedatives and analgesics during minor outpatient procedures should be very carefully warned about the risks of undertaking skilled tasks (e.g. driving) afterwards. For intravenous benzodiazepines the risk extends to **at least 24 hours** after administration. Responsible persons should be available to take patients home afterwards. The dangers of taking **alcohol** should be emphasised.

● MEDICINAL FORMS
There can be variation in the licensing of different medicines containing the same drug. Forms available from special-order manufacturers include: oral suspension, oral solution, solution for injection

Solution for injection
EXCIPIENTS: May contain Benzyl alcohol, propylene glycol
> Ativan (Pfizer Ltd)
Lorazepam 4 mg per 1 ml Ativan 4mg/1ml solution for injection ampoules | 10 ampoule ⟦PoM⟧ £3.54 ⟦CD4-1⟧

Oral solution
CAUTIONARY AND ADVISORY LABELS 2, 19
EXCIPIENTS: May contain Ethanol
> Lorazepam (Non-proprietary)
Lorazepam 1 mg per 1 ml Lorazepam 1mg/ml oral solution sugar free sugar-free | 150 ml ⟦PoM⟧ £103.62 DT = £103.62 ⟦CD4-1⟧

Tablet
CAUTIONARY AND ADVISORY LABELS 2, 19
> Lorazepam (Non-proprietary)
Lorazepam 1 mg Lorazepam 1mg tablets | 28 tablet ⟦PoM⟧ £6.59 DT = £3.83 ⟦CD4-1⟧
Lorazepam 2.5 mg Lorazepam 2.5mg tablets | 28 tablet ⟦PoM⟧ £11.43 DT = £9.14 ⟦CD4-1⟧

⟦⚑ 339⟧

Midazolam
21-Mar-2018

● INDICATIONS AND DOSE

Status epilepticus | Febrile convulsions
▶ BY BUCCAL ADMINISTRATION
> Child 1-2 months: 300 micrograms/kg (max. per dose 2.5 mg), then 300 micrograms/kg after 10 minutes (max. per dose 2.5 mg) if required
> Child 3-11 months: 2.5 mg, then 2.5 mg after 10 minutes if required
> Child 1-4 years: 5 mg, then 5 mg after 10 minutes if required
> Child 5-9 years: 7.5 mg, then 7.5 mg after 10 minutes if required
> Child 10-17 years: 10 mg, then 10 mg after 10 minutes if required
> Adult: 10 mg, then 10 mg after 10 minutes if required

Conscious sedation for procedures
▶ BY SLOW INTRAVENOUS INJECTION
> Adult: Initially 2–2.5 mg, to be administered 5–10 minutes before procedure at a rate of approximately 2 mg/minute, increased in steps of 1 mg if required, usual total dose is 3.5–5 mg; maximum 7.5 mg per course

▸ **Elderly:** Initially 0.5–1 mg, to be administered 5–10 minutes before procedure at a rate of approximately 2 mg/minute, increased in steps of 0.5–1 mg if required; maximum 3.5 mg per course

Sedative in combined anaesthesia
▸ INITIALLY BY INTRAVENOUS INJECTION
▸ **Adult:** 30–100 micrograms/kg, repeated if necessary, alternatively (by continuous intravenous infusion) 30–100 micrograms/kg/hour
▸ **Elderly:** Lower doses needed

Premedication
▸ BY DEEP INTRAMUSCULAR INJECTION
▸ **Adult:** 70–100 micrograms/kg, to be administered 20–60 minutes before induction, for debilitated patients, use elderly dose
▸ **Elderly:** 25–50 micrograms/kg, to be administered 20–60 minutes before induction
▸ BY INTRAVENOUS INJECTION
▸ **Adult:** 1–2 mg, repeated if necessary, to be administered 5–30 minutes before procedure, for debilitated patients, use elderly dose
▸ **Elderly:** 0.5 mg, repeated if necessary, initial dose to be administered 5–30 minutes before procedure, repeat dose slowly as required

Induction of anaesthesia (but rarely used)
▸ BY SLOW INTRAVENOUS INJECTION
▸ **Adult:** 150–200 micrograms/kg daily in divided doses (max. per dose 5 mg), dose to be given at intervals of 2 minutes, maximum total dose 600 micrograms/kg, for debilitated patients, use elderly dose
▸ **Elderly:** 50–150 micrograms/kg daily in divided doses (max. per dose 5 mg), dose to be given at intervals of 2 minutes, maximum total dose 600 micrograms/kg

Sedation of patient receiving intensive care
▸ INITIALLY BY SLOW INTRAVENOUS INJECTION
▸ **Adult:** Initially 30–300 micrograms/kg, dose to be given in steps of 1–2.5 mg every 2 minutes, then (by slow intravenous injection or by continuous intravenous infusion) 30–200 micrograms/kg/hour, reduce dose (or reduce or omit initial dose) in hypovolaemia, vasoconstriction, or hypothermia, lower doses may be adequate if opioid analgesic also used

Confusion and restlessness in palliative care (adjunct to antipsychotic)
▸ BY SUBCUTANEOUS INFUSION
▸ **Adult:** Initially 10–20 mg/24 hours, adjusted according to response; usual dose 20–60 mg/24 hours

Convulsions in palliative care
▸ BY CONTINUOUS SUBCUTANEOUS INFUSION
▸ **Adult:** Initially 20–40 mg/24 hours

● UNLICENSED USE Oromucosal solution not licensed for use in children under 3 months. Oromucosal solution not licensed for use in adults over 18 years. Unlicensed oromucosal formulations are also available and may have different doses—refer to product literature.

> IMPORTANT SAFETY INFORMATION
> ANAESTHESIA
> Benzodiazepines should only be administered for anaesthesia by, or under the direct supervision of, personnel experienced in their use, with adequate training in anaesthesia and airway management.
>
> PRESCRIBING OF MIDAZOLAM IN PALLIATIVE CARE
> The use of high-strength midazolam (5 mg/mL in 2 mL and 10 mL ampoules, or 2 mg/mL in 5 mL ampoules) should be considered in palliative care and other situations where a higher strength may be more

appropriate to administer the prescribed dose, and where the risk of overdosage has been assessed. It is advised that flumazenil is available when midazolam is used, to reverse the effects if necessary.

● CONTRA-INDICATIONS CNS depression · compromised airway · severe respiratory depression
● CAUTIONS Cardiac disease · children (particularly if cardiovascular impairment) · concentration of midazolam in children under 15 kg not to exceed 1 mg/mL · debilitated patients (reduce dose)(in children) · hypothermia · hypovolaemia (risk of severe hypotension) · neonates · risk of airways obstruction and hypoventilation in children under 6 months (monitor respiratory rate and oxygen saturation) · vasoconstriction

CAUTIONS, FURTHER INFORMATION
▸ Recovery when used for sedation Midazolam has a fast onset of action, recovery is faster than for other benzodiazepines such as diazepam, but may be significantly longer in the elderly, in patients with a low cardiac output, or after repeated dosing.

● INTERACTIONS → Appendix 1: midazolam
● SIDE-EFFECTS
GENERAL SIDE-EFFECTS
▸ **Common or very common** Level of consciousness decreased · vomiting
▸ **Uncommon** Skin reactions
▸ **Rare or very rare** Apnoea · bradycardia · cardiac arrest · constipation · dry mouth · dyspnoea · euphoric mood · hiccups · hostility · movement disorders · physical assault · respiratory disorders · vasodilation
▸ **Frequency not known** Appetite increased · disinhibition (severe; with sedative and peri-operative use) (in children) · embolism and thrombosis · fall · saliva altered

SPECIFIC SIDE-EFFECTS
▸ **With parenteral use** Angioedema · drug abuse · drug tolerance · drug withdrawal seizure

SIDE-EFFECTS, FURTHER INFORMATION Higher doses are associated with prolonged sedation and risk of hypoventilation. The co-administration of midazolam with other sedative, hypnotic, or CNS-depressant drugs results in increased sedation. Midazolam accumulates in adipose tissue, which can significantly prolong sedation, especially in patients with obesity, hepatic impairment or renal impairment.

Overdose There have been reports of overdosage when high strength midazolam has been used for conscious sedation. The use of high-strength midazolam (5mg/mL in 2mL and 10mL ampoules, or 2mg/mL in 5mL ampoules) should be restricted to general anaesthesia, intensive care, palliative care, or other situations where the risk has been assessed. It is advised that flumazenil is available when midazolam is used, to reverse the effects if necessary.

● BREAST FEEDING Small amount present in milk—avoid breast-feeding for 24 hours after administration (although amount probably too small to be harmful after single doses).

● HEPATIC IMPAIRMENT Use with caution particularly in sedative doses; can precipitate coma. For status epilepticus and febrile convulsions: use with caution in mild to moderate impairment; avoid in severe impairment.

● RENAL IMPAIRMENT Use with caution in chronic renal failure.

● DIRECTIONS FOR ADMINISTRATION For *intravenous infusion* (Hypnovel®), give continuously *in* Glucose 5% *or* Sodium chloride 0.9%.

- **PRESCRIBING AND DISPENSING INFORMATION**

Palliative care For further information on the use of midazolam in palliative care, see www.palliativedrugs.com/formulary/en/midazolam.html.

- **PATIENT AND CARER ADVICE** Patients or carers should be given advice on how to administer midazolam oromucosal solution.

Patients given sedatives and analgesics during minor outpatient procedures should be very carefully warned about the risks of undertaking skilled tasks (e.g. driving) afterwards. For intravenous benzodiazepines the risk extends to **at least 24 hours** after administration. Responsible persons should be available to take patients home afterwards. The dangers of taking **alcohol** should be emphasised.

Medicines for Children leaflet: Midazolam for stopping seizures www.medicinesforchildren.org.uk/midazolam-for-stopping-seizures

- **NATIONAL FUNDING/ACCESS DECISIONS**

EPISTATUS OROMUCOSAL SOLUTION

Scottish Medicines Consortium (SMC) Decisions
The *Scottish Medicines Consortium* has advised (November 2017) that midazolam oromucosal solution (*Epistatus®*) is accepted for use within NHS Scotland for the treatment of prolonged, acute, convulsive seizures in patients aged 10 years to less than 18 years.

- **MEDICINAL FORMS**
There can be variation in the licensing of different medicines containing the same drug. Forms available from special-order manufacturers include: oromucosal solution, solution for injection, infusion, solution for infusion

Solution for injection
▸ Midazolam (Non-proprietary)
Midazolam (as Midazolam hydrochloride) 1 mg per 1 ml Midazolam 5mg/5ml solution for injection ampoules | 10 ampoule [PoM] £16.89 DT = £8.18 [CD3]
Midazolam 2mg/2ml solution for injection ampoules | 10 ampoule [PoM] £5.00 DT = £5.00 [CD3]
Midazolam (as Midazolam hydrochloride) 2 mg per 1 ml Midazolam 10mg/5ml solution for injection ampoules | 10 ampoule [PoM] £6.75 DT = £6.89 (Hospital only) [CD3] | 10 ampoule [PoM] £6.94 DT = £6.89 [CD3]
Midazolam (as Midazolam hydrochloride) 5 mg per 1 ml Midazolam 50mg/10ml solution for injection ampoules | 10 ampoule [PoM] £33.77 DT = £29.41 [CD3]
Midazolam 10mg/2ml solution for injection ampoules | 10 ampoule [PoM] £7.65 DT = £6.02 [CD3]
▸ Hypnovel (Roche Products Ltd)
Midazolam (as Midazolam hydrochloride) 5 mg per 1 ml Hypnovel 10mg/2ml solution for injection ampoules | 10 ampoule [PoM] £7.11 DT = £6.02 [CD3]

Solution for infusion
▸ Midazolam (Non-proprietary)
Midazolam (as Midazolam hydrochloride) 1 mg per 1 ml Midazolam 50mg/50ml solution for infusion vials | 1 vial [PoM] £9.56–£11.00 [CD3]
Midazolam (as Midazolam hydrochloride) 2 mg per 1 ml Midazolam 100mg/50ml solution for infusion vials | 1 vial [PoM] £9.05–£12.50 [CD3]

Oromucosal solution
CAUTIONARY AND ADVISORY LABELS 2
EXCIPIENTS: May contain Ethanol
▸ Buccolam (Shire Pharmaceuticals Ltd)
Midazolam (as Midazolam hydrochloride) 5 mg per 1 ml Buccolam 7.5mg/1.5ml oromucosal solution pre-filled oral syringes sugar-free | 4 unit dose [PoM] £89.00 DT = £89.00 [CD3]
Buccolam 10mg/2ml oromucosal solution pre-filled oral syringes sugar-free | 4 unit dose [PoM] £91.50 DT = £91.50 [CD3]
Buccolam 5mg/1ml oromucosal solution pre-filled oral syringes sugar-free | 4 unit dose [PoM] £85.50 DT = £85.50 [CD3]
Buccolam 2.5mg/0.5ml oromucosal solution pre-filled oral syringes sugar-free | 4 unit dose [PoM] £82.00 DT = £82.00 [CD3]

▸ Epistatus (Special Products Ltd)
Midazolam (as Midazolam maleate) 10 mg per 1 ml Epistatus 10mg/1ml oromucosal solution pre-filled oral syringes sugar-free | 1 unit dose [PoM] £45.76 DT = £45.76 [CD3]

3   Mental health disorders
3.1   Anxiety

> **Other drugs used for Anxiety** Duloxetine, p. 364 · Escitalopram, p. 361 · Lorazepam, p. 335 · Moclobemide, p. 359 · Oxprenolol hydrochloride, p. 149 · Paroxetine, p. 363 · Pericyazine, p. 384 · Perphenazine, p. 384 · Pregabalin, p. 322 · Trazodone hydrochloride, p. 366 · Trifluoperazine, p. 387 · Venlafaxine, p. 365

ANTIDEPRESSANTS 〉 SEROTONIN RECEPTOR AGONISTS

Buspirone hydrochloride

- **INDICATIONS AND DOSE**

Anxiety (short-term use)
▸ BY MOUTH
▸ Adult: 5 mg 2–3 times a day, increased if necessary up to 45 mg daily, dose to be increased at intervals of 2–3 days; usual dose 15–30 mg daily in divided doses

DOSE ADJUSTMENTS DUE TO INTERACTIONS
▸ Manufacturer advises reduce dose to 2.5 mg twice daily with concurrent use of potent inhibitors of CYP3A4.

- **CONTRA-INDICATIONS** Epilepsy
- **CAUTIONS** Does not alleviate symptoms of benzodiazepine withdrawal

CAUTIONS, FURTHER INFORMATION A patient taking a benzodiazepine still needs to have the benzodiazepine withdrawn gradually; it is advisable to do this before starting buspirone.

- **INTERACTIONS** → Appendix 1: buspirone
- **SIDE-EFFECTS**
▸ **Common or very common** Abdominal pain · anger · anxiety · chest pain · cold sweat · concentration impaired · confusion · constipation · depression · diarrhoea · dizziness · drowsiness · dry mouth · fatigue · headache · laryngeal pain · movement disorders · musculoskeletal pain · nasal congestion · nausea · paraesthesia · skin reactions · sleep disorders · tachycardia · tinnitus · tremor · vision disorders · vomiting
▸ **Rare or very rare** Depersonalisation · emotional lability · galactorrhoea · hallucination · memory loss · parkinsonism · psychotic disorder · seizure · serotonin syndrome · syncope · urinary retention
- **PREGNANCY** Avoid.
- **BREAST FEEDING** Avoid.
- **HEPATIC IMPAIRMENT** Avoid in severe disease.
Dose adjustments Reduce dose in mild to moderate disease.
- **RENAL IMPAIRMENT** Avoid if eGFR less than 20 mL/minute/1.73 m^2.
Dose adjustments Reduce dose.
- **PATIENT AND CARER ADVICE**
Driving and skilled tasks May affect performance of skilled tasks (e.g. driving); effects of alcohol may be enhanced.

- MEDICINAL FORMS
There can be variation in the licensing of different medicines containing the same drug. Forms available from special-order manufacturers include: oral suspension, oral solution
Tablet
▸ Buspirone hydrochloride (Non-proprietary)
Buspirone hydrochloride 5 mg Buspirone 5mg tablets |
30 tablet PoM £13.30 DT = £4.92
Buspirone hydrochloride 10 mg Buspirone 10mg tablets |
30 tablet PoM £15.62 DT = £4.27

HYPNOTICS, SEDATIVES AND ANXIOLYTICS ›
BENZODIAZEPINES

Benzodiazepines

- CONTRA-INDICATIONS Acute pulmonary insufficiency · marked neuromuscular respiratory weakness · sleep apnoea syndrome · unstable myasthenia gravis
- CAUTIONS Avoid prolonged use (and abrupt withdrawal thereafter) · debilitated patients (reduce dose)(in adults) · elderly (reduce dose) · history of alcohol dependence or abuse · history of drug dependence or abuse · myasthenia gravis · personality disorder (within the fearful group—dependent, avoidant, obsessive-compulsive) may increase risk of dependence · respiratory disease
  CAUTIONS, FURTHER INFORMATION
▸ Paradoxical effects A paradoxical increase in hostility and aggression may be reported by patients taking benzodiazepines. The effects range from talkativeness and excitement to aggressive and antisocial acts. Adjustment of the dose (up or down) sometimes attenuates the impulses. Increased anxiety and perceptual disorders are other paradoxical effects.
- SIDE-EFFECTS
▸ **Common or very common** Alertness decreased · anxiety · ataxia (more common in elderly) · confusion (more common in elderly) · depression · dizziness · drowsiness · dysarthria · fatigue · gastrointestinal disorder · headache · hypotension · mood altered · muscle weakness · nausea · sleep disorders · suicidal ideation · tremor · vertigo · vision disorders · withdrawal syndrome
▸ **Uncommon** Agitation (more common in children and elderly) · anterograde amnesia · behaviour abnormal · hallucination · libido disorder · rash · urinary disorders
▸ **Rare or very rare** Aggression (more common in children and elderly) · blood disorder · delusions · jaundice · paradoxical drug reaction · psychosis · respiratory depression (particularly with high dose and intravenous use - facilities for its treatment are essential) · restlessness (frequency not known in children, with sedative and peri-operative use)
▸ **Frequency not known** Drug dependence
  Overdose Benzodiazepines taken alone cause drowsiness, ataxia, dysarthria, nystagmus, and occasionally respiratory depression, and coma. For details on the management of poisoning, see Benzodiazepines, under Emergency treatment of poisoning p. 1319.
- PREGNANCY Risk of neonatal withdrawal symptoms when used during pregnancy. Avoid regular use and use only if there is a clear indication such as seizure control. High doses administered during late pregnancy or labour may cause neonatal hypothermia, hypotonia, and respiratory depression.
- RENAL IMPAIRMENT Increased cerebral sensitivity to benzodiazepines.
- PATIENT AND CARER ADVICE
  Driving and skilled tasks Drowsiness may persist the next day and affect performance of skilled tasks (e.g. driving); effects of alcohol enhanced.

For information on 2015 legislation regarding driving whilst taking certain controlled drugs, including benzodiazepines, see *Drugs and driving* under Guidance on prescribing p. 1.

⏎ above

Alprazolam
20-Jul-2017

- INDICATIONS AND DOSE
Short-term use in anxiety
▸ BY MOUTH
▸ **Adult:** 250–500 micrograms 3 times a day, increased if necessary up to 3 mg daily, for debilitated patients, use elderly dose
▸ **Elderly:** 250 micrograms 2–3 times a day, increased if necessary up to 3 mg daily

- CONTRA-INDICATIONS Chronic psychosis · hyperkinesis · not for use alone to treat depression (or anxiety associated with depression) · obsessional states · phobic states · respiratory depression
- CAUTIONS Muscle weakness · organic brain changes
- INTERACTIONS → Appendix 1: alprazolam
- SIDE-EFFECTS
▸ **Common or very common** Appetite decreased · concentration impaired · constipation · dermatitis · disorientation · dry mouth · hypersomnia · lethargy · memory loss · movement disorders · nervousness · sexual dysfunction · vision blurred · weight changes
▸ **Uncommon** Menstruation irregular · mood altered
▸ **Frequency not known** Angioedema · autonomic dysfunction · drug tolerance · hepatic disorders · hostility · hyperprolactinaemia · peripheral oedema · photosensitivity reaction · suicide · thinking abnormal
- BREAST FEEDING Benzodiazepines are present in milk, and should be avoided if possible during breast-feeding.
- HEPATIC IMPAIRMENT Can precipitate coma. If treatment is necessary, benzodiazepines with shorter half-lives (such as temazepam or oxazepam) are safer. Avoid in severe impairment.
  Dose adjustments Start with smaller initial doses or reduce dose.
- RENAL IMPAIRMENT
  Dose adjustments Start with small doses in severe impairment.
- PATIENT AND CARER ADVICE
  Driving and skilled tasks May impair judgement and increase reaction time, and so affect ability to drive or operate machinery; they increase the effects of alcohol. Moreover the hangover effects of a night dose may impair driving on the following day.
- NATIONAL FUNDING/ACCESS DECISIONS
  NHS restrictions Alprazolam tablets are not prescribable in NHS primary care.
- MEDICINAL FORMS
There can be variation in the licensing of different medicines containing the same drug.
Tablet
CAUTIONARY AND ADVISORY LABELS 2
▸ Xanax (Pfizer Ltd)
Alprazolam 250 microgram Xanax 250microgram tablets |
60 tablet PoM £3.18 CD4-1
Alprazolam 500 microgram Xanax 500microgram tablets |
60 tablet PoM £6.09 CD4-1

4

Nervous system

⬛ 339

Chlordiazepoxide hydrochloride 20-Jul-2017

● **INDICATIONS AND DOSE**

Short-term use in anxiety

▸ BY MOUTH

▸ Adult: 10 mg 3 times a day, increased if necessary to 60–100 mg daily in divided doses, for debilitated patients, use elderly dose

▸ Elderly: 5 mg 3 times a day, increased if necessary to 30–50 mg daily in divided doses

Treatment of alcohol withdrawal in moderate dependence

▸ BY MOUTH

▸ Adult: 10–30 mg 4 times a day, dose to be gradually reduced over 5–7 days, consult local protocols for titration regimens

Treatment of alcohol withdrawal in severe dependence

▸ BY MOUTH

▸ Adult: 10–50 mg 4 times a day and 10–40 mg as required for the first 2 days, dose to be gradually reduced over 7–10 days, consult local protocols for titration regimens; maximum 250 mg per day

● CONTRA-INDICATIONS Chronic psychosis · hyperkinesis · not for use alone to treat depression (or anxiety associated with depression) · obsessional states · phobic states · respiratory depression

● CAUTIONS Muscle weakness · organic brain changes

● INTERACTIONS → Appendix 1: chlordiazepoxide

● SIDE-EFFECTS

▸ **Common or very common** Movement disorders

▸ **Rare or very rare** Abdominal distress · agranulocytosis · bone marrow disorders · erectile dysfunction · leucopenia · menstrual disorder · skin eruption · thrombocytopenia

▸ **Frequency not known** Appetite increased · gait abnormal · increased risk of fall · level of consciousness decreased · memory loss · psychotic disorder · saliva altered · suicide attempt

● BREAST FEEDING Benzodiazepines are present in milk, and should be avoided if possible during breast-feeding.

● HEPATIC IMPAIRMENT Can precipitate coma. If treatment is necessary, benzodiazepines with shorter half-lives (such as temazepam or oxazepam) are safer. Avoid in severe impairment.
Dose adjustments Start with smaller initial doses or reduce dose.

● RENAL IMPAIRMENT
Dose adjustments Start with small doses in severe impairment.

● PATIENT AND CARER ADVICE
Driving and skilled tasks May impair judgement and increase reaction time, and so affect ability to drive or operate machinery; chlordiazepoxide increases the effects of alcohol. Moreover the hangover effects of a night dose may impair driving on the following day.

● NATIONAL FUNDING/ACCESS DECISIONS
NHS restrictions *Librium*® is not prescribable in NHS primary care.

● MEDICINAL FORMS
There can be variation in the licensing of different medicines containing the same drug. Forms available from special-order manufacturers include: oral suspension, oral solution

Tablet
CAUTIONARY AND ADVISORY LABELS 2
▸ Chlordiazepoxide hydrochloride (Non-proprietary)
Chlordiazepoxide (as Chlordiazepoxide hydrochloride)
10 mg Chlordiazepoxide 10mg tablets | 100 tablet [PoM] £49.50 DT = £49.50 [CD4-1]

Capsule
CAUTIONARY AND ADVISORY LABELS 2
▸ Chlordiazepoxide hydrochloride (Non-proprietary)
Chlordiazepoxide hydrochloride 5 mg Chlordiazepoxide 5mg capsules | 100 capsule [PoM] £11.50 DT = £11.50 [CD4-1]
Chlordiazepoxide hydrochloride 10 mg Chlordiazepoxide 10mg capsules | 100 capsule [PoM] £17.80 DT = £17.80 [CD4-1]
▸ Librium (Meda Pharmaceuticals Ltd)
Chlordiazepoxide hydrochloride 5 mg Librium 5mg capsules | 100 capsule [PoM] £5.38 DT = £11.50 [CD4-1]
Chlordiazepoxide hydrochloride 10 mg Librium 10mg capsules | 100 capsule [PoM] £7.46 DT = £17.80 [CD4-1]

⬛ 339

Diazepam 21-Nov-2016

● **INDICATIONS AND DOSE**

Muscle spasm of varied aetiology

▸ BY MOUTH

▸ Adult: 2–15 mg daily in divided doses, then increased if necessary to 60 mg daily, adjusted according to response, dose only increased in spastic conditions

Acute muscle spasm

▸ BY INTRAMUSCULAR INJECTION, OR BY SLOW INTRAVENOUS INJECTION

▸ Adult: 10 mg, then 10 mg after 4 hours if required, intravenous injection to be administered into a large vein at a rate of no more than 5 mg/minute

Tetanus

▸ BY INTRAVENOUS INJECTION

▸ Child: 100–300 micrograms/kg every 1–4 hours

▸ Adult: 100–300 micrograms/kg every 1–4 hours

▸ BY INTRAVENOUS INFUSION, OR BY NASODUODENAL TUBE

▸ Child: 3–10 mg/kg, adjusted according to response, to be given over 24 hours

▸ Adult: 3–10 mg/kg, adjusted according to response, to be given over 24 hours

Muscle spasm in cerebral spasticity or in postoperative skeletal muscle spasm

▸ BY MOUTH

▸ Child 1-11 months: Initially 250 micrograms/kg twice daily

▸ Child 1-4 years: Initially 2.5 mg twice daily

▸ Child 5-11 years: Initially 5 mg twice daily

▸ Child 12-17 years: Initially 10 mg twice daily; maximum 40 mg per day

Anxiety

▸ BY MOUTH

▸ Adult: 2 mg 3 times a day, then increased if necessary to 15–30 mg daily in divided doses, for debilitated patients, use elderly dose

▸ Elderly: 1 mg 3 times a day, then increased if necessary to 7.5–15 mg daily in divided doses

Insomnia associated with anxiety

▸ BY MOUTH

▸ Adult: 5–15 mg daily, to be taken at bedtime

Severe acute anxiety | Control of acute panic attacks | Acute alcohol withdrawal

▸ BY INTRAMUSCULAR INJECTION, OR BY SLOW INTRAVENOUS INJECTION

▸ Adult: 10 mg, then 10 mg after at least 4 hours if required, intravenous injection to be administered into a large vein, at a rate of no more than 5 mg/minute

Acute drug-induced dystonic reactions

▸ BY INTRAVENOUS INJECTION

▸ Adult: 5–10 mg, then 5–10 mg after at least 10 minutes as required, to be administered into a large vein, at a rate of not more than 5 mg/minute

Acute anxiety and agitation
▸ BY RECTUM
▸ Adult: 500 micrograms/kg, then 500 micrograms/kg after 12 hours as required
▸ Elderly: 250 micrograms/kg, then 250 micrograms/kg after 12 hours as required

Premedication
▸ BY MOUTH
▸ Adult: 5–10 mg, to be given 1–2 hours before procedure, for debilitated patients, use elderly dose
▸ Elderly: 2.5–5 mg, to be given 1–2 hours before procedure
▸ BY INTRAVENOUS INJECTION
▸ Adult: 100–200 micrograms/kg, to be administered into a large vein at a rate of not more than 5 mg/minute, immediately before procedure

Sedation in dental procedures carried out in hospital
▸ BY MOUTH
▸ Adult: Up to 20 mg, to be given 1–2 hours before procedure

Conscious sedation for procedures, and in conjunction with local anaesthesia
▸ BY MOUTH
▸ Adult: 5–10 mg, to be given 1–2 hours before procedure, for debilitated patients, use elderly dose
▸ Elderly: 2.5–5 mg, to be given 1–2 hours before procedure

Sedative cover for minor surgical and medical procedures
▸ BY INTRAVENOUS INJECTION
▸ Adult: 10–20 mg, to be administered into a large vein over 2–4 minutes, immediately before procedure

Status epilepticus | Febrile convulsions | Convulsions due to poisoning
▸ BY INTRAVENOUS INJECTION
▸ Neonate: 300–400 micrograms/kg, then 300–400 micrograms/kg after 10 minutes if required, to be given over 3–5 minutes.
▸ Child 1 month–11 years: 300–400 micrograms/kg (max. per dose 10 mg), then 300–400 micrograms/kg after 10 minutes if required, to be given over 3–5 minutes
▸ Child 12–17 years: 10 mg, then 10 mg after 10 minutes if required, to be given over 3–5 minutes
▸ Adult: 10 mg, then 10 mg after 10 minutes if required, administered at a rate of 1 mL (5 mg) per minute
▸ BY RECTUM
▸ Neonate: 1.25–2.5 mg, then 1.25–2.5 mg after 10 minutes if required.
▸ Child 1 month–1 year: 5 mg, then 5 mg after 10 minutes if required
▸ Child 2–11 years: 5–10 mg, then 5–10 mg after 10 minutes if required
▸ Child 12–17 years: 10–20 mg, then 10–20 mg after 10 minutes if required
▸ Adult: 10–20 mg, then 10–20 mg after 10–15 minutes if required
▸ Elderly: 10 mg, then 10 mg after 10–15 minutes if required

Life-threatening acute drug-induced dystonic reactions
▸ BY INTRAVENOUS INJECTION
▸ Child 1 month–11 years: 100 micrograms/kg, repeated if necessary, to be given over 3–5 minutes
▸ Child 12–17 years: 5–10 mg, repeated if necessary, to be given over 3–5 minutes

Dyspnoea associated with anxiety in palliative care
▸ BY MOUTH
▸ Adult: 5–10 mg daily

Pain of muscle spasm in palliative care
▸ BY MOUTH
▸ Adult: 5–10 mg daily

● UNLICENSED USE *Diazepam Desitin*®, *Diazepam Rectubes*®, and *Stesolid Rectal Tubes*® not licensed for use in children under 1 year.

> **IMPORTANT SAFETY INFORMATION**
> ANAESTHESIA
> Benzodiazepines should only be administered for anaesthesia by, or under the direct supervision of, personnel experienced in their use, with adequate training in anaesthesia and airway management.

● CONTRA-INDICATIONS Avoid injections containing benzyl alcohol in neonates · chronic psychosis (in adults) · CNS depression · compromised airway · hyperkinesis · not for use alone to treat depression (or anxiety associated with depression) (in adults) · obsessional states · phobic states · respiratory depression
● CAUTIONS
  GENERAL CAUTIONS Muscle weakness · organic brain changes · parenteral administration (close observation required until full recovery from sedation)
  SPECIFIC CAUTIONS
▸ With intravenous use high risk of venous thrombophlebitis with intravenous use (reduced by using an emulsion formulation)
  CAUTIONS, FURTHER INFORMATION
▸ Special precautions for intravenous injection When given intravenously facilities for reversing respiratory depression with mechanical ventilation must be immediately available.
● INTERACTIONS → Appendix 1: diazepam
● SIDE-EFFECTS
  GENERAL SIDE-EFFECTS
▸ **Common or very common** Appetite abnormal · movement disorders · muscle spasms · palpitations · sensory disorder
▸ **Uncommon** Concentration impaired · constipation · diarrhoea · hypersalivation · skin reactions · speech slurred · vomiting
▸ **Rare or very rare** Bradycardia · bronchial secretion increased · cardiac arrest · dry mouth · gynaecomastia · heart failure · leucopenia · loss of consciousness · memory loss · psychiatric disorder · respiratory arrest · sexual dysfunction · syncope
▸ **Frequency not known** Apnoea · nystagmus · vision blurred
  SPECIFIC SIDE-EFFECTS
▸ With intramuscular use Chest pain · embolism and thrombosis · fall · increased risk of dementia · rebound effect
● PREGNANCY Women who have seizures in the second half of pregnancy should be assessed for eclampsia before any change is made to antiepileptic treatment. Status epilepticus should be treated according to the standard protocol.
  Epilepsy and Pregnancy Register All pregnant women with epilepsy, whether taking medication or not, should be encouraged to notify the UK Epilepsy and Pregnancy Register (Tel: 0800 389 1248).
● BREAST FEEDING Present in milk, and should be avoided if possible during breast-feeding.
● HEPATIC IMPAIRMENT Can precipitate coma. If treatment is necessary, benzodiazepines with shorter half lives are safer, such as temazepam or oxazepam. Avoid in severe impairment.
  Dose adjustments Start with smaller initial doses or reduce dose.
● RENAL IMPAIRMENT
  Dose adjustments Start with small doses in severe impairment.

4
Nervous system

Nervous system

4

- DIRECTIONS FOR ADMINISTRATION
‣ With intravenous use Diazepam is adsorbed by plastics of infusion bags and giving sets. Emulsion formulation preferred for intravenous injection.
‣ With intravenous use in children For *continuous intravenous infusion* of diazepam emulsion, dilute to a concentration of max. 400 micrograms/mL with Glucose 5% or 10%; max. 6 hours between addition and completion of infusion. For *continuous intravenous infusion* of diazepam solution, dilute to a concentration of max. 50 micrograms/mL with Glucose 5% or Sodium Chloride 0.9%.
‣ With intravenous use in adults For *intravenous infusion* (solution) (*Diazepam*, Wockhardt), give continuously *in* Glucose 5% or Sodium chloride 0.9%. Dilute to a concentration of not more than 10 mg in 200 mL. For *intravenous infusion* (emulsion) (*Diazemuls* ®), give continuously *in* Glucose 5% or 10%. May be diluted to a max. concentration of 200 mg in 500 mL; max. 6 hours between addition and completion of administration. May be given *via* drip tubing *in* Glucose 5% or 10% or Sodium chloride 0.9%.
‣ With intramuscular use or intravenous use in adults Solution for injection should not be diluted, except for intravenous infusion.
‣ With intramuscular use in adults Only use intramuscular route when oral and intravenous routes not possible.
- PRESCRIBING AND DISPENSING INFORMATION
Palliative care For further information on the use of diazepam in palliative care, see www.palliativedrugs.com/formulary/en/diazepam.html.
- PATIENT AND CARER ADVICE
Medicines for Children leaflet: Diazepam (rectal) for stopping seizures www.medicinesforchildren.org.uk/diazepam-rectal-stopping-seizures-0
Medicines for Children leaflet: Diazepam for muscle spasm www.medicinesforchildren.org.uk/diazepam-for-muscle-spasm

Driving and skilled tasks May impair judgement and increase reaction time, and so affect ability to drive or perform skilled tasks; they increase the effects of alcohol. Moreover the hangover effects of a night dose may impair performance on the following day.

Patients given sedatives and analgesics during minor outpatient procedures should be very carefully warned about the risks of undertaking skilled tasks (e.g. driving) afterwards. For intravenous benzodiazepines the risk extends to **at least 24 hours** after administration. Responsible persons should be available to take patients home afterwards. The dangers of taking **alcohol** should be emphasised.
- PROFESSION SPECIFIC INFORMATION
Dental practitioners' formulary
Diazepam Tablets may be prescribed.
Diazepam Oral Solution 2 mg/5 mL may be prescribed.
- MEDICINAL FORMS
There can be variation in the licensing of different medicines containing the same drug. Forms available from special-order manufacturers include: oral suspension, oral solution, suppository
Tablet
CAUTIONARY AND ADVISORY LABELS 2, 19
‣ Diazepam (Non-proprietary)
Diazepam 2 mg Diazepam 2mg tablets | 28 tablet [PoM] £1.10 DT = £0.33 [CD4-1] | 1000 tablet [PoM] £160.71 [CD4-1]
Diazepam 5 mg Diazepam 5mg tablets | 28 tablet [PoM] £1.12 DT = £0.37 [CD4-1] | 1000 tablet [PoM] £210.71 [CD4-1]
Diazepam 10 mg Diazepam 10mg tablets | 28 tablet [PoM] £4.99 DT = £0.43 [CD4-1] | 500 tablet [PoM] £113.04 [CD4-1]
Emulsion for injection
‣ Diazemuls (Accord Healthcare Ltd)
Diazepam 5 mg per 1 ml Diazemuls 10mg/2ml emulsion for injection ampoules | 10 ampoule [PoM] £9.05 [CD4-1]

Solution for injection
EXCIPIENTS: May contain Benzyl alcohol, ethanol, propylene glycol
‣ Diazepam (Non-proprietary)
Diazepam 5 mg per 1 ml Diazepam 10mg/2ml solution for injection ampoules | 10 ampoule [PoM] £5.50 DT = £5.50 [CD4-1]
Oral suspension
‣ Diazepam (Non-proprietary)
Diazepam 400 microgram per 1 ml Diazepam 2mg/5ml oral suspension | 100 ml [PoM] £31.75–£38.33 DT = £31.75 [CD4-1]
Oral solution
CAUTIONARY AND ADVISORY LABELS 2, 19
‣ Diazepam (Non-proprietary)
Diazepam 400 microgram per 1 ml Diazepam 2mg/5ml oral solution sugar free sugar-free | 100 ml [PoM] £31.75 DT = £31.75 [CD4-1]
Enema
CAUTIONARY AND ADVISORY LABELS 2, 19
‣ Diazepam (Non-proprietary)
Diazepam 2 mg per 1 ml Diazepam 2.5mg/1.25ml rectal solution tube | 5 tube [PoM] [⚠] [CD4-1]
Diazepam 5mg/2.5ml rectal solution tube | 5 tube [PoM] £5.85 DT = £5.85 [CD4-1]
Diazepam 4 mg per 1 ml Diazepam 10mg/2.5ml rectal solution tube | 5 tube [PoM] £7.35 DT = £7.35 [CD4-1]
‣ Stesolid (Actavis UK Ltd)
Diazepam 2 mg per 1 ml Stesolid 5mg rectal tube | 5 tube [PoM] £6.89 DT = £5.85 [CD4-1]

▸ 339

Oxazepam

- INDICATIONS AND DOSE
Anxiety (short-term use)
▸ BY MOUTH
▸ Adult: 15–30 mg 3–4 times a day, for debilitated patients, use elderly dose
▸ Elderly: 10–20 mg 3–4 times a day
Insomnia associated with anxiety
▸ BY MOUTH
▸ Adult: 15–25 mg once daily (max. per dose 50 mg), dose to be taken at bedtime

- CONTRA-INDICATIONS Chronic psychosis · hyperkinesis · not for use alone to treat depression (or anxiety associated with depression) · obsessional states · phobic states · respiratory depression
- CAUTIONS Muscle weakness · organic brain changes
CAUTIONS, FURTHER INFORMATION
▸ Paradoxical effects A paradoxical increase in hostility and aggression may be reported by patients taking benzodiazepines. The effects range from talkativeness and excitement to aggressive and antisocial acts. Adjustment of the dose (up or down) sometimes attenuates the impulses. Increased anxiety and perceptual disorders are other paradoxical effects.
- INTERACTIONS → Appendix 1: oxazepam
- SIDE-EFFECTS Disorientation · dreaming excessive · fever · lethargy · leucopenia · memory loss · oedema · saliva altered · skin reactions · speech slurred · syncope · vision blurred
- BREAST FEEDING Benzodiazepines are present in milk, and should be avoided if possible during breast-feeding.
- HEPATIC IMPAIRMENT Can precipitate coma. If treatment is necessary, benzodiazepines with shorter half-lives are safer. Avoid in severe impairment.
Dose adjustments Start with smaller initial doses or reduce dose.
- RENAL IMPAIRMENT
Dose adjustments Start with small doses in severe impairment.
- PATIENT AND CARER ADVICE
Driving and skilled tasks May impair judgement and increase reaction time, and so affect ability to drive or

operate machinery; they increase the effects of alcohol. Moreover the hangover effects of a night dose may impair driving on the following day.

● MEDICINAL FORMS
There can be variation in the licensing of different medicines containing the same drug. Forms available from special-order manufacturers include: oral suspension

Tablet
CAUTIONARY AND ADVISORY LABELS 2
▸ Oxazepam (Non-proprietary)
Oxazepam 10 mg Oxazepam 10mg tablets | 28 tablet PoM £15.85
DT = £15.85 CD4-1
Oxazepam 15 mg Oxazepam 15mg tablets | 28 tablet PoM £15.43
DT = £15.43 CD4-1

HYPNOTICS, SEDATIVES AND ANXIOLYTICS ＞
NON-BENZODIAZEPINE HYPNOTICS AND SEDATIVES

Meprobamate
06-Feb-2018

● INDICATIONS AND DOSE

Short-term use in anxiety—not recommended
▸ BY MOUTH
▸ Adult: 400 mg 3–4 times a day
▸ Elderly: Up to 200 mg 3–4 times a day

IMPORTANT SAFETY INFORMATION
MHRA/CHM ADVICE: MEPROBAMATE: LICENCE TO BE CANCELLED (APRIL 2016)
Following an EU-wide review of meprobamate, the UK licence holder has ceased manufacturing and the licence is due to be cancelled by December 2016. No new stock will be released into the normal distribution chain after 31 December 2016, although existing stock placed on the market before that date is likely to be dispensed until the products approach their expiry date.
   Prescribers should review the treatment of any patient who is currently receiving a meprobamate-containing medicine with a view to switching them to an alternative treatment, and not start any new patients on medicines that contain meprobamate.

● CONTRA-INDICATIONS Acute porphyrias p. 1025 · acute pulmonary insufficiency · respiratory depression
● CAUTIONS Abrupt withdrawal (may precipitate convulsions) · avoid prolonged use · debilitated · elderly · emotionally unstable personality (if taken over long periods)—increased risk of dependence · epilepsy (may induce seizures) · history of alcohol dependence · history of drug dependence · muscle weakness · respiratory disease
● INTERACTIONS → Appendix 1: meprobamate
● SIDE-EFFECTS Agitation · agranulocytosis · anal inflammation · ataxia · blood disorder · bone marrow disorders · dizziness · drowsiness · hypersensitivity · hypotension · nausea · paraesthesia · purpura non-thrombocytopenic · skin reactions · Stevens-Johnson syndrome · stomatitis · thrombocytopenia · vomiting · withdrawal syndrome
● PREGNANCY Avoid if possible.
● BREAST FEEDING Avoid. Concentration in milk may exceed maternal plasma concentrations fourfold and may cause drowsiness in infant.
● HEPATIC IMPAIRMENT Can precipitate coma.
● RENAL IMPAIRMENT Increased cerebral sensitivity.
Dose adjustments Start with small doses in severe impairment.

● PATIENT AND CARER ADVICE
Driving and skilled tasks Drowsiness may affect performance of skilled tasks (e.g. driving); effects of alcohol enhanced.
● LESS SUITABLE FOR PRESCRIBING Meprobamate is less suitable for prescribing.
● MEDICINAL FORMS
There can be variation in the licensing of different medicines containing the same drug. Forms available from special-order manufacturers include: oral suspension, oral solution

Tablet
CAUTIONARY AND ADVISORY LABELS 2
▸ Meprobamate (Non-proprietary)
Meprobamate 400 mg Meprobamate 400mg tablets | 84 tablet PoM £197.63 DT = £197.63 CD3

3.2 Attention deficit hyperactivity disorder

Attention deficit hyperactivity disorder
01-Sep-2017

Description of condition
Attention deficit hyperactivity disorder (ADHD) is a behavioural syndrome characterised by hyperactivity, impulsivity and inattention, which can lead to psychological, social, educational or occupational impairment. While these symptoms tend to co-exist, some people are predominantly hyperactive and impulsive, while others are principally inattentive. Symptoms typically appear in children 3–7 years of age, but may not be recognised until after 7 years of age, especially if the predominant trait is inattention.
   ADHD is usually a persisting disorder. Most older children with a sustained diagnosis will go on to have difficulties in adulthood, which may include continuing ADHD, personality disorders, emotional and social difficulties, and substance misuse.

Aims of treatment
The aims of treatment are to reduce functional impairment and the severity of symptoms, and to improve quality of life.

Drug treatment
EvGr Drug treatment, started by a specialist prescriber, is the first-line treatment for adults with ADHD with either moderate or severe levels of impairment. Methylphenidate hydrochloride p. 345 is the first-line drug. Psychological interventions without drug treatment may be effective for some patients with moderate impairment, but there are insufficient data to support this recommendation. If there is residual impairment despite some benefit from drug treatment, or there is no response to drug treatment, cognitive behavioural therapy (CBT) can be considered.
   Atomoxetine p. 344 or dexamfetamine sulfate p. 347 should be considered in patients unresponsive or intolerant to methylphenidate (adequate trial should usually be about 6 weeks). Where there may be concern about the potential for drug misuse and diversion, atomoxetine p. 344 may be used as first line. Further options for treatment include higher doses of methylphenidate hydrochloride p. 345 or atomoxetine p. 344; further or alternative psychological treatments; or referral to regional specialists for alternative drug treatment.
   When starting drug treatment, patients should be monitored for side-effects. In particular, patients treated with atomoxetine p. 344 should be observed for agitation, irritability, suicidal thinking and self-harming behaviour, and unusual changes in behaviour, particularly during the

Nervous system

4

initial months of treatment, or after a change in dose. They should also be warned of potential liver damage in rare cases. Patients aged 30 years or younger should also be warned of the potential of atomoxetine below to increase agitation, anxiety, suicidal thinking and self-harming behaviour in some people, especially during the first few weeks of treatment.

For patients with ADHD stabilised on drug treatment but with persisting functional impairment associated with the disorder, or where there has been no response to drug treatment, a course of either group or individual CBT to address the patient's functional impairment should be considered.

Following an adequate response, drug treatment for ADHD should be continued for as long as it is clinically effective. Treatment should be reviewed annually. ◁

Related drugs

Other drugs used for attention deficit hyperactivity disorder: guanfacine p. 349, imipramine hydrochloride p. 372, lisdexamfetamine mesilate p. 348.

Useful Resources

Attention deficit hyperactivity disorder: diagnosis and management. National Institute for Health and Care Excellence. Clinical guideline 72. September 2008 (updated February 2016).
www.nice.org.uk/guidance/CG72

CNS STIMULANTS ⟩ CENTRALLY ACTING SYMPATHOMIMETICS

Atomoxetine

28-Sep-2016

● **INDICATIONS AND DOSE**

Attention deficit hyperactivity disorder (initiated by a specialist)

▸ BY MOUTH

▸ Child 6-17 years (body-weight up to 70 kg): Initially 500 micrograms/kg daily for 7 days, dose is increased according to response; maintenance 1.2 mg/kg daily, total daily dose may be given either as a single dose in the morning or in 2 divided doses with last dose no later than early evening, high daily doses to be given under the direction of a specialist; maximum 1.8 mg/kg per day; maximum 120 mg per day

▸ Child 6-17 years (body-weight 70 kg and above): Initially 40 mg daily for 7 days, dose is increased according to response; maintenance 80 mg daily, total daily dose may be given as a single dose in the morning or in 2 divided doses with last dose no later than early evening, high daily doses to be given under the direction of a specialist; maximum 120 mg per day

▸ Adult (body-weight up to 70 kg): Initially 500 micrograms/kg daily for 7 days, dose is increased according to response; maintenance 1.2 mg/kg daily, total daily dose may be given either as a single dose in the morning or in 2 divided doses with last dose no later than early evening, high daily doses to be given under the direction of a specialist; maximum 1.8 mg/kg per day; maximum 120 mg per day

▸ Adult (body-weight 70 kg and above): Initially 40 mg daily for 7 days, dose is increased according to response; maintenance 80-100 mg daily, total daily dose may be given either as a single dose in the morning or in 2 divided doses with last dose no later than early evening, high daily doses to be given under the direction of a specialist; maximum 120 mg per day

● UNLICENSED USE Atomoxetine doses in BNF may differ from those in product literature.

▸ In children Doses above 100 mg daily not licensed.

▸ In adults Dose maximum of 120 mg not licensed.

● CONTRA-INDICATIONS Phaeochromocytoma · severe cardiovascular disease · severe cerebrovascular disease

● CAUTIONS QT-interval prolongation · aggressive behaviour · cardiovascular disease · cerebrovascular disease · emotional lability · history of seizures · hostility · hypertension · mania · psychosis · structural cardiac abnormalities · susceptibility to angle-closure glaucoma · tachycardia

● INTERACTIONS → Appendix 1: atomoxetine

● SIDE-EFFECTS

▸ **Common or very common** Anxiety · appetite decreased · arrhythmias (uncommon in children) · asthenia · chills (in adults) · constipation · depression · dizziness · drowsiness · dry mouth (in adults) · feeling jittery (in adults) · flatulence (in adults) · gastrointestinal discomfort · genital pain (rare in children) · headaches · hyperhidrosis (uncommon in children) · menstrual cycle irregularities (in adults) · mood altered · mydriasis (in children) · nausea · palpitations (uncommon in children) · prostatitis (in adults) · sensation abnormal (uncommon in children) · sexual dysfunction (rare in children) · skin reactions · sleep disorders · taste altered (in adults) · thirst (in adults) · tremor (uncommon in children) · urinary disorders (rare in children) · vasodilation (in adults) · vomiting · weight decreased

▸ **Uncommon** Behaviour abnormal · chest pain (very common in children) · dyspnoea · feeling cold (in adults) · hypersensitivity · muscle spasms (in adults) · peripheral coldness (in adults) · QT interval prolongation · suicidal behaviour · syncope · tic (very common in children) · vision blurred

▸ **Rare or very rare** Hallucination (uncommon in children) · hepatic disorders · psychosis (uncommon in children) · Raynaud's phenomenon · seizure (uncommon in children)

▸ **Frequency not known** Sudden cardiac death

● PREGNANCY Manufacturer advises avoid unless potential benefit outweighs risk.

● BREAST FEEDING Avoid-present in milk in *animal* studies.

● HEPATIC IMPAIRMENT

Dose adjustments Halve dose in moderate impairment. Quarter dose in severe impairment.

● MONITORING REQUIREMENTS

▸ Monitor for appearance or worsening of anxiety, depression or tics.

▸ Pulse, blood pressure, psychiatric symptoms, appetite, weight and height should be recorded at initiation of therapy, following each dose adjustment, and at least every 6 months thereafter.

● PATIENT AND CARER ADVICE

Medicines for Children leaflet: Atomoxetine for attention deficit hyperactivity disorder (ADHD) www.medicinesforchildren.org.uk/atomoxetine-attention-deficit-hyperactivity-disorder-adhd

Suicidal ideation Following reports of suicidal thoughts and behaviour, patients and their carers should be informed about the risk and told to report clinical worsening, suicidal thoughts or behaviour, irritability, agitation, or depression.

Hepatic impairment Following rare reports of hepatic disorders, patients and carers should be advised of the risk and be told how to recognise symptoms; prompt medical attention should be sought in case of abdominal pain, unexplained nausea, malaise, darkening of the urine, or jaundice.

● NATIONAL FUNDING/ACCESS DECISIONS

NICE decisions

▶ Methylphenidate, atomoxetine and dexamfetamine for attention deficit hyperactivity disorder (ADHD) (March 2006) NICE TA98

Atomoxetine is recommended, within its licensed indications, as an option for the management of ADHD in children and adolescents.

www.nice.org.uk/TA98

Scottish Medicines Consortium (SMC) Decisions

The *Scottish Medicines Consortium* has advised (December 2015) that atomoxetine oral solution (*Strattera®*) is accepted for restricted use, within its licensed indications, for treating patients who are unable to swallow capsules.

● MEDICINAL FORMS

There can be variation in the licensing of different medicines containing the same drug. Forms available from special-order manufacturers include: oral suspension, oral solution

Oral solution

CAUTIONARY AND ADVISORY LABELS 3

▶ Strattera (Eli Lilly and Company Ltd)

Atomoxetine (as Atomoxetine hydrochloride) 4 mg per 1 ml Strattera 4mg/1ml oral solution sugar-free | 300 ml PoM £85.00 DT = £85.00

Capsule

CAUTIONARY AND ADVISORY LABELS 3

▶ Strattera (Eli Lilly and Company Ltd)

Atomoxetine (as Atomoxetine hydrochloride) 10 mg Strattera 10mg capsules | 7 capsule PoM £13.28 | 28 capsule PoM £53.09 DT = £53.09

Atomoxetine (as Atomoxetine hydrochloride) 18 mg Strattera 18mg capsules | 7 capsule PoM £13.28 | 28 capsule PoM £53.09 DT = £53.09

Atomoxetine (as Atomoxetine hydrochloride) 25 mg Strattera 25mg capsules | 7 capsule PoM £13.28 | 28 capsule PoM £53.09 DT = £53.09

Atomoxetine (as Atomoxetine hydrochloride) 40 mg Strattera 40mg capsules | 7 capsule PoM £13.28 | 28 capsule PoM £53.09 DT = £53.09

Atomoxetine (as Atomoxetine hydrochloride) 60 mg Strattera 60mg capsules | 28 capsule PoM £53.09 DT = £53.09

Atomoxetine (as Atomoxetine hydrochloride) 80 mg Strattera 80mg capsules | 28 capsule PoM £70.79 DT = £70.79

Atomoxetine (as Atomoxetine hydrochloride) 100 mg Strattera 100mg capsules | 28 capsule PoM £70.79 DT = £70.79

Methylphenidate hydrochloride   03-Oct-2017

● INDICATIONS AND DOSE

Attention deficit hyperactivity disorder (initiated under specialist supervision)

▶ BY MOUTH USING IMMEDIATE-RELEASE MEDICINES

▶ Child 6-17 years: Initially 5 mg 1–2 times a day, increased in steps of 5–10 mg daily if required, at weekly intervals, increased if necessary up to 60 mg daily in 2–3 divided doses, increased if necessary up to 2.1 mg/kg daily in 2–3 divided doses, the licensed maximum dose is 60 mg daily in 2–3 doses, higher dose (up to a maximum of 90 mg daily) under the direction of a specialist, discontinue if no response after 1 month, if effect wears off in evening (with rebound hyperactivity) a dose at bedtime may be appropriate (establish need with trial bedtime dose). Treatment may be started using a modified-release preparation

▶ Adult: Initially 5 mg 2–3 times a day, dose is increased if necessary at weekly intervals according to response, increased if necessary up to 100 mg daily in 2–3 divided doses, if effect wears off in evening (with rebound hyperactivity) a dose at bedtime may be appropriate (establish need with trial bedtime dose). Treatment may be started using a modified-release preparation

Narcolepsy

▶ BY MOUTH USING IMMEDIATE-RELEASE MEDICINES

▶ Adult: 10–60 mg daily in divided doses; usual dose 20–30 mg daily in divided doses, dose to be taken before meals

DOSE EQUIVALENCE AND CONVERSION

▶ When switching from *immediate-release* preparations to *modified-release* preparations—consult product literature.

CONCERTA® XL

Attention deficit hyperactivity disorder

▶ BY MOUTH

▶ Child 6-17 years: Initially 18 mg once daily, dose to be taken in the morning, increased in steps of 18 mg every week, adjusted according to response; increased if necessary up to 2.1 mg/kg daily, licensed max. dose is 54 mg once daily, to be increased to higher dose only under direction of specialist; discontinue if no response after 1 month; maximum 108 mg per day

▶ Adult: Initially 18 mg once daily, dose to be taken in the morning; adjusted at weekly intervals according to response; maximum 108 mg per day

DOSE EQUIVALENCE AND CONVERSION

▶ Total daily dose of 15 mg of standard-release formulation is considered equivalent to *Concerta®* XL 18 mg once daily.

DELMOSART® PROLONGED-RELEASE TABLET

Attention deficit hyperactivity disorder (under expert supervision)

▶ BY MOUTH

▶ Child 6-17 years: Initially 18 mg once daily, dose to be taken in the morning, then increased in steps of 18 mg every week if required, discontinue if no response after 1 month; maximum 54 mg per day

▶ Adult: Initially 18 mg once daily, dose to be taken in the morning, then increased in steps of 18 mg every week if required, discontinue if no response after 1 month; maximum 54 mg per day

DOSE EQUIVALENCE AND CONVERSION

▶ Total daily dose of 15 mg of standard-release formulation is considered equivalent to *Delmosart®* 18 mg once daily.

EQUASYM® XL

Attention deficit hyperactivity disorder

▶ BY MOUTH

▶ Child 6-17 years: Initially 10 mg once daily, dose to be taken in the morning before breakfast; increased gradually at weekly intervals if necessary; increased if necessary up to 2.1 mg/kg daily, licensed max. dose is 60 mg daily, to be increased to higher dose only under direction of specialist; discontinue if no response after 1 month; maximum 90 mg per day

▶ Adult: Initially 10 mg once daily, dose to be taken in the morning before breakfast; increased gradually at weekly intervals if necessary; maximum 100 mg per day

MEDIKINET® XL

Attention deficit hyperactivity disorder

▶ BY MOUTH

▶ Child 6-17 years: Initially 10 mg once daily, dose to be taken in the morning with breakfast; adjusted at weekly intervals according to response; increased if necessary up to 2.1 mg/kg daily, licensed max. dose is 60 mg daily, to be increased to higher dose only under direction of specialist; discontinue if no response after 1 month; maximum 90 mg per day

▶ Adult: Initially 10 mg once daily, dose to be taken in the morning with breakfast; adjusted at weekly intervals according to response; maximum 100 mg per day

continued →

4

Nervous system

XAGGITIN ® XL

Attention deficit hyperactivity disorder (under expert supervision)

▶ BY MOUTH

▶ **Child 6–17 years:** Initially 18 mg once daily, dose to be taken in the morning, increased in steps of 18 mg every week, adjusted according to response, discontinue if no response after 1 month; maximum 54 mg per day

▶ **Adult:** Initially 18 mg once daily, dose to be taken in the morning, increased in steps of 18 mg every week, adjusted according to response, discontinue if no response after 1 month; maximum 54 mg per day

DOSE EQUIVALENCE AND CONVERSION

▶ Total daily dose of 15 mg of standard-release formulation is considered equivalent to *Xaggitin* ® XL 18 mg once daily.

● UNLICENSED USE Doses over 60 mg daily not licensed; doses of *Concerta XL* over 54 mg daily not licensed. Not licensed for use in narcolepsy. Not licensed for use in adults for attention deficit hyperactivity disorder.

● CONTRA-INDICATIONS Anorexia nervosa · arrhythmias · cardiomyopathy · cardiovascular disease · cerebrovascular disorders · heart failure · hyperthyroidism · phaeochromocytoma · psychosis · severe depression · severe hypertension · structural cardiac abnormalities · suicidal ideation · uncontrolled bipolar disorder · vasculitis

● CAUTIONS Agitation · alcohol dependence · anxiety · drug dependence · epilepsy (discontinue if increased seizure frequency) · family history of Tourette syndrome · susceptibility to angle-closure glaucoma · tics

CONCERTA ® XL, DELMOSART ® PROLONGED-RELEASE TABLET Dysphagia (dose form not appropriate) · restricted gastro-intestinal lumen (dose form not appropriate)

XAGGITIN ® XL Dysphagia (dose form not appropriate)

● INTERACTIONS → Appendix 1: methylphenidate

● SIDE-EFFECTS

▶ **Common or very common** Alopecia · anxiety · appetite decreased · arrhythmias · arthralgia · behaviour abnormal · cough · depression · diarrhoea · dizziness · drowsiness · dry mouth · fever · gastrointestinal discomfort · growth retardation (in children) · headaches · hypertension · laryngeal pain · mood altered · movement disorders · nasopharyngitis · nausea · palpitations · sleep disorders · vomiting · weight decreased

▶ **Uncommon** Chest discomfort · constipation · dyspnoea · fatigue · haematuria · hallucinations · muscle complaints · psychotic disorder · suicidal tendencies · tic · tremor · vision disorders

▶ **Rare or very rare** Anaemia · angina pectoris · cardiac arrest · cerebrovascular insufficiency · confusion · gynaecomastia · hepatic coma · hyperfocus · hyperhidrosis · leucopenia · mydriasis · myocardial infarction · neuroleptic malignant syndrome · peripheral coldness · Raynaud's phenomenon · seizures · sexual dysfunction · skin reactions · sudden cardiac death · thinking abnormal · thrombocytopenia

▶ **Frequency not known** Delusions · drug dependence · hyperpyrexia · intracranial haemorrhage · logorrhea · pancytopenia · vasculitis

● PREGNANCY Limited experience—avoid unless potential benefit outweighs risk.

● BREAST FEEDING Limited information available—avoid.

● MONITORING REQUIREMENTS

▶ Monitor for psychiatric disorders.

▶ Pulse, blood pressure, psychiatric symptoms, appetite, weight and height should be recorded at initiation of therapy, following each dose adjustment, and at least every 6 months thereafter.

● TREATMENT CESSATION Avoid abrupt withdrawal.

● DIRECTIONS FOR ADMINISTRATION

MEDIKINET ® XL Contents of capsule can be sprinkled on a tablespoon of apple sauce or yoghurt (then swallowed immediately without chewing).

EQUASYM ® XL Contents of capsule can be sprinkled on a tablespoon of apple sauce (then swallowed immediately without chewing).

● PRESCRIBING AND DISPENSING INFORMATION Different versions of modified-release preparations may not have the same clinical effect. To avoid confusion between these different formulations of methylphenidate, prescribers should specify the brand to be dispensed.

CONCERTA ® XL Consists of an immediate-release component (22% of the dose) and a modified-release component (78% of the dose).

MEDIKINET ® XL Consists of an immediate-release component (50% of the dose) and a modified-release component (50% of the dose).

EQUASYM ® XL Consists of an immediate-release component (30% of the dose) and a modified-release component (70% of the dose).

● PATIENT AND CARER ADVICE

Driving and skilled tasks

Drugs and Driving Prescribers and other healthcare professionals should advise patients if treatment is likely to affect their ability to perform skilled tasks (e.g. driving). This applies especially to drugs with sedative effects; patients should be warned that these effects are increased by alcohol. General information about a patient's fitness to drive is available from the Driver and Vehicle Licensing Agency at www.dvla.gov.uk.

2015 legislation regarding driving whilst taking certain drugs, may also apply to methylphenidate, see *Drugs and driving* under Guidance on prescribing p. 1.

CONCERTA ® XL Tablet membrane may pass through gastro-intestinal tract unchanged.

DELMOSART ® PROLONGED-RELEASE TABLET Manufacturer advises tablet membrane may pass through gastro-intestinal tract unchanged.

● NATIONAL FUNDING/ACCESS DECISIONS

NICE decisions

▶ **Methylphenidate, atomoxetine and dexamfetamine for attention deficit hyperactivity disorder (ADHD) (March 2006)** NICE TA98

▶ In children Methylphenidate is recommended, within its licensed indications, as an option for the management of ADHD in children and adolescents.

www.nice.org.uk/TA98

● MEDICINAL FORMS

There can be variation in the licensing of different medicines containing the same drug. Forms available from special-order manufacturers include: oral suspension, oral solution

Modified-release tablet

CAUTIONARY AND ADVISORY LABELS 25

▶ Concerta XL (Janssen-Cilag Ltd)

Methylphenidate hydrochloride 18 mg Concerta XL 18mg tablets | 30 tablet [PoM] £31.19 DT = £31.19 [CD2]

Methylphenidate hydrochloride 27 mg Concerta XL 27mg tablets | 30 tablet [PoM] £36.81 DT = £36.81 [CD2]

Methylphenidate hydrochloride 36 mg Concerta XL 36mg tablets | 30 tablet [PoM] £42.45 DT = £42.45 [CD2]

Methylphenidate hydrochloride 54 mg Concerta XL 54mg tablets | 30 tablet [PoM] £73.62 DT = £36.80 [CD2]

▶ Delmosart (Actavis UK Ltd)

Methylphenidate hydrochloride 18 mg Delmosart 18mg modified-release tablets | 30 tablet [PoM] £15.59 DT = £31.19 [CD2]

Methylphenidate hydrochloride 27 mg Delmosart 27mg modified-release tablets | 30 tablet [PoM] £18.41 DT = £36.81 [CD2]

Methylphenidate hydrochloride 36 mg Delmosart 36mg modified-release tablets | 30 tablet [PoM] £21.23 DT = £42.45 [CD2]

Methylphenidate hydrochloride 54 mg Delmosart 54mg modified-release tablets | 30 tablet [PoM] £36.81 DT = £36.80 [CD2]
▸ Xaggitin XL (Ethypharm UK Ltd)
Methylphenidate hydrochloride 18 mg Xaggitin XL 18mg tablets | 30 tablet [PoM] £15.58 DT = £31.19 [CD2]
Methylphenidate hydrochloride 27 mg Xaggitin XL 27mg tablets | 30 tablet [PoM] £18.40 DT = £36.81 [CD2]
Methylphenidate hydrochloride 36 mg Xaggitin XL 36mg tablets | 30 tablet [PoM] £21.22 DT = £42.45 [CD2]
Methylphenidate hydrochloride 54 mg Xaggitin XL 54mg tablets | 30 tablet [PoM] £36.80 DT = £36.80 [CD2]

Tablet
▸ Methylphenidate hydrochloride (Non-proprietary)
Methylphenidate hydrochloride 5 mg Methylphenidate 5mg tablets | 30 tablet [PoM] £3.03 DT = £3.03 [CD2]
Methylphenidate hydrochloride 10 mg Methylphenidate 10mg tablets | 30 tablet [PoM] £5.29 DT = £3.76 [CD2]
Methylphenidate hydrochloride 20 mg Methylphenidate 20mg tablets | 30 tablet [PoM] £10.92 DT = £10.92 [CD2]
▸ Medikinet (Flynn Pharma Ltd)
Methylphenidate hydrochloride 5 mg Medikinet 5mg tablets | 30 tablet [PoM] £3.03 DT = £3.03 [CD2]
Methylphenidate hydrochloride 10 mg Medikinet 10mg tablets | 30 tablet [PoM] £5.49 DT = £3.76 [CD2]
Methylphenidate hydrochloride 20 mg Medikinet 20mg tablets | 30 tablet [PoM] £10.92 DT = £10.92 [CD2]
▸ Ritalin (Novartis Pharmaceuticals UK Ltd)
Methylphenidate hydrochloride 10 mg Ritalin 10mg tablets | 30 tablet [PoM] £6.68 DT = £3.76 [CD2]
▸ Tranquilyn (Genesis Pharmaceuticals Ltd)
Methylphenidate hydrochloride 5 mg Tranquilyn 5mg tablets | 30 tablet [PoM] £3.03 DT = £3.03 [CD2]
Methylphenidate hydrochloride 10 mg Tranquilyn 10mg tablets | 30 tablet [PoM] £3.76 DT = £3.76 [CD2]
Methylphenidate hydrochloride 20 mg Tranquilyn 20mg tablets | 30 tablet [PoM] £10.92 DT = £10.92 [CD2]

Modified-release capsule
CAUTIONARY AND ADVISORY LABELS 25
▸ Equasym XL (Shire Pharmaceuticals Ltd)
Methylphenidate hydrochloride 10 mg Equasym XL 10mg capsules | 30 capsule [PoM] £25.00 DT = £25.00 [CD2]
Methylphenidate hydrochloride 20 mg Equasym XL 20mg capsules | 30 capsule [PoM] £30.00 DT = £30.00 [CD2]
Methylphenidate hydrochloride 30 mg Equasym XL 30mg capsules | 30 capsule [PoM] £35.00 DT = £35.00 [CD2]
▸ Medikinet XL (Flynn Pharma Ltd)
Methylphenidate hydrochloride 5 mg Medikinet XL 5mg capsules | 30 capsule [PoM] £24.04 [CD2]
Methylphenidate hydrochloride 10 mg Medikinet XL 10mg capsules | 30 capsule [PoM] £24.04 DT = £25.00 [CD2]
Methylphenidate hydrochloride 20 mg Medikinet XL 20mg capsules | 30 capsule [PoM] £28.86 DT = £30.00 [CD2]
Methylphenidate hydrochloride 30 mg Medikinet XL 30mg capsules | 30 capsule [PoM] £33.66 DT = £35.00 [CD2]
Methylphenidate hydrochloride 40 mg Medikinet XL 40mg capsules | 30 capsule [PoM] £57.72 DT = £57.72 [CD2]
Methylphenidate hydrochloride 50 mg Medikinet XL 50mg capsules | 30 capsule [PoM] £62.52 [CD2]
Methylphenidate hydrochloride 60 mg Medikinet XL 60mg capsules | 30 capsule [PoM] £67.32 [CD2]

CNS STIMULANTS > CENTRALLY ACTING SYMPATHOMIMETICS > AMFETAMINES

Dexamfetamine sulfate

(Dexamphetamine sulfate)

● **INDICATIONS AND DOSE**

Narcolepsy
▸ BY MOUTH
▸ Adult: Initially 10 mg daily in divided doses, increased in steps of 10 mg every week, maintenance dose to be given in 2–4 divided doses; maximum 60 mg per day
▸ Elderly: Initially 5 mg daily in divided doses, increased in steps of 5 mg every week, maintenance dose to be given in 2–4 divided doses; maximum 60 mg per day

Refractory attention deficit hyperactivity disorder (initiated under specialist supervision)
▸ BY MOUTH
▸ Child 6–17 years: Initially 2.5 mg 2–3 times a day, increased in steps of 5 mg once weekly if required, increased if necessary up to 1 mg/kg daily, maintenance dose to be given in 2–4 divided doses, up to 20 mg daily (40 mg daily has been required in some children)
▸ Adult: Initially 5 mg twice daily, dose is increased at weekly intervals according to response, maintenance dose to be given in 2–4 divided doses; maximum 60 mg per day

● UNLICENSED USE Not licensed for use in adults for refractory attention deficit hyperactivity disorder.

● CONTRA-INDICATIONS Advanced arteriosclerosis (in adults) · agitated states · cardiovascular disease · history of alcohol abuse · history of drug abuse · hyperexcitability · hyperthyroidism · moderate hypertension · severe hypertension · structural cardiac abnormalities

● CAUTIONS Anorexia · bipolar disorder · history of epilepsy (discontinue if seizures occur) · mild hypertension · psychosis · susceptibility to angle-closure glaucoma · tics · Tourette syndrome

CAUTIONS, FURTHER INFORMATION
▸ Tics and Tourette syndrome Discontinue use if tics occur.
▸ Growth restriction in children Monitor height and weight as growth restriction may occur during prolonged therapy (drug-free periods may allow catch-up in growth but withdraw slowly to avoid inducing depression or renewed hyperactivity).

● INTERACTIONS → Appendix 1: amfetamines

● SIDE-EFFECTS
▸ **Common or very common** Abdominal pain · anxiety · appetite decreased · arrhythmias · arthralgia · behaviour abnormal · depression · dry mouth · headache · mood altered · movement disorders · muscle cramps · nausea · palpitations · poor weight gain · sleep disorders · vertigo · vomiting · weight decreased
▸ **Rare or very rare** Anaemia · angina pectoris · cardiac arrest · cerebrovascular insufficiency · fatigue · growth retardation · hallucination · hepatic coma · hepatic function abnormal · intracranial haemorrhage · leucopenia · mydriasis · psychosis · seizure · skin reactions · suicidal tendencies · thrombocytopenia · tic (in those at risk) · vasculitis cerebral · vision disorders
▸ **Frequency not known** Acidosis · alopecia · cardiomyopathy · chest pain · circulatory collapse · colitis ischaemic · concentration impaired · confusion · diarrhoea · dizziness · drug dependence · drug tolerance · hyperhidrosis · hypermetabolism · hyperpyrexia · kidney injury · myocardial infarction · neuroleptic malignant syndrome · obsessive-compulsive disorder · reflexes increased · rhabdomyolysis · sexual dysfunction · sudden death · taste altered · tremor

Overdose Amfetamines cause wakefulness, excessive activity, paranoia, hallucinations, and hypertension followed by exhaustion, convulsions, hyperthermia, and coma. See Stimulants under Emergency treatment of poisoning p. 1319.

● PREGNANCY Avoid (retrospective evidence of uncertain significance suggesting possible embryotoxicity).

● BREAST FEEDING Significant amount in milk—avoid.

● RENAL IMPAIRMENT Use with caution.

● MONITORING REQUIREMENTS
▸ Monitor growth in children.
▸ Monitor for aggressive behaviour or hostility during initial treatment.

4

Nervous system

4

Nervous system

- Pulse, blood pressure, psychiatric symptoms, appetite, weight and height should be recorded at initiation of therapy, following each dose adjustment, and at least every 6 months thereafter.
- TREATMENT CESSATION Avoid abrupt withdrawal.
- DIRECTIONS FOR ADMINISTRATION
- In children Tablets can be halved.
- PRESCRIBING AND DISPENSING INFORMATION Data on safety and efficacy of long-term use not complete.
- PATIENT AND CARER ADVICE
  Driving and skilled tasks
  Drugs and Driving Prescribers and other healthcare professionals should advise patients if treatment is likely to affect their ability to perform skilled tasks (e.g. driving). This applies especially to drugs with sedative effects; patients should be warned that these effects are increased by alcohol. General information about a patient's fitness to drive is available from the Driver and Vehicle Licensing Agency at www.dvla.gov.uk.
  For information on 2015 legislation regarding driving whilst taking certain controlled drugs, including amfetamines, see *Drugs and driving* under Guidance on prescribing p. 1.
- NATIONAL FUNDING/ACCESS DECISIONS
  NICE decisions
- Methylphenidate, atomoxetine and dexamfetamine for attention deficit hyperactivity disorder (ADHD) (March 2006) NICE TA98
- In children Dexamfetamine is recommended, within its licensed indications, as an option for the management of ADHD in children and adolescents.
  www.nice.org.uk/TA98

- MEDICINAL FORMS
  There can be variation in the licensing of different medicines containing the same drug. Forms available from special-order manufacturers include: modified-release capsule, oral suspension, oral solution
  Oral solution
  ▸ Dexamfetamine sulfate (Non-proprietary)
  Dexamfetamine sulfate 1 mg per 1 ml Dexamfetamine 5mg/5ml oral solution sugar free sugar-free | 150 ml [PoM] £29.44-£34.35 [CD2] sugar-free | 500 ml [PoM] £114.49 DT = £114.49 [CD2]
  Modified-release capsule
  ▸ Dexedrine Spansules (Imported (United States))
  Dexamfetamine sulfate 5 mg Dexedrine 5mg Spansules | 100 capsule [PoM] [圖][CD2]
  Dexamfetamine sulfate 10 mg Dexedrine 10mg Spansules | 100 capsule [PoM] [圖][CD2]
  Dexamfetamine sulfate 15 mg Dexedrine 15mg Spansules | 100 capsule [PoM] [圖][CD2]
  Tablet
  ▸ Dexamfetamine sulfate (Non-proprietary)
  Dexamfetamine sulfate 5 mg Dexamfetamine 5mg tablets | 28 tablet [PoM] £24.75 DT = £24.13 [CD2]
  ▸ Amfexa (Flynn Pharma Ltd)
  Dexamfetamine sulfate 5 mg Amfexa 5mg tablets | 30 tablet [PoM] £19.89 [CD2]
  Dexamfetamine sulfate 10 mg Amfexa 10mg tablets | 30 tablet [PoM] £39.78 DT = £39.78 [CD2]
  Dexamfetamine sulfate 20 mg Amfexa 20mg tablets | 30 tablet [PoM] £79.56 [CD2]

Lisdexamfetamine mesilate
23-Jan-2018

- DRUG ACTION Lisdexamfetamine is a prodrug of dexamfetamine.

- INDICATIONS AND DOSE
  Attention deficit hyperactivity disorder (initiated by a specialist)
  ▸ BY MOUTH
  ▸ Child 6-17 years: Initially 30 mg once daily, alternatively initially 20 mg once daily, increased in steps of 10-20 mg every week if required, dose to be taken in the morning, discontinue if response insufficient after 1 month; maximum 70 mg per day
  ▸ Adult: Initially 30 mg once daily, increased in steps of 20 mg every week if required, dose to be taken in the morning, discontinue if response insufficient after 1 month; maximum 70 mg per day

- CONTRA-INDICATIONS Advanced arteriosclerosis · agitated states · hyperthyroidism · moderate hypertension · severe hypertension · symptomatic cardiovascular disease
- CAUTIONS Bipolar disorder · history of cardiovascular disease · history of substance abuse · may lower seizure threshold (discontinue if seizures occur) · psychotic disorders · susceptibility to angle-closure glaucoma · tics · Tourette syndrome
  CAUTIONS, FURTHER INFORMATION
  ▸ Cardiovascular disease Manufacturer advises caution in patients with underlying conditions that might be compromised by increases in blood pressure or heart rate; see also *Contra-indications*.
- INTERACTIONS → Appendix 1: amfetamines
- SIDE-EFFECTS
  ▸ **Common or very common** Abdominal pain upper · anxiety · appetite decreased · behaviour abnormal · constipation · diarrhoea · dizziness · dry mouth · dyspnoea · fatigue · feeling jittery · headache · hyperhidrosis (uncommon in children) · insomnia · mood altered · movement disorders (uncommon in children) · nausea · palpitations · sexual dysfunction (uncommon in children) · tachycardia · tremor · weight decreased
  ▸ **Uncommon** Depression (very common in children) · drowsiness (very common in children) · fever (very common in children) · logorrhea · psychiatric disorders (very common in children) · skin reactions (very common in children) · taste altered · vision blurred · vomiting (very common in children)
  ▸ **Frequency not known** Angioedema · cardiomyopathy (uncommon in children) · drug dependence · drug tolerance · hallucination (uncommon in children) · hepatitis allergic · mydriasis (uncommon in children) · psychotic disorder · Raynaud's phenomenon (uncommon in children) · seizure · Stevens-Johnson syndrome

  Overdose Amfetamines cause wakefulness, excessive activity, paranoia, hallucinations, and hypertension followed by exhaustion, convulsions, hyperthermia, and coma. See Stimulants under Emergency treatment of poisoning p. 1319.
- PREGNANCY Manufacturer advises use only if potential benefit outweighs risk.
- BREAST FEEDING Manufacturer advises avoid—present in human milk.
- RENAL IMPAIRMENT
  Dose adjustments Manufacturer advises max. dose 50 mg daily in severe impairment.
- MONITORING REQUIREMENTS
  ▸ Manufacturer advises monitor for aggressive behaviour or hostility during initial treatment.
  ▸ Manufacturer advises monitor pulse, blood pressure, and for psychiatric symptoms before treatment initiation,

following each dose adjustment, and at least every 6 months thereafter. Monitor weight in adults before treatment initiation and during treatment; in children, height and weight should be recorded before treatment initiation, and height, weight and appetite monitored at least every 6 months during treatment.

● TREATMENT CESSATION Avoid abrupt withdrawal.

● DIRECTIONS FOR ADMINISTRATION Manufacturer advises swallow whole or mix contents of capsule with soft food such as yoghurt or in a glass of water or orange juice; contents should be dispersed completely and consumed immediately.

● PATIENT AND CARER ADVICE Patients and carers should be counselled on the administration of capsules.
Driving and skilled tasks
Drugs and Driving Prescribers and other healthcare professionals should advise patients if treatment is likely to affect their ability to perform skilled tasks (e.g. driving). This applies especially to drugs with sedative effects; patients should be warned that these effects are increased by alcohol. General information about a patient's fitness to drive is available from the Driver and Vehicle Licensing Agency at www.dvla.gov.uk.

For information on 2015 legislation regarding driving whilst taking certain controlled drugs, including amfetamines, see *Drugs and driving* under Guidance on prescribing p. 1.

● NATIONAL FUNDING/ACCESS DECISIONS

Scottish Medicines Consortium (SMC) Decisions
The *Scottish Medicines Consortium* has advised (May 2013) that lisdexamfetamine dimesylate (*Elvanse* ®) is accepted for use within NHS Scotland as part of a comprehensive treatment programme for attention deficit hyperactivity disorder (ADHD) in children aged 6 years and over when response to previous methylphenidate treatment is considered clinically inadequate.

The *Scottish Medicines Consortium* has advised (September 2015) that lisdexamfetamine dimesylate (*Elvanse Adult* ®) is accepted for use within NHS Scotland as part of a comprehensive treatment programme for attention deficit hyperactivity disorder (ADHD) in adults. Based on clinical judgment, patients should have ADHD of at least moderate severity.

All Wales Medicines Strategy Group (AWMSG) Decisions
The *All Wales Medicines Strategy Group* has advised (December 2013) that lisdexamfetamine dimesylate (*Elvanse* ®) is recommended as an option for use within NHS Wales as part of a comprehensive treatment programme for attention deficit hyperactivity disorder (ADHD) in children aged six years and over when response to previous methylphenidate treatment is considered clinically inadequate. Treatment must be under the supervision of a specialist in childhood and/or adolescent behavioural disorders.

The *All Wales Medicines Strategy Group* has advised (October 2015) that lisdexamfetamine dimesylate (*Elvanse Adult* ®) is recommended as an option for use within NHS Wales as part of a comprehensive treatment programme for attention deficit hyperactivity disorder (ADHD) in adults.

● MEDICINAL FORMS
There can be variation in the licensing of different medicines containing the same drug.
Capsule
CAUTIONARY AND ADVISORY LABELS 3, 25
▸ Elvanse (Shire Pharmaceuticals Ltd) ▼
Lisdexamfetamine dimesylate 20 mg Elvanse 20mg capsules | 28 capsule [PoM] £54.62 DT = £54.62 [CD2]
Lisdexamfetamine dimesylate 30 mg Elvanse Adult 30mg capsules | 28 capsule [PoM] £58.24 DT = £58.24 [CD2]
Elvanse 30mg capsules | 28 capsule [PoM] £58.24 DT = £58.24 [CD2]

Lisdexamfetamine dimesylate 40 mg Elvanse 40mg capsules | 28 capsule [PoM] £62.82 DT = £62.82 [CD2]
Lisdexamfetamine dimesylate 50 mg Elvanse Adult 50mg capsules | 28 capsule [PoM] £68.60 DT = £68.60 [CD2]
Elvanse 50mg capsules | 28 capsule [PoM] £68.60 DT = £68.60 [CD2]
Lisdexamfetamine dimesylate 60 mg Elvanse 60mg capsules | 28 capsule [PoM] £75.18 DT = £75.18 [CD2]
Lisdexamfetamine dimesylate 70 mg Elvanse 70mg capsules | 28 capsule [PoM] £83.16 DT = £83.16 [CD2]
Elvanse Adult 70mg capsules | 28 capsule [PoM] £83.16 DT = £83.16 [CD2]

SYMPATHOMIMETICS ⟩ ALPHA₂-ADRENOCEPTOR AGONISTS

Guanfacine
26-May-2016

● INDICATIONS AND DOSE

Attention deficit hyperactivity disorder in children for whom stimulants are not suitable, not tolerated or ineffective (initiated under specialist supervision)
▸ BY MOUTH
  ▸ Child 6–12 years (body-weight 25 kg and above): Initially 1 mg once daily; adjusted in steps of 1 mg every week if necessary and if tolerated; maintenance 0.05–0.12 mg/kg once daily (max. per dose 4 mg), for optimal weight-adjusted dose titrations, consult product literature
  ▸ Child 13–17 years (body-weight 34–41.4 kg): Initially 1 mg once daily; adjusted in steps of 1 mg every week if necessary and if tolerated; maintenance 0.05–0.12 mg/kg once daily (max. per dose 4 mg), for optimal weight-adjusted dose titrations, consult product literature
  ▸ Child 13–17 years (body-weight 41.5–49.4 kg): Initially 1 mg once daily; adjusted in steps of 1 mg every week if necessary and if tolerated; maintenance 0.05–0.12 mg/kg once daily (max. per dose 5 mg), for optimal weight-adjusted dose titrations, consult product literature
  ▸ Child 13–17 years (body-weight 49.5–58.4 kg): Initially 1 mg once daily; adjusted in steps of 1 mg every week if necessary and if tolerated; maintenance 0.05–0.12 mg/kg once daily (max. per dose 6 mg), for optimal weight-adjusted dose titrations, consult product literature
  ▸ Child 13–17 years (body-weight 58.5 kg and above): Initially 1 mg once daily; adjusted in steps of 1 mg every week if necessary and if tolerated; maintenance 0.05–0.12 mg/kg once daily (max. per dose 7 mg), for optimal weight-adjusted dose titrations, consult product literature

DOSE ADJUSTMENTS DUE TO INTERACTIONS
▸ Manufacturer advises reduce dose by half with concurrent use of moderate and potent inhibitors of CYP3A4.
▸ Manufacturer advises increase dose up to max. 7 mg daily with concurrent use of potent inducers of CYP3A4—no specific recommendation made for children.

● CAUTIONS Bradycardia (risk of torsade de pointes) · heart block (risk of torsade de pointes) · history of cardiovascular disease · history of QT-interval prolongation · hypokalaemia (risk of torsade de pointes)

● INTERACTIONS → Appendix 1: guanfacine

● SIDE-EFFECTS
▸ **Common or very common** Anxiety · appetite decreased · arrhythmias · asthenia · constipation · depression · diarrhoea · dizziness · drowsiness · dry mouth · gastrointestinal discomfort · headache · hypotension · mood altered · nausea · skin reactions · sleep disorders · urinary disorders · vomiting · weight increased

▶ **Uncommon** Asthma · atrioventricular block · chest pain · hallucination · loss of consciousness · pallor · seizure · syncope

▶ **Rare or very rare** Hypertension · hypertensive encephalopathy · malaise

▶ **Frequency not known** Erectile dysfunction

SIDE-EFFECTS, FURTHER INFORMATION Somnolence and sedation may occur, predominantly during the first 2-3 weeks of treatment and with dose increases; manufacturer advises to consider dose reduction or discontinuation of treatment if symptoms are clinically significant or persistent.

Overdose Features may include hypotension, initial hypertension, bradycardia, lethargy, and respiratory depression. Manufacturer advises that patients who develop lethargy should be observed for development of more serious toxicity for up to 24 hours.

● CONCEPTION AND CONTRACEPTION Manufacturer recommends effective contraception in females of childbearing potential.

● PREGNANCY Manufacturer advises avoid—toxicity in *animal* studies.

● BREAST FEEDING Manufacturer advises avoid—present in milk in *animal* studies.

● HEPATIC IMPAIRMENT
Dose adjustments Manufacturer advises consider dose reduction.

● RENAL IMPAIRMENT
Dose adjustments Manufacturer advises consider dose reduction in severe impairment and end-stage renal disease.

● MONITORING REQUIREMENTS

▶ Manufacturer advises to conduct a baseline evaluation to identify patients at risk of somnolence, sedation, hypotension, bradycardia, QT-prolongation, and arrhythmia; this should include assessment of cardiovascular status. Monitor for signs of these adverse effects weekly during dose titration and then every 3 months during the first year of treatment, and every 6 months thereafter. Monitor BMI prior to treatment and then every 3 months for the first year of treatment, and every 6 months thereafter. More frequent monitoring is advised following dose adjustments.

▶ Monitor blood pressure and pulse during dose downward titration and following discontinuation of treatment.

● TREATMENT CESSATION Manufacturer advises avoid abrupt withdrawal; consider dose tapering to minimise potential withdrawal effects.

● DIRECTIONS FOR ADMINISTRATION Manufacturer advises avoid administration with high fat meals (may increase absorption).

● PATIENT AND CARER ADVICE Patients or carers should be counselled on administration of guanfacine modified-release tablets.
Missed doses Manufacturer advises that patients and carers should inform their prescriber if more than one dose is missed; consider dose re-titration.
Driving and skilled tasks Manufacturer advises patients and carers should be counselled about the effects on driving and performance of skilled tasks—increased risk of dizziness and syncope.

● MEDICINAL FORMS
There can be variation in the licensing of different medicines containing the same drug.
Modified-release tablet
CAUTIONARY AND ADVISORY LABELS 2, 25
▶ Intuniv (Shire Pharmaceuticals Ltd) ▼
Guanfacine (as Guanfacine hydrochloride) 1 mg Intuniv 1mg modified-release tablets | 28 tablet [PoM] £56.00

Guanfacine (as Guanfacine hydrochloride) 2 mg Intuniv 2mg modified-release tablets | 28 tablet [PoM] £58.52
Guanfacine (as Guanfacine hydrochloride) 3 mg Intuniv 3mg modified-release tablets | 28 tablet [PoM] £65.52
Guanfacine (as Guanfacine hydrochloride) 4 mg Intuniv 4mg modified-release tablets | 28 tablet [PoM] £76.16

3.3 Bipolar disorder and mania

Mania and hypomania
08-Jun-2018

Overview
Antimanic drugs are used to control acute attacks and to prevent recurrence of episodes of mania or hypomania. Long-term treatment of bipolar disorder should continue for at least two years from the last manic episode and up to five years if the patient has risk factors for relapse.

An antidepressant drug may also be required for the treatment of co-existing depression, but should be avoided in patients with rapid-cycling bipolar disorder, a recent history of hypomania, or with rapid mood fluctuations.

Benzodiazepines
Use of benzodiazepines (such as lorazepam p. 335) may be helpful in the initial stages of treatment for behavioural disturbance or agitation; they should not be used for long periods because of the risk of dependence.

Antipsychotic drugs
Antipsychotic drugs (normally olanzapine p. 394, quetiapine p. 397, or risperidone p. 398) are useful in acute episodes of mania and hypomania; if the response to antipsychotic drugs is inadequate, lithium or valproate may be added. An antipsychotic drug may be used concomitantly with lithium or valproate in the initial treatment of severe acute mania. See *Important safety information*, *Conception and contraception*, and *Pregnancy* in the valproic acid p. 351 and sodium valproate p. 325 monographs.

Olanzapine can be used for the long-term management of bipolar disorder in patients whose manic episode responded to olanzapine therapy. It can be given either as monotherapy, or in combination with lithium or valproate if the patient has frequent relapses or continuing functional impairment.

Asenapine p. 352, a second-generation antipsychotic, is licensed for the treatment of moderate to severe manic episodes associated with bipolar disorder.

When discontinuing antipsychotics, the dose should be reduced gradually over at least 4 weeks if the patient is continuing with other antimanic drugs; if the patient is not continuing with other antimanic drugs or if there is a history of manic relapse, a withdrawal period of up to 3 months should be considered.

Carbamazepine
Carbamazepine p. 309 may be used under specialist supervision for the prophylaxis of bipolar disorder (manic-depressive disorder) in patients unresponsive to a combination of other prophylactic drugs; it is used in patients with rapid-cycling manic-depressive illness (4 or more affective episodes per year). The dose of carbamazepine should not normally be increased if an acute episode of mania occurs.

Valproate
Valproate (valproic acid (as the semisodium salt) and sodium valproate) is used for the treatment of manic episodes associated with bipolar disorder. It must be started and supervised by a specialist experienced in managing bipolar disorder. Valproate (valproic acid and sodium valproate) is also used for the prophylaxis of bipolar disorder. Because of its high teratogenic risk, valproate must not be used in females of childbearing potential unless the conditions of

the Pregnancy Prevention Programme are met and alternative treatments are ineffective or not tolerated. Valproic acid and sodium valproate must not be used during pregnancy in bipolar disorder. The benefit and risk of valproate therapy should be carefully reconsidered at regular treatment reviews. For further information, see *Important safety information*, *Conception and contraception*, and *Pregnancy* in the valproic acid and sodium valproate monographs.

In patients with frequent relapse or continuing functional impairment, consider switching therapy to lithium or olanzapine, or adding lithium or olanzapine to valproate. If a patient taking valproate experiences an acute episode of mania that is not ameliorated by increasing the valproate dose, consider concomitant therapy with olanzapine, quetiapine, or risperidone.

Lithium

Lithium salts are used in the prophylaxis and treatment of mania, hypomania and depression in bipolar disorder (manic-depressive disorder), and in the prophylaxis and treatment of recurrent unipolar depression. Lithium is also used as concomitant therapy with antidepressant medication in patients who have had an incomplete response to treatment for acute bipolar depression and to augment other antidepressants in patients with treatment-resistant depression [unlicensed indication]. It is also licensed for the treatment of aggressive or self-harming behaviour.

The decision to give prophylactic lithium requires specialist advice, and must be based on careful consideration of the likelihood of recurrence in the individual patient, and the benefit of treatment weighed against the risks. The full prophylactic effect of lithium may not occur for six to twelve months after the initiation of therapy. Olanzapine or valproate (given alone or as adjunctive therapy with lithium) are alternative prophylactic treatments in patients who experience frequent relapses or continued functional impairment.

Other drugs used for Bipolar disorder and mania
Aripiprazole, p. 391 · Chlorpromazine hydrochloride, p. 381 · Haloperidol, p. 382 · Lamotrigine, p. 316 · Paliperidone, p. 395 · Perphenazine, p. 384 · Prochlorperazine, p. 385 · Zuclopenthixol acetate, p. 387

ANTIEPILEPTICS

Valproic acid
24-Apr-2018

● INDICATIONS AND DOSE

Treatment of manic episodes associated with bipolar disorder

▶ BY MOUTH
▶ Adult: Initially 750 mg daily in 2–3 divided doses, then increased to 1–2 g daily, adjusted according to response, doses greater than 45 mg/kg daily require careful monitoring

Migraine prophylaxis

▶ BY MOUTH
▶ Adult: Initially 250 mg twice daily, then increased if necessary to 1 g daily in divided doses

DOSE EQUIVALENCE AND CONVERSION
▶ Semisodium valproate comprises equimolar amounts of sodium valproate and valproic acid.

CONVULEX ®

Epilepsy

▶ BY MOUTH
▶ Adult: Initially 600 mg daily in 2–4 divided doses, increased in steps of 150–300 mg every 3 days; usual maintenance 1–2 g daily in 2–4 divided doses, max. 2.5 g daily in 2–4 divided doses

DOSE EQUIVALENCE AND CONVERSION
▶ *Convulex*® has a 1:1 dose relationship with products containing sodium valproate, but nevertheless care is needed if switching or making changes.

● UNLICENSED USE Not licensed for migraine prophylaxis.

IMPORTANT SAFETY INFORMATION
MHRA/CHM ADVICE: VALPROATE MEDICINES: CONTRA-INDICATED IN WOMEN AND GIRLS OF CHILDBEARING POTENTIAL UNLESS CONDITIONS OF PREGNANCY PREVENTION PROGRAMME ARE MET (APRIL 2018)

Valproate is highly teratogenic and evidence supports that use in pregnancy leads to neurodevelopmental disorders (approx. 30–40% risk) and congenital malformations (approx. 10% risk).

Valproate must not be used in women and girls of childbearing potential unless the conditions of the Pregnancy Prevention Programme are met (see *Conception and contraception*) and only if other treatments are ineffective or not tolerated, as judged by an experienced specialist.

Use of valproate in pregnancy is contra-indicated for migraine prophylaxis [unlicensed] and bipolar disorder; it must only be considered for epilepsy if there is no suitable alternative treatment (see *Pregnancy*).

Women and girls (and their carers) must be fully informed of the risks and the need to avoid exposure to valproate medicines in pregnancy; supporting materials have been provided to use in the implementation of the Pregnancy Prevention Programme (see *Prescribing and dispensing information*). The MHRA advises that:

● GPs must recall all women and girls who may be of childbearing potential, provide the Patient Guide, check they have been reviewed by a specialist in the last year and are on highly effective contraception;

● Specialists must book in review appointments at least annually with women and girls under the Pregnancy Prevention Programme, re-evaluate treatment as necessary, explain clearly the conditions as outlined in the supporting materials and complete and sign the Risk Acknowledgement Form—copies of the form must be given to the patient or carer and sent to their GP;

● Pharmacists must ensure valproate medicines are dispensed in whole packs whenever possible—all packs dispensed to women and girls of childbearing potential should have a warning label either on the carton or via a sticker. They must also discuss risks in pregnancy with female patients each time valproate medicines are dispensed, ensure they have the Patient Guide and have seen their GP or specialist to discuss their treatment and the need for contraception.

● CONTRA-INDICATIONS Acute porphyrias p. 1025 · known or suspected mitochondrial disorders (higher rate of acute liver failure and liver-related deaths) · personal or family history of severe hepatic dysfunction

● CAUTIONS Systemic lupus erythematosus
CAUTIONS, FURTHER INFORMATION
▶ Liver toxicity Liver dysfunction (including fatal hepatic failure) has occurred in association with valproate (especially in children under 3 years and in those with metabolic or degenerative disorders, organic brain disease or severe seizure disorders associated with mental retardation) usually in first 6 months and usually involving multiple antiepileptic therapy. Raised liver enzymes during valproate treatment are usually transient but patients should be reassessed clinically and liver function (including prothrombin time) monitored until return to normal—discontinue if abnormally prolonged prothrombin time (particularly in association with other relevant abnormalities).

Consider vitamin D supplementation in patients who are immobilised for long periods or who have inadequate sun exposure or dietary intake of calcium.

● INTERACTIONS → Appendix 1: antiepileptics

● SIDE-EFFECTS Abdominal pain · alertness increased · alopecia (regrowth may be curly) · anaemia · behaviour abnormal · bone disorders · bone fracture · cerebral atrophy · coma · confusion · consciousness impaired · dementia · diarrhoea · drowsiness · encephalopathy · fine postural tremor · gastrointestinal disorder · gynaecomastia · haemorrhage · hallucination · hearing loss · hepatic disorders · hirsutism · hyperammonaemia · leucopenia · menstrual cycle irregularities · movement disorders · nail disorder · nausea · obesity · pancreatitis · pancytopenia · parkinsonism · peripheral oedema · seizure · severe cutaneous adverse reactions (SCARs) · skin reactions · thrombocytopenia · urine abnormalities · vasculitis · vomiting · weight increased

SIDE-EFFECTS, FURTHER INFORMATION

Hepatic dysfunction Withdraw treatment immediately if persistent vomiting and abdominal pain, anorexia, jaundice, oedema, malaise, drowsiness, or loss of seizure control.

Pancreatitis Discontinue treatment if symptoms of pancreatitis develop.

● CONCEPTION AND CONTRACEPTION The MHRA advises that all women and girls of childbearing potential being treated with valproate medicines must be supported on a Pregnancy Prevention Programme—pregnancy should be excluded before treatment initiation and highly effective contraception must be used during treatment.

● PREGNANCY For *migraine prophylaxis* [unlicensed] and *bipolar disorder*, the MHRA advises that valproate must not be used. For *epilepsy*, the MHRA advises valproate must not be used unless there is no suitable alternative treatment; in such cases, access to counselling about the risks should be provided (see Healthcare Professional Guide for more information) and a Risk Acknowledgement Form signed by both specialist and patient. If valproate is to be used during pregnancy, the lowest effective dose should be prescribed in divided doses to avoid peaks in plasma-valproate concentrations; doses greater than 1 g daily are associated with an increased risk of teratogenicity. Neonatal bleeding (related to hypofibrinaemia). Neonatal hepatotoxicity also reported. **Monitoring** Specialist prenatal monitoring should be instigated when valproate has been taken in pregnancy.

The dose should be monitored carefully during pregnancy and after birth, and adjustments made on a clinical basis.

● BREAST FEEDING Present in milk—risk of haematological disorders in breast-fed newborns and infants.

● HEPATIC IMPAIRMENT Avoid if possible—hepatotoxicity and hepatic failure may occasionally occur (usually in first 6 months). Avoid in active liver disease.

● RENAL IMPAIRMENT
Dose adjustments Reduce dose.

● MONITORING REQUIREMENTS
▶ Monitor closely if dose greater than 45 mg/kg daily.
▶ Monitor liver function before therapy and during first 6 months especially in patients most at risk.
▶ Measure full blood count and ensure no undue potential for bleeding before starting and before surgery.

● EFFECT ON LABORATORY TESTS False-positive urine tests for ketones.

● TREATMENT CESSATION [EvGr] In bipolar disorder, avoid abrupt withdrawal; if treatment with valproate is stopped, reduce the dose gradually over at least 4 weeks. Ⓐ

● PRESCRIBING AND DISPENSING INFORMATION The Pregnancy Prevention Programme is supported by the

following materials provided by the manufacturer: *Patient Guide*, *Guide for Healthcare Professionals*, *Risk Acknowledgement Form*, and for pharmacists, *Patient Cards* and *Stickers with warning symbols*; the MHRA has also produced a patient information sheet providing advice for women and girls taking valproate medicines.

CONVULEX ® Patients being treated for epilepsy may need to be maintained on a specific manufacturer's branded or generic oral valproic acid product.

● PATIENT AND CARER ADVICE
Valproate use by women and girls The MHRA advises women and girls should **not** stop taking valproate without first discussing it with their doctor.
Blood or hepatic disorders Patients or their carers should be told how to recognise signs and symptoms of blood or liver disorders and advised to seek immediate medical attention if symptoms develop.
Pancreatitis Patients or their carers should be told how to recognise signs and symptoms of pancreatitis and advised to seek immediate medical attention if symptoms such as abdominal pain, nausea, or vomiting develop.
Pregnancy Prevention Programme Pharmacists must ensure that female patients have a patient card—see also *Important safety information*.

● MEDICINAL FORMS
There can be variation in the licensing of different medicines containing the same drug. Forms available from special-order manufacturers include: oral suspension, oral solution

Gastro-resistant capsule
CAUTIONARY AND ADVISORY LABELS 8, 10, 21, 25
▶ Convulex (Pfizer Ltd) ▼
Valproic acid 150 mg Convulex 150mg gastro-resistant capsules | 100 capsule [PoM] £3.68
Valproic acid 300 mg Convulex 300mg gastro-resistant capsules | 100 capsule [PoM] £7.35
Valproic acid 500 mg Convulex 500mg gastro-resistant capsules | 100 capsule [PoM] £12.25

Gastro-resistant tablet
CAUTIONARY AND ADVISORY LABELS 10, 21, 25
▶ Depakote (Sanofi) ▼
Valproic acid (as Valproate semisodium) 250 mg Depakote 250mg gastro-resistant tablets | 90 tablet [PoM] £17.08 DT = £17.08
Valproic acid (as Valproate semisodium) 500 mg Depakote 500mg gastro-resistant tablets | 90 tablet [PoM] £34.11 DT = £34.11

ANTIPSYCHOTICS > SECOND-GENERATION

⬛ 380

Asenapine

● INDICATIONS AND DOSE

Monotherapy for the treatment of moderate to severe manic episodes associated with bipolar disorder
▶ BY MOUTH
▶ Adult: Initially 10 mg twice daily, reduced to 5 mg twice daily, adjusted according to response

Combination therapy for the treatment of moderate to severe manic episodes associated with bipolar disorder
▶ BY MOUTH
▶ Adult: Initially 5 mg twice daily, increased if necessary to 10 mg twice daily, adjusted according to response

● CAUTIONS Dementia with Lewy Bodies
● INTERACTIONS → Appendix 1: asenapine
● SIDE-EFFECTS
▶ Common or very common Anxiety · appetite increased · fatigue · muscle rigidity · nausea · oral disorders · sedation · taste altered
▶ Uncommon Arrhythmias · bundle branch block · dysarthria · dysphagia · movement disorders · postural hypotension · sexual dysfunction · syncope
▶ Rare or very rare Accommodation disorder · rhabdomyolysis

- PREGNANCY Use only if potential benefit outweighs risk—toxicity in *animal* studies.
- BREAST FEEDING Avoid—no information available.
- HEPATIC IMPAIRMENT Use with caution in moderate impairment. Avoid in severe impairment.
- RENAL IMPAIRMENT Use with caution if eGFR less than 15 mL/minute/1.73 m² — no information available.
- PATIENT AND CARER ADVICE Patient or carer should be given advice on how to administer asenapine sublingual tablet.

- MEDICINAL FORMS
There can be variation in the licensing of different medicines containing the same drug.
Sublingual tablet
CAUTIONARY AND ADVISORY LABELS 2, 26
▸ Sycrest (Lundbeck Ltd)
Asenapine (as Asenapine maleate) 5 mg Sycrest 5mg sublingual tablets sugar-free | 60 tablet [PoM] £102.60 DT = £102.60
Asenapine (as Asenapine maleate) 10 mg Sycrest 10mg sublingual tablets sugar-free | 60 tablet [PoM] £102.60 DT = £102.60

ANTIPSYCHOTICS › LITHIUM SALTS

Lithium salts

- CONTRA-INDICATIONS Addison's disease · cardiac insufficiency · dehydration · family history of Brugada syndrome · low sodium diets · personal history of Brugada syndrome · rhythm disorder · untreated hypothyroidism
- CAUTIONS Avoid abrupt withdrawal · cardiac disease · concurrent ECT (may lower seizure threshold) · diuretic treatment (risk of toxicity) · elderly (reduce dose) · epilepsy (may lower seizure threshold) · myasthenia gravis · psoriasis (risk of exacerbation) · QT interval prolongation · review dose as necessary in diarrhoea · review dose as necessary in intercurrent infection (especially if sweating profusely) · review dose as necessary in vomiting · surgery
CAUTIONS, FURTHER INFORMATION
▸ Long-term use Long-term use of lithium has been associated with thyroid disorders and mild cognitive and memory impairment. Long-term treatment should therefore be undertaken only with careful assessment of risk and benefit, and with monitoring of thyroid function every 6 months (more often if there is evidence of deterioration).
The need for continued therapy should be assessed regularly and patients should be maintained on lithium after 3–5 years only if benefit persists.

- SIDE-EFFECTS
▸ Rare or very rare Nephropathy
▸ Frequency not known Abdominal discomfort · alopecia · angioedema · appetite decreased · arrhythmias · atrioventricular block · cardiomyopathy · cerebellar syndrome · circulatory collapse · coma · delirium · diarrhoea · dizziness · dry mouth · electrolyte imbalance · encephalopathy · folliculitis · gastritis · goitre · hyperglycaemia · hyperparathyroidism · hypersalivation · hypotension · hypothyroidism · idiopathic intracranial hypertension · leucocytosis · memory loss · movement disorders · muscle weakness · myasthenia gravis · nausea · neoplasms · nystagmus · peripheral neuropathy · peripheral oedema · polydipsia · polyuria · QT interval prolongation · reflexes abnormal · renal disorders · renal impairment · rhabdomyolysis · seizure · sexual dysfunction · skin reactions · skin ulcer · speech impairment · taste altered · thyrotoxicosis · tremor · vertigo · vision disorders · vomiting · weight increased

Overdose Signs of intoxication require withdrawal of treatment and include increasing gastro-intestinal disturbances (vomiting, diarrhoea), visual disturbances, polyuria, muscle weakness, fine tremor increasing to coarse tremor, CNS disturbances (confusion and drowsiness increasing to lack of coordination, restlessness, stupor); abnormal reflexes, myoclonus, incontinence, hypernatraemia. With severe overdosage serious, cardiac arrhythmias (including sino-atrial block, bradycardia and first-degree heart block), blood pressure changes, circulatory failure, renal failure, coma and sudden death reported.
For details on the management of poisoning, see Lithium, under Emergency treatment of poisoning p. 1319.

- CONCEPTION AND CONTRACEPTION Manufacturer advises effective contraception during treatment for women of child bearing potential.
- PREGNANCY Avoid if possible, particularly in the first trimester (risk of teratogenicity, including cardiac abnormalities).
Dose adjustments Dose requirements increased during the second and third trimesters (but on delivery return abruptly to normal).
Monitoring Close monitoring of serum-lithium concentration advised in pregnancy (risk of toxicity in neonate).
- BREAST FEEDING Present in milk and risk of toxicity in infant—avoid.
- RENAL IMPAIRMENT Caution in mild to moderate impairment. Avoid in severe impairment.
Monitoring In renal impairment monitor serum-lithium concentration closely and adjust dose accordingly.
- MONITORING REQUIREMENTS
▸ Serum concentrations Lithium salts have a narrow therapeutic/toxic ratio and should therefore not be prescribed unless facilities for monitoring serum-lithium concentrations are available.
Samples should be taken 12 hours after the dose to achieve a serum-lithium concentration of 0.4–1 mmol/litre (lower end of the range for maintenance therapy and elderly patients).
A target serum-lithium concentration of 0.8–1 mmol/litre is recommended for acute episodes of mania, and for patients who have previously relapsed or have sub-syndromal symptoms. It is important to determine the optimum range for each individual patient.
Routine serum-lithium monitoring should be performed weekly after initiation and after each dose change until concentrations are stable, then every 3 months thereafter. Additional serum-lithium measurements should be made if a patient develops significant intercurrent disease or if there is a significant change in a patient's sodium or fluid intake.
▸ Manufacturer advises to assess renal, cardiac, and thyroid function before treatment initiation. [EvGr] An ECG is recommended in patients with cardiovascular disease or risk factors for it. Body-weight or BMI, serum electrolytes, and a full blood count should also be measured before treatment initiation.
▸ Monitor body-weight or BMI, serum electrolytes, eGFR, and thyroid function every 6 months during treatment, and more often if there is evidence of impaired renal or thyroid function, or raised calcium levels. Ⓐ
Manufacturer also advises to monitor cardiac function regularly.
- TREATMENT CESSATION While there is no clear evidence of withdrawal or rebound psychosis, abrupt discontinuation of lithium increases the risk of relapse. If lithium is to be discontinued, the dose should be reduced gradually over a period of at least 4 weeks (preferably over a period of up to 3 months). Patients and their carers should be warned of the risk of relapse if lithium is discontinued abruptly. If lithium is stopped or is to be discontinued abruptly,

consider changing therapy to an atypical antipsychotic or valproate.

- PATIENT AND CARER ADVICE Patients should be advised to report signs and symptoms of lithium toxicity, hypothyroidism, renal dysfunction (including polyuria and polydipsia), and benign intracranial hypertension (persistent headache and visual disturbance). Maintain adequate fluid intake and avoid dietary changes which reduce or increase sodium intake.

Lithium treatment packs A lithium treatment pack should be given to patients on initiation of treatment with lithium. The pack consists of a patient information booklet, lithium alert card, and a record book for tracking serum-lithium concentration. Packs may be purchased from
3M
0845 610 1112
nhsforms@mmm.uk.com
Driving and skilled tasks May impair performance of skilled tasks (e.g. driving, operating machinery).

F 353

Lithium carbonate

- INDICATIONS AND DOSE

Treatment and prophylaxis of mania | Treatment and prophylaxis of bipolar disorder | Treatment and prophylaxis of recurrent depression | Treatment and prophylaxis of aggressive or self-harming behaviour
- BY MOUTH
- Adult: Dose adjusted according to serum-lithium concentration, doses are initially divided throughout the day, but once daily administration is preferred when serum-lithium concentration stabilised

DOSE EQUIVALENCE AND CONVERSION
- **Preparations vary widely in bioavailability;** changing the preparation requires the same precautions as initiation of treatment.

CAMCOLIT® IMMEDIATE-RELEASE TABLET

Treatment of mania | Treatment of bipolar disorder | Treatment of recurrent depression | Treatment of aggressive or self-harming behaviour
- BY MOUTH
- Adult: Initially 1–1.5 g daily, dose adjusted according to serum-lithium concentration, doses are initially divided throughout the day, but once daily administration is preferred when serum-lithium concentration stabilised
- Elderly: Reduce initial dose, dose adjusted according to serum-lithium concentration, doses are initially divided throughout the day, but once daily administration is preferred when serum-lithium concentration stabilised

Prophylaxis of mania | Prophylaxis of bipolar disorder | Prophylaxis of recurrent depression | Prophylaxis of aggressive or self-harming behaviour
- BY MOUTH
- Adult: Initially 300–400 mg daily, dose adjusted according to serum-lithium concentration, doses are initially divided throughout the day, but once daily administration is preferred when serum-lithium concentration stabilised

CAMCOLIT® MODIFIED-RELEASE TABLET

Treatment of mania | Treatment of bipolar disorder | Treatment of recurrent depression | Treatment of aggressive or self-harming behaviour
- BY MOUTH
- Adult: Initially 1–1.5 g daily, dose adjusted according to serum-lithium concentration, doses are initially divided throughout the day, but once daily

administration is preferred when serum-lithium concentration stabilised
- Elderly: Reduce initial dose, dose adjusted according to serum-lithium concentration, doses are initially divided throughout the day, but once daily administration is preferred when serum-lithium concentration stabilised

Prophylaxis of mania | Prophylaxis of bipolar disorder | Prophylaxis of recurrent depression | Prophylaxis of aggressive or self-harming behaviour
- BY MOUTH
- Adult: Initially 300–400 mg daily, dose adjusted according to serum-lithium concentration, doses are initially divided throughout the day, but once daily administration is preferred when serum-lithium concentration stabilised

LISKONUM®

Treatment of mania | Treatment of bipolar disorder | Treatment of recurrent depression | Treatment of aggressive or self-harming behaviour
- BY MOUTH
- Adult: Initially 450–675 mg twice daily, dose adjusted according to serum-lithium concentration, doses are initially divided throughout the day, but once daily administration is preferred when serum-lithium concentration stabilised
- Elderly: Initially 225 mg twice daily, dose adjusted according to serum-lithium concentration, doses are initially divided throughout the day, but once daily administration is preferred when serum-lithium concentration stabilised

Prophylaxis of mania | Prophylaxis of bipolar disorder | Prophylaxis of recurrent depression | Prophylaxis of aggressive or self-harming behaviour
- BY MOUTH
- Adult: Initially 450 mg twice daily, dose adjusted according serum-lithium concentration, doses are initially divided throughout the day, but once daily administration is preferred when serum-lithium concentration stabilised
- Elderly: Initially 225 mg twice daily, dose adjusted according to serum-lithium concentration, doses are initially divided throughout the day, but once daily administration is preferred when serum-lithium concentration stabilised

PRIADEL® TABLETS

Treatment and prophylaxis of mania | Treatment and prophylaxis of bipolar disorder | Treatment and prophylaxis of recurrent depression | Treatment and prophylaxis of aggressive or self-harming behaviour
- BY MOUTH
- Adult (body-weight up to 50 kg): Initially 200–400 mg daily, dose adjusted according to serum-lithium concentration, doses are initially divided throughout the day, but once daily administration is preferred when serum-lithium concentration stabilised
- Adult (body-weight 50 kg and above): Initially 0.4–1.2 g once daily, alternatively initially 0.4–1.2 g daily in 2 divided doses, dose adjusted according to serum-lithium concentration, doses are initially divided throughout the day, but once daily administration is preferred when serum-lithium concentration stabilised
- Elderly: Initially 200–400 mg daily, dose adjusted according to serum-lithium concentration, doses are initially divided throughout the day, but once daily administration is preferred when serum-lithium concentration stabilised

- INTERACTIONS → Appendix 1: lithium

- MEDICINAL FORMS
There can be variation in the licensing of different medicines containing the same drug. Forms available from special-order manufacturers include: oral suspension

Modified-release tablet

CAUTIONARY AND ADVISORY LABELS 10, 25
- Lithium carbonate (Non-proprietary)
  Lithium carbonate 400 mg Lithium carbonate 400mg modified-release tablets | 100 tablet [PoM] [℥] DT = £4.02
- Camcolit (Essential Pharma Ltd)
  Lithium carbonate 400 mg Camcolit 400 modified-release tablets | 100 tablet [PoM] £48.18 DT = £4.02
- Liskonum (Teofarma)
  Lithium carbonate 450 mg Liskonum 450mg modified-release tablets | 60 tablet [PoM] £11.84 DT = £11.84
- Priadel (lithium carbonate) (Sanofi)
  Lithium carbonate 200 mg Priadel 200mg modified-release tablets | 100 tablet [PoM] £2.76 DT = £2.76
  Lithium carbonate 400 mg Priadel 400mg modified-release tablets | 100 tablet [PoM] £4.02 DT = £4.02

Tablet

CAUTIONARY AND ADVISORY LABELS 10
- Lithium carbonate (Non-proprietary)
  Lithium carbonate 250 mg Lithium carbonate 250mg tablets | 100 tablet [PoM] £87.00 DT = £87.00

☞ 353

Lithium citrate

- INDICATIONS AND DOSE

Treatment and prophylaxis of mania | Treatment and prophylaxis of bipolar disorder | Treatment and prophylaxis of recurrent depression | Treatment and prophylaxis of aggressive or self-harming behaviour
▸ BY MOUTH
- Adult: Dose adjusted according to serum-lithium concentration; doses are initially divided throughout the day, but once daily administration is preferred when serum-lithium concentration stabilised

DOSE EQUIVALENCE AND CONVERSION
▸ **Preparations vary widely in bioavailability**; changing the preparation requires the same precautions as initiation of treatment.

LI-LIQUID ®

Treatment and prophylaxis of mania | Treatment and prophylaxis of bipolar disorder | Treatment and prophylaxis of recurrent depression | Treatment and prophylaxis of aggressive or self-harming behaviour
▸ BY MOUTH
- Adult (body-weight up to 50 kg): Initially 509 mg daily in 2 divided doses, dose adjusted according to serum-lithium concentration
- Adult (body-weight 50 kg and above): Initially 1.018–3.054 g daily in 2 divided doses, dose adjusted according to serum-lithium concentration
- Elderly: Initially 509 mg daily in 2 divided doses, dose adjusted according to serum-lithium concentration

DOSE EQUIVALENCE AND CONVERSION
▸ For *Li-Liquid* ®: Lithium citrate tetrahydrate 509 mg is equivalent to lithium carbonate 200 mg.

PRIADEL ® LIQUID

Treatment and prophylaxis of mania | Treatment and prophylaxis of bipolar disorder | Treatment and prophylaxis of recurrent depression | Treatment and prophylaxis of aggressive or self-harming behaviour
▸ BY MOUTH
- Adult (body-weight up to 50 kg): Initially 520 mg twice daily, dose adjusted according to serum-lithium concentration, doses are initially divided throughout the day, but once daily administration is preferred when serum-lithium concentration stabilised

- Adult (body-weight 50 kg and above): Initially 1.04–3.12 g daily in 2 divided doses, dose adjusted according to serum-lithium concentration, doses are initially divided throughout the day, but once daily administration is preferred when serum-lithium concentration stabilised
- Elderly: Initially 520 mg twice daily, dose adjusted according to serum-lithium concentration, doses are initially divided throughout the day, but once daily administration is preferred when serum-lithium concentration stabilised

DOSE EQUIVALENCE AND CONVERSION
▸ For *Priadel* ® *liquid*: Lithium citrate tetrahydrate 520 mg is equivalent to lithium carbonate 204 mg.

- INTERACTIONS → Appendix 1: lithium

- MEDICINAL FORMS
There can be variation in the licensing of different medicines containing the same drug.

Oral solution

CAUTIONARY AND ADVISORY LABELS 10
- Lithium citrate (Non-proprietary)
  Lithium citrate 101.8 mg per 1 ml Lithium citrate 509mg/5ml oral solution | 150 ml [PoM] [℥] DT = £5.79
  Lithium citrate 104 mg per 1 ml Lithium citrate 520mg/5ml oral solution sugar free sugar-free | 150 ml [PoM] [℥]
  Lithium citrate 203.6 mg per 1 ml Lithium citrate 1.018g/5ml oral solution | 150 ml [PoM] [℥] DT = £11.58
- Li-Liquid (Rosemont Pharmaceuticals Ltd)
  Lithium citrate 101.8 mg per 1 ml Li-Liquid 509mg/5ml oral solution | 150 ml [PoM] £5.79 DT = £5.79
  Lithium citrate 203.6 mg per 1 ml Li-Liquid 1.018g/5ml oral solution | 150 ml [PoM] £11.58 DT = £11.58
- Priadel (lithium citrate) (Sanofi)
  Lithium citrate 104 mg per 1 ml Priadel 520mg/5ml liquid sugar-free | 150 ml [PoM] £6.73

3.4 Depression

Antidepressant drugs

Overview

Antidepressant drugs are effective for treating moderate to severe depression associated with psychomotor and physiological changes such as loss of appetite and sleep disturbance; improvement in sleep is usually the first benefit of therapy. Ideally, patients with moderate to severe depression should be treated with psychological therapy in addition to drug therapy. Antidepressant drugs are also effective for dysthymia (lower grade chronic depression (typically of at least 2 years duration)).

Antidepressant drugs should not be used routinely in mild depression, and psychological therapy should be considered initially; however, a trial of antidepressant therapy may be considered in cases refractory to psychological treatments or in those associated with psychosocial or medical problems. Drug treatment of mild depression may also be considered in patients with a history of moderate or severe depression.

Choice

The major classes of antidepressant drugs include the tricyclic and related antidepressants, the selective serotonin re-uptake inhibitors (SSRIs), and the monoamine oxidase inhibitors (MAOIs). A number of antidepressant drugs cannot be accommodated easily into this classification.

There is little to choose between the different classes of antidepressant drugs in terms of efficacy, so choice should be based on the individual patient's requirements, including the presence of concomitant disease, existing therapy, suicide risk, and previous response to antidepressant therapy. Since there may be an interval of 2 weeks before the antidepressant action takes place, electroconvulsive treatment may be required in severe depression when delay is hazardous or intolerable. During the first few weeks of treatment, there is an increased potential for agitation, anxiety, and suicidal ideation.

SSRIs are better tolerated and are safer in overdose than other classes of antidepressants and should be considered first-line for treating depression. In patients with unstable angina or who have had a recent myocardial infarction, sertraline p. 364 has been shown to be safe.

Tricyclic antidepressants have similar efficacy to SSRIs but are more likely to be discontinued because of side-effects; toxicity in overdosage is also a problem. SSRIs are less sedating and have fewer antimuscarinic and cardiotoxic effects than tricyclic antidepressants.

MAOIs have dangerous interactions with some foods and drugs, and should be reserved for use by specialists.

Although anxiety is often present in depressive illness (and may be the presenting symptom), the use of an antipsychotic or an anxiolytic may mask the true diagnosis. Anxiolytics or antipsychotic drugs should therefore be used with caution in depression but they are useful adjuncts in agitated patients. Augmenting antidepressants with antipsychotics under specialist supervision may also be necessary in patients who have depression with psychotic symptoms.

St John's wort (*Hypericum perforatum*) is a popular herbal remedy on sale to the public for treating mild depression. It should not be prescribed or recommended for depression because St John's wort can induce drug metabolising enzymes and a number of important interactions with conventional drugs, including conventional antidepressants, have been identified. Furthermore, the amount of active ingredient varies between different preparations of St John's wort and switching from one to another can change the degree of enzyme induction. If a patient stops taking St John's wort, the concentration of interacting drugs may increase, leading to toxicity.

Management
Patients should be reviewed every 1–2 weeks at the start of antidepressant treatment. Treatment should be continued for at least 4 weeks (6 weeks in the elderly) before considering whether to switch antidepressant due to lack of efficacy. In cases of partial response, continue for a further 2–4 weeks (elderly patients may take longer to respond).

Following remission, antidepressant treatment should be continued at the same dose for at least 6 months (about 12 months in the elderly), or for at least 12 months in patients receiving treatment for generalised anxiety disorder (as the likelihood of relapse is high). Patients with a history of recurrent depression should receive maintenance treatment for at least 2 years.

Hyponatraemia and antidepressant therapy
Hyponatraemia (usually in the elderly and possibly due to inappropriate secretion of antidiuretic hormone) has been associated with all types of antidepressants; however, it has been reported more frequently with SSRIs than with other antidepressants. Hyponatraemia should be considered in all patients who develop drowsiness, confusion, or convulsions while taking an antidepressant.

Suicidal behaviour and antidepressant therapy
The use of antidepressants has been linked with suicidal thoughts and behaviour; children, young adults, and patients with a history of suicidal behaviour are particularly at risk. Where necessary patients should be monitored for suicidal behaviour, self-harm, or hostility, particularly at the beginning of treatment or if the dose is changed.

Serotonin syndrome
Serotonin syndrome or serotonin toxicity is a relatively uncommon adverse drug reaction caused by excessive central and peripheral serotonergic activity. Onset of symptoms, which range from mild to lifethreatening, can occur within hours or days following the initiation, dose escalation, or overdose of a serotonergic drug, the addition of a new serotonergic drug, or the replacement of one serotonergic drug by another without allowing a long enough washout period in-between, particularly when the first drug is an irreversible MAOI or a drug with a long half-life. Severe toxicity, which is a medical emergency, usually occurs with a combination of serotonergic drugs, one of which is generally an MAOI.

The characteristic symptoms of serotonin syndrome fall into 3 main areas, although features from each group may not be seen in all patients—neuromuscular hyperactivity (such as tremor, hyperreflexia, clonus, myoclonus, rigidity), autonomic dysfunction (tachycardia, blood pressure changes, hyperthermia, diaphoresis, shivering, diarrhoea), and altered mental state (agitation, confusion, mania).

Treatment consists of withdrawal of the serotonergic medication and supportive care; specialist advice should be sought.

Failure to respond
Failure to respond to initial treatment with an SSRI may require an increase in the dose, or switching to a different SSRI or mirtazapine p. 368. Other second-line choices include lofepramine p. 373, moclobemide p. 359, and reboxetine p. 360. Other tricyclic antidepressants and venlafaxine p. 365 should be considered for more severe forms of depression; irreversible MAOIs should only be prescribed by specialists. Failure to respond to a second antidepressant may require the addition of another antidepressant of a different class, or use of an augmenting agent (such as lithium, aripiprazole p. 391 [unlicensed], olanzapine p. 394 [unlicensed], quetiapine p. 397, or risperidone p. 398 [unlicensed]), but such adjunctive treatment should be initiated only by doctors with special experience of these combinations. Electroconvulsive therapy may be initiated in severe refractory depression.

Anxiety disorders and obsessive-compulsive disorder
Management of acute anxiety generally involves the use of a benzodiazepine or buspirone hydrochloride p. 338. For chronic anxiety (of longer than 4 weeks' duration) it may be appropriate to use an antidepressant. Combined therapy with a benzodiazepine may be required until the antidepressant takes effect. Patients with *generalised anxiety disorder*, a form of chronic anxiety, should be offered psychological treatment before initiating an antidepressant. If drug treatment is needed, an SSRI such as escitalopram p. 361, paroxetine p. 363, or sertraline p. 364 [unlicensed], can be used. Duloxetine p. 364 and venlafaxine p. 365 (serotonin and noradrenaline reuptake inhibitors) are also recommended for the treatment of generalised anxiety disorder; if the patient cannot tolerate SSRIs or serotonin and noradrenaline reuptake inhibitors (or if treatment has failed to control symptoms), pregabalin p. 322 can be considered.

Panic disorder, obsessive-compulsive disorder, post-traumatic stress disorder, and phobic states such as *social anxiety disorder* are treated with SSRIs. Clomipramine hydrochloride p. 370 or imipramine hydrochloride p. 372 can be used second-line in panic disorder [unlicensed]; clomipramine hydrochloride can also be used second-line for obsessive-compulsive disorder. Moclobemide p. 359 is licensed for the treatment of social anxiety disorder.

Tricyclic and related antidepressant drugs
Choice
Tricyclic and related antidepressants block the re-uptake of both serotonin and noradrenaline, although to different extents. For example, clomipramine hydrochloride is more selective for serotonergic transmission, and imipramine hydrochloride is more selective for noradrenergic transmission. Tricyclic and related antidepressant drugs can

be roughly divided into those with additional sedative properties and those that are less sedating. Agitated and anxious patients tend to respond best to the sedative compounds, whereas withdrawn and apathetic patients will often obtain most benefit from the less sedating ones. Those with **sedative** properties include amitriptyline hydrochloride p. 369, clomipramine hydrochloride, dosulepin hydrochloride p. 371, doxepin p. 372, mianserin hydrochloride p. 367, trazodone hydrochloride p. 366, and trimipramine p. 375. Those with **less sedative** properties include imipramine hydrochloride, lofepramine p. 373, and nortriptyline p. 374.

Tricyclic and related antidepressants also have varying degrees of antimuscarinic side-effects and cardiotoxicity in overdosage, which may be important in individual patients. Lofepramine has a lower incidence of side-effects and is less dangerous in overdosage but is infrequently associated with hepatic toxicity. Imipramine hydrochloride is also well established, but has more marked antimuscarinic side-effects than other tricyclic and related antidepressants. Amitriptyline hydrochloride and dosulepin hydrochloride are effective but they are particularly dangerous in overdosage and are not recommended for the treatment of depression; dosulepin hydrochloride should be initiated by a specialist.

Dosage

About 10 to 20% of patients fail to respond to tricyclic and related antidepressant drugs and inadequate dosage may account for some of these failures. It is important to use doses that are sufficiently high for effective treatment but not so high as to cause toxic effects. Low doses should be used for initial treatment in the **elderly**. In most patients the long half-life of tricyclic antidepressant drugs allows **once-daily** administration, usually at night; the use of modified-release preparations is therefore unnecessary.

Some tricyclic antidepressants are used in the management of *panic* and other *anxiety disorders*. Some tricyclic antidepressants may also have a role in some forms of *neuralgia* and in *nocturnal enuresis* in children.

Children and adolescents

Studies have shown that tricyclic antidepressants are not effective for treating depression in children.

Monoamine-oxidase inhibitors

Monoamine-oxidase inhibitors are used much less frequently than tricyclic and related antidepressants, or SSRIs and related antidepressants because of the dangers of dietary and drug interactions and the fact that it is easier to prescribe MAOIs when tricyclic antidepressants have been unsuccessful than vice versa.

Tranylcypromine p. 359 has a greater stimulant action than phenelzine p. 359 or isocarboxazid p. 358 and is more likely to cause a hypertensive crisis. Isocarboxazid and phenelzine are more likely to cause hepatotoxicity than tranylcypromine.

Moclobemide should be reserved as a second line treatment.

Phobic patients and depressed patients with atypical, hypochondriacal, or hysterical features are said to respond best to MAOIs. However, MAOIs should be tried in any patients who are refractory to treatment with other antidepressants as there is occasionally a dramatic response. Response to treatment may be delayed for 3 weeks or more and may take an additional 1 or 2 weeks to become maximal.

Interactions

Other antidepressants should not be started for 2 weeks after treatment with MAOIs has been stopped (3 weeks if starting clomipramine or imipramine). Conversely, an MAOI should not be started until:
- at least 2 weeks after a previous MAOI has been stopped (then started at a reduced dose)
- at least 7–14 days after a tricyclic or related antidepressant (3 weeks in the case of clomipramine or imipramine) has been stopped
- at least a week after an SSRI or related antidepressant (at least 5 weeks in the case of fluoxetine) has been stopped

Other antidepressant drugs

The thioxanthene flupentixol p. 382 (Fluanxol®) has antidepressant properties when given by mouth in low doses. Flupentixol is also used for the treatment of psychoses.

Vortioxetine p. 376, an antidepressant thought to directly modulate serotonergic receptor activity and inhibit the re-uptake of serotonin, is recommended in patients whose condition has responded inadequately to 2 antidepressants within the current episode.

Tryptophan is licensed for use in treatment-resistant depression, used as monotherapy and as an adjunct to other antidepressant drugs; it should be initiated by hospital specialists.

> **Other drugs used for Depression** Lithium carbonate, p. 354 · Lithium citrate, p. 355

ANTIDEPRESSANTS > MELATONIN RECEPTOR AGONISTS

Agomelatine
07-Feb-2017

- **DRUG ACTION** A melatonin receptor agonist and a selective serotonin-receptor antagonist; it does not affect the uptake of serotonin, noradrenaline, or dopamine.

- **INDICATIONS AND DOSE**
Major depression
▶ BY MOUTH
▸ Adult: 25 mg daily, dose to be taken at bedtime, dose to be increased if necessary after 2 weeks, increased if necessary to 50 mg daily, dose to be taken at bedtime

- **CONTRA-INDICATIONS** Dementia · patients over 75 years of age
- **CAUTIONS** Alcoholism · bipolar disorder · diabetes · excessive alcohol consumption · hypomania · mania · non-alcoholic fatty liver disease · obesity
- **INTERACTIONS** → Appendix 1: agomelatine
- **SIDE-EFFECTS**
▶ **Common or very common** Abdominal pain · anxiety · back pain · constipation · diarrhoea · dizziness · drowsiness · fatigue · headaches · nausea · sleep disorders · vomiting · weight changes
▶ **Uncommon** Aggression · confusion · hyperhidrosis · mood altered · movement disorders · paraesthesia · skin reactions · suicidal tendencies · tinnitus · vision blurred
▶ **Rare or very rare** Angioedema · face oedema · hallucination · hepatic disorders · urinary retention
SIDE-EFFECTS, FURTHER INFORMATION The use of antidepressants has been linked with suicidal thoughts and behaviour; children, young adults, and patients with a history of suicidal behaviour are particularly at risk. Where necessary patients should be monitored for suicidal behaviour, self-harm, or hostility, particularly at the beginning of treatment or if the dose is changed.
- **PREGNANCY** Manufacturer advises avoid.
- **BREAST FEEDING** Avoid—present in milk in *animal* studies.
- **HEPATIC IMPAIRMENT** Manufacturer advises avoid in impairment (or if baseline serum transaminases exceed 3 times the upper limit of reference range).
- **RENAL IMPAIRMENT** Caution in moderate to severe impairment.

- **MONITORING REQUIREMENTS** Test liver function before treatment and after 3, 6, 12 and 24 weeks of treatment, and then regularly thereafter when clinically indicated (restart monitoring schedule if dose increased); discontinue if serum transaminases exceed 3 times the upper limit of reference range or symptoms of liver disorder.
- **PATIENT AND CARER ADVICE**
  Hepatotoxicity Patients should be told how to recognise signs of liver disorder, and advised to seek immediate medical attention if symptoms such as dark urine, light coloured stools, jaundice, bruising, fatigue, abdominal pain, or pruritus develop.

  Patients should be given a booklet with more information on the risk of hepatic side-effects.

- **MEDICINAL FORMS**
  There can be variation in the licensing of different medicines containing the same drug.
  Tablet
  ▸ Valdoxan (Servier Laboratories Ltd)
  Agomelatine 25 mg Valdoxan 25mg tablets | 28 tablet [PoM] £30.00 DT = £30.00

ANTIDEPRESSANTS > MONOAMINE-OXIDASE INHIBITORS

Monoamine-oxidase inhibitors ●

- **DRUG ACTION** MAOIs inhibit monoamine oxidase, thereby causing an accumulation of amine neurotransmitters.
- **CONTRA-INDICATIONS** Cerebrovascular disease · not indicated in manic phase · phaeochromocytoma
- **CAUTIONS** Acute porphyrias p. 1025 · avoid in agitated patients · blood disorders · cardiovascular disease · concurrent electroconvulsive therapy · diabetes mellitus · elderly (great caution) · epilepsy · severe hypertensive reactions to certain drugs and foods · surgery
- **SIDE-EFFECTS**
- ▸ **Rare or very rare** Hepatic disorders
- ▸ **Frequency not known** Anxiety · appetite increased · arrhythmias · asthenia · behaviour abnormal · blood disorder · cardiovascular insufficiency · chest pain · confusion · constipation · delirium · diarrhoea · dizziness · drowsiness · drug dependence · dry mouth · dysuria · electrolyte imbalance · eye disorders · feeling jittery · fever · flushing · gastrointestinal disorder · glaucoma · granulocytopenia · hallucination · headaches · hyperhidrosis · hypermetabolism · hypertension · impaired driving ability · intracranial haemorrhage · lupus-like syndrome · malaise · mood altered · movement disorders · muscle tone increased · muscle twitching · nausea · neuroleptic malignant syndrome · oedema · pain · pallor · paraesthesia · peripheral neuritis · postural hypotension (more common in elderly) · reflexes increased · respiratory disorders · schizophrenia · seizure · sexual dysfunction · shock-like coma · skin reactions · sleep disorders · speech repetitive · suicidal tendencies · tremor · vision disorders · vomiting · weight increased
  SIDE-EFFECTS, FURTHER INFORMATION Risk of postural hypotension and hypertensive responses. Discontinue if palpitations or frequent headaches occur.
- **PREGNANCY** Increased risk of neonatal malformations—manufacturer advises avoid unless there are compelling reasons.
- **HEPATIC IMPAIRMENT** MAOIs may cause idiosyncratic hepatotoxicity if used in patients with hepatic impairment.
- **MONITORING REQUIREMENTS** Monitor blood pressure (risk of postural hypotension and hypertensive responses).
- **TREATMENT CESSATION**
  Withdrawal If possible avoid abrupt withdrawal.

MAOIs are associated with withdrawal symptoms on cessation of therapy. Symptoms include agitation, irritability, ataxia, movement disorders, insomnia, drowsiness, vivid dreams, cognitive impairment, and slowed speech. Withdrawal symptoms occasionally experienced when discontinuing MAOIs include hallucinations and paranoid delusions. If possible MAOIs should be withdrawn slowly.

Withdrawal effects may occur within 5 days of stopping treatment with antidepressant drugs; they are usually mild and self-limiting, but in some cases may be severe. The risk of withdrawal symptoms is increased if the antidepressant is stopped suddenly after regular administration for 8 weeks or more. The dose should preferably be reduced gradually over about 4 weeks, or longer if withdrawal symptoms emerge (6 months in patients who have been on long-term maintenance treatment).

- **PATIENT AND CARER ADVICE** Patients should be advised to eat only fresh foods and avoid food that is suspected of being stale or 'going off'. This is especially important with meat, fish, poultry or offal; game should be avoided. The danger of interaction persists for up to 2 weeks after treatment with MAOIs is discontinued. Patients should also be advised to avoid alcoholic drinks or de-alcoholised (low alcohol) drinks.
  Driving and skilled tasks Drowsiness may affect performance of skilled tasks (e.g. driving).

ANTIDEPRESSANTS > MONOAMINE-OXIDASE A AND B INHIBITORS, IRREVERSIBLE

◤ above

Isocarboxazid

- **INDICATIONS AND DOSE**
  Depressive illness
  ▸ BY MOUTH
  ▸ Adult: Initially 30 mg daily until improvement occurs, initial dose may be given in single or divided doses, dose may be increased if necessary after 4 weeks, increased to 60 mg daily for 4–6 weeks, dose to be increased under close supervision only, then reduced to 10–20 mg daily, usual maintenance dose, but up to 40 mg daily may be required
  ▸ Elderly: 5–10 mg daily

- **INTERACTIONS** → Appendix 1: monoamine-oxidase A and B inhibitors, irreversible
- **BREAST FEEDING** Avoid.
- **HEPATIC IMPAIRMENT** Avoid in hepatic impairment.
- **RENAL IMPAIRMENT** Use with caution.
- **LESS SUITABLE FOR PRESCRIBING** Less suitable for prescribing.

- **MEDICINAL FORMS**
  There can be variation in the licensing of different medicines containing the same drug. Forms available from special-order manufacturers include: oral suspension
  Tablet
  CAUTIONARY AND ADVISORY LABELS 3, 10
  ▸ Isocarboxazid (Non-proprietary)
  Isocarboxazid 10 mg Isocarboxazid 10mg tablets | 56 tablet [PoM] £217.75 DT = £217.75

Phenelzine

F 358

INDICATIONS AND DOSE

Depressive illness

▸ BY MOUTH

▸ Adult: Initially 15 mg 3 times a day, response is usually seen within first week; dose may be increased if necessary after 2 weeks if response is not evident, increased if necessary to 15 mg 4 times a day, doses up to 30 mg three times a day may be used in hospital patients; response may not become apparent for up to 4 weeks; once satisfactory response has been achieved, reduce dose gradually to lowest suitable maintenance dose (15 mg on alternate days may be adequate)

● INTERACTIONS → Appendix 1: monoamine-oxidase A and B inhibitors, irreversible

● BREAST FEEDING Avoid—no information available.

● HEPATIC IMPAIRMENT Avoid in hepatic impairment or if abnormal liver function tests.

● LESS SUITABLE FOR PRESCRIBING Less suitable for prescribing.

● MEDICINAL FORMS
There can be variation in the licensing of different medicines containing the same drug.

Tablet

CAUTIONARY AND ADVISORY LABELS 3, 10

▸ Nardil (Kyowa Kirin Ltd)
Phenelzine (as Phenelzine sulfate) 15 mg Nardil 15mg tablets | 100 tablet [PoM] £22.50 DT = £22.50

Tranylcypromine

F 358

INDICATIONS AND DOSE

Depressive illness

▸ BY MOUTH

▸ Adult: Initially 10 mg twice daily, dose to be taken at a time no later than 3 p.m, dose may be increased if necessary after 1 week, increased if necessary to 10 mg daily, dose to be taken in the morning and 20 mg daily, dose to be taken in the afternoon, doses above 30 mg daily, under close supervision only; maintenance 10 mg daily

● CONTRA-INDICATIONS Congestive heart failure · history of hepatic disease · hyperthyroidism

● INTERACTIONS → Appendix 1: monoamine-oxidase A and B inhibitors, irreversible

● BREAST FEEDING Present in milk in *animal* studies.

● HEPATIC IMPAIRMENT Avoid if history of hepatic disease or if abnormal liver function tests.

● LESS SUITABLE FOR PRESCRIBING Less suitable for prescribing.

● MEDICINAL FORMS
There can be variation in the licensing of different medicines containing the same drug.

Tablet

CAUTIONARY AND ADVISORY LABELS 3, 10

▸ Tranylcypromine (Non-proprietary)
Tranylcypromine (as Tranylcypromine sulfate)
10 mg Tranylcypromine 10mg tablets | 28 tablet [PoM] £270.00 DT = £241.50

ANTIDEPRESSANTS > MONOAMINE-OXIDASE A INHIBITORS, REVERSIBLE

Moclobemide

● DRUG ACTION Moclobemide is reported to act by reversible inhibition of monoamine oxidase type A (it is therefore termed a RIMA).

INDICATIONS AND DOSE

Depressive illness

▸ BY MOUTH

▸ Adult: Initially 300 mg daily in divided doses, adjusted according to response; usual dose 150–600 mg daily, dose to be taken after food

Social anxiety disorder

▸ BY MOUTH

▸ Adult: Initially 300 mg daily for 3 days, then increased to 600 mg daily in 2 divided doses continued for 8–12 weeks to assess efficacy

DOSE ADJUSTMENTS DUE TO INTERACTIONS

▸ Manufacturer advises reduce dose to half or one-third of the usual dose with concurrent use of cimetidine.

● CONTRA-INDICATIONS Acute confusional states · phaeochromocytoma

● CAUTIONS Avoid in agitated or excited patients (or give with sedative for up to 2–3 weeks) · may provoke manic episodes in bipolar disorders · thyrotoxicosis

● INTERACTIONS → Appendix 1: moclobemide

● SIDE-EFFECTS

▸ Common or very common Anxiety · constipation · diarrhoea · dizziness · dry mouth · headache · hypotension · irritability · nausea · paraesthesia · skin reactions · sleep disorder · vomiting

▸ Uncommon Asthenia · confusion · flushing · oedema · suicidal tendencies · taste altered · visual impairment

▸ Rare or very rare Appetite decreased · delusions · hyponatraemia · serotonin syndrome

● PREGNANCY Safety in pregnancy has not been established—manufacturer advises avoid unless there are compelling reasons.

● BREAST FEEDING Amount too small to be harmful, but patient information leaflet advises avoid.

● HEPATIC IMPAIRMENT
Dose adjustments Reduce dose in severe hepatic disease.

● TREATMENT CESSATION Withdrawal effects may occur within 5 days of stopping treatment with antidepressant drugs; they are usually mild and self-limiting, but in some cases may be severe. The risk of withdrawal symptoms is increased if the antidepressant is stopped suddenly after regular administration for 8 weeks or more. The dose should preferably be reduced gradually over about 4 weeks, or longer if withdrawal symptoms emerge (6 months in patients who have been on long-term maintenance treatment).

● PATIENT AND CARER ADVICE Moclobemide is claimed to cause less potentiation of the pressor effect of tyramine than the traditional (irreversible) MAOIs, but patients should avoid consuming large amounts of tyramine-rich food (such as mature cheese, yeast extracts and fermented soya bean products).

4

Nervous system

4

Nervous system

- **MEDICINAL FORMS**
  There can be variation in the licensing of different medicines containing the same drug. Forms available from special-order manufacturers include: oral suspension

  Tablet
  CAUTIONARY AND ADVISORY LABELS 10, 21
  ▸ Moclobemide (Non-proprietary)
  Moclobemide 150 mg Moclobemide 150mg tablets | 30 tablet [PoM] £22.12 DT = £22.10
  Moclobemide 300 mg Moclobemide 300mg tablets | 30 tablet [PoM] £15.00 DT = £13.99
  ▸ Manerix (Meda Pharmaceuticals Ltd)
  Moclobemide 150 mg Manerix 150mg tablets | 30 tablet [PoM] £9.33 DT = £22.10
  Moclobemide 300 mg Manerix 300mg tablets | 30 tablet [PoM] £13.99 DT = £13.99

ANTIDEPRESSANTS ⟩ NORADRENALINE REUPTAKE INHIBITORS

Reboxetine

- **DRUG ACTION** Reboxetine is a selective inhibitor of noradrenaline re-uptake.

- **INDICATIONS AND DOSE**

  Major depression
  ▸ BY MOUTH
  ▸ Adult: 4 mg twice daily for 3–4 weeks, then increased if necessary to 10 mg daily in divided doses; maximum 12 mg per day

- **CAUTIONS** Bipolar disorder · history of cardiovascular disease · history of epilepsy · prostatic hypertrophy · susceptibility to angle-closure glaucoma · urinary retention

- **INTERACTIONS** → Appendix 1: reboxetine

- **SIDE-EFFECTS**
  ▸ **Common or very common** Accommodation disorder · akathisia · anxiety · appetite decreased · chills · constipation · dizziness · dry mouth · headache · hyperhidrosis · hypertension · hypotension · insomnia · nausea · palpitations · paraesthesia · sexual dysfunction · skin reactions · tachycardia · taste altered · urinary disorders · urinary tract infection · vasodilation · vomiting
  ▸ **Uncommon** Mydriasis · vertigo
  ▸ **Rare or very rare** Glaucoma
  ▸ **Frequency not known** Aggression · hallucination · hyponatraemia · irritability · peripheral coldness · potassium depletion (long term use) · Raynaud's phenomenon · suicidal tendencies · testicular pain

- **PREGNANCY** Use only if potential benefit outweighs risk—limited information available.

- **BREAST FEEDING** Small amount present in milk—use only if potential benefit outweighs risk.

- **HEPATIC IMPAIRMENT**
  Dose adjustments Initial dose 2 mg twice daily, increased according to tolerance.

- **RENAL IMPAIRMENT**
  Dose adjustments Initial dose 2 mg twice daily, increased according to tolerance.

- **TREATMENT CESSATION** Caution— avoid abrupt withdrawal.

- **PATIENT AND CARER ADVICE**
  Driving and skilled tasks Counselling advised.

- **MEDICINAL FORMS**
  There can be variation in the licensing of different medicines containing the same drug.

  Tablet
  ▸ Edronax (Pfizer Ltd)
  Reboxetine (as Reboxetine mesilate) 4 mg Edronax 4mg tablets | 60 tablet [PoM] £18.91 DT = £18.91

Selective serotonin re-uptake inhibitors

- **DRUG ACTION** Selectively inhibit the re-uptake of serotonin (5-hydroxytryptamine, 5-HT).

- **CONTRA-INDICATIONS** Poorly controlled epilepsy · SSRIs should not be used if the patient enters a manic phase.

- **CAUTIONS** Cardiac disease · concurrent electroconvulsive therapy · diabetes mellitus · epilepsy (discontinue if convulsions develop) · history of bleeding disorders (especially gastro-intestinal bleeding) · history of mania · susceptibility to angle-closure glaucoma

- **SIDE-EFFECTS**
  ▸ **Common or very common** Anxiety · appetite abnormal · arrhythmias · arthralgia · asthenia · concentration impaired · confusion · constipation · depersonalisation · diarrhoea · dizziness · drowsiness · dry mouth · fever · gastrointestinal discomfort · haemorrhage · headache · hyperhidrosis · malaise · memory loss · menstrual cycle irregularities · myalgia · mydriasis · nausea (dose-related) · palpitations · paraesthesia · QT interval prolongation · sexual dysfunction · skin reactions · sleep disorders (uncommon in children) · taste altered · tinnitus · tremor · urinary disorders · visual impairment · vomiting · weight changes · yawning
  ▸ **Uncommon** Alopecia · angioedema · behaviour abnormal · hallucination · mania (very common in children) · movement disorders · photosensitivity reaction · postural hypotension · seizure · suicidal tendencies · syncope
  ▸ **Rare or very rare** Galactorrhoea · hepatitis · hyperprolactinaemia · hyponatraemia · serotonin syndrome · severe cutaneous adverse reactions (SCARs) · SIADH · thrombocytopenia
  ▸ **Frequency not known** Withdrawal syndrome

  Overdose Symptoms of poisoning by selective serotonin re-uptake inhibitors include nausea, vomiting, agitation, tremor, nystagmus, drowsiness, and sinus tachycardia; convulsions may occur. Rarely, severe poisoning results in the serotonin syndrome, with marked neuropsychiatric effects, neuromuscular hyperactivity, and autonomic instability; hyperthermia, rhabdomyolysis, renal failure, and coagulopathies may develop.
  For details on the management of poisoning, see Selective serotonin re-uptake inhibitors, under Emergency treatment of poisoning p. 1319.

- **PREGNANCY** Manufacturers advise avoid during pregnancy unless the potential benefit outweighs the risk. There is a small increased risk of congenital heart defects when taken during early pregnancy. If used during the third trimester there is a risk of neonatal withdrawal symptoms, and persistent pulmonary hypertension in the newborn has been reported.

- **TREATMENT CESSATION** Gastro-intestinal disturbances, headache, anxiety, dizziness, paraesthesia, electric shock sensation in the head, neck, and spine, tinnitus, sleep disturbances, fatigue, influenza-like symptoms, and sweating are the most common features of abrupt withdrawal of an SSRI or marked reduction of the dose; palpitation and visual disturbances can occur less commonly. The dose should be tapered over at least a few weeks to avoid these effects. For some patients, it may be necessary to withdraw treatment over a longer period; consider obtaining specialist advice if symptoms persist.
  Withdrawal effects may occur within 5 days of stopping treatment with antidepressant drugs; they are usually mild and self-limiting, but in some cases may be severe. The risk of withdrawal symptoms is increased if the

antidepressant is stopped suddenly after regular administration for 8 weeks or more.

● PATIENT AND CARER ADVICE
Driving and skilled tasks May also impair performance of skilled tasks (e.g. driving, operating machinery).

F 360

Citalopram

● INDICATIONS AND DOSE
Depressive illness
▸ BY MOUTH USING TABLETS
▸ Adult: 20 mg once daily, increased in steps of 20 mg daily if required, dose to be increased at intervals of 3–4 weeks; maximum 40 mg per day
▸ Elderly: 10–20 mg once daily; maximum 20 mg per day
▸ BY MOUTH USING ORAL DROPS
▸ Adult: 16 mg once daily, increased in steps of 16 mg daily if required, dose to be increased at intervals of 3–4 weeks; maximum 32 mg per day
▸ Elderly: 8–16 mg daily; maximum 16 mg per day

Panic disorder
▸ BY MOUTH USING TABLETS
▸ Adult: Initially 10 mg daily, increased in steps of 10 mg daily if required, dose to be increased gradually; usual dose 20–30 mg daily; maximum 40 mg per day
▸ Elderly: Initially 10 mg daily, increased in steps of 10 mg daily if required, dose to be increased gradually; maximum 20 mg per day
▸ BY MOUTH USING ORAL DROPS
▸ Adult: Initially 8 mg once daily, increased in steps of 8 mg if required, dose to be increased gradually; usual dose 16–24 mg daily; maximum 32 mg per day
▸ Elderly: Initially 8 mg once daily, increased in steps of 8 mg if required, dose to be increased gradually; maximum 16 mg per day

DOSE EQUIVALENCE AND CONVERSION
▸ 4 oral drops (8 mg) is equivalent in therapeutic effect to 10 mg tablet.

● CONTRA-INDICATIONS QT-interval prolongation
● CAUTIONS Susceptibility to QT-interval prolongation
● INTERACTIONS → Appendix 1: SSRIs
● SIDE-EFFECTS
▸ **Common or very common** Acute angle closure glaucoma · apathy · flatulence · hypersalivation · migraine · rhinitis
▸ **Uncommon** Oedema
▸ **Rare or very rare** Cough · generalised tonic-clonic seizure · haemorrhage
▸ **Frequency not known** Hypokalaemia
● BREAST FEEDING Present in milk—use with caution.
● HEPATIC IMPAIRMENT
Dose adjustments Use doses at lower end of range; for *tablets* up to maximum 20 mg; for *oral solution* up to maximum 16 mg.
● RENAL IMPAIRMENT No information available for eGFR less than 20 mL/minute/1.73 m².
● TREATMENT CESSATION The dose should preferably be reduced gradually over about 4 weeks, or longer if withdrawal symptoms emerge (6 months in patients who have been on long-term maintenance treatment).
● DIRECTIONS FOR ADMINISTRATION *Cipramil* ® oral drops should be mixed with water, orange juice, or apple juice before taking.
● PATIENT AND CARER ADVICE Counselling on administration of oral drops is advised.
Driving and skilled tasks Patients should be advised of the effects of citalopram on driving and skilled tasks.

● MEDICINAL FORMS
There can be variation in the licensing of different medicines containing the same drug.
Oral drops
EXCIPIENTS: May contain Alcohol
▸ Citalopram (Non-proprietary)
Citalopram (as Citalopram hydrochloride) 40 mg per 1 ml Citalopram 40mg/ml oral drops sugar free sugar-free | 15 ml PoM £20.16 DT = £4.10
▸ Cipramil (Lundbeck Ltd)
Citalopram (as Citalopram hydrochloride) 40 mg per 1 ml Cipramil 40mg/ml drops sugar-free | 15 ml PoM £10.08 DT = £4.10
Tablet
▸ Citalopram (Non-proprietary)
Citalopram (as Citalopram hydrobromide) 10 mg Citalopram 10mg tablets | 28 tablet PoM £8.90 DT = £1.51
Citalopram (as Citalopram hydrobromide) 20 mg Citalopram 20mg tablets | 28 tablet PoM £15.99 DT = £2.34
Citalopram (as Citalopram hydrobromide) 40 mg Citalopram 40mg tablets | 28 tablet PoM £27.00 DT = £2.37
▸ Cipramil (Lundbeck Ltd)
Citalopram (as Citalopram hydrobromide) 20 mg Cipramil 20mg tablets | 28 tablet PoM £8.95 DT = £2.34

F 360

Escitalopram

● DRUG ACTION Escitalopram is the active enantiomer of citalopram.

● INDICATIONS AND DOSE
Depressive illness | Generalised anxiety disorder | Obsessive-compulsive disorder
▸ BY MOUTH
▸ Adult: 10 mg once daily; increased if necessary up to 20 mg daily
▸ Elderly: Initially 5 mg once daily; maximum 10 mg per day

Panic disorder
▸ BY MOUTH
▸ Adult: Initially 5 mg once daily for 7 days, then increased to 10 mg daily; maximum 20 mg per day
▸ Elderly: Initially 2.5 mg once daily; maximum 10 mg per day

Social anxiety disorder
▸ BY MOUTH
▸ Adult: Initially 10 mg once daily for 2–4 weeks, dose to be adjusted after 2-4 weeks of treatment; usual dose 5–20 mg daily

● CONTRA-INDICATIONS QT-interval prolongation
● CAUTIONS Susceptibility to QT-interval prolongation
● INTERACTIONS → Appendix 1: SSRIs
● SIDE-EFFECTS
▸ **Common or very common** Sinusitis
▸ **Uncommon** Oedema
● BREAST FEEDING Present in breast milk; avoid.
● HEPATIC IMPAIRMENT
Dose adjustments Initial dose 5 mg daily for 2 weeks, thereafter increased to max. 10 mg daily according to response; particular caution in severe impairment.
● RENAL IMPAIRMENT Caution if eGFR less than 30 mL/minute/1.73m².
● TREATMENT CESSATION The dose should preferably be reduced gradually over about 4 weeks, or longer if withdrawal symptoms emerge (6 months in patients who have been on long-term maintenance treatment).
● DIRECTIONS FOR ADMINISTRATION Oral drops can be mixed with water, orange juice, or apple juice before taking.
● PATIENT AND CARER ADVICE Counselling on administration of oral drops advised.

Driving and skilled tasks Patients should be counselled about the effects on driving.

● MEDICINAL FORMS
There can be variation in the licensing of different medicines containing the same drug.

Oral drops

▸ Cipralex (Lundbeck Ltd)
Escitalopram (as Escitalopram oxalate) 20 mg per 1 ml Cipralex 20mg/ml oral drops sugar-free | 15 ml [PoM] £20.16 DT = £20.16

Tablet

▸ Escitalopram (Non-proprietary)
Escitalopram (as Escitalopram oxalate) 5 mg Escitalopram 5mg tablets | 28 tablet [PoM] £8.52 DT = £0.95
Escitalopram (as Escitalopram oxalate) 10 mg Escitalopram 10mg tablets | 28 tablet [PoM] £14.55 DT = £1.00
Escitalopram (as Escitalopram oxalate) 20 mg Escitalopram 20mg tablets | 28 tablet [PoM] £23.94 DT = £1.43

▸ Cipralex (Lundbeck Ltd)
Escitalopram (as Escitalopram oxalate) 5 mg Cipralex 5mg tablets | 28 tablet [PoM] £8.97 DT = £0.95
Escitalopram (as Escitalopram oxalate) 10 mg Cipralex 10mg tablets | 28 tablet [PoM] £14.91 DT = £1.00
Escitalopram (as Escitalopram oxalate) 20 mg Cipralex 20mg tablets | 28 tablet [PoM] £25.20 DT = £1.43

⚑ 360

Fluoxetine

19-Jul-2017

● INDICATIONS AND DOSE

Major depression

▸ BY MOUTH

▸ **Adult:** Initially 20 mg daily, dose is increased after 3–4 weeks if necessary, and at appropriate intervals thereafter, daily dose may be administered as a single or divided dose; maximum 60 mg per day

▸ **Elderly:** Initially 20 mg daily, dose is increased after 3–4 weeks if necessary, and at appropriate intervals thereafter, daily dose may be administered as a single or divided dose, usual maximum dose is 40 mg daily but doses up to 60 mg daily can be used

Bulimia nervosa

▸ BY MOUTH

▸ **Adult:** 60 mg daily, daily dose may be administered as a single or divided dose

▸ **Elderly:** Up to 40 mg daily, daily dose may be administered as a single or divided dose, usual maximum dose is 40 mg daily but doses up to 60 mg daily can be used

Obsessive-compulsive disorder

▸ BY MOUTH

▸ **Adult:** 20 mg daily, increased if necessary up to 60 mg daily, daily dose may be administered as a single or divided dose, dose to be increased gradually, review treatment if inadequate response after 10 weeks; maximum 60 mg per day

▸ **Elderly:** 20 mg daily, increased if necessary up to 40 mg daily, daily dose may be administered as a single or divided dose, dose to be increased gradually, review treatment if inadequate response after 10 weeks, usual maximum dose is 40 mg daily but doses up to 60 mg daily can be used

Menopausal symptoms, particularly hot flushes, in women with breast cancer (except those taking tamoxifen)

▸ BY MOUTH

▸ **Adult:** 20 mg once daily

PHARMACOKINETICS

▸ Consider the long half-life of fluoxetine when adjusting dosage (or in overdosage).

● UNLICENSED USE [EvGr] Not licensed for menopausal symptoms. ⑧

● INTERACTIONS → Appendix 1: SSRIs

● SIDE-EFFECTS

▸ **Common or very common** Chills · feeling abnormal · haemorrhage · postmenopausal haemorrhage · uterine disorder · vasodilation · vision blurred

▸ **Uncommon** Cold sweat · dysphagia · dyspnoea · dysuria · hypotension · mood altered · muscle twitching · self-injurious behaviour · temperature sensation altered · thinking abnormal

▸ **Rare or very rare** Leucopenia · neutropenia · oral disorders · pharyngitis · respiratory disorders · serum sickness · speech disorder · vasculitis

▸ **Frequency not known** Bone fracture

● BREAST FEEDING Present in milk—avoid.

● HEPATIC IMPAIRMENT
Dose adjustments Reduce dose or increase dose interval.

● DIRECTIONS FOR ADMINISTRATION Dispersible tablets can be dispersed in water for administration or swallowed whole with plenty of water.

● PATIENT AND CARER ADVICE Patients and carers should be counselled on the administration of dispersible tablets.
Driving and skilled tasks Patients should be counselled about the effects on driving and skilled tasks.

● MEDICINAL FORMS
There can be variation in the licensing of different medicines containing the same drug. Forms available from special-order manufacturers include: oral suspension, oral solution

Tablet

▸ Fluoxetine (Non-proprietary)
Fluoxetine (as Fluoxetine hydrochloride) 10 mg Fluoxetine 10mg tablets | 30 tablet [PoM] £44.00 DT = £44.00

Dispersible tablet

CAUTIONARY AND ADVISORY LABELS 10

▸ Olena (AMCo)
Fluoxetine (as Fluoxetine hydrochloride) 20 mg Olena 20mg dispersible tablets sugar-free | 28 tablet [PoM] £3.44 DT = £3.44

Oral solution

▸ Fluoxetine (Non-proprietary)
Fluoxetine (as Fluoxetine hydrochloride) 4 mg per 1 ml Fluoxetine 20mg/5ml oral solution | 70 ml [PoM] £12.75 DT = £2.78
Fluoxetine 20mg/5ml oral solution sugar free sugar-free | 70 ml [PoM] £12.95 DT = £12.95

▸ Prozac (Eli Lilly and Company Ltd)
Fluoxetine (as Fluoxetine hydrochloride) 4 mg per 1 ml Prozac 20mg/5ml liquid | 70 ml [PoM] £11.12 DT = £2.78

▸ Prozep (Chemidex Pharma Ltd)
Fluoxetine (as Fluoxetine hydrochloride) 4 mg per 1 ml Prozep 20mg/5ml oral solution sugar-free | 70 ml [PoM] £12.95 DT = £12.95

Capsule

▸ Fluoxetine (Non-proprietary)
Fluoxetine (as Fluoxetine hydrochloride) 10 mg Fluoxetine 10mg capsules | 30 capsule [PoM] £55.00–£58.50 DT = £58.11
Fluoxetine (as Fluoxetine hydrochloride) 20 mg Fluoxetine 20mg capsules | 30 capsule [PoM] £20.00 DT = £0.58
Fluoxetine (as Fluoxetine hydrochloride) 30 mg Fluoxetine 30mg capsules | 30 capsule [PoM] £1.80 DT = £1.80
Fluoxetine (as Fluoxetine hydrochloride) 40 mg Fluoxetine 40mg capsules | 30 capsule [PoM] £1.80–£2.16 DT = £2.16
Fluoxetine (as Fluoxetine hydrochloride) 60 mg Fluoxetine 60mg capsules | 30 capsule [PoM] £54.36 DT = £3.72

▸ Oxactin (Discovery Pharmaceuticals)
Fluoxetine (as Fluoxetine hydrochloride) 20 mg Oxactin 20mg capsules | 30 capsule [PoM] £0.57 DT = £0.58

▸ Prozac (Eli Lilly and Company Ltd)
Fluoxetine (as Fluoxetine hydrochloride) 20 mg Prozac 20mg capsules | 30 capsule [PoM] £1.50 DT = £0.58

Fluvoxamine maleate

▶ 360

● INDICATIONS AND DOSE

Depressive illness
▶ BY MOUTH
▷ **Adult:** Initially 50–100 mg daily, dose to be taken in the evening, dose to be increased gradually, increased if necessary up to 300 mg daily, doses over 150 mg daily are given in divided doses; maintenance 100 mg daily

Obsessive-compulsive disorder
▶ BY MOUTH
▷ **Adult:** Initially 50 mg daily, dose to be taken in the evening, dose is increased gradually if necessary after several weeks, increased if necessary up to 300 mg daily; maintenance 100–300 mg daily, doses over 150 mg daily are given in divided doses, if no improvement in obsessive-compulsive disorder within 10 weeks, treatment should be reconsidered

● INTERACTIONS → Appendix 1: SSRIs

● SIDE-EFFECTS
▶ **Uncommon** Allergic dermatitis · ataxia
▶ **Rare or very rare** Hepatic function abnormal (discontinue)
▶ **Frequency not known** Bone fracture · glaucoma · haemorrhage · neuroleptic malignant-like syndrome · urinary disorders

● BREAST FEEDING Present in milk—avoid.

● HEPATIC IMPAIRMENT
Dose adjustments Start with low dose.

● RENAL IMPAIRMENT
Dose adjustments Start with low dose.

● TREATMENT CESSATION The dose should preferably be reduced gradually over about 4 weeks, or longer if withdrawal symptoms emerge (6 months in patients who have been on long-term maintenance treatment).

● PATIENT AND CARER ADVICE
Driving and skilled tasks Patients should be counselled about the effects on driving and skilled tasks.

● MEDICINAL FORMS
There can be variation in the licensing of different medicines containing the same drug. Forms available from special-order manufacturers include: oral suspension

Tablet
▶ Fluvoxamine maleate (Non-proprietary)
  Fluvoxamine maleate 50 mg Fluvoxamine 50mg tablets | 60 tablet [PoM] £20.98 DT = £18.32
  Fluvoxamine maleate 100 mg Fluvoxamine 100mg tablets | 30 tablet [PoM] £20.98 DT = £18.32
▶ Faverin (Mylan)
  Fluvoxamine maleate 50 mg Faverin 50mg tablets | 60 tablet [PoM] £17.10 DT = £18.32
  Fluvoxamine maleate 100 mg Faverin 100mg tablets | 30 tablet [PoM] £17.10 DT = £18.32

Paroxetine

▶ 360

19-Jul-2017

● INDICATIONS AND DOSE

Major depression | Social anxiety disorder | Post-traumatic stress disorder | Generalised anxiety disorder
▶ BY MOUTH
▷ **Adult:** 20 mg daily, dose to be taken in the morning, no evidence of greater efficacy at higher doses; maximum 50 mg per day
▷ **Elderly:** 20 mg daily, dose to be taken in the morning, no evidence of greater efficacy at higher doses; maximum 40 mg per day

Obsessive-compulsive disorder
▶ BY MOUTH
▷ **Adult:** Initially 20 mg daily, dose to be taken in the morning, increased in steps of 10 mg, dose to be increased gradually, increased to 40 mg daily, no evidence of greater efficacy at higher doses; maximum 60 mg per day
▷ **Elderly:** Initially 20 mg daily, dose to be taken in the morning, increased in steps of 10 mg, dose to be increased gradually; maximum 40 mg per day

Panic disorder
▶ BY MOUTH
▷ **Adult:** Initially 10 mg daily, dose to be taken in the morning, increased in steps of 10 mg, dose to be increased gradually, increased to 40 mg daily, no evidence of greater efficacy at higher doses; maximum 60 mg per day
▷ **Elderly:** Initially 10 mg daily, dose to be taken in the morning, increased in steps of 10 mg, dose to be increased gradually; maximum 40 mg per day

Menopausal symptoms, particularly hot flushes, in women with breast cancer (except those taking tamoxifen).
▶ BY MOUTH
▷ **Adult:** 10 mg once daily

● UNLICENSED USE [EvGr] Not licensed for menopausal symptoms. Ⓑ

● CAUTIONS Achlorhydria · high gastric pH
CAUTIONS, FURTHER INFORMATION
▶ Achlorhydria or high gastric pH Causes reduced absorption of the oral suspension.

● INTERACTIONS → Appendix 1: SSRIs

● SIDE-EFFECTS
▶ **Common or very common** Vision blurred
▶ **Uncommon** Diabetic control impaired · sinus tachycardia
▶ **Rare or very rare** Acute glaucoma · erythema multiforme · hepatic disorders · peripheral oedema · restless legs

● PREGNANCY Increased risk of congenital malformations, especially if used in the first trimester.

● BREAST FEEDING Present in milk but amount too small to be harmful.

● HEPATIC IMPAIRMENT
Dose adjustments Reduce dose.

● RENAL IMPAIRMENT
Dose adjustments Reduce dose if eGFR less than 30 mL/minute/1.73 m^2.

● TREATMENT CESSATION Associated with a higher risk of withdrawal reactions. The dose should preferably be reduced gradually over about 4 weeks, or longer if withdrawal symptoms emerge (6 months in patients who have been on long-term maintenance treatment).

● PATIENT AND CARER ADVICE
Driving and skilled tasks Patients should be counselled about the effect on driving.

● MEDICINAL FORMS
There can be variation in the licensing of different medicines containing the same drug. Forms available from special-order manufacturers include: oral suspension, oral solution

Oral suspension
CAUTIONARY AND ADVISORY LABELS 5, 21
▶ Seroxat (GlaxoSmithKline UK Ltd)
  Paroxetine (as Paroxetine hydrochloride) 2 mg per 1 ml Seroxat 20mg/10ml liquid sugar-free | 150 ml [PoM] £9.12 DT = £9.12

Tablet
CAUTIONARY AND ADVISORY LABELS 21
▶ Paroxetine (Non-proprietary)
  Paroxetine (as Paroxetine hydrochloride) 10 mg Paroxetine 10mg tablets | 28 tablet [PoM] £17.03 DT = £9.43
  Paroxetine (as Paroxetine hydrochloride) 20 mg Paroxetine 20mg tablets | 30 tablet [PoM] £12.18 DT = £1.10

4

Nervous system

Paroxetine (as Paroxetine hydrochloride) 30 mg Paroxetine 30mg tablets | 30 tablet [PoM] £2.65 DT = £1.34
Paroxetine (as Paroxetine hydrochloride) 40 mg Paroxetine 40mg tablets | 28 tablet [PoM] £16.99–£17.03 | 30 tablet [PoM] £25.07
▸ Seroxat (GlaxoSmithKline UK Ltd)
Paroxetine (as Paroxetine hydrochloride) 10 mg Seroxat 10mg tablets | 28 tablet [PoM] £14.21 DT = £9.43
Paroxetine (as Paroxetine hydrochloride) 20 mg Seroxat 20mg tablets | 30 tablet [PoM] £15.23 DT = £1.10
Paroxetine (as Paroxetine hydrochloride) 30 mg Seroxat 30mg tablets | 30 tablet [PoM] £26.74 DT = £1.34

Sertraline

⬛ 360

19-Mar-2018

● **INDICATIONS AND DOSE**

Depressive illness
▸ BY MOUTH
  ▸ Adult: Initially 50 mg daily, then increased in steps of 50 mg at intervals of at least 1 week if required; maintenance 50 mg daily; maximum 200 mg per day

Obsessive-compulsive disorder
▸ BY MOUTH
  ▸ Adult: Initially 50 mg daily, then increased in steps of 50 mg at intervals of at least 1 week if required; maximum 200 mg per day

Panic disorder | Post-traumatic stress disorder | Social anxiety disorder
▸ BY MOUTH
  ▸ Adult: Initially 25 mg daily for 1 week, then increased to 50 mg daily, then increased in steps of 50 mg at intervals of at least 1 week if required, increase only if response is partial and if drug is tolerated; maximum 200 mg per day

● **INTERACTIONS** → Appendix 1: SSRIs

● **SIDE-EFFECTS**
▸ **Common or very common** Chest pain · depression · gastrointestinal disorders · increased risk of infection · neuromuscular dysfunction · vasodilation
▸ **Uncommon** Back pain · burping · chills · cold sweat · dizziness postural · dysphagia · dyspnoea · ear pain · haemorrhage · hypertension · hypothyroidism · migraine · mood altered · movement disorders · muscle complaints · muscle weakness · oedema · oral disorders · osteoarthritis · periorbital oedema · respiratory disorders · sensation abnormal · skin reactions · speech disorder · thinking abnormal · thirst · urinary disorders
▸ **Rare or very rare** Balanoposthitis · bone disorder · cardiac disorder · coma · conversion disorder · diabetes mellitus · drug dependence · drug tolerance decreased · dysphonia · eye disorders · gait abnormal · genital discharge · glaucoma · hair texture abnormal · hepatic disorders · hiccups · hypercholesterolaemia · hypoglycaemia · injury · lymphadenopathy · myocardial infarction · neoplasms · oliguria · paranoia · peripheral ischaemia · psychotic disorder · sleep walking · vision disorders · vulvovaginal atrophy
▸ **Frequency not known** Cerebrovascular insufficiency · gynaecomastia · hyperglycaemia · leucopenia · neuroleptic malignant syndrome · pancreatitis · severe cutaneous adverse reactions (SCARs)

● **BREAST FEEDING** Not known to be harmful but consider discontinuing breast-feeding.

● **HEPATIC IMPAIRMENT** Avoid in severe impairment.
Dose adjustments Reduce dose or increase dose interval in mild or moderate impairment.

● **RENAL IMPAIRMENT** Use with caution.

● **TREATMENT CESSATION** The dose should preferably be reduced gradually over about 4 weeks, or longer if withdrawal symptoms emerge (6 months in patients who have been on long-term maintenance treatment).

● **PATIENT AND CARER ADVICE**
Driving and skilled tasks Patients should be counselled on the effects on driving and skilled tasks.

● **MEDICINAL FORMS**
There can be variation in the licensing of different medicines containing the same drug. Forms available from special-order manufacturers include: oral suspension
Tablet
▸ Sertraline (Non-proprietary)
Sertraline (as Sertraline hydrochloride) 50 mg Sertraline 50mg tablets | 28 tablet [PoM] £19.25 DT = £0.67
Sertraline (as Sertraline hydrochloride) 100 mg Sertraline 100mg tablets | 28 tablet [PoM] £29.09 DT = £0.91
▸ Lustral (Pfizer Ltd)
Sertraline (as Sertraline hydrochloride) 50 mg Lustral 50mg tablets | 28 tablet [PoM] £17.82 DT = £0.67
Sertraline (as Sertraline hydrochloride) 100 mg Lustral 100mg tablets | 28 tablet [PoM] £29.16 DT = £0.91

ANTIDEPRESSANTS 〉 SEROTONIN AND NORADRENALINE RE-UPTAKE INHIBITORS

Duloxetine

● **DRUG ACTION** Inhibits the re-uptake of serotonin and noradrenaline.

● **INDICATIONS AND DOSE**

Major depressive disorder
▸ BY MOUTH
  ▸ Adult: 60 mg once daily

Generalised anxiety disorder
▸ BY MOUTH
  ▸ Adult: Initially 30 mg once daily, increased if necessary to 60 mg once daily; maximum 120 mg per day

Diabetic neuropathy
▸ BY MOUTH
  ▸ Adult: 60 mg once daily, discontinue if inadequate response after 2 months; review treatment at least every 3 months, maximum dose to be given in divided doses; maximum 120 mg per day

Moderate to severe stress urinary incontinence
▸ BY MOUTH
  ▸ Adult (female): 40 mg twice daily, patient should be assessed for benefit and tolerability after 2–4 weeks, alternatively initially 20 mg twice daily for 2 weeks, this can minimise side effects, then increased to 40 mg twice daily, the patient should be assessed for benefit and tolerability after 2–4 weeks.

● **CAUTIONS** Bleeding disorders · cardiac disease · elderly · history of mania · history of seizures · hypertension (avoid if uncontrolled) · raised intra-ocular pressure · susceptibility to angle-closure glaucoma

● **INTERACTIONS** → Appendix 1: duloxetine

● **SIDE-EFFECTS**
▸ **Common or very common** Anxiety · appetite decreased · constipation · diarrhoea · dizziness · drowsiness · dry mouth · fall · fatigue · flushing · gastrointestinal discomfort · gastrointestinal disorders · headache · muscle complaints · nausea · pain · palpitations · paraesthesia · sexual dysfunction · skin reactions · sleep disorders · sweat changes · tinnitus · tremor · urinary disorders · vision disorders · vomiting · weight changes · yawning
▸ **Uncommon** Apathy · arrhythmias · behaviour abnormal · burping · chills · concentration impaired · disorientation · dysphagia · ear pain · feeling abnormal · gait abnormal · haemorrhage · hepatic disorders · hyperglycaemia · increased risk of infection · malaise · menstrual disorder · movement disorders · mydriasis · peripheral coldness · photosensitivity reaction · postural hypotension · syncope

· taste altered · temperature sensation altered · testicular pain · thirst · throat tightness · vertigo
▸ **Rare or very rare** Angioedema · cutaneous vasculitis · dehydration · galactorrhoea · glaucoma · hallucination · hyperprolactinaemia · hypertensive crisis · hyponatraemia · hypothyroidism · mania · menopausal symptoms · oral disorders · seizure · serotonin syndrome · SIADH · Stevens-Johnson syndrome · urine odour abnormal

● PREGNANCY Toxicity in *animal* studies—avoid in patients with stress urinary incontinence; in other conditions use only if potential benefit outweighs risk. Risk of neonatal withdrawal symptoms if used near term.

● BREAST FEEDING Present in milk—manufacturer advises avoid.

● HEPATIC IMPAIRMENT Manufacturer advises avoid.

● RENAL IMPAIRMENT Avoid if eGFR less than 30 mL/minute/1.73 m^2.

● TREATMENT CESSATION Nausea, vomiting, headache, anxiety, dizziness, paraesthesia, sleep disturbances, and tremor are the most common features of abrupt withdrawal or marked reduction of the dose; dose should be reduced over at least 1–2 weeks.

● NATIONAL FUNDING/ACCESS DECISIONS
CYMBALTA ®

Scottish Medicines Consortium (SMC) Decisions
The *Scottish Medicines Consortium* has advised (September 2006) that duloxetine (*Cymbalta*®) should be restricted for use by specialists when other treatments for diabetic peripheral neuropathic pain are unsuitable or inadequate.

● MEDICINAL FORMS
There can be variation in the licensing of different medicines containing the same drug.

Gastro-resistant capsule
CAUTIONARY AND ADVISORY LABELS 2
▸ Duloxetine (Non-proprietary)
Duloxetine (as Duloxetine hydrochloride) 20 mg Duloxetine 20mg gastro-resistant capsules | 28 capsule [PoM] £18.48 DT = £6.46
Duloxetine (as Duloxetine hydrochloride) 30 mg Duloxetine 30mg gastro-resistant capsules | 28 capsule [PoM] £22.40 DT = £7.74
Duloxetine (as Duloxetine hydrochloride) 40 mg Duloxetine 40mg gastro-resistant capsules | 56 capsule [PoM] £36.96 DT = £13.39
Duloxetine (as Duloxetine hydrochloride) 60 mg Duloxetine 60mg gastro-resistant capsules | 28 capsule [PoM] £27.72 DT = £11.57
▸ Cymbalta (Eli Lilly and Company Ltd)
Duloxetine (as Duloxetine hydrochloride) 30 mg Cymbalta 30mg gastro-resistant capsules | 28 capsule [PoM] £22.40 DT = £7.74
Duloxetine (as Duloxetine hydrochloride) 60 mg Cymbalta 60mg gastro-resistant capsules | 28 capsule [PoM] £27.72 DT = £11.57
▸ Depalta (Disposable Medical Equipment Ltd)
Duloxetine (as Duloxetine hydrochloride) 30 mg Depalta 30mg gastro-resistant capsules | 28 capsule [PoM] £5.95 DT = £7.74
Duloxetine (as Duloxetine hydrochloride) 60 mg Depalta 60mg gastro-resistant capsules | 28 capsule [PoM] £8.95 DT = £11.57
▸ Duciltia (Aristo Pharma Ltd)
Duloxetine (as Duloxetine hydrochloride) 30 mg Duciltia 30mg gastro-resistant capsules | 28 capsule [PoM] £22.40 DT = £7.74
Duloxetine (as Duloxetine hydrochloride) 60 mg Duciltia 60mg gastro-resistant capsules | 28 capsule [PoM] £27.72 DT = £11.57
▸ Yentreve (Eli Lilly and Company Ltd)
Duloxetine (as Duloxetine hydrochloride) 20 mg Yentreve 20mg gastro-resistant capsules | 28 capsule [PoM] £18.48 DT = £6.46
Duloxetine (as Duloxetine hydrochloride) 40 mg Yentreve 40mg gastro-resistant capsules | 56 capsule [PoM] £36.96 DT = £13.39

Venlafaxine
26-Jul-2017

● DRUG ACTION A serotonin and noradrenaline re-uptake inhibitor.

● INDICATIONS AND DOSE
Major depression
▸ BY MOUTH USING IMMEDIATE-RELEASE MEDICINES
▸ Adult: Initially 75 mg daily in 2 divided doses, then increased if necessary up to 375 mg daily, dose to be increased if necessary at intervals of at least 2 weeks, faster dose titration may be necessary in some patients; maximum 375 mg per day
▸ BY MOUTH USING MODIFIED-RELEASE MEDICINES
▸ Adult: Initially 75 mg once daily, increased if necessary up to 375 mg once daily, dose to be increased if necessary at intervals of at least 2 weeks, faster dose titration may be necessary in some patients; maximum 375 mg per day

Generalised anxiety disorder
▸ BY MOUTH USING MODIFIED-RELEASE MEDICINES
▸ Adult: 75 mg once daily, increased if necessary up to 225 mg once daily, dose to be increased at intervals of at least 2 weeks; maximum 225 mg per day

Social anxiety disorder
▸ BY MOUTH USING MODIFIED-RELEASE MEDICINES
▸ Adult: 75 mg once daily, there is no evidence of greater efficacy at higher doses, increased if necessary up to 225 mg once daily, dose to be increased if necessary at intervals of at least 2 weeks; maximum 225 mg per day

Menopausal symptoms, particularly hot flushes, in women with breast cancer
▸ BY MOUTH USING MODIFIED-RELEASE MEDICINES
▸ Adult: 37.5 mg once daily for one week, then increased if necessary to 75 mg once daily

● UNLICENSED USE [EvGr] Not licensed for menopausal symptoms. Ⓐ

● CONTRA-INDICATIONS Conditions associated with high risk of cardiac arrhythmia · uncontrolled hypertension

● CAUTIONS Diabetes · heart disease (monitor blood pressure) · history of bleeding disorders · history of epilepsy · history or family history of mania · susceptibility to angle-closure glaucoma

● INTERACTIONS → Appendix 1: venlafaxine

● SIDE-EFFECTS
▸ **Common or very common** Anxiety · appetite decreased · arrhythmias · asthenia · chills · confusion · constipation · depersonalisation · diarrhoea · dizziness · dry mouth · dyspnoea · headache · hot flush · hypertension · menstrual cycle irregularities · movement disorders · muscle tone increased · mydriasis · nausea · palpitations · paraesthesia · sedation · sexual dysfunction · skin reactions · sleep disorders · sweat changes · taste altered · tinnitus · tremor · urinary disorders · vision disorders · vomiting · weight changes · yawning
▸ **Uncommon** Alopecia · angioedema · apathy · behaviour abnormal · derealisation · haemorrhage · hallucination · hypotension · mood altered · photosensitivity reaction · syncope
▸ **Rare or very rare** Agranulocytosis · angle closure glaucoma · bone marrow disorders · delirium · hepatitis · hyponatraemia · neuroleptic malignant syndrome · neutropenia · pancreatitis · QT interval prolongation · respiratory disorders · rhabdomyolysis · seizure · serotonin syndrome · severe cutaneous adverse reactions (SCARs) · SIADH · thrombocytopenia
▸ **Frequency not known** Suicidal tendencies · vertigo · withdrawal syndrome

Nervous system

4

- PREGNANCY Avoid unless potential benefit outweighs risk—toxicity in *animal* studies. Risk of withdrawal effects in neonate.
- BREAST FEEDING Present in milk—avoid.
- HEPATIC IMPAIRMENT
  Dose adjustments Consider reducing dose by 50% in mild or moderate impairment; use with caution and reduce dose by at least 50% in severe impairment.
- RENAL IMPAIRMENT Use with caution.
  Dose adjustments Use half normal dose (immediate-release tablets may be given once daily) if eGFR less than 30 mL/minute/1.73 m^2.
- TREATMENT CESSATION Associated with a higher risk of withdrawal effects compared with other antidepressants.
  Gastro-intestinal disturbances, headache, anxiety, dizziness, paraesthesia, tremor, sleep disturbances, and sweating are most common features of withdrawal if treatment stopped abruptly or if dose reduced markedly; dose should be reduced over several weeks.
- PATIENT AND CARER ADVICE
  Driving and skilled tasks May affect performance of skilled tasks (e.g. driving).

- MEDICINAL FORMS
  There can be variation in the licensing of different medicines containing the same drug. Forms available from special-order manufacturers include: oral suspension, oral solution

Modified-release tablet
CAUTIONARY AND ADVISORY LABELS 3, 21, 25
- Sunveniz XL (Sun Pharmaceuticals UK Ltd)
  Venlafaxine (as Venlafaxine hydrochloride) 75 mg Sunveniz XL 75mg tablets | 30 tablet [PoM] £11.14 DT = £2.60
  Venlafaxine (as Venlafaxine hydrochloride) 150 mg Sunveniz XL 150mg tablets | 30 tablet [PoM] £18.64 DT = £3.90
- Venladex XL (Dexcel-Pharma Ltd)
  Venlafaxine (as Venlafaxine hydrochloride) 75 mg Venladex XL 75mg tablets | 28 tablet [PoM] £11.20
  Venlafaxine (as Venlafaxine hydrochloride) 150 mg Venladex XL 150mg tablets | 28 tablet [PoM] £18.70
- Venlalic XL (Ethypharm UK Ltd)
  Venlafaxine (as Venlafaxine hydrochloride) 37.5 mg Venlalic XL 37.5mg tablets | 30 tablet [PoM] £6.60 DT = £6.60
  Venlafaxine (as Venlafaxine hydrochloride) 75 mg Venlalic XL 75mg tablets | 30 tablet [PoM] £2.60 DT = £2.60
  Venlafaxine (as Venlafaxine hydrochloride) 150 mg Venlalic XL 150mg tablets | 30 tablet [PoM] £3.90 DT = £3.90
  Venlafaxine (as Venlafaxine hydrochloride) 225 mg Venlalic XL 225mg tablets | 30 tablet [PoM] £33.60 DT = £33.60
- ViePax XL (Dexcel-Pharma Ltd)
  Venlafaxine (as Venlafaxine hydrochloride) 75 mg ViePax XL 75mg tablets | 28 tablet [PoM] £2.60
  Venlafaxine (as Venlafaxine hydrochloride) 150 mg ViePax XL 150mg tablets | 28 tablet [PoM] £3.90

Tablet
CAUTIONARY AND ADVISORY LABELS 3
- Venlafaxine (Non-proprietary)
  Venlafaxine (as Venlafaxine hydrochloride) 37.5 mg Venlafaxine 37.5mg tablets | 56 tablet [PoM] £6.99 DT = £1.97
  Venlafaxine (as Venlafaxine hydrochloride) 75 mg Venlafaxine 75mg tablets | 56 tablet [PoM] £6.06 DT = £1.94
- ViePax (Dexcel-Pharma Ltd)
  Venlafaxine (as Venlafaxine hydrochloride) 37.5 mg ViePax 37.5mg tablets | 56 tablet [PoM] £21.07 DT = £1.97
  Venlafaxine (as Venlafaxine hydrochloride) 75 mg ViePax 75mg tablets | 56 tablet [PoM] £35.13 DT = £1.94

Modified-release capsule
CAUTIONARY AND ADVISORY LABELS 3, 21, 25
- Venlafaxine (Non-proprietary)
  Venlafaxine (as Venlafaxine hydrochloride) 75 mg Venlafaxine 75mg modified-release capsules | 28 capsule [PoM] [⃰] DT = £2.60
  Venlafaxine (as Venlafaxine hydrochloride) 150 mg Venlafaxine 150mg modified-release capsules | 28 capsule [PoM] [⃰] DT = £3.90
  Venlafaxine (as Venlafaxine hydrochloride) 225 mg Venlafaxine 225mg modified-release capsules | 30 capsule [PoM] £44.75

- Alventa XL (Consilient Health Ltd)
  Venlafaxine (as Venlafaxine hydrochloride) 75 mg Alventa XL 75mg capsules | 28 capsule [PoM] £19.12 DT = £2.60
  Venlafaxine (as Venlafaxine hydrochloride) 150 mg Alventa XL 150mg capsules | 28 capsule [PoM] £31.88 DT = £3.90
- Depefex XL (Chiesi Ltd)
  Venlafaxine (as Venlafaxine hydrochloride) 75 mg Depefex XL 75mg capsules | 28 capsule [PoM] £10.40 DT = £2.60
  Venlafaxine (as Venlafaxine hydrochloride) 150 mg Depefex XL 150mg capsules | 28 capsule [PoM] £17.40 DT = £3.90
- Efexor XL (Pfizer Ltd)
  Venlafaxine (as Venlafaxine hydrochloride) 75 mg Efexor XL 75mg capsules | 28 capsule [PoM] £22.08 DT = £2.60
  Venlafaxine (as Venlafaxine hydrochloride) 150 mg Efexor XL 150mg capsules | 28 capsule [PoM] £36.81 DT = £3.90
  Venlafaxine (as Venlafaxine hydrochloride) 225 mg Efexor XL 225mg capsules | 28 capsule [PoM] £47.11 DT = £47.11
- Politid XL (Actavis UK Ltd)
  Venlafaxine (as Venlafaxine hydrochloride) 75 mg Politid XL 75mg capsules | 28 capsule [PoM] £23.41 DT = £2.60
  Venlafaxine (as Venlafaxine hydrochloride) 150 mg Politid XL 150mg capsules | 28 capsule [PoM] £39.03 DT = £3.90
- Rodomel XL (Teva UK Ltd)
  Venlafaxine (as Venlafaxine hydrochloride) 75 mg Rodomel XL 75mg capsules | 28 capsule [PoM] £17.91 DT = £2.60
  Venlafaxine (as Venlafaxine hydrochloride) 150 mg Rodomel XL 150mg capsules | 28 capsule [PoM] £29.85 DT = £3.90
- Tonpular XL (Wockhardt UK Ltd)
  Venlafaxine (as Venlafaxine hydrochloride) 75 mg Tonpular XL 75mg capsules | 28 capsule [PoM] £7.00 DT = £2.60
  Venlafaxine (as Venlafaxine hydrochloride) 150 mg Tonpular XL 150mg capsules | 28 capsule [PoM] £12.00 DT = £3.90
- Venaxx XL (AMCo)
  Venlafaxine (as Venlafaxine hydrochloride) 75 mg Venaxx XL 75mg capsules | 28 capsule [PoM] £10.40 DT = £2.60
  Venlafaxine (as Venlafaxine hydrochloride) 150 mg Venaxx XL 150mg capsules | 28 capsule [PoM] £17.40 DT = £3.90
- Vencarm XL (Aspire Pharma Ltd)
  Venlafaxine (as Venlafaxine hydrochloride) 37.5 mg Vencarm XL 37.5mg capsules | 28 capsule [PoM] £3.30 DT = £5.25
  Venlafaxine (as Venlafaxine hydrochloride) 75 mg Vencarm XL 75mg capsules | 28 capsule [PoM] £2.59 DT = £2.60
  Venlafaxine (as Venlafaxine hydrochloride) 150 mg Vencarm XL 150mg capsules | 28 capsule [PoM] £3.89 DT = £3.90
  Venlafaxine (as Venlafaxine hydrochloride) 225 mg Vencarm XL 225mg capsules | 28 capsule [PoM] £9.90 DT = £47.11
- Venlablue XL (Creo Pharma Ltd)
  Venlafaxine (as Venlafaxine hydrochloride) 37.5 mg Venlablue XL 37.5mg capsules | 28 capsule [PoM] £5.25 DT = £5.25
  Venlafaxine (as Venlafaxine hydrochloride) 75 mg Venlablue XL 75mg capsules | 28 capsule [PoM] £6.95 DT = £2.60
  Venlafaxine (as Venlafaxine hydrochloride) 150 mg Venlablue XL 150mg capsules | 28 capsule [PoM] £9.95 DT = £3.90
- Venlasov XL (Sovereign Medical Ltd)
  Venlafaxine (as Venlafaxine hydrochloride) 75 mg Venlasov XL 75mg capsules | 28 capsule [PoM] £2.45 DT = £2.60
  Venlafaxine (as Venlafaxine hydrochloride) 150 mg Venlasov XL 150mg capsules | 28 capsule [PoM] £3.75 DT = £3.90
- Vensir XL (Morningside Healthcare Ltd)
  Venlafaxine (as Venlafaxine hydrochloride) 75 mg Vensir XL 75mg capsules | 28 capsule [PoM] £2.60 DT = £2.60
  Venlafaxine (as Venlafaxine hydrochloride) 150 mg Vensir XL 150mg capsules | 28 capsule [PoM] £3.90 DT = £3.90
  Venlafaxine (as Venlafaxine hydrochloride) 225 mg Vensir XL 225mg capsules | 28 capsule [PoM] £21.90 DT = £47.11

ANTIDEPRESSANTS > SEROTONIN UPTAKE INHIBITORS

Trazodone hydrochloride

- INDICATIONS AND DOSE

Depressive illness (particularly where sedation is required)
- BY MOUTH
- Adult: Initially 150 mg daily in divided doses, dose to be taken after food, alternatively initially 150 mg once

daily, dose to be taken at bedtime, increased if necessary to 300 mg daily; increased if necessary to 600 mg daily in divided doses, higher dose for use in hospital patients only
▸ Elderly: Initially 100 mg daily in divided doses, dose to be taken after food, alternatively initially 100 mg once daily, dose to be taken at bedtime, increased if necessary to 300 mg daily; increased if necessary to 600 mg daily in divided doses, higher dose for use in hospital patients only

Anxiety
▸ BY MOUTH
▸ Adult: 75 mg daily, increased if necessary to 300 mg daily

● CONTRA-INDICATIONS Arrhythmias · during the manic phase of bipolar disorder · heart block · immediate recovery period after myocardial infarction
● CAUTIONS Cardiovascular disease · chronic constipation · diabetes · epilepsy · history of bipolar disorder · history of psychosis · hyperthyroidism (risk of arrhythmias) · increased intra-ocular pressure · patients with a significant risk of suicide · phaeochromocytoma (risk of arrhythmias) · prostatic hypertrophy · susceptibility to angle-closure glaucoma · urinary retention
CAUTIONS, FURTHER INFORMATION Treatment should be stopped if the patient enters a manic phase.
Elderly patients are particularly susceptible to many of the side-effects of tricyclic antidepressants; low initial doses should be used, with close monitoring, particularly for psychiatric and cardiac side-effects.
● INTERACTIONS → Appendix 1: trazodone
● SIDE-EFFECTS Aggression · agranulocytosis · alertness decreased · anaemia · anxiety · aphasia · appetite abnormal · arrhythmias · arthralgia · asthenia · blood disorder · chest pain · confusion · constipation · delirium · delusions · diarrhoea · dizziness · drowsiness · dry mouth · dyspnoea · eosinophilia · fever · gastroenteritis · gastrointestinal discomfort · hallucination · headache · hepatic disorders · hyperhidrosis · hypersalivation · hypertension · hyponatraemia · influenza like illness · leucopenia · libido decreased · mania · memory loss · movement disorders · myalgia · nasal congestion · nausea · neuroleptic malignant syndrome · oedema · pain · palpitations · paraesthesia · paralytic ileus · postural hypotension · priapism (discontinue) · QT interval prolongation · seizure · serotonin syndrome · SIADH · skin reactions · sleep disorders · suicidal tendencies · syncope · taste altered · thrombocytopenia · tremor · urinary disorder · vertigo · vision blurred · vomiting · weight decreased · withdrawal syndrome
SIDE-EFFECTS, FURTHER INFORMATION The risk of side-effects is reduced by titrating slowly to the minimum effective dose (every 2–3 days). Consider using a lower starting dose in elderly patients.
Overdose The tricyclic-related antidepressant drugs may be associated with a lower risk of cardiotoxicity in overdosage.
Tricyclic and related antidepressants cause dry mouth, coma of varying degree, hypotension, hypothermia, hyperreflexia, extensor plantar responses, convulsions, respiratory failure, cardiac conduction defects, and arrhythmias. Dilated pupils and urinary retention also occur. For details on the management of poisoning see Tricyclic and related antidepressants under Emergency treatment of pcisoning p. 1319.
● PREGNANCY Avoid during first trimester—limited information available. Monitor infant for signs of withdrawal if used until delivery.
● BREAST FEEDING The amount secreted into breast milk is too small to be harmful.

● HEPATIC IMPAIRMENT Sedative effects are increased in hepatic impairment. Avoid in severe liver disease.
● RENAL IMPAIRMENT Use with caution in severe impairment.
● TREATMENT CESSATION Withdrawal effects may occur within 5 days of stopping treatment with antidepressant drugs; they are usually mild and self-limiting, but in some cases may be severe. The risk of withdrawal symptoms is increased if the antidepressant is stopped suddenly after regular administration for 8 weeks or more. The dose should preferably be reduced gradually over about 4 weeks, or longer if withdrawal symptoms emerge (6 months in patients who have been on long-term maintenance treatment). If possible tricyclic and related antidepressants should be withdrawn slowly.
● PRESCRIBING AND DISPENSING INFORMATION Limited quantities of tricyclic antidepressants should be prescribed at any one time because their cardiovascular and epileptogenic effects are dangerous in overdosage.
● PATIENT AND CARER ADVICE
Driving and skilled tasks Drowsiness may affect the performance of skilled tasks (e.g. driving).
Effects of alcohol enhanced.

● MEDICINAL FORMS
There can be variation in the licensing of different medicines containing the same drug. Forms available from special-order manufacturers include: oral suspension, oral solution
Oral solution
CAUTIONARY AND ADVISORY LABELS 2, 21
▸ Trazodone hydrochloride (Non-proprietary)
Trazodone hydrochloride 10 mg per 1 ml Trazodone 50mg/5ml oral solution sugar free sugar-free | 120 ml [PoM] £180.00 DT = £109.20
Trazodone hydrochloride 20 mg per 1 ml Trazodone 100mg/5ml oral solution sugar free sugar-free | 120 ml [PoM] £163.00-£195.60
Tablet
CAUTIONARY AND ADVISORY LABELS 2, 21
▸ Trazodone hydrochloride (Non-proprietary)
Trazodone hydrochloride 150 mg Trazodone 150mg tablets | 28 tablet [PoM] £36.15 DT = £7.46
▸ Molipaxin (Zentiva)
Trazodone hydrochloride 150 mg Molipaxin 150mg tablets | 28 tablet [PoM] £16.08 DT = £7.46
Capsule
CAUTIONARY AND ADVISORY LABELS 2, 21
▸ Trazodone hydrochloride (Non-proprietary)
Trazodone hydrochloride 50 mg Trazodone 50mg capsules | 84 capsule [PoM] £36.20 DT = £7.11
Trazodone hydrochloride 100 mg Trazodone 100mg capsules | 56 capsule [PoM] £52.10 DT = £7.59
▸ Molipaxin (Zentiva)
Trazodone hydrochloride 50 mg Molipaxin 50mg capsules | 84 capsule [PoM] £23.92 DT = £7.11
Trazodone hydrochloride 100 mg Molipaxin 100mg capsules | 56 capsule [PoM] £28.14 DT = £7.59

ANTIDEPRESSANTS ⟩ TETRACYCLIC ANTIDEPRESSANTS

Mianserin hydrochloride

● INDICATIONS AND DOSE
Depressive illness (particularly where sedation is required)
▸ BY MOUTH
▸ Adult: Initially 30–40 mg daily in divided doses, alternatively initially 30–40 mg once daily, dose to be taken at bedtime, increase dose gradually as necessary; usual dose 30–90 mg
▸ Elderly: Initially 30 mg daily in divided doses, alternatively initially 30 mg once daily, dose to be taken at bedtime, increase dose gradually as necessary; usual dose 30–90 mg

- CONTRA-INDICATIONS Acute porphyrias p. 1025 · arrhythmias · during the manic phase of bipolar disorder · heart block · immediate recovery period after myocardial infarction
- CAUTIONS Cardiovascular disease · chronic constipation · diabetes · epilepsy · history of bipolar disorder · history of psychosis · hyperthyroidism (risk of arrhythmias) · increased intra-ocular pressure · patients with a significant risk of suicide · phaeochromocytoma (risk of arrhythmias) · prostatic hypertrophy · susceptibility to angle-closure glaucoma · urinary retention

  CAUTIONS, FURTHER INFORMATION Treatment should be stopped if the patient enters a manic phase.

  Elderly patients are particularly susceptible to many of the side-effects of tricyclic antidepressants; low initial doses should be used, with close monitoring, particularly for psychiatric and cardiac side-effects.
- INTERACTIONS → Appendix 1: mianserin
- SIDE-EFFECTS Agranulocytosis · arthritis · bone marrow disorders · breast abnormalities · dizziness · granulocytopenia · gynaecomastia · hepatic disorders · hyperhidrosis · hyponatraemia · joint disorders · lactation in absence of pregnancy · leucopenia · mood altered · neuromuscular irritability · oedema · paranoid delusions · postural hypotension · psychosis · rash · seizure · sexual dysfunction · suicidal tendencies · tremor · withdrawal syndrome

  SIDE-EFFECTS, FURTHER INFORMATION The risk of side-effects is reduced by titrating slowly to the minimum effective dose (every 2–3 days). Consider using a lower starting dose in elderly patients.

  Overdose The tricyclic-related antidepressant drugs may be associated with a lower risk of cardiotoxicity in overdosage.

  Tricyclic and related antidepressants cause dry mouth, coma of varying degree, hypotension, hypothermia, hyperreflexia, extensor plantar responses, convulsions, respiratory failure, cardiac conduction defects, and arrhythmias. Dilated pupils and urinary retention also occur. For details on the management of poisoning see Tricyclic and related antidepressants under Emergency treatment of poisoning p. 1319.
- PREGNANCY Avoid.
- BREAST FEEDING The amount secreted into breast milk is too small to be harmful.
- HEPATIC IMPAIRMENT Sedative effects are increased in hepatic impairment. Avoid in severe liver disease.
- RENAL IMPAIRMENT
  Dose adjustments Caution in renal impairment.
- MONITORING REQUIREMENTS A full **blood count** is recommended every 4 weeks during the first 3 months of treatment; clinical monitoring should continue subsequently and treatment should be stopped and a full blood count obtained if *fever, sore throat, stomatitis,* or other signs of infection develop.
- TREATMENT CESSATION Withdrawal effects may occur within 5 days of stopping treatment with antidepressant drugs; they are usually mild and self-limiting, but in some cases may be severe. The risk of withdrawal symptoms is increased if the antidepressant is stopped suddenly after regular administration for 8 weeks or more. The dose should preferably be reduced gradually over about 4 weeks, or longer if withdrawal symptoms emerge (6 months in patients who have been on long-term maintenance treatment). If possible tricyclic and related antidepressants should be withdrawn slowly.
- PRESCRIBING AND DISPENSING INFORMATION Limited quantities of tricyclic antidepressants should be prescribed at any one time because their cardiovascular and epileptogenic effects are dangerous in overdosage.

- PATIENT AND CARER ADVICE
  Driving and skilled tasks Drowsiness may affect the performance of skilled tasks (e.g. driving). Effects of alcohol enhanced.

- MEDICINAL FORMS
  There can be variation in the licensing of different medicines containing the same drug. Forms available from special-order manufacturers include: oral suspension, oral solution

  Tablet
  CAUTIONARY AND ADVISORY LABELS 2, 25
  ▶ Mianserin hydrochloride (Non-proprietary)
    Mianserin hydrochloride 10 mg Mianserin 10mg tablets | 28 tablet PoM £8.58 DT = £8.58
    Mianserin hydrochloride 30 mg Mianserin 30mg tablets | 28 tablet PoM £23.39 DT = £18.34

Mirtazapine

- DRUG ACTION Mirtazapine is a presynaptic alpha$_2$-adrenoreceptor antagonist which increases central noradrenergic and serotonergic neurotransmission.

- INDICATIONS AND DOSE
  Major depression
  ▶ BY MOUTH
    ▶ **Adult:** Initially 15–30 mg daily for 2–4 weeks, dose to be taken at bedtime, then adjusted according to response to up to 45 mg once daily, alternatively up to 45 mg daily in 2 divided doses

- CAUTIONS Cardiac disorders · diabetes mellitus · elderly · history of bipolar depression · history of seizures · history of urinary retention · hypotension · psychoses (may aggravate psychotic symptoms) · susceptibility to angle-closure glaucoma
- INTERACTIONS → Appendix 1: mirtazapine
- SIDE-EFFECTS
  ▶ **Common or very common** Anxiety · appetite increased · arthralgia · back pain · confusion · constipation · diarrhoea · dizziness · drowsiness · dry mouth · fatigue · headache (on discontinuation) · myalgia · nausea · oedema · postural hypotension · sleep disorders · tremor · vomiting · weight increased
  ▶ **Uncommon** Hallucination · mania · movement disorders · oral disorders · syncope
  ▶ **Rare or very rare** Aggression · pancreatitis
  ▶ **Frequency not known** Agranulocytosis · arrhythmias · bone marrow disorders · dysarthria · eosinophilia · granulocytopenia · hyponatraemia · QT interval prolongation · rhabdomyolysis · seizure · serotonin syndrome · severe cutaneous adverse reactions (SCARs) · SIADH · skin reactions · sudden death · suicidal tendencies · thrombocytopenia · urinary retention · withdrawal syndrome
- PREGNANCY Use with caution—limited experience; monitor neonate for withdrawal effects.
- BREAST FEEDING Present in milk; use only if potential benefit outweighs risk.
- HEPATIC IMPAIRMENT Use with caution. Discontinue if jaundice occurs.
- RENAL IMPAIRMENT Clearance reduced by 30% if eGFR less than 40 mL/minute/1.73 m^2; clearance reduced by 50% if eGFR less than 10 mL/minute/1.73 m^2.
- TREATMENT CESSATION Nausea, vomiting, dizziness, agitation, anxiety, and headache are most common features of withdrawal if treatment stopped abruptly or if dose reduced markedly; dose should be reduced over several weeks.
- DIRECTIONS FOR ADMINISTRATION Orodispersible tablet (*Zispin SolTab*®) should be placed on the tongue, allowed to disperse and swallowed.

• PATIENT AND CARER ADVICE Counselling on administration of orodispersible tablet advised.
Blood Disorders Patients should be advised to report any fever, sore throat, stomatitis or other signs of infection during treatment. Blood count should be performed and the drug stopped immediately if blood dyscrasia suspected.

• MEDICINAL FORMS
There can be variation in the licensing of different medicines containing the same drug. Forms available from special-order manufacturers include: capsule, oral suspension, oral solution

Tablet
CAUTIONARY AND ADVISORY LABELS 2, 25
▸ Mirtazapine (Non-proprietary)
Mirtazapine 15 mg Mirtazapine 15mg tablets | 28 tablet [PoM]
£4.60 DT = £2.28
Mirtazapine 30 mg Mirtazapine 30mg tablets | 28 tablet [PoM]
£17.50 DT = £1.04
Mirtazapine 45 mg Mirtazapine 45mg tablets | 28 tablet [PoM]
£4.95 DT = £2.32

Oral solution
CAUTIONARY AND ADVISORY LABELS 2
▸ Mirtazapine (Non-proprietary)
Mirtazapine 15 mg per 1 ml Mirtazapine 15mg/ml oral solution sugar free sugar-free | 66 ml [PoM] £49.51 DT = £49.51

Orodispersible tablet
CAUTIONARY AND ADVISORY LABELS 2
EXCIPIENTS: May contain Aspartame
▸ Mirtazapine (Non-proprietary)
Mirtazapine 15 mg Mirtazapine 15mg orodispersible tablets | 30 tablet [PoM] £19.19 DT = £1.00
Mirtazapine 30 mg Mirtazapine 30mg orodispersible tablets | 30 tablet [PoM] £19.19 DT = £1.17
Mirtazapine 45 mg Mirtazapine 45mg orodispersible tablets | 30 tablet [PoM] £19.19 DT = £1.68
▸ Zispin SolTab (Merck Sharp & Dohme Ltd)
Mirtazapine 15 mg Zispin SolTab 15mg orodispersible tablets | 30 tablet [PoM] £15.06 DT = £1.00
Mirtazapine 30 mg Zispin SolTab 30mg orodispersible tablets | 30 tablet [PoM] £15.06 DT = £1.17
Mirtazapine 45 mg Zispin SolTab 45mg orodispersible tablets | 30 tablet [PoM] £15.06 DT = £1.68

ANTIDEPRESSANTS › TRICYCLIC ANTIDEPRESSANTS

Amitriptyline hydrochloride

• INDICATIONS AND DOSE

Abdominal pain or discomfort (in patients who have not responded to laxatives, loperamide, or antispasmodics)
▸ BY MOUTH
▸ Adult: Initially 5–10 mg daily, to be taken at night; increased in steps of 10 mg at least every 2 weeks as required; maximum 30 mg per day

Major depressive disorder [not recommended—increased risk of fatality in overdose]
▸ BY MOUTH
▸ Adult: Initially 50 mg daily in 2 divided doses, then increased in steps of 25 mg once daily on alternate days if required, maximum 150 mg daily in 2 divided doses
▸ Elderly: Initially 10–25 mg daily, increased if necessary up to 100–150 mg daily in 2 divided doses, dose increases dependent on individual patient response and tolerability—doses above 100 mg should be used with caution

Major depressive disorder in patients with cardiovascular disease [not recommended—increased risk of fatality in overdose]
▸ BY MOUTH
▸ Adult: Initially 10–25 mg daily, increased if necessary up to 100–150 mg daily in 2 divided doses, dose increases dependent on individual patient response and tolerability—doses above 100 mg should be used with caution

Neuropathic pain | Migraine prophylaxis | Chronic tension-type headache prophylaxis
▸ BY MOUTH
▸ Adult: Initially 10–25 mg daily, dose to be taken in the evening, then increased, if tolerated, in steps of 10–25 mg every 3–7 days in 1–2 divided doses; usual dose 25–75 mg daily, dose to be taken in the evening, doses above 100 mg should be used with caution (doses above 75 mg should be used with caution in the elderly and in patients with cardiovascular disease); maximum per dose 75 mg

• UNLICENSED USE Not licensed for use in abdominal pain or discomfort in patients who have not responded to laxatives, loperamide, or antispasmodics.

• CONTRA-INDICATIONS Arrhythmias · during manic phase of bipolar disorder · heart block · immediate recovery period after myocardial infarction

• CAUTIONS Cardiovascular disease · chronic constipation · diabetes · epilepsy · history of bipolar disorder · history of psychosis · hyperthyroidism (risk of arrhythmias) · increased intra-ocular pressure · patients with a significant risk of suicide · phaeochromocytoma (risk of arrhythmias) · prostatic hypertrophy · susceptibility to angle-closure glaucoma · urinary retention
CAUTIONS, FURTHER INFORMATION Treatment should be stopped if the patient enters a manic phase.
Elderly patients are particularly susceptible to many of the side-effects of tricyclic antidepressants; low initial doses should be used, with close monitoring, particularly for psychiatric and cardiac side-effects.

• INTERACTIONS → Appendix 1: tricyclic antidepressants

• SIDE-EFFECTS
▸ **Common or very common** Anticholinergic syndrome · drowsiness · QT interval prolongation
▸ **Frequency not known** Agranulocytosis · alopecia · anxiety · appetite abnormal · arrhythmias · asthenia · bone marrow depression · breast enlargement · cardiac conduction disorders · coma · concentration impaired · confusion · constipation · delirium · delusions · diarrhoea · dizziness · dry mouth · dysarthria · eosinophilia · epigastric distress · face oedema · galactorrhoea · gynaecomastia · hallucination · headache · hepatic disorders · hyperhidrosis · hyperpyrexia · hypertension · hyponatraemia · hypotension · leucopenia · mood altered · movement disorders · mydriasis · myocardial infarction · nausea · neuroleptic malignant syndrome · oral disorders · palpitations · paralytic ileus · peripheral neuropathy · photosensitivity reaction · seizure · sensation abnormal · sexual dysfunction · SIADH · skin reactions · sleep disorders · stroke · sudden cardiac death · suicidal tendencies · syncope · taste altered · testicular swelling · thrombocytopenia · tinnitus · tremor · urinary disorders · urinary tract dilation · vision disorders · vomiting · weight changes · withdrawal syndrome
SIDE-EFFECTS, FURTHER INFORMATION The risk of side-effects is reduced by titrating slowly to the minimum effective dose (every 2–3 days). Consider using a lower starting dose in elderly patients.
Overdose Overdosage with amitriptyline is associated with a relatively high rate of fatality. Symptoms of overdosage may include dry mouth, coma of varying degree, hypotension, hypothermia, hyperreflexia, extensor plantar responses, convulsions, respiratory failure, cardiac conduction defects, and arrhythmias. Dilated pupils and urinary retention also occur. For details on the management of poisoning, see Tricyclic and related antidepressants, under Emergency treatment of poisoning p. 1319.

• PREGNANCY Use only if potential benefit outweighs risk.

- BREAST FEEDING The amount secreted into breast milk is too small to be harmful.
- HEPATIC IMPAIRMENT Sedative effects are increased in hepatic impairment. Avoid in severe liver disease.
- TREATMENT CESSATION Withdrawal effects may occur within 5 days of stopping treatment with antidepressant drugs; they are usually mild and self-limiting, but in some cases may be severe. The risk of withdrawal symptoms is increased if the antidepressant is stopped suddenly after regular administration for 8 weeks or more. The dose should preferably be reduced gradually over about 4 weeks, or longer if withdrawal symptoms emerge (6 months in patients who have been on long-term maintenance treatment). If possible tricyclic and related antidepressants should be withdrawn slowly.
- PRESCRIBING AND DISPENSING INFORMATION Limited quantities of tricyclic antidepressants should be prescribed at any one time because their cardiovascular and epileptogenic effects are dangerous in overdosage.
- PATIENT AND CARER ADVICE
  Driving and skilled tasks Drowsiness may affect the performance of skilled tasks (e.g. driving). Effects of alcohol enhanced.
- LESS SUITABLE FOR PRESCRIBING Amitriptyline hydrochloride is less suitable for prescribing, see Tricyclic and related antidepressant drugs in Antidepressant drugs p. 355.

- MEDICINAL FORMS
  There can be variation in the licensing of different medicines containing the same drug. Forms available from special-order manufacturers include: oral suspension, oral solution
  Oral solution
  CAUTIONARY AND ADVISORY LABELS 2
  ▸ Amitriptyline hydrochloride (Non-proprietary)
    Amitriptyline hydrochloride 2 mg per 1 ml Amitriptyline 10mg/5ml oral solution sugar free sugar-free | 150 ml [PoM] £122.76 DT = £111.96
    Amitriptyline hydrochloride 5 mg per 1 ml Amitriptyline 25mg/5ml oral solution sugar free sugar-free | 150 ml [PoM] £18.00 DT = £18.00
    Amitriptyline hydrochloride 10 mg per 1 ml Amitriptyline 50mg/5ml oral solution sugar free sugar-free | 150 ml [PoM] £24.00 DT = £19.20
  Tablet
  CAUTIONARY AND ADVISORY LABELS 2
  ▸ Amitriptyline hydrochloride (Non-proprietary)
    Amitriptyline hydrochloride 10 mg Amitriptyline 10mg tablets | 28 tablet [PoM] £1.50 DT = £0.97
    Amitriptyline hydrochloride 25 mg Amitriptyline 25mg tablets | 28 tablet [PoM] £1.75 DT = £0.74
    Amitriptyline hydrochloride 50 mg Amitriptyline 50mg tablets | 28 tablet [PoM] £5.99 DT = £2.46

Amitriptyline with perphenazine

The properties listed below are those particular to the combination only. For the properties of the components please consider, amitriptyline hydrochloride p. 369, perphenazine p. 384.

- **INDICATIONS AND DOSE**
  Depression with anxiety
  ▸ BY MOUTH
  ▸ Adult: 1 tablet 3 times a day, an additional tablet may be taken at bedtime when required

- INTERACTIONS → Appendix 1: phenothiazines · tricyclic antidepressants
- LESS SUITABLE FOR PRESCRIBING Less suitable for prescribing.

- MEDICINAL FORMS
  No licensed medicines listed.

Clomipramine hydrochloride

- **INDICATIONS AND DOSE**
  Depressive illness
  ▸ BY MOUTH
  ▸ Adult: Initially 10 mg daily, then increased if necessary to 30–150 mg daily in divided doses, dose to be increased gradually, alternatively increased if necessary to 30–150 mg once daily, dose to be taken at bedtime; maximum 250 mg per day
  ▸ Elderly: Initially 10 mg daily, then increased to 30–75 mg daily, dose to be increased carefully over approximately 10 days
  Phobic and obsessional states
  ▸ BY MOUTH
  ▸ Adult: Initially 25 mg daily, then increased to 100–150 mg daily, dose to be increased gradually over 2 weeks; maximum 250 mg per day
  ▸ Elderly: Initially 10 mg daily, then increased to 100–150 mg daily, dose to be increased gradually over 2 weeks; maximum 250 mg per day
  Adjunctive treatment of cataplexy associated with narcolepsy
  ▸ BY MOUTH
  ▸ Adult: Initially 10 mg daily, dose to be gradually increased until satisfactory response; increased if necessary to 10–75 mg daily

- CONTRA-INDICATIONS Acute porphyrias p. 1025 · arrhythmias · during the manic phase of bipolar disorder · heart block · immediate recovery period after myocardial infarction
- CAUTIONS Cardiovascular disease · chronic constipation · diabetes · epilepsy · history of bipolar disorder · history of psychosis · hyperthyroidism (risk of arrhythmias) · increased intra-ocular pressure · patients with a significant risk of suicide · phaeochromocytoma (risk of arrhythmias) · prostatic hypertrophy · susceptibility to angle-closure glaucoma · urinary retention
  CAUTIONS, FURTHER INFORMATION Treatment should be stopped if the patient enters a manic phase.
    Elderly patients are particularly susceptible to many of the side-effects of tricyclic antidepressants; low initial doses should be used, with close monitoring, particularly for psychiatric and cardiac side-effects.
- INTERACTIONS → Appendix 1: tricyclic antidepressants
- SIDE-EFFECTS
  ▸ Common or very common Aggression · anxiety · arrhythmias · breast enlargement · concentration impaired · confusion · constipation · delirium · depersonalisation · depression exacerbated · diarrhoea · dizziness · drowsiness · dry mouth · fatigue · galactorrhoea · gastrointestinal disorder · hallucination · headache · hot flush · hyperhidrosis · hypotension · memory loss · mood altered · movement disorders · muscle tone increased · muscle weakness · mydriasis · nausea · palpitations · paraesthesia · photosensitivity reaction · sexual dysfunction · skin reactions · sleep disorders · speech disorder · taste altered · tinnitus · tremor · urinary disorders · vision disorders · vomiting · weight increased · yawning
  ▸ Uncommon Psychosis · seizure
  ▸ Rare or very rare Agranulocytosis · alopecia · cardiac conduction disorders · eosinophilia · glaucoma · hepatic disorders · hyperpyrexia · leucopenia · neuroleptic malignant syndrome · oedema · QT interval prolongation · respiratory disorders · thrombocytopenia · vaginal haemorrhage
  ▸ Frequency not known Rhabdomyolysis · serotonin syndrome · suicidal tendencies · withdrawal syndrome
  SIDE-EFFECTS, FURTHER INFORMATION The patient should be encouraged to persist with treatment as some tolerance

to these side-effects seems to develop. The risk of side-effects is reduced by titrating slowly to the minimum effective dose (every 2–3 days). Consider using a lower starting dose in elderly patients.

Overdose Tricyclic and related antidepressants cause dry mouth, coma of varying degree, hypotension, hypothermia, hyperreflexia, extensor plantar responses, convulsions, respiratory failure, cardiac conduction defects, and arrhythmias. Dilated pupils and urinary retention also occur. For details on the management of poisoning see Tricyclic and related antidepressants under Emergency treatment of poisoning p. 1319.

- PREGNANCY Neonatal withdrawal symptoms reported if used during third trimester.
- BREAST FEEDING The amount secreted into breast milk is too small to be harmful.
- HEPATIC IMPAIRMENT Sedative effects are increased in hepatic impairment. Avoid in severe liver disease.
- TREATMENT CESSATION Withdrawal effects may occur within 5 days of stopping treatment with antidepressant drugs; they are usually mild and self-limiting, but in some cases may be severe. The risk of withdrawal symptoms is increased if the antidepressant is stopped suddenly after regular administration for 8 weeks or more. The dose should preferably be reduced gradually over about 4 weeks, or longer if withdrawal symptoms emerge (6 months in patients who have been on long-term maintenance treatment). If possible tricyclic and related antidepressants should be withdrawn slowly.
- PRESCRIBING AND DISPENSING INFORMATION Limited quantities of tricyclic antidepressants should be prescribed at any one time because their cardiovascular and epileptogenic effects are dangerous in overdosage.
- PATIENT AND CARER ADVICE
  Driving and skilled tasks Drowsiness may affect the performance of skilled tasks (e.g. driving). Effects of alcohol enhanced.

- MEDICINAL FORMS
  There can be variation in the licensing of different medicines containing the same drug. Forms available from special-order manufacturers include: oral suspension, oral solution
  Capsule
  CAUTIONARY AND ADVISORY LABELS 2
  ▸ Clomipramine hydrochloride (Non-proprietary)
  Clomipramine hydrochloride 10 mg Clomipramine 10mg capsules
  | 28 capsule [PoM] £6.72 DT = £1.22
  Clomipramine hydrochloride 25 mg Clomipramine 25mg capsules
  | 28 capsule [PoM] £9.36 DT = £1.48
  Clomipramine hydrochloride 50 mg Clomipramine 50mg capsules
  | 28 capsule [PoM] £11.76 DT = £1.88

Dosulepin hydrochloride

(Dothiepin hydrochloride)

- INDICATIONS AND DOSE

Depressive illness, particularly where sedation is required (not recommended—increased risk of fatality in overdose) (initiated by a specialist)
▸ BY MOUTH
▸ Adult: Initially 75 mg daily in divided doses, alternatively initially 75 mg once daily, dose to be taken at bedtime, increased if necessary to 150 mg daily, doses to be increased gradually; up to 225 mg daily in some circumstances (e.g. hospital use)
▸ Elderly: Initially 50–75 mg daily in divided doses, alternatively initially 50–75 mg once daily, dose to be taken at bedtime, increased if necessary to 75–150 mg daily, doses to be increased gradually; up to 225 mg daily in some circumstances (e.g. hospital use)

- CONTRA-INDICATIONS Acute porphyrias p. 1025 · arrhythmias · during the manic phase of bipolar disorder · heart block · immediate recovery period after myocardial infarction
- CAUTIONS Cardiovascular disease · chronic constipation · diabetes · epilepsy · history of bipolar disorder · history of psychosis · hyperthyroidism (risk of arrhythmias) · increased intra-ocular pressure · patients with a significant risk of suicide · phaeochromocytoma (risk of arrhythmias) · prostatic hypertrophy · susceptibility to angle-closure glaucoma · urinary retention

  CAUTIONS, FURTHER INFORMATION Treatment should be stopped if the patient enters a manic phase.
  Elderly patients are particularly susceptible to many of the side-effects of tricyclic antidepressants; low initial doses should be used, with close monitoring, particularly for psychiatric and cardiac side-effects.

- INTERACTIONS → Appendix 1: tricyclic antidepressants
- SIDE-EFFECTS Accommodation disorder · agranulocytosis · alveolitis · anticholinergic syndrome · appetite abnormal · arrhythmias · asthenia · bone marrow depression · cardiac conduction disorder · confusion · constipation · dizziness · drowsiness · dry mouth · endocrine disorder · eosinophilia · epigastric discomfort · galactorrhoea · gynaecomastia · hepatic disorders · hyperhidrosis · hypertension · hyponatraemia · hypotension · increased risk of fracture · leucopenia · mood altered · movement disorders · nausea · nervousness · paranoid delusions · photosensitivity reaction · psychosis · seizures · sexual dysfunction · SIADH · skin reactions · speech disorder · suicidal tendencies · testicular hypertrophy · thrombocytopenia · tremor · urinary hesitation · vomiting · weight changes · withdrawal syndrome

  SIDE-EFFECTS, FURTHER INFORMATION The risk of side-effects is reduced by titrating slowly to the minimum effective dose (every 2–3 days). Consider using a lower starting dose in elderly patients.

Overdose Overdosage with dosulepin is associated with a relatively high rate of fatality.
  Tricyclic and related antidepressants cause dry mouth, coma of varying degree, hypotension, hypothermia, hyperreflexia, extensor plantar responses, convulsions, respiratory failure, cardiac conduction defects, and arrhythmias. Dilated pupils and urinary retention also occur. For details on the management of poisoning see Tricyclic and related antidepressants under Emergency treatment of poisoning p. 1319.

- PREGNANCY Use only if potential benefit outweighs risk.
- BREAST FEEDING The amount secreted into breast milk is too small to be harmful.
- HEPATIC IMPAIRMENT Sedative effects are increased in hepatic impairment. Avoid in severe liver disease.
- TREATMENT CESSATION Withdrawal effects may occur within 5 days of stopping treatment with antidepressant drugs; they are usually mild and self-limiting, but in some cases may be severe. The risk of withdrawal symptoms is increased if the antidepressant is stopped suddenly after regular administration for 8 weeks or more. The dose should preferably be reduced gradually over about 4 weeks, or longer if withdrawal symptoms emerge. (6 months in patients who have been on long-term maintenance treatment). If possible tricyclic and related antidepressants should be withdrawn slowly.
- PRESCRIBING AND DISPENSING INFORMATION Limited quantities of tricyclic antidepressants should be prescribed at any one time because their cardiovascular and epileptogenic effects are dangerous in overdosage.
  A maximum prescription equivalent to 2 weeks' supply of 75 mg daily should be considered in patients with increased risk factors for suicide at initiation of

4 Nervous system

treatment, during any dose adjustment, and until improvement occurs.

- PATIENT AND CARER ADVICE
Driving and skilled tasks Drowsiness may affect the performance of skilled tasks (e.g. driving).
Effects of alcohol enhanced.

- LESS SUITABLE FOR PRESCRIBING Dosulepin hydrochloride is less suitable for prescribing, see Tricyclic and related antidepressant drugs in Antidepressant drugs p. 355.

- MEDICINAL FORMS
There can be variation in the licensing of different medicines containing the same drug. Forms available from special-order manufacturers include: oral suspension, oral solution
Tablet
CAUTIONARY AND ADVISORY LABELS 2
▸ Dosulepin hydrochloride (Non-proprietary)
Dosulepin hydrochloride 75 mg Dosulepin 75mg tablets | 28 tablet [PoM] £1.70 DT = £1.20
▸ Prothiaden (Teofarma)
Dosulepin hydrochloride 75 mg Prothiaden 75mg tablets | 28 tablet [PoM] £2.97 DT = £1.20
Capsule
CAUTIONARY AND ADVISORY LABELS 2
▸ Dosulepin hydrochloride (Non-proprietary)
Dosulepin hydrochloride 25 mg Dosulepin 25mg capsules | 28 capsule [PoM] £3.00 DT = £0.90
▸ Prothiaden (Teofarma)
Dosulepin hydrochloride 25 mg Prothiaden 25mg capsules | 28 capsule [PoM] £1.70 DT = £0.90

Doxepin

- INDICATIONS AND DOSE
Depressive illness (particularly where sedation is required)
▸ BY MOUTH
▸ Adult: Initially 75 mg daily in divided doses, alternatively 75 mg once daily, adjusted according to response, dose to taken at bedtime; maintenance 25–300 mg daily, doses above 100 mg given in 3 divided doses
▸ Elderly: Start with lower doses and adjust according to response

- CONTRA-INDICATIONS Acute porphyrias p. 1025 · arrhythmias · during manic phase of bipolar disorder · heart block · immediate recovery period after myocardial infarction

- CAUTIONS Cardiovascular disease · chronic constipation · diabetes · epilepsy · history of bipolar disorder · history of psychosis · hyperthyroidism (risk of arrhythmias) · increased intra-ocular pressure · patients with significant risk of suicide · phaeochromocytoma (risk of arrhythmias) · prostatic hypertrophy · susceptibility to angle-closure glaucoma · urinary retention
CAUTIONS, FURTHER INFORMATION Treatment should be stopped if the patient enters a manic phase.
Elderly patients are particularly susceptible to many of the side-effects of tricyclic antidepressants; low initial doses should be used, with close monitoring, particularly for psychiatric and cardiac side-effects.

- INTERACTIONS → Appendix 1: tricyclic antidepressants

- SIDE-EFFECTS Agitation · agranulocytosis · alopecia · anticholinergic syndrome · appetite decreased · asthenia · asthma exacerbated · bone marrow depression · breast enlargement · cardiovascular effects · chills · confusion · constipation · diarrhoea · dizziness · drowsiness · dry mouth · dyspepsia · eosinophilia · face oedema · flushing · galactorrhoea · gynaecomastia · haemolytic anaemia · hallucination · headache · hyperhidrosis · hyperpyrexia ·

increased risk of fracture · jaundice · leucopenia · mania · movement disorders · nausea · oral ulceration · paranoid delusions · photosensitivity reaction · postural hypotension · psychosis · seizure · sensation abnormal · sexual dysfunction · SIADH · skin reactions · sleep disorders · suicidal tendencies · tachycardia · taste altered · testicular swelling · thrombocytopenia · tinnitus · tremor · urinary retention · vision blurred · vomiting · weight increased

SIDE-EFFECTS, FURTHER INFORMATION The risk of side-effects is reduced by titrating slowly to the minimum effective dose (every 2–3 days). Consider using a lower starting dose in elderly patients.

Overdose Tricyclic and related antidepressants cause dry mouth, coma of varying degree, hypotension, hypothermia, hyperreflexia, extensor plantar responses, convulsions, respiratory failure, cardiac conduction defects, and arrhythmias. Dilated pupils and urinary retention also occur. For details on the management of poisoning see Tricyclic and related antidepressants under Emergency treatment of poisoning p. 1319.

- PREGNANCY Use with caution—limited information available.

- BREAST FEEDING The amount secreted into breast milk is too small to be harmful. Accumulation of metabolite may cause sedation and respiratory depression in neonate.

- HEPATIC IMPAIRMENT Sedative effects are increased in hepatic impairment. Avoid in severe liver disease.

- RENAL IMPAIRMENT Use with caution.

- TREATMENT CESSATION Withdrawal effects may occur within 5 days of stopping treatment with antidepressant drugs; they are usually mild and self-limiting, but in some cases may be severe. The risk of withdrawal symptoms is increased if the antidepressant is stopped suddenly after regular administration for 8 weeks or more. The dose should preferably be reduced gradually over about 4 weeks, or longer if withdrawal symptoms emerge (6 months in patients who have been on long-term maintenance treatment). If possible tricyclic and related antidepressants should be withdrawn slowly.

- PRESCRIBING AND DISPENSING INFORMATION Limited quantities of tricyclic antidepressants should be prescribed at any one time because their cardiovascular and epileptogenic effects are dangerous in overdosage.

- PATIENT AND CARER ADVICE
Driving and skilled tasks Drowsiness may affect performance of skilled tasks (e.g. driving).
Effects of alcohol enhanced.

- MEDICINAL FORMS
There can be variation in the licensing of different medicines containing the same drug. Forms available from special-order manufacturers include: capsule, oral suspension, oral solution
Capsule
CAUTIONARY AND ADVISORY LABELS 2
▸ Doxepin (Non-proprietary)
Doxepin (as Doxepin hydrochloride) 25 mg Doxepin 25mg capsules | 28 capsule [PoM] £97.00 DT = £97.00
Doxepin (as Doxepin hydrochloride) 50 mg Doxepin 50mg capsules | 28 capsule [PoM] £154.00 DT = £154.00

Imipramine hydrochloride

- INDICATIONS AND DOSE
Depressive illness
▸ BY MOUTH
▸ Adult: Initially up to 75 mg daily in divided doses, then increased to 150–200 mg daily, up to 150 mg may be given as a single dose at bedtime, dose to be increased gradually

‣ **Elderly:** Initially 10 mg daily, increased to 30–50 mg daily, dose to be increased gradually

Depressive illness in hospital patients

▶ BY MOUTH

‣ **Adult:** Initially up to 75 mg daily in divided doses, dose to be increased gradually, increased to up to 300 mg daily in divided doses

Nocturnal enuresis

▶ BY MOUTH

‣ **Child 6-7 years:** 25 mg once daily, to be taken at bedtime, initial period of treatment (including gradual withdrawal) 3 months—full physical examination before further course

‣ **Child 8-10 years:** 25–50 mg once daily, to be taken at bedtime, initial period of treatment (including gradual withdrawal) 3 months—full physical examination before further course

‣ **Child 11-17 years:** 50–75 mg once daily, to be taken at bedtime, initial period of treatment (including gradual withdrawal) 3 months—full physical examination before further course

● CONTRA-INDICATIONS Acute porphyrias p. 1025 · arrhythmia · during the manic phase of bipolar disorder · heart block · immediate recovery period after myocardial infarction (in adults)

● CAUTIONS Cardiovascular disease · chronic constipation · diabetes · epilepsy · history of bipolar disorder · history of psychosis · hyperthyroidism (risk of arrhythmias) · increased intra-ocular pressure (in adults) · patients with a significant risk of suicide · phaeochromocytoma (risk of arrhythmias) · prostatic hypertrophy (in adults) · susceptibility to angle-closure glaucoma · urinary retention

CAUTIONS, FURTHER INFORMATION Treatment should be stopped if the patient enters a manic phase.

Elderly patients are particularly susceptible to many of the side-effects of tricyclic antidepressants; low initial doses should be used, with close monitoring, particularly for psychiatric and cardiac side-effects.

● INTERACTIONS → Appendix 1: tricyclic antidepressants

● SIDE-EFFECTS

▶ **Common or very common** Anxiety · appetite decreased · arrhythmias · asthenia · cardiac conduction disorders · confusion · delirium · depression · dizziness · drowsiness · epilepsy · hallucination · headache · hepatic disorders · hypotension · mood altered · nausea · palpitations · paraesthesia · sexual dysfunction · skin reactions · sleep disorder · tremor · vomiting · weight changes

▶ **Uncommon** Psychosis

▶ **Rare or very rare** Aggression · agranulocytosis · alopecia · bone marrow depression · enlarged mammary gland · eosinophilia · fever · galactorrhoea · gastrointestinal disorders · glaucoma · heart failure · leucopenia · movement disorders · mydriasis · oedema · oral disorders · peripheral vasospastic reaction · photosensitivity reaction · respiratory disorders · SIADH · speech disorder · thrombocytopenia

▶ **Frequency not known** Anticholinergic syndrome · cardiovascular effects · drug fever · hyponatraemia · increased risk of fracture · neurological effects · paranoid delusions exacerbated · psychiatric disorder · suicidal tendencies · tinnitus · urinary disorder · withdrawal syndrome

SIDE-EFFECTS, FURTHER INFORMATION The risk of side-effects is reduced by titrating slowly to the minimum effective dose (every 2–3 days). Consider using a lower starting dose in elderly patients.

Overdose Tricyclic and related antidepressants cause dry mouth, coma of varying degree, hypotension, hypothermia, hyperreflexia, extensor plantar responses, convulsions, respiratory failure, cardiac conduction defects, and arrhythmias. Dilated pupils and urinary retention also occur. For details on the management of poisoning see Tricyclic and related antidepressants under Emergency treatment of poisoning p. 1319.

● PREGNANCY Colic, tachycardia, dyspnoea, irritability, muscle spasms, respiratory depression and withdrawal symptoms reported in neonates when used in the third trimester.

● BREAST FEEDING The amount secreted into breast milk is too small to be harmful.

● HEPATIC IMPAIRMENT Sedative effects are increased in hepatic impairment. Avoid in severe liver disease.

● RENAL IMPAIRMENT Use with caution in severe impairment.

● TREATMENT CESSATION Withdrawal effects may occur within 5 days of stopping treatment with antidepressant drugs; they are usually mild and self-limiting, but in some cases may be severe. The risk of withdrawal symptoms is increased if the antidepressant is stopped suddenly after regular administration for 8 weeks or more. The dose should preferably be reduced gradually over about 4 weeks, or longer if withdrawal symptoms emerge (6 months in patients who have been on long-term maintenance treatment). If possible tricyclic antidepressants should be withdrawn slowly.

● PRESCRIBING AND DISPENSING INFORMATION Limited quantities of tricyclic antidepressants should be prescribed at any one time because their cardiovascular and epileptogenic effects are dangerous in overdosage.

● PATIENT AND CARER ADVICE

Medicines for Children leaflet: Imipramine www.medicinesforchildren.org.uk/imipramine

Driving and skilled tasks Drowsiness may affect the performance of skilled tasks (e.g. driving).

Effects of alcohol enhanced.

● MEDICINAL FORMS

There can be variation in the licensing of different medicines containing the same drug. Forms available from special-order manufacturers include: oral suspension, oral solution

Oral solution

CAUTIONARY AND ADVISORY LABELS 2

▸ Imipramine hydrochloride (Non-proprietary)

Imipramine hydrochloride 5 mg per 1 ml Imipramine 25mg/5ml oral solution sugar free sugar-free | 150 ml [PoM] £42.00 DT = £42.00

Tablet

CAUTIONARY AND ADVISORY LABELS 2

▸ Imipramine hydrochloride (Non-proprietary)

Imipramine hydrochloride 10 mg Imipramine 10mg tablets | 28 tablet [PoM] £0.81 DT = £0.58

Imipramine hydrochloride 25 mg Imipramine 25mg tablets | 28 tablet [PoM] £0.81 DT = £0.61

Lofepramine

● INDICATIONS AND DOSE

Depressive illness

▶ BY MOUTH

‣ **Adult:** 140–210 mg daily in divided doses

‣ **Elderly:** May respond to lower doses

● CONTRA-INDICATIONS Acute porphyrias p. 1025 · arrhythmias · during the manic phase of bipolar disorder · heart block · immediate recovery period after myocardial infarction

● CAUTIONS Cardiovascular disease · chronic constipation · diabetes · epilepsy · history of bipolar disorder · history of psychosis · hyperthyroidism (risk of arrhythmias) · increased intra-ocular pressure · patients with a significant risk of suicide · phaeochromocytoma (risk of arrhythmias) ·

4

Nervous system

Nervous system

4

prostatic hypertrophy · susceptibility to angle-closure glaucoma · urinary retention

CAUTIONS, FURTHER INFORMATION Treatment should be stopped if the patient enters a manic phase.

Elderly patients are particularly susceptible to many of the side-effects of tricyclic antidepressants; low initial doses should be used, with close monitoring, particularly for psychiatric and cardiac side-effects.

- INTERACTIONS → Appendix 1: tricyclic antidepressants
- SIDE-EFFECTS Accommodation disorder · agitation · agranulocytosis · arrhythmias · bone marrow disorders · cardiac conduction disorder · confusion · constipation · coordination abnormal · dizziness · drowsiness · dry mouth · eosinophilia · face oedema · galactorrhoea · glaucoma · granulocytopenia · gynaecomastia · hallucination · headache · heart failure aggravated · hepatic disorders · hyperhidrosis (on discontinuation) · hyponatraemia · hypotension · increased risk of fracture · leucopenia · malaise · mood altered · mucositis · nausea · paraesthesia · paranoid delusions · photosensitivity reaction · psychosis · respiratory depression · seizure · sexual dysfunction · SIADH · skin haemorrhage · skin reactions · sleep disorder · suicidal tendencies · taste altered · testicular disorders · thrombocytopenia · tinnitus · tremor · urinary disorders · vomiting · withdrawal syndrome

SIDE-EFFECTS, FURTHER INFORMATION The risk of side-effects is reduced by titrating slowly to the minimum effective dose (every 2–3 days). Consider using a lower starting dose in elderly patients.

Overdose Tricyclic and related antidepressants cause dry mouth, coma of varying degree, hypotension, hypothermia, hyperreflexia, extensor plantar responses, convulsions, respiratory failure, cardiac conduction defects, and arrhythmias. Dilated pupils and urinary retention also occur. Lofepramine is associated with the lowest risk of fatality in overdosage, in comparison with other tricyclic antidepressant drugs. For details on the management of poisoning see Tricyclic and related antidepressants under Emergency treatment of poisoning p. 1319.

- PREGNANCY Neonatal withdrawal symptoms and respiratory depression reported if used during third trimester.
- BREAST FEEDING The amount secreted into breast milk is too small to be harmful.
- HEPATIC IMPAIRMENT Sedative effects are increased in hepatic impairment. Avoid in severe liver disease.
- RENAL IMPAIRMENT Avoid in severe impairment.
- TREATMENT CESSATION Withdrawal effects may occur within 5 days of stopping treatment with antidepressant drugs; they are usually mild and self-limiting, but in some cases may be severe. The risk of withdrawal symptoms is increased if the antidepressant is stopped suddenly after regular administration for 8 weeks or more. The dose should preferably be reduced gradually over about 4 weeks, or longer if withdrawal symptoms emerge (6 months in patients who have been on long-term maintenance treatment). If possible tricyclic and related antidepressants should be withdrawn slowly.
- PRESCRIBING AND DISPENSING INFORMATION Limited quantities of tricyclic antidepressants should be prescribed at any one time because their cardiovascular and epileptogenic effects are dangerous in overdosage.
- PATIENT AND CARER ADVICE
  Driving and skilled tasks Drowsiness may affect the performance of skilled tasks (e.g. driving).
  Effects of alcohol enhanced.

- MEDICINAL FORMS
There can be variation in the licensing of different medicines containing the same drug. Forms available from special-order manufacturers include: oral suspension, oral solution

Oral suspension
CAUTIONARY AND ADVISORY LABELS 2
▸ Lofepramine (Non-proprietary)
  Lofepramine (as Lofepramine hydrochloride) 14 mg per 1 ml Lofepramine 70mg/5ml oral suspension sugar free sugar-free | 150 ml PoM £27.22 DT = £27.22

Tablet
CAUTIONARY AND ADVISORY LABELS 2
▸ Lofepramine (Non-proprietary)
  Lofepramine (as Lofepramine hydrochloride) 70 mg Lofepramine 70mg tablets | 56 tablet PoM £59.97 DT = £9.31

Nortriptyline

- INDICATIONS AND DOSE

Depressive illness
▸ BY MOUTH
▸ Adult: To be initiated at a low dose, then increased if necessary to 75–100 mg daily in divided doses, alternatively increased if necessary to 75–100 mg once daily; maximum 150 mg per day
▸ Elderly: To be initiated at a low dose, then increased if necessary to 30–50 mg daily in divided doses

Neuropathic pain
▸ BY MOUTH
▸ Adult: Initially 10 mg once daily, to be taken at night, increased if necessary to 75 mg daily, dose to be increased gradually; higher doses to be given under specialist supervision

- UNLICENSED USE Not licensed for use in neuropathic pain.
- CONTRA-INDICATIONS Arrhythmias · during the manic phase of bipolar disorder · heart block · immediate recovery period after myocardial infarction
- CAUTIONS Cardiovascular disease · chronic constipation · diabetes · epilepsy · history of bipolar disorder · history of psychosis · hyperthyroidism (risk of arrhythmias) · increased intra-ocular pressure · patients with a significant risk of suicide · phaeochromocytoma (risk of arrhythmias) · prostatic hypertrophy · susceptibility to angle-closure glaucoma · urinary retention

CAUTIONS, FURTHER INFORMATION Treatment should be stopped if the patient enters a manic phase.

Elderly patients are particularly susceptible to many of the side-effects of tricyclic antidepressants; low initial doses should be used, with close monitoring, particularly for psychiatric and cardiac side-effects.

- INTERACTIONS → Appendix 1: tricyclic antidepressants
- SIDE-EFFECTS Agranulocytosis · alopecia · anxiety · appetite decreased · arrhythmias · asthenia · atrioventricular block · bone marrow disorders · breast enlargement · confusion · constipation · delusions · diarrhoea · dizziness · drowsiness · drug cross-reactivity · drug fever · dry mouth · eosinophilia · fever · flushing · galactorrhoea · gastrointestinal discomfort · gynaecomastia · hallucination · headache · hepatic disorders · hyperhidrosis · hypertension · hypomania · hypotension · increased risk of fracture · increased risk of infection · malaise · movement disorders · mydriasis · myocardial infarction · nausea · oedema · oral disorders · palpitations · paralytic ileus · peripheral neuropathy · photosensitivity reaction · psychosis exacerbated · seizure · sensation abnormal · sexual dysfunction · SIADH · skin reactions · sleep disorders · stroke · suicidal tendencies · taste altered · testicular swelling · thrombocytopenia · tinnitus · tremor · urinary disorders · urinary tract dilation · vision disorders · vomiting · weight changes

SIDE-EFFECTS, FURTHER INFORMATION The risk of side-effects is reduced by titrating slowly to the minimum effective dose (every 2–3 days). Consider using a lower starting dose in elderly patients.

Overdose Tricyclic and related antidepressants cause dry mouth, coma of varying degree, hypotension, hypothermia, hyperreflexia, extensor plantar responses, convulsions, respiratory failure, cardiac conduction defects, and arrhythmias. Dilated pupils and urinary retention also occur. For details on the management of poisoning see Tricyclic and related antidepressants under Emergency treatment of poisoning p. 1319.

● PREGNANCY Use only if potential benefit outweighs risk.

● BREAST FEEDING The amount secreted into breast milk is too small to be harmful.

● HEPATIC IMPAIRMENT Sedative effects are increased in hepatic impairment. Avoid in severe liver disease.

● MONITORING REQUIREMENTS
▸ Manufacturer advises plasma-nortriptyline concentration monitoring if dose above 100 mg daily, but evidence of practical value uncertain.

● TREATMENT CESSATION Withdrawal effects may occur within 5 days of stopping treatment with antidepressant drugs; they are usually mild and self-limiting, but in some cases may be severe. The risk of withdrawal symptoms is increased if the antidepressant is stopped suddenly after regular administration for 8 weeks or more. The dose should preferably be reduced gradually over about 4 weeks, or longer if withdrawal symptoms emerge (6 months in patients who have been on long-term maintenance treatment). If possible tricyclic and related antidepressants should be withdrawn slowly.

● PRESCRIBING AND DISPENSING INFORMATION Limited quantities of tricyclic antidepressants should be prescribed at any one time because their cardiovascular and epileptogenic effects are dangerous in overdosage.

● PATIENT AND CARER ADVICE Drowsiness may affect the performance of skilled tasks (e.g. driving). Effects of alcohol enhanced.

● MEDICINAL FORMS
There can be variation in the licensing of different medicines containing the same drug. Forms available from special-order manufacturers include: oral suspension, oral solution

Tablet
CAUTIONARY AND ADVISORY LABELS 2
▸ Nortriptyline (Non-proprietary)
  Nortriptyline (as Nortriptyline hydrochloride) 10 mg Nortriptyline 10mg tablets | 30 tablet PoM £6.87-£11.79 | 100 tablet PoM £68.41 DT = £9.57
  Nortriptyline (as Nortriptyline hydrochloride) 25 mg Nortriptyline 25mg tablets | 30 tablet PoM £6.81-£12.43 | 100 tablet PoM £111.06 DT = £11.57
  Nortriptyline (as Nortriptyline hydrochloride) 50 mg Nortriptyline 50mg tablets | 30 tablet PoM £24.86 DT = £24.86

Trimipramine

● INDICATIONS AND DOSE

Depressive illness (particularly where sedation required)
▸ BY MOUTH
▸ Adult: Initially 50–75 mg daily in divided doses, alternatively initially 50–75 mg once daily, dose to be taken at bedtime, increased if necessary to 150–300 mg daily
▸ Elderly: Initially 10–25 mg 3 times a day, maintenance 75–150 mg daily

● CONTRA-INDICATIONS Acute porphyrias p. 1025 · arrhythmias · during the manic phase of bipolar disorder ·

heart block · immediate recovery period after myocardial infarction

● CAUTIONS Cardiovascular disease · chronic constipation · diabetes · epilepsy · history of bipolar disorder · history of psychosis · hyperthyroidism (risk of arrhythmias) · increased intra-ocular pressure · patients with a significant risk of suicide · phaeochromocytoma (risk of arrhythmias) · prostatic hypertrophy · susceptibility to angle-closure glaucoma · urinary retention

CAUTIONS, FURTHER INFORMATION Treatment should be stopped if the patient enters a manic phase.
Elderly patients are particularly susceptible to many of the side-effects of tricyclic antidepressants; low initial doses should be used, with close monitoring, particularly for psychiatric and cardiac side-effects.

● INTERACTIONS → Appendix 1: tricyclic antidepressants

● SIDE-EFFECTS Accommodation disorder · agitation · agranulocytosis · anticholinergic syndrome · arrhythmias · bone fracture · bone marrow depression · constipation · drowsiness · dry mouth · hyperglycaemia · hyperhidrosis · hypotension · jaundice cholestatic · mood altered · paranoid delusions · peripheral neuropathy · rash · respiratory depression · seizure · sexual dysfunction · suicidal tendencies · tremor · urinary hesitation · withdrawal syndrome

SIDE-EFFECTS, FURTHER INFORMATION The risk of side-effects is reduced by titrating slowly to the minimum effective dose (every 2–3 days). Consider using a lower starting dose in elderly patients.

Overdose Tricyclic and related antidepressants cause dry mouth, coma of varying degree, hypotension, hypothermia, hyperreflexia, extensor plantar responses, convulsions, respiratory failure, cardiac conduction defects, and arrhythmias. Dilated pupils and urinary retention also occur. For details on the management of poisoning see Tricyclic and related antidepressants under Emergency treatment of poisoning p. 1319.

● PREGNANCY Use only if potential benefit outweighs risk.

● BREAST FEEDING The amount secreted into breast milk is too small to be harmful.

● HEPATIC IMPAIRMENT Sedative effects are increased in hepatic impairment. Avoid in severe liver disease.

● TREATMENT CESSATION Withdrawal effects may occur within 5 days of stopping treatment with antidepressant drugs; they are usually mild and self-limiting, but in some cases may be severe. The risk of withdrawal symptoms is increased if the antidepressant is stopped suddenly after regular administration for 8 weeks or more. The dose should preferably be reduced gradually over about 4 weeks, or longer if withdrawal symptoms emerge (6 months in patients who have been on long-term maintenance treatment). If possible tricyclic and related antidepressants should be withdrawn slowly.

● PRESCRIBING AND DISPENSING INFORMATION Limited quantities of tricyclic antidepressants should be prescribed at any one time because their cardiovascular and epileptogenic effects are dangerous in overdosage.

● PATIENT AND CARER ADVICE
Driving and skilled tasks Drowsiness may affect the performance of skilled tasks (e.g. driving).
Effects of alcohol enhanced.

4

Nervous system

Nervous system

4

- **MEDICINAL FORMS**
  There can be variation in the licensing of different medicines containing the same drug. Forms available from special-order manufacturers include: oral suspension, oral solution
  Tablet
  CAUTIONARY AND ADVISORY LABELS 2
  ▸ Trimipramine (Non-proprietary)
  Trimipramine (as Trimipramine maleate) 10 mg Trimipramine 10mg tablets | 28 tablet [PoM] £197.18 DT = £179.15
  Trimipramine (as Trimipramine maleate) 25 mg Trimipramine 25mg tablets | 28 tablet [PoM] £205.44 DT = £200.50
  Capsule
  CAUTIONARY AND ADVISORY LABELS 2
  ▸ Trimipramine (Non-proprietary)
  Trimipramine (as Trimipramine maleate) 50 mg Trimipramine 50mg capsules | 28 capsule [PoM] £190.00 DT = £190.00

OTHER ANTIDEPRESSANTS

Tryptophan

04-Oct-2017

(L-Tryptophan)

- **DRUG ACTION** Tryptophan is an essential dietary amino acid, and is a precursor of serotonin; it re-establishes the inhibitory action of serotonin on the amygdaloid nuclei, thereby reducing feelings of anxiety and depression.

- **INDICATIONS AND DOSE**
  Treatment-resistant depression (used alone or as adjunct to other antidepressant drugs) (initiated under direction of hospital consultant)
  ▸ BY MOUTH
  ▸ Adult: 1 g 3 times a day; maximum 6 g per day

- **CONTRA-INDICATIONS** History of eosinophilia myalgia syndrome following use of tryptophan
- **INTERACTIONS** → Appendix 1: tryptophan
- **SIDE-EFFECTS** Asthenia · dizziness · drowsiness · eosinophilia myalgia syndrome · headache · myalgia · myopathy · nausea · oedema · suicidal tendencies
  SIDE-EFFECTS, FURTHER INFORMATION If patients experience any symptoms of eosinophilia myalgia syndrome (EMS), manufacturer advises to withhold treatment until possibility of EMS is excluded.
- **PREGNANCY** Manufacturer advises caution—no information available.
- **BREAST FEEDING** Manufacturer advises avoid—no information available.
- **MONITORING REQUIREMENTS** Manufacturer advises close monitoring for signs of suicidal thoughts, particularly in patients at high risk and during early treatment and dose changes.
- **PATIENT AND CARER ADVICE** Manufacturer advises patients and carers should be advised to seek medical advice immediately if any clinical worsening, suicidal thoughts, or unusual behaviour develops.
  Driving and skilled tasks Manufacturer advises patients should be counselled on the effects on driving and performance of skilled tasks—increased risk of drowsiness.

- **MEDICINAL FORMS**
  There can be variation in the licensing of different medicines containing the same drug. Forms available from special-order manufacturers include: capsule
  Capsule
  ▸ Optimax (Intrapharm Laboratories Ltd)
  Tryptophan 500 mg Optimax 500mg capsules | 84 capsule [PoM] £30.00

Vortioxetine

17-May-2016

- **DRUG ACTION** Vortioxetine inhibits the re-uptake of serotonin (5-HT) and is an antagonist at 5-HT$_3$ and an agonist at 5-HT$_{1A}$ receptors. This multimodal activity appears to be associated with antidepressant and anxiolytic-like effects.

- **INDICATIONS AND DOSE**
  Major depression
  ▸ BY MOUTH
  ▸ Adult: Initially 10 mg once daily; adjusted according to response to 5–20 mg once daily
  ▸ Elderly: Initially 5 mg once daily; increased if necessary up to 20 mg once daily

- **CAUTIONS** Bleeding disorders · cirrhosis of the liver (risk of hyponatraemia) · elderly (risk of hyponatraemia) · history of mania (discontinue if patient entering manic phase) · history of seizures · unstable epilepsy
  CAUTIONS, FURTHER INFORMATION
  ▸ Seizures Discontinue treatment in patients who develop seizures or if there is an increase in seizure frequency.
  ▸ Elderly Manufacturer advises caution when treating elderly patients with doses over 10 mg daily—limited information.
- **INTERACTIONS** → Appendix 1: vortioxetine
- **SIDE-EFFECTS**
- **Common or very common** Abnormal dreams · constipation · diarrhoea · dizziness · nausea · pruritus · vomiting
- **Uncommon** Flushing · night sweats
- **Frequency not known** Hyponatraemia · neuroleptic malignant syndrome (discontinue—potentially fatal) · serotonin syndrome
- **PREGNANCY** Manufacturer advises avoid unless potential benefit outweighs risk—toxicity in *animal* studies. If used during the later stages of pregnancy, there is a risk of neonatal withdrawal symptoms and persistent pulmonary hypertension in the newborn.
- **BREAST FEEDING** Manufacturer advises avoid—present in milk in *animal* studies.
- **HEPATIC IMPAIRMENT** Manufacturer advises caution in severe impairment—no information available.
- **RENAL IMPAIRMENT** Manufacturer advises caution in severe impairment—limited information available.
- **TREATMENT CESSATION** Manufacturer advises treatment can be stopped abruptly, without need for gradual dose reduction.
- **PATIENT AND CARER ADVICE**
  Driving and skilled tasks Manufacturer advises patients and carers should be counselled on the effects on driving and performance of skilled tasks, especially when starting treatment or changing the dose.
- **NATIONAL FUNDING/ACCESS DECISIONS**
  NICE decisions
  ▸ **Vortioxetine for treating major depressive episodes (November 2015)** NICE TA367
  Vortioxetine is recommended as an option for treating major depressive episodes in adults whose condition has responded inadequately to 2 antidepressants within the current episode.
  Patients currently receiving vortioxetine whose disease does not meet the above criteria should be able to continue treatment until they and their clinician consider it appropriate to stop.
  www.nice.org.uk/TA367

- **MEDICINAL FORMS**
There can be variation in the licensing of different medicines containing the same drug.

Tablet

▸ Brintellix (Lundbeck Ltd) ▼

   Vortioxetine (as Vortioxetine hydrobromide) 5 mg Brintellix 5mg tablets | 28 tablet P○M £27.72 DT = £27.72

   Vortioxetine (as Vortioxetine hydrobromide) 10 mg Brintellix 10mg tablets | 28 tablet P○M £27.72 DT = £27.72

   Vortioxetine (as Vortioxetine hydrobromide) 20 mg Brintellix 20mg tablets | 28 tablet P○M £27.72 DT = £27.72

3.5 Inappropriate sexual behaviour

ANTIPSYCHOTICS ❯ FIRST-GENERATION

⚑ 380

Benperidol

- **INDICATIONS AND DOSE**

Control of deviant antisocial sexual behaviour

▸ BY MOUTH

▸ Adult: 0.25–1.5 mg daily in divided doses, adjusted according to response, for debilitated patients, use elderly dose

▸ Elderly: Initially 0.125–0.75 mg daily in divided doses, adjusted according to response

- **CONTRA-INDICATIONS** CNS depression · comatose states · phaeochromocytoma

- **CAUTIONS** Risk factors for stroke

- **INTERACTIONS** → Appendix 1: benperidol

- **SIDE-EFFECTS** Appetite decreased · blood disorder · cardiac arrest · depression · dyspepsia · granulocytopenia · headache · hepatic disorders · hyperhidrosis · hypersalivation · hypertension · movement disorders · muscle rigidity · nausea · oculogyric crisis · oedema · oligomenorrhoea · paradoxical drug reaction · psychiatric disorder · skin reactions · temperature regulation disorders · vomiting · weight change

- **PREGNANCY** Extrapyramidal effects and withdrawal syndrome have been reported occasionally in the neonate when antipsychotic drugs are taken during the third trimester of pregnancy. Following maternal use of antipsychotic drugs in the third trimester, neonates should be monitored for symptoms including agitation, hypertonia, hypotonia, tremor, drowsiness, feeding problems, and respiratory distress.

- **BREAST FEEDING** There is limited information available on the short- and long-term effects of antipsychotic drugs on the breast-fed infant. *Animal* studies indicate possible adverse effects of antipsychotic medicines on the developing nervous system. Chronic treatment with antipsychotic drugs whilst breast-feeding should be avoided unless absolutely necessary.

- **HEPATIC IMPAIRMENT** Can precipitate coma.

- **RENAL IMPAIRMENT**

   Dose adjustments Start with small doses in severe renal impairment because of increased cerebral sensitivity.

- **MONITORING REQUIREMENTS** Manufacturer advises regular blood counts and liver function tests during long-term treatment.

- **PRESCRIBING AND DISPENSING INFORMATION** The proprietary name *Benquil®* has been used for benperidol tablets.

- **MEDICINAL FORMS**
There can be variation in the licensing of different medicines containing the same drug. Forms available from special-order manufacturers include: oral suspension

Tablet

CAUTIONARY AND ADVISORY LABELS 2

▸ Benperidol (Non-proprietary)

   Benperidol 250 microgram Benperidol 250microgram tablets | 112 tablet P○M £117.31 DT = £117.31

▸ Anquil (Kyowa Kirin Ltd)

   Benperidol 250 microgram Anquil 250microgram tablets | 112 tablet P○M £117.31 DT = £117.31

3.6 Psychoses and schizophrenia

Psychoses and related disorders

06-Mar-2017

Advice of Royal College of Psychiatrists on doses of antipsychotic drugs above BNF upper limit

Unless otherwise stated, doses in the BNF are licensed doses—any higher dose is therefore **unlicensed**

- Consider alternative approaches including adjuvant therapy and newer or second-generation antipsychotic drugs such as clozapine.
- Bear in mind risk factors, including obesity; particular caution is indicated in older patients, especially those over 70.
- Consider potential for drug interactions—see interactions: Appendix 1 (antipsychotics).
- Carry out ECG to exclude untoward abnormalities such as prolonged QT interval; repeat ECG periodically and reduce dose if prolonged QT interval or other adverse cardiac abnormality develops.
- Increase dose slowly and not more often than once weekly.
- Carry out regular pulse, blood pressure, and temperature checks; ensure that patient maintains adequate fluid intake.
- Consider high-dose therapy to be for limited period and review regularly; abandon if no improvement after 3 months (return to standard dosage).

Important: When prescribing an antipsychotic for administration on an emergency basis, the intramuscular dose should be **lower** than the corresponding oral dose (owing to absence of first-pass effect), particularly if the patient is very active (increased blood flow to muscle considerably increases the rate of absorption). The prescription should specify the dose for **each route** and should **not** imply that the same dose can be given by mouth or by intramuscular injection. The dose of antipsychotic for emergency use should be reviewed at least **daily**.

Antipsychotic drugs

Antipsychotic drugs are also known as 'neuroleptics' and (misleadingly) as 'major tranquillisers'.

In the short term they are used to calm disturbed patients whatever the underlying psychopathology, which may be schizophrenia, brain damage, mania, toxic delirium, or agitated depression. Antipsychotic drugs are used to alleviate severe anxiety but this too should be a short-term measure.

Schizophrenia

The aim of treatment is to alleviate the suffering of the patient (and carer) and to improve social and cognitive functioning. Many patients require life-long treatment with antipsychotic medication. Antipsychotic drugs relieve positive psychotic symptoms such as thought disorder, hallucinations, and delusions, and prevent relapse; they are usually less effective on negative symptoms such as apathy and social withdrawal. In many patients, negative symptoms persist between episodes of treated positive symptoms, but earlier treatment of psychotic illness may protect against the development of negative symptoms over time. Patients with acute schizophrenia generally respond better than those with chronic symptoms.

Long-term treatment of a patient with a definitive diagnosis of schizophrenia is usually required after the first episode of illness in order to prevent relapses. Doses that are effective in acute episodes should generally be continued as prophylaxis.

First-generation antipsychotic drugs

The first-generation antipsychotic drugs act predominantly by blocking dopamine D_2 receptors in the brain. First-generation antipsychotic drugs are not selective for any of the four dopamine pathways in the brain and so can cause a range of side-effects, particularly extrapyramidal symptoms and elevated prolactin. The **phenothiazine** derivatives can be divided into 3 main groups:

- *Group* 1: chlorpromazine hydrochloride p. 381, levomepromazine p. 435, and promazine hydrochloride p. 401, generally characterised by pronounced sedative effects and moderate antimuscarinic and extrapyramidal side-effects.
- *Group* 2: pericyazine p. 384, generally characterised by moderate sedative effects, but fewer extrapyramidal side-effects than groups 1 or 3.
- *Group* 3: fluphenazine decanoate p. 389, perphenazine p. 384, prochlorperazine p. 385, and trifluoperazine p. 387, generally characterised by fewer sedative and antimuscarinic effects, but more pronounced extrapyramidal side-effects than groups 1 and 2.

Butyrophenones (benperidol p. 377 and haloperidol p. 382) resemble the group 3 phenothiazines in their clinical properties. **Thioxanthenes** (flupentixol p. 382 and zuclopenthixol p. 387) have moderate sedative, antimuscarinic effects, and extrapyramidal effects. **Diphenylbutylpiperidines** (pimozide p. 385) and the **substituted benzamides** (sulpiride p. 386) have reduced sedative, antimuscarinic, and extrapyramidal effects.

Second-generation antipsychotic drugs

The second-generation antipsychotic drugs (sometimes referred to as atypical antipsychotic drugs) act on a range of receptors in comparison to first-generation antipsychotic drugs and have more distinct clinical profiles, particularly with regard to side-effects.

Prescribing for the elderly

The balance of risks and benefit should be considered before prescribing antipsychotic drugs for elderly patients. In elderly patients with dementia, antipsychotic drugs are associated with a small increased risk of mortality and an increased risk of stroke or transient ischaemic attack (see Dementia p. 299). Furthermore, elderly patients are particularly susceptible to postural hypotension and to hyper- and hypothermia in hot or cold weather.

It is recommended that:

- Antipsychotic drugs should not be used in elderly patients to treat mild to moderate psychotic symptoms.
- Initial doses of antipsychotic drugs in elderly patients should be reduced (to half the adult dose or less), taking into account factors such as the patient's weight, co-morbidity, and concomitant medication.
- Treatment should be reviewed regularly.

Prescribing of antipsychotic drugs in patients with learning disabilities

EvGr When prescribing for patients with learning disabilities who are prescribed antipsychotic drugs and who are not experiencing psychotic symptoms, the following considerations should be taken into account:

- a reduction in dose or the discontinuation of long-term antipsychotic treatment;
- review of the patient's condition after dose reduction or discontinuation of an antipsychotic drug;
- referral to a psychiatrist experienced in working with patients who have learning disabilities and mental health problems;
- annual documentation of the reasons for continuing a prescription if the antipsychotic is not reduced in dose or discontinued Ⓐ.

Side effects of antipsychotic drugs

Side-effects caused by antipsychotic drugs are common and contribute significantly to non-adherence to therapy.

Extrapyramidal symptoms

Extrapyramidal symptoms occur most frequently with the piperazine phenothiazines (fluphenazine, perphenazine, prochlorperazine, and trifluoperazine), the butyrophenones (benperidol and haloperidol), and the first-generation depot preparations. They are easy to recognise but cannot be predicted accurately because they depend on the dose, the type of drug, and on individual susceptibility.

Extrapyramidal symptoms consist of:

- *parkinsonian symptoms* (including tremor), which may occur more commonly in adults or the elderly and may appear gradually;
- *dystonia* (abnormal face and body movements) and *dyskinesia*, which occur more commonly in children or young adults and appear after only a few doses;
- *akathisia* (restlessness), which characteristically occurs after large initial doses and may resemble an exacerbation of the condition being treated;
- *tardive dyskinesia* (rhythmic, involuntary movements of tongue, face, and jaw), which usually develops on long-term therapy or with high dosage, but it may develop on short-term treatment with low doses—short-lived tardive dyskinesia may occur after withdrawal of the drug.

Parkinsonian symptoms remit if the drug is withdrawn and may be suppressed by the administration of antimuscarinic drugs. However, routine administration of such drugs is not justified because not all patients are affected and they may unmask or worsen tardive dyskinesia.

Tardive dyskinesia is the most serious manifestation of extrapyramidal symptoms; it is of particular concern because it may be irreversible on withdrawing therapy and treatment is usually ineffective. In children, tardive dyskinesia is more likely to occur when the antipsychotic drug is withdrawn. However, some manufacturers suggest that drug withdrawal at the earliest signs of tardive dyskinesia (fine vermicular movements of the tongue) may halt its full development. Tardive dyskinesia occurs fairly frequently, especially in the elderly, and treatment must be carefully and regularly reviewed.

Hyperprolactinaemia

Most antipsychotic drugs, both first- and second-generation, increase prolactin concentration to some extent because dopamine inhibits prolactin release. Aripiprazole reduces prolactin because it is a dopamine-receptor partial agonist. Risperidone, amisulpride, and first-generation antipsychotic drugs are most likely to cause symptomatic hyperprolactinaemia. The clinical symptoms of hyperprolactinaemia include sexual dysfunction, reduced bone mineral density, menstrual disturbances, breast enlargement, and galactorrhoea.

Sexual dysfunction

Sexual dysfunction is one of the main causes of non-adherence to antipsychotic medication; physical illness, psychiatric illness, and substance misuse are contributing factors. Antipsychotic-induced sexual dysfunction is caused by more than one mechanism. Reduced dopamine transmission and hyperprolactinaemia decrease libido; antimuscarinic effects can cause disorders of arousal; and alpha$_1$-adrenoceptor antagonists are associated with erection and ejaculation problems in men. Risperidone and haloperidol commonly cause sexual dysfunction. If sexual dysfunction is thought to be antipsychotic-induced, dose reduction or switching medication should be considered.

Cardiovascular side-effects
Antipsychotic drugs have been associated with cardiovascular side-effects such as tachycardia, arrhythmias, and hypotension. QT-interval prolongation is a particular concern with pimozide and haloperidol. There is also a higher probability of QT-interval prolongation in patients using any intravenous antipsychotic drug, or any antipsychotic drug or combination of antipsychotic drugs with doses exceeding the recommended maximum. Cases of sudden death have occurred.

Hyperglycaemia and weight gain
Hyperglycaemia, and sometimes diabetes, can occur with antipsychotic drugs, particularly clozapine, olanzapine, quetiapine, and risperidone. All antipsychotic drugs may cause weight gain, but the risk and extent varies. Clozapine and olanzapine commonly cause weight gain.

Hypotension and interference with temperature regulation
Hypotension and interference with temperature regulation are dose-related side-effects that are liable to cause dangerous falls and hypothermia or hyperthermia in the elderly. Clozapine, chlorpromazine, lurasidone, and quetiapine can cause postural hypotension (especially during initial dose titration) which may be associated with syncope or reflex tachycardia in some patients.

Neuroleptic malignant syndrome
Neuroleptic malignant syndrome (hyperthermia, fluctuating level of consciousness, muscle rigidity, and autonomic dysfunction with pallor, tachycardia, labile blood pressure, sweating, and urinary incontinence) is a rare but potentially fatal side-effect of all antipsychotic drugs. Discontinuation of the antipsychotic drug is essential because there is no proven effective treatment, but bromocriptine and dantrolene have been used. The syndrome, which usually lasts for 5–7 days after drug discontinuation, may be unduly prolonged if depot preparations have been used.

Blood dyscrasias
Perform blood counts if unexplained infection or fever develops.

Choice
There is little meaningful difference in efficacy between each of the antipsychotic drugs (other than clozapine p. 392), and response and tolerability to each antipsychotic drug varies. There is no first-line antipsychotic drug which is suitable for all patients. Choice of antipsychotic medication is influenced by the patient's medication history, the degree of sedation required (although tolerance to this usually develops), and consideration of individual patient factors such as risk of extrapyramidal side-effects, weight gain, impaired glucose tolerance, QT-interval prolongation, or the presence of negative symptoms.

Negative symptoms
Second generation antipsychotic drugs may be better at treating the negative symptoms of schizophrenia.

Extrapyramidal side-effects
Second-generation antipsychotic drugs should be prescribed if extrapyramidal side-effects are a particular concern. Of these, aripiprazole p. 391, clozapine, olanzapine p. 394, and quetiapine p. 397 are least likely to cause extrapyramidal side-effects. Although amisulpride p. 390 is a dopamine-receptor antagonist, extrapyramidal side-effects are less common than with the first-generation antipsychotic drugs because amisulpride selectively blocks mesolimbic dopamine receptors, and extrapyramidal symptoms are caused by blockade of the striatal dopamine pathway.

QT interval
Aripiprazole has negligible effect on the QT interval. Other antipsychotic drugs with a reduced tendency to prolong QT interval include amisulpride, clozapine, flupentixol p. 382, fluphenazine decanoate p. 389, olanzapine, perphenazine p. 384, prochlorperazine p. 385, risperidone p. 398, and sulpiride p. 386.

Diabetes
Schizophrenia is associated with insulin resistance and diabetes; the risk of diabetes is increased in patients with schizophrenia who take antipsychotic drugs. First-generation antipsychotic drugs are less likely to cause diabetes than second-generation antipsychotic drugs, and of the first-generation antipsychotic drugs, fluphenazine decanoate and haloperidol p. 382 are lowest risk. Amisulpride and aripiprazole have the lowest risk of diabetes of the second-generation antipsychotic drugs. Amisulpride, aripiprazole, haloperidol, sulpiride, and trifluoperazine p. 387 are least likely to cause weight gain.

Sexual dysfunction and prolactin
The antipsychotic drugs with the lowest risk of sexual dysfunction are aripiprazole and quetiapine. Olanzapine may be considered if sexual dysfunction is judged to be secondary to hyperprolactinaemia. Hyperprolactinaemia is usually not clinically significant with aripiprazole, clozapine, olanzapine, and quetiapine treatment. When changing from other antipsychotic drugs, a reduction in prolactin concentration may increase fertility.

Patients should receive an antipsychotic drug for 4–6 weeks before it is deemed ineffective. Prescribing more than one antipsychotic drug at a time should be avoided except in exceptional circumstances (e.g. clozapine augmentation or when changing medication during titration) because of the increased risk of adverse effects such as extrapyramidal symptoms, QT-interval prolongation, and sudden cardiac death.

Clozapine is licensed for the treatment of schizophrenia in patients unresponsive to, or intolerant of, other antipsychotic drugs. Clozapine should be introduced if schizophrenia is not controlled despite the sequential use of two or more antipsychotic drugs (one of which should be a second-generation antipsychotic drug), each for at least 6–8 weeks. If symptoms do not respond adequately to an optimised dose of clozapine, plasma-clozapine concentration should be checked before adding a second antipsychotic drug to augment clozapine; allow 8–10 weeks' treatment to assess response. Patients must be registered with a clozapine patient monitoring service.

Monitoring
Full blood count, urea and electrolytes, and liver function test monitoring is required at the start of therapy with antipsychotic drugs, and then annually thereafter.

Blood lipids and weight should be measured at baseline, at 3 months (weight should be measured at frequent intervals during the first 3 months), and then yearly.

Fasting blood glucose should be measured at baseline, at 4–6 months, and then yearly.

Before initiating antipsychotic drugs, an ECG may be required, particularly if physical examination identifies cardiovascular risk factors, if there is a personal history of cardiovascular disease, or if the patient is being admitted as an inpatient.

Blood pressure monitoring is advised before starting therapy and frequently during dose titration of antipsychotic drugs.

Other uses
Some antipsychotic drugs can be used for the treatment of nausea and vomiting, choreas, and motor tics. Chlorpromazine hydrochloride p. 381 and haloperidol p. 382 can be used for intractable hiccup. Benperidol p. 377 is used

4

Nervous system

in deviant antisocial sexual behaviour but its value is not established.

Psychomotor agitation should be investigated for an underlying cause; it can be managed with low doses of chlorpromazine hydrochloride or haloperidol used for short periods. Antipsychotic drugs can be used with caution for the short-term treatment of severe agitation and restlessness in the elderly.

Equivalent doses of oral antipsychotics

These equivalences are intended **only** as an approximate guide; individual dosage instructions should **also** be checked; patients should be carefully monitored after **any** change in medication. Equivalent daily dose of antipsychotic drug:

- Chlorpromazine 100 mg
- Clozapine 50 mg
- Haloperidol 2–3 mg
- Pimozide 2 mg
- Risperidone 0.5–1 mg
- Sulpiride 200 mg
- Trifluoperazine 5 mg

Important: These equivalences must **not** be extrapolated beyond the maximum dose for the drug. Higher doses require careful titration in specialist units and the equivalences shown here may not be appropriate.

Dosage

After an initial period of stabilisation, in most patients, the total daily oral dose can be given as a single dose. The Royal College of Psychiatrists has published advice on doses of antipsychotic drugs above BNF upper limit.

Antipsychotic depot injections

Long-acting depot injections are used for maintenance therapy especially when compliance with oral treatment is unreliable. However, depot injections of conventional antipsychotics may give rise to a higher incidence of extrapyramidal reactions than oral preparations; extrapyramidal reactions occur less frequently with second-generation antipsychotic depot preparations, such as risperidone p. 398 and olanzapine embonate p. 399.

Choice

There is no clear-cut division in the use of the conventional antipsychotics, but zuclopenthixol p. 387 may be suitable for the treatment of agitated or aggressive patients whereas flupentixol decanoate p. 388 can cause over-excitement in such patients. Zuclopenthixol decanoate p. 390 may be more effective in preventing relapses than other conventional antipsychotic depot preparations. The incidence of extrapyramidal reactions is similar for the conventional antipsychotics.

Dosage

Individual responses to neuroleptic drugs are variable and to achieve optimum effect, dosage and dosage interval must be titrated according to the patient's response.

Equivalent doses of depot antipsychotics

Antipsychotic drug/interval	Dosage (mg)
Flupentixol decanoate / 2 weeks	40
Fluphenazine decanoate / 2 weeks	25
Haloperidol (as decanoate) / 4 weeks	100
Zuclopenthixol decanoate / 2 weeks	200

Important: These equivalences must **not** be extrapolated beyond the maximum dose for the drug

These equivalences are intended **only** as an approximate guide; individual dosage instructions should also be checked; patients should be carefully monitored after any change in medication.

ANTIPSYCHOTICS

Antipsychotic drugs

- **CAUTIONS** Blood dyscrasias · cardiovascular disease · conditions predisposing to seizures · depression · diabetes (may raise blood glucose) · epilepsy · history of jaundice · myasthenia gravis · Parkinson's disease (may be exacerbated) · photosensitisation (may occur with higher dosages) · prostatic hypertrophy (in adults) · severe respiratory disease · susceptibility to angle-closure glaucoma

  CAUTIONS, FURTHER INFORMATION
  ▸ Cardiovascular disease An ECG may be required, particularly if physical examination identifies cardiovascular risk factors, personal history of cardiovascular disease, or if the patient is being admitted as an inpatient.

- **SIDE-EFFECTS**
  ▸ **Common or very common** Agitation · amenorrhoea · arrhythmias · constipation · dizziness · drowsiness · dry mouth · galactorrhoea · gynaecomastia · hyperglycaemia · hyperprolactinaemia · hypotension (dose-related) · insomnia · leucopenia · movement disorders · neutropenia · parkinsonism · QT interval prolongation · rash · seizure · sexual dysfunction · tremor · urinary retention · weight increased
  ▸ **Uncommon** Agranulocytosis · confusion · embolism and thrombosis · neuroleptic malignant syndrome (discontinue—potentially fatal)
  ▸ **Rare or very rare** Sudden death

  SIDE-EFFECTS, FURTHER INFORMATION For depot antipsychotics—side-effects may persist until the drug has been cleared from its depot site.

  Overdose Phenothiazines cause less depression of consciousness and respiration than other sedatives. Hypotension, hypothermia, sinus tachycardia, and arrhythmias may complicate poisoning. For details on the management of poisoning see Antipsychotics under Emergency treatment of poisoning p. 1319.

- **PREGNANCY** Extrapyramidal effects and withdrawal syndrome have been reported occasionally in the neonate when antipsychotic drugs are taken during the third trimester of pregnancy. Following maternal use of antipsychotic drugs in the third trimester, neonates should be monitored for symptoms including agitation, hypertonia, hypotonia, tremor, drowsiness, feeding problems, and respiratory distress.

- **BREAST FEEDING** There is limited information available on the short- and long-term effects of antipsychotic drugs on the breast-fed infant. *Animal studies* indicate possible adverse effects of antipsychotic medicines on the developing nervous system. Chronic treatment with antipsychotic drugs whilst breast-feeding should be avoided unless absolutely necessary. Phenothiazine derivatives are sometimes used in breast-feeding women for short-term treatment of nausea and vomiting.

- **MONITORING REQUIREMENTS**
  ▸ It is advisable to monitor prolactin concentration at the start of therapy, at 6 months, and then yearly. Patients taking antipsychotic drugs not normally associated with symptomatic hyperprolactinaemia should be considered for prolactin monitoring if they show symptoms of hyperprolactinaemia (such as breast enlargement and galactorrhoea).
  ▸ Patients with schizophrenia should have physical health monitoring (including cardiovascular disease risk assessment) at least once per year.
  ▸ In children Regular clinical monitoring of endocrine function should be considered when children are taking an antipsychotic drug known to increase prolactin levels; this

includes measuring weight and height, assessing sexual maturation, and monitoring menstrual function.

- **TREATMENT CESSATION** There is a high risk of relapse if medication is stopped after 1–2 years. Withdrawal of antipsychotic drugs after long-term therapy should always be gradual and closely monitored to avoid the risk of acute withdrawal syndromes or rapid relapse. Patients should be monitored for 2 years after withdrawal of antipsychotic medication for signs and symptoms of relapse.
- **PATIENT AND CARER ADVICE** As photosensitisation may occur with higher dosages, patients should avoid direct sunlight.
  Driving and skilled tasks Drowsiness may affect performance of skilled tasks (e.g. driving or operating machinery), especially at start of treatment; effects of alcohol are enhanced.

ANTIPSYCHOTICS > FIRST-GENERATION

☞ 380

Chlorpromazine hydrochloride

- **INDICATIONS AND DOSE**

Schizophrenia and other psychoses | Mania | Short-term adjunctive management of severe anxiety | Psychomotor agitation, excitement, and violent or dangerously impulsive behaviour
- ▸ BY MOUTH
- ▸ Adult: Initially 25 mg 3 times a day, adjusted according to response, alternatively initially 75 mg once daily, adjusted according to response, dose to be taken at night; maintenance 75–300 mg daily, increased if necessary up to 1 g daily, this dose may be required in psychoses; use a third to half adult dose in the elderly or debilitated patients
- ▸ BY RECTUM
- ▸ Adult: 100 mg every 6–8 hours, dose expressed as chlorpromazine base

Intractable hiccup
- ▸ BY MOUTH
- ▸ Adult: 25–50 mg 3–4 times a day

Relief of acute symptoms of psychoses (under expert supervision)
- ▸ BY DEEP INTRAMUSCULAR INJECTION
- ▸ Adult: 25–50 mg every 6–8 hours

Nausea and vomiting of terminal illness (where other drugs have failed or are not available)
- ▸ BY MOUTH
- ▸ Child 1–5 years: 500 micrograms/kg every 4–6 hours; maximum 40 mg per day
- ▸ Child 6–11 years: 500 micrograms/kg every 4–6 hours; maximum 75 mg per day
- ▸ Child 12–17 years: 10–25 mg every 4–6 hours
- ▸ Adult: 10–25 mg every 4–6 hours
- ▸ BY DEEP INTRAMUSCULAR INJECTION
- ▸ Child 1–5 years: 500 micrograms/kg every 6–8 hours; maximum 40 mg per day
- ▸ Child 6–11 years: 500 micrograms/kg every 6–8 hours; maximum 75 mg per day
- ▸ Child 12–17 years: Initially 25 mg, then 25–50 mg every 3–4 hours until vomiting stops
- ▸ Adult: Initially 25 mg, then 25–50 mg every 3–4 hours until vomiting stops
- ▸ BY RECTUM
- ▸ Adult: 100 mg every 6–8 hours

DOSE EQUIVALENCE AND CONVERSION
- ▸ For equivalent therapeutic effect 100 mg chlorpromazine base given *rectally* as a suppository ≡ 20–25 mg chlorpromazine hydrochloride *by intramuscular injection* ≡ 40–50 mg of chlorpromazine base or hydrochloride given *by mouth*.

- **UNLICENSED USE** Rectal route is not licensed.
- **CONTRA-INDICATIONS** CNS depression · comatose states · hypothyroidism · phaeochromocytoma
- **INTERACTIONS** → Appendix 1: phenothiazines
- **SIDE-EFFECTS**
  GENERAL SIDE-EFFECTS
- ▸ **Common or very common** Anxiety · glucose tolerance impaired · mood altered · muscle tone increased · postural hypotension
- ▸ **Frequency not known** Accommodation disorder · angioedema · atrioventricular block · cardiac arrest · eye deposit · eye disorders · gastrointestinal disorders · hepatic disorders · hypertriglyceridaemia · hyponatraemia · photosensitivity reaction · respiratory disorders · SIADH · skin reactions · systemic lupus erythematosus (SLE) · temperature regulation disorder · trismus
  SPECIFIC SIDE-EFFECTS
- ▸ With intramuscular use Muscle rigidity · nasal congestion
  SIDE-EFFECTS, FURTHER INFORMATION Acute dystonic reactions may occur; children are particularly susceptible.
- **HEPATIC IMPAIRMENT** Can precipitate coma; phenothiazines are hepatotoxic.
- **RENAL IMPAIRMENT**
  Dose adjustments Start with small doses in severe renal impairment because of increased cerebral sensitivity.
- **MONITORING REQUIREMENTS**
- ▸ With intramuscular use Patients should remain supine, with blood pressure monitoring for 30 minutes after intramuscular injection.
- **HANDLING AND STORAGE** Owing to the risk of contact sensitisation, pharmacists, nurses, and other health workers should avoid direct contact with chlorpromazine; tablets should not be crushed and solutions should be handled with care.

- **MEDICINAL FORMS**
  There can be variation in the licensing of different medicines containing the same drug. Forms available from special-order manufacturers include: tablet, capsule, oral suspension, oral solution, suppository
  Tablet
  CAUTIONARY AND ADVISORY LABELS 2, 11
- ▸ Chlorpromazine hydrochloride (Non-proprietary)
  Chlorpromazine hydrochloride 25 mg Chlorpromazine 25mg tablets | 28 tablet [PoM] £42.00 DT = £37.13
  Chlorpromazine hydrochloride 50 mg Chlorpromazine 50mg tablets | 28 tablet [PoM] £42.00 DT = £28.09
  Chlorpromazine hydrochloride 100 mg Chlorpromazine 100mg tablets | 28 tablet [PoM] £42.00 DT = £37.51
  Solution for injection
- ▸ Largactil (Sanofi)
  Chlorpromazine hydrochloride 25 mg per 1 ml Largactil 50mg/2ml solution for injection ampoules | 10 ampoule [PoM] £7.51
  Oral solution
  CAUTIONARY AND ADVISORY LABELS 2, 11
- ▸ Chlorpromazine hydrochloride (Non-proprietary)
  Chlorpromazine hydrochloride 5 mg per 1 ml Chlorpromazine 25mg/5ml syrup | 150 ml [PoM] £2.35 DT = £2.35
  Chlorpromazine 25mg/5ml oral solution sugar free sugar-free | 150 ml [PoM] £2.35 DT = £2.35
  Chlorpromazine 25mg/5ml oral solution | 150 ml [PoM] £2.35 DT = £2.35
  Chlorpromazine hydrochloride 20 mg per 1 ml Chlorpromazine 100mg/5ml oral solution | 150 ml [PoM] £5.50 DT = £5.50

Flupentixol

(Flupenthixol)

F 380

● INDICATIONS AND DOSE

Schizophrenia and other psychoses, particularly with apathy and withdrawal but not mania or psychomotor hyperactivity
▸ BY MOUTH
▸ Adult: Initially 3–9 mg twice daily, adjusted according to response, for debilitated patients, use elderly dose; maximum 18 mg per day
▸ Elderly: Initially 0.75–4.5 mg twice daily, adjusted according to response

Depressive illness
▸ BY MOUTH
▸ Adult: Initially 1 mg once daily, dose to be taken in the morning, increased if necessary to 2 mg after 1 week, doses above 2 mg to be given in divided doses, last dose to be taken before 4 pm; discontinue if no response after 1 week at maximum dosage; maximum 3 mg per day
▸ Elderly: Initially 500 micrograms daily, dose to be taken in the morning, then increased if necessary to 1 mg after 1 week, doses above 1 mg to be given in divided doses, last dose to be taken before 4 pm; discontinue if no response after 1 week at maximum dosage; maximum 1.5 mg per day

● CONTRA-INDICATIONS Circulatory collapse · CNS depression · comatose states · excitable patients · impaired consciousness · overactive patients · phaeochromocytoma
● CAUTIONS Cardiac disorders · cardiovascular disease · cerebral arteriosclerosis · elderly · hyperthyroidism · hypothyroidism · parkinsonism · QT-interval prolongation · senile confusional states
● INTERACTIONS → Appendix 1: flupentixol
● SIDE-EFFECTS
▸ **Common or very common** Appetite abnormal · asthenia · concentration impaired · depression · diarrhoea · dyspnoea · gastrointestinal discomfort · headache · hyperhidrosis · hypersalivation · muscle complaints · nervousness · palpitations · skin reactions · urinary disorder · vision disorders · vomiting
▸ **Uncommon** Flatulence · hot flush · nausea · oculogyration · photosensitivity reaction · speech disorder
▸ **Rare or very rare** Glucose tolerance impaired · jaundice · thrombocytopenia
▸ **Frequency not known** Suicidal tendencies
● PREGNANCY Avoid unless potential benefit outweighs risk.
● BREAST FEEDING Present in breast milk—avoid.
● HEPATIC IMPAIRMENT Can precipitate coma.
Monitoring Consider serum-flupentixol concentration monitoring in hepatic impairment.
● RENAL IMPAIRMENT Manufacturer advises caution in renal failure.
Dose adjustments Start with small doses of antipsychotic drugs in severe renal impairment because of increased cerebral sensitivity.
● PATIENT AND CARER ADVICE Although drowsiness may occur, can also have an alerting effect so should not be taken in the evening.

● MEDICINAL FORMS
There can be variation in the licensing of different medicines containing the same drug. Forms available from special-order manufacturers include: oral suspension, oral solution
Tablet
CAUTIONARY AND ADVISORY LABELS 2
▸ Depixol (Lundbeck Ltd)
Flupentixol (as Flupentixol dihydrochloride) 3 mg Depixol 3mg tablets | 100 tablet [PoM] £13.92 DT = £13.92
▸ Fluanxol (Lundbeck Ltd)
Flupentixol (as Flupentixol dihydrochloride) 500 microgram Fluanxol 500microgram tablets | 60 tablet [PoM] £2.88 DT = £2.88
Flupentixol (as Flupentixol dihydrochloride) 1 mg Fluanxol 1mg tablets | 60 tablet [PoM] £4.86 DT = £4.86

Haloperidol

F 380

18-May-2018

● INDICATIONS AND DOSE

Nausea and vomiting
▸ BY INTRAMUSCULAR INJECTION
▸ Adult: 1–2 mg

Nausea and vomiting in palliative care
▸ BY MOUTH
▸ Adult: Initially 1.5 mg 1–2 times a day, increased if necessary to 5–10 mg daily in divided doses
▸ BY SUBCUTANEOUS INFUSION
▸ Adult: 2.5–10 mg/24 hours

Schizophrenia | Psychoses | Mania and hypomania | Organic brain damage (depending on symptoms)
▸ BY MOUTH
▸ Adult: Initially 2–20 mg once daily, alternatively initially 2–20 mg daily in divided doses; maintenance 1–3 mg 3 times a day, adjusted according to response, daily maximum to be given in divided doses, for debilitated patients, use elderly dose; maximum 20 mg per day
▸ Elderly: Initially 1–10 mg once daily, alternatively initially 1–10 mg daily in divided doses; maintenance 1–3 mg 3 times a day, adjusted according to response, daily maximum to be given in divided doses; maximum 20 mg per day
▸ BY INTRAMUSCULAR INJECTION
▸ Adult: Initially 2–5 mg, repeated if necessary, repeated dose given according to response and tolerability, for debilitated patients, use elderly dose; maximum 12 mg per day
▸ Elderly: Initially 1–2.5 mg, repeated if necessary, repeated dose given according to response and tolerability; maximum 12 mg per day

Agitation and restlessness in the elderly
▸ BY MOUTH
▸ Elderly: Initially 0.75–1.5 mg 2–3 times a day, adjusted according to response, if necessary

Management of mental or behavioural problems such as aggression, hyperactivity and self-mutilation in patients with intellectual disabilities and in patients with organic brain damage (depending on symptoms) | Gilles de la Tourette syndrome | Severe tics | Intractable hiccup | Adjunct to short-term management of moderate to severe psychomotor agitation, excitement and, violent or dangerously impulsive behaviour
▸ BY MOUTH
▸ Adult: Initially 1.5–3 mg 2–3 times a day, alternatively initially 3–5 mg 2–3 times a day, higher dose in severely affected or resistant patients; maintenance 0.5–1 mg 3 times a day, increased if necessary to 2–3 mg 3 times a day, once symptoms are controlled, gradually reduce dose to the lowest effective maintenance dose, for debilitated patients, use elderly dose

▸ **Elderly:** Initially 0.75–1.5 mg 2–3 times a day, alternatively initially 1.5–2.5 mg 2–3 times a day, higher dose in severely affected or resistant patients; maintenance 0.5–1 mg 3 times a day, increased if necessary to 2–3 mg 3 times a day, once symptoms are controlled, gradually reduce dose to the lowest effective maintenance dose

Restlessness and confusion in palliative care
▸ BY MOUTH
▸ Adult: 2 mg, then 2 mg every 2 hours if required
▸ BY SUBCUTANEOUS INJECTION
▸ Adult: 2.5 mg, then 2.5 mg every 2 hours if required
▸ BY SUBCUTANEOUS INFUSION
▸ Adult: 5–15 mg/24 hours

● UNLICENSED USE BNF doses for schizophrenia, psychoses, mania, hypomania, and organic brain damage differ from those in product literature.

IMPORTANT SAFETY INFORMATION
When prescribing, dispensing or administering, check that this injection is the correct preparation—this preparation is usually used in hospital for the rapid control of an *acute episode* and should **not** be confused with depot preparations which are usually used in the community or clinics for *maintenance* treatment.

● CONTRA-INDICATIONS CNS depression · comatose states · congenital long QT syndrome · dementia with Lewy bodies · history of torsade de pointes · history of ventricular arrhythmia · Parkinson's disease · progressive supranuclear palsy · QTc-interval prolongation · recent acute myocardial infarction · uncompensated heart failure · uncorrected hypokalaemia

● CAUTIONS Bradycardia · electrolyte disturbances (correct before treatment initiation) · family history of QTc-interval prolongation · history of heavy alcohol exposure · hyperthyroidism · hypotension (including orthostatic hypotension) · prolactin-dependent tumours · prolactinaemia · risk factors for stroke

● INTERACTIONS → Appendix 1: haloperidol

● SIDE-EFFECTS
▸ **Common or very common** Depression · eye disorders · headache · hypersalivation · nausea · neuromuscular dysfunction · postural hypotension · psychotic disorder · vision disorders · vomiting · weight decreased
▸ **Uncommon** Breast abnormalities · dyspnoea · gait abnormal · hepatic disorders · hyperhidrosis · menstrual cycle irregularities · muscle complaints · musculoskeletal stiffness · oedema · photosensitivity reaction · restlessness · sedation · skin reactions · temperature regulation disorders
▸ **Rare or very rare** Respiratory disorders · trismus
▸ **Frequency not known** Angioedema · extrasystole · hypersensitivity vasculitis · hypertension · hypoglycaemia · pancytopenia · parkinsonism · rhabdomyolysis · severe cutaneous adverse reactions (SCARs) · SIADH · thrombocytopenia

SIDE-EFFECTS, FURTHER INFORMATION Haloperiol is a less sedating antipsychotic.

● PREGNANCY Manufacturer advises it is preferable to avoid—moderate amount of data indicate no malformative or fetal/neonatal toxicity, however there are isolated case reports of birth defects following fetal exposure, mostly in combination with other drugs; reproductive toxicity shown in *animal* studies.

● HEPATIC IMPAIRMENT Manufacturer advises use with caution.
Dose adjustments Manufacturer advises halve initial dose and then adjust if necessary with smaller increments and at longer intervals.

● RENAL IMPAIRMENT Manufacturer advises use with caution.
Dose adjustments Manufacturer advises consider lower initial dose in severe impairment and then adjust if necessary with smaller increments and at longer intervals.

● MONITORING REQUIREMENTS
▸ Manufacturer advises monitor electrolytes before treatment initiation and periodically during treatment.
▸ Manufacturer advises perform ECG before treatment initiation and assess need for further ECGs during treatment on an individual basis; continuous ECG monitoring is recommended for repeated *intramuscular* doses, and for up to 6 hours after administration of *intramuscular* doses for prophylaxis or treatment of postoperative nausea and vomiting.

● PRESCRIBING AND DISPENSING INFORMATION
Palliative care For further information on the use of haloperidol in palliative care, see www.palliativedrugs.com/formulary/en/haloperidol.html.

● MEDICINAL FORMS
There can be variation in the licensing of different medicines containing the same drug. Forms available from special-order manufacturers include: oral suspension, oral solution

Tablet
CAUTIONARY AND ADVISORY LABELS 2
▸ Haloperidol (Non-proprietary)
Haloperidol **500 microgram** Haloperidol 500microgram tablets | 28 tablet [PoM] £22.05 DT = £22.05
Haloperidol **1.5 mg** Haloperidol 1.5mg tablets | 28 tablet [PoM] £15.00 DT = £12.91
Haloperidol **5 mg** Haloperidol 5mg tablets | 28 tablet [PoM] £18.00 DT = £14.95
Haloperidol **10 mg** Haloperidol 10mg tablets | 28 tablet [PoM] £27.00 DT = £22.25

Solution for injection
▸ Haloperidol (Non-proprietary)
Haloperidol **5 mg per 1 ml** Haloperidol 5mg/1ml solution for injection ampoules | 10 ampoule [PoM] £35.00 DT = £35.00

Oral solution
CAUTIONARY AND ADVISORY LABELS 2
▸ Haloperidol (Non-proprietary)
Haloperidol **1 mg per 1 ml** Haloperidol 5mg/5ml oral solution sugar free sugar-free | 100 ml [PoM] £35.99 DT = £6.47 sugar-free | 500 ml [PoM] £32.35
Haloperidol **2 mg per 1 ml** Haloperidol 10mg/5ml oral solution sugar free sugar-free | 100 ml [PoM] £46.75 DT = £7.10 sugar-free | 500 ml [PoM] £35.50
▸ Haldol (Janssen-Cilag Ltd)
Haldol **2 mg per 1 ml** Haldol 2mg/ml oral solution sugar-free | 100 ml [PoM] £4.45 DT = £7.10

Capsule
CAUTIONARY AND ADVISORY LABELS 2
▸ Serenace (Teva UK Ltd)
Haloperidol **500 microgram** Serenace 500microgram capsules | 30 capsule [PoM] £1.18 DT = £1.18

4

Nervous system

⬛ F 380

Loxapine

25-Apr-2017

● DRUG ACTION Loxapine is a dopamine D_2 and serotonin 5-HT_{2A} receptor antagonist. It also binds to noradrenergic, histaminergic, and cholinergic receptors.

● **INDICATIONS AND DOSE**

Rapid control of mild-to-moderate agitation in patients with schizophrenia or bipolar disorder (specialist supervision in hospital)

▸ BY INHALATION
▸ Adult: 9.1 mg as a single dose, followed by 9.1 mg after 2 hours if required, alternatively 4.5 mg as a single dose, followed by 4.5 mg after 2 hours if required, lower dose may be given if more appropriate or if the higher dose not previously tolerated

● CONTRA-INDICATIONS Acute respiratory symptoms · asthma · cardiovascular disease · cerebrovascular disease · chronic obstructive pulmonary disease · dehydration—risk of hypotension · elderly patients (especially those with dementia-related psychosis) · hypovolaemia—risk of hypotension

● CAUTIONS Bronchodilator treatment should be available for treatment of possible severe respiratory side-effects (bronchospasm) · history of extrapyramidal symptoms · risk factors for hypoventilation

● INTERACTIONS → Appendix 1: loxapine

● SIDE-EFFECTS
▸ **Common or very common** Fatigue · sedation · taste altered · throat irritation
▸ **Uncommon** Bronchospasm · oculogyration · restlessness
▸ **Frequency not known** Dry eye · hypertension · postural hypotension · syncope · vision blurred

● PREGNANCY Manufacturer advises use only if potential benefit outweighs risk.

● BREAST FEEDING Manufacturer advises to avoid for 48 hours after dose (express and discard milk produced during this time)—present in milk in *animal* studies.

● MONITORING REQUIREMENTS Manufacturer advises to observe patient during the first hour after each dose for signs and symptoms of bronchospasm.

● DIRECTIONS FOR ADMINISTRATION Manufacturer advises remove pull-tab and wait for green light to turn on (product must be used within 15 minutes of pulling tab); instruct patient to inhale through mouthpiece and then hold breath briefly. When green light turns off, this indicates the dose has been delivered.

● PRESCRIBING AND DISPENSING INFORMATION Educational risk minimisation materials are available for health care professionals.
Adasuve® 4.5 mg inhalation powder may be difficult to obtain.

● MEDICINAL FORMS
There can be variation in the licensing of different medicines containing the same drug.
Inhalation powder
▸ Adasuve (Galen Ltd)
Loxapine 9.1 mg Adasuve 9.1mg/dose inhalation powder | 1 dose PoM £58.30 (Hospital only)

⬛ F 380

Pericyazine

(Periciazine)

● **INDICATIONS AND DOSE**

Schizophrenia | Psychoses
▸ BY MOUTH
▸ Adult: Initially 75 mg daily in divided doses, then increased in steps of 25 mg every week, adjusted according to response; maximum 300 mg per day
▸ Elderly: Initially 15–30 mg daily in divided doses, then increased in steps of 25 mg every week, adjusted according to response; maximum 300 mg per day

Short-term adjunctive management of severe anxiety, psychomotor agitation, and violent or dangerously impulsive behaviour
▸ BY MOUTH
▸ Adult: Initially 15–30 mg daily in 2 divided doses, adjusted according to response, larger dose to be taken at bedtime
▸ Elderly: Initially 5–10 mg daily in 2 divided doses, adjusted according to response, larger dose to be taken at bedtime

● CONTRA-INDICATIONS CNS depression · comatose states · phaeochromocytoma

● CAUTIONS Hypothyroidism

● INTERACTIONS → Appendix 1: phenothiazines

● SIDE-EFFECTS Atrioventricular block · cardiac arrest · consciousness impaired · contact dermatitis · glucose tolerance impaired · hepatic disorders · hyperthermia · nasal congestion · postural hypotension · priapism · respiratory depression

● HEPATIC IMPAIRMENT Can precipitate coma; phenothiazines are hepatotoxic.

● RENAL IMPAIRMENT Avoid in renal impairment.

● MEDICINAL FORMS
There can be variation in the licensing of different medicines containing the same drug. Forms available from special-order manufacturers include: oral suspension, oral solution
Oral solution
CAUTIONARY AND ADVISORY LABELS 2
▸ Pericyazine (Non-proprietary)
Pericyazine 2 mg per 1 ml Pericyazine 10mg/5ml oral solution | 100 ml PoM £55.20 DT = £55.20
Tablet
CAUTIONARY AND ADVISORY LABELS 2
▸ Pericyazine (Non-proprietary)
Pericyazine 2.5 mg Pericyazine 2.5mg tablets | 84 tablet PoM £18.60 DT = £18.60
Pericyazine 10 mg Pericyazine 10mg tablets | 84 tablet PoM £48.00 DT = £48.00

⬛ F 380

Perphenazine

● **INDICATIONS AND DOSE**

Schizophrenia and other psychoses | Mania | Short-term adjunctive management of anxiety | Severe psychomotor agitation, excitement, and violent or dangerously impulsive behaviour | Severe nausea and vomiting unresponsive to other anti-emetics
▸ BY MOUTH
▸ Adult: Initially 4 mg 3 times a day, adjusted according to response; maximum 24 mg per day
▸ Elderly: Initially 1–2 mg 3 times a day; maximum 12 mg per day

● CONTRA-INDICATIONS Agitation in the elderly · CNS depression · comatose states · phaeochromocytoma · restlessness in the elderly

- CAUTIONS Hypothyroidism
- INTERACTIONS → Appendix 1: phenothiazines
- SIDE-EFFECTS Cardiac arrest · consciousness impaired · epilepsy · eye deposits · fatigue · headache · hepatic disorders · hyperhidrosis · menstruation with decreased bleeding · nasal congestion · nausea · oculogyric crisis · oedema · paralytic ileus · photosensitivity reaction · pigmented retinopathy · reflexes increased · saliva altered · systemic lupus erythematosus (SLE) · temperature regulation disorder · urinary hesitation · vision disorders

  SIDE-EFFECTS, FURTHER INFORMATION Acute dystonias are more common with potent first-generation antipsychotics. The risk is increased in men, young adults, children, antipsychotic-naïve patients, rapid dose escalation, and abrupt treatment discontinuation.
- HEPATIC IMPAIRMENT Can precipitate coma; phenothiazines are hepatotoxic.
- RENAL IMPAIRMENT
  Dose adjustments Start with small doses in severe renal impairment because of increased cerebral sensitivity.
- MEDICINAL FORMS
  Forms available from special-order manufacturers include: tablet, oral suspension

  ⚑ 380

Pimozide

- INDICATIONS AND DOSE
  Schizophrenia
  ▸ BY MOUTH
  ▸ Adult: Initially 2 mg daily, adjusted according to response, then increased in steps of 2–4 mg at intervals of not less than 1 week; usual dose 2–20 mg daily
  ▸ Elderly: Initially 1 mg daily, adjusted according to response, increased in steps of 2–4 mg at intervals of not less than 1 week; usual dose 2–20 mg daily

  Monosymptomatic hypochondriacal psychosis | Paranoid psychosis
  ▸ BY MOUTH
  ▸ Adult: Initially 4 mg daily, adjusted according to response, then increased in steps of 2–4 mg at intervals of not less than 1 week; maximum 16 mg per day
  ▸ Elderly: Initially 2 mg daily, adjusted according to response, increased in steps of 2–4 mg at intervals of not less than 1 week; maximum 16 mg per day

- CONTRA-INDICATIONS CNS depression · comatose states · history of arrhythmias · history or family history of congenital QT prolongation · phaeochromocytoma
- INTERACTIONS → Appendix 1: pimozide
- SIDE-EFFECTS
  ▸ **Common or very common** Appetite decreased · depression · fatigue · headache · hyperhidrosis · hypersalivation · lethargy · muscle complaints · restlessness · sebaceous gland overactivity · urinary disorders · vision blurred · vomiting
  ▸ **Uncommon** Cogwheel rigidity · dysarthria · face oedema · oculogyric crisis · skin reactions
  ▸ **Frequency not known** Cardiac arrest · generalised tonic-clonic seizure · glycosuria · hyponatraemia · libido decreased · neck stiffness · temperature regulation disorders
- HEPATIC IMPAIRMENT Can precipitate coma.
- RENAL IMPAIRMENT
  Dose adjustments Start with small doses in severe renal impairment because of increased cerebral sensitivity.
- MONITORING REQUIREMENTS
  ▸ ECG monitoring Following reports of sudden unexplained death, an ECG is recommended before treatment. It is also recommended that patients taking pimozide should have

an annual ECG (if the QT interval is prolonged, treatment should be reviewed and either withdrawn or dose reduced under close supervision) and that pimozide should not be given with other antipsychotic drugs (including depot preparations), tricyclic antidepressants or other drugs which prolong the QT interval, such as certain antimalarials, antiarrhythmic drugs and certain antihistamines and should not be given with drugs which cause electrolyte disturbances (especially diuretics).

- MEDICINAL FORMS
  There can be variation in the licensing of different medicines containing the same drug. Forms available from special-order manufacturers include: oral suspension
  Tablet
  CAUTIONARY AND ADVISORY LABELS 2
  ▸ Pimozide (Non-proprietary)
    Pimozide 4 mg Pimozide 4mg tablets | 100 tablet [PoM] Ⓢ DT = £40.31
  ▸ Orap (Eumedica Pharmaceuticals)
    Pimozide 4 mg Orap 4mg tablets | 100 tablet [PoM] £40.31 DT = £40.31

  ⚑ 380

Prochlorperazine

- INDICATIONS AND DOSE
  Schizophrenia and other psychoses | Mania
  ▸ BY MOUTH
  ▸ Adult: 12.5 mg twice daily for 7 days, dose to be adjusted at intervals of 4–7 days according to response; usual dose 75–100 mg daily
  ▸ BY DEEP INTRAMUSCULAR INJECTION
  ▸ Adult: 12.5–25 mg 2–3 times a day

  Short-term adjunctive management of severe anxiety
  ▸ BY MOUTH
  ▸ Adult: 15–20 mg daily in divided doses; maximum 40 mg per day

  Nausea and vomiting, acute attack
  ▸ BY MOUTH
  ▸ Adult: Initially 20 mg, then 10 mg after 2 hours
  ▸ BY DEEP INTRAMUSCULAR INJECTION
  ▸ Adult: 12.5 mg as required, to be followed if necessary after 6 hours by an oral dose

  Nausea and vomiting, prevention
  ▸ BY MOUTH
  ▸ Adult: 5–10 mg 2–3 times a day
  ▸ BY DEEP INTRAMUSCULAR INJECTION
  ▸ Adult: 12.5 mg as required, to be followed if necessary after 6 hours by an oral dose

  Prevention and treatment of nausea and vomiting
  ▸ BY MOUTH
  ▸ Child 1–11 years (body-weight 10 kg and above): 250 micrograms/kg 2–3 times a day
  ▸ Child 12–17 years: 5–10 mg up to 3 times a day if required
  ▸ BY INTRAMUSCULAR INJECTION
  ▸ Child 2–4 years: 1.25–2.5 mg up to 3 times a day if required
  ▸ Child 5–11 years: 5–6.25 mg up to 3 times a day if required
  ▸ Child 12–17 years: 12.5 mg up to 3 times a day if required

  Labyrinthine disorders
  ▸ BY MOUTH
  ▸ Adult: 5 mg 3 times a day, increased if necessary to 30 mg daily in divided doses, dose to be increased gradually, then reduced to 5–10 mg daily, dose is reduced after several weeks   continued →

4

Nervous system

Nausea and vomiting in previously diagnosed migraine
▶ BY MOUTH USING BUCCAL TABLET
▶ Child 12–17 years: 3–6 mg twice daily, tablets to be placed high between upper lip and gum and left to dissolve
▶ Adult: 3–6 mg twice daily, tablets to be placed high between upper lip and gum and left to dissolve

DOSE EQUIVALENCE AND CONVERSION
▶ Doses are expressed as prochlorperazine maleate or mesilate; 1 mg prochlorperazine maleate ≡ 1 mg prochlorperazine mesilate.

● UNLICENSED USE Injection not licensed for use in children. *Buccastem M*® tablets not licensed for use in children.
● CONTRA-INDICATIONS Avoid oral route in child under 10 kg · children (in psychotic disorders) · CNS depression · comatose states · phaeochromocytoma
● CAUTIONS Elderly · hypotension (more likely after intramuscular injection) · hypothyroidism (in adults)
● INTERACTIONS → Appendix 1: phenothiazines
● SIDE-EFFECTS

GENERAL SIDE-EFFECTS
▶ **Rare or very rare** Glucose tolerance impaired · hyponatraemia · SIADH
▶ **Frequency not known** Photosensitivity reaction · postural hypotension · skin reactions

SPECIFIC SIDE-EFFECTS
▶ **Rare or very rare**
▶ With buccal use Blood disorder · hepatic disorders
▶ **Frequency not known**
▶ With buccal use Oral disorders
▶ With intramuscular or oral use Atrioventricular block · cardiac arrest · consciousness impaired · eye disorders · hyperthermia · jaundice · muscle rigidity · nasal congestion · oculogyric crisis · postural hypotension · respiratory depression

SIDE-EFFECTS, FURTHER INFORMATION Acute dystonias are more common with potent first-generation antipsychotics. The risk is increased in men, young adults, children, antipsychotic-naïve patients, rapid dose escalation, and abrupt treatment discontinuation.

● HEPATIC IMPAIRMENT Can precipitate coma; phenothiazines are hepatotoxic.
● RENAL IMPAIRMENT
Dose adjustments Start with small doses in severe renal impairment because of increased cerebral sensitivity.
● DIRECTIONS FOR ADMINISTRATION
▶ With buccal use Buccal tablets are placed high between upper lip and gum and left to dissolve.
● PATIENT AND CARER ADVICE
▶ With buccal use Patients or carers should be given advice on how to administer prochlorperazine buccal tablets.

● MEDICINAL FORMS
There can be variation in the licensing of different medicines containing the same drug.
Tablet
CAUTIONARY AND ADVISORY LABELS 2
▶ Prochlorperazine (Non-proprietary)
Prochlorperazine maleate 5 mg Prochlorperazine 5mg tablets | 28 tablet [PoM] £0.72 DT = £0.50 | 84 tablet [PoM] £1.50–£2.16
▶ Stemetil (Sanofi)
Prochlorperazine maleate 5 mg Stemetil 5mg tablets | 28 tablet [PoM] £1.98 DT = £0.50 | 84 tablet [PoM] £5.94
Solution for injection
▶ Stemetil (Sanofi)
Prochlorperazine mesilate 12.5 mg per 1 ml Stemetil 12.5mg/1ml solution for injection ampoules | 10 ampoule [PoM] £5.23 DT = £5.23

Buccal tablet
CAUTIONARY AND ADVISORY LABELS 2
▶ Prochlorperazine (Non-proprietary)
Prochlorperazine maleate 3 mg Prochlorperazine 3mg buccal tablets | 50 tablet [PoM] £35.94–£51.75 DT = £51.75
▶ Buccastem (Alliance Pharmaceuticals Ltd)
Prochlorperazine maleate 3 mg Buccastem M 3mg tablets | 8 tablet [P] £4.01
Oral solution
CAUTIONARY AND ADVISORY LABELS 2
▶ Stemetil (Sanofi)
Prochlorperazine mesilate 1 mg per 1 ml Stemetil 5mg/5ml syrup | 100 ml [PoM] £3.34 DT = £3.34

F 380

Sulpiride

● INDICATIONS AND DOSE
Schizophrenia with predominantly negative symptoms
▶ BY MOUTH
▶ Adult: 200–400 mg twice daily; maximum 800 mg per day
▶ Elderly: Lower initial dose to be given, increased gradually according to response
Schizophrenia with mainly positive symptoms
▶ BY MOUTH
▶ Adult: 200–400 mg twice daily; maximum 2.4 g per day
▶ Elderly: Lower initial dose to be given, increased gradually according to response

● CONTRA-INDICATIONS CNS depression · comatose states · phaeochromocytoma
● CAUTIONS Aggressive patients (even low doses may aggravate symptoms) · agitated patients (even low doses may aggravate symptoms) · excited patients (even low doses may aggravate symptoms)
● INTERACTIONS → Appendix 1: sulpiride
● SIDE-EFFECTS
▶ **Common or very common** Breast abnormalities · sedation · skin reactions
▶ **Uncommon** Hypersalivation · muscle tone increased · postural hypotension
▶ **Rare or very rare** Oculogyric crisis
▶ **Frequency not known** Cardiac arrest · dyspnoea · hyponatraemia · SIADH · trismus
● HEPATIC IMPAIRMENT Can precipitate coma.
● RENAL IMPAIRMENT
Dose adjustments Start with small doses in severe renal impairment because of increased cerebral sensitivity.
● MONITORING REQUIREMENTS Sulpiride does not affect blood pressure to the same extent as other antipsychotic drugs and so blood pressure monitoring is not mandatory for this drug.
● PRESCRIBING AND DISPENSING INFORMATION Flavours of oral liquid formulations may include lemon and aniseed.

● MEDICINAL FORMS
There can be variation in the licensing of different medicines containing the same drug. Forms available from special-order manufacturers include: oral suspension, oral solution
Oral solution
CAUTIONARY AND ADVISORY LABELS 2
▶ Sulpiride (Non-proprietary)
Sulpiride 40 mg per 1 ml Sulpiride 200mg/5ml oral solution sugar free sugar-free | 150 ml [PoM] £28.00 DT = £28.00
Tablet
CAUTIONARY AND ADVISORY LABELS 2
▶ Sulpiride (Non-proprietary)
Sulpiride 200 mg Sulpiride 200mg tablets | 30 tablet [PoM] £9.49 DT = £4.40
Sulpiride 400 mg Sulpiride 400mg tablets | 30 tablet [PoM] £18.80 DT = £18.80
▶ Dolmatil (Sanofi)
Sulpiride 200 mg Dolmatil 200mg tablets | 100 tablet [PoM] £6.00
Sulpiride 400 mg Dolmatil 400mg tablets | 100 tablet [PoM] £19.00

Trifluoperazine ⟆ 380

- **INDICATIONS AND DOSE**

Schizophrenia and other psychoses | Short-term adjunctive management of psychomotor agitation, excitement, and violent or dangerously impulsive behaviour
▸ BY MOUTH
  ▸ Adult: Initially 5 mg twice daily, increased by 5 mg daily after 1 week, then at intervals of 3 days, according to response
  ▸ Elderly: Initially up to 2.5 mg twice daily, increased by 5 mg daily after 1 week, then at intervals of 3 days, according to response

Short-term adjunctive management of severe anxiety
▸ BY MOUTH
  ▸ Adult: 2–4 mg daily in divided doses, increased if necessary to 6 mg daily
  ▸ Elderly: Up to 2 mg daily in divided doses, increased if necessary to 6 mg daily

Severe nausea and vomiting
▸ BY MOUTH
  ▸ Adult: 2–4 mg daily in divided doses; maximum 6 mg per day

- **CONTRA-INDICATIONS** CNS depression · comatose states · phaeochromocytoma
- **INTERACTIONS** → Appendix 1: phenothiazines
- **SIDE-EFFECTS** Alertness decreased · anxiety · appetite decreased · blood disorder · cardiac arrest · fatigue · hyperpyrexia · jaundice cholestatic · lens opacity · muscle weakness · oedema · pancytopenia · photosensitivity reaction · postural hypotension (dose-related) · skin reactions · thrombocytopenia · urinary hesitation · vision blurred · withdrawal syndrome
  SIDE-EFFECTS, FURTHER INFORMATION Extrapyramidal symptoms are more frequent at doses exceeding 6mg daily. Acute dystonias are more common with potent first-generation antipsychotics. The risk is increased in men, young adults, children, antipsychotic-naïve patients, rapid dose escalation, and abrupt treatment discontinuation.
- **HEPATIC IMPAIRMENT** Can precipitate coma; phenothiazines are hepatotoxic.
- **RENAL IMPAIRMENT**
  Dose adjustments Start with small doses in severe renal impairment because of increased cerebral sensitivity.
- **MONITORING REQUIREMENTS** Trifluoperazine does not affect blood pressure to the same extent as other antipsychotic drugs and so blood pressure monitoring is not mandatory for this drug.
- **MEDICINAL FORMS**
  There can be variation in the licensing of different medicines containing the same drug.
  Oral solution
  CAUTIONARY AND ADVISORY LABELS 2
  ▸ Trifluoperazine (Non-proprietary)
    Trifluoperazine (as Trifluoperazine hydrochloride)
    200 microgram per 1 ml Trifluoperazine 1mg/5ml oral solution sugar free sugar-free | 200 ml PoM £112.25 DT = £112.25
    Trifluoperazine (as Trifluoperazine hydrochloride) 1 mg per 1 ml Trifluoperazine 5mg/5ml oral solution sugar free sugar-free | 150 ml PoM £25.50 DT = £25.50
  Tablet
  CAUTIONARY AND ADVISORY LABELS 2
  ▸ Trifluoperazine (Non-proprietary)
    Trifluoperazine (as Trifluoperazine hydrochloride)
    1 mg Trifluoperazine 1mg tablets | 112 tablet PoM £59.12–£99.80 DT = £59.12
    Trifluoperazine (as Trifluoperazine hydrochloride)
    5 mg Trifluoperazine 5mg tablets | 112 tablet PoM £134.89–£165.00 DT = £134.89

Zuclopenthixol ⟆ 380

- **INDICATIONS AND DOSE**

Schizophrenia and other psychoses
▸ BY MOUTH
  ▸ Adult: Initially 20–30 mg daily in divided doses, increased if necessary up to 150 mg daily; usual maintenance 20–50 mg daily (max. per dose 40 mg), for debilitated patients, use elderly dose
  ▸ Elderly: Initially 5–15 mg daily in divided doses, increased if necessary up to 150 mg daily; usual maintenance 20–50 mg daily (max. per dose 40 mg)

- **CONTRA-INDICATIONS** Apathetic states · CNS depression · comatose states · phaeochromocytoma · withdrawn states
- **CAUTIONS** Hyperthyroidism · hypothyroidism
- **INTERACTIONS** → Appendix 1: zuclopenthixol
- **SIDE-EFFECTS** Anxiety · appetite abnormal · asthenia · concentration impaired · depression · diarrhoea · dyspnoea · eye disorders · fever · flatulence · gait abnormal · gastrointestinal discomfort · glucose tolerance impaired · headaches · hepatic disorders · hot flush · hyperacusia · hyperhidrosis · hyperlipidaemia · hypersalivation · hypothermia · malaise · memory loss · muscle complaints · nasal congestion · nausea · neuromuscular dysfunction · pain · palpitations · paraesthesia · photosensitivity reaction · reflexes increased · seborrhoea · skin reactions · sleep disorders · speech disorder · syncope · thirst · thrombocytopenia · tinnitus · urinary disorders · vertigo · vision disorders · vomiting · vulvovaginal dryness · weight decreased · withdrawal syndrome
- **HEPATIC IMPAIRMENT** Can precipitate coma.
  Dose adjustments Halve dose.
  Monitoring Consider serum-level monitoring in patients with hepatic impairment.
- **RENAL IMPAIRMENT**
  Dose adjustments Halve dose in renal failure; smaller starting doses used in severe renal impairment because of increased cerebral sensitivity.
- **MEDICINAL FORMS**
  There can be variation in the licensing of different medicines containing the same drug.
  Tablet
  CAUTIONARY AND ADVISORY LABELS 2
  ▸ Clopixol (Lundbeck Ltd)
    Zuclopenthixol (as Zuclopenthixol dihydrochloride) 2 mg Clopixol 2mg tablets | 100 tablet PoM £3.14 DT = £3.14
    Zuclopenthixol (as Zuclopenthixol dihydrochloride)
    10 mg Clopixol 10mg tablets | 100 tablet PoM £8.06 DT = £8.06
    Zuclopenthixol (as Zuclopenthixol dihydrochloride)
    25 mg Clopixol 25mg tablets | 100 tablet PoM £16.13 DT = £16.13

Zuclopenthixol acetate ⟆ 380

- **INDICATIONS AND DOSE**

Short-term management of acute psychosis | Short-term management of mania | Short-term management of exacerbation of chronic psychosis
▸ BY DEEP INTRAMUSCULAR INJECTION
  ▸ Adult: 50–150 mg, then 50–150 mg after 2–3 days if required, (1 additional dose may be needed 1–2 days after the first injection); maximum cumulative dose 400 mg in 2 weeks and maximum 4 injections; maximum duration of treatment 2 weeks—if maintenance treatment necessary change to an oral antipsychotic 2–3 days after last injection, or to a longer acting antipsychotic depot injection given concomitantly with last injection of continued →

zuclopenthixol acetate; to be administered into the gluteal muscle or lateral thigh
▸ Elderly: 50–100 mg, then 50–100 mg after 2–3 days if required, (1 additional dose may be needed 1–2 days after the first injection); maximum cumulative dose 400 mg in 2 weeks and maximum 4 injections; maximum duration of treatment 2 weeks—if maintenance treatment necessary change to an oral antipsychotic 2–3 days after last injection, or to a longer acting antipsychotic depot injection given concomitantly with last injection of zuclopenthixol acetate; to be administered into the gluteal muscle or lateral thigh

---

IMPORTANT SAFETY INFORMATION
When prescribing, dispensing, or administering, check that this is the correct preparation—this preparation is usually used in hospital for an *acute episode* and should **not** be confused with depot preparations which are usually used in the community or clinics for *maintenance* treatment.

SAFE PRACTICE
Zuclopenthixol acetate has been confused with zuclopenthixol decanoate; care must be taken to ensure the correct drug is prescribed and dispensed.

● **CONTRA-INDICATIONS** CNS depression · comatose states · phaeochromocytoma
● **CAUTIONS** Hyperthyroidism · hypothyroidism
● **INTERACTIONS** → Appendix 1: zuclopenthixol
● **SIDE-EFFECTS** Anxiety · appetite abnormal · asthenia · concentration impaired · depression · diarrhoea · dyspnoea · eye disorders · fever · flatulence · gait abnormal · gastrointestinal discomfort · glucose tolerance impaired · headaches · hepatic disorders · hot flush · hyperacusia · hyperhidrosis · hyperlipidaemia · hypersalivation · hypothermia (dose-related) · malaise · memory loss · muscle complaints · nasal congestion · nausea · neuromuscular dysfunction · pain · palpitations · paraesthesia · photosensitivity reaction · reflexes increased · seborrhoea · sexual dysfunction · skin reactions · sleep disorders · speech disorder · syncope · thirst · thrombocytopenia · tinnitus · urinary disorders · vertigo · vision disorders · vomiting · vulvovaginal dryness · weight decreased · withdrawal syndrome
● **HEPATIC IMPAIRMENT** Can precipitate coma.
● **RENAL IMPAIRMENT**
Dose adjustments Start with small doses in severe renal impairment because of increased cerebral sensitivity.

● **MEDICINAL FORMS**
There can be variation in the licensing of different medicines containing the same drug.
Solution for injection
▸ Clopixol Acuphase (Lundbeck Ltd)
Zuclopenthixol acetate 50 mg per 1 ml Clopixol Acuphase 50mg/1ml solution for injection ampoules | 5 ampoule PoM £24.21 DT = £24.21

ANTIPSYCHOTICS > FIRST-GENERATION (DEPOT INJECTIONS)

◸ 380

▍Flupentixol decanoate
(Flupenthixol Decanoate)

● **INDICATIONS AND DOSE**
Maintenance in schizophrenia and other psychoses
▸ BY DEEP INTRAMUSCULAR INJECTION
▸ Adult: Test dose 20 mg, dose to be injected into the upper outer buttock or lateral thigh, then 20–40 mg after at least 7 days, then 20–40 mg every 2–4 weeks, adjusted according to response, usual maintenance dose 50 mg every 4 weeks to 300 mg every 2 weeks; maximum 400 mg per week
▸ Elderly: Dose is initially quarter to half adult dose

● **CONTRA-INDICATIONS** Children · CNS depression · comatose states · excitable patients · overactive patients · phaeochromocytoma
● **CAUTIONS** An alternative antipsychotic may be necessary if symptoms such as aggression or agitation appear · hyperthyroidism · hypothyroidism · when transferring from oral to depot therapy, the dose by mouth should be reduced gradually
● **INTERACTIONS** → Appendix 1: flupentixol
● **SIDE-EFFECTS**
▸ **Common or very common** Appetite abnormal · asthenia · concentration impaired · depression · diarrhoea · dyspnoea · gastrointestinal discomfort · headache · hyperhidrosis · hypersalivation · muscle complaints · nervousness · palpitations · skin reactions · urinary disorder · vision disorders · vomiting
▸ **Uncommon** Flatulence · hot flush · nausea · oculogyration · photosensitivity reaction · speech disorder
▸ **Rare or very rare** Glucose tolerance impaired · jaundice · thrombocytopenia
▸ **Frequency not known** Suicidal tendencies
● **HEPATIC IMPAIRMENT** Can precipitate coma.
● **RENAL IMPAIRMENT**
Dose adjustments Start with small doses in severe renal impairment because of increased cerebral sensitivity.
● **MONITORING REQUIREMENTS** Treatment requires careful monitoring for optimum effect.
● **DIRECTIONS FOR ADMINISTRATION** In general not more than 2–3mL of oily injection should be administered at any one site. Correct injection technique (including use of z-track technique) and rotation of injection sites are essential. When initiating therapy with sustained-release preparations of conventional antipsychotics, patients should first be given a small test-dose as undesirable side-effects are prolonged.

● **MEDICINAL FORMS**
There can be variation in the licensing of different medicines containing the same drug.
Solution for injection
▸ Flupentixol decanoate (Non-proprietary)
Flupentixol decanoate 100 mg per 1 ml Flupentixol 100mg/1ml solution for injection ampoules | 10 ampoule PoM Ⓢ DT = £62.51
▸ Depixol (Lundbeck Ltd)
Flupentixol decanoate 20 mg per 1 ml Depixol 40mg/2ml solution for injection ampoules | 10 ampoule PoM £25.39 DT = £25.39
Depixol 20mg/1ml solution for injection ampoules | 10 ampoule PoM £15.17 DT = £15.17
Flupentixol decanoate 100 mg per 1 ml Depixol Conc 100mg/1ml solution for injection ampoules | 10 ampoule PoM £62.51 DT = £62.51
Flupentixol decanoate 200 mg per 1 ml Depixol Low Volume 200mg/1ml solution for injection ampoules | 5 ampoule PoM £97.59 DT = £97.59

▸ Psytixol (Mylan)
Flupentixol decanoate 20 mg per 1 ml Psytixol 40mg/2ml solution for injection ampoules | 10 ampoule [PoM] £25.38 DT = £25.39
Psytixol 20mg/1ml solution for injection ampoules |
10 ampoule [PoM] £15.16 DT = £15.17
Flupentixol decanoate 100 mg per 1 ml Psytixol 50mg/0.5ml solution for injection ampoules | 10 ampoule [PoM] £34.12 DT = £34.12
Psytixol 100mg/1ml solution for injection ampoules |
10 ampoule [PoM] £62.50 DT = £62.51
Flupentixol decanoate 200 mg per 1 ml Psytixol 200mg/1ml solution for injection ampoules | 5 ampoule [PoM] £97.58 DT = £97.59

F 380

Fluphenazine decanoate

● **INDICATIONS AND DOSE**
Maintenance in schizophrenia and other psychoses
▸ BY DEEP INTRAMUSCULAR INJECTION
▸ **Adult:** Test dose 12.5 mg, dose to be administered into the gluteal muscle, then 12.5–100 mg after 4–7 days, then 12.5–100 mg every 14–35 days, adjusted according to response
▸ **Elderly:** Test dose 6.25 mg, dose to be administered into the gluteal muscle, then 12.5–100 mg after 4–7 days, then 12.5–100 mg every 14–35 days, adjusted according to response

● CONTRA-INDICATIONS Children · CNS depression · comatose states · marked cerebral atherosclerosis · phaeochromocytoma
● CAUTIONS Hypothyroidism · QT-interval prolongation · when transferring from oral to depot therapy, the dose by mouth should be reduced gradually
● INTERACTIONS → Appendix 1: phenothiazines
● SIDE-EFFECTS Acute kidney injury · arrhythmia · blood disorder · cognitive impairment · epileptiform seizure · headache · hepatic disorders · hyponatraemia · lens opacity · lethargy · leucocytosis · nasal congestion · oculogyric crisis · oedema · oligomenorrhoea · opisthotonus · SIADH · skin pigmentation change · systemic lupus erythematosus (SLE) · temperature regulation disorder · thrombocytopenia · urinary disorders · vision blurred · vomiting
● HEPATIC IMPAIRMENT Avoid in hepatic failure. Can precipitate coma; phenothiazines are hepatotoxic.
● RENAL IMPAIRMENT Manufacturer advises caution. Avoid in renal failure.
Dose adjustments Start with small doses of antipsychotic drugs in severe renal impairment because of increased cerebral sensitivity.
● MONITORING REQUIREMENTS Treatment requires careful monitoring for optimum effect.
● DIRECTIONS FOR ADMINISTRATION In general not more than 2–3 mL of oily injection should be administered at any one site. Correct injection technique (including use of z-track technique) and rotation of injection sites are essential. When initiating therapy with sustained-release preparations of conventional antipsychotics, patients should first be given a small test-dose as undesirable side-effects are prolonged.

● MEDICINAL FORMS
There can be variation in the licensing of different medicines containing the same drug.
Solution for injection
EXCIPIENTS: May contain Sesame oil
▸ Modecate (Sanofi)
Fluphenazine decanoate 25 mg per 1 ml Modecate 50mg/2ml solution for injection ampoules | 5 ampoule [PoM] £22.22
Modecate 25mg/1ml solution for injection ampoules |
10 ampoule [PoM] £22.55 DT = £22.55

Fluphenazine decanoate 100 mg per 1 ml Modecate Concentrate 100mg/1ml solution for injection ampoules | 5 ampoule [PoM] £43.73 DT = £43.73
Modecate Concentrate 50mg/0.5ml solution for injection ampoules | 10 ampoule [PoM] £44.73

F 380

Haloperidol decanoate

18-May-2018

● **INDICATIONS AND DOSE**
Maintenance in schizophrenia and other psychoses
▸ BY DEEP INTRAMUSCULAR INJECTION
▸ **Adult:** Initially 50 mg every 4 weeks, increased in steps of 50 mg if required, increased if necessary up to 300 mg every 4 weeks, higher doses may be needed in some patients, dose to be administered into gluteal muscle, if 2-weekly administration preferred, doses should be halved
▸ **Elderly:** Initially 12.5–25 mg every 4 weeks, if 2-weekly administration preferred, doses should be halved

IMPORTANT SAFETY INFORMATION
When prescribing, dispensing or administering, check that this is the correct preparation—this preparation is used for *maintenance* treatment and should **not** be used for the rapid control of an *acute episode*.

● CONTRA-INDICATIONS Children · CNS depression · comatose states · congenital long QT syndrome · dementia with Lewy bodies · history of torsade de pointes · history of ventricular arrhythmia · Parkinson's disease · progressive supranuclear palsy · QT-interval prolongation · recent acute myocardial infarction · uncompensated heart failure · uncorrected hypokalaemia
● CAUTIONS Bradycardia · electrolyte disturbances (correct before treatment initiation) · family history of QTc-interval prolongation · history of heavy alcohol exposure · hyperthyroidism · hypotension (including orthostatic hypotension) · prolactin-dependent tumours · prolactinaemia · risk factors for stroke · when transferring from oral to depot therapy, the dose by mouth should be reduced gradually
● INTERACTIONS → Appendix 1: haloperidol
● SIDE-EFFECTS
▸ **Common or very common** Depression · hypersalivation · muscle complaints · sedation
▸ **Uncommon** Eye disorders · headache · neuromuscular dysfunction · vision disorders
▸ **Frequency not known** Angioedema · breast abnormalities · cardiac arrest · dyspnoea · extrasystole · gait abnormal · hepatic disorders · hyperhidrosis · hypersensitivity vasculitis · hypoglycaemia · menstrual cycle irregularities · musculoskeletal stiffness · nausea · oedema · pancytopenia · photosensitivity reaction · postural hypotension · psychotic disorder · respiratory disorders · restlessness · rhabdomyolysis · SIADH · skin reactions · temperature regulation disorder · thrombocytopenia · trismus · vomiting · weight decreased
SIDE-EFFECTS, FURTHER INFORMATION Haloperiol is a less sedating antipsychotic.
● PREGNANCY Manufacturer advises it is preferable to avoid—moderate amount of data indicate no malformative or fetal/neonatal toxicity, however there are isolated case reports of birth defects following fetal exposure, mostly in combination with other drugs; reproductive toxicity shown in *animal* studies.
● HEPATIC IMPAIRMENT Manufacturer advises use with caution.
Dose adjustments Manufacturer advises halve initial dose and then adjust if necessary with smaller increments and at longer intervals.

4

Nervous system

- **RENAL IMPAIRMENT** Manufacturer advises use with caution.
  Dose adjustments Manufacturer advises consider lower initial dose in severe impairment and then adjust if necessary with smaller increments and at longer intervals.
- **MONITORING REQUIREMENTS**
- ▶ Manufacturer advises perform ECG before treatment initiation and assess need for further ECGs during treatment on an individual basis.
- ▶ Manufacturer advises monitor electrolytes before treatment initiation and periodically during treatment.
- **DIRECTIONS FOR ADMINISTRATION** In general not more than 2–3 mL of oily injection should be administered at any one site. Correct injection technique (including use of z-track technique) and rotation of injection sites are essential. When initiating therapy with sustained-release preparations of conventional antipsychotics, patients should first be given a small test-dose as undesirable side-effects are prolonged.

- **MEDICINAL FORMS**
  There can be variation in the licensing of different medicines containing the same drug.
  Solution for injection
  EXCIPIENTS: May contain Benzyl alcohol, sesame oil
- ▶ Haldol decanoate (Janssen-Cilag Ltd)
  Haloperidol (as Haloperidol decanoate) 50 mg per 1 ml Haldol decanoate 50mg/1ml solution for injection ampoules | 5 ampoule [PoM] £19.06
  Haloperidol (as Haloperidol decanoate) 100 mg per 1 ml Haldol decanoate 100mg/1ml solution for injection ampoules | 5 ampoule [PoM] £25.26

⌖ 380

Zuclopenthixol decanoate

- **INDICATIONS AND DOSE**

Maintenance in schizophrenia and paranoid psychoses
- ▶ BY DEEP INTRAMUSCULAR INJECTION
- ▶ Adult: Test dose 100 mg, dose to be administered into the upper outer buttock or lateral thigh, followed by 200–500 mg after at least 7 days, then 200–500 mg every 1–4 weeks, adjusted according to response, higher doses of more than 500mg can be used; do not exceed 600 mg weekly
- ▶ Elderly: A quarter to half usual starting dose to be used

---

IMPORTANT SAFETY INFORMATION
When prescribing, dispensing, or administering, check that this is the correct preparation—this preparation is used for *maintenance* treatment and should **not** be used for the short-term management of an *acute episode*.

SAFE PRACTICE
Zuclopenthixol decanoate has been confused with zuclopenthixol acetate; care must be taken to ensure the correct drug is prescribed and dispensed.

- **CONTRA-INDICATIONS** Children · CNS depression · comatose states · phaeochromocytoma
- **CAUTIONS** Hyperthyroidism · hypothyroidism · QT interval prolongation · when transferring from oral to depot therapy, the dose by mouth should be reduced gradually
- **INTERACTIONS** → Appendix 1: zuclopenthixol
- **SIDE-EFFECTS** Anxiety · appetite abnormal · asthenia · concentration impaired · depression · diarrhoea · dyspnoea · eye disorders · fever · flatulence · gait abnormal · gastrointestinal discomfort · glucose tolerance impaired · headaches · hepatic disorders · hot flush · hyperacusia · hyperhidrosis · hyperlipidaemia · hypersalivation · hypothermia · malaise · memory loss · muscle complaints · nasal congestion · nausea · neuromuscular dysfunction · pain · palpitations · paraesthesia · photosensitivity reaction

· reflexes increased · seborrhoea · skin reactions · sleep disorders · speech disorder · syncope · thirst · thrombocytopenia · tinnitus · urinary disorders · vertigo · vision disorders · vomiting · vulvovaginal dryness · weight decreased · withdrawal syndrome

- **HEPATIC IMPAIRMENT** Can precipitate coma.
- **RENAL IMPAIRMENT**
  Dose adjustments Start with small doses in severe renal impairment because of increased cerebral sensitivity.
- **MONITORING REQUIREMENTS** Treatment requires careful monitoring for optimum effect.
- **DIRECTIONS FOR ADMINISTRATION** In general not more than 2–3 mL of oily injection should be administered at any one site. Correct injection technique (including use of z-track technique) and rotation of injection sites are essential. When initiating therapy with sustained-release preparations of conventional antipsychotics, patients should first be given a small test-dose as undesirable side-effects are prolonged.

- **MEDICINAL FORMS**
  There can be variation in the licensing of different medicines containing the same drug.
  Solution for injection
- ▶ Clopixol (Lundbeck Ltd)
  Zuclopenthixol decanoate 200 mg per 1 ml Clopixol 200mg/1ml solution for injection ampoules | 10 ampoule [PoM] £31.51 DT = £31.51
  Zuclopenthixol decanoate 500 mg per 1 ml Clopixol Conc 500mg/1ml solution for injection ampoules | 5 ampoule [PoM] £37.18 DT = £37.18

ANTIPSYCHOTICS > SECOND-GENERATION

⌖ 380

Amisulpride

- **DRUG ACTION** Amisulpride is a selective dopamine receptor antagonist with high affinity for mesolimbic D_2 and D_3 receptors.

- **INDICATIONS AND DOSE**

Acute psychotic episode in schizophrenia
- ▶ BY MOUTH
- ▶ Adult: 400–800 mg daily in 2 divided doses, adjusted according to response; maximum 1.2 g per day

Schizophrenia with predominantly negative symptoms
- ▶ BY MOUTH
- ▶ Adult: 50–300 mg daily

- **CONTRA-INDICATIONS** CNS depression · comatose states · phaeochromocytoma · prolactin-dependent tumours
- **INTERACTIONS** → Appendix 1: amisulpride
- **SIDE-EFFECTS**
- ▶ Common or very common Anxiety · breast pain · hypersalivation · muscle rigidity · nausea · oculogyric crisis · trismus · vomiting
- ▶ Uncommon Bradycardia
- ▶ Frequency not known Angioedema · bone disorders · cardiac arrest · dyslipidaemia · hyponatraemia · nasal congestion · neoplasms · SIADH · urticaria · vision blurred
- **PREGNANCY** Avoid.
- **BREAST FEEDING** Avoid—no information available.
- **RENAL IMPAIRMENT** No information available if eGFR less than 10 mL/minute/1.73 m².
  Dose adjustments Halve dose if eGFR 30–60 mL/minute/1.73 m².
  Use one-third dose if eGFR 10–30 mL/minute/1.73 m².
- **MONITORING REQUIREMENTS** Amisulpride does not affect blood pressure to the same extent as other antipsychotic drugs and so blood pressure monitoring is not mandatory for this drug.

- **PRESCRIBING AND DISPENSING INFORMATION** Flavours of oral liquid formulations may include caramel.

- **MEDICINAL FORMS**
There can be variation in the licensing of different medicines containing the same drug. Forms available from special-order manufacturers include: oral suspension, oral solution

Oral solution
CAUTIONARY AND ADVISORY LABELS 2
▸ Amisulpride (Non-proprietary)
Amisulpride 100 mg per 1 ml Amisulpride 100mg/ml oral solution sugar free sugar-free | 60 ml [PoM] £36.00 DT = £36.00
▸ Solian (Sanofi)
Amisulpride 100 mg per 1 ml Solian 100mg/ml oral solution sugar-free | 60 ml [PoM] £33.76 DT = £36.00

Tablet
CAUTIONARY AND ADVISORY LABELS 2
▸ Amisulpride (Non-proprietary)
Amisulpride 50 mg Amisulpride 50mg tablets | 60 tablet [PoM] £22.76 DT = £1.61
Amisulpride 100 mg Amisulpride 100mg tablets | 60 tablet [PoM] £39.48 DT = £3.24
Amisulpride 200 mg Amisulpride 200mg tablets | 60 tablet [PoM] £66.00 DT = £5.59
Amisulpride 400 mg Amisulpride 400mg tablets | 60 tablet [PoM] £132.00 DT = £35.21
▸ Solian (Sanofi)
Amisulpride 50 mg Solian 50 tablets | 60 tablet [PoM] £22.76 DT = £1.61
Amisulpride 100 mg Solian 100 tablets | 60 tablet [PoM] £35.29 DT = £3.24
Amisulpride 200 mg Solian 200 tablets | 60 tablet [PoM] £58.99 DT = £5.59
Amisulpride 400 mg Solian 400 tablets | 60 tablet [PoM] £117.97 DT = £35.21

◀ 380

Aripiprazole

- **DRUG ACTION** Aripiprazole is a dopamine D_2 partial agonist with weak 5-HT$_{1a}$ partial agonism and 5-HT$_{2A}$ receptor antagonism.

● INDICATIONS AND DOSE

Maintenance in schizophrenia in patients stabilised with oral aripiprazole
▸ INITIALLY BY INTRAMUSCULAR INJECTION
▸ Adult: 400 mg every month, to be injected into the gluteal muscle, minimum of 26 days between injections, for dose adjustment due to side effects—consult product literature and (by mouth) 10–20 mg daily continued for 14 consecutive days after the first injection, for missed depot doses consult product literature

Schizophrenia
▸ BY MOUTH
▸ Adult: 10–15 mg once daily; usual dose 15 mg once daily (max. per dose 30 mg once daily)

Treatment and recurrence prevention of mania
▸ BY MOUTH
▸ Adult: 15 mg once daily, increased if necessary up to 30 mg once daily

Control of agitation and disturbed behaviour in schizophrenia
▸ BY INTRAMUSCULAR INJECTION
▸ Adult: Initially 5.25–15 mg for 1 dose, alternatively usual dose 9.75 mg for 1 dose, followed by 5.25–15 mg after 2 hours if required, maximum 3 injections daily; maximum daily combined oral and parenteral dose 30 mg

DOSE ADJUSTMENTS DUE TO INTERACTIONS
▸ With oral use Manufacturer advises double the dose with concurrent use of potent inducers of CYP3A4. Manufacturer advises reduce dose by half with

concurrent use of potent inhibitors of CYP3A4 or CYP2D6.
▸ With intramuscular use For dose adjustments due to concurrent use of interacting drugs—consult product literature.

IMPORTANT SAFETY INFORMATION
When prescribing, dispensing, or administering, check that the correct preparation is used—the preparation usually used in hospital for the rapid control of an *acute episode* (solution for injection containing aripiprazole 7.5 mg/mL) should **not** be confused with depot preparations (aripiprazole 400-mg vial with solvent), which are usually used in the community or clinics for *maintenance treatment*.

- **CONTRA-INDICATIONS** CNS depression · comatose state · phaeochromocytoma

- **CAUTIONS**
GENERAL CAUTIONS Cerebrovascular disease · elderly (reduce initial dose)
SPECIFIC CAUTIONS
▸ With intramuscular use When transferring from oral to depot therapy, the dose by mouth should be reduced gradually

- **INTERACTIONS** → Appendix 1: aripiprazole

- **SIDE-EFFECTS**
▸ **Common or very common** Anxiety · appetite abnormal · diabetes mellitus · extrapyramidal symptoms · fatigue · gastrointestinal discomfort · headache · hypersalivation · nausea · postural hypotension · sedation · vision disorders · vomiting
▸ **Uncommon** Depression · hiccups
▸ **Frequency not known** Aggression · alopecia · bradycardia · cardiac arrest · chest pain · diabetic hyperosmolar coma · diarrhoea · dysphagia · generalised tonic-clonic seizure · hepatic disorders · hyperhidrosis · hypertension · hyponatraemia · laryngospasm · musculoskeletal stiffness · myalgia · oropharyngeal spasm · pancreatitis · pathological gambling · peripheral oedema · photosensitivity reaction · pneumonia aspiration · rhabdomyolysis · serotonin syndrome · speech disorder · suicidal tendencies · syncope · temperature regulation disorder · thrombocytopenia · urinary incontinence · weight decreased

- **PREGNANCY** Use only if potential benefit outweighs risk.

- **BREAST FEEDING** Manufacturer advises avoid—present in milk.

- **HEPATIC IMPAIRMENT** Use with caution in severe impairment (oral treatment preferred to intramuscular administration).

- **MONITORING REQUIREMENTS**
▸ Aripiprazole does not affect blood pressure to the same extent as other antipsychotic drugs and so blood pressure monitoring is not mandatory for this drug.
▸ With intramuscular use Treatment requires careful monitoring for optimum effect.

- **DIRECTIONS FOR ADMINISTRATION**
▸ With oral use Orodispersible tablets should be placed on the tongue and allowed to dissolve, or be dispersed in water and swallowed.
▸ With intramuscular use Correct injection technique (including the use of z-track technique) and rotation of injection sites are essential.

- **PATIENT AND CARER ADVICE** Patients or carers should be given advice on how to administer aripiprazole orodispersible tablets.

● MEDICINAL FORMS
There can be variation in the licensing of different medicines containing the same drug. Forms available from special-order manufacturers include: oral solution

Tablet

CAUTIONARY AND ADVISORY LABELS 2
▸ Aripiprazole (Non-proprietary)
Aripiprazole 5 mg Aripiprazole 5mg tablets | 28 tablet [PoM] £96.04 DT = £2.37
Aripiprazole 10 mg Aripiprazole 10mg tablets | 28 tablet [PoM] £96.04 DT = £1.99
Aripiprazole 15 mg Aripiprazole 15mg tablets | 28 tablet [PoM] £96.04 DT = £2.75
Aripiprazole 30 mg Aripiprazole 30mg tablets | 28 tablet [PoM] £192.08 DT = £10.71

Solution for injection

▸ Abilify (Otsuka Pharmaceuticals (U.K.) Ltd)
Aripiprazole 7.5 mg per 1 ml Abilify 9.75mg/1.3ml solution for injection vials | 1 vial [PoM] £3.43

Oral solution

CAUTIONARY AND ADVISORY LABELS 2
▸ Aripiprazole (Non-proprietary)
Aripiprazole 1 mg per 1 ml Aripiprazole 1mg/ml oral solution | 150 ml [PoM] £102.90 DT = £99.66
▸ Abilify (Otsuka Pharmaceuticals (U.K.) Ltd)
Aripiprazole 1 mg per 1 ml Abilify 1mg/ml oral solution | 150 ml [PoM] £102.90 DT = £99.66

Powder and solvent for suspension for injection

▸ Abilify Maintena (Otsuka Pharmaceuticals (U.K.) Ltd)
Aripiprazole 400 mg Abilify Maintena 400mg powder and solvent for prolonged-release suspension for injection pre-filled syringes | 1 pre-filled disposable injection [PoM] £220.41
Abilify Maintena 400mg powder and solvent for prolonged-release suspension for injection vials | 1 vial [PoM] £220.41

Orodispersible tablet

CAUTIONARY AND ADVISORY LABELS 2
EXCIPIENTS: May contain Aspartame
▸ Aripiprazole (Non-proprietary)
Aripiprazole 10 mg Aripiprazole 10mg orodispersible tablets sugar free sugar-free | 28 tablet [PoM] £91.24 DT = £78.01
Aripiprazole 15 mg Aripiprazole 15mg orodispersible tablets sugar free sugar-free | 28 tablet [PoM] £91.24 DT = £78.01

🏴 380

Clozapine
27-Nov-2017

● DRUG ACTION Clozapine is a dopamine D_1, dopamine D_2, 5-HT_{2A}, alpha$_1$-adrenoceptor, and muscarinic-receptor antagonist.

● INDICATIONS AND DOSE

Schizophrenia in patients unresponsive to, or intolerant of, conventional antipsychotic drugs

▸ BY MOUTH
▸ Adult 18-59 years: 12.5 mg 1–2 times a day for day 1, then 25–50 mg for day 2, then increased, if tolerated, in steps of 25–50 mg daily, dose to be increased gradually over 14–21 days, increased to up to 300 mg daily in divided doses, larger dose to be taken at night, up to 200 mg daily may be taken as a single dose at bedtime; increased in steps of 50–100 mg 1–2 times a week if required, it is preferable to increase once a week; usual dose 200–450 mg daily, max. 900 mg per day, if restarting after interval of more than 48 hours, 12.5 mg once or twice on first day (but may be feasible to increase more quickly than on initiation)—extreme caution if previous respiratory or cardiac arrest with initial dosing
▸ Adult 60 years and over: 12.5 mg once daily for day 1, then increased to 25–37.5 mg for day 2, then increased, if tolerated, in steps of up to 25 mg daily, dose to be increased gradually over 14–21 days, increased to up to 300 mg daily in divided doses, larger dose to be taken at night, up to 200 mg daily may be taken as a single dose at bedtime; increased in steps of 50–100 mg 1–2 times

a week if required, it is preferable to increase once a week; usual dose 200–450 mg daily, max. 900 mg per day, if restarting after interval of more than 48 hours, 12.5 mg once or twice on first day (but may be feasible to increase more quickly than on initiation)—extreme caution if previous respiratory or cardiac arrest with initial dosing

Psychosis in Parkinson's disease

▸ BY MOUTH
▸ Adult: 12.5 mg once daily, dose to be taken at bedtime, then increased in steps of 12.5 mg up to twice weekly, adjusted according to response; usual dose 25–37.5 mg once daily, dose to be taken at bedtime; increased in steps of 12.5 mg once weekly, this applies only in exceptional cases, increased if necessary up to 100 mg daily in 1–2 divided doses; Usual maximum 50 mg/24 hours

---

IMPORTANT SAFETY INFORMATION

MHRA/CHM ADVICE: CLOZAPINE: REMINDER OF POTENTIALLY FATAL RISK OF INTESTINAL OBSTRUCTION, FAECAL IMPACTION, AND PARALYTIC ILEUS (OCTOBER 2017)
Clozapine has been associated with varying degrees of impairment of intestinal peristalsis—see Cautions and Contra-indications for further information. Patients and their carers should be advised to seek immediate medical advice before taking the next dose of clozapine if constipation develops.

● CONTRA-INDICATIONS Alcoholic and toxic psychoses · bone-marrow disorders · coma · drug intoxication · history of agranulocytosis · history of circulatory collapse · history of neutropenia · paralytic ileus · severe cardiac disorders (e.g. myocarditis) · severe CNS depression · uncontrolled epilepsy

● CAUTIONS Age over 60 years · prostatic hypertrophy · susceptibility to angle-closure glaucoma · taper off other antipsychotics before starting

CAUTIONS, FURTHER INFORMATION
▸ Agranulocytosis Neutropenia and potentially fatal agranulocytosis reported. Leucocyte and differential blood counts must be normal before starting; monitor counts every week for 18 weeks then at least every 2 weeks and if clozapine continued and blood count stable after 1 year at least every 4 weeks (and 4 weeks after discontinuation); if leucocyte count below 3000 /mm^3 or if absolute neutrophil count below 1500 /mm^3 discontinue permanently and refer to haematologist. Patients who have a low white blood cell count because of benign ethnic neutropenia may be started on clozapine with the agreement of a haematologist. Avoid drugs which depress leucopoiesis; patients should report immediately symptoms of infection, especially influenza-like illness.
▸ Myocarditis and cardiomyopathy Fatal myocarditis (most commonly in first 2 months) and cardiomyopathy reported.
● Perform physical examination and take full medical history before starting
● Specialist examination required if cardiac abnormalities or history of heart disease found—clozapine initiated only in absence of severe heart disease and if benefit outweighs risk
● Persistent tachycardia especially in first 2 months should prompt observation for other indicators for myocarditis or cardiomyopathy
● If myocarditis or cardiomyopathy suspected clozapine should be stopped and patient evaluated urgently by cardiologist
● Discontinue permanently in clozapine-induced myocarditis or cardiomyopathy

▸ Intestinal obstruction Impairment of intestinal peristalsis, including constipation, intestinal obstruction, faecal impaction, and paralytic ileus, (including fatal cases) reported. Clozapine should be used with caution in patients receiving drugs that may cause constipation (e.g. antimuscarinic drugs) or in those with a history of colonic disease or lower abdominal surgery. It is essential that constipation is recognised and actively treated.

● INTERACTIONS → Appendix 1: clozapine

● SIDE-EFFECTS

▸ **Common or very common** Appetite decreased · eosinophilia · fatigue · fever · headache · hypertension · leucocytosis · muscle complaints · nausea · oral disorders · postural hypotension (dose-related) · sedation · speech impairment · sweating abnormal · syncope · temperature regulation disorders · urinary disorders · vision blurred · vomiting

▸ **Rare or very rare** Anaemia · cardiac arrest · cardiac inflammation · cardiomyopathy · circulatory collapse · delirium · diabetes mellitus · dyslipidaemia · dysphagia · gastrointestinal disorders · glucose tolerance impaired · hepatic disorders · increased risk of infection · intestinal obstruction (including fatal cases) · ketoacidosis · nephritis tubulointerstitial · obsessive-compulsive disorder · pancreatitis · pericardial effusion · respiratory disorders · restlessness · skin reactions · thrombocytopenia · thrombocytosis

▸ **Frequency not known** Angina pectoris · angioedema · chest pain · cholinergic syndrome · diarrhoea · gastrointestinal discomfort · hypersensitivity vasculitis · muscle weakness · myocardial infarction · nasal congestion · pseudophaeochromocytoma · renal failure · systemic lupus erythematosus (SLE)

SIDE-EFFECTS, FURTHER INFORMATION Hypersalivation associated with clozapine therapy can be treated with hyoscine hydrobromide [unlicensed indication], provided that the patient is not at particular risk from the additive antimuscarinic side-effects of hyoscine and clozapine.

● PREGNANCY Use with caution.

● BREAST FEEDING Avoid.

● HEPATIC IMPAIRMENT Avoid in symptomatic liver disease. Avoid in progressive liver disease. Avoid in hepatic failure. **Monitoring** Monitor hepatic function regularly.

● RENAL IMPAIRMENT Avoid in severe impairment.

● MONITORING REQUIREMENTS

▸ Monitor leucocyte and differential blood counts. Clozapine requires differential white blood cell monitoring weekly for 18 weeks, then fortnightly for up to one year, and then monthly as part of the clozapine patient monitoring service.

▸ Close medical supervision during initiation (risk of collapse because of hypotension and convulsions).

▸ Blood lipids and weight should be measured at baseline, at 3 months (weight should be measured at frequent intervals during the first 3 months), and then yearly with antipsychotics. Patients taking clozapine require more frequent monitoring of these parameters: every 3 months for the first year, then yearly.

▸ Fasting blood glucose should be measured at baseline, at 4–6 months, and then yearly. Patients taking clozapine should have fasting blood glucose tested at baseline, after one months' treatment, then every 4–6 months.

▸ Patient, prescriber, and supplying pharmacist must be registered with the appropriate Patient Monitoring Service—it takes several days to do this.

● TREATMENT CESSATION On planned withdrawal reduce dose over 1–2 weeks to avoid risk of rebound psychosis. If abrupt withdrawal necessary observe patient carefully.

● DIRECTIONS FOR ADMINISTRATION Shake oral suspension well for 90 seconds when dispensing or if visibly settled

and stand for 24 hours before use; otherwise shake well for 10 seconds before use. May be diluted with water.

● PRESCRIBING AND DISPENSING INFORMATION Clozapine has been used for psychosis in Parkinson's disease in children aged 16 years and over.

● PATIENT AND CARER ADVICE Patients or carers should be given advice on how to administer clozapine oral suspension.

● MEDICINAL FORMS
There can be variation in the licensing of different medicines containing the same drug. Forms available from special-order manufacturers include: oral suspension, oral solution

Oral suspension
CAUTIONARY AND ADVISORY LABELS 2, 10
▸ Denzapine (Britannia Pharmaceuticals Ltd)
Clozapine 50 mg per 1 ml Denzapine 50mg/ml oral suspension sugar-free | 100 ml [PoM] £39.60

Tablet
CAUTIONARY AND ADVISORY LABELS 2, 10
▸ Clozaril (Mylan)
Clozapine 25 mg Clozaril 25mg tablets | 28 tablet [PoM] £3.02 | 84 tablet [PoM] £8.40 (Hospital only) | 100 tablet [PoM] £10.00 (Hospital only)
Clozapine 100 mg Clozaril 100mg tablets | 28 tablet [PoM] £12.07 | 84 tablet [PoM] £33.60 (Hospital only) | 100 tablet [PoM] £39.00 (Hospital only)

▸ Denzapine (Britannia Pharmaceuticals Ltd)
Clozapine 25 mg Denzapine 25mg tablets | 84 tablet [PoM] £16.64 | 100 tablet [PoM] £19.80
Clozapine 50 mg Denzapine 50mg tablets | 100 tablet [PoM] £39.60
Clozapine 100 mg Denzapine 100mg tablets | 84 tablet [PoM] £66.53 | 100 tablet [PoM] £79.20
Clozapine 200 mg Denzapine 200mg tablets | 100 tablet [PoM] £158.40

▸ Zaponex (Leyden Delta B.V.)
Clozapine 25 mg Zaponex 25mg tablets | 84 tablet [PoM] £8.28 | 500 tablet [PoM] £48.39
Clozapine 100 mg Zaponex 100mg tablets | 84 tablet [PoM] £33.88 | 500 tablet [PoM] £196.43

━━━━━━━━━━━━━━━━━━━━━━━━━━━━━ ⚑ 380

Lurasidone hydrochloride

● DRUG ACTION Lurasidone is a dopamine D_2, $5\text{-}HT_{2A}$, $5\text{-}HT_7$, $alpha_{2A}$- and $alpha_{2C}$- adrenoceptor antagonist, and is a partial agonist at $5\text{-}HT_{1a}$ receptors.

● INDICATIONS AND DOSE
Schizophrenia
▸ BY MOUTH
▸ Adult: Initially 37 mg once daily, increased if necessary up to 148 mg once daily

Schizophrenia when given with concomitant moderate CYP3A4 inhibitors (e.g. diltiazem, erythromycin, fluconazole, and verapamil)
▸ BY MOUTH
▸ Adult: Initially 18.5 mg once daily (max. per dose 74 mg once daily)

● CAUTIONS High doses in elderly · susceptibility to QT-interval prolongation

● INTERACTIONS → Appendix 1: lurasidone

● SIDE-EFFECTS

▸ **Common or very common** Anxiety · cogwheel rigidity · drooling · drowsiness · fatigue · gastrointestinal discomfort · muscle complaints · musculoskeletal stiffness · nausea · oculogyric crisis · oral disorders · pain · psychiatric disorders · sleep disorders · vomiting

▸ **Uncommon** Appetite decreased · dysarthria · dysuria · gait abnormal · gastrointestinal disorders · hot flush · hyperhidrosis · hypertension · joint stiffness · nasopharyngitis · postural hypotension · vision blurred

▸ **Rare or very rare** Eosinophilia · rhabdomyolysis

4

Nervous system

▸ **Frequency not known** Anaemia · angina pectoris · angioedema · atrioventricular block · bradycardia · breast abnormalities · diarrhoea · dysmenorrhoea · dysphagia · pruritus · renal failure · Stevens-Johnson syndrome · suicidal behaviour · vertigo
● PREGNANCY Use only if potential benefit outweighs risk— limited information available.
● HEPATIC IMPAIRMENT
 Dose adjustments Initially 18.5 mg once daily, up to max. 74 mg once daily in moderate impairment.
  Use with caution in severe impairment—initially 18.5 mg once daily, up to max. 37 mg once daily.
● RENAL IMPAIRMENT Manufacturer advises use only if potential benefit outweighs risk if eGFR less than 15 mL/minute/1.73 m^2.
 Dose adjustments Initially 18.5 mg once daily, up to max. 74 mg once daily if eGFR less than 50 mL/minute/1.73 m^2.
● DIRECTIONS FOR ADMINISTRATION Patients on doses higher than 111 mg once daily whose treatment is interrupted for longer than 3 days should restart on 111 mg once daily and titrate to usual dose; for all other doses, restart on usual dose.

● MEDICINAL FORMS
 There can be variation in the licensing of different medicines containing the same drug.
 Tablet
 CAUTIONARY AND ADVISORY LABELS 2, 21, 25
 ▸ Latuda (Sunovion Pharmaceuticals Europe Ltd) ▼
 Lurasidone (as Lurasidone hydrochloride) 18.5 mg Latuda 18.5mg tablets | 28 tablet [PoM] £90.72 DT = £90.72
 Lurasidone (as Lurasidone hydrochloride) 37 mg Latuda 37mg tablets | 28 tablet [PoM] £90.72 DT = £90.72
 Lurasidone (as Lurasidone hydrochloride) 74 mg Latuda 74mg tablets | 28 tablet [PoM] £90.72 DT = £90.72

◤ 380

Olanzapine

● DRUG ACTION Olanzapine is a dopamine D_1, D_2, D_4, 5-HT$_2$, histamine- 1-, and muscarinic-receptor antagonist.

● INDICATIONS AND DOSE

Schizophrenia | Combination therapy for mania
 ▸ BY MOUTH
 ▸ Adult: 10 mg daily, adjusted according to response, usual dose 5–20 mg daily, doses greater than 10 mg daily only after reassessment, when one or more factors present that might result in slower metabolism (e.g. female gender, elderly, non-smoker) consider lower initial dose and more gradual dose increase; maximum 20 mg per day

Preventing recurrence in bipolar disorder
 ▸ BY MOUTH
 ▸ Adult: 10 mg daily, adjusted according to response, usual dose 5–20 mg daily, doses greater than 10 mg daily only after reassessment, when one or more factors present that might result in slower metabolism (e.g. female gender, elderly, non-smoker) consider lower initial dose and more gradual dose increase; maximum 20 mg per day

Monotherapy for mania
 ▸ BY MOUTH
 ▸ Adult: 15 mg daily, adjusted according to response, usual dose 5–20 mg daily, doses greater than 15 mg daily only after reassessment, when one or more factors present that might result in slower metabolism (e.g. female gender, elderly, non-smoker) consider lower initial dose and more gradual dose increase; maximum 20 mg per day

Control of agitation and disturbed behaviour in schizophrenia or mania
 ▸ BY INTRAMUSCULAR INJECTION
 ▸ Adult: Initially 5–10 mg for 1 dose; usual dose 10 mg for 1 dose, followed by 5–10 mg after 2 hours if required, maximum 3 injections daily for 3 days; maximum daily combined oral and parenteral dose 20 mg, when one or more factors present that might result in slower metabolism (e.g. female gender, elderly, non-smoker) consider lower initial dose and more gradual dose increase
 ▸ Elderly: Initially 2.5–5 mg, followed by 2.5–5 mg after 2 hours if required, maximum 3 injections daily for 3 days; maximum daily combined oral and parenteral dose 20 mg, when one or more factors present that might result in slower metabolism (e.g. female gender, elderly, non-smoker) consider lower initial dose and more gradual dose increase

● CONTRA-INDICATIONS
 ▸ With intramuscular use Acute myocardial infarction · bradycardia · recent heart surgery · severe hypotension · sick sinus syndrome · unstable angina
● CAUTIONS Bone-marrow depression · hypereosinophilic disorders · low leucocyte count · low neutrophil count · myeloproliferative disease · paralytic ileus
 CAUTIONS, FURTHER INFORMATION
 ▸ CNS and respiratory depression
 ▸ With intramuscular use Blood pressure, pulse and respiratory rate should be monitored for at least 4 hours after intramuscular injection, particularly in those also receiving a benzodiazepine or another antipsychotic (leave at least one hour between administration of olanzapine intramuscular injection and parenteral benzodiazepines).
● INTERACTIONS → Appendix 1: olanzapine
● SIDE-EFFECTS
 GENERAL SIDE-EFFECTS
 ▸ **Common or very common** Appetite increased · arthralgia · oedema
 ▸ **Uncommon** Alopecia · epistaxis · memory loss
 ▸ **Rare or very rare** Hepatic disorders · pancreatitis · rhabdomyolysis
 SPECIFIC SIDE-EFFECTS
 ▸ **Common or very common**
 ▸ With intramuscular use Dyslipidaemia · malaise
 ▸ With oral use Anticholinergic syndrome · asthenia · drowsiness · eosinophilia · fever · glycosuria · hypersomnia · postural hypotension
 ▸ **Uncommon**
 ▸ With oral use Abdominal distension · bradycardia · breast enlargement · diabetes mellitus · diabetic coma · dysarthria · ketoacidosis · oculogyration · photosensitivity reaction · thromboembolism · urinary disorders
 ▸ **Rare or very rare**
 ▸ With oral use Hypothermia · thrombocytopenia
 ▸ **Frequency not known**
 ▸ With intramuscular use Hypoventilation
● PREGNANCY Use only if potential benefit outweighs risk; neonatal lethargy, tremor, and hypertonia reported when used in third trimester.
● BREAST FEEDING Avoid—present in milk.
● HEPATIC IMPAIRMENT
 Dose adjustments Consider initial dose of 5 mg daily.
● RENAL IMPAIRMENT
 Dose adjustments Consider initial dose of 5 mg daily.
● MONITORING REQUIREMENTS
 ▸ Blood lipids and weight should be measured at baseline, at 3 months (weight should be measured at frequent intervals during the first 3 months), and then yearly with antipsychotic drugs. Patients taking olanzapine require

more frequent monitoring of these parameters: every 3 months for the first year, then yearly.

▸ Fasting blood glucose should be measured at baseline, at 4–6 months, and then yearly. Patients taking olanzapine should have fasting blood glucose tested at baseline, after one months' treatment, then every 4–6 months.

● DIRECTIONS FOR ADMINISTRATION Olanzapine orodispersible tablet may be placed on the tongue and allowed to dissolve, or dispersed in water, orange juice, apple juice, milk, or coffee.

● PRESCRIBING AND DISPENSING INFORMATION
▸ With intramuscular use When prescribing, dispensing, or administering, check that this injection is the correct preparation—this preparation is usually used in hospital for the rapid control of an *acute episode* and should **not** be confused with depot preparations which are usually used in the community or clinics for *maintenance* treatment.

● PATIENT AND CARER ADVICE Patients or carers should be given advice on how to administer orodispersible tablets.

● MEDICINAL FORMS
There can be variation in the licensing of different medicines containing the same drug. Forms available from special-order manufacturers include: oral suspension, oral solution

Tablet
CAUTIONARY AND ADVISORY LABELS 2
▸ Olanzapine (Non-proprietary)
Olanzapine 2.5 mg Olanzapine 2.5mg tablets | 28 tablet PoM £21.85 DT = £5.03
Olanzapine 5 mg Olanzapine 5mg tablets | 28 tablet PoM £43.70 DT = £10.72
Olanzapine 7.5 mg Olanzapine 7.5mg tablets | 28 tablet PoM £62.27 DT = £29.71 | 56 tablet PoM £12.10–£131.10
Olanzapine 10 mg Olanzapine 10mg tablets | 28 tablet PoM £87.40 DT = £18.98
Olanzapine 15 mg Olanzapine 15mg tablets | 28 tablet PoM £119.18 DT = £24.58
Olanzapine 20 mg Olanzapine 20mg tablets | 28 tablet PoM £158.90 DT = £36.83
▸ Zalasta (Consilient Health Ltd)
Olanzapine 2.5 mg Zalasta 2.5mg tablets | 28 tablet PoM £18.57 DT = £5.03
Olanzapine 5 mg Zalasta 5mg tablets | 28 tablet PoM £37.14 DT = £10.72
Olanzapine 7.5 mg Zalasta 7.5mg tablets | 56 tablet PoM £111.43
Olanzapine 10 mg Zalasta 10mg tablets | 28 tablet PoM £74.29 DT = £18.98
Olanzapine 15 mg Zalasta 15mg tablets | 28 tablet PoM £101.30 DT = £24.58
Olanzapine 20 mg Zalasta 20mg tablets | 28 tablet PoM £135.06 DT = £36.83
▸ Zyprexa (Eli Lilly and Company Ltd)
Olanzapine 2.5 mg Zyprexa 2.5mg tablets | 28 tablet PoM £21.85 DT = £5.03
Olanzapine 5 mg Zyprexa 5mg tablets | 28 tablet PoM £43.70 DT = £10.72
Olanzapine 7.5 mg Zyprexa 7.5mg tablets | 56 tablet PoM £131.10
Olanzapine 10 mg Zyprexa 10mg tablets | 28 tablet PoM £87.40 DT = £18.98
Olanzapine 15 mg Zyprexa 15mg tablets | 28 tablet PoM £119.18 DT = £24.58
Olanzapine 20 mg Zyprexa 20mg tablets | 28 tablet PoM £158.90 DT = £36.83

Oral lyophilisate
▸ Zyprexa (Eli Lilly and Company Ltd)
Olanzapine 5 mg Zyprexa 5mg Velotabs sugar-free | 28 tablet PoM £48.07 DT = £48.07
Olanzapine 10 mg Zyprexa 10mg Velotabs sugar-free | 28 tablet PoM £87.40 DT = £87.40
Olanzapine 15 mg Zyprexa 15mg Velotabs sugar-free | 28 tablet PoM £131.10 DT = £131.10
Olanzapine 20 mg Zyprexa 20mg Velotabs sugar-free | 28 tablet PoM £174.79 DT = £174.79

Orodispersible tablet
CAUTIONARY AND ADVISORY LABELS 2
EXCIPIENTS: May contain Aspartame
▸ Olanzapine (Non-proprietary)
Olanzapine 5 mg Olanzapine 5mg orodispersible tablets sugar free | 28 tablet PoM £15.27–£27.03 DT = £21.53
Olanzapine 5mg orodispersible tablets | 28 tablet PoM £30.00 DT = £25.63
Olanzapine 10 mg Olanzapine 10mg orodispersible tablets | 28 tablet PoM £50.00 DT = £43.25
Olanzapine 10mg orodispersible tablets sugar free sugar-free | 28 tablet PoM £27.37–£49.74 DT = £34.53
Olanzapine 15 mg Olanzapine 15mg orodispersible tablets sugar free | 28 tablet PoM £30.86–£66.76 DT = £36.60
Olanzapine 15mg orodispersible tablets | 28 tablet PoM £50.00 DT = £44.33
Olanzapine 20 mg Olanzapine 20mg orodispersible tablets sugar free sugar-free | 28 tablet PoM £47.19–£96.14 DT = £78.52
Olanzapine 20mg orodispersible tablets | 28 tablet PoM £80.00 DT = £70.23
▸ Zalasta (Consilient Health Ltd)
Olanzapine 5 mg Zalasta 5mg orodispersible tablets sugar-free | 28 tablet PoM £40.85 DT = £21.53
Olanzapine 10 mg Zalasta 10mg orodispersible tablets sugar-free | 28 tablet PoM £74.29 DT = £34.53
Olanzapine 15 mg Zalasta 15mg orodispersible tablets sugar-free | 28 tablet PoM £111.43 DT = £36.60
Olanzapine 20 mg Zalasta 20mg orodispersible tablets sugar-free | 28 tablet PoM £148.57 DT = £78.52

🏳 380

Paliperidone
15-Jun-2017

● DRUG ACTION Paliperidone is a metabolite of risperidone.

● INDICATIONS AND DOSE

Schizophrenia | Psychotic or manic symptoms of schizoaffective disorder
▸ BY MOUTH
▸ Adult: 6 mg once daily, dose to be taken in the morning, then adjusted in steps of 3 mg if required, dose to be adjusted over at least 5 days; usual dose 3–12 mg daily

TREVICTA® PRE-FILLED SYRINGES

Maintenance of schizophrenia in patients who are clinically stable on once-monthly intramuscular paliperidone
▸ BY DEEP INTRAMUSCULAR INJECTION
▸ Adult: Initially 175–525 mg every 3 months, adjusted according to response, to be administered into the deltoid or gluteal muscle, dose is based on previous once-monthly intramuscular paliperidone and should be initiated in place of the next scheduled dose—consult product literature

XEPLION® PRE-FILLED SYRINGES

Maintenance in schizophrenia in patients previously responsive to paliperidone or risperidone
▸ BY DEEP INTRAMUSCULAR INJECTION
▸ Adult: 150 mg for 1 dose on day 1, then 100 mg for 1 dose on day 8, to be injected into the deltoid muscle, dose subsequently adjusted at monthly intervals according to response; maintenance 75 mg once a month, alternatively maintenance 25–150 mg once a month, following the second dose, monthly maintenance doses can be administered into either the deltoid or gluteal muscle

● CONTRA-INDICATIONS
▸ With intramuscular use Children

● CAUTIONS
GENERAL CAUTIONS Cataract surgery (risk of intraoperative floppy iris syndrome) · dementia with Lewy bodies · elderly patients with dementia · elderly patients with risk factors for stroke · predisposition to gastro-intestinal obstruction · prolactin-dependent tumours

4

Nervous system

SPECIFIC CAUTIONS When transferring from oral to depot therapy, the dose by mouth should be reduced gradually

● INTERACTIONS → Appendix 1: paliperidone
● SIDE-EFFECTS
GENERAL SIDE-EFFECTS
● **Common or very common** Anxiety · appetite abnormal · arrhythmias · asthenia · cardiac conduction disorders · cough · depression · diarrhoea · fever · gastrointestinal discomfort · headache · hypertension · increased risk of infection · joint disorders · laryngeal pain · nasal congestion · nausea · oral disorders · pain · postural hypotension · sedation · skin reactions · vision disorders · vomiting
▸ **Uncommon** Alopecia · anaemia · breast abnormalities · chest discomfort · chills · conjunctivitis · cystitis · dizziness postural · dry eye · dysarthria · dysphagia · dyspnoea · ear pain · epistaxis · fall · gait abnormal · gastrointestinal disorders · generalised tonic-clonic seizure · hypoglycaemia · malaise · menstrual cycle irregularities · mood altered · muscle spasms · muscle weakness · oedema · palpitations · respiratory disorders · sensation abnormal · sleep disorders · syncope · taste altered · thirst · thrombocytopenia · tinnitus · urinary disorders · vertigo
▸ **Rare or very rare** Angioedema · cerebrovascular insufficiency · coma · consciousness impaired · dandruff · dysphonia · eye disorders · flushing · glaucoma · head titubation · hypothermia · ischaemia · jaundice · pancreatitis · polydipsia · posture abnormal · rhabdomyolysis · SIADH · sleep apnoea · vaginal discharge · water intoxication · withdrawal syndrome
SPECIFIC SIDE-EFFECTS
▸ **Common or very common**
▸ With oral use Weight decreased
▸ **Uncommon**
▸ With oral use Concentration impaired · diabetes mellitus
▸ **Rare or very rare**
▸ With parenteral use Diabetic ketoacidosis
● PREGNANCY Use only if potential benefit outweighs risk—toxicity in *animal* studies; if discontinuation during pregnancy is necessary, withdraw gradually.
TREVICTA ® PRE-FILLED SYRINGES Manufacturer advises to consider long-acting nature of formulation—paliperidone detected in plasma up to 18 months after single dose.
● BREAST FEEDING Manufacturer advises avoid—present in milk.
TREVICTA ® PRE-FILLED SYRINGES Manufacturer advises to consider long-acting nature of formulation—paliperidone detected in plasma up to 18 months after single dose.
● HEPATIC IMPAIRMENT Caution in severe impairment—no information available.
● RENAL IMPAIRMENT
▸ With oral use Manufacturer advises avoid if creatinine clearance less than 10 mL/minute.
▸ With intramuscular use Manufacturer advises avoid if creatinine clearance less than 50 mL/minute.
Dose adjustments ▸ With oral use Manufacturer advises reduce initial dose to 3 mg once daily if creatinine clearance 50–80 mL/minute (max. 6 mg once daily). Manufacturer advises reduce initial dose to 1.5 mg once daily if creatinine clearance 10–50 mL/minute (max. 3 mg once daily).
TREVICTA ® PRE-FILLED SYRINGES Manufacturer advises dose should be adjusted and stabilised using once-monthly injectable paliperidone before switching to three-monthly injectable paliperidone, if creatinine clearance 50–80 mL/minute.
XEPLION ® PRE-FILLED SYRINGES Manufacturer advises initial dose 100 mg on day 1 and then 75 mg on day 8 if creatinine clearance 50–80 mL/minute; recommended

maintenance dose 50 mg (range 25–100 mg) monthly if creatinine clearance 50–80 mL/minute.
● MONITORING REQUIREMENTS
▸ With intramuscular use Treatment requires careful monitoring for optimum effect.
● DIRECTIONS FOR ADMINISTRATION
▸ With intramuscular use Correct injection technique (including the use of z-track technique) and rotation of injection sites are essential.
▸ With oral use Always take with breakfast or always take on an empty stomach.
● PATIENT AND CARER ADVICE
▸ With oral use Patients or carers should be given advice on how to administer paliperidone tablets.
Missed doses ▸ With intramuscular use For missed doses see product literature.
● NATIONAL FUNDING/ACCESS DECISIONS
TREVICTA ® PRE-FILLED SYRINGES
Scottish Medicines Consortium (SMC) Decisions
The *Scottish Medicines Consortium* has advised (September 2016) that paliperidone palmitate (*Trevicta* ®) is accepted for use within NHS Scotland for the maintenance treatment of schizophrenia in patients who are clinically stable on one-monthly paliperidone palmitate injectable product.

● MEDICINAL FORMS
There can be variation in the licensing of different medicines containing the same drug.
Prolonged-release suspension for injection
▸ Trevicta (Janssen-Cilag Ltd)
Paliperidone (as Paliperidone palmitate) 200 mg per 1 ml Trevicta 175mg/0.875ml prolonged-release suspension for injection pre-filled syringes | 1 pre-filled disposable injection PoM £551.76
Trevicta 263mg/1.315ml prolonged-release suspension for injection pre-filled syringes | 1 pre-filled disposable injection PoM £734.70
Trevicta 350mg/1.75ml prolonged-release suspension for injection pre-filled syringes | 1 pre-filled disposable injection PoM £942.21
Trevicta 525mg/2.625ml prolonged-release suspension for injection pre-filled syringes | 1 pre-filled disposable injection PoM £1,177.77
Modified-release tablet
CAUTIONARY AND ADVISORY LABELS 2, 25
▸ Paliperidone (Non-proprietary)
Paliperidone 3 mg Paliperidone 3mg modified-release tablets | 28 tablet PoM 🅂
Paliperidone 6 mg Paliperidone 6mg modified-release tablets | 28 tablet PoM 🅂
Paliperidone 9 mg Paliperidone 9mg modified-release tablets | 28 tablet PoM 🅂
▸ Invega (Janssen-Cilag Ltd)
Paliperidone 3 mg Invega 3mg modified-release tablets | 28 tablet PoM £97.28
Paliperidone 6 mg Invega 6mg modified-release tablets | 28 tablet PoM £97.28
Paliperidone 9 mg Invega 9mg modified-release tablets | 28 tablet PoM £145.92
Suspension for injection
▸ Xeplion (Janssen-Cilag Ltd)
Paliperidone (as Paliperidone palmitate) 100 mg per 1 ml Xeplion 150mg/1.5ml suspension for injection pre-filled syringes | 1 pre-filled disposable injection PoM £392.59 DT = £392.59
Xeplion 75mg/0.75ml suspension for injection pre-filled syringes | 1 pre-filled disposable injection PoM £244.90 DT = £244.90
Xeplion 100mg/1ml suspension for injection pre-filled syringes | 1 pre-filled disposable injection PoM £314.07 DT = £314.07
Xeplion 50mg/0.5ml suspension for injection pre-filled syringes | 1 pre-filled disposable injection PoM £183.92 DT = £183.92

Quetiapine

▶ 380

- **DRUG ACTION** Quetiapine is a dopamine D_1, dopamine D_2, 5-HT_2, alpha$_1$-adrenoceptor, and histamine-1 receptor antagonist.

- **INDICATIONS AND DOSE**

Schizophrenia
▶ BY MOUTH USING IMMEDIATE-RELEASE MEDICINES
▶ Adult: 25 mg twice daily for day 1, then 50 mg twice daily for day 2, then 100 mg twice daily for day 3, then 150 mg twice daily for day 4, then, adjusted according to response, usual dose 300–450 mg daily in 2 divided doses, the rate of dose titration may need to be slower and the daily dose lower in elderly patients; maximum 750 mg per day
▶ BY MOUTH USING MODIFIED-RELEASE MEDICINES
▶ Adult: 300 mg once daily for day 1, then 600 mg once daily for day 2, then, adjusted according to response, usual dose 600 mg once daily, maximum dose under specialist supervision; maximum 800 mg per day
▶ Elderly: Initially 50 mg once daily, adjusted according to response. adjusted in steps of 50 mg daily

Treatment of mania in bipolar disorder
▶ BY MOUTH USING IMMEDIATE-RELEASE MEDICINES
▶ Adult: 50 mg twice daily for day 1, then 100 mg twice daily for day 2, then 150 mg twice daily for day 3, then 200 mg twice daily for day 4, then adjusted in steps of up to 200 mg daily, adjusted according to response, usual dose 400–800 mg daily in 2 divided doses, the rate of dose titration may need to be slower and the daily dose lower in elderly patients; maximum 800 mg per day
▶ BY MOUTH USING MODIFIED-RELEASE MEDICINES
▶ Adult: 300 mg once daily for day 1, then 600 mg once daily for day 2, then, adjusted according to response, usual dose 400–800 mg once daily
▶ Elderly: Initially 50 mg once daily, adjusted according to response. adjusted in steps of 50 mg daily

Treatment of depression in bipolar disorder
▶ BY MOUTH USING IMMEDIATE-RELEASE MEDICINES
▶ Adult: 50 mg once daily for day 1, dose to be taken at bedtime, then 100 mg once daily for day 2, then 200 mg once daily for day 3, then 300 mg once daily for day 4, then, adjusted according to response; usual dose 300 mg once daily, the rate of dose titration may need to be slower and the daily dose lower in elderly patients; maximum 600 mg per day
▶ BY MOUTH USING MODIFIED-RELEASE MEDICINES
▶ Adult: 50 mg once daily for day 1, dose to be taken at bedtime, then 100 mg once daily for day 2, then 200 mg once daily for day 3, then 300 mg once daily for day 4, then, adjusted according to response; usual dose 300 mg once daily; maximum 600 mg per day

Prevention of mania and depression in bipolar disorder
▶ BY MOUTH USING IMMEDIATE-RELEASE MEDICINES
▶ Adult: Continue at the dose effective for treatment of bipolar disorder and adjust to lowest effective dose; usual dose 300–800 mg daily in 2 divided doses
▶ BY MOUTH USING MODIFIED-RELEASE MEDICINES
▶ Adult: Continue at the dose effective for treatment of bipolar disorder and adjust to lowest effective dose; usual dose 300–800 mg once daily

Adjunctive treatment of major depression
▶ BY MOUTH USING MODIFIED-RELEASE MEDICINES
▶ Adult: 50 mg once daily for 2 days, dose to be taken at bedtime, then 150 mg once daily for 2 days, then, adjusted according to response, usual dose 150–300 mg once daily

▶ Elderly: Initially 50 mg once daily for 3 days, then increased if necessary to 100 mg once daily for 4 days, then adjusted in steps of 50 mg, adjusted according to response, usual dose 50–300 mg once daily, dose of 300 mg should not be reached before day 22 of treatment

DOSE EQUIVALENCE AND CONVERSION
▶ Patients can be switched from immediate-release to modified-release tablets at the equivalent daily dose; to maintain clinical response, dose titration may be required.

- **CAUTIONS** Cerebrovascular disease · elderly · patients at risk of aspiration pneumonia · treatment of depression in patients under 25 years (increased risk of suicide)
- **INTERACTIONS** → Appendix 1: quetiapine
- **SIDE-EFFECTS**
▶ **Common or very common** Appetite increased · asthenia · dysarthria · dyspepsia · dyspnoea · fever · headache · irritability · palpitations · peripheral oedema · postural hypotension · rhinitis · sleep disorders · suicidal behaviour (particularly on initiation) · suicidal ideation (particularly on initiation) · syncope · vision blurred · vomiting · withdrawal syndrome
▶ **Uncommon** Anaemia · bradycardia · diabetes mellitus · dysphagia · hyponatraemia · hypothyroidism · sexual dysfunction · skin reactions · thrombocytopenia
▶ **Rare or very rare** Angioedema · breast swelling · gastrointestinal disorders · hepatic disorders · hypothermia · menstrual disorder · metabolic syndrome · pancreatitis · rhabdomyolysis · severe cutaneous adverse reactions (SCARs) · SIADH

- **PREGNANCY** Use only if potential benefit outweighs risk.
- **BREAST FEEDING** Manufacturer advises avoid.
- **HEPATIC IMPAIRMENT**
Dose adjustments For *immediate-release tablets*, initially 25 mg daily, increased daily in steps of 25–50 mg.
For *modified-release tablets*, initially 50 mg daily, increased daily in steps of 50 mg.

- **MEDICINAL FORMS**
There can be variation in the licensing of different medicines containing the same drug. Forms available from special-order manufacturers include: oral suspension, oral solution, powder
Modified-release tablet
CAUTIONARY AND ADVISORY LABELS 2, 23, 25
▶ Atrolak XL (Accord Healthcare Ltd)
Quetiapine (as Quetiapine fumarate) 50 mg Atrolak XL 50mg tablets | 60 tablet [PoM] £67.65 DT = £67.66
Quetiapine (as Quetiapine fumarate) 150 mg Atrolak XL 150mg tablets | 60 tablet [PoM] £107.45 DT = £113.10
Quetiapine (as Quetiapine fumarate) 200 mg Atrolak XL 200mg tablets | 60 tablet [PoM] £113.10 DT = £113.10
Quetiapine (as Quetiapine fumarate) 300 mg Atrolak XL 300mg tablets | 60 tablet [PoM] £169.99 DT = £170.00
Quetiapine (as Quetiapine fumarate) 400 mg Atrolak XL 400mg tablets | 60 tablet [PoM] £226.19 DT = £226.20
▶ Biquelle XL (Aspire Pharma Ltd)
Quetiapine (as Quetiapine fumarate) 50 mg Biquelle XL 50mg tablets | 60 tablet [PoM] £29.45 DT = £67.66
Quetiapine (as Quetiapine fumarate) 150 mg Biquelle XL 150mg tablets | 60 tablet [PoM] £49.45 DT = £113.10
Quetiapine (as Quetiapine fumarate) 200 mg Biquelle XL 200mg tablets | 60 tablet [PoM] £49.45 DT = £113.10
Quetiapine (as Quetiapine fumarate) 300 mg Biquelle XL 300mg tablets | 60 tablet [PoM] £74.45 DT = £170.00
Quetiapine (as Quetiapine fumarate) 400 mg Biquelle XL 400mg tablets | 60 tablet [PoM] £98.95 DT = £226.20
▶ Brancico XL (Zentiva)
Quetiapine (as Quetiapine fumarate) 50 mg Brancico XL 50mg tablets | 60 tablet [PoM] £12.00 DT = £67.66
Quetiapine (as Quetiapine fumarate) 150 mg Brancico XL 150mg tablets | 60 tablet [PoM] £26.00 DT = £113.10
Quetiapine (as Quetiapine fumarate) 200 mg Brancico XL 200mg tablets | 60 tablet [PoM] £26.00 DT = £113.10

4

Nervous system

Quetiapine (as Quetiapine fumarate) 300 mg Brancico XL 300mg
tablets | 60 tablet [PoM] £45.00 DT = £170.00
Quetiapine (as Quetiapine fumarate) 400 mg Brancico XL 400mg
tablets | 60 tablet [PoM] £60.00 DT = £226.20
▸ Mintreleq XL (Aristo Pharma Ltd)
Quetiapine (as Quetiapine fumarate) 50 mg Mintreleq XL 50mg
tablets | 60 tablet [PoM] £14.99 DT = £67.66
Quetiapine (as Quetiapine fumarate) 150 mg Mintreleq XL 150mg
tablets | 60 tablet [PoM] £29.99 DT = £113.10
Quetiapine (as Quetiapine fumarate) 200 mg Mintreleq XL 200mg
tablets | 60 tablet [PoM] £29.99 DT = £113.10
Quetiapine (as Quetiapine fumarate) 300 mg Mintreleq XL 300mg
tablets | 60 tablet [PoM] £49.99 DT = £170.00
Quetiapine (as Quetiapine fumarate) 400 mg Mintreleq XL 400mg
tablets | 60 tablet [PoM] £64.99 DT = £226.20
▸ Seroquel XL (AstraZeneca UK Ltd)
Quetiapine (as Quetiapine fumarate) 50 mg Seroquel XL 50mg
tablets | 60 tablet [PoM] £67.66 DT = £67.66
Quetiapine (as Quetiapine fumarate) 150 mg Seroquel XL 150mg
tablets | 60 tablet [PoM] £113.10 DT = £113.10
Quetiapine (as Quetiapine fumarate) 200 mg Seroquel XL 200mg
tablets | 60 tablet [PoM] £113.10 DT = £113.10
Quetiapine (as Quetiapine fumarate) 300 mg Seroquel XL 300mg
tablets | 60 tablet [PoM] £170.00 DT = £170.00
Quetiapine (as Quetiapine fumarate) 400 mg Seroquel XL 400mg
tablets | 60 tablet [PoM] £226.20 DT = £226.20
▸ Sondate XL (Teva UK Ltd)
Quetiapine (as Quetiapine fumarate) 50 mg Sondate XL 50mg
tablets | 60 tablet [PoM] £14.98 DT = £67.66
Quetiapine (as Quetiapine fumarate) 150 mg Sondate XL 150mg
tablets | 60 tablet [PoM] £29.98 DT = £113.10
Quetiapine (as Quetiapine fumarate) 200 mg Sondate XL 200mg
tablets | 60 tablet [PoM] £29.98 DT = £113.10
Quetiapine (as Quetiapine fumarate) 300 mg Sondate XL 300mg
tablets | 60 tablet [PoM] £49.98 DT = £170.00
Quetiapine (as Quetiapine fumarate) 400 mg Sondate XL 400mg
tablets | 60 tablet [PoM] £64.98 DT = £226.20
▸ Zaluron XL (Fontus Health Ltd)
Quetiapine (as Quetiapine fumarate) 50 mg Zaluron XL 50mg
tablets | 60 tablet [PoM] £27.96 DT = £67.66
Quetiapine (as Quetiapine fumarate) 150 mg Zaluron XL 150mg
tablets | 60 tablet [PoM] £46.96 DT = £113.10
Quetiapine (as Quetiapine fumarate) 200 mg Zaluron XL 200mg
tablets | 60 tablet [PoM] £46.96 DT = £113.10
Quetiapine (as Quetiapine fumarate) 300 mg Zaluron XL 300mg
tablets | 60 tablet [PoM] £70.71 DT = £170.00
Quetiapine (as Quetiapine fumarate) 400 mg Zaluron XL 400mg
tablets | 60 tablet [PoM] £93.98 DT = £226.20

Tablet
CAUTIONARY AND ADVISORY LABELS 2
▸ Quetiapine (Non-proprietary)
Quetiapine (as Quetiapine fumarate) 25 mg Quetiapine 25mg
tablets | 60 tablet [PoM] £38.05 DT = £11.16
Quetiapine (as Quetiapine fumarate) 100 mg Quetiapine 100mg
tablets | 60 tablet [PoM] £107.45 DT = £43.54
Quetiapine (as Quetiapine fumarate) 150 mg Quetiapine 150mg
tablets | 60 tablet [PoM] £107.45 DT = £51.42
Quetiapine (as Quetiapine fumarate) 200 mg Quetiapine 200mg
tablets | 60 tablet [PoM] £107.45 DT = £43.69
Quetiapine (as Quetiapine fumarate) 300 mg Quetiapine 300mg
tablets | 60 tablet [PoM] £161.50 DT = £72.57
▸ Seroquel (AstraZeneca UK Ltd)
Quetiapine (as Quetiapine fumarate) 25 mg Seroquel 25mg tablets
| 60 tablet [PoM] £48.60 DT = £11.16
Quetiapine (as Quetiapine fumarate) 100 mg Seroquel 100mg
tablets | 60 tablet [PoM] £135.72 DT = £43.54
Quetiapine (as Quetiapine fumarate) 200 mg Seroquel 200mg
tablets | 60 tablet [PoM] £135.72 DT = £43.69
Quetiapine (as Quetiapine fumarate) 300 mg Seroquel 300mg
tablets | 60 tablet [PoM] £204.00 DT = £72.57

Oral suspension
▸ Quetiapine (Non-proprietary)
Quetiapine (as Quetiapine fumarate) 20 mg per 1 ml Quetiapine
20mg/ml oral suspension sugar free sugar-free | 150 ml [PoM] £95.00
DT = £95.00

Risperidone
⚑ 380
07-Feb-2018

● DRUG ACTION Risperidone is a dopamine D_2, $5\text{-}HT_{2A}$, alpha$_1$-adrenoceptor, and histamine-1 receptor antagonist.

● INDICATIONS AND DOSE

Schizophrenia and other psychoses in patients tolerant to risperidone by mouth and taking oral risperidone up to 4 mg daily
▸ BY DEEP INTRAMUSCULAR INJECTION
▸ Adult: Initially 25 mg every 2 weeks, to be administered into the deltoid or gluteal muscle, adjusted in steps of 12.5 mg (max. per dose 50 mg every 2 weeks) at intervals of at least 4 weeks, during initiation risperidone by mouth may need to be continued for 4–6 weeks; risperidone by mouth may also be used during dose adjustment of depot injection

Schizophrenia and other psychoses in patients tolerant to risperidone by mouth and taking oral risperidone over 4 mg daily
▸ BY DEEP INTRAMUSCULAR INJECTION
▸ Adult: Initially 37.5 mg every 2 weeks, adjusted in steps of 12.5 mg (max. per dose 50 mg every 2 weeks) at intervals of at least 4 weeks, during initiation risperidone by mouth may need to be continued for 4–6 weeks; risperidone by mouth may also be used during dose adjustment of depot injection

Acute and chronic psychosis
▸ BY MOUTH
▸ Adult: 2 mg daily in 1–2 divided doses for day 1, then 4 mg daily in 1–2 divided doses for day 2, slower titration is appropriate in some patients, usual dose 4–6 mg daily, doses above 10 mg daily only if benefit considered to outweigh risk; maximum 16 mg per day
▸ Elderly: Initially 500 micrograms twice daily, then increased in steps of 500 micrograms twice daily, increased to 1–2 mg twice daily

Mania
▸ BY MOUTH
▸ Adult: Initially 2 mg once daily, then increased in steps of 1 mg daily if required; usual dose 1–6 mg daily
▸ Elderly: Initially 500 micrograms twice daily, then increased in steps of 500 micrograms twice daily, increased to 1–2 mg twice daily

Short-term treatment (up to 6 weeks) of persistent aggression in patients with moderate to severe Alzheimer's dementia unresponsive to non-pharmacological interventions and when there is a risk of harm to self or others
▸ BY MOUTH
▸ Adult: Initially 250 micrograms twice daily, then increased in steps of 250 micrograms twice a day on alternate days, adjusted according to response; usual dose 500 micrograms twice daily (max. per dose 1 mg twice daily)

> IMPORTANT SAFETY INFORMATION
> SAFE PRACTICE
> Risperidone has been confused with ropinirole; care must be taken to ensure the correct drug is prescribed and dispensed.

● CONTRA-INDICATIONS
▸ With intramuscular use Children
● CAUTIONS
GENERAL CAUTIONS Avoid in Acute porphyrias p. 1025 · cataract surgery (risk of intra-operative floppy iris syndrome) · dehydration · dementia with Lewy bodies · prolactin-dependent tumours

SPECIFIC CAUTIONS When transferring from oral to depot therapy, the dose by mouth should be reduced gradually

- INTERACTIONS → Appendix 1: risperidone
- SIDE-EFFECTS
- **Common or very common** Anaemia · anxiety · appetite abnormal · asthenia · chest discomfort · conjunctivitis · cough · depression · diarrhoea · dyspnoea · epistaxis · fall · fever · gastrointestinal discomfort · headache · hypertension · increased risk of infection · joint disorders · laryngeal pain · muscle spasms · nasal congestion · nausea · oedema · oral disorders · pain · sedation · skin reactions · sleep disorders · urinary disorders · vision disorders · vomiting · weight decreased
- **Uncommon** Alopecia · arrhythmias · breast abnormalities · cardiac conduction disorders · cerebrovascular insufficiency · chills · coma · concentration impaired · consciousness impaired · cystitis · diabetes mellitus · dizziness postural · dry eye · dysarthria · dysphagia · dysphonia · ear pain · eye disorders · feeling abnormal · flushing · gait abnormal · gastrointestinal disorders · malaise · menstrual cycle irregularities · mood altered · muscle weakness · palpitations · polydipsia · postural hypotension · posture abnormal · respiratory disorders · sensation abnormal · syncope · taste altered · thirst · thrombocytopenia · tinnitus · vaginal discharge · vertigo
- **Rare or very rare** Angioedema · dandruff · eyelid crusting · glaucoma · head titubation · hypoglycaemia · hypothermia · jaundice · pancreatitis · peripheral coldness · rhabdomyolysis · SIADH · sleep apnoea · water intoxication · withdrawal syndrome
- **Frequency not known** Cardiac arrest
- PREGNANCY Use only if potential benefit outweighs risk.
- BREAST FEEDING Use only if potential benefit outweighs risk—small amount present in milk.
- HEPATIC IMPAIRMENT
  Dose adjustments ▸ With intramuscular use If an oral dose of at least 2 mg daily tolerated, 25 mg as a depot injection can be given every 2 weeks.
  ▸ With oral use Initial and subsequent oral doses should be halved.
- RENAL IMPAIRMENT
  Dose adjustments Initial and subsequent oral doses should be halved.
- MONITORING REQUIREMENTS
  ▸ With intramuscular use Treatment requires careful monitoring for optimum effect.
- DIRECTIONS FOR ADMINISTRATION
  ▸ With oral use Orodispersible tablets should be placed on the tongue, allowed to dissolve and swallowed. Oral liquid may be diluted with any non-alcoholic drink, except tea.
  ▸ With intramuscular use Correct injection technique (including the use of z-track technique) and rotation of injection sites are essential.
- PATIENT AND CARER ADVICE Patients or carers should be given advice on how to administer risperidone orodispersible tablets and oral liquid (counselling on use of dose syringe advised).

- MEDICINAL FORMS
  There can be variation in the licensing of different medicines containing the same drug. Forms available from special-order manufacturers include: oral solution

  Oral solution
  CAUTIONARY AND ADVISORY LABELS 2
  ▸ Risperidone (Non-proprietary)
  Risperidone 1 mg per 1 ml Risperidone 1mg/ml oral solution sugar free sugar-free | 100 ml PoM £58.22 DT = £3.87
  ▸ Risperdal (Janssen-Cilag Ltd)
  Risperidone 1 mg per 1 ml Risperdal 1mg/ml oral solution sugar-free | 100 ml PoM £37.01 DT = £3.87

Orodispersible tablet
CAUTIONARY AND ADVISORY LABELS 2
EXCIPIENTS: May contain Aspartame
▸ Risperidone (Non-proprietary)
Risperidone 500 microgram Risperidone 500microgram orodispersible tablets sugar free sugar-free | 28 tablet PoM £23.88 DT = £23.86
Risperidone 1 mg Risperidone 1mg orodispersible tablets sugar free sugar-free | 28 tablet PoM £23.51 DT = £22.99
Risperidone 2 mg Risperidone 2mg orodispersible tablets sugar free sugar-free | 28 tablet PoM £42.95 DT = £42.40
Risperidone 3 mg Risperidone 3mg orodispersible tablets sugar free sugar-free | 28 tablet PoM £43.50 DT = £43.50
Risperidone 4 mg Risperidone 4mg orodispersible tablets sugar free sugar-free | 28 tablet PoM £50.35 DT = £50.35

Powder and solvent for suspension for injection
▸ Risperdal Consta (Janssen-Cilag Ltd)
Risperidone 25 mg Risperdal Consta 25mg powder and solvent for suspension for injection vials | 1 vial PoM £79.69 DT = £79.69
Risperidone 37.5 mg Risperdal Consta 37.5mg powder and solvent for suspension for injection vials | 1 vial PoM £111.32 DT = £111.32
Risperidone 50 mg Risperdal Consta 50mg powder and solvent for suspension for injection vials | 1 vial PoM £142.76 DT = £142.76

Tablet
CAUTIONARY AND ADVISORY LABELS 2
▸ Risperidone (Non-proprietary)
Risperidone 500 microgram Risperidone 500microgram tablets | 20 tablet PoM £6.95 DT = £0.40
Risperidone 1 mg Risperidone 1mg tablets | 20 tablet PoM £0.84 DT = £0.41 | 60 tablet PoM £1.23–£25.07
Risperidone 2 mg Risperidone 2mg tablets | 60 tablet PoM £60.10 DT = £1.36
Risperidone 3 mg Risperidone 3mg tablets | 60 tablet PoM £88.38 DT = £1.57
Risperidone 4 mg Risperidone 4mg tablets | 60 tablet PoM £116.67 DT = £1.83
Risperidone 6 mg Risperidone 6mg tablets | 28 tablet PoM £82.50 DT = £2.76
▸ Risperdal (Janssen-Cilag Ltd)
Risperidone 500 microgram Risperdal 500microgram tablets | 20 tablet PoM £5.08 DT = £0.40
Risperidone 1 mg Risperdal 1mg tablets | 20 tablet PoM £8.36 DT = £0.41 | 60 tablet PoM £17.56
Risperidone 2 mg Risperdal 2mg tablets | 60 tablet PoM £34.62 DT = £1.36
Risperidone 3 mg Risperdal 3mg tablets | 60 tablet PoM £50.91 DT = £1.57
Risperidone 4 mg Risperdal 4mg tablets | 60 tablet PoM £67.20 DT = £1.83
Risperidone 6 mg Risperdal 6mg tablets | 28 tablet PoM £67.88 DT = £2.76

ANTIPSYCHOTICS > SECOND-GENERATION (DEPOT INJECTIONS)

F 380

Olanzapine embonate
(Olanzapine pamoate)

- INDICATIONS AND DOSE

Maintenance in schizophrenia in patients tolerant to olanzapine by mouth (patients taking 10 mg oral olanzapine daily)
▸ BY DEEP INTRAMUSCULAR INJECTION
▸ Adult 18-75 years: Initially 210 mg every 2 weeks, alternatively initially 405 mg every 4 weeks, then maintenance 150 mg every 2 weeks, alternatively maintenance 300 mg every 4 weeks, maintenance dose to be started after 2 months of initial treatment, dose to be administered into the gluteal muscle, consult product literature if supplementation with oral olanzapine required continued →

Maintenance in schizophrenia in patients tolerant to olanzapine by mouth (patients taking 15 mg oral olanzapine daily)

▶ BY DEEP INTRAMUSCULAR INJECTION

▶ Adult 18-75 years: Initially 300 mg every 2 weeks, then maintenance 210 mg every 2 weeks, alternatively maintenance 405 mg every 4 weeks, maintenance dose to be started after 2 months of initial treatment, dose to be administered into the gluteal muscle, consult product literature if supplementation with oral olanzapine required

Maintenance in schizophrenia in patients tolerant to olanzapine by mouth (patients taking 20 mg oral olanzapine daily)

▶ BY DEEP INTRAMUSCULAR INJECTION

▶ Adult: Initially 300 mg every 2 weeks, then maintenance 300 mg every 2 weeks (max. per dose 300 mg every 2 weeks), adjusted according to response, dose to be administered into the gluteal muscle, consult product literature if supplementation with oral olanzapine required

---

IMPORTANT SAFETY INFORMATION
When prescribing, dispensing or administering, check that this is the correct preparation—this preparation is used for *maintenance* treatment and should **not** be used for the rapid control of an *acute* episode.

● CONTRA-INDICATIONS Children

● CAUTIONS Bone-marrow depression · hypereosinophilic disorders · low leucocyte count · low neutrophil count · myeloproliferative disease · paralytic ileus · when transferring from oral to depot therapy, the dose by mouth should be reduced gradually

● INTERACTIONS → Appendix 1: olanzapine

● SIDE-EFFECTS

▶ **Common or very common** Anticholinergic syndrome · appetite increased · arthralgia · asthenia · eosinophilia · fever · glycosuria · oedema · postural hypotension

▶ **Uncommon** Abdominal distension · alopecia · bradycardia · breast enlargement · diabetes mellitus · diabetic coma · dysarthria · epistaxis · ketoacidosis · memory loss · oculogyration · photosensitivity reaction · restless legs · urinary disorders

▶ **Rare or very rare** Drug reaction with eosinophilia and systemic symptoms (DRESS) · hepatic disorders · hypothermia · pancreatitis · rhabdomyolysis · thrombocytopenia

▶ **Frequency not known** Erythema · gait abnormal · increased risk of fall · lethargy · pneumonia · visual hallucinations

Overdose Post-injection reactions have been reported leading to signs and symptoms of overdose.

● PREGNANCY Use only if potential benefit outweighs risk; neonatal lethargy, tremor, and hypertonia reported when used in third trimester.

● BREAST FEEDING Avoid—present in milk.

● HEPATIC IMPAIRMENT Initially 150 mg every 4 weeks; increase with caution in moderate impairment.

● RENAL IMPAIRMENT
Dose adjustments Initially 150 mg every 4 weeks.

● MONITORING REQUIREMENTS

▶ Observe patient for at least 3 hours after injection.

▶ Treatment requires careful monitoring for optimum effect.

▶ Blood lipids and weight should be measured at baseline, at 3 months (weight should be measured at frequent intervals during the first 3 months), and then yearly with antipsychotic drugs. Patients taking olanzapine require more frequent monitoring of these parameters: every 3 months for the first year, then yearly.

▶ Fasting blood glucose should be measured at baseline, at 4–6 months, and then yearly. Patients taking olanzapine should have fasting blood glucose tested at baseline, after one months' treatment, then every 4–6 months.

● DIRECTIONS FOR ADMINISTRATION Correct injection technique (including use of z-track technique) and rotation of injection sites are essential.

● MEDICINAL FORMS
There can be variation in the licensing of different medicines containing the same drug.

Powder and solvent for suspension for injection

▶ Zypadhera (Eli Lilly and Company Ltd)
Olanzapine (as Olanzapine embonate monohydrate)
210 mg Zypadhera 210mg powder and solvent for suspension for injection vials | 1 vial [PoM] £142.76 (Hospital only)
Olanzapine (as Olanzapine embonate monohydrate)
300 mg Zypadhera 300mg powder and solvent for suspension for injection vials | 1 vial [PoM] £222.64 (Hospital only)
Olanzapine (as Olanzapine embonate monohydrate)
405 mg Zypadhera 405mg powder and solvent for suspension for injection vials | 1 vial [PoM] £285.52 (Hospital only)

4 Movement disorders

Motor neurone disease

17-May-2017

Description of condition

Motor neurone disease is a neurodegenerative condition affecting the brain and spinal cord. Degeneration of motor neurones leads to progressive muscle weakness; resulting symptoms include muscle cramps, wasting and stiffness, loss of dexterity, reduced respiratory function and cognitive dysfunction. The most common form is amyotrophic lateral sclerosis.

[EvGr] Patients suspected of having developed motor neurone disease should be referred to a neurologist without delay. Ⓐ

Aims of treatment

As there is no cure, treatment focuses on maintaining functional ability and managing symptoms.

Non-drug treatment

Non-drug treatment includes nutrition, psychosocial support, physiotherapy, exercise programmes and use of special equipment or mobility aids.

Management of symptoms

Muscular symptoms

[EvGr] Quinine p. 608 [unlicensed indication] is recommended as first line treatment for muscle cramps. If quinine is ineffective, not tolerated or contra-indicated, baclofen p. 1092 [unlicensed indication] should be considered as second line treatment. Subsequent treatment options include tizanidine p. 1094 [unlicensed indication], dantrolene sodium p. 1307 [unlicensed indication] or gabapentin p. 314 [unlicensed indication].

Symptoms of muscle stiffness, spasticity or increased tone can be managed with baclofen, tizanidine, dantrolene sodium or gabapentin [unlicensed indication]. Treatment of severe spasticity may require specialist referral. Ⓐ

Saliva problems

[EvGr] A trial of an antimuscarinic drug [unlicensed indication] can be considered for excessive drooling of saliva. Glycopyrronium bromide p. 246 is recommended in patients who have cognitive impairment as it has fewer central nervous system side-effects. If initial treatment is ineffective, not tolerated or contra-indicated, referral for specialist administration of botulinum toxin type A p. 403 [unlicensed indication] may be required.

Humidification, nebulisers and carbocisteine p. 290 can be used to treat patients with thick, tenacious saliva. ⟨Å⟩

Respiratory symptoms

EvGr Reversible causes of worsening respiratory impairment (such as respiratory tract infections or secretion problems) should be treated before considering other options.

Patients experiencing breathlessness can be treated with opioids [unlicensed indication], or benzodiazepines [unlicensed indication] if the patient's symptoms are exacerbated by anxiety. Non-invasive ventilation should be considered in patients with respiratory impairment. ⟨Å⟩

Amyotrophic lateral sclerosis

Riluzole p. 1089 is licensed for use in patients with amyotrophic lateral sclerosis to extend life or to extend the time to mechanical ventilation—see *National funding/access decisions* under riluzole.

Useful Resources

Motor neurone disease: assessment and management. National Institute for Health and Care Excellence. Clinical guideline NG42. February 2016. www.nice.org.uk/guidance/ng42

4.1 Dystonias and other involuntary movements

Essential tremor, chorea, tics, and related disorders

Drugs used in essential tremor, chorea, tics, and related disorders

Tetrabenazine p. 402 is mainly used to control movement disorders in Huntington's chorea and related disorders. Tetrabenazine can also be prescribed for the treatment of tardive dyskinesia if switching or withdrawing the causative antipsychotic drug is not effective. It acts by depleting nerve endings of dopamine. It is effective in only a proportion of patients and its use may be limited by the development of depression.

Haloperidol p. 382 [unlicensed indication], olanzapine p. 394 [unlicensed indication], risperidone p. 398 [unlicensed indication], and quetiapine p. 397 [unlicensed indication], can also be used to suppress chorea in Huntington's disease.

Haloperidol can also improve motor tics and symptoms of Tourette syndrome and related choreas. Other treatments for Tourette syndrome include pimozide p. 385 [unlicensed indication] (**important**: ECG monitoring required), clonidine hydrochloride p. 144 [unlicensed indication], and sulpiride p. 386 [unlicensed indication]. Trihexyphenidyl hydrochloride p. 407 in high dosage can also improve some movement disorders; it is sometimes necessary to build the dose up over many weeks. Chlorpromazine hydrochloride p. 381 and haloperidol are used to relieve intractable hiccup.

Propranolol hydrochloride p. 149 or another beta-adrenoceptor blocking drug may be useful in treating essential tremor or tremors associated with anxiety or thyrotoxicosis.

Primidone p. 332 in some cases provides relief from benign essential tremor; the dose is increased slowly to reduce side-effects.

Piracetam p. 402 is used as an adjunctive treatment for myoclonus of cortical origin. After an acute episode, attempts should be made every 6 months to decrease or discontinue treatment.

Riluzole p. 1089 is used to extend life in patients with motor neurone disease who have amyotrophic lateral sclerosis.

Torsion dystonia and other involuntary movements

Treatment with botulinum toxin type A p. 403 can be considered after an acquired non-progressive brain injury if rapid-onset spasticity causes postural or functional difficulties.

> **Other drugs used for Dystonias and other involuntary movements** Clozapine, p. 392 · Diazepam, p. 340 · Orphenadrine hydrochloride, p. 406 · Pericyazine, p. 384 · Pramipexole, p. 417 · Prochlorperazine, p. 385 · Procyclidine hydrochloride, p. 406 · Ropinirole, p. 419 · Rotigotine, p. 421 · Trifluoperazine, p. 387

ANTIPSYCHOTICS ⟩ FIRST-GENERATION

⌖ 380

Promazine hydrochloride

● **INDICATIONS AND DOSE**

Short-term adjunctive management of psychomotor agitation
▸ BY MOUTH
▸ Adult: 100–200 mg 4 times a day

Agitation and restlessness in elderly
▸ BY MOUTH
▸ Elderly: 25–50 mg 4 times a day

● CONTRA-INDICATIONS CNS depression · comatose states · phaeochromocytoma

● CAUTIONS Cerebral arteriosclerosis

● INTERACTIONS → Appendix 1: phenothiazines

● SIDE-EFFECTS Apathy · autonomic dysfunction · cardiac arrest · cardiovascular effects · consciousness impaired · corneal opacity · epilepsy · eye discolouration · gastrointestinal disorder · glaucoma · haemolytic anaemia · headache · hepatic disorders · hyperpyrexia · hypersensitivity · hyperthermia (dose-related) · hypothermia (dose-related) · lens opacity · menstrual disorder · muscle rigidity · nasal congestion · photosensitivity reaction · sedation · skin reactions · urinary hesitation · vision blurred · withdrawal syndrome

● HEPATIC IMPAIRMENT Can precipitate coma; phenothiazines are hepatotoxic.

● RENAL IMPAIRMENT
Dose adjustments Start with small doses in severe renal impairment because of increased cerebral sensitivity.

● LESS SUITABLE FOR PRESCRIBING Promazine hydrochloride is less suitable for prescribing.

● MEDICINAL FORMS
There can be variation in the licensing of different medicines containing the same drug. Forms available from special-order manufacturers include: oral suspension, oral solution

Oral solution
CAUTIONARY AND ADVISORY LABELS 2
▸ Promazine hydrochloride (Non-proprietary)
  Promazine hydrochloride 5 mg per 1 ml Promazine 25mg/5ml syrup | 150 ml PoM £13.00 DT = £13.01
  Promazine 25mg/5ml oral solution | 150 ml PoM £13.01 DT = £13.01
  Promazine hydrochloride 10 mg per 1 ml Promazine 50mg/5ml syrup | 150 ml PoM £15.00 DT = £15.01
  Promazine 50mg/5ml oral solution | 150 ml PoM £15.01 DT = £15.01

Tablet
CAUTIONARY AND ADVISORY LABELS 2
▸ Promazine hydrochloride (Non-proprietary)
  Promazine hydrochloride 25 mg Promazine 25mg tablets | 100 tablet PoM £49.99 DT = £49.07
  Promazine hydrochloride 50 mg Promazine 50mg tablets | 100 tablet PoM £76.49 DT = £76.34

CNS STIMULANTS

Piracetam

● **INDICATIONS AND DOSE**

Adjunctive treatment of cortical myoclonus
▶ BY MOUTH
▶ Adult: Initially 7.2 g daily in 2–3 divided doses, then increased in steps of 4.8 g every 3–4 days, adjusted according to response, subsequently, attempts should be made to reduce dose of concurrent therapy; maximum 24 g per day

● CONTRA-INDICATIONS Cerebral haemorrhage · Huntington's chorea

● CAUTIONS Gastric ulcer · history of haemorrhagic stroke · increased risk of bleeding · major surgery · underlying disorders of haemostasis

● SIDE-EFFECTS
▶ **Common or very common** Anxiety · movement disorders · weight increased
▶ **Uncommon** Asthenia · depression · drowsiness
▶ **Frequency not known** Angioedema · confusion · diarrhoea · epilepsy exacerbated · gastrointestinal discomfort · haemorrhagic disorder · hallucination · headache · insomnia · nausea · skin reactions · vertigo · vomiting

● PREGNANCY Avoid.

● BREAST FEEDING Avoid.

● HEPATIC IMPAIRMENT
Dose adjustments Adjust dose if both hepatic and renal impairment.

● RENAL IMPAIRMENT Avoid if eGFR less than 20 mL/minute/1.73 m^2.
Dose adjustments Use two-thirds of normal dose if eGFR 50–80 mL/minute/1.73 m^2; use one-third of normal dose in 2 divided doses if eGFR 30–50 mL/minute/1.73 m^2; use one-sixth of normal dose as a single dose if eGFR 20–30 mL/minute/1.73 m^2.

● TREATMENT CESSATION Avoid abrupt withdrawal.

● DIRECTIONS FOR ADMINISTRATION Follow the oral solution with a glass of water (or soft drink) to reduce bitter taste.

● PRESCRIBING AND DISPENSING INFORMATION Piracetam has been used in children 16 years and over as adjunctive treatment for cortical myoclonus.

● MEDICINAL FORMS
There can be variation in the licensing of different medicines containing the same drug.

Oral solution
CAUTIONARY AND ADVISORY LABELS 3
▶ Piracetam (Non-proprietary)
  Piracetam 333.3 mg per 1 ml Piracetam 333.3mg/ml oral solution sugar free sugar-free | 300 ml [PoM] ⟲
▶ Nootropil (UCB Pharma Ltd)
  Piracetam 333.3 mg per 1 ml Nootropil 33% oral solution sugar-free | 300 ml [PoM] £16.31

Tablet
CAUTIONARY AND ADVISORY LABELS 3
▶ Nootropil (UCB Pharma Ltd)
  Piracetam 800 mg Nootropil 800mg tablets | 90 tablet [PoM] £11.75
  Piracetam 1.2 gram Nootropil 1200mg tablets | 60 tablet [PoM] £10.97

MONOAMINE DEPLETING DRUGS

Tetrabenazine

● **INDICATIONS AND DOSE**

Movement disorders due to Huntington's chorea, hemiballismus, senile chorea, and related neurological conditions
▶ BY MOUTH
▶ Adult: Initially 25 mg 3 times a day, then increased, if tolerated, in steps of 25 mg every 3–4 days; maximum 200 mg per day
▶ Elderly: Lower initial dose may be necessary
Moderate to severe tardive dyskinesia
▶ BY MOUTH
▶ Adult: Initially 12.5 mg daily, dose to be gradually increased according to response

● CONTRA-INDICATIONS Depression · parkinsonism · phaeochromocytoma · prolactin-dependent tumours

● CAUTIONS Susceptibility to QT-interval prolongation

● INTERACTIONS → Appendix 1: tetrabenazine

● SIDE-EFFECTS
▶ **Common or very common** Anxiety · confusion · constipation · depression · diarrhoea · drowsiness · hypotension · insomnia · nausea · parkinsonism · vomiting
▶ **Uncommon** Consciousness impaired · hyperthermia
▶ **Rare or very rare** Neuroleptic malignant syndrome · skeletal muscle damage
▶ **Frequency not known** Bradycardia · dizziness · dry mouth · epigastric pain · suicidal ideation

● PREGNANCY Avoid unless essential—toxicity in *animal* studies.

● BREAST FEEDING Avoid.

● HEPATIC IMPAIRMENT Use with caution in severe impairment.
Dose adjustments Use half initial dose and slower dose titration in mild to moderate impairment.

● RENAL IMPAIRMENT Use with caution.

● TREATMENT CESSATION Avoid abrupt withdrawal.

● PATIENT AND CARER ADVICE
Driving and skilled tasks May affect performance of skilled tasks (e.g. driving).

● MEDICINAL FORMS
There can be variation in the licensing of different medicines containing the same drug. Forms available from special-order manufacturers include: oral suspension
Tablet
CAUTIONARY AND ADVISORY LABELS 2
▶ Tetrabenazine (Non-proprietary)
  Tetrabenazine 25 mg Tetrabenazine 25mg tablets | 112 tablet [PoM] £100.00 DT = £100.00
▶ Tardiben (AOP Orphan Pharmaceuticals AG)
  Tetrabenazine 25 mg Tardiben 25mg tablets | 112 tablet [PoM] £100.00 DT = £100.00
▶ Xenazine (Alliance Pharmaceuticals Ltd)
  Tetrabenazine 25 mg Xenazine 25 tablets | 112 tablet [PoM] £100.00 DT = £100.00

MUSCLE RELAXANTS > PERIPHERALLY ACTING > NEUROTOXINS (BOTULINUM TOXINS)

Botulinum toxin type A   24-Apr-2017

● **INDICATIONS AND DOSE**

Treatment of focal spasticity (including hand and wrist disability associated with stroke) (specialist use only) | Blepharospasm (specialist use only) | Hemifacial spasm (specialist use only) | Spasmodic torticollis (specialist use only) | Severe hyperhidrosis of the axillae (specialist use only) | Prophylaxis of headaches in adults with chronic migraine (specialist use only) | Temporary improvement of moderate to severe wrinkles between the eyebrows in adults under 65 years (specialist use only) | Ankle disability due to lower limb spasticity associated with stroke (specialist use only) | Management of bladder dysfunctions (specialist use only) | Temporary improvement of moderate to severe crow's feet (specialist use only)

▸ BY SUBCUTANEOUS INJECTION, OR BY INTRADERMAL INJECTION, OR BY INTRAMUSCULAR INJECTION
▸ Adult: (consult product literature)

DOSE EQUIVALENCE AND CONVERSION
▸ **Important**: information is specific to each individual preparation.

● **CONTRA-INDICATIONS** Acute urinary retention (specific to use in bladder disorders only) · catheterisation difficulties (specific to use in bladder disorders only) · generalised disorders of muscle activity · infection at injection site · myasthenia gravis · presence of bladder calculi (specific to use in bladder disorders only) · urinary tract infection (specific to use in bladder disorders only)

● **CAUTIONS**
GENERAL CAUTIONS Atrophy in target muscle · chronic respiratory disorder · elderly · excessive weakness in target muscle · history of aspiration · history of dysphagia · inflammation in target muscle · neurological disorders · neuromuscular disorders · off-label use (fatal adverse events reported)
SPECIFIC CAUTIONS
▸ When used for blepharospasm or hemifacial spasm Risk of angle-closure glaucoma

CAUTIONS, FURTHER INFORMATION Neuromuscular or neurological disorders can lead to increased sensitivity and exaggerated muscle weakness including dysphagia and respiratory compromise.
▸ Blepharospasm or hemifacial spasm When used for blepharospasm and hemifacial spasm, reduced blinking can lead to corneal exposure, persistent epithelial defect and corneal ulceration (especially in those with VIIth nerve disorders)—careful testing of corneal sensation in previously operated eyes, avoidance of injection in lower lid area to avoid ectropion, and vigorous treatment of epithelial defect needed.

● **INTERACTIONS** → Appendix 1: botulinum toxin type A
● **SIDE-EFFECTS**
▸ **Common or very common** Alopecia · asthenia · autonomic dysreflexia · bladder diverticulum · constipation · dizziness · drowsiness · dry eye · dry mouth · dysphagia (most common after injection into sternomastoid muscle) · ecchymosis (minimised by applying gentle pressure at injection site immediately after injection) · eye discomfort · eye disorders · eye inflammation · fall · fever · gait abnormal · haematuria · headaches · hot flush · increased risk of infection · influenza like illness · insomnia · joint disorders · leukocyturia · malaise · muscle complaints · muscle weakness · musculoskeletal stiffness · nausea · neuromuscular dysfunction · oedema · pain · paresis ·

sensation abnormal · skin reactions · urinary disorders · vision disorders
▸ **Uncommon** Anxiety · coordination abnormal · depression · dysphonia · dyspnoea · facial paralysis · memory loss · oral paraesthesia · photosensitivity reaction · postural hypotension · vertigo
▸ **Frequency not known** Abdominal pain · angioedema · angle closure glaucoma · appetite decreased · arrhythmia · diarrhoea · dysarthria · hearing impairment · hypersensitivity · myocardial infarction · myopathy · nerve disorders · respiratory disorders · seizure · syncope · vomiting

● CONCEPTION AND CONTRACEPTION Avoid in women of child-bearing age unless using effective contraception.
● PREGNANCY Avoid unless essential—toxicity in *animal* studies (manufacturer of *Botox*® advise avoid).
● BREAST FEEDING Low risk of systemic absorption but avoid unless essential.
● PRESCRIBING AND DISPENSING INFORMATION Preparations are not interchangeable.
● PATIENT AND CARER ADVICE Patients and carers should be warned of the signs and symptoms of toxin spread, such as muscle weakness and breathing difficulties; they should be advised to seek immediate medical attention if swallowing, speech or breathing difficulties occur.
● NATIONAL FUNDING/ACCESS DECISIONS

NICE decisions
▸ **Botulinum toxin type A for the prevention of headaches in adults with chronic migraine (June 2012)** NICE TA260
Botulinum toxin type A is recommended as an option for the prophylaxis of headaches in adults with chronic migraine, (defined as headaches on at least 15 days per month, of which at least 8 days are with migraine), that has not responded to at least three prior pharmacological prophylaxis therapies and whose condition is appropriately managed for medication overuse.
www.nice.org.uk/TA260

Scottish Medicines Consortium (SMC) Decisions
The *Scottish Medicines Consortium* has advised that *Azzalure*® and *Vistabel*® (December 2010), and *Bocouture*® (February 2011) are **not** recommended for use within NHS Scotland.
   The *Scottish Medicines Consortium* has advised (February 2017) that botulinum toxin type A (*Botox*®) is accepted for restricted use within NHS Scotland for the prophylaxis of headaches in adults with chronic migraine, (defined as headaches on at least 15 days per month, of which at least 8 days are with migraine), that has not responded to at least three prior oral pharmacological prophylaxis therapies and whose condition is appropriately managed for medication overuse.

● MEDICINAL FORMS
There can be variation in the licensing of different medicines containing the same drug.
Powder for solution for injection
▸ Azzalure (Galderma (UK) Ltd)
   Botulinum toxin type A 125 unit Azzalure 125unit powder for solution for injection vials | 1 vial [PoM] £64.00 | 2 vial [PoM] £128.00
▸ Bocouture (Merz Pharma UK Ltd)
   Botulinum toxin type A 50 unit Bocouture 50unit powder for solution for injection vials | 1 vial [PoM] £72.00
   Botulinum toxin type A 100 unit Bocouture 100unit powder for solution for injection vials | 1 vial [PoM] £229.90
▸ Botox (Allergan Ltd)
   Botulinum toxin type A 50 unit Botox 50unit powder for solution for injection vials | 1 vial [PoM] £77.50
   Botulinum toxin type A 100 unit Botox 100unit powder for solution for injection vials | 1 vial [PoM] £138.20
   Botulinum toxin type A 200 unit Botox 200unit powder for solution for injection vials | 1 vial [PoM] £276.40

4

Nervous system

Nervous system

4

- Dysport (Ipsen Ltd)
  Botulinum toxin type A 300 unit Dysport 300unit powder for
  solution for injection vials | 1 vial [PoM] £92.40
  Botulinum toxin type A 500 unit Dysport 500unit powder for
  solution for injection vials | 2 vial [PoM] £308.00
- Xeomin (Merz Pharma UK Ltd)
  Botulinum toxin type A 50 unit Xeomin 50unit powder for solution
  for injection vials | 1 vial [PoM] £72.00
  Botulinum toxin type A 100 unit Xeomin 100unit powder for
  solution for injection vials | 1 vial [PoM] £129.90
  Botulinum toxin type A 200 unit Xeomin 200unit powder for
  solution for injection vials | 1 vial [PoM] £259.80 (Hospital only)

Botulinum toxin type B

- **INDICATIONS AND DOSE**

**Spasmodic torticollis (cervical dystonia) (specialist use
only)**
  - BY INTRAMUSCULAR INJECTION
  - Adult: Initially 5000–10 000 units, adjusted according
    to response, dose to be divided between 2–4 most
    affected muscles
  DOSE EQUIVALENCE AND CONVERSION
  - **Important**: information specific to each individual
    preparation.

- CONTRA-INDICATIONS Neuromuscular disorders ·
  neuromuscular junctional disorders
- CAUTIONS History of dysphagia or aspiration · off-label
  use (risk of toxin spread) · tolerance may occur
- INTERACTIONS → Appendix 1: botulinum toxin type B
- SIDE-EFFECTS
- **Common or very common** Dry mouth · dysphagia ·
  dysphonia · headache · influenza like illness · muscle
  weakness · neck pain · taste altered · vision disorders
- **Frequency not known** Angioedema · asthenia · constipation
  · dyspnoea · pneumonia aspiration · ptosis · skin reactions ·
  vomiting
- PREGNANCY Low risk of systemic absorption but avoid
  unless essential.
- BREAST FEEDING Low risk of systemic absorption but
  avoid unless essential.
- DIRECTIONS FOR ADMINISTRATION Injection may be
  diluted with sodium chloride 0.9%.
- PRESCRIBING AND DISPENSING INFORMATION **Important**:
  not interchangeable with other botulinum toxin
  preparations.
- PATIENT AND CARER ADVICE Patients should be warned of
  the signs and symptoms of toxin spread, such as muscle
  weakness and breathing difficulties; they should be
  advised to seek immediate medical attention if swallowing,
  speech or breathing difficulties occur.

- MEDICINAL FORMS
  There can be variation in the licensing of different medicines
  containing the same drug.
  Solution for injection
  - NeuroBloc (Eisai Ltd)
    Botulinum toxin type B 5000 unit per 1 ml NeuroBloc
    5,000units/1ml solution for injection vials | 1 vial [PoM] £148.27
    (Hospital only)
    NeuroBloc 10,000units/2ml solution for injection vials | 1 vial [PoM]
    £197.69 (Hospital only)
    NeuroBloc 2,500units/0.5ml solution for injection vials | 1 vial [PoM]
    £111.20 (Hospital only)

NEUROPROTECTIVE DRUGS

Tafamidis

- **INDICATIONS AND DOSE**

**Treatment of transthyretin familial amyloid
polyneuropathy (TTR-FAP) in patients with stage 1
symptomatic polyneuropathy to delay peripheral
neurological impairment (initiated under specialist
supervision)**
  - BY MOUTH
  - Adult: 20 mg once daily

- SIDE-EFFECTS
- **Common or very common** Abdominal pain upper · diarrhoea
  · increased risk of infection
- CONCEPTION AND CONTRACEPTION Exclude pregnancy
  before treatment and ensure effective contraception
  during and for one month after stopping treatment.
- PREGNANCY Avoid (toxicity in *animal* studies).
- BREAST FEEDING Avoid—present in milk in *animal* studies.
- HEPATIC IMPAIRMENT Caution in severe impairment—no
  information available.
- PRESCRIBING AND DISPENSING INFORMATION Tafamidis
  should be prescribed in addition to standard treatment,
  but before liver transplantation; it should be discontinued
  in patients who undergo liver transplantation.

- MEDICINAL FORMS
  There can be variation in the licensing of different medicines
  containing the same drug.
  Capsule
  CAUTIONARY AND ADVISORY LABELS 25
  - Vyndaqel (Pfizer Ltd) ▼
    Tafamidis 20 mg Vyndaqel 20mg capsules | 30 capsule [PoM]
    £10,685.00 (Hospital only)

4.2 Parkinson's disease

Parkinson's disease   11-Aug-2017

Description of condition

Parkinson's disease is a progressive neurodegenerative
condition resulting from the death of dopaminergic cells of
the substantia nigra in the brain.

Patients with Parkinson's disease classically present with
motor-symptoms including hypokinesia, bradykinesia,
rigidity, rest tremor, and postural instability.

Non-motor symptoms include dementia, depression, sleep
disturbances, bladder and bowel dysfunction, speech and
language changes, swallowing problems and weight loss.

[EvGr] Patients with suspected Parkinson's disease should
be referred to a specialist and reviewed every 6 to 12 months.
When Parkinson's disease diagnosis is confirmed, patients
should be advised to inform the DVLA and their car insurer.
Ⓐ

Aims of treatment

Parkinson's disease is an incurable progressive condition,
and the aim of treatment is to control the symptoms and to
improve the patient's quality of life.

Non-drug treatment

[EvGr] Parkinson's disease patients should be offered
physiotherapy if balance or motor function problems are
present, speech and language therapy if they develop
communication, swallowing or saliva problems, and
occupational therapy if they experience difficulties with their
daily activities. Dietitian referral should be considered. Ⓐ

Drug treatment

Drug management of motor symptoms in Parkinson's disease

First-line treatment

[EvGr] In early stages of Parkinson's disease, patients whose motor symptoms decrease their quality of life should be offered *levodopa* combined with *carbidopa* (co-careldopa p. 410) or *benserazide* (co-beneldopa p. 409).

Parkinson's disease patients whose motor symptoms *do not* affect their quality of life, could be prescribed a choice of *levodopa*, *non-ergot-derived dopamine-receptor agonists* (pramipexole p. 417, ropinirole p. 419 or rotigotine p. 421) or *monoamine-oxidase-B inhibitors* (rasagiline p. 422 or selegiline hydrochloride p. 423).

Before starting antiparkinsonian treatment, the patient's individual circumstances, including symptoms, comorbidities and preferences, should be discussed together with the potential benefits and harms from the different drugs available.

Patients and their carers should be informed about the risk of adverse reactions from antiparkinsonian drugs, including psychotic symptoms, excessive sleepiness and sudden onset of sleep with dopamine-receptor agonists, and impulse control disorders with all dopaminergic therapy (especially *dopamine-receptor agonists*). For further information *see Impulse control disorders*. ⟨A⟩

Levodopa treatment is associated with motor complications, including response fluctuations and dyskinesias. Response fluctuations are characterised by large variations in motor performance, with normal function during the 'on' period, and weakness and restricted mobility during the 'off' period. 'End-of-dose' deterioration with progressively shorter duration of benefit can also occur. Modified-release preparations may help with 'end-of-dose' deterioration or nocturnal immobility.

The overall improvement in motor performance is more noticeable with *levodopa* than with *dopamine-receptor agonists*, and motor complications are less likely to occur with *dopamine-receptor agonists* when used alone long-term. Conversely, excessive sleepiness, hallucinations, and impulse control disorders are more likely to occur with *dopamine-receptor agonists* than with *levodopa*.

[EvGr] To avoid the potential for acute akinesia or neuroleptic malignant syndrome, antiparkinsonian drug concentrations should not be allowed to fall suddenly due to poor absorption or abrupt withdrawal. ⟨A⟩

Adjuvant therapy

[EvGr] If a patient with Parkinson's disease develops dyskinesia or motor fluctuations, specialist advice should be sought before modifying antiparkinsonian drug therapy.

Patients who develop dyskinesia or motor fluctuations despite optimal *levodopa* therapy should be offered a choice of *non-ergotic dopamine-receptor agonists* (pramipexole, ropinirole, rotigotine), *monoamine oxidase B inhibitors* (rasagiline or selegiline hydrochloride) or COMT inhibitors (entacapone p. 407 or tolcapone p. 408) as an adjunct to *levodopa*.

An *ergot-derived dopamine-receptor agonist* (bromocriptine p. 414, cabergoline p. 415 or pergolide p. 417) should **only** be considered as an adjunct to *levodopa* if symptoms are not adequately controlled with a *non-ergot-derived dopamine-receptor agonist*.

If dyskinesia is not adequately managed by modifying existing therapy, amantadine hydrochloride p. 412 should be considered. ⟨A⟩

Drug management of non-motor symptoms in Parkinson's disease

Daytime sleepiness and sudden onset of sleep

[EvGr] Patients who experience daytime sleepiness or sudden onset of sleep, should have their Parkinson's drug treatment adjusted under specialist medical guidance. If reversible pharmacological and physical causes have been excluded,

modafinil p. 485 should be considered to treat excessive daytime sleepiness, and treatment should be reviewed at least every 12 months.

Patients with Parkinson's disease who have daytime sleepiness or sudden onset of sleep should be advised not to drive, to inform the DVLA about their symptoms, and to think about any occupational hazards. ⟨A⟩

Nocturnal akinesia

[EvGr] When treating nocturnal akinesia in patients with Parkinson's disease, *levodopa* or oral *dopamine-receptor agonists* should be considered as first-line options and rotigotine p. 421 as second-line (if both *levodopa* or oral *dopamine-receptor agonists* are ineffective). ⟨A⟩

Postural hypotension

[EvGr] Patients with Parkinson's disease who develop postural hypotension should have their drug treatment reviewed to address any pharmacological cause. If drug therapy is required, midodrine hydrochloride p. 187 should be considered as the first option and fludrocortisone acetate p. 661 [unlicensed indication] as an alternative. ⟨A⟩

Depression

See Antidepressant drugs p. 355.

Psychotic symptoms

[EvGr] Hallucinations and delusions need not be treated if they are well tolerated. Otherwise, the dosage of any antiparkinsonism drugs that might have triggered hallucinations or delusions should be reduced, taking into account the severity of symptoms and possible withdrawal effects. Specialist advice should be sought before modifying drug treatment.

In Parkinson's disease patients with no cognitive impairment, quetiapine p. 397 [unlicensed indication] can be considered to treat hallucinations and delusions. If standard treatment is not effective, clozapine p. 392 should be offered to treat hallucinations and delusions in patients with Parkinson's disease. ⟨A⟩ It is important to acknowledge that other antipsychotic medicines (such as phenothiazines and butyrophenones) can worsen the motor features of Parkinson's disease.

Rapid eye movement sleep behaviour disorder

[EvGr] Clonazepam p. 334 [unlicensed indication] or melatonin p. 482 [unlicensed indication] should be considered to treat rapid eye movement sleep behaviour disorder in Parkinson's patients once possible pharmacological causes have been addressed. ⟨A⟩

Drooling of saliva

[EvGr] Drug treatment for drooling of saliva in patients with Parkinson's disease should only be considered if non-drug treatment such as speech and language therapy is not available or is ineffective.

Glycopyrronium bromide p. 246 [unlicensed indication] should be considered as first-line treatment and botulinum toxin type A p. 403 [unlicensed indication] as second-line.

Other antimuscarinic drugs, should only be considered if the risk of cognitive adverse effects is thought to be minimal; topical preparations, such as *atropine*[unlicensed indication], should be used if possible to reduce the risk of adverse events. ⟨A⟩

Parkinson's disease dementia

[EvGr] A cholinesterase inhibitor should be offered to patients with mild-to-moderate Parkinson's disease dementia and considered for patients with severe Parkinson's disease dementia [unlicensed indications apart from rivastigmine p. 302 capsules for the treatment of mild-to-moderate dementia in patients with Parkinson's disease]. If cholinesterase inhibitors are not tolerated or contra-indicated, memantine hydrochloride p. 303 [unlicensed indication] should be considered. ⟨A⟩ For further information *see* Dementia p. 299

Advanced Parkinson's disease

EvGr Patients with advanced Parkinson's disease can be offered apomorphine hydrochloride p. 413 as intermittent injections or continuous subcutaneous infusions. To control nausea and vomiting associated with *apomorphine*, administration of domperidone p. 426 is usually started two days before *apomorphine* therapy, and then discontinued as soon as possible. To reduce the risk of serious arrhythmia due to QT prolongation associated to the concomitant use of domperidone p. 426 and apomorphine hydrochloride p. 413, the MHRA recommends an assessment of cardiac risk factors and ECG monitoring and to ensure that the benefits outweighs the risks when initiating treatment. Ⓐ

Levodopa-carbidopa intestinal gel is used for the treatment of advanced levodopa-responsive Parkinson's disease with severe motor fluctuations and hyperkinesia or dyskinesia. The gel is administered with a portable pump directly into the duodenum or upper jejunum.

EvGr Deep brain stimulation should *only* be considered for patients with advanced Parkinson's disease whose symptoms are *not* adequately controlled by best drug therapy. Ⓐ

Impulse control disorders

Impulse control disorders (compulsive gambling, hypersexuality, binge eating, or obsessive shopping) can develop in a person with Parkinson's disease who is on any dopaminergic therapy at any stage in the disease course particularly if the patient has a history of previous impulsive behaviours, alcohol consumption, or smoking. EvGr Patients should be informed about the different types of impulse control disorders and that dopamine-receptor agonist therapy may be reduced or stopped if problematic impulse control disorders develop.

When managing impulse control disorders, dopamine-receptor agonist doses should be reduced gradually and patients should be monitored for symptoms of dopamine agonist withdrawal. Specialist cognitive behavioural therapy should be offered if modifying dopaminergic therapy is not effective. Ⓐ

Useful Resources

Parkinson's disease in adults. National Institute for Health and Care Excellence. NICE guideline 71. July 2017. www.nice.org.uk/guidance/NG71

ANTIMUSCARINICS

Orphenadrine hydrochloride

● DRUG ACTION Orphenadrine exerts its antiparkinsonian action by reducing the effects of the relative central cholinergic excess that occurs as a result of dopamine deficiency.

● INDICATIONS AND DOSE

Parkinsonism | Drug-induced extrapyramidal symptoms (but not tardive dyskinesia)
▸ BY MOUTH
▸ Adult: Initially 150 mg daily in divided doses, then increased in steps of 50 mg every 2–3 days, adjusted according to response; usual dose 150–300 mg daily in divided doses; maximum 400 mg per day
▸ Elderly: Preferably dose at lower end of range

● CONTRA-INDICATIONS Acute porphyrias p. 1025 · gastro-intestinal obstruction · myasthenia gravis
● CAUTIONS Cardiovascular disease · elderly · hypertension · in patients susceptible to angle-closure glaucoma · liable to abuse · prostatic hypertrophy · psychotic disorders · pyrexia
● INTERACTIONS → Appendix 1: orphenadrine

● SIDE-EFFECTS
▸ Common or very common Accommodation disorder · anxiety · dizziness · dry mouth · gastrointestinal disorder · nausea
▸ Uncommon Confusion · constipation · coordination abnormal · euphoric mood · hallucination · insomnia · sedation · seizure · tachycardia · urinary retention
▸ Rare or very rare Memory loss
● PREGNANCY Caution.
● BREAST FEEDING Caution.
● HEPATIC IMPAIRMENT Use with caution.
● RENAL IMPAIRMENT Use with caution.
● TREATMENT CESSATION Avoid abrupt withdrawal in patients taking long-term treatment.
● PATIENT AND CARER ADVICE
Driving and skilled tasks May affect performance of skilled tasks (e.g. driving).

● MEDICINAL FORMS
There can be variation in the licensing of different medicines containing the same drug. Forms available from special-order manufacturers include: oral solution
Oral solution
▸ Orphenadrine hydrochloride (Non-proprietary)
Orphenadrine hydrochloride 10 mg per 1 ml Orphenadrine 50mg/5ml oral solution sugar free sugar-free | 150 ml PoM £37.50 DT = £37.50

Procyclidine hydrochloride

● DRUG ACTION Procyclidine exerts its antiparkinsonian action by reducing the effects of the relative central cholinergic excess that occurs as a result of dopamine deficiency.

● INDICATIONS AND DOSE

Parkinsonism | Extrapyramidal symptoms (but not tardive dyskinesia)
▸ BY MOUTH
▸ Adult: 2.5 mg 3 times a day, then increased in steps of 2.5–5 mg daily if required; increased if necessary up to 30 mg daily in 2–4 divided doses, to be increased at 2–3 day intervals. Maximum daily dose only to be used in exceptional circumstances; maximum 60 mg per day
▸ Elderly: Lower end of range preferable

Acute dystonia
▸ BY INTRAMUSCULAR INJECTION, OR BY INTRAVENOUS INJECTION
▸ Adult: 5–10 mg, occasionally, more than 10 mg, dose usually effective in 5–10 minutes but may need 30 minutes for relief
▸ Elderly: Lower end of range preferable

● CONTRA-INDICATIONS Gastro-intestinal obstruction · myasthenia gravis
● CAUTIONS Cardiovascular disease · elderly · hypertension · liable to abuse · prostatic hypertrophy · psychotic disorders · pyrexia · those susceptible to angle-closure glaucoma
● INTERACTIONS → Appendix 1: procyclidine
● SIDE-EFFECTS
▸ Common or very common Constipation · dry mouth · urinary retention · vision blurred
▸ Uncommon Anxiety · cognitive impairment · confusion · dizziness · gingivitis · hallucination · memory loss · nausea · rash · vomiting
▸ Rare or very rare Psychotic disorder
● PREGNANCY Use only if potential benefit outweighs risk.
● BREAST FEEDING No information available.
● HEPATIC IMPAIRMENT Use with caution.
● RENAL IMPAIRMENT Use with caution.

- TREATMENT CESSATION Avoid abrupt withdrawal in patients taking long-term treatment.
- PATIENT AND CARER ADVICE
Driving and skilled tasks May affect performance of skilled tasks (e.g. driving).

- MEDICINAL FORMS
There can be variation in the licensing of different medicines containing the same drug. Forms available from special-order manufacturers include: oral suspension, oral solution
Solution for injection
▸ Procyclidine hydrochloride (Non-proprietary)
Procyclidine hydrochloride 5 mg per 1 ml Procyclidine 10mg/2ml solution for injection ampoules | 5 ampoule [PoM] £60.00–£78.75 DT = £72.50
Oral solution
▸ Procyclidine hydrochloride (Non-proprietary)
Procyclidine hydrochloride 500 microgram per 1 ml Procyclidine 2.5mg/5ml oral solution sugar free sugar-free | 150 ml [PoM] £8.22–£10.49 DT = £10.49
Procyclidine hydrochloride 1 mg per 1 ml Procyclidine 5mg/5ml oral solution sugar free sugar-free | 150 ml [PoM] £14.54–£18.54 DT = £18.54
Tablet
▸ Procyclidine hydrochloride (Non-proprietary)
Procyclidine hydrochloride 5 mg Procyclidine 5mg tablets | 28 tablet [PoM] £12.65 DT = £5.91 | 100 tablet [PoM] £8.94–£21.11 | 500 tablet [PoM] £44.63–£105.54
▸ Kemadrin (Aspen Pharma Trading Ltd)
Procyclidine hydrochloride 5 mg Kemadrin 5mg tablets | 100 tablet [PoM] £4.72 | 500 tablet [PoM] £23.62

Trihexyphenidyl hydrochloride

(Benzhexol hydrochloride)

- DRUG ACTION Trihexyphenidyl exerts its effects by reducing the effects of the relative central cholinergic excess that occurs as a result of dopamine deficiency.

- INDICATIONS AND DOSE

Parkinson's disease (if used in combination with co-careldopa or co-beneldopa)
▸ BY MOUTH
▸ Adult: Maintenance 2–6 mg daily in divided doses, use not recommended because of toxicity in the elderly and the risk of aggravating dementia
Parkinsonism | Drug-induced extrapyramidal symptoms (but not tardive dyskinesia)
▸ BY MOUTH
▸ Adult: 1 mg daily, then increased in steps of 2 mg every 3–5 days, adjusted according to response; maintenance 5–15 mg daily in 3–4 divided doses, not recommended for use in Parkinson's disease because of toxicity in the elderly and the risk of aggravating dementia; maximum 20 mg per day
▸ Elderly: Lower end of range preferable, not recommended for use in Parkinson's disease because of toxicity in the elderly and the risk of aggravating dementia

- CONTRA-INDICATIONS Gastro-intestinal obstruction · myasthenia gravis
- CAUTIONS Cardiovascular disease · elderly · hypertension · liable to abuse · prostatic hypertrophy · psychotic disorders · pyrexia · those susceptible to angle-closure glaucoma
- INTERACTIONS → Appendix 1: trihexyphenidyl
- SIDE-EFFECTS Anxiety · bronchial secretion decreased · confusion · constipation · delusions · dizziness · dry mouth · dysphagia · euphoric mood · fever · flushing · hallucination · insomnia · memory loss · myasthenia gravis aggravated · mydriasis · nausea · skin reactions · tachycardia · thirst · urinary disorders · vision disorders · vomiting

- PREGNANCY Use only if potential benefit outweighs risk.
- BREAST FEEDING Avoid.
- HEPATIC IMPAIRMENT Use with caution.
- RENAL IMPAIRMENT Use with caution.
- TREATMENT CESSATION Avoid abrupt withdrawal in patients taking long-term treatment.
- DIRECTIONS FOR ADMINISTRATION Tablets should be taken with or after food.
- PATIENT AND CARER ADVICE
Driving and skilled tasks May affect performance of skilled tasks (e.g. driving).

- MEDICINAL FORMS
There can be variation in the licensing of different medicines containing the same drug. Forms available from special-order manufacturers include: oral suspension, oral solution
Oral solution
EXCIPIENTS: May contain Propylene glycol
▸ Trihexyphenidyl hydrochloride (Non-proprietary)
Trihexyphenidyl hydrochloride 1 mg per 1 ml Trihexyphenidyl 5mg/5ml oral solution | 200 ml [PoM] £22.00 DT = £22.00
Tablet
▸ Trihexyphenidyl hydrochloride (Non-proprietary)
Trihexyphenidyl hydrochloride 2 mg Trihexyphenidyl 2mg tablets | 84 tablet [PoM] £4.20 DT = £3.28
Trihexyphenidyl hydrochloride 5 mg Trihexyphenidyl 5mg tablets | 84 tablet [PoM] £17.91 DT = £17.91

DOPAMINERGIC DRUGS > CATECHOL-O-METHYLTRANSFERASE INHIBITORS

Entacapone

- DRUG ACTION Entacapone prevents the peripheral breakdown of levodopa, by inhibiting catechol-*O*-methyltransferase, allowing more levodopa to reach the brain.

- INDICATIONS AND DOSE

Adjunct to co-beneldopa or co-careldopa in Parkinson's disease with 'end-of-dose' motor fluctuations (under expert supervision)
▸ BY MOUTH
▸ Adult: 200 mg, dose to be given with each dose of levodopa with dopa-decarboxylase inhibitor; maximum 2 g per day

- CONTRA-INDICATIONS History of neuroleptic malignant syndrome · history of non-traumatic rhabdomyolysis · phaeochromocytoma
- CAUTIONS Concurrent levodopa dose may need to be reduced by about 10–30% · ischaemic heart disease
- INTERACTIONS → Appendix 1: entacapone
- SIDE-EFFECTS
▸ **Common or very common** Abdominal pain · confusion · constipation · diarrhoea · dizziness · dry mouth · fall · fatigue · hallucination · hyperhidrosis · ischaemic heart disease · movement disorders · nausea · sleep disorders · urine discolouration · vomiting
▸ **Uncommon** Myocardial infarction
▸ **Rare or very rare** Agitation · appetite decreased · skin reactions · weight decreased
▸ **Frequency not known** Colitis · hair colour changes · hepatic disorders · impulse-control disorder · nail discolouration · neuroleptic malignant syndrome · rhabdomyolysis
- PREGNANCY Avoid—no information available.
- BREAST FEEDING Avoid—present in milk in *animal* studies.
- HEPATIC IMPAIRMENT Avoid.
- TREATMENT CESSATION Avoid abrupt withdrawal.

• PATIENT AND CARER ADVICE Patient counselling is advised (may colour urine reddish-brown, concomitant iron containing products).

• MEDICINAL FORMS
There can be variation in the licensing of different medicines containing the same drug. Forms available from special-order manufacturers include: oral suspension, oral solution

Tablet
CAUTIONARY AND ADVISORY LABELS 14
▸ Entacapone (Non-proprietary)
Entacapone 200 mg Entacapone 200mg tablets | 30 tablet [PoM] £16.38 DT = £4.13 | 100 tablet [PoM] £13.77–£54.58
▸ Comtess (Orion Pharma (UK) Ltd)
Entacapone 200 mg Comtess 200mg tablets | 30 tablet [PoM] £17.24 DT = £4.13 | 100 tablet [PoM] £57.45

Combinations available: *Levodopa with carbidopa and entacapone*, p. 412

Opicapone

11-Apr-2017

• DRUG ACTION Opicapone prevents the peripheral breakdown of levodopa, by inhibiting catechol- *O*-methyltransferase, allowing more levodopa to reach the brain.

• INDICATIONS AND DOSE

Adjunct to co-beneldopa or co-careldopa in Parkinson's disease with 'end-of-dose' motor fluctuations (under expert supervision)
▸ BY MOUTH
▸ Adult: 50 mg once daily, dose to be taken at bedtime, at least one hour before or after levodopa combinations

• CONTRA-INDICATIONS Catecholamine-secreting neoplasms · history of neuroleptic malignant syndrome · history of non-traumatic rhabdomyolysis · paraganglioma · phaeochromocytoma

• CAUTIONS Concurrent levodopa dose may need to be reduced · elderly over 85 years (limited information available)

• INTERACTIONS → Appendix 1: opicapone

• SIDE-EFFECTS
▸ Common or very common Constipation · dizziness · drowsiness · dry mouth · hallucinations · headache · hypotension · movement disorders · muscle complaints · sleep disorders · vomiting
▸ Uncommon Anxiety · appetite decreased · depression · dry eye · dyspnoea · ear congestion · gastrointestinal discomfort · hypertension · hypertriglyceridaemia · musculoskeletal stiffness · nocturia · pain in extremity · palpitations · syncope · taste altered · urine discolouration · weight decreased

SIDE-EFFECTS, FURTHER INFORMATION Manufacturer advises consider liver function tests in patients who experience progressive anorexia, asthenia and weight decrease within a relatively short period of time.

• PREGNANCY Manufacturer advises avoid—limited information available.

• BREAST FEEDING Manufacturer advises avoid—no information available.

• HEPATIC IMPAIRMENT Manufacturer advises avoid in severe impairment.
Dose adjustments Manufacturer advises use with caution in moderate impairment—dose adjustment may be necessary.

• MEDICINAL FORMS
There can be variation in the licensing of different medicines containing the same drug.
Capsule
▸ Ongentys (BIAL Pharma UK Ltd) ▼
Opicapone 50 mg Ongentys 50mg capsules | 30 capsule [PoM] £93.90 DT = £93.90

Tolcapone

• DRUG ACTION Tolcapone prevents the peripheral breakdown of levodopa, by inhibiting catechol- *O*-methyltransferase, allowing more levodopa to reach the brain.

• INDICATIONS AND DOSE

Adjunct to co-beneldopa or co-careldopa in Parkinson's disease with 'end-of-dose' motor fluctuations if another inhibitor of peripheral catechol-O-methyltransferase inappropriate (under expert supervision)
▸ BY MOUTH
▸ Adult: 100 mg 3 times a day (max. per dose 200 mg 3 times a day) continuing beyond 3 weeks **only** if substantial improvement, leave 6 hours between each dose; first daily dose should be taken at the same time as levodopa with dopa-decarboxylase inhibitor, dose maximum only in exceptional circumstances

• CONTRA-INDICATIONS Phaeochromocytoma · previous history of hyperthermia · previous history of neuroleptic malignant syndrome · previous history of rhabdomyolysis · severe dyskinesia

• CAUTIONS Most patients receiving more than 600 mg levodopa daily require reduction of levodopa dose by about 30%
CAUTIONS, FURTHER INFORMATION
▸ Hepatotoxicity Potentially life-threatening hepatotoxicity including fulminant hepatitis reported rarely, usually in women and during the first 6 months, but late-onset liver injury also reported; discontinue if abnormal liver function tests or symptoms of liver disorder; do not re-introduce tolcapone once discontinued.

• INTERACTIONS → Appendix 1: tolcapone

• SIDE-EFFECTS
▸ Common or very common Appetite decreased · chest pain · confusion · constipation · diarrhoea · dizziness · drowsiness · dry mouth · gastrointestinal discomfort · hallucination · headache · hyperhidrosis · influenza like illness · movement disorders · nausea · postural hypotension · sleep disorders · syncope · upper respiratory tract infection · urine discolouration · vomiting
▸ Uncommon Hepatocellular injury
▸ Rare or very rare Eating disorders · neuroleptic malignant syndrome (reported on dose reduction or withdrawal) · pathological gambling · psychiatric disorders · sexual dysfunction

• PREGNANCY Toxicity in *animal* studies—use only if potential benefit outweighs risk.

• BREAST FEEDING Avoid—present in milk in *animal* studies.

• HEPATIC IMPAIRMENT Avoid.

• RENAL IMPAIRMENT Caution if eGFR less than 30 mL/minute/1.73 m^2.

• MONITORING REQUIREMENTS Test liver function before treatment, and monitor every 2 weeks for first year, every 4 weeks for next 6 months and then every 8 weeks thereafter (restart monitoring schedule if dose increased).

• TREATMENT CESSATION Avoid abrupt withdrawal.

• PATIENT AND CARER ADVICE Patients should be told how to recognise signs of liver disorder and advised to seek immediate medical attention if symptoms such as anorexia, nausea, vomiting, fatigue, abdominal pain, dark urine, or pruritus develop.

● MEDICINAL FORMS
There can be variation in the licensing of different medicines containing the same drug.

Tablet
CAUTIONARY AND ADVISORY LABELS 14, 25
▸ Tasmar (Meda Pharmaceuticals Ltd)
  Tolcapone 100 mg Tasmar 100mg tablets | 100 tablet [PoM] £95.20

DOPAMINERGIC DRUGS ❭ DOPAMINE PRECURSORS

Co-beneldopa

● INDICATIONS AND DOSE

Parkinson's disease
▸ BY MOUTH USING IMMEDIATE-RELEASE MEDICINES
▸ Adult: Initially 50 mg 3–4 times a day, then increased in steps of 100 mg daily, dose to be increased once or twice weekly according to response; maintenance 400–800 mg daily in divided doses
▸ Elderly: Initially 50 mg 1–2 times a day, then increased in steps of 50 mg daily, dose to be increased every 3–4 days according to response

Parkinson's disease (in advanced disease)
▸ BY MOUTH USING IMMEDIATE-RELEASE MEDICINES
▸ Adult: Initially 100 mg 3 times a day, then increased in steps of 100 mg daily, dose to be increased once or twice weekly according to response; maintenance 400–800 mg daily in divided doses

Parkinson's disease (patients not taking levodopa/dopa-decarboxylase inhibitor therapy)
▸ BY MOUTH USING MODIFIED-RELEASE MEDICINES
▸ Adult: Initially 1 capsule 3 times a day; maximum 6 capsules per day

Parkinson's disease (patients transferring from immediate-release levodopa/dopa-decarboxylase inhibitor preparations)
▸ BY MOUTH USING MODIFIED-RELEASE MEDICINES
▸ Adult: Initially 1 capsule substituted for every 100 mg of levodopa and given at same dosage frequency, increased every 2–3 days according to response; average increase of 50% needed over previous levodopa dose and titration may take up to 4 weeks; supplementary dose of immediate-release *Madopar*® may be needed with first morning dose; if response still poor to total daily dose of *Madopar*® CR plus *Madopar*® corresponding to 1.2 g levodopa—consider alternative therapy.

DOSE EQUIVALENCE AND CONVERSION
▸ Dose is expressed as levodopa.

IMPORTANT SAFETY INFORMATION
IMPULSE CONTROL DISORDERS
Treatment with levodopa is associated with impulse control disorders, including pathological gambling, binge eating, and hypersexuality. Patients and their carers should be informed about the risk of impulse control disorders. If the patient develops an impulse control disorder, levodopa should be withdrawn or the dose reduced until the symptoms resolve.

● CAUTIONS Cushing's syndrome · diabetes mellitus · endocrine disorders · history of convulsions · history of myocardial infarction with residual arrhythmia · history of peptic ulcer · hyperthyroidism · osteomalacia · phaeochromocytoma · psychiatric illness (avoid if severe and discontinue if deterioration) · severe cardiovascular

disease · severe pulmonary disease · susceptibility to angle-closure glaucoma

● INTERACTIONS → Appendix 1: levodopa

● SIDE-EFFECTS
▸ **Common or very common** Anxiety · appetite decreased · arrhythmia · depression · diarrhoea · hallucination · movement disorders · nausea · parkinsonism · postural hypotension · sleep disorders · taste altered · vomiting
▸ **Rare or very rare** Leucopenia
▸ **Frequency not known** Aggression · confusion · delusions · drowsiness · eating disorders · euphoric mood · flushing · gastrointestinal haemorrhage · haemolytic anaemia · hyperhidrosis · oral disorders · pathological gambling · psychiatric disorders · psychosis · sexual dysfunction · skin reactions · thrombocytopenia · urine discolouration

● PREGNANCY Caution in pregnancy—toxicity has occurred in *animal* studies.

● BREAST FEEDING May suppress lactation; present in milk—avoid.

● HEPATIC IMPAIRMENT Use with caution.

● RENAL IMPAIRMENT Use with caution.

● EFFECT ON LABORATORY TESTS False positive tests for urinary ketones have been reported.

● TREATMENT CESSATION Avoid abrupt withdrawal (risk of neuroleptic malignant syndrome and rhabdomyolysis).

● DIRECTIONS FOR ADMINISTRATION The dispersible tablets can be dispersed in water or orange squash (not orange juice) or swallowed whole.

● PRESCRIBING AND DISPENSING INFORMATION Co-beneldopa is a mixture of benserazide hydrochloride and levodopa in mass proportions corresponding to 1 part of benserazide and 4 parts of levodopa.
  When transferring patients from another levodopa/dopa-decarboxylase inhibitor preparation, the previous preparation should be discontinued 12 hours before (although interval can be shorter).
  When switching from modified-release levodopa to dispersible co-beneldopa, reduce dose by approximately 30%.
  When administered as an adjunct to other antiparkinsonian drugs, once therapeutic effect apparent, the other drugs may be reduced or withdrawn.

● PATIENT AND CARER ADVICE Patients or carers should be given advice on how to administer co-beneldopa dispersible tablets.
Driving and skilled tasks
Sudden onset of sleep Excessive daytime sleepiness and sudden onset of sleep can occur with co-beneldopa.
  Patients starting treatment with these drugs should be warned of the risk and of the need to exercise caution when driving or operating machinery. Those who have experienced excessive sedation or sudden onset of sleep should refrain from driving or operating machines until these effects have stopped occurring.
  Management of excessive daytime sleepiness should focus on the identification of an underlying cause, such as depression or concomitant medication. Patients should be counselled on improving sleep behaviour.

● MEDICINAL FORMS
There can be variation in the licensing of different medicines containing the same drug. Forms available from special-order manufacturers include: oral suspension, oral solution
Dispersible tablet
CAUTIONARY AND ADVISORY LABELS 10, 14, 21
▸ Madopar (Roche Products Ltd)
  Benserazide (as Benserazide hydrochloride) 12.5 mg, Levodopa 50 mg Madopar 50mg/12.5mg dispersible tablets sugar-free | 100 tablet [PoM] £5.90 DT = £5.90

Benserazide (as Benserazide hydrochloride) 25 mg, Levodopa 100 mg Madopar 100mg/25mg dispersible tablets sugar-free | 100 tablet [PoM] £10.45 DT = £10.45

Modified-release capsule

CAUTIONARY AND ADVISORY LABELS 5, 10, 14, 25

▶ Madopar CR (Roche Products Ltd)

Benserazide (as Benserazide hydrochloride) 25 mg, Levodopa 100 mg Madopar CR capsules | 100 capsule [PoM] £12.77 DT = £12.77

Capsule

CAUTIONARY AND ADVISORY LABELS 10, 14, 21

▶ Co-beneldopa (Non-proprietary)

Benserazide (as Benserazide hydrochloride) 12.5 mg, Levodopa 50 mg Co-beneldopa 12.5mg/50mg capsules | 100 capsule [PoM] £4.71–£4.96 DT = £4.96

Benserazide (as Benserazide hydrochloride) 25 mg, Levodopa 100 mg Co-beneldopa 25mg/100mg capsules | 100 capsule [PoM] £6.56–£6.91 DT = £6.91

Benserazide (as Benserazide hydrochloride) 50 mg, Levodopa 200 mg Co-beneldopa 50mg/200mg capsules | 100 capsule [PoM] £11.19–£11.78 DT = £11.78

▶ Madopar (Roche Products Ltd)

Benserazide (as Benserazide hydrochloride) 12.5 mg, Levodopa 50 mg Madopar 50mg/12.5mg capsules | 100 capsule [PoM] £4.96 DT = £4.96

Benserazide (as Benserazide hydrochloride) 25 mg, Levodopa 100 mg Madopar 100mg/25mg capsules | 100 capsule [PoM] £6.91 DT = £6.91

Benserazide (as Benserazide hydrochloride) 50 mg, Levodopa 200 mg Madopar 200mg/50mg capsules | 100 capsule [PoM] £11.78 DT = £11.78

Co-careldopa

01-May-2018

● INDICATIONS AND DOSE

Parkinson's disease

▶ BY MOUTH

▶ Adult: Initially 25/100 mg 3 times a day, then increased in steps of 12.5/50 mg once or alternate days, alternatively increased in steps of 25/100 mg once daily or on alternate days, dose to be adjusted according to response; dose increased until 800 mg levodopa (with 200 mg carbidopa) daily in divided doses is reached, then maintenance up to 200/2000 mg daily in divided doses, adjusted according to response, when co-careldopa is used, the total daily dose of carbidopa should be at least 70 mg. A lower dose may not achieve full inhibition of extracerebral dopa-decarboxylase, with a resultant increase in side-effects

Parkinson's disease—alternative regimen

▶ BY MOUTH

▶ Adult: Initially 12.5/50 mg 3–4 times a day, alternatively initially 10/100 mg 3–4 times a day, then increased in steps of 12.5/50 mg once daily or on alternate days, adjusted according to response, alternatively increased in steps of 10/100 mg once daily or on alternate days, adjusted according to response, dose increased until 800 mg levodopa (with up to 200 mg carbidopa) daily in divided doses is reached, then maintenance up to 200/2000 mg daily in divided doses, adjusted according to response, when co-careldopa is used, the total daily dose of carbidopa should be at least 70 mg. A lower dose may not achieve full inhibition of extracerebral dopa-decarboxylase, with a resultant increase in side-effects

DOSE EQUIVALENCE AND CONVERSION

▶ The proportions are expressed in the form x/y where x and y are the strengths in milligrams of carbidopa and levodopa respectively.

▶ 2 tablets *Sinemet* ® 12.5 mg/50 mg is equivalent to 1 tablet *Sinemet* ® Plus 25 mg/100 mg.

CARAMET ® CR

Parkinson's disease (patients not receiving levodopa/dopa-decarboxylase inhibitor preparations, expressed as levodopa)

▶ BY MOUTH USING MODIFIED-RELEASE TABLETS

▶ Adult: Initially 100–200 mg twice daily, dose to be given at least 6 hours apart; dose adjusted according to response at intervals of at least 2 days

Parkinson's disease (patients transferring from immediate-release levodopa/dopa-decarboxylase inhibitor preparations)

▶ BY MOUTH USING MODIFIED-RELEASE TABLETS

▶ Adult: Discontinue previous preparation at least 12 hours before first dose of *Caramet* ® CR; substitute *Caramet* ® CR to provide a similar amount of levodopa daily and extend dosing interval by 30–50%; dose then adjusted according to response at intervals of at least 2 days.

DUODOPA ®

Severe Parkinson's disease inadequately controlled by other preparations

▶ Adult: Administered as intestinal gel, for use with enteral tube (consult product literature)

HALF SINEMET ® CR

Parkinson's disease (for fine adjustment of Sinemet ® CR dose)

▶ BY MOUTH

▶ Adult: (consult product literature)

SINEMET ® CR

Parkinson's disease (patients not receiving levodopa/dopa-decarboxylase inhibitor therapy)

▶ BY MOUTH

▶ Adult: Initially 1 tablet twice daily, both dose and interval then adjusted according to response at intervals of not less than 3 days

Parkinson's disease (patients transferring from immediate-release levodopa/dopa-decarboxylase inhibitor preparations)

▶ BY MOUTH

▶ Adult: 1 tablet twice daily, dose can be substituted for a daily dose of levodopa 300–400 mg in immediate-release *Sinemet* ® tablets (substitute *Sinemet* ® CR to provide approximately 10% more levodopa per day and extend dosing interval by 30–50%); dose and interval then adjusted according to response at intervals of not less than 3 days.

IMPORTANT SAFETY INFORMATION

IMPULSE CONTROL DISORDERS

Treatment with levodopa is associated with impulse control disorders, including pathological gambling, binge eating, and hypersexuality. Patients and their carers should be informed about the risk of impulse control disorders. If the patient develops an impulse control disorder, levodopa should be withdrawn or the dose reduced until the symptoms resolve.

● CAUTIONS Cushing's syndrome · diabetes mellitus · endocrine disorders · history of convulsions · history of myocardial infarction with residual arrhythmia · history of peptic ulcer · hyperthyroidism · osteomalacia · phaeochromocytoma · psychiatric illness (avoid if severe and discontinue if deterioration) · severe cardiovascular disease · severe pulmonary disease · susceptibility to angle-closure glaucoma

● INTERACTIONS →Appendix 1: carbidopa · levodopa

● SIDE-EFFECTS

▶ Rare or very rare Drowsiness · seizure · sleep disorders

▶ **Frequency not known** Agranulocytosis · alertness decreased · alopecia · anaemia · angioedema · anxiety · appetite decreased · asthenia · cardiac disorder · chest pain · compulsions · confusion · constipation · delusions · dementia · depression · diarrhoea · dizziness · dry mouth · dyskinesia · dysphagia · dyspnoea · eating disorders · euphoric mood · eye disorders · fall · focal tremor · gait abnormal · gastrointestinal discomfort · gastrointestinal disorders · gastrointestinal haemorrhage · haemolytic anaemia · hallucination · headache · Henoch-Schönlein purpura · hiccups · hoarseness · Horner's syndrome exacerbated · hypertension · hypotension · leucopenia · malaise · malignant melanoma · movement disorders · muscle complaints · nausea · neuroleptic malignant syndrome (on abrupt discontinuation) · oedema · on and off phenomenon · oral disorders · palpitations · pathological gambling · postural disorders · psychotic disorder · respiration abnormal · sensation abnormal · sexual dysfunction · skin reactions · suicidal ideation · sweat changes · syncope · taste bitter · teeth grinding · thrombocytopenia · trismus · urinary disorders · urine dark · vasodilation · vision disorders · vomiting · weight changes

● PREGNANCY Use with caution—toxicity has occurred in *animal* studies.

● BREAST FEEDING May suppress lactation; present in milk—avoid.

● HEPATIC IMPAIRMENT Use with caution.

● RENAL IMPAIRMENT Use with caution.

● EFFECT ON LABORATORY TESTS False positive tests for urinary ketones have been reported.

● TREATMENT CESSATION Avoid abrupt withdrawal (risk of neuroleptic malignant syndrome and rhabdomyolysis).

● PRESCRIBING AND DISPENSING INFORMATION Co-careldopa is a mixture of carbidopa and levodopa; the proportions are expressed in the form x/y where x and y are the strengths in milligrams of carbidopa and levodopa respectively.

When transferring patients from another levodopa/dopa-decarboxylase inhibitor preparation, the previous preparation should be discontinued at least 12 hours before.

Co-careldopa 25/100 provides an adequate dose of carbidopa when low doses of levodopa are needed.

● PATIENT AND CARER ADVICE
Driving and skilled tasks
Sudden onset of sleep Excessive daytime sleepiness and sudden onset of sleep can occur with co-careldopa.

Patients starting treatment with these drugs should be warned of the risk and of the need to exercise caution when driving or operating machinery. Those who have experienced excessive sedation or sudden onset of sleep should refrain from driving or operating machines until these effects have stopped occurring.

Management of excessive daytime sleepiness should focus on the identification of an underlying cause, such as depression or concomitant medication. Patients should be counselled on improving sleep behaviour.

● NATIONAL FUNDING/ACCESS DECISIONS
DUODOPA ®

Scottish Medicines Consortium (SMC) Decisions
SMC No. 316/06
The *Scottish Medicines Consortium* has advised (June 2016) that co-careldopa (*Duodopa®*) intestinal gel is accepted for restricted use within NHS Scotland, for the treatment of advanced levodopa-responsive Parkinson's disease with severe motor fluctuations and hyper-/dyskinesia when available combinations of Parkinson medicinal products have not given satisfactory results, only in patients not eligible for deep brain stimulation. This advice is contingent upon the continuing availability of the Patient Access Scheme in NHS Scotland or a list price that is equivalent or lower.

All Wales Medicines Strategy Group (AWMSG) Decisions
AWMSG No. 3397
The *All Wales Medicines Strategy Group* has advised (March 2018) that *Duodopa®* intestinal gel is recommended as an option for restricted use within NHS Wales, for the treatment of advanced levodopa-responsive Parkinson's disease with severe motor fluctuations and hyper-/dyskinesia when available combinations of Parkinson medicinal products have not given satisfactory results, only in patients not eligible for deep brain stimulation. This recommendation applies only in circumstances where the approved Wales Patient Access Scheme (WPAS) is utilised or where the list/contract price is equivalent or lower than the WPAS price.

● MEDICINAL FORMS
There can be variation in the licensing of different medicines containing the same drug. Forms available from special-order manufacturers include: oral suspension, oral solution

Modified-release tablet
CAUTIONARY AND ADVISORY LABELS 10, 14, 25
▶ Co-careldopa (Non-proprietary)
Carbidopa (as Carbidopa monohydrate) 25 mg, Levodopa 100 mg Co-careldopa 25mg/100mg modified-release tablets | 60 tablet [PoM] 🚫 DT = £11.60
Carbidopa (as Carbidopa monohydrate) 50 mg, Levodopa 200 mg Co-careldopa 50mg/200mg modified-release tablets | 60 tablet [PoM] 🚫 DT = £11.60
▶ Caramet CR (Teva UK Ltd)
Carbidopa (as Carbidopa monohydrate) 25 mg, Levodopa 100 mg Caramet 25mg/100mg CR tablets | 60 tablet [PoM] £11.47 DT = £11.60
Carbidopa (as Carbidopa monohydrate) 50 mg, Levodopa 200 mg Caramet 50mg/200mg CR tablets | 60 tablet [PoM] £11.47 DT = £11.60
▶ Half Sinemet CR (Merck Sharp & Dohme Ltd)
Carbidopa (as Carbidopa monohydrate) 25 mg, Levodopa 100 mg Half Sinemet CR 25mg/100mg tablets | 60 tablet [PoM] £11.60 DT = £11.60
▶ Sinemet CR (Merck Sharp & Dohme Ltd)
Carbidopa (as Carbidopa monohydrate) 50 mg, Levodopa 200 mg Sinemet CR 50mg/200mg tablets | 60 tablet [PoM] £11.60 DT = £11.60

Tablet
CAUTIONARY AND ADVISORY LABELS 10, 14
▶ Co-careldopa (Non-proprietary)
Carbidopa (as Carbidopa monohydrate) 12.5 mg, Levodopa 50 mg Co-careldopa 12.5mg/50mg tablets | 90 tablet [PoM] £6.28 DT = £6.28
Carbidopa (as Carbidopa monohydrate) 10 mg, Levodopa 100 mg Co-careldopa 10mg/100mg tablets | 100 tablet [PoM] £10.74 DT = £8.95
Carbidopa (as Carbidopa monohydrate) 25 mg, Levodopa 100 mg Co-careldopa 25mg/100mg tablets | 90 tablet [PoM] £8.14 | 100 tablet [PoM] £26.99 DT = £9.04
Carbidopa (as Carbidopa monohydrate) 25 mg, Levodopa 250 mg Co-careldopa 25mg/250mg tablets | 100 tablet [PoM] £35.00 DT = £34.98
▶ Sinemet 110 (Merck Sharp & Dohme Ltd)
Carbidopa (as Carbidopa monohydrate) 10 mg, Levodopa 100 mg Sinemet 10mg/100mg tablets | 100 tablet [PoM] £7.30 DT = £8.95
▶ Sinemet 275 (Merck Sharp & Dohme Ltd)
Carbidopa (as Carbidopa monohydrate) 25 mg, Levodopa 250 mg Sinemet 25mg/250mg tablets | 100 tablet [PoM] £18.29 DT = £34.98
▶ Sinemet 62.5 (Merck Sharp & Dohme Ltd)
Carbidopa (as Carbidopa monohydrate) 12.5 mg, Levodopa 50 mg Sinemet 12.5mg/50mg tablets | 90 tablet [PoM] £6.28 DT = £6.28
▶ Sinemet Plus (Merck Sharp & Dohme Ltd)
Carbidopa (as Carbidopa monohydrate) 25 mg, Levodopa 100 mg Sinemet Plus 25mg/100mg tablets | 100 tablet [PoM] £12.88 DT = £9.04

4

Nervous system

Gel

CAUTIONARY AND ADVISORY LABELS 10, 14

▸ Duodopa (AbbVie Ltd)

Carbidopa (as Carbidopa monohydrate) 5 mg per 1 ml, Levodopa 20 mg per 1 ml Duodopa intestinal gel 100ml cassette | 1 bag [PoM] £77.00

Levodopa with carbidopa and entacapone

The properties listed below are those particular to the combination only. For the properties of the components please consider, co-careldopa p. 410, entacapone p. 407.

● INDICATIONS AND DOSE

STALEVO ® 100/25/200

Parkinson's disease and end-of-dose motor fluctuations not adequately controlled with levodopa and dopa-decarboxylase inhibitor treatment

▸ BY MOUTH

▸ Adult: 1 tablet for each dose; maximum 10 tablets per day

STALEVO ® 125/31.25/200

Parkinson's disease and end-of-dose motor fluctuations not adequately controlled with levodopa and dopa-decarboxylase inhibitor treatment

▸ BY MOUTH

▸ Adult: 1 tablet for each dose; maximum 10 tablets per day

STALEVO ® 150/37.5/200

Parkinson's disease and end-of-dose motor fluctuations not adequately controlled with levodopa and dopa-decarboxylase inhibitor treatment

▸ BY MOUTH

▸ Adult: 1 tablet for each dose; maximum 10 tablets per day

STALEVO ® 175/43.75/200

Parkinson's disease and end-of-dose motor fluctuations not adequately controlled with levodopa and dopa-decarboxylase inhibitor treatment

▸ BY MOUTH

▸ Adult: 1 tablet for each dose; maximum 8 tablets per day

STALEVO ® 200/50/200

Parkinson's disease and end-of-dose motor fluctuations not adequately controlled with levodopa and dopa-decarboxylase inhibitor treatment

▸ BY MOUTH

▸ Adult: 1 tablet for each dose; maximum 7 tablets per day

STALEVO ® 50/12.5/200

Parkinson's disease and end-of-dose motor fluctuations not adequately controlled with levodopa and dopa-decarboxylase inhibitor treatment

▸ BY MOUTH

▸ Adult: 1 tablet for each dose; maximum 10 tablets per day

STALEVO ® 75/18.75/200

Parkinson's disease and end-of-dose motor fluctuations not adequately controlled with levodopa and dopa-decarboxylase inhibitor treatment

▸ BY MOUTH

▸ Adult: 1 tablet for each dose; maximum 10 tablets per day

● INTERACTIONS → Appendix 1: carbidopa · entacapone · levodopa

● PRESCRIBING AND DISPENSING INFORMATION Patients receiving standard-release co-careldopa or co-beneldopa alone, initiate *Stalevo* ® at a dose that provides similar (or slightly lower) amount of levodopa.

Patients with dyskinesia or receiving more than 800 mg levodopa daily, introduce entacapone before transferring to *Stalevo* ® (levodopa dose may need to be reduced by 10–30% initially).

Patients receiving entacapone and standard-release co-careldopa or co-beneldopa, initiate *Stalevo* ® at a dose that provides similar (or slightly higher) amount of levodopa.

● PATIENT AND CARER ADVICE

Driving and skilled tasks

Sudden onset of sleep Excessive daytime sleepiness and sudden onset of sleep can occur with carbidopa with entacapone and levodopa.

Patients starting treatment with these drugs should be warned of the risk and of the need to exercise caution when driving or operating machinery. Those who have experienced excessive sedation or sudden onset of sleep should refrain from driving or operating machines until these effects have stopped occurring.

Management of excessive daytime sleepiness should focus on the identification of an underlying cause, such as depression or concomitant medication. Patients should be counselled on improving sleep behaviour.

● MEDICINAL FORMS

There can be variation in the licensing of different medicines containing the same drug.

Tablet

CAUTIONARY AND ADVISORY LABELS 10, 14(urine reddish-brown), 25

▸ Stalevo (Orion Pharma (UK) Ltd)

Carbidopa 25 mg, Levodopa 100 mg, Entacapone 200 mg Stalevo 100mg/25mg/200mg tablets | 30 tablet [PoM] £20.79 DT = £20.79 | 100 tablet [PoM] £69.31 DT = £69.31

Carbidopa 18.75 mg, Levodopa 75 mg, Entacapone 200 mg Stalevo 75mg/18.75mg/200mg tablets | 30 tablet [PoM] £20.79 DT = £20.79 | 100 tablet [PoM] £69.31 DT = £69.31

Carbidopa 37.5 mg, Levodopa 150 mg, Entacapone 200 mg Stalevo 150mg/37.5mg/200mg tablets | 30 tablet [PoM] £20.79 DT = £20.79 | 100 tablet [PoM] £69.31 DT = £69.31

Carbidopa 12.5 mg, Levodopa 50 mg, Entacapone 200 mg Stalevo 50mg/12.5mg/200mg tablets | 30 tablet [PoM] £20.79 DT = £20.79 | 100 tablet [PoM] £69.31 DT = £69.31

Carbidopa 31.25 mg, Levodopa 125 mg, Entacapone 200 mg Stalevo 125mg/31.25mg/200mg tablets | 30 tablet [PoM] £20.79 DT = £20.79 | 100 tablet [PoM] £69.31 DT = £69.31

Carbidopa 43.75 mg, Levodopa 175 mg, Entacapone 200 mg Stalevo 175mg/43.75mg/200mg tablets | 30 tablet [PoM] £20.79 DT = £20.79 | 100 tablet [PoM] £69.31 DT = £69.31

Carbidopa 50 mg, Entacapone 200 mg, Levodopa 200 mg Stalevo 200mg/50mg/200mg tablets | 30 tablet [PoM] £20.79 DT = £20.79 | 100 tablet [PoM] £69.31 DT = £69.31

DOPAMINERGIC DRUGS > DOPAMINE RECEPTOR AGONISTS

Amantadine hydrochloride

● DRUG ACTION Amantadine is a weak dopamine agonist with modest antiparkinsonian effects.

● INDICATIONS AND DOSE

Parkinson's disease

▸ BY MOUTH

▸ Adult: 100 mg daily for 1 week, then increased to 100 mg twice daily, usually administered in conjunction with other treatment. Some patients may require higher doses; maximum 400 mg per day

▸ Elderly: 100 mg daily, adjusted according to response

Post-herpetic neuralgia
▸ BY MOUTH
▸ Adult: 100 mg twice daily for 14 days (continued for another 14 days if necessary)

Treatment of influenza A (but not recommended)
▸ BY MOUTH
▸ Adult: 100 mg daily 4–5 days

Prophylaxis of influenza A (but not recommended)
▸ BY MOUTH
▸ Adult: 100 mg daily usually for 6 weeks or with influenza vaccination for 2–3 weeks after vaccination

● CONTRA-INDICATIONS Epilepsy · history of gastric ulceration
● CAUTIONS Confused or hallucinatory states · congestive heart disease (may exacerbate oedema) · elderly · tolerance to the effects of amantadine may develop in Parkinson's disease
● INTERACTIONS → Appendix 1: dopamine receptor agonists
● SIDE-EFFECTS
▸ Common or very common Anxiety · appetite decreased · concentration impaired · confusion · constipation · depression · dizziness · dry mouth · hallucination · headache · hyperhidrosis · lethargy · mood altered · movement disorders · myalgia · nausea · palpitations · peripheral oedema · postural hypotension · skin reactions · sleep disorders · speech slurred · vision disorders · vomiting
▸ Uncommon Neuroleptic malignant-like syndrome · psychosis · seizure · tremor
▸ Rare or very rare Cardiovascular insufficiency · diarrhoea · eye disorders · eye inflammation · heart failure · leucopenia · photosensitivity reaction · urinary disorders
▸ Frequency not known Delirium
● PREGNANCY Avoid; toxicity in *animal* studies.
● BREAST FEEDING Avoid; present in milk; toxicity in infant reported.
● HEPATIC IMPAIRMENT Use with caution.
● RENAL IMPAIRMENT Avoid if eGFR less than 15 mL/minute/1.73 m^2.
  Dose adjustments Reduce dose.
● TREATMENT CESSATION Avoid abrupt withdrawal in Parkinson's disease.
● PATIENT AND CARER ADVICE
  Driving and skilled tasks May affect performance of skilled tasks (e.g. driving).
● NATIONAL FUNDING/ACCESS DECISIONS
  NICE decisions
▸ **Oseltamivir, zanamivir, and amantadine for prophylaxis of influenza (September 2008)** NICE TA158
  Amantadine is **not** recommended for prophylaxis of influenza.
  www.nice.org.uk/TA158
▸ **Oseltamivir, zanamivir, and amantadine for treatment of influenza (February 2009)** NICE TA168
  Amantadine is **not** recommended for treatment of influenza.
  www.nice.org.uk/TA168

● MEDICINAL FORMS
  There can be variation in the licensing of different medicines containing the same drug. Forms available from special-order manufacturers include: tablet
  Oral solution
▸ Amantadine hydrochloride (Non-proprietary)
  Amantadine hydrochloride 10 mg per 1 ml Amantadine 50mg/5ml oral solution sugar free sugar-free | 150 ml PoM £118.00-£140.00 DT = £129.54

Capsule
▸ Amantadine hydrochloride (Non-proprietary)
  Amantadine hydrochloride 100 mg Amantadine 100mg capsules | 14 capsule PoM £10.00-£10.25 | 56 capsule PoM £40.98-£41.00 DT = £40.95

Apomorphine hydrochloride

● INDICATIONS AND DOSE

Refractory motor fluctuations in Parkinson's disease ('off' episodes) inadequately controlled by co-beneldopa or co-careldopa or other dopaminergics (for capable and motivated patients) (under expert supervision)
▸ BY SUBCUTANEOUS INJECTION
▸ Adult: Initially 1 mg, dose to be administered at the first sign of 'off' episode, then 2 mg after 30 minutes, dose to be given if inadequate or no response following initial dose, thereafter increase dose at minimum 40-minute intervals until satisfactory response obtained, this determines threshold dose; usual dose 3–30 mg daily in divided doses (max. per dose 10 mg), subcutaneous infusion may be preferable in those requiring division of injections into more than 10 doses; maximum 100 mg per day

Refractory motor fluctuations in Parkinson's disease ('off' episodes) inadequately controlled by co-beneldopa or co-careldopa or other dopaminergics (in patients requiring division into more than 10 injections daily) (under expert supervision)
▸ BY CONTINUOUS SUBCUTANEOUS INFUSION
▸ Adult: Initially 1 mg/hour, adjusted according to response, then increased in steps of up to 500 micrograms/hour, dose to be increased at intervals not more often than every 4 hours; usual dose 1–4 mg/hour, alternatively usual dose 15–60 micrograms/kg/hour, change infusion site every 12 hours and give during waking hours only (tolerance may occur unless there is a 4-hour treatment-free period at night—24-hour infusions not recommended unless severe night time symptoms); intermittent bolus doses may be needed; maximum 100 mg per day

---

IMPORTANT SAFETY INFORMATION
IMPULSE CONTROL DISORDERS
Treatment with dopamine-receptor agonists are associated with impulse control disorders, including pathological gambling, binge eating, and hypersexuality. Patients and their carers should be informed about the risk of impulse control disorders. There is no evidence that ergot- and non-ergot-derived dopamine-receptor agonists differ in their propensity to cause impulse control disorders, so switching between dopamine-receptor agonists to control these side-effects is not recommended. If the patient develops an impulse control disorder, the dopamine-receptor agonist or levodopa should be withdrawn or the dose reduced until the symptoms resolve.

● CONTRA-INDICATIONS Avoid if 'on' response to levodopa marred by severe dyskinesia or dystonia · dementia · psychosis · respiratory depression
● CAUTIONS Cardiovascular disease · history of postural hypotension (special care on initiation) · neuropsychiatric conditions · pulmonary disease · susceptibility to QT-interval prolongation
● INTERACTIONS → Appendix 1: dopamine receptor agonists
● SIDE-EFFECTS
▸ Common or very common Confusion · dizziness · drowsiness · hallucinations · nausea · psychiatric disorders · vomiting · yawning

4

Nervous system

▶ **Uncommon** Dyskinesia (may require discontinuation) · dyspnoea · haemolytic anaemia · postural hypotension · skin reactions · sudden onset of sleep · thrombocytopenia
▶ **Rare or very rare** Bronchospasm · eosinophilia · hypersensitivity
▶ **Frequency not known** Aggression · agitation · eating disorders · pathological gambling · peripheral oedema · sexual dysfunction · syncope

● ALLERGY AND CROSS-SENSITIVITY Contra-indicated if history of hypersensitivity to opioids.
● PREGNANCY Avoid unless clearly necessary.
● BREAST FEEDING No information available; may suppress lactation.
● HEPATIC IMPAIRMENT Avoid.
● RENAL IMPAIRMENT Use with caution.
● MONITORING REQUIREMENTS
▶ Monitor hepatic, haemopoietic, renal, and cardiovascular function.
▶ *With concomitant levodopa* test initially and every 6 months for haemolytic anaemia and thrombocytopenia (development calls for specialist haematological care with dose reduction and possible discontinuation).
● TREATMENT CESSATION Antiparkinsonian drug therapy should never be stopped abruptly as this carries a small risk of neuroleptic malignant syndrome.
● PATIENT AND CARER ADVICE
Driving and skilled tasks
Sudden onset of sleep Excessive daytime sleepiness and sudden onset of sleep can occur with dopamine-receptor agonists.

Patients starting treatment with these drugs should be warned of the risk and of the need to exercise caution when driving or operating machinery. Those who have experienced excessive sedation or sudden onset of sleep should refrain from driving or operating machines until these effects have stopped occurring.

Management of excessive daytime sleepiness should focus on the identification of an underlying cause, such as depression or concomitant medication. Patients should be counselled on improving sleep behaviour.
Drugs and driving Prescribers and other healthcare professionals should advise patients if treatment is likely to affect their ability to perform skilled tasks (e.g. driving). This applies especially to drugs with sedative effects; patients should be warned that these effects are increased by alcohol. General information about a patient's fitness to drive is available from the Driver and Vehicle Licensing Agency at www.dvla.gov.uk.

2015 legislation regarding driving whilst taking certain drugs, may also apply to apomorphine, see *Drugs and driving* under Guidance on prescribing p. 1.
Hypotensive reactions Hypotensive reactions can occur in some patients taking dopamine-receptor agonists; these can be particularly problematic during the first few days of treatment and care should be exercised when driving or operating machinery.

● MEDICINAL FORMS
There can be variation in the licensing of different medicines containing the same drug. Forms available from special-order manufacturers include: solution for injection, solution for infusion
Solution for injection
CAUTIONARY AND ADVISORY LABELS 10
EXCIPIENTS: May contain Sulfites
▶ APO-go (Britannia Pharmaceuticals Ltd)
Apomorphine hydrochloride 10 mg per 1 ml APO-go 50mg/5ml solution for injection ampoules | 5 ampoule [PoM] £73.11 DT = £73.11
▶ APO-go Pen (Britannia Pharmaceuticals Ltd)
Apomorphine hydrochloride 10 mg per 1 ml APO-go PEN 30mg/3ml solution for injection | 5 pre-filled disposable injection [PoM] £123.91 DT = £123.91

Solution for infusion
CAUTIONARY AND ADVISORY LABELS 10
EXCIPIENTS: May contain Sulfites
▶ APO-go PFS (Britannia Pharmaceuticals Ltd)
Apomorphine hydrochloride 5 mg per 1 ml APO-go PFS 50mg/10ml solution for infusion pre-filled syringes | 5 pre-filled disposable injection [PoM] £73.11 DT = £73.11

Bromocriptine

● DRUG ACTION Bromocriptine is a stimulant of dopamine receptors in the brain; it also inhibits release of prolactin by the pituitary.

● INDICATIONS AND DOSE
Prevention of lactation
▶ BY MOUTH
▶ **Adult:** Initially 2.5 mg daily for 1 day, then 2.5 mg twice daily for 14 days
Suppression of lactation
▶ BY MOUTH
▶ **Adult:** Initially 2.5 mg daily for 2–3 days, then 2.5 mg twice daily for 14 days
Hypogonadism | Galactorrhoea | Infertility
▶ BY MOUTH
▶ **Adult:** Initially 1–1.25 mg daily, dose to be taken at bedtime, increase dose gradually; usual dose 7.5 mg daily in divided doses, increased if necessary up to 30 mg daily, usual dose in infertility without hyperprolactinaemia is 2.5 mg twice daily
Acromegaly
▶ BY MOUTH
▶ **Adult:** Initially 1–1.25 mg daily, dose to be taken at bedtime, then increased to 5 mg every 6 hours, increase dose gradually
Prolactinoma
▶ BY MOUTH
▶ **Adult:** Initially 1–1.25 mg daily, dose to be taken at bedtime, then increased to 5 mg every 6 hours, increase dose gradually. Occasionally patients may require up to 30 mg daily
Parkinson's disease
▶ BY MOUTH
▶ **Adult:** Initially 1–1.25 mg daily for 1 week, dose to be taken at night, then 2–2.5 mg daily for 1 week, dose to be taken at night, then 2.5 mg twice daily for 1 week, then 2.5 mg 3 times a day for 1 week, then increased in steps of 2.5 mg every 3–14 days, adjusted according to response; maintenance 10–30 mg daily

IMPORTANT SAFETY INFORMATION
FIBROTIC REACTIONS
Bromocriptine has been associated with pulmonary, retroperitoneal, and pericardial fibrotic reactions.

Exclude cardiac valvulopathy with echocardiography before starting treatment with these ergot derivatives for Parkinson's disease or chronic endocrine disorders (excludes suppression of lactation); it may also be appropriate to measure the erythrocyte sedimentation rate and serum creatinine and to obtain a chest X-ray. Patients should be monitored for dyspnoea, persistent cough, chest pain, cardiac failure, and abdominal pain or tenderness. If long-term treatment is expected, then lung-function tests may also be helpful.

IMPULSE CONTROL DISORDERS
Treatment with dopamine-receptor agonists is associated with impulse control disorders, including pathological gambling, binge eating, and hypersexuality. Patients and their carers should be informed about the risk of impulse control disorders. There is no evidence that ergot- and non-ergot-derived dopamine-receptor

agonists differ in their propensity to cause impulse control disorders, so switching between dopamine-receptor agonists to control these side-effects is not recommended. If the patient develops an impulse control disorder, the dopamine-receptor agonist should be withdrawn or the dose reduced until the symptoms resolve.

● CONTRA-INDICATIONS Avoid in pre-eclampsia · cardiac valvulopathy (exclude before treatment) · hypertension in postpartum women or in puerperium

CONTRA-INDICATIONS, FURTHER INFORMATION
▸ Postpartum or puerperium Should not be used postpartum or in puerperium in women with high blood pressure, coronary artery disease, or symptoms (or history) of serious mental disorder; monitor blood pressure carefully (especially during first few days) in postpartum women. Very rarely hypertension, myocardial infarction, seizures or stroke (both sometimes preceded by severe headache or visual disturbances), and mental disorders have been reported in postpartum women given bromocriptine for lactation suppression—caution with antihypertensive therapy and avoid other ergot alkaloids. Discontinue immediately if hypertension, unremitting headache, or signs of CNS toxicity develop.

● CAUTIONS Cardiovascular disease · history of peptic ulcer (particularly in acromegalic patients) · history of serious mental disorders (especially psychotic disorders) · Raynaud's syndrome

CAUTIONS, FURTHER INFORMATION
▸ Hyperprolactinemic patients In hyperprolactinaemic patients, the source of the hyperprolactinaemia should be established (i.e. exclude pituitary tumour before treatment).

● INTERACTIONS → Appendix 1: dopamine receptor agonists

● SIDE-EFFECTS
▸ Common or very common Constipation · drowsiness · headache · nasal congestion · nausea
▸ Uncommon Allergic dermatitis · alopecia · confusion · dizziness · dry mouth · fatigue · hallucination · hypotension · leg cramps · movement disorders · vomiting
▸ Rare or very rare Abdominal pain · arrhythmias · cardiac valvulopathy · diarrhoea · dyspnoea · gastrointestinal disorders · gastrointestinal haemorrhage · neuroleptic malignant-like syndrome · pallor · paraesthesia · pericardial effusion · pericarditis · peripheral oedema · psychotic disorder · respiratory disorders · sleep disorders · tinnitus · vision disorders
▸ Frequency not known Eating disorders · hypertension · myocardial infarction · pathological gambling · psychiatric disorders · seizure · sexual dysfunction · stroke

SIDE-EFFECTS, FURTHER INFORMATION Treatment should be withdrawn if gastro-intestinal bleeding occurs.

● ALLERGY AND CROSS-SENSITIVITY Bromocriptine should not be used in patients with hypersensitivity to ergot alkaloids.

● CONCEPTION AND CONTRACEPTION Caution—provide contraceptive advice if appropriate (oral contraceptives may increase prolactin concentration).

● BREAST FEEDING Suppresses lactation; avoid breast feeding for about 5 days if lactation prevention fails.

● HEPATIC IMPAIRMENT
Dose adjustments Dose reduction may be necessary.

● MONITORING REQUIREMENTS
▸ Specialist evaluation—monitor for pituitary enlargement, particularly during pregnancy; monitor visual field to detect secondary field loss in macroprolactinoma.
▸ Monitor for fibrotic disease.
▸ Monitor blood pressure for a few days after starting treatment and following dosage increase.

● TREATMENT CESSATION Antiparkinsonian drug therapy should never be stopped abruptly as this carries a small risk of neuroleptic malignant syndrome.

● PATIENT AND CARER ADVICE
Driving and skilled tasks
Sudden onset of sleep Excessive daytime sleepiness and sudden onset of sleep can occur with dopamine-receptor agonists.

Patients starting treatment with these drugs should be warned of the risk and of the need to exercise caution when driving or operating machinery. Those who have experienced excessive sedation or sudden onset of sleep should refrain from driving or operating machines until these effects have stopped occurring.

Management of excessive daytime sleepiness should focus on the identification of an underlying cause, such as depression or concomitant medication. Patients should be counselled on improving sleep behaviour.
Hypotensive reactions Hypotensive reactions can occur in some patients taking dopamine-receptor agonists; these can be particularly problematic during the first few days of treatment and care should be exercised when driving or operating machinery.

● MEDICINAL FORMS
There can be variation in the licensing of different medicines containing the same drug. Forms available from special-order manufacturers include: oral suspension
Tablet
CAUTIONARY AND ADVISORY LABELS 10, 21
▸ Bromocriptine (Non-proprietary)
Bromocriptine (as Bromocriptine mesilate) 1 mg Bromocriptine 1mg tablets | 100 tablet [PoM] £67.62 DT = £67.62
Bromocriptine (as Bromocriptine mesilate) 2.5 mg Bromocriptine 2.5mg tablets | 30 tablet [PoM] £74.97 DT = £74.97
Capsule
CAUTIONARY AND ADVISORY LABELS 10, 21
▸ Parlodel (Meda Pharmaceuticals Ltd)
Bromocriptine (as Bromocriptine mesilate) 5 mg Parlodel 5mg capsules | 100 capsule [PoM] £37.57 DT = £37.57
Bromocriptine (as Bromocriptine mesilate) 10 mg Parlodel 10mg capsules | 100 capsule [PoM] £69.50 DT = £69.50

Cabergoline

● DRUG ACTION Cabergoline is a stimulant of dopamine receptors in the brain and it also inhibits release of prolactin by the pituitary.

● INDICATIONS AND DOSE
Prevention of lactation
▸ BY MOUTH
▸ Adult: 1 mg, to be taken as a single dose on the first day postpartum
Suppression of established lactation
▸ BY MOUTH
▸ Adult: 250 micrograms every 12 hours for 2 days
Hyperprolactinaemic disorders
▸ BY MOUTH
▸ Adult: Initially 500 micrograms once weekly, dose may be taken as a single dose or as 2 divided doses on separate days, then increased in steps of 500 micrograms every month until optimal therapeutic response reached, increase dose following monthly monitoring of serum prolactin levels; usual dose 0.25–2 mg once weekly, usually 1 mg weekly; reduce initial dose and increase more gradually if patient intolerant, doses over 1 mg weekly to be given as divided dose; maximum 4.5 mg per week continued →

Alone or as adjunct to co-beneldopa or co-careldopa in Parkinson's disease where dopamine-receptor agonists other than ergot derivative not appropriate
▶ BY MOUTH
▶ Adult: Initially 1 mg daily, then increased in steps of 0.5–1 mg every 7–14 days, concurrent dose of levodopa may be decreased gradually while dose of cabergoline is increased; maximum 3 mg per day

IMPORTANT SAFETY INFORMATION
FIBROTIC REACTIONS
Cabergoline has been associated with pulmonary, retroperitoneal, and pericardial fibrotic reactions.
  Exclude cardiac valvulopathy with echocardiography before starting treatment with these ergot derivatives for Parkinson's disease or chronic endocrine disorders (excludes suppression of lactation); it may also be appropriate to measure the erythrocyte sedimentation rate and serum creatinine and to obtain a chest X-ray. Patients should be monitored for dyspnoea, persistent cough, chest pain, cardiac failure, and abdominal pain or tenderness. If long-term treatment is expected, then lung-function tests may also be helpful. Patients taking cabergoline should be regularly monitored for cardiac fibrosis by echocardiography (within 3–6 months of initiating treatment and subsequently at 6–12 month intervals).
IMPULSE CONTROL DISORDERS
Treatment with dopamine-receptor agonists are associated with impulse control disorders, including pathological gambling, binge eating, and hypersexuality. Patients and their carers should be informed about the risk of impulse control disorders. There is no evidence that ergot- and non-ergot-derived dopamine-receptor agonists differ in their propensity to cause impulse control disorders, so switching between dopamine-receptor agonists to control these side-effects is not recommended. If the patient develops an impulse control disorder, the dopamine-receptor agonist should be withdrawn or the dose reduced until the symptoms resolve.

● CONTRA-INDICATIONS Avoid in pre-eclampsia · cardiac valvulopathy (exclude before treatment) · history of pericardial fibrotic disorders · history of puerperal psychosis · history of pulmonary fibrotic disorders · history of retroperitoneal fibrotic disorders
● CAUTIONS Cardiovascular disease · history of peptic ulcer (particularly in acromegalic patients) · history of serious mental disorders (especially psychotic disorders) · Raynaud's syndrome
CAUTIONS, FURTHER INFORMATION
▶ Hyperprolactinemic patients In hyperprolactinaemic patients, the source of the hyperprolactinaemia should be established (i.e. exclude pituitary tumour before treatment).
● INTERACTIONS → Appendix 1: dopamine receptor agonists
● SIDE-EFFECTS
▶ Common or very common Angina pectoris · asthenia · cardiac valvulopathy · confusion · constipation · dizziness · drowsiness · dyspepsia · dyspnoea · gastritis · hallucination · headache · hypotension · movement disorders · nausea · oedema · pericardial effusion · pericarditis · sexual dysfunction · sleep disorders · vertigo · vomiting
▶ Uncommon Delusions · erythromelalgia · hepatic function abnormal · psychotic disorder · rash · respiratory disorders
▶ Rare or very rare Fibrosis
▶ Frequency not known Aggression · alopecia · chest pain · digital vasospasm · leg cramps · pathological gambling · syncope · tremor · visual impairment

● ALLERGY AND CROSS-SENSITIVITY Cabergoline should not be used in patients with hypersensitivity to ergot alkaloids.
● CONCEPTION AND CONTRACEPTION Exclude pregnancy before starting and perform monthly pregnancy tests during the amenorrhoeic period. Caution—advise non-hormonal contraception if pregnancy not desired. Discontinue 1 month before intended conception (ovulatory cycles persist for 6 months).
● PREGNANCY Discontinue if pregnancy occurs during treatment (specialist advice needed).
● BREAST FEEDING Suppresses lactation; avoid breast-feeding if lactation prevention fails.
● HEPATIC IMPAIRMENT
Dose adjustments Reduce dose in severe hepatic impairment.
● MONITORING REQUIREMENTS
▶ Monitor for fibrotic disease.
▶ Monitor blood pressure for a few days after starting treatment and following dosage increase.
● TREATMENT CESSATION Antiparkinsonian drug therapy should never be stopped abruptly as this carries a small risk of neuroleptic malignant syndrome.
● PRESCRIBING AND DISPENSING INFORMATION Dispense in original container (contains desiccant).
● PATIENT AND CARER ADVICE
Driving and skilled tasks
Sudden onset of sleep Excessive daytime sleepiness and sudden onset of sleep can occur with dopamine-receptor agonists.
  Patients starting treatment with these drugs should be warned of the risk and of the need to exercise caution when driving or operating machinery. Those who have experienced excessive sedation or sudden onset of sleep should refrain from driving or operating machines until these effects have stopped occurring.
  Management of excessive daytime sleepiness should focus on the identification of an underlying cause, such as depression or concomitant medication. Patients should be counselled on improving sleep behaviour.
Hypotensive reactions Hypotensive reactions can occur in some patients taking dopamine-receptor agonists; these can be particularly problematic during the first few days of treatment and care should be exercised when driving or operating machinery.

● MEDICINAL FORMS
There can be variation in the licensing of different medicines containing the same drug.
Tablet
CAUTIONARY AND ADVISORY LABELS 10, 21
▶ Cabergoline (Non-proprietary)
  Cabergoline 500 microgram Cabergoline 500microgram tablets | 8 tablet [PoM] £34.99 DT = £34.97
  Cabergoline 1 mg Cabergoline 1mg tablets | 20 tablet [PoM] £66.00 DT = £64.25
  Cabergoline 2 mg Cabergoline 2mg tablets | 20 tablet [PoM] £73.14 DT = £73.12
▶ Cabaser (Pfizer Ltd)
  Cabergoline 1 mg Cabaser 1mg tablets | 20 tablet [PoM] £83.00 DT = £64.25
  Cabergoline 2 mg Cabaser 2mg tablets | 20 tablet [PoM] £83.00 DT = £73.12
▶ Dostinex (Pfizer Ltd)
  Cabergoline 500 microgram Dostinex 500microgram tablets | 8 tablet [PoM] £30.04 DT = £34.97

Pergolide

- **INDICATIONS AND DOSE**

Monotherapy in Parkinson's disease where dopamine-receptor agonists other than ergot derivative not appropriate
▶ BY MOUTH
▶ Adult: Initially 50 micrograms once daily for day 1, dose to be taken at bedtime, then 50 micrograms twice daily for days 2–4, then increased in steps of 100–250 micrograms daily, dose to be increased at intervals of 3–4 days, increased to 1.5 mg daily in 3 divided doses at day 28, then increased in steps of up to 250 micrograms every 3–4 days, this increase to be started after day 30; maintenance 2.1–2.5 mg daily; maximum 3 mg per day

Adjunctive therapy with co-beneldopa or co-careldopa in Parkinson's disease where dopamine-receptor agonists other than ergot derivative not appropriate
▶ BY MOUTH
▶ Adult: Initially 50 micrograms daily for 2 days, then increased in steps of 100–150 micrograms every 3 days, dose to be adjusted over next 12 days following initial dose and usually given in 3 divided doses, then increased in steps of 250 micrograms every 3 days, during pergolide titration, levodopa dose may be reduced cautiously; maximum 3 mg per day

> **IMPORTANT SAFETY INFORMATION**
> FIBROTIC REACTIONS
> Pergolide has been associated with pulmonary, retroperitoneal, and pericardial fibrotic reactions.
> Exclude cardiac valvulopathy with echocardiography before starting treatment with pergolide; it may also be appropriate to measure the erythrocyte sedimentation rate and serum creatinine and to obtain a chest X-ray. Patients should be monitored for dyspnoea, persistent cough, chest pain, cardiac failure, and abdominal pain or tenderness. If long-term treatment is expected, then lung-function tests may also be helpful. Patients taking pergolide should be regularly monitored for cardiac fibrosis by echocardiography (within 3–6 months of initiating treatment and subsequently at 6–12 month intervals).
> IMPULSE CONTROL DISORDERS
> Treatment with dopamine-receptor agonists is associated with impulse control disorders, including pathological gambling, binge eating, and hypersexuality. Patients and their carers should be informed about the risk of impulse control disorders. There is no evidence that ergot- and non-ergot-derived dopamine-receptor agonists differ in their propensity to cause impulse control disorders, so switching between dopamine-receptor agonists to control these side-effects is not recommended. If the patient develops an impulse control disorder, the dopamine-receptor agonist or levodopa should be withdrawn or the dose reduced until the symptoms resolve.

- **CONTRA-INDICATIONS** Cardiac valvulopathy (exclude before treatment) · history of fibrotic disorders
- **CAUTIONS** Acute porphyrias p. 1025 · arrhythmias · dyskinesia (may exacerbate) · hallucinations · history of confusion · psychosis · underlying cardiac disease
- **INTERACTIONS** → Appendix 1: dopamine receptor agonists
- **SIDE-EFFECTS** Cardiac valve disorders · compulsions · confusion · constipation · diarrhoea · diplopia · dizziness · drowsiness · dyskinesia · dyspnoea · eating disorders · erythromelalgia · gastrointestinal discomfort · hallucination · hiccups · nausea · neuroleptic malignant

syndrome · pain · palpitations · pathological gambling · pericardial effusion · pericarditis · postural hypotension · pulmonary hypertension · rash · Raynaud's phenomenon · respiratory disorders · retroperitoneal fibrosis · rhinitis · sexual dysfunction · sleep disorders · syncope · vomiting
- **PREGNANCY** Use only if potential benefit outweighs risk.
- **BREAST FEEDING** May suppress lactation.
- **TREATMENT CESSATION** Antiparkinsonian drug therapy should never be stopped abruptly as this carries a small risk of neuroleptic malignant syndrome.
- **PATIENT AND CARER ADVICE**
Driving and skilled tasks
Sudden onset of sleep Excessive daytime sleepiness and sudden onset of sleep can occur with dopamine-receptor agonists.
  Patients starting treatment with these drugs should be warned of the risk and of the need to exercise caution when driving or operating machinery. Those who have experienced excessive sedation or sudden onset of sleep should refrain from driving or operating machines until these effects have stopped occurring.
  Management of excessive daytime sleepiness should focus on the identification of an underlying cause, such as depression or concomitant medication. Patients should be counselled on improving sleep behaviour.
Hypotensive reactions Hypotensive reactions can occur in some patients taking dopamine-receptor agonists; these can be particularly problematic during the first few days of treatment and care should be exercised when driving or operating machinery.

- **MEDICINAL FORMS**
There can be variation in the licensing of different medicines containing the same drug.
Tablet
CAUTIONARY AND ADVISORY LABELS 10
▶ Pergolide (Non-proprietary)
  Pergolide (as Pergolide mesilate) 250 microgram Pergolide 250microgram tablets | 100 tablet [PoM] £36.26 DT = £36.17
  Pergolide (as Pergolide mesilate) 1 mg Pergolide 1mg tablets | 100 tablet [PoM] £125.00–£135.00 DT = £131.66

Pramipexole

- **INDICATIONS AND DOSE**

Parkinson's disease, used alone or as an adjunct to co-beneldopa or co-careldopa
▶ BY MOUTH USING IMMEDIATE-RELEASE MEDICINES
▶ Adult: Initially 88 micrograms 3 times a day, if tolerated dose to be increased by doubling dose every 5–7 days, increased to 350 micrograms 3 times a day, then increased in steps of 180 micrograms 3 times a day if required, dose to be increased at weekly intervals, during dose titration and maintenance, levodopa dose may be reduced, maximum daily dose to be given in 3 divided doses; maximum 3.3 mg per day
▶ BY MOUTH USING MODIFIED-RELEASE MEDICINES
▶ Adult: Initially 260 micrograms once daily, dose to be increased by doubling dose every 5–7 days, increased to 1.05 mg once daily, then increased in steps of 520 micrograms every week if required, during dose titration and maintenance, levodopa dose may be reduced according to response; maximum 3.15 mg per day

Moderate to severe restless legs syndrome
▶ BY MOUTH USING IMMEDIATE-RELEASE MEDICINES
▶ Adult: Initially 88 micrograms once daily, dose to be taken 2–3 hours before bedtime, dose to be increased by doubling dose every 4–7 days if necessary, repeat dose titration if restarting treatment after continued →

4

Nervous system

an interval of more than a few days; maximum 540 micrograms per day

DOSE EQUIVALENCE AND CONVERSION
▸ Doses and strengths are stated in terms of pramipexole (base).
▸ Equivalent strengths of pramipexole (base) in terms of pramipexole dihydrochloride monohydrate (salt) for immediate-release preparations are as follows:
▸ 88 micrograms base ≡ 125 micrograms salt;
▸ 180 micrograms base ≡ 250 micrograms salt;
▸ 350 micrograms base ≡ 500 micrograms salt;
▸ 700 micrograms base ≡ 1 mg salt.
▸ Equivalent strengths of pramipexole (base) in terms of pramipexole dihydrochloride monohydrate (salt) for modified-release preparations are as follows:
▸ 260 micrograms base ≡ 375 micrograms salt;
▸ 520 micrograms base ≡ 750 micrograms salt;
▸ 1.05 mg base ≡ 1.5 mg salt;
▸ 1.57 mg base ≡ 2.25 mg salt;
▸ 2.1 mg base ≡ 3 mg salt;
▸ 2.62 mg base ≡ 3.75 mg salt;
▸ 3.15 mg base ≡ 4.5 mg salt.

IMPORTANT SAFETY INFORMATION
IMPULSE CONTROL DISORDERS
Treatment with dopamine-receptor agonists is associated with impulse control disorders, including pathological gambling, binge eating, and hypersexuality. Patients and their carers should be informed about the risk of impulse control disorders. There is no evidence that ergot- and non-ergot-derived dopamine-receptor agonists differ in their propensity to cause impulse control disorders, so switching between dopamine-receptor agonists to control these side-effects is not recommended. If the patient develops an impulse control disorder, the dopamine-receptor agonist should be withdrawn or the dose reduced until the symptoms resolve.

● CAUTIONS Psychotic disorders · risk of visual disorders (ophthalmological testing recommended) · severe cardiovascular disease
● INTERACTIONS → Appendix 1: dopamine receptor agonists
● SIDE-EFFECTS
▸ **Common or very common** Appetite abnormal · behaviour abnormal · confusion · constipation · dizziness · drowsiness · fatigue · hallucination · headache · hypotension · movement disorders · nausea · peripheral oedema · psychiatric disorders · sleep disorders · vision disorders · vomiting · weight changes
▸ **Uncommon** Anxiety · binge eating · delirium · delusions · dyspnoea · heart failure · hiccups · mania · memory loss · pathological gambling · pneumonia · sexual dysfunction · SIADH · skin reactions · syncope
▸ **Frequency not known** Depression · dopamine agonist withdrawal syndrome · generalised pain · sweating abnormal
● PREGNANCY Use only if potential benefit outweighs risk—no information available.
● BREAST FEEDING May suppress lactation; avoid—present in milk in *animal* studies.
● RENAL IMPAIRMENT For *modified-release* tablets, avoid if eGFR less than 30 mL/minute/1.73 m². **Dose adjustments** For *immediate-release* tablets in Parkinson's disease, initially 88 micrograms twice daily (max. 1.57 mg daily in 2 divided doses) if eGFR 20–50 mL/minute/1.73 m²; initially 88 micrograms once daily (max. 1.1 mg once daily) if eGFR less than 20 mL/minute/1.73 m². If renal function declines during

treatment, reduce dose by the same percentage as the decline in eGFR.
For *immediate-release* tablets in restless legs syndrome, reduce dose if eGFR less than 20 mL/minute/1.73 m².
For *modified-release* tablets, initially 260 micrograms on alternate days if eGFR 30–50 mL/minute/1.73 m², increased to 260 micrograms once daily after 1 week, further increased if necessary by 260 micrograms daily at weekly intervals to max. 1.57 mg daily.
● MONITORING REQUIREMENTS Risk of postural hypotension (especially on initiation)—monitor blood pressure.
● TREATMENT CESSATION Antiparkinsonian drug therapy should never be stopped abruptly as this carries a small risk of neuroleptic malignant syndrome.
● PATIENT AND CARER ADVICE
Driving and skilled tasks
Sudden onset of sleep Excessive daytime sleepiness and sudden onset of sleep can occur with dopamine-receptor agonists.
Patients starting treatment with these drugs should be warned of the risk and of the need to exercise caution when driving or operating machinery. Those who have experienced excessive sedation or sudden onset of sleep should refrain from driving or operating machines until these effects have stopped occurring.
Management of excessive daytime sleepiness should focus on the identification of an underlying cause, such as depression or concomitant medication. Patients should be counselled on improving sleep behaviour.
Hypotensive reactions Hypotensive reactions can occur in some patients taking dopamine-receptor agonists; these can be particularly problematic during the first few days of treatment and care should be exercised when driving or operating machinery.

● MEDICINAL FORMS
There can be variation in the licensing of different medicines containing the same drug.
Modified-release tablet
CAUTIONARY AND ADVISORY LABELS 10, 25
▸ Pramipexole (Non-proprietary)
Pramipexole (as Pramipexole dihydrochloride monohydrate)
260 microgram Pramipexole 260microgram modified-release tablets | 30 tablet [PoM] £8.50–£30.87 DT = £14.77
Pramipexole (as Pramipexole dihydrochloride monohydrate)
520 microgram Pramipexole 520microgram modified-release tablets | 30 tablet [PoM] £20.00–£61.73 DT = £30.74
Pramipexole (as Pramipexole dihydrochloride monohydrate)
1.05 mg Pramipexole 1.05mg modified-release tablets | 30 tablet [PoM] £28.00–£123.46 DT = £56.68
Pramipexole (as Pramipexole dihydrochloride monohydrate)
1.57 mg Pramipexole 1.57mg modified-release tablets | 30 tablet [PoM] £80.94–£192.24 DT = £126.82
Pramipexole (as Pramipexole dihydrochloride monohydrate)
2.1 mg Pramipexole 2.1mg modified-release tablets | 30 tablet [PoM] £50.00–£246.91 DT = £110.97
Pramipexole (as Pramipexole dihydrochloride monohydrate)
2.62 mg Pramipexole 2.62mg modified-release tablets | 30 tablet [PoM] £134.95–£320.41 DT = £222.06
Pramipexole (as Pramipexole dihydrochloride monohydrate)
3.15 mg Pramipexole 3.15mg modified-release tablets | 30 tablet [PoM] £155.95–£370.38 DT = £210.46
▸ Mirapexin (Boehringer Ingelheim Ltd)
Pramipexole (as Pramipexole dihydrochloride monohydrate)
260 microgram Mirapexin 0.26mg modified-release tablets | 30 tablet [PoM] £32.49 DT = £14.77
Pramipexole (as Pramipexole dihydrochloride monohydrate)
520 microgram Mirapexin 0.52mg modified-release tablets | 30 tablet [PoM] £64.98 DT = £30.74
Pramipexole (as Pramipexole dihydrochloride monohydrate)
1.05 mg Mirapexin 1.05mg modified-release tablets | 30 tablet [PoM] £129.96 DT = £56.68
Pramipexole (as Pramipexole dihydrochloride monohydrate)
1.57 mg Mirapexin 1.57mg modified-release tablets | 30 tablet [PoM] £202.36 DT = £126.82

Pramipexole (as Pramipexole dihydrochloride monohydrate)
2.1 mg Mirapexin 2.1mg modified-release tablets | 30 tablet [PoM]
£259.91 DT = £110.97

Pramipexole (as Pramipexole dihydrochloride monohydrate)
2.62 mg Mirapexin 2.62mg modified-release tablets |
30 tablet [PoM] £337.27 DT = £222.06

Pramipexole (as Pramipexole dihydrochloride monohydrate)
3.15 mg Mirapexin 3.15mg modified-release tablets | 30 tablet [PoM]
£389.87 DT = £210.46

▸ Oprymea (Consilient Health Ltd)

Pramipexole (as Pramipexole dihydrochloride monohydrate)
260 microgram Oprymea 0.26mg modified-release tablets |
30 tablet [PoM] £25.56 DT = £14.77

Pramipexole (as Pramipexole dihydrochloride monohydrate)
520 microgram Oprymea 0.52mg modified-release tablets |
30 tablet [PoM] £51.14 DT = £30.74

Pramipexole (as Pramipexole dihydrochloride monohydrate)
1.05 mg Oprymea 1.05mg modified-release tablets | 30 tablet [PoM]
£102.28 DT = £56.68

Pramipexole (as Pramipexole dihydrochloride monohydrate)
1.57 mg Oprymea 1.57mg modified-release tablets | 30 tablet [PoM]
£159.26 DT = £126.82

Pramipexole (as Pramipexole dihydrochloride monohydrate)
2.1 mg Oprymea 2.1mg modified-release tablets | 30 tablet [PoM]
£204.56 DT = £110.97

Pramipexole (as Pramipexole dihydrochloride monohydrate)
2.62 mg Oprymea 2.62mg modified-release tablets | 30 tablet [PoM]
£337.27 DT = £222.06

Pramipexole (as Pramipexole dihydrochloride monohydrate)
3.15 mg Oprymea 3.15mg modified-release tablets | 30 tablet [PoM]
£389.87 DT = £210.46

▸ Pipexus (Ethypharm UK Ltd)

Pramipexole (as Pramipexole dihydrochloride monohydrate)
260 microgram Pipexus 0.26mg modified-release tablets |
30 tablet [PoM] £16.25 DT = £14.77

Pramipexole (as Pramipexole dihydrochloride monohydrate)
520 microgram Pipexus 0.52mg modified-release tablets |
30 tablet [PoM] £32.49 DT = £30.74

Pramipexole (as Pramipexole dihydrochloride monohydrate)
1.05 mg Pipexus 1.05mg modified-release tablets | 30 tablet [PoM]
£64.98 DT = £56.68

Pramipexole (as Pramipexole dihydrochloride monohydrate)
1.57 mg Pipexus 1.57mg modified-release tablets | 30 tablet [PoM]
£101.18 DT = £126.82

Pramipexole (as Pramipexole dihydrochloride monohydrate)
2.1 mg Pipexus 2.1mg modified-release tablets | 30 tablet [PoM]
£129.96 DT = £110.97

Pramipexole (as Pramipexole dihydrochloride monohydrate)
2.62 mg Pipexus 2.62mg modified-release tablets | 30 tablet [PoM]
£168.64 DT = £222.06

Pramipexole (as Pramipexole dihydrochloride monohydrate)
3.15 mg Pipexus 3.15mg modified-release tablets | 30 tablet [PoM]
£194.94 DT = £210.46

Tablet

CAUTIONARY AND ADVISORY LABELS 10

▸ Pramipexole (Non-proprietary)

Pramipexole (as Pramipexole dihydrochloride monohydrate)
88 microgram Pramipexole 88microgram tablets | 30 tablet [PoM]
£8.60 DT = £8.39

Pramipexole (as Pramipexole dihydrochloride monohydrate)
180 microgram Pramipexole 180microgram tablets |
30 tablet [PoM] £17.19 DT = £1.69 | 100 tablet [PoM] £5.53–£5.63

Pramipexole (as Pramipexole dihydrochloride monohydrate)
350 microgram Pramipexole 350microgram tablets |
30 tablet [PoM] £34.38 DT = £13.65 | 100 tablet [PoM] £45.50–£46.50

Pramipexole (as Pramipexole dihydrochloride monohydrate)
700 microgram Pramipexole 700microgram tablets |
30 tablet [PoM] £68.76 DT = £2.80 | 100 tablet [PoM] £9.33–£10.30

▸ Mirapexin (Boehringer Ingelheim Ltd)

Pramipexole (as Pramipexole dihydrochloride monohydrate)
88 microgram Mirapexin 0.088mg tablets | 30 tablet [PoM] £11.24
DT = £8.39

Pramipexole (as Pramipexole dihydrochloride monohydrate)
180 microgram Mirapexin 0.18mg tablets | 30 tablet [PoM] £22.49
DT = £1.69 | 100 tablet [PoM] £74.95

Pramipexole (as Pramipexole dihydrochloride monohydrate)
350 microgram Mirapexin 0.35mg tablets | 30 tablet [PoM] £44.97
DT = £13.65 | 100 tablet [PoM] £149.90

Pramipexole (as Pramipexole dihydrochloride monohydrate)
700 microgram Mirapexin 0.7mg tablets | 30 tablet [PoM] £89.94
DT = £2.80 | 100 tablet [PoM] £299.82

▸ Oprymea (Consilient Health Ltd)

Pramipexole (as Pramipexole dihydrochloride monohydrate)
88 microgram Oprymea 0.088mg tablets | 30 tablet [PoM] £3.23 DT
= £8.39

Pramipexole (as Pramipexole dihydrochloride monohydrate)
180 microgram Oprymea 0.18mg tablets | 30 tablet [PoM] £6.09 DT
= £1.69 | 100 tablet [PoM] £15.46

Pramipexole (as Pramipexole dihydrochloride monohydrate)
350 microgram Oprymea 0.35mg tablets | 30 tablet [PoM] £32.47
DT = £13.65 | 100 tablet [PoM] £108.23

Pramipexole (as Pramipexole dihydrochloride monohydrate)
700 microgram Oprymea 0.7mg tablets | 30 tablet [PoM] £18.26 DT
= £2.80 | 100 tablet [PoM] £117.63

Ropinirole

● INDICATIONS AND DOSE

Parkinson's disease, either used alone or as adjunct to co-beneldopa or co-careldopa

▸ BY MOUTH USING IMMEDIATE-RELEASE MEDICINES

▸ Adult: Initially 750 micrograms daily in 3 divided doses, then increased in steps of 750 micrograms daily, dose to be increased at weekly intervals, increased to 3 mg daily in 3 divided doses, then increased in steps of 1.5–3 mg daily, adjusted according to response, dose to be increased at weekly intervals; usual dose 9–16 mg daily in 3 divided doses, higher doses may be required if used with levodopa, when administered as adjunct to levodopa, concurrent dose of levodopa may be reduced by approx. 20%, daily maximum dose to be given in 3 divided doses; maximum 24 mg per day

▸ BY MOUTH USING MODIFIED-RELEASE MEDICINES

▸ Adult: Initially 2 mg once daily for 1 week, then 4 mg once daily, increased in steps of 2 mg at intervals of at least 1 week, adjusted according to response, increased to up to 8 mg once daily, dose to be increased further if still no response; increased in steps of 2–4 mg at intervals of at least 2 weeks if required, consider slower titration in patients over 75 years, when administered as adjunct to levodopa, concurrent dose of levodopa may gradually be reduced by approx. 30%; maximum 24 mg per day

Parkinson's disease in patients transferring from ropinirole immediate-release tablets

▸ BY MOUTH USING MODIFIED-RELEASE MEDICINES

▸ Adult: Initially ropinirole modified-release once daily substituted for total daily dose equivalent of ropinirole immediate-release tablets; if control not maintained after switching, titrate dose as above

Moderate to severe restless legs syndrome

▸ BY MOUTH USING IMMEDIATE-RELEASE MEDICINES

▸ Adult: Initially 250 micrograms once daily for 2 days, increased if tolerated to 500 micrograms once daily for 5 days, then increased if tolerated to 1 mg once daily for 7 days, then increased in steps of 500 micrograms daily, adjusted according to response, dose to be increased at weekly intervals; usual dose 2 mg once daily, doses to be taken at night; maximum 4 mg per day

● UNLICENSED USE Doses in the BNF may differ from those in product literature.

IMPORTANT SAFETY INFORMATION
SAFE PRACTICE
Ropinirole has been confused with risperidone; care must be taken to ensure the correct drug is prescribed and dispensed.

4

Nervous system

IMPULSE CONTROL DISORDERS
Treatment with dopamine-receptor agonists is associated with impulse control disorders, including pathological gambling, binge eating, and hypersexuality. Patients and their carers should be informed about the risk of impulse control disorders. There is no evidence that ergot- and non-ergot-derived dopamine-receptor agonists differ in their propensity to cause impulse control disorders, so switching between dopamine-receptor agonists to control these side-effects is not recommended. If the patient develops an impulse control disorder, the dopamine-receptor agonist should be withdrawn or the dose reduced until the symptoms resolve.

● CAUTIONS Elderly · major psychotic disorders · severe cardiovascular disease (risk of hypotension—monitor blood pressure)

● INTERACTIONS → Appendix 1: dopamine receptor agonists

● SIDE-EFFECTS
▶ **Common or very common** Confusion · dizziness · drowsiness · early morning awakening · fatigue · gastrointestinal discomfort · hallucination · movement disorders · nausea · nervousness · peripheral oedema · syncope · vertigo · vomiting
▶ **Uncommon** Hypotension · sexual dysfunction
▶ **Rare or very rare** Hepatic reaction
▶ **Frequency not known** Behaviour abnormal · delirium · delusions · eating disorders · pathological gambling · psychiatric disorders · psychotic disorder

● PREGNANCY Avoid unless potential benefit outweighs risk—toxicity in *animal* studies.

● BREAST FEEDING May suppress lactation—avoid.

● HEPATIC IMPAIRMENT Avoid—no information available.

● RENAL IMPAIRMENT Avoid if eGFR less than 30 mL/minute/1.73 m^2.

● TREATMENT CESSATION Antiparkinsonian drug therapy should never be stopped abruptly as this carries a small risk of neuroleptic malignant syndrome.

● PATIENT AND CARER ADVICE
Missed doses ▶ When used for Parkinson's disease Manufacturer advises if treatment is interrupted for one day or more, re-initiation by dose titration should be considered—consult product literature.
▶ When used for Moderate to severe restless legs syndrome Manufacturer advises if treatment is interrupted for more than a few days, re-initiation by dose titration is recommended.
Driving and skilled tasks
Sudden onset of sleep Excessive daytime sleepiness and sudden onset of sleep can occur with dopamine-receptor agonists.
　　Patients starting treatment with these drugs should be warned of the risk and of the need to exercise caution when driving or operating machinery. Those who have experienced excessive sedation or sudden onset of sleep should refrain from driving or operating machines until these effects have stopped occurring.
　　Management of excessive daytime sleepiness should focus on the identification of an underlying cause, such as depression or concomitant medication. Patients should be counselled on improving sleep behaviour.
Hypotensive reactions Hypotensive reactions can occur in some patients taking dopamine-receptor agonists; these can be particularly problematic during the first few days of treatment and care should be exercised when driving or operating machinery.

● NATIONAL FUNDING/ACCESS DECISIONS
Scottish Medicines Consortium (SMC) Decisions
The Scottish Medicines Consortium has advised (June 2006) that *Adartrel*® should be restricted for use in patients with a baseline score of 24 points or more on the International Restless Legs Scale.

● MEDICINAL FORMS
There can be variation in the licensing of different medicines containing the same drug. Forms available from special-order manufacturers include: oral suspension, oral solution

Modified-release tablet
CAUTIONARY AND ADVISORY LABELS 10, 25
▶ Ropinirole (Non-proprietary)
　Ropinirole (as Ropinirole hydrochloride) 2 mg Ropinirole 2mg modified-release tablets | 28 tablet [PoM] £10.66 DT = £12.54
　Ropinirole (as Ropinirole hydrochloride) 4 mg Ropinirole 4mg modified-release tablets | 28 tablet [PoM] £21.33 DT = £25.09
　Ropinirole (as Ropinirole hydrochloride) 8 mg Ropinirole 8mg modified-release tablets | 28 tablet [PoM] £35.79 DT = £42.11
▶ Eppinix XL (Ethypharm UK Ltd)
　Ropinirole (as Ropinirole hydrochloride) 2 mg Ipinnia XL 2mg tablets | 28 tablet [PoM] £5.64 DT = £12.54
　Ropinirole (as Ropinirole hydrochloride) 3 mg Ipinnia XL 3mg tablets | 28 tablet [PoM] £8.46 DT = £8.46
　Ropinirole (as Ropinirole hydrochloride) 4 mg Ipinnia XL 4mg tablets | 28 tablet [PoM] £11.29 DT = £25.09
　Ropinirole (as Ropinirole hydrochloride) 6 mg Ipinnia XL 6mg tablets | 28 tablet [PoM] £15.32 DT = £15.32
　Ropinirole (as Ropinirole hydrochloride) 8 mg Ipinnia XL 8mg tablets | 28 tablet [PoM] £18.95 DT = £42.11
▶ Ralnea XL (Consilient Health Ltd)
　Ropinirole (as Ropinirole hydrochloride) 2 mg Ralnea XL 2mg tablets | 28 tablet [PoM] £10.65 DT = £12.54
　Ropinirole (as Ropinirole hydrochloride) 4 mg Ralnea XL 4mg tablets | 28 tablet [PoM] £21.32 DT = £25.09
　Ropinirole (as Ropinirole hydrochloride) 8 mg Ralnea XL 8mg tablets | 28 tablet [PoM] £35.79 DT = £42.11
▶ Raponer XL (Actavis UK Ltd)
　Ropinirole (as Ropinirole hydrochloride) 2 mg Raponer XL 2mg tablets | 28 tablet [PoM] £12.54 DT = £12.54
　Ropinirole (as Ropinirole hydrochloride) 4 mg Raponer XL 4mg tablets | 28 tablet [PoM] £25.09 DT = £25.09
　Ropinirole (as Ropinirole hydrochloride) 8 mg Raponer XL 8mg tablets | 28 tablet [PoM] £42.11 DT = £42.11
▶ ReQuip XL (GlaxoSmithKline UK Ltd)
　Ropinirole (as Ropinirole hydrochloride) 2 mg ReQuip XL 2mg tablets | 28 tablet [PoM] £12.54 DT = £12.54
　Ropinirole (as Ropinirole hydrochloride) 4 mg ReQuip XL 4mg tablets | 28 tablet [PoM] £25.09 DT = £25.09
　Ropinirole (as Ropinirole hydrochloride) 8 mg ReQuip XL 8mg tablets | 28 tablet [PoM] £42.11 DT = £42.11
▶ Repinex XL (Aspire Pharma Ltd)
　Ropinirole (as Ropinirole hydrochloride) 2 mg Repinex XL 2mg tablets | 28 tablet [PoM] £6.20 DT = £12.54
　Ropinirole (as Ropinirole hydrochloride) 4 mg Repinex XL 4mg tablets | 28 tablet [PoM] £12.50 DT = £25.09
　Ropinirole (as Ropinirole hydrochloride) 8 mg Repinex XL 8mg tablets | 28 tablet [PoM] £21.00 DT = £42.11
▶ Ropilynz XL (Lupin Healthcare (UK) Ltd)
　Ropinirole (as Ropinirole hydrochloride) 2 mg Ropilynz XL 2mg tablets | 28 tablet [PoM] £10.65 DT = £12.54
　Ropinirole (as Ropinirole hydrochloride) 4 mg Ropilynz XL 4mg tablets | 28 tablet [PoM] £21.32 DT = £25.09
　Ropinirole (as Ropinirole hydrochloride) 8 mg Ropilynz XL 8mg tablets | 28 tablet [PoM] £35.79 DT = £42.11
▶ Ropiqual XL (Milpharm Ltd)
　Ropinirole (as Ropinirole hydrochloride) 2 mg Ropiqual XL 2mg tablets | 28 tablet [PoM] £17.22 DT = £12.54
　Ropinirole (as Ropinirole hydrochloride) 4 mg Ropiqual XL 4mg tablets | 28 tablet [PoM] £25.09 DT = £25.09
　Ropinirole (as Ropinirole hydrochloride) 8 mg Ropiqual XL 8mg tablets | 28 tablet [PoM] £42.11 DT = £42.11
▶ Spiroco XL (Teva UK Ltd)
　Ropinirole (as Ropinirole hydrochloride) 2 mg Spiroco XL 2mg tablets | 28 tablet [PoM] £5.63 DT = £12.54
　Ropinirole (as Ropinirole hydrochloride) 4 mg Spiroco XL 4mg tablets | 28 tablet [PoM] £11.28 DT = £25.09

Ropinirole (as Ropinirole hydrochloride) 8 mg Spiroco XL 8mg tablets | 28 tablet PoM £18.94 DT = £42.11

Tablet

CAUTIONARY AND ADVISORY LABELS 10, 21

▸ Ropinirole (Non-proprietary)

Ropinirole (as Ropinirole hydrochloride)
250 microgram Ropinirole 250microgram tablets | 12 tablet PoM £15.00 DT = £3.65

Ropinirole (as Ropinirole hydrochloride)
500 microgram Ropinirole 500microgram tablets | 28 tablet PoM £25.00 DT = £8.70

Ropinirole (as Ropinirole hydrochloride) 1 mg Ropinirole 1mg tablets | 84 tablet PoM £56.71 DT = £56.71

Ropinirole (as Ropinirole hydrochloride) 2 mg Ropinirole 2mg tablets | 28 tablet PoM £21.25–£49.99 DT = £20.18 | 84 tablet PoM £33.35–£60.54

Ropinirole (as Ropinirole hydrochloride) 5 mg Ropinirole 5mg tablets | 84 tablet PoM £165.00 DT = £165.00

▸ Adartrel (GlaxoSmithKline UK Ltd)

Ropinirole (as Ropinirole hydrochloride) 250 microgram Adartrel 250microgram tablets | 12 tablet PoM £3.94 DT = £3.65

Ropinirole (as Ropinirole hydrochloride) 500 microgram Adartrel 500microgram tablets | 28 tablet PoM £15.75 DT = £8.70

Ropinirole (as Ropinirole hydrochloride) 2 mg Adartrel 2mg tablets | 28 tablet PoM £31.51 DT = £20.18

▸ ReQuip (GlaxoSmithKline UK Ltd)

Ropinirole (as Ropinirole hydrochloride) 250 microgram ReQuip 250microgram tablets | 21 tablet PoM £5.70

Ropinirole (as Ropinirole hydrochloride) 1 mg ReQuip 1mg tablets | 84 tablet PoM £56.71 DT = £56.71

Ropinirole (as Ropinirole hydrochloride) 2 mg ReQuip 2mg tablets | 84 tablet PoM £113.44

Ropinirole (as Ropinirole hydrochloride) 5 mg ReQuip 5mg tablets | 84 tablet PoM £195.92 DT = £165.00

| Rotigotine   05-Jun-2017

● **INDICATIONS AND DOSE**

Monotherapy in Parkinson's disease
▸ BY TRANSDERMAL APPLICATION USING PATCHES
▸ **Adult:** Initially 2 mg/24 hours, then increased in steps of 2 mg/24 hours every week if required; maximum 8 mg/24 hours per day

Adjunctive therapy with co-beneldopa or co-careldopa in Parkinson's disease
▸ BY TRANSDERMAL APPLICATION USING PATCHES
▸ **Adult:** Initially 4 mg/24 hours, then increased in steps of 2 mg/24 hours every week if required; maximum 16 mg/24 hours per day

Moderate to severe restless legs syndrome
▸ BY TRANSDERMAL APPLICATION USING PATCHES
▸ **Adult:** Initially 1 mg/24 hours, then increased in steps of 1 mg/24 hours every week if required; maximum 3 mg/24 hours per day

---

IMPORTANT SAFETY INFORMATION

IMPULSE CONTROL DISORDERS

Treatment with dopamine-receptor agonists is associated with impulse control disorders, including pathological gambling, binge eating, and hypersexuality. Patients and their carers should be informed about the risk of impulse control disorders. There is no evidence that ergot- and non-ergot-derived dopamine-receptor agonists differ in their propensity to cause impulse control disorders, so switching between dopamine-receptor agonists to control these side-effects is not recommended. If the patient develops an impulse control disorder, the dopamine-receptor agonist should be withdrawn or the dose reduced until the symptoms resolve.

● CAUTIONS Avoid exposure of patch to heat · remove patch (aluminium-containing) before magnetic resonance imaging or cardioversion

● INTERACTIONS → Appendix 1: dopamine receptor agonists

● SIDE-EFFECTS

▸ **Common or very common** Asthenia · behaviour abnormal · constipation · dizziness · drowsiness · dry mouth · dyskinesia · eating disorders · fall · gastrointestinal discomfort · hallucinations · headache · hiccups · hyperhidrosis · hypertension · hypotension · loss of consciousness · malaise · nausea · palpitations · pathological gambling · perception altered · peripheral oedema · psychiatric disorders · skin reactions · sleep disorders · syncope · vertigo · vomiting · weight changes

▸ **Uncommon** Agitation · angioedema · arrhythmias · confusion · sexual dysfunction · vision disorders

▸ **Rare or very rare** Delirium · delusions · irritability · psychotic disorder · seizure

● PREGNANCY Avoid—no information available.

● BREAST FEEDING May suppress lactation; avoid—present in milk in *animal* studies.

● HEPATIC IMPAIRMENT Caution in severe impairment— no information available.

● MONITORING REQUIREMENTS Ophthalmic testing recommended.

● TREATMENT CESSATION Antiparkinsonian drug therapy should never be stopped abruptly as this carries a small risk of neuroleptic malignant syndrome.

● DIRECTIONS FOR ADMINISTRATION Manufacturer advises apply patch to dry, non-irritated skin on torso, thigh, or upper arm by pressing the patch firmly against the skin for 20–30 seconds. Patches should be removed after 24 hours and the replacement patch applied on a different area (avoid using the same area for 14 days)—consult product literature for further information.

● PATIENT AND CARER ADVICE

Driving and skilled tasks

Sudden onset of sleep Excessive daytime sleepiness and sudden onset of sleep can occur with dopamine-receptor agonists.

Patients starting treatment with these drugs should be warned of the risk of and of the need to exercise caution when driving or operating machinery. Those who have experienced excessive sedation or sudden onset of sleep should refrain from driving or operating machines until these effects have stopped occurring.

Management of excessive daytime sleepiness should focus on the identification of an underlying cause, such as depression or concomitant medication. Patients should be counselled on improving sleep behaviour.

Hypotensive reactions Hypotensive reactions can occur in some patients taking dopamine-receptor agonists; these can be particularly problematic during the first few days of treatment and care should be exercised when driving or operating machinery.

● NATIONAL FUNDING/ACCESS DECISIONS

Scottish Medicines Consortium (SMC) Decisions

The *Scottish Medicines Consortium* has advised that *Neupro®* is accepted for restricted use for the treatment of advanced Parkinson's disease in combination with levodopa where the transdermal route would facilitate treatment (July 2007).

The *Scottish Medicines Consortium* has advised that *Neupro®* is accepted as monotherapy for the treatment of early-stage idiopathic Parkinson's disease (June 2007).

The *Scottish Medicines Consortium* has advised (April 2009) that rotigotine (*Neupro®*) is accepted for restricted use within NHS Scotland for the symptomatic treatment of moderate to severe idiopathic restless legs syndrome in

Nervous system

4

adults with a baseline score of 15 points or more on the International Restless Legs Scale.

● MEDICINAL FORMS
There can be variation in the licensing of different medicines containing the same drug.
Transdermal patch
CAUTIONARY AND ADVISORY LABELS 10
▸ Neupro (UCB Pharma Ltd)
Rotigotine 1 mg per 24 hour Neupro 1mg/24hours transdermal patches | 28 patch [PoM] £77.24
Rotigotine 2 mg per 24 hour Neupro 2mg/24hours transdermal patches | 28 patch [PoM] £81.10 DT = £81.10
Rotigotine 3 mg per 24 hour Neupro 3mg/24hours transdermal patches | 28 patch [PoM] £102.35
Rotigotine 4 mg per 24 hour Neupro 4mg/24hours transdermal patches | 28 patch [PoM] £123.60 DT = £123.60
Rotigotine 6 mg per 24 hour Neupro 6mg/24hours transdermal patches | 28 patch [PoM] £149.93 DT = £149.93
Rotigotine 8 mg per 24 hour Neupro 8mg/24hours transdermal patches | 28 patch [PoM] £149.93 DT = £149.93

DOPAMINERGIC DRUGS > MONOAMINE-OXIDASE B INHIBITORS

Rasagiline

● DRUG ACTION Rasagiline is a monoamine-oxidase B inhibitor.

● INDICATIONS AND DOSE

Parkinson's disease, used alone or as adjunct to co-beneldopa or co-careldopa for 'end-of-dose' fluctuations
▸ BY MOUTH
▸ Adult: 1 mg daily

● INTERACTIONS → Appendix 1: monoamine-oxidase B inhibitors

● SIDE-EFFECTS
▸ **Common or very common** Abdominal pain · abnormal dreams · angina pectoris · arthralgia · arthritis · conjunctivitis · depression · dermatitis · dry mouth · fall · fever · flatulence · hallucination · headache · increased risk of infection · leucopenia · malaise · nausea · neoplasms · pain · postural hypotension · urinary urgency · vertigo · vomiting · weight decreased
▸ **Uncommon** Appetite decreased · confusion
▸ **Frequency not known** Eating disorders · pathological gambling · psychiatric disorders · sexual dysfunction

● PREGNANCY Use with caution.

● BREAST FEEDING Use with caution—may suppress lactation.

● HEPATIC IMPAIRMENT Use with caution in mild impairment. Avoid in moderate to severe impairment.

● TREATMENT CESSATION Avoid abrupt withdrawal.

● MEDICINAL FORMS
There can be variation in the licensing of different medicines containing the same drug. Forms available from special-order manufacturers include: oral suspension, oral solution
Tablet
▸ Rasagiline (Non-proprietary)
Rasagiline 1 mg Rasagiline 1mg tablets | 28 tablet [PoM] £70.72 DT = £5.29
▸ Azilect (Teva UK Ltd)
Rasagiline 1 mg Azilect 1mg tablets | 28 tablet [PoM] £70.72 DT = £5.29

Safinamide

18-Jul-2017

● DRUG ACTION Safinamide is a monoamine-oxidase-B inhibitor.

● INDICATIONS AND DOSE

Parkinson's disease, as an adjunct to levodopa alone or in combination with other antiparkinsonian drugs, for mid- to late-stage fluctuations
▸ BY MOUTH
▸ Adult: 50 mg once daily, increased if necessary to 100 mg once daily

● CONTRA-INDICATIONS Active retinopathy · albinism · family history of hereditary retinal disease · retinal degeneration · uveitis

● CAUTIONS Hypertension (may raise blood pressure) · may exacerbate pre-existing dyskinesia (requiring levodopa dose reduction)

● INTERACTIONS → Appendix 1: monoamine-oxidase B inhibitors

● SIDE-EFFECTS
▸ **Common or very common** Cataract · dizziness · drowsiness · headache · hypotension · injury · nausea · sleep disorders
▸ **Uncommon** Anaemia · anxiety · appetite abnormal · arrhythmias · asthenia · cognitive disorder · confusion · constipation · cough · decreased leucocytes · depression · diarrhoea · dry mouth · dysarthria · dyslipidaemia · dyspnoea · emotional lability · eye disorders · eye inflammation · gastrointestinal discomfort · gastrointestinal disorders · glaucoma · hallucination · hyperglycaemia · hypertension · increased risk of infection · joint disorders · movement disorders · muscle complaints · muscle weakness · neoplasms · oral disorders · pain · palpitations · peripheral oedema · photosensitivity reaction · psychotic disorder · QT interval prolongation · red blood cell abnormality · rhinorrhoea · sensation abnormal · sensation of pressure · sexual dysfunction · skin reactions · sweat changes · syncope · temperature sensation altered · urinary disorders · varicose veins · vertigo · vision disorders · vomiting · weight changes
▸ **Rare or very rare** Alopecia · arterial spasm · atherosclerosis · benign prostatic hyperplasia · breast abnormalities · bronchospasm · cachexia · concentration impaired · delirium · diabetic retinopathy · drug effect decreased · dysphonia · eosinophilia · eye pain · fat embolism · fever · gambling · haemorrhage · hyperbilirubinaemia · hyperkalaemia · illusion · malaise · myocardial infarction · oropharyngeal complaints · osteoarthritis · paranoia · psychiatric disorders · pyuria · reflexes decreased · suicidal ideation · taste altered

● PREGNANCY Manufacturer advises avoid—toxicity in *animal* studies.

● BREAST FEEDING Manufacturer advises avoid—present in milk in *animal* studies.

● HEPATIC IMPAIRMENT Manufacturer advises caution in moderate impairment; avoid in severe impairment.
Dose adjustments Manufacturer advises max. daily dose should not exceed 50 mg daily in moderate impairment.

● MEDICINAL FORMS
There can be variation in the licensing of different medicines containing the same drug.
Tablet
▸ Xadago (Profile Pharma Ltd) ▼
Safinamide (as Safinamide methansulfonate) 50 mg Xadago 50mg tablets | 30 tablet [PoM] £69.00 DT = £69.00
Safinamide (as Safinamide methansulfonate) 100 mg Xadago 100mg tablets | 30 tablet [PoM] £69.00 DT = £69.00

Selegiline hydrochloride

● DRUG ACTION   Selegiline is a monoamine-oxidase-B inhibitor.

● INDICATIONS AND DOSE

Parkinson's disease, used alone or as adjunct to co-beneldopa or co-careldopa to reduce 'end of dose' deterioration | Symptomatic parkinsonism
▸ BY MOUTH USING IMMEDIATE-RELEASE MEDICINES
▸ Adult: Initially 5 mg once daily for 2–4 weeks, then increased if tolerated to 10 mg daily, dose to be taken in the morning
▸ BY MOUTH USING ORAL LYOPHILISATE
▸ Adult: 1.25 mg once daily, dose to be taken before breakfast
DOSE EQUIVALENCE AND CONVERSION
▸ 1.25-mg oral lyophilisate is equivalent to 10-mg tablet.
▸ Patients receiving 10 mg conventional selegiline hydrochloride tablets can be switched to oral lyophilisates (*Zelapar*®) 1.25 mg.

● CONTRA-INDICATIONS   Active duodenal ulceration · active gastric ulceration · avoid or use with great caution in postural hypotension (when used in combination with levodopa)
● CAUTIONS   Angina · arrhythmias · duodenal ulceration · gastric ulceration · history of hepatic dysfunction · patients predisposed to confusion and psychosis · psychosis · uncontrolled hypertension
● INTERACTIONS   → Appendix 1: monoamine-oxidase B inhibitors
● SIDE-EFFECTS
▸ **Common or very common** Arrhythmias · arthralgia · back pain · confusion · constipation · depression · diarrhoea · dizziness · dry mouth · fall · fatigue · hallucination · headache · hyperhidrosis · hypertension · hypotension · movement disorders · muscle cramps · nasal congestion · nausea · oral disorders · sleep disorders · throat pain · tremor · vertigo
▸ **Uncommon** Alopecia · angina pectoris · anxiety · appetite decreased · chest pain · dyspnoea · leucopenia · mood altered · myopathy · palpitations · peripheral oedema · pharyngitis · psychosis · skin eruption · thrombocytopenia · urinary disorders · vision blurred
▸ **Frequency not known** Hypersexuality
SIDE-EFFECTS, FURTHER INFORMATION   Side-effects of levodopa may be increased—concurrent levodopa dosage can be reduced by 10–30% in steps of 10% every 3–4 days.
● PREGNANCY   Avoid—no information available.
● BREAST FEEDING   Avoid—no information available.
● HEPATIC IMPAIRMENT   Use with caution in severe impairment.
● RENAL IMPAIRMENT   Use with caution in severe impairment.
● TREATMENT CESSATION   Avoid abrupt withdrawal.
● DIRECTIONS FOR ADMINISTRATION   Oral lyophilisates should be placed on the tongue and allowed to dissolve. Advise patient not to drink, rinse, or wash mouth out for 5 minutes after taking the tablet.
● PATIENT AND CARER ADVICE   Patients or carers should be advised on how to administer selegiline hydrochloride oral lyophilisates.
Driving and skilled tasks
Drugs and driving Prescribers and other healthcare professionals should advise patients if treatment is likely to affect their ability to perform skilled tasks (e.g. driving). This applies especially to drugs with sedative effects; patients should be warned that these effects are increased by alcohol. General information about a patient's fitness to drive is available from the Driver and Vehicle Licensing Agency at www.dvla.gov.uk.
2015 legislation regarding driving whilst taking certain drugs, may also apply to selegiline, see *Drugs and driving* under Guidance on prescribing p. 1.

● MEDICINAL FORMS
There can be variation in the licensing of different medicines containing the same drug. Forms available from special-order manufacturers include: oral solution
Tablet
▸ Selegiline hydrochloride (Non-proprietary)
  Selegiline hydrochloride 5 mg Selegiline 5mg tablets | 60 tablet [PoM] £28.08
  Selegiline hydrochloride 10 mg Selegiline 10mg tablets | 30 tablet [PoM] £27.20
▸ Eldepryl (Orion Pharma (UK) Ltd)
  Selegiline hydrochloride 5 mg Eldepryl 5mg tablets | 100 tablet [PoM] £16.52 DT = £16.52
  Selegiline hydrochloride 10 mg Eldepryl 10mg tablets | 100 tablet [PoM] £32.23 DT = £32.23
Oral lyophilisate
EXCIPIENTS: May contain Aspartame
▸ Zelapar (Teva UK Ltd)
  Selegiline hydrochloride 1.25 mg Zelapar 1.25mg oral lyophilisates sugar-free | 30 tablet [PoM] £43.16 DT = £43.16

5   Nausea and labyrinth disorders

Nausea and labyrinth disorders

Drug treatment

Antiemetics should be prescribed only when the cause of vomiting is known because otherwise they may delay diagnosis, particularly in children. Antiemetics are unnecessary and sometimes harmful when the cause can be treated, such as in diabetic ketoacidosis, or in digoxin p. 109 or antiepileptic overdose.

If antiemetic drug treatment is indicated, the drug is chosen according to the aetiology of vomiting.

Antihistamines are effective against nausea and vomiting resulting from many underlying conditions. There is no evidence that any one antihistamine is superior to another but their duration of action and incidence of adverse effects (drowsiness and antimuscarinic effects) differ.

The **phenothiazines** are dopamine antagonists and act centrally by blocking the chemoreceptor trigger zone. They are of considerable value for the prophylaxis and treatment of nausea and vomiting associated with diffuse neoplastic disease, radiation sickness, and the emesis caused by drugs such as opioids, general anaesthetics, and cytotoxics. Prochlorperazine p. 385, perphenazine p. 384, and trifluoperazine p. 387 are less sedating than chlorpromazine hydrochloride p. 381; severe dystonic reactions sometimes occur with phenothiazines, especially in children. Some phenothiazines are available as rectal suppositories, which can be useful in patients with persistent vomiting or with severe nausea; prochlorperazine can also be administered as a buccal tablet which is placed between the upper lip and the gum.

Other antipsychotic drugs including haloperidol p. 382 and levomepromazine p. 435 are used for the relief of nausea and vomiting in terminal illness.

Metoclopramide hydrochloride p. 426 is an effective antiemetic and its activity closely resembles that of the phenothiazines. Metoclopramide hydrochloride also acts directly on the gastro-intestinal tract and it may be superior to the phenothiazines for emesis associated with gastroduodenal, hepatic, and biliary disease.

Domperidone p. 426 acts at the chemoreceptor trigger zone; it is licensed only for the relief of nausea and vomiting. It has the advantage over metoclopramide hydrochloride and the phenothiazines of being less likely to cause central effects such as sedation and dystonic reactions because it does not readily cross the blood-brain barrier. In Parkinson's disease, it can be used to treat nausea caused by dopaminergic drugs.

Granisetron p. 429 and ondansetron p. 430 are of value in the management of nausea and vomiting in patients receiving cytotoxics and in postoperative nausea and vomiting. Palonosetron p. 431 is licensed for prevention of nausea and vomiting associated with moderately or highly emetogenic cytotoxic chemotherapy. Palonosetron is also available in combination with netupitant, a neurokinin 1-receptor antagonist, for the prevention of acute and delayed nausea and vomiting associated with moderately emetogenic chemotherapy and highly emetogenic cisplatin-based chemotherapy.

Dexamethasone p. 660 has antiemetic effects and it is used in vomiting associated with cancer chemotherapy. It can be used alone or with metoclopramide hydrochloride, prochlorperazine, lorazepam p. 335, or a 5HT$_3$-receptor antagonist.

Aprepitant p. 427, fosaprepitant p. 428, and rolapitant p. 428 are neurokinin 1-receptor antagonists. Aprepitant is licensed for the prevention of nausea and vomiting associated with highly and moderately emetogenic chemotherapy; fosaprepitant is licensed for the prevention of acute and delayed nausea and vomiting associated with highly emetogenic cisplatin-based chemotherapy and the prevention of nausea and vomiting associated with moderately emetogenic chemotherapy; rolapitant is licensed for the prevention of delayed nausea and vomiting associated with highly and moderately emetogenic chemotherapy. These drugs are given with dexamethasone and a 5HT$_3$-receptor antagonist.

Nabilone p. 425 is a synthetic cannabinoid with antiemetic properties. It may be used for nausea and vomiting caused by cytotoxic chemotherapy that is unresponsive to conventional antiemetics.

Vomiting during pregnancy

Nausea in the first trimester of pregnancy is generally mild and does not require drug therapy. On rare occasions if vomiting is severe, short-term treatment with an antihistamine, such as **promethazine**, may be required. Prochlorperazine or metoclopramide hydrochloride are alternatives. If symptoms do not settle in 24 to 48 hours then specialist opinion should be sought. Hyperemesis gravidarum is a more serious condition, which requires regular antiemetic therapy, intravenous fluid and electrolyte replacement and sometimes nutritional support. Supplementation with thiamine p. 1048 must be considered in order to reduce the risk of Wernicke's encephalopathy.

Postoperative nausea and vomiting

The incidence of postoperative nausea and vomiting depends on many factors including the anaesthetic used, and the type and duration of surgery. Other risk factors include female sex, non-smokers, a history of postoperative nausea and vomiting or motion sickness, and intraoperative and postoperative use of opioids. Therapy to prevent postoperative nausea and vomiting should be based on the assessed risk of postoperative nausea and vomiting in each patient. Drugs used include **5HT$_3$-receptor antagonists**, droperidol p. 434, dexamethasone, some **phenothiazines** (e.g. prochlorperazine), and **antihistamines** (e.g. cyclizine below). A combination of two or more antiemetic drugs that have different mechanisms of action is often indicated in those at high risk of postoperative nausea and vomiting or where postoperative vomiting presents a particular danger (e.g. in some types of surgery). When a prophylactic

antiemetic drug has failed, postoperative nausea and vomiting should be treated with one or more drugs from a different class.

Motion sickness

Antiemetics should be given to prevent motion sickness rather than after nausea or vomiting develop. The most effective drug for the prevention of motion sickness is hyoscine hydrobromide p. 433. The sedating antihistamines are slightly less effective against motion sickness, but are generally better tolerated than hyoscine. If a sedative effect is desired **promethazine** is useful, but generally a slightly less sedating antihistamine such as cyclizine or cinnarizine p. 432 is preferred. Domperidone, metoclopramide hydrochloride, 5HT$_3$-receptor antagonists, and the phenothiazines (except the antihistamine phenothiazine promethazine) are **ineffective** in motion sickness.

Other vestibular disorders

Management of vestibular diseases is aimed at treating the underlying cause as well as treating symptoms of the balance disturbance and associated nausea and vomiting. Vertigo and nausea associated with Ménière's disease and middle-ear surgery can be difficult to treat.

Betahistine dihydrochloride p. 435 is an analogue of histamine and is claimed to reduce endolymphatic pressure by improving the microcirculation. Betahistine dihydrochloride is licensed for vertigo, tinnitus, and hearing loss associated with Ménière's disease.

A **diuretic** alone or combined with salt restriction may provide some benefit in vertigo associated with Ménière's disease; **antihistamines** (such as cinnarizine), and **phenothiazines** (such as prochlorperazine) are also used. Where possible, prochlorperazine should be reserved for the treatment of acute symptoms.

Nausea caused by cytotoxic chemotherapy, palliative care, and migraine

Antiemetics have a role in the management of nausea and vomiting induced by cytotoxic chemotherapy, in palliative care, and associated with migraine.

> **Other drugs used for Nausea and labyrinth disorders**
> Paracetamol with metoclopramide, p. 469 · Promethazine hydrochloride, p. 286

ANTIEMETICS AND ANTINAUSEANTS >
ANTIHISTAMINES

Cyclizine

● **INDICATIONS AND DOSE**

Nausea | Vomiting | Vertigo | Motion sickness | Labyrinthine disorders
▸ BY MOUTH
▸ Adult: 50 mg up to 3 times a day, for motion sickness, take 1–2 hours before departure
▸ BY INTRAVENOUS INJECTION, OR BY INTRAMUSCULAR INJECTION
▸ Adult: 50 mg 3 times a day

Nausea and vomiting of known cause | Nausea and vomiting associated with vestibular disorders and palliative care
▸ BY MOUTH, OR BY INTRAVENOUS INJECTION
▸ Child 1 month-5 years: 0.5–1 mg/kg up to 3 times a day (max. per dose 25 mg), intravenous injection to be given over 3–5 minutes, for motion sickness, take 1–2 hours before departure

▸ **Child 6-11 years:** 25 mg up to 3 times a day, intravenous injection to be given over 3-5 minutes, for motion sickness, take 1-2 hours before departure
▸ **Child 12-17 years:** 50 mg up to 3 times a day, intravenous injection to be given over 3-5 minutes, for motion sickness, take 1-2 hours before departure
▸ BY RECTUM
▸ **Child 2-5 years:** 12.5 mg up to 3 times a day
▸ **Child 6-11 years:** 25 mg up to 3 times a day
▸ **Child 12-17 years:** 50 mg up to 3 times a day
▸ BY CONTINUOUS INTRAVENOUS INFUSION, OR BY SUBCUTANEOUS INFUSION
▸ **Child 1-23 months:** 3 mg/kg, dose to be given over 24 hours
▸ **Child 2-5 years:** 50 mg, dose to be given over 24 hours
▸ **Child 6-11 years:** 75 mg, dose to be given over 24 hours
▸ **Child 12-17 years:** 150 mg, dose to be given over 24 hours

Nausea and vomiting associated with palliative care
▸ BY SUBCUTANEOUS INFUSION
▸ **Adult:** 150 mg, dose to be given over 24 hours
▸ BY MOUTH
▸ **Adult:** 50 mg up to 3 times a day

● UNLICENSED USE Tablets not licensed for use in children under 6 years. Injection not licensed for use in children.
● CAUTIONS Epilepsy · glaucoma (in children) · may counteract haemodynamic benefits of opioids · neuromuscular disorders—increased risk of transient paralysis with intravenous use · prostatic hypertrophy (in adults) · pyloroduodenal obstruction · severe heart failure—may cause fall in cardiac output and associated increase in heart rate, mean arterial pressure and pulmonary wedge pressure · susceptibility to angle-closure glaucoma (in adults) · urinary retention
● INTERACTIONS → Appendix 1: antihistamines, sedating
● SIDE-EFFECTS
GENERAL SIDE-EFFECTS
▸ **Rare or very rare** Angle closure glaucoma · depression
▸ **Frequency not known** Abdominal pain · agranulocytosis · angioedema · anxiety · apnoea · appetite decreased · arrhythmias · asthenia · bronchospasm · constipation · diarrhoea · disorientation · dizziness · drowsiness · dry mouth · dry throat · euphoric mood · haemolytic anaemia · hallucinations · headache · hepatic disorders · hypertension · hypotension · increased gastric reflux · insomnia · leucopenia · movement disorders · muscle complaints · nasal dryness · nausea · oculogyric crisis · palpitations · paraesthesia · photosensitivity reaction · seizure · skin reactions · speech disorder · thrombocytopenia · tinnitus · tremor · urinary retention · vision blurred · vomiting
SPECIFIC SIDE-EFFECTS
▸ **Rare or very rare**
▸ With oral use Agitation (more common with high doses in children and elderly)
▸ **Frequency not known**
▸ With oral use Level of consciousness decreased
▸ With parenteral use Chills · consciousness impaired · pain · paralysis · sensation of pressure
● PREGNANCY Manufacturer advises avoid; however, there is no evidence of teratogenicity. The use of sedating antihistamines in the latter part of the third trimester may cause adverse effects in neonates such as irritability, paradoxical excitability, and tremor.
● BREAST FEEDING No information available. Most antihistamines are present in breast milk in varying amounts; although not known to be harmful, most manufacturers advise avoiding their use in mothers who are breast-feeding.

● HEPATIC IMPAIRMENT Avoid in severe liver disease—increased risk of coma.
● DIRECTIONS FOR ADMINISTRATION For administration *by mouth*, tablets may be crushed.
Mixing and compatibility for the use of syringe drivers in palliative care Cyclizine may precipitate at concentrations above 10 mg/mL or in the presence of sodium chloride 0.9% *or* as the concentration of diamorphine relative to cyclizine increases; mixtures of diamorphine and cyclizine are also likely to precipitate after 24 hours.
● PATIENT AND CARER ADVICE
Driving and skilled tasks Drowsiness may affect performance of skilled tasks (e.g. cycling, driving); effects of alcohol enhanced.

● MEDICINAL FORMS
There can be variation in the licensing of different medicines containing the same drug. Forms available from special-order manufacturers include: oral suspension, oral solution, suppository
Tablet
CAUTIONARY AND ADVISORY LABELS 2
▸ Cyclizine (Non-proprietary)
  Cyclizine hydrochloride 50 mg Cyclizine 50mg tablets | 30 tablet P £2.24-£5.00 | 100 tablet P £13.64 DT = £7.47
Solution for injection
▸ Cyclizine (Non-proprietary)
  Cyclizine lactate 50 mg per 1 ml Cyclizine 50mg/1ml solution for injection ampoules | 5 ampoule PoM £13.54 DT = £13.54

ANTIEMETICS AND ANTINAUSEANTS ›
CANNABINOIDS

Nabilone

● INDICATIONS AND DOSE
Nausea and vomiting caused by cytotoxic chemotherapy, unresponsive to conventional antiemetics (preferably in hospital setting) (under close medical supervision)
▸ BY MOUTH
▸ **Adult:** Initially 1 mg twice daily, increased if necessary to 2 mg twice daily throughout each cycle of cytotoxic therapy and, if necessary, for 48 hours after the last dose of each cycle, the first dose should be taken the night before initiation of cytotoxic treatment and the second dose 1-3 hours before the first dose of cytotoxic drug, daily dose maximum should be given in 3 divided doses; maximum 6 mg per day

● CAUTIONS Adverse effects on mental state can persist for 48-72 hours after stopping · elderly · heart disease · history of psychiatric disorder · hypertension
● INTERACTIONS → Appendix 1: nabilone
● SIDE-EFFECTS Abdominal pain · appetite decreased · concentration impaired · confusion · depression · dizziness · drowsiness · drug use disorders · dry mouth · euphoric mood · feeling of relaxation · hallucination · headache · hypotension · movement disorders · nausea · psychosis · sleep disorder · tachycardia · tremor · vertigo · visual impairment
SIDE-EFFECTS, FURTHER INFORMATION Drowsiness and dizziness occur frequently with standard doses.
● PREGNANCY Avoid unless essential.
● BREAST FEEDING Avoid—no information available.
● HEPATIC IMPAIRMENT Avoid in severe impairment.
● PATIENT AND CARER ADVICE
Behavioural effects Patients should be made aware of possible changes of mood and other adverse behavioural effects.
Driving and skilled tasks Drowsiness may affect performance of skilled tasks (e.g. driving).

4

Nervous system

Effects of alcohol enhanced.

For information on 2015 legislation regarding driving whilst taking certain controlled drugs, including nabilone, see *Drugs and driving* under Guidance on prescribing p. 1.

● MEDICINAL FORMS
There can be variation in the licensing of different medicines containing the same drug. Forms available from special-order manufacturers include: capsule

Capsule
CAUTIONARY AND ADVISORY LABELS 2
▶ Nabilone (Non-proprietary)
  Nabilone 250 microgram Nabilone 250microgram capsules | 20 capsule PoM £150.00 DT = £150.00 CD2
  Nabilone 1 mg Nabilone 1mg capsules | 20 capsule PoM £196.00 DT = £196.00 CD2

ANTIEMETICS AND ANTINAUSEANTS ›
DOPAMINE RECEPTOR ANTAGONISTS

Domperidone

17-Oct-2016

● INDICATIONS AND DOSE
Relief of nausea and vomiting
▶ BY MOUTH
▶ Child (body-weight up to 35 kg): 250 micrograms/kg up to 3 times a day; maximum 750 micrograms/kg per day
▶ Child 12-17 years (body-weight 35 kg and above): 10 mg up to 3 times a day; maximum 30 mg per day
▶ Adult (body-weight 35 kg and above): 10 mg up to 3 times a day; maximum 30 mg per day

Gastro-intestinal pain in palliative care
▶ BY MOUTH
▶ Adult: 10 mg 3 times a day, before meals

IMPORTANT SAFETY INFORMATION
MHRA/CHM ADVICE—DOMPERIDONE: RISK OF CARDIAC SIDE-EFFECTS—RESTRICTED INDICATION, NEW CONTRA-INDICATIONS, REDUCED DOSE AND DURATION OF USE
The benefits and risks of domperidone have been reviewed. As domperidone is associated with a small increased risk of serious cardiac side-effects, the following restrictions to indication, dose and duration of treatment have been made, and new contra-indications added:

• Domperidone should only be used for the relief of the symptoms of nausea and vomiting;
• Domperidone should be used at the lowest effective dose for the shortest possible duration (max. treatment duration should not normally exceed 1 week);
• Domperidone is contra-indicated for use in conditions where cardiac conduction is, or could be impaired, or where there is underlying cardiac disease, when administered concomitantly with drugs that prolong the QT interval or potent CYP3A4 inhibitors, and in severe hepatic impairment;
• The recommended dose in adults and adolescents over 12 years and over 35 kg is 10 mg up to 3 times daily;
• The recommended dose in children under 35 kg is 250 micrograms/kg up to 3 times daily;
• Oral liquid formulations should be given via an appropriately designed, graduated oral syringe to ensure dose accuracy.
This advice does not apply to unlicensed uses of domperidone (e.g. palliative care).

● CONTRA-INDICATIONS Cardiac disease · conditions where cardiac conduction is, or could be, impaired (in adults) · gastro-intestinal haemorrhage (in children) · if increased gastrointestinal motility harmful (in adults) · mechanical obstruction (in children) · mechanical perforation (in

children) · predisposition to cardiac conduction disorders (in children) · prolactinoma
● CAUTIONS Children · if there are cardiac concerns, obtain ECG before and during treatment (in children) · patients over 60 years—increased risk of ventricular arrhythmia
● INTERACTIONS → Appendix 1: domperidone
● SIDE-EFFECTS
▶ **Common or very common** Dry mouth
▶ **Uncommon** Anxiety · asthenia · breast abnormalities · diarrhoea · drowsiness · headache · lactation disorders · libido loss
▶ **Frequency not known** Arrhythmias · depression · gynaecomastia · menstrual cycle irregularities · movement disorders · oculogyric crisis · QT interval prolongation · seizure · sudden cardiac death · urinary retention
● PREGNANCY Use only if potential benefit outweighs risk.
● BREAST FEEDING Amount too small to be harmful.
● HEPATIC IMPAIRMENT Avoid in moderate or severe impairment.
● RENAL IMPAIRMENT
Dose adjustments Reduce frequency.
● PRESCRIBING AND DISPENSING INFORMATION
Palliative care For further information on the use of domperidone in palliative care, see www.palliativedrugs.com/formulary/en/domperidone.html.
● PATIENT AND CARER ADVICE
Arrhythmia Patients and their carers should be told how to recognise signs of arrhythmia and advised to seek medical attention if symptoms such as palpitation or syncope develop.

● MEDICINAL FORMS
There can be variation in the licensing of different medicines containing the same drug. Forms available from special-order manufacturers include: oral suspension

Oral suspension
CAUTIONARY AND ADVISORY LABELS 22
▶ Domperidone (non-proprietary) ▼
  Domperidone 1 mg per 1 ml Domperidone 1mg/ml oral suspension sugar free sugar-free | 200 ml PoM £13.43 DT = £13.43

Tablet
CAUTIONARY AND ADVISORY LABELS 22
▶ Domperidone (non-proprietary) ▼
  Domperidone (as Domperidone maleate) 10 mg Domperidone 10mg tablets | 30 tablet PoM £2.71 DT = £0.79 | 100 tablet PoM £9.04 DT = £2.63
▶ Motilium (Zentiva) ▼
  Domperidone (as Domperidone maleate) 10 mg Motilium 10mg tablets | 30 tablet PoM £2.71 DT = £0.79 | 100 tablet PoM £9.04 DT = £2.63

Metoclopramide hydrochloride

21-Nov-2016

● INDICATIONS AND DOSE
Symptomatic treatment of nausea and vomiting including that associated with acute migraine | Delayed (but not acute) chemotherapy-induced nausea and vomiting | Radiotherapy-induced nausea and vomiting | Prevention of postoperative nausea and vomiting
▶ BY MOUTH, OR BY INTRAMUSCULAR INJECTION, OR BY SLOW INTRAVENOUS INJECTION
▶ Adult (body-weight up to 60 kg): Up to 500 micrograms/kg daily in 3 divided doses, when administered by slow intravenous injection, to be given over at least 3 minutes
▶ Adult (body-weight 60 kg and above): 10 mg up to 3 times a day, when administered by slow intravenous injection, to be given over at least 3 minutes

Hiccup in palliative care
▸ BY MOUTH, OR BY INTRAMUSCULAR INJECTION, OR BY
  SUBCUTANEOUS INJECTION
▸ Adult: 10 mg every 6–8 hours

Nausea and vomiting in palliative care
▸ BY MOUTH
▸ Adult: 10 mg 3 times a day
▸ BY SUBCUTANEOUS INFUSION
▸ Adult: 30–100 mg/24 hours

IMPORTANT SAFETY INFORMATION

MHRA/CHM ADVICE—METOCLOPRAMIDE: RISK OF NEUROLOGICAL
ADVERSE EFFECTS—RESTRICTED DOSE AND DURATION OF USE
(AUGUST 2013)

The benefits and risks of metoclopramide have been
reviewed by the European Medicines Agency's
Committee on Medicinal Products for Human Use, which
concluded that the risk of neurological effects such as
extrapyramidal disorders and tardive dyskinesia
outweigh the benefits in long-term or high-dose
treatment. To help minimise the risk of potentially
serious neurological adverse effects, the following
restrictions to indications, dose, and duration of use
have been made:

• In adults over 18 years, metoclopramide should only
  be used for prevention of postoperative nausea and
  vomiting, radiotherapy-induced nausea and vomiting,
  delayed (but not acute) chemotherapy-induced nausea
  and vomiting, and symptomatic treatment of nausea
  and vomiting, including that associated with acute
  migraine (where it may also be used to improve
  absorption of oral analgesics);
• Metoclopramide should only be prescribed for short-
  term use (up to 5 days);
• Usual dose is 10 mg, repeated up to 3 times daily; max.
  daily dose is 500 micrograms/kg;
• Intravenous doses should be administered as a slow
  bolus over at least 3 minutes;
• Oral liquid formulations should be given via an
  appropriately designed, graduated oral syringe to
  ensure dose accuracy.

This advice does not apply to unlicensed uses of
metoclopramide (e.g. palliative care).

• **CONTRA-INDICATIONS** 3–4 days after gastrointestinal
  surgery · gastro-intestinal haemorrhage · gastro-intestinal
  obstruction · gastro-intestinal perforation ·
  phaeochromocytoma
• **CAUTIONS** Asthma · atopic allergy · bradycardia · cardiac
  conduction disturbances · children · elderly · epilepsy · may
  mask underlying disorders such as cerebral irritation ·
  Parkinson's disease · uncorrected electrolyte imbalance ·
  young adults (15–19 years old)
• **INTERACTIONS** → Appendix 1: metoclopramide
• **SIDE-EFFECTS**

  GENERAL SIDE-EFFECTS
▸ **Common or very common** Asthenia · depression · diarrhoea
  · drowsiness · hypotension · menstrual cycle irregularities ·
  movement disorders · parkinsonism
▸ **Uncommon** Arrhythmias · hallucination ·
  hyperprolactinaemia · level of consciousness decreased
▸ **Rare or very rare** Confusion · galactorrhoea · seizure
▸ **Frequency not known** Atrioventricular block · blood
  disorders · cardiac arrest · gynaecomastia · hypertension ·
  neuroleptic malignant syndrome · QT interval
  prolongation · shock · syncope

  SPECIFIC SIDE-EFFECTS
▸ **Frequency not known**
▸ With parenteral use Anxiety · dizziness · dyspnoea · oedema ·
  skin reactions · tremor · visual impairment

SIDE-EFFECTS, FURTHER INFORMATION Metoclopramide
can induce acute dystonic reactions involving facial and
skeletal muscle spasms and oculogyric crises. These
dystonic effects are more common in the young (especially
girls and young women) and the very old; they usually
occur shortly after starting treatment with
metoclopramide and subside within 24 hours of stopping
it. Injection of an antiparkinsonian drug such as
procyclidine will abort dystonic attacks.

• **PREGNANCY** Not known to be harmful.
• **BREAST FEEDING** Small amount present in milk; avoid.
• **HEPATIC IMPAIRMENT**
  Dose adjustments Reduce dose.
• **RENAL IMPAIRMENT**
  Dose adjustments Avoid or use small dose in severe
  impairment; increased risk of extrapyramidal reactions.
• **DIRECTIONS FOR ADMINISTRATION** Oral liquid preparation
  to be given via a graduated oral dosing syringe.
• **PRESCRIBING AND DISPENSING INFORMATION**
  Palliative care For further information on the use of
  metoclopramide hydrochloride in palliative care, see
  www.palliativedrugs.com/formulary/en/metoclopramide.html.
• **PATIENT AND CARER ADVICE** Counselling on use of pipette
  advised with oral solution.

• **MEDICINAL FORMS**
  There can be variation in the licensing of different medicines
  containing the same drug. Forms available from special-order
  manufacturers include: oral solution

  Solution for injection
▸ Metoclopramide hydrochloride (Non-proprietary)
  Metoclopramide hydrochloride 5 mg per 1 ml Metoclopramide
  10mg/2ml solution for injection ampoules | 5 ampoule [PoM] £1.31 |
  10 ampoule [PoM] £3.30 DT = £3.30
▸ Maxolon (AMCo)
  Metoclopramide hydrochloride 5 mg per 1 ml Maxolon 10mg/2ml
  solution for injection ampoules | 12 ampoule [PoM] £3.21
  Maxolon High Dose 100mg/20ml solution for injection ampoules |
  10 ampoule [PoM] £26.68

  Oral solution
▸ Metoclopramide hydrochloride (Non-proprietary)
  Metoclopramide hydrochloride 1 mg per 1 ml Metoclopramide
  5mg/5ml oral solution sugar free sugar-free | 150 ml [PoM] £19.77 DT
  = £19.77

  Tablet
▸ Metoclopramide hydrochloride (Non-proprietary)
  Metoclopramide hydrochloride 10 mg Metoclopramide 10mg
  tablets | 28 tablet [PoM] £1.40 DT = £0.33
▸ Maxolon (AMCo)
  Metoclopramide hydrochloride 10 mg Maxolon 10mg tablets |
  84 tablet [PoM] £5.24

  Combinations available: *Paracetamol with metoclopramide,*
  p. 469

ANTIEMETICS AND ANTINAUSEANTS ›
NEUROKININ RECEPTOR ANTAGONISTS

Aprepitant   13-Sep-2017

• **INDICATIONS AND DOSE**

  **Adjunct treatment to prevent nausea and vomiting
  associated with moderately and highly emetogenic
  chemotherapy**
▸ BY MOUTH
▸ Adult: Initially 125 mg, dose to be taken 1 hour before
  chemotherapy, then 80 mg once daily for 2 days,
  consult product literature for dose of concomitant
  dexamethasone and $5HT_3$-antagonist

• **CONTRA-INDICATIONS** Acute porphyrias p. 1025
• **INTERACTIONS** → Appendix 1: aprepitant

- SIDE-EFFECTS
▶ **Common or very common** Appetite decreased · asthenia · constipation · gastrointestinal discomfort · headache · hiccups
▶ **Uncommon** Anaemia · anxiety · burping · dizziness · drowsiness · dry mouth · febrile neutropenia · gastrointestinal disorders · hot flush · malaise · nausea · palpitations · skin reactions · urinary disorders · vomiting
▶ **Rare or very rare** Bradycardia · cardiovascular disorder · chest discomfort · cognitive disorder · conjunctivitis · cough · disorientation · euphoric mood · gait abnormal · hyperhidrosis · increased risk of infection · muscle spasms · muscle weakness · oedema · oropharyngeal pain · photosensitivity reaction · polydipsia · seborrhoea · severe cutaneous adverse reactions (SCARs) · sneezing · stomatitis · taste altered · throat irritation · tinnitus · weight decreased
▶ **Frequency not known** Dysarthria · dyspnoea · insomnia · miosis · sensation abnormal · visual acuity decreased · wheezing
- CONCEPTION AND CONTRACEPTION Manufacturer advises effectiveness of hormonal contraceptives may be reduced—alternative non-hormonal methods of contraception necessary during treatment and for 2 months after stopping aprepitant.
- PREGNANCY Manufacturer advises avoid unless clearly necessary—no information available.
- BREAST FEEDING Manufacturer advises avoid—present in milk in *animal* studies.
- HEPATIC IMPAIRMENT Manufacturer advises caution in moderate-to-severe impairment—limited information available.
- MEDICINAL FORMS
There can be variation in the licensing of different medicines containing the same drug. Forms available from special-order manufacturers include: oral suspension
Capsule
▶ Emend (Merck Sharp & Dohme Ltd)
Aprepitant 80 mg Emend 80mg capsules | 2 capsule [PoM] £31.61
Aprepitant 125 mg Emend 125mg capsules | 5 capsule [PoM] £79.03

Fosaprepitant

- DRUG ACTION Fosaprepitant is a prodrug of aprepitant.

- INDICATIONS AND DOSE
Adjunct to dexamethasone and a 5HT3-receptor antagonist in preventing nausea and vomiting associated with moderately and highly emetogenic chemotherapy
▶ BY INTRAVENOUS INFUSION
▶ Adult: 150 mg, dose to be administered over 20–30 minutes and given 30 minutes before chemotherapy on day 1 of cycle only, consult product literature for dose of concomitant corticosteroid and 5HT3-receptor antagonist

- CONTRA-INDICATIONS Acute porphyrias p. 1025
- INTERACTIONS → Appendix 1: fosaprepitant
- SIDE-EFFECTS
▶ **Common or very common** Appetite decreased · asthenia · constipation · gastrointestinal discomfort · headache · hiccups
▶ **Uncommon** Anaemia · anxiety · burping · dizziness · drowsiness · dry mouth · febrile neutropenia · gastrointestinal disorders · hot flush · malaise · nausea · palpitations · skin reactions · thrombophlebitis · urinary disorders · vomiting
▶ **Rare or very rare** Bradycardia · cardiovascular disorder · chest discomfort · cognitive disorder · conjunctivitis · cough · disorientation · euphoric mood · gait abnormal · hyperhidrosis · increased risk of infection · muscle spasms ·

muscle weakness · oedema · oropharyngeal pain · photosensitivity reaction · polydipsia · seborrhoea · severe cutaneous adverse reactions (SCARs) · sneezing · stomatitis · taste altered · throat irritation · tinnitus · weight decreased
▶ **Frequency not known** Dysarthria · dyspnoea · insomnia · miosis · sensation abnormal · visual acuity decreased · wheezing
- CONCEPTION AND CONTRACEPTION Effectiveness of hormonal contraceptives reduced—effective non-hormonal methods of contraception necessary during treatment and for 2 months after stopping fosaprepitant.
- PREGNANCY Avoid unless potential benefit outweighs risk—no information available.
- BREAST FEEDING Avoid—present in milk in *animal* studies.
- HEPATIC IMPAIRMENT Caution in moderate to severe impairment.
- DIRECTIONS FOR ADMINISTRATION For *intravenous infusion* (Ivemend®), give intermittently *in* Sodium chloride 0.9%; reconstitute each 150-mg vial with 5 mL sodium chloride 0.9% gently without shaking to avoid foaming, then dilute in 145 mL infusion fluid; give over 20–30 minutes.
- NATIONAL FUNDING/ACCESS DECISIONS
Scottish Medicines Consortium (SMC) Decisions
The *Scottish Medicines Consortium* has advised (January 2011) that fosaprepitant (*Ivemend®*) is accepted for restricted use within NHS Scotland for the prevention of acute and delayed nausea and vomiting associated with highly emetogenic cisplatin-based chemotherapy.

- MEDICINAL FORMS
There can be variation in the licensing of different medicines containing the same drug.
Powder for solution for infusion
▶ Ivemend (Merck Sharp & Dohme Ltd)
Fosaprepitant (as Fosaprepitant dimeglumine) 150 mg Ivemend 150mg powder for solution for infusion vials | 1 vial [PoM] £47.42

Rolapitant

26-Oct-2017

- INDICATIONS AND DOSE
Adjunct to dexamethasone and a 5HT3-receptor antagonist in preventing delayed nausea and vomiting associated with moderately and highly emetogenic chemotherapy
▶ BY MOUTH
▶ Adult: 180 mg as a single dose, dose should be administered up to 2 hours before chemotherapy. Interval between repeated doses must be at least 2 weeks, consult product literature for dose of concomitant corticosteroid and 5HT3-antagonist

- INTERACTIONS → Appendix 1: rolapitant
- SIDE-EFFECTS
▶ **Common or very common** Asthenia · constipation · headache
▶ **Uncommon** Appetite decreased · concentration impaired · diarrhoea · dizziness · drowsiness · gastrointestinal discomfort · hiccups · increased risk of infection · insomnia · myalgia · nausea · neutropenia · stomatitis · taste altered
▶ **Rare or very rare** Alopecia · angioedema · anxiety · arthralgia · back pain · dehydration · dry mouth · dyspnoea · gait abnormal · gastrointestinal disorders · hearing impairment · hypertension · hypomagnesaemia · leucopenia · movement disorders · muscle weakness · rhabdomyolysis · skin reactions · syncope · teeth grinding · thrombocytopenia · vision blurred · vomiting
- PREGNANCY Manufacturer advises avoid unless potential benefit outweighs risk—limited information available.

- **BREAST FEEDING** Manufacturer advises avoid—present in milk in *animal* studies.
- **HEPATIC IMPAIRMENT** Manufacturer advises use with caution in severe impairment—no information available.
- **RENAL IMPAIRMENT** Manufacturer advises use with caution in severe impairment—limited information available.
- **NATIONAL FUNDING/ACCESS DECISIONS**
Scottish Medicines Consortium (SMC) Decisions
SMC No. 1266/17
The *Scottish Medicines Consortium* has advised (September 2017) that rolapitant (*Varuby*®) is accepted for restricted use within NHS Scotland as a first-line option for the prevention of delayed nausea and vomiting in adults undergoing highly emetogenic chemotherapy. This advice is contingent upon the continuing availability of the patient access scheme in NHS Scotland or a list price that is equivalent or lower.

All Wales Medicines Strategy Group (AWMSG) Decisions
AWMSG No. 1303
The *All Wales Medicines Strategy Group* has advised (March 2018) that rolapitant (*Varuby*®) is **not** recommended for use within NHS Wales for the prevention of delayed nausea and vomiting associated with highly and moderately emetogenic cancer chemotherapy in adults. The case for cost-effectiveness has not been proven.

- **MEDICINAL FORMS**
There can be variation in the licensing of different medicines containing the same drug.
Tablet
CAUTIONARY AND ADVISORY LABELS 3
EXCIPIENTS: May contain Polysorbates
▸ Varuby (Tesaro UK Ltd) ▼
Rolapitant (as Rolapitant hydrochloride monohydrate)
90 mg Varuby 90mg tablets | 2 tablet [PoM] £47.42

ANTIEMETICS AND ANTINAUSEANTS ›
SEROTONIN (5HT₃) RECEPTOR ANTAGONISTS

Granisetron

- **DRUG ACTION** Granisetron is a specific 5HT₃-receptor antagonist which blocks 5HT₃ receptors in the gastro-intestinal tract and in the CNS.

- **INDICATIONS AND DOSE**
Nausea and vomiting induced by cytotoxic chemotherapy for planned duration of 3–5 days where oral antiemetics cannot be used
▸ BY TRANSDERMAL APPLICATION USING PATCHES
▸ Adult: Apply 3.1 mg/24 hours, apply patch to clean, dry, non-irritated, non-hairy skin on upper arm (or abdomen if upper arm cannot be used) 24–48 hours before treatment, patch may be worn for up to 7 days; remove at least 24 hours after completing chemotherapy

Prevention of postoperative nausea and vomiting
▸ BY INTRAVENOUS INJECTION
▸ Adult: 1 mg, to be administered before induction of anaesthesia, dose to be diluted to 5 mL and given over 30 seconds

Treatment of postoperative nausea and vomiting
▸ BY INTRAVENOUS INJECTION
▸ Adult: 1 mg, dose to be diluted to 5 mL and given over 30 seconds; maximum 3 mg per day

Management of nausea and vomiting induced by cytotoxic chemotherapy or radiotherapy
▸ BY MOUTH
▸ Adult: 1–2 mg, to be taken within 1 hour before start of treatment, then 2 mg daily in 1–2 divided doses for up

to 1 week following treatment, when intravenous route also used, maximum combined total dose 9 mg in 24 hours
▸ BY INTRAVENOUS INJECTION, OR BY INTRAVENOUS INFUSION
▸ Adult: 10–40 micrograms/kg (max. per dose 3 mg), to be given 5 minutes before start of treatment, dose may be repeated if necessary, further maintenance doses must not be given less than 10 minutes apart, for intravenous injection, each 1 mg granisetron diluted to 5 mL and given over not less than 30 seconds, for intravenous infusion, to be given over 5 minutes; maximum 9 mg per day

- **CAUTIONS** Subacute intestinal obstruction · susceptibility to QT-interval prolongation (including electrolyte disturbances)
- **INTERACTIONS** → Appendix 1: granisetron
- **SIDE-EFFECTS**
GENERAL SIDE-EFFECTS
▸ **Common or very common** Constipation · headache
SPECIFIC SIDE-EFFECTS
▸ **Common or very common**
▸ With intravenous use or with oral use Diarrhoea · insomnia
▸ **Uncommon**
▸ With intravenous use or with oral use Extrapyramidal symptoms · QT interval prolongation · serotonin syndrome
▸ With transdermal use Appetite decreased · arthralgia · dry mouth · flushing · generalised oedema · nausea · vertigo · vomiting
▸ **Rare or very rare**
▸ With transdermal use Dystonia
- **PREGNANCY** Manufacturer advises avoid.
- **BREAST FEEDING** Avoid—no information available.
- **HEPATIC IMPAIRMENT** Manufacturer advises use with caution.
- **DIRECTIONS FOR ADMINISTRATION** For *intravenous infusion*, give intermittently in Glucose 5% or Sodium Chloride 0.9%; dilute up to 3 mL in 20–50 mL infusion fluid; give over 5 minutes.
- **PATIENT AND CARER ADVICE**
▸ With transdermal use Patients should be advised not to expose the site of the patch to sunlight during use and for 10 days after removal.

- **MEDICINAL FORMS**
There can be variation in the licensing of different medicines containing the same drug.
Solution for injection
▸ Granisetron (Non-proprietary)
Granisetron (as Granisetron hydrochloride) 1 mg per 1 ml Granisetron 3mg/3ml concentrate for solution for injection ampoules | 5 ampoule [PoM] £24.00
Granisetron 1mg/1ml concentrate for solution for injection ampoules | 5 ampoule [PoM] £8.00
Tablet
▸ Granisetron (Non-proprietary)
Granisetron (as Granisetron hydrochloride) 1 mg Granisetron 1mg tablets | 10 tablet [PoM] £51.20 DT = £40.79
Granisetron (as Granisetron hydrochloride) 2 mg Granisetron 2mg tablets | 5 tablet [PoM] [⬇] DT = £52.39
▸ Kytril (Atnahs Pharma UK Ltd)
Granisetron (as Granisetron hydrochloride) 1 mg Kytril 1mg tablets | 10 tablet [PoM] £52.39 DT = £40.79
Granisetron (as Granisetron hydrochloride) 2 mg Kytril 2mg tablets | 5 tablet [PoM] £52.39 DT = £52.39
Transdermal patch
▸ Sancuso (Kyowa Kirin Ltd)
Granisetron 3.1 mg per 24 hour Sancuso 3.1mg/24hours transdermal patches | 1 patch [PoM] £56.00

4

Nervous system

Ondansetron

- DRUG ACTION Ondansetron is a specific 5HT$_3$-receptor antagonist which blocks 5HT$_3$ receptors in the gastro-intestinal tract and in the CNS.

- **INDICATIONS AND DOSE**

Moderately emetogenic chemotherapy or radiotherapy
- BY MOUTH
- Adult: Initially 8 mg, dose to be taken 1–2 hours before treatment, then 8 mg every 12 hours for up to 5 days
- BY RECTUM
- Adult: Initially 16 mg, dose to be taken 1–2 hours before treatment, then 16 mg daily for up to 5 days
- INITIALLY BY INTRAMUSCULAR INJECTION, OR BY SLOW INTRAVENOUS INJECTION
- Adult: Initially 8 mg, dose to be administered immediately before treatment, then (by mouth) 8 mg every 12 hours for up to 5 days, alternatively (by rectum) 16 mg daily for up to 5 days
- INITIALLY BY INTRAMUSCULAR INJECTION, OR BY INTRAVENOUS INFUSION
- Elderly: Initially 8 mg, dose to be administered immediately before treatment, intravenous infusion to be given over at least 15 minutes, then (by mouth) 8 mg every 12 hours for up to 5 days, alternatively (by rectum) 16 mg daily for up to 5 days

Severely emetogenic chemotherapy (consult product literature for dose of concomitant corticosteroid)
- BY MOUTH
- Adult: 24 mg, dose to be taken 1–2 hours before treatment, then 8 mg every 12 hours for up to 5 days
- BY RECTUM
- Adult: 16 mg, dose to be administered 1–2 hours before treatment, then 16 mg daily for up to 5 days
- INITIALLY BY INTRAMUSCULAR INJECTION, OR BY SLOW INTRAVENOUS INJECTION
- Adult: Initially 8 mg, dose to be administered immediately before treatment, followed by (by intramuscular injection or by slow intravenous injection) 8 mg every 4 hours if required for 2 doses, alternatively, followed by (by continuous intravenous infusion) 1 mg/hour for up to 24 hours, then (by mouth) 8 mg every 12 hours for up to 5 days, alternatively (by rectum) 16 mg daily for up to 5 days
- INITIALLY BY INTRAMUSCULAR INJECTION
- Adult 65–74 years: Initially 8 mg, to be given immediately before treatment, followed by (by intramuscular injection) 8 mg every 4 hours if required for 2 doses, alternatively, followed by (by continuous intravenous infusion) 1 mg/hour for up to 24 hours, then (by mouth) 8 mg every 12 hours for up to 5 days, alternatively (by rectum) 16 mg daily for up to 5 days
- INITIALLY BY INTRAVENOUS INFUSION
- Adult: Initially 16 mg, immediately before treatment (over at least 15 minutes), followed by (by intramuscular injection or by slow intravenous injection) 8 mg every 4 hours if required for 2 doses, then (by mouth) 8 mg every 12 hours for up to 5 days, alternatively (by rectum) 16 mg daily for up to 5 days
- Adult 65–74 years: Initially 8–16 mg, immediately before treatment (over at least 15 minutes), followed by (by intramuscular injection or by intravenous infusion) 8 mg every 4 hours if required for 2 doses, then (by mouth) 8 mg every 12 hours for up to 5 days, alternatively (by rectum) 16 mg daily for up to 5 days
- Adult 75 years and over: Initially 8 mg, immediately before treatment (over at least 15 minutes), followed by (by intravenous infusion) 8 mg every 4 hours if required for 2 doses, then (by mouth) 8 mg every 12 hours for up to 5 days, alternatively (by rectum) 16 mg daily for up to 5 days

Prevention of postoperative nausea and vomiting
- INITIALLY BY MOUTH
- Adult: 16 mg, dose to be taken 1 hour before anaesthesia, alternatively (by intramuscular injection or by slow intravenous injection) 4 mg, dose to be administered at induction of anaesthesia

Treatment of postoperative nausea and vomiting
- BY INTRAMUSCULAR INJECTION, OR BY SLOW INTRAVENOUS INJECTION
- Adult: 4 mg for 1 dose

- CONTRA-INDICATIONS Congenital long QT syndrome
- CAUTIONS Adenotonsillar surgery · subacute intestinal obstruction · susceptibility to QT-interval prolongation (including electrolyte disturbances)
- INTERACTIONS → Appendix 1: ondansetron
- SIDE-EFFECTS
- **Common or very common** Constipation · feeling hot · headache · sensation abnormal
- **Uncommon** Arrhythmias · chest pain · hiccups · hypotension · movement disorders · oculogyric crisis · seizure
- **Rare or very rare** Dizziness · QT interval prolongation · vision disorders
- PREGNANCY No information available; avoid unless potential benefit outweighs risk.
- BREAST FEEDING Present in milk in *animal* studies—avoid.
- HEPATIC IMPAIRMENT
  Dose adjustments Maximum 8 mg daily in moderate or severe impairment.
- DIRECTIONS FOR ADMINISTRATION
- With intravenous use For *intravenous infusion (Zofran®)*, give continuously or intermittently in Glucose 5% or Glucose 5% with Potassium chloride 0.3% or Sodium chloride 0.9% or Sodium chloride 0.9% with Potassium chloride 0.3% or Mannitol 10% or Ringers solution; for intermittent infusion, dilute the required dose in 50–100 mL of infusion fluid and give over at least 15 minutes.
- With oral use Orodispersible films and lyophilisates should be placed on the tongue, allowed to disperse and swallowed.
- PRESCRIBING AND DISPENSING INFORMATION Flavours of oral liquid formulations may include strawberry.
- PATIENT AND CARER ADVICE Patients or carers should be given advice on how to administer orodispersible films and lyophilisates.

- MEDICINAL FORMS
There can be variation in the licensing of different medicines containing the same drug. Forms available from special-order manufacturers include: oral suspension, oral solution

Tablet
- Ondansetron (Non-proprietary)
  Ondansetron (as Ondansetron hydrochloride) 4 mg Ondansetron 4mg tablets | 10 tablet [PoM] £0.81–£25.46 DT = £0.62 | 30 tablet [PoM] £1.86–£76.38
  Ondansetron (as Ondansetron hydrochloride) 8 mg Ondansetron 8mg tablets | 10 tablet [PoM] £47.99 DT = £1.73
- Ondemet (Alliance Pharmaceuticals Ltd)
  Ondansetron (as Ondansetron hydrochloride) 4 mg Ondemet 4mg tablets | 30 tablet [PoM] £81.15
  Ondansetron (as Ondansetron hydrochloride) 8 mg Ondemet 8mg tablets | 10 tablet [PoM] £54.36 DT = £1.73 (Hospital only)
- Zofran (Novartis Pharmaceuticals UK Ltd)
  Ondansetron (as Ondansetron hydrochloride) 4 mg Zofran 4mg tablets | 30 tablet [PoM] £107.91
  Ondansetron (as Ondansetron hydrochloride) 8 mg Zofran 8mg tablets | 10 tablet [PoM] £71.94 DT = £1.73

Suppository
- Zofran (Novartis Pharmaceuticals UK Ltd)
  Ondansetron 16 mg Zofran 16mg suppositories | 1 suppository [PoM] £14.39

Solution for injection

▸ Ondansetron (Non-proprietary)

Ondansetron (as Ondansetron hydrochloride) 2 mg per 1 ml Ondansetron 8mg/4ml solution for injection ampoules | 5 ampoule PoM £2.00–£58.45 DT = £59.95
Ondansetron 4mg/2ml solution for injection ampoules | 5 ampoule PoM £1.50–£29.97 DT = £29.97 | 10 ampoule PoM £7.50 DT = £7.50

▸ Zofran Flexi-amp (Novartis Pharmaceuticals UK Ltd)

Ondansetron (as Ondansetron hydrochloride) 2 mg per 1 ml Zofran Flexi-amp 8mg/4ml solution for injection | 5 ampoule PoM £59.95 DT = £59.95
Zofran Flexi-amp 4mg/2ml solution for injection | 5 ampoule PoM £29.97 DT = £29.97

Oral solution

▸ Ondansetron (Non-proprietary)

Ondansetron (as Ondansetron hydrochloride) 800 microgram per 1 ml Ondansetron 4mg/5ml oral solution sugar free sugar-free | 50 ml PoM £38.22 DT = £38.21

▸ Zofran (Novartis Pharmaceuticals UK Ltd)

Ondansetron (as Ondansetron hydrochloride) 800 microgram per 1 ml Zofran 4mg/5ml syrup sugar-free | 50 ml PoM £35.97 DT = £38.21

Orodispersible film

▸ Setofilm (Norgine Pharmaceuticals Ltd)

Ondansetron 4 mg Setofilm 4mg orodispersible films sugar-free | 10 film PoM £28.50
Ondansetron 8 mg Setofilm 8mg orodispersible films sugar-free | 10 film PoM £57.00

Oral lyophilisate

EXCIPIENTS: May contain Aspartame

▸ Zofran Melt (Novartis Pharmaceuticals UK Ltd)

Ondansetron 4 mg Zofran Melt 4mg oral lyophilisates sugar-free | 10 tablet PoM £35.97 DT = £35.97
Ondansetron 8 mg Zofran Melt 8mg oral lyophilisates sugar-free | 10 tablet PoM £71.94 DT = £71.94

Orodispersible tablet

▸ Ondansetron (Non-proprietary)

Ondansetron 4 mg Ondansetron 4mg orodispersible tablets | 10 tablet PoM £43.46 DT = £43.46
Ondansetron 8 mg Ondansetron 8mg orodispersible tablets | 10 tablet PoM £85.43 DT = £85.43

Palonosetron

● DRUG ACTION Palonosetron is a specific 5HT$_3$-receptor antagonist which blocks 5HT$_3$ receptors in the gastro-intestinal tract and in the CNS.

● INDICATIONS AND DOSE

Moderately emetogenic chemotherapy

▸ INITIALLY BY MOUTH

▸ Adult: 500 micrograms, dose to be taken 1 hour before treatment, alternatively (by intravenous injection) 250 micrograms for 1 dose, dose to be administered over 30 seconds, 30 minutes before treatment

Severely emetogenic chemotherapy

▸ BY INTRAVENOUS INJECTION

▸ Adult: 250 micrograms for 1 dose, dose to be administered over 30 seconds, 30 minutes before treatment

● CAUTIONS History of constipation · intestinal obstruction · susceptibility to QT-interval prolongation (including electrolyte disturbances)

● INTERACTIONS → Appendix 1: palonosetron

● SIDE-EFFECTS

GENERAL SIDE-EFFECTS

▸ **Common or very common** Constipation · headache
▸ **Uncommon** Dyspnoea

SPECIFIC SIDE-EFFECTS

▸ **Common or very common**
▸ With intravenous use Diarrhoea · dizziness · electrolyte imbalance · metabolic disorder

▸ **Uncommon**
▸ With intravenous use Amblyopia · anxiety · appetite decreased · arrhythmias · arthralgia · asthenia · drowsiness · dry mouth · dyspepsia · euphoric mood · eye irritation · feeling hot · fever · flatulence · glycosuria · hiccups · hyperbilirubinaemia · hyperglycaemia · hypertension · hypotension · influenza like illness · motion sickness · myocardial ischaemia · paraesthesia · peripheral neuropathy · QT interval prolongation · skin reactions · sleep disorders · tinnitus · urinary retention · vasodilation · vein discolouration
▸ With oral use Atrioventricular block · eye swelling · insomnia · myalgia
▸ **Rare or very rare**
▸ With intravenous use Shock

● PREGNANCY Avoid—no information available.

● BREAST FEEDING Avoid—no information available.

● PATIENT AND CARER ADVICE

Driving and skilled tasks Dizziness or drowsiness may affect performance of skilled tasks (e.g. driving).

● MEDICINAL FORMS

There can be variation in the licensing of different medicines containing the same drug.

Solution for injection

▸ Palonosetron (Non-proprietary)

Palonosetron (as Palonosetron hydrochloride) 50 microgram per 1 ml Palonosetron 250micrograms/5ml solution for injection vials | 1 vial PoM £53.10–£55.89

▸ Aloxi (Sinclair IS Pharma Plc)

Palonosetron (as Palonosetron hydrochloride) 50 microgram per 1 ml Aloxi 250micrograms/5ml solution for injection vials | 1 vial PoM £55.89

Capsule

▸ Aloxi (Sinclair IS Pharma Plc)

Palonosetron (as Palonosetron hydrochloride) 500 microgram Aloxi 500microgram capsules | 1 capsule PoM £55.89

Palonosetron with netupitant   20-Jun-2016

The properties listed below are those particular to the combination only. For the properties of the components please consider, palonosetron above.

● INDICATIONS AND DOSE

Moderately emetogenic chemotherapy | Highly emetogenic cisplatin-based chemotherapy

▸ BY MOUTH

▸ Adult: 1 capsule, to be taken approximately 1 hour before the start of each chemotherapy cycle

● CAUTIONS Patients over 75 years

● INTERACTIONS → Appendix 1: netupitant · palonosetron

● SIDE-EFFECTS

▸ **Common or very common** Asthenia · constipation · headache
▸ **Uncommon** Alopecia · cardiac conduction disorders · cardiomyopathy · diarrhoea · dizziness · flatulence · gastrointestinal discomfort · hiccups · hypertension · increased leucocytes · neutropenia · QT interval prolongation · sleep disorders · urticaria · vertigo
▸ **Rare or very rare** Acute psychosis · arrhythmias · conjunctivitis · cystitis · dysphagia · feeling hot · hypokalaemia · hypotension · leucopenia · mitral valve incompetence · mood altered · myocardial ischaemia · numbness · pain · tongue coated · vision blurred

● CONCEPTION AND CONTRACEPTION Manufacturer recommends exclude pregnancy before treatment in females of childbearing age; ensure effective contraception during treatment and for one month after treatment.

- **PREGNANCY** Manufacturer advises avoid—toxicity in *animal* studies.
- **BREAST FEEDING** Manufacturer advises avoid during treatment and for 1 month after last dose—no information available.
- **HEPATIC IMPAIRMENT** Manufacturer advises caution in severe impairment.
- **NATIONAL FUNDING/ACCESS DECISIONS**
  Scottish Medicines Consortium (SMC) Decisions
  The *Scottish Medicines Consortium* (December 2015) has advised that palonosetron in combination with netupitant (*Akynzeo*®) is accepted for restricted use within NHS Scotland for the prevention of acute and delayed nausea and vomiting associated with highly emetogenic cisplatin-based cancer chemotherapy.
- **MEDICINAL FORMS**
  There can be variation in the licensing of different medicines containing the same drug.
  Capsule
  CAUTIONARY AND ADVISORY LABELS 25
  ▸ Akynzeo (Chugai Pharma UK Ltd) ▼
  Palonosetron (as Palonosetron hydrochloride) 500 microgram, Netupitant 300 mg Akynzeo 300mg/0.5mg capsules | 1 capsule [PoM] £69.00 (Hospital only)

ANTIHISTAMINES > SEDATING

Cinnarizine

- **INDICATIONS AND DOSE**
  Relief of symptoms of vestibular disorders, such as vertigo, tinnitus, nausea, and vomiting in Ménière's disease
  ▸ BY MOUTH
  ▸ Child 5–11 years: 15 mg 3 times a day
  ▸ Child 12–17 years: 30 mg 3 times a day
  ▸ Adult: 30 mg 3 times a day
  Motion sickness
  ▸ BY MOUTH
  ▸ Child 5–11 years: Initially 15 mg, dose to be taken 2 hours before travel, then 7.5 mg every 8 hours if required, dose to be taken during journey
  ▸ Child 12–17 years: Initially 30 mg, dose to be taken 2 hours before travel, then 15 mg every 8 hours if required, dose to be taken during journey
  ▸ Adult: Initially 30 mg, dose to be taken 2 hours before travel, then 15 mg every 8 hours if required, dose to be taken during journey

- **CONTRA-INDICATIONS** Avoid in Acute porphyrias p. 1025
- **CAUTIONS** Epilepsy · glaucoma (in children) · Parkinson's disease · prostatic hypertrophy (in adults) · pyloroduodenal obstruction · susceptibility to angle-closure glaucoma (in adults) · urinary retention
- **INTERACTIONS** → Appendix 1: antihistamines, sedating
- **SIDE-EFFECTS**
  ▸ **Common or very common** Drowsiness · gastrointestinal discomfort · nausea · weight increased
  ▸ **Uncommon** Fatigue · hyperhidrosis · vomiting
  ▸ **Frequency not known** Dry mouth · gastrointestinal disorder · headache · jaundice cholestatic · movement disorders · muscle rigidity · parkinsonism · skin reactions · subacute cutaneous lupus erythematosus · tremor
- **PREGNANCY** Manufacturer advises avoid; however, there is no evidence of teratogenicity. The use of sedating antihistamines in the latter part of the third trimester may cause adverse effects in neonates such as irritability, paradoxical excitability, and tremor.
- **BREAST FEEDING** Most antihistamines are present in breast milk in varying amounts; although not known to be

harmful, most manufacturers advise avoiding their use in mothers who are breast-feeding.
- **HEPATIC IMPAIRMENT** Avoid in severe liver disease—increased risk of coma.
- **RENAL IMPAIRMENT** Use with caution—no information available.
- **PATIENT AND CARER ADVICE**
  Driving and skilled tasks Drowsiness may affect performance of skilled tasks (e.g. cycling, driving); sedating effects enhanced by alcohol.
- **MEDICINAL FORMS**
  There can be variation in the licensing of different medicines containing the same drug. Forms available from special-order manufacturers include: oral suspension
  Tablet
  CAUTIONARY AND ADVISORY LABELS 2
  ▸ Cinnarizine (Non-proprietary)
  Cinnarizine 15 mg Cinnarizine 15mg tablets | 84 tablet [P] £15.40 DT = £5.29
  ▸ Stugeron (McNeil Products Ltd, Janssen-Cilag Ltd)
  Cinnarizine 15 mg Stugeron 15mg tablets | 15 tablet [P] £2.21 | 100 tablet [P] £4.18

Cinnarizine with dimenhydrinate

The properties listed below are those particular to the combination only. For the properties of the components please consider, cinnarizine above.

- **INDICATIONS AND DOSE**
  Vertigo
  ▸ BY MOUTH
  ▸ Adult: 1 tablet 3 times a day
- **INTERACTIONS** → Appendix 1: antihistamines, sedating · dimenhydrinate
- **MEDICINAL FORMS**
  There can be variation in the licensing of different medicines containing the same drug.
  Tablet
  CAUTIONARY AND ADVISORY LABELS 2, 21
  ▸ Arlevert (Hampton Pharmaceuticals Ltd)
  Cinnarizine 20 mg, Dimenhydrinate 40 mg Arlevert tablets | 100 tablet [PoM] £24.00

Promethazine teoclate

- **INDICATIONS AND DOSE**
  Nausea | Vomiting | Labyrinthine disorders
  ▸ BY MOUTH
  ▸ Child 5–9 years: 12.5–37.5 mg daily
  ▸ Child 10–17 years: 25–75 mg daily; maximum 100 mg per day
  ▸ Adult: 25–75 mg daily; maximum 100 mg per day
  Motion sickness prevention (acts longer than promethazine hydrochloride)
  ▸ BY MOUTH
  ▸ Child 5–9 years: 12.5 mg once daily, dose to be taken at bedtime on night before travel or 1–2 hours before travel
  ▸ Child 10–17 years: 25 mg once daily, dose to be taken at bedtime on night before travel or 1–2 hours before travel
  ▸ Adult: 25 mg once daily, dose to be taken at bedtime on night before travel or 1–2 hours before travel

Motion sickness treatment (acts longer than promethazine hydrochloride)

▶ BY MOUTH
- Child 5–9 years: 12.5 mg, dose to be taken at onset of motion sickness, then 12.5 mg daily for 2 days, dose to be taken at bedtime
- Child 10–17 years: 25 mg, dose to be taken at onset of motion sickness, then 25 mg once daily for 2 days, dose to be taken at bedtime
- Adult: 25 mg, dose to be taken at onset of motion sickness, then 25 mg once daily for 2 days, dose to be taken at bedtime

IMPORTANT SAFETY INFORMATION

MHRA/CHM ADVICE (MARCH 2008 AND FEBRUARY 2009) OVER-THE-COUNTER COUGH AND COLD MEDICINES FOR CHILDREN

Children under 6 years should not be given over-the-counter cough and cold medicines containing promethazine.

- CONTRA-INDICATIONS Should not be given to children under 2 years, except on specialist advice, because the safety of such use has not been established
- CAUTIONS Asthma · bronchiectasis · bronchitis · epilepsy · prostatic hypertrophy (in adults) · pyloroduodenal obstruction · Reye's syndrome · severe coronary artery disease · susceptibility to angle-closure glaucoma · urinary retention
- INTERACTIONS → Appendix 1: antihistamines, sedating
- SIDE-EFFECTS Anticholinergic syndrome · anxiety · appetite decreased · arrhythmia · blood disorder · bronchial secretion viscosity increased · confusion · dizziness · drowsiness · dry mouth · epigastric discomfort · fatigue · haemolytic anaemia · headache · hypotension · jaundice · movement disorders · muscle spasms · nightmare · palpitations · photosensitivity reaction · urinary retention · vision blurred

  SIDE-EFFECTS, FURTHER INFORMATION Elderly patients are more susceptible to anticholinergic side-effects.
   In children paradoxical stimulation may occur, especially with high doses.
- PREGNANCY Most manufacturers of antihistamines advise avoiding their use during pregnancy; however, there is no evidence of teratogenicity. Use in the latter part of the third trimester may cause adverse effects in neonates such as irritability, paradoxical excitability, and tremor.
- BREAST FEEDING Most antihistamines are present in breast milk in varying amounts; although not known to be harmful, most manufacturers advise avoiding their use in mothers who are breast-feeding.
- HEPATIC IMPAIRMENT Avoid in severe liver disease—increased risk of coma.
- RENAL IMPAIRMENT Use with caution.
- PATIENT AND CARER ADVICE
  Driving and skilled tasks Drowsiness may affect performance of skilled tasks (e.g. cycling or driving); sedating effects enhanced by alcohol.
- MEDICINAL FORMS
  There can be variation in the licensing of different medicines containing the same drug.
  Tablet
  CAUTIONARY AND ADVISORY LABELS 2
  ▶ Avomine (Manx Healthcare Ltd)
    Promethazine teoclate 25 mg Avomine 25mg tablets | 10 tablet ℗ £1.13 | 28 tablet ℗ £3.13 DT = £3.13

📖 759

Hyoscine hydrobromide

17-Oct-2016

(Scopolamine hydrobromide)

● INDICATIONS AND DOSE

Motion sickness
▶ BY MOUTH
- Child 4–9 years: 75–150 micrograms, dose to be taken up to 30 minutes before the start of journey, then 75–150 micrograms every 6 hours if required; maximum 450 micrograms per day
- Child 10–17 years: 150–300 micrograms, dose to be taken up to 30 minutes before the start of journey, then 150–300 micrograms every 6 hours if required; maximum 900 micrograms per day
- Adult: 150–300 micrograms, dose to be taken up to 30 minutes before the start of journey, then 150–300 micrograms every 6 hours if required; maximum 900 micrograms per day
▶ BY TRANSDERMAL APPLICATION
- Child 10–17 years: Apply 1 patch, apply behind ear 5–6 hours before journey, then apply 1 patch after 72 hours if required, remove old patch and site replacement patch behind the other ear
- Adult: Apply 1 patch, apply behind ear 5–6 hours before journey, then apply 1 patch after 72 hours if required, remove old patch and site replacement patch behind the other ear

Hypersalivation associated with clozapine therapy
▶ BY MOUTH
- Adult: 300 micrograms up to 3 times a day; maximum 900 micrograms per day

Excessive respiratory secretion (in palliative care)
▶ BY SUBCUTANEOUS INJECTION
- Adult: 400 micrograms every 4 hours as required, hourly use is occasionally necessary, particularly in excessive respiratory secretions
▶ BY CONTINUOUS SUBCUTANEOUS INFUSION
- Adult: 1.2–2 mg/24 hours

Bowel colic in palliative care
▶ BY SUBCUTANEOUS INJECTION
- Adult: 400 micrograms every 4 hours as required, hourly use is occasionally necessary
▶ BY SUBCUTANEOUS INFUSION
- Adult: 1.2–2 mg/24 hours

Bowel colic pain in palliative care
▶ BY MOUTH USING SUBLINGUAL TABLETS
- Adult: 300 micrograms 3 times a day, as *Kwells*®.

Premedication
▶ BY SUBCUTANEOUS INJECTION, OR BY INTRAMUSCULAR INJECTION
- Adult: 200–600 micrograms, to be administered 30–60 minutes before induction of anaesthesia

● UNLICENSED USE Not licensed for hypersalivation associated with clozapine therapy.

IMPORTANT SAFETY INFORMATION
Antimuscarininc drugs used for premedication to general anaesthesia should only be administered by, or under the direct supervision of, personnel experienced in their use.

● CAUTIONS Epilepsy
CAUTIONS, FURTHER INFORMATION
▶ Anticholinergic syndrome In some patients, especially the elderly, hyoscine may cause the central anticholinergic syndrome (excitement, ataxia, hallucinations, behavioural abnormalities, and drowsiness).

Nervous system   4

- INTERACTIONS → Appendix 1: hyoscine
- SIDE-EFFECTS
  GENERAL SIDE-EFFECTS
- **Common or very common** Skin reactions
  SPECIFIC SIDE-EFFECTS
- **Common or very common**
- With transdermal use Eye disorders · eyelid irritation · myopia
- **Rare or very rare**
- With transdermal use Concentration impaired · disorientation · glaucoma · hallucinations · memory loss · restlessness
- **Frequency not known**
- With oral use Asthma · cardiovascular disorders · central nervous system stimulation · gastrointestinal disorder · hallucination · hypersensitivity · hyperthermia · hypohidrosis · mydriasis · oedema · respiratory tract reaction · restlessness · sedation · seizure
- With parenteral use Agitation · angle closure glaucoma · arrhythmias · delirium · dysphagia · dyspnoea · epilepsy exacerbated · hallucination · hypersensitivity · idiosyncratic drug reaction · loss of consciousness · mydriasis · neuroleptic malignant syndrome · photophobia · psychotic disorder · thirst
- With transdermal use Balance impaired
- PREGNANCY Use only if potential benefit outweighs risk. Injection may depress neonatal respiration.
- BREAST FEEDING Amount too small to be harmful.
- HEPATIC IMPAIRMENT Use with caution.
- RENAL IMPAIRMENT Use with caution.
- DIRECTIONS FOR ADMINISTRATION
- With transdermal use in children *Patch* applied to hairless area of skin behind ear; if less than whole patch required **either** cut with scissors along full thickness ensuring membrane is not peeled away **or** cover portion to prevent contact with skin.
- With oral use in children For administration by *mouth*, injection solution may be given orally.
- PRESCRIBING AND DISPENSING INFORMATION Flavours of chewable tablet formulations may include raspberry.
  Palliative care For further information on the use of hyoscine hydrobromide in palliative care, see www.palliativedrugs.com/formulary/en/hyoscine-hydrobromide.html.
- PATIENT AND CARER ADVICE
- With transdermal use Explain accompanying instructions to patient and in particular emphasise advice to wash hands after handling and to wash application site after removing, and to use one patch at a time.
  Driving and skilled tasks ▸ With transdermal use Drowsiness may persist for up to 24 hours or longer after removal of patch; effects of alcohol enhanced.

- MEDICINAL FORMS
  There can be variation in the licensing of different medicines containing the same drug. Forms available from special-order manufacturers include: oral suspension, oral solution, eye drops
  Tablet
  CAUTIONARY AND ADVISORY LABELS 2
  ▸ Hyoscine hydrobromide (Non-proprietary)
  Hyoscine hydrobromide 300 microgram Hyoscine hydrobromide 300microgram tablets | 12 tablet ℗ Ⓢ DT = £1.67
  ▸ Kwells (Bayer Plc)
  Hyoscine hydrobromide 150 microgram Kwells Kids 150microgram tablets | 12 tablet ℗ £1.67 DT = £1.67
  Hyoscine hydrobromide 300 microgram Kwells 300microgram tablets | 12 tablet ℗ £1.67 DT = £1.67
  ▸ Travel Calm (The Boots Company Plc)
  Hyoscine hydrobromide 300 microgram Travel Calm 300microgram tablets | 12 tablet ℗ Ⓢ DT = £1.67

Solution for injection
▸ Hyoscine hydrobromide (Non-proprietary)
Hyoscine hydrobromide 400 microgram per 1 ml Hyoscine hydrobromide 400micrograms/1ml solution for injection ampoules | 10 ampoule ℗ᵒᴹ £25.00–£47.21 DT = £47.21
Hyoscine hydrobromide 600 microgram per 1 ml Hyoscine hydrobromide 600micrograms/1ml solution for injection ampoules | 10 ampoule ℗ᵒᴹ £53.93 DT = £53.93
Transdermal patch
CAUTIONARY AND ADVISORY LABELS 19
▸ Scopoderm (GlaxoSmithKline Consumer Healthcare)
Hyoscine 1 mg per 72 hour Scopoderm 1.5mg patches | 2 patch ℗ £12.87 DT = £12.87
Chewable tablet
CAUTIONARY AND ADVISORY LABELS 2, 24
▸ Joy-Rides (Forest Laboratories UK Ltd)
Hyoscine hydrobromide 150 microgram Joy-rides 150microgram chewable tablets sugar-free | 12 tablet ℗ £1.55

ANTIPSYCHOTICS ⟩ FIRST-GENERATION

F 380

Droperidol

- DRUG ACTION Droperidol is a butyrophenone, structurally related to haloperidol, which blocks dopamine receptors in the chemoreceptor trigger zone.

- INDICATIONS AND DOSE
  Prevention and treatment of postoperative nausea and vomiting
  ▸ BY INTRAVENOUS INJECTION
  ▸ Adult: 0.625–1.25 mg, dose to be given 30 minutes before end of surgery, then 0.625–1.25 mg every 6 hours as required
  ▸ Elderly: 625 micrograms, dose to be given 30 minutes before end of surgery, then 625 micrograms every 6 hours as required
  Prevention of nausea and vomiting caused by opioid analgesics in postoperative patient-controlled analgesia (PCA)
  ▸ BY INTRAVENOUS INJECTION
  ▸ Adult: 15–50 micrograms of droperidol for every 1 mg of morphine in PCA, reduce dose in elderly; maximum 5 mg per day

- CONTRA-INDICATIONS Bradycardia · CNS depression · comatose states · hypokalaemia · hypomagnesaemia · phaeochromocytoma · QT-interval prolongation
- CAUTIONS Chronic obstructive pulmonary disease · electrolyte disturbances · history of alcohol abuse · respiratory failure
- INTERACTIONS → Appendix 1: droperidol
- SIDE-EFFECTS
- **Uncommon** Anxiety · oculogyration
- **Rare or very rare** Arrhythmia · blood disorder · cardiac arrest · dysphoria · movement disorders
- **Frequency not known** Coma · epilepsy · hallucination · oligomenorrhoea · respiratory disorders · SIADH · syncope
- BREAST FEEDING Limited information available—avoid repeated administration.
- HEPATIC IMPAIRMENT
  Dose adjustments In postoperative nausea and vomiting, max. 625 micrograms repeated every 6 hours as required.
  For nausea and vomiting caused by opioid analgesics in postoperative patient-controlled analgesia, reduce dose.
- RENAL IMPAIRMENT
  Dose adjustments In postoperative nausea and vomiting, max. 625 micrograms repeated every 6 hours as required.
  For nausea and vomiting caused by opioid analgesics in postoperative patient-controlled analgesia, reduce dose.

● MONITORING REQUIREMENTS Continuous pulse oximetry required if risk of ventricular arrhythmia—continue for 30 minutes following administration.

● MEDICINAL FORMS
There can be variation in the licensing of different medicines containing the same drug.
Solution for injection
▸ Droperidol (Non-proprietary)
  Droperidol 2.5 mg per 1 ml Droperidol 2.5mg/1ml solution for injection ampoules | 10 ampoule [PoM] [S]
▸ Xomolix (Kyowa Kirin Ltd)
  Droperidol 2.5 mg per 1 ml Xomolix 2.5mg/1ml solution for injection ampoules | 10 ampoule [PoM] £39.40

⚑ 380

Levomepromazine
12-Dec-2016
(Methotrimeprazine)

● INDICATIONS AND DOSE
Pain in palliative care (reserved for distressed patients with severe pain unresponsive to other measures)
▸ BY CONTINUOUS SUBCUTANEOUS INFUSION, OR BY INTRAMUSCULAR INJECTION, OR BY INTRAVENOUS INJECTION
▸ Adult: Seek specialist advice

Restlessness and confusion in palliative care
▸ BY CONTINUOUS SUBCUTANEOUS INFUSION
▸ Child 1-11 years: 0.35–3 mg/kg, to be administered over 24 hours
▸ Child 12-17 years: 12.5–200 mg, to be administered over 24 hours
▸ BY MOUTH
▸ Adult: 6 mg every 2 hours as required
▸ BY SUBCUTANEOUS INJECTION
▸ Adult: 6.25 mg every 2 hours as required
▸ BY SUBCUTANEOUS INFUSION
▸ Adult: Initially 12.5–50 mg/24 hours, titrated according to response (doses greater than 100 mg/24 hours should be given under specialist supervision)

Nausea and vomiting in palliative care
▸ BY CONTINUOUS INTRAVENOUS INFUSION, OR BY SUBCUTANEOUS INFUSION
▸ Child 1 month-11 years: 100–400 micrograms/kg, to be administered over 24 hours
▸ Child 12-17 years: 5–25 mg, to be administered over 24 hours
▸ BY MOUTH
▸ Adult: 6 mg once daily, dose to be taken at bedtime, increased if necessary to 12.5–25 mg twice daily
▸ BY SUBCUTANEOUS INJECTION
▸ Adult: 6.25 mg once daily, dose to be given at bedtime, increased if necessary to 12.5–25 mg twice daily
▸ BY SUBCUTANEOUS INFUSION
▸ Adult: 5–25 mg/24 hours, sedation can limit the dose

Schizophrenia (bed patients)
▸ BY MOUTH
▸ Adult: Initially 100–200 mg daily in 3 divided doses, increased if necessary to 1 g daily

Schizophrenia
▸ BY MOUTH
▸ Adult: Initially 25–50 mg daily in divided doses, dose can be increased as necessary

● CONTRA-INDICATIONS CNS depression · comatose states · phaeochromocytoma
● CAUTIONS Patients receiving large initial doses should remain supine
  CAUTIONS, FURTHER INFORMATION
▸ In adults Risk of postural hypotension; not recommended for ambulant patients over 50 years unless risk of hypotensive reaction assessed.

● INTERACTIONS → Appendix 1: phenothiazines
● SIDE-EFFECTS
▸ **Common or very common** Asthenia · heat stroke
▸ **Rare or very rare** Arrhythmia · cardiac arrest · hepatic disorders
▸ **Frequency not known** Allergic dermatitis · delirium · gastrointestinal disorders · glucose tolerance impaired · hyponatraemia · photosensitivity reaction · priapism · SIADH · sudden cardiac death
● HEPATIC IMPAIRMENT Can precipitate coma; phenothiazines are hepatotoxic.
● RENAL IMPAIRMENT
  Dose adjustments Start with small doses in severe renal impairment because of increased cerebral sensitivity.
● DIRECTIONS FOR ADMINISTRATION
▸ With subcutaneous use in children For administration by *subcutaneous infusion* dilute with a suitable volume of Sodium Chloride 0.9%.
● PRESCRIBING AND DISPENSING INFORMATION
  Palliative care For further information on the use of levomepromazine in palliative care, see www.palliativedrugs.com/formulary/en/levomepromazine.html.

● MEDICINAL FORMS
There can be variation in the licensing of different medicines containing the same drug. Forms available from special-order manufacturers include: tablet, oral suspension, oral solution
Solution for injection
▸ Levomepromazine (Non-proprietary)
  Levomepromazine hydrochloride 25 mg per 1 ml Levomepromazine 25mg/1ml solution for injection ampoules | 10 ampoule [PoM] £20.13 DT = £20.13
▸ Nozinan (Sanofi)
  Levomepromazine hydrochloride 25 mg per 1 ml Nozinan 25mg/1ml solution for injection ampoules | 10 ampoule [PoM] £20.13 DT = £20.13
Tablet
CAUTIONARY AND ADVISORY LABELS 2
▸ Levinan (Kyowa Kirin Ltd)
  Levomepromazine maleate 6 mg Levinan 6mg tablets | 28 tablet [PoM] [S]
▸ Nozinan (Sanofi)
  Levomepromazine maleate 25 mg Nozinan 25mg tablets | 84 tablet [PoM] £20.26 DT = £20.26

5.1 Ménière's disease

HISTAMINE ANALOGUES

Betahistine dihydrochloride

● INDICATIONS AND DOSE
Vertigo, tinnitus and hearing loss associated with Ménière's disease
▸ BY MOUTH
▸ Adult: Initially 16 mg 3 times a day, dose preferably taken with food; maintenance 24–48 mg daily

● CONTRA-INDICATIONS Phaeochromocytoma
● CAUTIONS Asthma · history of peptic ulcer
● INTERACTIONS → Appendix 1: betahistine
● SIDE-EFFECTS
▸ **Common or very common** Gastrointestinal discomfort · headache · nausea
▸ **Frequency not known** Allergic dermatitis · vomiting
● PREGNANCY Avoid unless clearly necessary—no information available.
● BREAST FEEDING Use only if potential benefit outweighs risk—no information available.

Nervous system 4

4

Nervous system

● MEDICINAL FORMS
There can be variation in the licensing of different medicines containing the same drug. Forms available from special-order manufacturers include: oral suspension, oral solution

Tablet

CAUTIONARY AND ADVISORY LABELS 21

▸ Betahistine dihydrochloride (Non-proprietary)
  Betahistine dihydrochloride 8 mg Betahistine 8mg tablets |
  84 tablet [PoM] £10.50 DT = £3.12 | 120 tablet [PoM] £3.71–£13.50
  Betahistine dihydrochloride 16 mg Betahistine 16mg tablets |
  84 tablet [PoM] £17.19 DT = £5.50
▸ Serc (Mylan)
  Betahistine dihydrochloride 8 mg Serc 8mg tablets |
  120 tablet [PoM] £9.04
  Betahistine dihydrochloride 16 mg Serc 16mg tablets |
  84 tablet [PoM] £12.65 DT = £5.50

6 Pain

Analgesics

Pain relief

The non-opioid drugs, paracetamol p. 438 and aspirin p. 121 (and other NSAIDs), are particularly suitable for pain in musculoskeletal conditions, whereas the opioid analgesics are more suitable for moderate to severe pain, particularly of visceral origin.

Pain in sickle-cell disease

The pain of mild sickle-cell crises is managed with paracetamol, a NSAID, codeine phosphate p. 448, or dihydrocodeine tartrate p. 450. Severe crises may require the use of morphine p. 456 or diamorphine hydrochloride p. 449; concomitant use of a NSAID may potentiate analgesia and allow lower doses of the opioid to be used. Pethidine hydrochloride p. 463 should be avoided if possible because accumulation of a neurotoxic metabolite can precipitate seizures; the relatively short half-life of pethidine hydrochloride necessitates frequent injections.

Dental and orofacial pain

Analgesics should be used judiciously in dental care as a **temporary** measure until the cause of the pain has been dealt with.

Dental pain of inflammatory origin, such as that associated with pulpitis, apical infection, localised osteitis or pericoronitis is usually best managed by treating the infection, providing drainage, restorative procedures, and other local measures. Analgesics provide temporary relief of pain (usually for about 1 to 7 days) until the causative factors have been brought under control. In the case of pulpitis, intra-osseous infection or abscess, reliance on analgesics alone is usually inappropriate.

Similarly the pain and discomfort associated with acute problems of the oral mucosa (e.g. acute herpetic gingivostomatitis, erythema multiforme) may be relieved by benzydamine hydrochloride p. 1180 mouthwash or spray until the cause of the mucosal disorder has been dealt with. However, where a patient is febrile, the antipyretic action of paracetamol or ibuprofen p. 1106 is often helpful.

The *choice* of an analgesic for dental purposes should be based on its suitability for the patient. Most dental pain is relieved effectively by non-steroidal anti-inflammatory drugs (NSAIDs). NSAIDs that are used for dental pain include ibuprofen, diclofenac sodium p. 1101, and aspirin. Paracetamol has analgesic and antipyretic effects but no anti-inflammatory effect.

Opioid analgesics such as dihydrocodeine tartrate act on the central nervous system and are traditionally used for *moderate to severe pain*. However, opioid analgesics are relatively ineffective in dental pain and their side-effects can be unpleasant. Paracetamol, ibuprofen, or aspirin are adequate for most cases of dental pain and an opioid is rarely required.

Combining a non-opioid with an opioid analgesic can provide greater relief of pain than either analgesic given alone. However, this applies only when an adequate dose of each analgesic is used. Most combination analgesic preparations have not been shown to provide greater relief of pain than an adequate dose of the non-opioid component given alone. Moreover, combination preparations have the disadvantage of an increased number of side-effects.

Any analgesic given before a dental procedure should have a low risk of increasing postoperative bleeding. In the case of pain after the dental procedure, taking an analgesic before the effect of the local anaesthetic has worn off can improve control. Postoperative analgesia with ibuprofen or aspirin is usually continued for about 24 to 72 hours.

Temporomandibular dysfunction can be related to anxiety in some patients who may clench or grind their teeth (bruxism) during the day or night. The muscle spasm (which appears to be the main source of pain) may be treated empirically with an overlay appliance which provides a free sliding occlusion and may also interfere with grinding. In addition, diazepam p. 340, which has muscle relaxant as well as anxiolytic properties, may be helpful but it should only be prescribed on a short-term basis during the acute phase. Analgesics such as aspirin or ibuprofen may also be required.

Dysmenorrhoea

Use of an oral contraceptive prevents the pain of dysmenorrhoea which is generally associated with ovulatory cycles. If treatment is necessary paracetamol or a NSAID will generally provide adequate relief of pain. The vomiting and severe pain associated with dysmenorrhoea in women with endometriosis may call for an antiemetic (in addition to an analgesic). Antispasmodics (such as alverine citrate p. 86) have been advocated for dysmenorrhoea but the antispasmodic action does not generally provide significant relief.

Non-opioid analgesics and compound analgesic preparations

Aspirin is indicated for headache, transient musculoskeletal pain, dysmenorrhoea, and pyrexia. In inflammatory conditions, most physicians prefer anti-inflammatory treatment with another NSAID which may be better tolerated and more convenient for the patient. Aspirin is used increasingly for its antiplatelet properties. Aspirin tablets or dispersible aspirin tablets are adequate for most purposes as they act rapidly.

Gastric irritation may be a problem; it is minimised by taking the dose after food. Enteric-coated preparations are available, but have a slow onset of action and are therefore unsuitable for single-dose analgesic use (though their prolonged action may be useful for night pain).

Aspirin interacts significantly with a number of other drugs and its interaction with warfarin sodium p. 139 is a **special hazard**.

Paracetamol is similar in efficacy to aspirin, but has no demonstrable anti-inflammatory activity; it is less irritant to the stomach and for that reason is now generally preferred to aspirin, particularly in the elderly. **Overdosage** with paracetamol is particularly dangerous as it may cause hepatic damage which is sometimes not apparent for 4 to 6 days.

Nefopam hydrochloride p. 440 may have a place in the relief of persistent pain unresponsive to other non-opioid analgesics. It causes little or no respiratory depression, but sympathomimetic and antimuscarinic side-effects may be troublesome.

Non-steroidal anti-inflammatory analgesics (NSAIDs) are particularly useful for the treatment of patients with chronic disease accompanied by pain and inflammation. Some of them are also used in the short-term treatment of mild to moderate pain including transient musculoskeletal pain but paracetamol is now often preferred, particularly in the elderly. They are also suitable for the relief of pain in *dysmenorrhoea* and to treat pain caused by *secondary bone tumours*, many of which produce lysis of bone and release prostaglandins. Selective inhibitors of cyclo-oxygenase-2 may be used in preference to non-selective NSAIDs for patients at high risk of developing serious gastro-intestinal side-effects. Several NSAIDs are also used for postoperative analgesia.

A non-opioid analgesic administered by intrathecal infusion (**ziconotide** (*Prialt®*), available from Eisai) is licensed for the treatment of chronic severe pain; ziconotide can be used by a hospital specialist as an adjunct to opioid analgesics.

Compound analgesic preparations

Compound analgesic preparations that contain a simple analgesic (such as aspirin or paracetamol p. 438) with an opioid component reduce the scope for effective titration of the individual components in the management of pain of varying intensity.

Compound analgesic preparations containing paracetamol or aspirin p. 121 with a *low dose* of an opioid analgesic (e.g. 8 mg of codeine phosphate p. 448 per compound tablet) are commonly used, but the advantages have not been substantiated. The low dose of the opioid may be enough to cause opioid side-effects (in particular, constipation) and can complicate the treatment of **overdosage** yet may not provide significant additional relief of pain.

A *full dose* of the opioid component (e.g. 60 mg codeine phosphate) in compound analgesic preparations effectively augments the analgesic activity but is associated with the full range of opioid side-effects (including nausea, vomiting, severe constipation, drowsiness, respiratory depression, and risk of dependence on long-term administration). **Important**: the elderly are particularly susceptible to opioid side-effects and should receive lower doses.

In general, when assessing pain, it is necessary to weigh up carefully whether there is a need for a non-opioid and an opioid analgesic to be taken simultaneously.

Caffeine is a weak stimulant that is often included, in small doses, in analgesic preparations. It is claimed that the addition of caffeine may enhance the analgesic effect, but the alerting effect, mild habit-forming effect and possible provocation of headache may not always be desirable. Moreover, in excessive dosage or on withdrawal caffeine may itself induce headache.

Co-proxamol tablets (dextropropoxyphene in combination with paracetamol) are no longer licensed because of safety concerns, particularly toxicity in overdose. Co-proxamol tablets [unlicensed] may still be prescribed for patients who find it difficult to change, because alternatives are not effective or suitable.

Opioid analgesics and dependence

Opioid analgesics are usually used to relieve moderate to severe pain particularly of visceral origin. Repeated administration may cause dependence and tolerance, but this is no deterrent in the control of pain in terminal illness. Regular use of a potent opioid may be appropriate for certain cases of chronic non-malignant pain; treatment should be supervised by a specialist and the patient should be assessed at regular intervals.

Strong opioids

Morphine p. 456 remains the most valuable opioid analgesic for severe pain although it frequently causes nausea and vomiting. It is the standard against which other opioid analgesics are compared. In addition to relief of pain, morphine also confers a state of euphoria and mental detachment.

Morphine is the opioid of choice for the oral treatment of *severe pain in palliative care*. It is given regularly every 4 hours (or every 12 or 24 hours as modified-release preparations).

Buprenorphine p. 442 has both opioid agonist and antagonist properties and may precipitate withdrawal symptoms, including pain, in patients dependent on other opioids. It has abuse potential and may itself cause dependence. It has a much longer duration of action than morphine and sublingually is an effective analgesic for 6 to 8 hours. Unlike most opioid analgesics, the effects of buprenorphine are only partially reversed by naloxone hydrochloride p. 1329.

Dipipanone hydrochloride used alone is less sedating than morphine but the only preparation available contains an antiemetic and is therefore not suitable for regular regimens in palliative care.

Diamorphine hydrochloride p. 449 (heroin) is a powerful opioid analgesic. It may cause less nausea and hypotension than morphine. In *palliative care* the greater solubility of diamorphine hydrochloride allows effective doses to be injected in smaller volumes and this is important in the emaciated patient.

Alfentanil p. 1304, fentanyl p. 451 and remifentanil p. 1304 are used by injection for intra-operative analgesia; fentanyl is available in a transdermal drug delivery system as a self-adhesive patch which is changed every 72 hours.

Methadone hydrochloride p. 495 is less sedating than morphine and acts for longer periods. In prolonged use, methadone hydrochloride should not be administered more often than twice daily to avoid the risk of accumulation and opioid overdosage. Methadone hydrochloride may be used instead of morphine in the occasional patient who experiences excitation (or exacerbation of pain) with morphine.

Oxycodone hydrochloride p. 459 has an efficacy and side-effect profile similar to that of morphine. It is used primarily for control of *pain in palliative care*.

Papaveretum p. 462 is rarely used; morphine is easier to prescribe and less prone to error with regard to the strength and dose.

Pentazocine p. 462 has both agonist and antagonist properties and precipitates withdrawal symptoms, including pain in patients dependent on other opioids. By injection it is more potent than dihydrocodeine tartrate p. 450 or codeine phosphate, but hallucinations and thought disturbances may occur. It is not recommended and, in particular, should be avoided after myocardial infarction as it may increase pulmonary and aortic blood pressure as well as cardiac work.

Pethidine hydrochloride p. 463 produces prompt and short-lasting analgesia; it is less constipating than morphine, but even in high doses is a less potent analgesic. It is not suitable for severe continuing pain. It is used for analgesia in labour; however, other opioids, such as morphine or diamorphine hydrochloride, are often preferred for obstetric pain.

Tapentadol p. 464 produces analgesia by two mechanisms. It is an opioid-receptor agonist and it also inhibits noradrenaline reuptake. Nausea, vomiting, and constipation are less likely to occur with tapentadol than with other strong opioid analgesics.

Tramadol hydrochloride p. 464 produces analgesia by two mechanisms: an opioid effect and an enhancement of serotonergic and adrenergic pathways. It has fewer of the typical opioid side-effects (notably, less respiratory depression, less constipation and less addiction potential); psychiatric reactions have been reported.

Weak opioids

Codeine phosphate can be used for the relief of mild to moderate pain where other painkillers such as paracetamol or ibuprofen p. 1106 have proved ineffective.

Dihydrocodeine tartrate has an analgesic efficacy similar to that of codeine phosphate. Higher doses may provide some additional pain relief but this may be at the cost of more nausea and vomiting.

Meptazinol p. 456 is claimed to have a low incidence of repiratory depression. It has a reported length of action of 2 to 7 hours with onset within 15 minutes.

Postoperative analgesia

A combination of opioid and non-opioid analgesics is used to treat postoperative pain. The use of intra-operative opioids affects the prescribing of postoperative analgesics. A postoperative opioid analgesic should be given with care since it may potentiate any residual respiratory depression.

Morphine is used most widely. Tramadol hydrochloride is not as effective in severe pain as other opioid analgesics. Buprenorphine may antagonise the analgesic effect of previously administered opioids and is generally not recommended. Pethidine hydrochloride is generally not recommended for postoperative pain because it is metabolised to norpethidine which may accumulate, particularly in renal impairment; norpethidine stimulates the central nervous system and may cause convulsions.

Opioids are also given epidurally [unlicensed route] in the postoperative period but are associated with side-effects such as pruritus, urinary retention, nausea and vomiting; respiratory depression can be delayed, particularly with morphine p. 456.

Patient-controlled analgesia (PCA) can be used to relieve postoperative pain—consult individual hospital protocols.

Pain management and opioid dependence

Although caution is necessary, patients who are dependent on opioids or have a history of drug dependence may be treated with opioid analgesics when there is a clinical need. Treatment with opioid analgesics in this patient group should normally be carried out with the advice of specialists. However, doctors do not require a special licence to prescribe opioid analgesics to patients with opioid dependence for relief of pain due to organic disease or injury.

Other drugs used for Pain Dexibuprofen, p. 1098 · Diclofenac potassium, p. 1100 · Fenoprofen, p. 1105 · Levomepromazine, p. 435 · Mefenamic acid, p. 1111

ANAESTHETICS, GENERAL > VOLATILE LIQUID ANAESTHETICS

Methoxyflurane

30-Jan-2018

● **INDICATIONS AND DOSE**

Moderate-to-severe pain associated with trauma (under close medical supervision)

▸ BY INHALATION
▸ Adult: 3–6 mL as required, avoid administration on consecutive days; administer using inhaler device; maximum 15 mL per week

IMPORTANT SAFETY INFORMATION
Manufacturer advises methoxyflurane should only be self-administered under the supervision of personnel experienced in its use, using a hand-held *Penthrox*® inhaler device.

● CONTRA-INDICATIONS Cardiovascular disease · history of liver damage associated with use of methoxyflurane or other halogenated anaesthetics · impaired consciousness · respiratory depression · susceptibility to malignant hyperthermia

● CAUTIONS Elderly—increased risk of hypotension · repeated administration more than once every 3 months—increased risk of hepatic injury · risk factors for hepatic impairment · risk factors for renal impairment

● INTERACTIONS → Appendix 1: volatile halogenated anaesthetics

● SIDE-EFFECTS
▸ **Common or very common** Anxiety · cough · depression · dizziness · drowsiness · dry mouth · dysarthria · headache · hyperhidrosis · hypotension · memory loss · mood altered · nausea · neuropathy sensory · taste altered
▸ **Uncommon** Appetite increased · chills · fatigue · oral discomfort · paraesthesia · vision disorders
▸ **Rare or very rare** Hepatic disorders
▸ **Frequency not known** Consciousness impaired · disorientation · dissociation · hypoxia · nystagmus · renal failure · vomiting

● ALLERGY AND CROSS-SENSITIVITY Contra-indicated in patients with hypersensitivity to fluorinated anaesthetics.

● PREGNANCY Manufacturer advises use with caution—limited information available.

● BREAST FEEDING Manufacturer advises use with caution—limited information available.

● HEPATIC IMPAIRMENT Manufacturer advises caution.

● RENAL IMPAIRMENT Manufacturer advises avoid.

● PRESCRIBING AND DISPENSING INFORMATION The manufacturer of *Penthrox*® has provided an *Administration Checklist* and an *Administration Guide* for healthcare professionals.

● HANDLING AND STORAGE Manufacturer advises exposure of healthcare professionals to methoxyflurane should be minimised—risk of serious side-effects.

● PATIENT AND CARER ADVICE Manufacturer advises that patients should given advice on appropriate inhaler technique.

A patient alert card should be provided.

Driving and skilled tasks Manufacturer advises patients and carers should be counselled on the effects on driving and performance of skilled tasks—increased risk of dizziness and drowsiness.

● MEDICINAL FORMS
There can be variation in the licensing of different medicines containing the same drug.

Inhalation vapour
EXCIPIENTS: May contain Butylated hydroxytoluene
▸ Penthrox (Galen Ltd) ▼
Methoxyflurane 999 mg per 1 gram Penthrox inhalation vapour 3ml bottles with device | 1 bottle PoM £17.89 (Hospital only)

ANALGESICS > NON-OPIOID

Paracetamol

05-May-2016

(Acetaminophen)

● **INDICATIONS AND DOSE**

Mild to moderate pain | Pyrexia
▸ BY MOUTH
▸ Adult: 0.5–1 g every 4–6 hours; maximum 4 g per day
▸ BY INTRAVENOUS INFUSION
▸ Adult (body-weight up to 50 kg): 15 mg/kg every 4–6 hours, dose to be administered over 15 minutes; maximum 60 mg/kg per day
▸ Adult (body-weight 50 kg and above): 1 g every 4–6 hours, dose to be administered over 15 minutes; maximum 4 g per day
▸ BY RECTUM
▸ Adult: 0.5–1 g every 4–6 hours; maximum 4 g per day

Mild to moderate pain in patients with risk factors for hepatotoxicity | Pyrexia in patients with risk factors for hepatotoxicity
▸ BY INTRAVENOUS INFUSION
▹ Adult (body-weight up to 50 kg): 15 mg/kg every 4–6 hours, dose to be administered over 15 minutes; maximum 60 mg/kg per day
▹ Adult (body-weight 50 kg and above): 1 g every 4–6 hours, dose to be administered over 15 minutes; maximum 3 g per day

Pain | Pyrexia with discomfort
▸ BY MOUTH
▹ Child 3–5 months: 60 mg every 4–6 hours; maximum 4 doses per day
▹ Child 6 months–1 year: 120 mg every 4–6 hours; maximum 4 doses per day
▹ Child 2–3 years: 180 mg every 4–6 hours; maximum 4 doses per day
▹ Child 4–5 years: 240 mg every 4–6 hours; maximum 4 doses per day
▹ Child 6–7 years: 240–250 mg every 4–6 hours; maximum 4 doses per day
▹ Child 8–9 years: 360–375 mg every 4–6 hours; maximum 4 doses per day
▹ Child 10–11 years: 480–500 mg every 4–6 hours; maximum 4 doses per day
▹ Child 12–15 years: 480–750 mg every 4–6 hours; maximum 4 doses per day
▹ Child 16–17 years: 0.5–1 g every 4–6 hours; maximum 4 doses per day
▸ BY RECTUM
▹ Child 3–11 months: 60–125 mg every 4–6 hours as required; maximum 4 doses per day
▹ Child 1–4 years: 125–250 mg every 4–6 hours as required; maximum 4 doses per day
▹ Child 5–11 years: 250–500 mg every 4–6 hours as required; maximum 4 doses per day
▹ Child 12–17 years: 500 mg every 4–6 hours

Prophylaxis of post-immunisation pyrexia following immunisation with meningococcal group B vaccine (Bexsero ®) given as part of the routine immunisation schedule
▸ BY MOUTH
▹ Child 2 months: 60 mg, first dose to be given at the time of vaccination, then 60 mg after 4–6 hours, then 60 mg after 4–6 hours, use weight-based doses for preterm infants born at less than 32 weeks gestation and currently weighing less than 4 kg—see oral doses for pain and pyrexia with discomfort
▹ Child 4 months: 60 mg, first dose to be given at the time of vaccination, then 60 mg after 4–6 hours, then 60 mg after 4–6 hours, use weight-based doses for preterm infants born at less than 32 weeks gestation and currently weighing less than 4 kg—see oral doses for pain and pyrexia with discomfort

Post-immunisation pyrexia in infants
▸ BY MOUTH
▹ Child 2–3 months: 60 mg for 1 dose, then 60 mg after 4–6 hours if required
▹ Child 4 months: 60 mg for 1 dose, then 60 mg after 4–6 hours; maximum 4 doses per day

● UNLICENSED USE Paracetamol oral suspension 500 mg/5 mL not licensed for use in children under 16 years. [EvGr] Not licensed for use as prophylaxis of post-immunisation pyrexia following immunisation with meningococcal group B vaccine. ⟨E⟩
● CAUTIONS Before administering, check when paracetamol last administered and cumulative paracetamol dose over previous 24 hours · body-weight under 50 kg · chronic alcohol consumption · chronic dehydration · chronic

malnutrition · hepatocellular insufficiency · long-term use (especially in those who are malnourished)

CAUTIONS, FURTHER INFORMATION [EvGr] Some patients may be at increased risk of experiencing toxicity at therapeutic doses, particularly those with a body-weight under 50 kg and those with risk factors for hepatotoxicity. Clinical judgement should be used to adjust the dose of oral and intravenous paracetamol in these patients.
  Co-administration of enzyme-inducing antiepileptic medications may increase toxicity; doses should be reduced. ⟨E⟩

● INTERACTIONS → Appendix 1: paracetamol
● SIDE-EFFECTS
GENERAL SIDE-EFFECTS
▸ Rare or very rare Thrombocytopenia
SPECIFIC SIDE-EFFECTS
▸ Common or very common
▹ With rectal use Anorectal erythema
▸ Rare or very rare
▹ With intravenous use Hypersensitivity · hypotension · leucopenia · malaise · neutropenia
▹ With rectal use Angioedema · liver injury · skin reactions
▸ Frequency not known
▹ With intravenous use Flushing · skin reactions · tachycardia
▹ With oral use Agranulocytosis · bronchospasm · hepatic function abnormal · severe cutaneous adverse reactions (SCARs)
▹ With rectal use Agranulocytosis · blood disorder

Overdose Important: liver damage and less frequently renal damage can occur following overdose.
  Nausea and vomiting, the only early features of poisoning, usually settle within 24 hours. Persistence beyond this time, often associated with the onset of right subcostal pain and tenderness, usually indicates development of hepatic necrosis.
  For specific details on the management of poisoning, see Paracetamol, under Emergency treatment of poisoning p. 1319.

● PREGNANCY Not known to be harmful.
● BREAST FEEDING Amount too small to be harmful.
● HEPATIC IMPAIRMENT Dose-related toxicity—avoid large doses.
● RENAL IMPAIRMENT
Dose adjustments Increase infusion dose interval to every 6 hours if eGFR less than 30 mL/minute/1.73 m^2.
● DIRECTIONS FOR ADMINISTRATION For *intravenous infusion* (Perfalgan ®), give in Glucose 5% or Sodium Chloride 0.9%; dilute to a concentration of not less than 1 mg/mL and use within an hour; may also be given undiluted. For children under 33 kg, use 50 mL-vial.
● PRESCRIBING AND DISPENSING INFORMATION BP directs that when Paediatric Paracetamol Oral Suspension or Paediatric Paracetamol Mixture is prescribed Paracetamol Oral Suspension 120 mg/5 mL should be dispensed.
● PATIENT AND CARER ADVICE
Medicines for Children leaflet: Paracetamol for mild-to-moderate pain www.medicinesforchildren.org.uk/paracetamol-for-mildtomoderate-pain
● PROFESSION SPECIFIC INFORMATION
Dental practitioners' formulary
Paracetamol Tablets may be prescribed.
Paracetamol Soluble Tablets 500 mg may be prescribed.
Paracetamol Oral Suspension may be prescribed.
● EXCEPTIONS TO LEGAL CATEGORY Paracetamol capsules or tablets can be sold to the public provided packs contain no more than 32 capsules or tablets; pharmacists can sell multiple packs up to a total quantity of 100 capsules or tablets in justifiable circumstances.

Nervous system

4

● MEDICINAL FORMS
There can be variation in the licensing of different medicines containing the same drug. Forms available from special-order manufacturers include: oral suspension, oral solution, suppository, powder

Tablet
CAUTIONARY AND ADVISORY LABELS 29, 30
▸ Paracetamol (Non-proprietary)
Paracetamol 500 mg Paracetamol 500mg caplets | 100 tablet [PoM] £3.05 DT = £0.97
Paracetamol 500mg tablets | 100 tablet [PoM] £2.13 DT = £0.97 | 1000 tablet [PoM] £9.69–£9.70
Paracetamol 1 gram Paracetamol 1g tablets | 100 tablet [PoM] £1.80
▸ Mandanol (M & A Pharmachem Ltd)
Paracetamol 500 mg Mandanol 500mg caplets | 100 tablet [PoM] £1.45 DT = £0.97
Mandanol 500mg tablets | 100 tablet [PoM] £1.45 DT = £0.97
▸ Paravict (Ecogen Europe Ltd)
Paracetamol 500 mg Paravict 500mg tablets | 100 tablet [PoM] £1.62 DT = £0.97

Suppository
CAUTIONARY AND ADVISORY LABELS 30
▸ Paracetamol (Non-proprietary)
Paracetamol 80 mg Paracetamol 80mg suppositories | 10 suppository [P] £10.00
Paracetamol 120 mg Paracetamol 120mg suppositories | 10 suppository [P] £12.39 DT = £12.39
Paracetamol 125 mg Paracetamol 125mg suppositories | 10 suppository [P] £15.00 DT = £13.80
Paracetamol 240 mg Paracetamol 240mg suppositories | 10 suppository [P] £22.01 DT = £22.01
Paracetamol 250 mg Paracetamol 250mg suppositories | 10 suppository [P] £24.15 DT = £27.60
Paracetamol 500 mg Paracetamol 500mg suppositories | 10 suppository [P] £36.50 DT = £36.50
Paracetamol 1 gram Paracetamol 1g suppositories | 10 suppository [P] £59.50 DT = £59.50
▸ Alvedon (Intrapharm Laboratories Ltd)
Paracetamol 60 mg Alvedon 60mg suppositories | 10 suppository [P] £11.95 DT = £11.95
Paracetamol 125 mg Alvedon 125mg suppositories | 10 suppository [P] £13.80 DT = £13.80
Paracetamol 250 mg Alvedon 250mg suppositories | 10 suppository [P] £27.60 DT = £27.60

Oral suspension
CAUTIONARY AND ADVISORY LABELS 30
▸ Paracetamol (Non-proprietary)
Paracetamol 24 mg per 1 ml Paracetamol 120mg/5ml oral suspension paediatric | 100 ml [P] £0.60–£1.26 | 500 ml [P] £4.57 DT = £4.57
Paracetamol 120mg/5ml oral suspension paediatric sugar free sugar-free | 100 ml [P] £1.19 DT = £1.19 sugar-free | 200 ml [P] £2.38 sugar-free | 500 ml [P] £5.95 sugar-free | 1000 ml [P] £11.90
Paracetamol 50 mg per 1 ml Paracetamol 250mg/5ml oral suspension | 100 ml [P] £1.25 DT = £1.25 | 500 ml [P] £3.50–£6.25
Paracetamol 250mg/5ml oral suspension sugar free sugar-free | 100 ml [P] £1.14–£1.19 sugar-free | 200 ml [P] £2.28 DT = £2.28 sugar-free | 500 ml [P] £5.70 sugar-free | 1000 ml [P] £11.40
Paracetamol 100 mg per 1 ml Paracetamol 500mg/5ml oral suspension sugar free sugar-free | 150 ml [PoM] £24.00 DT = £24.00
▸ Calpol (McNeil Products Ltd)
Paracetamol 24 mg per 1 ml Calpol Infant 120mg/5ml oral suspension | 200 ml [P] £3.78
Calpol Infant 120mg/5ml oral suspension sugar-free | 200 ml [P] £3.78
Paracetamol 50 mg per 1 ml Calpol Six Plus 250mg/5ml oral suspension | 200 ml [P] £4.40
Calpol Six Plus 250mg/5ml oral suspension sugar-free | 100 ml [P] £2.64 sugar-free | 200 ml [P] £4.40 DT = £2.28

Effervescent tablet
CAUTIONARY AND ADVISORY LABELS 29, 30
▸ Paracetamol (Non-proprietary)
Paracetamol 500 mg Paracetamol 500mg soluble tablets | 60 tablet [PoM] £5.00 | 100 tablet [PoM] £8.33 DT = £7.29
Paracetamol 500mg effervescent tablets sugar-free | 24 tablet [PoM] £1.88 sugar-free | 60 tablet [PoM] £4.25–£4.38 sugar-free | 100 tablet [PoM] £7.08–£7.29

Solution for infusion
▸ Paracetamol (Non-proprietary)
Paracetamol 10 mg per 1 ml Paracetamol 100mg/10ml solution for infusion ampoules | 20 ampoule [PoM] £12.00
Paracetamol 1g/100ml solution for infusion bottles | 10 bottle [PoM] [剤]
Paracetamol 1g/100ml solution for infusion vials | 10 vial [PoM] £12.00
▸ Perfalgan (Bristol-Myers Squibb Pharmaceuticals Ltd)
Paracetamol 10 mg per 1 ml Perfalgan 1g/100ml solution for infusion vials | 12 vial [PoM] £14.96
Perfalgan 500mg/50ml solution for infusion vials | 12 vial [PoM] £13.60

Oral solution
CAUTIONARY AND ADVISORY LABELS 30
▸ Paracetamol (Non-proprietary)
Paracetamol 24 mg per 1 ml Paracetamol 120mg/5ml oral solution paediatric sugar free sugar-free | 2000 ml [P] £23.80 DT = £23.80
Paracetamol 100 mg per 1 ml Paracetamol 500mg/5ml oral solution sugar free sugar-free | 150 ml [PoM] £24.00 sugar-free | 200 ml [PoM] £18.00 DT = £18.00

Powder
▸ Paracetamol (Non-proprietary)
Paracetamol 1 gram Paracetamol 1g oral powder sachets | 10 sachet [GSL] £1.11
▸ Brands may include Abdine Cold Relief

Capsule
CAUTIONARY AND ADVISORY LABELS 29, 30
▸ Paracetamol (Non-proprietary)
Paracetamol 500 mg Paracetamol 500mg capsules | 100 capsule [PoM] £3.84 DT = £1.88

Orodispersible tablet
CAUTIONARY AND ADVISORY LABELS 30
▸ Calpol Fastmelts (McNeil Products Ltd)
Paracetamol 250 mg Calpol Six Plus Fastmelts 250mg tablets sugar-free | 24 tablet [P] £4.12

Combinations available: *Co-codamol,* p. 447 · *Dihydrocodeine with paracetamol,* p. 450

ANALGESICS 〉 NON-OPIOID, CENTRALLY ACTING

Nefopam hydrochloride

● **INDICATIONS AND DOSE**
Moderate pain
▸ BY MOUTH
▸ **Adult:** Initially 60 mg 3 times a day, adjusted according to response; usual dose 30–90 mg 3 times a day
▸ **Elderly:** Initially 30 mg 3 times a day, adjusted according to response; usual dose 30–90 mg 3 times a day

● CONTRA-INDICATIONS Convulsive disorders · not indicated for myocardial infarction
● CAUTIONS Elderly · urinary retention
● INTERACTIONS → Appendix 1: nefopam
● SIDE-EFFECTS
▸ **Uncommon** Coma · drowsiness · headache · hyperhidrosis · insomnia · tachycardia · vision blurred · vomiting
▸ **Rare or very rare** Urine red
▸ **Frequency not known** Abdominal pain · angioedema · confusion · diarrhoea · dizziness · dry mouth · gastrointestinal disorder · hallucination · hypotension · nausea · nervousness · palpitations · paraesthesia · seizure · syncope · tremor · urinary retention
● PREGNANCY No information available—avoid unless no safer treatment.
● HEPATIC IMPAIRMENT Caution.
● RENAL IMPAIRMENT Caution.

- **MEDICINAL FORMS**
There can be variation in the licensing of different medicines containing the same drug. Forms available from special-order manufacturers include: oral suspension

Tablet
CAUTIONARY AND ADVISORY LABELS 2, 14
▸ Nefopam hydrochloride (Non-proprietary)
  Nefopam hydrochloride 30 mg Nefopam 30mg tablets |
  90 tablet [PoM] £68.39 DT = £16.41

ANALGESICS > NON-STEROIDAL ANTI-INFLAMMATORY DRUGS

Aspirin with codeine

The properties listed below are those particular to the combination only. For the properties of the components please consider, aspirin p. 121, codeine phosphate p. 448.

- **INDICATIONS AND DOSE**
Mild to moderate pain | Pyrexia
  ▸ BY MOUTH
  ▸ Adult: 1–2 tablets every 4–6 hours as required, dose to be dispersed in water; maximum 8 tablets per day

- **INTERACTIONS** → Appendix 1: aspirin · opioids

- **PRESCRIBING AND DISPENSING INFORMATION** When co-codaprin tablets or dispersible tablets are prescribed and no strength is stated, tablets or dispersible tablets, respectively, containing codeine phosphate 8 mg and aspirin 400 mg should be dispensed.

- **LESS SUITABLE FOR PRESCRIBING** Aspirin with codeine is less suitable for prescribing.

- **EXCEPTIONS TO LEGAL CATEGORY** Aspirin with codeine can be sold to the public provided packs contain no more than 32 capsules or tablets; pharmacists can sell multiple packs up to a total quantity of 100 capsules or tablets in justifiable circumstances.

- **MEDICINAL FORMS**
There can be variation in the licensing of different medicines containing the same drug.
  Dispersible tablet
  CAUTIONARY AND ADVISORY LABELS 13, 21, 32
  ▸ Aspirin with codeine (Non-proprietary)
    Codeine phosphate 8 mg, Aspirin 400 mg Co-codaprin
    8mg/400mg dispersible tablets | 100 tablet [PoM] £97.55 DT =
    £92.19 [CD5]
  ▸ Codis (Reckitt Benckiser Healthcare (UK) Ltd)
    Codeine phosphate 8 mg, Aspirin 500 mg Codis 500 dispersible
    tablets sugar-free | 32 tablet [P] £3.23 [CD5]
  Tablet
  ▸ Aspirin with codeine (Non-proprietary)
    Codeine phosphate 8 mg, Aspirin 400 mg Aspirin and Codeine
    tablets | 32 tablet [P] [⚠] [CD5]

ANALGESICS > OPIOIDS

Opioids

- **CONTRA-INDICATIONS** Acute respiratory depression · comatose patients · head injury (opioid analgesics interfere with pupillary responses vital for neurological assessment) · raised intracranial pressure (opioid analgesics interfere with pupillary responses vital for neurological assessment) · risk of paralytic ileus

- **CAUTIONS** Adrenocortical insufficiency (reduced dose is recommended) · asthma (avoid during an acute attack) · convulsive disorders · debilitated patients (reduced dose is recommended) (in adults) · diseases of the biliary tract · elderly (reduced dose is recommended) · hypotension · hypothyroidism (reduced dose is recommended) · impaired respiratory function (avoid in chronic obstructive pulmonary disease) · inflammatory bowel disorders ·

myasthenia gravis · obstructive bowel disorders · prostatic hypertrophy (in adults) · shock · urethral stenosis (in adults)

CAUTIONS, FURTHER INFORMATION
▸ **Dependence** Repeated use of opioid analgesics is associated with the development of psychological and physical dependence; although this is rarely a problem with therapeutic use, caution is advised if prescribing for patients with a history of drug dependence.
▸ **Palliative care** In the control of pain in terminal illness, the cautions listed should not necessarily be a deterrent to the use of opioid analgesics.

- **SIDE-EFFECTS**
▸ **Common or very common** Arrhythmias · confusion · constipation · dizziness · drowsiness (uncommon in children) · dry mouth · euphoric mood · flushing · hallucination · headache (uncommon in children) · hyperhidrosis · hypotension (with high doses) · miosis · nausea (more common on initiation) · palpitations · respiratory depression (frequency not known in children, with high doses) · skin reactions · urinary retention · vertigo · visual impairment (uncommon in children) · vomiting (more common on initiation)
▸ **Uncommon** Drug dependence · drug tolerance · dysphoria · withdrawal syndrome

SIDE-EFFECTS, FURTHER INFORMATION
Respiratory depression Respiratory depression is a major concern with opioid analgesics and it may be treated by artificial ventilation or be reversed by naloxone.
Dependence and withdrawal Psychological dependence rarely occurs when opioids are used therapeutically (e.g. for pain relief), but tolerance can develop during long-term treatment.
Overdose Opioids (narcotic analgesics) cause coma, respiratory depression, and pinpoint pupils. For details on the management of poisoning, see Opioids, under Emergency treatment of poisoning p. 1319 and consider the specific antidote, naloxone hydrochloride.

- **PREGNANCY** Respiratory depression and withdrawal symptoms can occur in the neonate if opioid analgesics are used during delivery; also gastric stasis and inhalation pneumonia has been reported in the mother if opioid analgesics are used during labour.

- **HEPATIC IMPAIRMENT** Avoid use or reduce dose; may precipitate coma in patients with hepatic impairment.

- **TREATMENT CESSATION** Avoid abrupt withdrawal after long-term treatment; they should be withdrawn gradually to avoid abstinence symptoms.

- **PRESCRIBING AND DISPENSING INFORMATION** The *Faculty of Pain Medicine* has produced resources for healthcare professionals around opioid prescribing: www.fpm.ac.uk/faculty-of-pain-medicine/opioids-aware

- **PATIENT AND CARER ADVICE**
Driving and skilled tasks Drowsiness may affect performance of skilled tasks (e.g. driving); effects of alcohol enhanced. Driving at the start of therapy with opioid analgesics, and following dose changes, should be avoided.

  For information on 2015 legislation regarding driving whilst taking certain controlled drugs, including opioids, see *Drugs and driving* under Guidance on prescribing p. 1.

Nervous system

4

Buprenorphine
F 441
19-Oct-2017

- **DRUG ACTION** Buprenorphine is an opioid-receptor partial agonist (it has opioid agonist and antagonist properties).

- **INDICATIONS AND DOSE**

Moderate to severe pain
▸ BY SUBLINGUAL ADMINISTRATION
▸ Child (body-weight 16-25 kg): 100 micrograms every 6-8 hours
▸ Child (body-weight 25-37.5 kg): 100-200 micrograms every 6-8 hours
▸ Child (body-weight 37.5-50 kg): 200-300 micrograms every 6-8 hours
▸ Child (body-weight 50 kg and above): 200-400 micrograms every 6-8 hours
▸ Adult: 200-400 micrograms every 6-8 hours
▸ BY INTRAMUSCULAR INJECTION, OR BY SLOW INTRAVENOUS INJECTION
▸ Child 6 months-11 years: 3-6 micrograms/kg every 6-8 hours (max. per dose 9 micrograms/kg)
▸ Child 12-17 years: 300-600 micrograms every 6-8 hours
▸ Adult: 300-600 micrograms every 6-8 hours

Premedication
▸ BY SUBLINGUAL ADMINISTRATION
▸ Adult: 400 micrograms
▸ BY INTRAMUSCULAR INJECTION
▸ Adult: 300 micrograms

Intra-operative analgesia
▸ BY SLOW INTRAVENOUS INJECTION
▸ Adult: 300-450 micrograms

Adjunct in the treatment of opioid dependence
▸ BY SUBLINGUAL ADMINISTRATION USING SUBLINGUAL TABLETS
▸ Adult: Initially 0.8-4 mg for 1 dose on the first day, adjusted in steps of 2-4 mg daily if required; usual dose 12-24 mg daily; maximum 32 mg per day
▸ BY MOUTH USING ORAL LYOPHILISATE
▸ Adult: Initially 2 mg daily, followed by 2-4 mg if required on day one, adjusted in steps of 2-6 mg daily if required, for adjustment of dosing interval following stabilisation, consult product literature; maximum 18 mg per day

DOSE EQUIVALENCE AND CONVERSION
▸ For opioid substitution therapy, in patients taking methadone who want to switch to buprenorphine, the dose of methadone should be reduced to a maximum of 30 mg daily before starting buprenorphine treatment—consult product literature. For *sublingual tablets*, if the dose of methadone is over 10 mg daily, buprenorphine can be started at a dose of 4 mg daily and titrated according to requirements; if the methadone dose is below 10 mg daily, buprenorphine can be started at a dose of 2 mg daily.

BUTRANS ®
Moderate, non-malignant pain unresponsive to non-opioid analgesics
▸ BY TRANSDERMAL APPLICATION USING PATCHES
▸ Adult: Initially 5 micrograms/hour up to every 7 days, dose adjustments—when starting, analgesic effect should not be evaluated until the system has been worn for 72 hours (to allow for gradual increase in plasma-buprenorphine concentration)—if necessary, dose should be adjusted at intervals of at least 3 days using a patch of the next strength or a combination of 2 patches applied in different places (applied at *same time* to avoid confusion). Maximum 2 patches can be used at any one time

BUPEAZE ®
Moderate to severe chronic cancer pain in patients who have not previously received strong opioid analgesic | Severe pain unresponsive to non-opioid analgesics in patients who have not previously received strong opioid analgesic
▸ BY TRANSDERMAL APPLICATION USING PATCHES
▸ Adult: Initially 35 micrograms/hour up to every 96 hours, dose adjustment—when starting, analgesic effect should not be evaluated until the system has been worn for 24 hours (to allow for gradual increase in plasma-buprenorphine concentration)—if necessary, dose should be adjusted at intervals of no longer than 96 hours using a patch of the next strength or using 2 patches of the same strength (applied at *same time* to avoid confusion). Maximum 2 patches can be used at any one time

Moderate to severe chronic cancer pain in patients who have previously received strong opioid analgesic | Severe pain unresponsive to non-opioid analgesics in patients who have previously received strong opioid analgesic
▸ BY TRANSDERMAL APPLICATION USING PATCHES
▸ Adult: The initial dose should be based on previous 24-hour opioid requirement, consult product literature, dose adjustment—when starting, analgesic effect should not be evaluated until the system has been worn for 24 hours (to allow for gradual increase in plasma-buprenorphine concentration)—if necessary, dose should be adjusted at intervals of no longer than 96 hours using a patch of the next strength or using 2 patches of the same strength (applied at *same time* to avoid confusion). Maximum 2 patches can be used at any one time

PHARMACOKINETICS
▸ For *Bupeaze*®: it may take approximately 30 hours for the plasma-buprenorphine concentration to decrease by 50% after patch is removed.

BUPLAST ®
Moderate to severe chronic cancer pain in patients who have not previously received strong opioid analgesic | Severe pain unresponsive to non-opioid analgesics in patients who have not previously received strong opioid analgesic
▸ BY TRANSDERMAL APPLICATION USING PATCHES
▸ Adult: Initially 35 micrograms/hour up to every 96 hours, dose adjustment—when starting, analgesic effect should not be evaluated until the system has been worn for 24 hours (to allow for gradual increase in plasma-buprenorphine concentration)—if necessary, dose should be adjusted at intervals of no longer than 96 hours using a patch of the same strength or using 2 patches of the same strength (applied at *same time* to avoid confusion). Maximum 2 patches can be used at any one time

Moderate to severe chronic cancer pain in patients who have previously received strong opioid analgesic | Severe pain unresponsive to non-opioid analgesics in patients who have previously received strong opioid analgesic
▸ BY TRANSDERMAL APPLICATION USING PATCHES
▸ Adult: The initial dose should be based on previous 24-hour opioid requirement, consult product literature, dose adjustment—when starting, analgesic effect should not be evaluated until the system has been worn for 24 hours (to allow for gradual increase in plasma-buprenorphine concentration)—if necessary, dose should be adjusted at intervals of no longer than 96 hours using a patch of the next strength or using 2 patches of the same strength (applied at *same time* to avoid confusion). Maximum 2 patches can be used at any one time

PHARMACOKINETICS
- For *Buplast*®: it may take approximately 30 hours for the plasma-buprenorphine concentration to decrease by 50% after patch is removed.

BUPRAMYL ®

Moderate, non-malignant pain unresponsive to non-opioid analgesics
- BY TRANSDERMAL APPLICATION USING PATCHES
- Adult: Initially 5 micrograms/hour up to every 7 days, dose adjustments—when starting, analgesic effect should not be evaluated until the system has been worn for 72 hours (to allow for gradual increase in plasma-buprenorphine concentration)—if necessary, dose should be adjusted at intervals of at least 3 days using a patch of the next strength or a combination of 2 patches applied in different places (applied at *same time* to avoid confusion). Maximum 2 patches can be used at any one time

PHARMACOKINETICS
- For *Bupramyl*®: it may take approximately 12 hours for the plasma-buprenorphine concentration to decrease by 50% after patch is removed.

BUTEC ®

Moderate, non-malignant pain unresponsive to non-opioid analgesics
- BY TRANSDERMAL APPLICATION USING PATCHES
- Adult: Initially 5 micrograms/hour up to every 7 days, dose adjustments—when starting, analgesic effect should not be evaluated until the system has been worn for 72 hours (to allow for gradual increase in plasma-buprenorphine concentration)—if necessary, dose should be adjusted at intervals of at least 3 days using a patch of the next strength or a combination of 2 patches applied in different places (applied at *same time* to avoid confusion). Maximum 2 patches can be used at any one time

PHARMACOKINETICS
- For *Butec*®: it may take approximately 12 hours for the plasma-buprenorphine concentration to decrease by 50% after patch is removed.

HAPOCTASIN ®

Moderate to severe chronic cancer pain in patients who have not previously received strong opioid analgesic | Severe pain unresponsive to non-opioid analgesics in patients who have not previously received strong opioid analgesic
- BY TRANSDERMAL APPLICATION USING PATCHES
- Adult: Initially 35 micrograms/hour up to every 72 hours, dose adjustment—when starting, analgesic effect should not be evaluated until the system has been worn for 24 hours (to allow for gradual increase in plasma-buprenorphine concentration)—if necessary, dose should be adjusted at intervals of no longer than 72 hours using a patch of the next strength or using 2 patches of the same strength (applied at *same time* to avoid confusion). Maximum 2 patches can be used at any one time, for breakthrough pain, consider 200–400 micrograms buprenorphine sublingually

Moderate to severe chronic cancer pain in patients who have previously received strong opioid analgesic | Severe pain unresponsive to non-opioid analgesics in patients who have previously received strong opioid analgesic
- BY TRANSDERMAL APPLICATION USING PATCHES
- Adult: The initial dose should be based on previous 24-hour opioid requirement, consult product literature, dose adjustment—when starting, analgesic effect should not be evaluated until the system has been worn for 24 hours (to allow for gradual increase in plasma-buprenorphine concentration)—if necessary,

dose should be adjusted at intervals of no longer than 72 hours using a patch of the next strength or using 2 patches of the same strength (applied at *same time* to avoid confusion). Maximum 2 patches can be used at any one time, for breakthrough pain, consider 200–400 micrograms buprenorphine sublingually

PHARMACOKINETICS
- For *Hapoctasin*®: it may take approximately 25 hours for the plasma-buprenorphine concentration to decrease by 50% after patch is removed.

PANITAZ ®

Moderate, non-malignant pain unresponsive to non-opioid analgesics
- BY TRANSDERMAL APPLICATION USING PATCHES
- Adult: Initially 5 micrograms/hour up to every 7 days, dose adjustments—when starting, analgesic effect should not be evaluated until the system has been worn for 72 hours (to allow for gradual increase in plasma-buprenorphine concentration)—if necessary, dose should be adjusted at intervals of at least 3 days using a patch of the next strength or a combination of 2 patches applied in different places (applied at *same time* to avoid confusion). Maximum 2 patches can be used at any one time

PHARMACOKINETICS
- For *Panitaz*®: it may take approximately 12 hours for the plasma-buprenorphine concentration to decrease by 50% after patch is removed.

PRENOTRIX ®

Moderate to severe chronic cancer pain in patients who have not previously received strong opioid analgesic | Severe pain unresponsive to non-opioid analgesics in patients who have not previously received strong opioid analgesic
- BY TRANSDERMAL APPLICATION USING PATCHES
- Adult: Initially 35 micrograms/hour up to every 72 hours, dose adjustment—when starting, analgesic effect should not be evaluated until the system has been worn for 24 hours (to allow for gradual increase in plasma-buprenorphine concentration)—if necessary, dose should be adjusted at intervals of no longer than 72 hours using a patch of the next strength or using 2 patches of the same strength (applied at *same time* to avoid confusion). Maximum 2 patches can be used at any one time

Moderate to severe chronic cancer pain in patients who have previously received strong opioid analgesic | Severe pain unresponsive to non-opioid analgesics in patients who have previously received strong opioid analgesic
- BY TRANSDERMAL APPLICATION USING PATCHES
- Adult: The initial dose should be based on previous 24-hour opioid requirement, consult product literature, dose adjustment—when starting, analgesic effect should not be evaluated until the system has been worn for 24 hours (to allow for gradual increase in plasma-buprenorphine concentration)—if necessary, dose should be adjusted at intervals of no longer than 72 hours using a patch of the next strength or using 2 patches of the same strength (applied at *same time* to avoid confusion). Maximum 2 patches can be used at any one time

PHARMACOKINETICS
- For *Prenotrix*®: it may take approximately 25 hours for the plasma-buprenorphine concentration to decrease by 50% after patch is removed. continued →

RELETRANS ®

Moderate, non-malignant pain unresponsive to non-opioid analgesics

▸ BY TRANSDERMAL APPLICATION USING PATCHES

▸ Adult: Initially 5 micrograms/hour up to every 7 days, dose adjustments—when starting, analgesic effect should not be evaluated until the system has been worn for 72 hours (to allow for gradual increase in plasma-buprenorphine concentration)—if necessary, dose should be adjusted at intervals of at least 3 days using a patch of the next strength or a combination of 2 patches applied in different places (applied at *same time* to avoid confusion). Maximum 2 patches can be used at any one time

PHARMACOKINETICS

▸ For *Reletrans®*: it may take approximately 12 hours for the plasma-buprenorphine concentration to decrease by 50% after patch is removed.

RELEVTEC ®

Moderate to severe chronic cancer pain in patients who have not previously received strong opioid analgesic | Severe pain unresponsive to non-opioid analgesics in patients who have not previously received strong opioid analgesic

▸ BY TRANSDERMAL APPLICATION USING PATCHES

▸ Adult: Initially 35 micrograms/hour up to every 96 hours, dose adjustment—when starting, analgesic effect should not be evaluated until the system has been worn for 24 hours (to allow for gradual increase in plasma-buprenorphine concentration)—if necessary, dose should be adjusted at intervals of no longer than 96 hours using a patch of the next strength or using 2 patches of the same strength (applied at *same time* to avoid confusion). Maximum 2 patches can be used at any one time

Moderate to severe chronic cancer pain in patients who have previously received strong opioid analgesic | Severe pain unresponsive to non-opioid analgesics in patients who have previously received strong opioid analgesic

▸ BY TRANSDERMAL APPLICATION USING PATCHES

▸ Adult: The initial dose should be based on previous 24-hour opioid requirement, consult product literature, dose adjustment—when starting, analgesic effect should not be evaluated until the system has been worn for 24 hours (to allow for gradual increase in plasma-buprenorphine concentration)—if necessary, dose should be adjusted at intervals of no longer than 96 hours using a patch of the next strength or using 2 patches of the same strength (applied at *same time* to avoid confusion). Maximum 2 patches can be used at any one time

PHARMACOKINETICS

▸ For *Relevtec®*: it may take approximately 30 hours for the plasma-buprenorphine concentration to decrease by 50% after patch is removed.

SEVODYNE ®

Moderate, non-malignant pain unresponsive to non-opioid analgesics

▸ BY TRANSDERMAL APPLICATION USING PATCHES

▸ Adult: Initially 5 micrograms/hour up to every 7 days, dose adjustments—when starting, analgesic effect should not be evaluated until the system has been worn for 72 hours (to allow for gradual increase in plasma-buprenorphine concentration)—if necessary, dose should be adjusted at intervals of at least 3 days using a patch of the next strength or a combination of 2 patches applied in different places (applied at *same time* to avoid confusion). Maximum 2 patches can be used at any one time

PHARMACOKINETICS

▸ For *Sevodyne®*: it may take approximately 12 hours for the plasma-buprenorphine concentration to decrease by 50% after patch is removed.

TRANSTEC ®

Moderate to severe chronic cancer pain in patients who have not previously received strong opioid analgesic | Severe pain unresponsive to non-opioid analgesics in patients who have not previously received strong opioid analgesic

▸ BY TRANSDERMAL APPLICATION USING PATCHES

▸ Adult: Initially 35 micrograms/hour up to every 96 hours, dose adjustment—when starting, analgesic effect should not be evaluated until the system has been worn for 24 hours (to allow for gradual increase in plasma-buprenorphine concentration)—if necessary, dose should be adjusted at intervals of no longer than 96 hours using a patch of the next strength or using 2 patches of the same strength (applied at *same time* to avoid confusion). Maximum 2 patches can be used at any one time, for breakthrough pain, consider 200–400 micrograms buprenorphine sublingually

Moderate to severe chronic cancer pain in patients who have previously received strong opioid analgesic | Severe pain unresponsive to non-opioid analgesics in patients who have previously received strong opioid analgesic

▸ BY TRANSDERMAL APPLICATION USING PATCHES

▸ Adult: The initial dose should be based on previous 24-hour opioid requirement, consult product literature, dose adjustment—when starting, analgesic effect should not be evaluated until the system has been worn for 24 hours (to allow for gradual increase in plasma-buprenorphine concentration)—if necessary, dose should be adjusted at intervals of no longer than 96 hours using a patch of the next strength or using 2 patches of the same strength (applied at *same time* to avoid confusion). Maximum 2 patches can be used at any one time, for breakthrough pain, consider 200–400 micrograms buprenorphine sublingually

PHARMACOKINETICS

▸ For *Transtec®*: it may take approximately 30 hours for the plasma-buprenorphine concentration to decrease by 50% after patch is removed.

● UNLICENSED USE Sublingual tablets not licensed for use in children under 6 years.

IMPORTANT SAFETY INFORMATION
Do not confuse the formulations of transdermal patches which are available as 72-hourly, 96-hourly and 7-day patches, see *Prescribing and dispensing information*.

● CAUTIONS

GENERAL CAUTIONS Impaired consciousness

SPECIFIC CAUTIONS

▸ With transdermal use Fever or external heat · other opioids should not be administered within 24 hours of patch removal (long duration of action)

▸ When used for adjunct in the treatment of opioid dependence Hepatitis B infection · hepatitis C infection · pre-existing liver enzyme abnormalities

CAUTIONS, FURTHER INFORMATION

▸ Fever or external heat Manufacturer advises monitor patients using patches for increased side-effects if fever present (increased absorption possible); avoid exposing application site to external heat (may also increase absorption).

● INTERACTIONS → Appendix 1: opioids

● **SIDE-EFFECTS**
▶ **Common or very common**
▶ With sublingual use Fatigue · postural hypotension · sleep disorders
▶ With transdermal use Anxiety · appetite decreased · asthenia · depression · diarrhoea · dyspnoea · gastrointestinal discomfort · muscle weakness · oedema · sleep disorders · tremor
▶ **Uncommon**
▶ With sublingual use Anxiety · apnoea · appetite decreased · atrioventricular block · coma · conjunctivitis · coordination abnormal · cyanosis · depersonalisation · depression · diarrhoea · diplopia · disorientation · dyspepsia · dyspnoea · hypertension · pallor · paraesthesia · psychosis · seizure · speech slurred · tinnitus · tremor · urinary disorder
▶ With transdermal use Aggression · chest pain · chills · circulatory collapse · concentration impaired · cough · dry eye · fever · gastrointestinal disorders · hiccups · hypertension · injury · memory loss · migraine · mood altered · movement disorders · muscle complaints · respiratory disorders · sensation abnormal · sexual dysfunction · speech impairment · syncope · taste altered · tinnitus · urinary disorders · vision blurred · weight decreased
▶ **Rare or very rare**
▶ With sublingual use Angioedema · bronchospasm
▶ With transdermal use Angina pectoris · asthma exacerbated · dehydration · dysphagia · ear pain · eyelid oedema · increased risk of infection · influenza like illness · muscle contractions involuntary · postural hypotension · psychotic disorder · vasodilation
▶ **Frequency not known**
▶ With parenteral use Angioedema · bronchospasm · hepatic disorders · psychotic disorder · vision blurred
▶ With sublingual use Cerebrospinal fluid pressure increased · circulation impaired · haemorrhagic diathesis · hepatic disorders · oral disorders · syncope
▶ With transdermal use Biliary colic · depersonalisation · seizure

Overdose The effects of buprenorphine are only partially reversed by naloxone.

● **BREAST FEEDING** Present in low levels in breast milk. **Monitoring** Neonates should be monitored for drowsiness, adequate weight gain, and developmental milestones.

● **RENAL IMPAIRMENT** Avoid use or reduce dose; opioid effects increased and prolonged; increased cerebral sensitivity.

● **PRE-TREATMENT SCREENING** Documentation of viral hepatitis status is recommended before commencing therapy for opioid dependence.

● **MONITORING REQUIREMENTS** Monitor liver function; when used in opioid dependence baseline liver function test is recommended before commencing therapy, and regular liver function tests should be performed throughout treatment.

● **DIRECTIONS FOR ADMINISTRATION**
▶ In children Sublingual tablets may be halved.
▶ In adults Manufacturer advises oral lyophilisates should be placed on the tongue and allowed to dissolve. Patients should be advised not to swallow for 2 minutes and not to consume food or drink for at least 5 minutes after administration.
   BUTRANS ® Apply patch to dry, non-irritated, non-hairy skin on upper torso, removing after 7 days and siting replacement patch on a different area (avoid same area for at least 3 weeks).
   PRENOTRIX ® Manufacturer advises apply patch to dry, non-irritated, non-hairy skin on upper torso, removing after no longer than 72 hours and siting replacement patch on a different area (avoid same area for at least 7 days).

HAPOCTASIN ® Apply patch to dry, non-irritated, non-hairy skin on upper torso, removing after no longer than 72 hours and siting replacement patch on a different area (avoid same area for at least 7 days).
BUPRAMYL ®, BUTEC ®, PANITAZ ®, RELETRANS ®, SEVODYNE ® Manufacturer advises apply patch to dry, non-irritated, non-hairy skin on upper torso or upper outer arm, removing after 7 days and siting replacement patch on a different area (avoid same area for at least 3 weeks).
TRANSTEC ® Apply patch to dry, non-irritated, non-hairy skin on upper torso, removing after no longer than 96 hours and siting replacement patch on a different area (avoid same area for at least 6 days).
BUPEAZE ®, BUPLAST ®, RELEVTEC ® Manufacturer advises apply patch to dry, non-irritated, non-hairy skin on upper torso, removing after no longer than 96 hours and siting replacement patch on a different area (avoid same area for at least 7 days).

● **PRESCRIBING AND DISPENSING INFORMATION** Transdermal buprenorphine patches are not suitable for acute pain or in those patients whose analgesic requirements are changing rapidly because the long time to steady state prevents rapid titration of the dose. Transdermal patches are available as 72-hourly, 96-hourly and 7-day formulations; prescribers and dispensers must ensure that the correct preparation is prescribed and dispensed. Preparations that should be applied up to every 72 hours include Hapoctasin® and Prenotrix®. Preparations that should be applied up to every 96 hours include Bupeaze®, Buplast®, Relevtec®, and Transtec®. Preparations that should be applied up to every 7 days include Bupramyl®, Butec®, BuTrans®, Panitaz®, Reletrans®, and Sevodyne®. Espranor® oral lyophilisate has different bioavailability to other buprenorphine products and is not interchangeable with them—consult product literature before switching between products.

● **PATIENT AND CARER ADVICE** Patients or carers should be given advice on how to administer buprenorphine products.

● **NATIONAL FUNDING/ACCESS DECISIONS**

NICE decisions
▶ **Methadone and buprenorphine for the management of opioid dependence (January 2007)** NICE TA114
Oral methadone and buprenorphine are recommended for maintenance therapy in the management of opioid dependence. Patients should be committed to a supportive care programme including a flexible dosing regimen administered under supervision for at least 3 months, until compliance is assured. Selection of methadone or buprenorphine should be made on a case-by-case basis, but methadone should be prescribed if both drugs are equally suitable.
www.nice.org.uk/guidance/TA114

Scottish Medicines Consortium (SMC) Decisions
The Scottish Medicines Consortium has advised (June 2017) that buprenorphine oral lyophilisate (Espranor®) is accepted for restricted use within NHS Scotland as substitution treatment for opioid dependence for patients in whom methadone is not suitable. This advice is contingent upon the continuing availability of the patient access scheme in NHS Scotland or a list price that is equivalent or lower.

BUTEC ®

Scottish Medicines Consortium (SMC) Decisions
The Scottish Medicines Consortium has advised (January 2017) that buprenorphine transdermal patches (Butec®) are accepted for restricted use within NHS Scotland for the treatment of chronic non-malignant pain of moderate

intensity when an opioid is necessary for obtaining adequate analgesia in elderly patients (over 65 years).

● MEDICINAL FORMS
There can be variation in the licensing of different medicines containing the same drug.

Solution for injection

▸ Temgesic (Indivior UK Ltd)

Buprenorphine (as Buprenorphine hydrochloride)
300 microgram per 1 ml Temgesic 300micrograms/1ml solution for injection ampoules | 5 ampoule [PoM] £2.46 [CD3]

Sublingual tablet

CAUTIONARY AND ADVISORY LABELS 2, 26

▸ Buprenorphine (Non-proprietary)

Buprenorphine (as Buprenorphine hydrochloride)
200 microgram Buprenorphine 200microgram sublingual tablets sugar free sugar-free | 50 tablet [PoM] £5.04 DT = £5.04 [CD3]
Buprenorphine (as Buprenorphine hydrochloride)
400 microgram Buprenorphine 400microgram sublingual tablets sugar free sugar-free | 7 tablet [PoM] £1.60 DT = £1.60 [CD3] sugar-free | 50 tablet [PoM] £10.07 DT = £10.07 [CD3]
Buprenorphine (as Buprenorphine hydrochloride)
2 mg Buprenorphine 2mg sublingual tablets sugar free sugar-free | 7 tablet [PoM] £8.35 DT = £0.93 [CD3]
Buprenorphine (as Buprenorphine hydrochloride)
8 mg Buprenorphine 8mg sublingual tablets sugar free sugar-free | 7 tablet [PoM] £22.50 DT = £1.81 [CD3]

▸ Natzon (Morningside Healthcare Ltd)

Buprenorphine (as Buprenorphine hydrochloride)
400 microgram Natzon 0.4mg sublingual tablets sugar-free | 7 tablet [PoM] £1.60 DT = £1.60 [CD3]
Buprenorphine (as Buprenorphine hydrochloride) 2 mg Natzon 2mg sublingual tablets sugar-free | 7 tablet [PoM] £6.35 DT = £0.93 [CD3]
Buprenorphine (as Buprenorphine hydrochloride) 8 mg Natzon 8mg sublingual tablets sugar-free | 7 tablet [PoM] £19.05 DT = £1.81 [CD3]

▸ Prefibin (Sandoz Ltd)

Buprenorphine (as Buprenorphine hydrochloride)
400 microgram Prefibin 0.4mg sublingual tablets sugar-free | 7 tablet [PoM] £1.60 DT = £1.60 [CD3]
Buprenorphine (as Buprenorphine hydrochloride) 2 mg Prefibin 2mg sublingual tablets sugar-free | 7 tablet [PoM] £5.38 DT = £0.93 [CD3]
Buprenorphine (as Buprenorphine hydrochloride) 8 mg Prefibin 8mg sublingual tablets sugar-free | 7 tablet [PoM] £16.15 DT = £1.81 [CD3]

▸ Subutex (Indivior UK Ltd)

Buprenorphine (as Buprenorphine hydrochloride)
400 microgram Subutex 0.4mg sublingual tablets sugar-free | 7 tablet [PoM] £1.60 DT = £1.60 [CD3]
Buprenorphine (as Buprenorphine hydrochloride) 2 mg Subutex 2mg sublingual tablets sugar-free | 7 tablet [PoM] £6.35 DT = £0.93 [CD3]
Buprenorphine (as Buprenorphine hydrochloride) 8 mg Subutex 8mg sublingual tablets sugar-free | 7 tablet [PoM] £19.05 DT = £1.81 [CD3]

▸ Temgesic (Indivior UK Ltd)

Buprenorphine (as Buprenorphine hydrochloride)
200 microgram Temgesic 200microgram sublingual tablets sugar-free | 50 tablet [PoM] £5.04 DT = £5.04 [CD3]
Buprenorphine (as Buprenorphine hydrochloride)
400 microgram Temgesic 400microgram sublingual tablets sugar-free | 50 tablet [PoM] £10.07 DT = £10.07 [CD3]

▸ Tephine (Sandoz Ltd)

Buprenorphine (as Buprenorphine hydrochloride)
200 microgram Tephine 200microgram sublingual tablets sugar-free | 50 tablet [PoM] £4.27 DT = £5.04 [CD3]
Buprenorphine (as Buprenorphine hydrochloride)
400 microgram Tephine 400microgram sublingual tablets sugar-free | 50 tablet [PoM] £8.54 DT = £10.07 [CD3]

Oral lyophilisate

CAUTIONARY AND ADVISORY LABELS 2
EXCIPIENTS: May contain Aspartame, gelatin

▸ Espranor (Martindale Pharmaceuticals Ltd)

Buprenorphine (as Buprenorphine hydrochloride) 2 mg Espranor 2mg oral lyophilisates sugar-free | 7 tablet [PoM] £6.35 [CD3]
Buprenorphine (as Buprenorphine hydrochloride) 8 mg Espranor 8mg oral lyophilisates sugar-free | 7 tablet [PoM] £19.05 [CD3]

Transdermal patch

CAUTIONARY AND ADVISORY LABELS 2

▸ BuTrans (Napp Pharmaceuticals Ltd)

Buprenorphine 5 microgram per 1 hour BuTrans 5micrograms/hour transdermal patches | 4 patch [PoM] £17.60 DT = £17.60 [CD3]
Buprenorphine 10 microgram per 1 hour BuTrans 10micrograms/hour transdermal patches | 4 patch [PoM] £31.55 DT = £31.55 [CD3]
Buprenorphine 15 microgram per 1 hour BuTrans 15micrograms/hour transdermal patches | 4 patch [PoM] £49.15 DT = £49.15 [CD3]
Buprenorphine 20 microgram per 1 hour BuTrans 20micrograms/hour transdermal patches | 4 patch [PoM] £57.46 DT = £57.46 [CD3]

▸ Bupeaze (Dr Reddy's Laboratories (UK) Ltd)

Buprenorphine 35 microgram per 1 hour Bupeaze 35micrograms/hour transdermal patches | 4 patch [PoM] £11.85 DT = £15.80 [CD3]
Buprenorphine 52.5 microgram per 1 hour Bupeaze 52.5micrograms/hour transdermal patches | 4 patch [PoM] £17.78 DT = £23.71 [CD3]
Buprenorphine 70 microgram per 1 hour Bupeaze 70micrograms/hour transdermal patches | 4 patch [PoM] £23.70 DT = £31.60 [CD3]

▸ Buplast (Mylan)

Buprenorphine 35 microgram per 1 hour Buplast 35micrograms/hour transdermal patches | 4 patch [PoM] £15.80 DT = £15.80 [CD3]
Buprenorphine 52.5 microgram per 1 hour Buplast 52.5micrograms/hour transdermal patches | 4 patch [PoM] £23.71 DT = £23.71 [CD3]
Buprenorphine 70 microgram per 1 hour Buplast 70micrograms/hour transdermal patches | 4 patch [PoM] £31.60 DT = £31.60 [CD3]

▸ Bupramyl (Mylan)

Buprenorphine 5 microgram per 1 hour Bupramyl 5micrograms/hour transdermal patches | 4 patch [PoM] £7.04 DT = £17.60 [CD3]
Buprenorphine 10 microgram per 1 hour Bupramyl 10micrograms/hour transdermal patches | 4 patch [PoM] £12.62 DT = £31.55 [CD3]
Buprenorphine 20 microgram per 1 hour Bupramyl 20micrograms/hour transdermal patches | 4 patch [PoM] £22.98 DT = £57.46 [CD3]

▸ Butec (Qdem Pharmaceuticals Ltd)

Buprenorphine 5 microgram per 1 hour Butec 5micrograms/hour transdermal patches | 4 patch [PoM] £7.92 DT = £17.60 [CD3]
Buprenorphine 10 microgram per 1 hour Butec 10micrograms/hour transdermal patches | 4 patch [PoM] £14.20 DT = £31.55 [CD3]
Buprenorphine 15 microgram per 1 hour Butec 15micrograms/hour transdermal patches | 4 patch [PoM] £22.12 DT = £49.15 [CD3]
Buprenorphine 20 microgram per 1 hour Butec 20micrograms/hour transdermal patches | 4 patch [PoM] £25.86 DT = £57.46 [CD3]

▸ Hapoctasin (Actavis UK Ltd)

Buprenorphine 35 microgram per 1 hour Hapoctasin 35micrograms/hour transdermal patches | 4 patch [PoM] £9.48 DT = £15.80 [CD3]
Buprenorphine 52.5 microgram per 1 hour Hapoctasin 52.5micrograms/hour transdermal patches | 4 patch [PoM] £14.23 DT = £23.71 [CD3]
Buprenorphine 70 microgram per 1 hour Hapoctasin 70micrograms/hour transdermal patches | 4 patch [PoM] £18.96 DT = £31.60 [CD3]

▸ Panitaz (Dr Reddy's Laboratories (UK) Ltd)

Buprenorphine 5 microgram per 1 hour Panitaz 5micrograms/hour transdermal patches | 4 patch [PoM] £7.04 DT = £17.60 [CD3]
Buprenorphine 10 microgram per 1 hour Panitaz 10micrograms/hour transdermal patches | 4 patch [PoM] £12.62 DT = £31.55 [CD3]
Buprenorphine 20 microgram per 1 hour Panitaz 20micrograms/hour transdermal patches | 4 patch [PoM] £22.98 DT = £57.46 [CD3]

▸ Reletrans (Sandoz Ltd)

Buprenorphine 5 microgram per 1 hour Reletrans 5micrograms/hour transdermal patches | 4 patch [PoM] £7.92 DT = £17.60 [CD3]

Buprenorphine 10 microgram per 1 hour Reletrans
10micrograms/hour transdermal patches | 4 patch [PoM] £14.20 DT =
£31.55 [CD3]
Buprenorphine 15 microgram per 1 hour Reletrans
15micrograms/hour transdermal patches | 4 patch [PoM] £22.12 DT =
£49.15 [CD3]
Buprenorphine 20 microgram per 1 hour Reletrans
20micrograms/hour transdermal patches | 4 patch [PoM] £25.86 DT =
£57.46 [CD3]
▸ Relevtec (Sandoz Ltd)
Buprenorphine 35 microgram per 1 hour Relevtec
35micrograms/hour transdermal patches | 4 patch [PoM] £11.06 DT =
£15.80 [CD3]
Buprenorphine 52.5 microgram per 1 hour Relevtec
52.5micrograms/hour transdermal patches | 4 patch [PoM] £16.60 DT
= £23.71 [CD3]
Buprenorphine 70 microgram per 1 hour Relevtec
70micrograms/hour transdermal patches | 4 patch [PoM] £22.12 DT =
£31.60 [CD3]
▸ Sevodyne (Aspire Pharma Ltd)
Buprenorphine 5 microgram per 1 hour Sevodyne
5micrograms/hour transdermal patches | 4 patch [PoM] £7.92 DT =
£17.60 [CD3]
Buprenorphine 10 microgram per 1 hour Sevodyne
10micrograms/hour transdermal patches | 4 patch [PoM] £14.20 DT =
£31.55 [CD3]
Buprenorphine 20 microgram per 1 hour Sevodyne
20micrograms/hour transdermal patches | 4 patch [PoM] £25.86 DT =
£57.46 [CD3]
▸ Transtec (Napp Pharmaceuticals Ltd)
Buprenorphine 35 microgram per 1 hour Transtec
35micrograms/hour transdermal patches | 4 patch [PoM] £15.80 DT =
£15.80 [CD3]
Buprenorphine 52.5 microgram per 1 hour Transtec
52.5micrograms/hour transdermal patches | 4 patch [PoM] £23.71 DT
= £23.71 [CD3]
Buprenorphine 70 microgram per 1 hour Transtec
70micrograms/hour transdermal patches | 4 patch [PoM] £31.60 DT =
£31.60 [CD3]

⟋ 441

Co-codamol

The properties listed below are those particular to the
combination only. For the properties of the components
please consider, paracetamol p. 438.

● **INDICATIONS AND DOSE**

**Moderate pain (using co-codamol 8/500 preparations
only)**
▸ BY MOUTH
▸ Adult: 8/500–16/1000 mg every 4–6 hours as required;
  maximum 64/4000 mg per day
**Moderate pain (using co-codamol 15/500 preparations
only)**
▸ BY MOUTH
▸ Adult: 15/500–30/1000 mg every 4–6 hours as required;
  maximum 120/4000 mg per day
**Moderate to severe pain (using co-codamol 30/500
preparations only)**
▸ BY MOUTH
▸ Adult: 30/500–60/1000 mg every 4–6 hours as required;
  maximum 240/4000 mg per day

KAPAKE ® 15/500

Mild to moderate pain
▸ BY MOUTH
▸ Adult: 2 tablets every 4–6 hours as required; maximum
  8 tablets per day

SOLPADOL ® CAPLETS

Severe pain
▸ BY MOUTH
▸ Adult: 2 tablets every 4–6 hours as required; maximum
  8 tablets per day

SOLPADOL ® CAPSULES

Severe pain
▸ BY MOUTH
▸ Adult: 2 capsules every 4–6 hours as required;
  maximum 8 capsules per day

SOLPADOL ® EFFERVESCENT TABLETS

Severe pain
▸ BY MOUTH USING EFFERVESCENT TABLETS
▸ Adult: 2 tablets every 4–6 hours as required, tablets to
  be dispersed in water; maximum 8 tablets per day

● CONTRA-INDICATIONS Acute ulcerative colitis · antibiotic-
  associated colitis · conditions where abdominal distention
  develops · conditions where inhibition of peristalsis should
  be avoided · known ultra-rapid codeine metabolisers
● CAUTIONS Acute abdomen · alcohol dependence · avoid
  abrupt withdrawal after long-term treatment · cardiac
  arrhythmias · chronic alcoholism · chronic dehydration ·
  chronic malnutrition · convulsive disorders · gallstones ·
  hepatocellular insufficiency
  CAUTIONS, FURTHER INFORMATION
▸ Variation in metabolism The capacity to metabolise codeine
  to morphine can vary considerably between individuals;
  there is a marked increase in morphine toxicity in patients
  who are ultra-rapid codeine metabolisers (CYP2D6 ultra-
  rapid metabolisers) and a reduced therapeutic effect in
  poor codeine metabolisers.
● INTERACTIONS → Appendix 1: opioids · paracetamol
● SIDE-EFFECTS Abdominal pain · addiction ·
  agranulocytosis · blood disorder · irritability · pancreatitis ·
  restlessness · severe cutaneous adverse reactions (SCARs) ·
  thrombocytopenia
  Overdose   Important: liver damage (and less frequently
  renal damage) following overdosage with paracetamol.
● BREAST FEEDING Avoid—although amount of codeine
  usually too small to be harmful, mothers vary considerably
  in their capacity to metabolise codeine—risk of morphine
  overdose in infant.
● HEPATIC IMPAIRMENT
  Dose adjustments Dose-related toxicity with
  paracetamol—avoid large doses.
● RENAL IMPAIRMENT Reduce dose or avoid codeine;
  increased and prolonged effect; increased cerebral
  sensitivity.
● PRESCRIBING AND DISPENSING INFORMATION Co-codamol
  is a mixture of codeine phosphate and paracetamol; the
  proportions are expressed in the form x/y, where x and y
  are the strengths in milligrams of codeine phosphate and
  paracetamol respectively.
     When co-codamol tablets, dispersible (or effervescent)
  tablets, or capsules are prescribed and **no strength is
  stated**, tablets, dispersible (or effervescent) tablets, or
  capsules, respectively, containing codeine phosphate 8 mg
  and paracetamol 500 mg should be dispensed.
     The Drug Tariff allows tablets of co-codamol labelled
  'dispersible' to be dispensed against an order for
  'effervescent' and *vice versa*.
● LESS SUITABLE FOR PRESCRIBING Co-codamol is less
  suitable for prescribing.
● EXCEPTIONS TO LEGAL CATEGORY Co-codamol 8/500 can
  be sold to the public in certain circumstances; for
  exemptions see *Medicines, Ethics and Practice,* London,
  Pharmaceutical Press (always consult latest edition).

● MEDICINAL FORMS
There can be variation in the licensing of different medicines containing the same drug. Forms available from special-order manufacturers include: oral suspension, oral solution

Tablet
CAUTIONARY AND ADVISORY LABELS 2(does not apply to the 8/500 tablet), 29, 30
▸ Co-codamol (Non-proprietary)
  Codeine phosphate 8 mg, Paracetamol 500 mg Co-codamol 8mg/500mg tablets | 100 tablet [PoM] £2.70 DT = £1.97 [CD5] | 500 tablet [PoM] £5.70–£9.85 [CD5] | 1000 tablet [PoM] £19.70 [CD5] Co-codamol 8mg/500mg caplets | 32 tablet [P] £0.95 [CD5]
  Codeine phosphate 15 mg, Paracetamol 500 mg Co-codamol 15mg/500mg tablets | 100 tablet [PoM] DT = £4.93 [CD5]
  Codeine phosphate 30 mg, Paracetamol 500 mg Co-codamol 30mg/500mg caplets | 100 tablet [PoM] DT = £2.83 [CD5] Co-codamol 30mg/500mg tablets | 30 tablet [PoM] £1.17 DT = £0.85 [CD5] | 100 tablet [PoM] £7.53 DT = £2.83 [CD5]
  Codeine phosphate 60 mg, Paracetamol 1 gram Co-codamol 60mg/1000mg tablets | 100 tablet [PoM] £11.50 [CD5]
▸ Codipar (AMCo)
  Codeine phosphate 15 mg, Paracetamol 500 mg Codipar 15mg/500mg tablets | 100 tablet [PoM] £8.25 DT = £4.93 [CD5]
▸ Kapake (Galen Ltd)
  Codeine phosphate 30 mg, Paracetamol 500 mg Kapake 30mg/500mg tablets | 100 tablet [PoM] £7.10 DT = £2.83 [CD5]
▸ Migraleve Yellow (McNeil Products Ltd)
  Codeine phosphate 8 mg, Paracetamol 500 mg Migraleve Yellow tablets | 16 tablet [PoM] [Ⓢ] [CD5]
▸ Panadol Ultra (GlaxoSmithKline Consumer Healthcare)
  Codeine phosphate 12.8 mg, Paracetamol 500 mg Panadol Ultra 12.8mg/500mg tablets | 20 tablet [P] £2.61 DT = £3.61 [CD5]
▸ Solpadeine Max (Omega Pharma Ltd)
  Codeine phosphate 12.8 mg, Paracetamol 500 mg Solpadeine Max 12.8mg/500mg tablets | 20 tablet [P] £3.61 = £3.61 [CD5] | 30 tablet [P] £4.65 DT = £4.65 [CD5]
▸ Solpadol (Sanofi)
  Codeine phosphate 30 mg, Paracetamol 500 mg Solpadol 30mg/500mg caplets | 30 tablet [PoM] £2.02 DT = £0.85 [CD5] | 100 tablet [PoM] £6.74 DT = £2.83 [CD5]
▸ Zapain (AMCo)
  Codeine phosphate 30 mg, Paracetamol 500 mg Zapain 30mg/500mg tablets | 100 tablet [PoM] £3.11 DT = £2.83 [CD5]

Effervescent tablet
CAUTIONARY AND ADVISORY LABELS 2(does not apply to the 8/500 tablet), 13, 29, 30
EXCIPIENTS: May contain Aspartame
ELECTROLYTES: May contain Sodium
▸ Co-codamol (Non-proprietary)
  Codeine phosphate 8 mg, Paracetamol 500 mg Co-codamol 8mg/500mg effervescent tablets | 100 tablet [PoM] £8.75 DT = £7.00 [CD5]
  Codeine phosphate 30 mg, Paracetamol 500 mg Co-codamol 30mg/500mg effervescent tablets | 32 tablet [PoM] £5.40 DT = £2.29 [CD5] | 100 tablet [PoM] £19.20 DT = £7.16 [CD5]
▸ Codipar (AMCo)
  Codeine phosphate 15 mg, Paracetamol 500 mg Codipar 15mg/500mg effervescent tablets sugar-free | 100 tablet [PoM] £8.25 DT = £8.25 [CD5]
▸ Paracodol (Bayer Plc)
  Codeine phosphate 8 mg, Paracetamol 500 mg Paracodol 8mg/500mg effervescent tablets | 32 tablet [P] [Ⓢ] DT = £2.24 [CD5]
▸ Solpadol (Sanofi)
  Codeine phosphate 30 mg, Paracetamol 500 mg Solpadol 30mg/500mg effervescent tablets | 32 tablet [PoM] £2.59 DT = £2.29 [CD5] | 100 tablet [PoM] £8.90 DT = £7.16 [CD5]

Capsule
CAUTIONARY AND ADVISORY LABELS 2(does not apply to the 8/500 capsule), 29, 30
EXCIPIENTS: May contain Sulfites
▸ Co-codamol (Non-proprietary)
  Codeine phosphate 8 mg, Paracetamol 500 mg Co-codamol 8mg/500mg capsules | 100 capsule [PoM] £14.48 DT = £14.23 [CD5]
  Codeine phosphate 15 mg, Paracetamol 500 mg Co-codamol 15mg/500mg capsules | 100 capsule [PoM] £7.25–£8.85 DT = £8.13 [CD5]
  Codeine phosphate 30 mg, Paracetamol 500 mg Co-codamol 30mg/500mg capsules | 100 capsule [PoM] £7.01 DT = £3.88 [CD5]

▸ Codipar (AMCo)
  Codeine phosphate 15 mg, Paracetamol 500 mg Codipar 15mg/500mg capsules | 100 capsule [PoM] £7.85 DT = £8.13 [CD5]
▸ Kapake (Galen Ltd)
  Codeine phosphate 30 mg, Paracetamol 500 mg Kapake 30mg/500mg capsules | 100 capsule [PoM] £7.10 DT = £3.88 [CD5]
▸ Solpadol (Sanofi)
  Codeine phosphate 30 mg, Paracetamol 500 mg Solpadol 30mg/500mg capsules | 100 capsule [PoM] £6.74 DT = £3.88 [CD5]
▸ Tylex (UCB Pharma Ltd)
  Codeine phosphate 30 mg, Paracetamol 500 mg Tylex 30mg/500mg capsules | 100 capsule [PoM] £7.93 DT = £3.88 [CD5]
▸ Zapain (AMCo)
  Codeine phosphate 30 mg, Paracetamol 500 mg Zapain 30mg/500mg capsules | 100 capsule [PoM] £3.85 DT = £3.88 [CD5]

▸ F 441

Codeine phosphate

● INDICATIONS AND DOSE
Acute diarrhoea
▸ BY MOUTH
▸ Child 12–17 years: 30 mg 3–4 times a day; usual dose 15–60 mg 3–4 times a day
▸ Adult: 30 mg 3–4 times a day; usual dose 15–60 mg 3–4 times a day
Mild to moderate pain
▸ BY MOUTH
▸ Adult: 30–60 mg every 4 hours if required; maximum 240 mg per day
▸ BY INTRAMUSCULAR INJECTION
▸ Adult: 30–60 mg every 4 hours if required
Short-term treatment of acute moderate pain
▸ BY MOUTH, OR BY INTRAMUSCULAR INJECTION
▸ Child 12–17 years: 30–60 mg every 6 hours if required for maximum 3 days; maximum 240 mg per day
Dry or painful cough
▸ BY MOUTH USING LINCTUS
▸ Adult: 15–30 mg 3–4 times a day

IMPORTANT SAFETY INFORMATION
MHRA/CHM ADVICE (JULY 2013) CODEINE FOR ANALGESIA: RESTRICTED USE IN CHILDREN DUE TO REPORTS OF MORPHINE TOXICITY
Codeine should only be used to relieve acute moderate pain in children older than 12 years and only if it cannot be relieved by other painkillers such as paracetamol or ibuprofen alone. A significant risk of serious and life-threatening adverse reactions has been identified in children with obstructive sleep apnoea who received codeine after tonsillectomy or adenoidectomy:
• in children aged 12–18 years, the maximum daily dose of codeine should not exceed 240 mg. Doses may be taken up to four times a day at intervals of no less than 6 hours. The lowest effective dose should be used and duration of treatment should be limited to 3 days
• codeine is contra-indicated in all children (under 18 years) who undergo the removal of tonsils or adenoids for the treatment of obstructive sleep apnoea
• codeine is not recommended for use in children whose breathing may be compromised, including those with neuromuscular disorders, severe cardiac or respiratory conditions, respiratory infections, multiple trauma or extensive surgical procedures
• codeine is contra-indicated in patients of any age who are known to be ultra-rapid metabolisers of codeine (CYP2D6 ultra-rapid metabolisers)
• codeine should not be used in breast-feeding mothers because it can pass to the baby through breast milk
• parents and carers should be advised on how to recognise signs and symptoms of morphine toxicity, and to stop treatment and seek medical attention if signs or symptoms of toxicity occur (including reduced

consciousness, lack of appetite, somnolence, constipation, respiratory depression, 'pin-point' pupils, nausea, vomiting)

MHRA/CHM ADVICE (APRIL 2015) CODEINE FOR COUGH AND COLD: RESTRICTED USE IN CHILDREN

Do not use codeine in children under 12 years as it is associated with a risk of respiratory side effects. Codeine is not recommended for adolescents (12–18 years) who have problems with breathing. When prescribing or dispensing codeine-containing medicines for cough and cold, consider that codeine is contra-indicated in:
- children younger than 12 years old
- patients of any age known to be CYP2D6 ultra-rapid metabolisers
- breastfeeding mothers

- **CONTRA-INDICATIONS** Acute ulcerative colitis · antibiotic-associated colitis · children under 18 years who undergo the removal of tonsils or adenoids for the treatment of obstructive sleep apnoea · conditions where abdominal distension develops · conditions where inhibition of peristalsis should be avoided · known ultra-rapid codeine metabolisers

- **CAUTIONS** Acute abdomen · cardiac arrhythmias · gallstones · not recommended for adolescents aged 12–18 years with breathing problems

  CAUTIONS, FURTHER INFORMATION
  ▸ Variation in metabolism The capacity to metabolise codeine to morphine can vary considerably between individuals; there is a marked increase in morphine toxicity in patients who are ultra-rapid codeine metabolisers (CYP2D6 ultra-rapid metabolisers) and a reduced therapeutic effect in poor codeine metabolisers.

- **INTERACTIONS** → Appendix 1: opioids

- **SIDE-EFFECTS**

  GENERAL SIDE-EFFECTS Biliary spasm · hypothermia · mood altered · postural hypotension · sexual dysfunction · ureteral spasm

  SPECIFIC SIDE-EFFECTS
  ▸ With oral use Abdominal cramps · addiction · appetite decreased · depression · drug reaction with eosinophilia and systemic symptoms (DRESS) · dyskinesia · dyspnoea · face oedema · fatigue · fever · hyperglycaemia · hypersensitivity · intracranial pressure increased · lymphadenopathy · malaise · muscle rigidity (with high doses) · nightmare · pancreatitis · restlessness · seizure · splenomegaly · urinary disorders · vision disorders
  ▸ With parenteral use Dysuria

- **BREAST FEEDING** Avoid—although amount usually too small to be harmful, mothers vary considerably in their capacity to metabolise codeine—risk of morphine overdose in infant.

- **RENAL IMPAIRMENT** Avoid use or reduce dose; opioid effects increased and prolonged and increased cerebral sensitivity occurs.

- **PRESCRIBING AND DISPENSING INFORMATION** BP directs that when Diabetic Codeine Linctus is prescribed, Codeine Linctus formulated with a vehicle appropriate for administration to diabetics, whether or not labelled 'Diabetic Codeine Linctus', shall be dispensed or supplied.

- **PATIENT AND CARER ADVICE**
  Medicines for Children leaflet: Codeine phosphate for pain www.medicinesforchildren.org.uk/codeine-phosphate-pain-0

- **MEDICINAL FORMS**
  There can be variation in the licensing of different medicines containing the same drug. Forms available from special-order manufacturers include: oral suspension, oral solution, solution for injection

  Tablet
  CAUTIONARY AND ADVISORY LABELS 2
  ▸ Codeine phosphate (Non-proprietary)
  Codeine phosphate 15 mg Codeine 15mg tablets | 28 tablet PoM £1.40 DT = £0.65 CD5 | 100 tablet PoM £2.32 DT = £2.32 CD5
  Codeine phosphate 30 mg Codeine 30mg tablets | 28 tablet PoM £1.59 DT = £0.76 CD5 | 100 tablet PoM £5.68 DT = £2.71 CD5
  Codeine phosphate 60 mg Codeine 60mg tablets | 28 tablet PoM £5.95 DT = £1.32 CD5

  Solution for injection
  ▸ Codeine phosphate (Non-proprietary)
  Codeine phosphate 60 mg per 1 ml Codeine 60mg/1ml solution for injection ampoules | 10 ampoule PoM £24.10–£24.18 DT = £24.18 CD2

  Oral solution
  CAUTIONARY AND ADVISORY LABELS 2
  ▸ Codeine phosphate (Non-proprietary)
  Codeine phosphate 3 mg per 1 ml Codeine 15mg/5ml linctus sugar free sugar-free | 200 ml P £1.90 DT = £1.62 CD5 sugar-free | 2000 ml P £16.20 CD5
  Codeine 15mg/5ml linctus | 200 ml P £1.90 DT = £1.90 CD5
  Codeine phosphate 5 mg per 1 ml Codeine 25mg/5ml oral solution | 500 ml PoM £6.46 DT = £6.46 CD5
  ▸ Galcodine (Thornton & Ross Ltd)
  Codeine phosphate 3 mg per 1 ml Galcodine 15mg/5ml linctus sugar-free | 2000 ml P £9.90 CD5

  Combinations available: *Aspirin with codeine*, p. 441

📖 441

Diamorphine hydrochloride   10-Jun-2016

(Heroin hydrochloride)

- **INDICATIONS AND DOSE**

Acute pain
▸ BY INTRAMUSCULAR INJECTION, OR BY SUBCUTANEOUS INJECTION
▸ Adult: 5 mg every 4 hours if required
▸ BY SLOW INTRAVENOUS INJECTION
▸ Adult: 1.25–2.5 mg every 4 hours if required

Acute pain (heavier, well-muscled patients)
▸ BY INTRAMUSCULAR INJECTION, OR BY SUBCUTANEOUS INJECTION
▸ Adult: Up to 10 mg every 4 hours if required
▸ BY SLOW INTRAVENOUS INJECTION
▸ Adult: 2.5–5 mg every 4 hours if required

Chronic pain not currently treated with a strong opioid analgesic
▸ BY SUBCUTANEOUS INJECTION, OR BY INTRAMUSCULAR INJECTION
▸ Adult: Initially 2.5–5 mg every 4 hours, adjusted according to response
▸ BY SUBCUTANEOUS INFUSION
▸ Adult: Initially 5–10 mg, adjusted according to response, dose to be administered over 24 hours

Acute pulmonary oedema
▸ BY SLOW INTRAVENOUS INJECTION
▸ Adult: 2.5–5 mg, dose to be administered at a rate of 1 mg/minute

Myocardial infarction
▸ BY SLOW INTRAVENOUS INJECTION
▸ Adult: 5 mg, followed by 2.5–5 mg if required, dose to be administered at a rate of 1–2 mg/minute
▸ Elderly: 2.5 mg, followed by 1.25–2.5 mg if required, dose to be administered at a rate of 1–2 mg/minute

Myocardial infarction (frail patients)
▸ BY SLOW INTRAVENOUS INJECTION
▸ Adult: 2.5 mg, followed by 1.25–2.5 mg if required, dose to be administered at a rate of 1–2 mg/minute

- CONTRA-INDICATIONS Delayed gastric emptying · phaeochromocytoma
- CAUTIONS CNS depression · severe cor pulmonale · severe diarrhoea · toxic psychosis
- INTERACTIONS → Appendix 1: opioids
- SIDE-EFFECTS Biliary spasm · circulatory depression · intracranial pressure increased · mood altered · postural hypotension
- BREAST FEEDING Therapeutic doses unlikely to affect infant; withdrawal symptoms in infants of dependent mothers; breast-feeding not best method of treating dependence in offspring.
- RENAL IMPAIRMENT Avoid use or reduce dose; opioid effects increased and prolonged; increased cerebral sensitivity.

- MEDICINAL FORMS
There can be variation in the licensing of different medicines containing the same drug. Forms available from special-order manufacturers include: solution for injection, powder for solution for injection

Powder for solution for injection
- Diamorphine hydrochloride (Non-proprietary)
  Diamorphine hydrochloride 5 mg Diamorphine 5mg powder for solution for injection ampoules | 5 ampoule [PoM] £11.36 DT = £11.36 [CD2]
  Diamorphine hydrochloride 10 mg Diamorphine 10mg powder for solution for injection ampoules | 5 ampoule [PoM] £12.95–£16.56 DT = £12.95 [CD2]
  Diamorphine hydrochloride 30 mg Diamorphine 30mg powder for solution for injection ampoules | 5 ampoule [PoM] £13.80–£16.52 DT = £11.22 [CD2]
  Diamorphine hydrochloride 100 mg Diamorphine 100mg powder for solution for injection ampoules | 5 ampoule [PoM] £42.39 DT = £42.39 [CD2]
  Diamorphine hydrochloride 500 mg Diamorphine 500mg powder for solution for injection ampoules | 5 ampoule [PoM] £187.70 DT = £187.70 [CD2]

☞ 441

Dihydrocodeine tartrate

- INDICATIONS AND DOSE

Moderate to severe pain
- BY MOUTH USING IMMEDIATE-RELEASE MEDICINES
- Child 4–11 years: 0.5–1 mg/kg every 4–6 hours (max. per dose 30 mg)
- Child 12–17 years: 30 mg every 4–6 hours
- Adult: 30 mg every 4–6 hours as required
- BY DEEP SUBCUTANEOUS INJECTION, OR BY INTRAMUSCULAR INJECTION
- Adult: Up to 50 mg every 4–6 hours if required

Chronic severe pain
- BY MOUTH USING MODIFIED-RELEASE MEDICINES
- Child 12–17 years: 60–120 mg every 12 hours
- Adult: 60–120 mg every 12 hours

DF118 FORTE ®
Severe pain
- BY MOUTH
- Child 12–17 years: 40–80 mg 3 times a day; maximum 240 mg per day
- Adult: 40–80 mg 3 times a day; maximum 240 mg per day

- UNLICENSED USE Most preparations not licensed for use in children under 4 years.
- CAUTIONS Pancreatitis · severe cor pulmonale
- INTERACTIONS → Appendix 1: opioids
- SIDE-EFFECTS
  GENERAL SIDE-EFFECTS Dysuria · mood altered · postural hypotension

SPECIFIC SIDE-EFFECTS
- With oral use Biliary spasm · bronchospasm · hypothermia · sexual dysfunction · ureteral spasm
- BREAST FEEDING Use only if potential benefit outweighs risk.
- RENAL IMPAIRMENT Avoid use or reduce dose; opioid effects increased and prolonged and increased cerebral sensitivity occurs.
- PROFESSION SPECIFIC INFORMATION
  Dental practitioners' formulary
  Dihydrocodeine tablets 30 mg may be prescribed.

- MEDICINAL FORMS
There can be variation in the licensing of different medicines containing the same drug. Forms available from special-order manufacturers include: oral suspension, oral solution

Modified-release tablet
CAUTIONARY AND ADVISORY LABELS 2, 25
- DHC Continus (Napp Pharmaceuticals Ltd)
  Dihydrocodeine tartrate 60 mg DHC Continus 60mg tablets | 56 tablet [PoM] £5.20 DT = £5.20 [CD5]
  Dihydrocodeine tartrate 90 mg DHC Continus 90mg tablets | 56 tablet [PoM] £8.66 DT = £8.66 [CD5]
  Dihydrocodeine tartrate 120 mg DHC Continus 120mg tablets | 56 tablet [PoM] £10.95 DT = £10.95 [CD5]

Tablet
CAUTIONARY AND ADVISORY LABELS 2
- Dihydrocodeine tartrate (Non-proprietary)
  Dihydrocodeine tartrate 30 mg Dihydrocodeine 30mg tablets | 28 tablet [PoM] £1.09 DT = £0.72 [CD5] | 30 tablet [PoM] £0.77–£1.56 [CD5] | 100 tablet [PoM] £3.89 DT = £2.57 [CD5] | 500 tablet [PoM] £12.85 [CD5]
- DF 118 (Martindale Pharmaceuticals Ltd)
  Dihydrocodeine tartrate 40 mg DF 118 Forte 40mg tablets | 100 tablet [PoM] £11.51 DT = £11.51 [CD5]

Solution for injection
- Dihydrocodeine tartrate (Non-proprietary)
  Dihydrocodeine tartrate 50 mg per 1 ml Dihydrocodeine 50mg/1ml solution for injection ampoules | 10 ampoule [PoM] £105.27 DT = £105.27 [CD2]

Oral solution
CAUTIONARY AND ADVISORY LABELS 2
- Dihydrocodeine tartrate (Non-proprietary)
  Dihydrocodeine tartrate 2 mg per 1 ml Dihydrocodeine 10mg/5ml oral solution | 150 ml [PoM] £8.94 DT = £8.94 [CD5]

☞ 441

Dihydrocodeine with paracetamol

18-Jan-2018

The properties listed below are those particular to the combination only. For the properties of the components please consider, paracetamol p. 438.

- INDICATIONS AND DOSE

Mild to moderate pain (using 10/500 preparations only)
- BY MOUTH
- Adult: 10/500–20/1000 mg every 4–6 hours as required; maximum 80/4000 mg per day

Severe pain (using 20/500 preparations only)
- BY MOUTH
- Adult: 20/500–40/1000 mg every 4–6 hours as required; maximum 160/4000 mg per day

Severe pain (using 30/500 preparations only)
- BY MOUTH
- Adult: 30/500–60/1000 mg every 4–6 hours as required; maximum 240/4000 mg per day

DOSE EQUIVALENCE AND CONVERSION
- A mixture of dihydrocodeine tartrate and paracetamol; the proportions are expressed in the form x/y, where x

and y are the strengths in milligrams of dihydrocodeine and paracetamol respectively.

> IMPORTANT SAFETY INFORMATION
> MHRA/CHM ADVICE: DIHYDROCODEINE WITH PARACETAMOL (CO-DYDRAMOL): PRESCRIBE AND DISPENSE BY STRENGTH TO MINIMISE RISK OF MEDICATION ERROR (JANUARY 2018)
> The MHRA has advised that dihydrocodeine with paracetamol preparations are prescribed and dispensed by strength to minimise dispensing errors and the risk of accidental opioid overdose—see Prescribing and dispensing information.

- CAUTIONS Alcohol dependence · before administering, check when paracetamol last administered and cumulative paracetamol dose over previous 24 hours · chronic alcoholism · chronic dehydration · chronic malnutrition · hepatocellular insufficiency · pancreatitis · severe cor pulmonale
- INTERACTIONS → Appendix 1: opioids · paracetamol
- SIDE-EFFECTS Abdominal pain · blood disorder · leucopenia · malaise · neutropenia · pancreatitis · paraesthesia · paralytic ileus · severe cutaneous adverse reactions (SCARs) · thrombocytopenia

  Overdose Important liver damage (and less frequently renal damage) following overdosage with paracetamol
- BREAST FEEDING Amount of dihydrocodeine too small to be harmful but use only if potential benefit outweighs risk.
- HEPATIC IMPAIRMENT Dose-related toxicity with paracetamol—avoid large doses.
- RENAL IMPAIRMENT Reduce dose or avoid dihydrocodeine; increased and prolonged effect; increased cerebral sensitivity.
- PRESCRIBING AND DISPENSING INFORMATION The MHRA advises when prescribing dihydrocodeine with paracetamol, the tablet strength and dose must be clearly indicated; when dispensing dihydrocodeine with paracetamol, ensure the prescribed strength is supplied—contact the prescriber if in doubt.

  The BP defines *Co-dydramol* Tablets as containing dihydrocodeine tartrate 10 mg and paracetamol 500 mg.
- LESS SUITABLE FOR PRESCRIBING Dihydrocodeine with paracetamol is less suitable for prescribing.

- MEDICINAL FORMS
There can be variation in the licensing of different medicines containing the same drug. Forms available from special-order manufacturers include: oral suspension, oral solution
Tablet
CAUTIONARY AND ADVISORY LABELS 2, 29, 30
> Dihydrocodeine with paracetamol (Non-proprietary)
Dihydrocodeine tartrate 10 mg, Paracetamol 500 mg Co-dydramol 10mg/500mg tablets | 30 tablet PoM £1.14 DT = £0.59 CD5 | 100 tablet PoM £3.00 DT = £1.97 CD5 | 500 tablet PoM £9.85 CD5
Dihydrocodeine tartrate 20 mg, Paracetamol 500 mg Co-dydramol 20mg/500mg tablets | 56 tablet PoM £5.57-£5.87 CD5 | 112 tablet PoM £11.13 DT = £11.13 CD5
Dihydrocodeine tartrate 30 mg, Paracetamol 500 mg Co-dydramol 30mg/500mg tablets | 56 tablet PoM £6.82 DT = £6.82 CD5
> Eroset (M & A Pharmachem Ltd)
Dihydrocodeine tartrate 10 mg, Paracetamol 500 mg Eroset 500mg/10mg tablets | 30 tablet PoM £0.68 DT = £0.59 CD5 | 100 tablet PoM £2.27 DT = £1.97 CD5
> Remedeine (Crescent Pharma Ltd)
Dihydrocodeine tartrate 20 mg, Paracetamol 500 mg Remedeine tablets | 56 tablet PoM £5.87 CD5 | 112 tablet PoM £11.13 DT = £11.13 CD5
Dihydrocodeine tartrate 30 mg, Paracetamol 500 mg Remedeine Forte tablets | 56 tablet PoM £6.82 DT = £6.82 CD5

F 441

Dipipanone hydrochloride with cyclizine

- INDICATIONS AND DOSE
Acute pain
> BY MOUTH
> Adult: Initially 1 tablet every 6 hours, then increased if necessary up to 3 tablets every 6 hours, dose to be increased gradually

- CAUTIONS Diabetes mellitus · palliative care (not recommended) · phaeochromocytoma
- INTERACTIONS → Appendix 1: antihistamines, sedating · opioids
- SIDE-EFFECTS Agranulocytosis · anxiety · biliary spasm · consciousness impaired · disorientation · dry throat · dysuria · hallucinations · hepatic disorders · insomnia · intracranial pressure increased · mood altered · movement disorders · muscle complaints · nasal dryness · psychosis · renal spasm · seizure · skin reactions · speech disorder · tremor · vision blurred
- BREAST FEEDING No information available.
- RENAL IMPAIRMENT Avoid use or reduce dose; opioid effects increased and prolonged and increased cerebral sensitivity occurs.

- MEDICINAL FORMS
There can be variation in the licensing of different medicines containing the same drug.
Tablet
> Dipipanone hydrochloride with cyclizine (Non-proprietary)
Dipipanone hydrochloride 10 mg, Cyclizine hydrochloride 30 mg Dipipanone 10mg / Cyclizine 30mg tablets | 50 tablet PoM £386.53 DT = £386.53 CD2

F 441

Fentanyl

21-May-2018

- INDICATIONS AND DOSE
Chronic intractable pain not currently treated with a strong opioid analgesic
> BY TRANSDERMAL APPLICATION
> Child 16–17 years: Initially 12 micrograms/hour every 72 hours, alternatively initially 25 micrograms/hour every 72 hours, when starting, evaluation of the analgesic effect should not be made before the system has been worn for 24 hours (to allow for the gradual increase in plasma-fentanyl concentration)—previous analgesic therapy should be phased out gradually from time of first patch application, dose should be adjusted at 48–72 hour intervals in steps of 12–25 micrograms/hour if necessary, more than one patch may be used at a time (but applied at the same time to avoid confusion)—consider additional or alternative analgesic therapy if dose required exceeds 300 micrograms/hour (important: it takes 17 hours or more for the plasma-fentanyl concentration to decrease by 50%— replacement opioid therapy should be initiated at a low dose and increased gradually)
> Adult: Initially 12 micrograms/hour every 72 hours, alternatively initially 25 micrograms/hour every 72 hours, when starting, evaluation of the analgesic effect should not be made before the system has been worn for 24 hours (to allow for the gradual increase in plasma-fentanyl concentration)—previous analgesic therapy should be phased out gradually from time of first patch application, dose should be adjusted at 48–72 hour intervals in steps of 12–25 micrograms/hour if necessary, more than one patch may be used at a time (but applied at continued →

4

Nervous system

the same time to avoid confusion)—consider additional or alternative analgesic therapy if dose required exceeds 300 micrograms/hour (important: it takes 17 hours or more for the plasma-fentanyl concentration to decrease by 50%— replacement opioid therapy should be initiated at a low dose and increased gradually)

Chronic intractable pain currently treated with a strong opioid analgesic
▸ BY TRANSDERMAL APPLICATION
▸ Child 2-17 years: Initial dose based on previous 24-hour opioid requirement (consult product literature), for evaluating analgesic efficacy and dose increments, see under *Chronic intractable pain not currently treated with a strong opioid analgesic*, for conversion from long term oral morphine to transdermal fentanyl, see *Pain management with opioids* under Prescribing in palliative care p. 23.
▸ Adult: Initial dose based on previous 24-hour opioid requirement (consult product literature), for evaluating analgesic efficacy and dose increments, see under *Chronic intractable pain not currently treated with a strong opioid analgesic*, for conversion from long term oral morphine to transdermal fentanyl, see *Pain management with opioids* under Prescribing in palliative care p. 23.

Spontaneous respiration: analgesia and enhancement of anaesthesia, during operation
▸ BY SLOW INTRAVENOUS INJECTION
▸ Adult: Initially 50–100 micrograms (max. per dose 200 micrograms), dose maximum on specialist advice, then 25–50 micrograms as required
▸ BY INTRAVENOUS INFUSION
▸ Adult: 3–4.8 micrograms/kg/hour, adjusted according to response

Assisted ventilation: analgesia and enhancement of anaesthesia during operation
▸ BY SLOW INTRAVENOUS INJECTION
▸ Adult: Initially 300–3500 micrograms, then 100–200 micrograms as required
▸ BY INTRAVENOUS INFUSION
▸ Adult: Initially 10 micrograms/kg, dose to be given over 10 minutes, then 6 micrograms/kg/hour, adjusted according to response, may require up to 180 micrograms/kg/hour during cardiac surgery

Assisted ventilation: analgesia and respiratory depression in intensive care
▸ BY SLOW INTRAVENOUS INJECTION
▸ Adult: Initially 300–3500 micrograms, then 100–200 micrograms as required
▸ BY INTRAVENOUS INFUSION
▸ Adult: Initially 10 micrograms/kg, dose to be given over 10 minutes, then 6 micrograms/kg/hour, adjusted according to response, may require up to 180 micrograms/kg/hour during cardiac surgery

Breakthrough pain in patients receiving opioid therapy for chronic cancer pain
▸ BY BUCCAL ADMINISTRATION USING LOZENGES
▸ Child 16-17 years: Initially 200 micrograms, dose to be given over 15 minutes, then 200 micrograms after 15 minutes if required, no more than 2 dose units for each pain episode; if adequate pain relief not achieved with 1 dose unit for consecutive breakthrough pain episodes, increase the strength of the dose unit until adequate pain relief achieved with 4 lozenges or less daily, if more than 4 episodes of breakthrough pain each day, adjust background analgesia
▸ Adult: Initially 200 micrograms, dose to be given over 15 minutes, then 200 micrograms after 15 minutes if required, no more than 2 dose units for each pain episode; if adequate pain relief not achieved with

1 dose unit for consecutive breakthrough pain episodes, increase the strength of the dose unit until adequate pain relief achieved with 4 lozenges or less daily, if more than 4 episodes of breakthrough pain each day, adjust background analgesia
▸ BY BUCCAL ADMINISTRATION USING BUCCAL FILMS
▸ Adult: Initially 200 micrograms, adjusted according to response, consult product literature for information on dose adjustments, maximum 1.2 mg per episode of breakthrough pain; leave at least 4 hours between treatment of episodes of breakthrough pain, if more than 4 episodes of breakthrough pain each day occur on more than 4 consecutive days, adjust background analgesia

DOSE EQUIVALENCE AND CONVERSION
▸ Fentanyl films are **not bioequivalent** to other fentanyl preparations.
▸ Fentanyl preparations for the treatment of breakthrough pain are not interchangeable; if patients are switched from another fentanyl-containing preparation, a new dose titration is required.

DOSES AT EXTREMES OF BODY-WEIGHT
▸ To avoid excessive dosage in obese patients, weight-based doses may need to be calculated on the basis of ideal bodyweight.

ABSTRAL ®
Breakthrough pain in patients receiving opioid therapy for chronic cancer pain
▸ BY MOUTH USING SUBLINGUAL TABLETS
▸ Adult: Initially 100 micrograms, then 100 micrograms after 15–30 minutes if required, dose to be adjusted according to response—consult product literature, no more than 2 dose units 15–30 minutes apart, for each pain episode; max. 800 micrograms per episode of breakthrough pain; leave at least 2 hours between treatment of episodes of breakthrough pain, if more than 4 episodes of breakthrough pain each day, adjust background analgesia

EFFENTORA ®
Breakthrough pain in patients receiving opioid therapy for chronic cancer pain
▸ BY MOUTH USING SUBLINGUAL TABLETS
▸ Adult: Initially 100 micrograms, then 100 micrograms after 30 minutes if required, dose to be adjusted according to response—consult product literature, no more than 2 dose units for each pain episode; max. 800 micrograms per episode of breakthrough pain; leave at least 4 hours between treatment of episodes of breakthrough pain during titration

INSTANYL ®
Breakthrough pain in patients receiving opioid therapy for chronic cancer pain
▸ BY INTRANASAL ADMINISTRATION
▸ Adult: Initially 50 micrograms, dose to be administered into one nostril, then 50 micrograms after 10 minutes if required, dose to be adjusted according to response, maximum 2 sprays for each pain episode and minimum 4 hours between treatment of each pain episode, if more than 4 breakthrough pain episodes daily, adjust background analgesia

PECFENT ®
Breakthrough pain in patients receiving opioid therapy for chronic cancer pain
▸ BY INTRANASAL ADMINISTRATION
▸ Adult: Initially 100 micrograms, adjusted according to response, dose to be administered into one nostril only, maximum 2 sprays for each pain episode and minimum 4 hours between treatment of each pain

episode, if more than 4 breakthrough pain episodes daily, adjust background analgesia

RECIVIT ® SUBLINGUAL TABLETS

Breakthrough pain in patients receiving opioid therapy for chronic cancer pain

▸ BY MOUTH
▸ Adult: Initially 133 micrograms, then 133 micrograms after 15–30 minutes (max. per dose 800 micrograms), dose to be repeated only if necessary. Consult product literature for dose adjustments, no more than 2 dose units, 15-30 minutes apart, for each pain episode, maximum of 800 micrograms per episode of breakthrough pain, if more than 4 episodes of breakthrough pain each day, adjust background analgesia; maximum 4 doses per day

● CAUTIONS
GENERAL CAUTIONS Cerebral tumour · diabetes mellitus (with *Actiq* ® lozenges) · impaired consciousness
SPECIFIC CAUTIONS
▸ With buccal use mucositis—absorption from oral preparations may be increased, caution during dose titration (in adults)
CAUTIONS, FURTHER INFORMATION
▸ With transdermal use Transdermal fentanyl patches are not suitable for acute pain or in those patients whose analgesic requirements are changing rapidly because the long time to steady state prevents rapid titration of the dose. Risk of fatal respiratory depression, particularly in patients not previously treated with a strong opioid analgesic; manufacturer recommends use only in opioid tolerant patients.
▸ With intravenous use Repeated intra-operative doses should be given with care since the resulting respiratory depression can persist postoperatively and occasionally it may become apparent for the first time postoperatively when monitoring of the patient might be less intensive.

● INTERACTIONS → Appendix 1: opioids

● SIDE-EFFECTS
▸ **Common or very common**
▸ With parenteral use Allergic dermatitis · apnoea · arrhythmia · hypertension · movement disorders · muscle rigidity · respiratory disorders · vascular disorders
▸ With transdermal use Anxiety · appetite decreased · asthenia · depression · diarrhoea · dyspnoea · gastrointestinal discomfort · hypertension · insomnia · malaise · muscle complaints · peripheral oedema · sensation abnormal · skin reactions · temperature sensation altered · tremor
▸ **Uncommon**
▸ With parenteral use Airway complication of anaesthesia · chills · hiccups · hypothermia
▸ With transdermal use Consciousness impaired · cyanosis · disorientation · fever · gastrointestinal disorders · influenza like illness · memory loss · respiratory disorders · seizures · sexual dysfunction · vision blurred
▸ **Rare or very rare**
▸ With transdermal use Apnoea
▸ **Frequency not known**
▸ With intranasal use Circulatory depression · diarrhoea · epistaxis · fall · fatigue · fever · hot flush · insomnia · malaise · motion sickness · myoclonus · nasal complaints · peripheral oedema · seizure · sensation abnormal · shock · skin pain · stomatitis · taste altered · throat irritation
▸ With buccal use or oral use Adrenal insufficiency (long term use) · androgen deficiency · anxiety · appetite decreased · asthenia · circulatory depression · coma · depersonalisation · depression · diarrhoea · dyspnoea · emotional lability · fever · gait abnormal · gastrointestinal discomfort · gastrointestinal disorders · gingival haemorrhage · gingivitis · hypotension exacerbated · injury · loss of consciousness · malaise · movement disorders · oral

disorders · peripheral oedema · seizure · sensation abnormal · shock · sleep disorders · speech slurred · taste altered · thinking abnormal · throat oedema · ulcer · vasodilation · vision disorders · weight decreased
▸ With parenteral use Biliary spasm · cardiac arrest · cough · hyperalgesia · loss of consciousness · seizure
▸ With transdermal use Myoclonus
SIDE-EFFECTS, FURTHER INFORMATION
Muscle rigidity Intravenous administration of fentanyl can cause muscle rigidity, which may involve the thoracic muscles. Manufacturer advises administration by slow intravenous injection to avoid; higher doses may require premedication with benzodiazepines and muscle relaxants.
Transdermal use Monitor patients using patches for increased side-effects if fever is present (increased absorption possible); avoid exposing application site to external heat, for example a hot bath or sauna (may also increase absorption).

● BREAST FEEDING
▸ With buccal use or intranasal use or sublingual use Manufacturer advises avoid during treatment and for 5 days after last administration—present in milk.
▸ With intravenous use Manufacturer advises avoid during treatment and for 24 hours after last administration—present in milk.
▸ With transdermal use Manufacturer advises avoid during treatment and for 72 hours after removal of patch—present in milk.

● RENAL IMPAIRMENT Avoid use or reduce dose; opioid effects increased and prolonged and increased cerebral sensitivity occurs.

● DIRECTIONS FOR ADMINISTRATION
▸ With transdermal use For *patches*, apply to dry, non-irritated, non-irradiated, non-hairy skin on torso or upper arm, removing after 72 hours and siting replacement patch on a different area (avoid using the same area for several days).
▸ With intravenous use For *intravenous infusion* (*Sublimaze*), give continuously or intermittently in Glucose 5% or Sodium Chloride 0.9%.
▸ With buccal use in adults For buccal films, moisten mouth, place film on inner lining of cheek (pink side to cheek), hold for at least 5 seconds until it sticks, and leave to dissolve (15–30 minutes); if more than 1 film required do not overlap, but use another area of the mouth. Avoid liquids for 5 minutes after application; avoid food until the film has dissolved.
▸ With buccal use Patients should be advised to place the lozenge in the mouth against the cheek and move it around the mouth using the applicator; each lozenge should be sucked over a 15 minute period. In patients with a dry mouth, water may be used to moisten the buccal mucosa. Patients with diabetes should be advised each lozenge contains approximately 2 g glucose.
INSTANYL ® Patient should sit or stand during administration.
EFFENTORA ® Place tablet between cheek and gum and leave to dissolve; if more than 1 tablet required, place second tablet on the other side of the mouth; tablet may alternatively be placed under the tongue (sublingually).

● PRESCRIBING AND DISPENSING INFORMATION
Prescriptions for fentanyl patches can be written to show the strength in terms of the release rate and it is acceptable to write '*Fentanyl 25 patches*' to prescribe patches that release fentanyl 25 micrograms per hour. The dosage should be expressed in terms of the interval between applying a patch and replacing it with a new one, e.g. '*one patch to be applied every 72 hours*'. The total quantity of patches to be supplied should be written in words and figures.

Nervous system

● PATIENT AND CARER ADVICE

Medicines for Children leaflet: Fentanyl lozenges for pain
www.medicinesforchildren.org.uk/fentanyl-lozenges-for-pain
Medicines for Children leaflet: Fentanyl patches for pain
www.medicinesforchildren.org.uk/fentanyl-patches-for-pain
▸ With transdermal use Patients and carers should be
informed about safe use, including correct administration
and disposal, strict adherence to dosage instructions, and
the symptoms and signs of opioid overdosage. Patches
should be removed immediately in case of breathing
difficulties, marked drowsiness, confusion, dizziness, or
impaired speech, and patients and carers should seek
prompt medical attention.
▸ In adults Patients or carers should be given advice on how
to administer fentanyl buccal films or fentanyl lozenges.
Patients or carers should be given advice on how to
administer fentanyl nasal spray.
PECFENT ® Avoid concomitant use of other nasal
preparations.
   Patients or carers should be given advice on how to
administer *PecFent*® spray.
INSTANYL ® Avoid concomitant use of other nasal
preparations.
   Patients or carers should be given advice on how to
administer *Instanyl*® spray.
EFFENTORA ® Patients or carers should be given advice on
how to administer *Effentora*® buccal tablets.
   Patients should be advised not to eat or drink until the
tablet is completely dissolved; after 30 minutes, if any
remnants remain, they may be swallowed with a glass of
water. Patients with a dry mouth should be advised to
drink water to moisten the buccal mucosa before
administration of the tablets; if appropriate effervescence
does not occur, a switch of therapy may be advised.
ABSTRAL ® Patients should be advised not to eat or drink
until the tablet is completely dissolved.
   In patients with a dry mouth, the buccal mucosa may be
moistened with water before administration of tablet.
RECIVIT ® SUBLINGUAL TABLETS Patients should be
advised not to eat or drink until the tablet is completely
dissolved; after 30 minutes, if any remnants remain, they
may be swallowed. In patients with a dry mouth, the
buccal mucosa may be moistened with water before
administration of tablet.

● NATIONAL FUNDING/ACCESS DECISIONS
PECFENT ®

Scottish Medicines Consortium (SMC) Decisions
The *Scottish Medicines Consortium* has advised (September
2008) that *PecFent*® nasal spray should be restricted for
use within NHS Scotland for the management of
breakthrough pain in adult patients using opioid therapy
for chronic cancer pain, when other short-acting opioids
are unsuitable.
INSTANYL ®

Scottish Medicines Consortium (SMC) Decisions
The *Scottish Medicines Consortium* has advised that
Instanyl® nasal spray should be restricted for use within
NHS Scotland for the management of breakthrough pain in
adult patients using opioid therapy for chronic cancer
pain, when other short-acting opioids are unsuitable.
EFFENTORA ®

Scottish Medicines Consortium (SMC) Decisions
The *Scottish Medicines Consortium* has advised that
Effentora® buccal tablets should be restricted for the
management of breakthrough pain in adult patients using
opioid therapy for chronic cancer pain, when other short
acting opioids are unsuitable.

ABSTRAL ®

Scottish Medicines Consortium (SMC) Decisions
The *Scottish Medicines Consortium* has advised (January
2009) that *Abstral*® sublingual tablets should be restricted
for the management of breakthrough pain in adult
patients using opioid therapy for chronic cancer pain,
when other short acting opioids are unsuitable.

● MEDICINAL FORMS
There can be variation in the licensing of different medicines
containing the same drug. Forms available from special-order
manufacturers include: solution for injection, infusion,
solution for infusion.

Solution for injection
▸ Fentanyl (Non-proprietary)
  Fentanyl (as Fentanyl citrate) 50 microgram per 1 ml Fentanyl
  100micrograms/2ml solution for injection ampoules |
  10 ampoule [PoM] £7.50–£13.95 [CD2]
  Fentanyl 500micrograms/10ml solution for injection ampoules |
  10 ampoule [PoM] £12.50–£16.15 [CD2]
▸ Sublimaze (Piramal Critical Care Ltd)
  Fentanyl (as Fentanyl citrate) 50 microgram per 1 ml Sublimaze
  500micrograms/10ml solution for injection ampoules |
  5 ampoule [PoM] £6.53 [CD2]

Spray
CAUTIONARY AND ADVISORY LABELS 2
▸ Instanyl (Takeda UK Ltd)
  Fentanyl (as Fentanyl citrate) 50 microgram per 1 dose Instanyl
  50micrograms/dose nasal spray | 6 dose [PoM] £35.70 [CD2] |
  10 dose [PoM] £59.50 [CD2] | 20 dose [PoM] £119.00 [CD2]
  Fentanyl (as Fentanyl citrate) 100 microgram per 1 dose Instanyl
  100micrograms/dose nasal spray | 6 dose [PoM] £35.70 [CD2] |
  10 dose [PoM] £59.50 [CD2] | 20 dose [PoM] £119.00 [CD2]
  Fentanyl (as Fentanyl citrate) 200 microgram per 1 dose Instanyl
  200micrograms/dose nasal spray | 6 dose [PoM] £35.70 [CD2] |
  10 dose [PoM] £59.50 [CD2] | 20 dose [PoM] £119.00 [CD2]
▸ PecFent (Kyowa Kirin Ltd)
  Fentanyl (as Fentanyl citrate) 100 microgram per 1 dose PecFent
  100micrograms/dose nasal spray | 8 dose [PoM] £36.48 [CD2] |
  32 dose [PoM] £145.92 [CD2]
  Fentanyl (as Fentanyl citrate) 400 microgram per 1 dose PecFent
  400micrograms/dose nasal spray | 8 dose [PoM] £36.48 [CD2] |
  32 dose [PoM] £145.92 [CD2]

Buccal tablet
CAUTIONARY AND ADVISORY LABELS 2
ELECTROLYTES: May contain Sodium
▸ Effentora (Teva UK Ltd)
  Fentanyl (as Fentanyl citrate) 100 microgram Effentora
  100microgram buccal tablets sugar-free | 4 tablet [PoM] £19.96 [CD2]
  sugar-free | 28 tablet [PoM] £139.72 DT = £139.72 [CD2]
  Fentanyl (as Fentanyl citrate) 200 microgram Effentora
  200microgram buccal tablets sugar-free | 4 tablet [PoM] £19.96 [CD2]
  sugar-free | 28 tablet [PoM] £139.72 DT = £139.72 [CD2]
  Fentanyl (as Fentanyl citrate) 400 microgram Effentora
  400microgram buccal tablets sugar-free | 4 tablet [PoM] £19.96 [CD2]
  sugar-free | 28 tablet [PoM] £139.72 DT = £139.72 [CD2]
  Fentanyl (as Fentanyl citrate) 600 microgram Effentora
  600microgram buccal tablets sugar-free | 4 tablet [PoM] £19.96 [CD2]
  sugar-free | 28 tablet [PoM] £139.72 DT = £139.72 [CD2]
  Fentanyl (as Fentanyl citrate) 800 microgram Effentora
  800microgram buccal tablets sugar-free | 4 tablet [PoM] £19.96 [CD2]
  sugar-free | 28 tablet [PoM] £139.72 DT = £139.72 [CD2]

Solution for infusion
▸ Fentanyl (Non-proprietary)
  Fentanyl (as Fentanyl citrate) 50 microgram per 1 ml Fentanyl
  2.5mg/50ml solution for infusion vials | 1 vial [PoM] £5.00 [CD2]

Sublingual tablet
CAUTIONARY AND ADVISORY LABELS 2, 26
▸ Abstral (Kyowa Kirin Ltd)
  Fentanyl (as Fentanyl citrate) 100 microgram Abstral
  100microgram sublingual tablets sugar-free | 10 tablet [PoM]
  £49.99 [CD2] sugar-free | 30 tablet [PoM] £149.70 [CD2]
  Fentanyl (as Fentanyl citrate) 200 microgram Abstral
  200microgram sublingual tablets sugar-free | 10 tablet [PoM]
  £49.99 [CD2] sugar-free | 30 tablet [PoM] £149.70 [CD2]
  Fentanyl (as Fentanyl citrate) 300 microgram Abstral
  300microgram sublingual tablets sugar-free | 10 tablet [PoM]
  £49.99 [CD2] sugar-free | 30 tablet [PoM] £149.70 [CD2]

Fentanyl (as Fentanyl citrate) 400 microgram Abstral
400microgram sublingual tablets sugar-free | 10 tablet [PoM]
£49.99 [CD2] sugar-free | 30 tablet [PoM] £149.70 [CD2]
Fentanyl (as Fentanyl citrate) 600 microgram Abstral
600microgram sublingual tablets sugar-free | 30 tablet [PoM]
£149.70 [CD2]
Fentanyl (as Fentanyl citrate) 800 microgram Abstral
800microgram sublingual tablets sugar-free | 30 tablet [PoM]
£149.70 [CD2]

Transdermal patch
CAUTIONARY AND ADVISORY LABELS 2
▶ Fentanyl (Non-proprietary)
Fentanyl 12 microgram per 1 hour Fentanyl 12micrograms/hour
transdermal patches | 5 patch [PoM] [⊠] DT = £12.59 [CD2]
Fentanyl 25 microgram per 1 hour Fentanyl 25micrograms/hour
transdermal patches | 5 patch [PoM] [⊠] DT = £17.99 [CD2]
Fentanyl 50 microgram per 1 hour Fentanyl 50micrograms/hour
transdermal patches | 5 patch [PoM] [⊠] DT = £33.66 [CD2]
Fentanyl 75 microgram per 1 hour Fentanyl 75micrograms/hour
transdermal patches | 5 patch [PoM] [⊠] DT = £46.99 [CD2]
Fentanyl 100 microgram per 1 hour Fentanyl 100micrograms/hour
transdermal patches | 5 patch [PoM] [⊠] DT = £57.86 [CD2]
▶ Durogesic DTrans (Janssen-Cilag Ltd)
Fentanyl 12 microgram per 1 hour Durogesic DTrans 12micrograms
transdermal patches | 5 patch [PoM] £12.59 DT = £12.59 [CD2]
Fentanyl 25 microgram per 1 hour Durogesic DTrans 25micrograms
transdermal patches | 5 patch [PoM] £17.99 DT = £17.99 [CD2]
Fentanyl 50 microgram per 1 hour Durogesic DTrans 50micrograms
transdermal patches | 5 patch [PoM] £33.66 DT = £33.66 [CD2]
Fentanyl 75 microgram per 1 hour Durogesic DTrans 75micrograms
transdermal patches | 5 patch [PoM] £46.99 DT = £46.99 [CD2]
Fentanyl 100 microgram per 1 hour Durogesic DTrans
100micrograms transdermal patches | 5 patch [PoM] £57.86 DT =
£57.86 [CD2]
▶ Fencino (Ethypharm UK Ltd)
Fentanyl 12 microgram per 1 hour Fencino 12micrograms/hour
transdermal patches | 5 patch [PoM] £8.46 DT = £12.59 [CD2]
Fentanyl 25 microgram per 1 hour Fencino 25micrograms/hour
transdermal patches | 5 patch [PoM] £12.10 DT = £17.99 [CD2]
Fentanyl 50 microgram per 1 hour Fencino 50micrograms/hour
transdermal patches | 5 patch [PoM] £22.62 DT = £33.66 [CD2]
Fentanyl 75 microgram per 1 hour Fencino 75micrograms/hour
transdermal patches | 5 patch [PoM] £31.54 DT = £46.99 [CD2]
Fentanyl 100 microgram per 1 hour Fencino 100micrograms/hour
transdermal patches | 5 patch [PoM] £38.88 DT = £57.86 [CD2]
▶ Fentalis (Sandoz Ltd)
Fentanyl 25 microgram per 1 hour Fentalis Reservoir
25micrograms/hour transdermal patches | 5 patch [PoM] £22.89 =
£17.99 [CD2]
Fentanyl 50 microgram per 1 hour Fentalis Reservoir
50micrograms/hour transdermal patches | 5 patch [PoM] £42.77 DT =
£33.66 [CD2]
Fentanyl 75 microgram per 1 hour Fentalis Reservoir
75micrograms/hour transdermal patches | 5 patch [PoM] £59.62 DT =
£46.99 [CD2]
Fentanyl 100 microgram per 1 hour Fentalis Reservoir
100micrograms/hour transdermal patches | 5 patch [PoM] £73.49 DT
= £57.86 [CD2]
▶ Matrifen (Teva UK Ltd)
Fentanyl 12 microgram per 1 hour Matrifen 12micrograms/hour
transdermal patches | 5 patch [PoM] £7.52 DT = £12.59 [CD2]
Fentanyl 25 microgram per 1 hour Matrifen 25micrograms/hour
transdermal patches | 5 patch [PoM] £10.76 DT = £17.99 [CD2]
Fentanyl 50 microgram per 1 hour Matrifen 50micrograms/hour
transdermal patches | 5 patch [PoM] £20.12 DT = £33.66 [CD2]
Fentanyl 75 microgram per 1 hour Matrifen 75micrograms/hour
transdermal patches | 5 patch [PoM] £28.06 DT = £46.99 [CD2]
Fentanyl 100 microgram per 1 hour Matrifen 100micrograms/hour
transdermal patches | 5 patch [PoM] £34.59 DT = £57.86 [CD2]
▶ Mezolar Matrix (Sandoz Ltd)
Fentanyl 12 microgram per 1 hour Mezolar Matrix
12micrograms/hour transdermal patches | 5 patch [PoM] £7.53 DT =
£12.59 [CD2]
Fentanyl 25 microgram per 1 hour Mezolar Matrix
25micrograms/hour transdermal patches | 5 patch [PoM] £10.77 =
£17.99 [CD2]
Fentanyl 37.5 microgram per 1 hour Mezolar Matrix
37.5microgram/hour transdermal patches | 5 patch [PoM]
£15.46 [CD2]

Fentanyl 50 microgram per 1 hour Mezolar Matrix
50micrograms/hour transdermal patches | 5 patch [PoM] £20.13 DT =
£33.66 [CD2]
Fentanyl 75 microgram per 1 hour Mezolar Matrix
75micrograms/hour transdermal patches | 5 patch [PoM] £28.07 DT =
£46.99 [CD2]
Fentanyl 100 microgram per 1 hour Mezolar Matrix
100micrograms/hour transdermal patches | 5 patch [PoM] £34.60 DT
= £57.86 [CD2]
▶ Opiodur (RX Farma)
Fentanyl 12 microgram per 1 hour Opiodur 12micrograms/hour
transdermal patches | 5 patch [PoM] £7.14 DT = £12.59 [CD2]
Fentanyl 25 microgram per 1 hour Opiodur 25micrograms/hour
transdermal patches | 5 patch [PoM] £10.22 DT = £17.99 [CD2]
Fentanyl 50 microgram per 1 hour Opiodur 50micrograms/hour
transdermal patches | 5 patch [PoM] £19.11 DT = £33.66 [CD2]
Fentanyl 75 microgram per 1 hour Opiodur 75micrograms/hour
transdermal patches | 5 patch [PoM] £26.66 DT = £46.99 [CD2]
Fentanyl 100 microgram per 1 hour Opiodur 100micrograms/hour
transdermal patches | 5 patch [PoM] £32.84 DT = £57.86 [CD2]
▶ Osmanil (Zentiva)
Fentanyl 12 microgram per 1 hour Osmanil 12micrograms/hour
transdermal patches | 5 patch [PoM] £18.11 DT = £12.59 [CD2]
Fentanyl 25 microgram per 1 hour Osmanil 25micrograms/hour
transdermal patches | 5 patch [PoM] £26.94 DT = £17.99 [CD2]
Fentanyl 50 microgram per 1 hour Osmanil 50micrograms/hour
transdermal patches | 5 patch [PoM] £50.32 DT = £33.66 [CD2]
Fentanyl 75 microgram per 1 hour Osmanil 75micrograms/hour
transdermal patches | 5 patch [PoM] £70.15 DT = £46.99 [CD2]
Fentanyl 100 microgram per 1 hour Osmanil 100micrograms/hour
transdermal patches | 5 patch [PoM] £86.46 DT = £57.86 [CD2]
▶ Tilofyl (Tillomed Laboratories Ltd)
Fentanyl 25 microgram per 1 hour Tilofyl 25micrograms/hour
transdermal patches | 5 patch [PoM] £27.00 DT = £17.99 [CD2]
Fentanyl 50 microgram per 1 hour Tilofyl 50micrograms/hour
transdermal patches | 5 patch [PoM] £51.00 DT = £33.66 [CD2]
Fentanyl 75 microgram per 1 hour Tilofyl 75micrograms/hour
transdermal patches | 5 patch [PoM] £71.00 DT = £46.99 [CD2]
Fentanyl 100 microgram per 1 hour Tilofyl 100micrograms/hour
transdermal patches | 5 patch [PoM] £88.00 DT = £57.86 [CD2]
▶ Victanyl (Actavis UK Ltd)
Fentanyl 12 microgram per 1 hour Victanyl 12micrograms/hour
transdermal patches | 5 patch [PoM] £12.58 DT = £12.59 [CD2]
Fentanyl 25 microgram per 1 hour Victanyl 25micrograms/hour
transdermal patches | 5 patch [PoM] £25.89 DT = £17.99 [CD2]
Fentanyl 50 microgram per 1 hour Victanyl 50micrograms/hour
transdermal patches | 5 patch [PoM] £48.36 DT = £33.66 [CD2]
Fentanyl 75 microgram per 1 hour Victanyl 75micrograms/hour
transdermal patches | 5 patch [PoM] £67.41 DT = £46.99 [CD2]
Fentanyl 100 microgram per 1 hour Victanyl 100micrograms/hour
transdermal patches | 5 patch [PoM] £83.09 DT = £57.86 [CD2]
▶ Yemex (Sandoz Ltd)
Fentanyl 12 microgram per 1 hour Yemex 12micrograms/hour
transdermal patches | 5 patch [PoM] £12.59 DT = £12.59 [CD2]
Fentanyl 25 microgram per 1 hour Yemex 25micrograms/hour
transdermal patches | 5 patch [PoM] £17.99 DT = £17.99 [CD2]
Fentanyl 50 microgram per 1 hour Yemex 50micrograms/hour
transdermal patches | 5 patch [PoM] £33.66 DT = £33.66 [CD2]
Fentanyl 75 microgram per 1 hour Yemex 75micrograms/hour
transdermal patches | 5 patch [PoM] £46.99 DT = £46.99 [CD2]
Fentanyl 100 microgram per 1 hour Yemex 100micrograms/hour
transdermal patches | 5 patch [PoM] £57.86 DT = £57.86 [CD2]

Lozenge
CAUTIONARY AND ADVISORY LABELS 2
EXCIPIENTS: May contain Propylene glycol
▶ Actiq (Teva UK Ltd)
Fentanyl (as Fentanyl citrate) 200 microgram Actiq
200microgram lozenges with integral oromucosal applicator |
3 lozenge [PoM] £21.05 DT = £21.05 [CD2] | 30 lozenge [PoM] £210.41
DT = £210.41 [CD2]
Fentanyl (as Fentanyl citrate) 400 microgram Actiq
400microgram lozenges with integral oromucosal applicator |
3 lozenge [PoM] £21.05 DT = £21.05 [CD2] | 30 lozenge [PoM] £210.41
DT = £210.41 [CD2]
Fentanyl (as Fentanyl citrate) 600 microgram Actiq
600microgram lozenges with integral oromucosal applicator |
3 lozenge [PoM] £21.05 DT = £21.05 [CD2] | 30 lozenge [PoM] £210.41
DT = £210.41 [CD2]
Fentanyl (as Fentanyl citrate) 800 microgram Actiq
800microgram lozenges with integral oromucosal applicator |

3 lozenge PoM £21.05 DT = £21.05 CD2 | 30 lozenge PoM £210.41 DT = £210.41 CD2
Fentanyl (as Fentanyl citrate) 1.2 mg Actiq 1.2mg lozenges with integral oromucosal applicator | 3 lozenge PoM £21.05 DT = £21.05 CD2 | 30 lozenge PoM £210.41 DT = £210.41 CD2
Fentanyl (as Fentanyl citrate) 1.6 mg Actiq 1.6mg lozenges with integral oromucosal applicator | 3 lozenge PoM £21.05 CD2 | 30 lozenge PoM £210.41 CD2

F 441

Hydromorphone hydrochloride

INDICATIONS AND DOSE

Severe pain in cancer
▸ BY MOUTH USING IMMEDIATE-RELEASE MEDICINES
▸ Child 12-17 years: 1.3 mg every 4 hours, dose to be increased if necessary according to severity of pain
▸ Adult: 1.3 mg every 4 hours, dose to be increased if necessary according to severity of pain
▸ BY MOUTH USING MODIFIED-RELEASE MEDICINES
▸ Child 12-17 years: 4 mg every 12 hours, dose to be increased if necessary according to severity of pain
▸ Adult: 4 mg every 12 hours, dose to be increased if necessary according to severity of pain

● CONTRA-INDICATIONS Acute abdomen
● CAUTIONS Pancreatitis · toxic psychosis
● INTERACTIONS → Appendix 1: opioids
● SIDE-EFFECTS
▸ **Common or very common** Anxiety · appetite decreased · asthenia · gastrointestinal discomfort · sleep disorders
▸ **Uncommon** Depression · diarrhoea · dyspnoea · malaise · movement disorders · paraesthesia · peripheral oedema · sexual dysfunction · taste altered · tremor
▸ **Rare or very rare** Bronchospasm · lethargy
▸ **Frequency not known** Hyperalgesia · paralytic ileus · seizure
● BREAST FEEDING Avoid—no information available.
● RENAL IMPAIRMENT Avoid use or reduce dose; opioid effects increased and prolonged and increased cerebral sensitivity occurs.
● DIRECTIONS FOR ADMINISTRATION For *immediate-release* capsules, swallow whole capsule or sprinkle contents on soft food. For *modified-release* capsules, swallow whole or open capsule and sprinkle contents on soft cold food (swallow the pellets within the capsule whole; do not crush or chew).
● PATIENT AND CARER ADVICE Patients or carers should be given advice on how to administer hydromorphone hydrochloride capsules and modified-release capsules.

● MEDICINAL FORMS
There can be variation in the licensing of different medicines containing the same drug. Forms available from special-order manufacturers include: oral solution
Modified-release capsule
CAUTIONARY AND ADVISORY LABELS 2
▸ Palladone SR (Napp Pharmaceuticals Ltd)
Hydromorphone hydrochloride 2 mg Palladone SR 2mg capsules | 56 capsule PoM £20.98 CD2
Hydromorphone hydrochloride 4 mg Palladone SR 4mg capsules | 56 capsule PoM £28.75 CD2
Hydromorphone hydrochloride 8 mg Palladone SR 8mg capsules | 56 capsule PoM £56.08 CD2
Hydromorphone hydrochloride 16 mg Palladone SR 16mg capsules | 56 capsule PoM £106.53 CD2
Hydromorphone hydrochloride 24 mg Palladone SR 24mg capsules | 56 capsule PoM £159.82 CD2
Capsule
CAUTIONARY AND ADVISORY LABELS 2
▸ Palladone (Napp Pharmaceuticals Ltd)
Hydromorphone hydrochloride 1.3 mg Palladone 1.3mg capsules | 56 capsule PoM £8.82 CD2
Hydromorphone hydrochloride 2.6 mg Palladone 2.6mg capsules | 56 capsule PoM £17.64 CD2

F 441

Meptazinol

INDICATIONS AND DOSE

Moderate to severe pain, including post-operative pain and renal colic
▸ BY MOUTH
▸ Adult: 200 mg every 3–6 hours as required
▸ BY INTRAMUSCULAR INJECTION
▸ Adult: 75–100 mg every 2–4 hours if required
▸ BY SLOW INTRAVENOUS INJECTION
▸ Adult: 50–100 mg every 2–4 hours if required
Obstetric analgesia
▸ BY INTRAMUSCULAR INJECTION
▸ Adult: 2 mg/kg, usual dose 100–150 mg

● CONTRA-INDICATIONS Myocardial infarction · phaeochromocytoma
● INTERACTIONS → Appendix 1: opioids
● SIDE-EFFECTS
▸ **Common or very common** Diarrhoea · gastrointestinal discomfort
Overdose Effects only partially reversed by naloxone.
● BREAST FEEDING Use only if potential benefit outweighs risk.
● RENAL IMPAIRMENT Avoid use or reduce dose; opioid effects increased and prolonged and increased cerebral sensitivity occurs.

● MEDICINAL FORMS
There can be variation in the licensing of different medicines containing the same drug.
Solution for injection
▸ Meptid (Almirall Ltd)
Meptazinol (as Meptazinol hydrochloride) 100 mg per 1 ml Meptid 100mg/1ml solution for injection ampoules | 10 ampoule PoM £19.21
Tablet
CAUTIONARY AND ADVISORY LABELS 2
▸ Meptid (Almirall Ltd)
Meptazinol (as Meptazinol hydrochloride) 200 mg Meptid 200mg tablets | 112 tablet PoM £22.11 DT = £22.11

F 441

Morphine

12-Dec-2016

INDICATIONS AND DOSE

Pain
▸ BY SUBCUTANEOUS INJECTION
▸ Child 1-5 months: Initially 100–200 micrograms/kg every 6 hours, adjusted according to response
▸ Child 6 months-1 year: Initially 100–200 micrograms/kg every 4 hours, adjusted according to response
▸ Child 2-11 years: Initially 200 micrograms/kg every 4 hours, adjusted according to response
▸ Child 12-17 years: Initially 2.5–10 mg every 4 hours, adjusted according to response
▸ INITIALLY BY INTRAVENOUS INJECTION
▸ Child 1-5 months: 100 micrograms/kg every 6 hours, adjusted according to response, dose to be administered over at least 5 minutes, alternatively (by intravenous injection) initially 100 micrograms/kg, dose to be administered over at least 5 minutes, followed by (by continuous intravenous infusion) 10–30 micrograms/kg/hour, adjusted according to response
▸ Child 6 months-11 years: 100 micrograms/kg every 4 hours, adjusted according to response, dose to be administered over at least 5 minutes, alternatively (by intravenous injection) initially 100 micrograms/kg, dose to be administered over at least 5 minutes,

followed by (by continuous intravenous infusion) 20–30 micrograms/kg/hour, adjusted according to response
- Child 12-17 years: 5 mg every 4 hours, adjusted according to response, dose to be administered over at least 5 minutes, alternatively (by intravenous injection) initially 5 mg, dose to be administered over at least 5 minutes, followed by (by continuous intravenous infusion) 20–30 micrograms/kg/hour, adjusted according to response
▸ BY MOUTH, OR BY RECTUM
- Child 1-2 months: Initially 50–100 micrograms/kg every 4 hours, adjusted according to response
- Child 3-5 months: 100–150 micrograms/kg every 4 hours, adjusted according to response
- Child 6-11 months: 200 micrograms/kg every 4 hours, adjusted according to response
- Child 1 year: Initially 200–300 micrograms/kg every 4 hours, adjusted according to response
- Child 2-11 years: Initially 200–300 micrograms/kg every 4 hours (max. per dose 10 mg), adjusted according to response
- Child 12-17 years: Initially 5–10 mg every 4 hours, adjusted according to response

Acute pain
▸ BY MOUTH, OR BY SUBCUTANEOUS INJECTION, OR BY INTRAMUSCULAR INJECTION
- Adult: Initially 10 mg every 4 hours, adjusted according to response, subcutaneous injection not suitable for oedematous patients, dose can be given more frequently during titration, use dose for elderly in frail patients
- Elderly: Initially 5 mg every 4 hours, adjusted according to response, subcutaneous injection not suitable for oedematous patients, dose can be given more frequently during titration
▸ BY SLOW INTRAVENOUS INJECTION
- Adult: Initially 5 mg every 4 hours, adjusted according to response, dose can be adjusted more frequently during titration, reduced dose recommended in frail and elderly patients

Chronic pain
▸ BY MOUTH, OR BY SUBCUTANEOUS INJECTION, OR BY INTRAMUSCULAR INJECTION
- Adult: Initially 5–10 mg every 4 hours, adjusted according to response, subcutaneous injection not suitable for oedematous patients
▸ BY RECTUM
- Adult: Initially 15–30 mg every 4 hours, adjusted according to response

Pain (with modified-release 12-hourly preparations)
▸ BY MOUTH USING MODIFIED-RELEASE MEDICINES
- Adult: Every 12 hours, dose adjusted according to daily morphine requirements, dosage requirements should be reviewed if the brand is altered

Pain (with modified-release 24-hourly preparations)
▸ BY MOUTH USING MODIFIED-RELEASE MEDICINES
- Adult: Every 24 hours, dose adjusted according to daily morphine requirements, dosage requirements should be reviewed if the brand is altered

Pain management in palliative care (starting dose for opioid-naïve patients)
▸ BY MOUTH
- Adult: 20–30 mg daily in divided doses, using immediate-release preparation 4-hourly or a 12-hourly modified-release preparation, for management of breakthrough pain and other general advice, see *Pain management with opioids* under Prescribing in palliative care p. 23.

Pain management in palliative care (starting dose for patients being switched from a regular weak opioid)
▸ BY MOUTH
- Adult: 40–60 mg daily in divided doses, using immediate-release preparation 4-hourly or 12-hourly modified-release preparation, for management of breakthrough pain and other general advice, see *Pain management with opioids* under Prescribing in palliative care p. 23.

Pain in palliative care (following initial titration)
▸ BY MOUTH USING IMMEDIATE-RELEASE MEDICINES
- Adult: Usual dose 30 mg every 4 hours; up to 200 mg every 4 hours, higher dose may be required for some patients (occasionally more is needed); for management of breakthrough pain and other general advice, see *Pain management with opioids* under p. 23.
▸ BY MOUTH USING MODIFIED-RELEASE MEDICINES
- Adult: Usual dose 100 mg every 12 hours; up to 600 mg every 12 hours, higher dose may be required for some patients (occasionally more is needed); for management of breakthrough pain and other general advice, see *Pain management with opioids* under p. 23.

Cough in terminal disease
▸ BY MOUTH
- Adult: Initially 5 mg every 4 hours

Premedication
▸ BY SUBCUTANEOUS INJECTION, OR BY INTRAMUSCULAR INJECTION
- Adult: Up to 10 mg, dose to be administered 60–90 minutes before operation

Patient controlled analgesia (PCA)
▸ BY INTRAVENOUS INFUSION
- Adult: (consult local protocol)

Myocardial infarction
▸ BY SLOW INTRAVENOUS INJECTION
- Adult: 5–10 mg, followed by 5–10 mg if required, dose to be administered at a rate of 1–2 mg/minute, use dose for elderly in frail patients
- Elderly: 2.5–5 mg, followed by 2.5–5 mg if required, dose to be administered at a rate of 1–2 mg/minute

Acute pulmonary oedema
▸ BY SLOW INTRAVENOUS INJECTION
- Adult: 5–10 mg, dose to be administered at a rate of 2 mg/minute, use dose for elderly in frail patients
- Elderly: 2.5–5 mg, dose to be administered at a rate of 2 mg/minute

Dyspnoea at rest in palliative care
▸ BY MOUTH
- Adult: Initially 5 mg every 4 hours, to be given in carefully titrated doses

DOSE EQUIVALENCE AND CONVERSION
▸ The doses stated refer equally to morphine hydrochloride and sulfate.

● UNLICENSED USE *Oramorph* ® solution and *MXL* ® capsules not licensed for use in children under 1 year. *Sevredol* ® tablets not licensed for use in children under 3 years. *Oramorph* ® unit dose vials and *Filnarine* ® SR tablets not licensed for use in children under 6 years. *MST Continus* ® preparations licensed to treat children with cancer pain (age-range not specified by manufacturer). Suppositories are not licensed for use in children.

IMPORTANT SAFETY INFORMATION
Do not confuse modified-release 12-hourly preparations with 24-hourly preparations, see *Prescribing and dispensing information.*

● CONTRA-INDICATIONS Acute abdomen · delayed gastric emptying · heart failure secondary to chronic lung disease · phaeochromocytoma

- CAUTIONS Cardiac arrhythmias · pancreatitis · severe cor pulmonale
- INTERACTIONS → Appendix 1: opioids
- SIDE-EFFECTS
► Common or very common
► With oral use Appetite decreased · asthenic conditions · gastrointestinal discomfort · insomnia · neuromuscular dysfunction
► Uncommon
► With oral use Agitation · bronchospasm · ileus · mood altered · myoclonus · paraesthesia · peripheral oedema · pulmonary oedema · seizure · syncope · taste altered
► Frequency not known
► With oral use Amenorrhoea · biliary pain · cough decreased · hyperalgesia · hypertension · pancreatitis exacerbated · sexual dysfunction · thinking abnormal · ureteral spasm
► With parenteral use Alertness decreased · bile duct disorders · contact dermatitis · mood altered · myoclonus · postural hypotension · sexual dysfunction · ureteral spasm · urinary disorders · vision disorders
- BREAST FEEDING Therapeutic doses unlikely to affect infant.
- RENAL IMPAIRMENT Avoid use or reduce dose; opioid effects increased and prolonged; increased cerebral sensitivity.
- DIRECTIONS FOR ADMINISTRATION
► With intravenous use in children For *continuous intravenous infusion*, dilute with Glucose 5% or 10% or Sodium Chloride 0.9%.
► With oral use For *modified release capsules*—swallow whole or open capsule and sprinkle contents on soft food.
- PRESCRIBING AND DISPENSING INFORMATION Modified-release preparations are available as 12-hourly or 24-hourly formulations; prescribers must ensure that the correct preparation is prescribed. Preparations that should be given 12-hourly include *Filnarine® SR, MST Continus®, Morphgesic® SR* and *Zomorph®*. Preparations that should be given 24-hourly include *MXL®*.
  Prescriptions must specify the 'form'.
► With rectal use Both the strength of the suppositories and the morphine salt contained in them must be specified by the prescriber.

  Palliative care For further information on the use of morphine in palliative care, see www.palliativedrugs.com/formulary/en/morphine.html.
- PATIENT AND CARER ADVICE Patients or carers should be given advice on how to administer morphine modified-release capsules.
  Medicines for Children leaflet: Morphine for pain www.medicinesforchildren.org.uk/morphine-for-pain
- EXCEPTIONS TO LEGAL CATEGORY
  Morphine Oral Solutions Prescription-only medicines or schedule 2 controlled drug. The proportion of morphine hydrochloride may be altered when specified by the prescriber; if above 13 mg per 5 mL the solution becomes a schedule 2 controlled drug. It is usual to adjust the strength so that the dose volume is 5 or 10 mL.
  Oral solutions of morphine can be prescribed by writing the formula:
  Morphine hydrochloride 5 mg
  Chloroform water to 5 mL

- MEDICINAL FORMS
  There can be variation in the licensing of different medicines containing the same drug. Forms available from special-order manufacturers include: capsule, oral solution, solution for injection, infusion, suppository
  Modified-release tablet
  CAUTIONARY AND ADVISORY LABELS 2, 25
  ► MST Continus (Napp Pharmaceuticals Ltd)
  Morphine sulfate 5 mg MST Continus 5mg tablets | 60 tablet [PoM] £3.29 DT = £3.29 [CD2]

Morphine sulfate 10 mg MST Continus 10mg tablets | 60 tablet [PoM] £5.20 DT = £5.20 [CD2]
Morphine sulfate 15 mg MST Continus 15mg tablets | 60 tablet [PoM] £9.10 DT = £9.10 [CD2]
Morphine sulfate 30 mg MST Continus 30mg tablets | 60 tablet [PoM] £12.47 DT = £12.47 [CD2]
Morphine sulfate 60 mg MST Continus 60mg tablets | 60 tablet [PoM] £24.32 DT = £24.32 [CD2]
Morphine sulfate 100 mg MST Continus 100mg tablets | 60 tablet [PoM] £38.50 DT = £38.50 [CD2]
Morphine sulfate 200 mg MST Continus 200mg tablets | 60 tablet [PoM] £81.34 DT = £81.34 [CD2]
► Morphgesic SR (AMCo)
Morphine sulfate 10 mg Morphgesic SR 10mg tablets | 60 tablet [PoM] £3.85 DT = £5.20 [CD2]
Morphine sulfate 30 mg Morphgesic SR 30mg tablets | 60 tablet [PoM] £9.24 DT = £12.47 [CD2]
Morphine sulfate 60 mg Morphgesic SR 60mg tablets | 60 tablet [PoM] £18.04 DT = £24.32 [CD2]
Morphine sulfate 100 mg Morphgesic SR 100mg tablets | 60 tablet [PoM] £28.54 DT = £38.50 [CD2]

Tablet
CAUTIONARY AND ADVISORY LABELS 2
► Sevredol (Napp Pharmaceuticals Ltd)
Morphine sulfate 10 mg Sevredol 10mg tablets | 56 tablet [PoM] £5.31 DT = £5.31 [CD2]
Morphine sulfate 20 mg Sevredol 20mg tablets | 56 tablet [PoM] £10.61 DT = £10.61 [CD2]
Morphine sulfate 50 mg Sevredol 50mg tablets | 56 tablet [PoM] £28.02 DT = £28.02 [CD2]

Suppository
CAUTIONARY AND ADVISORY LABELS 2
► Morphine (Non-proprietary)
Morphine sulfate 10 mg Morphine sulfate 10mg suppositories | 12 suppository [PoM] £19.45 DT = £19.45 [CD2]

Solution for injection
► Morphine (Non-proprietary)
Morphine sulfate 1 mg per 1 ml Morphine sulfate 5mg/5ml solution for injection ampoules | 10 ampoule [PoM] £39.60 [CD2]
Morphine sulfate 1mg/1ml solution for injection ampoules | 10 ampoule [PoM] £28.70 [CD2]
Morphine sulfate 10mg/10ml solution for injection ampoules | 10 ampoule [PoM] £13.50–£15.00 [CD2]
Morphine sulfate 10 mg per 1 ml Morphine sulfate 10mg/1ml solution for injection ampoules | 10 ampoule [PoM] £10.30 DT = £9.36 [CD2]
Morphine sulfate 15 mg per 1 ml Morphine sulfate 15mg/1ml solution for injection ampoules | 10 ampoule [PoM] £10.74 DT = £10.74 [CD2]
Morphine sulfate 20 mg per 1 ml Morphine sulfate 20mg/1ml solution for injection ampoules | 10 ampoule [PoM] £59.70 DT = £59.70 [CD2]
Morphine sulfate 30 mg per 1 ml Morphine sulfate 30mg/1ml solution for injection ampoules | 10 ampoule [PoM] £11.49 DT = £11.49 [CD2]
Morphine sulfate 60mg/2ml solution for injection ampoules | 5 ampoule [PoM] £10.07 DT = £10.07 [CD2]

Modified-release capsule
CAUTIONARY AND ADVISORY LABELS 2
► MXL (Napp Pharmaceuticals Ltd)
Morphine sulfate 30 mg MXL 30mg capsules | 28 capsule [PoM] £10.91 [CD2]
Morphine sulfate 60 mg MXL 60mg capsules | 28 capsule [PoM] £14.95 [CD2]
Morphine sulfate 90 mg MXL 90mg capsules | 28 capsule [PoM] £22.04 = £22.04 [CD2]
Morphine sulfate 120 mg MXL 120mg capsules | 28 capsule [PoM] £29.15 = £29.15 [CD2]
Morphine sulfate 150 mg MXL 150mg capsules | 28 capsule [PoM] £36.43 DT = £36.43 [CD2]
Morphine sulfate 200 mg MXL 200mg capsules | 28 capsule [PoM] £46.15 [CD2]
► Zomorph (Ethypharm UK Ltd)
Morphine sulfate 10 mg Zomorph 10mg modified-release capsules | 60 capsule [PoM] £3.47 DT = £3.47 [CD2]
Morphine sulfate 30 mg Zomorph 30mg modified-release capsules | 60 capsule [PoM] £8.30 DT = £8.30 [CD2]
Morphine sulfate 60 mg Zomorph 60mg modified-release capsules | 60 capsule [PoM] £16.20 DT = £16.20 [CD2]

Morphine sulfate 100 mg Zomorph 100mg modified-release capsules | 60 capsule [PoM] £21.80 DT = £21.80 [CD2]
Morphine sulfate 200 mg Zomorph 200mg modified-release capsules | 60 capsule [PoM] £43.60 DT = £43.60 [CD2]

Solution for infusion

▶ Morphine (Non-proprietary)
Morphine sulfate 1 mg per 1 ml Morphine sulfate 50mg/50ml solution for infusion vials | 1 vial [PoM] £5.78 DT = £5.78 [CD2] | 10 vial [PoM] £38.70 [CD2]
Morphine sulfate 2 mg per 1 ml Morphine sulfate 100mg/50ml solution for infusion vials | 1 vial [PoM] £6.48 [CD2] | 10 vial [PoM] £64.80 [CD2]

Oral solution

CAUTIONARY AND ADVISORY LABELS 2

▶ Morphine (Non-proprietary)
Morphine sulfate 2 mg per 1 ml Morphine sulfate 10mg/5ml oral solution | 100 ml [PoM] £1.68-£1.82 [CD5] | 300 ml [PoM] £5.45 DT = £5.45 [CD5] | 500 ml [PoM] £7.10-£9.10 [CD5]

▶ Oramorph (Boehringer Ingelheim Ltd)
Morphine sulfate 2 mg per 1 ml Oramorph 10mg/5ml oral solution | 100 ml [PoM] £1.89 [CD5] | 300 ml [PoM] £5.45 DT = £5.45 [CD5] | 500 ml [PoM] £8.50 [CD5]
Morphine sulfate 20 mg per 1 ml Oramorph 20mg/ml concentrated oral solution sugar-free | 30 ml [PoM] £4.98 [CD2] sugar-free | 120 ml [PoM] £19.50 DT = £19.50 [CD2]

Modified-release granules

CAUTIONARY AND ADVISORY LABELS 2, 13

▶ MST Continus (Napp Pharmaceuticals Ltd)
Morphine sulfate 20 mg MST Continus Suspension 20mg granules sachets sugar-free | 30 sachet [PoM] £24.58 [CD2]
Morphine sulfate 30 mg MST Continus Suspension 30mg granules sachets sugar-free | 30 sachet [PoM] £25.54 [CD2]
Morphine sulfate 60 mg MST Continus Suspension 60mg granules sachets sugar-free | 30 sachet [PoM] £51.09 [CD2]
Morphine sulfate 100 mg MST Continus Suspension 100mg granules sachets sugar-free | 30 sachet [PoM] £85.15 [CD2]
Morphine sulfate 200 mg MST Continus Suspension 200mg granules sachets sugar-free | 30 sachet [PoM] £170.30 [CD2]

Morphine with cyclizine

The properties listed below are those particular to the combination only. For the properties of the components please consider, morphine p. 456, cyclizine p. 424.

● INDICATIONS AND DOSE

CYCLIMORPH-10 ®

Moderate to severe pain (short-term use only)

▶ BY SUBCUTANEOUS INJECTION, OR BY INTRAMUSCULAR INJECTION, OR BY INTRAVENOUS INJECTION

▶ Adult: 1 mL, do not repeat dose more often than every 4 hours; maximum 3 doses per day

CYCLIMORPH-15 ®

Moderate to severe pain (short-term use only)

▶ BY SUBCUTANEOUS INJECTION, OR BY INTRAMUSCULAR INJECTION, OR BY INTRAVENOUS INJECTION

▶ Adult: 1 mL, do not repeat dose more often than every 4 hours; maximum 3 doses per day

● CAUTIONS Myocardial infarction (cyclizine may aggravate severe heart failure and counteract the haemodynamic benefits of opioids) · not recommended in palliative care

● INTERACTIONS → Appendix 1: antihistamines, sedating · opioids

● MEDICINAL FORMS
There can be variation in the licensing of different medicines containing the same drug.

Solution for injection

▶ Cyclimorph (AMCo)
Morphine tartrate 15 mg per 1 ml, Cyclizine tartrate 50 mg per 1 ml Cyclimorph 15 solution for injection 1ml ampoules | 5 ampoule [PoM] £9.12 [CD2]

Morphine tartrate 10 mg per 1 ml, Cyclizine tartrate 50 mg per 1 ml Cyclimorph 10 solution for injection 1ml ampoules | 5 ampoule [PoM] £8.77 [CD2]

F 441

Oxycodone hydrochloride   19-May-2017

● INDICATIONS AND DOSE

Postoperative pain | Severe pain | Moderate to severe pain in palliative care

▶ BY MOUTH USING IMMEDIATE-RELEASE MEDICINES

▶ Adult: Initially 5 mg every 4–6 hours, dose to be increased if necessary according to severity of pain, some patients may require higher doses than the maximum daily dose; maximum 400 mg per day

▶ BY MOUTH USING MODIFIED-RELEASE MEDICINES

▶ Adult: Initially 10 mg every 12 hours (max. per dose 200 mg every 12 hours), dose to be increased if necessary according to severity of pain, some patients might require higher doses than the maximum daily dose, use 12-hourly modified-release preparations for this dose; see Prescribing and dispensing information

▶ BY SLOW INTRAVENOUS INJECTION

▶ Adult: 1–10 mg every 4 hours as required

▶ BY INTRAVENOUS INFUSION

▶ Adult: Initially 2 mg/hour, adjusted according to response

▶ BY SUBCUTANEOUS INJECTION

▶ Adult: Initially 5 mg every 4 hours as required

▶ BY SUBCUTANEOUS INFUSION

▶ Adult: Initially 7.5 mg/24 hours, adjusted according to response

Patient controlled analgesia (PCA)

▶ BY INTRAVENOUS INFUSION

▶ Adult: (consult local protocol)

DOSE EQUIVALENCE AND CONVERSION

▶ 2 mg oral oxycodone is approximately equivalent to 1 mg parenteral oxycodone.

ONEXILA XL ®

Severe pain

▶ BY MOUTH

▶ Adult: Initially 10 mg every 24 hours, dose to be increased if necessary according to severity of pain, some patients may require higher doses than the maximum daily dose; maximum 400 mg per day

IMPORTANT SAFETY INFORMATION
Do not confuse modified-release 12-hourly preparations with 24-hourly preparations, see Prescribing and dispensing information.

● CONTRA-INDICATIONS Acute abdomen · chronic constipation · cor pulmonale · delayed gastric emptying

● CAUTIONS Pancreatitis · toxic psychosis

● INTERACTIONS → Appendix 1: opioids

● SIDE-EFFECTS

GENERAL SIDE-EFFECTS

▶ Common or very common Anxiety · appetite abnormal · asthenia · bronchospasm · depression · diarrhoea · dyspnoea · gastrointestinal discomfort · hiccups · lethargy · mood altered · skin reactions · tremor

▶ Uncommon Biliary colic · burping · chills · dehydration · dysphagia · gastrointestinal disorders · malaise · memory loss · neuromuscular dysfunction · oedema · seizure · sensation abnormal · sexual dysfunction · speech disorder · supraventricular tachycardia · syncope · taste altered · thirst · vasodilation

▶ Rare or very rare Postural hypotension

▶ Frequency not known Aggression · amenorrhoea · cholestasis

4

Nervous system

Nervous system

4

SPECIFIC SIDE-EFFECTS
▶ **Common or very common**
▶ With oral use Cognitive impairment · insomnia · movement disorders · perception altered · psychiatric disorders · urinary frequency increased
▶ With parenteral use Cough decreased · sleep disorders · thinking abnormal
▶ **Uncommon**
▶ With oral use Chest pain · cough · hyperacusia · increased risk of infection · injury · lacrimation disorder · migraine · oral disorders · pain · SIADH · voice alteration
▶ With parenteral use Disorientation · fever · hypogonadism · ureteral spasm
▶ **Rare or very rare**
▶ With oral use Haemorrhage · lymphadenopathy · muscle spasms · photosensitivity reaction · weight changes
▶ **Frequency not known**
▶ With parenteral use Dental caries · hyperalgesia
● BREAST FEEDING Present in milk—avoid.
● HEPATIC IMPAIRMENT Avoid in moderate to severe impairment.
  Dose adjustments Max. initial dose 2.5 mg every 6 hours in patients not currently treated with an opioid with mild impairment.
● RENAL IMPAIRMENT Opioid effects increased and prolonged and increased cerebral sensitivity occurs. Avoid if eGFR less than 10 mL/minute/1.73 m².
  Dose adjustments Max. initial dose 2.5 mg every 6 hours in patients not currently treated with an opioid with mild to moderate impairment.
● DIRECTIONS FOR ADMINISTRATION For intravenous infusion (*Oxynorm* ®), give continuously *or* intermittently in Glucose 5% or Sodium chloride 0.9%; dilute to a concentration of 1 mg/mL.
● PRESCRIBING AND DISPENSING INFORMATION Modified-release preparations are available as 12-hourly or 24-hourly formulations. Preparations that should be given 12-hourly include *Abtard* ®, *Carexil* ®, *Leveraxo* ®, *Longtec* ®, *Oxeltra* ®, *OxyContin* ®, *Oxylan* ®, *Reltebon* ®, and *Zomestine* ®. Preparations that should be given 24-hourly include *Onexila* ® XL.
  Palliative care For further information on the use of oxycodone in palliative care, see www.palliativedrugs.com/formulary/en/oxycodone.html.
● NATIONAL FUNDING/ACCESS DECISIONS
  Scottish Medicines Consortium (SMC) Decisions
  The *Scottish Medicines Consortium* has advised (October 2004 and November 2010) that *OxyNorm* ® injection is restricted for use within NHS Scotland for patients with cancer who have difficulty in tolerating morphine or diamorphine.

● MEDICINAL FORMS
  There can be variation in the licensing of different medicines containing the same drug. Forms available from special-order manufacturers include: oral solution, solution for infusion

Modified-release tablet
CAUTIONARY AND ADVISORY LABELS 2, 25
▶ Oxycodone hydrochloride (Non-proprietary)
  Oxycodone hydrochloride 15 mg Oxycodone 15mg modified-release tablets | 56 tablet [PoM] £38.12 DT = £38.12 [CD2]
  Oxycodone hydrochloride 30 mg Oxycodone 30mg modified-release tablets | 56 tablet [PoM] £76.23 DT = £76.23 [CD2]
  Oxycodone hydrochloride 60 mg Oxycodone 60mg modified-release tablets | 56 tablet [PoM] £152.49 DT = £152.49 [CD2]
▶ Abtard (Ethypharm UK Ltd)
  Oxycodone hydrochloride 5 mg Abtard 5mg modified-release tablets | 28 tablet [PoM] £6.26 DT = £12.52 [CD2]
  Oxycodone hydrochloride 10 mg Abtard 10mg modified-release tablets | 56 tablet [PoM] £12.52 DT = £25.04 [CD2]
  Oxycodone hydrochloride 15 mg Abtard 15mg modified-release tablets | 56 tablet [PoM] £19.06 DT = £38.12 [CD2]

Oxycodone hydrochloride 20 mg Abtard 20mg modified-release tablets | 56 tablet [PoM] £25.04 DT = £50.08 [CD2]
Oxycodone hydrochloride 30 mg Abtard 30mg modified-release tablets | 56 tablet [PoM] £38.11 DT = £76.23 [CD2]
Oxycodone hydrochloride 40 mg Abtard 40mg modified-release tablets | 56 tablet [PoM] £50.09 DT = £100.19 [CD2]
Oxycodone hydrochloride 60 mg Abtard 60mg modified-release tablets | 56 tablet [PoM] £76.24 DT = £152.49 [CD2]
Oxycodone hydrochloride 80 mg Abtard 80mg modified-release tablets | 56 tablet [PoM] £100.19 DT = £200.39 [CD2]
▶ Carexil (Sandoz Ltd)
Oxycodone hydrochloride 5 mg Carexil 5mg modified-release tablets | 28 tablet [PoM] £6.26 DT = £12.52 [CD2]
Oxycodone hydrochloride 10 mg Carexil 10mg modified-release tablets | 56 tablet [PoM] £12.52 DT = £25.04 [CD2]
Oxycodone hydrochloride 20 mg Carexil 20mg modified-release tablets | 56 tablet [PoM] £25.04 DT = £50.08 [CD2]
Oxycodone hydrochloride 40 mg Carexil 40mg modified-release tablets | 56 tablet [PoM] £60.11 DT = £100.19 [CD2]
Oxycodone hydrochloride 80 mg Carexil 80mg modified-release tablets | 56 tablet [PoM] £120.23 DT = £200.39 [CD2]
▶ Leveraxo (Mylan)
Oxycodone hydrochloride 5 mg Leveraxo 5mg modified-release tablets | 28 tablet [PoM] £12.39 DT = £12.52 [CD2]
Oxycodone hydrochloride 10 mg Leveraxo 10mg modified-release tablets | 56 tablet [PoM] £24.79 DT = £25.04 [CD2]
Oxycodone hydrochloride 20 mg Leveraxo 20mg modified-release tablets | 56 tablet [PoM] £49.58 DT = £50.08 [CD2]
Oxycodone hydrochloride 30 mg Leveraxo 30mg modified-release tablets | 56 tablet [PoM] £75.47 DT = £76.23 [CD2]
Oxycodone hydrochloride 40 mg Leveraxo 40mg modified-release tablets | 56 tablet [PoM] £99.19 DT = £100.19 [CD2]
Oxycodone hydrochloride 60 mg Leveraxo 60mg modified-release tablets | 56 tablet [PoM] £150.97 DT = £152.49 [CD2]
Oxycodone hydrochloride 80 mg Leveraxo 80mg modified-release tablets | 56 tablet [PoM] £198.39 DT = £200.39 [CD2]
▶ Longtec (Qdem Pharmaceuticals Ltd)
Oxycodone hydrochloride 5 mg Longtec 5mg modified-release tablets | 28 tablet [PoM] £6.26 DT = £12.52 [CD2]
Oxycodone hydrochloride 10 mg Longtec 10mg modified-release tablets | 56 tablet [PoM] £12.52 DT = £25.04 [CD2]
Oxycodone hydrochloride 15 mg Longtec 15mg modified-release tablets | 56 tablet [PoM] £19.06 DT = £38.12 [CD2]
Oxycodone hydrochloride 20 mg Longtec 20mg modified-release tablets | 56 tablet [PoM] £25.04 DT = £50.08 [CD2]
Oxycodone hydrochloride 30 mg Longtec 30mg modified-release tablets | 56 tablet [PoM] £38.11 DT = £76.23 [CD2]
Oxycodone hydrochloride 40 mg Longtec 40mg modified-release tablets | 56 tablet [PoM] £50.09 DT = £100.19 [CD2]
Oxycodone hydrochloride 60 mg Longtec 60mg modified-release tablets | 56 tablet [PoM] £76.24 DT = £152.49 [CD2]
Oxycodone hydrochloride 80 mg Longtec 80mg modified-release tablets | 56 tablet [PoM] £100.19 DT = £200.39 [CD2]
Oxycodone hydrochloride 120 mg Longtec 120mg modified-release tablets | 56 tablet [PoM] £152.51 DT = £305.02 [CD2]
▶ Onexila XL (Aspire Pharma Ltd)
Oxycodone hydrochloride 10 mg Onexila XL 10mg tablets | 28 tablet [PoM] £12.52 [CD2]
Oxycodone hydrochloride 20 mg Onexila XL 20mg tablets | 28 tablet [PoM] £12.52 [CD2]
Oxycodone hydrochloride 40 mg Onexila XL 40mg tablets | 28 tablet [PoM] £25.04 [CD2]
Oxycodone hydrochloride 80 mg Onexila XL 80mg tablets | 28 tablet [PoM] £50.09 [CD2]
▶ Oxeltra (Wockhardt UK Ltd)
Oxycodone hydrochloride 5 mg Oxeltra 5mg modified-release tablets | 28 tablet [PoM] £11.27 DT = £12.52 [CD2]
Oxycodone hydrochloride 10 mg Oxeltra 10mg modified-release tablets | 56 tablet [PoM] £22.54 DT = £25.04 [CD2]
Oxycodone hydrochloride 15 mg Oxeltra 15mg modified-release tablets | 56 tablet [PoM] £34.31 DT = £38.12 [CD2]
Oxycodone hydrochloride 20 mg Oxeltra 20mg modified-release tablets | 56 tablet [PoM] £45.07 DT = £50.08 [CD2]
Oxycodone hydrochloride 30 mg Oxeltra 30mg modified-release tablets | 56 tablet [PoM] £68.61 DT = £76.23 [CD2]
Oxycodone hydrochloride 40 mg Oxeltra 40mg modified-release tablets | 56 tablet [PoM] £90.17 DT = £100.19 [CD2]
Oxycodone hydrochloride 60 mg Oxeltra 60mg modified-release tablets | 56 tablet [PoM] £137.24 DT = £152.49 [CD2]

Oxycodone hydrochloride 80 mg Oxeltra 80mg modified-release tablets | 56 tablet [PoM] £180.35 DT = £200.39 [CD2]
▸ OxyContin (Napp Pharmaceuticals Ltd)
Oxycodone hydrochloride 5 mg OxyContin 5mg modified-release tablets | 28 tablet [PoM] £12.52 DT = £12.52 [CD2]
Oxycodone hydrochloride 10 mg OxyContin 10mg modified-release tablets | 56 tablet [PoM] £25.04 DT = £25.04 [CD2]
Oxycodone hydrochloride 15 mg OxyContin 15mg modified-release tablets | 56 tablet [PoM] £38.12 DT = £38.12 [CD2]
Oxycodone hydrochloride 20 mg OxyContin 20mg modified-release tablets | 56 tablet [PoM] £50.08 DT = £50.08 [CD2]
Oxycodone hydrochloride 30 mg OxyContin 30mg modified-release tablets | 56 tablet [PoM] £76.23 DT = £76.23 [CD2]
Oxycodone hydrochloride 40 mg OxyContin 40mg modified-release tablets | 56 tablet [PoM] £100.19 DT = £100.19 [CD2]
Oxycodone hydrochloride 60 mg OxyContin 60mg modified-release tablets | 56 tablet [PoM] £152.49 DT = £152.49 [CD2]
Oxycodone hydrochloride 80 mg OxyContin 80mg modified-release tablets | 56 tablet [PoM] £200.39 DT = £200.39 [CD2]
Oxycodone hydrochloride 120 mg OxyContin 120mg modified-release tablets | 56 tablet [PoM] £305.02 DT = £305.02 [CD2]
▸ Oxylan (Chanelle Medical UK Ltd)
Oxycodone hydrochloride 5 mg Oxylan 5mg modified-release tablets | 28 tablet [PoM] £12.50 DT = £12.52 [CD2]
Oxycodone hydrochloride 10 mg Oxylan 10mg modified-release tablets | 56 tablet [PoM] £24.99 DT = £25.04 [CD2]
Oxycodone hydrochloride 20 mg Oxylan 20mg modified-release tablets | 56 tablet [PoM] £49.98 DT = £50.08 [CD2]
Oxycodone hydrochloride 40 mg Oxylan 40mg modified-release tablets | 56 tablet [PoM] £99.98 DT = £100.19 [CD2]
Oxycodone hydrochloride 80 mg Oxylan 80mg modified-release tablets | 56 tablet [PoM] £199.97 DT = £200.39 [CD2]
▸ Reltebon (Actavis UK Ltd)
Oxycodone hydrochloride 5 mg Reltebon 5mg modified-release tablets | 28 tablet [PoM] £6.26 DT = £12.52 [CD2]
Oxycodone hydrochloride 10 mg Reltebon 10mg modified-release tablets | 56 tablet [PoM] £12.52 DT = £25.04 [CD2]
Oxycodone hydrochloride 15 mg Reltebon 15mg modified-release tablets | 56 tablet [PoM] £19.06 DT = £38.12 [CD2]
Oxycodone hydrochloride 20 mg Reltebon 20mg modified-release tablets | 56 tablet [PoM] £25.04 DT = £50.08 [CD2]
Oxycodone hydrochloride 30 mg Reltebon 30mg modified-release tablets | 56 tablet [PoM] £38.11 DT = £76.23 [CD2]
Oxycodone hydrochloride 40 mg Reltebon 40mg modified-release tablets | 56 tablet [PoM] £50.09 DT = £100.19 [CD2]
Oxycodone hydrochloride 60 mg Reltebon 60mg modified-release tablets | 56 tablet [PoM] £76.24 DT = £152.49 [CD2]
Oxycodone hydrochloride 80 mg Reltebon 80mg modified-release tablets | 56 tablet [PoM] £100.19 DT = £200.39 [CD2]
▸ Zomestine (Accord Healthcare Ltd)
Oxycodone hydrochloride 5 mg Zomestine 5mg modified-release tablets | 28 tablet [PoM] £11.89 DT = £12.52 [CD2]
Oxycodone hydrochloride 10 mg Zomestine 10mg modified-release tablets | 56 tablet [PoM] £23.79 DT = £25.04 [CD2]
Oxycodone hydrochloride 20 mg Zomestine 20mg modified-release tablets | 56 tablet [PoM] £47.58 DT = £50.08 [CD2]
Oxycodone hydrochloride 40 mg Zomestine 40mg modified-release tablets | 56 tablet [PoM] £95.18 DT = £100.19 [CD2]
Oxycodone hydrochloride 80 mg Zomestine 80mg modified-release tablets | 56 tablet [PoM] £190.37 DT = £200.39 [CD2]

Solution for injection
▸ Oxycodone hydrochloride (Non-proprietary)
Oxycodone hydrochloride 10 mg per 1 ml Oxycodone 20mg/2ml solution for injection ampoules | 5 ampoule [PoM] £16.00 DT = £16.00 [CD2]
Oxycodone 10mg/1ml solution for injection ampoules | 5 ampoule [PoM] £8.00 DT = £8.00 [CD2]
Oxycodone hydrochloride 50 mg per 1 ml Oxycodone 50mg/1ml solution for injection ampoules | 5 ampoule [PoM] £70.10 DT = £70.10 [CD2]
▸ OxyNorm (Napp Pharmaceuticals Ltd)
Oxycodone hydrochloride 10 mg per 1 ml OxyNorm 20mg/2ml solution for injection ampoules | 5 ampoule [PoM] £16.00 DT = £16.00 [CD2]
OxyNorm 10mg/1ml solution for injection ampoules | 5 ampoule [PoM] £8.00 DT = £8.00 [CD2]
Oxycodone hydrochloride 50 mg per 1 ml OxyNorm 50mg/1ml solution for injection ampoules | 5 ampoule [PoM] £70.10 DT = £70.10 [CD2]

▸ Shortec (Qdem Pharmaceuticals Ltd)
Oxycodone hydrochloride 10 mg per 1 ml Shortec 20mg/2ml solution for injection ampoules | 5 ampoule [PoM] £13.60 DT = £16.00 [CD2]
Shortec 10mg/1ml solution for injection ampoules | 5 ampoule £6.80 DT = £8.00 [CD2]
Oxycodone hydrochloride 50 mg per 1 ml Shortec 50mg/1ml solution for injection ampoules | 5 ampoule [PoM] £59.59 DT = £70.10 [CD2]

Oral solution
CAUTIONARY AND ADVISORY LABELS 2
▸ Oxycodone hydrochloride (Non-proprietary)
Oxycodone hydrochloride 1 mg per 1 ml Oxycodone 5mg/5ml oral solution sugar free sugar-free | 250 ml [PoM] £9.71 DT = £9.71 [CD2]
Oxycodone hydrochloride 10 mg per 1 ml Oxycodone 10mg/ml oral solution sugar-free | 120 ml [PoM] £46.63 DT = £46.63 [CD2]
▸ OxyNorm (Napp Pharmaceuticals Ltd)
Oxycodone hydrochloride 1 mg per 1 ml OxyNorm liquid 5mg/5ml oral solution sugar-free | 250 ml [PoM] £9.71 DT = £9.71 [CD2]
Oxycodone hydrochloride 10 mg per 1 ml OxyNorm 10mg/ml concentrate oral solution sugar-free | 120 ml [PoM] £46.63 DT = £46.63 [CD2]
▸ Shortec (Qdem Pharmaceuticals Ltd)
Oxycodone hydrochloride 1 mg per 1 ml Shortec liquid 5mg/5ml oral solution sugar-free | 250 ml [PoM] £8.25 DT = £9.71 [CD2]
Oxycodone hydrochloride 10 mg per 1 ml Shortec 10mg/ml concentrate oral solution sugar-free | 120 ml [PoM] £39.64 DT = £46.63 [CD2]

Capsule
CAUTIONARY AND ADVISORY LABELS 2
▸ Lynlor (Actavis UK Ltd)
Oxycodone hydrochloride 5 mg Lynlor 5mg capsules | 56 capsule [PoM] £6.86 DT = £11.43 [CD2]
Oxycodone hydrochloride 10 mg Lynlor 10mg capsules | 56 capsule [PoM] £13.72 DT = £22.86 [CD2]
Oxycodone hydrochloride 20 mg Lynlor 20mg capsules | 56 capsule [PoM] £27.43 DT = £45.71 [CD2]
▸ OxyNorm (Napp Pharmaceuticals Ltd)
Oxycodone hydrochloride 5 mg OxyNorm 5mg capsules | 56 capsule [PoM] £11.43 DT = £11.43 [CD2]
Oxycodone hydrochloride 10 mg OxyNorm 10mg capsules | 56 capsule [PoM] £22.86 DT = £22.86 [CD2]
Oxycodone hydrochloride 20 mg OxyNorm 20mg capsules | 56 capsule [PoM] £45.71 DT = £45.71 [CD2]
▸ Shortec (Qdem Pharmaceuticals Ltd)
Oxycodone hydrochloride 5 mg Shortec 5mg capsules | 56 capsule [PoM] £6.86 DT = £11.43 [CD2]
Oxycodone hydrochloride 10 mg Shortec 10mg capsules | 56 capsule [PoM] £13.72 DT = £22.86 [CD2]
Oxycodone hydrochloride 20 mg Shortec 20mg capsules | 56 capsule [PoM] £27.43 DT = £45.71 [CD2]

Oxycodone with naloxone

The properties listed below are those particular to the combination only. For the properties of the components please consider, oxycodone hydrochloride p. 459, naloxone hydrochloride p. 1329.

● INDICATIONS AND DOSE

Severe pain requiring opioid analgesia in patients not currently treated with opioid analgesics
▸ BY MOUTH
▸ Adult: Initially 10/5 mg every 12 hours (max. per dose 40/20 mg every 12 hours), dose to be increased according to response; patients already receiving opioid analgesics can start with a higher dose

Second-line treatment of symptomatic severe to very severe idiopathic restless legs syndrome after failure of dopaminergic therapy
▸ BY MOUTH
▸ Adult: Initially 5/2.5 mg every 12 hours, adjusted weekly according to response, usual dose 10/5 mg every 12 hours; maximum 60/30 mg per day   continued →

DOSE EQUIVALENCE AND CONVERSION
‣ Dose quantities are expressed in the form x/y where x and y are the strengths in milligrams of oxycodone and naloxone respectively.

● INTERACTIONS → Appendix 1: opioids

● MEDICINAL FORMS
There can be variation in the licensing of different medicines containing the same drug. Forms available from special-order manufacturers include: oral suspension
Modified-release tablet
CAUTIONARY AND ADVISORY LABELS 2, 25
‣ Targinact (Napp Pharmaceuticals Ltd)
Naloxone hydrochloride 2.5 mg, Oxycodone hydrochloride 5 mg Targinact 5mg/2.5mg modified-release tablets | 28 tablet PoM £21.16 DT = £21.16 CD2
Naloxone hydrochloride 5 mg, Oxycodone hydrochloride 10 mg Targinact 10mg/5mg modified-release tablets | 56 tablet PoM £42.32 DT = £42.32 CD2
Naloxone hydrochloride 10 mg, Oxycodone hydrochloride 20 mg Targinact 20mg/10mg modified-release tablets | 56 tablet PoM £84.62 DT = £84.62 CD2
Naloxone hydrochloride 20 mg, Oxycodone hydrochloride 40 mg Targinact 40mg/20mg modified-release tablets | 56 tablet PoM £169.28 DT = £169.28 CD2

Ϝ 441

Papaveretum
14-Mar-2018

● INDICATIONS AND DOSE
Postoperative analgesia | Severe chronic pain
‣ BY SUBCUTANEOUS INJECTION, OR BY INTRAMUSCULAR INJECTION
‣ Adult: 7.7–15.4 mg every 4 hours if required
‣ Elderly: Initially 7.7 mg every 4 hours if required
‣ BY INTRAVENOUS INJECTION
‣ Adult: Use 25 to 50% of the corresponding subcutaneous/intramuscular dose
Premedication
‣ BY SUBCUTANEOUS INJECTION, OR BY INTRAMUSCULAR INJECTION
‣ Adult: 7.7–15.4 mg
‣ Elderly: 7.7 mg

IMPORTANT SAFETY INFORMATION
Do **not** confuse with papaverine.

● CONTRA-INDICATIONS Heart failure secondary to chronic lung disease · phaeochromocytoma
● CAUTIONS Supraventricular tachycardia
● INTERACTIONS → Appendix 1: opioids
● SIDE-EFFECTS Biliary spasm · dysuria · hypothermia · mood altered · postural hypotension · sexual dysfunction · ureteral spasm
● BREAST FEEDING Therapeutic doses unlikely to affect infant.
● RENAL IMPAIRMENT Avoid use or reduce dose; opioid effects increased and prolonged and increased cerebral sensitivity occurs.
● PRESCRIBING AND DISPENSING INFORMATION The name *Omnopon*® was formerly used for papaveretum preparations.
Papaveretum is a mixture of 253 parts of morphine hydrochloride, 23 parts of papaverine hydrochloride and 20 parts of codeine hydrochloride.
● LESS SUITABLE FOR PRESCRIBING Papaveretum is less suitable for prescribing.

● MEDICINAL FORMS
There can be variation in the licensing of different medicines containing the same drug. Forms available from special-order manufacturers include: solution for injection
Solution for injection
‣ Papaveretum (Non-proprietary)
Papaveretum 15.4 mg per 1 ml Papaveretum 15.4mg/1ml solution for injection ampoules | 10 ampoule PoM £48.96 CD2

Ϝ 441

Pentazocine

● INDICATIONS AND DOSE
Moderate to severe pain
‣ BY MOUTH
‣ Adult: 50 mg every 3–4 hours, dose to be taken preferably after food, usual dose 25–100 mg every 3–4 hours; maximum 600 mg per day
Moderate pain
‣ BY SUBCUTANEOUS INJECTION, OR BY INTRAMUSCULAR INJECTION, OR BY INTRAVENOUS INJECTION
‣ Adult: 30 mg every 3–4 hours as required; maximum 360 mg per day
Severe pain
‣ BY SUBCUTANEOUS INJECTION, OR BY INTRAMUSCULAR INJECTION, OR BY INTRAVENOUS INJECTION
‣ Adult: 45–60 mg every 3–4 hours as required; maximum 360 mg per day

● CONTRA-INDICATIONS Acute porphyrias p. 1025 · heart failure secondary to chronic lung disease · patients dependent on opioids (can precipitate withdrawal)
● CAUTIONS Arterial hypertension · cardiac arrhythmias · myocardial infarction · pancreatitis · phaeochromocytoma · pulmonary hypertension
● INTERACTIONS → Appendix 1: opioids
● SIDE-EFFECTS Biliary spasm · blood disorders · chills · circulatory depression · dermatitis · disorientation · face oedema · facial plethora · generalised tonic-clonic seizure · hypertension · hypothermia · intracranial pressure increased · mood altered · myalgia · paraesthesia · sexual dysfunction · sleep disorders · syncope · toxic epidermal necrolysis · tremor · ureteral spasm
Overdose Effects only partially reversed by naloxone.
● BREAST FEEDING Use with caution—limited information available.
● RENAL IMPAIRMENT Avoid use or reduce dose; opioid effects increased and prolonged and increased cerebral sensitivity occurs.
● LESS SUITABLE FOR PRESCRIBING Pentazocine is less suitable for prescribing.

● MEDICINAL FORMS
There can be variation in the licensing of different medicines containing the same drug.
Tablet
CAUTIONARY AND ADVISORY LABELS 2, 21
‣ Pentazocine (Non-proprietary)
Pentazocine hydrochloride 25 mg Pentazocine 25mg tablets | 28 tablet PoM £24.27 DT = £24.27 CD3
Capsule
CAUTIONARY AND ADVISORY LABELS 2, 21
‣ Pentazocine (Non-proprietary)
Pentazocine hydrochloride 50 mg Pentazocine 50mg capsules | 28 capsule PoM £28.50 DT = £28.50 CD3

4

F 441

Pethidine hydrochloride

(Meperidine)

● **INDICATIONS AND DOSE**

Acute pain
▸ BY MOUTH
  ▸ Adult: 50–150 mg every 4 hours
▸ BY SUBCUTANEOUS INJECTION, OR BY INTRAMUSCULAR INJECTION
  ▸ Adult: 25–100 mg, then 25–100 mg after 4 hours, for debilitated patients use dose described for elderly patients
  ▸ Elderly: Initially 25 mg, then 25–100 mg after 4 hours
▸ BY SLOW INTRAVENOUS INJECTION
  ▸ Adult: 25–50 mg, then 25–50 mg after 4 hours, for debilitated patients use dose described for elderly patients
  ▸ Elderly: Initially 25 mg, then 25–50 mg after 4 hours

Obstetric analgesia
▸ BY SUBCUTANEOUS INJECTION, OR BY INTRAMUSCULAR INJECTION
  ▸ Adult: 50–100 mg, then 50–100 mg after 1–3 hours if required; maximum 400 mg per day

Premedication
▸ BY INTRAMUSCULAR INJECTION
  ▸ Adult: 25–100 mg, dose to be given 1 hour before operation, for debilitated patients use dose described for elderly patients
  ▸ Elderly: 25 mg, dose to be given 1 hour before operation

Postoperative pain
▸ BY SUBCUTANEOUS INJECTION, OR BY INTRAMUSCULAR INJECTION
  ▸ Adult: 25–100 mg every 2–3 hours if required, for debilitated patients use dose described for elderly patients
  ▸ Elderly: Initially 25 mg every 2–3 hours if required

● CONTRA-INDICATIONS Phaeochromocytoma
● CAUTIONS Accumulation of metabolites may result in neurotoxicity · cardiac arrhythmias · not suitable for severe continuing pain · severe cor pulmonale
● INTERACTIONS → Appendix 1: opioids
● SIDE-EFFECTS
  GENERAL SIDE-EFFECTS Biliary spasm · dysuria · hypothermia
  SPECIFIC SIDE-EFFECTS
▸ With oral use Agitation · mood altered · muscle rigidity · postural hypotension · sexual dysfunction · ureteral spasm
▸ With parenteral use Anxiety · asthenia · coordination abnormal · delirium · seizure · syncope · tremor
  Overdose Convulsions reported in overdosage.
● BREAST FEEDING Present in milk but not known to be harmful.
● RENAL IMPAIRMENT Avoid use or reduce dose; opioid effects increased and prolonged and increased cerebral sensitivity occurs.

● MEDICINAL FORMS
There can be variation in the licensing of different medicines containing the same drug. Forms available from special-order manufacturers include: capsule, oral solution, solution for injection
Tablet
CAUTIONARY AND ADVISORY LABELS 2
▸ Pethidine hydrochloride (Non-proprietary)
  Pethidine hydrochloride 50 mg Pethidine 50mg tablets | 50 tablet PoM £49.92 DT = £49.92 CD2

Solution for injection
▸ Pethidine hydrochloride (Non-proprietary)
  Pethidine hydrochloride 10 mg per 1 ml Pethidine 50mg/5ml solution for injection ampoules | 10 ampoule PoM £52.91 CD2
  Pethidine hydrochloride 50 mg per 1 ml Pethidine 50mg/1ml solution for injection ampoules | 10 ampoule PoM £5.11 DT = £5.11 CD2
  Pethidine 100mg/2ml solution for injection ampoules | 10 ampoule PoM £4.66 DT = £4.66 CD2

F 441

Sufentanil

27-Feb-2017

● DRUG ACTION Sufentanil is a potent, highly-selective μ-opioid receptor agonist.

● **INDICATIONS AND DOSE**

Acute moderate-to-severe post-operative pain
▸ BY SUBLINGUAL ADMINISTRATION
  ▸ Adult (specialist supervision in hospital): 15 micrograms every 20 minutes if required for a maximum of 72 hours

● CAUTIONS Brain tumour · head injury · history of bradyarrhythmias (increased risk of bradycardia) · increased susceptibility to cerebral effects of CO_2 retention (including increased intracranial pressure and impaired consciousness)
● INTERACTIONS → Appendix 1: opioids
● SIDE-EFFECTS
▸ **Common or very common** Dyspepsia · fever · muscle complaints
▸ **Uncommon** Apnoea · asthenia · chills · paraesthesia
▸ **Frequency not known** Apathy · biliary spasm · coma · movement disorders · nervousness · reflexes increased · respiratory arrest · seizure · skin reactions
● PREGNANCY Manufacturer advises avoid—toxicity in *animal* studies.
● BREAST FEEDING Manufacturer advises avoid—risk of opioid effects or toxicity in the infant.
● RENAL IMPAIRMENT Manufacturer advises caution and close monitoring in severe impairment—limited information available.
● DIRECTIONS FOR ADMINISTRATION Manufacturer advises doses should be administered using patient controlled analgesia administration device—consult product literature.
● PATIENT AND CARER ADVICE Manufacturer advises patients should avoid eating and drinking, and minimise talking, for 10 minutes after each dose. Patients should be instructed on appropriate use of the patient controlled analgesia administration device—consult product literature.
  Driving and skilled tasks Manufacturer advises patients should be counselled on the effects on driving and skilled tasks—increased risk of dizziness and visual disturbances.

● MEDICINAL FORMS
There can be variation in the licensing of different medicines containing the same drug.
Sublingual tablet
CAUTIONARY AND ADVISORY LABELS 3, 26
▸ Zalviso (Grunenthal Ltd)
  Sufentanil (as Sufentanil citrate) 15 microgram Zalviso 15microgram sublingual tablets sugar-free | 800 tablet PoM (Hospital only) CD2

4

Nervous system

Tapentadol

F 441

- ● INDICATIONS AND DOSE

Moderate to severe acute pain which can be managed only with opioid analgesics

▸ BY MOUTH USING IMMEDIATE-RELEASE MEDICINES

▸ Adult: Initially 50 mg every 4–6 hours, adjusted according to response, maximum 700 mg in the first 24 hours, during the first 24 hours of treatment, an additional dose of 50 mg may be taken 1 hour after the initial dose, if pain control not achieved; maximum 600 mg per day

Severe chronic pain

▸ BY MOUTH USING MODIFIED-RELEASE MEDICINES

▸ Adult: Initially 50 mg every 12 hours, adjusted according to response; maximum 500 mg per day

- ● INTERACTIONS → Appendix 1: opioids
- ● SIDE-EFFECTS

▸ **Common or very common** Anxiety · appetite decreased · asthenia · diarrhoea · feeling of body temperature change · gastrointestinal discomfort · muscle spasms · sleep disorders · tremor

▸ **Uncommon** Concentration impaired · depressed mood · disorientation · dysarthria · dyspnoea · feeling abnormal · irritability · memory loss · movement disorders · muscle contractions involuntary · oedema · presyncope · sensation abnormal · urinary disorders

▸ **Rare or very rare** Angioedema · impaired gastric emptying · level of consciousness decreased · seizure · thinking abnormal

- ● BREAST FEEDING Avoid—no information available.

- ● HEPATIC IMPAIRMENT

Dose adjustments For *immediate-release tablets*, initial max. daily dose 150 mg; for *modified-release tablets*, initial max. daily dose 50 mg.

- ● RENAL IMPAIRMENT Avoid in severe impairment; opioid effects increased and prolonged and increased cerebral sensitivity occurs.

Dose adjustments Manufacturer advises no dose adjustment needed in mild or moderate impairment.

- ● NATIONAL FUNDING/ACCESS DECISIONS

Scottish Medicines Consortium (SMC) Decisions
The *Scottish Medicines Consortium* has advised (May 2011) that tapentadol (*Palexia* ® *SR*) is accepted for restricted use within NHS Scotland for the management of severe chronic pain in adult patients, which can be adequately managed only with opioid analgesics, when morphine sulfate modified-release has failed to provide adequate pain control or is not tolerated.

- ● MEDICINAL FORMS
There can be variation in the licensing of different medicines containing the same drug.

Oral solution
CAUTIONARY AND ADVISORY LABELS 2
EXCIPIENTS: May contain Propylene glycol
▸ Palexia (Grunenthal Ltd)
  Tapentadol (as Tapentadol hydrochloride) 20 mg per 1 ml Palexia 20mg/ml oral solution sugar-free | 100 ml [PoM] £17.80 DT = £17.80 [CD2] sugar-free | 200 ml [PoM] £35.60 [CD2]

Modified-release tablet
CAUTIONARY AND ADVISORY LABELS 2, 25
▸ Palexia SR (Grunenthal Ltd)
  Tapentadol (as Tapentadol hydrochloride) 50 mg Palexia SR 50mg tablets | 28 tablet [PoM] £12.46 DT = £12.46 [CD2] | 56 tablet [PoM] £24.91 [CD2]
  Tapentadol (as Tapentadol hydrochloride) 100 mg Palexia SR 100mg tablets | 56 tablet [PoM] £49.82 DT = £49.82 [CD2]
  Tapentadol (as Tapentadol hydrochloride) 150 mg Palexia SR 150mg tablets | 56 tablet [PoM] £74.73 DT = £74.73 [CD2]

  Tapentadol (as Tapentadol hydrochloride) 200 mg Palexia SR 200mg tablets | 56 tablet [PoM] £99.64 DT = £99.64 [CD2]
  Tapentadol (as Tapentadol hydrochloride) 250 mg Palexia SR 250mg tablets | 56 tablet [PoM] £124.55 DT = £124.55 [CD2]

Tablet
CAUTIONARY AND ADVISORY LABELS 2
▸ Palexia (Grunenthal Ltd)
  Tapentadol (as Tapentadol hydrochloride) 50 mg Palexia 50mg tablets | 28 tablet [PoM] £12.46 DT = £12.46 [CD2] | 56 tablet [PoM] £24.91 [CD2]
  Tapentadol (as Tapentadol hydrochloride) 75 mg Palexia 75mg tablets | 28 tablet [PoM] £18.68 DT = £18.68 [CD2] | 56 tablet [PoM] £37.37 [CD2]

F 441

Tramadol hydrochloride

- ● INDICATIONS AND DOSE

Moderate to severe pain

▸ BY INTRAMUSCULAR INJECTION, OR BY INTRAVENOUS INJECTION, OR BY INTRAVENOUS INFUSION

▸ Adult: 50–100 mg every 4–6 hours, intravenous injection to be given over 2–3 minutes

Moderate to severe acute pain

▸ BY MOUTH USING IMMEDIATE-RELEASE MEDICINES

▸ Child 12–17 years: Initially 100 mg, then 50–100 mg every 4–6 hours; Usual maximum 400 mg/24 hours

▸ Adult: Initially 100 mg, then 50–100 mg every 4–6 hours; Usual maximum 400 mg/24 hours

Moderate to severe chronic pain

▸ BY MOUTH USING IMMEDIATE-RELEASE MEDICINES

▸ Child 12–17 years: Initially 50 mg, then, adjusted according to response; Usual maximum 400 mg/24 hours

▸ Adult: Initially 50 mg, then, adjusted according to response; Usual maximum 400 mg/24 hours

Postoperative pain

▸ BY INTRAVENOUS INJECTION

▸ Adult: Initially 100 mg, then 50 mg every 10–20 minutes if required to total maximum 250 mg (including initial dose) in first hour, then 50–100 mg every 4–6 hours, intravenous injection to be given over 2–3 minutes; maximum 600 mg per day

Moderate to severe pain (with modified-release 12-hourly preparations)

▸ BY MOUTH USING MODIFIED-RELEASE MEDICINES

▸ Child 12–17 years: 50–100 mg twice daily, increased if necessary to 150–200 mg twice daily, doses exceeding the usual maximum not generally required; Usual maximum 400 mg/24 hours

▸ Adult: 50–100 mg twice daily, increased if necessary to 150–200 mg twice daily, doses exceeding the usual maximum not generally required; Usual maximum 400 mg/24 hours

Moderate to severe pain (with modified-release 24-hourly preparations)

▸ BY MOUTH USING MODIFIED-RELEASE MEDICINES

▸ Child 12–17 years: Initially 100–150 mg once daily, increased if necessary up to 400 mg once daily; Usual maximum 400 mg/24 hours

▸ Adult: Initially 100–150 mg once daily, increased if necessary up to 400 mg once daily; Usual maximum 400 mg/24 hours

ZYDOL® XL

Moderate to severe pain

▸ BY MOUTH USING MODIFIED-RELEASE TABLETS

▸ Child 12–17 years: Initially 150 mg once daily, increased if necessary up to 400 mg once daily

▸ **Adult:** Initially 150 mg once daily, increased if necessary up to 400 mg once daily

---

IMPORTANT SAFETY INFORMATION
Do not confuse modified-release 12-hourly preparations with 24-hourly preparations, see *Prescribing and dispensing information*.

● CONTRA-INDICATIONS Acute intoxication with alcohol · acute intoxication with analgesics · acute intoxication with hypnotics · acute intoxication with opioids · not suitable for narcotic withdrawal treatment · uncontrolled epilepsy

● CAUTIONS Excessive bronchial secretions · history of epilepsy—use tramadol only if compelling reasons · impaired consciousness · not suitable as a substitute in opioid-dependent patients · not suitable in some types of general anaesthesia · susceptibility to seizures—use tramadol only if compelling reasons

CAUTIONS, FURTHER INFORMATION
▸ General anaesthesia Not recommended for analgesia during potentially light planes of general anaesthesia (possibly increased intra-operative recall reported).

● INTERACTIONS → Appendix 1: opioids

● SIDE-EFFECTS

GENERAL SIDE-EFFECTS
▸ **Common or very common** Fatigue
▸ **Uncommon** Postural hypotension
▸ **Rare or very rare** Dyspnoea · epileptiform seizure · respiratory disorders · sleep disorders · vision blurred
▸ **Frequency not known** Asthma exacerbated · hypoglycaemia

SPECIFIC SIDE-EFFECTS
▸ **Uncommon**
▸ With parenteral use Circulatory collapse · gastrointestinal discomfort · skin eruption
▸ **Rare or very rare**
▸ With parenteral use Angioedema · appetite change · behaviour abnormal · cognitive disorder · dysuria · hypersensitivity · mood altered · movement disorders · muscle weakness · perception disorders · psychiatric disorder · sensation abnormal
▸ **Frequency not known**
▸ With oral use Anxiety · blood disorder · gastrointestinal disorder · hyperkinesia · hypertension · paraesthesia · syncope · tremor · urinary disorder

● PREGNANCY Embryotoxic in *animal* studies—manufacturers advise avoid.

● BREAST FEEDING Amount probably too small to be harmful, but manufacturer advises avoid.

● HEPATIC IMPAIRMENT Caution (avoid for *oral drops*) in severe impairment.

● RENAL IMPAIRMENT Avoid use or reduce dose; opioid effects increased and prolonged and increased cerebral sensitivity occurs. Caution (avoid for *oral drops*) in severe impairment.

● DIRECTIONS FOR ADMINISTRATION Tramadol hydrochloride *orodispersible tablets* should be sucked and then swallowed. May also be dispersed in water. Some tramadol hydrochloride modified-release capsule preparations may be opened and the contents swallowed immediately without chewing—check individual preparations.

For *intravenous infusion*, dilute in Glucose 5% or Sodium Chloride 0.9%.

● PRESCRIBING AND DISPENSING INFORMATION Modified-release preparations are available as 12-hourly or 24-hourly formulations. Non-proprietary preparations of modified-release tramadol may be available as either 12-hourly or 24-hourly formulations; prescribers and dispensers must ensure that the correct formulation is prescribed and dispensed. Branded preparations that should be given 12-hourly include *Invodol® SR, Mabron®, Maneo®, Marol®, Maxitram® SR, Oldaram®, Tilodol® SR, Tramquel® SR, Tramulief® SR, Zamadol® SR, Zeridame® SR* and *Zydol SR®*. Preparations that should be given 24-hourly include *Tradorec XL®, Zamadol® 24hr,* and *Zydol XL®*.

● PATIENT AND CARER ADVICE Patients or carers should be given advice on how to administer tramadol hydrochloride orodispersible tablets.
Medicines for Children leaflet: Tramadol for pain www.medicinesforchildren.org.uk/tramadol-for-pain

● MEDICINAL FORMS
There can be variation in the licensing of different medicines containing the same drug. Forms available from special-order manufacturers include: oral suspension

Modified-release tablet
CAUTIONARY AND ADVISORY LABELS 2, 25
▸ Tramadol hydrochloride (Non-proprietary)
   Tramadol hydrochloride 50 mg Tramadol 50mg modified-release tablets | 60 tablet [PoM] Ⓢ DT = £4.60 [CD3]
   Tramadol hydrochloride 100 mg Tramadol 100mg modified-release tablets | 60 tablet [PoM] £6.95–£44.80 [CD3]
   Tramadol hydrochloride 150 mg Tramadol 150mg modified-release tablets | 60 tablet [PoM] £10.40–£57.85 [CD3]
   Tramadol hydrochloride 200 mg Tramadol 200mg modified-release tablets | 60 tablet [PoM] £14.20–£69.60 [CD3]
   Tramadol hydrochloride 300 mg Tramadol 300mg modified-release tablets | 30 tablet [PoM] Ⓢ [CD3]
   Tramadol hydrochloride 400 mg Tramadol 400mg modified-release tablets | 28 tablet [PoM] Ⓢ [CD3]
▸ Brimisol PR (Bristol Laboratories Ltd)
   Tramadol hydrochloride 100 mg Brimisol PR 100mg tablets | 60 tablet [PoM] £18.00 [CD3]
▸ Invodol SR (Ennogen Healthcare Ltd)
   Tramadol hydrochloride 100 mg Invodol SR 100mg tablets | 60 tablet [PoM] £14.61 [CD3]
   Tramadol hydrochloride 150 mg Invodol SR 150mg tablets | 60 tablet [PoM] £21.91 [CD3]
   Tramadol hydrochloride 200 mg Invodol SR 200mg tablets | 60 tablet [PoM] £29.22 [CD3]
▸ Mabron (Teva UK Ltd, Morningside Healthcare Ltd)
   Tramadol hydrochloride 100 mg Mabron 100mg modified-release tablets | 60 tablet [PoM] £15.52 [CD3]
   Tramadol hydrochloride 150 mg Mabron 150mg modified-release tablets | 60 tablet [PoM] £23.28 [CD3]
   Tramadol hydrochloride 200 mg Mabron 200mg modified-release tablets | 60 tablet [PoM] £31.04 [CD3]
▸ Maneo (Mylan)
   Tramadol hydrochloride 100 mg Maneo 100mg modified-release tablets | 60 tablet [PoM] £6.95 [CD3]
   Tramadol hydrochloride 150 mg Maneo 150mg modified-release tablets | 60 tablet [PoM] £10.40 [CD3]
   Tramadol hydrochloride 200 mg Maneo 200mg modified-release tablets | 60 tablet [PoM] £14.20 [CD3]
▸ Marol (Teva UK Ltd)
   Tramadol hydrochloride 100 mg Marol 100mg modified-release tablets | 60 tablet [PoM] £6.94 [CD3]
   Tramadol hydrochloride 150 mg Marol 150mg modified-release tablets | 60 tablet [PoM] £10.39 [CD3]
   Tramadol hydrochloride 200 mg Marol 200mg modified-release tablets | 60 tablet [PoM] £14.19 [CD3]
▸ Tilodol SR (Sandoz Ltd)
   Tramadol hydrochloride 100 mg Tilodol SR 100mg tablets | 60 tablet [PoM] £15.52 [CD3]
   Tramadol hydrochloride 150 mg Tilodol SR 150mg tablets | 60 tablet [PoM] £23.28 [CD3]
   Tramadol hydrochloride 200 mg Tilodol SR 200mg tablets | 60 tablet [PoM] £31.04 [CD3]
▸ Tradorec XL (Endo Ventures Ltd)
   Tramadol hydrochloride 100 mg Tradorec XL 100mg tablets | 30 tablet [PoM] £14.10 [CD3]
   Tramadol hydrochloride 200 mg Tradorec XL 200mg tablets | 30 tablet [PoM] £14.98 [CD3]
   Tramadol hydrochloride 300 mg Tradorec XL 300mg tablets | 30 tablet [PoM] £22.47 [CD3]

Nervous system

4

▸ Tramulief SR (AMCo)
Tramadol hydrochloride 100 mg Tramulief SR 100mg tablets |
60 tablet [PoM] £6.98 [CD3]
Tramadol hydrochloride 150 mg Tramulief SR 150mg tablets |
60 tablet [PoM] £10.48 [CD3]
Tramadol hydrochloride 200 mg Tramulief SR 200mg tablets |
60 tablet [PoM] £14.28 [CD3]
▸ Zamadol 24hr (Meda Pharmaceuticals Ltd)
Tramadol hydrochloride 150 mg Zamadol 24hr 150mg modified-
release tablets | 28 tablet [PoM] £10.70 [CD3]
Tramadol hydrochloride 200 mg Zamadol 24hr 200mg modified-
release tablets | 28 tablet [PoM] £14.26 [CD3]
Tramadol hydrochloride 300 mg Zamadol 24hr 300mg modified-
release tablets | 28 tablet [PoM] £21.39 [CD3]
Tramadol hydrochloride 400 mg Zamadol 24hr 400mg modified-
release tablets | 28 tablet [PoM] £28.51 [CD3]
▸ Zeridame SR (Actavis UK Ltd)
Tramadol hydrochloride 100 mg Zeridame SR 100mg tablets |
60 tablet [PoM] £17.21 [CD3]
Tramadol hydrochloride 150 mg Zeridame SR 150mg tablets |
60 tablet [PoM] £25.82 [CD3]
Tramadol hydrochloride 200 mg Zeridame SR 200mg tablets |
60 tablet [PoM] £34.43 [CD3]
▸ Zydol SR (Grunenthal Ltd)
Tramadol hydrochloride 50 mg Zydol SR 50mg tablets |
60 tablet [PoM] £4.60 DT = £4.60 [CD3]
Tramadol hydrochloride 100 mg Zydol SR 100mg tablets |
60 tablet [PoM] £17.22 [CD3]
Tramadol hydrochloride 150 mg Zydol SR 150mg tablets |
60 tablet [PoM] £25.83 [CD3]
Tramadol hydrochloride 200 mg Zydol SR 200mg tablets |
60 tablet [PoM] £34.40 [CD3]
▸ Zydol XL (Grunenthal Ltd)
Tramadol hydrochloride 150 mg Zydol XL 150mg tablets |
30 tablet [PoM] £12.18 [CD3]
Tramadol hydrochloride 200 mg Zydol XL 200mg tablets |
30 tablet [PoM] £17.98 [CD3]
Tramadol hydrochloride 300 mg Zydol XL 300mg tablets |
30 tablet [PoM] £24.94 [CD3]
Tramadol hydrochloride 400 mg Zydol XL 400mg tablets |
30 tablet [PoM] £32.47 [CD3]
▸ Zytram SR (Qdem Pharmaceuticals Ltd)
Tramadol hydrochloride 75 mg Zytram SR 75mg tablets |
60 tablet [PoM] £5.15 [CD3]
Tramadol hydrochloride 100 mg Zytram SR 100mg tablets |
60 tablet [PoM] £6.94 [CD3]
Tramadol hydrochloride 150 mg Zytram SR 150mg tablets |
60 tablet [PoM] £10.39 [CD3]
Tramadol hydrochloride 200 mg Zytram SR 200mg tablets |
60 tablet [PoM] £14.19 [CD3]

Soluble tablet
CAUTIONARY AND ADVISORY LABELS 2, 13
▸ Zydol (Grunenthal Ltd)
Tramadol hydrochloride 50 mg Zydol 50mg soluble tablets sugar-
free | 20 tablet [PoM] £2.79 Schedule 3 (CD No Register Exempt Safe
Custody) sugar-free | 100 tablet [PoM] £13.33 DT = £13.33 [CD3]

Solution for injection
CAUTIONARY AND ADVISORY LABELS 2, 13
▸ Tramadol hydrochloride (Non-proprietary)
Tramadol hydrochloride 50 mg per 1 ml Tramadol 100mg/2ml
solution for injection ampoules | 5 ampoule [PoM] £4.90 [CD3] |
10 ampoule [PoM] £10.00 [CD3]
▸ Zamadol (Meda Pharmaceuticals Ltd)
Tramadol hydrochloride 50 mg per 1 ml Zamadol 100mg/2ml
solution for injection ampoules | 5 ampoule [PoM] £5.49 [CD3]
▸ Zydol (Grunenthal Ltd)
Tramadol hydrochloride 50 mg per 1 ml Zydol 100mg/2ml solution
for injection ampoules | 5 ampoule [PoM] £4.00 [CD3]

Modified-release capsule
CAUTIONARY AND ADVISORY LABELS 2, 25
▸ Tramadol hydrochloride (Non-proprietary)
Tramadol hydrochloride 50 mg Tramadol 50mg modified-release
capsules | 60 capsule [PoM] £7.24 DT = £7.24 [CD3]
Tramadol hydrochloride 100 mg Tramadol 100mg modified-release
capsules | 60 capsule [PoM] £14.47 DT = £14.47 [CD3]
Tramadol hydrochloride 150 mg Tramadol 150mg modified-release
capsules | 60 capsule [PoM] £21.10 DT = £21.71 [CD3]
Tramadol hydrochloride 200 mg Tramadol 200mg modified-release
capsules | 60 capsule [PoM] £28.93 DT = £28.93 [CD3]

▸ Maxitram SR (Chiesi Ltd)
Tramadol hydrochloride 50 mg Maxitram SR 50mg capsules |
60 capsule [PoM] £4.55 DT = £7.24 [CD3]
Tramadol hydrochloride 100 mg Maxitram SR 100mg capsules |
60 capsule [PoM] £12.14 DT = £14.47 [CD3]
Tramadol hydrochloride 150 mg Maxitram SR 150mg capsules |
60 capsule [PoM] £18.21 DT = £21.71 [CD3]
Tramadol hydrochloride 200 mg Maxitram SR 200mg capsules |
60 capsule [PoM] £24.28 DT = £28.93 [CD3]
▸ Tramquel SR (Beechmere Pharmaceuticals Ltd)
Tramadol hydrochloride 50 mg Tramquel SR 50mg capsules |
60 capsule [PoM] £7.24 DT = £7.24 [CD3]
Tramadol hydrochloride 100 mg Tramquel SR 100mg capsules |
60 capsule [PoM] £14.47 DT = £14.47 [CD3]
Tramadol hydrochloride 150 mg Tramquel SR 150mg capsules |
60 capsule [PoM] £21.71 DT = £21.71 [CD3]
Tramadol hydrochloride 200 mg Tramquel SR 200mg capsules |
60 capsule [PoM] £28.93 DT = £28.93 [CD3]
▸ Zamadol SR (Meda Pharmaceuticals Ltd)
Tramadol hydrochloride 50 mg Zamadol SR 50mg capsules |
60 capsule [PoM] £7.24 DT = £7.24 [CD3]
Tramadol hydrochloride 100 mg Zamadol SR 100mg capsules |
60 capsule [PoM] £14.47 DT = £14.47 [CD3]
Tramadol hydrochloride 150 mg Zamadol SR 150mg capsules |
60 capsule [PoM] £21.71 DT = £21.71 [CD3]
Tramadol hydrochloride 200 mg Zamadol SR 200mg capsules |
60 capsule [PoM] £28.93 DT = £28.93 [CD3]

Oral drops
CAUTIONARY AND ADVISORY LABELS 2, 13
▸ Tramadol hydrochloride (Non-proprietary)
Tramadol (as Tramadol hydrochloride) 100 mg per 1 ml Tramadol
100mg/ml oral drops | 10 ml [PoM] £3.50 DT = £3.50 [CD3]

Capsule
CAUTIONARY AND ADVISORY LABELS 2
▸ Tramadol hydrochloride (Non-proprietary)
Tramadol hydrochloride 50 mg Tramadol 50mg capsules |
30 capsule [PoM] £4.71 DT = £0.66 [CD3] | 100 capsule [PoM] £14.40
DT = £2.20 [CD3]
▸ Zamadol (Meda Pharmaceuticals Ltd)
Tramadol hydrochloride 50 mg Zamadol 50mg capsules |
100 capsule [PoM] £8.00 DT = £2.20 [CD3]
▸ Zydol (Grunenthal Ltd)
Tramadol hydrochloride 50 mg Zydol 50mg capsules |
30 capsule [PoM] £2.29 DT = £0.66 [CD3] | 100 capsule [PoM] £7.63 DT
= £2.20 [CD3]

Orodispersible tablet
CAUTIONARY AND ADVISORY LABELS 2
▸ Tramadol hydrochloride (Non-proprietary)
Tramadol hydrochloride 50 mg Tramadol 50mg orodispersible
tablets sugar free sugar-free | 60 tablet [PoM] [Ⓝ] [CD3]
▸ Zamadol Melt (Meda Pharmaceuticals Ltd)
Tramadol hydrochloride 50 mg Zamadol Melt 50mg tablets sugar-
free | 60 tablet [PoM] £7.12 [CD3]

Combinations available: *Tramadol with paracetamol,* p. 467

Tramadol with dexketoprofen

24-Apr-2018

The properties listed below are those particular to the
combination only. For the properties of the components
please consider, tramadol hydrochloride p. 464,
dexketoprofen p. 1099.

● INDICATIONS AND DOSE

Moderate to severe acute pain
▸ BY MOUTH
▸ Adult: 75/25 mg every 8 hours as required for up to
5 days
▸ Elderly: 75/25 mg every 8 hours as required for up to
5 days; Usual maximum 150/50 mg/24 hours

DOSE EQUIVALENCE AND CONVERSION
▸ Dose expressed as x/y mg of tramadol/dexketoprofen.

● INTERACTIONS → Appendix 1: NSAIDs · opioids

● MEDICINAL FORMS
There can be variation in the licensing of different medicines containing the same drug.

Tablet
CAUTIONARY AND ADVISORY LABELS 2, 22
▸ Skudexa (A. Menarini Farmaceutica Internazionale SRL)
Dexketoprofen 25 mg, Tramadol hydrochloride 75 mg Skudexa 75mg/25mg tablets | 10 tablet [PoM] £3.68 [CD3] | 20 tablet [PoM] £5.52 [CD3]

Tramadol with paracetamol   22-Feb-2018

The properties listed below are those particular to the combination only. For the properties of the components please consider, paracetamol p. 438, tramadol hydrochloride p. 464.

● **INDICATIONS AND DOSE**

Moderate to severe pain
▸ BY MOUTH
  ▸ Child 12-17 years: 75/650 mg every 6 hours as required
  ▸ Adult: 75/650 mg every 6 hours as required

DOSE EQUIVALENCE AND CONVERSION
▸ The proportions are expressed in the form x/y, where x and y are the strengths in milligrams of tramadol and paracetamol respectively.

● INTERACTIONS → Appendix 1: opioids · paracetamol

● MEDICINAL FORMS
There can be variation in the licensing of different medicines containing the same drug.

Effervescent tablet
CAUTIONARY AND ADVISORY LABELS 2, 13, 29, 30
ELECTROLYTES: May contain Sodium
▸ Tramacet (Grunenthal Ltd)
  Tramadol hydrochloride 37.5 mg, Paracetamol 325 mg Tramacet 37.5mg/325mg effervescent tablets sugar-free | 60 tablet [PoM] £9.68 DT = £9.68 [CD3]

Tablet
CAUTIONARY AND ADVISORY LABELS 2, 25, 29, 30
▸ Tramadol with paracetamol (Non-proprietary)
  Tramadol hydrochloride 37.5 mg, Paracetamol 325 mg Tramadol 37.5mg / Paracetamol 325mg tablets | 60 tablet [PoM] £3.02-£9.68 DT = £3.02 [CD3]
  Tramadol hydrochloride 75 mg, Paracetamol 650 mg Tramadol 75mg / Paracetamol 650mg tablets | 30 tablet [PoM] £19.50 DT = £19.50 [CD3]
▸ Tramacet (Grunenthal Ltd)
  Tramadol hydrochloride 37.5 mg, Paracetamol 325 mg Tramacet 37.5mg/325mg tablets | 60 tablet [PoM] £9.68 DT = £3.02 [CD3]

6.1   Headache

Other drugs used for Headache Clonidine hydrochloride, p. 144 · Sumatriptan, p. 474 · Verapamil hydrochloride, p. 163

ANTIHISTAMINES > SEDATING

Pizotifen

● **INDICATIONS AND DOSE**

Prevention of vascular headache | Prevention of classical migraine | Prevention of common migraine | Prevention of cluster headache
▸ BY MOUTH
  ▸ Adult: Initially 500 micrograms once daily, then increased to 1.5 mg once daily, dose to be increased gradually and taken at night, alternatively increased to 1.5 mg daily in 3 divided doses, doses to be increased gradually; increased if necessary up to 4.5 mg daily (max. per dose 3 mg), this dose is rarely necessary

Prophylaxis of migraine
▸ BY MOUTH
  ▸ Child 5-17 years: Initially 500 micrograms once daily, dose to be taken at night, then increased to up to 1.5 mg daily in divided doses, dose to be increased gradually, max. single dose (at night) 1 mg

● UNLICENSED USE 1.5 mg tablets not licensed for use in children.

● CONTRA-INDICATIONS Acute porphyrias p. 1025

● CAUTIONS Avoid abrupt withdrawal · history of epilepsy · susceptibility to angle-closure glaucoma · urinary retention

● INTERACTIONS → Appendix 1: antihistamines, sedating

● SIDE-EFFECTS
▸ **Common or very common** Appetite increased · dizziness · drowsiness · dry mouth · fatigue · nausea · weight increased
▸ **Uncommon** Constipation
▸ **Rare or very rare** Aggression · anxiety · arthralgia · central nervous system stimulation · depression · hallucination · muscle complaints · paraesthesia · seizure · skin reactions · sleep disorders
▸ **Frequency not known** Hepatic disorders

● PREGNANCY Avoid unless potential benefit outweighs risk.

● BREAST FEEDING Amount probably too small to be harmful, but manufacturer advises avoid.

● HEPATIC IMPAIRMENT Use with caution.

● RENAL IMPAIRMENT Use with caution.

● PATIENT AND CARER ADVICE
Medicines for Children leaflet: Pizotifen to prevent migraine headaches www.medicinesforchildren.org.uk/pizotifen-to-prevent-migraine-headaches
Driving and skilled tasks Drowsiness may affect performance of skilled tasks (e.g. driving); effects of alcohol enhanced.

● MEDICINAL FORMS
There can be variation in the licensing of different medicines containing the same drug. Forms available from special-order manufacturers include: oral solution

Tablet
CAUTIONARY AND ADVISORY LABELS 2
▸ Pizotifen (Non-proprietary)
  Pizotifen (as Pizotifen hydrogen malate)
  500 microgram Pizotifen 500microgram tablets | 28 tablet [PoM] £8.50 DT = £1.10 | 60 tablet [PoM] £27.00
  Pizotifen (as Pizotifen hydrogen malate) 1.5 mg Pizotifen 1.5mg tablets | 28 tablet [PoM] £8.50 DT = £1.20

6.1a Migraine

Migraine   08-Jun-2018

Treatment of acute migraine

Treatment of a migraine attack should be guided by response to previous treatment and the severity of the attacks. A **simple analgesic** such as aspirin p. 121, paracetamol p. 438 (preferably in a soluble or dispersible form) or a NSAID is often effective; concomitant **antiemetic** treatment may be required. If treatment with an analgesic is inadequate, an attack may be treated with a specific antimigraine compound such as a **5HT$_1$-receptor agonist** ('triptan'). **Ergot alkaloids** are rarely required now; oral preparations are associated with many side-effects and should be avoided in cerebrovascular or cardiovascular disease.

Excessive use of acute treatments for migraine (opioid and non-opioid analgesics, 5HT$_1$-receptor agonists, and ergotamine) is associated with medication-overuse headache (analgesic-induced headache); therefore, increasing consumption of these medicines needs careful management.

Analgesics
Most migraine headaches respond to analgesics such as aspirin or paracetamol but because peristalsis is often reduced during migraine attacks the medication may not be sufficiently well absorbed to be effective; dispersible or effervescent preparations are therefore preferred. Compound preparations containing analgesics and antiemetics are available.

The NSAID tolfenamic acid p. 469 is licensed specifically for the treatment of an acute attack of migraine; diclofenac potassium p. 1100, flurbiprofen p. 1106, and ibuprofen p. 1106 are also licensed for use in migraine.

5HT₁-receptor agonists
A 5HT$_1$-receptor agonist is of considerable value in the treatment of an acute migraine attack. The 5HT$_1$-receptor agonists ('triptans') act on the 5HT (serotonin) 1B/1D receptors and they are therefore sometimes referred to as 5HT$_{1B/1D}$-receptor agonists. A 5HT$_1$-receptor agonist may be used during the established headache phase of an attack and is the preferred treatment in those who fail to respond to conventional analgesics. 5HT$_1$-receptor agonists are **not** indicated for the treatment of hemiplegic, basilar, or opthalmoplegic migraine.

The 5HT$_1$-receptor agonists available for treating migraine are almotriptan p. 471, eletriptan p. 471, frovatriptan p. 472, naratriptan p. 473, rizatriptan p. 473, sumatriptan p. 474, and zolmitriptan p. 475. If a patient does not respond to one 5HT$_1$-receptor agonist, an alternative 5HT1-receptor agonist should be tried. For patients who have prolonged attacks that frequently recur despite treatment with a 5HT1-receptor agonist, combination therapy with a NSAID such as naproxen can be considered. Sumatriptan or zolmitriptan are also used to treat cluster headache.

Ergot Alkaloids
The value of ergotamine tartrate p. 470 for migraine is limited by difficulties in absorption and by its side-effects, particularly nausea, vomiting, abdominal pain, and muscular cramps; it is best avoided. The recommended doses of ergotamine tartrate preparations should **not** be exceeded and treatment should **not** be repeated at intervals of less than 4 days.

To avoid habituation the frequency of administration of ergotamine tartrate should be limited to **no more than** twice a month. It should **never** be prescribed prophylactically but in the management of cluster headache a low dose is occasionally given for 1 to 2 weeks [unlicensed indication].

Antiemetics
Antiemetics, such as metoclopramide hydrochloride p. 426 or domperidone p. 426, or phenothiazine and antihistamine antiemetics, relieve the nausea associated with migraine attacks. Antiemetics may be given by intramuscular injection or rectally if vomiting is a problem. Metoclopramide hydrochloride and domperidone have the added advantage of promoting gastric emptying and normal peristalsis; a single dose should be given at the onset of symptoms. Oral analgesic preparations containing metoclopramide hydrochloride are a convenient alternative.

Prophylaxis of migraine
Where migraine attacks are frequent, possible provoking factors such as stress, irregular life-style (e.g. lack of sleep), or chemical triggers (e.g. alcohol and nitrates) should be sought; combined oral contraceptives may also provoke migraine.

Preventive treatment for migraine should be considered for patients who:
- suffer at least two attacks a month;
- suffer an increasing frequency of headaches;
- suffer significant disability despite suitable treatment for migraine attacks;
- cannot take suitable treatment for migraine attacks.

Prophylaxis is also necessary in some rare migraine subtypes and those at risk of migrainous infarction.

The beta-blockers propranolol hydrochloride p. 149, atenolol p. 151, metoprolol tartrate p. 154, nadolol p. 148, and timolol maleate p. 150 are all effective. Propranolol hydrochloride is the most commonly used.

Tricyclic antidepressants [unlicensed indication], gabapentin p. 314 [unlicensed indication], topiramate p. 328, sodium valproate p. 325 [unlicensed indication], and valproic acid p. 351 [unlicensed indication] are also effective for preventing migraine. See *Conception and contraception*, and *Pregnancy* in the topiramate drug monograph for information on use in females of childbearing potential and pregnancy.

Valproic acid and sodium valproate are highly teratogenic. They must not be used in females of childbearing potential unless the conditions of the Pregnancy Prevention Programme are met and alternative treatments are ineffective or not tolerated, and must not be used during pregnancy for migraine prophylaxis. For further information see *Important safety information*, *Conception and contraception*, and *Pregnancy* in the valproic acid and sodium valproate drug monographs.

Pizotifen p. 467 is an antihistamine and a serotonin-receptor antagonist, structurally related to the tricyclic antidepressants. It is of limited value and may cause weight gain.

Botulinum toxin type A p. 403 is licensed for the prophylaxis of headaches in adults with chronic migraine.

Cluster headache and the trigeminal autonomic cephalalgias
Cluster headache rarely responds to standard analgesics. Sumatriptan given by subcutaneous injection is the drug of choice for the *treatment* of cluster headache. If an injection is unsuitable, sumatriptan nasal spray or zolmitriptan nasal spray [both unlicensed use] may be used. Alternatively, 100% oxygen at a rate of 10–15 litres/minute for 10–20 minutes is useful in aborting an attack.

Prophylaxis of cluster headache is considered if the attacks are frequent, last over 3 weeks, or if they cannot be treated effectively. Verapamil hydrochloride p. 163 or lithium [both unlicensed use] are used for prophylaxis.

Prednisolone p. 664 can be used for short-term prophylaxis of episodic cluster headache [unlicensed use] either as monotherapy, or in combination with verapamil hydrochloride during verapamil titration.

Ergotamine tartrate, used on an intermittent basis is an alternative for patients with short bouts, but it should not be used for prolonged periods.

The other trigeminal autonomic cephalalgias, paroxysmal hemicrania (sensitive to indometacin p. 1109), and short-lasting unilateral neuralgiform headache attacks with conjunctival injection and tearing, are seen rarely and are best managed by a specialist.

Other drugs used for Migraine Amitriptyline hydrochloride, p. 369 · Clonidine hydrochloride, p. 144 · Cyclizine, p. 424 · Trifluoperazine, p. 387

ANALGESICS > NON-OPIOID

Paracetamol with isometheptene

The properties listed below are those particular to the combination only. For the properties of the components please consider, paracetamol p. 438.

- **INDICATIONS AND DOSE**

Treatment of acute attacks of migraine
▶ BY MOUTH
▶ Adult: 2 capsules, dose to be taken at onset of attack, followed by 1 capsule every 1 hour if required, maximum of 5 capsules in 12 hours

- **CONTRA-INDICATIONS** Acute porphyrias p. 1025
- **INTERACTIONS** → Appendix 1: paracetamol · sympathomimetics, vasoconstrictor
- **PATIENT AND CARER ADVICE** Patient counselling is advised (dosage).
- **LESS SUITABLE FOR PRESCRIBING** Isometheptene with paracetamol is less suitable for prescribing (more effective treatments available).

- **MEDICINAL FORMS**
There can be variation in the licensing of different medicines containing the same drug.
Capsule
CAUTIONARY AND ADVISORY LABELS 30
▶ Midrid (DHP Healthcare Ltd)
Isometheptene mucate 65 mg, Paracetamol 325 mg Midrid 325mg/65mg capsules | 30 capsule PoM £7.50

Paracetamol with metoclopramide

The properties listed below are those particular to the combination only. For the properties of the components please consider, paracetamol p. 438, metoclopramide hydrochloride p. 426.

- **INDICATIONS AND DOSE**

Acute migraine
▶ BY MOUTH USING TABLETS
▶ Adult: 2 tablets, to be taken at the onset of attack, followed by 2 tablets every 4 hours if required; maximum 6 tablets per day
▶ BY MOUTH USING EFFERVESCENT POWDER SACHETS
▶ Adult: 2 sachets, to be taken at the onset of attack, followed by 2 sachets every 4 hours if required, sachets to be dissolved in a quarter tumblerful of water; maximum 6 sachets per day

IMPORTANT SAFETY INFORMATION
Metoclopramide can cause **severe extrapyramidal effects**, particularly in young adults.

- **CAUTIONS** Treatment should not exceed 3 months due to risk of tardive dyskinesia
- **INTERACTIONS** → Appendix 1: metoclopramide · paracetamol

- **MEDICINAL FORMS**
There can be variation in the licensing of different medicines containing the same drug.
Effervescent powder
CAUTIONARY AND ADVISORY LABELS 13, 17, 30
▶ Paramax (Zentiva)
Metoclopramide hydrochloride 5 mg, Paracetamol 500 mg Paramax sachets sugar-free | 42 sachet PoM £12.52 DT = £12.52

Tablet
CAUTIONARY AND ADVISORY LABELS 17, 30
▶ Paramax (Zentiva)
Metoclopramide hydrochloride 5 mg, Paracetamol 500 mg Paramax tablets | 42 tablet PoM £9.64 DT = £9.64

ANALGESICS > NON-STEROIDAL ANTI-INFLAMMATORY DRUGS

Aspirin with metoclopramide

The properties listed below are those particular to the combination only. For the properties of the components please consider, aspirin p. 121, metoclopramide hydrochloride p. 426.

- **INDICATIONS AND DOSE**

Acute migraine
▶ BY MOUTH
▶ Adult: 1 sachet, sachet to be mixed in water, and dose to be taken at the start of the attack, then 1 sachet after 2 hours if required; maximum 3 sachets per day

IMPORTANT SAFETY INFORMATION
Metoclopramide can cause **severe extrapyramidal effects**, particularly in children and young adults.

- **CAUTIONS** Treatment should not exceed 3 months due to risk of tardive dyskinesia
- **INTERACTIONS** → Appendix 1: aspirin · metoclopramide
- **PRESCRIBING AND DISPENSING INFORMATION** Flavours of oral powder formulations may include lemon.

- **MEDICINAL FORMS**
There can be variation in the licensing of different medicines containing the same drug.
Powder
CAUTIONARY AND ADVISORY LABELS 13, 21, 32
EXCIPIENTS: May contain Aspartame
▶ MigraMax (Zentiva)
Metoclopramide hydrochloride 10 mg, Aspirin DL-Lysine 900 mg MigraMax oral powder sachets sugar-free | 6 sachet PoM £6.61 DT = £6.61

Tolfenamic acid

- **INDICATIONS AND DOSE**

Treatment of acute migraine
▶ BY MOUTH
▶ Adult: 200 mg, dose to be taken at onset, then 200 mg after 1–2 hours if required

- **CONTRA-INDICATIONS** Active gastro-intestinal bleeding · active gastro-intestinal ulceration · history of gastro-intestinal bleeding related to previous NSAID therapy · history of gastro-intestinal haemorrhage (two or more distinct episodes) · history of gastro-intestinal perforation related to previous NSAID therapy · history of recurrent gastro-intestinal ulceration (two or more distinct episodes) · severe heart failure
- **CAUTIONS** Allergic disorders · cardiac impairment (NSAIDs may impair renal function) · cerebrovascular disease · coagulation defects · connective-tissue disorders · Crohn's disease (may be exacerbated) · elderly (risk of serious side-effects and fatalities) · heart failure · ischaemic heart disease · peripheral arterial disease · risk factors for cardiovascular events · ulcerative colitis (may be exacerbated) · uncontrolled hypertension
- **INTERACTIONS** → Appendix 1: NSAIDs
- **SIDE-EFFECTS** Agranulocytosis · angioedema · aplastic anaemia · asthma · confusion · constipation · Crohn's

4

Nervous system

disease aggravated · depression · diarrhoea · dizziness · drowsiness · dyspnoea · dysuria (most common in men) · euphoric mood · fatigue · fertility decreased female · gastrointestinal discomfort · gastrointestinal disorders · haemolytic anaemia · haemorrhage · hallucination · headache · heart failure · hepatic disorders · hypersensitivity · hypertension · increased risk of arterial thromboembolism · malaise · meningitis aseptic (patients with connective-tissue disorders such as systemic lupus erythematosus may be especially susceptible) · nausea · nephritis tubulointerstitial · nephropathy · neutropenia · oedema · optic neuritis · oral ulceration · pancreatitis · paraesthesia · photosensitivity reaction · renal failure (more common in patients with pre-existing renal impairment) · respiratory disorders · severe cutaneous adverse reactions (SCARs) · skin reactions · thrombocytopenia · tinnitus · tremor · vertigo · visual impairment · vomiting

SIDE-EFFECTS, FURTHER INFORMATION For information about cardiovascular and gastrointestinal side-effects, and a possible exacerbation of symptoms in asthma, see Non-steroidal anti-inflammatory drugs p. 1094.

● ALLERGY AND CROSS-SENSITIVITY Contra-indicated in patients with a history of hypersensitivity to aspirin or any other NSAID—which includes those in whom attacks of asthma, angioedema, urticaria or rhinitis have been precipitated by aspirin or any other NSAID.

● CONCEPTION AND CONTRACEPTION Caution—long-term use of some NSAIDs is associated with reduced female fertility, which is reversible on stopping treatment.

● PREGNANCY Avoid unless the potential benefit outweighs the risk. Avoid during the third trimester (risk of closure of fetal ductus arteriosus *in utero* and possibly persistent pulmonary hypertension of the newborn); onset of labour may be delayed and duration may be increased.

● BREAST FEEDING Amount too small to be harmful. Use with caution during breast-feeding.

● HEPATIC IMPAIRMENT Use with caution; there is an increased risk of gastro-intestinal bleeding and fluid retention. Avoid in severe liver disease.

● RENAL IMPAIRMENT Avoid if possible or use with caution. **Dose adjustments** The lowest effective dose should be used for the shortest possible duration.
Monitoring In renal impairment monitor renal function; sodium and water retention may occur and renal function may deteriorate, possibly leading to renal failure.

● MEDICINAL FORMS
There can be variation in the licensing of different medicines containing the same drug.
Tablet
CAUTIONARY AND ADVISORY LABELS 21
▸ Tolfenamic acid (Non-proprietary)
 Tolfenamic acid 200 mg Tolfenamic acid 200mg tablets | 10 tablet PoM £24.62-£25.22 DT = £24.92
▸ Clotam Rapid (Galen Ltd)
 Tolfenamic acid 200 mg Clotam Rapid 200mg tablets | 10 tablet PoM £12.75 DT = £24.92

ANTIHISTAMINES ⟩ SEDATING

Paracetamol with buclizine hydrochloride and codeine phosphate

The properties listed below are those particular to the combination only. For the properties of the components please consider, paracetamol p. 438, codeine phosphate p. 448.

● INDICATIONS AND DOSE
MIGRALEVE ®
Acute migraine
▸ BY MOUTH
▸ Child 12–14 years: Initially 1 tablet, (pink tablet) to be taken at onset of attack, or if it is imminent, followed by 1 tablet every 4 hours if required, (yellow tablet) to be taken following initial dose; maximum 1 pink and 3 yellow tablets in 24 hours
▸ Child 15–17 years: Initially 2 tablets, (pink tablets) to be taken at onset of attack or if it is imminent, followed by 2 tablets every 4 hours if required, (yellow tablets) to be taken following initial dose; maximum 2 pink and 6 yellow tablets in 24 hours
▸ Adult: Initially 2 tablets, (pink tablets) to be taken at onset of attack or if it is imminent, followed by 2 tablets every 4 hours if required, (yellow tablets) to be taken following initial dose; maximum 2 pink and 6 yellow tablets in 24 hours

● INTERACTIONS → Appendix 1: antihistamines, sedating · opioids · paracetamol

● LESS SUITABLE FOR PRESCRIBING
MIGRALEVE ® *Migraleve*® is less suitable for prescribing.

● MEDICINAL FORMS
There can be variation in the licensing of different medicines containing the same drug.
Tablet
CAUTIONARY AND ADVISORY LABELS 2, 17, 30
▸ Migraleve Pink (McNeil Products Ltd)
 Buclizine hydrochloride 6.25 mg, Codeine phosphate 8 mg, Paracetamol 500 mg Migraleve Pink tablets | 12 tablet P £3.79 CD5 | 24 tablet P £6.08 CD5 | 48 tablet PoM £3.97 CD5
▸ Migraleve Yellow (McNeil Products Ltd)
 Codeine phosphate 8 mg, Paracetamol 500 mg Migraleve Yellow tablets | 16 tablet P 🗶 CD5

ERGOT ALKALOIDS

Ergotamine tartrate

● INDICATIONS AND DOSE
Management of cluster headache
▸ BY MOUTH USING TABLETS
▸ Adult: 1 mg once daily for 6 nights in 7; occasionally given for 1–2 weeks, dose to be taken at night

● UNLICENSED USE Not licensed for the management of cluster headache.

● CONTRA-INDICATIONS Acute porphyrias p. 1025 · coronary heart disease · hyperthyroidism · inadequately controlled hypertension · obliterative vascular disease · peripheral vascular disease · Raynaud's syndrome · sepsis · severe hypertension · temporal arteritis

● CAUTIONS Anaemia · cardiac disease · dependence · elderly · risk of peripheral vasospasm

● INTERACTIONS → Appendix 1: ergotamine

● SIDE-EFFECTS
▸ **Common or very common** Abdominal pain · dizziness · nausea · vomiting

▸ **Uncommon** Cyanosis · diarrhoea · muscle weakness · pain in extremity · sensation abnormal · vasoconstriction
▸ **Rare or very rare** Arrhythmias · cardiac valve fibrosis · dyspnoea · ergot poisoning (including absence of pulse and numbness in extremities) · gangrene · intestinal ischaemia · myalgia · myocardial infarction · myocardial ischaemia · skin reactions
▸ **Frequency not known** Anxiety · arthralgia · blood disorder · cerebral ischaemia · confusion · constipation · depression · drowsiness · dry mouth · extrapyramidal symptoms · hallucination · renal artery spasm · seizure · sleep disorder · thrombosis · tremor · urinary retention · vision blurred
● PREGNANCY Avoid; oxytocic effect on the uterus.
● BREAST FEEDING Avoid; ergotism may occur in infant; repeated doses may inhibit lactation.
● HEPATIC IMPAIRMENT Avoid in severe impairment—risk of toxicity increased.
● RENAL IMPAIRMENT Avoid; risk of renal vasoconstriction.
● PATIENT AND CARER ADVICE
Peripheral vasospasm Warn patient to stop treatment immediately if numbness or tingling of extremities develops and to contact doctor.
● LESS SUITABLE FOR PRESCRIBING Ergotamine tartrate is less suitable for prescribing.

● MEDICINAL FORMS
No licensed medicines listed

Ergotamine tartrate with caffeine hydrate and cyclizine hydrochloride

The properties listed below are those particular to the combination only. For the properties of the components please consider, ergotamine tartrate p. 470, cyclizine p. 424.

● INDICATIONS AND DOSE

Treatment of acute migraine and migraine variants unresponsive to analgesics
▸ BY MOUTH
▸ Adult: 1 tablet, to be taken at onset, followed by 0.5–1 tablet after 30 minutes, then 0.5–1 tablet every 30 minutes if required, max. 3 tablets in 24 hours, max. 4 tablets per attack, max. 6 tablets in one week

● INTERACTIONS → Appendix 1: antihistamines, sedating · ergotamine
● PATIENT AND CARER ADVICE Patient counselling is advised for cyclizine hydrochloride with caffeine hydrate and ergotamine tartrate tablets (dosage).
● LESS SUITABLE FOR PRESCRIBING Cyclizine hydrochloride with caffeine hydrate and ergotamine tartrate (Migril®) is less suitable for prescribing.

● MEDICINAL FORMS
There can be variation in the licensing of different medicines containing the same drug.
Tablet
CAUTIONARY AND ADVISORY LABELS 2, 18
▸ Migril (Wockhardt UK Ltd)
Ergotamine tartrate 2 mg, Cyclizine hydrochloride 50 mg, Caffeine hydrate 100 mg Migril tablets | 100 tablet [PoM] £51.00

TRIPTANS

Almotriptan

● INDICATIONS AND DOSE

Treatment of acute migraine
▸ BY MOUTH
▸ Adult: 12.5 mg, dose to be taken as soon as possible after onset, followed by 12.5 mg after 2 hours if required, dose to be taken only if migraine recurs (patient not responding to initial dose should not take second dose for same attack); maximum 25 mg per day

● UNLICENSED USE Not licensed for use in elderly.
● CONTRA-INDICATIONS Coronary vasospasm · ischaemic heart disease · peripheral vascular disease · previous cerebrovascular accident · previous myocardial infarction · previous transient ischaemic attack · Prinzmetal's angina · severe hypertension · uncontrolled hypertension
● CAUTIONS Conditions which predispose to coronary artery disease · elderly
● INTERACTIONS → Appendix 1: almotriptan
● SIDE-EFFECTS
▸ **Common or very common** Asthenia · dizziness · drowsiness · nausea · vomiting
▸ **Uncommon** Bone pain · chest pain · diarrhoea · dry mouth · dyspepsia · headache · myalgia · palpitations · paraesthesia · throat tightness · tinnitus
▸ **Rare or very rare** Coronary vasospasm · myocardial infarction · tachycardia
▸ **Frequency not known** Intestinal ischaemia · seizure · vision disorders
SIDE-EFFECTS, FURTHER INFORMATION Discontinue if symptoms of heat, heaviness, pressure or tightness (including throat and chest) occur.
● ALLERGY AND CROSS-SENSITIVITY Caution in patients with sensitivity to sulfonamides.
● PREGNANCY There is limited experience of using 5HT$_1$-receptor agonists during pregnancy; manufacturers advise that they should be avoided unless the potential benefit outweighs the risk.
● BREAST FEEDING Present in milk in *animal* studies—withhold breast-feeding for 24 hours.
● HEPATIC IMPAIRMENT Caution in mild to moderate impairment. Avoid in severe impairment.
● RENAL IMPAIRMENT
Dose adjustments Max. 12.5 mg in 24 hours if eGFR less than 30 mL/minute/1.73 m^2.

● MEDICINAL FORMS
There can be variation in the licensing of different medicines containing the same drug.
Tablet
CAUTIONARY AND ADVISORY LABELS 3
▸ Almotriptan (Non-proprietary)
Almotriptan (as Almotriptan hydrogen malate)
12.5 mg Almotriptan 12.5mg tablets | 3 tablet [PoM] £6.65–£9.07 | 6 tablet [PoM] £18.14 DT = £18.14 | 9 tablet [PoM] £21.75–£27.21
▸ Almogran (Almirall Ltd)
Almotriptan (as Almotriptan hydrogen malate) 12.5 mg Almogran 12.5mg tablets | 3 tablet [PoM] £9.07 | 6 tablet [PoM] £18.14 DT = £18.14

Eletriptan

● INDICATIONS AND DOSE

Treatment of acute migraine
▸ BY MOUTH
▸ Adult: 40 mg, followed by 40 mg after 2 hours if required, dose to be taken only if migraine continued →

4

Nervous system

recurs (patient not responding to initial dose should not take second dose for same attack); increased if necessary to 80 mg, dose to be taken for subsequent attacks if 40 mg dose inadequate; maximum 80 mg per day

- UNLICENSED USE Not licensed for use in elderly.
- CONTRA-INDICATIONS Arrhythmias · coronary vasospasm · heart failure · ischaemic heart disease · peripheral vascular disease · previous cerebrovascular accident · previous myocardial infarction · previous transient ischaemic attack · Prinzmetal's angina · severe hypertension · uncontrolled hypertension
- CAUTIONS Conditions which predispose to coronary artery disease · elderly
- INTERACTIONS → Appendix 1: eletriptan
- SIDE-EFFECTS
  ▶ **Common or very common** Arrhythmias · asthenia · chest discomfort · chills · dizziness · drowsiness · dry mouth · feeling hot · flushing · gastrointestinal discomfort · headache · hyperhidrosis · increased risk of infection · muscle complaints · muscle tone increased · muscle weakness · nausea · pain · palpitations · sensation abnormal · throat tightness · vertigo
  ▶ **Uncommon** Agitation · appetite decreased · arthralgia · arthritis · confusion · depersonalisation · depression · diarrhoea · dyspnoea · ear pain · eye pain · insomnia · lacrimation disorder · malaise · mood altered · movement disorders · oedema · oral disorders · peripheral vascular disease · respiratory disorder · skin reactions · speech disorder · stupor · taste altered · thinking abnormal · thirst · tinnitus · tremor · urinary disorders · urinary tract disorder · vision disorders · yawning
  ▶ **Rare or very rare** Asthma · breast pain · burping · conjunctivitis · constipation · gastrointestinal disorders · hyperbilirubinaemia · lymphadenopathy · menorrhagia · myopathy · shock · voice alteration
  ▶ **Frequency not known** Coronary vasospasm · hypertension · myocardial infarction · myocardial ischaemia · serotonin syndrome · stroke · syncope · vomiting

  SIDE-EFFECTS, FURTHER INFORMATION Discontinue if symptoms of heat, heaviness, pressure or tightness (including throat and chest) occur.
- PREGNANCY There is limited experience of using 5HT$_1$-receptor agonists during pregnancy; manufacturers advise that they should be avoided unless the potential benefit outweighs the risk.
- BREAST FEEDING Present in milk—avoid breast-feeding for 24 hours.
- HEPATIC IMPAIRMENT Avoid in severe impairment.
- RENAL IMPAIRMENT Avoid if eGFR less than 30 mL/minute/1.73 m^2.
  Dose adjustments Reduce initial dose to 20 mg; maximum 40 mg in 24 hours.

- MEDICINAL FORMS
  There can be variation in the licensing of different medicines containing the same drug.
  Tablet
  CAUTIONARY AND ADVISORY LABELS 3
  ▶ Relpax (Pfizer Ltd)
  Eletriptan (as Eletriptan hydrobromide) 20 mg Relpax 20mg tablets | 6 tablet [PoM] £22.50 DT = £22.50
  Eletriptan (as Eletriptan hydrobromide) 40 mg Relpax 40mg tablets | 6 tablet [PoM] £22.50 DT = £22.50

Frovatriptan

- INDICATIONS AND DOSE
  Treatment of acute migraine
  ▶ BY MOUTH
  ▶ Adult: 2.5 mg, dose to be taken as soon as possible after onset, followed by 2.5 mg after 2 hours if required, dose to be taken only if migraine recurs (patient not responding to initial dose should not take second dose for same attack); maximum 5 mg per day

- UNLICENSED USE Not licensed for use in elderly.
- CONTRA-INDICATIONS Coronary vasospasm · ischaemic heart disease · peripheral vascular disease · previous cerebrovascular attack · previous myocardial infarction · previous transient ischaemic attack · Prinzmetal's angina · severe hypertension · uncontrolled hypertension
- CAUTIONS Conditions which predispose to coronary artery disease · elderly
- INTERACTIONS → Appendix 1: frovatriptan
- SIDE-EFFECTS
  ▶ **Common or very common** Chest discomfort · dizziness · drowsiness · dry mouth · flushing · gastrointestinal discomfort · headache · hyperhidrosis · nausea · sensation abnormal · throat complaints · vision disorders
  ▶ **Uncommon** Anxiety · arrhythmias · arthralgia · concentration impaired · confusion · dehydration · depression · diarrhoea · dysphagia · ear discomfort · eye discomfort · gastrointestinal disorders · hypertension · increased risk of infection · malaise · musculoskeletal stiffness · neuromuscular dysfunction · pain · palpitations · peripheral coldness · psychiatric disorders · skin reactions · sleep disorders · taste altered · temperature sensation altered · thirst · tinnitus · tremor · urinary disorders · vertigo
  ▶ **Rare or very rare** Breast tenderness · burping · constipation · ear disorder · epistaxis · fever · hiccups · hyperacusia · hypoglycaemia · irritable bowel syndrome · lymphadenopathy · memory loss · movement disorder · oral disorders · piloerection · reflexes decreased · renal pain · respiratory disorders · self mutilation
  ▶ **Frequency not known** Angioedema · coronary vasospasm · hypersensitivity · myocardial infarction

  SIDE-EFFECTS, FURTHER INFORMATION Discontinue if symptoms of heat, heaviness, pressure or tightness (including throat and chest) occur.
- PREGNANCY There is limited experience of using 5HT$_1$-receptor agonists during pregnancy; manufacturers advise that they should be avoided unless the potential benefit outweighs the risk.
- BREAST FEEDING Present in milk in *animal* studies—withhold breast-feeding for 24 hours.
- HEPATIC IMPAIRMENT Avoid in severe impairment.

- MEDICINAL FORMS
  There can be variation in the licensing of different medicines containing the same drug.
  Tablet
  CAUTIONARY AND ADVISORY LABELS 3
  ▶ Frovatriptan (Non-proprietary)
  Frovatriptan (as Frovatriptan succinate monohydrate)
  2.5 mg Frovatriptan 2.5mg tablets | 6 tablet [PoM] £8.50–£16.67 DT = £8.81
  ▶ Migard (A. Menarini Farmaceutica Internazionale SRL)
  Frovatriptan (as Frovatriptan succinate monohydrate)
  2.5 mg Migard 2.5mg tablets | 6 tablet [PoM] £16.67 DT = £8.81
  ▶ Mylatrip (Mylan)
  Frovatriptan (as Frovatriptan succinate monohydrate)
  2.5 mg Mylatrip 2.5mg tablets | 6 tablet [PoM] £16.50 DT = £8.81

Naratriptan

- **INDICATIONS AND DOSE**
Treatment of acute migraine
  ▶ BY MOUTH
  ▶ Adult: 2.5 mg, followed by 2.5 mg after at least 4 hours if required, to be taken only if migraine recurs (patient not responding to initial dose should not take second dose for same attack); maximum 5 mg per day

- **UNLICENSED USE** Not licensed for use in elderly.
- **CONTRA-INDICATIONS** Coronary vasospasm · ischaemic heart disease · moderate or severe hypertension · peripheral vascular disease · previous cerebrovascular accident · previous myocardial infarction · previous transient ischaemic attack · Prinzmetal's angina · uncontrolled hypertension
- **CAUTIONS** Conditions which predispose to coronary artery disease · elderly
- **INTERACTIONS** → Appendix 1: naratriptan
- **SIDE-EFFECTS**
  ▶ **Common or very common** Dizziness · drowsiness · fatigue · feeling hot · malaise · nausea · paraesthesia · vomiting
  ▶ **Uncommon** Arrhythmias · feeling abnormal · pain · palpitations · visual impairment
  ▶ **Rare or very rare** Angina pectoris · colitis ischaemic · coronary vasospasm · face oedema · myocardial infarction · peripheral vascular disease · skin reactions
  SIDE-EFFECTS, FURTHER INFORMATION Discontinue if symptoms of heat, heaviness, pressure or tightness (including throat and chest) occur.
- **ALLERGY AND CROSS-SENSITIVITY** Caution in patients with sensitivity to sulfonamides.
- **PREGNANCY** There is limited experience of using 5HT$_1$-receptor agonists during pregnancy; manufacturers advise that they should be avoided unless the potential benefit outweighs the risk.
- **BREAST FEEDING** Withhold breast-feeding for 24 hours.
- **HEPATIC IMPAIRMENT** Avoid if severe.
  Dose adjustments Max. 2.5 mg in 24 hours in moderate impairment.
- **RENAL IMPAIRMENT** Avoid if eGFR less than 15 mL/minute/1.73 m^2.
  Dose adjustments Max. 2.5 mg in 24 hours.
- **PATIENT AND CARER ADVICE**
  Driving and skilled tasks Drowsiness may affect performance of skilled tasks (e.g. driving).

- **MEDICINAL FORMS**
There can be variation in the licensing of different medicines containing the same drug.
  Tablet
  CAUTIONARY AND ADVISORY LABELS 3
  ▶ Naratriptan (Non-proprietary)
    Naratriptan (as Naratriptan hydrochloride) 2.5 mg Naratriptan 2.5mg tablets | 6 tablet [PoM] £24.55 DT = £12.43 | 12 tablet [PoM] £30.00-£46.00
  ▶ Naramig (GlaxoSmithKline UK Ltd)
    Naratriptan (as Naratriptan hydrochloride) 2.5 mg Naramig 2.5mg tablets | 6 tablet [PoM] £24.55 DT = £12.43

Rizatriptan

- **INDICATIONS AND DOSE**
Treatment of acute migraine
  ▶ BY MOUTH
  ▶ Adult: 10 mg, dose to be taken as soon as possible after onset, followed by 10 mg after 2 hours if required, dose to be taken only if migraine recurs (patient not

responding to initial dose should not take second dose for same attack); maximum 20 mg per day
  DOSE ADJUSTMENTS DUE TO INTERACTIONS
  ▶ Manufacturer advises reduce dose to 5 mg with concurrent use of propranolol.

- **UNLICENSED USE** Not licensed for use in elderly.
- **CONTRA-INDICATIONS** Coronary vasospasm · ischaemic heart disease · peripheral vascular disease · previous cerebrovascular accident · previous myocardial infarction · previous transient ischaemic attack · Prinzmetal's angina · severe hypertension · uncontrolled hypertension
- **CAUTIONS** Conditions which predispose to coronary artery disease · elderly
- **INTERACTIONS** → Appendix 1: rizatriptan
- **SIDE-EFFECTS**
  ▶ **Common or very common** Alertness decreased · asthenia · diarrhoea · dizziness · drowsiness · dry mouth · feeling abnormal · headache · insomnia · musculoskeletal stiffness · nausea · pain · palpitations · sensation abnormal · throat complaints · vasodilation · vomiting
  ▶ **Uncommon** Angioedema · arrhythmias · ataxia · disorientation · dyspnoea · face oedema · hyperhidrosis · hypertension · muscle weakness · myalgia · nervousness · skin reactions · syncope · taste altered · thirst · tongue swelling · tremor · vertigo · vision blurred
  ▶ **Rare or very rare** Hypersensitivity · stroke · wheezing
  ▶ **Frequency not known** Colitis ischaemic · myocardial infarction · myocardial ischaemia · peripheral vascular disease · seizure · serotonin syndrome · toxic epidermal necrolysis
  SIDE-EFFECTS, FURTHER INFORMATION Discontinue if symptoms of heat, heaviness, pressure or tightness (including throat and chest) occur.
- **PREGNANCY** There is limited experience of using 5HT$_1$-receptor agonists during pregnancy; manufacturers advise that they should be avoided unless the potential benefit outweighs the risk.
- **BREAST FEEDING** Present in milk in *animal* studies—withhold breast-feeding for 24 hours.
- **HEPATIC IMPAIRMENT** Avoid in severe impairment.
  Dose adjustments Reduce dose to 5 mg in mild to moderate impairment.
- **RENAL IMPAIRMENT** Avoid in severe impairment.
  Dose adjustments Reduce dose to 5 mg in mild to moderate impairment.
- **DIRECTIONS FOR ADMINISTRATION** Rizatriptan orodispersible tablets should be placed on the tongue, allowed to disperse and swallowed. Rizatriptan oral lyophilisates should be placed on the tongue and allowed to dissolve.
- **PATIENT AND CARER ADVICE** Patients or carers should be given advice on how to administer rizatriptan orodispersible tablets and oral lyophilisates.
  Driving and skilled tasks Drowsiness may affect performance of skilled tasks (e.g. driving).

- **MEDICINAL FORMS**
There can be variation in the licensing of different medicines containing the same drug.
  Orodispersible tablet
  CAUTIONARY AND ADVISORY LABELS 3
  EXCIPIENTS: May contain Aspartame
  ▶ Rizatriptan (Non-proprietary)
    Rizatriptan (as Rizatriptan benzoate) 10 mg Rizatriptan 10mg orodispersible tablets sugar free sugar-free | 3 tablet [PoM] £14.90 DT = £14.63 sugar-free | 6 tablet [PoM] £3.60-£29.80

Tablet

CAUTIONARY AND ADVISORY LABELS 3
▶ Rizatriptan (Non-proprietary)
Rizatriptan (as Rizatriptan benzoate) 5 mg Rizatriptan 5mg tablets
| 3 tablet [PoM] £13.37 | 6 tablet [PoM] £26.74 DT = £26.74
Rizatriptan (as Rizatriptan benzoate) 10 mg Rizatriptan 10mg
tablets | 3 tablet [PoM] £13.37 DT = £9.33 | 6 tablet [PoM] £16.52-
£26.74
▶ Maxalt (Merck Sharp & Dohme Ltd)
Rizatriptan (as Rizatriptan benzoate) 5 mg Maxalt 5mg tablets |
6 tablet [PoM] £26.74 DT = £26.74
Rizatriptan (as Rizatriptan benzoate) 10 mg Maxalt 10mg tablets
| 3 tablet [PoM] £13.37 DT = £9.33 | 6 tablet [PoM] £26.74

Oral lyophilisate

CAUTIONARY AND ADVISORY LABELS 3
EXCIPIENTS: May contain Aspartame
▶ Maxalt Melt (Merck Sharp & Dohme Ltd)
Rizatriptan (as Rizatriptan benzoate) 10 mg Maxalt Melt 10mg
oral lyophilisates sugar-free | 3 tablet [PoM] £13.37 DT = £13.37
sugar-free | 6 tablet [PoM] £26.74 DT = £26.74 sugar-free |
12 tablet [PoM] £53.48

Sumatriptan

● **INDICATIONS AND DOSE**

Treatment of acute migraine

▶ BY MOUTH
▶ **Adult:** Initially 50–100 mg for 1 dose, followed by
50–100 mg after at least 2 hours if required, to be taken
only if migraine recurs (patient not responding to
initial dose should not take second dose for same
attack); maximum 300 mg per day
▶ BY SUBCUTANEOUS INJECTION
▶ **Adult:** Initially 6 mg for 1 dose, followed by 6 mg after
at least 1 hour if required, to be taken only if migraine
recurs (patient not responding to initial dose should
not take second dose for same attack), dose to be
administered using an auto-injector; not for
intravenous injection which may cause coronary
vasospasm and angina; maximum 12 mg per day
▶ BY INTRANASAL ADMINISTRATION
▶ **Adult 18-65 years:** Initially 10–20 mg, to be
administered into one nostril, followed by 10–20 mg
after at least 2 hours if required, to be taken only if
migraine recurs (patient not responding to initial dose
should not take second dose for same attack);
maximum 40 mg per day

Treatment of acute cluster headache

▶ BY SUBCUTANEOUS INJECTION
▶ **Adult:** Initially 6 mg for 1 dose, followed by 6 mg after
at least 1 hour if required, to be taken only if headache
recurs (patient not responding to initial dose should
not take second dose for same attack), dose to be
administered using an auto-injector; not for
intravenous injection which may cause coronary
vasospasm and angina; maximum 12 mg per day
▶ BY INTRANASAL ADMINISTRATION
▶ **Adult 18-65 years:** Initially 10–20 mg, dose to be
administered into one nostril, followed by 10–20 mg
after at least 2 hours if required, to be taken only if
headache recurs (patient not responding to initial dose
should not take second dose for same attack);
maximum 40 mg per day

● UNLICENSED USE Not licensed for use in elderly.
● CONTRA-INDICATIONS Coronary vasospasm · ischaemic
heart disease · mild uncontrolled hypertension · moderate
and severe hypertension · peripheral vascular disease ·
previous cerebrovascular accident · previous myocardial
infarction · previous transient ischaemic attack ·
Prinzmetal's angina
● CAUTIONS Conditions which predispose to coronary artery
disease · elderly · history of seizures · mild, controlled

hypertension · pre-existing cardiac disease · risk factors for
seizures
● INTERACTIONS → Appendix 1: sumatriptan
● SIDE-EFFECTS

GENERAL SIDE-EFFECTS
▶ **Common or very common** Asthenia · dizziness · drowsiness ·
dyspnoea · feeling abnormal · flushing · myalgia · nausea ·
pain · sensation abnormal · temperature sensation altered ·
vomiting
▶ **Rare or very rare** Hypersensitivity
▶ **Frequency not known** Angina pectoris · anxiety ·
arrhythmias · arthralgia · colitis ischaemic · coronary
vasospasm · diarrhoea · dystonia · hyperhidrosis ·
hypotension · myocardial infarction · nystagmus ·
palpitations · Raynaud's phenomenon · seizure · tremor ·
vision disorders

SPECIFIC SIDE-EFFECTS
▶ **Common or very common**
▶ With intranasal use Epistaxis · nasal irritation · taste altered ·
throat irritation
▶ With subcutaneous use Haemorrhage · skin reactions ·
swelling
▶ **Frequency not known**
▶ With intranasal use Skin reactions
▶ With oral use Allergic dermatitis

SIDE-EFFECTS, FURTHER INFORMATION Discontinue if
symptoms of heat, heaviness, pressure or tightness
(including throat and chest) occur.
● ALLERGY AND CROSS-SENSITIVITY Caution in patients with
sensitivity to sulfonamides.
● PREGNANCY There is limited experience of using 5HT$_1$-
receptor agonists during pregnancy; manufacturers advise
that they should be avoided unless the potential benefit
outweighs the risk.
● BREAST FEEDING Present in milk but amount probably too
small to be harmful; withhold breast-feeding for 12 hours
after treatment.
● HEPATIC IMPAIRMENT Avoid in severe impairment.
Dose adjustments Reduce oral dose to 25–50 mg.
● RENAL IMPAIRMENT Use with caution.
● PATIENT AND CARER ADVICE
Driving and skilled tasks Drowsiness may affect
performance of skilled tasks (e.g. driving).
● EXCEPTIONS TO LEGAL CATEGORY Sumatriptan 50 mg
tablets can be sold to the public to treat previously
diagnosed migraine; max. daily dose 100 mg.

● MEDICINAL FORMS
There can be variation in the licensing of different medicines
containing the same drug.
Solution for injection
CAUTIONARY AND ADVISORY LABELS 3, 10
▶ Sumatriptan (Non-proprietary)
**Sumatriptan (as Sumatriptan succinate) 12 mg per
1 ml** Sumatriptan 6mg/0.5ml solution for injection pre-filled pen |
2 pre-filled disposable injection [PoM] £39.50 DT = £39.50
▶ Imigran Subject (GlaxoSmithKline UK Ltd)
Sumatriptan (as Sumatriptan succinate) 12 mg per 1 ml Imigran
Subject 6mg/0.5ml solution for injection syringe refill pack | 2 pre-
filled disposable injection [PoM] £40.41 DT = £40.41
Imigran Subject 6mg/0.5ml solution for injection pre-filled syringes
with device | 2 pre-filled disposable injection [PoM] £50.96 DT =
£50.96
Spray
CAUTIONARY AND ADVISORY LABELS 3, 10
▶ Imigran (GlaxoSmithKline UK Ltd)
Sumatriptan 100 mg per 1 ml Imigran 10mg nasal spray | 2 unit
dose [PoM] £11.80 DT = £11.80
Sumatriptan 200 mg per 1 ml Imigran 20mg nasal spray | 2 unit
dose [PoM] £14.16 | 6 unit dose [PoM] £42.47 DT = £42.47

Tablet
CAUTIONARY AND ADVISORY LABELS 3, 10
- Sumatriptan (Non-proprietary)
  Sumatriptan (as Sumatriptan succinate) 50 mg Sumatriptan 50mg tablets | 6 tablet [PoM] £31.00 DT = £6.94
  Sumatriptan (as Sumatriptan succinate) 100 mg Sumatriptan 100mg tablets | 6 tablet [PoM] £40.18 DT = £6.82
- Imigran (GlaxoSmithKline UK Ltd, Forest Laboratories UK Ltd)
  Sumatriptan (as Sumatriptan succinate) 50 mg Imigran Radis 50mg tablets | 6 tablet [PoM] £23.90 DT = £6.94
  Imigran 50mg tablets | 6 tablet [PoM] £31.85 DT = £6.94
  Imigran Recovery 50mg tablets | 2 tablet [P] £4.76
  Sumatriptan (as Sumatriptan succinate) 100 mg Imigran 100mg tablets | 6 tablet [PoM] £51.48 DT = £6.82
  Imigran Radis 100mg tablets | 6 tablet [PoM] £42.90 DT = £6.82
- Migraitan (Bristol Laboratories Ltd)
  Sumatriptan (as Sumatriptan succinate) 50 mg Migraitan 50mg tablets | 2 tablet [P] £4.44

Zolmitriptan

- **INDICATIONS AND DOSE**
Treatment of acute migraine
- BY MOUTH
- Adult: 2.5 mg, followed by 2.5 mg after at least 2 hours if required, dose to be taken only if migraine recurs, then increased if necessary to 5 mg, dose to be taken only for subsequent attacks in patients not achieving satisfactory relief with 2.5 mg dose; maximum 10 mg per day
- BY INTRANASAL ADMINISTRATION
- Adult: 5 mg, dose to be administered as soon as possible after onset into one nostril only, followed by 5 mg after at least 2 hours if required, dose to be administered only if migraine recurs; maximum 10 mg per day

Treatment of acute cluster headache
- BY INTRANASAL ADMINISTRATION
- Adult: 5 mg, dose to be administered as soon as possible after onset into one nostril only, followed by 5 mg after at least 2 hours if required, dose to be administered only if migraine recurs; maximum 10 mg per day

DOSE ADJUSTMENTS DUE TO INTERACTIONS
- Manufacturer advises max. dose 5 mg in 24 hours with concurrent use of moderate and potent inhibitors of CYP1A2, cimetidine and moclobemide.

DOSE EQUIVALENCE AND CONVERSION
- 1 spray of *Zomig*® nasal spray = 5 mg zolmitriptan.

- **UNLICENSED USE** Not licensed for use in elderly. Not licensed for treatment of cluster headaches.
- **CONTRA-INDICATIONS** Arrhythmias associated with accessory cardiac conduction pathways · coronary vasospasm · ischaemic heart disease · moderate to severe hypertension · peripheral vascular disease · previous cerebrovascular accident · previous myocardial infarction · Prinzmetal's angina · transient ischaemic attack · uncontrolled hypertension · Wolff-Parkinson-White syndrome
- **CAUTIONS** Conditions which predispose to coronary artery disease · elderly · should not be taken within 24 hours of any other 5HT$_1$-receptor agonist
- **INTERACTIONS** → Appendix 1: zolmitriptan
- **SIDE-EFFECTS**
  GENERAL SIDE-EFFECTS
- **Common or very common** Abdominal pain · asthenia · chest discomfort · dizziness · drowsiness · dry mouth · dysphagia · feeling hot · headache · limb discomfort · muscle weakness · nausea · pain · palpitations · sensation · vomiting
- **Uncommon** Tachycardia · urinary disorders

- **Rare or very rare** Angina pectoris · angioedema · coronary vasospasm · gastrointestinal disorders · gastrointestinal infarction · hypersensitivity · myocardial infarction · splenic infarction · urticaria
  SPECIFIC SIDE-EFFECTS
- **Common or very common**
- With intranasal use Feeling abnormal · haemorrhage · myalgia · nasal discomfort · taste altered · throat pain
- With oral use Muscle complaints · sensation of pressure · throat complaints
- **Rare or very rare**
- With oral use Diarrhoea
  SIDE-EFFECTS, FURTHER INFORMATION Discontinue if symptoms of heat, heaviness, pressure or tightness (including throat and chest) occur.
- **PREGNANCY** There is limited experience of using 5HT$_1$-receptor agonists during pregnancy; manufacturers advise that they should be avoided unless the potential benefit outweighs the risk.
- **BREAST FEEDING** Use with caution—present in milk in *animal* studies.
- **HEPATIC IMPAIRMENT**
  Dose adjustments Max. 5 mg in 24 hours in moderate or severe impairment.
- **DIRECTIONS FOR ADMINISTRATION** Zolmitriptan orodispersible tablets should be placed on the tongue, allowed to disperse and swallowed.
- **PATIENT AND CARER ADVICE** Patients or carers should be given advice on how to administer zolmitriptan orodispersible tablets.

- **MEDICINAL FORMS**
  There can be variation in the licensing of different medicines containing the same drug.
  Spray
- Zomig (AstraZeneca UK Ltd)
  Zolmitriptan 50 mg per 1 ml Zomig 5mg/0.1ml nasal spray 0.1ml unit dose | 6 unit dose [PoM] £36.50 DT = £36.50
  Orodispersible tablet
  EXCIPIENTS: May contain Aspartame
- Zolmitriptan (Non-proprietary)
  Zolmitriptan 2.5 mg Zolmitriptan 2.5mg orodispersible tablets sugar free sugar-free | 6 tablet [PoM] £20.35 DT = £14.84
  Zolmitriptan 5 mg Zolmitriptan 5mg orodispersible tablets sugar free sugar-free | 6 tablet [PoM] £20.35 DT = £13.79
- Zomig Rapimelt (AstraZeneca UK Ltd)
  Zolmitriptan 2.5 mg Zomig Rapimelt 2.5mg orodispersible tablets sugar-free | 6 tablet [PoM] £23.99 DT = £14.84
  Zolmitriptan 5 mg Zomig Rapimelt 5mg orodispersible tablets sugar-free | 6 tablet [PoM] £23.94 DT = £13.79
  Tablet
- Zolmitriptan (Non-proprietary)
  Zolmitriptan 2.5 mg Zolmitriptan 2.5mg tablets | 6 tablet [PoM] £15.78 DT = £15.78 | 12 tablet [PoM] £31.56
  Zolmitriptan 5 mg Zolmitriptan 5mg tablets | 6 tablet [PoM] £3.60 DT = £3.60 | 12 tablet [PoM] £7.20
- Zomig (AstraZeneca UK Ltd)
  Zolmitriptan 2.5 mg Zomig 2.5mg tablets | 6 tablet [PoM] £23.94 DT = £15.78

6.2 Neuropathic pain

Neuropathic pain

Overview and management

Neuropathic pain, which occurs as a result of damage to neural tissue, includes *phantom limb pain, compression neuropathies, peripheral neuropathies* (e.g. due to Diabetic complications p. 674, chronic excessive alcohol intake, HIV infection p. 628, chemotherapy, idiopathic neuropathy), *trauma, central pain* (e.g. pain following stroke, spinal cord injury, and syringomyelia), and *postherpetic neuralgia* (peripheral nerve damage following acute herpes zoster infection (shingles)). The pain may occur in an area of sensory deficit and is sometimes accompanied by pain that is evoked by a non-noxious stimulus (allodynia).

Trigeminal neuralgia is also caused by dysfunction of neural tissue, but its management is distinct from other forms of neuropathic pain.

Neuropathic pain is generally managed with a **tricyclic antidepressant** or with certain **antiepileptic drugs**. Amitriptyline hydrochloride p. 369 [unlicensed indication] and pregabalin p. 322 are effective treatments for neuropathic pain. Amitriptyline hydrochloride and pregabalin can be used in combination if the patient has an inadequate response to either drug at the maximum tolerated dose.

Nortriptyline p. 374 [unlicensed indication] may be better tolerated than amitriptyline hydrochloride.

Gabapentin p. 314 is also effective for the treatment of neuropathic pain.

Neuropathic pain may respond to **opioid analgesics**. There is evidence of efficacy for tramadol hydrochloride p. 464, morphine p. 456, and oxycodone hydrochloride p. 459; however, treatment with morphine or oxycodone hydrochloride should be initiated only under specialist supervision. Tramadol hydrochloride can be prescribed when other treatments have been unsuccessful, while the patient is waiting for assessment by a specialist.

Patients with localised pain who are unable to take oral medicines may benefit from **topical local anaesthetic preparations**, such as lidocaine hydrochloride p. 1312 medicated plasters, while awaiting specialist review.

Capsaicin below is licensed for neuropathic pain (but the intense burning sensation during initial treatment may limit use). Capsaicin 0.075% cream is licensed for the symptomatic relief of *postherpetic neuralgia*. A self-adhesive patch containing capsaicin 8% is licensed for the treatment of peripheral neuropathic pain in non-diabetic patients. It should be used under specialist supervision.

A corticosteroid may help to relieve pressure in compression neuropathy and thereby reduce pain.

Neuromodulation by spinal cord stimulation may be of benefit in some patients. Many patients with chronic neuropathic pain require multidisciplinary management, including physiotherapy and psychological support.

Trigeminal neuralgia
Surgery may be the treatment of choice in many patients; a neurological assessment will identify those who stand to benefit. Carbamazepine p. 309 taken during the acute stages of trigeminal neuralgia, reduces the frequency and severity of attacks. It is very effective for the severe pain associated with trigeminal neuralgia and (less commonly) glossopharyngeal neuralgia. Blood counts and electrolytes should be monitored when high doses are given. Small doses should be used initially to reduce the incidence of side-effects e.g. dizziness. Some cases respond to phenytoin p. 321; the drug may be given by intravenous infusion (possibly as fosphenytoin sodium p. 313) in a crisis (specialist use only).

Chronic facial pain
Chronic oral and facial pain including *persistent idiopathic facial pain* (also termed 'atypical facial pain') and *temporomandibular dysfunction* (previously termed temporomandibular joint pain dysfunction syndrome) may call for prolonged use of analgesics or for other drugs. **Tricyclic antidepressants** may be useful for facial pain [unlicensed indication], but are not on the Dental Practitioners' List. Disorders of this type require specialist referral and psychological support to accompany drug treatment. Patients on long-term therapy need to be monitored both for progress and for side-effects.

Other drugs used for Neuropathic pain Amantadine hydrochloride, p. 412

ANALGESICS > PLANT ALKALOIDS

Capsaicin

● **INDICATIONS AND DOSE**

AXSAIN ®

Post-herpetic neuralgia
▸ TO THE SKIN
▸ Adult: Apply 3–4 times a day, dose to be applied sparingly; **important; after** lesions have healed, not more often than every 4 hours

Painful diabetic neuropathy (under expert supervision)
▸ TO THE SKIN
▸ Adult: Apply 3–4 times a day for 8 weeks then review, dose to be applied sparingly, not more often than every 4 hours

QUTENZA ®

Peripheral neuropathic pain in non-diabetic patients (under the supervision of a physician)
▸ BY TRANSDERMAL APPLICATION USING PATCHES
▸ Adult: (consult product literature)

ZACIN ®

Symptomatic relief in osteoarthritis
▸ TO THE SKIN
▸ Adult: Apply 4 times a day, dose to be applied sparingly, not more often than every 4 hours

● **CAUTIONS**

GENERAL CAUTIONS Avoid contact with broken skin · avoid contact with inflamed skin
SPECIFIC CAUTIONS
▸ With topical use Avoid contact with eyes · avoid hot shower or bath just before or after application (burning sensation enhanced) · avoid inhalation of vapours · not to be used under tight bandages
▸ With transdermal use avoid contact with the face, scalp or in proximity to mucous membranes · avoid holding near eyes or mucous membranes · recent cardiovascular events · uncontrolled hypertension

● **SIDE-EFFECTS**

GENERAL SIDE-EFFECTS
▸ Uncommon Cough
SPECIFIC SIDE-EFFECTS
▸ Common or very common
▸ With transdermal use Sensation abnormal
▸ Uncommon
▸ With transdermal use Atrioventricular block · eye irritation · muscle spasms · nausea · palpitations · peripheral oedema · skin reactions · tachycardia · taste altered · throat irritation
▸ Rare or very rare
▸ With topical use Sneezing · watering eye
▸ Frequency not known
▸ With topical use Asthma exacerbated · dyspnoea · skin burning sensation (particularly if too much used or if administered more than 4 times daily) · skin irritation

● **MONITORING REQUIREMENTS**
▸ With transdermal use Monitor blood pressure during treatment procedure.

● **HANDLING AND STORAGE**
▸ With topical use Wash hands immediately after use (or wash hands 30 minutes after application if hands treated).
▸ With transdermal use Nitrile gloves to be worn while handling patches and cleaning treatment areas (latex gloves do not provide adequate protection).

4

Nervous system

● NATIONAL FUNDING/ACCESS DECISIONS
QUTENZA ®

Scottish Medicines Consortium (SMC) Decisions
The *Scottish Medicines Consortium* has advised (January 2011) that capsaicin 179 mg (8%) patch (*Qutenza*®) is accepted for restricted use within NHS Scotland for the treatment of postherpetic neuralgia in patients who have not achieved adequate pain relief from, or who have not tolerated conventional first and second line treatments. Treatment should be under the supervision of a specialist in pain management.

● MEDICINAL FORMS
There can be variation in the licensing of different medicines containing the same drug.

Cutaneous patch
EXCIPIENTS: May contain Butylated hydroxyanisole
▸ Qutenza (Grunenthal Ltd)
　Capsaicin 179 mg Qutenza 179mg cutaneous patches |
　1 patch [PoM] £210.00

Cream
EXCIPIENTS: May contain Benzyl alcohol, cetostearyl alcohol (including cetyl and stearyl alcohol)
▸ Axsain (Teva UK Ltd)
　Capsaicin 750 microgram per 1 gram Axsain 0.075% cream |
　45 gram [PoM] £14.58 DT = £14.58
▸ Zacin (Teva UK Ltd)
　Capsaicin 250 microgram per 1 gram Zacin 0.025% cream |
　45 gram [PoM] £17.71 DT = £17.71

7　Sleep disorders

7.1　Insomnia

Hypnotics and anxiolytics

Overview

Most anxiolytics ('sedatives') will induce sleep when given at night and most hypnotics will sedate when given during the day. Prescribing of these drugs is widespread but dependence (both physical and psychological) and tolerance occur. This may lead to difficulty in withdrawing the drug after the patient has been taking it regularly for more than a few weeks. Hypnotics and anxiolytics should therefore be reserved for short courses to alleviate acute conditions after causal factors have been established.

Benzodiazepines are the most commonly used anxiolytics and hypnotics; they act at benzodiazepine receptors which are associated with gamma-aminobutyric acid (GABA) receptors. Older drugs such as meprobamate p. 343 and barbiturates are **not** recommended—they have more side-effects and interactions than benzodiazepines and are much more dangerous in overdosage.

Benzodiazepine indications

● Benzodiazepines are indicated for the short-term relief (two to four weeks only) of anxiety that is severe, disabling, or causing the patient unacceptable distress, occurring alone or in association with insomnia or short-term psychosomatic, organic, or psychotic illness.
● The use of benzodiazepines to treat short-term 'mild' anxiety is inappropriate.
● Benzodiazepines should be used to treat insomnia only when it is severe, disabling, or causing the patient extreme distress.

Dependence and withdrawal

Withdrawal of a benzodiazepine should be gradual because abrupt withdrawal may produce confusion, toxic psychosis, convulsions, or a condition resembling delirium tremens.

The benzodiazepine withdrawal syndrome may develop at any time up to 3 weeks after stopping a long-acting benzodiazepine, but may occur within a day in the case of a short-acting one. It is characterised by insomnia, anxiety, loss of appetite and of body-weight, tremor, perspiration, tinnitus, and perceptual disturbances. Some symptoms may be similar to the original complaint and encourage further prescribing; some symptoms may continue for weeks or months after stopping benzodiazepines.

Benzodiazepine withdrawal should be flexible and carried out at a reduction rate that is tolerable for the patient. The rate should depend on the initial dose of benzodiazepine, duration of use, and the patient's clinical response. Short-term users of benzodiazepines (2–4 weeks only) can usually taper off within 2–4 weeks. However, long-term users should be withdrawn over a much longer period of several months or more.

A suggested protocol for withdrawal for prescribed long-term benzodiazepine patients is as follows:

● Transfer patient stepwise, one dose at a time over about a week, to an equivalent daily dose of diazepam preferably taken at night.
● Reduce diazepam dose, usually by 1–2 mg every 2–4 weeks (in patients taking high doses of benzodiazepines, initially it may be appropriate to reduce the dose by up to one-tenth every 1–2 weeks). If uncomfortable withdrawal symptoms occur, maintain this dose until symptoms lessen.
● Reduce diazepam dose further, if necessary in smaller steps; steps of 500 micrograms may be appropriate towards the end of withdrawal. Then stop completely.
● For long-term patients, the period needed for complete withdrawal may vary from several months to a year or more.

Approximate equivalent doses, diazepam 5 mg
　≡ alprazolam 250 micrograms
　≡ clobazam 10 mg
　≡ clonazepam 250 micrograms
　≡ flurazepam 7.5–15 mg
　≡ chlordiazepoxide 12.5 mg
　≡ loprazolam 0.5–1 mg
　≡ lorazepam 500 micrograms
　≡ lormetazepam 0.5–1 mg
　≡ nitrazepam 5 mg
　≡ oxazepam 10 mg
　≡ temazepam 10 mg

Withdrawal symptoms for long-term users usually resolve within 6–18 months of the last dose. Some patients will recover more quickly, others may take longer. The addition of beta-blockers, antidepressants and antipsychotics should be avoided where possible.

Counselling can be of considerable help both during and after the taper.

Hypnotics

Before a hypnotic is prescribed the cause of the insomnia should be established and, where possible, underlying factors should be treated. However, it should be noted that some patients have unrealistic sleep expectations, and others understate their alcohol consumption which is often the cause of the insomnia. Short-acting hypnotics are preferable in patients with sleep onset insomnia, when sedation the following day is undesirable, or when prescribing for elderly patients. Long-acting hypnotics are indicated in patients with poor sleep maintenance (e.g. early morning waking) that causes daytime effects, when an anxiolytic effect is needed during the day, or when sedation the following day is acceptable.

Transient insomnia may occur in those who normally sleep well and may be due to extraneous factors such as noise, shift work, and jet lag. If a hypnotic is indicated one that is rapidly eliminated should be chosen, and only one or two doses should be given.

Short-term insomnia is usually related to an emotional problem or serious medical illness. It may last for a few weeks and may recur; a hypnotic can be useful but should not be given for more than three weeks (preferably only one week). Intermittent use is desirable with omission of some doses. A short-acting drug is usually appropriate.

Chronic insomnia is rarely benefited by hypnotics and is sometimes due to mild dependence caused by injudicious prescribing of hypnotics. Psychiatric disorders such as anxiety, depression, and abuse of drugs and alcohol are common causes. Sleep disturbance is very common in depressive illness and early wakening is often a useful pointer. The underlying psychiatric complaint should be treated, adapting the drug regimen to alleviate insomnia. For example, clomipramine hydrochloride p. 370 or mirtazapine p. 368 prescribed for depression will also help to promote sleep if taken at night. Other causes of insomnia include daytime cat-napping and physical causes such as pain, pruritus, and dyspnoea.

Hypnotics should **not** be prescribed indiscriminately and routine prescribing is undesirable. They should be reserved for short courses in the acutely distressed. Tolerance to their effects develops within 3 to 14 days of continuous use and long-term efficacy cannot be assured. A major drawback of long-term use is that withdrawal can cause rebound insomnia and a withdrawal syndrome.

Where prolonged administration is unavoidable hypnotics should be discontinued as soon as feasible and the patient warned that sleep may be disturbed for a few days before normal rhythm is re-established; broken sleep with vivid dreams may persist for several weeks.

Elderly
Benzodiazepines and the Z–drugs should be avoided in the elderly, because the elderly are at greater risk of becoming ataxic and confused, leading to falls and injury.

Dental patients
Some anxious patients may benefit from the use of hypnotics during dental procedures such as temazepam p. 481 or diazepam p. 340. Temazepam is preferred when it is important to minimise any residual effect the following day.

Benzodiazepines
Benzodiazepines used as hypnotics include nitrazepam p. 480 and flurazepam p. 479 which have a prolonged action and may give rise to residual effects on the following day; repeated doses tend to be cumulative.

Loprazolam p. 479, lormetazepam p. 480, and temazepam act for a shorter time and they have little or no hangover effect. Withdrawal phenomena are more common with the short-acting benzodiazepines.

If insomnia is associated with daytime anxiety then the use of a long-acting benzodiazepine anxiolytic such as diazepam given as a single dose at night may effectively treat both symptoms.

Zaleplon, zolpidem, and zopiclone
Zaleplon p. 483, zolpidem tartrate p. 483 and zopiclone p. 484 are non-benzodiazepine hypnotics (sometimes referred to as Z-drugs), but they act at the benzodiazepine receptor. They are not licensed for long-term use; dependence has been reported in a small number of patients. Zolpidem tartrate and zopiclone have a short duration of action; zaleplon is very short acting.

Chloral and derivatives
There is no convincing evidence that they are particularly useful in the elderly and their role as hypnotics is now very limited.

Clomethiazole
Clomethiazole p. 482 may be a useful hypnotic for elderly patients because of its freedom from hangover but, as with all hypnotics, routine administration is undesirable and dependence occurs.

Antihistamines
Some **antihistamines** such as promethazine hydrochloride p. 286 are on sale to the public for occasional insomnia; their prolonged duration of action can often cause drowsiness the following day. The sedative effect of antihistamines may diminish after a few days of continued treatment; antihistamines are associated with headache, psychomotor impairment and antimuscarinic effects.

Alcohol
Alcohol is a poor hypnotic because the diuretic action interferes with sleep during the latter part of the night. Alcohol also disturbs sleep patterns, and so can worsen sleep disorders.

Melatonin
Melatonin p. 482 is a pineal hormone; it is licensed for the short-term treatment of insomnia in adults over 55 years.

Anxiolytics

Benzodiazepine anxiolytics can be effective in alleviating anxiety states. Although these drugs are sometimes prescribed for stress-related symptoms, unhappiness, or minor physical disease, their use in such conditions is inappropriate. Benzodiazepine anxiolytics should not be used as sole treatment for chronic anxiety, and they are not appropriate for treating depression or chronic psychosis. In bereavement, psychological adjustment may be inhibited by benzodiazepines.

Anxiolytic benzodiazepine treatment should be limited to the lowest possible dose for the shortest possible time. Dependence is particularly likely in patients with a history of alcohol or drug abuse and in patients with marked personality disorders.

Some antidepressant drugs are licensed for use in anxiety and related disorders. Some antipsychotic drugs, in low doses, are also sometimes used in severe anxiety for their sedative action, but long-term use should be avoided because of the risk of adverse effects. The use of antihistamines (e.g. hydroxyzine hydrochloride p. 284) for their sedative effect in anxiety is not appropriate.

Beta-adrenoceptor blocking drugs do not affect psychological symptoms of anxiety, such as worry, tension, and fear, but they do reduce autonomic symptoms, such as palpitation and tremor; they do not reduce non-autonomic symptoms, such as muscle tension. Beta-blockers are therefore indicated for patients with predominantly somatic symptoms; this, in turn, may prevent the onset of worry and fear.

Benzodiazepines
Benzodiazepines are indicated for the *short-term relief of severe anxiety*; long-term use should be avoided. Diazepam, alprazolam p. 339, chlordiazepoxide hydrochloride p. 340, and clobazam p. 333 have a sustained action. Shorter-acting compounds such as lorazepam p. 335 and oxazepam p. 342 may be preferred in patients with hepatic impairment but they carry a greater risk of withdrawal symptoms.

In *panic disorders* (with or without agoraphobia) resistant to antidepressant therapy, a benzodiazepine may be used; alternatively, a benzodiazepine may be used as short-term adjunctive therapy at the start of antidepressant treatment to prevent the initial worsening of symptoms.

Diazepam or lorazepam are very occasionally administered intravenously for the *control of panic attacks*. This route is the most rapid but the procedure is not without risk and should be used only when alternative measures have failed. The intramuscular route has no advantage over the oral route.

Buspirone

Buspirone hydrochloride p. 338 is thought to act at specific serotonin ($5HT_{1A}$) receptors. Response to treatment may take up to 2 weeks. It does not alleviate the symptoms of benzodiazepine withdrawal. Therefore a patient taking a benzodiazepine still needs to have the benzodiazepine withdrawn gradually; it is advisable to do this before starting buspirone hydrochloride. The dependence and abuse potential of buspirone hydrochloride is low; it is, however, licensed for short-term use only (but specialists occasionally use it for several months).

Meprobamate

Meprobamate p. 343 is **less effective** than the benzodiazepines, more hazardous in overdosage, and can also induce dependence. It is **not** recommended.

Barbiturates

The intermediate-acting **barbiturates** have a place only in the treatment of severe intractable insomnia in patients **already taking** barbiturates; they should be **avoided** in the elderly. Intermediate-acting barbiturate preparations containing amobarbital sodium, butobarbital, and secobarbital sodium are available on a named patient basis.

The long-acting barbiturate phenobarbital is still sometimes of value in epilepsy but its use as a sedative is unjustified.

The very short-acting barbiturate thiopental sodium p. 335 is used in anaesthesia.

Increased hostility and aggression after barbiturates and alcohol usually indicates intoxication.

HYPNOTICS, SEDATIVES AND ANXIOLYTICS > BENZODIAZEPINES

Flurazepam

20-Jul-2017

● **INDICATIONS AND DOSE**

Insomnia (short-term use)

▸ BY MOUTH
  ▸ Adult: 15–30 mg once daily, dose to be taken at bedtime, for debilitated patients, use elderly dose
  ▸ Elderly: 15 mg once daily, dose to be taken at bedtime

● CONTRA-INDICATIONS Not for use alone to treat chronic psychosis · not for use alone to treat depression (or anxiety associated with depression) · respiratory depression

● CAUTIONS Acute porphyrias p. 1025 · hypoalbuminaemia · muscle weakness

  CAUTIONS, FURTHER INFORMATION

▸ Paradoxical effects A paradoxical increase in hostility and aggression may be reported by patients taking benzodiazepines. The effects range from talkativeness and excitement to aggressive and antisocial acts. Adjustment of the dose (up or down) sometimes attenuates the impulses. Increased anxiety and perceptual disorders are other paradoxical effects.

● INTERACTIONS → Appendix 1: flurazepam

● SIDE-EFFECTS

▸ **Common or very common** Taste altered
▸ **Rare or very rare** Abdominal discomfort · skin eruption
▸ **Frequency not known** Agranulocytosis · extrapyramidal symptoms · leucopenia · pancytopenia · psychotic disorder · rebound effect · suicide attempt · thrombocytopenia

● BREAST FEEDING Benzodiazepines are present in milk, and should be avoided if possible during breast-feeding.

● HEPATIC IMPAIRMENT Can precipitate coma. If treatment is necessary, benzodiazepines with shorter half-lives (such as temazepam or oxazepam) are safer. Avoid in severe impairment.

Dose adjustments Start with smaller initial doses or reduce dose.

● RENAL IMPAIRMENT
  Dose adjustments Start with small doses in severe impairment.

● PATIENT AND CARER ADVICE
  Driving and skilled tasks May impair judgement and increase reaction time, and so affect ability to drive or operate machinery; they increase the effects of alcohol. Moreover the hangover effects of a night dose may impair driving on the following day.

● NATIONAL FUNDING/ACCESS DECISIONS
  NHS restrictions Flurazepam capsules are not prescribable in NHS primary care.

● MEDICINAL FORMS
  There can be variation in the licensing of different medicines containing the same drug.

  Capsule
  CAUTIONARY AND ADVISORY LABELS 19
  ▸ Dalmane (Meda Pharmaceuticals Ltd)
    Flurazepam (as Flurazepam hydrochloride) **15 mg** Dalmane 15mg capsules | 30 capsule [PoM] £6.73 [CD4-1]
    Flurazepam (as Flurazepam hydrochloride) **30 mg** Dalmane 30mg capsules | 30 capsule [PoM] £8.63 [CD4-1]

Loprazolam

● **INDICATIONS AND DOSE**

Insomnia (short-term use)

▸ BY MOUTH
  ▸ Adult: 1 mg once daily, then increased to 1.5–2 mg once daily if required, dose to be taken at bedtime, for debilitated patients, use elderly dose
  ▸ Elderly: 0.5–1 mg once daily, dose to be taken at bedtime

● CONTRA-INDICATIONS Not for use alone to treat chronic psychosis · not for use alone to treat depression (or anxiety associated with depression) · respiratory depression

● CAUTIONS Acute porphyrias p. 1025 · hypoalbuminaemia · muscle weakness

  CAUTIONS, FURTHER INFORMATION

▸ Paradoxical effects A paradoxical increase in hostility and aggression may be reported by patients taking benzodiazepines. The effects range from talkativeness and excitement to aggressive and antisocial acts. Adjustment of the dose (up or down) sometimes attenuates the impulses. Increased anxiety and perceptual disorders are other paradoxical effects.

● INTERACTIONS → Appendix 1: loprazolam

● SIDE-EFFECTS Adjustment disorder · cognitive disorder · muscle tone decreased · speech disorder · vision blurred

● BREAST FEEDING Benzodiazepines are present in milk, and should be avoided if possible during breast-feeding.

● HEPATIC IMPAIRMENT Can precipitate coma. If treatment is necessary, benzodiazepines with shorter half-lives (such as temazepam or oxazepam) are safer. Avoid in severe impairment.
  Dose adjustments Start with smaller initial doses or reduce dose.

● RENAL IMPAIRMENT
  Dose adjustments Start with small doses in severe impairment.

● PATIENT AND CARER ADVICE
  Driving and skilled tasks May impair judgement and increase reaction time, and so affect ability to drive or operate machinery; they increase the effects of alcohol. Moreover the hangover effects of a night dose may impair driving on the following day.

● MEDICINAL FORMS
There can be variation in the licensing of different medicines containing the same drug.

Tablet
CAUTIONARY AND ADVISORY LABELS 19
▸ Loprazolam (Non-proprietary)
 Loprazolam (as Loprazolam mesilate) 1 mg Loprazolam 1mg tablets | 28 tablet [PoM] £18.00 DT = £18.00 [CD4-1]

⚑ 339

Lormetazepam

● INDICATIONS AND DOSE

Insomnia (short-term use)
▸ BY MOUTH
▸ **Adult:** 0.5–1.5 mg once daily, dose to be taken at bedtime, for debilitated patients, use elderly dose
▸ **Elderly:** 500 micrograms once daily, dose to be taken at bedtime

● CONTRA-INDICATIONS Not for use alone to treat chronic psychosis · not for use alone to treat depression (or anxiety associated with depression) · respiratory depression
● CAUTIONS Acute porphyrias p. 1025 · hypoalbuminaemia · muscle weakness
 CAUTIONS, FURTHER INFORMATION
▸ Paradoxical effects A paradoxical increase in hostility and aggression may be reported by patients taking benzodiazepines. The effects range from talkativeness and excitement to aggressive and antisocial acts. Adjustment of the dose (up or down) sometimes attenuates the impulses. Increased anxiety and perceptual disorders are other paradoxical effects.
● INTERACTIONS → Appendix 1: lormetazepam
● SIDE-EFFECTS
▸ **Common or very common** Asthenia
▸ **Rare or very rare** Agranulocytosis · allergic dermatitis · apnoea · appetite change · coma · constipation · disinhibition · euphoric mood · extrapyramidal symptoms · hyponatraemia · hypothermia · leucopenia · memory loss · obstructive pulmonary disease exacerbated · pancytopenia · saliva altered · sexual dysfunction · SIADH · speech slurred · thrombocytopenia · vision blurred
▸ **Frequency not known** Suicide attempt
● BREAST FEEDING Benzodiazepines are present in milk, and should be avoided if possible during breast-feeding.
● HEPATIC IMPAIRMENT Can precipitate coma. If treatment is necessary, benzodiazepines with shorter half-lives (such as temazepam or oxazepam) are safer. Avoid in severe impairment.
 Dose adjustments Start with smaller initial doses or reduce dose.
● RENAL IMPAIRMENT
 Dose adjustments Start with small doses in severe impairment.
● PATIENT AND CARER ADVICE
 Driving and skilled tasks May impair judgement and increase reaction time, and so affect ability to drive or operate machinery; they increase the effects of alcohol. Moreover the hangover effects of a night dose may impair driving on the following day.
● MEDICINAL FORMS
There can be variation in the licensing of different medicines containing the same drug. Forms available from special-order manufacturers include: oral suspension

Tablet
CAUTIONARY AND ADVISORY LABELS 19
▸ Lormetazepam (Non-proprietary)
 Lormetazepam 500 microgram Lormetazepam 500microgram tablets | 30 tablet [PoM] £64.17 DT = £8.98 [CD4-1]

Lormetazepam 1 mg Lormetazepam 1mg tablets | 30 tablet [PoM] £12.38 DT = £4.91 [CD4-1]

⚑ 339

Nitrazepam

● INDICATIONS AND DOSE

Insomnia (short-term use)
▸ BY MOUTH
▸ **Adult:** 5–10 mg daily, dose to be taken at bedtime, for debilitated patients, use elderly dose
▸ **Elderly:** 2.5–5 mg daily, dose to be taken at bedtime

● CONTRA-INDICATIONS Not for use alone to treat chronic psychosis · not for use alone to treat depression (or anxiety associated with depression) · respiratory depression
● CAUTIONS Acute porphyrias p. 1025 · hypoalbuminaemia · muscle weakness
 CAUTIONS, FURTHER INFORMATION
▸ Paradoxical effects A paradoxical increase in hostility and aggression may be reported by patients taking benzodiazepines. The effects range from talkativeness and excitement to aggressive and antisocial acts. Adjustment of the dose (up or down) sometimes attenuates the impulses. Increased anxiety and perceptual disorders are other paradoxical effects.
● INTERACTIONS → Appendix 1: nitrazepam
● SIDE-EFFECTS
▸ **Common or very common** Movement disorders
▸ **Uncommon** Concentration impaired
▸ **Rare or very rare** Abdominal distress · muscle cramps · psychiatric disorder · skin reactions · Stevens-Johnson syndrome
▸ **Frequency not known** Drug abuse
● BREAST FEEDING Benzodiazepines are present in milk, and should be avoided if possible during breast-feeding.
● HEPATIC IMPAIRMENT Can precipitate coma. If treatment is necessary, benzodiazepines with shorter half-lives (such as temazepam or oxazepam) are safer. Avoid in severe impairment.
 Dose adjustments Start with smaller initial doses or reduce dose.
● RENAL IMPAIRMENT
 Dose adjustments Start with small doses in severe impairment.
● PATIENT AND CARER ADVICE
 Driving and skilled tasks May impair judgement and increase reaction time, and so affect ability to drive or operate machinery; they increase the effects of alcohol. Moreover the hangover effects of a night dose may impair driving on the following day.

● MEDICINAL FORMS
There can be variation in the licensing of different medicines containing the same drug. Forms available from special-order manufacturers include: oral suspension
Oral suspension
CAUTIONARY AND ADVISORY LABELS 19
▸ Nitrazepam (Non-proprietary)
 Nitrazepam 500 microgram per 1 ml Nitrazepam 2.5mg/5ml oral suspension | 70 ml [PoM] £114.00 DT = £114.00 [CD4-1]
Tablet
CAUTIONARY AND ADVISORY LABELS 19
▸ Nitrazepam (Non-proprietary)
 Nitrazepam 5 mg Nitrazepam 5mg tablets | 28 tablet [PoM] £5.00 DT = £0.61 [CD4-1] | 500 tablet [PoM] £13.93 [CD4-1]
▸ Mogadon (Meda Pharmaceuticals Ltd)
 Nitrazepam 5 mg Mogadon 5mg tablets | 30 tablet [PoM] £5.76 [CD4-1]

F 339

Temazepam

- **INDICATIONS AND DOSE**

Insomnia (short-term use)
▶ BY MOUTH
▶ Adult: 10–20 mg once daily, alternatively 30–40 mg once daily, higher dose range only to be administered in exceptional circumstances, dose to be taken at bedtime, for debilitated patients, use elderly dose
▶ Elderly: 10 mg once daily, alternatively 20 mg once daily, higher dose only to be administered in exceptional circumstances, dose to be taken at bedtime

Conscious sedation for dental procedures
▶ BY MOUTH
▶ Adult: 15–30 mg, to be administered 30–60 minutes before procedure

Premedication before surgery or investigatory procedures
▶ BY MOUTH
▶ Adult: 10–20 mg, to be taken 1–2 hours before procedure, alternatively 30 mg, to be taken 1–2 hours before procedure, higher alternate dose only administered in exceptional circumstances
▶ Elderly: 10 mg, to be taken 1–2 hours before procedure, alternatively 20 mg, to be taken 1–2 hours before procedure, higher alternate dose only administered in exceptional circumstances

- **UNLICENSED USE** Temazepam doses in BNF may differ from those in product literature.
  Not licensed for conscious sedation for dental procedures.
- **CONTRA-INDICATIONS** CNS depression · compromised airway · hyperkinesis · not for use alone to treat chronic psychosis · not for use alone to treat depression (or anxiety associated with depression) · obsessional state · phobic states · respiratory depression
- **CAUTIONS** Hypoalbuminaemia · muscle weakness · organic brain changes
  CAUTIONS, FURTHER INFORMATION
  ▶ Paradoxical effects A paradoxical increase in hostility and aggression may be reported by patients taking benzodiazepines. The effects range from talkativeness and excitement to aggressive and antisocial acts. Adjustment of the dose (up or down) sometimes attenuates the impulses. Increased anxiety and perceptual disorders are other paradoxical effects.
- **INTERACTIONS** → Appendix 1: temazepam
- **SIDE-EFFECTS** Dreaming excessive · drug abuse · dry mouth · hypersalivation · speech slurred
- **BREAST FEEDING** Benzodiazepines are present in milk, and should be avoided if possible during breast-feeding.
- **HEPATIC IMPAIRMENT** Can precipitate coma. Avoid in severe impairment. If treatment is necessary, benzodiazepines with shorter half-lives are safer.
  Dose adjustments Start with smaller initial doses or reduce dose.
- **RENAL IMPAIRMENT**
  Dose adjustments Start with small doses in severe impairment.
- **PATIENT AND CARER ADVICE**
  Driving and skilled tasks May impair judgement and increase reaction time, and so affect ability to drive or operate machinery; they increase the effects of alcohol. Moreover, the hangover effects of a night dose may impair driving on the following day.
  Patients given sedatives and analgesics during minor outpatient procedures should be very carefully warned about the risks of undertaking skilled tasks (e.g. driving) afterwards. Responsible persons should be available to

take patients home afterwards. The dangers of taking **alcohol** should be emphasised.

- **PROFESSION SPECIFIC INFORMATION**
  Dental practitioners' formulary
  Temazepam Tablets and Oral Solution may be prescribed.
- **MEDICINAL FORMS**
  There can be variation in the licensing of different medicines containing the same drug. Forms available from special-order manufacturers include: oral suspension, oral solution
  Oral solution
  CAUTIONARY AND ADVISORY LABELS 19
  ▶ Temazepam (Non-proprietary)
  Temazepam 2 mg per 1 ml Temazepam 10mg/5ml oral solution sugar free sugar-free | 300 ml [PoM] £184.50 DT = £169.44 [CD3]
  Tablet
  CAUTIONARY AND ADVISORY LABELS 19
  ▶ Temazepam (Non-proprietary)
  Temazepam 10 mg Temazepam 10mg tablets | 28 tablet [PoM] £35.00 DT = £1.36 [CD3] | 500 tablet [PoM] £24.29–£624.82 [CD3]
  Temazepam 20 mg Temazepam 20mg tablets | 28 tablet [PoM] £35.00 DT = £1.43 [CD3] | 250 tablet [PoM] £12.77–£307.94 [CD3]

HYPNOTICS, SEDATIVES AND ANXIOLYTICS ›
NON-BENZODIAZEPINE HYPNOTICS AND SEDATIVES

Chloral hydrate

- **INDICATIONS AND DOSE**

Insomnia (short-term use) using Chloral Mixture, BP 2000
▶ BY MOUTH USING ORAL SOLUTION
▶ Adult: 0.5–2 g daily, dose to be taken at bedtime

Insomnia (short-term use), using chloral hydrate 143.3 mg/5 mL oral solution
▶ BY MOUTH USING ORAL SOLUTION
▶ Adult: 430–860 mg once daily (max. per dose 2 g), dose to be taken with water or milk at bedtime

Insomnia (short-term use), using chloral betaine 707 mg (≡ 414 mg chloral hydrate) tablets
▶ BY MOUTH USING TABLETS
▶ Adult: 1–2 tablets, alternatively 414–828 mg once daily, dose to be taken with water or milk at bedtime; maximum 4 tablets per day; maximum 2 g per day

- **CONTRA-INDICATIONS** Acute porphyrias p. 1025 · gastritis · severe cardiac disease
- **CAUTIONS** Avoid contact with mucous membranes · avoid contact with skin · avoid prolonged use (and abrupt withdrawal thereafter) · reduce dose in debilitated · reduce dose in elderly
- **INTERACTIONS** → Appendix 1: chloral hydrate
- **SIDE-EFFECTS** Agitation · allergic dermatitis · ataxia · confusion · delirium (more common on abrupt discontinuation) · drug tolerance · drug use disorders · gastrointestinal discomfort · gastrointestinal disorders · headache · injury · ketonuria · kidney injury
- **PREGNANCY** Avoid.
- **BREAST FEEDING** Risk of sedation in infant—avoid.
- **HEPATIC IMPAIRMENT** Can precipitate coma. Avoid in severe impairment.
  Dose adjustments Reduce dose in mild to moderate impairment.
- **RENAL IMPAIRMENT** Avoid in severe impairment.
- **DIRECTIONS FOR ADMINISTRATION** For administration by mouth dilute liquid with plenty of water or juice to mask unpleasant taste.
- **PRESCRIBING AND DISPENSING INFORMATION** Flavours of oral liquid formulations may include black currant.

Nervous system

4

When prepared extemporaneously, the BP states Chloral Mixture, BP 2000 consists of chloral hydrate 500 mg/5 mL in a suitable vehicle.

● PATIENT AND CARER ADVICE
Driving and skilled tasks Drowsiness may persist the next day and affect performance of skilled tasks (e.g. driving); effects of alcohol enhanced.

● LESS SUITABLE FOR PRESCRIBING Chloral hydrate is less suitable for prescribing in insomnia.

● MEDICINAL FORMS
There can be variation in the licensing of different medicines containing the same drug. Forms available from special-order manufacturers include: oral suspension, oral solution
Tablet
CAUTIONARY AND ADVISORY LABELS 19, 27
▸ Chloral hydrate (Non-proprietary)
Chloral betaine 707 mg Cloral betaine 707mg tablets | 30 tablet PoM £138.59 DT = £138.59
Oral solution
CAUTIONARY AND ADVISORY LABELS 1(paediatric solution only), 19 (solution other than paediatric only), 27
▸ Chloral hydrate (Non-proprietary)
Chloral hydrate 28.66 mg per 1 ml Chloral hydrate 143.3mg/5ml oral solution BP | 150 ml PoM £244.25 DT = £244.25

Clomethiazole

(Chlormethiazole)

● INDICATIONS AND DOSE

Severe insomnia (short-term use)
▸ BY MOUTH USING CAPSULES
▸ Elderly: 192–384 mg once daily, dose to be taken at bedtime
▸ BY MOUTH USING ORAL SOLUTION
▸ Elderly: 5–10 mL once daily, dose to be taken at bedtime

Restlessness and agitation
▸ BY MOUTH USING CAPSULES
▸ Elderly: 192 mg 3 times a day
▸ BY MOUTH USING ORAL SOLUTION
▸ Elderly: 5 mL 3 times a day

Alcohol withdrawal
▸ BY MOUTH USING CAPSULES
▸ Adult: Initially 2–4 capsules, to be repeated if necessary after some hours. 9–12 capsules daily in 3–4 divided doses on day 1 (first 24 hours), then 6–8 capsules daily in 3–4 divided doses on day 2, then 4–6 capsules daily in 3–4 divided doses on day 3, dose then to be gradually reduced over days 4–6, total duration of treatment for no more than 9 days
▸ BY MOUTH USING ORAL SOLUTION
▸ Adult: Initially 10–20 mL, to be repeated if necessary after some hours, then 45–60 mL daily in 3–4 divided doses on day 1 (first 24 hours), then 30–40 mL daily in 3–4 divided doses on day 2, then 20–30 mL daily in 3–4 divided doses on day 3, dose then to be gradually reduced over days 4–6, total duration of treatment for no more than 9 days

● CONTRA-INDICATIONS Acute pulmonary insufficiency · alcohol-dependent patients who continue to drink

● CAUTIONS Avoid prolonged use (and abrupt withdrawal thereafter) · cardiac disease (confusional state may indicate hypoxia) · chronic pulmonary insufficiency · elderly · excessive sedation may occur (particularly with higher doses); · history of drug abuse · marked personality disorder · respiratory disease (confusional state may indicate hypoxia) · sleep apnoea syndrome

● INTERACTIONS → Appendix 1: clomethiazole

● SIDE-EFFECTS Agitation · bronchial secretion increased · confusion · conjunctival irritation · drug dependence · drug tolerance · excessive sedation · gastrointestinal disorder · hangover · nasal complaints · skin reactions · upper airway secretion increased

● PREGNANCY Avoid if possible—especially during the first and third trimesters.

● BREAST FEEDING Use only if benefit outweighs risk—present in breast milk but effects unknown.

● HEPATIC IMPAIRMENT Can precipitate coma.
Dose adjustments Reduce dose.

● RENAL IMPAIRMENT Increased cerebral sensitivity.
Dose adjustments Start with small doses in severe impairment.

● PATIENT AND CARER ADVICE
Driving and skilled tasks Drowsiness may persist the next day and affect performance of skilled tasks (e.g. driving); effects of alcohol enhanced.

● MEDICINAL FORMS
There can be variation in the licensing of different medicines containing the same drug.
Oral solution
CAUTIONARY AND ADVISORY LABELS 19
EXCIPIENTS: May contain Alcohol
▸ Clomethiazole (Non-proprietary)
Clomethiazole (as Clomethiazole edisilate) 50 mg per 1 ml Clomethiazole 31.5mg/ml oral solution sugar free sugar-free | 300 ml PoM £30.00
Capsule
CAUTIONARY AND ADVISORY LABELS 19
▸ Clomethiazole (Non-proprietary)
Clomethiazole 192 mg Clomethiazole 192mg capsules | 60 capsule PoM £30.00–£32.80 DT = £32.80

Melatonin

● INDICATIONS AND DOSE

Insomnia (short-term use)
▸ BY MOUTH USING MODIFIED-RELEASE TABLETS
▸ Adult 55 years and over: 2 mg once daily for up to 13 weeks, dose to be taken 1–2 hours before bedtime

● CAUTIONS Autoimmune disease (manufacturer advises avoid—no information available)

● INTERACTIONS → Appendix 1: melatonin

● SIDE-EFFECTS
▸ **Common or very common** Arthralgia · headaches · increased risk of infection · pain
▸ **Uncommon** Anxiety · asthenia · chest pain · dizziness · drowsiness · dry mouth · gastrointestinal discomfort · hyperbilirubinaemia · hypertension · menopausal symptoms · mood altered · movement disorders · nausea · night sweats · oral disorders · skin reactions · sleep disorders · urine abnormalities · weight increased
▸ **Rare or very rare** Aggression · angina pectoris · arthritis · concentration impaired · crying · depression · disorientation · electrolyte imbalance · excessive tearing · gastrointestinal disorders · haematuria · hot flush · hypertriglyceridaemia · leucopenia · memory loss · muscle complaints · nail disorder · palpitations · paraesthesia · partial complex seizure · prostatitis · sexual dysfunction · syncope · thirst · thrombocytopenia · urinary disorders · vertigo · vision disorders · vomiting
▸ **Frequency not known** Angioedema · galactorrhoea

● PREGNANCY No information available—avoid.

● BREAST FEEDING Present in milk—avoid.

● HEPATIC IMPAIRMENT Clearance reduced—avoid.

● RENAL IMPAIRMENT No information available—use with caution.

- MEDICINAL FORMS
There can be variation in the licensing of different medicines
containing the same drug. Forms available from special-order
manufacturers include: modified-release tablet
Modified-release tablet
CAUTIONARY AND ADVISORY LABELS 2, 21, 25
  ▸ Melatonin (Non-proprietary)
    Melatonin 3 mg Melatonin 3mg modified-release tablets |
    120 tablet PoM �S
  ▸ Circadin (Flynn Pharma Ltd)
    Melatonin 2 mg Circadin 2mg modified-release tablets |
    30 tablet PoM £15.39 DT = £15.39

Zaleplon

- INDICATIONS AND DOSE
Insomnia (short-term use)
  ▸ BY MOUTH
  ▸ Adult: 10 mg daily for up to 2 weeks, dose to be taken at
    bedtime or after going to bed if difficulty falling asleep
  ▸ Elderly: 5 mg daily for up to 2 weeks, dose to be taken
    at bedtime or after going to bed if difficulty falling
    asleep

- CONTRA-INDICATIONS Marked neuromuscular respiratory
weakness · sleep apnoea syndrome · unstable myasthenia
gravis
- CAUTIONS Avoid prolonged use (risk of tolerance and
withdrawal symptoms) · depression (risk of suicidal
ideation) · history of alcohol abuse · history of drug abuse ·
muscle weakness · myasthenia gravis · respiratory
insufficiency (avoid if severe)
- INTERACTIONS → Appendix 1: zaleplon
- SIDE-EFFECTS
  ▸ **Common or very common** Drowsiness · dysmenorrhoea ·
    memory loss · paraesthesia
  ▸ **Uncommon** Altered smell sensation · appetite decreased ·
    asthenia · concentration impaired · confusion ·
    coordination abnormal · depersonalisation · depression ·
    dizziness · hallucination · hearing impairment · nausea ·
    photosensitivity reaction · speech disorder · visual
    impairment
  ▸ **Frequency not known** Paradoxical drug reaction · sleep
    walking
  SIDE-EFFECTS, FURTHER INFORMATION A paradoxical
  increase in hostility, anxiety and aggression has been
  reported. The effects range from talkativeness and
  excitement to aggression.
- PREGNANCY Use only if necessary and restrict to
occasional short-term use. Risk of withdrawal symptoms
in neonate if used in late pregnancy.
- BREAST FEEDING Present in milk but amount probably too
small to be harmful.
- HEPATIC IMPAIRMENT Can precipitate coma. Avoid if
severe impairment.
  Dose adjustments Reduce dose to 5 mg.
- RENAL IMPAIRMENT Avoid in severe impairment.
- PATIENT AND CARER ADVICE Patients should be advised
not to take a second dose during a single night.
- NATIONAL FUNDING/ACCESS DECISIONS
NICE decisions
  ▸ **Zaleplon, zolpidem, and zopiclone for the short-term
    management of insomnia (April 2004)** NICE TA77
    Zaleplon is recommended for the short-term management
    of severe insomnia that interferes with normal daily life,
    and should be prescribed for short periods of time only.
    www.nice.org.uk/TA77
- MEDICINAL FORMS
No licensed medicines listed.

Zolpidem tartrate

- INDICATIONS AND DOSE
Insomnia (short-term use)
  ▸ BY MOUTH
  ▸ Adult: 10 mg daily for up to 4 weeks, dose to be taken at
    bedtime, for debilitated patients, use elderly dose
  ▸ Elderly: 5 mg daily for up to 4 weeks, dose to be taken
    at bedtime

- CONTRA-INDICATIONS Acute respiratory depression ·
marked neuromuscular respiratory weakness · obstructive
sleep apnoea · psychotic illness · severe respiratory
depression · unstable myasthenia gravis
- CAUTIONS Avoid prolonged use (and abrupt withdrawal
thereafter) · depression · elderly · history of alcohol abuse ·
history of drug abuse · muscle weakness · myasthenia
gravis
- INTERACTIONS → Appendix 1: zolpidem
- SIDE-EFFECTS
  ▸ **Common or very common** Abdominal pain · anterograde
    amnesia · anxiety · back pain · diarrhoea · dizziness · fatigue
    · hallucination · headache · increased risk of infection ·
    nausea · sleep disorders · vomiting
  ▸ **Uncommon** Confusion · diplopia · irritability
  ▸ **Frequency not known** Angioedema · behaviour abnormal ·
    concentration impaired · delusions · depression · drug
    dependence · drug tolerance · fall · gait abnormal · hepatic
    disorders · hyperhidrosis · level of consciousness decreased
    · libido disorder · muscle weakness · psychosis · respiratory
    depression · skin reactions · speech disorder · withdrawal
    syndrome
- PREGNANCY Avoid regular use (risk of neonatal
withdrawal symptoms); high doses during late pregnancy
or labour may cause neonatal hypothermia, hypotonia,
and respiratory depression.
- BREAST FEEDING Small amounts present in milk—avoid.
- HEPATIC IMPAIRMENT Can precipitate coma. Avoid if
severe impairment.
  Dose adjustments Reduce dose to 5 mg.
- RENAL IMPAIRMENT Use with caution.
- PATIENT AND CARER ADVICE
Driving and skilled tasks Drowsiness may persist the next
day—leave at least 8 hours between taking zolpidem and
performing skilled tasks (e.g. driving, or operating
machinery); effects of alcohol and other CNS depressants
enhanced.
- NATIONAL FUNDING/ACCESS DECISIONS
NICE decisions
  ▸ **Zaleplon, zolpidem, and zopiclone for the short-term
    management of insomnia (April 2004)** NICE TA77
    Zolpidem is recommended for the short-term
    management of severe insomnia that interferes with
    normal daily life, and should be prescribed for short
    periods of time only.
    www.nice.org.uk/TA77
- MEDICINAL FORMS
There can be variation in the licensing of different medicines
containing the same drug.
Tablet
CAUTIONARY AND ADVISORY LABELS 19
  ▸ Zolpidem tartrate (Non-proprietary)
    Zolpidem tartrate 5 mg Zolpidem 5mg tablets | 28 tablet PoM
    £3.08 DT = £0.75 CD4–1
    Zolpidem tartrate 10 mg Zolpidem 10mg tablets | 28 tablet PoM
    £4.48 DT = £0.78 CD4–1 | 30 tablet PoM £4.48 CD4–1
  ▸ Stilnoct (Sanofi)
    Zolpidem tartrate 5 mg Stilnoct 5mg tablets | 28 tablet PoM £1.10
    DT = £0.75 CD4–1
    Zolpidem tartrate 10 mg Stilnoct 10mg tablets | 28 tablet PoM
    £1.00 DT = £0.78 CD4–1

4

Nervous system

Zopiclone

- **INDICATIONS AND DOSE**

Insomnia (short-term use)
▶ BY MOUTH
- ▶ **Adult:** 7.5 mg once daily for up to 4 weeks, dose to be taken at bedtime
- ▶ **Elderly:** Initially 3.75 mg once daily for up to 4 weeks, dose to be taken at bedtime, increased if necessary to 7.5 mg daily

Insomnia (short-term use) in patients with chronic pulmonary insufficiency
▶ BY MOUTH
- ▶ **Adult:** Initially 3.75 mg once daily for up to 4 weeks, dose to be taken at bedtime, increased if necessary to 7.5 mg daily

- **CONTRA-INDICATIONS** Marked neuromuscular respiratory weakness · respiratory failure · severe sleep apnoea syndrome · unstable myasthenia gravis
- **CAUTIONS** Avoid prolonged use (risk of tolerance and withdrawal symptoms) · chronic pulmonary insufficiency (increased risk of respiratory depression) · elderly · history of drug abuse · muscle weakness · myasthenia gravis (avoid if unstable) · psychiatric illness
- **INTERACTIONS** → Appendix 1: zopiclone
- **SIDE-EFFECTS**
- ▶ **Common or very common** Dry mouth · taste bitter
- ▶ **Uncommon** Anxiety · dizziness · fatigue · headache · nausea · sleep disorders · vomiting
- ▶ **Rare or very rare** Behaviour abnormal · confusion · dyspnoea · fall · hallucination · irritability · libido disorder · memory impairment · skin reactions
- ▶ **Frequency not known** Cognitive disorder · concentration impaired · delusions · depressed mood · diplopia · drug dependence · dyspepsia · movement disorders · muscle weakness · paraesthesia · respiratory depression · speech disorder · withdrawal syndrome
- **PREGNANCY** Not recommended (risk of neonatal withdrawal symptoms). Use during late pregnancy or labour may cause neonatal hypothermia, hypotonia, and respiratory depression.
- **BREAST FEEDING** Present in milk—avoid.
- **HEPATIC IMPAIRMENT** Avoid in severe impairment—can precipitate encephalopathy.
  Dose adjustments Reduce dose to 3.75 mg in mild to moderate impairment, dose can be increased with caution if necessary.
- **RENAL IMPAIRMENT** Increased cerebral sensitivity.
  Dose adjustments Start with reduced dose of 3.75 mg.
- **PATIENT AND CARER ADVICE**
  Driving and skilled tasks Drowsiness may persist the next day and affect performance of skilled tasks (e.g. driving); effects of alcohol enhanced.
- **NATIONAL FUNDING/ACCESS DECISIONS**

  NICE decisions
- ▶ **Zaleplon, zolpidem and zopiclone for the short-term management of insomnia (April 2004)** NICE TA77
  Zopiclone is recommended for the short-term management of severe insomnia that interferes with normal daily life, and should be prescribed for short periods of time only.
  www.nice.org.uk/TA77

- **MEDICINAL FORMS**
  There can be variation in the licensing of different medicines containing the same drug. Forms available from special-order manufacturers include: oral suspension, oral solution

Tablet
CAUTIONARY AND ADVISORY LABELS 19, 25
- ▶ Zopiclone (Non-proprietary)
  Zopiclone 3.75 mg Zopiclone 3.75mg tablets | 28 tablet [PoM] £2.49 DT = £0.66 [CD4-1]
  Zopiclone 7.5 mg Zopiclone 7.5mg tablets | 28 tablet [PoM] £3.75 DT = £0.69 [CD4-1]
- ▶ Zimovane (Sanofi)
  Zopiclone 3.75 mg Zimovane LS 3.75mg tablets | 28 tablet [PoM] £2.24 DT = £0.66 [CD4-1]
  Zopiclone 7.5 mg Zimovane 7.5mg tablets | 28 tablet [PoM] £3.26 DT = £0.69 [CD4-1]

7.2 Narcolepsy

Other drugs used for Narcolepsy Dexamfetamine sulfate, p. 347 · Methylphenidate hydrochloride, p. 345

CENTRAL NERVOUS SYSTEM DEPRESSANTS

Sodium oxybate

- **DRUG ACTION** A central nervous system depressant.

- **INDICATIONS AND DOSE**

Narcolepsy with cataplexy (under expert supervision)
▶ BY MOUTH
- ▶ **Adult:** Initially 2.25 g daily, dose to be taken on retiring and 2.25 g after 2.5–4 hours, then increased in steps of 1.5 g daily in 2 divided doses, dose adjusted according to response at intervals of 1–2 weeks; dose titration should be repeated if restarting after interval of more than 14 days, maximum 9 g daily in 2 divided doses

DOSE ADJUSTMENTS DUE TO INTERACTIONS
- ▶ Manufacturer advises reduce dose by 20 % with concurrent use of sodium valproate or valproic acid.

- **CONTRA-INDICATIONS** Major depression · succinic semi-aldehyde dehydrogenase deficiency
- **CAUTIONS** Body mass index of 40 kg/m^2 or greater (higher risk of sleep apnoea) · elderly · epilepsy · heart failure (high sodium content) · history of depression · history of drug abuse · hypertension (high sodium content) · respiratory disorders · risk of discontinuation effects including rebound cataplexy and withdrawal symptoms
- **INTERACTIONS** → Appendix 1: sodium oxybate
- **SIDE-EFFECTS**
- ▶ **Common or very common** Abdominal pain upper · anxiety · appetite abnormal · arthralgia · asthenia · back pain · concentration impaired · confusion · depression · diarrhoea · dizziness · dyspnoea · fall · feeling drunk · headache · hyperhidrosis · hypertension · increased risk of infection · movement disorders · muscle spasms · nasal congestion · nausea · palpitations · peripheral oedema · sedation · sensation abnormal · skin reactions · sleep disorders · sleep paralysis · snoring · taste altered · tremor · urinary disorders · vertigo · vision blurred · vomiting · weight decreased
- ▶ **Uncommon** Behaviour abnormal · faecal incontinence · hallucination · memory loss · psychosis · suicidal tendencies · thinking abnormal
- ▶ **Frequency not known** Angioedema · dehydration · delusions · dry mouth · homicidal ideation · loss of consciousness · mood altered · respiratory depression · seizure · sleep apnoea
- **PREGNANCY** Avoid.

- **HEPATIC IMPAIRMENT**
  Dose adjustments Halve initial dose.
- **RENAL IMPAIRMENT** Caution—contains 3.96 mmol Na⁺ per mL.
- **DIRECTIONS FOR ADMINISTRATION** Dilute each dose with 60 mL water; prepare both doses before retiring. Observe the same time interval (2–3 hours) each night between the last meal and the first dose.
- **PATIENT AND CARER ADVICE** Patients or carers should be given advice on how to administer sodium oxybate oral solution.
  Driving and skilled tasks Leave at least 6 hours between taking sodium oxybate and performing skilled tasks (e.g. driving or operating machinery); effects of alcohol and other CNS depressants enhanced.

- **MEDICINAL FORMS**
  There can be variation in the licensing of different medicines containing the same drug.
  Oral solution
  CAUTIONARY AND ADVISORY LABELS 13, 19
  ELECTROLYTES: May contain Sodium
  ▸ Xyrem (UCB Pharma Ltd)
    Sodium oxybate 500 mg per 1 ml Xyrem 500mg/ml oral solution sugar-free | 180 ml [PoM] £360.00 DT = £360.00 [CD2]

CNS STIMULANTS

Pitolisant   11-Apr-2017

- **DRUG ACTION** Pitolisant is a histamine H₃-receptor antagonist which enhances the activity of brain histaminergic neurons.

- **INDICATIONS AND DOSE**

  Narcolepsy with or without cataplexy (initiated by a specialist)
  ▸ BY MOUTH
  ▸ Adult: Initially 9 mg once daily for 1 week, then increased if necessary to 18 mg once daily for 1 week, then increased if necessary to 36 mg once daily, dose to be taken in the morning with breakfast, dose can be decreased (down to 4.5 mg per day) or increased (up to 36 mg per day) according to response and tolerance

- **CAUTIONS** Acid-related gastric disorders · epilepsy · history of psychiatric disorders · severe anorexia · severe obesity
- **INTERACTIONS** → Appendix 1: pitolisant
- **SIDE-EFFECTS**
  ▸ **Common or very common** Anxiety · asthenia · depression · dizziness · gastrointestinal discomfort · headaches · mood altered · nausea · sleep disorders · tremor · vertigo · vomiting
  ▸ **Uncommon** Appetite abnormal · arrhythmias · arthralgia · blepharospasm · chest pain · concentration impaired · constipation · diarrhoea · drowsiness · dry mouth · epilepsy · feeling abnormal · fluid retention · gastrointestinal disorders · hallucinations · hot flush · hypertension · hypotension · malaise · metrorrhagia · movement disorders · muscle complaints · muscle weakness · oedema · on and off phenomenon · oral paraesthesia · pain · paraesthesia · QT interval prolongation · sexual dysfunction · skin reactions · sweat changes · tinnitus · urinary frequency increased · visual acuity decreased · weight changes (review treatment if significant) · yawning
  ▸ **Rare or very rare** Behaviour abnormal · cognitive impairment · confusion · loss of consciousness · memory loss · obsessive thoughts · photosensitivity reaction · sense of oppression · swallowing difficulty
- **CONCEPTION AND CONTRACEPTION** Manufacturer advises effective contraception in women of childbearing potential

for at least 21 days after treatment discontinuation— pitolisant may reduce the effectiveness of hormonal contraceptives.
- **PREGNANCY** Manufacturer advises avoid unless potential benefit outweighs risk—toxicity in *animal* studies.
- **BREAST FEEDING** Manufacturer advises avoid—present in milk in *animal* studies.
- **HEPATIC IMPAIRMENT** Manufacturer advises caution in moderate impairment; avoid in severe impairment.
  Dose adjustments Manufacturer advises initial dose may be increased after two weeks in moderate impairment— maximum daily dose should not exceed 18 mg.
- **RENAL IMPAIRMENT**
  Dose adjustments Manufacturer advises use with caution; maximum daily dose should not exceed 18 mg.

- **MEDICINAL FORMS**
  There can be variation in the licensing of different medicines containing the same drug.
  Tablet
  ▸ Wakix (Lincoln Medical Ltd) ▼
    Pitolisant (as Pitolisant hydrochloride) 4.5 mg Wakix 4.5mg tablets | 30 tablet [PoM] £310.00
    Pitolisant (as Pitolisant hydrochloride) 18 mg Wakix 18mg tablets | 30 tablet [PoM] £310.00

CNS STIMULANTS > CENTRALLY ACTING SYMPATHOMIMETICS

Modafinil

- **INDICATIONS AND DOSE**

  Excessive sleepiness associated with narcolepsy with or without cataplexy
  ▸ BY MOUTH
  ▸ Adult: Initially 200 mg daily in 2 divided doses, dose to be taken in the morning and at noon, alternatively initially 200 mg once daily, dose to be taken in the morning, adjusted according to response to 200–400 mg daily in 2 divided doses, alternatively adjusted according to response to 200–400 mg once daily
  ▸ Elderly: Initially 100 mg daily

- **CONTRA-INDICATIONS** Arrhythmia · history of clinically significant signs of CNS stimulant-induced mitral valve prolapse (including ischaemic ECG changes, chest pain and arrhythmias) · history of cor pulmonale · history of left ventricular hypertrophy · moderate uncontrolled hypertension · severe uncontrolled hypertension
- **CAUTIONS** History of alcohol abuse · history of depression · history of drug abuse · history of mania · history of psychosis · possibility of dependence
- **INTERACTIONS** → Appendix 1: modafinil
- **SIDE-EFFECTS**
  ▸ **Common or very common** Anxiety · appetite abnormal · arrhythmias · asthenia · chest pain · confusion · constipation · depression · diarrhoea · dizziness · drowsiness · dry mouth · gastrointestinal discomfort · headaches · mood altered · nausea · palpitations · sensation abnormal · sleep disorders · thinking abnormal · vasodilation · vision disorders
  ▸ **Uncommon** Allergic rhinitis · arthralgia · asthma · behaviour abnormal · central nervous system stimulation · cough aggravated · diabetes mellitus · dry eye · dysphagia · dyspnoea · eosinophilia · epistaxis · gastrointestinal disorders · hypercholesterolaemia · hyperglycaemia · hyperhidrosis · hypertension · hypotension · increased risk of infection · leucopenia · libido decreased · memory loss · menstrual disorder · movement disorders · muscle complaints · muscle tone increased · muscle weakness ·

Nervous system

4

oral disorders · pain · peripheral oedema · psychiatric disorders · skin reactions · speech disorder · suicidal ideation · taste altered · thirst · tremor · urinary frequency increased · urine abnormal · vertigo · vomiting · weight changes

▶ **Rare or very rare** Hallucination · psychosis
▶ **Frequency not known** Angioedema · delusions · fever · hypersensitivity · lymphadenopathy · severe cutaneous adverse reactions (SCARs)

SIDE-EFFECTS, FURTHER INFORMATION Discontinue treatment if rash develops.
Discontinue treatment if psychiatric symptoms develop.

● PREGNANCY Avoid.

● BREAST FEEDING Avoid—present in milk in *animal* studies.

● HEPATIC IMPAIRMENT
Dose adjustments Halve dose in severe impairment.

● RENAL IMPAIRMENT Use with caution—limited information available.

● PRE-TREATMENT SCREENING ECG required before initiation.

● MONITORING REQUIREMENTS Monitor blood pressure and heart rate in hypertensive patients.

● MEDICINAL FORMS
There can be variation in the licensing of different medicines containing the same drug. Forms available from special-order manufacturers include: oral suspension, oral solution

Tablet
▶ Modafinil (Non-proprietary)
Modafinil 100 mg Modafinil 100mg tablets | 30 tablet PoM £52.60 DT = £4.39
Modafinil 200 mg Modafinil 200mg tablets | 30 tablet PoM £105.21 DT = £9.89
▶ Provigil (Teva UK Ltd)
Provigil 100 mg Provigil 100mg tablets | 30 tablet PoM £52.60 DT = £4.39
Provigil 200 mg Provigil 200mg tablets | 30 tablet PoM £105.21 DT = £9.89

8   Substance dependence

Substance dependence

Guidance on treatment of drug misuse

The UK health departments have produced guidance on the treatment of drug misuse in the UK. *Drug Misuse and Dependence: UK Guidelines on Clinical Management* (2007) is available at www.nta.nhs.uk/uploads/clinical_guidelines_2007.pdf.

Alcohol dependence

See Alcohol dependence p. 488.

Nicotine dependence

Smoking cessation interventions are a cost-effective way of reducing ill health and prolonging life. Smokers should be advised to stop and offered help with follow-up when appropriate. If possible, smokers should have access to smoking cessation services for behavioural support.

Therapy to aid smoking cessation is chosen according to the smoker's likely adherence, availability of counselling and support, previous experience of smoking-cessation aids, contra-indications and adverse effects of the preparations, and the smoker's preferences. **Nicotine p. 492 replacement therapy**, bupropion hydrochloride p. 491, and varenicline p. 494 are effective aids to smoking cessation. The use of nicotine replacement therapy in an individual who is already accustomed to nicotine introduces few new risks and it is

widely accepted that there are no circumstances in which it is safer to smoke than to use nicotine replacement therapy.

Some patients benefit from having more than one type of nicotine replacement therapy prescribed, such as a combination of transdermal and oral preparations. The combination of nicotine replacement therapy with varenicline or bupropion hydrochloride is not recommended.

Concomitant medication
Cigarette smoking increases the metabolism of some medicines by stimulating the hepatic enzyme CYP1A2. When smoking is discontinued, the dose of these drugs, in particular theophylline, cinacalcet, ropinirole, and some antipsychotics (including clozapine, olanzapine, chlorpromazine hydrochloride, and haloperidol, may need to be reduced. Regular monitoring for adverse effects is advised.

Bupropion hydrochloride has been used as an antidepressant. Its mode of action in smoking cessation is not clear and may involve an effect on noradrenaline and dopamine neurotransmission.

Nicotine replacement therapy
Nicotine replacement therapy can be used in place of cigarettes after abrupt cessation of smoking, or alternatively to reduce the amount of cigarettes used in advance of making a quit attempt. Nicotine replacement therapy can also be used to minimise passive smoking, and to treat cravings and reduce compensatory smoking after enforced abstinence in smoke-free environments. Smokers who find it difficult to achieve abstinence should consult a healthcare professional for advice.

Choice
Nicotine patches are a prolonged-release formulation and are applied for 16 hours (with the patch removed overnight) or for 24 hours. If patients experience strong cravings for cigarettes on waking, a 24-hour patch may be more suitable. Immediate-release nicotine preparations (gum, lozenges, sublingual tablets, inhalator, nasal spray, and oral spray) are used whenever the urge to smoke occurs or to prevent cravings.

The choice of nicotine replacement preparation depends largely on patient preference, and should take into account what preparations, if any, have been tried before. Patients with a high level of nicotine dependence, or who have failed with nicotine replacement therapy previously, may benefit from using a combination of an immediate-release preparation and patches to achieve abstinence.

Side-effects of specific nicotine preparations
Mild local reactions at the beginning of treatment are common because of the irritant effect of nicotine. Oral preparations and *inhalation cartridges* can cause irritation of the throat, *gum*, *lozenges*, and *oral spray* can cause increased salivation, and *patches* can cause minor skin irritation. The *nasal spray* commonly causes coughing, nasal irritation, epistaxis, sneezing, and watery eyes; the *oral spray* can cause watery eyes and blurred vision.

Gastro-intestinal disturbances are common and may be caused by swallowed nicotine. Nausea, vomiting, dyspepsia, and hiccup occur most frequently. Ulcerative stomatitis has also been reported. Dry mouth is a common side-effect of *lozenges*, *patches*, *oral spray*, and *sublingual tablets*. *Lozenges* cause diarrhoea, constipation, dysphagia, oesophagitis, gastritis, mouth ulcers, bloating, flatulence, and less commonly, taste disturbance, thirst, gingival bleeding, and halitosis. The *oral spray* may also cause abdominal pain, flatulence, and taste disturbance.

Palpitations may occur with nicotine replacement therapy and rarely *patches* and *oral spray* can cause arrhythmia. *Patches*, *lozenges*, and *oral spray* can cause chest pain. The *inhalator* can very rarely cause reversible atrial fibrillation.

Paraesthesia is a common side-effect of *oral spray*. Abnormal dreams can occur with *patches*; removal of the patch before bed may help. *Lozenges* and *oral spray* may cause rash and hot flushes. Sweating and myalgia can occur with *patches* and *oral spray*; the *patches* can also cause arthralgia.

Opioid dependence

The management of opioid dependence requires medical, social, and psychological treatment; access to a multidisciplinary team is recommended. Treatment for opioid dependence should be initiated under the supervision of an appropriately qualified prescriber.

Untreated heroin dependence shows early withdrawal symptoms within 8 hours, with peak symptoms at 36–72 hours; symptoms subside substantially after 5 days. Methadone hydrochloride p. 495 or buprenorphine p. 442 withdrawal occurs later, with longer-lasting symptoms.

Opioid substitution therapy

Methadone hydrochloride and buprenorphine are used as substitution therapy in opioid dependence. Substitute medication should be commenced with a short period of stabilisation, followed by either a withdrawal regimen or by maintenance treatment. Maintenance treatment enables patients to achieve stability, reduces drug use and crime, and improves health; it should be regularly reviewed to ensure the patient continues to derive benefit. The prescriber should monitor for signs of toxicity, and the patient should be told to be aware of warning signs of toxicity on initiation and during titration.

A withdrawal regimen after stabilisation with methadone hydrochloride or buprenorphine should be attempted only after careful consideration. Enforced withdrawal is ineffective for sustained abstinence, and it increases the risk of patients relapsing and subsequently overdosing because of loss of tolerance. Complete withdrawal from opioids usually takes up to 4 weeks in an inpatient or residential setting, and up to 12 weeks in a community setting. If abstinence is not achieved, illicit drug use is resumed, or the patient cannot tolerate withdrawal, the withdrawal regimen should be stopped and maintenance therapy should be resumed at the optimal dose. Following successful withdrawal treatment, further support and monitoring to maintain abstinence should be provided for a period of at least 6 months.

Missed doses

Patients who miss 3 days or more of their regular prescribed dose of opioid maintenance therapy are at risk of overdose because of loss of tolerance. Consider reducing the dose in these patients.

If the patient misses 5 or more days of treatment, an assessment of illicit drug use is also recommended before restarting substitution therapy; this is particularly important for patients taking buprenorphine p. 442 because of the risk of precipitated withdrawal.

Buprenorphine

Buprenorphine is preferred by some patients because it is less sedating than methadone hydrochloride p. 495; for this reason it may be more suitable for employed patients or those undertaking other skilled tasks such as driving. Buprenorphine is safer than methadone hydrochloride when used in conjunction with other sedating drugs, and has fewer drug interactions. Dose reductions may be easier than with methadone hydrochloride because the withdrawal symptoms are milder, and patients generally require fewer adjunctive medications; there is also a lower risk of overdose. Buprenorphine can be given on alternate days in higher doses and it requires a shorter drug-free period than methadone hydrochloride before induction with naltrexone hydrochloride p. 491 for prevention of relapse.

Patients dependent on high doses of opioids may be at increased risk of precipitated withdrawal. Precipitated withdrawal can occur in any patient if buprenorphine is administered when other opioid agonist drugs are in circulation. Precipitated opioid withdrawal, if it occurs, starts within 1–3 hours of the first buprenorphine dose and peaks at around 6 hours. Non-opioid adjunctive therapy, such as lofexidine hydrochloride p. 497, may be required if symptoms are severe.

To reduce the risk of precipitated withdrawal, the first dose of buprenorphine should be given when the patient is exhibiting signs of withdrawal, or 6–12 hours after the last use of heroin (or other short-acting opioid), or 24–48 hours after the last dose of methadone hydrochloride. It is possible to titrate the dose of buprenorphine within one week—more rapidly than with methadone hydrochloride therapy—but care is still needed to avoid toxicity or precipitated withdrawal; dividing the dose on the first day may be useful.

A combination preparation containing buprenorphine with naloxone p. 496 (Suboxone ®) can be prescribed for patients when there is a risk of dose diversion for parenteral administration; the naloxone hydrochloride p. 1329 component precipitates withdrawal if the preparation is injected, but it has little effect when the preparation is taken sublingually.

Methadone

Methadone hydrochloride, a long-acting opioid agonist, is usually administered in a single daily dose as methadone hydrochloride oral solution 1 mg/mL. Patients with a long history of opioid misuse, those who typically abuse a variety of sedative drugs and alcohol, and those who experience increased anxiety during withdrawal of opioids may prefer methadone hydrochloride to buprenorphine because it has a more pronounced sedative effect.

Methadone hydrochloride is initiated at least 8 hours after the last heroin dose, provided that there is objective evidence of withdrawal symptoms. A supplementary dose on the first day may be considered if there is evidence of persistent opioid withdrawal symptoms. Because of the long half-life, plasma concentrations progressively rise during initial treatment even if the patient remains on the same daily dose (it takes 3–10 days for plasma concentrations to reach steady-state in patients on a stable dose); a dose tolerated on the first day of treatment may become a toxic dose on the third day as cumulative toxicity develops. Thus, titration to the optimal dose in methadone hydrochloride maintenance treatment may take several weeks.

Opioid substitution during pregnancy

Acute withdrawal of opioids should be avoided in pregnancy because it can cause fetal death. Opioid substitution therapy is recommended during pregnancy because it carries a lower risk to the fetus than continued use of illicit drugs. If a woman who is stabilised on methadone hydrochloride or buprenorphine for treatment of opioid dependence becomes pregnant, therapy should be continued [buprenorphine is not licensed for use in pregnancy]. Many pregnant patients choose a withdrawal regimen, but withdrawal during the first trimester should be avoided because it is associated with an increased risk of spontaneous miscarriage. Withdrawal of methadone hydrochloride or buprenorphine should be undertaken gradually during the second trimester, with dose reductions made every 3–5 days. If illicit drug use occurs, the patient should be re-stabilised at the optimal maintenance dose and consideration should be given to stopping the withdrawal regimen.

Further withdrawal of methadone hydrochloride or buprenorphine in the third trimester is not recommended because maternal withdrawal, even if mild, is associated with fetal distress, stillbirth, and the risk of neonatal mortality. Drug metabolism can be increased in the third trimester; it may be necessary to either increase the dose of methadone hydrochloride or change to twice-daily consumption (or a combination of both strategies) to prevent withdrawal symptoms from developing.

Nervous system

4

The neonate should be monitored for respiratory depression and signs of withdrawal if the mother is prescribed high doses of opioid substitute.

Signs of neonatal withdrawal from opioids usually develop 24–72 hours after delivery but symptoms may be delayed for up to 14 days, so monitoring may be required for several weeks. Symptoms include a high-pitched cry, rapid breathing, hungry but ineffective suckling, and excessive wakefulness; severe, but rare symptoms include hypertonicity and convulsions.

Opioid substitution during breastfeeding
Doses of methadone and buprenorphine should be kept as low as possible in breast-feeding mothers. Increased sleepiness, breathing difficulties, or limpness in breast-fed babies of mothers taking opioid substitutes should be reported urgently to a healthcare professional.

Adjunctive therapy and symptomatic treatment
Adjunctive therapy may be required for the management of opioid withdrawal symptoms. Loperamide hydrochloride p. 66 may be used for the control of diarrhoea; mebeverine hydrochloride p. 86 for controlling stomach cramps; paracetamol p. 438 and **non-steroidal anti-inflammatory drugs** for muscular pains and headaches; metoclopramide hydrochloride p. 426 or prochlorperazine p. 385 may be useful for nausea or vomiting. Topical **rubefacients** can be helpful for relieving muscle pain associated with methadone hydrochloride withdrawal. If a patient is suffering from insomnia, short-acting **benzodiazepines** or zopiclone p. 484 may be prescribed, but because of the potential for abuse, prescriptions should be limited to a short course of a few days only. If anxiety or agitation is severe, specialist advice should be sought.

Lofexidine
Lofexidine hydrochloride may alleviate some of the physical symptoms of opioid withdrawal by attenuating the increase in adrenergic neurotransmission that occurs during opioid withdrawal. Lofexidine hydrochloride can be prescribed as an adjuvant to opioid substitution therapy, initiated either at the same time as the opioid substitute or during withdrawal of the opioid substitute. Alternatively, lofexidine hydrochloride may be prescribed instead of an opioid substitute in patients who have mild or uncertain dependence (including young people), and those with a short history of illicit drug use.

Opioid-receptor antagonists
Patients dependant on opioids can be given a supply of naloxone hydrochloride p. 1329 to be used in case of accidental overdose.

Naltrexone hydrochloride p. 491 precipitates withdrawal symptoms in opioid-dependent subjects. Because the effects of opioid-receptor agonists are blocked by naltrexone hydrochloride, it is prescribed as an aid to prevent relapse in formerly opioid-dependent patients.

Opioid dependence in children
In younger patients (under 18 years), the harmful effects of drug misuse are more often related to acute intoxication than to dependence, so substitution therapy is usually inappropriate. Maintenance treatment with opioid substitution therapy is therefore controversial in young people; however, it may be useful for the older adolescent who has a history of opioid use to undergo a period of stabilisation with buprenorphine p. 442 or methadone hydrochloride p. 495 before starting a withdrawal regimen.

8.1 Alcohol dependence

Alcohol dependence
01-Sep-2017

Description of condition
Alcohol dependence is a cluster of behavioural, cognitive and physiological factors that typically include a strong desire to drink alcohol, tolerance to its effects, and difficulties controlling its use. Someone who is alcohol-dependent may persist in drinking, despite harmful consequences, such as physical or mental health problems.

In severely dependent patients who have been drinking excessively for a prolonged period of time, an abrupt reduction in alcohol intake may result in the development of an alcohol withdrawal syndrome, which, in the absence of medical management, can lead to seizures, delirium tremens, and death.

Assisted alcohol withdrawal
[EvGr] Patients with mild alcohol dependence usually do not need assisted alcohol withdrawal. Patients with moderate dependence can generally be treated in a community setting unless they are at high risk of developing alcohol withdrawal seizures or delirium tremens; individuals with severe dependence should undergo withdrawal in an inpatient setting. Patients with decompensated liver disease should be treated under specialist supervision.

A long-acting benzodiazepine, such as chlordiazepoxide hydrochloride p. 340 or diazepam p. 340, is recommended to attenuate alcohol withdrawal symptoms; local clinical protocols should be followed.

In primary care, *fixed-dose reducing regimens* are used. This involves using a standard, initial dose (determined by the severity of alcohol dependence or level of alcohol consumption), followed by dose reduction to zero, usually over 7–10 days. In inpatient or residential settings, a *fixed-dose regimen* or a *symptom-triggered regimen* can be used. A symptom-triggered approach involves tailoring the drug regimen according to the severity of withdrawal and any complications in an individual patient; adequate monitoring facilities should be available. The patient should be monitored on a regular basis and treatment only continued as long as there are withdrawal symptoms.

Carbamazepine p. 309 [unlicensed indication] can be used as an alternative treatment in acute alcohol withdrawal.

Clomethiazole p. 482 may be considered as an alternative to a benzodiazepine or carbamazepine p. 309. It should only be used in an inpatient setting and should not be prescribed if the patient is liable to continue drinking alcohol. ⚠Note: Alcohol combined with clomethiazole p. 482, particularly in patients with cirrhosis, can lead to fatal respiratory depression even with short-term use.

[EvGr] When managing withdrawal from **co-existing** benzodiazepine and alcohol dependence, the dose of benzodiazepine used for withdrawal should be increased. The initial daily dose is calculated, based on the requirements for alcohol withdrawal plus the equivalent regularly used daily dose of benzodiazepine. A single benzodiazepine (chlordiazepoxide hydrochloride p. 340 or diazepam p. 340) should be used rather than multiple benzodiazepines. Inpatient withdrawal regimens should last for 2–3 weeks or longer, depending on the severity of benzodiazepine dependence. When withdrawal is managed in the community, or where there is a high level of benzodiazepine dependence, or both, the regimen should last for a minimum of 3 weeks (according to the patient's symptoms).

If alcohol withdrawal seizures occur, a fast-acting benzodiazepine (such as lorazepam p. 335 [unlicensed indication]) should be prescribed to reduce the likelihood of further seizures. If alcohol withdrawal seizures develop in a person during treatment for acute alcohol withdrawal, review their withdrawal drug regimen. ⒶⒶ

Delirium tremens

EvGr Delirium tremens is a medical emergency that requires specialist inpatient care. In patients with delirium tremens (characterised by agitation, confusion, paranoia, and visual and auditory hallucinations), oral lorazepam p. 335 should be used as first-line treatment. If symptoms persist or oral medication is declined, parenteral lorazepam p. 335 [unlicensed], or haloperidol p. 382 [unlicensed] can be given as adjunctive therapy. If delirium tremens develops during treatment for acute alcohol withdrawal, the withdrawal drug regimen should also be reviewed. ⒶⒶ

Alcohol dependence

EvGr In harmful drinkers or patients with mild alcohol dependence, a psychological intervention (such as cognitive behavioural therapy) should be offered. In those who have not responded to psychological interventions alone or who have specifically requested a pharmacological treatment, acamprosate calcium p. 490 or oral naltrexone hydrochloride p. 491 can be used in combination with a psychological intervention.

Acamprosate calcium p. 490 or oral naltrexone hydrochloride p. 491 in combination with a psychological intervention are recommended for relapse prevention in patients with moderate and severe alcohol dependence, to start after successful assisted withdrawal. Disulfiram below is an alternative for patients in whom acamprosate calcium p. 490 and oral naltrexone hydrochloride p. 491 are not suitable, or if the patient prefers disulfiram below and understands the risks of taking the drug.

Nalmefene p. 490 is recommended for the reduction of alcohol consumption in patients with alcohol dependence who have a high drinking risk level, without physical withdrawal symptoms, and who do not require immediate detoxification (see *National funding/access decisions* for nalmefene p. 490).

Patients with severe alcohol-related hepatitis with a discriminant function of 32 or more can be given corticosteroids but only after any active infection or gastro-intestinal bleeding is treated, any renal impairment is controlled, and following discussion of the potential benefits and risks of treatment. Corticosteroid treatment has been shown to improve survival in the short term (1 month) but not over a longer term (3 months to 1 year). It has also been shown to increase the risk of serious infections within the first 3 months of starting treatment.

Patients with chronic alcohol-related pancreatitis should be offered nutritional support; those who have symptoms of steatorrhoea or who have poor nutritional status due to Exocrine pancreatic insufficiency p. 95 should be prescribed pancreatic enzyme supplements; supplements are not indicated when pain is the only symptom. ⒶⒶ

Wernicke's encephalopathy

EvGr Patients with alcohol dependence are at risk of developing Wernicke's encephalopathy; patients at high risk are those who are malnourished, at risk of malnourishment, or have decompensated liver disease. Parenteral thiamine p. 1048, followed by oral thiamine p. 1048, should be given to patients with suspected Wernicke's encephalopathy, those who are malnourished or at risk of malnourishment, those who have decompensated liver disease or who are attending hospital for acute treatment. Prophylactic oral thiamine p. 1048 should also be given to harmful or dependent drinkers if they are in acute withdrawal, or before and during assisted alcohol withdrawal. ⒶⒶ. Parenteral thiamine is available as part of a vitamin B substances with ascorbic acid p. 1048 preparation.

Useful Resources

Alcohol-use disorders: diagnosis, assessment and management of harmful drinking and alcohol dependence. National Institute for Health and Care Excellence. Clinical guideline 115. February 2011.
www.nice.org.uk/guidance/cg115

Alcohol-use disorders: diagnosis and management of physical complications. National Institute for Health and Care Excellence. Clinical guideline 100. June 2010 (updated April 2017).
www.nice.org.uk/guidance/cg100

ALDEHYDE DEHYDROGENASE INHIBITORS

Disulfiram

● **INDICATIONS AND DOSE**

Adjunct in the treatment of alcohol dependence (under expert supervision)
▶ BY MOUTH
▶ Adult: 200 mg daily, increased if necessary up to 500 mg daily

● **UNLICENSED USE** Disulfiram doses in BNF may differ from those in product literature.

● **CONTRA-INDICATIONS** Cardiac failure · coronary artery disease · history of cerebrovascular accident · hypertension · psychosis · severe personality disorder · suicide risk

● **CAUTIONS** Alcohol challenge **not** recommended on routine basis (if considered essential—specialist units only with resuscitation facilities) · avoid in Acute porphyrias p. 1025 · diabetes mellitus · epilepsy · respiratory disease

● **INTERACTIONS** → Appendix 1: disulfiram

● **SIDE-EFFECTS** Allergic dermatitis · breath odour · depression · drowsiness · encephalopathy · fatigue · hepatocellular injury · libido decreased · mania · nausea · nerve disorders · paranoia · schizophrenia · vomiting

● **PREGNANCY** High concentrations of acetaldehyde which occur in presence of alcohol may be teratogenic; avoid in first trimester.

● **BREAST FEEDING** Avoid—no information available.

● **HEPATIC IMPAIRMENT** Use with caution.

● **RENAL IMPAIRMENT** Use with caution.

● **PRE-TREATMENT SCREENING** Before initiating disulfiram, prescribers should evaluate the patient's suitability for treatment, because some patient factors, for example memory impairment or social circumstances, make compliance to treatment or abstinence from alcohol difficult.

● **MONITORING REQUIREMENTS** During treatment with disulfiram, patients should be monitored at least every 2 weeks for the first 2 months, then each month for the following 4 months, and at least every 6 months thereafter.

● **PATIENT AND CARER ADVICE** Manufacturer advises patients and their carers should be counselled on the disulfiram-alcohol reaction—reactions may occur following exposure to small amounts of alcohol found in perfume, aerosol sprays, or low alcohol and "non-alcohol" beers and wines; symptoms may be severe and life-threatening and can include nausea, flushing, palpitations, arrhythmias, hypotension, respiratory depression, and coma. EvGr Patients and their carers should be counselled on the signs of hepatotoxicity—patients should discontinue treatment and seek immediate medical attention if they feel unwell or symptoms such as fever or jaundice develop. ⒶⒶ

4

Nervous system

● MEDICINAL FORMS
There can be variation in the licensing of different medicines
containing the same drug.

Tablet
CAUTIONARY AND ADVISORY LABELS 2
▸ Disulfiram (Non-proprietary)
   Disulfiram 200 mg Disulfiram 200mg tablets | 50 tablet [PoM]
   £91.73 DT = £91.73

GAMMA-AMINOBUTYRIC ACID ANALOGUES AND DERIVATIVES

Acamprosate calcium

● INDICATIONS AND DOSE
Maintenance of abstinence in alcohol-dependent patients
▸ BY MOUTH
▸ Adult 18–65 years (body-weight up to 60 kg): 666 mg once
   daily at breakfast and 333 mg twice daily at midday and
   at night
▸ Adult 18–65 years (body-weight 60 kg and above): 666 mg
   3 times a day

● CAUTIONS Continued alcohol abuse (risk of treatment
failure)

● SIDE-EFFECTS
Common or very common Abdominal pain · diarrhoea ·
flatulence · nausea · sexual dysfunction · skin reactions ·
vomiting

● PREGNANCY Manufacturer advises avoid unless potential
benefit outweighs risk.

● BREAST FEEDING Avoid.

● HEPATIC IMPAIRMENT Avoid if severe.

● RENAL IMPAIRMENT Avoid if serum-creatinine greater
than 120 micromol/litre.

● PRESCRIBING AND DISPENSING INFORMATION
Acamprosate calcium has been used for the maintenance
of abstinence in alcohol dependence in children aged
16 years and over.

● MEDICINAL FORMS
There can be variation in the licensing of different medicines
containing the same drug.

Gastro-resistant tablet
CAUTIONARY AND ADVISORY LABELS 5, 21, 25
ELECTROLYTES: May contain Calcium
▸ Acamprosate calcium (Non-proprietary)
   Acamprosate calcium 333 mg Acamprosate 333mg gastro-resistant
   tablets | 168 tablet [PoM] £33.75 DT = £33.75
▸ Campral EC (Merck Serono Ltd)
   Acamprosate calcium 333 mg Campral EC 333mg tablets |
   168 tablet [PoM] £28.80 DT = £33.75

OPIOID RECEPTOR ANTAGONISTS

Nalmefene

● INDICATIONS AND DOSE
**Reduction of alcohol consumption in patients with alcohol
dependence who have a high drinking risk level without
physical withdrawal symptoms, and who do not require
immediate detoxification**
▸ BY MOUTH
▸ Adult: 18 mg daily if required, taken on each day there
   is a risk of drinking alcohol, preferably taken 1–2 hours
   before the anticipated time of drinking, if a dose has
   not been taken before drinking alcohol, 1 dose should
   be taken as soon as possible; maximum 18 mg per day

● CONTRA-INDICATIONS Recent history of acute alcohol
withdrawal syndrome · recent or current opioid use

● CAUTIONS Continued treatment for more than 1 year ·
history of seizure disorders (including alcohol withdrawal
seizures) · psychiatric illness

● INTERACTIONS → Appendix 1: nalmefene

● SIDE-EFFECTS
▸ **Common or very common** Appetite decreased · asthenia ·
concentration impaired · confusion · diarrhoea · dizziness ·
drowsiness · dry mouth · feeling abnormal · headache ·
hyperhidrosis · libido decreased · malaise · muscle spasms ·
nausea · palpitations · restlessness · sensation abnormal ·
sleep disorders · tachycardia · tremor · vomiting · weight
decreased
▸ **Frequency not known** Dissociation · hallucinations

● PREGNANCY Manufacturer advises avoid—toxicity in
animal studies.

● BREAST FEEDING Manufacturer advises avoid—present in
milk in *animal* studies.

● HEPATIC IMPAIRMENT Use with caution—avoid in severe
impairment.

● RENAL IMPAIRMENT Use with caution—avoid in severe
impairment.

● PRE-TREATMENT SCREENING Before initiating treatment,
prescribers should evaluate the patient's clinical status,
alcohol dependence, and level of alcohol consumption.
Nalmefene should only be prescribed for patients who
continue to have a high drinking risk level two weeks after
the initial assessment.

● MONITORING REQUIREMENTS During treatment, patients
should be monitored regularly and the need for continued
treatment assessed.

● NATIONAL FUNDING/ACCESS DECISIONS

NICE decisions
▸ **Nalmefene for reducing alcohol consumption in people with
alcohol dependence (November 2014)** NICE TA325
Nalmefene is recommended within its marketing
authorisation, as an option for reducing alcohol
consumption, for patients with alcohol dependence:
● who have a high drinking risk level (defined as alcohol
consumption of more than 60 g per day for men and
more than 40 g per day for women, according to the
World Health Organization's drinking risk levels)
without physical withdrawal symptoms, **and**
● who do not require immediate detoxification.
The marketing authorisation states that nalmefene
should:
● only be prescribed in conjunction with continuous
psychosocial support focused on treatment adherence
and reducing alcohol consumption, **and**
● be initiated only in patients who continue to have a high
drinking risk level 2 weeks after initial assessment.
www.nice.org.uk/TA325

● MEDICINAL FORMS
There can be variation in the licensing of different medicines
containing the same drug.

Tablet
CAUTIONARY AND ADVISORY LABELS 25
▸ Selincro (Lundbeck Ltd)
   Nalmefene (as Nalmefene hydrochloride) 18 mg Selincro 18mg
   tablets | 14 tablet [PoM] £42.42 DT = £42.42 | 28 tablet [PoM] £84.84

Naltrexone hydrochloride

17-Aug-2017

● **DRUG ACTION** Naltrexone is an opioid-receptor antagonist.

● **INDICATIONS AND DOSE**

Adjunct to prevent relapse in formerly opioid-dependent patients (who have remained opioid-free for at least 7–10 days) (initiated under specialist supervision)
▸ BY MOUTH
▸ Adult: Initially 25 mg daily, then increased to 50 mg daily, total weekly dose may be divided and given on 3 days of the week for improved compliance (e.g. 100 mg on Monday and Wednesday, and 150 mg on Friday); maximum 350 mg per week

Adjunct to prevent relapse in formerly alcohol-dependent patients (initiated under specialist supervision)
▸ BY MOUTH
▸ Adult: 25 mg once daily on the first day, then increased if tolerated to 50 mg daily

● **UNLICENSED USE** 25 mg dose for adjunct to prevent relapse in formerly alcohol-dependent patients is an unlicensed dose.

● **CONTRA-INDICATIONS** Patients currently dependent on opioids

● **CAUTIONS** Concomitant use of opioids

CAUTIONS, FURTHER INFORMATION
▸ Concomitant use of opioids Concomitant use of opioids should be avoided but increased dose of opioid analgesic may be required for pain—manufacturer advises to monitor for opioid intoxication.

● **INTERACTIONS** → Appendix 1: naltrexone

● **SIDE-EFFECTS**
▸ **Common or very common** Abdominal pain · anxiety · appetite abnormal · arthralgia · asthenia · chest pain · chills · constipation · diarrhoea · dizziness · eye disorders · headache · hyperhidrosis · mood altered · myalgia · nausea · palpitations · sexual dysfunction · skin reactions · sleep disorders · tachycardia · thirst · vomiting
▸ **Uncommon** Alopecia · confusion · cough · depression · drowsiness · dry mouth · dysphonia · dyspnoea · ear discomfort · eye discomfort · eye swelling · feeling hot · fever · flatulence · flushing · hallucination · hepatic disorders · lymphadenopathy · nasal complaints · oropharyngeal pain · pain · paranoia · peripheral coldness · seborrhoea · sinus disorder · sputum increased · tinnitus · tremor · ulcer · urinary disorders · vertigo · vision disorders · weight changes · yawning
▸ **Rare or very rare** Immune thrombocytopenic purpura · rhabdomyolysis · suicidal tendencies
▸ **Frequency not known** Withdrawal syndrome

● **PREGNANCY** Use only if benefit outweighs risk.

● **BREAST FEEDING** Avoid—potential toxicity.

● **HEPATIC IMPAIRMENT** Avoid in acute hepatitis, hepatic failure, or severe impairment.

● **RENAL IMPAIRMENT** Avoid in severe impairment.

● **PRE-TREATMENT SCREENING** Test for opioid dependence with naloxone before treatment.

● **MONITORING REQUIREMENTS** Liver function tests needed before and during treatment.

● **PATIENT AND CARER ADVICE** Patients should be warned that an attempt to overcome the blockade of opioid receptors by overdosing could result in acute opioid intoxication.

● **NATIONAL FUNDING/ACCESS DECISIONS**
NICE decisions
▸ Naltrexone for the management of opioid dependence (January 2007) NICE TA115
Naltrexone is recommended for the prevention of relapse in formerly opioid-dependent patients who are motivated to remain in a supportive care abstinence programme. Naltrexone should be administered under supervision and its effectiveness in preventing opioid misuse reviewed regularly.
www.nice.org.uk/TA115

● **MEDICINAL FORMS**
There can be variation in the licensing of different medicines containing the same drug. Forms available from special-order manufacturers include: capsule, oral suspension, oral solution
Tablet
▸ Naltrexone hydrochloride (Non-proprietary)
Naltrexone hydrochloride 50 mg Naltrexone 50mg tablets |
28 tablet [PoM] £23.00 DT = £22.34
▸ Adepend (AOP Orphan Pharmaceuticals AG)
Naltrexone hydrochloride 50 mg Adepend 50mg tablets |
28 tablet [PoM] £47.43 DT = £22.34
▸ Nalorex (Bristol-Myers Squibb Pharmaceuticals Ltd)
Naltrexone hydrochloride 50 mg Nalorex 50mg tablets |
28 tablet [PoM] £22.34 DT = £22.34

8.2 Nicotine dependence

ANTIDEPRESSANTS 〉 SEROTONIN AND NORADRENALINE RE-UPTAKE INHIBITORS

Bupropion hydrochloride

07-Sep-2017

(Amfebutamone hydrochloride)

● **INDICATIONS AND DOSE**

To aid smoking cessation in combination with motivational support in nicotine-dependent patients
▸ BY MOUTH
▸ Adult: Initially 150 mg daily for 6 days, then 150 mg twice daily (max. per dose 150 mg), minimum 8 hours between doses; period of treatment 7–9 weeks, start treatment 1–2 weeks before target stop date, discontinue if abstinence not achieved at 7 weeks, consider maximum 150 mg daily in patients with risk factors for seizures; maximum 300 mg per day
▸ Elderly: 150 mg daily for 7–9 weeks, start treatment 1–2 weeks before target stop date, discontinue if abstinence not achieved at 7 weeks; maximum 150 mg per day

● **CONTRA-INDICATIONS** Acute alcohol withdrawal · acute benzodiazepine withdrawal · bipolar disorder · CNS tumour · eating disorders · history of seizures · severe hepatic cirrhosis

● **CAUTIONS** Alcohol abuse · diabetes · elderly · history of head trauma · predisposition to seizures (prescribe only if benefit clearly outweighs risk)

● **INTERACTIONS** → Appendix 1: bupropion

● **SIDE-EFFECTS**
▸ **Common or very common** Abdominal pain · anxiety · concentration impaired · constipation · dizziness · dry mouth · fever · gastrointestinal disorder · headache · hyperhidrosis · hypersensitivity · insomnia (reduced by avoiding dose at bedtime) · nausea · skin reactions · taste altered · tremor · vomiting
▸ **Uncommon** Appetite decreased · asthenia · chest pain · confusion · tachycardia · tinnitus · vasodilation · visual impairment
▸ **Rare or very rare** Angioedema · arthralgia · behaviour abnormal · bronchospasm · delusions · depersonalisation ·

4

Nervous system

dyspnoea · hallucination · hepatic disorders · irritability · memory loss · movement disorders · muscle complaints · palpitations · paraesthesia · parkinsonism · postural hypotension · seizure · sleep disorders · Stevens-Johnson syndrome · syncope · urinary disorders

‣ **Frequency not known** Anaemia · hyponatraemia · leucopenia · psychosis · suicidal tendencies · thrombocytopenia

● **PREGNANCY** Avoid—no information available.

● **BREAST FEEDING** Present in milk—avoid.

● **HEPATIC IMPAIRMENT** Avoid in severe hepatic cirrhosis.
Dose adjustments Reduce dose to 150 mg daily.

● **RENAL IMPAIRMENT**
Dose adjustments Reduce dose to 150 mg daily.

● **MONITORING REQUIREMENTS** Manufacturer advises monitor blood pressure before and during treatment.

● **PATIENT AND CARER ADVICE** Manufacturer advises patients and carers should be instructed to report any clinical worsening of depression, suicidal behaviour or thoughts and unusual changes in behaviour.
Driving and skilled tasks Manufacturer advises patients and carers should be counselled on the effects on driving and performance of skilled tasks—increased risk of dizziness and light-headedness.

● **MEDICINAL FORMS**
There can be variation in the licensing of different medicines containing the same drug.
Modified-release tablet
CAUTIONARY AND ADVISORY LABELS 25
‣ Zyban (GlaxoSmithKline UK Ltd)
Bupropion hydrochloride 150 mg Zyban 150mg modified-release tablets | 60 tablet [PoM] £41.76 DT = £41.76

NICOTINIC RECEPTOR AGONISTS

▌Nicotine

● **INDICATIONS AND DOSE**

Nicotine replacement therapy in individuals who smoke fewer than 20 cigarettes each day

‣ BY MOUTH USING CHEWING GUM

‣ **Adult:** 2 mg as required, chew 1 piece of gum when the urge to smoke occurs or to prevent cravings, if attempting smoking cessation, treatment should continue for 3 months before reducing the dose

‣ BY SUBLINGUAL ADMINISTRATION USING SUBLINGUAL TABLETS

‣ **Adult:** 1 tablet every 1 hour, increased to 2 tablets every 1 hour if required, if attempting smoking cessation, treatment should continue for up to 3 months before reducing the dose; maximum 40 tablets per day

Nicotine replacement therapy in individuals who smoke more than 20 cigarettes each day or who require more than 15 pieces of 2-mg strength gum each day

‣ BY MOUTH USING CHEWING GUM

‣ **Adult:** 4 mg as required, chew 1 piece of gum when the urge to smoke occurs or to prevent cravings, individuals should not exceed 15 pieces of 4-mg strength gum daily, if attempting smoking cessation, treatment should continue for 3 months before reducing the dose

Nicotine replacement therapy in individuals who smoke more than 20 cigarettes each day

‣ BY SUBLINGUAL ADMINISTRATION USING SUBLINGUAL TABLETS

‣ **Adult:** 2 tablets every 1 hour, if attempting smoking cessation, treatment should continue for up to 3 months before reducing the dose; maximum 40 tablets per day

Nicotine replacement therapy

‣ BY INHALATION USING INHALATOR

‣ **Adult:** As required, the cartridges can be used when the urge to smoke occurs or to prevent cravings, individuals should not exceed 12 cartridges of the 10-mg strength daily, or 6 cartridges of the 15-mg strength daily

‣ BY MOUTH USING LOZENGES

‣ **Adult:** 1 lozenge every 1–2 hours as required, one lozenge should be used when the urge to smoke occurs, individuals who smoke less than 20 cigarettes each day should usually use the lower-strength lozenges; individuals who smoke more than 20 cigarettes each day and those who fail to stop smoking with the low-strength lozenges should use the higher-strength lozenges; If attempting smoking cessation, treatment should continue for 6–12 weeks before attempting a reduction in dose; maximum 15 lozenges per day

‣ BY MOUTH USING OROMUCOSAL SPRAY

‣ **Adult:** 1–2 sprays as required, individuals can spray in the mouth when the urge to smoke occurs or to prevent cravings, individuals should not exceed 2 sprays per episode (up to 4 sprays every hour); maximum 64 sprays per day

‣ BY INTRANASAL ADMINISTRATION USING NASAL SPRAY

‣ **Adult:** 1 spray as required, individuals can spray into each nostril when the urge to smoke occurs, up to twice every hour for 16 hours daily, if attempting smoking cessation, treatment should continue for 8 weeks before reducing the dose; maximum 64 sprays per day

‣ BY TRANSDERMAL APPLICATION USING PATCHES

‣ **Adult:** Individuals who smoke more than 10 cigarettes daily should apply a high-strength patch daily for 6–8 weeks, followed by the medium-strength patch for 2 weeks, and then the low-strength patch for the final 2 weeks; individuals who smoke fewer than 10 cigarettes daily can usually start with the medium-strength patch for 6–8 weeks, followed by the low-strength patch for 2–4 weeks; a slower titration schedule can be used in individuals who are not ready to quit but want to reduce cigarette consumption before a quit attempt; if abstinence is not achieved, or if withdrawal symptoms are experienced, the strength of the patch used should be maintained or increased until the patient is stabilised; individuals using the high-strength patch who experience excessive side-effects, that do not resolve within a few days, should change to a medium-strength patch for the remainder of the initial period and then use the low-strength patch for 2–4 weeks

● **CAUTIONS**
GENERAL CAUTIONS Diabetes mellitus—blood-glucose concentration should be monitored closely when initiating treatment · haemodynamically unstable patients hospitalised with cerebrovascular accident · haemodynamically unstable patients hospitalised with myocardial infarction · haemodynamically unstable patients hospitalised with severe arrhythmias · phaeochromocytoma · uncontrolled hyperthyroidism
SPECIFIC CAUTIONS
‣ When used by inhalation Bronchospastic disease · chronic throat disease · obstructive lung disease
‣ With intranasal use Bronchial asthma (may exacerbate)
‣ With oral use *Gum* may also stick to and damage dentures · gastritis (can be aggravated by swallowed nicotine) · oesophagitis (can be aggravated by swallowed nicotine) · peptic ulcers (can be aggravated by swallowed nicotine)
‣ With transdermal use *Patches* should not be placed on broken skin · patients with skin disorders
CAUTIONS, FURTHER INFORMATION Most warnings for nicotine replacement therapy also apply to continued

cigarette smoking, but the risk of continued smoking outweighs any risks of using nicotine preparations.

Specific cautions for individual preparations are usually related to the local effect of nicotine.

- SIDE-EFFECTS
  GENERAL SIDE-EFFECTS
  ▸ **Common or very common** Dizziness · headache · hyperhidrosis · nausea · palpitations · skin reactions · vomiting
  ▸ **Uncommon** Flushing
  SPECIFIC SIDE-EFFECTS
  ▸ **Common or very common**
  ▸ When used by inhalation Asthenia · cough · dry mouth · flatulence · gastrointestinal discomfort · hiccups · hypersensitivity · nasal complaints · oral disorders · taste altered · throat complaints
  ▸ With intranasal use Chest discomfort · cough · dyspnoea · epistaxis · nasal complaints · paraesthesia · throat irritation
  ▸ With oral use Anxiety · appetite abnormal · burping · diarrhoea · dyspepsia (may be caused by swallowed nicotine) · gastrointestinal disorders · hiccups · increased risk of infection · mood altered · oral disorders · sleep disorders
  ▸ With sublingual use Asthenia · cough · dry mouth · flatulence · gastrointestinal discomfort · hiccups · hypersensitivity · oral disorders · rhinitis · taste altered · throat complaints
  ▸ **Uncommon**
  ▸ When used by inhalation Abnormal dreams · arrhythmias · bronchospasm · burping · chest discomfort · dysphonia · dyspnoea · hypertension · malaise
  ▸ With intranasal use Abnormal dreams · asthenia · hypertension · malaise
  ▸ With oral use Anger · asthma exacerbated · cough · dyspepsia aggravated · dysphagia · haemorrhage · laryngospasm · nasal complaints · nocturia · numbness · overdose · pain · palpitations exacerbated · peripheral oedema · tachycardia · taste altered · throat complaints · vascular disorders
  ▸ With sublingual use Abnormal dreams · arrhythmias · bronchospasm · burping · chest discomfort · dysphonia · dyspnoea · hypertension · malaise · nasal complaints
  ▸ With transdermal use Arrhythmias · asthenia · chest discomfort · dyspnoea · hypertension · malaise · myalgia · paraesthesia
  ▸ **Rare or very rare**
  ▸ When used by inhalation Dysphagia
  ▸ With intranasal use Arrhythmias
  ▸ With oral use Coagulation disorder · platelet disorder
  ▸ With sublingual use Dysphagia
  ▸ With transdermal use Abdominal discomfort · angioedema · pain in extremity
  ▸ **Frequency not known**
  ▸ When used by inhalation Angioedema · excessive tearing · vision blurred
  ▸ With intranasal use Abdominal discomfort · angioedema · excessive tearing · oropharyngeal complaints
  ▸ With sublingual use Excessive tearing · muscle tightness · vision blurred
  SIDE-EFFECTS, FURTHER INFORMATION Some systemic effects occur on initiation of therapy, particularly if the patient is using high-strength preparations; however, the patient may confuse side-effects of the nicotine-replacement preparation with nicotine withdrawal symptoms. Common symptoms of nicotine withdrawal include malaise, headache, dizziness, sleep disturbance, coughing, influenza–like symptoms, depression, irritability, increased appetite, weight gain, restlessness, anxiety, drowsiness, aphthous ulcers, decreased heart rate, and impaired concentration.
- PREGNANCY The use of nicotine replacement therapy in pregnancy is preferable to the continuation of smoking,

but should be used only if smoking cessation without nicotine replacement fails. Intermittent therapy is preferable to patches but avoid liquorice-flavoured nicotine products. Patches are useful, however, if the patient is experiencing pregnancy-related nausea and vomiting. If patches are used, they should be removed before bed.

- BREAST FEEDING Nicotine is present in milk; however, the amount to which the infant is exposed is small and less hazardous than second-hand smoke. Intermittent therapy is preferred.
- HEPATIC IMPAIRMENT Use with caution in moderate to severe hepatic impairment.
- RENAL IMPAIRMENT Use with caution in severe renal impairment.
- DIRECTIONS FOR ADMINISTRATION Acidic beverages, such as coffee or fruit juice, may decrease the absorption of nicotine through the buccal mucosa and should be avoided for 15 minutes before the use of oral nicotine replacement therapy.
  Administration by transdermal patch Patches should be applied on waking to dry, non-hairy skin on the hip, trunk, or upper arm and held in position for 10–20 seconds to ensure adhesion; place next patch on a different area and avoid using the same site for several days.
  Administration by nasal spray Initially 1 spray should be used in both nostrils but when withdrawing from therapy, the dose can be gradually reduced to 1 spray in 1 nostril.
  Administration by oral spray The oral spray should be released into the mouth, holding the spray as close to the mouth as possible and avoiding the lips. The patient should not inhale while spraying and avoid swallowing for a few seconds after use. If using the oral spray for the first time, or if unit not used for 2 or more days, prime the unit before administration.
  Administration by sublingual tablet Each tablet should be placed under the tongue and allowed to dissolve.
  Administration by lozenge Slowly allow each lozenge to dissolve in the mouth; periodically move the lozenge from one side of the mouth to the other. Lozenges last for 10–30 minutes, depending on their size.
  Administration by inhalation Insert the cartridge into the device and draw in air through the mouthpiece; each session can last for approximately 5 minutes. The amount of nicotine from 1 puff of the cartridge is less than that from a cigarette, therefore it is necessary to inhale more often than when smoking a cigarette. A single 10 mg cartridge lasts for approximately 20 minutes of intense use; a single 15 mg cartridge lasts for approximately 40 minutes of intense use.
  Administration by medicated chewing gum Chew the gum until the taste becomes strong, then rest it between the cheek and gum; when the taste starts to fade, repeat this process. One piece of gum lasts for approximately 30 minutes.
- PRESCRIBING AND DISPENSING INFORMATION Flavours of chewing gum and lozenges may include mint, freshfruit, freshmint, icy white, or cherry.
- PATIENT AND CARER ADVICE Patient or carers should be given advice on how to administer nicotine chewing gum, inhalators, lozenges, sublingual tablets, oral spray, nasal spray and patches.

- MEDICINAL FORMS
  There can be variation in the licensing of different medicines containing the same drug.
  Spray
  EXCIPIENTS: May contain Ethanol
  ▸ Nicorette (McNeil Products Ltd)
  Nicotine 500 microgram per 1 actuation Nicorette 500micrograms/dose nasal spray | 10 ml GSL £16.18 DT = £14.84

Nervous system

4

▸ Nicorette QuickMist (McNeil Products Ltd)

Nicotine 1 mg per 1 actuation Nicorette QuickMist 1mg/dose mouthspray sugar-free | 13.2 ml GSL £13.03 DT = £13.03 sugar-free | 26.4 ml GSL £20.58

Sublingual tablet

CAUTIONARY AND ADVISORY LABELS 26

▸ Nicorette Microtab (McNeil Products Ltd)

Nicotine (as Nicotine cyclodextrin complex) 2 mg Nicorette Microtab 2mg sublingual tablets sugar-free | 100 tablet GSL £15.23 DT = £14.10

Transdermal patch

▸ NiQuitin (Omega Pharma Ltd)

Nicotine 7 mg per 24 hour NiQuitin 7mg patches | 7 patch GSL £9.97

Nicotine 14 mg per 24 hour NiQuitin 14mg patches | 7 patch GSL £9.97

Nicotine 21 mg per 24 hour NiQuitin 21mg patches | 7 patch GSL £9.97 DT = £9.97 | 14 patch GSL £18.79

▸ NiQuitin Clear (Omega Pharma Ltd)

Nicotine 7 mg per 24 hour NiQuitin Clear 7mg patches | 7 patch GSL £9.97

Nicotine 14 mg per 24 hour NiQuitin Clear 14mg patches | 7 patch GSL £9.97

Nicotine 21 mg per 24 hour NiQuitin Clear 21mg patches | 7 patch GSL £9.97 DT = £9.97 | 14 patch GSL £18.79
NiQuitin Pre-Quit Clear 21mg patches | 7 patch GSL £9.97 DT = £9.97

▸ Nicorette invisi (McNeil Products Ltd)

Nicotine 10 mg per 16 hour Nicorette invisi 10mg/16hours patches | 7 patch GSL £10.99 DT = £10.99

Nicotine 15 mg per 16 hour Nicorette invisi 15mg/16hours patches | 7 patch GSL £11.10 DT = £11.10

Nicotine 25 mg per 16 hour Nicorette invisi 25mg/16hours patches | 7 patch GSL £11.15 DT = £11.15 | 14 patch GSL £18.28

▸ Nicotinell TTS (GlaxoSmithKline Consumer Healthcare)

Nicotine 7 mg per 24 hour Nicotinell TTS 10 patches | 7 patch GSL £9.12

Nicotine 14 mg per 24 hour Nicotinell TTS 20 patches | 7 patch GSL £9.40

Nicotine 21 mg per 24 hour Nicotinell TTS 30 patches | 7 patch GSL £9.97 DT = £9.97 | 21 patch GSL £24.51

Medicated chewing-gum

▸ NiQuitin (Omega Pharma Ltd)

Nicotine 2 mg NiQuitin Fresh Mint 2mg medicated chewing gum sugar-free | 12 piece GSL £1.71 sugar-free | 24 piece GSL £2.85 sugar-free | 96 piece GSL £8.55 DT = £8.26
NiQuitin Extra Fresh Mint 2mg medicated chewing gum sugar-free | 30 piece GSL £5.16 sugar-free | 100 piece GSL £11.82 sugar-free | 200 piece GSL £20.69

Nicotine 4 mg NiQuitin Extra Fresh Mint 4mg medicated chewing gum sugar-free | 30 piece GSL £5.16 sugar-free | 100 piece GSL £11.82 sugar-free | 200 piece GSL £20.69
NiQuitin Fresh Mint 4mg medicated chewing gum sugar-free | 12 piece GSL £1.71 sugar-free | 24 piece GSL £2.85 sugar-free | 96 piece GSL £8.55 DT = £10.26

▸ Nicorette (McNeil Products Ltd)

Nicotine 2 mg Nicorette Freshmint 2mg medicated chewing gum sugar-free | 25 piece GSL £3.52 sugar-free | 105 piece GSL £10.27 sugar-free | 210 piece GSL £16.42
Nicorette Fruitfusion 2mg medicated chewing gum sugar-free | 105 piece GSL £10.27
Nicorette Original 2mg medicated chewing gum sugar-free | 105 piece GSL £10.27 sugar-free | 210 piece GSL £16.42

Nicotine 4 mg Nicorette Fruitfusion 4mg medicated chewing gum sugar-free | 105 piece GSL £12.57
Nicorette Original 4mg medicated chewing gum sugar-free | 105 piece GSL £12.56 sugar-free | 210 piece GSL £20.28
Nicorette Freshmint 4mg medicated chewing gum sugar-free | 25 piece GSL £3.53 sugar-free | 105 piece GSL £12.56 sugar-free | 210 piece GSL £20.28

Nicotine 6 mg Nicorette Fruitfusion 6mg medicated chewing gum sugar-free | 105 piece GSL £12.97 DT = £12.97 sugar-free | 210 piece GSL £20.81 DT = £20.81

▸ Nicorette Icy White (McNeil Products Ltd)

Nicotine 2 mg Nicorette Icy White 2mg medicated chewing gum sugar-free | 25 piece GSL £3.52 sugar-free | 105 piece GSL £10.26 sugar-free | 210 piece GSL £16.41

Nicotine 4 mg Nicorette Icy White 4mg medicated chewing gum sugar-free | 105 piece GSL £12.55

▸ Nicotinell (GlaxoSmithKline Consumer Healthcare)

Nicotine 2 mg Nicotinell Liquorice 2mg medicated chewing gum sugar-free | 96 piece GSL £8.26 DT = £8.26
Nicotinell Mint 2mg medicated chewing gum sugar-free | 96 piece GSL £8.26 DT = £8.26 sugar-free | 204 piece GSL £14.23
Nicotinell Fruit 2mg medicated chewing gum sugar-free | 96 piece GSL £8.26 DT = £8.26 sugar-free | 204 piece GSL £14.23

Nicotine 4 mg Nicotinell Liquorice 4mg medicated chewing gum sugar-free | 96 piece GSL £10.26 DT = £10.26
Nicotinell Mint 4mg medicated chewing gum sugar-free | 96 piece GSL £10.26 DT = £10.26
Nicotinell Fruit 4mg medicated chewing gum sugar-free | 96 piece GSL £10.26 DT = £10.26

Lozenge

EXCIPIENTS: May contain Aspartame
ELECTROLYTES: May contain Sodium

▸ NiQuitin (Omega Pharma Ltd)

Nicotine 1.5 mg NiQuitin Minis Mint 1.5mg lozenges sugar-free | 20 lozenge GSL £3.82 sugar-free | 60 lozenge GSL £10.21 DT = £10.21

Nicotine 2 mg NiQuitin Mint 2mg lozenges sugar-free | 36 lozenge GSL £5.91 sugar-free | 72 lozenge GSL £7.40 DT = £7.40
NiQuitin 2mg lozenges original menthol mint sugar-free | 36 lozenge GSL £5.91 sugar-free | 72 lozenge GSL £7.40 DT = £7.40

Nicotine 4 mg NiQuitin Mint 4mg lozenges sugar-free | 36 lozenge GSL £5.91 sugar-free | 72 lozenge GSL £7.40 DT = £7.40
NiQuitin Minis Mint 4mg lozenges sugar-free | 20 lozenge GSL £3.82 sugar-free | 60 lozenge GSL £10.21
NiQuitin Pre-Quit Mint 4mg lozenges sugar-free | 36 lozenge GSL £5.91
NiQuitin 4mg lozenges original menthol mint sugar-free | 36 lozenge GSL £5.91 sugar-free | 72 lozenge GSL £7.40 DT = £7.40

▸ Nicorette (McNeil Products Ltd)

Nicotine 2 mg Nicorette Cools 2mg lozenges sugar-free | 20 lozenge GSL £3.34 sugar-free | 80 lozenge GSL £12.05

Nicotine 4 mg Nicorette Cools 4mg lozenges sugar-free | 80 lozenge GSL £12.17

▸ Nicotinell (GlaxoSmithKline Consumer Healthcare)

Nicotine (as Nicotine bitartrate) 1 mg Nicotinell 1mg lozenges sugar-free | 12 lozenge GSL £1.59 sugar-free | 72 lozenge GSL £8.03 sugar-free | 96 lozenge GSL £9.12 DT = £9.12 sugar-free | 144 lozenge GSL £13.59

Nicotine (as Nicotine bitartrate) 2 mg Nicotinell 2mg lozenges sugar-free | 72 lozenge GSL £9.41 sugar-free | 96 lozenge GSL £10.60 sugar-free | 144 lozenge GSL £15.88

Inhalation vapour

▸ Nicorette (McNeil Products Ltd)

Nicotine 15 mg Nicorette 15mg Inhalator | 4 cartridge GSL £4.87 DT = £4.59 | 20 cartridge GSL £17.78 DT = £16.24 | 36 cartridge GSL £28.28 DT = £25.83

Varenicline

● **DRUG ACTION** Varenicline is a selective nicotine-receptor partial agonist.

● **INDICATIONS AND DOSE**

To aid smoking cessation

▸ BY MOUTH

▸ **Adult:** Initially 500 micrograms once daily for 3 days, increased to 500 micrograms twice daily for 4 days, then 1 mg twice daily for 11 weeks; reduced if not tolerated to 500 micrograms twice daily, usually to be started 1–2 weeks before target stop date but can be started up to a maximum of 5 weeks before target stop date, 12-week course can be repeated in abstinent individuals to reduce risk of relapse

IMPORTANT SAFETY INFORMATION

MHRA/CHM ADVICE: SUICIDAL BEHAVIOUR AND VARENICLINE
Patients should be advised to discontinue treatment and seek prompt medical advice if they develop agitation, depressed mood, or suicidal thoughts. Patients with a

history of psychiatric illness should be monitored closely while taking varenicline.

- CAUTIONS Conditions that may lower seizure threshold · history of cardiovascular disease · history of psychiatric illness (may exacerbate underlying illness including depression) · predisposition to seizures
- SIDE-EFFECTS
- **Common or very common** Appetite abnormal · asthenia · chest discomfort · constipation · diarrhoea · dizziness · drowsiness · dry mouth · gastrointestinal discomfort · gastrointestinal disorders · headache · joint disorders · muscle complaints · nausea · oral disorders · pain · skin reactions · sleep disorders · vomiting · weight increased
- **Uncommon** Allergic rhinitis · anxiety · arrhythmias · behaviour abnormal · burping · conjunctivitis · depression · eye pain · fever · fungal infection · haemorrhage · hallucination · hot flush · hyperglycaemia · influenza like illness · malaise · menorrhagia · mood swings · numbness · palpitations · seizure · sexual dysfunction · suicidal ideation · sweat changes · thinking abnormal · tinnitus · tremor · urinary disorders
- **Rare or very rare** Angioedema · bradyphrenia · coordination abnormal · costochondritis · cyst · diabetes mellitus · dysarthria · eye disorders · feeling cold · glycosuria · muscle tone increased · polydipsia · psychosis · scleral discolouration · severe cutaneous adverse reactions (SCARs) · snoring · vaginal discharge · vision disorders
- PREGNANCY Avoid—toxicity in *animal* studies.
- BREAST FEEDING Avoid—present in milk in *animal* studies.
- RENAL IMPAIRMENT
  Dose adjustments If eGFR less than 30 mL/minute/1.73 m^2, initial dose 500 micrograms once daily, increased after 3 days to 1 mg once daily.
- TREATMENT CESSATION Risk of relapse, irritability, depression, and insomnia on discontinuation; consider dose tapering on completion of 12-week course.
- NATIONAL FUNDING/ACCESS DECISIONS
  NICE decisions
- Varenicline for smoking cessation (July 2007) NICE TA123 Varenicline is recommended, within its licensed indications, as an option for smokers who have expressed a desire to quit smoking; it should normally be prescribed only as part of a programme of behavioural support. www.nice.org.uk/TA123
- MEDICINAL FORMS
  There can be variation in the licensing of different medicines containing the same drug.
  Tablet
  CAUTIONARY AND ADVISORY LABELS 3
  - Champix (Pfizer Ltd)
    Varenicline (as Varenicline tartrate) 500 microgram Champix 0.5mg tablets | 56 tablet [PoM] £54.60 DT = £54.60
    Varenicline (as Varenicline tartrate) 1 mg Champix 1mg tablets | 28 tablet [PoM] £27.30 DT = £27.30 | 56 tablet [PoM] £54.60
    Champix 0.5mg/1mg 2 week treatment initiation pack | 25 tablet [PoM] £27.30 DT = £27.30
    Champix 0.5mg/1mg 4 week treatment initiation pack | 53 tablet [PoM] £54.60

8.3 Opioid dependence

Other drugs used for Opioid dependence Buprenorphine, p. 442 · Naltrexone hydrochloride, p. 491

ANALGESICS > OPIOIDS

▶ 441

Methadone hydrochloride

- INDICATIONS AND DOSE
  Severe pain
- ▶ BY MOUTH, OR BY SUBCUTANEOUS INJECTION, OR BY INTRAMUSCULAR INJECTION
- ▶ Adult: 5–10 mg every 6–8 hours, adjusted according to response, on prolonged use not to be given more frequently than every 12 hours

Adjunct in treatment of opioid dependence
- ▶ BY MOUTH USING ORAL SOLUTION
- ▶ Adult: Initially 10–30 mg daily, increased in steps of 5–10 mg daily if required until no signs of withdrawal nor evidence of intoxication, dose to be increased in the first week, then increased every few days as necessary up to usual dose, maximum weekly dose increase of 30 mg; usual dose 60–120 mg daily

Adjunct in treatment of opioid dependence if tolerance low or not known
- ▶ BY MOUTH USING ORAL SOLUTION
- ▶ Adult: Initially 10–20 mg daily, increased in steps of 5–10 mg daily if required until no signs of withdrawal nor evidence of intoxication, dose to be increased in the first week, then increased every few days as necessary up to usual dose, maximum weekly dose increase of 30 mg; usual dose 60–120 mg daily

Adjunct in treatment of opioid dependence if tolerance high (under expert supervision)
- ▶ BY MOUTH USING ORAL SOLUTION
- ▶ Adult: Initially up to 40 mg daily, increased in steps of 5–10 mg daily if required until no signs of withdrawal nor evidence of intoxication, dose to be increased in the first week, then increased every few days as necessary up to usual dose, maximum weekly dose increase of 30 mg; usual dose 60–120 mg daily

Cough in terminal disease
- ▶ INITIALLY BY MOUTH USING LINCTUS
- ▶ Adult: 1–2 mg every 4–6 hours, (by mouth) reduced to 1–2 mg twice daily, use twice daily frequency if prolonged use

DOSE EQUIVALENCE AND CONVERSION
- ▶ See buprenorphine p. 442 for dose adjustments in opioid substitution therapy, for patients taking methadone who want to switch to buprenorphine.

- UNLICENSED USE Methadone hydrochloride doses for opioid dependence in the BNF may differ from those in the product literature.

> IMPORTANT SAFETY INFORMATION
> Methadone oral solution 1 mg/mL is 2½ times the strength of Methadone Linctus (2 mg/5mL). Many preparations of Methadone oral solution are licensed for opioid drug addiction only but some are also licensed for analgesia in severe pain.

- CONTRA-INDICATIONS Phaeochromocytoma
- CAUTIONS Family history of sudden death (ECG monitoring recommended) · history of cardiac conduction abnormalities
  CAUTIONS, FURTHER INFORMATION
- ▶ QT-interval prolongation Patients with the following risk factors for QT-interval prolongation should be carefully monitored while taking methadone: heart or liver disease, electrolyte abnormalities, or concomitant treatment with drugs that can prolong QT interval; patients requiring more than 100 mg daily should also be monitored.
- INTERACTIONS → Appendix 1: opioids

4

Nervous system

- SIDE-EFFECTS

  GENERAL SIDE-EFFECTS Asthma exacerbated · dry eye · dysuria · hyperprolactinaemia · hypothermia · menstrual cycle irregularities · mood altered · nasal dryness · postural hypotension · QT interval prolongation · torsade de pointes

  SPECIFIC SIDE-EFFECTS

- With oral use Galactorrhoea · intracranial pressure increased

- With parenteral use Biliary spasm · muscle rigidity · oedema · restlessness · sexual dysfunction · sleep disorder · ureteral spasm

  SIDE-EFFECTS, FURTHER INFORMATION Methadone is a long-acting opioid therefore effects may be cumulative.
  Methadone, even in low doses is a special hazard for children; non-dependent adults are also at risk of toxicity; dependent adults are at risk if tolerance is incorrectly assessed during induction.

  Overdose Methadone has a very long duration of action; patients may need to be monitored for long periods following large overdoses.

- BREAST FEEDING Withdrawal symptoms in infant; breast-feeding permissible during maintenance but dose should be as low as possible and infant monitored to avoid sedation (high doses of methadone carry an increased risk of sedation and respiratory depression in the neonate).

- RENAL IMPAIRMENT Avoid use or reduce dose; opioid effects increased and prolonged and increased cerebral sensitivity occurs.

- TREATMENT CESSATION Avoid abrupt withdrawal.

- DIRECTIONS FOR ADMINISTRATION Syrup preserved with hydroxybenzoate (parabens) esters may be incompatible with methadone hydrochloride.

- PRESCRIBING AND DISPENSING INFORMATION Flavours of oral liquid formulations may include tolu.

  METHADOSE ® The final strength of the methadone mixture to be dispensed to the patient must be specified on the prescription.
  Important—care is required in prescribing and dispensing the **correct strength** since any confusion could lead to an overdose; this preparation should be dispensed only **after dilution** as appropriate with *Methadose* ® Diluent (life of diluted solution 3 months) and is for drug dependent persons.

- NATIONAL FUNDING/ACCESS DECISIONS

  NICE decisions

- **Methadone and buprenorphine for the management of opioid dependence (January 2007)** NICE TA114
  Oral methadone and buprenorphine are recommended for maintenance therapy in the management of opioid dependence. Patients should be committed to a supportive care programme including a flexible dosing regimen administered under supervision for at least 3 months, until compliance is assured. Selection of methadone or buprenorphine should be made on a case-by-case basis, but methadone should be prescribed if both drugs are equally suitable.
  www.nice.org.uk/TA114

- LESS SUITABLE FOR PRESCRIBING Methadone linctus is less suitable for prescribing for cough in terminal disease (has a tendency to accumulate).

- MEDICINAL FORMS
  There can be variation in the licensing of different medicines containing the same drug. Forms available from special-order manufacturers include: tablet, capsule, oral suspension, oral solution, solution for injection

  Tablet
  CAUTIONARY AND ADVISORY LABELS 2
  ▶ Physeptone (Martindale Pharmaceuticals Ltd)
    Methadone hydrochloride 5 mg Physeptone 5mg tablets | 50 tablet [PoM] £2.84 DT = £2.84 [CD2]

  Solution for injection
  ▶ Methadone hydrochloride (Non-proprietary)
    Methadone hydrochloride 10 mg per 1 ml Methadone 35mg/3.5ml solution for injection ampoules | 10 ampoule [PoM] £13.92 DT = £12.87 [CD2]
    Methadone hydrochloride 50 mg per 1 ml Methadone 50mg/1ml solution for injection ampoules | 10 ampoule [PoM] 🛇 [CD2]
  ▶ Physeptone (Martindale Pharmaceuticals Ltd)
    Methadone hydrochloride 10 mg per 1 ml Physeptone 35mg/3.5ml solution for injection ampoules | 10 ampoule [PoM] £12.87 DT = £12.87 [CD2]
    Physeptone 50mg/5ml solution for injection ampoules | 10 ampoule [PoM] £16.33 DT = £16.33 [CD2]
    Physeptone 20mg/2ml solution for injection ampoules | 10 ampoule [PoM] £13.15 DT = £13.15 [CD2]
    Physeptone 10mg/1ml solution for injection ampoules | 10 ampoule [PoM] £7.63 DT = £7.63 [CD2] | 100 ampoule [PoM] £73.05 [CD2]
    Methadone hydrochloride 25 mg per 1 ml Physeptone 50mg/2ml solution for injection ampoules | 10 ampoule [PoM] £17.72 [CD2]
    Methadone hydrochloride 50 mg per 1 ml Physeptone 50mg/1ml solution for injection ampoules | 10 ampoule [PoM] £17.72 [CD2]

  Oral solution
  CAUTIONARY AND ADVISORY LABELS 2
  ▶ Methadone hydrochloride (Non-proprietary)
    Methadone hydrochloride 1 mg per 1 ml Methadone 1mg/ml oral solution | 100 ml [PoM] £0.91–£1.00 DT = £0.64 [CD2] | 500 ml [PoM] £6.18 DT = £3.20 [CD2] | 2500 ml [PoM] £16.00–£32.10 [CD2]
    Methadone 1mg/ml oral solution sugar-free sugar-free | 50 ml [PoM] £1.04 DT = £1.04 [CD2] sugar-free | 100 ml [PoM] £2.08 DT = £2.08 [CD2] sugar-free | 500 ml [PoM] £6.30 DT = £6.30 [CD2] sugar-free | 2500 ml [PoM] £31.50–£32.50 [CD2]
  ▶ Methadose (Rosemont Pharmaceuticals Ltd)
    Methadone hydrochloride 10 mg per 1 ml Methadose 10mg/ml oral solution concentrate sugar-free | 150 ml [PoM] £12.01 [CD2]
    Methadone hydrochloride 20 mg per 1 ml Methadose 20mg/ml oral solution concentrate sugar-free | 150 ml [PoM] £24.02 [CD2]
  ▶ Metharose (Rosemont Pharmaceuticals Ltd)
    Methadone hydrochloride 1 mg per 1 ml Metharose 1mg/ml oral solution sugar free sugar-free | 500 ml [PoM] £6.82 DT = £6.30 [CD2]
  ▶ Physeptone (Martindale Pharmaceuticals Ltd)
    Methadone hydrochloride 1 mg per 1 ml Physeptone 1mg/ml mixture | 100 ml [PoM] £1.08 DT = £0.64 [CD2] | 500 ml [PoM] £5.46 DT = £3.20 [CD2] | 2500 ml [PoM] £27.29 [CD2]
    Physeptone 1mg/ml oral solution sugar free sugar-free | 100 ml [PoM] £1.08 DT = £2.08 [CD2] sugar-free | 500 ml [PoM] £5.46 DT = £6.30 [CD2] sugar-free | 2500 ml [PoM] £27.29 [CD2]

OPIOID RECEPTOR ANTAGONISTS

Buprenorphine with naloxone

The properties listed below are those particular to the combination only. For the properties of the components please consider, buprenorphine p. 442, naloxone hydrochloride p. 1329.

- INDICATIONS AND DOSE

  Adjunct in the treatment of opioid dependence (dose expressed as buprenorphine)
  ▶ BY SUBLINGUAL ADMINISTRATION
  ▶ Adult: Initially 2–4 mg once daily, an additional dose of 2–4 mg may be administered on day 1 depending on the individual patient's requirement, increased in steps of 2–8 mg, adjusted according to response, total weekly dose may be divided and given on alternate days or 3 times weekly; maximum 24 mg per day

● INTERACTIONS → Appendix 1: opioids

● NATIONAL FUNDING/ACCESS DECISIONS

Scottish Medicines Consortium (SMC) Decisions
The *Scottish Medicines Consortium* has advised (February 2007) that Suboxone ® should be restricted for use in patients in whom methadone is not suitable.

● MEDICINAL FORMS
There can be variation in the licensing of different medicines containing the same drug.

Sublingual tablet
CAUTIONARY AND ADVISORY LABELS 2, 26
▸ Suboxone (Indivior UK Ltd)
  Naloxone (as Naloxone hydrochloride) 500 microgram, Buprenorphine (as Buprenorphine hydrochloride) 2 mg Suboxone 2mg/500microgram sublingual tablets sugar-free | 28 tablet [PoM] £25.40 DT = £25.40 [CD3]
  Naloxone (as Naloxone hydrochloride) 2 mg, Buprenorphine (as Buprenorphine hydrochloride) 8 mg Suboxone 8mg/2mg sublingual tablets sugar-free | 28 tablet [PoM] £76.19 DT = £76.19 [CD3]
  Naloxone (as Naloxone hydrochloride) 4 mg, Buprenorphine (as Buprenorphine hydrochloride) 16 mg Suboxone 16mg/4mg sublingual tablets sugar-free | 28 tablet [PoM] £152.38 [CD3]

SYMPATHOMIMETICS › ALPHA$_2$-ADRENOCEPTOR AGONISTS

Lofexidine hydrochloride

● DRUG ACTION Lofexidine is an alpha$_2$-adrenergic agonist.

● INDICATIONS AND DOSE

Management of symptoms of opioid withdrawal
▸ BY MOUTH
▸ Adult: Initially 800 micrograms daily in divided doses, increased in steps of 400–800 micrograms daily (max. per dose 800 micrograms) as required recommended duration of treatment 7–10 days if no opioid use (but longer may be required); maximum 2.4 mg per day

● CAUTIONS Bradycardia · cerebrovascular disease · depression · history of QT prolongation · hypotension (monitor pulse rate and blood pressure) · metabolic disturbances · recent myocardial infarction · severe coronary insufficiency

● INTERACTIONS → Appendix 1: lofexidine

● SIDE-EFFECTS
▸ Common or very common Bradycardia · dizziness · drowsiness · hypotension · mucosal dryness
▸ Frequency not known QT interval prolongation

● PREGNANCY Use only if benefit outweighs risk—no information available.

● BREAST FEEDING Use only if benefit outweighs risk—no information available.

● RENAL IMPAIRMENT Caution in chronic impairment.

● MONITORING REQUIREMENTS Monitoring of blood pressure and pulse rate is recommended on initiation, for at least 72 hours or until a stable dose is achieved, and on discontinuation.

● TREATMENT CESSATION Treatment should be withdrawn gradually over 2–4 days (or longer) to reduce the risk of rebound hypertension and associated symptoms.

● PRESCRIBING AND DISPENSING INFORMATION Lofexidine has been used in children over 12 years in the management of symptoms of opioid withdrawal.

● PATIENT AND CARER ADVICE The patient should take part of the dose at bedtime to offset insomnia associated with opioid withdrawal.

● MEDICINAL FORMS
There can be variation in the licensing of different medicines containing the same drug.

Tablet
CAUTIONARY AND ADVISORY LABELS 2
▸ BritLofex (Britannia Pharmaceuticals Ltd)
  Lofexidine hydrochloride 200 microgram BritLofex 200microgram tablets | 60 tablet [PoM] £61.79

Chapter 5
Infection

CONTENTS

1 Amoebic infection

Other drugs used for Amoebic infection Metronidazole, p. 533 · Tinidazole, p. 534

ANTIPROTOZOALS

Diloxanide furoate

● **INDICATIONS AND DOSE**

Chronic amoebiasis | Acute amoebiasis as adjunct to metronidazole or tinidazole

▶ BY MOUTH
▶ Child 12–17 years: 500 mg 3 times a day for 10 days
▶ Adult: 500 mg 3 times a day for 10 days

● UNLICENSED USE Not licensed for use in children under 25 kg body-weight.
● SIDE-EFFECTS Abdominal cramps · appetite decreased · diarrhoea · dizziness · flatulence · headache · nausea · skin reactions · vomiting
● PREGNANCY Manufacturer advises avoid—no information available.
● BREAST FEEDING Manufacturer advises avoid.
● MEDICINAL FORMS There can be variation in the licensing of different medicines containing the same drug. Forms available from special-order manufacturers include: oral suspension, oral solution

Tablet
CAUTIONARY AND ADVISORY LABELS 9
▶ Diloxanide furoate (Non-proprietary)
Diloxanide furoate 500 mg Diloxanide 500mg tablets | 30 tablet [PoM] £93.50

Mepacrine hydrochloride

● **INDICATIONS AND DOSE**

Giardiasis

▶ BY MOUTH
▶ Adult: 100 mg every 8 hours for 5–7 days

● UNLICENSED USE Not licensed for use in giardiasis.
● CAUTIONS Avoid in psoriasis · elderly · history of psychosis
● INTERACTIONS → Appendix 1: mepacrine
● SIDE-EFFECTS Aplastic anaemia (long term use) · central nervous system stimulation (with high doses) · corneal deposits · dermatosis (long term use) · dizziness · exfoliative dermatitis (severe; long term use) · gastrointestinal disorder · headache · hepatitis (long term use) · nail discolouration · nausea (with high doses) · oral discolouration · skin discolouration (long term use) · toxic psychosis (transient; with high doses) · urine discolouration (long term use) · visual impairment · vomiting (with high doses)
● HEPATIC IMPAIRMENT Use with caution.
● MEDICINAL FORMS Forms available from special-order manufacturers include: tablet

2 Bacterial infection

Antibacterials, principles of therapy
07-Mar-2017

Antibacterial drug choice

Before selecting an antibacterial the clinician must first consider two factors— the patient and the known or likely causative organism. Factors related to the patient which must be considered include history of allergy, renal and hepatic function, susceptibility to infection (i.e. whether immunocompromised), ability to tolerate drugs by mouth, severity of illness, ethnic origin, age, whether taking other medication and, if female, whether pregnant, breast-feeding or taking an oral contraceptive.

The known or likely organism and its antibacterial sensitivity, in association with the above factors, will suggest one or more antibacterials, the final choice depending on the microbiological, pharmacological, and toxicological properties.

An example of a rational approach to the selection of an antibacterial is treatment of a urinary-tract infection in a patient complaining of nausea and symptoms of a urinary-tract infection in early pregnancy. The organism is reported as being resistant to ampicillin p. 540 but sensitive to nitrofurantoin p. 579 (can cause nausea), gentamicin p. 510 (can be given only by injection and best avoided in pregnancy), tetracycline p. 557 (causes dental discoloration) and trimethoprim p. 563 (folate antagonist therefore theoretical teratogenic risk), and cefalexin p. 516. The safest antibiotics in pregnancy are the penicillins and cephalosporins; therefore, cefalexin would be indicated for this patient.

The principles involved in selection of an antibacterial must allow for a number of variables including changing renal and hepatic function, increasing bacterial resistance, and information on side-effects. Duration of therapy, dosage, and route of administration depend on site, type and severity of infection and response.

Antibacterial policies

Local policies often limit the antibacterials that may be used to achieve reasonable economy consistent with adequate cover, and to reduce the development of resistant organisms. A policy may indicate a range of drugs for general use, and permit other drugs only on the advice of the microbiologist or physician responsible for the control of infectious diseases.

Antibacterials, considerations before starting therapy

The following precepts should be considered before starting:

- Viral infections should not be treated with antibacterials. However, antibacterials may be used to treat secondary bacterial infection (e.g. bacterial pneumonia secondary to influenza);
- Samples should be taken for culture and sensitivity testing; ' **blind**' antibacterial prescribing for unexplained pyrexia usually leads to further difficulty in establishing the diagnosis;
- Knowledge of **prevalent organisms** and their current sensitivity is of great help in choosing an antibacterial before bacteriological confirmation is available. Generally, narrow-spectrum antibacterials are preferred to broad-spectrum antibacterials unless there is a clear clinical indication (e.g. life-threatening sepsis);
- The **dose** of an antibacterial varies according to a number of factors including age, weight, hepatic function, renal function, and severity of infection. The prescribing of the so-called 'standard' dose in serious infections may result in failure of treatment or even death of the patient; therefore it is important to prescribe a dose appropriate to the condition. An inadequate dose may also increase the likelihood of antibacterial resistance. On the other hand, for an antibacterial with a narrow margin between the toxic and therapeutic dose (e.g. an aminoglycoside) it is also important to avoid an excessive dose and the concentration of the drug in the plasma may need to be monitored;
- The **route** of administration of an antibacterial often depends on the severity of the infection. Life-threatening infections require intravenous therapy. Antibacterials that are well absorbed may be given by mouth even for some serious infections. Parenteral administration is also appropriate when the oral route cannot be used (e.g. because of vomiting) or if absorption is inadequate. Whenever possible, painful intramuscular injections should be avoided in children;
- **Duration** of therapy depends on the nature of the infection and the response to treatment. Courses should not be unduly prolonged because they encourage resistance, they may lead to side-effects and they are

costly. However, in certain infections such as tuberculosis or osteomyelitis it may be necessary to treat for prolonged periods. Conversely a single dose of an antibacterial may cure uncomplicated urinary-tract infections. The prescription for an antibacterial should specify the duration of treatment or the date when treatment is to be reviewed.

Superinfection

In general, broad-spectrum antibacterial drugs such as the cephalosporins are more likely to be associated with adverse reactions related to the selection of resistant organisms e.g. *fungal infections* or *antibiotic-associated colitis* (pseudomembranous colitis); other problems associated with superinfection include vaginitis and pruritus ani.

Antibacterial therapy

When the pathogen has been isolated treatment may be changed to a more appropriate antibacterial if necessary. If no bacterium is cultured the antibacterial can be continued or stopped on clinical grounds.

Notifiable diseases

Doctors must notify the Proper Officer of the local authority (usually the consultant in communicable disease control) when attending a patient suspected of suffering from any of the diseases listed below; a form is available from the Proper Officer.

Anthrax	Mumps
Botulism	Paratyphoid fever
Brucellosis	Plague
Cholera	Poliomyelitis, acute
Diarrhoea (infectious bloody)	Rabies
Diphtheria	Rubella
Encephalitis, acute	SARS
Food poisoning	Scarlet fever
Haemolytic uraemic syndrome	Smallpox
Haemorrhagic fever (viral)	Streptococcal disease (Group A, invasive)
Hepatitis, viral	
Legionnaires' disease	Tetanus
Leprosy	Tuberculosis
Malaria	Typhoid fever
Measles	Typhus
Meningitis	Whooping cough
Meningococcal septicaemia	Yellow fever

Note It is good practice for doctors to also inform the consultant in communicable disease control of instances of other infections (e.g. psittacosis) where there could be a public health risk.

Sepsis, early management

[EvGr] Patients identified as being at high risk of severe illness or death due to suspected sepsis should be given a broad-spectrum antibacterial at the maximum recommended dose without delay (ideally within one hour). Microbiological samples and blood cultures must be taken prior to administration of antibiotics; the prescription should be adjusted subsequently according to susceptibility results.

A thorough clinical examination should be carried out to identify sources of infection. If the source of infection is identified, treat in line with local antibacterial guidance or susceptibility results.

Patients who require empirical intravenous treatment for a suspected infection, but who have no confirmed diagnosis, should be treated with an intravenous antibiotic from the local formulary and in line with national guidelines.

The need for intravenous fluids, inotropes, vasopressors and oxygen should also be assessed without delay, taking into consideration the patient's lactate concentration, systolic blood pressure, and their risk of severe illness or death. Patients at high risk should be monitored continuously if possible, and no less than every 30 minutes.

Patients with suspected sepsis who are not immediately deemed to be at high risk of severe illness or death, should be re-assessed regularly for the need for empirical treatment, taking into consideration all risk factors including lactate concentration and evidence of acute kidney injury. Ⓐ

Antibacterials, use for prophylaxis

16-Mar-2017

Rheumatic fever: prevention of recurrence

- Phenoxymethylpenicillin p. 538 *or* sulfadiazine p. 553.

Invasive group A streptococcal infection: prevention of secondary cases

- Phenoxymethylpenicillin.

Patients who are penicillin allergic, *either* erythromycin p. 530 *or* azithromycin p. 528 [unlicensed indication].

For details of those who should receive chemoprophylaxis contact a consultant in communicable disease control (or a consultant in infectious diseases or the local Public Health England Laboratory).

Meningococcal meningitis: prevention of secondary cases

- Ciprofloxacin p. 548 *or* rifampicin p. 571 *or* i/m ceftriaxone p. 520 [unlicensed indication].

For details of those who should receive chemoprophylaxis contact a consultant in communicable disease control (or a consultant in infectious diseases or the local Public Health England laboratory). Unless there has been direct exposure of the mouth or nose to infectious droplets from a patient with meningococcal disease who has received less than 24 hours of antibacterial treatment, healthcare workers do not generally require chemoprophylaxis.

Haemophilus influenzae type b disease: prevention of secondary cases

- Rifampicin *or* (if rifampicin cannot be used) i/m or i/v ceftriaxone [unlicensed indication].

For details of those who should receive chemoprophylaxis contact a consultant in communicable disease control (or a consultant in infectious diseases or the local Public Health England laboratory). Unless there has been direct exposure of the mouth or nose to infectious droplets from a patient with meningococcal disease who has received less than 24 hours of antibacterial treatment, healthcare workers do not generally require chemoprophylaxis.

Within 4 weeks of illness onset in an index case with confirmed or suspected invasive *Haemophilus influenzae* type b disease, give antibacterial prophylaxis to all household contacts if there is a vulnerable individual in the household. Also, give antibacterial prophylaxis to the index case if they are in contact with vulnerable household contacts or if they are under 10 years of age. Vulnerable individuals include the immunocompromised, those with asplenia, or children under 10 years of age. If there are 2 or more cases of invasive *Haemophilus influenzae* type b disease within 120 days in a pre-school or primary school, antibacterial prophylaxis should also be given to all room contacts (including staff). Also see immunisation against *Haemophilus influenzae* type b disease.

Diphtheria in non-immune patients: prevention of secondary cases

- Erythromycin (*or* another macrolide e.g. azithromycin *or* clarithromycin p. 529).

Treat for further 10 days if nasopharyngeal swabs positive after first 7 days' treatment.

Pertussis, antibacterial prophylaxis

- Clarithromycin (*or* azithromycin *or* erythromycin).

Within 3 weeks of onset of cough in the index case, give antibacterial prophylaxis to all close contacts if amongst them there is at least one unimmunised or partially immunised child under 1 year of age, *or* if there is at least one individual who has not received a pertussis-containing vaccine more than 1 week and less than 5 years ago (so long as that individual lives or works with children under 4 months of age, is pregnant at over 32 weeks gestation, or is a healthcare worker who works with children under 1 year of age or with pregnant women).

Pneumococcal infection in asplenia or in patients with sickle-cell disease, antibacterial prophylaxis

- Phenoxymethylpenicillin.

If penicillin-allergic, erythromycin.

Antibacterial prophylaxis is not fully reliable. Antibacterial prophylaxis may be discontinued in children over 5 years of age with sickle-cell disease who have received pneumococcal immunisation and who do not have a history of severe pneumococcal infection.

Tuberculosis antibacterial prophylaxis in susceptible close contacts or those who have become tuberculin positive

- See *Close contacts* and *Chemoprophylaxis for latent tuberculosis* under Tuberculosis p. 567.

Animal and human bites, antibacterial prophylaxis

- Co-amoxiclav p. 542 alone (*or* doxycycline p. 555 + metronidazole p. 533 if penicillin-allergic).

Cleanse wound thoroughly. For tetanus-prone wound, give human tetanus immunoglobulin p. 1257 (with a tetanus-containing vaccine if necessary, according to immunisation history and risk of infection).

Consider rabies prophylaxis for bites from animals in endemic countries. Assess risk of blood-borne viruses (including HIV, hepatitis B and C) and give appropriate prophylaxis to prevent viral spread.

Antibacterial prophylaxis recommended for wounds less than 48–72 hours old when the risk of infection is high (e.g. bites from humans or cats; bites to the hand, foot, face, or genital area; bites involving oedema, crush or puncture injury, or other moderate to severe injury; wounds that cannot be debrided adequately; patients with diabetes mellitus, cirrhosis, asplenia, prosthetic joints or valves, or those who are immunocompromised). Give antibacterial prophylaxis for up to 5 days.

Early-onset neonatal infection, antibacterial prophylaxis

- i/v benzylpenicillin sodium p. 537 (or i/v clindamycin p. 526 if history of allergy to penicillins).

Give intrapartum prophylaxis to women with group B streptococcal colonisation, bacteriuria, or infection in the current pregnancy, or to women who had a previous baby with an invasive group B streptococcal infection. Consider prophylaxis for women in preterm labour if there is prelabour rupture of membranes or if intrapartum rupture of membranes lasting more than 18 hours is suspected.

Gastro-intestinal procedures, antibacterial prophylaxis

Operations on stomach or oesophagus

- Single dose of i/v gentamicin p. 510 *or* i/v cefuroxime p. 518 *or* i/v co-amoxiclav (additional intra-operative or postoperative doses may be given for prolonged procedures or if there is major blood loss).

Intravenous antibacterial prophylaxis should be given up to 30 minutes before the procedure.

Add i/v teicoplanin p. 524 (*or* vancomycin p. 525) if high risk of meticillin-resistant *Staphylococcus aureus*.

Open biliary surgery

- Single dose of i/v cefuroxime + i/v metronidazole *or* i/v gentamicin + i/v metronidazole *or* i/v co-amoxiclav alone (additional intra-operative or postoperative doses may be given for prolonged procedures or if there is major blood loss).

Intravenous antibacterial prophylaxis should be given up to 30 minutes before the procedure.

Where i/v metronidazole is suggested, it may alternatively be given by suppository but to allow adequate absorption, it should be given 2 hours before surgery.

Add i/v teicoplanin (*or* vancomycin) if high risk of meticillin-resistant *Staphylococcus aureus*.

Resections of colon and rectum for carcinoma, and resections in inflammatory bowel disease, and appendicectomy

- Single dose of i/v gentamicin + i/v metronidazole *or* i/v cefuroxime + i/v metronidazole *or* i/v co-amoxiclav alone (additional intra-operative or postoperative doses may be given for prolonged procedures or if there is major blood loss).

Intravenous antibacterial prophylaxis should be given up to 30 minutes before the procedure.

Where i/v metronidazole is suggested, it may alternatively be given by suppository but to allow adequate absorption, it should be given 2 hours before surgery.

Add i/v teicoplanin (*or* vancomycin) if high risk of meticillin-resistant *Staphylococcus aureus*.

Endoscopic retrograde cholangiopancreatography

- Single dose of i/v gentamicin p. 510 *or* oral *or* i/v ciprofloxacin p. 548.

Intravenous antibacterial prophylaxis should be given up to 30 minutes before the procedure.

Prophylaxis recommended if pancreatic pseudocyst, immunocompromised, history of liver transplantation, or risk of incomplete biliary drainage. For biliary complications following liver transplantation, add i/v amoxicillin p. 539 or i/v teicoplanin p. 524 (*or* vancomycin p. 525).

Percutaneous endoscopic gastrostomy or jejunostomy

- Single dose of i/v co-amoxiclav p. 542 *or* i/v cefuroxime p. 518.

Intravenous antibacterial prophylaxis should be given up to 30 minutes before the procedure.

Use single dose of i/v teicoplanin (*or* vancomycin) if history of allergy to penicillins or cephalosporins, or if high risk of meticillin-resistant *Staphylococcus aureus*.

Orthopaedic surgery, antibacterial prophylaxis

Joint replacement including hip and knee

- Single dose of i/v cefuroxime alone *or* i/v flucloxacillin p. 544+ i/v gentamicin (additional intra-operative or postoperative doses may be given for prolonged procedures or if there is major blood loss).

Intravenous antibacterial prophylaxis should be given up to 30 minutes before the procedure.

If history of allergy to penicillins or to cephalosporins or if high risk of meticillin-resistant *Staphylococcus aureus*, use single dose of i/v teicoplanin (*or* vancomycin) + i/v gentamicin (additional intra-operative or postoperative doses may be given for prolonged procedures or if there is major blood loss).

Closed fractures

- Single dose of i/v cefuroxime *or* i/v flucloxacillin (additional intra-operative or postoperative doses may be given for prolonged procedures or if there is major blood loss).

Intravenous antibacterial prophylaxis should be given up to 30 minutes before the procedure.

If history of allergy to penicillins or to cephalosporins or if high risk of meticillin-resistant *Staphylococcus aureus*, use single dose of i/v teicoplanin (*or* vancomycin) (additional intra-operative or postoperative doses may be given for prolonged procedures or if there is major blood loss).

Open fractures

- Use i/v co-amoxiclav alone *or* i/v cefuroxime + i/v metronidazole p. 533 (*or* i/v clindamycin p. 526 alone if history of allergy to penicillins or to cephalosporins).

Add i/v teicoplanin (*or* vancomycin) if high risk of meticillin-resistant *Staphylococcus aureus*. Start prophylaxis within 3 hours of injury and continue until soft tissue closure (max. 72 hours).

At first debridement also use a single dose of i/v cefuroxime + i/v metronidazole + i/v gentamicin *or* i/v co-amoxiclav + i/v gentamicin (*or* i/v clindamycin + i/v gentamicin if history of allergy to penicillins or to cephalosporins).

At time of skeletal stabilisation and definitive soft tissue closure use a single dose of i/v gentamicin + i/v teicoplanin (*or* vancomycin) (intravenous antibacterial prophylaxis should be given up to 30 minutes before the procedure).

High lower-limb amputation

- Use i/v co-amoxiclav alone *or* i/v cefuroxime + i/v metronidazole.

Intravenous antibacterial prophylaxis should be given up to 30 minutes before the procedure.

Continue antibacterial prophylaxis for at least 2 doses after procedure (max. duration of prophylaxis 5 days). If history of allergy to penicillin or to cephalosporins, or if high risk of meticillin-resistant *Staphylococcus aureus*, use i/v teicoplanin (*or* vancomycin) + i/v gentamicin + i/v metronidazole.

Where i/v metronidazole is suggested, it may alternatively be given by suppository but to allow adequate absorption, it should be given 2 hours before surgery.

Urological procedures, antibacterial prophylaxis

Transrectal prostate biopsy

- Single dose of oral ciprofloxacin + oral metronidazole *or* i/v gentamicin + i/v metronidazole (additional intra-operative or postoperative doses may be given for prolonged procedures or if there is major blood loss).

Intravenous antibacterial prophylaxis should be given up to 30 minutes before the procedure.

Use single dose of i/v gentamicin + i/v metronidazole if high risk of meticillin-resistant *Staphylococcus aureus* (additional intra-operative or postoperative doses of antibacterial may be given for prolonged procedures or if there is major blood loss).

Where i/v metronidazole is suggested, it may alternatively be given by suppository but to allow adequate absorption, it should be given 2 hours before surgery.

Transurethral resection of prostate

- Single dose of oral ciprofloxacin *or* i/v gentamicin *or* i/v cefuroxime (additional intra-operative or postoperative doses may be given for prolonged procedures or if there is major blood loss).

502 Bacterial infection

BNF 76

Intravenous antibacterial prophylaxis should be given up to 30 minutes before the procedure.

Use single dose of i/v gentamicin if high risk of meticillin-resistant *Staphylococcus aureus* (additional intra-operative or postoperative doses may be given for prolonged procedures or if there is major blood loss).

Obstetric and gynaecological surgery, antibacterial prophylaxis

Caesarean section

- Single dose of i/v cefuroxime (additional intra-operative or postoperative doses may be given for prolonged procedures or if there is major blood loss).

Intravenous antibacterial prophylaxis should be given up to 30 minutes before the procedure.

Substitute i/v clindamycin if history of allergy to penicillins or cephalosporins. Add i/v teicoplanin (*or* vancomycin) if high risk of meticillin-resistant *Staphylococcus aureus*.

Hysterectomy

- Single dose of i/v cefuroxime + i/v metronidazole *or* i/v gentamicin + i/v metronidazole *or* i/v co-amoxiclav alone (additional intra-operative or postoperative doses may be given for prolonged procedures or if there is major blood loss).

Intravenous antibacterial prophylaxis should be given up to 30 minutes before the procedure.

Use single dose of i/v gentamicin + i/v metronidazole or add i/v teicoplanin (*or* vancomycin) to other regimens if high risk of meticillin-resistant *Staphylococcus aureus* (additional intra-operative or postoperative doses may be given for prolonged procedures or if there is major blood loss).

Where i/v metronidazole is suggested, it may alternatively be given by suppository but to allow adequate absorption, it should be given 2 hours before surgery.

Termination of pregnancy

- Single dose of oral metronidazole (additional intra-operative or postoperative doses may be given for prolonged procedures or if there is major blood loss).

If genital chlamydial infection cannot be ruled out, give doxycycline p. 555 postoperatively.

Cardiology procedures, antibacterial prophylaxis

Cardiac pacemaker insertion

- Single dose of i/v cefuroxime alone *or* i/v flucloxacillin + i/v gentamicin *or* i/v teicoplanin (*or* vancomycin) + i/v gentamicin (additional intra-operative or postoperative doses may be given for prolonged procedures or if there is major blood loss).

Intravenous antibacterial prophylaxis should be given up to 30 minutes before the procedure.

Use single dose of i/v teicoplanin (*or* vancomycin) + i/v cefuroxime *or* i/v teicoplanin (*or* vancomycin) + i/v gentamicin if high risk of meticillin-resistant *Staphylococcus aureus* (additional intra-operative or postoperative doses may be given for prolonged procedures or if there is major blood loss).

Vascular surgery, antibacterial prophylaxis

Reconstructive arterial surgery of abdomen, pelvis or legs

- Single dose of i/v cefuroxime alone *or* i/v flucloxacillin + i/v gentamicin p. 510 (additional intra-operative or postoperative doses may be given for prolonged procedures or if there is major blood loss).

Intravenous antibacterial prophylaxis should be given up to 30 minutes before the procedure.

Add i/v metronidazole p. 533 for patients at risk from anaerobic infections including those with diabetes, gangrene, or undergoing amputation. Use single dose of i/v

teicoplanin p. 524 (*or* vancomycin p. 525) + i/v gentamicin if history of allergy to penicillins or cephalosporins, or if high risk of meticillin-resistant *Staphylococcus aureus* (additional intra-operative or postoperative doses may be given for prolonged procedures or if there is major blood loss).

Infective endocarditis, antibacterial prophylaxis

NICE guidance: Antimicrobial prophylaxis against infective endocarditis in adults and children undergoing interventional procedures (March 2008, updated 2016)

- Chlorhexidine mouthwash is **not** recommended for the prevention of infective endocarditis in at risk patients undergoing dental procedures.

Antibacterial prophylaxis is **not** *routinely* recommended for the prevention of infective endocarditis in patients undergoing the following procedures:

▸ dental;
▸ upper and lower respiratory tract (including ear, nose, and throat procedures and bronchoscopy);
▸ genito-urinary tract (including urological, gynaecological, and obstetric procedures);
▸ upper and lower gastro-intestinal tract.

Whilst these procedures can cause bacteraemia, there is no clear association with the development of infective endocarditis. Prophylaxis may expose patients to the adverse effects of antimicrobials when the evidence of benefit has not been proven.

Any infection in patients at risk of endocarditis should be investigated promptly and treated appropriately to reduce the risk of endocarditis.

If patients at risk of endocarditis are undergoing a gastro-intestinal or genito-urinary tract procedure at a site where infection is suspected, they should receive appropriate antibacterial therapy that includes cover against organisms that cause infective endocarditis.

Patients at risk of infective endocarditis should be:

▸ advised to maintain good oral hygiene;
▸ told how to recognise signs of infective endocarditis, and advised when to seek expert advice.

Patients at risk of infective endocarditis include those with valve replacement, acquired valvular heart disease with stenosis or regurgitation, structural congenital heart disease (including surgically corrected or palliated structural conditions, but excluding isolated atrial septal defect, fully repaired ventricular septal defect, fully repaired patent ductus arteriosus, and closure devices considered to be endothelialised), hypertrophic cardiomyopathy, or a previous episode of infective endocarditis.

Dermatological procedures

- Advice of a Working Party of the British Society for Antimicrobial Chemotherapy is that patients who undergo dermatological procedures do not require antibacterial prophylaxis against endocarditis.

The British Association of Dermatologists Therapy Guidelines and Audit Subcommittee advise that such dermatological procedures include skin biopsies and excision of moles or of malignant lesions.

Joint prostheses and dental treatment, antibacterial prophylaxis

- Advice of a Working Party of the British Society for Antimicrobial Chemotherapy is that patients with prosthetic joint implants (including total hip replacements) do not require antibiotic prophylaxis for dental treatment. The Working Party considers that it is unacceptable to expose patients to the adverse effects of antibiotics when there is no evidence that such prophylaxis is of any benefit, but that those who develop any intercurrent infection require prompt treatment with antibiotics to which the infecting organisms are sensitive.

The Working Party has commented that joint infections have rarely been shown to follow dental procedures and are even more rarely caused by oral streptococci.

Immunosuppression and indwelling intraperitoneal catheters

Advice of a Working Party of the British Society for Antimicrobial Chemotherapy is that patients who are immunosuppressed (including transplant patients) and patients with indwelling intraperitoneal catheters do not require antibiotic prophylaxis for dental treatment provided there is no other indication for prophylaxis.

The Working Party has commented that there is little evidence that dental treatment is followed by infection in immunosuppressed and immunodeficient patients nor is there evidence that dental treatment is followed by infection in patients with indwelling intraperitoneal catheters.

Blood infections, antibacterial therapy

Septicaemia (community-acquired)

- A broad-spectrum antipseudomonal penicillin (e.g. piperacillin with tazobactam p. 536, ticarcillin with clavulanic acid p. 537) *or* a broad-spectrum cephalosporin (e.g. cefuroxime p. 518)
▸ If meticillin-resistant *Staphylococcus aureus* suspected, add vancomycin p. 525 (*or* teicoplanin p. 524).
▸ If anaerobic infection suspected, add metronidazole p. 533 to broad-spectrum cephalosporin.
▸ If other resistant micro-organisms suspected, use a more broad-spectrum beta-lactam antibacterial (e.g. meropenem p. 514).

Septicaemia (hospital-acquired)

- A broad-spectrum antipseudomonal beta-lactam antibacterial (e.g. piperacillin with tazobactam, ticarcillin with clavulanic acid, ceftazidime p. 519, imipenem with cilastatin p. 514, *or* meropenem)
▸ If meticillin-resistant *Staphylococcus aureus* suspected, add vancomycin (*or* teicoplanin).
▸ If anaerobic infection suspected, add metronidazole to broad-spectrum cephalosporin

Septicaemia related to vascular catheter

- Vancomycin (*or* teicoplanin)
▸ If Gram-negative sepsis suspected, especially in the immunocompromised, add a broad-spectrum antipseudomonal beta-lactam.
▸ Consider removing vascular catheter, particularly if infection caused by *Staphylococcus aureus*, pseudomonas, or *Candida* species.

Meningococcal septicaemia

If meningococcal disease suspected, a single dose of benzylpenicillin sodium p. 537 should be given before urgent transfer to hospital, so long as this does not delay the transfer; cefotaxime p. 519 may be an alternative in penicillin allergy; chloramphenicol p. 558 may be used if history of immediate hypersensitivity reaction to penicillin or to cephalosporins.

- Benzylpenicillin sodium or cefotaxime (*or* ceftriaxone p. 520)
- *If history of immediate hypersensitivity reaction to penicillin or to cephalosporins*, chloramphenicol

To eliminate nasopharyngeal carriage, ciprofloxacin p. 548, or rifampicin p. 571, or ceftriaxone may be used.

Cardiovascular system infections, antibacterial therapy

Endocarditis: initial 'blind' therapy

- *Native valve endocarditis*, amoxicillin p. 539 (*or* ampicillin p. 540)
▸ Consider adding low-dose gentamicin p. 510
▸ If penicillin-allergic, or if meticillin-resistant *Staphylococcus aureus* suspected, or if severe sepsis, use vancomycin p. 525 + low-dose gentamicin
▸ If severe sepsis with risk factors for Gram-negative infection, use vancomycin + meropenem p. 514
- *If prosthetic valve endocarditis*, vancomycin + rifampicin p. 571+ low-dose gentamicin

Endocarditis (native valve) caused by staphylococci

- Flucloxacillin p. 544
▸ *Suggested duration of treatment* 4 weeks (at least 6 weeks if secondary lung abscess or osteomyelitis also present)
- *If penicillin-allergic or if meticillin-resistant Staphylococcus aureus*, vancomycin + rifampicin
▸ *Suggested duration of treatment* 4 weeks (at least 6 weeks if secondary lung abscess or osteomyelitis also present)

Endocarditis (prosthetic valve) caused by staphylococci

- Flucloxacillin + rifampicin + low-dose gentamicin
▸ *Suggested duration of treatment* at least 6 weeks; review need to continue gentamicin at 2 weeks—seek specialist advice if gentamicin considered necessary beyond 2 weeks
- *If penicillin-allergic or if meticillin-resistant Staphylococcus aureus*, vancomycin + rifampicin + low-dose gentamicin
▸ *Suggested duration of treatment* at least 6 weeks; review need to continue gentamicin at 2 weeks—seek specialist advice if gentamicin considered necessary beyond 2 weeks

Endocarditis caused by fully-sensitive streptococci

- Benzylpenicillin sodium p. 537
▸ *Suggested duration of treatment* 4–6 weeks (6 weeks for prosthetic valve endocarditis)
- *If penicillin-allergic*, vancomycin (*or* teicoplanin p. 524) + low-dose gentamicin
▸ *Suggested duration of treatment* 4–6 weeks (stop gentamicin after 2 weeks)

Endocarditis caused by less-sensitive streptococci

- Benzylpenicillin sodium + low-dose gentamicin
▸ *Suggested duration of treatment* 4–6 weeks (6 weeks for prosthetic valve endocarditis); review need to continue gentamicin at 2 weeks—seek specialist advice if gentamicin considered necessary beyond 2 weeks; stop gentamicin at 2 weeks if micro-organisms moderately sensitive to penicillin
- *If penicillin-allergic or highly penicillin-resistant*, vancomycin (*or* teicoplanin) + low-dose gentamicin
▸ *Suggested duration of treatment* 4–6 weeks (6 weeks for prosthetic valve endocarditis); review need to continue gentamicin at 2 weeks—seek specialist advice if gentamicin considered necessary beyond 2 weeks; stop gentamicin at 2 weeks if micro-organisms moderately sensitive to penicillin

Endocarditis caused by enterococci

- Amoxicillin (*or* ampicillin) + low dose gentamicin *or* benzylpenicillin sodium + low-dose gentamicin
▸ *Suggested duration of treatment* 4–6 weeks (6 weeks for prosthetic valve endocarditis); review need to continue

gentamicin at 2 weeks—seek specialist advice if gentamicin considered necessary beyond 2 weeks

- If *penicillin-allergic or penicillin-resistant*, vancomycin (*or* teicoplanin) + low-dose gentamicin
▸ *Suggested duration of treatment* 4–6 weeks (6 weeks for prosthetic valve endocarditis); review need to continue gentamicin at 2 weeks—seek specialist advice if gentamicin considered necessary beyond 2 weeks
- If gentamicin resistant, amoxicillin (*or* ampicillin)
▸ Add streptomycin p. 512 (if susceptible) for 2 weeks
▸ *Suggested duration of treatment* at least 6 weeks

Endocarditis caused by *Haemophilus, Actinobacillus, Cardiobacterium, Eikenella*, and *Kingella* species ('HACEK' micro-organisms)

- Amoxicillin (*or* ampicillin) + low-dose gentamicin
▸ *Suggested duration of treatment* 4 weeks (6 weeks for prosthetic valve endocarditis); stop gentamicin after 2 weeks
▸ If amoxicillin-*resistant*, ceftriaxone p. 520 (*or* cefotaxime p. 519) + low-dose gentamicin
▸ *Suggested duration of treatment* 4 weeks (6 weeks for prosthetic valve endocarditis); stop gentamicin after 2 weeks

Central nervous system infections, antibacterial therapy

Meningitis: initial empirical therapy

- Transfer patient to hospital urgently.
- If *meningococcal disease* (meningitis with non-blanching rash or meningococcal septicaemia) suspected, benzylpenicillin sodium p. 537 should be given before transfer to hospital, so long as this does not delay the transfer. If a patient with suspected bacterial meningitis without non-blanching rash cannot be transferred to hospital urgently, benzylpenicillin sodium should be given before the transfer. Cefotaxime p. 519 may be an alternative in penicillin allergy; chloramphenicol p. 558 may be used if history of immediate hypersensitivity reaction to penicillin or to cephalosporins.
- In hospital, consider adjunctive treatment with dexamethasone p. 660 (particularly if pneumococcal meningitis suspected in adults), preferably starting before or with first dose of antibacterial, but no later than 12 hours after starting antibacterial; avoid dexamethasone in septic shock, meningococcal septicaemia, or if immunocompromised, or in meningitis following surgery.

In hospital, if aetiology unknown:

- *Adult and child* 3 *months–50 years,* cefotaxime (*or* ceftriaxone p. 520)
▸ Consider adding vancomycin p. 525 if prolonged or multiple use of other antibacterials in the last 3 months, or if travelled, in the last 3 months, to areas outside the UK with highly penicillin- and cephalosporin-resistant pneumococci.
▸ *Suggested duration of treatment* at least 10 days
- *Adult over 50 years* cefotaxime (*or* ceftriaxone) + amoxicillin p. 539 (*or* ampicillin p. 540)
▸ Consider adding vancomycin if prolonged or multiple use of other antibacterials in the last 3 months, or if travelled, in the last 3 months, to areas outside the UK with highly penicillin- and cephalosporin-resistant pneumococci.
▸ *Suggested duration of treatment* at least 10 days

Meningitis caused by meningococci

- Benzylpenicillin sodium *or* cefotaxime (*or* ceftriaxone)

▸ *Suggested duration of treatment* 7 days.
- If history of immediate hypersensitivity reaction to penicillin or to cephalosporins, chloramphenicol
▸ *Suggested duration of treatment* 7 days.

Meningitis caused by pneumococci

- Cefotaxime (*or* ceftriaxone)
▸ Consider adjunctive treatment with dexamethasone, preferably starting before or with first dose of antibacterial, but no later than 12 hours after starting antibacterial (may reduce penetration of vancomycin into cerebrospinal fluid).
▸ If micro-organism penicillin-sensitive, replace cefotaxime with benzylpenicillin sodium.
▸ If micro-organism highly penicillin- and cephalosporin-resistant, add vancomycin and if necessary rifampicin p. 571.
▸ *Suggested duration of antibacterial treatment* 14 days

Meningitis caused by *Haemophilus influenzae*

- Cefotaxime (*or* ceftriaxone)
▸ Consider adjunctive treatment with dexamethasone, preferably starting before or with first dose of antibacterial, but no later than 12 hours after starting antibacterial.
▸ *Suggested duration of antibacterial treatment* 10 days.
▸ For *H. influenzae* type b give rifampicin for 4 days before hospital discharge to those under 10 years of age or to those in contact with vulnerable household contacts
- *If history of immediate hypersensitivity reaction to penicillin or to cephalosporins, or if micro-organism resistant to* cefotaxime, chloramphenicol
▸ Consider adjunctive treatment with dexamethasone, preferably starting before or with first dose of antibacterial, but no later than 12 hours after starting antibacterial.
▸ *Suggested duration of antibacterial treatment* 10 days.
▸ For *H. influenzae* type b give rifampicin for 4 days before hospital discharge to those under 10 years of age or to those in contact with vulnerable household contacts

Meningitis caused by Listeria

- Amoxicillin (*or* ampicillin) + gentamicin p. 510
▸ *Suggested duration of treatment* 21 days.
▸ Consider stopping gentamicin after 7 days.
▸ If history of immediate hypersensitivity reaction to penicillin, co-trimoxazole p. 552
▸ *Suggested duration of treatment* 21 days.

Ear infections, antibacterial therapy

Otitis externa

- For topical treatments, consider *Otitis externa*, under Ear p. 1159.
Consider systemic antibacterial if spreading cellulitis or patient systemically unwell.
- Flucloxacillin p. 544
▸ If *penicillin-allergic*, clarithromycin p. 529 (*or* azithromycin p. 528 *or* erythromycin p. 530)
▸ If *pseudomonas suspected*, ciprofloxacin p. 548 (*or* an aminoglycoside)

Otitis media

- Many infections are caused by viruses. Most uncomplicated cases resolve without antibacterial treatment. In children without systemic features, antibacterial treatment may be started after 72 hours if no improvement. Consider earlier treatment if deterioration, if systemically unwell, if at high risk of serious complications (e.g. in immunosuppression, cystic fibrosis), if mastoiditis present, or in children under 2 years of age with bilateral otitis media.

- Amoxicillin p. 539 (*or* ampicillin p. 540)
- Consider co-amoxiclav p. 542 if no improvement after 48 hours.
- In severe infection, initial parenteral therapy with co-amoxiclav or cefuroxime p. 518.
- *Suggested duration of treatment* 5 days (longer if severely ill).
- *If penicillin-allergic*, clarithromycin (*or* azithromycin *or* erythromycin)
- *Suggested duration of treatment* 5 days (longer if severely ill)

Eye infections, antibacterial therapy

Conjunctivitis (purulent)

- Chloramphenicol p. 558 eye drops.

Gastro-intestinal system infections, antibacterial therapy

Gastro-enteritis

- Frequently self-limiting and may not be bacterial.
- Antibacterial not usually indicated

Campylobacter enteritis

- Frequently self-limiting; treat if immunocompromised or if severe infection.
- Clarithromycin p. 529 (*or* azithromycin p. 528 *or* erythromycin p. 530)
- *Alternative*, ciprofloxacin p. 548
- Strains with decreased sensitivity to ciprofloxacin isolated frequently

Salmonella (non-typhoid)

- Treat invasive or severe infection. Do not treat less severe infection unless there is a risk of developing invasive infection (e.g. immunocompromised patients, those with haemoglobinopathy, or children under 6 months of age).
- Ciprofloxacin *or* cefotaxime p. 519

Shigellosis

- Antibacterial not indicated for mild cases.
- Ciprofloxacin *or* azithromycin
- *Alternatives if micro-organism sensitive*, amoxicillin p. 539 *or* trimethoprim p. 563

Typhoid fever

- Infections from Middle-East, South Asia, and South-East Asia may be multiple-antibacterial-resistant and sensitivity should be tested.
- Cefotaxime (*or* ceftriaxone p. 520)
- azithromycin may be an alternative in mild or moderate disease caused by multiple-antibacterial-resistant organisms.
- *Alternative if micro-organism sensitive*, ciprofloxacin

Clostridium difficile infection

- *Clostridium difficile* infection is caused by colonisation of the colon with *Clostridium difficile* and production of toxin. It often follows antibiotic therapy and is usually of acute onset, but may become chronic. It is a particular hazard of

ampicillin p. 540, amoxicillin, co-amoxiclav p. 542, second- and third-generation cephalosporins, clindamycin p. 526, and quinolones, but few antibiotics are free of this side-effect. Treatment options include metronidazole p. 533, vancomycin p. 525, and fidaxomicin p. 560.

- *For first episode of mild to moderate infection*, oral metronidazole
- *Suggested duration of treatment* 10–14 days
- *For second or subsequent episode of infection, for severe infection, for infection not responding to* metronidazole*, or in patients intolerant of* metronidazole, oral vancomycin
- For severe infection in patients with multiple co-morbidities who are receiving treatment with other antibacterials, or for second or subsequent episode of infection, fidaxomicin can replace vancomycin
- *Suggested duration of treatment* 10–14 days
- *For infection not responding to* vancomycin *or* fidaxomicin, *for life-threatening infection, or in patients with ileus*, oral vancomycin + i/v metronidazole
- For infection not responding to vancomycin in patients without life-threatening infection or ileus, fidaxomicin can be used instead of vancomycin + metronidazole
- *Suggested duration of treatment* 10–14 days

Biliary-tract infection

- Ciprofloxacin *or* gentamicin p. 510 *or* a cephalosporin

Peritonitis

- A cephalosporin + metronidazole *or* gentamicin + metronidazole *or* gentamicin + clindamycin *or* piperacillin with tazobactam p. 536 alone

Peritonitis: peritoneal dialysis-associated

- Vancomycin (*or* teicoplanin p. 524) + ceftazidime p. 519 added to dialysis fluid *or* vancomycin added to dialysis fluid + ciprofloxacin by mouth
- *Suggested duration of treatment* 14 days or longer

Genital system infections, antibacterial therapy

Bacterial vaginosis

- Oral metronidazole p. 533
- *Suggested duration of treatment* 5–7 days (or high-dose metronidazole as a single dose)
- *Alternatively*, topical metronidazole for 5 days *or* topical clindamycin p. 526 for 7 days

Uncomplicated genital chlamydial infection, non-gonococcal urethritis, and non-specific genital infection

- Contact tracing recommended.
- Azithromycin p. 528 *or* doxycycline p. 555
- *Suggested duration of treatment* azithromycin as a single dose or doxycycline for 7 days
- *Alternatively*, erythromycin p. 530.
- *Suggested duration of treatment* 14 days

Gonorrhoea: uncomplicated

- Contact tracing recommended. Consider chlamydia co-infection. Choice of alternative antibacterial regimen depends on locality where infection acquired.
- Azithromycin + i/m ceftriaxone p. 520
- *Suggested duration of treatment* is a single-dose of each antibacterial

- *Alternatively, when parenteral administration is not possible,* cefixime p. 518 + azithromycin
▸ *Suggested duration of treatment* is a single-dose of each antibacterial
▸ *Alternatively, if micro-organism is sensitive to a quinolone,* ciprofloxacin p. 548 + azithromycin
▸ *Suggested duration of treatment* is a single-dose of each antibacterial
- *Pharyngeal infection,* azithromycin + i/m ceftriaxone
▸ *Suggested duration of treatment* is a single-dose of each antibacterial

Pelvic inflammatory disease

- Contact tracing recommended.
- Doxycycline + metronidazole + single-dose of i/m ceftriaxone *or* ofloxacin p. 551 + metronidazole
▸ *Suggested duration of treatment* 14 days (except i/m ceftriaxone).
▸ In severely ill patients initial treatment with doxycycline + i/v ceftriaxone + i/v metronidazole, then switch to oral treatment with doxycycline + metronidazole to complete 14 days' treatment

Early syphilis (infection of less than 2 years)

- Contact tracing recommended.
- Benzathine benzylpenicillin [unlicensed]
▸ *Suggested duration of treatment* single-dose (repeat dose after 7 days for women in the third trimester of pregnancy)
- *Alternatively,* doxycycline or erythromycin
▸ *Suggested duration of treatment* 14 days

Late latent syphilis (asymptomatic infection of more than 2 years)

- Contact tracing recommended.
- Benzathine benzylpenicillin [unlicensed]
▸ *Suggested duration of treatment* once weekly for 2 weeks
- *Alternatively,* doxycycline
▸ *Suggested duration of treatment* 28 days

Asymptomatic contacts of patients with infectious syphilis

- Doxycycline
- *Suggested duration of treatment* 14 days

Musculoskeletal system infections, antibacterial therapy

Osteomyelitis

- Seek specialist advice if chronic infection or prostheses present.
▸ Flucloxacillin p. 544
▸ Consider adding fusidic acid p. 561 or rifampicin p. 571 for initial 2 weeks
▸ *Suggested duration of treatment* 6 weeks for acute infection
- *If penicillin-allergic,* clindamycin p. 526
▸ Consider adding fusidic acid or rifampicin for initial 2 weeks.
▸ *Suggested duration of treatment* 6 weeks for acute infection
- *If meticillin-resistant Staphylococcus aureus suspected,* vancomycin p. 525 (*or* teicoplanin p. 524)
▸ Consider adding fusidic acid or rifampicin for initial 2 weeks.
▸ *Suggested duration of treatment* 6 weeks for acute infection

Septic arthritis

- Seek specialist advice if prostheses present.
- Flucloxacillin
▸ *Suggested duration of treatment* 4–6 weeks (longer if infection complicated).
- *If penicillin-allergic,* clindamycin
▸ *Suggested duration of treatment* 4–6 weeks (longer if infection complicated).
- *If meticillin-resistant Staphylococcus aureus suspected,* vancomycin (*or* teicoplanin)
▸ *Suggested duration of treatment* 4–6 weeks (longer if infection complicated).
- *If gonococcal arthritis or Gram-negative infection suspected,* cefotaxime p. 519 (*or* ceftriaxone p. 520)
▸ *Suggested duration of treatment* 4–6 weeks (longer if infection complicated; treat gonococcal infection for 2 weeks).

Nose infections, antibacterial therapy
31-Oct-2017

Sinusitis (acute)

Acute sinusitis is generally triggered by a viral infection, although occasionally it may become complicated by a bacterial infection caused by *Streptococcus pneumoniae,* *Haemophilus influenzae, Moraxella catarrhalis,* or *Staphylococcus aureus.* For further information *see* Sinusitis (acute) p. 1168.

Treatment

EvGr Antibacterial therapy should *only* be offered to patients with acute sinusitis who are systemically very unwell, have signs and symptoms of a more serious illness, those who are at high-risk of complications due to pre-existing comorbidities, or whenever bacterial sinusitis is suspected.

Patients presenting with symptoms for around 10 days or more with no improvement may be prescribed a back-up antibiotic prescription, which can be used if symptoms do not improve within 7 days or if they worsen significantly at any time. A For further information *see,* Sinusitis (acute) p. 1168.

Choice of antibacterial therapy
No penicillin allergy

- EvGr *First line:*
▸ Non-life threatening symptoms: phenoxymethylpenicillin p. 538.
▸ Systemically very unwell, signs and symptoms of a more serious illness, or at high-risk of complications: co-amoxiclav p. 542.
- *Second line* (worsening symptoms despite 2 or 3 days of antibiotic treatment):
▸ Non-life threatening symptoms: co-amoxiclav.
▸ Systemically very unwell, signs and symptoms of a more serious illness or at high-risk of complications: consult local microbiologist. A
Penicillin allergy or intolerance
- EvGr *First line:* doxycycline p. 555 or clarithromycin p. 529 (erythromycin p. 530 in pregnancy).
- *Second line* (worsening symptoms despite 2 or 3 days of antibiotic treatment): consult local microbiologist. A

Useful Resources

Sinusitis (acute): antimicrobial prescribing. National Institute for Health and Care Excellence. NICE guideline 79. October 2017.
www.nice.org.uk/guidance/ng79

Oral bacterial infections

Antibacterial drugs

Antibacterial drugs should only be prescribed for the *treatment* of oral infections on the basis of defined need. They may be used in conjunction with (but not as an alternative to) other appropriate measures, such as providing drainage or extracting a tooth.

The 'blind' prescribing of an antibacterial for unexplained pyrexia, cervical lymphadenopathy, or facial swelling can lead to difficulty in establishing the diagnosis. In severe oral infections, a sample should always be taken for bacteriology.

Oral infections which may require antibacterial treatment include acute periapical or periodontal abscess, cellulitis, acutely created oral-antral communication (and acute sinusitis), severe pericoronitis, localised osteitis, acute necrotising ulcerative gingivitis, and destructive forms of chronic periodontal disease. Most of these infections are readily resolved by the early establishment of drainage and removal of the cause (typically an infected necrotic pulp). Antibacterials may be required if treatment has to be delayed, in immunocompromised patients, or in those with conditions such as diabetes or Paget's disease. Certain rarer infections including bacterial sialadenitis, osteomyelitis, actinomycosis, and infections involving fascial spaces such as Ludwig's angina, require antibiotics and specialist hospital care.

Antibacterial drugs may also be useful after dental surgery in some cases of spreading infection. Infection may spread to involve local lymph nodes, to fascial spaces (where it can cause airway obstruction), or into the bloodstream (where it can lead to cavernous sinus thrombosis and other serious complications). Extension of an infection can also lead to maxillary sinusitis; osteomyelitis is a complication, which usually arises when host resistance is reduced.

If the oral infection fails to respond to antibacterial treatment within 48 hours the antibacterial should be changed, preferably on the basis of bacteriological investigation. Failure to respond may also suggest an incorrect diagnosis, lack of essential additional measures (such as drainage), poor host resistance, or poor patient compliance.

Combination of a penicillin (or a macrolide) with metronidazole p. 533 may sometimes be helpful for the treatment of severe oral infections or oral infections that have not responded to initial antibacterial treatment.

Penicillins

Phenoxymethylpenicillin p. 538 is effective for dentoalveolar abscess.

Broad-spectrum penicillins

Amoxicillin p. 539 is as effective as phenoxymethylpenicillin but is better absorbed; however, it may encourage emergence of resistant organisms.

Like phenoxymethylpenicillin, amoxicillin is ineffective against bacteria that produce beta-lactamases.

Amoxicillin may be useful for short course oral regimens.

Co-amoxiclav p. 542 is active against beta-lactamase-producing bacteria that are resistant to amoxicillin. Co-amoxiclav may be used for severe dental infection with spreading cellulitis or dental infection not responding to first-line antibacterial treatment.

Cephalosporins

The cephalosporins offer little advantage over the penicillins in dental infections, often being less active against anaerobes. Infections due to oral streptococci (often termed viridans streptococci) which become resistant to penicillin are usually also resistant to cephalosporins. This is of importance in the case of patients who have had rheumatic fever and are on long-term penicillin therapy. Cefalexin

p. 516 and cefradine p. 516 have been used in the treatment of oral infections.

Tetracyclines

In adults, tetracyclines can be effective against oral anaerobes but the development of resistance (especially by oral streptococci) has reduced their usefulness for the treatment of acute oral infections; they may still have a role in the treatment of destructive (refractory) forms of periodontal disease. Doxycycline p. 555 has a longer duration of action than tetracycline p. 557 or oxytetracycline p. 557 and need only be given once daily; it is reported to be more active against anaerobes than some other tetracyclines.

Doxycycline may have a role in the treatment of recurrent aphthous ulceration, or as an adjunct to gingival scaling and root planing for periodontitis.

Macrolides

The macrolides are an alternative for oral infections in penicillin-allergic patients or where a beta-lactamase producing organism is involved. However, many organisms are now resistant to macrolides or rapidly develop resistance; their use should therefore be limited to short courses.

Clindamycin

Clindamycin p. 526 should not be used routinely for the treatment of oral infections because it may be no more effective than penicillins against anaerobes and there may be cross-resistance with erythromycin-resistant bacteria. Clindamycin can be used for the treatment of dentoalveolar abscess that has not responded to penicillin or to metronidazole.

Metronidazole and tinidazole

Metronidazole is an alternative to a penicillin for the treatment of many oral infections where the patient is allergic to penicillin or the infection is due to beta-lactamase-producing anaerobes. It is the drug of first choice for the treatment of acute necrotising ulcerative gingivitis (Vincent's infection) and pericoronitis; amoxicillin is a suitable alternative. For these purposes metronidazole for 3 days is sufficient, but the duration of treatment may need to be longer in pericoronitis. Tinidazole p. 534 is licensed for the treatment of acute ulcerative gingivitis.

Respiratory system infections, antibacterial therapy

Epiglottitis (*Haemophilus influenzae*)

- Cefotaxime p. 519 (*or* ceftriaxone p. 520)
- ▸ *If history of immediate hypersensitivity reaction to penicillin or to cephalosporins*, chloramphenicol p. 558

Chronic bronchitis: acute exacerbations

- Treat if increase in sputum purulence accompanied by an increase in sputum volume or increase in dyspnoea.
- ▸ Amoxicillin p. 539 (*or* ampicillin p. 540) *or* a tetracycline p. 557
- ▸ Some pneumococci and *Haemophilus influenzae* strains tetracycline-resistant; approx. 20% *H. influenzae* strains amoxicillin-resistant
- ▸ *Suggested duration of treatment* 5 days; longer treatment may be necessary in severely ill patients
- ▸ *Alternative*, clarithromycin p. 529 (*or* azithromycin p. 528 *or* erythromycin p. 530)
- ▸ *Suggested duration of treatment* 5 days; longer treatment may be necessary in severely ill patients

Community-acquired pneumonia: low-severity

- Amoxicillin (or ampicillin)
▸ Pneumococci with decreased penicillin sensitivity being isolated, but not yet common in UK.
▸ If atypical pathogens suspected, add clarithromycin (or azithromycin or erythromycin).
▸ If staphylococci suspected (e. g. in influenza or measles), add flucloxacillin p. 544.
▸ *Suggested duration of treatment* 7 days (14–21 days for infections caused by staphylococci)
▸ *Alternatives*, doxycycline p. 555 or clarithromycin (or azithromycin or erythromycin)
▸ *Suggested duration of treatment* 7 days (14–21 days for infections caused by staphylococci)

Community-acquired pneumonia: moderate-severity

- Amoxicillin (or ampicillin) + clarithromycin (or azithromycin or erythromycin) or doxycycline alone
▸ Pneumococci with decreased penicillin sensitivity being isolated, but not yet common in UK.
▸ If meticillin-resistant *Staphylococcus aureus* suspected, add vancomycin p. 525 (or teicoplanin p. 524).
▸ *Suggested duration of treatment* 7 days (14–21 days for infections caused by staphylococci)

Community-acquired pneumonia: high-severity

- Benzylpenicillin sodium p. 537 + clarithromycin (or azithromycin or erythromycin) or benzylpenicillin sodium + doxycycline
▸ If meticillin-resistant *Staphylococcus aureus* suspected, add vancomycin (or teicoplanin).
▸ *Suggested duration of treatment* 7–10 days (may extend treatment to 14–21 days in some cases e.g. if staphylococci suspected)
▸ *If life-threatening infection, or if Gram-negative infection suspected, or if co-morbidities present, or if living in long-term residential or nursing home*, co-amoxiclav p. 542 + clarithromycin (or azithromycin or erythromycin)
▸ If meticillin-resistant *Staphylococcus aureus* suspected, add vancomycin (or teicoplanin).
▸ *Suggested duration of treatment* 7–10 days (may extend treatment to 14–21 days in some cases e.g. if staphylococci or Gram-negative enteric bacilli suspected)
▸ *Alternatives if life-threatening infection, or if Gram-negative infection suspected, or if co-morbidities present, or if living in long-term residential or nursing home*, cefuroxime p. 518 + clarithromycin (or azithromycin or erythromycin) or cefotaxime (or ceftriaxone) + clarithromycin (or azithromycin or erythromycin)
▸ If meticillin-resistant *Staphylococcus aureus* suspected, add vancomycin (or teicoplanin).
▸ *Suggested duration of treatment* 7–10 days (may extend treatment to 14–21 days in some cases e.g. if staphylococci or Gram-negative enteric bacilli suspected)

Pneumonia possibly caused by atypical pathogens

- Clarithromycin (or azithromycin or erythromycin)
▸ If high-severity Legionella infection, add rifampicin p. 571 for the first few days.
▸ *Suggested duration of treatment* 14 days (usually 7–10 days for Legionella)
▸ *Alternative if Legionella infection suspected*, a quinolone
▸ If high-severity Legionella infection, add clarithromycin (or azithromycin or erythromycin) or rifampicin for the first few days.
▸ *Suggested duration of treatment* usually 7–10 days
▸ *Alternative for chlamydial or mycoplasma infections*, doxycycline
▸ *Suggested duration of treatment* 14 days

Hospital-acquired pneumonia

- *Early-onset infection* less than 5 days after admission to hospital), co-amoxiclav or cefuroxime
▸ If life-threatening infection, or if history of antibacterial treatment in the last 3 months, or if resistant micro-organisms suspected, treat as for late-onset hospital-acquired pneumonia.
▸ *Suggested duration of treatment* 7 days
▸ *Late-onset infection* (more than 5 days after admission to hospital), an antipseudomonal penicillin (e.g. piperacillin with tazobactam p. 536) or a broad-spectrum cephalosporin (e.g. ceftazidime p. 519) or another antipseudomonal beta-lactam or a quinolone (e.g. ciprofloxacin p. 548)
▸ If meticillin-resistant *Staphylococcus aureus* suspected, add vancomycin.
▸ For severe illness caused by *Pseudomonas aeruginosa*, consider adding an aminoglycoside.
▸ *Suggested duration of treatment* 7 days (longer if *Pseudomonas aeruginosa* confirmed)

Skin infections, antibacterial therapy

Impetigo: small areas of skin infected

- Seek local microbiology advice before using topical treatment in hospital.
▸ Topical fusidic acid p. 561
▸ *Suggested duration of treatment* 7 days is usually adequate (max. 10 days).
▸ Alternatively, if meticillin-resistant *Staphylococcus aureus*, topical mupirocin p. 1168
▸ *Suggested duration of treatment* 7 days is usually adequate (max. 10 days).

Impetigo: widespread infection

- Oral flucloxacillin p. 544
▸ If streptococci suspected in severe infection, add phenoxymethylpenicillin p. 538.
▸ *Suggested duration of treatment* 7 days.
- *If penicillin-allergic*, oral clarithromycin p. 529 (or azithromycin p. 528 or erythromycin p. 530)
▸ *Suggested duration of treatment* 7 days.

Erysipelas

- Phenoxymethylpenicillin or benzylpenicillin sodium p. 537
- If severe infection, replace phenoxymethylpenicillin or benzylpenicillin sodium with high-dose flucloxacillin
▸ *Suggested duration of treatment* at least 7 days.
- *If penicillin-allergic*, clindamycin p. 526 or clarithromycin (or azithromycin or erythromycin)
▸ *Suggested duration of treatment* at least 7 days

Cellulitis

- Flucloxacillin (high-dose)
▸ If streptococcal infection confirmed, replace flucloxacillin with phenoxymethylpenicillin or benzylpenicillin sodium
▸ If Gram-negative bacteria or anaerobes suspected, use broad-spectrum antibacterials
- *If penicillin-allergic*, clindamycin or clarithromycin (or azithromycin or erythromycin) or vancomycin p. 525 (or teicoplanin p. 524)
▸ If Gram-negative bacteria suspected, use broad-spectrum antibacterials.

Animal and human bites

- Cleanse wound thoroughly. For tetanus-prone wound, give human tetanus immunoglobulin p. 1257 (with a tetanus-containing vaccine if necessary, according to immunisation history and risk of infection). Consider rabies prophylaxis for bites from animals in endemic countries. Assess risk of blood-borne viruses (including HIV, hepatitis B and C) and give appropriate prophylaxis to prevent viral spread.
- Co-amoxiclav p. 542
- If *penicillin-allergic*, doxycycline p. 555 + metronidazole p. 533

Mastitis during breast-feeding

- Treat if severe, if systemically unwell, if nipple fissure present, if symptoms do not improve after 12–24 hours of effective milk removal, or if culture indicates infection. Continue breast-feeding or expressing milk during treatment.

Flucloxacillin
▸ *Suggested duration of treatment* 10–14 days.
- If *penicillin-allergic*, erythromycin
- *Suggested duration of treatment* 10–14 days.

ANTIBACTERIALS > AMINOGLYCOSIDES

Aminoglycosides

Overview

These include amikacin p. 510, gentamicin p. 510, neomycin sulfate p. 511, streptomycin p. 512, and tobramycin p. 512. All are bactericidal and active against some Gram-positive and many Gram-negative organisms. Amikacin, gentamicin, and tobramycin are also active against *Pseudomonas aeruginosa*; streptomycin is active against *Mycobacterium tuberculosis* and is now almost entirely reserved for tuberculosis.

The aminoglycosides are not absorbed from the gut (although there is a risk of absorption in inflammatory bowel disease and liver failure) and must therefore be given by injection for systemic infections.

Gentamicin is the aminoglycoside of choice in the UK and is used widely for the treatment of serious infections. It has a broad spectrum but is inactive against anaerobes and has poor activity against haemolytic streptococci and pneumococci. When used for the 'blind' therapy of undiagnosed serious infections it is usually given in conjunction with a penicillin or metronidazole p. 533 (or both). Gentamicin is used together with another antibiotic for the treatment of endocarditis. Streptomycin may be used as an alternative in gentamicin-resistant enterococcal endocarditis.

Loading and maintenance doses of gentamicin may be calculated on the basis of the patient's weight and renal function (e.g. using a nomogram); adjustments are then made according to serum-gentamicin concentrations. High doses are occasionally indicated for serious infections, especially in the neonate, in the patient with cystic fibrosis, or in the immunocompromised patient. Whenever possible treatment should not exceed 7 days.

Amikacin is more stable than gentamicin to enzyme inactivation. Amikacin is used in the treatment of serious infections caused by gentamicin-resistant Gram-negative bacilli.

Tobramycin has similar activity to gentamicin. It is slightly more active against *Ps. aeruginosa* but shows less activity against certain other Gram-negative bacteria. Tobramycin can be administered by nebuliser or by inhalation of powder on a cyclical basis (28 days of tobramycin followed by a 28-day tobramycin-free interval) for the treatment of

chronic pulmonary *Ps. aeruginosa* infection in cystic fibrosis; however, resistance may develop and some patients do not respond to treatment.

Neomycin sulfate is too toxic for parenteral administration and can only be used for infections of the skin or mucous membranes or to reduce the bacterial population of the colon prior to bowel surgery or in hepatic failure. Oral administration may lead to malabsorption. Small amounts of neomycin sulfate may be absorbed from the gut in patients with hepatic failure and, as these patients may also be uraemic, cumulation may occur with resultant ototoxicity.

Once daily dosage

Once daily administration of aminoglycosides is more convenient, provides adequate serum concentrations, and in many cases has largely superseded *multiple daily dose regimens* (given in 2–3 divided doses during the 24 hours). Local guidelines on dosage and serum concentrations should be consulted. A once-daily, high-dose regimen of an aminoglycoside should be avoided in patients with endocarditis due to Gram-positive bacteria, HACEK endocarditis, burns of more than 20% of the total body surface area, or creatinine clearance less than 20 mL/minute. There is insufficient evidence to recommend a once daily, high-dose regimen of an aminoglycoside in pregnancy.

Serum concentrations

Serum concentration monitoring avoids both excessive and subtherapeutic concentrations thus preventing toxicity and ensuring efficacy. Serum-aminoglycoside concentrations should be monitored in patients receiving parenteral aminoglycosides and **must** be determined in the elderly, in obesity, and in cystic fibrosis, or if high doses are being given, or if there is renal impairment.

Aminoglycosides (by injection)

- CONTRA-INDICATIONS Myasthenia gravis (aminoglycosides may impair neuromuscular transmission)
- CAUTIONS Care must be taken with dosage (the main side-effects of the aminoglycosides are dose-related) · conditions characterised by muscular weakness (aminoglycosides may impair neuromuscular transmission) · if possible, dehydration should be corrected before starting an aminoglycoside · whenever possible, parenteral treatment should not exceed 7 days
- SIDE-EFFECTS
▸ **Common or very common** Hearing impairment
▸ **Uncommon** Nausea · skin reactions (very common in children) · vomiting
▸ **Rare or very rare** Anaemia · eosinophilia · fever · headache · hypomagnesaemia · paraesthesia · renal impairment
▸ **Frequency not known** Bronchospasm · confusion · lethargy · nephrotoxicity

  SIDE-EFFECTS, FURTHER INFORMATION Nephrotoxicity occurs most commonly in patients with renal impairment, who require reduced doses; monitoring is particularly important in the elderly.

- PREGNANCY There is a risk of auditory or vestibular nerve damage in the infant when aminoglycosides are used in the second and third trimesters of pregnancy. The risk is greatest with streptomycin. The risk is probably very small with gentamicin and tobramycin, but their use should be avoided unless essential.
  Monitoring If given during pregnancy, serum-aminoglycoside concentration monitoring is essential.
- RENAL IMPAIRMENT Excretion of aminoglycosides is principally via the kidney and accumulation occurs in renal impairment. Ototoxicity and nephrotoxicity occur commonly in patients with renal failure.

5

Infection

▸ **In adults** A once-daily, high-dose regimen of an aminoglycoside should be avoided in patients with a creatinine clearance less than 20 mL/minute.
▸ **In children** A once-daily, high-dose regimen of an aminoglycoside should be avoided in children over 1 month of age with a creatinine clearance less than 20 mL/minute/1.73 m².
Dose adjustments If there is impairment of renal function, the interval between doses must be increased; if the renal impairment is severe, the dose itself should be reduced as well.
Monitoring Serum-aminoglycoside concentrations **must** be monitored in patients with renal impairment; earlier and more frequent measurement of aminoglycoside concentration may be required.

● MONITORING REQUIREMENTS
▸ **Serum concentrations** Serum concentration monitoring avoids both excessive and subtherapeutic concentrations thus preventing toxicity and ensuring efficacy. Serum-aminoglycoside concentrations should be measured in all patients receiving parenteral aminoglycosides and **must** be determined in obesity, if high doses are being given and in cystic fibrosis.
▸ **In adults** Serum aminoglycoside concentrations **must** be determined in the elderly. In patients with normal renal function, aminoglycoside concentrations should be measured after 3 or 4 doses of a multiple daily dose regimen and after a dose change. For multiple daily dose regimens, blood samples should be taken approximately 1 hour after intramuscular or intravenous administration ('peak' concentration) and also just before the next dose ('trough' concentration). If the pre-dose ('trough') concentration is high, the interval between doses must be increased; if the post-dose ('peak') concentration is high, the dose must be decreased. For once daily dose regimens, consult local guidelines on serum concentration monitoring.
▸ **In children** In children with normal renal function, aminoglycoside concentrations should be measured after 3 or 4 doses of a multiple daily dose regimen. Blood samples should be taken just before the next dose is administered ('trough' concentration). If the pre-dose ('trough') concentration is high, the interval between doses must be increased. For multiple daily dose regimens, blood samples should also be taken approximately 1 hour after intramuscular or intravenous administration ('peak' concentration). If the post-dose ('peak') concentration is high, the dose must be decreased.
▸ Renal function should be assessed before starting an aminoglycoside and during treatment.
▸ Auditory and vestibular function should also be monitored during treatment.

⬛ 509

Amikacin

● INDICATIONS AND DOSE
Serious Gram-negative infections resistant to gentamicin (multiple daily dose regimen)
▸ BY INTRAMUSCULAR INJECTION, OR BY SLOW INTRAVENOUS INJECTION, OR BY INTRAVENOUS INFUSION
▸ Adult: 15 mg/kg daily in 2 divided doses, increased to 22.5 mg/kg daily in 3 divided doses for up to 10 days, higher dose to be used in severe infections; maximum 1.5 g per day; maximum 15 g per course
Serious Gram-negative infections resistant to gentamicin (once daily dose regimen)
▸ BY INTRAVENOUS INFUSION
▸ Adult: Initially 15 mg/kg (max. per dose 1.5 g once daily), dose to be adjusted according to serum-amikacin concentration; maximum 15 g per course

DOSES AT EXTREMES OF BODY-WEIGHT
▸ To avoid excessive dosage in obese patients, use ideal weight for height to calculate dose and monitor serum-amikacin concentration closely

● INTERACTIONS → Appendix 1: aminoglycosides
● SIDE-EFFECTS
▸ **Uncommon** Superinfection
▸ **Rare or very rare** Albuminuria · arthralgia · azotaemia · balance impaired · hypotension · muscle twitching · tremor
▸ **Frequency not known** Apnoea · neuromuscular blockade · paralysis
● MONITORING REQUIREMENTS
▸ With intravenous use *Multiple daily dose regimen*: one-hour ('peak') serum concentration should not exceed 30 mg/litre; pre-dose ('trough') concentration should be less than 10 mg/litre. *Once daily dose regimen*: pre-dose ('trough') concentration should be less than 5 mg/litre.
● DIRECTIONS FOR ADMINISTRATION For *intravenous infusion* (*Amikin*®); intermittent in Glucose 5% *or* Sodium chloride 0.9%. To be given over 30 minutes.
● PRESCRIBING AND DISPENSING INFORMATION Once daily dose regimen not to be used for endocarditis, febrile neutropenia, or meningitis. Consult local guidelines.

● MEDICINAL FORMS
There can be variation in the licensing of different medicines containing the same drug. Forms available from special-order manufacturers include: solution for injection
Solution for injection
▸ Amikacin (Non-proprietary)
Amikacin (as Amikacin sulfate) 250 mg per 1 ml Amikacin 500mg/2ml solution for injection vials | 5 vial [PoM] £60.00 (Hospital only)
▸ Amikacin (Bristol-Myers Squibb Pharmaceuticals Ltd)
Amikacin (as Amikacin sulfate) 50 mg per 1 ml Amikin 100mg/2ml solution for injection vials | 5 vial [PoM] £10.33

⬛ 509

Gentamicin

11-Dec-2017

● INDICATIONS AND DOSE
Gram-positive bacterial endocarditis or HACEK endocarditis (in combination with other antibacterials)
▸ BY INTRAMUSCULAR INJECTION, OR BY SLOW INTRAVENOUS INJECTION, OR BY INTRAVENOUS INFUSION
▸ Adult: 1 mg/kg every 12 hours, intravenous injection to be administered over at least 3 minutes, to be given in a multiple daily dose regimen
Septicaemia | Meningitis and other CNS infections | Biliary-tract infection | Acute pyelonephritis | Endocarditis | Pneumonia in hospital patients | Adjunct in listerial meningitis | Prostatitis
▸ BY INTRAVENOUS INFUSION, OR BY SLOW INTRAVENOUS INJECTION, OR BY INTRAMUSCULAR INJECTION
▸ Adult: 3–5 mg/kg daily in 3 divided doses, to be given in a multiple daily dose regimen, divided doses to be given every 8 hours, intravenous injection to be administered over at least 3 minutes
▸ BY INTRAVENOUS INFUSION
▸ Adult: Initially 5–7 mg/kg, subsequent doses adjusted according to serum-gentamicin concentration, to be given in a once daily dose regimen
CNS infections (administered on expert advice)
▸ BY INTRATHECAL INJECTION
▸ Adult: 1 mg daily, increased if necessary to 5 mg daily, seek specialist advice
Surgical prophylaxis
▸ BY SLOW INTRAVENOUS INJECTION
▸ Adult: 1.5 mg/kg, intravenous injection to be administered over at least 3 minutes, administer dose up to 30 minutes before the procedure, dose may be

repeated every 8 hours for high-risk procedures; up to 3 further doses may be given

Surgical prophylaxis in joint replacement surgery

▸ BY INTRAVENOUS INFUSION

▸ Adult: 5 mg/kg for 1 dose, administer dose up to 30 minutes before the procedure

DOSES AT EXTREMES OF BODY-WEIGHT

▸ With intramuscular use or intravenous use

▸ To avoid excessive dosage in obese patients, use ideal weight for height to calculate parenteral dose and monitor serum-gentamicin concentration closely.

IMPORTANT SAFETY INFORMATION

MHRA/CHM ADVICE: POTENTIAL FOR HISTAMINE-RELATED ADVERSE DRUG REACTIONS WITH SOME BATCHES (NOVEMBER 2017)

Following reports that some batches of gentamicin sulphate active pharmaceutical ingredient (API) used to manufacture gentamicin may contain higher than expected levels of histamine, which is a residual from the manufacturing process, the MHRA advise to monitor patients for signs of histamine-related adverse reactions; particular caution is required in patients taking concomitant drugs known to cause histamine release, in children, and in patients with severe renal impairment.

● INTERACTIONS → Appendix 1: aminoglycosides

● SIDE-EFFECTS Antibiotic associated colitis · blood disorder · depression · encephalopathy · hallucination · hepatic reaction · neurotoxicity · peripheral neuropathy · purpura · seizure · stomatitis · vestibular damage

● MONITORING REQUIREMENTS

▸ With intramuscular use or intravenous use For multiple daily dose regimen, one-hour ('peak') serum concentration should be 5–10 mg/litre; pre-dose ('trough') concentration should be less than 2 mg/litre.
For multiple daily dose regimen in endocarditis, one-hour ('peak') serum concentration should be 3–5 mg/litre; pre-dose ('trough') concentration should be less than 1 mg/litre. Serum-gentamicin concentration should be measured after 3 or 4 doses, then at least every 3 days and after a dose change (more frequently in renal impairment).

▸ With intravenous use For once-daily dose regimen, consult local guidelines on monitoring serum-gentamicin concentration.

● DIRECTIONS FOR ADMINISTRATION

▸ With intrathecal use For *intrathecal* injection, use preservative-free intrathecal preparations only.

▸ With intravenous use For *intravenous infusion (Cidomycin®); Gentamicin paediatric injection,* Beacon; *Gentamicin injection* Hospira), give intermittently *or* via drip tubing in Glucose 5% or Sodium Chloride 0.9%. Suggested volume for intermittent infusion 50–100 ml given over 20–30 minutes (given over 60 minutes for once daily dose regimen).

● PRESCRIBING AND DISPENSING INFORMATION

▸ With intravenous use Local guidelines may vary in the dosing advice provided for once daily administration.

▸ With intrathecal use Only preservative-free intrathecal preparation should be used.

● MEDICINAL FORMS
There can be variation in the licensing of different medicines containing the same drug.

Solution for injection

▸ Gentamicin (Non-proprietary)
Gentamicin (as Gentamicin sulfate) 5 mg per 1 ml Gentamicin Intrathecal 5mg/1ml solution for injection ampoules | 5 ampoule PoM £36.28 (Hospital only)
Gentamicin (as Gentamicin sulfate) 10 mg per 1 ml Gentamicin 20mg/2ml solution for injection ampoules | 5 ampoule PoM £11.25

Gentamicin Paediatric 20mg/2ml solution for injection vials | 5 vial PoM £11.25 DT = £11.25
Gentamicin (as Gentamicin sulfate) 40 mg per 1 ml Gentamicin 80mg/2ml solution for injection vials | 5 vial PoM £20.00 (Hospital only)
Gentamicin 80mg/2ml solution for injection ampoules | 5 ampoule PoM £6.88 | 10 ampoule PoM £10.00

▸ Cidomycin (Sanofi)
Gentamicin (as Gentamicin sulfate) 40 mg per 1 ml Cidomycin Adult Injectable 80mg/2ml solution for injection vials | 5 vial PoM £6.88
Cidomycin Adult Injectable 80mg/2ml solution for injection ampoules | 5 ampoule PoM £6.88

Infusion

▸ Gentamicin (Non-proprietary)
Gentamicin (as Gentamicin sulfate) 1 mg per 1 ml Gentamicin 80mg/80ml infusion bags | 20 bag PoM £40.17
Gentamicin (as Gentamicin sulfate) 3 mg per 1 ml Gentamicin 240mg/80ml infusion bags | 20 bag PoM £122.57-£122.58
Gentamicin 360mg/120ml infusion bags | 20 bag PoM £174.07

Neomycin sulfate

● **INDICATIONS AND DOSE**

Bowel sterilisation before surgery

▸ BY MOUTH

▸ Adult: 1 g every 1 hour for 4 hours, then 1 g every 4 hours for 2–3 days

Hepatic coma

▸ BY MOUTH

▸ Adult: Up to 4 g daily in divided doses usually for 5–7 days

● CONTRA-INDICATIONS Intestinal obstruction · myasthenia gravis (aminoglycosides may impair neuromuscular transmission)

● CAUTIONS Avoid prolonged use
CAUTIONS, FURTHER INFORMATION Although neomycin is associated with the same cautions as other aminoglycosides it is generally considered too toxic for systemic use.

● INTERACTIONS → Appendix 1: neomycin

● SIDE-EFFECTS Blood disorder · confusion · diarrhoea · drug cross-reactivity · electrolyte imbalance · gastrointestinal disorders · haemolytic anaemia · nausea · nephrotoxicity · nystagmus · oral disorders · ototoxicity · paraesthesia · superinfection · vomiting
SIDE-EFFECTS, FURTHER INFORMATION Although neomycin is associated with the same side effects as other aminoglycosides, it is poorly absorbed after oral administration.

● PREGNANCY There is a risk of auditory or vestibular nerve damage in the infant when aminoglycosides are used in the second and third trimesters of pregnancy.

● HEPATIC IMPAIRMENT Absorbed from gastro-intestinal tract in liver disease—increased risk of ototoxicity.

● RENAL IMPAIRMENT Avoid—risk of ototoxicity and nephrotoxicity.

● MONITORING REQUIREMENTS

▸ Renal function should be assessed before starting an aminoglycoside and during treatment.

▸ Auditory and vestibular function should also be monitored during treatment.

● MEDICINAL FORMS
There can be variation in the licensing of different medicines containing the same drug. Forms available from special-order manufacturers include: oral solution

Tablet

▸ Neomycin sulfate (Non-proprietary)
Neomycin sulfate 500 mg Neomycin 500mg tablets | 100 tablet PoM £34.69 DT = £34.69

Streptomycin

⌦ 509

● INDICATIONS AND DOSE

Tuberculosis, resistant to other treatment, in combination with other drugs
▶ BY DEEP INTRAMUSCULAR INJECTION
▸ Adult: 15 mg/kg daily (max. per dose 1 g), reduce dose in those under 50 kg and those over 40 years

Adjunct to doxycycline in brucellosis (administered on expert advice)
▶ BY DEEP INTRAMUSCULAR INJECTION
▸ Adult: (consult local protocol)

Enterococcal endocarditis
▸ Adult: (consult local protocol)

● UNLICENSED USE Use in tuberculosis is an unlicensed indication.

> IMPORTANT SAFETY INFORMATION
> Side-effects increase after a cumulative dose of 100 g, which should only be exceeded in exceptional circumstances.

● INTERACTIONS → Appendix 1: aminoglycosides

● SIDE-EFFECTS Hypersensitivity · oral paraesthesia

● RENAL IMPAIRMENT
Dose adjustments Should preferably be avoided. If essential, use with great care and consider dose reduction.

● MONITORING REQUIREMENTS
▸ One-hour ('peak') concentration should be 15–40 mg/litre; pre-dose ('trough') concentration should be less than 5 mg/litre (less than 1 mg/litre in renal impairment or in those over 50 years).

● MEDICINAL FORMS
Forms available from special-order manufacturers include: powder for solution for injection

Tobramycin

⌦ 509

28-Nov-2016

● INDICATIONS AND DOSE

Septicaemia | Meningitis and other CNS infections | Biliary-tract infection | Acute pyelonephritis or prostatitis | Pneumonia in hospital patients
▶ BY INTRAMUSCULAR INJECTION, OR BY SLOW INTRAVENOUS INJECTION, OR BY INTRAVENOUS INFUSION
▸ Adult: 3 mg/kg daily in 3 divided doses; increased if necessary up to 5 mg/kg daily in 3–4 divided doses, increased dose used in severe infection; dose to be reduced back to 3 mg/kg daily as soon as clinically indicated

Urinary-tract infection
▶ BY INTRAMUSCULAR INJECTION
▸ Adult: 2–3 mg/kg for 1 dose

Chronic Pseudomonas aeruginosa infection in patients with cystic fibrosis
▶ BY INHALATION OF NEBULISED SOLUTION
▸ Adult: 300 mg every 12 hours for 28 days, subsequent courses repeated after 28-day interval without tobramycin nebuliser solution
▶ BY INHALATION OF POWDER
▸ Adult: 112 mg every 12 hours for 28 days, subsequent courses repeated after 28-day interval without tobramycin inhalation powder

DOSES AT EXTREMES OF BODY-WEIGHT
▸ To avoid excessive dosage in obese patients, use ideal weight for height to calculate parenteral dose and monitor serum-tobramycin concentration closely.

VANTOBRA® NEBULISER SOLUTION

Chronic pulmonary Pseudomonas aeruginosa infection in patients with cystic fibrosis
▶ BY INHALATION OF NEBULISED SOLUTION
▸ Adult: 170 mg every 12 hours for 28 days, subsequent courses repeated after 28-day interval without tobramycin nebuliser solution

● CAUTIONS
▸ When used by inhalation Conditions characterised by muscular weakness—may impair neuromuscular transmission · history of prolonged previous or concomitant intravenous aminoglycosides—increased risk of ototoxicity · renal impairment—limited information available · severe haemoptysis—risk of further haemorrhage

● INTERACTIONS → Appendix 1: aminoglycosides

● SIDE-EFFECTS
▶ Common or very common
▸ When used by inhalation Dysphonia · increased risk of infection · malaise · respiratory disorder · sputum discolouration
▶ Frequency not known
▸ When used by inhalation Aphonia · oropharyngeal pain · taste altered
▸ With parenteral use Diarrhoea · disorientation · dizziness · exfoliative dermatitis · granulocytopenia · leucocytosis · leucopenia · nerve disorders · thrombocytopenia · urine abnormalities · vertigo

SIDE-EFFECTS, FURTHER INFORMATION Manufacturer advises to monitor serum-tobramycin concentration in patients with known or suspected signs of auditory dysfunction; if ototoxicity develops—discontinue treatment until serum concentration falls below 2 mg/litre.

● RENAL IMPAIRMENT
▸ When used by inhalation Manufacturer advises monitor serum-tobramycin concentration; if nephrotoxicity develops—discontinue treatment until serum concentration falls below 2 mg/litre.

● MONITORING REQUIREMENTS
▸ With intramuscular use or intravenous use One-hour ('peak') serum concentration should not exceed 10 mg/litre; pre-dose ('trough') concentration should be less than 2 mg/litre.
▸ When used by inhalation Measure lung function before and after initial dose of tobramycin and monitor for bronchospasm; if bronchospasm occurs in a patient not using a bronchodilator, repeat test using bronchodilator. Manufacturer advises monitor renal function before treatment and then annually.

● DIRECTIONS FOR ADMINISTRATION
▸ With intravenous use For intravenous infusion (Nebcin®); intermittent or via drip tubing in Glucose 5% or Sodium chloride 0.9%. For adult intermittent infusion suggested volume 50–100 mL given over 20–60 minutes.
▸ When used by inhalation Other inhaled drugs should be administered before tobramycin.

● PATIENT AND CARER ADVICE
▸ When used by inhalation Patient counselling is advised for Tobramycin dry powder for inhalation (administration).
VANTOBRA® NEBULISER SOLUTION Manufacturer advises if a dose is more than 6 hours late, the missed dose should not be taken and the next dose should be taken at the normal time.

● NATIONAL FUNDING/ACCESS DECISIONS
NICE decisions
▸ Tobramycin by dry powder inhalation for pseudomonal lung infection in cystic fibrosis (March 2013) NICE TA276
▸ When used by inhalation Tobramycin dry powder for inhalation is recommended for chronic pulmonary

infection caused by *Pseudomonas aeruginosa* in patients with cystic fibrosis only if there is an inadequate response to colistimethate sodium, or if colistimethate sodium cannot be used because of contra-indications or intolerance. The manufacturer must provide tobramycin dry powder for inhalation at the discount agreed as part of the patient access scheme to primary, secondary and tertiary care in the NHS. Patients currently receiving tobramycin dry powder for inhalation can continue treatment until they and their clinician consider it appropriate to stop.
www.nice.org.uk/TA276

● MEDICINAL FORMS
There can be variation in the licensing of different medicines containing the same drug.

Solution for injection
▸ Tobramycin (Non-proprietary)
Tobramycin (as Tobramycin sulfate) 40 mg per 1 ml Tobramycin 80mg/2ml solution for injection vials | 5 vial PoM £20.80
Tobramycin 240mg/6ml solution for injection vials | 1 vial PoM £19.20
▸ Nebcin (Flynn Pharma Ltd)
Tobramycin (as Tobramycin sulfate) 40 mg per 1 ml Nebcin 80mg/2ml solution for injection vials | 1 vial PoM £5.37

Inhalation powder
▸ Tobi Podhaler (Novartis Pharmaceuticals UK Ltd)
Tobramycin 28 mg Tobi Podhaler 28mg inhalation powder capsules with device | 56 capsule PoM £447.50 | 224 capsule PoM £1,790.00

Nebuliser liquid
▸ Tobramycin (Non-proprietary)
Tobramycin 60 mg per 1 ml Tobramycin 300mg/5ml nebuliser liquid ampoules | 56 ampoule PoM £1,187.00 DT = £1,305.92
▸ Bramitob (Chiesi Ltd)
Tobramycin 75 mg per 1 ml Bramitob 300mg/4ml nebuliser solution 4ml ampoules | 56 ampoule PoM £1,187.00
▸ TOBI (Novartis Pharmaceuticals UK Ltd)
Tobramycin 60 mg per 1 ml Tobi 300mg/5ml nebuliser solution 5ml ampoules | 56 ampoule PoM £1,305.92 DT = £1,305.92
▸ Tymbrineb (Teva UK Ltd)
Tobramycin 60 mg per 1 ml Tymbrineb 300mg/5ml nebuliser solution 5ml ampoules | 56 ampoule PoM £780.00 DT = £1,305.92
▸ Vantobra (Pari Medical Ltd)
Tobramycin 100 mg per 1 ml Vantobra 170mg/1.7ml nebuliser solution 1.7ml ampoules | 56 ampoule PoM £1,305.00

ANTIBACTERIALS > CARBAPENEMS

Carbapenems

Overview

The carbapenems are beta-lactam antibacterials with a broad-spectrum of activity which includes many Gram-positive and Gram-negative bacteria, and anaerobes; **imipenem** (imipenem with cilastatin p. 514) and meropenem p. 514 have good activity against *Pseudomonas aeruginosa*. The carbapenems are not active against meticillin-resistant *Staphylococcus aureus* and *Enterococcus faecium*.

Imipenem (imipenem with cilastatin) and meropenem are used for the treatment of severe hospital-acquired infections and polymicrobial infections including septicaemia, hospital-acquired pneumonia, intra-abdominal infections, skin and soft-tissue infections, and complicated urinary-tract infections.

Ertapenem below is licensed for treating abdominal and gynaecological infections and for community-acquired pneumonia, but it is not active against atypical respiratory pathogens and it has limited activity against penicillin-resistant pneumococci. It is also licensed for treating foot infections of the skin and soft tissue in patients with diabetes. Unlike the other carbapenems, ertapenem is not active against *Pseudomonas* or against *Acinetobacter spp*.

Imipenem is partially inactivated in the kidney by enzymatic activity and is therefore administered in combination with **cilastatin** (imipenem with cilastatin), a specific enzyme inhibitor, which blocks its renal metabolism. Meropenem and ertapenem are stable to the renal enzyme which inactivates imipenem and therefore can be given without cilastatin.

Side-effects of imipenem with cilastatin are similar to those of other beta-lactam antibiotics. Meropenem has less seizure-inducing potential and can be used to treat central nervous system infection.

Ertapenem

● INDICATIONS AND DOSE

Abdominal infections | Acute gynaecological infections | Community-acquired pneumonia
▸ BY INTRAVENOUS INFUSION
▸ Adult: 1 g once daily

Diabetic foot infections of the skin and soft-tissue
▸ BY INTRAVENOUS INFUSION
▸ Adult: 1 g once daily

Surgical prophylaxis, colorectal surgery
▸ BY INTRAVENOUS INFUSION
▸ Adult: 1 g for 1 dose, dose to be completed within 1 hour before surgery

● CAUTIONS CNS disorders—risk of seizures · elderly
● INTERACTIONS → Appendix 1: carbapenems
● SIDE-EFFECTS
▸ **Common or very common** Diarrhoea · headache · nausea · vomiting
▸ **Uncommon** Appetite decreased · arrhythmias · asthenia · confusion · constipation · dizziness · drowsiness · dry mouth · gastrointestinal discomfort · gastrointestinal disorders · hypotension · increased risk of infection · insomnia · oedema · pseudomembranous enterocolitis · seizure · skin reactions · swelling · taste altered · throat discomfort
▸ **Rare or very rare** Anxiety · cholecystitis · depression · dysphagia · eye disorder · haemorrhage · hepatic disorders · hypersensitivity · hypoglycaemia · malaise · muscle cramps · nasal congestion · neutropenia · renal impairment · shoulder pain · syncope · thrombocytopenia · tremor
▸ **Frequency not known** Aggression · delirium · drug reaction with eosinophilia and systemic symptoms (DRESS) · gait abnormal · hallucination · level of consciousness decreased · movement disorders · muscle weakness · psychiatric disorder · tooth discolouration

● ALLERGY AND CROSS-SENSITIVITY Avoid if history of **immediate hypersensitivity** reaction to beta-lactam antibacterials.
Use with caution in patients with sensitivity to beta-lactam antibacterials.

● PREGNANCY Manufacturer advises avoid unless potential benefit outweighs risk.

● BREAST FEEDING Present in milk—manufacturer advises avoid.

● RENAL IMPAIRMENT
Dose adjustments Risk of seizures; max. 500 mg daily if eGFR less than 30 mL/minute/1.73 m².

● DIRECTIONS FOR ADMINISTRATION For *intravenous infusion* (*Invanz*®), give intermittently *in* Sodium chloride 0.9%. Reconstitute 1 g with 10 mL Water for injections *or* Sodium chloride 0.9%; dilute requisite dose in infusion fluid to a final concentration not exceeding 20 mg/mL; give over 30 minutes; incompatible with glucose solutions.

5

Infection

- MEDICINAL FORMS
There can be variation in the licensing of different medicines containing the same drug.

Powder for solution for infusion
ELECTROLYTES: May contain Sodium
▸ Invanz (Merck Sharp & Dohme Ltd)
Ertapenem (as Ertapenem sodium) 1 gram Invanz 1g powder for solution for infusion vials | 1 vial [PoM] £31.65

Imipenem with cilastatin

- INDICATIONS AND DOSE

Aerobic and anaerobic Gram-positive and Gram-negative infections (not indicated for CNS infections) | Hospital-acquired septicaemia
▸ BY INTRAVENOUS INFUSION
▸ Adult: 500 mg every 6 hours, alternatively 1 g every 8 hours

Infection caused by *Pseudomonas* or other less sensitive organisms | Empirical treatment of infection in febrile patients with neutropenia | Life-threatening infection
▸ BY INTRAVENOUS INFUSION
▸ Adult: 1 g every 6 hours

DOSE EQUIVALENCE AND CONVERSION
▸ Dose expressed in terms of imipenem.

- CAUTIONS CNS disorders · epilepsy
- INTERACTIONS → Appendix 1: carbapenems
- SIDE-EFFECTS
▸ **Common or very common** Diarrhoea · eosinophilia · nausea · skin reactions · vomiting
▸ **Uncommon** Bone marrow disorders · confusion · dizziness · drowsiness · hallucination · hypotension · leucopenia · movement disorders · psychiatric disorder · seizure · thrombocytopenia · thrombocytosis
▸ **Rare or very rare** Agranulocytosis · anaphylactic reaction · angioedema · chest discomfort · colitis haemorrhagic · cyanosis · dyspnoea · encephalopathy · flushing · focal tremor · gastrointestinal discomfort · haemolytic anaemia · headache · hearing impairment · hepatic disorders · hyperhidrosis · hyperventilation · increased risk of infection · myasthenia gravis aggravated · oral disorders · palpitations · paraesthesia · polyarthralgia · polyuria · pseudomembranous enterocolitis · renal impairment · severe cutaneous adverse reactions (SCARs) · spinal pain · tachycardia · taste altered · urine discolouration · vertigo
▸ **Frequency not known** Agitation
- ALLERGY AND CROSS-SENSITIVITY Avoid if history of **immediate hypersensitivity** reaction to beta-lactam antibacterials.
  Use with caution in patients with sensitivity to beta-lactam antibacterials.
- PREGNANCY Manufacturer advises avoid unless potential benefit outweighs risk (toxicity in *animal* studies).
- BREAST FEEDING Present in milk but unlikely to be absorbed.
- RENAL IMPAIRMENT
Dose adjustments Risk of CNS side-effects; reduce dose if eGFR less than 70 mL/minute/1.73 m^2— consult product literature.
- EFFECT ON LABORATORY TESTS Positive Coombs' test.
- DIRECTIONS FOR ADMINISTRATION For *intravenous infusion* dilute to a concentration of 5 mg (as imipenem)/mL in Sodium chloride 0.9%; give up to 500 mg (as imipenem) over 20–30 minutes, give dose greater than 500 mg (as imipenem) over 40–60 minutes.

- MEDICINAL FORMS
There can be variation in the licensing of different medicines containing the same drug.

Powder for solution for infusion
ELECTROLYTES: May contain Sodium
▸ Imipenem with cilastatin (Non-proprietary)
Cilastatin (as Cilastatin sodium) 500 mg, Imipenem (as Imipenem monohydrate) 500 mg Imipenem 500mg / Cilastatin 500mg powder for solution for infusion vials | 1 vial [PoM] £12.00 (Hospital only) | 5 vial [PoM] £60.00 (Hospital only)
▸ Primaxin I.V. (Merck Sharp & Dohme Ltd)
Cilastatin (as Cilastatin sodium) 500 mg, Imipenem (as Imipenem monohydrate) 500 mg Primaxin IV 500mg powder for solution for infusion vials | 1 vial [PoM] £12.00

Meropenem

- INDICATIONS AND DOSE

Aerobic and anaerobic Gram-positive and Gram-negative infections | Hospital-acquired septicaemia
▸ BY INTRAVENOUS INFUSION, OR BY INTRAVENOUS INJECTION
▸ Adult: 0.5–1 g every 8 hours

Exacerbations of chronic lower respiratory-tract infection in cystic fibrosis
▸ BY INTRAVENOUS INFUSION, OR BY INTRAVENOUS INJECTION
▸ Adult: 2 g every 8 hours

Meningitis
▸ BY INTRAVENOUS INFUSION, OR BY INTRAVENOUS INJECTION
▸ Adult: 2 g every 8 hours

Endocarditis (in combination with another antibacterial)
▸ BY INTRAVENOUS INFUSION, OR BY INTRAVENOUS INJECTION
▸ Adult: 2 g every 8 hours

- UNLICENSED USE Not licensed for use in endocarditis.
- INTERACTIONS → Appendix 1: carbapenems
- SIDE-EFFECTS
▸ **Common or very common** Abdominal pain · diarrhoea · headache · inflammation · nausea · pain · skin reactions · thrombocytosis · vomiting
▸ **Uncommon** Agranulocytosis · antibiotic associated colitis · eosinophilia · haemolytic anaemia · increased risk of infection · leucopenia · neutropenia · paraesthesia · severe cutaneous adverse reactions (SCARs) · thrombocytopenia
▸ **Rare or very rare** Seizure
- ALLERGY AND CROSS-SENSITIVITY Avoid if history of **immediate hypersensitivity** reaction to beta-lactam antibacterials.
  Use with caution in patients with sensitivity to beta-lactam antibacterials.
- PREGNANCY Use only if potential benefit outweighs risk— no information available.
- BREAST FEEDING Unlikely to be absorbed (however, manufacturer advises avoid).
- HEPATIC IMPAIRMENT
Monitoring Monitor liver function in hepatic impairment.
- RENAL IMPAIRMENT
Dose adjustments Use normal dose every 12 hours if eGFR 26–50 mL/minute/1.73 m^2.
  Use half normal dose every 12 hours if eGFR 10–25 mL/minute/1.73 m^2.
  Use half normal dose every 24 hours if eGFR less than 10 mL/minute/1.73 m^2.
- EFFECT ON LABORATORY TESTS Positive Coombs' test.
- DIRECTIONS FOR ADMINISTRATION *Intravenous injection* to be administered over 5 minutes.
  For *intravenous infusion* (*Meronem*®), give intermittently in Glucose 5% *or* Sodium chloride 0.9%.
  Dilute dose in infusion fluid to a final concentration of 1–20 mg/mL; give over 15–30 minutes.

- MEDICINAL FORMS
  There can be variation in the licensing of different medicines containing the same drug.

Powder for solution for injection
ELECTROLYTES: May contain Sodium

▸ Meropenem (Non-proprietary)

Meropenem (as Meropenem trihydrate) 500 mg Meropenem 500mg powder for solution for injection vials | 10 vial [PoM] £84.70–£103.14 DT = £84.70 | 10 vial [PoM] £83.00 DT = £84.70 (Hospital only)

Meropenem (as Meropenem trihydrate) 1 gram Meropenem 1g powder for solution for injection vials | 10 vial [PoM] £169.30–£206.30 DT = £169.30 | 10 vial [PoM] £160.00–£206.28 DT = £169.30 (Hospital only)

▸ Meronem (Pfizer Ltd)

Meropenem (as Meropenem trihydrate) 500 mg Meronem 500mg powder for solution for injection vials | 10 vial [PoM] £103.14 DT = £84.70

Meropenem (as Meropenem trihydrate) 1 gram Meronem 1g powder for solution for injection vials | 10 vial [PoM] £206.28 DT = £169.30

ANTIBACTERIALS > CEPHALOSPORINS

Cephalosporins

Overview

The cephalosporins are broad-spectrum antibiotics which are used for the treatment of septicaemia, pneumonia, meningitis, biliary-tract infections, peritonitis, and urinary-tract infections. The pharmacology of the cephalosporins is similar to that of the penicillins, excretion being principally renal. Cephalosporins penetrate the cerebrospinal fluid poorly unless the meninges are inflamed; cefotaxime p. 519 and ceftriaxone p. 520 are suitable cephalosporins for infections of the CNS (e.g meningitis).

The principal side-effect of the cephalosporins is hypersensitivity and about 0.5–6.5% of penicillin-sensitive patients will also be allergic to the cephalosporins. If a cephalosporin is essential in patients with a history of immediate hypersensitivity to penicillin, because a suitable alternative antibacterial is not available, then cefixime p. 518, cefotaxime, ceftazidime p. 519, ceftriaxone, or cefuroxime p. 518 can be used with caution; cefaclor p. 517, cefadroxil below, cefalexin p. 516, cefradine p. 516, and ceftaroline fosamil p. 522 should be avoided.

The orally active 'first generation' cephalosporins, cefalexin, cefradine, and cefadroxil and the 'second generation' cephalosporin, cefaclor, have a similar antimicrobial spectrum. They are useful for urinary-tract infections which do not respond to other drugs or which occur in pregnancy, respiratory-tract infections, otitis media, and skin and soft-tissue infections. Cefaclor has good activity against *H. influenzae*. Cefadroxil has a long duration of action and can be given twice daily; it has poor activity against *H. influenzae*. **Cefuroxime axetil**, an ester of the 'second generation' cephalosporin cefuroxime, has the same antibacterial spectrum as the parent compound; it is poorly absorbed and needs to be given with food to maximise absorption.

Cefixime is an orally active 'third generation' cephalosporin. It has a longer duration of action than the other cephalosporins that are active by mouth. It is only licensed for acute infections.

Cefuroxime is a 'second generation' cephalosporin that is less susceptible than the earlier cephalosporins to inactivation by beta-lactamases. It is, therefore, active against certain bacteria which are resistant to the other drugs and has greater activity against *Haemophilus influenzae*.

Cefotaxime, ceftazidime and ceftriaxone are 'third generation' cephalosporins with greater activity than the 'second generation' cephalosporins against certain Gram-negative bacteria. However, they are less active than

cefuroxime against Gram-positive bacteria, most notably *Staphylococcus aureus*. Their broad antibacterial spectrum may encourage superinfection with resistant bacteria or fungi.

Ceftazidime has good activity against pseudomonas. It is also active against other Gram-negative bacteria.

Ceftriaxone has a longer half-life and therefore needs to be given only once daily. Indications include serious infections such as septicaemia, pneumonia, and meningitis. The calcium salt of ceftriaxone forms a precipitate in the gall bladder which may rarely cause symptoms but these usually resolve when the antibiotic is stopped.

Ceftaroline fosamil is a 'fifth generation' cephalosporin with bactericidal activity similar to cefotaxime; however, ceftaroline fosamil has an extended spectrum of activity against Gram-positive bacteria that includes meticillin-resistant *Staphylococcus aureus* and multi-drug resistant *Streptococcus pneumoniae*. Ceftaroline fosamil is licensed for the treatment of community-acquired pneumonia and complicated skin and soft-tissue infections, but there is no experience of its use in pneumonia caused by meticillin-resistant *S. aureus*.

Cephalosporins

- **DRUG ACTION** Cephalosporins are antibacterials that attach to penicillin binding proteins to interrupt cell wall biosynthesis, leading to bacterial cell lysis and death.
- SIDE-EFFECTS
- ▸ **Common or very common** Abdominal pain · diarrhoea · dizziness · eosinophilia · fungal infection · headache · leucopenia · nausea · neutropenia · skin reactions · thrombocytopenia · vomiting
- ▸ **Uncommon** Anaphylactic reaction · antibiotic associated colitis
- ▸ **Rare or very rare** Agranulocytosis · angioedema · haemolytic anaemia · nephritis tubulointerstitial (reversible) · severe cutaneous adverse reactions (SCARs)
- **ALLERGY AND CROSS-SENSITIVITY** Contra-indicated in patients with cephalosporin hypersensitivity.
- Cross-sensitivity with other beta-lactam antibacterials About 0.5–6.5% of penicillin-sensitive patients will also be allergic to the cephalosporins. Patients with a history of **immediate hypersensitivity** to penicillin and other beta-lactams should not receive a cephalosporin. Cephalosporins should be used with caution in patients with sensitivity to penicillin and other beta-lactams.
- **EFFECT ON LABORATORY TESTS** False positive urinary glucose (if tested for reducing substances). False positive Coombs' test.

ANTIBACTERIALS > CEPHALOSPORINS, FIRST-GENERATION

☞ above

Cefadroxil

- INDICATIONS AND DOSE

Susceptible infections due to sensitive Gram-positive and Gram-negative bacteria

▸ BY MOUTH
▸ Child 6–17 years (body-weight up to 40 kg): 0.5 g twice daily
▸ Child 6–17 years (body-weight 40 kg and above): 0.5–1 g twice daily
▸ Adult: 0.5–1 g twice daily

continued →

Skin infections | Soft-tissue infections | Uncomplicated urinary-tract infections
▶ BY MOUTH
▸ Child 6-17 years (body-weight 40 kg and above): 1 g once daily
▸ Adult: 1 g daily

● INTERACTIONS → Appendix 1: cephalosporins
● SIDE-EFFECTS
▶ Common or very common Dyspepsia · glossitis
▶ Rare or very rare Arthralgia · drug fever · fatigue · hepatic disorders · insomnia · nervousness · serum sickness-like reaction
● PREGNANCY Not known to be harmful.
● BREAST FEEDING Present in milk in low concentration, but appropriate to use.
● RENAL IMPAIRMENT
Dose adjustments ▸ In adults 1 g initially, then 500 mg every 12 hours if eGFR 26–50 mL/minute/1.73 m^2. 1 g initially, then 500 mg every 24 hours if eGFR 11–26 mL/minute/1.73 m^2. 1 g initially, then 500 mg every 36 hours if eGFR less than 11 mL/minute/1.73 m^2.
▸ In children Reduce dose if estimated glomerular filtration rate less than 50 mL/minute/1.73 m^2.

● MEDICINAL FORMS
There can be variation in the licensing of different medicines containing the same drug.
Capsule
CAUTIONARY AND ADVISORY LABELS 9
▶ Cefadroxil (Non-proprietary)
Cefadroxil (as Cefadroxil monohydrate) 500 mg Cefadroxil 500mg capsules | 20 capsule [PoM] £22.38 DT = £15.24 | 100 capsule [PoM] £26.22–£111.90

▸ 515

Cefalexin

(Cephalexin)

● INDICATIONS AND DOSE

Susceptible infections due to sensitive Gram-positive and Gram-negative bacteria
▶ BY MOUTH
▶ Child 1-11 months: 12.5 mg/kg twice daily, alternatively 125 mg twice daily
▶ Child 1-4 years: 12.5 mg/kg twice daily, alternatively 125 mg 3 times a day
▶ Child 5-11 years: 12.5 mg/kg twice daily, alternatively 250 mg 3 times a day
▶ Child 12-17 years: 500 mg 2–3 times a day
▶ Adult: 250 mg every 6 hours, alternatively 500 mg every 8–12 hours; increased to 1–1.5 g every 6–8 hours, increased dose to be used for severe infections

Serious susceptible infections due to sensitive Gram-positive and Gram-negative bacteria
▶ BY MOUTH
▶ Child 1 month-11 years: 25 mg/kg 2–4 times a day (max. per dose 1 g 4 times a day)
▶ Child 12-17 years: 1–1.5 g 3–4 times a day

Prophylaxis of recurrent urinary-tract infection
▶ BY MOUTH
▶ Child: 12.5 mg/kg once daily (max. per dose 125 mg), dose to be taken at night
▶ Adult: 125 mg once daily, dose to be taken at night

● INTERACTIONS → Appendix 1: cephalosporins
● SIDE-EFFECTS Agitation · arthritis · confusion · fatigue · gastrointestinal discomfort · genital pruritus · hallucination · hepatitis (transient) · hypersensitivity · jaundice cholestatic (transient) · joint disorders · vaginal discharge

● PREGNANCY Not known to be harmful.
● BREAST FEEDING Present in milk in low concentration, but appropriate to use.
● RENAL IMPAIRMENT
Dose adjustments ▸ In adults Max. 3 g daily if eGFR 40–50 mL/minute/1.73 m^2. Max. 1.5 g daily if eGFR 10–40 mL/minute/1.73 m^2. Max. 750 mg daily if eGFR less than 10 mL/minute/1.73 m^2.
▸ In children Reduce dose in moderate impairment.

● PATIENT AND CARER ADVICE
Medicines for Children leaflet: Cefalexin for bacterial infections www.medicinesforchildren.org.uk/cefalexin-bacterial-infections-0

● PROFESSION SPECIFIC INFORMATION
Dental practitioners' formulary
Cefalexin Capsules may be prescribed.
  Cefalexin Tablets may be prescribed.
  Cefalexin Oral Suspension may be prescribed.

● MEDICINAL FORMS
There can be variation in the licensing of different medicines containing the same drug.
Oral suspension
CAUTIONARY AND ADVISORY LABELS 9
▶ Cefalexin (Non-proprietary)
Cefalexin 25 mg per 1 ml Cefalexin 125mg/5ml oral suspension sugar free sugar-free | 100 ml [PoM] £0.84
Cefalexin 125mg/5ml oral suspension | 100 ml [PoM] £4.90 DT = £0.84
Cefalexin 50 mg per 1 ml Cefalexin 250mg/5ml oral suspension sugar free sugar-free | 100 ml [PoM] £1.72–£1.90
Cefalexin 250mg/5ml oral suspension | 100 ml [PoM] £5.25 DT = £1.90
Cefalexin 100 mg per 1 ml Cefalexin 500mg/5ml oral suspension | 100 ml [PoM] 🚫
▶ Keflex (Flynn Pharma Ltd)
Cefalexin 25 mg per 1 ml Keflex 125mg/5ml oral suspension | 100 ml [PoM] £0.84 DT = £0.84
Cefalexin 50 mg per 1 ml Keflex 250mg/5ml oral suspension | 100 ml [PoM] £1.40 DT = £1.90
Tablet
CAUTIONARY AND ADVISORY LABELS 9
▶ Cefalexin (Non-proprietary)
Cefalexin 250 mg Cefalexin 250mg tablets | 28 tablet [PoM] £5.02 DT = £1.50
Cefalexin 500 mg Cefalexin 500mg tablets | 21 tablet [PoM] £5.88 DT = £1.84
▶ Keflex (Flynn Pharma Ltd)
Cefalexin 250 mg Keflex 250mg tablets | 28 tablet [PoM] £1.60 DT = £1.50
Cefalexin 500 mg Keflex 500mg tablets | 21 tablet [PoM] £2.08 DT = £1.84
Capsule
CAUTIONARY AND ADVISORY LABELS 9
▶ Cefalexin (Non-proprietary)
Cefalexin 250 mg Cefalexin 250mg capsules | 28 capsule [PoM] £4.01 DT = £1.46
Cefalexin 500 mg Cefalexin 500mg capsules | 21 capsule [PoM] £4.45 DT = £1.79 | 100 capsule [PoM] £9.43
▶ Keflex (Flynn Pharma Ltd)
Cefalexin 250 mg Keflex 250mg capsules | 28 capsule [PoM] £1.46 DT = £1.46
Cefalexin 500 mg Keflex 500mg capsules | 21 capsule [PoM] £1.98 DT = £1.79

▸ 515

Cefradine

(Cephradine)

● INDICATIONS AND DOSE

Susceptible infections due to sensitive Gram-positive and Gram-negative bacteria | Surgical prophylaxis
▶ BY MOUTH
▶ Child 7-11 years: 25–50 mg/kg daily in 2–4 divided doses

▶ Child 12-17 years: 250–500 mg 4 times a day, alternatively 0.5–1 g twice daily; increased if necessary up to 1 g 4 times a day, increased dose may be used in severe infections

▶ Adult: 250–500 mg 4 times a day, alternatively 0.5–1 g twice daily; increased if necessary up to 1 g 4 times a day, increased dose may be used in severe infections

● INTERACTIONS → Appendix 1: cephalosporins

● SIDE-EFFECTS Akathisia · aplastic anaemia · arthralgia · blood disorder · chest tightness · confusion · gastrointestinal discomfort · glossitis · hepatitis (transient) · hypersensitivity · jaundice cholestatic · muscle tone increased · nervousness · oedema · sleep disorder

● PREGNANCY Not known to be harmful.

● BREAST FEEDING Present in milk in low concentration, but appropriate to use.

● RENAL IMPAIRMENT
Dose adjustments ▶ In adults Use half normal dose if eGFR 5–20 mL/minute/1.73 m^2. Use one-quarter normal dose if eGFR less than 5 mL/minute/1.73 m^2.
▶ In children Reduce dose if estimated glomerular filtration rate less than 20 mL/minute/1.73 m^2.

● PROFESSION SPECIFIC INFORMATION
Dental practitioners' formulary
Cefradine Capsules may be prescribed.

● MEDICINAL FORMS
There can be variation in the licensing of different medicines containing the same drug.
Capsule
CAUTIONARY AND ADVISORY LABELS 9
▶ Cefradine (Non-proprietary)
Cefradine 250 mg Cefradine 250mg capsules | 20 capsule PoM £6.00 DT = £2.25
Cefradine 500 mg Cefradine 500mg capsules | 20 capsule PoM £8.75 DT = £3.33
▶ Nicef (Strides Shasun (UK) Ltd)
Cefradine 250 mg Nicef 250mg capsules | 20 capsule PoM £3.55 DT = £2.25 | 100 capsule PoM £9.39
Cefradine 500 mg Nicef 500mg capsules | 20 capsule PoM £5.58 DT = £3.33 | 100 capsule PoM £33.72

ANTIBACTERIALS ⟩ CEPHALOSPORINS, SECOND-GENERATION

◀ 515

Cefaclor

● INDICATIONS AND DOSE
Susceptible infections due to sensitive Gram-positive and Gram-negative bacteria
▶ BY MOUTH USING IMMEDIATE-RELEASE MEDICINES
▶ Child 1-11 months: 20 mg/kg daily in 3 divided doses, alternatively 62.5 mg 3 times a day
▶ Child 1-4 years: 20 mg/kg daily in 3 divided doses, alternatively 125 mg 3 times a day
▶ Child 5-11 years: 20 mg/kg daily in 3 divided doses, usual max. 1 g daily, alternatively 250 mg 3 times a day
▶ Child 12-17 years: 250 mg 3 times a day; maximum 4 g per day
▶ Adult: 250 mg 3 times a day; maximum 4 g per day
▶ BY MOUTH USING MODIFIED-RELEASE MEDICINES
▶ Child 12-17 years: 375 mg every 12 hours, dose to be taken with food
▶ Adult: 375 mg every 12 hours, dose to be taken with food

Severe susceptible infections due to sensitive Gram-positive and Gram-negative bacteria
▶ BY MOUTH USING IMMEDIATE-RELEASE MEDICINES
▶ Child 1-11 months: 40 mg/kg daily in 3 divided doses, usual max. 1 g daily, alternatively 125 mg 3 times a day

▶ Child 1-4 years: 40 mg/kg daily in 3 divided doses, usual max. 1 g daily, alternatively 250 mg 3 times a day
▶ Child 5-11 years: 40 mg/kg daily in 3 divided doses, usual max. 1 g daily
▶ Child 12-17 years: 500 mg 3 times a day; maximum 4 g per day
▶ Adult: 500 mg 3 times a day; maximum 4 g per day
Pneumonia
▶ BY MOUTH USING MODIFIED-RELEASE TABLETS
▶ Child 12-17 years: 750 mg every 12 hours, dose to be taken with food
▶ Adult: 750 mg every 12 hours, dose to be taken with food
Lower urinary-tract infections
▶ BY MOUTH USING MODIFIED-RELEASE MEDICINES
▶ Child 12-17 years: 375 mg every 12 hours, dose to be taken with food
▶ Adult: 375 mg every 12 hours, dose to be taken with food
Asymptomatic carriage of *Haemophilus influenzae* or mild exacerbations in cystic fibrosis
▶ BY MOUTH USING IMMEDIATE-RELEASE MEDICINES
▶ Child 1-11 months: 125 mg every 8 hours
▶ Child 1-6 years: 250 mg 3 times a day
▶ Child 7-17 years: 500 mg 3 times a day

● INTERACTIONS → Appendix 1: cephalosporins

● SIDE-EFFECTS Akathisia · anxiety · aplastic anaemia · arthralgia · arthritis · asthenia · colitis · confusion · drowsiness · dyspnoea · fever · genital pruritus · hallucination · hepatitis (transient) · hypersensitivity · insomnia · jaundice cholestatic (transient) · lymphadenopathy · lymphocytosis · muscle tone increased · oedema · paraesthesia · proteinuria · syncope · vasodilation

SIDE-EFFECTS, FURTHER INFORMATION Cefaclor is associated with protracted skin reactions, especially in children.

● PREGNANCY Not known to be harmful.

● BREAST FEEDING Present in milk in low concentration, but appropriate to use.

● RENAL IMPAIRMENT Manufacturer advises caution.
Dose adjustments No dose adjustment required.

● MEDICINAL FORMS
There can be variation in the licensing of different medicines containing the same drug.
Oral suspension
CAUTIONARY AND ADVISORY LABELS 9
▶ Cefaclor (Non-proprietary)
Cefaclor (as Cefaclor monohydrate) 25 mg per 1 ml Cefaclor 125mg/5ml oral suspension | 100 ml PoM Ⓢ
Cefaclor (as Cefaclor monohydrate) 50 mg per 1 ml Cefaclor 250mg/5ml oral suspension | 100 ml PoM Ⓢ
▶ Distaclor (Flynn Pharma Ltd)
Cefaclor (as Cefaclor monohydrate) 25 mg per 1 ml Distaclor 125mg/5ml oral suspension | 100 ml PoM £4.13
Cefaclor (as Cefaclor monohydrate) 50 mg per 1 ml Distaclor 250mg/5ml oral suspension | 100 ml PoM £8.26
▶ Keftid (Strides Shasun (UK) Ltd)
Cefaclor (as Cefaclor monohydrate) 25 mg per 1 ml Keftid 125mg/5ml oral suspension sugar-free | 100 ml PoM £5.16 DT = £5.16
Cefaclor (as Cefaclor monohydrate) 50 mg per 1 ml Keftid 250mg/5ml oral suspension sugar-free | 100 ml PoM £10.32 DT = £10.32
Modified-release tablet
CAUTIONARY AND ADVISORY LABELS 9, 21, 25
▶ Distaclor MR (Flynn Pharma Ltd)
Cefaclor (as Cefaclor monohydrate) 375 mg Distaclor MR 375mg tablets | 14 tablet PoM £9.10 DT = £9.10

5

Infection

5

Infection

Capsule
CAUTIONARY AND ADVISORY LABELS 9
- Cefaclor (Non-proprietary)
  Cefaclor (as Cefaclor monohydrate) 250 mg Cefaclor 250mg capsules | 21 capsule [PoM] ⓢ DT = £6.80
- Distaclor (Flynn Pharma Ltd)
  Cefaclor (as Cefaclor monohydrate) 500 mg Distaclor 500mg capsules | 21 capsule [PoM] £7.50 DT = £7.50
- Keftid (Strides Shasun (UK) Ltd)
  Cefaclor (as Cefaclor monohydrate) 250 mg Keftid 250mg capsules | 21 capsule [PoM] £6.80 DT = £6.80
  Cefaclor (as Cefaclor monohydrate) 500 mg Keftid 500mg capsules | 50 capsule [PoM] £31.99

F 515

Cefuroxime
17-Mar-2017

- **INDICATIONS AND DOSE**

Susceptible infections due to Gram-positive and Gram-negative bacteria
- BY MOUTH
- Child 3 months-1 year: 10 mg/kg twice daily (max. per dose 125 mg)
- Child 2-11 years: 15 mg/kg twice daily (max. per dose 250 mg)
- Child 12-17 years: 250 mg twice daily, dose may be doubled in severe lower respiratory-tract infections or if pneumonia is suspected
- Adult: 250 mg twice daily, dose may be doubled in severe lower respiratory-tract infections or if pneumonia is suspected
- BY INTRAVENOUS INFUSION, OR BY INTRAVENOUS INJECTION, OR BY INTRAMUSCULAR INJECTION
- Child: 20 mg/kg every 8 hours (max. per dose 750 mg); increased to 50-60 mg/kg every 6-8 hours (max. per dose 1.5 g), increased dose used for severe infection and cystic fibrosis
- Adult: 750 mg every 6-8 hours; increased if necessary up to 1.5 g every 6-8 hours, increased dose used for severe infections

Lyme disease
- BY MOUTH
- Adult: 500 mg twice daily for 14-21 days (for 28 days in Lyme arthritis)

Lower urinary-tract infection
- BY MOUTH
- Child 12-17 years: 125 mg twice daily
- Adult: 125 mg twice daily

Pyelonephritis
- BY MOUTH
- Adult: 250 mg twice daily

Surgical prophylaxis
- INITIALLY BY INTRAVENOUS INJECTION
- Adult: 1.5 g, to be administered up to 30 minutes before the procedure, then (by intravenous injection or by intramuscular injection) 750 mg every 8 hours if required for up to 3 doses (in high risk procedures)

Open fractures, prophylaxis
- BY INTRAVENOUS INFUSION, OR BY INTRAVENOUS INJECTION
- Adult: 1.5 g every 8 hours until soft tissue closure (maximum duration 72 hours)

- UNLICENSED USE Duration of treatment in Lyme disease is unlicensed.
- INTERACTIONS → Appendix 1: cephalosporins
- SIDE-EFFECTS
- Uncommon
- With parenteral use Gastrointestinal disorder
- Frequency not known
- With oral use Drug fever · hepatic disorders · Jarisch-Herxheimer reaction · serum sickness
- With parenteral use Cutaneous vasculitis · drug fever

- PREGNANCY Not known to be harmful.
- BREAST FEEDING Present in milk in low concentration, but appropriate to use.
- RENAL IMPAIRMENT
  Dose adjustments - In adults Use parenteral dose of 750 mg twice daily if eGFR 10-20 mL/minute/1.73 m². Use parenteral dose of 750 mg once daily if eGFR less than 10 mL/minute/1.73 m².
  - In children Reduce parenteral dose if estimated glomerular filtration rate less than 20 mL/minute/1.73 m².
- DIRECTIONS FOR ADMINISTRATION Single doses over 750 mg should be administered by the intravenous route only.
- With intravenous use in children Displacement value may be significant when reconstituting injection, consult local guidelines. For intermittent intravenous infusion, dilute reconstituted solution further in glucose 5% or sodium chloride 0.9%; give over 30 minutes.
- With intravenous use in adults For *intravenous infusion* (*Zinacef®*), give intermittently or via drip tubing in *Glucose* 5% or Sodium chloride 0.9%. Dissolve initially in water for injections (at least 2 mL for each 250 mg,15 mL for 1.5 g); suggested volume 50-100 mL given over 30 minutes.

- MEDICINAL FORMS
There can be variation in the licensing of different medicines containing the same drug. Forms available from special-order manufacturers include: solution for injection, infusion

Tablet
CAUTIONARY AND ADVISORY LABELS 9, 21, 25
- Cefuroxime (Non-proprietary)
  Cefuroxime (as Cefuroxime axetil) 250 mg Cefuroxime 250mg tablets | 14 tablet [PoM] £17.72 DT = £17.72
- Zinnat (GlaxoSmithKline UK Ltd)
  Cefuroxime (as Cefuroxime axetil) 125 mg Zinnat 125mg tablets | 14 tablet [PoM] £4.56 DT = £4.56
  Cefuroxime (as Cefuroxime axetil) 250 mg Zinnat 250mg tablets | 14 tablet [PoM] £9.11 DT = £17.72

Powder for injection
ELECTROLYTES: May contain Sodium
- Cefuroxime (Non-proprietary)
  Cefuroxime (as Cefuroxime sodium) 250 mg Cefuroxime 250mg powder for injection vials | 10 vial [PoM] £9.25
  Cefuroxime (as Cefuroxime sodium) 750 mg Cefuroxime 750mg powder for injection vials | 1 vial [PoM] £2.52 | 10 vial [PoM] £25.20
  Cefuroxime (as Cefuroxime sodium) 1.5 gram Cefuroxime 1.5g powder for injection vials | 1 vial [PoM] £5.05 | 10 vial [PoM] £50.50
- Zinacef (GlaxoSmithKline UK Ltd)
  Cefuroxime (as Cefuroxime sodium) 250 mg Zinacef 250mg powder for injection vials | 5 vial [PoM] £4.70
  Cefuroxime (as Cefuroxime sodium) 750 mg Zinacef 750mg powder for injection vials | 5 vial [PoM] £11.72 (Hospital only)
  Cefuroxime (as Cefuroxime sodium) 1.5 gram Zinacef 1.5g powder for injection vials | 1 vial [PoM] £4.70

Oral suspension
CAUTIONARY AND ADVISORY LABELS 9, 21
EXCIPIENTS: May contain Aspartame, sucrose
- Zinnat (GlaxoSmithKline UK Ltd)
  Cefuroxime (as Cefuroxime axetil) 25 mg per 1 ml Zinnat 125mg/5ml oral suspension | 70 ml [PoM] £5.20 DT = £5.20

ANTIBACTERIALS > CEPHALOSPORINS, THIRD-GENERATION

F 515

Cefixime

- **INDICATIONS AND DOSE**

Acute infections due to sensitive Gram-positive and Gram-negative bacteria
- BY MOUTH
- Child 6-11 months: 75 mg daily
- Child 1-4 years: 100 mg daily
- Child 5-9 years: 200 mg daily

- ▸ Child 10–17 years: 200–400 mg daily, alternatively 100–200 mg twice daily
- ▸ Adult: 200–400 mg daily in 1–2 divided doses

Uncomplicated gonorrhoea
- ▸ BY MOUTH
- ▸ Adult: 400 mg for 1 dose

- ● UNLICENSED USE Use of cefixime for uncomplicated gonorrhoea is an unlicensed indication.
- ● INTERACTIONS → Appendix 1: cephalosporins
- ● SIDE-EFFECTS Acute kidney injury · arthralgia · drug fever · drug reaction with eosinophilia and systemic symptoms (DRESS) · dyspepsia · dyspnoea · face oedema · flatulence · genital pruritus · granulocytopenia · hypereosinophilia · jaundice · serum sickness-like reaction · thrombocytosis
- ● PREGNANCY Not known to be harmful.
- ● BREAST FEEDING Manufacturer advises avoid unless essential—no information available.
- ● RENAL IMPAIRMENT

  Dose adjustments ▸ In adults Reduce dose if eGFR less than 20 mL/minute/1.73 m^2 (max. 200 mg once daily).

  ▸ In children Reduce dose if estimated glomerular filtration rate less than 20 mL/minute/1.73 m^2.

- ● MEDICINAL FORMS
  There can be variation in the licensing of different medicines containing the same drug.

  Tablet
  CAUTIONARY AND ADVISORY LABELS 9
  - ▸ Cefixime (Non-proprietary)
    Cefixime 400 mg Cefixime 400mg tablets | 7 tablet [PoM] £16.87
  - ▸ Suprax (Sanofi)
    Cefixime 200 mg Suprax 200mg tablets | 7 tablet [PoM] £13.23 DT = £13.23

▸ 515

Cefotaxime

- ● INDICATIONS AND DOSE

Uncomplicated gonorrhoea
- ▸ BY INTRAMUSCULAR INJECTION
- ▸ Adult: 500 mg for 1 dose

Infections due to sensitive Gram-positive and Gram-negative bacteria | Surgical prophylaxis | Haemophilus epiglottitis
- ▸ BY INTRAMUSCULAR INJECTION, OR BY INTRAVENOUS INJECTION, OR BY INTRAVENOUS INFUSION
- ▸ Adult: 1 g every 12 hours

Severe susceptible infections due to sensitive Gram-positive and Gram-negative bacteria | Meningitis
- ▸ BY INTRAMUSCULAR INJECTION, OR BY INTRAVENOUS INJECTION, OR BY INTRAVENOUS INFUSION
- ▸ Adult: 8 g daily in 4 divided doses, increased if necessary to 12 g daily in 3–4 divided doses, intramuscular doses over 1 g should be divided between more than one site

Emergency treatment of suspected bacterial meningitis or meningococcal disease, before urgent transfer to hospital, in patients who cannot be given benzylpenicillin (e.g. because of an allergy)
- ▸ BY INTRAVENOUS INJECTION, OR BY INTRAMUSCULAR INJECTION
- ▸ Child 1 month–11 years: 50 mg/kg for 1 dose
- ▸ Child 12–17 years: 1 g for 1 dose
- ▸ Adult: 1 g for 1 dose

- ● INTERACTIONS → Appendix 1: cephalosporins
- ● SIDE-EFFECTS
- ▸ **Uncommon** Drug fever · Jarisch-Herxheimer reaction · renal impairment · seizure

- ▸ **Frequency not known** Arrhythmia (following rapid injection) · bronchospasm · encephalopathy · granulocytopenia · hepatic disorders
- ● PREGNANCY Not known to be harmful.
- ● BREAST FEEDING Present in milk in low concentration, but appropriate to use.
- ● RENAL IMPAIRMENT

  Dose adjustments ▸ In adults If eGFR less than 5 mL/minute/1.73 m^2, initial dose of 1 g then use half normal dose.

  ▸ In children Usual initial dose, then use half normal dose if estimated glomerular filtration rate less than 5 mL/minute/1.73 m^2.

- ● DIRECTIONS FOR ADMINISTRATION
- ▸ With intravenous use in children Displacement value may be significant, consult local guidelines. For intermittent *intravenous infusion* dilute in glucose 5% *or* sodium chloride 0.9%; administer over 20–60 minutes; incompatible with alkaline solutions.
- ▸ With intravenous use in adults For *intravenous infusion*, give intermittently *in* Glucose 5% *or* Sodium chloride 0.9%. Suggested volume 40–100 mL given over 20–60 minutes; incompatible with alkaline solutions.

- ● MEDICINAL FORMS
  There can be variation in the licensing of different medicines containing the same drug.

  Powder for solution for injection
  - ▸ Cefotaxime (Non-proprietary)
    Cefotaxime (as Cefotaxime sodium) 500 mg Cefotaxime 500mg powder for solution for injection vials | 10 vial [PoM] £21.00–£30.00
    Cefotaxime (as Cefotaxime sodium) 1 gram Cefotaxime 1g powder for solution for injection vials | 10 vial [PoM] £35.00–£42.00
    Cefotaxime (as Cefotaxime sodium) 2 gram Cefotaxime 2g powder for solution for injection vials | 10 vial [PoM] £37.50

▸ 515

Ceftazidime
02-Aug-2017

- ● INDICATIONS AND DOSE

Prophylaxis for transurethral resection of prostate
- ▸ BY INTRAVENOUS INJECTION, OR BY INTRAVENOUS INFUSION, OR BY DEEP INTRAMUSCULAR INJECTION
- ▸ Adult: 1 g, single dose to be administered up to 30 minutes before procedure and may be repeated if necessary when catheter removed

Pseudomonal lung infection in cystic fibrosis
- ▸ BY INTRAVENOUS INFUSION, OR BY INTRAVENOUS INJECTION, OR BY DEEP INTRAMUSCULAR INJECTION
- ▸ Adult: 100–150 mg/kg daily in 3 divided doses; maximum 9 g per day

Complicated urinary-tract infection
- ▸ BY INTRAVENOUS INJECTION, OR BY INTRAVENOUS INFUSION, OR BY DEEP INTRAMUSCULAR INJECTION
- ▸ Adult: 1–2 g every 8–12 hours

Septicaemia | Hospital-acquired pneumonia
- ▸ BY INTRAVENOUS INFUSION, OR BY INTRAVENOUS INJECTION
- ▸ Adult: 2 g every 8 hours

Febrile neutropenia
- ▸ BY INTRAVENOUS INFUSION, OR BY INTRAVENOUS INJECTION
- ▸ Adult: 2 g every 8 hours

Meningitis
- ▸ BY INTRAVENOUS INFUSION, OR BY INTRAVENOUS INJECTION
- ▸ Adult: 2 g every 8 hours

Susceptible infections due to sensitive Gram-positive and Gram-negative bacteria
- ▸ BY INTRAVENOUS INFUSION, OR BY INTRAVENOUS INJECTION, OR BY DEEP INTRAMUSCULAR INJECTION
- ▸ Adult: 1–2 g every 8 hours

- ● INTERACTIONS → Appendix 1: cephalosporins

5

Infection

- SIDE-EFFECTS
- ▶ Common or very common Thrombocytosis
- ▶ Rare or very rare Acute kidney injury
- ▶ Frequency not known Coma · drug reaction with eosinophilia and systemic symptoms (DRESS) · encephalopathy · jaundice · lymphocytosis · myoclonus · neurological effects · paraesthesia · seizure · taste altered · tremor
- PREGNANCY Not known to be harmful.
- BREAST FEEDING Present in milk in low concentration, but appropriate to use.
- HEPATIC IMPAIRMENT Manufacturer advises caution in severe impairment.
- RENAL IMPAIRMENT
  Dose adjustments Manufacturer advises reduce dose if creatinine clearance 50 mL/minute or less—consult product literature.
- DIRECTIONS FOR ADMINISTRATION Intramuscular administration used when intravenous administration not possible; single doses over 1 g by intravenous route only.
- ▶ With intravenous use For *intravenous infusion* give intermittently *or via* drip tubing *in* Glucose 5% or 10% *or* Sodium chloride 0.9%. Dissolve 2 g initially in 10 mL (3 g in 15 mL) infusion fluid. For *Fortum*® dilute further to a concentration of 40 mg/mL. For *Kefadim*® dilute further to a concentration of 20 mg/mL. Give over up to 30 minutes.

- MEDICINAL FORMS
  There can be variation in the licensing of different medicines containing the same drug. Forms available from special-order manufacturers include: infusion, solution for infusion
  Powder for solution for injection
  ELECTROLYTES: May contain Sodium
  - ▶ Ceftazidime (Non-proprietary)
    Ceftazidime (as Ceftazidime pentahydrate) 500 mg Ceftazidime 500mg powder for solution for injection vials | 1 vial PoM £4.25
    Ceftazidime (as Ceftazidime pentahydrate) 1 gram Ceftazidime 1g powder for solution for injection vials | 10 vial PoM £13.90–£79.10
    Ceftazidime (as Ceftazidime pentahydrate) 2 gram Ceftazidime 2g powder for solution for injection vials | 5 vial PoM £79.15 | 10 vial PoM £27.70
  - ▶ Fortum (GlaxoSmithKline UK Ltd)
    Ceftazidime (as Ceftazidime pentahydrate) 500 mg Fortum 500mg powder for solution for injection vials | 1 vial PoM £4.40 (Hospital only)
    Ceftazidime (as Ceftazidime pentahydrate) 1 gram Fortum 1g powder for solution for injection vials | 1 vial PoM £8.79 (Hospital only)
    Ceftazidime (as Ceftazidime pentahydrate) 2 gram Fortum 2g powder for solution for injection vials | 1 vial PoM £17.59 (Hospital only)
    Ceftazidime (as Ceftazidime pentahydrate) 3 gram Fortum 3g powder for solution for injection vials | 1 vial PoM £25.76 (Hospital only)

  Combinations available: *Ceftazidime with avibactam*, p. 521

Ceftriaxone

▶ 515

15-Jun-2016

- INDICATIONS AND DOSE
Community-acquired pneumonia | Hospital-acquired pneumonia | Intra-abdominal infections | Complicated urinary-tract infections | Acute exacerbations of chronic obstructive pulmonary disease
  - ▶ BY INTRAVENOUS INFUSION, OR BY INTRAVENOUS INJECTION, OR BY DEEP INTRAMUSCULAR INJECTION
  - ▶ Adult: 1–2 g once daily, 2 g dose to be used for hospital-acquired pneumonia and severe cases

Complicated skin and soft tissue infections | Infections of bones and joints
  - ▶ BY INTRAVENOUS INFUSION, OR BY INTRAVENOUS INJECTION, OR BY DEEP INTRAMUSCULAR INJECTION
  - ▶ Adult: 2 g once daily

Suspected bacterial infection in neutropenic patients
  - ▶ BY INTRAVENOUS INFUSION, OR BY INTRAVENOUS INJECTION, OR BY DEEP INTRAMUSCULAR INJECTION
  - ▶ Adult: 2–4 g daily, doses at the higher end of the recommended range used in severe cases

Bacterial meningitis | Bacterial endocarditis
  - ▶ BY INTRAVENOUS INFUSION, OR BY INTRAVENOUS INJECTION, OR BY DEEP INTRAMUSCULAR INJECTION
  - ▶ Adult: 2–4 g daily, doses at the higher end of the recommended range used in severe cases
  - ▶ BY INTRAVENOUS INFUSION
  - ▶ Child 1 month–11 years (body-weight up to 50 kg): 80–100 mg/kg once daily, 100 mg/kg once daily dose should be used for bacterial endocarditis; maximum 4 g per day
  - ▶ Child 9–11 years (body-weight 50 kg and above): 2–4 g once daily, doses at the higher end of the recommended range used in severe cases
  - ▶ Child 12–17 years: 2–4 g once daily, doses at the higher end of the recommended range used in severe cases
  - ▶ BY INTRAVENOUS INJECTION
  - ▶ Child 9–11 years (body-weight 50 kg and above): 2–4 g once daily, doses at the higher end of the recommended range used in severe cases; doses of 50 mg/kg or more should be given by infusion
  - ▶ Child 12–17 years: 2–4 g once daily, doses at the higher end of the recommended range used in severe cases
  - ▶ BY DEEP INTRAMUSCULAR INJECTION
  - ▶ Child 1 month–11 years (body-weight up to 50 kg): 80–100 mg/kg daily, 100 mg/kg daily dose should be used for bacterial endocarditis; maximum 4 g per day
  - ▶ Child 9–11 years (body-weight 50 kg and above): 2–4 g daily, doses at the higher end of the recommended range used in severe cases
  - ▶ Child 12–17 years: 2–4 g daily, doses at the higher end of the recommended range used in severe cases

Surgical prophylaxis
  - ▶ BY INTRAVENOUS INFUSION, OR BY INTRAVENOUS INJECTION, OR BY DEEP INTRAMUSCULAR INJECTION
  - ▶ Adult: 2 g for 1 dose, dose to be administered 30–90 minutes before procedure

Uncomplicated gonorrhoea | Pelvic inflammatory disease
  - ▶ BY DEEP INTRAMUSCULAR INJECTION
  - ▶ Adult: 500 mg for 1 dose

Syphilis
  - ▶ BY INTRAVENOUS INFUSION, OR BY INTRAVENOUS INJECTION, OR BY DEEP INTRAMUSCULAR INJECTION
  - ▶ Adult: 0.5–1 g once daily for 10–14 days, dose increased to 2 g once daily for neurosyphilis

Disseminated Lyme borreliosis (early [Stage II] and late [Stage III])
  - ▶ BY INTRAVENOUS INFUSION, OR BY INTRAVENOUS INJECTION, OR BY DEEP INTRAMUSCULAR INJECTION
  - ▶ Adult: 2 g once daily for 14–21 days, the recommended treatment durations vary and national or local guidelines should be taken into consideration

Prevention of secondary case of meningococcal meningitis
  - ▶ BY INTRAMUSCULAR INJECTION
  - ▶ Adult: 250 mg for 1 dose

Prevention of secondary case of *Haemophilus influenzae* type b disease
  - ▶ BY INTRAMUSCULAR INJECTION, OR BY INTRAVENOUS INJECTION, OR BY INTRAVENOUS INFUSION
  - ▶ Adult: 1 g daily for 2 days

Acute otitis media
  - ▶ BY DEEP INTRAMUSCULAR INJECTION
  - ▶ Adult: 1–2 g for 1 dose, dose can be given for 3 days if severely ill or previous therapy failed

- UNLICENSED USE [EvGr] Not licensed for prophylaxis of *Haemophilus influenzae* type b disease. [E] Not licensed for prophylaxis of meningococcal meningitis. [EvGr] Dose not licensed for treatment of pelvic inflammatory disease in adults over 18 years. [A]
- CAUTIONS
  GENERAL CAUTIONS History of hypercalciuria · history of kidney stones
  SPECIFIC CAUTIONS
- With intravenous use Concomitant treatment with intravenous calcium (including total parenteral nutrition containing calcium) (in adults)
- INTERACTIONS → Appendix 1: cephalosporins
- SIDE-EFFECTS
- **Uncommon** Anaemia · coagulation disorder · granulocytopenia
- **Rare or very rare** Bronchospasm · glycosuria · haematuria · oedema
- **Frequency not known** Acute generalised exanthematous pustulosis (AGEP) · cholelithiasis · hypersensitivity · nephrolithiasis · oliguria · oral disorders · pancreatitis · seizure · vertigo
  SIDE-EFFECTS, FURTHER INFORMATION Precipitates of calcium ceftriaxone can occur in the gall bladder and urine (particularly in very young, dehydrated or those who are immobilised)—consider discontinuation if symptomatic.
- PREGNANCY Manufacturer advises use only if benefit outweighs risk—limited data available but not known to be harmful in *animal* studies. [EvGr] Specialist sources indicate suitable for use in pregnancy. [D]
- BREAST FEEDING [EvGr] Specialist sources advise ceftriaxone is compatible with breastfeeding—present in milk in low concentration but limited effects to breast-fed infant. [D]
- RENAL IMPAIRMENT
  Dose adjustments Manufacturer advises reduce dose and monitor efficacy in patients with severe renal impairment in combination with hepatic impairment—no information available.
  - In adults Manufacturer advises reduce dose if eGFR less than 10 mL/minute/1.73 m^2 (max. 2 g daily).
  - In children Manufacturer advises reduce dose if estimated glomerular filtration rate less than 10 mL/minute/1.73 m^2 max. 50 mg/kg daily or max. 2 g daily).
- MONITORING REQUIREMENTS Manufacturer advises to monitor full blood count regularly during prolonged treatment.
- DIRECTIONS FOR ADMINISTRATION
- With intramuscular use or intravenous use Twice daily dosing may be considered for doses greater than 2 g daily.
- With intravenous use in children For *intravenous infusion* (preferred route), dilute reconstituted solution with Glucose 5% (or 10% in neonates) *or* Sodium Chloride 0.9%; give over at least 30 minutes (60 minutes in neonates—may displace bilirubin from serum albumin). Not to be given simultaneously with parenteral nutrition or infusion fluids containing calcium, even by different infusion lines; in children, may be infused sequentially with infusion fluids containing calcium if infusion lines at different sites are used, or if the infusion lines are replaced or thoroughly flushed between infusions with Sodium Chloride 0.9% to avoid precipitation—consult product literature. Displacement value may be significant, consult local guidelines. For *intravenous injection*, give over 5 minutes.
- With intramuscular use in children For *intramuscular injection*, may be mixed with 1% Lidocaine Hydrochloride Injection to reduce pain at intramuscular injection site. Intramuscular injection should only be considered when the intravenous route is not possible or less appropriate. If administered by intramuscular injection, the lower end of

the dose range should be used for the shortest time possible; volume depends on the age and size of the child, but doses over 1 g must be divided between more than one site. Displacement value may be significant, consult local guidelines. The maximum single intramuscular dose is 2 g, doses greater than 2 g must be given in divided doses or by intravenous administration (see above).
- With intravenous use in adults For *intravenous infusion* (preferred route) (*Rocephin*®; *Ceftriaxone Injection*, Genus), give intermittently *or via* drip tubing *in* Glucose 5% or 10% or Sodium Chloride 0.9%. Reconstitute 2-g vial with 40 mL infusion fluid. Give by intermittent infusion over at least 30 minutes. Not to be given simultaneously with total parenteral nutrition or infusion fluids containing calcium, even by different infusion lines. May be infused sequentially with infusion fluids containing calcium if infusion lines at different sites are used, or if the infusion lines are replaced or thoroughly flushed between infusions with Sodium Chloride 0.9% to avoid precipitation—consult product literature. For *intravenous injection*, give over 5 minutes.
- With intramuscular use in adults For *intramuscular injection*, doses over 1 g must be divided between more than one site. Displacement value may be significant, consult local guidelines. The maximum single intramuscular dose is 2 g, doses greater than 2 g must be given in divided doses or by intravenous administration.

- MEDICINAL FORMS
  There can be variation in the licensing of different medicines containing the same drug. Forms available from special-order manufacturers include: infusion
  Powder for solution for injection
  ELECTROLYTES: May contain Sodium
  - Ceftriaxone (Non-proprietary)
    Ceftriaxone (as Ceftriaxone sodium) 250 mg Ceftriaxone 250mg powder for solution for injection vials | 1 vial [PoM] £2.30 DT = £2.40
    Ceftriaxone (as Ceftriaxone sodium) 1 gram Ceftriaxone 1g powder for solution for injection vials | 1 vial [PoM] [⊠] DT = £9.58 | 10 vial [PoM] £91.50-£95.80
    Ceftriaxone (as Ceftriaxone sodium) 2 gram Ceftriaxone 2g powder for solution for injection vials | 1 vial [PoM] £18.30 DT = £19.18 | 10 vial [PoM] £191.80
    Ceftriaxone 2g powder for solution for infusion vials | 1 vial [PoM] £19.18 DT = £19.18
  - Rocephin (Roche Products Ltd)
    Ceftriaxone (as Ceftriaxone sodium) 250 mg Rocephin 250mg powder for solution for injection vials | 1 vial [PoM] £2.40 DT = £2.40
    Ceftriaxone (as Ceftriaxone sodium) 1 gram Rocephin 1g powder for solution for injection vials | 1 vial [PoM] £9.58 DT = £9.58
    Ceftriaxone (as Ceftriaxone sodium) 2 gram Rocephin 2g powder for solution for injection vials | 1 vial [PoM] £19.18 DT = £19.18

ANTIBACTERIALS > CEPHALOSPORINS, THIRD-GENERATION WITH BETA-LACTAMASE INHIBITOR

☞ 515

Ceftazidime with avibactam   27-Jul-2017

The properties listed below are those particular to the combination only. For the properties of the components please consider, ceftazidime p. 519.

- INDICATIONS AND DOSE
  Complicated intra-abdominal infection
  ▶ BY INTRAVENOUS INFUSION
  ▶ Adult: 2/0.5 g every 8 hours for 5–14 days
  Complicated urinary tract infection, including pyelonephritis
  ▶ BY INTRAVENOUS INFUSION
  ▶ Adult: 2/0.5 g every 8 hours for 5–10 days   continued →

5

Infection

Hospital-acquired pneumonia, including ventilator-associated pneumonia
▶ BY INTRAVENOUS INFUSION
▶ Adult: 2/0.5 g every 8 hours for 7–14 days

Infections due to Gram-negative bacteria with limited treatment options
▶ BY INTRAVENOUS INFUSION
▶ Adult: 2/0.5 g every 8 hours, duration of treatment guided by infection severity, pathogen, and response

DOSE EQUIVALENCE AND CONVERSION
▶ Dose expressed as *x/y* g ceftazidime/avibactam

● INTERACTIONS → Appendix 1: cephalosporins
● SIDE-EFFECTS
▶ **Common or very common** Thrombocytosis
▶ **Uncommon** Acute kidney injury · lymphocytosis · paraesthesia · taste altered
▶ **Frequency not known** Coma · drug reaction with eosinophilia and systemic symptoms (DRESS) · encephalopathy · jaundice · myoclonus · neurological effects · seizures · tremor
● PREGNANCY Manufacturer advises avoid unless potential benefit outweighs risk—toxicity in *animal* studies.
● BREAST FEEDING Manufacturer advises avoid—presence of avibactam in milk unknown.
● DIRECTIONS FOR ADMINISTRATION Manufacturer advises for *intravenous infusion* (Zavicefta ®) give in Glucose 5%, *or* Sodium Chloride 0.9%, *or* Sodium Chloride 0.45% with Glucose 2.5% combination *or* Lactated Ringer's solution. Reconstitute each 2 g/0.5 g vial with 10 mL water for injections; dilute requisite dose in an appropriate infusion bag and give over 120 minutes.
● PATIENT AND CARER ADVICE
Driving and skilled tasks Manufacturer advises patients and carers should be counselled on the effects on driving and performance of skilled tasks—risk of dizziness.

● MEDICINAL FORMS
There can be variation in the licensing of different medicines containing the same drug.
Powder for solution for infusion
ELECTROLYTES: May contain Sodium
▶ Zavicefta (Pfizer Ltd) ▼
Avibactam (as Avibactam sodium) 500 mg, Ceftazidime (as Ceftazidime pentahydrate) 2 gram Zavicefta 2g/0.5g powder for concentrate for solution for infusion vials | 10 vial [PoM] £857.00 (Hospital only)

Ceftolozane with tazobactam
09-Mar-2017

● INDICATIONS AND DOSE

Complicated intra-abdominal infection (in combination with metronidazole when anaerobic pathogens suspected)
▶ BY INTRAVENOUS INFUSION
▶ Adult: 1/0.5 g every 8 hours for 4–14 days

Complicated urinary tract infection | Acute pyelonephritis
▶ BY INTRAVENOUS INFUSION
▶ Adult: 1/0.5 g every 8 hours for 7 days

DOSE EQUIVALENCE AND CONVERSION
▶ Dose expressed as *x/y* g where x and y are ceftolozane and tazobactam respectively.

● INTERACTIONS → Appendix 1: cephalosporins
● SIDE-EFFECTS
▶ **Common or very common** Anxiety · constipation · electrolyte imbalance · hypotension · insomnia · thrombocytosis
▶ **Uncommon** Anaemia · angina pectoris · arrhythmias · dyspnoea · gastrointestinal discomfort · gastrointestinal

disorders · hyperglycaemia · ischaemic stroke · renal impairment · venous thrombosis
● PREGNANCY Manufacturer advises to use only if potential benefit outweighs risk—toxicity in *animal* studies with tazobactam.
● BREAST FEEDING Manufacturer advises avoid—no information available.
● RENAL IMPAIRMENT Manufacturer advises monitor for changes in renal function.
Dose adjustments Manufacturer advises reduce dose to 500/250 mg every 8 hours if eGFR 30–50 mL/minute/1.73 m^2 and 250/125 mg every 8 hours if eGFR 15–29 mL/minute/1.73 m^2.
● DIRECTIONS FOR ADMINISTRATION For *intravenous infusion* (Zerbaxa ®), give intermittently in Glucose 5% or Sodium chloride 0.9%; reconstitute initially each vial with 10 mL Water for Injections or Sodium chloride 0.9% to give a final volume of 11.4 mL; dilute requisite dose in 100 mL of Glucose 5% or Sodium chloride 0.9%; give over 1 hour.
● HANDLING AND STORAGE Manufacturer advises store in a refrigerator at 2°C–8°C.
● PATIENT AND CARER ADVICE
Driving and skilled tasks Manufacturer advises ceftolozane with tazobactam may influence driving and performance of skilled tasks—increased risk of dizziness.
● NATIONAL FUNDING/ACCESS DECISIONS
Scottish Medicines Consortium (SMC) Decisions
The *Scottish Medicines Consortium* has advised (May 2016) that ceftolozane with tazobactam (Zerbaxa ®) is not recommended for use within NHS Scotland for the treatment of complicated intra-abdominal infections, complicated urinary tract infections, and acute pyelonephritis.

● MEDICINAL FORMS
There can be variation in the licensing of different medicines containing the same drug.
Powder for solution for infusion
ELECTROLYTES: May contain Sodium
▶ Zerbaxa (Merck Sharp & Dohme Ltd) ▼
Tazobactam (as Tazobactam sodium) 500 mg, Ceftolozane (as Ceftolozane sulfate) 1 gram Zerbaxa 1g/0.5g powder for concentrate for solution for infusion vials | 10 vial [PoM] £670.30 (Hospital only)

ANTIBACTERIALS 〉 CEPHALOSPORINS, OTHER

▶ 515

Ceftaroline fosamil

● INDICATIONS AND DOSE

Community-acquired pneumonia
▶ BY INTRAVENOUS INFUSION
▶ Adult: 600 mg every 12 hours for 5–7 days

Complicated skin infections | Complicated soft-tissue infections
▶ BY INTRAVENOUS INFUSION
▶ Adult: 600 mg every 12 hours for 5–14 days

● CAUTIONS Seizure disorders
● INTERACTIONS → Appendix 1: cephalosporins
● SIDE-EFFECTS
▶ **Uncommon** Anaemia · hypersensitivity
● PREGNANCY Manufacturer advises avoid unless essential—no information available.
● BREAST FEEDING Manufacturer advises avoid—no information available.
● RENAL IMPAIRMENT Manufacturer advises avoid if eGFR less than 30 mL/minute/1.73 m^2.

Dose adjustments 400 mg every 12 hours if eGFR 30–50 mL/minute/1.73 m^2.

- DIRECTIONS FOR ADMINISTRATION For *intravenous infusion*, give intermittently in Glucose 5% or Sodium chloride 0.9%. Reconstitute 600 mg with 20 mL water for injections, then dilute with 250 mL infusion fluid (in fluid restriction, may be diluted with 50–100 mL infusion fluid); give over 60 minutes.
- NATIONAL FUNDING/ACCESS DECISIONS

Scottish Medicines Consortium (SMC) Decisions

The *Scottish Medicines Consortium*, has advised (Dec 2012) that ceftaroline fosamil (*Zinforo* ®) is accepted for restricted use within NHS Scotland when meticillin–resistant *S. aureus* is suspected in complicated skin and soft-tissue infection and vancomycin cannot be used.

- MEDICINAL FORMS

There can be variation in the licensing of different medicines containing the same drug.

Powder for solution for infusion

▶ Zinforo (Pfizer Ltd)

Ceftaroline fosamil (as Ceftaroline fosamil acetic acid solvate monohydrate) 600 mg Zinforo 600mg powder for concentrate for solution for infusion vials | 10 vial [PoM] £375.00 (Hospital only)

🏴 515

Ceftobiprole

12-Dec-2016

- INDICATIONS AND DOSE

Hospital-acquired pneumonia (excluding ventilator-associated pneumonia) | Community-acquired pneumonia

▶ BY INTRAVENOUS INFUSION

▶ Adult: 500 mg every 8 hours

- CAUTIONS Pre-existing seizure disorder—increased risk of seizures · supra-normal creatinine clearance

CAUTIONS, FURTHER INFORMATION

▶ Supra-normal creatinine clearance Manufacturer advises to measure baseline renal function and increase duration of infusion if creatinine clearance greater than 150 mL/minute.

- INTERACTIONS → Appendix 1: cephalosporins
- SIDE-EFFECTS

▶ Common or very common Drowsiness · dyspepsia · electrolyte imbalance · hypersensitivity · pruritic rash · taste altered

▶ Uncommon Anaemia · anxiety · asthma · dyspnoea · laryngeal pain · muscle spasms · peripheral oedema · renal failure · sleep disorders · thrombocytosis

▶ Frequency not known Seizure

- PREGNANCY Manufacturer advises avoid unless essential—no information available.
- BREAST FEEDING Manufacturer advises avoid—present in milk in *animal* studies.
- RENAL IMPAIRMENT Manufacturer advises use with caution in severe impairment—limited information available.

Dose adjustments Reduce dose to 500 mg every 12 hours in moderate impairment and 250 mg every 12 hours in severe impairment.

- DIRECTIONS FOR ADMINISTRATION Manufacturer advises for *intravenous infusion* (*Zevtera* ®), give intermittently in Glucose 5%, or Sodium Chloride 0.9%, or Lactated Ringer's solution; reconstitute each 500 mg with 10 mL Water for injections or Glucose 5%; dilute in 250 mL infusion fluid and give over 2 hours (increased to 4 hours if creatinine clearance greater than 150 mL/minute). Do not mix with calcium-containing solutions (except Lactated Ringer's solution) in the same intravenous line—precipitation may occur.

- HANDLING AND STORAGE Manufacturer advises store in a refrigerator (2–8°C)—consult product literature for storage after reconstitution and dilution.
- PATIENT AND CARER ADVICE

Driving and skilled tasks Manufacturer advises patients and carers should be counselled on the effects on driving and performance of skilled tasks—increased risk of dizziness.

- MEDICINAL FORMS

There can be variation in the licensing of different medicines containing the same drug.

Powder for solution for infusion

ELECTROLYTES: May contain Sodium

▶ Zevtera (Basilea Pharmaceutica International Ltd) ▼

Ceftobiprole (as Ceftobiprole medocaril sodium) 500 mg Zevtera 500mg powder for concentrate for solution for infusion vials | 10 vial [PoM] £396.30 (Hospital only)

ANTIBACTERIALS > GLYCOPEPTIDE ANTIBACTERIALS

Dalbavancin

18-Jul-2017

- DRUG ACTION Dalbavancin is a glycopeptide antibacterial; it has bactericidal activity against Gram-positive bacteria including various staphylococci. However, there are reports of *Staphylococcus aureus* with reduced susceptibility to glycopeptides and increasing reports of glycopeptide-resistant enterococci.

- INDICATIONS AND DOSE

Acute bacterial skin and skin structure infections

▶ BY INTRAVENOUS INFUSION

▶ Adult: 1500 mg for 1 dose, alternatively 1000 mg, then 500 mg after 1 week

- SIDE-EFFECTS

▶ Common or very common Diarrhoea · headache · nausea

▶ Uncommon Anaemia · antibiotic associated colitis · appetite decreased · constipation · cough · dizziness · eosinophilia · flushing · gastrointestinal discomfort · increased risk of infection · infusion related reaction · insomnia · leucopenia · neutropenia · skin reactions · taste altered · thrombocytosis · vomiting · vulvovaginal pruritus

▶ Rare or very rare Bronchospasm

▶ Frequency not known Ototoxicity

- ALLERGY AND CROSS-SENSITIVITY Manufacturer advises use with caution in patients with other glycopeptide sensitivity.
- PREGNANCY

Dose adjustments Manufacturer advises avoid unless essential—toxicity in *animal* studies.

- BREAST FEEDING

Dose adjustments Manufacturer advises avoid—present in milk in *animal* studies.

- HEPATIC IMPAIRMENT Manufacturer advises caution in moderate-to-severe impairment—no information available.
- RENAL IMPAIRMENT

Dose adjustments Manufacturer advises reduce dose to 1000 mg as a single infusion or reduce dose to 750 mg followed one week later by 375 mg if creatinine clearance <30 mL/minute.

- DIRECTIONS FOR ADMINISTRATION Manufacturer advises for *intravenous infusion* (*Xydalba* ®), reconstitute each 500 mg vial to produce a 20 mg/mL solution with 25 mL water for injections. Dilute reconstituted solution to a concentration of 1–5 mg/mL with Glucose 5%; give intermittently over 30 minutes (avoid rapid infusion—risk of 'red man' syndrome).

5

Infection

● NATIONAL FUNDING/ACCESS DECISIONS

Scottish Medicines Consortium (SMC) Decisions
The *Scottish Medicines Consortium* has advised (January 2017) that dalbavancin (*Xydalba*®) is accepted for restricted use within NHS Scotland for the treatment of acute bacterial skin and skin structure infections (ABSSSI), only if:
● used as second-line treatment, or
● meticillin-resistant *Staphylococcus aureus* infection is suspected, or
● under local microbiologist or infectious diseases specialist advice; **and**
● the patient is initially hospitalised due to ABSSSI requiring intravenous antibiotics but is eligible for early discharge as soon as their medical condition does not require further inpatient treatment.

● MEDICINAL FORMS
There can be variation in the licensing of different medicines containing the same drug.
Powder for solution for infusion
▸ Xydalba (Cardiome UK Ltd) ▼
Dalbavancin (as Dalbavancin hydrochloride) 500 mg Xydalba 500mg powder for concentrate for solution for infusion vials | 1 vial [PoM] £558.70 (Hospital only)

| Teicoplanin

27-Nov-2017

● DRUG ACTION The glycopeptide antibiotic teicoplanin has bactericidal activity against aerobic and anaerobic Gram-positive bacteria including multi-resistant staphylococci. However, there are reports of *Staphylococcus aureus* with reduced susceptibility to glycopeptides and increasing reports of glycopeptide-resistant enterococci. Teicoplanin is similar to vancomycin, but has a significantly longer duration of action, allowing once daily administration after the loading dose.

● INDICATIONS AND DOSE

***Clostridium difficile* infection**
▸ BY MOUTH
▸ Adult: 100–200 mg twice daily for 7–14 days

Serious infections caused by Gram-positive bacteria (e.g. complicated skin and soft-tissue infections, pneumonia, complicated urinary tract infections)
▸ BY INTRAVENOUS INJECTION, OR BY INTRAVENOUS INFUSION, OR BY INTRAMUSCULAR INJECTION
▸ Adult: Initially 6 mg/kg every 12 hours for 3 doses, then 6 mg/kg once daily

Streptococcal or enterococcal endocarditis (in combination with another antibacterial) | Bone and joint infections
▸ INITIALLY BY INTRAVENOUS INJECTION, OR BY INTRAVENOUS INFUSION
▸ Adult: 12 mg/kg every 12 hours for 3–5 doses, then (by intravenous injection or by intravenous infusion or by intramuscular injection) 12 mg/kg once daily

Surgical prophylaxis
▸ BY INTRAVENOUS INJECTION
▸ Adult: 400 mg, to be administered up to 30 minutes before the procedure

Surgical prophylaxis in open fractures
▸ BY INTRAVENOUS INFUSION
▸ Adult: 800 mg, to be administered up to 30 minutes before skeletal stabilisation and definitive soft-tissue closure

Peritonitis associated with peritoneal dialysis (added to dialysis fluid)
▸ BY INTRAPERITONEAL INFUSION
▸ Adult: (consult local protocol)

PHARMACOKINETICS
▸ Teicoplanin should **not** be given by mouth for systemic infections because it is not absorbed significantly.

● UNLICENSED USE Not licensed for surgical prophylaxis.
● INTERACTIONS → Appendix 1: teicoplanin
● SIDE-EFFECTS
▸ **Common or very common** Fever · pain · skin reactions
▸ **Uncommon** Bronchospasm · diarrhoea · dizziness · eosinophilia · headache · hearing impairment · hypersensitivity · leucopenia · nausea · thrombocytopenia · vomiting
▸ **Rare or very rare** Abscess · red man syndrome
▸ **Frequency not known** Agranulocytosis · angioedema · chills · neutropenia · overgrowth of nonsusceptible organisms · renal impairment · seizure · severe cutaneous adverse reactions (SCARs)
SIDE-EFFECTS, FURTHER INFORMATION Teicoplanin is associated with a lower incidence of nephrotoxicity than vancomycin.

● ALLERGY AND CROSS-SENSITIVITY Caution if history of vancomycin sensitivity.
● PREGNANCY Manufacturer advises use only if potential benefit outweighs risk.
● BREAST FEEDING No information available.
● RENAL IMPAIRMENT
Dose adjustments Use normal dose regimen on days 1–4, then use normal maintenance dose every 48 hours if eGFR 30–80 mL/minute/1.73 m^2 and use normal maintenance dose every 72 hours if eGFR less than 30 mL/minute/1.73 m^2.
Monitoring Monitor renal and auditory function during prolonged treatment in renal impairment.

● MONITORING REQUIREMENTS
▸ With intramuscular use or intravenous use Manufacturer advises monitor serum-teicoplanin trough concentration at steady state after completion of loading dose and during maintenance treatment—consult product literature.
▸ Blood counts and liver and kidney function tests required.
▸ Manufacturer advises monitoring for adverse reactions when doses of 12 mg/kg twice daily are administered.

● DIRECTIONS FOR ADMINISTRATION
▸ With intravenous use For intravenous infusion (*Targocid*®), give intermittently in Glucose 5% *or* Sodium chloride 0.9%; reconstitute initially with water for injections provided; infuse over 30 minutes. Continuous infusion not usually recommended.
▸ With oral use Injection can be used to prepare solution for oral administration.

● MEDICINAL FORMS
There can be variation in the licensing of different medicines containing the same drug. Forms available from special-order manufacturers include: solution for injection
Powder and solvent for solution for injection
ELECTROLYTES: May contain Sodium
▸ Targocid (Sanofi) ▼
Teicoplanin 200 mg Targocid 200mg powder and solvent for solution for injection vials | 1 vial [PoM] £3.93
Teicoplanin 400 mg Targocid 400mg powder and solvent for solution for injection vials | 1 vial [PoM] £7.32

Telavancin

- **DRUG ACTION** Telavancin is a glycopeptide antibacterial; it has bactericidal activity against aerobic and anaerobic Gram-positive bacteria including multi-resistant staphylococci. However, there are reports of *Staphylococcus aureus* with reduced susceptibility to glycopeptides. There are increasing reports of glycopeptide-resistant enterococci.

- **INDICATIONS AND DOSE**

Hospital-acquired pneumonia, known or suspected to be caused by meticillin-resistant *Staphylococcus aureus* when other antibacterials cannot be used
- ▸ BY INTRAVENOUS INFUSION
- ▸ Adult: 10 mg/kg once daily for 7–21 days

- **CAUTIONS** Conditions that predispose to renal impairment · predisposition to QT interval prolongation (including electrolyte disturbances, congenital long QT syndrome, uncompensated heart failure, severe left ventricular hypertrophy)

- **INTERACTIONS** → Appendix 1: telavancin

- **SIDE-EFFECTS**

- **Common or very common** Asthenia · constipation · diarrhoea · dizziness · headaches · increased risk of infection · insomnia · nausea · renal impairment · skin reactions · taste altered · urine abnormalities · vomiting

- **Uncommon** Altered smell sensation · anaemia · angina pectoris · anxiety · appetite decreased · arrhythmias · arthralgia · confusion · congestive heart failure · depression · drowsiness · dry mouth · dyspnoea · electrolyte imbalance · eye irritation · flatulence · flushing · gastrointestinal discomfort · haematuria · hearing impairment · hepatitis · hiccups · hyperglycaemia · hyperhidrosis · hypertension · hypoglycaemia · hypotension · laryngeal pain · leucopenia · muscle complaints · nasal congestion · oedema · oral hypoaesthesia · pain · palpitations · paraesthesia · QT interval prolongation · red man syndrome · thrombocytopenia · thrombocytosis · tremor · urinary disorders · vision blurred

- **ALLERGY AND CROSS-SENSITIVITY** Use with caution in patients with vancomycin or teicoplanin sensitivity.

- **CONCEPTION AND CONTRACEPTION** Effective contraception required during treatment.

- **PREGNANCY** Avoid (teratogenic in *animal* studies).

- **BREAST FEEDING** Manufacturer advises avoid unless potential benefit outweighs risk—no information available.

- **HEPATIC IMPAIRMENT** Manufacturer advises caution in severe impairment—no information available.

- **RENAL IMPAIRMENT** Avoid in acute renal failure—risk of mortality increased. In chronic renal failure, avoid if eGFR less than 30 mL/minute/1.73 m^2.
  Dose adjustments In chronic renal failure, use 7.5 mg/kg once daily if eGFR 30–50 mL/minute/1.73 m^2.

- **MONITORING REQUIREMENTS** Monitor renal function daily for at least the first 3–5 days, then every 2–3 days thereafter.

- **DIRECTIONS FOR ADMINISTRATION** For *intravenous infusion* (*Vibativ*®). Avoid rapid infusion (can cause 'red man' syndrome). Give intermittently *in* Glucose 5% *or* Sodium chloride 0.9%; reconstitute each 750 mg with 45 mL glucose 5%, sodium chloride 0.9%, or water for injections to produce a 15 mg/mL solution; for doses of 150–800 mg, dilute requisite dose in 100 to 250 mL infusion fluid; for doses outside this range, dilute to a final concentration of 0.6–8 mg/mL; give over at least 60 minutes.

- **MEDICINAL FORMS**
There can be variation in the licensing of different medicines containing the same drug.
Powder for solution for infusion
- ▸ Vibativ (Clinigen Healthcare Ltd) ▼
  Telavancin (as Telavancin hydrochloride) 750 mg Vibativ 750mg powder for solution for infusion vials | 1 vial [PoM] £645.00 (Hospital only)

Vancomycin

11-May-2018

- **DRUG ACTION** The glycopeptide antibiotic vancomycin has bactericidal activity against aerobic and anaerobic Gram-positive bacteria including multi-resistant staphylococci. However, there are reports of *Staphylococcus aureus* with reduced susceptibility to glycopeptides. There are increasing reports of glycopeptide-resistant enterococci. Penetration into cerebrospinal fluid is poor.

- **INDICATIONS AND DOSE**

***Clostridium difficile* infection [first episode]**
- ▸ BY MOUTH
- ▸ Adult: 125 mg every 6 hours for 10 days; increased if necessary to 500 mg every 6 hours for 10 days, increased dose if severe or complicated infection

***Clostridium difficile* infection [multiple recurrences]**
- ▸ BY MOUTH
- ▸ Adult: 125 mg every 6 hours for 10 days, followed by, either tapering the dose (gradually reducing until 125 mg daily) or a pulse regimen (125–500 mg every 2–3 days for at least 3 weeks)

Complicated skin and soft tissue infections | Bone infections | Joint infections | Community-acquired pneumonia | Hospital-acquired pneumonia [including ventilator-associated pneumonia] | Infective endocarditis | Acute bacterial meningitis | Bacteraemia [occurring in association with or suspected to be associated with the licensed indications]
- ▸ BY INTRAVENOUS INFUSION
- ▸ Adult: 15–20 mg/kg every 8–12 hours (max. per dose 2 g) adjusted according to plasma-concentration monitoring, duration should be tailored to type and severity of infection and the individual clinical response—consult product literature for further information, in seriously ill patients, a loading dose of 25–30 mg/kg (usual max. 2 g) can be used to facilitate rapid attainment of the target trough serum-vancomycin concentration

Perioperative prophylaxis of bacterial endocarditis [in patients at high risk of developing bacterial endocarditis when undergoing major surgical procedures]
- ▸ BY INTRAVENOUS INFUSION
- ▸ Adult: 15 mg/kg, to be given prior to induction of anaesthesia, a second dose may be required depending on duration of surgery

Surgical prophylaxis (when high risk of MRSA)
- ▸ BY INTRAVENOUS INFUSION
- ▸ Adult: 1 g for 1 dose

Peritonitis associated with peritoneal dialysis
- ▸ BY INTRAPERITONEAL ADMINISTRATION
- ▸ Adult: (consult local protocol)

PHARMACOKINETICS
- ▸ Vancomycin should **not** be given by mouth for systemic infections because it is not absorbed significantly.

- **UNLICENSED USE** Vancomycin doses in BNF publications may differ from those in product literature. Use of vancomycin (added to dialysis fluid) for the treatment of peritonitis associated with peritoneal dialysis is an unlicensed route.

5

Infection

5

Infection

● CONTRA-INDICATIONS
▸ With intravenous use Previous hearing loss
● CAUTIONS
▸ With oral use Systemic absorption may be enhanced in patients with inflammatory disorders of the intestinal mucosa or with *Clostridium difficile*-induced pseudomembranous colitis (increased risk of adverse reactions)
● INTERACTIONS → Appendix 1: vancomycin
● SIDE-EFFECTS

GENERAL SIDE-EFFECTS Agranulocytosis · dizziness · drug fever · eosinophilia · hypersensitivity · nausea · nephritis tubulointerstitial · neutropenia (more common after 1 week or cumulative dose of 25g) · renal failure · severe cutaneous adverse reactions (SCARs) · skin reactions · thrombocytopenia · tinnitus (discontinue) · vasculitis · vertigo

SPECIFIC SIDE-EFFECTS
▸ With intravenous use Back pain · bradycardia · cardiac arrest (on rapid intravenous injection) · cardiogenic shock (on rapid intravenous injection) · chest pain · dyspnoea · hearing loss · hypotension · muscle complaints · pseudomembranous enterocolitis · red man syndrome · wheezing

SIDE-EFFECTS, FURTHER INFORMATION Vancomycin is associated with a higher incidence of nephrotoxicity than teicoplanin.

● ALLERGY AND CROSS-SENSITIVITY Caution if teicoplanin sensitivity.
● PREGNANCY Manufacturer advises use only if potential benefit outweighs risk.
Monitoring Plasma-vancomycin concentration monitoring essential to reduce risk of fetal toxicity.
● BREAST FEEDING Present in milk—significant absorption following oral administration unlikely.
● RENAL IMPAIRMENT Manufacturer advises serial monitoring of renal function.
▸ With intravenous use Manufacturer advises use with caution—increased risk of toxic effects with prolonged high blood concentration.
Dose adjustments ▸ With oral use Manufacturer advises dose adjustment is unlikely to be required unless substantial oral absorption occurs in inflammatory disorders of the intestinal mucosa or with *Clostridium difficile*-induced pseudomembranous colitis, see *Monitoring*.
▸ With intravenous use Manufacturer advises initial dose must not be reduced—consult product literature.
● MONITORING REQUIREMENTS
▸ With intravenous use Manufacturer advises initial doses should be based on body-weight; subsequent dose adjustments should be based on serum-vancomycin concentrations to achieve targeted therapeutic concentrations. All patients require serum-vancomycin measurement (on the second day of treatment, immediately before the next dose if renal function normal, earlier if renal impairment—consult product literature). Frequency of monitoring depends on the clinical situation and response to treatment; regular monitoring indicated in high-dose therapy and longer-term use, particularly in patients with impaired renal function, impaired hearing, or concurrent use of nephrotoxic or ototoxic drugs. Manufacturer advises pre-dose ('trough') concentration should normally be 10–20 mg/litre depending on the site of infection and the susceptibility of the pathogen; trough concentration of 15–20 mg/litre is usually recommended to cover susceptible pathogens with MIC greater than or equal to 1 mg/litre—consult product literature.
▸ Manufacturer advises periodic testing of auditory function.

▸ Manufacturer advises monitor blood counts, urinalysis, hepatic and renal function periodically in all patients; monitor leucocyte count regularly in patients receiving long-term vancomycin or if given concurrently with other drugs that may cause neutropenia or agranulocytosis.
▸ Manufacturer advises monitor vestibular and auditory function during and after treatment in the elderly; avoid concurrent or sequential use of other ototoxic drugs.
▸ With oral use Manufacturer advises monitoring serum-vancomycin concentration in inflammatory intestinal disorders.
● DIRECTIONS FOR ADMINISTRATION
▸ With intravenous use Avoid rapid infusion (risk of anaphylactoid reactions) and rotate infusion sites.
  For *intravenous infusion*, give intermittently in Glucose 5% or Sodium chloride 0.9%; reconstitute each 500 mg with 10 mL water for injections and dilute with infusion fluid to a concentration of up to 5 mg/mL (10 mg/mL in fluid restriction but increased risk of infusion-related effects); give over at least 60 minutes (rate not to exceed 10 mg/minute for doses over 500 mg); use continuous infusion only if intermittent not feasible.
▸ With oral use Injection can be used to prepare solution for oral administration—consult product literature.

● MEDICINAL FORMS
There can be variation in the licensing of different medicines containing the same drug. Forms available from special-order manufacturers include: oral suspension, oral solution, solution for injection, infusion

Powder for solution for infusion
▸ Vancomycin (Non-proprietary)
  Vancomycin (as Vancomycin hydrochloride) 500 mg Vancomycin 500mg powder for solution for infusion vials | 1 vial [PoM] £7.25 | 10 vial [PoM] £62.50
  Vancomycin 500mg powder for concentrate for solution for infusion vials | 1 vial [PoM] £8.50 (Hospital only) | 1 vial [PoM] £5.49 | 10 vial [PoM] £62.50
  Vancomycin (as Vancomycin hydrochloride) 1 gram Vancomycin 1g powder for solution for infusion vials | 1 vial [PoM] £14.50 | 10 vial [PoM] £125.00
  Vancomycin 1g powder for concentrate for solution for infusion vials | 1 vial [PoM] £17.25 (Hospital only) | 1 vial [PoM] £11.25 | 10 vial [PoM] £125.00
▸ Vancocin (Flynn Pharma Ltd)
  Vancomycin (as Vancomycin hydrochloride) 500 mg Vancocin 500mg powder for solution for infusion vials | 1 vial [PoM] £6.25
  Vancomycin (as Vancomycin hydrochloride) 1 gram Vancocin 1g powder for solution for infusion vials | 1 vial [PoM] £12.50

Capsule
CAUTIONARY AND ADVISORY LABELS 9
▸ Vancomycin (Non-proprietary)
  Vancomycin (as Vancomycin hydrochloride) 125 mg Vancomycin 125mg capsules | 28 capsule [PoM] £132.47 DT = £132.47
  Vancomycin (as Vancomycin hydrochloride) 250 mg Vancomycin 250mg capsules | 28 capsule [PoM] £140.08 DT = £140.08
▸ Vancocin Matrigel (Flynn Pharma Ltd)
  Vancomycin (as Vancomycin hydrochloride) 125 mg Vancocin Matrigel 125mg capsules | 28 capsule [PoM] £88.31 DT = £132.47

ANTIBACTERIALS ⟩ LINCOSAMIDES

Clindamycin

● DRUG ACTION Clindamycin is active against Gram-positive cocci, including streptococci and penicillin-resistant staphylococci, and also against many anaerobes, especially *Bacteroides fragilis*. It is well concentrated in bone and excreted in bile and urine.

● **INDICATIONS AND DOSE**

Staphylococcal bone and joint infections such as osteomyelitis | Peritonitis | Intra-abdominal sepsis | Meticillin-resistant *Staphylococcus aureus* (MRSA) in bronchiectasis, bone and joint infections, and skin and soft-tissue infections | Erysipelas or cellulitis in penicillin-allergic patients (alternative to macrolides)
▸ BY MOUTH
  ▸ Child: 3–6 mg/kg 4 times a day (max. per dose 450 mg)
  ▸ Adult: 150–300 mg every 6 hours; increased if necessary up to 450 mg every 6 hours if required, increased dose used in severe infection
▸ BY DEEP INTRAMUSCULAR INJECTION, OR BY INTRAVENOUS INFUSION
  ▸ Adult: 0.6–2.7 g daily in 2–4 divided doses; increased if necessary up to 4.8 g daily, increased dose used in life-threatening infection, single doses above 600 mg to be administered by intravenous infusion only, single doses by intravenous infusion not to exceed 1.2 g

Treatment of mild to moderate pneumocystis pneumonia (in combination with primaquine)
▸ BY MOUTH
  ▸ Adult: 600 mg every 8 hours

Treatment of falciparum malaria (to be given with or following quinine)
▸ BY MOUTH
  ▸ Child: 7–13 mg/kg every 8 hours (max. per dose 450 mg) for 7 days
  ▸ Adult: 450 mg every 8 hours for 7 days

● UNLICENSED USE Not licensed for treatment of mild to moderate pneumocystis infection. Not licensed for treatment of falciparum malaria.
● CONTRA-INDICATIONS Diarrhoeal states
● CAUTIONS Avoid in Acute porphyrias p. 1025 · middle-aged and elderly women, especially after an operation (antibiotic-associated colitis more common)
● INTERACTIONS → Appendix 1: clindamycin
● SIDE-EFFECTS
  GENERAL SIDE-EFFECTS
▸ **Common or very common** Abdominal pain · antibiotic associated colitis · diarrhoea (discontinue) · skin reactions
▸ **Uncommon** Nausea · vomiting
▸ **Frequency not known** Agranulocytosis · angioedema · eosinophilia · jaundice · leucopenia · neutropenia · severe cutaneous adverse reactions (SCARs) · taste altered · thrombocytopenia · vulvovaginal infection
  SPECIFIC SIDE-EFFECTS
▸ **Frequency not known**
  ▸ With oral use Gastrointestinal disorders
  ▸ With parenteral use Cardiac arrest · hypotension
  SIDE-EFFECTS, FURTHER INFORMATION Clindamycin has been associated with antibiotic-associated colitis, which may be fatal. Although antibiotic-associated colitis can occur with most antibacterials, it occurs more frequently with clindamycin. If *C. difficile* infection is suspected or confirmed, discontinue the antibiotic if appropriate. Seek specialist advice if the antibiotic cannot be stopped and the diarrhoea is severe.
● PREGNANCY Not known to be harmful.
● BREAST FEEDING Amount probably too small to be harmful but bloody diarrhoea reported in 1 infant.
● MONITORING REQUIREMENTS Monitor liver and renal function if treatment exceeds 10 days.
  ▸ In children Monitor liver and renal function in neonates and infants.
● DIRECTIONS FOR ADMINISTRATION Avoid rapid intravenous administration.
  For *intravenous infusion* (*Dalacin® C Phosphate*), give continuously *or* intermittently *in* Glucose 5% *or* Sodium

Chloride 0.9%; dilute to not more than 18 mg/mL and give over 10–60 minutes at a rate not exceeding 30 mg/minute (1.2 g over at least 60 minutes; higher doses by continuous infusion).
● PATIENT AND CARER ADVICE Capsules should be swallowed with a glass of water. Patients and their carers should be advised to discontinue immediately and contact doctor if diarrhoea develops.
● PROFESSION SPECIFIC INFORMATION
  Dental practitioners' formulary
  Clindamycin capsules may be prescribed.

● MEDICINAL FORMS
  There can be variation in the licensing of different medicines containing the same drug. Forms available from special-order manufacturers include: oral suspension, oral solution

Solution for injection
EXCIPIENTS: May contain Benzyl alcohol
  ▸ Clindamycin (Non-proprietary)
    Clindamycin (as Clindamycin phosphate) 150 mg per 1 ml Clindamycin 600mg/4ml solution for injection ampoules | 5 ampoule [PoM] £59.00–£61.75
    Clindamycin 300mg/2ml solution for injection ampoules | 5 ampoule [PoM] £29.50–£31.01
  ▸ Dalacin C (Pfizer Ltd)
    Clindamycin (as Clindamycin phosphate) 150 mg per 1 ml Dalacin C Phosphate 300mg/2ml solution for injection ampoules | 5 ampoule [PoM] £31.01 (Hospital only)
    Dalacin C Phosphate 600mg/4ml solution for injection ampoules | 5 ampoule [PoM] £61.75 (Hospital only)

Capsule
CAUTIONARY AND ADVISORY LABELS 9, 27
  ▸ Clindamycin (Non-proprietary)
    Clindamycin (as Clindamycin hydrochloride) 150 mg Clindamycin 150mg capsules | 24 capsule [PoM] £18.29 DT = £3.79 | 100 capsule [PoM] £15.16–£76.20
    Clindamycin (as Clindamycin hydrochloride) 300 mg Clindamycin 300mg capsules | 30 capsule [PoM] £46.00 DT = £38.45
  ▸ Dalacin C (Pfizer Ltd)
    Clindamycin (as Clindamycin hydrochloride) 75 mg Dalacin C 75mg capsules | 24 capsule [PoM] £7.45 DT = £7.45
    Clindamycin (as Clindamycin hydrochloride) 150 mg Dalacin C 150mg capsules | 24 capsule [PoM] £13.72 DT = £3.79 | 100 capsule [PoM] £55.08

ANTIBACTERIALS > MACROLIDES

Macrolides

Overview

The macrolides have an antibacterial spectrum that is similar but not identical to that of penicillin; they are thus an alternative in penicillin-allergic patients. They are active against many-penicillin-resistant staphylococci, but some are now also resistant to the macrolides.

Indications for the macrolides include campylobacter enteritis, respiratory infections (including pneumonia, whooping cough, Legionella, chlamydia, and mycoplasma infection), and skin infections.

Erythromycin p. 530 is also used in the treatment of early syphilis, uncomplicated genital chlamydial infection, and non-gonococcal urethritis. Erythromycin has poor activity against *Haemophilus influenzae*. Erythromycin causes nausea, vomiting, and diarrhoea in some patients; in mild to moderate infections this can be avoided by giving a lower dose, but if a more serious infection, such as Legionella pneumonia, is suspected higher doses are needed.

Azithromycin p. 528 is a macrolide with slightly less activity than erythromycin against Gram-positive bacteria, but enhanced activity against some Gram-negative organisms including *H. influenzae*. Plasma concentrations are very low, but tissue concentrations are much higher. It has a long tissue half-life and once daily dosage is recommended. Azithromycin is also used in the treatment of uncomplicated genital chlamydial infection, non-gonococcal urethritis, uncomplicated gonorrhoea, typhoid [unlicensed indication], and trachoma [unlicensed indication].

Clarithromycin p. 529 is an erythromycin derivative with slightly greater activity than the parent compound. Tissue concentrations are higher than with erythromycin. It is given twice daily. Clarithromycin is also used in regimens for *Helicobacter pylori* eradication.

Erythromycin, azithromycin, and clarithromycin have a role in the treatment of Lyme disease p. 567.

Spiramycin is also a macrolide which is used for the treatment of toxoplasmosis.

Macrolides

- CAUTIONS Electrolyte disturbances (predisposition to QT interval prolongation) · may aggravate myasthenia gravis · predisposition to QT interval prolongation
- SIDE-EFFECTS
- **Common or very common** Appetite decreased · arthralgia · diarrhoea · dizziness · eye discomfort · gastrointestinal discomfort · gastrointestinal disorders · headache · hearing impairment · nausea · pancreatitis · sensation abnormal · skin reactions · sleep disorders · taste altered · vasodilation · vision disorders · vomiting
- **Uncommon** Angioedema · anxiety · arrhythmias · burping · candida infection · cardiac arrest · chest pain · constipation · drowsiness · dry mouth · eosinophilia · eye allergy · haemorrhage · hepatic disorders · leucopenia · loss of consciousness · movement disorders · muscle complaints · neutropenia · oedema · oral disorders · palpitations · photosensitivity reaction · pulmonary embolism · QT interval prolongation · severe cutaneous adverse reactions (SCARs) · thrombocytosis · tremor · vertigo
- **Rare or very rare** Antibiotic associated colitis · hearing loss (can occur after large doses) · myasthenia gravis · nephritis tubulointerstitial
- **Frequency not known** Aggression · agranulocytosis · atrioventricular block · cerebral impairment · depersonalisation · depression · haemolytic anaemia · hallucination · hypotension · mania · myopathy · psychotic disorder · renal impairment · seizure · smell altered · syncope · thrombocytopenia · urine discolouration

Azithromycin

- INDICATIONS AND DOSE

Prevention of secondary case of invasive group A streptococcal infection in patients who are allergic to penicillin
- BY MOUTH
- Child 6 months–11 years: 12 mg/kg once daily (max. per dose 500 mg) for 5 days
- Child 12–17 years: 500 mg once daily for 5 days
- Adult: 500 mg once daily for 5 days

Respiratory-tract infections, otitis media, skin and soft-tissue infections
- BY MOUTH
- Child 6 months–17 years: 10 mg/kg once daily (max. per dose 500 mg) for 3 days
- Child 6 months–17 years (body-weight 15-25 kg): 200 mg once daily for 3 days
- Child 6 months–17 years (body-weight 26-35 kg): 300 mg once daily for 3 days
- Child 6 months–17 years (body-weight 36-45 kg): 400 mg once daily for 3 days
- Child 6 months–17 years (body-weight 46 kg and above): 500 mg once daily for 3 days

- Adult: 500 mg once daily for 3 days, alternatively initially 500 mg once daily for 1 day, then 250 mg once daily for 4 days

Uncomplicated genital chlamydial infections | Non-gonococcal urethritis
- BY MOUTH
- Child 12–17 years: 1 g for 1 dose
- Adult: 1 g for 1 dose

Uncomplicated gonorrhoea
- BY MOUTH
- Adult: 1 g for 1 dose

Lyme disease (under expert supervision)
- BY MOUTH
- Adult: 500 mg once daily for 7–10 days

Mild to moderate typhoid due to multiple-antibacterial resistant organisms
- BY MOUTH
- Adult: 500 mg once daily for 7 days

Community-acquired pneumonia, low to moderate severity
- BY MOUTH
- Adult: 500 mg once daily for 3 days, alternatively initially 500 mg once daily for 1 day, then 250 mg once daily for 4 days

Community-acquired pneumonia, high severity
- INITIALLY BY INTRAVENOUS INFUSION
- Adult: Initially 500 mg once daily for at least 2 days, then (by mouth) 500 mg once daily for a total duration of 7–10 days

Antibacterial prophylaxis for insertion of intra-uterine device
- BY MOUTH
- Adult: 1 g for 1 dose

- UNLICENSED USE
- In children Not licensed for prophylaxis of group A streptococcal infection.
- In adults Oral azithromycin not licensed for trachoma which results from chronic infection with *Chlamydia trachomatis*. Not licensed for uncomplicated gonorrhoea, mild or moderate typhoid due to multiple-antibacterial-resistant organisms, Lyme disease, or prophylaxis of group A streptococcal infection. Not licensed for community-acquired pneumonia (high severity) when oral treatment continues for more than 3 days.

- INTERACTIONS → Appendix 1: macrolides
- PREGNANCY Manufacturers advise use only if adequate alternatives not available.
- BREAST FEEDING Present in milk; use only if no suitable alternatives.
- HEPATIC IMPAIRMENT Manufacturers advise avoid in severe liver disease—no information available.
- RENAL IMPAIRMENT
  Dose adjustments ► In adults Use with caution if eGFR less than 10 mL/minute/1.73 m².
  ► In children Use with caution if estimated glomerular filtration rate less than 10 mL/minute/1.73 m².
- DIRECTIONS FOR ADMINISTRATION For *intravenous infusion* (*Zedbac*®), give intermittently *in* Glucose 5% *or* Sodium Chloride 0.9%. Reconstitute 500 mg with 4.8 mL water for injections to produce a 100 mg/mL solution, then dilute 5 mL of solution with infusion fluid to a final concentration of 1 or 2 mg/mL; give the 1 mg/mL solution over 3 hours *or* give the 2 mg/mL solution over 1 hour.
- PRESCRIBING AND DISPENSING INFORMATION Flavours of oral liquid formulations may include cherry or banana.

5

Infection

● PATIENT AND CARER ADVICE
Medicines for Children leaflet: Azithromycin for bacterial infections www.medicinesforchildren.org.uk/azithromycin-bacterial-infections-0

● PROFESSION SPECIFIC INFORMATION
Dental practitioners' formulary
Azithromycin Capsules may be prescribed.
Azithromycin Tablets may be prescribed.
Azithromycin Oral Suspension 200 mg/5 mL may be prescribed.

● EXCEPTIONS TO LEGAL CATEGORY Azithromycin tablets can be sold to the public for the treatment of confirmed, asymptomatic *Chlamydia trachomatis* genital infection in those over 16 years of age, and for the epidemiological treatment of their sexual partners, subject to maximum single dose of 1 g, maximum daily dose 1 g, and a pack size of 1 g.

● MEDICINAL FORMS
There can be variation in the licensing of different medicines containing the same drug. Forms available from special-order manufacturers include: oral suspension

Tablet
CAUTIONARY AND ADVISORY LABELS 5, 9
▸ Azithromycin (Non-proprietary)
Azithromycin 250 mg Azithromycin 250mg tablets | 4 tablet PoM £10.11 DT = £1.12 | 6 tablet PoM £2.04–£14.46
Azithromycin 500 mg Azithromycin 500mg tablets | 3 tablet PoM £9.80 DT = £0.88

Oral suspension
CAUTIONARY AND ADVISORY LABELS 5, 9
▸ Azithromycin (Non-proprietary)
Azithromycin 40 mg per 1 ml Azithromycin 200mg/5ml oral suspension | 15 ml PoM £6.18 DT = £4.06 | 30 ml PoM £11.04 DT = £11.04
▸ Zithromax (Pfizer Ltd)
Azithromycin 40 mg per 1 ml Zithromax 200mg/5ml oral suspension | 15 ml PoM £4.06 DT = £4.06 | 22.5 ml PoM £6.10 = £6.10 | 30 ml PoM £11.04 DT = £11.04

Powder for solution for infusion
ELECTROLYTES: May contain Sodium
▸ Zedbac (Aspire Pharma Ltd)
Azithromycin (as Azithromycin dihydrate) 500 mg Zedbac 500mg powder for solution for infusion vials | 1 vial PoM £9.50 (Hospital only)

Capsule
CAUTIONARY AND ADVISORY LABELS 5, 9, 23
▸ Azithromycin (Non-proprietary)
Azithromycin (as Azithromycin dihydrate) 250 mg Azithromycin 250mg capsules | 4 capsule PoM £3.59–£10.10 | 6 capsule PoM £15.15 DT = £5.39
▸ Zithromax (Pfizer Ltd)
Azithromycin (as Azithromycin dihydrate) 250 mg Zithromax 250mg capsules | 4 capsule PoM £7.16 | 6 capsule PoM £10.74 DT = £5.39

F 528

Clarithromycin

● INDICATIONS AND DOSE
Respiratory-tract infections | Mild to moderate skin and soft-tissue infections | Otitis media
▸ BY MOUTH USING IMMEDIATE-RELEASE MEDICINES
▹ Child 1 month–11 years (body-weight up to 8 kg): 7.5 mg/kg twice daily
▹ Child 1 month–11 years (body-weight 8-11 kg): 62.5 mg twice daily
▹ Child 1 month–11 years (body-weight 12-19 kg): 125 mg twice daily
▹ Child 1 month–11 years (body-weight 20-29 kg): 187.5 mg twice daily
▹ Child 1 month–11 years (body-weight 30-40 kg): 250 mg twice daily

▹ Child 12–17 years: 250 mg twice daily usually for 7–14 days, increased to 500 mg twice daily, if required in severe infections (e.g. pneumonia)
▹ Adult: 250 mg twice daily usually for 7–14 days, increased to 500 mg twice daily, if required in severe infections (e.g. pneumonia)
▸ BY MOUTH USING MODIFIED-RELEASE MEDICINES
▹ Child 12–17 years: 500 mg once daily usually for 7–14 days, increased to 1 g once daily, if required in severe infections (e.g. pneumonia)
▹ Adult: 500 mg once daily usually for 7–14 days, increased to 1 g once daily, if required in severe infections (e.g. pneumonia)
▸ BY INTRAVENOUS INFUSION
▹ Adult: 500 mg every 12 hours maximum duration 5 days, switch to oral route when appropriate, to be administered into a large proximal vein

Lyme disease
▸ BY MOUTH
▹ Child 12–17 years: 500 mg twice daily for 14–21 days
▹ Adult: 500 mg twice daily for 14–21 days

Prevention of pertussis
▸ BY MOUTH
▹ Child 1 month–11 years (body-weight up to 8 kg): 7.5 mg/kg twice daily for 7 days
▹ Child 1 month–11 years (body-weight 8-11 kg): 62.5 mg twice daily for 7 days
▹ Child 1 month–11 years (body-weight 12-19 kg): 125 mg twice daily for 7 days
▹ Child 1 month–11 years (body-weight 20-29 kg): 187.5 mg twice daily for 7 days
▹ Child 1 month–11 years (body-weight 30-40 kg): 250 mg twice daily for 7 days
▹ Child 12–17 years: 500 mg twice daily for 7 days
▹ Adult: 500 mg twice daily for 7 days

Helicobacter pylori **eradication in combination with a proton pump inhibitor and amoxicillin**
▸ BY MOUTH
▹ Adult: 500 mg twice daily

Helicobacter pylori **eradication in combination with a proton pump inhibitor and metronidazole**
▸ BY MOUTH
▹ Adult: 250 mg twice daily

Acute sinusitis
▸ BY MOUTH
▹ Adult: 500 mg twice daily for 5 days

● UNLICENSED USE EvGr Duration of treatment and child age ranges for acute sinusitis differ from product literature and adhere to national guidelines. ⚠ See Sinusitis (acute) p. 1168 for further information. Tablets not licensed for use in children under 12 years; oral suspension not licensed for use in infants under 6 months.

● INTERACTIONS → Appendix 1: macrolides

● PREGNANCY Manufacturer advises avoid, particularly in the first trimester, unless potential benefit outweighs risk.

● BREAST FEEDING Manufacturer advises avoid unless potential benefit outweighs risk—present in milk.

● HEPATIC IMPAIRMENT Avoid in severe impairment if renal impairment also present.

● RENAL IMPAIRMENT Avoid if severe hepatic impairment also present.
▹ With oral use in adults Avoid *Klaricid XL*® or clarithromycin m/r preparations if eGFR less than 30 mL/minute/1.73 m².
▹ With oral use in children Avoid *Klaricid XL*® or clarithromyin m/r preparations if estimated glomerular filtration rate less than 30 mL/minute/1.73 m².
Dose adjustments ▸ In adults Use half normal dose if eGFR less than 30 mL/minute/1.73 m², max. duration 14 days.

5

Infection

▸ In children Use half normal dose if estimated glomerular filtration rate less than 30 mL/minute/1.73 m², max. duration 14 days.

● DIRECTIONS FOR ADMINISTRATION For *intravenous infusion* (*Klaricid® I.V.*), give intermittently in Glucose 5% or Sodium Chloride 0.9%; dissolve initially in water for injections (500 mg in 10 mL) then dilute to a concentration of 2 mg/mL; give over 60 minutes.

● PATIENT AND CARER ADVICE
Medicines for Children leaflet: Clarithromycin for bacterial infections www.medicinesforchildren.org.uk/clarithromycin-bacterial-infections

● PROFESSION SPECIFIC INFORMATION

Dental practitioners' formulary
Clarithromycin Tablets may be prescribed.
Clarithromycin Oral Suspension may be prescribed.

● MEDICINAL FORMS
There can be variation in the licensing of different medicines containing the same drug. Forms available from special-order manufacturers include: infusion

Modified-release tablet
CAUTIONARY AND ADVISORY LABELS 9, 21, 25
▸ Clarie XL (Teva UK Ltd)
Clarithromycin 500 mg Clarie XL 500mg tablets | 7 tablet [PoM]
£6.72 DT = £6.72 | 14 tablet [PoM] £13.23
▸ Klaricid XL (Mylan)
Clarithromycin 500 mg Klaricid XL 500mg tablets | 7 tablet [PoM]
£6.72 DT = £6.72 | 14 tablet [PoM] £13.23
▸ Xetinin XL (Morningside Healthcare Ltd)
Clarithromycin 500 mg Xetinin XL 500mg tablets | 7 tablet [PoM]
£6.72 DT = £6.72 | 14 tablet [PoM] £13.23

Granules
CAUTIONARY AND ADVISORY LABELS 9, 13
▸ Klaricid (Mylan)
Clarithromycin 250 mg Klaricid Adult 250mg granules sachets | 14 sachet [PoM] £11.68

Tablet
CAUTIONARY AND ADVISORY LABELS 9
▸ Clarithromycin (Non-proprietary)
Clarithromycin 250 mg Clarithromycin 250mg tablets | 14 tablet [PoM] £10.50 DT = £1.07
Clarithromycin 500 mg Clarithromycin 500mg tablets | 14 tablet [PoM] £21.50 DT = £1.95

Oral suspension
CAUTIONARY AND ADVISORY LABELS 9
▸ Clarithromycin (Non-proprietary)
Clarithromycin 25 mg per 1 ml Clarithromycin 125mg/5ml oral suspension | 70 ml [PoM] £3.75 DT = £3.39
Clarithromycin 50 mg per 1 ml Clarithromycin 250mg/5ml oral suspension | 70 ml [PoM] £5.25 DT = £4.60
▸ Klaricid (Mylan)
Clarithromycin 25 mg per 1 ml Klaricid Paediatric 125mg/5ml oral suspension | 70 ml [PoM] £5.26 DT = £3.39 | 100 ml [PoM] £9.04
Clarithromycin 50 mg per 1 ml Klaricid Paediatric 250mg/5ml oral suspension | 70 ml [PoM] £10.51 DT = £4.60

Powder for solution for infusion
ELECTROLYTES: May contain Sodium
▸ Clarithromycin (Non-proprietary)
Clarithromycin 500 mg Clarithromycin 500mg powder for solution for infusion vials | 1 vial [PoM] £11.25 DT = £9.45
Clarithromycin 500mg powder for concentrate for solution for infusion vials | 1 vial [PoM] £8.98 DT = £9.45
▸ Klaricid (Mylan)
Clarithromycin 500 mg Klaricid IV 500mg powder for solution for infusion vials | 1 vial [PoM] £9.45 DT = £9.45

◤ 528

Erythromycin

● INDICATIONS AND DOSE

Susceptible infections in patients with penicillin hypersensitivity (e.g. respiratory-tract infections (including Legionella infection), skin and oral infections, and campylobacter enteritis)
▸ BY MOUTH
▸ Child 1 month-1 year: 125 mg 4 times a day, total daily dose may alternatively be given in two divided doses, increased to 250 mg 4 times a day, dose increase may be used in severe infections
▸ Child 2-7 years: 250 mg 4 times a day, total daily dose may alternatively be given in two divided doses, increased to 500 mg 4 times a day, dose increase may be used in severe infections
▸ Child 8-17 years: 250–500 mg 4 times a day, total daily dose may alternatively be given in two divided doses, increased to 500–1000 mg 4 times a day, dose increase may be used in severe infections
▸ Adult: 250–500 mg 4 times a day, total daily dose may alternatively be given in two divided doses, increased to 500–1000 mg 4 times a day, dose increase may be used in severe infections
▸ BY INTRAVENOUS INFUSION
▸ Child: 12.5 mg/kg every 6 hours (max. per dose 1 g)
▸ Adult: 6.25 mg/kg every 6 hours, for mild infections when oral treatment not possible. increased to 12.5 mg/kg every 6 hours, dose increase may be used in severe infections

Lyme disease (under expert supervision)
▸ BY MOUTH
▸ Adult: 500 mg 4 times a day for 14–21 days

Early syphilis
▸ BY MOUTH
▸ Adult: 500 mg 4 times a day for 14 days

Uncomplicated genital chlamydia | Non-gonococcal urethritis
▸ BY MOUTH
▸ Adult: 500 mg twice daily for 14 days

Chronic prostatitis
▸ BY MOUTH
▸ Adult: 250–500 mg 4 times a day, total daily dose may alternatively be given in two divided doses, increased to 4 g daily in divided doses, dose increase may be used in severe infections
▸ BY INTRAVENOUS INFUSION
▸ Adult: 6.25 mg/kg every 6 hours, for mild infections when oral treatment is not possible, increased to 12.5 mg/kg every 6 hours, dose increase may be used in severe infections

Prevention and treatment of pertussis
▸ BY MOUTH
▸ Child 1 month-1 year: 125 mg 4 times a day, total daily dose may alternatively be given in two divided doses, increased to 250 mg 4 times a day, dose increase may be used in severe infections
▸ Child 2-7 years: 250 mg 4 times a day, total daily dose may alternatively be given in two divided doses, increased to 500 mg 4 times a day, dose increase may be used in severe infections
▸ Child 8-17 years: 250–500 mg 4 times a day, total daily dose may alternatively be given in two divided doses, increased to 500–1000 mg 4 times a day, dose increase may be used in severe infections
▸ Adult: (consult local protocol)

Prevention of secondary case of diphtheria in non-immune patient

▶ BY MOUTH
▶ Child 1 month-1 year: 125 mg every 6 hours for 7 days, treat for further 10 days if nasopharyngeal swabs positive after first 7 days' treatment
▶ Child 2-7 years: 250 mg every 6 hours for 7 days, treat for further 10 days if nasopharyngeal swabs positive after first 7 days' treatment
▶ Child 8-17 years: 500 mg every 6 hours for 7 days, treat for further 10 days if nasopharyngeal swabs positive after first 7 days' treatment
▶ Adult: 500 mg every 6 hours for 7 days, treat for further 10 days if nasopharyngeal swabs positive after first 7 days' treatment

Prevention of secondary case of invasive group A streptococcal infection in penicillin allergic patients

▶ BY MOUTH
▶ Child 1 month-1 year: 125 mg every 6 hours for 10 days
▶ Child 2-7 years: 250 mg every 6 hours for 10 days
▶ Child 8-17 years: 250–500 mg every 6 hours for 10 days
▶ Adult: 250–500 mg every 6 hours for 10 days

Prevention of pneumococcal infection in asplenia or in patients with sickle-cell disease (if penicillin-allergic)

▶ BY MOUTH
▶ Child 1 month-1 year: 125 mg twice daily, antibiotic prophylaxis is not fully reliable
▶ Child 2-7 years: 250 mg twice daily, antibiotic prophylaxis is not fully reliable. It may be discontinued in those over 5 years of age with sickle-cell disease who have received pneumococcal immunisation and who do not have a history of severe pneumococcal infection
▶ Child 8-17 years: 500 mg twice daily, antibiotic prophylaxis is not fully reliable. It may be discontinued in those with sickle-cell disease who have received pneumococcal immunisation and who do not have a history of severe pneumococcal infection
▶ Adult: 500 mg twice daily, antibiotic prophylaxis is not fully reliable. It may be discontinued in those with sickle-cell disease who have received pneumococcal immunisation and who do not have a history of severe pneumococcal infection

Prevention of recurrence of rheumatic fever

▶ BY MOUTH
▶ Child 1 month-1 year: 125 mg twice daily
▶ Child 2-17 years: 250 mg twice daily

Rosacea

▶ BY MOUTH
▶ Adult: 500 mg twice daily courses usually last 6–12 weeks and are repeated intermittently

Acne

▶ BY MOUTH
▶ Adult: 500 mg twice daily

● CAUTIONS Avoid in Acute porphyrias p. 1025
● INTERACTIONS → Appendix 1: macrolides
● PREGNANCY Not known to be harmful.
● BREAST FEEDING Only small amounts in milk—not known to be harmful.
● HEPATIC IMPAIRMENT May cause idiosyncratic hepatotoxicity.
● RENAL IMPAIRMENT
Dose adjustments ▶ In adults Max. 1.5 g daily in severe renal impairment (ototoxicity).
▶ In children Reduce dose in severe renal impairment (ototoxicity).
● DIRECTIONS FOR ADMINISTRATION
▶ With intravenous use in children Dilute reconstituted solution further in glucose 5% (neutralised with Sodium bicarbonate) or sodium chloride 0.9% to a concentration of 1–5 mg/mL; give over 20–60 minutes. Concentration of up to 10 mg/mL may be used in fluid-restriction if administered via a central venous catheter.
▶ With intravenous use in adults For *intravenous infusion* (as lactobionate), give intermittently *in* Glucose 5% (neutralised with sodium bicarbonate) *or* Sodium chloride 0.9%; dissolve initially in water for injections (1 g in 20 mL) then dilute to a concentration of 1–5 mg/mL; give over 20–60 minutes.

● PRESCRIBING AND DISPENSING INFORMATION Flavours of oral liquid formulations may include banana.

● PATIENT AND CARER ADVICE
Medicines for Children leaflet: Erythromycin for bacterial infections www.medicinesforchildren.org.uk/erythromycin-for-bacterial-infections

● PROFESSION SPECIFIC INFORMATION

Dental practitioners' formulary
Erythromycin tablets e/c may be prescribed. Erythromycin ethyl succinate oral suspension may be prescribed. Erythromycin stearate tablets may be prescribed. Erythromycin ethyl succinate tablets may be prescribed.

● MEDICINAL FORMS
There can be variation in the licensing of different medicines containing the same drug.

Gastro-resistant tablet
CAUTIONARY AND ADVISORY LABELS 5, 9, 25
▶ Erythromycin (Non-proprietary)
Erythromycin 250 mg Erythromycin 250mg gastro-resistant tablets | 28 tablet [PoM] £2.25 DT = £1.28 | 500 tablet [PoM] £22.86–£27.20

Tablet
CAUTIONARY AND ADVISORY LABELS 9
▶ Erythromycin (Non-proprietary)
Erythromycin (as Erythromycin ethyl succinate)
500 mg Erythromycin ethyl succinate 500mg tablets | 28 tablet [PoM] £15.95 DT = £10.78
▶ Erythrocin (AMCo)
Erythromycin (as Erythromycin stearate) 250 mg Erythrocin 250 tablets | 100 tablet [PoM] £18.20 DT = £18.20
Erythromycin (as Erythromycin stearate) 500 mg Erythrocin 500 tablets | 100 tablet [PoM] £36.40 DT = £36.40
▶ Erythrolar (Ennogen Pharma Ltd)
Erythromycin (as Erythromycin stearate) 250 mg Erythrolar 250mg tablets | 100 tablet [PoM] £22.80 DT = £18.20
Erythromycin (as Erythromycin stearate) 500 mg Erythrolar 500mg tablets | 100 tablet [PoM] £45.60 DT = £36.40
▶ Erythroped A (AMCo)
Erythromycin (as Erythromycin ethyl succinate)
500 mg Erythroped A 500mg tablets | 28 tablet [PoM] £10.78 DT = £10.78

Oral suspension
CAUTIONARY AND ADVISORY LABELS 9
▶ Erythromycin (Non-proprietary)
Erythromycin (as Erythromycin ethyl succinate) 25 mg per 1 ml Erythromycin ethyl succinate 125mg/5ml oral suspension | 100 ml [PoM] £4.80 DT = £4.75
Erythromycin ethyl succinate 125mg/5ml oral suspension sugar-free | 100 ml [PoM] £4.99 DT = £3.61
Erythromycin (as Erythromycin ethyl succinate) 50 mg per 1 ml Erythromycin ethyl succinate 250mg/5ml oral suspension | 100 ml [PoM] £8.18 DT = £8.14
Erythromycin ethyl succinate 250mg/5ml oral suspension sugar-free | 100 ml [PoM] £7.43 DT = £6.22
Erythromycin (as Erythromycin ethyl succinate) 100 mg per 1 ml Erythromycin ethyl succinate 500mg/5ml oral suspension | 100 ml [PoM] £14.54 DT = £14.54
Erythromycin ethyl succinate 500mg/5ml oral suspension sugar-free | 100 ml [PoM] [S]
▶ Erythroped (AMCo)
Erythromycin (as Erythromycin ethyl succinate) 25 mg per 1 ml Erythroped PI SF 125mg/5ml oral suspension sugar-free | 140 ml [PoM] £3.06
Erythromycin (as Erythromycin ethyl succinate) 50 mg per 1 ml Erythroped SF 250mg/5ml oral suspension sugar-free | 140 ml [PoM] £5.95

Erythromycin (as Erythromycin ethyl succinate) 100 mg per
1 ml Erythroped Forte SF 500mg/5ml oral suspension sugar-free |
140 ml [PoM] £10.56 DT = £10.56

Powder for solution for infusion
▸ Erythromycin (Non-proprietary)
Erythromycin (as Erythromycin lactobionate)
1 gram Erythromycin 1g powder for solution for infusion vials |
1 vial [PoM] £18.45-£22.92

ANTIBACTERIALS > MONOBACTAMS

Aztreonam

- DRUG ACTION Aztreonam is a monocyclic beta-lactam
  ('monobactam') antibiotic with an antibacterial spectrum
  limited to Gram-negative aerobic bacteria including
  Pseudomonas aeruginosa, *Neisseria meningitidis*, and
  Haemophilus influenzae; it should not be used alone for
  'blind' treatment since it is not active against Gram-
  positive organisms. Aztreonam is also effective against
  Neisseria gonorrhoeae (but not against concurrent
  chlamydial infection).

- INDICATIONS AND DOSE

**Gram-negative infections including *Pseudomonas
aeruginosa*, *Haemophilus influenzae*, and *Neisseria
meningitidis***
▸ BY DEEP INTRAMUSCULAR INJECTION, OR BY INTRAVENOUS
  INFUSION, OR BY INTRAVENOUS INJECTION
▸ Adult: 1 g every 8 hours, alternatively 2 g every
  12 hours, single doses over 1 g intravenous route only

**Severe gram-negative infections including *Pseudomonas
aeruginosa*, *Haemophilus influenzae*, *Neisseria
meningitidis*, and lung infections in cystic fibrosis**
▸ BY INTRAVENOUS INFUSION, OR BY INTRAVENOUS INJECTION
▸ Adult: 2 g every 6-8 hours

Gonorrhoea | Cystitis
▸ BY INTRAMUSCULAR INJECTION
▸ Adult: 1 g for 1 single dose

Urinary-tract infections
▸ BY DEEP INTRAMUSCULAR INJECTION, OR BY INTRAVENOUS
  INFUSION, OR BY INTRAVENOUS INJECTION
▸ Adult: 0.5-1 g every 8-12 hours

**Chronic pulmonary *Pseudomonas aeruginosa* infection in
patients with cystic fibrosis**
▸ BY INHALATION OF NEBULISED SOLUTION
▸ Adult: 75 mg 3 times a day for 28 days, doses to be
  administered at least 4 hours apart, subsequent courses
  repeated after 28-day interval without aztreonam
  nebuliser solution

- CAUTIONS
▸ When used by inhalation Haemoptysis— risk of further
  haemorrhage

- SIDE-EFFECTS
  GENERAL SIDE-EFFECTS
▸ **Common or very common** Dyspnoea · respiratory disorders
  SPECIFIC SIDE-EFFECTS
▸ **Common or very common**
▸ When used by inhalation Cough · haemoptysis · joint
  disorders · laryngeal pain · nasal complaints · rash
▸ **Rare or very rare**
▸ With parenteral use Anaemia · asthenia · breast tenderness ·
  chest pain · confusion · diplopia · dizziness · eosinophilia ·
  haemorrhage · headache · hepatic disorders · hypotension ·
  insomnia · leucocytosis · myalgia · nasal congestion ·
  neutropenia · oral disorders · pancytopenia · paraesthesia ·
  pseudomembranous enterocolitis · seizure ·
  thrombocytopenia · thrombocytosis · tinnitus · vertigo ·
  vulvovaginal candidiasis

▸ **Frequency not known**
▸ With parenteral use Abdominal pain · angioedema ·
  diarrhoea · nausea · skin reactions · taste altered · toxic
  epidermal necrolysis · vomiting

- ALLERGY AND CROSS-SENSITIVITY Contra-indicated in
  aztreonam hypersensitivity.
    Use with caution in patients with hypersensitivity to
  other beta-lactam antibiotics (although aztreonam may be
  less likely than other beta-lactams to cause
  hypersensitivity in penicillin-sensitive patients).

- PREGNANCY
▸ With systemic use No information available; manufacturer
  of injection advises avoid.
▸ When used by inhalation No information available;
  manufacturer of powder for nebuliser solution advises
  avoid unless essential.

- BREAST FEEDING Amount in milk probably too small to be
  harmful.

- HEPATIC IMPAIRMENT
▸ With systemic use Use injection with caution.
  Monitoring ▸ With systemic use Monitor liver function.

- RENAL IMPAIRMENT
  Dose adjustments ▸ With systemic use If eGFR
  10-30 mL/minute/1.73 m^2, usual initial dose of injection,
  then half normal dose. If eGFR less than
  10 mL/minute/1.73 m^2, usual initial dose of injection, then
  one-quarter normal dose.

- MONITORING REQUIREMENTS
▸ When used by inhalation Measure lung function before and
  after initial dose of aztreonam and monitor for
  bronchospasm.

- DIRECTIONS FOR ADMINISTRATION For *intravenous
  injection*, give over 3-5 minutes. For *intravenous infusion*
  (*Azactam*®), give intermittently in Glucose 5% or Sodium
  chloride 0.9%. Dissolve initially in water for injections (1 g
  per 3 mL) then dilute to a concentration of less than
  20 mg/mL; to be given over 20-60 minutes.
▸ When used by inhalation Other inhaled drugs should be
  administered before aztreonam; a bronchodilator should
  be administered before each dose.

- NATIONAL FUNDING/ACCESS DECISIONS
  Scottish Medicines Consortium (SMC) Decisions
  The *Scottish Medicines Consortium* has advised (December
  2014) that aztreonam powder for nebuliser solution
  (*Cayston*®) is accepted for restricted use within NHS
  Scotland when inhaled colistimethate sodium and inhaled
  tobramycin are not tolerated or are not providing
  satisfactory therapeutic benefit (measured as ≥2% decline
  in forced expiratory volume in 1 second).

- MEDICINAL FORMS
  There can be variation in the licensing of different medicines
  containing the same drug.
  Powder and solvent for nebuliser solution
▸ Cayston (Gilead Sciences International Ltd)
  Aztreonam (as Aztreonam lysine) 75 mg Cayston 75mg powder
  and solvent for nebuliser solution vials with Altera Nebuliser Handset
  | 84 vial [PoM] £2,181.53
  Powder for solution for injection
▸ Azactam (Bristol-Myers Squibb Pharmaceuticals Ltd)
  Aztreonam 1 gram Azactam 1g powder for solution for injection vials
  | 1 vial [PoM] £9.40 (Hospital only)
  Aztreonam 2 gram Azactam 2g powder for solution for injection vials
  | 1 vial [PoM] £18.82 (Hospital only)

ANTIBACTERIALS ⟩ NITROIMIDAZOLE DERIVATIVES

Metronidazole

- DRUG ACTION Metronidazole is an antimicrobial drug with high activity against anaerobic bacteria and protozoa.

- INDICATIONS AND DOSE

Anaerobic infections
▶ BY MOUTH
- Child 1 month: 7.5 mg/kg every 12 hours usually treated for 7 days (for 10–14 days in *Clostridium difficile* infection)
- Child 2 months–11 years: 7.5 mg/kg every 8 hours (max. per dose 400 mg) usually treated for 7 days (for 10–14 days in *Clostridium difficile* infection)
- Child 12–17 years: 400 mg every 8 hours usually treated for 7 days (for 10–14 days in *Clostridium difficile* infection)
- Adult: 400 mg every 8 hours, alternatively 500 mg every 8 hours usually treated for 7 days (for 10–14 days in *Clostridium difficile* infection)
▶ BY RECTUM
- Child 1–11 months: 125 mg 3 times a day for 3 days, then 125 mg twice daily, for usual total treatment duration of 7 days
- Child 1–4 years: 250 mg 3 times a day for 3 days, then 250 mg twice daily, for usual total treatment duration of 7 days
- Child 5–9 years: 500 mg 3 times a day for 3 days, then 500 mg twice daily, for usual total treatment duration of 7 days
- Child 10–17 years: 1 g 3 times a day for 3 days, then 1 g twice daily, for usual total treatment duration of 7 days
- Adult: 1 g 3 times a day for 3 days, then 1 g twice daily, for usual total treatment duration of 7 days
▶ BY INTRAVENOUS INFUSION
- Adult: 500 mg every 8 hours usually treated for 7 days (for 10–14 days in *Clostridium difficile* infection), to be given over 20 minutes

***Helicobacter pylori* eradication; in combination with clarithromycin and esomeprazole; or in combination with clarithromycin and lansoprazole; or in combination with amoxicillin and lansoprazole; or in combination with clarithromycin and omeprazole; or in combination with clarithromycin and pantoprazole; or in combination with clarithromycin and rabeprazole**
▶ BY MOUTH
- Adult: 400 mg twice daily

***Helicobacter pylori* eradication; in combination with amoxicillin and omeprazole**
▶ BY MOUTH
- Adult: 400 mg 3 times a day

Fistulating Crohn's disease
▶ BY MOUTH
- Adult: 10–20 mg/kg daily in divided doses, usual dose 400–500 mg 3 times a day usually given for 1 month but no longer than 3 months because of concerns about peripheral neuropathy

Leg ulcers and pressure sores
▶ BY MOUTH
- Adult: 400 mg every 8 hours for 7 days

Bacterial vaginosis (notably *Gardnerella vaginalis* infection)
▶ BY MOUTH
- Adult: 400–500 mg twice daily for 5–7 days, alternatively 2 g for 1 dose

Bacterial vaginosis
▶ BY VAGINA USING VAGINAL GEL
- Adult: 1 applicatorful daily for 5 days, dose to be administered at night

DOSE EQUIVALENCE AND CONVERSION
▶ 1 applicator full delivers a 5 g dose of metronidazole 0.75%.

Pelvic inflammatory disease
▶ BY MOUTH
- Adult: 400 mg twice daily for 14 days

Acute ulcerative gingivitis
▶ BY MOUTH
- Child 1–2 years: 50 mg every 8 hours for 3 days
- Child 3–6 years: 100 mg every 12 hours for 3 days
- Child 7–9 years: 100 mg every 8 hours for 3 days
- Child 10–17 years: 200–250 mg every 8 hours for 3 days
- Adult: 400 mg every 8 hours for 3 days

Acute oral infections
▶ BY MOUTH
- Child 1–2 years: 50 mg every 8 hours for 3–7 days
- Child 3–6 years: 100 mg every 12 hours for 3–7 days
- Child 7–9 years: 100 mg every 8 hours for 3–7 days
- Child 10–17 years: 200–250 mg every 8 hours for 3–7 days
- Adult: 400 mg every 8 hours for 3–7 days

Surgical prophylaxis
▶ BY MOUTH
- Adult: 400–500 mg, to be administered 2 hours before surgery, then 400–500 mg every 8 hours if required for up to 3 doses (in high-risk procedures)
▶ BY RECTUM
- Adult: 1 g, to be administered 2 hours before surgery, then 1 g every 8 hours if required for up to 3 doses (in high-risk procedures)
▶ BY INTRAVENOUS INFUSION
- Adult: 500 mg, to be administered up to 30 minutes before the procedure (if rectal administration inappropriate), then 500 mg every 8 hours if required for up to 3 further doses (in high-risk procedures)

Invasive intestinal amoebiasis | Extra-intestinal amoebiasis (including liver abscess)
▶ BY MOUTH
- Child 1–2 years: 200 mg 3 times a day for 5 days in intestinal infection (for 5–10 days in extra-intestinal infection)
- Child 3–6 years: 200 mg 4 times a day for 5 days in intestinal infection (for 5–10 days in extra-intestinal infection)
- Child 7–9 years: 400 mg 3 times a day for 5 days in intestinal infection (for 5–10 days in extra-intestinal infection)
- Child 10–17 years: 800 mg 3 times a day for 5 days in intestinal infection (for 5–10 days in extra-intestinal infection)
- Adult: 800 mg 3 times a day for 5 days in intestinal infection (for 5–10 days in extra-intestinal infection)

Urogenital trichomoniasis
▶ BY MOUTH
- Child 1–2 years: 50 mg 3 times a day for 7 days
- Child 3–6 years: 100 mg twice daily for 7 days
- Child 7–9 years: 100 mg 3 times a day for 7 days
- Child 10–17 years: 200 mg 3 times a day for 5–7 days, alternatively 400–500 mg twice daily for 5–7 days, alternatively 2 g for 1 dose
- Adult: 200 mg 3 times a day for 7 days, alternatively 400–500 mg twice daily for 5–7 days, alternatively 2 g for 1 dose

continued →

5

Infection

Giardiasis

▶ BY MOUTH
▶ Child 1–2 years: 500 mg once daily for 3 days
▶ Child 3–6 years: 600–800 mg once daily for 3 days
▶ Child 7–9 years: 1 g once daily for 3 days
▶ Child 10–17 years: 2 g once daily for 3 days, alternatively 400 mg 3 times a day for 5 days, alternatively 500 mg twice daily for 7–10 days
▶ Adult: 2 g once daily for 3 days, alternatively 400 mg 3 times a day for 5 days, alternatively 500 mg twice daily for 7–10 days

Established case of tetanus

▶ BY INTRAVENOUS INFUSION
▶ Adult: (consult product literature)

● UNLICENSED USE
▶ With systemic use in adults Metronidazole doses in the BNF may differ from those in product literature.

● CAUTIONS
▶ With vaginal use Not recommended during menstruation · some systemic absorption may occur with vaginal gel

● INTERACTIONS → Appendix 1: metronidazole

● SIDE-EFFECTS
▶ **Common or very common**
▶ With systemic use Dry mouth · myalgia · nausea · oral disorders · taste altered · vomiting
▶ With vaginal use Pelvic discomfort · vulvovaginal candidiasis · vulvovaginal disorders
▶ **Uncommon**
▶ With systemic use Asthenia · headache · leucopenia (with long term or intensive therapy)
▶ With vaginal use Menstrual cycle irregularities · vaginal haemorrhage
▶ **Rare or very rare**
▶ With systemic use Agranulocytosis · angioedema · appetite decreased · ataxia · confusion · diarrhoea · dizziness · drowsiness · encephalopathy · epigastric pain · epileptiform seizure (with long term or intensive therapy) · hallucination · hepatic disorders · meningitis aseptic · mucositis · neutropenia · optic neuropathy · pancreatitis · pancytopenia · peripheral neuropathy (with long term or intensive therapy) · psychotic disorder · severe cutaneous adverse reactions (SCARs) · skin reactions · thrombocytopenia · urine dark · vision disorders
▶ **Frequency not known**
▶ With systemic use Depressed mood · hearing impairment

● PREGNANCY
▶ With systemic use Manufacturer advises avoidance of high-dose regimens; use only if potential benefit outweighs risk.

● BREAST FEEDING
▶ With systemic use Significant amount in milk; manufacturer advises avoid large single doses though otherwise compatible; may give milk a bitter taste.

● HEPATIC IMPAIRMENT
▶ With systemic use Use with caution in hepatic encephalopathy.
Dose adjustments ▶ With systemic use In severe liver disease reduce total daily dose to one-third, and give once daily.

● MONITORING REQUIREMENTS
▶ With systemic use Clinical and laboratory monitoring advised if treatment exceeds 10 days.

● DIRECTIONS FOR ADMINISTRATION For *intravenous infusion*, give over 20–30 minutes.

● PRESCRIBING AND DISPENSING INFORMATION Metronidazole is well absorbed orally and the intravenous route is normally reserved for severe infections. Metronidazole by the rectal route is an effective alternative to the intravenous route when oral administration is not possible.

● PATIENT AND CARER ADVICE Medicines for Children leaflet: Metronidazole for bacterial infections www.medicinesforchildren.org.uk/metronidazole-bacterial-infections

● PROFESSION SPECIFIC INFORMATION
Dental practitioners' formulary
Metronidazole Tablets may be prescribed. Metronidazole Oral Suspension may be prescribed.

● MEDICINAL FORMS There can be variation in the licensing of different medicines containing the same drug. Forms available from special-order manufacturers include: oral suspension, oral solution, suppository, gel

Tablet
CAUTIONARY AND ADVISORY LABELS 4, 9, 21, 25, 27
▶ Metronidazole (Non-proprietary)
Metronidazole 200 mg Metronidazole 200mg tablets | 21 tablet [PoM] £4.99 DT = £4.03 | 250 tablet [PoM] £20.00
Metronidazole 400 mg Metronidazole 400mg tablets | 21 tablet [PoM] £7.95 DT = £4.30
Metronidazole 500 mg Metronidazole 500mg tablets | 21 tablet [PoM] £37.82 DT = £37.82
▶ Flagyl (Zentiva)
Metronidazole 200 mg Flagyl 200mg tablets | 21 tablet [PoM] £4.49 DT = £4.03
Metronidazole 400 mg Flagyl 400mg tablets | 14 tablet [PoM] £6.34

Suppository
CAUTIONARY AND ADVISORY LABELS 4, 9
▶ Flagyl (Zentiva)
Metronidazole 500 mg Flagyl 500mg suppositories | 10 suppository [PoM] £15.18
Metronidazole 1 gram Flagyl 1g suppositories | 10 suppository [PoM] £23.06

Oral suspension
CAUTIONARY AND ADVISORY LABELS 4, 9
▶ Metronidazole (Non-proprietary)
Metronidazole (as Metronidazole benzoate) 40 mg per 1 ml Metronidazole 200mg/5ml oral suspension | 100 ml [PoM] £32.93 DT = £32.93

Infusion
ELECTROLYTES: May contain Sodium
▶ Metronidazole (Non-proprietary)
Metronidazole 5 mg per 1 ml Metronidazole 500mg/100ml infusion 100ml Macoflex bags | 1 bag [PoM] [Ⓢ]
Metronidazole 500mg/100ml infusion 100ml bags | 20 bag [PoM] £63.86

Vaginal gel
EXCIPIENTS: May contain Disodium edetate, hydroxybenzoates (parabens), propylene glycol
▶ Metronidazole (Non-proprietary)
Metronidazole 7.5 mg per 1 gram Metronidazole 0.75% vaginal gel | 40 gram [PoM] [Ⓢ] DT = £4.31
▶ Zidoval (Meda Pharmaceuticals Ltd)
Metronidazole 7.5 mg per 1 gram Zidoval 0.75% vaginal gel | 40 gram [PoM] £4.31 DT = £4.31

Tinidazole

● DRUG ACTION Tinidazole is an antimicrobial drug with high activity against anaerobic bacteria and protozoa; it has a longer duration of action than metronidazole.

● INDICATIONS AND DOSE
Anaerobic infections
▶ BY MOUTH
▶ Adult: Initially 2 g, followed by 1 g daily usually for 5–6 days, alternatively 500 mg twice daily usually for 5–6 days

Bacterial vaginosis | Acute ulcerative gingivitis
▶ BY MOUTH
▶ Adult: 2 g for 1 single dose

Abdominal surgery prophylaxis
▸ BY MOUTH
▸ Adult: 2 g for 1 single dose, to be administered approximately 12 hours before surgery

Intestinal amoebiasis
▸ BY MOUTH
▸ Child 1 month-11 years: 50–60 mg/kg once daily (max. per dose 2 g) for 3 days
▸ Child 12-17 years: 2 g once daily for 2–3 days
▸ Adult: 2 g once daily for 2–3 days

Amoebic involvement of liver
▸ BY MOUTH
▸ Child 1 month-11 years: 50–60 mg/kg once daily (max. per dose 2 g) for 5 days
▸ Child 12-17 years: 1.5–2 g once daily for 3–6 days
▸ Adult: 1.5–2 g once daily for 3–6 days

Urogenital trichomoniasis | Giardiasis
▸ BY MOUTH
▸ Child 1 month-11 years: 50–75 mg/kg (max. per dose 2 g) for 1 single dose, dose may be repeated once if necessary
▸ Child 12-17 years: 2 g for 1 single dose, dose may be repeated once if necessary
▸ Adult: 2 g for 1 single dose

Helicobacter pylori eradication
▸ BY MOUTH
▸ Adult: (consult local protocol)

● INTERACTIONS → Appendix 1: tinidazole
● SIDE-EFFECTS
▸ **Common or very common** Abdominal pain · appetite decreased · diarrhoea · headache · nausea · skin reactions · vertigo · vomiting
▸ **Frequency not known** Angioedema · ataxia · dizziness · fatigue · flushing · leucopenia · oral disorders · peripheral neuropathy · seizure · sensation abnormal · taste altered · urine discolouration
● PREGNANCY Manufacturer advises avoid in first trimester.
● BREAST FEEDING Present in milk—manufacturer advises avoid breast-feeding during and for 3 days after stopping treatment.
● MONITORING REQUIREMENTS Clinical and laboratory monitoring advised if treatment exceeds 10 days.

● MEDICINAL FORMS
There can be variation in the licensing of different medicines containing the same drug.
Tablet
CAUTIONARY AND ADVISORY LABELS 4, 9, 21, 25
▸ Fasigyn (Pfizer Ltd)
Tinidazole 500 mg Fasigyn 500mg tablets | 16 tablet [PoM] £11.04
DT = £11.04

ANTIBACTERIALS > PENICILLINS

Penicillins

Benzylpenicillin and phenoxymethylpenicillin

Benzylpenicillin sodium p. 537 (Penicillin G) remains an important and useful antibiotic but is inactivated by bacterial beta-lactamases. It is effective for many streptococcal (including pneumococcal), gonococcal, and meningococcal infections and also for anthrax, diphtheria, gas-gangrene, leptospirosis, and treatment of Lyme disease. Pneumococci, meningococci, and gonococci which have decreased sensitivity to penicillin have been isolated; benzylpenicillin sodium is no longer the drug of first choice for pneumococcal meningitis. Although benzylpenicillin sodium is effective in the treatment of tetanus, metronidazole p. 533 is preferred. Benzylpenicillin is inactivated by gastric acid and absorption from the gastro-intestinal tract is low; therefore it must be given by injection.

Benzathine benzylpenicillin is used for the treatment of early syphilis and late latent syphilis; it is given by intramuscular injection.

Phenoxymethylpenicillin p. 538 (Penicillin V) has a similar antibacterial spectrum to benzylpenicillin sodium, but is less active. It is gastric acid-stable, so is suitable for oral administration. It should not be used for serious infections because absorption can be unpredictable and plasma concentrations variable. It is indicated principally for respiratory-tract infections in children, for streptococcal tonsillitis, and for continuing treatment after one or more injections of benzylpenicillin sodium when clinical response has begun. It should not be used for meningococcal or gonococcal infections. Phenoxymethylpenicillin is used for prophylaxis against streptococcal infections following rheumatic fever and against pneumococcal infections following splenectomy or in sickle-cell disease.

Penicillinase-resistant penicillins

Most staphylococci are now resistant to benzylpenicillin because they produce penicillinases. Flucloxacillin p. 544, however, is not inactivated by these enzymes and is thus effective in infections caused by penicillin-resistant staphylococci, which is the sole indication for its use. Flucloxacillin is acid-stable and can, therefore, be given by mouth as well as by injection. Flucloxacillin is well absorbed from the gut.

Temocillin p. 545 is active against Gram-negative bacteria and is stable against a wide range of beta-lactamases. It should be reserved for the treatment of infections caused by beta-lactamase-producing strains of Gram-negative bacteria, including those resistant to third-generation cephalosporins. Temocillin is not active against *Pseudomonas aeruginosa* or *Acinetobacter* spp.

Broad-spectrum penicillins

Ampicillin p. 540 is active against certain Gram-positive and Gram-negative organisms but is inactivated by penicillinases including those produced by *Staphylococcus aureus* and by common Gram-negative bacilli such as *Escherichia coli*. Almost all staphylococci, approx. 60% of *E. coli* strains and approx. 20% of *Haemophilus influenzae* strains are now resistant. The likelihood of resistance should therefore be considered before using ampicillin for the 'blind' treatment of infections; in particular, it should not be used for hospital patients without checking sensitivity.

Ampicillin is well excreted in the bile and urine. It is principally indicated for the treatment of exacerbations of chronic bronchitis and middle ear infections, both of which may be due to *Streptococcus pneumoniae* and *H. influenzae*, and for urinary-tract infections.

Ampicillin can be given by mouth but less than half the dose is absorbed, and absorption is further decreased by the presence of food in the gut.

Maculopapular rashes commonly occur with ampicillin (and amoxicillin p. 539) but are not usually related to true penicillin allergy. They almost always occur in patients with glandular fever; broad-spectrum penicillins should not therefore be used for 'blind' treatment of a sore throat. The risk of rash is also increased in patients with acute or chronic lymphocytic leukaemia or in cytomegalovirus infection.

Amoxicillin is a derivative of ampicillin and has a similar antibacterial spectrum. It is better absorbed than ampicillin when given by mouth, producing higher plasma and tissue concentrations; unlike ampicillin, absorption is not affected by the presence of food in the stomach. Amoxicillin may also be used for the treatment of Lyme disease [not licensed].

Co-amoxiclav p. 542 consists of amoxicillin with the betalactamase inhibitor clavulanic acid. Clavulanic acid itself has no significant antibacterial activity but, by inactivating

5

Infection

beta-lactamases, it makes the combination active against beta-lactamase-producing bacteria that are resistant to amoxicillin. These include resistant strains of *Staph. aureus*, *E. coli*, and *H. influenzae*, as well as many *Bacteroides* and *Klebsiella* spp. Co-amoxiclav should be reserved for infections likely, or known, to be caused by amoxicillin-resistant beta-lactamase-producing strains.

A combination of ampicillin with flucloxacillin (as co-fluampicil p. 541 is available to treat infections involving either streptococci or staphylococci (e.g. cellulitis).

Antipseudomonal penicillins

Piperacillin, a ureidopenicillin, is only available in combination with the beta-lactamase inhibitor tazobactam. **Ticarcillin**, a carboxypenicillin, is only available in combination with the beta-lactamase inhibitor clavulanic acid. Both preparations have a broad spectrum of activity against a range of Gram-positive and Gram-negative bacteria, and anaerobes. Piperacillin with tazobactam below has activity against a wider range of Gram-negative organisms than ticarcillin with clavulanic acid p. 537 and it is more active against *Pseudomonas aeruginosa*. These antibacterials are not active against MRSA. They are used in the treatment of septicaemia, hospital-acquired pneumonia, and complicated infections involving the urinary tract, skin and soft tissues, or intra-abdomen. For severe pseudomonas infections these antipseudomonal penicillins can be given with an aminoglycoside (e.g. gentamicin p. 510) since they have a synergistic effect.

Mecillinams

Pivmecillinam hydrochloride p. 544 has significant activity against many Gram-negative bacteria including *Escherichia coli*, klebsiella, enterobacter, and salmonellae. It is not active against *Pseudomonas aeruginosa* or enterococci. Pivmecillinam hydrochloride is hydrolysed to mecillinam, which is the active drug.

Penicillins

- **DRUG ACTION** The penicillins are bactericidal and act by interfering with bacterial cell wall synthesis. They diffuse well into body tissues and fluids, but penetration into the cerebrospinal fluid is poor except when the meninges are inflamed. They are excreted in the urine in therapeutic concentrations.
- **CAUTIONS** History of allergy
- **SIDE-EFFECTS**
- **Common or very common** Diarrhoea · hypersensitivity · nausea · skin reactions · thrombocytopenia · vomiting
- **Uncommon** Antibiotic associated colitis · leucopenia
- **Rare or very rare** Agranulocytosis · angioedema · haemolytic anaemia · hepatic disorders · nephritis tubulointerstitial · neutropenia · seizure · severe cutaneous adverse reactions (SCARs)

SIDE-EFFECTS, FURTHER INFORMATION Diarrhoea frequently occurs during oral penicillin therapy. It is most common with broad-spectrum penicillins, which can cause antibiotic-associated colitis.

- **ALLERGY AND CROSS-SENSITIVITY** The most important side-effect of the penicillins is hypersensitivity which causes rashes and anaphylaxis and can be fatal. Allergic reactions to penicillins occur in 1–10% of exposed individuals; anaphylactic reactions occur in fewer than 0.05% of treated patients. Patients with a history of atopic allergy (e.g. asthma, eczema, hay fever) are at a higher risk of anaphylactic reactions to penicillins. Individuals with a history of anaphylaxis, urticaria, or rash immediately after penicillin administration are at risk of immediate hypersensitivity to a penicillin; these individuals should not receive a penicillin. Individuals with a history of a

minor rash (i.e. non-confluent, non-pruritic rash restricted to a small area of the body) or a rash that occurs more than 72 hours after penicillin administration are probably not allergic to penicillin and in these individuals a penicillin should not be withheld unnecessarily for serious infections; the possibility of an allergic reaction should, however, be borne in mind. Other beta-lactam antibiotics (including cephalosporins) can be used in these patients.

Patients who are allergic to one penicillin will be allergic to all because the hypersensitivity is related to the basic penicillin structure. Patients with a history of immediate hypersensitivity to penicillins may also react to the cephalosporins and other beta-lactam antibiotics, they should not receive these antibiotics. If a penicillin (or another beta-lactam antibiotic) is essential in an individual with immediate hypersensitivity to penicillin then specialist advice should be sought on hypersensitivity testing or using a beta-lactam antibiotic with a different structure to the penicillin that caused the hypersensitivity.

ANTIBACTERIALS > PENICILLINS, ANTIPSEUDOMONAL WITH BETA-LACTAMASE INHIBITOR

above

Piperacillin with tazobactam

- **INDICATIONS AND DOSE**

Hospital-acquired pneumonia | Septicaemia | Complicated infections involving the urinary-tract | Complicated infections involving the skin | Complicated infections involving the soft-tissues
- BY INTRAVENOUS INFUSION
- Adult: 4.5 g every 8 hours; increased if necessary to 4.5 g every 6 hours, increased frequency may be used for severe infections

Infections in neutropenic patients
- BY INTRAVENOUS INFUSION
- Adult: 4.5 g every 6 hours

- **CAUTIONS** High doses may lead to hypernatraemia (owing to sodium content of preparations)
- **INTERACTIONS** → Appendix 1: penicillins
- **SIDE-EFFECTS**
- **Common or very common** Anaemia · candida infection · constipation · gastrointestinal discomfort · headache · insomnia
- **Uncommon** Arthralgia · flushing · hypokalaemia · hypotension · myalgia
- **Rare or very rare** Epistaxis · stomatitis
- **Frequency not known** Eosinophilia · pancytopenia · pneumonia eosinophilic · renal failure · thrombocytosis
- **PREGNANCY** Manufacturers advise use only if potential benefit outweighs risk.
- **BREAST FEEDING** Trace amount in milk, but appropriate to use.
- **RENAL IMPAIRMENT**
Dose adjustments Max. 4.5 g every 8 hours if eGFR 20–40 mL/minute/1.73 m^2.
Max. 4.5 g every 12 hours if eGFR less than 20 mL/minute/1.73 m^2.
- **EFFECT ON LABORATORY TESTS** False-positive urinary glucose (if tested for reducing substances).
- **DIRECTIONS FOR ADMINISTRATION** For *intravenous infusion*, give intermittently in Glucose 5% or Sodium chloride 0.9%. Reconstitute initially (2.25 g in 10 mL, 4.5 g in 20 mL) with water for injections, or glucose 5% (*Tazocin*® brand only), or sodium chloride 0.9%, then dilute to 50–150 mL with infusion fluid; give over 30 minutes.

- PRESCRIBING AND DISPENSING INFORMATION Dose expressed as a combination of piperacillin and tazobactam (both as sodium salts) in a ratio of 8:1.

- MEDICINAL FORMS
There can be variation in the licensing of different medicines containing the same drug. Forms available from special-order manufacturers include: infusion
Powder for solution for injection
ELECTROLYTES: May contain Sodium
▶ Piperacillin with tazobactam (Non-proprietary)
Tazobactam (as Tazobactam sodium) 250 mg, Piperacillin (as Piperacillin sodium) 2 gram Piperacillin 2g / Tazobactam 250mg powder for solution for injection vials | 1 vial [PoM] £9.55 DT = £7.65 (Hospital only)
Piperacillin 2g / Tazobactam 250mg powder for solution for infusion vials | 1 vial [PoM] £7.85 DT = £7.65
▶ Tazocin (Pfizer Ltd)
Tazobactam (as Tazobactam sodium) 250 mg, Piperacillin (as Piperacillin sodium) 2 gram Tazocin 2.25g powder for solution for injection vials | 1 vial [PoM] £7.65 DT = £7.65

F 536

Ticarcillin with clavulanic acid

- INDICATIONS AND DOSE

Infections due to *Pseudomonas* and *Proteus* spp.
▶ BY INTRAVENOUS INFUSION
▶ Adult: 3.2 g every 6–8 hours; increased if necessary to 3.2 g every 4 hours, increased frequency used for more severe infections

- CAUTIONS High doses may lead to hypernatraemia (owing to sodium content of preparations)
CAUTIONS, FURTHER INFORMATION
▶ Cholestatic jaundice Cholestatic jaundice is possibly associated with clavulanic acid. An epidemiological study has shown that the risk of acute liver toxicity was about 6 times greater with co-amoxiclav (amoxicillin, clavulanic acid) than with amoxicillin. Cholestatic jaundice is more common in patients above the age of 65 years and in men; these reactions have only rarely been reported in children. Jaundice is usually self-limiting and very rarely fatal. The duration of treatment should be appropriate to the indication and should not usually exceed 14 days.
- INTERACTIONS → Appendix 1: clavulanic acid · penicillins
- SIDE-EFFECTS Bullous dermatitis · eosinophilia · haemorrhage · hypokalaemia
- PREGNANCY Not known to be harmful.
- BREAST FEEDING Trace amounts in milk, but appropriate to use.
- HEPATIC IMPAIRMENT Manufacturer advises caution in severe impairment.
- RENAL IMPAIRMENT Accumulation of electrolytes contained in preparation can occur in patients with renal failure.
Dose adjustments Reduce dose to 3.2 g every eight hours if eGFR 30–60 mL/minute/1.73 m^2; 1.6 g every eight hours if eGFR 10–30 mL/minute/1.73 m^2; 1.6 g every twelve hours if eGFR less than 10 mL/minute/1.73 m^2.
- EFFECT ON LABORATORY TESTS False-positive urinary glucose (if tested for reducing substances).
- DIRECTIONS FOR ADMINISTRATION For *intravenous infusion* (*Timentin*®), give intermittently *in* Glucose 5%. Suggested volume (depending on dose) 100–150 mL; give over 30–40 minutes.
- PRESCRIBING AND DISPENSING INFORMATION Dose is expressed as a combination of ticarcillin (as sodium salt) and clavulanic acid (as potassium salt) in a ratio of 15:1.

- MEDICINAL FORMS
There can be variation in the licensing of different medicines containing the same drug.
Powder for solution for infusion
ELECTROLYTES: May contain Potassium, sodium
▶ Timentin (GlaxoSmithKline UK Ltd)
Clavulanic acid (as Potassium clavulanate) 200 mg, Ticarcillin (as Ticarcillin sodium) 3 gram Timentin 3.2g powder for solution for infusion vials | 4 vial [PoM] £21.32

ANTIBACTERIALS > PENICILLINS, BETA-LACTAMASE SENSITIVE

F 536

Benzylpenicillin sodium

(Penicillin G)

- INDICATIONS AND DOSE

Mild to moderate susceptible infections | Throat infections | Otitis media | Cellulitis | Pneumonia
▶ BY INTRAMUSCULAR INJECTION, OR BY SLOW INTRAVENOUS INJECTION, OR BY INTRAVENOUS INFUSION
▶ Adult: 0.6–1.2 g every 6 hours, dose may be increased if necessary in more serious infections (consult product literature), single doses over 1.2 g to be given by intravenous route only

Endocarditis (in combination with other antibacterial if necessary)
▶ BY SLOW INTRAVENOUS INJECTION, OR BY INTRAVENOUS INFUSION
▶ Adult: 1.2 g every 4 hours, increased if necessary to 2.4 g every 4 hours, dose may be increased in infections such as enterococcal endocarditis

Anthrax (in combination with other antibacterials)
▶ BY SLOW INTRAVENOUS INJECTION, OR BY INTRAVENOUS INFUSION
▶ Adult: 2.4 g every 4 hours

Intrapartum prophylaxis against group B streptococcal infection
▶ BY SLOW INTRAVENOUS INJECTION, OR BY INTRAVENOUS INFUSION
▶ Adult: Initially 3 g for 1 dose, then 1.5 g every 4 hours until delivery

Meningitis | Meningococcal disease
▶ BY SLOW INTRAVENOUS INJECTION, OR BY INTRAVENOUS INFUSION
▶ Adult: 2.4 g every 4 hours
▶ BY INTRAVENOUS INFUSION
▶ Neonate up to 7 days: 50 mg/kg every 12 hours.
▶ Neonate 7 days to 28 days: 50 mg/kg every 8 hours.
▶ Child: 50 mg/kg every 4–6 hours (max. per dose 2.4 g every 4 hours)

Suspected meningococcal disease (meningitis with non-blanching rash or meningococcal septicaemia) prior to urgent transfer to hospital
▶ BY INTRAVENOUS INJECTION, OR BY INTRAMUSCULAR INJECTION
▶ Child 1–11 months: 300 mg, administer as single dose prior to urgent transfer to hospital so long as does not delay transfer
▶ Child 1–9 years: 600 mg, administer as single dose prior to urgent transfer to hospital so long as does not delay transfer
▶ Child 10–17 years: 1.2 g, administer as single dose prior to urgent transfer to hospital so long as does not delay transfer
▶ Adult: 1.2 g, administer as single dose prior to urgent transfer to hospital so long as does not delay transfer

continued →

Suspected bacterial meningitis without non-blanching rash where patient cannot be transferred to hospital urgently

▶ BY INTRAVENOUS INJECTION, OR BY INTRAMUSCULAR INJECTION
  ▸ Child 1-11 months: 300 mg, administer as single dose prior to transfer to hospital
  ▸ Child 1-9 years: 600 mg, administer as single dose prior to transfer to hospital
  ▸ Child 10-17 years: 1.2 g, administer as single dose prior to transfer to hospital
  ▸ Adult: 1.2 g, administer as single dose prior to transfer to hospital

● UNLICENSED USE Benzylpenicillin doses in the BNF may differ from those in product literature.

> IMPORTANT SAFETY INFORMATION
> Intrathecal injection of benzylpenicillin is **not** recommended.

● CAUTIONS Accumulation of sodium from injection can occur with high doses
● INTERACTIONS → Appendix 1: penicillins
● SIDE-EFFECTS
  ▶ **Common or very common** Fever · Jarisch-Herxheimer reaction
  ▶ **Rare or very rare** Neurotoxicity
  ▶ **Frequency not known** Coma
● PREGNANCY Not known to be harmful.
● BREAST FEEDING Trace amounts in milk, but appropriate to use.
● RENAL IMPAIRMENT Accumulation of sodium from injection can occur in renal failure. High doses may cause neurotoxicity, including cerebral irritation, convulsions, or coma.
  Dose adjustments ▸ In adults Reduce dose—consult product literature.
    ▸ In children Estimated glomerular filtration rate 10–50 mL/minute/1.73 m^2, use normal dose every 8–12 hours. Estimated glomerular filtration rate less than 10 mL/minute/1.73 m^2 use normal dose every 12 hours.
● EFFECT ON LABORATORY TESTS False-positive urinary glucose (if tested for reducing substances).
● DIRECTIONS FOR ADMINISTRATION
  ▶ With intravenous use in children Intravenous route recommended in neonates and infants. For *intravenous infusion*, dilute with Glucose 5% or Sodium Chloride 0.9%; give over 15–30 minutes. Longer administration time is particularly important when using doses of 50 mg/kg (or greater) to avoid CNS toxicity.
  ▶ With intravenous use in adults For *intravenous infusion* (Crystapen ®), give intermittently in Glucose 5% or Sodium chloride 0.9%; suggested volume 100 mL given over 30–60 minutes. Continuous infusion not usually recommended.

● MEDICINAL FORMS
There can be variation in the licensing of different medicines containing the same drug. Forms available from special-order manufacturers include: infusion
Powder for solution for injection
ELECTROLYTES: May contain Sodium
  ▸ Benzylpenicillin sodium (Non-proprietary)
    Benzylpenicillin sodium 600 mg Benzylpenicillin 600mg powder for solution for injection vials | 2 vial PoM £5.46 DT = £5.46 | 25 vial PoM £68.25–£68.29
    Benzylpenicillin sodium 1.2 gram Benzylpenicillin 1.2g powder for solution for injection vials | 25 vial PoM £92.01–£92.03 DT = £92.02

▶ 536
Phenoxymethylpenicillin
(Penicillin V)

● INDICATIONS AND DOSE
Oral infections | Tonsillitis | Otitis media | Erysipelas | Cellulitis
▶ BY MOUTH
  ▸ Child 1-11 months: 62.5 mg 4 times a day; increased if necessary up to 12.5 mg/kg 4 times a day
  ▸ Child 1-5 years: 125 mg 4 times a day; increased if necessary up to 12.5 mg/kg 4 times a day
  ▸ Child 6-11 years: 250 mg 4 times a day; increased if necessary up to 12.5 mg/kg 4 times a day
  ▸ Child 12-17 years: 500 mg 4 times a day; increased if necessary up to 1 g 4 times a day
  ▸ Adult: 500 mg every 6 hours, increased if necessary up to 1 g every 6 hours

Prevention of recurrence of rheumatic fever
▶ BY MOUTH
  ▸ Child 1 month-5 years: 125 mg twice daily
  ▸ Child 6-17 years: 250 mg twice daily
  ▸ Adult: 250 mg twice daily

Prevention of secondary case of invasive group A streptococcal infection
▶ BY MOUTH
  ▸ Child 1-11 months: 62.5 mg every 6 hours for 10 days
  ▸ Child 1-5 years: 125 mg every 6 hours for 10 days
  ▸ Child 6-11 years: 250 mg every 6 hours for 10 days
  ▸ Child 12-17 years: 250–500 mg every 6 hours for 10 days
  ▸ Adult: 250–500 mg every 6 hours for 10 days

Prevention of pneumococcal infection in asplenia or in patients with sickle-cell disease
▶ BY MOUTH
  ▸ Child 1-11 months: 62.5 mg twice daily
  ▸ Child 1-4 years: 125 mg twice daily
  ▸ Child 5-17 years: 250 mg twice daily
  ▸ Adult: 250 mg twice daily

Acute sinusitis
▶ BY MOUTH
  ▸ Child 1-11 months: 62.5 mg 4 times a day for 5 days
  ▸ Child 1-5 years: 125 mg 4 times a day for 5 days
  ▸ Child 6-11 years: 250 mg 4 times a day for 5 days
  ▸ Child 12-17 years: 500 mg 4 times a day for 5 days
  ▸ Adult: 500 mg 4 times a day for 5 days

● UNLICENSED USE EvGr Duration of treatment for acute sinusitis adheres to national guidelines. ◬ See Sinusitis (acute) p. 1168 for further information.
  Phenoxymethylpenicillin doses in the BNF may differ from product literature.
● INTERACTIONS → Appendix 1: penicillins
● SIDE-EFFECTS Arthralgia · circulatory collapse · coagulation disorder · eosinophilia · exfoliative dermatitis · faeces soft · fever · increased risk of infection · neurotoxicity · oral disorders · paraesthesia
● PREGNANCY Not known to be harmful.
● BREAST FEEDING Trace amounts in milk, but appropriate to use.
● EFFECT ON LABORATORY TESTS False-positive urinary glucose (if tested for reducing substances).
● PATIENT AND CARER ADVICE
Medicines for Children leaflet: Penicillin V for bacterial infections www.medicinesforchildren.org.uk/penicillin-v-for-bacterial-infections
Medicines for Children leaflet: Penicillin V for prevention of pneumococcal infection www.medicinesforchildren.org.uk/penicillin-v-for-prevention-of-pneumococcal-infection

● PROFESSION SPECIFIC INFORMATION

Dental practitioners' formulary

Phenoxymethylpenicillin Tablets may be prescribed.
Phenoxymethylpenicillin Oral Solution may be prescribed.

● MEDICINAL FORMS

There can be variation in the licensing of different medicines
containing the same drug.

Oral solution

CAUTIONARY AND ADVISORY LABELS 9, 23

▸ Phenoxymethylpenicillin (Non-proprietary)

Phenoxymethylpenicillin (as Phenoxymethylpenicillin potassium)
25 mg per 1 ml Phenoxymethylpenicillin 125mg/5ml oral solution |
100 ml [PoM] £34.00 DT = £4.97
Phenoxymethylpenicillin 125mg/5ml oral solution sugar free sugar-
free | 100 ml [PoM] £25.00 DT = £8.10
Phenoxymethylpenicillin (as Phenoxymethylpenicillin potassium)
50 mg per 1 ml Phenoxymethylpenicillin 250mg/5ml oral solution |
100 ml [PoM] £35.00 DT = £7.34
Phenoxymethylpenicillin 250mg/5ml oral solution sugar free sugar-
free | 100 ml [PoM] £35.00 DT = £7.99

Tablet

CAUTIONARY AND ADVISORY LABELS 9, 23

▸ Phenoxymethylpenicillin (Non-proprietary)

Phenoxymethylpenicillin (as Phenoxymethylpenicillin potassium)
250 mg Phenoxymethylpenicillin 250mg tablets | 28 tablet [PoM]
£5.00 DT = £0.71

ANTIBACTERIALS > PENICILLINS, BROAD-SPECTRUM

⌕ 536

Amoxicillin

(Amoxycillin)

● INDICATIONS AND DOSE

Susceptible infections (including urinary-tract infections, otitis media, sinusitis, uncomplicated community acquired pneumonia, salmonellosis, oral infections)

▸ BY MOUTH

▸ Child 1-11 months: 125 mg 3 times a day; increased if
necessary up to 30 mg/kg 3 times a day

▸ Child 1-4 years: 250 mg 3 times a day; increased if
necessary up to 30 mg/kg 3 times a day

▸ Child 5-11 years: 500 mg 3 times a day; increased if
necessary up to 30 mg/kg 3 times a day (max. per dose
1 g)

▸ Child 12-17 years: 500 mg 3 times a day; increased if
necessary up to 1 g 3 times a day, use increased dose in
severe infections

▸ Adult: 500 mg every 8 hours, increased if necessary to
1 g every 8 hours, increased dose used in severe
infections

▸ BY INTRAMUSCULAR INJECTION

▸ Adult: 500 mg every 8 hours

▸ BY INTRAVENOUS INJECTION, OR BY INTRAVENOUS INFUSION

▸ Adult: 500 mg every 8 hours, increased to 1 g every
6 hours, use increased dose in severe infections

Lyme disease (under expert supervision)

▸ BY MOUTH

▸ Child 5-17 years: 500 mg 3 times a day for 14-21 days
(for 28 days in Lyme arthritis)

▸ Adult: 500 mg 3 times a day for 14-21 days (for 28 days
in Lyme arthritis)

Anthrax (treatment and post-exposure prophylaxis)

▸ BY MOUTH

▸ Child (body-weight up to 20 kg): 80 mg/kg daily in
3 divided doses

▸ Child (body-weight 20 kg and above): 500 mg 3 times a
day

▸ Adult: 500 mg 3 times a day

Dental abscess (short course)

▸ BY MOUTH

▸ Adult: 3 g, then 3 g after 8 hours

Urinary-tract infections (short course)

▸ BY MOUTH

▸ Adult: 3 g, then 3 g after 10-12 hours

Listerial meningitis (in combination with another antibiotic)

▸ BY INTRAVENOUS INFUSION

▸ Adult: 2 g every 4 hours

Endocarditis (in combination with another antibiotic if necessary)

▸ BY INTRAVENOUS INFUSION

▸ Adult: 2 g every 4 hours

Prevention of pneumococcal infection in asplenia or in patients with sickle-cell disease—if cover also needed for *Haemophilus influenzae*

▸ BY MOUTH

▸ Child 1 month-4 years: 125 mg twice daily

▸ Child 5-11 years: 250 mg twice daily

▸ Child 12-17 years: 500 mg twice daily

***Helicobacter pylori* eradication in combination with metronidazole and omeprazole**

▸ BY MOUTH

▸ Adult: 500 mg 3 times a day

***Helicobacter pylori* eradication in combination with clarithromycin and esomeprazole; or in combination with clarithromycin and lansoprazole; or in combination with metronidazole and lansoprazole; or in combination with clarithromycin and omeprazole; or in combination with clarithromycin and pantoprazole; or in combination with clarithromycin and rabeprazole**

▸ BY MOUTH

▸ Adult: 1 g twice daily

● UNLICENSED USE Amoxicillin doses in BNF Publications
may differ from those in product literature.

● CAUTIONS

GENERAL CAUTIONS Acute lymphocytic leukaemia
(increased risk of erythematous rashes) · chronic
lymphocytic leukaemia (increased risk of erythematous
rashes) · cytomegalovirus infection (increased risk of
erythematous rashes) · glandular fever (erythematous
rashes common) · maintain adequate hydration with high
doses (particularly during parenteral therapy)

SPECIFIC CAUTIONS

▸ With intravenous use Accumulation of sodium can occur
with high parenteral doses

● INTERACTIONS → Appendix 1: penicillins

● SIDE-EFFECTS

GENERAL SIDE-EFFECTS

▸ **Rare or very rare** Acute generalised exanthematous
pustulosis (AGEP) · colitis haemorrhagic · crystalluria ·
dizziness · hyperkinesia · hypersensitivity vasculitis ·
mucocutaneous candidiasis

▸ **Frequency not known** Jarisch-Herxheimer reaction

SPECIFIC SIDE-EFFECTS

▸ **Rare or very rare**

▸ With oral use Black hairy tongue

● PREGNANCY Not known to be harmful.

● BREAST FEEDING Trace amount in milk, but appropriate to
use.

● RENAL IMPAIRMENT Risk of crystalluria with high doses
(particularly during parenteral therapy). Accumulation of
sodium from injection can occur in patients with renal
failure.

5

Infection

Dose adjustments Reduce dose in severe impairment; rashes more common.

- DIRECTIONS FOR ADMINISTRATION For *intravenous infusion* (*Amoxil®*), give intermittently *in* Glucose 5% *or* Sodium chloride 0.9%. Reconstituted solutions diluted and given without delay; suggested volume 100 mL given over 30–60 minutes or *give via* drip tubing *in* Glucose 5% *or* Sodium chloride 0.9%; continuous infusion not usually recommended.
- PRESCRIBING AND DISPENSING INFORMATION Flavours of oral liquid formulations and sachets may include peach, strawberry, or lemon.
- PATIENT AND CARER ADVICE Patient counselling is advised for Amoxicillin (*Amoxil®*) paediatric suspension (use of pipette).
  Medicines for Children leaflet: Amoxicillin for bacterial infections www.medicinesforchildren.org.uk/amoxicillin-bacterial-infections-0
- PROFESSION SPECIFIC INFORMATION

Dental practitioners' formulary
Amoxicillin capsules may be prescribed. Amoxicillin sachets may be prescribed as Amoxicillin Oral Powder. Amoxicillin Oral Suspension may be prescribed.

- MEDICINAL FORMS
  There can be variation in the licensing of different medicines containing the same drug.
  Powder for solution for injection
  ELECTROLYTES: May contain Sodium
  - Amoxicillin (Non-proprietary)
    Amoxicillin (as Amoxicillin sodium) 250 mg Amoxicillin 250mg powder for solution for injection vials | 10 vial [PoM] £4.50–£4.80
    Amoxicillin (as Amoxicillin sodium) 500 mg Amoxicillin 500mg powder for solution for injection vials | 10 vial [PoM] £9.60–£12.00 DT = £5.48
    Amoxicillin (as Amoxicillin sodium) 1 gram Amoxicillin 1g powder for solution for injection vials | 1 vial [PoM] £1.92 | 10 vial [PoM] £16.50 DT = £10.96
  - Amoxil (GlaxoSmithKline UK Ltd)
    Amoxicillin (as Amoxicillin sodium) 500 mg Amoxil 500mg powder for solution for injection vials | 10 vial [PoM] £5.48 DT = £5.48
    Amoxicillin (as Amoxicillin sodium) 1 gram Amoxil 1g powder for solution for injection vials | 10 vial [PoM] £10.96 DT = £10.96

Oral suspension
CAUTIONARY AND ADVISORY LABELS 9
EXCIPIENTS: May contain Sucrose
- Amoxicillin (Non-proprietary)
  Amoxicillin (as Amoxicillin trihydrate) 25 mg per 1 ml Amoxicillin 125mg/5ml oral suspension sugar free sugar-free | 100 ml [PoM] £25.00 DT = £0.99
  Amoxicillin 125mg/5ml oral suspension | 100 ml [PoM] £25.00 DT = £1.17
  Amoxicillin (as Amoxicillin trihydrate) 50 mg per 1 ml Amoxicillin 250mg/5ml oral suspension sugar free sugar-free | 100 ml [PoM] £35.00 DT = £1.24
  Amoxicillin 250mg/5ml oral suspension | 100 ml [PoM] £35.00 DT = £1.35
- Amoxil (GlaxoSmithKline UK Ltd)
  Amoxicillin (as Amoxicillin trihydrate) 100 mg per 1 ml Amoxil 125mg/1.25ml paediatric oral suspension | 20 ml [PoM] £3.18 DT = £3.18

Powder
CAUTIONARY AND ADVISORY LABELS 9, 13
- Amoxicillin (Non-proprietary)
  Amoxicillin (as Amoxicillin trihydrate) 3 gram Amoxicillin 3g oral powder sachets sugar free sugar-free | 2 sachet [PoM] £15.00 DT = £9.98

Capsule
CAUTIONARY AND ADVISORY LABELS 9
- Amoxicillin (Non-proprietary)
  Amoxicillin (as Amoxicillin trihydrate) 250 mg Amoxicillin 250mg capsules | 15 capsule [PoM] £5.00 DT = £0.43 | 21 capsule [PoM] £8.99 DT = £0.60 | 500 capsule [PoM] £14.29–£120.00
  Amoxicillin (as Amoxicillin trihydrate) 500 mg Amoxicillin 500mg capsules | 15 capsule [PoM] £7.50 DT = £0.56 | 21 capsule [PoM] £15.00 DT = £0.78 | 100 capsule [PoM] £3.71–£75.00

- Amoxil (GlaxoSmithKline UK Ltd)
  Amoxicillin (as Amoxicillin trihydrate) 250 mg Amoxil 250mg capsules | 21 capsule [PoM] £0.92 DT = £0.60
  Amoxicillin (as Amoxicillin trihydrate) 500 mg Amoxil 500mg capsules | 21 capsule [PoM] £0.89 DT = £0.78

Combinations available: *Co-amoxiclav*, p. 542

⟩ 536

Ampicillin

- INDICATIONS AND DOSE

Susceptible infections (including bronchitis, urinary-tract infections, otitis media, sinusitis, uncomplicated community-acquired pneumonia, salmonellosis)
▸ BY MOUTH
▸ Child 1–11 months: 125 mg 4 times a day; increased if necessary up to 30 mg/kg 4 times a day
▸ Child 1–4 years: 250 mg 4 times a day; increased if necessary up to 30 mg/kg 4 times a day
▸ Child 5–11 years: 500 mg 4 times a day; increased if necessary up to 30 mg/kg 4 times a day (max. per dose 1 g)
▸ Child 12–17 years: 500 mg 4 times a day; increased if necessary to 1 g 4 times a day, use increased dose in severe infection
▸ Adult: 0.5–1 g every 6 hours
▸ BY INTRAVENOUS INJECTION, OR BY INTRAVENOUS INFUSION
▸ Adult: 500 mg every 4–6 hours
▸ BY INTRAMUSCULAR INJECTION
▸ Adult: 500 mg every 4–6 hours

Endocarditis (in combination with another antibiotic if necessary) | Listerial meningitis (in combination with another antibiotic)
▸ BY INTRAVENOUS INFUSION
▸ Adult: 2 g every 4 hours

- UNLICENSED USE Ampicillin doses in BNF may differ from those in product literature.
- CAUTIONS
  GENERAL CAUTIONS Acute lymphocytic leukaemia (increased risk of erythematous rashes) · chronic lymphocytic leukaemia (increased risk of erythematous rashes) · cytomegalovirus infection (increased risk of erythematous rashes) · glandular fever (erythematous rashes common)
  SPECIFIC CAUTIONS
  - With intravenous use Accumulation of electrolytes contained in parenteral preparations can occur with high doses
- INTERACTIONS → Appendix 1: penicillins
- SIDE-EFFECTS Colitis haemorrhagic · purpura
- PREGNANCY Not known to be harmful.
- BREAST FEEDING Trace amounts in milk, but appropriate to use.
- RENAL IMPAIRMENT Accumulation of electrolytes contained in parenteral preparations can occur in patients with renal failure.
  Dose adjustments ▸ In adults Reduce dose if eGFR less than 10 mL/minute/1.73 m²; rashes more common.
  ▸ In children If estimated glomerular filtration rate less than 10 mL/minute/1.73 m² reduce dose or frequency; rashes more common.
- DIRECTIONS FOR ADMINISTRATION
  - With oral use Administer at least 30 minutes before food.
  - With intravenous use For *intravenous infusion* (*Penbritin®*), give intermittently *in* Glucose 5% *or* Sodium chloride 0.9%. Reconstituted solutions diluted and given without delay; suggested volume 100 mL given over 30–60 minutes *via* drip tubing *in* Glucose 5% *or* Sodium chloride 0.9%. Continuous infusion not usually recommended.

● PATIENT AND CARER ADVICE
Medicines for Children leaflet: Ampicillin for bacterial
infection www.medicinesforchildren.org.uk/ampicillin-
bacterial-infection

● MEDICINAL FORMS
There can be variation in the licensing of different medicines
containing the same drug.

Oral suspension
CAUTIONARY AND ADVISORY LABELS 9, 23
▸ Ampicillin (Non-proprietary)
　Ampicillin 25 mg per 1 ml Ampicillin 125mg/5ml oral suspension |
　100 ml [PoM] £29.86 DT = £29.86
　Ampicillin 50 mg per 1 ml Ampicillin 250mg/5ml oral suspension |
　100 ml [PoM] £38.86 DT = £38.86

Capsule
CAUTIONARY AND ADVISORY LABELS 9, 23
▸ Ampicillin (Non-proprietary)
　Ampicillin 250 mg Ampicillin 250mg capsules | 28 capsule [PoM]
　£20.50 DT = £20.50
　Ampicillin 500 mg Ampicillin 500mg capsules | 28 capsule [PoM]
　£40.30 DT = £40.30

Powder for solution for injection
▸ Ampicillin (Non-proprietary)
　Ampicillin (as Ampicillin sodium) 500 mg Ampicillin 500mg
　powder for solution for injection vials | 10 vial [PoM] £78.30 DT =
　£78.30

⚑ 536

Co-fluampicil

● INDICATIONS AND DOSE

**Mixed infections involving beta-lactamase-producing
staphylococci**
▸ BY MOUTH
　▸ Child 1 month-9 years: 125/125 mg every 6 hours
　▸ Child 10-17 years: 250/250 mg every 6 hours
　▸ Adult: 250/250 mg every 6 hours
▸ BY INTRAMUSCULAR INJECTION, OR BY SLOW INTRAVENOUS
　INJECTION, OR BY INTRAVENOUS INFUSION
　▸ Adult: 250/250 mg every 6 hours

**Severe mixed infections involving beta-lactamase-
producing staphylococci**
▸ BY MOUTH
　▸ Child 1 month-9 years: 250/250 mg every 6 hours
　▸ Adult: 500/500 mg every 6 hours
▸ BY INTRAMUSCULAR INJECTION, OR BY SLOW INTRAVENOUS
　INJECTION, OR BY INTRAVENOUS INFUSION
　▸ Adult: 500/500 mg every 6 hours

IMPORTANT SAFETY INFORMATION
HEPATIC DISORDERS
Cholestatic jaundice and hepatitis may occur very rarely,
up to two months after treatment with flucloxacillin has
been stopped. Administration for more than 2 weeks and
increasing age are risk factors. Healthcare professionals
are reminded that:
● flucloxacillin should not be used in patients with a
　history of hepatic dysfunction associated with
　flucloxacillin;
● flucloxacillin should be used with caution in patients
　with hepatic impairment;
● careful enquiry should be made about hypersensitivity
　reactions to beta-lactam antibacterials.

● CAUTIONS
GENERAL CAUTIONS Acute lymphocytic leukaemia
(increased risk of erythematous rashes) · chronic
lymphocytic leukaemia (increased risk of erythematous
rashes) · cytomegalovirus infection (increased risk of
erythematous rashes) · glandular fever (erythematous
rashes common)

SPECIFIC CAUTIONS
▸ With intravenous use Accumulation of electrolytes
contained in parenteral preparations can occur with high
doses

● INTERACTIONS → Appendix 1: penicillins

● SIDE-EFFECTS Arthralgia · bronchospasm · coma ·
dyspnoea · electrolyte imbalance · eosinophilia · erythema
nodosum · gastrointestinal disorder · hallucination ·
Jarisch-Herxheimer reaction · myalgia · purpura non-
thrombocytopenic · vasculitis

● PREGNANCY Not known to be harmful.

● BREAST FEEDING Trace amount in milk, but appropriate to
use.

● HEPATIC IMPAIRMENT Use with caution.

● RENAL IMPAIRMENT Accumulation of electrolytes
contained in parenteral preparations can occur in patients
with renal failure.
Dose adjustments ▸ In adults Reduce dose if eGFR less than
$10 \, mL/minute/1.73 \, m^2$; rashes more common.
▸ In children Reduce dose or frequency if estimated
glomerular filtration rate less than $10 \, mL/minute/1.73 \, m^2$;
rashes more common.

● EFFECT ON LABORATORY TESTS False-positive urinary
glucose (if tested for reducing substances).

● DIRECTIONS FOR ADMINISTRATION For *intravenous infusion*
(*Magnapen®*), give intermittently *in* Glucose 5% *or* Sodium
chloride 0.9%. Reconstituted solutions diluted and given
without delay; suggested volume 100 mL given over
30-60 minutes. *Via* drip tubing *in* Glucose 5% *or* Sodium
chloride 0.9%.

● PRESCRIBING AND DISPENSING INFORMATION Dose
expressed as a combination of equal parts by mass of
flucloxacillin and ampicillin.

● MEDICINAL FORMS
There can be variation in the licensing of different medicines
containing the same drug.

Oral suspension
CAUTIONARY AND ADVISORY LABELS 9, 22
▸ Co-fluampicil (Non-proprietary)
　**Ampicillin (as Ampicillin trihydrate) 25 mg per 1 ml, Flucloxacillin
　(as Flucloxacillin magnesium) 25 mg per 1 ml** Co-fluampicil
　125mg/125mg/5ml oral suspension | 100 ml [PoM] £23.93 DT =
　£23.93

Powder for solution for injection
ELECTROLYTES: May contain Sodium
▸ Co-fluampicil (Non-proprietary)
　**Ampicillin (as Ampicillin sodium) 250 mg, Flucloxacillin (as
　Flucloxacillin sodium) 250 mg** Co-fluampicil 250mg/250mg powder
　for solution for injection vials | 10 vial [PoM] £13.33

Capsule
CAUTIONARY AND ADVISORY LABELS 9, 22
▸ Co-fluampicil (Non-proprietary)
　**Ampicillin (as Ampicillin trihydrate) 250 mg, Flucloxacillin (as
　Flucloxacillin sodium) 250 mg** Co-fluampicil 250mg/250mg
　capsules | 28 capsule [PoM] £2.27 DT = £1.97 | 100 capsule [PoM]
　£8.11

ANTIBACTERIALS > PENICILLINS, BROAD-SPECTRUM WITH BETA-LACTAMASE INHIBITOR

⟋ 536

Co-amoxiclav

● INDICATIONS AND DOSE

Infections due to beta-lactamase-producing strains (where amoxicillin alone not appropriate), including respiratory tract infections, bone and joint infections, genito-urinary and abdominal infections, cellulitis and animal bites
▸ BY MOUTH USING TABLETS
▸ Child 12–17 years: 250/125 mg every 8 hours; increased to 500/125 mg every 8 hours, increased dose used for severe infection
▸ Adult: 250/125 mg every 8 hours; increased to 500/125 mg every 8 hours, increased dose used for severe infection
▸ BY INTRAVENOUS INJECTION, OR BY INTRAVENOUS INFUSION
▸ Child 1–2 months: 30 mg/kg every 12 hours
▸ Child 3 months–17 years: 30 mg/kg every 8 hours (max. per dose 1.2 g every 8 hours)
▸ Adult: 1.2 g every 8 hours

Infections due to beta-lactamase-producing strains (where amoxicillin alone not appropriate) including respiratory-tract infections, bone and joint infections, genito-urinary and abdominal infections, cellulitis, animal bites (doses for 125/31 suspension)
▸ BY MOUTH USING ORAL SUSPENSION
▸ Child 1–11 months: 0.25 mL/kilogram 3 times a day, dose doubled in severe infection
▸ Child 1–5 years: 0.25 mL/kilogram 3 times a day, alternatively 5 mL 3 times a day, dose doubled in severe infection

Infections due to beta-lactamase-producing strains (where amoxicillin alone not appropriate) including respiratory-tract infections, bone and joint infections, genito-urinary and abdominal infections, cellulitis, animal bites (doses for 250/62 suspension)
▸ BY MOUTH USING ORAL SUSPENSION
▸ Child 6–11 years: 0.15 mL/kilogram 3 times a day, alternatively 5 mL 3 times a day, dose doubled in severe infection

Infections due to beta-lactamase-producing strains (where amoxicillin alone not appropriate) including respiratory-tract infections, bone and joint infections, genito-urinary and abdominal infections, cellulitis, animal bites (doses for 400/57 suspension)
▸ BY MOUTH USING ORAL SUSPENSION
▸ Child 2 months–1 year: 0.15 mL/kilogram twice daily, doubled in severe infection
▸ Child 2–6 years (body-weight 13–21 kg): 2.5 mL twice daily, doubled in severe infection
▸ Child 7–12 years (body-weight 22–40 kg): 5 mL twice daily, doubled in severe infection
▸ Child 12–17 years (body-weight 41 kg and above): 10 mL twice daily; increased if necessary to 10 mL 3 times a day, increased frequency to be used in severe infection
▸ Adult: 10 mL twice daily; increased if necessary to 10 mL 3 times a day, increased frequency to be used in severe infection

Severe dental infection with spreading cellulitis | Dental infection not responding to first-line antibacterial
▸ BY MOUTH USING TABLETS
▸ Child 12–17 years: 250/125 mg every 8 hours for 5 days
▸ Adult: 250/125 mg every 8 hours for 5 days

Surgical prophylaxis
▸ BY INTRAVENOUS INJECTION, OR BY INTRAVENOUS INFUSION
▸ Adult: 1.2 g, to be administered up to 30 minutes before the procedure, then 1.2 g every 8 hours for up to 2–3 further doses in high risk procedures

Acute sinusitis (doses for 125/31 suspension)
▸ BY MOUTH USING ORAL SUSPENSION
▸ Child 1–11 months: 0.25 mL/kilogram 3 times a day for 5 days
▸ Child 1–5 years: 5 mL 3 times a day for 5 days, alternatively 0.25 mL/kilogram 3 times a day for 5 days

Acute sinusitis (doses for 250/62 suspension)
▸ BY MOUTH USING ORAL SUSPENSION
▸ Child 6–11 years: 5 mL 3 times a day for 5 days, alternatively 0.15 mL/kilogram 3 times a day for 5 days

Acute sinusitis
▸ BY MOUTH
▸ Child 12–17 years: 250/125 mg 3 times a day for 5 days, alternatively 500/125 mg 3 times a day for 5 days
▸ Adult: 500/125 mg 3 times a day for 5 days

DOSE EQUIVALENCE AND CONVERSION
▸ Doses are expressed as co-amoxiclav.
▸ A mixture of amoxicillin (as the trihydrate or as the sodium salt) and clavulanic acid (as potassium clavulanate); the proportions are expressed in the form x/y where x and y are the strengths in milligrams of amoxicillin and clavulanic acid respectively.

● UNLICENSED USE EvGr Doses and duration of treatment for acute sinusitis in BNF Publications differ from product literature and adhere to national guidelines. ⒶSee Sinusitis (acute) p. 1168 for further information.
● CONTRA-INDICATIONS History of co-amoxiclav-associated jaundice or hepatic dysfunction · history of penicillin-associated jaundice or hepatic dysfunction
● CAUTIONS
GENERAL CAUTIONS Acute lymphocytic leukaemia (increased risk of erythematous rashes) · chronic lymphocytic leukaemia (increased risk of erythematous rashes) · cytomegalovirus infection (increased risk of erythematous rashes) · glandular fever (erythematous rashes common) · maintain adequate hydration with high doses (particularly during parental therapy)
SPECIFIC CAUTIONS
▸ With intravenous use Accumulation of electrolytes contained in parenteral preparations can occur with high doses
CAUTIONS, FURTHER INFORMATION
▸ Cholestatic jaundice Cholestatic jaundice can occur either during or shortly after the use of co-amoxiclav. An epidemiological study has shown that the risk of acute liver toxicity was about 6 times greater with co-amoxiclav than with amoxicillin. Cholestatic jaundice is more common in patients above the age of 65 years and in men; these reactions have only rarely been reported in children. Jaundice is usually self-limiting and very rarely fatal. The duration of treatment should be appropriate to the indication and should not usually exceed 14 days.
● INTERACTIONS → Appendix 1: clavulanic acid · penicillins
● SIDE-EFFECTS
GENERAL SIDE-EFFECTS
▸ Common or very common Increased risk of infection
▸ Uncommon Dizziness · dyspepsia · headache
▸ Frequency not known Acute generalised exanthematous pustulosis (AGEP) · colitis haemorrhagic · crystalluria · hypersensitivity vasculitis · meningitis aseptic
SPECIFIC SIDE-EFFECTS
▸ With oral use Akathisia · black hairy tongue
● PREGNANCY Not known to be harmful.

- **BREAST FEEDING** Trace amount in milk, but appropriate to use.
- **HEPATIC IMPAIRMENT**
  Monitoring Monitor liver function in liver disease.
- **RENAL IMPAIRMENT** Risk of crystalluria with high doses (particularly during parenteral therapy).
  ‣ With intravenous use Accumulation of electrolytes contained in parenteral preparations can occur in patients with renal failure.
  Dose adjustments ‣ With oral use in adults *Co-amoxiclav 250/125 tablets or 500/125 tablets*: if eGFR 10–30 mL/minute/1.73 m², one 250/125 strength tablet every 12 hours or one 500/125 strength tablet every 12 hours; if eGFR less than 10 mL/minute/1.73 m², one 250/125 strength tablet every 24 hours or one 500/125 strength tablet every 24 hours.
  Co-amoxiclav 400/57 suspension: avoid if eGFR less than 30 mL/minute/1.73 m².
  ‣ With intravenous use in adults *Co-amoxiclav injection* (expressed as co-amoxiclav): if eGFR 10–30 mL/minute/1.73 m², 1.2 g initially, then 600 mg every 12 hours; if eGFR less than 10 mL/minute/1.73 m², 1.2 g initially, then 600 mg every 24 hours.
  ‣ With oral use in children *Co-amoxiclav 125/31 suspension, 250/62 suspension, 250/125 tablets, or 500/125 tablets*: use normal dose every 12 hours if estimated glomerular filtration rate 10–30 mL/minute/1.73 m². Use the normal dose recommended for mild or moderate infections every 12 hours if estimated glomerular filtration rate less than 10 mL/minute/1.73 m².
  Co-amoxiclav 400/57 suspension: avoid if estimated glomerular filtration rate less than 30 mL/minute/1.73 m².
  ‣ With intravenous use in children *Co-amoxiclav injection*: use normal initial dose and then use half normal dose every 12 hours if estimated glomerular filtration rate 10–30 mL/minute/1.73 m²; use normal initial dose and then use half normal dose every 24 hours if estimated glomerular filtration rate less than 10 mL/minute/1.73 m².
- **DIRECTIONS FOR ADMINISTRATION**
  ‣ With intravenous use in children For *intravenous infusion*, dilute reconstituted solution to a concentration of 10 mg/mL with Sodium Chloride 0.9%; give intermittently over 30–40 minutes. For *intravenous injection*, administer over 3–4 minutes.
  ‣ With intravenous use in adults For *intravenous infusion* (*Augmentin®*), give intermittently in Sodium chloride 0.9%. Reconstitute 600 mg initially with 10 mL water for injections, then dilute with 50 mL infusion fluid; reconstitute 1.2 g initially with 20 mL water for injections, then dilute with 100 mL infusion fluid; give over 30–40 minutes. For *intravenous injection*, administer over 3–4 minutes. *Via* drip tubing *in* Sodium chloride 0.9%.
- **PRESCRIBING AND DISPENSING INFORMATION** Doses are expressed as co-amoxiclav: a mixture of amoxicillin (as the trihydrate or as the sodium salt) and clavulanic acid (as potassium clavulanate); the proportions are expressed in the form x/y where x and y are the strengths in milligrams of amoxicillin and clavulanic acid respectively.
  ‣ With oral use Flavours of oral liquid formulations may include raspberry and orange.
- **PATIENT AND CARER ADVICE**
  Medicines for Children leaflet: Co-amoxiclav for bacterial infections www.medicinesforchildren.org.uk/co-amoxiclav-bacterial-infections-0
- **PROFESSION SPECIFIC INFORMATION**
  Dental practitioners' formulary
  Co-amoxiclav 250/125 Tablets may be prescribed.
  Co-amoxiclav 125/31 Suspension may be prescribed.
  Co-amoxiclav 250/62 Suspension may be prescribed.

- **MEDICINAL FORMS**
  There can be variation in the licensing of different medicines containing the same drug. Forms available from special-order manufacturers include: infusion

Oral suspension
CAUTIONARY AND ADVISORY LABELS 9
EXCIPIENTS: May contain Aspartame
‣ Co-amoxiclav (Non-proprietary)
  Clavulanic acid (as Potassium clavulanate) 6.25 mg per 1 ml, Amoxicillin (as Amoxicillin trihydrate) 25 mg per 1 ml Co-amoxiclav 125mg/31mg/5ml oral suspension | 100 ml PoM £5.00 DT = £5.00
  Co-amoxiclav 125mg/31mg/5ml oral suspension sugar free sugar-free | 100 ml PoM £1.95 DT = £1.95
  Clavulanic acid (as Potassium clavulanate) 12.5 mg per 1 ml, Amoxicillin (as Amoxicillin trihydrate) 50 mg per 1 ml Co-amoxiclav 250mg/62mg/5ml oral suspension | 100 ml PoM £5.00 DT = £5.00
  Co-amoxiclav 250mg/62mg/5ml oral suspension sugar free sugar-free | 100 ml PoM £1.68 DT = £1.51
  Clavulanic acid (as Potassium clavulanate) 11.4 mg per 1 ml, Amoxicillin (as Amoxicillin trihydrate) 80 mg per 1 ml Co-amoxiclav 400mg/57mg/5ml oral suspension sugar free sugar-free | 35 ml PoM £4.13 DT = £4.13 sugar-free | 70 ml PoM £6.97 DT = £5.79
‣ Augmentin (GlaxoSmithKline UK Ltd)
  Clavulanic acid (as Potassium clavulanate) 6.25 mg per 1 ml, Amoxicillin (as Amoxicillin trihydrate) 25 mg per 1 ml Augmentin 125/31 SF oral suspension sugar-free | 100 ml PoM £3.54 DT = £1.95
  Clavulanic acid (as Potassium clavulanate) 12.5 mg per 1 ml, Amoxicillin (as Amoxicillin trihydrate) 50 mg per 1 ml Augmentin 250/62 SF oral suspension sugar-free | 100 ml PoM £3.60 DT = £1.51
‣ Augmentin-Duo (GlaxoSmithKline UK Ltd)
  Clavulanic acid (as Potassium clavulanate) 11.4 mg per 1 ml, Amoxicillin (as Amoxicillin trihydrate) 80 mg per 1 ml Augmentin-Duo 400/57 oral suspension sugar-free | 35 ml PoM £4.13 DT = £4.13 sugar-free | 70 ml PoM £5.79 DT = £5.79

Tablet
CAUTIONARY AND ADVISORY LABELS 9
‣ Co-amoxiclav (Non-proprietary)
  Clavulanic acid (as Potassium clavulanate) 125 mg, Amoxicillin (as Amoxicillin trihydrate) 250 mg Co-amoxiclav 250mg/125mg tablets | 21 tablet PoM £6.00 DT = £1.67
  Clavulanic acid (as Potassium clavulanate) 125 mg, Amoxicillin (as Amoxicillin trihydrate) 500 mg Co-amoxiclav 500mg/125mg tablets | 21 tablet PoM £15.00 DT = £1.84
  Clavulanic acid (as Potassium clavulanate) 125 mg, Amoxicillin (as Amoxicillin trihydrate) 875 mg Co-amoxiclav 875mg/125mg tablets | 14 tablet PoM £18.00 DT = £18.00
‣ Augmentin (GlaxoSmithKline UK Ltd)
  Clavulanic acid (as Potassium clavulanate) 125 mg, Amoxicillin (as Amoxicillin trihydrate) 250 mg Augmentin 375mg tablets | 21 tablet PoM £5.03 DT = £1.67
  Clavulanic acid (as Potassium clavulanate) 125 mg, Amoxicillin (as Amoxicillin trihydrate) 500 mg Augmentin 625mg tablets | 21 tablet PoM £9.60 DT = £1.84

Powder for solution for injection
ELECTROLYTES: May contain Potassium, sodium
‣ Co-amoxiclav (Non-proprietary)
  Clavulanic acid (as Potassium clavulanate) 100 mg, Amoxicillin (as Amoxicillin sodium) 500 mg Co-amoxiclav 500mg/100mg powder for solution for injection vials | 10 vial PoM £13.50–£14.90
  Clavulanic acid (as Potassium clavulanate) 200 mg, Amoxicillin (as Amoxicillin sodium) 1000 mg Co-amoxiclav 1000mg/200mg powder for solution for injection vials | 10 vial PoM £27.50–£29.70
‣ Augmentin Intravenous (GlaxoSmithKline UK Ltd)
  Clavulanic acid (as Potassium clavulanate) 100 mg, Amoxicillin (as Amoxicillin sodium) 500 mg Augmentin Intravenous 600mg powder for solution for injection vials | 10 vial PoM £10.60
  Clavulanic acid (as Potassium clavulanate) 200 mg, Amoxicillin (as Amoxicillin sodium) 1000 mg Augmentin Intravenous 1.2g powder for solution for injection vials | 10 vial PoM £10.60

⊩ 536

ANTIBACTERIALS ⟩ PENICILLINS, MECILLINAM-TYPE

Pivmecillinam hydrochloride

● **INDICATIONS AND DOSE**

Acute uncomplicated cystitis
▶ BY MOUTH
▶ Child (body-weight 40 kg and above): Initially 400 mg for 1 dose, then 200 mg every 8 hours for 3 days
▶ Adult (body-weight 40 kg and above): Initially 400 mg for 1 dose, then 200 mg every 8 hours for 3 days

Chronic or recurrent bacteriuria
▶ BY MOUTH
▶ Child (body-weight 40 kg and above): 400 mg every 6–8 hours
▶ Adult (body-weight 40 kg and above): 400 mg every 6–8 hours

Urinary-tract infections
▶ BY MOUTH
▶ Child (body-weight up to 40 kg): 5–10 mg/kg every 6 hours, alternatively 20–40 mg/kg daily in 3 divided doses

● **UNLICENSED USE** Not licensed for use in children under 3 months.
● **CONTRA-INDICATIONS** Carnitine deficiency · gastrointestinal obstruction · infants under 3 months · oesophageal strictures
● **CAUTIONS** Avoid in Acute porphyrias p. 1025
● **INTERACTIONS** → Appendix 1: penicillins
● **SIDE-EFFECTS**
▶ **Common or very common** Vulvovaginal fungal infection
▶ **Uncommon** Dizziness · fatigue · gastrointestinal discomfort · gastrointestinal disorders · headache · hepatic function abnormal · oral ulceration · vertigo
● **PREGNANCY** Not known to be harmful, but manufacturer advises avoid.
● **BREAST FEEDING** Trace amount in milk, but appropriate to use.
● **MONITORING REQUIREMENTS** Liver and renal function tests required in long-term use.
● **EFFECT ON LABORATORY TESTS** False-positive urinary glucose (if tested for reducing substances).
● **DIRECTIONS FOR ADMINISTRATION** Tablets should be swallowed whole with plenty of fluid during meals while sitting or standing.
● **PATIENT AND CARER ADVICE** Patient counselling is advised on administration of pivmecillinam hydrochloride tablets (posture).

● **MEDICINAL FORMS** There can be variation in the licensing of different medicines containing the same drug.

Tablet
CAUTIONARY AND ADVISORY LABELS 9, 21, 27
▶ Pivmecillinam hydrochloride (Non-proprietary)
Pivmecillinam hydrochloride 200 mg Pivmecillinam 200mg tablets | 10 tablet [PoM] £5.40 DT = £5.40
▶ Selexid (LEO Pharma)
Pivmecillinam hydrochloride 200 mg Selexid 200mg tablets | 10 tablet [PoM] £5.40 DT = £5.40 | 18 tablet [PoM] £9.72

ANTIBACTERIALS ⟩ PENICILLINS, PENICILLINASE-RESISTANT

Flucloxacillin

● **INDICATIONS AND DOSE**

Infections due to beta-lactamase-producing staphylococci including otitis externa | Adjunct in pneumonia | Adjunct in impetigo | Adjunct in cellulitis
▶ BY MOUTH
▶ Child 1 month-1 year: 62.5–125 mg 4 times a day
▶ Child 2–9 years: 125–250 mg 4 times a day
▶ Child 10–17 years: 250–500 mg 4 times a day
▶ Adult: 250–500 mg 4 times a day
▶ BY INTRAMUSCULAR INJECTION
▶ Adult: 250–500 mg every 6 hours
▶ BY SLOW INTRAVENOUS INJECTION, OR BY INTRAVENOUS INFUSION
▶ Adult: 0.25–2 g every 6 hours

Endocarditis (in combination with other antibacterial if necessary)
▶ BY SLOW INTRAVENOUS INJECTION, OR BY INTRAVENOUS INFUSION
▶ Adult (body-weight up to 85 kg): 8 g daily in 4 divided doses
▶ Adult (body-weight 85 kg and above): 12 g daily in 6 divided doses

Osteomyelitis
▶ BY SLOW INTRAVENOUS INJECTION, OR BY INTRAVENOUS INFUSION
▶ Adult: Up to 8 g daily in 3–4 divided doses

Surgical prophylaxis
▶ INITIALLY BY SLOW INTRAVENOUS INJECTION, OR BY INTRAVENOUS INFUSION
▶ Adult: 1–2 g, to be administered up to 30 minutes before the procedure, then (by mouth or by intramuscular injection or by slow intravenous injection or by intravenous infusion) 500 mg every 6 hours if required for up to 4 further doses in high risk procedures

Staphylococcal lung infection in cystic fibrosis
▶ BY MOUTH
▶ Child: 25 mg/kg 4 times a day (max. per dose 1 g), alternatively 100 mg/kg daily in 3 divided doses; maximum 4 g per day

Prevention of *Staphylococcus aureus* lung infection in cystic fibrosis—primary prevention
▶ BY MOUTH
▶ Child 1 month-3 years: 125 mg twice daily

Prevention of *Staphylococcus aureus* lung infection in cystic fibrosis—secondary prevention
▶ BY MOUTH
▶ Child: 50 mg/kg twice daily (max. per dose 1 g twice daily)

● **UNLICENSED USE** Flucloxacillin doses in the BNF may differ from those in product literature.

IMPORTANT SAFETY INFORMATION
HEPATIC DISORDERS
Cholestatic jaundice and hepatitis may occur very rarely, up to two months after treatment with flucloxacillin has been stopped. Administration for more than 2 weeks and increasing age are risk factors. Healthcare professionals are reminded that:
● flucloxacillin should not be used in patients with a history of hepatic dysfunction associated with flucloxacillin
● flucloxacillin should be used with caution in patients with hepatic impairment

- careful enquiry should be made about hypersensitivity reactions to beta-lactam antibacterials

- CAUTIONS
▶ With intravenous use Accumulation of electrolytes can occur with high doses
- INTERACTIONS → Appendix 1: penicillins
- SIDE-EFFECTS
GENERAL SIDE-EFFECTS
▶ Rare or very rare Arthralgia · fever
SPECIFIC SIDE-EFFECTS
▶ Common or very common
▶ With oral use Gastrointestinal disorder
▶ Uncommon
▶ With oral use Purpura
▶ Rare or very rare
▶ With oral use Eosinophilia · myalgia
▶ Frequency not known
▶ With parenteral use Acute generalised exanthematous pustulosis (AGEP) · bronchospasm · bullous pemphigoid · coma · dyspnoea · electrolyte imbalance · erythema nodosum · hallucination · Jarisch-Herxheimer reaction · nephropathy · neurotoxicity · oral candidiasis · platelet dysfunction · purpura non-thrombocytopenic · vasculitis
- PREGNANCY Not known to be harmful.
- BREAST FEEDING Trace amounts in milk, but appropriate to use.
- HEPATIC IMPAIRMENT Use with caution.
- RENAL IMPAIRMENT
▶ With intravenous use Accumulation of electrolytes can occur in patients with renal failure.
Dose adjustments ▶ In adults Reduce dose if eGFR less than 10 mL/minute/1.73 m^2.
▶ In children Use normal dose every 8 hours if estimated glomerular filtration rate less than 10 mL/minute/1.73 m^2.
- EFFECT ON LABORATORY TESTS False-positive urinary glucose (if tested for reducing substances).
- DIRECTIONS FOR ADMINISTRATION For *intravenous infusion* (*Floxapen*®), give intermittently *in* Glucose 5% *or* Sodium chloride 0.9%; suggested volume 100 mL given over 30–60 minutes. *Via* drip tubing *in* Glucose 5% *or* Sodium chloride 0.9%; continuous infusion not usually recommended.
- PATIENT AND CARER ADVICE
Medicines for Children leaflet: Flucloxacillin for bacterial infections www.medicinesforchildren.org.uk/flucloxacillin-for-bacterial-infections

- MEDICINAL FORMS
There can be variation in the licensing of different medicines containing the same drug. Forms available from special-order manufacturers include: infusion
Oral solution
CAUTIONARY AND ADVISORY LABELS 9, 23
▶ Flucloxacillin (Non-proprietary)
Flucloxacillin (as Flucloxacillin sodium) 25 mg per 1 ml Flucloxacillin 125mg/5ml oral solution | 100 ml [PoM] £20.99 DT = £6.93
Flucloxacillin 125mg/5ml oral solution sugar free sugar-free | 100 ml [PoM] £30.08 DT = £23.26
Flucloxacillin (as Flucloxacillin sodium) 50 mg per 1 ml Flucloxacillin 250mg/5ml oral solution sugar free sugar-free | 100 ml [PoM] £36.27 DT = £27.88
Flucloxacillin 250mg/5ml oral solution | 100 ml [PoM] £30.22 DT = £28.44
Capsule
CAUTIONARY AND ADVISORY LABELS 9, 23
▶ Flucloxacillin (Non-proprietary)
Flucloxacillin (as Flucloxacillin sodium) 250 mg Flucloxacillin 250mg capsules | 20 capsule [PoM] £3.58 | 28 capsule [PoM] £5.00 DT = £1.11 | 100 capsule [PoM] £3.96–£17.80

Flucloxacillin (as Flucloxacillin sodium) 500 mg Flucloxacillin 500mg capsules | 20 capsule [PoM] £7.50 | 28 capsule [PoM] £10.50 DT = £1.94 | 100 capsule [PoM] £6.93–£37.50
Powder for solution for injection
▶ Flucloxacillin (Non-proprietary)
Flucloxacillin (as Flucloxacillin sodium) 250 mg Flucloxacillin 250mg powder for solution for injection vials | 10 vial [PoM] £8.60–£12.25
Flucloxacillin (as Flucloxacillin sodium) 500 mg Flucloxacillin 500mg powder for solution for injection vials | 10 vial [PoM] £17.20–£24.50
Flucloxacillin (as Flucloxacillin sodium) 1 gram Flucloxacillin 1g powder for solution for injection vials | 10 vial [PoM] £34.50–£49.00
Flucloxacillin (as Flucloxacillin sodium) 2 gram Flucloxacillin 2g powder for solution for injection vials | 1 vial [PoM] £6.00

Combinations available: *Co-fluampicil*, p. 541

F 536

Temocillin

29-May-2018

- INDICATIONS AND DOSE

Septicaemia | Urinary-tract infections | Lower respiratory-tract infections caused by susceptible Gram-negative bacteria
▶ BY INTRAMUSCULAR INJECTION, OR BY SLOW INTRAVENOUS INJECTION, OR BY INTRAVENOUS INFUSION
▶ Adult: 2 g every 12 hours, alternatively 2 g every 8 hours, higher daily dose to be used in critically ill patients
▶ BY CONTINUOUS INTRAVENOUS INFUSION
▶ Adult: (consult product literature)

- CAUTIONS Accumulation of sodium from injection can occur with high doses
- INTERACTIONS → Appendix 1: penicillins
- SIDE-EFFECTS Arthralgia · fever · myalgia · nervous system disorder
- PREGNANCY Not known to be harmful.
- BREAST FEEDING Trace amounts in milk.
- RENAL IMPAIRMENT Accumulation of sodium from injection can occur in patients with renal failure.
Dose adjustments Manufacturer advises reduce usual dose to 1 g every 12 hours if creatinine clearance 30–60 mL/minute; reduce usual dose to 1 g every 24 hours if creatinine clearance 10–30 mL/minute; reduce usual dose to 1 g every 48 hours *or* 500 mg every 24 hours if creatinine clearance less than 10 mL/minute; no information available to recommend dose adjustments with higher daily dose for use in critically ill patients.
- EFFECT ON LABORATORY TESTS False-positive urinary glucose (if tested for reducing substances).
- DIRECTIONS FOR ADMINISTRATION Manufacturer advises for *intramuscular injection*, reconstitute 1 g with 2 mL water for injections *or* Sodium chloride 0.9% (*or* 0.5 or 1% lidocaine solution, if pain is experienced at injection site). Manufacturer advises for *slow intravenous injection*, reconstitute 1 g with 10 mL water for injections *or* Sodium chloride 0.9%; give over 3–4 minutes. Manufacturer advises for *intermittent intravenous infusion*, give in Glucose 5% or 10% *or* Sodium chloride 0.9% *or* Ringer's solution *or* Lactated Ringer's solution. Reconstitute 1 g with 10 mL water for injections *or* infusion fluid, then dilute in up to 150 mL infusion fluid; give over 30–40 minutes. For *continuous intravenous infusion*, consult product literature.

- MEDICINAL FORMS
There can be variation in the licensing of different medicines containing the same drug.
Powder for solution for injection
ELECTROLYTES: May contain Sodium
▶ Negaban (Eumedica Pharmaceuticals)
Temocillin (as Temocillin sodium) 1 gram Negaban 1g powder for solution for injection vials | 1 vial [PoM] £25.45

5

Infection

Colistimethate sodium

18-Dec-2016

(Colistin sulfomethate sodium)

- **DRUG ACTION** The polymyxin antibiotic, colistimethate sodium (colistin sulfomethate sodium), is active against Gram-negative organisms including *Pseudomonas aeruginosa*, *Acinetobacter baumanii*, and *Klebsiella pneumoniae*. It is not absorbed by mouth and thus needs to be given by injection for a systemic effect.

- **INDICATIONS AND DOSE**

Gram-negative infections resistant to other antibacterials, including those caused by *Pseudomonas aeruginosa*, *Acinetobacter baumanii* and *Klebsiella pneumoniae*

▸ BY SLOW INTRAVENOUS INJECTION, OR BY INTRAVENOUS INFUSION

▸ Adult (body-weight up to 60 kg): 50 000–75 000 units/kg daily in 3 divided doses, to be administered into a totally implantable venous access device when giving via slow intravenous injection

▸ Adult (body-weight 60 kg and above): 1–2 million units every 8 hours, to be administered into a totally implantable venous access device when giving via slow intravenous injection; maximum 6 million units per day

Adjunct to standard antibacterial therapy for *Pseudomonas aeruginosa* infection in cystic fibrosis

▸ BY INHALATION OF NEBULISED SOLUTION

▸ Adult: 1–2 million units twice daily, adjusted according to response, increased to 2 million units 3 times daily for subsequent respiratory isolates of *Pseudomonas aeruginosa*

▸ BY INHALATION OF POWDER

▸ Adult: 1.66 million units twice daily

PROMIXIN ® INJECTION

Gram-negative infections resistant to other antibacterials, including those caused by *Pseudomonas aeruginosa*, *Acinetobacter baumanii* , *Klebsiella pneumoniae*

▸ BY SLOW INTRAVENOUS INJECTION, OR BY INTRAVENOUS INFUSION

▸ Adult: 9 million units daily in 2–3 divided doses, to be administered into a totally implantable venous access device when giving via slow intravenous injection, an initial loading dose of 9 million units (up to max. 12 million units, if adequate renal function) should be used in those who are critically ill, consult product literature for details

PROMIXIN ® NEBULISER SOLUTION

Management of chronic pulmonary infections due to *Pseudomonas aeruginosa* in patients with cystic fibrosis

▸ BY INHALATION OF NEBULISED SOLUTION

▸ Child 2-17 years: 1–2 million units 2–3 times a day, for specific advice on administration using nebulisers—consult product literature; maximum 6 million units per day

▸ Adult: 1–2 million units 2–3 times a day, for specific advice on administration using nebulisers—consult product literature; maximum 6 million units per day

- **CONTRA-INDICATIONS** Myasthenia gravis
- **CAUTIONS**
▸ When used by inhalation Severe haemoptysis—risk of further haemorrhage
- **INTERACTIONS** → Appendix 1: colistimethate

- **SIDE-EFFECTS**
▸ **Common or very common**
▸ When used by inhalation Arthralgia · asthenia · asthma · balance impaired · chest discomfort · cough · dysphonia · dyspnoea · fever · haemorrhage · headache · lower respiratory tract infection · nausea · respiratory disorders · taste altered · throat complaints · tinnitus · vomiting
▸ **Uncommon**
▸ When used by inhalation Anxiety · appetite decreased · diarrhoea · drowsiness · ear congestion · flatulence · oral disorders · proteinuria · seizure · sputum purulent · thirst · weight change
▸ **Rare or very rare**
▸ With parenteral use Confusion · nephrotoxicity · presyncope · psychosis · speech slurred · visual impairment
▸ **Frequency not known**
▸ With parenteral use Apnoea · neurological effects · neurotoxicity · renal disorder · sensory disorder
SIDE-EFFECTS, FURTHER INFORMATION Neurotoxicity and nephrotoxicity are dose-related.

- **PREGNANCY**
▸ When used by inhalation Clinical use suggests probably safe.
▸ With intravenous use Use only if potential benefit outweighs risk.

- **BREAST FEEDING** Present in milk but poorly absorbed from gut; manufacturers advise avoid (or use only if potential benefit outweighs risk).

- **RENAL IMPAIRMENT**
Dose adjustments ▸ With intravenous use Reduce dose.
Monitoring ▸ With intravenous use In renal impairment, monitor plasma colistimethate sodium concentration during parenteral treatment—consult product literature. Recommended 'peak' plasma colistimethate sodium concentration (approx. 1 hour after intravenous injection or infusion) 5–15 mg/litre; pre-dose ('trough') concentration 2–6 mg/litre.

- **MONITORING REQUIREMENTS**
▸ With intravenous use Monitor renal function.
▸ When used by inhalation Measure lung function before and after initial dose of colistimethate sodium and monitor for bronchospasm; if bronchospasm occurs in a patient not using a bronchodilator, repeat test using a bronchodilator before the dose of colistimethate sodium.

- **DIRECTIONS FOR ADMINISTRATION**
▸ When used by inhalation Other inhaled drugs should be administered before colistimethate sodium. For *nebulisation* administer required dose in 2–4 mL of sodium chloride 0.9% (or water for injections) or a 1:1 mixture of sodium chloride 0.9% and water for injection.
▸ With intravenous use For *intravenous infusion (Colomycin®, Promixin®)*, give intermittently in Sodium chloride 0.9% (or Glucose 5% for Promixin® brand only); dilute with 50 mL infusion fluid and give over 30 minutes.
COLOMYCIN ® *Colomycin®* Injection may be used for nebulisation; administer required dose in 2–4 mL of sodium chloride 0.9%, (or water for injections) or a 1:1 mixture of sodium chloride 0.9% and water for injection.

- **PRESCRIBING AND DISPENSING INFORMATION**
Colistimethate sodium is included in some preparations for topical application.

- **PATIENT AND CARER ADVICE**
▸ When used by inhalation Patient should be advised to rinse mouth with water after each dose of dry powder inhalation. Patients or carers should be given advice on how to administer colistimethate sodium; first dose should be given under medical supervision.
Driving and skilled tasks Manufacturer advises patients and carers should be counselled on the effects on driving and performance of skilled tasks—increased risk of dizziness, confusion and visual disturbances.

● NATIONAL FUNDING/ACCESS DECISIONS

NICE decisions

▸ Colistimethate sodium by dry powder inhalation for pseudomonal lung infection in cystic fibrosis (March 2013)
NICE TA276
Colistimethate sodium dry powder for inhalation is recommended for chronic pulmonary infection caused by *Pseudomonas aeruginosa* in patients with cystic fibrosis who would benefit from continued treatment, but do not tolerate the drug in its nebulised form. The manufacturer must provide colistimethate sodium dry powder for inhalation at the discount agreed as part of the patient access scheme to primary, secondary and tertiary care in the NHS. Patients currently receiving colistimethate sodium dry powder for inhalation can continue treatment until they and their clinician consider it appropriate to stop.
www.nice.org.uk/TA276

● MEDICINAL FORMS
There can be variation in the licensing of different medicines containing the same drug.

Powder for solution for injection
ELECTROLYTES: May contain Sodium
▸ Colistimethate sodium (Non-proprietary)
Colistimethate sodium 1000000 unit Colistimethate 1million unit powder for solution for injection vials | 10 vial [PoM] £18.00 DT = £18.00 | 10 vial [PoM] £18.00 DT = £18.00 (Hospital only)
▸ Colomycin (Teva UK Ltd)
Colistimethate sodium 1000000 unit Colomycin 1million unit powder for solution for injection vials | 10 vial [PoM] £18.00 DT = £18.00
Colistimethate sodium 2000000 unit Colomycin 2million unit powder for solution for injection vials | 10 vial [PoM] £32.40 DT = £32.40
▸ Promixin (Profile Pharma Ltd)
Colistimethate sodium 1000000 unit Promixin 1million unit powder for solution for injection vials | 10 vial [PoM] £30.00 DT = £18.00 (Hospital only)

Inhalation powder
▸ Colobreathe (Teva UK Ltd)
Colistimethate sodium 1662500 unit Colobreathe 1,662,500unit inhalation powder capsules | 56 capsule [PoM] £968.80

Powder for nebuliser solution
▸ ColiFin (Pari Medical Ltd)
Colistimethate sodium 1000000 unit ColiFin 1 MIU powder for nebuliser solution unit dose vials | 56 unit dose [PoM] £180.53
Colistimethate sodium 2000000 unit ColiFin 2 MIU powder for nebuliser solution unit dose vials | 56 unit dose [PoM] £261.72
▸ Promixin (Profile Pharma Ltd)
Colistimethate sodium 1000000 unit Promixin 1million unit powder for nebuliser solution unit dose vials | 30 unit dose [PoM] £168.00 DT = £168.00

ANTIBACTERIALS > QUINOLONES

Quinolones

31-Oct-2017

Overview
Nalidixic acid and norfloxacin p. 551 are effective in uncomplicated urinary-tract infections.

Ciprofloxacin p. 548 is active against both Gram-positive and Gram-negative bacteria. It is particularly active against Gram-negative bacteria, including *Salmonella*, *Shigella*, *Campylobacter*, *Neisseria*, and *Pseudomonas*. Ciprofloxacin has only moderate activity against Gram-positive bacteria such as *Streptococcus pneumoniae* and *Enterococcus faecalis*; it should not be used for pneumococcal pneumonia. It is active against *Chlamydia* and some mycobacteria. Most anaerobic organisms are not susceptible. Ciprofloxacin can be used for respiratory tract infections (but not for pneumococcal pneumonia), urinary-tract infections, infections of the gastro-intestinal system (including typhoid

fever), bone and joint infections, gonorrhoea and septicaemia caused by sensitive organisms.

Ofloxacin p. 551 is used for urinary-tract infections, lower respiratory-tract infections, gonorrhoea, and non-gonococcal urethritis and cervicitis.

Levofloxacin p. 549 is active against Gram-positive and Gram-negative organisms. It has greater activity against *Pneumococci* than ciprofloxacin.

Many *Staphylococci* are resistant to quinolones and their use should be avoided in MRSA infections.

Moxifloxacin p. 550 is active against Gram-positive and Gram-negative organisms. It has greater activity against Gram-positive organisms, including *Pneumococci*, than ciprofloxacin. Moxifloxacin is not active against *Pseudomonas aeruginosa* or meticillin-resistant *Staphylococcus aureus* (MRSA).

Quinolones

IMPORTANT SAFETY INFORMATION
The CSM has warned that quinolones may induce **convulsions** in patients with or without a history of convulsions; taking NSAIDs at the same time may also induce them.

TENDON DAMAGE
Tendon damage (including rupture) has been reported rarely in patients receiving quinolones. Tendon rupture may occur within 48 hours of starting treatment; cases have also been reported several months after stopping a quinolone. Healthcare professionals are reminded that:
• quinolones are contra-indicated in patients with a history of tendon disorders related to quinolone use;
• patients over 60 years of age are more prone to tendon damage;
• the risk of tendon damage is increased by the concomitant use of corticosteroids;
• if tendinitis is suspected, the quinolone should be discontinued immediately.

● CONTRA-INDICATIONS History of tendon disorders related to quinolone use

● CAUTIONS Can prolong the QT interval · children or adolescents (arthropathy has developed in weight-bearing joints in young *animals*) · conditions that predispose to seizures · diabetes (may affect blood glucose) · exposure to excessive sunlight should be avoided (discontinue if photosensitivity occurs) · G6PD deficiency · history of epilepsy · myasthenia gravis (risk of exacerbation)
CAUTIONS, FURTHER INFORMATION
▸ Use in children Quinolones cause arthropathy in the weight-bearing joints of immature *animals* and are therefore generally not recommended in children and growing adolescents. However, the significance of this effect in humans is uncertain and in some specific circumstances short-term use of ciprofloxacin may be justified in children.

● SIDE-EFFECTS
▸ Common or very common Appetite decreased · arthralgia · asthenia · constipation · diarrhoea · dizziness · dyspnoea · eye discomfort · eye disorders · fever · gastrointestinal discomfort · headache · hearing impairment · hepatic disorders · myalgia · nausea · QT interval prolongation · rhabdomyolysis · skin reactions · sleep disorders · taste altered · vision disorders · vomiting
▸ Uncommon Anaemia · anxiety · arrhythmias · chest pain · confusion · depression · drowsiness · dry eye · eosinophilia · eye inflammation · flatulence · hallucination · hyperhidrosis · hypersensitivity · hypotension · leucopenia · neutropenia · pain · paraesthesia · renal failure · seizure ·

smell altered · tendon disorders · thrombocytopenia · tremor · vertigo

▸ **Rare or very rare** Agranulocytosis · angioedema · arthritis · coordination abnormal · haemolytic anaemia · hyperglycaemia · hypoglycaemia · muscle weakness · myasthenia gravis aggravated · nephritis tubulointerstitial · pancreatitis · photosensitivity reaction · polyneuropathy · pseudomembranous enterocolitis · psychotic disorder · severe cutaneous adverse reactions (SCARs) · stomatitis · suicidal tendencies · syncope · vasculitis

▸ **Frequency not known** Peripheral neuropathy (sometimes irreversible)

SIDE-EFFECTS, FURTHER INFORMATION The drug should be discontinued if psychiatric, neurological, or hypersensitivity reactions (including severe rash) occur.

● ALLERGY AND CROSS-SENSITIVITY Use of quinolones contra-indicated in quinolone hypersensitivity.

● PREGNANCY Avoid in pregnancy—shown to cause arthropathy in *animal* studies; safer alternatives are available.

Ciprofloxacin

26-Apr-2018

▸ **F 547**

● **INDICATIONS AND DOSE**

Fistulating Crohn's disease
▸ BY MOUTH
▸ Adult: 500 mg twice daily

Respiratory-tract infections
▸ BY MOUTH
▸ Adult: 500–750 mg twice daily
▸ BY INTRAVENOUS INFUSION
▸ Adult: 400 mg every 8–12 hours, to be given over 60 minutes

Pseudomonal lower respiratory-tract infection in cystic fibrosis
▸ BY MOUTH
▸ Adult: 750 mg twice daily

Urinary-tract infections
▸ BY MOUTH
▸ Adult: 250–750 mg twice daily
▸ BY INTRAVENOUS INFUSION
▸ Adult: 400 mg every 8–12 hours, to be given over 60 minutes

Acute uncomplicated cystitis in women
▸ BY MOUTH
▸ Adult: 250 mg twice daily for 3 days

Acute or chronic prostatitis
▸ BY MOUTH
▸ Adult: 500 mg twice daily for 28 days
▸ BY INTRAVENOUS INFUSION
▸ Adult: 400 mg every 8–12 hours, to be given over 60 minutes

Gonorrhoea
▸ BY MOUTH
▸ Adult: 500 mg for 1 dose

Most other infections
▸ BY MOUTH
▸ Adult: Initially 500 mg twice daily; increased to 750 mg twice daily, in severe or deep-seated infection
▸ BY INTRAVENOUS INFUSION
▸ Adult: 400 mg every 8–12 hours, to be given over 60 minutes

Surgical prophylaxis
▸ BY MOUTH
▸ Adult: 750 mg, to be taken 60 minutes before procedure

Anthrax (treatment and post-exposure prophylaxis)
▸ BY MOUTH
▸ Adult: 500 mg twice daily

▸ BY INTRAVENOUS INFUSION
▸ Adult: 400 mg every 12 hours, to be given over 60 minutes

Prevention of secondary case of meningococcal meningitis
▸ BY MOUTH
▸ Child 1 month–4 years: 30 mg/kg (max. per dose 125 mg) for 1 dose
▸ Child 5–11 years: 250 mg for 1 dose
▸ Child 12–17 years: 500 mg for 1 dose
▸ Adult: 500 mg for 1 dose

● UNLICENSED USE Not licensed for use in children for prophylaxis of meningococcal meningitis.

● CAUTIONS Acute myocardial infarction (risk factor for QT interval prolongation) · avoid excessive alkalinity of urine (risk of crystalluria) · bradycardia (risk factor for QT interval prolongation) · congenital long QT syndrome (risk factor for QT interval prolongation) · electrolyte disturbances (risk factor for QT interval prolongation) · ensure adequate fluid intake (risk of crystalluria) · heart failure with reduced left ventricular ejection fraction (risk factor for QT interval prolongation) · history of symptomatic arrhythmias (risk factor for QT interval prolongation)

● INTERACTIONS → Appendix 1: quinolones

● SIDE-EFFECTS
▸ **Common or very common** Arthropathy (in children)
▸ **Uncommon** Akathisia · fungal superinfection · musculoskeletal pain · oedema · renal impairment · sensation abnormal · thrombocytosis · vasodilation
▸ **Rare or very rare** Antibiotic associated colitis · asthma · bone marrow disorders · crystalluria · erythema nodosum · gait abnormal · haematuria · intracranial pressure increased · leucocytosis · migraine · muscle cramps · muscle tone increased · olfactory nerve disorder · petechiae · status epilepticus
▸ **Frequency not known** Mood altered

● PREGNANCY A single dose of ciprofloxacin may be used for the prevention of a secondary case of meningococcal meningitis.

● BREAST FEEDING Amount too small to be harmful but manufacturer advises avoid.

● RENAL IMPAIRMENT
Dose adjustments ▸ With oral use in adults Give 250–500 mg every 12 hours if eGFR 30–60 mL/minute/1.73 m^2 (every 24 hours if eGFR less than 30 mL/minute/1.73 m^2).
▸ With intravenous use in adults Give (200 mg over 30 minutes), 200–400 mg every 12 hours if eGFR 30–60 mL/minute/1.73m^2 (every 24 hours if eGFR less than 30 mL/minute/1.73 m^2).
▸ In children Reduce dose if estimated glomerular filtration rate less than 30 mL/minute/1.73 m^2—consult product literature.

● PRESCRIBING AND DISPENSING INFORMATION Flavours of oral liquid formulations may include strawberry.

● PATIENT AND CARER ADVICE
Medicines for Children leaflet: Ciprofloxacin for bacterial infections www.medicinesforchildren.org.uk/ciprofloxacin-bacterial-infections-0
Driving and skilled tasks May impair performance of skilled tasks (e.g. driving); effects enhanced by alcohol.

- **MEDICINAL FORMS**
  There can be variation in the licensing of different medicines containing the same drug. Forms available from special-order manufacturers include: oral suspension

Tablet
CAUTIONARY AND ADVISORY LABELS 7, 9, 25
- Ciprofloxacin (Non-proprietary)
  Ciprofloxacin (as Ciprofloxacin hydrochloride)
  100 mg Ciprofloxacin 100mg tablets | 6 tablet [PoM] £4.50 DT = £1.97
  Ciprofloxacin (as Ciprofloxacin hydrochloride)
  250 mg Ciprofloxacin 250mg tablets | 10 tablet [PoM] £7.25 DT = £0.39 | 20 tablet [PoM] £0.78–£11.20 | 100 tablet [PoM] £5.90
  Ciprofloxacin (as Ciprofloxacin hydrochloride)
  500 mg Ciprofloxacin 500mg tablets | 10 tablet [PoM] £14.00 DT = £0.71 | 20 tablet [PoM] £1.42–£21.23 | 100 tablet [PoM] £8.20
  Ciprofloxacin (as Ciprofloxacin hydrochloride)
  750 mg Ciprofloxacin 750mg tablets | 10 tablet [PoM] £20.00 DT = £8.00
- Ciproxin (Bayer Plc)
  Ciprofloxacin (as Ciprofloxacin hydrochloride) 500 mg Ciproxin 500mg tablets | 10 tablet [PoM] £12.49 DT = £0.71
  Ciprofloxacin (as Ciprofloxacin hydrochloride) 750 mg Ciproxin 750mg tablets | 10 tablet [PoM] £17.78 DT = £8.00

Oral suspension
CAUTIONARY AND ADVISORY LABELS 7, 9, 25
- Ciproxin (Bayer Plc)
  Ciprofloxacin 50 mg per 1 ml Ciproxin 250mg/5ml oral suspension | 100 ml [PoM] £21.29 DT = £21.29

Solution for infusion
ELECTROLYTES: May contain Sodium
- Ciprofloxacin (Non-proprietary)
  Ciprofloxacin (as Ciprofloxacin lactate) 2 mg per 1 ml Ciprofloxacin 200mg/100ml solution for infusion vials | 1 vial [PoM] £2.00–£5.00
  Ciprofloxacin 200mg/100ml solution for infusion bottles | 10 bottle [PoM] £14.45
  Ciprofloxacin 100mg/50ml solution for infusion vials | 1 vial [PoM] £2.25–£7.20
  Ciprofloxacin 400mg/200ml solution for infusion bottles | 1 bottle [PoM] £6.00 | 10 bottle [PoM] £195.90
  Ciprofloxacin 400mg/200ml solution for infusion vials | 1 vial [PoM] £2.50
- Ciproxin (Bayer Plc)
  Ciprofloxacin (as Ciprofloxacin lactate) 2 mg per 1 ml Ciproxin Infusion 100mg/50ml solution for infusion bottles | 1 bottle [PoM] £7.61 (Hospital only)
  Ciproxin Infusion 400mg/200ml solution for infusion bottles | 5 bottle [PoM] £114.23 (Hospital only)
  Ciproxin Infusion 200mg/100ml solution for infusion bottles | 5 bottle [PoM] £75.06 (Hospital only)

Infusion
- Ciprofloxacin (Non-proprietary)
  Ciprofloxacin (as Ciprofloxacin lactate) 2 mg per 1 ml Ciprofloxacin 200mg/100ml infusion bags | 5 bag [PoM] £60.00 (Hospital only)
  Ciprofloxacin 400mg/200ml infusion bags | 5 bag [PoM] £85.00 | 10 bag [PoM] £200.00 (Hospital only)

◀ 547

Levofloxacin

13-Jul-2017

- **INDICATIONS AND DOSE**

Acute sinusitis
- BY MOUTH
- Adult: 500 mg once daily for 10–14 days

Acute exacerbation of chronic bronchitis
- BY MOUTH
- Adult: 500 mg once daily for 7–10 days

Community-acquired pneumonia
- BY MOUTH
- Adult: 500 mg 1–2 times a day for 7–14 days
- BY INTRAVENOUS INFUSION
- Adult: 500 mg 1–2 times a day, to be given over at least 60 minutes

Urinary-tract infections
- BY MOUTH
- Adult: 500 mg once daily for 7–14 days

Urinary-tract infections (uncomplicated infection)
- BY MOUTH
- Adult: 250 mg once daily for 3 days

Complicated urinary-tract infections
- BY INTRAVENOUS INFUSION
- Adult: 500 mg once daily, to be given over at least 60 minutes

Chronic prostatitis
- BY MOUTH
- Adult: 500 mg once daily for 28 days
- BY INTRAVENOUS INFUSION
- Adult: 500 mg once daily, to be given over at least 60 minutes

Complicated skin infections | Complicated soft-tissue infections
- BY MOUTH
- Adult: 500 mg 1–2 times a day for 7–14 days
- BY INTRAVENOUS INFUSION
- Adult: 500 mg 1–2 times a day, to be given over at least 60 minutes

Inhalation of anthrax (treatment and post-exposure prophylaxis)
- BY MOUTH
- Adult: 500 mg once daily for 8 weeks
- BY INTRAVENOUS INFUSION
- Adult: 500 mg once daily, to be given over at least 60 minutes

Chronic pulmonary infections due to *Pseudomonas aeruginosa* in cystic fibrosis
- BY INHALATION OF NEBULISED SOLUTION
- Adult: 240 mg twice daily for 28 days, subsequent courses repeated after 28-day interval without levofloxacin nebuliser solution

- **CAUTIONS** History of psychiatric illness · risk factors for QT interval prolongation (e.g. electrolyte disturbances, acute myocardial infarction, heart failure with reduced left ventricular ejection fraction, bradycardia, congenital long QT syndrome, history of symptomatic arrhythmias)
- **INTERACTIONS** → Appendix 1: quinolones
- **SIDE-EFFECTS**
- **Common or very common**
- When used by inhalation Bronchial secretion changes · cough · dysphonia · exercise tolerance decreased · haemoptysis · increased risk of infection · respiratory disorders · weight decreased
- **Uncommon**
- When used by inhalation Costochondritis · hyperbilirubinaemia · joint stiffness
- With intravenous use or oral use Increased risk of infection
- **Rare or very rare**
- With intravenous use or oral use Acute kidney injury · nightmare · palpitations
- **Frequency not known**
- With intravenous use or oral use Anosmia · cardiac arrest · diarrhoea haemorrhagic · hypersensitivity vasculitis · hypoglycaemic coma · idiopathic intracranial hypertension · ligament rupture · movement disorders · muscle rupture · pancytopenia · respiratory disorders · uveitis · ventricular tachycardia · vision loss

SIDE-EFFECTS, FURTHER INFORMATION Systemic side-effects may occur with nebulised levofloxacin.
Bronchospasm Manufacturer advises if acute symptomatic bronchospasm occurs after receiving nebulised levofloxacin, patients may benefit from the use of a short-acting inhaled bronchodilator at least 15 minutes to 4 hours prior to subsequent doses.

Infection

5

- BREAST FEEDING Manufacturer advises avoid.
- RENAL IMPAIRMENT
  Dose adjustments ▸ With intravenous use or oral use Usual initial dose, then use half normal dose if eGFR 20–50 mL/minute/1.73 m²; consult product literature if eGFR less than 20 mL/minute/1.73 m².
  ▸ When used by inhalation Manufacturer advises avoid if creatinine clearance less than 20 mL/minute.
- PATIENT AND CARER ADVICE
- ▸ When used by inhalation Manufacturer advises patients and carers should be given advice on how to administer levofloxacin.
  Missed doses ▸ When used by inhalation Manufacturer advises if a dose is more than 4 hours late, the missed dose should not be taken and the next dose should be taken at the normal time.
  Driving and skilled tasks May impair performance of skilled tasks (e.g. driving).
- NATIONAL FUNDING/ACCESS DECISIONS
  Scottish Medicines Consortium (SMC) Decisions
  The *Scottish Medicines Consortium* has advised (August 2016) that levofloxacin (*Quinsair®*) is accepted for restricted use within NHS Scotland for the management of chronic pulmonary infections due to *Pseudomonas aeruginosa* in patients with cystic fibrosis, as a third-line treatment option after colistimethate sodium (first line) and tobramycin (second line). This advice is contingent upon the continuing availability of the Patient Access Scheme in NHS Scotland or a list price that is equivalent or lower.

  All Wales Medicines Strategy Group (AWMSG) Decisions
  The *All Wales Medicines Strategy Group* has advised (November 2016) that levofloxacin (*Quinsair®*) is recommended as an option for restricted use within NHS Wales as third-line therapy for the management of chronic pulmonary infections due to *Pseudomonas aeruginosa* in patients with cystic fibrosis, who do not respond to, or are intolerant of, second-line treatment with tobramycin, only if the approved Wales Patient Access Scheme (WPAS) is used or where the list price is equivalent or lower.

- MEDICINAL FORMS
  There can be variation in the licensing of different medicines containing the same drug.

  Tablet
  CAUTIONARY AND ADVISORY LABELS 6, 9, 25
  ▸ Levofloxacin (Non-proprietary)
    Levofloxacin (as Levofloxacin hemihydrate) 250 mg Levofloxacin 250mg tablets | 5 tablet [PoM] £1.90–£7.23 | 10 tablet [PoM] £10.94 DT = £6.37
    Levofloxacin (as Levofloxacin hemihydrate) 500 mg Levofloxacin 500mg tablets | 5 tablet [PoM] £7.90–£12.93 | 10 tablet [PoM] £25.85 DT = £20.92

  Solution for infusion
  ELECTROLYTES: May contain Sodium
  ▸ Levofloxacin (Non-proprietary)
    Levofloxacin (as Levofloxacin hemihydrate) 5 mg per 1 ml Levofloxacin 500mg/100ml solution for infusion vials | 1 vial [PoM] £25.00
    Levofloxacin 500mg/100ml solution for infusion bottles | 1 bottle [PoM] £4.00

  Nebuliser liquid
  ▸ Quinsair (Chiesi Ltd) ▼
    Levofloxacin (as Levofloxacin hemihydrate) 100 mg per 1 ml Quinsair 240mg nebuliser solution ampoules | 56 ampoule [PoM] £2,181.53

  Infusion
  ▸ Levofloxacin (Non-proprietary)
    Levofloxacin (as Levofloxacin hemihydrate) 5 mg per 1 ml Levofloxacin 500mg/100ml infusion bags | 20 bag [PoM] £502.00 (Hospital only)

▶ 547

Moxifloxacin

- INDICATIONS AND DOSE
  Sinusitis
  ▸ BY MOUTH
  ▸ **Adult:** 400 mg once daily for 7 days
  Community-acquired pneumonia
  ▸ BY MOUTH
  ▸ **Adult:** 400 mg once daily for 7–14 days
  ▸ BY INTRAVENOUS INFUSION
  ▸ **Adult:** 400 mg once daily for 7–14 days, to be given over 60 minutes
  Exacerbations of chronic bronchitis
  ▸ BY MOUTH
  ▸ **Adult:** 400 mg once daily for 5–10 days
  Mild to moderate pelvic inflammatory disease
  ▸ BY MOUTH
  ▸ **Adult:** 400 mg once daily for 14 days
  Complicated skin and soft-tissue infections which have failed to respond to other antibacterials or for patients who cannot be treated with other antibacterials
  ▸ BY MOUTH
  ▸ **Adult:** 400 mg once daily for 7–21 days
  ▸ BY INTRAVENOUS INFUSION
  ▸ **Adult:** 400 mg once daily for 7–21 days, to be given over 60 minutes

- CONTRA-INDICATIONS Acute myocardial infarction (risk factor for QT interval prolongation) · bradycardia (risk factor for QT interval prolongation) · congenital long QT syndrome (risk factor for QT interval prolongation) · electrolyte disturbances (risk factor for QT interval prolongation) · heart failure with reduced left ventricular ejection fraction (risk factor for QT interval prolongation) · history of symptomatic arrhythmias (risk factor for QT interval prolongation)

- INTERACTIONS → Appendix 1: quinolones

- SIDE-EFFECTS
- ▸ **Common or very common** Increased risk of infection
- ▸ **Uncommon** Akathisia · angina pectoris · antibiotic associated colitis · dehydration · dry skin · gastritis · hyperlipidaemia · malaise · oedema · palpitations · renal impairment · respiratory disorders · thrombocytosis · vasodilation
- ▸ **Rare or very rare** Allergic oedema · cardiac arrest · concentration impaired · depersonalisation · dysphagia · emotional lability · gait abnormal · hypertension · hyperuricaemia · memory loss · muscle complaints · sensation abnormal · speech disorder · vision loss

- BREAST FEEDING Manufacturer advises avoid—present in milk in *animal* studies.

- HEPATIC IMPAIRMENT Manufacturer advises avoid in severe impairment.

- PATIENT AND CARER ADVICE
  Driving and skilled tasks May impair performance of skilled tasks (e.g. driving).

- MEDICINAL FORMS
  There can be variation in the licensing of different medicines containing the same drug.

  Tablet
  CAUTIONARY AND ADVISORY LABELS 6, 9
  ▸ Moxifloxacin (Non-proprietary)
    Moxifloxacin (as Moxifloxacin hydrochloride) 400 mg Moxifloxacin 400mg tablets | 5 tablet [PoM] £13.15 DT = £9.55
  ▸ Avelox (Bayer Plc)
    Moxifloxacin (as Moxifloxacin hydrochloride) 400 mg Avelox 400mg tablets | 5 tablet [PoM] £12.43 DT = £9.55

Solution for infusion
ELECTROLYTES: May contain Sodium
▸ Avelox (Bayer Plc)
Moxifloxacin (as Moxifloxacin hydrochloride) 1.6 mg per
1 ml Avelox 400mg/250ml solution for infusion bottles |
1 bottle PoM £39.95 (Hospital only) | 5 bottle PoM £199.75
(Hospital only)

┌──────────────────────────── ℉ 547 ─┐

Norfloxacin

● INDICATIONS AND DOSE

Lower urinary-tract infections
▸ BY MOUTH
▸ Adult: 400 mg twice daily for 7–10 days (for 3 days for
uncomplicated infections in women)

Chronic relapsing lower urinary-tract infections
▸ BY MOUTH
▸ Adult: 400 mg twice daily for up to 12 weeks; reduced
to 400 mg once daily, if adequate suppression within
first 4 weeks

Chronic prostatitis
▸ BY MOUTH
▸ Adult: 400 mg twice daily for 28 days

● CAUTIONS Acute myocardial infarction (risk factor for QT
interval prolongation) · bradycardia (risk factor for QT
interval prolongation) · congenital long QT syndrome (risk
factor for QT interval prolongation) · electrolyte
disturbances (risk factor for QT interval prolongation) ·
heart failure with reduced left ventricular ejection fraction
(risk factor for QT interval prolongation) · history of
symptomatic arrhythmias (risk factor for QT interval
prolongation)

● INTERACTIONS → Appendix 1: quinolones

● SIDE-EFFECTS
▸ **Common or very common** Hepatitis cholestatic
▸ **Uncommon** Abdominal cramps · crystalluria
▸ **Rare or very rare** Guillain-Barre syndrome · mood altered ·
psychiatric disorder · tenosynovitis · vulvovaginal
candidiasis

● BREAST FEEDING No information available—manufacturer
advises avoid.

● RENAL IMPAIRMENT
Dose adjustments Use 400 mg once daily if eGFR less than
30 mL/minute/1.73 m².

● PATIENT AND CARER ADVICE
Driving and skilled tasks May impair performance of skilled
tasks (e.g. driving).

● MEDICINAL FORMS
There can be variation in the licensing of different medicines
containing the same drug.
Tablet
CAUTIONARY AND ADVISORY LABELS 7, 9, 23
▸ Norfloxacin (Non-proprietary)
Norfloxacin 400 mg Norfloxacin 400mg tablets | 14 tablet PoM ⊠

┌──────────────────────────── ℉ 547 ─┐

Ofloxacin

● INDICATIONS AND DOSE

Urinary-tract infections
▸ BY MOUTH
▸ Adult: 200–400 mg daily, preferably taken in the
morning; increased if necessary to 400 mg twice daily,
in upper urinary tract infections

Complicated urinary-tract infection
▸ BY INTRAVENOUS INFUSION
▸ Adult: 200 mg daily, increased if necessary to 400 mg
twice daily, dose increased for severe or complicated

infections, to be given over at least 30 minutes for each
200 mg

Acute or chronic prostatitis
▸ BY MOUTH
▸ Adult: 200 mg twice daily for 28 days

Lower respiratory-tract infections
▸ BY MOUTH
▸ Adult: 400 mg daily, dose preferably taken in the
morning, then increased if necessary to 400 mg twice
daily
▸ BY INTRAVENOUS INFUSION
▸ Adult: 200 mg twice daily, increased to 400 mg twice
daily, dose to be increased for severe or complicated
infections, to be given over at least 30 minutes for each
200 mg

Skin and soft-tissue infections
▸ BY MOUTH
▸ Adult: 400 mg twice daily
▸ BY INTRAVENOUS INFUSION
▸ Adult: 400 mg twice daily, to be given over at least
30 minutes for each 200 mg

Uncomplicated gonorrhoea
▸ BY MOUTH
▸ Adult: 400 mg as a single dose

**Uncomplicated genital chlamydial infection | Non-
gonococcal urethritis**
▸ BY MOUTH
▸ Adult: 400 mg daily for 7 days, dose may be taken as a
single daily dose or in divided doses

Pelvic inflammatory disease
▸ BY MOUTH
▸ Adult: 400 mg twice daily for 14 days

Septicaemia
▸ BY INTRAVENOUS INFUSION
▸ Adult: 200 mg twice daily, increased if necessary to
400 mg twice daily, dose to be increased for severe or
complicated infections, to be given over at least
30 minutes for each 200 mg

● CAUTIONS Acute myocardial infarction (risk factor for QT
interval prolongation) · bradycardia (risk factor for QT
interval prolongation) · congenital long QT syndrome (risk
factor for QT interval prolongation) · electrolyte
disturbances (risk factor for QT interval prolongation) ·
heart failure with reduced left ventricular ejection fraction
(risk factor for QT interval prolongation) · history of
psychiatric illness · history of symptomatic arrhythmias
(risk factor for QT interval prolongation)

● INTERACTIONS → Appendix 1: quinolones

● SIDE-EFFECTS
▸ **Uncommon** Cough · increased risk of infection
▸ **Rare or very rare** Acute kidney injury · enterocolitis · hot
flush · hypersensitivity · movement disorders · nightmare ·
respiratory disorders
▸ **Frequency not known** Acute generalised exanthematous
pustulosis (AGEP) · bone marrow failure · hypoglycaemic
coma · ligament rupture · muscle rupture · myopathy ·
nephritis acute interstitial · uveitis

● BREAST FEEDING Amount probably too small to be
harmful but manufacturer advises avoid.

● HEPATIC IMPAIRMENT Use with caution; elimination may
be reduced in severe impairment.

● RENAL IMPAIRMENT
Dose adjustments Usual initial dose, then use half normal
dose if eGFR 20–50 mL/minute/1.73 m²; 100 mg every
24 hours if eGFR less than 20 mL/minute/1.73 m²

● PATIENT AND CARER ADVICE
Driving and skilled tasks May affect performance of skilled
tasks (e.g. driving); effects enhanced by alcohol.

5

Infection

Infection

5

● MEDICINAL FORMS
There can be variation in the licensing of different medicines containing the same drug. Forms available from special-order manufacturers include: oral suspension, oral solution

Tablet
CAUTIONARY AND ADVISORY LABELS 6, 9, 11
▸ Ofloxacin (Non-proprietary)
Ofloxacin 200 mg Ofloxacin 200mg tablets | 10 tablet [PoM] £6.75
DT = £6.73
Ofloxacin 400 mg Ofloxacin 400mg tablets | 5 tablet [PoM] £12.80
DT = £12.78 | 10 tablet [PoM] £4.59–£25.56
▸ Tarivid (Sanofi)
Ofloxacin 400 mg Tarivid 400mg tablets | 10 tablet [PoM] £14.99

Solution for infusion
▸ Tarivid (Sanofi)
Ofloxacin (as Ofloxacin hydrochloride) 2 mg per 1 ml Tarivid 200mg/100ml solution for infusion bottles | 1 bottle [PoM] £16.16

ANTIBACTERIALS > SULFONAMIDES

Co-trimoxazole

● DRUG ACTION Sulfamethoxazole and trimethoprim are used in combination (as co-trimoxazole) because of their synergistic activity (the importance of the sulfonamides has decreased as a result of increasing bacterial resistance and their replacement by antibacterials which are generally more active and less toxic).

● **INDICATIONS AND DOSE**

Treatment of susceptible infections
▸ BY MOUTH
▸ Child 6 weeks–5 months: 120 mg twice daily, alternatively 24 mg/kg twice daily
▸ Child 6 months–5 years: 240 mg twice daily, alternatively 24 mg/kg twice daily
▸ Child 6–11 years: 480 mg twice daily, alternatively 24 mg/kg twice daily
▸ Child 12–17 years: 960 mg twice daily
▸ Adult: 960 mg twice daily
▸ BY INTRAVENOUS INFUSION
▸ Adult: 960 mg every 12 hours, increased to 1.44 g every 12 hours, increased dose used in severe infection

Treatment of *Pneumocystis jirovecii* (*Pneumocystis carinii*) infections (undertaken where facilities for appropriate monitoring available—consult microbiologist and product literature)
▸ BY MOUTH, OR BY INTRAVENOUS INFUSION
▸ Child: 120 mg/kg daily in 2–4 divided doses for 14–21 days, oral route preferred for children
▸ Adult: 120 mg/kg daily in 2–4 divided doses for 14–21 days

Prophylaxis of *Pneumocystis jirovecii* (*Pneumocystis carinii*) infections
▸ BY MOUTH
▸ Child: 450 mg/m^2 twice daily (max. per dose 960 mg twice daily) for 3 days of the week (either consecutively or on alternate days), dose regimens may vary, consult local guidelines
▸ Adult: 960 mg once daily, reduced if not tolerated to 480 mg once daily, alternatively 960 mg once daily on alternate days, alternate day dose to be given 3 times weekly, alternatively 960 mg twice a day on alternate days, alternate day dose to be given 3 times weekly

DOSE EQUIVALENCE AND CONVERSION
▸ 480 mg of co-trimoxazole consists of sulfamethoxazole 400 mg and trimethoprim 80 mg.

● UNLICENSED USE Not licensed for *Burkholderia cepacia* infections in cystic fibrosis. Not licensed for

Stenotrophomonas maltophilia infections. Not licensed for use in children under 6 weeks.

IMPORTANT SAFETY INFORMATION
RESTRICTIONS ON THE USE OF CO-TRIMOXAZOLE
Co-trimoxazole is the drug of choice in the prophylaxis and treatment of *Pneumocystis jirovecii* (*Pneumocystis carinii*) pneumonia; it is also indicated for nocardiasis, *Stenotrophomonas maltophilia* infection [unlicensed indication], and toxoplasmosis. It should only be considered for use in acute exacerbations of chronic bronchitis and infections of the urinary tract when there is bacteriological evidence of sensitivity to co-trimoxazole and good reason to prefer this combination to a single antibacterial; similarly it should only be used in acute otitis media in children when there is good reason to prefer it. Co-trimoxazole is also used for the treatment of infections caused by *Burkholderia cepacia* in cystic fibrosis [unlicensed indication].

● CONTRA-INDICATIONS Acute porphyrias p. 1025
● CAUTIONS Asthma · avoid in blood disorders (unless under specialist supervision) · avoid in infants under 6 weeks (except for treatment or prophylaxis of pneumocystis pneumonia) because of the risk of kernicterus · elderly (increased risk of serious side-effects) · G6PD deficiency (risk of haemolytic anaemia) · maintain adequate fluid intake · predisposition to folate deficiency · predisposition to hyperkalaemia (in adults)
● INTERACTIONS → Appendix 1: sulfonamides · trimethoprim
● SIDE-EFFECTS
▸ **Common or very common** Diarrhoea · electrolyte imbalance · fungal overgrowth · headache · nausea · skin reactions
▸ **Uncommon** Vomiting
▸ **Rare or very rare** Agranulocytosis · angioedema · aplastic anaemia · appetite decreased · arthralgia · ataxia · cough · depression · dizziness · dyspnoea · eosinophilia · fever · haemolysis · haemolytic anaemia · hallucination · hepatic disorders · hypoglycaemia · leucopenia · lung infiltration · megaloblastic anaemia · meningitis aseptic · metabolic acidosis · methaemoglobinaemia · myalgia · myocarditis allergic · nephritis tubulointerstitial · neutropenia · oral disorders · pancreatitis · peripheral neuritis · photosensitivity reaction · pseudomembranous enterocolitis · renal impairment · renal tubular acidosis · seizure · serum sickness · severe cutaneous adverse reactions (SCARs) · systemic lupus erythematosus (SLE) · thrombocytopenia · tinnitus · uveitis · vasculitis · vertigo

SIDE-EFFECTS, FURTHER INFORMATION Co-trimoxazole is associated with rare but serious side effects. Discontinue immediately if blood disorders (including leucopenia, thrombocytopenia, megaloblastic anaemia, eosinophilia) or rash (including Stevens-Johnson syndrome or toxic epidermal necrolysis) develop.

● PREGNANCY Teratogenic risk in first trimester (trimethoprim a folate antagonist). Neonatal haemolysis and methaemoglobinaemia in third trimester; fear of increased risk of kernicterus in neonates appears to be unfounded.

● BREAST FEEDING Small risk of kernicterus in jaundiced infants and of haemolysis in G6PD-deficient infants (due to sulfamethoxazole).

● HEPATIC IMPAIRMENT Manufacturer advises avoid in severe liver disease.

● RENAL IMPAIRMENT
▸ In adults Avoid if eGFR less than 15 mL/minute/1.73 m^2 and if plasma-sulfamethoxazole concentration cannot be monitored.
▸ In children Avoid if estimated glomerular filtration rate less than 15 mL/minute/1.73 m^2 and if plasma-sulfamethoxazole concentration cannot be monitored.

Dose adjustments ▸ In adults Use half normal dose if eGFR 15–30 mL/minute/1.73 m^2.
  ▸ In children Use half normal dose if estimated glomerular filtration rate 15–30 mL/minute/1.73 m^2.

● MONITORING REQUIREMENTS
▸ In children Plasma concentration monitoring may be required with high doses; seek expert advice.
▸ Monitor blood counts on prolonged treatment.

● DIRECTIONS FOR ADMINISTRATION
▸ With intravenous use in children For intermittent *intravenous infusion*, may be further diluted in glucose 5% and 10% or sodium chloride 0.9%. Dilute contents of 1 ampoule (5 mL) to 125 mL, 2 ampoules (10 mL) to 250 mL or 3 ampoules (15 mL) to 500 mL; suggested duration of infusion 60–90 minutes (but may be adjusted according to fluid requirements); if fluid restriction necessary, 1 ampoule (5 mL) may be diluted with 75 mL glucose 5% and the required dose infused over max. 60 minutes; check container for haze or precipitant during administration. In severe fluid restriction may be given undiluted via a central venous line.
▸ With intravenous use in adults For *intravenous infusion* (*Septrin® for infusion*), give intermittently in Glucose 5% or 10% or Sodium chloride 0.9%. Dilute contents of 1 ampoule (5 mL) to 125 mL, 2 ampoules (10 mL) to 250 mL or 3 ampoules (15 mL) to 500 mL; suggested duration of infusion 60–90 minutes (but may be adjusted according to fluid requirements); if fluid restriction necessary, 1 ampoule (5 mL) may be diluted with 75 mL glucose 5% and infused over max. 60 minutes.

● PRESCRIBING AND DISPENSING INFORMATION
Co-trimoxazole is a mixture of trimethoprim and sulfamethoxazole (sulphamethoxazole) in the proportions of 1 part to 5 parts.
Flavours of oral liquid formulations may include banana, or vanilla.

● MEDICINAL FORMS
There can be variation in the licensing of different medicines containing the same drug.

Solution for infusion
EXCIPIENTS: May contain Alcohol, propylene glycol, sulfites
ELECTROLYTES: May contain Sodium
▸ Co-trimoxazole (Non-proprietary)
  Trimethoprim 16 mg per 1 ml, Sulfamethoxazole 80 mg per 1 ml Co-trimoxazole 80mg/400mg/5ml solution for infusion ampoules | 10 ampoule PoM £35.00
▸ Septrin (Aspen Pharma Trading Ltd)
  Trimethoprim 16 mg per 1 ml, Sulfamethoxazole 80 mg per 1 ml Septrin for Infusion 80mg/400mg/5ml solution for infusion ampoules | 10 ampoule PoM £17.76

Oral suspension
CAUTIONARY AND ADVISORY LABELS 9
▸ Co-trimoxazole (Non-proprietary)
  Trimethoprim 8 mg per 1 ml, Sulfamethoxazole 40 mg per 1 ml Co-trimoxazole 40mg/200mg/5ml oral suspension sugar free sugar-free | 100 ml PoM £9.95–£9.97 DT = £9.96
  Trimethoprim 16 mg per 1 ml, Sulfamethoxazole 80 mg per 1 ml Co-trimoxazole 80mg/400mg/5ml oral suspension | 100 ml PoM £10.95–£10.97 DT = £10.96

Tablet
CAUTIONARY AND ADVISORY LABELS 9
▸ Co-trimoxazole (Non-proprietary)
  Trimethoprim 80 mg, Sulfamethoxazole 400 mg Co-trimoxazole 80mg/400mg tablets | 28 tablet PoM £15.50 DT = £2.37 | 100 tablet PoM £8.46–£10.91
  Trimethoprim 160 mg, Sulfamethoxazole 800 mg Co-trimoxazole 160mg/800mg tablets | 100 tablet PoM £23.40–£23.46 DT = £23.46

Sulfadiazine
07-Feb-2018
(Sulphadiazine)

● DRUG ACTION Sulfadiazine is a short-acting sulphonamide with bacteriostatic activity against a broad spectrum of organisms. The importance of the sulfonamides has decreased as a result of increasing bacterial resistance and their replacement by antibacterials which are generally more active and less toxic.

● INDICATIONS AND DOSE
Prevention of rheumatic fever recurrence
▸ BY MOUTH
▸ Adult (body-weight up to 30 kg): 500 mg daily
▸ Adult (body-weight 30 kg and above): 1 g daily

IMPORTANT SAFETY INFORMATION
SAFE PRACTICE
Sulfadiazine has been confused with sulfasalazine; care must be taken to ensure the correct drug is prescribed and dispensed.

● CONTRA-INDICATIONS Acute porphyrias p. 1025
● CAUTIONS Asthma · avoid in blood disorders (unless under specialist supervision) · avoid in infants under 6 weeks (except for treatment or prophylaxis of *pneumocystis pneumonia*) because of the risk of kernicterus · elderly · G6PD deficiency (risk of haemolytic anaemia) · maintain adequate fluid intake · predisposition to folate deficiency · predisposition to hyperkalaemia
● INTERACTIONS → Appendix 1: sulfonamides
● SIDE-EFFECTS
▸ **Rare or very rare** Haemolytic anaemia
▸ **Frequency not known** Agranulocytosis · aplastic anaemia · appetite decreased · ataxia · back pain · blood disorders · cough · crystalluria · cyanosis · depression · diarrhoea · dizziness · drowsiness · dyspnoea · eosinophilia · erythema nodosum · fatigue · fever · haematuria · hallucination · headache · hepatic disorders · hypoglycaemia · hypoprothrombinaemia · hypothyroidism · idiopathic intracranial hypertension · insomnia · leucopenia · meningitis aseptic · myocarditis · nausea · nephritis tubulointerstitial · nephrotoxicity · nerve disorders · neurological effects · neutropenia · oral disorders · pancreatitis · photosensitivity reaction · pseudomembranous enterocolitis · psychosis · renal impairment · renal tubular necrosis · respiratory disorders · seizure · serum sickness-like reaction · severe cutaneous adverse reactions (SCARs) · skin reactions · systemic lupus erythematosus (SLE) · thrombocytopenia · tinnitus · vasculitis · vertigo · vomiting

SIDE-EFFECTS, FURTHER INFORMATION Discontinue immediately if blood disorders (including leucopenia, thrombocytopenia, megaloblastic anaemia, eosinophilia) or rash (including Stevens-Johnson syndrome or toxic epidermal necrolysis) develop.

● PREGNANCY Risk of neonatal haemolysis and methaemoglobinaemia in third trimester; fear of increased risk of kernicterus in neonates appears to be unfounded.

● BREAST FEEDING Small risk of kernicterus in jaundiced infants and of haemolysis in G6PD-deficient infants.

● HEPATIC IMPAIRMENT Use with caution in mild to moderate impairment; avoid in severe impairment.

● RENAL IMPAIRMENT Use with caution in mild to moderate impairment; avoid in severe impairment; high risk of crystalluria.

● MONITORING REQUIREMENTS Monitor blood counts on prolonged treatment.

- MEDICINAL FORMS
There can be variation in the licensing of different medicines containing the same drug. Forms available from special-order manufacturers include: oral suspension
Tablet
CAUTIONARY AND ADVISORY LABELS 9, 27
▸ Sulfadiazine (Non-proprietary)
Sulfadiazine 500 mg Sulfadiazine 500mg tablets | 56 tablet [PoM] £190.74 DT = £152.95

ANTIBACTERIALS ❯ TETRACYCLINES AND RELATED DRUGS

Tetracyclines

Overview

The tetracyclines are broad-spectrum antibiotics whose value has decreased owing to increasing bacterial resistance. They remain, however, the treatment of choice for infections caused by chlamydia (trachoma, psittacosis, salpingitis, urethritis, and lymphogranuloma venereum), rickettsia (including Q-fever), brucella (doxycycline p. 555 with either streptomycin p. 512 or rifampicin p. 571), and the spirochaete, *Borrelia burgdorferi* (See Lyme disease). They are also used in respiratory and genital mycoplasma infections, in acne, in destructive (refractory) periodontal disease, in exacerbations of chronic bronchitis (because of their activity against *Haemophilus influenzae*), and for leptospirosis in penicillin hypersensitivity (as an alternative to erythromycin p. 530).

Tetracyclines have a role in the management of meticillin-resistant *Staphylococcus aureus* (MRSA) infection.

Microbiologically, there is little to choose between the various tetracyclines, the only exception being minocycline p. 556 which has a broader spectrum; it is active against *Neisseria meningitidis* and has been used for meningococcal prophylaxis but is no longer recommended because of side-effects including dizziness and vertigo. Compared to other tetracyclines, minocycline is associated with a greater risk of lupus-erythematosus-like syndrome. Minocycline sometimes causes irreversible pigmentation.

Tetracyclines

- CONTRA-INDICATIONS Children under 12 years (deposition in growing bone and teeth, by binding to calcium, causes staining and occasionally dental hypoplasia)
- CAUTIONS Myasthenia gravis (muscle weakness may be increased) · systemic lupus erythematosus (may be exacerbated)
- SIDE-EFFECTS
▸ **Common or very common** Angioedema · diarrhoea · headache · Henoch-Schönlein purpura · hypersensitivity · nausea · pericarditis · photosensitivity reaction · skin reactions · systemic lupus erythematosus exacerbated · vomiting
▸ **Rare or very rare** Appetite decreased · discolouration of thyroid gland · dysphagia · eosinophilia · fontanelle bulging (in infants) · gastrointestinal disorders · haemolytic anaemia · hepatic disorders · idiopathic intracranial hypertension · increased risk of infection · neutropenia · oral disorders · pancreatitis · pseudomembranous enterocolitis · severe cutaneous adverse reactions (SCARs) · thrombocytopenia
▸ **Frequency not known** Dizziness
SIDE-EFFECTS, FURTHER INFORMATION Headache and visual disturbances may indicate benign intracranial hypertension (discontinue treatment if raised intracranial pressure develops).

- PREGNANCY Should **not** be given to pregnant women; effects on skeletal development have been documented in the first trimester in *animal* studies. Administration during the second or third trimester may cause discoloration of the child's teeth, and maternal hepatotoxicity has been reported with large parenteral doses.
- BREAST FEEDING Should **not** be given to women who are breast-feeding (although absorption and therefore discoloration of teeth in the infant is probably usually prevented by chelation with calcium in milk).
- HEPATIC IMPAIRMENT Should be avoided or used with caution in patients with hepatic impairment.

Demeclocycline hydrochloride

- INDICATIONS AND DOSE
Susceptible infections (e.g. chlamydia, rickettsia and mycoplasma)
▸ BY MOUTH
▸ Adult: 150 mg 4 times a day, alternatively 300 mg twice daily

Treatment of hyponatraemia resulting from inappropriate secretion of antidiuretic hormone, if fluid restriction alone does not restore sodium concentration or is not tolerable
▸ BY MOUTH
▸ Adult: Initially 0.9–1.2 g daily in divided doses, maintenance 600–900 mg daily

- CAUTIONS Photosensitivity more common than with other tetracyclines
- INTERACTIONS → Appendix 1: tetracyclines
- SIDE-EFFECTS
▸ **Rare or very rare** Agranulocytosis · aplastic anaemia · hearing impairment · nephritis
▸ **Frequency not known** Intracranial pressure increased · muscle weakness · nephrogenic diabetes insipidus · vision disorders
- HEPATIC IMPAIRMENT
Dose adjustments Max. 1 g daily in divided doses.
- RENAL IMPAIRMENT May exacerbate renal failure and should **not** be given to patients with renal impairment.
- PATIENT AND CARER ADVICE Patients should be advised to avoid exposure to sunlight or sun lamps.

- MEDICINAL FORMS
There can be variation in the licensing of different medicines containing the same drug. Forms available from special-order manufacturers include: tablet, oral suspension, oral solution
Tablet
▸ Demeclocycline hydrochloride (Non-proprietary)
Demeclocycline hydrochloride 150 mg Demeclocycline 150mg tablets | 100 tablet [PoM] 🔲
Capsule
CAUTIONARY AND ADVISORY LABELS 7, 9, 11, 23
▸ Demeclocycline hydrochloride (Non-proprietary)
Demeclocycline hydrochloride 150 mg Demeclocycline 150mg capsules | 28 capsule [PoM] £176.16 DT = £176.16

⬛ **5**

`▶ 554`

Doxycycline

● **INDICATIONS AND DOSE**

Susceptible infections (e.g. chlamydia, rickettsia and mycoplasma)
▸ BY MOUTH USING IMMEDIATE-RELEASE MEDICINES
▹ Child 12–17 years: Initially 200 mg daily for 1 dose, then maintenance 100 mg once daily
▹ Adult: Initially 200 mg daily for 1 dose, then maintenance 100 mg once daily

Acute sinusitis
▸ BY MOUTH USING IMMEDIATE-RELEASE MEDICINES
▹ Child 12–17 years: Initially 200 mg daily for 1 dose, then maintenance 100 mg once daily for 4 days
▹ Adult: Initially 200 mg daily for 1 dose, then maintenance 100 mg once daily for 4 days

Severe infections (including refractory urinary-tract infections)
▸ BY MOUTH USING IMMEDIATE-RELEASE MEDICINES
▹ Child 12–17 years: 200 mg daily
▹ Adult: 200 mg once daily

Acne
▸ BY MOUTH USING IMMEDIATE-RELEASE MEDICINES
▹ Child 12–17 years: 100 mg once daily
▹ Adult: 100 mg once daily

Rosacea
▸ BY MOUTH USING IMMEDIATE-RELEASE MEDICINES
▹ Adult: 100 mg once daily

Papulopustular facial rosacea (without ocular involvement)
▸ BY MOUTH USING MODIFIED-RELEASE MEDICINES
▹ Adult: 40 mg once daily for 16 weeks, dose to be taken in the morning, consider discontinuing treatment if no response after 6 weeks

Early syphilis
▸ BY MOUTH USING IMMEDIATE-RELEASE MEDICINES
▹ Child 12–17 years: 100 mg twice daily for 14 days
▹ Adult: 100 mg twice daily for 14 days

Late latent syphilis
▸ BY MOUTH USING IMMEDIATE-RELEASE MEDICINES
▹ Child 12–17 years: 100 mg twice daily for 28 days
▹ Adult: 100 mg twice daily for 28 days

Neurosyphilis
▸ BY MOUTH USING IMMEDIATE-RELEASE MEDICINES
▹ Adult: 200 mg twice daily for 28 days

Uncomplicated genital chlamydia | Non-gonococcal urethritis
▸ BY MOUTH USING IMMEDIATE-RELEASE MEDICINES
▹ Child 12–17 years: 100 mg twice daily for 7 days
▹ Adult: 100 mg twice daily for 7 days

Pelvic inflammatory disease
▸ BY MOUTH USING IMMEDIATE-RELEASE MEDICINES
▹ Child 12–17 years: 100 mg twice daily for 14 days
▹ Adult: 100 mg twice daily for 14 days

Lyme disease (under expert supervision)
▸ BY MOUTH USING IMMEDIATE-RELEASE MEDICINES
▹ Child 12–17 years: 100 mg twice daily for 10–14 days (for 28 days in Lyme arthritis)
▹ Adult: 100 mg twice daily for 10–14 days (for 28 days in Lyme arthritis)

Anthrax (treatment or post-exposure prophylaxis)
▸ BY MOUTH USING IMMEDIATE-RELEASE MEDICINES
▹ Child 12–17 years: 100 mg twice daily
▹ Adult: 100 mg twice daily

Prophylaxis of malaria
▸ BY MOUTH USING IMMEDIATE-RELEASE MEDICINES
▹ Child 12–17 years: 100 mg once daily, to be started 1–2 days before entering endemic area and continued for 4 weeks after leaving, can be used for up to 2 years
▹ Adult: 100 mg once daily, to be started 1–2 days before entering endemic area and continued for 4 weeks after leaving, can be used for up to 2 years

Adjunct to quinine in treatment of *Plasmodium falciparum* malaria
▸ BY MOUTH USING IMMEDIATE-RELEASE MEDICINES
▹ Child 12–17 years: 200 mg daily for 7 days
▹ Adult: 200 mg daily for 7 days

Periodontitis (as an adjunct to gingival scaling and root planing)
▸ BY MOUTH USING IMMEDIATE-RELEASE MEDICINES
▹ Child 12–17 years: 20 mg twice daily for 3 months
▹ Adult: 20 mg twice daily for 3 months

● UNLICENSED USE Doxycycline doses in BNF Publications may differ from those in product literature. Not licensed for malaria prophylaxis during pregnancy. Not licensed for treatment or post-exposure prophylaxis of anthrax. EvGr Duration of treatment for acute sinusitis adheres to national guidelines. ⓐ See Sinusitis (acute) p. 1168 for further information. Immediate-release doxycycline not licensed for treatment of rosacea.

● CAUTIONS Alcohol dependence

● INTERACTIONS → Appendix 1: tetracyclines

● SIDE-EFFECTS
▸ **Common or very common** Dyspnoea · hypotension · peripheral oedema · serum sickness · tachycardia
▸ **Uncommon** Gastritis · gastrointestinal discomfort
▸ **Rare or very rare** Antibiotic associated colitis · arthralgia · flushing · hepatic function abnormal · myalgia · photoonycholysis · tinnitus · vision disorders

● PREGNANCY When travel to malarious areas is unavoidable during pregnancy, doxycycline can be used for malaria prophylaxis if other regimens are unsuitable, and if the entire course of doxycycline can be completed before 15 weeks' gestation.

● RENAL IMPAIRMENT Use with caution (avoid excessive doses).

● MONITORING REQUIREMENTS When used for periodontitis, monitor for superficial fungal infection, particularly if predisposition to oral candidiasis.

● DIRECTIONS FOR ADMINISTRATION Capsules and Tablets should be swallowed whole with plenty of fluid, while sitting or standing. Capsules should be taken during meals.

● PATIENT AND CARER ADVICE Counselling on administration advised.
Photosensitivity Patients should be advised to avoid exposure to sunlight or sun lamps.

● PROFESSION SPECIFIC INFORMATION

Dental practitioners' formulary
Doxycycline Capsules 100 mg may be prescribed. Dispersible tablets may be prescribed as Dispersible Doxycycline Tablets. Tablets may be prescribed as Doxycycline Tablets 20 mg.

● MEDICINAL FORMS
There can be variation in the licensing of different medicines containing the same drug. Forms available from special-order manufacturers include: oral suspension, oral solution
Tablet
CAUTIONARY AND ADVISORY LABELS 6, 11, 27
▸ Periostat (Alliance Pharmaceuticals Ltd)
Doxycycline (as Doxycycline hyclate) 20 mg Periostat 20mg tablets | 56 tablet PoM £17.30 DT = £17.30

Dispersible tablet

CAUTIONARY AND ADVISORY LABELS 6, 9, 11, 13

▸ Vibramycin-D (Pfizer Ltd)

Doxycycline (as Doxycycline monohydrate) 100 mg Vibramycin-D 100mg dispersible tablets sugar-free | 8 tablet [PoM] £4.91 DT = £4.91

Modified-release capsule

CAUTIONARY AND ADVISORY LABELS 6, 11, 27

▸ Efracea (Galderma (UK) Ltd)

Doxycycline (as Doxycycline monohydrate) 40 mg Efracea 40mg modified-release capsules | 14 capsule [PoM] £7.99 DT = £7.99 | 56 capsule [PoM] £21.71

Capsule

CAUTIONARY AND ADVISORY LABELS 6, 9, 11, 27

▸ Doxycycline (Non-proprietary)

Doxycycline (as Doxycycline hyclate) 50 mg Doxycycline 50mg capsules | 28 capsule [PoM] £4.00 DT = £1.08

Doxycycline (as Doxycycline hyclate) 100 mg Doxycycline 100mg capsules | 8 capsule [PoM] £3.00 DT = £0.51 | 14 capsule [PoM] £5.25 | 50 capsule [PoM] £3.19–£19.00

▶ 554

Lymecycline

● **INDICATIONS AND DOSE**

Susceptible infections (e.g. chlamydia, rickettsia and mycoplasma)

▸ BY MOUTH

▸ Child 12–17 years: 408 mg twice daily, increased to 1.224–1.632 g daily, (in severe infection)

▸ Adult: 408 mg twice daily, increased to 1.224–1.632 g daily, (in severe infection)

Acne

▸ BY MOUTH

▸ Child 12–17 years: 408 mg daily for at least 8 weeks

▸ Adult: 408 mg daily for at least 8 weeks

● INTERACTIONS → Appendix 1: tetracyclines

● SIDE-EFFECTS

▸ **Common or very common** Gastrointestinal discomfort

▸ **Frequency not known** Visual impairment

● RENAL IMPAIRMENT May exacerbate renal failure and should **not** be given to patients with renal impairment.

● MEDICINAL FORMS
There can be variation in the licensing of different medicines containing the same drug.

Capsule

CAUTIONARY AND ADVISORY LABELS 6, 9

▸ Lymecycline (Non-proprietary)

Lymecycline 408 mg Lymecycline 408mg capsules | 28 capsule [PoM] £6.95 DT = £4.59 | 56 capsule [PoM] £9.18–£11.66

▸ Tetralysal (Galderma (UK) Ltd)

Lymecycline 408 mg Tetralysal 300 capsules | 28 capsule [PoM] £6.95 DT = £4.59 | 56 capsule [PoM] £11.53

▶ 554

Minocycline

● **INDICATIONS AND DOSE**

Susceptible infections (e.g. chlamydia, rickettsia and mycoplasma)

▸ BY MOUTH USING IMMEDIATE-RELEASE MEDICINES

▸ Child 12–17 years: 100 mg twice daily

▸ Adult: 100 mg twice daily

Acne

▸ BY MOUTH USING IMMEDIATE-RELEASE MEDICINES

▸ Child 12–17 years: 100 mg once daily, alternatively 50 mg twice daily

▸ Adult: 100 mg once daily, alternatively 50 mg twice daily

▸ BY MOUTH USING MODIFIED-RELEASE MEDICINES

▸ Child 12–17 years: 100 mg daily

▸ Adult: 100 mg daily

Prophylaxis of asymptomatic meningococcal carrier state (but no longer recommended)

▸ BY MOUTH USING IMMEDIATE-RELEASE MEDICINES

▸ Adult: 100 mg twice daily for 5 days, minocycline treatment is usually followed by administration of rifampicin

● CAUTIONS Systemic lupus erythematosus

● INTERACTIONS → Appendix 1: tetracyclines

● SIDE-EFFECTS

▸ **Rare or very rare** Acute kidney injury · hearing impairment · respiratory disorders

▸ **Frequency not known** Alopecia · antibiotic associated colitis · arthralgia · ataxia · breast secretion · conjunctival discolouration · dyspepsia · hyperbilirubinaemia · hyperhidrosis · polyarteritis nodosa · sensation abnormal · tear discolouration · vertigo

● RENAL IMPAIRMENT Use with caution (avoid excessive doses).

● MONITORING REQUIREMENTS If treatment continued for longer than 6 months, monitor every 3 months for hepatotoxicity, pigmentation and for systemic lupus erythematosus—discontinue if these develop or if pre-existing systemic lupus erythematosus worsens.

● DIRECTIONS FOR ADMINISTRATION Tablets or capsules should be swallowed whole with plenty of fluid while sitting or standing.

● PATIENT AND CARER ADVICE Counselling on administration advised (posture).

● LESS SUITABLE FOR PRESCRIBING Less suitable for prescribing (compared with other tetracyclines, minocycline is associated with a greater risk of lupus-erythematosus-like syndrome; it sometimes causes irreversible pigmentation).

● MEDICINAL FORMS
There can be variation in the licensing of different medicines containing the same drug. Forms available from special-order manufacturers include: oral suspension, oral solution

Tablet

CAUTIONARY AND ADVISORY LABELS 6, 9

▸ Minocycline (Non-proprietary)

Minocycline (as Minocycline hydrochloride) 50 mg Minocycline 50mg tablets | 28 tablet [PoM] £8.50 DT = £6.19

Minocycline (as Minocycline hydrochloride) 100 mg Minocycline 100mg tablets | 28 tablet [PoM] £14.50 DT = £14.01

Modified-release capsule

CAUTIONARY AND ADVISORY LABELS 6, 25

▸ Minocycline (Non-proprietary)

Minocycline (as Minocycline hydrochloride) 100 mg Minocycline 100mg modified-release capsules | 56 capsule [PoM] £20.08 DT = £20.08

▸ Acnamino MR (Dexcel-Pharma Ltd)

Minocycline (as Minocycline hydrochloride) 100 mg Acnamino MR 100mg capsules | 56 capsule [PoM] £21.14 DT = £20.08

▸ Minocin MR (Meda Pharmaceuticals Ltd)

Minocin (as Minocycline hydrochloride) 100 mg Minocin MR 100mg capsules | 56 capsule [PoM] £20.08 DT = £20.08

Capsule

CAUTIONARY AND ADVISORY LABELS 6, 9

▸ Aknemin (Almirall Ltd)

Minocycline (as Minocycline hydrochloride) 50 mg Aknemin 50 capsules | 56 capsule [PoM] £15.27 DT = £15.27

Minocycline (as Minocycline hydrochloride) 100 mg Aknemin 100mg capsules | 28 capsule [PoM] £13.09 DT = £13.09

Oxytetracycline

554

● INDICATIONS AND DOSE

Susceptible infections (e.g. chlamydia, rickettsia and mycoplasma)
▶ BY MOUTH
▶ Child 12–17 years: 250–500 mg 4 times a day
▶ Adult: 250–500 mg 4 times a day

Rosacea
▶ BY MOUTH
▶ Adult: 500 mg twice daily usually for 6–12 weeks (course may be repeated intermittently)

Acne
▶ BY MOUTH
▶ Child 12–17 years: 500 mg twice daily for at least 3 months, if there is no improvement after the first 3 months another oral antibacterial should be used, maximum improvement usually occurs after 4 to 6 months but in more severe cases treatment may need to be continued for 2 years or longer
▶ Adult: 500 mg twice daily for at least 3 months, if there is no improvement after the first 3 months another oral antibacterial should be used, maximum improvement usually occurs after 4 to 6 months but in more severe cases treatment may need to be continued for 2 years or longer

● INTERACTIONS → Appendix 1: tetracyclines

● SIDE-EFFECTS Gastrointestinal discomfort · hepatic steatosis · increased risk of infection · renal impairment

● RENAL IMPAIRMENT May exacerbate renal failure and should **not** be given to patients with renal impairment.

● PROFESSION SPECIFIC INFORMATION
Dental practitioners' formulary
Oxytetracycline Tablets may be prescribed.

● MEDICINAL FORMS
There can be variation in the licensing of different medicines containing the same drug. Forms available from special-order manufacturers include: oral suspension
Tablet
CAUTIONARY AND ADVISORY LABELS 7, 9, 23
▶ Oxytetracycline (Non-proprietary)
Oxytetracycline (as Oxytetracycline dihydrate)
250 mg Oxytetracycline 250mg tablets | 28 tablet [PoM] £0.79 DT = £0.47

Tetracycline

554

● INDICATIONS AND DOSE

Susceptible infections (e.g. chlamydia, rickettsia, mycoplasma)
▶ BY MOUTH
▶ Child 12–17 years: 250 mg 4 times a day, increased if necessary to 500 mg 3–4 times a day, increased dose used in severe infections
▶ Adult: 250 mg 4 times a day, increased if necessary to 500 mg 3–4 times a day, increased dose used in severe infections

Rosacea
▶ BY MOUTH
▶ Adult: 500 mg twice daily usually for 6–12 weeks (course may be repeated intermittently)

Acne
▶ BY MOUTH
▶ Child 12–17 years: 500 mg twice daily for at least 3 months, if there is no improvement after the first 3 months another oral antibacterial should be used, maximum improvement usually occurs after 4 to

6 months but in more severe cases treatment may need to be continued for 2 years or longer
▶ Adult: 500 mg twice daily for at least 3 months, if there is no improvement after the first 3 months another oral antibacterial should be used, maximum improvement usually occurs after 4 to 6 months but in more severe cases treatment may need to be continued for 2 years or longer

Diabetic diarrhoea in autonomic neuropathy
▶ BY MOUTH
▶ Adult: 250 mg for 2 or 3 doses

Non-gonococcal urethritis
▶ BY MOUTH
▶ Child 12–17 years: 500 mg 4 times a day for 7–14 days (21 days if failure or relapse after first course)
▶ Adult: 500 mg 4 times a day for 7–14 days (21 days if failure or relapse after first course)

● UNLICENSED USE Not licensed for treatment of diabetic diarrhoea in *autonomic neuropathy*.

● INTERACTIONS → Appendix 1: tetracyclines

● SIDE-EFFECTS
▶ **Rare or very rare** Agranulocytosis · aplastic anaemia · nephritis · renal impairment
▶ **Frequency not known** Gastrointestinal discomfort · hepatic steatosis · overgrowth of nonsusceptible organisms

● HEPATIC IMPAIRMENT
Dose adjustments Max. 1 g daily in divided doses.

● RENAL IMPAIRMENT May exacerbate renal failure and should **not** be given to patients with renal impairment.

● DIRECTIONS FOR ADMINISTRATION Tablets should be swallowed whole with plenty of fluid while sitting or standing.

● PATIENT AND CARER ADVICE Counselling on administration advised.

● PROFESSION SPECIFIC INFORMATION
Dental practitioners' formulary
Tetracycline Tablets may be prescribed.

● MEDICINAL FORMS
There can be variation in the licensing of different medicines containing the same drug. Forms available from special-order manufacturers include: capsule, oral solution
Tablet
CAUTIONARY AND ADVISORY LABELS 7, 9, 23
▶ Tetracycline (Non-proprietary)
Tetracycline hydrochloride 250 mg Tetracycline 250mg tablets | 28 tablet [PoM] £13.90 DT = £1.27

Tigecycline

● DRUG ACTION Tigecycline is a glycylcycline antibacterial structurally related to the tetracyclines. Tigecycline is active against Gram-positive and Gram-negative bacteria, including tetracycline-resistant organisms, and some anaerobes. It is also active against meticillin-resistant *Staphylococcus aureus* and vancomycin-resistant enterococci, but *Pseudomonas aeruginosa* and many strains of *Proteus spp* are resistant to tigecycline.

● INDICATIONS AND DOSE

Treatment of complicated skin and soft-tissue infections and complicated abdominal infections caused by multiple-antibacterial resistant organisms when other antibacterials cannot be used
▶ BY INTRAVENOUS INFUSION
▶ Adult: Initially 100 mg, then 50 mg every 12 hours for 5–14 days, not recommended for the treatment of foot infections in patients with diabetes

● CAUTIONS Cholestasis

● INTERACTIONS → Appendix 1: tetracyclines

● SIDE-EFFECTS

▶ **Common or very common** Abscess · appetite decreased · diarrhoea · dizziness · gastrointestinal discomfort · headache · healing impaired · hyperbilirubinaemia · hypoglycaemia · hypoproteinaemia · increased risk of infection · nausea · sepsis · skin reactions · vomiting

▶ **Uncommon** Hepatic disorders · pancreatitis · thrombocytopenia

▶ **Frequency not known** Acidosis · azotaemia · hyperphosphataemia · hypofibrinogenaemia · idiopathic intracranial hypertension · photosensitivity reaction · pseudomembranous enterocolitis · severe cutaneous adverse reactions (SCARs) · tooth discolouration
SIDE-EFFECTS, FURTHER INFORMATION Side-effects similar to those of the tetracyclines can potentially occur.

● ALLERGY AND CROSS-SENSITIVITY Contra-indicated in patients hypersensitive to tetracyclines.

● PREGNANCY Tetracyclines should **not** be given to pregnant women; effects on skeletal development have been documented in the first trimester in *animal* studies. Administration during the second or third trimester may cause discoloration of the child's teeth, and maternal hepatotoxicity has been reported with large parenteral doses.

● BREAST FEEDING Manufacturer advises caution—present in milk in *animal* studies.

● HEPATIC IMPAIRMENT
Dose adjustments Initially 100 mg then 25 mg every 12 hours in severe hepatic impairment.

● DIRECTIONS FOR ADMINISTRATION For *intravenous infusion* (*Tygacil*®), give intermittently in Glucose 5% *or* Sodium Chloride 0.9%. Reconstitute each vial with 5.3 mL infusion fluid to produce a 10 mg/mL solution; dilute requisite dose in 100 mL infusion fluid; give over 30–60 minutes.

● MEDICINAL FORMS
There can be variation in the licensing of different medicines containing the same drug.

Powder for solution for infusion
  ▸ Tigecycline (Non-proprietary)
  Tigecycline 50 mg Tigecycline 50mg powder for solution for infusion vials | 10 vial [PoM] £290.79 (Hospital only)
  ▸ Tygacil (Pfizer Ltd)
  Tigecycline 50 mg Tygacil 50mg powder for solution for infusion vials | 10 vial [PoM] £323.10 (Hospital only)

ANTIBACTERIALS > OTHER

Chloramphenicol

● DRUG ACTION Chloramphenicol is a potent broad-spectrum antibiotic.

● INDICATIONS AND DOSE
Life threatening infections particularly those caused by *Haemophilus influenzae* | Typhoid fever
  ▸ BY MOUTH, OR BY INTRAVENOUS INJECTION, OR BY INTRAVENOUS INFUSION
  ▸ Adult: 12.5 mg/kg every 6 hours, in exceptional cases dose can be doubled for severe infections such as septicaemia and meningitis, providing high doses reduced as soon as clinically indicated

● CONTRA-INDICATIONS Acute porphyrias p. 1025

● CAUTIONS Avoid repeated courses and prolonged treatment

● INTERACTIONS → Appendix 1: chloramphenicol

● SIDE-EFFECTS

▶ **Rare or very rare**
▶ With parenteral use Aplastic anaemia (reversible or irreversible, with reports of resulting leukaemia)

▶ **Frequency not known**
▶ With oral use Bone marrow disorders · circulatory collapse · diarrhoea · enterocolitis · nausea · optic neuritis · oral disorders · ototoxicity · vomiting
▶ With parenteral use Agranulocytosis · bone marrow disorders · depression · diarrhoea · dry mouth · fungal superinfection · headache · nausea · nerve disorders · thrombocytopenic purpura · urticaria · vision disorders · vomiting
SIDE-EFFECTS, FURTHER INFORMATION Associated with serious haematological side-effects when given systemically and should therefore be reserved for the treatment of life-threatening infections.

● PREGNANCY Manufacturer advises avoid; neonatal 'grey-baby syndrome' if used in third trimester.

● BREAST FEEDING Manufacturer advises avoid; use another antibiotic; may cause bone-marrow toxicity in infant; concentration in milk usually insufficient to cause 'grey syndrome'.

● HEPATIC IMPAIRMENT Avoid if possible—increased risk of bone-marrow depression.
Dose adjustments Reduce dose.
Monitoring Monitor plasma-chloramphenicol concentration in hepatic impairment.

● RENAL IMPAIRMENT Avoid in severe renal impairment unless no alternative; dose-related depression of haematopoiesis.

● MONITORING REQUIREMENTS
▶ Plasma concentration monitoring preferred in the elderly.
▶ Recommended peak plasma concentration (approx. 2 hours after administration by mouth, intravenous injection or infusion) 10–25 mg/litre; pre-dose ('trough') concentration should not exceed 15 mg/litre.
▶ Blood counts required before and periodically during treatment.

● DIRECTIONS FOR ADMINISTRATION For *intravenous infusion*, give intermittently or via drip tubing in Glucose 5% *or* Sodium chloride 0.9%.

● MEDICINAL FORMS
There can be variation in the licensing of different medicines containing the same drug.
Powder for solution for injection
ELECTROLYTES: May contain Sodium
  ▸ Chloramphenicol (Non-proprietary)
  Chloramphenicol (as Chloramphenicol sodium succinate)
  1 gram Chloramphenicol 1g powder for solution for injection vials | 1 vial [PoM] £22.00 DT = £22.00
Capsule
  ▸ Chloramphenicol (Non-proprietary)
  Chloramphenicol 250 mg Chloramphenicol 250mg capsules | 60 capsule [PoM] £377.00 DT = £377.00

Daptomycin

25-Apr-2018

● DRUG ACTION Daptomycin is a lipopeptide antibacterial with a spectrum of activity similar to vancomycin but its efficacy against enterococci has not been established. It needs to be given with other antibacterials for mixed infections involving Gram-negative bacteria and some anaerobes.

● INDICATIONS AND DOSE
Complicated skin and soft-tissue infections caused by Gram-positive bacteria
  ▸ BY INTRAVENOUS INFUSION
  ▸ Child 12-23 months: 10 mg/kg once daily for up to 14 days, alternatively 12 mg/kg once daily, higher dose only if associated with *Staphylococcus aureus* bacteraemia—duration of treatment in accordance with risk of complications in individual patients

5

▹ Child 2-6 years: 9 mg/kg once daily for up to 14 days, alternatively 12 mg/kg once daily, higher dose only if associated with *Staphylococcus aureus* bacteraemia— duration of treatment in accordance with risk of complications in individual patients

▹ Child 7-11 years: 7 mg/kg once daily for up to 14 days, alternatively 9 mg/kg once daily, higher dose only if associated with *Staphylococcus aureus* bacteraemia— duration of treatment in accordance with risk of complications in individual patients

▹ Child 12-17 years: 5 mg/kg once daily for up to 14 days, alternatively 7 mg/kg once daily, higher dose only if associated with *Staphylococcus aureus* bacteraemia— duration of treatment in accordance with risk of complications in individual patients

Complicated skin and soft-tissue infections caused by Gram-positive bacteria

▸ BY SLOW INTRAVENOUS INJECTION, OR BY INTRAVENOUS INFUSION

▹ Adult: 4 mg/kg once daily for 7–14 days or longer if necessary, alternatively 6 mg/kg once daily, higher dose only if associated with *Staphylococcus aureus* bacteraemia—duration of treatment may need to be longer than 14 days in accordance with risk of complications in individual patients

Right-sided infective endocarditis caused by *Staphylococcus aureus* (administered on expert advice)

▸ BY SLOW INTRAVENOUS INJECTION, OR BY INTRAVENOUS INFUSION

▹ Adult: 6 mg/kg once daily, duration of treatment in accordance with official recommendations

● CAUTIONS Obesity (limited information on safety and efficacy)

● INTERACTIONS → Appendix 1: daptomycin

● SIDE-EFFECTS

▸ **Common or very common** Anaemia · anxiety · asthenia · constipation · diarrhoea · dizziness · fever · flatulence · gastrointestinal discomfort · headache · hypertension · hypotension · increased risk of infection · insomnia · nausea · pain · skin reactions · vomiting

▸ **Uncommon** Appetite decreased · arrhythmias · arthralgia · electrolyte imbalance · eosinophilia · flushing · glossitis · hyperglycaemia · muscle weakness · myalgia · myopathy · paraesthesia · renal impairment · taste altered · thrombocytosis · tremor · vertigo

▸ **Rare or very rare** Jaundice

▸ **Frequency not known** Acute generalised exanthematous pustulosis (AGEP) · antibiotic associated colitis · chills · cough · infusion related reaction · peripheral neuropathy · respiratory disorders · syncope

SIDE-EFFECTS, FURTHER INFORMATION If unexplained muscle pain, tenderness, weakness, or cramps develop during treatment, measure creatine kinase every 2 days; discontinue if unexplained muscular symptoms and creatine elevated markedly.

● PREGNANCY Manufacturer advises use only if potential benefit outweighs risk—no information available.

● BREAST FEEDING Present in milk in small amounts, but absorption from gastrointestinal tract negligible.

● HEPATIC IMPAIRMENT Manufacturer advises caution in severe hepatic impairment—no information available.

● RENAL IMPAIRMENT

▹ In children Manufacturer advises the dosage regimen has not been established—use with caution and monitor renal function regularly.

▹ In adults Manufacturer advises use only when potential benefit outweighs risk—higher risk of developing myopathy; monitor renal function regularly.

Dose adjustments ▹ In adults Use normal dose every 48 hours if eGFR less than 30 mL/minute/1.73 m^2.

● MONITORING REQUIREMENTS

▸ Manufacturer advises monitor plasma creatine phosphokinase (CPK) before treatment and then at least weekly during treatment; monitor CPK more frequently in patients at higher risk of developing myopathy, including those with renal impairment, taking other drugs associated with myopathy, or if CPK elevated more than 5 times upper limit of normal before treatment.

▸ Manufacturer advises monitor renal function regularly during concomitant administration of potentially nephrotoxic drugs.

● EFFECT ON LABORATORY TESTS Interference with assay for prothrombin time and INR—take blood sample immediately before daptomycin dose.

● DIRECTIONS FOR ADMINISTRATION

▹ In children For *intravenous infusion*, manufacturer advises give intermittently in Sodium Chloride 0.9%; reconstitute with Sodium Chloride 0.9% (350 mg in 7 mL, 500 mg in 10 mL); gently rotate vial without shaking; allow to stand for at least 10 minutes then rotate gently to dissolve; dilute requisite dose in 50 mL infusion fluid and give over 60 minutes for children aged 1–6 years and over 30 minutes for children aged 7–17 years.

▹ In adults For *intravenous infusion*, manufacturer advises give intermittently in Sodium Chloride 0.9%; reconstitute with Sodium Chloride 0.9% (350 mg in 7 mL, 500 mg in 10 mL); gently rotate vial without shaking; allow to stand for at least 10 minutes then rotate gently to dissolve; dilute requisite dose in 50 mL infusion fluid and give over 30 minutes. For *intravenous injection*, give over 2 minutes.

● HANDLING AND STORAGE Manufacturer advises store in a refrigerator (2–8 °C)—consult product literature for further information regarding storage after reconstitution and dilution.

● NATIONAL FUNDING/ACCESS DECISIONS

Scottish Medicines Consortium (SMC) Decisions
SMC No. 248/06

▹ In adults The *Scottish Medicines Consortium* has advised (April 2006) that daptomycin (*Cubicin*®) is accepted for restricted use within NHS Scotland for treatment of complicated skin and soft tissue infections in patients with known or suspected methicillin resistant *Staphylococcus aureus* infection and on the advice of local microbiologists or specialists in infectious disease.
SMC No. 449/08

▹ In adults The *Scottish Medicines Consortium* has advised (March 2008) that daptomycin (*Cubicin*®) is accepted for restricted use within NHS Scotland for the treatment of *Staphylococcus aureus* bacteraemia associated with right-sided endocarditis or with complicated skin and soft-tissue infections in patients with known or suspected methicillin resistant infection and on the advice of local microbiologists or specialists in infectious disease.

● MEDICINAL FORMS
There can be variation in the licensing of different medicines containing the same drug.

Powder for solution for infusion

▹ Daptomycin (Non-proprietary)
Daptomycin 350 mg Daptomycin 350mg powder for solution for infusion vials | 1 vial [PoM] £60.00 (Hospital only)
Daptomycin 500 mg Daptomycin 500mg powder for solution for infusion vials | 1 vial [PoM] £88.00 (Hospital only)

▹ Cubicin (Merck Sharp & Dohme Ltd)
Daptomycin 350 mg Cubicin 350mg powder for concentrate for solution for infusion vials | 1 vial [PoM] £62.00
Daptomycin 500 mg Cubicin 500mg powder for concentrate for solution for infusion vials | 1 vial [PoM] £88.57 (Hospital only)

5

Infection

Fidaxomicin

- **DRUG ACTION** Fidaxomicin is a macrocyclic antibacterial that is poorly absorbed from the gastro-intestinal tract, and, therefore, it should not be used to treat systemic infections.

- **INDICATIONS AND DOSE**

Clostridium difficile infection

▸ BY MOUTH

▸ Adult: 200 mg every 12 hours for 10 days, limited clinical data is available on the use of fidaxomicin in severe or life-threatening *Clostridium difficile* infection

- **CAUTIONS** Inflammatory bowel disease · severe or life-threatening *C. difficile* infection

- **INTERACTIONS** → Appendix 1: fidaxomicin

- **SIDE-EFFECTS**
▸ **Common or very common** Constipation · nausea · vomiting
▸ **Uncommon** Abdominal distension · appetite decreased · dizziness · dry mouth · flatulence · headache · skin reactions · taste altered
▸ **Frequency not known** Angioedema · dyspnoea · hypersensitivity

- **ALLERGY AND CROSS-SENSITIVITY** Use with caution in macrolide hypersensitivity.

- **PREGNANCY** Manufacturer advises avoid—no information available.

- **BREAST FEEDING** Manufacturer advises avoid—no information available.

- **HEPATIC IMPAIRMENT** Manufacturer advises caution in moderate to severe impairment—no information available.

- **RENAL IMPAIRMENT** Manufacturer advises caution in severe impairment—no information available.

- **NATIONAL FUNDING/ACCESS DECISIONS**

Scottish Medicines Consortium (SMC) Decisions
The *Scottish Medicines Consortium* has advised (June 2012) that fidaxomicin (*Dificlir®*) is accepted for restricted use within NHS Scotland to treat the first recurrence of *C. difficile* infection, on the advice of a microbiologist or specialist in infectious diseases.

- **MEDICINAL FORMS**
There can be variation in the licensing of different medicines containing the same drug.
Tablet
CAUTIONARY AND ADVISORY LABELS 9
▸ Dificlir (Astellas Pharma Ltd)
Fidaxomicin 200 mg Dificlir 200mg tablets | 20 tablet [PoM]
£1,350.00

Fosfomycin

22-Mar-2017

- **DRUG ACTION** Fosfomycin, a phosphonic acid antibacterial, is active against a range of Gram-positive and Gram-negative bacteria including *Staphylococcus aureus* and Enterobacteriaceae.

- **INDICATIONS AND DOSE**

Acute uncomplicated lower urinary-tract infections

▸ BY MOUTH USING GRANULES
▸ Adult: 3 g for 1 dose

Prophylaxis of urinary-tract infections in transurethral surgical procedures

▸ BY MOUTH USING GRANULES
▸ Adult: 3 g, to be given 3 hours before surgery. Dose may be repeated once, 24 hours after surgery

Osteomyelitis when first-line treatments are inappropriate or ineffective | Hospital-acquired lower respiratory-tract infections when first-line treatments are inappropriate or ineffective

▸ BY INTRAVENOUS INFUSION
▸ Adult: 12–24 g daily in 2–3 divided doses (max. per dose 8 g), use the high-dose regimen in severe infection suspected or known to be caused by less sensitive organisms

Complicated urinary-tract infections when first-line treatment ineffective or inappropriate

▸ BY INTRAVENOUS INFUSION
▸ Adult: 12–16 g daily in 2–3 divided doses (max. per dose 8 g)

Bacterial meningitis when first-line treatment ineffective or inappropriate

▸ BY INTRAVENOUS INFUSION
▸ Adult: 16–24 g daily in 3–4 divided doses (max. per dose 8 g), use the high-dose regimen in severe infection suspected or known to be caused by less sensitive organisms

- **CAUTIONS**
▸ With intravenous use Cardiac insufficiency · elderly (high doses) · hyperaldosteronism · hypernatraemia · hypertension · pulmonary oedema

- **SIDE-EFFECTS**
GENERAL SIDE-EFFECTS
▸ **Common or very common** Abdominal pain · antibiotic associated colitis · diarrhoea · headache · nausea · vomiting
▸ **Uncommon** Skin reactions
SPECIFIC SIDE-EFFECTS
▸ **Common or very common**
▸ With oral use Dizziness · vulvovaginal infection
▸ **Uncommon**
▸ With parenteral use Appetite decreased · dyspnoea · electrolyte imbalance · fatigue · oedema · taste altered · vertigo
▸ **Rare or very rare**
▸ With parenteral use Bone marrow disorders · eosinophilia · hepatic disorders · visual impairment
▸ **Frequency not known**
▸ With parenteral use Agranulocytosis · asthmatic attack · confusion · leucopenia · neutropenia · pseudomembranous enterocolitis · tachycardia · thrombocytopenia

- **PREGNANCY** Manufacturer advises use only if potential benefit outweighs risk.

- **BREAST FEEDING** Manufacturer advises use only if potential benefit outweighs risk—present in milk.

- **RENAL IMPAIRMENT**
▸ With oral use Avoid *oral* treatment if eGFR less than 10 mL/minute/1.73 m².
▸ With intravenous use Use *intravenous* treatment with caution if eGFR 40–80 mL/minute/1.73 m² and consult product literature for dose if eGFR less than 40 mL/minute/1.73 m².

- **MONITORING REQUIREMENTS**
▸ With intravenous use Monitor electrolytes and fluid balance.

- **DIRECTIONS FOR ADMINISTRATION**
▸ With intravenous use For *intravenous infusion* (*Fomicyt®*), give intermittently *in* Glucose 5% *or* 10% *or* Water for Injections; reconstitute each 2-g vial with 50 mL infusion fluid; give 2 g over 15 minutes.
▸ With oral use Manufacturer advises granules should be taken on an empty stomach (about 2–3 hours before or after a meal), preferably before bedtime and after emptying the bladder. The granules should be dissolved into a glass of water and taken immediately.

- **PRESCRIBING AND DISPENSING INFORMATION** Doses expressed as fosfomycin base.

● NATIONAL FUNDING/ACCESS DECISIONS

Scottish Medicines Consortium (SMC) Decisions
The *Scottish Medicines Consortium* has advised (February 2015) that fosfomycin (*Fomicyt* ®) is accepted for restricted use within NHS Scotland; initiation should be restricted to microbiologists or infectious disease specialists.

The *Scottish Medicines Consortium* has advised (September 2016) that fosfomycin trometamol (*Monuril* ®) is accepted for use within NHS Scotland for the treatment of acute lower uncomplicated urinary tract infections, caused by pathogens sensitive to fosfomycin in adult and adolescent females and for prophylaxis in diagnostic and surgical transurethral procedures.

● MEDICINAL FORMS
There can be variation in the licensing of different medicines containing the same drug.
Powder for solution for infusion
ELECTROLYTES: May contain Sodium
▸ Fomicyt (Nordic Pharma Ltd)
  Fosfomycin (as Fosfomycin sodium) 2 gram Fomicyt 2g powder for solution for infusion vials | 10 vial [PoM] £150.00
  Fosfomycin (as Fosfomycin sodium) 4 gram Fomicyt 4g powder for solution for infusion vials | 10 vial [PoM] £300.00
Granules
CAUTIONARY AND ADVISORY LABELS 9, 13, 23
EXCIPIENTS: May contain Sucrose
▸ Fosfomycin (Non-proprietary)
  Fosfomycin (as Fosfomycin trometamol) 3 gram Fosfomycin 3g granules sachets | 1 sachet [PoM] £75.45 DT = £4.86
▸ Monuril (Zambon S.p.A.)
  Fosfomycin (as Fosfomycin trometamol) 3 gram Monuril 3g granules sachets | 1 sachet [PoM] £4.86 DT = £4.86

Fusidic acid
16-Jun-2017

● DRUG ACTION Fusidic acid and its salts are narrow-spectrum antibiotics used for staphylococcal infections.

● INDICATIONS AND DOSE

Staphylococcal skin infection
▸ BY MOUTH USING TABLETS
▸ Child 12–17 years: 250 mg every 12 hours for 5-10 days, dose expressed as sodium fusidate
▸ Adult: 250 mg every 12 hours for 5-10 days, dose expressed as sodium fusidate
▸ TO THE SKIN
▸ Child: Apply 3–4 times a day usually for 7 days
▸ Adult: Apply 3–4 times a day

Penicillin-resistant staphylococcal infection including osteomyelitis | Staphylococcal endocarditis in combination with other antibacterials
▸ BY MOUTH USING ORAL SUSPENSION
▸ Child 1–11 months: 15 mg/kg 3 times a day
▸ Child 1–4 years: 250 mg 3 times a day
▸ Child 5–11 years: 500 mg 3 times a day
▸ Child 12–17 years: 750 mg 3 times a day
▸ Adult: 750 mg 3 times a day
▸ BY MOUTH USING TABLETS
▸ Child 12–17 years: 500 mg every 8 hours, increased to 1 g every 8 hours, increased dose can be used for severe infections, dose expressed as sodium fusidate
▸ Adult: 500 mg every 8 hours, increased to 1 g every 8 hours, increased dose can be used for severe infections, dose expressed as sodium fusidate

Staphylococcal infections due to susceptible organisms
▸ BY INTRAVENOUS INFUSION
▸ Child (body-weight up to 50 kg): 6–7 mg/kg 3 times a day, dose expressed as sodium fusidate
▸ Child (body-weight 50 kg and above): 500 mg 3 times a day, dose expressed as sodium fusidate
▸ Adult (body-weight up to 50 kg): 6–7 mg/kg 3 times a day, dose expressed as sodium fusidate
▸ Adult (body-weight 50 kg and above): 500 mg 3 times a day, dose expressed as sodium fusidate
DOSE EQUIVALENCE AND CONVERSION
▸ With oral use
▸ Fusidic acid is incompletely absorbed and doses recommended for suspension are proportionately higher than those for sodium fusidate tablets.

● CAUTIONS
▸ With systemic use Impaired transport and metabolism of bilirubin
▸ With topical use Avoid contact of cream or ointment with eyes
CAUTIONS, FURTHER INFORMATION
▸ Avoiding resistance
▸ With topical use To avoid the development of resistance, fusidic acid should not be used for longer than 10 days and local microbiology advice should be sought before using it in hospital.

● INTERACTIONS → Appendix 1: fusidic acid

● SIDE-EFFECTS
GENERAL SIDE-EFFECTS
▸ **Common or very common** Dizziness · drowsiness · hepatic disorders · hyperbilirubinaemia
▸ **Uncommon** Appetite decreased · asthenia · headache · malaise · skin reactions
▸ **Frequency not known** Agranulocytosis · anaemia · leucopenia · neutropenia · pancytopenia · renal failure · rhabdomyolysis · thrombocytopenia
SPECIFIC SIDE-EFFECTS
▸ **Common or very common**
▸ With intravenous use Vascular pain (reduced if given via central vein)
▸ With oral use Diarrhoea · gastrointestinal discomfort · nausea · vomiting
SIDE-EFFECTS, FURTHER INFORMATION Elevated liver enzymes, hyperbilirubinaemia and jaundice can occur with systemic use—these effects are usually reversible following withdrawal of therapy.

● PREGNANCY
▸ With systemic use Not known to be harmful; manufacturer advises use only if potential benefit outweighs risk.

● BREAST FEEDING
▸ With systemic use Present in milk—manufacturer advises caution.

● HEPATIC IMPAIRMENT
▸ With systemic use Manufacturer advises caution—monitor liver function periodically during treatment.

● MONITORING REQUIREMENTS
▸ With systemic use Manufacturer advises monitor liver function with high doses or on prolonged therapy; monitoring also advised for patients with biliary tract obstruction, those taking potentially hepatotoxic medication, or those taking concurrent medication with a similar excretion pathway.

● DIRECTIONS FOR ADMINISTRATION Manufacturer advises *for intravenous infusion*, give intermittently in Sodium chloride 0.9% or Glucose 5%; reconstitute each vial with 10 mL buffer solution, then add contents of vial to 500 mL infusion fluid to give a solution containing approximately 1 mg/mL. Give requisite dose via a central line over

5

Infection

5

Infection

2 hours (give over at least 6 hours if administered via a large peripheral vein).

- PRESCRIBING AND DISPENSING INFORMATION Flavours of oral liquid formulations may include banana and orange.
- PROFESSION SPECIFIC INFORMATION

Dental practitioners' formulary
May be prescribed as Sodium Fusidate ointment.

- MEDICINAL FORMS
There can be variation in the licensing of different medicines containing the same drug.

Oral suspension
CAUTIONARY AND ADVISORY LABELS 9, 21
▸ Fucidin (LEO Pharma)
  Fusidic acid 50 mg per 1 ml Fucidin 250mg/5ml oral suspension | 50 ml [PoM] £6.73 DT = £6.73

Powder and solvent for solution for infusion
ELECTROLYTES: May contain Sodium
▸ Fusidic acid (Non-proprietary)
  Sodium fusidate 500 mg Sodium fusidate 500mg powder and solvent for solution for infusion vials | 1 vial [PoM] £38.00

Tablet
CAUTIONARY AND ADVISORY LABELS 9
▸ Fucidin (Sodium fusidate) (LEO Pharma)
  Sodium fusidate 250 mg Fucidin 250mg tablets | 10 tablet [PoM] £6.02 DT = £6.02 | 100 tablet [PoM] £54.99

Cream
EXCIPIENTS: May contain Butylated hydroxyanisole, cetostearyl alcohol (including cetyl and stearyl alcohol)
▸ Fusidic acid (Non-proprietary)
  Fusidic acid 20 mg per 1 gram Fusidic acid 2% cream | 15 gram [PoM] £1.92 DT = £1.46 | 30 gram [PoM] £5.00 DT = £2.92
▸ Fucidin (LEO Pharma)
  Fusidic acid 20 mg per 1 gram Fucidin 20mg/g cream | 15 gram [PoM] £1.92 DT = £1.46 | 30 gram [PoM] £3.59 DT = £2.92

Ointment
EXCIPIENTS: May contain Cetostearyl alcohol (including cetyl and stearyl alcohol), woolfat and related substances (including lanolin)
▸ Fucidin (LEO Pharma)
  Sodium fusidate 20 mg per 1 gram Fucidin 20mg/g ointment | 15 gram [PoM] £2.68 DT = £2.68 | 30 gram [PoM] £4.55 DT = £4.55

Linezolid

- DRUG ACTION Linezolid, an oxazolidinone antibacterial, is active against Gram-positive bacteria including meticillin-resistant *Staphylococcus aureus* (MRSA), and glycopeptide-resistant enterococci. Resistance to linezolid can develop with prolonged treatment or if the dose is less than that recommended. Linezolid is **not** active against common Gram-negative organisms; it must be given in combination with other antibacterials for mixed infections that also involve Gram-negative organisms.

- INDICATIONS AND DOSE

Pneumonia (when other antibacterials e.g. a glycopeptide, such as vancomycin, cannot be used) (initiated under specialist supervision) | Complicated skin and soft-tissue infections caused by Gram-positive bacteria, when other antibacterials cannot be used (initiated under specialist supervision)
▸ BY MOUTH
▸ Adult: 600 mg every 12 hours usually for 10–14 days (maximum duration of treatment 28 days)
▸ BY INTRAVENOUS INFUSION
▸ Adult: 600 mg every 12 hours

IMPORTANT SAFETY INFORMATION
CHM ADVICE (OPTIC NEUROPATHY)
Severe optic neuropathy may occur rarely, particularly if linezolid is used for longer than 28 days. The CHM recommends that:

- patients should be warned to report symptoms of visual impairment (including blurred vision, visual field defect, changes in visual acuity and colour vision) immediately;
- patients experiencing new visual symptoms (regardless of treatment duration) should be evaluated promptly, and referred to an ophthalmologist if necessary;
- visual function should be monitored regularly if treatment is required for longer than 28 days.

BLOOD DISORDERS
Haematopoietic disorders (including thrombocytopenia, anaemia, leucopenia, and pancytopenia) have been reported in patients receiving linezolid. It is recommended that full blood counts are monitored weekly. Close monitoring is recommended in patients who:

- receive treatment for more than 10–14 days;
- have pre-existing myelosuppression;
- are receiving drugs that may have adverse effects on haemoglobin, blood counts, or platelet function;
- have severe renal impairment.

If significant myelosuppression occurs, treatment should be stopped unless it is considered essential, in which case intensive monitoring of blood counts and appropriate management should be implemented.

- CAUTIONS Acute confusional states · bipolar depression · carcinoid tumour · elderly (increased risk of blood disorders) · history of seizures · phaeochromocytoma · schizophrenia · thyrotoxicosis · uncontrolled hypertension
CAUTIONS, FURTHER INFORMATION
▸ Close observation Unless close observation and blood pressure monitoring possible, linezolid should be avoided in uncontrolled hypertension, phaeochromocytoma, carcinoid tumour, thyrotoxicosis, bipolar depression, schizophrenia, or acute confusional states.
- INTERACTIONS → Appendix 1: linezolid
- SIDE-EFFECTS
▸ **Common or very common** Anaemia · constipation · diarrhoea · dizziness · gastrointestinal discomfort · headache · hypertension · increased risk of infection · insomnia · localised pain · nausea · skin reactions · taste altered · vomiting
▸ **Uncommon** Arrhythmia · chills · dry mouth · eosinophilia · fatigue · gastritis · hyperhidrosis · hyponatraemia · leucopenia · neutropenia · oral disorders · pancreatitis · polyuria · renal failure · seizure · sensation abnormal · thirst · thrombocytopenia · tinnitus · transient ischaemic attack · vision disorders · vulvovaginal disorder
▸ **Rare or very rare** Antibiotic associated colitis · bone marrow disorders
▸ **Frequency not known** Alopecia · angioedema · lactic acidosis · nerve disorders · serotonin syndrome · severe cutaneous adverse reactions (SCARs)
- PREGNANCY Manufacturer advises use only if potential benefit outweighs risk—no information available.
- BREAST FEEDING Manufacturer advises avoid—present in milk in *animal* studies.
- HEPATIC IMPAIRMENT In severe hepatic impairment manufacturer advises use only if potential benefit outweighs risk.
- RENAL IMPAIRMENT Manufacturer advises metabolites may accumulate if eGFR less than 30 mL/minute/1.73 m^2.
- MONITORING REQUIREMENTS Monitor full blood count (including platelet count) weekly.
- DIRECTIONS FOR ADMINISTRATION
▸ With intravenous use Infusion to be administered over 30–120 minutes.

- PRESCRIBING AND DISPENSING INFORMATION Flavours of oral liquid formulations may include orange.
- PATIENT AND CARER ADVICE Patients should be advised to read the patient information leaflet given with linezolid.

- MEDICINAL FORMS
There can be variation in the licensing of different medicines containing the same drug.

Infusion
EXCIPIENTS: May contain Glucose
ELECTROLYTES: May contain Sodium
▸ Linezolid (Non-proprietary)
  Linezolid 2 mg per 1 ml Linezolid 600mg/300ml infusion bags | 10 bag PoM £445.00 (Hospital only)
▸ Zyvox (Pfizer Ltd)
  Linezolid 2 mg per 1 ml Zyvox 600mg/300ml infusion bags | 10 bag PoM £445.00

Oral suspension
CAUTIONARY AND ADVISORY LABELS 9, 10
EXCIPIENTS: May contain Aspartame
▸ Zyvox (Pfizer Ltd)
  Linezolid 20 mg per 1 ml Zyvox 100mg/5ml granules for oral suspension | 150 ml PoM £222.50

Tablet
CAUTIONARY AND ADVISORY LABELS 9, 10
▸ Linezolid (Non-proprietary)
  Linezolid 600 mg Linezolid 600mg tablets | 10 tablet PoM £82.12-£445.00 DT = £335.35
▸ Zyvox (Pfizer Ltd)
  Linezolid 600 mg Zyvox 600mg tablets | 10 tablet PoM £445.00 DT = £335.35

Tedizolid

26-Sep-2016

- DRUG ACTION Tedizolid is an oxazolidinone antibacterial, which inhibits bacterial protein synthesis.

● INDICATIONS AND DOSE

Treatment of acute bacterial skin and skin structure infections
▸ BY INTRAVENOUS INFUSION, OR BY MOUTH
▸ Adult: 200 mg once daily for 6 days, patients should be switched from the intravenous to the oral route when clinically appropriate

- CAUTIONS Neutropenia—limited clinical experience · patients aged 75 years and over—limited clinical experience
- INTERACTIONS → Appendix 1: tedizolid
- SIDE-EFFECTS
  GENERAL SIDE-EFFECTS
▸ **Common or very common** Diarrhoea · dizziness · fatigue · headache · nausea · skin reactions · vomiting
▸ **Uncommon** Abscess · alopecia · antibiotic associated colitis · anxiety · arthralgia · bradycardia · chills · constipation · cough · dehydration · diabetic control impaired · drowsiness · dry mouth · fever · gastrointestinal discomfort · gastrointestinal disorders · haematochezia · hyperhidrosis · hyperkalaemia · increased risk of infection · infusion related reaction · irritability · limb discomfort · lymphadenopathy · muscle spasms · nasal dryness · pain · peripheral oedema · pulmonary congestion · sensation abnormal · sleep disorders · taste altered · tremor · urine odour abnormal · vasodilation · vision blurred · vitreous floater · vulvovaginal pruritus
- CONCEPTION AND CONTRACEPTION Manufacturer recommends effective contraception in women of childbearing potential; an additional method of contraception is advised in women taking hormonal contraceptives—effectiveness may be reduced.
- PREGNANCY Manufacturer advises avoid—fetal developmental toxicity in *animal* studies.
- BREAST FEEDING Manufacturer advises avoid—present in milk in *animal* studies.

- DIRECTIONS FOR ADMINISTRATION For *intravenous infusion* (*Sivextro*®) give intermittently in Sodium Chloride 0.9%; reconstitute each 200 mg vial with 4 mL Water for Injections, then dilute reconstituted solution in 250 mL sodium chloride 0.9%; give over approx. 1 hour.
- PATIENT AND CARER ADVICE
  Optic neuropathy Although neuropathy (peripheral and optic) has not been reported in patients treated with tedizolid, manufacturer advises patients and carers are warned to report symptoms of visual impairment (including blurred vision, visual field defect, changes in visual acuity and colour vision) immediately; patients should be evaluated promptly, and referred to an ophthalmologist if necessary.
  Missed doses Manufacturer advises that if a dose is more than 16 hours late, the missed dose should not be taken and the next dose should be taken at the normal time.
  Driving and skilled tasks Patients and carers should be counselled on the effects on driving and skilled tasks—increased risk of dizziness and fatigue.
- NATIONAL FUNDING/ACCESS DECISIONS
  Scottish Medicines Consortium (SMC) Decisions
  The *Scottish Medicines Consortium* has advised (August 2015) that tedizolid (*Sivextro*®) is accepted for restricted use within NHS Scotland as an alternative oxazolidinone antibacterial for the treatment of acute bacterial skin and skin structure infections caused by Gram-positive *Staphylococcus aureus* (specifically methicillin-resistant *Staphylococcus aureus* [MRSA] isolates), on the specific advice of local microbiologists or specialists in infectious disease.

- MEDICINAL FORMS
There can be variation in the licensing of different medicines containing the same drug.
Powder for solution for infusion
▸ Sivextro (Merck Sharp & Dohme Ltd) ▼
  Tedizolid phosphate 200 mg Sivextro 200mg powder for concentrate for solution for infusion vials | 6 vial PoM £862.00
Tablet
▸ Sivextro (Merck Sharp & Dohme Ltd) ▼
  Tedizolid phosphate 200 mg Sivextro 200mg tablets | 6 tablet PoM £862.00

Trimethoprim

● INDICATIONS AND DOSE

Urinary-tract infections | Respiratory tract infections
▸ BY MOUTH
▸ Child 4–5 weeks: 4 mg/kg twice daily (max. per dose 200 mg)
▸ Child 6 weeks–5 months: 4 mg/kg twice daily (max. per dose 200 mg), alternatively 25 mg twice daily
▸ Child 6 months–5 years: 4 mg/kg twice daily (max. per dose 200 mg), alternatively 50 mg twice daily
▸ Child 6–11 years: 4 mg/kg twice daily (max. per dose 200 mg), alternatively 100 mg twice daily
▸ Child 12–17 years: 200 mg twice daily
▸ Adult: 200 mg twice daily

Prophylaxis of urinary-tract infection (considered for recurrent infection, significant urinary-tract anomalies, or significant kidney damage)
▸ BY MOUTH
▸ Child 4–5 weeks: 2 mg/kg once daily (max. per dose 100 mg), dose to be taken at night
▸ Child 6 weeks–5 months: 2 mg/kg once daily (max. per dose 100 mg), dose to be taken at night, alternatively 12.5 mg once daily, dose to be taken at night
▸ Child 6 months–5 years: 2 mg/kg once daily (max. per dose 100 mg), dose to be taken at night, alternatively 25 mg once daily, dose to be taken at night continued →

Infection

5

- Child 6-11 years: 2 mg/kg once daily (max. per dose 100 mg), dose to be taken at night, alternatively 50 mg once daily, dose to be taken at night
- Child 12-17 years: 100 mg once daily, dose to be taken at night
- Adult: 100 mg once daily, dose to be taken at night

Treatment of mild to moderate _Pneumocystis jirovecii_ (_Pneumocystis carinii_) pneumonia in patients who cannot tolerate co-trimoxazole (in combination with dapsone)
- BY MOUTH
- Child: 5 mg/kg every 6–8 hours
- Adult: 5 mg/kg every 6–8 hours

Acne resistant to other antibacterials
- BY MOUTH
- Adult: 300 mg twice daily

Prostatitis
- BY MOUTH
- Adult: (consult product literature)

Shigellosis | Invasive salmonella infection
- BY MOUTH
- Adult: (consult product literature)

- UNLICENSED USE Not licensed for treatment of pneumocystis pneumonia. Not licensed for use in children under 6 weeks. Not licensed for treatment of acne resistant to other antibacterials.
- CONTRA-INDICATIONS Blood dyscrasias
- CAUTIONS Elderly · Acute porphyrias p. 1025 · predisposition to folate deficiency
- INTERACTIONS → Appendix 1: trimethoprim
- SIDE-EFFECTS
- Common or very common Diarrhoea · electrolyte imbalance · fungal overgrowth · headache · nausea · skin reactions · vomiting
- Rare or very rare Agranulocytosis · angioedema · anxiety · appetite decreased · arthralgia · behaviour abnormal · bone marrow disorders · confusion · constipation · cough · depression · dizziness · dyspnoea · eosinophilia · erythema nodosum · fever · haemolysis · haemolytic anaemia · haemorrhage · hallucination · hepatic disorders · hypoglycaemia · lethargy · leucopenia · meningitis aseptic · movement disorders · myalgia · neutropenia · oral disorders · pancreatitis · paraesthesia · peripheral neuritis · photosensitivity reaction · pseudomembranous enterocolitis · renal impairment · seizure · severe cutaneous adverse reactions (SCARs) · sleep disorders · syncope · systemic lupus erythematosus (SLE) · thrombocytopenia · tinnitus · tremor · uveitis · vasculitis · vertigo · wheezing
- Frequency not known Gastrointestinal disorder · megaloblastic anaemia · methaemoglobinaemia
- PREGNANCY Teratogenic risk in first trimester (folate antagonist). Manufacturers advise avoid during pregnancy.
- BREAST FEEDING Present in milk—short-term use not known to be harmful.
- RENAL IMPAIRMENT
  Dose adjustments ▸ In adults Use half normal dose after 3 days if eGFR 15–30 mL/minute/1.73 m². Use half normal dose if eGFR less than 15 mL/minute/1.73 m².
  ▸ In children Use half normal dose after 3 days if estimated glomerular filtration rate 15–30 mL/minute/1.73 m². Use half normal dose if estimated glomerular filtration rate less than 15 mL/minute/1.73 m².
  Monitoring Monitor plasma-trimethoprim concentration if eGFR less than 10 mL/minute/1.73 m².
- MONITORING REQUIREMENTS Manufacturer recommends blood counts on long-term therapy (but evidence of practical value unsatisfactory).

- PATIENT AND CARER ADVICE
  Blood disorders On long-term treatment, patients and their carers should be told how to recognise signs of blood disorders and advised to seek immediate medical attention if symptoms such as fever, sore throat, rash, mouth ulcers, purpura, bruising or bleeding develop.
  Medicines for Children leaflet: Trimethoprim for bacterial infections www.medicinesforchildren.org.uk/trimethoprim-for-bacterial-infections

- MEDICINAL FORMS
  There can be variation in the licensing of different medicines containing the same drug. Forms available from special-order manufacturers include: oral suspension, oral solution
  Oral suspension
  CAUTIONARY AND ADVISORY LABELS 9
  ▸ Trimethoprim (Non-proprietary)
    Trimethoprim 10 mg per 1 ml Trimethoprim 50mg/5ml oral suspension sugar free sugar-free | 100 ml [PoM] £5.24 DT = £2.30
  ▸ Monotrim (Chemidex Pharma Ltd)
    Trimethoprim 10 mg per 1 ml Monotrim 50mg/5ml oral suspension sugar-free | 100 ml [PoM] £1.77 DT = £2.30
  Tablet
  CAUTIONARY AND ADVISORY LABELS 9
  ▸ Trimethoprim (Non-proprietary)
    Trimethoprim 100 mg Trimethoprim 100mg tablets | 28 tablet [PoM] £9.99 DT = £0.86
    Trimethoprim 200 mg Trimethoprim 200mg tablets | 6 tablet [PoM] £2.15 DT = £0.31 | 14 tablet [PoM] £9.99 DT = £0.73

  Combinations available: _Co-trimoxazole_, p. 552

ANTIMYCOBACTERIALS > RIFAMYCINS

Rifabutin

- INDICATIONS AND DOSE
  Prophylaxis of _Mycobacterium avium_ complex infections in immunosuppressed patients with low CD4 count
  - BY MOUTH
  - Adult: 300 mg once daily, also consult product literature

  Treatment of non-tuberculous mycobacterial disease, in combination with other drugs
  - BY MOUTH
  - Adult: 450–600 mg once daily for up to 6 months after cultures negative

  Treatment of pulmonary tuberculosis, in combination with other drugs
  - BY MOUTH
  - Adult: 150–450 mg once daily for at least 6 months

- CAUTIONS Acute porphyrias p. 1025 · discolours soft contact lenses
- INTERACTIONS → Appendix 1: rifabutin
- SIDE-EFFECTS Agranulocytosis · anaemia · arthralgia · bronchospasm · chest pain · corneal deposits · decreased leucocytes · dyspnoea · eosinophilia · fever · haemolysis · hepatic disorders · influenza like illness · myalgia · nausea · neutropenia · pancytopenia · skin reactions · thrombocytopenia · urine discolouration · uveitis (more common following high doses or concomitant use with drugs that increase plasma concentration) · vomiting
- ALLERGY AND CROSS-SENSITIVITY Contra-indicated in patients with rifamycin hypersensitivity.
- CONCEPTION AND CONTRACEPTION
  Important Rifabutin induces hepatic enzymes and the effectiveness of hormonal contraceptives is reduced; alternative family planning advice should be offered.
- PREGNANCY Manufacturer advises avoid—no information available.
- BREAST FEEDING Manufacturer advises avoid—no information available.

- **HEPATIC IMPAIRMENT**
  Dose adjustments Reduce dose in severe impairment.
  Monitoring In patients with pre-existing liver disease or hepatic impairment monitor liver function regularly and particularly frequently in the first 2 months; blood counts should also be monitored in these patients.
- **RENAL IMPAIRMENT**
  Dose adjustments Use half normal dose if eGFR less than 30 mL/minute/1.73 m^2.
- **MONITORING REQUIREMENTS**
  ▶ *Renal function* should be checked before treatment.
  ▶ *Hepatic function* should be checked before treatment. If there is no evidence of liver disease (and pre-treatment liver function is normal), further checks are only necessary if the patient develops fever, malaise, vomiting, jaundice or unexplained deterioration during treatment. However, hepatic function should be monitored on prolonged therapy.
  ▶ Blood counts should be monitored on prolonged therapy.
  ▶ Those with alcohol dependence should have frequent checks of hepatic function, particularly in the first 2 months. Blood counts should also be monitored in these patients.
- **PRESCRIBING AND DISPENSING INFORMATION** If treatment interruption occurs, re-introduce with low dosage and increase gradually.
- **PATIENT AND CARER ADVICE**
  Soft contact lenses Patients or their carers should be advised that rifabutin discolours soft contact lenses.
  Hepatic disorders Patients or their carers should be told how to recognise signs of liver disorder, and advised to discontinue treatment and seek immediate medical attention if symptoms such as persistent nausea, vomiting, malaise or jaundice develop.
- **MEDICINAL FORMS**
  There can be variation in the licensing of different medicines containing the same drug. Forms available from special-order manufacturers include: oral suspension, oral solution
  Capsule
  CAUTIONARY AND ADVISORY LABELS 8, 14
  ▶ Mycobutin (Pfizer Ltd)
    Rifabutin 150 mg Mycobutin 150mg capsules | 30 capsule [PoM] £90.38

Rifaximin

- **DRUG ACTION** Rifaximin is a rifamycin that is poorly absorbed from the gastro-intestinal tract, and, therefore, should not be used to treat systemic infections.

- **INDICATIONS AND DOSE**
  Travellers' diarrhoea that is not associated with fever, bloody diarrhoea, blood or leucocytes in the stool, or 8 or more unformed stools in the previous 24 hours
  ▶ BY MOUTH
  ▶ Adult: 200 mg every 8 hours for 3 days
  Reduction in recurrence of hepatic encephalopathy
  ▶ BY MOUTH
  ▶ Adult: 550 mg twice daily

- **CONTRA-INDICATIONS** Intestinal obstruction
- **INTERACTIONS** → Appendix 1: rifaximin
- **SIDE-EFFECTS**
- **Common or very common** Arthralgia · ascites · constipation · depression · dizziness · dyspnoea · gastrointestinal discomfort · gastrointestinal disorders · headaches · muscle complaints · nausea · oedema · skin reactions · vomiting
- **Uncommon** Anaemia · anxiety · appetite decreased · asthenia · balance impaired · concentration impaired · confusion · cough · diplopia · drowsiness · dry lips · dry mouth · dry throat · ear pain · fall · haematuria · hot flush ·

hyperhidrosis · hyperkalaemia · increased risk of infection · lymphocytosis · memory loss · muscle weakness · nasal complaints · neutropenia · oropharyngeal pain · pain · palpitations · polymenorrhoea · respiratory disorders · seizure · sensation abnormal · sleep disorders · sunburn · taste altered · urinary disorders · urine abnormalities · vertigo
- **Rare or very rare** Hypertension · hypotension
- **Frequency not known** Angioedema · syncope · thrombocytopenia · urine discolouration
- **ALLERGY AND CROSS-SENSITIVITY** Contra-indicated if history of rifamycin hypersensitivity.
- **PREGNANCY** Manufacturer advises avoid—toxicity in *animal* studies.
- **BREAST FEEDING** Unlikely to be present in milk in significant amounts, but manufacturer advises avoid.
- **HEPATIC IMPAIRMENT** Manufacturer advises caution when used for hepatic encephalopathy in patients with severe hepatic impairment.
- **PRESCRIBING AND DISPENSING INFORMATION** Not recommended for diarrhoea associated with invasive organisms such as *Campylobacter* and *Shigella*.
- **NATIONAL FUNDING/ACCESS DECISIONS**
  NICE decisions
  ▶ Rifaximin for preventing episodes of overt hepatic encephalopathy (March 2015) NICE TA337
  Rifaximin is recommended, within its marketing authorisation, as an option for reducing the recurrence of episodes of overt hepatic encephalopathy in adults.
  www.nice.org.uk/TA337
- **MEDICINAL FORMS**
  There can be variation in the licensing of different medicines containing the same drug. Forms available from special-order manufacturers include: oral suspension
  Tablet
  CAUTIONARY AND ADVISORY LABELS 9 (Xifaxantan ® brand only), 14
  ▶ Targaxan (Norgine Pharmaceuticals Ltd)
    Rifaximin 550 mg Targaxan 550mg tablets | 56 tablet [PoM] £259.23 DT = £259.23
  ▶ Xifaxanta (Norgine Pharmaceuticals Ltd)
    Rifaximin 200 mg Xifaxanta 200mg tablets | 9 tablet [PoM] £15.15 DT = £15.15

2.1 Anthrax

Anthrax

Treatment and post-exposure prophylaxis

Inhalation or *gastro-intestinal anthrax* should be treated initially with either ciprofloxacin p. 548 or, in patients over 12 years, doxycycline p. 555 [unlicensed indication] combined with one or two other antibacterials (such as amoxicillin p. 539, benzylpenicillin sodium p. 537, chloramphenicol p. 558, clarithromycin p. 529, clindamycin p. 526, imipenem with cilastatin p. 514, rifampicin p. 571 [unlicensed indication], and vancomycin p. 525). When the condition improves and the sensitivity of the *Bacillus anthracis* strain is known, treatment may be switched to a single antibacterial. Treatment should continue for 60 days because germination may be delayed.

Cutaneous anthrax should be treated with either ciprofloxacin [unlicensed indication] or doxycycline [unlicensed indication] for 7 days. Treatment may be switched to amoxicillin if the infecting strain is susceptible. Treatment may need to be extended to 60 days if exposure is due to aerosol. A combination of antibacterials for 14 days is recommended for cutaneous anthrax with systemic features, extensive oedema, or lesions of the head or neck.

Ciprofloxacin or doxycycline may be given for *post-exposure prophylaxis*. If exposure is confirmed, antibacterial prophylaxis should continue for 60 days. Antibacterial prophylaxis may be switched to amoxicillin after 10–14 days if the strain of *B. anthracis* is susceptible. Vaccination against anthrax may allow the duration of antibacterial prophylaxis to be shortened.

2.2 Leprosy

Leprosy

Management
Advice from a member of the Panel of Leprosy Opinion is essential for the treatment of leprosy (Hansen's disease). Details can be obtained from the Hospital for Tropical Diseases, London (telephone (020) 3456 7890).

The World Health Organization has made recommendations to overcome the problem of dapsone below resistance and to prevent the emergence of resistance to other antileprotic drugs. Drugs recommended are dapsone, rifampicin p. 571, and clofazimine below. Other drugs with significant activity against *Mycobacterium leprae* include ofloxacin p. 551, minocycline p. 556 and clarithromycin p. 529, but none of these are as active as rifampicin; at present they should be reserved as second-line drugs for leprosy.

A three-drug regimen is recommended for *multibacillary leprosy* (lepromatous, borderline-lepromatous, and borderline leprosy) and a two-drug regimen for *paucibacillary leprosy* (borderline-tuberculoid, tuberculoid, and indeterminate).

Multibacillary leprosy should be treated with a combination of rifampicin, dapsone and clofazimine for at least 2 years. Treatment should be continued unchanged during both type I (reversal) or type II (erythema nodosum leprosum) reactions. During reversal reactions neuritic pain or weakness can herald the rapid onset of permanent nerve damage. Treatment with prednisolone p. 664 should be instituted at once. Mild type II reactions may respond to aspirin. Severe type II reactions may require corticosteroids; thalidomide p. 936 [unlicensed] is also useful in patients who have become corticosteroid dependent, but it should be used only under **specialist supervision**. Thalidomide is teratogenic and, therefore, contra-indicated in pregnancy; it must **not** be given to women of child-bearing potential unless they comply with a pregnancy prevention programme. Increased doses of clofazimine are also useful.

Paucibacillary leprosy should be treated with rifampicin and dapsone for 6 months. If treatment is interrupted the regimen should be recommenced where it was left off to complete the full course.

Neither the multibacillary nor the paucibacillary antileprosy regimen is sufficient to treat tuberculosis.

ANTIMYCOBACTERIALS

Clofazimine

● INDICATIONS AND DOSE

Multibacillary leprosy in combination with rifampicin and dapsone (3-drug regimen) (administered on expert advice)
▸ BY MOUTH
▸ Adult: 300 mg once a month, to be administered under supervision and 50 mg daily, to be self-administered, alternatively 300 mg once a month, to be administered under supervision and 100 mg once daily on alternate days, to be self-administered

Lepromatous lepra reactions (administered on expert advice)
▸ BY MOUTH
▸ Adult: 300 mg daily for max. 3 months

Severe type II (erythema nodosum leprosum) reactions (administered on expert advice)
▸ BY MOUTH
▸ Adult: 100 mg 3 times a day for one month, subsequent dose reductions are required, may take 4–6 weeks to attain full effect

● CAUTIONS Avoid if persistent abdominal pain and diarrhoea · may discolour soft contact lenses

● INTERACTIONS → Appendix 1: clofazimine

● SIDE-EFFECTS Abdominal pain · appetite decreased · dry eye · eye discolouration · fatigue · gastrointestinal disorders · hair colour changes (reversible) · headache · lymphadenopathy · nausea · photosensitivity reaction · red discolouration of body fluids · skin discolouration (including areas exposed to light) · skin reactions · splenic infarction · urine red · visual impairment · vomiting (hospitalise if persistent) · weight decreased

● PREGNANCY Use with caution.

● BREAST FEEDING May alter colour of milk; skin discoloration of infant.

● HEPATIC IMPAIRMENT Use with caution.

● RENAL IMPAIRMENT Use with caution.

● MEDICINAL FORMS There can be variation in the licensing of different medicines containing the same drug. Forms available from special-order manufacturers include: capsule

Dapsone

● INDICATIONS AND DOSE

Multibacillary leprosy in combination with rifampicin and clofazimine (3-drug regimen) | Paucibacillary leprosy in combination with rifampicin (2-drug regimen)
▸ BY MOUTH
▸ Adult (body-weight up to 35 kg): 50 mg daily, alternatively 1–2 mg/kg daily, may be self-administered
▸ Adult (body-weight 35 kg and above): 100 mg daily, may be self-administered

Dermatitis herpetiformis
▸ BY MOUTH
▸ Adult: (consult product literature or local protocols)

Treatment of mild to moderate *Pneumocystis jirovecii* (*Pneumocystis carinii*) pneumonia (in combination with trimethoprim)
▸ BY MOUTH
▸ Adult: 100 mg once daily

Prophylaxis of *Pneumocystis jirovecii* (*Pneumocystis carinii*) pneumonia
▸ BY MOUTH
▸ Adult: 100 mg daily

● UNLICENSED USE Not licensed for treatment of pneumocystis (*P. jirovecii*) pneumonia.

● CAUTIONS Anaemia (treat severe anaemia before starting) · avoid in Acute porphyrias p. 1025 · cardiac disease · G6PD deficiency · pulmonary disease · susceptibility to haemolysis

● INTERACTIONS → Appendix 1: dapsone

● SIDE-EFFECTS Agranulocytosis · appetite decreased · haemolysis · haemolytic anaemia · headache · hepatic disorders · hypoalbuminaemia · insomnia · lepra reaction · methaemoglobinaemia · motor loss · nausea · peripheral neuropathy · photosensitivity reaction · psychosis · severe cutaneous adverse reactions (SCARs) · skin reactions · tachycardia · vomiting

SIDE-EFFECTS, FURTHER INFORMATION Side-effects are dose-related.

If dapsone syndrome occurs (rash with fever and eosinophilia)—discontinue immediately (may progress to exfoliative dermatitis, hepatitis, hypoalbuminaemia, psychosis and death).

● PREGNANCY Folic acid p. 993 (higher dose) should be given to mother throughout pregnancy; neonatal haemolysis and methaemoglobinaemia reported in third trimester.

● BREAST FEEDING Haemolytic anaemia; although significant amount in milk, risk to infant very small unless infant is G6PD deficient.

● PATIENT AND CARER ADVICE
Blood disorders On long-term treatment, patients and their carers should be told how to recognise signs of blood disorders and advised to seek immediate medical attention if symptoms such as fever, sore throat, rash, mouth ulcers, purpura, bruising or bleeding develop.

● MEDICINAL FORMS
There can be variation in the licensing of different medicines containing the same drug. Forms available from special-order manufacturers include: oral suspension, oral solution

Tablet
CAUTIONARY AND ADVISORY LABELS 8
▸ Dapsone (Non-proprietary)
Dapsone 50 mg Dapsone 50mg tablets | 28 tablet PoM £38.04 DT = £38.04
Dapsone 100 mg Dapsone 100mg tablets | 28 tablet PoM £97.39 DT = £95.15

2.3 Lyme disease

Lyme disease

Treatment
Doxycycline p. 555, amoxicillin p. 539 [unlicensed indication] or cefuroxime p. 518 (as cefuroxime axetil) are the antibacterials of choice for *early Lyme disease* or *Lyme arthritis*. If these antibacterials are contra-indicated, a **macrolide** (e.g. clarithromycin p. 529) can be used for early Lyme disease. Intravenous administration of ceftriaxone p. 520, cefotaxime p. 519, or benzylpenicillin sodium p. 537 is recommended for Lyme disease associated with cardiac or neurological complications. The duration of treatment is usually 2–4 weeks; Lyme arthritis may require further treatment.

2.4 Methicillin-resistant *Staphylococcus aureus*

MRSA

Management
Infection from *Staphylococcus aureus* strains resistant to meticillin [now discontinued] (meticillin-resistant *Staph. aureus*, MRSA) and to flucloxacillin p. 544 can be difficult to manage. Treatment is guided by the sensitivity of the infecting strain.

Rifampicin p. 571 or fusidic acid p. 561 should **not** be used alone because resistance may develop rapidly. A **tetracycline** alone or a combination of rifampicin and fusidic acid can be used for *skin* and *soft-tissue infections*

caused by MRSA; clindamycin p. 526 alone is an alternative. A **glycopeptide** (e.g. vancomycin p. 525) can be used for severe skin and soft-tissue infections associated with MRSA; if a glycopeptide is unsuitable, linezolid p. 562 can be used on expert advice. As linezolid is **not** active against Gram-negative organisms, it can be used for mixed skin and soft-tissue infections only when other treatments are not available; linezolid must be given with other antibacterials if the infection also involves Gram-negative organisms. A combination of a glycopeptide and fusidic acid *or* a glycopeptide and rifampicin can be considered for skin and soft-tissue infections that have failed to respond to a single antibacterial.

Tigecycline p. 557 and daptomycin p. 558 are licensed for the treatment of complicated skin and soft-tissue infections involving MRSA.

A **tetracycline** or clindamycin can be used for *bronchiectasis* caused by MRSA. A **glycopeptide** can be used for *pneumonia* associated with MRSA; if a glycopeptide is unsuitable, linezolid can be used on expert advice. Linezolid must be given with other antibacterials if the infection also involves Gram-negative organisms.

A **tetracycline** can be used for *urinary-tract infections* caused by MRSA; trimethoprim p. 563 or nitrofurantoin p. 579 are alternatives. A **glycopeptide** can be used for urinary-tract infections that are severe or resistant to other antibacterials.

A **glycopeptide** can be used for *septicaemia* associated with MRSA.

See the management of *endocarditis, osteomyelitis,* or *septic arthritis* associated with MRSA.

Prophylaxis with vancomycin or teicoplanin p. 524 (alone or in combination with another antibacterial active against other pathogens) is appropriate for patients undergoing surgery if:

● there is a history of MRSA colonisation or infection without documented eradication;
● there is a risk that the patient's MRSA carriage has recurred;
● the patient comes from an area with a high prevalence of MRSA.

See eradication of nasal carriage of MRSA in Nose p. 1165.

2.5 Tuberculosis

Tuberculosis
16-Mar-2017

Treatment phases, overview
Active tuberculosis is treated in two phases—an *initial phase* using four drugs and a *continuation phase* using two drugs in fully sensitive cases. Treatment requires specialised knowledge and supervision, particularly where the disease involves resistant organisms or non-respiratory organs.

There are two regimens recommended for the treatment of tuberculosis in the UK; variations occur in other countries. Either the unsupervised regimen or the supervised regimen should be used; the two regimens should **not** be used concurrently. Compliance with therapy is a major determinant of its success.

Initial phase
The concurrent use of four drugs during the initial phase is designed to reduce the bacterial population as rapidly as possible and to prevent the emergence of drug-resistant bacteria. The drugs are best given as fixed-dose, combination preparations unless one of the components cannot be given because of resistance or intolerance. The treatment of choice for the initial phase is the daily use of rifampicin p. 571, ethambutol hydrochloride p. 575, pyrazinamide p. 577 and

isoniazid p. 576 (with pyridoxine hydrochloride p. 1047 for prophylaxis of isoniazid-induced neuropathy); modified according to drug susceptibility testing. Treatment should be started without waiting for culture results if clinical features or histology results are consistent with tuberculosis; treatment should be continued even if initial culture results are negative. The initial phase drugs should be continued for two months. Where a positive culture for *M. tuberculosis* has been obtained, but susceptibility results are not available after two months, treatment with rifampicin, ethambutol hydrochloride, isoniazid and pyrazinamide (with pyridoxine hydrochloride) should be continued until full susceptibility is confirmed, even if this is for longer than two months.

Streptomycin p. 512 is rarely used in the UK but it may be used in the initial phase of treatment if resistance to isoniazid has been established before therapy is commenced, or when patients cannot tolerate standard treatment.

Continuation phase

After the initial phase, daily treatment is continued for a further four months with rifampicin and isoniazid (preferably given as a combination preparation) with pyridoxine hydrochloride. Longer treatment is necessary for meningitis, direct spinal cord involvement, and for resistant organisms which may also require modification of the regimen.

Unsupervised treatment

The unsupervised treatment regimen should be used for patients who are likely to take antituberculosis drugs reliably **without supervision**. Patients who are unable or unlikely to comply with daily administration of therapy should be treated with the regimen described under *Supervised Treatment*.

Pregnancy and breast-feeding

The standard unsupervised six month treatment regimen may be used during pregnancy. Streptomycin should not be given in pregnancy.

The standard unsupervised six month treatment regimen may be used during breast-feeding.

Supervised treatment

Drug administration should be **fully supervised** (directly observed therapy, DOT) in patients who cannot comply reliably with the treatment regimen. If daily directly observed therapy is not possible, a supervised dosing schedule of three times a week should be considered. Regimens with a dosing schedule of fewer than three times a week should not be used.

Directly observed therapy should be offered to patients who:

- have a history of non-adherence;
- have previously been treated for tuberculosis;
- are in denial of the tuberculosis diagnosis;
- have multidrug-resistant tuberculosis;
- have a major psychiatric or cognitive disorder;
- have a history of homelessness, drug or alcohol misuse;
- are in prison, or have been in the past 5 years;
- are too ill to self-administer treatment;
- request directly observed therapy.

Immunocompromised patients

Multi-resistant *Mycobacterium tuberculosis* may be present in immunocompromised patients. The organism should always be cultured to confirm its type and drug sensitivity. Confirmed *M. tuberculosis* infection sensitive to first-line drugs should be treated with a standard six month regimen; after completing treatment, patients should be closely monitored. The regimen may need to be modified if infection is caused by resistant organisms, and specialist advice is needed.

Specialist advice should be sought about tuberculosis treatment or chemoprophylaxis for patients who are HIV-positive (see also *Latent tuberculosis* below); care is required in choosing the regimen and in avoiding potentially serious interactions. Starting antiretroviral treatment in the first two months of antituberculosis treatment increases the risk of immune reconstitution syndrome. Treatment for tuberculosis should not routinely exceed six months in patients who are HIV-positive, unless the tuberculosis has central nervous system involvement (in which case treatment should not routinely extend beyond twelve months).

Infection may also be caused by other mycobacteria e.g. *M. avium* complex, in which case specialist advice on management is needed.

Extrapulmonary tuberculosis

Central nervous system tuberculosis

Patients with active central nervous system tuberculosis should be offered treatment with rifampicin, ethambutol hydrochloride, isoniazid and pyrazinamide (with pyridoxine hydrochloride for prophylaxis of isoniazid-induced neuropathy) for two months. After completion of the initial treatment phase, rifampicin and isoniazid (with pyridoxine hydrochloride) should be continued for a further ten months. Treatment for tuberculosis meningitis should be offered if clinical signs and laboratory findings are consistent with the diagnosis, even if a rapid diagnostic test is negative.

An initial high dose of dexamethasone p. 660 or prednisolone p. 664 should be started at the same time as antituberculosis therapy, and then slowly withdrawn over 4–8 weeks.

Referral for surgery should be considered only in patients who have raised intracranial pressure.

Pericardial tuberculosis

An initial high dose of oral prednisolone should be offered to patients with active pericardial tuberculosis at the same time as initiation of antituberculosis therapy; it should then be slowly withdrawn over 2–3 weeks.

Latent tuberculosis

Clinicians should be aware that some patients with latent tuberculosis are at increased risk of developing active tuberculosis (such as patients who are HIV-positive, diabetic or receiving treatment with a tumour necrosis factor alpha inhibitor). These patients should be advised of the risks and symptoms of active tuberculosis.

Note: the risk of adverse events to chemoprophylaxis in patients aged over 35 years with a risk of hepatotoxicity is likely to be greater than the potential benefit of treating latent disease. *When indicated*, drug treatment should only be offered to patients aged 35–65 years if hepatotoxicity is not a concern. Treatment for latent tuberculosis is not usually indicated in patients over 65 years.

Close contacts

Anyone aged under 65 years who is a close contact (prolonged, frequent or intense contact, e.g. household contacts or partners) of a person with pulmonary or laryngeal tuberculosis should be tested for latent tuberculosis. Chemoprophylaxis should be offered to all patients aged younger than 65 years, with evidence of latent tuberculosis if the close contact has *suspected-infectious* or *confirmed-active* pulmonary or laryngeal drug-sensitive tuberculosis.

Immunocompromised

Patients who are immunocompromised, such as those with HIV or who have had a solid organ or allogeneic stem cell transplant, should be tested for latent tuberculosis using an appropriate method. Patients who test positive should then be assessed for active disease, and if negative, offered treatment for latent tuberculosis.

Recommended dosage for standard unsupervised 6-month treatment

Rifampicin with isoniazid and pyrazinamide	Adult: ▸ body-weight up to 40 kg 3 tablets daily for 2 months (initial phase), use *Rifater*® Tablets, preferably taken before breakfast; ▸ body-weight 40–49 kg 4 tablets daily for 2 months (initial phase), use *Rifater*® Tablets, preferably taken before breakfast; ▸ body-weight 50–64 kg 5 tablets daily for 2 months (initial phase), use *Rifater*® Tablets, preferably taken before breakfast; ▸ body-weight 65 kg and above 6 tablets daily for 2 months (initial phase), use *Rifater*® Tablets, preferably taken before breakfast
Ethambutol hydrochloride	Adult: 15 mg/kg once daily for 2 months (initial phase)
Rifampicin with isoniazid	Adult: ▸ body-weight up to 50 kg 450/300 mg daily for 4 months (continuation phase after 2-month initial phase), use *Rifinah*® *150/100* Tablets, preferably taken before breakfast; ▸ body-weight 50 kg and above 600/300 mg daily for 4 months (continuation phase after 2-month initial phase), use *Rifinah*® *300/150* Tablets, preferably taken before breakfast

or (if combination preparations not appropriate):

Isoniazid	Child: 10 mg/kg once daily (max. per dose 300 mg) for 6 months (initial and continuation phases) Adult: 300 mg daily for 6 months (initial and continuation phases)
Rifampicin	Child: ▸ body-weight up to 50 kg 15 mg/kg once daily for 6 months (initial and continuation phases); maximum 450 mg per day; ▸ body-weight 50 kg and above 15 mg/kg once daily for 6 months (initial and continuation phases); maximum 600 mg per day Adult: ▸ body-weight up to 50 kg 450 mg once daily for 6 months (initial and continuation phases); ▸ body-weight 50 kg and above 600 mg once daily for 6 months (initial and continuation phases)
Pyrazinamide	Child: ▸ body-weight up to 50 kg 35 mg/kg once daily for 2 months (initial phase); maximum 1.5 g per day; ▸ body-weight 50 kg and above 35 mg/kg once daily for 2 months (initial phase); maximum 2 g per day Adult: ▸ body-weight up to 50 kg 1.5 g once daily for 2 months (initial phase); ▸ body-weight 50 kg and above 2 g once daily for 2 months (initial phase)
Ethambutol hydrochloride	Child: 20 mg/kg once daily for 2 months (initial phase) Adult: 15 mg/kg once daily for 2 months (initial phase)

Recommended dosage for intermittent supervised 6-month treatment

Isoniazid	Child: 15 mg/kg 3 times a week (max. per dose 900 mg) for 6 months (initial and continuation phases) Adult: 15 mg/kg 3 times a week (max. per dose 900 mg) for 6 months (initial and continuation phases)
Rifampicin	Child: 15 mg/kg 3 times a week (max. per dose 900 mg) for 6 months (initial and continuation phases) Adult: 600–900 mg 3 times a week for 6 months (initial and continuation phases)
Pyrazinamide	Child: ▸ body-weight up to 50 kg 50 mg/kg 3 times a week (max. per dose 2 g 3 times a week) for 2 months (initial phase); ▸ body-weight 50 kg and above 50 mg/kg 3 times a week (max. per dose 2.5 g 3 times a week) for 2 months (initial phase) Adult: ▸ body-weight up to 50 kg 2 g 3 times a week for 2 months (initial phase); ▸ body-weight 50 kg and above 2.5 g 3 times a week for 2 months (initial phase)
Ethambutol hydrochloride	Child: 30 mg/kg 3 times a week for 2 months (initial phase) Adult: 30 mg/kg 3 times a week for 2 months (initial phase)

5

Infection

Healthcare workers

New NHS employees who are new entrants from a high incidence country should be offered appropriate testing for latent tuberculosis; those who are not new entrants from a high incidence country, but who will be in contact with patients or clinical materials should be offered appropriate testing for latent tuberculosis if prior BCG vaccination cannot be verified (see also *BCG vaccine* under Vaccines p. 1259).

Those who test positive should then be assessed for active disease, and if negative, offered treatment for latent tuberculosis.

For healthcare workers who are immunocompromised, follow standard advice for testing and treatment (see *Immunocompromised* above).

Chemoprophylaxis for latent tuberculosis

Chemoprophylaxis involves use of either isoniazid p. 576 (with pyridoxine hydrochloride p. 1047) alone for six months (recommended if interactions with rifamycins are a concern) **or** rifampicin p. 571 and isoniazid (with pyridoxine hydrochloride) for three months (recommended when hepatotoxicity is a concern).

Choice of regimen is dependent on clinical factors, including age, risk of hepatotoxicity and possible drug interactions. Testing for HIV, hepatitis B and hepatitis C should be offered before starting antituberculosis treatment as this may affect choice of therapy.

Patients with severe liver disease should be treated under the care of a specialist team; careful monitoring of liver function is necessary in patients with non-severe liver disease, abnormal liver function, or who misuse alcohol or drugs.

See advice on immunisation against tuberculosis under Vaccines p. 1259.

Treatment failure

Major causes of treatment failure are incorrect prescribing by the physician and inadequate compliance by the patient. Monthly tablet counts and urine examination (rifampicin imparts an orange-red coloration) may be useful indicators of compliance with treatment. Avoid both excessive and inadequate dosage. Treatment should be supervised by a specialist physician.

Treatment interruptions

A break in antituberculosis treatment of at least two weeks (during the initial phase) or missing more than 20 % of prescribed doses is classified as treatment interruption. Re-establishing treatment appropriately following interruptions is key to ensuring treatment success without relapse, drug resistance or further adverse events. If an adverse reaction recurs upon re-introducing a particular drug, do not give that drug in future regimens and consider extending the total regimen accordingly.

Treatment interruptions due to drug-induced hepatotoxicity

Following treatment interruption due to drug-induced hepatotoxicity, all potential causes of hepatotoxicity should be investigated. Once hepatic function has recovered, antituberculosis therapy should be sequentially re-introduced at previous full doses over a period of no more than ten days, initially with ethambutol hydrochloride p. 575 and either isoniazid (with pyridoxine hydrochloride) or rifampicin.

In patients with severe or highly infectious tuberculosis who need to interrupt the standard regimen, consider continuing treatment with at least two drugs with low risk of hepatotoxicity, such as ethambutol hydrochloride and streptomycin p. 512 (with or without a quinolone, such as levofloxacin p. 549 or moxifloxacin p. 550), with ongoing monitoring by a liver specialist.

Treatment interruptions due to cutaneous reactions

If a patient with severe or highly infectious tuberculosis has a cutaneous reaction, consider continuing treatment with a combination of at least two drugs with low risk for causing cutaneous reactions, such as ethambutol hydrochloride and streptomycin, with monitoring by a dermatologist.

Antituberculosis drugs

Isoniazid is cheap and highly effective. Like rifampicin it should always be included in any antituberculosis regimen unless there is a specific contra-indication.

Rifampicin, a rifamycin, is a key component of any antituberculosis regimen. Like isoniazid it should always be included unless there is a specific contra-indication.

During the first two months ('initial phase') of rifampicin administration transient disturbance of liver function with elevated serum transaminases is common but generally does not require interruption of treatment. Occasionally more serious liver toxicity requires a change of treatment particularly in those with pre-existing liver disease.

On intermittent treatment six toxicity syndromes have been recognised—influenza-like, abdominal, and respiratory symptoms, shock, renal failure, and thrombocytopenic purpura—and can occur in 20–30% of patients.

Rifabutin p. 564, another rifamycin, is indicated for *prophylaxis* against *M. avium* complex infections in patients with a low CD4 count; it is also licensed for the *treatment* of non-tuberculous mycobacterial disease and pulmonary tuberculosis.

Pyrazinamide p. 577 is a bactericidal drug only active against intracellular dividing forms of *Mycobacterium tuberculosis*; it exerts its main effect only in the first two or three months. It is particularly useful in tuberculous meningitis because of good meningeal penetration. It is not active against *M. bovis*.

Ethambutol hydrochloride is included in a treatment regimen if isoniazid resistance is suspected; it can be omitted if the risk of resistance is low.

Streptomycin [unlicensed] is now rarely used in the UK except for resistant organisms.

Drug-resistant tuberculosis

Drug-resistant tuberculosis should be treated by a specialist physician with experience in such cases, and where appropriate facilities for infection-control exist. Multidrug-resistant tuberculosis (*resistance to isoniazid and rifampicin, with or without any other resistance*) requires treatment with at least six antituberculosis drugs to which the mycobacterium is likely to be sensitive. Testing for resistance to second-line drugs is recommended and treatment should be modified according to susceptibility. The risk of resistance is minimised by ensuring therapy is administered in the correct dose and combination for the prescribed duration.

Second-line drugs available for infections caused by resistant organisms, or when first-line drugs cause unacceptable side-effects, include **aminosalicylic acid** p. 573, **amikacin** p. 510, **capreomycin** p. 574, **cycloserine** p. 575, newer macrolides (e.g. **azithromycin** p. 528 and **clarithromycin** p. 529), **moxifloxacin** and protionamide (prothionamide; no longer on UK market). **Bedaquiline** p. 574 and **delamanid** p. 575 are licensed for the treatment of multiple-drug resistant pulmonary tuberculosis. Bedaquiline has a long half-life.

Single drug-resistant tuberculosis

For single drug-resistance the following treatment regimens are recommended:

Resistance to isoniazid:

- First two months (initial phase): rifampicin, pyrazinamide and ethambutol hydrochloride

- Continue with (continuation phase): rifampicin and ethambutol hydrochloride for seven months (up to ten months for extensive disease)

Resistance to pyrazinamide:

- First two months (initial phase): rifampicin, ethambutol hydrochloride and isoniazid (with pyridoxine hydrochloride)
- Continue with (continuation phase): rifampicin and isoniazid (with pyridoxine hydrochloride) for seven months

Resistance to ethambutol hydrochloride:

- First two months (initial phase): rifampicin, pyrazinamide and isoniazid (with pyridoxine hydrochloride)
- Continue with (continuation phase): rifampicin and isoniazid (with pyridoxine hydrochloride) for four months

Resistance to rifampicin below:

- Offer treatment with at least six antituberculosis drugs to which the mycobacterium is likely to be sensitive.

Management of tuberculosis in children

Children are given isoniazid p. 576, rifampicin, pyrazinamide p. 577, and ethambutol hydrochloride p. 575 for the first two months followed by isoniazid and rifampicin during the next four months. However, care is needed in young children receiving ethambutol hydrochloride because of the difficulty in testing eyesight and in obtaining reports of visual symptoms.

ANTIMYCOBACTERIALS > RIFAMYCINS

Rifampicin

● **INDICATIONS AND DOSE**

Brucellosis in combination with other antibacterials | Legionnaires disease in combination with other antibacterials | Serious staphylococcal infections in combination with other antibacterials

▸ BY MOUTH, OR BY INTRAVENOUS INFUSION

▸ Child 1–11 months: 5–10 mg/kg twice daily
▸ Child 1–17 years: 10 mg/kg twice daily (max. per dose 600 mg)
▸ Adult: 0.6–1.2 g daily in 2–4 divided doses

Endocarditis in combination with other drugs

▸ BY MOUTH, OR BY INTRAVENOUS INFUSION

▸ Adult: 0.6–1.2 g daily in 2–4 divided doses

Tuberculosis, in combination with other drugs (intermittent supervised 6-month treatment) (under expert supervision)

▸ BY MOUTH

▸ Child: 15 mg/kg 3 times a week (max. per dose 900 mg) for 6 months (initial and continuation phases)
▸ Adult: 600–900 mg 3 times a week for 6 months (initial and continuation phases)

Tuberculosis, in combination with other drugs (standard unsupervised 6-month treatment)

▸ BY MOUTH

▸ Child (body-weight up to 50 kg): 15 mg/kg once daily for 6 months (initial and continuation phases); maximum 450 mg per day
▸ Child (body-weight 50 kg and above): 15 mg/kg once daily for 6 months (initial and continuation phases); maximum 600 mg per day
▸ Adult (body-weight up to 50 kg): 450 mg once daily for 6 months (initial and continuation phases)
▸ Adult (body-weight 50 kg and above): 600 mg once daily for 6 months (initial and continuation phases)

Prevention of tuberculosis in susceptible close contacts or those who have become tuberculin positive, in combination with isoniazid

▸ BY MOUTH

▸ Child 1 month–11 years (body-weight up to 50 kg): 15 mg/kg daily for 3 months; maximum 450 mg per day
▸ Child 1 month–11 years (body-weight 50 kg and above): 15 mg/kg daily for 3 months; maximum 600 mg per day
▸ Child 12–17 years (body-weight up to 50 kg): 450 mg daily for 3 months
▸ Child 12–17 years (body-weight 50 kg and above): 600 mg daily for 3 months
▸ Adult (body-weight up to 50 kg): 450 mg daily for 3 months
▸ Adult (body-weight 50 kg and above): 600 mg daily for 3 months

Prevention of tuberculosis in susceptible close contacts or those who have become tuberculin positive, who are isoniazid-resistant

▸ BY MOUTH

▸ Child 1 month–11 years (body-weight up to 50 kg): 15 mg/kg daily for 6 months; maximum 450 mg per day
▸ Child 1 month–11 years (body-weight 50 kg and above): 15 mg/kg daily for 6 months; maximum 600 mg per day
▸ Child 12–17 years (body-weight up to 50 kg): 450 mg daily for 6 months
▸ Child 12–17 years (body-weight 50 kg and above): 600 mg daily for 6 months

Prevention of tuberculosis in susceptible close contacts or those who have become tuberculin positive, who are isoniazid-resistant and under 35 years

▸ BY MOUTH

▸ Adult 18–34 years (body-weight up to 50 kg): 450 mg daily for 6 months
▸ Adult 18–34 years (body-weight 50 kg and above): 600 mg daily for 6 months

Prevention of secondary case of *Haemophilus influenzae* type b disease

▸ BY MOUTH

▸ Child 1–2 months: 10 mg/kg once daily for 4 days
▸ Child 3 months–11 years: 20 mg/kg once daily (max. per dose 600 mg) for 4 days
▸ Child 12–17 years: 600 mg once daily for 4 days
▸ Adult: 600 mg once daily for 4 days

Prevention of secondary case of meningococcal meningitis

▸ BY MOUTH

▸ Child 1–11 months: 5 mg/kg every 12 hours for 2 days
▸ Child 1–11 years: 10 mg/kg every 12 hours (max. per dose 600 mg), for 2 days
▸ Child 12–17 years: 600 mg every 12 hours for 2 days
▸ Adult: 600 mg every 12 hours for 2 days

Multibacillary leprosy in combination with dapsone and clofazimine (3-drug regimen) | Paucibacillary leprosy in combination with dapsone (2-drug regimen)

▸ BY MOUTH

▸ Adult (body-weight up to 35 kg): 450 mg once a month, supervised administration
▸ Adult (body-weight 35 kg and above): 600 mg once a month, supervised administration

● CONTRA-INDICATIONS Acute porphyrias p. 1025 · jaundice
● CAUTIONS Discolours soft contact lenses
● INTERACTIONS → Appendix 1: rifampicin

5

Infection

- **SIDE-EFFECTS**
  GENERAL SIDE-EFFECTS
  ‣ **Common or very common** Nausea · thrombocytopenia · vomiting
  ‣ **Uncommon** Diarrhoea · leucopenia
  ‣ **Frequency not known** Abdominal discomfort · acute kidney injury · adrenal insufficiency · agranulocytosis · appetite decreased · disseminated intravascular coagulation · dyspnoea · eosinophilia · flushing · haemolytic anaemia · hepatitis · hypersensitivity · influenza · intracranial haemorrhage · menstrual disorder · muscle weakness · myopathy · oedema · pseudomembranous enterocolitis · severe cutaneous adverse reactions (SCARs) · shock · skin reactions · sputum discolouration · sweat discolouration · tear discolouration · urine discolouration · vasculitis · wheezing
  SPECIFIC SIDE-EFFECTS
  ‣ **With intravenous use** Bone pain · gastrointestinal disorder · hyperbilirubinaemia · psychotic disorder
  ‣ **With oral use** Psychosis
  SIDE-EFFECTS, FURTHER INFORMATION Side-effects that mainly occur with intermittent therapy include influenza-like symptoms (with chills, fever, dizziness, bone pain), respiratory symptoms (including shortness of breath), collapse and shock, haemolytic anaemia, thrombocytopenic purpura, and acute renal failure. Discontinue if serious side-effects develop.

- **ALLERGY AND CROSS-SENSITIVITY** Contra-indicated in patients with rifamycin hypersensitivity.

- **CONCEPTION AND CONTRACEPTION**
  Important Effectiveness of hormonal contraceptives is reduced and alternative family planning advice should be offered.

- **PREGNANCY** Manufacturers advise very high doses teratogenic in *animal* studies in first trimester; risk of neonatal bleeding may be increased in third trimester.

- **BREAST FEEDING** Amount too small to be harmful.

- **HEPATIC IMPAIRMENT** Impaired elimination.
  Dose adjustments Avoid or do not exceed 8 mg/kg daily.
  Monitoring In patients with pre-existing liver disease or hepatic impairment, monitor liver function regularly and particularly frequently in the first 2 months; blood counts should also be monitored in these patients.

- **RENAL IMPAIRMENT**
  ‣ **In children** Use with caution if doses above 10 mg/kg daily.
  ‣ **In adults** Use with caution if dose above 600 mg daily.

- **MONITORING REQUIREMENTS**
  ‣ *Renal function* should be checked before treatment.
  ‣ *Hepatic function* should be checked before treatment. If there is no evidence of liver disease (and pre-treatment liver function is normal), further checks are only necessary if the patient develops fever, malaise, vomiting, jaundice or unexplained deterioration during treatment. However, liver function should be monitored on prolonged therapy.
  ‣ Blood counts should be monitored in patients on prolonged therapy.
  ‣ **In adults** Those with alcohol dependence should have frequent checks of hepatic function, particularly in the first 2 months. Blood counts should also be monitored in these patients.

- **DIRECTIONS FOR ADMINISTRATION**
  ‣ **With intravenous use in adults** For *intravenous infusion* (*Rifadin®*), give intermittently in Glucose 5% *or* Sodium chloride 0.9%; reconstitute with solvent provided then dilute with 500 mL infusion fluid; give over 2–3 hours.
  ‣ **With intravenous use in children** Displacement value may be significant, consult local reconstitution guidelines; reconstitute with solvent provided. May be further diluted with Glucose 5% *or* Sodium chloride 0.9% to a final concentration of 1.2 mg/mL. Infuse over 2–3 hours.

- **PRESCRIBING AND DISPENSING INFORMATION** If treatment interruption occurs, re-introduce with low dosage and increase gradually.
  Flavours of syrup may include raspberry.
  ‣ **With oral use in children** In general, doses should be rounded up to facilitate administration of suitable volumes of liquid or an appropriate strength of tablet. Doses may also need to be recalculated to allow for weight gain in younger children.

- **PATIENT AND CARER ADVICE**
  Soft contact lenses Patients or their carers should be advised that rifampicin discolours soft contact lenses.
  Hepatic disorders Patients or their carers should be told how to recognise signs of liver disorder, and advised to discontinue treatment and seek immediate medical attention if symptoms such as persistent nausea, vomiting, malaise or jaundice develop.
  Medicines for Children leaflet: Rifampicin for meningococcal prophylaxis www.medicinesforchildren.org.uk/rifampicin-meningococcal-prophylaxis
  Medicines for Children leaflet: Rifampicin for the treatment of tuberculosis www.medicinesforchildren.org.uk/rifampicin-treatment-tuberculosis

- **MEDICINAL FORMS**
  There can be variation in the licensing of different medicines containing the same drug. Forms available from special-order manufacturers include: oral suspension, oral solution

Oral suspension
CAUTIONARY AND ADVISORY LABELS 8, 14, 23
EXCIPIENTS: May contain Sucrose
‣ Rifadin (Sanofi)
  Rifampicin 20 mg per 1 ml Rifadin 100mg/5ml syrup | 120 ml [PoM] £4.27

Capsule
CAUTIONARY AND ADVISORY LABELS 8, 14, 23
‣ Rifampicin (Non-proprietary)
  Rifampicin 150 mg Rifampicin 150mg capsules | 100 capsule [PoM] £50.49 DT = £50.49
  Rifampicin 300 mg Rifampicin 300mg capsules | 100 capsule [PoM] £123.89 DT = £123.87
‣ Rifadin (Sanofi)
  Rifampicin 150 mg Rifadin 150mg capsules | 100 capsule [PoM] £18.32 DT = £50.49
  Rifampicin 300 mg Rifadin 300mg capsules | 100 capsule [PoM] £36.63 DT = £123.87
‣ Rimactane (Sandoz Ltd)
  Rifampicin 300 mg Rimactane 300mg capsules | 60 capsule [PoM] £21.98

Powder and solvent for solution for infusion
ELECTROLYTES: May contain Sodium
‣ Rifadin (Sanofi)
  Rifampicin 600 mg Rifadin 600mg powder and solvent for solution for infusion vials | 1 vial [PoM] £9.20

Rifampicin with ethambutol, isoniazid and pyrazinamide

The properties listed below are those particular to the combination only. For the properties of the components please consider, rifampicin p. 571, ethambutol hydrochloride p. 575, isoniazid p. 576, pyrazinamide p. 577.

- **INDICATIONS AND DOSE**
  Initial treatment of tuberculosis
  ‣ BY MOUTH
  ‣ Adult (body-weight 30–39 kg): 2 tablets daily for 2 months (initial phase)
  ‣ Adult (body-weight 40–54 kg): 3 tablets daily for 2 months (initial phase)
  ‣ Adult (body-weight 55–69 kg): 4 tablets daily for 2 months (initial phase)

5
Infection

▸ Adult (body-weight 70 kg and above): 5 tablets daily for 2 months (initial phase)

DOSE EQUIVALENCE AND CONVERSION
▸ Tablet quantities refer to the number of *Voractiv*® Tablets which should be taken. Each *Voractiv*® Tablet contains ethambutol hydrochloride 275 mg, isoniazid 75 mg, pyrazinamide 400 mg and rifampicin 150 mg.

● CAUTIONS
CAUTIONS, FURTHER INFORMATION
▸ Peripheral neuropathy The risk of peripheral neuropathy may be increased by high doses of isoniazid; pyridoxine should, therefore, be considered for those receiving *Voractiv*® 5 tablets daily.

● INTERACTIONS → Appendix 1: ethambutol · isoniazid · pyrazinamide · rifampicin

● MEDICINAL FORMS
There can be variation in the licensing of different medicines containing the same drug.
Tablet
CAUTIONARY AND ADVISORY LABELS 8, 14, 22
▸ Voractiv (Thornton & Ross Ltd)
Isoniazid 75 mg, Rifampicin 150 mg, Ethambutol hydrochloride 275 mg, Pyrazinamide 400 mg Voractiv tablets | 60 tablet [PoM] £39.50

Rifampicin with isoniazid

The properties listed below are those particular to the combination only. For the properties of the components please consider, rifampicin p. 571, isoniazid p. 576.

● INDICATIONS AND DOSE
Treatment of tuberculosis (continuation phase)
▸ BY MOUTH
▸ Adult (body-weight up to 50 kg): 450/300 mg daily for 4 months (continuation phase after 2-month initial phase), use *Rifinah*® 150/100 Tablets, preferably taken before breakfast.
▸ Adult (body-weight 50 kg and above): 600/300 mg daily for 4 months (continuation phase after 2-month initial phase), use *Rifinah*® 300/150 Tablets, preferably taken before breakfast.

DOSE EQUIVALENCE AND CONVERSION
▸ *Rifinah*® Tablets contain rifampicin and isoniazid; the proportions are expressed in the form x/y where x and y are the strengths in milligrams of rifampicin and isoniazid respectively.
▸ Each *Rifinah*® 150/100 Tablet contains rifampicin 150 mg and isoniazid 100 mg.
▸ Each *Rifinah*® 300/150 Tablet contains rifampicin 300 mg and isoniazid 150 mg.

● INTERACTIONS → Appendix 1: isoniazid · rifampicin

● MEDICINAL FORMS
There can be variation in the licensing of different medicines containing the same drug.
Tablet
CAUTIONARY AND ADVISORY LABELS 8, 14, 23
▸ Rifinah (Sanofi)
Isoniazid 100 mg, Rifampicin 150 mg Rifinah 150mg/100mg tablets | 84 tablet [PoM] £19.09
Isoniazid 150 mg, Rifampicin 300 mg Rifinah 300mg/150mg tablets | 56 tablet [PoM] £25.22

Rifampicin with isoniazid and pyrazinamide

The properties listed below are those particular to the combination only. For the properties of the components please consider, rifampicin p. 571, isoniazid p. 576, pyrazinamide p. 577.

● INDICATIONS AND DOSE
Initial unsupervised treatment of tuberculosis (in combination with ethambutol)
▸ BY MOUTH
▸ Adult (body-weight up to 40 kg): 3 tablets daily for 2 months (initial phase), use *Rifater*® Tablets, preferably taken before breakfast.
▸ Adult (body-weight 40–49 kg): 4 tablets daily for 2 months (initial phase), use *Rifater*® Tablets, preferably taken before breakfast.
▸ Adult (body-weight 50–64 kg): 5 tablets daily for 2 months (initial phase), use *Rifater*® Tablets, preferably taken before breakfast.
▸ Adult (body-weight 65 kg and above): 6 tablets daily for 2 months (initial phase), use *Rifater*® Tablets, preferably taken before breakfast.

DOSE EQUIVALENCE AND CONVERSION
▸ Tablet quantities refer to the number of *Rifater*® Tablets which should be taken. Each *Rifater*® Tablet contains isoniazid 50 mg, pyrazinamide 300 mg and rifampicin 120 mg.

● INTERACTIONS → Appendix 1: isoniazid · pyrazinamide · rifampicin

● MEDICINAL FORMS
There can be variation in the licensing of different medicines containing the same drug.
Tablet
CAUTIONARY AND ADVISORY LABELS 8, 14, 22
▸ Rifater (Sanofi)
Isoniazid 50 mg, Rifampicin 120 mg, Pyrazinamide 300 mg Rifater tablets | 100 tablet [PoM] £26.34

ANTIMYCOBACTERIALS ❭ OTHER

Aminosalicylic acid

● INDICATIONS AND DOSE
Multiple-drug resistant tuberculosis, in combination with other drugs
▸ BY MOUTH
▸ Adult: 4 g every 8 hours for a usual treatment duration of 24 months; maximum 12 g per day
Desensitisation regimen
▸ BY MOUTH
▸ Adult: (consult product literature)

● CAUTIONS Peptic ulcer
● INTERACTIONS → Appendix 1: aminosalicylic acid
● SIDE-EFFECTS
▸ **Common or very common** Diarrhoea · gastrointestinal discomfort · nausea · skin reactions · vestibular syndrome · vomiting
▸ **Uncommon** Appetite decreased
▸ **Rare or very rare** Agranulocytosis · anaemia · crystalluria · dizziness · gastrointestinal disorders · gastrointestinal haemorrhage · headache · hepatic disorders · hypoglycaemia · hypothyroidism · leucopenia · methaemoglobinaemia · peripheral neuropathy · taste metallic · tendon pain · thrombocytopenia · visual impairment · weight decreased
▸ **Frequency not known** Hypersensitivity

- PREGNANCY Manufacturer advises avoid unless essential—toxicity in *animal* studies (highest risk during first trimester).
- BREAST FEEDING Present in milk—manufacturer advises avoid.
- HEPATIC IMPAIRMENT Use with caution.
- RENAL IMPAIRMENT Use with caution in mild to moderate impairment. Avoid in severe impairment due to accumulation of inactive metabolites.
- MONITORING REQUIREMENTS
- ▶ Monitor for hypersensitivity reaction during the first 3 months of treatment—for desensitisation dosing regimen consult product literature.
- ▶ Monitor liver function—discontinue immediately if signs or symptoms of hepatic toxicity (including rash, fever and gastrointestinal disturbance).
- DIRECTIONS FOR ADMINISTRATION Disperse granules in orange or tomato juice and take immediately (granules will not dissolve, ensure all granules are swallowed). Granules can be sprinkled on apple sauce or yoghurt for administration.
- PATIENT AND CARER ADVICE Patients should be advised that the skeletons of the granules may be seen in the stools. Counselling advised on administration.

- MEDICINAL FORMS
  There can be variation in the licensing of different medicines containing the same drug.
  Gastro-resistant granules
  CAUTIONARY AND ADVISORY LABELS 9, 25
  ▶ Granupas (Lucane Pharma Ltd)
  Aminosalicylic acid 1 gram per 1 gram Granupas gastro-resistant granules 4g sachets sugar-free | 30 sachet [PoM] £331.00

Bedaquiline

- INDICATIONS AND DOSE

Multiple-drug resistant pulmonary tuberculosis, in combination with other drugs
- ▶ BY MOUTH
- ▶ Adult: Initially 400 mg once daily for 2 weeks, then 200 mg 3 times a week for 22 weeks, intervals of at least 48 hours between each dose, continue appropriate combination therapy after bedaquiline

- CONTRA-INDICATIONS QTc interval more than 500 milliseconds (derived using Fridericia's formula) · ventricular arrhythmia
- CAUTIONS Hypothyroidism · QTc interval (derived using Fridericia's formula) 450–500 milliseconds—discontinue if QTc interval more than 500 milliseconds · risk factors for QT interval prolongation (e.g. electrolyte disturbances, heart failure with reduced left ventricular ejection fraction, history of symptomatic arrhythmias (avoid if ventricular arrhythmia present), bradycardia, congenital long QT syndrome)
- INTERACTIONS → Appendix 1: bedaquiline
- SIDE-EFFECTS
- ▶ Common or very common Arthralgia · diarrhoea · dizziness · headache · hepatic function abnormal · myalgia · nausea · QT interval prolongation · vomiting
  SIDE-EFFECTS, FURTHER INFORMATION If syncope occurs, obtain ECG.
- PREGNANCY Manufacturer advises avoid unless potential benefit outweighs risk.
- BREAST FEEDING Manufacturer advises avoid—present in milk in *animal* studies.
- HEPATIC IMPAIRMENT Manufacturer advises caution in moderate impairment; avoid in severe impairment—no

information available. Avoid concomitant use of hepatotoxic drugs unless essential.
- RENAL IMPAIRMENT Manufacturer advises caution if eGFR less than 30 mL/minute/1.73 m^2.
- MONITORING REQUIREMENTS
- ▶ Determine serum potassium, calcium, and magnesium before starting treatment (correct if abnormal)—remeasure if QT prolongation occurs during treatment.
- ▶ Obtain ECG before starting treatment, and then at least monthly during treatment or more frequently if concomitant use with other drugs known to prolong the QT interval.
- ▶ Monitor liver function before starting treatment and then at least monthly during treatment—discontinue treatment if severe abnormalities in liver function tests.
- PATIENT AND CARER ADVICE
  Missed doses If a dose is missed during the first two weeks of treatment, the missed dose should not be taken and the next dose should be taken at the usual time; if a dose is missed during weeks 3–24 of treatment, the missed dose should be taken as soon as possible and then the usual regimen resumed.
  Driving and skilled tasks Dizziness may affect performance of skilled tasks (e.g. driving)

- MEDICINAL FORMS
  There can be variation in the licensing of different medicines containing the same drug.
  Tablet
  CAUTIONARY AND ADVISORY LABELS 4, 8, 21
  ▶ Sirturo (Janssen-Cilag Ltd) ▼
  Bedaquiline (as Bedaquiline fumarate) 100 mg Sirturo 100mg tablets | 188 tablet [PoM] £18,700.00

Capreomycin

- INDICATIONS AND DOSE

Tuberculosis resistant to first-line drugs, in combination with other drugs
- ▶ BY DEEP INTRAMUSCULAR INJECTION
- ▶ Adult: 1 g daily (max. per dose 20 mg/kg) for 2–4 months, then reduced to 1 g 2–3 times a week

- CAUTIONS Auditory impairment
- INTERACTIONS → Appendix 1: capreomycin
- SIDE-EFFECTS Eosinophilia · febrile disorders · hearing impairment · leucocytosis · leucopenia · nephrotoxicity · pain · pseudo-Bartter syndrome · skin reactions · thrombocytopenia · vertigo
- PREGNANCY Manufacturer advises use only if potential benefit outweighs risk—teratogenic in *animal* studies.
- BREAST FEEDING Manufacturer advises caution—no information available.
- HEPATIC IMPAIRMENT Use with caution.
- RENAL IMPAIRMENT Nephrotoxic; ototoxic.
  Dose adjustments Reduce dose—consult product literature.
- MONITORING REQUIREMENTS Monitor renal, hepatic, auditory, and vestibular function and electrolytes.

- MEDICINAL FORMS
  There can be variation in the licensing of different medicines containing the same drug.
  Powder for solution for injection
  ▶ Capreomycin (Non-proprietary)
  Capreomycin (as Capreomycin sulfate) 1 gram Capreomycin 1g powder for solution for injection vials | 1 vial [PoM] £31.47

5

Infection

Cycloserine

● **INDICATIONS AND DOSE**

Tuberculosis resistant to first-line drugs, in combination with other drugs

▶ BY MOUTH
▶ Adult: Initially 250 mg every 12 hours for 2 weeks, then increased if necessary up to 500 mg every 12 hours, dose to be increased according to blood concentration and response

PHARMACOKINETICS
▶ Cycloserine penetrates the CNS.

● CONTRA-INDICATIONS Alcohol dependence · depression · epilepsy · psychotic states · severe anxiety
● INTERACTIONS → Appendix 1: cycloserine
● SIDE-EFFECTS Behaviour abnormal · coma · confusion · congestive heart failure · drowsiness · dysarthria · headache · hyperirritability · megaloblastic anaemia · memory loss · neurological effects · paraesthesia · paresis · psychosis · rash · reflexes increased · seizures · suicidal ideation · tremor · vertigo

SIDE-EFFECTS, FURTHER INFORMATION

CNS toxicity Discontinue or reduce dose if symptoms of CNS toxicity occur.
Rashes or allergic dermatitis Discontinue or reduce dose if rashes or allergic dermatitis develops.

● PREGNANCY Manufacturer advises use only if potential benefit outweighs risk—crosses the placenta.
● BREAST FEEDING Present in milk—amount too small to be harmful.
● RENAL IMPAIRMENT
Dose adjustments Increase interval between doses if creatinine clearance less than 50 mL/minute.
Monitoring Monitor blood-cycloserine concentration if creatinine clearance less than 50 mL/minute.
● MONITORING REQUIREMENTS
▶ Blood concentration monitoring required especially in renal impairment or if dose exceeds 500 mg daily or if signs of toxicity; blood concentration should not exceed 30 mg/litre.
▶ Monitor haematological, renal, and hepatic function.

● MEDICINAL FORMS
There can be variation in the licensing of different medicines containing the same drug.
Capsule
CAUTIONARY AND ADVISORY LABELS 2, 8
▶ Cycloserine (Non-proprietary)
Cycloserine 250 mg Cycloserine 250mg capsules | 100 capsule [PoM] £442.89 DT = £442.89

Delamanid

● **INDICATIONS AND DOSE**

Multiple-drug resistant pulmonary tuberculosis, in combination with other drugs

▶ BY MOUTH
▶ Adult: 100 mg twice daily for 24 weeks, continue appropriate combination therapy after delamanid

● CONTRA-INDICATIONS QTc interval more than 500 milliseconds (derived using Fridericia's formula) · serum albumin less than 28 g/litre
● CAUTIONS Risk factors for QT interval prolongation (e.g. electrolyte disturbances, acute myocardial infarction, heart failure with reduced left ventricular ejection fraction, severe hypertension, left ventricular hypertrophy, bradycardia, congenital long QT syndrome, history of symptomatic arrhythmias)

● INTERACTIONS → Appendix 1: delamanid
● SIDE-EFFECTS
▶ **Common or very common** Anxiety · appetite decreased · asthenia · chest pain · cough · depression · dyslipidaemia · dyspnoea · ear pain · electrolyte imbalance · gastrointestinal discomfort · haemoptysis · headache · hyperhidrosis · hypertension · hypotension · malaise · muscle weakness · nausea · oropharyngeal pain · osteochondrosis · pain · palpitations · peripheral neuropathy · photophobia · psychotic disorder · QT interval prolongation · reticulocytosis · sensation abnormal · skin reactions · sleep disorders · throat irritation · tinnitus · tremor · vomiting
▶ **Uncommon** Aggression · atrioventricular block · balance impaired · dehydration · delusional disorder, persecutory type · dysphagia · extrasystole · hepatic function abnormal · increased risk of infection · lethargy · leucopenia · oral paraesthesia · psychiatric disorders · thrombocytopenia · urinary disorders
● CONCEPTION AND CONTRACEPTION Effective contraception required during treatment.
● PREGNANCY Manufacturer advises avoid—toxicity in *animal* studies.
● BREAST FEEDING Manufacturer advises avoid—present in milk in *animal* studies.
● HEPATIC IMPAIRMENT Manufacturer advises avoid in moderate to severe impairment.
● RENAL IMPAIRMENT Manufacturer advises avoid in severe impairment—no information available.
● MONITORING REQUIREMENTS
▶ Monitor serum albumin and electrolytes before starting treatment and then during treatment—discontinue treatment if serum albumin less than 28 g/litre.
▶ Obtain ECG before starting treatment and then monthly during treatment (more frequently if serum albumin 28–34 g/litre, or if concomitant use of potent CYP3A4 inhibitors, or if risk factors for QT interval prolongation, or if QTc interval 450–500 milliseconds in men or 470–500 milliseconds in women)—discontinue treatment if QTc interval more than 500 milliseconds (derived using Fridericia's formula).
● HANDLING AND STORAGE Dispense in original container (contains desiccant).

● MEDICINAL FORMS
There can be variation in the licensing of different medicines containing the same drug.
Tablet
CAUTIONARY AND ADVISORY LABELS 8, 21
▶ Deltyba (Otsuka Novel Products GmbH) ▼
Delamanid 50 mg Deltyba 50mg tablets | 48 tablet [PoM] £1,250.00

Ethambutol hydrochloride   19-Mar-2018

● **INDICATIONS AND DOSE**

Tuberculosis, in combination with other drugs (standard unsupervised 6-month treatment)

▶ BY MOUTH
▶ Child: 20 mg/kg once daily for 2 months (initial phase)
▶ Adult: 15 mg/kg once daily for 2 months (initial phase)

Tuberculosis, in combination with other drugs (intermittent supervised 6-month treatment) (under expert supervision)

▶ BY MOUTH
▶ Child: 30 mg/kg 3 times a week for 2 months (initial phase)
▶ Adult: 30 mg/kg 3 times a week for 2 months (initial phase)

● CONTRA-INDICATIONS Optic neuritis · poor vision

- CAUTIONS Elderly · young children

CAUTIONS, FURTHER INFORMATION

▸ **Understanding warnings** Patients who cannot understand warnings about visual side-effects should, if possible, be given an alternative drug. In particular, ethambutol should be used with caution in children until they are at least 5 years old and capable of reporting symptomatic visual changes accurately.

- INTERACTIONS → Appendix 1: ethambutol
- SIDE-EFFECTS
▸ **Common or very common** Hyperuricaemia · nerve disorders · visual impairment
▸ **Rare or very rare** Nephritis tubulointerstitial
▸ **Frequency not known** Alveolitis allergic · appetite decreased · asthenia · confusion · dizziness · eosinophilia · fever · flatulence · gastrointestinal discomfort · gout · hallucination · headache · jaundice · leucopenia · nausea · nephrotoxicity · neutropenia · photosensitive lichenoid eruption · sensation abnormal · severe cutaneous adverse reactions (SCARs) · skin reactions · taste metallic · thrombocytopenia · tremor · vomiting

SIDE-EFFECTS, FURTHER INFORMATION Ocular toxicity is more common where excessive dosage is used or if the patient's renal function is impaired. Early discontinuation of the drug is almost always followed by recovery of eyesight.

- PREGNANCY Not known to be harmful.
- BREAST FEEDING Amount too small to be harmful.
- RENAL IMPAIRMENT Risk of optic nerve damage. Should preferably be avoided in patients with renal impairment. **Dose adjustments** ▸ In adults If creatinine clearance less than 30 mL/minute, use 15–25 mg/kg (max. 2.5 g) 3 times a week.
  ▸ In children If creatinine clearance less than 30 mL/minute/1.73 m^2, use 15–25 mg/kg (max. 2.5 g) 3 times a week.
  Monitoring If creatinine clearance less than 30 mL/minute, monitor plasma-ethambutol concentration.
- MONITORING REQUIREMENTS
▸ 'Peak' concentration (2–2.5 hours after dose) should be 2–6 mg/litre (7–22 micromol/litre); 'trough' (pre-dose) concentration should be less than 1 mg/litre (4 micromol/litre).
▸ Renal function should be checked before treatment.
▸ Visual acuity should be tested by Snellen chart before treatment with ethambutol.
▸ In children In young children, routine ophthalmological monitoring recommended.
- PRESCRIBING AND DISPENSING INFORMATION The RCPCH and NPPG recommend that, when a liquid special of ethambutol is required, the following strength is used: 400 mg/5 mL.
- PATIENT AND CARER ADVICE
Ocular toxicity The earliest features of ocular toxicity are subjective and patients should be advised to discontinue therapy immediately if they develop deterioration in vision and promptly seek further advice.
Medicines for Children leaflet: Ethambutol for the treatment of tuberculosis www.medicinesforchildren.org.uk/ethambutol-for-the-treatment-of-tuberculosis

- MEDICINAL FORMS
There can be variation in the licensing of different medicines containing the same drug. Forms available from special-order manufacturers include: oral suspension, oral solution

Tablet

CAUTIONARY AND ADVISORY LABELS 8

▸ Ethambutol hydrochloride (Non-proprietary)
  Ethambutol hydrochloride 100 mg Ethambutol 100mg tablets | 56 tablet [PoM] £12.00 DT = £11.51
  Ethambutol hydrochloride 400 mg Ethambutol 400mg tablets | 56 tablet [PoM] £42.74 DT = £42.74

Combinations available: *Rifampicin with ethambutol, isoniazid and pyrazinamide*, p. 572

Isoniazid

- INDICATIONS AND DOSE

Tuberculosis, in combination with other drugs (standard unsupervised 6-month treatment)
▸ BY MOUTH, OR BY INTRAMUSCULAR INJECTION, OR BY INTRAVENOUS INJECTION
▸ Child: 10 mg/kg once daily (max. per dose 300 mg) for 6 months (initial and continuation phases)
▸ Adult: 300 mg daily for 6 months (initial and continuation phases)

Tuberculosis, in combination with other drugs (intermittent supervised 6-month treatment) (under expert supervision)
▸ BY MOUTH, OR BY INTRAMUSCULAR INJECTION, OR BY INTRAVENOUS INJECTION
▸ Child: 15 mg/kg 3 times a week (max. per dose 900 mg) for 6 months (initial and continuation phases)
▸ Adult: 15 mg/kg 3 times a week (max. per dose 900 mg) for 6 months (initial and continuation phases)

Prevention of tuberculosis in susceptible close contacts or those who have become tuberculin positive
▸ INITIALLY BY MOUTH, OR BY INTRAMUSCULAR INJECTION, OR BY INTRAVENOUS INJECTION
▸ Child 1 month–11 years: 10 mg/kg daily (max. per dose 300 mg) for 6 months, alternatively (by mouth) 10 mg/kg daily (max. per dose 300 mg) for 3 months, to be taken in combination with rifampicin
▸ Child 12–17 years: 300 mg daily for 6 months, alternatively (by mouth) 300 mg daily for 3 months, to be taken in combination with rifampicin
▸ Adult: 300 mg daily for 6 months, alternatively (by mouth) 300 mg daily for 3 months, to be taken in combination with rifampicin

- CONTRA-INDICATIONS Drug-induced liver disease
- CAUTIONS Acute porphyrias p. 1025 · alcohol dependence · diabetes mellitus · epilepsy · history of psychosis · HIV infection · malnutrition · slow acetylator status (increased risk of side-effects)

CAUTIONS, FURTHER INFORMATION

▸ **Peripheral neuropathy** Peripheral neuropathy is more likely to occur where there are pre-existing risk factors such as diabetes, alcohol dependence, chronic renal failure, pregnancy, malnutrition and HIV infection. In patients at increased risk of peripheral neuropathy, pyridoxine hydrochloride p. 1047 should be given prophylactically from the start of treatment.

- INTERACTIONS → Appendix 1: isoniazid
- SIDE-EFFECTS
▸ **Uncommon** Hepatic disorders
▸ **Rare or very rare** Severe cutaneous adverse reactions (SCARs)
▸ **Frequency not known** Agranulocytosis · alopecia · anaemia · aplastic anaemia · eosinophilia · fever · gynaecomastia · haemolytic anaemia · hyperglycaemia · lupus-like syndrome · nerve disorders · optic atrophy · pancreatitis ·

pellagra · psychosis · seizure · skin reactions · thrombocytopenia · vasculitis

SIDE-EFFECTS, FURTHER INFORMATION Hepatitis more common in those aged over 35 years and those with a daily alcohol intake.

● PREGNANCY Not known to be harmful; prophylactic pyridoxine recommended.

● BREAST FEEDING Theoretical risk of convulsions and neuropathy; prophylactic pyridoxine advisable in mother. **Monitoring** In breast-feeding, monitor infant for possible toxicity.

● HEPATIC IMPAIRMENT Use with caution. **Monitoring** In patients with pre-existing liver disease or hepatic impairment monitor liver function regularly and particularly frequently in the first 2 months.

● RENAL IMPAIRMENT Risk of ototoxicity and peripheral neuropathy; prophylactic pyridoxine hydrochloride p. 1047 recommended.

● MONITORING REQUIREMENTS
▸ *Renal function* should be checked before treatment.
▸ *Hepatic function* should be checked before treatment. If there is no evidence of liver disease (and pre-treatment liver function is normal), further checks are only necessary if the patient develops fever, malaise, vomiting, jaundice or unexplained deterioration during treatment.
▸ In adults Those with alcohol dependence should have frequent checks of hepatic function, particularly in the first 2 months.

● PRESCRIBING AND DISPENSING INFORMATION
▸ With oral use in children In general, doses should be rounded up to facilitate administration of suitable volumes of liquid or an appropriate strength of tablet. The RCPCH and NPPG recommend that, when a liquid special of isoniazid is required, the following strength is used: 50 mg/5 mL.
▸ In children Doses may need to be recalculated to allow for weight gain in younger children.

● PATIENT AND CARER ADVICE
Hepatic disorders Patients or their carers should be told how to recognise signs of liver disorder, and advised to discontinue treatment and seek immediate medical attention if symptoms such as persistent nausea, vomiting, malaise or jaundice develop.
Medicines for Children leaflet: Isoniazid for latent tuberculosis www.medicinesforchildren.org.uk/isoniazid-for-latent-tuberculosis
Medicines for Children leaflet: Isoniazid for treatment of tuberculosis www.medicinesforchildren.org.uk/isoniazid-treatment-tuberculosis

● MEDICINAL FORMS
There can be variation in the licensing of different medicines containing the same drug. Forms available from special-order manufacturers include: oral suspension, oral solution

Solution for injection
▸ Isoniazid (Non-proprietary)
  Isoniazid 25 mg per 1 ml Isoniazid 50mg/2ml solution for injection ampoules | 10 ampoule PoM £361.98

Tablet
CAUTIONARY AND ADVISORY LABELS 8, 22
▸ Isoniazid (Non-proprietary)
  Isoniazid 50 mg Isoniazid 50mg tablets | 56 tablet PoM £19.28 DT = £19.26
  Isoniazid 100 mg Isoniazid 100mg tablets | 28 tablet PoM £19.24 DT = £19.24
  Isoniazid 300 mg Isoniazid 300mg tablets | 30 tablet PoM 🛇

Combinations available: *Rifampicin with ethambutol, isoniazid and pyrazinamide,* p. 572 · *Rifampicin with isoniazid,* p. 573 · *Rifampicin with isoniazid and pyrazinamide,* p. 573

Pyrazinamide

● INDICATIONS AND DOSE

Tuberculosis, in combination with other drugs (standard unsupervised 6-month treatment)
▸ BY MOUTH
▸ Child (body-weight up to 50 kg): 35 mg/kg once daily for 2 months (initial phase); maximum 1.5 g per day
▸ Child (body-weight 50 kg and above): 35 mg/kg once daily for 2 months (initial phase); maximum 2 g per day
▸ Adult (body-weight up to 50 kg): 1.5 g once daily for 2 months (initial phase)
▸ Adult (body-weight 50 kg and above): 2 g once daily for 2 months (initial phase)

Tuberculosis, in combination with other drugs (intermittent supervised 6-month treatment) (under expert supervision)
▸ BY MOUTH
▸ Child (body-weight up to 50 kg): 50 mg/kg 3 times a week (max. per dose 2 g 3 times a week) for 2 months (initial phase)
▸ Child (body-weight 50 kg and above): 50 mg/kg 3 times a week (max. per dose 2.5 g 3 times a week) for 2 months (initial phase)
▸ Adult (body-weight up to 50 kg): 2 g 3 times a week for 2 months (initial phase)
▸ Adult (body-weight 50 kg and above): 2.5 g 3 times a week for 2 months (initial phase)

● CONTRA-INDICATIONS Acute attack of gout (in adults)

● CAUTIONS Diabetes · gout (in adults)

● INTERACTIONS → Appendix 1: pyrazinamide

● SIDE-EFFECTS Appetite decreased · arthralgia · dysuria · flushing · gout aggravated · hepatic disorders · malaise · nausea · peptic ulcer aggravated · photosensitivity reaction · sideroblastic anaemia · skin reactions · splenomegaly · vomiting

● PREGNANCY Manufacturer advises use only if potential benefit outweighs risk.

● BREAST FEEDING Amount too small to be harmful.

● HEPATIC IMPAIRMENT Idiosyncratic hepatotoxicity more common; avoid in severe hepatic impairment.
Monitoring In patients with pre-existing liver disease or hepatic impairment monitor liver function regularly and particularly frequently in the first 2 months.

● RENAL IMPAIRMENT
Dose adjustments ▸ In adults 25–30 mg/kg 3 times a week if eGFR less than 30 mL/minute/1.73 m^2.
▸ In children If estimated glomerular filtration rate less than 30 mL/minute/1.73 m^2, use 25–30 mg/kg 3 times a week.
Monitoring Monitor for gout in renal impairment.

● MONITORING REQUIREMENTS
▸ *Renal function* should be checked before treatment.
▸ *Hepatic function* should be checked before treatment. If there is no evidence of liver disease (and pre-treatment liver function is normal), further checks are only necessary if the patient develops fever, malaise, vomiting, jaundice or unexplained deterioration during treatment.
▸ In adults Those with alcohol dependence should have frequent checks of hepatic function, particularly in the first 2 months.

● PRESCRIBING AND DISPENSING INFORMATION
▸ In children In general, doses should be rounded up to facilitate administration of suitable volumes of liquid or an appropriate strength of tablet. Doses may also need to be recalculated to allow for weight gain in younger children. The RCPCH and NPPG recommend that, when a liquid special of pyrazinamide is required, the following strength is used: 500 mg/5 mL.

● PATIENT AND CARER ADVICE
Hepatic disorders Patients or their carers should be told how
to recognise signs of liver disorder, and advised to
discontinue treatment and seek immediate medical
attention if symptoms such as persistent nausea,
vomiting, malaise or jaundice develop.
Medicines for Children leaflet: Pyrazinamide for treatment of
tuberculosis www.medicinesforchildren.org.uk/pyrazinamide-
for-tuberculosis

● MEDICINAL FORMS
There can be variation in the licensing of different medicines
containing the same drug. Forms available from special-order
manufacturers include: oral suspension, oral solution

Tablet
CAUTIONARY AND ADVISORY LABELS 8
▶ Pyrazinamide (Non-proprietary)
Pyrazinamide 500 mg Pyrazinamide 500mg tablets |
30 tablet [PoM] £36.12 DT = £36.12
▶ Zinamide (Thornton & Ross Ltd)
Pyrazinamide 500 mg Zinamide 500mg tablets | 30 tablet [PoM]
£31.35 DT = £36.12

Combinations available: _Rifampicin with ethambutol,_
isoniazid and pyrazinamide, p. 572 · **_Rifampicin with isoniazid_**
and pyrazinamide, p. 573

2.6 Urinary tract infections

Urinary-tract infections

Overview
Urinary-tract infection is more common in women than in
men; when it occurs in men there is frequently an underlying
abnormality of the renal tract. Recurrent episodes of
infection are an indication for radiological investigation
especially in children in whom untreated pyelonephritis may
lead to permanent kidney damage.

Escherichia coli is the most common cause of urinary-tract
infection; _Staphylococcus saprophyticus_ is also common in
sexually active young women. Less common causes include
Proteus and _Klebsiella_ spp. _Pseudomonas aeruginosa_
infections usually occur in the hospital setting and may be
associated with functional or anatomical abnormalities of
the renal tract. _Staphylococcus epidermidis_ and _Enterococcus_
faecalis infection may complicate catheterisation or
instrumentation.

A specimen of urine should be collected for culture and
sensitivity testing before starting antibacterial therapy;

● in men;
● in pregnant women;
● in children under 3 years of age;
● in patients with suspected upper urinary-tract infection;
● complicated infection, or recurrent infection;
● if resistant organisms are suspected;
● if urine dipstick testing gives a single positive result for
  leucocyte esterase or nitrite;
● if clinical symptoms are not consistent with results of
  dipstick testing.

Treatment should not be delayed while waiting for results.
The antibacterial chosen should reflect current local
bacterial sensitivity to antibacterials.

Antibacterial therapy for lower urinary-tract
infections
Uncomplicated lower urinary-tract infections often respond to
trimethoprim p. 563 or nitrofurantoin p. 579, _or alternatively_,
amoxicillin p. 539, ampicillin p. 540 or oral cephalosporin.

Suggested duration of treatment is 7 days, but a short course
(e.g. 3 days) is usually adequate for uncomplicated urinary-
tract infections in women.

Infections caused by fully sensitive bacteria respond to
amoxicillin.

Widespread bacterial resistance to ampicillin, amoxicillin,
and trimethoprim has been reported. Alternatives for
resistant organisms include co-amoxiclav p. 542 (amoxicillin
with clavulanic acid), an oral cephalosporin, nitrofurantoin,
pivmecillinam hydrochloride p. 544, or a quinolone.

Fosfomycin p. 560 can be used, on the advice of a
microbiologist, for the treatment of acute uncomplicated
lower urinary-tract infections caused by organisms sensitive
to fosfomycin.

Long-term low dose therapy may be required in selected
patients to prevent _recurrence of infection_; indications
include frequent relapses and significant kidney damage.
Trimethoprim, nitrofurantoin and cefalexin p. 516 have been
recommended for long-term therapy.

Methenamine hippurate p. 579 (hexamine hippurate)
should **not** generally be used because it requires an acidic
urine for its antimicrobial activity and it is ineffective for
upper urinary-tract infections; it may, however, have a role
in the prophylaxis and treatment of chronic or recurrent
uncomplicated lower urinary-tract infections.

Antibacterial therapy for upper urinary-tract
infections
Acute pyelonephritis can lead to septicaemia and is treated
initially by injection of a broad-spectrum antibacterial such
as a cephalosporin (e.g. cefuroxime p. 518) or a quinolone if
the patient is severely ill; gentamicin p. 510 can also be used.

Suggested duration of treatment is 10–14 days (longer
treatment may be necessary in complicated pyelonephritis).

Prostatitis can be difficult to cure and requires treatment
for several weeks with an antibacterial which penetrates
prostatic tissue such as some of the quinolones
(ciprofloxacin p. 548 _or_ ofloxacin p. 551), or _alternatively_,
trimethoprim.

Suggested duration of treatment is 28 days.

Where infection is localised and associated with an
indwelling _catheter_, a bladder instillation is often effective.

Pregnancy
Urinary-tract infection in pregnancy may be asymptomatic
and requires prompt treatment to prevent progression to
acute pyelonephritis. Penicillins and cephalosporins are
suitable for treating urinary-tract infection during
pregnancy. Nitrofurantoin may also be used but it should be
avoided at term. Sulfonamides and quinolones should be
avoided during pregnancy; trimethoprim should also
preferably be avoided particularly in the first trimester.

Renal impairment
In renal failure antibacterials normally excreted by the
kidney accumulate with resultant toxicity unless the dose is
reduced. This applies especially to the aminoglycosides
which should be used with great caution; tetracyclines,
methenamine hippurate, and nitrofurantoin should be
avoided altogether.

ANTIBACTERIALS

Methenamine hippurate

(Hexamine hippurate)

- **INDICATIONS AND DOSE**

Prophylaxis and long-term treatment of chronic or recurrent uncomplicated lower urinary-tract infections
▸ BY MOUTH
 ▹ Adult: 1 g every 12 hours

Prophylaxis and long-term treatment of chronic or recurrent uncomplicated lower urinary-tract infections in patients with catheters
▸ BY MOUTH
 ▹ Adult: 1 g every 8–12 hours

- **CONTRA-INDICATIONS** Gout · metabolic acidosis · severe dehydration
- **INTERACTIONS** → Appendix 1: methenamine
- **SIDE-EFFECTS**
▸ **Uncommon** Epigastric discomfort · skin reactions
- **PREGNANCY** Use with caution.
- **BREAST FEEDING** Amount too small to be harmful.
- **HEPATIC IMPAIRMENT** Avoid.
- **RENAL IMPAIRMENT** Avoid if eGFR less than 10 mL/minute/1.73 m^2—risk of hippurate crystalluria.
- **LESS SUITABLE FOR PRESCRIBING** Methenamine (hexamine) hippurate should **not** generally be used because it requires an acidic urine for its antimicrobial activity and it is ineffective for upper urinary-tract infections; it may, however, have a role in the prophylaxis and treatment of chronic or recurrent uncomplicated lower urinary-tract infections. It is considered less suitable for prescribing.

- **MEDICINAL FORMS**
There can be variation in the licensing of different medicines containing the same drug.

Tablet
CAUTIONARY AND ADVISORY LABELS 9
 ▹ Hiprex (Meda Pharmaceuticals Ltd)
  Methenamine hippurate 1 gram Hiprex 1g tablets | 60 tablet ℗
  £19.74 DT = £19.74

Nitrofurantoin

- **INDICATIONS AND DOSE**

Acute uncomplicated urinary-tract infections
▸ BY MOUTH USING IMMEDIATE-RELEASE MEDICINES
 ▹ Child 3 months–11 years: 750 micrograms/kg 4 times a day for 3–7 days
 ▹ Child 12–17 years: 50 mg 4 times a day for 3–7 days
 ▹ Adult: 50 mg 4 times a day for 3–7 days, dose to be taken with food
▸ BY MOUTH USING MODIFIED-RELEASE MEDICINES
 ▹ Child 12–17 years: 100 mg twice daily, dose to be taken with food
 ▹ Adult: 100 mg twice daily, dose to be taken with food

Severe chronic recurrent urinary-tract infections
▸ BY MOUTH USING IMMEDIATE-RELEASE MEDICINES
 ▹ Child 12–17 years: 100 mg 4 times a day for 3–7 days
 ▹ Adult: 100 mg 4 times a day for 7 days, dose to be taken with food, reduce dose or discontinue treatment if severe nausea occurs

Prophylaxis of urinary-tract infection (considered for recurrent infection, significant urinary-tract anomalies, or significant kidney damage)
▸ BY MOUTH USING IMMEDIATE-RELEASE MEDICINES
 ▹ Child 3 months–11 years: 1 mg/kg once daily, dose to be taken at night
 ▹ Child 12–17 years: 50–100 mg once daily, dose to be taken at night
 ▹ Adult: 50–100 mg once daily, dose to be taken at night

Genito-urinary surgical prophylaxis
▸ BY MOUTH USING MODIFIED-RELEASE MEDICINES
 ▹ Adult: 100 mg twice daily on day of procedure and for 3 days after

- **CONTRA-INDICATIONS** Acute porphyrias p. 1025 · G6PD deficiency · infants less than 3 months old
- **CAUTIONS** Anaemia · diabetes mellitus · electrolyte imbalance · folate deficiency · pulmonary disease · susceptibility to peripheral neuropathy · urine may be coloured yellow or brown · vitamin B deficiency
- **INTERACTIONS** → Appendix 1: nitrofurantoin
- **SIDE-EFFECTS** Agranulocytosis · alopecia · anaemia · angioedema · aplastic anaemia · appetite decreased · arthralgia · asthenia · chest pain · chills · circulatory collapse · confusion · cough · cyanosis · depression · diarrhoea · dizziness · drowsiness · dyspnoea · eosinophilia · euphoric mood · fever · granulocytopenia · haemolytic anaemia · headache · hepatic disorders · idiopathic intracranial hypertension · increased risk of infection · leucopenia · lupus-like syndrome · nausea · nerve disorders · nystagmus · pancreatitis · psychotic disorder · pulmonary hypersensitivity · pulmonary reaction (possible association with lupus erythematosus-like syndrome) · respiratory disorders · skin reactions · Stevens-Johnson syndrome · thrombocytopenia · urine discolouration · vertigo · vomiting
- **PREGNANCY** Avoid at term—may produce neonatal haemolysis.
- **BREAST FEEDING** Avoid; only small amounts in milk but enough to produce haemolysis in G6PD-deficient infants.
- **HEPATIC IMPAIRMENT** Use with caution; cholestatic jaundice and chronic active hepatitis reported.
- **RENAL IMPAIRMENT** Risk of peripheral neuropathy; antibacterial efficacy depends on renal secretion of the drug into urinary tract.
 ▹ In adults Avoid if eGFR less than 45 mL/minute/1.73 m^2; may be used with caution if eGFR 30–44 mL/minute/1.73 m^2 as a short-course only (3 to 7 days), to treat uncomplicated lower urinary-tract infection caused by suspected or proven multidrug resistant bacteria and only if potential benefit outweighs risk.
 ▹ In children Avoid if estimated glomerular filtration rate less than 45 mL/minute/1.73 m^2; may be used with caution if estimated glomerular filtration rate 30–44 mL/minute/1.73 m^2 as a short-course only (3 to 7 days), to treat uncomplicated lower urinary-tract infection caused by suspected or proven multidrug resistant bacteria and only if potential benefit outweighs risk.
- **MONITORING REQUIREMENTS** On long-term therapy, monitor liver function and monitor for pulmonary symptoms, especially in the elderly (discontinue if deterioration in lung function).
- **EFFECT ON LABORATORY TESTS** False positive urinary glucose (if tested for reducing substances).
- **PATIENT AND CARER ADVICE**
Medicines for Children leaflet: Nitrofurantoin for urinary tract infections www.medicinesforchildren.org.uk/nitrofurantoin-for-urinary-tract-infections

5

Infection

5

Infection

● MEDICINAL FORMS
There can be variation in the licensing of different medicines containing the same drug. Forms available from special-order manufacturers include: oral suspension, oral solution

Tablet

CAUTIONARY AND ADVISORY LABELS 9, 14, 21
▸ Nitrofurantoin (Non-proprietary)
Nitrofurantoin 50 mg Nitrofurantoin 50mg tablets | 28 tablet PoM £35.00 DT = £11.36 | 100 tablet PoM £40.57-£111.89
Nitrofurantoin 100 mg Nitrofurantoin 100mg tablets | 28 tablet PoM £12.99 DT = £8.13 | 100 tablet PoM £22.14-£29.04
▸ Genfura (Genesis Pharmaceuticals Ltd)
Nitrofurantoin 50 mg Genfura 50mg tablets | 28 tablet PoM £8.00 DT = £11.36 | 100 tablet PoM £28.57
Nitrofurantoin 100 mg Genfura 100mg tablets | 28 tablet PoM £8.50 DT = £8.13 | 100 tablet PoM £30.36

Oral suspension

CAUTIONARY AND ADVISORY LABELS 9, 14, 21
▸ Nitrofurantoin (Non-proprietary)
Nitrofurantoin 5 mg per 1 ml Nitrofurantoin 25mg/5ml oral suspension sugar free sugar-free | 300 ml PoM £446.95 DT = £446.95

Modified-release capsule

CAUTIONARY AND ADVISORY LABELS 9, 14, 21, 25
▸ Macrobid (AMCo)
Nitrofurantoin 100 mg Macrobid 100mg modified-release capsules | 14 capsule PoM £9.50 DT = £9.50

Capsule

CAUTIONARY AND ADVISORY LABELS 9, 14, 21
▸ Nitrofurantoin (Non-proprietary)
Nitrofurantoin 50 mg Nitrofurantoin 50mg capsules | 30 capsule PoM £15.42 DT = £15.42
Nitrofurantoin 100 mg Nitrofurantoin 100mg capsules | 30 capsule PoM £10.42 DT = £10.42

3 Fungal infection

Antifungals, systemic use

Fungal infections

The systemic treatment of common fungal infections is outlined below; specialist treatment is required in most forms of systemic or disseminated fungal infections. Local treatment is suitable for a number of fungal infections (genital, bladder, eye, ear, oropharynx, and skin).

Aspergillosis

Aspergillosis most commonly affects the respiratory tract but in severely immunocompromised patients, invasive forms can affect the heart, brain, and skin. Voriconazole p. 588 is the treatment of choice for aspergillosis; liposomal amphotericin p. 583 is an alternative first-line treatment when voriconazole cannot be used. Caspofungin p. 582, or itraconazole p. 586, can be used in patients who are refractory to, or intolerant of voriconazole and liposomal amphotericin. Itraconazole is also used for the treatment of chronic pulmonary aspergillosis or as an adjunct in the treatment of allergic bronchopulmonary aspergillosis [unlicensed indication]. Posaconazole p. 587 is licensed for use in patients with invasive aspergillosis who are refractory to, or intolerant of itraconazole or amphotericin.

Candidiasis

Many superficial candidal infections including infections of the skin are treated locally; widespread or intractable infection requires systemic antifungal treatment. Vaginal candidiasis may be treated with locally acting antifungals or with fluconazole p. 584 given by mouth; for resistant organisms in adults, itraconazole can be given by mouth.

Oropharyngeal candidiasis generally responds to topical therapy; fluconazole is given by mouth for unresponsive infections; it is effective and is reliably absorbed. Itraconazole may be used for infections that do not respond

to fluconazole. Topical therapy may not be adequate in immunocompromised patients and an oral triazole antifungal is preferred.

For *invasive or disseminated candidiasis*, an **echinocandin** can be used. Fluconazole is an alternative for *Candida albicans* infection in clinically stable patients who have not received an azole antifungal recently. Amphotericin is an alternative when an echinocandin or fluconazole cannot be used, however, amphotericin should be considered for the initial treatment of CNS candidiasis. Voriconazole can be used for infections caused by fluconazole-resistant *Candida* spp. when oral therapy is required, or in patients intolerant of amphotericin or an echinocandin. In refractory cases, flucytosine p. 590 can be used with intravenous amphotericin.

Cryptococcosis

Cryptococcosis is uncommon but infection in the immunocompromised, especially in HIV-positive patients, can be life-threatening; cryptococcal meningitis is the most common form of fungal meningitis. The treatment of choice in cryptococcal meningitis is amphotericin by intravenous infusion and flucytosine by intravenous infusion for 2 weeks, followed by fluconazole by mouth for 8 weeks or until cultures are negative. In cryptococcosis, fluconazole is sometimes given alone as an alternative in HIV-positive patients with mild, localised infections or in those who cannot tolerate amphotericin. Following successful treatment, fluconazole can be used for prophylaxis against relapse until immunity recovers.

Histoplasmosis

Histoplasmosis is rare in temperate climates; it can be life-threatening, particularly in HIV-infected persons. Itraconazole can be used for the treatment of immunocompetent patients with indolent non-meningeal infection, including chronic pulmonary histoplasmosis. Amphotericin by intravenous infusion is used for the initial treatment of fulminant or severe infections, followed by a course of itraconazole by mouth. Following successful treatment, itraconazole can be used for prophylaxis against relapse until immunity recovers.

Skin and nail infections

Mild localised fungal infections of the skin (including tinea corporis, tinea cruris, and tinea pedis) respond to topical therapy. Systemic therapy is appropriate if topical therapy fails, if many areas are affected, or if the site of infection is difficult to treat such as in infections of the nails (onychomycosis) and of the scalp (tinea capitis). Oral imidazole or triazole antifungals (particularly itraconazole) and terbinafine p. 1200 are used more frequently than griseofulvin p. 590 because they have a broader spectrum of activity and require a shorter duration of treatment.

Tinea capitis is treated systemically; additional topical application of an antifungal may reduce transmission. Griseofulvin is used for tinea capitis in adults and children; it is effective against infections caused by *Trichophyton tonsurans* and *Microsporum spp.* Terbinafine is used for tinea capitis caused by *T. tonsurans* [unlicensed indication]. The role of terbinafine in the management of *Microsporum* infections is uncertain.

Pityriasis versicolor may be treated with itraconazole by mouth if topical therapy is ineffective; fluconazole by mouth is an alternative. Oral terbinafine is **not** effective for pityriasis versicolor.

Antifungal treatment may not be necessary in asymptomatic patients with tinea infection of the nails. If treatment is necessary, a systemic antifungal is more effective than topical therapy. Terbinafine and itraconazole have largely replaced griseofulvin for the systemic treatment of *onychomycosis*, particularly of the toenail; terbinafine is considered to be the drug of choice. Itraconazole can be administered as intermittent 'pulse' therapy. Topical antifungals also have a role in the treatment of onychomycosis.

Immunocompromised patients

Immunocompromised patients are at particular risk of fungal infections and may receive antifungal drugs prophylactically; oral triazole antifungals are the drugs of choice for prophylaxis. Fluconazole is more reliably absorbed than itraconazole, but fluconazole is not effective against *Aspergillus* spp. Itraconazole is preferred in patients at risk of invasive aspergillosis. Posaconazole can be used for prophylaxis in patients who are undergoing haematopoietic stem cell transplantation or receiving chemotherapy for acute myeloid leukaemia or myelodysplastic syndrome. Micafungin p. 582 can be used for prophylaxis of candidiasis in patients undergoing haematopoietic stem cell transplantation when fluconazole, itraconazole or posaconazole cannot be used.

Amphotericin by intravenous infusion or caspofungin is used for the empirical *treatment* of serious fungal infections; caspofungin is not effective against fungal infections of the CNS.

Triazole antifungals

Triazole antifungal drugs have a role in the prevention and systemic treatment of fungal infections.

Fluconazole is very well absorbed after oral administration. It also achieves good penetration into the cerebrospinal fluid to treat fungal meningitis. Fluconazole is excreted largely unchanged in the urine and can be used to treat candiduria.

Itraconazole is active against a wide range of dermatophytes. Itraconazole capsules require an acid environment in the stomach for optimal absorption. Itraconazole has been associated with liver damage and should be avoided or used with caution in patients with liver disease; fluconazole is less frequently associated with hepatotoxicity.

Posaconazole is licensed for the treatment of invasive fungal infections unresponsive to conventional treatment.

Voriconazole is a broad-spectrum antifungal drug which is licensed for use in life-threatening infections.

Imidazole antifungals

The imidazole antifungals include clotrimazole p. 810, econazole nitrate p. 811, ketoconazole p. 666, and tioconazole p. 1199. They are used for the local treatment of vaginal candidiasis and for dermatophyte infections. Miconazole p. 811 can be used locally for oral infections; it is also effective in intestinal infections. Systemic absorption may follow use of miconazole oral gel and may result in significant drug interactions.

Polyene antifungals

The polyene antifungals include amphotericin p. 583 and nystatin p. 1184; neither drug is absorbed when given by mouth. Nystatin is used for oral, oropharyngeal, and perioral infections by local application in the mouth. Nystatin is also used for *Candida albicans* infection of the skin.

Amphotericin by intravenous infusion is used for the treatment of systemic fungal infections and is active against most fungi and yeasts. It is highly protein bound and penetrates poorly into body fluids and tissues. When given parenterally amphotericin is toxic and side-effects are common. Lipid formulations of amphotericin (*Abelcet*® and *AmBisome*®) are significantly less toxic and are recommended when the conventional formulation of amphotericin is contra-indicated because of toxicity, especially nephrotoxicity or when response to conventional amphotericin is inadequate; lipid formulations are more expensive.

Echinocandin antifungals

The echinocandin antifungals include anidulafungin below, caspofungin p. 582 and micafungin p. 582. They are only active against *Aspergillus* spp. and *Candida* spp.; however, anidulafungin and micafungin are not used for the treatment of aspergillosis. Echinocandins are not effective against fungal infections of the CNS.

Other antifungals

Flucytosine p. 590 is used with amphotericin in a synergistic combination. Bone marrow depression can occur which limits its use, particularly in HIV-positive patients; weekly blood counts are necessary during prolonged therapy. Resistance to flucytosine can develop during therapy and sensitivity testing is essential before and during treatment. Flucytosine has a role in the treatment of systemic candidiasis and cryptococcal meningitis.

Griseofulvin p. 590 is effective for widespread or intractable dermatophyte infections but has been superseded by newer antifungals, particularly for nail infections. It is the drug of choice for trichophyton infections in children. Duration of therapy is dependent on the site of the infection and may extend to a number of months.

Terbinafine p. 1200 is the drug of choice for fungal nail infections and is also used for ringworm infections where oral treatment is considered appropriate.

ANTIFUNGALS > ECHINOCANDIN ANTIFUNGALS

Anidulafungin

- ● **INDICATIONS AND DOSE**

Invasive candidiasis
- ▶ BY INTRAVENOUS INFUSION
  - ▶ **Adult:** Initially 200 mg once daily for 1 day, then 100 mg once daily

- ● SIDE-EFFECTS
- ▶ **Common or very common** Bronchospasm · cholestasis · diarrhoea · dyspnoea · headache · hyperglycaemia · hypertension · hypokalaemia · hypotension · nausea · seizure · skin reactions · vomiting
- ▶ **Uncommon** Abdominal pain upper · coagulation disorder · vasodilation

- ● PREGNANCY Manufacturer advises avoid—no information available.

- ● BREAST FEEDING Manufacturer advises avoid unless potential benefit outweighs risk—present in milk in *animal* studies.

- ● DIRECTIONS FOR ADMINISTRATION For *intravenous infusion* (*Ecalta*®), give intermittently in Glucose 5% *or* Sodium chloride 0.9%. Reconstitute each 100 mg with 30 mL water for injections and allow up to 5 minutes for reconstitution; dilute dose in infusion fluid to a concentration of 770 micrograms/mL; give at a rate not exceeding 1.1 mg/minute. Follow product information if using stock supplied with ethanol solvent.

- ● MEDICINAL FORMS
There can be variation in the licensing of different medicines containing the same drug.
Powder for solution for infusion
- ▶ Ecalta (Pfizer Ltd)
  Anidulafungin 100 mg Ecalta 100mg powder for concentrate for solution for infusion vials | 1 vial PoM £299.99 (Hospital only)

5

Infection

Caspofungin

● INDICATIONS AND DOSE

Invasive aspergillosis | Invasive candidiasis | Empirical treatment of systemic fungal infections in patients with neutropenia
▶ BY INTRAVENOUS INFUSION
▶ Adult (body-weight up to 81 kg): 70 mg once daily for 1 day, then 50 mg once daily
▶ Adult (body-weight 81 kg and above): 70 mg once daily

DOSE ADJUSTMENTS DUE TO INTERACTIONS
▶ Manufacturer advises increase dose to 70 mg daily with concurrent use of some enzyme inducers (such as carbamazepine, dexamethasone, phenytoin, and rifampicin); no dose adjustment required for patients already on 70 mg daily.

● INTERACTIONS → Appendix 1: caspofungin
● SIDE-EFFECTS
▶ **Common or very common** Arthralgia · diarrhoea · dyspnoea · electrolyte imbalance · fever · headache · hyperhidrosis · nausea · skin reactions · vomiting
▶ **Uncommon** Anaemia · anxiety · appetite decreased · arrhythmias · ascites · chest discomfort · coagulation disorder · congestive heart failure · constipation · cough · disorientation · dizziness · drowsiness · dry mouth · dysphagia · excessive tearing · eyelid oedema · fatigue · flatulence · fluid overload · flushing · gastrointestinal discomfort · haematuria · hepatic disorders · hyperbilirubinaemia · hyperglycaemia · hypertension · hypotension · hypoxia · insomnia · laryngeal pain · leucopenia · malaise · metabolic acidosis · muscle weakness · myalgia · nasal congestion · oedema · pain · palpitations · renal impairment · respiratory disorders · sensation abnormal · taste altered · thrombocytopenia · tremor · vision blurred
▶ **Frequency not known** Severe cutaneous adverse reactions (SCARs)

● PREGNANCY Manufacturer advises avoid unless essential—toxicity in *animal* studies.
● BREAST FEEDING Present in milk in *animal* studies— manufacturer advises avoid.
● HEPATIC IMPAIRMENT No information available for severe impairment.
Dose adjustments 70 mg on first day then 35 mg once daily in moderate impairment.
● DIRECTIONS FOR ADMINISTRATION For *intravenous infusion* (*Cancidas*®), give intermittently *in* Sodium chloride 0.9%. Allow vial to reach room temperature; initially reconstitute each vial with 10.5 mL water for injections, mixing gently to dissolve then dilute requisite dose in 250 mL infusion fluid (35- or 50-mg doses may be diluted in 100 ml infusion fluid if necessary); give over 60 minutes; incompatible with glucose solutions.

● MEDICINAL FORMS
There can be variation in the licensing of different medicines containing the same drug.
Powder for solution for infusion
▶ Caspofungin (Non-proprietary)
Caspofungin (as Caspofungin acetate) 50 mg Caspofungin 50mg powder for concentrate for solution for infusion vials | 1 vial [PoM] £81.92–£327.67
Caspofungin (as Caspofungin acetate) 70 mg Caspofungin 70mg powder for concentrate for solution for infusion vials | 1 vial [PoM] £104.20–£416.78
▶ Cancidas (Merck Sharp & Dohme Ltd)
Caspofungin (as Caspofungin acetate) 50 mg Cancidas 50mg powder for solution for infusion vials | 1 vial [PoM] £327.67
Caspofungin (as Caspofungin acetate) 70 mg Cancidas 70mg powder for solution for infusion vials | 1 vial [PoM] £416.78

Micafungin

● INDICATIONS AND DOSE

Invasive candidiasis
▶ BY INTRAVENOUS INFUSION
▶ Adult (body-weight up to 40 kg): 2 mg/kg once daily for at least 14 days; increased if necessary to 4 mg/kg once daily, increase dose if response inadequate
▶ Adult (body-weight 40 kg and above): 100 mg once daily for at least 14 days; increased if necessary to 200 mg once daily, increase dose if response inadequate

Oesophageal candidiasis
▶ BY INTRAVENOUS INFUSION
▶ Adult (body-weight up to 40 kg): 3 mg/kg once daily
▶ Adult (body-weight 40 kg and above): 150 mg once daily

Prophylaxis of candidiasis in patients undergoing bone-marrow transplantation or who are expected to become neutropenic for over 10 days
▶ BY INTRAVENOUS INFUSION
▶ Adult (body-weight up to 40 kg): 1 mg/kg once daily continue for at least 7 days after neutrophil count is in desirable range
▶ Adult (body-weight 40 kg and above): 50 mg once daily continue for at least 7 days after neutrophil count is in desirable range

● INTERACTIONS → Appendix 1: micafungin
● SIDE-EFFECTS Anaemia · anxiety · appetite decreased · arrhythmias · confusion · constipation · diarrhoea · disseminated intravascular coagulation · dizziness · drowsiness · dyspnoea · electrolyte imbalance · eosinophilia · flushing · gastrointestinal discomfort · haemolysis · haemolytic anaemia · headache · hepatic disorders · hepatic failure (potentially life-threatening) · hyperbilirubinaemia · hyperhidrosis · hypersensitivity · hypertension · hypoalbuminaemia · hypotension · insomnia · leucopenia · nausea · neutropenia · palpitations · pancytopenia · peripheral oedema · renal impairment · severe cutaneous adverse reactions (SCARs) · shock · skin reactions · taste altered · thrombocytopenia · tremor · vomiting

● PREGNANCY Manufacturer advises avoid unless essential—toxicity in *animal* studies.
● BREAST FEEDING Manufacturer advises use only if potential benefit outweighs risk—present in milk in *animal* studies.
● HEPATIC IMPAIRMENT Use with caution in mild to moderate impairment. Avoid in severe impairment.
● RENAL IMPAIRMENT Use with caution; renal function may deteriorate.
● MONITORING REQUIREMENTS
▶ Monitor renal function.
▶ Monitor liver function—discontinue if significant and persistent abnormalities in liver function tests develop.
● DIRECTIONS FOR ADMINISTRATION For *intravenous infusion* (*Mycamine*®), give intermittenly *in* Glucose 5% or Sodium chloride 0.9%. Reconstitute each vial with 5 mL infusion fluid; gently rotate vial, without shaking, to dissolve; dilute requisite dose with infusion fluid to 100 mL (final concentration of 0.5–2 mg/mL); protect infusion from light; give over 60 minutes.

● MEDICINAL FORMS
There can be variation in the licensing of different medicines containing the same drug.
Powder for solution for infusion
▶ Mycamine (Astellas Pharma Ltd)
Micafungin (as Micafungin sodium) 50 mg Mycamine 50mg powder for solution for infusion vials | 1 vial [PoM] £196.08
Micafungin (as Micafungin sodium) 100 mg Mycamine 100mg powder for solution for infusion vials | 1 vial [PoM] £341.00

ANTIFUNGALS > POLYENE ANTIFUNGALS

Amphotericin
(Amphotericin B)

- **INDICATIONS AND DOSE**

ABELCET ®

Severe invasive candidiasis | Severe systemic fungal infections in patients not responding to conventional amphotericin or to other antifungal drugs or where toxicity or renal impairment precludes conventional amphotericin, including invasive aspergillosis, cryptococcal meningitis and disseminated cryptococcosis in HIV patients

▸ BY INTRAVENOUS INFUSION
▸ Adult: Test dose 1 mg, to be given over 15 minutes, then 5 mg/kg once daily for at least 14 days

AMBISOME ®

Severe systemic or deep mycoses where toxicity (particularly nephrotoxicity) precludes use of conventional amphotericin | Suspected or proven infection in febrile neutropenic patients unresponsive to broad-spectrum antibacterials

▸ BY INTRAVENOUS INFUSION
▸ Adult: Test dose 1 mg, to be given over 10 minutes, then 3 mg/kg once daily; maximum 5 mg/kg per day

Aspergillosis

▸ BY INTRAVENOUS INFUSION
▸ Adult: Test dose 1 mg, to be given over 10 minutes, then 3 mg/kg once daily; maximum 5 mg/kg per day

Visceral leishmaniasis (unresponsive to the antimonial alone)

▸ BY INTRAVENOUS INFUSION
▸ Adult: 1–3 mg/kg daily for 10–21 days to a cumulative dose of 21–30 mg/kg, alternatively 3 mg/kg for 5 consecutive days, followed by 3 mg/kg after 6 days for 1 dose

FUNGIZONE ®

Systemic fungal infections

▸ BY INTRAVENOUS INFUSION
▸ Adult: Test dose 1 mg, to be given over 20–30 minutes, then 250 micrograms/kg daily, gradually increased over 2–4 days, increased if tolerated to 1 mg/kg daily, max. (severe infection) 1.5 mg/kg daily or on alternate days. Prolonged treatment usually necessary; if interrupted for longer than 7 days recommence at 250 micrograms/kg daily and increase gradually

- **UNLICENSED USE** AMBISOME ® Use at the maximum dose of 5 mg/kg once daily is an unlicensed dose.
- **CAUTIONS** Avoid rapid infusion (risk of arrhythmias) · when given parenterally, toxicity common (close supervision necessary and close observation required for at least 30 minutes after test dose)

CAUTIONS, FURTHER INFORMATION
▸ Anaphylaxis Anaphylaxis can occur with any intravenous amphotericin product and a test dose is advisable before the first infusion; the patient should be carefully observed for at least 30 minutes after the test dose. Prophylactic antipyretics or hydrocortisone should only be used in patients who have previously experienced acute adverse reactions (in whom continued treatment with amphotericin is essential).

- **INTERACTIONS** → Appendix 1: amphotericin
- **SIDE-EFFECTS**
▸ Common or very common Anaemia · appetite decreased · azotaemia · chills · diarrhoea · dyspnoea · electrolyte imbalance · fever · headache · hepatic function abnormal

(discontinue) · hyposthenuria · hypotension · nausea · nephrocalcinosis · renal impairment · renal tubular acidosis · skin reactions · vomiting

▸ **Uncommon** Agranulocytosis · arrhythmias · flushing · gastrointestinal discomfort · hepatic disorders · leucopenia · myalgia · peripheral neuropathy · respiratory disorders · thrombocytopenia

▸ **Rare or very rare** Arthralgia · cardiac arrest · coagulation disorder · encephalopathy · eosinophilia · haemorrhage · hearing impairment · heart failure · hypersensitivity · hypertension · malaise · nephrogenic diabetes insipidus · pain · pulmonary oedema non-cardiogenic · seizure · severe cutaneous adverse reactions (SCARs) · shock · vertigo · vision disorders · weight decreased

- **PREGNANCY** Not known to be harmful but manufacturers advise avoid unless potential benefit outweighs risk.
- **BREAST FEEDING** No information available.
- **RENAL IMPAIRMENT** Use only if no alternative; nephrotoxicity may be reduced with use of lipid formulation.
- **MONITORING REQUIREMENTS** Hepatic and renal function tests, blood counts, and plasma electrolyte (including plasma-potassium and magnesium concentration) monitoring required.
- **DIRECTIONS FOR ADMINISTRATION**

ABELCET ® **Amphotericin (lipid complex)**
For *intravenous infusion*, give intermittently *in* Glucose 5%. Allow suspension to reach room temperature, shake gently to ensure no yellow settlement, withdraw requisite dose (using 17-19 gauge needle) into one or more 20-mL syringes; replace needle on syringe with a 5-micron filter needle provided (fresh needle for each syringe) and dilute to a concentration of 1 mg/mL (2 mg/mL can be used in fluid restriction and in children); preferably give *via* an infusion pump at a rate of 2.5 mg/kg/hour (initial test dose of 1 mg over 15 minutes) may be used; do not use sodium chloride or other electrolyte solutions, flush existing intravenous line with glucose 5% or use separate line.

AMBISOME ® **Amphotericin (liposomal)**
For *intravenous infusion (AmBisome®)*, give intermittently *in* Glucose 5% or 10%. Reconstitute each vial with 12 mL water for injections and shake vigorously to produce a preparation containing 4 mg/mL; withdraw requisite dose from vial and introduce into infusion fluid through the 5 micron filter provided to produce a final concentration of 0.2–2 mg/mL; infuse over 30–60 minutes, or if non-anaphylactic infusion-related reactions occur infuse over 2 hours (initial test dose of 1 mg over 10 minutes); an in-line filter (pore size no less than 1 micron) may be used; incompatible with sodium chloride solutions, flush existing intravenous line with glucose 5% or 10%, or use separate line.

FUNGIZONE ® **Amphotericin (as sodium deoxycholate complex)**
For *intravenous infusion (Fungizone®)*, give intermittently *in* Glucose 5%. Reconstitute each vial with 10 mL water of injections and shake immediately to produce a 5 mg/mL colloidal solution; dilute further in infusion fluid to a concentration of 100 micrograms/mL; pH of the glucose must not be below 4.2 (check each container—consult product literature for details of the buffer); infuse over 2–4 hours, or longer if not tolerated (initial test dose of 1 mg over 20–30 minutes); begin infusion immediately after dilution; protect from light; incompatible with sodium chloride solutions, flush existing intravenous line with glucose 5% or use separate line; an in-line filter (pore size no less than 1 micron) may be used.

- **PRESCRIBING AND DISPENSING INFORMATION** Different preparations of intravenous amphotericin vary in their pharmacodynamics, pharmacokinetics, dosage, and

5

Infection

administration; these preparations should **not** be considered interchangeable. To avoid confusion, prescribers should specify the brand to be dispensed.

- MEDICINAL FORMS
There can be variation in the licensing of different medicines containing the same drug.

Suspension for infusion
ELECTROLYTES: May contain Sodium
‣ Abelcet (Teva UK Ltd)
Amphotericin B (as Amphotericin B phospholipid complex) 5 mg per 1 ml Abelcet 100mg/20ml concentrate for suspension for infusion vials | 10 vial [PoM] £775.04 (Hospital only)

Powder for solution for infusion
EXCIPIENTS: May contain Sucrose
ELECTROLYTES: May contain Sodium
‣ AmBisome (Gilead Sciences International Ltd)
Amphotericin B liposomal 50 mg AmBisome 50mg powder for solution for infusion vials | 10 vial [PoM] £821.87
‣ Fungizone (Bristol-Myers Squibb Pharmaceuticals Ltd)
Amphotericin B 50 mg Fungizone Intravenous 50mg powder for solution for infusion vials | 1 vial [PoM] £3.88

ANTIFUNGALS › TRIAZOLE ANTIFUNGALS

Fluconazole

- INDICATIONS AND DOSE
Candidal balanitis
▸ BY MOUTH
▸ Child 16–17 years: 150 mg for 1 dose
▸ Adult: 150 mg for 1 dose
Vaginal candidiasis
▸ BY MOUTH
▸ Child 16–17 years: 150 mg for 1 dose
▸ Adult: 150 mg for 1 dose
Vulvovaginal candidiasis (recurrent)
▸ BY MOUTH
▸ Adult: Initially 150 mg every 72 hours for 3 doses, then 150 mg once weekly for 6 months
Mucosal candidiasis (except genital)
▸ BY MOUTH, OR BY INTRAVENOUS INFUSION
▸ Child 1 month–11 years: 3–6 mg/kg, dose to be given on first day, then 3 mg/kg daily (max. per dose 100 mg) for 7–14 days in oropharyngeal candidiasis (max. 14 days except in severely immunocompromised patients); for 14–30 days in other mucosal infections (e.g. oesophagitis, candiduria, non-invasive bronchopulmonary infections)
▸ Child 12–17 years: 50 mg daily for 7–14 days in oropharyngeal candidiasis (max. 14 days except in severely immunocompromised patients); for 14–30 days in other mucosal infections (e.g. oesophagitis, candiduria, non-invasive bronchopulmonary infections); increased to 100 mg daily, increased dose only for unusually difficult infections
▸ BY MOUTH
▸ Adult: 50 mg daily given for 7–14 days in oropharyngeal candidiasis (max. 14 days except in severely immunocompromised patients); for 14 days in atrophic oral candidiasis associated with dentures; for 14–30 days in other mucosal infections (e.g. oesophagitis, candiduria, non-invasive bronchopulmonary infections); increased to 100 mg daily, increased dose only for unusually difficult infections
Tinea pedis, corporis, cruris, pityriasis versicolor | Dermal candidiasis
▸ BY MOUTH
▸ Adult: 50 mg daily for 2–4 weeks (for up to 6 weeks in tinea pedis); max. duration of treatment 6 weeks

Invasive candidal infections (including candidaemia and disseminated candidiasis) and cryptococcal infections (including meningitis)
▸ BY MOUTH, OR BY INTRAVENOUS INFUSION
▸ Child: 6–12 mg/kg daily (max. per dose 800 mg), treatment continued according to response (at least 8 weeks for cryptococcal meningitis)
▸ Adult: 400 mg, dose to be given on first day, then 200–400 mg daily (max. per dose 800 mg once daily), treatment continued according to response (at least 8 weeks for cryptococcal meningitis), maximum dose for use in severe infections

Prevention of fungal infections in immunocompromised patients
▸ BY MOUTH, OR BY INTRAVENOUS INFUSION
▸ Child: 3–12 mg/kg daily (max. per dose 400 mg), commence treatment before anticipated onset of neutropenia and continue for 7 days after neutrophil count in desirable range, dose given according to extent and duration of neutropenia
▸ Adult: 50–400 mg daily, commence treatment before anticipated onset of neutropenia and continue for 7 days after neutrophil count in desirable range, dose adjusted according to risk

Prevention of fungal infections in immunocompromised patients (for patients with high risk of systemic infections e.g. following bone-marrow transplantation)
▸ BY MOUTH, OR BY INTRAVENOUS INFUSION
▸ Adult: 400 mg daily, commence treatment before anticipated onset of neutropenia and continue for 7 days after neutrophil count in desirable range

Prevention of relapse of cryptococcal meningitis in HIV-infected patients after completion of primary therapy
▸ BY MOUTH, OR BY INTRAVENOUS INFUSION
▸ Adult: 200 mg daily

- CONTRA-INDICATIONS Acute porphyrias p. 1025
- CAUTIONS Susceptibility to QT interval prolongation
- INTERACTIONS → Appendix 1: antifungals, azoles
- SIDE-EFFECTS
GENERAL SIDE-EFFECTS
▸ **Common or very common** Diarrhoea · gastrointestinal discomfort · headache · nausea · skin reactions · vomiting
▸ **Uncommon** Dizziness · flatulence · hepatic disorders · seizure · taste altered
▸ **Rare or very rare** Agranulocytosis · alopecia · dyslipidaemia · hypokalaemia · leucopenia · neutropenia · QT interval prolongation · severe cutaneous adverse reactions (SCARs) · thrombocytopenia · torsade de pointes
SPECIFIC SIDE-EFFECTS
▸ **Uncommon**
▸ With parenteral use Anaemia · appetite decreased · asthenia · constipation · drowsiness · dry mouth · fever · hyperhidrosis · insomnia · malaise · myalgia · paraesthesia · vertigo
▸ **Rare or very rare**
▸ With parenteral use Angioedema · face oedema · tremor
▸ **Frequency not known**
▸ With oral use Cardio-respiratory distress · oedema
SIDE-EFFECTS, FURTHER INFORMATION If rash occurs, discontinue treatment (or monitor closely if infection invasive or systemic); severe cutaneous reactions are more likely in patients with AIDS.
- PREGNANCY Manufacturer advises avoid—multiple congenital abnormalities reported with long-term high doses.
- BREAST FEEDING Present in milk but amount probably too small to be harmful.
- HEPATIC IMPAIRMENT Toxicity with related drugs.

- **RENAL IMPAIRMENT**
Dose adjustments ▸ In adults Usual initial dose then halve subsequent doses if eGFR less than 50 mL/minute/1.73 m². ▸ In children Usual initial dose then halve subsequent doses if estimated glomerular filtration rate less than 50 mL/minute/1.73 m².

- **MONITORING REQUIREMENTS** Monitor liver function with high doses or extended courses—discontinue if signs or symptoms of hepatic disease (risk of hepatic necrosis).

- **DIRECTIONS FOR ADMINISTRATION**
▸ In children For *intravenous infusion*, give over 10–30 minutes; do not exceed an infusion rate of 5–10 mL/minute.

- **PRESCRIBING AND DISPENSING INFORMATION** Flavours of oral liquid formulations may include orange.

- **PROFESSION SPECIFIC INFORMATION**

Dental practitioners' formulary
Fluconazole Capsules 50 mg may be prescribed.
Fluconazole Oral Suspension 50 mg/5 mL may be prescribed.

- **EXCEPTIONS TO LEGAL CATEGORY** Fluconazole capsules can be sold to the public for vaginal candidiasis and associated candidal balanitis in those aged 16–60 years, in a container or packaging containing not more than 150 mg and labelled to show a max. dose of 150 mg.

- **MEDICINAL FORMS**
There can be variation in the licensing of different medicines containing the same drug.

Infusion
▸ Fluconazole (Non-proprietary)
Fluconazole 2 mg per 1 ml Fluconazole 200mg/100ml infusion bags | 5 bag PoM £19.45
Fluconazole 400mg/200ml infusion bags | 5 bag PoM £72.50

Solution for infusion
ELECTROLYTES: May contain Sodium
▸ Fluconazole (Non-proprietary)
Fluconazole 2 mg per 1 ml Fluconazole 200mg/100ml solution for infusion vials | 1 vial PoM £3.00–£29.28
Fluconazole 50mg/25ml solution for infusion vials | 1 vial PoM £7.31–£7.32
Fluconazole 200mg/100ml solution for infusion bottles | 5 bottle PoM £274.50
▸ Diflucan (Pfizer Ltd)
Fluconazole 2 mg per 1 ml Diflucan 200mg/100ml solution for infusion vials | 1 vial PoM £29.28 (Hospital only)

Oral suspension
CAUTIONARY AND ADVISORY LABELS 9
▸ Fluconazole (Non-proprietary)
Fluconazole 10 mg per 1 ml Fluconazole 50mg/5ml oral suspension | 35 ml PoM £20.51 DT = £20.51
▸ Diflucan (Pfizer Ltd)
Fluconazole 10 mg per 1 ml Diflucan 50mg/5ml oral suspension | 35 ml PoM £16.61 DT = £20.51
Fluconazole 40 mg per 1 ml Diflucan 200mg/5ml oral suspension | 35 ml PoM £66.42 DT = £66.42

Capsule
CAUTIONARY AND ADVISORY LABELS 9 (50 mg and 200 mg strengths only)
▸ Fluconazole (Non-proprietary)
Fluconazole 50 mg Fluconazole 50mg capsules | 7 capsule PoM £5.00 DT = £0.45
Fluconazole 150 mg Fluconazole 150mg capsules | 1 capsule PoM £8.50 DT = £0.39 | 1 capsule P Ⓢ DT = £0.39
Fluconazole 200 mg Fluconazole 200mg capsules | 7 capsule PoM £6.02 DT = £5.30
▸ Canesten (fluconazole) (Bayer Plc)
Fluconazole 150 mg Canesten Thrush Oral 150mg capsules | 1 capsule P £6.33 DT = £0.39
▸ Diflucan (Pfizer Ltd)
Fluconazole 50 mg Diflucan 50mg capsules | 7 capsule PoM £16.61 DT = £0.45
Fluconazole 150 mg Diflucan 150mg capsules | 1 capsule PoM £7.12 DT = £0.39
Fluconazole 200 mg Diflucan 200mg capsules | 7 capsule PoM £66.42 DT = £5.30

Isavuconazole

22-Mar-2017

- **DRUG ACTION** Isavuconazole is a triazole antifungal that blocks the synthesis of ergosterol, a key component of the fungal cell membrane.

- **INDICATIONS AND DOSE**

Invasive aspergillosis | Mucormycosis in patients for whom amphotericin B is inappropriate
▸ BY MOUTH, OR BY INTRAVENOUS INFUSION
▸ Adult: Loading dose 200 mg every 8 hours for 48 hours (6 administrations in total), then maintenance 200 mg once daily, maintenance dose to be started at least 12 hours after the last loading dose; long-term treatment should be reviewed after 6-months

- **CONTRA-INDICATIONS** Acute porphyrias p. 1025 · short QT syndrome

- **CAUTIONS** Elderly—limited information

- **INTERACTIONS** → Appendix 1: antifungals, azoles

- **SIDE-EFFECTS**
GENERAL SIDE-EFFECTS
▸ **Common or very common** Appetite decreased · asthenia · chest pain · delirium · diarrhoea · drowsiness · electrolyte imbalance · gastrointestinal discomfort · headache · hepatic disorders · nausea · skin reactions
▸ **Uncommon** Alopecia · anaemia · arrhythmias · back pain · circulatory collapse · confusion · constipation · depression · dizziness · dyspnoea · encephalopathy · haemorrhage · hypersensitivity · hypoalbuminaemia · hypoglycaemia · hypotension · insomnia · leucopenia · malaise · malnutrition · neutropenia · palpitations · pancytopenia · paraesthesia · peripheral neuropathy · renal failure · respiratory disorders · seizures · syncope · taste altered · thrombocytopenia · vertigo · vomiting

SPECIFIC SIDE-EFFECTS
▸ **Common or very common**
▸ With intravenous use Hyperbilirubinaemia
▸ **Uncommon**
▸ With intravenous use Peripheral oedema
SIDE-EFFECTS, FURTHER INFORMATION Infusion-related reactions have been reported, including hypotension, dyspnoea, dizziness, paraesthesia, nausea, and headache—manufacturer advises discontinue treatment if these reactions occur.

- **PREGNANCY** Manufacturer advises avoid unless severe or life-threatening infection—toxicity in *animal* studies.

- **BREAST FEEDING** Manufacturer advises avoid—present in milk in *animal* studies.

- **HEPATIC IMPAIRMENT** Manufacturer advises use with caution and monitor for toxicity in severe impairment—no information available.

- **DIRECTIONS FOR ADMINISTRATION** For *intravenous infusion*, reconstitute each 200 mg with 5 mL Water for Injection; dilute dose to concentration of 0.8 mg/mL with Glucose 5% or Sodium Chloride 0.9% and give via a 0.2–1.2 micron filter over at least 1 hour.

- **HANDLING AND STORAGE**
▸ With intravenous use Manufacturer advises store in a refrigerator (2–8°C)—consult product literature for storage after reconstitution or dilution.

- **PATIENT AND CARER ADVICE**
Driving and skilled tasks Manufacturer advises patients and carers should be cautioned on the effects on driving and performance of skilled tasks—increased risk of confusion, syncope and dizziness.

- **NATIONAL FUNDING/ACCESS DECISIONS**
All Wales Medicines Strategy Group (AWMSG) Decisions
The *All Wales Medicines Strategy Group* has advised (January 2017) that isavuconazole (*Cresemba*®) is

recommended as an option for use in adults within NHS Wales for the treatment of invasive aspergillosis, and the treatment of mucormycosis in patients for whom amphotericin B is inappropriate, only if the approved Wales Patient Access Scheme (WPAS) is used or where the list/contract price is equivalent or lower.

● MEDICINAL FORMS
There can be variation in the licensing of different medicines containing the same drug.

Powder for solution for infusion
CAUTIONARY AND ADVISORY LABELS 3
‣ Cresemba (Pfizer Ltd) ▼
Isavuconazole (as Isavuconazonium sulfate) 200 mg Cresemba 200mg powder for concentrate for solution for infusion vials | 1 vial [PoM] £297.84 (Hospital only)

Capsule
CAUTIONARY AND ADVISORY LABELS 3, 25
‣ Cresemba (Pfizer Ltd) ▼
Isavuconazole (as Isavuconazonium sulfate) 100 mg Cresemba 100mg capsules | 14 capsule [PoM] £599.28 (Hospital only)

Itraconazole

● INDICATIONS AND DOSE

Vulvovaginal candidiasis
▶ BY MOUTH
‣ Adult: 200 mg twice daily for 1 day

Vulvovaginal candidiasis (recurrent)
▶ BY MOUTH
‣ Adult: 50–100 mg daily for 6 months

Oral or oesophageal candidiasis that has not responded to fluconazole
▶ BY MOUTH USING ORAL SOLUTION
‣ Adult: 100–200 mg twice daily for 2 weeks (continue for another 2 weeks if no response; the higher dose should not be used for longer than 2 weeks if no signs of improvement)

Oral or oesophageal candidiasis in HIV-positive or other immunocompromised patients
▶ BY MOUTH USING ORAL SOLUTION
‣ Adult: 200 mg daily in 1–2 divided doses for 1 week (continue for another week if no response)

Systemic candidiasis where other antifungal drugs inappropriate or ineffective
▶ BY MOUTH
‣ Adult: 100–200 mg once daily
▶ BY INTRAVENOUS INFUSION
‣ Adult: 200 mg every 12 hours for 2 days, then 200 mg once daily for max. 12 days

Systemic candidiasis (invasive or disseminated) where other antifungal drugs inappropriate or ineffective
▶ BY MOUTH
‣ Adult: 200 mg twice daily

Pityriasis versicolor
▶ BY MOUTH
‣ Adult: 200 mg once daily for 7 days

Tinea pedis | Tinea manuum
▶ BY MOUTH
‣ Adult: 100 mg once daily for 30 days, alternatively 200 mg twice daily for 7 days

Tinea corporis | Tinea cruris
▶ BY MOUTH
‣ Adult: 100 mg once daily for 15 days, alternatively 200 mg once daily for 7 days

Onychomycosis
▶ BY MOUTH
‣ Adult: 200 mg once daily for 3 months, alternatively 200 mg twice daily for 7 days, subsequent courses repeated after 21-day intervals; fingernails 2 courses, toenails 3 courses

Aspergillosis
▶ BY MOUTH
‣ Adult: 200 mg twice daily

Systemic aspergillosis where other antifungal drugs inappropriate or ineffective
▶ BY INTRAVENOUS INFUSION
‣ Adult: 200 mg every 12 hours for 2 days, then 200 mg once daily for max. 12 days

Histoplasmosis
▶ BY MOUTH
‣ Adult: 200 mg 3 times a day for 3 days, then 200 mg 1–2 times a day
▶ BY INTRAVENOUS INFUSION
‣ Adult: 200 mg every 12 hours for 2 days, then 200 mg once daily for max. 12 days

Systemic cryptococcosis including cryptococcal meningitis where other antifungal drugs inappropriate or ineffective
▶ BY MOUTH
‣ Adult: 200 mg once daily, dose increased in invasive or disseminated disease and in cryptococcal meningitis, increased to 200 mg twice daily
▶ BY INTRAVENOUS INFUSION
‣ Adult: 200 mg every 12 hours for 2 days, then 200 mg once daily for max. 12 days

Maintenance in HIV-infected patients to prevent relapse of underlying fungal infection and prophylaxis in neutropenia when standard therapy inappropriate
▶ BY MOUTH
‣ Adult: 200 mg once daily, then increased to 200 mg twice daily, dose increased only if low plasma-itraconazole concentration

Prophylaxis of deep fungal infections (when standard therapy inappropriate) in patients with haematological malignancy or undergoing bone-marrow transplantation who are expected to become neutropenic
▶ BY MOUTH USING ORAL SOLUTION
‣ Adult: 5 mg/kg daily in 2 divided doses, to be started before transplantation or before chemotherapy (taking care to avoid interaction with cytotoxic drugs) and continued until neutrophil count recovers, safety and efficacy not established in elderly patients

DOSE ADJUSTMENTS DUE TO INTERACTIONS
▶ Manufacturer advises max. dose 200 mg daily with concurrent use of cobicistat.

● UNLICENSED USE Itraconazole doses in BNF may differ from those in product literature.

IMPORTANT SAFETY INFORMATION
HEART FAILURE
Following reports of heart failure, caution is advised when prescribing itraconazole to patients at high risk of heart failure. Those at risk include:
● patients receiving high doses and longer treatment courses;
● older adults and those with cardiac disease;
● patients with chronic lung disease (including chronic obstructive pulmonary disease) associated with pulmonary hypertension;
● patients receiving treatment with negative inotropic drugs, e.g. calcium channel blockers.

Itraconazole should be avoided in patients with ventricular dysfunction or a history of heart failure unless the infection is serious.

- CONTRA-INDICATIONS Acute porphyrias p. 1025
- CAUTIONS Active liver disease · history of hepatotoxicity with other drugs · susceptibility to congestive heart failure
- INTERACTIONS → Appendix 1: antifungals, azoles
- SIDE-EFFECTS
  GENERAL SIDE-EFFECTS
  ▸ **Common or very common** Alopecia · constipation · diarrhoea · dyspnoea · gastrointestinal discomfort · headache · heart failure · hepatic disorders · hyperbilirubinaemia · hypotension · nausea · oedema · pulmonary oedema · skin reactions · vision disorders · vomiting
  ▸ **Uncommon** Taste altered
  ▸ **Rare or very rare** Angioedema · hypersensitivity vasculitis · hypertriglyceridaemia · pancreatitis · photosensitivity reaction · severe cutaneous adverse reactions (SCARs)
  ▸ **Frequency not known** Peripheral neuropathy (discontinue)
  SPECIFIC SIDE-EFFECTS
  ▸ **Common or very common**
  ▸ With intravenous use Chest pain · confusion · cough · dizziness · drowsiness · electrolyte imbalance · fatigue · gastrointestinal disorder · granulocytopenia · hyperglycaemia · hyperhidrosis · hypersensitivity · hypertension · myalgia · pain · renal impairment · tachycardia · tremor · urinary incontinence
  ▸ **Uncommon**
  ▸ With intravenous use Dysphonia · hearing loss · numbness · thrombocytopenia
  ▸ With oral use Flatulence · menstrual disorder
  ▸ **Rare or very rare**
  ▸ With oral use Erectile dysfunction · hearing impairment · leucopenia · sensation abnormal · serum sickness · urinary frequency increased
  SIDE-EFFECTS, FURTHER INFORMATION Potentially life-threatening hepatotoxicity reported very rarely—discontinue if signs of hepatitis develop.
- CONCEPTION AND CONTRACEPTION Ensure effective contraception during treatment and until the next menstrual period following end of treatment.
- PREGNANCY Manufacturer advises use only in life-threatening situations (toxicity at high doses in *animal* studies).
- BREAST FEEDING Small amounts present in milk—may accumulate; manufacturer advises avoid.
- HEPATIC IMPAIRMENT Use only if potential benefit outweighs risk of hepatotoxicity.
  Dose adjustments Dose reduction may be necessary.
- RENAL IMPAIRMENT Risk of congestive heart failure.
  ▸ With oral use Bioavailability of oral formulations possibly reduced.
  ▸ With intravenous use Use intravenous infusion with caution if eGFR 30–80 mL/minute/1.73 m^2; avoid intravenous infusion if eGFR less than 30 mL/minute/1.73 m^2.
- MONITORING REQUIREMENTS
  ▸ Absorption reduced in AIDS and neutropenia (monitor plasma-itraconazole concentration and increase dose if necessary).
  ▸ Monitor liver function if treatment continues for longer than one month, if receiving other hepatotoxic drugs, if history of hepatotoxicity with other drugs, or in hepatic impairment.
- DIRECTIONS FOR ADMINISTRATION
  ▸ With intravenous use For *intravenous infusion (Sporanox®)*, give intermittently in Sodium Chloride 0.9%; dilute 250 mg in 50 mL infusion fluid and infuse only 60 mL through an in-line filter (0.2 micron) over 60 minutes.

▸ With oral use For *oral liquid*, do not take with food; swish around mouth and swallow, do not rinse afterwards.

- PRESCRIBING AND DISPENSING INFORMATION Flavours of oral liquid formulations may include cherry.
- PATIENT AND CARER ADVICE Patients should be told how to recognise signs of liver disorder and advised to seek prompt medical attention if symptoms such as anorexia, nausea, vomiting, fatigue, abdominal pain or dark urine develop.
  ▸ With oral use Patients or carers should be given advice on how to administer itraconazole oral liquid.

- MEDICINAL FORMS
  There can be variation in the licensing of different medicines containing the same drug. Forms available from special-order manufacturers include: oral suspension, oral solution

  Solution for infusion
  EXCIPIENTS: May contain Propylene glycol
  ▸ Sporanox (Janssen-Cilag Ltd)
    Itraconazole 10 mg per 1 ml Sporanox I.V. 250mg/25ml solution for infusion ampoules and diluent | 1 ampoule [PoM] £79.71

  Oral solution
  CAUTIONARY AND ADVISORY LABELS 9, 23
  ▸ Itraconazole (Non-proprietary)
    Itraconazole 10 mg per 1 ml Itraconazole 50mg/5ml oral solution sugar free sugar-free | 150 ml [PoM] £58.34 DT = £58.34
  ▸ Sporanox (Janssen-Cilag Ltd)
    Itraconazole 10 mg per 1 ml Sporanox 50mg/5ml oral solution sugar-free | 150 ml [PoM] £58.34 DT = £58.34

  Capsule
  CAUTIONARY AND ADVISORY LABELS 5, 9, 21, 25
  ▸ Itraconazole (Non-proprietary)
    Itraconazole 100 mg Itraconazole 100mg capsules | 15 capsule [PoM] £13.77 DT = £3.40 | 60 capsule [PoM] £13.60-£56.21
  ▸ Sporanox (Janssen-Cilag Ltd)
    Itraconazole 100 mg Sporanox-Pulse 100mg capsules | 28 capsule [PoM] £25.72
    Sporanox 100mg capsules | 4 capsule [PoM] £3.67 | 15 capsule [PoM] £13.77 DT = £3.40 | 60 capsule [PoM] £55.10

Posaconazole

10-Nov-2017

- INDICATIONS AND DOSE

Invasive aspergillosis either refractory to, or in patients intolerant of, itraconazole or amphotericin | Fusariosis either refractory to, or in patients intolerant of, amphotericin | Chromoblastomycosis and mycetoma either refractory to, or in patients intolerant of, itraconazole | Coccidioidomycosis either refractory to, or in patients intolerant of, amphotericin, itraconazole, or fluconazole
  ▸ BY MOUTH USING ORAL SUSPENSION
  ▸ Adult: 400 mg twice daily, to be taken with food, alternatively 200 mg 4 times a day, if unable to tolerate food
  ▸ BY MOUTH USING TABLETS, OR BY INTRAVENOUS INFUSION
  ▸ Adult: Loading dose 300 mg twice daily on first day, then 300 mg once daily, switch from intravenous to oral route when appropriate

Oropharyngeal candidiasis (severe infection or in immunocompromised patients only)
  ▸ BY MOUTH USING ORAL SUSPENSION
  ▸ Adult: Loading dose 200 mg on first day, then 100 mg once daily for 13 days, dose to be taken with food

continued →

5

Infection

Prophylaxis of invasive fungal infections in patients at high risk and undergoing high-dose immunosuppressive therapy for haematopoietic stem cell transplantation or receiving chemotherapy for acute myeloid leukaemia or myelodysplastic syndrome and expected to develop prolonged neutropenia
‣ BY MOUTH USING ORAL SUSPENSION
‣ Adult: 200 mg 3 times a day, dose to be taken with food, for chemotherapy patients, start several days before the expected onset of neutropenia and continue for 7 days after neutrophil count rises above 500 cells/mm^3
‣ BY MOUTH USING TABLETS, OR BY INTRAVENOUS INFUSION
‣ Adult: Loading dose 300 mg twice daily on first day, then 300 mg once daily, for chemotherapy patients, start several days before the expected onset of neutropenia and continue for 7 days after neutrophil count rises above 500 cells/mm^3, switch from intravenous to oral route when appropriate

DOSE EQUIVALENCE AND CONVERSION
‣ Posaconazole oral suspension is **not** interchangeable with tablets on a milligram-for-milligram basis.

PHARMACOKINETICS
‣ Posaconazole oral suspension should be taken with food (preferably a high fat meal) or nutritional supplement to ensure adequate exposure for systemic effects. Where possible, tablets should be used in preference to suspension because tablets have a higher bioavailability.

● CONTRA-INDICATIONS Acute porphyrias p. 1025
● CAUTIONS Administration by intravenous infusion, particularly by peripheral catheter—increased risk of QTc interval prolongation · body-weight over 120 kg—risk of treatment failure possibly increased · body-weight under 60 kg—risk of side effects increased · bradycardia · cardiomyopathy · history of QTc interval prolongation · symptomatic arrhythmias
● INTERACTIONS → Appendix 1: antifungals, azoles
● SIDE-EFFECTS
‣ **Common or very common** Appetite decreased · asthenia · constipation · diarrhoea · dizziness · drowsiness · dry mouth · electrolyte imbalance · gastrointestinal discomfort · gastrointestinal disorders · headache · hypertension · nausea · neutropenia · sensation abnormal · skin reactions · taste altered · vomiting
‣ **Uncommon** Alopecia · anaemia · aphasia · arrhythmias · burping · chest discomfort · confusion · cough · embolism and thrombosis · eosinophilia · feeling jittery · haemorrhage · hepatic disorders · hiccups · hyperglycaemia · hypoglycaemia · hypotension · leucopenia · lymphadenopathy · malaise · menstrual disorder · mucositis · nasal congestion · oedema · oral disorders · pain · palpitations · pancreatitis · peripheral neuropathy · QT interval prolongation · renal impairment · respiratory disorders · seizure · sleep disorders · splenic infarction · thrombocytopenia · tremor · vasculitis · vision disorders
‣ **Rare or very rare** Adrenal insufficiency · breast pain · cardiac arrest · coagulation disorder · depression · encephalopathy · haemolytic uraemic syndrome · hearing impairment · heart failure · myocardial infarction · nephritis tubulointerstitial · pancytopenia · psychotic disorder · pulmonary hypertension · renal tubular acidosis · Stevens-Johnson syndrome · stroke · sudden cardiac death · syncope
● CONCEPTION AND CONTRACEPTION Manufacturer recommends effective contraception during treatment.
● PREGNANCY Manufacturer advises avoid unless potential benefit outweighs risk; toxicity in *animal* studies.
● BREAST FEEDING Manufacturer advises avoid—present in milk in *animal* studies.

● HEPATIC IMPAIRMENT Manufacturer advises caution.
● RENAL IMPAIRMENT Manufacturer advises monitor efficacy in severe impairment—variable exposure expected.
‣ With intravenous use Manufacturer advises caution if eGFR less than 50 mL/minute/1.73 m^2—intravenous vehicle may accumulate.
● MONITORING REQUIREMENTS
‣ Monitor electrolytes (including potassium, magnesium, and calcium) before and during therapy.
‣ Monitor liver function before and during therapy.
● DIRECTIONS FOR ADMINISTRATION
‣ With intravenous use Manufacturer advises for *intravenous infusion* (*Noxafil®*), give continuously in Glucose 5% *or* Sodium Chloride 0.9%; dilute requisite dose in infusion fluid to produce a final concentration of 1–2 mg/mL; give via a central venous catheter or peripherally inserted central catheter over approx. 90 minutes (can give a single dose via peripheral venous catheter if central access not established—dilute to a final concentration of 2 mg/mL and give over approx. 30 minutes).
● PRESCRIBING AND DISPENSING INFORMATION Flavours of oral liquid formulations may include cherry.
● HANDLING AND STORAGE
‣ With intravenous use Manufacturer advises store in a refrigerator (2–8 °C).
● PATIENT AND CARER ADVICE
Driving and skilled tasks Manufacturer advises patients and carers should be counselled on the effects on driving and performance of skilled tasks—increased risk of dizziness and somnolence.

● MEDICINAL FORMS
There can be variation in the licensing of different medicines containing the same drug.
Solution for infusion
ELECTROLYTES: May contain Sodium
‣ Noxafil (Merck Sharp & Dohme Ltd)
   Posaconazole 18 mg per 1 ml Noxafil 300mg/16.7ml concentrate for solution for infusion vials | 1 vial [PoM] £211.00 (Hospital only)
Oral suspension
CAUTIONARY AND ADVISORY LABELS 3, 9, 21
‣ Noxafil (Merck Sharp & Dohme Ltd)
   Posaconazole 40 mg per 1 ml Noxafil 40mg/ml oral suspension | 105 ml [PoM] £491.20 (Hospital only)
Gastro-resistant tablet
CAUTIONARY AND ADVISORY LABELS 3, 9, 25
‣ Noxafil (Merck Sharp & Dohme Ltd)
   Posaconazole 100 mg Noxafil 100mg gastro-resistant tablets | 24 tablet [PoM] £596.96 | 96 tablet [PoM] £2,387.85

Voriconazole

● INDICATIONS AND DOSE
Invasive aspergillosis | Serious infections caused by *Scedosporium* spp., *Fusarium* spp., or invasive fluconazole-resistant *Candida* spp. (including *C. krusei*)
‣ BY MOUTH
‣ Adult (body-weight up to 40 kg): Initially 200 mg every 12 hours for 2 doses, then 100 mg every 12 hours, increased if necessary to 150 mg every 12 hours
‣ Adult (body-weight 40 kg and above): Initially 400 mg every 12 hours for 2 doses, then 200 mg every 12 hours, increased if necessary to 300 mg every 12 hours
‣ BY INTRAVENOUS INFUSION
‣ Adult: Initially 6 mg/kg every 12 hours for 2 doses, then 4 mg/kg every 12 hours; reduced if not tolerated to 3 mg/kg every 12 hours; for max. 6 months

DOSE ADJUSTMENTS DUE TO INTERACTIONS
▸ With intravenous use Manufacturer advises increase maintenance dose to 5 mg/kg every 12 hours with concurrent use of fosphenytoin, phenytoin or rifabutin.
▸ With oral use Manufacturer advises increase maintenance dose with concurrent use of fosphenytoin or phenytoin; 400 mg every 12 hours for patients of body-weight 40 kg and above; 200 mg every 12 hours for patients of body-weight less than 40 kg. Manufacturer advises if concurrent use of rifabutin is unavoidable, increase maintenance dose to 350 mg every 12 hours for patients of body-weight 40 kg and above; 200 mg every 12 hours for patients of body-weight less than 40 kg.

● CONTRA-INDICATIONS Acute porphyrias p. 1025
● CAUTIONS Avoid exposure to sunlight · bradycardia · cardiomyopathy · electrolyte disturbances · history of QT interval prolongation · patients at risk of pancreatitis · symptomatic arrhythmias
● INTERACTIONS → Appendix 1: antifungals, azoles
● SIDE-EFFECTS
▸ Common or very common Acute kidney injury · agranulocytosis · alopecia · anaemia · anxiety · arrhythmias · asthenia · bone marrow disorders · chest pain · chills · confusion · constipation · depression · diarrhoea · dizziness · drowsiness · dyspnoea · electrolyte imbalance · eye disorders · eye inflammation · fever · gastrointestinal discomfort · haemorrhage · hallucination · headache · hepatic disorders · hypoglycaemia · hypotension · increased risk of infection · insomnia · leucopenia · muscle tone increased · nausea · neutropenia · oedema · oral disorders · pain · pulmonary oedema · respiratory disorders · seizure · sensation abnormal · skin reactions · syncope · tetany · thrombocytopenia · tremor · vision disorders · vomiting
▸ Uncommon Adrenal insufficiency · arthritis · brain oedema · duodenitis · encephalopathy · eosinophilia · gallbladder disorders · hearing impairment · hypothyroidism · influenza like illness · lymphadenopathy · lymphangitis · movement disorders · nephritis · nerve disorders · pancreatitis · parkinsonism · phototoxicity · proteinuria · pseudomembranous enterocolitis · QT interval prolongation · renal tubular necrosis · severe cutaneous adverse reactions (SCARs) · taste altered · vertigo
▸ Rare or very rare Angioedema · cardiac conduction disorders · disseminated intravascular coagulation · hyperthyroidism
▸ Frequency not known Cutaneous lupus erythematosus · infusion related reaction · periostitis (more common in transplant patients) · squamous cell carcinoma (more common in presence of phototoxicity)

SIDE-EFFECTS, FURTHER INFORMATION
Hepatotoxicity Hepatitis, cholestasis, and acute hepatic failure have been reported; risk of hepatotoxicity increased in patients with haematological malignancy. Consider treatment discontinuation if severe abnormalities in liver function tests.
Phototoxicity Phototoxicity occurs uncommonly. If phototoxicity occurs, consider treatment discontinuation; if treatment is continued, monitor for pre-malignant skin lesions and squamous cell carcinoma, and discontinue treatment if they occur.

● CONCEPTION AND CONTRACEPTION Effective contraception required during treatment.
● PREGNANCY Toxicity in *animal* studies—manufacturer advises avoid unless potential benefit outweighs risk.
● BREAST FEEDING Manufacturer advises avoid—no information available.
● HEPATIC IMPAIRMENT
Dose adjustments In mild to moderate hepatic cirrhosis use usual initial dose then halve maintenance dose. No

information available for severe hepatic cirrhosis—manufacturer advises use only if potential benefit outweighs risk.
● RENAL IMPAIRMENT Intravenous vehicle may accumulate if eGFR less than 50 mL/minute/1.73 m² —use intravenous infusion only if potential benefit outweighs risk, and monitor renal function; alternatively, use tablets or oral suspension (no dose adjustment required).
● MONITORING REQUIREMENTS
▸ Monitor renal function.
▸ Monitor liver function before starting treatment, then at least weekly for 1 month, and then monthly during treatment.
● DIRECTIONS FOR ADMINISTRATION For *intravenous infusion*, reconstitute each 200 mg with 19 mL Water for Injections *or* Sodium Chloride 0.9% to produce a 10 mg/mL solution; dilute dose to concentration of 0.5–5 mg/mL with Glucose 5% or Sodium Chloride 0.9% and give intermittently at a rate not exceeding 3 mg/kg/hour.
● PRESCRIBING AND DISPENSING INFORMATION Flavours of oral liquid formulations may include orange.
● PATIENT AND CARER ADVICE Patients and their carers should be told how to recognise symptoms of liver disorder, and advised to seek immediate medical attention if symptoms such as persistent nausea, vomiting, malaise or jaundice develop.
  Patients and their carers should be advised that patients should avoid intense or prolonged exposure to direct sunlight, and to avoid the use of sunbeds. In sunlight, patients should cover sun-exposed areas of skin and use a sunscreen with a high sun protection factor. Patients should seek medical attention if they experience sunburn or a severe skin reaction following exposure to light or sun.
  Patients and their carers should be advised to keep the alert card with them at all times.

● MEDICINAL FORMS
There can be variation in the licensing of different medicines containing the same drug.

Tablet
CAUTIONARY AND ADVISORY LABELS 9, 11, 23
▸ Voriconazole (Non-proprietary)
 Voriconazole 50 mg Voriconazole 50mg tablets | 28 tablet [PoM] £45.43–£275.68 DT = £193.58
 Voriconazole 200 mg Voriconazole 200mg tablets | 28 tablet [PoM] £157.49–£1,102.74 DT = £766.96
▸ VFEND (Pfizer Ltd)
 Voriconazole 50 mg VFEND 50mg tablets | 28 tablet [PoM] £275.68 DT = £193.58
 Voriconazole 200 mg VFEND 200mg tablets | 28 tablet [PoM] £1,102.74 DT = £766.96

Oral suspension
CAUTIONARY AND ADVISORY LABELS 9, 11, 23
▸ VFEND (Pfizer Ltd)
 Voriconazole 40 mg per 1 ml VFEND 40mg/ml oral suspension | 75 ml [PoM] £551.37

Powder for solution for infusion
EXCIPIENTS: May contain Sulfobutylether beta cyclodextrin sodium
ELECTROLYTES: May contain Sodium
▸ Voriconazole (Non-proprietary)
 Voriconazole 200 mg Voriconazole 200mg powder for solution for infusion vials | 1 vial [PoM] £51.43–£77.14 (Hospital only)
▸ VFEND (Pfizer Ltd)
 Voriconazole 200 mg VFEND 200mg powder for solution for infusion vials | 1 vial [PoM] £77.14 (Hospital only)

Powder and solvent for solution for infusion
EXCIPIENTS: May contain Sulfobutylether beta cyclodextrin sodium
ELECTROLYTES: May contain Sodium
▸ VFEND (Pfizer Ltd)
 Voriconazole 200 mg VFEND 200mg powder and solvent for solution for infusion vials | 1 vial [PoM] £77.14 (Hospital only)

ANTIFUNGALS > OTHER

Flucytosine

- **INDICATIONS AND DOSE**

Systemic yeast and fungal infections | Adjunct to amphotericin in severe systemic candidiasis and in other severe or long-standing infections
- BY INTRAVENOUS INFUSION
- Adult: Usual dose 200 mg/kg daily in 4 divided doses usually for not more than 7 days, alternatively 100–150 mg/kg daily in 4 divided doses, lower dose may be sufficient for extremely sensitive organisms

Cryptococcal meningitis (adjunct to amphotericin)
- BY INTRAVENOUS INFUSION
- Adult: 100 mg/kg daily in 4 divided doses for 2 weeks

- UNLICENSED USE Use in cryptococcal meningitis for 2 weeks is an unlicensed duration.
- CAUTIONS Blood disorders · elderly
- INTERACTIONS → Appendix 1: flucytosine
- SIDE-EFFECTS Agranulocytosis · aplastic anaemia · blood disorder · cardiotoxicity · confusion · diarrhoea · hallucination · headache · hepatic disorders · leucopenia · nausea · rash · sedation · seizure · thrombocytopenia · toxic epidermal necrolysis · ventricular dysfunction · vertigo · vomiting
- PREGNANCY Teratogenic in *animal* studies; manufacturer advises use only if potential benefit outweighs risk.
- BREAST FEEDING Manufacturer advises avoid.
- RENAL IMPAIRMENT
  Dose adjustments Use 50 mg/kg every 12 hours if creatinine clearance 20–40 mL/minute; use 50 mg/kg every 24 hours if creatinine clearance 10–20 mL/minute; use initial dose of 50 mg/kg if creatinine clearance less than 10 mL/minute and then adjust dose according to plasma-flucytosine concentration.
  Monitoring In renal impairment liver- and kidney-function tests and blood counts required weekly.
- MONITORING REQUIREMENTS
- For plasma concentration monitoring, blood should be taken shortly before starting the next infusion; plasma concentration for optimum response 25–50 mg/litre (200–400 micromol/litre)—should not be allowed to exceed 80 mg/litre (620 micromol/litre).
- Liver- and kidney-function tests and blood counts required (weekly in blood disorders).
- DIRECTIONS FOR ADMINISTRATION For *intravenous infusion*, give over 20–40 minutes.

- MEDICINAL FORMS
  There can be variation in the licensing of different medicines containing the same drug.
  Solution for infusion
  ELECTROLYTES: May contain Sodium
  - Ancotil (Meda Pharmaceuticals Ltd)
    Flucytosine 10 mg per 1 ml Ancotil 2.5g/250ml solution for infusion bottles | 5 bottle [PoM] £151.67 (Hospital only)

Griseofulvin

- **INDICATIONS AND DOSE**

Dermatophyte infections of the skin, scalp, hair and nails where topical therapy has failed or is inappropriate
- BY MOUTH
- Adult: 500 mg daily, increased if necessary to 1 g daily, for severe infections; reduce dose when response occurs, daily dose may be taken once daily or in divided doses

Tinea capitis caused by *Trichophyton tonsurans*
- BY MOUTH
- Adult: 1 g once daily, alternatively 1 g daily in divided doses

- UNLICENSED USE Griseofulvin doses in BNF may differ from those in product literature.
- CONTRA-INDICATIONS Acute porphyrias p. 1025 · systemic lupus erythematosus (risk of exacerbation)
- INTERACTIONS → Appendix 1: griseofulvin
- SIDE-EFFECTS
- **Common or very common** Diarrhoea · epigastric discomfort · headache · nausea · vomiting
- **Uncommon** Appetite decreased · confusion · coordination abnormal · dizziness · drowsiness · insomnia · irritability · peripheral neuropathy · photosensitivity reaction · skin reactions · taste altered · toxic epidermal necrolysis
- **Rare or very rare** Anaemia · hepatic disorders · leucopenia · neutropenia · systemic lupus erythematosus (SLE)
- CONCEPTION AND CONTRACEPTION Effective contraception required during and for at least 1 month after administration to women (important: effectiveness of oral contraceptives may be reduced, additional contraceptive precautions e.g. barrier method, required). Men should avoid fathering a child during and for at least 6 months after administration
- PREGNANCY Avoid (fetotoxicity and teratogenicity in *animals*).
- BREAST FEEDING Avoid—no information available.
- HEPATIC IMPAIRMENT Avoid in severe liver disease.
- PATIENT AND CARER ADVICE
  Driving and skilled tasks May impair performance of skilled tasks (e.g. driving); effects of alcohol enhanced.

- MEDICINAL FORMS
  There can be variation in the licensing of different medicines containing the same drug. Forms available from special-order manufacturers include: oral suspension
  Tablet
  CAUTIONARY AND ADVISORY LABELS 9, 21
  - Griseofulvin (Non-proprietary)
    Griseofulvin 125 mg Griseofulvin 125mg tablets | 100 tablet [PoM] £96.67 DT = £96.67
    Griseofulvin 500 mg Griseofulvin 500mg tablets | 90 tablet £85.73 | 100 tablet [PoM] £90.34 DT = £92.80

3.1 Pneumocystis pneumonia

Pneumocystis pneumonia

Overview

Pneumonia caused by *Pneumocystis jirovecii* (*Pneumocystis carinii*) occurs in immunosuppressed patients; it is a common cause of pneumonia in AIDS. Pneumocystis pneumonia should generally be treated by those experienced in its management. Blood gas measurement is used to assess disease severity.

Treatment

Mild to moderate disease
Co-trimoxazole p. 552 in high dosage is the drug of choice for the treatment of mild to moderate pneumocystis pneumonia.

Atovaquone p. 591 is licensed for the treatment of mild to moderate pneumocystis infection in patients who cannot tolerate co-trimoxazole. A combination of dapsone p. 566 with trimethoprim p. 563 is given by mouth for the treatment of mild to moderate disease [unlicensed indication].

A combination of clindamycin p. 526 and primaquine p. 607 by mouth is used in the treatment of mild to moderate disease [unlicensed indication]; this combination is associated with considerable toxicity.

Severe disease
Co-trimoxazole in high dosage, given by mouth or by intravenous infusion, is the drug of choice for the treatment of severe pneumocystis pneumonia. Pentamidine isetionate below given by intravenous infusion is an alternative for patients who cannot tolerate co-trimoxazole, or who have not responded to it. Pentamidine isetionate is a potentially toxic drug that can cause severe hypotension during or immediately after infusion.

Corticosteroid treatment can be lifesaving in those with severe pneumocystis pneumonia.

Adjunctive therapy
In moderate to severe infections associated with HIV infection, prednisolone p. 664 is given by mouth for 5 days (alternatively, hydrocortisone p. 662 may be given parenterally); the dose is then reduced to complete 21 days of treatment. Corticosteroid treatment should ideally be started at the same time as the anti-pneumocystis therapy and certainly no later than 24–72 hours afterwards. The corticosteroid should be withdrawn before anti-pneumocystis treatment is complete.

Prophylaxis
Prophylaxis against pneumocystis pneumonia should be given to all patients with a history of the infection. Prophylaxis against pneumocystis pneumonia should also be considered for severely immunocompromised patients. Prophylaxis should continue until immunity recovers sufficiently. It should not be discontinued if the patient has oral candidiasis, continues to lose weight, or is receiving cytotoxic therapy or long-term immunosuppressant therapy.

Co-trimoxazole by mouth is the drug of choice for prophylaxis against pneumocystis pneumonia. It is given daily or on alternate days (3 times a week); the dose may be reduced to improve tolerance.

Inhaled pentamidine isetionate is better tolerated than parenteral pentamidine isetionate. Intermittent inhalation of pentamidine isetionate is used for prophylaxis against pneumocystis pneumonia in patients unable to tolerate co-trimoxazole. It is effective but patients may be prone to extrapulmonary infection. Alternatively, dapsone can be used. Atovaquone has also been used for prophylaxis [unlicensed indication].

ANTIPROTOZOALS

Atovaquone

● **INDICATIONS AND DOSE**

Treatment of mild to moderate *Pneumocystis jirovecii* (*Pneumocystis carinii*) **pneumonia in patients intolerant of co-trimoxazole**
▶ BY MOUTH
▸ Adult: 750 mg twice daily for 21 days, dose to be taken with food, particularly high fat food

Prophylaxis against pneumocystis pneumonia
▶ BY MOUTH
▸ Adult: 750 mg twice daily

● UNLICENSED USE Not licensed for prophylaxis against pneumocystis pneumonia.
● CAUTIONS Other causes of pulmonary disease should be sought and treated · elderly · initial diarrhoea and difficulty in taking with food may reduce absorption (and require alternative therapy)
● INTERACTIONS → Appendix 1: antimalarials

● SIDE-EFFECTS
▶ **Common or very common** Anaemia · angioedema · bronchospasm · diarrhoea · headache · hypersensitivity · hyponatraemia · insomnia · nausea · neutropenia · skin reactions · throat tightness · vomiting
▶ **Frequency not known** Stevens-Johnson syndrome
● PREGNANCY Manufacturer advises avoid unless potential benefit outweighs risk—no information available.
● BREAST FEEDING Manufacturer advises avoid.
● HEPATIC IMPAIRMENT Manufacturer advises caution. **Monitoring** Monitor more closely in hepatic impairment.
● RENAL IMPAIRMENT Manufacturer advises caution. **Monitoring** Monitor more closely in renal impairment.
● PRESCRIBING AND DISPENSING INFORMATION Flavours of oral liquid formulations may include tutti-frutti.

● MEDICINAL FORMS
There can be variation in the licensing of different medicines containing the same drug.
Oral suspension
CAUTIONARY AND ADVISORY LABELS 21
▸ Wellvone (GlaxoSmithKline UK Ltd)
Atovaquone 150 mg per 1 ml Wellvone 750mg/5ml oral suspension sugar-free | 226 ml [PoM] £486.37

Pentamidine isetionate

● **INDICATIONS AND DOSE**

Treatment of *Pneumocystis jirovecii* (*Pneumocystis carinii*) **pneumonia (specialist use only)**
▶ BY INTRAVENOUS INFUSION
▸ Adult: 4 mg/kg once daily for at least 14 days

Prophylaxis of *Pneumocystis jirovecii* (*Pneumocystis carinii*) **pneumonia (specialist use only)**
▶ BY INHALATION OF NEBULISED SOLUTION
▸ Adult: 300 mg every 4 weeks, alternatively 150 mg every 2 weeks, using suitable equipment—consult product literature

Visceral leishmaniasis (specialist use only)
▶ BY DEEP INTRAMUSCULAR INJECTION
▸ Adult: 3–4 mg/kg once daily on alternate days, maximum total of 10 injections, course may be repeated if necessary

Cutaneous leishmaniasis (specialist use only)
▶ BY DEEP INTRAMUSCULAR INJECTION
▸ Adult: 3–4 mg/kg 1–2 times a week until condition resolves

Trypanosomiasis (specialist use only)
▶ BY DEEP INTRAMUSCULAR INJECTION, OR BY INTRAVENOUS INFUSION
▸ Adult: 4 mg/kg once daily or on alternate days for a total of 7–10 injections

● UNLICENSED USE Not licensed for primary prevention of *Pneumocystis jirovecii* (*Pneumocystis carinii*) pneumonia by inhalation of nebulised solution.
● CAUTIONS Anaemia · bradycardia · coronary heart disease · history of ventricular arrhythmias · hyperglycaemia · hypertension · hypoglycaemia · hypokalaemia · hypomagnesaemia · hypotension · leucopenia · risk of severe hypotension following administration · thrombocytopenia
● INTERACTIONS → Appendix 1: pentamidine
● SIDE-EFFECTS
GENERAL SIDE-EFFECTS
▶ **Common or very common** Dizziness · hypoglycaemia (can be severe and sometimes fatal) · hypotension (can be severe and sometimes fatal) · local reaction · nausea · rash · taste altered
▶ **Rare or very rare** QT interval prolongation

5

Infection

▸ **Frequency not known** Pancreatitis acute (can be severe and sometimes fatal)

SPECIFIC SIDE-EFFECTS

▸ **Common or very common**

▸ When used by inhalation Cough · dyspnoea · respiratory disorders

▸ With parenteral use Acute kidney injury · anaemia · azotaemia · electrolyte imbalance · flushing · haematuria · hyperglycaemia · leucopenia · localised pain · myopathy · syncope · thrombocytopenia · vomiting

▸ **Rare or very rare**

▸ With parenteral use Arrhythmia (can be severe and sometimes fatal) · pancreatitis (can be severe and sometimes fatal)

▸ **Frequency not known**

▸ When used by inhalation Angioedema · appetite decreased · bradycardia · fatigue · renal failure

▸ With parenteral use Arrhythmias · perioral hypoaesthesia · sensation abnormal · Stevens-Johnson syndrome

● PREGNANCY Manufacturer advises avoid unless essential.

● BREAST FEEDING Manufacturer advises avoid unless essential—no information available.

● HEPATIC IMPAIRMENT Manufacturer advises caution.

● RENAL IMPAIRMENT
Dose adjustments Reduce intravenous dose for pneumocystis pneumonia if creatinine clearance less than 10 mL/minute: in *life-threatening infection*, use 4 mg/kg once daily for 7–10 days, then 4 mg/kg on alternate days to complete course of at least 14 doses; in *less severe infection*, use 4 mg/kg on alternate days for at least 14 doses.

● MONITORING REQUIREMENTS

▸ Monitor blood pressure before starting treatment, during administration, and at regular intervals, until treatment concluded.

▸ Carry out laboratory monitoring according to product literature.

● DIRECTIONS FOR ADMINISTRATION Patient should be lying down when receiving drug parenterally. Direct intravenous injection should be avoided whenever possible and **never** given rapidly; intramuscular injections should be deep and preferably given into the buttock. For *intravenous infusion*, reconstitute 300 mg with 3–5 mL Water for Injections (displacement value may be significant), then dilute required dose with 50–250 mL Glucose 5% *or* Sodium Chloride 0.9%; give over at least 60 minutes.
Powder for injection (dissolved in water for injection) may be used for nebulisation.

● HANDLING AND STORAGE Pentamidine isetionate is toxic and personnel should be adequately protected during handling and administration—consult product literature.

● MEDICINAL FORMS
There can be variation in the licensing of different medicines containing the same drug.
Powder for solution for injection
▸ Pentacarinat (Sanofi)
Pentamidine isetionate 300 mg Pentacarinat 300mg powder for solution for injection vials | 5 vial [PoM] £158.86

4   Helminth infection

Helminth infections

Specialist centres

Advice on prophylaxis and treatment of helminth infections is available from the following specialist centres:

Birmingham	(0121) 424 0357
Scotland	Contact local Infectious Diseases Unit
Liverpool	(0151) 705 3100
London	0845 155 5000 (treatment)

Threadworms

Anthelmintics are effective in threadworm (pinworms, *Enterobius vermicularis*) infections, but their use needs to be combined with hygienic measures to break the cycle of auto-infection. All members of the family require treatment.

Adult threadworms do not live for longer than 6 weeks and for development of fresh worms, ova must be swallowed and exposed to the action of digestive juices in the upper intestinal tract. Direct multiplication of worms does not take place in the large bowel. Adult female worms lay ova on the perianal skin which causes pruritus; scratching the area then leads to ova being transmitted on fingers to the mouth, often via food eaten with unwashed hands. Washing hands and scrubbing nails before each meal and after each visit to the toilet is essential. A bath taken immediately after rising will remove ova laid during the night.

Mebendazole p. 594 is the drug of choice for treating threadworm infection in patients of all ages over 6 months. It is given as a single dose; as reinfection is very common, a second dose may be given after 2 weeks.

Ascaricides (common roundworm infections)

Mebendazole is effective against *Ascaris lumbricoides* and is generally considered to be the drug of choice.

Levamisole p. 594 [unlicensed] (available from 'special-order' manufacturers or specialist importing companies) is an alternative when mebendazole cannot be used. It is very well tolerated.

Tapeworm infections

Taenicides

Niclosamide [unlicensed] (available from 'special-order' manufacturers or specialist importing companies) is the most widely used drug for tapeworm infections and side-effects are limited to occasional gastro-intestinal upset, lightheadedness, and pruritus; it is not effective against larval worms. Fears of developing cysticercosis in *Taenia solium* infections have proved unfounded. All the same, an antiemetic can be given before treatment and a laxative can be given 2 hours after niclosamide.

Praziquantel p. 594 [unlicensed] (available from 'special-order' manufacturers or specialist importing companies) is as effective as niclosamide.

Hydatid disease

Cysts caused by *Echinococcus granulosus* grow slowly and asymptomatic patients do not always require treatment. Surgical treatment remains the method of choice in many situations. Albendazole p. 593 [unlicensed] (available from 'special-order' manufacturers or specialist importing companies) is used in conjunction with surgery to reduce the risk of recurrence or as primary treatment in inoperable cases. Alveolar echinococcosis due to *E. multilocularis* is usually fatal if untreated. Surgical removal with albendazole cover is the treatment of choice, but where effective surgery is impossible, repeated cycles of albendazole (for a year or more) may help. Careful monitoring of liver function is particularly important during drug treatment.

Hookworms

Hookworms (ancylostomiasis, necatoriasis) live in the upper small intestine and draw blood from the point of their attachment to their host. An iron-deficiency anaemia may occur and, if present, effective treatment of the infection requires not only expulsion of the worms but treatment of the anaemia.

Mebendazole has a useful broad-spectrum activity, and is effective against hookworms. Albendazole [unlicensed] (available from 'special-order' manufacturers or specialist importing companies) is an alternative. Levamisole is also is also effective in children.

Schistosomicides (bilharziasis)

Adult *Schistosoma haematobium* worms live in the genito-urinary veins and adult *S. mansoni* in those of the colon and mesentery. *S. japonicum* is more widely distributed in veins of the alimentary tract and portal system.

Praziquantel [unlicensed] is available from Merck Serono (*Cysticide®*) and is effective against all human schistosomes. No serious adverse effects have been reported. Of all the available schistosomicides, it has the most attractive combination of effectiveness, broad-spectrum activity, and low toxicity.

Filaricides

Diethylcarbamazine [unlicensed] (available from 'special-order' manufacturers or specialist importing companies) is effective against microfilariae and adults of *Loa loa*, *Wuchereria bancrofti*, and *Brugia malayi*. To minimise reactions, treatment in adults and children over 1 month, is commenced with a dose of diethylcarbamazine citrate on the first day and increased gradually over 3 days. Length of treatment varies according to infection type, and usually gives a radical cure for these infections. Close medical supervision is necessary particularly in the early phase of treatment.

In heavy infections there may be a febrile reaction, and in heavy *Loa loa* infection there is a small risk of encephalopathy. In such cases specialist advice should be sought, and treatment must be given under careful in-patient supervision and stopped at the first sign of cerebral involvement.

Ivermectin below [unlicensed] (available from 'special-order' manufacturers or specialist importing companies) is very effective in *onchocerciasis* and it is now the drug of choice; reactions are usually slight. Diethylcarbamazine or suramin should no longer be used for *onchocerciasis* because of their toxicity.

Cutaneous larva migrans (creeping eruption)

Dog and cat hookworm larvae may enter human skin where they produce slowly extending itching tracks usually on the foot. Single tracks can be treated with topical tiabendazole (no commercial preparation available). Multiple infections respond to ivermectin, albendazole or **tiabendazole** (thiabendazole) by mouth [all unlicensed] (available from 'special-order' manufacturers or specialist importing companies).

Strongyloidiasis

Adult *Strongyloides stercoralis* live in the gut and produce larvae which penetrate the gut wall and invade the tissues, setting up a cycle of auto-infection. Ivermectin [unlicensed] (available from 'special-order' manufacturers or specialist importing companies) is the treatment of choice for chronic *Strongyloides* infection in adults and children over 5 years. Albendazole [unlicensed] (available from 'special order' manufacturers or specialist importing companies) is an alternative given to adults and children over 2 years.

ANTHELMINTICS

Albendazole

● **INDICATIONS AND DOSE**

Chronic *Strongyloides* infection
▸ BY MOUTH
  ▸ Adult: 400 mg twice daily for 3 days, dose may be repeated after 3 weeks if necessary

Hydatid disease, in conjunction with surgery to reduce the risk of recurrence or as primary treatment in inoperable cases
▸ BY MOUTH
  ▸ Adult: (consult product literature)

Hookworm infections
▸ BY MOUTH
  ▸ Adult: 400 mg for 1 dose

● UNLICENSED USE Albendazole is an unlicensed drug.

● INTERACTIONS → Appendix 1: albendazole

● MEDICINAL FORMS
There can be variation in the licensing of different medicines containing the same drug. Forms available from special-order manufacturers include: tablet, chewable tablet, oral suspension

Tablet
CAUTIONARY AND ADVISORY LABELS 9
▸ Eskazole (Imported (France))
  Albendazole 400 mg Eskazole 400mg tablets | 60 tablet PoM Ⓢ
Chewable tablet
CAUTIONARY AND ADVISORY LABELS 9
▸ Zentel (Imported)
  Albendazole 200 mg Zentel 200mg chewable tablets | 6 tablet PoM Ⓢ
  Albendazole 400 mg Zentel 400mg chewable tablets | 1 tablet PoM Ⓢ

Diethylcarbamazine

● **INDICATIONS AND DOSE**

***Wuchereria bancrofti* infections | *Brugia malayi* infections**
▸ BY MOUTH
  ▸ Adult: Initially 1 mg/kg daily on the first day, then increased to 6 mg/kg daily in divided doses, dose to be increased gradually over 3 days

***Loa loa* infections**
▸ BY MOUTH
  ▸ Adult: Initially 1 mg/kg daily on the first day, then increased to 6 mg/kg daily in divided doses, dose to be increased gradually over 3 days; maximum 9 mg/kg per day

● UNLICENSED USE Diethylcarbamazine is an unlicensed drug.

● MEDICINAL FORMS
No licensed medicines listed.

Ivermectin

17-May-2017

● **INDICATIONS AND DOSE**

Chronic *Strongyloides* infection
▸ BY MOUTH
  ▸ Adult: 200 micrograms/kg daily for 2 days

Onchocerciasis
▸ BY MOUTH
  ▸ Adult: 150 micrograms/kg for 1 dose, retreatment at intervals of 6 to 12 months, depending on symptoms, must be given until the adult worms die out continued →

5

Infection

Scabies, in combination with topical drugs, for the treatment of hyperkeratotic (crusted or 'Norwegian') scabies that does not respond to topical treatment alone
▶ BY MOUTH
▶ Adult: 200 micrograms/kg for 1 dose, further doses of 200 micrograms/kg may be required

● UNLICENSED USE Ivermectin is unlicensed.
● INTERACTIONS → Appendix 1: ivermectin
● SIDE-EFFECTS
▶ **Common or very common** Skin reactions (frequency not known in children)

● MEDICINAL FORMS
There can be variation in the licensing of different medicines containing the same drug. Forms available from special-order manufacturers include: tablet
Tablet
▶ Stromectol (Imported (France))
Ivermectin 3 mg Stromectol 3mg tablets | 4 tablet [PoM] [◻]

Levamisole

● INDICATIONS AND DOSE
Roundworm infections
▶ BY MOUTH
▶ Adult: 120–150 mg for 1 dose

● UNLICENSED USE Not licensed.
● CONTRA-INDICATIONS Blood disorders
● CAUTIONS Epilepsy · Sjögren's syndrome
● INTERACTIONS → Appendix 1: levamisole
● SIDE-EFFECTS Arthralgia (long term use) · blood disorder (long term use) · diarrhoea · dizziness · headache · influenza like illness (long term use) · insomnia (long term use) · myalgia (long term use) · nausea · rash (long term use) · seizure (long term use) · taste altered (long term use) · vasculitis (long term use) · vomiting
● PREGNANCY Embryotoxic in *animal* studies, avoid if possible.
● BREAST FEEDING No information available.
● HEPATIC IMPAIRMENT
Dose adjustments Use with caution—dose adjustment may be necessary.

● MEDICINAL FORMS
There can be variation in the licensing of different medicines containing the same drug. Forms available from special-order manufacturers include: tablet
Tablet
CAUTIONARY AND ADVISORY LABELS 4
▶ Ergamisol (Imported (Belgium))
Levamisole (as Levamisole hydrochloride) 50 mg Ergamisol 50mg tablets | 20 tablet [PoM] [◻]

Mebendazole

● INDICATIONS AND DOSE
Threadworm infections
▶ BY MOUTH
▶ Child 6 months–17 years: 100 mg for 1 dose, if reinfection occurs, second dose may be needed after 2 weeks
▶ Adult: 100 mg for 1 dose, if reinfection occurs, second dose may be needed after 2 weeks

Whipworm infections | Hookworm infections
▶ BY MOUTH
▶ Child 1–17 years: 100 mg twice daily for 3 days
▶ Adult: 100 mg twice daily for 3 days

Roundworm infections
▶ BY MOUTH
▶ Child 1 year: 100 mg twice daily for 3 days
▶ Child 2–17 years: 100 mg twice daily for 3 days, alternatively 500 mg for 1 dose
▶ Adult: 100 mg twice daily for 3 days, alternatively 500 mg for 1 dose

● UNLICENSED USE Not licensed for use as a single dose of 500 mg in roundworm infections. Not licensed for use in children under 2 years.
● INTERACTIONS → Appendix 1: mebendazole
● SIDE-EFFECTS
▶ **Common or very common** Gastrointestinal discomfort
▶ **Uncommon** Diarrhoea · flatulence
▶ **Rare or very rare** Alopecia · dizziness · hepatitis · neutropenia · seizure · severe cutaneous adverse reactions (SCARs) · skin reactions
● PREGNANCY Manufacturer advises avoid—toxicity in *animal* studies.
● BREAST FEEDING Amount present in milk too small to be harmful but manufacturer advises avoid.
● PRESCRIBING AND DISPENSING INFORMATION Flavours of oral liquid formulations may include banana.
● PATIENT AND CARER ADVICE
Medicines for Children leaflet: Mebendazole for worm infections www.medicinesforchildren.org.uk/mebendazole-for-worm-infections
● EXCEPTIONS TO LEGAL CATEGORY Mebendazole tablets can be sold to the public if supplied for oral use in the treatment of enterobiasis in adults and children over 2 years provided its container or package is labelled to show a max. single dose of 100 mg and it is supplied in a container or package containing not more than 800 mg.

● MEDICINAL FORMS
There can be variation in the licensing of different medicines containing the same drug.
Oral suspension
▶ Ovex (McNeil Products Ltd)
Mebendazole 20 mg per 1 ml Ovex 100mg/5ml oral suspension | 30 ml [P] £6.74 DT = £1.55
▶ Vermox (Janssen-Cilag Ltd)
Mebendazole 20 mg per 1 ml Vermox 100mg/5ml oral suspension | 30 ml [PoM] £1.55 DT = £1.55
Chewable tablet
▶ Ovex (McNeil Products Ltd)
Mebendazole 100 mg Ovex 100mg chewable tablets sugar-free | 1 tablet [P] £2.37 sugar-free | 4 tablet [P] £5.55
▶ Vermox (Janssen-Cilag Ltd)
Mebendazole 100 mg Vermox 100mg chewable tablets sugar-free | 6 tablet [PoM] £1.34 DT = £1.34

Praziquantel

● INDICATIONS AND DOSE
Tapeworm infections (*Taenia solium*)
▶ BY MOUTH
▶ Adult: 5–10 mg/kg for 1 dose, to be taken after a light breakfast

Tapeworm infections (*Hymenolepis nana*)
▶ BY MOUTH
▶ Adult: 25 mg/kg for 1 dose, to be taken after a light breakfast

***Schistosoma haematobium* worm infections | *Schistosoma mansoni* worm infections**
▶ BY MOUTH
▶ Adult: 20 mg/kg, followed by 20 mg/kg after 4–6 hours

***Schistosoma japonicum* worm infections**
▶ BY MOUTH
▶ Adult: 20 mg/kg 3 times a day for 1 day

- UNLICENSED USE Praziquantel is an unlicensed drug.
- INTERACTIONS → Appendix 1: praziquantel

- MEDICINAL FORMS
  There can be variation in the licensing of different medicines containing the same drug. Forms available from special-order manufacturers include: tablet

Tablet
▶ Cesol (Imported (Germany))
  Praziquantel 150 mg Praziquantel 150mg tablets | 6 tablet PoM Ⓢ
▶ Biltricide (Imported (Germany))
  Praziquantel 600 mg Praziquantel 600mg tablets | 6 tablet PoM Ⓢ
▶ Cysticide (Imported (Germany))
  Praziquantel 500 mg Cysticide 500mg tablets | 90 tablet PoM Ⓢ

5   Protozoal infection

Antiprotozoal drugs

Amoebicides

Metronidazole p. 533 is the drug of choice for *acute invasive amoebic dysentery* since it is very effective against vegetative forms of *Entamoeba histolytica* in ulcers. Tinidazole p. 534 is also effective. Metronidazole and tinidazole are also active against amoebae which may have migrated to the liver. Treatment with metronidazole (or tinidazole) is followed by a 10-day course of diloxanide furoate p. 498.

Diloxanide furoate is the drug of choice for asymptomatic patients with *E. histolytica* cysts in the faeces; metronidazole and tinidazole are relatively ineffective. Diloxanide furoate is relatively free from toxic effects and the usual course is of 10 days, given alone for chronic infections or following metronidazole or tinidazole treatment.

For *amoebic abscesses* of the liver metronidazole is effective; tinidazole is an alternative. Aspiration of the abscess is indicated where it is suspected that it may rupture or where there is no improvement after 72 hours of metronidazole; the aspiration may need to be repeated. Aspiration aids penetration of metronidazole and, for abscesses with more than 100 mL of pus, if carried out in conjunction with drug therapy, may reduce the period of disability.

Diloxanide furoate is not effective against hepatic amoebiasis, but a 10-day course should be given at the completion of metronidazole or tinidazole treatment to destroy any amoebae in the gut.

Trichomonacides

Metronidazole is the treatment of choice for *Trichomonas vaginalis* infection. Contact tracing is recommended and sexual contacts should be treated simultaneously. If metronidazole is ineffective, tinidazole may be tried.

Antigiardial drugs

Metronidazole is the treatment of choice for *Giardia lamblia* infections. Alternative treatments are tinidazole or mepacrine hydrochloride p. 498.

Leishmaniacides

Cutaneous leishmaniasis frequently heals spontaneously but if skin lesions are extensive or unsightly, treatment is indicated, as it is in visceral leishmaniasis (kala-azar). Leishmaniasis should be treated under specialist supervision.

Sodium stibogluconate below, an organic pentavalent antimony compound, is used for visceral leishmaniasis. The dosage varies with different geographical regions and expert advice should be obtained. Some early non-inflamed lesions of cutaneous leishmaniasis can be treated with intralesional injections of sodium stibogluconate under specialist supervision.

Amphotericin p. 583 is used with or after an antimony compound for visceral leishmaniasis unresponsive to the antimonial alone; side-effects may be reduced by using liposomal amphotericin (*AmBisome®*). *Abelcet®*, a lipid formulation of amphotericin, is also likely to be effective but less information is available.

Pentamidine isetionate p. 591 has been used in antimony-resistant visceral leishmaniasis, but although the initial response is often good, the relapse rate is high; it is associated with serious side-effects. Other treatments include paromomycin [unlicensed] (available from 'special-order' manufacturers or specialist importing companies).

Trypanocides

The prophylaxis and treatment of trypanosomiasis is difficult and differs according to the strain of organism. Expert advice should therefore be obtained.

Toxoplasmosis

Most infections caused by *Toxoplasma gondii* are self-limiting, and treatment is not necessary. Exceptions are patients with eye involvement (toxoplasma choroidoretinitis), and those who are immunosuppressed. Toxoplasmic encephalitis is a common complication of AIDS. The treatment of choice is a combination of pyrimethamine p. 609 and sulfadiazine p. 553, given for several weeks (expert advice **essential**). Pyrimethamine is a folate antagonist, and adverse reactions to this combination are relatively common (folinic acid supplements and weekly blood counts needed). Alternative regimens use combinations of pyrimethamine with clindamycin p. 526 or clarithromycin p. 529 or azithromycin p. 528. Long-term secondary prophylaxis is required after treatment of toxoplasmosis in immunocompromised patients; prophylaxis should continue until immunity recovers.

If toxoplasmosis is acquired in pregnancy, transplacental infection may lead to severe disease in the fetus; specialist advice should be sought on management. Spiramycin [unlicensed] (available from 'special-order' manufacturers or specialist importing companies) may reduce the risk of transmission of maternal infection to the fetus.

5.1   Leishmaniasis

> **Other drugs used for Leishmaniasis** Amphotericin, p. 583 · Pentamidine isetionate, p. 591

ANTIPROTOZOALS

Sodium stibogluconate

- **INDICATIONS AND DOSE**

Visceral leishmaniasis (specialist use only)
▶ BY INTRAVENOUS INJECTION, OR BY INTRAMUSCULAR INJECTION
  ▹ Adult: 20 mg/kg daily for 28 days

Cutaneous leishmaniasis (specialist use only)
▶ BY INTRAVENOUS INJECTION, OR BY INTRAMUSCULAR INJECTION
  ▹ Adult: 20 mg/kg daily for 20 days

- CAUTIONS Heart disease (withdraw if conduction disturbances occur) · mucocutaneous disease · predisposition to QT interval prolongation · treat intercurrent infection (e.g. pneumonia)

CAUTIONS, FURTHER INFORMATION
▶ Mucocutaneous disease Successful treatment of mucocutaneous leishmaniasis may induce severe

5

Infection

Infection

5

inflammation around the lesions (may be life-threatening if pharyngeal or tracheal involvement)—may require corticosteroid.

● INTERACTIONS → Appendix 1: sodium stibogluconate

● SIDE-EFFECTS
▸ **Common or very common** Abdominal pain · appetite decreased · arthralgia · diarrhoea · headache · lethargy · malaise · myalgia · nausea · vomiting
▸ **Rare or very rare** Chest pain · chills · fever · flushing · haemorrhage · hyperhidrosis · jaundice · skin reactions · vertigo
▸ **Frequency not known** Arrhythmias · cough · pain · pancreatitis · pneumonia · QT interval prolongation · thrombosis

● PREGNANCY Manufacturer advises use only if potential benefit outweighs risk.

● BREAST FEEDING Amount probably too small to be harmful.

● HEPATIC IMPAIRMENT Use with caution.

● RENAL IMPAIRMENT Avoid in significant impairment.

● MONITORING REQUIREMENTS Monitor ECG before and during treatment.

● DIRECTIONS FOR ADMINISTRATION Intravenous injections must be given slowly over 5 minutes (to reduce risk of local thrombosis) and stopped if coughing or substernal pain occur. Injection should be filtered immediately before administration using a filter of 5 microns or less.

● MEDICINAL FORMS
There can be variation in the licensing of different medicines containing the same drug.
Solution for injection
▸ Pentostam (GlaxoSmithKline UK Ltd)
Antimony pentavalent (as Sodium stibogluconate) 100 mg per 1 ml Pentostam 10g/100ml solution for injection vials | 1 vial [PoM] £66.43

5.2 Malaria

Antimalarials

23-Jan-2018

Artemether with lumefantrine

Artemether with lumefantrine p. 603 is licensed for the *treatment of acute non-complicated falciparum malaria*.

Chloroquine

Chloroquine p. 604 is used for the *prophylaxis of malaria* in areas of the world where the *risk of chloroquine-resistant falciparum malaria is still low*. It is also used with proguanil hydrochloride p. 607 when chloroquine-resistant falciparum malaria is present but this regimen may not give optimal protection (for details, see Recommended regimens for prophylaxis against malaria p. 598).

Guidelines for malaria prevention in travellers from the United Kingdom (2017) published by Public Health England state that patients already taking hydroxychloroquine sulfate p. 1062 for another indication, and for whom chloroquine would be an appropriate antimalarial, can remain on hydroxychloroquine sulfate.

Chloroquine is **no longer recommended** for the *treatment of falciparum malaria* owing to widespread resistance, nor is it recommended if the infective species is *not known* or if the infection is *mixed*; in these cases treatment should be with quinine p. 608, *Malarone®*, or *Riamet®*. It is still recommended for the *treatment of non-falciparum malaria*.

Mefloquine

Mefloquine p. 606 is used for the *prophylaxis of malaria* in areas of the world where there is a *high risk of chloroquine-*

resistant falciparum malaria (for details, see Recommended regimens for prophylaxis against malaria p. 598).

Mefloquine is now rarely used for the *treatment of falciparum malaria* because of increased resistance. It is rarely used for the *treatment of non-falciparum malaria* because better tolerated alternatives are available. Mefloquine should not be used for treatment if it has been used for prophylaxis.

Piperaquine with artenimol

Artenimol with piperaquine phosphate p. 603 is not recommended for the first-line treatment of acute uncomplicated falciparum malaria because there is limited experience of its use in travellers who usually reside in areas where malaria is not endemic. Piperaquine has a long half-life.

Primaquine

Primaquine p. 607 is used to eliminate the liver stages of *P. vivax* or *P. ovale* following chloroquine treatment.

Proguanil

Proguanil hydrochloride is used (usually *with chloroquine*, but occasionally *alone*) for the *prophylaxis of malaria*, (for details, see Recommended regimens for prophylaxis against malaria p. 598).

Proguanil hydrochloride used alone is not suitable for the *treatment of malaria*; however, *Malarone®* (a combination of atovaquone with proguanil hydrochloride p. 604) is licensed for the treatment of acute uncomplicated falciparum malaria. *Malarone®* is also used for the *prophylaxis of falciparum malaria* in areas of *widespread mefloquine or chloroquine resistance*. *Malarone®* is also used as an alternative to mefloquine or doxycycline p. 555. *Malarone®* is particularly suitable for short trips to highly chloroquine-resistant areas because it needs to be taken only for 7 days after leaving an endemic area.

Pyrimethamine

Pyrimethamine p. 609 should not be used alone, but is used with sulfadoxine.

Pyrimethamine with sulfadoxine is not recommended for the *prophylaxis of malaria*, but can be used in the *treatment of falciparum malaria with (or following) quinine*.

Quinine

Quinine is not suitable for the *prophylaxis of malaria*.

Quinine is used for the *treatment of falciparum malaria* or if the infective species is *not known* or if the infection is mixed (for details see Malaria, treatment p. 602).

Tetracyclines

Doxycycline is used in adults and children over 12 years for the *prophylaxis of malaria* in areas of *widespread mefloquine* or *chloroquine resistance*. Doxycycline is also used as an alternative to mefloquine or *Malarone®* (for details, see Recommended regimens for prophylaxis against malaria p. 598).

Malaria, prophylaxis

23-Jan-2018

Prophylaxis against malaria

The recommendations on prophylaxis reflect guidelines agreed by UK malaria specialists, published in the Public Health England Guidelines for malaria prevention in travellers from the United Kingdom, 2017. The advice is aimed at residents of the UK who travel to endemic areas.

For specialist centres offering advice on specific malaria-related problems, see Malaria, treatment p. 602. The choice of drug for a particular individual should take into account:

- risk of exposure to malaria
- extent of drug resistance
- efficacy of the recommended drugs
- side-effects of the drugs
- patient-related factors (e.g. age, pregnancy, renal or hepatic impairment, compliance with prophylactic regimen)

For more information on choice of drug, see also Antimalarials p. 596.

Protection against bites

Prophylaxis is not absolute, and breakthrough infection can occur with any of the drugs recommended. Personal protection against being bitten is very important and is recommended even in malaria-free areas as a preventive measure against other insect vector-borne diseases. Mosquito nets impregnated with permethrin p. 1203 provide the most effective barrier protection against insects; mats and vaporised insecticides are also useful. Diethyltoluamide (DEET) 20–50% (available as sprays, and modified-release polymer formulations) is safe and effective when applied to the skin of adults and children over 2 months of age. It can also be used during pregnancy and breast-feeding. However, ingestion should be avoided, therefore breast-feeding mothers should wash their hands and breast tissue before handling infants. The duration of protection varies according to the concentration of DEET and is longest for DEET 50%. When sunscreen is also required, DEET should be applied after the sunscreen. DEET reduces the SPF of sunscreen, so a sunscreen of SPF 30–50 should be applied. Long sleeves and trousers worn after dusk also provide protection against bites.

Length of prophylaxis

In order to determine tolerance and to establish habit, prophylaxis should generally be started one week (2–3 weeks in the case of mefloquine p. 606) before travel into an endemic area; *Malarone*® or doxycycline p. 555 prophylaxis should be started 1–2 days before travel. Prophylaxis should be continued for **4 weeks after leaving** (except for *Malarone*® prophylaxis which should be stopped 1 week after leaving). For extensive journeys across different regions, the traveller must be protected in all areas of risk.

In those requiring long-term prophylaxis, chloroquine p. 604 and proguanil hydrochloride p. 607 may be used. However there is considerable concern over the protective efficacy of the combination of chloroquine and proguanil hydrochloride in certain areas where it was previously useful. Mefloquine is licensed for up to 1 year (although, if it is tolerated in the short term, there is no evidence of harm when it is used for up to 3 years). Doxycycline can be used for up to 2 years. *Malarone*® can be used for up to 1 year. Prophylaxis with mefloquine, doxycycline, or *Malarone*® may be considered for longer durations if it is justified by the risk of exposure to malaria. Specialist advice should be sought for long-term prophylaxis.

Return from malarial region

It is important to be aware that **any illness** that occurs within 1 year and **especially within 3 months of return might be malaria** even if all recommended precautions against malaria were taken. Travellers should be **warned** of this and told that if they develop any illness **particularly within 3 months** of their return they should go **immediately** to a doctor and specifically mention their exposure to malaria.

Epilepsy

Both chloroquine and mefloquine are unsuitable for malaria prophylaxis in individuals with a history of epilepsy. In areas *without chloroquine resistance* proguanil hydrochloride alone is recommended; in areas *with chloroquine resistance*, doxycycline or *Malarone*® may be considered.

Asplenia

Asplenic individuals (or those with severe splenic dysfunction) are at particular risk of severe malaria. If travel to malarious areas is unavoidable, rigorous precautions are required against contracting the disease.

Pregnancy

Travel to malarious areas should be avoided during pregnancy; if travel is unavoidable, effective prophylaxis must be used. Chloroquine and proguanil hydrochloride can be given in the usual doses during pregnancy, but these drugs are not appropriate for most areas because their effectiveness has declined, particularly in Sub-Saharan Africa; in the case of proguanil hydrochloride, folic acid p. 993 (dosed as a pregnancy at 'high-risk' of neural tube defects) should be given for at least the first trimester. The centres listed (see Malaria, treatment p. 602) should be consulted for advice on prophylaxis in chloroquine-resistant areas. Although the manufacturer advises that mefloquine should not be used during pregnancy, particularly in the first trimester, unless the potential benefit outweighs the risk, studies of mefloquine in pregnancy (including use in the first trimester) indicate that it can be considered for travel to chloroquine-resistant areas. Doxycycline is contra-indicated during pregnancy; however, it can be used for malaria prophylaxis if other regimens are unsuitable, and if the entire course of doxycycline can be completed before 15 weeks' gestation [unlicensed]. *Malarone*® should be avoided during pregnancy, however, it can be considered during the second and third trimesters if there is no suitable alternative.

Breast-feeding

Prophylaxis is required in **breast-fed infants**; although antimalarials are present in milk, the amounts are too variable to give reliable protection.

Anticoagulants

Travellers taking warfarin sodium p. 139 should begin chemoprophylaxis 2–3 weeks before departure. The INR should be stable before departure. It should be measured before starting chemoprophylaxis, 7 days after starting, and after completing the course. For prolonged stays, the INR should be checked at regular intervals.

Standby treatment

Travellers visiting remote, malarious areas for prolonged periods should carry standby treatment if they are likely to be more than 24 hours away from medical care. Self-medication should be **avoided** if medical help is accessible.

In order to avoid excessive self-medication, the traveller should be provided with **written instructions** that urgent medical attention should be sought if fever (38°C or more) develops 7 days (or more) after arriving in a malarious area and that self-treatment is indicated if medical help is not available within 24 hours of fever onset.

In view of the continuing emergence of resistant strains and of the different regimens required for different areas expert advice should be sought on the best treatment course for an individual traveller. A drug used for chemoprophylaxis should not be considered for standby treatment for the same traveller.

Malaria prophylaxis, specific recommendations

Where a journey requires two regimens, the regimen for the higher risk area should be used for the whole journey. Those travelling to remote or little-visited areas may require expert advice. See *Recommended regimens for prophylaxis against malaria*.

Important

Settled immigrants (or long-term visitors) to the UK may be unaware that **any immunity they may have acquired while living in malarious areas is lost rapidly** after migration to

Key to recommended regimens for prophylaxis against malaria

Codes for regimens	Details of regimens for prophylaxis against malaria
-	No risk
1	Chemoprophylaxis not recommended, but avoid mosquito bites and consider malaria if fever presents
2	Chloroquine only
3	Chloroquine with proguanil
4	Atovaquone with proguanil hydrochloride or doxycycline or mefloquine

Specific recommendations

Country	Comments on risk of malaria and regional or seasonal variation	Codes for regimens
Afghanistan	Low risk below 2000 m from May–November	1
	Very low risk below 2000 m from December–April	1
Algeria	Very low risk in remote focus in Illizi department only	1
Andaman and Nicobar Islands (India)	Low risk	1
Angola	High risk	4
Argentina	Very low risk in low altitude areas of Salta provinces bordering Bolivia and in Chaco, Corrientes, and Misiones provinces close to border with Paraguay and Brazil	1
	No risk in Iguaçu Falls and areas other than those above	-
Armenia	No risk	1
Azerbaijan	Very low risk	1
Bangladesh	High risk in Chittagong Hill Tract districts (but not Chittagong city)	4
	Very low risk in Chittagong city and other areas, except Chittagong Hill Tract districts	1
Belize	Low risk in rural areas	1
	No risk in Belize district (including Belize city and islands)	-
Benin	High risk	4
Bhutan	Low risk in southern belt districts, along border with India: Chukha, Geyleg-phug, Samchi, Samdrup Jonkhar, and Shemgang	1
	No risk in areas other than those above	-
Bolivia	Low risk in Amazon basin	1
	Low risk in rural areas below 2500 m (other than above)	1
	No risk above 2500 m	-
Botswana	High risk from November–June in northern half, including Okavango Delta area	4
	Low risk from July–October in northern half	1
	Very low risk in southern half	1
Brazil	Low risk in Amazon basin, including city of Manaus	1
	Very low risk in areas other than those above	1
	No risk in Iguaçu Falls	-
Brunei Darussalam	Very low risk	1
Burkina Faso	High risk	4
Burundi	High risk	4
Cambodia	Low risk. Mefloquine resistance widespread in western provinces bordering Thailand	1
	Very low risk in Angkor Wat and Lake Tonle Sap, including Siem Reap	1
	No risk in Phnom Penh	-
Cameroon	High risk	4
Cape Verde	Very low risk on island of Santiago (Sao Tiago) and Boa Vista	1
Central African Republic	High risk	4
Chad	High risk	4
China	Low risk in Yunnan and Hainan provinces	1
	Very low risk in southern and some central provinces, including Anhui, Ghuizhou, Hena, Hubei, and Jiangsu below 1500 m	1
	Very low risk in areas other than those above and below	1
	No risk in Hong Kong	-

Country	Comments on risk of malaria and regional or seasonal variation	Codes for regimens
Colombia	Low risk in rural areas below 1600 m	1
	Very low risk above 1600 m and in Cartagena	1
Comoros	High risk	4
Congo	High risk	4
Costa Rica	Low risk in Limon province (but not city of Limon)	1
	Very low risk in areas other than those above	1
Cote d'Ivoire (Ivory Coast)	High risk	4
Democratic Republic of the Congo	High risk	4
Djibouti	High risk	4
Dominican Republic	Low risk	1
	No risk in cities of Santiago and Santo Domingo	-
East Timor (Timor-Leste)	Risk present	4
Ecuador	Low risk in areas below 1500 m including coastal provinces and Amazon basin	1
	No risk in Galapagos islands or city of Guayaquil	-
Egypt	No risk	1
El Salvador	Low risk in rural areas of Santa Ana, Ahuachapán, and La Unión provinces in western part of country; very low risk in other areas	1
Equatorial Guinea	High risk	4
Eritrea	High risk below 2200 m	4
Ethiopia	High risk below 2000 m	4
	No risk in Addis Ababa or in areas above 2000 m	-
French Guiana	Risk present (particularly in border areas) except city of Cayenne or Devil's Island (Ile du Diable)	4
	Low risk in city of Cayenne or Devil's Island (Ile du Diable)	1
Gabon	High risk	4
Gambia	High risk	4
Georgia	Very low risk in rural south east from June–October	1
Ghana	High risk	4
Guatemala	Low risk below 1500 m	1
	No risk in Guatemala City, Antigua, or Lake Atitlan and above 1500 m	-
Guinea	High risk	4
Guinea-Bissau	High risk	4
Guyana	Risk present in all interior regions	4
	Very low risk in Georgetown and coastal region	1
Haiti	Risk present	3
Honduras	Low risk below 1000 m and in Roatán and other Bay Islands	1
	No risk in San Pedro Sula or Tegucigalpa and areas above 1000 m	-
India	Risk present in states of Assam and Orissa, districts of East Godavari, Srikakulam, Vishakhapatnam, and Vizianagaram in the state of Andhra Pradesh, and districts of Balaghat, Dindori, Mandla, and Seoni in the state of Madhya Pradesh	4
	Low risk in areas other than those above or below (including Goa, Andaman and Nicobar islands)	1
	Exceptional circumstances in low risk areas (dependent on individual risk assessment)	3
	No risk in Lakshadweep islands	-
Indonesia	High risk in Irian Jaya (Papua)	4
	Low risk in Bali, Lombok and islands of Java and Sumatra	1
	No risk in city of Jakarta	-
Indonesia (Borneo)	Low risk	1
Iran	Low risk from March–November in rural south eastern provinces and in north, along Azerbaijan border in Ardabil, and near Turkmenistan border in North Khorasan	1
	Very low risk in areas other than those above	1
Iraq	Very low risk from May–November in rural northern area below 1500 m	1
	No risk in areas other than those above	-

5

Infection

Key to recommended regimens for prophylaxis against malaria

Codes for regimens	Details of regimens for prophylaxis against malaria
-	No risk
1	Chemoprophylaxis not recommended, but avoid mosquito bites and consider malaria if fever presents
2	Chloroquine only
3	Chloroquine with proguanil
4	Atovaquone with proguanil hydrochloride or doxycycline or mefloquine

Specific recommendations

Country	Comments on risk of malaria and regional or seasonal variation	Codes for regimens
Kenya	High risk (except city of Nairobi)	4
	Very low risk in the highlands above 2500 m and in city of Nairobi	1
Lao People's Democratic Republic (Laos)	Low risk	1
	Very low risk in city of Vientiane	1
Liberia	High risk	4
Libya	No risk	1
Madagascar	High risk	4
Malawi	High risk	4
Malaysia	Low risk in mainland Malaysia	1
Malaysia (Borneo)	Low risk in inland areas of Sabah and in inland, forested areas of Sarawak	1
	Very low risk in areas other than those above, including coastal areas of Sabah and Sarawak	1
Mali	High risk	4
Mauritania	High risk all year in southern provinces, and from July–October in the northern provinces	4
	Low risk from November–June in the northern provinces	1
Mauritius	No risk	1
Mayotte	Risk present	4
Mexico	Very low risk	1
Mozambique	High risk	4
Myanmar	Low risk	1
Namibia	High risk all year in regions of Caprivi Strip, Kavango, and Kunene river, and from November–June in northern third of country	4
	Very low risk in areas other than those above; low risk from July–October in northern third of country	1
Nepal	Low risk below 1500 m, including the Terai district	1
	No risk in city of Kathmandu and on typical Himalayan treks	-
Nicaragua	Low risk (except Managua)	1
	Very low risk in Managua	1
Niger	High risk	4
Nigeria	High risk	4
North Korea	Very low risk in some southern areas	1
Pakistan	Low risk below 2000 m	1
	Very low risk above 2000 m	1
Panama	Low risk east of Canal Zone	1
	Very low risk west of Canal Zone	1
	No risk in Panama City or Canal Zone itself	-
Papua New Guinea	High risk below 1800 m	4
	Very low risk above 1800 m	1
Paraguay	Very low risk	1
Peru	Low risk in Amazon basin along border with Brazil, particularly in Loreto province and in rural areas below 2000 m including the Amazon basin bordering Bolivia	1
	No risk in city of Lima and coastal region south of Chiclayo	-

Country	Comments on risk of malaria and regional or seasonal variation	Codes for regimens
Philippines	Low risk in rural areas below 600 m and on islands of Luzon, Mindanao, Mindoro, and Palawan	1
	No risk in cities or on islands of Boracay, Bohol, Catanduanes, Cebu, or Leyte	-
Rwanda	High risk	4
São Tomé and Principe	High risk	4
Saudi Arabia	Low risk in south-western provinces along border with Yemen, including below 2000 m in Asir province	1
	No risk in cities of Jeddah, Makkah (Mecca), Medina, Riyadh, or Ta'if, or above 2000 m in Asir province	-
Senegal	High risk	4
Sierra Leone	High risk	4
Solomon Islands	High risk	4
Somalia	High risk	4
South Africa	Risk from September–May in low altitude areas of Mpumalanga and Limpopo, which border Mozambique and Zimbabwe (including Kruger National Park)	4
	Low risk in north-east KwaZulu-Natal	1
	Low risk in areas bordering those above	1
South Korea	Very low risk in northern areas, in Gangwon-do and Gyeonggi-do provinces, and Incheon city (towards Demilitarized Zone)	1
South Sudan	High risk	4
Sri Lanka	Low risk north of Vavuniya	1
	Very low risk in areas other than those above and below	1
	No risk in Colombo or Kandy	-
Sudan	High risk in central and southern areas; risk also present in rest of country (except Khartoum)	4
	Very low risk in Khartoum	1
Suriname	Risk present on the French Guiana border	4
	Low risk in areas other than above and below	1
	No risk in city of Paramaribo	-
Swaziland	Risk in northern and eastern regions bordering Mozambique and South Africa, including all of Lubombo district and Big Bend, Mhlume, Simunye, and Tshaneni regions	4
	Very low risk in the areas other than those above	1
Syria	Very low risk in small, remote foci of El Hasakah	1
Tajikistan	Very low risk	1
	No risk above 2000 m	-
Tanzania	High risk below 1800 m; risk also in Zanzibar	4
	No risk above 1800 m	-
Thailand	Mefloquine resistance present. Low risk in rural forested borders with Cambodia, Laos, and Myanmar	1
	Very low risk in areas other than those above, including Kanchanaburi (Kwai Bridge)	1
	No risk in cities of Bangkok, Chiang Mai, Chiang Rai, Koh Phangan, Koh Samui, and Pattaya	-
Togo	High risk	4
Turkey	Very low risk	1
Uganda	High risk	4
Uzbekistan	Very low risk in extreme south-east	1
Vanuatu	Risk present	4
Venezuela	Risk in all areas south of, and including, the Orinoco river and Angel Falls, rural areas of Apure, Monagas, Sucre, and Zulia states	1
	No risk in city of Caracas or on Margarita Island	-
Vietnam	Low risk in rural areas, and in southern provinces of Tay Ninh, Lam Dong, Dac Lac, Gia Lai, and Kon Tum	1
	No risk in large cities (including Ho Chi Minh City (Saigon) and Hanoi), the Red River delta, coastal areas north of Nha Trang and Phu Quoc Island	1
Western Sahara	No risk	1

5

Infection

5

Infection

Key to recommended regimens for prophylaxis against malaria

Codes for regimens	Details of regimens for prophylaxis against malaria
.	No risk
1	Chemoprophylaxis not recommended, but avoid mosquito bites and consider malaria if fever presents
2	Chloroquine only
3	Chloroquine with proguanil
4	Atovaquone with proguanil hydrochloride or doxycycline or mefloquine

Specific recommendations

Country	Comments on risk of malaria and regional or seasonal variation	Codes for regimens
Yemen	Risk below 2000 m	3
	Very low risk on Socrota Island; no risk above 2000 m, including Sana'a city	1
Zambia	High risk	4
Zimbabwe	High risk all year in Zambezi valley, and from November–June in areas below 1200 m	4
	Low risk from July–October in areas below 1200 m; very low risk all year in Harare and Bulawayo	1

the UK, or that any non-malarious areas where they lived previously **may now be malarious**.

Malaria, treatment

Advice for healthcare professionals

A number of specialist centres are able to provide advice on specific problems.

PHE (Public Health England) Malaria Reference Laboratory (020) 7637 0248 (fax) (prophylaxis only) www.malaria-reference.co.uk

National Travel Health Network and Centre 0845 602 6712

Monday and Friday: 9–11 a.m. and 1–2 p.m, Tuesday to Thursday: 9–11 a.m. and 1–3:30 p.m. https://travelhealthpro.org.uk/

Travel Medicine Team, Health Protection Scotland (registered users of Travax only) www.travax.nhs.uk (for registered users of the NHS Travax website only) (0141) 300 1100 (weekdays 2–4 p.m. only)
Birmingham (0121) 424 2358
Liverpool (0151) 705 3100
London 0845 155 5000 (treatment)
Oxford (01865) 225 430

Advice for travellers

Hospital for Tropical Diseases Travel Healthline (020) 7950 7799 www.fitfortravel.nhs.uk

WHO advice on international travel and health www.who.int/ith

National Travel Health Network and Centre (NaTHNaC) https://travelhealthpro.org.uk/

Treatment of malaria

Recommendations on the treatment of malaria reflect guidelines agreed by UK malaria specialists.

If the infective species is **not known**, or if the infection is **mixed**, initial treatment should be as for *falciparum malaria* with quinine p. 608, *Malarone*® (atovaquone with proguanil hydrochloride p. 604), or *Riamet*® (artemether with lumefantrine p. 603). Falciparum malaria can progress rapidly in unprotected individuals and antimalarial treatment should be considered in those with features of severe malaria and possible exposure, even if the initial blood tests for the organism are negative.

Falciparum malaria (treatment)

Falciparum malaria (malignant malaria) is caused by *Plasmodium falciparum*. In most parts of the world *P. falciparum* is now resistant to chloroquine p. 604 which should not therefore be given for treatment.

Quinine, *Malarone*® (atovaquone with proguanil hydrochloride), or *Riamet*® (artemether with lumefantrine) can be given *by mouth* if the patient can swallow and retain tablets and there are no serious manifestations (e.g. impaired consciousness); quinine should be given by *intravenous infusion* if the patient is seriously ill or unable to take tablets. Mefloquine p. 606 is now rarely used for treatment because of concerns about resistance.

Oral quinine is given by mouth for 5–7 days, together with or followed by either doxycycline p. 555 for 7 days or clindamycin p. 526 for 7 days [unlicensed].

If the parasite is likely to be sensitive, pyrimethamine with sulfadoxine as a single dose [unlicensed] may be given (instead of either clindamycin or doxycycline) together with, or after, a course of quinine.

Alternatively, *Malarone*®, or *Riamet*® may be given instead of quinine. It is not necessary to give clindamycin, doxycycline, or pyrimethamine with sulfadoxine after *Malarone*® or *Riamet*® treatment.

If the patient is seriously ill or unable to take tablets, or if more than 2% of red blood cell are parasitized, quinine should be given by *intravenous infusion* [unlicensed] (until patient can swallow tablets to complete the 7-day course *together with* or *followed by either* doxycycline or clindamycin).

Specialist advice should be sought in difficult cases (e.g. very high parasite count, deterioration on optimal doses of quinine, infection acquired in quinine-resistant areas of south east Asia) because intravenous **artesunate** may be available for 'named-patient' use.

Pregnancy
Falciparum malaria is particularly dangerous in pregnancy, especially in the last trimester. The adult treatment doses or oral and intravenous quinine (including the loading dose) can safely be given to pregnant women. Clindamycin should be given after quinine [unlicensed indication]. Doxycycline should be avoided in pregnancy (affects teeth and skeletal development); pyrimethamine with sulfadoxine, *Malarone*®, and *Riamet*® are also best avoided until more information is available. Specialist advice should be sought in difficult cases (e.g. very high parasite count, deterioration on optimal doses of quinine, infection acquired in quinine-resistant areas of

south east Asia) because intravenous artesunate may be available for 'named patient' use.

Non-falciparum malaria (treatment)

Non-falciparum malaria is usually caused by *Plasmodium vivax* and less commonly by *P. ovale* and *P. malariae.P. knowlesi* is also common in the Asia-Pacific region. Chloroquine is the drug of choice for the treatment of non-falciparum malaria (but chloroquine-resistant *P. vivax* has been reported in the Indonesian archipelago, the Malay Peninsula, including Myanmar, and eastward to Southern Vietnam).

For the treatment of chloroquine-resistant non-falciparum malaria, *Malarone®* [unlicensed indication], quinine, or *Riamet®* [unlicensed indication] can be used; as with chloroquine, primaquine p. 607 should be given for radical cure.

Chloroquine alone is adequate for *P. malariae* and *P. knowlesi* infections but in the case of *P. vivax* and *P. ovale*, a *radical cure* (to destroy parasites in the liver and thus prevent relapses) is required. This is achieved with primaquine [unlicensed] given after chloroquine, with the dose dependent on the infecting organism. For a radical cure, primaquine [unlicensed] is then given for 14 days, with the dose also dependent on the infecting organism.

Parenteral

Parenteral If the patient is unable to take oral therapy, quinine can be given by intravenous infusion [unlicensed], changed to oral chloroquine as soon as the patient's condition permits.

Pregnancy

The adult treatment doses of chloroquine can be given for non-falciparum malaria. In the case of *P. vivax* or *P. ovale*, however, the radical cure with primaquine should be **postponed** until the pregnancy is over; instead chloroquine should be continued, given weekly during the pregnancy.

ANTIPROTOZOALS > ANTIMALARIALS

Artemether with lumefantrine

● **INDICATIONS AND DOSE**

Treatment of acute uncomplicated falciparum malaria | **Treatment of chloroquine-resistant non-falciparum malaria**

▸ BY MOUTH

▸ Adult (body-weight 35 kg and above): Initially 4 tablets, followed by 4 tablets for 5 doses each given at 8, 24, 36, 48 and 60 hours (total 24 tablets over 60 hours)

● UNLICENSED USE Use in treatment of non-falciparum malaria is an unlicensed indication.

● CONTRA-INDICATIONS Family history of congenital QT interval prolongation · family history of sudden death · history of arrhythmias · history of clinically relevant bradycardia · history of congestive heart failure accompanied by reduced left ventricular ejection fraction

● CAUTIONS Avoid in Acute porphyrias p. 1025 · electrolyte disturbances

● INTERACTIONS → Appendix 1: antimalarials

● SIDE-EFFECTS

▸ **Common or very common** Abdominal pain · appetite decreased · arthralgia · asthenia · cough · diarrhoea · dizziness · gait abnormal · headache · movement disorders (uncommon in children) · myalgia · nausea · palpitations · QT interval prolongation · sensation abnormal · skin reactions · sleep disorders · vomiting

▸ **Uncommon** Drowsiness

▸ **Frequency not known** Angioedema

● PREGNANCY Toxicity in *animal* studies with artemether. Manufacturer advises use only if potential benefit outweighs risk.

● BREAST FEEDING Manufacturer advises avoid breastfeeding for at least 1 week after last dose. Present in milk in *animal* studies.

● HEPATIC IMPAIRMENT Manufacturer advises caution in severe impairment.

● RENAL IMPAIRMENT Manufacturer advises caution in severe impairment.
  Monitoring In severe renal impairment monitor ECG and plasma potassium concentration.

● MONITORING REQUIREMENTS Monitor patients unable to take food (greater risk of recrudescence).

● DIRECTIONS FOR ADMINISTRATION Tablets may be crushed just before administration.

● PATIENT AND CARER ADVICE
  Driving and skilled tasks Dizziness may affect performance of skilled tasks (e.g. driving).

● MEDICINAL FORMS
  There can be variation in the licensing of different medicines containing the same drug.

  Tablet
  CAUTIONARY AND ADVISORY LABELS 21
  ▸ Riamet (Novartis Pharmaceuticals UK Ltd)
     Artemether 20 mg, Lumefantrine 120 mg Riamet tablets | 24 tablet [PoM] £22.50

Artenimol with piperaquine phosphate

(Piperaquine tetraphosphate with dihydroartemisinin)

● **INDICATIONS AND DOSE**

Treatment of uncomplicated falciparum malaria

▸ BY MOUTH

▸ Child 6 months–17 years (body-weight 7–12 kg): 0.5 tablet once daily for 3 days, max. 2 courses in 12 months; second course given at least 2 months after first course

▸ Child 6 months–17 years (body-weight 13–23 kg): 1 tablet once daily for 3 days, max. 2 courses in 12 months; second course given at least 2 months after first course

▸ Child 6 months–17 years (body-weight 24–35 kg): 2 tablets once daily for 3 days, max. 2 courses in 12 months; second course given at least 2 months after first course

▸ Child 6 months–17 years (body-weight 36–74 kg): 3 tablets once daily for 3 days, max. 2 courses in 12 months; second course given at least 2 months after first course

▸ Child 6 months–17 years (body-weight 75–99 kg): 4 tablets once daily for 3 days, max. 2 courses in 12 months; second course given at least 2 months after first course

▸ Adult (body-weight 36–74 kg): 3 tablets once daily for 3 days, max. 2 courses in 12 months; second course given at least 2 months after first course

▸ Adult (body-weight 75–99 kg): 4 tablets once daily for 3 days, max. 2 courses in 12 months; second course given at least 2 months after first course

● CONTRA-INDICATIONS Acute myocardial infarction · bradycardia · congenital long QT syndrome · electrolyte disturbances · family history of sudden death · heart failure with reduced left ventricular ejection fraction · history of symptomatic arrhythmias · left ventricular hypertrophy · risk factors for QT interval prolongation · severe hypertension

● INTERACTIONS → Appendix 1: antimalarials

5

Infection

● SIDE-EFFECTS
▶ **Common or very common** Anaemia · arrhythmias (in adults) · asthenia · conjunctivitis (in children) · eosinophilia · fever · headache (uncommon in children) · leucocytosis (in children) · leucopenia (in children) · neutropenia (in children) · QT interval prolongation · thrombocytopenia (in children)
▶ **Uncommon** Abdominal pain (very common in children) · appetite decreased (very common in children) · arthralgia · cardiac conduction disorder · cough (very common in children) · diarrhoea (very common in children) · dizziness (in adults) · epistaxis (in children) · hepatic disorders · hypochromia (in children) · increased risk of infection (very common in children) · lymphadenopathy (in children) · myalgia (in adults) · nausea · rhinorrhoea (in children) · seizure · skin reactions (very common in children) · splenomegaly (in children) · stomatitis (in children) · thrombocytosis (in children) · vomiting (very common in children)
● PREGNANCY Teratogenic in *animal* studies—manufacturer advises use only if other antimalarials cannot be used.
● BREAST FEEDING Manufacturer advises avoid—present in milk in *animal* studies.
● HEPATIC IMPAIRMENT No information available in moderate to severe impairment.
  Monitoring Manufacturer advises monitor ECG and plasma-potassium concentration in moderate to severe hepatic impairment.
● RENAL IMPAIRMENT No information available in moderate to severe impairment.
  Monitoring Manufacturer advises monitor ECG and plasma-potassium concentration in moderate to severe renal impairment.
● MONITORING REQUIREMENTS
▶ Consider obtaining ECG in all patients before third dose and 4–6 hours after third dose. If QT$_C$ interval more than 500 milliseconds, discontinue treatment and monitor ECG for a further 24–48 hours.
▶ Obtain ECG as soon as possible after starting treatment then continue monitoring in those taking medicines that increase plasma-piperaquine concentration, in children who are vomiting, in females, or in the elderly.
● DIRECTIONS FOR ADMINISTRATION Tablets to be taken at least 3 hours before and at least 3 hours after food. Tablets may be crushed and mixed with water immediately before administration.
● PATIENT AND CARER ADVICE Patients or carers should be given advice on how to administer tablets containing piperaquine phosphate with artenimol.

● MEDICINAL FORMS
There can be variation in the licensing of different medicines containing the same drug.
Tablet
▶ Eurartesim (Logixx Pharma Solutions Ltd) ▼
  Artenimol 40 mg, Piperaquine phosphate 320 mg Eurartesim 320mg/40mg tablets | 12 tablet [PoM] £40.00

Atovaquone with proguanil hydrochloride

● INDICATIONS AND DOSE
MALARONE® 250 MG/100 MG
Prophylaxis of falciparum malaria, particularly where resistance to other antimalarial drugs suspected
▶ BY MOUTH
▶ Adult (body-weight 41 kg and above): 1 tablet daily, to be started 1–2 days before entering endemic area and continued for 1 week after leaving

Treatment of acute uncomplicated falciparum malaria | Treatment of non-falciparum malaria
▶ BY MOUTH
▶ Adult: 4 tablets once daily for 3 days

● UNLICENSED USE Not licensed for treatment of non-falciparum malaria.
● CAUTIONS Diarrhoea or vomiting (reduced absorption of atovaquone) · efficacy not evaluated in cerebral or complicated malaria (including hyperparasitaemia, pulmonary oedema or renal failure)
● INTERACTIONS → Appendix 1: antimalarials
● SIDE-EFFECTS
▶ **Common or very common** Abdominal pain · appetite decreased · cough · depression · diarrhoea · dizziness · fever · headache · nausea · skin reactions · sleep disorders · vomiting
▶ **Uncommon** Alopecia · anxiety · blood disorder · hyponatraemia · oral disorders · palpitations
▶ **Frequency not known** Hallucination · hepatic disorders · photosensitivity reaction · seizure · Stevens-Johnson syndrome · tachycardia · vasculitis
● PREGNANCY Manufacturer advises avoid unless essential.
● BREAST FEEDING Use only if no suitable alternative available.
● RENAL IMPAIRMENT Avoid for malaria prophylaxis (and if possible for malaria treatment) if eGFR less than 30 mL/minute/1.73m^2.
● PATIENT AND CARER ADVICE Warn travellers about **importance** of avoiding mosquito bites, **importance** of taking prophylaxis regularly, and **importance** of immediate visit to doctor if ill within 1 year and **especially** within 3 months of return.
● NATIONAL FUNDING/ACCESS DECISIONS
NHS restrictions Drugs for malaria prophylaxis are not prescribable in NHS primary care; health authorities may investigate circumstances under which antimalarials are prescribed.

● MEDICINAL FORMS
There can be variation in the licensing of different medicines containing the same drug.
Tablet
CAUTIONARY AND ADVISORY LABELS 21
▶ Malarone (GlaxoSmithKline UK Ltd)
  Proguanil hydrochloride 100 mg, Atovaquone 250 mg Malarone 250mg/100mg tablets | 12 tablet [PoM] £25.21 DT = £25.21

Chloroquine

● INDICATIONS AND DOSE
Active rheumatoid arthritis (administered on expert advice) | Systemic and discoid lupus erythematosus (administered on expert advice)
▶ BY MOUTH USING TABLETS
▶ Adult: 155 mg daily; maximum 2.5 mg/kg per day

Prophylaxis of malaria
▶ INITIALLY BY MOUTH USING SYRUP
▶ Child 4–5 weeks (body-weight up to 4.5 kg): 25 mg once weekly, started 1 week before entering endemic area and continued for 4 weeks after leaving
▶ Child 6 weeks–5 months (body-weight 4.5–7 kg): 50 mg once weekly, started 1 week before entering endemic area and continued for 4 weeks after leaving
▶ Child 6–11 months (body-weight 8–10 kg): 75 mg once weekly, started 1 week before entering endemic area and continued for 4 weeks after leaving

- Child 1–2 years (body-weight 11–14 kg): 100 mg once weekly, started 1 week before entering endemic area and continued for 4 weeks after leaving
- Child 3–4 years (body-weight 15–16.4 kg): 125 mg once weekly, started 1 week before entering endemic area and continued for 4 weeks after leaving
- Child 5–7 years (body-weight 16.5–24 kg): 150 mg once weekly, alternatively (by mouth using tablets) 155 mg once weekly, started 1 week before entering endemic area and continued for 4 weeks after leaving
- Child 8–13 years (body-weight 25–44 kg): 225 mg once weekly, alternatively (by mouth using tablets) 232.5 mg once weekly, started 1 week before entering endemic area and continued for 4 weeks after leaving
- INITIALLY BY MOUTH USING TABLETS
- Child 14–17 years (body-weight 45 kg and above): 310 mg once weekly, alternatively (by mouth using syrup) 300 mg once weekly, started 1 week before entering endemic area and continued for 4 weeks after leaving
- Adult (body-weight 45 kg and above): 310 mg once weekly, alternatively (by mouth using syrup) 300 mg once weekly, started 1 week before entering endemic area and continued for 4 weeks after leaving

Treatment of non-falciparum malaria
- BY MOUTH
- Child: Initially 10 mg/kg (max. per dose 620 mg), then 5 mg/kg after 6–8 hours (max. per dose 310 mg), then 5 mg/kg daily (max. per dose 310 mg) for 2 days
- Adult: Initially 620 mg, then 310 mg after 6–8 hours, then 310 mg daily for 2 days, approximate total cumulative dose of 25 mg/kg of base

***P. vivax* or *P. ovale* infection during pregnancy while radical cure is postponed**
- BY MOUTH
- Adult: 310 mg once weekly

DOSE EQUIVALENCE AND CONVERSION
- Doses expressed as chloroquine base.
- Each tablet contains 155 mg of chloroquine base (equivalent to 250 mg of chloroquine phosphate). Syrup contains 50 mg/5 mL of chloroquine base (equivalent to 80 mg/5 mL of chloroquine phosphate).

DOSES AT EXTREMES OF BODY-WEIGHT
- With oral use in adults In active rheumatoid arthritis and systemic and discoid lupus erythematosus, to avoid excessive dosage in obese patients, the daily maximum dose should be calculated on the basis of ideal body weight.

- UNLICENSED USE Chloroquine doses for the treatment and prophylaxis of malaria in BNF publications may differ from those in product literature.

> IMPORTANT SAFETY INFORMATION
> ▸ In adults
> Ocular toxicity is unlikely if the dose of chloroquine phosphate does not exceed 4 mg/kg daily (equivalent to chloroquine base approx. 2.5 mg/kg daily).

- CAUTIONS Acute porphyrias p. 1025 · diabetes (may lower blood glucose) · elderly · G6PD deficiency · long-term therapy (regular ophthalmic examination recommended by manufacturers) · may aggravate myasthenia gravis · may exacerbate psoriasis · neurological disorders, especially epilepsy (avoid for prophylaxis of malaria if history of epilepsy) · severe gastro-intestinal disorders

CAUTIONS, FURTHER INFORMATION
- Screening for ocular toxicity
- In adults A review group convened by the Royal College of Ophthalmologists has updated guidelines for screening to prevent ocular toxicity on long-term treatment with chloroquine and hydroxychloroquine (*Hydroxychloroquine and Ocular Toxicity: Recommendations on Screening* 2009).

Chloroquine should be considered (for treating chronic inflammatory conditions) **only** if other drugs have failed. All patients taking chloroquine should receive ocular examination according to a protocol arranged locally between the prescriber and the ophthalmologist.

- INTERACTIONS → Appendix 1: antimalarials
- SIDE-EFFECTS
- ▸ **Rare or very rare** Cardiomyopathy · hallucination · hepatitis
- ▸ **Frequency not known** Abdominal pain · agranulocytosis · alopecia · anxiety · atrioventricular block · bone marrow disorders · confusion · corneal deposits · depression · diarrhoea · eye disorders · gastrointestinal disorder · headache · hearing impairment · hypoglycaemia · hypotension · insomnia · interstitial lung disease · movement disorders · myopathy · nausea · neuromyopathy · neutropenia · personality change · photosensitivity reaction · psychotic disorder · QT interval prolongation · seizure · severe cutaneous adverse reactions (SCARs) · skin reactions · thrombocytopenia · tongue protrusion · vision disorders · vomiting

SIDE-EFFECTS, FURTHER INFORMATION Side-effects which occur at doses used in the prophylaxis or treatment of malaria are generally not serious.

Overdose Chloroquine is very toxic in overdosage; overdosage is extremely hazardous and difficult to treat. Urgent advice from the National Poisons Information Service is essential. Life-threatening features include arrhythmias (which can have a very rapid onset) and convulsions (which can be intractable).

- PREGNANCY Benefit of use in prophylaxis and treatment in malaria outweighs risk. For rheumatoid disease, it is not necessary to withdraw an antimalarial drug during pregnancy if the disease is well controlled.
- BREAST FEEDING Present in breast milk and breast-feeding should be avoided when used to treat rheumatic disease. Amount in milk probably too small to be harmful when used for malaria.
- HEPATIC IMPAIRMENT Use with caution in moderate to severe impairment.
- RENAL IMPAIRMENT Manufacturers advise caution. **Dose adjustments** Only partially excreted by the kidneys and reduction of the dose is not required for prophylaxis of malaria except in severe impairment.
  For rheumatoid arthritis and lupus erythematosus, reduce dose.
- MONITORING REQUIREMENTS
- In adults Manufacturers recommend regular ophthalmological examination but the evidence of practical value is unsatisfactory.
- In children Ophthalmic examination with long-term therapy.
- PATIENT AND CARER ADVICE Warn travellers going to malarious areas about **importance** of avoiding mosquito bites, **importance** of taking prophylaxis regularly, and **importance** of immediate visit to doctor if ill within 1 year and **especially** within 3 months of return.
- NATIONAL FUNDING/ACCESS DECISIONS
  NHS restrictions Drugs for malaria prophylaxis are not prescribable in NHS primary care; health authorities may investigate circumstances under which antimalarials are prescribed.
- EXCEPTIONS TO LEGAL CATEGORY Can be sold to the public provided it is licensed and labelled for the prophylaxis of malaria.

5

Infection

- MEDICINAL FORMS
  There can be variation in the licensing of different medicines
  containing the same drug.
  Oral solution
  CAUTIONARY AND ADVISORY LABELS 5
  ▸ Malarivon (Wallace Manufacturing Chemists Ltd)
    Chloroquine phosphate 16 mg per 1 ml Malarivon 80mg/5ml syrup
    | 75 ml [PoM] £30.00 DT = £30.00
  Tablet
  CAUTIONARY AND ADVISORY LABELS 5
  ▸ Avloclor (Alliance Pharmaceuticals Ltd)
    Chloroquine phosphate 250 mg Avloclor 250mg tablets |
    20 tablet [PoM] £8.59 DT = £8.59

Chloroquine with proguanil

The properties listed below are those particular to the
combination only. For the properties of the components
please consider, chloroquine p. 604, proguanil hydrochloride
p. 607.

- INDICATIONS AND DOSE
  Prophylaxis of malaria
  ▸ BY MOUTH
  ▸ Adult: (consult product literature)

- INTERACTIONS → Appendix 1: antimalarials

- EXCEPTIONS TO LEGAL CATEGORY Can be sold to the public
  provided it is licensed and labelled for the prophylaxis of
  malaria.

- MEDICINAL FORMS
  There can be variation in the licensing of different medicines
  containing the same drug.
  Tablet
  ▸ Paludrine/Avloclor (Alliance Pharmaceuticals Ltd)
    Paludrine/Avloclor tablets anti-malarial travel pack | 112 tablet [P]
    £13.50

Mefloquine

- INDICATIONS AND DOSE
  Treatment of malaria
  ▸ BY MOUTH
  ▸ Adult: (consult product literature)
  Prophylaxis of malaria
  ▸ BY MOUTH
  ▸ Child (body-weight 5–15 kg): 62.5 mg once weekly, dose
    to be started 2–3 weeks before entering endemic area
    and continued for 4 weeks after leaving
  ▸ Child (body-weight 16–24 kg): 125 mg once weekly, dose
    to be started 2–3 weeks before entering endemic area
    and continued for 4 weeks after leaving
  ▸ Child (body-weight 25–44 kg): 187.5 mg once weekly,
    dose to be started 2–3 weeks before entering endemic
    area and continued for 4 weeks after leaving
  ▸ Child (body-weight 45 kg and above): 250 mg once
    weekly, dose to be started 2–3 weeks before entering
    endemic area and continued for 4 weeks after leaving
  ▸ Adult (body-weight 45 kg and above): 250 mg once
    weekly, dose to be started 2–3 weeks before entering
    endemic area and continued for 4 weeks after leaving

- UNLICENSED USE Mefloquine doses in BNF Publications
  may differ from those in product literature. Not licensed
  for use in children under 5 kg body-weight and under
  3 months.

- CONTRA-INDICATIONS Avoid for prophylaxis if history of
  psychiatric disorders (including depression) or convulsions
  · avoid for standby treatment if history of convulsions ·
  history of blackwater fever

- CAUTIONS Cardiac conduction disorders · epilepsy (avoid
  for prophylaxis) · not recommended in infants under
  3 months (5 kg) · traumatic brain injury
  CAUTIONS, FURTHER INFORMATION
  ▸ Neuropsychiatric reactions Mefloquine is associated with
    potentially serious neuropsychiatric reactions. Abnormal
    dreams, insomnia, anxiety, and depression occur
    commonly. Psychosis, suicidal ideation, and suicide have
    also been reported. Psychiatric symptoms such as
    nightmares, acute anxiety, depression, restlessness, or
    confusion should be regarded as potentially prodromal for
    a more serious event. Adverse reactions may occur and
    persist up to several months after discontinuation because
    mefloquine has a long half-life. For a prescribing checklist,
    and further information on side-effects, particularly
    neuropsychiatric side-effects, which may be associated
    with the use of mefloquine for malaria prophylaxis, see the
    Guide for Healthcare Professionals provided by the
    manufacturer.

- INTERACTIONS → Appendix 1: antimalarials

- SIDE-EFFECTS
  ▸ **Common or very common** Anxiety · depression · diarrhoea ·
    dizziness · gastrointestinal discomfort · headache · nausea ·
    skin reactions · sleep disorders · vision disorders · vomiting
  ▸ **Frequency not known** Acute kidney injury · agranulocytosis
    · alopecia · aplastic anaemia · appetite decreased ·
    arrhythmias · arthralgia · asthenia · behaviour abnormal ·
    cardiac conduction disorders · cataract · chest pain · chills ·
    concentration impaired · confusion · cranial nerve
    paralysis · delusional disorder · depersonalisation ·
    drowsiness · dyspnoea · encephalopathy · eye disorder ·
    fever · flushing · gait abnormal · hallucination · hearing
    impairment · hepatic disorders · hyperacusia ·
    hyperhidrosis · hypertension · hypotension · leucocytosis ·
    leucopenia · malaise · memory loss · mood altered ·
    movement disorders · muscle complaints · muscle
    weakness · nephritis · nerve disorders · oedema ·
    palpitations · pancreatitis · paraesthesia · pneumonia ·
    pneumonitis · psychosis · seizure · self-endangering
    behaviour · speech disorder · Stevens-Johnson syndrome ·
    suicidal tendencies · syncope · thrombocytopenia · tremor ·
    vertigo

- ALLERGY AND CROSS-SENSITIVITY Contra-indicated in
  patients with hypersensitivity to quinine.

- CONCEPTION AND CONTRACEPTION Manufacturer advises
  adequate contraception during prophylaxis and for
  3 months after stopping (teratogenicity in *animal* studies).

- PREGNANCY Manufacturer advises avoid (particularly in
  the first trimester) unless the potential benefit outweighs
  the risk; however, studies of mefloquine in pregnancy
  (including use in the first trimester) indicate that it can be
  considered for travel to chloroquine-resistant areas.

- BREAST FEEDING Present in milk but risk to infant
  minimal.

- HEPATIC IMPAIRMENT Elimination may be prolonged;
  avoid in severe impairment.

- RENAL IMPAIRMENT Manufacturer advises caution.

- DIRECTIONS FOR ADMINISTRATION Tablet may be crushed
  and mixed with food such as jam or honey just before
  administration.

- PATIENT AND CARER ADVICE Manufacturer advises that
  patients receiving mefloquine for malaria prophylaxis
  should be informed to discontinue its use if
  neuropsychiatric symptoms occur and seek immediate
  medical advice so that mefloquine can be replaced with an
  alternative antimalarial. Travellers should also be warned
  about **importance** of avoiding mosquito bites,
  importance of taking prophylaxis regularly, and
  importance of immediate visit to doctor if ill within 1 year
  and especially within 3 months of return.

A patient alert card should be provided.

Driving and skilled tasks Dizziness or a disturbed sense of balance may affect performance of skilled tasks (e.g. driving); effects may occur and persist up to several months after stopping mefloquine.

● NATIONAL FUNDING/ACCESS DECISIONS
NHS restrictions Drugs for malaria prophylaxis are not prescribable in NHS primary care; health authorities may investigate circumstances under which antimalarials are prescribed.

● MEDICINAL FORMS
There can be variation in the licensing of different medicines containing the same drug.
Tablet
CAUTIONARY AND ADVISORY LABELS 10, 21, 27
▸ Lariam (Roche Products Ltd)
　Mefloquine (as Mefloquine hydrochloride) 250 mg Lariam 250mg tablets | 8 tablet PoM £14.53

Primaquine

● INDICATIONS AND DOSE
Adjunct in the treatment of non-falciparum malaria caused by P.vivax infection
▸ BY MOUTH
▸ Adult: 30 mg daily for 14 days

Adjunct in the treatment of non-falciparum malaria caused by P.ovale infection
▸ BY MOUTH
▸ Adult: 15 mg daily for 14 days

Adjunct in the treatment of non-falciparum malaria caused by P.vivax infection in patients with mild G6PD deficiency (administered on expert advice) | Adjunct in the treatment of non-falciparum malaria caused by P.ovale infection in patients with mild G6PD deficiency (administered on expert advice)
▸ BY MOUTH
▸ Adult: 45 mg once weekly for 8 weeks

Treatment of mild to moderate pneumocystis infection (in combination with clindamycin)
▸ BY MOUTH
▸ Adult: 30 mg daily, this combination is associated with considerable toxicity

● UNLICENSED USE Not licensed.

● CAUTIONS G6PD deficiency · systemic diseases associated with granulocytopenia (e.g. juvenile idiopathic arthritis, rheumatoid arthritis, lupus erythematosus)

● INTERACTIONS → Appendix 1: antimalarials

● SIDE-EFFECTS
▸ **Common or very common** Abdominal pain · appetite decreased · nausea · vomiting
▸ **Uncommon** Haemolytic anaemia (more common in G6PD deficiency) · leucopenia · methaemoglobinaemia

● PREGNANCY Risk of neonatal haemolysis and methaemoglobinaemia in third trimester.

● BREAST FEEDING No information available; theoretical risk of haemolysis in G6PD-deficient infants.

● PRE-TREATMENT SCREENING Before starting primaquine, blood should be tested for glucose-6-phosphate dehydrogenase (G6PD) activity since the drug can cause haemolysis in G6PD-deficient patients. Specialist advice should be obtained in G6PD deficiency.

● MEDICINAL FORMS
There can be variation in the licensing of different medicines containing the same drug. Forms available from special-order manufacturers include: oral suspension
Tablet
▸ Primaquine (Non-proprietary)
　Primaquine (as Primaquine phosphate) 7.5 mg Primaquine 7.5mg tablets | 100 tablet £189.36
　Primaquine (as Primaquine phosphate) 15 mg Primaquine 15mg tablets | 100 tablet PoM Ⓢ

Proguanil hydrochloride

● INDICATIONS AND DOSE
Prophylaxis of malaria
▸ BY MOUTH
▸ Child 4-11 weeks (body-weight up to 6 kg): 25 mg once daily, dose to be started 1 week before entering endemic area and continued for 4 weeks after leaving
▸ Child 3-11 months (body-weight 6-9 kg): 50 mg once daily, dose to be started 1 week before entering endemic area and continued for 4 weeks after leaving
▸ Child 1-3 years (body-weight 10-15 kg): 75 mg once daily, dose to be started 1 week before entering endemic area and continued for 4 weeks after leaving
▸ Child 4-7 years (body-weight 16-24 kg): 100 mg once daily, dose to be started 1 week before entering endemic area and continued for 4 weeks after leaving
▸ Child 8-12 years (body-weight 25-44 kg): 150 mg once daily, dose to be started 1 week before entering endemic area and continued for 4 weeks after leaving
▸ Child 13-17 years (body-weight 45 kg and above): 200 mg once daily, dose to be started 1 week before entering endemic area and continued for 4 weeks after leaving
▸ Adult: 200 mg once daily, dose to be started 1 week before entering endemic area and continued for 4 weeks after leaving

● UNLICENSED USE Proguanil doses in BNF Publications may differ from those in product literature.

● INTERACTIONS → Appendix 1: antimalarials

● SIDE-EFFECTS Alopecia · angioedema · bone marrow disorders · cholestasis · constipation · diarrhoea · fever · gastric disorder · megaloblastic anaemia · oral disorders · skin reactions · vasculitis

● PREGNANCY Benefit of prophylaxis in malaria outweighs risk. Adequate folate supplements should be given to mother.

● BREAST FEEDING Amount in milk probably too small to be harmful when used for malaria prophylaxis.

● RENAL IMPAIRMENT
Dose adjustments ▸ In children Use half normal dose if estimated glomerular filtration rate 20–60 mL/minute/1.73m^2. Use one-quarter normal dose on alternate days if estimated glomerular filtration rate 10–20 mL/minute/1.73m^2. Use one-quarter normal dose once weekly if estimated glomerular filtration rate less than 10 mL/minute/1.73m^2; increased risk of haematological toxicity in severe impairment.
▸ In adults 100 mg once daily if eGFR 20–60 mL/minute/1.73m^2. 50 mg on alternate days if eGFR 10–20 mL/minute/1.73m^2. 50 mg once weekly if eGFR less than 10 mL/minute/1.73m^2; increased risk of haematological toxicity in severe impairment.

● DIRECTIONS FOR ADMINISTRATION Tablet may be crushed and mixed with food such as milk, jam, or honey just before administration.

● PATIENT AND CARER ADVICE Warn travellers about **importance** of avoiding mosquito bites, **importance** of taking prophylaxis regularly, and **importance** of immediate visit to doctor if ill within 1 year and **especially** within 3 months of return.

5

Infection

5

Infection

- NATIONAL FUNDING/ACCESS DECISIONS
NHS restrictions Drugs for malaria prophylaxis are not prescribable in NHS primary care; health authorities may investigate circumstances under which antimalarials are prescribed.
- EXCEPTIONS TO LEGAL CATEGORY Can be sold to the public provided it is licensed and labelled for the prophylaxis of malaria.
- MEDICINAL FORMS
There can be variation in the licensing of different medicines containing the same drug. Forms available from special-order manufacturers include: oral suspension, oral solution
Tablet
CAUTIONARY AND ADVISORY LABELS 21
▸ Paludrine (Alliance Pharmaceuticals Ltd)
Proguanil hydrochloride 100 mg Paludrine 100mg tablets | 98 tablet [P] £11.95 DT = £11.95

Quinine

04-Dec-2017

- INDICATIONS AND DOSE
Nocturnal leg cramps
▸ BY MOUTH
▸ Adult: 200–300 mg once daily, to be taken at bedtime
Non-falciparum malaria
▸ BY INTRAVENOUS INFUSION
▸ Adult: 10 mg/kg every 8 hours (max. per dose 700 mg), infused over 4 hours, given if patient is unable to take oral therapy. Change to oral chloroquine as soon as the patient's condition permits, reduce dose to 5–7 mg/kg if parenteral treatment is required for more than 48 hours
Falciparum malaria
▸ BY MOUTH
▸ Child: 10 mg/kg every 8 hours (max. per dose 600 mg) for 7 days, to be given together with or followed by either doxycycline (in children over 12 years), or clindamycin
▸ Adult: 600 mg every 8 hours for 5–7 days, to be given together with or followed by either doxycycline or clindamycin
▸ BY INTRAVENOUS INFUSION
▸ Adult: Loading dose 20 mg/kg (max. per dose 1.4 g), infused over 4 hours, the loading dose of 20 mg/kg should **not** be used if the patient has received quinine or mefloquine during the previous 12 hours, then maintenance 10 mg/kg every 8 hours (max. per dose 700 mg) until patient can swallow tablets to complete the 7-day course, maintenance dose to be given 8 hours after the start of the loading dose and infused over 4 hours, to be given together with or followed by either doxycycline or clindamycin, reduce maintenance dose to 5–7 mg/kg if parenteral treatment is required for more than 48 hours
Falciparum malaria (in intensive care unit)
▸ BY INTRAVENOUS INFUSION
▸ Adult: Loading dose 7 mg/kg, infused over 30 minutes, followed immediately by 10 mg/kg, infused over 4 hours, then maintenance 10 mg/kg every 8 hours (max. per dose 700 mg) until patient can swallow tablets to complete the 7-day course, maintenance dose to be given 8 hours after the start of the loading dose and infused over 4 hours, to be given together with or followed by either doxycycline or clindamycin, reduce maintenance dose to 5–7 mg/kg if parenteral treatment is required for more than 48 hours
DOSE EQUIVALENCE AND CONVERSION
▸ When using quinine for malaria, doses are valid for quinine hydrochloride, dihydrochloride, and sulfate; they are **not valid** for quinine bisulfate which contains a correspondingly smaller amount of quinine.

▸ Quinine (anhydrous base) 100 mg = quinine bisulfate 169 mg; quinine dihydrochloride 122 mg; quinine hydrochloride 122 mg; and quinine sulfate 121 mg. Quinine bisulfate 300 mg tablets are available but provide less quinine than 300 mg of the dihydrochloride, hydrochloride, or sulfate.

- UNLICENSED USE Injection not licensed.

IMPORTANT SAFETY INFORMATION

MHRA/CHM ADVICE: REMINDER OF DOSE-DEPENDENT QT-PROLONGING EFFECTS (NOVEMBER 2017)
Quinine has been associated with dose-dependent QT-interval-prolonging effects and should be used with caution in patients with risk factors for QT prolongation or in those with atrioventricular block—see Cautions for further information.

- CONTRA-INDICATIONS Haemoglobinuria · myasthenia gravis · optic neuritis · tinnitus
- CAUTIONS Atrial fibrillation (monitor ECG during parenteral treatment) · cardiac disease (monitor ECG during parenteral treatment) · conduction defects (monitor ECG during parenteral treatment) · elderly (monitor ECG during parenteral treatment) · electrolyte disturbance · G6PD deficiency · heart block (monitor ECG during parenteral treatment)
- INTERACTIONS → Appendix 1: antimalarials
- SIDE-EFFECTS Abdominal pain · agitation · agranulocytosis · angioedema · asthma · atrioventricular conduction changes · bronchospasm · cardiotoxicity · cerebral impairment · coagulation disorders · coma · confusion · death · diarrhoea · dyspnoea · fever · flushing · gastrointestinal disorder · haemoglobinuria · haemolysis · haemolytic uraemic syndrome · headache · hearing impairment · hypersensitivity · loss of consciousness · muscle weakness · myasthenia gravis aggravated · nausea · ocular toxicity · oedema · pancytopenia · photosensitivity reaction · QT interval prolongation · renal impairment · skin reactions · thrombocytopenia · vertigo · vision disorders · vomiting

Overdose Quinine is very toxic in overdosage; life-threatening features include arrhythmias (which can have a very rapid onset) and convulsions (which can be intractable).
    For details on the management of poisoning, see Emergency treatment of poisoning p. 1319.
- PREGNANCY High doses are teratogenic in *first trimester*, but in malaria benefit of treatment outweighs risk.
- BREAST FEEDING Present in milk but not known to be harmful.
- HEPATIC IMPAIRMENT
Dose adjustments ▸ With intravenous use For treatment of malaria in severe impairment, reduce parenteral maintenance dose to 5–7 mg/kg of quinine salt.
- RENAL IMPAIRMENT
Dose adjustments ▸ With intravenous use For treatment of malaria in severe impairment, reduce parenteral maintenance dose to 5–7 mg/kg of quinine salt.
- MONITORING REQUIREMENTS
▸ With intravenous use Monitor blood glucose and electrolyte concentration during parenteral treatment.
▸ In adults Patients taking quinine for nocturnal leg cramps should be monitored closely during the early stages for adverse effects as well as for benefit.
- DIRECTIONS FOR ADMINISTRATION For *intravenous infusion*, give continuously in Glucose 5% or Sodium Chloride 0.9%. To be given over 4 hours.

● PRESCRIBING AND DISPENSING INFORMATION
▸ With intravenous use Intravenous injection of quinine is so
hazardous that it has been superseded by infusion.

● MEDICINAL FORMS
There can be variation in the licensing of different medicines
containing the same drug. Forms available from special-order
manufacturers include: capsule, oral suspension, oral solution,
solution for infusion

Tablet
▸ Quinine (Non-proprietary)
Quinine sulfate 200 mg Quinine sulfate 200mg tablets |
28 tablet PoM £2.90 DT = £1.43
Quinine bisulfate 300 mg Quinine bisulfate 300mg tablets |
28 tablet PoM £2.57 DT = £1.94
Quinine sulfate 300 mg Quinine sulfate 300mg tablets |
28 tablet PoM £2.83 DT = £1.96

5.3 Toxoplasmosis

ANTIPROTOZOALS

Pyrimethamine

● INDICATIONS AND DOSE

**Toxoplasmosis in pregnancy (in combination with
sulfadiazine and folinic acid)**
▸ BY MOUTH
▸ Adult: 50 mg once daily until delivery

● CAUTIONS History of seizures—avoid large loading doses ·
predisposition to folate deficiency

● INTERACTIONS → Appendix 1: antimalarials

● SIDE-EFFECTS
▸ **Common or very common** Anaemia · diarrhoea · dizziness ·
headache · leucopenia · nausea · skin reactions ·
thrombocytopenia · vomiting
▸ **Uncommon** Fever
▸ **Rare or very rare** Abdominal pain · oral ulceration ·
pancytopenia · pneumonia eosinophilic · seizure

● PREGNANCY Theoretical teratogenic risk in *first trimester*
(folate antagonist). Adequate folate supplements should
be given to the mother.

● BREAST FEEDING Significant amount in milk—avoid
administration of other folate antagonists to infant. Avoid
breast-feeding during toxoplasmosis treatment.

● HEPATIC IMPAIRMENT Manufacturer advises caution.

● RENAL IMPAIRMENT Manufacturer advises caution.

● MONITORING REQUIREMENTS Blood counts required with
prolonged treatment.

● MEDICINAL FORMS
There can be variation in the licensing of different medicines
containing the same drug. Forms available from special-order
manufacturers include: oral suspension

Tablet
▸ Daraprim (GlaxoSmithKline UK Ltd)
Pyrimethamine 25 mg Daraprim 25mg tablets | 30 tablet PoM
£13.00

6 Viral infection

6.1 Hepatitis

Hepatitis

Overview

Treatment for viral hepatitis should be initiated by a
specialist. The management of uncomplicated acute viral
hepatitis is largely symptomatic. Early treatment of acute

hepatitis C with interferon alfa p. 930 [unlicensed indication]
may reduce the risk of chronic infection. Hepatitis B and
hepatitis C viruses are major causes of chronic hepatitis.
Active or passive immunisation against hepatitis A and B
infections can be given.

Chronic hepatitis B

Peginterferon alfa p. 612 is an option for the initial
treatment of chronic hepatitis B and may be preferable to
interferon alfa. The use of peginterferon alfa and interferon
alfa is limited by a response rate of 30–40% and relapse is
frequent. Treatment should be discontinued if no
improvement occurs after 4 months. The manufacturers of
peginterferon alfa-2a and interferon alfa contraindicate use
in decompensated liver disease, but low doses can be used
with great caution in these patients. Although interferon alfa
is contra-indicated in patients receiving immunosuppressant
treatment (or who have received it recently), cautious use of
peginterferon alfa-2a may be justified in some cases.
Entecavir p. 610 or tenofovir disoproxil p. 641 are options
for the initial treatment of chronic hepatitis B. If the
response is inadequate after 6–9 months of treatment, a
change in treatment should be considered. Other drugs that
are licensed for the treatment of chronic hepatitis B include
adefovir dipivoxil p. 611, lamivudine p. 640, or telbivudine
p. 611.
Entecavir alone, tenofovir disoproxil alone, or a
combination of lamivudine with either adefovir dipivoxil or
tenofovir disoproxil can be used in patients with
decompensated liver disease.
If drug-resistant hepatitis B virus emerges during
treatment, another antiviral drug to which the virus is
sensitive should be added. Hepatitis B viruses with reduced
susceptibility to lamivudine have emerged following
extended therapy. Adefovir dipivoxil or tenofovir disoproxil
can be given with lamivudine in lamivudine-resistant
chronic hepatitis B; telbivudine or entecavir should not be
used because cross-resistance can occur.
If there is no toxicity or loss in efficacy, treatment with
adefovir dipivoxil, entecavir, lamivudine, telbivudine, or
tenofovir disoproxil is usually continued until 6 months after
adequate seroconversion has occurred. Treatment is usually
continued long-term in patients with decompensated liver
disease.
Tenofovir disoproxil, or a combination of tenofovir
disoproxil with either emtricitabine p. 638 or lamivudine
may be used with other antiretrovirals, as part of 'highly
active antiretroviral therapy' in patients who require
treatment for both HIV and chronic hepatitis B. If patients
infected with both HIV and chronic hepatitis B only require
treatment for chronic hepatitis B, they should receive
antivirals that are not active against HIV, such as
peginterferon alfa or adefovir dipivoxil. Treatment may be
continued long-term, even if adequate seroconversion
occurs. Management of these patients should be coordinated
between HIV and hepatology specialists.

Chronic hepatitis C

Before starting treatment, the genotype of the infecting
hepatitis C virus should be determined and the viral load
measured as this may affect the choice and duration of
treatment. A combination of ribavirin p. 615 and
peginterferon alfa is used for the treatment of chronic
hepatitis C. The combination of ribavirin and interferon alfa
is less effective than the combination of peginterferon alfa
and ribavirin. Peginterferon alfa alone should be used if
ribavirin is contra-indicated or not tolerated. Ribavirin
monotherapy is ineffective.
Daclatasvir p. 614 is licensed for use in combination with
sofosbuvir p. 618 for the treatment of chronic hepatitis C
infection of genotypes 1 or 4, with or without compensated
cirrhosis; the addition of ribavirin should be considered for

patients with advanced liver disease or with other negative prognostic factors, such as prior treatment experience. It is also licensed in combination with sofosbuvir and ribavirin for the treatment of chronic hepatitis C infection of genotype 3 in patients who are treatment experienced, with or without compensated cirrhosis, and in combination with peginterferon alfa and ribavirin for the treatment of chronic hepatitis C infection of genotype 4. Daclatasvir must not be given as monotherapy.

Ombitasvir with paritaprevir and ritonavir p. 615 (*Viekirax*®), is licensed for use in combination with dasabuvir p. 621, with or without ribavirin, for the treatment of chronic hepatitis C infection of genotype 1 in patients with or without compensated cirrhosis; it is also licensed for use in combination with ribavirin for the treatment of chronic hepatitis C infection of genotype 4 with or without compensated cirrhosis.

Ribavirin inhibits a wide range of DNA and RNA viruses. It is given by mouth for the treatment of chronic hepatitis C infection, in double therapy with peginterferon alfa, interferon alfa, or sofosbuvir, or in triple therapy with peginterferon alfa and one protease inhibitor (i.e. simeprevir p. 620) or sofosbuvir. Ribavirin is also effective in Lassa fever [unlicensed indication].

Sofosbuvir is a pro-drug of a nucleoside inhibitor that is effective against hepatitis C virus polymerase NS5B. It is licensed for use in combination with ribavirin, with or without peginterferon alfa, for the treatment of chronic hepatitis C infection of genotypes 1, 2, 3, 4, 5, or 6 in patients with compensated liver disease. Sofosbuvir monotherapy is not recommended because it is less effective than combination therapy.

Ledipasvir is licensed for use in combination with sofosbuvir (ledipasvir with sofosbuvir p. 617), with or without ribavirin, for the treatment of chronic hepatitis C infections of genotypes 1, 3, 4, 5 or 6.

Sofosbuvir with velpatasvir and voxilaprevir p. 619 is licensed for the treatment of chronic hepatitis C of all genotypes.

Simeprevir is licensed for use in combination with ribavirin and peginterferon alfa for the treatment of chronic hepatitis C infection of genotype 1 or 4; regimens containing peginterferon alfa-2b are less effective than those containing peginterferon alfa-2a. Simeprevir may also be used in combination with sofosbuvir, with or without ribavirin, for the urgent treatment of chronic hepatitis C infection of genotypes 1 or 4 only when peginterferon alfa cannot be used because of intolerance or contra-indications. Simeprevir monotherapy is not recommended.

6.2 Hepatitis infections
6.2a Chronic hepatitis B

> **Other drugs used for Chronic hepatitis B** Interferon alfa, p. 930 · Lamivudine, p. 640 · Tenofovir disoproxil, p. 641

ANTIVIRALS > NUCLEOSIDE ANALOGUES

Entecavir

- **INDICATIONS AND DOSE**

Chronic hepatitis B in patients with compensated liver disease (with evidence of viral replication, and histologically documented active liver inflammation or fibrosis) not previously treated with nucleoside analogues
▸ BY MOUTH
▸ Adult: 500 micrograms once daily

Chronic hepatitis B in patients with compensated liver disease (with evidence of viral replication, and histologically documented active liver inflammation or fibrosis) and lamivudine-resistance
▸ BY MOUTH
▸ Adult: 1 mg once daily, consider other treatment if inadequate response after 6 months

Chronic hepatitis B in patients with decompensated liver disease
▸ BY MOUTH
▸ Adult: 1 mg once daily

- **CAUTIONS** HIV infection—risk of HIV resistance in patients not receiving 'highly active antiretroviral therapy' · lamivudine-resistant chronic hepatitis B—risk of entecavir resistance
  CAUTIONS, FURTHER INFORMATION Discontinue if deterioration in liver function, hepatic steatosis, progressive hepatomegaly or unexplained lactic acidosis.
- **SIDE-EFFECTS**
▸ **Common or very common** Diarrhoea · dizziness · drowsiness · dyspepsia · fatigue · headache · insomnia · nausea · vomiting
▸ **Uncommon** Alopecia · rash
▸ **Frequency not known** Lactic acidosis
- **CONCEPTION AND CONTRACEPTION** Effective contraception required during treatment.
- **PREGNANCY** Toxicity in *animal* studies—manufacturer advises use only if potential benefit outweighs risk.
- **BREAST FEEDING** Manufacturer advises avoid—present in milk in *animal* studies.
- **RENAL IMPAIRMENT** Consult product literature.
  Dose adjustments Reduce dose if eGFR less than 50 mL/minute/1.73 m^2.
- **MONITORING REQUIREMENTS** Monitor liver function tests every 3 months, and viral markers for hepatitis B every 3–6 months during treatment (continue monitoring for at least 1 year after discontinuation—recurrent hepatitis may occur on discontinuation).
- **DIRECTIONS FOR ADMINISTRATION** To be taken at least 2 hours before or 2 hours after food.
- **PRESCRIBING AND DISPENSING INFORMATION** Flavours of oral liquid formulations may include orange.
- **PATIENT AND CARER ADVICE** Patients or carers should be counselled on the administration of entecavir tablets and oral solution.
- **NATIONAL FUNDING/ACCESS DECISIONS**
  NICE decisions
▸ **Entecavir for chronic hepatitis B (August 2008)** NICE TA153 Entecavir is an option for the treatment of chronic hepatitis B.
  www.nice.org.uk/TA153
- **MEDICINAL FORMS**
  There can be variation in the licensing of different medicines containing the same drug.
  Oral solution
▸ Baraclude (Bristol-Myers Squibb Pharmaceuticals Ltd)
  Entecavir (as Entecavir monohydrate) **50 microgram per 1 ml** Baraclude 0.05mg/ml oral solution sugar-free | 210 ml PoM £423.80 DT = £423.80
  Tablet
▸ Entecavir (Non-proprietary)
  Entecavir (as Entecavir monohydrate) **500 microgram** Entecavir 500microgram tablets | 30 tablet PoM £25.00–£363.26 DT = £363.26
  Entecavir (as Entecavir monohydrate) **1 mg** Entecavir 1mg tablets | 30 tablet PoM £35.00–£363.26 DT = £363.26
▸ Baraclude (Bristol-Myers Squibb Pharmaceuticals Ltd)
  Entecavir (as Entecavir monohydrate) **500 microgram** Baraclude 0.5mg tablets | 30 tablet PoM £363.26 DT = £363.26
  Entecavir (as Entecavir monohydrate) **1 mg** Baraclude 1mg tablets | 30 tablet PoM £363.26 DT = £363.26

Telbivudine

- ● **INDICATIONS AND DOSE**

  Chronic hepatitis B infection with compensated liver disease, evidence of viral replication, and histologically documented active liver inflammation or fibrosis, when other treatment is not appropriate
  - ▸ BY MOUTH
  - ▸ Adult: 600 mg once daily

- ● CAUTIONS Lamivudine-resistant chronic hepatitis B—risk of telbivudine resistance

  CAUTIONS, FURTHER INFORMATION Discontinue if deterioration in liver function, hepatic steatosis, progressive hepatomegaly or unexplained lactic acidosis.

- ● INTERACTIONS → Appendix 1: telbivudine
- ● SIDE-EFFECTS
  - ▸ **Common or very common** Abdominal pain · cough · diarrhoea · dizziness · fatigue · headache · nausea · rash
  - ▸ **Uncommon** Arthralgia · malaise · muscle complaints · nerve disorders · pain · sensation abnormal · taste altered
  - ▸ **Rare or very rare** Lactic acidosis
- ● PREGNANCY Manufacturer advises use only if potential benefit outweighs risk.
- ● BREAST FEEDING Manufacturer advises avoid—present in milk in *animal* studies.
- ● RENAL IMPAIRMENT

  Dose adjustments 600 mg every 48 hours if eGFR 30–49 mL/minute/1.73 m^2; 600 mg every 72 hours if eGFR less than 30 mL/minute/1.73 m^2.

- ● MONITORING REQUIREMENTS Monitor liver function tests every 3 months and viral markers of hepatitis B every 3–6 months during treatment (continue monitoring for at least 1 year after discontinuation—recurrent hepatitis may occur on discontinuation.
- ● PATIENT AND CARER ADVICE

  Muscle effects and peripheral neuropathy Patients should be advised to promptly report unexplained muscle pain, tenderness, or weakness, or numbness, tingling or burning sensations.

- ● NATIONAL FUNDING/ACCESS DECISIONS

  NICE decisions
  - ▸ **Telbivudine for chronic hepatitis B (August 2008)** NICE TA154 Telbivudine is not recommended for the treatment of chronic hepatitis B. Patients currently receiving telbivudine can continue treatment until they and their clinician consider it appropriate to stop.
  www.nice.org.uk/TA154

- ● MEDICINAL FORMS
  There can be variation in the licensing of different medicines containing the same drug.
  Tablet
  - ▸ Sebivo (Novartis Pharmaceuticals UK Ltd)
    Telbivudine 600 mg Sebivo 600mg tablets | 28 tablet PoM £290.33

ANTIVIRALS > NUCLEOSIDE REVERSE TRANSCRIPTASE INHIBITORS

⏳ 634

Tenofovir alafenamide

26-Feb-2018

- ● **INDICATIONS AND DOSE**

  Chronic hepatitis B (initiated by a specialist)
  - ▸ BY MOUTH
  - ▸ Adult: 25 mg once daily (for duration of treatment consult product literature)

- ● CAUTIONS Decompensated liver disease · HIV co-infection
- ● INTERACTIONS → Appendix 1: tenofovir alafenamide

- ● SIDE-EFFECTS
  - ▸ **Common or very common** Abdominal distension
  - ▸ **Frequency not known** Hepatitis aggravated (during or following treatment)
- ● BREAST FEEDING Manufacturer advises avoid—present in milk in *animal* studies.
- ● HEPATIC IMPAIRMENT Manufacturer advises monitor hepatic and renal function in decompensated liver disease—risk of adverse effects may be increased (no information available).
- ● PRE-TREATMENT SCREENING Manufacturer advises HIV antibody testing should be offered to those with unknown HIV-1 status before initiation of treatment.
- ● MONITORING REQUIREMENTS Manufacturer advises monitor liver function tests at repeated intervals during treatment and for at least 6 months after last dose—recurrent hepatitis may occur on discontinuation.
- ● PATIENT AND CARER ADVICE

  Missed doses Manufacturer advises if a dose is more than 18 hours late, the missed dose should not be taken and the next dose should be taken at the normal time.

- ● MEDICINAL FORMS
  There can be variation in the licensing of different medicines containing the same drug.
  Tablet
  CAUTIONARY AND ADVISORY LABELS 21
  - ▸ Vemlidy (Gilead Sciences International Ltd) ▼
    Tenofovir alafenamide (as Tenofovir alafenamide fumarate) 25 mg Vemlidy 25mg tablets | 30 tablet PoM £325.73

ANTIVIRALS > NUCLEOTIDE ANALOGUES

Adefovir dipivoxil

- ● **INDICATIONS AND DOSE**

  Chronic hepatitis B infection with either compensated liver disease with evidence of viral replication, and histologically documented active liver inflammation and fibrosis, when other treatment not appropriate or decompensated liver disease in combination with another antiviral for chronic hepatitis B that has no cross-resistance to adefovir
  - ▸ BY MOUTH
  - ▸ Adult: 10 mg once daily

- ● CAUTIONS Elderly

  CAUTIONS, FURTHER INFORMATION Discontinue if deterioration in liver function, hepatic steatosis, progressive hepatomegaly or unexplained lactic acidosis.

- ● INTERACTIONS → Appendix 1: adefovir
- ● SIDE-EFFECTS
  - ▸ **Common or very common** Asthenia · diarrhoea · flatulence · gastrointestinal discomfort · headache · nausea · renal impairment · skin reactions · vomiting
  - ▸ **Frequency not known** Bone fracture · bone pain · hypophosphataemia · myopathy · nephrotoxicity · osteomalacia · pancreatitis · proximal renal tubulopathy
- ● CONCEPTION AND CONTRACEPTION Effective contraception required during treatment.
- ● PREGNANCY Toxicity in *animal* studies—manufacturer advises use only if potential benefit outweighs risk.
- ● BREAST FEEDING Manufacturer advises avoid—no information available.
- ● RENAL IMPAIRMENT No information available if eGFR less than 10 mL/minute/1.73 m^2.

  Dose adjustments 10 mg every 48 hours if eGFR 30–50 mL/minute/1.73 m^2; 10 mg every 72 hours if eGFR 10–30 mL/minute/1.73 m^2.

  Monitoring Monitor renal function more frequently in patients with renal impairment.

5

Infection

- **MONITORING REQUIREMENTS**
- ▶ Monitor liver function tests every 3 months, and viral markers for hepatitis B every 3–6 months during treatment (continue monitoring for at least 1 year after discontinuation—recurrent hepatitis may occur on discontinuation).
- ▶ Monitor renal function before treatment then every 3 months, more frequently in patients receiving nephrotoxic drugs.

- **MEDICINAL FORMS**
  There can be variation in the licensing of different medicines containing the same drug.
  Tablet
  - ▶ Hepsera (Gilead Sciences International Ltd)
    Adefovir dipivoxil 10 mg Hepsera 10mg tablets | 30 tablet [PoM]
    £252.22

IMMUNOSTIMULANTS > INTERFERONS

Peginterferon alfa

- **DRUG ACTION** Polyethylene glycol-conjugated ('pegylated') derivatives of interferon alfa (**peginterferon alfa-2a** and **peginterferon alfa-2b**) are available; pegylation increases the persistence of the interferon in the blood.

- **INDICATIONS AND DOSE**
  PEGASYS ®

  Combined with ribavirin for chronic hepatitis C | Monotherapy for chronic hepatitis C if ribavirin not tolerated or contra-indicated | Monotherapy for chronic hepatitis B
  - ▶ BY SUBCUTANEOUS INJECTION
  - ▶ Adult: (consult product literature)

  VIRAFERONPEG ®

  Combined with ribavirin for chronic hepatitis C | Combined with ribavirin and boceprevir for chronic hepatitis C infection of genotype 1 in patients with compensated liver disease | Monotherapy for chronic hepatitis C if ribavirin not tolerated or contra-indicated
  - ▶ BY SUBCUTANEOUS INJECTION
  - ▶ Adult: (consult product literature)

- **CONTRA-INDICATIONS**
  CONTRA-INDICATIONS, FURTHER INFORMATION
  For contra-indications consult product literature.

- **CAUTIONS**
  CAUTIONS, FURTHER INFORMATION For cautions consult product literature.

- **INTERACTIONS** → Appendix 1: interferons

- **SIDE-EFFECTS**
- ▶ **Common or very common** Alopecia · anaemia · anxiety · appetite abnormal · arrhythmias · arthralgia · arthritis · asthenia · behaviour abnormal · breast pain · chest discomfort · chills · concentration impaired · confusion · constipation · cough · crying · dehydration · depression · diarrhoea · dizziness · drowsiness · dry eye · dry mouth · dysphagia · dysphonia · dyspnoea · ear pain · eye discomfort · eye disorders · eye inflammation · feeling abnormal · fever · gastrointestinal discomfort · gastrointestinal disorders · haemolytic anaemia · haemorrhage · hair texture abnormal · headaches · hearing impairment · hyperbilirubinaemia · hypertension · hyperthyroidism · hyperuricaemia · hypotension · hypothyroidism · increased risk of infection · influenza like illness · leucopenia · lymphadenopathy · malaise · memory loss · menstrual cycle irregularities · mood altered · movement disorders · muscle complaints · muscle weakness · nail disorder · nasal complaints · nausea · neuromuscular dysfunction · neutropenia · oedema · oral

disorders · ovarian disorder · pain · palpitations · photosensitivity reaction · prostatitis · respiratory disorders · sensation abnormal · sepsis · sexual dysfunction · skin reactions · sleep disorders · sweat changes · syncope · taste altered · thirst · throat complaints · thrombocytopenia · tremor · urinary disorders · urine abnormalities · vasodilation · vertigo · vision disorders · vomiting · vulvovaginal disorders · weight decreased
- ▶ **Uncommon** Diabetes mellitus · hallucination · hypersensitivity · hypertriglyceridaemia · myocardial infarction · nerve disorders · pancreatitis · psychosis · sarcoidosis · suicidal tendencies · thyroiditis
- ▶ **Rare or very rare** Angioedema · bone marrow disorders · cardiac inflammation · cardiomyopathy · cerebral ischaemia · CNS haemorrhage · coma · congestive heart failure · embolism and thrombosis · encephalopathy · facial paralysis · ischaemic heart disease · myopathy · renal failure · retinopathy · seizure (more common with high doses in the elderly) · severe cutaneous adverse reactions (SCARs) · systemic lupus erythematosus (SLE) · ulcerative colitis · vasculitis
- ▶ **Frequency not known** Homicidal ideation · pericardial effusion · peripheral ischaemia · pulmonary arterial hypertension · pure red cell aplasia · solid organ transplant rejection

- **CONCEPTION AND CONTRACEPTION** Effective contraception required during treatment—consult product literature.

- **PREGNANCY** Manufacturers recommend avoid unless potential benefit outweighs risk (toxicity in *animal* studies).

- **BREAST FEEDING** Manufacturers advise avoid—no information available.

- **HEPATIC IMPAIRMENT** Avoid in severe impairment.
  Monitoring Close monitoring required in mild to moderate hepatic impairment.

- **RENAL IMPAIRMENT** For further information on peginterferon alfa use in renal impairment consult product literature.
  Dose adjustments Reduce dose in moderate to severe impairment.
  Monitoring Close monitoring required in renal impairment.

- **MONITORING REQUIREMENTS** Monitoring of lipid concentration is recommended.

- **NATIONAL FUNDING/ACCESS DECISIONS**
  NICE decisions
- ▶ **Peginterferon alfa and ribavirin for mild chronic hepatitis C (August 2006 and September 2010)** NICE TA200
  The combination of peginterferon alfa and ribavirin can be used for treating mild chronic hepatitis C in patients over 18 years. Alternatively, treatment can be delayed until the disease has reached a moderate stage ('watchful waiting'). Peginterferon alfa alone can be used if ribavirin is contra-indicated or not tolerated.
  www.nice.org.uk/TA200
- ▶ **Peginterferon alfa, interferon alfa, and ribavirin for moderate to severe chronic hepatitis C (January 2004 and September 2010)** NICE TA200
  The combination of peginterferon alfa and ribavirin should be used for treating moderate to severe chronic hepatitis C in patients aged over 18 years:
  - not previously treated with interferon alfa or peginterferon alfa;
  - treated previously with interferon alfa alone or in combination with ribavirin;
  - whose condition did not respond to peginterferon alfa alone or to a combination of peginterferon alfa and ribavirin, or responded but subsequently relapsed;
  - co-infected with HIV.

Peginterferon alfa alone should be used if ribavirin is contra-indicated or not tolerated. Interferon alfa for either monotherapy or combined therapy should be used only if neutropenia and thrombocytopenia are a particular risk. Patients receiving interferon alfa may be switched to peginterferon alfa.
www.nice.org.uk/TA200

● MEDICINAL FORMS
There can be variation in the licensing of different medicines containing the same drug.

Solution for injection
EXCIPIENTS: May contain Benzyl alcohol
▸ Pegasys (Roche Products Ltd)
Peginterferon alfa-2a 180 microgram per 1 ml Pegasys 90micrograms/0.5ml solution for injection pre-filled syringes | 1 pre-filled disposable injection PoM £76.51
Peginterferon alfa-2a 270 microgram per 1 ml Pegasys 135micrograms/0.5ml solution for injection pre-filled syringes | 1 pre-filled disposable injection PoM £107.76 DT = £107.76
Peginterferon alfa-2a 360 microgram per 1 ml Pegasys 180micrograms/0.5ml solution for injection pre-filled syringes | 4 pre-filled disposable injection PoM £497.60

Powder and solvent for solution for injection
▸ ViraferonPeg (Merck Sharp & Dohme Ltd)
Peginterferon alfa-2b 50 microgram ViraferonPeg 50microgram powder and solvent for solution for injection pre-filled disposable devices CLEARCLICK | 1 pre-filled disposable injection PoM £66.46
Peginterferon alfa-2b 80 microgram ViraferonPeg 80microgram powder and solvent for solution for injection pre-filled disposable devices CLEARCLICK | 1 pre-filled disposable injection PoM £106.34
Peginterferon alfa-2b 100 microgram ViraferonPeg 100microgram powder and solvent for solution for injection pre-filled disposable devices CLEARCLICK | 1 pre-filled disposable injection PoM £132.92
Peginterferon alfa-2b 120 microgram ViraferonPeg 120microgram powder and solvent for solution for injection pre-filled disposable devices CLEARCLICK | 1 pre-filled disposable injection PoM £159.51
Peginterferon alfa-2b 150 microgram ViraferonPeg 150microgram powder and solvent for solution for injection pre-filled disposable devices CLEARCLICK | 1 pre-filled disposable injection PoM £199.38

6.2b Chronic hepatitis C

Other drugs used for Chronic hepatitis C Interferon alfa, p. 930 · Peginterferon alfa, p. 612

ANTIVIRALS 〉 HCV INHIBITORS

Elbasvir with grazoprevir   24-Apr-2017

● DRUG ACTION Elbasvir is an HCV NS5A inhibitor and grazoprevir is an HCV NS3/4A protease inhibitor; they reduce viral load by inhibiting hepatitis C virus RNA replication.

● INDICATIONS AND DOSE
Chronic hepatitis C infection of genotypes 1 or 4 (with or without ribavirin) (initiated by a specialist)
▸ BY MOUTH
▸ Adult: 50/100 mg once daily for 12 weeks (may extend to 16 weeks in some circumstances—consult product literature)
DOSE EQUIVALENCE AND CONVERSION
▸ Dose expressed as x/y mg elbasvir/grazoprevir.

IMPORTANT SAFETY INFORMATION
MHRA/CHM ADVICE: DIRECT-ACTING ANTIVIRALS TO TREAT CHRONIC HEPATITIS C: RISK OF INTERACTION WITH VITAMIN K ANTAGONISTS AND CHANGES IN INR (JANUARY 2017)
An EU-wide review has identified that changes in liver function, secondary to hepatitis C treatment with direct-acting antivirals, may affect the efficacy of vitamin K antagonists; the MHRA has advised that INR should be

monitored closely in patients receiving concomitant treatment.

MHRA/CHM ADVICE: DIRECT-ACTING ANTIVIRAL INTERFERON-FREE REGIMENS TO TREAT CHRONIC HEPATITIS C: RISK OF HEPATITIS B REACTIVATION (JANUARY 2017)
An EU-wide review has concluded that direct-acting antiviral interferon-free regimens for chronic hepatitis C can cause hepatitis B reactivation in patients co-infected with hepatitis B and C viruses; the MHRA recommends to screen patients for hepatitis B before starting treatment—patients infected with both hepatitis B and C viruses must be monitored and managed according to current clinical guidelines.

● CAUTIONS Hepatitis B co-infection · re-treatment following previous exposure to elbasvir with grazoprevir, or to drugs of the same classes (NS5A inhibitors or NS3/4A inhibitors other than telaprevir, simeprevir, boceprevir)—efficacy not demonstrated

● INTERACTIONS → Appendix 1: elbasvir · grazoprevir

● SIDE-EFFECTS
▸ Common or very common Alopecia · anxiety · appetite decreased · arthralgia · asthenia · constipation · depression · diarrhoea · dizziness · dry mouth · gastrointestinal discomfort · headache · insomnia · irritability · myalgia · nausea · pruritus · vomiting
▸ Uncommon Anaemia · transient ischaemic attack

● PREGNANCY Manufacturer advises use only if potential benefit outweighs risk.

● BREAST FEEDING Manufacturer advises avoid—present in milk in *animal* studies.

● HEPATIC IMPAIRMENT Manufacturer advises avoid in moderate-to-severe impairment.

● MONITORING REQUIREMENTS Manufacturer advises monitor liver function before treatment, at week 8 in all patients, at week 12 in patients receiving 16 weeks of treatment, and then as clinically indicated—consider discontinuing treatment if alanine aminotransferase (ALT) is greater than 10 times the upper limit of normal; discontinue treatment if ALT elevation is accompanied by signs or symptoms of hepatic impairment or inflammation.

● PATIENT AND CARER ADVICE
Hepatic effects Manufacturer advises that patients and their carers should consult a healthcare professional if signs and symptoms of hepatic dysfunction occur (including fatigue, weakness, lack of appetite, nausea and vomiting, jaundice or discoloured faeces).
Vomiting Manufacturer advises if vomiting occurs within 4 hours of a dose, an additional dose should be taken.
Missed doses Manufacturer advises if a dose is more than 16 hours late, the missed dose should not be taken and the next dose should be taken at the normal time.

● NATIONAL FUNDING/ACCESS DECISIONS
NICE decisions
▸ Elbasvir–grazoprevir for treating chronic hepatitis C (October 2016) NICE TA413
Elbasvir with grazoprevir is recommended, within its marketing authorisation, as an option for treating genotype 1 or 4 chronic hepatitis C infection:
● of genotype 1a—12 weeks' treatment (consider use in combination with ribavirin for 16 weeks in patients with a baseline hepatitis C virus RNA level of more than 800 000 IU/mL or specific NS5A polymorphisms causing at least a 5-fold reduction in activity of elbasvir);
● of genotype 1b—12 weeks' treatment;
● of genotype 4—12 weeks' treatment (consider use in combination with ribavirin for 16 weeks in patients with a baseline hepatitis C virus RNA level of more than 800 000 IU/mL).

This is contingent on the manufacturer providing the drug at the same price or lower than that agreed with the Commercial Medicines Unit.
www.nice.org.uk/guidance/ta413

Scottish Medicines Consortium (SMC) Decisions
The *Scottish Medicines Consortium* advises (December 2016) that *Zepatier*® (elbasvir with grazoprevir) is accepted for use within NHS Scotland for the treatment of chronic hepatitis C in adults with genotype 1a, 1b or 4; this advice is contingent upon the continuing availability of the Patient Access Scheme in NHS Scotland or a list price that is equivalent or lower.

● MEDICINAL FORMS
There can be variation in the licensing of different medicines containing the same drug.
Tablet
CAUTIONARY AND ADVISORY LABELS 3
ELECTROLYTES: May contain Sodium
▸ Zepatier (Merck Sharp & Dohme Ltd) ▼
  Elbasvir 50 mg, Grazoprevir 100 mg Zepatier 50mg/100mg tablets
  | 28 tablet [PoM] £12,166.67

ANTIVIRALS > NON-STRUCTURAL PROTEIN 5A INHIBITORS

Daclatasvir

11-May-2017

● DRUG ACTION Daclatasvir is an inhibitor of the multifunctional protein NS5A, which is an essential component of the hepatitis C virus replication process.

● INDICATIONS AND DOSE

In combination with sofosbuvir for the treatment of chronic hepatitis C infection of genotypes 1 or 4, with or without compensated cirrhosis | In combination with sofosbuvir and ribavirin for the treatment of chronic hepatitis C infection of genotype 3 in patients who are treatment experienced, with or without compensated cirrhosis | In combination with peginterferon alfa and ribavirin for the treatment of chronic hepatitis C infection of genotype 4
▸ BY MOUTH
▸ Adult: Usual dose 60 mg once daily (for duration of treatment consult product literature)
DOSE ADJUSTMENTS DUE TO INTERACTIONS
▸ Manufacturer advises reduce dose to 30 mg once daily with concurrent use of some of the potent CYP3A4 inhibitors—consult product literature.
▸ Manufacturer advises increase dose to 90 mg once daily with bosentan.

IMPORTANT SAFETY INFORMATION
MHRA/CHM ADVICE: DIRECT-ACTING ANTIVIRALS TO TREAT CHRONIC HEPATITIS C: RISK OF INTERACTION WITH VITAMIN K ANTAGONISTS AND CHANGES IN INR (JANUARY 2017)
An EU-wide review has identified that changes in liver function, secondary to hepatitis C treatment with direct-acting antivirals, may affect the efficacy of vitamin K antagonists; the MHRA has advised that INR should be monitored closely in patients receiving concomitant treatment.

MHRA/CHM ADVICE: DIRECT-ACTING ANTIVIRAL INTERFERON-FREE REGIMENS TO TREAT CHRONIC HEPATITIS C: RISK OF HEPATITIS B REACTIVATION (JANUARY 2017)
An EU-wide review has concluded that direct-acting antiviral interferon-free regimens for chronic hepatitis C can cause hepatitis B reactivation in patients co-infected with hepatitis B and C viruses; the MHRA recommends to screen patients for hepatitis B before starting treatment—patients infected with both hepatitis B and C

viruses must be monitored and managed according to current clinical guidelines.

● CAUTIONS Decompensated liver disease · hepatitis B virus co-infection · human immunodeficiency virus co-infection · organ transplant patients · retreatment—efficacy not established in patients with prior exposure to a NS5A inhibitor

● INTERACTIONS → Appendix 1: daclatasvir

● SIDE-EFFECTS
▸ **Common or very common** Abdominal pain · alopecia · anaemia · appetite decreased · arthralgia · constipation · cough · diarrhoea · dizziness · dry mouth · dyspnoea · fatigue · gastrointestinal disorders · headaches · hot flush · insomnia · irritability · myalgia · nasal congestion · nausea · skin reactions · vomiting
▸ **Frequency not known** Atrioventricular block · bradycardia
SIDE-EFFECTS, FURTHER INFORMATION Side-effects listed are reported when daclatasvir is used in combination with sofosbuvir with or without ribavirin or with ribavirin and peginterferon alfa.

● CONCEPTION AND CONTRACEPTION Highly effective contraception required during and for 5 weeks after treatment.

● PREGNANCY Manufacturer advises avoid (toxicity in *animal* studies).

● BREAST FEEDING Manufacturer advises avoid—present in milk in *animal* studies.

● PATIENT AND CARER ADVICE
Missed doses If a dose is more than 20 hours late, the missed dose should not be taken and the next dose should be taken at the normal time.
Driving and skilled tasks May affect performance of skilled tasks (e.g. driving).

● NATIONAL FUNDING/ACCESS DECISIONS
NICE decisions
▸ Daclatasvir for treating chronic hepatitis C (November 2015) NICE TA364
Daclatasvir in combination with sofosbuvir or peginterferon alfa, and with/without ribavirin, is recommended as an option for the treatment of chronic hepatitis C infection of genotypes 1, 3 or 4 in adults, depending on the level of fibrosis **and** only if the manufacturer provides daclatasvir at the same price or lower than agreed with the Commercial Medicines Unit.
www.nice.org.uk/TA364

Scottish Medicines Consortium (SMC) Decisions
The *Scottish Medicines Consortium* has advised (November 2014) that daclatasvir (*Daklinza*®) is accepted for restricted use within NHS Scotland for the treatment of chronic hepatitis C virus infection in patients with significant fibrosis (Metavir score F3–F4) or compensated cirrhosis.

● MEDICINAL FORMS
There can be variation in the licensing of different medicines containing the same drug.
Tablet
CAUTIONARY AND ADVISORY LABELS 25
▸ Daklinza (Bristol-Myers Squibb Pharmaceuticals Ltd) ▼
  Daclatasvir (as Daclatasvir dihydrochloride) 30 mg Daklinza 30mg tablets | 28 tablet [PoM] £8,172.61
  Daclatasvir (as Daclatasvir dihydrochloride) 60 mg Daklinza 60mg tablets | 28 tablet [PoM] £8,172.61

Ombitasvir with paritaprevir and ritonavir

14-Feb-2017

The properties listed below are those particular to the combination only. For the properties of the components please consider, ritonavir p. 646.

● **INDICATIONS AND DOSE**

Chronic hepatitis C of genotype 1 (in combination with dasabuvir, with or without ribavirin) | Chronic hepatitis C of genotype 4 (in combination with ribavirin)

▶ BY MOUTH
  ▸ Adult: 2 tablets once daily for duration of treatment consult product literature, to be taken with food

---

● **IMPORTANT SAFETY INFORMATION**

MHRA/CHM ADVICE: DIRECT-ACTING ANTIVIRALS TO TREAT CHRONIC HEPATITIS C: RISK OF INTERACTION WITH VITAMIN K ANTAGONISTS AND CHANGES IN INR (JANUARY 2017)

An EU-wide review has identified that changes in liver function, secondary to hepatitis C treatment with direct-acting antivirals, may affect the efficacy of vitamin K antagonists; the MHRA has advised that INR should be monitored closely in patients receiving concomitant treatment.

MHRA/CHM ADVICE: DIRECT-ACTING ANTIVIRAL INTERFERON-FREE REGIMENS TO TREAT CHRONIC HEPATITIS C: RISK OF HEPATITIS B REACTIVATION (JANUARY 2017)

An EU-wide review has concluded that direct-acting antiviral interferon-free regimens for chronic hepatitis C can cause hepatitis B reactivation in patients co-infected with hepatitis B and C viruses; the MHRA recommends to screen patients for hepatitis B before starting treatment—patients infected with both hepatitis B and C viruses must be monitored and managed according to current clinical guidelines.

● CONTRA-INDICATIONS HIV co-infection without suppressive antiretroviral therapy
● CAUTIONS Retreatment—efficacy not established
● INTERACTIONS → Appendix 1: HIV-protease inhibitors · ombitasvir · paritaprevir
● SIDE-EFFECTS
▶ **Common or very common** Anaemia · asthenia · insomnia · nausea · pruritus
▶ **Rare or very rare** Angioedema
▶ **Frequency not known** Depression · suicidal behaviour
  SIDE-EFFECTS, FURTHER INFORMATION Side-effects listed are reported when ombitasvir with paritaprevir and ritonavir is used in combination with dasabuvir, with or without ribavirin.
● CONCEPTION AND CONTRACEPTION For women of child-bearing potential, exclude pregnancy before initiation of treatment; effective contraception should be used during treatment.
● PREGNANCY Manufacturer advises avoid—toxicity in *animal* studies.
● BREAST FEEDING Manufacturer advises avoid—present in milk in *animal* studies.
● HEPATIC IMPAIRMENT Manufacturer advises avoid in moderate or severe impairment.
● PATIENT AND CARER ADVICE
  Missed doses If a dose is more than 12 hours late, the missed dose should not be taken and the next dose should be taken at the normal time.

● NATIONAL FUNDING/ACCESS DECISIONS

NICE decisions

▶ **Ombitasvir with paritaprevir and ritonavir with or without dasabuvir for treating chronic hepatitis C** NICE TA365
  Ombitasvir with paritaprevir and ritonavir with or without dasabuvir is recommended, within its marketing authorisation, as an option for treating genotype 1 or 4 chronic hepatitis C in adults, only if the manufacturer provides it with the discount agreed in the patient access scheme.
  www.nice.org.uk/guidance/ta365

● MEDICINAL FORMS
There can be variation in the licensing of different medicines containing the same drug.

Tablet
CAUTIONARY AND ADVISORY LABELS 21, 25
EXCIPIENTS: May contain Propylene glycol
▶ Viekirax (AbbVie Ltd) ▼
  Ombitasvir 12.5 mg, Ritonavir 50 mg, Paritaprevir 75 mg Viekirax 12.5mg/75mg/50mg tablets | 56 tablet [PoM] £10,733.33

ANTIVIRALS > NUCLEOSIDE ANALOGUES

Ribavirin

(Tribavirin)

● **INDICATIONS AND DOSE**

Bronchiolitis

▶ BY INHALATION OF AEROSOL, OR BY INHALATION OF NEBULISED SOLUTION
  ▸ Child 1–23 months: Inhale a solution containing 20 mg/mL for 12–18 hours for at least 3 days, maximum of 7 days, to be administered via small particle aerosol generator

Life-threatening RSV, parainfluenza virus, and adenovirus infection in immunocompromised children (administered on expert advice)

▶ BY INTRAVENOUS INFUSION
  ▸ Child: 33 mg/kg for 1 dose, to be administered over 15 minutes, then 16 mg/kg every 6 hours for 4 days, then 8 mg/kg every 8 hours for 3 days

COPEGUS® TABLETS

Chronic hepatitis C (in combination with direct acting antivirals, or interferon alfa 2a, or peginterferon alfa 2a with or without direct acting antivirals)

▶ BY MOUTH
  ▸ Adult (body-weight up to 75 kg): 400 mg, dose to be taken in the morning and 600 mg, dose to be taken in the evening
  ▸ Adult (body-weight 75 kg and above): 600 mg twice daily

Chronic hepatitis C (in combination with peginterferon alfa 2b with or without direct acting antivirals)

▶ BY MOUTH
  ▸ Adult (body-weight up to 65 kg): 400 mg twice daily
  ▸ Adult (body-weight 65–80 kg): 400 mg, to be taken in the morning and 600 mg, to be taken in the evening
  ▸ Adult (body-weight 81–105 kg): 600 mg twice daily
  ▸ Adult (body-weight 106 kg and above): 600 mg, to be taken in the morning and 800 mg, to be taken in the evening

Chronic hepatitis C genotype 2 or 3 (not previously treated), or patients infected with HIV and hepatitis C (in combination with peginterferon alfa)

▶ BY MOUTH
  ▸ Adult: Usual dose 400 mg twice daily

continued →

REBETOL ® CAPSULES

Chronic hepatitis C (in combination with interferon alfa 2b, or peginterferon alfa 2b with or without boceprevir)
▸ BY MOUTH
▸ Adult (body-weight up to 65 kg): 400 mg twice daily
▸ Adult (body-weight 65-80 kg): 400 mg, dose to be taken in the morning and 600 mg, dose to be taken in the evening
▸ Adult (body-weight 81-104 kg): 600 mg twice daily
▸ Adult (body-weight 105 kg and above): 600 mg, dose to be taken in the morning and 800 mg, dose to be taken in the evening

REBETOL ® ORAL SOLUTION

Chronic hepatitis C (in combination with interferon alfa 2b, or peginterferon alfa 2b with or without boceprevir)
▸ BY MOUTH
▸ Adult (body-weight up to 65 kg): 400 mg twice daily
▸ Adult (body-weight 65-80 kg): 400 mg daily, dose to be taken in the morning and 600 mg daily, dose to be taken in the evening
▸ Adult (body-weight 81-104 kg): 600 mg twice daily
▸ Adult (body-weight 105 kg and above): 600 mg daily, dose to be taken in the morning and 800 mg daily, dose to be taken in the evening

● **UNLICENSED USE** Inhalation licensed for use in children (age range not specified by manufacturer). Intravenous preparation not licensed.

● **CONTRA-INDICATIONS**
▸ With systemic use Active severe psychiatric condition (in children) · autoimmune disease (in children) · autoimmune hepatitis (in children) · consult product literature for specific contra-indications when ribavirin used in combination with other medicinal products · haemoglobinopathies · history of severe psychiatric condition (in children) · severe cardiac disease (in adults) · severe debilitating medical conditions · severe, uncontrolled cardiac disease in children with chronic hepatitis C · unstable or uncontrolled cardiac disease in previous 6 months (in adults)

● **CAUTIONS**
▸ When used by inhalation Maintain standard supportive respiratory and fluid management therapy
▸ With systemic use Anaemia (haemoglobin concentration should be monitored during the treatment and corrective action taken) (in adults) · cardiac disease (assessment including ECG recommended before and during treatment—discontinue if deterioration) · consult product literature for specific cautions when ribavirin used in combination with other medicinal products · gout (in adults) · haemolysis (haemoglobin concentration should be monitored during the treatment and corrective action taken) (in adults) · patients with a transplant—risk of rejection · risk of growth retardation in children, the reversibility of which is uncertain—if possible, consider starting treatment after pubertal growth spurt · severe dental disorders (in adults) · severe ocular disorders (in adults) · severe periodontal disorders (in adults) · severe psychiatric effects (in adults)

● **INTERACTIONS** → Appendix 1: ribavirin

● **SIDE-EFFECTS**
▸ **Common or very common** Alopecia · anaemia · anxiety · appetite decreased · arrhythmias · arthralgia · arthritis · asthenia · behaviour abnormal · chest pain · chills · concentration impaired · constipation · cough · depression · diarrhoea · dizziness · drowsiness · dry mouth · dysphagia · dyspnoea · ear pain · eye disorders · eye inflammation · eye pain · fever · gastrointestinal discomfort · gastrointestinal disorders · haemorrhage · headaches · hearing impairment · hyperthyroidism · hypotension · hypothyroidism · increased risk of infection · influenza like illness ·

lymphadenopathy · malaise · memory loss · mood altered · muscle complaints · muscle weakness · nasal congestion · nausea · neutropenia · oral disorders · pain · palpitations · peripheral oedema · photosensitivity reaction · respiratory disorders · sensation abnormal · sexual dysfunction · skin reactions · sleep disorders · sweat changes · syncope · taste altered · thirst · throat pain · thrombocytopenia · tremor · vasodilation · vertigo · vision disorders · vomiting · weight decreased
▸ **Uncommon** Dehydration · diabetes mellitus · hallucination · hepatic disorders · hypertension · nerve disorders · sarcoidosis · suicidal tendencies · thyroiditis
▸ **Rare or very rare** Angina pectoris · angioedema · bone marrow disorders · cardiac inflammation · cerebral ischaemia · cholangitis · coma · congestive heart failure · facial paralysis · hypersensitivity · intracranial haemorrhage · myocardial infarction · myopathy · pancreatitis · psychotic disorder · pulmonary embolism · retinopathy · seizure · severe cutaneous adverse reactions (SCARs) · systemic lupus erythematosus (SLE) · vasculitis
▸ **Frequency not known** Haemolytic anaemia · homicidal ideation · nephrotic syndrome · pure red cell aplasia · renal failure · solid organ transplant rejection · ulcerative colitis
SIDE-EFFECTS, FURTHER INFORMATION Side effects listed are reported when oral ribavirin is used in combination with peginterferon alfa or interferon alfa, consult product literature for details.

● **CONCEPTION AND CONTRACEPTION**
▸ With systemic use Exclude pregnancy before treatment in females of childbearing age. Effective contraception essential during treatment and for 4 months after treatment in females and for 7 months after treatment in males of childbearing age. Routine monthly pregnancy tests recommended. Condoms must be used if partner of male patient is pregnant (ribavirin excreted in semen).
▸ When used by inhalation Women planning pregnancy should avoid exposure to aerosol.

● **PREGNANCY** Avoid; teratogenicity in *animal* studies.
▸ When used by inhalation Pregnant women should avoid exposure to aerosol.

● **BREAST FEEDING** Avoid—no information available.

● **HEPATIC IMPAIRMENT** Avoid oral ribavirin in severe hepatic dysfunction or decompensated cirrhosis.
Dose adjustments No dosage adjustment required.

● **RENAL IMPAIRMENT** Plasma-ribavirin concentration increased.
▸ In adults Manufacturer advises avoid oral ribavirin unless essential if eGFR less than 50 mL/minute/1.73 m^2—monitor haemoglobin concentration closely.
▸ In children Manufacturer advises avoid oral ribavirin if estimated glomerular filtration rate less than 50 mL/minute/1.73 m^2—monitor haemoglobin concentration closely. Manufacturer advises use intravenous preparation with caution if estimated glomerular filtration rate less than 30 mL/minute/1.73 m^2.

● **MONITORING REQUIREMENTS**
▸ When used by inhalation Monitor electrolytes closely. Monitor equipment for precipitation.
▸ With systemic use in children Determine full blood count, platelets, electrolytes, serum creatinine, liver function tests and uric acid before starting treatment and then on weeks 2 and 4 of treatment, then as indicated clinically—adjust dose if adverse reactions or laboratory abnormalities develop (consult product literature).

Test thyroid function before treatment and then every 3 months.

- With systemic use in adults Determine full blood count, platelets, electrolytes, glucose, serum creatinine, liver function tests and uric acid before starting treatment and then on weeks 2 and 4 of treatment, then as indicated clinically—adjust dose if adverse reactions or laboratory abnormalities develop (consult product literature).
- PRESCRIBING AND DISPENSING INFORMATION Flavours of oral liquid formulations may include bubble-gum.
- NATIONAL FUNDING/ACCESS DECISIONS

NICE decisions
- Peginterferon alfa and ribavirin for mild chronic hepatitis C (August 2006 and September 2010) NICE TA200
The combination of peginterferon alfa and ribavirin can be used for treating mild chronic hepatitis C in patients over 18 years. Alternatively, treatment can be delayed until the disease has reached a moderate stage ('watchful waiting').
www.nice.org.uk/TA200
- Peginterferon alfa, interferon alfa, and ribavirin for moderate to severe chronic hepatitis C (January 2004 and September 2010) NICE TA200
The combination of peginterferon alfa and ribavirin should be used for treating moderate to severe chronic hepatitis C in patients aged over 18 years:
  - not previously treated with interferon alfa or peginterferon alfa;
  - treated previously with interferon alfa alone or in combination with ribavirin;
  - whose condition did not respond to peginterferon alfa alone or to a combination of peginterferon alfa and ribavirin, or responded but subsequently relapsed;
  - co-infected with HIV.
Peginterferon alfa alone should be used if ribavirin is contra-indicated or not tolerated. Interferon alfa for either monotherapy or combined therapy should be used only if neutropenia and thrombocytopenia are a particular risk. Patients receiving interferon alfa may be switched to peginterferon alfa.
www.nice.org.uk/TA200
- LESS SUITABLE FOR PRESCRIBING Ribavirin inhalation is less suitable for prescribing.

- MEDICINAL FORMS
There can be variation in the licensing of different medicines containing the same drug.
Solution for injection
- Virazole (Meda Pharmaceuticals Ltd)
Ribavirin 100 mg per 1 ml Virazole 1.2g/12ml solution for injection vials | 5 vial PoM £3,600.00
Oral solution
CAUTIONARY AND ADVISORY LABELS 21
- Rebetol (Merck Sharp & Dohme Ltd)
Ribavirin 40 mg per 1 ml Rebetol 40mg/ml oral solution | 100 ml PoM £67.08
Tablet
CAUTIONARY AND ADVISORY LABELS 21
- Copegus (Roche Products Ltd)
Ribavirin 200 mg Copegus 200mg tablets | 112 tablet PoM £233.58 | 168 tablet PoM £350.37
Ribavirin 400 mg Copegus 400mg tablets | 56 tablet PoM £233.58
Capsule
CAUTIONARY AND ADVISORY LABELS 21
- Rebetol (Merck Sharp & Dohme Ltd)
Ribavirin 200 mg Rebetol 200mg capsules | 84 capsule PoM £160.69 | 140 capsule PoM £267.81 | 168 capsule PoM £321.38

ANTIVIRALS > NUCLEOTIDE ANALOGUES

Ledipasvir with sofosbuvir 09-Nov-2017

The properties listed below are those particular to the combination only. For the properties of the components please consider, sofosbuvir p. 618.
- DRUG ACTION Sofosbuvir is a nucleotide analogue inhibitor and ledipasvir is an HCV inhibitor; they reduce viral load by inhibiting hepatitis C virus RNA replication.

- INDICATIONS AND DOSE
Chronic hepatitis C infection (initiated by a specialist)
- BY MOUTH
- Adult: 90/400 mg once daily, for duration of treatment consult product literature
DOSE ADJUSTMENTS DUE TO INTERACTIONS
- Manufacturer advises reduce dose of concurrent H_2-receptor antagonist if above a dose comparable to famotidine 40 mg twice daily.
- Manufacturer advises reduce dose of concurrent proton pump inhibitor if above a dose comparable to omeprazole 20 mg; take at the same time as sofosbuvir with ledipasvir.
DOSE EQUIVALENCE AND CONVERSION
- Dose expressed as x/y mg ledipasvir/sofosbuvir.

- CAUTIONS Retreatment following treatment failure—efficacy not established
- INTERACTIONS → Appendix 1: ledipasvir · sofosbuvir
- SIDE-EFFECTS
- **Common or very common** Fatigue · headache · rash
- **Frequency not known** Angioedema · arrhythmia
- PRESCRIBING AND DISPENSING INFORMATION Dispense in original container (contains desiccant).
- PATIENT AND CARER ADVICE
Vomiting If vomiting occurs within 5 hours of administration, an additional dose should be taken.
Missed doses If a dose is more than 18 hours late, the missed dose should not be taken and the next dose should be taken at the normal time.
- NATIONAL FUNDING/ACCESS DECISIONS

NICE decisions
- Ledipasvir with sofosbuvir for the treatment of chronic hepatitis C (November 2015) NICE TA363
Ledipasvir with sofosbuvir is recommended as an option for treating adults with chronic hepatitis C infection:
  - of genotype 1 without cirrhosis (treatment naive patients)—8 weeks' treatment
  - of genotype 1 or 4 with cirrhosis (treatment naive patients)—12 weeks' treatment
  - of genotype 1 or 4 without cirrhosis (or with cirrhosis but only if the person has a low risk of the disease getting worse) that has not responded adequately to previous treatment—12 weeks' treatment
In addition, ledipasvir with sofosbuvir is only recommended in patients with cirrhosis for the durations mentioned above if the following criteria are met:
  - Child-Pugh class A
  - platelet count of $75\,000/mm^3$ or more
  - no features of portal hypertension
  - no history of an HCV-associated decompensation episode
  - not previously treated with an NS5A inhibitor
Patients whose treatment with ledipasvir with sofosbuvir is not recommended in this NICE guidance, but was started within the NHS before this guidance was published, should be able to continue treatment until they and their clinician consider it appropriate to stop.
www.nice.org.uk/TA363

5

Infection

The *Scottish Medicines Consortium* has advised (March and September 2015) that *Harvoni®* (ledipasvir with sofosbuvir) is accepted for restricted use within NHS Scotland for the treatment of chronic hepatitis C infection of genotypes 1, 3 and 4 only, in patients who are ineligible for, or unable to tolerate, interferon.

● MEDICINAL FORMS
There can be variation in the licensing of different medicines containing the same drug.
Tablet
CAUTIONARY AND ADVISORY LABELS 25
▸ Harvoni (Gilead Sciences International Ltd) ▼
  Ledipasvir 90 mg, Sofosbuvir 400 mg Harvoni 90mg/400mg tablets | 28 tablet PoM £12,993.33

Sofosbuvir
09-Nov-2017

● INDICATIONS AND DOSE
Chronic hepatitis C infection
▸ BY MOUTH
▸ Adult: 400 mg once daily, for duration of treatment consult product literature

IMPORTANT SAFETY INFORMATION
MHRA/CHM ADVICE: DIRECT-ACTING ANTIVIRALS TO TREAT CHRONIC HEPATITIS C: RISK OF INTERACTION WITH VITAMIN K ANTAGONISTS AND CHANGES IN INR (JANUARY 2017)
An EU-wide review has identified that changes in liver function, secondary to hepatitis C treatment with direct-acting antivirals, may affect the efficacy of vitamin K antagonists; the MHRA has advised that INR should be monitored closely in patients receiving concomitant treatment.

MHRA/CHM ADVICE: DIRECT-ACTING ANTIVIRAL INTERFERON-FREE REGIMENS TO TREAT CHRONIC HEPATITIS C: RISK OF HEPATITIS B REACTIVATION (JANUARY 2017)
An EU-wide review has concluded that direct-acting antiviral interferon-free regimens for chronic hepatitis C can cause hepatitis B reactivation in patients co-infected with hepatitis B and C viruses; the MHRA recommends to screen patients for hepatitis B before starting treatment—patients infected with both hepatitis B and C viruses must be monitored and managed according to current clinical guidelines.

● CAUTIONS
CAUTIONS, FURTHER INFORMATION Manufacturer advises in chronic hepatitis C of genotype 1, 4, 5, or 6, only use sofosbuvir with ribavirin dual therapy in those with intolerance or contra-indications to peginterferon alfa who require urgent treatment.
● INTERACTIONS → Appendix 1: sofosbuvir
● SIDE-EFFECTS
▸ Common or very common Alopecia · anaemia · anxiety · appetite decreased · arthralgia · asthenia · chest pain · chills · concentration impaired · constipation · cough · depression · diarrhoea · dizziness · dry mouth · dyspnoea · fever · gastrointestinal discomfort · gastrooesophageal reflux disease · headaches · influenza like illness · insomnia · irritability · memory loss · muscle complaints · nasopharyngitis · nausea · neutropenia · pain · skin reactions · vision blurred · vomiting · weight decreased
▸ Frequency not known Arrhythmia
SIDE-EFFECTS, FURTHER INFORMATION Side-effects listed are reported when sofosbuvir is used in combination with ribavirin or with ribavirin and peginterferon alfa.

● PREGNANCY Manufacturer advises avoid—limited information available.
● BREAST FEEDING Manufacturer advises avoid—present in milk in *animal* studies.
● RENAL IMPAIRMENT Safety and efficacy not established if eGFR less than 30 mL/minute/1.73 m^2—accumulation may occur.
● PRESCRIBING AND DISPENSING INFORMATION Dispense in original container (contains desiccant).
● PATIENT AND CARER ADVICE
Missed doses Manufacturer advises if a dose is more than 18 hours late, the missed dose should not be taken and the next dose should be taken at the normal time.
● NATIONAL FUNDING/ACCESS DECISIONS
NICE decisions
▸ Sofosbuvir for treating chronic hepatitis C (February 2015) NICE TA330
Sofosbuvir in combination with peginterferon alfa and ribavirin is an option for treating adults with chronic hepatitis C infection:
● of genotype 1
● of genotype 3 with cirrhosis (treatment naive patients)
● of genotype 3 that has not adequately responded to interferon-based treatment
● of genotype 4, 5, or 6 with cirrhosis
Sofosbuvir in combination with ribavirin is an option for treating adults with chronic hepatitis C infection:
● of genotype 2 who are intolerant to or ineligible for interferon (treatment naive patients)
● of genotype 2 that has not adequately responded to interferon-based treatment
● of genotype 3 with cirrhosis who are intolerant to or ineligible for interferon (treatment naive patients)
● of genotype 3 with cirrhosis that has not adequately responded to interferon-based treatment
www.nice.org.uk/TA330
▸ Sofosbuvir for treating chronic hepatitis C (February 2015) NICE TA330
Sofosbuvir in combination with ribavirin is not recommended for the treatment of adults with chronic hepatitis C infection of genotypes 1, 4, 5, or 6.
www.nice.org.uk/TA330
Scottish Medicines Consortium (SMC) Decisions
The *Scottish Medicines Consortium* has advised (June 2014) that sofosbuvir (*Sovaldi®*) is accepted for use within NHS Scotland for the treatment of chronic hepatitis C infection of genotypes 1 to 6; its use in combination with ribavirin as dual therapy for chronic hepatitis C infection of either genotype 2 (in treatment naive patients) or genotype 3 is restricted to those who cannot use peginterferon alfa because of intolerance or contra-indications.

● MEDICINAL FORMS
There can be variation in the licensing of different medicines containing the same drug.
Tablet
CAUTIONARY AND ADVISORY LABELS 21, 25
▸ Sovaldi (Gilead Sciences International Ltd) ▼
  Sofosbuvir 400 mg Sovaldi 400mg tablets | 28 tablet PoM £11,660.98

Sofosbuvir with velpatasvir   24-Jul-2017

The properties listed below are those particular to the combination only. For the properties of the components please consider, sofosbuvir p. 618.

- **DRUG ACTION** Sofosbuvir is a nucleotide analogue inhibitor and velpatasvir is an HCV inhibitor; they reduce viral load by inhibiting hepatitis C virus RNA replication.

- **INDICATIONS AND DOSE**

Chronic hepatitis C infection, with or without ribavirin (initiated by a specialist)
▸ BY MOUTH
▸ Adult: 400/100 mg once daily for 12 weeks (may extend to 24 weeks in some circumstances—consult product literature)

DOSE ADJUSTMENTS DUE TO INTERACTIONS
▸ Manufacturer advises reduce dose of concurrent H_2-receptor antagonist if above a dose comparable to famotidine 40 mg twice daily.
▸ Manufacturer advises reduce dose of concurrent proton pump inhibitor if above a dose comparable to omeprazole 20 mg; take 4 hours after sofosbuvir with velpatasvir.

DOSE EQUIVALENCE AND CONVERSION
▸ Dose expressed as x/y mg sofosbuvir/velpatasvir.

- **CAUTIONS** Hepatitis B co-infection
- **INTERACTIONS** → Appendix 1: sofosbuvir · velpatasvir
- **SIDE-EFFECTS** Atrioventricular block · bradycardia · fatigue · headache · nausea
- **PATIENT AND CARER ADVICE**
Vomiting Manufacturer advises if vomiting occurs within 3 hours of administration, an additional dose should be taken.
- **NATIONAL FUNDING/ACCESS DECISIONS**

NICE decisions
▸ Sofosbuvir–velpatasvir for treating chronic hepatitis C (January 2017) NICE TA430
Sofosbuvir with velpatasvir is recommended as an option for treating chronic hepatitis C infection in adults, if the following criteria are met:
- of genotype 1, 3, 4, 5 or 6 with or without cirrhosis (previously treated or treatment naive patients);
- of genotype 2 with cirrhosis (previously treated or treatment naive patients);
- of genotype 2 without cirrhosis (treatment naive patients), only if interferon not suitable or not tolerated, or without cirrhosis (previously treated patients).
This is contingent on the manufacturer providing the drug with the discount agreed in the simple discount agreement.
    Patients whose treatment was started within the NHS before this guidance was published, should continue treatment until they and their clinician consider it appropriate to stop.
www.nice.org.uk/guidance/ta430
Scottish Medicines Consortium (SMC) Decisions
SMC No. 1195/16
The *Scottish Medicines Consortium* has advised (November 2016) that sofosbuvir with velpatasvir (*Epclusa* ®) is accepted for restricted use within NHS Scotland for the treatment of adults with chronic hepatitis C infection of genotype 3 only.
SMC No. 1271/17
    The *Scottish Medicines Consortium* has advised (October 2017) that sofosbuvir with velpatasvir (*Epclusa* ®) is accepted for restricted use within NHS Scotland for the treatment of chronic hepatitis C virus (HCV) infection in adults with genotype 2, 5 or 6 or decompensated cirrhosis, irrespective of chronic HCV genotype. This advice is

contingent upon the continuing availability of the patient access scheme in NHS Scotland or a list price that is equivalent or lower.
SMC No. 1271/17
    The *Scottish Medicines Consortium* has advised (April 2018) that sofosbuvir with velpatasvir (*Epclusa* ®) is accepted for restricted use within NHS Scotland for the treatment of chronic hepatitis C virus (HCV) infection in adults with genotype 1 or 4. This advice is contingent upon the continuing availability of the patient access scheme in NHS Scotland or a list price that is equivalent or lower.

- **MEDICINAL FORMS**
There can be variation in the licensing of different medicines containing the same drug.
Tablet
CAUTIONARY AND ADVISORY LABELS 25
▸ Epclusa (Gilead Sciences International Ltd) ▼
    Velpatasvir 100 mg, Sofosbuvir 400 mg Epclusa 400mg/100mg tablets | 28 tablet [PoM] £12,993.33

Sofosbuvir with velpatasvir and voxilaprevir   19-Mar-2018

The properties listed below are those particular to the combination only. For the properties of the components please consider, sofosbuvir p. 618.

- **INDICATIONS AND DOSE**

Chronic hepatitis C infection (specialist use only)
▸ BY MOUTH
▸ Adult: 1 tablet once daily, for duration of treatment, consult product literature

DOSE ADJUSTMENTS DUE TO INTERACTIONS
▸ Manufacturer advises reduce dose of concurrent H_2-receptor antagonist if above a dose comparable to famotidine 40 mg twice daily.
▸ Manufacturer advises reduce dose of concurrent proton pump inhibitor if above a dose comparable to omeprazole 20 mg.

- **CAUTIONS** Hepatitis B co-infection
- **INTERACTIONS** → Appendix 1: sofosbuvir · velpatasvir · voxilaprevir
- **HEPATIC IMPAIRMENT** Manufacturer advises avoid in moderate-to-severe impairment.
- **PATIENT AND CARER ADVICE**
Vomiting Manufacturer advises if vomiting occurs within 4 hours of administration, an additional dose should be taken.
- **NATIONAL FUNDING/ACCESS DECISIONS**

NICE decisions
▸ Sofosbuvir–velpatasvir–voxilaprevir for treating chronic hepatitis C (February 2018) NICE TA507
Sofosbuvir with velpatasvir and voxilaprevir is recommended as an option for treating adults with chronic hepatitis C infection:
- of genotype 1 to 6 with or without compensated cirrhosis (previously treated with direct-acting antivirals)—recommended for 12 weeks, *or*
- of genotype 3 with or without compensated cirrhosis (no treatment history with direct-acting antivirals)—recommended for 8 weeks, **and**
- the manufacturer provides the drug at the same price or lower than that agreed with the Commercial Medicines Unit.
Patients whose treatment was started within the NHS before this guidance was published should have the option to continue treatment, without change to their funding

arrangements, until they and their NHS clinician consider it appropriate to stop.
www.nice.org.uk/guidance/ta507

Scottish Medicines Consortium (SMC) Decisions
SMC No. 1317/18
The *Scottish Medicines Consortium* has advised (April 2018) that sofosbuvir with velpatasvir and voxilaprevir (*Vosevi*®) is accepted for restricted use within NHS Scotland for the treatment of chronic hepatitis C virus (HCV) infection in adults who:

- have failed to achieve a sustained virologic response (SVR) with a direct-acting anti-viral (DAA), **or**
- are DAA-naive, have genotype 3 (GT3) HCV infection, with or without cirrhosis, and are suitable for treatment with an eight-week course.

This advice is contingent upon the continuing availability of the patient access scheme in NHS Scotland or a list price that is equivalent or lower.

- MEDICINAL FORMS
There can be variation in the licensing of different medicines containing the same drug.
Tablet
CAUTIONARY AND ADVISORY LABELS 21, 25
▸ Vosevi (Gilead Sciences International Ltd) ▼
Velpatasvir 100 mg, Voxilaprevir 100 mg, Sofosbuvir 400 mg Vosevi 400mg/100mg/100mg tablets | 28 tablet PoM £14,942.33

ANTIVIRALS ⟩ PROTEASE INHIBITORS

Glecaprevir with pibrentasvir   25-Oct-2017

- INDICATIONS AND DOSE
Chronic hepatitis C (specialist use only)
▸ BY MOUTH
▸ Adult: 300/120 mg once daily, for duration of treatment, consult product literature
DOSE EQUIVALENCE AND CONVERSION
▸ Dose expressed as x/y mg glecaprevir/pibrentasvir.

IMPORTANT SAFETY INFORMATION
HEPATITIS B INFECTION
Cases of hepatitis B reactivation, sometimes fatal, have been reported in patients co-infected with hepatitis B and C viruses; manufacturer advises to assess patients for hepatitis B prior to initiation of therapy and manage according to current clinical guidelines.

- CAUTIONS Hepatitis B infection · post-liver transplant patients · re-treatment of patients with prior exposure to NS3/4A- or NS5A-inhibitors—efficacy not established
- INTERACTIONS → Appendix 1: glecaprevir · pibrentasvir
- SIDE-EFFECTS
▸ Common or very common Asthenia · diarrhoea · headache · nausea
▸ Frequency not known Pruritus · transient ischaemic attack
- PREGNANCY Manufacturer advises avoid—limited information available.
- BREAST FEEDING Manufacturer advises avoid—present in milk in *animal* studies.
- HEPATIC IMPAIRMENT Manufacturer advises avoid in moderate-to-severe impairment.
- PATIENT AND CARER ADVICE
Missed doses Manufacturer advises if a dose is more than 18 hours late, the missed dose should not be taken and the next dose should be taken at the normal time.

- NATIONAL FUNDING/ACCESS DECISIONS
NICE decisions
▸ Glecaprevir–pibrentasvir for treating chronic hepatitis C (January 2018) NICE TA499
Glecaprevir with pibrentasvir is recommended, within its marketing authorisation, as an option for treating chronic hepatitis C in adults, only if the manufacturer provides the drug at the same price or lower than that agreed with the Commercial Medicines Unit.
www.nice.org.uk/guidance/ta499

Scottish Medicines Consortium (SMC) Decisions
The *Scottish Medicines Consortium* has advised (November 2017) that glecaprevir with pibrentasvir (*Maviret*®) is accepted for use within NHS Scotland for the treatment of chronic hepatitis C virus (HCV) infection in adults. This advice is contingent upon the continuing availability of the patient access scheme in NHS Scotland or a list price that is equivalent or lower.

- MEDICINAL FORMS
There can be variation in the licensing of different medicines containing the same drug.
Tablet
CAUTIONARY AND ADVISORY LABELS 21, 25
▸ Maviret (AbbVie Ltd) ▼
Pibrentasvir 40 mg, Glecaprevir 100 mg Maviret 100mg/40mg tablets | 84 tablet PoM £12,993.66

Simeprevir   14-Feb-2017

- INDICATIONS AND DOSE
In combination with ribavirin and peginterferon alfa for chronic hepatitis C infection of genotype 1 or 4 | In combination with sofosbuvir (with or without ribavirin) for urgent treatment of chronic hepatitis C infection of genotype 1 or 4 when peginterferon alfa cannot be used because of intolerance or contra-indications
▸ BY MOUTH
▸ Adult: 150 mg once daily (for duration of treatment consult product literature)

IMPORTANT SAFETY INFORMATION
MHRA/CHM ADVICE: DIRECT-ACTING ANTIVIRALS TO TREAT CHRONIC HEPATITIS C: RISK OF INTERACTION WITH VITAMIN K ANTAGONISTS AND CHANGES IN INR (JANUARY 2017)
An EU-wide review has identified that changes in liver function, secondary to hepatitis C treatment with direct-acting antivirals, may affect the efficacy of vitamin K antagonists; the MHRA has advised that INR should be monitored closely in patients receiving concomitant treatment.

MHRA/CHM ADVICE: DIRECT-ACTING ANTIVIRAL INTERFERON-FREE REGIMENS TO TREAT CHRONIC HEPATITIS C: RISK OF HEPATITIS B REACTIVATION (JANUARY 2017)
An EU-wide review has concluded that direct-acting antiviral interferon-free regimens for chronic hepatitis C can cause hepatitis B reactivation in patients co-infected with hepatitis B and C viruses; the MHRA recommends to screen patients for hepatitis B before starting treatment—patients infected with both hepatitis B and C viruses must be monitored and managed according to current clinical guidelines.

- CAUTIONS Consider alternative treatment in presence of NS3 Q80K polymorphism—efficacy of simeprevir is reduced · patients of East Asian origin
- INTERACTIONS → Appendix 1: simeprevir
- SIDE-EFFECTS
▸ Common or very common Constipation · dyspnoea · nausea · photosensitivity reaction · skin reactions

SIDE-EFFECTS, FURTHER INFORMATION Monitor rash for deterioration if mild or moderate; discontinue if severe.

- CONCEPTION AND CONTRACEPTION Effective contraception essential during treatment.
- PREGNANCY Manufacturer advises use only if potential benefit outweighs risk—toxicity in *animal* studies.
- BREAST FEEDING Manufacturer advises avoid—present in plasma of breast-fed *animals*.
- HEPATIC IMPAIRMENT Manufacturer advises caution in moderate to severe impairment—elimination reduced in severe impairment. Manufacturer advises caution in decompensated cirrhosis—elimination reduced in severe impairment.
- RENAL IMPAIRMENT Manufacturer advises caution if eGFR less than 30 mL/minute/1.73 m² —elimination may be reduced.
- PRE-TREATMENT SCREENING Test for NS3 Q80K polymorphism before combination treatment with ribavirin and peginterferon alfa in patients with chronic hepatitis C infection of genotype 1a. Consider testing for NS3 Q80K polymorphism before combination treatment with sofosbuvir (with or without ribavirin) in patients with chronic hepatitis C infection of genotype 1a.
- PATIENT AND CARER ADVICE
  Missed doses If a dose is more than 12 hours late, the missed dose should not be taken and the next dose should be taken at the normal time.
- NATIONAL FUNDING/ACCESS DECISIONS
  NICE decisions
  ▶ **Simeprevir in combination with peginterferon alfa and ribavirin for treating genotypes 1 and 4 chronic hepatitis C (February 2015)** NICE TA331
  Simeprevir in combination with peginterferon alfa and ribavirin, is recommended within its marketing authorisation, as an option for the treatment of chronic hepatitis C infection of genotype 1 and 4 in adults.
  www.nice.org.uk/TA331

- MEDICINAL FORMS
  No licensed medicines listed.

ANTIVIRALS > OTHER

Dasabuvir

14-Feb-2017

- DRUG ACTION Dasabuvir is a non-nucleoside inhibitor of hepatitis C virus polymerase NS5B, which is an essential component of the hepatitis C virus replication process.

- **INDICATIONS AND DOSE**
  Chronic hepatitis C infection of genotype 1, in combination with other antiviral drugs (ombitasvir with paritaprevir and ritonavir, with or without ribavirin)
  ▶ BY MOUTH
  ▶ Adult: 250 mg twice daily for details of duration of treatment, consult product literature, dose to be taken in the morning and evening

  IMPORTANT SAFETY INFORMATION
  MHRA/CHM ADVICE: DIRECT-ACTING ANTIVIRALS TO TREAT CHRONIC HEPATITIS C: RISK OF INTERACTION WITH VITAMIN K ANTAGONISTS AND CHANGES IN INR (JANUARY 2017)
  A EU-wide review has identified that changes in liver function, secondary to hepatitis C treatment with direct-acting antivirals, may affect the efficacy of vitamin K antagonists; the MHRA has advised that INR should be monitored closely in patients receiving concomitant treatment.

MHRA/CHM ADVICE: DIRECT-ACTING ANTIVIRAL INTERFERON-FREE REGIMENS TO TREAT CHRONIC HEPATITIS C: RISK OF HEPATITIS B REACTIVATION (JANUARY 2017)
An EU-wide review has concluded that direct-acting antiviral interferon-free regimens for chronic hepatitis C can cause hepatitis B reactivation in patients co-infected with hepatitis B and C viruses; the MHRA recommends to screen patients for hepatitis B before starting treatment—patients infected with both hepatitis B and C viruses must be monitored and managed according to current clinical guidelines.

- CONTRA-INDICATIONS HIV co-infection without suppressive antiretroviral therapy
- CAUTIONS Retreatment—efficacy not established
- INTERACTIONS → Appendix 1: dasabuvir
- SIDE-EFFECTS
  ▶ **Common or very common** Anaemia · asthenia · insomnia · nausea · pruritus
  ▶ **Rare or very rare** Angioedema
  ▶ **Frequency not known** Depression · suicidal ideation
  SIDE-EFFECTS, FURTHER INFORMATION Side-effects listed are reported when dasabuvir is used in combination with Viekirax (ombitasvir with paritaprevir and ritonavir), with or without ribavirin.
- PREGNANCY Manufacturer advises avoid—no information available.
- BREAST FEEDING Manufacturer advises avoid—present in milk in *animal* studies.
- HEPATIC IMPAIRMENT Manufacturer advises avoid in moderate to severe impairment.
- PATIENT AND CARER ADVICE
  Missed doses If a dose is more than 6 hours late, the missed dose should not be taken and the next dose should be taken at the normal time.
- NATIONAL FUNDING/ACCESS DECISIONS
  NICE decisions
  ▶ **Ombitasvir with paritaprevir and ritonavir with or without dasabuvir for treating chronic hepatitis C (November 2015)** NICE TA365
  Dasabuvir, in combination with ombitasvir with paritaprevir and ritonavir p. 615, is recommended, within its marketing authorisation, as an option for treating genotype 1 or 4 chronic hepatitis C in adults only if the manufacturer provides it with the discount agreed in the patient access scheme.
  www.nice.org.uk/guidance/ta365

- MEDICINAL FORMS
  There can be variation in the licensing of different medicines containing the same drug.
  Tablet
  CAUTIONARY AND ADVISORY LABELS 3, 21, 25
  ▶ Exviera (AbbVie Ltd) ▼
    Dasabuvir (as Dasabuvir sodium monohydrate) 250 mg Exviera 250mg tablets | 56 tablet [PoM] £933.33

6.3 Herpesvirus infections

Herpesvirus infections

Herpes simplex and varicella–zoster infection

The two most important herpesvirus pathogens are herpes simplex virus (herpesvirus hominis) and varicella–zoster virus.

Herpes simplex infections

Herpes infection of the mouth and lips and in the eye is generally associated with herpes simplex virus serotype 1

(HSV-1); other areas of the skin may also be infected, especially in immunodeficiency. Genital infection is most often associated with HSV-2 and also HSV-1. Treatment of herpes simplex infection should start as early as possible and usually within 5 days of the appearance of the infection.

In individuals with good immune function, mild infection of the eye (ocular herpes) and of the lips (herpes labialis or cold sores) is treated with a topical antiviral drug. Primary herpetic gingivostomatitis is managed by changes to diet and with analgesics. Severe infection, neonatal herpes infection or infection in immunocompromised individuals requires treatment with a systemic antiviral drug. Primary or recurrent genital herpes simplex infection is treated with an antiviral drug given by mouth. Persistence of a lesion or recurrence in an immunocompromised patient may signal the development of resistance.

Specialist advice should be sought for systemic treatment of herpes simplex infection in pregnancy.

Varicella-zoster infections

Regardless of immune function and the use of any immunoglobulins, neonates with *chickenpox* should be treated with a parenteral antiviral to reduce the risk of severe disease. Oral therapy in children is not recommended as absorption is variable. Chickenpox in otherwise healthy children between 1 month and 12 years is usually mild and antiviral treatment is not usually required.

Chickenpox is more severe in adolescents and adults than in children; antiviral treatment started within 24 hours of the onset of rash may reduce the duration and severity of symptoms in otherwise healthy adults and adolescents. Antiviral treatment is generally recommended in immunocompromised patients and those at special risk (e.g. because of severe cardiovascular or respiratory disease or chronic skin disorder); in such cases, an antiviral is given for 10 days with at least 7 days of parenteral treatment.

Pregnant women who develop severe chickenpox may be at risk of complications, especially varicella pneumonia. Specialist advice should be sought for the treatment of chickenpox during pregnancy.

Those who have been exposed to chickenpox and are at special risk of complications may require prophylaxis with varicella-zoster immunoglobulin (see under Disease Specific Immunoglobulins).

In *herpes zoster* (shingles) systemic antiviral treatment can reduce the severity and duration of pain, reduce complications, and reduce viral shedding. Treatment with the antiviral should be started within 72 hours of the onset of rash and is usually continued for 7–10 days. Immunocompromised patients at high risk of disseminated or severe infection should be treated with a parenteral antiviral drug.

Chronic pain which persists after the rash has healed (postherpetic neuralgia) requires specific management.

Choice

Aciclovir p. 623 is active against herpesviruses but does not eradicate them. Uses of aciclovir include systemic treatment of varicella–zoster and the systemic and topical treatment of herpes simplex infections of the skin and mucous membranes. It is used by mouth for severe herpetic stomatitis. Aciclovir eye ointment is used for herpes simplex infections of the eye; it is combined with systemic treatment for ophthalmic zoster.

Famciclovir p. 625, a prodrug of penciclovir, is similar to aciclovir and is licensed for use in herpes zoster and genital herpes.

Valaciclovir p. 625 is an ester of aciclovir, licensed for herpes zoster and herpes simplex infections of the skin and mucous membranes (including genital herpes); it is also licensed for preventing cytomegalovirus disease following solid organ transplantation. Famciclovir or valaciclovir are suitable alternatives to aciclovir for oral lesions associated with herpes zoster. Valaciclovir once daily may reduce the risk of transmitting genital herpes to heterosexual partners—specialist advice should be sought.

Foscarnet sodium p. 628 is used for mucocutaneous herpes simplex virus infection unresponsive to aciclovir in immunocompromised patients; it is toxic and can cause renal impairment.

Inosine pranobex below has been used by mouth for herpes simplex infections; its effectiveness remains unproven.

Cytomegalovirus infection

Ganciclovir p. 626 is related to aciclovir but it is more active against cytomegalovirus (CMV); it is also much more toxic than aciclovir and should therefore be prescribed only when the potential benefit outweighs the risks. Ganciclovir is administered by intravenous infusion for the *initial treatment* of CMV infection. Ganciclovir causes profound myelosuppression when given with zidovudine p. 642; the two should not normally be given together particularly during initial ganciclovir therapy. The likelihood of ganciclovir resistance increases in patients with a high viral load or in those who receive the drug over a long duration.

Valaciclovir is licensed for prevention of cytomegalovirus disease following renal transplantation.

Valganciclovir p. 627 is an ester of ganciclovir which is licensed for the *initial treatment* and *maintenance treatment* of CMV retinitis in AIDS patients. Valganciclovir is also licensed for preventing CMV disease following solid organ transplantation from a cytomegalovirus-positive donor.

Foscarnet sodium is also active against cytomegalovirus; it is toxic and can cause renal impairment.

See local treatment of CMV retinitis.

ANTIVIRALS > INOSINE COMPLEXES

Inosine pranobex

(Inosine acedoben dimepranol)

● **INDICATIONS AND DOSE**

Mucocutaneous herpes simplex

▶ BY MOUTH
▶ Adult: 1 g 4 times a day for 7–14 days

Adjunctive treatment of genital warts

▶ BY MOUTH
▶ Adult: 1 g 3 times a day for 14–28 days

Subacute sclerosing panencephalitis

▶ BY MOUTH
▶ Adult: 50–100 mg/kg daily in 6 divided doses

● CAUTIONS History of gout · history of hyperuricaemia

● SIDE-EFFECTS Arthralgia · constipation · diarrhoea · drowsiness · epigastric discomfort · fatigue · headache · insomnia · malaise · nausea · nervousness · polyuria · skin reactions · vertigo · vomiting

● PREGNANCY Manufacturer advises avoid.

● RENAL IMPAIRMENT Manufacturer advises caution; metabolised to uric acid.

● LESS SUITABLE FOR PRESCRIBING Inosine pranobex is less suitable for prescribing.

● MEDICINAL FORMS
There can be variation in the licensing of different medicines containing the same drug.

Tablet

CAUTIONARY AND ADVISORY LABELS 9

▶ Imunovir (KoRa Healthcare)
  Inosine acedoben dimepranol 500 mg Imunovir 500mg tablets |
  100 tablet [PoM] £39.50

ANTIVIRALS > NUCLEOSIDE ANALOGUES

Aciclovir
(Acyclovir)

● INDICATIONS AND DOSE

Herpes simplex, suppression
▸ BY MOUTH
▸ Child 12-17 years: 400 mg twice daily, alternatively 200 mg 4 times a day; increased to 400 mg 3 times a day, dose may be increased if recurrences occur on standard suppressive therapy or for suppression of genital herpes during late pregnancy (from 36 weeks gestation), therapy interrupted every 6–12 months to reassess recurrence frequency—consider restarting after two or more recurrences
▸ Adult: 400 mg twice daily, alternatively 200 mg 4 times a day; increased to 400 mg 3 times a day, dose may be increased if recurrences occur on standard suppressive therapy or for suppression of genital herpes during late pregnancy (from 36 weeks gestation), therapy interrupted every 6–12 months to reassess recurrence frequency—consider restarting after two or more recurrences

Herpes simplex, prophylaxis in the immunocompromised
▸ BY MOUTH
▸ Child 1–23 months: 100–200 mg 4 times a day
▸ Child 2-17 years: 200–400 mg 4 times a day
▸ Adult: 200–400 mg 4 times a day
▸ BY INTRAVENOUS INFUSION
▸ Adult: 5 mg/kg every 8 hours

Herpes simplex, treatment (non-genital)
▸ BY MOUTH
▸ Adult: 200 mg 5 times a day usually for 5 days (longer if new lesions appear during treatment or if healing incomplete)

Herpes simplex, treatment (non-genital) in immunocompromised or if absorption impaired
▸ BY MOUTH
▸ Adult: 400 mg 5 times a day usually for 5 days (longer if new lesions appear during treatment or if healing incomplete)

Herpes simplex, treatment
▸ BY MOUTH
▸ Child 1-23 months: 100 mg 5 times a day usually for 5 days (longer if new lesions appear during treatment or if healing incomplete)
▸ Child 2-17 years: 200 mg 5 times a day usually for 5 days (longer if new lesions appear during treatment or if healing incomplete)

Herpes simplex, treatment, in immunocompromised or if absorption impaired
▸ BY MOUTH
▸ Child 1-23 months: 200 mg 5 times a day usually for 5 days (longer if new lesions appear during treatment or if healing incomplete)
▸ Child 2-17 years: 400 mg 5 times a day usually for 5 days (longer if new lesions appear during treatment or if healing incomplete)

Genital herpes simplex, treatment of first episode
▸ BY MOUTH
▸ Adult: 200 mg 5 times a day, alternatively 400 mg 3 times a day both courses usually for 5 days (longer if new lesions appear during treatment or if healing incomplete)

Genital herpes simplex, treatment of first episode, in immunocompromised or HIV-positive
▸ BY MOUTH
▸ Adult: 400 mg 5 times a day for 7–10 days (longer if new lesions appear during treatment or if healing incomplete)

Severe genital herpes simplex, treatment, initial infection | Treatment of herpes simplex in the immunocompromised
▸ BY INTRAVENOUS INFUSION
▸ Adult: Initially 5 mg/kg every 8 hours usually for 5 days, alternatively 10 mg/kg every 8 hours for at least 14 days in encephalitis (at least 21 days if also immunocompromised)—confirm cerebrospinal fluid negative for herpes simplex virus before stopping treatment, higher dose to be used only if resistant organisms suspected or in simplex encephalitis

Genital herpes simplex, treatment of recurrent infection
▸ BY MOUTH
▸ Adult: 800 mg 3 times a day for 2 days, alternatively 200 mg 5 times a day for 5 days, alternatively 400 mg 3 times a day for 3–5 days

Genital herpes simplex, treatment of recurrent infection in immunocompromised or HIV-positive patients
▸ BY MOUTH
▸ Adult: 400 mg 3 times a day for 5–10 days

Varicella zoster (chickenpox), treatment | Herpes zoster (shingles), treatment
▸ BY MOUTH
▸ Child 1–23 months: 200 mg 4 times a day for 5 days
▸ Child 2-5 years: 400 mg 4 times a day for 5 days
▸ Child 6–11 years: 800 mg 4 times a day for 5 days
▸ Child 12-17 years: 800 mg 5 times a day for 7 days
▸ Adult: 800 mg 5 times a day for 7 days
▸ BY INTRAVENOUS INFUSION
▸ Adult: 5 mg/kg every 8 hours usually for 5 days

Varicella zoster (chickenpox), treatment in immunocompromised | Herpes zoster (shingles), treatment in immunocompromised
▸ BY INTRAVENOUS INFUSION
▸ Adult: 10 mg/kg every 8 hours usually for 5 days

Herpes zoster (shingles), treatment in immunocompromised
▸ BY MOUTH
▸ Child 1–23 months: 200 mg 4 times a day continued for 2 days after crusting of lesions
▸ Child 2-5 years: 400 mg 4 times a day continued for 2 days after crusting of lesions
▸ Child 6-11 years: 800 mg 4 times a day continued for 2 days after crusting of lesions
▸ Child 12-17 years: 800 mg 5 times a day continued for 2 days after crusting of lesions
▸ Adult: 800 mg 5 times a day continued for 2 days after crusting of lesions

Herpes zoster, treatment in encephalitis | Varicella zoster, treatment in encephalitis
▸ BY INTRAVENOUS INFUSION
▸ Adult: 10 mg/kg every 8 hours given for 10–14 days in encephalitis, possibly longer if also immunocompromised or if severe infection

Varicella zoster (chickenpox), attenuation of infection if varicella–zoster immunoglobulin not indicated
▸ BY MOUTH
▸ Child: 10 mg/kg 4 times a day for 7 days, to be started 1 week after exposure
▸ Adult: 10 mg/kg 4 times a day for 7 days, to be started 1 week after exposure continued →

5

Infection

5

Infection

DOSES AT EXTREMES OF BODY-WEIGHT
▸ To avoid excessive dosage in obese patients parenteral dose should be calculated on the basis of ideal weight for height.

● **UNLICENSED USE** Tablets and suspension not licensed for suppression of herpes simplex or for treatment of herpes zoster in children (age range not specified by manufacturer).
▸ With oral use Aciclovir doses in BNF may differ from those in product literature. Attenuation of chickenpox is an unlicensed indication.

● **CAUTIONS**
▸ With systemic use Elderly (risk of neurological reactions) · maintain adequate hydration (especially with infusion or high doses)

● **INTERACTIONS** → Appendix 1: aciclovir

● **SIDE-EFFECTS**
▸ **Common or very common** Nausea · photosensitivity reaction · skin reactions · vomiting
▸ **Uncommon** Abdominal pain · anaemia · diarrhoea · dizziness · fatigue · fever · headache · leucopenia · thrombocytopenia
▸ **Rare or very rare** Alopecia · agitation · angioedema · ataxia · coma · confusion · drowsiness · dysarthria · dyspnoea · encephalopathy · hallucination · hepatic disorders · psychosis · renal impairment · renal pain · seizure · tremor
▸ **Frequency not known** Crystalluria

● **PREGNANCY** Not known to be harmful—manufacturers advise use only when potential benefit outweighs risk.

● **BREAST FEEDING** Significant amount in milk after systemic administration—not known to be harmful but manufacturer advises caution.

● **RENAL IMPAIRMENT** Risk of neurological reactions increased. Maintain adequate hydration (especially during renal impairment).
Dose adjustments ▸ With intravenous use Use normal intravenous dose every 12 hours if eGFR 25–50 mL/minute/1.73 m^2 (every 24 hours if eGFR 10–25 mL/minute/1.73 m^2). Consult product literature for intravenous dose if eGFR less than 10 mL/minute/1.73 m^2.
▸ With oral use in adults For *herpes zoster*, use normal oral dose every 8 hours if eGFR 10–25 mL/minute/1.73 m^2 (every 12 hours if eGFR less than 10 mL/minute/1.73 m^2). For *herpes simplex*, use normal oral dose every 12 hours if eGFR less than 10 mL/minute/1.73 m^2.
▸ With oral use in children For *herpes zoster*, use normal oral dose every 8 hours if estimated glomerular filtration rate 10–25 mL/minute/1.73 m^2 (every 12 hours if estimated glomerular filtration rate less than 10 mL/minute/1.73 m^2). For *herpes simplex*, use normal dose every 12 hours if estimated glomerular filtration rate less than 10 mL/minute/1.73 m^2.

● **DIRECTIONS FOR ADMINISTRATION** For *intravenous infusion Zovirax IV®*, *Aciclovir IV* (Genus), give intermittently *in* Sodium chloride 0.9% *or* Sodium chloride and glucose; initially reconstitute to 25 mg/mL in water for injection or sodium chloride 0.9% then dilute to not more than 5 mg/mL with the infusion fluid; to be given over 1 hour; alternatively, may be administered in a concentration of 25 mg/mL using a suitable infusion pump and given over 1 hour; for *Aciclovir IV* (Hospira) dilute to not more than 5 mg/mL with infusion fluid; give over 1 hour.

● **PRESCRIBING AND DISPENSING INFORMATION** Flavours of oral liquid preparations may include banana, or orange.

● **PATIENT AND CARER ADVICE**
Medicines for Children leaflet: Aciclovir (oral) for viral infections www.medicinesforchildren.org.uk/aciclovir-for-viral-infections

● **PROFESSION SPECIFIC INFORMATION**
Dental practitioners' formulary
Aciclovir Tablets 200 mg or 800 mg may be prescribed.
Aciclovir Oral Suspension 200 mg/5mL may be prescribed.

● **MEDICINAL FORMS**
There can be variation in the licensing of different medicines containing the same drug.

Tablet
CAUTIONARY AND ADVISORY LABELS 9
▸ Aciclovir (Non-proprietary)
Aciclovir 200 mg Aciclovir 200mg tablets | 25 tablet PoM £10.00 DT = £0.83
Aciclovir 400 mg Aciclovir 400mg tablets | 56 tablet PoM £15.00 DT = £2.39
Aciclovir 800 mg Aciclovir 800mg tablets | 35 tablet PoM £20.00 DT = £2.88

Dispersible tablet
CAUTIONARY AND ADVISORY LABELS 9
▸ Aciclovir (Non-proprietary)
Aciclovir 200 mg Aciclovir 200mg dispersible tablets | 25 tablet PoM £0.86 DT = £0.86
Aciclovir 400 mg Aciclovir 400mg dispersible tablets | 56 tablet PoM £20.00 DT = £11.98
Aciclovir 800 mg Aciclovir 800mg dispersible tablets | 35 tablet PoM £65.00 DT = £10.98
▸ Zovirax (GlaxoSmithKline UK Ltd)
Aciclovir 200 mg Zovirax 200mg dispersible tablets | 25 tablet PoM £2.85 DT = £0.86
Aciclovir 800 mg Zovirax 800mg dispersible tablets | 35 tablet PoM £10.50 DT = £10.98

Oral suspension
CAUTIONARY AND ADVISORY LABELS 9
▸ Aciclovir (Non-proprietary)
Aciclovir 40 mg per 1 ml Aciclovir 200mg/5ml oral suspension sugar free sugar-free | 125 ml PoM £35.76 DT = £35.76
Aciclovir 80 mg per 1 ml Aciclovir 400mg/5ml oral suspension sugar free sugar-free | 100 ml PoM £39.47 DT = £39.47
▸ Zovirax (GlaxoSmithKline UK Ltd)
Aciclovir 40 mg per 1 ml Zovirax 200mg/5ml oral suspension sugar-free | 125 ml PoM £29.56 DT = £35.76
Aciclovir 80 mg per 1 ml Zovirax Double Strength 400mg/5ml oral suspension sugar-free | 100 ml PoM £33.02 DT = £39.47

Solution for infusion
ELECTROLYTES: May contain Sodium
▸ Aciclovir (Non-proprietary)
Aciclovir (as Aciclovir sodium) 25 mg per 1 ml Aciclovir 1g/40ml solution for infusion vials | 1 vial PoM £40.00 (Hospital only)
Aciclovir 250mg/10ml concentrate for solution for infusion vials | 5 vial PoM £50.00 (Hospital only) | 5 vial PoM £9.00
Aciclovir 500mg/20ml solution for infusion vials | 5 vial PoM £100.00 (Hospital only) | 5 vial PoM £18.00
Aciclovir 500mg/20ml concentrate for solution for infusion vials | 5 vial PoM £18.00 (Hospital only)

Powder for solution for infusion
ELECTROLYTES: May contain Sodium
▸ Aciclovir (Non-proprietary)
Aciclovir (as Aciclovir sodium) 250 mg Aciclovir 250mg powder for solution for infusion vials | 5 vial PoM £49.30
▸ Zovirax I.V. (GlaxoSmithKline UK Ltd)
Aciclovir (as Aciclovir sodium) 250 mg Zovirax I.V. 250mg powder for solution for infusion vials | 5 vial PoM £16.70
Aciclovir (as Aciclovir sodium) 500 mg Zovirax I.V. 500mg powder for solution for infusion vials | 5 vial PoM £17.00

Famciclovir

- **INDICATIONS AND DOSE**

Herpes zoster infection, treatment
▸ BY MOUTH
▸ Adult: 500 mg 3 times a day for 7 days, alternatively 750 mg 1–2 times a day for 7 days

Herpes zoster infection, treatment in immunocompromised patients
▸ BY MOUTH
▸ Adult: 500 mg 3 times a day for 10 days, continue for 2 days after crusting of lesions

Genital herpes, suppression
▸ BY MOUTH
▸ Adult: 250 mg twice daily, therapy to be interrupted every 6–12 months to reassess recurrence frequency— consider restarting after two or more recurrences

Genital herpes, suppression in immunocompromised or HIV-positive patients
▸ BY MOUTH
▸ Adult: 500 mg twice daily, therapy to be interrupted every 6–12 months to reassess recurrence frequency— consider restarting after two or more recurrences

Genital herpes infection, treatment of first episode
▸ BY MOUTH
▸ Adult: 250 mg 3 times a day for 5 days or longer if new lesions appear during treatment or if healing incomplete

Genital herpes infection, treatment of first episode in immunocompromised or HIV-positive patients
▸ BY MOUTH
▸ Adult: 500 mg twice daily for 10 days

Genital herpes infection, treatment of recurrent infection
▸ BY MOUTH
▸ Adult: 125 mg twice daily for 5 days, alternatively 1 g twice daily for 1 day

Genital herpes infection, treatment of recurrent infections in immunocompromised or HIV-positive patients
▸ BY MOUTH
▸ Adult: 500 mg twice daily for 5–10 days

Herpes simplex infection (non-genital), treatment in immunocompromised patients
▸ BY MOUTH
▸ Adult: 500 mg twice daily for 7 days

- **UNLICENSED USE** Famciclovir doses in BNF may differ from those in product literature.
- **SIDE-EFFECTS**
▸ **Common or very common** Abdominal pain · diarrhoea · dizziness · headache · nausea · skin reactions · vomiting
▸ **Uncommon** Angioedema · confusion · drowsiness
▸ **Rare or very rare** Hallucination · jaundice cholestatic · palpitations · thrombocytopenia
- **PREGNANCY** Manufacturers advise avoid unless potential benefit outweighs risk.
- **BREAST FEEDING** No information available—present in milk in *animal* studies.
- **HEPATIC IMPAIRMENT** Usual dose in well compensated liver disease (information not available on decompensated).
- **RENAL IMPAIRMENT**
  Dose adjustments Reduce dose; consult product literature.
- **PRESCRIBING AND DISPENSING INFORMATION** Famciclovir is a pro-drug of penciclovir.

- **MEDICINAL FORMS**
There can be variation in the licensing of different medicines containing the same drug. Forms available from special-order manufacturers include: tablet

Tablet
CAUTIONARY AND ADVISORY LABELS 9
▸ Famciclovir (Non-proprietary)
  Famciclovir **125 mg** Famciclovir 125mg tablets | 10 tablet [PoM] £36.72 DT = £36.66
  Famciclovir **250 mg** Famciclovir 250mg tablets | 15 tablet [PoM] £88.53–£110.97 | 21 tablet [PoM] £155.87 DT = £155.28 | 56 tablet [PoM] £330.52–£414.29
  Famciclovir **500 mg** Famciclovir 500mg tablets | 14 tablet [PoM] £181.17 DT = £177.08 | 30 tablet [PoM] £265.54
▸ Famvir (Novartis Pharmaceuticals UK Ltd)
  Famciclovir **125 mg** Famvir 125mg tablets | 10 tablet [PoM] £53.45 DT = £36.66
  Famciclovir **250 mg** Famvir 250mg tablets | 15 tablet [PoM] £160.34 | 21 tablet [PoM] £187.04 DT = £155.28 | 56 tablet [PoM] £598.56
  Famciclovir **500 mg** Famvir 500mg tablets | 14 tablet [PoM] £249.43 DT = £177.08 | 30 tablet [PoM] £641.21

Valaciclovir

- **INDICATIONS AND DOSE**

Herpes zoster infection, treatment
▸ BY MOUTH
▸ Adult: 1 g 3 times a day for 7 days

Herpes zoster infection, treatment in immunocompromised patients
▸ BY MOUTH
▸ Adult: 1 g 3 times a day for at least 7 days and continued for 2 days after crusting of lesions

Herpes simplex, treatment of first infective episode
▸ BY MOUTH
▸ Adult: 500 mg twice daily for 5 days (longer if new lesions appear during treatment or healing is incomplete)

Herpes simplex infections treatment of first episode in immunocompromised or HIV-positive patients
▸ BY MOUTH
▸ Adult: 1 g twice daily for 10 days

Herpes simplex, treatment of recurrent infections
▸ BY MOUTH
▸ Adult: 500 mg twice daily for 3–5 days

Treatment of recurrent herpes simplex infections in immunocompromised or HIV-positive patients
▸ BY MOUTH
▸ Adult: 1 g twice daily for 5–10 days

Herpes labialis treatment
▸ BY MOUTH
▸ Child 12–17 years: Initially 2 g, then 2 g after 12 hours
▸ Adult: Initially 2 g, then 2 g after 12 hours

Herpes simplex, suppression of infections
▸ BY MOUTH
▸ Adult: 500 mg daily in 1–2 divided doses, therapy to be interrupted every 6–12 months to reassess recurrence frequency—consider restarting after two or more recurrences

Herpes simplex, suppression of infections in immunocompromised or HIV-positive patients
▸ BY MOUTH
▸ Adult: 500 mg twice daily, therapy to be interrupted every 6–12 months to reassess recurrence frequency— consider restarting after two or more recurrences

Genital herpes, reduction of transmission (administered on expert advice)
▸ BY MOUTH
▸ Adult: 500 mg once daily, to be taken by the infected partner continued →

5

Infection

5

Infection

Prevention of cytomegalovirus disease following solid organ transplantation when valganciclovir or ganciclovir cannot be used
▸ BY MOUTH
▸ Adult: 2 g 4 times a day usually for 90 days, preferably starting within 72 hours of transplantation

● CAUTIONS Elderly (risk of neurological reactions) · maintain adequate hydration (especially with high doses)
● INTERACTIONS → Appendix 1: valaciclovir
● SIDE-EFFECTS
▸ **Common or very common** Diarrhoea · dizziness · headache · nausea · photosensitivity reaction · skin reactions · vomiting
▸ **Uncommon** Abdominal discomfort · agitation · confusion · dyspnoea · haematuria · hallucination · leucopenia · level of consciousness decreased · renal pain · thrombocytopenia · tremor
▸ **Rare or very rare** Angioedema · ataxia · coma · delirium · dysarthria · encephalopathy · nephrolithiasis · psychosis · renal impairment · seizure
▸ **Frequency not known** Microangiopathic haemolytic anaemia

SIDE-EFFECTS, FURTHER INFORMATION Neurological reactions more frequent with higher doses.

● PREGNANCY Not known to be harmful—manufacturers advise use only when potential benefit outweighs risk.
● BREAST FEEDING Significant amount in milk after systemic administration—not known to be harmful but manufacturer advises caution.
● HEPATIC IMPAIRMENT Manufacturer advises caution with high doses used for herpes labialis and prevention of cytomegalovirus disease—no information available.
● RENAL IMPAIRMENT Maintain adequate hydration.
Dose adjustments ▸ In adults For *herpes zoster*, 1 g every 12 hours if eGFR 30–50 mL/minute/1.73 m^2 (1 g every 24 hours if eGFR 10– 30 mL/minute/1.73 m^2; 500 mg every 24 hours if eGFR less than 10 mL/minute/1.73 m^2). For *treatment of herpes simplex*, 500 mg (1 g in immunocompromised or HIV-positive patients) every 24 hours if eGFR less than 30 mL/minute/1.73 m^2. For *treatment of herpes labialis*, if eGFR 30–50 mL/minute/1.73 m^2, initially 1 g, then 1 g 12 hours after initial dose (if eGFR 10–30 mL/minute/1.73 m^2, initially 500 mg, then 500 mg 12 hours after initial dose; if eGFR less than 10 mL/minute/1.73 m^2, 500 mg as a single dose). For *suppression of herpes simplex*, 250 mg (500 mg in immunocompromised or HIV-positive patients) every 24 hours if eGFR less than 30 mL/minute/1.73 m^2. For *reduction of genital herpes transmission*, 250 mg every 24 hours if eGFR less than 15 mL/minute/1.73 m^2. Reduce dose according to eGFR for *cytomegalovirus prophylaxis* following solid organ transplantation (consult product literature).
▸ In children For *treatment of herpes labialis*, if estimated glomerular filtration rate 30–50 mL/minute/1.73 m^2, initially 1 g, then 1 g 12 hours after initial dose (if estimated glomerular filtration rate 10–30 mL/minute/1.73 m^2, initially 500 mg, then 500 mg 12 hours after initial dose; if estimated glomerular filtration rate less than 10 mL/minute/1.73 m^2, 500 mg as a single dose).
● PRESCRIBING AND DISPENSING INFORMATION Valaciclovir is a pro-drug of aciclovir.

● MEDICINAL FORMS
There can be variation in the licensing of different medicines containing the same drug. Forms available from special-order manufacturers include: oral suspension
Tablet
CAUTIONARY AND ADVISORY LABELS 9
▸ Valaciclovir (Non-proprietary)
  Valaciclovir (as Valaciclovir hydrochloride) 500 mg Valaciclovir 500mg tablets | 10 tablet P̲o̲M̲ £20.59 DT = £2.92 | 42 tablet P̲o̲M̲ £8.50–£86.30
▸ Valtrex (GlaxoSmithKline UK Ltd)
  Valaciclovir (as Valaciclovir hydrochloride) 250 mg Valtrex 250mg tablets | 60 tablet P̲o̲M̲ £123.28 DT = £123.28
  Valaciclovir (as Valaciclovir hydrochloride) 500 mg Valtrex 500mg tablets | 10 tablet P̲o̲M̲ £20.59 DT = £2.92 | 42 tablet P̲o̲M̲ £86.30

6.3a Cytomegalovirus infections

ANTIVIRALS ⟩ NUCLEOSIDE ANALOGUES

Ganciclovir

31-May-2018

● INDICATIONS AND DOSE
Prevention of cytomegalovirus disease [pre-emptive therapy in patients with drug-induced immunosuppression]
▸ BY INTRAVENOUS INFUSION
▸ Adult: Initially 5 mg/kg every 12 hours for 7–14 days, then maintenance 6 mg/kg once daily, on 5 days of the week, alternatively maintenance 5 mg/kg once daily
Prevention of cytomegalovirus disease [universal prophylaxis in patients with drug-induced immunosuppression]
▸ BY INTRAVENOUS INFUSION
▸ Adult: 6 mg/kg once daily, on 5 days of the week, alternatively 5 mg/kg once daily
Treatment of cytomegalovirus disease [in immunocompromised patients]
▸ BY INTRAVENOUS INFUSION
▸ Adult: Initially 5 mg/kg every 12 hours for 14–21 days, then maintenance 6 mg/kg once daily, on 5 days of the week, alternatively maintenance 5 mg/kg once daily, maintenance only for patients at risk of relapse; if disease progresses initial induction treatment may be repeated

● CONTRA-INDICATIONS Abnormally low haemoglobin count (consult product literature) · abnormally low neutrophil count (consult product literature) · abnormally low platelet count (consult product literature)
● CAUTIONS History of cytopenia · potential carcinogen (including long-term carcinogenicity) · potential teratogen (including long-term teratogenicity) · radiotherapy
● INTERACTIONS → Appendix 1: ganciclovir
● SIDE-EFFECTS
▸ **Common or very common** Anaemia · anxiety · appetite decreased · arthralgia · asthenia · bone marrow disorders · chest pain · chills · confusion · constipation · cough · depression · diarrhoea · dizziness · dysphagia · dyspnoea · ear pain · eye disorders · eye inflammation · eye pain · fever · flatulence · gastrointestinal discomfort · headache · hepatic function abnormal · increased risk of infection · insomnia · leucopenia · malaise · muscle complaints · nausea · neutropenia · night sweats · pain · peripheral neuropathy · renal impairment · seizure · sensation abnormal · sepsis · skin reactions · taste altered · thinking abnormal · thrombocytopenia · vomiting · weight decreased

- **Uncommon** Alopecia · arrhythmia · deafness · haematuria · hypotension · infertility male · oral ulceration · pancreatitis · psychotic disorder · tremor · visual impairment
- **Rare or very rare** Agranulocytosis · hallucination

- ALLERGY AND CROSS-SENSITIVITY Contra-indicated in patients hypersensitive to valganciclovir, aciclovir, or valaciclovir.

- CONCEPTION AND CONTRACEPTION Manufacturer advises women of childbearing potential should use effective contraception during and for at least 30 days after treatment; men with partners of childbearing potential should be advised to use barrier contraception during and for at least 90 days after treatment. Ganciclovir may cause temporary or permanent inhibition of spermatogenesis—impaired fertility observed in *animal* studies.

- PREGNANCY Manufacturer advises avoid unless potential benefit outweighs risk—teratogenicity in *animal* studies.

- BREAST FEEDING Manufacturer advises avoid—present in milk in *animal* studies.

- RENAL IMPAIRMENT
Dose adjustments Manufacturer advises reduce dose for patients receiving mg/kg dosing if creatinine clearance less than 70 mL/minute—consult product literature.

- MONITORING REQUIREMENTS Monitor full blood count closely (severe deterioration may require correction and possibly treatment interruption).

- DIRECTIONS FOR ADMINISTRATION Manufacturer advises, for *intravenous infusion*, give intermittently in Glucose 5% or Sodium Chloride 0.9%. Reconstitute with Water for Injections (500 mg/10 mL) then dilute requisite dose to a concentration of not more than 10 mg/mL with infusion fluid; give over 1 hour into a vein with adequate flow, preferably using a plastic cannula.

- HANDLING AND STORAGE
Caution in handling Ganciclovir is a potential teratogen and carcinogen. Manufacturer advises avoid inhalation of the powder or direct contact of the powder or reconstituted solution with the skin or mucous membranes; if contact occurs, wash thoroughly with soap and water; rinse eyes thoroughly with plain water.

- MEDICINAL FORMS
There can be variation in the licensing of different medicines containing the same drug.
Powder for solution for infusion
ELECTROLYTES: May contain Sodium
  - Ganciclovir (Non-proprietary)
    Ganciclovir (as Ganciclovir sodium) 500 mg Ganciclovir 500mg powder for concentrate for solution for infusion vials | 5 vial PoM £125.95
  - Cymevene (Roche Products Ltd)
    Ganciclovir (as Ganciclovir sodium) 500 mg Cymevene 500mg powder for solution for infusion vials | 5 vial PoM £148.83

Valganciclovir
31-May-2018

- INDICATIONS AND DOSE
Cytomegalovirus retinitis [induction and maintenance treatment in patients with AIDS]
  ▶ BY MOUTH
  ▶ Adult: Initially 900 mg twice daily for 21 days, then maintenance 900 mg daily, induction regimen may be repeated if retinitis progresses

Prevention of cytomegalovirus disease [following solid organ transplantation from a cytomegalovirus positive donor]
  ▶ BY MOUTH
  ▶ Adult: 900 mg daily for 100 days (for 100–200 days following kidney transplantation), to be started within 10 days of transplantation

DOSE EQUIVALENCE AND CONVERSION
  ▶ Oral valganciclovir 900 mg twice daily is equivalent to intravenous ganciclovir 5 mg/kg twice daily.

- CONTRA-INDICATIONS Abnormally low haemoglobin count (consult product literature) · abnormally low neutrophil count (consult product literature) · abnormally low platelet count (consult product literature)

- CAUTIONS History of cytopenia · potential carcinogen (including long-term carcinogenicity) · potential teratogen (including long-term teratogenicity) · radiotherapy

- INTERACTIONS → Appendix 1: valganciclovir

- SIDE-EFFECTS
- **Common or very common** Anaemia · anxiety · appetite decreased · arthralgia · asthenia · bone marrow disorders · chest pain · confusion · constipation · cough · depression · diarrhoea · dizziness · dysphagia · dyspnoea · ear pain · eye disorders · eye inflammation · eye pain · flatulence · gastrointestinal discomfort · headache · hepatic function abnormal · increased risk of infection · insomnia · leucopenia · malaise · muscle complaints · nausea · neutropenia · night sweats · pain · peripheral neuropathy · renal impairment · seizure · sensation abnormal · sepsis · skin reactions · taste altered · thinking abnormal · thrombocytopenia · vomiting · weight decreased
- **Uncommon** Alopecia · arrhythmia · deafness · haematuria · hallucination · hypotension · infertility male · oral ulceration · pancreatitis · psychotic disorder · tremor · visual impairment

- ALLERGY AND CROSS-SENSITIVITY Contra-indicated in patients hypersensitive to ganciclovir, aciclovir, or valaciclovir.

- CONCEPTION AND CONTRACEPTION Manufacturer advises women of childbearing potential should use effective contraception during and for at least 30 days after treatment; men with partners of childbearing potential should be advised to use barrier contraception during and for at least 90 days after treatment. *Ganciclovir* may cause temporary or permanent inhibition of spermatogenesis—impaired fertility observed in *animal* studies.

- PREGNANCY Manufacturer advises avoid unless potential benefit outweighs risk—teratogenicity observed with *ganciclovir* in *animal* studies.

- BREAST FEEDING Manufacturer advises avoid— *ganciclovir* present in milk in *animal* studies.

- RENAL IMPAIRMENT
Dose adjustments Manufacturer advises reduce dose if creatinine clearance less than 60 mL/minute—consult product literature.

- MONITORING REQUIREMENTS Monitor full blood count closely (severe deterioration may require correction and possibly treatment interruption).

- PRESCRIBING AND DISPENSING INFORMATION
Valganciclovir is a pro-drug of ganciclovir.
    Flavours of oral liquid formulations may include tutti-frutti.

- HANDLING AND STORAGE Manufacturer advises reconstituted powder for oral solution should be stored in a refrigerator (2–8°C) for up to 49 days.
Caution in handling Valganciclovir is a potential teratogen and carcinogen. Manufacturer advises caution when handling the powder, reconstituted solution, or broken tablets and avoid inhalation of powder; if contact with skin or mucous membranes occurs, wash thoroughly with soap and water; rinse eyes thoroughly with plain water.

5

Infection

- MEDICINAL FORMS
There can be variation in the licensing of different medicines containing the same drug. Forms available from special-order manufacturers include: oral solution

Oral solution

CAUTIONARY AND ADVISORY LABELS 21
▸ Valcyte (Roche Products Ltd)
Valganciclovir (as Valganciclovir hydrochloride) 50 mg per 1 ml Valcyte 50mg/ml oral solution sugar-free | 100 ml [PoM] £230.32

Tablet

CAUTIONARY AND ADVISORY LABELS 21
▸ Valganciclovir (Non-proprietary)
Valganciclovir (as Valganciclovir hydrochloride) 450 mg Valganciclovir 450mg tablets | 60 tablet [PoM] £865.17-£1,081.46
▸ Valcyte (Roche Products Ltd)
Valganciclovir (as Valganciclovir hydrochloride) 450 mg Valcyte 450mg tablets | 60 tablet [PoM] £1,081.46

ANTIVIRALS > OTHER

Foscarnet sodium

- INDICATIONS AND DOSE

Cytomegalovirus disease
▸ BY INTRAVENOUS INFUSION
▸ Adult: Initially 60 mg/kg every 8 hours for 2–3 weeks, alternatively initially 90 mg/kg every 12 hours for 2–3 weeks, then maintenance 60 mg/kg daily, then increased if tolerated to 90–120 mg/kg daily, if disease progresses on maintenance dose, repeat induction regimen

Mucocutaneous herpes simplex virus infections unresponsive to aciclovir in immunocompromised patients
▸ BY INTRAVENOUS INFUSION
▸ Adult: 40 mg/kg every 8 hours for 2–3 weeks or until lesions heal

- UNLICENSED USE Licensed for CMV retinitis in AIDS patients only. Foscarnet doses in BNF may differ from those in product literature.
- CAUTIONS Ensure adequate hydration
- INTERACTIONS → Appendix 1: foscarnet
- SIDE-EFFECTS
▸ **Common or very common** Aggression · anaemia · anxiety · appetite decreased · arrhythmias · asthenia · chest pain · chills · confusion · constipation · coordination abnormal · dehydration · depression · diarrhoea · dizziness · electrolyte imbalance · fever · gastrointestinal discomfort · genital discomfort (due to high concentrations excreted in urine) · genital ulceration (due to high concentrations excreted in urine) · haemorrhage · headache · hepatic function abnormal · hypertension · hypotension · leucopenia · malaise · muscle contractions involuntary · myalgia · nausea (reduce infusion rate) · neutropenia · numbness · oedema · palpitations · pancreatitis · paraesthesia (reduce infusion rate) · peripheral neuropathy · proteinuria · renal impairment · seizure · sepsis · skin reactions · thrombocytopenia · tremor · urinary disorders · vomiting
▸ **Uncommon** Acidosis · angioedema · glomerulonephritis · nephropathy · pancytopenia
▸ **Frequency not known** Anaphylactoid reaction · diabetes insipidus · muscle weakness · myopathy · oesophageal ulcer · QT interval prolongation · renal pain · renal tubular acidosis · severe cutaneous adverse reactions (SCARs)
- CONCEPTION AND CONTRACEPTION Men should avoid fathering a child during and for 6 months after treatment.
- PREGNANCY Manufacturer advises avoid.
- BREAST FEEDING Avoid—present in milk in *animal* studies.

- RENAL IMPAIRMENT
Dose adjustments Reduce dose; consult product literature.
- MONITORING REQUIREMENTS
▸ Monitor electrolytes, particularly calcium and magnesium.
▸ Monitor serum creatinine every second day during induction and every week during maintenance.
- DIRECTIONS FOR ADMINISTRATION Avoid rapid infusion. For *intravenous infusion* (Foscavir®), give intermittently *in* Glucose 5% or Sodium Chloride 0.9%; dilute to a concentration of 12 mg/mL for infusion into peripheral vein (undiluted solution *via* central venous line only); infuse over at least 1 hour (infuse doses greater than 60 mg/kg over 2 hours).

- MEDICINAL FORMS
There can be variation in the licensing of different medicines containing the same drug.

Solution for infusion
ELECTROLYTES: May contain Sodium
▸ Foscavir (Clinigen Healthcare Ltd)
Foscarnet sodium 24 mg per 1 ml Foscavir 6g/250ml solution for infusion bottles | 1 bottle [PoM] £119.85 (Hospital only)

6.4 HIV infection

HIV infection

02-Jun-2017

Overview

There is no cure for infection caused by the human immunodeficiency virus (HIV) but a number of drugs slow or halt disease progression. Drugs for HIV infection (antiretrovirals) may be associated with serious side-effects. Although antiretrovirals increase life expectancy considerably and decrease the risk of complications associated with premature ageing, mortality and morbidity remain slightly higher than in uninfected individuals. Treatment should be undertaken only by those experienced in their use.

Aims of treatment

Treatment aims to prevent the mortality and morbidity associated with chronic HIV infection whilst minimising drug toxicity. Although it should be started before the immune system is irreversibly damaged, the need for early drug treatment should be balanced against the risk of toxicity. Commitment to treatment and strict adherence over many years are required; the regimen chosen should take into account convenience and patient tolerance. The development of drug resistance is reduced by using a combination of drugs; such combinations should have synergistic or additive activity whilst ensuring that their toxicity is not additive. It is recommended that viral sensitivity to antiretroviral drugs is established before starting treatment or before switching drugs if the infection is not responding.

Treatment also reduces the risk of HIV transmission to sexual partners, but the risk is not eliminated completely; this risk and strategies to reduce HIV transmission should be discussed with patients and their sexual partners.

Initiation of treatment

The optimum time for initiating antiretroviral treatment depends primarily on the CD4 cell count. The timing and choice of treatment should also take account of clinical symptoms, comorbidities, and the possible effect of antiretroviral drugs on factors such as the risk of cardiovascular events. Treatment includes a combination of drugs known as 'highly active antiretroviral therapy'. Treatment of HIV-1 infection is initiated with 2 nucleoside reverse transcriptase inhibitors and *either* a non-nucleoside reverse transcriptase inhibitor, *or* a boosted protease inhibitor, *or* an integrase inhibitor; the regimens of choice contain tenofovir disoproxil p. 641 and emtricitabine p. 638 with *either* efavirenz p. 632 *or* ritonavir p. 646-boosted atazanavir p. 643, *or* ritonavir-boosted darunavir p. 643, *or* raltegravir p. 631. Alternative regimens contain abacavir p. 634 and lamivudine p. 640 with *either* lopinavir with ritonavir p. 645, *or* ritonavir-boosted fosamprenavir p. 645, *or* nevirapine p. 633, *or* rilpivirine p. 634. Patients who require treatment for both HIV and chronic hepatitis B should be treated with antivirals active against both diseases.

HIV infection, switching therapy

Deterioration of the condition (including clinical and virological changes) may require a change in therapy. The choice of an alternative regimen depends on factors such as the response to previous treatment, tolerance and the possibility of cross-resistance.

HIV infection in pregnancy

Treatment of HIV infection in pregnancy aims to reduce the risk of toxicity to the fetus (although information on the teratogenic potential of most antiretroviral drugs is limited), to minimise the viral load and disease progression in the mother, and to prevent transmission of infection to the neonate. **All treatment options require careful assessment by a specialist**. Combination antiretroviral therapy maximises the chance of preventing transmission and represents optimal therapy for the mother. However, it may be associated with a greater risk of preterm delivery. Pregnancies in HIV-positive women and babies born to them should be reported prospectively to the National Study of HIV in Pregnancy and Childhood at www.ucl.ac.uk/nshpc/ **and** to the Antiretroviral Pregnancy Registry at www.apregistry.com.

HIV infection and breast-feeding

Breast-feeding by HIV-positive mothers may cause HIV infection in the infant and should be avoided.

HIV infection, pre-exposure prophylaxis

The risk of acquiring HIV is increased in:
- men or transgender individuals who have unprotected anal intercourse with men;
- sexual partners of people who are HIV-positive with a detectable viral load;
- HIV-negative heterosexual individuals who have unprotected intercourse with a HIV-positive person, and are likely to repeat this with the same person or another person with a similar status.

Emtricitabine with tenofovir disoproxil p. 639 may be appropriate for pre-exposure prophylaxis to reduce the risk of sexually acquired HIV-1 infection in combination with safer sex practices in adults at high risk; recommendations developed by the British Association for Sexual Health and HIV are available at: www.bashh.org.

HIV infection, post-exposure prophylaxis

Prophylaxis with antiretroviral drugs [unlicensed indication] may be appropriate following exposure to HIV-contaminated material. Immediate expert advice should be sought in such cases; national guidelines on post-exposure prophylaxis for healthcare workers have been developed (by the Chief Medical Officer's Expert Advisory Group on AIDS), www.gov.uk/dh and local ones may also be available. Antiretrovirals for prophylaxis are chosen on the basis of efficacy and potential for toxicity. Prompt prophylaxis with antiretroviral drugs [unlicensed indication] is also appropriate following potential sexual exposure to HIV; recommendations have been developed by the British Association for Sexual Health and HIV, www.bashh.org.

Drug treatment

Zidovudine p. 642, a nucleoside reverse transcriptase inhibitor (or 'nucleoside analogue'), was the first anti-HIV drug to be introduced. Other nucleoside reverse transcriptase inhibitors include abacavir, didanosine p. 636, emtricitabine, lamivudine, stavudine p. 640, and tenofovir disoproxil.

The protease inhibitors include atazanavir, darunavir, fosamprenavir (a pro-drug of amprenavir), lopinavir (available as lopinavir with ritonavir), ritonavir, saquinavir p. 646, and tipranavir p. 646. Ritonavir in low doses boosts the activity of atazanavir, darunavir, fosamprenavir, lopinavir (available as lopinavir with ritonavir), saquinavir, and tipranavir increasing the persistence of plasma concentrations of these drugs; at such a low dose, ritonavir has no intrinsic antiviral activity. The protease inhibitors are metabolised by cytochrome P450 enzyme systems and therefore have a significant potential for drug interactions. Protease inhibitors are associated with lipodystrophy and metabolic effects.

The non-nucleoside reverse transcriptase inhibitors efavirenz, etravirine p. 633, nevirapine, and rilpivirine are used in the treatment of HIV-1 infection, but not against the subtype HIV-2, a subtype that is rare in the UK. Nevirapine is associated with a high incidence of rash (including Stevens-Johnson syndrome) and occasionally fatal hepatitis. Rash is also associated with efavirenz and etravirine but it is usually milder. Psychiatric or CNS disturbances are common with efavirenz; CNS disturbances are often self-limiting and can be reduced by taking the dose at bedtime (especially in the first 2–4 weeks of treatment). Efavirenz has also been associated with an increased plasma-cholesterol concentration. Etravirine is used in regimens containing a boosted protease inhibitor for HIV infection resistant to other non-nucleoside reverse transcriptase inhibitors and protease inhibitors.

Enfuvirtide p. 630, which inhibits the fusion of HIV to the host cell, is licensed for managing infection that has failed to respond to a regimen of other antiretroviral drugs; enfuvirtide should be combined with other potentially active antiretroviral drugs.

Maraviroc p. 647 is an antagonist of the CCR5 chemokine receptor. It is licensed for patients exclusively infected with CCR5-tropic HIV.

Dolutegravir p. 630, elvitegravir p. 631 and raltegravir p. 631 are inhibitors of HIV integrase. They are licensed for the treatment of HIV infection in combination with other antiretroviral drugs.

Cobicistat p. 647 is a pharmacokinetic enhancer that boosts the concentrations of other antiretrovirals, but it has no antiretroviral activity itself.

Immune reconstitution syndrome

Improvement in immune function as a result of antiretroviral treatment may provoke a marked inflammatory reaction against residual opportunistic organisms; these reactions may occur within the first few weeks or months of initiating treatment. Autoimmune disorders (such as Graves' disease) have also been reported many months after initiation of treatment.

Osteonecrosis

Osteonecrosis has been reported in patients with advanced HIV disease or following long-term exposure to combination antiretroviral therapy.

HIV infection in children

HIV disease in children has a different natural progression to adults. Children infected with HIV should be managed within a formal paediatric HIV clinical network by specialists with access to guidelines and information on antiretroviral drugs for children.

ANTIVIRALS › HIV-FUSION INHIBITORS

Enfuvirtide

- **DRUG ACTION** Enfuvirtide inhibits the fusion of HIV to the host cell.

- ● **INDICATIONS AND DOSE**

HIV infection in combination with other antiretroviral drugs for resistant infection or for patients intolerant to other antiretroviral regimens
▸ BY SUBCUTANEOUS INJECTION
▸ Adult: 90 mg twice daily

- ● **SIDE-EFFECTS**
▸ **Common or very common** Anxiety · appetite decreased · asthenia · concentration impaired · conjunctivitis · diabetes mellitus · gastrooesophageal reflux disease · haematuria · hypertriglyceridaemia · increased risk of infection · influenza like illness · irritability · lymphadenopathy · myalgia · nasal congestion · nephrolithiasis · nightmare · numbness · pancreatitis · peripheral neuropathy · skin papilloma · skin reactions · tremor · vertigo · weight decreased
▸ **Frequency not known** Diarrhoea · hypersensitivity · immune reconstitution inflammatory syndrome · nausea · osteonecrosis

SIDE-EFFECTS, FURTHER INFORMATION
Hypersensitivity Hypersensitivity reactions including rash, fever, nausea, vomiting, chills, rigors, low blood pressure, respiratory distress, glomerulonephritis, and raised liver enzymes reported; discontinue immediately if any signs or symptoms of systemic hypersensitivity develop and do not rechallenge.
Osteonecrosis Osteonecrosis has been reported in patients with advanced HIV disease or following long-term exposure to combination antiretroviral therapy.

- ● **PREGNANCY** Manufacturer advises use only if potential benefit outweighs risk.

- ● **HEPATIC IMPAIRMENT** Manufacturer advises caution— no information available; chronic hepatitis B or C (possibly greater risk of hepatic side-effects).

- ● **DIRECTIONS FOR ADMINISTRATION** For *subcutaneous injection*, reconstitute with 1.1 mL Water for Injections and allow to stand (for up to 45 minutes) to dissolve; do **not** shake or invert vial.

- ● **PATIENT AND CARER ADVICE**
Hypersensitivity reactions Patients or carers should be told how to recognise signs of hypersensitivity, and advised to discontinue treatment and seek immediate medical attention if symptoms develop.

- ● **MEDICINAL FORMS**
There can be variation in the licensing of different medicines containing the same drug.
Powder and solvent for solution for injection
ELECTROLYTES: May contain Sodium
▸ Fuzeon (Roche Products Ltd)
Enfuvirtide 108 mg Fuzeon 108mg powder and solvent for solution for injection vials | 60 vial [PoM] £1,081.57

ANTIVIRALS › HIV-INTEGRASE INHIBITORS

Dolutegravir

05-Jun-2018

- **DRUG ACTION** Dolutegravir is an inhibitor of HIV integrase.

- ● **INDICATIONS AND DOSE**

HIV infection without resistance to other inhibitors of HIV integrase, in combination with other antiretroviral drugs
▸ BY MOUTH
▸ Adult: 50 mg once daily

HIV infection in patients where resistance to other inhibitors of HIV integrase suspected, in combination with other antiretroviral drugs
▸ BY MOUTH
▸ Adult: 50 mg twice daily, dose to be taken with food

HIV infection in combination with other antiretroviral drugs (with concomitant carbamazepine, efavirenz, etravirine (without boosted protease inhibitors, but see also Interactions), fosphenytoin, phenobarbital, phenytoin, primidone, nevirapine, oxcarbazepine, St John's wort, rifampicin, or tipranavir)
▸ BY MOUTH
▸ Adult: 50 mg twice daily, avoid concomitant use with these drugs if resistance to other inhibitors of HIV integrase suspected

IMPORTANT SAFETY INFORMATION
MHRA/CHM ADVICE: *TIVICAY*® (DOLUTEGRAVIR), *TRIUMEQ*® (DOLUTEGRAVIR, ABACAVIR, LAMIVUDINE), *JULUCA*® (DOLUTEGRAVIR, RILPIVIRINE): NEURAL TUBE DEFECTS REPORTED IN INFANTS BORN TO WOMEN EXPOSED TO DOLUTEGRAVIR AT THE TIME OF CONCEPTION (MAY 2018)
In an ongoing birth outcome surveillance study conducted in Botswana, 4 cases of neural tube defects have been reported in 426 infants born to women who took dolutegravir as part of combined antiretroviral therapy at the time of conception. The manufacturer, in agreement with the European Medicines Agency, has recommended the following measures while this safety signal is being evaluated:
- Pregnancy testing should be performed and pregnancy excluded before initiation of treatment in females of childbearing potential; effective contraception should be used throughout treatment;
- Use of dolutegravir should be avoided in pregnancy; if pregnancy occurs and is confirmed in the first trimester, it is recommended to switch to an alternative treatment unless there is no suitable alternative.

- ● **INTERACTIONS** → Appendix 1: dolutegravir
- ● **SIDE-EFFECTS**
▸ **Common or very common** Depression · diarrhoea · dizziness · fatigue · flatulence · gastrointestinal discomfort · headache · nausea · skin reactions · sleep disorders · vomiting
▸ **Uncommon** Arthralgia · hepatitis · hypersensitivity · immune reconstitution inflammatory syndrome · myalgia · suicidal tendencies

SIDE-EFFECTS, FURTHER INFORMATION
Hypersensitivity Hypersensitivity reactions (including severe rash, or rash accompanied by fever, malaise, arthralgia, myalgia, blistering, oral lesions, conjunctivitis, angioedema, eosinophilia, or raised liver enzymes) reported uncommonly. Discontinue immediately if any sign or symptoms of hypersensitivity reactions develop.
Osteonecrosis Osteonecrosis has been reported in patients with advanced HIV disease or following long-term exposure to combination antiretroviral therapy.

- PREGNANCY Manufacturer advises avoid, see *Important Safety Information*.
- HEPATIC IMPAIRMENT Manufacturer advises caution in severe impairment—no information available.
- PATIENT AND CARER ADVICE Patients or carers should be given advice on how to administer dolutegravir tablets.
  Missed doses If a dose is more than 20 hours late on the once daily regimen (or more than 8 hours late on the twice daily regimen), the missed dose should not be taken and the next dose should be taken at the normal time.
- NATIONAL FUNDING/ACCESS DECISIONS
  Scottish Medicines Consortium (SMC) Decisions
  The *Scottish Medicines Consortium* has advised (May 2014) that dolutegravir (*Tivicay®*) is accepted for use within NHS Scotland when used in combination with other anti-retroviral medicines for the treatment of HIV infected adults. This advice is contingent upon the continuing availability of the patient access scheme in NHS Scotland or a list price that is equivalent or lower.
  All Wales Medicines Strategy Group (AWMSG) Decisions
  The *All Wales Medicines Strategy Group* has advised (October 2017) that dolutegravir (*Tivicay®*) is recommended as an option for use within NHS Wales in combination with other anti-retroviral medicinal products for the treatment of HIV infected adults. This recommendation applies only in circumstances where the approved Wales Patient Access Scheme (WPAS) is utilised or where the list/contract price is equivalent or lower than the WPAS price.

- MEDICINAL FORMS
  There can be variation in the licensing of different medicines containing the same drug.
  Tablet
  ▸ Tivicay (ViiV Healthcare UK Ltd) ▼
  Dolutegravir (as Dolutegravir sodium) 10 mg Tivicay 10mg tablets | 30 tablet PoM £99.75
  Dolutegravir (as Dolutegravir sodium) 25 mg Tivicay 25mg tablets | 30 tablet PoM £249.38
  Dolutegravir (as Dolutegravir sodium) 50 mg Tivicay 50mg tablets | 30 tablet PoM £498.75

  Combinations available: *Abacavir with dolutegravir and lamivudine,* p. 635

Elvitegravir
31-Jan-2017

- DRUG ACTION Elvitegravir is an inhibitor of HIV integrase, which is an enzyme required for viral replication.

- INDICATIONS AND DOSE

  HIV infection without resistance to other inhibitors of HIV integrase, in combination with low-dose ritonavir and atazanavir or lopinavir
  ▸ BY MOUTH
  ▸ Adult: 85 mg once daily, take at the same time as a once daily ritonavir-boosted regimen or with the first dose of a twice daily ritonavir-boosted regimen

  HIV infection without resistance to other inhibitors of HIV integrase, in combination with low-dose ritonavir and darunavir or fosamprenavir
  ▸ BY MOUTH
  ▸ Adult: 150 mg once daily, take with the first dose of a twice daily ritonavir-boosted regimen

- CAUTIONS Elderly—limited information available
- INTERACTIONS → Appendix 1: elvitegravir
- SIDE-EFFECTS
- **Common or very common** Diarrhoea · fatigue · headache · nausea · rash · vomiting
- **Uncommon** Depression · dizziness · drowsiness · flatulence · gastrointestinal discomfort · insomnia · paraesthesia ·

suicidal ideation (in patients with history of depression or psychiatric illness) · taste altered
▸ **Frequency not known** Hyperglycaemia · osteonecrosis · weight increased

SIDE-EFFECTS, FURTHER INFORMATION For further information regarding **osteonecrosis** see HIV infection p. 628.

- CONCEPTION AND CONTRACEPTION Manufacturer advises women of child-bearing potential should use effective contraception during treatment (if using a hormonal contraceptive, it must contain norgestimate as the progestogen and at least 30 micrograms ethinylestradiol).
- PREGNANCY Manufacturer advises avoid unless essential—limited data available.
- HEPATIC IMPAIRMENT Manufacturer advises use with caution in severe impairment—no information available. Use with caution in patients with chronic hepatitis B or C (greater risk of hepatic side-effects).
- PATIENT AND CARER ADVICE
  Missed doses Manufacturer advises if a dose is more than 18 hours late, the missed dose should not be taken and the next dose should be taken at the normal time. If vomiting occurs within 1 hour of taking a dose, a replacement dose should be taken.

- MEDICINAL FORMS
  No licensed medicines listed.

  Combinations available: *Elvitegravir with cobicistat, emtricitabine and tenofovir alafenamide,* p. 637 · *Elvitegravir with cobicistat, emtricitabine and tenofovir disoproxil,* p. 637

Raltegravir
10-May-2018

- DRUG ACTION Raltegravir is an inhibitor of HIV integrase.

- INDICATIONS AND DOSE

  HIV-1 infection (initiated by a specialist)
  ▸ BY MOUTH USING TABLETS
  ▸ Adult: 400 mg twice daily, alternatively 1200 mg once daily, once daily dosing for use in patients who are treatment naive or virologically suppressed on an initial regimen of 400 mg twice daily—use 600 mg tablets only

- CAUTIONS Psychiatric illness (may exacerbate underlying illness including depression) · risk factors for myopathy · risk factors for rhabdomyolysis
- INTERACTIONS → Appendix 1: raltegravir
- SIDE-EFFECTS
- **Common or very common** Akathisia · appetite abnormal · asthenia · behaviour abnormal · depression · diarrhoea · dizziness · fever · gastrointestinal discomfort · gastrointestinal disorders · headaches · nausea · skin reactions · sleep disorders · vertigo · vomiting
- **Uncommon** Alopecia · anaemia · anxiety · arrhythmias · arthralgia · arthritis · body fat disorder · burping · cachexia · chest discomfort · chills · cognitive disorder · concentration impaired · confusion · constipation · diabetes mellitus · drowsiness · dry mouth · dyslipidaemia · dysphonia · erectile dysfunction · feeling jittery · glossitis · gynaecomastia · haemorrhage · hepatic disorders · hot flush · hyperglycaemia · hypersensitivity · hypertension · immune reconstitution inflammatory syndrome · increased risk of infection · lipodystrophy · lymph node abscess · lymphatic abnormalities · malaise · memory loss · menopausal symptoms · mood altered · myalgia · myopathy · nasal congestion · nephritis · nephrolithiasis · nerve disorders · neutropenia · nocturia · odynophagia · oedema · osteopenia · pain · palpitations · pancreatitis acute · polydipsia · psychiatric disorder · renal cyst · renal impairment · sensation abnormal · severe cutaneous

adverse reactions (SCARs) · skin papilloma · submandibular mass · suicidal tendencies · sweat changes · taste altered · tendinitis · thrombocytopenia · tinnitus · tremor · visual impairment · weight increased

▶ **Frequency not known** Osteonecrosis

SIDE-EFFECTS, FURTHER INFORMATION Rash occurs commonly. Discontinue if severe rash or rash accompanied by fever, malaise, arthralgia, myalgia, blistering, mouth ulceration, conjunctivitis, angioedema, hepatitis, or eosinophilia.

For further information regarding **lipodystrophy** and **osteonecrosis** see HIV infection p. 628.

● PREGNANCY Manufacturer advises avoid—toxicity in *animal* studies.

● HEPATIC IMPAIRMENT Manufacturer advises caution in severe impairment—no information available. Use with caution in patients with chronic hepatitis B or C (at greater risk of hepatic side-effects).

● PRESCRIBING AND DISPENSING INFORMATION Dispense raltegravir chewable tablets in original container (contains desiccant).

● NATIONAL FUNDING/ACCESS DECISIONS

Scottish Medicines Consortium (SMC) Decisions
The *Scottish Medicines Consortium* has advised (May 2010) that raltegravir (*Isentress* ®) is accepted for restricted use within NHS Scotland for the treatment of HIV-1 infection when non-nucleoside reverse transcriptase inhibitors or protease inhibitors cannot be used because of intolerance, drug interactions, or resistance.

The *Scottish Medicines Consortium* has advised (November 2017) that raltegravir 600 mg film-coated tablets (*Isentress* ®) are accepted for restricted use within NHS Scotland for the treatment of HIV-1 infection in adults and paediatric patients weighing at least 40 kg when non-nucleoside reverse transcriptase inhibitors or protease inhibitors cannot be used because of intolerance, drug interactions, or resistance.

● MEDICINAL FORMS
There can be variation in the licensing of different medicines containing the same drug.

Tablet
CAUTIONARY AND ADVISORY LABELS 25
▶ Isentress (Merck Sharp & Dohme Ltd)
Raltegravir 400 mg Isentress 400mg tablets | 60 tablet PoM
£471.41
Raltegravir 600 mg Isentress 600mg tablets | 60 tablet PoM
£471.41

ANTIVIRALS › NON-NUCLEOSIDE REVERSE TRANSCRIPTASE INHIBITORS

Efavirenz

● INDICATIONS AND DOSE

HIV infection in combination with other antiretroviral drugs
▶ BY MOUTH USING CAPSULES
▶ Adult: 600 mg once daily
▶ BY MOUTH USING TABLETS
▶ Adult: 600 mg once daily
▶ BY MOUTH USING ORAL SOLUTION
▶ Adult: 720 mg once daily

DOSE EQUIVALENCE AND CONVERSION
▶ The bioavailability of *Sustiva* ® oral solution is lower than that of the capsules and tablets; the oral solution is **not** interchangeable with either capsules or tablets on a milligram-for-milligram basis.

● UNLICENSED USE Opening capsules and adding contents to food is an unlicensed method of administration.

● CAUTIONS Acute porphyrias p. 1025 · elderly · history of psychiatric disorders · history of seizures

● INTERACTIONS → Appendix 1: efavirenz

● SIDE-EFFECTS

▶ **Common or very common** Abdominal pain · anxiety · concentration impaired · depression · diarrhoea · dizziness · drowsiness · dyslipidaemia · fatigue · headache · movement disorders · nausea · skin reactions · sleep disorders · vomiting

▶ **Uncommon** Behaviour abnormal · confusion · flushing · gynaecomastia · hallucination · hepatic disorders · memory loss · mood altered · pancreatitis · psychosis · seizure · Stevens-Johnson syndrome · suicidal tendencies · thinking abnormal · tinnitus · tremor · vertigo · vision blurred

▶ **Rare or very rare** Delusions · photosensitivity reaction

▶ **Frequency not known** Immune reconstitution inflammatory syndrome · osteonecrosis

SIDE-EFFECTS, FURTHER INFORMATION For further information regarding **osteonecrosis, immune reconstitution syndrome** and **lipodystrophy,** see HIV infection p. 628.
Rash Rash, usually in the first 2 weeks, is the most common side-effect; discontinue if severe rash with blistering, desquamation, mucosal involvement or fever; if rash mild or moderate, may continue without interruption—usually resolves within 1 month.
CNS effects Administration at bedtime especially in first 2–4 weeks reduces CNS effects.

● PREGNANCY Reports of neural tube defects when used in first trimester.

● HEPATIC IMPAIRMENT Greater risk of hepatic side-effects in chronic hepatitis B or C. Avoid in moderate to severe impairment.
Monitoring In mild liver disease, monitor for dose related side-effects (e.g. CNS effects) and monitor liver function.

● RENAL IMPAIRMENT Manufacturer advises caution in severe renal failure—no information available.

● MONITORING REQUIREMENTS Monitor liver function if receiving other hepatotoxic drugs.

● DIRECTIONS FOR ADMINISTRATION Capsules may be opened and contents added to food (contents have a peppery taste).

● PRESCRIBING AND DISPENSING INFORMATION Flavours of oral liquid formulations may include strawberry and mint.

● PATIENT AND CARER ADVICE
Psychiatric disorders Patients or their carers should be advised to seek immediate medical attention if symptoms such as severe depression, psychosis or suicidal ideation occur.

● MEDICINAL FORMS
There can be variation in the licensing of different medicines containing the same drug.

Tablet
CAUTIONARY AND ADVISORY LABELS 23
▶ Efavirenz (Non-proprietary)
Efavirenz 600 mg Efavirenz 600mg tablets | 30 tablet PoM
£30.00-£452.94 | 30 tablet PoM £27.87 (Hospital only)
▶ Sustiva (Bristol-Myers Squibb Pharmaceuticals Ltd)
Efavirenz 600 mg Sustiva 600mg tablets | 30 tablet PoM £200.27
(Hospital only)

Capsule
CAUTIONARY AND ADVISORY LABELS 23
▶ Sustiva (Bristol-Myers Squibb Pharmaceuticals Ltd)
Efavirenz 50 mg Sustiva 50mg capsules | 30 capsule PoM £16.73
(Hospital only)
Efavirenz 100 mg Sustiva 100mg capsules | 30 capsule PoM
£33.41 (Hospital only)
Efavirenz 200 mg Sustiva 200mg capsules | 90 capsule PoM
£200.27 (Hospital only)

Combinations available: *Efavirenz with emtricitabine and tenofovir disoproxil,* p. 636

Etravirine

- **INDICATIONS AND DOSE**

HIV infection resistant to other non-nucleoside reverse transcriptase inhibitor and protease inhibitors in combination with other antiretroviral drugs (including a boosted protease inhibitor)
▶ BY MOUTH
▶ Adult: 200 mg twice daily, to be taken after food

- **CONTRA-INDICATIONS** Acute porphyrias p. 1025
- **INTERACTIONS** → Appendix 1: etravirine
- **SIDE-EFFECTS**
▶ **Common or very common** Diabetes mellitus · diarrhoea · headache · hyperglycaemia · myocardial infarction · nausea · skin reactions · vomiting
▶ **Uncommon** Angioedema · bronchospasm · dry mouth · dyslipidaemia · gynaecomastia · haematemesis · hepatic disorders · hyperhidrosis · hypersensitivity · hypersomnia · numbness · pancreatitis · sluggishness · vision blurred
▶ **Rare or very rare** Severe cutaneous adverse reactions (SCARs)
▶ **Frequency not known** Haemorrhagic stroke · osteonecrosis · weight increased

SIDE-EFFECTS, FURTHER INFORMATION For further information regarding **osteonecrosis, immune reconstitution syndrome** and **lipodystrophy,** see HIV infection p. 628.
Hypersensitivity reactions Rash, usually in the second week, is the most common side-effect and appears more frequently in females. Life-threatening hypersensitivity reactions reported usually during week 3 - 6 of treatment and characterised by rash, eosinophilia, and systemic symptoms (including fever, general malaise, myalgia, arthralgia, blistering, oral lesions, conjunctivitis, and hepatitis). Discontinue permanently if hypersensitivity reaction or severe rash develop. If rash mild or moderate (without signs of hypersensitivity reaction), may continue without interruption -usually resolves within 2 weeks.

- **HEPATIC IMPAIRMENT** Manufacturer advises caution in moderate impairment; avoid in severe impairment— no information available; greater risk of hepatic side-effects in chronic hepatitis B or C.
- **DIRECTIONS FOR ADMINISTRATION** Patients with swallowing difficulties may disperse tablets in a glass of water just before administration.
- **PRESCRIBING AND DISPENSING INFORMATION** Dispense in original container (contains desiccant).
- **PATIENT AND CARER ADVICE**
Hypersensitivity reactions Patients or carers should be told how to recognise hypersensitivity reactions and advised to seek immediate medical attention if hypersensitivity reaction or severe rash develop.
Missed doses If a dose is more than 6 hours late, the missed dose should not be taken and the next dose should be taken at the normal time.

- **MEDICINAL FORMS**
There can be variation in the licensing of different medicines containing the same drug.
Tablet
CAUTIONARY AND ADVISORY LABELS 21
▶ Intelence (Janssen-Cilag Ltd)
Etravirine 25 mg Intelence 25mg tablets | 120 tablet [PoM] £75.32
Etravirine 100 mg Intelence 100mg tablets | 120 tablet [PoM] £301.27
Etravirine 200 mg Intelence 200mg tablets | 60 tablet [PoM] £301.27

Nevirapine

- **INDICATIONS AND DOSE**

HIV infection in combination with other antiretroviral drugs (initial dose)
▶ BY MOUTH USING IMMEDIATE-RELEASE MEDICINES
▶ Adult: Initially 200 mg once daily for first 14 days, initial dose titration using 'immediate-release' preparation should not exceed 28 days; if rash occurs and is not resolved within 28 days, alternative treatment should be sought. If treatment interrupted for more than 7 days, restart using the lower dose of the 'immediate-release' preparation for the first 14 days as for new treatment

HIV infection in combination with other antiretroviral drugs (maintenance dose following initial dose titration if no rash present)
▶ BY MOUTH USING IMMEDIATE-RELEASE MEDICINES
▶ Adult: 200 mg twice daily
▶ BY MOUTH USING MODIFIED-RELEASE MEDICINES
▶ Adult: 400 mg once daily

- **CONTRA-INDICATIONS** Acute porphyrias p. 1025 · post-exposure prophylaxis
- **CAUTIONS** Females (at greater risk of hepatic side-effects) · high CD4 cell count (at greater risk of hepatic side-effects)
CAUTIONS, FURTHER INFORMATION
▶ **Hepatic effects** Patients with chronic hepatitis B or C, high CD4 cell count, and women are at increased risk of hepatic side-effects—if plasma HIV-1 RNA detectable, manufacturer advises avoid in women with CD4 cell count greater than 250 cells/mm^3 or in men with CD4 cell count greater than 400 cells/mm^3 unless potential benefit outweighs risk.

- **INTERACTIONS** → Appendix 1: nevirapine
- **SIDE-EFFECTS**
▶ **Common or very common** Abdominal pain · angioedema · diarrhoea · fatigue · fever · headache · hepatic disorders · hypersensitivity · hypertransaminasaemia · nausea · skin reactions · vomiting
▶ **Uncommon** Anaemia · arthralgia · myalgia · severe cutaneous adverse reactions (SCARs)
▶ **Frequency not known** Eosinophilia · osteonecrosis · weight increased

SIDE-EFFECTS, FURTHER INFORMATION
Hepatic effects Potentially life-threatening hepatotoxicity including fatal fulminant hepatitis reported usually in first 6 weeks; discontinue permanently if abnormalities in liver function tests accompanied by hypersensitivity reaction (rash, fever, arthralgia, myalgia, lymphadenopathy, hepatitis, renal impairment, eosinophilia, granulocytopenia); suspend if severe abnormalities in liver function tests but no hypersensitivity reaction—discontinue permanently if significant liver function abnormalities recur; monitor patient closely if mild to moderate abnormalities in liver function tests with no hypersensitivity reaction.
Rash Rash, usually in first 6 weeks, is most common side-effect; incidence reduced if introduced at low dose and dose increased gradually (after 14 days); Discontinue permanently if severe rash or if rash accompanied by blistering, oral lesions, conjunctivitis, facial oedema, general malaise or hypersensitivity reactions; if rash mild or moderate may continue without interruption but dose should not be increased until rash resolves.
Osteonecrosis Osteonecrosis has been reported in patients with advanced HIV disease or following long-term exposure to combination antiretroviral therapy.

- **HEPATIC IMPAIRMENT** Manufacturer advises avoid modified-release preparation—no information available; use 'immediate-release' preparation with caution in

5

Infection

moderate impairment and avoid in severe impairment. Use with caution in patients with chronic hepatitis B or C (at greater risk of hepatic side-effects).

● RENAL IMPAIRMENT Manufacturer advises avoid modified-release preparation—no information available.

● MONITORING REQUIREMENTS
▸ Hepatic disease Close monitoring of liver function required during first 18 weeks; monitor liver function before treatment then every 2 weeks for 2 months then after 1 month and then regularly.
▸ Rash Monitor closely for skin reactions during first 18 weeks.

● PATIENT AND CARER ADVICE
Hypersensitivity reactions Patients or carers should be told how to recognise hypersensitivity reactions and advised to discontinue treatment and seek immediate medical attention if severe skin reaction, hypersensitivity reactions, or symptoms of hepatitis develop.
Missed doses If a dose is more than 8 hours late with the 'immediate-release' preparation (or more than 12 hours late with the modified-release preparation), the missed dose should not be taken and the next dose should be taken at the usual time.

● MEDICINAL FORMS
There can be variation in the licensing of different medicines containing the same drug.
Oral suspension
▸ Viramune (Boehringer Ingelheim Ltd)
Nevirapine (as Nevirapine hemihydrate) 10 mg per 1 ml Viramune 50mg/5ml oral suspension | 240 ml [PoM] £50.40
Modified-release tablet
CAUTIONARY AND ADVISORY LABELS 25
▸ Nevirapine (Non-proprietary)
Nevirapine 400 mg Nevirapine 400mg modified-release tablets | 30 tablet [PoM] £23.00–£170.00
▸ Viramune (Boehringer Ingelheim Ltd)
Nevirapine 100 mg Viramune 100mg modified-release tablets | 90 tablet [PoM] £127.50 (Hospital only)
Nevirapine 400 mg Viramune 400mg modified-release tablets | 30 tablet [PoM] £170.00 (Hospital only)
Tablet
▸ Nevirapine (Non-proprietary)
Nevirapine 200 mg Nevirapine 200mg tablets | 14 tablet [PoM] £33.69 | 60 tablet [PoM] £21.45–£170.00
▸ Viramune (Boehringer Ingelheim Ltd)
Nevirapine 200 mg Viramune 200mg tablets | 60 tablet [PoM] £170.00

Rilpivirine

28-Sep-2016

● INDICATIONS AND DOSE
HIV infection in combination with other antiretroviral drugs in patients not previously treated with antiretroviral therapy and if plasma HIV-1 RNA concentration less than or equal to 100 000 copies/mL
▸ BY MOUTH
▸ Adult: 25 mg once daily

● CAUTIONS Acute porphyrias p. 1025
● INTERACTIONS → Appendix 1: rilpivirine
● SIDE-EFFECTS
▸ **Common or very common** Appetite decreased · depression · dizziness · drowsiness · dry mouth · fatigue · gastrointestinal discomfort · headache · nausea · rash · sleep disorders · vomiting
▸ **Uncommon** Immune reconstitution inflammatory syndrome
SIDE-EFFECTS, FURTHER INFORMATION For further information regarding lipodystrophy, see HIV infection p. 628.

● PREGNANCY Manufacturer advises avoid unless essential— no information available.

● HEPATIC IMPAIRMENT Manufacturer advises caution in moderate impairment; avoid in severe impairment— no information available; greater risk of hepatic side-effects in chronic hepatitis B or C.

● RENAL IMPAIRMENT Manufacturer advises caution in severe impairment.

● PATIENT AND CARER ADVICE Patients or carers should be given advice on how to administer rilpivirine tablets.
Missed doses If a dose is more than 12 hours late, the missed dose should not be taken and the next dose should be taken at the normal time.

● MEDICINAL FORMS
There can be variation in the licensing of different medicines containing the same drug.
Tablet
CAUTIONARY AND ADVISORY LABELS 21, 25
▸ Edurant (Janssen-Cilag Ltd)
Rilpivirine (as Rilpivirine hydrochloride) 25 mg Edurant 25mg tablets | 30 tablet [PoM] £200.27

Combinations available: *Emtricitabine with rilpivirine and tenofovir alafenamide*, p. 638 · *Emtricitabine with rilpivirine and tenofovir disoproxil*, p. 639

ANTIVIRALS > NUCLEOSIDE REVERSE TRANSCRIPTASE INHIBITORS

Nucleoside reverse transcriptase inhibitors

● SIDE-EFFECTS
▸ **Common or very common** Abdominal pain · anaemia (may require transfusion) · appetite decreased · asthenia · diarrhoea · dizziness · headache · myalgia · nausea · skin reactions · vomiting
▸ **Uncommon** Hepatic steatosis · lactic acidosis · pancreatitis · thrombocytopenia
▸ **Frequency not known** Immune reconstitution inflammatory syndrome · osteonecrosis · weight increased
SIDE-EFFECTS, FURTHER INFORMATION Osteonecrosis has been reported in patients with advanced HIV disease or following long-term exposure to combination antiretroviral therapy.

● PREGNANCY
Monitoring Mitochondrial dysfunction has been reported in infants exposed to nucleoside reverse transcriptase inhibitors in utero; the main effects include haematological, metabolic, and neurological disorders; all infants whose mothers received nucleoside reverse transcriptase inhibitors during pregnancy should be monitored for relevant signs or symptoms.

● HEPATIC IMPAIRMENT Use with caution in patients with chronic hepatitis B or C (greater risk of hepatic side-effects).

⬆ above

Abacavir

● INDICATIONS AND DOSE
HIV infection in combination with other antiretroviral drugs
▸ BY MOUTH
▸ Adult: 600 mg daily in 1–2 divided doses

● CAUTIONS HIV load greater than 100 000 copies/mL · patients at high risk of cardiovascular disease (especially if 10-year cardiovascular risk greater than 20%)

- INTERACTIONS → Appendix 1: abacavir
- SIDE-EFFECTS
- ▶ **Common or very common** Fever · lethargy
- ▶ **Rare or very rare** Erythema multiforme · severe cutaneous adverse reactions (SCARs)
- ▶ **Frequency not known** Hypersensitivity

  SIDE-EFFECTS, FURTHER INFORMATION Life-threatening hypersensitivity reactions have been reported-characterised by fever or rash and possibly nausea, vomiting, diarrhoea, abdominal pain, dyspnoea, cough, lethargy, malaise, headache, and myalgia; less frequently mouth ulceration, oedema, hypotension, sore throat, acute respiratory distress syndrome, anaphylaxis, paraesthesia, arthralgia, conjunctivitis, lymphadenopathy, lymphocytopenia and renal failure; rarely myolysis. Laboratory abnormalities may include raised liver function tests and creatine kinase; symptoms usually appear in the first 6 weeks, but may occur at any time. Discontinue immediately if any symptom of hypersensitivity develops and do not rechallenge (risk of more severe hypersensitivity reaction).

- ALLERGY AND CROSS-SENSITIVITY Caution—increased risk of hypersensitivity reaction in presence of HLA-B*5701 allele.
- HEPATIC IMPAIRMENT Monitor closely in mild impairment (combination preparations not recommended as reduced abacavir dose may be required). Avoid in moderate impairment unless essential—close monitoring recommended. Avoid in severe impairment.
- RENAL IMPAIRMENT Manufacturer advises avoid in end-stage renal disease.
- PRE-TREATMENT SCREENING Test for HLA-B*5701 allele before treatment or if restarting treatment and HLA-B*5701 status not known.
- MONITORING REQUIREMENTS Monitor for symptoms of hypersensitivity reaction every 2 weeks for 2 months.
- PRESCRIBING AND DISPENSING INFORMATION Flavours of oral liquid formulations may include banana, or strawberry.
- PATIENT AND CARER ADVICE Patients and their carers should be told the importance of regular dosing (intermittent therapy may increase the risk of sensitisation), how to recognise signs of hypersensitivity, and advised to seek immediate medical attention if symptoms develop or before re-starting treatment.
  Patients should be provided with an alert card and advised to keep it with them at all times.

- MEDICINAL FORMS
  There can be variation in the licensing of different medicines containing the same drug.
  Oral solution
  EXCIPIENTS: May contain Propylene glycol
  ▶ Ziagen (ViiV Healthcare UK Ltd)
  Abacavir (as Abacavir sulfate) 20 mg per 1 ml Ziagen 20mg/ml oral solution sugar-free | 240 ml PoM £55.72
  Tablet
  ▶ Ziagen (ViiV Healthcare UK Ltd)
  Abacavir (as Abacavir sulfate) 300 mg Ziagen 300mg tablets | 60 tablet PoM £208.95

Abacavir with dolutegravir and lamivudine

The properties listed below are those particular to the combination only. For the properties of the components please consider, abacavir p. 634, lamivudine p. 640, dolutegravir p. 630.

- INDICATIONS AND DOSE
  HIV infection
  ▶ BY MOUTH
  ▶ Adult (body-weight 40 kg and above): 1 tablet once daily

- INTERACTIONS → Appendix 1: abacavir · dolutegravir · lamivudine
- RENAL IMPAIRMENT Avoid *Triumeq*® if eGFR less than 50 mL/minute/1.73 m^2 (consult product literature).
- PATIENT AND CARER ADVICE
  Missed doses If a dose is more than 20 hours late, the missed dose should not be taken and the next dose should be taken at the normal time.

- MEDICINAL FORMS
  There can be variation in the licensing of different medicines containing the same drug.
  Tablet
  ▶ Triumeq (ViiV Healthcare UK Ltd) ▼
  Dolutegravir (as Dolutegravir sodium) 50 mg, Lamivudine 300 mg, Abacavir (as Abacavir sulfate) 600 mg Triumeq 50mg/600mg/300mg tablets | 30 tablet PoM £798.16

Abacavir with lamivudine

The properties listed below are those particular to the combination only. For the properties of the components please consider, abacavir p. 634, lamivudine p. 640.

- INDICATIONS AND DOSE
  HIV infection in combination with other antiretrovirals
  ▶ BY MOUTH
  ▶ Adult (body-weight 40 kg and above): 1 tablet once daily

- INTERACTIONS → Appendix 1: abacavir · lamivudine
- RENAL IMPAIRMENT Avoid *Kivexa*® if eGFR less than 50 mL/minute/1.73 m^2 (consult product literature).

- MEDICINAL FORMS
  There can be variation in the licensing of different medicines containing the same drug.
  Tablet
  ▶ Abacavir with lamivudine (Non-proprietary)
  Lamivudine 300 mg, Abacavir 600 mg Abacavir 600mg / Lamivudine 300mg tablets | 30 tablet PoM £150.83-£299.41 | 30 tablet PoM £224.56 (Hospital only)
  ▶ Kivexa (ViiV Healthcare UK Ltd)
  Lamivudine 300 mg, Abacavir 600 mg Kivexa 600mg/300mg tablets | 30 tablet PoM £352.25

Abacavir with lamivudine and zidovudine

The properties listed below are those particular to the combination only. For the properties of the components please consider, abacavir p. 634, lamivudine p. 640, zidovudine p. 642.

- INDICATIONS AND DOSE
  HIV infection (use only if patient is stabilised for 6-8 weeks on the individual components in the same proportions)
  ▶ BY MOUTH
  ▶ Adult: 1 tablet twice daily

- INTERACTIONS → Appendix 1: abacavir · lamivudine · zidovudine
- RENAL IMPAIRMENT Avoid *Trizivir®* if eGFR less than 50 mL/minute/1.73 m² (consult product literature).

- MEDICINAL FORMS
There can be variation in the licensing of different medicines containing the same drug.
Tablet
▸ Trizivir (ViiV Healthcare UK Ltd)
Lamivudine 150 mg, Abacavir (as Abacavir sulfate) 300 mg, Zidovudine 300 mg Trizivir tablets | 60 tablet [PoM] £509.06

▶ 634

Didanosine

01-Sep-2016

(ddI; DDI)

- INDICATIONS AND DOSE
HIV infection in combination with other antiretroviral drugs
▸ BY MOUTH
▸ Adult (body-weight up to 60 kg): 250 mg daily in 1–2 divided doses
▸ Adult (body-weight 60 kg and above): 400 mg daily in 1–2 divided doses

- CAUTIONS History of pancreatitis (preferably avoid, otherwise extreme caution) · hyperuricaemia · lactic acidosis · peripheral neuropathy
CAUTIONS, FURTHER INFORMATION
▸ Lactic acidosis Lactic acidosis associated with hepatomegaly and hepatic steatosis has been reported with didanosine. Use with caution in patients with hepatomegaly, hepatitis, or other risk factors for liver disease and hepatic steatosis (including obesity and alcohol abuse). Discontinue treatment if symptoms of hyperlactataemia, lactic acidosis, progressive hepatomegaly or rapid deterioration of liver function become apparent.

- INTERACTIONS → Appendix 1: didanosine

- SIDE-EFFECTS
▸ **Common or very common** Arthralgia · chills · dry mouth · fever · flatulence · gynaecomastia · hepatic disorders · pain · peripheral neuropathy (switch to another antiretroviral if develops)
▸ **Uncommon** Acute kidney injury · alopecia · diabetes mellitus · dry eye · haemodialysis · hyperglycaemia · hypoglycaemia · leucopenia · myopathy · optic neuritis · retinal discolouration · sialadenitis
▸ **Rare or very rare** Parotid gland enlargement
▸ **Frequency not known** Lipoatrophy
SIDE-EFFECTS, FURTHER INFORMATION
Pancreatitis Suspend treatment if serum lipase raised or if symptoms of pancreatitis develop; discontinue if pancreatitis confirmed. Whenever possible avoid concomitant treatment with other drugs known to cause pancreatic toxicity; monitor closely if concomitant therapy unavoidable. Since significant elevations of triglycerides cause pancreatitis monitor closely if elevated.
Lipodystrophy syndrome Metabolic effects may occur with didanosine; these include fat redistribution, insulin resistance, and dyslipidaemia—collectively termed lipodystrophy syndrome. Manufacturer advises monitoring of plasma lipids and blood-glucose.

- PREGNANCY Manufacturer advises use only if potential benefit outweighs risk.
- HEPATIC IMPAIRMENT Insufficient information.
Monitoring In hepatic impairment, monitor for toxicity.
- RENAL IMPAIRMENT
Dose adjustments Reduce dose if eGFR less than 60 mL/minute/1.73 m²; consult product literature.

- MONITORING REQUIREMENTS Ophthalmological examination (including visual acuity, colour vision, and dilated fundus examination) recommended annually or if visual changes occur.
- DIRECTIONS FOR ADMINISTRATION Capsules should be swallowed whole and taken at least 2 hours before or 2 hours after food.
With chewable tablets, to ensure sufficient antacid, each dose to be taken as at least 2 tablets chewed thoroughly, crushed or dispersed in water; clear apple juice may be added for flavouring; tablets to be taken 2 hours after lopinavir with ritonavir capsules and oral solution or atazanavir with ritonavir.
- PATIENT AND CARER ADVICE Patients or carers should be given advice on how to administer didanosine capsules and chewable tablets.

- MEDICINAL FORMS
There can be variation in the licensing of different medicines containing the same drug.
Gastro-resistant capsule
CAUTIONARY AND ADVISORY LABELS 25
▸ Videx EC (Bristol-Myers Squibb Pharmaceuticals Ltd)
Didanosine 125 mg Videx EC 125mg capsules | 30 capsule [PoM] £48.18 (Hospital only)
Didanosine 200 mg Videx EC 200mg capsules | 30 capsule [PoM] £77.09 (Hospital only)
Didanosine 250 mg Videx EC 250mg capsules | 30 capsule [PoM] £96.37 (Hospital only)
Didanosine 400 mg Videx EC 400mg capsules | 30 capsule [PoM] £154.19 (Hospital only)
Chewable tablet
CAUTIONARY AND ADVISORY LABELS 23
EXCIPIENTS: May contain Aspartame
▸ Videx (Bristol-Myers Squibb Pharmaceuticals Ltd)
Didanosine 25 mg Videx 25mg chewable dispersible tablets sugar-free | 60 tablet [PoM] £25.06 (Hospital only)

Efavirenz with emtricitabine and tenofovir disoproxil

The properties listed below are those particular to the combination only. For the properties of the components please consider, tenofovir disoproxil p. 641, efavirenz p. 632, emtricitabine p. 638.

- INDICATIONS AND DOSE
HIV infection stabilised on antiretroviral therapy for more than 3 months
▸ BY MOUTH
▸ Adult: 1 tablet once daily

- INTERACTIONS → Appendix 1: efavirenz · tenofovir disoproxil
- HEPATIC IMPAIRMENT Manufacturer of *Atripla®* advises caution in mild impairment; avoid *Atripla®* in moderate to severe impairment.
- RENAL IMPAIRMENT Avoid *Atripla®* if eGFR less than 50 mL/minute/1.73 m².
- PATIENT AND CARER ADVICE
Missed doses If a dose is more than 12 hours late, the missed dose should not be taken and the next dose should be taken at the normal time.

- **MEDICINAL FORMS**
  There can be variation in the licensing of different medicines
  containing the same drug.
  Tablet
  CAUTIONARY AND ADVISORY LABELS 23, 25
  - ▸ Efavirenz with emtricitabine and tenofovir disoproxil (Non-proprietary)
    Emtricitabine 200 mg, Tenofovir disoproxil (as Tenofovir disoproxil fumarate) 245 mg, Efavirenz 600 mg Efavirenz 600mg / Emtricitabine 200mg / Tenofovir disoproxil 245mg tablets | 30 tablet ᴘᴏᴍ £506.23–£532.87
  - ▸ Atripla (Gilead Sciences International Ltd)
    Emtricitabine 200 mg, Tenofovir disoproxil (as Tenofovir disoproxil fumarate) 245 mg, Efavirenz 600 mg Atripla 600mg/200mg/245mg tablets | 30 tablet ᴘᴏᴍ £532.87

Elvitegravir with cobicistat, emtricitabine and tenofovir alafenamide

03-May-2018

The properties listed below are those particular to the combination only. For the properties of the components please consider, emtricitabine p. 638, elvitegravir p. 631, cobicistat p. 647, tenofovir alafenamide p. 611.

- **INDICATIONS AND DOSE**
  HIV-1 infection (specialist use only)
  - ▸ BY MOUTH
  - ▸ Adult: 1 tablet once daily

- **INTERACTIONS** → Appendix 1: cobicistat · elvitegravir · tenofovir alafenamide

- **SIDE-EFFECTS**
  - ▸ **Common or very common** Abnormal dreams · diarrhoea · dizziness · fatigue · flatulence · gastrointestinal discomfort · headache · nausea · skin reactions · vomiting
  - ▸ **Uncommon** Anaemia · angioedema · depression
  - ▸ **Frequency not known** Nephrotoxicity · osteonecrosis · weight increased

- **CONCEPTION AND CONTRACEPTION** Manufacturer advises effective contraception in women of childbearing potential; if using a hormonal contraceptive, it must contain drospirenone or norgestimate as the progestogen and at least 30 micrograms ethinylestradiol.

- **HEPATIC IMPAIRMENT** Manufacturer advises use with caution in mild-to-moderate impairment (greater risk of hepatic side-effects); avoid in severe impairment—no information available.

- **RENAL IMPAIRMENT** Manufacturer advises avoid if creatinine clearance less than 30 mL/minute—limited information available.

- **PRESCRIBING AND DISPENSING INFORMATION** Dispense in original container—contains desiccant.

- **PATIENT AND CARER ADVICE**
  Missed doses Manufacturer advises if a dose is more than 18 hours late, the missed dose should not be taken and the next dose should be taken at the normal time.
  Driving and skilled tasks Manufacturer advises patients and carers should be counselled on the effects on driving and performance of skilled tasks—increased risk of dizziness.

- **NATIONAL FUNDING/ACCESS DECISIONS**
  Scottish Medicines Consortium (SMC) Decisions
  The *Scottish Medicines Consortium* has advised (May 2016) that elvitegravir with cobicistat, emtricitabine and tenofovir alafenamide (*Genvoya*®) is accepted for use within NHS Scotland for the treatment of human immunodeficiency virus type 1 (HIV-1), without known mutations associated with resistance to the integrase inhibitor class, emtricitabine or tenofovir. This advice is contingent upon the continuing availability of the patient access scheme in NHS Scotland or a list price that is equivalent or lower.

  All Wales Medicines Strategy Group (AWMSG) Decisions
  The *All Wales Medicines Strategy Group* has advised (July 2016) that elvitegravir with cobicistat, emtricitabine and tenofovir alafenamide (*Genvoya*®) is recommended as an option for use within NHS Wales for the treatment of human immunodeficiency virus type 1 (HIV-1), without known mutations associated with resistance to the integrase inhibitor class, emtricitabine or tenofovir. The recommendation applies only if the approved Wales Patient Access Scheme (WPAS) is used or where the list price is equivalent or lower.

- **MEDICINAL FORMS**
  There can be variation in the licensing of different medicines containing the same drug.
  Tablet
  CAUTIONARY AND ADVISORY LABELS 21
  - ▸ Genvoya (Gilead Sciences International Ltd) ▼
    Tenofovir alafenamide 10 mg, Cobicistat 150 mg, Elvitegravir 150 mg, Emtricitabine 200 mg Genvoya 150mg/150mg/200mg/10mg tablets | 30 tablet ᴘᴏᴍ £879.51

Elvitegravir with cobicistat, emtricitabine and tenofovir disoproxil

The properties listed below are those particular to the combination only. For the properties of the components please consider, tenofovir disoproxil p. 641, emtricitabine p. 638, cobicistat p. 647, elvitegravir p. 631.

- **INDICATIONS AND DOSE**
  HIV infection
  - ▸ BY MOUTH
  - ▸ Adult: 1 tablet once daily

- **INTERACTIONS** → Appendix 1: cobicistat · elvitegravir · tenofovir disoproxil

- **SIDE-EFFECTS**
  - ▸ **Common or very common** Appetite decreased · asthenia · constipation · diarrhoea · dizziness · electrolyte imbalance · flatulence · gastrointestinal discomfort · headache · hyperbilirubinaemia · hyperglycaemia · hypersensitivity · hypertriglyceridaemia · nausea · neutropenia · pain · rash pustular · skin reactions · sleep disorders · vomiting
  - ▸ **Uncommon** Anaemia · angioedema · depression (in patients with history of depression or psychiatric illness) · muscle weakness · myopathy · pancreatitis · proteinuria · renal failure · renal tubular disorders · suicidal ideation (in patients with history of depression or psychiatric illness)
  - ▸ **Rare or very rare** Acute tubular necrosis · hepatic disorders · lactic acidosis · nephritis · nephrogenic diabetes insipidus · osteomalacia
  - ▸ **Frequency not known** Autoimmune disorder · Grave's disease · inflammation · osteonecrosis · weight increased

- **CONCEPTION AND CONTRACEPTION** Women of child-bearing potential should use effective contraception during treatment (if using a hormonal contraceptive, it must contain norgestimate as the progestogen and at least 30 micrograms ethinylestradiol).

- **PREGNANCY** Manufacturer advises use only if potential benefit outweighs risk.

- **HEPATIC IMPAIRMENT** Avoid *Stribild*® in severe impairment.

- **RENAL IMPAIRMENT** If eGFR less than 90 mL/minute/1.73 m², only *initiate Stribild*® if other treatments cannot be used (avoid *initiating Stribild*® if eGFR less than 70 mL/minute/1.73 m²); if eGFR less than 70 mL/minute/1.73 m², only *continue Stribild*® if potential benefit outweighs risk (discontinue *Stribild* ® if eGFR less than 50 mL/minute/1.73 m²).

- MONITORING REQUIREMENTS Test urine glucose before treatment, then every 4 weeks for 1 year and then every 3 months.
- PRESCRIBING AND DISPENSING INFORMATION Dispense in original container (contains desiccant).
- PATIENT AND CARER ADVICE Patients or carers should be given advice on how to administer *Stribild* ®.
  Missed doses If a dose is more than 18 hours late, the missed dose should not be taken and the next dose should be taken at the normal time.

- MEDICINAL FORMS
  There can be variation in the licensing of different medicines containing the same drug.
  Tablet
  CAUTIONARY AND ADVISORY LABELS 21
  ▸ Stribild (Gilead Sciences International Ltd) ▼
    Cobicistat 150 mg, Elvitegravir 150 mg, Emtricitabine 200 mg, Tenofovir disoproxil (as Tenofovir disoproxil fumarate) **245 mg** Stribild 150mg/150mg/200mg/245mg tablets | 30 tablet [PoM] £879.51

⏻ 634

Emtricitabine

(FTC)

- INDICATIONS AND DOSE
  HIV infection in combination with other antiretroviral drugs
  ▸ BY MOUTH USING CAPSULES
  ▸ Adult: 200 mg once daily
  ▸ BY MOUTH USING ORAL SOLUTION
  ▸ Adult: 240 mg once daily
  DOSE EQUIVALENCE AND CONVERSION
  ▸ 240 mg oral solution ≡ 200 mg capsule; where appropriate the capsule may be used instead of the oral solution.

- SIDE-EFFECTS
- Common or very common Dyspepsia · hyperbilirubinaemia · hyperglycaemia · hypersensitivity · hypertriglyceridaemia · neutropenia · pain · rash pustular · sleep disorders
- Uncommon Angioedema

- HEPATIC IMPAIRMENT
  Monitoring On discontinuation, monitor patients with hepatitis B (risk of exacerbation of hepatitis).

- RENAL IMPAIRMENT
  Dose adjustments Reduce dose if eGFR less than 50 mL/minute/1.73 m²; consult product literature.

- PRESCRIBING AND DISPENSING INFORMATION Flavours of oral liquid formulations may include candy.

- PATIENT AND CARER ADVICE
  Missed doses If a dose is more than 12 hours late, the missed dose should not be taken and the next dose should be taken at the normal time.

- MEDICINAL FORMS
  There can be variation in the licensing of different medicines containing the same drug.
  Oral solution
  ELECTROLYTES: May contain Sodium
  ▸ Emtriva (Gilead Sciences International Ltd)
    Emtricitabine 10 mg per 1 ml Emtriva 10mg/ml oral solution sugar-free | 170 ml [PoM] £39.53
  Capsule
  ▸ Emtriva (Gilead Sciences International Ltd)
    Emtricitabine 200 mg Emtriva 200mg capsules | 30 capsule [PoM] £138.98

Combinations available: *Darunavir with cobicistat, emtricitabine and tenofovir alafenamide*, p. 644

Emtricitabine with rilpivirine and tenofovir alafenamide

05-Jun-2017

The properties listed below are those particular to the combination only. For the properties of the components please consider, emtricitabine above, rilpivirine p. 634, tenofovir alafenamide p. 611.

- INDICATIONS AND DOSE
  HIV infection in patients with plasma HIV-1 RNA concentration of 100 000 copies/mL or less (specialist use only)
  ▸ BY MOUTH
  ▸ Adult: 1 tablet once daily

- INTERACTIONS → Appendix 1: rilpivirine · tenofovir alafenamide

- SIDE-EFFECTS
- Common or very common Appetite decreased · depression · diarrhoea · dizziness · drowsiness · dry mouth · fatigue · flatulence · gastrointestinal discomfort · headache · nausea · skin reactions · sleep disorders · vomiting
- Uncommon Anaemia · angioedema · arthralgia · immune reconstitution inflammatory syndrome
- Frequency not known Conjunctivitis · drug reaction with eosinophilia and systemic symptoms (DRESS) · eosinophilia · fever · osteonecrosis · QT interval prolongation · weight increased

  SIDE-EFFECTS, FURTHER INFORMATION Systemic symptoms reported with severe skin reactions include fever, blisters, conjunctivitis, angioedema, elevated liver function tests, and eosinophilia.

- HEPATIC IMPAIRMENT Manufacturer advises use with caution in moderate impairment (greater risk of hepatic side-effects); avoid in severe impairment—no information available.

- RENAL IMPAIRMENT Manufacturer advises avoid if creatinine clearance less than 30 mL/minute—no information available.

- PATIENT AND CARER ADVICE
  Vomiting Manufacturer advises if vomiting occurs within 4 hours of taking a dose, a replacement dose should be taken.
  Driving and skilled tasks Manufacturer advises patients and carers should be counselled on the effects on driving and performance of skilled tasks—increased risk of dizziness.

- NATIONAL FUNDING/ACCESS DECISIONS
  Scottish Medicines Consortium (SMC) Decisions
  The *Scottish Medicines Consortium* has advised (October 2016) that emtricitabine with rilpivirine and tenofovir alafenamide (*Odefsey* ®) is accepted for use within NHS Scotland for the treatment of human immunodeficiency virus type 1 (HIV-1), without known mutations associated with resistance to the non-nucleoside reverse transcriptase inhibitor (NNRTI) class, tenofovir or emtricitabine, and with viral load HIV-1 RNA of 100 000 copies/mL or less.

  All Wales Medicines Strategy Group (AWMSG) Decisions
  The *All Wales Medicines Strategy Group* has advised (November 2016) that emtricitabine with rilpivirine and tenofovir alafenamide (*Odefsey* ®) is recommended as an option for use within NHS Wales for the treatment of human immunodeficiency virus type 1, without known mutations associated with resistance to the non-nucleoside reverse transcriptase inhibitor (NNRTI) class, tenofovir or emtricitabine, and with viral load HIV-1 RNA of 100 000 copies/mL or less.

● MEDICINAL FORMS
There can be variation in the licensing of different medicines containing the same drug.

Tablet
CAUTIONARY AND ADVISORY LABELS 3, 21
 ▸ Odefsey (Gilead Sciences International Ltd) ▼
   Rilpivirine (as Rilpivirine hydrochloride) 25 mg, Tenofovir alafenamide (as Tenofovir alafenamide fumarate) 25 mg, Emtricitabine 200 mg Odefsey 200mg/25mg/25mg tablets | 30 tablet PoM £525.95

Emtricitabine with rilpivirine and tenofovir disoproxil

The properties listed below are those particular to the combination only. For the properties of the components please consider, tenofovir disoproxil p. 641, emtricitabine p. 638, rilpivirine p. 634.

 ● INDICATIONS AND DOSE

HIV infection in patients with plasma HIV-1 RNA concentration less than 100 000 copies/mL
 ▸ BY MOUTH
 ▸ Adult: 1 tablet once daily

● INTERACTIONS → Appendix 1: rilpivirine · tenofovir disoproxil

● HEPATIC IMPAIRMENT Manufacturer of *Eviplera* ® advises caution in moderate impairment; avoid *Eviplera* ® in severe impairment.

● RENAL IMPAIRMENT Avoid *Eviplera* ® if eGFR less than 50 mL/minute/1.73 m^2.

● PATIENT AND CARER ADVICE Patients or carers should be given advice on how to administer *Eviplera* ®.
Missed doses If a dose is more than 12 hours late, the missed dose should not be taken and the next dose should be taken at the normal time.

● MEDICINAL FORMS
There can be variation in the licensing of different medicines containing the same drug.

Tablet
CAUTIONARY AND ADVISORY LABELS 21, 25
 ▸ Eviplera (Gilead Sciences International Ltd)
   Rilpivirine (as Rilpivirine hydrochloride) 25 mg, Emtricitabine 200 mg, Tenofovir disoproxil (as Tenofovir disoproxil fumarate) 245 mg Eviplera 200mg/25mg/245mg tablets | 30 tablet PoM £525.95

Emtricitabine with tenofovir alafenamide
05-Jun-2017

The properties listed below are those particular to the combination only. For the properties of the components please consider, emtricitabine p. 638, tenofovir alafenamide p. 611.

 ● INDICATIONS AND DOSE

HIV infection in combination with other antiretroviral drugs (specialist use only)
 ▸ BY MOUTH
 ▸ Adult: 200/10–200/25 mg once daily, dose is dependent on drug regimen—consult product literature

DOSE EQUIVALENCE AND CONVERSION
 ▸ Dose expressed as x/y mg emtricitabine/tenofovir alafenamide.

● INTERACTIONS → Appendix 1: tenofovir alafenamide

● SIDE-EFFECTS
 ▸ **Common or very common** Abnormal dreams · diarrhoea · dizziness · fatigue · flatulence · gastrointestinal discomfort · headache · nausea · skin reactions · vomiting
 ▸ **Uncommon** Anaemia · arthralgia
 ▸ **Frequency not known** Angioedema · osteonecrosis

● HEPATIC IMPAIRMENT Manufacturer advises use with caution (greater risk of hepatic side-effects).

● RENAL IMPAIRMENT Manufacturer advises avoid if creatinine clearance less than 30 mL/minute—limited information available.

● PATIENT AND CARER ADVICE
Driving and skilled tasks Manufacturer advises patients and carers should be counselled on the effects on driving and performance of skilled tasks—increased risk of dizziness.

● NATIONAL FUNDING/ACCESS DECISIONS
Scottish Medicines Consortium (SMC) Decisions
The *Scottish Medicines Consortium* has advised (August 2016) that emtricitabine with tenofovir alafenamide (*Descovy*®) is accepted for use within NHS Scotland for the treatment of human immunodeficiency virus type 1 in combination with other antiretroviral agents.

All Wales Medicines Strategy Group (AWMSG) Decisions
The *All Wales Medicines Strategy Group* has advised (September 2016) that emtricitabine with tenofovir alafenamide (*Descovy*®) is recommended as an option for use within NHS Wales for the treatment of human immunodeficiency virus type 1 in combination with other antiretroviral agents.

● MEDICINAL FORMS
There can be variation in the licensing of different medicines containing the same drug.

Tablet
 ▸ Descovy (Gilead Sciences International Ltd) ▼
   Tenofovir alafenamide (as Tenofovir alafenamide fumarate) 25 mg, Emtricitabine 200 mg Descovy 200mg/25mg tablets | 30 tablet PoM £355.73
   Tenofovir alafenamide (as Tenofovir alafenamide fumarate) 10 mg, Emtricitabine 200 mg Descovy 200mg/10mg tablets | 30 tablet PoM £355.73

Emtricitabine with tenofovir disoproxil
29-May-2018

The properties listed below are those particular to the combination only. For the properties of the components please consider, tenofovir disoproxil p. 641, emtricitabine p. 638.

 ● INDICATIONS AND DOSE

HIV-1 infection (initiated by a specialist)
 ▸ BY MOUTH
 ▸ Adult: 200/245 mg once daily

Pre-exposure prophylaxis of HIV-1 infection (initiated by a specialist)
 ▸ BY MOUTH
 ▸ Adult: 200/245 mg once daily

DOSE EQUIVALENCE AND CONVERSION
 ▸ Dose expressed as x/y mg emtricitabine/tenofovir disoproxil.

● INTERACTIONS → Appendix 1: tenofovir disoproxil

● RENAL IMPAIRMENT
 ▸ When used for HIV-1 infection Manufacturer advises avoid in severe impairment.
 ▸ When used for Pre-exposure prophylaxis of HIV-1 infection Manufacturer advises avoid if creatinine clearance less than 60 mL/minute.

5

Infection

Dose adjustments
- When used for HIV-1 infection Manufacturer advises use normal dose every 2 days in moderate impairment.
- DIRECTIONS FOR ADMINISTRATION Patients with swallowing difficulties may disperse tablet in half a glass of water, orange juice, or grape juice (but bitter taste).
- PATIENT AND CARER ADVICE Patients or carers should be given advice on how to administer emtricitabine with tenofovir tablets.
  Missed doses If a dose is more than 12 hours late, the missed dose should not be taken and the next dose should be taken at the normal time.
- NATIONAL FUNDING/ACCESS DECISIONS
  Scottish Medicines Consortium (SMC) Decisions
  The *Scottish Medicines Consortium* has advised (April 2017) that emtricitabine with tenofovir disoproxil (*Truvada®*) is accepted for use within NHS Scotland in combination with safer sex practices for pre-exposure prophylaxis of sexually acquired HIV-1 infection in adults at high risk.
  All Wales Medicines Strategy Group (AWMSG) Decisions
  The *All Wales Medicines Strategy Group* has advised (September 2017) that emtricitabine/tenofovir disoproxil (*Truvada®*) is not recommended for use within NHS Wales in combination with safer sex practices for pre-exposure prophylaxis to reduce the risk of sexually acquired HIV 1 infection in adults at high risk. The case for cost-effectiveness has not been proven.
  Subsequent to this AWMSG recommendation, *Truvada®* has been made available in Wales and is being provided through NHS Wales from 17 July 2017 for up to three years for use as pre-exposure prophylaxis. During this time, eligible patients will receive *Truvada®* and data will be collected to assess its effectiveness at preventing HIV and address some of the concerns of AWMSG in relation to cost-effectiveness.
- MEDICINAL FORMS
  There can be variation in the licensing of different medicines containing the same drug.
  Tablet
  CAUTIONARY AND ADVISORY LABELS 21
  - Emtricitabine with tenofovir disoproxil (Non-proprietary)
    Emtricitabine 200 mg, Tenofovir disoproxil (as Tenofovir disoproxil fumarate) 245 mg Emtricitabine 200mg / Tenofovir 245mg tablets | 30 tablet [PoM] £106.72–£355.73 | 30 tablet [PoM] £355.73 (Hospital only)
  - Truvada (Gilead Sciences International Ltd)
    Emtricitabine 200 mg, Tenofovir disoproxil (as Tenofovir disoproxil fumarate) 245 mg Truvada tablets | 30 tablet [PoM] £355.73

☞ 634

Lamivudine
(3TC)

- INDICATIONS AND DOSE
  EPIVIR® ORAL SOLUTION
  HIV infection in combination with other antiretroviral drugs
  - BY MOUTH
  - Adult: 150 mg every 12 hours, alternatively 300 mg once daily
  EPIVIR® TABLETS
  HIV infection in combination with other antiretroviral drugs
  - BY MOUTH
  - Adult: 150 mg every 12 hours, alternatively 300 mg once daily

ZEFFIX®
Chronic hepatitis B infection either with compensated liver disease (with evidence of viral replication and histology of active liver inflammation or fibrosis) when first-line treatments cannot be used, or (in combination with another antiviral drug without cross-resistance to lamivudine) with decompensated liver disease
- BY MOUTH
- Adult: 100 mg once daily, patients receiving lamivudine for concomitant HIV infection should continue to receive lamivudine in a dose appropriate for HIV infection

- CAUTIONS Recurrent hepatitis in patients with chronic hepatitis B may occur on discontinuation of lamivudine
- INTERACTIONS → Appendix 1: lamivudine
- SIDE-EFFECTS
  - Common or very common Hepatitis aggravated · muscle cramps · myopathy
  - Rare or very rare Angioedema
  - Frequency not known Abdominal discomfort · malaise · respiratory tract infection · throat complaints
- BREAST FEEDING Can be used with caution in women infected with chronic hepatitis B alone, providing that adequate measures are taken to prevent hepatitis B infection in infants.
- RENAL IMPAIRMENT
  Dose adjustments Reduce dose if eGFR less than 50 mL/minute/1.73 m^2; consult product literature.
- MONITORING REQUIREMENTS When treating chronic hepatitis B with lamivudine, monitor liver function tests every 3 months, and viral markers of hepatitis B every 3–6 months, more frequently in patients with advanced liver disease or following transplantation (monitoring to continue for at least 1 year after discontinuation—recurrent hepatitis may occur on discontinuation).
- PRESCRIBING AND DISPENSING INFORMATION Flavours of oral liquid formulations may include banana and strawberry.
- MEDICINAL FORMS
  There can be variation in the licensing of different medicines containing the same drug.
  Oral solution
  EXCIPIENTS: May contain Sucrose
  - Epivir (ViiV Healthcare UK Ltd)
    Lamivudine 10 mg per 1 ml Epivir 50mg/5ml oral solution | 240 ml [PoM] £39.01
  Tablet
  - Epivir (ViiV Healthcare UK Ltd)
    Lamivudine 150 mg Epivir 150mg tablets | 60 tablet [PoM] £143.32 DT = £121.82
    Lamivudine 300 mg Epivir 300mg tablets | 30 tablet [PoM] £157.51 DT = £133.89
  - Zeffix (GlaxoSmithKline UK Ltd)
    Lamivudine 100 mg Zeffix 100mg tablets | 28 tablet [PoM] £78.09 DT = £73.81

☞ 634

Stavudine
01-Sep-2016
(d4T)

- INDICATIONS AND DOSE
  HIV infection in combination with other antiretroviral drugs when no suitable alternative available and when prescribed for shortest period possible
  - BY MOUTH
  - Adult (body-weight up to 60 kg): 30 mg every 12 hours, to be taken preferably at least 1 hour before food
  - Adult (body-weight 60 kg and above): 40 mg every 12 hours, to be taken preferably at least 1 hour before food

- CAUTIONS Excessive alcohol intake · history of pancreatitis · history of peripheral neuropathy · lactic acidosis (especially when used in combination with didanosine)— use only if alternative regimens are not suitable

CAUTIONS, FURTHER INFORMATION
- Lactic acidosis Lactic acidosis associated with hepatomegaly and hepatic steatosis has been reported with stavudine. Use with caution in patients with hepatomegaly, hepatitis, or other risk factors for liver disease and hepatic steatosis (including obesity and alcohol abuse). Discontinue treatment if symptoms of hyperlactataemia, lactic acidosis, progressive hepatomegaly or rapid deterioration of liver function become apparent.

- INTERACTIONS → Appendix 1: stavudine
- SIDE-EFFECTS
- **Common or very common** Depression · drowsiness · dyspepsia · hyperlactacidaemia · lipoatrophy · nerve disorders · paraesthesia · peripheral neuropathy (switch to another antiretroviral if develops) · sleep disorders · thinking abnormal
- **Uncommon** Anxiety · arthralgia · emotional lability · gynaecomastia · hepatic disorders · urticaria
- **Rare or very rare** Diabetes mellitus · hyperglycaemia · muscle weakness · neutropenia

SIDE-EFFECTS, FURTHER INFORMATION Metabolic effects may occur with stavudine; plasma lipids and blood glucose concentrations should be measured routinely.

- PREGNANCY Manufacturer advises use only if potential benefit outweighs risk.
- RENAL IMPAIRMENT Risk of peripheral neuropathy.
Dose adjustments Use half normal dose every 12 hours if eGFR 25–50 mL/minute/1.73 m^2.
Use half normal dose every 24 hours if eGFR less than 25 mL/minute/1.73 m^2.

- PRESCRIBING AND DISPENSING INFORMATION Flavours of oral liquid formulations may include cherry.
- LESS SUITABLE FOR PRESCRIBING Stavudine (especially in combination with didanosine) is associated with a higher risk of lipoatrophy and should be used only if alternative regimens are not suitable; it is considered to be less suitable for prescribing.

- MEDICINAL FORMS
There can be variation in the licensing of different medicines containing the same drug.
Oral solution
- Zerit (Bristol-Myers Squibb Pharmaceuticals Ltd)
Stavudine 1 mg per 1 ml Zerit 1mg/ml oral solution | 200 ml PoM £22.94 (Hospital only)
Capsule
- Zerit (Bristol-Myers Squibb Pharmaceuticals Ltd)
Stavudine 20 mg Zerit 20mg capsules | 56 capsule PoM £139.46 (Hospital only)
Stavudine 30 mg Zerit 30mg capsules | 56 capsule PoM £146.25 (Hospital only)
Stavudine 40 mg Zerit 40mg capsules | 56 capsule PoM £150.66 (Hospital only)

Tenofovir disoproxil

- INDICATIONS AND DOSE
HIV infection in combination with other antiretroviral drugs | Chronic hepatitis B infection with compensated liver disease (with evidence of viral replication, and histologically documented active liver inflammation or fibrosis) | Chronic hepatitis B infection with decompensated liver disease
- BY MOUTH
- Adult: 245 mg once daily

DOSE EQUIVALENCE AND CONVERSION
- 7.5 scoops of granules contains approx. 245 mg tenofovir disoproxil (as fumarate).

- INTERACTIONS → Appendix 1: tenofovir disoproxil
- SIDE-EFFECTS
- **Common or very common** Abdominal distension · flatulence
- **Uncommon** Proximal renal tubulopathy
- **Rare or very rare** Acute tubular necrosis · angioedema · hepatitis · nephritis · nephrogenic diabetes insipidus · renal impairment
- RENAL IMPAIRMENT
Dose adjustments *Granules*: 132 mg once daily if eGFR 30–50 mL/minute/1.73 m^2; 66 mg once daily if eGFR 20–30 mL/minute/1.73 m^2; 33 mg once daily if eGFR 10–20 mL/minute/1.73 m^2.
Tablets: 245 mg every 2 days if eGFR 30–50 mL/minute/1.73 m^2; 245 mg every 3–4 days if eGFR 10–30 mL/minute/1.73 m^2.
Monitoring Monitor renal function—interrupt treatment if further deterioration.
- MONITORING REQUIREMENTS
- Test renal function and serum phosphate before treatment, then every 4 weeks (more frequently if at increased risk of renal impairment) for 1 year and then every 3 months, interrupt treatment if renal function deteriorates or serum phosphate decreases.
- When treating chronic hepatitis B with tenofovir, monitor liver function tests every 3 months and viral markers for hepatitis B every 3–6 months during treatment (continue monitoring for at least 1 year after discontinuation— recurrent hepatitis may occur on discontinuation).
- DIRECTIONS FOR ADMINISTRATION *Granules*: mix 1 scoop of granules with 1 tablespoon of soft food (e.g. yoghurt, apple sauce) and take immediately without chewing. Do **not** mix granules with liquids.
- PATIENT AND CARER ADVICE Patients or carers should be given advice on how to administer tenofovir granules.
Missed doses If a dose is more than 12 hours late, the missed dose should not be taken and the next dose should be taken at the normal time.
- NATIONAL FUNDING/ACCESS DECISIONS
NICE decisions
- **Tenofovir disoproxil for the treatment of chronic hepatitis B (July 2009)** NICE TA173
Tenofovir is an option for the treatment of chronic hepatitis B.
www.nice.org.uk/TA173
- MEDICINAL FORMS
There can be variation in the licensing of different medicines containing the same drug.
Granules
CAUTIONARY AND ADVISORY LABELS 21
- Viread (Gilead Sciences International Ltd)
Tenofovir disoproxil (as Tenofovir disoproxil fumarate) 33 mg per 1 gram Viread 33mg/g granules | 60 gram PoM £54.50
Tablet
CAUTIONARY AND ADVISORY LABELS 21
- Tenofovir disoproxil (Non-proprietary)
Tenofovir disoproxil 245 mg Tenofovir 245mg tablets | 30 tablet PoM £61.32–£204.39
- Viread (Gilead Sciences International Ltd)
Tenofovir disoproxil (as Tenofovir disoproxil fumarate) 123 mg Viread 123mg tablets | 30 tablet PoM £102.60
Tenofovir disoproxil (as Tenofovir disoproxil fumarate) 163 mg Viread 163mg tablets | 30 tablet PoM £135.98
Tenofovir disoproxil (as Tenofovir disoproxil fumarate) 204 mg Viread 204mg tablets | 30 tablet PoM £170.19
Tenofovir disoproxil 245 mg Viread 245mg tablets | 30 tablet PoM £204.39

5

Infection

Zidovudine

F 634

01-Sep-2016

(Azidothymidine; AZT)

● INDICATIONS AND DOSE

HIV infection in combination with other antiretroviral drugs
▸ BY MOUTH
  ▸ Adult: 250–300 mg twice daily
Prevention of maternal-fetal HIV transmission
▸ BY MOUTH, OR BY INTRAVENOUS INFUSION
  ▸ Adult: Seek specialist advice (combination therapy preferred) (consult local protocol)
HIV infection in combination with other antiretroviral drugs in patients temporarily unable to take zidovudine by mouth
▸ BY INTRAVENOUS INFUSION
  ▸ Adult: 0.8–1 mg/kg every 4 hours usually for not more than 2 weeks, dose approximating to 1.2–1.5 mg/kg every 4 hours by mouth

● CONTRA-INDICATIONS Abnormally low haemoglobin concentration (consult product literature) · abnormally low neutrophil counts (consult product literature)
● CAUTIONS Elderly · lactic acidosis · risk of haematological toxicity particularly with high dose and advanced disease · vitamin B$_{12}$ deficiency (increased risk of neutropenia)
  CAUTIONS, FURTHER INFORMATION
▸ Lactic acidosis Lactic acidosis associated with hepatomegaly and hepatic steatosis has been reported with zidovudine. Use with caution in patients with hepatomegaly, hepatitis, or other risk factors for liver disease and hepatic steatosis (including obesity and alcohol abuse). Discontinue treatment if symptoms of hyperlactataemia, lactic acidosis, progressive hepatomegaly or rapid deterioration of liver function become apparent.
● INTERACTIONS → Appendix 1: zidovudine
● SIDE-EFFECTS
▸ **Common or very common** Leucopenia · malaise · neutropenia
▸ **Uncommon** Bone marrow disorders · dyspnoea · fever · flatulence · generalised pain · myopathy
▸ **Rare or very rare** Alertness decreased · anxiety · cardiomyopathy · chest pain · chills · cough · depression · drowsiness · dyspepsia · gynaecomastia · hepatic disorders · hyperhidrosis · influenza like illness · insomnia · nail discolouration · oral discolouration · paraesthesia · pure red cell aplasia · seizure · taste altered · urinary frequency increased
▸ **Frequency not known** Lipoatrophy
  SIDE-EFFECTS, FURTHER INFORMATION
  Anaemia and myelosuppression If anaemia or myelosuppression occur, reduce dose or interrupt treatment according to product literature, or consider other treatment.
  Lipodystrophy syndrome Metabolic effects may occur with zidovudine; plasma lipids and blood glucose concentrations should be measured routinely.
● HEPATIC IMPAIRMENT Accumulation may occur.
● RENAL IMPAIRMENT
  Dose adjustments Reduce oral dose to 300–400 mg daily in divided doses or intravenous dose to 1 mg/kg 3–4 times daily if eGFR is less than 10 mL/minute/1.73 m^2.
● MONITORING REQUIREMENTS Monitor full blood count after 4 weeks of treatment, then every 3 months.
● DIRECTIONS FOR ADMINISTRATION For *intermittent intravenous infusion*, dilute to a concentration of 2 mg/mL or 4 mg/mL with Glucose 5% and give over 1 hour.

● PRESCRIBING AND DISPENSING INFORMATION The abbreviation AZT which is sometimes used for zidovudine has also been used for another drug.
● MEDICINAL FORMS
There can be variation in the licensing of different medicines containing the same drug.
Solution for infusion
▸ Retrovir (ViiV Healthcare UK Ltd)
  Zidovudine 10 mg per 1 ml Retrovir IV 200mg/20ml concentrate for solution for infusion vials | 5 vial [PoM] £52.48
Oral solution
▸ Retrovir (ViiV Healthcare UK Ltd)
  Zidovudine 10 mg per 1 ml Retrovir 50mg/5ml oral solution sugar-free | 200 ml [PoM] £20.91
Capsule
▸ Zidovudine (Non-proprietary)
  Zidovudine 100 mg Zidovudine 100mg capsules | 60 capsule [PoM] £53.31
  Zidovudine 250 mg Zidovudine 250mg capsules | 60 capsule [PoM] £13.32-£96.36
▸ Retrovir (ViiV Healthcare UK Ltd)
  Zidovudine 100 mg Retrovir 100mg capsules | 100 capsule [PoM] £104.54
  Zidovudine 250 mg Retrovir 250mg capsules | 40 capsule [PoM] £104.54

Zidovudine with lamivudine

The properties listed below are those particular to the combination only. For the properties of the components please consider, zidovudine above, lamivudine p. 640.

● INDICATIONS AND DOSE

HIV infection in combination with other antiretroviral drugs
▸ BY MOUTH
  ▸ Adult: 1 tablet twice daily

● INTERACTIONS → Appendix 1: lamivudine · zidovudine
● RENAL IMPAIRMENT Avoid if eGFR less than 50 mL/minute/1.73 m^2 (consult product literature).
● DIRECTIONS FOR ADMINISTRATION
  COMBIVIR® TABLETS Tablets may be crushed and mixed with semi-solid food or liquid just before administration.
● MEDICINAL FORMS
There can be variation in the licensing of different medicines containing the same drug.
Tablet
▸ Zidovudine with lamivudine (Non-proprietary)
  Lamivudine 150 mg, Zidovudine 300 mg Zidovudine 300mg / Lamivudine 150mg tablets | 60 tablet [PoM] £240.10-£255.10
▸ Combivir (ViiV Healthcare UK Ltd)
  Lamivudine 150 mg, Zidovudine 300 mg Combivir 150mg/300mg tablets | 60 tablet [PoM] £300.12

ANTIVIRALS 〉 PROTEASE INHIBITORS

Protease inhibitors

● CONTRA-INDICATIONS Acute porphyrias p. 1025
● CAUTIONS Haemophilia (increased risk of bleeding)
● SIDE-EFFECTS
▸ **Common or very common** Alopecia · anaemia · angioedema · anxiety · appetite abnormal · arthralgia · asthenia · diabetes mellitus · diarrhoea · dizziness · dry mouth · dyslipidaemia · dyspnoea · fever · gastrointestinal discomfort · gastrointestinal disorders · headache · hepatic disorders · hypersensitivity · hypertension · malaise · muscle complaints · nausea · neutropenia · oral ulceration · pancreatitis · peripheral neuropathy · seizure · skin reactions · sleep disorders · taste altered · vomiting

‣ **Uncommon** Drowsiness · immune reconstitution inflammatory syndrome · osteonecrosis · Stevens-Johnson syndrome · weight increased
● HEPATIC IMPAIRMENT Use with caution in patients with chronic hepatitis B or C (increased risk of hepatic side-effects).

▶ 642

Atazanavir

● **INDICATIONS AND DOSE**

HIV infection in combination with other antiretroviral drugs—with low-dose ritonavir
‣ BY MOUTH
 ‣ Adult: 300 mg once daily

HIV infection in combination with other antiretroviral drugs—with cobicistat
‣ BY MOUTH
 ‣ Adult: 300 mg daily

● CAUTIONS Cardiac conduction disorders · electrolyte disturbances · predisposition to QT interval prolongation
● INTERACTIONS → Appendix 1: HIV-protease inhibitors
● SIDE-EFFECTS
‣ **Uncommon** Abnormal dreams · chest pain · depression · disorientation · drug reaction with eosinophilia and systemic symptoms (DRESS) · gallbladder disorders · gastritis · gynaecomastia · haematuria · memory loss · myopathy · nephritis tubulointerstitial · nephrolithiasis · proteinuria · syncope · torsade de pointes · urinary frequency increased
‣ **Rare or very rare** Gait abnormal · oedema · palpitations · QT interval prolongation · renal pain · vasodilation
 SIDE-EFFECTS, FURTHER INFORMATION Mild to moderate rash occurs commonly, usually within the first 3 weeks of therapy. Severe rash occurs less frequently and may be accompanied by systemic symptoms. Discontinue if severe rash develops.
● PREGNANCY Theoretical risk of hyperbilirubinaemia in neonate if used at term.
 Monitoring In pregnancy, monitor viral load and plasma-atazanavir concentration during third trimester.
● HEPATIC IMPAIRMENT Manufacturer advises caution in mild impairment; avoid in moderate to severe impairment.

● MEDICINAL FORMS
There can be variation in the licensing of different medicines containing the same drug.
Capsule
CAUTIONARY AND ADVISORY LABELS 5, 21
 ‣ Reyataz (Bristol-Myers Squibb Pharmaceuticals Ltd)
 Atazanavir (as Atazanavir sulfate) 150 mg Reyataz 150mg capsules | 60 capsule PoM £303.38 (Hospital only)
 Atazanavir (as Atazanavir sulfate) 200 mg Reyataz 200mg capsules | 60 capsule PoM £303.38 (Hospital only)
 Atazanavir (as Atazanavir sulfate) 300 mg Reyataz 300mg capsules | 30 capsule PoM £303.38 (Hospital only)

Atazanavir with cobicistat   18-Apr-2017

The properties listed below are those particular to the combination only. For the properties of the components please consider, atazanavir above, cobicistat p. 647.

● **INDICATIONS AND DOSE**

HIV infection, in combination with other antiretroviral drugs (initiated by a specialist)
‣ BY MOUTH
 ‣ Adult: 300/150 mg once daily
 DOSE EQUIVALENCE AND CONVERSION
 ‣ Dose expressed as x/y mg of atazanavir/cobicistat.

● CONTRA-INDICATIONS Haemodialysis
● INTERACTIONS → Appendix 1: cobicistat · HIV-protease inhibitors

● MEDICINAL FORMS
There can be variation in the licensing of different medicines containing the same drug.
Tablet
CAUTIONARY AND ADVISORY LABELS 21
 ‣ Evotaz (Bristol-Myers Squibb Pharmaceuticals Ltd) ▼
 Cobicistat 150 mg, Atazanavir (as Atazanavir sulfate) 300 mg Evotaz 300mg/150mg tablets | 30 tablet PoM £323.38

▶ 642

Darunavir

● **INDICATIONS AND DOSE**

HIV infection in combination with other antiretroviral drugs in patients previously treated with antiretroviral therapy—with low-dose ritonavir
‣ BY MOUTH
 ‣ Adult: 600 mg twice daily, alternatively 800 mg once daily, once daily dose only to be used if no resistance to darunavir, if plasma HIV-RNA concentration less than 100 000 copies/mL, and if CD4 cell count greater than 100 cells × 10^6/ litre

HIV infection in combination with other antiretroviral drugs in patients previously treated with antiretroviral therapy—with cobicistat
‣ BY MOUTH
 ‣ Adult: 800 mg once daily, dose appropriate if no resistance to darunavir, if plasma HIV-RNA concentration less than 100 000 copies/mL, and if CD4 cell count greater than 100 cells × 10^6/litre

HIV infection in combination with other antiretroviral drugs in patients not previously treated with antiretroviral therapy—with low-dose ritonavir
‣ BY MOUTH
 ‣ Adult: 800 mg once daily

HIV infection in combination with other antiretroviral drugs in patients not previously treated with antiretroviral therapy—with cobicistat
‣ BY MOUTH
 ‣ Adult: 800 mg once daily

● INTERACTIONS → Appendix 1: HIV-protease inhibitors
● SIDE-EFFECTS
‣ **Common or very common** Hyperlipidaemia
‣ **Uncommon** Abdominal discomfort · angina pectoris · arrhythmias · burping · chest pain · concentration impaired · confusion · constipation · cough · depression · dry eye · eye erythema · feeling hot · flushing · gastritis · gout · gynaecomastia · haemorrhage · herpes simplex · hyperglycaemia · hypothyroidism · lethargy · leucopenia · memory loss · mood altered · muscle weakness · myocardial infarction · nail discolouration · nephrolithiasis · oral disorders · osteoporosis · pain · peripheral oedema · polydipsia · QT interval prolongation · renal impairment · sensation abnormal · sexual dysfunction · sweat changes · throat irritation · thrombocytopenia · urinary disorders · urine abnormalities · vertigo
‣ **Rare or very rare** Arthritis · chills · feeling abnormal · joint stiffness · musculoskeletal stiffness · palpitations · restlessness · rhinorrhoea · severe cutaneous adverse reactions (SCARs) · syncope · taste loss · visual impairment
 SIDE-EFFECTS, FURTHER INFORMATION Mild to moderate rash occurs commonly, usually within the first 4 weeks of therapy and resolves without stopping treatment. Severe skin rash (including Stevens-Johnson syndrome and toxic epidermal necrolysis) occurs less frequently and may be accompanied by fever, malaise, arthralgia, myalgia, oral

5

Infection

lesions, conjunctivitis, hepatitis, or eosinophilia; treatment should be stopped if this develops.

● ALLERGY AND CROSS-SENSITIVITY Use with caution in patients with sulfonamide sensitivity.

● PREGNANCY Manufacturer advises use only if potential benefit outweighs risk; if required, use the twice daily dose regimen.

● HEPATIC IMPAIRMENT Manufacturer advises caution in mild to moderate impairment; avoid in severe impairment—no information available.

● MONITORING REQUIREMENTS Monitor liver function before and during treatment.

● PRESCRIBING AND DISPENSING INFORMATION Flavours of oral liquid formulations may include strawberry.

● PATIENT AND CARER ADVICE

Missed doses If a dose is more than 6 hours late on the twice daily regimen (or more than 12 hours late on the once daily regimen), the missed dose should not be taken and the next dose should be taken at the normal time.

● MEDICINAL FORMS
There can be variation in the licensing of different medicines containing the same drug.
Oral suspension
CAUTIONARY AND ADVISORY LABELS 21
▸ Prezista (Janssen-Cilag Ltd)
  Darunavir (as Darunavir ethanolate) 100 mg per 1 ml Prezista 100mg/ml oral suspension sugar-free | 200 ml PoM £248.17
Tablet
CAUTIONARY AND ADVISORY LABELS 21
▸ Prezista (Janssen-Cilag Ltd)
  Darunavir (as Darunavir ethanolate) 75 mg Prezista 75mg tablets | 480 tablet PoM £446.70
  Darunavir (as Darunavir ethanolate) 150 mg Prezista 150mg tablets | 240 tablet PoM £446.70
  Darunavir (as Darunavir ethanolate) 400 mg Prezista 400mg tablets | 60 tablet PoM £297.80
  Darunavir (as Darunavir ethanolate) 600 mg Prezista 600mg tablets | 60 tablet PoM £446.70
  Darunavir (as Darunavir ethanolate) 800 mg Prezista 800mg tablets | 30 tablet PoM £297.80

Darunavir with cobicistat
14-Mar-2018

The properties listed below are those particular to the combination only. For the properties of the components please consider, cobicistat p. 647, darunavir p. 643.

● INDICATIONS AND DOSE

HIV infection, in combination with other antiretroviral drugs (initiated by a specialist)
▸ BY MOUTH
▸ Adult: 800/150 mg once daily, dosage should not be altered or therapy discontinued without instruction from the healthcare provider
DOSE EQUIVALENCE AND CONVERSION
▸ Dose expressed as x/y mg of darunavir/cobicistat.

● CONTRA-INDICATIONS Treatment-experienced patients with 1 or more darunavir resistance-associated mutations, plasma HIV-RNA concentration of 100 000 copies/mL or greater, or CD4 count less than 100 cells $\times 10^6$/litre

● CAUTIONS Elderly

● INTERACTIONS → Appendix 1: cobicistat · HIV-protease inhibitors

● PREGNANCY Manufacturer advises use only if potential benefit outweighs risk.

● NATIONAL FUNDING/ACCESS DECISIONS

Scottish Medicines Consortium (SMC) Decisions
SMC No. 1081/15

The *Scottish Medicines Consortium* has advised (August 2015) that darunavir with cobicistat (*Rezolsta*®) is accepted for use within NHS Scotland for the treatment of human immunodeficiency virus-1 (HIV-1) infection in adults, in combination with other antiretrovirals. Genotypic testing should guide its use.

● MEDICINAL FORMS
There can be variation in the licensing of different medicines containing the same drug.
Tablet
CAUTIONARY AND ADVISORY LABELS 21
▸ Rezolsta (Janssen-Cilag Ltd) ▼
  Cobicistat 150 mg, Darunavir (as Darunavir ethanolate) 800 mg Rezolsta 800mg/150mg tablets | 30 tablet PoM £317.24

Darunavir with cobicistat, emtricitabine and tenofovir alafenamide
06-Feb-2018

The properties listed below are those particular to the combination only. For the properties of the components please consider, darunavir p. 643, cobicistat p. 647, emtricitabine p. 638, tenofovir alafenamide p. 611.

● INDICATIONS AND DOSE

HIV infection (initiated by a specialist)
▸ BY MOUTH
▸ Adult: 1 tablet once daily

● INTERACTIONS → Appendix 1: cobicistat · HIV-protease inhibitors · tenofovir alafenamide

● PREGNANCY Manufacturer advises use only if potential benefit outweighs risk.

● RENAL IMPAIRMENT Manufacturer advises avoid if eGFR less than 30 mL/minute/1.73 m²—no information available.

● PATIENT AND CARER ADVICE
Driving and skilled tasks Manufacturer advises patients and carers should be counselled on the effects on driving and performance of skilled tasks—increased risk of dizziness.

● NATIONAL FUNDING/ACCESS DECISIONS

Scottish Medicines Consortium (SMC) Decisions
SMC No. 1290/18

The *Scottish Medicines Consortium* has advised (January 2018) that darunavir with cobicistat, emtricitabine and tenofovir alafenamide (*Symtuza*®) is accepted for use within NHS Scotland for the treatment of human immunodeficiency virus type 1 (HIV-1) infection in adults and adolescents (aged 12 years and older with body weight at least 40 kg).

All Wales Medicines Strategy Group (AWMSG) Decisions
AWMSG No. 2418

The *All Wales Medicines Strategy Group* has advised (March 2018) that darunavir with cobicistat, emtricitabine and tenofovir alafenamide (*Symtuza*®) is recommended as an option for use within NHS Wales for the treatment of human immunodeficiency virus type 1 (HIV-1) infection in adults and adolescents (aged 12 years and older with body weight at least 40 kg).

● MEDICINAL FORMS
There can be variation in the licensing of different medicines containing the same drug.
Tablet
CAUTIONARY AND ADVISORY LABELS 21
▸ Symtuza (Janssen-Cilag Ltd) ▼
  Tenofovir alafenamide (as Tenofovir alafenamide fumarate) 10 mg, Cobicistat 150 mg, Emtricitabine 200 mg, Darunavir (as Darunavir ethanolate) 800 mg Symtuza 800mg/150mg/200mg/10mg tablets | 30 tablet PoM £672.97

⚑ 642

Fosamprenavir

● DRUG ACTION Fosamprenavir is a pro-drug of amprenavir.

● **INDICATIONS AND DOSE**

HIV infection in combination with other antiretroviral drugs—with low-dose ritonavir

▶ BY MOUTH
▶ Adult: 700 mg twice daily

DOSE EQUIVALENCE AND CONVERSION
▶ 700 mg fosamprenavir is equivalent to approximately 600 mg amprenavir.

● INTERACTIONS → Appendix 1: HIV-protease inhibitors

● SIDE-EFFECTS
▶ **Common or very common** Oral paraesthesia
▶ **Frequency not known** Rash erythematous

SIDE-EFFECTS, FURTHER INFORMATION Rash may occur, usually in the second week of therapy; discontinue permanently if severe rash with systemic or allergic symptoms or, mucosal involvement; if rash mild or moderate, may continue without interruption—usually resolves and may respond to antihistamines.

● PREGNANCY Toxicity in *animal* studies; manufacturer advises use only if potential benefit outweighs risk.

● HEPATIC IMPAIRMENT Manufacturer advises caution in mild impairment.
Dose adjustments Reduce dose to 450 mg twice daily in moderate impairment; reduce dose to 300 mg twice daily in severe impairment.

● DIRECTIONS FOR ADMINISTRATION In adults, oral suspension should be taken on an empty stomach.

● PRESCRIBING AND DISPENSING INFORMATION Flavours of oral liquid formulations may include grape, bubblegum, or peppermint.

● PATIENT AND CARER ADVICE Patients or carers should be given advice on how to administer fosamprenavir oral suspension.

● MEDICINAL FORMS
There can be variation in the licensing of different medicines containing the same drug.
Oral suspension
EXCIPIENTS: May contain Propylene glycol
▶ Telzir (ViiV Healthcare UK Ltd)
Fosamprenavir (as Fosamprenavir calcium) 50 mg per 1 ml Telzir 50mg/ml oral suspension | 225 ml PoM £69.06
Tablet
▶ Telzir (ViiV Healthcare UK Ltd)
Fosamprenavir (as Fosamprenavir calcium) 700 mg Telzir 700mg tablets | 60 tablet PoM £258.97

⚑ 642

Lopinavir with ritonavir

19-Mar-2018

● **INDICATIONS AND DOSE**

HIV infection in combination with other antiretroviral drugs

▶ BY MOUTH USING TABLETS
▶ Adult: 400/100 mg twice daily, alternatively 800/200 mg once daily, once daily dose to be used only in adults with a HIV strain that has less than 3 mutations to protease inhibitors
▶ BY MOUTH USING ORAL SOLUTION
▶ Adult: 5 mL twice daily

DOSE EQUIVALENCE AND CONVERSION
▶ Oral solution contains 400 mg lopinavir, 100 mg ritonavir/5 mL (or 80 mg lopinavir, 20 mg ritonavir/mL).

● CAUTIONS Cardiac conduction disorders · pancreatitis · patients at high risk of cardiovascular disease (especially if

10-year cardiovascular risk greater than 20%) · structural heart disease

● INTERACTIONS → Appendix 1: HIV-protease inhibitors

● SIDE-EFFECTS
▶ **Common or very common** Increased risk of infection · leucopenia · lymphadenopathy · menstrual cycle irregularities · migraine · muscle weakness · myopathy · night sweats · pain · sexual dysfunction
▶ **Uncommon** Abnormal dreams · atherosclerosis · atrioventricular block · cholangitis · constipation · deep vein thrombosis · haemorrhage · hyperbilirubinaemia · hypogonadism · myocardial infarction · nephritis · stomatitis · stroke · taste loss · tinnitus · tremor · tricuspid valve incompetence · vasculitis · vertigo · visual impairment

SIDE-EFFECTS, FURTHER INFORMATION Signs and symptoms suggestive of pancreatitis (including raised serum lipase) should be evaluated—discontinue if pancreatitis diagnosed

● PREGNANCY Avoid oral solution due to high alcohol and propylene glycol content; use tablets only if potential benefit outweighs risk (toxicity in *animal* studies).

● HEPATIC IMPAIRMENT Avoid oral solution due to propylene glycol content; manufacturer advises avoid tablets in severe impairment.

● RENAL IMPAIRMENT Avoid oral solution due to high propylene glycol content. Use tablets with caution in severe impairment.

● MONITORING REQUIREMENTS
▶ Monitor liver function before and during treatment.
▶ With oral solution, monitor for signs of alcohol and propylene glycol toxicity (particularly in infants).

● PRESCRIBING AND DISPENSING INFORMATION With oral solution, manufacturer advises high alcohol (42 % v/v) and propylene glycol content—consider total amounts from all medicines that are to be given to infants in order to avoid toxicity; caution in patients for which consumption may be harmful.

● PATIENT AND CARER ADVICE Oral solution tastes bitter.

● NATIONAL FUNDING/ACCESS DECISIONS

Scottish Medicines Consortium (SMC) Decisions
SMC No. 326/06
The *Scottish Medicines Consortium* has advised (November 2006) that lopinavir with ritonavir tablet (*Kaletra*®) is accepted for use within NHS Scotland in combination with other antiretrovirals for the treatment of HIV-1 infected adults and children above the age of 2 years.

● MEDICINAL FORMS
There can be variation in the licensing of different medicines containing the same drug.
Oral solution
CAUTIONARY AND ADVISORY LABELS 21
EXCIPIENTS: May contain Alcohol, propylene glycol
▶ Kaletra (AbbVie Ltd)
Ritonavir 20 mg per 1 ml, Lopinavir 80 mg per 1 ml Kaletra 80mg/20mg/1ml oral solution | 120 ml PoM £122.96 | 300 ml PoM £307.39
Tablet
CAUTIONARY AND ADVISORY LABELS 25
▶ Kaletra (AbbVie Ltd)
Ritonavir 25 mg, Lopinavir 100 mg Kaletra 100mg/25mg tablets | 60 tablet PoM £76.85
Ritonavir 50 mg, Lopinavir 200 mg Kaletra 200mg/50mg tablets | 120 tablet PoM £285.41

Ritonavir

℉ 642

- **INDICATIONS AND DOSE**

HIV infection in combination with other antiretroviral drugs (high-dose ritonavir)
- ▸ BY MOUTH
- ▸ Adult: Initially 300 mg every 12 hours for 3 days, increased in steps of 100 mg every 12 hours over not longer than 14 days; increased to 600 mg every 12 hours

Low-dose booster to increase effect of other protease inhibitors
- ▸ BY MOUTH
- ▸ Adult: 100–200 mg 1–2 times a day

- **CAUTIONS** Cardiac conduction disorders · pancreatitis · structural heart disease
- **INTERACTIONS** → Appendix 1: HIV-protease inhibitors
- **SIDE-EFFECTS**
- ▸ **Common or very common** Back pain · concentration impaired · confusion · cough · dehydration · feeling hot · flushing · gastrointestinal discomfort · gastrointestinal haemorrhage · gout · hypotension · menorrhagia · myopathy · oedema · oral paraesthesia · oropharyngeal pain · paraesthesia · peripheral coldness · pharyngitis · renal impairment · syncope · thrombocytopenia · urinary frequency increased · vision blurred
- ▸ **Uncommon** Myocardial infarction
- ▸ **Rare or very rare** Hyperglycaemia · toxic epidermal necrolysis

  SIDE-EFFECTS, FURTHER INFORMATION Signs and symptoms suggestive of pancreatitis (including raised serum lipase) should be evaluated—discontinue if pancreatitis diagnosed.

- **PREGNANCY**
  Dose adjustments Only use low-dose booster to increase the effect of other protease inhibitors.
- **HEPATIC IMPAIRMENT** Avoid in decompensated liver disease; in severe impairment without decompensation, use 'booster' doses with caution (avoid treatment doses).
- **DIRECTIONS FOR ADMINISTRATION** Bitter taste of oral solution can be masked by mixing with chocolate milk; do not mix with water, measuring cup must be dry.
- **PATIENT AND CARER ADVICE** Patients or carers should be given advice on how to administer ritonavir oral solution.

- **MEDICINAL FORMS**
  There can be variation in the licensing of different medicines containing the same drug.
  Tablet
  CAUTIONARY AND ADVISORY LABELS 21, 25
  - ▸ Norvir (AbbVie Ltd)
    Ritonavir 100 mg Norvir 100mg tablets | 30 tablet [PoM] £19.44

Saquinavir

℉ 642

- **INDICATIONS AND DOSE**

HIV infection in combination with other antiretrovirals in patients previously treated with antiretroviral therapy—with low-dose ritonavir
- ▸ BY MOUTH
- ▸ Adult: 1 g every 12 hours

HIV infection in combination with other antiretrovirals in patients not previously treated with antiretroviral therapy—with low-dose ritonavir
- ▸ BY MOUTH
- ▸ Adult: 500 mg every 12 hours for 7 days, then increased to 1 g every 12 hours

- **CONTRA-INDICATIONS** Bradycardia · congenital QT prolongation · electrolyte disturbances · heart failure with reduced left ventricular ejection fraction · history of symptomatic arrhythmias · predisposition to cardiac arrhythmias
- **INTERACTIONS** → Appendix 1: HIV-protease inhibitors
- **SIDE-EFFECTS**
- ▸ **Common or very common** Abdominal pain upper · burping · constipation · dry lips · libido decreased · lipoatrophy · paraesthesia
- ▸ **Uncommon** Mucosal ulceration · renal impairment · visual impairment
- ▸ **Frequency not known** QT interval prolongation
- **HEPATIC IMPAIRMENT** Manufacturer advises caution in moderate impairment; avoid in decompensated liver disease.
- **RENAL IMPAIRMENT** Use with caution if eGFR less than 30 mL/minute/1.73 m^2.
- **MONITORING REQUIREMENTS** Monitor ECG before starting treatment (do not initiate treatment if QT interval over 450 milliseconds); if baseline QT interval less than 450 milliseconds, monitor ECG during treatment (particularly 10 days after starting treatment in patients not previously treated with antiretroviral therapy)—discontinue if QT interval increases over 480 milliseconds, if QT interval more than 20 milliseconds above baseline, if prolongation of PR interval, or if arrthymias occur.
- **PATIENT AND CARER ADVICE**
  Arrhythmias Patients should be told how to recognise signs of arrhythmia and advised to seek medical attention if symptoms such as palpitation or syncope develop.

- **MEDICINAL FORMS**
  There can be variation in the licensing of different medicines containing the same drug.
  Tablet
  CAUTIONARY AND ADVISORY LABELS 21
  - ▸ Invirase (Roche Products Ltd)
    Saquinavir (as Saquinavir mesilate) 500 mg Invirase 500mg tablets | 120 tablet [PoM] £251.26

Tipranavir

℉ 642

- **INDICATIONS AND DOSE**

HIV infection resistant to other protease inhibitors, in combination with other antiretroviral drugs in patients previously treated with antiretrovirals–with low-dose ritonavir
- ▸ BY MOUTH USING CAPSULES
- ▸ Adult: 500 mg twice daily

  DOSE EQUIVALENCE AND CONVERSION
  - ▸ The bioavailability of tipranavir oral solution is higher than that of the capsules; the oral solution is not interchangeable with the capsules on a milligram-for-milligram basis.

- **CAUTIONS** Patients at risk of increased bleeding from trauma, surgery or other pathological conditions
- **INTERACTIONS** → Appendix 1: HIV-protease inhibitors
- **SIDE-EFFECTS**
- ▸ **Common or very common** Hyperlipidaemia
- ▸ **Uncommon** Exanthema · hyperamylasaemia · hyperglycaemia · influenza like illness · renal failure · thrombocytopenia
- ▸ **Rare or very rare** Dehydration · hyperbilirubinaemia · intracranial haemorrhage
- ▸ **Frequency not known** Bleeding tendency

  SIDE-EFFECTS, FURTHER INFORMATION Potentially life-threatening hepatotoxicity reported. Discontinue if signs or symptoms of hepatitis develop or if liver-function abnormality develops (consult product literature).

● PREGNANCY Manufacturer advises use only if potential benefit outweighs risk—toxicity in *animal* studies.

● HEPATIC IMPAIRMENT Manufacturer advises caution in mild impairment; avoid in moderate or severe impairment—no information available.

● MONITORING REQUIREMENTS Monitor liver function before treatment then every 2 weeks for 1 month, then every 3 months.

● PRESCRIBING AND DISPENSING INFORMATION Flavours of oral liquid formulations may include toffee and mint.

● PATIENT AND CARER ADVICE Patients or carers should be told to observe the oral solution for crystallisation; the bottle should be replaced if more than a thin layer of crystals form (doses should continue to be taken at the normal time until the bottle is replaced).

● MEDICINAL FORMS
There can be variation in the licensing of different medicines containing the same drug.
Oral solution
CAUTIONARY AND ADVISORY LABELS 5, 21
EXCIPIENTS: May contain Vitamin e
  ▸ Aptivus (Boehringer Ingelheim Ltd)
  Tipranavir 100 mg per 1 ml Aptivus 100mg/ml oral solution sugar-free | 95 ml PoM £129.65
Capsule
CAUTIONARY AND ADVISORY LABELS 5, 21
EXCIPIENTS: May contain Ethanol
  ▸ Aptivus (Boehringer Ingelheim Ltd)
  Tipranavir 250 mg Aptivus 250mg capsules | 120 capsule PoM £441.00

ANTIVIRALS > OTHER

Maraviroc

● DRUG ACTION Maraviroc is an antagonist of the CCR5 chemokine receptor.

● INDICATIONS AND DOSE

CCR5-tropic HIV infection in combination with other antiretroviral drugs in patients previously treated with antiretrovirals
  ▸ BY MOUTH
  ▸ Adult: 300 mg twice daily

● CAUTIONS Cardiovascular disease

● INTERACTIONS → Appendix 1: maraviroc

● SIDE-EFFECTS
  ▸ **Common or very common** Abdominal pain · anaemia · appetite decreased · asthenia · depression · diarrhoea · flatulence · headache · insomnia · nausea · rash
  ▸ **Uncommon** Hyperbilirubinaemia · increased risk of infection · myopathy · postural hypotension · proteinuria · renal failure · seizure
  ▸ **Rare or very rare** Angina pectoris · granulocytopenia · hepatic disorders · metastases · neoplasms · pancytopenia · severe cutaneous adverse reactions (SCARs)
  ▸ **Frequency not known** Fever · hypersensitivity · immune reconstitution inflammatory syndrome · organ dysfunction · osteonecrosis

  SIDE-EFFECTS, FURTHER INFORMATION Osteonecrosis has been reported in patients with advanced HIV disease or following long-term exposure to combination antiretroviral therapy.

● PREGNANCY Manufacturer advises use only if potential benefit outweighs risk—toxicity in *animal* studies.

● HEPATIC IMPAIRMENT Manufacturer advises caution in hepatic impairment, including patients with chronic hepatitis B or C.

● RENAL IMPAIRMENT If eGFR less than 80 mL/minute/1.73 m^2, consult product literature.

● NATIONAL FUNDING/ACCESS DECISIONS
Scottish Medicines Consortium (SMC) Decisions
The *Scottish Medicines Consortium* has advised (March 2008) that maraviroc (*Celsentri*®) is **not** recommended for use within NHS Scotland.

● MEDICINAL FORMS
There can be variation in the licensing of different medicines containing the same drug.
Tablet
  ▸ Celsentri (ViiV Healthcare UK Ltd)
  Maraviroc 25 mg Celsentri 25mg tablets | 120 tablet PoM £147.09
  Maraviroc 75 mg Celsentri 75mg tablets | 120 tablet PoM £441.27
  Maraviroc 150 mg Celsentri 150mg tablets | 60 tablet PoM £519.14
  Maraviroc 300 mg Celsentri 300mg tablets | 60 tablet PoM £519.14

PHARMACOKINETIC ENHANCERS

Cobicistat

● INDICATIONS AND DOSE

Pharmacokinetic enhancer used to increase the effect of atazanavir or darunavir
  ▸ BY MOUTH
  ▸ Adult: 150 mg once daily

● INTERACTIONS → Appendix 1: cobicistat

● SIDE-EFFECTS
  ▸ **Common or very common** Appetite increased · asthenia · diarrhoea · dizziness · drowsiness · dry mouth · flatulence · gastrointestinal discomfort · headache · hepatic disorders · hyperbilirubinaemia · hyperglycaemia · nausea · skin reactions · sleep disorders · taste altered · vomiting
  ▸ **Uncommon** Depression · fever · haematuria · myalgia · nephrolithiasis · proteinuria

● PREGNANCY Manufacturer advises avoid unless essential.

● HEPATIC IMPAIRMENT Manufacturer advises avoid in severe impairment—no information available.

● RENAL IMPAIRMENT No dose adjustment required; inhibits tubular secretion of creatinine; when any co-administered drug requires dose adjustment based on renal function, avoid initiating cobicistat if eGFR less than 70 mL/minute/1.73 m^2.

● PRESCRIBING AND DISPENSING INFORMATION Dispense in original container (contains desiccant).

● PATIENT AND CARER ADVICE
Missed doses If a dose is more than 12 hours late, the missed dose should not be taken and the next dose should be taken at the normal time.

● MEDICINAL FORMS
There can be variation in the licensing of different medicines containing the same drug.
Tablet
CAUTIONARY AND ADVISORY LABELS 21
  ▸ Tybost (Gilead Sciences International Ltd) ▼
  Cobicistat 150 mg Tybost 150mg tablets | 30 tablet PoM £21.38

Combinations available: *Atazanavir with cobicistat,* p. 643 · *Darunavir with cobicistat,* p. 644 · *Darunavir with cobicistat, emtricitabine and tenofovir alafenamide,* p. 644 · *Elvitegravir with cobicistat, emtricitabine and tenofovir alafenamide,* p. 637 · *Elvitegravir with cobicistat, emtricitabine and tenofovir disoproxil,* p. 637

6.5 Influenza

Influenza

Management

Oseltamivir below and zanamivir p. 649 are most effective for the treatment of influenza if started within a few hours of the onset of symptoms; they are licensed for use within 48 hours of the first symptoms. In otherwise healthy individuals they reduce the duration of symptoms by about 1–1.5 days. Oseltamivir or zanamivir can reduce the risk of complications from influenza in the elderly and in patients with chronic disease.

Oseltamivir and zanamivir are licensed for post-exposure prophylaxis of influenza when influenza is circulating in the community. Oseltamivir should be given within 48 hours of exposure to influenza while zanamivir should be given within 36 hours of exposure to influenza. However, in patients with severe influenza or in those who are immunocompromised, antivirals may still be effective after this time if viral shedding continues [unlicensed use]. Oseltamivir and zanamivir are also licensed for use in exceptional circumstances (e.g. when vaccination does not cover the infecting strain) to prevent influenza in an epidemic.

There is evidence that some strains of influenza A virus have reduced susceptibility to oseltamivir, but may retain susceptibility to zanamivir. Resistance to oseltamivir may be greater in severely immunocompromised patients.

Zanamivir should be reserved for patients who are severely immunocompromised, or when oseltamivir cannot be used, or when resistance to oseltamivir is suspected. For those unable to use the dry powder for inhalation, zanamivir is available as a solution that can be administered by nebuliser or intravenously [unlicensed use].

Amantadine hydrochloride p. 412 is licensed for prophylaxis and treatment of influenza A but it is no longer recommended.

Information on pandemic influenza, avian influenza, and swine influenza may be found at www.gov.uk/phe.

Immunisation against influenza is recommended for persons at high risk, and to reduce transmission of infection.

Oseltamivir in children under 1 year of age

Data on the use of oseltamivir in children under 1 year of age is limited. Furthermore, oseltamivir may be ineffective in neonates because they may not be able to metabolise oseltamivir to its active form. However, oseltamivir can be used (under specialist supervision) for the treatment or post-exposure prophylaxis of influenza in children under 1 year of age. The Department of Health has advised (May 2009) that during a pandemic, treatment with oseltamivir can be overseen by healthcare professionals experienced in assessing children.

ANTIVIRALS > NEURAMINIDASE INHIBITORS

Oseltamivir

20-Jul-2017

- **DRUG ACTION** Reduces replication of influenza A and B viruses by inhibiting viral neuraminidase.

- **INDICATIONS AND DOSE**
  Prevention of influenza
  ▸ BY MOUTH
  ▸ Child 1–11 months: 3 mg/kg once daily for 10 days for post-exposure prophylaxis
  ▸ Child 1–12 years (body-weight 10–15 kg): 30 mg once daily for 10 days for post-exposure prophylaxis; for up to 6 weeks during an epidemic

▸ Child 1–12 years (body-weight 15–23 kg): 45 mg once daily for 10 days for post-exposure prophylaxis; for up to 6 weeks during an epidemic
▸ Child 1–12 years (body-weight 23–40 kg): 60 mg once daily for 10 days for post-exposure prophylaxis; for up to 6 weeks during an epidemic
▸ Child 1–12 years (body-weight 40 kg and above): 75 mg once daily for 10 days for post-exposure prophylaxis; for up to 6 weeks during an epidemic
▸ Child 13–17 years: 75 mg once daily for 10 days for post-exposure prophylaxis; for up to 6 weeks during an epidemic
▸ Adult: 75 mg once daily for 10 days for post-exposure prophylaxis; for up to 6 weeks during an epidemic

Treatment of influenza
▸ BY MOUTH
▸ Child 1–11 months: 3 mg/kg twice daily for 5 days
▸ Child 1–12 years (body-weight 10–15 kg): 30 mg twice daily for 5 days
▸ Child 1–12 years (body-weight 15–23 kg): 45 mg twice daily for 5 days
▸ Child 1–12 years (body-weight 23–40 kg): 60 mg twice daily for 5 days
▸ Child 1–12 years (body-weight 40 kg and above): 75 mg twice daily for 5 days
▸ Child 13–17 years: 75 mg twice daily for 5 days
▸ Adult: 75 mg twice daily for 5 days

- **UNLICENSED USE** Not licensed for use in premature infants.

- **SIDE-EFFECTS**
- ▸ **Common or very common** Dizziness (in adults) · dyspepsia · herpes simplex (in adults) · insomnia (in adults) · pain (in adults) · vertigo (in adults)
- ▸ **Uncommon** Arrhythmia (in adults) · consciousness impaired · seizure · skin reactions
- ▸ **Rare or very rare** Agitation (in adults) · angioedema (in adults) · anxiety · behaviour abnormal · confusion · delirium · delusions · haemorrhage (in adults) · hallucination · hepatic disorders (in adults) · nightmare · self-injurious behaviour (in adults) · severe cutaneous adverse reactions (SCARs) (in adults) · thrombocytopenia (in adults) · visual impairment (in adults)

  SIDE-EFFECTS, FURTHER INFORMATION Neurological and psychiatric disorders occur more commonly in children and adolescents.

- **PREGNANCY** Although safety data are limited, oseltamivir can be used in women who are pregnant when the potential benefit outweighs the risk (e.g. during a pandemic). Use only if potential benefit outweighs risk (e.g. during a pandemic).

- **BREAST FEEDING** Although safety data are limited, oseltamivir can be used in women who are breast-feeding when the potential benefit outweighs the risk (e.g. during a pandemic). Oseltamivir is the preferred drug in women who are breast-feeding. Amount probably too small to be harmful; use only if potential benefit outweighs risk (e.g. during a pandemic).

- **RENAL IMPAIRMENT**
- ▸ In adults Avoid for *treatment* and *prevention* if eGFR less than 10 mL/minute/1.73 m^2.
- ▸ In children Avoid for *treatment* and *prevention* if estimated glomerular filtration rate less than 10 mL/minute/1.73 m^2.
  Dose adjustments ▸ In adults For *treatment*, use 30 mg twice daily if eGFR 30–60 mL/minute/1.73 m^2 (30 mg once daily if eGFR 10–30 mL/minute/1.73 m^2). For *prevention*, use 30 mg once daily if eGFR 30–60 mL/minute/1.73 m^2 (30 mg every 48 hours if eGFR 10–30 mL/minute/1.73 m^2).
  ▸ In children For *treatment*, use 40% of normal dose twice daily if estimated glomerular filtration rate 30–60 mL/minute/1.73 m^2 (40% of normal dose once daily

if estimated glomerular filtration rate
10–30 mL/minute/1.73 m^2). For *prevention*, use 40% of
normal dose once daily if estimated glomerular filtration
rate 30–60 mL/minute/1.73 m^2 (40% of normal dose every
48 hours if estimated glomerular filtration rate
10–30 mL/minute/1.73 m^2).

- DIRECTIONS FOR ADMINISTRATION If suspension not
available, capsules can be opened and the contents mixed
with a small amount of sweetened food, such as sugar
water or chocolate syrup, just before administration.

- PRESCRIBING AND DISPENSING INFORMATION Flavours of
oral liquid formulations may include tutti-frutti.

- PATIENT AND CARER ADVICE
Medicines for Children leaflet: Oseltamivir for influenza (flu)
www.medicinesforchildren.org.uk/oseltamivir-for-influenza

- NATIONAL FUNDING/ACCESS DECISIONS

NICE decisions

▶ Oseltamivir, zanamivir, and amantadine for prophylaxis of
influenza (September 2008) NICE TA158
Oseltamivir is **not** a substitute for vaccination, which
remains the most effective way of preventing illness from
influenza.

- Oseltamivir is **not** recommended for seasonal
prophylaxis against influenza.
- When influenza is circulating in the community,
oseltamivir is an option recommended (in accordance
with UK licensing) for post-exposure prophylaxis in at-
risk patients who are not effectively protected by
influenza vaccine, and who have been in close contact
with someone suffering from influenza-like illness in the
same household or residential setting. Oseltamivir
should be given within 48 hours of exposure to
influenza. (National surveillance schemes, including
those run by Public Health England, should be used to
indicate when influenza is circulating in the
community.)
- During local outbreaks of influenza-like illness, when
there is a high level of certainty that influenza is
present, oseltamivir may be used for post-exposure
prophylaxis in at-risk patients (regardless of influenza
vaccination) living in long-term residential or nursing
homes.

At risk patients include those aged 65 years or older *or*
those who have one or more of the following conditions:

- chronic respiratory disease (including asthma and
chronic obstructive pulmonary disease);
- chronic heart disease;
- chronic renal disease;
- chronic liver disease;
- chronic neurological disease;
- immunosuppression;
- diabetes mellitus.

The Department of Health in England has advised
(November 2010 and April 2011) that 'at risk patients' also
includes patients under 65 years of age who are at risk of
developing medical complications from influenza
(treatment only) or women who are pregnant.

This guidance does not cover the circumstances of a
pandemic, an impending pandemic, or a widespread
epidemic of a new strain of influenza to which there is
little or no immunity in the community.
www.nice.org.uk/guidance/ta158

▶ Oseltamivir, zanamivir, and amantadine for treatment of
influenza (February 2009) NICE TA168
Oseltamivir is **not** a substitute for vaccination, which
remains the most effective way of preventing illness from
influenza.

- When influenza is circulating in the community,
oseltamivir is an option recommended (in accordance
with UK licensing) for the treatment of influenza in at-
risk patients who can start treatment within 48 hours of

the onset of symptoms. (National surveillance schemes,
including those run by Public Health England, should be
used to indicate when influenza is circulating in the
community.)

- During local outbreaks of influenza-like illness, when
there is a high level of certainty that influenza is
present, oseltamivir may be used for treatment in at-risk
patients living in long-term residential or nursing
homes.

At risk patients include those aged over 65 years *or* those
who have one or more of the following conditions:

- chronic respiratory disease (including asthma and
chronic obstructive pulmonary disease);
- chronic heart disease;
- chronic renal disease;
- chronic liver disease;
- chronic neurological disease;
- immunosuppression;
- diabetes mellitus.

The Department of Health in England has advised
(November 2010 and April 2011) that 'at risk patients' also
includes patients under 65 years of age who are at risk of
developing medical complications from influenza
(treatment only) or women who are pregnant.

This guidance does not cover the circumstances of a
pandemic, an impending pandemic, or a widespread
epidemic of a new strain of influenza to which there is
little or no immunity in the community.
www.nice.org.uk/guidance/ta168

NHS restrictions *Tamiflu*® is not prescribable in NHS
primary care except for the treatment and prophylaxis of
influenza as indicated in the NICE guidance; endorse
prescription 'SLS'.

- MEDICINAL FORMS
There can be variation in the licensing of different medicines
containing the same drug. Forms available from special-order
manufacturers include: oral suspension, oral solution

Oral solution
CAUTIONARY AND ADVISORY LABELS 9
▶ Oseltamivir (Non-proprietary)
  Oseltamivir (as Oseltamivir phosphate) 15 mg per
  1 ml Oseltamivir 15mg/ml oral solution sugar free sugar-free |
  20 ml PoM £10.00

Oral suspension
CAUTIONARY AND ADVISORY LABELS 9
EXCIPIENTS: May contain Sorbitol
▶ Tamiflu (Roche Products Ltd)
  Oseltamivir (as Oseltamivir phosphate) 6 mg per 1 ml Tamiflu
  6mg/ml oral suspension sugar-free | 65 ml PoM £10.27

Capsule
CAUTIONARY AND ADVISORY LABELS 9
▶ Tamiflu (Roche Products Ltd)
  Oseltamivir (as Oseltamivir phosphate) 30 mg Tamiflu 30mg
  capsules | 10 capsule PoM £7.71
  Oseltamivir (as Oseltamivir phosphate) 45 mg Tamiflu 45mg
  capsules | 10 capsule PoM £15.41
  Oseltamivir (as Oseltamivir phosphate) 75 mg Tamiflu 75mg
  capsules | 10 capsule PoM £15.41

Zanamivir

- DRUG ACTION Reduces replication of influenza A and B
viruses by inhibiting viral neuraminidase.

- INDICATIONS AND DOSE

Post-exposure prophylaxis of influenza
▶ BY INHALATION OF POWDER
▶ Child 5–17 years: 10 mg once daily for 10 days
▶ Adult: 10 mg once daily for 10 days   continued →

5

Infection

Prevention of influenza during an epidemic
▸ BY INHALATION OF POWDER
▸ Child 5-17 years: 10 mg once daily for up to 28 days
▸ Adult: 10 mg once daily for up to 28 days

Treatment of influenza
▸ BY INHALATION OF POWDER
▸ Child 5-17 years: 10 mg twice daily for 5 days (for up to 10 days if resistance to oseltamivir suspected)
▸ Adult: 10 mg twice daily for 5 days (for up to 10 days if resistance to oseltamivir suspected)

● UNLICENSED USE Use of zanamivir for up to 10 days if resistance to oseltamivir suspected is an unlicensed duration.

● CAUTIONS Asthma · chronic pulmonary disease · uncontrolled chronic illness
   CAUTIONS, FURTHER INFORMATION
▸ Asthma and chronic pulmonary disease Risk of bronchospasm—short-acting bronchodilator should be available.
   Avoid in severe asthma unless close monitoring possible and appropriate facilities available to treat bronchospasm.

● SIDE-EFFECTS
▸ **Common or very common** Skin reactions
▸ **Uncommon** Bronchospasm · dehydration · dyspnoea · oropharyngeal oedema · presyncope · severe cutaneous adverse reactions (SCARs) · throat tightness
▸ **Rare or very rare** Face oedema
▸ **Frequency not known** Behaviour abnormal · delirium · hallucination · level of consciousness decreased · psychiatric disorder · seizure
   SIDE-EFFECTS, FURTHER INFORMATION Neurological and psychiatric disorders occur more commonly in children and adolescents.

● PREGNANCY Although safety data are limited, zanamivir can be used in women who are pregnant when the potential benefit outweighs the risk (e.g. during a pandemic). Use only if potential benefit outweighs risk (e.g. during a pandemic).

● BREAST FEEDING Although safety data are limited, zanamivir can be used in women who are breast-feeding when the potential benefit outweighs the risk (e.g. during a pandemic). Amount probably too small to be harmful; use only if potential benefit outweighs risk (e.g. during a pandemic).

● DIRECTIONS FOR ADMINISTRATION Other inhaled drugs should be administered before zanamivir.

● PRESCRIBING AND DISPENSING INFORMATION Except for the treatment and prophylaxis of influenza as indicated in the NICE guidance; endorse prescription 'SLS'.

● NATIONAL FUNDING/ACCESS DECISIONS

NICE decisions
▸ **Oseltamivir, zanamivir, and amantadine for prophylaxis of influenza (September 2008)** NICE TA158
Zanamivir is **not** a substitute for vaccination, which remains the most effective way of preventing illness from influenza.
   ● Zanamivir is **not** recommended for seasonal prophylaxis against influenza.
   ● When influenza is circulating in the community, zanamivir is an option recommended (in accordance with UK licensing) for post-exposure prophylaxis in at-risk patients who are not effectively protected by influenza vaccine, and who have been in close contact with someone suffering from influenza-like illness in the same household or residential setting. Zanamivir should be given within 36 hours of exposure to influenza. (National surveillance schemes, including those run by Public Health England, should be used to indicate when influenza is circulating in the community).

● During local outbreaks of influenza-like illness, when there is a high level of certainty that influenza is present, zanamivir may be used for post-exposure prophylaxis in at-risk patients (regardless of influenza vaccination) living in long-term residential or nursing homes.
At risk patients include those aged over 65 years *or* those who have one or more of the following conditions:
● chronic respiratory disease (including asthma and chronic obstructive pulmonary disease);
● chronic heart disease;
● chronic renal disease;
● chronic liver disease;
● chronic neurological disease;
● immunosuppression;
● diabetes mellitus.
The Department of Health in England has advised (November 2010 and April 2011) that 'at risk patients' also includes patients under 65 years of age who are at risk of developing medical complications from influenza (treatment only) or women who are pregnant.
   This guidance does not cover the circumstances of a pandemic, an impending pandemic, or a widespread epidemic of a new strain of influenza to which there is little or no immunity in the community.
www.nice.org.uk/guidance/TA158

▸ **Oseltamivir, zanamivir, and amantadine for treatment of influenza (February 2009)** NICE TA168
Zanamivir is **not** a substitute for vaccination, which remains the most effective way of preventing illness from influenza.
   ● When influenza is circulating in the community, zanamivir is an option recommended (in accordance with UK licensing) for the treatment of influenza in at-risk patients who can start treatment within 48 hours (within 36 hours for zanamivir in children) of the onset of symptoms. (National surveillance schemes, including those run by Public Health England, should be used to indicate when influenza is circulating in the community.)
   ● During local outbreaks of influenza-like illness, when there is a high level of certainty that influenza is present, zanamivir may be used for treatment in at-risk patients living in long-term residential or nursing homes.
At risk patients include those aged over 65 years *or* those who have one or more of the following conditions:
● chronic respiratory disease (including asthma and chronic obstructive pulmonary disease);
● chronic heart disease;
● chronic renal disease;
● chronic liver disease;
● chronic neurological disease;
● immunosuppression;
● diabetes mellitus.
The Department of Health in England has advised (November 2010 and April 2011) that 'at risk patients' also includes patients under 65 years of age who are at risk of developing medical complications from influenza (treatment only) or women who are pregnant.
   This guidance does not cover the circumstances of a pandemic, an impending pandemic, or a widespread epidemic of a new strain of influenza to which there is little or no immunity in the community.
www.nice.org.uk/guidance/TA168

● MEDICINAL FORMS
There can be variation in the licensing of different medicines containing the same drug.

Inhalation powder
▸ Relenza (GlaxoSmithKline UK Ltd)
   Zanamivir 5 mg Relenza 5mg inhalation powder blisters with Diskhaler | 20 blister PoM £16.36

6.6 Respiratory syncytial virus

Respiratory syncytial virus

Management in children

Ribavirin p. 615 is licensed for administration by inhalation
for the treatment of severe bronchiolitis caused by the
respiratory syncytial virus (RSV) in infants, especially when
they have other serious diseases. However, there is no
evidence that ribavirin produces clinically relevant benefit in
RSV bronchiolitis.

Palivizumab below is a monoclonal antibody licensed for
preventing serious lower respiratory-tract disease caused by
respiratory syncytial virus in children at high risk of the
disease; it should be prescribed under specialist supervision
and on the basis of the likelihood of hospitalisation.
Palivizumab is recommended for:

- children under 9 months of age with chronic lung disease
  (defined as requiring oxygen for at least 28 days from
  birth) and who were born preterm;
- children under 6 months of age with haemodynamically
  significant, acyanotic congenital heart disease who were
  born preterm.

Palivizumab should be considered for:

- children under 2 years of age with severe combined
  immunodeficiency syndrome;
- children under 1 year of age who require long-term
  ventilation;
- children 1–2 years of age who require long-term
  ventilation and have an additional co-morbidity (including
  cardiac disease or pulmonary hypertension).

For details of the preterm age groups included in the
recommendations, see *Immunisation against Infectious
Disease* (2006), available at www.gov.uk/dh.

DRUGS FOR RESPIRATORY DISEASES ›
MONOCLONAL ANTIBODIES

Palivizumab

- **INDICATIONS AND DOSE**

**Prevention of serious lower respiratory-tract disease
caused by respiratory syncytial virus in children at high
risk of the disease (under expert supervision)**
- ▸ BY INTRAMUSCULAR INJECTION
- ▸ Child 1–23 months: 15 mg/kg once a month, preferably
  injected in the anterolateral thigh, to be administered
  during season of RSV risk, injection volume over 1 mL
  should be divided between 2 or more sites

**Prevention of serious lower respiratory-tract disease
caused by respiratory syncytial virus in children at high
risk of the disease and undergoing cardiac bypass
surgery (under expert supervision)**
- ▸ BY INTRAMUSCULAR INJECTION
- ▸ Child 1–23 months: Initially 15 mg/kg, to be
  administered as soon as stable after surgery, preferably
  in the anterolateral thigh, then 15 mg/kg once a
  month, preferably injected in the anterolateral thigh,
  to be administered during season of RSV risk, injection
  volume over 1 mL should be divided between 2 or more
  sites

- **UNLICENSED USE** Licensed for the prevention of serious
  lower respiratory-tract disease caused by respiratory
  syncytial virus (RSV) in children under 6 months of age (at
  the start of the RSV season) and born at less than 35 weeks
  corrected gestational age, or in children under 2 years of
  age who have received treatment for bronchopulmonary

dysplasia in the last 6 months, or in children under 2 years
of age with haemodynamically significant congenital heart
disease.

- **CAUTIONS** Moderate to severe acute infection · moderate
  to severe febrile illness · serum-palivizumab concentration
  may be reduced after cardiac surgery · thrombocytopenia

- **SIDE-EFFECTS**
- ▸ **Common or very common** Apnoea
- ▸ **Uncommon** Seizure · thrombocytopenia · urticaria
- ▸ **Frequency not known** Hypersensitivity

- **ALLERGY AND CROSS-SENSITIVITY** Hypersensitivity to
  humanised monoclonal antibodies.

- **MEDICINAL FORMS**
  There can be variation in the licensing of different medicines
  containing the same drug.
  Solution for injection
- ▸ Synagis (AbbVie Ltd)
  Palivizumab 100 mg per 1 ml Synagis 100mg/1ml solution for
  injection vials | 1 vial PoM £563.64
  Synagis 50mg/0.5ml solution for injection vials | 1 vial PoM £306.34

5

Infection

Chapter 6
Endocrine system

CONTENTS

1 Antidiuretic hormone disorders

Posterior pituitary hormones and antagonists

Posterior pituitary hormones

Diabetes insipidus

Vasopressin p. 655 (antidiuretic hormone, ADH) is used in the treatment of *pituitary* ('cranial') *diabetes insipidus* as is its analogue desmopressin p. 653. Dosage is tailored to produce a slight diuresis every 24 hours to avoid water intoxication. Treatment may be required for a limited period only in diabetes insipidus following trauma or pituitary surgery.

Desmopressin is more potent and has a longer duration of action than vasopressin; unlike vasopressin it has no vasoconstrictor effect. It is given by mouth or intranasally for maintenance therapy, and by injection in the postoperative period or in unconscious patients. Desmopressin is also used in the differential diagnosis of diabetes insipidus. Following a dose intramuscularly or intranasally, restoration of the ability to concentrate urine after water deprivation confirms a diagnosis of cranial diabetes insipidus. Failure to respond occurs in nephrogenic diabetes insipidus.

In *nephrogenic* and *partial pituitary diabetes insipidus* benefit may be gained from the paradoxical antidiuretic effect of thiazides.

Carbamazepine p. 309 is sometimes useful in partial pituitary diabetes insipidus [unlicensed]; it may act by sensitising the renal tubules to the action of remaining endogenous vasopressin.

Other uses

Desmopressin is also used to boost factor VIII concentration in mild to moderate haemophilia and in von Willebrand's disease; it is also used to test fibrinolytic response. Desmopressin may also have a role in nocturnal enuresis.

Vasopressin infusion is used to control variceal bleeding in portal hypertension, prior to more definitive treatment and with variable results. Terlipressin acetate, a derivative of vasopressin with reportedly less pressor and antidiuretic activity, is used similarly.

Oxytocin p. 804, another posterior pituitary hormone, is indicated in obstetrics.

Antidiuretic hormone antagonists

Demeclocycline hydrochloride p. 554 can be used in the treatment of hyponatraemia resulting from inappropriate secretion of antidiuretic hormone, if fluid restriction alone does not restore sodium concentration or is not tolerable. Demeclocycline hydrochloride is thought to act by directly blocking the renal tubular effect of antidiuretic hormone.

Tolvaptan p. 655 is a vasopressin V_2-receptor antagonist licensed for the treatment of hyponatraemia secondary to syndrome of inappropriate antidiuretic hormone secretion; treatment duration with tolvaptan is determined by the underlying disease and its treatment.

Rapid correction of hyponatraemia during tolvaptan therapy can cause osmotic demyelination, leading to serious neurological events; close monitoring of serum sodium concentration and fluid balance is essential.

1.1 Diabetes insipidus

> **Other drugs used for Diabetes insipidus** Chlortalidone, p. 229

PITUITARY AND HYPOTHALAMIC HORMONES AND ANALOGUES › VASOPRESSIN AND ANALOGUES

Desmopressin

09-Jun-2017

● **DRUG ACTION** Desmopressin is an analogue of vasopressin.

● **INDICATIONS AND DOSE**

Diabetes insipidus, treatment

▶ BY MOUTH
▸ **Child 1–23 months:** Initially 10 micrograms 2–3 times a day, adjusted according to response; usual dose 30–150 micrograms daily
▸ **Child 2–11 years:** Initially 50 micrograms 2–3 times a day, adjusted according to response; usual dose 100–800 micrograms daily
▸ **Child 12–17 years:** Initially 100 micrograms 2–3 times a day, adjusted according to response; usual dose 0.2–1.2 mg daily
▸ **Adult:** Initially 100 micrograms 3 times a day; maintenance 100–200 micrograms 3 times a day; usual dose 0.2–1.2 mg daily

▶ BY SUBLINGUAL ADMINISTRATION
▸ **Child 2–17 years:** Initially 60 micrograms 3 times a day, adjusted according to response; usual dose 40–240 micrograms 3 times a day
▸ **Adult:** Initially 60 micrograms 3 times a day, adjusted according to response; usual dose 40–240 micrograms 3 times a day

▶ BY INTRANASAL ADMINISTRATION
▸ **Child 1–23 months:** Initially 2.5–5 micrograms 1–2 times a day, adjusted according to response
▸ **Child 2–11 years:** Initially 5–20 micrograms 1–2 times a day, adjusted according to response
▸ **Child 12–17 years:** Initially 10–20 micrograms 1–2 times a day, adjusted according to response
▸ **Adult:** 10–40 micrograms daily in 1–2 divided doses

▶ BY SUBCUTANEOUS INJECTION, OR BY INTRAVENOUS INJECTION, OR BY INTRAMUSCULAR INJECTION
▸ **Adult:** 1–4 micrograms daily

Primary nocturnal enuresis

▶ BY MOUTH
▸ **Child 5–17 years:** 200 micrograms once daily, only increased to 400 micrograms if lower dose not effective; withdraw for at least 1 week for reassessment after 3 months, dose to be taken at bedtime, limit fluid intake from 1 hour before to 8 hours after administration
▸ **Adult 18–65 years:** 200 micrograms once daily, only increased to 400 micrograms if lower dose not effective; withdraw for at least 1 week for reassessment after 3 months, dose to be taken at bedtime, limit fluid intake from 1 hour before to 8 hours after administration

▶ BY SUBLINGUAL ADMINISTRATION
▸ **Child 5–17 years:** 120 micrograms once daily, increased if necessary to 240 micrograms once daily, dose to be taken at bedtime, limit fluid intake from 1 hour before to 8 hours after administration, dose to be increased only if lower dose not effective, reassess after 3 months by withdrawing treatment for at least 1 week
▸ **Adult 18–65 years:** 120 micrograms once daily, increased if necessary to 240 micrograms once daily, dose to be taken at bedtime, limit fluid intake from 1 hour before to 8 hours after administration, dose to be increased only if lower dose not effective, reassess after 3 months by withdrawing treatment for at least 1 week

Postoperative polyuria or polydipsia

▶ BY MOUTH
▸ **Adult:** Dose to be adjusted according to urine osmolality

Polyuria or polydipsia after hypophysectomy

▶ BY SUBLINGUAL ADMINISTRATION
▸ **Adult:** Dose to be adjusted according to urine osmolality

Idiopathic nocturnal polyuria in females

▶ BY SUBLINGUAL ADMINISTRATION
▸ **Adult:** 25 micrograms daily, to be taken 1 hour before bedtime

Idiopathic nocturnal polyuria in males

▶ BY SUBLINGUAL ADMINISTRATION
▸ **Adult:** 50 micrograms daily, to be taken 1 hour before bedtime

Diabetes insipidus, diagnosis (water deprivation test)

▶ BY INTRANASAL ADMINISTRATION
▸ **Adult:** 20 micrograms, limit fluid intake to 500 mL from 1 hour before to 8 hours after administration

▶ BY INTRAMUSCULAR INJECTION, OR BY SUBCUTANEOUS INJECTION
▸ **Adult:** 2 micrograms for 1 dose, limit fluid intake to 500 mL from 1 hour before to 8 hours after administration

Nocturia associated with multiple sclerosis (when other treatments have failed)

▶ BY INTRANASAL ADMINISTRATION
▸ **Adult 18–65 years:** 10–20 micrograms once daily, to be taken at bedtime, dose not to be repeated within 24 hours, limit fluid intake from 1 hour before to 8 hours after administration

Renal function testing

▶ BY INTRANASAL ADMINISTRATION
▸ **Adult:** 40 micrograms, empty bladder at time of administration and limit fluid intake to 500 mL from 1 hour before until 8 hours after administration to avoid fluid overload

▶ BY SUBCUTANEOUS INJECTION, OR BY INTRAMUSCULAR INJECTION
▸ **Adult:** 2 micrograms, empty bladder at time of administration and restrict fluid intake to 500 mL from 1 hour before until 8 hours after administration to avoid fluid overload

Mild to moderate haemophilia and von Willebrand's disease

▶ BY INTRANASAL ADMINISTRATION
▸ **Adult:** 300 micrograms every 12 hours if required, one 150 microgram spray into each nostril, 30 minutes before surgery or when bleeding, dose may alternatively be repeated at intervals of at least 3 days, if self-administered

▶ BY INTRAVENOUS INFUSION, OR BY SUBCUTANEOUS INJECTION
▸ **Adult:** 300 nanograms/kg for 1 dose, to be administered immediately before surgery or after trauma; may be repeated at intervals of 12 hours

Fibrinolytic response testing

▶ BY INTRANASAL ADMINISTRATION
▸ **Adult:** 300 micrograms, blood to be sampled after 1 hour for fibrinolytic activity, one 150 microgram spray to be administered into each nostril

▶ BY SUBCUTANEOUS INJECTION, OR BY INTRAVENOUS INJECTION
▸ **Adult:** 300 nanograms/kg for 1 dose, blood to be sampled after 20 minutes for fibrinolytic activity

Lumbar-puncture-associated headache

▶ BY INTRAMUSCULAR INJECTION, OR BY SUBCUTANEOUS INJECTION
▸ **Adult:** (consult product literature)

6

Endocrine system

- UNLICENSED USE Consult product literature for individual preparations. Oral use of *DDAVP* intravenous injection is not licensed.
- CONTRA-INDICATIONS Cardiac insufficiency · conditions treated with diuretics · history of hyponatraemia · polydipsia in alcohol dependence · psychogenic polydipsia · syndrome of inappropriate ADH secretion (in adults)
- CAUTIONS
  GENERAL CAUTIONS Asthma · avoid fluid overload · cardiovascular disease (not indicated for nocturnal enuresis or nocturia) · conditions which might be aggravated by water retention · cystic fibrosis · elderly (avoid for primary nocturnal enuresis and nocturia associated with multiple sclerosis in those over 65 years) · epilepsy · heart failure · hypertension (not indicated for nocturnal enuresis or nocturia) · migraine · nocturia—limit fluid intake to minimum from 1 hour before dose until 8 hours afterwards · nocturnal enuresis—limit fluid intake to minimum from 1 hour before dose until 8 hours afterwards
  SPECIFIC CAUTIONS
  ▸ With intranasal use Should not be given intranasally for nocturnal enuresis due to an increased incidence of side-effects
  CAUTIONS, FURTHER INFORMATION Elderly patients are at increased risk of hyponatraemia and renal impairment— manufacturer advises measure baseline serum sodium concentration, then monitor regularly during treatment; discontinue treatment if levels fall below the normal range. Review treatment if no therapeutic benefit after 3 months.
- INTERACTIONS → Appendix 1: desmopressin
- SIDE-EFFECTS
  GENERAL SIDE-EFFECTS
  ▸ **Common or very common** Hyponatraemia (on administration without restricting fluid intake) · nausea
  ▸ **Frequency not known** Abdominal pain · aggression (in children) · allergic dermatitis · emotional disorder · fluid retention · headache · hyponatraemic seizure · vomiting · weight increased
  SPECIFIC SIDE-EFFECTS
  ▸ With intranasal use Epistaxis · nasal congestion · rhinitis
  SIDE-EFFECTS, FURTHER INFORMATION Manufacturer advises avoiding concomitant use of drugs which increase secretion of vasopressin (e.g. tricyclic antidepressants)— increases risk of hyponatraemia.
- PREGNANCY Small oxytocic effect in third trimester; increased risk of pre-eclampsia.
- BREAST FEEDING Amount too small to be harmful.
- RENAL IMPAIRMENT Use with caution; antidiuretic effect may be reduced.
- MONITORING REQUIREMENTS In *nocturia*, periodic blood pressure and weight checks are needed to monitor for fluid overload.
- DIRECTIONS FOR ADMINISTRATION *DDAVP*® and *Desmotabs*® tablets may be crushed.
  DDAVP® intranasal solution may be diluted with Sodium Chloride 0.9% to a concentration of 10 micrograms/mL.
  DDAVP® injection may be administered orally.
  Desmopressin oral lyophilisates are for sublingual administration.
  ▸ With intravenous use in adults For *intravenous infusion* (*DDAVP*®, *Octim*®), give intermittently in Sodium chloride 0.9%; dilute with 50 mL and give over 20 minutes.
- PRESCRIBING AND DISPENSING INFORMATION Oral, intranasal, intravenous, subcutaneous and intramuscular doses are expressed as desmopressin acetate; sublingual doses are expressed as desmopressin base.

Children requiring an intranasal dose of less than 10 micrograms should be given *DDAVP*® intranasal solution.

- PATIENT AND CARER ADVICE
  Hyponatraemic convulsions Patients being treated for primary nocturnal enuresis should be warned to avoid fluid overload (including during swimming) and to stop taking desmopressin during an episode of vomiting or diarrhoea (until fluid balance normal).
  Medicines for Children leaflet: Desmopressin for bedwetting www.medicinesforchildren.org.uk/desmopressin-bedwetting-0
- NATIONAL FUNDING/ACCESS DECISIONS
  Scottish Medicines Consortium (SMC) Decisions
  The *Scottish Medicines Consortium* has advised (August 2017) that desmopressin oral lyophilisate (*Noqdirna*®) is accepted for restricted use within NHS Scotland for the symptomatic treatment of nocturia due to idiopathic nocturnal polyuria in patients aged 65 years and over.
  All Wales Medicines Strategy Group (AWMSG) Decisions
  The *All Wales Medicines Strategy Group* has advised (October 2017) that desmopressin acetate (*Noqdirna*®) is recommended for restricted use within NHS Wales for idiopathic nocturnal polyuria in adults aged over 65 years, for whom treatment options are currently limited.

- MEDICINAL FORMS
  There can be variation in the licensing of different medicines containing the same drug. Forms available from special-order manufacturers include: capsule, oral suspension, oral solution, spray, nasal drops

  Tablet
  ▸ Desmopressin (Non-proprietary)
    Desmopressin acetate 100 microgram Desmopressin 100microgram tablets | 90 tablet [PoM] £76.62 DT = £63.08
    Desmopressin acetate 200 microgram Desmopressin 200microgram tablets | 30 tablet [PoM] £35.23 DT = £9.09
  ▸ DDAVP (Ferring Pharmaceuticals Ltd)
    Desmopressin acetate 100 microgram DDAVP 0.1mg tablets | 90 tablet [PoM] £44.12 DT = £63.08
    Desmopressin acetate 200 microgram DDAVP 0.2mg tablets | 90 tablet [PoM] £88.23
  ▸ Desmotabs (Ferring Pharmaceuticals Ltd)
    Desmopressin acetate 200 microgram Desmotabs 0.2mg tablets | 30 tablet [PoM] £29.43 DT = £9.09

  Solution for injection
  ▸ DDAVP (Ferring Pharmaceuticals Ltd)
    Desmopressin acetate 4 microgram per 1 ml DDAVP 4micrograms/1ml solution for injection ampoules | 10 ampoule [PoM] £13.16
  ▸ Octim (Ferring Pharmaceuticals Ltd)
    Desmopressin acetate 15 microgram per 1 ml Octim 15micrograms/1ml solution for injection ampoules | 10 ampoule [PoM] £192.20

  Spray
  ▸ Desmopressin (Non-proprietary)
    Desmopressin acetate 10 microgram per 1 dose Desmopressin 10micrograms/dose nasal spray | 60 dose [PoM] £31.50 DT = £28.06
  ▸ Desmospray (Ferring Pharmaceuticals Ltd)
    Desmopressin acetate 2.5 microgram per 1 dose Desmospray 2.5micrograms/dose nasal spray | 50 dose [🔒]
    Desmopressin acetate 10 microgram per 1 dose Desmospray 10micrograms/dose nasal spray | 60 dose [PoM] £25.02 DT = £28.06
  ▸ Octim (Ferring Pharmaceuticals Ltd)
    Desmopressin acetate 150 microgram per 1 dose Octim 150micrograms/dose nasal spray | 25 dose [PoM] £576.60

  Oral lyophilisate
  CAUTIONARY AND ADVISORY LABELS 26
  ▸ DDAVP Melt (Ferring Pharmaceuticals Ltd)
    Desmopressin (as Desmopressin acetate) 60 microgram DDAVP Melt 60microgram oral lyophilisates sugar-free | 100 tablet [PoM] £50.53 DT = £50.53
    Desmopressin (as Desmopressin acetate) 120 microgram DDAVP Melt 120microgram oral lyophilisates sugar-free | 100 tablet [PoM] £101.07 DT = £101.07

Desmopressin (as Desmopressin acetate) 240 microgram DDAVP
Melt 240microgram oral lyophilisates sugar-free | 100 tablet PoM
£202.14
▸ **DesmoMelt** (Ferring Pharmaceuticals Ltd)
Desmopressin (as Desmopressin acetate)
120 microgram DesmoMelt 120microgram oral lyophilisates sugar-
free | 30 tablet PoM £30.34 DT = £30.34
Desmopressin (as Desmopressin acetate)
240 microgram DesmoMelt 240microgram oral lyophilisates sugar-
free | 30 tablet PoM £60.68 DT = £60.68
▸ **Noqdirna** (Ferring Pharmaceuticals Ltd)
Desmopressin (as Desmopressin acetate) 25 microgram Noqdirna
25microgram oral lyophilisates sugar-free | 30 tablet PoM £15.16 DT
= £15.16
Desmopressin (as Desmopressin acetate)
50 microgram Noqdirna 50microgram oral lyophilisates sugar-free
| 30 tablet PoM £15.16 DT = £15.16
Nasal drops
▸ **DDAVP** (Ferring Pharmaceuticals Ltd)
Desmopressin acetate 100 microgram per 1 ml DDAVP
100micrograms/ml intranasal solution | 2.5 ml PoM £9.72 DT = £9.72

Vasopressin

● **INDICATIONS AND DOSE**
Pituitary diabetes insipidus
▸ BY INTRAMUSCULAR INJECTION, OR BY SUBCUTANEOUS
  INJECTION
▸ Adult: 5–20 units every 4 hours
Initial control of oesophageal variceal bleeding
▸ BY INTRAVENOUS INFUSION
▸ Adult: 20 units, dose to be administered over
  15 minutes

● CONTRA-INDICATIONS Chronic nephritis (until reasonable
  blood nitrogen concentrations attained) · vascular disease
  (especially disease of coronary arteries) unless extreme
  caution
● CAUTIONS Asthma · avoid fluid overload · conditions which
  might be aggravated by water retention · epilepsy · heart
  failure · hypertension · migraine
● SIDE-EFFECTS Abdominal pain · angina pectoris ·
  bronchospasm · cardiac arrest · chest pain · diarrhoea ·
  flatulence · fluid imbalance · gangrene · headache ·
  hyperhidrosis · hypertension · musculoskeletal chest pain ·
  nausea · pallor · peripheral ischaemia · tremor · urticaria ·
  vertigo · vomiting
● PREGNANCY Oxytocic effect in third trimester.
● BREAST FEEDING Not known to be harmful.
● DIRECTIONS FOR ADMINISTRATION For *intravenous infusion*
  (argipressin), give intermittently in Glucose 5%; suggested
  concentration 20 units/100mL given over 15 minutes.

● MEDICINAL FORMS
  There can be variation in the licensing of different medicines
  containing the same drug.
  Solution for injection
  ▸ Vasopressin (Non-proprietary)
    Argipressin 20 unit per 1 ml Argipressin 20units/1ml solution for
    injection ampoules | 10 ampoule PoM £800.00 (Hospital only)

1.2 Syndrome of inappropriate antidiuretic hormone secretion

**Other drugs used for Syndrome of inappropriate
antidiuretic hormone secretion** Demeclocycline
hydrochloride, p. 554

DIURETICS ⟩ SELECTIVE VASOPRESSIN V$_2$-
RECEPTOR ANTAGONISTS

Tolvaptan

● DRUG ACTION Tolvaptan is a vasopressin V$_2$-receptor
  antagonist.

● **INDICATIONS AND DOSE**
JINARC ®
**Autosomal dominant polycystic kidney disease in adults
with CKD stage 1 to 3 at initiation of treatment with
evidence of rapidly progressing disease (initiated by a
specialist)**
▸ BY MOUTH
▸ Adult: Initially 60 mg daily in 2 divided doses for at
  least a week, 45 mg in the morning before breakfast,
  and then 15 mg taken 8 hours later; increased to 90 mg
  daily in 2 divided doses for at least a week, 60 mg in the
  morning before breakfast, and then 30 mg taken
  8 hours later, then increased if tolerated to 120 mg
  daily in 2 divided doses, 90 mg in the morning before
  breakfast, and then 30 mg taken 8 hours later, dose
  titration should be performed cautiously; patients may
  down-titrate to lower doses based on tolerability

SAMSCA ®
**Treatment of hyponatraemia secondary to syndrome of
inappropriate antidiuretic hormone secretion**
▸ BY MOUTH
▸ Adult: 15 mg once daily, increased if necessary up to
  60 mg daily; treatment duration is determined by the
  underlying disease and its treatment

● CONTRA-INDICATIONS Anuria · hypernatraemia ·
  hypovolaemic hyponatraemia · impaired perception of
  thirst · volume depletion
● CAUTIONS Alcoholism (increased risk of demyelination
  syndrome if rapid correction of hyponatraemia) · diabetes
  mellitus · ensure adequate fluid intake · hypoxia (increased
  risk of demyelination syndrome if rapid correction of
  hyponatraemia) · malnutrition (increased risk of
  demyelination syndrome if rapid correction of
  hyponatraemia) · pseudohyponatraemia associated with
  diabetes mellitus (exclude before treatment)
● INTERACTIONS → Appendix 1: tolvaptan
● SIDE-EFFECTS
▸ Common or very common Appetite decreased · asthenia ·
  constipation · dehydration · diarrhoea · dizziness · dry
  mouth · dyspnoea · gastrointestinal discomfort ·
  gastrooesophageal reflux disease · headache · hepatic
  function abnormal (discontinue) · hyperglycaemia ·
  hypernatraemia · hyperuricaemia · insomnia · muscle
  spasms · palpitations · polydipsia · skin reactions · thirst ·
  urinary disorders · weight decreased

  SIDE-EFFECTS, FURTHER INFORMATION Discontinue and
  perform liver-function tests promptly if symptoms of
  hepatic impairment (anorexia, nausea, vomiting, fatigue,
  abdominal pain, jaundice, dark urine, pruritus).
● PREGNANCY Avoid—toxicity in *animal* studies.
● BREAST FEEDING Avoid—present in milk in *animal* studies.
● HEPATIC IMPAIRMENT Use with caution in severe
  impairment—no information available.
● RENAL IMPAIRMENT No information available in severe
  impairment.
● MONITORING REQUIREMENTS
▸ Monitor for dehydration in patients who are fluid-
  restricted.
▸ Monitor serum-sodium concentration and fluid balance no
  later than 6 hours after initiating treatment and every
  6 hours during the first 1–2 days of treatment and until

dose stabilised. Discontinue if rapid rise in serum-sodium concentration (greater than 12 mmol/litre in 24 hours or 18 mmol/litre in 48 hours).

- **PATIENT AND CARER ADVICE** For *Jinarc*®, morning dose to be taken 30 minutes before food, second dose can be taken with or without food.

- **NATIONAL FUNDING/ACCESS DECISIONS**

  NICE decisions

  ▸ **Tolvaptan for treating autosomal dominant polycystic kidney disease (October 2015)** NICE TA358

  Tolvaptan (*Jinarc*®) is recommended as an option for the treatment of autosomal dominant polycystic kidney disease in adults if:

  - the patient has chronic kidney disease stage 2 or 3 at the start of treatment *and*
  - there is evidence of rapidly progressing disease
  - **and** the manufacturer provides tolvaptan with the discount agreed in the patient access scheme

  Patients currently receiving tolvaptan (*Jinarc*®) whose disease does not meet the above criteria should be able to continue treatment until they and their clinician consider it appropriate to stop.

  www.nice.org.uk/guidance/TA358

- **MEDICINAL FORMS**
  There can be variation in the licensing of different medicines containing the same drug.

  Tablet
  ▸ Jinarc (Otsuka Pharmaceuticals (U.K.) Ltd) ▼

Tolvaptan 15 mg	Jinarc 15mg tablets | 7 tablet [PoM]	£302.05
Tolvaptan 30 mg	Jinarc 30mg tablets | 7 tablet [PoM]	£302.05
Tolvaptan 45 mg	Jinarc 45mg tablets | 7 tablet [PoM] 🚫	
Tolvaptan 60 mg	Jinarc 60mg tablets | 7 tablet [PoM] 🚫	
Tolvaptan 90 mg	Jinarc 90mg tablets | 7 tablet [PoM] 🚫	

  ▸ Samsca (Otsuka Pharmaceuticals (U.K.) Ltd)

Tolvaptan 15 mg	Samsca 15mg tablets | 10 tablet [PoM]	£746.80
Tolvaptan 30 mg	Samsca 30mg tablets | 10 tablet [PoM]	£746.80

2   Corticosteroid responsive conditions

CORTICOSTEROIDS

Corticosteroids, general use

Overview

Dosages of corticosteroids vary widely in different diseases and in different patients. If the use of a corticosteroid can save or prolong life, as in exfoliative dermatitis, pemphigus, acute leukaemia or acute transplant rejection, high doses may need to be given, because the complications of therapy are likely to be less serious than the effects of the disease itself.

When long-term corticosteroid therapy is used in some chronic diseases, the adverse effects of treatment may become greater than the disabilities caused by the disease. To minimise side-effects the maintenance dose should be kept as low as possible.

When potentially less harmful measures are ineffective corticosteroids are used topically for the treatment of inflammatory conditions of the skin. Corticosteroids should be avoided or used only under specialist supervision in psoriasis.

Corticosteroids are used both topically (by rectum) and systemically (by mouth or intravenously) in the management of ulcerative colitis and Crohn's disease. They are also included in locally applied creams for haemorrhoids.

Use can be made of the mineralocorticoid activity of fludrocortisone acetate p. 661 to treat postural hypotension in autonomic neuropathy.

High-dose corticosteroids should be avoided for the management of septic shock. However, there is evidence that administration of lower doses of hydrocortisone p. 662 and fludrocortisone acetate is of benefit in adrenocortical insufficiency resulting from septic shock.

Dexamethasone p. 660 and betamethasone p. 660 have little if any mineralocorticoid action and their long duration of action makes them particularly suitable for suppressing corticotropin secretion in congenital adrenal hyperplasia where the dose should be tailored to clinical response and by measurement of adrenal androgens and 17-hydroxyprogesterone. In common with all glucocorticoids their suppressive action on the hypothalamic- pituitary-adrenal axis is greatest and most prolonged when they are given at night. In most individuals a single dose of dexamethasone at night, is sufficient to inhibit corticotropin secretion for 24 hours. This is the basis of the 'overnight dexamethasone suppression test' for diagnosing Cushing's syndrome.

Betamethasone and dexamethasone are also appropriate for conditions where water retention would be a disadvantage.

A corticosteroid may be used in the management of raised intracranial pressure or cerebral oedema that occurs as a result of malignancy (see Prescribing in palliative care p. 23); high doses of betamethasone or dexamethasone are generally used. However, a corticosteroid should not be used for the management of head injury or stroke because it is unlikely to be of benefit and may even be harmful.

In acute hypersensitivity reactions, such as angioedema of the upper respiratory tract and anaphylaxis, corticosteroids are indicated as an adjunct to emergency treatment with adrenaline/epinephrine p. 221. In such cases hydrocortisone (as sodium succinate) by intravenous injection may be required.

Corticosteroids are preferably used by inhalation in the management of asthma but systemic therapy in association with bronchodilators is required for the emergency treatment of severe acute asthma.

Corticosteroids may also be useful in conditions such as autoimmune hepatitis, rheumatoid arthritis and sarcoidosis; they may also lead to remissions of acquired haemolytic anaemia, and some cases of the nephrotic syndrome (particularly in children) and thrombocytopenic purpura.

Corticosteroids can improve the prognosis of serious conditions such as systemic lupus erythematosus, temporal arteritis, and polyarteritis nodosa; the effects of the disease process may be suppressed and symptoms relieved, but the underlying condition is not cured, although it may ultimately remit. It is usual to begin therapy in these conditions at fairly high dose, and then to reduce the dose to the lowest commensurate with disease control.

For other references to the use of corticosteroids see: Prescribing in Palliative Care, immunosuppression, rheumatic diseases, eye, otitis externa allergic rhinitis, and aphthous ulcers.

Side-effects

MHRA/CHM advice: Corticosteroids: rare risk of central serous chorioretinopathy with local as well as systemic administration (August 2017)

Central serous chorioretinopathy is a retinal disorder that has been linked to the systemic use of corticosteroids. Recently, it has also been reported after local administration of corticosteroids via inhaled and intranasal, epidural, intra-articular, topical dermal, and periocular routes. The MHRA recommends that patients should be advised to report any blurred vision or other visual disturbances with corticosteroid treatment given by any route; consider referral to an ophthalmologist for evaluation of possible causes if a patient presents with vision problems.

Overdosage or prolonged use can exaggerate some of the normal physiological actions of corticosteroids leading to mineralocorticoid and glucocorticoid side-effects.

Mineralocorticoid side effects

- hypertension
- sodium retention
- water retention
- potassium loss
- calcium loss

Mineralocorticoid side effects are most marked with fludrocortisone, but are significant with hydrocortisone, corticotropin, and tetracosactide. Mineralocorticoid actions are negligible with the high potency glucocorticoids, betamethasone and dexamethasone, and occur only slightly with methylprednisolone, prednisolone, and triamcinolone.

Glucocorticoid side effects

- diabetes
- osteoporosis, which is a danger, particularly in the elderly, as it can result in osteoporotic fractures for example of the hip or vertebrae;
- in addition high doses are associated with avascular necrosis of the femoral head.
- muscle wasting (proximal myopathy) can also occur.
- corticosteroid therapy is also weakly linked with peptic ulceration and perforation.
- psychiatric reactions may also occur.

Managing side-effects

Side-effects can be minimised by using lowest effective dose for minimum period possible. The suppressive action of a corticosteroid on cortisol secretion is least when it is given as a single dose in the morning. In an attempt to reduce pituitary-adrenal suppression further, the total dose for two days can sometimes be taken as a single dose on alternate days; alternate-day administration has not been very successful in the management of asthma. Pituitary-adrenal suppression can also be reduced by means of intermittent therapy with short courses. In some conditions it may be possible to reduce the dose of corticosteroid by adding a small dose of an immunosuppressive drug.

Whenever possible *local treatment* with creams, intra-articular injections, inhalations, eye-drops, or enemas should be used in preference to *systemic treatment*.

Inhaled corticosteroids have considerably fewer systemic effects than oral corticosteroids, but adverse effects including adrenal suppression have been reported. Use of other corticosteroid therapy (including topical) or concurrent use of drugs which inhibit corticosteroid metabolism should be taken into account when assessing systemic risk. In children, growth restriction associated with systemic corticosteroid therapy does not seem to occur with recommended doses of inhaled therapy; although initial growth velocity may be reduced, there appears to be no effect on achieving normal adult height. Large-volume spacer devices should be used for administering inhaled corticosteroids in children under 15 years; they are also useful in older children and adults, particularly if high doses are required. Spacer devices increase airway deposition and reduce oropharyngeal deposition.

Corticosteroids, replacement therapy

Overview

The adrenal cortex normally secretes hydrocortisone p. 662 (cortisol) which has glucocorticoid activity and weak mineralocorticoid activity. It also secretes the mineralocorticoid aldosterone.

In deficiency states, physiological replacement is best achieved with a combination of hydrocortisone and the mineralocorticoid fludrocortisone acetate p. 661; hydrocortisone alone does not usually provide sufficient mineralocorticoid activity for complete replacement.

In *Addison's disease* or following adrenalectomy, hydrocortisone by mouth is usually required. This is given in 2 doses, the larger in the morning and the smaller in the evening, mimicking the normal diurnal rhythm of cortisol secretion. The optimum daily dose is determined on the basis of clinical response. Glucocorticoid therapy is supplemented by fludrocortisone acetate.

In *acute adrenocortical insufficiency*, hydrocortisone is given intravenously (preferably as sodium succinate) every 6 to 8 hours in sodium chloride intravenous infusion 0.9% p. 1008.

In *hypopituitarism*, glucocorticoids should be given as in adrenocortical insufficiency, but since production of aldosterone is also regulated by the renin-angiotensin system a mineralocorticoid is not usually required. Additional replacement therapy with levothyroxine sodium p. 756 and sex hormones should be given as indicated by the pattern of hormone deficiency.

Glucocorticoid therapy

Glucocorticoid and mineralocorticoid activity

In comparing the relative potencies of corticosteroids in terms of their anti-inflammatory (glucocorticoid) effects it should be borne in mind that high glucocorticoid activity in itself is of no advantage unless it is accompanied by relatively low mineralocorticoid activity (see Disadvantages of Corticosteroids). The mineralocorticoid activity of fludrocortisone acetate p. 661 is so high that its anti-inflammatory activity is of no clinical relevance.

Equivalent anti-inflammatory doses of corticosteroids
This table takes no account of mineralocorticoid effects, nor does it take account of variations in duration of action
Prednisolone 5 mg
≡ Betamethasone 750 micrograms
≡ Deflazacort 6 mg
≡ Dexamethasone 750 micrograms
≡ Hydrocortisone 20 mg
≡ Methylprednisolone 4 mg
≡ Prednisone 5 mg
≡ Triamcinolone 4 mg

The relatively high mineralocorticoid activity of hydrocortisone p. 662, and the resulting fluid retention, makes it unsuitable for disease suppression on a long-term basis. However, hydrocortisone can be used for adrenal replacement therapy. Hydrocortisone is used on a short-term basis by intravenous injection for the emergency management of some conditions. The relatively moderate anti-inflammatory potency of hydrocortisone also makes it a useful topical corticosteroid for the management of inflammatory skin conditions because side-effects (both topical and systemic) are less marked.

Prednisolone p. 664 and prednisone p. 666 have predominantly glucocorticoid activity. Prednisolone is the corticosteroid most commonly used by mouth for long-term disease suppression.

6

Endocrine system

Betamethasone p. 660 and dexamethasone p. 660 have very high glucocorticoid activity in conjunction with insignificant mineralocorticoid activity. This makes them particularly suitable for high-dose therapy in conditions where fluid retention would be a disadvantage.

Betamethasone and dexamethasone also have a long duration of action and this, coupled with their lack of mineralocorticoid action makes them particularly suitable for conditions which require suppression of corticotropin (corticotrophin) secretion (e.g. congenital adrenal hyperplasia).

Some esters of betamethasone and of beclometasone dipropionate p. 43 (beclomethasone) exert a considerably more marked topical effect (e.g. on the skin or the lungs) than when given by mouth; use is made of this to obtain topical effects whilst minimising systemic side-effects (e.g. for skin applications and asthma inhalations).

Deflazacort p. 660 has a high glucocorticoid activity; it is derived from prednisolone.

Corticosteroids (systemic)

> **IMPORTANT SAFETY INFORMATION**
>
> MHRA/CHM ADVICE: CORTICOSTEROIDS: RARE RISK OF CENTRAL SEROUS CHORIORETINOPATHY WITH LOCAL AS WELL AS SYSTEMIC ADMINISTRATION (AUGUST 2017)
>
> Central serous chorioretinopathy is a retinal disorder that has been linked to the systemic use of corticosteroids. Recently, it has also been reported after local administration of corticosteroids via inhaled and intranasal, epidural, intra-articular, topical dermal, and periocular routes. The MHRA recommends that patients should be advised to report any blurred vision or other visual disturbances with corticosteroid treatment given by any route; consider referral to an ophthalmologist for evaluation of possible causes if a patient presents with vision problems.

● **CONTRA-INDICATIONS** Avoid injections containing benzyl alcohol in neonates (in neonates) · avoid live virus vaccines in those receiving immunosuppressive doses (serum antibody response diminished) · systemic infection (unless specific therapy given)

CONTRA-INDICATIONS, FURTHER INFORMATION For further information on contra-indications associated with intra-articular, intradermal and intralesional preparations, consult product literature.

● **CAUTIONS** Congestive heart failure · diabetes mellitus (including a family history of) · diverticulitis · epilepsy · glaucoma (including a family history of or susceptibility to) · history of steroid myopathy · history of tuberculosis or X-ray changes (frequent monitoring required) · hypertension · hypothyroidism · infection (particularly untreated) · myasthenia gravis · ocular herpes simplex (risk of corneal perforation) · osteoporosis (in children) · osteoporosis (post-menopausal women and the elderly at special risk) · peptic ulcer · psychiatric reactions · recent intestinal anastomoses · recent myocardial infarction (rupture reported) · severe affective disorders (particularly if history of steroid-induced psychosis) · should not be used long-term · thromboembolic disorders · ulcerative colitis

CAUTIONS, FURTHER INFORMATION For further information on cautions associated with intra-articular, intradermal and intralesional preparations, consult product literature.

● **SIDE-EFFECTS**

▶ **Common or very common** Adrenal suppression · anxiety · appetite increased · behaviour abnormal · cataract subcapsular · cognitive impairment · Cushing's syndrome · diabetic control impaired · electrolyte imbalance · fluid retention · gastrointestinal discomfort · glaucoma · headache · healing impaired · hirsutism · hypertension · increased risk of infection · leucocytosis · menstrual cycle irregularities · mood altered · nausea · osteoporosis · peptic ulcer · psychotic disorder · skin reactions · sleep disorders · telangiectasia · weight increased

▶ **Uncommon** Alkalosis hypokalaemic · bone fractures · haemorrhage · heart failure · hyperhidrosis · myopathy · oedema · osteonecrosis · pancreatitis · papilloedema · seizure · thromboembolism · tuberculosis reactivation · vertigo · vision blurred

▶ **Rare or very rare** Bruising · tendon rupture

▶ **Frequency not known** Chorioretinopathy · eye disorders · growth retardation (very common in children) · intracranial pressure increased with papilloedema (usually after withdrawal) (in children) · myocardial rupture (following recent myocardial infarction)

SIDE-EFFECTS, FURTHER INFORMATION

Adrenal suppression During prolonged therapy with corticosteroids, particularly with systemic use, adrenal atrophy develops and can persist for years after stopping. Abrupt withdrawal after a prolonged period can lead to acute adrenal insufficiency, hypotension, or death. To compensate for a diminished adrenocortical response caused by prolonged corticosteroid treatment, any significant intercurrent illness, trauma, or surgical procedure requires a temporary increase in corticosteroid dose, or if already stopped, a temporary reintroduction of corticosteroid treatment. Patients on long-term corticosteroid treatment should carry a steroid treatment card which gives guidance on minimising risk and provides details of prescriber, drug, dosage and duration of treatment.

Infections Prolonged courses of corticosteroids increase susceptibility to infections and severity of infections; clinical presentation of infections may also be atypical. Serious infections e.g. septicaemia and tuberculosis may reach an advanced stage before being recognised, and amoebiasis or strongyloidiasis may be activated or exacerbated (exclude before initiating a corticosteroid in those at risk or with suggestive symptoms). Fungal or viral ocular infections may also be exacerbated.

Chickenpox Unless they have had chickenpox, patients receiving oral or parenteral corticosteroids for purposes other than replacement should be regarded as being at risk of severe chickenpox. Manifestations of fulminant illness include pneumonia, hepatitis and disseminated intravascular coagulation; rash is not necessarily a prominent feature. Passive immunisation with varicella–zoster immunoglobulin is needed for exposed non–immune patients receiving systemic corticosteroids or for those who have used them within the previous 3 months. Confirmed chickenpox warrants specialist care and urgent treatment. Corticosteroids should not be stopped and dosage may need to be increased.

Measles Patients taking corticosteroids should be advised to take particular care to avoid exposure to measles and to seek immediate medical advice if exposure occurs. Prophylaxis with intramuscular normal immunoglobulin may be needed.

Psychiatric reactions Systemic corticosteroids, particularly in high doses, are linked to psychiatric reactions including euphoria, insomnia, irritability, mood lability, suicidal thoughts, psychotic reactions, and behavioural disturbances. These reactions frequently subside on reducing the dose or discontinuing the corticosteroid but they may also require specific management. Patients should be advised to seek medical advice if psychiatric symptoms (especially depression and suicidal thoughts) occur and they should also be alert to the rare possibility of such reactions during withdrawal of corticosteroid treatment. Systemic corticosteroids should be prescribed with care in those predisposed to psychiatric reactions, including those who have previously suffered corticosteroid–induced psychosis, or who have a personal or family history of psychiatric disorders.

● **PREGNANCY** The benefit of treatment with corticosteroids during pregnancy outweighs the risk. Corticosteroid cover is required during labour. Following a review of the data on the safety of systemic corticosteroids used in pregnancy and breast-feeding the CSM (May 1998) concluded that corticosteroids vary in their ability to cross the placenta but there is no convincing evidence that systemic corticosteroids increase the incidence of congenital abnormalities such as cleft palate or lip. When administration is prolonged or repeated during pregnancy, systemic corticosteroids increase the risk of intra-uterine growth restriction; there is no evidence of intra-uterine growth restriction following short-term treatment (e.g. prophylactic treatment for neonatal respiratory distress syndrome). Any adrenal suppression in the neonate following prenatal exposure usually resolves spontaneously after birth and is rarely clinically important. **Monitoring** Pregnant women with fluid retention should be monitored closely when given systemic corticosteroids.

● **BREAST FEEDING** The benefit of treatment with corticosteroids during breast-feeding outweighs the risk.

● **HEPATIC IMPAIRMENT** The plasma-drug concentration may be increased (particularly on systemic use). Oral and parenteral use should be undertaken with caution.

● **RENAL IMPAIRMENT** Use by oral and injectable routes should be undertaken with caution.

● **MONITORING REQUIREMENTS** The height and weight of children receiving prolonged treatment with corticosteroids should be monitored annually; if growth is slowed, referral to a paediatrician should be considered.

● **EFFECT ON LABORATORY TESTS** Suppression of skin test reactions.

● **TREATMENT CESSATION**

▶ In adults Abrupt withdrawal after a prolonged period can lead to acute adrenal insufficiency, hypotension or death. Withdrawal can also be associated with fever, myalgia, arthralgia, rhinitis, conjunctivitis, painful itchy skin nodules and weight loss. The magnitude and speed of dose reduction in corticosteroid withdrawal should be determined on a case-by-case basis, taking into consideration the underlying condition that is being treated, and individual patient factors such as the likelihood of relapse and the duration of corticosteroid treatment. *Gradual* withdrawal of systemic corticosteroids should be considered in those whose disease is unlikely to relapse and have:
- received more than 40 mg prednisolone (or equivalent) daily for more than 1 week;
- been given repeat doses in the evening;
- received more than 3 weeks' treatment;
- recently received repeated courses (particularly if taken for longer than 3 weeks);
- taken a short course within 1 year of stopping long-term therapy;
- other possible causes of adrenal suppression.

Systemic corticosteroids may be stopped abruptly in those whose disease is unlikely to relapse *and* who have received treatment for 3 weeks or less *and* who are not included in the patient groups described above.

During corticosteroid withdrawal the dose may be reduced rapidly down to physiological doses (equivalent to prednisolone 7.5 mg daily) and then reduced more slowly. Assessment of the disease may be needed during withdrawal to ensure that relapse does not occur.

▶ In children The magnitude and speed of dose reduction in corticosteroid withdrawal should be determined on a case-by-case basis, taking into consideration the underlying

condition that is being treated, and individual patient factors such as the likelihood of relapse and the duration of corticosteroid treatment. *Gradual* withdrawal of systemic corticosteroids should be considered in those whose disease is unlikely to relapse and have:
- received more than 40 mg prednisolone (or equivalent) daily for more than 1 week *or* 2 mg/kg daily for 1 week *or* 1 mg/kg daily for 1 month;
- been given repeat doses in the evening;
- received more than 3 weeks' treatment;
- recently received repeated courses (particularly if taken for longer than 3 weeks);
- taken a short course within 1 year of stopping long-term therapy;
- other possible causes of adrenal suppression.

Systemic corticosteroids may be stopped abruptly in those whose disease is unlikely to relapse *and* who have received treatment for 3 weeks or less *and* who are not included in the patient groups described above.

During corticosteroid withdrawal the dose may be reduced rapidly down to physiological doses (equivalent to prednisolone $2–2.5 \text{ mg/m}^2$ daily) and then reduced more slowly. Assessment of the disease may be needed during withdrawal to ensure that relapse does not occur.

● **PATIENT AND CARER ADVICE**

Advice for patients Patients on long-term corticosteroid treatment should carry a Steroid Treatment Card which gives guidance on minimising risk and provides details of prescriber, drug, dosage and duration of treatment.

A patient information leaflet should be supplied to every patient when a systemic corticosteroid is prescribed. Patients should especially be advised of the following:
- **Immunosuppression** Prolonged courses of corticosteroids can increase susceptibility to infection and serious infections can go unrecognised. Unless already immune, patients are at risk of severe **chickenpox** and should avoid close contact with people who have chickenpox or shingles. Similarly, precautions should also be taken against contracting **measles**;
- **Adrenal suppression** If the corticosteroid is given for longer than 3 weeks, treatment must not be stopped abruptly. Adrenal suppression can last for a year or more after stopping treatment and the patient must mention the course of corticosteroid when receiving treatment for any illness or injury;
- **Mood and behaviour changes** Corticosteroid treatment, especially with high doses, can alter mood and behaviour early in treatment—the patient can become confused, irritable and suffer from delusion and suicidal thoughts. These effects can also occur when corticosteroid treatment is being withdrawn. Medical advice should be sought if worrying psychological changes occur;
- **Other serious effects** Serious gastro-intestinal, musculoskeletal, and ophthalmic effects which require medical help can also occur.

Steroid treatment cards Steroid treatment cards should be issued where appropriate. Consider giving a 'steroid card' to support communication of the risks associated with treatment, and specific written advice to consider corticosteroid replacement during an episode of stress, such as severe intercurrent illness or an operation, to patients using greater than maximum licensed doses of inhaled corticosteroids. Steroid treatment cards are available for purchase from the NHS Print online ordering portal www.nhsforms.co.uk

GP practices can obtain supplies through Primary Care Support England. NHS Trusts can order supplies via the online ordering portal.

6

Endocrine system

In **Scotland**, steroid treatment cards can be obtained from APS Group Scotland by emailing stockorders.dppas@apsgroup.co.uk or by fax on 0131 629 9967.

Betamethasone

↞ 658

21-Dec-2017

● INDICATIONS AND DOSE

Suppression of inflammatory and allergic disorders | Congenital adrenal hyperplasia
▶ BY MOUTH
▸ Adult: Usual dose 0.5–5 mg daily
▶ BY INTRAMUSCULAR INJECTION, OR BY SLOW INTRAVENOUS INJECTION, OR BY INTRAVENOUS INFUSION
▸ Adult: 4–20 mg, repeated up to 4 times in 24 hours

● INTERACTIONS → Appendix 1: corticosteroids
● SIDE-EFFECTS Hiccups · malaise · Stevens-Johnson syndrome
● PREGNANCY Readily crosses the placenta. Transient effect on fetal movements and heart rate.
● DIRECTIONS FOR ADMINISTRATION For *intravenous infusion* (as sodium phosphate) (*Betnesol®*), give continuously or intermittently *or via* drip tubing *in* Glucose 5% *or* Sodium chloride 0.9%.
● PATIENT AND CARER ADVICE Patient counselling is advised for betamethasone soluble tablets (steroid card).

● MEDICINAL FORMS
There can be variation in the licensing of different medicines containing the same drug.
Soluble tablet
CAUTIONARY AND ADVISORY LABELS 10, 13, 21 (not for use as mouthwash for oral ulceration)
▸ Betamethasone (Non-proprietary)
 Betamethasone (as Betamethasone sodium phosphate)
 500 microgram Betamethasone 500microgram soluble tablets sugar free sugar-free | 100 tablet PoM £51.12 DT = £51.12
Solution for injection
CAUTIONARY AND ADVISORY LABELS 10
▸ Betamethasone (Non-proprietary)
 Betamethasone (as Betamethasone sodium phosphate) 4 mg per 1 ml Betamethasone 4mg/1ml solution for injection ampoules | 5 ampoule PoM £18.81 DT = £17.25

Deflazacort

↞ 658

21-Dec-2017

● INDICATIONS AND DOSE

Suppression of inflammatory and allergic disorders
▶ BY MOUTH
▸ Adult: Maintenance 3–18 mg daily

Suppression of inflammatory and allergic disorders (acute disorders)
▶ BY MOUTH
▸ Adult: Initially up to 120 mg daily

Inflammatory and allergic disorders
▶ BY MOUTH
▸ Child 1 month–11 years: 0.25–1.5 mg/kg once daily or on alternate days; increased if necessary up to 2.4 mg/kg daily (max. per dose 120 mg), in emergency situations
▸ Child 12–17 years: 3–18 mg once daily or on alternate days; increased if necessary up to 2.4 mg/kg daily (max. per dose 120 mg), in emergency situations

● INTERACTIONS → Appendix 1: corticosteroids
● SIDE-EFFECTS Hypotension
● PATIENT AND CARER ADVICE Patient counselling is advised for deflazacort tablets (steroid card).

● MEDICINAL FORMS
There can be variation in the licensing of different medicines containing the same drug. Forms available from special-order manufacturers include: tablet
Tablet
CAUTIONARY AND ADVISORY LABELS 5, 10
▸ Calcort (Sanofi)
 Deflazacort 6 mg Calcort 6mg tablets | 60 tablet PoM £15.82

Dexamethasone

↞ 658

21-Dec-2017

● INDICATIONS AND DOSE

Suppression of inflammatory and allergic disorders
▶ BY MOUTH
▸ Adult: 0.5–10 mg daily

Mild croup
▶ BY MOUTH
▸ Child: 150 micrograms/kg for 1 dose

Severe croup (or mild croup that might cause complications)
▶ INITIALLY BY MOUTH
▸ Child: Initially 150 micrograms/kg for 1 dose, to be given before transfer to hospital, then (by mouth or by intravenous injection) 150 micrograms/kg, then (by mouth or by intravenous injection) 150 micrograms/kg after 12 hours if required

Congenital adrenal hyperplasia (under expert supervision)
▶ BY MOUTH
▸ Adult: Consult specialist for advice on dosing
▶ BY INTRAMUSCULAR INJECTION, OR BY SLOW INTRAVENOUS INJECTION, OR BY INTRAVENOUS INFUSION
▸ Adult: Consult specialist for advice on dosing

Overnight dexamethasone suppression test
▶ BY MOUTH
▸ Adult: 1 mg for 1 dose, to be given at night

Adjunctive treatment of bacterial meningitis (starting before or with first dose of antibacterial)
▶ BY INTRAVENOUS INJECTION
▸ Adult: 8.3 mg every 6 hours for 4 days

Symptom control of anorexia (in palliative care)
▸ Adult: 2–4 mg daily

Obstruction due to tumour (dysphagia in palliative care)
▸ Adult: 8 mg daily

Bronchospasm or partial obstruction (dyspnoea in palliative care)
▸ Adult: 4–8 mg daily

Nausea and vomiting (adjunct in palliative care)
▶ BY MOUTH
▸ Adult: 8–16 mg daily

Headaches due to raised intracranial pressure (in palliative care)
▸ Adult: 16 mg daily for 4–5 days, then reduced to 4–6 mg daily, reduce dose if possible. To be given before 6pm to reduce the risk of insomnia

Pain due to nerve compression (in palliative care)
▸ Adult: 8 mg daily

Cerebral oedema associated with malignancy
▶ BY MOUTH
▸ Adult: 0.5–10 mg daily

Cerebral oedema
▶ INITIALLY BY INTRAVENOUS INJECTION
▸ Adult: Initially 8–16 mg for 1 dose, then (by intramuscular injection or by intravenous injection) 5 mg every 6 hours until adequate response achieved then taper-off gradually, use the 3.8 mg/mL injection preparation for this dose

Cerebral oedema associated with malignancy
▶ INITIALLY BY INTRAVENOUS INJECTION
▶ Adult: Initially 8.3 mg for 1 dose, then (by intramuscular injection) 3.3 mg every 6 hours as required for 2–4 days, subsequently, reduce dose gradually and stop over 5–7 days, use the 3.3 mg/mL injection preparation for this dose

● UNLICENSED USE
▶ With intravenous use Consult product literature; not licensed for use in bacterial meningitis.

● INTERACTIONS → Appendix 1: corticosteroids

● SIDE-EFFECTS
▶ With parenteral use Hypotension · perineal irritation (may occur following the intravenous injection of large doses of the phosphate ester)
▶ With oral use Exophthalmos · hiccups · hyperglycaemia · hypotension · malaise · protein catabolism

● PREGNANCY Dexamethasone readily crosses the placenta.

● DIRECTIONS FOR ADMINISTRATION
▶ With oral use in children For administration *by mouth* tablets may be dispersed in water or injection solution given by mouth.
▶ With intravenous use in adults For *intravenous infusion* (*Dexamethasone*, Hospira) give continuously *or* intermittently *or via* drip tubing *in* Glucose 5% *or* Sodium Chloride 0.9%.

● PRESCRIBING AND DISPENSING INFORMATION
▶ With systemic use Dexamethasone 3.8 mg/mL Injection has replaced Dexamethasone 4 mg/mL Injection. All dosage recommendations for intravenous, intramuscular, intrarticular use or local infiltration; are given in units of dexamethasone base.

● PATIENT AND CARER ADVICE Patient counselling is advised for dexamethasone tablet, oral solution and injection (steroid card).
Medicines for Children leaflet: Dexamethasone for croup
www.medicinesforchildren.org.uk/dexamethasone-croup-0

● MEDICINAL FORMS
There can be variation in the licensing of different medicines containing the same drug. Forms available from special-order manufacturers include: capsule, oral suspension, oral solution

Soluble tablet
▶ Dexamethasone (Non-proprietary)
Dexamethasone (as Dexamethasone sodium phosphate) 2 mg Dexamethasone 2mg soluble tablets sugar free sugar-free | 50 tablet [PoM] £30.00–£30.01 DT = £30.01
Dexamethasone (as Dexamethasone sodium phosphate) 4 mg Dexamethasone 4mg soluble tablets sugar free sugar-free | 50 tablet [PoM] £60.00–£60.01 DT = £60.01
Dexamethasone (as Dexamethasone sodium phosphate) 8 mg Dexamethasone 8mg soluble tablets sugar free sugar-free | 50 tablet [PoM] £120.00–£120.02 DT = £120.01
▶ Glensoludex (Glenmark Pharmaceuticals Europe Ltd)
Dexamethasone (as Dexamethasone sodium phosphate) 2 mg Glensoludex 2mg soluble tablets sugar-free | 50 tablet [PoM] £10.00 DT = £30.01
Dexamethasone (as Dexamethasone sodium phosphate) 4 mg Glensoludex 4mg soluble tablets sugar-free | 50 tablet [PoM] £20.00 DT = £60.01
Dexamethasone (as Dexamethasone sodium phosphate) 8 mg Glensoludex 8mg soluble tablets sugar-free | 50 tablet [PoM] £40.00 DT = £120.01

Tablet
CAUTIONARY AND ADVISORY LABELS 10, 21
▶ Dexamethasone (Non-proprietary)
Dexamethasone 500 microgram Dexamethasone 500microgram tablets | 28 tablet [PoM] £14.25–£54.24 DT = £16.22 | 30 tablet [PoM] £17.38–£64.82
Dexamethasone 2 mg Dexamethasone 2mg tablets | 50 tablet [PoM] £49.00 DT = £14.25 | 100 tablet [PoM] £28.50–£98.00 | 500 tablet [PoM] £490.00

Dexamethasone 4 mg Dexamethasone 4mg tablets | 50 tablet [PoM] £85.00 DT = £85.00
▶ Neofordex (Aspire Pharma Ltd)
Dexamethasone 40 mg Neofordex 40mg tablets | 10 tablet [PoM] £200.00 DT = £200.00

Solution for injection
CAUTIONARY AND ADVISORY LABELS 10
▶ Dexamethasone (Non-proprietary)
Dexamethasone (as Dexamethasone sodium phosphate) 3.3 mg per 1 ml Dexamethasone 6.6mg/2ml solution for injection vials | 5 vial [PoM] £24.00 DT = £24.00
Dexamethasone 6.6mg/2ml solution for injection ampoules | 5 ampoule [PoM] £11.00 DT = £11.00 | 10 ampoule [PoM] £22.00
Dexamethasone 3.3mg/1ml solution for injection ampoules | 5 ampoule [PoM] £12.00 | 10 ampoule [PoM] £12.00–£19.67 DT = £19.67
Dexamethasone (as Dexamethasone sodium phosphate) 3.8 mg per 1 ml Dexamethasone 3.8mg/1ml solution for injection vials | 10 vial [PoM] £19.99–£20.01 DT = £20.00

Oral solution
CAUTIONARY AND ADVISORY LABELS 10, 21
▶ Dexamethasone (Non-proprietary)
Dexamethasone (as Dexamethasone sodium phosphate) 400 microgram per 1 ml Dexamethasone 2mg/5ml oral solution sugar free sugar-free | 150 ml [PoM] £42.30 DT = £42.30
Dexamethasone (as Dexamethasone sodium phosphate) 2 mg per 1 ml Dexamethasone 10mg/5ml oral solution sugar free sugar-free | 50 ml [PoM] £24.50–£24.95 sugar-free | 150 ml [PoM] £101.40 DT = £94.44
Dexamethasone (as Dexamethasone sodium phosphate) 4 mg per 1 ml Dexamethasone 20mg/5ml oral solution sugar free sugar-free | 50 ml [PoM] £49.50 DT = £49.50
▶ Dexsol (Rosemont Pharmaceuticals Ltd)
Dexamethasone (as Dexamethasone sodium phosphate) 400 microgram per 1 ml Dexsol 2mg/5ml oral solution sugar-free | 75 ml [PoM] £21.15 sugar-free | 150 ml [PoM] £42.30 DT = £42.30
▶ Martapan (Martindale Pharmaceuticals Ltd)
Dexamethasone (as Dexamethasone sodium phosphate) 400 microgram per 1 ml Martapan 2mg/5ml oral solution sugar-free | 150 ml [PoM] £35.96 DT = £42.30

F 658

Fluordocortisone acetate

21-Dec-2017

● INDICATIONS AND DOSE

Neuropathic postural hypotension
▶ BY MOUTH
▶ Adult: 100–400 micrograms daily

Mineralocorticoid replacement in adrenocortical insufficiency
▶ BY MOUTH
▶ Adult: 50–300 micrograms once daily

Adrenocortical insufficiency resulting from septic shock (in combination with hydrocortisone)
▶ BY MOUTH
▶ Adult: 50 micrograms daily

● UNLICENSED USE Not licensed for use in neuropathic postural hypotension.

● INTERACTIONS → Appendix 1: corticosteroids

● SIDE-EFFECTS Conjunctivitis · exophthalmos · fatigue · idiopathic intracranial hypertension · muscle atrophy · muscle weakness · petechiae

● HEPATIC IMPAIRMENT
Monitoring Monitor patient closely in hepatic impairment.

● MEDICINAL FORMS
There can be variation in the licensing of different medicines containing the same drug. Forms available from special-order manufacturers include: capsule, oral suspension

Tablet
CAUTIONARY AND ADVISORY LABELS 10
▶ Fludrocortisone acetate (Non-proprietary)
Fludrocortisone acetate 100 microgram Fludrocortisone 100microgram tablets | 30 tablet [PoM] £13.60 DT = £13.60

6

Endocrine system

Hydrocortisone

📖 658

21-Dec-2017

● **INDICATIONS AND DOSE**

Thyrotoxic crisis (thyroid storm)
▶ BY INTRAVENOUS INJECTION
▸ Adult: 100 mg every 6 hours, to be administered as sodium succinate

Adrenocortical insufficiency resulting from septic shock
▶ BY INTRAVENOUS INJECTION
▸ Adult: 50 mg every 6 hours, given in combination with fludrocortisone

Acute hypersensitivity reactions such as angioedema of the upper respiratory tract and anaphylaxis (adjunct to adrenaline)
▶ BY INTRAVENOUS INJECTION
▸ Adult: 100–300 mg, to be administered as sodium succinate

Corticosteroid replacement, in patients who have taken more than 10 mg prednisolone daily (or equivalent) within 3 months of minor surgery under general anaesthesia
▶ BY INTRAVENOUS INJECTION, OR BY INTRAVENOUS INFUSION
▸ Adult: Initially 25–50 mg, to be administered at induction of surgery, the patient's usual oral corticosteroid dose is recommenced after surgery

Corticosteroid replacement, in patients who have taken more than 10 mg prednisolone daily (or equivalent) within 3 months of moderate or major surgery
▶ INITIALLY BY INTRAVENOUS INJECTION, OR BY INTRAVENOUS INFUSION
▸ Adult: Initially 25–50 mg, to be administered at induction of surgery (following usual oral corticosteroid dose on the morning of surgery), followed by (by intravenous injection) 25–50 mg 3 times a day for 24 hours after moderate surgery and for 48–72 hours after major surgery

Adrenocortical insufficiency in Addison's disease or following adrenalectomy
▶ BY MOUTH USING IMMEDIATE-RELEASE MEDICINES
▸ Adult: 20–30 mg daily in 2 divided doses, the larger dose to be given in the morning and the smaller in the evening, mimicking the normal diurnal rhythm of cortisol secretion, the optimum daily dose is determined on the basis of clinical response

Adrenocortical insufficiency
▶ BY INTRAMUSCULAR INJECTION, OR BY SLOW INTRAVENOUS INJECTION, OR BY INTRAVENOUS INFUSION
▸ Adult: 100–500 mg 3–4 times a day or when required

Severe inflammatory bowel disease
▶ BY SLOW INTRAVENOUS INJECTION, OR BY INTRAVENOUS INFUSION
▸ Adult: 100–500 mg 3–4 times a day or when required

Replacement in adrenocortical insufficiency
▶ BY MOUTH USING MODIFIED-RELEASE MEDICINES
▸ Adult: 20–30 mg once daily, adjusted according to response, dose to be taken in the morning
▶ BY MOUTH USING IMMEDIATE-RELEASE MEDICINES
▸ Adult: 20–30 mg daily in divided doses, adjusted according to response

Ulcerative colitis | Proctitis | Proctosigmoiditis
▶ BY RECTUM USING RECTAL FOAM
▸ Adult: Initially 1 metered application 1–2 times a day for 2–3 weeks, then reduced to 1 metered application once daily on alternate days, to be inserted into the rectum

Acute hypersensitivity reactions | Angioedema
▶ BY INTRAMUSCULAR INJECTION, OR BY INTRAVENOUS INJECTION
▸ Child 1–5 months: Initially 25 mg 3 times a day, adjusted according to response
▸ Child 6 months–5 years: Initially 50 mg 3 times a day, adjusted according to response
▸ Child 6–11 years: Initially 100 mg 3 times a day, adjusted according to response
▸ Child 12–17 years: Initially 200 mg 3 times a day, adjusted according to response

Severe acute asthma | Life-threatening acute asthma
▶ BY INTRAVENOUS INJECTION
▸ Child 1 month–1 year: 4 mg/kg every 6 hours (max. per dose 100 mg), alternatively 25 mg every 6 hours until conversion to oral prednisolone is possible, dose given, preferably, as sodium succinate
▸ Child 2–4 years: 4 mg/kg every 6 hours (max. per dose 100 mg), alternatively 50 mg every 6 hours until conversion to oral prednisolone is possible, dose given, preferably, as sodium succinate
▸ Child 5–11 years: 4 mg/kg every 6 hours (max. per dose 100 mg), alternatively 100 mg every 6 hours until conversion to oral prednisolone is possible, dose given, preferably, as sodium succinate
▸ Child 12–17 years: 4 mg/kg every 6 hours (max. per dose 100 mg), alternatively 100 mg every 6 hours until conversion to oral prednisolone is possible, dose given, preferably, as sodium succinate
▸ Adult: 100 mg every 6 hours until conversion to oral prednisolone is possible, dose given, preferably, as sodium succinate

DOSE EQUIVALENCE AND CONVERSION
▸ With oral use
▸ When switching from immediate-release hydrocortisone tablets to modified release *Plenadren*® use same total dose. Bioavailability of *Plenadren*® lower than immediate release tablets—monitor clinical response.

● **CONTRA-INDICATIONS**
▸ With rectal use Bowel perforation · extensive fistulas · intestinal obstruction · recent intestinal anastomoses

● **CAUTIONS**
▸ With rectal use Systemic absorption may occur

● **INTERACTIONS** → Appendix 1: corticosteroids

● **SIDE-EFFECTS**
▶ **Uncommon**
▸ With rectal use Skin discolouration
▶ **Frequency not known**
▸ With oral use Dyslipidaemia · fatigue · hypotension · malaise
▸ With parenteral use Exophthalmos · hiccups · Kaposi's sarcoma · lipomatosis · malaise

● **DIRECTIONS FOR ADMINISTRATION**
▸ With intravenous use in children For *intravenous administration*, dilute with Glucose 5% or Sodium Chloride 0.9%. For *intermittent infusion* give over 20–30 minutes.
▸ With intravenous use in adults For *intravenous infusion* (*SoluCortef*® or *Efcortesol*®), give continuously *or* intermittently *or via* drip tubing *in* Glucose 5% *or* Sodium chloride 0.9%.

● **PRESCRIBING AND DISPENSING INFORMATION**
▸ In children The RCPCH and NPPG recommend that, when a liquid special of hydrocortisone is required, the following strength is used: 5 mg/5 mL.

● **PATIENT AND CARER ADVICE** Patient counselling is advised for hydrocortisone tablets and injections (steroid card).

- NATIONAL FUNDING/ACCESS DECISIONS

Scottish Medicines Consortium (SMC) Decisions
The *Scottish Medicines Consortium* has advised (December 2016) that hydrocortisone modified release (*Plenadren*®) is **not** recommended for use within NHS Scotland for treatment of adrenal insufficiency in adults as there was insufficient evidence submitted.

- LESS SUITABLE FOR PRESCRIBING
- With intravenous use Hydrocortisone as the sodium phosphate is less suitable for prescribing as paraesthesia and pain (particularly in the perineal region) may follow intravenous injection.

- EXCEPTIONS TO LEGAL CATEGORY Prescription only medicine restriction does not apply where administration is for saving life in emergency.

- MEDICINAL FORMS
There can be variation in the licensing of different medicines containing the same drug. Forms available from special-order manufacturers include: capsule, oral suspension, oral solution

Modified-release tablet
CAUTIONARY AND ADVISORY LABELS 10, 22, 25
- Plenadren (Shire Pharmaceuticals Ltd)
  Hydrocortisone 5 mg Plenadren 5mg modified-release tablets | 50 tablet [PoM] £242.50 DT = £242.50
  Hydrocortisone 20 mg Plenadren 20mg modified-release tablets | 50 tablet [PoM] £400.00 DT = £400.00

Tablet
CAUTIONARY AND ADVISORY LABELS 10, 21
- Hydrocortisone (Non-proprietary)
  Hydrocortisone 10 mg Hydrocortisone 10mg tablets | 30 tablet [PoM] £101.76 DT = £32.79
  Hydrocortisone 20 mg Hydrocortisone 20mg tablets | 30 tablet [PoM] £147.26 DT = £83.26

Powder for solution for injection
- Solu-Cortef (Pfizer Ltd)
  Hydrocortisone (as Hydrocortisone sodium succinate) 100 mg Solu-Cortef 100mg powder for solution for injection vials | 10 vial [PoM] £9.17

Suspension for injection
- Hydrocortistab (AMCo)
  Hydrocortisone acetate 25 mg per 1 ml Hydrocortistab 25mg/1ml suspension for injection ampoules | 10 ampoule [PoM] £68.72 DT = £68.72

Powder and solvent for solution for injection
CAUTIONARY AND ADVISORY LABELS 10
- Solu-Cortef (Pfizer Ltd)
  Hydrocortisone (as Hydrocortisone sodium succinate) 100 mg Solu-Cortef 100mg powder and solvent for solution for injection vials | 1 vial [PoM] £1.16 DT = £1.16

Solution for injection
CAUTIONARY AND ADVISORY LABELS 10
- Hydrocortisone (Non-proprietary)
  Hydrocortisone (as Hydrocortisone sodium phosphate) 100 mg per 1 ml Hydrocortisone sodium phosphate 100mg/1ml solution for injection ampoules | 5 ampoule [PoM] £8.33 DT = £8.33

Foam
EXCIPIENTS: May contain Cetostearyl alcohol (including cetyl and stearyl alcohol), hydroxybenzoates (parabens), propylene glycol
- Colifoam (Meda Pharmaceuticals Ltd)
  Hydrocortisone acetate 100 mg per 1 gram Colifoam 10% aerosol | 14 dose [PoM] £9.33 DT = £9.33

⟩ 658

Methylprednisolone
03-Nov-2017

- INDICATIONS AND DOSE

Suppression of inflammatory and allergic disorders | Cerebral oedema associated with malignancy
- BY MOUTH
- Adult: Initially 2–40 mg daily
- BY INTRAMUSCULAR INJECTION, OR BY SLOW INTRAVENOUS INJECTION, OR BY INTRAVENOUS INFUSION
- Adult: Initially 10–500 mg

Treatment of graft rejection reactions
- BY INTRAVENOUS INFUSION
- Adult: Up to 1 g daily for up to 3 days

Treatment of relapse in multiple sclerosis
- BY MOUTH
- Adult: 500 mg once daily for 5 days

Treatment of relapse in multiple sclerosis (when oral steroids have failed or have not been tolerated, or in those who require hospital admission)
- BY INTRAVENOUS INFUSION
- Adult: 1 g once daily for 3–5 days

DEPO-MEDRONE ®

Suppression of inflammatory and allergic disorders
- BY DEEP INTRAMUSCULAR INJECTION
- Adult: 40–120 mg, then 40–120 mg after 2–3 weeks if required, to be injected into the gluteal muscle

- UNLICENSED USE [EvGr] Not licensed for use by mouth for the treatment of multiple sclerosis relapse. Not licensed for use by intravenous infusion for the treatment of multiple sclerosis relapse for durations longer than 3 days. ⓐ. Methylprednisolone doses in the BNF may differ from those in product literature.

> IMPORTANT SAFETY INFORMATION
> MHRA/CHM ADVICE: METHYLPREDNISOLONE INJECTABLE MEDICINE CONTAINING LACTOSE (*SOLU-MEDRONE*® 40 MG): DO NOT USE IN PATIENTS WITH COWS' MILK ALLERGY (OCTOBER 2017)
> - With intramuscular use or intravenous use
> An EU-wide review has concluded that *Solu-Medrone*® 40 mg may contain trace amounts of milk proteins and should not be used in patients with a known or suspected allergy to cows' milk. Serious allergic reactions, including bronchospasm and anaphylaxis, have been reported in patients allergic to cows' milk proteins. If a patient's symptoms worsen or new allergic symptoms occur, administration should be stopped and the patient treated accordingly.

- CAUTIONS Rapid intravenous administration of large doses associated with cardiovascular collapse

- INTERACTIONS → Appendix 1: corticosteroids

- SIDE-EFFECTS Diarrhoea · dizziness · dyslipidaemia · exophthalmos · fatigue · hiccups · hypotension · Kaposi's sarcoma · lipomatosis · malaise

- DIRECTIONS FOR ADMINISTRATION For *intravenous infusion* (as sodium succinate) (*Solu-Medrone*®), give continuously or intermittently or via drip tubing in Glucose 5% or Sodium chloride 0.9%. Reconstitute initially with water for injections; doses up to 250 mg should be given over at least 5 minutes, high doses over at least 30 minutes.

- PATIENT AND CARER ADVICE Patient counselling is advised for methylprednisolone tablets and injections (steroid card).

- MEDICINAL FORMS
There can be variation in the licensing of different medicines containing the same drug. Forms available from special-order manufacturers include: oral suspension

Powder and solvent for solution for injection
CAUTIONARY AND ADVISORY LABELS 10
- Methylprednisolone (Non-proprietary)
  Methylprednisolone (as Methylprednisolone sodium succinate) 500 mg Methylprednisolone sodium succinate 500mg powder and solvent for solution for injection vials | 1 vial [PoM] £9.60
  Methylprednisolone (as Methylprednisolone sodium succinate) 1 gram Methylprednisolone sodium succinate 1g powder and solvent for solution for injection vials | 1 vial [PoM] £17.30
- Solu-Medrone (Pfizer Ltd)
  Methylprednisolone (as Methylprednisolone sodium succinate) 40 mg Solu-Medrone 40mg powder and solvent for solution for injection vials | 1 vial [PoM] £1.58

6

Endocrine system

Methylprednisolone (as Methylprednisolone sodium succinate)
125 mg Solu-Medrone 125mg powder and solvent for solution for injection vials | 1 vial [PoM] £4.75

Methylprednisolone (as Methylprednisolone sodium succinate)
500 mg Solu-Medrone 500mg powder and solvent for solution for injection vials | 1 vial [PoM] £9.60

Methylprednisolone (as Methylprednisolone sodium succinate)
1 gram Solu-Medrone 1g powder and solvent for solution for injection vials | 1 vial [PoM] £17.30

Methylprednisolone (as Methylprednisolone sodium succinate)
2 gram Solu-Medrone 2g powder and solvent for solution for injection vials | 1 vial [PoM] £32.86

Tablet
CAUTIONARY AND ADVISORY LABELS 10, 21
▶ Medrone (Pfizer Ltd)
Methylprednisolone 2 mg Medrone 2mg tablets | 30 tablet [PoM] £3.88

Methylprednisolone 4 mg Medrone 4mg tablets | 30 tablet [PoM] £6.19

Methylprednisolone 16 mg Medrone 16mg tablets | 30 tablet [PoM] £17.17

Methylprednisolone 100 mg Medrone 100mg tablets | 20 tablet [PoM] £48.32

Suspension for injection
CAUTIONARY AND ADVISORY LABELS 10
▶ Depo-Medrone (Pfizer Ltd)
Methylprednisolone acetate 40 mg per 1 ml Depo-Medrone 40mg/1ml suspension for injection vials | 1 vial [PoM] £3.44 DT = £3.44 | 10 vial [PoM] £34.04
Depo-Medrone 80mg/2ml suspension for injection vials | 1 vial [PoM] £6.18 DT = £6.18 | 10 vial [PoM] £61.39
Depo-Medrone 120mg/3ml suspension for injection vials | 1 vial [PoM] £8.96 DT = £8.96 | 10 vial [PoM] £88.81

⚑ 658

Prednisolone
21-Dec-2017

● INDICATIONS AND DOSE

Acute exacerbation of chronic obstructive pulmonary disease (if increased breathlessness interferes with daily activities)
▶ BY MOUTH
▸ Adult: 30 mg daily for 7–14 days

Severe croup (before transfer to hospital) | Mild croup that might cause complications (before transfer to hospital)
▶ BY MOUTH
▸ Child: 1–2 mg/kg

Mild to moderate acute asthma (when oral corticosteroid taken for more than a few days) | Severe or life-threatening acute asthma (when oral corticosteroid taken for more than a few days)
▶ BY MOUTH
▸ Child 1 month-11 years: 2 mg/kg once daily (max. per dose 60 mg) for up to 3 days, longer if necessary

Mild to moderate acute asthma | Severe or life-threatening acute asthma
▶ BY MOUTH
▸ Child 1 month-11 years: 1–2 mg/kg once daily (max. per dose 40 mg) for up to 3 days, longer if necessary
▸ Child 12-17 years: 40–50 mg daily for at least 5 days
▸ Adult: 40–50 mg daily for at least 5 days

Suppression of inflammatory and allergic disorders
▶ BY MOUTH
▸ Adult: Initially 10–20 mg daily, dose preferably taken in the morning after breakfast, can often be reduced within a few days but may need to be continued for several weeks or months; maintenance 2.5–15 mg daily, higher doses may be needed; cushingoid side-effects increasingly likely with doses above 7.5 mg daily
▶ BY INTRAMUSCULAR INJECTION
▸ Adult: 25–100 mg 1–2 times a week, as prednisolone acetate

Suppression of inflammatory and allergic disorders (initial dose in severe disease)
▶ BY MOUTH
▸ Adult: Initially up to 60 mg daily, dose preferably taken in the morning after breakfast, can often be reduced within a few days but may need to be continued for several weeks or months

Idiopathic thrombocytopenic purpura
▶ BY MOUTH
▸ Adult: 1 mg/kg daily, gradually reduce dose over several weeks

Ulcerative colitis | Crohn's disease
▶ BY MOUTH
▸ Adult: Initially 20–40 mg daily until remission occurs, followed by reducing doses, up to 60 mg daily, may be used in some cases, doses preferably taken in the morning after breakfast

Neuritic pain or weakness heralding rapid onset of permanent nerve damage (during reversal reactions multibacillary leprosy)
▶ BY MOUTH
▸ Adult: Initially 40–60 mg daily, dose to be instituted at once

Generalised myasthenia gravis (when given on alternate days)
▶ BY MOUTH
▸ Adult: Initially 10 mg once daily on alternate days, then increased in steps of 10 mg once daily on alternate days, increased to 1–1.5 mg/kg once daily on alternate days (max. per dose 100 mg)

Generalised myasthenia gravis in ventilated patients (when given on alternate days)
▶ BY MOUTH
▸ Adult: Initially 1.5 mg/kg once daily on alternate days (max. per dose 100 mg)

Generalised myasthenia gravis (when giving daily)
▶ BY MOUTH
▸ Adult: Initially 5 mg daily, increased in steps of 5 mg daily. maintenance 60–80 mg daily, alternatively maintenance 0.75–1 mg/kg daily, ventilated patients may be started on 1.5 mg/kg (max. 100 mg) on alternate days

Ocular myasthenia
▶ BY MOUTH
▸ Adult: Usual dose 10–40 mg once daily on alternate days, reduce to minimum effective dose

Reduction in rate of joint destruction in moderate to severe rheumatoid arthritis of less than 2 years' duration
▶ BY MOUTH
▸ Adult: 7.5 mg daily

Polymyalgia rheumatica
▶ BY MOUTH
▸ Adult: 10–15 mg daily until remission of disease activity; maintenance 7.5–10 mg daily, reduce gradually to maintenance dose. Many patients require treatment for at least 2 years and in some patients it may be necessary to continue long term low-dose corticosteroid treatment

Giant cell (temporal) arteritis
▶ BY MOUTH
▸ Adult: 40–60 mg daily until remission of disease activity, the higher dose being used if visual symptoms occur; maintenance 7.5–10 mg daily, reduce gradually to maintenance dose. Many patients require treatment for at least 2 years and in some patients it may be necessary to continue long term low-dose corticosteroid treatment

Polyarteritis nodosa | Polymyositis | Systemic lupus erythematosus
▸ BY MOUTH
▸ Adult: Initially 60 mg daily, to be reduced gradually; maintenance 10–15 mg daily

Anorexia (symptom control in palliative care)
▸ BY MOUTH
▸ Adult: 15–30 mg daily

Pneumocystis pneumonia in moderate to severe infections associated with HIV infection
▸ BY MOUTH
▸ Adult: 50–80 mg daily for 5 days, the dose is then reduced to complete 21 days of treatment, corticosteroid treatment should ideally be started at the same time as the anti-pneumocystis therapy and certainly no later than 24–72 hours afterwards. The corticosteroid should be withdrawn before anti-pneumocystis treatment is complete

Short-term prophylaxis of episodic cluster headache as monotherapy or in combination with verapamil during verapamil titration
▸ BY MOUTH
▸ Adult: 60–100 mg once daily for 2–5 days, then reduced in steps of 10 mg every 2–3 days until prednisolone is discontinued

Proctitis
▸ BY RECTUM USING RECTAL FOAM
▸ Adult: 1 metered application 1–2 times a day for 2 weeks, continued for further 2 weeks if good response, to be inserted into the rectum, 1 metered application contains 20 mg prednisolone
▸ BY RECTUM USING SUPPOSITORIES
▸ Adult: 5 mg twice daily, to be inserted in to the rectum morning and night, after a bowel movement

Distal ulcerative colitis
▸ BY RECTUM USING RECTAL FOAM
▸ Adult: 1 metered application 1–2 times a day for 2 weeks, continued for further 2 weeks if good response, to be inserted into the rectum, 1 metered application contains 20 mg prednisolone

Rectal complications of Crohn's disease
▸ BY RECTUM USING SUPPOSITORIES
▸ Adult: 5 mg twice daily, to be inserted in to the rectum morning and night, after a bowel movement

Rectal and rectosigmoidal ulcerative colitis | Rectal and rectosigmoidal Crohn's disease
▸ BY RECTUM USING ENEMA
▸ Adult: 20 mg daily for 2–4 weeks, continued if response good, to be used at bedtime

---

IMPORTANT SAFETY INFORMATION

SAFE PRACTICE
Prednisolone has been confused with propranolol; care must be taken to ensure the correct drug is prescribed and dispensed.

● CONTRA-INDICATIONS
▸ With rectal use Bowel perforation · extensive fistulas · intestinal obstruction · recent intestinal anastomoses
● CAUTIONS
▸ With rectal use Systemic absorption may occur with rectal preparations
▸ With systemic use Duchenne's muscular dystrophy (possible transient rhabdomyolysis and myoglobinuria following strenuous physical activity)
● INTERACTIONS → Appendix 1: corticosteroids

● SIDE-EFFECTS
▸ With intramuscular use Diarrhoea · dizziness · exophthalmos · hiccups · hypotension · Kaposi's sarcoma · malaise vomiting
▸ With oral use Diarrhoea · dizziness · dyslipidaemia · exophthalmos · fatigue · lipomatosis · malaise · protein catabolism
● PREGNANCY As it crosses the placenta 88% of prednisolone is inactivated.
  Monitoring ▸ With systemic use Pregnant women with fluid retention should be monitored closely.
● BREAST FEEDING Prednisolone appears in small amounts in breast milk but maternal doses of up to 40 mg daily are unlikely to cause systemic effects in the infant.
  Monitoring ▸ With systemic use Infant should be monitored for adrenal suppression if mother is taking a dose higher than 40 mg.
● PATIENT AND CARER ADVICE Patient counselling is advised for prednisolone tablets (steroid card).
  Medicines for Children leaflet: Prednisolone for asthma
  www.medicinesforchildren.org.uk/prednisolone-for-asthma

● MEDICINAL FORMS
There can be variation in the licensing of different medicines containing the same drug. Forms available from special-order manufacturers include: oral suspension, oral solution, enema

Foam
▸ Prednisolone (Non-proprietary)
  Prednisolone (as Prednisolone sodium metasulfobenzoate)
  20 mg per 1 application Prednisolone 20mg/application foam enema | 14 dose [PoM] £187.00 DT = £187.00

Gastro-resistant tablet
CAUTIONARY AND ADVISORY LABELS 5, 10, 25
▸ Prednisolone (Non-proprietary)
  Prednisolone 1 mg Prednisolone 1mg gastro-resistant tablets | 30 tablet [PoM] £1.60-£1.92 DT = £1.92
  Prednisolone 2.5 mg Prednisolone 2.5mg gastro-resistant tablets | 28 tablet [PoM] £0.83 DT = £0.74 | 30 tablet [PoM] £0.79-£6.15
  Prednisolone 5 mg Prednisolone 5mg gastro-resistant tablets | 28 tablet [PoM] £0.76 DT = £0.76 | 30 tablet [PoM] £0.81-£6.29
▸ Deltacortril Enteric (Alliance Pharmaceuticals Ltd)
  Prednisolone 2.5 mg Deltacortril 2.5mg gastro-resistant tablets | 30 tablet [PoM] £1.16
  Prednisolone 5 mg Deltacortril 5mg gastro-resistant tablets | 30 tablet [PoM] £1.19
▸ Dilacort (Crescent Pharma Ltd, Teva UK Ltd)
  Prednisolone 2.5 mg Dilacort 2.5mg gastro-resistant tablets | 28 tablet [PoM] £1.14-£1.85 DT = £0.74
  Prednisolone 5 mg Dilacort 5mg gastro-resistant tablets | 28 tablet [PoM] £1.45-£1.85 DT = £0.76

Soluble tablet
CAUTIONARY AND ADVISORY LABELS 10, 13, 21
▸ Prednisolone (Non-proprietary)
  Prednisolone (as Prednisolone sodium phosphate)
  5 mg Prednisolone 5mg soluble tablets | 30 tablet [PoM] £53.48 DT = £21.47

Tablet
CAUTIONARY AND ADVISORY LABELS 10, 21
▸ Prednisolone (Non-proprietary)
  Prednisolone 1 mg Prednisolone 1mg tablets | 28 tablet [PoM] £4.00 DT = £0.37
  Prednisolone 2.5 mg Prednisolone 2.5mg tablets | 28 tablet [PoM] £1.33
  Prednisolone 5 mg Prednisolone 5mg tablets | 28 tablet [PoM] £9.86 DT = £0.47
  Prednisolone 10 mg Prednisolone 10mg tablets | 28 tablet [PoM] £1.77
  Prednisolone 20 mg Prednisolone 20mg tablets | 28 tablet [PoM] £3.55
  Prednisolone 25 mg Prednisolone 25mg tablets | 56 tablet [PoM] £75.00 DT = £75.00
  Prednisolone 30 mg Prednisolone 30mg tablets | 28 tablet [PoM] £8.15
▸ Pevanti (AMCo)
  Prednisolone 2.5 mg Pevanti 2.5mg tablets | 30 tablet [PoM] £1.42 DT = £1.42

6

Endocrine system

Prednisolone 5 mg Pevanti 5mg tablets | 30 tablet [PoM] £0.95
Prednisolone 10 mg Pevanti 10mg tablets | 30 tablet [PoM] £1.90
DT = £1.90
Prednisolone 20 mg Pevanti 20mg tablets | 30 tablet [PoM] £3.80
DT = £3.80
Prednisolone 25 mg Pevanti 25mg tablets | 56 tablet [PoM] £40.00
DT = £75.00

Suppository
▸ Prednisolone (Non-proprietary)
Prednisolone (as Prednisolone sodium phosphate)
5 mg Prednisolone sodium phosphate 5mg suppositories |
10 suppository [PoM] £55.61 DT = £50.98

Suspension for injection
▸ Deltastab (AMCo)
Prednisolone acetate 25 mg per 1 ml Deltastab 25mg/1ml
suspension for injection ampoules | 10 ampoule [PoM] £68.72

Oral solution
CAUTIONARY AND ADVISORY LABELS 10
▸ Prednisolone (Non-proprietary)
Prednisolone 1 mg per 1 ml Prednisolone 5mg/5ml oral solution unit
dose | 10 unit dose [PoM] £11.41 DT = £11.41
Prednisolone 10 mg per 1 ml Prednisolone 10mg/ml oral solution
sugar free sugar-free | 30 ml [PoM] £55.00–£55.50 DT = £55.50

Enema
▸ Predsol (RPH Pharmaceuticals AB)
Prednisolone sodium phosphate 200 microgram per 1 ml Predsol
20mg/100ml retention enema | 7 enema [PoM] £7.50 DT = £7.50

⟶ 658

Prednisone
21-Dec-2017

● **INDICATIONS AND DOSE**
Moderate to severe rheumatoid arthritis
▸ BY MOUTH USING MODIFIED-RELEASE MEDICINES
▸ Adult: 10–20 mg daily, adjusted according to response,
dose to be take at bedtime

● INTERACTIONS → Appendix 1: corticosteroids
● SIDE-EFFECTS Diarrhoea · dyslipidaemia · lipomatosis ·
vomiting
● HEPATIC IMPAIRMENT
Monitoring Monitor patient closely in hepatic impairment.
● PATIENT AND CARER ADVICE Patient counselling is advised
for prednisone tablets (steroid card).

● MEDICINAL FORMS
There can be variation in the licensing of different medicines
containing the same drug.
Modified-release tablet
CAUTIONARY AND ADVISORY LABELS 10, 21, 25
▸ Lodotra (Napp Pharmaceuticals Ltd)
Prednisone 1 mg Lodotra 1mg modified-release tablets |
30 tablet [PoM] £26.70
Prednisone 2 mg Lodotra 2mg modified-release tablets |
30 tablet [PoM] £26.70 | 100 tablet [PoM] £89.00
Prednisone 5 mg Lodotra 5mg modified-release tablets |
30 tablet [PoM] £26.70 | 100 tablet [PoM] £89.00

⟶ 658

Triamcinolone acetonide
21-Dec-2017

● **INDICATIONS AND DOSE**
Suppression of inflammatory and allergic disorders
▸ BY DEEP INTRAMUSCULAR INJECTION
▸ Adult: 40 mg (max. per dose 100 mg), repeated if
necessary, dose given for depot effect, to be
administered into gluteal muscle; repeated at intervals
according to patient's response

● CAUTIONS High dosage (may cause proximal myopathy),
avoid in chronic therapy
● INTERACTIONS → Appendix 1: corticosteroids
● SIDE-EFFECTS
▸ **Uncommon** Dizziness · exophthalmos · fatigue · flushing ·
hyperglycaemia · hypotension

● PATIENT AND CARER ADVICE Patient counselling is advised
for triamcinolone acetonide injection (steroid card).

● MEDICINAL FORMS
There can be variation in the licensing of different medicines
containing the same drug.
Suspension for injection
CAUTIONARY AND ADVISORY LABELS 10
EXCIPIENTS: May contain Benzyl alcohol
▸ Adcortyl Intra-articular / Intradermal (Bristol-Myers Squibb
Pharmaceuticals Ltd)
Triamcinolone acetonide 10 mg per 1 ml Adcortyl Intra-articular /
Intradermal 50mg/5ml suspension for injection vials | 1 vial [PoM]
£3.63
Adcortyl Intra-articular / Intradermal 10mg/1ml suspension for
injection ampoules | 5 ampoule [PoM] £4.47 DT = £4.47
▸ Kenalog (Bristol-Myers Squibb Pharmaceuticals Ltd)
Triamcinolone acetonide 40 mg per 1 ml Kenalog Intra-articular /
Intramuscular 40mg/1ml suspension for injection vials | 5 vial [PoM]
£7.45 DT = £7.45

2.1 Cushing's syndrome and disease

Cushing's Syndrome

Management
Most types of *Cushing's syndrome* are treated surgically, that
which occasionally accompanies carcinoma of the bronchus
is not usually amenable to surgery. Metyrapone p. 667 has
been found helpful in controlling the symptoms of the
disease; it is also used in other forms of Cushing's syndrome
to prepare the patient for surgery.
The dosages of metyrapone used are either low, and
tailored to cortisol production, or high, in which case
corticosteroid replacement therapy is also needed.
Ketoconazole below may have a direct effect on
corticotropic tumour cells in patients with Cushing's disease.
It is used under specialist supervision for treatment of
endogenous Cushing's syndrome.

Other drugs used for Cushing's syndrome and disease
Pasireotide, p. 925

ENZYME INHIBITORS

Ketoconazole
20-Jul-2017

● DRUG ACTION An imidazole derivative which acts as a
potent inhibitor of cortisol and aldosterone synthesis by
inhibiting the activity of 17α-hydroxylase,
11-hydroxylation steps and at higher doses the cholesterol
side-chain cleavage enzyme. It also inhibits the activity of
adrenal C17-20 lyase enzymes resulting in androgen
synthesis inhibition, and may have a direct effect on
corticotropic tumour cells in patients with Cushing's
disease.

● **INDICATIONS AND DOSE**
Endogenous Cushing's syndrome (specialist use only)
▸ BY MOUTH
▸ Adult: Initially 400–600 mg daily in 2–3 divided doses,
increased to 800–1200 mg daily; maintenance
400–800 mg daily in 2–3 divided doses, for dose
titrations in patients with established dose,
adjustments in adrenal insufficiency, or concomitant
corticosteroid replacement therapy, consult product
literature; maximum 1200 mg per day

DOSE ADJUSTMENTS DUE TO INTERACTIONS
▸ Manufacturer advises max. dose 200 mg daily with concurrent use of cobicistat.

> **IMPORTANT SAFETY INFORMATION**
> CHMP ADVICE: KETOCONAZOLE (JULY 2013)
> The CHMP has recommended that the marketing authorisation for oral ketoconazole to treat fungal infections should be suspended. The CHMP concluded that the risk of hepatotoxicity associated with oral ketoconazole is greater than the benefit in treating fungal infections. Doctors should review patients who are being treated with oral ketoconazole for fungal infections, with a view to stopping treatment or choosing an alternative treatment. Patients with a prescription of oral ketoconazole for fungal infections should be referred back to their doctors.
> Oral ketoconazole for Cushing's syndrome and topical products containing ketoconazole are not affected by this advice.

● CONTRA-INDICATIONS Acquired QTc prolongation · Acute porphyrias p. 1025 · avoid concomitant use of hepatotoxic drugs · congenital QTc prolongation
● CAUTIONS Risk of adrenal insufficiency
● INTERACTIONS → Appendix 1: antifungals, azoles
● SIDE-EFFECTS
▸ **Common or very common** Adrenal insufficiency · diarrhoea · gastrointestinal discomfort · nausea · skin reactions · vomiting
▸ **Uncommon** Allergic conditions · alopecia · angioedema · asthenia · dizziness · drowsiness · headache · thrombocytopenia
▸ **Rare or very rare** Fever · hepatic disorders · taste altered
▸ **Frequency not known** Alcohol intolerance · appetite abnormal · arthralgia · azoospermia · dry mouth · epistaxis · flatulence · fontanelle bulging · gynaecomastia · hot flush · insomnia · intracranial pressure increased · malaise · menstrual disorder · myalgia · nervousness · papilloedema · paraesthesia · peripheral oedema · photophobia · photosensitivity reaction · tongue discolouration
SIDE-EFFECTS, FURTHER INFORMATION Potentially life-threatening hepatotoxicity reported rarely with oral use.
● CONCEPTION AND CONTRACEPTION Effective contraception must be used in women of child-bearing potential.
● PREGNANCY Manufacturer advises avoid—teratogenic in *animal* studies.
● BREAST FEEDING Manufacturer advises avoid—present in breast milk.
● HEPATIC IMPAIRMENT Avoid in acute or chronic impairment. Do not initiate treatment if liver enzymes greater than 2 times the normal upper limit.
● MONITORING REQUIREMENTS
▸ Monitor ECG before and one week after initiation, and then as clinically indicated thereafter.
▸ Adrenal insufficiency Monitor adrenal function within one week of initiation, then regularly thereafter. When cortisol levels are normalised or close to target and effective dose established, monitor every 3–6 months as there is a risk of autoimmune disease development or exacerbation after normalisation of cortisol levels. If symptoms suggestive of adrenal insufficiency such as fatigue, anorexia, nausea, vomiting, hypotension, hyponatraemia, hyperkalaemia, and/or hypoglycaemia occur, measure cortisol levels and discontinue treatment temporarily (can be resumed thereafter at lower dose) or reduce dose and if necessary, initiate corticosteroid substitution.
▸ Hepatotoxicity Monitor liver function before initiation of treatment, then weekly for 1 month after initiation, then monthly for 6 months—more frequently if dose adjusted or abnormal liver function detected. Reduce dose if liver enzymes increase less than 3 times the normal upper limit—consult product literature; if liver enzymes are raised to 3 times or greater the normal upper limit, discontinue treatment permanently.
● PATIENT AND CARER ADVICE Patients or their carers should be told how to recognise signs of liver disorder, and advised to discontinue treatment and seek prompt medical attention if symptoms such as anorexia, nausea, vomiting, fatigue, jaundice, abdominal pain, or dark urine develop. Patients or their carers should also be told how to recognise signs of adrenal insufficiency.
Driving and skilled tasks Dizziness and somnolence may affect the performance of skilled tasks (e.g. driving).
● MEDICINAL FORMS
There can be variation in the licensing of different medicines containing the same drug. Forms available from special-order manufacturers include: oral suspension
Tablet
CAUTIONARY AND ADVISORY LABELS 2, 5, 21
▸ Ketoconazole (non-proprietary) ▼
Ketoconazole 200 mg Ketoconazole 200mg tablets |
60 tablet [PoM] £480.00

Metyrapone

● DRUG ACTION Metyrapone is a competitive inhibitor of 11β-hydroxylation in the adrenal cortex; the resulting inhibition of cortisol (and to a lesser extent aldosterone) production leads to an increase in ACTH production which, in turn, leads to increased synthesis and release of cortisol precursors. Metyrapone may be used as a test of anterior pituitary function.

● INDICATIONS AND DOSE
Differential diagnosis of ACTH-dependent Cushing's syndrome (specialist supervision in hospital)
▸ BY MOUTH
▸ Adult: 750 mg every 4 hours for 6 doses
Management of Cushing's syndrome (specialist supervision in hospital)
▸ BY MOUTH
▸ Adult: Usual dose 0.25–6 g daily, dose to be tailored to cortisol production, dose is either low, and tailored to cortisol production, or high, in which case corticosteroid replacement therapy is also needed
Resistant oedema due to increased aldosterone secretion in cirrhosis, nephrotic syndrome, and congestive heart failure (with glucocorticoid replacement therapy) (specialist supervision in hospital)
▸ BY MOUTH
▸ Adult: 3 g daily in divided doses

● CONTRA-INDICATIONS Adrenocortical insufficiency
● CAUTIONS Avoid in Acute porphyrias p. 1025 · gross hypopituitarism (risk of precipitating acute adrenal failure) · hypertension on long-term administration · hypothyroidism (delayed response)
● INTERACTIONS → Appendix 1: metyrapone
● SIDE-EFFECTS
▸ **Common or very common** Dizziness · headache · hypotension · nausea · sedation · vomiting
▸ **Rare or very rare** Abdominal pain · adrenal insufficiency · allergic dermatitis · hirsutism
▸ **Frequency not known** Alopecia · bone marrow failure · hypertension
● PREGNANCY Avoid (may impair biosynthesis of fetal-placental steroids).
● BREAST FEEDING Avoid—no information available.

6

Endocrine system

- HEPATIC IMPAIRMENT Use with caution in hepatic impairment (delayed response).
- PATIENT AND CARER ADVICE
  Driving and skilled tasks Drowsiness may affect the performance of skilled tasks (e.g. driving).

- MEDICINAL FORMS
  There can be variation in the licensing of different medicines containing the same drug.
  Capsule
  CAUTIONARY AND ADVISORY LABELS 21
  ▸ Metopirone (HRA Pharma UK Ltd)
  Metyrapone 250 mg Metopirone 250mg capsules |
  100 capsule [PoM] £363.66

---

3 Diabetes mellitus and hypoglycaemia

3.1 Diabetes mellitus

Diabetes

05-Jun-2017

Description of condition

Diabetes mellitus is a group of metabolic disorders in which persistent hyperglycaemia is caused by deficient insulin secretion or by resistance to the action of insulin. This leads to the abnormalities of carbohydrate, fat and protein metabolism that are characteristic of diabetes mellitus.

Type 1 diabetes mellitus p. 669 and Type 2 diabetes mellitus p. 671 are the two most common classifications of diabetes. Other common types of diabetes are gestational diabetes (develops during pregnancy and resolves after delivery) and secondary diabetes (may be caused by pancreatic damage, hepatic cirrhosis, or endocrine disease). Treatment with endocrine, antiviral, or antipsychotic drugs may also cause secondary diabetes.

Driving

Drivers with diabetes may be required to notify the Driver and Vehicle Licensing Agency (DVLA) of their condition depending on their treatment, the type of licence they hold, and whether they have diabetic complications (including episodes of hypoglycaemia). All drivers who are treated with insulin must inform the DVLA, with some exceptions for temporary treatment. Detailed guidance on notification requirements, eligibility to drive, and precautions required, is available from the DVLA at www.gov.uk/guidance/diabetes-mellitus-assessing-fitness-to-drive.

Advice from the DVLA

The DVLA recommends (2016) that drivers with diabetes need to be particularly careful to avoid hypoglycaemia and should be informed of the warning signs and actions to take. Drivers treated with insulin should always carry a glucose meter and blood-glucose strips when driving, and check their blood-glucose concentration no more than 2 hours before driving and every 2 hours while driving. More frequent self-monitoring may be required if, for any reason, there is a greater risk of hypoglycaemia, such as after physical activity or altered meal routine.

Blood-glucose should always be above 5 mmol/litre while driving. If blood-glucose falls to 5 mmol/litre or below, a snack should be taken. Drivers treated with insulin should ensure that a supply of fast-acting carbohydrate is always available in the vehicle. If blood-glucose is less than 4 mmol/Litre, or warning signs of hypoglycaemia develop, the driver should not drive. If already driving, the driver should:

- stop the vehicle in a safe place;

- switch off the engine, remove keys from the ignition, and move from the driver's seat;
- eat or drink a suitable source of sugar;
- wait until 45 minutes after blood-glucose has returned to normal, before continuing journey.

Drivers must not drive if hypoglycaemia awareness has been lost and the DVLA must be notified; driving may resume if a medical report confirms that awareness has been regained.

Depending on the type of licence, notification and monitoring may also be necessary for drivers taking oral antidiabetic drugs, particularly those which carry a risk of hypoglycaemia (e.g. sulfonylureas, nateglinide p. 686, repaglinide p. 687).

Note: additional criteria apply for drivers of large goods or passenger carrying vehicles—consult DVLA guidance.

Alcohol

Alcohol can make the signs of hypoglycaemia less clear, and can cause delayed hypoglycaemia; specialist sources recommend that patients with diabetes should drink alcohol only in moderation, and when accompanied by food.

Oral glucose tolerance tests

The oral glucose tolerance test is used mainly for diagnosis of impaired glucose tolerance; it is **not** recommended or necessary for routine diagnostic use when severe symptoms of hyperglycaemia are present. In patients who have less severe symptoms and a blood-glucose concentration that does not establish or exclude diabetes (e.g. impaired fasting glycaemia), an oral glucose tolerance test may be required. It is also used to establish the presence of gestational diabetes.

An oral glucose tolerance test involves measuring the blood-glucose concentration after fasting, and then 2 hours after drinking a standard anhydrous glucose drink. Anhydrous glucose may alternatively be given as the appropriate amount of *Polycal®* or as *Rapilose®* OGTT oral solution.

HbA1c measurement

Glycated haemoglobin (HbA1c) forms when red blood cells are exposed to glucose in the plasma. The HbA1c test reflects average plasma glucose over the previous 2 to 3 months and provides a good indicator of glycaemic control. Unlike the oral glucose tolerance test, an HbA1c test can be performed at any time of the day and does not require any special preparation such as fasting.

HbA1c values are expressed in *mmol of glycated haemoglobin per mol of haemoglobin (mmol/mol)*, a standardised unit specific for HbA1c created by the International Federation of Clinical Chemistry and Laboratory Medicine (IFCC). HbA1c values were previously aligned to the assay used in the Diabetes Control and Complications Trial (DCCT) and expressed as a percentage.

Equivalent values	
IFCC-HbA1c (mmol/mol)	DCCT-HbA1c (%)
42	6.0
48	6.5
53	7.0
59	7.5
64	8.0
69	8.5
75	9.0

Diagnosis

The HbA1c test is used for monitoring glycaemic control in both Type 1 diabetes p. 669 and Type 2 diabetes p. 671 and is now also used for diagnosis of type 2 diabetes. [EvGr] HbA1c should not be used for diagnosis in those with suspected type 1 diabetes, in children, during pregnancy, or in women who are up to two months postpartum. It should also not be used for patients who have:

- had symptoms of diabetes for less than 2 months;
- a high diabetes risk and are acutely ill;
- treatment with medication that may cause hyperglycaemia;
- Acute pancreatic damage;
- end-stage chronic kidney disease;
- HIV infection.

HbA1c used for diagnosis of diabetes should be interpreted with caution in patients with abnormal haemoglobin, anaemia, altered red cell lifespan, or who have had a recent blood transfusion. Ⓐ

Monitoring

ⒺⓋⒼⓇ HbA1c is also a reliable predictor of microvascular and macrovascular complications and mortality. Lower HbA1c is associated with a lower risk of long term vascular complications and patients should aim for an individualised HbA1c target (see Type 1 diabetes below and Type 2 diabetes p. 671).

HbA1c should usually be measured in patients with type 1 diabetes every 3 to 6 months, and more frequently if blood-glucose control is thought to be changing rapidly. Patients with type 2 diabetes should be monitored every 3 to 6 months until HbA1c and medication are stable when monitoring can be reduced to every 6 months. Ⓐ

HbA1c monitoring is invalid for patients with disturbed erythrocyte turnover or for patients with a lack of, or abnormal haemoglobin. In these cases, quality-controlled plasma glucose profiles, total glycated haemoglobin estimation (if there is abnormal haemoglobin), or fructosamine estimation can be used.

Laboratory measurement of fructosamine concentration measures the glycated fraction of all plasma proteins over the previous 14 to 21 days but is a less accurate measure of glycaemic control than HbA1c.

Type 1 diabetes

05-Jun-2017

Description of condition

Type 1 diabetes describes an absolute insulin deficiency in which there is little or no endogenous insulin secretory capacity due to destruction of insulin-producing beta-cells in the pancreatic islets of Langerhans. This form of the disease has an auto-immune basis in most cases, and it can occur at any age, but most commonly before adulthood.

Loss of insulin secretion results in hyperglycaemia and other metabolic abnormalities. If poorly managed, the resulting tissue damage has both short-term and long-term adverse effects on health; this can result in retinopathy, nephropathy, neuropathy, premature cardiovascular disease, and peripheral arterial disease.

Typical features in adult patients presenting with type 1 diabetes are hyperglycaemia (random plasma-glucose concentration above 11 mmol/litre), ketosis, rapid weight loss, a body mass index below 25 kg/m^2, age younger than 50 years, and a personal/family history of autoimmune disease (though not all features may be present).

Aims of treatment

Treatment is aimed at using insulin regimens to achieve as optimal a level of blood-glucose control as is feasible, while avoiding or reducing the frequency of hypoglycaemic episodes, in order to minimise the risk of long-term microvascular and macrovascular complications.

Disability from complications can often be prevented by early detection and active management of the disease (see Diabetic complications p. 674). ⒺⓋⒼⓇ The target for glycaemic control should be individualised for each patient,

considering factors such as daily activities, aspirations, likelihood of complications, adherence to treatment, comorbidities, occupation and history of hypoglycaemia.

A target HbA1c concentration of 48 mmol/mol (6.5 %) or lower is recommended in patients with type 1 diabetes. Blood-glucose concentration should be monitored at least four times a day, including before each meal and before bed. Ⓐ Patients should aim for:

- ⒺⓋⒼⓇ a fasting blood-glucose concentration of 5–7 mmol/litre on waking;
- a blood-glucose concentration of 4–7 mmol/litre before meals at other times of the day;
- a blood-glucose concentration of 5–9 mmol/litre at least 90 minutes after eating;
- a blood-glucose concentration of at least 5 mmol/litre when driving. Ⓐ

Overview

ⒺⓋⒼⓇ Type 1 diabetes requires insulin replacement, supported by active management of other cardiovascular risk factors, such as hypertension and high circulating lipids (see Diabetic complications p. 674). Ⓐ Insulin replacement therapy aims to recreate normal fluctuations in circulating insulin concentrations while supporting a flexible lifestyle with minimal restrictions. Flexible insulin therapy usually involves self-injecting multiple daily doses of insulin, with doses adjusted according to planned exercise, intended food intake and other factors, including current blood-glucose, which the patient needs to test on a regular basis.

ⒺⓋⒼⓇ Patients who have a BMI of 25 kg/m^2 or above (23 kg/m^2 or above for patients of South Asian or related ethnicity) who wish to improve their blood-glucose control while minimising their effective insulin dose, may benefit from metformin hydrochloride p. 678 [unlicensed indication] as an addition to insulin therapy.

Dietary control is important in both type 1 and type 2 diabetes and patients should receive advice from a dietitian. Dietary advice should include information on weight control, cardiovascular risk, hyperglycaemic effects of different foods and appropriate changes in insulin doses according to food intake. Healthy eating can reduce cardiovascular risk and dietary modifications may be recommended to account for various associated features of diabetes such as excess weight and obesity, low body-weight, eating disorders, hypertension and renal failure. Patients with type 1 diabetes should be offered carbohydrate-counting training as part of a structured education programme. Ⓐ

Management of type 1 diabetes with insulin

ⒺⓋⒼⓇ All patients with type 1 diabetes require insulin therapy (see also Insulin p. 670). Treatment should be initiated and managed by clinicians with relevant expertise; there are several different types of regimens. Ⓐ

Multiple daily injection basal-bolus insulin regimens

One or more separate daily injections of intermediate-acting insulin or long-acting insulin analogue as the basal insulin; alongside multiple bolus injections of short-acting insulin before meals. This regimen offers flexibility to tailor insulin therapy with the carbohydrate load of each meal.

Mixed (biphasic) regimen

One, two, or three insulin injections per day of short-acting insulin mixed with intermediate-acting insulin. The insulin preparations may be mixed by the patient at the time of injection, or a premixed product can be used.

Continuous subcutaneous insulin infusion (insulin pump)

A regular or continuous amount of insulin (usually in the form of a rapid-acting insulin analogue or soluble insulin), delivered by a programmable pump and insulin storage reservoir via a subcutaneous needle or cannula.

6

Endocrine system

Recommended insulin regimens

EvGr Patients with type 1 diabetes should be offered multiple daily injection basal-bolus insulin regimens as the **first-line choice**. Twice-daily insulin detemir p. 701 should be offered as the long-acting basal insulin therapy. Once-daily insulin glargine p. 701 may be prescribed if insulin detemir is not tolerated, or if a twice-daily regimen is not acceptable to the patient. Insulin detemir may also be offered as an alternative once-daily regimen.

Patients who are using alternative basal regimens may continue if agreed targets are being achieved; other basal insulin regimens should be considered only if the recommended regimens do not deliver agreed targets. Non-basal-bolus insulin regimens (e.g. twice-daily mixed [biphasic], basal-only, or bolus-only regimens) are **not** recommended for adults with *newly diagnosed* type 1 diabetes.

A rapid-acting insulin analogue is recommended as the bolus or mealtime insulin replacement, rather than soluble human insulin or animal insulin (rarely used). The rapid-acting insulin analogue should be injected before meals—routine use after meals should be discouraged. Patients who have a strong preference for an alternative mealtime insulin should be offered their preferred insulin.

Alternatively, if a multiple daily injection basal–bolus regimen is not possible, a twice-daily mixed insulin regimen should be considered if it is preferred.

In patients who are using a twice-daily *human* insulin mixed regimen and have hypoglycaemia that affects their quality of life, a trial of a twice-daily analogue mixed insulin regimen should be considered.

Continuous subcutaneous insulin infusion (insulin pump) therapy, should only be offered to adults who suffer disabling hypoglycaemia, or, who have high HbA1c concentrations (69 mmol/mol [8.5 %] or above) with multiple daily injection therapy (including, if appropriate, the use of long-acting insulin analogues) despite a high level of care. Insulin pump therapy should be initiated by a specialist team. A

Insulin requirements

EvGr The dosage of insulin must be determined individually for each patient and should be adjusted as necessary according to the results of regular monitoring of blood-glucose concentrations.

Persistent poor glucose control, leading to erratic insulin requirements or episodes of hypoglycaemia, may be due to many factors, including adherence, injection technique, injection site problems, blood-glucose monitoring skills, lifestyle issues (including diet, exercise and alcohol intake), psychological issues, and organic causes such as renal disease, thyroid disorders, coeliac disease, Addison's disease or gastroparesis. A

Infection, stress, accidental or surgical trauma can all increase the required insulin dose. Insulin requirements may be decreased (and therefore susceptibility to hypoglycaemia increased) by physical activity, intercurrent illness, reduced food intake, impaired renal function, and in certain endocrine disorders.

Risks of hypoglycaemia with insulin

EvGr Hypoglycaemia is an inevitable adverse effect of insulin treatment, and patients should be advised of the warning signs and actions to take (for guidance on management, see Hypoglycaemia p. 707).

Impaired awareness of hypoglycaemia can occur when the ability to recognise usual symptoms is lost, or when the symptoms are blunted or no longer present. Patients' awareness of hypoglycaemia should be assessed annually using the Gold score or the Clarke score. A

An increase in the frequency of hypoglycaemic episodes may reduce the warning symptoms experienced by the patient. Impaired awareness of symptoms below 3 mmol/litre is associated with a significantly increased risk of severe

hypoglycaemia. Beta-blockers can also blunt hypoglycaemic awareness, by reducing warning signs such as tremor.

Loss of warning of hypoglycaemia among insulin-treated patients can be a serious hazard, especially for drivers and those in dangerous occupations. Advice should be given in line with the Driver and Vehicle Licensing Agency (DVLA) guidance (see *Driving* under Diabetes p. 668).

EvGr To restore the warning signs, episodes of hypoglycaemia must be minimised. Insulin regimens, doses and blood-glucose targets should be reviewed and continuous subcutaneous insulin infusion therapy and real-time continuous blood-glucose monitoring should be considered. Patients should receive structured education to ensure they are following the principles of a flexible insulin regimen correctly, with additional education regarding avoiding and treating hypoglycaemia for those who continue to have impaired awareness. Relaxation of individualised blood-glucose targets should be avoided as a strategy to improve impaired awareness of symptoms. If recurrent severe episodes of hypoglycaemia continue despite appropriate interventions, the patient should be referred to a specialist centre. A

There is conflicting evidence regarding reports that some patients may experience loss of awareness of hypoglycaemia after transfer from animal to human insulin; clinical studies do not confirm that human insulin decreases hypoglycaemia awareness.

Manufacturers advise any switch between brands or formulation of insulin (including switching from animal to human insulin) should be done under strict supervision; a change in dose may be required.

Hypodermic equipment

EvGr Patients should be advised on the safe disposal of lancets, single-use syringes, and needles, and should be provided with suitable disposal containers. Arrangements should be made for the suitable disposal of these containers. A

Lancets, needles, syringes, and accessories are listed under Hypodermic Equipment in Part IXA of the Drug Tariff (Part III of the Northern Ireland Drug Tariff, Part 3 of the Scottish Drug Tariff). The drug Tariffs can be access online at:

- National Health Service Drug Tariff for England and Wales:
  www.nhsbsa.nhs.uk/pharmacies-gp-practices-and-appliance-contractors/drug-tariff

- Health and Personal Social Services for Northern Ireland Drug Tariff:
  www.hscbusiness.hscni.net/services/2034.htm

- Scottish Drug Tariff:
  www.isdscotland.org/Health-Topics/Prescribing-and-Medicines/Scottish-Drug-Tariff

Useful Resources

Type 1 diabetes in adults: diagnosis and management. National Institute for Health and Care Excellence. Clinical guideline NG17. August 2015.
www.nice.org.uk/guidance/ng17

Insulin

05-Jun-2017

Overview

For recommended insulin regimens see Type 1 diabetes p. 669 and Type 2 diabetes p. 671.

Insulin is a polypeptide hormone secreted by pancreatic beta-cells. Insulin increases glucose uptake by adipose tissue and muscles, and suppresses hepatic glucose release. The role of insulin is to lower blood-glucose concentrations in order to prevent hyperglycaemia and its associated microvascular, macrovascular and metabolic complications.

The natural profile of insulin secretion in the body consists of basal insulin (a low and steady secretion of background insulin that controls the glucose continuously released from the liver) and meal-time bolus insulin (secreted in response to glucose absorbed from food and drink).

Sources of insulin

Three types of insulin are available in the UK: human insulin, human insulin analogues, and animal insulin. Animal insulins are extracted and purified from animal sources (bovine or porcine insulin). Although widely used in the past, animal insulins are no longer initiated in people with diabetes but may still be used by some adult patients who cannot, or do not wish to, change to human insulins.

Human insulins are produced by recombinant DNA technology and have the same amino acid sequence as endogenous human insulin. Human insulin analogues are produced in the same way as human insulins, but the insulin is modified to produce a desired kinetic characteristic, such as an extended duration of action or faster absorption and onset of action.

Immunological resistance to insulin is uncommon and true insulin allergy is rare. Human insulin and insulin analogues are less immunogenic than animal insulins.

Administration of insulin

Insulin is inactivated by gastro-intestinal enzymes and must therefore be given by injection; the subcutaneous route is ideal in most circumstances. Insulin should be injected into a body area with plenty of subcutaneous fat—usually the abdomen (fastest absorption rate) or outer thighs/buttocks (slower absorption compared with the abdomen or inner thighs).

Absorption from a limb site can vary considerably (by as much as 20–40%) day-to-day, particularly in children. Local tissue reactions, changes in insulin sensitivity, injection site, blood flow, depth of injection, and the amount of insulin injected can all affect the rate of absorption. Increased blood flow around the injection site due to exercise can also increase insulin absorption.

EvGr Lipohypertrophy can occur due to repeatedly injecting into the same small area, and can cause erratic absorption of insulin, and contribute to poor glycaemic control. Patients should be advised not to use affected areas for further injection until the skin has recovered. Lipohypertrophy can be minimised by using different injection sites in rotation. Injection sites should be checked for signs of infection, swelling, bruising, and lipohypertrophy before administration. ◁A▷

Insulin preparations

Insulin preparations can be broadly categorised into three groups based on their time-action profiles: short-acting insulins (including soluble insulin and rapid-acting insulins), intermediate-acting insulins and long-acting insulins. The duration of action of each particular type of insulin varies considerably from one patient to another, and needs to be assessed individually.

Short-acting insulins

Short-acting insulins have a short duration and a relatively rapid onset of action, to replicate the insulin normally produced by the body in response to glucose absorbed from a meal. These are available as soluble insulin p. 670 (human and, bovine or porcine—both rarely used), and the rapid-acting insulin analogues (insulin aspart p. 696, insulin glulisine p. 697 and insulin lispro p. 698).

Soluble insulin
Soluble insulin is usually given subcutaneously but some preparations can be given intravenously and intramuscularly. For maintenance regimens, it is usual to inject the insulin 15 to 30 minutes before meals, depending on the insulin preparation used.

When injected subcutaneously, soluble insulin has a rapid onset of action (30 to 60 minutes), a peak action between 1 and 4 hours, and a duration of action of up to 9 hours.

When injected intravenously, soluble insulin has a short half-life of only a few minutes and its onset of action is instantaneous.

Soluble insulin administered intravenously is the most appropriate form of insulin for use in diabetic emergencies e.g. Diabetic ketoacidosis p. 674 and peri-operatively.

Rapid-acting insulin
Insulin aspart, insulin glulisine, and insulin lispro have a faster onset of action (within 15 minutes) and shorter duration of action (approximately 2–5 hours) than soluble insulin, and are usually given by subcutaneous injection.

EvGr For maintenance regimens, these insulins should ideally be injected immediately before meals. Rapid-acting insulin, administered before meals, has an advantage over short-acting soluble insulin in terms of improved glucose control, reduction of HbA1c, and reduction in the incidence of severe hypoglycaemia, including nocturnal hypoglycaemia.

The routine use of *post-meal* injections of rapid-acting insulin should be avoided—when given during or after meals, they are associated with poorer glucose control, an increased risk of high postprandial-glucose concentration, and subsequent hypoglycaemia. ◁A▷

Intermediate-acting insulin

Intermediate-acting insulins (isophane insulin p. 699) have an intermediate duration of action, designed to mimic the effect of endogenous basal insulin. When given by subcutaneous injection, they have an onset of action of approximately 1–2 hours, a maximal effect at 3–12 hours, and a duration of action of 11–24 hours.

Isophane insulin is a suspension of insulin with protamine; it may be given as one or more daily injections alongside separate meal-time short-acting insulin injections, or mixed with a short-acting (soluble or rapid-acting) insulin in the same syringe—for recommended insulin regimens see Type 1 diabetes p. 669 and Type 2 diabetes below. Isophane insulin may be mixed with a short-acting insulin by the patient, or a pre-mixed biphasic insulin can be supplied (biphasic isophane insulin p. 698, biphasic insulin aspart p. 699 and biphasic insulin lispro p. 700).

Biphasic insulins (biphasic isophane insulin, biphasic insulin aspart, biphasic insulin lispro) are pre-mixed insulin preparations containing various combinations of short-acting insulin (soluble insulin or rapid-acting analogue insulin) and an intermediate-acting insulin.

The percentage of short-acting insulin varies from 15% to 50%. These preparations should be administered by subcutaneous injection immediately before a meal.

Long-acting insulin

Like intermediate-acting insulins, the long-acting insulins (protamine zinc insulin p. 702, insulin zinc suspension p. 701, insulin detemir p. 701, insulin glargine p. 701, insulin degludec p. 700) mimic endogenous basal insulin secretion, but their duration of action may last up to 36 hours. They achieve a steady-state level after 2–4 days to produce a constant level of insulin.

Insulin glargine and insulin degludec are given once daily and insulin detemir is given once or twice daily according to individual requirements. The older long-acting insulins, (insulin zinc suspension and protamine zinc insulin) are now rarely prescribed.

Type 2 diabetes   05-Jun-2017

Description of condition

Type 2 diabetes is a chronic metabolic condition characterised by insulin resistance. Insufficient pancreatic insulin production also occurs progressively over time, resulting in hyperglycaemia.

It is commonly associated with obesity, physical inactivity, raised blood pressure, dyslipidaemia and a tendency to develop thrombosis; therefore it increases cardiovascular risk. It is associated with long-term microvascular and macrovascular complications, together with reduced quality of life and life expectancy.

Type 2 diabetes typically develops later in life but is increasingly diagnosed in children, despite previously being considered a disease of adulthood.

Aims of treatment

Treatment is aimed at minimising the risk of long-term microvascular and macrovascular complications by effective blood-glucose control and maintenance of HbA1c at or below the target value set for each individual patient.

Overview

EvGr Weight loss, smoking cessation and regular exercise can help to reduce hyperglycaemia and reduce cardiovascular risk, and should be encouraged (with input from a dietitian where appropriate). Antidiabetic drugs should be prescribed to augment lifestyle interventions, when these changes are not adequate to control blood-glucose alone. A

Antidiabetic drugs

There are several classes of non-insulin antidiabetic drugs available for the treatment of type 2 diabetes. EvGr The choice of drug should be based on effectiveness, safety, tolerability and should also take into consideration the patient's comorbidities and concomitant medication. For recommended treatment regimens and the place in therapy of each drug, see *Drug treatment, antidiabetic drugs* (below).
A

Metformin hydrochloride p. 678 has an anti-hyperglycaemic effect, lowering both basal and postprandial blood-glucose concentrations. It does not stimulate insulin secretion and therefore, when given alone, does not cause hypoglycaemia. EvGr The dose of standard-release metformin hydrochloride should be increased gradually to minimise the risk of gastro-intestinal side effects. Modified-release metformin hydrochloride should be offered if standard treatment is not tolerated. A

The **sulfonylureas** (glibenclamide p. 692, gliclazide p. 692, glimepiride p. 693, glipizide p. 693, tolbutamide p. 693) may cause hypoglycaemia; it is more likely with long-acting sulfonylureas such as glibenclamide, which have been associated with severe, prolonged and sometimes fatal cases of hypoglycaemia. Sulfonylureas are also associated with modest weight gain, probably due to increased plasma-insulin concentrations.

Acarbose p. 677 has a poorer anti-hyperglycaemic effect than many other antidiabetic drugs, including the sulfonylureas, metformin hydrochloride, and pioglitazone p. 694.

The meglitinides, nateglinide p. 686 and repaglinide p. 687, have a rapid onset of action and short duration of activity. These drugs can be used flexibly around mealtimes and adjusted to fit around individual eating habits which may be beneficial for some patients, but generally are a less preferred option than the sulfonylureas.

The thiazolidinedione, pioglitazone, is associated with several long-term risks and its ongoing benefit to the patient should be reviewed regularly and treatment stopped if response is insufficient (see *Important safety information* under pioglitazone).

The dipeptidylpeptidase-4 inhibitors (gliptins), alogliptin p. 679, linagliptin p. 680, sitagliptin p. 681, saxagliptin p. 680, and vildagliptin p. 682, do not appear to be associated

with weight gain and have less incidence of hypoglycaemia than the sulfonylureas.

The sodium glucose co-transporter 2 inhibitors, canagliflozin p. 687, dapagliflozin p. 689, and empagliflozin p. 690, may be suitable for some patients when first-line options are not appropriate; they are associated with a risk of diabetic ketoacidosis.

The glucagon-like peptide-1 receptor agonists, albiglutide p. 683, dulaglutide p. 683, exenatide p. 684, liraglutide p. 685 and lixisenatide p. 686, should be reserved for combination therapy when other treatment options have failed.

Polycystic ovary syndrome

EvGr Metformin hydrochloride (initiated by a specialist) is prescribed as an insulin sensitising drug in women with polycystic ovary syndrome who are not planning pregnancy [unlicensed indication] A. Long-term benefit or superiority over other treatment options has not been confirmed by good quality evidence. Metformin hydrochloride may improve short-term insulin sensitivity and reduce androgen concentrations, but there is insufficient supporting evidence that metformin improves weight gain, hirsutism, acne or regulation of the menstrual cycle. Treatment should only be initiated by a specialist. Metformin hydrochloride does not exert a hypoglycaemic action in non-diabetic patients except in overdose.

Drug treatment, antidiabetic drugs

EvGr Type 2 diabetes should initially be treated with a single oral antidiabetic drug. A target HbA1c concentration of 48 mmol/mol (6.5 %) is generally recommended when type 2 diabetes is managed by diet and lifestyle alone or when combined with a single antidiabetic drug not associated with hypoglycaemia (such as metformin hydrochloride). Adults prescribed a single drug associated with hypoglycaemia (such as a sulphonylurea), or two or more antidiabetic drugs in combination, should usually aim for an HbA1c concentration of 53 mmol/mol (7.0 %). Targets may differ and should be individualised and agreed with each patient.

Note: Consider relaxing the target HbA1c level on a case-by-case basis, with particular consideration for people who are older, frail, or where tight blood-glucose control is not appropriate or poses a high risk of the consequences of hypoglycaemia.

If HbA1c concentrations are poorly controlled despite treatment with a single drug (usually considered to be a rise of HbA1c to 58 mmol/mol (7.5 %) or higher), the drug treatment should be intensified, alongside reinforcement of advice regarding diet, lifestyle, and adherence to drug treatment.

When two or more antidiabetic drugs are prescribed, an HbA1c concentration target of 53 mmol/mol (7.0 %) is recommended for patients in which it is appropriate, but a relaxation of the target may be more appropriate in some individual cases (for example, those at high risk of the consequences of hypoglycaemia, poor life expectancy, or significant comorbidities). A

Initial treatment

EvGr Metformin hydrochloride is recommended as the first choice for initial treatment for all patients, due to its positive effect on weight loss, reduced risk of hypoglycaemic events and the additional long-term cardiovascular benefits associated with its use. A

If metformin is contra-indicated or not tolerated, see *Alternative non-metformin regimens* below.

First intensification of treatment

EvGr If metformin hydrochloride (alongside modification to diet) does not control HbA1c to below the agreed threshold, treatment should be intensified, and metformin hydrochloride combined with one of the following:

- a sulfonylurea (glibenclamide, gliclazide, glimepiride, glipizide, tolbutamide) ;

- Pioglitazone;
- a dipeptidylpeptidase-4 inhibitor (linagliptin, saxagliptin, sitagliptin, or vildagliptin);
- a sodium glucose co-transporter 2 inhibitor (canagliflozin, dapagliflozin or empagliflozin) only when sulfonylureas are contra-indicated or not tolerated, or if the patient is at significant risk of hypoglycaemia or its consequences. Ⓐ

ᴱᵛᴳʳ Elderly patients or those with renal impairment are at particular risk of hypoglycaemia; if a sulfonylurea is indicated, a shorter-acting sulfonylurea, such as gliclazide or tolbutamide should be prescribed. Ⓔ

The place in therapy of alogliptin (a dipeptidylpeptidase-4 inhibitor) is not yet known.

Second intensification of treatment

ᴱᵛᴳʳ If dual therapy is unsuccessful, treatment should be intensified again, and one of the following triple therapy regimens prescribed:

- Metformin hydrochloride p. 678 and a dipeptidylpeptidase-4 inhibitor and a sulfonylurea;
- Metformin hydrochloride and pioglitazone p. 694 and a sulfonylurea;
- Metformin hydrochloride and a sulfonylurea and one of the sodium glucose co-transporter 2 inhibitors;
- Metformin hydrochloride and pioglitazone and a sodium glucose co-transporter 2 inhibitor (canagliflozin p. 687 or empagliflozin p. 690; note that dapagliflozin is not recommended in a triple therapy regimen with pioglitazone).

Alternatively, it may be appropriate to start **insulin**-based treatment at this stage—see *Drug treatment, insulin.* Ⓐ

Glucagon-like peptide-1 receptor agonists

ᴱᵛᴳʳ If triple therapy with metformin hydrochloride and two other oral drugs is tried and is not effective, not tolerated or contra-indicated, a **glucagon-like peptide-1 receptor agonist** (exenatide p. 684, liraglutide p. 685 or lixisenatide p. 686) may be prescribed as part of a triple combination regimen with metformin hydrochloride and a sulfonylurea.

These should only be prescribed for patients who have a BMI of 35 kg/m² *or above* (adjusted for ethnicity) **and** who also have specific psychological or medical problems associated with obesity; **or** for those who have a BMI *lower* than 35 kg/m² but for whom insulin therapy would have significant occupational implications **or** if the weight loss associated with glucagon-like peptide-1 receptor agonists would benefit other significant obesity-related comorbidities.

After 6 months, the drug should be reviewed and only continued if there has been a beneficial metabolic response (a reduction of at least 11 mmol/mol [1.0 %] in HbA1c and a weight loss of at least 3 % of initial body-weight). Ⓐ

The place in therapy of the newer glucagon-like peptide-1 receptor agonists, albiglutide p. 683 and dulaglutide p. 683, is not yet known.

ᴱᵛᴳʳ Insulin should only be prescribed in combination with a glucagon-like peptide-1 receptor agonist under specialist care advice and with ongoing support from a consultant-led multidisciplinary team. Ⓐ

Alternative non-metformin regimens

ᴱᵛᴳʳ If metformin is contra-indicated or not tolerated, initial treatment should be single therapy with:

- a dipeptidyl peptidase-4 inhibitor (linagliptin p. 680, saxagliptin p. 680, sitagliptin p. 681, or vildagliptin p. 682), or
- Pioglitazone, or
- a sulfonylurea (glibenclamide p. 692, gliclazide p. 692, glimepiride p. 693, glipizide p. 693, or tolbutamide p. 693). Ⓐ

The **sodium glucose co-transporter 2 inhibitors** canagliflozin, dapagliflozin p. 689, or empagliflozin are also

options for **monotherapy** when metformin is contra-indicated or not tolerated, only if a dipeptidylpeptidase-4 inhibitor would otherwise be prescribed and neither a sulfonylurea nor pioglitazone is appropriate.

ᴱᵛᴳʳ Repaglinide p. 687 is also an effective alternative option for single therapy, but it has a limited role in treatment because, should an intensification of treatment be required, it is not licensed to be used in any combination other than with metformin hydrochloride; it would therefore require a complete change of treatment in those patients who have started it due to intolerance or contra-indication to metformin. Ⓐ

Intensification

ᴱᵛᴳʳ If the initial single drug does not control HbA1c to below the agreed threshold, treatment should be intensified and one of the following dual combinations prescribed:

- a dipeptidylpeptidase-4 inhibitor and pioglitazone;
- a dipeptidylpeptidase-4 inhibitor and a sulfonylurea; or
- pioglitazone and a sulfonylurea .

If dual therapy does not provide adequate glucose control, insulin-based treatment should be considered—see *Drug treatment, insulin.* Ⓐ

Drug treatment, insulin

ᴱᵛᴳʳ When indicated for intensification, insulin (see also, Insulin p. 670) should be started with a structured support programme covering insulin dose titration, injection technique, self-monitoring, and knowledge of dietary effects and glucose control. Metformin hydrochloride should be continued unless it is contra-indicated or not tolerated. Other antidiabetic drugs should be reviewed and stopped if necessary.

Recommended insulin regimens include:

- human isophane insulin p. 699 injected once or twice daily, according to requirements;
- a human isophane insulin in combination with a short-acting insulin, administered either separately or as a pre-mixed (biphasic) human insulin preparation (this may be particularly appropriate if HbA1c is 75 mmol/mol (9.0 %) or higher;
- Insulin detemir p. 701 or insulin glargine p. 701 as an alternative to human isophane insulin. This can be preferable if a *once daily* injection would be beneficial (for example if assistance is required to inject insulin), or if recurrent symptomatic hypoglycaemic episodes are problematic, or if the patient would otherwise need twice-daily human isophane insulin injections in combination with other glucose-lowering drugs. Also consider switching to insulin detemir or insulin glargine from human isophane insulin if significant hypoglycaemia is problematic, or in patients who cannot use the device needed to inject human isophane insulin;
- biphasic preparations (pre-mixed) that include a short-acting human *analogue* insulin (rather than short-acting human *soluble insulin*) can be preferable for patients who prefer injecting insulin immediately before a meal, or if hypoglycaemia is a problem, or if blood-glucose concentrations rise markedly after meals.

Patients who are prescribed a basal insulin regimen (human isophane insulin, insulin detemir or insulin glargine) should be monitored for the need for short-acting insulin before meals (or a biphasic insulin preparation).

Patients who are prescribed a biphasic insulin should be monitored for the need for a further injection of short-acting insulin before meals or for a change to a basal-bolus regimen with human isophane insulin or insulin detemir or insulin glargine if blood-glucose control remains inadequate. Ⓐ

Useful Resources

Type 2 diabetes in adults: management. National Institute for Health and Care Excellence. Clinical guideline NG28. December 2015.
www.nice.org.uk/guidance/ng28

Diabetic complications

See also

Diabetes p. 668
  Type 1 diabetes p. 669
  Type 2 diabetes p. 671

Diabetes and cardiovascular disease

Diabetes is a strong risk factor for cardiovascular disease. Other risk factors for cardiovascular disease such as smoking, hypertension, obesity, and hyperlipidaemia should be addressed. Cardiovascular risk in patients with diabetes can be further reduced by the use of an ACE inhibitor, low-dose aspirin p. 121 and a lipid-regulating drug.

Diabetic nephropathy

Regular review of diabetic patients should include an annual test for urinary protein (using *Albustix®*) and serum creatinine measurement. If the urinary protein test is negative, the urine should be tested for microalbuminuria (the earliest sign of nephropathy). If reagent strip tests (*Micral-Test II®* or *Microbumintest®*) are used and prove positive, the result should be confirmed by laboratory analysis of a urine sample. Provided there are no contra-indications, all diabetic patients with nephropathy causing proteinurea or with established microalbuminuria (at least 3 positive tests) should be treated with an ACE inhibitor or an angiotensin-II receptor antagonist even if the blood pressure is normal; in any case, to minimise the risk of renal deterioration, blood pressure should be carefully controlled. Patients with diabetic nephropathy are particularly susceptible to developing hyperkalaemia and should not be given an ACE inhibitor together with an angiotensin-II receptor antagonist.

ACE inhibitors can potentiate the hypoglycaemic effect of insulin and oral antidiabetic drugs; this effect is more likely during the first weeks of combined treatment and in patients with renal impairment.

See also treatment of hypertension in diabetes.

Diabetic neuropathy

Optimal diabetic control is beneficial for the management of *painful neuropathy* in patients with type 1 diabetes. Paracetamol p. 438 or a non-steroidal anti-inflammatory drug such as ibuprofen p. 1106 may relieve *mild to moderate pain*.

Duloxetine p. 364 is effective for the treatment of painful diabetic neuropathy; amitriptyline hydrochloride p. 369 [unlicensed use] can be used if duloxetine is ineffective or unsuitable. Nortriptyline p. 374 [unlicensed use] may be better tolerated than amitriptyline hydrochloride. If treatment with amitriptyline hydrochloride or duloxetine is inadequate, treatment with pregabalin p. 322 should be tried. Combination therapy of duloxetine or amitriptyline hydrochloride with pregabalin can be used if monotherapy at the maximum tolerated dose does not control symptoms.

Neuropathic pain may respond to opioid analgesics. There is evidence of efficacy for tramadol hydrochloride p. 464, morphine p. 456, and oxycodone hydrochloride p. 459; however treatment with morphine or oxycodone hydrochloride should be initiated only under specialist supervision. Tramadol hydrochloride can be prescribed while the patient is waiting for assessment by a specialist if other treatments have been unsuccessful.

Gabapentin p. 314 and carbamazepine p. 309 are sometimes used for the treatment of neuropathic pain. Capsaicin p. 476 cream 0.075% is licensed for painful diabetic neuropathy and may have some effect, but it produces an intense burning sensation during the initial treatment period.

In *autonomic neuropathy* diabetic diarrhoea can often be managed by tetracycline p. 557 [unlicensed use], otherwise codeine phosphate p. 448 is the best drug, but other antidiarrhoeal preparations can be tried. Erythromycin p. 530 (especially when given intravenously) may be beneficial for gastroparesis [unlicensed use] but this needs confirmation.

In *neuropathic postural hypotension* increased salt intake and the use of the mineralcorticoid fludrocortisone acetate p. 661 [unlicensed use] may help by increasing plasma volume, but uncomfortable oedema is a common side-effect. Fludrocortisone can also be combined with flurbiprofen p. 1106 and ephedrine hydrochloride p. 271 [both unlicensed]. Midodrine [unlicensed], an alpha agonist, may also be useful in postural hypotension.

Gustatory sweating can be treated with an antimuscarinic such as propantheline bromide p. 85; side-effects are common. See also, the management of hyperhidrosis (Hyperhidrosis p. 1228).

In some patients with *neuropathic oedema*, ephedrine hydrochloride [unlicensed use] offers effective relief.

See also the management of Erectile dysfunction p. 793.

Diabetic ketoacidosis

Management

The management of diabetic ketoacidosis involves the replacement of fluid and electrolytes and the administration of insulin. Guidelines for the Management of Diabetic Ketoacidosis in Adults, published by the Joint British Diabetes Societies Inpatient Care Group (available at www.diabetes.org.uk/Professionals/Position-statements-reports/Specialist-care-for-children-and-adults-and-complications/The-Management-of-Diabetic-Ketoacidosis-in-Adults/), should be followed.

- To restore circulating volume if systolic blood pressure is below 90 mmHg (adjusted for age, sex, and medication as appropriate), give 500 mL **sodium chloride 0.9%** by intravenous infusion over 10–15 minutes; repeat if blood pressure remains below 90 mmHg and seek senior medical advice.
- When blood pressure is over 90 mmHg, **sodium chloride 0.9%** should be given by intravenous infusion at a rate that replaces deficit and provides maintenance; see guideline or suggested regimen.
- Include **potassium chloride** in the fluids unless anuria is suspected; adjust according to plasma-potassium concentration (measure at 60 minutes, 2 hours, and 2 hourly thereafter; measure hourly if outside the normal range).
- Start an intravenous insulin infusion: **soluble insulin** should be diluted (and **mixed thoroughly**) with **sodium chloride 0.9%** intravenous infusion to a concentration of 1 unit/mL; infuse at a fixed rate of 0.1 units/kg/hour.
- Established subcutaneous therapy with long-acting insulin analogues (insulin detemir p. 701 or insulin glargine p. 701) should be continued during treatment of diabetic ketoacidosis.
- Monitor blood-ketone and blood-glucose concentrations hourly and adjust the insulin infusion rate accordingly. Blood-ketone concentration should fall by at least 0.5 mmol/litre/hour and blood-glucose concentration should fall by at least 3 mmol/litre/hour.
- Once blood-glucose concentration falls below 14 mmol/litre, **glucose 10%** should be given by

intravenous infusion (into a large vein through a large-gauge needle) at a rate of 125 mL/hour, in addition to the **sodium chloride 0.9% infusion**.

- Continue insulin infusion until blood-ketone concentration is below 0.3 mmol/litre, blood pH is above 7.3 *and* the patient is able to eat and drink; ideally give subcutaneous fast-acting insulin and a meal, and stop the insulin infusion 1 hour later.

The management of hyperosmolar hyperglycaemic state or hyperosmolar hyperglycaemic nonketotic coma is similar to that of diabetic ketoacidosis, although lower rates of insulin infusion are usually necessary and slower rehydration may be required.

Diabetes, surgery and medical illness
05-Jun-2017

Management of diabetes during surgery

Peri-operative management of blood-glucose concentrations depends on factors including the required duration of fasting, timing of surgery (morning or afternoon), usual treatment regimen (insulin, antidiabetic drugs or diet), prior glycaemic control, other co-morbidities, and the likelihood that the patient will be capable of self-managing their diabetes in the immediate post-operative period. EvGr All patients should have emergency treatment for hypoglycaemia written on their drug chart on admission. ⟨E⟩

Note: The following recommendations provide general guidance for the management of diabetes during surgery. **Local protocols and guidelines should be followed where they exist.**

Use of insulin during surgery
Elective surgery—minor procedures in patients with good glycaemic control

EvGr Patients usually treated with insulin who have good glycaemic control (HbA1c less than 69 mmol/mol or 8.5 %) and are undergoing *minor procedures*, can be managed during the operative period by adjustment of their usual insulin regimen, which should be adjusted depending on the type of insulin usually prescribed, following detailed local protocols (which should also include intravenous fluid management, monitoring and control of electrolytes and avoidance of hyperchloraemic metabolic acidosis). On the day before the surgery, the patient's usual insulin should be given as normal, other than once daily long-acting insulin analogues, which should be given at a dose reduced by 20 %. ⟨E⟩

Elective surgery—major procedures or poor glycaemic control

EvGr Patients usually treated with insulin, who are either undergoing *major procedures* (surgery requiring a long fasting period of more than one missed meal) or whose diabetes is poorly controlled, will usually require a variable rate intravenous insulin infusion (continued until the patient is eating/drinking and stabilised on their previous glucose-lowering medication).

The aim is to achieve and maintain glucose concentration within the usual target range (6–10 mmol/litre; but up to 12 mmol/litre is acceptable) by infusing a constant rate of glucose-containing fluid as a substrate, while also infusing insulin at a variable rate. Detailed local protocols should be consulted. In general, the following steps should be followed:

- on the *day before surgery*, once daily long-acting insulin analogues should be given at 80 % of the usual dose; otherwise the patient's usual insulin should be given as normal;
- on the *day of surgery and throughout the intra-operative period,* once daily long-acting insulin analogues should be continued at 80 % of the usual dose; all other insulin

should be stopped until the patient is eating and drinking again after surgery;
- on the *day of surgery*, start an intravenous substrate infusion of potassium chloride with glucose and sodium chloride p. 1007 (based on serum electrolytes which must be measured frequently), and infuse at a rate appropriate to the patient's fluid requirements. To prevent hypoglycaemia, this infusion must **not** be stopped while the insulin infusion is running;
- a variable rate intravenous insulin infusion of soluble human insulin p. 696 in sodium chloride 0.9 % p. 1008 (made either according to locally agreed protocols or using prefilled syringes) should be given via a syringe pump at an initial infusion rate determined by bedside capillary blood-glucose measurement. Hourly blood-glucose measurement should be taken to ensure that the intravenous insulin infusion rate is correct for at least the first 12 hours; the insulin infusion rate should be adjusted according to local protocol to maintain blood-glucose concentrations within the usual target range (6–10 mmol/litre; up to 12 mmol/litre is acceptable);
- intravenous glucose 20 % p. 1009 should be given if blood-glucose drops below 6 mmol/litre, and blood-glucose checked every hour, to prevent a drop below 4 mmol/litre. If blood-glucose drops below 4 mmol/litre, intravenous glucose 20 % should be adjusted and blood-glucose checked every 15 minutes, until blood-glucose is above 6 mmol/litre (testing can then revert to hourly). If blood-glucose rises above 12 mmol/litre, check ketones and consider other signs of diabetic ketoacidosis (see Diabetic ketoacidosis p. 674).

Conversion back to a subcutaneous insulin should not begin until the patient can eat and drink without nausea or vomiting. Once the patient's previous insulin regimen is re-started, the usual insulin dose may require adjustment, as insulin requirements can change due to post-operative stress, infection or altered food intake.

Previous subcutaneous basal-bolus regimens, should be restarted when the first postoperative meal-time insulin dose is due (e.g. with breakfast or lunch); doses may need adjustment due to postoperative stress, infection or altered food intake. The variable rate intravenous insulin infusion and intravenous fluids should be continued until 30–60 minutes **after** the first meal-time short-acting insulin dose. If the patient was previously on a **long-acting insulin analogue**, this should have been continued throughout the operative period at 80 % of the normal dose, and should now just continue at that same dose until the patient leaves hospital; only the short-acting insulin needs to be restarted as above.

Previous subcutaneous twice-daily mixed insulin regimens, should be restarted before breakfast or an evening meal (not at any other time). The variable rate intravenous insulin infusion should be maintained for 30–60 minutes after the first subcutaneous insulin dose has been given.

Patients who were **previously managed with a continuous subcutaneous insulin infusion** should be referred to a specialist team. The subcutaneous infusion should be restarted at the normal basal rate, not at bedtime, and the insulin infusion continued until the next meal bolus has been given.

Patients **not previously prescribed insulin**, who are to start a subcutaneous insulin regimen post-surgery, should have an insulin dose calculated with advice from a specialist diabetes team, considering the patient's sensitivity to insulin, degree of glycaemic control, weight, age, and the average hourly insulin dose used in the peri-operative period. ⟨E⟩

Emergency surgery

EvGr Patients with diabetes (type 1 and 2) requiring emergency surgery, should always have their blood-glucose,

6

Endocrine system

blood or urinary ketone concentration, serum electrolytes and serum bicarbonate checked before surgery. If ketones are high or bicarbonate is low, blood gases should also be checked. If ketoacidosis is present, recommendations for Diabetic ketoacidosis p. 674 should be followed immediately, and surgery delayed if possible. If there is no acidosis, intravenous fluids and an insulin infusion should be started and managed as for *major elective surgery* (above). ⒺⒼⓇ

Use of antidiabetic drugs during surgery

EvGr Manipulation of antidiabetic drug may **not** be appropriate for all surgery or for all patients; particularly when fasting time is more than one missed meal, in patients with poor glycaemic control, and when there is risk of renal injury. In these cases, a *variable rate intravenous insulin infusion* p. 696 should be used as for *major elective surgery* (above), and usual antidiabetic medication adjusted in the peri-operative period. Insulin is almost always required in medical and surgical emergencies.

When insulin is required and given during surgery, acarbose p. 677, meglitinides, sulfonylureas, pioglitazone p. 694, dipeptidyl peptidase-4 inhibitors (gliptins) and sodium glucose co-transporter 2 inhibitors should be stopped once the insulin infusion is commenced and not restarted until the patient is eating and drinking normally. Glucagon-like peptide-1 receptor agonists can be continued as normal during the insulin infusion.

If elective *minor surgical procedures* only require a short-fasting period (just one missed meal), it may be possible to adjust antidiabetic drugs to avoid a switch to a variable rate intravenous insulin infusion; normal drug treatment can continue.

In suitable cases, acarbose, nateglinide p. 686 and repaglinide p. 687 can be continued with just the dose omitted on the morning of surgery if fasting (the morning dose may be given if the patient is not fasting and surgery is in the afternoon).

Pioglitazone, **dipeptidylpeptidase-4 inhibitors (gliptins)** and **glucagon-like peptide-1 receptor agonists** can be taken as normal during the whole peri-operative period.

Sodium glucose co-transporter 2 inhibitors should be omitted on the day of surgery and not restarted until the patient is stable; their use during periods of dehydration and acute illness is associated with an increased risk of developing diabetic ketoacidosis.

Sulfonylureas are associated with hypoglycaemia in the fasted state and therefore should always be omitted on the day of surgery until the patient is eating and drinking again. Capillary blood-glucose should be checked hourly. If hyperglycaemia occurs, an appropriate dose of subcutaneous rapid-acting insulin may be given. A second dose may be given 2 hours later, and a variable rate intravenous insulin infusion considered if hyperglycaemia persists.

Metformin hydrochloride p. 678 is renally excreted; renal impairment may lead to accumulation and lactic acidosis during surgery. If only one meal will be missed during surgery, and the patient has an eGFR greater than 60 mL/minute/1.73m² and a low risk of acute kidney injury (and the procedure does not involve administration of contrast media), it may be possible to continue metformin hydrochloride throughout the peri-operative period—just the lunchtime dose should be omitted if the usual dose is prescribed three times a day.

If the patient will miss more than one meal or there is significant risk of the patient developing acute kidney injury, metformin hydrochloride should be stopped when the pre-operative fast begins. A variable rate intravenous insulin infusion should be started if the metformin hydrochloride dose is more than once daily. Otherwise insulin should only be started if blood-glucose concentration is greater than 12 mmol/litre on two consecutive occasions. Metformin

should not be recommenced until the patient is eating and drinking again, and normal renal function has been assured.

There is no need to stop metformin hydrochloride after contrast medium in patients missing only one meal or who have an eGFR greater than 60 mL/minute/1.73m². If contrast medium is to be used, and eGFR is less than 60 mL/minute/1.73m², metformin should be omitted on the day of the procedure and for the following 48 hours. ⒺⒼⓇ

Use of antidiabetic drugs during medical illness

Manufacturers of some antidiabetic drugs recommend that they may need to be replaced temporarily with insulin during intercurrent illness when the drug is unlikely to control hyperglycaemia (such as myocardial infarction, coma, severe infection, trauma and other medical emergencies). Consult individual product literature.

Sodium glucose co-transporter 2 inhibitors are associated with increased risk of developing diabetic ketoacidosis during periods of dehydration, stress, surgery, trauma, acute medical illness or any other catabolic state, and should be used with caution during these times. The MHRA has advised (2016) that these drugs should be temporarily stopped in patients who are hospitalised for acute serious illness until the patient is medically stable.

Diabetes, pregnancy and breast-feeding

01-Aug-2017

Description of condition

Diabetes in pregnancy is associated with increased risks to the woman (such as pre-eclampsia and rapidly worsening retinopathy), and to the developing fetus, compared with pregnancy in non-diabetic women. Effective blood-glucose control before conception and throughout pregnancy reduces (but does not eliminate) the risk of adverse outcomes such as miscarriage, congenital malformation, stillbirth, and neonatal death.

Management of pre-existing diabetes

EvGr Women with pre-existing diabetes who are planning on becoming pregnant should aim to keep their HbA1c level below 48 mmol/mol (6.5%) if possible without causing problematic hypoglycaemia. Any reduction towards this target is likely to reduce the risk of congenital malformations in the newborn.

Women with pre-existing diabetes who are planning to become pregnant should be advised to take folic acid at the dose for women who are at high-risk of conceiving a child with a neural tube defect, see folic acid p. 993. Ⓐ

Overview

Oral antidiabetic drugs

EvGr All oral antidiabetic drugs, except metformin hydrochloride p. 678, should be discontinued before pregnancy (or as soon as an unplanned pregnancy is identified) and substituted with insulin therapy. Women with diabetes may be treated with metformin hydrochloride p. 678 [unlicensed in type 1 diabetes] as an adjunct or alternative to insulin in the preconception period and during pregnancy, when the likely benefits from improved blood-glucose control outweigh the potential for harm. Metformin hydrochloride p. 678 can be continued, or glibenclamide p. 692 resumed, immediately after birth and during breast-feeding for those with pre-existing Type 2 diabetes p. 671. All other antidiabetic drugs should be avoided while breast-feeding. Ⓐ

Insulin

Limited evidence suggests that the rapid-acting insulin analogues (insulin aspart p. 696 and insulin lispro p. 698) can be associated with fewer episodes of hypoglycaemia, a reduction in postprandial glucose excursions and an improvement in overall glycaemic control compared with regular human insulin.

EvGr Isophane insulin p. 699 is the first-choice for long-acting insulin during pregnancy, however in women who have good blood-glucose control before pregnancy with the long-acting insulin analogues (insulin detemir p. 701 or insulin glargine p. 701), it may be appropriate to continue using them throughout pregnancy.

Continuous subcutaneous insulin p. 696 infusion (insulin pump therapy) may be appropriate for pregnant women who have difficulty achieving glycaemic control with multiple daily injections of insulin p. 696 without significant disabling hypoglycaemia.

All women treated with insulin p. 696 during pregnancy should be aware of the risks of hypoglycaemia, particularly in the first trimester, and should be advised to always carry a fast-acting form of glucose, such as dextrose tablets or a glucose-containing drink. Pregnant women with Type 1 diabetes p. 669 should also be prescribed glucagon p. 707 for use if needed.

Women with pre-existing diabetes treated with insulin p. 696 during pregnancy are at increased risk of hypoglycaemia in the postnatal period and should reduce their insulin immediately after birth. Blood-glucose levels should be monitored carefully to establish the appropriate dose. (A)

Medication for diabetic complications

EvGr Angiotensin-converting enzyme inhibitors and angiotensin II receptor antagonists should be discontinued and replaced with an alternative antihypertensive suitable for use in pregnancy before conception or as soon as pregnancy is confirmed (see *Hypertension in pregnancy* under Hypertension p. 139). Statins should not be prescribed during pregnancy and should be discontinued before a planned pregnancy. (A)

Gestational diabetes

EvGr Women with gestational diabetes who have a fasting plasma glucose below 7 mmol/litre at diagnosis, should first attempt a change in diet and exercise alone in order to reduce blood-glucose. If blood-glucose targets are not met within 1 to 2 weeks, metformin hydrochloride p. 678 may be prescribed [unlicensed use]. Insulin p. 696 may be prescribed if metformin is contra-indicated or not acceptable, and may also be added to treatment if metformin is not effective alone. (A)

EvGr Women who have a fasting plasma glucose above 7 mmol/litre at diagnosis should be treated with insulin p. 696 immediately, with or without metformin hydrochloride p. 678, in addition to a change in diet and exercise.

Women who have a fasting plasma glucose between 6 and 6.9 mmol/litre alongside complications such as macrosomia or hydramnios should be considered for immediate insulin p. 696 treatment, with or without metformin hydrochloride p. 678.

Glibenclamide p. 692 [unlicensed use] may be considered for women from 11 weeks gestation (after organogenesis) who cannot tolerate metformin, or for those in whom metformin is not effective and do not wish to have insulin therapy.

Women with gestational diabetes should discontinue hypoglycaemic treatment immediately after giving birth. (A)

Useful Resources

Diabetes in pregnancy: management from preconception to the postnatal period. National Institute for Health and Care Excellence. Clinical guideline NG3. February 2015.
www.nice.org.uk/guidance/ng3

BLOOD GLUCOSE LOWERING DRUGS > ALPHA GLUCOSIDASE INHIBITORS

Acarbose

● **DRUG ACTION** Acarbose, an inhibitor of intestinal alpha glucosidases, delays the digestion and absorption of starch and sucrose; it has a small but significant effect in lowering blood glucose.

● **INDICATIONS AND DOSE**

Diabetes mellitus inadequately controlled by diet or by diet with oral antidiabetic drugs

▶ BY MOUTH
▸ Adult: Initially 50 mg daily, then increased to 50 mg 3 times a day for 6–8 weeks, then increased if necessary to 100 mg 3 times a day (max. per dose 200 mg 3 times a day)

● **CONTRA-INDICATIONS** Hernia · inflammatory bowel disease · predisposition to partial intestinal obstruction · previous abdominal surgery

● **CAUTIONS** May enhance hypoglycaemic effects of insulin and sulfonylureas (hypoglycaemic episodes may be treated with oral glucose but not with sucrose)

● **INTERACTIONS** → Appendix 1: acarbose

● **SIDE-EFFECTS**
▸ **Common or very common** Diarrhoea (may need to reduce dose) · gastrointestinal discomfort · gastrointestinal disorders
▸ **Uncommon** Nausea · vomiting
▸ **Rare or very rare** Hepatic disorders · oedema
▸ **Frequency not known** Acute generalised exanthematous pustulosis (AGEP) · thrombocytopenia

SIDE-EFFECTS, FURTHER INFORMATION Antacids containing magnesium and aluminium salts unlikely to be beneficial for treating side-effects.

● **PREGNANCY** Avoid.

● **BREAST FEEDING** Avoid.

● **HEPATIC IMPAIRMENT** Avoid.

● **RENAL IMPAIRMENT** Avoid if eGFR less than 25 mL/minute/1.73 m^2.

● **MONITORING REQUIREMENTS** Monitor liver function.

● **DIRECTIONS FOR ADMINISTRATION** Tablets should be chewed with first mouthful of food or swallowed whole with a little liquid immediately before food.

● **PATIENT AND CARER ADVICE** Antacids unlikely to be beneficial for treating side-effects. To counteract possible hypoglycaemia, patients receiving insulin or a sulfonylurea as well as acarbose need to carry glucose (not sucrose—acarbose interferes with sucrose absorption). Patients should be given advice on how to administer acarbose tablets.

● MEDICINAL FORMS
There can be variation in the licensing of different medicines containing the same drug.
Tablet
▸ Acarbose (Non-proprietary)
   Acarbose 50 mg Acarbose 50mg tablets | 90 tablet PoM £11.51 DT = £11.51
   Acarbose 100 mg Acarbose 100mg tablets | 90 tablet PoM £19.03 DT = £19.03
▸ Glucobay (Bayer Plc)
   Acarbose 50 mg Glucobay 50mg tablets | 90 tablet PoM £7.35 DT = £11.51
   Acarbose 100 mg Glucobay 100mg tablets | 90 tablet PoM £13.50 DT = £19.03

6

Endocrine system

6

Endocrine system

BLOOD GLUCOSE LOWERING DRUGS ›
BIGUANIDES

Metformin hydrochloride
06-Jun-2017

- **DRUG ACTION** Metformin exerts its effect mainly by decreasing gluconeogenesis and by increasing peripheral utilisation of glucose; since it acts only in the presence of endogenous insulin it is effective only if there are some residual functioning pancreatic islet cells.

- **INDICATIONS AND DOSE**

Type 2 diabetes mellitus [monotherapy or in combination with other antidiabetic drugs (including insulin)]
  ▶ BY MOUTH USING IMMEDIATE-RELEASE MEDICINES
  ▶ Child 10–17 years (specialist use only): Initially 500 mg once daily, dose to be adjusted according to response at intervals of at least 1 week, maximum daily dose to be given in 2–3 divided doses; maximum 2 g per day
  ▶ Adult: Initially 500 mg once daily for at least 1 week, dose to be taken with breakfast, then 500 mg twice daily for at least 1 week, dose to be taken with breakfast and evening meal, then 500 mg 3 times a day, dose to be taken with breakfast, lunch and evening meal; maximum 2 g per day
  ▶ BY MOUTH USING MODIFIED-RELEASE MEDICINES
  ▶ Adult: Initially 500 mg once daily, then increased if necessary up to 2 g once daily, dose increased gradually, every 10–15 days, dose to be taken with evening meal, alternatively increased to 1 g twice daily, dose to be taken with meals, alternative dose only to be used if control not achieved with once daily dose regimen. If control still not achieved then change to standard release tablets

Type 2 diabetes mellitus [reduction in risk or delay of onset]
  ▶ BY MOUTH USING MODIFIED-RELEASE MEDICINES
  ▶ Adult 18–74 years: Initially 500 mg once daily, then increased if necessary up to 2 g once daily, dose increased gradually, every 10–15 days, dose to be taken with evening meal, for further information on risk factors—consult product literature

Polycystic ovary syndrome
  ▶ BY MOUTH USING IMMEDIATE-RELEASE MEDICINES
  ▶ Adult: Initially 500 mg once daily for 1 week, dose to be taken with breakfast, then 500 mg twice daily for 1 week, dose to be taken with breakfast and evening meal, then 1.5–1.7 g daily in 2–3 divided doses

- **UNLICENSED USE**
  ▶ In adults [EvGr] Based on clinical experience of increased side-effects, maximum dose for metformin immediate-release medicines in BNF Publications differs from product licence. [E] Not licensed for polycystic ovary syndrome.

- **CONTRA-INDICATIONS** Acute metabolic acidosis (including lactic acidosis and diabetic ketoacidosis)

- **CAUTIONS** Risk factors for lactic acidosis

  CAUTIONS, FURTHER INFORMATION
  ▶ Risk factors for lactic acidosis Manufacturer advises caution in chronic stable heart failure (monitor cardiac function), and concomitant use of drugs that can acutely impair renal function; interrupt treatment if dehydration occurs, and avoid in conditions that can acutely worsen renal function, or cause tissue hypoxia.

- **INTERACTIONS** → Appendix 1: metformin

- **SIDE-EFFECTS**
  ▶ **Common or very common** Abdominal pain · appetite decreased · diarrhoea (usually transient) · gastrointestinal disorder · nausea · taste altered · vomiting
  ▶ **Rare or very rare** Hepatitis · lactic acidosis (discontinue) · skin reactions · vitamin B12 absorption decreased

SIDE-EFFECTS, FURTHER INFORMATION Gastro-intestinal side-effects are initially common with metformin, and may persist in some patients, particularly when very high doses are given. A slow increase in dose may improve tolerability.

- **PREGNANCY** Can be used in pregnancy for both pre-existing and gestational diabetes. Women with gestational diabetes should discontinue treatment after giving birth.

- **BREAST FEEDING** May be used during breast-feeding in women with pre-existing diabetes.

- **HEPATIC IMPAIRMENT** Withdraw if tissue hypoxia likely.

- **RENAL IMPAIRMENT**
  ▶ In adults Manufacturer advises avoid if eGFR is less than 30 mL/minute/1.73 m^2.
  ▶ In children Manufacturer advises avoid if estimated glomerular filtration rate is less than 30 mL/minute/1.73 m^2.
  Dose adjustments ▶ In children Manufacturer advises consider dose reduction in moderate impairment.
  ▶ In adults Manufacturer advises reduce dose in moderate impairment—consult product literature.

- **MONITORING REQUIREMENTS** Determine renal function before treatment and at least annually (at least twice a year in patients with additional risk factors for renal impairment, or if deterioration suspected).

- **PRESCRIBING AND DISPENSING INFORMATION**
  ▶ In adults Patients taking up to 2 g daily of the standard-release metformin may start with the same daily dose of metformin modified release; not suitable if dose of standard-release tablets more than 2 g daily.

- **PATIENT AND CARER ADVICE** Manufacturer advises that patients and their carers should be informed of the risk of lactic acidosis and told to seek immediate medical attention if symptoms such as dyspnoea, muscle cramps, abdominal pain, hypothermia, or asthenia occur. Medicines for Children leaflet: Metformin for diabetes www.medicinesforchildren.org.uk/metformin-diabetes

- **NATIONAL FUNDING/ACCESS DECISIONS**
  GLUCOPHAGE ® SR
  Scottish Medicines Consortium (SMC) Decisions
  The *Scottish Medicines Consortium* has advised (September 2009) that *Glucophage® SR* is accepted for restricted use within NHS Scotland for the treatment of type 2 diabetes mellitus in adult patients who are intolerant of standard-release metformin, and in whom the prolonged-release tablet allows the use of a dose of metformin not previously tolerated, or in patients for whom a once daily preparation offers a clinically significant benefit.

- **MEDICINAL FORMS**
  There can be variation in the licensing of different medicines containing the same drug. Forms available from special-order manufacturers include: capsule, oral suspension, oral solution
  Modified-release tablet
  CAUTIONARY AND ADVISORY LABELS 21, 25
  ▶ Metformin hydrochloride (Non-proprietary)
    Metformin hydrochloride 500 mg Metformin 500mg modified-release tablets | 28 tablet [PoM] £3.20 | 56 tablet [PoM] £6.40 DT = £5.32
    Metformin hydrochloride 1 gram Metformin 1g modified-release tablets | 56 tablet [PoM] [S] DT = £8.52
  ▶ Bolamyn SR (Teva UK Ltd)
    Metformin hydrochloride 500 mg Bolamyn SR 500mg tablets | 28 tablet [PoM] £3.20 | 56 tablet [PoM] £6.40 DT = £5.32
    Metformin hydrochloride 1 gram Bolamyn SR 1000mg tablets | 28 tablet [PoM] £5.06 | 56 tablet [PoM] £10.13 DT = £8.52
  ▶ Glucient SR (Consilient Health Ltd)
    Metformin hydrochloride 500 mg Glucient SR 500mg tablets | 28 tablet [PoM] £2.51 | 56 tablet [PoM] £5.03 DT = £5.32
    Metformin hydrochloride 750 mg Glucient SR 750mg tablets | 28 tablet [PoM] £3.20
    Metformin hydrochloride 1 gram Glucient SR 1000mg tablets | 28 tablet [PoM] £4.26 | 56 tablet [PoM] £8.52 DT = £8.52

- Glucophage SR (Merck Serono Ltd)
  Metformin hydrochloride 500 mg Glucophage SR 500mg tablets |
  28 tablet [PoM] £2.66 | 56 tablet [PoM] £5.32 DT = £5.32
  Metformin hydrochloride 750 mg Glucophage SR 750mg tablets |
  28 tablet [PoM] £3.20 | 56 tablet [PoM] £6.40 DT = £6.40
  Metformin hydrochloride 1 gram Glucophage SR 1000mg tablets |
  28 tablet [PoM] £4.26 | 56 tablet [PoM] £8.52 DT = £8.52
- Meijumet (Medreich Plc)
  Metformin hydrochloride 500 mg Meijumet 500mg modified-
  release tablets | 28 tablet [PoM] £2.66 | 56 tablet [PoM] £5.32 DT =
  £5.32
  Metformin hydrochloride 750 mg Meijumet 750mg modified-
  release tablets | 28 tablet [PoM] £3.20 | 56 tablet [PoM] £6.40 DT =
  £6.40
  Metformin hydrochloride 1 gram Meijumet 1000mg modified-
  release tablets | 28 tablet [PoM] £4.26 | 56 tablet [PoM] £8.52 DT =
  £8.52
- Metabet SR (Morningside Healthcare Ltd, Actavis UK Ltd)
  Metformin hydrochloride 500 mg Metabet SR 500mg tablets |
  28 tablet [PoM] £2.61–£2.66 | 56 tablet [PoM] £5.22–£5.32 DT = £5.32
  Metformin hydrochloride 1 gram Metabet SR 1000mg tablets |
  28 tablet [PoM] £4.53 | 56 tablet [PoM] £9.06 DT = £8.52
- Sukkarto SR (Morningside Healthcare Ltd)
  Metformin hydrochloride 500 mg Sukkarto SR 500mg tablets |
  56 tablet [PoM] £3.46 DT = £5.32
  Metformin hydrochloride 1 gram Sukkarto SR 1000mg tablets |
  56 tablet [PoM] £5.54 DT = £8.52

Tablet
CAUTIONARY AND ADVISORY LABELS 21
- Metformin hydrochloride (Non-proprietary)
  Metformin hydrochloride 500 mg Metformin 500mg tablets |
  28 tablet [PoM] £1.55 DT = £0.90 | 84 tablet [PoM] £2.16–£2.70 |
  500 tablet [PoM] £16.07
  Metformin hydrochloride 850 mg Metformin 850mg tablets |
  56 tablet [PoM] £2.56 DT = £1.17 | 300 tablet [PoM] £6.27–£7.13
- Glucophage (Merck Serono Ltd)
  Metformin hydrochloride 500 mg Glucophage 500mg tablets |
  84 tablet [PoM] £2.88
  Metformin hydrochloride 850 mg Glucophage 850mg tablets |
  56 tablet [PoM] £3.20 DT = £1.17

Oral solution
CAUTIONARY AND ADVISORY LABELS 21
- Metformin hydrochloride (Non-proprietary)
  Metformin hydrochloride 100 mg per 1 ml Metformin 500mg/5ml
  oral solution sugar free sugar-free | 100 ml [PoM] £5.85–£10.50
  sugar-free | 150 ml [PoM] £60.00 DT = £8.78
  Metformin hydrochloride 170 mg per 1 ml Metformin 850mg/5ml
  oral solution sugar free sugar-free | 150 ml [PoM] £19.95 DT = £19.95
  Metformin hydrochloride 200 mg per 1 ml Metformin 1g/5ml oral
  solution sugar free sugar-free | 150 ml [PoM] £23.48–£24.00 DT =
  £24.00

Powder
- Metformin hydrochloride (Non-proprietary)
  Metformin hydrochloride 1 gram Metformin 1g oral powder sachets
  sugar free sugar-free | 30 sachet [PoM] [S]

Combinations available: *Alogliptin with metformin*, p. 680 ·
Canagliflozin with metformin, p. 688 · *Dapagliflozin with
metformin*, p. 690 · *Empagliflozin with metformin*, p. 691 ·
Linagliptin with metformin, p. 680 · *Pioglitazone with
metformin*, p. 695 · *Saxagliptin with metformin*, p. 681 ·
Sitagliptin with metformin, p. 682 · *Vildagliptin with
metformin*, p. 683

BLOOD GLUCOSE LOWERING DRUGS ›
DIPEPTIDYLPEPTIDASE-4 INHIBITORS (GLIPTINS)

Alogliptin
30-Aug-2017

- **DRUG ACTION** Inhibits dipeptidylpeptidase-4 to increase
  insulin secretion and lower glucagon secretion.

- **INDICATIONS AND DOSE**

  **Type 2 diabetes mellitus in combination with other
  antidiabetic drugs (including insulin) if existing
  treatment fails to achieve adequate glycaemic control**
  - BY MOUTH
  - Adult: 25 mg once daily, for further information on use
    with other antidiabetic drugs—consult product
    literature

  DOSE ADJUSTMENTS DUE TO INTERACTIONS
  - Dose of concomitant sulfonylurea or insulin may need
    to be reduced.
  - Caution with use in combination with both metformin
    and pioglitazone—risk of hypoglycaemia (dose of
    metformin or pioglitazone may need to be reduced).

- **CONTRA-INDICATIONS** Ketoacidosis

- **CAUTIONS** History of pancreatitis · not recommended in
  moderate to severe heart failure (limited experience)

- **INTERACTIONS** → Appendix 1: alogliptin

- **SIDE-EFFECTS**
- **Common or very common** Abdominal pain ·
  gastrooesophageal reflux disease · headache · increased
  risk of infection · skin reactions
- **Frequency not known** Angioedema · hepatic function
  abnormal · pancreatitis acute · Stevens-Johnson syndrome
  SIDE-EFFECTS, FURTHER INFORMATION Discontinue if
  symptoms of acute pancreatitis occur such as persistent,
  severe abdominal pain.

- **ALLERGY AND CROSS-SENSITIVITY** Contra-indicated if
  history of serious hypersensitivity to dipeptidylpeptidase-
  4 inhibitors.

- **PREGNANCY** Manufacturer advises avoid—no information
  available.

- **BREAST FEEDING** Avoid—present in milk in *animal* studies.

- **HEPATIC IMPAIRMENT** Manufacturer advises avoid in
  severe impairment—no information available.

- **RENAL IMPAIRMENT** Use with caution if eGFR less than
  30 mL/minute/1.73 m^2.
  Dose adjustments Reduce dose to 12.5 mg once daily if
  eGFR 30–50 mL/minute/1.73 m^2.
      Reduce dose to 6.25 mg once daily if eGFR less than
  30 mL/minute/1.73 m^2.

- **MONITORING REQUIREMENTS** Determine renal function
  before treatment and periodically thereafter.

- **MEDICINAL FORMS**
  There can be variation in the licensing of different medicines
  containing the same drug.
  Tablet
  - Vipidia (Takeda UK Ltd) ▼
    Alogliptin (as Alogliptin benzoate) 6.25 mg Vipidia 6.25mg tablets
    | 28 tablet [PoM] £26.60 DT = £26.60
    Alogliptin (as Alogliptin benzoate) 12.5 mg Vipidia 12.5mg tablets
    | 28 tablet [PoM] £26.60 DT = £26.60
    Alogliptin (as Alogliptin benzoate) 25 mg Vipidia 25mg tablets |
    28 tablet [PoM] £26.60 DT = £26.60

6

Endocrine system

6

Endocrine system

Alogliptin with metformin

The properties listed below are those particular to the combination only. For the properties of the components please consider, alogliptin p. 679, metformin hydrochloride p. 678.

● **INDICATIONS AND DOSE**

Type 2 diabetes mellitus not controlled by metformin alone or by metformin in combination with either pioglitazone or insulin
▶ BY MOUTH
▶ Adult: 1 tablet twice daily, based on patient's current metformin dose

● INTERACTIONS → Appendix 1: alogliptin · metformin

● **MEDICINAL FORMS**
There can be variation in the licensing of different medicines containing the same drug.
Tablet
CAUTIONARY AND ADVISORY LABELS 21
▶ Vipdomet (Takeda UK Ltd) ▼
 Alogliptin (as Alogliptin benzoate) 12.5 mg, Metformin hydrochloride 1 gram Vipdomet 12.5mg/1000mg tablets | 56 tablet [PoM] £26.60 DT = £26.60

Linagliptin

19-Sep-2017

● **DRUG ACTION** Inhibits dipeptidylpeptidase-4 to increase insulin secretion and lower glucagon secretion.

● **INDICATIONS AND DOSE**

Type 2 diabetes mellitus as monotherapy (if metformin inapproriate), or in combination with other antidiabetic drugs (including insulin) if existing treatment fails to achieve adequate glycaemic control
▶ BY MOUTH
▶ Adult: 5 mg once daily, for further information on use with other antidiabetic drugs—consult product literature
DOSE ADJUSTMENTS DUE TO INTERACTIONS
▶ Dose of concomitant sulfonylurea or insulin may need to be reduced.

● INTERACTIONS → Appendix 1: linagliptin

● SIDE-EFFECTS
▶ **Uncommon** Cough · nasopharyngitis
▶ **Rare or very rare** Angioedema · skin reactions
▶ **Frequency not known** Pancreatitis

SIDE-EFFECTS, FURTHER INFORMATION Discontinue if symptoms of acute pancreatitis occur such as persistent, severe abdominal pain.

● PREGNANCY Avoid—no information available.

● BREAST FEEDING Avoid—present in milk in *animal* studies.

● **NATIONAL FUNDING/ACCESS DECISIONS**
Scottish Medicines Consortium (SMC) Decisions
The *Scottish Medicines Consortium* has advised that linagliptin (*Trajenta* ®) is accepted for restricted use within NHS Scotland for the treatment of type 2 diabetes mellitus as monotherapy when both metformin and a sulfonylurea are inappropriate (January 2013), and in combination with metformin when addition of a sulfonylurea is inappropriate (December 2011).

● **MEDICINAL FORMS**
There can be variation in the licensing of different medicines containing the same drug.
Tablet
▶ Trajenta (Boehringer Ingelheim Ltd)
 Linagliptin 5 mg Trajenta 5mg tablets | 28 tablet [PoM] £33.26 DT = £33.26

Linagliptin with metformin

The properties listed below are those particular to the combination only. For the properties of the components please consider, linagliptin above, metformin hydrochloride p. 678.

● **INDICATIONS AND DOSE**

Type 2 diabetes mellitus not controlled by metformin alone or by metformin in combination with either a sulfonylurea or insulin
▶ BY MOUTH
▶ Adult: 1 tablet twice daily, based on patient's current metformin dose

● INTERACTIONS → Appendix 1: linagliptin · metformin

● **NATIONAL FUNDING/ACCESS DECISIONS**
Scottish Medicines Consortium (SMC) Decisions
The *Scottish Medicines Consortium* has advised (May 2015) that linagliptin plus metformin combination tablets (*Jentadueto* ®) are accepted for restricted use within NHS Scotland for the treatment of adult patients with type 2 diabetes mellitus in combination with insulin, as an adjunct to diet and exercise to improve glycaemic control when a combination of insulin and metformin alone is inadequate. It is restricted to use in the treatment of patients for whom a combination of linagliptin and metformin is an appropriate choice of therapy and the fixed doses are considered appropriate.

● **MEDICINAL FORMS**
There can be variation in the licensing of different medicines containing the same drug.
Tablet
CAUTIONARY AND ADVISORY LABELS 21
▶ Jentadueto (Boehringer Ingelheim Ltd)
 Linagliptin 2.5 mg, Metformin hydrochloride 850 mg Jentadueto 2.5mg/850mg tablets | 56 tablet [PoM] £33.26 DT = £33.26
 Linagliptin 2.5 mg, Metformin hydrochloride 1000 mg Jentadueto 2.5mg/1000mg tablets | 56 tablet [PoM] £33.26 DT = £33.26

Saxagliptin

19-Sep-2017

● **DRUG ACTION** Inhibits dipeptidylpeptidase-4 to increase insulin secretion and lower glucagon secretion.

● **INDICATIONS AND DOSE**

Type 2 diabetes mellitus as monotherapy (if metformin inapproriate), or in combination with other antidiabetic drugs (including insulin) if existing treatment fails to achieve adequate glycaemic control
▶ BY MOUTH
▶ Adult: 5 mg once daily, for further information on use with other antidiabetic drugs—consult product literature
DOSE ADJUSTMENTS DUE TO INTERACTIONS
▶ Dose of concomitant sulfonylurea or insulin may need to be reduced.

● CAUTIONS Elderly · history of pancreatitis

● INTERACTIONS → Appendix 1: saxagliptin

● SIDE-EFFECTS
▶ **Common or very common** Abdominal pain · dizziness · fatigue · headache · increased risk of infection · skin reactions · vomiting
▶ **Uncommon** Pancreatitis
▶ **Rare or very rare** Angioedema
▶ **Frequency not known** Constipation · nausea

SIDE-EFFECTS, FURTHER INFORMATION Discontinue if symptoms of acute pancreatitis occur such as persistent, severe abdominal pain.

- **ALLERGY AND CROSS-SENSITIVITY** Contra-indicated if patient has a history of serious hypersensitivity to dipeptidylpeptidase-4 inhibitors.
- **PREGNANCY** Avoid unless essential—toxicity in *animal* studies.
- **BREAST FEEDING** Avoid—present in milk in *animal* studies.
- **HEPATIC IMPAIRMENT** Use with caution in moderate impairment. Avoid in severe impairment.
- **RENAL IMPAIRMENT** Use with caution in severe impairment.
  Dose adjustments Reduce dose to 2.5 mg once daily in moderate to severe impairment.
- **MONITORING REQUIREMENTS** Determine renal function before treatment and periodically thereafter.
- **NATIONAL FUNDING/ACCESS DECISIONS**
  Scottish Medicines Consortium (SMC) Decisions
  The *Scottish Medicines Consortium* has advised that saxagliptin (*Onglyza*®) is accepted for restricted use within NHS Scotland for the treatment of type 2 diabetes mellitus as triple therapy in combination with metformin and a sulfonylurea, as an alternative to existing dipeptidyl peptidase-4 inhibitors, when treatment with metformin and a sulfonylurea is inadequate (November 2013).

- **MEDICINAL FORMS**
  There can be variation in the licensing of different medicines containing the same drug.
  Tablet
  ▸ Onglyza (AstraZeneca UK Ltd)
  Saxagliptin (as Saxagliptin hydrochloride) 2.5 mg Onglyza 2.5mg tablets | 28 tablet PoM £31.60 DT = £31.60
  Saxagliptin (as Saxagliptin hydrochloride) 5 mg Onglyza 5mg tablets | 28 tablet PoM £31.60 DT = £31.60

Saxagliptin with dapagliflozin   19-Jul-2017

The properties listed below are those particular to the combination only. For the properties of the components please consider, saxagliptin p. 680, dapagliflozin p. 689.

- **INDICATIONS AND DOSE**
  Type 2 diabetes mellitus not controlled by metformin and/or a sulfonylurea with either saxagliptin or dapagliflozin
  ▸ BY MOUTH
  ▸ Adult 18–74 years: 5/10 mg once daily
  ▸ Adult 75 years and over: Initiation not recommended
  DOSE ADJUSTMENTS DUE TO INTERACTIONS
  ▸ Dose of concomitant sulfonylurea may need to be reduced.
  DOSE EQUIVALENCE AND CONVERSION
  ▸ Dose expressed as x/y mg saxagliptin/dapagliflozin.

- **INTERACTIONS** → Appendix 1: dapagliflozin · saxagliptin
- **HEPATIC IMPAIRMENT** Manufacturer advises use with caution in moderate impairment; avoid in severe impairment.
- **RENAL IMPAIRMENT**
  Dose adjustments Manufacturer advises avoid if eGFR less than 60 mL/minute/1.73 m² (ineffective).
- **PATIENT AND CARER ADVICE**
  Missed doses Manufacturer advises if a dose is more than 12 hours late, the missed dose should not be taken and the next dose should be taken at the normal time.
- **NATIONAL FUNDING/ACCESS DECISIONS**
  Scottish Medicines Consortium (SMC) Decisions
  The *Scottish Medicines Consortium* has advised (July 2017) that saxagliptin with dapagliflozin 5 mg/10 mg (*Qtern*®) is accepted for restricted use within NHS Scotland for the treatment of patients with type 2 diabetes mellitus in

combination with metformin when the use of a sulfonylurea is inappropriate, only if:
- metformin and/or a sulfonylurea, in combination with dapagliflozin or saxagliptin, do not provide adequate glycaemic control; or
- the patient is already being treated with the free combination of dapagliflozin and saxagliptin.

- **MEDICINAL FORMS**
  There can be variation in the licensing of different medicines containing the same drug.
  Tablet
  ▸ Qtern (AstraZeneca UK Ltd) ▼
  Saxagliptin (as Saxagliptin hydrochloride) 5 mg, Dapagliflozin (as Dapagliflozin propanediol monohydrate) 10 mg Qtern 5mg/10mg tablets | 28 tablet PoM £49.56 DT = £49.56

Saxagliptin with metformin

The properties listed below are those particular to the combination only. For the properties of the components please consider, saxagliptin p. 680, metformin hydrochloride p. 678.

- **INDICATIONS AND DOSE**
  Type 2 diabetes mellitus not controlled by metformin alone or by metformin in combination with either a sulfonylurea or insulin
  ▸ BY MOUTH
  ▸ Adult: 1 tablet twice daily, based on patient's current metformin dose

- **INTERACTIONS** → Appendix 1: metformin · saxagliptin
- **NATIONAL FUNDING/ACCESS DECISIONS**
  Scottish Medicines Consortium (SMC) Decisions
  The *Scottish Medicines Consortium* has advised (May 2013) that *Komboglyze*® is accepted for restricted use within NHS Scotland for the treatment of type 2 diabetes mellitus in patients unable to achieve adequate glycaemic control with metformin alone and when the addition of a sulfonylurea is inappropriate.

- **MEDICINAL FORMS**
  There can be variation in the licensing of different medicines containing the same drug.
  Tablet
  CAUTIONARY AND ADVISORY LABELS 21
  ▸ Komboglyze (AstraZeneca UK Ltd)
  Saxagliptin (as Saxagliptin hydrochloride) 2.5 mg, Metformin hydrochloride 850 mg Komboglyze 2.5mg/850mg tablets | 56 tablet PoM £31.60 DT = £31.60
  Saxagliptin (as Saxagliptin hydrochloride) 2.5 mg, Metformin hydrochloride 1 gram Komboglyze 2.5mg/1000mg tablets | 56 tablet PoM £31.60 DT = £31.60

Sitagliptin

- **DRUG ACTION** Inhibits dipeptidylpeptidase-4 to increase insulin secretion and lower glucagon secretion.

- **INDICATIONS AND DOSE**
  Type 2 diabetes mellitus as monotherapy (if metformin inappropriate), or in combination with other antidiabetic drugs (including insulin) if existing treatment fails to achieve adequate glycaemic control
  ▸ BY MOUTH
  ▸ Adult: 100 mg once daily, for further information on use with other antidiabetic drugs—consult product literature
  DOSE ADJUSTMENTS DUE TO INTERACTIONS
  ▸ Dose of concomitant sulfonylurea or insulin may need to be reduced.

6

Endocrine system

- CONTRA-INDICATIONS Ketoacidosis
- INTERACTIONS → Appendix 1: sitagliptin
- SIDE-EFFECTS
▶ **Common or very common** Headache
▶ **Uncommon** Constipation · dizziness · skin reactions
▶ **Frequency not known** Angioedema · back pain · cutaneous vasculitis · interstitial lung disease · joint disorders · myalgia · pancreatitis acute · renal impairment · Stevens-Johnson syndrome · vomiting
  SIDE-EFFECTS, FURTHER INFORMATION Discontinue if symptoms of acute pancreatitis occur such as persistent, severe abdominal pain.
- PREGNANCY Avoid—toxicity in *animal* studies.
- BREAST FEEDING Avoid—present in milk in *animal* studies.
- RENAL IMPAIRMENT
  Dose adjustments Reduce dose to 50 mg once daily if eGFR 30–50 mL/minute/1.73 m^2.
  Reduce dose to 25 mg once daily if eGFR less than 30 mL/minute/1.73 m^2.
- NATIONAL FUNDING/ACCESS DECISIONS
  Scottish Medicines Consortium (SMC) Decisions
  The *Scottish Medicines Consortium* has advised (June 2010) that *Januvia* ® is accepted for restricted use within NHS Scotland as monotherapy, to improve glycaemic control in patients with type 2 diabetes mellitus, for whom both metformin and sulfonylureas are not appropriate.

- MEDICINAL FORMS
  There can be variation in the licensing of different medicines containing the same drug.
  Tablet
  ▶ Januvia (Merck Sharp & Dohme Ltd)
    Sitagliptin (as Sitagliptin phosphate) **25 mg** Januvia 25mg tablets | 28 tablet [PoM] £33.26 DT = £33.26
    Sitagliptin (as Sitagliptin phosphate) **50 mg** Januvia 50mg tablets | 28 tablet [PoM] £33.26 DT = £33.26
    Sitagliptin (as Sitagliptin phosphate) **100 mg** Januvia 100mg tablets | 28 tablet [PoM] £33.26 DT = £33.26

Sitagliptin with metformin

The properties listed below are those particular to the combination only. For the properties of the components please consider, sitagliptin p. 681, metformin hydrochloride p. 678.

- INDICATIONS AND DOSE
  Type 2 diabetes mellitus not controlled by metformin alone or by metformin in combination with either a sulfonylurea or pioglitazone or insulin
  ▶ BY MOUTH
  ▶ Adult: 1 tablet twice daily

- INTERACTIONS → Appendix 1: metformin · sitagliptin
- NATIONAL FUNDING/ACCESS DECISIONS
  Scottish Medicines Consortium (SMC) Decisions
  The *Scottish Medicines Consortium* has advised (July 2008) that *Janumet* ® is accepted for restricted use within NHS Scotland for the treatment of type 2 diabetes mellitus when the addition of a sulfonylurea to metformin is not appropriate; it is also accepted for use in NHS Scotland in combination with a sulfonylurea in patients inadequately controlled on maximum tolerated doses of metformin and a sulfonylurea.

- MEDICINAL FORMS
  There can be variation in the licensing of different medicines containing the same drug.
  Tablet
  CAUTIONARY AND ADVISORY LABELS 21
  ▶ Janumet (Merck Sharp & Dohme Ltd)
    Sitagliptin (as Sitagliptin phosphate) **50 mg, Metformin hydrochloride 1 gram** Janumet 50mg/1000mg tablets | 56 tablet [PoM] £33.26 DT = £33.26

Vildagliptin

19-Sep-2017

- DRUG ACTION Inhibits dipeptidylpeptidase-4 to increase insulin secretion and lower glucagon secretion.

- INDICATIONS AND DOSE
  Type 2 diabetes mellitus as monotherapy (if metformin inappropriate), or in combination with other antidiabetic drugs (including insulin) if existing treatment fails to achieve adequate glycaemic control
  ▶ BY MOUTH
  ▶ Adult: 50 mg twice daily, reduce dose to 50 mg once daily in the morning when used in dual combination with a sulfonylurea. For further information on use with other antidiabetic drugs—consult product literature
  DOSE ADJUSTMENTS DUE TO INTERACTIONS
  ▶ Dose of concomitant sulfonylurea or insulin may need to be reduced.

- CONTRA-INDICATIONS Ketoacidosis
- CAUTIONS Manufacturer advises avoid in severe heart failure—no information available
- INTERACTIONS → Appendix 1: vildagliptin
- SIDE-EFFECTS
▶ **Common or very common** Dizziness
▶ **Uncommon** Arthralgia · constipation · headache · hypoglycaemia · peripheral oedema
▶ **Rare or very rare** Increased risk of infection
▶ **Frequency not known** Hepatitis · myalgia · pancreatitis · skin reactions
  SIDE-EFFECTS, FURTHER INFORMATION
  Pancreatitis Discontinue if symptoms of acute pancreatitis occur, such as persistent severe abdominal pain.
  Liver toxicity Rare reports of liver dysfunction; discontinue if jaundice or other signs of liver dysfunction occur.
- PREGNANCY Avoid—toxicity in *animal* studies.
- BREAST FEEDING Avoid—present in milk in *animal* studies.
- HEPATIC IMPAIRMENT Avoid.
- RENAL IMPAIRMENT
  Dose adjustments Reduce dose to 50 mg once daily if eGFR less than 50 mL/minute/1.73 m^2.
- MONITORING REQUIREMENTS Monitor liver function before treatment and every 3 months for first year and periodically thereafter.
- PATIENT AND CARER ADVICE
  Liver toxicity Patients should be advised to seek prompt medical attention if symptoms such as nausea, vomiting, abdominal pain, fatigue, and dark urine develop.
- NATIONAL FUNDING/ACCESS DECISIONS
  Scottish Medicines Consortium (SMC) Decisions
  The *Scottish Medicines Consortium* has advised that vildagliptin (*Galvus* ®) is accepted for restricted use within NHS Scotland for the treatment of type 2 diabetes mellitus as monotherapy when treatment with metformin or a sulfonylurea is inappropriate (December 2012), and in combination with metformin when addition of a sulfonylurea is inappropriate (March 2008), and in

combination with a sulfonylurea if metformin is inappropriate (September 2009), and also as triple therapy in combination with metformin and a sulfonylurea, as an alternative to existing dipeptidyl peptidase-4 inhibitors, when treatment with metformin and a sulfonylurea is inadequate (November 2013).

- MEDICINAL FORMS
  There can be variation in the licensing of different medicines containing the same drug.
  Tablet
  ▸ Galvus (Novartis Pharmaceuticals UK Ltd)
  Vildagliptin 50 mg Galvus 50mg tablets | 56 tablet PoM £33.35 DT = £33.35

Vildagliptin with metformin

The properties listed below are those particular to the combination only. For the properties of the components please consider, vildagliptin p. 682, metformin hydrochloride p. 678.

- INDICATIONS AND DOSE

  Type 2 diabetes mellitus not controlled by metformin alone or by metformin in combination with either a sulfonylurea or insulin
  ▸ BY MOUTH
  ▸ Adult: 1 tablet twice daily, based on patient's current metformin dose

- INTERACTIONS → Appendix 1: metformin · vildagliptin
- NATIONAL FUNDING/ACCESS DECISIONS

  Scottish Medicines Consortium (SMC) Decisions
  The *Scottish Medicines Consortium* has advised (June 2008) that *Eucreas*® is accepted for restricted use within NHS Scotland for the treatment of type 2 diabetes mellitus in patients unable to achieve adequate glycaemic control with metformin alone or those already treated with vildagliptin and metformin as separate tablets.

- MEDICINAL FORMS
  There can be variation in the licensing of different medicines containing the same drug.
  Tablet
  CAUTIONARY AND ADVISORY LABELS 21
  ▸ Eucreas (Novartis Pharmaceuticals UK Ltd)
  Vildagliptin 50 mg, Metformin hydrochloride 850 mg Eucreas 50mg/850mg tablets | 60 tablet PoM £35.68 DT = £35.68
  Vildagliptin 50 mg, Metformin hydrochloride 1 gram Eucreas 50mg/1000mg tablets | 60 tablet PoM £35.68 DT = £35.68

BLOOD GLUCOSE LOWERING DRUGS ⟩
GLUCAGON-LIKE PEPTIDE-1 RECEPTOR AGONISTS

Albiglutide   01-Jun-2016

- DRUG ACTION Albiglutide is a GLP-1 (glucagon-like peptide-1) receptor agonist that augments glucose-dependent insulin secretion, and slows gastric emptying.

- INDICATIONS AND DOSE

  Type 2 diabetes mellitus as monotherapy when treatment with metformin is considered inappropriate | Type 2 diabetes mellitus in combination with basal insulin and other oral glucose lowering agents
  ▸ BY SUBCUTANEOUS INJECTION
  ▸ Adult: 30 mg once weekly, increased if necessary up to 50 mg once weekly, to be administered on the same day each week

  DOSE ADJUSTMENTS DUE TO INTERACTIONS
  ▸ Dose of concomitant insulin or drugs that stimulate insulin secretion may need to be reduced.

- CONTRA-INDICATIONS Severe gastrointestinal disease—no information available
- CAUTIONS History of pancreatitis · moderate to severe heart failure—no information available
- INTERACTIONS → Appendix 1: albiglutide
- SIDE-EFFECTS
  ▸ **Common or very common** Arrhythmias · constipation · diarrhoea · dyspepsia · gastrointestinal disorders · hypoglycaemia · nausea · pneumonia · vomiting
  ▸ **Uncommon** Pancreatitis (discontinue)
  ▸ **Frequency not known** Appetite decreased
- CONCEPTION AND CONTRACEPTION Manufacturer recommends effective contraception in women of childbearing potential. Discontinue treatment at least one month before a planned pregnancy.
- PREGNANCY Manufacturer advises avoid—toxicity in *animal* studies.
- BREAST FEEDING Manufacturer advises avoid—no information available.
- RENAL IMPAIRMENT Manufacturer advises avoid if eGFR less than 30 mL/minute/1.73 m².
- HANDLING AND STORAGE Store at 2–8°C. May be stored at temperatures up to 30°C for up to 4 weeks.
- PATIENT AND CARER ADVICE Patients or carers should be given advice on how to administer albiglutide injection.
  Acute pancreatitis Patients should be told how to recognise signs and symptoms of acute pancreatitis and advised to seek medical attention if symptoms such as persistent, severe abdominal pain develop.
  Missed doses If a dose is missed it should be administered as soon as possible within 3 days; if more than 3 days have passed, the missed dose should not be taken and the next dose should be taken at the normal time.
- NATIONAL FUNDING/ACCESS DECISIONS

  Scottish Medicines Consortium (SMC) Decisions
  The *Scottish Medicines Consortium* has advised (January 2016) that albiglutide (*Eperzan*®) is accepted for restricted use for treating adults with type 2 diabetes to improve glycaemic control in combination with other glucose-lowering medicines when these, together with diet and exercise, do not provide adequate glycaemic control. It is restricted to use as an alternative once weekly GLP-1 mimetic for use in combination with oral anti-diabetic agents as a third-line pre-insulin treatment option.

- MEDICINAL FORMS
  There can be variation in the licensing of different medicines containing the same drug.
  Powder and solvent for solution for injection
  ▸ Eperzan (GlaxoSmithKline UK Ltd) ▼
  Albiglutide 30 mg Eperzan 30mg powder and solvent for solution for injection pre-filled pen | 4 pre-filled disposable injection PoM £71.00
  Albiglutide 50 mg Eperzan 50mg powder and solvent for solution for injection pre-filled pen | 4 pre-filled disposable injection PoM £71.00

Dulaglutide   14-Jun-2016

- DRUG ACTION Dulaglutide is a long-acting glucagon-like peptide 1 (GLP-1) receptor agonist that augments glucose-dependent insulin secretion, and slows gastric emptying.

- INDICATIONS AND DOSE

  Type 2 diabetes mellitus as monotherapy if metformin inappropriate
  ▸ BY SUBCUTANEOUS INJECTION
  ▸ Adult: 0.75 mg once weekly

continued →

Type 2 diabetes mellitus in combination with insulin or other antidiabetic drugs (if existing treatment fails to achieve adequate glycaemic control)
▶ BY SUBCUTANEOUS INJECTION
  ▶ Adult: 1.5 mg once weekly
  DOSE ADJUSTMENTS DUE TO INTERACTIONS
  ▶ Dose of concomitant insulin or drugs that stimulate insulin secretion may need to be reduced.

● CONTRA-INDICATIONS Severe gastro-intestinal disease— no information available
● CAUTIONS Congestive heart failure—no information available
● INTERACTIONS → Appendix 1: dulaglutide
● SIDE-EFFECTS
  ▶ **Common or very common** Appetite decreased · atrioventricular block · burping · constipation · diarrhoea · fatigue · gastrointestinal discomfort · gastrointestinal disorders · hypoglycaemia · nausea · sinus tachycardia · vomiting
  ▶ **Rare or very rare** Anaphylactic reaction · angioedema · pancreatitis acute (discontinue)
● PREGNANCY Manufacturer advises avoid—toxicity in *animal* studies.
● BREAST FEEDING Manufacturer advises avoid— no information available.
● RENAL IMPAIRMENT Manufacturer advises avoid in severe impairment and end stage renal disease—no information available.
● HANDLING AND STORAGE **Refrigerated storage** is usually necessary (2 °C – 8 °C). Once in use, may be stored unrefrigerated for up to 14 days at a temperature not above 30 °C.
● PATIENT AND CARER ADVICE Patients or carers should be given advice on how to administer dulaglutide injection. Acute pancreatitis Patients should be told how to recognise signs and symptoms of acute pancreatitis and advised to seek medical attention if symptoms such as persistent, severe abdominal pain develop.
  Missed doses If a dose is missed, it should be administered as soon as possible only if there are at least 3 days until the next scheduled dose; if less than 3 days remain before the next scheduled dose, the missed dose should not be taken and the next dose should be taken at the normal time.
● NATIONAL FUNDING/ACCESS DECISIONS
  Scottish Medicines Consortium (SMC) Decisions
  The *Scottish Medicines Consortium* has advised (January 2016) that dulaglutide (*Trulicity*®) is accepted for restricted use for treating adults with type 2 diabetes to improve glycaemic control as add-on therapy in combination with other glucose-lowering medicines, when these, together with diet and exercise, do not provide adequate glycaemic control. It is restricted to use as part of a triple therapy in people with inadequate glycaemic control on 2 oral anti-diabetic medicines, as an alternative GLP-1 mimetic option.

● MEDICINAL FORMS
  There can be variation in the licensing of different medicines containing the same drug.
  Solution for injection
  ▶ Trulicity (Eli Lilly and Company Ltd) ▼
    Dulaglutide 1.5 mg per 1 ml Trulicity 0.75mg/0.5ml solution for injection pre-filled pen | 4 pre-filled disposable injection PoM £73.25
    DT = £73.25
    Dulaglutide 3 mg per 1 ml Trulicity 1.5mg/0.5ml solution for injection pre-filled pen | 4 pre-filled disposable injection PoM £73.25
    DT = £73.25

Exenatide

● DRUG ACTION Binds to, and activates, the GLP-1 (glucagon-like peptide-1) receptor to increase insulin secretion, suppresses glucagon secretion, and slows gastric emptying.

● INDICATIONS AND DOSE
  Type 2 diabetes mellitus in combination with metformin or a sulfonylurea, or both, or with pioglitazone, or with both metformin and pioglitazone, in patients who have not achieved adequate glycaemic control with these drugs alone or in combination
  ▶ BY SUBCUTANEOUS INJECTION USING IMMEDIATE-RELEASE MEDICINES
    ▶ Adult: Initially 5 micrograms twice daily for at least 1 month, then increased if necessary up to 10 micrograms twice daily, dose to be taken within 1 hour before 2 main meals (at least 6 hours apart)
  ▶ BY SUBCUTANEOUS INJECTION USING MODIFIED-RELEASE MEDICINES
    ▶ Adult: 2 mg once weekly
  Type 2 diabetes mellitus in combination with basal insulin alone or with metformin or pioglitazone (or both)
  ▶ BY SUBCUTANEOUS INJECTION USING IMMEDIATE-RELEASE MEDICINES
    ▶ Adult: Initially 5 micrograms twice daily for at least 1 month, then increased if necessary up to 10 micrograms twice daily, dose to be taken within 1 hour before 2 main meals (at least 6 hours apart)
  DOSE ADJUSTMENTS DUE TO INTERACTIONS
  ▶ Dose of concomitant sulfonylurea may need to be reduced.
  PHARMACOKINETICS
  ▶ Effect of *modified-release* exenatide injection (*Bydureon*®) may persist for 10 weeks after discontinuation.

● CONTRA-INDICATIONS Ketoacidosis · severe gastro-intestinal disease
● CAUTIONS Elderly · may cause weight loss greater than 1.5 kg weekly · pancreatitis
● INTERACTIONS → Appendix 1: exenatide
● SIDE-EFFECTS
  ▶ **Common or very common** Appetite decreased · asthenia · constipation · diarrhoea · dizziness · gastrointestinal discomfort · gastrointestinal disorders · headache · nausea · skin reactions · vomiting
  ▶ **Uncommon** Alopecia · burping · drowsiness · hyperhidrosis · renal impairment · taste altered
  ▶ **Frequency not known** Angioedema · pancreatitis acute
  SIDE-EFFECTS, FURTHER INFORMATION Severe pancreatitis (sometimes fatal), including haemorrhagic or necrotising pancreatitis, has been reported rarely; discontinue permanently if diagnosed.
● CONCEPTION AND CONTRACEPTION Women of child-bearing age should use effective contraception during treatment with modified-release exenatide and for 12 weeks after discontinuation.
● PREGNANCY Avoid—toxicity in *animal* studies.
● BREAST FEEDING Avoid—no information available.
● RENAL IMPAIRMENT For *standard-release* injection, use with caution if eGFR 30–50 mL/minute/1.73 m². For *standard-release* injection, avoid if eGFR less than 30 mL/minute/1.73 m². For *modified-release* injection, avoid if eGFR less than 50 mL/minute/1.73 m².
● PATIENT AND CARER ADVICE Patients changing from standard-release to modified-release exenatide formulation may experience initial transient increase in blood glucose. Some oral medications should be taken at

least 1 hour before or 4 hours after exenatide injection—consult product literature for details. Patients or their carers should be told how to recognise signs and symptoms of pancreatitis and advised to seek prompt medical attention if symptoms such as abdominal pain, nausea, and vomiting develop.

Missed doses If a dose of the immediate-release medicine is missed, continue with the next scheduled dose—do not administer **after** a meal.

● NATIONAL FUNDING/ACCESS DECISIONS

Scottish Medicines Consortium (SMC) Decisions

The *Scottish Medicines Consortium* has advised (June 2007) that standard-release exenatide (*Byetta*®) is accepted for restricted use within NHS Scotland for the treatment of type 2 diabetes in combination with metformin or sulfonylurea (or both), as an alternative to treatment with insulin in patients where treatment with metformin or sulfonylurea (or both) at maximally tolerated doses has been inadequate, and treatment with insulin would be the next option.

The *Scottish Medicines Consortium* has also advised (February 2011) that standard-release exenatide (*Byetta*®) is accepted for restricted use within NHS Scotland for the treatment of type 2 diabetes in combination with metformin and pioglitazone as a third-line pre-insulin treatment option.

The *Scottish Medicines Consortium* has advised (December 2011) that modified-release exenatide (*Bydureon*®) is accepted for restricted use within NHS Scotland for the treatment of type 2 diabetes as a third-line treatment option.

● MEDICINAL FORMS

There can be variation in the licensing of different medicines containing the same drug.

Solution for injection

CAUTIONARY AND ADVISORY LABELS 10

▸ Byetta (AstraZeneca UK Ltd)

Exenatide 250 microgram per 1 ml Byetta 10micrograms/0.04ml solution for injection 2.4ml pre-filled disposable devices | 1 pre-filled disposable injection [PoM] £81.89 DT = £81.89
Byetta 5micrograms/0.02ml solution for injection 1.2ml pre-filled disposable devices | 1 pre-filled disposable injection [PoM] £81.89 DT = £81.89

Powder and solvent for prolonged-release suspension for inj

CAUTIONARY AND ADVISORY LABELS 10

▸ Bydureon (AstraZeneca UK Ltd)

Exenatide 2 mg Bydureon 2mg powder and solvent for prolonged-release suspension for injection pre-filled pen | 4 pre-filled disposable injection [PoM] £73.36 DT = £73.36

Liraglutide

19-Jan-2018

● DRUG ACTION Liraglutide binds to, and activates, the GLP-1 (glucagon-like peptide-1) receptor to increase insulin secretion, suppresses glucagon secretion, and slows gastric emptying.

● INDICATIONS AND DOSE

SAXENDA®

Adjunct in weight management [in conjunction with dietary measures and increased physical activity in individuals with a body mass index (BMI) of 30 kg/m^2 or more, or in individuals with a BMI of 27 kg/m^2 or more in the presence of at least one weight-related co-morbidity]

▸ BY SUBCUTANEOUS INJECTION

▸ Adult: Initially 0.6 mg once daily, then increased in steps of 0.6 mg, dose to be increased at intervals of at least 1 week; consider discontinuation if escalation to the next dose is not tolerated for 2 consecutive weeks.

Discontinue if at least 5% of initial body-weight has not been lost after 12 weeks at maximum dose; maximum 3 mg per day

VICTOZA®

Type 2 diabetes mellitus [monotherapy (if metformin inappropriate), or in combination with other antidiabetic drugs]

▸ BY SUBCUTANEOUS INJECTION

▸ Adult: Initially 0.6 mg once daily for at least 1 week, then increased to 1.2 mg once daily for at least 1 week, then increased if necessary to 1.8 mg once daily, for information on use with other antidiabetic drugs—consult product literature

DOSE ADJUSTMENTS DUE TO INTERACTIONS

▸ Dose of concomitant insulin or sulfonylurea may need to be reduced.

● CONTRA-INDICATIONS Diabetic gastroparesis · inflammatory bowel disease · severe congestive heart failure—no information available

SAXENDA® Concomitant use with other products for weight management · elderly 75 years or over (limited information) · obesity secondary to endocrinological or eating disorders

VICTOZA® Diabetic ketoacidosis

● CAUTIONS Thyroid disease

● INTERACTIONS → Appendix 1: liraglutide

● SIDE-EFFECTS

▸ Common or very common Asthenia · burping · constipation · diarrhoea · dizziness · dry mouth · gallbladder disorders · gastrointestinal discomfort · gastrointestinal disorders · insomnia · nausea · taste altered · vomiting

▸ Uncommon Malaise · pancreatitis · tachycardia · urticaria

▸ Rare or very rare Renal impairment

SIDE-EFFECTS, FURTHER INFORMATION Discontinue if symptoms of acute pancreatitis occur, such as persistent, severe abdominal pain.

● PREGNANCY Manufacturer advises avoid—toxicity in *animal* studies (recommendation also supported by tertiary sources).

● BREAST FEEDING Manufacturer advises avoid—no information available; *animal* studies suggest that transfer into milk is low, but excretion into human milk not known (a tertiary source confirms lack of information in human lactation, but also states that risk to infants appears to be negligible. [EvGr] Blood glucose monitoring of the infant should be considered) ⬦.

● HEPATIC IMPAIRMENT

SAXENDA® Manufacturer advises use with caution in mild-to-moderate impairment; avoid in severe impairment.

VICTOZA® Manufacturer advises avoid in severe impairment.

● RENAL IMPAIRMENT

SAXENDA® Manufacturer advises avoid if creatinine clearance less than 30 mL/minute.

● HANDLING AND STORAGE Manufacturer advises store in a refrigerator (2–8°C)—after first use can also be stored below 30°C and used within 1 month; keep cap on pen to protect from light.

● PATIENT AND CARER ADVICE Manufacturer advises patients and their carers should be told how to recognise signs and symptoms of acute pancreatitis and advised to seek immediate medical attention if symptoms develop. Manufacturer advises patients and their carers should be informed of the potential risk of dehydration in relation to gastro-intestinal side-effects and advised to take precautions to avoid fluid depletion; they should also be informed of the symptoms of cholelithiasis and cholecystitis, and of increased heart rate.

SAXENDA ® **Missed doses** Manufacturer advises if a dose is more than 12 hours late, the missed dose should not be taken and the next dose should be taken at the normal time.

● MEDICINAL FORMS
There can be variation in the licensing of different medicines containing the same drug.
Solution for injection
▸ Saxenda (Novo Nordisk Ltd) ▼
   Liraglutide 6 mg per 1 ml Saxenda 6mg/ml solution for injection 3ml pre-filled pen | 5 pre-filled disposable injection PoM £196.20
▸ Victoza (Novo Nordisk Ltd)
   Liraglutide 6 mg per 1 ml Victoza 6mg/ml solution for injection 3ml pre-filled pen | 2 pre-filled disposable injection PoM £78.48 DT = £78.48 | 3 pre-filled disposable injection PoM £117.72

Combinations available: *Insulin degludec with liraglutide,* p. 700

Lixisenatide

● DRUG ACTION Binds to, and activates, the GLP-1 (glucagon-like peptide-1) receptor to increase insulin secretion, suppresses glucagon secretion, and slows gastric emptying.

● INDICATIONS AND DOSE

Type 2 diabetes mellitus in combination with oral antidiabetic drugs (e.g. metformin, pioglitazone, or a sulfonylurea) or basal insulin, or both, when adequate glycaemic control has not been achieved with these drugs
   ▸ BY SUBCUTANEOUS INJECTION
   ▸ Adult: Initially 10 micrograms once daily for 14 days, then increased to 20 micrograms once daily, dose to be taken within 1 hour before the first meal of the day or the evening meal

DOSE ADJUSTMENTS DUE TO INTERACTIONS
   ▸ Dose of concomitant sulfonylurea or insulin may need to be reduced.

● CONTRA-INDICATIONS Ketoacidosis · severe gastro-intestinal disease
● INTERACTIONS → Appendix 1: lixisenatide
● SIDE-EFFECTS
▸ **Common or very common** Back pain · cystitis · diarrhoea · dizziness · drowsiness · dyspepsia · headache · increased risk of infection · nausea · vomiting
▸ **Uncommon** Urticaria

SIDE-EFFECTS, FURTHER INFORMATION Discontinue if symptoms of acute pancreatitis occur, such as persistent, severe abdominal pain.

● CONCEPTION AND CONTRACEPTION Women of child-bearing age should use effective contraception.
● PREGNANCY Avoid—toxicity in *animal* studies.
● BREAST FEEDING Avoid—no information available.
● RENAL IMPAIRMENT Use with caution if eGFR 30–50 mL/minute/1.73 m^2. Avoid if eGFR less than 30 mL/minute/1.73 m^2—no information available.
● PATIENT AND CARER ADVICE Some oral medications should be taken at least 1 hour before or 4 hours after lixisenatide injection—consult product literature for details.
Missed doses If a dose is missed, inject within 1 hour before the next meal—do not administer **after** a meal.
● NATIONAL FUNDING/ACCESS DECISIONS

Scottish Medicines Consortium (SMC) Decisions
The *Scottish Medicines Consortium* has advised (August 2013) that lixisenatide (*Lyxumia ®*) is accepted for restricted use within NHS Scotland for the treatment of

type 2 diabetes in combination with oral antidiabetic drugs or basal insulin (or both), when adequate glycaemic control has not been achieved with these drugs; use is restricted to patients in whom a GLP-1 agonist is appropriate, as an alternative to an existing GLP-1 agonist (exenatide or liraglutide).

● MEDICINAL FORMS
There can be variation in the licensing of different medicines containing the same drug.
Solution for injection
CAUTIONARY AND ADVISORY LABELS 10
▸ Lyxumia (Sanofi)
   Lixisenatide 50 microgram per 1 ml Lyxumia 10micrograms/0.2ml solution for injection 3ml pre-filled pen | 1 pre-filled disposable injection PoM £31.67 DT = £31.67
   Lixisenatide 100 microgram per 1 ml Lyxumia 20micrograms/0.2ml solution for injection 3ml pre-filled pen | 2 pre-filled disposable injection PoM £57.93 DT = £57.93

BLOOD GLUCOSE LOWERING DRUGS ⟩
MEGLITINIDES

Nateglinide

● DRUG ACTION Nateglinide stimulates insulin secretion.

● INDICATIONS AND DOSE

Type 2 diabetes mellitus in combination with metformin when metformin alone inadequate
   ▸ BY MOUTH
   ▸ Adult: Initially 60 mg 3 times a day (max. per dose 180 mg), adjusted according to response, to be taken within 30 minutes before main meals

● CONTRA-INDICATIONS Ketoacidosis
● CAUTIONS Debilitated patients · elderly · malnourished patients

CAUTIONS, FURTHER INFORMATION Substitute insulin during intercurrent illness (such as myocardial infarction, coma, infection, and trauma) and during surgery (omit nateglinide on morning of surgery and recommence when eating and drinking normally).

● INTERACTIONS → Appendix 1: nateglinide
● SIDE-EFFECTS
▸ **Common or very common** Diarrhoea · gastrointestinal discomfort · hypoglycaemia · nausea
▸ **Uncommon** Vomiting
▸ **Rare or very rare** Skin reactions
▸ **Frequency not known** Appetite increased · dizziness · fatigue · muscle weakness · palpitations · sweating abnormal · tremor

● PREGNANCY Avoid—toxicity in *animal* studies.
● BREAST FEEDING Avoid—present in milk in *animal* studies.
● HEPATIC IMPAIRMENT Caution in moderate hepatic impairment. Avoid in severe impairment—no information available.
● PATIENT AND CARER ADVICE
Driving and skilled tasks Drivers need to be particularly careful to avoid hypoglycaemia and should be warned of the problems.

● MEDICINAL FORMS
There can be variation in the licensing of different medicines containing the same drug.
Tablet
▸ Starlix (Novartis Pharmaceuticals UK Ltd)
   Nateglinide 60 mg Starlix 60mg tablets | 84 tablet PoM £26.12 DT = £26.12
   Nateglinide 120 mg Starlix 120mg tablets | 84 tablet PoM £29.76 DT = £29.76
   Nateglinide 180 mg Starlix 180mg tablets | 84 tablet PoM £29.76 DT = £29.76

Repaglinide

● DRUG ACTION Repaglinide stimulates insulin secretion.

● **INDICATIONS AND DOSE**

Type 2 diabetes mellitus (as monotherapy or in combination with metformin when metformin alone inadequate)

▶ BY MOUTH
▸ Adult 18–74 years: Initially 500 micrograms (max. per dose 4 mg), adjusted according to response, dose to be taken within 30 minutes before main meals and adjusted at intervals of 1–2 weeks; maximum 16 mg per day
▸ Adult 75 years and over: Not recommended

Type 2 diabetes mellitus (as monotherapy or in combination with metformin when metformin alone inadequate), if transferring from another oral antidiabetic drug

▶ BY MOUTH
▸ Adult 18–74 years: Initially 1 mg (max. per dose 4 mg), adjusted according to response, dose to be taken within 30 minutes before main meals and adjusted at intervals of 1–2 weeks; maximum 16 mg per day
▸ Adult 75 years and over: Not recommended

● CONTRA-INDICATIONS Ketoacidosis

● CAUTIONS Debilitated patients · malnourished patients
  CAUTIONS, FURTHER INFORMATION Substitute insulin during intercurrent illness (such as myocardial infarction, coma, infection, and trauma) and during surgery.

● INTERACTIONS → Appendix 1: repaglinide

● SIDE-EFFECTS
▶ **Common or very common** Abdominal pain · diarrhoea · hypoglycaemia
▶ **Rare or very rare** Cardiovascular disease · constipation · hepatic function abnormal · vasculitis · vision disorders · vomiting
▶ **Frequency not known** Acute coronary syndrome · hypoglycaemic coma · nausea · skin reactions

● PREGNANCY Avoid.

● BREAST FEEDING Avoid—present in milk in *animal* studies.

● HEPATIC IMPAIRMENT Avoid in severe liver disease.

● RENAL IMPAIRMENT Use with caution.

● PATIENT AND CARER ADVICE
  Driving and skilled tasks Drivers need to be particularly careful to avoid hypoglycaemia and should be warned of the problems.

● MEDICINAL FORMS
  There can be variation in the licensing of different medicines containing the same drug.

Tablet
▶ Repaglinide (Non-proprietary)
  Repaglinide 500 microgram Repaglinide 500microgram tablets | 30 tablet [PoM] £3.01–£3.92 | 90 tablet [PoM] £11.76 DT = £9.03
  Repaglinide 1 mg Repaglinide 1mg tablets | 30 tablet [PoM] £3.33–£3.92 | 90 tablet [PoM] £11.76 DT = £10.36
  Repaglinide 2 mg Repaglinide 2mg tablets | 90 tablet [PoM] £28.00 DT = £5.88
▶ Enyglid (Consilient Health Ltd)
  Repaglinide 500 microgram Enyglid 0.5mg tablets | 30 tablet [PoM] £3.33 | 90 tablet [PoM] £9.99 DT = £9.03
  Repaglinide 1 mg Enyglid 1mg tablets | 30 tablet [PoM] £3.33 | 90 tablet [PoM] £9.99 DT = £10.36
  Repaglinide 2 mg Enyglid 2mg tablets | 90 tablet [PoM] £9.99 DT = £5.88
▶ Prandin (Novo Nordisk Ltd)
  Repaglinide 500 microgram Prandin 0.5mg tablets | 30 tablet [PoM] £3.92
  Repaglinide 1 mg Prandin 1mg tablets | 30 tablet [PoM] £3.92
  Repaglinide 2 mg Prandin 2mg tablets | 90 tablet [PoM] £11.76 DT = £5.88

BLOOD GLUCOSE LOWERING DRUGS > SODIUM GLUCOSE CO-TRANSPORTER 2 INHIBITORS

Canagliflozin

11-Apr-2017

● DRUG ACTION Reversibly inhibits sodium-glucose co-transporter 2 (SGLT2) in the renal proximal convoluted tubule to reduce glucose reabsorption and increase urinary glucose excretion.

● **INDICATIONS AND DOSE**

Type 2 diabetes mellitus as monotherapy (if metformin inappropriate) | Type 2 diabetes mellitus in combination with insulin or other antidiabetic drugs (if existing treatment fails to achieve adequate glycaemic control)

▶ BY MOUTH
▸ Adult: 100 mg once daily; increased if tolerated to 300 mg once daily if required, dose to be taken preferably before breakfast

DOSE ADJUSTMENTS DUE TO INTERACTIONS
▸ Manufacturer advises increase dose if tolerated to 300 mg once daily with concurrent use of rifampicin.

IMPORTANT SAFETY INFORMATION
MHRA/CHM ADVICE (UPDATED MARCH 2017): INCREASED RISK OF LOWER-LIMB AMPUTATION (MAINLY TOES)
Canagliflozin may increase the risk of lower-limb amputation (mainly toes) in patients with type 2 diabetes. Preventive foot care is important for all patients with diabetes. The MHRA has issued the following advice while clinical trials are ongoing:
● consider stopping canagliflozin if a patient develops a significant lower limb complication (e.g. skin ulcer, osteomyelitis, or gangrene)
● carefully monitor patients who have risk factors for amputation (e.g. previous amputations, existing peripheral vascular disease, or neuropathy)
● monitor all patients for signs and symptoms of water or salt loss; ensure patients stay sufficiently hydrated to prevent volume depletion in line with the manufacturer's recommendations
● advise patients to stay well hydrated, carry out routine preventive foot care, and seek medical advice promptly if they develop skin ulceration, discolouration, or new pain or tenderness
● start treatment for foot problems (e.g. ulceration, infection, or new pain or tenderness) as early as possible
● continue to follow standard treatment guidelines for routine preventive foot care for people with diabetes.

MHRA/CHM ADVICE (UPDATED APRIL 2016): RISK OF DIABETIC KETOACIDOSIS WITH SODIUM-GLUCOSE CO-TRANSPORTER 2 (SGLT2) INHIBITORS (CANAGLIFLOZIN, DAPAGLIFLOZIN OR EMPAGLIFLOZIN)
A review by the European Medicines Agency has concluded that serious, life-threatening, and fatal cases of diabetic ketoacidosis (DKA) have been reported rarely in patients taking an SGLT2 inhibitor. In several cases, the presentation of DKA was atypical with patients having only moderately elevated blood glucose levels, and some of them occurred during off-label use.
  To minimise the risk of such effects when treating patients with a SGLT2 inhibitor, the European Medicines Agency has issued the following advice:
● inform patients of the signs and symptoms of DKA, (including rapid weight loss, nausea or vomiting, abdominal pain, fast and deep breathing, sleepiness, a sweet smell to the breath, a sweet or metallic taste in the mouth, or a different odour to urine or sweat), and advise them to seek immediate medical advice if they develop any of these

- test for raised ketones in patients with signs and symptoms of DKA, even if plasma glucose levels are near-normal
- use canagliflozin with caution in patients with risk factors for DKA, (including a low beta cell reserve, conditions leading to restricted food intake or severe dehydration, sudden reduction in insulin, increased insulin requirements due to acute illness, surgery or alcohol abuse), and discuss these risk factors with patients
- discontinue treatment if DKA is suspected or diagnosed
- do not restart treatment with any SGLT2 inhibitor in patients who experienced DKA during use, unless another cause for DKA was identified and resolved
- interrupt SGLT2 treatment in patients who are hospitalised for major surgery or acute serious illnesses; treatment may be restarted once the patient's condition has stabilised

- CONTRA-INDICATIONS Ketoacidosis
- CAUTIONS Cardiovascular disease (risk of hypotension) · elderly (risk of hypotension) · elevated haematocrit · history of hypotension

  CAUTIONS, FURTHER INFORMATION
  ▸ Volume depletion Correct hypovolaemia before starting treatment.
- INTERACTIONS → Appendix 1: canagliflozin
- SIDE-EFFECTS
  ▸ **Common or very common** Balanoposthitis · constipation · dyslipidaemia · hypoglycaemia (in combination with insulin or sulphonylurea) · increased risk of infection · nausea · thirst · urinary disorders · urosepsis
  ▸ **Uncommon** Dehydration · dizziness postural · hypotension · lower limb amputations · renal failure · skin reactions · syncope
  ▸ **Rare or very rare** Anaphylactic reaction · angioedema · diabetic ketoacidosis

  SIDE-EFFECTS, FURTHER INFORMATION Consider interrupting treatment if volume depletion occurs.
- PREGNANCY Avoid—toxicity in *animal* studies.
- BREAST FEEDING Avoid—present in milk in *animal* studies.
- HEPATIC IMPAIRMENT Manufacturer advises avoid in severe impairment—no information available.
- RENAL IMPAIRMENT Avoid initiation if eGFR less than 60 mL/minute/1.73 m^2. Avoid if eGFR less than 45 mL/minute/1.73 m^2.
  Dose adjustments Reduce dose to 100 mg once daily if eGFR falls persistently below 60 mL/minute/1.73 m^2 and existing canagliflozin treatment tolerated.
  Monitoring Monitor renal function at least twice a year in moderate impairment.
- MONITORING REQUIREMENTS Determine renal function before treatment and at least annually thereafter, and before initiation of concomitant drugs that reduce renal function and periodically thereafter.
- PATIENT AND CARER ADVICE Patients should be advised to report symptoms of volume depletion including postural hypotension and dizziness. Patients should be informed of the signs and symptoms of diabetic ketoacidosis, see MHRA advice.
- NATIONAL FUNDING/ACCESS DECISIONS
  NICE decisions
  ▸ **Canagliflozin, dapagliflozin and empagliflozin as monotherapies for treating type 2 diabetes (May 2016)** NICE TA390
  Canagliflozin as monotherapy is recommended as an option for treating type 2 diabetes in adults for whom metformin is contra-indicated or not tolerated, only if a dipeptidyl peptidase-4 (DPP-4) inhibitor would otherwise be prescribed **and** a sulfonylurea or pioglitazone is not appropriate.
  Patients currently receiving canagliflozin whose disease does not meet the above criteria should be able to continue treatment until they and their clinician consider it appropriate to stop.
  www.nice.org.uk/TA390
  ▸ **Canagliflozin in combination therapy for treating type 2 diabetes (June 2014)** NICE TA315
  Canagliflozin in a dual therapy regimen in combination with metformin is recommended for the treatment of type 2 diabetes, only if a sulfonylurea is contra-indicated or not tolerated *or* the patient has a significant risk of hypoglycaemia.
  Canagliflozin in a triple therapy regimen is an option for the treatment of type 2 diabetes in combination with metformin and a sulfonylurea *or* metformin and a thiazolidinedione.
  Canagliflozin in combination with insulin (alone or with other antidiabetic drugs) is an option for the treatment of type 2 diabetes.
  Patients currently receiving canagliflozin in a dual or triple therapy regimen that is not recommended according to the above criteria should have the option to continue treatment until they and their clinician consider it appropriate to stop.
  www.nice.org.uk/TA315

- MEDICINAL FORMS
  There can be variation in the licensing of different medicines containing the same drug.
  Tablet
  ▸ Invokana (Napp Pharmaceuticals Ltd) ▼
    Canagliflozin (as Canagliflozin hemihydrate) 100 mg Invokana 100mg tablets | 30 tablet [PoM] £39.20 DT = £39.20
    Canagliflozin (as Canagliflozin hemihydrate) 300 mg Invokana 300mg tablets | 30 tablet [PoM] £39.20 DT = £39.20

Canagliflozin with metformin

The properties listed below are those particular to the combination only. For the properties of the components please consider, canagliflozin p. 687, metformin hydrochloride p. 678.

- INDICATIONS AND DOSE

  Type 2 diabetes mellitus not controlled by metformin alone or by metformin in combination with insulin or other antidiabetic drugs
  ▸ BY MOUTH
  ▸ Adult: 1 tablet twice daily, dose based on patient's current metformin dose, daily dose of metformin should not exceed 2 g

  DOSE ADJUSTMENTS DUE TO INTERACTIONS
  ▸ Dose of concomitant insulin or drugs that stimulate insulin secretion may need to be reduced.

- INTERACTIONS → Appendix 1: canagliflozin · metformin
- RENAL IMPAIRMENT Avoid if eGFR less than 60 mL/minute/1.73 m^2.
- NATIONAL FUNDING/ACCESS DECISIONS
  Scottish Medicines Consortium (SMC) Decisions
  The *Scottish Medicines Consortium* has advised (December 2014) that *Vokanamet*® is accepted for restricted use within NHS Scotland in patients with type 2 diabetes mellitus for whom a combination of canagliflozin and metformin is an appropriate choice of therapy.

- MEDICINAL FORMS
There can be variation in the licensing of different medicines containing the same drug.

Tablet

CAUTIONARY AND ADVISORY LABELS 21

▸ Vokanamet (Napp Pharmaceuticals Ltd) ▼

Canagliflozin (as Canagliflozin hemihydrate) 50 mg, Metformin hydrochloride 850 mg Vokanamet 50mg/850mg tablets | 60 tablet [PoM] £39.20 DT = £39.20

Canagliflozin (as Canagliflozin hemihydrate) 50 mg, Metformin hydrochloride 1 gram Vokanamet 50mg/1000mg tablets | 60 tablet [PoM] £39.20 DT = £39.20

Dapagliflozin

18-May-2017

- DRUG ACTION Reversibly inhibits sodium-glucose co-transporter 2 (SGLT2) in the renal proximal convoluted tubule to reduce glucose reabsorption and increase urinary glucose excretion.

- INDICATIONS AND DOSE

Type 2 diabetes mellitus as monotherapy (if metformin inappropriate) | Type 2 diabetes mellitus in combination with insulin or other antidiabetic drugs (if existing treatment fails to achieve adequate glycaemic control)

▸ BY MOUTH

▸ Adult 18–74 years: 10 mg once daily

▸ Adult 75 years and over: Initiation not recommended

DOSE ADJUSTMENTS DUE TO INTERACTIONS

▸ Dose of concomitant insulin or drugs that stimulate insulin secretion may need to be reduced.

IMPORTANT SAFETY INFORMATION

MHRA/CHM ADVICE (UPDATED APRIL 2016): RISK OF DIABETIC KETOACIDOSIS WITH SODIUM-GLUCOSE CO-TRANSPORTER 2 (SGLT2) INHIBITORS (CANAGLIFLOZIN, DAPAGLIFLOZIN OR EMPAGLIFLOZIN)

A review by the European Medicines Agency has concluded that serious, life-threatening, and fatal cases of diabetic ketoacidosis (DKA) have been reported rarely in patients taking an SGLT2 inhibitor. In several cases, the presentation of DKA was atypical with patients having only moderately elevated blood glucose levels, and some of them occurred during off-label use.

To minimise the risk of such effects when treating patients with a SGLT2 inhibitor, the European Medicines Agency has issued the following advice:

- inform patients of the signs and symptoms of DKA, (including rapid weight loss, nausea or vomiting, abdominal pain, fast and deep breathing, sleepiness, a sweet smell to the breath, a sweet or metallic taste in the mouth, or a different odour to urine or sweat), and advise them to seek immediate medical advice if they develop any of these

- test for raised ketones in patients with signs and symptoms of DKA, even if plasma glucose levels are near-normal

- use dapagliflozin with caution in patients with risk factors for DKA, (including a low beta cell reserve, conditions leading to restricted food intake or severe dehydration, sudden reduction in insulin, increased insulin requirements due to acute illness, surgery or alcohol abuse), and discuss these risk factors with patients

- discontinue treatment if DKA is suspected or diagnosed

- do not restart treatment with any SGLT2 inhibitor in patients who experienced DKA during use, unless another cause for DKA was identified and resolved

- interrupt SGLT2 treatment in patients who are hospitalised for major surgery or acute serious illnesses; treatment may be restarted once the patient's condition has stabilised

- CONTRA-INDICATIONS Ketoacidosis

- CAUTIONS Cardiovascular disease (risk of hypotension) · elderly (risk of hypotension) · electrolyte disturbances · hypotension · raised haematocrit

CAUTIONS, FURTHER INFORMATION

▸ Volume depletion Correct hypovolaemia before starting treatment.

- INTERACTIONS → Appendix 1: dapagliflozin

- SIDE-EFFECTS

▸ **Common or very common** Back pain · balanoposthitis · dizziness · dyslipidaemia · hypoglycaemia (in combination with insulin or sulphonylurea) · increased risk of infection · rash · urinary disorders

▸ **Uncommon** Constipation · dry mouth · genital pruritus · hypovolaemia · renal impairment · thirst · vulvovaginal pruritus · weight decreased

▸ **Rare or very rare** Diabetic ketoacidosis

SIDE-EFFECTS, FURTHER INFORMATION Interrupt treatment if volume depletion occurs.

- PREGNANCY Avoid—toxicity in *animal* studies.

- BREAST FEEDING Avoid—present in milk in *animal* studies.

- HEPATIC IMPAIRMENT

Dose adjustments Initial dose 5 mg daily in severe impairment, increased according to response.

- RENAL IMPAIRMENT Avoid if eGFR less than 60 mL/minute/1.73 m^2 (ineffective).

- MONITORING REQUIREMENTS Determine renal function before treatment and at least annually thereafter.

- PATIENT AND CARER ADVICE Patients should be informed of the signs and symptoms of diabetic ketoacidosis, see MHRA advice.

- NATIONAL FUNDING/ACCESS DECISIONS

NICE decisions

▸ **Dapagliflozin in combination therapy for treating type 2 diabetes (updated November 2016)** NICE TA288

Dapagliflozin in a dual therapy regimen in combination with metformin is recommended for the treatment of type 2 diabetes, only if the patient is at significant risk of hypoglycaemia or its consequences, *or* if a sulfonylurea is contra-indicated or not tolerated.

Dapagliflozin in combination with insulin (alone or with other antidiabetic drugs) is an option for the treatment of type 2 diabetes.

Patients currently receiving dapagliflozin in a dual therapy regimen that is not recommended according to the above criteria should have the option to continue treatment until they and their clinician consider it appropriate to stop.

www.nice.org.uk/TA288

▸ **Canagliflozin, dapagliflozin and empagliflozin as monotherapies for treating type 2 diabetes (May 2016)** NICE TA390

Dapagliflozin as monotherapy is recommended as an option for treating type 2 diabetes in adults for whom metformin is contra-indicated or not tolerated, only if a dipeptidyl peptidase-4 (DPP-4) inhibitor would otherwise be prescribed **and** a sulfonylurea or pioglitazone is not appropriate.

Patients currently receiving dapagliflozin whose disease does not meet the above criteria should be able to continue treatment until they and their clinician consider it appropriate to stop.

www.nice.org.uk/TA390

6

Endocrine system

▸ **Dapagliflozin in triple therapy for treating type 2 diabetes (November 2016)** NICE TA418

Dapagliflozin in a triple therapy regimen is recommended as an option for treating type 2 diabetes in adults, only in combination with metformin and a sulfonylurea.

Patients currently receiving dapagliflozin in other triple therapy regimens, whose treatment was started within the NHS before this guidance was published should have the option to continue treatment, without change to their funding arrangements, until they and their clinician consider it appropriate to stop.
www.nice.org.uk/TA418

Scottish Medicines Consortium (SMC) Decisions
The *Scottish Medicines Consortium* has advised that dapagliflozin (*Forxiga* ®) is accepted for restricted use within NHS Scotland for the treatment of type 2 diabetes in combination with metformin, when treatment with metformin alone is inadequate and a sulfonylurea is inappropriate (December 2012), or in combination with insulin when treatment with insulin alone is inadequate (February 2014).

● **MEDICINAL FORMS**
There can be variation in the licensing of different medicines containing the same drug.

Tablet
▸ Forxiga (AstraZeneca UK Ltd)
Dapagliflozin 5 mg Forxiga 5mg tablets | 28 tablet [PoM] £36.59 DT = £36.59
Dapagliflozin 10 mg Forxiga 10mg tablets | 28 tablet [PoM] £36.59 DT = £36.59

Combinations available: *Saxagliptin with dapagliflozin*, p. 681

Dapagliflozin with metformin

The properties listed below are those particular to the combination only. For the properties of the components please consider, dapagliflozin p. 689, metformin hydrochloride p. 678.

● **INDICATIONS AND DOSE**

Type 2 diabetes mellitus not controlled by metformin alone or by metformin in combination with insulin or other antidiabetic drugs
▸ BY MOUTH
▸ **Adult 18-74 years:** 1 tablet twice daily, based on patient's current metformin dose
▸ **Adult 75 years and over:** Initiation not recommended

● **INTERACTIONS** → Appendix 1: dapagliflozin · metformin

● **HEPATIC IMPAIRMENT** Avoid.

● **NATIONAL FUNDING/ACCESS DECISIONS**
Scottish Medicines Consortium (SMC) Decisions
The *Scottish Medicines Consortium* has advised (July 2014) that dapagliflozin plus metformin (*Xigduo* ®) is accepted for restricted use within NHS Scotland in patients for whom a combination of dapagliflozin and metformin is an appropriate choice of therapy i.e when metformin alone does not provide adequate glycaemic control and a sulfonylurea is inappropriate, *or* in combination with insulin, when insulin and metformin does not provide adequate control, *or* in combination with a sulphonylurea, when a sulfonylurea and metformin does not provide adequate control.

● **MEDICINAL FORMS**
There can be variation in the licensing of different medicines containing the same drug.

Tablet
CAUTIONARY AND ADVISORY LABELS 21
▸ Xigduo (AstraZeneca UK Ltd) ▼
Dapagliflozin 5 mg, Metformin hydrochloride 850 mg Xigduo 5mg/850mg tablets | 56 tablet [PoM] £36.59 DT = £36.59
Dapagliflozin 5 mg, Metformin hydrochloride 1 gram Xigduo 5mg/1000mg tablets | 56 tablet [PoM] £36.59 DT = £36.59

Empagliflozin

18-May-2017

● **DRUG ACTION** Reversibly inhibits sodium-glucose co-transporter 2 (SGLT2) in the renal proximal convoluted tubule to reduce glucose reabsorption and increase urinary glucose excretion.

● **INDICATIONS AND DOSE**

Type 2 diabetes mellitus as monotherapy (if metformin inappropriate) | Type 2 diabetes mellitus in combination with insulin or other antidiabetic drugs (if existing treatment fails to achieve adequate glycaemic control)
▸ BY MOUTH
▸ **Adult 18-84 years:** 10 mg once daily, increased to 25 mg once daily if necessary and if tolerated
▸ **Adult 85 years and over:** Initiation not recommended

DOSE ADJUSTMENTS DUE TO INTERACTIONS
▸ Dose of concomitant insulin or drugs that stimulate insulin secretion may need to be reduced.

IMPORTANT SAFETY INFORMATION

MHRA/CHM ADVICE (UPDATED APRIL 2016): RISK OF DIABETIC KETOACIDOSIS WITH SODIUM-GLUCOSE CO-TRANSPORTER 2 (SGLT2) INHIBITORS (CANAGLIFLOZIN, DAPAGLIFLOZIN OR EMPAGLIFLOZIN)

A review by the European Medicines Agency has concluded that serious, life-threatening, and fatal cases of diabetic ketoacidosis (DKA) have been reported rarely in patients taking an SGLT2 inhibitor. In several cases, the presentation of DKA was atypical with patients having only moderately elevated blood glucose levels, and some of them occurred during off-label use.

To minimise the risk of such effects when treating patients with a SGLT2 inhibitor, the European Medicines Agency has issued the following advice:
● inform patients of the signs and symptoms of DKA, (including rapid weight loss, nausea or vomiting, abdominal pain, fast and deep breathing, sleepiness, a sweet smell to the breath, a sweet or metallic taste in the mouth, or a different odour to urine or sweat), and advise them to seek immediate medical advice if they develop any of these
● test for raised ketones in patients with signs and symptoms of DKA, even if plasma glucose levels are near-normal
● use empagliflozin with caution in patients with risk factors for DKA, (including a low beta cell reserve, conditions leading to restricted food intake or severe dehydration, sudden reduction in insulin, increased insulin requirements due to acute illness, surgery or alcohol abuse), and discuss these risk factors with patients
● discontinue treatment if DKA is suspected or diagnosed
● do not restart treatment with any SGLT2 inhibitor in patients who experienced DKA during use, unless another cause for DKA was identified and resolved
● interrupt SGLT2 treatment in patients who are hospitalised for major surgery or acute serious

illnesses; treatment may be restarted once the patient's condition has stabilised

- **CONTRA-INDICATIONS** Diabetic ketoacidosis
- **CAUTIONS** Cardiovascular disease (increased risk of volume depletion) · complicated urinary tract infections— consider temporarily interrupting treatment · concomitant antihypertensive therapy (increased risk of volume depletion) · elderly patients aged over 75 years (increased risk of volume depletion) · heart failure · history of hypotension (increased risk of volume depletion) · patients at increased risk of volume depletion · predisposition to fluid disturbances e.g. gastro-intestinal illness, concomitant use of diuretics (increased risk of volume depletion)

  CAUTIONS, FURTHER INFORMATION
  ▸ Volume depletion Correct hypovolaemia before starting treatment. Consider interrupting treatment if volume depletion occurs.
- **INTERACTIONS** → Appendix 1: empagliflozin
- **SIDE-EFFECTS**
  ▸ **Common or very common** Balanoposthitis · hypoglycaemia (in combination with insulin or sulphonylurea) · increased risk of infection · pruritus generalised · thirst · urinary disorders
  ▸ **Uncommon** Hypovolaemia
  ▸ **Rare or very rare** Diabetic ketoacidosis
- **PREGNANCY** Manufacturer advises avoid—toxicity in *animal* studies.
- **BREAST FEEDING** Manufacturer advises avoid—present in milk in *animal* studies.
- **HEPATIC IMPAIRMENT** Manufacturer advises avoid in severe impairment—no information available.
- **RENAL IMPAIRMENT** Avoid initiation if eGFR below 60 mL/minute/1.73 m². Avoid if eGFR is persistently below 45 mL/minute/1.73 m².
  Dose adjustments Reduce dose to 10 mg once daily if eGFR falls persistently below 60 mL/minute/1.73 m².
- **MONITORING REQUIREMENTS** Determine renal function before treatment and before initiation of concomitant drugs that may reduce renal function, then at least annually thereafter.
- **PATIENT AND CARER ADVICE** Patients should be informed of the signs and symptoms of diabetic ketoacidosis, see MHRA advice.
- **NATIONAL FUNDING/ACCESS DECISIONS**
  NICE decisions
  ▸ **Canagliflozin, dapagliflozin and empagliflozin as monotherapy for treating type 2 diabetes (May 2016)** NICE TA390
  Empagliflozin as monotherapy is recommended as an option for treating type 2 diabetes in adults for whom metformin is contra-indicated or not tolerated, only if a dipeptidyl peptidase-4 (DPP-4) inhibitor would otherwise be prescribed **and** a sulfonylurea or pioglitazone is not appropriate.
  Patients currently receiving empagliflozin whose disease does not meet the above criteria should be able to continue treatment until they and their clinician consider it appropriate to stop.
  www.nice.org.uk/TA390
  ▸ **Empagliflozin in combination therapy for treating type 2 diabetes (March 2015)** NICE TA336
  Empagliflozin in a dual therapy regimen in combination with metformin is an option for the treatment of type 2 diabetes, only if:
  - a sulfonylurea is contra-indicated or not tolerated, **or**
  - the patient is at significant risk of hypoglycaemia or its consequences.

Empagliflozin in a triple therapy regimen is an option for the treatment of type 2 diabetes in combination with:
- metformin and a sulfonylurea **or**
- metformin and a thiazolidinedione.

Empagliflozin in combination with insulin with or without other antidiabetic drugs is an option for the treatment of type 2 diabetes.

Patients currently receiving empagliflozin whose disease does not meet the above criteria should have the option to continue treatment until they and their clinician consider it appropriate to stop.
www.nice.org.uk/TA336

- **MEDICINAL FORMS**
  There can be variation in the licensing of different medicines containing the same drug.
  Tablet
  ▸ Jardiance (Boehringer Ingelheim Ltd) ▼
  Empagliflozin 10 mg Jardiance 10mg tablets | 28 tablet [PoM] £36.59 DT = £36.59
  Empagliflozin 25 mg Jardiance 25mg tablets | 28 tablet [PoM] £36.59 DT = £36.59

Empagliflozin with metformin   25-Apr-2016

The properties listed below are those particular to the combination only. For the properties of the components please consider, empagliflozin p. 690, metformin hydrochloride p. 678.

- **INDICATIONS AND DOSE**
  Type 2 diabetes mellitus not controlled by metformin alone or by metformin in combination with other antidiabetic drugs or insulin
  ▸ **BY MOUTH**
  ▸ Adult 18-84 years: 5/850–5/1000 mg twice daily, based on patient's current metformin dose, increased if necessary to 12.5/850–12.5/1000 mg twice daily
  ▸ **BY MOUTH**
  ▸ Adult 85 years and over: Initiation not recommended

  DOSE ADJUSTMENTS DUE TO INTERACTIONS
  ▸ Dose of concomitant insulin or drugs that stimulate insulin secretion may need to be reduced.

  DOSE EQUIVALENCE AND CONVERSION
  ▸ The proportions are expressed in the form "x"/"y" where "x" and "y" are the strengths in milligrams of empagliflozin and metformin respectively.

- **INTERACTIONS** → Appendix 1: empagliflozin · metformin
- **NATIONAL FUNDING/ACCESS DECISIONS**
  Scottish Medicines Consortium (SMC) Decisions
  The *Scottish Medicines Consortium* has advised (October 2015) that *Synjardy®* (empagliflozin with metformin) is accepted for restricted use within NHS Scotland in patients for whom a fixed dose combination of empagliflozin and metformin is an appropriate choice of therapy *or* when use of a sulfonylurea is considered inappropriate.

- **MEDICINAL FORMS**
  There can be variation in the licensing of different medicines containing the same drug.
  Tablet
  CAUTIONARY AND ADVISORY LABELS 21
  ▸ Synjardy (Boehringer Ingelheim Ltd) ▼
  Empagliflozin 12.5 mg, Metformin hydrochloride 850 mg Synjardy 12.5mg/850mg tablets | 56 tablet [PoM] £36.59 DT = £36.59
  Empagliflozin 5 mg, Metformin hydrochloride 850 mg Synjardy 5mg/850mg tablets | 56 tablet [PoM] £36.59 DT = £36.59
  Empagliflozin 12.5 mg, Metformin hydrochloride 1 gram Synjardy 12.5mg/1000mg tablets | 56 tablet [PoM] £36.59 DT = £36.59
  Empagliflozin 5 mg, Metformin hydrochloride 1 gram Synjardy 5mg/1000mg tablets | 56 tablet [PoM] £36.59 DT = £36.59

6

Endocrine system

6

Endocrine system

BLOOD GLUCOSE LOWERING DRUGS ›
SULFONYLUREAS

Sulfonylureas

- **DRUG ACTION** The sulfonylureas act mainly by augmenting insulin secretion and consequently are effective only when some residual pancreatic beta-cell activity is present; during long-term administration they also have an extrapancreatic action.

- **CONTRA-INDICATIONS** Presence of ketoacidosis

- **CAUTIONS** Can encourage weight gain (should be prescribed only if poor control and symptoms persist despite adequate attempts at dieting) · elderly · G6PD deficiency

- **SIDE-EFFECTS**
  ▶ **Common or very common** Diarrhoea · gastrointestinal discomfort · hypoglycaemia · nausea
  ▶ **Uncommon** Hepatic disorders · vomiting
  ▶ **Rare or very rare** Agranulocytosis · erythropenia · granulocytopenia · haemolytic anaemia · leucopenia · pancytopenia · thrombocytopenia
  ▶ **Frequency not known** Allergic dermatitis (usually in the first 6–8 weeks of therapy) · constipation · visual impairment

- **HEPATIC IMPAIRMENT** Jaundice may occur.
  Dose adjustments Sulfonylureas should be avoided or a reduced dose should be used in severe hepatic impairment, because there is an increased risk of hypoglycaemia.

- **RENAL IMPAIRMENT** Sulfonylureas should be used with care in those with mild to moderate renal impairment, because of the hazard of hypoglycaemia. Care is required to use the lowest dose that adequately controls blood glucose. Avoid where possible in severe renal impairment.

- **PATIENT AND CARER ADVICE** The risk of hypoglycaemia associated with sulfonylureas should be discussed with the patient, especially when concomitant glucose-lowering drugs are prescribed.
  Driving and skilled tasks Drivers need to be particularly careful to avoid hypoglycaemia and should be warned of the problems.

⬆ above

Glibenclamide

- **INDICATIONS AND DOSE**

Type 2 diabetes mellitus
  ▶ BY MOUTH
  ▶ Adult: Initially 5 mg daily, adjusted according to response, dose to be taken with or immediately after breakfast; maximum 15 mg per day

- **UNLICENSED USE** Not licensed for use in breast feeding women with pre-existing diabetes. Not licensed for use in gestational diabetes.

- **CONTRA-INDICATIONS** Avoid where possible in Acute porphyrias p. 1025

- **INTERACTIONS** → Appendix 1: sulfonylureas

- **SIDE-EFFECTS** Appetite decreased · SIADH · taste metallic

- **PREGNANCY** The use of sulfonylureas in pregnancy should generally be avoided because of the risk of neonatal hypoglycaemia; however, glibenclamide can be used during the second and third trimesters of pregnancy in women with gestational diabetes.

- **BREAST FEEDING** Glibenclamide can be used during breast-feeding in women with pre-existing diabetes.

- **MEDICINAL FORMS**
  There can be variation in the licensing of different medicines containing the same drug. Forms available from special-order manufacturers include: oral suspension, oral solution
  Tablet
  ▶ Glibenclamide (Non-proprietary)
    Glibenclamide 2.5 mg Glibenclamide 2.5mg tablets | 28 tablet [PoM] £11.78 DT = £10.49
    Glibenclamide 5 mg Glibenclamide 5mg tablets | 28 tablet [PoM] £14.72 DT = £3.16

⬆ above

Gliclazide

- **INDICATIONS AND DOSE**

Type 2 diabetes mellitus
  ▶ BY MOUTH USING IMMEDIATE-RELEASE MEDICINES
  ▶ Adult: Initially 40–80 mg daily, adjusted according to response, increased if necessary up to 160 mg once daily, dose to be taken with breakfast, doses higher than 160 mg to be given in divided doses; maximum 320 mg per day
  ▶ BY MOUTH USING MODIFIED-RELEASE MEDICINES
  ▶ Adult: Initially 30 mg daily, dose to be taken with breakfast, adjust dose according to response every 4 weeks (after 2 weeks if no decrease in blood glucose); maximum 120 mg per day

  DOSE EQUIVALENCE AND CONVERSION
  ▶ Gliclazide modified release 30 mg may be considered to be approximately equivalent in therapeutic effect to standard formulation gliclazide 80 mg.

- **CONTRA-INDICATIONS** Avoid where possible in Acute porphyrias p. 1025

- **INTERACTIONS** → Appendix 1: sulfonylureas

- **SIDE-EFFECTS** Anaemia · angioedema · dyspepsia · gastrointestinal disorder · hypersensitivity vasculitis · hyponatraemia · severe cutaneous adverse reactions (SCARs) · skin reactions

- **PREGNANCY** The use of sulfonylureas in pregnancy should generally be avoided because of the risk of neonatal hypoglycaemia.

- **BREAST FEEDING** Avoid—theoretical possibility of hypoglycaemia in the infant.

- **RENAL IMPAIRMENT** If necessary, gliclazide which is principally metabolised in the liver, can be used in renal impairment but careful monitoring of blood-glucose concentration is essential.

- **MEDICINAL FORMS**
  There can be variation in the licensing of different medicines containing the same drug. Forms available from special-order manufacturers include: oral suspension
  Modified-release tablet
  CAUTIONARY AND ADVISORY LABELS 25
  ▶ Gliclazide (Non-proprietary)
    Gliclazide 30 mg Gliclazide 30mg modified-release tablets | 28 tablet [PoM] [🔺] DT = £2.81
  ▶ Bilxona (Actavis UK Ltd)
    Gliclazide 30 mg Bilxona 30mg modified-release tablets | 28 tablet [PoM] £1.63 DT = £2.81 | 56 tablet [PoM] £3.27
    Gliclazide 60 mg Bilxona 60mg modified-release tablets | 28 tablet [PoM] £3.27 DT = £4.77 | 56 tablet [PoM] £6.55
  ▶ Dacadis MR (Mylan)
    Gliclazide 30 mg Dacadis MR 30mg tablets | 28 tablet [PoM] £2.81 DT = £2.81
  ▶ Diamicron MR (Servier Laboratories Ltd)
    Gliclazide 30 mg Diamicron 30mg MR tablets | 28 tablet [PoM] £2.81 DT = £2.81 | 56 tablet [PoM] £5.62
  ▶ Edicil MR (Teva UK Ltd)
    Gliclazide 30 mg Edicil MR 30mg tablets | 28 tablet [PoM] £2.62 DT = £2.81 | 56 tablet [PoM] £5.24

▸ Laaglyda MR (Consilient Health Ltd)
Gliclazide 60 mg Laaglyda MR 60mg tablets | 28 tablet [PoM] £4.77 DT = £4.77
▸ Nazdol MR (Consilient Health Ltd)
Gliclazide 30 mg Nazdol MR 30mg tablets | 28 tablet [PoM] £2.35 DT = £2.81 | 56 tablet [PoM] £4.92
▸ Vamju (AMCo)
Gliclazide 30 mg Vamju 30mg modified-release tablets | 28 tablet [PoM] £1.64 DT = £2.81 | 56 tablet [PoM] £3.28
Gliclazide 60 mg Vamju 60mg modified-release tablets | 28 tablet [PoM] £3.28 DT = £4.77
▸ Ziclaseg (Lupin Healthcare (UK) Ltd)
Gliclazide 30 mg Ziclaseg 30mg modified-release tablets | 28 tablet [PoM] £2.38 DT = £2.81 | 56 tablet [PoM] £4.77
▸ Zicron PR (Bristol Laboratories Ltd)
Gliclazide 30 mg Zicron PR 30mg tablets | 28 tablet [PoM] £1.95 DT = £2.81 | 56 tablet [PoM] £3.90

Tablet
▸ Gliclazide (Non-proprietary)
Gliclazide 40 mg Gliclazide 40mg tablets | 28 tablet [PoM] £3.19 DT = £3.04
Gliclazide 80 mg Gliclazide 80mg tablets | 28 tablet [PoM] £7.22 DT = £0.92 | 60 tablet [PoM] £0.81–£9.32
▸ Diamicron (Servier Laboratories Ltd)
Gliclazide 80 mg Diamicron 80mg tablets | 60 tablet [PoM] £4.38
▸ Zicron (Bristol Laboratories Ltd)
Gliclazide 40 mg Zicron 40mg tablets | 28 tablet [PoM] £3.36 DT = £3.04

F 692

Glimepiride

● **INDICATIONS AND DOSE**
Type 2 diabetes mellitus
▸ BY MOUTH
▸ Adult: Initially 1 mg daily, adjusted according to response, then increased in steps of 1 mg every 1–2 weeks, increased to 4 mg daily, dose to be taken shortly before or with first main meal, the daily dose may be increased further, in exceptional circumstances; maximum 6 mg per day

● CAUTIONS
CAUTIONS, FURTHER INFORMATION
▸ Porphyria Sulfonylureas should be avoided where possible in Acute porphyrias p. 1025 but glimepiride is thought to be safe.

● INTERACTIONS → Appendix 1: sulfonylureas

● SIDE-EFFECTS
▸ **Rare or very rare** Hypersensitivity vasculitis
▸ **Frequency not known** Drug cross-reactivity · rash · thrombocytopenic purpura

● PREGNANCY The use of sulfonylureas in pregnancy should generally be avoided because of the risk of neonatal hypoglycaemia.

● BREAST FEEDING Avoid—theoretical possibility of hypoglycaemia in the infant.

● MONITORING REQUIREMENTS Manufacturer recommends regular hepatic and haematological monitoring but limited evidence of clinical value.

● MEDICINAL FORMS
There can be variation in the licensing of different medicines containing the same drug. Forms available from special-order manufacturers include: oral suspension, oral solution
Tablet
▸ Glimepiride (Non-proprietary)
Glimepiride 1 mg Glimepiride 1mg tablets | 30 tablet [PoM] £5.00 DT = £1.63
Glimepiride 2 mg Glimepiride 2mg tablets | 30 tablet [PoM] £7.13 DT = £2.54
Glimepiride 3 mg Glimepiride 3mg tablets | 30 tablet [PoM] £10.75 DT = £3.65
Glimepiride 4 mg Glimepiride 4mg tablets | 30 tablet [PoM] £14.24 DT = £4.74

▸ Amaryl (Zentiva)
Glimepiride 3 mg Amaryl 3mg tablets | 30 tablet [PoM] £10.75 DT = £3.65

F 692

Glipizide

● **INDICATIONS AND DOSE**
Type 2 diabetes mellitus
▸ BY MOUTH
▸ Adult: Initially 2.5–5 mg daily, adjusted according to response, dose to be taken shortly before breakfast or lunch, doses up to 15 mg may be given as a single dose, higher doses to be given in divided doses; maximum 20 mg per day

● CAUTIONS
CAUTIONS, FURTHER INFORMATION
▸ Porphyria Sulfonylureas should be avoided where possible in Acute porphyrias p. 1025 but glipizide is thought to be safe.

● INTERACTIONS → Appendix 1: sulfonylureas

● SIDE-EFFECTS
▸ **Uncommon** Dizziness · drowsiness · skin reactions · tremor · vision disorders
▸ **Frequency not known** Confusion · headache · hyponatraemia · malaise · photosensitivity reaction

● PREGNANCY The use of sulfonylureas in pregnancy should generally be avoided because of the risk of neonatal hypoglycaemia.

● BREAST FEEDING Avoid—theoretical possibility of hypoglycaemia in the infant.

● HEPATIC IMPAIRMENT Avoid if the patient has both renal and hepatic impairment.

● RENAL IMPAIRMENT Avoid if the patient has both renal and hepatic impairment.

● MEDICINAL FORMS
There can be variation in the licensing of different medicines containing the same drug.
Tablet
▸ Glipizide (Non-proprietary)
Glipizide 5 mg Glipizide 5mg tablets | 28 tablet [PoM] £3.00 DT = £1.46 | 56 tablet [PoM] £2.92–£6.00
▸ Minodiab (Pfizer Ltd)
Glipizide 5 mg Minodiab 5mg tablets | 28 tablet [PoM] £1.26 DT = £1.46

F 692

Tolbutamide

● **INDICATIONS AND DOSE**
Type 2 diabetes mellitus
▸ BY MOUTH
▸ Adult: 0.5–1.5 g daily in divided doses, dose to be taken with or immediately after meals, alternatively 0.5–1.5 g once daily, dose to be taken with or immediately after breakfast; maximum 2 g per day

● CONTRA-INDICATIONS Avoid where possible in Acute porphyrias p. 1025

● INTERACTIONS → Appendix 1: sulfonylureas

● SIDE-EFFECTS
▸ **Rare or very rare** Aplastic anaemia · blood disorder
▸ **Frequency not known** Alcohol intolerance · appetite abnormal · erythema multiforme (usually in the first 6–8 weeks of therapy) · exfoliative dermatitis (usually in the first 6–8 weeks of therapy) · fever (usually in the first 6–8 weeks of therapy) · headache · hypersensitivity (usually in the first 6–8 weeks of therapy) · paraesthesia · photosensitivity reaction · tinnitus · weight increased

- PREGNANCY The use of sulfonylureas in pregnancy should generally be avoided because of the risk of neonatal hypoglycaemia.
- BREAST FEEDING The use of sulfonylureas in breast-feeding should be avoided because there is a theoretical possibility of hypoglycaemia in the infant.
- RENAL IMPAIRMENT If necessary, the short-acting drug tolbutamide can be used in renal impairment but careful monitoring of blood-glucose concentration is essential.

- MEDICINAL FORMS
There can be variation in the licensing of different medicines containing the same drug. Forms available from special-order manufacturers include: oral suspension

Tablet
▸ Tolbutamide (Non-proprietary)
   Tolbutamide 500 mg Tolbutamide 500mg tablets | 28 tablet PoM
   £34.88 DT = £4.56 | 112 tablet PoM £17.60–£18.24

BLOOD GLUCOSE LOWERING DRUGS ›
THIAZOLIDINEDIONES

Pioglitazone

- DRUG ACTION The thiazolidinedione, pioglitazone, reduces peripheral insulin resistance, leading to a reduction of blood-glucose concentration.

- ● INDICATIONS AND DOSE

Type 2 diabetes mellitus (alone or combined with metformin or a sulfonylurea, or with both, or with insulin)
▸ BY MOUTH
▸ Adult: Initially 15–30 mg once daily, adjusted according to response to 45 mg once daily, in elderly patients, initiate with lowest possible dose and increase gradually; review treatment after 3–6 months and regularly thereafter

DOSE ADJUSTMENTS DUE TO INTERACTIONS
▸ Dose of concomitant sulfonylurea or insulin may need to be reduced.

IMPORTANT SAFETY INFORMATION
MHRA/CHM ADVICE: PIOGLITAZONE CARDIOVASCULAR SAFETY (DECEMBER 2007 AND JANUARY 2011)
Incidence of heart failure is increased when pioglitazone is combined with insulin especially in patients with predisposing factors e.g. previous myocardial infarction. Patients who take pioglitazone should be closely monitored for signs of heart failure; treatment should be discontinued if any deterioration in cardiac status occurs.
   Pioglitazone should not be used in patients with heart failure or a history of heart failure.

PIOGLITAZONE: RISK OF BLADDER CANCER (JULY 2011)
The European Medicines Agency has advised that there is a small increased risk of bladder cancer associated with pioglitazone use. However, in patients who respond adequately to treatment, the benefits of pioglitazone continue to outweigh the risks.
   Pioglitazone should not be used in patients with active bladder cancer or a past history of bladder cancer, or in those who have uninvestigated macroscopic haematuria. Pioglitazone should be used with caution in elderly patients as the risk of bladder cancer increases with age.
   Before initiating treatment with pioglitazone, patients should be assessed for risk factors of bladder cancer (including age, smoking status, exposure to certain occupational or chemotherapy agents, or previous radiation therapy to the pelvic region) and any macroscopic haematuria should be investigated. The safety and efficacy of pioglitazone should be reviewed

after 3–6 months and pioglitazone should be stopped in patients who do not respond adequately to treatment.
   Patients already receiving treatment with pioglitazone should be assessed for risk factors of bladder cancer and treatment should be reviewed after 3–6 months, as above.
   Patients should be advised to report promptly any haematuria, dysuria, or urinary urgency during treatment.

- CONTRA-INDICATIONS History of heart failure · previous or active bladder cancer · uninvestigated macroscopic haematuria
- CAUTIONS Cardiovascular disease or in combination with insulin (risk of heart failure) · elderly (increased risk of heart failure, fractures, and bladder cancer) · increased risk of bone fractures, particularly in women · risk factors for bladder cancer
   CAUTIONS, FURTHER INFORMATION Substitute insulin during peri-operative period.
- INTERACTIONS → Appendix 1: pioglitazone
- SIDE-EFFECTS
▸ **Common or very common** Bone fracture · increased risk of infection · numbness · visual impairment · weight increased
▸ **Uncommon** Bladder cancer · insomnia
▸ **Frequency not known** Macular oedema
   SIDE-EFFECTS, FURTHER INFORMATION Rare reports of liver dysfunction; discontinue if jaundice occurs.
- PREGNANCY Avoid—toxicity in *animal* studies.
- BREAST FEEDING Avoid—present in milk in *animal* studies.
- HEPATIC IMPAIRMENT Avoid.
- MONITORING REQUIREMENTS Monitor liver function before treatment and periodically thereafter.
- PATIENT AND CARER ADVICE
Liver toxicity Patients should be advised to seek immediate medical attention if symptoms such as nausea, vomiting, abdominal pain, fatigue and dark urine develop.
- NATIONAL FUNDING/ACCESS DECISIONS
Scottish Medicines Consortium (SMC) Decisions
The *Scottish Medicines Consortium* accepts use of pioglitazone (February 2007) with metformin and a sulfonylurea, for patients (especially if overweight) whose glycaemic control is inadequate despite the use of 2 oral hypoglycaemic drugs and who are unable or unwilling to take insulin; treatment should be initiated and monitored by an experienced diabetes physician.

- MEDICINAL FORMS
There can be variation in the licensing of different medicines containing the same drug. Forms available from special-order manufacturers include: oral suspension

Tablet
▸ Pioglitazone (Non-proprietary)
   Pioglitazone (as Pioglitazone hydrochloride) 15 mg Pioglitazone 15mg tablets | 28 tablet PoM £25.83 DT = £0.50
   Pioglitazone (as Pioglitazone hydrochloride) 30 mg Pioglitazone 30mg tablets | 28 tablet PoM £35.89 DT = £0.92
   Pioglitazone (as Pioglitazone hydrochloride) 45 mg Pioglitazone 45mg tablets | 28 tablet PoM £39.55 DT = £0.66
▸ Actos (Takeda UK Ltd)
   Pioglitazone (as Pioglitazone hydrochloride) 15 mg Actos 15mg tablets | 28 tablet PoM £25.83 DT = £0.50
   Pioglitazone (as Pioglitazone hydrochloride) 30 mg Actos 30mg tablets | 28 tablet PoM £35.89 DT = £0.92
   Pioglitazone (as Pioglitazone hydrochloride) 45 mg Actos 45mg tablets | 28 tablet PoM £39.55 DT = £0.66
▸ Diabiom (Tillomed Laboratories Ltd)
   Pioglitazone (as Pioglitazone hydrochloride) 15 mg Diabiom 15mg tablets | 28 tablet PoM £26.00 DT = £0.50
   Pioglitazone (as Pioglitazone hydrochloride) 30 mg Diabiom 30mg tablets | 28 tablet PoM £36.00 DT = £0.92

Pioglitazone (as Pioglitazone hydrochloride) **45 mg** Diabiom
45mg tablets | 28 tablet [PoM] £40.00 DT = £0.66
▸ Glidipion (Actavis UK Ltd)
Pioglitazone (as Pioglitazone hydrochloride) **15 mg** Glidipion
15mg tablets | 28 tablet [PoM] £25.83 DT = £0.50
Pioglitazone (as Pioglitazone hydrochloride) **30 mg** Glidipion
30mg tablets | 28 tablet [PoM] £35.89 DT = £0.92
Pioglitazone (as Pioglitazone hydrochloride) **45 mg** Glidipion
45mg tablets | 28 tablet [PoM] £39.55 DT = £0.66

Pioglitazone with metformin

The properties listed below are those particular to the
combination only. For the properties of the components
please consider, pioglitazone p. 694, metformin
hydrochloride p. 678.

● **INDICATIONS AND DOSE**

Type 2 diabetes not controlled by metformin alone
▸ BY MOUTH
▸ Adult: 1 tablet twice daily, titration with the individual
  components (pioglitazone and metformin) desirable
  before initiation

● INTERACTIONS → Appendix 1: metformin · pioglitazone

● MEDICINAL FORMS
There can be variation in the licensing of different medicines
containing the same drug.
Tablet
CAUTIONARY AND ADVISORY LABELS 21
▸ Competact (Takeda UK Ltd)
  Pioglitazone (as Pioglitazone hydrochloride) **15 mg**, Metformin
  hydrochloride **850 mg** Competact 15mg/850mg tablets |
  56 tablet [PoM] £35.89 DT = £35.89

INSULINS

Insulins

IMPORTANT SAFETY INFORMATION
NHS IMPROVEMENT PATIENT SAFETY ALERT: RISK OF SEVERE
HARM AND DEATH DUE TO WITHDRAWING INSULIN FROM PEN
DEVICES (NOVEMBER 2016)
Insulin should not be extracted from insulin pen devices.
   The strength of insulin in pen devices can vary by
multiples of 100 units/mL. Insulin syringes have
graduations only suitable for calculating doses of
standard 100 units/mL. If insulin extracted from a pen or
cartridge is of a higher strength, and that is not
considered in determining the volume required, it can
lead to a significant and potentially fatal overdose.

● SIDE-EFFECTS
▸ **Common or very common** Oedema
▸ **Uncommon** Lipodystrophy · skin reactions
SIDE-EFFECTS, FURTHER INFORMATION
Overdose Overdose causes hypoglycaemia.

● PREGNANCY
Dose adjustments During pregnancy, insulin requirements
may alter and doses should be assessed frequently by an
experienced diabetes physician.
   The dose of insulin generally needs to be increased in
the second and third trimesters of pregnancy.

● BREAST FEEDING
Dose adjustments During breast-feeding, insulin
requirements may alter and doses should be assessed
frequently by an experienced diabetes physician.

● HEPATIC IMPAIRMENT
Dose adjustments Insulin requirements may be decreased
in patients with hepatic impairment.

● RENAL IMPAIRMENT The compensatory response to
hypoglycaemia is impaired in renal impairment.
Dose adjustments Insulin requirements may decrease in
patients with renal impairment and therefore dose
reduction may be necessary.

● MONITORING REQUIREMENTS
▸ Many patients now monitor their own blood-glucose
concentrations; all carers and children need to be trained
to do this.
▸ Since blood-glucose concentration varies substantially
throughout the day, 'normoglycaemia' cannot always be
achieved throughout a 24-hour period without causing
damaging hypoglycaemia.
▸ In adults It is therefore best to recommend that patients
should maintain a blood-glucose concentration of between
4 and 9 mmol/litre for most of the time (4–7 mmol/litre
before meals and less than 9 mmol/litre after meals).
▸ In children It is therefore best to recommend that children
should maintain a blood-glucose concentration of between
4 and 10 mmol/litre for most of the time (4–8 mmol/litre
before meals and less than 10 mmol/litre after meals).
▸ While accepting that on occasions, for brief periods, the
blood-glucose concentration will be above these values;
strenuous efforts should be made to prevent it from falling
below 4 mmol/litre. Patients using multiple injection
regimens should understand how to adjust their insulin
dose according to their carbohydrate intake. With fixed-
dose insulin regimens, the carbohydrate intake needs to be
regulated, and should be distributed throughout the day to
match the insulin regimen. The intake of energy and of
simple and complex carbohydrates should be adequate to
allow normal growth and development but obesity must be
avoided.

● DIRECTIONS FOR ADMINISTRATION Insulin is generally
given by *subcutaneous injection*; the injection site should
be rotated to prevent lipodystrophy. Injection devices
('pens'), which hold the insulin in a cartridge and meter
the required dose, are convenient to use. Insulin syringes
(for use with needles) are required for insulins not
available in cartridge form, but are less popular with
children and carers. For intensive insulin regimens
multiple subcutaneous injections (3 or more times daily)
are usually recommended.

● PRESCRIBING AND DISPENSING INFORMATION Show
container to patient or carer and confirm the expected
version is dispensed.
Units The word 'unit' should **not** be abbreviated.

● PATIENT AND CARER ADVICE
Hypoglycaemia Hypoglycaemia is a potential problem with
insulin therapy. All patients must be carefully instructed
on how to avoid it; this involves appropriate adjustment of
insulin type, dose and frequency together with suitable
timing and quantity of meals and snacks.
Insulin Passport Insulin Passports and patient information
booklets should be offered to patients receiving insulin.
The Insulin Passport provides a record of the patient's
current insulin preparations and contains a section for
emergency information. The patient information booklet
provides advice on the safe use of insulin. They are
available for purchase from:
3M Security Print and Systems Limited
Gorse Street, Chadderton
Oldham
OL9 9QH
Tel: 0845 610 1112
   GP practices can obtain supplies through their Local
Area Team stores.
   NHS Trusts can order supplies from www.nhsforms.co.uk/
or by emailing nhsforms@mmm.com. Further information
is available at www.npsa.nhs.uk.

6

Endocrine system

Driving and skilled tasks Drivers need to be particularly careful to avoid hypoglycaemia and should be warned of the problems.

INSULINS › RAPID-ACTING

Insulin

▶ 695

(Insulin Injection; Neutral Insulin; Soluble Insulin—short acting)

- **INDICATIONS AND DOSE**

Diabetes mellitus
▶ BY SUBCUTANEOUS INJECTION, OR BY INTRAMUSCULAR INJECTION, OR BY INTRAVENOUS INJECTION, OR BY INTRAVENOUS INFUSION
▶ Adult: According to requirements

Diabetic ketoacidosis | Diabetes during surgery
▶ BY INTRAVENOUS INFUSION
▶ Adult: (consult local protocol)

- **INTERACTIONS** → Appendix 1: insulins
- **SIDE-EFFECTS**
▶ **Rare or very rare** Refraction disorder
- **DIRECTIONS FOR ADMINISTRATION** Short-acting injectable insulins can be given by continuous subcutaneous infusion using a portable infusion pump. This device delivers a continuous basal insulin infusion and patient-activated bolus doses at meal times. This technique can be useful for patients who suffer recurrent hypoglycaemia or marked morning rise in blood-glucose concentration despite optimised multiple-injection regimens. Patients on subcutaneous insulin infusion must be highly motivated, able to monitor their blood-glucose concentration, and have expert training, advice and supervision from an experienced healthcare team. Some insulin preparations are not recommended for use in subcutaneous insulin infusion pumps—may precipitate in catheter or needle—consult product literature.
▶ With intravenous use For *intravenous infusion* give continuously in Sodium chloride 0.9%. Adsorbed to some extent by plastic infusion set; ensure insulin is not injected into 'dead space' of injection port of the infusion bag.
- **PRESCRIBING AND DISPENSING INFORMATION** A sterile solution of insulin (i.e. bovine or porcine) or of human insulin; pH 6.6–8.0.
- **NATIONAL FUNDING/ACCESS DECISIONS**

NICE decisions
▶ **Continuous subcutaneous insulin infusion for the treatment of diabetes mellitus (type 1) (July 2008)** NICE TA151
Continuous subcutaneous insulin infusion is recommended as an option in adults and children over 12 years with type 1 diabetes:
  • who suffer repeated or unpredictable hypoglycaemia, whilst attempting to achieve optimal glycaemic control with multiple-injection regimens, **or**
  • whose glycaemic control remains inadequate (HbA$_{1c}$ over 8.5% [69 mmol/mol]) despite optimised multiple-injection regimens (including the use of long-acting insulin analogues where appropriate).
Continuous subcutaneous insulin infusion is also recommended as an option for children under 12 years with type 1 diabetes for whom multiple-injection regimens are considered impractical or inappropriate. Children on insulin pumps should undergo a trial of multiple-injection therapy between the ages of 12 and 18 years.
www.nice.org.uk/TA151

- **MEDICINAL FORMS**
There can be variation in the licensing of different medicines containing the same drug. Forms available from special-order manufacturers include: solution for injection, solution for infusion

Solution for injection
▶ Actrapid (Novo Nordisk Ltd)
  Insulin human (as Insulin soluble human) 100 unit per 1 ml Actrapid 100units/ml solution for injection 10ml vials | 1 vial PoM £7.48
▶ Humulin S (Eli Lilly and Company Ltd)
  Insulin human (as Insulin soluble human) 100 unit per 1 ml Humulin S 100units/ml solution for injection 10ml vials | 1 vial PoM £15.68
  Humulin S 100units/ml solution for injection 3ml cartridges | 5 cartridge PoM £19.08 DT = £19.08
▶ Hypurin Bovine Neutral (Wockhardt UK Ltd)
  Insulin bovine (as Insulin soluble bovine) 100 unit per 1 ml Hypurin Bovine Neutral 100units/ml solution for injection 10ml vials | 1 vial PoM £27.72
  Hypurin Bovine Neutral 100units/ml solution for injection 3ml cartridges | 5 cartridge PoM £41.58
▶ Hypurin Porcine Neutral (Wockhardt UK Ltd)
  Insulin porcine (as Insulin soluble porcine) 100 unit per 1 ml Hypurin Porcine Neutral 100units/ml solution for injection 10ml vials | 1 vial PoM £31.30
  Hypurin Porcine Neutral 100units/ml solution for injection 3ml cartridges | 5 cartridge PoM £46.95
▶ Insuman Infusat (Sanofi)
  Insulin human 100 unit per 1 ml Insuman Infusat 100units/ml solution for injection 3.15ml cartridges | 5 cartridge PoM £250.00
  Insuman Infusat 100units/ml solution for injection 10ml vials | 3 vial PoM £250.00
▶ Insuman Rapid (Sanofi)
  Insulin human (as Insulin soluble human) 100 unit per 1 ml Insuman Rapid 100units/ml solution for injection 3ml cartridges | 5 cartridge PoM £17.50 DT = £19.08

▶ 695

Insulin aspart

18-Jul-2017

(Recombinant human insulin analogue—short acting)

- **INDICATIONS AND DOSE**

FIASP®
Diabetes mellitus
▶ BY SUBCUTANEOUS INJECTION, OR BY INTRAVENOUS INFUSION, OR BY CONTINUOUS SUBCUTANEOUS INFUSION
▶ Adult: According to requirements

NOVORAPID®
Diabetes mellitus
▶ BY SUBCUTANEOUS INJECTION
▶ Child 2-17 years: Administer immediately before meals or when necessary shortly after meals, according to requirements
▶ Adult: Administer immediately before meals or when necessary shortly after meals, according to requirements
▶ BY SUBCUTANEOUS INFUSION, OR BY INTRAVENOUS INFUSION, OR BY INTRAVENOUS INJECTION
▶ Child 2-17 years: According to requirements
▶ Adult: According to requirements

- **INTERACTIONS** → Appendix 1: insulins
- **SIDE-EFFECTS**
▶ **Uncommon** Refraction disorder
- **PREGNANCY** Not known to be harmful—may be used during pregnancy.
- **BREAST FEEDING** Not known to be harmful—may be used during lactation.
- **DIRECTIONS FOR ADMINISTRATION** Short-acting injectable insulins can be given by continuous subcutaneous infusion using a portable infusion pump. This device delivers a

continuous basal insulin infusion and patient-activated bolus doses at meal times. This technique can be useful for patients who suffer recurrent hypoglycaemia or marked morning rise in blood-glucose concentration despite optimised multiple-injection regimens. Patients on subcutaneous insulin infusion must be highly motivated, able to monitor their blood-glucose concentration, and have expert training, advice and supervision from an experienced healthcare team.

▸ With intravenous use in adults For *intravenous infusion*, give continuously in Glucose 5% or Sodium chloride 0.9%; dilute to 0.05-1 unit/mL with infusion fluid; adsorbed to some extent by plastics of infusion set.

▸ With intravenous use in children For *intravenous infusion*, dilute to a concentration of 0.05–1 unit/mL with Glucose 5% or Sodium Chloride 0.9% and mix thoroughly; insulin may be adsorbed by plastics, flush giving set with 5 mL of infusion fluid containing insulin.

● NATIONAL FUNDING/ACCESS DECISIONS

NICE decisions

▸ **Continuous subcutaneous insulin infusion for the treatment of diabetes mellitus (type 1) (July 2008)** NICE TA151
Continuous subcutaneous insulin infusion is recommended as an option in adults and children over 12 years with type 1 diabetes:

• who suffer repeated or unpredictable hypoglycaemia, whilst attempting to achieve optimal glycaemic control with multiple-injection regimens, **or**

• whose glycaemic control remains inadequate (HbA$_{1c}$ over 8.5% [69 mmol/mol]) despite optimised multiple-injection regimens (including the use of long-acting insulin analogues where appropriate).

Continuous subcutaneous insulin infusion is also recommended as an option for children under 12 years with type 1 diabetes for whom multiple-injection regimens are considered impractical or inappropriate. Children on insulin pumps should undergo a trial of multiple-injection therapy between the ages of 12 and 18 years.
www.nice.org.uk/TA151

Scottish Medicines Consortium (SMC) Decisions
The *Scottish Medicines Consortium* has advised (April 2017) that insulin aspart (*Fiasp*®) is accepted for use within NHS Scotland for the treatment of diabetes mellitus in adults.

● MEDICINAL FORMS
There can be variation in the licensing of different medicines containing the same drug.

Solution for injection

▸ Fiasp (Novo Nordisk Ltd) ▼
Insulin aspart 100 unit per 1 ml Fiasp 100units/ml solution for injection 10ml vials | 1 vial [PoM] £14.08 DT = £14.08

▸ Fiasp FlexTouch (Novo Nordisk Ltd) ▼
Insulin aspart 100 unit per 1 ml Fiasp FlexTouch 100units/ml solution for injection 3ml pre-filled pen | 5 pre-filled disposable injection [PoM] £30.60 DT = £30.60

▸ Fiasp Penfill (Novo Nordisk Ltd) ▼
Insulin aspart 100 unit per 1 ml Fiasp Penfill 100units/ml solution for injection 3ml cartridges | 5 cartridge [PoM] £28.31 DT = £28.31

▸ NovoRapid (Novo Nordisk Ltd)
Insulin aspart 100 unit per 1 ml NovoRapid 100units/ml solution for injection 10ml vials | 1 vial [PoM] £14.08 DT = £14.08

▸ NovoRapid FlexPen (Novo Nordisk Ltd)
Insulin aspart 100 unit per 1 ml NovoRapid FlexPen 100units/ml solution for injection 3ml pre-filled pen | 5 pre-filled disposable injection [PoM] £30.60 DT = £30.60

▸ NovoRapid FlexTouch (Novo Nordisk Ltd)
Insulin aspart 100 unit per 1 ml NovoRapid FlexTouch 100units/ml solution for injection 3ml pre-filled pen | 5 pre-filled disposable injection [PoM] £32.13 DT = £30.60

▸ NovoRapid Penfill (Novo Nordisk Ltd)
Insulin aspart 100 unit per 1 ml NovoRapid Penfill 100units/ml solution for injection 3ml cartridges | 5 cartridge [PoM] £28.31 DT = £28.31

▸ NovoRapid PumpCart (Novo Nordisk Ltd)
Insulin aspart 100 unit per 1 ml NovoRapid PumpCart 100units/ml solution for injection 1.6ml cartridges | 5 cartridge [PoM] £15.10 DT = £15.10

F 695

Insulin glulisine

(Recombinant human insulin analogue–short acting)

● INDICATIONS AND DOSE

Diabetes mellitus

▸ BY SUBCUTANEOUS INJECTION

▸ Child: Administer immediately before meals or when necessary shortly after meals, according to requirements

▸ Adult: Administer immediately before meals or when necessary shortly after meals, according to requirements

▸ BY SUBCUTANEOUS INFUSION, OR BY INTRAVENOUS INFUSION

▸ Child: According to requirements

▸ Adult: According to requirements

● UNLICENSED USE Not licensed for children under 6 years.

● INTERACTIONS → Appendix 1: insulins

● DIRECTIONS FOR ADMINISTRATION Short-acting injectable insulins can be given by continuous subcutaneous infusion using a portable infusion pump. This device delivers a continuous basal insulin infusion and patient-activated bolus doses at meal times. This technique can be useful for patients who suffer recurrent hypoglycaemia or marked morning rise in blood-glucose concentration despite optimised multiple-injection regimens. Patients on subcutaneous insulin infusion must be highly motivated, able to monitor their blood-glucose concentration, and have expert training, advice and supervision from an experienced healthcare team.

▸ With intravenous use in adults For *intravenous infusion* (*Apidra*®), give continuously in Sodium chloride 0.9%; dilute to 1 unit/mL with infusion fluid; use a co-extruded polyolefin/polyamide plastic infusion bag with a dedicated infusion line.

● NATIONAL FUNDING/ACCESS DECISIONS

NICE decisions

▸ **Continuous subcutaneous insulin infusion for the treatment of diabetes mellitus (type 1) (July 2008)** NICE TA151
Continuous subcutaneous insulin infusion is recommended as an option in adults and children over 12 years with type 1 diabetes:

• who suffer repeated or unpredictable hypoglycaemia, whilst attempting to achieve optimal glycaemic control with multiple-injection regimens, **or**

• whose glycaemic control remains inadequate (HbA$_{1c}$ over 8.5% [69 mmol/mol]) despite optimised multiple-injection regimens (including the use of long-acting insulin analogues where appropriate).

Continuous subcutaneous insulin infusion is also recommended as an option for children under 12 years with type 1 diabetes for whom multiple-injection regimens are considered impractical or inappropriate. Children on insulin pumps should undergo a trial of multiple-injection therapy between the ages of 12 and 18 years.
www.nice.org.uk/TA151

Scottish Medicines Consortium (SMC) Decisions
The *Scottish Medicines Consortium* has advised (October 2008) that *Apidra*® is accepted for restricted use within NHS Scotland for the treatment of adults and children over 6 years with diabetes mellitus in whom the use of a short-acting insulin analogue is appropriate.

6

Endocrine system

- MEDICINAL FORMS
There can be variation in the licensing of different medicines containing the same drug.
Solution for injection
▸ Apidra (Sanofi)
Insulin glulisine 100 unit per 1 ml Apidra 100units/ml solution for injection 3ml cartridges | 5 cartridge PoM £28.30
Apidra 100units/ml solution for injection 10ml vials | 1 vial PoM £16.00
▸ Apidra SoloStar (Sanofi)
Insulin glulisine 100 unit per 1 ml Apidra 100units/ml solution for injection 3ml pre-filled SoloStar pen | 5 pre-filled disposable injection PoM £28.30 DT = £28.30

⊩ 695

Insulin lispro

21-Feb-2018

(Recombinant human insulin analogue—short acting)

- INDICATIONS AND DOSE
Diabetes mellitus
▸ BY SUBCUTANEOUS INJECTION
▸ Child 2-17 years: Administer shortly before meals or when necessary shortly after meals, according to requirements
▸ Adult: Administer shortly before meals or when necessary shortly after meals, according to requirements
▸ BY SUBCUTANEOUS INFUSION, OR BY INTRAVENOUS INFUSION, OR BY INTRAVENOUS INJECTION
▸ Child 2-17 years: According to requirements
▸ Adult: According to requirements

- CAUTIONS Children under 12 years (use only if benefit likely compared to soluble insulin)
- INTERACTIONS → Appendix 1: insulins
- PREGNANCY Not known to be harmful—may be used during pregnancy.
- BREAST FEEDING Not known to be harmful—may be used during lactation.
- DIRECTIONS FOR ADMINISTRATION Short-acting injectable insulins can be given by continuous subcutaneous infusion using a portable infusion pump. This device delivers a continuous basal insulin infusion and patient-activated bolus doses at meal times. This technique can be useful for patients who suffer recurrent hypoglycaemia or marked morning rise in blood-glucose concentration despite optimised multiple-injection regimens (see also NICE guidance, below). Patients on subcutaneous insulin infusion must be highly motivated, able to monitor their blood-glucose concentration, and have expert training, advice and supervision from an experienced healthcare team.
▸ With intravenous use in adults For *intravenous infusion* give continuously in Glucose 5% or Sodium chloride 0.9%. Adsorbed to some extent by plastics of infusion set.
▸ With intravenous use in children For *intravenous infusion*, dilute to a concentration of 0.1–1 unit/mL with Glucose 5% or Sodium Chloride 0.9% and mix thoroughly; insulin may be adsorbed by plastics, flush giving set with 5 mL of infusion fluid containing insulin.
- PRESCRIBING AND DISPENSING INFORMATION Insulin lispro is a biological medicine. Biological medicines must be prescribed and dispensed by brand name, see *Biological medicines* and *Biosimilar medicines*, under Guidance on prescribing p. 1.

- NATIONAL FUNDING/ACCESS DECISIONS
NICE decisions
▸ **Continuous subcutaneous insulin infusion for the treatment of diabetes mellitus (type 1) (July 2008)** NICE TA151
Continuous subcutaneous insulin infusion is recommended as an option in adults and children over 12 years with type 1 diabetes:
  • who suffer repeated or unpredictable hypoglycaemia, whilst attempting to achieve optimal glycaemic control with multiple-injection regimens, **or**
  • whose glycaemic control remains inadequate (HbA$_{1c}$ over 8.5% [69 mmol/mol]) despite optimised multiple-injection regimens (including the use of long-acting insulin analogues where appropriate).
Continuous subcutaneous insulin infusion is also recommended as an option for children under 12 years with type 1 diabetes for whom multiple-injection regimens are considered impractical or inappropriate. Children on insulin pumps should undergo a trial of multiple-injection therapy between the ages of 12 and 18 years.
www.nice.org.uk/TA151

- MEDICINAL FORMS
There can be variation in the licensing of different medicines containing the same drug.
Solution for injection
▸ Humalog (Eli Lilly and Company Ltd)
Insulin lispro 100 unit per 1 ml Humalog 100units/ml solution for injection 10ml vials | 1 vial PoM £16.61 DT = £16.61
Humalog 100units/ml solution for injection 3ml cartridges | 5 cartridge PoM £28.31 DT = £28.31
▸ Humalog Junior KwikPen (Eli Lilly and Company Ltd)
Insulin lispro 100 unit per 1 ml Humalog Junior KwikPen 100units/ml solution for injection 3ml pre-filled pen | 5 pre-filled disposable injection PoM £29.46 DT = £29.46
▸ Humalog KwikPen (Eli Lilly and Company Ltd)
Insulin lispro 100 unit per 1 ml Humalog KwikPen 100units/ml solution for injection 3ml pre-filled pen | 5 pre-filled disposable injection PoM £29.46 DT = £29.46
Insulin lispro 200 unit per 1 ml Humalog KwikPen 200units/ml solution for injection 3ml pre-filled pen | 5 pre-filled disposable injection PoM £58.92

INSULINS ⟩ INTERMEDIATE-ACTING

⊩ 695

Biphasic isophane insulin

(Biphasic Isophane Insulin Injection— intermediate acting)

- INDICATIONS AND DOSE
Diabetes mellitus
▸ BY SUBCUTANEOUS INJECTION
▸ Child: According to requirements
▸ Adult: According to requirements

- INTERACTIONS → Appendix 1: insulins
- SIDE-EFFECTS
▸ **Rare or very rare** Angioedema
▸ **Frequency not known** Hypokalaemia · weight increased
- PRESCRIBING AND DISPENSING INFORMATION A sterile buffered suspension of either porcine or human insulin complexed with protamine sulfate (or another suitable protamine) in a solution of insulin of the same species.
  Check product container—the proportions of the two components should be checked carefully (the order in which the proportions are stated may not be the same in other countries).

● MEDICINAL FORMS
There can be variation in the licensing of different medicines containing the same drug.
Suspension for injection
▸ Humulin M3 (Eli Lilly and Company Ltd)
Insulin human (as Insulin soluble human) 30 unit per 1 ml, Insulin human (as Insulin isophane human) 70 unit per 1 ml Humulin M3 100units/ml suspension for injection 3ml cartridges | 5 cartridge PoM £19.08 DT = £19.08
Humulin M3 100units/ml suspension for injection 10ml vials | 1 vial PoM £15.68
▸ Humulin M3 KwikPen (Eli Lilly and Company Ltd)
Insulin human (as Insulin soluble human) 30 unit per 1 ml, Insulin human (as Insulin isophane human) 70 unit per 1 ml Humulin M3 KwikPen 100units/ml suspension for injection 3ml pre-filled pen | 5 pre-filled disposable injection PoM £21.70 DT = £21.70
▸ Hypurin Porcine 30/70 Mix (Wockhardt UK Ltd)
Insulin porcine (as Insulin soluble porcine) 30 unit per 1 ml, Insulin porcine (as Insulin isophane porcine) 70 unit per 1 ml Hypurin Porcine 30/70 Mix 100units/ml suspension for injection 3ml cartridges | 5 cartridge PoM £46.95
Hypurin Porcine 30/70 Mix 100units/ml suspension for injection 10ml vials | 1 vial PoM £31.30
▸ Insuman Comb 15 (Sanofi)
Insulin human (as Insulin soluble human) 15 unit per 1 ml, Insulin human (as Insulin isophane human) 85 unit per 1 ml Insuman Comb 15 100units/ml suspension for injection 3ml cartridges | 5 cartridge PoM £17.50
▸ Insuman Comb 25 (Sanofi)
Insulin human (as Insulin soluble human) 25 unit per 1 ml, Insulin human (as Insulin isophane human) 75 unit per 1 ml Insuman Comb 25 100units/ml suspension for injection 5ml vials | 1 vial PoM £5.61
Insuman Comb 25 100units/ml suspension for injection 3ml pre-filled SoloStar pen | 5 pre-filled disposable injection PoM £19.80
Insuman Comb 25 100units/ml suspension for injection 3ml cartridges | 5 cartridge PoM £17.50
▸ Insuman Comb 50 (Sanofi)
Insulin human (as Insulin soluble human) 50 unit per 1 ml, Insulin human (as Insulin isophane human) 50 unit per 1 ml Insuman Comb 50 100units/ml suspension for injection 3ml cartridges | 5 cartridge PoM £17.50

F 695

Isophane insulin

(Isophane Insulin Injection; Isophane Protamine Insulin Injection; Isophane Insulin (NPH)–intermediate acting)

● INDICATIONS AND DOSE
Diabetes mellitus
▸ BY SUBCUTANEOUS INJECTION
▸ Child: According to requirements
▸ Adult: According to requirements

● INTERACTIONS → Appendix 1: insulins

● PREGNANCY Recommended where longer-acting insulins are needed.

● PRESCRIBING AND DISPENSING INFORMATION A sterile suspension of bovine or porcine insulin or of human insulin in the form of a complex obtained by the addition of protamine sulfate or another suitable protamine.

● MEDICINAL FORMS
There can be variation in the licensing of different medicines containing the same drug.
Suspension for injection
▸ Humulin I (Eli Lilly and Company Ltd)
Insulin human (as Insulin isophane human) 100 unit per 1 ml Humulin I 100units/ml suspension for injection 10ml vials | 1 vial PoM £15.68
Humulin I 100units/ml suspension for injection 3ml cartridges | 5 cartridge PoM £19.08 DT = £19.08

▸ Humulin I KwikPen (Eli Lilly and Company Ltd)
Insulin human (as Insulin isophane human) 100 unit per 1 ml Humulin I KwikPen 100units/ml suspension for injection 3ml pre-filled pen | 5 pre-filled disposable injection PoM £21.70 DT = £21.70
▸ Hypurin Bovine Isophane (Wockhardt UK Ltd)
Insulin bovine (as Insulin isophane bovine) 100 unit per 1 ml Hypurin Bovine Isophane 100units/ml suspension for injection 10ml vials | 1 vial PoM £27.72
▸ Hypurin Porcine Isophane (Wockhardt UK Ltd)
Insulin porcine (as Insulin isophane porcine) 100 unit per 1 ml Hypurin Porcine Isophane 100units/ml suspension for injection 3ml cartridges | 5 cartridge PoM £46.95
Hypurin Porcine Isophane 100units/ml suspension for injection 10ml vials | 1 vial PoM £31.30
▸ Insulatard (Novo Nordisk Ltd)
Insulin human (as Insulin isophane human) 100 unit per 1 ml Insulatard 100units/ml suspension for injection 10ml vials | 1 vial PoM £7.48
▸ Insulatard InnoLet (Novo Nordisk Ltd)
Insulin human (as Insulin isophane human) 100 unit per 1 ml Insulatard InnoLet 100units/ml suspension for injection 3ml pre-filled pen | 5 pre-filled disposable injection PoM £20.40 DT = £21.70
▸ Insulatard Penfill (Novo Nordisk Ltd)
Insulin human (as Insulin isophane human) 100 unit per 1 ml Insulatard Penfill 100units/ml suspension for injection 3ml cartridges | 5 cartridge PoM £22.90 DT = £19.08
▸ Insuman Basal (Sanofi)
Insulin human (as Insulin isophane human) 100 unit per 1 ml Insuman Basal 100units/ml suspension for injection 5ml vials | 1 vial PoM £5.61
Insuman Basal 100units/ml suspension for injection 3ml cartridges | 5 cartridge PoM £17.50 DT = £19.08
▸ Insuman Basal SoloStar (Sanofi)
Insulin human (as Insulin isophane human) 100 unit per 1 ml Insuman Basal 100units/ml suspension for injection 3ml pre-filled SoloStar pen | 5 pre-filled disposable injection PoM £19.80 DT = £21.70

INSULINS › INTERMEDIATE-ACTING COMBINED WITH RAPID-ACTING

F 695

Biphasic insulin aspart

(Intermediate-acting insulin)

● INDICATIONS AND DOSE
Diabetes mellitus
▸ BY SUBCUTANEOUS INJECTION
▸ Child: Administer up to 10 minutes before or soon after a meal, according to requirements
▸ Adult: Administer up to 10 minutes before or soon after a meal, according to requirements

● INTERACTIONS → Appendix 1: insulins

● PRESCRIBING AND DISPENSING INFORMATION Check product container—the proportions of the two components should be checked carefully (the order in which the proportions are stated may not be the same in other countries).

● MEDICINAL FORMS
There can be variation in the licensing of different medicines containing the same drug.
Suspension for injection
▸ NovoMix 30 FlexPen (Novo Nordisk Ltd)
Insulin aspart 30 unit per 1 ml, Insulin aspart (as Insulin aspart protamine) 70 unit per 1 ml NovoMix 30 FlexPen 100units/ml suspension for injection 3ml pre-filled pen | 5 pre-filled disposable injection PoM £29.89 DT = £29.89
▸ NovoMix 30 Penfill (Novo Nordisk Ltd)
Insulin aspart 30 unit per 1 ml, Insulin aspart (as Insulin aspart protamine) 70 unit per 1 ml NovoMix 30 Penfill 100units/ml suspension for injection 3ml cartridges | 5 cartridge PoM £28.79 DT = £28.79

6

Endocrine system

Endocrine system

6

Biphasic insulin lispro

▶ 695

(Intermediate-acting insulin)

- **INDICATIONS AND DOSE**

Diabetes mellitus
▶ BY SUBCUTANEOUS INJECTION
▶ Child: Administer up to 15 minutes before or soon after a meal, according to requirements
▶ Adult: Administer up to 15 minutes before or soon after a meal, according to requirements

- **CAUTIONS** Children under 12 years (use only if benefit likely compared to soluble insulin)
- **INTERACTIONS** → Appendix 1: insulins
- **PRESCRIBING AND DISPENSING INFORMATION** Check product container—the proportions of the two components should be checked carefully (the order in which the proportions are stated may not be the same in other countries).

- **MEDICINAL FORMS**
There can be variation in the licensing of different medicines containing the same drug.
Suspension for injection
▶ Humalog Mix25 (Eli Lilly and Company Ltd)
 Insulin lispro 25 unit per 1 ml, Insulin lispro (as Insulin lispro protamine) 75 unit per 1 ml Humalog Mix25 100units/ml suspension for injection 10ml vials | 1 vial ⟨PoM⟩ £16.61
 Humalog Mix25 100units/ml suspension for injection 3ml cartridges | 5 cartridge ⟨PoM⟩ £29.46 DT = £29.46
▶ Humalog Mix25 KwikPen (Eli Lilly and Company Ltd)
 Insulin lispro 25 unit per 1 ml, Insulin lispro (as Insulin lispro protamine) 75 unit per 1 ml Humalog Mix25 KwikPen 100units/ml suspension for injection 3ml pre-filled pen | 5 pre-filled disposable injection ⟨PoM⟩ £30.98 DT = £30.98
▶ Humalog Mix50 (Eli Lilly and Company Ltd)
 Insulin lispro 50 unit per 1 ml, Insulin lispro (as Insulin lispro protamine) 50 unit per 1 ml Humalog Mix50 100units/ml suspension for injection 3ml cartridges | 5 cartridge ⟨PoM⟩ £29.46 DT = £29.46
▶ Humalog Mix50 KwikPen (Eli Lilly and Company Ltd)
 Insulin lispro 50 unit per 1 ml, Insulin lispro (as Insulin lispro protamine) 50 unit per 1 ml Humalog Mix50 KwikPen 100units/ml suspension for injection 3ml pre-filled pen | 5 pre-filled disposable injection ⟨PoM⟩ £30.98 DT = £30.98

INSULINS > LONG-ACTING

▶ 695

Insulin degludec

14-Mar-2017

(Recombinant human insulin analogue—long acting)

- **INDICATIONS AND DOSE**

Diabetes mellitus
▶ BY SUBCUTANEOUS INJECTION
▶ Child 1-17 years: Dose to be given according to requirements
▶ Adult: Dose to be given according to requirements

- **INTERACTIONS** → Appendix 1: insulins
- **SIDE-EFFECTS**
▶ **Uncommon** Peripheral oedema
- **PREGNANCY** Evidence of the safety of long-acting insulin analogues in pregnancy is limited, therefore isophane insulin is recommended where longer-acting insulins are needed; insulin detemir may also be considered.
- **PRESCRIBING AND DISPENSING INFORMATION** Insulin degludec (*Tresiba*®) is available in strengths of 100 units/mL (allows 1-unit dose adjustment) and 200 units/mL (allows 2-unit dose adjustment)—ensure correct strength prescribed.

- **NATIONAL FUNDING/ACCESS DECISIONS**
All Wales Medicines Strategy Group (AWMSG) Decisions
▶ In adults The *All Wales Medicines Strategy Group* has advised (October 2016) that insulin degludec (*Tresiba*®) is recommended as an option for restricted use within NHS Wales for the treatment of diabetes mellitus in adult patients where treatment with a basal insulin analogue is considered appropriate.
▶ In children The *All Wales Medicines Strategy Group* has advised (October 2016) that insulin degludec (*Tresiba*®) is **not** recommended for use within NHS Wales for the treatment of diabetes mellitus in adolescents and children from the age of 1 year.

- **MEDICINAL FORMS**
There can be variation in the licensing of different medicines containing the same drug.
Solution for injection
▶ Tresiba FlexTouch (Novo Nordisk Ltd)
 Insulin human (as Insulin degludec) 100 unit per 1 ml Tresiba FlexTouch 100units/ml solution for injection 3ml pre-filled pen | 5 pre-filled disposable injection ⟨PoM⟩ £46.60 DT = £46.60
 Insulin human (as Insulin degludec) 200 unit per 1 ml Tresiba FlexTouch 200units/ml solution for injection 3ml pre-filled pen | 3 pre-filled disposable injection ⟨PoM⟩ £55.92 DT = £55.92
▶ Tresiba Penfill (Novo Nordisk Ltd)
 Insulin human (as Insulin degludec) 100 unit per 1 ml Tresiba Penfill 100units/ml solution for injection 3ml cartridges | 5 cartridge ⟨PoM⟩ £46.60 DT = £46.60

Insulin degludec with liraglutide

02-Jun-2016

The properties listed below are those particular to the combination only. For the properties of the components please consider, insulin degludec above, liraglutide p. 685.

- **INDICATIONS AND DOSE**

As add-on to oral antidiabetics in type 2 diabetes mellitus not controlled by oral antidiabetics alone
▶ BY SUBCUTANEOUS INJECTION
▶ Adult: Initially 10 dose-steps once daily, adjusted according to response; maximum 50 dose-steps per day

When transferring from basal insulin in type 2 diabetes mellitus not controlled by oral antidiabetics in combination with basal insulin
▶ BY SUBCUTANEOUS INJECTION
▶ Adult: Initially 16 dose-steps once daily, adjusted according to response; maximum 50 dose-steps per day

- **INTERACTIONS** → Appendix 1: insulins · liraglutide
- **PATIENT AND CARER ADVICE** Counselling advised on administration. Show container to patient and confirm that patient is expecting the version dispensed.
- **NATIONAL FUNDING/ACCESS DECISIONS**
Scottish Medicines Consortium (SMC) Decisions
The *Scottish Medicines Consortium* has advised (October 2015) that insulin degludec with liraglutide (*Xultophy*®) is accepted for restricted use within NHS Scotland for the treatment of type 2 diabetes mellitus to improve glycaemic control in combination with oral glucose-lowering medicinal products when these alone or combined with a GLP-1 receptor agonist or with basal insulin do not provide adequate glycaemic control.

- **MEDICINAL FORMS**
There can be variation in the licensing of different medicines containing the same drug.
Solution for injection
▶ Xultophy (Novo Nordisk Ltd) ▼
 Liraglutide 3.6 mg per 1 ml, Insulin human (as Insulin degludec) 100 unit per 1 ml Xultophy 100units/ml / 3.6mg/ml solution for injection 3ml pre-filled pen | 3 pre-filled disposable injection ⟨PoM⟩ £95.53 DT = £95.53

6

⬛ 695

Insulin detemir

(Recombinant human insulin analogue—long acting)

● **INDICATIONS AND DOSE**

Diabetes mellitus
▸ BY SUBCUTANEOUS INJECTION
▸ Child 2-17 years: According to requirements
▸ Adult: According to requirements

● INTERACTIONS → Appendix 1: insulins
● SIDE-EFFECTS
▸ **Uncommon** Refraction disorder
● PREGNANCY Evidence of the safety of long-acting insulin analogues in pregnancy is limited, therefore isophane insulin p. 699 is recommended where longer-acting insulins are needed; insulin detemir may also be considered where longer-acting insulins are needed.

● MEDICINAL FORMS
There can be variation in the licensing of different medicines containing the same drug.
Solution for injection
▸ Levemir FlexPen (Novo Nordisk Ltd)
 Insulin human (as Insulin detemir) 100 unit per 1 ml Levemir FlexPen 100units/ml solution for injection 3ml pre-filled pen | 5 pre-filled disposable injection PoM £42.00 DT = £42.00
▸ Levemir InnoLet (Novo Nordisk Ltd)
 Insulin human (as Insulin detemir) 100 unit per 1 ml Levemir InnoLet 100units/ml solution for injection 3ml pre-filled pen | 5 pre-filled disposable injection PoM £44.85 DT = £42.00
▸ Levemir Penfill (Novo Nordisk Ltd)
 Insulin human (as Insulin detemir) 100 unit per 1 ml Levemir Penfill 100units/ml solution for injection 3ml cartridges | 5 cartridge PoM £42.00 DT = £42.00

⬛ 695

Insulin glargine

(Recombinant human insulin analogue—long acting)

● **INDICATIONS AND DOSE**

Diabetes mellitus
▸ BY SUBCUTANEOUS INJECTION
▸ Child 2-17 years: According to requirements
▸ Adult: According to requirements

TOUJEO ®

Diabetes mellitus
▸ BY SUBCUTANEOUS INJECTION
▸ Adult: According to requirements

● INTERACTIONS → Appendix 1: insulins
● SIDE-EFFECTS
▸ **Rare or very rare** Myalgia · sodium retention · taste altered
● PREGNANCY Evidence of the safety of long-acting insulin analogues in pregnancy is limited, therefore isophane insulin is recommended where longer-acting insulins are needed; insulin detemir may also be considered.

● PRESCRIBING AND DISPENSING INFORMATION Insulin glargine is a biological medicine. Biological medicines must be prescribed and dispensed by brand name, see *Biological medicines* and *Biosimilar medicines*, under Guidance on prescribing p. 1. Dose adjustments and close metabolic monitoring is recommended if switching between insulin glargine preparations.

● NATIONAL FUNDING/ACCESS DECISIONS
Scottish Medicines Consortium (SMC) Decisions
The *Scottish Medicines Consortium* has advised that *Lantus* ® preparations (April 2013) and *Toujeo* ® (August

2015) are accepted for restricted use within NHS Scotland for the treatment of type 1 diabetes:
● in those who are at risk of or experience unacceptable frequency or severity of nocturnal hypoglycaemia on attempting to achieve better hypoglycaemic control during treatment with other insulins
● as a once daily insulin therapy for patients who require a carer to administer their insulin
It is **not** recommended for routine use in patients with type 2 diabetes unless they suffer from recurrent episodes of hypoglycaemia or require assistance with their insulin injections.

● MEDICINAL FORMS
There can be variation in the licensing of different medicines containing the same drug.
Solution for injection
▸ Abasaglar (Eli Lilly and Company Ltd) ▼
 Insulin human (as Insulin glargine) 100 unit per 1 ml Abasaglar 100units/ml solution for injection 3ml cartridges | 5 cartridge PoM £35.28 DT = £37.77
▸ Abasaglar KwikPen (Eli Lilly and Company Ltd) ▼
 Insulin human (as Insulin glargine) 100 unit per 1 ml Abasaglar KwikPen 100units/ml solution for injection 3ml pre-filled pen | 5 pre-filled disposable injection PoM £35.28 DT = £37.77
▸ Lantus (Sanofi)
 Insulin human (as Insulin glargine) 100 unit per 1 ml Lantus 100units/ml solution for injection 3ml cartridges | 5 cartridge PoM £37.77 DT = £37.77
 Lantus 100units/ml solution for injection 3ml pre-filled SoloStar pen | 5 pre-filled disposable injection PoM £37.77 DT = £37.77
 Lantus 100units/ml solution for injection 10ml vials | 1 vial PoM £27.92 DT = £27.92
▸ Toujeo (Sanofi)
 Insulin human (as Insulin glargine) 300 unit per 1 ml Toujeo 300units/ml solution for injection 1.5ml pre-filled SoloStar pen | 3 pre-filled disposable injection PoM £33.13 DT = £33.13

⬛ 695

Insulin zinc suspension

(Insulin zinc suspension (mixed)—long acting)

● **INDICATIONS AND DOSE**

Diabetes mellitus
▸ BY SUBCUTANEOUS INJECTION
▸ Child: According to requirements
▸ Adult: According to requirements

● INTERACTIONS → Appendix 1: insulins
● SIDE-EFFECTS Hypokalaemia · weight increased
● PREGNANCY Evidence of the safety of long-acting insulin analogues in pregnancy is limited, therefore isophane insulin p. 699 is recommended where longer-acting insulins are needed; insulin detemir above may also be considered.
● PRESCRIBING AND DISPENSING INFORMATION A sterile neutral suspension of bovine and/or porcine insulin or of human insulin in the form of a complex obtained by the addition of a suitable zinc salt; consists of rhombohedral crystals (10–40 microns) and of particles of no uniform shape (not exceeding 2 microns).

● MEDICINAL FORMS
There can be variation in the licensing of different medicines containing the same drug.
Suspension for injection
▸ Hypurin Bovine Lente (Wockhardt UK Ltd)
 Insulin bovine (as Insulin zinc suspension mixed bovine) 100 unit per 1 ml Hypurin Bovine Lente 100units/ml suspension for injection 10ml vials | 1 vial PoM £27.72

Protamine zinc insulin

▶ 695

(Protamine zinc insulin injection—long acting)

● INDICATIONS AND DOSE

Diabetes mellitus
▶ BY SUBCUTANEOUS INJECTION
▶ Child: According to requirements
▶ Adult: According to requirements

● INTERACTIONS → Appendix 1: insulins

● SIDE-EFFECTS Hypokalaemia

● PREGNANCY Evidence of the safety of long-acting insulin analogues in pregnancy is limited, therefore isophane insulin p. 699 is recommended where longer-acting insulins are needed; insulin detemir p. 701 may also be considered.

● PRESCRIBING AND DISPENSING INFORMATION A sterile suspension of insulin in the form of a complex obtained by the addition of a suitable protamine and zinc chloride; this preparation was included in BP 1980 but is not included in BP 1988.

● MEDICINAL FORMS
There can be variation in the licensing of different medicines containing the same drug.
Suspension for injection
▶ Hypurin Bovine Protamine Zinc (Wockhardt UK Ltd)
   Insulin bovine (as Insulin protamine zinc bovine) 100 unit per 1 ml Hypurin Bovine Protamine Zinc 100units/ml suspension for injection 10ml vials | 1 vial [PoM] £27.72

3.1a Diabetes, diagnosis and monitoring

Diabetes mellitus, diagnostic and monitoring devices

Urinalysis: urinary glucose

Reagent strips are available for measuring for glucose in the urine. Tests for ketones by patients are rarely required unless they become unwell—see Blood Monitoring.
   Microalbuminuria can be detected with *Micral-Test II*® but this should be followed by confirmation in the laboratory, since false positive results are common.

Blood glucose monitoring

Blood glucose monitoring using a meter gives a direct measure of the glucose concentration at the time of the test and can detect hypoglycaemia as well as hyperglycaemia. Patients should be properly trained in the use of blood glucose monitoring systems and to take appropriate action on the results obtained. Inadequate understanding of the normal fluctuations in blood glucose can lead to confusion and inappropriate action.
   Patients using multiple injection regimens should understand how to adjust their insulin dose according to their carbohydrate intake. With fixed-dose insulin regimens, the carbohydrate intake needs to be regulated, and should be distributed throughout the day to match the insulin regimen.
   Self-monitoring of blood-glucose concentration is appropriate for patients with type 2 diabetes:

● who are treated with insulin;
● who are treated with oral hypoglycaemic drugs e.g. sulfonylureas, to provide information on hypoglycaemia;
● to monitor changes in blood-glucose concentration resulting from changes in lifestyle or medication, and during intercurrent illness;

● to ensure safe blood-glucose concentration during activities, including driving.

In the UK blood-glucose concentration is expressed in mmol/litre and Diabetes UK advises that these units should be used for self-monitoring of blood glucose. In other European countries units of mg/100 mL (or mg/dL) are commonly used.
   It is advisable to check that the meter is pre-set in the correct units.
   If the patient is unwell and diabetic ketoacidosis is suspected, blood **ketones** should be measured according to local guidelines. Patients and their carers should be trained in the use of blood ketone monitoring systems and to take appropriate action on the results obtained, including when to seek medical attention.

Other drugs used for Diabetes, diagnosis and monitoring
Glucose, p. 1009

Blood glucose testing strips

● BLOOD GLUCOSE TESTING STRIPS

Accu-Chek Inform II testing strips (Roche Diagnostics Ltd)
50 strip · No NHS indicative price available · Drug Tariff (Part IXr)

Active testing strips (Roche Diabetes Care Ltd)
50 strip · NHS indicative price = £9.95 · Drug Tariff (Part IXr)

Advocate Redi-Code+ testing strips (Diabetes Care Technology Ltd)
50 strip · NHS indicative price = £9.95 · Drug Tariff (Part IXr)

AutoSense testing strips (Advance Diagnostic Products (NI) Ltd)
25 strip · NHS indicative price = £4.50 · Drug Tariff (Part IXr)

Aviva testing strips (Roche Diabetes Care Ltd)
50 strip · NHS indicative price = £16.09 · Drug Tariff (Part IXr)

BGStar testing strips (Sanofi)
50 strip · NHS indicative price = £14.73 · Drug Tariff (Part IXr)

Betachek C50 cassette (National Diagnostic Products)
100 device · NHS indicative price = £29.98 · Drug Tariff (Part IXr)

Betachek G5 testing strips (National Diagnostic Products)
50 strip · NHS indicative price = £14.19 · Drug Tariff (Part IXr)

Betachek Visual testing strips (National Diagnostic Products)
50 strip · NHS indicative price = £6.80 · Drug Tariff (Part IXr)

Breeze 2 testing discs (Bayer Plc)
50 strip · NHS indicative price = £15.00 · Drug Tariff (Part IXr)

CareSens N testing strips (Spirit Healthcare Ltd)
50 strip · NHS indicative price = £12.75 · Drug Tariff (Part IXr)

CareSens PRO testing strips (Spirit Healthcare Ltd)
50 strip · NHS indicative price = £9.95 · Drug Tariff (Part IXr)

Compact testing strips (Roche Diabetes Care Ltd)
51 strip · NHS indicative price = £16.53 · Drug Tariff (Part IXr)

Contour Next testing strips (Bayer Diagnostics Manufacturing Ltd)
50 strip · NHS indicative price = £15.04 · Drug Tariff (Part IXr)

Contour TS testing strips (Bayer Diagnostics Manufacturing Ltd)
50 strip · NHS indicative price = £9.50 · Drug Tariff (Part IXr)

Contour testing strips (Bayer Diagnostics Manufacturing Ltd)
50 strip · NHS indicative price = £9.95 · Drug Tariff (Part IXr)

Dario Lite testing strips (LabStyle Innovations Ltd)
50 strip · NHS indicative price = £9.95 · Drug Tariff (Part IXr)

Dario testing strips (LabStyle Innovations Ltd)
50 strip · NHS indicative price = £14.95 · Drug Tariff (Part IXr)

Diastix testing strips (Bayer Diagnostics Manufacturing Ltd)
50 strip · NHS indicative price = £2.89 · Drug Tariff (Part IXr)

Element testing strips (Neon Diagnostics Ltd)
50 strip · NHS indicative price = £9.89 · Drug Tariff (Part IXr)

Finetest Lite testing strips (Neon Diagnostics Ltd)
50 strip · NHS indicative price = £5.95 · Drug Tariff (Part IXr)

FreeStyle Lite testing strips (Abbott Laboratories Ltd)
50 strip · NHS indicative price = £16.10 · Drug Tariff (Part IXr)

FreeStyle Optium H testing strips (Abbott Laboratories Ltd)
100 strip · No NHS indicative price available · Drug Tariff (Part IXr)

FreeStyle Optium testing strips (Abbott Laboratories Ltd)
50 strip · NHS indicative price = £16.00 · Drug Tariff (Part IXr)

Meters and test strips

Meter (all NHS)	Type of monitoring	Compatible test strips	Test strip net price	Sensitivity range (mmol/litre)	Manufacturer
Accu-Chek® Active	Blood glucose	Active®	50 strip= £9.95	0.6– 33.3 mmol/litre	Roche Diabetes Care Ltd
Accu-Chek® Advantage Meter no longer available	Blood glucose	Advantage Plus®	50 strip= £0.00	0.6– 33.3 mmol/litre	Roche Diabetes Care Ltd
Accu-Chek® Aviva	Blood glucose	Aviva®	50 strip= £16.09	0.6– 33.3 mmol/litre	Roche Diabetes Care Ltd
Accu-Chek® Aviva Expert	Blood glucose	Aviva®	50 strip= £16.09	0.6– 33.3 mmol/litre	Roche Diabetes Care Ltd
Accu-Chek® Compact Plus Meter no longer available	Blood glucose	Compact®	3 × 17 strips= £16.53	0.6– 33.3 mmol/litre	Roche Diabetes Care Ltd
Accu-Chek® Mobile	Blood glucose	Mobile®	100 device= £0.00	0.3– 33.3 mmol/litre	Roche Diabetes Care Ltd
Accu-Chek® Aviva Nano	Blood glucose	Aviva®	50 strip= £16.09	0.6– 33.3 mmol/litre	Roche Diabetes Care Ltd
BGStar® Free of charge from diabetes healthcare professionals	Blood glucose	BGStar®	50 strip £14.73	1.1– 33.3 mmol/litre	Sanofi
Breeze 2®	Blood glucose	Breeze 2®	50 strip= £15.00	0.6– 33.3 mmol/litre	Bayer Plc
CareSens N® Free of charge from diabetes healthcare professionals	Blood glucose	CareSens N®	50 strip= £12.75	1.1– 33.3 mmol/litre	Spirit Healthcare Ltd
Contour®	Blood glucose	Contour®	50 strip= £9.95	0.6– 33.3 mmol/litre	Bayer Diagnostics Manufacturing Ltd
Contour® XT	Blood glucose	Contour® Next	50 strip= £15.04	0.6– 33.3 mmol/litre	Bayer Diagnostics Manufacturing Ltd
Element®	Blood glucose	Element®	50 strip= £9.89	0.55– 33.3 mmol/litre	Neon Diagnostics Ltd
FreeStyle® Meter no longer available	Blood glucose	FreeStyle®	50 strip= £16.10	1.1– 27.8 mmol/litre	Abbott Laboratories Ltd
FreeStyle Freedom® Meter no longer available	Blood glucose	FreeStyle®	50 strip= £16.10	1.1– 27.8 mmol/litre	Abbott Laboratories Ltd
FreeStyle Freedom Lite®	Blood glucose	FreeStyle Lite®	50 strip= £16.10	1.1– 27.8 mmol/litre	Abbott Laboratories Ltd
FreeStyle InsuLinx®	Blood glucose	FreeStyle Lite®	50 strip= £16.10	1.1– 27.8 mmol/litre	Abbott Laboratories Ltd
FreeStyle Lite®	Blood glucose	FreeStyle Lite®	50 strip= £16.10	1.1– 27.8 mmol/litre	Abbott Laboratories Ltd
FreeStyle Mini® Meter no longer available	Blood glucose	FreeStyle®	50 strip= £16.10	1.1– 27.8 mmol/litre	Abbott Laboratories Ltd
FreeStyle Optium®	Blood glucose	FreeStyle Optium®	50 strip= £16.00	1.1– 27.8 mmol/litre	Abbott Laboratories Ltd
FreeStyle Optium®	Blood ketones	FreeStyle Optium® β-ketone	10 strip= £21.53	0– 8.0 mmol/litre	Abbott Laboratories Ltd
FreeStyle Optium Neo®	Blood glucose	FreeStyle Optium®	50 strip= £16.00	1.1– 27.8 mmol/litre	Abbott Laboratories Ltd
FreeStyle Optium Neo®	Blood ketones	FreeStyle Optium® β-ketone	10 strip= £21.53	0– 8.0 mmol/litre	Abbott Laboratories Ltd
GlucoDock® module	Blood glucose	GlucoDock®	50 strip= £14.90	1.1– 33.3 mmol/litre For use with iPhone®, iPod touch®, and iPad®	Medisana Healthcare (UK) Ltd
GlucoLab®	Blood glucose	GlucoLab®	50 strip= £9.89	0.55– 33.3 mmol/litre	Neon Diagnostics Ltd
GlucoMen® GM	Blood glucose	GlucoMen® GM	50 strip= £9.95	0.6– 33.3 mmol/litre	

6

Endocrine system

Meter (all NHS)	Type of monitoring	Compatible test strips	Test strip net price	Sensitivity range (mmol/litre)	Manufacturer
					A. Menarini Diagnostics Ltd
GlucoMen® LX	Blood glucose	GlucoMen® LX Sensor	50 strip= £15.76	1.1- 33.3 mmol/litre	A. Menarini Diagnostics Ltd
GlucoMen® LX Plus	Blood glucose	GlucoMen® LX Sensor	50 strip= £15.76	1.1- 33.3 mmol/litre	A. Menarini Diagnostics Ltd
GlucoMen® LX Plus	Blood ketones	GlucoMen® LX Ketone	10 strip= £21.06	0- 0.8 mmol/litre	A. Menarini Diagnostics Ltd
GlucoMen® Visio	Blood glucose	GlucoMen® Visio Sensor	50 strip= £0.00	1.1- 33.3 mmol/litre	A. Menarini Diagnostics Ltd
GlucoRx® Free of charge from diabetes healthcare professionals	Blood glucose	GlucoRx®	50 strip= £5.45	1.1- 33.3 mmol/litre	GlucoRx Ltd
GlucoRx Nexus® Free of charge from diabetes healthcare professionals	Blood glucose	GlucoRx Nexus®	50 strip= £9.95	1.1- 33.3 mmol/litre	GlucoRx Ltd
Glucotrend® Meter no longer available	Blood glucose	Active®	50 strip= £9.95	0.6- 33.3 mmol/litre	Roche Diabetes Care Ltd
iBGStar®	Blood glucose	BGStar®	50 strip= £14.73	1.1- 33.3 mmol/litre	Sanofi
IME-DC®	Blood glucose	IME-DC®	50 strip= £14.10	1.1- 33.3 mmol/litre	Arctic Medical Ltd
Mendor Discreet®	Blood glucose	Mendor Discreet®	50 strip= £14.75	1.1- 33.3 mmol/litre	SpringMed Solutions Ltd
Microdot®+ Free of charge from diabetes healthcare professionals	Blood glucose	Microdot®+	50 strip= £9.49	1.1- 29.2 mmol/litre	Cambridge Sensors Ltd
MyGlucoHealth®	Blood glucose	MyGlucoHealth®	50 strip= £15.50	0.6- 33.3 mmol/litre	Entra Health Systems Ltd
Omnitest® 3	Blood glucose	Omnitest® 3	50 strip= £9.89	0.6- 33.3 mmol/litre	B.Braun Medical Ltd
One Touch Ultra® Meter no longer available	Blood glucose	One Touch Ultra®	50 strip= £9.99	1.1- 33.3 mmol/litre	LifeScan
One Touch Ultra 2® Free of charge from diabetes healthcare professionals	Blood glucose	One Touch Ultra®	50 strip= £9.99	1.1- 33.3 mmol/litre	LifeScan
One Touch UltraEasy® Free of charge from diabetes healthcare professionals	Blood glucose	One Touch Ultra®	50 strip= £9.99	1.1- 33.3 mmol/litre	LifeScan
One Touch UltraSmart® Free of charge from diabetes healthcare professionals	Blood glucose	One Touch Ultra®	50 strip= £9.99	1.1- 33.3 mmol/litre	LifeScan
One Touch® VerioPro Free of charge from diabetes healthcare professionals	Blood glucose	One Touch® Verio	50 strip= £15.12	1.1- 33.3 mmol/litre	LifeScan
One Touch® Vita Free of charge from diabetes healthcare professionals	Blood glucose	One Touch® Vita	50 strip= £15.07	1.1- 33.3 mmol/litre	LifeScan
SD CodeFree®	Blood glucose	SD CodeFree®	50 strip= £6.99	0.6- 33.3 mmol/litre	SD Biosensor Inc
Sensocard Plus® Meter no longer available	Blood glucose	Sensocard®	50 strip= £16.30	1.1- 33.3 mmol/litre	BBI Healthcare Ltd

Meter (all NHS)	Type of monitoring	Compatible test strips	Test strip net price	Sensitivity range (mmol/litre)	Manufacturer
SuperCheck2® Free of charge from diabetes healthcare professionals	Blood glucose	SuperCheck2®	50 strip= £8.49	1.1- 33.3 mmol/litre	Apollo Medical Technologies Ltd
TRUEone® All-in-one test strips and meter	Blood glucose	TRUEone®	50 strip= £0.00	1.1- 33.3 mmol/litre	Nipro Diagnostics (UK) Ltd
TRUEresult® Free of charge from diabetes healthcare professionals	Blood glucose	TRUEresult®	50 strip= £14.99	1.1- 33.3 mmol/litre	Nipro Diagnostics (UK) Ltd
TRUEresult twist® Free of charge from diabetes healthcare professionals	Blood glucose	TRUEresult®	50 strip= £14.99	1.1- 33.3 mmol/litre	Nipro Diagnostics (UK) Ltd
TRUEtrack® Free of charge from diabetes healthcare professionals	Blood glucose	TRUEtrack®	50 strip= £14.99	1.1- 33.3 mmol/litre	Nipro Diagnostics (UK) Ltd
TRUEyou mini®	Blood glucose	TRUEyou®	50 strip= £9.92	1.1- 33.3 mmol/litre	Nipro Diagnostics (UK) Ltd
WaveSense JAZZ® Free of charge from diabetes healthcare professionals	Blood glucose	WaveSense JAZZ®	50 strip= £8.74	1.1- 33.3 mmol/litre	AgaMatrix Europe Ltd

6

Endocrine system

FreeStyle Precision Pro testing strips (Abbott Laboratories Ltd)
100 strip • No NHS indicative price available • Drug Tariff (Part IXr)

FreeStyle testing strips (Abbott Laboratories Ltd)
50 strip • NHS indicative price = £16.10 • Drug Tariff (Part IXr)

GluNEO testing strips (Neon Diagnostics Ltd)
50 strip • NHS indicative price = £9.89 • Drug Tariff (Part IXr)

GlucoDock testing strips (Medisana Healthcare (UK) Ltd)
50 strip • NHS indicative price = £14.90 • Drug Tariff (Part IXr)

GlucoLab testing strips (Neon Diagnostics Ltd)
50 strip • NHS indicative price = £9.89 • Drug Tariff (Part IXr)

GlucoMen GM testing strips (A. Menarini Diagnostics Ltd)
50 strip • NHS indicative price = £9.95 • Drug Tariff (Part IXr)

GlucoMen LX Sensor testing strips (A. Menarini Diagnostics Ltd)
50 strip • NHS indicative price = £15.76 • Drug Tariff (Part IXr)

GlucoMen areo Sensor testing strips (A. Menarini Diagnostics Ltd)
50 strip • NHS indicative price = £9.95 • Drug Tariff (Part IXr)

GlucoRx GO Professional testing strips (GlucoRx Ltd)
50 strip • NHS indicative price = £9.95 • Drug Tariff (Part IXr)

GlucoRx GO testing strips (GlucoRx Ltd)
50 strip • NHS indicative price = £9.95 • Drug Tariff (Part IXr)

GlucoRx HCT Glucose testing strips (GlucoRx Ltd)
50 strip • NHS indicative price = £9.95 • Drug Tariff (Part IXr)

GlucoRx Nexus testing strips (GlucoRx Ltd)
50 strip • NHS indicative price = £9.95 • Drug Tariff (Part IXr)

GlucoRx Q testing strips (GlucoRx Ltd)
50 strip • NHS indicative price = £5.45 • Drug Tariff (Part IXr)

GlucoZen.auto testing strips (GlucoZen Ltd)
50 strip • NHS indicative price = £7.64 • Drug Tariff (Part IXr)100 strip •
NHS indicative price = £10.85 • Drug Tariff (Part IXr)

Glucoflex-R testing strips (Bio-Diagnostics Ltd)
50 strip • NHS indicative price = £6.75 • Drug Tariff (Part IXr)

IME-DC testing strips (Arctic Medical Ltd)
50 strip • NHS indicative price = £14.10 • Drug Tariff (Part IXr)

MODZ testing strips (Modz Oy)
50 strip • NHS indicative price = £14.00 • Drug Tariff (Part IXr)

Medi-Test Glucose testing strips (BHR Pharmaceuticals Ltd)
50 strip • NHS indicative price = £2.33 • Drug Tariff (Part IXr)

MediSense SoftSense testing strips (Abbott Laboratories Ltd)
50 strip • NHS indicative price = £15.05 • Drug Tariff (Part IXr)

MediTouch 2 testing strips (Medisana Healthcare (UK) Ltd)
50 strip • NHS indicative price = £12.49 • Drug Tariff (Part IXr)

MediTouch testing strips (Medisana Healthcare (UK) Ltd)
50 strip • NHS indicative price = £14.90 • Drug Tariff (Part IXr)

Mendor Discreet testing strips (SpringMed Solutions Ltd)
50 strip • NHS indicative price = £14.75 • Drug Tariff (Part IXr)

Microdot+ testing strips (Cambridge Sensors Ltd)
50 strip • NHS indicative price = £9.49 • Drug Tariff (Part IXr)

Mobile cassette (Roche Diabetes Care Ltd)
50 device • NHS indicative price = £9.99 • Drug Tariff (Part IXr)

Myglucohealth testing strips (Entra Health Systems Ltd)
50 strip • NHS indicative price = £15.50 • Drug Tariff (Part IXr)

Mylife Pura testing strips (Ypsomed Ltd)
50 strip • NHS indicative price = £9.50 • Drug Tariff (Part IXr)

Mylife Unio testing strips (Ypsomed Ltd)
50 strip • NHS indicative price = £9.50 • Drug Tariff (Part IXr)

Omnitest 3 testing strips (B.Braun Medical Ltd)
50 strip • NHS indicative price = £9.89 • Drug Tariff (Part IXr)

Omnitest 5 testing strips (B.Braun Medical Ltd)
50 strip • NHS indicative price = £9.89 • Drug Tariff (Part IXr)

On-Call Advanced testing strips (Point Of Care Testing Ltd)
50 strip • NHS indicative price = £13.65 • Drug Tariff (Part IXr)

OneTouch Select Plus testing strips (LifeScan)
50 strip • NHS indicative price = £9.99 • Drug Tariff (Part IXr)

OneTouch Ultra testing strips (LifeScan)
50 strip • NHS indicative price = £9.99 • Drug Tariff (Part IXr)

OneTouch Verio testing strips (LifeScan)
50 strip • NHS indicative price = £15.12 • Drug Tariff (Part IXr)

OneTouch Vita testing strips (LifeScan)
50 strip • NHS indicative price = £15.07 • Drug Tariff (Part IXr)

Performa testing strips (Roche Diabetes Care Ltd)
50 strip • NHS indicative price = £9.95 • Drug Tariff (Part IXr)

SD CodeFree testing strips (SD Biosensor Inc)
50 strip • NHS indicative price = £6.99 • Drug Tariff (Part IXr)

SURESIGN Resure testing strips (Ciga Healthcare Ltd)
50 strip • NHS indicative price = £8.49 • Drug Tariff (Part IXr)

Sensocard testing strips (BBI Healthcare Ltd)
50 strip • NHS indicative price = £16.30 • Drug Tariff (Part IXr)

StatStrip testing strips (Nova Biomedical)
50 strip • No NHS indicative price available • Drug Tariff (Part IXr)

TEE2 testing strips (Spirit Healthcare Ltd)
50 strip • NHS indicative price = £7.75 • Drug Tariff (Part IXr)

Endocrine system 6

TRUEresult testing strips (Nipro Diagnostics (UK) Ltd)
50 strip · NHS indicative price = £14.99 · Drug Tariff (Part IXr)

TRUEyou testing strips (Nipro Diagnostics (UK) Ltd)
50 strip · NHS indicative price = £9.92 · Drug Tariff (Part IXr)

True Metrix testing strips (Trividia Health UK Ltd)
50 strip · NHS indicative price = £9.90 · Drug Tariff (Part IXr)

TrueTrack System testing strips (Nipro Diagnostics (UK) Ltd)
50 strip · NHS indicative price = £14.99 · Drug Tariff (Part IXr)

VivaChek Ino testing strips (JR Biomedical Ltd)
50 strip · NHS indicative price = £8.99 · Drug Tariff (Part IXr)

WaveSense JAZZ Duo testing strips (AgaMatrix Europe Ltd)
50 strip · NHS indicative price = £8.74 · Drug Tariff (Part IXr)

WaveSense JAZZ testing strips (AgaMatrix Europe Ltd)
50 strip · NHS indicative price = £8.74 · Drug Tariff (Part IXr)

Xceed Precision Pro testing strips (Abbott Laboratories Ltd)
10 strip · No NHS indicative price available 50 strip · No NHS indicative
price available · Drug Tariff (Part IXr) 100 strip · No NHS indicative price
available · Drug Tariff (Part IXr)

eBchek testing strips (IRASCO Ltd)
50 strip · NHS indicative price = £15.89 · Drug Tariff (Part IXr)

iHealth testing strips (Technomed Ltd)
50 strip · NHS indicative price = £9.49 · Drug Tariff (Part IXr)

palmdoc iCare Advanced Solo testing strips (Palmdoc Ltd)
50 strip · NHS indicative price = £13.50 · Drug Tariff (Part IXr)

palmdoc iCare Advanced testing strips (Palmdoc Ltd)
50 strip · NHS indicative price = £9.70 · Drug Tariff (Part IXr)

palmdoc testing strips (Palmdoc Ltd)
50 strip · NHS indicative price = £9.40 · Drug Tariff (Part IXr)

Blood ketones testing strips

● BLOOD KETONES TESTING STRIPS

FreeStyle Optium H beta-ketone testing strips (Abbott
Laboratories Ltd) | 10 strip · No NHS indicative price available · Drug
Tariff (Part IXr)

FreeStyle Optium beta-ketone testing strips (Abbott Laboratories
Ltd) | 10 strip · NHS indicative price = £21.53 · Drug Tariff (Part IXr)

FreeStyle Precision Pro beta-ketone testing strips (Abbott
Laboratories Ltd) | 50 strip · No NHS indicative price available

GlucoMen LX beta-ketone testing strips (A. Menarini Diagnostics
Ltd) | 10 strip · NHS indicative price = £21.06 · Drug Tariff (Part IXr)

GlucoMen areo Ketone Sensor testing strips (A. Menarini
Diagnostics Ltd) | 10 strip · NHS indicative price = £9.95 · Drug Tariff
(Part IXr)

GlucoRx HCT Ketone testing strips (GlucoRx Ltd) | 10 strip · NHS
indicative price = £9.95 · Drug Tariff (Part IXr)

KetoSens testing strips (Spirit Healthcare Ltd) | 10 strip · NHS
indicative price = £9.95 · Drug Tariff (Part IXr)

StatStrip beta-ketone testing strips (Nova Biomedical) | 50 strip ·
No NHS indicative price available

Xceed Precision Pro beta-ketone testing strips (Abbott
Laboratories Ltd) | 10 strip · No NHS indicative price available · Drug
Tariff (Part IXr) | 50 strip · No NHS indicative price available | 100 strip ·
No NHS indicative price available

Hypodermic insulin injection pens

● HYPODERMIC INSULIN INJECTION PENS
AUTOPEN ® 24
Autopen ® 24 (for use with Sanofi- Aventis 3-mL insulin
cartridges), allowing 1-unit dosage adjustment, max.
21 units (single-unit version) or 2-unit dosage adjustment,
max. 42 units (2- unit version).

**Autopen 24 hypodermic insulin injection pen reusable for 3ml
cartridge 1 unit dial up / range 1-21 units** (Owen Mumford Ltd)
1 device · NHS indicative price = £16.71 · Drug Tariff (Part IXa)

**Autopen 24 hypodermic insulin injection pen reusable for 3ml
cartridge 2 unit dial up / range 2-42 units** (Owen Mumford Ltd)
1 device · NHS indicative price = £16.71 · Drug Tariff (Part IXa)

AUTOPEN ® CLASSIC
Autopen ® *Classic* (for use with Lilly and Wockhardt 3-mL
insulin cartridges), allowing 1-unit dosage adjustment,
max. 21 units (single-version) or 2-unit dosage
adjustment, max. 42 units (2-unit version).

**Autopen Classic hypodermic insulin injection pen reusable for
3ml cartridge 1 unit dial up / range 1-21 units** (Owen Mumford Ltd)
1 device · NHS indicative price = £16.96 · Drug Tariff (Part IXa)

**Autopen Classic hypodermic insulin injection pen reusable for
3ml cartridge 2 unit dial up / range 2-42 units** (Owen Mumford
Ltd)
1 device · NHS indicative price = £16.96 · Drug Tariff (Part IXa)

CLIKSTAR ®
For use with *Lantus* ®, *Apidra* ®, and *Insuman* ® 3-mL
insulin cartridges; allowing 1-unit dose adjustment, max.
80 units.

HUMAPEN ® LUXURA HD
For use with *Humulin* ® and *Humalog* ® 3-mL cartridges;
allowing 0.5-unit dosage adjustment, max. 30 units.

**HumaPen Luxura HD hypodermic insulin injection pen
reusable for 3ml cartridge 0.5 unit dial up / range 1-30 units**
(Eli Lilly and Company Ltd)
1 device · NHS indicative price = £27.01 · Drug Tariff (Part IXa)

NOVOPEN ® 4
For use with *Penfill* ® 3-mL insulin cartridges; allowing
1-unit dosage adjustment, max. 60 units.

**NovoPen 4 hypodermic insulin injection pen reusable for 3ml
cartridge 1 unit dial up / range 1-60 units** (Novo Nordisk Ltd)
1 device · NHS indicative price = £26.86 · Drug Tariff (Part IXa)

**NovoPen 4 hypodermic insulin injection pen reusable for 3ml
cartridge 1 unit dial up / range 1-60 units** (Novo Nordisk Ltd)
1 device · NHS indicative price = £26.86 · Drug Tariff (Part IXa)

Needle free insulin delivery systems

● NEEDLE FREE INSULIN DELIVERY SYSTEMS
INSUJET ®
For use with any 10-mL vial or 3-mL cartridge of insulin,
allowing 1-unit dosage adjustment, max 40 units.
Available as *starter set* (*InsuJet* ® device, nozzle cap, nozzle
and piston, 1 × 10-mL adaptor, 1 × 3-mL adaptor,
1 cartridge cap removal key), *nozzle pack* (15 nozzles),
cartridge adaptor pack (15 adaptors), or *vial adaptor pack*
(15 adaptors).

InsuJet starter set (Spirit Healthcare Ltd)
1 pack · NHS indicative price = £90.00 · Drug Tariff (Part IXa)

Urine glucose testing strips

● URINE GLUCOSE TESTING STRIPS

Diastix testing strips (Bayer Diagnostics Manufacturing Ltd)
50 strip · NHS indicative price = £2.89 · Drug Tariff (Part IXr)

Medi-Test Glucose testing strips (BHR Pharmaceuticals Ltd)
50 strip · NHS indicative price = £2.33 · Drug Tariff (Part IXr)

Urine ketone testing strips

● URINE KETONES TESTING STRIPS

GlucoRx KetoRx Sticks 2GK testing strips (GlucoRx Ltd)
50 strip · NHS indicative price = £2.25 · Drug Tariff (Part IXr)

Ketostix testing strips (Bayer Diagnostics Manufacturing Ltd)
50 strip · NHS indicative price = £3.06 · Drug Tariff (Part IXr)

Urine protein testing strips

● URINE PROTEIN TESTING STRIPS

Albustix testing strips (Siemens Medical Solutions Diagnostics Ltd)
50 strip · NHS indicative price = £4.10 · Drug Tariff (Part IXr)

Medi-Test Protein 2 testing strips (BHR Pharmaceuticals Ltd)
50 strip · NHS indicative price = £3.27 · Drug Tariff (Part IXr)

3.2 Hypoglycaemia

Hypoglycaemia

02-Jun-2017

Treatment of hypoglycaemia

Initially glucose 10–20 g is given by mouth either in liquid form or as granulated sugar or sugar lumps. If necessary this may be repeated after 10–15 minutes. After initial treatment, a snack providing sustained availability of carbohydrate (e.g. a sandwich, fruit, milk, or biscuits) or the next meal (if it is due) can prevent blood-glucose concentration from falling again.

Proprietary products of quick-acting carbohydrate (e.g. *GlucoGel*®, *Dextrogel*®, *GSF-Syrup*®, *Rapilose*® gel) are available on prescription for patients to keep on hand in case of hypoglycaemia.

Alternatively, approximately 10 g of glucose is available from 2 teaspoons of sugar, or from 3 sugar lumps, and also from non-diet versions of the following soft drinks: 110 mL of *Lucozade*® *Energy Original* (also, see note below), 100 mL of *Coca-Cola*®, 19 mL of *Ribena*® *Blackcurrant* (to be diluted).

Note: the carbohydrate content of some commercially available glucose-containing drinks is currently subject to change—individual product labels should be checked . Patients should be aware that for a time, both old and new bottles and cans may be available—individual product labels should be checked.

Hypoglycaemia which causes unconsciousness is an emergency. Glucagon below, a polypeptide hormone produced by the alpha cells of the islets of Langerhans, increases plasma-glucose concentration by mobilising glycogen stored in the liver. In hypoglycaemia, if sugar cannot be given by mouth, glucagon can be given by injection. Carbohydrates should be given as soon as possible to restore liver glycogen; glucagon is not appropriate for chronic hypoglycaemia. Glucagon may be issued to close relatives of insulin-treated patients for emergency use in hypoglycaemic attacks. It is often advisable to prescribe on an 'if necessary' basis to hospitalised insulin-treated patients, so that it may be given rapidly by the nurses during an hypoglycaemic emergency. If not effective in 10 minutes intravenous glucose should be given.

Alternatively, glucose **intravenous infusion 20%** p. 1009 may be given intravenously into a large vein through a large-gauge needle; care is required since this concentration is irritant especially if extravasation occurs. Glucose intravenous infusion 10% may also be used but larger volumes are needed. Glucose intravenous infusion 50% is not recommended because of the higher risk of extravasation injury and because administration is difficult. Close monitoring is necessary in the case of an overdose with a long-acting insulin because further administration of glucose may be required. Patients whose hypoglycaemia is caused by an oral antidiabetic drug should be transferred to hospital because the hypoglycaemic effects of these drugs may persist for many hours.

See also, emergency management of hypoglycaemia in dental practice for further advice.

Chronic hypoglycaemia

Diazoxide p. 708, administered by mouth, is useful in the management of patients with chronic hypoglycaemia from excess endogenous insulin secretion, either from an islet cell tumour or islet cell hyperplasia. It has no place in the management of acute hypoglycaemia.

GLYCOGENOLYTIC HORMONES

❚ Glucagon

- ● **INDICATIONS AND DOSE**

Insulin-induced hypoglycaemia
- ▶ BY SUBCUTANEOUS INJECTION, OR BY INTRAMUSCULAR INJECTION
- ▸ Child 1 month-1 year: 500 micrograms
- ▸ Child 2-17 years (body-weight up to 25 kg): 500 micrograms, if no response within 10 minutes intravenous glucose must be given
- ▸ Child 2-17 years (body-weight 25 kg and above): 1 mg, if no response within 10 minutes intravenous glucose must be given
- ▸ Adult: 1 mg, if no response within 10 minutes intravenous glucose must be given

Beta-blocker poisoning (cardiogenic shock unresponsive to atropine)
- ▶ INITIALLY BY INTRAVENOUS INJECTION
- ▸ Child: 50–150 micrograms/kg (max. per dose 10 mg), to be administered in glucose 5% (with precautions to protect the airway in case of vomiting), followed by (by intravenous infusion) 50 micrograms/kg/hour
- ▸ Adult: 2–10 mg, to be administered in glucose 5% (with precautions to protect the airway in case of vomiting), followed by (by intravenous infusion) 50 micrograms/kg/hour

Diagnostic aid
- ▶ BY INTRAVENOUS INJECTION, OR BY INTRAMUSCULAR INJECTION
- ▸ Adult: (consult product literature)

DOSE EQUIVALENCE AND CONVERSION
- ▸ 1 unit of glucagon = 1 mg of glucagon.

- ● UNLICENSED USE Dose and indication for cardiogenic shock unresponsive to atropine in beta-blocker overdose not licensed.

- ● CONTRA-INDICATIONS Phaeochromocytoma

- ● CAUTIONS Glucagonoma · ineffective in chronic hypoglycaemia, starvation, and adrenal insufficiency · insulinoma · when used in the diagnosis of growth hormone secretion, delayed hypoglycaemia may result—deaths reported (ensure a meal is eaten before discharge) (in children)

- ● INTERACTIONS → Appendix 1: glucagon

- ● SIDE-EFFECTS
- ▶ **Common or very common** Nausea
- ▶ **Uncommon** Vomiting
- ▶ **Rare or very rare** Abdominal pain · hypertension · hypotension · tachycardia

- ● DIRECTIONS FOR ADMINISTRATION
- ▶ With intravenous use in children When administered by *continuous intravenous infusion*, do not add to infusion fluids containing calcium—precipitation may occur.

- ● PATIENT AND CARER ADVICE
Medicines for Children leaflet: Glucagon for hypoglycaemia
www.medicinesforchildren.org.uk/glucagon-for-hypoglycaemia

- ● EXCEPTIONS TO LEGAL CATEGORY Prescription-only medicine restriction does not apply where administration is for saving life in emergency.

- ● MEDICINAL FORMS
There can be variation in the licensing of different medicines containing the same drug.

Powder and solvent for solution for injection
- ▸ GlucaGen Hypokit (Novo Nordisk Ltd)
  Glucagon hydrochloride 1 mg GlucaGen Hypokit 1mg powder and solvent for solution for injection | 1 vial PoM £11.52 DT = £11.52

3.2a Chronic hypoglycaemia

GLYCOGENOLYTIC HORMONES

Diazoxide

- **INDICATIONS AND DOSE**

Chronic intractable hypoglycaemia
  ▸ BY MOUTH
  ▸ **Adult:** Initially 5 mg/kg daily in 2–3 divided doses, adjusted according to response; maintenance 3–8 mg/kg daily in 2–3 divided doses

- CAUTIONS Aortic coarctation · aortic stenosis · arteriovenous shunt · heart failure · hyperuricaemia · impaired cardiac circulation · impaired cerebral circulation
- INTERACTIONS → Appendix 1: diazoxide
- SIDE-EFFECTS Abdominal pain · albuminuria · appetite decreased (long term use) · arrhythmia · azotaemia · cardiomegaly · cataract · constipation · diabetic hyperosmolar coma · diarrhoea · dizziness · dyspnoea · eosinophilia · extrapyramidal symptoms · fever · fluid retention · galactorrhoea · haemorrhage · headache · heart failure · hirsutism · hyperglycaemia · hyperuricaemia (long term use) · hypogammaglobulinaemia · hypotension · ileus · ketoacidosis · leucopenia · libido decreased · musculoskeletal pain · nausea · nephritic syndrome · oculogyric crisis · pancreatitis · parkinsonism · pulmonary hypertension · skin reactions · sodium retention · taste altered · thrombocytopenia · tinnitus · vision disorders · voice alteration (long term use) · vomiting
- PREGNANCY Use only if essential; alopecia and hypertrichosis reported in neonates with prolonged use; may inhibit uterine activity during labour.
- BREAST FEEDING Manufacturer advises avoid—no information available.
- RENAL IMPAIRMENT
Dose adjustments Dose reduction may be required.
- MONITORING REQUIREMENTS
  ▸ Monitor blood pressure.
  ▸ Monitor white cell and platelet count during prolonged use.
- MEDICINAL FORMS
There can be variation in the licensing of different medicines containing the same drug. Forms available from special-order manufacturers include: capsule, oral suspension, oral solution

Tablet
  ▸ Eudemine (RPH Pharmaceuticals AB)
    Diazoxide 50 mg Eudemine 50mg tablets | 100 tablet [PoM] £46.45

Capsule
  ▸ Diazoxide (Non-proprietary)
    Diazoxide 25 mg Proglycem 25 capsules | 100 capsule [PoM] 🚫

---

4 Disorders of bone metabolism

Osteoporosis

20-Oct-2017

Description of condition

Osteoporosis is a progressive bone disease characterised by low bone mass measured by bone mineral density (BMD), and microarchitectural deterioration of bone tissue. This leads to an increased risk of fragility fractures as a result. Osteoporosis is considered severe if there have been one or more fragility fractures.

Osteoporosis occurs most commonly in postmenopausal women, men over 50 years, and in patients taking long-term oral corticosteroids (glucocorticoids). Risk factors for osteoporosis include age, low body mass index (BMI), cigarette smoking, excess alcohol intake, lack of physical activity, vitamin D deficiency and low calcium intake, family history of hip fractures, a previous fracture at a site characteristic of osteoporotic fractures and early menopause. Some diseases are also known to be associated with osteoporosis such as rheumatoid arthritis and diabetes.

Aims of treatment

A combination of lifestyle changes and drug treatment aims to prevent bone fractures in patients with osteoporosis.

Lifestyle changes

[EvGr] Patients should be encouraged to increase their level of physical activity, stop smoking, maintain a normal BMI level (between 20–25 kg/m^2), and reduce their alcohol intake to improve their bone health and reduce the risk of fragility fractures.

Patients at risk of osteoporosis should also ensure an adequate intake of calcium and vitamin D, preferably through increasing dietary intake.

Elderly patients, especially those who are housebound or live in residential or nursing homes, are at increased risk of calcium and vitamin D deficiency and can benefit from supplements. Ⓐ Elderly patients also have an increased risk of falls (see Prescribing in the elderly p. 28).

Drug treatment

Postmenopausal osteoporosis

The therapeutic options for the prevention and treatment of osteoporosis in postmenopausal women are the same.

[EvGr] Oral bisphosphonates, alendronic acid p. 710 and risedronate sodium p. 713 are considered as first-line choices for most patients with postmenopausal osteoporosis due to their broad spectrum of anti-fracture efficacy. Alendronic acid and risedronate sodium have been shown to reduce occurrence of vertebral, non-vertebral and hip fractures. Intravenous bisphosphonates (ibandronic acid p. 711 or zoledronic acid p. 715), denosumab p. 717, or raloxifene hydrochloride p. 736 are alternative options in women who are intolerant of oral bisphosphonates or in whom they are contra-indicated.

Hormone replacement therapy (HRT) is an additional option. The use of HRT for osteoporosis is generally restricted to younger postmenopausal women with menopausal symptoms who are at high risk of fractures. This is due to the risk of adverse effects such as cardiovascular disease and cancer in older postmenopausal women and women on long-term HRT therapy.

Teriparatide p. 716 is reserved for postmenopausal women with severe osteoporosis at very high risk for vertebral fractures. Its duration of treatment is limited to 24 months. Ⓐ

Glucocorticoid-induced osteoporosis

Glucocorticoid therapy is associated with bone loss and increased risk of fractures. The greatest rate of bone loss occurs early after initiation of glucocorticoids and increases with dose and duration of therapy. [EvGr] Bone-protection treatment should be started at the onset of therapy in patients who are at a high risk of fracture.

If glucocorticoid therapy is stopped, the need to continue bone-protection treatment should be reviewed. However, bone-protection treatment should be continued with long-term glucocorticoid therapy. Complex cases of glucocorticoid-induced osteoporosis should be referred to a specialist.

Women aged 70 years or over, or with a previous fragility fracture, or taking large doses of glucocorticoids (prednisolone ≥7.5 mg daily or equivalent) are at high risk of fractures and should be assessed for prophylactic bone-protection. Some younger patients, particularly those with a previous history of fracture or receiving high doses of glucocorticoids can also be considered for bone-protection treatment.

The therapeutic options for prophylaxis and treatment of glucocorticoid-induced osteoporosis are the same; oral bisphosphonates, alendronic acid, or risedronate sodium are first-line options. Intravenous zoledronic acid or teriparatide are alternatives in patients intolerant of oral bisphosphonates or in whom they are contra-indicated. ⟨A⟩

Osteoporosis in men

[EvGr] Oral bisphosphonates, alendronic acid or risedronate sodium are recommended as first-line treatments for osteoporosis in men. Intravenous zoledronic acid or denosumab are alternatives in men who are intolerant of oral bisphosphonates or in whom they are contra-indicated; teriparatide is an additional option. ⟨A⟩

Men having long-term androgen deprivation therapy for prostate cancer have an increased fracture risk. [EvGr] Fracture risk should be assessed when starting this therapy. A bisphosphonate can be offered to men with confirmed osteoporosis; denosumab is an alternative if bisphosphonates are contra-indicated or not tolerated. ⟨A⟩

Bisphosphonates: treatment duration

[EvGr] There is some evidence to suggest that patients can benefit from a bisphosphonate-free perioid as their therapeutic effects last for some time after cessation of treatment.

Bisphosphonate treatment should be reviewed after 5 years of treatment with alendronic acid, risedronate sodium or ibandronic acid, and after 3 years of treatment with zoledronic acid. Patients over 75 years of age, or with a history of previous hip or vertebral fracture, or patients who have had one or more fragility fractures during treatment, or who are taking long-term glucocorticoid therapy can continue bisphosphonates beyond this period. ⟨A⟩

> **Other drugs used for Disorders of bone metabolism**
> Calcitriol, p. 1050

ANABOLIC STEROIDS

Nandrolone

- **INDICATIONS AND DOSE**

Osteoporosis in postmenopausal women (but not recommended)
▶ BY DEEP INTRAMUSCULAR INJECTION
▶ Adult (female): 50 mg every 3 weeks.

- CONTRA-INDICATIONS Acute porphyrias p. 1025 · male breast cancer · prostate cancer
- CAUTIONS Cardiac impairment · diabetes mellitus · epilepsy · hypertension · migraine · skeletal metastases (risk of hypercalcaemia)
- INTERACTIONS → Appendix 1: nandrolone
- SIDE-EFFECTS Clitoris enlarged · dysphonia · hepatic disorders · hepatic neoplasm · hirsutism · hypertension · libido increased · nausea · oedema · skin reactions · sodium retention · urine flow decreased · virilism (with high doses including voice changes - sometimes irreversible)
- HEPATIC IMPAIRMENT Use in severe hepatic impairment only if benefit outweighs risk.
- RENAL IMPAIRMENT Use with caution—may cause sodium and water retention.
- MONITORING REQUIREMENTS Monitor skeletal maturation in young patients.

- LESS SUITABLE FOR PRESCRIBING Nandrolone injection is less suitable for prescribing.

- MEDICINAL FORMS
There can be variation in the licensing of different medicines containing the same drug.
Solution for injection
EXCIPIENTS: May contain Arachis (peanut) oil, benzyl alcohol
▶ Deca-Durabolin (Aspen Pharma Trading Ltd)
Nandrolone decanoate 50 mg per 1 ml Deca-Durabolin 50mg/1ml solution for injection ampoules | 1 ampoule [PoM] £3.17 [CD4-2]

BISPHOSPHONATES

Bisphosphonates ▣

- DRUG ACTION Bisphosphonates are adsorbed onto hydroxyapatite crystals in bone, slowing both their rate of growth and dissolution, and therefore reducing the rate of bone turnover.

> IMPORTANT SAFETY INFORMATION
> MHRA/CHM ADVICE: BISPHOSPHONATES: ATYPICAL FEMORAL FRACTURES (JUNE 2011)
> Atypical femoral fractures have been reported rarely with bisphosphonate treatment, mainly in patients receiving long-term treatment for osteoporosis.
> The need to continue bisphosphonate treatment for osteoporosis should be re-evaluated periodically based on an assessment of the benefits and risks of treatment for individual patients, particularly after 5 or more years of use.
> Patients should be advised to report any thigh, hip, or groin pain during treatment with a bisphosphonate.
> Discontinuation of bisphosphonate treatment in patients suspected to have an atypical femoral fracture should be considered after an assessment of the benefits and risks of continued treatment.
>
> MHRA/CHM ADVICE: BISPHOSPHONATES: OSTEONECROSIS OF THE JAW (NOVEMBER 2009) AND INTRAVENOUS BISPHOSPHONATES: OSTEONECROSIS OF THE JAW—FURTHER MEASURES TO MINIMISE RISK (JULY 2015)
> The risk of osteonecrosis of the jaw is substantially greater for patients receiving intravenous bisphosphonates in the treatment of cancer than for patients receiving oral bisphosphonates for osteoporosis or Paget's disease.
> Risk factors for developing osteonecrosis of the jaw that should be considered are: potency of bisphosphonate (highest for zoledronate), route of administration, cumulative dose, duration and type of malignant disease, concomitant treatment, smoking, comorbid conditions, and history of dental disease.
> All patients should have a dental check-up (and any necessary remedial work should be performed) before bisphosphonate treatment, or as soon as possible after starting treatment. Patients should also maintain good oral hygiene, receive routine dental check-ups, and report any oral symptoms such as dental mobility, pain, or swelling, non-healing sores or discharge to a doctor and dentist during treatment.
> Before prescribing an intravenous bisphosphonate, patients should be given a patient reminder card and informed of the risk of osteonecrosis of the jaw. Advise patients to tell their doctor if they have any problems with their mouth or teeth before starting treatment, and if the patient wears dentures, they should make sure their dentures fit properly. Patients should tell their doctor and dentist that they are receiving an intravenous bisphosphonate if they need dental treatment or dental surgery.
> Guidance for dentists in primary care is included in *Oral Health Management of Patients Prescribed*

Endocrine system

6

Bisphosphonates: Dental Clinical Guidance, Scottish Dental Clinical Effectiveness Programme, April 2011 (available at www.sdcep.org.uk).

MHRA/CHM ADVICE: BISPHOSPHONATES: OSTEONECROSIS OF THE EXTERNAL AUDITORY CANAL (DECEMBER 2015)
Benign idiopathic osteonecrosis of the external auditory canal has been reported very rarely with bisphosphonate treatment, mainly in patients receiving long-term therapy (2 years or longer).

The possibility of osteonecrosis of the external auditory canal should be considered in patients receiving bisphosphonates who present with ear symptoms, including chronic ear infections, or suspected cholesteatoma.

Risk factors for developing osteonecrosis of the external auditory canal include: steroid use, chemotherapy, infection, an ear operation, or cotton-bud use.

Patients should be advised to report any ear pain, discharge from the ear, or an ear infection during treatment with a bisphosphonate.

● SIDE-EFFECTS
▸ **Common or very common** Alopecia · anaemia · arthralgia · asthenia · constipation · diarrhoea · dizziness · dysphagia · electrolyte imbalance · eye inflammation · fever · gastritis · gastrointestinal discomfort · headache · influenza like illness · malaise · myalgia · nausea · oesophageal ulcer (discontinue) · oesophagitis (discontinue) · pain · peripheral oedema · renal impairment · skin reactions · taste altered · vomiting
▸ **Uncommon** Anaphylactic reaction · angioedema · bronchospasm · oesophageal stenosis (discontinue) · osteonecrosis
▸ **Rare or very rare** Atypical femur fracture · Stevens-Johnson syndrome
● PATIENT AND CARER ADVICE
Atypical femoral fractures Patients should be advised to report any thigh, hip, or groin pain during treatment with a bisphosphonate.
Osteonecrosis of the jaw During bisphosphonate treatment patients should maintain good oral hygiene, receive routine dental check-ups, and report any oral symptoms.
Osteonecrosis of the external auditory canal Patients should be advised to report any ear pain, discharge from ear or an ear infection during treatment with a bisphosphonate.

▸ 709

Alendronic acid

14-Sep-2017

(Alendronate)

● INDICATIONS AND DOSE
Treatment of postmenopausal osteoporosis
▸ BY MOUTH
▸ Adult (female): 10 mg daily, alternatively 70 mg once weekly.
Treatment of osteoporosis in men
▸ BY MOUTH
▸ Adult (male): 10 mg daily.
Prevention and treatment of corticosteroid-induced osteoporosis in postmenopausal women not receiving hormone replacement therapy
▸ BY MOUTH
▸ Adult (female): 10 mg daily.

● CONTRA-INDICATIONS Abnormalities of oesophagus · hypocalcaemia · other factors which delay emptying (e.g. stricture or achalasia)
● CAUTIONS Active gastro-intestinal bleeding · atypical femoral fractures · duodenitis · dysphagia · exclude other causes of osteoporosis · gastritis · history (within 1 year) of

ulcers · surgery of the upper gastro-intestinal tract · symptomatic oesophageal disease · ulcers · upper gastro-intestinal disorders
● INTERACTIONS → Appendix 1: bisphosphonates
● SIDE-EFFECTS
▸ **Common or very common** Abdominal distension · gastrointestinal disorders · joint swelling · vertigo
▸ **Uncommon** Erythema · eye inflammation · haemorrhage
▸ **Rare or very rare** Femoral stress fracture · oropharyngeal ulceration · photosensitivity reaction · severe cutaneous adverse reactions (SCARs)
SIDE-EFFECTS, FURTHER INFORMATION Severe oesophageal reactions (oesophagitis, oesophageal ulcers, oesophageal stricture and oesophageal erosions) have been reported; patients should be advised to stop taking the tablets and to seek medical attention if they develop symptoms of oesophageal irritation such as dysphagia, new or worsening heartburn, pain on swallowing or retrosternal pain.
● PREGNANCY Avoid.
● BREAST FEEDING Manufacturer advises avoid—no information available.
● RENAL IMPAIRMENT Avoid if eGFR less than 35 mL/minute/1.73 m^2.
● MONITORING REQUIREMENTS Correct disturbances of calcium and mineral metabolism (e.g. vitamin-D deficiency, hypocalcaemia) before starting treatment. Monitor serum-calcium concentration during treatment.
● DIRECTIONS FOR ADMINISTRATION Tablets should be swallowed whole and oral solution should be swallowed as a single 100 mL dose. Doses should be taken with plenty of water while sitting or standing, on an empty stomach at least 30 minutes before breakfast (or another oral medicine); patient should stand or sit upright for at least 30 minutes after administration.
● PATIENT AND CARER ADVICE Patients or their carers should be given advice on how to administer alendronic acid tablets and oral solution.
Oesophageal reactions Patients (or their carers) should be advised to stop taking alendronic acid and to seek medical attention if they develop symptoms of oesophageal irritation such as dysphagia, new or worsening heartburn, pain on swallowing or retrosternal pain.
● NATIONAL FUNDING/ACCESS DECISIONS
NICE decisions
▸ **Bisphosphonates for treating osteoporosis (updated February 2018)** NICE TA464
This technology appraisal guidance should be applied clinically in conjunction with:
● NICE guideline on assessing the risk of fragility fractures (CG146), which defines who is eligible for osteoporotic fracture risk assessment.
● NICE quality standard on osteoporosis (QS149), which defines the clinical intervention thresholds for the 10-year fracture probability of a major osteoporotic fracture, in those patients who have undergone fracture risk assessment.
Alendronic acid is recommended as an option for treating osteoporosis in patients, only if:
● the person is eligible for risk assessment as defined in the full NICE guideline on osteoporosis, **and**
● the 10-year probability of osteoporotic fragility fracture is at least 1%.
Patients whose treatment was started within the NHS before this guidance was published should have the option to continue treatment, without change to their funding arrangements, until they and their NHS clinician consider it appropriate to stop.
www.nice.org.uk/guidance/ta464

Scottish Medicines Consortium (SMC) Decisions
The *Scottish Medicines Consortium* has advised (April 2016)
that alendronic acid (*Binosto*®) is accepted for restricted
use within NHS Scotland for the treatment of
postmenopausal osteoporosis where alendronic acid is the
appropriate treatment choice, but the patient is unable to
swallow tablets.

● MEDICINAL FORMS
There can be variation in the licensing of different medicines
containing the same drug. Forms available from special-order
manufacturers include: oral solution

Oral solution
▸ Alendronic acid (Non-proprietary)
  Alendronic acid 700 microgram per 1 ml Alendronic acid
  70mg/100ml oral solution unit dose sugar free sugar-free | 4 unit
  dose PoM £28.56 DT = £28.56

Effervescent tablet
▸ Binosto (Internis Pharmaceuticals Ltd)
  Alendronic acid (as Alendronate sodium) 70 mg Binosto 70mg
  effervescent tablets sugar-free | 4 tablet PoM £22.80 DT = £22.80

Tablet
▸ Alendronic acid (Non-proprietary)
  Alendronic acid (as Alendronate sodium) 10 mg Alendronic acid
  10mg tablets | 28 tablet PoM £3.25 DT = £1.38
  Alendronic acid (as Alendronate sodium) 70 mg Alendronic acid
  70mg tablets | 4 tablet PoM £22.80 DT = £0.41
▸ Fosamax Once Weekly (Merck Sharp & Dohme Ltd)
  Alendronic acid (as Alendronate sodium) 70 mg Fosamax Once
  Weekly 70mg tablets | 4 tablet PoM £22.80 DT = £0.41

Alendronic acid with colecalciferol

The properties listed below are those particular to the
combination only. For the properties of the components
please consider, alendronic acid p. 710, colecalciferol
p. 1051.

● INDICATIONS AND DOSE
**Treatment of postmenopausal osteoporosis in women at
risk of vitamin D deficiency**
▸ BY MOUTH
▸ Adult (female): 1 tablet once weekly.

● INTERACTIONS → Appendix 1: bisphosphonates · vitamin D
substances

● DIRECTIONS FOR ADMINISTRATION Tablets should be
swallowed whole with plenty of water while sitting or
standing; to be taken on an empty stomach at least
30 minutes before breakfast (or another oral medicine);
patient should stand or sit upright for at least 30 minutes
after taking tablet.

● PATIENT AND CARER ADVICE Patients or carers should be
given advice on how to administer alendronic acid with
colecalciferol tablets.

● MEDICINAL FORMS
There can be variation in the licensing of different medicines
containing the same drug.

Tablet
▸ Alendronic acid with colecalciferol (Non-proprietary)
  **Colecalciferol 70 microgram, Alendronic acid (as Alendronate
  sodium) 70 mg** Alendronic acid 70mg / Colecalciferol 70microgram
  tablets | 4 tablet PoM £22.80 DT = £22.80
▸ Fosavance (Merck Sharp & Dohme Ltd)
  **Colecalciferol 70 microgram, Alendronic acid (as Alendronate
  sodium) 70 mg** Fosavance tablets | 4 tablet PoM £22.80 DT =
  £22.80

Ibandronic acid
⚑ 709
28-Sep-2017

● INDICATIONS AND DOSE
**Reduction of bone damage in bone metastases in breast
cancer**
▸ INITIALLY BY MOUTH
▸ Adult: 50 mg daily, alternatively (by intravenous
  infusion) 6 mg every 3–4 weeks
Hypercalcaemia of malignancy
▸ BY INTRAVENOUS INFUSION
▸ Adult: 2–4 mg as a single infusion, dose to be adjusted
  according to serum calcium concentration
Treatment of postmenopausal osteoporosis
▸ INITIALLY BY MOUTH
▸ Adult (female): 150 mg once a month, alternatively (by
  intravenous injection) 3 mg every 3 months, to be
  administered over 15–30 seconds.

● CONTRA-INDICATIONS
GENERAL CONTRA-INDICATIONS Hypocalcaemia
SPECIFIC CONTRA-INDICATIONS
▸ With oral use Abnormalities of the oesophagus · other
  factors which delay emptying (e.g. stricture or achalasia)
● CAUTIONS Atypical femoral fractures · cardiac disease
  (avoid fluid overload)
● INTERACTIONS → Appendix 1: bisphosphonates
● SIDE-EFFECTS
GENERAL SIDE-EFFECTS
▸ **Common or very common** Face oedema
▸ **Uncommon** Asthma exacerbated
▸ **Rare or very rare** Eye inflammation
SPECIFIC SIDE-EFFECTS
▸ **Common or very common**
▸ With intravenous use Bundle branch block · cataract ·
  increased risk of infection · joint disorder · oral disorders ·
  osteoarthritis · parathyroid disorder · thirst
▸ With oral use Acute phase reaction · muscle cramps ·
  musculoskeletal stiffness
▸ **Uncommon**
▸ With intravenous use Acrochordon · affective disorder ·
  altered smell sensation · anxiety · blood disorder ·
  cardiovascular disorder · cerebrovascular disorder ·
  cholelithiasis · cystitis · deafness · hyperaesthesia ·
  hypothermia · injury · memory loss · migraine · muscle tone
  increased · myocardial ischaemia · neuralgia · palpitations ·
  pelvic pain · pulmonary oedema · radiculopathy · renal cyst
  · sleep disorder · stridor · urinary retention · weight
  decreased
▸ **Rare or very rare**
▸ With intravenous use Hypersensitivity
● PREGNANCY Avoid.
● BREAST FEEDING Avoid—present in milk in *animal* studies.
● RENAL IMPAIRMENT When used for postmenopausal
  osteoporosis, avoid if eGFR less than
  30 mL/minute/1.73 m^2.
  Dose adjustments ▸ With intravenous use When used for
  bone metastases, if eGFR 30–50 mL/minute/1.73 m^2
  reduce dose to 4 mg and infuse over 1 hour; if eGFR less
  than 30 mL/minute/1.73 m^2 reduce dose to 2 mg and infuse
  over 1 hour.
  ▸ With oral use When used for bone metastases, if eGFR
  30–50 mL/minute/1.73 m^2 reduce dose to 50 mg on
  alternative days; if eGFR less than 30 mL/minute/1.73 m^2
  reduce dose to 50 mg once weekly.
● MONITORING REQUIREMENTS Monitor renal function and
  serum calcium, phosphate and magnesium.
● DIRECTIONS FOR ADMINISTRATION Tablets should be
  swallowed whole with plenty of water while sitting or

6

Endocrine system

6

Endocrine system

standing; to be taken on an empty stomach at least 30 minutes (for most ibandronic acid tablets, 50 mg) or 1 hour (for *Bonviva* ® tablets, 150 mg) before first food or drink (other than water) of the day, or another oral medicine; patient should stand or sit upright for at least 1 hour after taking tablet.

For *intravenous infusion* (*Bondronat* ®), give intermittently in Glucose 5% or Sodium chloride 0.9%; dilute requisite dose in 500 mL infusion fluid and give over 1–2 hours.

● PATIENT AND CARER ADVICE Patients or carers should be given advice on how to administer ibandronic acid tablets. Oesophageal reactions Patients and carers should be advised to stop tablets and seek medical attention for symptoms of oesophageal irritation such as dysphagia, pain on swallowing, retrosternal pain, or heartburn.

A patient reminder card should be provided to patients receiving intravenous ibandronic acid (risk of osteonecrosis of the jaw).

● NATIONAL FUNDING/ACCESS DECISIONS

NICE decisions

▸ **Bisphosphonates for treating osteoporosis (updated February 2018)** NICE TA464

This technology appraisal guidance should be applied clinically in conjunction with:
● NICE guideline on assessing the risk of fragility fractures (CG146), which defines who is eligible for osteoporotic fracture risk assessment.
● NICE quality standard on osteoporosis (QS149), which defines the clinical intervention thresholds for the 10-year fracture probability of a major osteoporotic fracture, in those patients who have undergone fracture risk assessment.

With oral use ibandronic acid is recommended as an option for treating osteoporosis in patients, only if:
● the person is eligible for risk assessment as defined in the full NICE guideline on osteoporosis, **and**
● the 10-year probability of osteoporotic fragility fracture is at least 1%.

With intravenous use ibandronic acid is recommended as an option for treating osteoporosis in patients, only if:
● the person is eligible for risk assessment as defined in the full NICE guideline on osteoporosis, **and**
● the 10-year probability of osteoporotic fragility fracture is at least 10%, **or**
● the 10-year probability of osteoporotic fragility fracture is at least 1% and the person has difficulty taking oral bisphosphonates (alendronic acid, ibandronic acid or risedronate sodium) or these drugs are contra-indicated or not tolerated.

Patients whose treatment was started within the NHS before this guidance was published should have the option to continue treatment, without change to their funding arrangements, until they and their NHS clinician consider it appropriate to stop.

www.nice.org.uk/guidance/ta464

● MEDICINAL FORMS
There can be variation in the licensing of different medicines containing the same drug.

Solution for injection

▸ Ibandronic acid (Non-proprietary)
Ibandronic acid (as Ibandronic sodium monohydrate) 1 mg per 1 ml Ibandronic acid 3mg/3ml solution for injection pre-filled syringes | 1 pre-filled disposable injection PoM £65.20–£68.64

▸ Bonviva (Roche Products Ltd)
Ibandronic acid (as Ibandronic sodium monohydrate) 1 mg per 1 ml Bonviva 3mg/3ml solution for injection pre-filled syringes | 1 pre-filled disposable injection PoM £68.64

Solution for infusion

▸ Ibandronic acid (Non-proprietary)
Ibandronic acid (as Ibandronic sodium monohydrate) 1 mg per 1 ml Ibandronic acid 6mg/6ml concentrate for solution for infusion vials | 1 vial PoM £130.42 (Hospital only)
Ibandronic acid 2mg/2ml concentrate for solution for infusion vials | 1 vial PoM £43.47 (Hospital only)

▸ Bondronat (Roche Products Ltd)
Ibandronic acid (as Ibandronic sodium monohydrate) 1 mg per 1 ml Bondronat 2mg/2ml concentrate for solution for infusion vials | 1 vial PoM £89.36 (Hospital only)
Bondronat 6mg/6ml concentrate for solution for infusion vials | 1 vial PoM £183.69

Tablet

▸ Ibandronic acid (Non-proprietary)
Ibandronic acid (as Ibandronic sodium monohydrate)
50 mg Ibandronic acid 50mg tablets | 28 tablet PoM £13.49 DT = £6.25
Ibandronic acid (as Ibandronic sodium monohydrate)
150 mg Ibandronic acid 150mg tablets | 1 tablet PoM £15.64 DT = £0.83 | 3 tablet PoM £2.49–£52.44

▸ Bondronat (Roche Products Ltd)
Ibandronic acid (as Ibandronic sodium monohydrate)
50 mg Bondronat 50mg tablets | 28 tablet PoM £183.69 DT = £6.25

▸ Bonviva (Roche Products Ltd)
Ibandronic acid (as Ibandronic sodium monohydrate)
150 mg Bonviva 150mg tablets | 1 tablet PoM £18.40 DT = £0.83

▸ Iasibon (Aspire Pharma Ltd)
Ibandronic acid (as Ibandronic sodium monohydrate)
50 mg Iasibon 50mg tablets | 28 tablet PoM £174.50 DT = £6.25

▸ Quodixor (Aspire Pharma Ltd)
Ibandronic acid (as Ibandronic sodium monohydrate)
150 mg Quodixor 150mg tablets | 1 tablet PoM £18.40 DT = £0.83

F 709

Pamidronate disodium

(Formerly called aminohydroxypropylidenediphosphonate disodium (APD))

● INDICATIONS AND DOSE

Hypercalcaemia of malignancy
▸ BY INTRAVENOUS INFUSION
▸ Adult: 15–60 mg, to be given (via cannula in a relatively large vein) as a single infusion or in divided doses over 2–4 days, dose adjusted according to serum calcium concentration; maximum 90 mg per course

Osteolytic lesions and bone pain in bone metastases associated with breast cancer or multiple myeloma
▸ BY INTRAVENOUS INFUSION
▸ Adult: 90 mg every 4 weeks, to be administered via cannula in a relatively large vein, dose may alternatively be administered every 3 weeks, to coincide with chemotherapy in breast cancer

Paget's disease of bone
▸ BY INTRAVENOUS INFUSION
▸ Adult: 30 mg every week for a 6 week course (total dose 180 mg), alternatively initially 30 mg once weekly for 1 week, then increased to 60 mg every 2 weeks (max. per dose 60 mg) for a 6 week course (total dose 210 mg), to be administered via cannula in a relatively large vein, course may be repeated every 6 months; maximum 360 mg per course

● CAUTIONS Atypical femoral fractures · cardiac disease (especially in elderly) · ensure adequate hydration · previous thyroid surgery (risk of hypocalcaemia)

● INTERACTIONS → Appendix 1: bisphosphonates

● SIDE-EFFECTS
▸ Common or very common Appetite decreased · chills · decreased leucocytes · drowsiness · electrolyte imbalance · flushing · hypertension · insomnia · paraesthesia · tetany · thrombocytopenia

▸ **Uncommon** Agitation · dyspnoea · eye inflammation · hypotension · muscle cramps · osteonecrosis · seizure

▸ **Rare or very rare** Confusion · glomerulonephritis · haematuria · heart failure · nephritis tubulointerstitial · nephrotic syndrome · oedema · pulmonary oedema · reactivation of infections · renal disorder exacerbated · renal tubular disorder · respiratory disorders · visual hallucinations · xanthopsia

▸ **Frequency not known** Atrial fibrillation

SIDE-EFFECTS, FURTHER INFORMATION Oral supplements are advised to minimise potential risk of hypocalcaemia for those with mainly lytic bone metastases or multiple myeloma at risk of calcium or vitamin D deficiency (e.g. through malabsorption or lack of exposure to sunlight) and in those with Paget's disease.

● PREGNANCY Avoid—toxicity in *animal* studies.

● BREAST FEEDING Avoid.

● HEPATIC IMPAIRMENT Caution in severe hepatic impairment—no information available.

● RENAL IMPAIRMENT
Dose adjustments Max. infusion rate 20 mg/hour. Avoid if eGFR less than 30 mL/minute/1.73 m^2, except in life-threatening hypercalcaemia if benefit outweighs risk.
    If renal function deteriorates in patients with bone metastases, withhold dose until serum creatinine returns to within 10% of baseline value.

● MONITORING REQUIREMENTS
▸ Monitor serum electrolytes, calcium and phosphate—possibility of convulsions due to electrolyte changes.
▸ Assess renal function before each dose.

● DIRECTIONS FOR ADMINISTRATION For *slow intravenous infusion* (Aredia®; *Pamidronate disodium*, Hospira, Medac, Wockhardt), give intermittently in Glucose 5% or Sodium chloride 0.9%; give at a rate not exceeding 1 mg/minute; not to be given with infusion fluids containing calcium. For *Aredia*®, reconstitute initially with water for injections (15 mg in 5 mL, 30 mg or 90 mg in 10 mL), then dilute with infusion fluid to a concentration of not more than 90 mg in 250 mL. For *Pamidronate disodium* (Medac, Hospira, Wockhardt) dilute with infusion fluid to a concentration of not more than 90 mg in 250 mL

● PATIENT AND CARER ADVICE A patient reminder card should be provided (risk of osteonecrosis of the jaw).
Driving and skilled tasks Patients should be warned against performing skilled tasks (e.g. cycling, driving or operating machinery) immediately after treatment (somnolence or dizziness can occur).

● MEDICINAL FORMS
There can be variation in the licensing of different medicines containing the same drug.

Solution for infusion

▸ Pamidronate disodium (Non-proprietary)
Pamidronate disodium 3 mg per 1 ml Pamidronate disodium 15mg/5ml solution for infusion vials | 1 vial PoM £27.50 (Hospital only) | 5 vial PoM £149.15 (Hospital only)
Pamidronate disodium 30mg/10ml solution for infusion vials | 1 vial PoM £55.00-£59.66 (Hospital only)
Pamidronate disodium 60mg/20ml solution for infusion vials | 1 vial PoM £110.00 (Hospital only)
Pamidronate disodium 90mg/30ml solution for infusion vials | 1 vial PoM £165.00 (Hospital only)
Pamidronate disodium 9 mg per 1 ml Pamidronate disodium 90mg/10ml solution for infusion vials | 1 vial PoM £170.45 (Hospital only)
Pamidronate disodium 15 mg per 1 ml Pamidronate disodium 60mg/4ml solution for infusion ampoules | 1 ampoule PoM £119.32
Pamidronate disodium 15mg/1ml solution for infusion ampoules | 4 ampoule PoM £119.32
Pamidronate disodium 90mg/6ml solution for infusion ampoules | 1 ampoule PoM £170.46
Pamidronate disodium 30mg/2ml solution for infusion ampoules | 2 ampoule PoM £119.32

⌐ 709

Risedronate sodium
28-Sep-2017

● INDICATIONS AND DOSE

Paget's disease of bone
▸ BY MOUTH
▸ Adult: 30 mg daily for 2 months, course may be repeated if necessary after at least 2 months

Treatment of postmenopausal osteoporosis to reduce risk of vertebral or hip fractures
▸ BY MOUTH
▸ Adult (female): 5 mg daily, alternatively 35 mg once weekly.

Prevention of osteoporosis (including corticosteroid-induced osteoporosis) in postmenopausal women
▸ BY MOUTH
▸ Adult (female): 5 mg daily.

Treatment of osteoporosis in men at high risk of fractures
▸ BY MOUTH
▸ Adult (male): 35 mg once weekly.

● CONTRA-INDICATIONS Hypocalcaemia

● CAUTIONS Atypical femoral fractures · oesophageal abnormalities · other factors which delay transit or emptying (e.g. stricture or achalasia

● INTERACTIONS → Appendix 1: bisphosphonates

● SIDE-EFFECTS
▸ **Uncommon** Gastrointestinal disorders · iritis
▸ **Rare or very rare** Glossitis
▸ **Frequency not known** Amblyopia · apnoea · chest pain · corneal lesion · dry eye · hypersensitivity · hypersensitivity vasculitis · increased risk of infection · leg cramps · liver disorder · muscle weakness · neoplasms · nocturia · pain · tinnitus · toxic epidermal necrolysis · weight decreased

● PREGNANCY Avoid.

● BREAST FEEDING Avoid.

● RENAL IMPAIRMENT Avoid if eGFR less than 30 mL/minute/1.73 m^2.

● MONITORING REQUIREMENTS
▸ Correct hypocalcaemia before starting.
▸ Correct other disturbances of bone and mineral metabolism (e.g. vitamin-D deficiency) at onset of treatment.

● DIRECTIONS FOR ADMINISTRATION Swallow tablets whole with full glass of water; on rising, take on an empty stomach at least 30 minutes before first food or drink of the day **or**, if taking at any other time of the day, avoid food and drink for at least 2 hours before or after risedronate (particularly avoid calcium-containing products e.g. milk; also avoid iron and mineral supplements and antacids); stand or sit upright for at least 30 minutes; do not take tablets at bedtime or before rising.

● PATIENT AND CARER ADVICE Patients or carers should be given advice on how to administer risedronate sodium tablets.
Oesophageal reactions Patients should be advised to stop taking the tablets and seek medical attention if they develop symptoms of oesophageal irritation such as dysphagia, pain on swallowing, retrosternal pain, or heartburn.

● NATIONAL FUNDING/ACCESS DECISIONS

NICE decisions
▸ **Bisphosphonates for treating osteoporosis (updated February 2018)** NICE TA464
This technology appraisal guidance should be applied clinically in conjunction with:
● NICE guideline on assessing the risk of fragility fractures (CG146), which defines who is eligible for osteoporotic fracture risk assessment.

6

Endocrine system

6

Endocrine system

- NICE quality standard on osteoporosis (QS149), which defines the clinical intervention thresholds for the 10-year fracture probability of a major osteoporotic fracture, in those patients who have undergone fracture risk assessment.

Risedronate sodium is recommended as an option for treating osteoporosis in patients, only if:
- the person is eligible for risk assessment as defined in the full NICE guideline on osteoporosis, **and**
- the 10-year probability of osteoporotic fragility fracture is at least 1%.

Patients whose treatment was started within the NHS before this guidance was published should have the option to continue treatment, without change to their funding arrangements, until they and their NHS clinician consider it appropriate to stop.
www.nice.org.uk/guidance/ta464

- **MEDICINAL FORMS** There can be variation in the licensing of different medicines containing the same drug. Forms available from special-order manufacturers include: oral suspension, oral solution

Tablet
- Risedronate sodium (Non-proprietary)
  Risedronate sodium 5 mg Risedronate sodium 5mg tablets | 28 tablet [PoM] £24.78 DT = £18.85
  Risedronate sodium 30 mg Risedronate sodium 30mg tablets | 28 tablet [PoM] £143.95 DT = £143.83
  Risedronate sodium 35 mg Risedronate sodium 35mg tablets | 4 tablet [PoM] £19.12 DT = £0.58
- Actonel (Warner Chilcott UK Ltd, Teva UK Ltd)
  Risedronate sodium 5 mg Actonel 5mg tablets | 28 tablet [PoM] £17.99 DT = £18.85
  Risedronate sodium 30 mg Actonel 30mg tablets | 28 tablet [PoM] £143.95 DT = £143.83
  Risedronate sodium 35 mg Actonel Once a Week 35mg tablets | 4 tablet [PoM] £19.12 DT = £0.58
  Actonel 35mg tablets | 4 tablet [PoM] [🔬] DT = £0.58

Risedronate with calcium carbonate and colecalciferol

The properties listed below are those particular to the combination only. For the properties of the components please consider, risedronate sodium p. 713, calcium carbonate p. 1013, colecalciferol p. 1051.

- **INDICATIONS AND DOSE**

Treatment of postmenopausal osteoporosis to reduce risk of vertebral or hip fractures
- BY MOUTH
- Adult: 1 tablet once weekly on day 1 of the weekly cycle, followed by 1 sachet daily on days 2–6 of the weekly cycle

- **INTERACTIONS** → Appendix 1: bisphosphonates · calcium salts · vitamin D substances
- **DIRECTIONS FOR ADMINISTRATION** Tablets should be swallowed whole with plenty of water while sitting or standing; to be taken on an empty stomach at least 30 minutes before breakfast (or another oral medicine); patient should stand or sit upright for at least 30 minutes after taking tablet. Granules should be stirred into a glass of water and after dissolution complete taken immediately.
- **PRESCRIBING AND DISPENSING INFORMATION** *Actonel Combi*® effervescent granules contain calcium carbonate 2.5 g (calcium 1 g or Ca²⁺ 25 mmol) and colecalciferol 22 micrograms (880 units)/sachet.
- **PATIENT AND CARER ADVICE** Patients or carers should be given advice on how to administer calcium carbonate with colecalciferol and risedronate tablets and granules.

- **MEDICINAL FORMS** There can be variation in the licensing of different medicines containing the same drug.

Tablet/granules
- Actonel Combi (Teva UK Ltd)
  Actonel Combi 35mg tablets and 1000mg/880unit effervescent granules sachets | 4 week supply [PoM] £19.12

▸ 709

Sodium clodronate

- **INDICATIONS AND DOSE**

Osteolytic lesions, hypercalcaemia and bone pain associated with skeletal metastases in patients with breast cancer or multiple myeloma
- BY MOUTH
- Adult: 1.6 g daily in 1–2 divided doses, then increased if necessary up to 3.2 g daily in 2 divided doses

LORON 520®

Osteolytic lesions, hypercalcaemia and bone pain associated with skeletal metastases in patients with breast cancer or multiple myeloma
- BY MOUTH
- Adult: Initially 2 tablets daily in 1–2 divided doses, increased if necessary up to 4 tablets daily

- **CONTRA-INDICATIONS** Acute gastro-intestinal inflammatory conditions
- **CAUTIONS** Atypical femoral fractures · maintain adequate fluid intake during treatment
- **INTERACTIONS** → Appendix 1: bisphosphonates
- **SIDE-EFFECTS** Proteinuria · respiratory disorder
- **PREGNANCY** Avoid.
- **BREAST FEEDING** Manufacturer advises avoid—no information available.
- **RENAL IMPAIRMENT** Avoid if eGFR less than 10 mL/minute/1.73 m².
  Dose adjustments Max. initial dose 1200 mg daily if eGFR 30–50 mL/minute/1.73m².
  Use half normal dose if eGFR 10–30 mL/minute/1.73 m².
- **MONITORING REQUIREMENTS** Monitor renal function, serum calcium and serum phosphate before and during treatment.
- **DIRECTIONS FOR ADMINISTRATION** Avoid food for 2 hours before and 1 hour after treatment, particularly calcium-containing products e.g. milk; also avoid iron and mineral supplements and antacids; maintain adequate fluid intake.
- **PATIENT AND CARER ADVICE** Patients or carers should be given advice on how to administer sodium clodronate capsules and tablets.

- **MEDICINAL FORMS** There can be variation in the licensing of different medicines containing the same drug.

Tablet
CAUTIONARY AND ADVISORY LABELS 10
- Sodium clodronate (Non-proprietary)
  Sodium clodronate 800 mg Sodium clodronate 800mg tablets | 60 tablet [PoM] £116.72 DT = £146.43
- Bonefos (Bayer Plc)
  Sodium clodronate 800 mg Bonefos 800mg tablets | 60 tablet [PoM] £146.43 DT = £146.43
- Loron (Intrapharm Laboratories Ltd)
  Sodium clodronate 520 mg Loron 520mg tablets | 60 tablet [PoM] £114.44 DT = £114.44

Capsule
- Sodium clodronate (Non-proprietary)
  Sodium clodronate 400 mg Sodium clodronate 400mg capsules | 30 capsule [PoM] £34.96 | 120 capsule [PoM] £139.83 DT = £139.83
- Bonefos (Bayer Plc)
  Sodium clodronate 400 mg Bonefos 400mg capsules | 120 capsule [PoM] £139.83 DT = £139.83

6

▸ Clasteon (Kent Pharmaceuticals Ltd)
Sodium clodronate 400 mg Clasteon 400mg capsules |
30 capsule PoM £34.96 | 120 capsule PoM £139.83 DT = £139.83

F 709

Zoledronic acid

28-Sep-2017

● **INDICATIONS AND DOSE**

ACLASTA ®

Treatment of Paget's disease of bone

▸ BY INTRAVENOUS INFUSION

▸ Adult: 5 mg as a single dose, to be administered over at least 15 minutes, at least 500 mg elemental calcium twice daily (with vitamin D) for at least 10 days is recommended following infusion

Treatment of postmenopausal osteoporosis and osteoporosis in men (including corticosteroid-induced osteoporosis)

▸ BY INTRAVENOUS INFUSION

▸ Adult: 5 mg once yearly as a single dose, to be administered over at least 15 minutes, in patients with a recent low-trauma hip fracture, the dose should be given 2 or more weeks following hip fracture repair; before first infusion give 50 000–125 000 units of vitamin D

ZOMETA ® INFUSION

Reduction of bone damage in advanced malignancies involving bone

▸ BY INTRAVENOUS INFUSION

▸ Adult: 4 mg every 3–4 weeks, to be administered over at least 15 minutes, calcium 500 mg daily and vitamin D 400 units daily should also be taken

Hypercalcaemia of malignancy

▸ BY INTRAVENOUS INFUSION

▸ Adult: 4 mg for 1 dose, to be administered over at least 15 minutes

● **CAUTIONS** Atypical femoral fractures · cardiac disease (avoid fluid overload) · concomitant medicines that affect renal function

● **INTERACTIONS** → Appendix 1: bisphosphonates

● **SIDE-EFFECTS**

▸ **Common or very common** Appetite decreased · chills · flushing

▸ **Uncommon** Anxiety · arrhythmias · chest pain · circulatory collapse · cough · drowsiness · dry mouth · dyspnoea · electrolyte imbalance · haematuria · hyperhidrosis · hypertension · hypotension · leucopenia · muscle spasms · orbital inflammation · proteinuria · respiratory disorders · sensation abnormal · sleep disorder · stomatitis · syncope · thrombocytopenia · tremor · vision blurred · weight increased

▸ **Rare or very rare** Confusion · Fanconi syndrome acquired · osteonecrosis · pancytopenia

▸ **Frequency not known** Acute phase reaction

SIDE-EFFECTS, FURTHER INFORMATION Renal impairment and renal failure have been reported; ensure patient is hydrated before each dose and assess renal function.

● **CONCEPTION AND CONTRACEPTION** Contra-indicated in women of child-bearing potential.

● **PREGNANCY** Avoid—toxicity in *animal* studies.

● **BREAST FEEDING** Avoid—no information available.

● **HEPATIC IMPAIRMENT** Caution in severe hepatic impairment—limited information available.

● **RENAL IMPAIRMENT** Avoid in tumour-induced hypercalcaemia if serum creatinine above 400 micromol/litre. Avoid in advanced malignancies involving bone if eGFR less than 30 mL/minute/1.73 m² (or if serum creatinine greater than 265 micromol/litre). Avoid in Paget's disease, treatment of postmenopausal

osteoporosis and osteoporosis in men if eGFR less than 35 mL/minute/1.73 m².

Dose adjustments In advanced malignancies involving bone, if eGFR 50–60 mL/minute/1.73 m² reduce dose to 3.5 mg every 3–4 weeks; if eGFR 40–50 mL/minute/1.73 m² reduce dose to 3.3 mg every 3–4 weeks; if eGFR 30–40 mL/minute/1.73 m² reduce dose to 3 mg every 3–4 weeks; if renal function deteriorates in patients with bone metastases, withhold dose until serum creatinine returns to within 10% of baseline value.

● **MONITORING REQUIREMENTS**

▸ Correct disturbances of calcium metabolism (e.g. vitamin D deficiency, hypocalcaemia) before starting. Monitor serum electrolytes, calcium, phosphate and magnesium.

▸ Monitor renal function in patients at risk, such as those with pre-existing renal impairment, those of advanced age, those taking concomitant nephrotoxic drugs or diuretics, or those who are dehydrated.

● **DIRECTIONS FOR ADMINISTRATION** For *intravenous infusion* (*Zometa*®), give intermittently in Glucose 5% *or* Sodium chloride 0.9%; dilute requisite dose according to product literature; infuse over at least 15 minutes; administer as a single intravenous solution in a separate infusion line.

● **PATIENT AND CARER ADVICE** A patient reminder card should be provided (risk of osteonecrosis of the jaw).

● **NATIONAL FUNDING/ACCESS DECISIONS**

NICE decisions

▸ Bisphosphonates for treating osteoporosis (updated February 2018) NICE TA464

This technology appraisal guidance should be applied clinically in conjunction with:

● NICE guideline on assessing the risk of fragility fractures (CG146), which defines who is eligible for osteoporotic fracture risk assessment.

● NICE quality standard on osteoporosis (QS149), which defines the clinical intervention thresholds for the 10-year fracture probability of a major osteoporotic fracture, in those patients who have undergone fracture risk assessment.

Zoledronic acid is recommended as an option for treating osteoporosis in patients, only if:

● the person is eligible for risk assessment as defined in the full NICE guideline on osteoporosis, **and**

● the 10-year probability of osteoporotic fragility fracture is at least 10%, **or**

● the 10-year probability of osteoporotic fragility fracture is at least 1% and the person has difficulty taking oral bisphosphonates (alendronic acid, ibandronic acid or risedronate sodium) or these drugs are contra-indicated or not tolerated.

Patients whose treatment was started within the NHS before this guidance was published should have the option to continue treatment, without change to their funding arrangements, until they and their NHS clinician consider it appropriate to stop.

www.nice.org.uk/guidance/ta464

ACLASTA ®

Scottish Medicines Consortium (SMC) Decisions

The *Scottish Medicines Consortium* has advised (February 2008) that in postmenopausal women *Aclasta*® is accepted for restricted use within the NHS Scotland for the treatment of osteoporosis in those for whom oral treatment options for osteoporosis are inappropriate and when initiated by a specialist.

ZOMETA ® INFUSION

Scottish Medicines Consortium (SMC) Decisions

The *Scottish Medicines Consortium* has advised (May 2003) that for the prevention of skeletal related events *Zometa*® is accepted for restricted use within NHS Scotland for the treatment of patients with breast cancer and multiple myeloma if prescribed by an oncologist.

6

Endocrine system

● MEDICINAL FORMS
There can be variation in the licensing of different medicines containing the same drug.

Infusion
▸ Aclasta (Novartis Pharmaceuticals UK Ltd)
Zoledronic acid (as Zoledronic acid monohydrate) 50 microgram per 1 ml Aclasta 5mg/100ml infusion bottles | 1 bottle $\boxed{\text{PoM}}$ £253.38
▸ Zometa (Novartis Pharmaceuticals UK Ltd)
Zoledronic acid (as Zoledronic acid monohydrate) 40 microgram per 1 ml Zometa 4mg/100ml infusion bottles | 1 bottle $\boxed{\text{PoM}}$ £174.14

CALCIUM REGULATING DRUGS › BONE RESORPTION INHIBITORS

Calcitonin (salmon)

(Salcatonin)

● INDICATIONS AND DOSE

Hypercalcaemia of malignancy
▸ BY SUBCUTANEOUS INJECTION, OR BY INTRAMUSCULAR INJECTION
▸ Adult: 100 units every 6–8 hours (max. per dose 400 units every 6–8 hours), adjusted according to response
▸ BY INTRAVENOUS INFUSION
▸ Adult: Up to 10 units/kg, in severe or emergency cases, to be administered by slow intravenous infusion over at least 6 hours

Paget's disease of bone
▸ BY SUBCUTANEOUS INJECTION, OR BY INTRAMUSCULAR INJECTION
▸ Adult: 100 units daily, adjusted according to response for maximum 3 months (6 months in exceptional circumstances), a minimum dosage regimen of 50 units three times a week has been shown to achieve clinical and biochemical improvement

Prevention of acute bone loss due to sudden immobility
▸ BY SUBCUTANEOUS INJECTION, OR BY INTRAMUSCULAR INJECTION
▸ Adult: Initially 100 units daily in 1–2 divided doses, then reduced to 50 units daily at the start of mobilisation, usual duration of treatment is 2 weeks; maximum 4 weeks

● CONTRA-INDICATIONS Hypocalcaemia

● CAUTIONS Heart failure · history of allergy (skin test advised) · risk of malignancy—avoid prolonged use (use lowest effective dose for shortest possible time)

● INTERACTIONS → Appendix 1: calcitonin (salmon)

● SIDE-EFFECTS
▸ Common or very common Abdominal pain · arthralgia · diarrhoea · dizziness · fatigue · flushing · headache · musculoskeletal pain · nausea · secondary malignancy (long term use) · taste altered · vomiting
▸ Uncommon Hypersensitivity · hypertension · influenza like illness · oedema · polyuria · skin reactions · visual impairment
▸ Rare or very rare Bronchospasm · throat swelling · tongue swelling
▸ Frequency not known Hypocalcaemia · tremor

● PREGNANCY Avoid unless potential benefit outweighs risk (toxicity in *animal* studies).

● BREAST FEEDING Avoid; inhibits lactation in *animals*.

● RENAL IMPAIRMENT Use with caution.

● DIRECTIONS FOR ADMINISTRATION For *intravenous infusion*, give intermittently in Sodium chloride 0.9%. Diluted solution given without delay. Dilute in 500 mL give over at least 6 hours; glass or hard plastic containers

should not be used; some loss of potency on dilution and administration.

● MEDICINAL FORMS
There can be variation in the licensing of different medicines containing the same drug.

Solution for injection
▸ Calcitonin (salmon) (Non-proprietary)
Calcitonin (salmon) 50 unit per 1 ml Calcitonin (salmon) 50units/1ml solution for injection ampoules | 5 ampoule $\boxed{\text{PoM}}$ £167.50
Calcitonin (salmon) 100 unit per 1 ml Calcitonin (salmon) 100units/1ml solution for injection ampoules | 5 ampoule $\boxed{\text{PoM}}$ £220.00
Calcitonin (salmon) 200 unit per 1 ml Calcitonin (salmon) 400units/2ml solution for injection vials | 1 vial $\boxed{\text{PoM}}$ £352.00

CALCIUM REGULATING DRUGS › PARATHYROID HORMONES AND ANALOGUES

Teriparatide   21-Feb-2018

● INDICATIONS AND DOSE

Treatment of osteoporosis in postmenopausal women and in men at increased risk of fractures | Treatment of corticosteroid-induced osteoporosis
▸ BY SUBCUTANEOUS INJECTION
▸ Adult: 20 micrograms daily for maximum duration of treatment 24 months (course not to be repeated)

● CONTRA-INDICATIONS Bone metastases · hyperparathyroidism · metabolic bone diseases · Paget's disease · pre-existing hypercalcaemia · previous radiation therapy to the skeleton · skeletal malignancies · unexplained raised alkaline phosphatase

● SIDE-EFFECTS
▸ Common or very common Anaemia · asthenia · chest pain · gastrointestinal disorders · headache · hypercholesterolaemia · hyperhidrosis · hypotension · muscle complaints · palpitations · sciatica · skin reactions · syncope · vomiting
▸ Uncommon Arthralgia · back pain · emphysema · hypercalcaemia · hyperuricaemia · nephrolithiasis · tachycardia · urinary disorders · weight increased
▸ Rare or very rare Oedema · renal impairment

● PREGNANCY Avoid.

● BREAST FEEDING Avoid.

● RENAL IMPAIRMENT Caution in moderate impairment; avoid if severe.

● PRESCRIBING AND DISPENSING INFORMATION Teriparatide is a biological medicine. Biological medicines must be prescribed and dispensed by brand name, see *Biological medicines* and *Biosimilar medicines*, under Guidance on prescribing p. 1.

● NATIONAL FUNDING/ACCESS DECISIONS

NICE decisions
▸ **Raloxifene and teriparatide for the secondary prevention of osteoporotic fragility fractures in postmenopausal women (updated February 2018)** NICE TA161
Teriparatide is recommended as an alternative treatment option for the secondary prevention of osteoporotic fragility fractures in postmenopausal women:
● who are unable to take alendronate and risedronate, or have a contra-indication to or are intolerant of alendronate and risedronate, or have had an unsatisfactory response to treatment with alendronate or risedronate, **and**
● who are 65 years or older and have a T-score of -4 standard deviations (SD) or below, or a T-score of -3.5 SD or below plus more than two fractures, or who are aged 55-64 years and have a T-score of -4 SD or below plus more than two fractures.

Women who are currently receiving treatment, but for whom treatment would not have been recommended, should have the option to continue treatment until they and their NHS clinician consider it appropriate to stop.
www.nice.org.uk/guidance/ta161

● MEDICINAL FORMS
There can be variation in the licensing of different medicines containing the same drug.
Solution for injection
▸ Forsteo (Eli Lilly and Company Ltd)
  Teriparatide 250 microgram per 1 ml Forsteo 20micrograms/80microlitres solution for injection 2.4ml pre-filled disposable devices | 1 pre-filled disposable injection PoM £271.88

DRUGS AFFECTING BONE STRUCTURE AND MINERALISATION ⟩ MONOCLONAL ANTIBODIES

Denosumab

● DRUG ACTION Denosumab is a human monoclonal antibody that inhibits osteoclast formation, function, and survival, thereby decreasing bone resorption.

● INDICATIONS AND DOSE

PROLIA ®

Treatment of osteoporosis in postmenopausal women and in men at increased risk of fractures | Treatment of bone loss associated with hormone ablation in men with prostate cancer at increased risk of fractures
▸ BY SUBCUTANEOUS INJECTION
▸ Adult: 60 mg every 6 months, supplement with calcium and vitamin D

XGEVA ®

Prevention of skeletal related events in patients with bone metastases from solid tumours
▸ BY SUBCUTANEOUS INJECTION
▸ Adult: 120 mg every 4 weeks, supplementation of at least Calcium 500 mg and vitamin D 400 units daily should also be taken unless hypercalcaemia is present

Treatment of giant cell tumour of bone that is unresectable or where surgical resection is likely to result in severe morbidity in adults and skeletally mature adolescents
▸ BY SUBCUTANEOUS INJECTION
▸ Adult: 120 mg every 4 weeks, give additional dose on days 8 and 15 of the first month of treatment only, supplementation of at least Calcium 500 mg and vitamin D 400 units daily should also be taken unless hypercalcaemia is present

---

IMPORTANT SAFETY INFORMATION

MHRA/CHM ADVICE: DENOSUMAB: ATYPICAL FEMORAL FRACTURES (FEBRUARY 2013)
Atypical femoral fractures have been reported rarely in patients receiving denosumab for the long-term treatment (2.5 or more years) of postmenopausal osteoporosis.
  Patients should be advised to report any new or unusual thigh, hip, or groin pain during treatment with denosumab.
  Discontinuation of denosumab in patients suspected to have an atypical femoral fracture should be considered after an assessment of the benefits and risks of continued treatment.

MHRA/CHM ADVICE: DENOSUMAB: MINIMISING THE RISK OF OSTEONECROSIS OF THE JAW; MONITORING FOR HYPOCALCAEMIA—UPDATED RECOMMENDATIONS (SEPTEMBER 2014) AND DENOSUMAB: OSTEONECROSIS OF THE JAW—FURTHER MEASURES TO MINIMISE RISK (JULY 2015)
Denosumab is associated with a risk of osteonecrosis of the jaw (ONJ) and with a risk of hypocalcaemia.

Osteonecrosis of the jaw
Osteonecrosis of the jaw is a well-known and common side-effect in patients receiving denosumab 120 mg for cancer. Risk factors include smoking, old age, poor oral hygiene, invasive dental procedures (including tooth extractions, dental implants, oral surgery), comorbidity (including dental disease, anaemia, coagulopathy, infection), advanced cancer, previous treatment with bisphosphonates, and concomitant treatments (including chemotherapy, anti-angiogenic biologics, corticosteroids, and radiotherapy to head and neck). The following precautions are now recommended to reduce the risk of ONJ:
Denosumab 120 mg (cancer indication)
● A dental examination and appropriate preventative dentistry before starting treatment are now recommended for all patients
● Do not start denosumab in patients with a dental or jaw condition requiring surgery, or in patients who have unhealed lesions from dental or oral surgery
Denosumab 60 mg (osteoporosis indication)
● Check for ONJ risk factors before starting treatment. A dental examination and appropriate preventative dentistry are now recommended for patients with risk factors
All patients should be given a patient reminder card and informed of the risk of ONJ. Advise patients to tell their doctor if they have any problems with their mouth or teeth before starting treatment, if they wear dentures they should make sure their dentures fit properly before starting treatment, to maintain good oral hygiene, receive routine dental check-ups during treatment, and immediately report any oral symptoms such as dental mobility, pain, swelling, non-healing sores or discharge to a doctor and dentist. Patients should tell their doctor and dentist that they are receiving denosumab if they need dental treatment or dental surgery.

Hypocalcaemia
Denosumab is associated with a risk of hypocalcaemia. This risk increases with the degree of renal impairment. Hypocalcaemia usually occurs in the first weeks of denosumab treatment, but it can also occur later in treatment.
  Plasma-calcium concentration monitoring is recommended for denosumab 120 mg (cancer indication):
● before the first dose
● within two weeks after the initial dose
● if suspected symptoms of hypocalcaemia occur
● consider monitoring more frequently in patients with risk factors for hypocalcaemia (e.g. severe renal impairment, creatinine clearance less than 30 mL/minute)
Plasma-calcium concentration monitoring is recommended for denosumab 60 mg (osteoporosis indication):
● before each dose
● within two weeks after the initial dose in patients with risk factors for hypocalcaemia (e.g. severe renal impairment, creatinine clearance less than 30 mL/minute)
● if suspected symptoms of hypocalcaemia occur
All patients should be advised to report symptoms of hypocalcaemia to their doctor (e.g. muscle spasms, twitches, cramps, numbness or tingling in the fingers, toes, or around the mouth).

MHRA/CHM ADVICE: DENOSUMAB: REPORTS OF OSTEONECROSIS OF THE EXTERNAL AUDITORY CANAL (JUNE 2017)
Osteonecrosis of the external auditory canal has been reported with denosumab and this should be considered in patients who present with ear symptoms including chronic ear infections or in those with suspected

cholesteatoma. Possible risk factors include steroid use and chemotherapy, with or without local risk factors such as infection or trauma. The MHRA recommends advising patients to report any ear pain, discharge from the ear, or an ear infection during denosumab treatment.

- CONTRA-INDICATIONS Hypocalcaemia
  XGEVA® Unhealed lesions from dental or oral surgery
- CAUTIONS Atypical femoral fractures · hypocalcaemia · osteonecrosis of the jaw—consider temporary interruption of treatment if occurs
- SIDE-EFFECTS
- ▶ **Common or very common** Abdominal discomfort · cataract · constipation · increased risk of infection · pain · sciatica · skin reactions
- ▶ **Uncommon** Cellulitis (seek prompt medical attention)
- ▶ **Rare or very rare** Atypical femur fracture · hypocalcaemia · osteonecrosis
- CONCEPTION AND CONTRACEPTION Ensure effective contraception in women of child-bearing potential, during treatment and for at least 5 months after stopping treatment.
- PREGNANCY Avoid—toxicity in *animal* studies; risk of toxicity increases with each trimester—advise women who become pregnant during treatment to enrol in the manufacturer's Pregnancy Surveillance Programme (consult product literature).
- BREAST FEEDING Avoid (if women do decide to breast-feed during treatment, they should enrol in the manufacturer's Lactation Surveillance Programme—consult product literature.
- RENAL IMPAIRMENT Increased risk of hypocalcaemia if eGFR less than 30 mL/minute/1.73 m^2.
- MONITORING REQUIREMENTS Correct hypocalcaemia and vitamin D deficiency before starting. Monitor plasma-calcium concentration during therapy.
- PATIENT AND CARER ADVICE
  Atypical femoral fractures Patients should be advised to report any new or unusual thigh, hip, or groin pain during treatment with denosumab.
  Osteonecrosis of the jaw All patients should be informed to maintain good oral hygiene, receive routine dental check-ups, and immediately report any oral symptoms such as dental mobility, pain, or swelling to a doctor and dentist.
  Hypocalaemia All patients should be advised to report symptoms of hypocalcaemia to their doctor (e.g. muscle spasms, twitches, cramps, numbness or tingling in the fingers, toes, or around the mouth).
  A patient reminder card should be provided (risk of osteonecrosis of the jaw).
- NATIONAL FUNDING/ACCESS DECISIONS
  NICE decisions
- ▶ **Denosumab for the prevention of osteoporotic fractures in postmenopausal women (October 2010)** NICE TA204
  Denosumab is recommended as a treatment option for the *primary prevention* of osteoporotic fragility fractures in postmenopausal women at increased risk of fractures:
  - who are unable to comply with the special instructions for administering alendronate and risedronate, or have an intolerance of, or a contra-indication to, those treatments **and**
  - who comply with particular combinations of bone mineral density measurement, age, and independent risk factors for fracture, as indicated in the full NICE guidance.
  Denosumab is recommended as a treatment option for the *secondary prevention* of osteoporotic fragility fractures only in postmenopausal women at increased risk of fractures who are unable to comply with the special instructions for

administering alendronate and risedronate, or have an intolerance of, or a contra-indication to, those treatments. www.nice.org.uk/TA204

- ▶ **Denosumab for the prevention of skeletal-related events in adults with bone metastases from solid tumours (October 2012)** NICE TA265
  Denosumab is recommended for the prevention of skeletal-related events in adults with bone metastases from breast cancer and from solid tumours other than prostate if:
  - bisphosphonates would otherwise be prescribed, **and**
  - the manufacturer provides denosumab with the discount agreed in the patient access scheme.
  Denosumab is **not** recommended for preventing skeletal-related events in adults with bone metastases from prostate cancer.
  Patients with bone metastases from solid tumours currently receiving denosumab whose disease does not meet the above criteria can continue treatment until they and their clinician consider it appropriate to stop. www.nice.org.uk/TA265
  PROLIA®
  Scottish Medicines Consortium (SMC) Decisions
  The *Scottish Medicines Consortium* has advised (November 2010) that denosumab (*Prolia*®) is accepted for restricted use within NHS Scotland for the treatment of osteoporosis in postmenopausal women at increased risk of fractures who have a bone mineral density T-score <-2.5 and ≥ -4.0 and for whom bisphosphonates are unsuitable.

- MEDICINAL FORMS
  There can be variation in the licensing of different medicines containing the same drug.
  Solution for injection
  ▶ Prolia (Amgen Ltd)
    Denosumab 60 mg per 1 ml Prolia 60mg/1ml solution for injection pre-filled syringes | 1 pre-filled disposable injection [PoM] £183.00 DT = £183.00
  ▶ Xgeva (Amgen Ltd) ▼
    Denosumab 70 mg per 1 ml Xgeva 120mg/1.7ml solution for injection vials | 1 vial [PoM] £309.86

5 Dopamine responsive conditions

DOPAMINERGIC DRUGS ⟩ DOPAMINE RECEPTOR AGONISTS

Dopamine-receptor agonists

Overview

Bromocriptine p. 414 is used for the treatment of galactorrhoea, and for the treatment of prolactinomas (when it reduces both plasma prolactin concentration and tumour size). Bromocriptine also inhibits the release of growth hormone and is sometimes used in the treatment of acromegaly, but somatostatin analogues (such as octreotide p. 924) are more effective.

Cabergoline p. 415 has similar side-effects to bromocriptine, however patients intolerant of bromocriptine may be able to tolerate cabergoline (and *vice versa*).

Quinagolide p. 719 has actions and uses similar to those of ergot-derived dopamine agonists, but its side-effects differ slightly.

Suppression of lactation

Although bromocriptine and cabergoline are licensed to suppress lactation, they are **not** recommended for routine suppression (or for the relief of symptoms of postpartum pain and engorgement) that can be adequately treated with simple analgesics and breast support. If a dopamine-receptor agonist is required, cabergoline is preferred. Quinagolide is not licensed for the suppression of lactation.

Quinagolide

● DRUG ACTION Quinagolide is a non-ergot dopamine D_2 agonist.

● INDICATIONS AND DOSE
Hyperprolactinaemia
▶ BY MOUTH
▶ Adult: Initially 25 micrograms once daily for 3 days, dose to be taken at bedtime, increased in steps of 25 micrograms every 3 days; usual dose 75–150 micrograms daily, for doses higher than 300 micrograms daily increase in steps of 75–150 micrograms at intervals of not less than 4 weeks

● UNLICENSED USE Not licensed for the suppression of lactation.
● CAUTIONS Acute porphyrias p. 1025 · history of psychotic illness · history of serious mental disorders
 CAUTIONS, FURTHER INFORMATION In hyperprolactinaemic patients, the source of the hyperprolactinaemia should be established (i.e. exclude pituitary tumour before treatment).
● INTERACTIONS → Appendix 1: dopamine receptor agonists
● SIDE-EFFECTS
▶ Common or very common Abdominal pain · appetite decreased · constipation · diarrhoea · dizziness · fatigue · flushing · headache · hypotension · insomnia · nasal congestion · nausea · oedema · syncope · vomiting
▶ Rare or very rare Acute psychosis · drowsiness
● ALLERGY AND CROSS-SENSITIVITY Quinagolide should not be used in patients with hypersensitivity to quinagolide (does not apply to hypersensitivity to ergot alkaloids).
● CONCEPTION AND CONTRACEPTION Advise non-hormonal contraception if pregnancy not desired.
● PREGNANCY Discontinue when pregnancy confirmed unless medical reason for continuing (specialist advice needed).
● BREAST FEEDING Suppresses lactation.
● HEPATIC IMPAIRMENT Avoid—no information available.
● RENAL IMPAIRMENT Avoid—no information available.
● MONITORING REQUIREMENTS Monitor blood pressure for a few days after starting treatment and following dosage increase.
● PATIENT AND CARER ADVICE
 Driving and skilled tasks
 Sudden onset of sleep Excessive daytime sleepiness and sudden onset of sleep can occur with dopamine-receptor agonists.
  Patients starting treatment with these drugs should be warned of the risk and of the need to exercise caution when driving or operating machinery. Those who have experienced excessive sedation or sudden onset of sleep should refrain from driving or operating machines until these effects have stopped occurring.
  Management of excessive daytime sleepiness should focus on the identification of an underlying cause, such as depression or concomitant medication. Patients should be counselled on improving sleep behaviour.
 Hypotensive reactions Hypotensive reactions can be disturbing in some patients during the first few days of treatment with dopamine-receptor agonists, particular care should be exercised when driving or operating machinery.

● MEDICINAL FORMS
There can be variation in the licensing of different medicines containing the same drug.
Tablet
CAUTIONARY AND ADVISORY LABELS 10, 21
▶ Quinagolide (Non-proprietary)
 Quinagolide (as Quinagolide hydrochloride)
 25 microgram Quinagolide 25microgram tablets | 3 tablet PoM ⦸
 Quinagolide (as Quinagolide hydrochloride)
 50 microgram Quinagolide 50microgram tablets | 3 tablet PoM ⦸
 Quinagolide (as Quinagolide hydrochloride)
 75 microgram Quinagolide 75microgram tablets | 30 tablet PoM £75.00 DT = £75.00
 Quinagolide 50microgram tablets and Quinagolide 25microgram tablets | 6 tablet PoM £30.00–£37.50
▶ Norprolac (Ferring Pharmaceuticals Ltd)
 Quinagolide (as Quinagolide hydrochloride)
 25 microgram Norprolac 25microgram tablets | 3 tablet PoM ⦸
 Quinagolide (as Quinagolide hydrochloride)
 50 microgram Norprolac 50microgram tablets | 3 tablet PoM ⦸

6   Gonadotrophin responsive conditions

Gonadotrophins

Gonadotrophin-affecting drugs

Danazol p. 725 is licensed for the treatment of *endometriosis* and for the relief of severe pain and tenderness in *benign fibrocystic breast disease* where other measures have proved unsatisfactory. It may also be effective in the long-term management of *hereditary angioedema* [unlicensed indication].
  Cetrorelix p. 720 and ganirelix p. 720 are luteinising hormone releasing hormone antagonists, which inhibit the release of gonadotrophins (luteinising hormone and follicle stimulating hormone). They are used in the treatment of infertility by assisted reproductive techniques.

Gonadorelin analogues
Gonadorelin analogues are used in the treatment of endometriosis, precocious puberty, infertility, male hypersexuality with severe sexual deviation, anaemia due to uterine fibroids (together with iron supplementation), breast cancer, prostate cancer and before intra-uterine surgery. Use of leuprorelin acetate and triptorelin for 3 to 4 months before surgery reduces the uterine volume, fibroid size and associated bleeding. For women undergoing hysterectomy or myomectomy, a vaginal procedure is made more feasible following the use of a gonadorelin analogue.

Breast pain (mastalgia)
Once any serious underlying cause for breast pain has been ruled out, most women will respond to reassurance and reduction in dietary fat; withdrawal of an oral contraceptive or of hormone replacement therapy may help to resolve the pain.
  Mild, non-cyclical breast pain is treated with simple analgesics; moderate to severe pain, cyclical pain or symptoms that persist for longer than 6 months may require specific drug treatment.
  Danazol is licensed for the relief of severe pain and tenderness in benign fibrocystic breast disease which has not responded to other treatment.
  Tamoxifen p. 927 may be a useful adjunct in the treatment of mastalgia [unlicensed indication] especially when symptoms can definitely be related to cyclic oestrogen production; it may be given on the days of the cycle when symptoms are predicted.
  Treatment for breast pain should be reviewed after 6 months and continued if necessary. Symptoms recur in

about 50% of women within 2 years of withdrawal of therapy but may be less severe.

PITUITARY AND HYPOTHALAMIC HORMONES AND ANALOGUES > ANTI-GONADOTROPHIN-RELEASING HORMONES

Cetrorelix

● INDICATIONS AND DOSE

Adjunct in the treatment of female infertility (initiated under specialist supervision)
▸ BY SUBCUTANEOUS INJECTION
▸ Adult (female): 250 micrograms once daily, dose to be administered in the morning, starting on day 5 or 6 of ovarian stimulation with gonadotrophins (or each evening starting on day 5 of ovarian stimulation), continue throughout administration of gonadotrophin including day of ovulation induction (or evening before ovulation induction), dose to be injected into the lower abdominal wall.

● SIDE-EFFECTS
▸ **Common or very common** Ovarian hyperstimulation syndrome
▸ **Uncommon** Headache · hypersensitivity · nausea
● PREGNANCY Avoid in confirmed pregnancy.
● BREAST FEEDING Avoid.
● HEPATIC IMPAIRMENT Avoid in moderate or severe liver impairment.
● RENAL IMPAIRMENT Avoid in moderate or severe renal impairment.

● MEDICINAL FORMS
There can be variation in the licensing of different medicines containing the same drug.
Powder and solvent for solution for injection
▸ Cetrotide (Merck Serono Ltd)
Cetrorelix (as Cetrorelix acetate) 250 microgram Cetrotide 250microgram powder and solvent for solution for injection vials | 1 vial [PoM] £22.61

Ganirelix

● INDICATIONS AND DOSE

Adjunct in the treatment of female infertility (initiated under specialist supervision)
▸ BY SUBCUTANEOUS INJECTION
▸ Adult: 250 micrograms once daily, dose to be administered in the morning (or each afternoon) starting on day 5 or day 6 of ovarian stimulation with gonadotrophins, continue throughout administration of gonadotrophins including day of ovulation induction (if administering in afternoon, give last dose in afternoon before ovulation induction), dose to be injected preferably into the upper leg (rotate injection sites to prevent lipoatrophy)

● SIDE-EFFECTS
▸ **Common or very common** Skin reactions
▸ **Uncommon** Headache · malaise · nausea
▸ **Rare or very rare** Dyspnoea · facial swelling · hypersensitivity
▸ **Frequency not known** Abdominal distension · ovarian hyperstimulation syndrome · pelvic pain
● PREGNANCY Avoid in confirmed pregnancy—toxicity in *animal* studies.
● BREAST FEEDING Avoid—no information available.
● HEPATIC IMPAIRMENT Avoid in moderate or severe hepatic impairment.

● RENAL IMPAIRMENT Avoid in moderate to severe renal impairment.

● MEDICINAL FORMS
There can be variation in the licensing of different medicines containing the same drug.
Solution for injection
▸ Fyremadel (Ferring Pharmaceuticals Ltd)
Ganirelix 500 microgram per 1 ml Fyremadel 250micrograms/0.5ml solution for injection pre-filled syringes | 1 pre-filled disposable injection [PoM] [S]
▸ Orgalutran (Merck Sharp & Dohme Ltd)
Ganirelix 500 microgram per 1 ml Orgalutran 250micrograms/0.5ml solution for injection pre-filled syringes | 1 pre-filled disposable injection [PoM] £21.48

PITUITARY AND HYPOTHALAMIC HORMONES AND ANALOGUES > GONADOTROPHIN-RELEASING HORMONES

Buserelin

● DRUG ACTION Administration of gonadorelin analogues produces an initial phase of stimulation; continued administration is followed by down-regulation of gonadotrophin-releasing hormone receptors, thereby reducing the release of gonadotrophins (follicle stimulating hormone and luteinising hormone) which in turn leads to inhibition of androgen and oestrogen production.

● INDICATIONS AND DOSE

Endometriosis
▸ BY INTRANASAL ADMINISTRATION
▸ Adult: 300 micrograms 3 times a day maximum duration of treatment 6 months (do not repeat), to be started on days 1 or 2 of menstruation; administer one 150 microgram spray into each nostril

Pituitary desensitisation before induction of ovulation by gonadotrophins for in vitro fertilisation (under expert supervision)
▸ BY SUBCUTANEOUS INJECTION
▸ Adult: 200–500 micrograms once daily, increased if necessary up to 500 micrograms twice daily, starting in early follicular phase (day 1) or, after exclusion of pregnancy, in midluteal phase (day 21) and continued until down-regulation achieved (usually 1–3 weeks) then maintained during gonadotrophin administration (stopping gonadotrophin and buserelin on administration of chorionic gonadotrophin at appropriate stage of follicular development)
▸ BY INTRANASAL ADMINISTRATION
▸ Adult: 150–300 micrograms 4 times a day, (150 micrograms equivalent to one spray), to be administered during waking hours. Start in early follicular phase (day 1) or, after exclusion of pregnancy, in the midluteal phase (day 21) and continued until down-regulation achieved (usually about 2–3 weeks) then maintained during gonadotrophin administration (stopping gonadotrophin and buserelin on administration of chorionic gonadotrophin at appropriate stage of follicular development)

Advanced prostate cancer
▸ INITIALLY BY SUBCUTANEOUS INJECTION
▸ Adult: 500 micrograms every 8 hours for 7 days, then (by intranasal administration) 200 micrograms 6 times a day, (a single 100 microgram spray to be administered into each nostril)

- CONTRA-INDICATIONS
- When used for endometriosis Hormone dependent tumours · undiagnosed vaginal bleeding · use longer than 6 months (do not repeat)
- When used for pituitary desensitisation Hormone dependent tumours · undiagnosed vaginal bleeding
- CAUTIONS Depression · diabetes · hypertension · patients with metabolic bone disease (decrease in bone mineral density can occur) · polycystic ovarian disease
- SIDE-EFFECTS
  GENERAL SIDE-EFFECTS
- Common or very common Depression · mood altered
- Rare or very rare Hearing impairment · hypotension · leucopenia · pituitary tumour benign · thrombocytopenia
- Frequency not known Alopecia · anxiety · appetite change · breast abnormalities · broken nails · concentration impaired · constipation · diarrhoea · dizziness · drowsiness · dry eye · dysuria · embolism and thrombosis · fatigue · feeling of pressure behind the eyes · follicle recruitment increased · galactorrhoea · gastrointestinal discomfort · gynaecomastia · hair changes · headache · hot flush · hydronephrosis · hyperhidrosis · increased risk of fracture · lymphostasis · memory loss · menopausal symptoms · menstrual cycle irregularities · muscle weakness in legs · musculoskeletal discomfort · nausea · oedema · osteoporosis · ovarian and fallopian tube disorders · pain · painful sexual intercourse · palpitations · paraesthesia · QT interval prolongation · sexual dysfunction · shock · skin reactions · sleep disorder · testicular atrophy · thirst · tumour activation temporary · uterine leiomyoma degeneration · vision disorders · vomiting · vulvovaginal disorders · weight changes
  SPECIFIC SIDE-EFFECTS
- With intranasal use Altered smell sensation · epistaxis · hoarseness · nasal irritation · taste altered
  SIDE-EFFECTS, FURTHER INFORMATION During the initial stage (1–2 weeks) increased production of testosterone may be associated with progression of prostate cancer. In susceptible patients this tumour 'flare' may cause spinal cord compression, ureteric obstruction or increased bone pain.
- CONCEPTION AND CONTRACEPTION Non-hormonal, barrier methods of contraception should be used during entire treatment period. Pregnancy should be excluded before treatment, the first injection should be given during menstruation or shortly afterwards or use barrier contraception for 1 month beforehand.
- PREGNANCY Avoid.
- BREAST FEEDING Avoid.
- DIRECTIONS FOR ADMINISTRATION
- With intranasal use Avoid use of nasal decongestants before and for at least 30 minutes after treatment.
- With subcutaneous use Rotate injection site to prevent atrophy and nodule formation.
- PATIENT AND CARER ADVICE Patients or carers should be given advice on how to administer buserelin nasal spray.

- MEDICINAL FORMS
  There can be variation in the licensing of different medicines containing the same drug.
  Solution for injection
- Suprecur (Sanofi)
  Buserelin (as Buserelin acetate) 1 mg per 1 ml Suprecur 5.5mg/5.5ml solution for injection vials | 2 vial [PoM] £33.02
- Suprefact (Sanofi)
  Buserelin (as Buserelin acetate) 1 mg per 1 ml Suprefact 5.5mg/5.5ml solution for injection vials | 2 vial [PoM] £34.37
  Spray
- Suprecur (Sanofi)
  Buserelin (as Buserelin acetate) 150 microgram per 1 dose Suprecur 150micrograms/dose nasal spray | 168 dose [PoM] £105.16

- Suprefact (Sanofi)
  Buserelin (as Buserelin acetate) 100 microgram per 1 dose Suprefact 100micrograms/dose nasal spray | 336 dose [PoM] £122.24

Goserelin

- DRUG ACTION Administration of gonadorelin analogues produces an initial phase of stimulation; continued administration is followed by down-regulation of gonadotrophin-releasing hormone receptors, thereby reducing the release of gonadotrophins (follicle stimulating hormone and luteinising hormone) which in turn leads to inhibition of androgen and oestrogen production.

- INDICATIONS AND DOSE
  ZOLADEX LA ®
  Locally advanced prostate cancer as an alternative to surgical castration | Adjuvant treatment to radiotherapy or radical prostatectomy in patients with high-risk localised or locally advanced prostate cancer | Neoadjuvant treatment prior to radiotherapy in patients with high-risk localised or locally advanced prostate cancer | Metastatic prostate cancer
- BY SUBCUTANEOUS INJECTION
- Adult: 10.8 mg every 12 weeks, to be administered into the anterior abdominal wall
  ZOLADEX ®
  Locally advanced prostate cancer as an alternative to surgical castration | Adjuvant treatment to radiotherapy or radical prostatectomy in patients with high-risk localised or locally advanced prostate cancer | Neoadjuvant treatment prior to radiotherapy in patients with high-risk localised or locally advanced prostate cancer | Metastatic prostate cancer | Advanced breast cancer | Oestrogen-receptor-positive early breast cancer
- BY SUBCUTANEOUS INJECTION
- Adult: 3.6 mg every 28 days, to be administered into the anterior abdominal wall
  Endometriosis
- BY SUBCUTANEOUS INJECTION
- Adult: 3.6 mg every 28 days maximum duration of treatment 6 months (do not repeat), to be administered into the anterior abdominal wall
  Endometrial thinning before intra-uterine surgery
- BY SUBCUTANEOUS INJECTION
- Adult: 3.6 mg, dose may be repeated after 28 days if uterus is large or to allow flexible surgical timing, to be administered into the anterior abdominal wall
  Before surgery in women who have anaemia due to uterine fibroids
- BY SUBCUTANEOUS INJECTION
- Adult: 3.6 mg every 28 days maximum duration of treatment 3 months, to be given with supplementary iron, to be administered into the anterior abdominal wall
  Pituitary desensitisation before induction of ovulation by gonadotrophins for in vitro fertilisation (after exclusion of pregnancy) (under expert supervision)
- BY SUBCUTANEOUS INJECTION
- Adult: 3.6 mg, dose given to achieve pituitary down-regulation (usually 1–3 weeks) then gonadotrophin is administered (stopping gonadotrophin on administration of chorionic gonadotrophin at appropriate stage of follicular development), to be administered into the anterior abdominal wall

- CONTRA-INDICATIONS Undiagnosed vaginal bleeding · use longer than 6 months in endometriosis (do not repeat)

6

Endocrine system

- CAUTIONS Depression · diabetes · hypertension · patients with metabolic bone disease (decrease in bone mineral density can occur) · polycystic ovarian disease · risk of spinal cord compression in men · risk of ureteric obstruction in men
- SIDE-EFFECTS
- ▶ **Common or very common** Alopecia · arthralgia · bone pain · breast abnormalities · depression · glucose tolerance impaired · gynaecomastia · headache · heart failure · hot flush · hyperhidrosis · mood altered · myocardial infarction · neoplasm complications · paraesthesia · sexual dysfunction · skin reactions · spinal cord compression · vulvovaginal disorders · weight increased
- ▶ **Uncommon** Hypercalcaemia (in women) · ureteral obstruction
- ▶ **Rare or very rare** Ovarian and fallopian tube disorders · pituitary haemorrhage · pituitary tumour · psychotic disorder
- ▶ **Frequency not known** Abdominal cramps · body hair change · constipation · diarrhoea · fatigue · hepatic function abnormal · interstitial pneumonia · muscle complaints · nausea · nervousness · peripheral oedema (when used for gynaecological conditions) · premature menopause · pulmonary embolism · QT interval prolongation · sleep disorder · uterine leiomyoma degeneration · voice alteration · vomiting · vulvovaginal infection · withdrawal bleed

  SIDE-EFFECTS, FURTHER INFORMATION Tumour flare can occur when androgen deprivation therapy is initiated.
- CONCEPTION AND CONTRACEPTION Non-hormonal, barrier methods of contraception should be used during entire treatment period. Pregnancy should be excluded before treatment, the first injection should be given during menstruation or shortly afterwards or use barrier contraception for 1 month beforehand.
- PREGNANCY Avoid.
- BREAST FEEDING Avoid.
- MONITORING REQUIREMENTS Men at risk of tumour 'flare' should be monitored closely during the first month of therapy for prostate cancer.
- DIRECTIONS FOR ADMINISTRATION Rotate injection site to prevent atrophy and nodule formation.

- MEDICINAL FORMS
  There can be variation in the licensing of different medicines containing the same drug.
  Implant
  - ▶ Zoladex (AstraZeneca UK Ltd)
    Goserelin (as Goserelin acetate) 3.6 mg Zoladex 3.6mg implant SafeSystem pre-filled syringes | 1 pre-filled disposable injection [PoM] £65.00 DT = £65.00
  - ▶ Zoladex LA (AstraZeneca UK Ltd)
    Goserelin (as Goserelin acetate) 10.8 mg Zoladex LA 10.8mg implant SafeSystem pre-filled syringes | 1 pre-filled disposable injection [PoM] £235.00 DT = £235.00

Leuprorelin acetate

- DRUG ACTION Administration of gonadorelin analogues produces an initial phase of stimulation; continued administration is followed by down-regulation of gonadotrophin-releasing hormone receptors, thereby reducing the release of gonadotrophins (follicle stimulating hormone and luteinising hormone) which in turn leads to inhibition of androgen and oestrogen production.

- INDICATIONS AND DOSE
  PROSTAP 3 DCS ®
  Locally advanced prostate cancer as an alternative to surgical castration | Adjuvant treatment to radiotherapy or radical prostatectomy in patients with high-risk localised or locally advanced prostate cancer | Metastatic prostate cancer
  - ▶ BY SUBCUTANEOUS INJECTION
  - ▶ Adult: 11.25 mg every 3 months
  Endometriosis
  - ▶ BY INTRAMUSCULAR INJECTION
  - ▶ Adult: Initially 11.25 mg for 1 dose, dose to be given as a single dose in first 5 days of menstrual cycle, then 11.25 mg every 3 months for maximum 6 months (course not to be repeated)
  PROSTAP SR DCS ®
  Locally advanced prostate cancer as an alternative to surgical castration | Adjuvant treatment to radiotherapy or radical prostatectomy in patients with high-risk localised or locally advanced prostate cancer | Metastatic prostate cancer
  - ▶ BY SUBCUTANEOUS INJECTION, OR BY INTRAMUSCULAR INJECTION
  - ▶ Adult: 3.75 mg every month
  Endometriosis
  - ▶ BY SUBCUTANEOUS INJECTION, OR BY INTRAMUSCULAR INJECTION
  - ▶ Adult: Initially 3.75 mg for 1 dose, dose to be given as a single dose in first 5 days of menstrual cycle, then 3.75 mg every month for maximum 6 months (course not to be repeated)
  Endometrial thinning before intra-uterine surgery
  - ▶ BY SUBCUTANEOUS INJECTION, OR BY INTRAMUSCULAR INJECTION
  - ▶ Adult: Initially 3.75 mg for 1 dose, dose to be given as a single dose between day 3 and 5 of menstrual cycle, 5–6 weeks before surgery
  Reduction of size of uterine fibroids and of associated bleeding before surgery
  - ▶ BY SUBCUTANEOUS INJECTION, OR BY INTRAMUSCULAR INJECTION
  - ▶ Adult: Initially 3.75 mg every month usually for 3–4 months (maximum 6 months)

- CONTRA-INDICATIONS
  GENERAL CONTRA-INDICATIONS Undiagnosed vaginal bleeding
  SPECIFIC CONTRA-INDICATIONS
  - ▶ When used for endometriosis Use longer than 6 months (do not repeat)
- CAUTIONS Diabetes · family history of osteoporosis · patients with metabolic bone disease (decrease in bone mineral density can occur) · risk of spinal cord compression in men with prostate cancer · risk of ureteric obstruction in men with prostate cancer
- SIDE-EFFECTS
- ▶ **Common or very common** Appetite decreased · arthralgia · bone pain · breast abnormalities · depression · dizziness · fatigue · gynaecomastia · headache · hepatic disorders · hot flush · hyperhidrosis · insomnia · mood altered · muscle weakness · nausea · paraesthesia · peripheral oedema · sexual dysfunction · testicular atrophy · vulvovaginal disorders · weight change
- ▶ **Uncommon** Alopecia · diarrhoea · fever · myalgia · palpitations · visual impairment · vomiting
- ▶ **Rare or very rare** Haemorrhage
- ▶ **Frequency not known** Anaemia · glucose tolerance impaired · hypertension · hypotension · leucopenia · paralysis · pulmonary embolism · QT interval prolongation · seizure ·

spinal fracture · thrombocytopenia · urinary tract obstruction

SIDE-EFFECTS, FURTHER INFORMATION In prostate cancer, during the initial stage (1–2 weeks) increased production of testosterone may be associated with progression of prostate cancer. In susceptible patients this tumour 'flare' may cause spinal cord compression, ureteric obstruction or increased bone pain.

● CONCEPTION AND CONTRACEPTION Non-hormonal, barrier methods of contraception should be used during entire treatment period. Pregnancy should be excluded before treatment, the first injection should be given during menstruation or shortly afterwards or use barrier contraception for 1 month beforehand.

● PREGNANCY Avoid—teratogenic in *animal* studies.

● BREAST FEEDING Avoid.

● MONITORING REQUIREMENTS
▶ Monitor liver function.
▶ Men at risk of tumour 'flare' should be monitored closely during the first month of therapy.

● DIRECTIONS FOR ADMINISTRATION Rotate injection site to prevent atrophy and nodule formation.

● MEDICINAL FORMS
There can be variation in the licensing of different medicines containing the same drug.

Powder and solvent for suspension for injection
▶ Prostap 3 DCS (Takeda UK Ltd)
Leuprorelin acetate 11.25 mg Prostap 3 DCS 11.25mg powder and solvent for suspension for injection pre-filled syringes | 1 pre-filled disposable injection PoM £225.72 DT = £225.72
▶ Prostap SR DCS (Takeda UK Ltd)
Leuprorelin acetate 3.75 mg Prostap SR DCS 3.75mg powder and solvent for suspension for injection pre-filled syringes | 1 pre-filled disposable injection PoM £75.24 DT = £75.24

Nafarelin

● DRUG ACTION Administration of gonadorelin analogues produces an initial phase of stimulation; continued administration is followed by down-regulation of gonadotrophin-releasing hormone receptors, thereby reducing the release of gonadotrophins (follicle stimulating hormone and luteinising hormone) which in turn leads to inhibition of androgen and oestrogen production.

● INDICATIONS AND DOSE

Endometriosis
▶ BY INTRANASAL ADMINISTRATION
▶ Adult (female): 200 micrograms twice daily for maximum 6 months (do not repeat), one spray in one nostril in the morning, and one spray in the other nostril in the evening (starting on days 2–4 of menstruation).

Pituitary desensitisation before induction of ovulation by gonadotrophins for in vitro fertilisation (under expert supervision)
▶ BY INTRANASAL ADMINISTRATION
▶ Adult: 400 micrograms twice daily, one spray in each nostril, to be started in early follicular phase (day 2) or, after exclusion of pregnancy, in midluteal phase (day 21) and continued until down regulation achieved (usually within 4 weeks) then maintained (usually for 8–12 days) during gonadotrophin administration (stopping gonadotrophin and nafarelin on administration of chorionic gonadotrophin at follicular maturity), discontinue if down-regulation not achieved within 12 weeks

● CONTRA-INDICATIONS Undiagnosed vaginal bleeding · use longer than 6 months in the treatment of endometriosis (do not repeat)

● CAUTIONS Patients with metabolic bone disease (decrease in bone mineral density can occur)

● SIDE-EFFECTS
▶ **Common or very common** Artificial menopause · breast abnormalities · chest pain · depression · dyspnoea · emotional lability · headaches · hirsutism · hot flush · hypersensitivity · hypertension · hypotension · insomnia · myalgia · oedema · oestrogen deficiency · paraesthesia · rhinitis · seborrhoea · sexual dysfunction · skin reactions · uterine haemorrhage · vulvovaginal dryness · weight changes
▶ **Uncommon** Alopecia · arthralgia · ovarian cyst (may require discontinuation)
▶ **Frequency not known** Ovarian hyperstimulation syndrome · palpitations · vision blurred

● CONCEPTION AND CONTRACEPTION Non-hormonal, barrier methods of contraception should be used during entire treatment period. Pregnancy should be excluded before treatment, the first dose should be given during menstruation or shortly afterwards or use barrier contraception for 1 month beforehand.

● PREGNANCY Avoid.

● BREAST FEEDING Avoid.

● DIRECTIONS FOR ADMINISTRATION Avoid use of nasal decongestants before and for at least 30 minutes after treatment; repeat dose if sneezing occurs during or immediately after administration.

● PATIENT AND CARER ADVICE Patients or carers should be given advice on how to administer nafarelin nasal spray.

● MEDICINAL FORMS
There can be variation in the licensing of different medicines containing the same drug.

Spray
CAUTIONARY AND ADVISORY LABELS 10
▶ Synarel (Pfizer Ltd)
Nafarelin (as Nafarelin acetate) 200 microgram per 1 dose Synarel 200micrograms/dose nasal spray | 60 dose PoM £52.43

Triptorelin   27-Apr-2017

● DRUG ACTION Administration of gonadorelin analogues produces an initial phase of stimulation; continued administration is followed by down-regulation of gonadotrophin-releasing hormone receptors, thereby reducing the release of gonadotrophins (follicle stimulating hormone and luteinising hormone) which in turn leads to inhibition of androgen and oestrogen production.

● INDICATIONS AND DOSE

DECAPEPTYL® SR 11.25MG

Locally advanced non-metastatic prostate cancer as an alternative to surgical castration | Metastatic prostate cancer | Adjuvant treatment to radiotherapy in high-risk localised or locally advanced prostate cancer | Neoadjuvant treatment prior to radiotherapy in patients with high-risk localised or locally advanced prostate cancer | Adjuvant treatment to radical prostatectomy in patients with locally advanced prostate cancer at high risk of disease progression
▶ BY INTRAMUSCULAR INJECTION
▶ Adult: 11.25 mg every 3 months   continued →

6

Endocrine system

Endometriosis

▶ BY INTRAMUSCULAR INJECTION

▶ Adult: 11.25 mg every 3 months for maximum 6 months (not to be repeated), to be started during first 5 days of menstrual cycle

DECAPEPTYL ® SR 22.5MG

Locally advanced non-metastatic prostate cancer as an alternative to surgical castration | Metastatic prostate cancer | Adjuvant treatment to radiotherapy in high-risk localised or locally advanced prostate cancer | Neoadjuvant treatment prior to radiotherapy in patients with high-risk localised or locally advanced prostate cancer | Adjuvant treatment to radical prostatectomy in patients with locally advanced prostate cancer at high risk of disease progression

▶ BY INTRAMUSCULAR INJECTION

▶ Adult: 22.5 mg every 6 months

DECAPEPTYL ® SR 3MG

Locally advanced non-metastatic prostate cancer as an alternative to surgical castration | Metastatic prostate cancer | Adjuvant treatment to radiotherapy in high-risk localised or locally advanced prostate cancer | Neoadjuvant treatment prior to radiotherapy in patients with high-risk localised or locally advanced prostate cancer | Adjuvant treatment to radical prostatectomy in patients with locally advanced prostate cancer at high risk of disease progression

▶ BY INTRAMUSCULAR INJECTION

▶ Adult: 3 mg every 4 weeks

Endometriosis

▶ BY INTRAMUSCULAR INJECTION

▶ Adult: 3 mg every 4 weeks maximum duration of 6 months (not to be repeated), to be started during first 5 days of menstrual cycle

Reduction in size of uterine fibroids

▶ BY INTRAMUSCULAR INJECTION

▶ Adult: 3 mg every 4 weeks for at least 3 months, maximum duration of treatment 6 months (not to be repeated), to be started during first 5 days of menstrual cycle

GONAPEPTYL DEPOT ®

Advanced prostate cancer

▶ BY SUBCUTANEOUS INJECTION, OR BY DEEP INTRAMUSCULAR INJECTION

▶ Adult: 3.75 mg every 4 weeks

Endometriosis | Reduction in size of uterine fibroids

▶ BY SUBCUTANEOUS INJECTION, OR BY DEEP INTRAMUSCULAR INJECTION

▶ Adult: 3.75 mg every 4 weeks maximum duration of 6 months (not to be repeated), to be started during first 5 days of menstrual cycle

SALVACYL ®

Male hypersexuality with severe sexual deviation

▶ BY INTRAMUSCULAR INJECTION

▶ Adult: 11.25 mg every 12 weeks

● CONTRA-INDICATIONS In endometriosis do not use for longer than 6 months (do not repeat) · undiagnosed vaginal bleeding

SALVACYL ® Severe osteoporosis

● CAUTIONS

GENERAL CAUTIONS Patients with metabolic bone disease (decrease in bone mineral density can occur)

SPECIFIC CAUTIONS

▶ When used for prostate cancer Risk factors for osteoporosis · risk of spinal cord compression in men · risk of ureteric obstruction in men

SALVACYL ® Increased risk of sensitivity to restored testosterone if treatment interrupted—consider administration of an antiandrogen before stopping treatment · transient increase in serum testosterone occurs on initiation—consider administration of an anti-androgen

● SIDE-EFFECTS

▶ **Common or very common** Asthenia · depression · dizziness · dysuria · gastrointestinal discomfort · gynaecomastia · haemorrhage · headache · hot flush · hyperhidrosis · hypersensitivity · joint disorders · menstrual cycle irregularities · mood altered · muscle complaints · nausea · oedema · ovarian and fallopian tube disorders · pain · painful sexual intercourse · paraesthesia · pelvic pain · sexual dysfunction · sleep disorders · vulvovaginal disorders

▶ **Uncommon** Alopecia · appetite abnormal · asthma exacerbated · breast pain · chills · constipation · diarrhoea · drowsiness · dry mouth · dyspnoea · embolism · gout · hypertension · muscle weakness · skin reactions · testicular disorders · tinnitus · vision disorders · vomiting · weight changes

▶ **Rare or very rare** Abnormal sensation in eye · chest pain · confusion · diabetes mellitus · difficulty standing · fever · flatulence · hypotension · influenza like illness · memory loss · musculoskeletal stiffness · nasopharyngitis · orthopnoea · osteoarthritis · taste altered · vertigo

▶ **Frequency not known** Angioedema · anxiety · bone disorders · malaise · QT interval prolongation

SIDE-EFFECTS, FURTHER INFORMATION During the initial stage increased production of testosterone may be associated with progression of prostate cancer. In susceptible patients this tumour 'flare' may cause spinal cord compression, ureteric obstruction or increased pain.

● CONCEPTION AND CONTRACEPTION Non-hormonal, barrier methods of contraception should be used during entire treatment period. Pregnancy should be excluded before treatment, the first injection should be given during menstruation or shortly afterwards or use barrier contraception for 1 month beforehand.

● PREGNANCY Avoid.

● BREAST FEEDING Avoid.

● MONITORING REQUIREMENTS

▶ When used for Prostate cancer Men at risk of tumour 'flare' should be monitored closely during the first month of therapy.

● DIRECTIONS FOR ADMINISTRATION Rotate injection site to prevent atrophy and nodule formation.

● PRESCRIBING AND DISPENSING INFORMATION

DECAPEPTYL ® SR 22.5MG Each vial includes an overage to allow accurate administration of a 22.5 mg dose.

DECAPEPTYL ® SR 3MG Each vial includes an overage to allow accurate administration of 3 mg dose.

DECAPEPTYL ® SR 11.25MG Each vial includes an overage to allow accurate administration of an 11.25 mg dose.

● NATIONAL FUNDING/ACCESS DECISIONS

All Wales Medicines Strategy Group (AWMSG) Decisions

The *All Wales Medicines Strategy Group* has advised (March 2017) that triptorelin (*Decapeptyl® SR*) is recommended as an option for use within NHS Wales as an adjuvant treatment to radiotherapy and as a neoadjuvant treatment prior to radiotherapy, in patients with high-risk localised or locally advanced prostate cancer.

- MEDICINAL FORMS
  There can be variation in the licensing of different medicines containing the same drug.

  Powder and solvent for suspension for injection
  - Decapeptyl SR (Ipsen Ltd)
    Triptorelin (as Triptorelin acetate) 3 mg Decapeptyl SR 3mg powder and solvent for suspension for injection vials | 1 vial [PoM] £69.00 DT = £69.00
    Triptorelin 11.25 mg Decapeptyl SR 11.25mg powder and solvent for suspension for injection vials | 1 vial [PoM] £207.00 DT = £207.00
    Triptorelin (as Triptorelin embonate) 22.5 mg Decapeptyl SR 22.5mg powder and solvent for suspension for injection vials | 1 vial [PoM] £414.00 DT = £414.00
  - Gonapeptyl Depot (Ferring Pharmaceuticals Ltd)
    Triptorelin (as Triptorelin acetate) 3.75 mg Gonapeptyl Depot 3.75mg powder and solvent for suspension for injection pre-filled disposable devices | 1 pre-filled disposable injection [PoM] £81.69
  - Salvacyl (Ipsen Ltd)
    Triptorelin 11.25 mg Salvacyl 11.25mg powder and solvent for injection vials | 1 vial [PoM] £248.00 DT = £207.00

6.1 Hereditary angioedema

PITUITARY AND HYPOTHALAMIC HORMONES AND ANALOGUES > ANTI-GONADOTROPHIN-RELEASING HORMONES

Danazol

- DRUG ACTION Danazol inhibits pituitary gonadotrophins; it combines androgenic activity with antioestrogenic and antiprogestogenic activity.

- INDICATIONS AND DOSE
  Endometriosis
  - BY MOUTH
  - Adult: 200–800 mg daily in up to 4 divided doses usually for 3–6 months, dose to be adjusted to achieve amenorrhoea, in women of child-bearing potential, treatment should start during menstruation, preferably on day 1

  Severe pain and tenderness in benign fibrocystic breast disease not responding to other treatment
  - BY MOUTH
  - Adult: 300 mg daily in divided doses usually for 3–6 months, in women of child-bearing potential, treatment should start during menstruation, preferably on day 1

  Hereditary angioedema
  - BY MOUTH
  - Adult: Initially 100–200 mg daily, dose to be reduced according to response, in women of child-bearing potential, treatment should start during menstruation, preferably on day 1

- UNLICENSED USE Not licensed for use in hereditary angioedema.

- CONTRA-INDICATIONS Acute porphyrias p. 1025 · androgen-dependent tumours · thromboembolic disease · undiagnosed genital bleeding

- CAUTIONS Cardiac impairment (avoid if severe) · diabetes mellitus · elderly · epilepsy · history of thrombosis or thromboembolic disease · hypertension · lipoprotein disorder · migraine · polycythaemia

- INTERACTIONS → Appendix 1: danazol

- SIDE-EFFECTS Alopecia · aminolevulinic acid synthetase induction · anxiety · appetite increased · breast atrophy · carpal tunnel syndrome · clitoris enlarged · contact lens intolerance · cutaneous lupus erythematosus · depressed mood · dizziness · embolism and thrombosis · emotional lability · eosinophilia · epigastric pain · epilepsy

exacerbated · face oedema · fatigue · fever · fluid retention · flushing · glucose tolerance impaired · haematuria · headaches · hepatic disorders · hirsutism · hypertension · idiopathic intracranial hypertension · insulin resistance · joint disorders · leucopenia · libido disorder · menstrual cycle irregularities · muscle contractions involuntary · muscle cramps · myocardial infarction · nausea · neoplasms · pain · palpitations · pancreatitis · photosensitivity reaction · polycythaemia · respiratory disorders · seborrhoea · skin reactions · speech pitch disorder · spermatogenesis reduced · splenic peliosis · tachycardia · throat pain · thrombocytopenia · tremor · vertigo · vision disorders · voice alteration · vulvovaginal disorders · weight increased

SIDE-EFFECTS, FURTHER INFORMATION Withdraw if virilisation effects occur—may be irreversible on continued use.

- CONCEPTION AND CONTRACEPTION Ensure patients with amenorrhoea are not pregnant. Non-hormonal contraceptive methods should be used, if appropriate.

- PREGNANCY Avoid; has weak androgenic effects and virilisation of female fetus reported.

- BREAST FEEDING No data available but avoid because of possible androgenic effects in infant.

- HEPATIC IMPAIRMENT Caution in hepatic impairment (avoid if severe).

- RENAL IMPAIRMENT Caution in renal impairment (avoid if severe).

- MEDICINAL FORMS
  There can be variation in the licensing of different medicines containing the same drug. Forms available from special-order manufacturers include: capsule

  Capsule
  - Danazol (Non-proprietary)
    Danazol 100 mg Danazol 100mg capsules | 28 capsule [PoM] £7.64-£18.40 [CD4-2]
    Danazol 200 mg Danazol 200mg capsules | 56 capsule [PoM] £30.27-£66.20 [CD4-2]
  - Danol (Sanofi)
    Danazol 100 mg Danol 100mg capsules | 60 capsule [PoM] £16.38 DT = £16.38 [CD4-2]
    Danazol 200 mg Danol 200mg capsules | 60 capsule [PoM] £32.43 DT = £32.43 [CD4-2]

7 Hypothalamic and anterior pituitary hormone related disorders

Hypothalamic and anterior pituitary hormones

Anterior pituitary hormones

Corticotrophins
Tetracosactide p. 726 (tetracosactrin), an analogue of corticotropin (ACTH), is used to test adrenocortical function; failure of the plasma cortisol concentration to rise after administration of tetracosactide indicates adrenocortical insufficiency.

Both corticotropin and tetracosactide were formerly used as alternatives to corticosteroids in conditions such as Crohn's disease or rheumatoid arthritis; their value was limited by the variable and unpredictable therapeutic response and by the waning of their effect with time.

Gonadotrophins
Follicle-stimulating hormone (FSH) and luteinising hormone (LH) together, follicle-stimulating hormone alone (as in

6

Endocrine system

follitropin), or chorionic gonadotrophin p. 727, are used in the treatment of infertility in women with proven hypopituitarism or who have not responded to clomifene citrate p. 750, or in superovulation treatment for assisted conception (such as *in vitro* fertilisation).

The gonadotrophins are also occasionally used in the treatment of hypogonadotrophic hypogonadism and associated oligospermia. There is no justification for their use in primary gonadal failure.

Chorionic gonadotrophin has also been used in delayed puberty in the male to stimulate endogenous testosterone production, but has little advantage over testosterone.

Growth hormone

Growth hormone is used to treat deficiency of the hormone in children and in adults. In children it is used in Prader-Willi syndrome, Turner syndrome, chronic renal insufficiency, short children considered small for gestational age at birth, and short stature homeobox-containing gene (SHOX) deficiency.

Growth hormone of human origin (HGH; somatotrophin) has been replaced by a growth hormone of human sequence, somatropin p. 731, produced using recombinant DNA technology.

Mecasermin, a human insulin-like growth factor-I (rhIGF-I), is licensed to treat growth failure in children and adolescents with severe primary insulin-like growth factor-I deficiency.

Hypothalamic hormones

Gonadorelin p. 727 when injected intravenously in normal subjects leads to a rapid rise in plasma concentrations of both luteinising hormone (LH) and follicle-stimulating hormone (FSH). It has not proved to be very helpful, however, in distinguishing hypothalamic from pituitary lesions. **Gonadorelin analogues** are indicated in endometriosis and infertility and in breast and prostate cancer.

7.1 Adrenocortical function testing

PITUITARY AND HYPOTHALAMIC HORMONES AND ANALOGUES ❭ CORTICOTROPHINS

Tetracosactide

(Tetracosactrin)

● **INDICATIONS AND DOSE**

Diagnosis of adrenocortical insufficiency (diagnostic 30-minute test)

▸ BY INTRAVENOUS INJECTION, OR BY INTRAMUSCULAR INJECTION

▸ Adult: 250 micrograms for 1 dose

Diagnosis of adrenocortical insufficiency (diagnostic 5-hour test)

▸ BY INTRAMUSCULAR INJECTION USING DEPOT INJECTION

▸ Adult: 1 mg for 1 dose

Alternative to corticosteroids in conditions such as Crohn's disease or rheumatoid arthritis (formerly used but value was limited by the variable and unpredictable therapeutic response and by the waning of effect with time)

▸ BY INTRAMUSCULAR INJECTION USING DEPOT INJECTION

▸ Adult: Initially 1 mg daily, alternatively initially 1 mg every 12 hours, (in acute cases), then reduced to 1 mg every 2–3 days, followed by 1 mg once weekly, alternatively 500 micrograms every 2–3 days

● **CONTRA-INDICATIONS** Acute psychosis · adrenogenital syndrome · allergic disorders · asthma · avoid injections containing benzyl alcohol in neonates · Cushing's syndrome · infectious diseases · peptic ulcer · primary adrenocortical insufficiency · refractory heart failure

● **CAUTIONS** Active infectious diseases (should not be used unless adequate disease-specific therapy is being given) · active systemic diseases (should not be used unless adequate disease-specific therapy is being given) · diabetes mellitus · diverticulitis · history of asthma · history of atopic allergy · history of eczema · history of hayfever · history of hypersensitivity · hypertension · latent amoebiasis (may become activated) · latent tuberculosis (may become activated) · myasthenia gravis · ocular herpes simplex · osteoporosis · predisposition to thromboembolic · psychological disturbances may be triggered · recent intestinal anastomosis · reduced immune response (should not be used unless adequate disease-specific therapy is being given) · ulcerative colitis

CAUTIONS, FURTHER INFORMATION

▸ **Risk of anaphylaxis** Should only be administered under medical supervision. Consult product literature.

▸ **Hypertension** Patients already receiving medication for moderate to severe hypertension must have their dosage adjusted if treatment started.

▸ **Diabetes mellitus** Patients already receiving medication for diabetes mellitus must have their dosage adjusted if treatment started.

● **SIDE-EFFECTS** Abdominal distension · abscess · adrenocortical unresponsiveness · angioedema · appetite increased · bone fractures · congestive heart failure · Cushing's syndrome · diabetes mellitus exacerbated · dizziness · dyspnoea · electrolyte imbalance · exophthalmos · fluid retention · flushing · gastrointestinal disorders · glaucoma · growth retardation · haemorrhage · headache · healing impaired · hirsutism · hyperglycaemia · hyperhidrosis · hypersensitivity (may be more severe in patients susceptible to allergies, especially asthma) · hypertension · idiopathic intracranial hypertension exacerbated · increased risk of infection · leucocytosis · malaise · menstruation irregular · muscle weakness · myopathy · nausea · osteonecrosis · osteoporosis · pancreatitis · papilloedema · pituitary unresponsiveness · posterior subcapsular cataract · protein catabolism · psychiatric disorder · seizure · skin reactions · tendon rupture · thromboembolism · vasculitis necrotising · vertigo · vomiting · weight increased

● **ALLERGY AND CROSS-SENSITIVITY** Contra-indicated in patients with history of hypersensitivity to tetracosactide/corticotrophins or excipients.

● **PREGNANCY** Avoid (but may be used diagnostically if essential).

● **BREAST FEEDING** Avoid (but may be used diagnostically if essential).

● **HEPATIC IMPAIRMENT** An enhanced effect of tetracosactide therapy may occur in patients with cirrhosis of the liver. Use with caution in hepatic impairment. **Monitoring** Monitor hepatic function closely during treatment.

● **RENAL IMPAIRMENT** Use with caution in patients with renal impairment.

● **EFFECT ON LABORATORY TESTS** May suppress skin test reactions.

Post administration total plasma cortisol levels during 30-minute test for diagnosis of adrenocotical insufficiency might be misleading due to altered cortisol binding globulin levels in some special clinical situations including, patients on oral contraceptives, post-operative patients, critical illness, severe liver disease and nephrotic syndrome.

- **MEDICINAL FORMS**
  There can be variation in the licensing of different medicines containing the same drug.
  Solution for injection
  ▸ Synacthen (Mallinckrodt Specialty Pharmaceuticals Ireland Ltd)
    Tetracosactide acetate 250 microgram per 1 ml Synacthen 250micrograms/1ml solution for injection ampoules | 1 ampoule [PoM] £38.00
  Suspension for injection
  EXCIPIENTS: May contain Benzyl alcohol
  ▸ Synacthen Depot (Mallinckrodt Specialty Pharmaceuticals Ireland Ltd)
    Tetracosactide acetate 1 mg per 1 ml Synacthen Depot 1mg/1ml suspension for injection ampoules | 1 ampoule [PoM] £346.28

7.2 Assessment of pituitary function

PITUITARY AND HYPOTHALAMIC HORMONES AND ANALOGUES > GONADOTROPIN-RELEASING HORMONES

Gonadorelin

(Gonadotrophin-releasing hormone; GnRH; LH–RH)

- **INDICATIONS AND DOSE**
  Assessment of pituitary function
  ▸ BY SUBCUTANEOUS INJECTION, OR BY INTRAVENOUS INJECTION
  ▸ Adult: 100 micrograms for 1 dose

- **CAUTIONS** Pituitary adenoma
- **SIDE-EFFECTS**
- ▸ **Uncommon** Pain · skin reactions · swelling
- ▸ **Rare or very rare** Abdominal discomfort · bronchospasm · dizziness · eye erythema · flushing · headache · nausea · tachycardia
- ▸ **Frequency not known** Menorrhagia · sepsis
- **PREGNANCY** Avoid.
- **BREAST FEEDING** Avoid.

- **MEDICINAL FORMS**
  There can be variation in the licensing of different medicines containing the same drug.
  Powder and solvent for solution for injection
  EXCIPIENTS: May contain Benzyl alcohol
  ▸ Gonadorelin (Non-proprietary)
    Gonadorelin (as Gonadorelin hydrochloride)
    100 microgram Gonadorelin 100microgram powder and solvent for solution for injection vials | 1 vial [PoM] £75.00 (Hospital only)

7.3 Gonadotrophin replacement therapy

GONADOTROPHINS

Choriogonadotropin alfa

(Human chorionic gonadotropin)

- **INDICATIONS AND DOSE**
  Treatment of infertility in women with proven hypopituitarism or who have not responded to clomifene | Superovulation treatment for assisted conception (such as in vitro fertilisation)
  ▸ BY SUBCUTANEOUS INJECTION
  ▸ Adult (female): Adjusted according to response.

- **CONTRA-INDICATIONS** Active thromboembolic disorders · ectopic pregnancy in previous 3 months · hypothalamus malignancy · mammary malignancy · ovarian enlargement or cyst (unless caused by polycystic ovarian disease) · ovarian malignancy · pituitary malignancy · uterine malignancy
- **CAUTIONS** Acute porphyrias p. 1025
- **SIDE-EFFECTS**
- ▸ **Common or very common** Abdominal pain · fatigue · headache · nausea · ovarian hyperstimulation syndrome · vomiting
- ▸ **Uncommon** Breast pain · depression · diarrhoea · irritability · restlessness
- ▸ **Rare or very rare** Rash · shock · thromboembolism

- **MEDICINAL FORMS**
  There can be variation in the licensing of different medicines containing the same drug.
  Solution for injection
  ▸ Ovitrelle (Merck Serono Ltd)
    Choriogonadotropin alfa 500 microgram per 1 ml Ovitrelle 250micrograms/0.5ml solution for injection pre-filled syringes | 1 pre-filled disposable injection [PoM] £31.38 [CD4-2]
    Ovitrelle 250micrograms/0.5ml solution for injection pre-filled pen | 1 pre-filled disposable injection [PoM] £31.38 [CD4-2]

Chorionic gonadotrophin

(Human chorionic gonadotrophin; HCG)

- **DRUG ACTION** A preparation of a glycoprotein fraction secreted by the placenta and obtained from the urine of pregnant women having the action of the pituitary luteinising hormone.

- **INDICATIONS AND DOSE**
  Treatment of infertility in women with proven hypopituitarism or who have not responded to clomifene | Superovulation treatment for assisted conception (such as in vitro fertilisation)
  ▸ BY INTRAMUSCULAR INJECTION, OR BY SUBCUTANEOUS INJECTION
  ▸ Adult (female): Adjusted according to response.

- **CONTRA-INDICATIONS** Androgen-dependent tumours
- **CAUTIONS** Asthma · cardiac impairment · epilepsy · migraine
- **SIDE-EFFECTS** Fatigue · fever · fluid retention · gynaecomastia · headache · hypersensitivity · mood altered · oedema · ovarian hyperstimulation syndrome · skin reactions · sodium retention
- **RENAL IMPAIRMENT** Use with caution.

- **MEDICINAL FORMS**
  There can be variation in the licensing of different medicines containing the same drug.
  Powder and solvent for solution for injection
  ▸ Pregnyl (Merck Sharp & Dohme Ltd)
    Chorionic gonadotrophin human 1500 unit Pregnyl 1,500unit powder and solvent for solution for injection ampoules | 1 ampoule [PoM] £2.12 [CD4-2]
    Chorionic gonadotrophin human 5000 unit Pregnyl 5,000unit powder and solvent for solution for injection ampoules | 1 ampoule [PoM] £3.15 [CD4-2]

Corifollitropin alfa

- **INDICATIONS AND DOSE**
  Controlled ovarian stimulation in combination with a gonadotrophin-releasing hormone antagonist
  ▸ BY SUBCUTANEOUS INJECTION
  ▸ Adult (body-weight up to 60 kg): 100 micrograms
  ▸ Adult (body-weight 60 kg and above): 150 micrograms

- **CONTRA-INDICATIONS** History of ovarian hyperstimulation syndrome · ovarian enlargement or cyst · polycystic ovarian syndrome · tumours of breast · tumours of hypothalamus · tumours of ovaries · tumours of pituitary · tumours of uterus · vaginal bleeding of unknown cause
- **CAUTIONS** Acute porphyrias p. 1025 · risk factors for thromboembolism · risk of ovarian hyperstimulation syndrome
- **SIDE-EFFECTS**
- **Common or very common** Breast abnormalities · fatigue · headache · nausea · ovarian and fallopian tube disorders · pelvic disorders
- **Uncommon** Abdominal distension · back pain · constipation · diarrhoea · dizziness · hot flush · mood altered · premature ovulation · uterine pain · vomiting
- **Frequency not known** Rash
- **BREAST FEEDING** Avoid.
- **RENAL IMPAIRMENT** Avoid.

- **MEDICINAL FORMS**
There can be variation in the licensing of different medicines containing the same drug.
Solution for injection
  ▸ Elonva (Merck Sharp & Dohme Ltd)
    Corifollitropin alfa 200 microgram per 1 ml Elonva 100micrograms/0.5ml solution for injection pre-filled syringes | 1 pre-filled disposable injection PoM £638.00
    Corifollitropin alfa 300 microgram per 1 ml Elonva 150micrograms/0.5ml solution for injection pre-filled syringes | 1 pre-filled disposable injection PoM £638.00

Follitropin alfa

(Recombinant human follicle stimulating hormone)

- **INDICATIONS AND DOSE**

Infertility in women with proven hypopituitarism or who have not responded to clomifene | Superovulation treatment for assisted conception (such as in vitro fertilisation)
  ▸ BY SUBCUTANEOUS INJECTION
  ▸ Adult (female): Adjusted according to response.
Hypogonadotrophic hypogonadism
  ▸ BY SUBCUTANEOUS INJECTION
  ▸ Adult (male): (consult product literature).

- **CONTRA-INDICATIONS** Ovarian cysts (not caused by polycystic ovarian syndrome) · ovarian enlargement (not caused by polycystic ovarian syndrome) · tumours of breast · tumours of hypothalamus · tumours of ovaries · tumours of pituitary · tumours of prostate · tumours of testes · tumours of uterus · vaginal bleeding of unknown cause
- **CAUTIONS** Acute porphyrias p. 1025 · history of tubal disease
- **SIDE-EFFECTS**
- **Common or very common** Acne · diarrhoea · gastrointestinal discomfort · gynaecomastia · headache · nausea · ovarian and fallopian tube disorders · varicocele · vomiting · weight increased
- **Rare or very rare** Asthma exacerbated · thromboembolism
- **PREGNANCY** Avoid.
- **BREAST FEEDING** Avoid.
- **PRESCRIBING AND DISPENSING INFORMATION** Follitropin alfa is a biological medicine. Biological medicines must be prescribed and dispensed by brand name, see *Biological medicines* and *Biosimilar medicines*, under Guidance on prescribing p. 1.

- **PATIENT AND CARER ADVICE**
Conception and contraception Patients planning to conceive should be warned that there is a risk of multiple pregnancy.

- **MEDICINAL FORMS**
There can be variation in the licensing of different medicines containing the same drug.
Solution for injection
  ▸ Bemfola (Gedeon Richter (UK) Ltd) ▼
    Follitropin alfa 600 unit per 1 ml Bemfola 225units/0.375ml solution for injection pre-filled pen | 1 pre-filled disposable injection £70.50
    Bemfola 300units/0.5ml solution for injection pre-filled pen | 1 pre-filled disposable injection PoM £94.00
    Bemfola 150units/0.25ml solution for injection pre-filled pen | 1 pre-filled disposable injection PoM £47.00
    Bemfola 75units/0.125ml solution for injection pre-filled pen | 1 pre-filled disposable injection PoM £23.50
    Bemfola 450units/0.75ml solution for injection pre-filled pen | 1 pre-filled disposable injection PoM £141.00
  ▸ Gonal-f (Merck Serono Ltd)
    Follitropin alfa 600 unit per 1 ml Gonal-f 900units/1.5ml solution for injection pre-filled pen | 1 pre-filled disposable injection PoM £282.00
    Gonal-f 300units/0.5ml solution for injection pre-filled pen | 1 pre-filled disposable injection PoM £94.00
    Gonal-f 450units/0.75ml solution for injection pre-filled pen | 1 pre-filled disposable injection PoM £141.00
  ▸ Ovaleap (Teva UK Ltd) ▼
    Follitropin alfa 600 unit per 1 ml Ovaleap 450units/0.75ml solution for injection cartridges | 1 cartridge PoM £112.80
    Ovaleap 900units/1.5ml solution for injection cartridges | 1 cartridge PoM £225.60
    Ovaleap 300units/0.5ml solution for injection cartridges | 1 cartridge PoM £75.20
Powder and solvent for solution for injection
  ▸ Gonal-f (Merck Serono Ltd)
    Follitropin alfa 75 unit Gonal-f 75unit powder and solvent for solution for injection vials | 1 vial PoM £21.02
    Follitropin alfa 450 unit Gonal-f 450unit powder and solvent for solution for injection vials | 1 vial PoM £126.10
    Follitropin alfa 1050 unit Gonal-f 1,050unit powder and solvent for solution for injection vials | 1 vial PoM £294.22

Follitropin alfa with lutropin alfa

The properties listed below are those particular to the combination only. For the properties of the components please consider, follitropin alfa above, lutropin alfa p. 730.

- **INDICATIONS AND DOSE**

Infertility in women with proven hypopituitarism or who have not responded to clomifene | Superovulation treatment for assisted conception (such as in vitro fertilisation)
  ▸ BY SUBCUTANEOUS INJECTION
  ▸ Adult (female): Adjusted according to response.

- **MEDICINAL FORMS**
There can be variation in the licensing of different medicines containing the same drug.
Powder and solvent for solution for injection
ELECTROLYTES: May contain Sodium
  ▸ Pergoveris (Merck Serono Ltd)
    Lutropin alfa 75 unit, Follitropin alfa 150 unit Pergoveris 150unit/75unit powder and solvent for solution for injection vials | 1 vial PoM £60.29

Follitropin beta

(Recombinant human follicle stimulating hormone)

- **INDICATIONS AND DOSE**

Infertility in women with proven hypopituitarism or who have not responded to clomifene | Superovulation treatment for assisted conception (such as in vitro fertilisation)
  - ▶ BY INTRAMUSCULAR INJECTION, OR BY SUBCUTANEOUS INJECTION
  - ▶ Adult (female): Adjusted according to response.

Hypogonadotrophic hypogonadism
  - ▶ BY INTRAMUSCULAR INJECTION, OR BY SUBCUTANEOUS INJECTION
  - ▶ Adult (male): (consult product literature).

- **CONTRA-INDICATIONS** Ovarian cysts (not caused by polycystic ovarian syndrome) · ovarian enlargement (not caused by polycystic ovarian syndrome) · tumours of breast · tumours of hypothalamus · tumours of ovaries · tumours of pituitary · tumours of prostate · tumours of testes · tumours of uterus · vaginal bleeding of unknown cause
- **CAUTIONS** Acute porphyrias p. 1025 · history of tubal disease
- **SIDE-EFFECTS**
  - ▶ **Common or very common** Epididymal cyst · gastrointestinal discomfort · gynaecomastia · headache · ovarian and fallopian tube disorders · pelvic pain · skin reactions
  - ▶ **Uncommon** Breast abnormalities · constipation · diarrhoea · metrorrhagia · nausea · uterine enlargement · vaginal haemorrhage
  - ▶ **Frequency not known** Thromboembolism
- **PREGNANCY** Avoid.
- **BREAST FEEDING** Avoid.
- **DIRECTIONS FOR ADMINISTRATION** Cartridges and vials are used for subcutaneous administration; vials are used for intramuscular injection.
- **PATIENT AND CARER ADVICE**

Conception and contraception Patients planning to conceive should be warned that there is a risk of multiple pregnancy.

- **MEDICINAL FORMS**
There can be variation in the licensing of different medicines containing the same drug.

Solution for injection
EXCIPIENTS: May contain Neomycin, streptomycin
  - ▶ Puregon (Merck Sharp & Dohme Ltd)
    Follitropin beta 100 unit per 1 ml Puregon 50units/0.5ml solution for injection vials | 1 vial [PoM] £18.03
    Follitropin beta 200 unit per 1 ml Puregon 100units/0.5ml solution for injection vials | 1 vial [PoM] £36.06
    Follitropin beta 833 unit per 1 ml Puregon 900units/1.08ml solution for injection cartridges | 1 cartridge [PoM] £292.23
    Puregon 600units/0.72ml solution for injection cartridges | 1 cartridge [PoM] £194.82
    Puregon 300units/0.36ml solution for injection cartridges | 1 cartridge [PoM] £97.41

Follitropin delta

06-Sep-2017

- **DRUG ACTION** Follitropin delta is a recombinant human follicle stimulating hormone, which causes development of multiple mature follicles.

- **INDICATIONS AND DOSE**

Superovulation treatment for assisted conception (such as in vitro fertilisation) (initiated under specialist supervision)
  - ▶ BY SUBCUTANEOUS INJECTION
  - ▶ Adult (female): Initial dosing based on serum anti-Müllerian hormone concentration and body-weight—consult product literature.

- **CONTRA-INDICATIONS** Ovarian cysts (not caused by polycystic ovarian syndrome) · ovarian enlargement (not caused by polycystic ovarian syndrome) · tumours of breast · tumours of hypothalamus · tumours of ovaries · tumours of pituitary · tumours of uterus · vaginal bleeding of unknown cause
- **CAUTIONS** Acute porphyrias p. 1025 · history of tubal disease (increased risk of ectopic pregnancy)
- **SIDE-EFFECTS**
  - ▶ **Common or very common** Fatigue · headache · nausea · ovarian and fallopian tube disorders · pelvic disorders · uterine pain
  - ▶ **Uncommon** Abdominal discomfort · breast abnormalities · constipation · diarrhoea · dizziness · drowsiness · mood swings · vaginal haemorrhage · vomiting
  - ▶ **Rare or very rare** Thromboembolism

  SIDE-EFFECTS, FURTHER INFORMATION If ovarian hyperstimulation syndrome occurs, the patient should be advised to withhold hCG and avoid intercourse or use barrier contraceptive methods for at least 4 days.
- **PREGNANCY** Manufacturer advises avoid—not indicated during pregnancy.
- **BREAST FEEDING** Manufacturer advises avoid—not indicated during breastfeeding.
- **MONITORING REQUIREMENTS** Manufacturer advises regular monitoring of ovarian response with ultrasound alone, or in combination with serum estradiol levels. Frequent monitoring of follicular development is required to reduce the risk of ovarian hyperstimulation syndrome during treatment, and for at least 2 weeks after triggering of final follicular maturation—consult product literature.
- **DIRECTIONS FOR ADMINISTRATION** Manufacturer recommends the cartridge should be used with the *Rekovelle*® injection pen. The first injection should be performed under direct medical supervision; self-administration should only be performed by patients who are well motivated, adequately trained and have access to expert advice.
- **PRESCRIBING AND DISPENSING INFORMATION** Follitropin delta is a biological medicine. Biological medicines must be prescribed and dispensed by brand name, see *Biological medicines* and *Biosimilar medicines*, under Guidance on prescribing p. 1.
- **HANDLING AND STORAGE** Manufacturer advises store in a refrigerator (2–8 °C)—consult product literature for further information regarding storage conditions outside refrigerator.
- **PATIENT AND CARER ADVICE**

Conception and contraception Manufacturer advises that patients planning to conceive should be warned that there is a risk of multiple pregnancy.

6

Endocrine system

● **MEDICINAL FORMS**
There can be variation in the licensing of different medicines containing the same drug.
Solution for injection
▸ Rekovelle (Ferring Pharmaceuticals Ltd) ▼
 Follitropin delta 33.33 microgram per 1 ml Rekovelle 12micrograms/0.36ml solution for injection cartridges | 1 cartridge [PoM] £118.31
 Rekovelle 36micrograms/1.08ml solution for injection cartridges | 1 cartridge [PoM] £354.94
 Rekovelle 72micrograms/2.16ml solution for injection cartridges | 1 cartridge [PoM] £709.89

Lutropin alfa

(Recombinant human luteinising hormone)

● **INDICATIONS AND DOSE**
Treatment of infertility in women with proven hypopituitarism or who have not responded to clomifene (in conjunction with follicle-stimulating hormone) | Superovulation treatment for assisted conception (such as in vitro fertilisation) (in conjunction with follicle-stimulating hormone)
▸ BY SUBCUTANEOUS INJECTION
▸ Adult (female): Adjusted according to response.

● **CONTRA-INDICATIONS** Mammary carcinoma · ovarian carcinoma · ovarian enlargement or cyst (unless caused by polycystic ovarian disease) · tumours of hypothalamus · tumours of pituitary · undiagnosed vaginal bleeding · uterine carcinoma
● **CAUTIONS** Acute porphyrias p. 1025
● **SIDE-EFFECTS**
▸ **Common or very common** Breast pain · diarrhoea · gastrointestinal discomfort · headache · nausea · ovarian and fallopian tube disorders · pelvic pain · vomiting
▸ **Rare or very rare** Thromboembolism

● **MEDICINAL FORMS**
There can be variation in the licensing of different medicines containing the same drug.
Powder and solvent for solution for injection
▸ Luveris (Merck Serono Ltd)
 Lutropin alfa 75 unit Luveris 75unit powder and solvent for solution for injection vials | 1 vial [PoM] £31.38

Menotrophin

● **INDICATIONS AND DOSE**
Infertility in women with proven hypopituitarism or who have not responded to clomifene | Superovulation treatment for assisted conception (such as in vitro fertilisation)
▸ BY SUBCUTANEOUS INJECTION, OR BY DEEP INTRAMUSCULAR INJECTION
▸ Adult (female): Adjusted according to response.
Hypogonadotrophic hypogonadism
▸ BY DEEP INTRAMUSCULAR INJECTION, OR BY SUBCUTANEOUS INJECTION
▸ Adult (male): (consult product literature).

● **CONTRA-INDICATIONS** Ovarian cysts (not caused by polycystic ovarian syndrome) · ovarian enlargement (not caused by polycystic ovarian syndrome) · tumours of breast · tumours of hypothalamus · tumours of ovaries · tumours of pituitary · tumours of prostate · tumours of testes · tumours of uterus · vaginal bleeding of unknown cause
● **CAUTIONS** Acute porphyrias p. 1025 · history of tubal disease

● **SIDE-EFFECTS**
▸ **Common or very common** Gastrointestinal discomfort · headache · nausea · ovarian hyperstimulation syndrome · pelvic pain · vomiting
▸ **Uncommon** Deep vein thrombosis
● **PREGNANCY** Avoid.
● **BREAST FEEDING** Avoid.
● **PRESCRIBING AND DISPENSING INFORMATION**
Menotrophin is purified extract of human post-menopausal urine containing follicle-stimulating hormone (FSH) and luteinising hormone (LH) in a ratio of 1:1
● **PATIENT AND CARER ADVICE**
Conception and contraception Patients planning to conceive should be warned that there is a risk of multiple pregnancy.

● **MEDICINAL FORMS**
There can be variation in the licensing of different medicines containing the same drug.
Powder and solvent for solution for injection
▸ Menopur (Ferring Pharmaceuticals Ltd)
 Menotrophin 75 unit Menopur 75unit powder and solvent for solution for injection vials | 1 vial [PoM] £18.02 | 10 vial [PoM] £180.18
 Menotrophin 150 unit Menopur 150unit powder and solvent for solution for injection vials | 1 vial [PoM] £360.36
 Menotrophin 600 unit Menopur 600unit powder and solvent for solution for injection vials | 1 vial [PoM] £144.14
 Menotrophin 1200 unit Menopur 1,200unit powder and solvent for solution for injection vials | 1 vial [PoM] £288.29
▸ Meriofert (Pharmasure Ltd) ▼
 Menotrophin 75 unit Meriofert 75unit powder and solvent for solution for injection vials | 10 vial [PoM] £279.00
 Menotrophin 150 unit Meriofert 150unit powder and solvent for solution for injection vials | 10 vial [PoM] £558.00
▸ Merional (IBSA Farmaceutici Italia Srl)
 Menotrophin 75 unit Merional 75unit powder and solvent for solution for injection vials | 10 vial [PoM] £279.00
 Menotrophin 150 unit Merional 150unit powder and solvent for solution for injection vials | 10 vial [PoM] £558.00

Urofollitropin

● **INDICATIONS AND DOSE**
Infertility in women with proven hypopituitarism or who have not responded to clomifene | Superovulation treatment for assisted conception (such as in vitro fertilisation)
▸ BY SUBCUTANEOUS INJECTION, OR BY DEEP INTRAMUSCULAR INJECTION
▸ Adult (female): Adjusted according to response.

● **CONTRA-INDICATIONS** Ovarian cysts (not caused by polycystic ovarian syndrome) · tumours of breast · tumours of hypothalamus · tumours of ovaries · tumours of pituitary · tumours of prostate · tumours of testes · tumours of uterus · vaginal bleeding of unknown cause
● **CAUTIONS** Acute porphyrias p. 1025
● **SIDE-EFFECTS**
▸ **Common or very common** Breast tenderness · constipation · diarrhoea · gastrointestinal discomfort · headache · hot flush · increased risk of infection · muscle spasms · nausea · ovarian hyperstimulation syndrome · pain · pelvic pain · rash · vaginal discharge · vaginal haemorrhage · vomiting
● **PREGNANCY** Avoid.
● **BREAST FEEDING** Avoid.
● **PRESCRIBING AND DISPENSING INFORMATION**
Urofollitropin is purified extract of human post-menopausal urine containing follicle-stimulating hormone (FSH).

- **PATIENT AND CARER ADVICE**
Conception and contraception Patients planning to conceive should be warned that there is a risk of multiple pregnancy.

- **MEDICINAL FORMS**
There can be variation in the licensing of different medicines containing the same drug.
Powder and solvent for solution for injection
  ‣ Bravelle (Ferring Pharmaceuticals Ltd)
  Follicle stimulating hormone human (as Urofollitropin)
  75 unit Bravelle 75unit powder and solvent for solution for injection vials | 10 vial PoM £270.00
  ‣ Fostimon (IBSA Farmaceutici Italia Srl)
  Follicle stimulating hormone human (as Urofollitropin)
  75 unit Fostimon 75unit powder and solvent for solution for injection vials | 10 vial PoM £279.00
  Follicle stimulating hormone human (as Urofollitropin)
  150 unit Fostimon 150unit powder and solvent for solution for injection vials | 10 vial PoM £558.00

7.4   Growth hormone disorders

> **Other drugs used for Growth hormone disorders**
> Pasireotide, p. 925

PITUITARY AND HYPOTHALAMIC HORMONES AND ANALOGUES 〉 GROWTH HORMONE RECEPTOR ANTAGONISTS

Pegvisomant   19-Dec-2017

- **DRUG ACTION** Pegvisomant is a genetically modified analogue of human growth hormone and is a highly selective growth hormone receptor antagonist.

- **INDICATIONS AND DOSE**
Treatment of acromegaly in patients with inadequate response to surgery, radiation, or both, and to treatment with somatostatin analogues (initiated by a specialist)
  ▸ BY SUBCUTANEOUS INJECTION
  ▸ Adult: Initially 80 mg for 1 dose, followed by 10 mg daily, then increased in steps of 5 mg daily, adjusted according to response; maximum 30 mg per day

- **CAUTIONS** Diabetes mellitus (adjustment of antidiabetic therapy may be necessary) · liver disease

- **SIDE-EFFECTS**
  ▸ **Common or very common** Arthralgia · arthritis · asthenia · constipation · diarrhoea · dizziness · drowsiness · dyslipidaemia · dyspnoea · eye pain · fever · gastrointestinal discomfort · gastrointestinal disorders · haemorrhage · headaches · hyperglycaemia · hypertension · hypoglycaemia · influenza like illness · lipohypertrophy · myalgia · nausea · numbness · oedema · skin reactions · sleep disorders · sweat changes · tremor · vomiting · weight increased
  ▸ **Uncommon** Apathy · confusion · dry mouth · eye strain · feeling abnormal · healing impaired · hunger · leucocytosis · leucopenia · libido increased · memory loss · Meniere's disease · oral disorders · panic attack · polyuria · proteinuria · renal impairment · taste altered · thrombocytopenia
  ▸ **Frequency not known** Anger · angioedema · laryngospasm
  SIDE-EFFECTS, FURTHER INFORMATION Rotate injection sites to avoid lipohypertrophy.

- **CONCEPTION AND CONTRACEPTION** Possible increase in female fertility.

- **PREGNANCY** Avoid.

- **BREAST FEEDING** Avoid.

- **MONITORING REQUIREMENTS** Monitor liver enzymes every 4–6 weeks for 6 months or if symptoms of hepatitis develop.

- **NATIONAL FUNDING/ACCESS DECISIONS**
Scottish Medicines Consortium (SMC) Decisions
The *Scottish Medicines Consortium* has advised (November 2017) that pegvisomant (Somavert®) is accepted for use within NHS Scotland for the treatment of patients with acromegaly who have had an inadequate response to surgery and/or radiation therapy and in whom an appropriate medical treatment with somatostatin analogues did not normalise IGF-1 [insulin-like growth factor 1] concentrations or was not tolerated. This advice is contingent upon the continuing availability of the patient access scheme in NHS Scotland or a list price that is equivalent or lower.

All Wales Medicines Strategy Group (AWMSG) Decisions
The *All Wales Medicines Strategy Group* has advised (November 2017) that pegvisomant (Somavert®) is recommended as an option for use within NHS Wales for the treatment of patients with acromegaly who have had an inadequate response to surgery and/or radiation therapy and in whom an appropriate medical treatment with somatostatin analogues did not normalise insulin-like growth factor-1 (IGF-1) concentrations or was not tolerated. This recommendation applies only in circumstances where the approved Wales Patient Access Scheme (WPAS) is utilised or where the list/contract price is equivalent or lower than the WPAS price.

- **MEDICINAL FORMS**
There can be variation in the licensing of different medicines containing the same drug.
Powder and solvent for solution for injection
  ‣ Somavert (Pfizer Ltd)
  Pegvisomant 10 mg Somavert 10mg powder and solvent for solution for injection vials | 30 vial PoM £1,500.00 (Hospital only)
  Pegvisomant 15 mg Somavert 15mg powder and solvent for solution for injection vials | 30 vial PoM £2,250.00 (Hospital only)
  Pegvisomant 20 mg Somavert 20mg powder and solvent for solution for injection vials | 1 vial PoM £100.00 (Hospital only) | 30 vial PoM £3,000.00 (Hospital only)
  Pegvisomant 25 mg Somavert 25mg powder and solvent for solution for injection vials | 30 vial PoM £3,750.00 (Hospital only)
  Pegvisomant 30 mg Somavert 30mg powder and solvent for solution for injection vials | 30 vial PoM £4,500.00 (Hospital only)

PITUITARY AND HYPOTHALAMIC HORMONES AND ANALOGUES 〉 HUMAN GROWTH HORMONES

Somatropin

(Recombinant Human Growth Hormone)

- **INDICATIONS AND DOSE**
Gonadal dysgenesis (Turner syndrome)
  ▸ BY SUBCUTANEOUS INJECTION
  ▸ Adult: 1.4 mg/m^2 daily, alternatively 45–50 micrograms/kg daily
Deficiency of growth hormone
  ▸ BY SUBCUTANEOUS INJECTION
  ▸ Adult: Initially 150–300 micrograms daily, then increased if necessary up to 1 mg daily, dose to be increased gradually, use minimum effective dose (requirements may decrease with age)
  DOSE EQUIVALENCE AND CONVERSION
  ▸ Dose formerly expressed in units; somatropin 1 mg ≡ 3 units.

- **CONTRA-INDICATIONS** Evidence of tumour activity (complete antitumour therapy and ensure intracranial lesions inactive before starting) · not to be used after renal

6

Endocrine system

transplantation · severe obesity in Prader-Willi syndrome · severe respiratory impairment in Prader-Willi syndrome

● CAUTIONS Diabetes mellitus (adjustment of antidiabetic therapy may be necessary) · disorders of the epiphysis of the hip (monitor for limping) · history of malignant disease · hypothyroidism—manufacturers recommend periodic thyroid function tests but limited evidence of clinical value · initiation of treatment close to puberty not recommended in child born small for corrected gestational age · papilloedema · relative deficiencies of other pituitary hormones · resolved intracranial hypertension (monitor closely) · Silver-Russell syndrome

● INTERACTIONS → Appendix 1: somatropin

● SIDE-EFFECTS

▶ **Common or very common** Carpal tunnel syndrome · fluid retention · headache · joint disorders · lipoatrophy · myalgia · paraesthesia

▶ **Uncommon** Gynaecomastia · idiopathic intracranial hypertension

▶ **Rare or very rare** Hyperglycaemia · hyperinsulinism · hypothyroidism · osteonecrosis of femur · pancreatitis · slipped capital femoral epiphysis

▶ **Frequency not known** Leukaemia · musculoskeletal stiffness · oedema

SIDE-EFFECTS, FURTHER INFORMATION Funduscopy for papilloedema recommended if severe or recurrent headache, visual problems, nausea and vomiting occur—if papilloedema confirmed consider benign intracranial hypertension (rare cases reported).

● PREGNANCY Discontinue if pregnancy occurs—no information available.

● BREAST FEEDING No information available. Absorption from milk unlikely.

● DIRECTIONS FOR ADMINISTRATION Rotate subcutaneous injection sites to prevent lipoatrophy.

SAIZEN ® SOLUTION FOR INJECTION For use by subcutaneous injection.

NORDITROPIN ® PREPARATIONS For use by subcutaneous injection.

OMNITROPE ® For use by subcutaneous injection.

NUTROPINAQ ® For use by subcutaneous injection.

HUMATROPE ® Cartridges for use by subcutaneous injection.

Powder for reconstitution for use by subcutaneous or intramuscular injection.

ZOMACTON ® For use by subcutaneous injection.

SAIZEN ® POWDER AND SOLVENT FOR SOLUTION FOR INJECTION For use by subcutaneous injection.

GENOTROPIN ® PREPARATIONS For use by subcutaneous injection.

● PRESCRIBING AND DISPENSING INFORMATION Somatropin is a biological medicine. Biological medicines must be prescribed and dispensed by brand name, see *Biological medicines* and *Biosimilar medicines*, under Guidance on prescribing p. 1.

SAIZEN ® SOLUTION FOR INJECTION For use with *cool.click* ® needle-free autoinjector device or *easypod* ® autoinjector device (non-NHS but available free of charge from clinics).

NORDITROPIN ® PREPARATIONS Cartridges are for use with appropriate *NordiPen* ® device (non-NHS but available free of charge from clinics).

Multidose disposable prefilled pens for use with *NovoFine* ® or *NovoTwist* ® needles.

OMNITROPE ® For use with *Omnitrope Pen 5* ® and *Omnitrope Pen 10* ® devices (non-NHS but available free of charge from clinics).

NUTROPINAQ ® For use with *NutropinAq* ® Pen device (non-NHS but available free of charge from clinics).

ZOMACTON ® 4 mg vial for use with *ZomaJet 2* ® *Vision* needle-free device (non-NHS but available free of charge from clinics) or with needles and syringes.

10 mg vial for use with *ZomaJet Vision X* ® needle-free device (non-NHS but available free of charge from clinics) or with needles and syringes.

SAIZEN ® POWDER AND SOLVENT FOR SOLUTION FOR INJECTION For use with *one. click* ® autoinjector device or *cool.click* ® needle-free autoinjector device or *easypod* ® autoinjector device (non-NHS but available free of charge from clinics).

GENOTROPIN ® PREPARATIONS Cartridges are for use with *Genotropin* ® Pen device (non-NHS but available free of charge from clinics).

● NATIONAL FUNDING/ACCESS DECISIONS

NICE decisions

▶ **Somatropin for the treatment of growth failure in children (May 2010) NICE TA188**
Somatropin is recommended for children with growth failure who:
● have growth-hormone deficiency
● have Turner syndrome
● have Prader-Willi syndrome
● have chronic renal insufficiency
● are born small for gestational age with subsequent growth failure at 4 years of age or later
● have short stature homeobox-containing gene (SHOX) deficiency.
Treatment should be discontinued if growth velocity increases by less than 50% from baseline in the first year of treatment.
www.nice.org.uk/TA188

▶ **Somatropin for adults with growth hormone deficiency (August 2003) NICE TA64**
Somatropin is recommended in adults **only** if the following 3 criteria are fulfilled:
● Severe growth hormone deficiency, established by an appropriate method,
● Impaired quality of life, measured by means of a specific questionnaire,
● Already receiving treatment for another pituitary hormone deficiency.
Somatropin treatment should be discontinued if the quality of life has not improved sufficiently by 9 months.

Severe growth hormone deficiency developing after linear growth is complete but before the age of 25 years should be treated with growth hormone; treatment should continue until adult peak bone mass has been achieved. Treatment for adult-onset growth hormone deficiency should be stopped only when the patient and the patient's physician consider it appropriate.

Treatment with somatropin should be initiated and managed by a physician with expertise in growth hormone disorders; maintenance treatment can be prescribed in the community under a shared-care protocol.
www.nice.org.uk/TA64

● MEDICINAL FORMS
There can be variation in the licensing of different medicines containing the same drug.

Solution for injection
EXCIPIENTS: May contain Benzyl alcohol

▶ Norditropin NordiFlex (Novo Nordisk Ltd)
Somatropin (epr) 3.3 mg per 1 ml Norditropin NordiFlex 5mg/1.5ml solution for injection pre-filled pen | 1 pre-filled disposable injection [PoM] £115.90 [CD4-2]
Somatropin (epr) 6.7 mg per 1 ml Norditropin NordiFlex 10mg/1.5ml solution for injection pre-filled pen | 1 pre-filled disposable injection [PoM] £231.80 [CD4-2]

Somatropin (epr) 10 mg per 1 ml Norditropin NordiFlex 15mg/1.5ml solution for injection pre-filled pen | 1 pre-filled disposable injection [PoM] £347.70 [CD4-2]

▸ Norditropin SimpleXx (Novo Nordisk Ltd)

Somatropin (epr) 3.3 mg per 1 ml Norditropin SimpleXx 5mg/1.5ml solution for injection cartridges | 1 cartridge [PoM] £106.35 DT = £106.35 [CD4-2]

Somatropin (epr) 6.7 mg per 1 ml Norditropin SimpleXx 10mg/1.5ml solution for injection cartridges | 1 cartridge [PoM] £212.70 DT = £212.70 [CD4-2]

Somatropin (epr) 10 mg per 1 ml Norditropin SimpleXx 15mg/1.5ml solution for injection cartridges | 1 cartridge [PoM] £319.05 [CD4-2]

▸ NutropinAq (Ipsen Ltd)

Somatropin (rbe) 5 mg per 1 ml NutropinAq 10mg/2ml solution for injection cartridges | 1 cartridge [PoM] £203.00 [CD4-2] | 3 cartridge [PoM] £609.00 [CD4-2]

▸ Omnitrope SurePal (Sandoz Ltd)

Somatropin (rbe) 3.333 mg per 1 ml Omnitrope SurePal 5 5mg/1.5ml solution for injection cartridges | 5 cartridge [PoM] £368.74 [CD4-2]

Somatropin (rbe) 6.667 mg per 1 ml Omnitrope SurePal 10 10mg/1.5ml solution for injection cartridges | 5 cartridge [PoM] £737.49 [CD4-2]

Somatropin (rbe) 10 mg per 1 ml Omnitrope SurePal 15 15mg/1.5ml solution for injection cartridges | 5 cartridge [PoM] £1,106.22 [CD4-2]

▸ Saizen (Merck Serono Ltd)

Somatropin (rmc) 5.825 mg per 1 ml Saizen 6mg/1.03ml solution for injection cartridges | 1 cartridge [PoM] £139.08 DT = £139.08 [CD4-2]

Somatropin (rmc) 8 mg per 1 ml Saizen 20mg/2.5ml solution for injection cartridges | 1 cartridge [PoM] £463.60 DT = £463.60 [CD4-2] Saizen 12mg/1.5ml solution for injection cartridges | 1 cartridge [PoM] £278.16 DT = £278.16 [CD4-2]

Powder and solvent for solution for injection
EXCIPIENTS: May contain Benzyl alcohol

▸ Genotropin (Pfizer Ltd)

Somatropin (rbe) 5.3 mg Genotropin 5.3mg powder and solvent for solution for injection cartridges | 1 cartridge [PoM] £92.15 DT = £92.15 [CD4-2]

Somatropin (rbe) 12 mg Genotropin 12mg powder and solvent for solution for injection cartridges | 1 cartridge [PoM] £208.65 DT = £208.65 [CD4-2]

▸ Genotropin GoQuick (Pfizer Ltd)

Somatropin (rbe) 5.3 mg Genotropin GoQuick 5.3mg powder and solvent for solution for injection pre-filled disposable devices | 1 pre-filled disposable injection [PoM] £92.15 DT = £92.15 [CD4-2]

Somatropin (rbe) 12 mg Genotropin GoQuick 12mg powder and solvent for solution for injection pre-filled disposable devices | 1 pre-filled disposable injection [PoM] £208.65 [CD4-2]

▸ Genotropin MiniQuick (Pfizer Ltd)

Somatropin (rbe) 200 microgram Genotropin MiniQuick 200microgram powder and solvent for solution for injection pre-filled disposable devices | 7 pre-filled disposable injection [PoM] £24.35 DT = £24.35 [CD4-2]

Somatropin (rbe) 400 microgram Genotropin MiniQuick 400microgram powder and solvent for solution for injection pre-filled disposable devices | 7 pre-filled disposable injection [PoM] £48.68 DT = £48.68 [CD4-2]

Somatropin (rbe) 600 microgram Genotropin MiniQuick 600microgram powder and solvent for solution for injection pre-filled disposable devices | 7 pre-filled disposable injection [PoM] £73.03 DT = £73.03 [CD4-2]

Somatropin (rbe) 800 microgram Genotropin MiniQuick 800microgram powder and solvent for solution for injection pre-filled disposable devices | 7 pre-filled disposable injection [PoM] £97.37 DT = £97.37 [CD4-2]

Somatropin (rbe) 1 mg Genotropin MiniQuick 1mg powder and solvent for solution for injection pre-filled disposable devices | 7 pre-filled disposable injection [PoM] £121.71 DT = £121.71 [CD4-2]

Somatropin (rbe) 1.2 mg Genotropin MiniQuick 1.2mg powder and solvent for solution for injection pre-filled disposable devices | 7 pre-filled disposable injection [PoM] £146.06 DT = £146.06 [CD4-2]

Somatropin (rbe) 1.4 mg Genotropin MiniQuick 1.4mg powder and solvent for solution for injection pre-filled disposable devices | 7 pre-filled disposable injection [PoM] £170.39 DT = £170.39 [CD4-2]

Somatropin (rbe) 1.6 mg Genotropin MiniQuick 1.6mg powder and solvent for solution for injection pre-filled disposable devices | 7 pre-filled disposable injection [PoM] £194.74 DT = £194.74 [CD4-2]

Somatropin (rbe) 1.8 mg Genotropin MiniQuick 1.8mg powder and solvent for solution for injection pre-filled disposable devices | 7 pre-filled disposable injection [PoM] £219.08 DT = £219.08 [CD4-2]

Somatropin (rbe) 2 mg Genotropin MiniQuick 2mg powder and solvent for solution for injection pre-filled disposable devices | 7 pre-filled disposable injection [PoM] £243.42 DT = £243.42 [CD4-2]

▸ Humatrope (Eli Lilly and Company Ltd)

Somatropin (rbe) 6 mg Humatrope 6mg powder and solvent for solution for injection cartridges | 1 cartridge [PoM] £108.00 [CD4-2]

Somatropin (rbe) 12 mg Humatrope 12mg powder and solvent for solution for injection cartridges | 1 cartridge [PoM] £216.00 DT = £208.65 [CD4-2]

Somatropin (rbe) 24 mg Humatrope 24mg powder and solvent for solution for injection cartridges | 1 cartridge [PoM] £432.00 [CD4-2]

▸ Saizen (Merck Serono Ltd)

Somatropin (rmc) 8 mg Saizen 8mg click.easy powder and solvent for solution for injection vials | 1 vial [PoM] £185.44 DT = £185.44 [CD4-2]

▸ Zomacton (Ferring Pharmaceuticals Ltd)

Somatropin (rbe) 4 mg Zomacton 4mg powder and solvent for solution for injection vials | 1 vial [PoM] £68.28 DT = £68.28 [CD4-2]

Somatropin (rbe) 10 mg Zomacton 10mg powder and solvent for solution for injection vials | 1 vial [PoM] £170.70 DT = £170.70 [CD4-2]

8   Sex hormone responsive conditions

Endometriosis

19-Sep-2017

Description of condition

Endometriosis is the growth of endometrial-like tissue outside the uterus. Endometriosis is a condition affecting women mainly of reproductive age and, although its exact cause is unknown, it is an oestrogen-dependent condition and is associated with menstruation. Endometriosis is typically associated with symptoms such as pelvic pain, painful periods and subfertility. Women with endometriosis report pain, which can be frequent, chronic and severe, as well as tiredness, more sick days, and a significant physical, sexual, psychological and social impact. Endometriosis is an important cause of subfertility and this can also have a significant effect on quality of life.

Women may also have endometriosis without symptoms, so it is difficult to know how common the disease is in the population. It is also unclear whether endometriosis is always progressive or can remain stable or improve with time.

Aims of treatment

The aim of treatment is to reduce the severity of symptoms, improve the quality of life, and to improve fertility if this is affected.

Drug treatment

Management options for endometriosis include drug treatment and surgery. Most drug treatments for endometriosis work by suppressing ovarian function and are contraceptive. Surgical treatment aims to remove or destroy endometriotic lesions. The choice of treatment depends on the woman's preferences and priorities in terms of pain management and fertility.

[EvGr] A short trial (such as 3 months) of paracetamol or an NSAID alone or in combination should be considered for first-line management of endometriosis-related pain. If pain relief is inadequate, consider other forms of pain management and referral for further assessment.

Hormonal treatment (with a combined oral contraceptive or a progestogen) should be offered to women with suspected, confirmed or recurrent endometriosis. The patient should be informed that hormonal treatment for endometriosis can reduce pain and has no permanent negative effect on subsequent fertility. If initial hormonal treatment for endometriosis is not effective, not tolerated or is contra-indicated, the woman should be referred to a gynaecologist or specialist endometriosis service for possible further treatment, which could include other hormonal treatments or surgery. Ⓐ For use of drugs to treat neuropathic pain, see Neuropathic pain.

Surgery

EvGr Women with suspected or confirmed endometriosis should be asked about their symptoms, preferences and priorities with respect to pain and fertility, to guide surgical decision-making. For deep endometriosis involving the bowel, bladder or ureter, gonadotropin-releasing hormones given for 3 months before surgery should be considered. Excision rather than ablation should be considered to treat endometriomas, taking into account the woman's desire for fertility and her ovarian reserve. After laparoscopic excision or ablation of endometriosis, consider hormonal treatment (with, for example, a combined hormonal contraceptive), to prolong the benefits of surgery and manage symptoms.

A hysterectomy may be indicated if, for example, the woman has adenomyosis or heavy menstrual bleeding that has not responded to other treatments. Ⓐ

Surgical management if fertility is a priority

EvGr If fertility is a priority, the management of endometriosis-related subfertility should have multidisciplinary involvement with input from a fertility specialist. Women with endometriosis who are trying to conceive should not be offered hormonal treatment, because it does not improve spontaneous pregnancy rates. Ⓐ

Useful Resources

Endometriosis: diagnosis and management. National Institute for Health and Care Excellence. NICE guidance 73. February 2017.
www.nice.org.uk/guidance/ng73

Sex hormones

Oestrogens and HRT

Oestrogens are necessary for the development of female secondary sexual characteristics; they also stimulate myometrial hypertrophy with endometrial hyperplasia.

In terms of oestrogenic activity *natural oestrogens* (estradiol p. 738 (oestradiol), estrone (oestrone), and estriol p. 813 (oestriol)) have a more appropriate profile for hormone replacement therapy (HRT) than *synthetic oestrogens* (ethinylestradiol p. 742 (ethinyloestradiol) and mestranol). Tibolone p. 743 has oestrogenic, progestogenic and weak androgenic activity.

Oestrogen therapy is given cyclically or continuously for a number of gynaecological conditions. If long-term therapy is required in women with a uterus, a progestogen should normally be added to reduce the risk of cystic hyperplasia of the endometrium (or of endometriotic foci in women who have had a hysterectomy) and possible transformation to cancer.

Oestrogens are no longer used to suppress lactation because of their association with thromboembolism.

Hormone replacement therapy

Hormone replacement therapy (HRT) with small doses of an oestrogen (together with a progestogen in women with a uterus) is appropriate for alleviating menopausal symptoms such as vaginal atrophy or vasomotor instability. Oestrogen given systemically in the perimenopausal and postmenopausal period or tibolone given in the postmenopausal period also diminish postmenopausal osteoporosis but other drugs are preferred. Menopausal

atrophic vaginitis may respond to a short course of a topical vaginal oestrogen preparation used for a few weeks and repeated if necessary.

Systemic therapy with an oestrogen or drugs with oestrogenic properties alleviates the symptoms of oestrogen deficiency such as vasomotor symptoms. Tibolone combines oestrogenic and progestogenic activity with weak androgenic activity; it is given continuously, without cyclical progestogen.

HRT may be used in women with early natural or surgical menopause (before age 45 years), since they are at high risk of osteoporosis. For early menopause, HRT can be given until the approximate age of natural menopause (i.e. until age 50 years). Alternatives to HRT should be considered if osteoporosis is the main concern.

Clonidine hydrochloride p. 144 may be used to reduce vasomotor symptoms in women who cannot take an oestrogen, but clonidine hydrochloride may cause unacceptable side-effects.

HRT increases the risk of venous thromboembolism, stroke, endometrial cancer (reduced by a progestogen), breast cancer, and ovarian cancer; there is an increased risk of coronary heart disease in women who start combined HRT more than 10 years after menopause. For details of these risks see HRT Risk table.

The minimum effective dose of HRT should be used for the shortest duration. Treatment should be reviewed at least annually and for osteoporosis alternative treatments considered. HRT does not prevent coronary heart disease or protect against a decline in cognitive function and it should not be prescribed for these purposes. Experience of treating women over 65 years with HRT is limited.

For the treatment of menopausal symptoms the benefits of short-term HRT outweigh the risks in the majority of women, especially in those aged under 60 years.

Risk of breast cancer

It is estimated that using all types of HRT, including tibolone, increases the risk of breast cancer within 1–2 years of initiating treatment. The increased risk is related to the duration of HRT use (but not to the age at which HRT is started) and this excess risk disappears within 5 years of stopping. Radiological detection of breast cancer can be made more difficult as mammographic density can increase with HRT use; tibolone has only a limited effect on mammographic density.

Risk of endometrial cancer

The increased risk of endometrial cancer depends on the dose and duration of oestrogen-only HRT. In women with a uterus, the addition of a progestogen cyclically (for at least 10 days per 28-day cycle) reduces the additional risk of endometrial cancer; this additional risk is eliminated if a progestogen is given continuously. However, this should be weighed against the increased risk of breast cancer.

Risk of ovarian cancer

Long-term use of combined HRT or oestrogen-only HRT is associated with a small increased risk of ovarian cancer; this excess risk disappears within a few years of stopping.

Risk of venous thromboembolism

Women using combined or oestrogen-only HRT are at an increased risk of deep vein thrombosis and of pulmonary embolism especially in the first year of use. In women who have predisposing factors (such as a personal or family history of deep vein thrombosis or pulmonary embolism, severe varicose veins, obesity, trauma, or prolonged bed-rest) it is prudent to review the need for HRT, as in some cases the risks of HRT may exceed the benefits. Travel involving prolonged immobility further increases the risk of deep vein thrombosis.

HRT Risks

Risk	Age range (years)	Background incidence per 1000 women in Europe not using HRT		Additional cases per 1000 women using oestrogen only HRT (estimated)		Additional cases per 1000 women using combined (oestrogen-progesterone) HRT (estimated)	
		Over 5 years	Over 10 years	For 5 years' use	For 10 years' use	For 5 years' use	For 10 years' use
Breast cancer[1]	50–59	10	20	2	6	6	24
	60–69	15	30	3	9	9	36
Endometrial cancer[2,3]	50–59	2	4	4	32	NS	NS
	60–69	3	6	6	48	NS	NS
Ovarian cancer	50–59	2	4	<1	1	<1	1
	60–69	3	6	<1	2	<1	2
Venous thromboembolism[4,5]	50–59	5	–	2	–	7	–
	60–69	8	–	2	–	10	–
Stroke[6]	50–59	4	–	1	–	1	–
	60–69	9	–	3	–	3	–
Coronary heart disease[7,8]	70–79	29–44	–	NS	–	15	–

Where background incidence or additional cases have not been included in the table, this indicates a lack of available data. NS indicates a non-significant difference. Taken from MHRA/CHM (*Drug Safety* 2007; 1 (2): 2-6) available at www.gov.uk/drug-safety-update

1 Tibolone increases the risk of breast cancer but to a lesser extent than with combined HRT.

2 Evidence suggests an increased risk of endometrial cancer with tibolone. After 2.7 years of use (in women of average age 68 years), 1 extra case of endometrial hyperplasia and 4 extra cases of endometrial cancer were diagnosed compared with placebo users.

3 The risk of endometrial cancer cannot be reliably estimated in those using combined HRT because the addition of progestogen for at least 10 days per 28-day cycle greatly reduces the additional risk, and addition of a daily progestogen eliminates the additional risk. The risk of endometrial cancer in women who have not used HRT increases with body mass index (BMI); the increased risk of endometrial cancer in users of oestrogen-only HRT or tibolone is more apparent in women who are not overweight.

4 Limited data does not suggest an increased risk of thromboembolism with tibolone compared with combined HRT or women not taking HRT.

5 Although the level of risk of thromboembolism associated with non-oral routes of administration of HRT has not been established, it may be lower for the transdermal route.

6 Tibolone increases the risk of stroke about 2.2 times from the first year of treatment; risk of stroke is age-dependent and therefore the absolute risk of stroke with tibolone increases with age.

7 Increased risk of coronary heart disease in women who start combined HRT more than 10 years after menopause.

8 There is insufficient data to draw a conclusion on the risk of coronary heart disease with tibolone.

Risk of stroke
Risk of stroke increases with age, therefore older women have a greater absolute risk of stroke. Combined HRT or oestrogen-only HRT slightly increases the risk of stroke. Tibolone increases the risk of stroke about 2.2 times from the first year of treatment.

Risk of coronary heart disease
HRT does not prevent coronary heart disease and should not be prescribed for this purpose. There is an increased risk of coronary heart disease in women who start combined HRT more than 10 years after menopause. Although very little information is available on the risk of coronary heart disease in younger women who start HRT close to the menopause, studies suggest a lower relative risk compared with older women.

Choice
The choice of HRT for an individual depends on an overall balance of indication, risk, and convenience. A woman with a uterus normally requires oestrogen with cyclical progestogen for the last 12 to 14 days of the cycle or a preparation which involves continuous administration of an oestrogen and a progestogen (or one which provides both oestrogenic and progestogenic activity in a single preparation). Continuous combined preparations or tibolone are **not suitable** for use in the perimenopause or within 12 months of the last menstrual period; women who use such preparations may bleed irregularly in the early stages of treatment—if bleeding continues endometrial abnormality should be ruled out and consideration given to changing to cyclical HRT.

An oestrogen alone is suitable for continuous use in women without a uterus. However, in endometriosis, endometrial foci may remain despite hysterectomy and the addition of a progestogen should be considered in these circumstances.

An oestrogen may be given by mouth or by transdermal administration, which avoids first-pass metabolism.

Surgery
Major surgery under general anaesthesia, including orthopaedic and vascular leg surgery, is a predisposing factor for venous thromboembolism and it may be prudent to stop HRT 4–6 weeks before surgery; it should be restarted only after full mobilisation. If HRT is continued or if discontinuation is not possible (e.g. in non-elective surgery), prophylaxis with unfractionated or low molecular weight heparin and graduated compression hosiery is advised.

Reasons to stop HRT
Hormone replacement therapy should be stopped (pending investigation and treatment), if any of the following occur:

* sudden severe chest pain (even if not radiating to left arm);
* sudden breathlessness (or cough with blood-stained sputum);
* unexplained swelling or severe pain in calf of one leg;
* severe stomach pain;
* serious neurological effects including unusual severe, prolonged headache especially if first time or getting progressively worse or sudden partial or complete loss of vision or sudden disturbance of hearing or other perceptual disorders or dysphasia or bad fainting attack or collapse or first unexplained epileptic seizure or weakness,

6

Endocrine system

motor disturbances, very marked numbness suddenly affecting one side or one part of body;
- hepatitis, jaundice, liver enlargement;
- blood pressure above systolic 160 mmHg or diastolic 95 mmHg;
- prolonged immobility after surgery or leg injury;
- detection of a risk factor which contra-indicates treatment

Ethinylestradiol

Ethinylestradiol p. 742 (ethinyloestradiol) is licensed for short-term treatment of symptoms of oestrogen deficiency, for osteoporosis prophylaxis if other drugs cannot be used and for the treatment of female hypogonadism and menstrual disorders.

Ethinylestradiol is occasionally used under **specialist supervision** for the management of *hereditary haemorrhagic telangiectasia* (but evidence of benefit is limited). It is also used licensed for the palliative treatment of prostate cancer.

Raloxifene

Raloxifene hydrochloride below is licensed for the treatment and prevention of *postmenopausal osteoporosis*; unlike hormone replacement therapy, raloxifene hydrochloride does not reduce menopausal vasomotor symptoms.

Progestogens and progesterone receptor modulators

There are two main groups of progestogen, progesterone and its analogues (dydrogesterone and medroxyprogesterone acetate p. 791) and testosterone analogues (norethisterone p. 747 and norgestrel). The newer progestogens (desogestrel p. 786, norgestimate, and gestodene) are all derivatives of norgestrel; levonorgestrel p. 787 is the active isomer of norgestrel and has twice its potency. Progesterone p. 748 and its analogues are less androgenic than the testosterone derivatives and neither progesterone nor dydrogesterone causes virilisation.

Where endometriosis requires drug treatment, it may respond to a progestogen, e.g. norethisterone, administered on a continuous basis. Danazol p. 725 and gonadorelin analogues are also available.

Although oral progestogens have been used widely for menorrhagia they are relatively ineffective compared with tranexamic acid p. 110 or, particularly where dysmenorrhoea is also a factor, mefenamic acid p. 1111; the levonorgestrel-releasing intra-uterine system may be particularly useful for women also requiring contraception. Oral progestogens have also been used for severe dysmenorrhoea, but where contraception is also required in younger women the best choice is a combined oral contraceptive.

Progestogens have also been advocated for the alleviation of premenstrual symptoms, but no convincing physiological basis for such treatment has been shown.

Progestogens have been used for the prevention of miscarriage in women with a history of recurrent miscarriage but there is no evidence of benefit and they are **not** recommended for this purpose. In pregnant women with antiphospholipid antibody syndrome who have suffered recurrent miscarriage, administration of low-dose aspirin p. 121 and a prophylactic dose of a low molecular weight heparin may decrease the risk of fetal loss (use under specialist supervision only).

Hormone replacement therapy

In women with a uterus a progestogen needs to be added to long-term oestrogen therapy for hormone replacement, to prevent cystic hyperplasia of the endometrium and possible transformation to cancer; it can be added on a cyclical or a continuous basis. Combined packs incorporating suitable progestogen tablets are available.

Oral contraception

Desogestrel, gestodene, levonorgestrel, norethisterone, and norgestimate are used in combined oral contraceptives and in progestogen-only contraceptives.

Cancer

Progestogens also have a role in neoplastic disease.

Progesterone receptor modulators

Ulipristal acetate p. 785 is a progesterone receptor modulator with a partial progesterone antagonist effect. Ulipristal acetate is used in the pre-operative treatment of moderate to severe symptoms of uterine fibroids; it is also used as an hormonal emergency contraceptive.

Heavy menstrual bleeding

EvGr Ulipristal acetate (up to four courses) is recommended in patients with heavy menstrual bleeding associated with uterine fibroids of a diameter of 3 cm or more, and a haemoglobin level of 102 g/litre or below; ulipristal acetate may also be considered if the haemoglobin level is greater than 102 g/litre. A

8.1 Female sex hormone responsive conditions

CALCIUM REGULATING DRUGS > BONE RESORPTION INHIBITORS

Raloxifene hydrochloride

28-Sep-2017

- **INDICATIONS AND DOSE**

Treatment and prevention of postmenopausal osteoporosis
▶ BY MOUTH
- Adult: 60 mg once daily

Breast cancer [chemoprevention in postmenopausal women at moderate to high risk] (initiated under specialist supervision)
▶ BY MOUTH
- Adult: 60 mg once daily for 5 years

- UNLICENSED USE Not licensed for chemoprevention of breast cancer in the UK. Licensed for this indication in USA.

- CONTRA-INDICATIONS Cholestasis · endometrial cancer · history of venous thromboembolism · undiagnosed uterine bleeding

- CAUTIONS Avoid in Acute porphyrias p. 1025 · breast cancer (manufacturer advises avoid during treatment for breast cancer) · history of oestrogen-induced hypertriglyceridaemia (monitor serum triglycerides) · risk factors for stroke · risk factors for venous thromboembolism (discontinue if prolonged immobilisation)

- INTERACTIONS → Appendix 1: raloxifene

- SIDE-EFFECTS
  ▶ Common or very common Influenza · leg cramps · peripheral oedema · vasodilation
  ▶ Uncommon Embolism and thrombosis
  ▶ Rare or very rare Breast abnormalities · gastrointestinal discomfort · gastrointestinal disorder · headaches · nausea · rash · thrombocytopenia · vomiting

- HEPATIC IMPAIRMENT Avoid.

- RENAL IMPAIRMENT Caution in mild to moderate impairment. Avoid in severe impairment.

● NATIONAL FUNDING/ACCESS DECISIONS

NICE decisions

▶ Raloxifene for the primary prevention of osteoporotic fragility fractures in postmenopausal women (updated February 2018) NICE TA160

Raloxifene is **not** recommended as a treatment option for the primary prevention of osteoporotic fragility fractures in postmenopausal women.

Women who are currently receiving treatment, but for whom treatment would not have been recommended, should have the option to continue treatment until they and their NHS clinician consider it appropriate to stop. www.nice.org.uk/guidance/ta160

▶ Raloxifene and teriparatide for the secondary prevention of osteoporotic fragility fractures in postmenopausal women (updated February 2018) NICE TA161

Raloxifene is recommended as an alternative treatment option for the secondary prevention of osteoporotic fragility fractures in postmenopausal women:

- who are unable to comply with the special instructions for the administration of alendronate and risedronate, or have a contra-indication to or are intolerant of alendronate and risedronate, **and**
- have a combination of T-score, age and number of independent clinical risk factors for fracture, as indicated in the full NICE guidance.

Women who are currently receiving treatment, but for whom treatment would not have been recommended, should have the option to continue treatment until they and their NHS clinician consider it appropriate to stop. www.nice.org.uk/guidance/ta161

● MEDICINAL FORMS

There can be variation in the licensing of different medicines containing the same drug.

Tablet

▶ Raloxifene hydrochloride (Non-proprietary)
  Raloxifene hydrochloride 60 mg Raloxifene 60mg tablets |
  28 tablet [PoM] £17.06 DT = £3.42 | 84 tablet [PoM] £11.10–£56.61
▶ Evirex (Somex Pharma)
  Raloxifene hydrochloride 60 mg Evirex 60mg tablets |
  28 tablet [PoM] £5.10 DT = £3.42
▶ Evista (Daiichi Sankyo UK Ltd)
  Raloxifene hydrochloride 60 mg Evista 60mg tablets |
  28 tablet [PoM] £17.06 DT = £3.42
▶ Ostiral (Lupin Healthcare (UK) Ltd)
  Raloxifene hydrochloride 60 mg Ostiral 60mg tablets |
  28 tablet [PoM] £14.50 DT = £3.42
▶ Razylan (Aspire Pharma Ltd)
  Raloxifene hydrochloride 60 mg Razylan 60mg tablets |
  28 tablet [PoM] £17.06 DT = £3.42

OESTROGENS

Conjugated oestrogens (equine)

10-May-2018

● INDICATIONS AND DOSE

PREMARIN ® TABLETS

Menopausal symptoms
▶ BY MOUTH
  ▶ Adult: 0.3–1.25 mg daily continuously; with cyclical progestogen for 12–14 days of each cycle in women with a uterus

Postmenopausal osteoporosis prophylaxis
▶ BY MOUTH
  ▶ Adult: 0.625–1.25 mg daily continuously; with cyclical progestogen for 12–14 days of each cycle in women with a uterus

● CONTRA-INDICATIONS Active arterial thromboembolic disease (e.g. angina or myocardial infarction) · active thrombophlebitis · Dubin-Johnson syndromes (or monitor

closely) · history of breast cancer · history of recurrent venous thromboembolism (unless already on anticoagulant treatment) · liver disease (where liver function tests have failed to return to normal) · oestrogen-dependent cancer · recent arterial thromboembolic disease (e.g. angina or myocardial infarction) · Rotor syndromes (or monitor closely) · thrombophilic disorder · undiagnosed vaginal bleeding · untreated endometrial hyperplasia · venous thromboembolism

● CAUTIONS Acute porphyrias p. 1025 · diabetes (increased risk of heart disease) · factors predisposing to thromboembolism · history of breast nodules (closely monitor breast status—risk of breast cancer) · history of endometrial hyperplasia · history of fibrocystic disease (closely monitor breast status—risk of breast cancer) · hypophyseal tumours · increased risk of gall-bladder disease reported · migraine · migraine-like headaches · presence of antiphospholipid antibodies (increased risk of thrombotic events) · risk factors for oestrogen-dependent tumours (e.g. breast cancer in first-degree relative) · risk of breast cancer

CAUTIONS, FURTHER INFORMATION

▶ Risk of breast cancer It is estimated that using *all* types of HRT, including tibolone, increases the risk of breast cancer within 1–2 years of initiating treatment. The increased risk is related to the duration of HRT use (but not to the age at which HRT is started) and this excess risk disappears within 5 years of stopping.

Radiological detection of breast cancer can be made more difficult as mammographic density can increase with HRT use.

▶ Risk of endometrial cancer The increased risk of endometrial cancer depends on the dose and duration of oestrogen-only HRT.

In women with a uterus, the addition of a progestogen cyclically (for at least 10 days per 28-day cycle) reduces the additional risk of endometrial cancer; this additional risk is eliminated if a progestogen is given continuously. However, this should be weighed against the increased risk of breast cancer.

▶ Risk of ovarian cancer Long-term use of combined HRT or oestrogen-only HRT is associated with a small increased risk of ovarian cancer. This excess risk disappears within a few years of stopping.

▶ Risk of venous thromboembolism Women using combined or oestrogen-only HRT are at an increased risk of deep vein thrombosis and of pulmonary embolism especially in the first year of use.

In *women who have predisposing factors* (such as a personal or family history of deep vein thrombosis or pulmonary embolism, severe varicose veins, obesity, trauma, or prolonged bed-rest) it is prudent to review the need for HRT, as in some cases the risks of HRT may exceed the benefits.

Travel involving prolonged immobility further increases the risk of deep vein thrombosis.

▶ Risk of stroke Risk of stroke increases with age, therefore older women have a greater absolute risk of stroke. Combined HRT or oestrogen-only HRT slightly increases the risk of stroke.

▶ Risk of coronary heart disease HRT does not prevent coronary heart disease and should not be prescribed for this purpose. There is an increased risk of coronary heart disease in women who start combined HRT more than 10 years after menopause. Although very little information is available on the risk of coronary heart disease in younger women who start HRT close to the menopause, studies suggest a lower relative risk compared with older women.

▶ Other conditions The product literature advises caution in other conditions including hypertension, renal disease, asthma, epilepsy, sickle-cell disease, melanoma,

6

Endocrine system

otosclerosis, multiple sclerosis, and systemic lupus erythematosus (but care required if antiphospholipid antibodies present). Evidence for caution in these conditions is unsatisfactory and many women with these conditions may stand to benefit from HRT.

- INTERACTIONS → Appendix 1: hormone replacement therapy
- SIDE-EFFECTS
  ▸ **Common or very common** Alopecia · arthralgia · breast abnormalities · depression · leg cramps · menstrual cycle irregularities · vaginal discharge · weight changes
  ▸ **Uncommon** Anxiety · cervical abnormalities · contact lens intolerance · dizziness · embolism and thrombosis · gallbladder disorder · gastrointestinal discomfort · headaches · hirsutism · libido disorder · mood altered · nausea · oedema · skin reactions · vulvovaginal candidiasis
  ▸ **Rare or very rare** Angioedema · asthma exacerbated · cerebrovascular insufficiency · chorea exacerbated · colitis ischaemic · epilepsy exacerbated · galactorrhoea · glucose tolerance impaired · hypocalcaemia · jaundice cholestatic · myocardial infarction · neoplasms · pancreatitis · pelvic pain · vomiting
  ▸ **Frequency not known** Endometrial hyperplasia · erythema nodosum

  SIDE-EFFECTS, FURTHER INFORMATION Cyclical HRT (where a progestogen is taken for 12–14 days of each 28-day oestrogen treatment cycle) usually results in regular withdrawal bleeding towards the end of the progestogen. Continuous combined HRT commonly produces irregular breakthrough bleeding in the first 4–6 months of treatment. Bleeding beyond 6 months or after a spell of amenorrhoea requires further investigation to exclude serious gynaecological pathology.

- CONCEPTION AND CONTRACEPTION HRT does **not** provide contraception and a woman is considered potentially fertile for 2 years after her last menstrual period if she is under 50 years, and for 1 year if she is over 50 years. A woman who is under 50 years and free of all risk factors for venous and arterial disease can use a low-oestrogen combined oral contraceptive pill to provide both relief of menopausal symptoms and contraception; it is recommended that the oral contraceptive be stopped at 50 years of age since there are more suitable alternatives. If any potentially fertile woman needs HRT, non-hormonal contraceptive measures (such as condoms) are necessary. Measurement of follicle-stimulating hormone can help to determine fertility, but high measurements alone (particularly in women aged under 50 years) do not necessarily preclude the possibility of becoming pregnant.

- PREGNANCY Manufacturer advises avoid—not indicated during pregnancy.

- BREAST FEEDING Avoid until weaning or for 6 months after birth (adverse effects on lactation).

- HEPATIC IMPAIRMENT Avoid in active liver disease including disorders of hepatic excretion (e.g. Dubin-Johnson or Rotor syndromes), infective hepatitis (until liver function returns to normal), and liver tumours.

- MEDICINAL FORMS
  There can be variation in the licensing of different medicines containing the same drug.
  Tablet
  ▸ Premarin (Pfizer Ltd)
  Conjugated oestrogens 300 microgram Premarin 0.3mg tablets | 84 tablet [PoM] £6.07 DT = £6.07
  Conjugated oestrogens 625 microgram Premarin 0.625mg tablets | 84 tablet [PoM] £4.02 DT = £4.02
  Conjugated oestrogens 1.25 mg Premarin 1.25mg tablets | 84 tablet [PoM] £3.58 DT = £3.58

  Combinations available: *Conjugated oestrogens with medroxyprogesterone*, p. 743

Conjugated oestrogens with bazedoxifene acetate

28-Mar-2017

The properties listed below are those particular to the combination only. For the properties of the components please consider, conjugated oestrogens (equine) p. 737.

- INDICATIONS AND DOSE
  Menopausal symptoms (in women with at least 12 months since last menses for whom treatment with progestogen-containing therapy is not appropriate)
  ▸ BY MOUTH
  ▸ Adult: 0.45/20 mg daily continuously
  DOSE EQUIVALENCE AND CONVERSION
  ▸ Dose expressed as x/y mg conjugated oestrogens/bazedoxifene.

- INTERACTIONS → Appendix 1: hormone replacement therapy
- SIDE-EFFECTS
  ▸ **Common or very common** Abdominal pain · constipation · diarrhoea · drowsiness · dry mouth · hot flush · muscle complaints · nausea · peripheral oedema · skin reactions · vulvovaginal candidiasis
  ▸ **Uncommon** Cholecystitis
  ▸ **Rare or very rare** Embolism and thrombosis
  ▸ **Frequency not known** Dry eye · eye disorders · eye inflammation · eye pain · palpitations · vision disorders

- MEDICINAL FORMS
  There can be variation in the licensing of different medicines containing the same drug.
  Modified-release tablet
  CAUTIONARY AND ADVISORY LABELS 3, 25
  ▸ Duavive (Pfizer Ltd)
  Conjugated oestrogens 450 microgram, Bazedoxifene (as Bazedoxifene acetate) 20 mg Duavive 0.45mg/20mg modified-release tablets | 28 tablet [PoM] £15.00 DT = £15.00

Estradiol

- INDICATIONS AND DOSE
  BEDOL ®
  Menopausal symptoms | Osteoporosis prophylaxis
  ▸ BY MOUTH
  ▸ Adult: 2 mg daily, started on day 1–5 of menstruation (or at any time if cycles have ceased or are infrequent), to be taken with cyclical progestogen for 12–14 days of each cycle in women with a uterus

  CLIMAVAL ®
  Menopausal symptoms (if patient has had a hysterectomy)
  ▸ BY MOUTH
  ▸ Adult: 1–2 mg daily

  ELLESTE SOLO ® MX
  Menopausal symptoms
  ▸ BY TRANSDERMAL APPLICATION
  ▸ Adult: Apply 1 patch twice weekly continuously, started within 5 days of onset of menstruation (or at any time if cycles have ceased or are infrequent), to be used with cyclical progestogen for 12–14 days of each cycle in women with a uterus, initiate therapy with *MX* 40, subsequently adjust according to response

  Osteoporosis prophylaxis
  ▸ BY TRANSDERMAL APPLICATION
  ▸ Adult: Apply 1 patch twice weekly continuously, started within 5 days of onset of menstruation (or at any time if cycles have ceased or are infrequent), to be used with cyclical progestogen for 12–14 days of each

cycle in women with a uterus, initiate therapy with *MX* 80, subsequently adjust according to response

ELLESTE-SOLO ® 1-MG

Menopausal symptoms

▶ BY MOUTH
▶ Adult: 1 mg daily, starting on day 1 of menstruation (or at any time if cycles have ceased or are infrequent), to be taken with cyclical progestogen for 12–14 days of each cycle in women with a uterus

ELLESTE-SOLO ® 2-MG

Menopausal symptoms not controlled with lower strength | Osteoporosis prophylaxis

▶ BY MOUTH
▶ Adult: 2 mg daily, started on day 1 of menstruation (or at any time if cycles have ceased or are infrequent), to be given with cyclical progestogen for 12–14 days of each cycle in women with a uterus

ESTRADERM MX ®

Menopausal symptoms

▶ BY TRANSDERMAL APPLICATION
▶ Adult: Apply 1 patch twice weekly continuously, started within 5 days of onset of menstruation (or at any time if cycles have ceased or are infrequent), to be used with cyclical progestogen for at least 12 days of each cycle in women with a uterus, initiate therapy with *MX*25 for first 3 months; subsequently adjust according to response

Osteoporosis prophylaxis

▶ BY TRANSDERMAL APPLICATION
▶ Adult: Apply 1 patch twice weekly continuously, started within 5 days of onset of menstruation (or at any time if cycles have ceased or are infrequent), to be used with cyclical progestogen for at least 12 days of each cycle in women with a uterus, initiate therapy with *MX*50; subsequently adjust according to response

ESTRADOT ®

Menopausal symptoms

▶ BY TRANSDERMAL APPLICATION
▶ Adult: Apply 1 patch twice weekly continuously, to be used with cyclical progestogen for 12–14 days of each cycle in women with a uterus, initiate therapy with 25 *patch* for 3 months; subsequently adjust according to response

Osteoporosis prophylaxis

▶ BY TRANSDERMAL APPLICATION
▶ Adult: Apply 1 patch twice weekly continuously, to be used with cyclical progestogen for 12–14 days of each cycle in women with a uterus, initiate therapy with 50 *patch*; subsequently adjust according to response

EVOREL ®

Menopausal symptoms | Osteoporosis prophylaxis

▶ BY TRANSDERMAL APPLICATION
▶ Adult: Apply 1 patch twice weekly continuously, started within 5 days of onset of menstruation (or at any time if cycles have ceased or are infrequent), to be used with cyclical progestogen for 12–14 days of each cycle in women with a uterus, therapy should be initiated with *Evorel* 50 patch; subsequently adjust according to response; dose may be reduced to *Evorel* 25 patch after first month if necessary for menopausal symptoms **only**

FEMSEVEN ®

Menopausal symptoms | Osteoporosis prophylaxis

▶ BY TRANSDERMAL APPLICATION
▶ Adult: Apply 1 patch once weekly continuously, to be used with cyclical progestogen for 12–14 days of each cycle in women with a uterus, initiate therapy with *FemSeven* 50 patches for the first few months, subsequently adjust according to response

OESTROGEL ®

Menopausal symptoms

▶ TO THE SKIN
▶ Adult: Apply 1.5 mg once daily continuously, increased if necessary up to 3 mg after 1 month continuously, to be applied over an area twice that of the template provided, starting within 5 days of menstruation (or anytime if cycles have ceased or are infrequent), to be used with cyclical progestogen for at least 12 days of each cycle in women with a uterus

Osteoporosis prophylaxis

▶ TO THE SKIN
▶ Adult: Apply 1.5 mg once daily continuously, to be applied over an area twice that of the template provided, starting within 5 days of menstruation (or anytime if cycles have ceased or are infrequent), to be used with cyclical progestogen for at least 12 days of each cycle in women with a uterus

DOSE EQUIVALENCE AND CONVERSION
▶ For *Oestrogel*®: 2 measures is equivalent to estradiol 1.5 mg.

PROGYNOVA ®

Menopausal symptoms

▶ BY MOUTH
▶ Adult: 1–2 mg daily continuously, to be started on day 1 of menstruation (or at any time if cycles have ceased or are infrequent), to be taken with cyclical progestogen for 12–14 days of each cycle in women with a uterus

Osteoporosis prophylaxis

▶ BY MOUTH
▶ Adult: 2 mg daily continuously, to be taken with cyclical progestogen for 12–14 days of each cycle in women with a uterus

PROGYNOVA ® TS

Menopausal symptoms | Osteoporosis prophylaxis

▶ BY TRANSDERMAL APPLICATION
▶ Adult: Apply 1 patch once weekly continuously, alternatively apply 1 patch once weekly for 3 weeks, followed by a 7-day patch-free interval (cyclical), to be used with cyclical progestogen for 12–14 days of each cycle in women with a uterus, initiate therapy with *Progynova TS* 50, subsequently adjust according to response, women receiving *Progynova TS* 100 patches for menopausal symptoms may continue with this strength for osteoporosis prophylaxis

SANDRENA ®

Menopausal symptoms

▶ TO THE SKIN
▶ Adult: Apply 1 mg once daily, to be applied over area 1–2 times size of hand; with cyclical progestogen for 12–14 days of each cycle in women with a uterus, dose may be adjusted after 2–3 cycles to lowest effective dose; usual dose 0.5–1.5 mg daily

ZUMENON ®

Menopausal symptoms

▶ BY MOUTH
▶ Adult: Initially 1 mg daily, to be started within 5 days of onset of menstruation (or any time if cycles have ceased or are infrequent), increased if necessary to 2 mg daily, to be taken with a cyclical progestogen for 12–14 days of each cycle in women with a uterus

Osteoporosis prophylaxis

▶ BY MOUTH
▶ Adult: 2 mg daily, to be taken with a cyclical progestogen for 12–14 days of each cycle in women with a uterus

● CONTRA-INDICATIONS Active arterial thromboembolic disease (e.g. angina or myocardial infarction) · active thrombophlebitis · Dubin-Johnson syndrome (or monitor closely) · history of breast cancer · history of recurrent venous thromboembolism (unless already on anticoagulant treatment) · oestrogen-dependent cancer · recent arterial thromboembolic disease (e.g. angina or myocardial infarction) · Rotor syndrome (or monitor closely) · thrombophilic disorder · undiagnosed vaginal bleeding · untreated endometrial hyperplasia · venous thromboembolism

● CAUTIONS Acute porphyrias p. 1025 · diabetes (increased risk of heart disease) · history of breast nodules—closely monitor breast status (risk of breast cancer) · history of endometrial hyperplasia · factors predisposing to thromboembolism · history of fibrocystic disease—closely monitor breast status (risk of breast cancer) · hypophyseal tumours · increased risk of gall-bladder disease · migraine (or migraine-like headaches) · presence of antiphospholipid antibodies (increased risk of thrombotic events) · prolonged exposure to unopposed oestrogens may increase risk of developing endometrial cancer · risk factors for oestrogen-dependent tumours (e.g. breast cancer in first-degree relative) · symptoms of endometriosis may be exacerbated · uterine fibroids may increase in size

CAUTIONS, FURTHER INFORMATION
▸ Risk of breast cancer It is estimated that using *all* types of HRT increases the risk of breast cancer within 1–2 years of initiating treatment. The increased risk is related to the duration of HRT use (but not to the age at which HRT is started) and this excess risk disappears within 5 years of stopping.

Radiological detection of breast cancer can be made more difficult as mammographic density can increase with HRT use.
▸ Risk of endometrial cancer The increased risk of endometrial cancer depends on the dose and duration of oestrogen-only HRT.

In women with a uterus, the addition of a progestogen cyclically (for at least 10 days per 28-day cycle) reduces the additional risk of endometrial cancer; this additional risk is eliminated if a progestogen is given continuously. However, this should be weighed against the increased risk of breast cancer.
▸ Risk of ovarian cancer Long-term use of combined HRT or oestrogen-only HRT is associated with a small increased risk of ovarian cancer. This excess risk disappears within a few years of stopping.
▸ Risk of venous thromboembolism Women using combined or oestrogen-only HRT are at an increased risk of deep vein thrombosis and of pulmonary embolism especially in the first year of use.

In *women who have predisposing factors* (such as a personal or family history of deep vein thrombosis or pulmonary embolism, severe varicose veins, obesity, trauma, or prolonged bed-rest) it is prudent to review the need for HRT, as in some cases the risks of HRT may exceed the benefits.

Travel involving prolonged immobility further increases the risk of deep vein thrombosis.
▸ Risk of stroke Risk of stroke increases with age, therefore older women have a greater absolute risk of stroke. Combined HRT or oestrogen-only HRT slightly increases the risk of stroke.
▸ Risk of coronary heart disease HRT does not prevent coronary heart disease and should not be prescribed for this purpose. There is an increased risk of coronary heart disease in women who start combined HRT more than 10 years after menopause. Although very little information is available on the risk of coronary heart disease in younger women who start HRT close to the menopause,

studies suggest a lower relative risk compared with older women.
▸ Other conditions The product literature advises caution in other conditions including hypertension, renal disease, asthma, epilepsy, sickle-cell disease, melanoma, otosclerosis, multiple sclerosis, and systemic lupus erythematosus (but care required if antiphospholipid antibodies present). Evidence for caution in these conditions is unsatisfactory and many women with these conditions may stand to benefit from HRT.

● INTERACTIONS → Appendix 1: hormone replacement therapy

● SIDE-EFFECTS
GENERAL SIDE-EFFECTS
▸ Common or very common Headaches · nausea · skin reactions
▸ Uncommon Hypertension
SPECIFIC SIDE-EFFECTS
▸ Common or very common
▸ With oral use Asthenia · gastrointestinal discomfort · gastrointestinal disorders · haemorrhage · menstrual cycle irregularities · muscle complaints · pelvic pain · weight changes
▸ With transdermal use Abdominal pain · breast abnormalities · menstrual cycle irregularities · uterine disorders · vaginal discharge · weight changes
▸ Uncommon
▸ With oral use Anxiety · back pain · breast abnormalities · cervical abnormalities · cystitis-like symptom · depression · dizziness · embolism and thrombosis · erythema nodosum · gallbladder disorder · oedema · palpitations · peripheral vascular disease · tumour growth · visual impairment · vulvovaginal candidiasis
▸ With transdermal use Asthenia · breast neoplasm benign · depression · flatulence · increased risk of infection · leiomyoma · mood swings · venous thromboembolism · vertigo · vomiting
▸ Rare or very rare
▸ With oral use Angioedema · cerebrovascular insufficiency · chorea · contact lens intolerance · haemolytic anaemia · hepatic disorders · hirsutism · malaise · myocardial infarction · sexual dysfunction · steepening of corneal curvature · vaginal discharge · vomiting
▸ With transdermal use Epilepsy exacerbated · galactorrhoea · glucose tolerance impaired · libido disorder
▸ Frequency not known
▸ With oral use Carbohydrate metabolism change · epilepsy exacerbated · hypertriglyceridaemia · increased risk of coronary artery disease · neoplasms · pancreatitis · systemic lupus erythematosus (SLE)

SIDE-EFFECTS, FURTHER INFORMATION Cyclical HRT (where a progestogen is taken for 12–14 days of each 28-day oestrogen treatment cycle) usually results in regular withdrawal bleeding towards the end of the progestogen. Continuous combined HRT commonly produces irregular breakthrough bleeding in the first 4–6 months of treatment. Bleeding beyond 6 months or after a spell of amenorrhoea requires further investigation to exclude serious gynaecological pathology.

● CONCEPTION AND CONTRACEPTION HRT does **not** provide contraception and a woman is considered potentially fertile for 2 years after her last menstrual period if she is under 50 years, and for 1 year if she is over 50 years. A woman who is under 50 years and free of all risk factors for venous and arterial thromboembolism can use a low-oestrogen combined oral contraceptive pill to provide both relief of menopausal symptoms and contraception; it is recommended that the oral contraceptive be stopped at 50 years of age since there are more suitable alternatives. If any potentially fertile woman needs HRT, non-hormonal contraceptive measures (such as condoms) are necessary.

Measurement of follicle-stimulating hormone can help to determine fertility, but high measurements alone (particularly in women aged under 50 years) do not necessarily preclude the possibility of becoming pregnant.

● PREGNANCY Not known to be harmful.

● BREAST FEEDING Avoid; adverse effects on lactation.

● HEPATIC IMPAIRMENT Avoid in active liver disease including disorders of hepatic excretion (e.g. Dubin-Johnson or Rotor syndromes), infective hepatitis (until liver function returns to normal), and liver tumours.

● MONITORING REQUIREMENTS
▶ History of breast nodules or fibrocystic disease—closely monitor breast status (risk of breast cancer).
▶ The endometrial safety of long-term or repeated use of topical vaginal oestrogens is uncertain; treatment should be reviewed at least annually, with special consideration given to any symptoms of endometrial hyperplasia or carcinoma.

● DIRECTIONS FOR ADMINISTRATION
▶ With transdermal use Patch should be removed after 3–4 days (or once a week in case of 7-day patch) and replaced with fresh patch on slightly different site; recommended sites: clean, dry, unbroken areas of skin on trunk below waistline; not to be applied on or near breasts or under waistband. If patch falls off in bath allow skin to cool before applying new patch.

● PATIENT AND CARER ADVICE
▶ With transdermal use Patient counselling is advised for estradiol patches (administration).
▶ With topical use Patient counselling is advised for estradiol gels (administration).

OESTROGEL ® Apply gel to clean, dry, intact skin such as arms, shoulders or inner thighs and allow to dry for 5 minutes before covering with clothing. Not to be applied on or near breasts or on vulval region. Avoid skin contact with another person (particularly male) and avoid other skin products or washing the area for at least 1 hour after application.

SANDRENA ® Apply gel to intact areas of skin such as lower trunk or thighs, using right and left sides on alternate days. Wash hands after application. Not to be applied on the breasts or face and avoid contact with eyes. Allow area of application to dry for 5 minutes and do not wash area for at least 1 hour.

● MEDICINAL FORMS
There can be variation in the licensing of different medicines containing the same drug. Forms available from special-order manufacturers include: implant

Tablet
▶ Bedol (ReSource Medical UK Ltd)
Estradiol 2 mg Bedol 2mg tablets | 84 tablet [PoM] £5.07 DT = £5.06
▶ Elleste Solo (Meda Pharmaceuticals Ltd)
Estradiol 1 mg Elleste Solo 1mg tablets | 84 tablet [PoM] £5.06 DT = £5.06
Estradiol 2 mg Elleste Solo 2mg tablets | 84 tablet [PoM] £5.06 DT = £5.06
▶ Progynova (Bayer Plc)
Estradiol valerate 1 mg Progynova 1mg tablets | 84 tablet [PoM] £7.30 DT = £7.30
Estradiol valerate 2 mg Progynova 2mg tablets | 84 tablet [PoM] £7.30 DT = £7.30
▶ Zumenon (Mylan)
Estradiol 1 mg Zumenon 1mg tablets | 84 tablet [PoM] £6.89 DT = £5.06
Estradiol 2 mg Zumenon 2mg tablets | 84 tablet [PoM] £6.89 DT = £5.06

Transdermal patch
▶ Elleste Solo MX (Meda Pharmaceuticals Ltd)
Estradiol 40 microgram per 24 hour Elleste Solo MX 40 transdermal patches | 8 patch [PoM] £5.19
Estradiol 80 microgram per 24 hour Elleste Solo MX 80 transdermal patches | 8 patch [PoM] £5.99

▶ Estraderm MX (Merus Labs Luxco S.a R.L.)
Estradiol 25 microgram per 24 hour Estraderm MX 25 patches | 8 patch [PoM] £5.50 | 24 patch [PoM] £16.46
Estradiol 50 microgram per 24 hour Estraderm MX 50 patches | 8 patch [PoM] £5.51 | 24 patch [PoM] £16.46
Estradiol 75 microgram per 24 hour Estraderm MX 75 patches | 8 patch [PoM] £6.42 DT = £4.12 | 24 patch [PoM] £19.27
Estradiol 100 microgram per 24 hour Estraderm MX 100 patches | 8 patch [PoM] £6.66 | 24 patch [PoM] £19.99
▶ Estradot (Novartis Pharmaceuticals UK Ltd)
Estradiol 25 microgram per 24 hour Estradot 25micrograms/24hours patches | 8 patch [PoM] £5.99
Estradiol 37.5 microgram per 24 hour Estradot 37.5micrograms/24hours patches | 8 patch [PoM] £6.00
Estradiol 50 microgram per 24 hour Estradot 50micrograms/24hours patches | 8 patch [PoM] £6.02
Estradiol 75 microgram per 24 hour Estradot 75micrograms/24hours patches | 8 patch [PoM] £7.00 DT = £4.12
Estradiol 100 microgram per 24 hour Estradot 100micrograms/24hours patches | 8 patch [PoM] £7.27
▶ Evorel (Janssen-Cilag Ltd)
Estradiol 25 microgram per 24 hour Evorel 25 patches | 8 patch [PoM] £3.42
Estradiol 50 microgram per 24 hour Evorel 50 patches | 8 patch [PoM] £3.88 | 24 patch [PoM] £11.66
Estradiol 75 microgram per 24 hour Evorel 75 patches | 8 patch [PoM] £4.12 DT = £4.12
Estradiol 100 microgram per 24 hour Evorel 100 patches | 8 patch [PoM] £4.28
▶ FemSeven (Teva UK Ltd)
Estradiol 50 microgram per 24 hour FemSeven 50 patches | 4 patch [PoM] £6.04 | 12 patch [PoM] £18.02
Estradiol 75 microgram per 24 hour FemSeven 75 patches | 4 patch [PoM] £6.98
Estradiol 100 microgram per 24 hour FemSeven 100 patches | 4 patch [PoM] £7.28
▶ Progynova TS (Bayer Plc)
Estradiol 50 microgram per 24 hour Progynova TS 50micrograms/24hours transdermal patches | 12 patch [PoM] £18.90
Estradiol 100 microgram per 24 hour Progynova TS 100micrograms/24hours transdermal patches | 12 patch [PoM] £20.70

Gel
EXCIPIENTS: May contain Propylene glycol
▶ Oestrogel (Besins Healthcare (UK) Ltd)
Estradiol 600 microgram per 1 gram Oestrogel Pump-Pack 0.06% gel | 80 gram [PoM] £4.80 DT = £4.80
▶ Sandrena (Orion Pharma (UK) Ltd)
Estradiol (as Estradiol hemihydrate) 500 microgram Sandrena 500microgram gel sachets | 28 sachet [PoM] £5.08 DT = £5.08
Estradiol (as Estradiol hemihydrate) 1 mg Sandrena 1mg gel sachets | 28 sachet [PoM] £5.85 DT = £5.85 | 91 sachet [PoM] £17.57

Combinations available: *Estradiol with drospirenone,* p. 744 · *Estradiol with dydrogesterone,* p. 744 · *Estradiol with levonorgestrel,* p. 745 · *Estradiol with medroxyprogesterone,* p. 745 · *Estradiol with norethisterone,* p. 745 · *Estradiol with norgestrel,* p. 747

Estradiol with estriol and estrone

The properties listed below are those particular to the combination only. For the properties of the components please consider, estradiol p. 738, estriol p. 813.

● INDICATIONS AND DOSE

Menopausal symptoms | Osteoporosis prophylaxis
▶ BY MOUTH
▶ Adult: 1–2 tablets daily continuously or cyclically (21 days out of 28), started within 5 days of onset of menstruation (or at any time if cycles have ceased or are infrequent), to be taken with cyclical progestogen for 12–14 days of each cycle in women with a uterus

● INTERACTIONS → Appendix 1: hormone replacement therapy

● MEDICINAL FORMS
No licensed medicines listed.

Ethinylestradiol

(Ethinyloestradiol)

● INDICATIONS AND DOSE

Short-term treatment of symptoms of oestrogen deficiency | Osteoporosis prophylaxis if other drugs cannot be used
▸ BY MOUTH
▸ Adult (female): 10–50 micrograms daily for 21 days, repeated after 7-day tablet-free period, to be given with progestogen for 12–14 days per cycle in women with intact uterus.

Female hypogonadism
▸ BY MOUTH
▸ Adult (female): 10–50 micrograms daily usually on cyclical basis, initial oestrogen therapy should be followed by combined oestrogen and progestogen therapy.

Menstrual disorders
▸ BY MOUTH
▸ Adult (female): 20–50 micrograms daily from day 5 to 25 of each cycle, to be given with progestogen, added either throughout the cycle or from day 15 to 25.

Palliative treatment of prostate cancer
▸ BY MOUTH
▸ Adult (male): 0.15–1.5 mg daily.

● CONTRA-INDICATIONS Active or recent arterial thromboembolic disease (e.g. angina or myocardial infarction) · active thrombophlebitis · Acute porphyrias p. 1025 · Dubin-Johnson and Rotor syndromes (or monitor closely) · gallstones · heart disease associated with pulmonary hypertension · heart disease associated with risk of embolus · history during pregnancy of cholestatic jaundice · history during pregnancy of chorea · history during pregnancy of pemphigoid gestationis · history during pregnancy of pruritus · history of breast cancer · history of haemolytic uraemic syndrome · liver disease (where liver function tests have failed to return to normal) · migraine with aura · oestrogen-dependent cancer · sclerosing treatment for varicose veins · severe or multiple risk factors for arterial disease · severe or multiple risk factors for venous thromboembolism · systemic lupus erythematosus with (or unknown) antiphospholipid antibodies · thrombophilic disorder · transient cerebral ischaemic attacks without headaches · undiagnosed vaginal bleeding · untreated endometrial hyperplasia · venous thromboembolism, or history of recurrent venous thromboembolism (unless already on anticoagulant treatment)

● CAUTIONS Active trophoblastic disease (until return to normal of urine- and plasma-gonadotrophin concentration)—seek specialist advice · cardiovascular disease (sodium retention with oedema, thromboembolism) · Crohn's disease · diabetes (increased risk of heart disease) · gene mutations associated with breast cancer (e.g. BRCA 1) · history of breast nodules or fibrocystic disease—closely monitor breast status (risk of breast cancer) · history of endometrial hyperplasia · history of severe depression (especially if induced by hormonal contraceptive) · hyperprolactinaemia (seek specialist advice) · hypophyseal tumours · increased risk of gall-bladder disease · inflammatory bowel disease · migraine (migraine-like headaches) · personal or family history of hypertriglyceridaemia (increased risk of pancreatitis) · presence of antiphospholipid antibodies (increased risk of thrombotic events) · prolonged exposure to unopposed

oestrogens may increase risk of developing endometrial cancer · risk factors for arterial disease · risk factors for migraine · risk factors for oestrogen-dependent tumours (e.g. breast cancer in first-degree relative) · risk factors for venous thromboembolism · sickle-cell disease · undiagnosed breast mass

CAUTIONS, FURTHER INFORMATION
▸ Other conditions The product literature advises caution in other conditions including hypertension, renal disease, asthma, epilepsy, sickle-cell disease, melanoma, otosclerosis, multiple sclerosis, and systemic lupus erythematosus (but care required if antiphospholipid antibodies present, see above). Evidence for caution in these conditions is unsatisfactory and many women with these conditions may stand to benefit from HRT.
▸ Risk of venous thromboembolism Use with **caution** if any of following factors present but **avoid** if two or more factors present:
  ● *family history of venous thromboembolism* in first-degree relative aged under 45 years (avoid if known prothrombotic coagulation abnormality e.g. factor V Leiden or antiphospholipid antibodies (including lupus anticoagulant));
  ● *obesity*—body mass index ≥30 kg/m² (avoid if body mass index ≥35 kg/m² unless no suitable alternative); (In adolescents, caution if obese according to BMI (adjusted for age and gender); in those who are markedly obese, avoid unless no suitable alternative);
  ● *long-term immobilisation* e.g. in a wheelchair (avoid if confined to bed or leg in plaster cast);
  ● *history of superficial thrombophlebitis;*
  ● *age* over 35 years (avoid if over 50 years);
  ● *smoking.*
▸ Risk factors for arterial disease Use with **caution** if any one of following factors present but **avoid** if two or more factors present:
  ● *family history of arterial disease* in first degree relative aged under 45 years (avoid if atherogenic lipid profile);
  ● *diabetes mellitus* (avoid if diabetes complications present);
  ● *hypertension*—blood pressure above *systolic* 140 *mmHg* or *diastolic* 90 *mmHg* (avoid if blood pressure above *systolic* 160 *mmHg* or *diastolic* 95 *mmHg*); (In adolescents, avoid if blood pressure very high);
  ● *smoking* (avoid if smoking 40 or more cigarettes daily);
  ● *age* over 35 years (avoid if over 50 years);
  ● *obesity* (avoid if body mass index ≥35 kg/m² unless no suitable alternative); (In adolescents, caution if obese according to BMI (adjusted for age and gender); in those who are markedly obese, avoid unless no suitable alternative);
  ● *migraine without aura* (avoid if *migraine with aura* (focal symptoms), *or* severe migraine frequently lasting over 72 hours despite treatment, *or* migraine treated with ergot derivatives).
▸ Migraine Women should report any increase in headache frequency or onset of focal symptoms (discontinue immediately and refer urgently to neurology expert if focal neurological symptoms not typical of aura persist for more than 1 hour).

● INTERACTIONS → Appendix 1: hormone replacement therapy

● SIDE-EFFECTS Breast abnormalities · cervical mucus increased · cholelithiasis · contact lens intolerance · depression · electrolyte imbalance · embolism and thrombosis · erythema nodosum · feminisation · fluid retention · headaches · hypertension · jaundice cholestatic · metrorrhagia · mood altered · myocardial infarction · nausea · neoplasms · skin reactions · stroke · uterine disorders · vomiting · weight change

SIDE-EFFECTS, FURTHER INFORMATION Cyclical HRT (where a progestogen is taken for 12–14 days of each

28-day oestrogen treatment cycle) usually results in regular withdrawal bleeding towards the end of the progestogen. Continuous combined HRT commonly produces irregular breakthrough bleeding in the first 4–6 months of treatment. Bleeding beyond 6 months or after a spell of amenorrhoea requires further investigation to exclude serious gynaecological pathology.

- PREGNANCY Not known to be harmful.
- BREAST FEEDING Avoid until weaning or for 6 months after birth (adverse effects on lactation).
- HEPATIC IMPAIRMENT Avoid.

- MEDICINAL FORMS
There can be variation in the licensing of different medicines containing the same drug. Forms available from special-order manufacturers include: tablet, capsule, oral suspension
Tablet
‣ Ethinylestradiol (Non-proprietary)
Ethinylestradiol 2 microgram Ethinylestradiol 2microgram tablets | 100 tablet [PoM] £200.00
Ethinylestradiol 10 microgram Ethinylestradiol 10microgram tablets | 21 tablet [PoM] £200.00 DT = £200.00
Ethinylestradiol 50 microgram Ethinylestradiol 50microgram tablets | 21 tablet [PoM] £200.00 DT = £200.00
Ethinylestradiol 1 mg Ethinylestradiol 1mg tablets | 28 tablet [PoM] £200.00 DT = £200.00

Tibolone

- INDICATIONS AND DOSE
Short-term treatment of symptoms of oestrogen deficiency (including women being treated with gonadotrophin releasing hormone analogues) | Osteoporosis prophylaxis in women at high risk of fractures when other prophylaxis contra-indicated or not tolerated
‣ BY MOUTH
‣ Adult: 2.5 mg daily

- CONTRA-INDICATIONS Active or recent arterial thromboembolic disease (e.g. angina or myocardial infarction) · active thrombophlebitis · Acute porphyrias p. 1025 · Dubin-Johnson and Rotor syndrome (or monitor closely) · history of breast cancer · history of cardiovascular disease · history of cerebrovascular disease · history of recurrent venous thromboembolism (unless already on anticoagulant treatment) · history of thromboembolism · history of thrombophlebitis · hormone-dependent tumours · liver disease (where liver function tests have failed to return to normal) · oestrogen-dependent cancer · thrombophilic disorder · uninvestigated or undiagnosed vaginal bleeding · untreated endometrial hyperplasia · venous thromboembolism

- CAUTIONS Diabetes (increased risk of heart disease) · epilepsy · factors predisposing to thromboembolism · history of breast nodules—closely monitor breast status (risk of breast cancer) · history of endometrial hyperplasia · history of fibrocystic disease—closely monitor breast status (risk of breast cancer) · history of liver disease · hypertriglyceridaemia · hypophyseal tumours · migraine (or migraine-like headaches) · presence of antiphospholipid antibodies (increased risk of thrombotic events) · prolonged exposure to unopposed oestrogens may increase risk of developing endometrial cancer · risk factors for oestrogen-dependent tumours (e.g. breast cancer in first-degree relative) · risk of stroke
CAUTIONS, FURTHER INFORMATION
‣ Other conditions The product literature advises caution in other conditions including hypertension, renal disease, asthma, epilepsy, sickle-cell disease, melanoma, otosclerosis, multiple sclerosis, and systemic lupus erythematosus (but care required if antiphospholipid

antibodies present). Evidence for caution in these conditions is unsatisfactory and many women with these conditions may stand to benefit from HRT.

- INTERACTIONS → Appendix 1: tibolone
- SIDE-EFFECTS
▸ **Common or very common** Breast abnormalities · cervical dysplasia · endometrial thickening · gastrointestinal discomfort · genital abnormalities · hair growth abnormal · increased risk of infection · pelvic pain · postmenopausal haemorrhage · vaginal discharge · vaginal haemorrhage · weight increased
▸ **Uncommon** Oedema · skin reactions
▸ **Frequency not known** Arthralgia · dementia · depression · dizziness · erythema nodosum · gallbladder disorder · headaches · increased risk of ischaemic stroke · myalgia · neoplasms · vision disorders
SIDE-EFFECTS, FURTHER INFORMATION
Vaginal bleeding Investigate for endometrial cancer if bleeding continues beyond 6 months or after stopping treatment.
Reasons to withdraw treatment Withdraw treatment if signs of thromboembolic disease, abnormal liver function tests, or signs of cholestatic jaundice.

- PREGNANCY Avoid; toxicity in *animal* studies.
- BREAST FEEDING Avoid.
- HEPATIC IMPAIRMENT Avoid in acute liver disease or if history of liver disease and liver function tests not returned to normal.
- RENAL IMPAIRMENT
Monitoring Patients with renal impairment should be closely monitored (risk of fluid retention).
- PRESCRIBING AND DISPENSING INFORMATION Unsuitable for use in the premenopause (unless being treated with gonadotrophin-releasing hormone analogue) and as (or with) an oral contraceptive.
Also unsuitable for use within 12 months of last menstrual period (may cause irregular bleeding).
If transferring from cyclical HRT, start at end of regimen; if transferring from continuous-combined HRT, start at any time.

- MEDICINAL FORMS
There can be variation in the licensing of different medicines containing the same drug.
Tablet
‣ Tibolone (Non-proprietary)
Tibolone 2.5 mg Tibolone 2.5mg tablets | 28 tablet [PoM] £10.36 DT = £10.36 | 84 tablet [PoM] £31.08
‣ Livial (Merck Sharp & Dohme Ltd)
Tibolone 2.5 mg Livial 2.5mg tablets | 28 tablet [PoM] £10.36 DT = £10.36 | 84 tablet [PoM] £31.08

OESTROGENS COMBINED WITH PROGESTOGENS

Conjugated oestrogens with medroxyprogesterone

The properties listed below are those particular to the combination only. For the properties of the components please consider, conjugated oestrogens (equine) p. 737, medroxyprogesterone acetate p. 791.

- INDICATIONS AND DOSE
PREMIQUE ® LOW DOSE TABLETS
Menopausal symptoms in women with a uterus
‣ BY MOUTH
‣ Adult: 1 tablet daily continuously

- INTERACTIONS → Appendix 1: hormone replacement therapy

6

Endocrine system

- MEDICINAL FORMS
  There can be variation in the licensing of different medicines containing the same drug.
  Modified-release tablet
  ▸ Premique (Pfizer Ltd)
    Conjugated oestrogens 300 microgram, Medroxyprogesterone acetate 1.5 mg Premique Low Dose 0.3mg/1.5mg modified-release tablets | 84 tablet PoM £6.52 DT = £6.52

Estradiol with drospirenone

The properties listed below are those particular to the combination only. For the properties of the components please consider, estradiol p. 738.

- INDICATIONS AND DOSE
  Menopausal symptoms in women with a uterus whose last menstrual period occurred over 12 months previously | Osteoporosis prophylaxis in women with a uterus whose last menstrual period occurred over 12 months previously
  ▸ BY MOUTH
  ▸ Adult: 1 tablet daily continuously, if changing from cyclical HRT begin treatment the day after finishing oestrogen plus progestogen phase

- CAUTIONS Use with care if an increased concentration of potassium might be hazardous
- INTERACTIONS → Appendix 1: hormone replacement therapy
- SIDE-EFFECTS
  ▸ **Common or very common** Anxiety · asthenia · breast abnormalities · depression · emotional lability · gastrointestinal discomfort · headaches · menstrual disorder · nausea · neoplasms · oedema · vulvovaginal disorders
  ▸ **Uncommon** Alopecia · appetite abnormal · arthralgia · cervix disorder · chest pain · concentration impaired · constipation · diarrhoea · dizziness · dry mouth · dyspnoea · embolism and thrombosis · eye disorder · gastrointestinal disorders · hair changes · hyperhidrosis · hyperlipidaemia · hypertension · increased risk of infection · libido decreased · malaise · muscle complaints · ovarian disorder · pain · palpitations · paraesthesia · pelvic pain · skin reactions · sleep disorder · taste altered · urinary tract disorder · uterine disorders · varicose veins · visual impairment · vomiting · weight changes
  ▸ **Rare or very rare** Anaemia · chills · cholelithiasis · galactorrhoea · tinnitus · vertigo
  ▸ **Frequency not known** Atrial flutter · cardiomegaly · erythema nodosum · heart failure · hyperkalaemia · QT interval prolongation
- RENAL IMPAIRMENT Avoid if eGFR less than 30 mL/minute/1.73 m^2.

- MEDICINAL FORMS
  There can be variation in the licensing of different medicines containing the same drug.
  Tablet
  ▸ Angeliq (Bayer Plc)
    Estradiol (as Estradiol hemihydrate) 1 mg, Drospirenone 2 mg Angeliq 1mg/2mg tablets | 84 tablet PoM £31.90 DT = £31.90

Estradiol with dydrogesterone

The properties listed below are those particular to the combination only. For the properties of the components please consider, estradiol p. 738.

- INDICATIONS AND DOSE
  FEMOSTON ® 1 MG/10 MG
  Menopausal symptoms in women with a uterus
  ▸ BY MOUTH
  ▸ Adult: 1 tablet daily for 14 days, white tablet to be taken and started within 5 days of onset of menstruation (or any time if cycles have ceased or are infrequent), then 1 tablet daily for 14 days, grey tablet to be taken, subsequent courses repeated without interval, Femoston ® 1 mg/10 mg given initially and Femoston ® 2 mg/10 mg substituted if symptoms not controlled
  Osteoporosis prophylaxis in women with a uterus
  ▸ BY MOUTH
  ▸ Adult: 1 tablet daily for 14 days, white tablet to be taken and started within 5 days of onset of menstruation (or any time if cycles have ceased or are infrequent), then 1 tablet daily for 14 days, grey tablet to be taken, subsequent courses repeated without interval

  FEMOSTON ® 2 MG/10 MG
  Menopausal symptoms in women with a uterus
  ▸ BY MOUTH
  ▸ Adult: 1 tablet daily for 14 days, red tablet to be taken and started within 5 days of onset of menstruation (or any time if cycles have ceased or are infrequent), then 1 tablet daily for 14 days, yellow tablet to be taken, subsequent courses repeated without interval, Femoston ® 1 mg/10 mg given initially and Femoston ® 2 mg/10 mg substituted if symptoms not controlled
  Osteoporosis prophylaxis in women with a uterus
  ▸ BY MOUTH
  ▸ Adult: 1 tablet daily for 14 days, red tablet to be taken and started within 5 days of onset of menstruation (or any time if cycles have ceased or are infrequent), then 1 tablet daily for 14 days, yellow tablet to be taken, subsequent courses repeated without interval

  FEMOSTON ®-CONTI 0.5 MG/2.5MG
  Menopausal symptoms in women with a uterus whose last menstrual period occurred over 12 months previously
  ▸ BY MOUTH
  ▸ Adult: 1 tablet daily continuously, if changing from cyclical HRT begin treatment the day after finishing oestrogen plus progestogen phase

  FEMOSTON ®-CONTI 1 MG/5MG
  Menopausal symptoms in women with a uterus whose last menstrual period occurred over 12 months previously | Osteoporosis prophylaxis in women with a uterus whose last menstrual period occurred over 12 months previously
  ▸ BY MOUTH
  ▸ Adult: 1 tablet daily continuously, if changing from cyclical HRT begin treatment the day after finishing oestrogen plus progestogen phase

- CONTRA-INDICATIONS Acute porphyrias p. 1025 · genital or breast cancer · history during pregnancy of idiopathic jaundice, severe pruritus, or pemphigoid gestationis · history of liver tumours · severe arterial disease · undiagnosed vaginal bleeding
- CAUTIONS Conditions that may worsen with fluid retention e.g. epilepsy, hypertension, migraine, asthma, or cardiac dysfunction · diabetes (progestogens can decrease glucose tolerance) · history of depression · in those

susceptible to thromboembolism (particular caution with high dose)

- **INTERACTIONS** → Appendix 1: hormone replacement therapy
- **SIDE-EFFECTS**
- **Common or very common** Asthenia · breast abnormalities · cervical abnormalities · depression · dizziness · flatulence · gastrointestinal discomfort · headaches · malaise · menstrual cycle irregularities · nausea · nervousness · pain · pelvic pain · peripheral oedema · postmenopausal haemorrhage · skin reactions · vomiting · vulvovaginal candidiasis · weight changes
- **Uncommon** Cystitis-like symptom · embolism and thrombosis · gallbladder disorder · hepatic function abnormal · hypertension · libido disorder · peripheral vascular disease · tumour growth · varicose veins
- **Rare or very rare** Angioedema · myocardial infarction
- **Frequency not known** Chorea · contact lens intolerance · dementia · epilepsy exacerbated · erythema nodosum · haemolytic anaemia · hypertriglyceridaemia · leg cramps · neoplasms · pancreatitis · steepening of corneal curvature · systemic lupus erythematosus (SLE) · urinary incontinence
- **HEPATIC IMPAIRMENT** Avoid.
- **RENAL IMPAIRMENT** Use with caution.

- **MEDICINAL FORMS**
There can be variation in the licensing of different medicines containing the same drug.
  Tablet
  - Femoston 1/10 (Mylan)
  Femoston 1/10mg tablets | 84 tablet [PoM] £16.16
  - Femoston 2/10 (Mylan)
  Femoston 2/10mg tablets | 84 tablet [PoM] £16.16
  - Femoston-conti (Mylan)
  Estradiol 500 microgram, Dydrogesterone 2.5 mg Femoston-conti 0.5mg/2.5mg tablets | 84 tablet [PoM] £24.43 DT = £24.43
  Estradiol 1 mg, Dydrogesterone 5 mg Femoston-conti 1mg/5mg tablets | 84 tablet [PoM] £24.43 DT = £24.43

Estradiol with levonorgestrel

The properties listed below are those particular to the combination only. For the properties of the components please consider, estradiol p. 738, levonorgestrel p. 787.

- **INDICATIONS AND DOSE**
  FEMSEVEN CONTI ®
  Menopausal symptoms in women with a uterus whose last menstrual period occurred over 12 months previously
  - BY TRANSDERMAL APPLICATION
  - Adult: Apply 1 patch once weekly continuously
  FEMSEVEN SEQUI ®
  Menopausal symptoms in women with a uterus
  - BY TRANSDERMAL APPLICATION
  - Adult: Apply 1 patch once weekly for 2 weeks, phase 1 patches to be applied, then apply 1 patch once weekly for 2 weeks, phase 2 patches to be applied, subsequent courses are repeated without interval

- **INTERACTIONS** → Appendix 1: hormone replacement therapy
- **PATIENT AND CARER ADVICE** Patient counselling is advised for estradiol with levonorgestrel patches (application).

- **MEDICINAL FORMS**
There can be variation in the licensing of different medicines containing the same drug.
  Transdermal patch
  - FemSeven Conti (Teva UK Ltd)
  Levonorgestrel 7 microgram per 24 hour, Estradiol 50 microgram per 24 hour FemSeven Conti patches | 4 patch [PoM] £15.48 | 12 patch [PoM] £44.12
  - FemSeven Sequi (Teva UK Ltd)
  FemSeven Sequi patches | 4 patch [PoM] £13.18 | 12 patch [PoM] £37.54

Estradiol with medroxyprogesterone

The properties listed below are those particular to the combination only. For the properties of the components please consider, estradiol p. 738, medroxyprogesterone acetate p. 791.

- **INDICATIONS AND DOSE**
  INDIVINA ® TABLETS
  Menopausal symptoms in women with a uterus whose last menstrual period occurred over 3 years previously | Osteoporosis prophylaxis in women with a uterus whose last menstrual period occurred over 3 years previously
  - BY MOUTH
  - Adult: Initially 1/2.5 mg daily taken continuously, adjust according to response, to be started at end of scheduled bleed if changing from cyclical HRT
  TRIDESTRA ®
  Menopausal symptoms in women with a uterus | Osteoporosis prophylaxis in women with a uterus
  - BY MOUTH
  - Adult: 1 tablet daily for 70 days, white tablet to be taken, then 1 tablet daily for 14 days, blue tablet to be taken, then 1 tablet daily for 7 days, yellow tablet to be taken, subsequent courses are repeated without interval

- **INTERACTIONS** → Appendix 1: hormone replacement therapy

- **MEDICINAL FORMS**
There can be variation in the licensing of different medicines containing the same drug.
  Tablet
  - Indivina (Orion Pharma (UK) Ltd)
  Estradiol valerate 1 mg, Medroxyprogesterone acetate 2.5 mg Indivina 1mg/2.5mg tablets | 84 tablet [PoM] £20.58 DT = £20.58
  Estradiol valerate 2 mg, Medroxyprogesterone acetate 5 mg Indivina 2mg/5mg tablets | 84 tablet [PoM] £20.58 DT = £20.58
  Estradiol valerate 1 mg, Medroxyprogesterone acetate 5 mg Indivina 1mg/5mg tablets | 84 tablet [PoM] £20.58 DT = £20.58
  - Tridestra (Orion Pharma (UK) Ltd)
  Tridestra tablets | 91 tablet [PoM] £20.49

Estradiol with norethisterone

The properties listed below are those particular to the combination only. For the properties of the components please consider, estradiol p. 738, norethisterone p. 747.

- **INDICATIONS AND DOSE**
  CLIMAGEST ® 1-MG
  Menopausal symptoms
  - BY MOUTH
  - Adult: 1 tablet daily for 16 days, grey tablet to be taken and started on day 1 of menstruation (or at any time if cycles have ceased or are infrequent), then 1 tablet daily for 12 days, white tablet to be taken, subsequent courses are repeated without interval continued →

CLIMAGEST ® 2-MG

Menopausal symptoms (if symptoms not controlled with lower strength)
▸ BY MOUTH
▸ Adult: 1 tablet daily for 16 days, blue tablet to be taken and started on day 1 of menstruation (or at any time if cycles have ceased or are infrequent), then 1 tablet daily for 12 days, white tablet to be taken, subsequent courses are repeated without interval

CLIMESSE ®

Menopausal symptoms in women with a uterus whose last menstrual period occurred over 12 months previously | Osteoporosis prophylaxis in women with a uterus whose last menstrual period occurred over 12 months previously
▸ BY MOUTH
▸ Adult: 1 tablet daily continuously

CLINORETTE ®

Menopausal symptoms in women with a uterus | Osteoporosis prophylaxis in women with a uterus
▸ BY MOUTH
▸ Adult: 1 tablet daily for 16 days, white tablets to be taken, starting on day 5 of menstruation (or at any time if cycles have ceased or are infrequent), then 1 tablet daily for 12 days, pink tablets to be taken, subsequent courses repeated without interval

ELLESTE-DUET ® 1-MG

Menopausal symptoms
▸ BY MOUTH
▸ Adult: 1 tablet daily for 16 days, white tablet to be taken and started on day 1 of menstruation (or at any time if cycles have ceased or are infrequent), then 1 tablet daily for 12 days, green tablets to be taken, subsequent courses are repeated without interval

ELLESTE-DUET ® 2-MG

Menopausal symptoms | Osteoporosis prophylaxis
▸ BY MOUTH
▸ Adult: 1 tablet daily for 16 days, orange tablet to be taken, to be started on day 1 of menstruation (or at any time if cycles have ceased or are infrequent), then 1 tablet daily for 12 days, grey tablet to be taken, subsequent courses are repeated without interval

ELLESTE-DUET ® CONTI

Menopausal symptoms in women with a uterus whose last menstrual period occurred over 12 months previously | Osteoporosis prophylaxis in women with a uterus whose last menstrual period occurred over 12 months previously
▸ BY MOUTH
▸ Adult: 1 tablet daily continuous basis, if changing from cyclical HRT begin treatment at the end of scheduled bleed

EVOREL ® CONTI

Menopausal symptoms in women with a uterus | Osteoporosis prophylaxis in women with a uterus
▸ BY TRANSDERMAL APPLICATION
▸ Adult: Apply 1 patch twice weekly continuously

EVOREL ® SEQUI

Menopausal symptoms in women with a uterus | Osteoporosis prophylaxis in women with a uterus
▸ BY TRANSDERMAL APPLICATION
▸ Adult: Apply 1 patch twice weekly for 2 weeks, *Evorel* ® 50 patch to be applied and started within 5 days of onset of menstruation (or at any time if cycles have ceased or are infrequent), then apply 1 patch twice weekly, *Evorel* ® Conti patch to be applied, subsequent courses are repeated without interval.

KLIOFEM ®

Menopausal symptoms in women with a uterus whose last menstrual period occurred over 12 months previously | Osteoporosis prophylaxis in women with a uterus whose last menstrual period occurred over 12 months previously
▸ BY MOUTH
▸ Adult: 1 tablet daily continuously, to be started at end of scheduled bleed if changing from cyclical HRT

KLIOVANCE ®

Menopausal symptoms in women with a uterus whose last menstrual period occurred over 12 months previously | Osteoporosis prophylaxis in women with a uterus whose last menstrual period occurred over 12 months previously
▸ BY MOUTH
▸ Adult: 1 tablet daily continuously, to be started at end of scheduled bleed if changing from cyclical HRT

NOVOFEM ®

Menopausal symptoms in women with a uterus | Osteoporosis prophylaxis in women with a uterus
▸ BY MOUTH
▸ Adult: 1 tablet daily for 16 days, red tablets to be taken, then 1 tablet daily for 12 days, white tablets to be taken, subsequent courses are repeated without interval; start treatment with red tablet at any time or if changing from cyclical HRT, start treatment the day after finishing oestrogen plus progestogen phase

NUVELLE ® CONTINUOUS

Menopausal symptoms in women with a uterus whose last menstrual period occurred over 12 months previously | Osteoporosis prophylaxis in women with a uterus whose last menstrual period occurred over 12 months previously
▸ BY MOUTH
▸ Adult: 1 tablet daily continuously, if changing from cyclical HRT, start treatment the day after finishing oestrogen plus progestogen phase

TRISEQUENS ®

Menopausal symptoms in women with a uterus | Osteoporosis prophylaxis in women with a uterus
▸ BY MOUTH
▸ Adult: 1 tablet daily for 12 days, blue tablets to be taken, followed by 1 tablet daily for 10 days, white tablet to be taken, then 1 tablet daily for 6 days, red tablet to be taken, subsequent courses are repeated without interval

● INTERACTIONS → Appendix 1: hormone replacement therapy

● PATIENT AND CARER ADVICE
EVOREL ® SEQUI Patients and carers should be advised on the application of *Evorel* ® Sequi patches.

● MEDICINAL FORMS
There can be variation in the licensing of different medicines containing the same drug.

Tablet
▸ Clinorette (ReSource Medical UK Ltd)
Clinorette tablets | 84 tablet [PoM] £9.23
▸ Elleste Duet (Meda Pharmaceuticals Ltd)
Elleste Duet 1mg tablets | 84 tablet [PoM] £9.20
Elleste Duet 2mg tablets | 84 tablet [PoM] £9.20
▸ Elleste Duet Conti (Meda Pharmaceuticals Ltd)
Norethisterone acetate 1 mg, Estradiol 2 mg Elleste Duet Conti tablets | 84 tablet [PoM] £17.02 DT = £17.02
▸ Kliofem (Novo Nordisk Ltd)
Norethisterone acetate 1 mg, Estradiol 2 mg Kliofem tablets | 84 tablet [PoM] £11.43 DT = £17.02
▸ Kliovance (Novo Nordisk Ltd)
Norethisterone acetate 500 microgram, Estradiol 1 mg Kliovance tablets | 84 tablet [PoM] £13.20 DT = £13.20

- Novofem (Novo Nordisk Ltd)
  Novofem tablets | 84 tablet [PoM] £11.43
- Nuvelle Continuous (Bayer Plc)
  Norethisterone acetate 1 mg, Estradiol 2 mg Nuvelle Continuous tablets | 84 tablet [PoM] £19.00 DT = £17.02
- Trisequens (Novo Nordisk Ltd)
  Trisequens tablets | 84 tablet [PoM] £11.10

Transdermal patch

- Evorel Conti (Janssen-Cilag Ltd)
  Estradiol 50 microgram per 24 hour, Norethisterone acetate 170 microgram per 24 hour Evorel Conti patches | 8 patch [PoM] £13.00 | 24 patch [PoM] £37.22 DT = £37.22
- Evorel Sequi (Janssen-Cilag Ltd)
  Evorel Sequi patches | 8 patch [PoM] £11.09

Estradiol with norgestrel

The properties listed below are those particular to the combination only. For the properties of the components please consider, estradiol p. 738.

● **INDICATIONS AND DOSE**

CYCLO-PROGYNOVA ® 2MG TABLETS

Menopausal symptoms in women with a uterus | Osteoporosis prophylaxis in women with a uterus

▶ BY MOUTH
▶ Adult: 1 tablet daily for 11 days, white tablet to be taken; start on day 5 of menstruation (or at any time if cycles have ceased or are infrequent), then 1 tablet daily for 10 days, brown tablet to be taken, followed by a 7-day tablet free interval

● **INTERACTIONS** → Appendix 1: hormone replacement therapy

● **SIDE-EFFECTS**

▶ **Common or very common** Gastrointestinal discomfort · haemorrhage · headaches · menstrual cycle irregularities · nausea · skin reactions · weight changes
▶ **Uncommon** Breast abnormalities · depressed mood · dizziness · erythema nodosum · oedema · palpitations · visual impairment
▶ **Rare or very rare** Anxiety · contact lens intolerance · fatigue · hirsutism · muscle cramps · sexual dysfunction · vaginal discharge · vomiting
▶ **Frequency not known** Angioedema · dementia · gallbladder disorder · myocardial infarction · neoplasms · stroke · venous thromboembolism

● **MEDICINAL FORMS**
There can be variation in the licensing of different medicines containing the same drug.

Tablets

▶ Cyclo-Progynova (Meda Pharmaceuticals Ltd)
  Cyclo-Progynova 2mg tablets | 21 tablet [PoM] £3.11

PROGESTOGENS

Norethisterone

● **INDICATIONS AND DOSE**

Endometriosis

▶ BY MOUTH
▶ Adult: 10–15 mg daily for 4–6 months or longer, to be started on day 5 of cycle; increased to 20–25 mg daily if required, dose only increased if spotting occurs and reduced once bleeding has stopped

Dysfunctional uterine bleeding (to arrest bleeding) | Menorrhagia (to arrest bleeding)

▶ BY MOUTH
▶ Adult: 5 mg 3 times a day for 10 days

Dysfunctional uterine bleeding (to prevent bleeding) | Menorrhagia (to prevent bleeding)

▶ BY MOUTH
▶ Adult: 5 mg twice daily, to be taken from day 19 to day 26 of cycle

Dysmenorrhoea

▶ BY MOUTH
▶ Adult: 5 mg 3 times a day for 3–4 cycles, to be taken from day 5–24 of cycle

Premenstrual syndrome (but not recommended)

▶ BY MOUTH
▶ Adult: 5 mg 2–3 times a day for several cycles, to be taken from day 19–26 of cycle

Postponement of menstruation

▶ BY MOUTH
▶ Females of childbearing potential: 5 mg 3 times a day, to be started 3 days before expected onset (menstruation occurs 2–3 days after stopping)

Breast cancer

▶ BY MOUTH
▶ Adult: 40 mg daily, increased if necessary to 60 mg daily

Short-term contraception

▶ BY DEEP INTRAMUSCULAR INJECTION
▶ Females of childbearing potential: 200 mg, to be administered within first 5 days of cycle or immediately after parturition (duration 8 weeks). To be injected into the gluteal muscle, then 200 mg after 8 weeks if required

Contraception

▶ BY MOUTH
▶ Females of childbearing potential: 350 micrograms daily, dose to be taken at same time each day, starting on day 1 of cycle then continuously, if administration delayed for 3 hours or more it should be regarded as a 'missed pill'

● **CONTRA-INDICATIONS**

GENERAL CONTRA-INDICATIONS Avoid in patients with a history of liver tumours · breast cancer (unless progestogens are being used in the management of this condition) · genital cancer (unless progestogens are being used in the management of this condition) · history during pregnancy of idiopathic jaundice · history during pregnancy of pemphigoid gestationis (non-contraceptive indications) · history during pregnancy of severe pruritus (non-contraceptive indications) · when used as a contraceptive, history of breast cancer (can be used after 5 years if no evidence of disease and non-hormonal contraceptive methods unacceptable)

SPECIFIC CONTRA-INDICATIONS
▶ With oral use Acute porphyrias p. 1025 · severe arterial disease · undiagnosed vaginal bleeding

● **CAUTIONS**

GENERAL CAUTIONS Asthma · cardiac dysfunction · conditions that may worsen with fluid retention · diabetes (progestogens can decrease glucose tolerance—monitor patient closely) · epilepsy · history of depression · hypertension · migraine · susceptibility to thromboembolism (particular caution with high dose)

SPECIFIC CAUTIONS
▶ When used for contraception Active trophoblastic disease (until return to normal of urine- and plasma-gonadotrophin concentration)—seek specialist advice · arterial disease · functional ovarian cysts · history of jaundice in pregnancy · malabsorption syndromes · past ectopic pregnancy · sex-steroid dependent cancer · systemic lupus erythematosus with positive (or unknown) anti-phospholipid antibodies

Endocrine system

6

▸ With intramuscular use for contraception Disturbances of lipid metabolism · history during pregnancy of deterioration of otosclerosis · history during pregnancy of pruritus · possible risk of breast cancer

CAUTIONS, FURTHER INFORMATION

▸ Use as a contraceptive in co-morbidities The product literature advises caution in patients with history of thromboembolism, hypertension, diabetes mellitus and migraine; evidence for caution in these conditions is unsatisfactory.

▸ Breast cancer risk with contraceptive use There is a small increase in the risk of having breast cancer diagnosed in women using, or who have recently used, a progestogen-only contraceptive pill; this relative risk may be due to an earlier diagnosis. The most important risk factor appears to be the age at which the contraceptive is stopped rather than the duration of use; the risk disappears gradually during the 10 years after stopping and there is no excess risk by 10 years. A possible small increase in the risk of breast cancer should be weighed against the benefits.

● INTERACTIONS → Appendix 1: norethisterone

● SIDE-EFFECTS

GENERAL SIDE-EFFECTS

▸ **Common or very common** Menstrual cycle irregularities
▸ **Uncommon** Breast tenderness · depression
▸ **Frequency not known** Hepatic cancer · skin reactions · thromboembolism · weight change

SPECIFIC SIDE-EFFECTS

▸ **Common or very common**
▸ With intramuscular use Dizziness · haemorrhage · headache · hypersensitivity · nausea
▸ **Uncommon**
▸ With intramuscular use Abdominal distension
▸ **Frequency not known**
▸ With oral use Appetite change · fatigue · gastrointestinal disorder · headaches · hypertension · libido disorder · nervousness

● PREGNANCY

▸ With oral use Masculinisation of female fetuses and other defects reported with non-contraceptive use.

● BREAST FEEDING Progestogen-only contraceptives do not affect lactation. Higher doses (used in malignant conditions) may suppress lactation and alter milk composition—use lowest effective dose.

▸ With intramuscular use Withhold breast-feeding for neonates with severe or persistent jaundice requiring medical treatment.

● HEPATIC IMPAIRMENT When used as a contraceptive; caution in severe liver disease and recurrent cholestatic jaundice, avoid in liver tumour. Avoid in non-contraceptive indications.

● RENAL IMPAIRMENT Use with caution in non-contraceptive indications.

● PATIENT AND CARER ADVICE

Diarrhoea and vomiting with oral contraceptives Vomiting and persistent, severe diarrhoea can interfere with the absorption of oral progestogen-only contraceptives. If vomiting occurs within 2 hours of taking an oral progestogen-only contraceptive, another pill should be taken as soon as possible. If a replacement pill is not taken within 3 hours of the normal time for taking the progestogen-only pill, or in cases of persistent vomiting or very severe diarrhoea, additional precautions should be used during illness and for 2 days after recovery.

Starting routine for oral contraceptives One tablet daily, on a continuous basis, starting on day 1 of cycle and taken at the same time each day (if delayed by longer than 3 hours contraceptive protection may be lost). Additional contraceptive precautions are not required if norethisterone is started up to and including day 5 of the menstrual cycle; if started after this time, additional contraceptive precautions are required for 2 days.

Changing from a combined oral contraceptive Start on the day following completion of the combined oral contraceptive course without a break (or in the case of ED tablets omitting the inactive ones).

After childbirth Oral progestogen-only contraceptives can be started up to and including day 21 postpartum without the need for additional contraceptive precautions. If started more than 21 days postpartum, additional contraceptive precautions are required for 2 days.

Contraceptives by injection Full counselling backed by *patient information leaflet* required before administration— likelihood of menstrual disturbance and the potential for a delay in return to full fertility. Delayed return of fertility and irregular cycles may occur after discontinuation of treatment but there is no evidence of permanent infertility.

Missed oral contraceptive pill The following advice is recommended: 'If you forget a pill, take it as soon as you remember and carry on with the next pill at the right time. If the pill was more than 3 hours overdue you are not protected. Continue normal pill-taking but you must also use another method, such as the condom, for the next 2 days.'

The Faculty of Sexual and Reproductive Healthcare recommends emergency contraception if one or more progestogen-only contraceptive tablets are missed or taken more than 3 hours late and unprotected intercourse has occurred before 2 further tablets have been correctly taken.

● MEDICINAL FORMS

There can be variation in the licensing of different medicines containing the same drug. Forms available from special-order manufacturers include: oral suspension

Solution for injection

▸ Noristerat (Bayer Plc)
Norethisterone enantate 200 mg per 1 ml Noristerat 200mg/1ml solution for injection ampoules | 1 ampoule [PoM] £4.05

Tablet

▸ Norethisterone (Non-proprietary)
Norethisterone 5 mg Norethisterone 5mg tablets | 30 tablet [PoM] £2.23 DT = £2.06
▸ Noriday (Pfizer Ltd)
Norethisterone 350 microgram Noriday 350microgram tablets | 84 tablet [PoM] £2.10 DT = £2.10
▸ Primolut N (Bayer Plc)
Norethisterone 5 mg Primolut N 5mg tablets | 30 tablet [PoM] £2.26 DT = £2.06
▸ Utovlan (Pfizer Ltd)
Norethisterone 5 mg Utovlan 5mg tablets | 30 tablet [PoM] £1.40 DT = £2.06 | 90 tablet [PoM] £4.21

Combinations available: *Estradiol with norethisterone*, p. 745

Progesterone

06-Jun-2017

● INDICATIONS AND DOSE

CRINONE® VAGINAL GEL

Infertility due to inadequate luteal phase

▸ BY VAGINA
▸ Adult: 1 applicatorful daily, to be started either after documented ovulation or on day 18–21 of cycle, in vitro fertilisation, daily application continued for 30 days after laboratory evidence of pregnancy

CYCLOGEST® PESSARIES

Premenstrual syndrome | Post-natal depression

▸ BY VAGINA, OR BY RECTUM
▸ Adult: 200–800 mg daily, doses above 200 mg to be given in 2 divided doses, for premenstrual syndrome start on day 12–14 and continue until onset of

menstruation (but not recommended); rectally if barrier methods of contraception are used, in patients who have recently given birth or in those who suffer from vaginal infection or recurrent cystitis

GESTONE ® SOLUTION FOR INJECTION
Dysfunctional uterine bleeding
▸ BY DEEP INTRAMUSCULAR INJECTION
▸ Adult: 5–10 mg daily for 5–10 days until 2 days before expected onset of menstruation, to be administered into buttocks

Recurrent miscarriage due to inadequate luteal phase (but not recommended) or following in vitro fertilisation or gamete intra-fallopian transfer
▸ BY DEEP INTRAMUSCULAR INJECTION
▸ Adult: 25–100 mg 2–7 times a week from day 15, or day of embryo or gamete transfer, until 8–16 weeks of pregnancy, to be administered into buttocks; maximum 200 mg per day

LUBION ®
Supplementation of luteal phase during assisted reproductive technology (ART) treatment in women for whom vaginal preparations are inappropriate
▸ BY SUBCUTANEOUS INJECTION, OR BY INTRAMUSCULAR INJECTION
▸ Adult: 25 mg once daily from day of oocyte retrieval up to week 12 of pregnancy

LUTIGEST ®
Luteal support as part of an Assisted Reproductive Technology (ART) treatment programme
▸ BY VAGINA
▸ Adult: 100 mg 3 times a day, to be started the day after oocyte retrieval, and continued for 30 days once pregnancy is confirmed

UTROGESTAN ® CAPSULES
Progestogenic opposition of oestrogen HRT
▸ BY MOUTH
▸ Adult: 200 mg once daily on days 15–26 of each 28-day oestrogen HRT cycle, alternatively 100 mg once daily on days 1–25 of each 28-day oestrogen HRT cycle

UTROGESTAN ® VAGINAL CAPSULES
Supplementation of luteal phase during assisted reproductive technology (ART) cycles
▸ BY VAGINA
▸ Adult: 1 capsule 3 times a day from day of embryo transfer until at least week 7 of pregnancy up to week 12 of pregnancy

● CONTRA-INDICATIONS Acute porphyrias p. 1025 · avoid in patients with a history of liver tumours · breast cancer (unless progestogens are being used in the management of this condition) · genital cancer (unless progestogens are being used in the management of this condition) · history during pregnancy of idiopathic jaundice · history during pregnancy of pemphigoid gestationis · history during pregnancy of severe pruritus · history of thromboembolism · incomplete miscarriage · missed miscarriage · severe arterial disease · thrombophlebitis · undiagnosed vaginal bleeding

● CAUTIONS Asthma · cardiac dysfunction · conditions that may worsen with fluid retention · diabetes (progestogens can decrease glucose tolerance—monitor patient closely) · epilepsy · history of depression · hypertension · migraine · susceptibility to thromboembolism (particular caution with high dose)

● SIDE-EFFECTS
GENERAL SIDE-EFFECTS
▸ **Common or very common** Drowsiness · menstrual cycle irregularities

SPECIFIC SIDE-EFFECTS
▸ **Common or very common**
▸ With oral use Headache
▸ With vaginal use Breast pain · gastrointestinal discomfort
▸ **Uncommon**
▸ With oral use Breast pain · constipation · diarrhoea · dizziness · jaundice cholestatic · skin reactions · vomiting
▸ **Rare or very rare**
▸ With oral use Depression · nausea
▸ **Frequency not known**
▸ With intramuscular use Alopecia · breast changes · cervical abnormalities · depression · fever · hirsutism · insomnia · jaundice cholestatic · nausea · oedema · protein catabolism · skin reactions · weight increased
▸ With rectal use Diarrhoea · flatulence
▸ With vaginal use Leakage of the pessary base · vulvovaginal pain

● PREGNANCY Not known to be harmful.
● BREAST FEEDING Avoid—present in milk.
● HEPATIC IMPAIRMENT Avoid in hepatic impairment. Avoid in active liver disease including disorders of hepatic excretion (e.g. Dublin-Johnson or Rotor Syndromes), infective hepatitis (until liver function returns to normal) and liver tumours.
● RENAL IMPAIRMENT Use with caution.
● DIRECTIONS FOR ADMINISTRATION
▸ With oral use Capsules should be taken at bedtime on an empty stomach.
● PATIENT AND CARER ADVICE
▸ With oral use Patient counselling is advised for progesterone capsules (administration).

● NATIONAL FUNDING/ACCESS DECISIONS
LUTIGEST ®
Scottish Medicines Consortium (SMC) Decisions
The *Scottish Medicines Consortium* has advised (October 2016) that progesterone (*Lutigest®*) is accepted for use within NHS Scotland for luteal support as part of an assisted reproductive technology (ART) treatment program for infertile women. This advice is contingent upon the continuing availability of the Patient Access Scheme (PAS) in NHS Scotland or a list price that is equivalent or lower.
UTROGESTAN ® VAGINAL CAPSULES
Scottish Medicines Consortium (SMC) Decisions
The *Scottish Medicines Consortium* has advised (May 2017) that micronised progesterone (*Utrogestan Vaginal®*) is accepted for use within NHS Scotland for supplementation of the luteal phase during Assisted Reproductive Technology cycles in women. This advice is contingent upon the continuing availability of the Patient Access Scheme in Scotland or a list price that is equivalent or lower.

● LESS SUITABLE FOR PRESCRIBING Progesterone pessaries are less suitable for prescribing.

● MEDICINAL FORMS
There can be variation in the licensing of different medicines containing the same drug. Forms available from special-order manufacturers include: solution for injection
Pessary
▸ Cyclogest (Teva UK Ltd)
Progesterone 200 mg Cyclogest 200mg pessaries | 15 pessary PoM £8.95 DT = £8.95
Progesterone 400 mg Cyclogest 400mg pessaries | 15 pessary PoM £12.96 DT = £12.96
▸ Lutigest (Ferring Pharmaceuticals Ltd)
Progesterone 100 mg Lutigest 100mg vaginal tablets | 21 pessary PoM £19.50 DT = £19.50

Endocrine system
6

Solution for injection

▸ Gestone (Nordic Pharma Ltd)

Progesterone 50 mg per 1 ml Gestone 50mg/1ml solution for injection ampoules | 10 ampoule [PoM] £45.00

Gestone 100mg/2ml solution for injection ampoules | 10 ampoule [PoM] £45.00

Vaginal gel

▸ Crinone (Merck Serono Ltd)

Progesterone 80 mg per 1 gram Crinone 8% progesterone vaginal gel | 15 unit dose [PoM] £30.83

Capsule

EXCIPIENTS: May contain Arachis (peanut) oil

▸ Utrogestan (Besins Healthcare (UK) Ltd)

Progesterone 100 mg Utrogestan 100mg capsules | 30 capsule [PoM] £5.13 DT = £5.13

Progesterone 200 mg Utrogestan 200mg vaginal capsules with applicators | 21 capsule [PoM] £21.00 DT = £21.00

8.1a Anti-oestrogens

OVULATION STIMULANTS

Clomifene citrate

08-Feb-2018

(Clomiphene citrate)

● **DRUG ACTION** Anti-oestrogen which induces gonadotrophin release by occupying oestrogen receptors in the hypothalamus, thereby interfering with feedback mechanisms; chorionic gonadotrophin is sometimes used as an adjunct.

● **INDICATIONS AND DOSE**

Female infertility due to ovulatory dysfunction

▸ BY MOUTH

▸ Adult (female): 50 mg once daily for 5 days, to be started at any time if no recent uterine bleeding or on or around the fifth day of cycle if progestogen-induced bleeding is planned or if spontaneous uterine bleeding occurs, then 100 mg once daily if required for 5 days, this second course to be given at least 30 days after the first course, only in the absence of ovulation; most patients who are going to respond will do so to first course, 3 courses should constitute adequate therapeutic trial; long-term cyclical therapy not recommended (beyond a total of 6 cycles).

> **IMPORTANT SAFETY INFORMATION**
> The CSM has recommended that clomifene should not normally be used for longer than 6 cycles (possibly increased risk of ovarian cancer).

● **CONTRA-INDICATIONS** Abnormal uterine bleeding of undetermined cause · hormone-dependent tumours · ovarian cysts

● **CAUTIONS** Ectopic pregnancy · incidence of multiple births increased (consider ultrasound monitoring) · ovarian hyperstimulation syndrome · polycystic ovary syndrome (cysts may enlarge during treatment, also risk of exaggerated response to usual doses) · uterine fibroids

● **SIDE-EFFECTS** Abdominal distension · after images · alopecia · angioedema · anxiety · breast tenderness · cataract · cerebral thrombosis · depression · disorientation · dizziness · fatigue · headache · hot flush · hypertriglyceridaemia · insomnia · jaundice cholestatic · menstrual cycle irregularities · mood altered · nausea · neoplasms · nervous system disorders · optic neuritis · ovarian and fallopian tube disorders · palpitations · pancreatitis · paraesthesia · psychosis · seizure · skin reactions · speech disorder · stroke · syncope · tachycardia · uterine disorders · vertigo · vision disorders (discontinue and initiate ophthalmological examination) · vomiting

● **CONCEPTION AND CONTRACEPTION** Exclude pregnancy before treatment.

● **PREGNANCY** Possible effects on fetal development.

● **BREAST FEEDING** May inhibit lactation.

● **HEPATIC IMPAIRMENT** Avoid in severe liver disease.

● **PATIENT AND CARER ADVICE**

Conception and contraception Patients planning to conceive should be warned that there is a risk of multiple pregnancy (*rarely* more than twins).

● **MEDICINAL FORMS**
There can be variation in the licensing of different medicines containing the same drug.

Tablet

▸ Clomifene citrate (Non-proprietary)

Clomifene citrate 50 mg Clomifene 50mg tablets | 30 tablet [PoM] £10.15 DT = £10.15

▸ Clomid (Sanofi)

Clomifene citrate 50 mg Clomid 50mg tablets | 30 tablet [PoM] £10.15 DT = £10.15

8.2 Male sex hormone responsive conditions

Androgens, anti-androgens and anabolic steroids

Androgens

Androgens cause masculinisation; they may be used as replacement therapy in castrated adults and in those who are hypogonadal due to either pituitary or testicular disease. In the normal male they inhibit pituitary gonadotrophin secretion and depress spermatogenesis. Androgens also have an anabolic action which led to the development of anabolic steroids.

Androgens are useless as a treatment of impotence and impaired spermatogenesis unless there is associated hypogonadism; they should not be given until the hypogonadism has been properly investigated. Treatment should be under expert supervision.

When given to patients with hypopituitarism they can lead to normal sexual development and potency but not to fertility. If fertility is desired, the usual treatment is with gonadotrophins or pulsatile gonadotrophin-releasing hormone which will stimulate spermatogenesis as well as androgen production.

Intramuscular depot preparations of **testosterone esters** are preferred for replacement therapy. Testosterone enantate, propionate or undecanoate, or alternatively *Sustanon®*, which consists of a mixture of testosterone esters and has a longer duration of action, may be used.

Anti-androgens

Cyproterone acetate

Cyproterone acetate p. 753 is an anti-androgen used in the treatment of severe hypersexuality and sexual deviation in the male. It inhibits spermatogenesis and produces reversible infertility (but is not a male contraceptive); abnormal sperm forms are produced. Fully informed consent is recommended and an initial spermatogram. As hepatic tumours have been produced in *animal* studies, careful consideration should be given to the risk/benefit ratio before treatment. Cyproterone acetate is also licensed for use alone in patients with metastatic prostate cancer refractory to gonadorelin analogue therapy and has been used as an adjunct in prostatic cancer and in the treatment of acne and hirsutism in women.

Dutasteride and finasteride

Dutasteride p. 769 and finasteride p. 769 are alternatives to alpha-blockers particularly in men with a significantly enlarged prostate. Finasteride is also licensed for use with doxazosin p. 765 in the management of benign prostatic hyperplasia.

A low strength of finasteride is licensed for treating male-pattern baldness in men.

Anabolic steroids

Anabolic steroids have some androgenic activity but they cause less virilisation than androgens in women. They are used in the treatment of some *aplastic anaemias*. Anabolic steroids have been given for osteoporosis in women but they are no longer advocated for this purpose.

The protein-building properties of anabolic steroids have not proved beneficial in the clinical setting. Their use as body builders or tonics is unjustified; some athletes abuse them.

ANDROGENS

Androgens

- **CONTRA-INDICATIONS** Breast cancer in males · history of liver tumours · hypercalcaemia · prostate cancer
- **CAUTIONS** Cardiac impairment · diabetes mellitus · elderly · epilepsy · hypertension · ischaemic heart disease · migraine · pre-pubertal boys (fusion of epiphyses is hastened and may result in short stature)—statural growth and sexual development should be monitored · skeletal metastases—risk of hypercalcaemia or hypercalciuria (if this occurs, treat appropriately and restart treatment once normal serum calcium concentration restored) · sleep apnoea · stop treatment or reduce dose if severe polycythaemia occurs · tumours—risk of hypercalcaemia or hypercalciuria (if this occurs, treat appropriately and restart treatment once normal serum calcium concentration restored)
- **SIDE-EFFECTS**
- **Common or very common** Headache · skin reactions
- **Uncommon** Alopecia · gynaecomastia · nausea
- **Frequency not known** Fluid retention · jaundice · sexual dysfunction

  SIDE-EFFECTS, FURTHER INFORMATION Stop treatment or reduce dose if severe polycythaemia occurs.
- **PREGNANCY** Avoid—causes masculinisation of female fetus.
- **BREAST FEEDING** Avoid.
- **HEPATIC IMPAIRMENT** Avoid if possible—fluid retention and dose-related toxicity.
- **RENAL IMPAIRMENT** Caution—potential for fluid retention.
- **MONITORING REQUIREMENTS**
- Monitor haematocrit and haemoglobulin before treatment, every three months for the first year, and yearly thereafter.
- Monitor prostate and PSA in men over 45 years.
- **PATIENT AND CARER ADVICE**
  Androgenic effects in women Women should be advised to report any signs of virilisation e.g. deepening of the voice or hirsutism.

Mesterolone

- **INDICATIONS AND DOSE**

Androgen deficiency | Male infertility associated with hypogonadism
- ▶ BY MOUTH
- ▶ Adult: 25 mg 3–4 times a day for several months, then maintenance 50–75 mg daily in divided doses

---

- **MEDICINAL FORMS**
There can be variation in the licensing of different medicines containing the same drug.

Tablet
- ▶ Pro-Viron (Bayer Plc)
  Mesterolone 25 mg Pro-Viron 25mg tablets | 30 tablet [PoM]
  £4.19 [CD4-2]

Testosterone   19-Apr-2018

- **INDICATIONS AND DOSE**

TESTIM ®

Hypogonadism due to testosterone deficiency in men
- ▶ BY TRANSDERMAL APPLICATION
- ▶ Adult: Apply 50 mg once daily, subsequent application adjusted according to response; maximum 100 mg per day

DOSE EQUIVALENCE AND CONVERSION
- ▶ For *Testim*®: one tube of 5 g contains 50 mg testosterone.

TESTOGEL ® 16.2MG/G

Hypogonadism due to androgen deficiency in men
- ▶ BY TRANSDERMAL APPLICATION
- ▶ Adult: Apply 40.5 mg once daily; increased in steps of 20.25 mg, adjusted according to response; maximum 81 mg per day

DOSE EQUIVALENCE AND CONVERSION
- ▶ For *Testogel*® 16.2mg/g: one pump actuation delivers 1.25 g of gel containing 20.25 mg of testosterone.

TESTOGEL ® 50MG/5G

Hypogonadism due to androgen deficiency in men
- ▶ BY TRANSDERMAL APPLICATION
- ▶ Adult: Apply 50 mg once daily; increased in steps of 25 mg, adjusted according to response; maximum 100 mg per day

DOSE EQUIVALENCE AND CONVERSION
- ▶ For *Testogel*® 50mg/5g: one sachet of 5 g contains 50 mg of testosterone.

TOSTRAN ®

Hypogonadism due to testosterone deficiency in men
- ▶ BY TRANSDERMAL APPLICATION
- ▶ Adult: Apply 60 mg once daily, subsequent application adjusted according to response; maximum 80 mg per day

DOSE EQUIVALENCE AND CONVERSION
- ▶ For *Tostran*®: 1 g of gel contains 20 mg testosterone.

- **CAUTIONS** Thrombophilia—increased risk of thrombosis
- **SIDE-EFFECTS**
- **Common or very common** Hypertension
- **Uncommon** Peripheral oedema · vasodilation
- **Rare or very rare** Azoospermia
- **Frequency not known** Anxiety · electrolyte imbalance · emotional lability · hirsutism · muscle cramps · paraesthesia · priapism · prostate abnormalities · prostate cancer · seborrhoea · weight increased
- **DIRECTIONS FOR ADMINISTRATION** Avoid skin contact with gel application sites to prevent testosterone transfer to

6

Endocrine system

other people, especially pregnant women and children—consult product literature.

TESTIM ® Squeeze entire content of tube on to one palm and apply as a thin layer on clean, dry, healthy skin of shoulder or upper arm, preferably in the morning after washing or bathing (if 2 tubes required use 1 per shoulder or upper arm); rub in and allow to dry before putting on clothing to cover site; wash hands with soap after application; avoid washing application site for at least 6 hours.

TESTOGEL ® 16.2MG/G Apply thin layer of gel on clean, dry, healthy skin over right and left upper arms and shoulders. Not to be applied on genital area as high alcohol content may cause local irritation. Allow to dry for 3–5 minutes before dressing. Wash hands with soap and water after applying gel, and cover the site with clothing once gel dried; avoid shower or bath for at least 2 hours.

TESTOGEL ® 50MG/5G Apply thin layer of gel on clean, dry, healthy skin such as shoulders, arms or abdomen, immediately after sachet is opened. Not to be applied on genital area as high alcohol content may cause local irritation. Allow to dry for 3–5 minutes before dressing. Wash hands with soap and water after applying gel, avoid shower or bath for at least 6 hours.

TOSTRAN ® Apply gel on clean, dry, intact skin of abdomen or both inner thighs, preferably in the morning. Gently rub in with a finger until dry before dressing. Wash hands with soap and water after applying gel; avoid washing application site for at least 2 hours. Not to be applied on genital area.

● PATIENT AND CARER ADVICE Patient or carer should be given advice on how to administer testosterone gel.

● MEDICINAL FORMS
There can be variation in the licensing of different medicines containing the same drug.
Gel
EXCIPIENTS: May contain Butylated hydroxytoluene, propylene glycol
▸ Testim (Ferring Pharmaceuticals Ltd)
Testosterone 50 mg Testim 50mg/5g gel | 30 tube [PoM] £32.00 DT = £32.00 [CD4-2]
▸ Testogel (Besins Healthcare (UK) Ltd)
Testosterone 50 mg Testogel 50mg/5g gel sachets | 30 sachet [PoM] £31.11 DT = £31.11 [CD4-2]
Testosterone 16.2 mg per 1 gram Testogel 16.2mg/g gel | 88 gram [PoM] £31.11 [CD4-2]
▸ Tostran (Kyowa Kirin Ltd)
Testosterone 20 mg per 1 gram Tostran 2% gel | 60 gram [PoM] £28.67 DT = £28.67 [CD4-2]

Testosterone decanoate, isocaproate, phenylpropionate and propionate

The properties listed below are those particular to the combination only. For the properties of the components please consider, testosterone propionate below.

● INDICATIONS AND DOSE
Androgen deficiency
▸ BY DEEP INTRAMUSCULAR INJECTION
▸ Adult: 1 mL every 3 weeks

● MEDICINAL FORMS
There can be variation in the licensing of different medicines containing the same drug.
Solution for injection
EXCIPIENTS: May contain Arachis (peanut) oil, benzyl alcohol
▸ Sustanon (Aspen Pharma Trading Ltd)
Testosterone propionate 30 mg per 1 ml, Testosterone isocaproate 60 mg per 1 ml, Testosterone phenylpropionate 60 mg per 1 ml, Testosterone decanoate 100 mg per 1 ml Sustanon 250mg/1ml solution for injection ampoules | 1 ampoule [PoM] £2.45 [CD4-2]

F 751

Testosterone enantate

● INDICATIONS AND DOSE
Hypogonadism
▸ BY SLOW INTRAMUSCULAR INJECTION
▸ Adult: Initially 250 mg every 2–3 weeks; maintenance 250 mg every 3–6 weeks

Breast cancer
▸ BY SLOW INTRAMUSCULAR INJECTION
▸ Adult: 250 mg every 2–3 weeks

● UNLICENSED USE Not licensed for use in breast cancer.
● CAUTIONS Thrombophilia—increased risk of thrombosis
● SIDE-EFFECTS Androgenetic alopecia · anxiety · asthenia · bone disorders · circulatory system disorder · depression · gastrointestinal disorder · gastrointestinal haemorrhage · hepatomegaly · hypercalcaemia · libido increased · neoplasms · oedema · paraesthesia · polycythaemia · precocious puberty · prostatic disorder · spermatogenesis abnormal · urticaria

● MEDICINAL FORMS
There can be variation in the licensing of different medicines containing the same drug.
Solution for injection
▸ Testosterone enantate (Non-proprietary)
Testosterone enantate 250 mg per 1 ml Testosterone enantate 250mg/1ml solution for injection ampoules | 3 ampoule [PoM] £83.74–£87.73 DT = £85.74 [CD4-2]

F 751

Testosterone propionate

● INDICATIONS AND DOSE
Androgen deficiency
▸ BY INTRAMUSCULAR INJECTION
▸ Adult: 50 mg 2–3 times a week

Delayed puberty in males
▸ BY INTRAMUSCULAR INJECTION
▸ Adult: 50 mg once weekly

Breast cancer in women
▸ BY INTRAMUSCULAR INJECTION
▸ Adult: 100 mg 2–3 times a week

● CAUTIONS Thrombophilia—increased risk of thrombosis
● SIDE-EFFECTS
▸ Rare or very rare Pulmonary oil microembolism

● MEDICINAL FORMS
Forms available from special-order manufacturers include: solution for injection

F 751

Testosterone undecanoate

● INDICATIONS AND DOSE
Androgen deficiency
▸ BY MOUTH
▸ Adult: 120–160 mg daily for 2–3 weeks; maintenance 40–120 mg daily

Hypogonadism
▸ BY DEEP INTRAMUSCULAR INJECTION
▸ Adult (male): 1 g every 10–14 weeks, to be given over 2 minutes, if necessary, second dose may be given after 6 weeks to achieve rapid steady state plasma testosterone levels and then every 10–14 weeks.

● CAUTIONS Thrombophilia—increased risk of thrombosis
● SIDE-EFFECTS
GENERAL SIDE-EFFECTS
▸ Common or very common Polycythaemia

▶ **Uncommon** Depression · diarrhoea · hypertension · mood altered
SPECIFIC SIDE-EFFECTS
▶ **Common or very common**
▶ With intramuscular use Hot flush · prostate abnormalities · weight increased
▶ **Uncommon**
▶ With intramuscular use Anxiety · appetite increased · arthralgia · asthenia · behaviour abnormal · breast abnormalities · cardiovascular disorder · cough · dizziness · dysphonia · dyspnoea · hypercholesterolaemia · increased risk of infection · insomnia · migraine · muscle complaints · musculoskeletal stiffness · pain in extremity · snoring · sweat changes · testicular disorders · tremor · urinary disorders · urinary tract disorder
▶ **Rare or very rare**
▶ With intramuscular use Pulmonary oil microembolism
▶ **Frequency not known**
▶ With intramuscular use Hair growth increased · oedema · seborrhoea · sleep apnoea · spermatogenesis reduced
▶ With oral use Benign prostatic hyperplasia · fluid imbalance · gastrointestinal discomfort · hepatic function abnormal · lipid metabolism change · myalgia · nervousness · prostate cancer · sperm abnormalities · urinary tract obstruction

● MEDICINAL FORMS
There can be variation in the licensing of different medicines containing the same drug.
Solution for injection
▶ Nebido (Bayer Plc)
Testosterone undecanoate 250 mg per 1 ml Nebido 1000mg/4ml solution for injection vials | 1 vial [PoM] £87.11 DT = £87.11 [CD4-2]
Capsule
CAUTIONARY AND ADVISORY LABELS 21, 25
▶ Restandol (Merck Sharp & Dohme Ltd)
Testosterone undecanoate 40 mg Restandol 40mg Testocaps | 30 capsule [PoM] £8.55 [CD4-2] | 60 capsule [PoM] £17.10 DT = £17.10 [CD4-2]

8.2a Male sex hormone antagonism

ANTI-ANDROGENS

Cyproterone acetate

● INDICATIONS AND DOSE
Hyper-sexuality in males | Sexual deviation in males
▶ BY MOUTH
▶ Adult: 50 mg twice daily, to be taken after food
Prevention of tumour flare with initial gonadorelin analogue therapy
▶ BY MOUTH
▶ Adult (male): 200 mg daily in 2–3 divided doses for 5–7 days before initiation of gonadorelin analogue, followed by 200 mg daily in 2–3 divided doses for 3–4 weeks after initiation of gonadorelin analogue; maximum 300 mg per day.
Long-term palliative therapy where gonadorelin analogues or orchidectomy contra-indicated, not tolerated, or where oral therapy preferred
▶ BY MOUTH
▶ Adult (male): 200–300 mg daily in 2–3 divided doses.
Hot flushes with gonadorelin analogue therapy or after orchidectomy
▶ BY MOUTH
▶ Adult (male): Initially 50 mg daily, then adjusted according to response to 50–150 mg daily in 1–3 divided doses.

● CONTRA-INDICATIONS In hypersexuality, Dubin-Johnson syndrome · in hypersexuality, history of thromboembolic disorders · in hypersexuality, liver-disease · in hypersexuality, malignant diseases · in hypersexuality, previous or existing liver tumours · in hypersexuality, Rotor syndrome · in hypersexuality, severe depression · in hypersexuality, severe diabetes (with vascular changes) · in hypersexuality, sickle-cell anaemia · in hypersexuality, wasting diseases · meningioma or history of meningioma
● CAUTIONS Diabetes mellitus · in prostate cancer, severe depression · in prostate cancer, sickle-cell anaemia · ineffective for male hypersexuality in chronic alcoholism (relevance to prostate cancer not known)
● SIDE-EFFECTS
▶ **Common or very common** Depressed mood · dyspnoea · fatigue · gynaecomastia · hepatic disorders · hot flush · hyperhidrosis · nipple pain · restlessness · weight change
▶ **Uncommon** Skin reactions
▶ **Rare or very rare** Galactorrhoea · neoplasms
▶ **Frequency not known** Adrenocortical suppression · anaemia · azoospermia · hair changes · hypotrichosis · osteoporosis · sebaceous gland underactivity (may clear acne) · thromboembolism
SIDE-EFFECTS, FURTHER INFORMATION Direct hepatic toxicity including jaundice, hepatitis and hepatic failure have been reported (fatalities reported, usually after several months, at dosages of 100mg and above). If hepatotoxicity is confirmed, cyproterone should normally be withdrawn unless the hepatotoxicity can be explained by another cause such as metastatic disease (in which case cyproterone should be continued only if the perceived benefit exceeds the risk).
● HEPATIC IMPAIRMENT Avoid (unless used for prostate cancer)—dose-related toxicity.
● MONITORING REQUIREMENTS
▶ Monitor blood counts initially and throughout treatment.
▶ Monitor adrenocortical function regularly.
▶ Monitor hepatic function regularly—liver function tests should be performed before and regularly during treatment and whenever symptoms suggestive of hepatotoxicity occur.
● PATIENT AND CARER ADVICE
Driving and skilled tasks Fatigue and lassitude may impair performance of skilled tasks (e.g. driving).

● MEDICINAL FORMS
There can be variation in the licensing of different medicines containing the same drug. Forms available from special-order manufacturers include: tablet, capsule, oral suspension, oral solution
Tablet
CAUTIONARY AND ADVISORY LABELS 21
▶ Cyproterone acetate (Non-proprietary)
Cyproterone acetate 50 mg Cyproterone 50mg tablets | 56 tablet [PoM] £48.95 DT = £29.00 | 168 tablet [PoM] £87.00
Cyproterone acetate 100 mg Cyproterone 100mg tablets | 84 tablet [PoM] £132.57 DT = £55.19
▶ Androcur (Bayer Plc)
Cyproterone acetate 50 mg Androcur 50mg tablets | 60 tablet [PoM] £31.34
▶ Cyprostat (Bayer Plc)
Cyproterone acetate 50 mg Cyprostat 50mg tablets | 160 tablet [PoM] £82.86
Cyproterone acetate 100 mg Cyprostat 100mg tablets | 80 tablet [PoM] £82.86

6

Endocrine system

9 Thyroid disorders

PITUITARY AND HYPOTHALAMIC HORMONES AND ANALOGUES >THYROID STIMULATING HORMONES

Thyrotropin alfa

(Recombinant human thyroid stimulating hormone; rhTSH)

- DRUG ACTION Thyrotropin alfa is a recombinant form of thyrotrophin (thyroid stimulating hormone).

- INDICATIONS AND DOSE

  Detection of thyroid remnants and thyroid cancer in post-thyroidectomy patients, together with serum thyroglobulin testing (with or without radioiodine imaging) | To increase radio-iodine uptake for the ablation of thyroid remnant tissue in suitable post-thyroidectomy patients
  ▶ BY INTRAMUSCULAR INJECTION
  ▶ Adult: 900 micrograms every 24 hours for 2 doses, dose to be administered into the gluteal muscle, consult product literature for further information on indications and dose

- CAUTIONS Presence of thyroglobulin autoantibodies may give false negative results
- SIDE-EFFECTS
  ▶ Common or very common Asthenia · dizziness · headache · nausea · vomiting
  ▶ Uncommon Chills · diarrhoea · feeling hot · fever · flushing · hypersensitivity · influenza · influenza like illness · pain · paraesthesia · pulmonary reaction · skin reactions · taste altered
  ▶ Rare or very rare Atrial fibrillation · hyperthyroidism
  ▶ Frequency not known Arthralgia · dyspnoea · goitre · hyperhidrosis · myalgia · neoplasm complications · palpitations · residual metastases enlarged · stroke · tremor
- ALLERGY AND CROSS-SENSITIVITY Contra-indicated if previous hypersensitivity to bovine or human thyrotrophin.
- PREGNANCY Avoid.
- BREAST FEEDING Avoid.

- MEDICINAL FORMS
  There can be variation in the licensing of different medicines containing the same drug.
  Powder for solution for injection
  ▶ Thyrogen (Genzyme Therapeutics Ltd)
  Thyrotropin alfa 900 microgram Thyrogen 900microgram powder for solution for injection vials | 2 vial [PoM] £583.04

9.1 Hyperthyroidism

Antithyroid drugs

Overview

Antithyroid drugs are used for hyperthyroidism either to prepare patients for thyroidectomy or for long-term management. In the UK carbimazole below is the most commonly used drug. Propylthiouracil p. 755 should be reserved for patients who are intolerant of carbimazole or for those who experience sensitivity reactions to carbimazole (sensitivity is not necessarily displayed to both drugs), and for whom other treatments are inappropriate. Both drugs act primarily by interfering with the synthesis of thyroid hormones.

Over-treatment with antithyroid drugs can result in the rapid development of hypothyroidism and should be avoided particularly during pregnancy because it can cause fetal goitre.

A combination of carbimazole with levothyroxine sodium p. 756 daily, may be used in a *blocking-replacement regimen*; therapy is usually given for 18 months. The blocking-replacement regimen is **not** suitable during pregnancy.

Iodine has been used as an adjunct to antithyroid drugs for 10 to 14 days before partial thyroidectomy; however, there is little evidence of a beneficial effect. Iodine should not be used for long-term treatment because its antithyroid action tends to diminish.

Radioactive sodium iodide (^{131} I) solution is used increasingly for the treatment of thyrotoxicosis at all ages, particularly where medical therapy or compliance is a problem, in patients with cardiac disease, and in patients who relapse after thyroidectomy.

Propranolol hydrochloride p. 149 is useful for rapid relief of thyrotoxic symptoms and may be used in conjunction with antithyroid drugs or as an adjunct to radioactive iodine. Beta-blockers are also useful in neonatal thyrotoxicosis and in supraventricular arrhythmias due to hyperthyroidism. Propranolol hydrochloride has been used in conjunction with iodine to prepare mildly thyrotoxic patients for surgery but it is preferable to make the patient euthyroid with carbimazole. Laboratory tests of thyroid function are not altered by beta-blockers. Most experience in treating thyrotoxicosis has been gained with propranolol hydrochloride but nadolol p. 148 is also used.

Thyrotoxic crisis ('thyroid storm') requires emergency treatment with intravenous administration of fluids, propranolol hydrochloride and hydrocortisone p. 662 (as sodium succinate), as well as oral iodine solution and carbimazole or propylthiouracil which may need to be administered by nasogastric tube.

Antithyroid drugs in pregnancy

Radioactive iodine therapy is contra-indicated during pregnancy. Propylthiouracil and carbimazole can be given but the blocking-replacement regimen is **not** suitable. Rarely, carbimazole has been associated with congenital defects, including aplasia cutis of the neonate, therefore propylthiouracil remains the drug of choice during the first trimester of pregnancy. In the second trimester, consider switching to carbimazole because of the potential risk of hepatotoxicity with propylthiouracil. Both propylthiouracil and carbimazole cross the placenta and in high doses may cause fetal goitre and hypothyroidism—the lowest dose that will control the hyperthyroid state should be used (requirements in Graves' disease tend to fall during pregnancy).

> **Other drugs used for Hyperthyroidism** Metoprolol tartrate, p. 154

ANTITHYROID DRUGS >SULFUR-CONTAINING IMIDAZOLES

Carbimazole

- INDICATIONS AND DOSE

  Hyperthyroidism
  ▶ BY MOUTH
  ▶ Adult: 15–40 mg daily continue until the patient becomes euthyroid, usually after 4 to 8 weeks, higher doses should be prescribed under specialist supervision only, then reduced to 5–15 mg daily, reduce dose gradually, therapy usually given for 12 to 18 months

6

Hyperthyroidism (blocking-replacement regimen) in combination with levothyroxine
▶ BY MOUTH
▶ Adult: 40–60 mg daily, therapy usually given for 18 months

DOSE EQUIVALENCE AND CONVERSION
▶ When substituting, carbimazole 1 mg is considered equivalent to propylthiouracil 10 mg but the dose may need adjusting according to response.

> IMPORTANT SAFETY INFORMATION
> NEUTROPENIA AND AGRANULOCYTOSIS
> Doctors are reminded of the importance of recognising bone marrow suppression induced by carbimazole and the need to stop treatment promptly.
> • Patient should be asked to report symptoms and signs suggestive of infection, especially sore throat.
> • A white blood cell count should be performed if there is any clinical evidence of infection.
> • Carbimazole should be stopped promptly if there is clinical or laboratory evidence of neutropenia.

● CONTRA-INDICATIONS Severe blood disorders
● INTERACTIONS → Appendix 1: carbimazole
● SIDE-EFFECTS
▶ **Rare or very rare** Bone marrow disorders · haemolytic anaemia · severe cutaneous adverse reactions (SCARs) · thrombocytopenia
▶ **Frequency not known** Agranulocytosis · alopecia · angioedema · dyspepsia · eosinophilia · fever · gastrointestinal disorder · generalised lymphadenopathy · haemorrhage · headache · hepatic disorders · insulin autoimmune syndrome · leucopenia · malaise · myopathy · nausea · nerve disorders · neutropenia · salivary gland enlargement · skin reactions · taste loss
● PREGNANCY Carbimazole can be given but the blocking-replacement regimen is **not** suitable. Rarely, carbimazole has been associated with congenital defects, including aplasia cutis of the neonate. Carbimazole cross the placenta and in high doses may cause fetal goitre and hypothyroidism—the lowest dose that will control the hyperthyroid state should be used (requirements in Graves' disease tend to fall during pregnancy).
● BREAST FEEDING Present in breast milk but this does not preclude breast-feeding as long as neonatal development is closely monitored and the lowest effective dose is used. Amount in milk may be sufficient to affect neonatal thyroid function therefore lowest effective dose should be used.
● HEPATIC IMPAIRMENT Use with caution in mild to moderate impairment. Avoid in severe impairment.
● PATIENT AND CARER ADVICE Warn patient or carers to tell doctor **immediately** if sore throat, mouth ulcers, bruising, fever, malaise, or non-specific illness develops.

● MEDICINAL FORMS
There can be variation in the licensing of different medicines containing the same drug. Forms available from special-order manufacturers include: capsule, oral suspension, oral solution
Tablet
▶ Carbimazole (Non-proprietary)
  Carbimazole 5 mg Carbimazole 5mg tablets | 100 tablet PoM £84.80 DT = £43.74
  Carbimazole 10 mg Carbimazole 10mg tablets | 100 tablet PoM £81.32
  Carbimazole 15 mg Carbimazole 15mg tablets | 100 tablet PoM £115.98
  Carbimazole 20 mg Carbimazole 20mg tablets | 100 tablet PoM £208.17 DT = £144.47

ANTITHYROID DRUGS > THIOURACILS

Propylthiouracil

● INDICATIONS AND DOSE
Hyperthyroidism
▶ BY MOUTH
▶ Adult: Initially 200–400 mg daily in divided doses until the patient becomes euthyroid, then reduced to 50–150 mg daily in divided doses, initial dose should be gradually reduced to the maintenance dose

DOSE EQUIVALENCE AND CONVERSION
▶ When substituting, carbimazole 1 mg is considered equivalent to propylthiouracil 10 mg but the dose may need adjusting according to response.

● INTERACTIONS → Appendix 1: propylthiouracil
● SIDE-EFFECTS
▶ **Rare or very rare** Agranulocytosis · bone marrow disorders · glomerulonephritis acute · hearing impairment · leucopenia · thrombocytopenia · vomiting
▶ **Frequency not known** Alopecia · arthralgia · arthritis · encephalopathy · fever · gastrointestinal disorder · haemorrhage · headache · hepatic disorders · hypoprothrombinaemia · interstitial pneumonitis · lupus-like syndrome · lymphadenopathy · myopathy · nausea · nephritis · skin reactions · taste altered · vasculitis

SIDE-EFFECTS, FURTHER INFORMATION Severe hepatic reactions have been reported, including fatal cases and cases requiring liver transplant—discontinue if significant liver-enzyme abnormalities develop.

● PREGNANCY Propylthiouracil can be given but the blocking-replacement regimen is **not** suitable. Propylthiouracil crosses the placenta and in high doses may cause fetal goitre and hypothyroidism—the lowest dose that will control the hyperthyroid state should be used (requirements in Graves' disease tend to fall during pregnancy).
● BREAST FEEDING Present in breast milk but this does not preclude breast-feeding as long as neonatal development is closely monitored and the lowest effective dose is used. Amount in milk probably too small to affect infant; high doses may affect neonatal thyroid function.
Monitoring Monitor infant's thyroid status.
● HEPATIC IMPAIRMENT
Dose adjustments Reduce dose.
● RENAL IMPAIRMENT
Dose adjustments Use three-quarters normal dose if eGFR 10–50 mL/minute/1.73 m^2.
  Use half normal dose if eGFR less than 10 mL/minute/1.73 m^2.
● MONITORING REQUIREMENTS Monitor for hepatotoxicity.
● PATIENT AND CARER ADVICE Patients should be told how to recognise signs of liver disorder and advised to seek prompt medical attention if symptoms such as anorexia, nausea, vomiting, fatigue, abdominal pain, jaundice, dark urine, or pruritus develop.

● MEDICINAL FORMS
There can be variation in the licensing of different medicines containing the same drug. Forms available from special-order manufacturers include: oral suspension, oral solution
Tablet
▶ Propylthiouracil (Non-proprietary)
  Propylthiouracil 50 mg Propylthiouracil 50mg tablets | 56 tablet PoM £57.58 DT = £55.21 | 100 tablet PoM £98.59–£115.98

VITAMINS AND TRACE ELEMENTS

Iodide with iodine

- **INDICATIONS AND DOSE**
Thyrotoxicosis (pre-operative)
▸ BY MOUTH USING ORAL SOLUTION
▸ Adult: 0.1–0.3 mL 3 times a day

- CAUTIONS Children · not for long-term treatment
- SIDE-EFFECTS Conjunctivitis · depression (long term use) · erectile dysfuncton (long term use) · excessive tearing · headache · hypersensitivity · increased risk of infection · influenza-like illness · insomnia (long term use) · rash · salivary gland pain
- PREGNANCY Neonatal goitre and hypothyroidism.
- BREAST FEEDING Stop breast-feeding. Danger of neonatal hypothyroidism or goitre. Appears to be concentrated in milk.
- DIRECTIONS FOR ADMINISTRATION For oral solution, dilute well with milk or water.

- MEDICINAL FORMS
No licensed medicines listed.

9.2 Hypothyroidism

Thyroid hormones

Overview

Thyroid hormones are used in hypothyroidism (myxoedema), and also in diffuse non-toxic goitre, Hashimoto's thyroiditis (lymphadenoid goitre), and thyroid carcinoma. Neonatal hypothyroidism requires prompt treatment for normal development. Levothyroxine sodium below (thyroxine sodium) is the treatment of choice for *maintenance* therapy.

In infants and children with congenital hypothyroidism and juvenile myxoedema, the dose of levothyroxine sodium should be titrated according to clinical response, growth assessment, and measurements of plasma thyroxine and thyroid-stimulating hormone.

Liothyronine sodium p. 757 has a similar action to levothyroxine sodium but is more rapidly metabolised and has a more rapid effect. Its effects develop after a few hours and disappear within 24 to 48 hours of discontinuing treatment. It may be used in *severe hypothyroid states* when a rapid response is desired.

Liothyronine sodium by intravenous injection is the treatment of choice in *hypothyroid coma*. Adjunctive therapy includes intravenous fluids, hydrocortisone p. 662, and treatment of infection; assisted ventilation is often required.

THYROID HORMONES

Levothyroxine sodium

(Thyroxine sodium)

- **INDICATIONS AND DOSE**
Hypothyroidism
▸ BY MOUTH
▸ Adult 18–49 years: Initially 50–100 micrograms once daily; adjusted in steps of 25–50 micrograms every 3–4 weeks, adjusted according to response; maintenance 100–200 micrograms once daily, dose to be taken preferably at least 30 minutes before breakfast, caffeine-containing liquids (e.g. coffee, tea), or other medication
▸ Adult 50 years and over: Initially 25 micrograms once daily; adjusted in steps of 25 micrograms every 4 weeks, adjusted according to response; maintenance 50–200 micrograms once daily, dose to be taken preferably at least 30 minutes before breakfast, caffeine-containing liquids (e.g. coffee, tea), or other medication

Hypothyroidism in patients with cardiac disease | Severe hypothyroidism
▸ BY MOUTH
▸ Adult: Initially 25 micrograms once daily; adjusted in steps of 25 micrograms every 4 weeks, adjusted according to response; maintenance 50–200 micrograms once daily, dose to be taken preferably at least 30 minutes before breakfast, caffeine-containing liquids (e.g. coffee, tea), or other medication

Hyperthyroidism (blocking-replacement regimen) in combination with carbimazole
▸ BY MOUTH
▸ Adult: 50–150 micrograms daily therapy usually given for 18 months

- CONTRA-INDICATIONS Thyrotoxicosis
- CAUTIONS Cardiovascular disorders · diabetes insipidus · diabetes mellitus (dose of antidiabetic drugs including insulin may need to be increased) · elderly · hypertension · long-standing hypothyroidism · myocardial infarction · myocardial insufficiency · panhypopituitarism (initiate corticosteroid therapy before starting levothyroxine) · predisposition to adrenal insufficiency (initiate corticosteroid therapy before starting levothyroxine)
CAUTIONS, FURTHER INFORMATION
▸ Cardiovascular disorders Baseline ECG is valuable because changes induced by hypothyroidism can be confused with ischaemia.

- INTERACTIONS → Appendix 1: thyroid hormones
- SIDE-EFFECTS Angina pectoris · anxiety · arrhythmias · arthralgia · diarrhoea · dyspnoea · fever · flushing · headache · hyperhidrosis · insomnia · malaise · menstruation irregular · muscle spasms · muscle weakness · oedema · palpitations · skin reactions · thyrotoxic crisis · tremor · vomiting · weight decreased

SIDE-EFFECTS, FURTHER INFORMATION Initial dosage in patients with cardiovascular disorders—if metabolism increases too rapidly (causing diarrhoea, nervousness, rapid pulse, insomnia, tremors and sometimes anginal pain where there is latent myocardial ischaemia), reduce dose or withhold for 1–2 days and start again at a lower dose.

- PREGNANCY Levothyroxine may cross the placenta. Excessive or insufficient maternal thyroid hormones can be detrimental to fetus.
Dose adjustments Levothyroxine requirement may increase during pregnancy.
Monitoring Assess maternal thyroid function before conception (if possible), at diagnosis of pregnancy, at antenatal booking, during both the second and third trimesters, and after delivery (more frequent monitoring required on initiation or adjustment of levothyroxine).
- BREAST FEEDING Amount too small to affect tests for neonatal hypothyroidism.

- MEDICINAL FORMS
There can be variation in the licensing of different medicines containing the same drug. Forms available from special-order manufacturers include: capsule, oral suspension, oral solution
Tablet
▸ Levothyroxine sodium (Non-proprietary)
  Levothyroxine sodium anhydrous 12.5 microgram Levothyroxine sodium 12.5microgram tablets | 28 tablet [PoM] £2.80–£14.00 DT = £13.60

Levothyroxine sodium anhydrous 25 microgram Levothyroxine
sodium 25microgram tablets | 28 tablet [PoM] £3.05 DT = £1.87 |
500 tablet [PoM] £41.61–£56.25
Levothyroxine sodium 25microgram tablets lactose free |
100 tablet [PoM] [S̶]
Levothyroxine sodium anhydrous 50 microgram Levothyroxine
sodium 50microgram tablets lactose free | 100 tablet [PoM] [S̶]
Levothyroxine sodium 50microgram tablets | 28 tablet [PoM] £1.50
DT = £0.97 | 1000 tablet [PoM] £38.93–£55.71
Levothyroxine sodium anhydrous 75 microgram Levothyroxine
sodium 75microgram tablets | 28 tablet [PoM] £2.10–£4.00 DT = £2.73
Levothyroxine sodium anhydrous 100 microgram Levothyroxine
sodium 100microgram tablets lactose free | 100 tablet [PoM] [S̶]
Levothyroxine sodium 100microgram tablets | 28 tablet [PoM] £1.50
DT = £0.96 | 1000 tablet [PoM] £38.93–£56.07
‣ Eltroxin (AMCo)
Levothyroxine sodium anhydrous 25 microgram Eltroxin
25microgram tablets | 28 tablet [PoM] £2.54 DT = £1.87
Levothyroxine sodium anhydrous 50 microgram Eltroxin
50microgram tablets | 28 tablet [PoM] £1.77 DT = £0.97
Levothyroxine sodium anhydrous 100 microgram Eltroxin
100microgram tablets | 28 tablet [PoM] £1.78 DT = £0.96

Oral solution
‣ Levothyroxine sodium (Non-proprietary)
Levothyroxine sodium anhydrous 5 microgram per
1 ml Levothyroxine sodium 25micrograms/5ml oral solution sugar
free sugar-free | 100 ml [PoM] £118.63 DT = £94.94
Levothyroxine sodium anhydrous 10 microgram per
1 ml Levothyroxine sodium 50micrograms/5ml oral solution sugar
free sugar-free | 100 ml [PoM] £91.22 DT = £89.66
Levothyroxine sodium anhydrous 20 microgram per
1 ml Levothyroxine sodium 100micrograms/5ml oral solution sugar
free sugar-free | 100 ml [PoM] £165.00 DT = £164.88

Capsule
‣ Levothyroxine sodium (Non-proprietary)
Levothyroxine sodium anhydrous 25 microgram Tirosint
25microgram capsules | 28 capsule [PoM] [S̶]
Levothyroxine sodium anhydrous 50 microgram Tirosint
50microgram capsules | 28 capsule [PoM] [S̶]
Levothyroxine sodium anhydrous 100 microgram Tirosint
100microgram capsules | 28 capsule [PoM] [S̶]

Liothyronine sodium

(L-Tri-iodothyronine sodium)

● **INDICATIONS AND DOSE**

Hypothyroidism
▸ BY MOUTH
▸ Adult: Initially 10–20 micrograms daily; increased to
60 micrograms daily in 2–3 divided doses, dose should
be increased gradually, smaller initial doses given for
the elderly

Hypothyroid coma
▸ BY SLOW INTRAVENOUS INJECTION
▸ Adult: 5–20 micrograms every 12 hours, increased to
5–20 micrograms every 4 hours if required,
alternatively initially 50 micrograms for 1 dose, then
25 micrograms every 8 hours, reduced to
25 micrograms twice daily

DOSE EQUIVALENCE AND CONVERSION
▸ 20–25 micrograms of liothyronine sodium is equivalent
to approximately 100 micrograms of levothyroxine
sodium.
▸ Brands without a UK licence may not be bioequivalent
and dose adjustment may be necessary.

● CONTRA-INDICATIONS Thyrotoxicosis

● CAUTIONS Cardiovascular disorders · diabetes insipidus ·
diabetes mellitus (dose of antidiabetic drugs including
insulin may need to be increased) · elderly · hypertension ·
long-standing hypothyroidism · myocardial infarction ·
myocardial insufficiency · panhypopituitarism (initiate
corticosteroid therapy before starting liothyronine) ·

predisposition to adrenal insufficiency (initiate
corticosteroid therapy before starting liothyronine)

CAUTIONS, FURTHER INFORMATION
▸ Cardiovascular disorders Baseline ECG is valuable because
changes induced by hypothyroidism can be confused with
ischaemia.

● INTERACTIONS → Appendix 1: thyroid hormones

● SIDE-EFFECTS

GENERAL SIDE-EFFECTS
▸ **Rare or very rare** Alopecia · angina pectoris (more common
at excessive dosage) · arrhythmia (more common at
excessive dosage) · diarrhoea (more common at excessive
dosage) · heat intolerance · muscle cramps · muscle
weakness · palpitations (more common at excessive
dosage) · tachycardia (more common at excessive dosage) ·
vomiting (more common at excessive dosage)
▸ **Frequency not known** Agitation · fever · flushing · headache
· hyperhidrosis · insomnia (more common at excessive
dosage) · oedema · restlessness (more common at excessive
dosage) · skin reactions · tremor (more common at
excessive dosage) · weight decreased

SPECIFIC SIDE-EFFECTS
▸ **Rare or very rare**
▸ With intravenous use Menstruation irregular

SIDE-EFFECTS, FURTHER INFORMATION Initial dosage in
patients with cardiovascular disorders —if metabolism
increases too rapidly (causing diarrhoea, nervousness,
rapid pulse, insomnia, tremors and sometimes anginal
pain where there is latent myocardial ischaemia), reduce
dose or withhold for 1–2 days and start again at a lower
dose.

● PREGNANCY Does not cross the placenta in significant
amounts. Excessive or insufficient maternal thyroid
hormones can be detrimental to fetus.
Dose adjustments Liothyronine requirement may increase
during pregnancy.
Monitoring Assess maternal thyroid function before
conception (if possible), at diagnosis of pregnancy, at
antenatal booking, during both the second and third
trimesters, and after delivery (more frequent monitoring
required on initiation or adjustment of liothyronine).

● BREAST FEEDING Amount too small to affect tests for
neonatal hypothyroidism.

● PRESCRIBING AND DISPENSING INFORMATION
Switching to a different brand Patients switched to a different
brand should be monitored (particularly if pregnant or if
heart disease present) as brands without a UK licence may
not be bioequivalent. Pregnant women or those with heart
disease should undergo an early review of thyroid status,
and other patients should have thyroid function assessed if
experiencing a significant change in symptoms. If
liothyronine is continued long-term, thyroid function tests
should be repeated 1–2 months after any change in brand.

● MEDICINAL FORMS
There can be variation in the licensing of different medicines
containing the same drug. Forms available from special-order
manufacturers include: tablet, capsule, oral suspension, oral
solution, solution for injection
Tablet
▸ Liothyronine sodium (Non-proprietary)
Liothyronine sodium 20 microgram Liothyronine 20microgram
tablets | 28 tablet [PoM] £258.20 DT = £246.69
▸ Iraksin (Morningside Healthcare Ltd)
Liothyronine sodium 20 microgram Iraksin 20microgram tablets |
28 tablet [PoM] £249.98 DT = £246.69
Powder for solution for injection
▸ Liothyronine sodium (Non-proprietary)
Liothyronine sodium 20 microgram Liothyronine 20microgram
powder for solution for injection vials | 5 vial [PoM] £1,425.00

Chapter 7
Genito-urinary system

CONTENTS

1 Bladder and urinary disorders

1.1 Urinary frequency, enuresis, and incontinence

Urinary frequency, enuresis and incontinence

Urinary frequency and incontinence

Incontinence in adults which arises from detrusor instability is managed by combining drug therapy with conservative methods for managing urge incontinence such as pelvic floor exercises and bladder training; stress incontinence is generally managed by non-drug methods. Duloxetine p. 364 can be added and is licensed for the treatment of moderate to severe stress incontinence in women; it may be more effective when used as an adjunct to pelvic floor exercises.

Antimuscarinic drugs reduce symptoms of urgency and urge incontinence and increase bladder capacity. Oxybutynin hydrochloride p. 760 also has a direct relaxant effect on urinary smooth muscle. Side-effects limit the use of oxybutynin hydrochloride, but they may be reduced by starting at a lower dose. A modified-release preparation of oxybutynin hydrochloride is effective and has fewer side-effects; a transdermal patch is also available. The efficacy and side-effects of tolterodine tartrate p. 762 are comparable to those of modified-release oxybutynin hydrochloride. Flavoxate hydrochloride p. 760 has less marked side-effects but it is also less effective. Darifenacin p. 759, fesoterodine fumarate p. 759, propiverine hydrochloride p. 762, solifenacin succinate p. 761, and trospium chloride p. 761 are newer antimuscarinic drugs licensed for urinary frequency, urgency, and incontinence. The need for continuing antimuscarinic drug therapy should be reviewed every 4–6 weeks until symptoms stabilise, and then every 6–12 months.

Propantheline bromide p. 85 and tricyclic antidepressants were used for urge incontinence but they are little used now because of their side-effects. The use of imipramine hydrochloride p. 372 is limited by its potential to cause cardiac side-effects.

Mirabegron p. 763, a selective beta$_3$ agonist, is licensed for the treatment of urinary frequency, urgency, and urge incontinence associated with overactive bladder syndrome.

Purified bovine collagen implant (*Contigen*®, Bard) is indicated for *urinary incontinence* caused by intrinsic sphincter deficiency (poor or non-functioning bladder outlet mechanism). The implant should be inserted only by surgeons or physicians trained in the technique for injection of the implant.

See also Nocturnal enuresis in children below.

Nocturnal enuresis in children

23-May-2017

Description of condition

Nocturnal enuresis is the involuntary discharge of urine during sleep, which is common in young children. Children are generally expected to be dry by a developmental age of 5 years, and historically it has been common practice to consider children for treatment only when they reach 7 years; however, symptoms may still persist in a small proportion by the age of 10 years.

Treatment

Children under 5 years

EvGr For children under 5 years, treatment is usually unnecessary as the condition is likely to resolve spontaneously. Reassurance and advice can be useful for some families. ⒶⒸ

Non Drug Treatment

EvGr Initially, advice should be given on fluid intake, diet, toileting behaviour, and use of reward systems. For children who do not respond to this advice (more than 1–2 wet beds per week), an enuresis alarm should be the recommended treatment for motivated, well-supported children. Alarms in children under 7 years should be considered depending on the child's maturity, motivation and understanding of the alarm. Alarms have a lower relapse rate than drug treatment when discontinued.

Treatment using an alarm should be reviewed after 4 weeks and continued until a minimum of 2 weeks' uninterrupted dry nights have been achieved. If complete dryness is not achieved after 3 months but the condition is still improving and the child remains motivated to use the alarm, it is recommended to continue the treatment. Combined treatment with desmopressin p. 653, or the use of desmopressin alone, is recommended if the initial alarm treatment is unsuccessful or it is no longer appropriate or desirable. Ⓐ

Drug Treatment

EvGr Treatment with oral or sublingual desmopressin is recommended for children over 5 years of age when alarm use is inappropriate or undesirable, or when rapid or short-term results are the priority (for example, to cover periods away from home). Desmopressin alone can also be used if there has been a partial response to a combination of desmopressin and an alarm following initial treatment with an alarm alone. Treatment should be assessed after 4 weeks and continued for 3 months if there are signs of response. Repeated courses of desmopressin can be used in responsive children who experience repeated recurrences of bedwetting, but should be withdrawn **gradually** at regular intervals (for 1 week every 3 months) for full reassessment.

Under specialist supervision, nocturnal enuresis associated with daytime symptoms (overactive bladder) can be managed with desmopressin alone or in combination with an antimuscarinic drug (such as oxybutynin hydrochloride p. 760 or tolterodine tartrate p. 762 [unlicensed indication]). Treatment should be continued for 3 months; the course can be repeated if necessary.

The tricyclic antidepressant imipramine hydrochloride p. 372 can be considered for children who have not responded to all other treatments and have undergone specialist assessment, however relapse is common after withdrawal and children and their carers should be aware of the dangers of overdose. Initial treatment should continue for 3 months; further courses can be considered following a medical review every 3 months. Tricyclic antidepressants should be withdrawn gradually. Ⓐ

Useful Resources

Bedwetting in under 19s. National Institute for Health and Care Excellence. Clinical guideline CG111. October 2010. www.nice.org.uk/guidance/cg111

ANTIMUSCARINICS

Antimuscarinics (systemic) ⊖

- **CONTRA-INDICATIONS** Gastro-intestinal obstruction · intestinal atony · myasthenia gravis (but some antimuscarinics may be used to decrease muscarinic side-effects of anticholinesterases) · paralytic ileus · prostatic enlargement (in adults) · pyloric stenosis · severe ulcerative colitis · significant bladder outflow obstruction · toxic megacolon · urinary retention
- **CAUTIONS** Acute myocardial infarction (in adults) · arrhythmias (may be worsened) · autonomic neuropathy · cardiac insufficiency (due to association with tachycardia) · cardiac surgery (due to association with tachycardia) · children (increased risk of side-effects) · conditions characterised by tachycardia · congestive heart failure (may be worsened) · coronary artery disease (may be worsened) · diarrhoea · elderly (especially if frail) · gastro-oesophageal reflux disease · hiatus hernia with reflux oesophagitis · hypertension · hyperthyroidism (due to association with tachycardia) · individuals susceptible to

angle-closure glaucoma · prostatic hyperplasia (in adults) · pyrexia · ulcerative colitis

- **SIDE-EFFECTS**
- ▸ **Common or very common** Constipation · dizziness · drowsiness · dry mouth · dyspepsia · flushing · headache · nausea · palpitations · skin reactions · tachycardia · urinary disorders · vision disorders · vomiting
- ▸ **Uncommon** Angioedema
- ▸ **Rare or very rare** Confusion (more common in elderly)
- **PATIENT AND CARER ADVICE**
  Driving and skilled tasks Antimuscarinics can affect the performance of skilled tasks (e.g. driving).

ANTIMUSCARINICS ⟩ URINARY
⏍ above

Darifenacin

- **INDICATIONS AND DOSE**

  Urinary frequency | Urinary urgency | Incontinence
  - ▸ BY MOUTH
  - ▸ Adult: Initially 7.5 mg once daily, increased if necessary to 15 mg after 2 weeks

- **INTERACTIONS** → Appendix 1: darifenacin
- **SIDE-EFFECTS**
- ▸ **Common or very common** Abdominal pain · dry eye · nasal dryness
- ▸ **Uncommon** Asthenia · bladder pain · cough · diarrhoea · dyspnoea · erectile dysfunction · flatulence · hyperhidrosis · hypertension · increased risk of infection · injury · insomnia · oedema · oral ulceration · pruritus · taste altered · thinking abnormal · urinary tract disorder · visual impairment
- **PREGNANCY** Manufacturer advises avoid—toxicity in *animal* studies.
- **BREAST FEEDING** Present in milk in *animal* studies—manufacturer advises caution.
- **HEPATIC IMPAIRMENT** Avoid in severe impairment.
  Dose adjustments Max. 7.5 mg daily in moderate impairment.
- **PRESCRIBING AND DISPENSING INFORMATION** The need for continuing therapy for urinary incontinence should be reviewed every 4–6 weeks until symptoms stabilise, and then every 6–12 months.

- **MEDICINAL FORMS**
  There can be variation in the licensing of different medicines containing the same drug.
  Modified-release tablet
  CAUTIONARY AND ADVISORY LABELS 3, 25
  - ▸ Emselex (Merus Labs Luxco S.a R.L.)
    Darifenacin (as Darifenacin hydrobromide) 7.5 mg Emselex 7.5mg modified-release tablets | 28 tablet [PoM] £25.48 DT = £25.48
    Darifenacin (as Darifenacin hydrobromide) 15 mg Emselex 15mg modified-release tablets | 28 tablet [PoM] £25.48
⏍ above

Fesoterodine fumarate
08-May-2017

- **INDICATIONS AND DOSE**

  Urinary frequency | Urinary urgency | Urge incontinence
  - ▸ BY MOUTH
  - ▸ Adult: 4 mg once daily, increased if necessary up to 8 mg once daily

  DOSE ADJUSTMENTS DUE TO INTERACTIONS
  - ▸ Manufacturer advises max. 4 mg daily with concurrent use of potent inhibitors of CYP3A4; avoid concurrent use in patients who also have hepatic or renal impairment.
continued →

7

Genito-urinary system

▸ For dose adjustments with concurrent use of moderate inhibitors of CYP3A4 in patients with hepatic or renal impairment, consult product literature.

● INTERACTIONS → Appendix 1: fesoterodine
● SIDE-EFFECTS
▸ **Common or very common** Diarrhoea · dry eye · gastrointestinal discomfort · insomnia · throat complaints
▸ **Uncommon** Cough · fatigue · gastrointestinal disorders · nasal dryness · taste altered · urinary disorders · urinary tract infection · vertigo
● PREGNANCY Manufacturer advises avoid—toxicity in *animal* studies.
● BREAST FEEDING Manufacturer advises avoid—no information available.
● HEPATIC IMPAIRMENT Manufacturer advises avoid in severe impairment.
Dose adjustments Manufacturer advises increase dose cautiously in mild impairment; max. 4 mg daily in moderate impairment.
● RENAL IMPAIRMENT
Dose adjustments Increase dose cautiously if eGFR 30–80 mL/minute/1.73m^2; max. 4 mg daily if eGFR less than 30 mL/minute/1.73m^2.
● PRESCRIBING AND DISPENSING INFORMATION The need for continuing therapy for urinary incontinence should be reviewed every 4–6 weeks until symptoms stabilise, and then every 6–12 months.
● NATIONAL FUNDING/ACCESS DECISIONS
Scottish Medicines Consortium (SMC) Decisions
The *Scottish Medicines Consortium* has advised (June 2008) that fesoterodine (*Toviaz*®) is accepted for restricted use within NHS Scotland as a second-line treatment for overactive bladder syndrome.
● MEDICINAL FORMS
There can be variation in the licensing of different medicines containing the same drug.
Modified-release tablet
CAUTIONARY AND ADVISORY LABELS 3, 25
▸ Toviaz (Pfizer Ltd)
Fesoterodine fumarate 4 mg Toviaz 4mg modified-release tablets | 28 tablet [PoM] £25.78 DT = £25.78
Fesoterodine fumarate 8 mg Toviaz 8mg modified-release tablets | 28 tablet [PoM] £25.78 DT = £25.78

▶ 759

Flavoxate hydrochloride

● INDICATIONS AND DOSE
Urinary frequency | Urinary incontinence | Dysuria | Urinary urgency | Bladder spasm due to catheterisation, cytoscopy, or surgery
▸ BY MOUTH
▸ Adult: 200 mg 3 times a day

● CONTRA-INDICATIONS Gastro-intestinal haemorrhage
● INTERACTIONS → Appendix 1: flavoxate
● SIDE-EFFECTS Diarrhoea · dysphagia · eosinophilia · fatigue · hyperpyrexia · hypersensitivity · leucopenia · nervousness · vertigo
● PREGNANCY Manufacturer advises avoid unless no safer alternative.
● BREAST FEEDING Manufacturer advises caution—no information available.
● PRESCRIBING AND DISPENSING INFORMATION The need for continuing therapy for urinary incontinence should be reviewed every 4–6 weeks until symptoms stabilise, and then every 6–12 months.

● MEDICINAL FORMS
There can be variation in the licensing of different medicines containing the same drug. Forms available from special-order manufacturers include: oral suspension, oral solution
Tablet
CAUTIONARY AND ADVISORY LABELS 3
▸ Urispas (Recordati Pharmaceuticals Ltd)
Flavoxate hydrochloride 200 mg Urispas 200 tablets | 90 tablet [PoM] £11.67 DT = £11.67

▶ 759

Oxybutynin hydrochloride

● INDICATIONS AND DOSE
Urinary frequency | Urinary urgency | Urinary incontinence | Neurogenic bladder instability
▸ BY MOUTH USING IMMEDIATE-RELEASE MEDICINES
▸ Child 5–11 years: Initially 2.5–3 mg twice daily, increased to 5 mg 2–3 times a day
▸ Child 12–17 years: Initially 5 mg 2–3 times a day, increased if necessary up to 5 mg 4 times a day
▸ Adult: Initially 5 mg 2–3 times a day, increased if necessary up to 5 mg 4 times a day
▸ Elderly: Initially 2.5–3 mg twice daily, increased if tolerated to 5 mg twice daily, adjusted according to response
▸ BY MOUTH USING MODIFIED-RELEASE TABLETS
▸ Child 5–17 years: Initially 5 mg once daily, adjusted in steps of 5 mg every week, adjusted according to response; maximum 15 mg per day
▸ Adult: Initially 5 mg once daily, increased in steps of 5 mg every week, adjusted according to response; maximum 20 mg per day

Urinary frequency | Urinary urgency | Urinary incontinence
▸ BY TRANSDERMAL APPLICATION USING PATCHES
▸ Adult: Apply 1 patch twice weekly, patch is to be applied to clean, dry unbroken skin on abdomen, hip or buttock. Patch should be removed every 3–4 days and site replacement patch on a different area. The same area should be avoided for 7 days

Nocturnal enuresis associated with overactive bladder
▸ BY MOUTH USING IMMEDIATE-RELEASE MEDICINES
▸ Child 5–17 years: 2.5–3 mg twice daily, increased to 5 mg 2–3 times a day, last dose to be taken before bedtime
▸ BY MOUTH USING MODIFIED-RELEASE TABLETS
▸ Child 5–17 years: Initially 5 mg once daily, adjusted in steps of 5 mg every week, adjusted according to response; maximum 15 mg per day

DOSE EQUIVALENCE AND CONVERSION
▸ Patients taking immediate-release oxybutynin may be transferred to the nearest equivalent daily dose of *Lyrinel*® XL

● CAUTIONS Acute porphyrias p. 1025
● INTERACTIONS → Appendix 1: oxybutynin
● SIDE-EFFECTS
GENERAL SIDE-EFFECTS
▸ **Common or very common** Diarrhoea
▸ **Uncommon** Urticaria
SPECIFIC SIDE-EFFECTS
▸ **Common or very common**
▸ With oral use Dry eye
▸ With transdermal use Gastrointestinal discomfort · increased risk of infection
▸ **Uncommon**
▸ With oral use Abdominal discomfort · appetite decreased · dysphagia
▸ With transdermal use Back pain · hot flush · injury

▶ **Frequency not known**
▶ With oral use Anxiety · arrhythmia · cognitive disorder · depressive symptom · disorientation · drug dependence · gastrointestinal disorders · glaucoma · hallucination · heat stroke · hypohidrosis · mydriasis · nightmare · paranoia · photosensitivity reaction · seizure · urinary tract infection

● PREGNANCY Manufacturers advise avoid unless essential—toxicity in *animal* studies.

● BREAST FEEDING Manufacturers advise avoid—present in milk in *animal* studies.

● HEPATIC IMPAIRMENT Manufacturer advises caution.

● RENAL IMPAIRMENT Manufacturer advises caution.

● DIRECTIONS FOR ADMINISTRATION Apply patches to clean, dry, unbroken skin on abdomen, hip or buttock, remove after every 3–4 days and site replacement patch on a different area (avoid using same area for 7 days).

● PRESCRIBING AND DISPENSING INFORMATION
▶ In adults The need for continuing therapy for urinary incontinence should be reviewed every 4–6 weeks until symptoms stabilise, and then every 6–12 months.
▶ In children The need for therapy for urinary indications should be reviewed soon after it has been commenced and then at regular intervals; a response usually occurs within 6 months but may take longer.

● PATIENT AND CARER ADVICE
Medicines for Children leaflet: Oxybutynin for daytime urinary symptoms www.medicinesforchildren.org.uk/oxybutynin-for-daytime-urinary-symptoms
Patients or carers should be given advice on how to administer oxybutynin transdermal patches.

● NATIONAL FUNDING/ACCESS DECISIONS
Scottish Medicines Consortium (SMC) Decisions
The *Scottish Medicines Consortium* has advised (July 2005) that *Kentera*® should be restricted for use in patients who benefit from oral oxybutynin but cannot tolerate its side-effects.

● MEDICINAL FORMS
There can be variation in the licensing of different medicines containing the same drug. Forms available from special-order manufacturers include: oral suspension, oral solution

Modified-release tablet
CAUTIONARY AND ADVISORY LABELS 3, 25
▶ Lyrinel XL (Janssen-Cilag Ltd)
Oxybutynin hydrochloride 5 mg Lyrinel XL 5mg tablets |
30 tablet PoM £13.77 DT = £13.77
Oxybutynin hydrochloride 10 mg Lyrinel XL 10mg tablets |
30 tablet PoM £27.54 DT = £27.54

Tablet
CAUTIONARY AND ADVISORY LABELS 3
▶ Oxybutynin hydrochloride (Non-proprietary)
Oxybutynin hydrochloride 2.5 mg Oxybutynin 2.5mg tablets |
56 tablet PoM £14.40 DT = £0.84 | 84 tablet PoM £3.84-£21.60
Oxybutynin hydrochloride 3 mg Oxybutynin 3mg tablets |
56 tablet PoM £16.80 DT = £16.80
Oxybutynin hydrochloride 5 mg Oxybutynin 5mg tablets |
56 tablet PoM £23.40 DT = £1.19 | 84 tablet PoM £4.75-£20.77
▶ Cystrin (Zentiva)
Oxybutynin hydrochloride 5 mg Cystrin 5mg tablets |
84 tablet PoM £21.99
▶ Ditropan (Sanofi)
Oxybutynin hydrochloride 2.5 mg Ditropan 2.5mg tablets |
84 tablet PoM £1.60
Oxybutynin hydrochloride 5 mg Ditropan 5mg tablets |
84 tablet PoM £2.90

Oral solution
CAUTIONARY AND ADVISORY LABELS 3
▶ Oxybutynin hydrochloride (Non-proprietary)
Oxybutynin hydrochloride 500 microgram per 1 ml Oxybutynin 2.5mg/5ml oral solution sugar free sugar-free | 150 ml PoM £154.50-£214.85 DT = £184.68
Oxybutynin hydrochloride 1 mg per 1 ml Oxybutynin 5mg/5ml oral solution sugar free sugar-free | 150 ml PoM £199.20 DT = £199.20

Transdermal patch
CAUTIONARY AND ADVISORY LABELS 3
▶ Kentera (Orion Pharma (UK) Ltd)
Oxybutynin 3.9 mg per 24 hour Kentera 3.9mg/24hours patches |
8 patch PoM £27.20 DT = £27.20

⚑ 759

Solifenacin succinate

● INDICATIONS AND DOSE
Urinary frequency | Urinary urgency | Urinary incontinence
▶ BY MOUTH
▶ Adult: 5 mg once daily, increased if necessary to 10 mg once daily
DOSE ADJUSTMENTS DUE TO INTERACTIONS
▶ Manufacturer advises max. dose 5 mg daily with concurrent use of potent inhibitors of CYP3A4; avoid concurrent use in patients who also have moderate hepatic impairment or severe renal impairment.

● CONTRA-INDICATIONS Narrow-angle glaucoma
● CAUTIONS Neurogenic bladder disorder · susceptibility to QT-interval prolongation
● INTERACTIONS → Appendix 1: solifenacin
● SIDE-EFFECTS
▶ **Common or very common** Gastrointestinal discomfort
▶ **Uncommon** Cystitis · dry eye · dry throat · fatigue · gastrointestinal disorders · nasal dryness · peripheral oedema · taste altered · urinary tract infection
▶ **Rare or very rare** Hallucination · skin reactions
▶ **Frequency not known** Anaphylactic reaction · appetite decreased · arrhythmias · delirium · dysphonia · glaucoma · hyperkalaemia · liver disorder · muscle weakness · QT interval prolongation · renal impairment

● PREGNANCY Manufacturer advises caution—no information available.

● BREAST FEEDING Manufacturer advises avoid—present in milk in *animal* studies.

● HEPATIC IMPAIRMENT Avoid in severe impairment.
Dose adjustments Max. 5 mg daily in moderate impairment.

● RENAL IMPAIRMENT
Dose adjustments Max. 5 mg daily if eGFR less than 30 mL/minute/1.73 m^2.

● PRESCRIBING AND DISPENSING INFORMATION The need for continuing therapy for urinary incontinence should be reviewed every 4–6 weeks until symptoms stabilise, and then every 6–12 months.

● MEDICINAL FORMS
There can be variation in the licensing of different medicines containing the same drug. Forms available from special-order manufacturers include: oral suspension, oral solution

Tablet
CAUTIONARY AND ADVISORY LABELS 3
▶ Vesicare (Astellas Pharma Ltd)
Solifenacin succinate 5 mg Vesicare 5mg tablets | 30 tablet PoM £27.62 DT = £27.62
Solifenacin succinate 10 mg Vesicare 10mg tablets | 30 tablet PoM £35.91 DT = £35.91

⚑ 759

Trospium chloride   11-May-2018

● INDICATIONS AND DOSE
Urinary frequency | Urinary urgency | Urge incontinence
▶ BY MOUTH USING IMMEDIATE-RELEASE MEDICINES
▶ Adult: 20 mg twice daily, to be taken before food
▶ BY MOUTH USING MODIFIED-RELEASE MEDICINES
▶ Adult: 60 mg once daily

● INTERACTIONS → Appendix 1: trospium

7

Genito-urinary system

- SIDE-EFFECTS
- ► **Common or very common** Abdominal pain
- ► **Uncommon** Chest pain · diarrhoea · flatulence
- ► **Rare or very rare** Arthralgia · asthenia · dyspnoea · myalgia · urinary disorder · vision disorder
- ► **Frequency not known** Agitation · anaphylactic reaction · hallucination · severe cutaneous adverse reactions (SCARs)
- PREGNANCY Manufacturer advises caution.
- BREAST FEEDING Manufacturer advises caution.
- HEPATIC IMPAIRMENT Manufacturer advises caution in mild to moderate impairment. Avoid in severe impairment.
- RENAL IMPAIRMENT Use with caution. Avoid *Regurin* ® XL.
  Dose adjustments Reduce dose to 20 mg once daily or 20 mg on alternate days if eGFR 10–30 mL/minute/1.73m^2.
- PRESCRIBING AND DISPENSING INFORMATION The need for continuing therapy for urinary incontinence should be reviewed every 4–6 weeks until symptoms stabilise, and then every 6–12 months.
- MEDICINAL FORMS
  There can be variation in the licensing of different medicines containing the same drug. Forms available from special-order manufacturers include: oral solution
  Modified-release capsule
  CAUTIONARY AND ADVISORY LABELS 23, 25
  ► Trospium chloride (Non-proprietary)
    Trospium chloride 60 mg Trospium chloride 60mg modified-release capsules | 28 capsule [PoM] [Ⓢ] DT = £23.05
  ► Regurin XL (Speciality European Pharma Ltd)
    Trospium chloride 60 mg Regurin XL 60mg capsules | 28 capsule [PoM] £23.05 DT = £23.05
  Tablet
  CAUTIONARY AND ADVISORY LABELS 23
  ► Trospium chloride (Non-proprietary)
    Trospium chloride 20 mg Trospium chloride 20mg tablets | 60 tablet [PoM] £9.00 DT = £8.26
  ► Flotros (Galen Ltd)
    Trospium chloride 20 mg Flotros 20mg tablets | 60 tablet [PoM] £18.20 DT = £8.26
  ► Regurin (Speciality European Pharma Ltd)
    Trospium chloride 20 mg Regurin 20mg tablets | 60 tablet [PoM] £26.00 DT = £8.26
  ► Uraplex (Speciality European Pharma Ltd)
    Trospium chloride 20 mg Uraplex 20mg tablets | 60 tablet [PoM] £26.00 DT = £8.26

ANTIMUSCARINICS > OTHER

Propiverine hydrochloride   F 759

- INDICATIONS AND DOSE
  Urinary frequency, urgency and incontinence associated with overactive bladder
  ► BY MOUTH USING IMMEDIATE-RELEASE MEDICINES
  ► Adult: 15 mg 1–2 times a day, increased if necessary up to 15 mg 3 times a day
  ► BY MOUTH USING MODIFIED-RELEASE CAPSULES
  ► Adult: 30 mg once daily
  Urinary frequency, urgency and incontinence associated with neurogenic bladder instability
  ► BY MOUTH USING IMMEDIATE-RELEASE MEDICINES
  ► Adult: 15 mg 3 times a day

- INTERACTIONS → Appendix 1: propiverine
- SIDE-EFFECTS
- ► **Common or very common** Abdominal pain · fatigue · visual impairment
- ► **Uncommon** Taste altered · tremor
- ► **Rare or very rare** Restlessness
- ► **Frequency not known** Hallucination
- PREGNANCY Manufacturer advises avoid (restriction of skeletal development in *animals*).

- BREAST FEEDING Manufacturer advises avoid—present in milk in *animal* studies.
- HEPATIC IMPAIRMENT Avoid in moderate to severe impairment.
- RENAL IMPAIRMENT Manufacturer advises caution in mild or moderate impairment.
  Dose adjustments Max. daily dose 30 mg if eGFR less than 30 mL/minute/1.73m^2.
- PRESCRIBING AND DISPENSING INFORMATION The need for continuing therapy for urinary incontinence should be reviewed every 4–6 weeks until symptoms stabilise, and then every 6–12 months.
- MEDICINAL FORMS
  There can be variation in the licensing of different medicines containing the same drug.
  Modified-release capsule
  CAUTIONARY AND ADVISORY LABELS 3, 25
  ► Detrunorm XL (AMCo)
    Propiverine hydrochloride 30 mg Detrunorm XL 30mg capsules | 28 capsule [PoM] £26.90 DT = £26.90
    Propiverine hydrochloride 45 mg Detrunorm XL 45mg capsules | 28 capsule [PoM] £29.70 DT = £29.70
  Tablet
  CAUTIONARY AND ADVISORY LABELS 3
  ► Detrunorm (AMCo)
    Propiverine hydrochloride 15 mg Detrunorm 15mg tablets | 56 tablet [PoM] £19.80 DT = £19.80

Tolterodine tartrate   F 759

- INDICATIONS AND DOSE
  Urinary frequency | Urinary urgency | Urinary incontinence
  ► BY MOUTH USING IMMEDIATE-RELEASE MEDICINES
  ► Adult: 2 mg twice daily, reduced if not tolerated to 1 mg twice daily
  ► BY MOUTH USING MODIFIED-RELEASE CAPSULES
  ► Adult: 4 mg once daily
  DOSE EQUIVALENCE AND CONVERSION
  ► Children stabilised on immediate-release tolterodine tartrate 2 mg twice daily may be transferred to modified-release tolterodine tartrate 4 mg once daily.

- CAUTIONS History of QT-interval prolongation
- INTERACTIONS → Appendix 1: tolterodine
- SIDE-EFFECTS
- ► **Common or very common** Abdominal pain · bronchitis · chest pain · diarrhoea · dry eye · fatigue · gastrointestinal disorders · paraesthesia · peripheral oedema · vertigo · visual impairment · weight increased
- ► **Uncommon** Arrhythmia · heart failure · memory loss · nervousness
- ► **Frequency not known** Disorientation · hallucination
- PREGNANCY Manufacturer advises avoid—toxicity in *animal* studies.
- BREAST FEEDING Manufacturer advises avoid—no information available.
- HEPATIC IMPAIRMENT Avoid modified-release preparations.
  Dose adjustments Reduce dose to 1 mg twice daily.
- RENAL IMPAIRMENT Avoid modified-release preparations if eGFR less than 30 mL/minute/1.73m^2.
  Dose adjustments Reduce dose to 1 mg twice daily if eGFR less than 30 mL/minute/1.73m^2.
- PRESCRIBING AND DISPENSING INFORMATION The need for continuing therapy for urinary incontinence should be reviewed every 4–6 weeks until symptoms stabilise, and then every 6–12 months.

● MEDICINAL FORMS
There can be variation in the licensing of different medicines containing the same drug. Forms available from special-order manufacturers include: oral suspension, oral solution

Tablet
CAUTIONARY AND ADVISORY LABELS 3
▸ Tolterodine tartrate (Non-proprietary)
Tolterodine tartrate 1 mg Tolterodine 1mg tablets | 56 tablet [PoM]
£29.03 DT = £1.79
Tolterodine tartrate 2 mg Tolterodine 2mg tablets | 56 tablet [PoM]
£30.56 DT = £2.09
▸ Detrusitol (Pfizer Ltd)
Tolterodine tartrate 1 mg Detrusitol 1mg tablets | 56 tablet [PoM]
£29.03 DT = £1.79
Tolterodine tartrate 2 mg Detrusitol 2mg tablets | 56 tablet [PoM]
£30.56 DT = £2.09

Modified-release capsule
CAUTIONARY AND ADVISORY LABELS 3, 25
▸ Tolterodine tartrate (Non-proprietary)
Tolterodine tartrate 2 mg Tolterodine 2mg modified-release capsules | 28 capsule [PoM] [🚗] DT = £11.60
▸ Blerone XL (Zentiva)
Tolterodine tartrate 4 mg Blerone XL 4mg capsules | 28 capsule [PoM] £25.78 DT = £25.78
▸ Detrusitol XL (Pfizer Ltd)
Tolterodine tartrate 4 mg Detrusitol XL 4mg capsules | 28 capsule [PoM] £25.78 DT = £25.78
▸ Efflosomyl XL (Mylan)
Tolterodine tartrate 4 mg Efflosomyl XL 4mg capsules | 28 capsule [PoM] £20.62 DT = £25.78
▸ Inconex XL (Sandoz Ltd)
Tolterodine tartrate 4 mg Inconex XL 4mg capsules | 28 capsule [PoM] £21.91 DT = £25.78
▸ Mariosea XL (Teva UK Ltd)
Tolterodine tartrate 2 mg Mariosea XL 2mg capsules | 28 capsule [PoM] £11.59 DT = £11.60
Tolterodine tartrate 4 mg Mariosea XL 4mg capsules | 28 capsule [PoM] £12.88 DT = £25.78
▸ Neditol XL (Aspire Pharma Ltd)
Tolterodine tartrate 2 mg Neditol XL 2mg capsules | 28 capsule [PoM] £11.60 DT = £11.60
Tolterodine tartrate 4 mg Neditol XL 4mg capsules | 28 capsule [PoM] £12.89 DT = £25.78
▸ Preblacon XL (Actavis UK Ltd)
Tolterodine tartrate 4 mg Preblacon XL 4mg capsules | 28 capsule [PoM] £25.78 DT = £25.78
▸ Santizor XL (Pfizer Ltd)
Tolterodine tartrate 4 mg Santizor XL 4mg capsules | 28 capsule [PoM] £25.78 DT = £25.78

BETA₃-ADRENOCEPTOR AGONISTS

Mirabegron

● INDICATIONS AND DOSE
Urinary frequency, urgency, and urge incontinence
▸ BY MOUTH
▸ **Adult:** 50 mg once daily
DOSE ADJUSTMENTS DUE TO INTERACTIONS
▸ Manufacturer advises reduce dose to 25 mg once daily in patients with mild hepatic impairment with concurrent use of potent inhibitors of CYP3A4; avoid in moderate impairment.
▸ Manufacturer advises reduce dose to 25 mg once daily if eGFR 30–89 mL/minute/1.73 m² with concurrent use of potent inhibitors of CYP3A4; avoid if eGFR less than 30 mL/minute/1.73 m².

● CONTRA-INDICATIONS Severe uncontrolled hypertension (systolic blood pressure ≥180 mmHg or diastolic blood pressure ≥110 mmHg)
● CAUTIONS History of QT-interval prolongation · stage 2 hypertension
● INTERACTIONS → Appendix 1: mirabegron

● SIDE-EFFECTS
▸ **Common or very common** Arrhythmias · constipation · diarrhoea · dizziness · headache · increased risk of infection · nausea
▸ **Uncommon** Cystitis · dyspepsia · gastritis · joint swelling · palpitations · skin reactions · vulvovaginal pruritus
▸ **Rare or very rare** Angioedema · eyelid oedema · hypersensitivity vasculitis · hypertensive crisis · lip swelling · urinary retention
▸ **Frequency not known** Insomnia
● CONCEPTION AND CONTRACEPTION Contraception advised in women of child-bearing potential.
● PREGNANCY Avoid—toxicity in *animal* studies.
● BREAST FEEDING Avoid—present in milk in *animal* studies.
● HEPATIC IMPAIRMENT Avoid in severe impairment—no information available.
Dose adjustments Reduce dose to 25 mg once daily in moderate impairment.
● RENAL IMPAIRMENT Avoid if eGFR less than 15 mL/minute/1.73 m²—no information available.
Dose adjustments Reduce dose to 25 mg once daily if eGFR 15–29 mL/minute/1.73 m².
● MONITORING REQUIREMENTS Blood pressure should be monitored before starting treatment and regularly during treatment, especially in patients with pre-existing hypertension.
● NATIONAL FUNDING/ACCESS DECISIONS
NICE decisions
▸ **Mirabegron for treating symptoms of overactive bladder (June 2013)** NICE TA290
Mirabegron is recommended as an option only for patients in whom antimuscarinic drugs are ineffective, contra-indicated, or not tolerated; patients currently receiving mirabegron who do not meet these criteria should have the option to continue until they and their clinician consider it appropriate to stop.
www.nice.org.uk/TA290

● MEDICINAL FORMS
There can be variation in the licensing of different medicines containing the same drug.
Modified-release tablet
CAUTIONARY AND ADVISORY LABELS 25
▸ Betmiga (Astellas Pharma Ltd)
Mirabegron 25 mg Betmiga 25mg modified-release tablets | 30 tablet [PoM] £29.00 DT = £29.00
Mirabegron 50 mg Betmiga 50mg modified-release tablets | 30 tablet [PoM] £29.00 DT = £29.00

1.2 Urinary retention

Urinary retention

31-May-2017

Description of condition

Urinary retention is the inability to voluntarily urinate. It may be secondary to urethral blockage, drug treatment (such as use of antimuscarinic drugs, sympathomimetics, tricyclic antidepressants), conditions that reduce detrusor contractions or interfere with relaxation of the urethra, neurogenic causes, or it may occur postpartum or postoperatively.

Acute urinary retention is a medical emergency characterised by the abrupt development of the inability to pass urine (over a period of hours).

Chronic urinary retention is the gradual (over months or years) development of the inability to empty the bladder completely, characterised by a residual volume greater than one litre or associated with the presence of a distended or palpable bladder.

Urinary retention due to benign prostatic hyperplasia
The most common cause of urinary retention in men is benign prostatic hyperplasia. Men with an enlarged prostate can have lower urinary tract symptoms associated with obstruction, such as urinary retention (acute or chronic), frequency, urgency or nocturia.

Treatment
Treatment of urinary retention depends on the underlying condition. Catheterisation is used to relieve acute painful urinary retention or when no cause can be found. Surgical procedures or dilatation are often used to correct mechanical outflow obstructions.

Acute urinary retention
[EvGr] Acute retention is painful and requires immediate treatment by catheterisation. Before the catheter is removed an alpha-adrenoceptor blocker (such as alfuzosin hydrochloride below, doxazosin p. 765, tamsulosin hydrochloride p. 767, prazosin p. 766, indoramin p. 766 or terazosin p. 768) should be given for at least two days to manage acute urinary retention ⚠.

Chronic urinary retention
[EvGr] In patients with chronic urinary retention, intermittent bladder catheterisation should be offered before an indwelling catheter. Catheters may be used as a long-term solution where persistent urinary retention is causing incontinence, infection, or renal dysfunction and a surgical solution is not feasible. ⚠ Their use is associated with an increased risk of adverse events including recurrent urinary infections, trauma to the urethra, pain, and stone formation.

[EvGr] In men who have symptoms that are bothersome, drug treatment should only be offered when other conservative management options have failed. Men with moderate-to-severe symptoms should be offered an alpha-adrenoceptor blocker (alfuzosin hydrochloride, doxazosin, tamsulosin hydrochloride or terazosin). Treatment should initially be reviewed after 4–6 weeks and then every 6–12 months. ⚠

The parasympathomimetic bethanechol chloride p. 768 increases detrusor muscle contraction. It is licensed for acute postoperative, postpartum and neurogenic urinary retention but its use has largely been superseded by catheterisation.

Urinary retention due to benign prostatic hyperplasia
In patients with benign prostatic hyperplasia, treatment is influenced by the severity of symptoms and their effect on the patient's quality of life. [EvGr] Watchful waiting is suitable for men with symptoms that are not troublesome and in those who have not yet developed complications of benign prostatic hyperplasia such as renal impairment, urinary retention or recurrent infection.

The recommended treatment of benign prostatic hyperplasia is usually an alpha-adrenoceptor blocker. The alpha$_1$-selective adrenoceptor blockers relax smooth muscle in benign prostatic hyperplasia producing an increase in urinary flow-rate and an improvement in obstructive symptoms.

In patients with an enlarged prostate, a raised prostate specific antigen concentration, and who are considered to be at high risk of progression (such as the elderly), a 5α-reductase inhibitor (such as finasteride p. 769 or dutasteride p. 769) should be used. A combination of an alpha-adrenoceptor blocker and a 5α-reductase inhibitor can be offered if symptoms remain a problem.

Surgery is recommended for men with more severe symptoms that do not respond to drug therapy, or who have complications such as acute urinary retention, haematuria, renal failure, bladder calculi or recurrent urinary-tract infection. ⚠

Related drugs
Other drugs used for urinary retention: neostigmine p. 1090, pyridostigmine bromide p. 1091.

Useful Resources
Lower urinary tract symptoms in men. National Institute for Health and Care Excellence. Clinical guideline CG97. May 2010 (updated June 2015).
www.nice.org.uk/guidance/cg97

ALPHA-ADRENOCEPTOR BLOCKERS

Alfuzosin hydrochloride

- ● **INDICATIONS AND DOSE**
  Benign prostatic hyperplasia
  - ▶ BY MOUTH USING IMMEDIATE-RELEASE MEDICINES
    - ▸ Adult: 2.5 mg 3 times a day; maximum 10 mg per day
    - ▸ Elderly: Initially 2.5 mg twice daily, adjusted according to response; maximum 10 mg per day
  - ▶ BY MOUTH USING MODIFIED-RELEASE MEDICINES
    - ▸ Adult: 10 mg once daily

  Acute urinary retention associated with benign prostatic hyperplasia
  - ▶ BY MOUTH USING MODIFIED-RELEASE TABLETS
    - ▸ Elderly: 10 mg once daily for 2–3 days during catheterisation and for one day after removal; max. 4 days

- ● CONTRA-INDICATIONS Avoid if history micturition syncope · avoid if history of postural hypotension

- ● CAUTIONS Acute heart failure · concomitant antihypertensives (reduced dosage and specialist supervision may be required) · discontinue if angina worsens · elderly · history of QT-interval prolongation · patients undergoing cataract surgery (risk of intra-operative floppy iris syndrome)

- ● INTERACTIONS → Appendix 1: alpha blockers

- ● SIDE-EFFECTS
  - ▶ **Common or very common** Asthenia · diarrhoea · dizziness · dry mouth · headache · malaise · nausea · postural hypotension · vertigo · vomiting
  - ▶ **Uncommon** Abdominal pain · arrhythmias · chest pain · drowsiness · flushing · oedema · palpitations · rhinitis · skin reactions · syncope · visual impairment
  - ▶ **Rare or very rare** Angina pectoris · angioedema
  - ▶ **Frequency not known** Cerebral ischaemia · floppy iris syndrome · hepatic disorders · neutropenia · priapism · thrombocytopenia

  SIDE-EFFECTS, FURTHER INFORMATION First dose may cause collapse due to hypotensive effect (therefore should be taken on retiring to bed). Patient should be warned to lie down if symptoms such as dizziness, fatigue or sweating develop, and to remain lying down until they abate completely.

- ● HEPATIC IMPAIRMENT Avoid modified-release preparations.
  Dose adjustments Initial dose 2.5 mg once daily, adjusted according to response to 2.5 mg twice daily in mild to moderate impairment—avoid if severe.

- ● RENAL IMPAIRMENT Manufacturers advise avoid use of modified-release preparations if eGFR less than 30 mL/minute/1.73 m^2 as limited experience.
  Dose adjustments Initial dose 2.5 mg twice daily and adjust according to response.

- ● PATIENT AND CARER ADVICE Patient should be counselled on the first dose effect.
  Driving and skilled tasks May affect performance of skilled tasks e.g. driving.

● MEDICINAL FORMS
There can be variation in the licensing of different medicines containing the same drug. Forms available from special-order manufacturers include: oral solution

Modified-release tablet
CAUTIONARY AND ADVISORY LABELS 21, 25
‣ Alfuzosin hydrochloride (Non-proprietary)
Alfuzosin hydrochloride 10 mg Alfuzosin 10mg modified-release tablets | 30 tablet [PoM] [Ⓢ] DT = £12.51
‣ Besavar XL (Zentiva)
Alfuzosin hydrochloride 10 mg Besavar XL 10mg tablets | 30 tablet [PoM] £12.51 DT = £12.51
‣ Fuzatal XL (Teva UK Ltd)
Alfuzosin hydrochloride 10 mg Fuzatal XL 10mg tablets | 30 tablet [PoM] £12.76 DT = £12.51
‣ Vasran XL (Ranbaxy (UK) Ltd)
Alfuzosin hydrochloride 10 mg Vasran XL 10mg tablets | 30 tablet [PoM] £11.48 DT = £12.51
‣ Xatral XL (Sanofi)
Alfuzosin hydrochloride 10 mg Xatral XL 10mg tablets | 30 tablet [PoM] £12.51 DT = £12.51
‣ Zochek (Aurobindo Pharma Ltd)
Alfuzosin hydrochloride 10 mg Zochek 10mg modified-release tablets | 30 tablet [PoM] £1.47 DT = £12.51

Tablet
‣ Alfuzosin hydrochloride (Non-proprietary)
Alfuzosin hydrochloride 2.5 mg Alfuzosin 2.5mg tablets | 60 tablet [PoM] £21.20 DT = £1.54
‣ Xatral (Sanofi)
Alfuzosin hydrochloride 2.5 mg Xatral 2.5mg tablets | 60 tablet [PoM] £20.37 DT = £1.54

Doxazosin

● INDICATIONS AND DOSE

Hypertension
‣ BY MOUTH USING IMMEDIATE-RELEASE MEDICINES
‣ Adult: Initially 1 mg once daily for 1–2 weeks, then increased to 2 mg once daily, then increased if necessary to 4 mg once daily; maximum 16 mg per day
‣ BY MOUTH USING MODIFIED-RELEASE MEDICINES
‣ Adult: Initially 4 mg once daily, dose can be adjusted after 4 weeks, then increased if necessary to 8 mg once daily

Benign prostatic hyperplasia
‣ BY MOUTH USING IMMEDIATE-RELEASE MEDICINES
‣ Adult: Initially 1 mg daily, dose may be doubled at intervals of 1–2 weeks according to response; usual maintenance 2–4 mg daily; maximum 8 mg per day
‣ BY MOUTH USING MODIFIED-RELEASE MEDICINES
‣ Adult: Initially 4 mg once daily, dose can be adjusted after 4 weeks, then increased if necessary to 8 mg once daily

DOSE EQUIVALENCE AND CONVERSION
‣ Patients stabilised on immediate-release doxazosin can be transferred to the equivalent dose of modified-release doxazosin.

● CONTRA-INDICATIONS History of micturition syncope (in patients with benign prostatic hypertrophy) · history of postural hypotension · monotherapy in patients with overflow bladder or anuria
● CAUTIONS Care with initial dose (postural hypotension) · cataract surgery (risk of intra-operative floppy iris syndrome) · elderly · heart failure · pulmonary oedema due to aortic or mitral stenosis
● INTERACTIONS → Appendix 1: alpha blockers
● SIDE-EFFECTS
‣ Common or very common Arrhythmias · asthenia · chest pain · cough · cystitis · dizziness · drowsiness · dry mouth · dyspnoea · gastrointestinal discomfort · headache · hypotension · increased risk of infection · influenza like

illness · muscle complaints · nausea · oedema · pain · palpitations · skin reactions · urinary disorders · vertigo
‣ Uncommon Angina pectoris · anxiety · appetite abnormal · arthralgia · constipation · depression · diarrhoea · gastrointestinal disorders · gout · haemorrhage · insomnia · myocardial infarction · sensation abnormal · sexual dysfunction · stroke · syncope · tinnitus · tremor · vomiting · weight increased
‣ Rare or very rare Alopecia · bronchospasm · flushing · gynaecomastia · hepatic disorders · leucopenia · malaise · muscle weakness · thrombocytopenia · vision blurred
‣ Frequency not known Floppy iris syndrome
● PREGNANCY No evidence of teratogenicity; manufacturers advise use only when potential benefit outweighs risk.
● BREAST FEEDING Accumulates in milk in *animal* studies—manufacturer advises avoid.
● HEPATIC IMPAIRMENT Use with caution. Manufacturer advises avoid in severe impairment—no information available.
● PATIENT AND CARER ADVICE Patient counselling is advised for doxazosin tablets (initial dose).
Driving and skilled tasks May affect performance of skilled tasks e.g. driving.

● MEDICINAL FORMS
There can be variation in the licensing of different medicines containing the same drug. Forms available from special-order manufacturers include: capsule, oral suspension, oral solution

Modified-release tablet
CAUTIONARY AND ADVISORY LABELS 25
‣ Cardura XL (Pfizer Ltd)
Doxazosin (as Doxazosin mesilate) 4 mg Cardura XL 4mg tablets | 28 tablet [PoM] £5.00 DT = £5.00
Doxazosin (as Doxazosin mesilate) 8 mg Cardura XL 8mg tablets | 28 tablet [PoM] £9.98 DT = £9.98
‣ Doxadura XL (Discovery Pharmaceuticals)
Doxazosin (as Doxazosin mesilate) 4 mg Doxadura XL 4mg tablets | 28 tablet [PoM] £4.75 DT = £5.00
‣ Larbex XL (Teva UK Ltd)
Doxazosin (as Doxazosin mesilate) 4 mg Larbex XL 4mg tablets | 28 tablet [PoM] £6.08 DT = £5.00
‣ Raporsin XL (Actavis UK Ltd)
Doxazosin (as Doxazosin mesilate) 4 mg Raporsin XL 4mg tablets | 28 tablet [PoM] £5.70 DT = £5.00
‣ Slocinx XL (Zentiva)
Doxazosin (as Doxazosin mesilate) 4 mg Slocinx XL 4mg tablets | 28 tablet [PoM] £5.96 DT = £5.00

Tablet
‣ Doxazosin (Non-proprietary)
Doxazosin (as Doxazosin mesilate) 1 mg Doxazosin 1mg tablets | 28 tablet [PoM] £10.56 DT = £0.44
Doxazosin (as Doxazosin mesilate) 2 mg Doxazosin 2mg tablets | 28 tablet [PoM] £14.08 DT = £0.50
Doxazosin (as Doxazosin mesilate) 4 mg Doxazosin 4mg tablets | 28 tablet [PoM] £14.08 DT = £0.60
‣ Cardura (Pfizer Ltd)
Doxazosin (as Doxazosin mesilate) 1 mg Cardura 1mg tablets | 28 tablet [PoM] £10.56 DT = £0.44
Doxazosin (as Doxazosin mesilate) 2 mg Cardura 2mg tablets | 28 tablet [PoM] £14.08 DT = £0.50
‣ Doxadura (Discovery Pharmaceuticals)
Doxazosin (as Doxazosin mesilate) 1 mg Doxadura 1mg tablets | 28 tablet [PoM] £0.43 DT = £0.44
Doxazosin (as Doxazosin mesilate) 2 mg Doxadura 2mg tablets | 28 tablet [PoM] £0.49 DT = £0.50
Doxazosin (as Doxazosin mesilate) 4 mg Doxadura 4mg tablets | 28 tablet [PoM] £0.59 DT = £0.60

7

Genito-urinary system

Indoramin

- **INDICATIONS AND DOSE**

Hypertension
▶ BY MOUTH
▹ Adult: Initially 25 mg twice daily, increased in steps of 25–50 mg every 2 weeks, maximum daily dose should be given in divided doses; maximum 200 mg per day

Benign prostatic hyperplasia
▶ BY MOUTH
▹ Adult: 20 mg twice daily, increased in steps of 20 mg every 2 weeks if required, increased if necessary up to 100 mg daily in divided doses
▹ Elderly: 20 mg daily may be adequate, dose to be taken at night

DOSE ADJUSTMENTS DUE TO INTERACTIONS
▶ Caution with concomitant antihypertensives in benign prostatic hyperplasia—reduced dosage and specialist supervision may be required.

- **CONTRA-INDICATIONS** Established heart failure · history micturition syncope (when used for benign prostatic hyperplasia) · history of postural hypotension (when used for benign prostatic hyperplasia)
- **CAUTIONS** Cataract surgery (risk of intra-operative floppy iris syndrome) · control incipient heart failure before initiating indoramin · elderly · epilepsy (convulsions in *animal* studies) · history of depression · Parkinson's disease (extrapyramidal disorders reported)
- **INTERACTIONS** → Appendix 1: alpha blockers
- **SIDE-EFFECTS**
▶ **Rare or very rare** Parkinson's disease exacerbated
▶ **Frequency not known** Depression · dizziness · drowsiness · dry mouth · ejaculation failure · fatigue · headache · nasal congestion · weight increased
- **PREGNANCY** No evidence of teratogenicity; manufacturers advise use only when potential benefit outweighs risk.
- **BREAST FEEDING** No information available.
- **HEPATIC IMPAIRMENT** Manufacturer advises caution.
- **RENAL IMPAIRMENT** Manufacturer advises caution.
- **PATIENT AND CARER ADVICE**
Driving and skilled tasks Drowsiness may affect performance of skilled tasks (e.g. driving); effects of alcohol may be enhanced.

- **MEDICINAL FORMS**
There can be variation in the licensing of different medicines containing the same drug.
Tablet
CAUTIONARY AND ADVISORY LABELS 2
▶ Indoramin (Non-proprietary)
Indoramin hydrochloride 20 mg Indoramin 20mg tablets | 60 tablet [PoM] £61.00 DT = £8.49
Indoramin (as Indoramin hydrochloride) 25 mg Indoramin 25mg tablets | 84 tablet [PoM] £60.26 DT = £60.26
▶ Doralese Tiltab (Chemidex Pharma Ltd)
Indoramin hydrochloride 20 mg Doralese Tiltab 20mg tablets | 60 tablet [PoM] £11.44 DT = £8.49

Prazosin

- **INDICATIONS AND DOSE**

Hypertension
▶ BY MOUTH
▹ Adult: Initially 500 micrograms 2–3 times a day for 3–7 days, the initial dose should be taken on retiring to bed at night to avoid collapse, increased to 1 mg 2–3 times a day for a further 3–7 days, then increased if necessary up to 20 mg daily in divided doses

Congestive heart failure (rarely used)
▶ BY MOUTH
▹ Adult: 500 micrograms 2–4 times a day, initial dose to be taken at bedtime, then increased to 4 mg daily in divided doses; maintenance 4–20 mg daily in divided doses

Raynaud's syndrome (but efficacy not established)
▶ BY MOUTH
▹ Adult: Initially 500 micrograms twice daily, initial dose to be taken at bedtime, dose may be increased after 3–7 days, then increased if necessary to 1–2 mg twice daily

Benign prostatic hyperplasia
▶ BY MOUTH
▹ Adult: Initially 500 micrograms twice daily for 3–7 days, subsequent doses should be adjusted according to response, maintenance 2 mg twice daily, initiate with lowest possible dose in elderly patients

DOSE ADJUSTMENTS DUE TO INTERACTIONS
▶ Caution with concomitant antihypertensives in benign prostatic hyperplasia—reduced dosage and specialist supervision may be required.

- **CONTRA-INDICATIONS** History of micturition syncope · history of postural hypotension · not recommended for congestive heart failure due to mechanical obstruction (e.g. aortic stenosis)
- **CAUTIONS** Cataract surgery (risk of intra-operative floppy iris syndrome) · elderly · first dose hypotension
- **INTERACTIONS** → Appendix 1: alpha blockers
- **SIDE-EFFECTS**
▶ **Common or very common** Asthenia · constipation · depression · diarrhoea · dizziness · drowsiness · dry mouth · dyspnoea · headache · nasal congestion · nausea · nervousness · oedema · palpitations · postural hypotension · sexual dysfunction · skin reactions · syncope · urinary disorders · vertigo · vision blurred · vomiting
▶ **Uncommon** Angina pectoris · arrhythmias · arthralgia · epistaxis · eye pain · eye redness · gastrointestinal discomfort · hyperhidrosis · paraesthesia · sleep disorders · tinnitus
▶ **Rare or very rare** Alopecia · fever · flushing · gynaecomastia · hallucination · hepatic function abnormal · pain · pancreatitis · vasculitis
- **PREGNANCY** No evidence of teratogenicity; manufacturers advise use only when potential benefit outweighs risk.
- **BREAST FEEDING** Present in milk, amount probably too small to be harmful; manufacturer advises use with caution.
- **HEPATIC IMPAIRMENT**
Dose adjustments Initially 500 micrograms daily; increased with caution.
- **RENAL IMPAIRMENT**
Dose adjustments Initially 500 micrograms daily in moderate to severe impairment; increased with caution.
- **PATIENT AND CARER ADVICE**
First dose effect First dose may cause collapse due to hypotensive effect (therefore should be taken on retiring to bed). Patients should be warned to lie down if symptoms such as dizziness, fatigue or sweating develop, and to remain lying down until they abate completely.
Driving and skilled tasks May affect performance of skilled tasks e.g. driving.

- **MEDICINAL FORMS**
  There can be variation in the licensing of different medicines containing the same drug. Forms available from special-order manufacturers include: tablet, oral suspension, oral solution

Tablet
▸ Hypovase (Pfizer Ltd)
  Prazosin (as Prazosin hydrochloride) 500 microgram Hypovase 500microgram tablets | 60 tablet [PoM] £2.69 DT = £2.69
  Prazosin (as Prazosin hydrochloride) 1 mg Hypovase 1mg tablets | 60 tablet [PoM] £3.46 DT = £3.46

Tamsulosin hydrochloride

- **INDICATIONS AND DOSE**

Benign prostatic hyperplasia
▸ BY MOUTH USING MODIFIED-RELEASE MEDICINES
▸ Adult: 400 micrograms once daily

- **CONTRA-INDICATIONS** History of micturition syncope · history of postural hypotension
- **CAUTIONS** Cataract surgery (risk of intra-operative floppy iris syndrome) · concomitant antihypertensives (reduced dosage and specialist supervision may be required) · elderly
- **INTERACTIONS** → Appendix 1: alpha blockers
- **SIDE-EFFECTS**
▸ **Common or very common** Dizziness · sexual dysfunction
▸ **Uncommon** Asthenia · constipation · diarrhoea · headache · nausea · palpitations · postural hypotension · rhinitis · skin reactions · vomiting
▸ **Rare or very rare** Angioedema · Stevens-Johnson syndrome · syncope
▸ **Frequency not known** Dry mouth · epistaxis · vision disorders
- **HEPATIC IMPAIRMENT** Avoid in severe impairment.
- **RENAL IMPAIRMENT** Use with caution if eGFR less than 10 mL/minute/1.73 m^2.
- **PATIENT AND CARER ADVICE**
  Driving and skilled tasks May affect performance of skilled tasks e.g. driving.
- **EXCEPTIONS TO LEGAL CATEGORY** Tamsulosin hydrochloride 400 microgram capsules can be sold to the public for the treatment of functional symptoms of benign prostatic hyperplasia in men aged 45–75 years to be taken for up to 6 weeks before clinical assessment by a doctor.

- **MEDICINAL FORMS**
  There can be variation in the licensing of different medicines containing the same drug. Forms available from special-order manufacturers include: oral solution

Modified-release tablet
CAUTIONARY AND ADVISORY LABELS 25
▸ Tamsulosin hydrochloride (Non-proprietary)
  Tamsulosin hydrochloride 400 microgram Tamsulosin 400microgram modified-release tablets | 30 tablet [PoM] £10.47 DT = £10.47
▸ Cositam XL (Consilient Health Ltd)
  Tamsulosin hydrochloride 400 microgram Cositam XL 400microgram tablets | 30 tablet [PoM] £8.89 DT = £10.47
▸ Faramsil (Sandoz Ltd)
  Tamsulosin hydrochloride 400 microgram Faramsil 400microgram modified-release tablets | 30 tablet [PoM] £8.89 DT = £10.47
▸ Flectone XL (Teva UK Ltd)
  Tamsulosin hydrochloride 400 microgram Flectone XL 400microgram tablets | 30 tablet [PoM] £9.95 DT = £10.47
▸ Flomaxtra XL (Astellas Pharma Ltd)
  Tamsulosin hydrochloride 400 microgram Flomaxtra XL 400microgram tablets | 30 tablet [PoM] £10.47 DT = £10.47

Modified-release capsule
CAUTIONARY AND ADVISORY LABELS 25
▸ Tamsulosin hydrochloride (Non-proprietary)
  Tamsulosin hydrochloride 400 microgram Tamsulosin 400microgram modified-release capsules | 30 capsule [PoM] £5.07 DT = £3.87
▸ Contiflo XL (Ranbaxy (UK) Ltd)
  Tamsulosin hydrochloride 400 microgram Contiflo XL 400microgram capsules | 30 capsule [PoM] £7.44 DT = £3.87
▸ Diffundox XL (Zentiva)
  Tamsulosin hydrochloride 400 microgram Diffundox XL 400microgram capsules | 30 capsule [PoM] £9.55 DT = £3.87
▸ Flomax MR (Sanofi)
  Tamsulosin hydrochloride 400 microgram Flomax Relief MR 400microgram capsules | 14 capsule [P] £5.58 | 28 capsule [P] £10.55
▸ Pamsvax XL (Almus Pharmaceuticals Ltd, Actavis UK Ltd)
  Tamsulosin hydrochloride 400 microgram Pamsvax XL 400microgram capsules | 30 capsule [PoM] £1.28 DT = £3.87
▸ Petyme MR (Teva UK Ltd)
  Tamsulosin hydrochloride 400 microgram Petyme 400microgram MR capsules | 30 capsule [PoM] £4.06 DT = £3.87
▸ Pinexel PR (Wockhardt UK Ltd)
  Tamsulosin hydrochloride 400 microgram Pinexel PR 400microgram capsules | 30 capsule [PoM] £2.50 DT = £3.87
▸ Prosurin XL (Mylan)
  Tamsulosin hydrochloride 400 microgram Prosurin XL 400microgram capsules | 30 capsule [PoM] £4.28 DT = £3.87
▸ Tabphyn MR (Thornton & Ross Ltd)
  Tamsulosin hydrochloride 400 microgram Tabphyn MR 400microgram capsules | 30 capsule [PoM] £4.45 DT = £3.87
▸ Tamfrex XL (Milpharm Ltd)
  Tamsulosin hydrochloride 400 microgram Tamfrex XL 400microgram capsules | 30 capsule [PoM] £3.87 DT = £3.87
▸ Tamurex (Somex Pharma)
  Tamsulosin hydrochloride 400 microgram Tamurex 400microgram modified-release capsules | 30 capsule [PoM] £3.50 DT = £3.87

Tamsulosin with dutasteride

The properties listed below are those particular to the combination only. For the properties of the components please consider, tamsulosin hydrochloride above, dutasteride p. 769.

- **INDICATIONS AND DOSE**

Benign prostatic hyperplasia
▸ BY MOUTH
▸ Adult (male): 1 capsule daily.

- **INTERACTIONS** → Appendix 1: alpha blockers · dutasteride
- **PATIENT AND CARER ADVICE**
  Driving and skilled tasks May affect performance of skilled tasks e.g. driving.

- **MEDICINAL FORMS**
  There can be variation in the licensing of different medicines containing the same drug.

Capsule
CAUTIONARY AND ADVISORY LABELS 25
▸ Combodart (GlaxoSmithKline UK Ltd)
  Tamsulosin hydrochloride 400 microgram, Dutasteride 500 microgram Combodart 0.5mg/0.4mg capsules | 30 capsule [PoM] £19.80 DT = £19.80

7

Genito-urinary system

Tamsulosin with solifenacin

The properties listed below are those particular to the combination only. For the properties of the components please consider, tamsulosin hydrochloride p. 767, solifenacin succinate p. 761.

- **INDICATIONS AND DOSE**

Moderate to severe urinary frequency, urgency, and obstructive symptoms associated with benign prostatic hyperplasia when monotherapy ineffective
  ▸ BY MOUTH
  ▸ Adult (male): 1 tablet daily.
  DOSE ADJUSTMENTS DUE TO INTERACTIONS
  ▸ Manufacturer advises max. 1 *Vesomni*® tablet daily with concurrent use of potent inhibitors of CYP3A4; avoid concurrent use in patients who also have moderate hepatic impairment, severe renal impairment, are poor metabolisers of CYP2D6, or in patients also taking a potent inhibitor of CYP2D6.

- **INTERACTIONS** → Appendix 1: alpha blockers · solifenacin
- **HEPATIC IMPAIRMENT**
  Dose adjustments Max. 1 *Vesomni*® tablet daily in moderate impairment.
- **RENAL IMPAIRMENT**
  Dose adjustments Max. 1 *Vesomni*® tablet daily if eGFR less than 30 mL/minute/1.73 m².

- **MEDICINAL FORMS**
  There can be variation in the licensing of different medicines containing the same drug.
  Modified-release tablet
  CAUTIONARY AND ADVISORY LABELS 3, 25
  ▸ Vesomni (Astellas Pharma Ltd)
  Tamsulosin hydrochloride 400 microgram, Solifenacin succinate 6 mg Vesomni 6mg/0.4mg modified-release tablets | 30 tablet PoM £27.62 DT = £27.62

Terazosin

- **INDICATIONS AND DOSE**

Mild to moderate hypertension
  ▸ BY MOUTH
  ▸ Adult: 1 mg daily for 7 days, then increased if necessary to 2 mg daily, dose should be taken at bedtime; maintenance 2–10 mg once daily, doses above 20 mg rarely improve efficacy

Benign prostatic hyperplasia
  ▸ BY MOUTH
  ▸ Adult: Initially 1 mg daily, dose should be taken at bedtime, if necessary dose may be doubled at intervals of 1–2 weeks according to response; maintenance 5–10 mg daily; maximum 10 mg per day

- **CONTRA-INDICATIONS** History of micturition syncope (in benign prostatic hyperplasia) · history of postural hypotension (in benign prostatic hyperplasia)
- **CAUTIONS** Cataract surgery (risk of intra-operative floppy iris syndrome) · elderly · first dose
  CAUTIONS, FURTHER INFORMATION First dose may cause collapse due to hypotension within 30–90 minutes, therefore should be taken on retiring to bed; may also occur with rapid dose increase.
- **INTERACTIONS** → Appendix 1: alpha blockers
- **SIDE-EFFECTS** Angioedema · anxiety · arrhythmias · arthritis · asthenia · chest pain · conjunctivitis · constipation · cough · depression · diarrhoea · dizziness · drowsiness · dry mouth · dyspnoea · epistaxis · fever · flatulence · gastrointestinal discomfort · gout · headache · hyperhidrosis · increased risk of infection · insomnia · joint

disorders · myalgia · nasal congestion · nausea · oedema · pain · palpitations · paraesthesia · postural hypotension · sexual dysfunction · skin reactions · syncope · thrombocytopenia · tinnitus · urinary disorders · vasodilation · vertigo · vision disorders · vomiting · weight increased

- **PREGNANCY** No evidence of teratogenicity; manufacturers advise use only when potential benefit outweighs risk.
- **BREAST FEEDING** No information available.
- **PATIENT AND CARER ADVICE** Patient counselling is advised for terazosin tablets (initial dose).
  First dose effect First dose may cause collapse due to hypotensive effect (therefore should be taken on retiring to bed). Patient should be warned to lie down if symptoms such as dizziness, fatigue or sweating develop, and to remain lying down until they abate completely.
  Driving and skilled tasks May affect performance of skilled tasks e.g. driving.

- **MEDICINAL FORMS**
  There can be variation in the licensing of different medicines containing the same drug.
  Tablet
  ▸ Terazosin (Non-proprietary)
  Terazosin (as Terazosin hydrochloride) 2 mg Terazosin 2mg tablets | 28 tablet PoM £2.70 DT = £1.49
  Terazosin (as Terazosin hydrochloride) 5 mg Terazosin 5mg tablets | 28 tablet PoM £3.34 DT = £1.18
  Terazosin (as Terazosin hydrochloride) 10 mg Terazosin 10mg tablets | 28 tablet PoM £7.87-£8.11 DT = £7.87
  ▸ Benph (Mylan)
  Terazosin (as Terazosin hydrochloride) 2 mg Benph 2mg tablets | 28 tablet PoM £1.87 DT = £1.49
  ▸ Hytrin (AMCo)
  Terazosin (as Terazosin hydrochloride) 1 mg Hytrin 1mg tablets | 7 tablet PoM ▨
  Terazosin (as Terazosin hydrochloride) 2 mg Hytrin 2mg tablets | 28 tablet PoM £2.20 DT = £1.49
  Terazosin (as Terazosin hydrochloride) 5 mg Hytrin 5mg tablets | 28 tablet PoM £4.13 DT = £1.18
  Terazosin (as Terazosin hydrochloride) 10 mg Hytrin 10mg tablets | 28 tablet PoM £7.87 DT = £7.87
  Hytrin BPH tablets starter pack | 28 tablet PoM £10.97
  Hytrin tablets starter pack | 28 tablet PoM £13.00

CHOLINE ESTERS

Bethanechol chloride

- **INDICATIONS AND DOSE**

Urinary retention
  ▸ BY MOUTH
  ▸ Adult: 10–25 mg 3–4 times a day, to be taken 30 minutes before food

- **CONTRA-INDICATIONS** Bradycardia · cardiovascular disorders · conditions where increased motility of the gastro-intestinal tract could be harmful · conditions where increased motility of the urinary tract could be harmful · epilepsy · heart block · hyperthyroidism · hypotension · intestinal obstruction · obstructive airways disease · parkinsonism · peptic ulcer · recent myocardial infarction · urinary obstruction
- **CAUTIONS** Autonomic neuropathy (use lower initial dose)
- **SIDE-EFFECTS** Abdominal pain · hyperhidrosis · nausea · vomiting
- **PREGNANCY** Manufacturer advises avoid—no information available.
- **BREAST FEEDING** Manufacturer advises avoid; gastrointestinal disturbances in infant reported.
- **LESS SUITABLE FOR PRESCRIBING** Less suitable for prescribing.

● **MEDICINAL FORMS**
There can be variation in the licensing of different medicines containing the same drug. Forms available from special-order manufacturers include: oral suspension, oral solution

Tablet
CAUTIONARY AND ADVISORY LABELS 22
▸ Myotonine (Glenwood GmbH)
   Bethanechol chloride 10 mg Myotonine 10mg tablets |
   100 tablet [PoM] £18.51
   Bethanechol chloride 25 mg Myotonine 25mg tablets |
   100 tablet [PoM] £27.26

5α-REDUCTASE INHIBITORS

Dutasteride

● **DRUG ACTION** A specific inhibitor of the enzyme 5α-reductase, which metabolises testosterone into the more potent androgen, dihydrotestosterone.

● **INDICATIONS AND DOSE**
Benign prostatic hyperplasia
▸ BY MOUTH
▸ Adult: 500 micrograms daily, review treatment at 3–6 months and then every 6–12 months (may require several months treatment before benefit is obtained)

● INTERACTIONS → Appendix 1: dutasteride

● SIDE-EFFECTS
▸ **Common or very common** Breast disorder · sexual dysfunction
▸ **Uncommon** Alopecia · hypertrichosis
▸ **Frequency not known** Angioedema · depressed mood · hypersensitivity · localised oedema · skin reactions · testicular disorders

● **CONCEPTION AND CONTRACEPTION** Dutasteride is excreted in semen and use of a condom is recommended if sexual partner is pregnant or likely to become pregnant.

● **HEPATIC IMPAIRMENT** Avoid in severe impairment—no information available.

● **MONITORING REQUIREMENTS** Manufacturer advises that patients should be regularly evaluated for prostate cancer.

● **EFFECT ON LABORATORY TESTS** May decrease serum concentration of prostate cancer markers such as prostate-specific antigen; reference values may need adjustment.

● **HANDLING AND STORAGE** Women of childbearing potential should avoid handling leaking capsules of dutasteride.

● **PATIENT AND CARER ADVICE** Cases of male breast cancer have been reported. Patients or their carers should be told to promptly report to their doctor any changes in breast tissue such as lumps, pain, or nipple discharge.

● **MEDICINAL FORMS**
There can be variation in the licensing of different medicines containing the same drug. Forms available from special-order manufacturers include: oral solution

Capsule
CAUTIONARY AND ADVISORY LABELS 25
▸ Dutasteride (Non-proprietary)
   Dutasteride 500 microgram Dutasteride 500microgram capsules |
   30 capsule [PoM] £5.00–£14.60 DT = £11.75
▸ Avodart (GlaxoSmithKline UK Ltd)
   Dutasteride 500 microgram Avodart 500microgram capsules |
   30 capsule [PoM] £14.60 DT = £11.75

Combinations available: *Tamsulosin with dutasteride,* p. 767

Finasteride   20-Jul-2017

● **DRUG ACTION** A specific inhibitor of the enzyme 5α-reductase, which metabolises testosterone into the more potent androgen, dihydrotestosterone.

● **INDICATIONS AND DOSE**
Benign prostatic hyperplasia
▸ BY MOUTH
▸ Adult: 5 mg daily, review treatment at 3–6 months and then every 6–12 months (may require several months treatment before benefit is obtained)
Androgenetic alopecia in men
▸ BY MOUTH
▸ Adult: 1 mg daily

> **IMPORTANT SAFETY INFORMATION**
> MHRA/CHM ADVICE: RARE REPORTS OF DEPRESSION AND SUICIDAL THOUGHTS (MAY 2017)
> The MHRA has received reports of depression and, in rare cases, suicidal thoughts in men taking finasteride (*Propecia*®) for male pattern hair loss; depression is also associated with *Proscar*® for benign prostatic hyperplasia. Patients should be advised to stop finasteride immediately and inform a healthcare professional if they develop depression.

● CAUTIONS Obstructive uropathy

● SIDE-EFFECTS
▸ **Common or very common** Sexual dysfunction
▸ **Uncommon** Breast abnormalities · skin reactions
▸ **Frequency not known** Angioedema · depression · infertility male · palpitations · testicular pain

● **CONCEPTION AND CONTRACEPTION** Finasteride is excreted in semen and use of a condom is recommended if sexual partner is pregnant or likely to become pregnant.

● **EFFECT ON LABORATORY TESTS** Decreases serum concentration of prostate cancer markers such as prostate-specific antigen; reference values may need adjustment.

● **HANDLING AND STORAGE** Women of childbearing potential should avoid handling crushed or broken tablets of finasteride.

● **PATIENT AND CARER ADVICE** Cases of male breast cancer have been reported. Patients or their carers should be told to promptly report to their doctor any changes in breast tissue such as lumps, pain, or nipple discharge.

● **NATIONAL FUNDING/ACCESS DECISIONS**
NHS restrictions Finasteride is not prescribable in NHS primary care for the treatment of androgenetic alopecia in men.

● **MEDICINAL FORMS**
There can be variation in the licensing of different medicines containing the same drug. Forms available from special-order manufacturers include: oral suspension

Tablet
CAUTIONARY AND ADVISORY LABELS 25
▸ Finasteride (Non-proprietary)
   Finasteride 1 mg Finasteride 1mg tablets | 28 tablet [PoM] [Ⓢ]
   Finasteride 5 mg Finasteride 5mg tablets | 28 tablet [PoM] £11.85
   DT = £0.89
▸ Aindeem (Actavis UK Ltd)
   Finasteride 1 mg Aindeem 1mg tablet | 28 tablet [PoM] £33.68 |
   84 tablet [PoM] £88.40
▸ Propecia (Merck Sharp & Dohme Ltd)
   Finasteride 1 mg Propecia 1mg tablets | 28 tablet [PoM] £33.68 |
   84 tablet [PoM] £88.40
▸ Proscar (Merck Sharp & Dohme Ltd)
   Finasteride 5 mg Proscar 5mg tablets | 28 tablet [PoM] £13.94 DT =
   £0.89

1.3 Urological pain

Urological pain

Treatment

The acute pain of *ureteric colic* may be relieved with pethidine hydrochloride p. 463. **Diclofenac** by injection or as suppositories is also effective and compares favourably with pethidine hydrochloride; other non-steroidal anti-inflammatory drugs are occasionally given by injection.

Lidocaine hydrochloride gel is a useful topical application in *urethral pain* or to relieve the discomfort of catheterisation.

Alkalinisation of urine

Alkalinisation of urine can be undertaken with potassium citrate. The alkalinising action may relieve the discomfort of *cystitis* caused by lower urinary tract infections. Sodium bicarbonate p. 1006 is used as a urinary alkalinising agent in some metabolic and renal disorders.

ALKALISING DRUGS

Citric acid with potassium citrate

● **INDICATIONS AND DOSE**

Relief of discomfort in mild urinary-tract infections | Alkalinisation of urine
▶ BY MOUTH USING ORAL SOLUTION
▶ Adult: 10 mL 3 times a day, diluted well with water

● CAUTIONS Cardiac disease · elderly
● INTERACTIONS → Appendix 1: potassium citrate
● SIDE-EFFECTS Hyperkalaemia · nausea · vomiting
● RENAL IMPAIRMENT Avoid in severe impairment.
   Monitoring Close monitoring required in renal impairment—high risk of hyperkalaemia.
● PRESCRIBING AND DISPENSING INFORMATION When prepared extemporaneously, the BP states Potassium Citrate Mixture BP consists of potassium citrate 30%, citric acid monohydrate 5% in a suitable vehicle with a lemon flavour. Extemporaneous preparations should be recently prepared according to the following formula: potassium citrate 3 g, citric acid monohydrate 500 mg, syrup 2.5 mL, quillaia tincture 0.1 mL, lemon spirit 0.05 mL, double-strength chloroform water 3 mL, water to 10 mL. Contains about 28 mmol K^+/10 mL.
● EXCEPTIONS TO LEGAL CATEGORY Proprietary brands of potassium citrate are on sale to the public for the relief of discomfort in mild urinary-tract infections.

● MEDICINAL FORMS
There can be variation in the licensing of different medicines containing the same drug.
Oral solution
CAUTIONARY AND ADVISORY LABELS 27
▶ Citric acid with potassium citrate (Non-proprietary)
   Citric acid monohydrate 50 mg per 1 ml, Potassium citrate 300 mg per 1 ml Potassium citrate mixture | 200 ml [GSL] £1.36–£1.38 DT = £1.36 | 200 ml [P] £1.38 DT = £1.36

Sodium citrate

● **INDICATIONS AND DOSE**

Bladder washouts
▶ Adult: (consult product literature)

Relief of discomfort in mild urinary-tract infections
▶ BY MOUTH
▶ Adult: (consult product literature)

MICOLETTE ®

Constipation
▶ BY RECTUM
▶ Child 3–17 years: 5–10 mL for 1 dose
▶ Adult: 5–10 mL for 1 dose

MICRALAX ®

Constipation
▶ BY RECTUM
▶ Child 3–17 years: 5 mL for 1 dose
▶ Adult: 5 mL for 1 dose

RELAXIT ®

Constipation
▶ BY RECTUM
▶ Child 1 month-2 years: 5 mL for 1 dose, insert only half the nozzle length
▶ Child 3–17 years: 5 mL for 1 dose
▶ Adult: 5 mL for 1 dose

● CONTRA-INDICATIONS
▶ With rectal use Acute gastro-intestinal conditions
● CAUTIONS
▶ With oral use Cardiac disease (in adults) · elderly · hypertension (in adults) · patients on a sodium-restricted diet (in adults)
▶ With rectal use Debilitated patients (in adults) · sodium and water retention in susceptible individuals
● INTERACTIONS → Appendix 1: sodium citrate
● SIDE-EFFECTS Polyuria
● PREGNANCY
▶ With oral use Use with caution.
● RENAL IMPAIRMENT
▶ With oral use In patients with fluid retention, avoid antacids containing large amounts of sodium.
● PRESCRIBING AND DISPENSING INFORMATION Sodium citrate 300 mmol/litre (88.2 mg/mL) oral solution is licensed for use before general anaesthesia for caesarean section (available from Viridian).
● EXCEPTIONS TO LEGAL CATEGORY Proprietary brands of sodium citrate are on sale to the public for the relief of discomfort in mild urinary-tract infections.

● MEDICINAL FORMS
There can be variation in the licensing of different medicines containing the same drug. Forms available from special-order manufacturers include: oral solution
Granules
▶ Sodium citrate (Non-proprietary)
   Sodium citrate 4 gram Sodium citrate 4g oral granules sachets | 6 sachet [GSL] £2.38
▶ Brands may include Cymalon (sodium citrate), Cystocalm
Oral solution
▶ Sodium citrate (Non-proprietary)
   Sodium citrate 88.23 mg per 1 ml Sodium citrate 0.3M oral solution | 30 ml [PoM] £4.50
   Sodium citrate 441.17mg/5ml oral solution | 30 ml [PoM] [N]
Powder
▶ Sodium citrate (Non-proprietary)
   Sodium citrate 4 gram Sodium citrate 4g oral powder sachets | 6 sachet [GSL] £1.65 DT = £1.65
Irrigation solution
▶ Sodium citrate (Non-proprietary)
   Sodium citrate 3% irrigation solution 1litre bags | 1 bag [N]
Enema
▶ Sodium citrate (Non-proprietary)
   Sodium citrate 90 mg per 1 ml Sodium citrate compound 5ml enema | 12 enema [P] [N]

▸ Micolette Micro-enema (Pinewood Healthcare)
Sodium citrate 90 mg per 1 ml Micolette Micro-enema 5ml |
12 enema Ⓟ £4.50
▸ Micralax Micro-enema (RPH Pharmaceuticals AB)
Sodium citrate 90 mg per 1 ml Micralax Micro-enema 5ml |
12 enema Ⓟ £4.87
▸ Relaxit (Supra Enterprises Ltd)
Sodium citrate 90 mg per 1 ml Relaxit Micro-enema 5ml |
12 enema £5.21

TERPENES

Anethol with borneol, camphene, cineole, fenchone and pinene

● **INDICATIONS AND DOSE**
Urolithiasis for the expulsion of calculi
▸ BY MOUTH
▸ Adult: 1–2 capsules 3–4 times a day, to be taken before food

● **LESS SUITABLE FOR PRESCRIBING** Preparation is less suitable for prescribing.

● **MEDICINAL FORMS**
There can be variation in the licensing of different medicines containing the same drug.
Capsule
CAUTIONARY AND ADVISORY LABELS 25
▸ Rowatinex (Meadow Laboratories Ltd)
Cineole 3 mg, Anethol 4 mg, Fenchone 4 mg, Borneol 10 mg, Camphene 15 mg, Pinene 31 mg Rowatinex capsules |
50 capsule PoM £7.35

2   Bladder instillations and urological surgery

Bladder instillations and urological surgery

Bladder infection
Various solutions are available as irrigations or washouts.
Aqueous chlorhexidine p. 1175 can be used in the management of common infections of the bladder but it is ineffective against most *Pseudomonas spp*. Solutions containing chlorhexidine 1 in 5000 (0.02%) are used but they may irritate the mucosa and cause burning and haematuria (in which case they should be discontinued); sterile sodium chloride solution 0.9% p. 1008 (physiological saline) is usually adequate and is preferred as a mechanical irrigant.
Continuous bladder irrigation with amphotericin 50 micrograms/mL p. 583 may be of value in mycotic infections in adults.

Dissolution of blood clots
Clot retention is usually treated by irrigation with sterile sodium chloride solution 0.9% but sterile sodium citrate solution for bladder irrigation 3% p. 770 may also be helpful.

Bladder cancer
Bladder instillations of doxorubicin hydrochloride p. 876 and mitomycin p. 895 are used for recurrent superficial bladder tumours. Such instillations reduce systemic side-effects; adverse effects on the bladder (e.g. micturition disorders and reduction in bladder capacity) may occur.
Instillation of epirubicin hydrochloride p. 877 is used for treatment and prophylaxis of certain forms of superficial bladder cancer; instillation of doxorubicin hydrochloride is also used for some papillary tumours.

Instillation of **BCG** (Bacillus Calmette-Guérin p. 932), a live attenuated strain derived from *Mycobacterium bovis* is licensed for the treatment of primary or recurrent bladder carcinoma *in-situ* and for the prevention of recurrence following transurethral resection.

Urological surgery
Glycine irrigation solution 1.5% below is the irrigant of choice for transurethral resection of the prostate gland and bladder tumours; sterile sodium chloride solution 0.9% (physiological saline) is used for percutaneous renal surgery.

Maintenance of indwelling urinary catheters
The deposition which occurs in catheterised patients is usually chiefly composed of phosphate and to minimise this the catheter (if latex) should be changed at least as often as every 6 weeks. If the catheter is to be left for longer periods a silicone catheter should be used together with the appropriate use of catheter maintenance solutions. Repeated blockage usually indicates that the catheter needs to be changed.

ANTISEPTICS AND DISINFECTANTS

Chlorhexidine with lidocaine
The properties listed below are those particular to the combination only. For the properties of the components please consider, chlorhexidine p. 1175, lidocaine hydrochloride p. 1312.

● **INDICATIONS AND DOSE**
Urethral sounding and catheterisation
▸ BY URETHRAL APPLICATION
▸ Adult: 6–11 mL
Cystoscopy
▸ BY URETHRAL APPLICATION
▸ Adult: 11 mL, then 6–11 mL if required

● **INTERACTIONS** → Appendix 1: antiarrhythmics

● **MEDICINAL FORMS**
There can be variation in the licensing of different medicines containing the same drug.
Gel
EXCIPIENTS: May contain Hydroxybenzoates (parabens)
▸ Instillagel (CliniMed Ltd)
Chlorhexidine gluconate 500 microgram per 1 ml, Lidocaine hydrochloride 20 mg per 1 ml Instillagel gel | 60 ml Ⓟ £14.05 DT = £14.05 | 110 ml Ⓟ £15.76 DT = £15.76

IRRIGATING SOLUTIONS

Glycine

● **INDICATIONS AND DOSE**
Bladder irrigation during urological surgery | Irrigation for transurethral resection of the prostate gland and bladder tumours
▸ Adult: (consult product literature)

● **CAUTIONS**
CAUTIONS, FURTHER INFORMATION
▸ Urological surgery There is a high risk of fluid absorption from the irrigant used in endoscopic surgery within the urinary tract.
● **SIDE-EFFECTS** Cardiovascular disorder · electrolyte depletion · fluid overload · pulmonary disorder · seizure · vision blurred

• MEDICINAL FORMS
There can be variation in the licensing of different medicines containing the same drug.

Irrigation solution

▸ Glycine (Non-proprietary)
Glycine 1.5% irrigation solution 3litre Easyflow bags | 1 bag 🅢
Glycine 1.5% irrigation solution 1litre Flowfusor bottles | 1 bottle 🅢
Glycine 1.5% irrigation solution 1litre Easyflow bags | 1 bag 🅢
Glycine 1.5% irrigation solution 2litre Flowfusor bottles | 1 bottle 🅢

Catheter maintenance solutions

• CATHETER MAINTENANCE SOLUTIONS

OptiFlo R citric acid 6% catheter maintenance solution (Bard Ltd)
50 ml · NHS indicative price = £3.63 · Drug Tariff (Part IXa)
100 ml · NHS indicative price = £3.63 · Drug Tariff (Part IXa)

Uro-Tainer Twin Solutio R citric acid 6% catheter maintenance solution (B.Braun Medical Ltd)
60 ml · NHS indicative price = £4.85 · Drug Tariff (Part IXa)

OptiFlo S saline 0.9% catheter maintenance solution (Bard Ltd)
Sodium chloride 9 mg per 1 ml
50 ml · NHS indicative price = £3.42 · Drug Tariff (Part IXa)
100 ml · NHS indicative price = £3.42 · Drug Tariff (Part IXa)

Uro-Tainer M sodium chloride 0.9% catheter maintenance solution (B.Braun Medical Ltd) Sodium chloride 9 mg per 1 ml
50 ml · No NHS indicative price available · Drug Tariff (Part IXa)
100 ml · No NHS indicative price available · Drug Tariff (Part IXa)

Uro-Tainer sodium chloride 0.9% catheter maintenance solution (B.Braun Medical Ltd) Sodium chloride 9 mg per 1 ml
50 ml · NHS indicative price = £3.54 · Drug Tariff (Part IXa)
100 ml · NHS indicative price = £3.54 · Drug Tariff (Part IXa)

3   Contraception

Contraceptives, hormonal

Overview

The Fraser Guidelines (Department of Health Guidance (July 2004): Best practice guidance for doctors and other health professionals on the provision of advice and treatment to young people under 16 on contraception, sexual and reproductive health, available at www.tinyurl.com/bpg16) should be followed when prescribing contraception for women under 16 years. The UK Medical Eligibility Criteria for Contraceptive Use (available at www.fsrh.org) is published by the Faculty of Sexual and Reproductive Healthcare; it categorises the risks of using contraceptive methods with pre-existing medical conditions.

Hormonal contraception is the most effective method of fertility control, but can have major and minor side-effects, especially for certain groups of women. Hormonal contraception should only be used by adolescents after menarche.

Intra-uterine devices are a highly effective method of contraception but may produce undesirable local side-effects. They may be used in women of all ages irrespective of parity, but are less appropriate for those with an increased risk of pelvic inflammatory disease.

Barrier methods alone (condoms, diaphragms, and caps) are less effective but can be reliable for well-motivated couples if used in conjunction with a **spermicide**. Occasionally sensitivity reactions occur. A female condom (*Femidom* ®) is also available; it is pre-lubricated but does not contain a spermicide.

Combined hormonal contraceptives

Oral contraceptives containing an oestrogen and a progestogen ('combined oral contraceptives') are effective preparations for general use. Advantages of combined oral contraceptives include:

• reliable and reversible;
• reduced dysmenorrhoea and menorrhagia;
• reduced incidence of premenstrual tension;
• less symptomatic fibroids and functional ovarian cysts;
• less benign breast disease;
• reduced risk of ovarian and endometrial cancer;
• reduced risk of pelvic inflammatory disease.

Combined oral contraceptives containing a fixed amount of an oestrogen and a progestogen in each active tablet are termed 'monophasic'; those with varying amounts of the two hormones are termed 'phasic'. A transdermal patch and a vaginal ring, both containing an oestrogen with a progestogen, are also available.

Combined Oral Contraceptives Monophasic 21-day preparations

Oestrogen content	Progestogen content	Brand
Ethinylestradiol 20 micrograms	Desogestrel 150 micrograms	Gedarel® 20/150
Ethinylestradiol 20 micrograms	Desogestrel 150 micrograms	Mercilon®
Ethinylestradiol 20 micrograms	Gestodene 75 micrograms	Femodette®
Ethinylestradiol 20 micrograms	Gestodene 75 micrograms	Millinette® 20/75
Ethinylestradiol 20 micrograms	Gestodene 75 micrograms	Sunya® 20/75
Ethinylestradiol 20 micrograms	Norethisterone acetate 1 mg	Loestrin® 20
Ethinylestradiol 30 micrograms	Desogestrel 150 micrograms	Gedarel® 30/150
Ethinylestradiol 30 micrograms	Desogestrel 150 micrograms	Marvelon®
Ethinylestradiol 30 micrograms	Drospirenone 3 mg	Yasmin®
Ethinylestradiol 30 micrograms	Gestodene 75 micrograms	Femodene®
Ethinylestradiol 30 micrograms	Gestodene 75 micrograms	Katya® 30/75
Ethinylestradiol 30 micrograms	Gestodene 75 micrograms	Millinette® 30/75
Ethinylestradiol 30 micrograms	Levonorgestrel 150 micrograms	Levest®
Ethinylestradiol 30 micrograms	Levonorgestrel 150 micrograms	Microgynon® 30
Ethinylestradiol 30 micrograms	Levonorgestrel 150 micrograms	Ovranette®
Ethinylestradiol 30 micrograms	Levonorgestrel 150 micrograms	Rigevidon®
Ethinylestradiol 30 micrograms	Norethisterone acetate 1.5 mg	Loestrin® 30
Ethinylestradiol 35 micrograms	Norgestimate 250 micrograms	Cilest®
Ethinylestradiol 35 micrograms	Norethisterone 500 micrograms	Brevinor®
Ethinylestradiol 35 micrograms	Norethisterone 1 mg	Norimin®
Mestranol 50 micrograms	Norethisterone 1 mg	Norinyl-1®

Combined Oral Contraceptives Monophasic 28-day preparations

Oestrogen content	Progestogen content	Brand
Ethinylestradiol 30 micrograms	Gestodene 75 micrograms	Femodene® ED
Ethinylestradiol 30 micrograms	Levonorgestrel 150 micrograms	Microgynon® 30 ED
Estradiol (as hemihydrate) 1.5 mg	Nomegestrol acetate 2.5 mg	Zoely®

Combined Oral Contraceptives Phasic 21-day preparations

Oestrogen content	Progestogen content	Brand
Ethinylestradiol 30 micrograms	Gestodene 50 micrograms	
Ethinylestradiol 40 micrograms	Gestodene 70 micrograms	Triadene®
Ethinylestradiol 30 micrograms	Gestodene 100 micrograms	
Ethinylestradiol 30 micrograms	Levonorgestrel 50 micrograms	
Ethinylestradiol 40 micrograms	Levonorgestrel 75 micrograms	Logynon®
Ethinylestradiol 30 micrograms	Levonorgestrel 125 micrograms	
Ethinylestradiol 30 micrograms	Levonorgestrel 50 micrograms	
Ethinylestradiol 40 micrograms	Levonorgestrel 75 micrograms	TriRegol®
Ethinylestradiol 30 micrograms	Levonorgestrel 125 micrograms	
Ethinylestradiol 35 micrograms	Norethisterone 500 micrograms	
Ethinylestradiol 35 micrograms	Norethisterone 1 mg	Synphase®
Ethinylestradiol 35 micrograms	Norethisterone 500 micrograms	

Combined Oral Contraceptives Phasic 28-day preparations

Oestrogen content	Progestogen content	Brand
Ethinylestradiol 30 micrograms	Levonorgestrel 50 micrograms	
Ethinylestradiol 40 micrograms	Levonorgestrel 75 micrograms	Logynon® ED
Ethinylestradiol 30 micrograms	Levonorgestrel 125 micrograms	
Estradiol valerate 3 mg		
Estradiol valerate 2 mg	Dienogest 2 mg	
Estradiol valerate 2 mg	Dienogest 3 mg	Qlaira®
Estradiol valerate 1 mg		

Choice

The majority of combined oral contraceptives contain ethinylestradiol as the oestrogen component; mestranol and estradiol are also used. The ethinylestradiol content of combined oral contraceptives ranges from 20 to 40 micrograms. Generally a preparation with the lowest oestrogen and progestogen content which gives good cycle control and minimal side-effects in the individual woman is chosen. It is recommended that combined hormonal contraceptives are not continued beyond 50 years of age since more suitable alternatives exist.

- *Low strength preparations* (containing ethinylestradiol 20 micrograms) are particularly appropriate for women with risk factors for circulatory disease, provided a combined oral contraceptive is otherwise suitable.
- *Standard strength preparations* (containing ethinylestradiol 30 or 35 micrograms or in 30–40 microgram *phased* preparations) are appropriate for standard use. Phased preparations are generally reserved for women who *either* do not have withdrawal bleeding or who have breakthrough bleeding with monophasic products.

The progestogens ethinylestradiol with desogestrel p. 779, ethinylestradiol with drospirenone p. 780, and ethinylestradiol with gestodene p. 780 may be considered for women who have side-effects (such as acne, headache, depression, breast symptoms, and breakthrough bleeding) with other progestogens. Drospirenone, a derivative of spironolactone, has anti-androgenic and anti-mineralocorticoid activity; it should be used with care if an increased plasma-potassium concentration might be hazardous.

Dienogest with estradiol valerate p. 778 is in the combined oral contraceptive *Qlaira®*. Nomegestrol is the progestogen contained in the combined oral contraceptive *Zoely®*, in combination with estradiol.

The progestogen norelgestromin is combined with ethinylestradiol in a transdermal patch (*Evra®*). The vaginal contraceptive ring contains the progestogen etonogestrel combined with ethinylestradiol (*NuvaRing®*).

Surgery

Oestrogen-containing contraceptives should preferably be discontinued (and adequate alternative contraceptive arrangements made) 4 weeks before major elective surgery and all surgery to the legs or surgery which involves prolonged immobilisation of a lower limb; they should normally be recommenced at the first menses occurring at least 2 weeks after full mobilisation. A progestogen-only contraceptive may be offered as an alternative and the oestrogen-containing contraceptive restarted after mobilisation. When discontinuation of an oestrogen-containing contraceptive is not possible, e.g. after trauma or if a patient admitted for an elective procedure is still on an oestrogen-containing contraceptive, thromboprophylaxis (with unfractionated or low molecular weight heparin and graduated compression hosiery) is advised. These recommendations do not apply to minor surgery with short duration of anaesthesia, e.g. laparoscopic sterilisation or tooth extraction, or to women using oestrogen-free hormonal contraceptives.

Reason to stop immediately

Combined hormonal contraceptives or hormone replacement therapy (HRT) should be stopped (pending investigation and treatment), if any of the following occur:

- sudden severe chest pain (even if not radiating to left arm);
- sudden breathlessness (or cough with blood-stained sputum);
- unexplained swelling or severe pain in calf of one leg;
- severe stomach pain;
- serious neurological effects including unusual severe, prolonged headache especially if first time or getting

progressively worse *or* sudden partial *or* complete loss of vision *or* sudden disturbance of hearing or other perceptual disorders *or* dysphasia *or* bad fainting attack or collapse *or* first unexplained epileptic seizure *or* weakness, motor disturbances, very marked numbness suddenly affecting one side or one part of body;

- hepatitis, jaundice, liver enlargement;
- blood pressure above systolic 160 mmHg or diastolic 95 mmHg; (in adolescents stop if blood pressure very high);
- prolonged immobility after surgery or leg injury;
- detection of a risk factor which contra-indicates treatment.

Progestogen-only contraceptives

Oral progestogen-only contraceptives

Oral progestogen-only preparations alter cervical mucus to prevent sperm penetration and may inhibit ovulation in some women; oral desogestrel-only preparations consistently inhibit ovulation and this is their primary mechanism of action. There is insufficient clinical trial evidence to compare the efficacy of oral progestogen-only contraceptives with each other or with combined hormonal contraceptives. Progestogen-only contraceptives offer a suitable alternative to combined hormonal contraceptives when oestrogens are contra-indicated (including those with venous thrombosis or a past history or predisposition to venous thrombosis, heavy smokers, those with hypertension above systolic 160 mmHg or diastolic 95 mmHg, valvular heart disease, diabetes mellitus with complications, and migraine with aura).

Parenteral progestogen-only contraceptives

Medroxyprogesterone acetate p. 791 (*Depo-Provera®*, *SAYANA PRESS®*) is a long-acting progestogen given by injection; it is at least as effective as the combined oral preparations but because of its prolonged action it should never be given without *full counselling backed by the patient information leaflet*. It may be used as a short-term or long-term contraceptive for women who have been counselled about the likelihood of menstrual disturbance and the potential for a delay in return to full fertility. Delayed return of fertility and irregular cycles may occur after discontinuation of treatment but there is no evidence of permanent infertility. Troublesome bleeding has been reported in patients given medroxyprogesterone acetate in the immediate puerperium; delaying the first injection until 6 weeks after birth may minimise bleeding problems. If the woman is not breast-feeding, the first injection may be given within 5 days postpartum (she should be warned that the risk of troublesome bleeding may be increased).

- In adolescents, medroxyprogesterone acetate (*Depo-Provera®, SAYANA PRESS®*) should be used only when other methods of contraception are inappropriate;
- in all women, the benefits of using medroxyprogesterone acetate beyond 2 years should be evaluated against the risks;
- in women with risk factors for osteoporosis, a method of contraception other than medroxyprogesterone acetate should be considered.

Norethisterone enantate (*Noristerat®*) is a long-acting progestogen given as an oily injection which provides contraception for 8 weeks; it is used as short-term interim contraception e.g. before vasectomy becomes effective.

An **etonogestrel-releasing implant** (*Nexplanon®*) is also available. It is a highly effective long-acting contraceptive, consisting of a single flexible rod that is inserted subdermally into the lower surface of the upper arm and provides contraception for up to 3 years. The manufacturer advises that in heavier women, blood-etonogestrel concentrations are lower and therefore the implant may not provide effective contraception during the third year; they advise that earlier replacement may be considered in such

patients—however, evidence to support this recommendation is lacking. Local reactions such as bruising and itching can occur at the insertion site. The contraceptive effect of etonogestrel is rapidly reversed on removal of the implant.

Intra-uterine progestogen-only device

The progestogen-only intra-uterine systems *Mirena®*, *Jaydess®* and *Levosert®* release levonorgestrel p. 787 directly into the uterine cavity. *Mirena®* is licensed for use as a contraceptive, for the treatment of primary menorrhagia and for the prevention of endometrial hyperplasia during oestrogen replacement therapy. *Jaydess®* and *Levosert®* are licensed for contraception, and *Levosert®* is additionally licensed for the treatment of menorrhagia. These may therefore be a contraceptive method of choice for women who have excessively heavy menses.

The effects of the progestogen-only intra-uterine system are mainly local and hormonal including prevention of endometrial proliferation, thickening of cervical mucus, and suppression of ovulation in some women (in some cycles). In addition to the progestogenic activity, the intra-uterine system itself may contribute slightly to the contraceptive effect. Return of fertility after removal is rapid and appears to be complete.

Advantages of the progestogen-only intra-uterine system over copper intra-uterine devices are that there may be an improvement in any dysmenorrhoea and a reduction in blood loss; there is also evidence that the frequency of pelvic inflammatory disease may be reduced (particularly in the youngest age groups who are most at risk).

In primary menorrhagia, menstrual bleeding is reduced significantly within 3–6 months of inserting the progestogen-only intra-uterine system, probably because it prevents endometrial proliferation. Another treatment should be considered if menorrhagia does not improve within this time.

Surgery

All progestogen-only contraceptives (including those given by injection) are suitable for use as an alternative to combined hormonal contraceptives before major elective surgery, before all surgery to the legs, or before surgery which involves prolonged immobilisation of a lower limb.

Contraceptives, non-hormonal

Spermicidal contraceptives

Spermicidal contraceptives are useful additional safeguards but do **not** give adequate protection if used alone unless fertility is already significantly diminished. They have two components: a spermicide and a vehicle which itself may have some inhibiting effect on sperm activity. They are suitable for use with barrier methods, such as diaphragms or caps; however, spermicidal contraceptives are not generally recommended for use with condoms, as there is no evidence of any additional protection compared with non-spermicidal lubricants.

Spermicidal contraceptives are not suitable for use in those with or at high risk of sexually transmitted infections (including HIV); high frequency use of the spermicide nonoxinol '9' p. 793 has been associated with genital lesions, which may increase the risk of acquiring these infections.

Contraceptive devices

Intra-uterine devices

The intra-uterine device (IUD) is a suitable contraceptive for women of all ages irrespective of parity; however, it is less appropriate for those with an increased risk of pelvic inflammatory disease e.g. women under 25 years.

The most effective intra-uterine devices have at least 380 mm^2 of copper and have banded copper on the arms.

Smaller devices have been introduced to minimise side-effects; these consist of a plastic carrier wound with copper wire or fitted with copper bands; some also have a central core of silver to prevent fragmentation of the copper.

Fertility declines with age and therefore a copper intra-uterine device which is fitted in a woman over the age of 40, may remain in the uterus until menopause.

A frameless, copper-bearing intra-uterine device (*Gyne Fix®*) is also available. It consists of a knotted, polypropylene thread with 6 copper sleeves; the device is anchored in the uterus by inserting the knot into the uterine fundus.

Caution with oil-based lubricants

Products such as petroleum jelly (*Vaseline®*), baby oil and oil-based vaginal and rectal preparations are likely to damage condoms and contraceptive diaphragms made from latex rubber, and may render them less effective as a barrier method of contraception and as a protection from sexually transmitted infections (including HIV).

Emergency contraception   01-Sep-2017

Overview

EvGr Emergency contraception is intended for occasional use, to reduce the risk of pregnancy after unprotected sexual intercourse. It does not replace effective regular contraception.

Women who do not wish to conceive should be offered emergency contraception after unprotected sexual intercourse that has taken place on any day of a natural menstrual cycle. Emergency contraception should also be offered after unprotected intercourse from day 21 after childbirth (unless the criteria for lactational amenorrhoea are met), and from day 5 after abortion, miscarriage, ectopic pregnancy or uterine evacuation for gestational trophoblastic disease.

Emergency contraception should also be offered to women if their regular contraception has been compromised or has been used incorrectly. Ⓐ

Emergency contraceptive methods

Copper intra-uterine devices

EvGr Insertion of a copper intra-uterine device (see intra-uterine contraceptive devices (copper) p. 784) is the most effective form of emergency contraception and should be offered (if appropriate) to all women who have had unprotected sexual intercourse and do not want to conceive. A copper intra-uterine contraceptive device can be inserted up to 120 hours (5 days) after unprotected intercourse or up to 5 days after the earliest likely calculated ovulation (i.e. within the minimum period before implantation), regardless of the number of episodes of unprotected intercourse earlier in the cycle. Antibacterial cover should be considered for copper intra-uterine contraceptive device insertion if there is a significant risk of sexually transmitted infection that could be associated with ascending pelvic infection.

A copper intra-uterine device is not known to be affected by body mass index (BMI) or body-weight or by other drugs. Ⓐ

Hormonal methods

EvGr Hormonal emergency contraceptives (includes levonorgestrel p. 787 and ulipristal acetate p. 785) should be offered as soon as possible after unprotected intercourse if a copper intra-uterine device is not appropriate or is not acceptable to the patient; either drug should be taken as soon as possible after unprotected intercourse to increase efficacy. Hormonal emergency contraception administered after ovulation is ineffective.

Levonorgestrel is effective if taken within 72 hours (3 days) of unprotected intercourse and may also be used

between 72 and 96 hours after unprotected intercourse [unlicensed use], but efficacy decreases with time. Ulipristal acetate is effective if taken within 120 hours (5 days) of unprotected intercourse. Ulipristal acetate has been demonstrated to be more effective than levonorgestrel for emergency contraception.

It is possible that a higher body-weight or BMI could reduce the effectiveness of oral emergency contraception, particularly levonorgestrel; if BMI is greater than 26 kg/m^2 or body-weight is greater than 70 kg, it is recommended that either ulipristal acetate or a double dose of levonorgestrel [unlicensed indication] (see *Emergency contraception* under levonorgestrel) is given. It is unknown which is more effective.

Ulipristal acetate should be considered as the first-line hormonal emergency contraceptive for a woman who has had unprotected intercourse 96–120 hours ago (even if she has also had unprotected intercourse within the last 96 hours). It should also be considered first line for a woman who has had unprotected sexual intercourse within the last 5 days if it is likely to have taken place during the 5 days before the estimated day of ovulation. Ⓐ

Hormonal emergency contraception interactions
See Contraceptives, interactions below.

Starting hormonal contraception after emergency hormonal contraception

Emergency hormonal contraception methods do **not** provide ongoing contraception. EvGr After taking levonorgestrel, women should start suitable hormonal contraception immediately. They must use condoms reliably or abstain from intercourse until contraception becomes effective.

Women should wait 5 days after taking ulipristal acetate before starting suitable hormonal contraception. Women must use condoms reliably or abstain from intercourse during the 5 day waiting period and also until their contraceptive method is effective. Ⓐ

The copper intra-uterine device immediately provides effective ongoing contraception.

Useful Resources

Emergency Contraception. The Faculty of Sexual and Reproductive Healthcare. Clinical guidance. March 2017.
www.fsrh.org/standards-and-guidance/documents/ceu-clinical-guidance-emergency-contraception-march-2017

Contraceptives, interactions   06-Jun-2017

Overview

The effectiveness of *combined* oral contraceptives, *progestogen-only* oral contraceptives, contraceptive patches, vaginal rings, and emergency hormonal contraception can be considerably reduced by interaction with drugs that induce hepatic enzyme activity (e.g. carbamazepine p. 309, eslicarbazepine acetate, nevirapine p. 633, oxcarbazepine p. 319, phenytoin p. 321, phenobarbital p. 331, primidone p. 332, ritonavir p. 646, St John's Wort, topiramate p. 328 and, above all, rifabutin p. 564 and rifampicin p. 571) and possibly also griseofulvin p. 590. EvGr A condom together with a long-acting method (such as an injectable contraceptive) may be more suitable for patients with HIV infection or at risk of HIV infection; advice on the possibility of interaction with antiretroviral drugs should be sought from HIV specialists. Ⓐ

Combined hormonal contraceptives interactions

EvGr Women using combined hormonal contraceptive patches, vaginal rings or oral tablets who require enzyme-inducing drugs or griseofulvin should be advised to change to a reliable contraceptive method that is unaffected by enzyme-inducers, such as some parenteral progestogen-only contraceptives (medroxyprogesterone acetate p. 791 and

7

Genito-urinary system

norethisterone p. 747) or intra-uterine devices (levonorgestrel p. 787; see also Contraceptives, non-hormonal p. 774). This should be continued for the duration of treatment and for four weeks after stopping. If a change in contraceptive method is undesirable or inappropriate the following options should be discussed: Ⓐ

Short course (2 months or less) of an enzyme-inducing drug
EvGr Continuing the combined hormonal contraceptive method may be appropriate if used in combination with consistent and careful use of condoms for the duration of treatment and for four weeks after stopping the enzyme-inducing drug. Ⓐ

Long-term course (over 2 months) of an enzyme-inducing drug (except rifampicin or rifabutin) or a course of griseofulvin
EvGr Use a monophasic combined oral contraceptive at a dose of ethinylestradiol 50 micrograms or more daily [unlicensed use] and use either an extended or a 'tricycling' regimen (i.e. taking three packets of monophasic tablets without a break followed by a shortened tablet-free interval of four days [unlicensed use]); continue for the duration of treatment with the interacting drug and for four weeks after stopping.

If breakthrough bleeding occurs (and all other causes are ruled out) it is recommended that the dose of ethinylestradiol is increased by increments of 10 micrograms up to a maximum of 70 micrograms daily [unlicensed use] on specialist advice, or to use additional precautions, or to change to a method unaffected by the interacting drugs.

Use of contraceptive patches and vaginal rings (including concurrent use of two patches or two vaginal rings) is not recommended for women taking enzyme-inducing drugs over a long period. Ⓐ

Long-term course (over 2 months) of rifampicin or rifabutin
An alternative method of contraception (such as an IUD) is **always** recommended because they are such potent enzyme-inducing drugs; the alternative method of contraception should be continued for four weeks after stopping the enzyme-inducing drug.

Antibacterials that do not induce liver enzymes
EvGr It is recommended that no additional contraceptive precautions are required when *combined* oral contraceptives, contraceptive patches or vaginal rings are used with antibacterials that do not induce liver enzymes, unless diarrhoea or vomiting occur. These recommendations should be discussed with the woman.

There had been concerns that some antibacterials that do not induce liver enzymes (e.g. ampicillin p. 540, doxycycline p. 555) reduce the efficacy of *combined* oral contraceptives by impairing the bacterial flora responsible for recycling ethinylestradiol from the large bowel. However, there is a lack of evidence to support this interaction.

Oral progestogen-only contraceptives interactions
Effectiveness of oral progestogen-only preparations is not affected by antibacterials that do not induce liver enzymes. EvGr The efficacy of oral progestogen-only preparations is, however, reduced by enzyme-inducing drugs or griseofulvin and an alternative contraceptive method, unaffected by the interacting drug, is recommended during treatment with an interacting drug and for at least 4 weeks afterwards.

For a short course of an enzyme-inducing drug (less than two months), continuing the progestogen-only oral method may be appropriate if used in combination with consistent and careful use of condoms for the duration of treatment and for four weeks after stopping the enzyme-inducing drug. Ⓐ

Parenteral progestogen-only contraceptives interactions
Effectiveness of parenteral progestogen-only contraceptives is not affected by antibacterials that do not induce liver enzymes. EvGr The effectiveness of intramuscular norethisterone injection and intramuscular and subcutaneous medroxyprogesterone acetate injections is not

affected by enzyme-inducing drugs and they may be continued as normal during courses of these drugs.

Effectiveness of the etonogestrel-releasing implant p. 790 may be reduced by enzyme-inducing drugs or griseofulvin and an alternative contraceptive method, unaffected by the interacting drug, is recommended during treatment with the interacting drug and for at least 4 weeks after stopping.

For a short course of an enzyme-inducing drug, if a change in contraceptive method is undesirable or inappropriate, continued contraception with the implant may be appropriate if used in combination with consistent and careful use of condoms for the duration of treatment and for 4 weeks after stopping the enzyme-inducing drug. Ⓐ

Hormonal emergency contraception interactions
The effectiveness of levonorgestrel and ulipristal acetate p. 785 is reduced in women taking enzyme-inducing drugs or griseofulvin (and for at least 4 weeks after stopping). EvGr A copper intra-uterine device can be offered instead. If the copper intra-uterine device is declined or unsuitable, the dose of levonorgestrel should be increased (See *Dose adjustments due to interactions* under levonorgestrel). There is no need to increase the dose for emergency contraception if the patient is taking antibacterials that are not enzyme inducers. Ⓐ

The effectiveness of ulipristal acetate for emergency contraception in women using drugs that increase gastric pH has not been studied. EvGr Levonorgestrel or a copper intra-uterine device should be considered as alternatives.

Hormonal contraception should not be newly initiated in a patient until five days after administration of ulipristal acetate as emergency hormonal contraception—the contraceptive effect of ulipristal acetate will be reduced. Consistent and careful use of condoms is recommended.

Ulipristal acetate can be used as emergency hormonal contraception more than once in the same cycle. Ⓐ Conversely, manufacturer advises that use of levonorgestrel as emergency contraception more than once in the same cycle is not advisable due to increased risk of side-effects (such as menstrual irregularities).

EvGr Levonorgestrel should not be used (as emergency hormonal contraception) within 5 days of administration of ulipristal acetate (as emergency hormonal contraception), as the contraceptive effect of ulipristal acetate may be reduced by progestogens.

Ulipristal acetate is not recommend for use in women who have severe asthma treated by oral corticosteroids, due to the antiglucocorticoid effect of ulipristal acetate. Ⓐ

Useful Resources

Drug interactions with hormonal contraception. The Faculty of Sexual and Reproductive Healthcare. Clinical guidance. January 2018.
www.fsrh.org/standards-and-guidance/current-clinical-guidance/drug-interactions

3.1 Contraception, combined

OESTROGENS COMBINED WITH PROGESTOGENS

Combined hormonal contraceptives

- **CONTRA-INDICATIONS** Acute porphyrias p. 1025 · gallstones · heart disease associated with pulmonary hypertension or risk of embolus · history during pregnancy of cholestatic jaundice · history during pregnancy of chorea · history during pregnancy of pemphigoid gestationis · history during pregnancy of pruritus · history of breast cancer (but can be used after 5 years if no evidence of disease and non-hormonal methods unacceptable) · history of haemolytic uraemic syndrome · migraine with aura · personal history of venous or arterial thrombosis · sclerosing treatment for varicose veins · severe or multiple risk factors for arterial disease · severe or multiple risk factors for venous thromboembolism · systemic lupus erythematosus with (or unknown) antiphospholipid antibodies · transient cerebral ischaemic attacks without headaches · undiagnosed vaginal bleeding

● CAUTIONS Active trophoblastic disease (until return to normal of urine- and plasma-gonadotrophin concentration)—seek specialist advice · Crohn's disease · gene mutations associated with breast cancer (e.g. BRCA 1) · history of severe depression especially if induced by hormonal contraceptive · hyperprolactinaemia (seek specialist advice) · inflammatory bowel disease · migraine · personal or family history of hypertriglyceridaemia (increased risk of pancreatitis) · risk factors for arterial disease · risk factors for venous thromboembolism · sickle-cell disease · undiagnosed breast mass

CAUTIONS, FURTHER INFORMATION

▸ Risk of venous thromboembolism There is an increased risk of venous thromboembolic disease in users of combined hormonal contraceptives particularly during the first year and possibly after restarting combined hormonal contraceptives following a break of four weeks or more. This risk is considerably smaller than that associated with pregnancy (about 60 cases of venous thromboembolic disease per 100 000 pregnancies). In all cases the risk of venous thromboembolism increases with age and in the presence of other risk factors, such as obesity. The risk also varies depending on the type of progestogen.

Provided that women are informed of the relative risks of venous thromboembolism and accept them, the choice of oral contraceptive is for the woman together with the prescriber jointly to make in light of her individual medical history and any contra-indications.

Combined hormonal contraceptives also slightly increase the risk of *arterial* thromboembolism; however, there is no evidence to suggest that this risk varies between different preparations.

▸ Risk factors for venous thromboembolism Use with **caution** if any of following factors present but **avoid** if two or more factors present:
  ● *family history of venous thromboembolism* in first-degree relative aged under 45 years (avoid contraceptive containing desogestrel or gestodene, *or* avoid if known prothrombotic coagulation abnormality e.g. factor V Leiden or antiphospholipid antibodies (including lupus anticoagulant));
  ● *obesity*; body mass index $\geq$ 30 kg/m^2 (avoid if body mass index $\geq$ 35 kg/m^2 unless no suitable alternative); (in adolescents, caution if obese according to BMI (adjusted for age and gender); in those who are markedly obese, avoid unless no suitable alternative);
  ● *long-term immobilisation* e.g. in a wheelchair (avoid if confined to bed or leg in plaster cast);
  ● *history of superficial thrombophlebitis;*
  ● *age* over 35 years (avoid if over 50 years);
  ● *smoking.*

Combined Hormonal Contraception and Risk of Venous Thromboembolism

Progestogen in Combined Hormonal Contraceptive	Estimated incidence per 10 000 women per year of use
Non-pregnant, not using combined hormonal contraception	2
Levonorgestrel[1]	5–7
Norgestimate[1]	5–7
Norethisterone[1]	5–7
Etonogestrel[1]	6–12
Norelgestromin[1]	6–12
Gestodene[1]	9–12
Desogestrel[1]	9–12
Drospirenone[1]	9–12
Dienogest[2]	Not known—insufficient data
Nomegestrol[2]	Not known—insufficient data

[1] Combined with ethinylestradiol [2] Combined with estradiol

▸ Risk factors for arterial disease Use with **caution** if any one of following factors present but **avoid** if two or more factors present:
  ● *family history of arterial disease* in first degree relative aged under 45 years (avoid if atherogenic lipid profile);
  ● *diabetes mellitus* (avoid if diabetes complications present);
  ● *hypertension*; blood pressure above *systolic* 140 *mmHg* or *diastolic* 90 *mmHg* (avoid if blood pressure above *systolic* 160 *mmHg* or *diastolic* 95 *mmHg*); (in adolescents, avoid if blood pressure very high);
  ● *smoking* (avoid if smoking 40 or more cigarettes daily);
  ● *age* over 35 years (avoid if over 50 years);
  ● *obesity* (avoid if body mass index $\geq$ 35 kg/m^2 unless no suitable alternative); (in adolescents, caution if obese according to BMI (adjusted for age and gender); in those who are markedly obese, avoid unless no suitable alternative);
  ● *migraine without aura* (avoid if *migraine with aura* (focal symptoms), *or* severe migraine frequently lasting over 72 hours despite treatment, *or* migraine treated with ergot derivatives).

▸ Migraine Women should report any increase in headache frequency or onset of focal symptoms (discontinue immediately and refer urgently to neurology expert if focal neurological symptoms not typical of aura persist for more than 1 hour).

Combined hormonal contraceptives should be stopped (pending investigation and treatment), if serious neurological effects occur, including unusual severe, prolonged headache especially if first time or getting progressively worse *or* sudden partial or complete loss of vision *or* sudden disturbance of hearing or other perceptual disorders *or* dysphasia *or* bad fainting attack or collapse *or* first unexplained epileptic seizure *or* weakness, motor disturbances, very marked numbness suddenly affecting one side or one part of body.

● SIDE-EFFECTS
▸ **Common or very common** Acne · fluid retention · headaches · menstrual cycle irregularities · nausea · weight increased
▸ **Uncommon** Alopecia · hypertension
▸ **Rare or very rare** Venous thromboembolism

SIDE-EFFECTS, FURTHER INFORMATION
Breast cancer There is a small increase in the risk of having breast cancer diagnosed in women taking the combined oral contraceptive pill; this relative risk may be due to an earlier diagnosis. In users of combined oral contraceptive pills the cancers are more likely to be

localised to the breast. The most important factor for diagnosing breast cancer appears to be the age at which the contraceptive is stopped rather than the duration of use; any increase in the rate of diagnosis diminishes gradually during the 10 years after stopping and disappears by 10 years.

Cervical cancer Use of combined oral contraceptives for 5 years or longer is associated with a small increased risk of cervical cancer; the risk diminishes after stopping and disappears by about 10 years. The possible small increase in the risk of breast cancer and cervical cancer should be weighed against the protective effect against cancers of the ovary and endometrium.

- PREGNANCY Not known to be harmful.
- BREAST FEEDING Avoid until weaning or for 6 months after birth (adverse effects on lactation).
- HEPATIC IMPAIRMENT Avoid in active liver disease including disorders of hepatic excretion (e.g. Dubin-Johnson or Rotor syndromes), infective hepatitis (until liver function returns to normal), liver tumours.
- DIRECTIONS FOR ADMINISTRATION
‣ With oral use Each tablet should be taken at approximately same time each day; if delayed, contraceptive protection may be lost. 21-*day combined preparations*, 1 tablet daily for 21 days; subsequent courses repeated after a 7-day interval (during which withdrawal bleeding occurs); if reasonably certain woman is not pregnant, first course can be started on any day of cycle—if starting on day 6 of cycle or later, additional precautions (barrier methods) necessary during first 7 days. *Every day (ED) combined preparations*, 1 *active* tablet daily for 21 days, followed by 1 *inactive* tablet daily for 7 days; subsequent courses repeated without interval (withdrawal bleeding occurs when *inactive* tablets being taken); if reasonably certain woman is not pregnant, first course can be started on any day of cycle—if starting on day 6 of cycle or later, additional precautions (barrier methods) necessary during first 7 days.

Changing to combined preparation containing different progestogen If previous contraceptive used correctly, or pregnancy can reasonably be excluded, start the first active tablet of new brand immediately. See individual monographs for requirements of specific preparations.
Changing from progestogen-only tablet If previous contraceptive used correctly, or pregnancy can reasonably be excluded, start new brand immediately, additional precautions (barrier methods) necessary for first 7 days.
Secondary amenorrhoea (exclude pregnancy) Start any day, additional precautions (barrier methods) necessary during first 7 days (9 days for *Qlaira*®).
After childbirth (not breast-feeding) Start 3 weeks after birth (increased risk of thrombosis if started earlier); later than 3 weeks postpartum additional precautions (barrier methods) necessary for first 7 days (9 days for *Qlaira*®).
After abortion or miscarriage Start same day.

- PATIENT AND CARER ADVICE
Travel Women taking oral contraceptives are at an increased risk of deep vein thrombosis during travel involving long periods of immobility (over 3 hours). The risk may be reduced by appropriate exercise during the journey and possibly by wearing graduated compression hosiery.
Diarrhoea and vomiting Vomiting and persistent, severe diarrhoea can interfere with the absorption of combined oral contraceptives. If vomiting occurs within 2 hours of taking a combined oral contraceptive another pill should be taken as soon as possible. In cases of persistent vomiting or severe diarrhoea lasting more than 24 hours, additional precautions should be used during and for 7 days after recovery. If the vomiting and diarrhoea occurs during the last 7 tablets, the next pill-free interval should

be omitted (in the case of ED tablets the inactive ones should be omitted).
Missed doses The critical time for loss of contraceptive protection is when a pill is omitted at the *beginning* or *end* of a cycle (which lengthens the pill-free interval).
If a woman forgets to take a pill, it should be taken as soon as she remembers, and the next one taken at the normal time (even if this means taking 2 pills together). A missed pill is one that is 24 or more hours late. If a woman misses only one pill, she should take an active pill as soon as she remembers and then resume normal pill-taking. No additional precautions are necessary.
If a woman misses 2 or more pills (especially from the first 7 in a packet), she may not be protected. She should take an active pill as soon as she remembers and then resume normal pill-taking. In addition, she must either abstain from sex or use an additional method of contraception such as a condom for the next 7 days. If these 7 days run beyond the end of the packet, the next packet should be started at once, omitting the pill-free interval (or, in the case of *everyday* (ED) pills, omitting the 7 inactive tablets).
Emergency contraception is recommended if 2 or more combined oral contraceptive tablets are missed from the first 7 tablets in a packet and unprotected intercourse has occurred since finishing the last packet.

F 776

Dienogest with estradiol valerate

- INDICATIONS AND DOSE

Contraception with 28-day combined preparations | Menstrual symptoms with 28-day combined preparations
‣ BY MOUTH
‣ Females of childbearing potential: 1 active tablet once daily for 26 days, followed by 1 inactive tablet daily for 2 days, withdrawal bleeding may occur during the 2-day interval of *inactive* tablets, tablets should be taken at approximately the same time each day

- INTERACTIONS → Appendix 1: combined hormonal contraceptives
- SIDE-EFFECTS
‣ **Common or very common** Breast abnormalities · gastrointestinal discomfort · headaches · increased risk of infection
‣ **Uncommon** Appetite increased · cervical abnormalities · crying · depression · diarrhoea · dizziness · fatigue · haemorrhage · hot flush · hyperhidrosis · mood altered · muscle spasms · neoplasms · oedema · ovarian and fallopian tube disorders · painful sexual intercourse · pelvic disorders · sexual dysfunction · skin reactions · sleep disorders · uterine cramps · vomiting · vulvovaginal disorders · weight decreased
‣ **Rare or very rare** Aggression · anxiety · arterial thromboembolism · asthma · chest pain · cholecystitis chronic · concentration impaired · constipation · contact lens intolerance · dry eye · dry mouth · dyspnoea · eye swelling · fever · galactorrhoea · gastrooesophageal reflux disease · genital discharge · hair changes · hypertriglyceridaemia · hypotension · lymphadenopathy · malaise · myocardial infarction · pain · palpitations · paraesthesia · seborrhoea · sensation of pressure · urinary tract pain · vascular disorders · vertigo
- DIRECTIONS FOR ADMINISTRATION
Changing to *Qlaira*® Start the first active *Qlaira*® tablet on the day after taking the last active tablet of the previous brand.

7

Genito-urinary system

PATIENT AND CARER ADVICE
Diarrhoea and vomiting In cases of persistent vomiting or severe diarrhoea lasting more than 12 hours in women taking *Qlaira®*, refer to product literature.
Missed doses A missed pill for a patient taking *Qlaira®* is one that is 12 hours or more late; for information on how to manage missed pills in women taking *Qlaira®*, refer to product literature.

MEDICINAL FORMS
There can be variation in the licensing of different medicines containing the same drug.

Tablet
▸ Dienogest with estradiol valerate (Non-proprietary)
  Dienogest 2 mg, Estradiol valerate 2 mg Estradiol valerate 2mg / Dienogest 2mg tablets | 15 tablet [PoM] Ⓢ
  Estradiol valerate 2 mg, Dienogest 3 mg Estradiol valerate 2mg / Dienogest 3mg tablets | 51 tablet [PoM] Ⓢ
▸ Qlaira (Bayer Plc)
  Qlaira tablets | 84 tablet [PoM] £25.18

F 776

Estradiol with nomegestrol

INDICATIONS AND DOSE

Contraception
▸ BY MOUTH
▸ Females of childbearing potential: 1 active tablet daily for 24 days, followed by 1 inactive tablet daily for 4 days, to be started on day 1 of cycle with first active tablet (withdrawal bleeding occurs when inactive tablets being taken); subsequent courses repeated without interval

INTERACTIONS → Appendix 1: combined hormonal contraceptives

SIDE-EFFECTS
▸ **Common or very common** Breast abnormalities · depression · mood altered · pelvic pain · sexual dysfunction
▸ **Uncommon** Abdominal distension · appetite abnormal · galactorrhoea · hot flush · hyperhidrosis · oedema · painful sexual intercourse · seborrhoea · sensation of pressure · skin reactions · uterine cramps · vulvovaginal disorders
▸ **Rare or very rare** Cerebrovascular insufficiency · concentration impaired · contact lens intolerance · dry eye · dry mouth · gallbladder disorders · hypertrichosis

PREGNANCY Toxicity in *animal* studies.

DIRECTIONS FOR ADMINISTRATION *Zoely®* (every day (ED) combined (monophasic) preparation), 1 *active* tablet daily for 24 days, followed by 1 *inactive* tablet daily for 4 days, starting on day 1 of cycle with first *active* tablet; subsequent courses repeated without interval (withdrawal bleeding occurs when *inactive* tablets being taken). Changing to *Zoely®* Start the first active *Zoely®* tablet on the day after taking the last active tablet of the previous brand or, at the latest, the day after the tablet-free or inactive tablet interval of the previous brand.

PATIENT AND CARER ADVICE
Diarrhoea and vomiting In cases of persistent vomiting or severe diarrhoea lasting more than 12 hours in women taking *Zoely®*, refer to product literature.
Missed doses A missed pill for a patient taking *Zoely®* is one that is 12 hours or more late; for information on how to manage missed pills in women taking *Zoely®*, refer to product literature.

MEDICINAL FORMS
There can be variation in the licensing of different medicines containing the same drug.

Tablet
▸ Zoely (Merck Sharp & Dohme Ltd) ▼
  Estradiol (as Estradiol hemihydrate) 1.5 mg, Nomegestrol acetate 2.5 mg Zoely 2.5mg/1.5mg tablets | 84 tablet [PoM] £19.80 DT = £19.80

F 776

Ethinylestradiol with desogestrel

INDICATIONS AND DOSE

Contraception with 21-day combined preparations | Menstrual symptoms with 21-day combined preparations
▸ BY MOUTH
▸ Females of childbearing potential: 1 tablet once daily for 21 days; subsequent courses repeated after 7-day interval, withdrawal bleeding occurs during the 7-day interval, if reasonably certain woman is not pregnant, first course can be started on any day of cycle—if starting on day 6 of cycle or later, additional precautions (barrier methods) necessary during first 7 days, tablets should be taken at approximately the same time each day

INTERACTIONS → Appendix 1: combined hormonal contraceptives

MEDICINAL FORMS
There can be variation in the licensing of different medicines containing the same drug.

Tablet
▸ Ethinylestradiol with desogestrel (Non-proprietary)
  Ethinylestradiol 20 microgram, Desogestrel 150 microgram Ethinylestradiol 20microgram / Desogestrel 150microgram tablets | 63 tablet [PoM] Ⓢ DT = £5.08
  Ethinylestradiol 30 microgram, Desogestrel 150 microgram Ethinylestradiol 30microgram / Desogestrel 150microgram tablets | 63 tablet [PoM] Ⓢ DT = £4.19
▸ Alenvona (Teva UK Ltd)
  Ethinylestradiol 30 microgram, Desogestrel 150 microgram Alenvona 150microgram/30microgram tablets | 63 tablet [PoM] £6.13 DT = £4.19
▸ Bimizza (Morningside Healthcare Ltd)
  Ethinylestradiol 20 microgram, Desogestrel 150 microgram Bimizza 150microgram/20microgram tablets | 63 tablet [PoM] £5.04 DT = £5.08
▸ Cimizt (Morningside Healthcare Ltd)
  Ethinylestradiol 30 microgram, Desogestrel 150 microgram Cimizt 30microgram/150microgram tablets | 63 tablet [PoM] £3.80 DT = £4.19
▸ Gedarel (Consilient Health Ltd)
  Ethinylestradiol 20 microgram, Desogestrel 150 microgram Gedarel 20microgram/150microgram tablets | 63 tablet [PoM] £5.08 DT = £5.08
  Ethinylestradiol 30 microgram, Desogestrel 150 microgram Gedarel 30microgram/150microgram tablets | 63 tablet [PoM] £4.19 DT = £4.19
▸ Marvelon (Merck Sharp & Dohme Ltd)
  Ethinylestradiol 30 microgram, Desogestrel 150 microgram Marvelon tablets | 63 tablet [PoM] £7.10 DT = £4.19
▸ Mercilon (Merck Sharp & Dohme Ltd)
  Ethinylestradiol 20 microgram, Desogestrel 150 microgram Mercilon 150microgram/20microgram tablets | 63 tablet [PoM] £8.44 DT = £5.08
▸ Munalea (Lupin Healthcare (UK) Ltd)
  Ethinylestradiol 20 microgram, Desogestrel 150 microgram Munalea 150microgram/20microgram tablets | 63 tablet [PoM] £5.07 DT = £5.08
  Ethinylestradiol 30 microgram, Desogestrel 150 microgram Munalea 150microgram/30microgram tablets | 63 tablet [PoM] £4.18 DT = £4.19

7

Genito-urinary system

Ethinylestradiol with drospirenone

F 776

● INDICATIONS AND DOSE

Contraception with 21-day combined preparations | Menstrual symptoms with 21-day combined preparations
▸ BY MOUTH
▸ Females of childbearing potential: 1 tablet once daily for 21 days; subsequent courses repeated after 7-day interval, withdrawal bleeding occurs during the 7-day interval

● INTERACTIONS → Appendix 1: combined hormonal contraceptives

● SIDE-EFFECTS
▸ **Common or very common** Breast abnormalities · depressed mood · increased risk of infection · vaginal discharge
▸ **Uncommon** Diarrhoea · hypotension · sexual dysfunction · skin reactions · vomiting · weight decreased
▸ **Rare or very rare** Arterial thromboembolism · asthma · erythema nodosum · hearing impairment

● PATIENT AND CARER ADVICE
Pill-free interval Withdrawal bleeding can occur during the 7-day tablet-free interval.

● MEDICINAL FORMS
There can be variation in the licensing of different medicines containing the same drug.
Tablet
▸ Ethinylestradiol with drospirenone (Non-proprietary)
Ethinylestradiol 30 microgram, Drospirenone 3 mg Ethinylestradiol 30microgram / Drospirenone 3mg tablets | 63 tablet [PoM] [⬛] DT = £14.70
▸ Daylette (Consilient Health Ltd)
Ethinylestradiol 20 microgram, Drospirenone 3 mg Daylette 0.02mg/3mg tablets | 84 tablet [PoM] £10.50 DT = £14.70
▸ Dretine (Teva UK Ltd)
Ethinylestradiol 30 microgram, Drospirenone 3 mg Dretine 0.03mg/3mg tablets | 63 tablet [PoM] £8.30 DT = £14.70
▸ ELOINE (Bayer Plc)
Ethinylestradiol 20 microgram, Drospirenone 3 mg Eloine 0.02mg/3mg tablets | 84 tablet [PoM] £14.70 DT = £14.70
▸ Lucette (Consilient Health Ltd)
Ethinylestradiol 30 microgram, Drospirenone 3 mg Lucette 0.03mg/3mg tablets | 63 tablet [PoM] £9.35 DT = £14.70
▸ Yacella (Morningside Healthcare Ltd)
Ethinylestradiol 30 microgram, Drospirenone 3 mg Yacella 0.03mg/3mg tablets | 63 tablet [PoM] £8.30 DT = £14.70
▸ Yasmin (Bayer Plc)
Ethinylestradiol 30 microgram, Drospirenone 3 mg Yasmin tablets | 63 tablet [PoM] £14.70 DT = £14.70
▸ Yiznell (Lupin Healthcare (UK) Ltd)
Ethinylestradiol 30 microgram, Drospirenone 3 mg Yiznell 0.03mg/3mg tablets | 63 tablet [PoM] £8.30 DT = £14.70

Ethinylestradiol with etonogestrel

F 776

● INDICATIONS AND DOSE

Contraception | Menstrual symptoms
▸ BY VAGINA
▸ Females of childbearing potential: 1 unit, insert the ring into the vagina on day 1 of cycle and leave in for 3 weeks; remove ring on day 22; subsequent courses repeated after 7-day ring free interval (during which withdrawal bleeding occurs)

● INTERACTIONS → Appendix 1: combined hormonal contraceptives

● DIRECTIONS FOR ADMINISTRATION
Changing method of contraception to vaginal ring
Changing from combined hormonal contraception Insert ring at the latest on the day after the usual tablet-free, patch-free, or inactive-tablet interval. If previous contraceptive used

correctly, or pregnancy can reasonably be excluded, can switch to ring on any day of cycle.
Changing from progestogen-only method From an implant or intra-uterine progestogen-only device, insert ring on the day implant or intra-uterine progestogen-only device removed; from an injection, insert ring when next injection due; from oral preparation, first ring may be inserted on any day after stopping pill. For all methods additional precautions (barrier methods) should be used concurrently for first 7 days.

● PATIENT AND CARER ADVICE Patients or carers should be given advice on how to administer vaginal ring.
Counselling The presence of the ring should be checked regularly.
Missed doses
Expulsion, delayed insertion or removal, or broken vaginal ring If the vaginal ring is expelled for *less than* 3 *hours*, rinse the ring with cool water and reinsert immediately; no additional contraception is needed.

If the ring remains outside the vagina for *more than* 3 *hours* or if the user does not know when the ring was expelled, contraceptive protection may be reduced:
• If ring expelled during week 1 or 2 of cycle, rinse ring with cool water and reinsert; use additional precautions (barrier methods) for next 7 days;
• If ring expelled during week 3 of cycle, either insert a new ring to start a new cycle *or* allow a withdrawal bleed and insert a new ring no later than 7 days after ring was expelled; latter option only available if ring was used continuously for at least 7 days before expulsion.
If insertion of a new ring at the start of a new cycle is delayed, contraceptive protection is lost. A new ring should be inserted as soon as possible; additional precautions (barrier methods) should be used for the first 7 days of the new cycle. If intercourse occurred during the extended ring-free interval, pregnancy should be considered.

No additional contraception is required if removal of the ring is delayed by up to 1 week (4 weeks of continuous use). The 7-day ring-free interval should be observed and subsequently a new ring should be inserted. Contraceptive protection may be reduced with continuous use of the ring for more than 4 weeks—pregnancy should be ruled out before inserting a new ring.

If the ring breaks during use, remove it and insert a new ring immediately; additional precautions (barrier methods) should be used for the first 7 days of the new cycle.

● MEDICINAL FORMS
There can be variation in the licensing of different medicines containing the same drug.
Vaginal delivery system
▸ Ethinylestradiol with etonogestrel (Non-proprietary)
Ethinylestradiol 2.7 mg, Etonogestrel 11.7 mg Ethinylestradiol 2.7mg / Etonogestrel 11.7mg vaginal delivery system | 3 system [PoM] [⬛] DT = £29.70
▸ NuvaRing (Merck Sharp & Dohme Ltd)
Ethinylestradiol 2.7 mg, Etonogestrel 11.7 mg NuvaRing 0.12mg/0.015mg per day vaginal delivery system | 3 system [PoM] £29.70 DT = £29.70

Ethinylestradiol with gestodene

F 776

● INDICATIONS AND DOSE

Contraception with 21-day combined preparations | Menstrual symptoms with 21-day combined preparations
▸ BY MOUTH
▸ Females of childbearing potential: 1 tablet once daily for 21 days; subsequent courses repeated after 7-day interval, withdrawal bleeding occurs during the 7-day

interval, if reasonably certain woman is not pregnant, first course can be started on any day of cycle—if starting on day 6 of cycle or later, additional precautions (barrier methods) necessary during first 7 days, tablets should be taken at approximately the same time each day

Contraception with 28-day combined preparations | Menstrual symptoms with 28-day combined preparations

▸ BY MOUTH

▸ Females of childbearing potential: 1 active tablet once daily for 21 days, followed by 1 inactive tablet daily for 7 days; subsequent courses repeated without interval, withdrawal bleeding occurs during the 7-day interval of *inactive* tablets being taken, if reasonably certain woman is not pregnant, first course can be started on any day of cycle—if starting on day 6 of cycle or later, additional precautions (barrier methods) necessary during first 7 days, tablets should be taken at approximately the same time each day

● INTERACTIONS → Appendix 1: combined hormonal contraceptives

● SIDE-EFFECTS

▸ **Common or very common** Abdominal pain · breast abnormalities · depression · dizziness · increased risk of infection · mood swings · nervousness · vaginal discharge
▸ **Uncommon** Appetite abnormal · diarrhoea · hirsutism · hypertriglyceridaemia · sexual dysfunction · skin reactions · vomiting
▸ **Rare or very rare** Angioedema · chorea exacerbated · ear disorders · embolism and thrombosis · erythema nodosum · eye irritation · gallbladder disorders · gastrointestinal disorders · haemolytic uraemic syndrome · hepatic disorders · hypersensitivity · inflammatory bowel disease · neoplasms · optic neuritis · pancreatitis · systemic lupus erythematosus exacerbated · varicose veins exacerbated · weight decreased

● MEDICINAL FORMS
There can be variation in the licensing of different medicines containing the same drug.

Tablet
▸ Ethinylestradiol with gestodene (Non-proprietary)
Ethinylestradiol 30 microgram, Gestodene
50 microgram Ethinylestradiol 30microgram / Gestodene 50microgram tablets | 18 tablet PoM 🅂
Ethinylestradiol 40 microgram, Gestodene
70 microgram Ethinylestradiol 40microgram / Gestodene 70microgram tablets | 15 tablet PoM 🅂
Ethinylestradiol 20 microgram, Gestodene
75 microgram Ethinylestradiol 20microgram / Gestodene 75microgram tablets | 63 tablet PoM 🅂 DT = £8.85
Ethinylestradiol 30 microgram, Gestodene
75 microgram Ethinylestradiol 30microgram / Gestodene 75microgram tablets | 63 tablet PoM 🅂 DT = £6.73
Ethinylestradiol 30 microgram, Gestodene
100 microgram Ethinylestradiol 30microgram / Gestodene 100microgram tablets | 30 tablet PoM 🅂
▸ Aidulan (Lupin Healthcare (UK) Ltd)
Ethinylestradiol 30 microgram, Gestodene 75 microgram Aidulan 30microgram/75microgram tablets | 63 tablet PoM £4.11 DT = £6.73
Ethinylestradiol 20 microgram, Gestodene 75 microgram Aidulan 20microgram/75microgram tablets | 63 tablet PoM £5.40 DT = £8.85
▸ Femodene (Bayer Plc)
Ethinylestradiol 30 microgram, Gestodene
75 microgram Femodene tablets | 63 tablet PoM £6.73 DT = £6.73
▸ Femodette (Bayer Plc)
Ethinylestradiol 20 microgram, Gestodene
75 microgram Femodette tablets | 63 tablet PoM £8.85 DT = £8.85
▸ Juliperla (Actavis UK Ltd)
Ethinylestradiol 20 microgram, Gestodene
75 microgram Juliperla 75microgram/20microgram tablets | 63 tablet PoM £5.41 DT = £8.85

▸ Katya (Stragen UK Ltd)
Ethinylestradiol 30 microgram, Gestodene 75 microgram Katya 30/75 tablets | 63 tablet PoM £5.03 DT = £6.73
▸ Millinette (Consilient Health Ltd)
Ethinylestradiol 30 microgram, Gestodene
75 microgram Millinette 30microgram/75microgram tablets | 63 tablet PoM £4.12 DT = £6.73
Ethinylestradiol 20 microgram, Gestodene
75 microgram Millinette 20microgram/75microgram tablets | 63 tablet PoM £5.41 DT = £8.85
▸ Sofiperla (Actavis UK Ltd)
Ethinylestradiol 30 microgram, Gestodene
75 microgram Sofiperla 75microgram/30microgram tablets | 63 tablet PoM £4.12 DT = £6.73
▸ Sunya (Stragen UK Ltd)
Ethinylestradiol 20 microgram, Gestodene 75 microgram Sunya 20/75 tablets | 63 tablet PoM £4.86 DT = £8.85

F 776

Ethinylestradiol with levonorgestrel

● INDICATIONS AND DOSE

Contraception with 21-day combined preparations | Menstrual symptoms with 21-day combined preparations

▸ BY MOUTH

▸ Females of childbearing potential: 1 tablet once daily for 21 days; subsequent courses repeated after 7-day interval, withdrawal bleeding occurs during the 7-day interval, if reasonably certain woman is not pregnant, first course can be started on any day of cycle—if starting on day 6 of cycle or later, additional precautions (barrier methods) necessary during first 7 days, tablets should be taken at approximately the same time each day

Contraception with 28-day combined preparations | Menstrual symptoms with 28-day combined preparations

▸ BY MOUTH

▸ Females of childbearing potential: 1 active tablet once daily for 21 days, followed by 1 inactive tablet once daily for 7 days, withdrawal bleeding occurs during the 7-day interval of *inactive* tablets being taken, if reasonably certain woman is not pregnant, first course can be started on any day of cycle—if starting on day 6 of cycle or later, additional precautions (barrier methods) necessary during first 7 days, tablets should be taken at approximately the same time each day. Subsequent courses repeated without interval

● INTERACTIONS → Appendix 1: combined hormonal contraceptives

● MEDICINAL FORMS
There can be variation in the licensing of different medicines containing the same drug.

Tablet
▸ Ethinylestradiol with levonorgestrel (Non-proprietary)
Ethinylestradiol 30 microgram, Levonorgestrel
50 microgram Ethinylestradiol 30microgram / Levonorgestrel 50microgram tablets | 6 tablet PoM 🅂
Ethinylestradiol 40 microgram, Levonorgestrel
75 microgram Ethinylestradiol 40microgram / Levonorgestrel 75microgram tablets | 5 tablet PoM 🅂
Ethinylestradiol 30 microgram, Levonorgestrel
125 microgram Ethinylestradiol 30microgram / Levonorgestrel 125microgram tablets | 10 tablet PoM 🅂
▸ Elevin (MedRx Licences Ltd)
Ethinylestradiol 30 microgram, Levonorgestrel
150 microgram Elevin 150microgram/30microgram tablets | 63 tablet PoM £29.25 DT = £2.82
▸ Erlibelle (Actavis UK Ltd)
Ethinylestradiol 30 microgram, Levonorgestrel
150 microgram Erlibelle 30microgram/150microgram tablets | 63 tablet PoM £2.82 DT = £2.82

▸ Leandra (Genesis Pharmaceuticals Ltd)
**Ethinylestradiol 30 microgram, Levonorgestrel
150 microgram** Leandra 30microgram/150microgram tablets |
63 tablet PoM £2.82 DT = £2.82
▸ Levest (Morningside Healthcare Ltd)
**Ethinylestradiol 30 microgram, Levonorgestrel
150 microgram** Levest 150/30 tablets | 21 tablet PoM £0.85
(Hospital only) | 63 tablet PoM £1.80 DT = £2.82
▸ Maexeni (Lupin Healthcare (UK) Ltd)
**Ethinylestradiol 30 microgram, Levonorgestrel
150 microgram** Maexeni 150microgram/30microgram tablets |
63 tablet PoM £1.88 DT = £2.82
▸ Microgynon 30 (Bayer Plc)
**Ethinylestradiol 30 microgram, Levonorgestrel
150 microgram** Microgynon 30 tablets | 63 tablet PoM £2.82 DT =
£2.82
▸ Ovranette (Pfizer Ltd)
**Ethinylestradiol 30 microgram, Levonorgestrel
150 microgram** Ovranette 150microgram/30microgram tablets |
63 tablet PoM £2.20 DT = £2.82
▸ Rigevidon (Consilient Health Ltd)
**Ethinylestradiol 30 microgram, Levonorgestrel
150 microgram** Rigevidon tablets | 63 tablet PoM £1.89 DT = £2.82

☞ 776

Ethinylestradiol with norelgestromin

● **INDICATIONS AND DOSE**

Contraception | Menstrual symptoms
▸ BY TRANSDERMAL APPLICATION
▸ Females of childbearing potential: Apply 1 patch once
weekly for 3 weeks, apply first patch on day 1 of cycle,
change patch on days 8 and 15; remove third patch on
day 22 and apply new patch after 7-day patch-free
interval to start subsequent contraceptive cycle,
subsequent courses repeated after a 7-day patch free
interval (during which withdrawal bleeding occurs)

● INTERACTIONS → Appendix 1: combined hormonal
contraceptives

● SIDE-EFFECTS
▸ **Common or very common** Anxiety · breast abnormalities ·
diarrhoea · dizziness · fatigue · gastrointestinal discomfort ·
increased risk of infection · malaise · mood altered · muscle
spasms · skin reactions · uterine cramps · vaginal
haemorrhage · vomiting · vulvovaginal disorders
▸ **Uncommon** Appetite increased · dyslipidaemia · insomnia ·
lactation disorders · oedema · photosensitivity reaction ·
sexual dysfunction
▸ **Rare or very rare** Embolism and thrombosis · gallbladder
disorders · genital discharge · neoplasms · stroke · swelling
▸ **Frequency not known** Anger · angioedema · cervical
dysplasia · colitis · contact lens intolerance · erythema
nodosum · hepatic disorders · hyperglycaemia ·
hypertensive crisis · intracranial haemorrhage · myocardial
infarction · pulmonary artery thrombosis · taste altered

● DIRECTIONS FOR ADMINISTRATION Adhesives or bandages
should not be used to hold patch in place. If no longer
sticky do not reapply but use a new patch.
Changing to a transdermal combined hormonal contraceptive
Changing from combined oral contraception
Apply patch on the first day of withdrawal bleeding; if no
withdrawal bleeding within 5 days of taking last *active*
tablet, rule out pregnancy before applying first patch.
Unless patch is applied on first day of withdrawal bleeding,
additional precautions (barrier methods) should be used
concurrently for first 7 days.
Changing from progestogen-only method
● from an implant, apply first patch on the day implant
removed
● from an injection, apply first patch when next injection
due
● from oral progestogen, first patch may be applied on any
day after stopping pill

For all methods additional precautions (barrier methods)
should be used concurrently for first 7 days.
After childbirth (not breast-feeding) Start 4 weeks
after birth; if started later than 4 weeks after birth
additional precautions (barrier methods) should be used
for first 7 days.
After abortion or miscarriage Before 20 weeks'
gestation start immediately; no additional contraception
required if started immediately. After 20 weeks' gestation
start on day 21 after abortion or on the first day of first
spontaneous menstruation; additional precautions (barrier
methods) should be used for first 7 days after applying the
patch.

● PATIENT AND CARER ADVICE Patients and carers should be
given advice on how to administer patches.
Travel Women using patches are at an increased risk of
deep vein thrombosis during travel involving long periods
of immobility (over 3 hours). The risk may be reduced by
appropriate exercise during the journey and possibly by
wearing graduated compression hosiery.
Missed doses
Delayed application or detached patch If a patch is partly
detached for less than 24 hours, reapply to the same site or
replace with a new patch immediately; no additional
contraception is needed and the next patch should be
applied on the usual 'change day'. If a patch remains
detached for more than 24 hours or if the user is not aware
when the patch became detached, then stop the current
contraceptive cycle and start a new cycle by applying a new
patch, giving a new 'Day 1'; an additional non-hormonal
contraceptive must be used concurrently for the first
7 days of the new cycle.
If application of a new patch at the start of a new cycle is
delayed, contraceptive protection is lost. A new patch
should be applied as soon as remembered giving a new
'Day 1'; additional non-hormonal methods of
contraception should be used for the first 7 days of the new
cycle. If application of a patch in the middle of the cycle is
delayed (i.e. the patch is not changed on day 8 or day 15):
● for up to 48 hours, apply a new patch immediately; next
patch 'change day' remains the same and no additional
contraception is required;
● for more than 48 hours, contraceptive protection may
have been lost. Stop the current cycle and start a new
4-week cycle immediately by applying a new patch
giving a new 'Day 1'; additional non-hormonal
contraception should be used for the first 7 days of the
new cycle.
If the patch is not removed at the end of the cycle (day 22),
remove it as soon as possible and start the next cycle on
the usual 'change day', the day after day 28; no additional
contraception is required.

● NATIONAL FUNDING/ACCESS DECISIONS

Scottish Medicines Consortium (SMC) Decisions
The *Scottish Medicines Consortium* has advised (September
2003) that *Evra®* patches should be restricted for use in
women who are likely to comply poorly with combined oral
contraceptives.

● MEDICINAL FORMS
There can be variation in the licensing of different medicines
containing the same drug.

Transdermal patch
▸ Evra (Janssen-Cilag Ltd)
**Ethinylestradiol 33.9 microgram per 24 hour, Norelgestromin
203 microgram per 24 hour** Evra transdermal patches |
9 patch PoM £19.51 DT = £19.51

Ethinylestradiol with norethisterone

● **INDICATIONS AND DOSE**

Contraception with 21-day combined preparations | Menstrual symptoms with 21-day combined preparations

▸ BY MOUTH

▸ Females of childbearing potential: 1 tablet once daily for 21 days; subsequent courses repeated after 7-day interval, withdrawal bleeding occurs during the 7-day interval, if reasonably certain woman is not pregnant, first course can be started on any day of cycle—if starting on day 6 of cycle or later, additional precautions (barrier methods) necessary during first 7 days, tablets should be taken at approximately the same time each day

● **INTERACTIONS** → Appendix 1: combined hormonal contraceptives

● **MEDICINAL FORMS**
There can be variation in the licensing of different medicines containing the same drug.

Tablet
▸ Ethinylestradiol with norethisterone (Non-proprietary)
  Ethinylestradiol 35 microgram, Norethisterone
  500 microgram Ethinylestradiol 35microgram / Norethisterone 500microgram tablets | 5 tablet [PoM] [S̶]
  Ethinylestradiol 35 microgram, Norethisterone
  750 microgram Ethinylestradiol 35microgram / Norethisterone 750microgram tablets | 21 tablet [PoM] [S̶]
  Ethinylestradiol 35 microgram, Norethisterone
  1 mg Ethinylestradiol 35microgram / Norethisterone 1mg tablets | 9 tablet [PoM] [S̶]
▸ Brevinor (Pfizer Ltd)
  Ethinylestradiol 35 microgram, Norethisterone
  500 microgram Brevinor 500microgram/35microgram tablets | 63 tablet [PoM] £1.99 DT = £1.99
▸ Loestrin 20 (Galen Ltd)
  Ethinylestradiol 20 microgram, Norethisterone acetate
  1 mg Loestrin 20 tablets | 63 tablet [PoM] £2.70 DT = £2.70
▸ Loestrin 30 (Galen Ltd)
  Ethinylestradiol 30 microgram, Norethisterone acetate
  1.5 mg Loestrin 30 tablets | 63 tablet [PoM] £3.90 DT = £3.90
▸ Norimin (Pfizer Ltd)
  Ethinylestradiol 35 microgram, Norethisterone 1 mg Norimin 1mg/35microgram tablets | 63 tablet [PoM] £2.28 DT = £2.28

Ethinylestradiol with norgestimate

● **INDICATIONS AND DOSE**

Contraception with 21-day combined preparations | Menstrual symptoms with 21-day combined preparations

▸ BY MOUTH

▸ Females of childbearing potential: 1 tablet once daily for 21 days; subsequent courses repeated after 7-day interval, withdrawal bleeding occurs during the 7-day interval, if reasonably certain woman is not pregnant, first course can be started on any day of cycle—if starting on day 6 of cycle or later, additional precautions (barrier methods) necessary during first 7 days, tablets should be taken at approximately the same time each day

● **INTERACTIONS** → Appendix 1: combined hormonal contraceptives

● **SIDE-EFFECTS**
▸ **Common or very common** Anxiety · asthenic conditions · breast abnormalities · chest pain · constipation · depression · diarrhoea · dizziness · gastrointestinal discomfort · gastrointestinal disorders · genital discharge · hypersensitivity · increased risk of infection · insomnia ·

mood altered · muscle complaints · oedema · pain · skin reactions · vomiting
▸ **Uncommon** Appetite abnormal · cervical dysplasia · dry eye · dyspnoea · embolism and thrombosis · hirsutism · hot flush · libido disorder · ovarian cyst · palpitations · paraesthesia · syncope · visual impairment · vulvovaginal disorders · weight changes
▸ **Rare or very rare** Hepatic disorders · pancreatitis · photosensitivity reaction · sweat changes · tachycardia · vertigo
▸ **Frequency not known** Angioedema · contact lens intolerance · dyslipidaemia · erythema nodosum · neoplasms · seizure · suppressed lactation

● **MEDICINAL FORMS**
There can be variation in the licensing of different medicines containing the same drug.

Tablet
▸ Ethinylestradiol with norgestimate (Non-proprietary)
  Ethinylestradiol 35 microgram, Norgestimate
  250 microgram Ethinylestradiol 35microgram / Norgestimate 250microgram tablets | 63 tablet [PoM] [S̶] DT = £7.16
▸ Cilest (Janssen-Cilag Ltd)
  Ethinylestradiol 35 microgram, Norgestimate
  250 microgram Cilest 35microgram/250microgram tablets | 63 tablet [PoM] £7.16 DT = £7.16 | 126 tablet [PoM] £14.32
▸ Cilique (Consilient Health Ltd)
  Ethinylestradiol 35 microgram, Norgestimate
  250 microgram Cilique 250microgram/35microgram tablets | 63 tablet [PoM] £4.65 DT = £7.16
▸ Lizinna (Morningside Healthcare Ltd)
  Ethinylestradiol 35 microgram, Norgestimate
  250 microgram Lizinna 250microgram/35microgram tablets | 63 tablet [PoM] £5.37 DT = £7.16

Norethisterone with mestranol

● **INDICATIONS AND DOSE**

Contraception | Menstrual symptoms

▸ BY MOUTH

▸ Females of childbearing potential: 1 tablet once daily for 21 days; subsequent courses repeated after 7-day interval, withdrawal bleeding can occur during the 7-day interval, if reasonably certain woman is not pregnant, first course can be started on any day of cycle—if starting on day 6 of cycle or later, additional precautions (barrier methods) necessary during first 7 days, tablets should be taken at the same time each day

● **INTERACTIONS** → Appendix 1: combined hormonal contraceptives

● **SIDE-EFFECTS** Appetite change · breast tenderness · depression · gastrointestinal disorder · libido disorder · metabolic disorders · uterine leiomyoma exacerbated

● **MEDICINAL FORMS**
There can be variation in the licensing of different medicines containing the same drug.

Tablet
▸ Norinyl-1 (Pfizer Ltd)
  Mestranol 50 microgram, Norethisterone 1 mg Norinyl-1 tablets | 63 tablet [PoM] £2.19 DT = £2.19

3.2 Contraception, devices

Other drugs used for Contraception, devices
Levonorgestrel, p. 787

CONTRACEPTIVE DEVICES

Intra-uterine contraceptive devices (copper)

- INDICATIONS AND DOSE

Contraception

▶ BY INTRA-UTERINE ADMINISTRATION

▶ Females of childbearing potential: (consult product literature)

IMPORTANT SAFETY INFORMATION

MHRA/CHM ADVICE (JUNE 2015) INTRA-UTERINE CONTRACEPTION: UTERINE PERFORATION—UPDATED INFORMATION ON RISK FACTORS

Uterine perforation most often occurs during insertion, but might not be detected until sometime later. The risk of uterine perforation is increased when the device is inserted up to 36 weeks postpartum or in patients who are breastfeeding. Before inserting an intra-uterine contraceptive device, inform patients that perforation occurs in approximately 1 in every 1000 insertions and signs and symptoms include:

- severe pelvic pain after insertion (worse than period cramps);
- pain or increased bleeding after insertion which continues for more than a few weeks;
- sudden changes in periods;
- pain during intercourse;
- unable to feel the threads.

Patients should be informed on how to check their threads and to arrange a check-up if threads cannot be felt, especially if they also have significant pain. Partial perforation may occur even if the threads can be seen; consider this if there is severe pain following insertion and perform an ultrasound.

- CONTRA-INDICATIONS Active trophoblastic disease (until return to normal of urine and plasma-gonadotrophin concentration) · distorted uterine cavity · established or marked immunosuppression · genital malignancy · medical diathermy · pelvic inflammatory disease · recent sexually transmitted infection (if not fully investigated and treated) · severe anaemia · small uterine cavity · unexplained uterine bleeding · Wilson's disease

- CAUTIONS Anaemia · anticoagulant therapy (avoid if possible) · diabetes · disease-induced immunosuppression (risk of infection—avoid if marked immunosuppression) · drug-induced immunosuppression (risk of infection—avoid if marked immunosuppression) · endometriosis · epilepsy (risk of seizure at time of insertion) · fertility problems · history of pelvic inflammatory disease · increased risk of expulsion if inserted before uterine involution · menorrhagia (progestogen intra-uterine system might be preferable) · nulliparity · severe cervical stenosis · severe primary dysmenorrhoea · severely scarred uterus (including after endometrial resection) · young age

CAUTIONS, FURTHER INFORMATION

▶ Risk of infection The main excess risk of infection occurs in the first 20 days after insertion and is believed to be related to existing carriage of a sexually transmitted infection. Women are considered to be at a higher risk of sexually transmitted infections if:
- they are under 25 years old *or*
- they are over 25 years old *and*
  - have a new partner *or*
  - have had more than one partner in the past year *or*
  - their regular partner has other partners.

In these women, pre-insertion screening (for chlamydia and, depending on sexual history and local prevalence of disease, *Neisseria gonorrhoeae*) should be performed. If results are unavailable at the time of fitting an intra-uterine device for emergency contraception, appropriate prophylactic antibacterial cover should be given. The woman should be advised to attend *as an emergency* if she experiences sustained pain during the next 20 days.

An intra-uterine device should not be removed in mid-cycle unless an additional contraceptive was used for the previous 7 days. If removal is essential post-coital contraception should be considered.

- SIDE-EFFECTS Device complications · epilepsy (on insertion) · haemorrhage (on insertion) · hypersensitivity · menstrual cycle irregularities · pain (on insertion—alleviated by NSAID such as ibuprofen 30 minutes before insertion) · pelvic infection exacerbated · presyncope (on insertion) · uterine injuries

SIDE-EFFECTS, FURTHER INFORMATION Advise the patient to seek medical attention promptly in case of significant symptoms—very small risk of uterine perforation, ectopic pregnancy and pelvic inflammatory disease.

- ALLERGY AND CROSS-SENSITIVITY Contra-indicated if patient has a copper allergy.

- PREGNANCY If an intra-uterine device fails and the woman wishes to continue to full-term the device should be removed in the first trimester if possible. Remove device; if pregnancy occurs, increased likelihood that it may be ectopic.

- BREAST FEEDING Not known to be harmful.

- MONITORING REQUIREMENTS Gynaecological examination before insertion, 6–8 weeks after insertion, then annually.

- DIRECTIONS FOR ADMINISTRATION The timing and technique of fitting an intra-uterine device are critical for its subsequent performance. *The healthcare professional inserting (or removing) the device should be fully trained in the technique and should provide full counselling backed, where available, by the patient information leaflet.* Devices should not be fitted during the heavy days of the period; they are best fitted after the end of menstruation and before the calculated time of implantation.

- PRESCRIBING AND DISPENSING INFORMATION

TT380 ® SLIMLINE For uterine length 6.5–9 cm; replacement every 10 years.

LOAD ® 375 For uterine length over 7 cm; replacement every 5 years.

NOVAPLUS T 380 ® AG ' *Mini*' size for minimum uterine length 5 cm; ' *Normal*' size for uterine length 6.5–9 cm; replacement every 5 years.

MULTILOAD ® CU375 For uterine length 6–9 cm; replacement every 5 years.

GYNEFIX ® Suitable for all uterine sizes; replacement every 5 years.

UT380 STANDARD ® For uterine length 6.5–9 cm; replacement every 5 years.

UT380 SHORT ® For uterine length 5–7 cm; replacement every 5 years.

MULTI-SAFE ® 375 For uterine length 6–9 cm; replacement every 5 years.

ANCORA ® 375 CU For uterine length over 6.5 cm; replacement every 5 years.

T-SAFE ® 380A QL For uterine length 6.5–9 cm; replacement every 10 years.

NEO-SAFE ® T380 For uterine length 6.5–9 cm; replacement every 5 years.

MINI TT380 ® SLIMLINE For minimum uterine length 5 cm; replacement every 5 years.

COPPER T380 A ® For uterine length 6.5–9 cm; replacement every 10 years.

NOVAPLUS T 380 ® CU '*Mini*' size for minimum uterine length 5 cm; '*Normal*' size for uterine length 6.5–9 cm; replacement every 5 years.

NOVA-T ® 380 For uterine length 6.5–9 cm; replacement every 5 years.

FLEXI-T ®+ 380 For uterine length over 6 cm; replacement every 5 years.

FLEXI-T ® 300 For uterine length over 5 cm; replacement every 5 years.

● MEDICINAL FORMS
There can be variation in the licensing of different medicines containing the same drug.

Intra-uterine contraceptive devices
▸ Intra-uterine contraceptive devices (R.F. Medical Supplies Ltd, Farla Medical Ltd, Durbin Plc, Williams Medical Supplies Ltd, Bayer Plc, Organon Laboratories Ltd)
Copper T380 A intra-uterine contraceptive device | 1 device £8.95
Steriload intra-uterine contraceptive device | 1 device £9.65
Load 375 intra-uterine contraceptive device | 1 device £8.52
Novaplus T 380 Ag intra-uterine contraceptive device mini | 1 device £12.50
T-Safe 380A QL intra-uterine contraceptive device | 1 device £10.55
UT380 Standard intra-uterine contraceptive device | 1 device £11.22
Nova-T 380 intra-uterine contraceptive device | 1 device £15.20
Flexi-T+ 380 intra-uterine contraceptive device | 1 device £10.06
Mini TT380 Slimline intra-uterine contraceptive device | 1 device £12.46
Flexi-T 300 intra-uterine contraceptive device | 1 device £9.47
Multi-Safe 375 intra-uterine contraceptive device | 1 device £8.96
Multiload Cu375 intra-uterine contraceptive device | 1 device £9.24
Optima TCu 380A intra-uterine contraceptive device | 1 device £9.65
Novaplus T 380 Ag intra-uterine contraceptive device normal | 1 device £12.50
GyneFix intra-uterine contraceptive device | 1 device £27.11
Novaplus T 380 Cu intra-uterine contraceptive device mini | 1 device £10.95
TT380 Slimline intra-uterine contraceptive device | 1 device £12.46
Ancora 375 Cu intra-uterine contraceptive device | 1 device £7.95
Novaplus T 380 Cu intra-uterine contraceptive device normal | 1 device £10.95
Neo-Safe T380 intra-uterine contraceptive device | 1 device £13.40
UT380 Short intra-uterine contraceptive device | 1 device £11.22

Silicone contraceptive diaphragms

● SILICONE CONTRACEPTIVE DIAPHRAGMS
Milex arcing spring silicone diaphragm 60mm (Durbin Plc)
1 device · NHS indicative price = £10.21 · Drug Tariff (Part IXa)

Milex arcing spring silicone diaphragm 65mm (Durbin Plc)
1 device · NHS indicative price = £10.21 · Drug Tariff (Part IXa)

Milex arcing spring silicone diaphragm 70mm (Durbin Plc)
1 device · NHS indicative price = £10.21 · Drug Tariff (Part IXa)

Milex arcing spring silicone diaphragm 75mm (Durbin Plc)
1 device · NHS indicative price = £10.21 · Drug Tariff (Part IXa)

Milex arcing spring silicone diaphragm 80mm (Durbin Plc)
1 device · NHS indicative price = £10.21 · Drug Tariff (Part IXa)

Milex arcing spring silicone diaphragm 85mm (Durbin Plc)
1 device · NHS indicative price = £10.21 · Drug Tariff (Part IXa)

Milex arcing spring silicone diaphragm 90mm (Durbin Plc)
1 device · NHS indicative price = £10.21 · Drug Tariff (Part IXa)

Milex omniflex coil spring silicone diaphragm 60mm (Durbin Plc)
1 device · NHS indicative price = £10.21 · Drug Tariff (Part IXa)

Milex omniflex coil spring silicone diaphragm 65mm (Durbin Plc)
1 device · NHS indicative price = £10.21 · Drug Tariff (Part IXa)

Milex omniflex coil spring silicone diaphragm 70mm (Durbin Plc)
1 device · NHS indicative price = £10.21 · Drug Tariff (Part IXa)

Milex omniflex coil spring silicone diaphragm 75mm (Durbin Plc)
1 device · NHS indicative price = £10.21 · Drug Tariff (Part IXa)

Milex omniflex coil spring silicone diaphragm 80mm (Durbin Plc)
1 device · NHS indicative price = £10.21 · Drug Tariff (Part IXa)

Milex omniflex coil spring silicone diaphragm 85mm (Durbin Plc)
1 device · NHS indicative price = £10.21 · Drug Tariff (Part IXa)

Milex omniflex coil spring silicone diaphragm 90mm (Durbin Plc)
1 device · NHS indicative price = £10.21 · Drug Tariff (Part IXa)

Silicone contraceptive pessaries

● SILICONE CONTRACEPTIVE PESSARIES
FemCap 22mm (Durbin Plc)
1 device · NHS indicative price = £15.29 · Drug Tariff (Part IXa)

FemCap 26mm (Durbin Plc)
1 device · NHS indicative price = £15.29 · Drug Tariff (Part IXa)

FemCap 30mm (Durbin Plc)
1 device · NHS indicative price = £15.29 · Drug Tariff (Part IXa)

3.3 Contraception, emergency

Other drugs used for Contraception, emergency Intra-uterine contraceptive devices (copper), p. 784 · Levonorgestrel, p. 787

PROGESTERONE RECEPTOR MODULATORS

Ulipristal acetate
12-Apr-2018

● DRUG ACTION Ulipristal acetate is a progesterone receptor modulator with a partial progesterone antagonist effect.

● INDICATIONS AND DOSE

Pre-operative and intermittent treatment of moderate to severe symptoms of uterine fibroids
▸ BY MOUTH
▸ Adult: 5 mg once daily for up to 3 months starting during the first week of menstruation, courses may be repeated if necessary, re-treatment should start no sooner than during the first week of the second menstruation following completion of the first course; max. 4 courses

Emergency contraception
▸ BY MOUTH
▸ Females of childbearing potential: 30 mg for 1 dose, to be taken as soon as possible after coitus, but no later than after 120 hours

---

IMPORTANT SAFETY INFORMATION
MHRA/CHM ADVICE: *ESMYA* ® (ULIPRISTAL ACETATE) FOR UTERINE FIBROIDS: DO NOT INITIATE OR RE-START TREATMENT; MONITOR LIVER FUNCTION IN CURRENT AND RECENT USERS (MARCH 2018)
Temporary safety measures are in place while an EU review investigates the link between cases of serious liver injury, including 4 cases requiring liver transplantation, and *Esmya* ® for uterine fibroids.
The MHRA recommends the following until the EU review is completed:
● do not initiate new treatment courses, including in women who have completed prior courses;
● perform liver function tests at least once a month in women currently taking *Esmya* ® and again 2–4 weeks after stopping;
● check transaminase levels immediately in current or recent users who present with signs or symptoms suggestive of liver injury and stop treatment in any woman who develops transaminase levels more than 2 times the upper limit of normal—closely monitor and

refer for specialist hepatology evaluation as clinically indicated;
- advise women using *Esmya*® about the signs and symptoms of liver injury and tell them to seek immediate medical attention if they occur.

- CONTRA-INDICATIONS
  ‣ When used for uterine fibroids Breast cancer · cervical cancer · ovarian cancer · undiagnosed vaginal bleeding · uterine cancer · vaginal bleeding not caused by uterine fibroids
- CAUTIONS Uncontrolled severe asthma
- INTERACTIONS → Appendix 1: ulipristal
- SIDE-EFFECTS
  ‣ **Common or very common** Back pain · breast tenderness · dizziness · fatigue · gastrointestinal discomfort · headaches · menstrual cycle irregularities · mood altered · myalgia · nausea · pelvic pain · vomiting
  ‣ **Uncommon** Anxiety · appetite disorder · chills · concentration impaired · diarrhoea · drowsiness · dry mouth · fever · flatulence · hot flush · increased risk of infection · insomnia · libido disorder · malaise · skin reactions · vision disorders · vulvovaginal disorders
  ‣ **Rare or very rare** Abnormal sensation in eye · disorientation · dry throat · eye erythema · genital pruritus · ovarian cyst ruptured · painful sexual intercourse · syncope · taste altered · thirst · tremor · vertigo
- CONCEPTION AND CONTRACEPTION When ulipristal is given as an emergency contraceptive the effectiveness of combined hormonal and progestogen-only contraceptives may be reduced—additional precautions (barrier methods) required for 14 days for combined and parenteral progestogen-only hormonal contraceptives (16 days for *Qlaira*®) and 9 days for oral progestogen-only contraceptives. When ulipristal is given for uterine fibroids non-hormonal contraceptive methods (barrier methods or intra-uterine device) should be used both during treatment and for 12 days after stopping, if required.
- PREGNANCY Limited information available when used as an emergency contraceptive. Manufacturer advises avoid for uterine fibroids—no information available.
- BREAST FEEDING In emergency contraception manufacturer advises avoid for 1 week after administration—present in milk. When used for uterine fibroids, manufacturer advises avoid—no information available.
- HEPATIC IMPAIRMENT
  ‣ When used for Emergency contraception Manufacturer advises avoid in severe impairment—no information available.
  ‣ When used for Uterine fibroids MHRA advises avoid—see Important safety information for further information.
- RENAL IMPAIRMENT
  ‣ When used for uterine fibroids Manufacturer advises avoid in severe impairment unless patient is closely monitored—no information available.
- MONITORING REQUIREMENTS
  ‣ When used for uterine fibroids Manufacturer advises to perform liver function tests at least monthly during treatment—discontinue if serum transaminases exceed 2 times the upper limit of normal; an additional test, 2–4 weeks after treatment has stopped, is also advised. Manufacturer advises periodic monitoring of the endometrium following repeated intermittent treatment.
- PATIENT AND CARER ADVICE
  ‣ When used for Emergency contraception If vomiting occurs within 3 hours of taking a dose, a replacement dose should be given. When prescribing or supplying hormonal emergency contraception, women should be advised:
    - that their next period may be early or late;
    - that a barrier method of contraception needs to be used until the next period;

- to seek medical attention promptly if any lower abdominal pain occurs because this could signify an ectopic pregnancy;
- to return in 3 to 4 weeks if the subsequent menstrual bleed is abnormally light, heavy or brief, or absent, or if she is otherwise concerned (if there is any doubt as to whether menstruation has occurred, a pregnancy test should be performed at least 3 weeks after unprotected intercourse).

Treatment free intervals
  ‣ When used for Uterine fibroids The prescriber should explain the requirement for treatment free intervals.

Missed doses
  ‣ When used for Uterine fibroids If a dose is more than 12 hours late, the missed dose should not be taken and the next dose should be taken at the normal time.

- MEDICINAL FORMS
  There can be variation in the licensing of different medicines containing the same drug.

Tablet
  ‣ Ellaone (HRA Pharma UK Ltd)
    Ulipristal acetate 30 mg EllaOne 30mg tablets | 1 tablet Ⓟ £14.05 DT = £14.05
  ‣ Esmya (Gedeon Richter (UK) Ltd)
    Ulipristal acetate 5 mg Esmya 5mg tablets | 28 tablet PoM £114.13 DT = £114.13

3.4 Contraception, oral progestogen-only

Other drugs used for Contraception, oral progestogen-only Norethisterone, p. 747

PROGESTOGENS

Desogestrel

- INDICATIONS AND DOSE
Contraception
  ‣ BY MOUTH
  ‣ Females of childbearing potential: 75 micrograms daily, dose to be taken at same time each day, starting on day 1 of cycle then continuously, if administration delayed for 12 hours or more it should be regarded as a 'missed pill'

- CONTRA-INDICATIONS Acute porphyrias p. 1025 · history of breast cancer but can be used after 5 years if no evidence of disease and non-hormonal contraceptive methods unacceptable · severe arterial disease · undiagnosed vaginal bleeding
- CAUTIONS Active trophoblastic disease (until return to normal of urine- and plasma-gonadotrophin concentration)—seek specialist advice · arterial disease · functional ovarian cysts · history of jaundice in pregnancy · malabsorption syndromes · past ectopic pregnancy · sex-steroid dependent cancer · systemic lupus erythematosus with positive (or unknown) antiphospholipid antibodies
  CAUTIONS, FURTHER INFORMATION
  ‣ Other conditions The product literature advises caution in patients with history of thromboembolism, hypertension, diabetes mellitus and migraine; evidence for caution in these conditions is unsatisfactory.
- INTERACTIONS → Appendix 1: desogestrel
- SIDE-EFFECTS
  ‣ **Common or very common** Breast abnormalities · depressed mood · headache · libido decreased · menstrual cycle

irregularities · mood altered · nausea · skin reactions · weight increased
▶ **Uncommon** Alopecia · contact lens intolerance · fatigue · ovarian cyst · vomiting · vulvovaginal infection
▶ **Rare or very rare** Erythema nodosum
▶ **Frequency not known** Angioedema · embolism and thrombosis · neoplasms

SIDE-EFFECTS, FURTHER INFORMATION The benefits of using progestogen-only contraceptives (POCs), such as desogestrel, should be weighed against the possible risks for each individual woman.

There is a small increase in the risk of having breast cancer diagnosed in women using a combined oral contraceptive pill (COC); this relative risk may be due to an earlier diagnosis, biological effects of the pill or a combination of both. This increased risk is related to the age of the woman using the COC rather than the duration of use and disappears gradually within 10 years after discontinuation.

The risk of breast cancer in users of POCs is possibly of similar magnitude to that associated with COCs, however the evidence is less conclusive.

Available evidence does not support an association between the use of a progestegen-only contraceptive pill and breast cancer. Any increased risk is likely to be small and reduces gradually during the 10 years after stopping; there is no excess risk 10 years after stopping. The older age at which the contraceptive is stopped appears to have a greater influence on increased risk rather than the duration of use.

● PREGNANCY Not known to be harmful.

● BREAST FEEDING Progestogen-only contraceptives do not affect lactation.

● HEPATIC IMPAIRMENT Caution in severe liver disease and recurrent cholestatic jaundice. Avoid in liver tumour.

● PATIENT AND CARER ADVICE
Surgery All progestogen-only contraceptives are suitable for use as an alternative to combined hormonal contraceptives before major elective surgery, before all surgery to the legs, or before surgery which involves prolonged immobilisation of a lower limb.
Starting routine One tablet daily, on a continuous basis, starting on day 1 of cycle and taken at the same time each day (if delayed by longer than 12 hours contraceptive protection may be lost). Additional contraceptive precautions are not required if desogestrel is started up to and including day 5 of the menstrual cycle; if started after this time, additional contraceptive precautions are required for 2 days.
Changing from a combined oral contraceptive Start on the day following completion of the combined oral contraceptive course without a break (or in the case of ED tablets omitting the inactive ones).
After childbirth Oral progestogen-only contraceptives can be started up to and including day 21 postpartum without the need for additional contraceptive precautions. If started more than 21 days postpartum, additional contraceptive precautions are required for 2 days.
Diarrhoea and vomiting Vomiting and persistent, severe diarrhoea can interfere with the absorption of oral progestogen-only contraceptives. If vomiting occurs within 2 hours of taking desogestrel, another pill should be taken as soon as possible. If a replacement pill is not taken within 12 hours of the normal time for taking desogestrel, or in cases of persistent vomiting or very severe diarrhoea, additional precautions should be used during illness and for 2 days after recovery.
Missed doses The following advice is recommended: 'If you forget a pill, take it as soon as you remember and carry on with the next pill at the right time. If the pill was more than 12 hours overdue you are not protected. Continue

normal pill-taking but you must also use another method, such as the condom, for the next 2 days'.

The Faculty of Sexual and Reproductive Healthcare recommends emergency contraception if one or more tablets are missed or taken more than 12 hours late and unprotected intercourse has occurred before 2 further tablets have been correctly taken.

● NATIONAL FUNDING/ACCESS DECISIONS
Scottish Medicines Consortium (SMC) Decisions
The *Scottish Medicines Consortium* has advised (September 2003) that *Cerazette*® should be restricted for use in women who cannot tolerate oestrogen-containing contraceptives or in whom such preparations are contra-indicated.

● MEDICINAL FORMS
There can be variation in the licensing of different medicines containing the same drug.

Tablet
▶ Desogestrel (Non-proprietary)
Desogestrel 75 microgram Desogestrel 75microgram tablets | 84 tablet [PoM] £9.55 DT = £2.95
▶ Aizea (Besins Healthcare (UK) Ltd)
Desogestrel 75 microgram Aizea 75microgram tablets | 84 tablet [PoM] £5.21 DT = £2.95
▶ Cerazette (Merck Sharp & Dohme Ltd)
Desogestrel 75 microgram Cerazette 75microgram tablets | 84 tablet [PoM] £9.55 DT = £2.95
▶ Cerelle (Consilient Health Ltd)
Desogestrel 75 microgram Cerelle 75microgram tablets | 84 tablet [PoM] £3.50 DT = £2.95
▶ Desomono (MedRx Licences Ltd)
Desogestrel 75 microgram Desomono 75microgram tablets | 84 tablet [PoM] £6.50 DT = £2.95
▶ Desorex (Somex Pharma)
Desogestrel 75 microgram Desorex 75microgram tablets | 84 tablet [PoM] £2.99 DT = £2.95
▶ Feanolla (Lupin Healthcare (UK) Ltd)
Desogestrel 75 microgram Feanolla 75microgram tablets | 84 tablet [PoM] £3.49 DT = £2.95
▶ Zelleta (Morningside Healthcare Ltd)
Desogestrel 75 microgram Zelleta 75microgram tablets | 84 tablet [PoM] £2.98 DT = £2.95

Levonorgestrel
16-Apr-2018

● INDICATIONS AND DOSE
Emergency contraception
▶ BY MOUTH
▶ Females of childbearing potential: 1.5 mg for 1 dose, taken as soon as possible after coitus, preferably within 12 hours and no later than after 72 hours (may also be used between 72–96 hours after coitus but efficacy decreases with time), alternatively 3 mg for 1 dose, taken as soon as possible after coitus, preferably within 12 hours and no later than after 72 hours (may also be used between 72–96 hours after coitus but efficacy decreases with time). Higher dose should be considered for patients with body-weight over 70 kg or BMI over 26 kg/m^2

Contraception
▶ BY MOUTH
▶ Females of childbearing potential: 30 micrograms daily starting on day 1 of the cycle then continuously, dose is to be taken at the same time each day, if administration delayed for 3 hours or more it should be regarded as a "missed pill"

JAYDESS® 13.5MG INTRA-UTERINE DEVICE
Contraception
▶ BY INTRA-UTERINE ADMINISTRATION
▶ Females of childbearing potential: Insert into uterine cavity within 7 days of onset of continued →

7

Genito-urinary system

menstruation, or any time if replacement, or immediately after first-trimester termination; postpartum insertions should be delayed until at least 6 weeks after delivery (12 weeks if uterus involution is substantially delayed); effective for 3 years

KYLEENA ® 19.5MG INTRA-UTERINE DEVICE

Contraception
▶ BY INTRA-UTERINE ADMINISTRATION
▶ Females of childbearing potential: Insert into uterine cavity within 7 days of onset of menstruation, or any time if replacement, or immediately after first-trimester termination; postpartum insertions should be delayed until at least 6 weeks after delivery and not before uterus is fully involuted; effective for 5 years

LEVOSERT ® 20MICROGRAMS/24HOURS INTRA-UTERINE DEVICE

Contraception | Menorrhagia
▶ BY INTRA-UTERINE ADMINISTRATION
▶ Females of childbearing potential: Insert into uterine cavity within 7 days of onset of menstruation, or any time if replacement, or immediately after first-trimester abortion; postpartum insertions should be delayed until at least 6 weeks after delivery and not before uterus is fully involuted; effective for 4 years

MIRENA ® 20MICROGRAMS/24HOURS INTRA-UTERINE DEVICE

Contraception | Menorrhagia
▶ BY INTRA-UTERINE ADMINISTRATION
▶ Females of childbearing potential: Insert into uterine cavity within 7 days of onset of menstruation, or any time if replacement, or any time if reasonably certain woman is not pregnant and there is no risk of conception (additional precautions (e.g. barrier methods) necessary for next 7 days), or immediately after first-trimester termination by curettage; postpartum insertions should be delayed until at least 4 weeks after delivery; effective for 5 years

Prevention of endometrial hyperplasia during oestrogen replacement therapy
▶ BY INTRA-UTERINE ADMINISTRATION
▶ Females of childbearing potential: Insert during last days of menstruation or withdrawal bleeding or at any time if amenorrhoeic; effective for 4 years

● UNLICENSED USE [EvGr] Dose for emergency contraception in patients with body-weight over 70 kg or BMI over 26 kg/m^2 differs from product licence. Use for emergency contraception between 72–96 hours after coitus differs from product licence. ⒶⒷ
▶ With oral use in children Consult product literature for licensing status of individual preparations.
▶ With vaginal use in children Not licensed for use in women under 18 years.

IMPORTANT SAFETY INFORMATION

MHRA/CHM ADVICE (JUNE 2015) INTRA-UTERINE CONTRACEPTION: UTERINE PERFORATION—UPDATED INFORMATION ON RISK FACTORS

Uterine perforation most often occurs during insertion, but might not be detected until sometime later. The risk of uterine perforation is increased when the device is inserted up to 36 weeks postpartum or in patients who are breastfeeding. Before inserting an intra-uterine contraceptive device, inform patients that perforation occurs in approximately 1 in every 1000 insertions and signs and symptoms include:
● severe pelvic pain after insertion (worse than period cramps);
● pain or increased bleeding after insertion which continues for more than a few weeks;
● sudden changes in periods;
● pain during intercourse;

● unable to feel the threads.
Patients should be informed on how to check their threads and to arrange a check-up if threads cannot be felt, especially if they also have significant pain. Partial perforation may occur even if the threads can be seen; consider this if there is severe pain following insertion and perform an ultrasound.

● CONTRA-INDICATIONS
▶ With intra-uterine use Active trophoblastic disease (until return to normal of urine- and plasma-gonadotrophin concentration) · acute cervicitis · acute malignancies affecting the blood (use with caution in remission) · acute vaginitis · distorted uterine cavity · history of breast cancer but can be considered for a woman in long-term remission who has menorrhagia and requires effective contraception · increased risk factors for pelvic infections · infected abortion during the previous three months · not suitable for emergency contraception · pelvic inflammatory disease · postpartum endometritis · unexplained uterine bleeding · unresolved cervical intraepithelial neoplasia · uterine or cervical malignancy
▶ With oral use Acute porphyrias p. 1025
▶ When used for contraception with oral use History of breast cancer but can be used after 5 years if no evidence of disease and non-hormonal contraceptive methods unacceptable · severe arterial disease · undiagnosed vaginal bleeding

● CAUTIONS
GENERAL CAUTIONS Risk factors for ectopic pregnancy (including previous ectopic pregnancy, tubal surgery or pelvic infection)
SPECIFIC CAUTIONS
▶ With intra-uterine use Disease-induced immunosuppression (risk of infection—avoid if marked immunosuppression) · acute venous thromboembolism (consider removal) · anaemia · anticoagulant therapy (avoid if possible) · diabetes · drug-induced immunosuppression (risk of infection—avoid if marked immunosuppression) · endometriosis · epilepsy (risk of seizure at time of insertion) · fertility problems · history of pelvic inflammatory disease · increased risk of expulsion if inserted before uterine involution · jaundice (consider removal) · marked increase of blood pressure (consider removal) · menorrhagia (progestogen intra-uterine system might be preferable) · migraine (consider removal) · nulliparity · severe arterial disease (consider removal) · severe cervical stenosis · severe headache (consider removal) · severe primary dysmenorrhoea · severely scarred uterus (including after endometrial resection) · young age
▶ When used for contraception with oral use Active trophoblastic disease (until return to normal of urine- and plasma-gonadotrophin concentration)—seek specialist advice · arterial disease · functional ovarian cysts · history of jaundice in pregnancy · malabsorption syndromes · past ectopic pregnancy · sex-steroid dependent cancer · systemic lupus erythematosus with positive (or unknown) antiphospholipid antibodies
▶ When used for emergency contraception with oral use Active trophoblastic disease (until return to normal of urine- and plasma-gonadotrophin concentration)—seek specialist advice · past ectopic pregnancy · severe malabsorption syndromes

CAUTIONS, FURTHER INFORMATION An intra-uterine device should not be removed in mid-cycle unless an additional contraceptive was used for the previous 7 days. If removal is essential post-coital contraception should be considered.
▶ Risk of infection with intra-uterine devices The main excess risk of infection occurs in the first 20 days after insertion and is believed to be related to existing carriage of a sexually

transmitted infection. Women are considered to be at a higher risk of sexually transmitted infections if:

- they are under 25 years old *or*
- they are over 25 years old *and*
  - have a new partner *or*
  - have had more than one partner in the past year *or*
  - their regular partner has other partners.

In these women, pre-insertion screening (for chlamydia and, depending on sexual history and local prevalence of disease, *Neisseria gonorrhoeae*) should be performed. If results are unavailable at the time of fitting an intra-uterine device for emergency contraception, appropriate prophylactic antibacterial cover should be given. The woman should be advised to attend *as an emergency* if she experiences sustained pain during the next 20 days.

‣ Use as a contraceptive in co-morbidities
‣ With oral use The product literature advises caution in patients with history of thromboembolism, hypertension, diabetes mellitus and migraine; evidence for caution in these conditions is unsatisfactory.

MIRENA ® 20MICROGRAMS/24HOURS INTRA-UTERINE DEVICE Advanced uterine atrophy

● INTERACTIONS → Appendix 1: levonorgestrel

● SIDE-EFFECTS
‣ **Common or very common**
‣ With intra-uterine use Back pain · breast abnormalities · depression · device expulsion · gastrointestinal discomfort · headaches · hirsutism · increased risk of infection · libido decreased · menstrual cycle irregularities · nausea · nervousness · ovarian cyst · pelvic disorders · skin reactions · uterine haemorrhage (on insertion) · vaginal haemorrhage (on insertion) · vulvovaginal disorders · weight increased
‣ With oral use Breast tenderness · diarrhoea · dizziness · fatigue · gastrointestinal discomfort · haemorrhage · headaches · menstrual cycle irregularities · nausea · vomiting
‣ **Uncommon**
‣ With intra-uterine use Alopecia · endometritis · oedema · uterine rupture
‣ **Rare or very rare**
‣ With oral use Face oedema · pelvic pain · skin reactions
‣ **Frequency not known**
‣ With oral use Cerebrovascular insufficiency · depressed mood · diabetes mellitus · embolism and thrombosis · neoplasms · sexual dysfunction · weight changes

SIDE-EFFECTS, FURTHER INFORMATION
Breast cancer There is a small increase in the risk of having breast cancer diagnosed in women using, or who have recently used, a progestogen-only contraceptive pill; this relative risk may be due to an earlier diagnosis. The most important risk factor appears to be the age at which the contraceptive is stopped rather than the duration of use; the risk disappears gradually during the 10 years after stopping and there is no excess risk by 10 years. A possible small increase in the risk of breast cancer should be weighed against the benefits.
With intra-uterine use There is no evidence of an association between the levonorgestrel intra-uterine system and breast cancer. The levonorgestrel intra-uterine system should be avoided in patients with a history of breast cancer; any consideration of it's use should be by a specialist in contraception and in consultation with the patients cancer specialist.

Patients should be informed about the device that has been inserted and when it should be removed or replaced (including refering them to a patient information leaflet and other sources of information).

Patients may experience irregular, prolonged or infrequent menstrual bleeding in the 3–6 months following insertion; bleeding pattern improves with time but persists in some patients.

Progestogenic side-effects resolve with time (after the first few months).

● PREGNANCY
‣ With oral use Not known to be harmful.
‣ With vaginal use If an intra-uterine device fails and the woman wishes to continue to full-term the device should be removed in the first trimester if possible. Avoid; if pregnancy occurs remove intra-uterine system.

● BREAST FEEDING Progestogen-only contraceptives do not affect lactation.

● HEPATIC IMPAIRMENT
‣ With intra-uterine use or oral use for Contraception Manufacturer advises avoid in liver tumour.
‣ With oral use for Contraception or Emergency contraception Manufacturer advises avoid in severe impairment.
‣ With intra-uterine use Manufacturer advises avoid in severe impairment—no information available; avoid in acute hepatic disease.

● MONITORING REQUIREMENTS
‣ With intra-uterine use Gynaecological examination before insertion, 4–6 weeks after insertion, then annually.

● DIRECTIONS FOR ADMINISTRATION
‣ With intra-uterine use *The doctor or nurse administering (or removing) the system should be fully trained in the technique and should provide full counselling reinforced by the patient information leaflet.*

● PRESCRIBING AND DISPENSING INFORMATION
Levonorgestrel-releasing intra-uterine devices vary in licensed indication, duration of use and insertion technique—the MHRA recommends to prescribe and dispense by brand name to avoid inadvertent switching.

MIRENA ® 20MICROGRAMS/24HOURS INTRA-UTERINE DEVICE When system is removed (and not immediately replaced) and pregnancy is not desired, remove during the first few days of menstruation, otherwise additional precautions (e.g. barrier methods) should be used for at least 7 days before removal.

JAYDESS ® 13.5MG INTRA-UTERINE DEVICE When system is removed (and not immediately replaced) and pregnancy is not desired, remove within 7 days of the onset of menstruation; additional precautions (e.g. barrier methods) should be used if the system is removed at some other time during the cycle and there is intercourse within 7 days.

KYLEENA ® 19.5MG INTRA-UTERINE DEVICE When system is removed (and not immediately replaced) and pregnancy is not desired, remove within 7 days of the onset of menstruation; additional precautions (e.g. barrier methods) should be used if the system is removed at some other time during the cycle, or in case of irregular menses, and if there is intercourse within 7 days.

LEVONELLE ® ONE STEP Can be sold to women over 16 years; when supplying emergency contraception to the public, pharmacists should refer to guidance issued by the Royal Pharmaceutical Society.

● PATIENT AND CARER ADVICE
Diarrhoea and vomiting with use as an oral contraceptive Vomiting and persistent, severe diarrhoea can interfere with the absorption of oral progestogen-only contraceptives. If vomiting occurs within 2 hours of taking an oral progestogen-only contraceptive, another pill should be taken as soon as possible. If a replacement pill is not taken within 3 hours of the normal time for taking the progestogen-only pill, or in cases of persistent vomiting or very severe diarrhoea, additional precautions should be used during illness and for 2 days after recovery.
Starting routine
‣ With oral use for Contraception One tablet daily, on a continuous basis, starting on day 1 of cycle and taken at the same time each day (if delayed by longer than 3 hours

contraceptive protection may be lost). Additional contraceptive precautions are not required if levonorgestrel is started up to and including day 5 of the menstrual cycle; if started after this time, additional contraceptive precautions are required for 2 days.

Changing from a combined oral contraceptive Start on the day following completion of the combined oral contraceptive course without a break (or in the case of ED tablets omitting the inactive ones).

After childbirth Oral progestogen-only contraceptives can be started up to and including day 21 postpartum without the need for additional contraceptive precautions. If started more than 21 days postpartum, additional contraceptive precautions are required for 2 days.

▸ **With oral use for Emergency contraception** Manufacturer advises if vomiting occurs within 3 hours of taking levonorgestrel, a replacement dose should be taken immediately.

When prescribing or supplying hormonal emergency contraception, women should be advised:

- that their next period may be early or late;
- that a barrier method of contraception needs to be used until the next period;
- to seek medical attention promptly if any lower abdominal pain occurs because this could signify an ectopic pregnancy;
- to return in 3 to 4 weeks if the subsequent menstrual bleed is abnormally light, heavy or brief, or is absent, or if she is otherwise concerned (if there is any doubt as to whether menstruation has occurred, a pregnancy test should be performed at least 3 weeks after unprotected intercourse).

▸ **With intra-uterine use** Counsel women on the signs, symptoms and risks of perforation and ectopic pregnancy.

Missed doses When used as an oral contraceptive, the following advice is recommended 'If you forget a pill, take it as soon as you remember and carry on with the next pill at the right time. If the pill was more than 3 hours overdue you are not protected. Continue normal pill-taking but you must also use another method, such as the condom, for the next 2 days'.

The Faculty of Sexual and Reproductive Healthcare recommends emergency contraception if one or more progestogen-only contraceptive tablets are missed or taken more than 3 hours late and unprotected intercourse has occurred before 2 further tablets have been correctly taken.

● **NATIONAL FUNDING/ACCESS DECISIONS**

KYLEENA ® 19.5MG INTRA-UTERINE DEVICE

Scottish Medicines Consortium (SMC) Decisions
The *Scottish Medicines Consortium* has advised (February 2018) that levonorgestrel (*Kyleena ®*) is accepted for use within NHS Scotland as a contraceptive device for up to 5 years.

● **EXCEPTIONS TO LEGAL CATEGORY** *Levonelle ® One Step* can be sold to women over 16 years; when supplying emergency contraception to the public, pharmacists should refer to guidance issued by the Royal Pharmaceutical Society.

● **MEDICINAL FORMS**
There can be variation in the licensing of different medicines containing the same drug.

Intra-uterine device
▸ Jaydess (Bayer Plc) ▼
Levonorgestrel 13.5 mg Jaydess 13.5mg intra-uterine device | 1 device PoM £69.22
▸ Kyleena (Bayer Plc)
Levonorgestrel 19.5 mg Kyleena 19.5mg intra-uterine device | 1 device PoM £76.00

▸ Levosert (Gedeon Richter (UK) Ltd)
Levonorgestrel 20 microgram per 24 hour Levosert 20micrograms/24hours intra-uterine device | 1 device PoM £66.00 DT = £88.00
▸ Mirena (Bayer Plc)
Levonorgestrel 20 microgram per 24 hour Mirena 20micrograms/24hours intra-uterine device | 1 device PoM £88.00 DT = £88.00

Tablet
▸ Levonorgestrel (Non-proprietary)
Levonorgestrel 1.5 mg Levonorgestrel 1.5mg tablets | 1 tablet P £13.83 DT = £5.20 | 1 tablet PoM £3.74–£5.20 DT = £5.20
▸ Emerres (Morningside Healthcare Ltd)
Levonorgestrel 1.5 mg Emerres Una 1.5mg tablets | 1 tablet P £13.83 DT = £5.20
Emerres 1.5mg tablets | 1 tablet PoM £3.65 DT = £5.20
▸ Ezinelle (Mylan)
Levonorgestrel 1.5 mg Ezinelle 1.5mg tablets | 1 tablet PoM £9.64 DT = £5.20
▸ Levonelle (Bayer Plc)
Levonorgestrel 1.5 mg Levonelle 1500microgram tablets | 1 tablet PoM £5.20 DT = £5.20
▸ Levonelle One Step (Bayer Plc)
Levonorgestrel 1.5 mg Levonelle One Step 1.5mg tablets | 1 tablet P £13.83 DT = £5.20
▸ Norgeston (Bayer Plc)
Levonorgestrel 30 microgram Norgeston 30microgram tablets | 35 tablet PoM £0.92 DT = £0.92
▸ Upostelle (Consilient Health Ltd)
Levonorgestrel 1.5 mg Upostelle 1500microgram tablets | 1 tablet PoM £3.75 DT = £5.20

3.5 Contraception, parenteral progestogen-only

Other drugs used for Contraception, parenteral progestogen-only Norethisterone, p. 747

PROGESTOGENS

Etonogestrel

27-Sep-2016

● **INDICATIONS AND DOSE**

Contraception (no hormonal contraceptive use in previous month)
▸ BY SUBDERMAL IMPLANTATION
▸ Females of childbearing potential: 1 implant inserted during first 5 days of cycle, implant should be removed within 3 years of insertion

Contraception (postpartum)
▸ BY SUBDERMAL IMPLANTATION
▸ Females of childbearing potential: 1 implant to be inserted 21–28 days after delivery (delay until 28 days postpartum if breast-feeding), implant should be removed within 3 years of insertion

Contraception following abortion or miscarriage in the second trimester
▸ BY SUBDERMAL IMPLANTATION
▸ Females of childbearing potential: 1 implant to be inserted 21–28 days after abortion or miscarriage, implant should be removed within 3 years of insertion

Contraception following abortion or miscarriage in the first trimester
▸ BY SUBDERMAL IMPLANTATION
▸ Females of childbearing potential: 1 implant to be inserted within 5 days after abortion or miscarriage, implant should be removed within 3 years of insertion

Contraception (changing from other hormonal contraceptive)

▶ BY SUBDERMAL IMPLANTATION
▸ Females of childbearing potential: Implant should be removed within 3 years of insertion (consult product literature)

● UNLICENSED USE *Nexplanon*® not licensed for use in females outside of the age range 18–40 years.

> **IMPORTANT SAFETY INFORMATION**
> MHRA/CHM ADVICE (JUNE 2016): *NEXPLANON*® (ETONOGESTREL) CONTRACEPTIVE IMPLANTS: REPORTS OF DEVICE IN VASCULATURE AND LUNG
> There have been rare reports of *Nexplanon*® implants reaching the lung via the pulmonary artery. An implant that cannot be palpated at its insertion site should be located and removed as soon as possible; if unable to locate implant within the arm, the MHRA recommends using chest imaging. Correct subdermal insertion reduces the risk of these events.

● CONTRA-INDICATIONS Acute porphyrias p. 1025 · history of breast cancer but can be used after 5 years if no evidence of disease and non-hormonal contraceptive methods unacceptable · severe arterial disease · undiagnosed vaginal bleeding
● CAUTIONS Active trophoblastic disease (until return to normal of urine- and plasma-gonadotrophin concentration)—seek specialist advice · arterial disease · disturbances of lipid metabolism · history during pregnancy of deterioration of otosclerosis · history during pregnancy of pruritus · history of jaundice in pregnancy · malabsorption syndromes · possible risk of breast cancer · sex-steroid dependent cancer · systemic lupus erythematosus with positive (or unknown) antiphospholipid antibodies
● INTERACTIONS → Appendix 1: etonogestrel
● SIDE-EFFECTS
▶ Common or very common Abdominal pain · alopecia · anxiety · appetite increased · breast abnormalities · depressed mood · dizziness · emotional lability · fatigue · flatulence · headaches · hot flush · increased risk of infection · influenza like illness · libido decreased · menstrual cycle irregularities · nausea · ovarian cyst · pain · skin reactions · weight changes
▶ Uncommon Arthralgia · constipation · diarrhoea · drowsiness · dysuria · fever · galactorrhoea · genital abnormalities · hypertrichosis · insomnia · myalgia · oedema · vomiting · vulvovaginal discomfort
▶ Frequency not known Abscess · angioedema · embolism and thrombosis · haemorrhage · insulin resistance · neoplasms · paraesthesia · seborrhoea

SIDE-EFFECTS, FURTHER INFORMATION The benefits of using progestogen-only contraceptives (POCs), such as etonogestrel, should be weighed against the possible risks for each individual woman.
  There is a small increase in the risk of having breast cancer diagnosed in women using a combined oral contraceptive pill (COC); this relative risk may be due to an earlier diagnosis, biological effects of the pill or a combination of both. This increased risk is related to the age of the woman using the COC rather than the duration of use and disappears gradually within 10 years after discontinuation.
  The risk of breast cancer in users of POCs is possibly of similar magnitude as that associated with COCs, however the evidence is less conclusive.

● PREGNANCY Not known to be harmful, remove implant if pregnancy occurs.

● BREAST FEEDING Progestogen-only contraceptives do not affect lactation.
● DIRECTIONS FOR ADMINISTRATION The doctor or nurse administering (or removing) the system should be fully trained in the technique and should provide full counselling reinforced by the patient information leaflet.
● PATIENT AND CARER ADVICE Full counselling backed by patient information leaflet required before administration.

● MEDICINAL FORMS
There can be variation in the licensing of different medicines containing the same drug.
Implant
▸ Etonogestrel (Non-proprietary)
  Etonogestrel 68 mg Etonogestrel 68mg implant | 1 device PoM ℥ DT = £83.43
▸ Nexplanon (Merck Sharp & Dohme Ltd)
  Etonogestrel 68 mg Nexplanon 68mg implant | 1 device PoM £83.43 DT = £83.43

Medroxyprogesterone acetate   24-May-2017

● INDICATIONS AND DOSE
Dysfunctional uterine bleeding
▶ BY MOUTH
▸ Adult: 2.5–10 mg daily for 5–10 days, repeated for 2 cycles, begin treatment on day 16–21 of cycle
Secondary amenorrhoea
▶ BY MOUTH
▸ Adult: 2.5–10 mg daily for 5–10 days, repeated for 3 cycles, begin treatment on day 16–21 of cycle
Mild to moderate endometriosis
▶ BY MOUTH
▸ Adult: 10 mg 3 times a day for 90 consecutive days, begin treatment on day 1 of cycle
Progestogenic opposition of oestrogen HRT
▶ BY MOUTH
▸ Adult: 10 mg daily for the last 14 days of each 28-day oestrogen HRT cycle
Endometrial cancer | Renal cell cancer
▶ BY MOUTH
▸ Adult: 200–600 mg daily
Breast cancer
▶ BY MOUTH
▸ Adult: 0.4–1.5 g daily
Contraception
▶ BY DEEP INTRAMUSCULAR INJECTION
▸ Females of childbearing potential: 150 mg, to be administered within the first 5 days of cycle or within first 5 days after parturition (delay until 6 weeks after parturition if breast-feeding)
▶ BY SUBCUTANEOUS INJECTION
▸ Females of childbearing potential: 104 mg, to be administered within first 5 days of cycle or within 5 days postpartum (delay until 6 weeks postpartum if breast-feeding), injected into anterior thigh or abdomen, dose only suitable if no hormonal contraceptive use in previous month
Long-term contraception
▶ BY DEEP INTRAMUSCULAR INJECTION
▸ Females of childbearing potential: 150 mg every 12 weeks, first dose to be administered within the first 5 days of cycle or within 5 days after parturition (delay until 6 weeks after parturition if breast-feeding)
▶ BY SUBCUTANEOUS INJECTION
▸ Females of childbearing potential: 104 mg every 13 weeks, first dose to be administered within first 5 days of cycle or within 5 days postpartum (delay until 6 weeks postpartum if breast-feeding), continued →

injected into anterior thigh or abdomen, dose only suitable if no hormonal contraceptive use in previous month

Contraception (when patient changing from other hormonal contraceptive)
‣ BY SUBCUTANEOUS INJECTION
‣ Females of childbearing potential: (consult product literature)

Hot flushes caused by long-term androgen suppression in men with prostate cancer
‣ BY MOUTH
‣ Adult: 20 mg once daily initially for 10 weeks, evaluate effect at the end of the treatment period

● UNLICENSED USE EvGr Not licensed for the treatment of hot flushes caused by long-term androgen suppression in men. Ⓐ

● CONTRA-INDICATIONS
  GENERAL CONTRA-INDICATIONS Acute porphyrias p. 1025 · severe arterial disease · undiagnosed vaginal bleeding
  SPECIFIC CONTRA-INDICATIONS
‣ With intramuscular use or subcutaneous use History of breast cancer but can be used after 5 years if no evidence of disease and non-hormonal contraceptive methods unacceptable
‣ With oral use Breast cancer (unless progestogens are being used in the management of this condition) · genital cancer (unless progestogens are being used in the management of this condition) · history of liver tumours

● CAUTIONS
  GENERAL CAUTIONS Possible risk of breast cancer
  SPECIFIC CAUTIONS
‣ With intramuscular use or subcutaneous use History during pregnancy in disturbances of lipid metabolism · history during pregnancy of deterioration of otosclerosis · history during pregnancy of pruritus
‣ With oral use Asthma · cardiac dysfunction · conditions that may worsen with fluid retention · diabetes (progestogens can decrease glucose tolerance—monitor patient closely) · epilepsy · history of depression · hypertension · migraine · susceptibility to thromboembolism (particular caution with high dose)

● INTERACTIONS → Appendix 1: medroxyprogesterone

● SIDE-EFFECTS
  GENERAL SIDE-EFFECTS
▸ **Common or very common** Alopecia · breast abnormalities · depression · dizziness · fluid retention · insomnia · menstrual cycle irregularities · nausea · sexual dysfunction · skin reactions · weight changes
▸ **Uncommon** Drowsiness · embolism and thrombosis · fever · galactorrhoea · hirsutism · muscle spasms · tachycardia
  SPECIFIC SIDE-EFFECTS
▸ **Common or very common**
‣ With oral use Appetite increased · cervical abnormalities · constipation · fatigue · headache · hyperhidrosis · hypersensitivity · nervousness · oedema · tremor · vomiting
‣ With parenteral use Anxiety · asthenia · gastrointestinal discomfort · headaches · mood altered · pain · vulvovaginal infection
▸ **Uncommon**
‣ With oral use Congestive heart failure · corticoid-like effects · diabetes mellitus exacerbated · diarrhoea · dry mouth · euphoric mood · hypercalcaemia
‣ With parenteral use Appetite abnormal · arthralgia · hot flush · hypertension · ovarian cyst · painful sexual intercourse · uterine haemorrhage · varicose veins · vertigo · vulvovaginal disorders
▸ **Rare or very rare**
‣ With oral use Cerebral infarction · jaundice · malaise · myocardial infarction

‣ With parenteral use Breast cancer · lipodystrophy
▸ **Frequency not known**
‣ With oral use Adrenergic-like effects · cataract diabetic · concentration impaired · confusion · glycosuria · palpitations · visual impairment (discontinue if papilloedema or retinal vascular lesions)
‣ With parenteral use Hepatic disorders · osteoporosis · osteoporotic fractures · seizure
  SIDE-EFFECTS, FURTHER INFORMATION
  With oral use In general, side effects may be more common with high doses such as those used in malignant disease.
  With parenteral use Reduction in bone mineral density is greater with increasing duration of use. The loss is mostly recovered on discontinuation.

● CONCEPTION AND CONTRACEPTION
‣ With intramuscular use If interval between dose is greater than 12 weeks and 5 days (in long-term contraception), rule out pregnancy before next injection and advise patient to use additional contraceptive measures (e.g. barrier) for 14 days after the injection.
‣ With subcutaneous use If interval between dose is greater than 13 weeks and 7 days (in long-term contraception), rule out pregnancy before next injection.

● PREGNANCY
‣ With oral use Avoid—genital malformations and cardiac defects reported.
‣ With intramuscular use or subcutaneous use Not known to be harmful.

● BREAST FEEDING Present in milk—no adverse effects reported. Progestogen-only contraceptives do not affect lactation.
‣ With intramuscular use or subcutaneous use The manufacturers advise that in women who are breast-feeding, the first dose should be delayed until 6 weeks after birth; however, evidence suggests no harmful effect to infant if given earlier. The benefits of using medroxyprogesterone acetate in breast-feeding women outweigh any risks.

● HEPATIC IMPAIRMENT Avoid in liver tumour.
‣ With oral use Avoid in hepatic impairment.
‣ With intramuscular use or subcutaneous use Caution in severe liver disease and recurrent cholestatic jaundice.

● RENAL IMPAIRMENT
‣ When used for Mild to moderate endometriosis or Progestogenic opposition of oestrogen HRT or Dysfunctional uterine bleeding or Secondary amenorrhoea Use with caution.

● PATIENT AND CARER ADVICE
‣ With intramuscular use or subcutaneous use Full counselling backed by *patient information leaflet* required before administration—likelihood of menstrual disturbance and the potential for a delay in return to full fertility. Delayed return of fertility and irregular cycles may occur after discontinuation of treatment but there is no evidence of permanent infertility.

● MEDICINAL FORMS
There can be variation in the licensing of different medicines containing the same drug. Forms available from special-order manufacturers include: oral suspension, oral solution

Tablet
▸ Climanor (ReSource Medical UK Ltd)
  Medroxyprogesterone acetate 5 mg Climanor 5mg tablets | 28 tablet PoM £3.27
▸ Provera (Pfizer Ltd)
  Medroxyprogesterone acetate 2.5 mg Provera 2.5mg tablets | 30 tablet PoM £1.84 DT = £1.84
  Medroxyprogesterone acetate 5 mg Provera 5mg tablets | 10 tablet PoM £1.23 DT = £1.23 | 100 tablet PoM £12.32
  Medroxyprogesterone acetate 10 mg Provera 10mg tablets | 10 tablet PoM £2.47 | 90 tablet PoM £22.16 DT = £22.16 | 100 tablet PoM £24.73

Medroxyprogesterone acetate 100 mg Provera 100mg tablets |
60 tablet [PoM] £29.98 | 100 tablet [PoM] £49.94 DT = £49.94
Medroxyprogesterone acetate 200 mg Provera 200mg tablets |
30 tablet [PoM] £29.65 DT = £29.65
Medroxyprogesterone acetate 400 mg Provera 400mg tablets |
30 tablet [PoM] £58.67 DT = £58.67

Suspension for injection
▸ Depo-Provera (Pfizer Ltd)
Medroxyprogesterone acetate 150 mg per 1 ml Depo-Provera
150mg/1ml suspension for injection pre-filled syringes | 1 pre-filled
disposable injection [PoM] £6.01 DT = £6.01
▸ Sayana Press (Pfizer Ltd)
Medroxyprogesterone acetate 160 mg per 1 ml Sayana Press
104mg/0.65 ml suspension for injection pre-filled disposable devices
| 1 pre-filled disposable injection [PoM] £6.90

3.6 Contraception, spermicidal

SPERMICIDALS

Nonoxinol

- **INDICATIONS AND DOSE**

Spermicidal contraceptive in conjunction with barrier methods of contraception such as diaphragms or caps
▸ BY VAGINA
▸ Females of childbearing potential: (consult product literature)

- SIDE-EFFECTS Genital erosion · increased risk of HIV infection · pain · paraesthesia · skin reactions · vaginal redness
  SIDE-EFFECTS, FURTHER INFORMATION High frequency use of the spermicide nonoxinol-9 has been associated with genital lesions, which may increase the risk of acquiring sexually transmitted infections.
- CONCEPTION AND CONTRACEPTION No evidence of harm to latex condoms and diaphragms.
- PREGNANCY Toxicity in *animal* studies.
- BREAST FEEDING Present in milk in *animal* studies.

- MEDICINAL FORMS
  There can be variation in the licensing of different medicines containing the same drug.
  Gel
  EXCIPIENTS: May contain Hydroxybenzoates (parabens), propylene glycol, sorbic acid
  ▸ Gygel (Marlborough Pharmaceuticals Ltd)
  Nonoxinol-9 20 mg per 1 ml Gygel 2% contraceptive jelly |
  30 gram [GSL] £4.25 | 81 gram [GSL] £11.00

4 Erectile and ejaculatory conditions

4.1 Erectile dysfunction

Erectile dysfunction
06-Mar-2017

Description of condition
Erectile dysfunction (impotence) is the persistent inability to attain and maintain an erection that is sufficient to permit satisfactory sexual performance. It can have physical or psychological causes. Erectile dysfunction can also be a side-effect of drugs such as antihypertensives, antidepressants, antipsychotics, cytotoxic drugs and recreational drugs (including alcohol).
Risk factors for erectile dysfunction include sedentary lifestyle, obesity, smoking, hypercholesterolaemia and metabolic syndrome. Erectile dysfunction increases the risk of cardiovascular disease. All men with unexplained erectile dysfunction should be evaluated for the presence of cardiovascular risk factors and any identified risk should be addressed.

Drug treatment
[EvGr] The recommended approach for the management of erectile dysfunction is a combination of drug treatment and lifestyle changes (including regular exercise, reduction in body mass index, smoking cessation, and reduced alcohol consumption).
An oral phosphodiesterase type-5 inhibitor is the first-line drug treatment for erectile dysfunction, regardless of the cause. Ⓐ These drugs act by increasing the blood flow to the penis. They do not initiate an erection—sexual stimulation is required.
The choice of oral phosphodiesterase type-5 inhibitor depends on the frequency of intercourse and response to treatment. [EvGr] Avanafil p. 794, sildenafil p. 794 and vardenafil p. 797 are short-acting drugs and are suitable for occasional use as required. Tadalafil p. 796 is a longer-acting drug. It can be used as required, but can also be used as a regular lower daily dose to allow for spontaneous (rather than scheduled) sexual activity or in those who have frequent sexual activity. A patient with erectile dysfunction should receive six doses of an individual phosphodiesterase type-5 inhibitor at the maximum dose (with sexual stimulation) before being classified as a non-responder. Patients who fail to respond to the maximum dose of at least two different phosphodiesterase type-5 inhibitors should be referred to a specialist.
Intracavernosal, intraurethral or topical application of alprostadil p. 798 (prostaglandin E$_1$) is recommended as second-line therapy under careful medical supervision. Intracavernosal or intraurethral preparations can also be used to aid diagnosis. ◇Ⓐ

Priapism associated with alprostadil
Manufacturers advise that patients should seek medical help if a prolonged erection lasting four hours or more occurs; application of an ice pack to the upper-inner thigh (alternating between the left and right thighs every two minutes for up to ten minutes) may result in reflex opening of the venous valves.
If priapism has lasted more than six hours, treatment should not be delayed; manufacturer advises management as follows:
- Initial therapy by penile aspiration: using aseptic technique, 20–50mL of blood should be aspirated using a 19–21 gauge butterfly needle inserted into the *corpus cavernosum*; if necessary the procedure may be repeated on the opposite side;
- Lavage: if initial aspiration is unsuccessful, a second 19–21 gauge butterfly needle can be inserted into the opposite *corpus cavernosum*; sterile physiological saline can be injected through the first needle and drained through the second;
- If aspiration and lavage of are unsuccessful, intracavernosal injection of a sympathomimetic with action on alpha-adrenergic receptors can be given, with continuous monitoring of blood pressure and pulse— see phenylephrine hydrochloride p. 800 [unlicensed indication], adrenaline/epinephrine p. 799 [unlicensed indication], and metaraminol p. 187 [unlicensed indication]. Extreme **caution** is required in patients with coronary heart disease, hypertension, cerebral ischaemia and in patients taking a monoamine-oxidase inhibitor (facilities for managing hypertensive crisis should be available when administered to patients taking MAOIs);
- If necessary the sympathomimetic injections can be followed by further aspiration of blood through the same butterfly needle;

Genito-urinary system

7

- If administration of a sympathomimetic drug is unsuccessful, urgent referral for surgical management is required.

Prescribing on the NHS
Some drug treatments for erectile dysfunction may only be prescribed on the NHS under certain circumstances; for details see the criteria listed in part XVIIIB of the Drug Tariff (Part XIb of the Northern Ireland Drug Tariff, Part 12 of the Scottish Drug Tariff). The Drug Tariffs can be accessed online at:
National Health Service Drug Tariff for England and Wales: www.nhsbsa.nhs.uk/pharmacies-gp-practices-and-appliance-contractors/drug-tariff.
Health and Personal Social Services for Northern Ireland Drug Tariff: www.hscbusiness.hscni.net/services/2034.htm.
Scottish Drug Tariff: www.isdscotland.org/Health-Topics/Prescribing-and-Medicines/Scottish-Drug-Tariff/.

Related drugs
Other drugs used for Erectile dysfunction: aviptadil with phentolamine mesilate p. 800.

PHOSPHODIESTERASE TYPE-5 INHIBITORS

Avanafil

22-Feb-2017

- **INDICATIONS AND DOSE**

Erectile dysfunction
▶ BY MOUTH
▶ Adult: Initially 100 mg, to be taken approximately 15–30 minutes before sexual activity, then adjusted according to response to 50–200 mg (max. per dose 200 mg), to be taken as a single dose as needed; maximum 1 dose per day

Erectile dysfunction in patients on alpha-blocker therapy
▶ BY MOUTH
▶ Adult: Initially 50 mg, to be taken approximately 15–30 minutes before sexual activity, then adjusted according to response to 50–200 mg (max. per dose 200 mg), to be taken as a single dose as needed; maximum 1 dose per day

DOSE ADJUSTMENTS DUE TO INTERACTIONS
▶ Manufacturer advises max. 100 mg once every 48 hours with concurrent use of moderate inhibitors of CYP3A4.

- CONTRA-INDICATIONS Avoid if systolic blood pressure below 90 mmHg (no information available) · blood pressure >170/100 mmHg · hereditary degenerative retinal disorders · history of non-arteritic anterior ischaemic optic neuropathy · life-threatening arrhythmia in previous 6 months · mild to severe heart failure · patients in whom vasodilation or sexual activity are inadvisable · recent history of myocardial infarction · recent history of stroke · recent unstable angina
- CAUTIONS Active peptic ulceration · anatomical deformation of the penis (e.g. angulation, cavernosal fibrosis, Peyronie's disease) · bleeding disorders · cardiovascular disease · left ventricular outflow obstruction · predisposition to priapism (e.g. in sickle-cell disease, multiple myeloma, or leukaemia)
- INTERACTIONS → Appendix 1: phosphodiesterase type-5 inhibitors
- SIDE-EFFECTS
▶ **Common or very common** Headaches · nasal complaints · vasodilation
▶ **Uncommon** Asthenia · dizziness · drowsiness · dyspnoea exertional · gastrointestinal discomfort · muscle complaints · nausea · pain · palpitations · respiratory disorders · vision blurred · vomiting
▶ **Rare or very rare** Akathisia · angina pectoris · chest pain · diarrhoea · dry mouth · emotional disorder · gastritis ·

genital pruritus · gout · haematuria · hypertension · increased risk of infection · influenza like illness · insomnia · penis disorder · peripheral oedema · rash · seasonal allergy · sexual dysfunction · tachycardia · urinary frequency increased · weight increased

- HEPATIC IMPAIRMENT Manufacturer advises avoid in severe impairment—no information available.
  Dose adjustments Use lowest effective initial dose in mild to moderate impairment, adjusted according to response.
- RENAL IMPAIRMENT Avoid if eGFR less than 30 mL/minute/1.73 m^2.
- PATIENT AND CARER ADVICE Onset of effect may be delayed if taken with food.
- NATIONAL FUNDING/ACCESS DECISIONS

Scottish Medicines Consortium (SMC) Decisions
The *Scottish Medicines Consortium* has advised (September 2015) that avanafil (*Spedra®*) is **not** recommended for use within NHS Scotland, for treatment of erectile dysfunction in men as the clinical and economic analysis presented was not sufficiently robust.

All Wales Medicines Strategy Group (AWMSG) Decisions
The *All Wales Medicines Strategy Group* has advised (July 2015) that avanafil (*Spedra®*) is recommended as an option for use within NHS Wales for the treatment of erectile dysfunction in men.
NHS restrictions *Spedra®* is not prescribable in NHS primary care for the treatment of erectile dysfunction except in men who meet the criteria listed in part XVIIIB of the Drug Tariff (Part XIb of the Northern Ireland Drug Tariff, Part 12 of the Scottish Drug Tariff). The prescription must be endorsed 'SLS'. For more information see *Prices in the BNF*, under How to use the BNF.

- MEDICINAL FORMS
There can be variation in the licensing of different medicines containing the same drug.

Tablet
▶ Spedra (A. Menarini Farmaceutica Internazionale SRL) ▼
Avanafil 50 mg Spedra 50mg tablets | 4 tablet [PoM] £10.94 DT = £10.94 | 8 tablet [PoM] £19.70 DT = £19.70
Avanafil 100 mg Spedra 100mg tablets | 4 tablet [PoM] £14.08 DT = £14.08 | 8 tablet [PoM] £26.26 DT = £26.26
Avanafil 200 mg Spedra 200mg tablets | 4 tablet [PoM] £21.90 DT = £21.90 | 8 tablet [PoM] £39.40 DT = £39.40

Sildenafil

20-Jul-2017

- **INDICATIONS AND DOSE**

Pulmonary arterial hypertension (initiated under specialist supervision)
▶ BY MOUTH
▶ Adult: 20 mg 3 times a day
▶ BY INTRAVENOUS INJECTION
▶ Adult: 10 mg 3 times a day, use intravenous route when the oral route is not appropriate

Erectile dysfunction
▶ BY MOUTH
▶ Adult: Initially 50 mg, to be taken approximately 1 hour before sexual activity, adjusted according to response to 25–100 mg (max. per dose 100 mg) as required, to be taken as a single dose; maximum 1 dose per day

Digital ulcers [associated with systemic sclerosis]
▶ BY MOUTH
▶ Adult: 25 mg 3 times a day, increased to 50 mg 3 times a day

DOSE ADJUSTMENTS DUE TO INTERACTIONS
▶ When used for Erectile dysfunction Manufacturer advises a starting dose of 25 mg with concurrent use of moderate and potent inhibitors of CYP3A4. Manufacturer advises

if concurrent use of ritonavir is unavoidable, the max. dose should not exceed 25 mg within 48 hours.

▸ With oral use for Pulmonary arterial hypertension Manufacturer advises reduce dose to 20 mg twice daily with concurrent use of moderate inhibitors of CYP3A4. Manufacturer advises reduce dose to 20 mg once daily with concurrent use of some potent inhibitors of CYP3A4 (avoid with ketoconazole, itraconazole and ritonavir).

▸ With intravenous use for Pulmonary arterial hypertension Manufacturer advises reduce dose to 10 mg twice daily with concurrent use of moderate inhibitors of CYP3A4. Manufacturer advises reduce dose to 10 mg once daily with concurrent use of some potent inhibitors of CYP3A4 (avoid with ketoconazole, itraconazole and ritonavir).

● UNLICENSED USE [EvGr] Sildenafil is used for the treatment of digital ulcer, ⒺⒸ but is not licensed for this indication.

● CONTRA-INDICATIONS

GENERAL CONTRA-INDICATIONS Hereditary degenerative retinal disorders · history of non-arteritic anterior ischaemic optic neuropathy · recent history of myocardial infarction · recent history of stroke

SPECIFIC CONTRA-INDICATIONS

▸ When used for erectile dysfunction Avoid if systolic blood pressure below 90 mmHg (no information available) · patients in whom vasodilation or sexual activity are inadvisable · recent unstable angina

▸ When used for pulmonary arterial hypertension Sickle-cell anaemia

● CAUTIONS

GENERAL CAUTIONS Active peptic ulceration · bleeding disorders · cardiovascular disease · left ventricular outflow obstruction

SPECIFIC CAUTIONS

▸ When used for erectile dysfunction Anatomical deformation of the penis (e.g. angulation, cavernosal fibrosis, Peyronie's disease) · predisposition to priapism (e.g. in sickle-cell disease, multiple myeloma, or leukaemia)

▸ When used for pulmonary arterial hypertension Anatomical deformation of the penis · autonomic dysfunction · hypotension (avoid if systolic blood pressure below 90 mmHg) · intravascular volume depletion · predisposition to priapism · pulmonary veno-occlusive disease

● INTERACTIONS → Appendix 1: phosphodiesterase type-5 inhibitors

● SIDE-EFFECTS

GENERAL SIDE-EFFECTS

▸ Common or very common Dry mouth · eye discomfort · gastrointestinal discomfort · haemorrhage · myalgia · vertigo · vision disorders

▸ Uncommon Haematospermia · hypotension

▸ Rare or very rare Optic neuropathy (discontinue if sudden visual impairment occurs) · retinal occlusion

SPECIFIC SIDE-EFFECTS

▸ Common or very common

▸ With intravenous use Alopecia · anaemia · anxiety · cough · diarrhoea · eye erythema · fever · flushing · gastrointestinal disorders · headaches · increased risk of infection · insomnia · nasal congestion · night sweats · pain · sensation abnormal · skin reactions · tremor

▸ With oral use Dizziness · headache · nasal complaints · nausea · vasodilation

▸ Uncommon

▸ With intravenous use Gynaecomastia

▸ With oral use Arrhythmias · chest pain · drowsiness · dry eye · eye disorders · eye inflammation · fatigue · feeling hot · gastroesophageal reflux disease · hearing impairment ·

hypertension · numbness · pain in extremity · palpitations · rash · rhinitis · sinus congestion · vomiting

▸ Rare or very rare

▸ With oral use Acute coronary syndrome · arteriosclerotic retinopathy · cerebrovascular insufficiency · glaucoma · irritability · oral hypoaesthesia · priapism · scleral discolouration · seizure · severe cutaneous adverse reactions (SCARs) · sudden cardiac death · syncope · throat tightness

▸ Frequency not known

▸ With intravenous use Sexual dysfunction · sudden hearing loss

● PREGNANCY Use only if potential benefit outweighs risk— no evidence of harm in *animal* studies.

● BREAST FEEDING Manufacturer advises avoid—no information available.

● HEPATIC IMPAIRMENT Manufacturer advises avoid in severe impairment.

Dose adjustments In pulmonary arterial hypertension, if usual dose not tolerated, reduce *oral* dose to 20 mg twice daily and *intravenous* dose to 10 mg twice daily.

For erectile dysfunction, use initial dose of 25 mg.

● RENAL IMPAIRMENT

Dose adjustments Use initial dose of 25 mg in erectile dysfunction if eGFR less than 30 mL/minute/1.73 m².

In pulmonary hypertension, if usual dose not tolerated, reduce *oral* dose to 20 mg twice daily and *intravenous* dose to 10 mg twice daily.

● TREATMENT CESSATION

▸ When used for Pulmonary arterial hypertension Consider gradual withdrawal.

● PATIENT AND CARER ADVICE

▸ When used for Erectile dysfunction Onset of effect may be delayed if taken with food.

● NATIONAL FUNDING/ACCESS DECISIONS

Scottish Medicines Consortium (SMC) Decisions
The *Scottish Medicines Consortium* has advised (February 2010) that sildenafil tablets (*Revatio®*) is accepted for restricted use within NHS Scotland and should be initiated for patients with pulmonary arterial hypertension only by specialists in the Scottish Pulmonary Vascular Unit or other similar specialists.

The *Scottish Medicines Consortium* has advised (March 2011) that sildenafil injection (*Revatio®*) is accepted for restricted use within NHS Scotland for patients with pulmonary arterial hypertension who are currently prescribed oral sildenafil and are temporarily unable to take oral medicine, and should be prescribed only on the advice of specialists in the Scottish Pulmonary Vascular Unit or the Scottish Adult Congenital Cardiac Service.

NHS restrictions *Viagra®* is not prescribable in NHS primary care for treatment of erectile dysfunction except in men who meet the criteria listed in part XVIIIB of the Drug Tariff (Part XIb of the Northern Ireland Drug Tariff, Part 12 of the Scottish Drug Tariff). The prescription must be endorsed 'SLS'. For more information see *Prices in the BNF*, under How to use the BNF.

● MEDICINAL FORMS
There can be variation in the licensing of different medicines containing the same drug. Forms available from special-order manufacturers include: oral suspension, oral solution

Tablet
▸ Sildenafil (Non-proprietary)
   Sildenafil (as Sildenafil citrate) 20 mg Sildenafil 20mg tablets | 90 tablet [PoM] £379.38–£424.01 DT = £446.33
   Sildenafil (as Sildenafil citrate) 25 mg Sildenafil 25mg tablets | 4 tablet [PoM] £16.59 DT = £0.37 | 8 tablet [PoM] £0.74–£33.19
   Sildenafil (as Sildenafil citrate) 50 mg Sildenafil 50mg tablets | 4 tablet [PoM] £21.27 DT = £0.42 | 8 tablet [PoM] £0.84–£42.54

7

Genito-urinary system

Sildenafil (as Sildenafil citrate) 100 mg Sildenafil 100mg tablets |
4 tablet [PoM] £23.50 DT = £0.59 | 8 tablet [PoM] £1.18–£46.99 |
12 tablet [PoM] £3.69

▸ Granpidam (Accord Healthcare Ltd)

Sildenafil (as Sildenafil citrate) 20 mg Granpidam 20mg tablets |
90 tablet [PoM] £424.01 DT = £446.33

▸ Revatio (Pfizer Ltd)

Sildenafil (as Sildenafil citrate) 20 mg Revatio 20mg tablets |
90 tablet [PoM] £446.33 DT = £446.33

▸ Viagra (Pfizer Ltd)

Sildenafil (as Sildenafil citrate) 25 mg Viagra 25mg tablets |
4 tablet [PoM] £16.59 DT = £0.37 | 8 tablet [PoM] £33.19
Sildenafil (as Sildenafil citrate) 50 mg Viagra 50mg tablets |
4 tablet [PoM] £21.27 DT = £0.42 | 8 tablet [PoM] £42.54
Sildenafil (as Sildenafil citrate) 100 mg Viagra 100mg tablets |
4 tablet [PoM] £23.50 DT = £0.59 | 8 tablet [PoM] £46.99

▸ Vizarsin (Consilient Health Ltd)

Sildenafil (as Sildenafil citrate) 25 mg Vizarsin 25mg tablets |
4 tablet [PoM] £14.10 DT = £0.37
Sildenafil (as Sildenafil citrate) 50 mg Vizarsin 50mg tablets |
4 tablet [PoM] £18.07 DT = £0.42
Sildenafil (as Sildenafil citrate) 100 mg Vizarsin 100mg tablets |
4 tablet [PoM] £19.97 DT = £0.59

Solution for injection

▸ Revatio (Pfizer Ltd)

Sildenafil (as Sildenafil citrate).8 mg per 1 ml Revatio
10mg/12.5ml solution for injection vials | 1 vial [PoM] £45.28
(Hospital only)

Oral suspension

▸ Revatio (Pfizer Ltd)

Sildenafil (as Sildenafil citrate) 10 mg per 1 ml Revatio 10mg/ml
oral suspension sugar-free | 112 ml [PoM] £186.75

Tadalafil

20-Jul-2017

● INDICATIONS AND DOSE

**Pulmonary arterial hypertension (initiated under
specialist supervision)**

▸ BY MOUTH

▸ Adult: 40 mg once daily

Erectile dysfunction

▸ BY MOUTH

▸ Adult: Initially 10 mg (max. per dose 20 mg), to be
taken at least 30 minutes before sexual activity,
subsequent doses adjusted according to response, the
effect of intermittent dosing may persist for longer
than 24 hours, continuous daily use not recommended;
maximum 1 dose per day

**Erectile dysfunction; for patients who anticipate sexual
activity at least twice a week**

▸ BY MOUTH

▸ Adult: 5 mg once daily, reduced to 2.5 mg once daily,
adjusted according to response

Benign prostatic hyperplasia

▸ BY MOUTH

▸ Adult: 5 mg once daily

● CONTRA-INDICATIONS

GENERAL CONTRA-INDICATIONS History of non-arteritic
anterior ischaemic optic neuropathy

SPECIFIC CONTRA-INDICATIONS

▸ When used for benign prostatic hyperplasia or erectile
dysfunction Hypotension (avoid if systolic blood pressure
below 90 mmHg) · mild to severe heart failure · myocardial
infarction · patients in whom vasodilation or sexual
activity are inadvisable · recent stroke · uncontrolled
arrhythmias · uncontrolled hypertension · unstable angina

▸ When used for pulmonary arterial hypertension Acute
myocardial infarction in past 90 days

● CAUTIONS

▸ When used for benign prostatic hyperplasia or erectile
dysfunction Anatomical deformation of the penis (e.g.
angulation, cavernosal fibrosis, Peyronie's disease) ·

cardiovascular disease · left ventricular outflow
obstruction · predisposition to priapism (e.g. in sickle-cell
disease, multiple myeloma, or leukaemia)

▸ When used for pulmonary arterial hypertension Anatomical
deformation of the penis · aortic and mitral valve disease ·
congestive cardiomyopathy · coronary artery disease ·
hereditary degenerative retinal disorders · hypotension
(avoid if systolic blood pressure below 90 mmHg) · left
ventricular dysfunction · life-threatening arrhythmias ·
pericardial constriction · predisposition to priapism ·
pulmonary veno-occlusive disease · uncontrolled
hypertension

● INTERACTIONS → Appendix 1: phosphodiesterase type-5
inhibitors

● SIDE-EFFECTS

▸ **Common or very common** Flushing · gastrointestinal
discomfort · headaches · myalgia · nasal congestion · pain

▸ **Uncommon** Arrhythmias · chest pain · dizziness · dyspnoea
· eye pain · fatigue · gastrooesophageal reflux disease ·
haemorrhage · hypertension · hypotension · nausea ·
oedema · palpitations · skin reactions · tinnitus · vision
disorders · vomiting

▸ **Rare or very rare** Acute coronary syndrome · angioedema ·
cerebrovascular insufficiency · eye erythema · eye swelling
· haematospermia · hyperhidrosis · memory loss · optic
neuropathy (discontinue if sudden visual impairment
occurs) · priapism · retinal occlusion · seizure · Stevens-
Johnson syndrome · sudden cardiac death · sudden hearing
loss (discontinue drug and seek medical advice) · syncope

● PREGNANCY Manufacturer advises avoid.

● BREAST FEEDING Manufacturer advises avoid—present in
milk in *animal* studies.

● HEPATIC IMPAIRMENT

▸ When used for Pulmonary arterial hypertension Manufacturer
advises use with caution in mild-to-moderate impairment;
avoid in severe impairment.

▸ When used for Benign prostatic hyperplasia or Erectile
dysfunction Manufacturer advises caution in severe impairment and
for regular once-daily dosing—no information available.

Dose adjustments

▸ When used for Pulmonary arterial hypertension Manufacturer
advises use initial dose of 20 mg once daily in mild-to-
moderate impairment.

▸ When used for Erectile dysfunction Manufacturer advises
maximum dose of 10 mg for intermittent use.

● RENAL IMPAIRMENT

▸ When used for Pulmonary arterial hypertension Manufacturer
advises avoid in severe impairment.

▸ When used for Erectile dysfunction or Benign prostatic hyperplasia
Manufacturer advises avoid regular once-daily dosing in
severe impairment.

Dose adjustments

▸ When used for Pulmonary arterial hypertension Manufacturer
advises initial dose of 20 mg once daily in mild-to-
moderate impairment; dose may be increased to 40 mg
once daily if tolerated.

▸ When used for Erectile dysfunction Manufacturer advises
maximum dose of 10 mg for intermittent use in severe
impairment.

● NATIONAL FUNDING/ACCESS DECISIONS

Scottish Medicines Consortium (SMC) Decisions
The *Scottish Medicines Consortium* has advised (July 2012)
that tadalafil (*Adcirca* ®) is accepted for restricted use
within NHS Scotland for adults with pulmonary arterial
hypertension and should be initiated only by specialists in
the Scottish Pulmonary Vascular Unit or other similar
specialists. This advice is contingent upon the continuing
availability of the Patient Access Scheme in NHS Scotland.
NHS restrictions   *Cialis* ® is not prescribable in NHS
primary care for the treatment of erectile dysfunction
except in men who meet the criteria listed in part XVIIIB of

the Drug Tariff (Part XIb of the Northern Ireland Drug Tariff, Part 12 of the Scottish Drug Tariff). The prescription must be endorsed 'SLS'. For more information see *Prices in the BNF*, under How to use the BNF.

● MEDICINAL FORMS
There can be variation in the licensing of different medicines containing the same drug.
Tablet
▸ Tadalafil (Non-proprietary)
  Tadalafil 2.5 mg Tadalafil 2.5mg tablets | 28 tablet [PoM] £5.50–£54.99 DT = £54.99
  Tadalafil 5 mg Tadalafil 5mg tablets | 28 tablet [PoM] £5.50–£54.99 DT = £8.55
  Tadalafil 10 mg Tadalafil 10mg tablets | 4 tablet [PoM] £2.13–£28.88 DT = £2.13
  Tadalafil 20 mg Tadalafil 20mg tablets | 4 tablet [PoM] £2.89–£54.99 DT = £3.17 | 8 tablet [PoM] £5.18–£109.98 | 56 tablet [PoM] £392.98–£466.66
▸ Adcirca (Eli Lilly and Company Ltd)
  Tadalafil 20 mg Adcirca 20mg tablets | 56 tablet [PoM] £491.22
▸ Cialis (Eli Lilly and Company Ltd)
  Tadalafil 2.5 mg Cialis 2.5mg tablets | 28 tablet [PoM] £54.99 DT = £54.99
  Tadalafil 5 mg Cialis 5mg tablets | 28 tablet [PoM] £54.99 DT = £8.55
  Tadalafil 10 mg Cialis 10mg tablets | 4 tablet [PoM] £28.88 DT = £2.13
  Tadalafil 20 mg Cialis 20mg tablets | 4 tablet [PoM] £28.88 DT = £3.17 | 8 tablet [PoM] £57.76
▸ Talmanco (Mylan)
  Tadalafil 20 mg Talmanco 20mg tablets | 56 tablet [PoM] £417.54 (Hospital only)

Vardenafil

20-Jul-2017

● INDICATIONS AND DOSE
Erectile dysfunction
▸ BY MOUTH USING TABLETS
▸ Adult: Initially 10 mg (max. per dose 20 mg), to be taken approximately 25–60 minutes before sexual activity, subsequent doses adjusted according to response, onset of effect may be delayed if taken with high-fat meal; maximum 1 dose per day
▸ BY MOUTH USING ORODISPERSIBLE TABLET
▸ Adult: 10 mg, to be taken approximately 25–60 minutes before sexual activity; maximum 10 mg per day

Erectile dysfunction (patients on alpha-blocker therapy)
▸ BY MOUTH USING TABLETS
▸ Adult: Initially 5 mg (max. per dose 20 mg), to be taken approximately 25–60 minutes before sexual activity, subsequent doses adjusted according to response, onset of effect may be delayed if taken with high-fat meal; maximum 1 dose per day

DOSE EQUIVALENCE AND CONVERSION
▸ *Levitra* ® 10 mg *orodispersible tablets* and *Levitra* ® 10 mg *film coated tablets* are **not** bioequivalent.

● CONTRA-INDICATIONS Avoid if systolic blood pressure below 90 mmHg · hereditary degenerative retinal disorders · myocardial infarction · patients in whom vasodilation or sexual activity are inadvisable · previous history of non-arteritic anterior ischaemic optic neuropathy · recent stroke · unstable angina
● CAUTIONS Active peptic ulceration · anatomical deformation of the penis (e.g. angulation, cavernosal fibrosis, Peyronie's disease) · bleeding disorders · cardiovascular disease · elderly · left ventricular outflow obstruction · predisposition to priapism (e.g. in sickle-cell disease, multiple myeloma, or leukaemia) · susceptibility to prolongation of QT interval
● INTERACTIONS → Appendix 1: phosphodiesterase type-5 inhibitors

● SIDE-EFFECTS
▸ **Common or very common** Dizziness · flushing · gastrointestinal discomfort · headache · nasal congestion
▸ **Uncommon** Allergic oedema · angioedema · arrhythmias · back pain · diarrhoea · drowsiness · dry mouth · dyspnoea · eye discomfort · eye disorders · gastrointestinal disorders · hearing impairment · malaise · muscle complaints · muscle tone increased · nausea · palpitations · sensation abnormal · sinus congestion · skin reactions · sleep disorder · vertigo · vision disorders · vomiting
▸ **Rare or very rare** Angina pectoris · anxiety · chest pain · conjunctivitis · haemorrhage · hypertension · hypotension · memory loss · myocardial infarction · photosensitivity reaction · priapism · seizure · syncope
▸ **Frequency not known** Haematospermia · optic neuropathy (discontinue if sudden visual impairment occurs) · QT interval prolongation

● HEPATIC IMPAIRMENT Manufacturer advises avoid in severe impairment. Orodispersible tablets not suitable for patients with moderate hepatic impairment.
Dose adjustments Initial dose 5 mg in mild to moderate impairment, increased subsequently according to response (max. 10 mg in moderate impairment).

● RENAL IMPAIRMENT Orodispersible tablets not suitable if eGFR less than 30 mL/minute/1.73 m^2.
Dose adjustments Initial dose 5 mg if eGFR less than 30 mL/minute/1.73 m^2.

● PRESCRIBING AND DISPENSING INFORMATION
Orodispersible tablets not suitable for initiation of therapy in patients taking alpha-blockers.

● NATIONAL FUNDING/ACCESS DECISIONS
Scottish Medicines Consortium (SMC) Decisions
The *Scottish Medicines Consortium* has advised (October 2011) that vardenafil orodispersible tablets (*Levitra* ®) are accepted for restricted use within NHS Scotland for treatment of erectile dysfunction in men for whom an orodispersible tablet is an appropriate formulation.
NHS restrictions *Levitra* ® is not prescribable in NHS primary care for the treatment of erectile dysfunction except in men who meet the criteria listed in part XVIIIB of the Drug Tariff (Part XIb of the Northern Ireland Drug Tariff, Part 12 of the Scottish Drug Tariff). The prescription must be endorsed 'SLS'. For more information see *Prices in the BNF*, under How to use the BNF.

LEVITRA ® ORODISPERSIBLE TABLETS
Scottish Medicines Consortium (SMC) Decisions
The *Scottish Medicines Consortium* has advised (September 2011) that vardenafil orodispersible tablets (*Levitra* ®) are accepted for restricted use within NHS Scotland for men for whom an orodispersible tablet is an appropriate formulation.

● MEDICINAL FORMS
There can be variation in the licensing of different medicines containing the same drug.
Orodispersible tablet
EXCIPIENTS: May contain Aspartame
▸ Levitra (Bayer Plc)
  Vardenafil (as Vardenafil hydrochloride trihydrate) 10 mg Levitra 10mg orodispersible tablets sugar-free | 4 tablet [PoM] £19.67 DT = £19.67
Tablet
▸ Levitra (Bayer Plc)
  Vardenafil (as Vardenafil hydrochloride trihydrate) 5 mg Levitra 5mg tablets | 4 tablet [PoM] £8.32 DT = £8.32 | 8 tablet [PoM] £16.63
  Vardenafil (as Vardenafil hydrochloride trihydrate) 10 mg Levitra 10mg tablets | 4 tablet [PoM] £14.78 DT = £14.78 | 8 tablet [PoM] £29.57
  Vardenafil (as Vardenafil hydrochloride trihydrate) 20 mg Levitra 20mg tablets | 4 tablet [PoM] £24.30 DT = £24.30 | 8 tablet [PoM] £48.60

7

Genito-urinary system

PROSTAGLANDIN ANALOGUES AND PROSTAMIDES > PROSTAGLANDINS

Alprostadil

20-Jul-2017

● INDICATIONS AND DOSE

Erectile dysfunction (initiated under specialist supervision)

▶ BY URETHRAL APPLICATION

▸ Adult: Initially 250 micrograms, adjusted according to response; usual dose 0.125–1 mg; maximum 2 doses per day; maximum 7 doses per week

Aid to diagnosis of erectile dysfunction

▶ BY URETHRAL APPLICATION

▸ Adult: 500 micrograms for 1 dose

Erectile dysfunction

▶ TO THE SKIN

▸ Adult: Apply 300 micrograms, to the tip of the penis, 5–30 minutes before sexual activity; max 1 dose in 24 hours not more than 2–3 times per week

CAVERJECT ®

Erectile dysfunction

▶ BY INTRACAVERNOSAL INJECTION

▸ Adult: Initially 2.5 micrograms for 1 dose (first dose), followed by 5 micrograms for 1 dose (second dose), to be given if some response to first dose, alternatively 7.5 micrograms for 1 dose (second dose), to be given if no response to first dose, then increased in steps of 5–10 micrograms, to obtain a dose suitable for producing erection lasting not more than 1 hour; if no response to dose then next higher dose can be given within 1 hour, if there is a response the next dose should not be given for at least 24 hours; usual dose 5–20 micrograms (max. per dose 60 micrograms), maximum frequency of injection not more than 3 times per week with at least 24 hour interval between injections

Erectile dysfunction associated with neurological dysfunction

▶ BY INTRACAVERNOSAL INJECTION

▸ Adult: Initially 1.25 micrograms for 1 dose (first dose), then 2.5 micrograms for 1 dose (second dose), then 5 micrograms for 1 dose (third dose), increased in steps of 5–10 micrograms, to obtain a dose suitable for producing erection lasting not more than 1 hour; if no response to dose then next higher dose can be given within 1 hour, if there is a response the next dose should not be given for at least 24 hours; usual dose 5–20 micrograms (max. per dose 60 micrograms), maximum frequency of injection not more than 3 times per week with at least 24 hour interval between injections

Aid to diagnosis

▶ BY INTRACAVERNOSAL INJECTION

▸ Adult: 10–20 micrograms for 1 dose (consult product literature)

Aid to diagnosis where evidence of neurological dysfunction

▶ BY INTRACAVERNOSAL INJECTION

▸ Adult: Initially 5 micrograms (max. per dose 10 micrograms) for 1 dose, (consult product literature)

CAVERJECT ® DUAL CHAMBER

Erectile dysfunction

▶ BY INTRACAVERNOSAL INJECTION

▸ Adult: Initially 2.5 micrograms for 1 dose (first dose), followed by 5 micrograms for 1 dose (second dose), to be given if some response to first dose, alternatively 7.5 micrograms for 1 dose (second dose), to be given if no response to first dose, then increased in steps of 5–10 micrograms, to obtain a dose suitable for producing erection lasting not more than 1 hour; if no response to dose then next higher dose can be given within 1 hour, if there is a response the next dose should not be given for at least 24 hours; usual dose 5–20 micrograms (max. per dose 60 micrograms), maximum frequency of injection not more than 3 times per week with at least 24 hour interval between injections

Erectile dysfunction associated with neurological dysfunction

▶ BY INTRACAVERNOSAL INJECTION

▸ Adult: Initially 1.25 micrograms for 1 dose (first dose), then 2.5 micrograms for 1 dose (second dose), then 5 micrograms for 1 dose (third dose), increased in steps of 5–10 micrograms, to obtain a dose suitable for producing erection lasting not more than 1 hour; if no response to dose then next higher dose can be given within 1 hour, if there is a response the next dose should not be given for at least 24 hours; usual dose 5–20 micrograms (max. per dose 60 micrograms), maximum frequency of injection not more than 3 times per week with at least 24 hour interval between injections

Aid to diagnosis

▶ BY INTRACAVERNOSAL INJECTION

▸ Adult: 10–20 micrograms for 1 dose (consult product literature)

Aid to diagnosis where evidence of neurological dysfunction

▶ BY INTRACAVERNOSAL INJECTION

▸ Adult: Initially 5 micrograms (max. per dose 10 micrograms) for 1 dose, (consult product literature)

VIRIDAL ® DUO

Neurogenic erectile dysfunction

▶ BY INTRACAVERNOSAL INJECTION

▸ Adult: Initially 1.25 micrograms, increased in steps of 2.5–5 micrograms, to obtain dose suitable for producing erection not lasting more than 1 hour; usual dose 10–20 micrograms (max. per dose 40 micrograms), maximum frequency of injection not more than 3 times per week with at least 24 hour interval between injections; reduce dose if erection lasts longer than 2 hours

Erectile dysfunction

▶ BY INTRACAVERNOSAL INJECTION

▸ Adult: Initially 2.5 micrograms, increased in steps of 2.5–5 micrograms, to obtain dose suitable for producing erection not lasting more than 1 hour; usual dose 10–20 micrograms (max. per dose 40 micrograms), maximum frequency of injection not more than 3 times per week with at least 24 hour interval between injections; reduce dose if erection lasts longer than 2 hours

● CONTRA-INDICATIONS

GENERAL CONTRA-INDICATIONS Not for use in patients with penile implants or when sexual activity medically inadvisable (e.g. orthostatic hypotension, myocardial infarction, and syncope) · not for use with other agents for erectile dysfunction · predisposition to prolonged erection (as in thrombocythemia, polycythemia, sickle cell anaemia, multiple myeloma or leukaemia) · urethral application contra-indicated in balanitis · urethral application contra-indicated in severe curvature · urethral application contra-indicated in severe hypospadia · urethral application contra-indicated in urethral stricture · urethral application contra-indicated in urethritis

SPECIFIC CONTRA-INDICATIONS

▸ With topical use Balanitis · severe curvature · severe hypospadia · urethral stricture · urethritis

- CAUTIONS Anatomical deformations of penis (painful erection more likely)—follow up regularly to detect signs of penile fibrosis (consider discontinuation if angulation, cavernosal fibrosis or Peyronie's disease develop) · priapism (patients should be instructed to report any erection lasting 4 hours or longer)
- INTERACTIONS → Appendix 1: alprostadil
- SIDE-EFFECTS
  ▸ **Common or very common**
  ▸ With intracavernosal use Haemorrhage · muscle spasms · penile disorders · sexual dysfunction · skin reactions
  ▸ With topical use Balanoposthitis · genital abnormalities · penile disorders · rash · sexual dysfunction · urinary tract pain
  ▸ With urethral use Dizziness · haemorrhage · headache · hypotension · muscle spasms · penile disorders · sexual dysfunction · urethral burning
  ▸ **Uncommon**
  ▸ With intracavernosal use Asthenia · balanoposthitis · dry mouth · extrasystole · hyperhidrosis · hypotension · increased risk of infection · inflammation · mydriasis · nausea · oedema · pelvic pain · peripheral vascular disease · presyncope · scrotal disorders · sensation abnormal · spermatocele · testicular disorders · urinary disorders · vascular disorders · vasodilation
  ▸ With topical use Dizziness · hyperaesthesia · hypotension · muscle rigidity · pain in extremity · scrotal pain · syncope · urinary tract disorders
  ▸ With urethral use Balanoposthitis · hyperhidrosis · increased risk of infection · leg pain · nausea · pelvic pain · perineal pain · peripheral vascular disease · scrotal disorders · sensation abnormal · skin reactions · spermatocele · syncope · testicular disorders · urinary disorders · vascular disorders · vasodilation
  ▸ **Frequency not known**
  ▸ With intracavernosal use Myocardial ischaemia · stroke
- CONCEPTION AND CONTRACEPTION
  ▸ With urethral use If partner is pregnant, barrier contraception should be used. No evidence of harm to latex condoms and diaphragms.
  ▸ With topical use Condoms should be used to avoid exposure to women of child-bearing age, pregnant or lactating women. No evidence of harm to latex condoms.
- DIRECTIONS FOR ADMINISTRATION
  ▸ With intracavernosal use The first dose of the intracavernosal injection must be given by medically trained personnel; self-administration may only be undertaken after proper training.
  ▸ With urethral use During initiation of treatment the urethral application should be used under medical supervision; self-administration may only be undertaken after proper training.
- PATIENT AND CARER ADVICE Patients should be instructed to report any erection lasting 4 hours or longer.
  ▸ With topical use Counsel patients that condoms should be used to avoid local reactions and exposure of alprostadil to women of childbearing age, pregnant, or lactating women.
- NATIONAL FUNDING/ACCESS DECISIONS
  NHS restrictions *Caverject*®, *Viridal*® *Duo*, *Vitaros*® and *MUSE*® are not prescribable in NHS primary care for the treatment of erectile dysfunction except in men who meet the criteria listed in part XVIIIB of the Drug Tariff (Part XIb of the Northern Ireland Drug Tariff, Part 12 of the Scottish Drug Tariff). The prescription must be endorsed 'SLS'. For more information see *Prices in the BNF*, under *How to use BNF publications*.

- MEDICINAL FORMS
  There can be variation in the licensing of different medicines containing the same drug.

Stick
  ▸ Muse (Meda Pharmaceuticals Ltd)
    Alprostadil 250 microgram Muse 250microgram urethral sticks | 1 applicator PoM £11.30 DT = £11.30 | 6 applicator PoM £67.79
    Alprostadil 500 microgram Muse 500microgram urethral sticks | 1 applicator PoM £11.30 DT = £11.30 | 6 applicator PoM £67.79
    Alprostadil 1 mg Muse 1000microgram urethral sticks | 1 applicator PoM £11.56 DT = £11.56 | 6 applicator PoM £65.67

Cream
  ▸ Vitaros (Ferring Pharmaceuticals Ltd)
    Alprostadil 3 mg per 1 gram Vitaros 3mg/g cream | 4 applicator PoM £40.00

Powder and solvent for solution for injection
  ▸ Caverject (Pfizer Ltd)
    Alprostadil 10 microgram Caverject 10microgram powder and solvent for solution for injection vials | 1 vial PoM £9.24 DT = £9.24
    Caverject Dual Chamber 10microgram powder and solvent for solution for injection | 2 pre-filled disposable injection PoM £14.70
    Alprostadil 20 microgram Caverject Dual Chamber 20microgram powder and solvent for solution for injection | 2 pre-filled disposable injection PoM £19.00
    Caverject 20microgram powder and solvent for solution for injection vials | 1 vial PoM £11.94 DT = £11.94
    Alprostadil 40 microgram Caverject 40microgram powder and solvent for solution for injection vials | 1 vial PoM £21.58 DT = £21.58
  ▸ Viridal (UCB Pharma Ltd)
    Alprostadil 10 microgram Viridal Duo Starter Pack 10microgram powder and solvent for solution for injection cartridges with device | 2 cartridge PoM £20.13 (Hospital only)
    Viridal Duo Continuation Pack 10microgram powder and solvent for solution for injection cartridges | 2 cartridge PoM £16.55
    Alprostadil 20 microgram Viridal Duo Starter Pack 20microgram powder and solvent for solution for injection cartridges with device | 2 cartridge PoM £24.54 (Hospital only)
    Viridal Duo Continuation Pack 20microgram powder and solvent for solution for injection cartridges | 2 cartridge PoM £21.39
    Alprostadil 40 microgram Viridal Duo Starter Pack 40microgram powder and solvent for solution for injection cartridges with device | 2 cartridge PoM £29.83 (Hospital only)
    Viridal Duo Continuation Pack 40microgram powder and solvent for solution for injection cartridges | 2 cartridge PoM £27.22

SYMPATHOMIMETICS > VASOCONSTRICTOR

Adrenaline/epinephrine   27-Sep-2017

- DRUG ACTION Acts on both alpha and beta receptors and increases both heart rate and contractility (beta$_1$ effects); it can cause peripheral vasodilation (a beta$_2$ effect) or vasoconstriction (an alpha effect).

- INDICATIONS AND DOSE
  Priapism associated with alprostadil, if aspiration and lavage of corpora are unsuccessful (alternative to phenylephrine or metaraminol)
  ▸ BY INTRACAVERNOSAL INJECTION
  ▸ Adult: 10–20 micrograms every 5–10 minutes, using a 20 microgram/mL solution, **Important:** if suitable strength of adrenaline not available may be specially prepared by diluting 0.1 mL of the adrenaline 1 in 1000 (1 mg/mL) injection to 5 mL with sodium chloride 0.9%, continuously monitor blood pressure and pulse; maximum 100 micrograms per course

- UNLICENSED USE The use of adrenaline for the treatment of priapism is an unlicensed indication.
- CAUTIONS Arteriosclerosis · arrhythmias · cerebrovascular disease · cor pulmonale · diabetes mellitus · elderly · hypercalcaemia · hyperreflexia · hypertension · hyperthyroidism · hypokalaemia · ischaemic heart disease · obstructive cardiomyopathy · occlusive vascular disease · organic brain damage · phaeochromocytoma · prostate

7

Genito-urinary system

disorders · psychoneurosis · severe angina · susceptibility to angle-closure glaucoma

CAUTIONS, FURTHER INFORMATION Cautions listed are only for non-life-threatening situations.

● INTERACTIONS → Appendix 1: sympathomimetics, vasoconstrictor

● SIDE-EFFECTS Angina pectoris · angle closure glaucoma · anxiety · appetite decreased · arrhythmias · asthenia · confusion · dizziness · dry mouth · dyspnoea · headache · hepatic necrosis · hyperglycaemia · hyperhidrosis · hypersalivation · hypertension (increased risk of cerebral haemorrhage) · hypokalaemia · insomnia · intestinal necrosis · metabolic acidosis · mydriasis · myocardial infarction · nausea · pallor · palpitations · peripheral coldness · psychosis · pulmonary oedema (on excessive dosage or extreme sensitivity) · renal necrosis · soft tissue necrosis · tremor · urinary disorders · vomiting

● RENAL IMPAIRMENT Manufacturers advise use with caution in severe impairment.

● MONITORING REQUIREMENTS Monitor blood pressure and ECG.

● MEDICINAL FORMS
There can be variation in the licensing of different medicines containing the same drug. Forms available from special-order manufacturers include: solution for injection
Solution for injection
EXCIPIENTS: May contain Sulfites
▸ Adrenaline/epinephrine (Non-proprietary)
Adrenaline 1 mg per 1 ml Adrenaline (base) 10mg/10ml (1 in 1,000) solution for injection ampoules | 10 ampoule PoM £87.62
Adrenaline (base) for anaphylaxis 1mg/1ml (1 in 1,000) solution for injection pre-filled syringes | 1 pre-filled disposable injection PoM £10.40
Adrenaline (base) 1mg/1ml (1 in 1,000) solution for injection pre-filled syringes | 1 pre-filled disposable injection PoM £10.40
Adrenaline (as Adrenaline acid tartrate) 1 mg per 1 ml Adrenaline (base) 5mg/5ml (1 in 1,000) solution for injection ampoules | 10 ampoule PoM £85.07
Adrenaline (base) 500micrograms/0.5ml (1 in 1,000) solution for injection ampoules | 10 ampoule PoM £67.72 DT = £67.72
Adrenaline (base) 1mg/1ml (1 in 1,000) solution for injection ampoules | 10 ampoule PoM £6.01 DT = £6.01

Metaraminol

● INDICATIONS AND DOSE
Priapism (alternative to intracavernosal injections of phenylephrine and adrenaline)
▸ BY INTRACAVERNOSAL INJECTION
▸ Adult: 1 mg every 15 minutes

● UNLICENSED USE Use for priapism is an unlicensed indication.

● CONTRA-INDICATIONS Hypertension

● CAUTIONS Associated with fatal hypertensive crises · cirrhosis · coronary vascular thrombosis · diabetes mellitus · elderly · extravasation at injection site may cause necrosis · following myocardial infarction · hypercapnia · hyperthyroidism · hypoxia · mesenteric vascular thrombosis · peripheral vascular thrombosis · Prinzmetal's variant angina · uncorrected hypovolaemia

● INTERACTIONS → Appendix 1: sympathomimetics, vasoconstrictor

● SIDE-EFFECTS
▸ **Common or very common** Headache · hypertension
▸ **Rare or very rare** Skin exfoliation · soft tissue necrosis
▸ **Frequency not known** Abscess · arrhythmias · nausea · palpitations · peripheral ischaemia

● MONITORING REQUIREMENTS Monitor blood pressure and rate of flow frequently.

● DIRECTIONS FOR ADMINISTRATION For *intracavernosal injection*, dilute 1 mg (0.1 mL of 10 mg/mL) metaraminol injection to 50 mL with Sodium chloride injection 0.9% and give carefully by slow injection into the corpora in 5 mL injections.

● MEDICINAL FORMS
There can be variation in the licensing of different medicines containing the same drug. Forms available from special-order manufacturers include: solution for injection
Solution for injection
▸ Metaraminol (Non-proprietary)
Metaraminol (as Metaraminol tartrate) 10 mg per 1 ml Metaraminol 10mg/1ml solution for injection ampoules | 10 ampoule PoM £39.40

Phenylephrine hydrochloride

● INDICATIONS AND DOSE
Priapism associated with alprostodil, if aspiration and lavage of the corpora are unsuccessful (alternative to adrenaline or metaraminol)
▸ BY INTRACAVERNOSAL INJECTION
▸ Adult: 100–200 micrograms every 5–10 minutes, dose to be administered using a 200 micrograms/mL solution; maximum 1 mg per course

● UNLICENSED USE Use of phenylephrine hydrochloride injection in priapism is an unlicensed indication.

● CONTRA-INDICATIONS Hypertension

● INTERACTIONS → Appendix 1: sympathomimetics, vasoconstrictor

● SIDE-EFFECTS Angle closure glaucoma · anxiety · appetite decreased · arrhythmias · asthenia · confusion · dyspnoea · headache · hypertension · hypoxia · insomnia · nausea · palpitations · peripheral ischaemia · psychosis · tremor · urinary retention · vomiting

● DIRECTIONS FOR ADMINISTRATION For *intracavernosal injection*, if suitable strength of phenylephrine injection is not available, it may be specially prepared by diluting 0.1 mL of the phenylephrine 1% (10 mg/mL) injection to 5 mL with sodium chloride 0.9%.

● MEDICINAL FORMS
There can be variation in the licensing of different medicines containing the same drug. Forms available from special-order manufacturers include: solution for injection
Solution for injection
▸ Phenylephrine hydrochloride (Non-proprietary)
Phenylephrine hydrochloride 10 mg per 1 ml Phenylephrine 10mg/1ml solution for injection ampoules | 10 ampoule PoM £99.12

VASODILATORS > PERIPHERAL VASODILATORS

Aviptadil with phentolamine mesilate
13-Sep-2017

● DRUG ACTION Phentolamine is a short-acting alpha-adrenoceptor antagonist that acts directly on vascular smooth muscle, resulting in vasodilatation; aviptadil is a vasoactive intestinal polypeptide that acts as a smooth muscle relaxant.

● INDICATIONS AND DOSE
Erectile dysfunction
▸ BY INTRACAVERNOSAL INJECTION
▸ Adult: 25/2000 micrograms, frequency of injection should not exceed once daily or three times weekly, duration of erection should not exceed 1 hour

DOSE EQUIVALENCE AND CONVERSION
▹ Dose expressed as x/y micrograms of aviptadil/phentolamine.

- **CONTRA-INDICATIONS** Anatomical deformation of the penis (e.g. angulation, cavernosal fibrosis, Peyronie's disease) · not for use with other agents for erectile dysfunction · patients for whom sexual activity is inadvisable · penile implants · predisposition to priapism (e.g. in sickle cell anaemia or trait, multiple myeloma, or leukemia)
- **CAUTIONS** Concomitant treatment with anticoagulants (potential increased risk of bleeding) · history of psychiatric disorder or addiction (potential for abuse) · severe cardiovascular disease · severe cerebrovascular disease
- **SIDE-EFFECTS**
- ▶ **Common or very common** Bruising · flushing
- ▶ **Uncommon** Dizziness · haematoma · headache · palpitations · tachycardia
- ▶ **Rare or very rare** Angina pectoris · myocardial infarction · penile fibrosis (following multiple injections) · penile nodules · sexual dysfunction
- **MONITORING REQUIREMENTS** Manufacturer advises monitor regularly (e.g. every 3 months), particularly in the initial stages of self-injection therapy; careful examination of the penis is recommended to detect signs of penile fibrosis or Peyronie's disease—discontinue treatment in patients who develop penile angulation, cavernosal fibrosis, or Peyronie's disease.
- **DIRECTIONS FOR ADMINISTRATION** Manufacturer advises that the initial injections of *Invicorp*® must be administered by medically trained personnel; self-administration may only be undertaken after proper training.
- **HANDLING AND STORAGE** Manufacturer advises store in a refrigerator (2–8°C).
- **PATIENT AND CARER ADVICE** Manufacturer advises that patients should be instructed to report any erection lasting 4 hours or longer.
- **NATIONAL FUNDING/ACCESS DECISIONS**
  Scottish Medicines Consortium (SMC) Decisions
  The *Scottish Medicines Consortium* has advised (December 2017) that aviptadil with phentolamine (*Invicorp*®) is accepted for restricted use within NHS Scotland for the symptomatic treatment of erectile dysfunction due to neurogenic, vasculogenic, psychogenic, or mixed aetiology in adult males who have failed on oral therapies (oral phosphodiesterase type-5 inhibitors) and other non-injectable formulations of erectile dysfunction medications.

  All Wales Medicines Strategy Group (AWMSG) Decisions
  The *All Wales Medicines Strategy Group* has advised (July 2017) that aviptadil with phentolamine (*Invicorp*®) is recommended as an option for the symptomatic treatment of erectile dysfunction in adult males due to neurogenic, vasculogenic, psychogenic, or mixed aetiology that has not responded to oral phosphodiesterase type-5 inhibitor therapy.

- **MEDICINAL FORMS**
  There can be variation in the licensing of different medicines containing the same drug.

  Solution for injection
  ▶ Invicorp (Evolan Pharma AB)
   Aviptadil 71.43 microgram per 1 ml, Phentolamine mesilate 5.71 mg per 1 ml Invicorp 25micrograms/2mg/0.35ml solution for injection ampoules | 2 ampoule [PoM] £19.00 | 5 ampoule [PoM] £47.50

4.2 Premature ejaculation

Premature ejaculation
01-Aug-2017

Description of condition
Premature ejaculation is a common male sexual disorder characterised by brief ejaculatory latency, loss of control, and psychological distress.

Treatment
[EvGr] Non-drug treatment (including psychosexual counselling, education, and behavioural treatments) are recommended in patients for whom premature ejaculation causes few (if any) problems or in patients who prefer not to take drug treatment. These techniques can also be used in addition to a drug treatment.

For patients with life-long premature ejaculation, drug treatment is the recommended approach. ⟨A⟩ Dapoxetine below, a short-acting selective serotonin re-uptake inhibitor, is licensed to be used when required for this condition (not continuous daily use).

[EvGr] Other selective serotonin re-uptake inhibitors (citalopram p. 361, fluoxetine p. 362, fluvoxamine maleate p. 363, escitalopram p. 361, paroxetine p. 363, sertraline p. 364 [unlicensed indications]) and the tricyclic antidepressant clomipramine [unlicensed indication] have been widely used as regular, daily treatment. Caution is suggested in prescribing selective serotonin re-uptake inhibitors for young adolescents with premature ejaculation, and to men who also have a depressive disorder, particularly when associated with suicidal ideation. Ejaculation delay may start a few days after the start of treatment, but it is more evident after 1 to 2 weeks, since receptor desensitisation requires time to occur.

If premature ejaculation is secondary to Erectile dysfunction p. 793, the erectile dysfunction should be treated first. ⟨A⟩

Topical anaesthetic preparations for the management of premature ejaculation are available without prescription.

SELECTIVE SEROTONIN RE-UPTAKE INHIBITORS

Dapoxetine

- **DRUG ACTION** Dapoxetine is a short-acting selective serotonin re-uptake inhibitor.

- **INDICATIONS AND DOSE**
  Premature ejaculation in men who meet all the following criteria: poor control over ejaculation, a history of premature ejaculation over the past 6 months, marked distress or interpersonal difficulty as a consequence of premature ejaculation, and an intravaginal ejaculatory latency time of less than two minutes
  ▶ BY MOUTH
  ▶ Adult: Initially 30 mg, to be taken approximately 1–3 hours before sexual activity, subsequent doses adjusted according to response; review treatment after 4 weeks (or 6 doses) and at least every 6 months thereafter, not recommended for adults 65 years and over; maximum 1 dose per day; maximum 60 mg per day

  DOSE ADJUSTMENTS DUE TO INTERACTIONS
  ▶ Manufacturer advises max. dose 30 mg with concurrent use of moderate inhibitors of CYP3A4 except in patients verified to be extensive CYP2D6 metabolisers where manufacturer recommends max. dose 60 mg.

continued →

Genito-urinary system

7

▸ Manufacturer advises avoid with concurrent use of potent inhibitors of CYP3A4 except in patients verified to be extensive CYP2D6 metabolisers where manufacturer recommends max. dose 30 mg.

- CONTRA-INDICATIONS History of bipolar disorder · history of mania · history of severe depression · history of syncope · significant cardiac disease · uncontrolled epilepsy
- CAUTIONS Bleeding disorders · epilepsy (discontinue if convulsions develop) · susceptibility to angle-closure glaucoma
- INTERACTIONS → Appendix 1: SSRIs
- SIDE-EFFECTS
  ▸ **Common or very common** Anxiety · asthenia · concentration impaired · constipation · diarrhoea · dizziness · drowsiness · dry mouth · gastrointestinal discomfort · gastrointestinal disorders · headache · hypotension · mood altered · nausea · paraesthesia · sexual dysfunction · sinus congestion · sleep disorders · sweat changes · syncope · tinnitus · tremor · vasodilation · vision blurred · vomiting · yawning
  ▸ **Uncommon** Akathisia · arrhythmias · behaviour abnormal · confusion · depression · eye pain · feeling abnormal · feeling hot · hypertension · level of consciousness decreased · mydriasis · pruritus · taste altered · thinking abnormal · vertigo

  SIDE-EFFECTS, FURTHER INFORMATION Discontinue if psychiatric disorder develops.

- HEPATIC IMPAIRMENT Avoid in moderate to severe impairment.
- RENAL IMPAIRMENT Use with caution if eGFR 30–80 mL/minute/1.73 m^2; avoid if eGFR less than 30 mL/minute/1.73 m^2.
- PRE-TREATMENT SCREENING Test for postural hypotension before starting treatment.
- TREATMENT CESSATION The dose should preferably be reduced gradually over about 4 weeks, or longer if withdrawal symptoms emerge (6 months in patients who have been on long-term maintenance treatment).
- PATIENT AND CARER ADVICE
  Postural hypotension and syncope Patients should be advised to maintain hydration and to sit or lie down until prodromal symptoms such as nausea, dizziness, and sweating abate.

- MEDICINAL FORMS
  There can be variation in the licensing of different medicines containing the same drug.
  Tablet
  CAUTIONARY AND ADVISORY LABELS 2, 25
  ▸ Priligy (A. Menarini Farmaceutica Internazionale SRL)
  Dapoxetine 30 mg Priligy 30mg tablets | 3 tablet [PoM] £14.71 DT = £14.71 | 6 tablet [PoM] £26.48 DT = £26.48
  Dapoxetine 60 mg Priligy 60mg tablets | 3 tablet [PoM] £19.12 DT = £19.12 | 6 tablet [PoM] £34.42 DT = £34.42

5 Obstetrics

Obstetrics

20-Sep-2017

Prostaglandins and oxytocics

Prostaglandins and oxytocics are used to induce abortion or induce or augment labour and to minimise blood loss from the placental site. They include oxytocin p. 804, carbetocin p. 805, ergometrine maleate p. 805, and the prostaglandins. All induce uterine contractions with varying degrees of pain according to the strength of contractions induced.

Induction of abortion

Gemeprost p. 807, a prostaglandin administered vaginally as pessaries, is suitable for the medical induction of late therapeutic abortion; gemeprost is also used to ripen the cervix before surgical abortion, particularly in primigravidas. The prostaglandin misoprostol p. 807 is given by mouth, buccally, sublingually, or vaginally, to induce medical abortion [unlicensed indication]; intravaginal use ripens the cervix before surgical abortion [unlicensed indication]. Extra-amniotic dinoprostone is rarely used nowadays.

Pre-treatment with mifepristone p. 806 can facilitate the process of medical abortion. It sensitises the uterus to subsequent administration of a prostaglandin and, therefore, abortion occurs in a shorter time and with a lower dose of prostaglandin.

Induction and augmentation of labour

Dinoprostone is available as vaginal tablets, pessaries and vaginal gels for the induction of labour. The intravenous solution is rarely used; it is associated with more side-effects.

Oxytocin (*Syntocinon*®) is administered by slow intravenous infusion, using an infusion pump, to induce and augment labour, usually in conjunction with amniotomy. Uterine activity must be monitored carefully and hyperstimulation avoided. Large doses of oxytocin may result in excessive fluid retention.

Misoprostol is given orally [unlicensed route] or vaginally for the induction of labour.

NICE Guidance, Induction of labour (updated July 2008), available at www.nice.org.uk/guidance/CG70.

Prevention and treatment of haemorrhage

Bleeding due to incomplete miscarriage or abortion can be controlled with ergometrine maleate and oxytocin (*Syntometrine*®) given intramuscularly, the dose is adjusted according to the patient's condition and blood loss. This is commonly used before surgical evacuation of the uterus, particularly when surgery is delayed. Oxytocin and ergometrine maleate combined are more effective in early pregnancy than either drug alone.

Active management of the third stage of labour reduces the risk of postpartum haemorrhage; oxytocin is given by intramuscular injection [unlicensed] on delivery of the anterior shoulder or, at the latest, immediately after the baby is delivered. Alternatively, ergometrine maleate with oxytocin (*Syntometrine*®) can be given by intramuscular injection in the absence of hypertension; oxytocin alone causes less nausea, vomiting, and hypertension than when given with ergometrine maleate.

In excessive uterine bleeding, any placental products remaining in the uterus should be removed. Oxytocic drugs are used to treat postpartum haemorrhage caused by uterine atony; treatment options are as follows:

- oxytocin by slow intravenous injection, followed in severe cases by intravenous infusion of oxytocin at a rate that controls uterine atony *or*
- ergometrine by intramuscular injection *or*
- ergometrine by slow intravenous injection (use with caution—risk of hypertension) *or*
- ergometrine with oxytocin (*Syntometrine*®) by intramuscular injection

Carboprost p. 805 has an important role in severe postpartum haemorrhage unresponsive to ergometrine maleate and oxytocin.

Misoprostol [unlicensed] can be used in postpartum haemorrhage when oxytocin, ergometrine maleate, and carboprost are not available or are inappropriate.

Mifepristone

For termination of pregnancy, a single dose of mifepristone is followed by administration of a prostaglandin (gemeprost or misoprostol [unlicensed]).

Guidelines of the Royal College of Obstetricians and Gynaecologists (November 2011) include [unlicensed] regimens for inducing medical abortion.

Ectopic pregnancy

Systemic methotrexate p. 888 [unlicensed indication] is used for the management of ectopic pregnancy.

Myometrial relaxants

Tocolytic drugs postpone *premature labour* and they are used with the aim of reducing harm to the child. However, there is no satisfactory evidence that the use of these drugs reduces mortality. The greatest benefit is gained by using the delay to administer corticosteroid therapy or to implement other measures which improve perinatal health (including transfer to a unit with neonatal intensive care facility).

The oxytocin receptor antagonist, atosiban p. 806, is licensed for the inhibition of uncomplicated premature labour *between* 24 *and* 33 *weeks* of gestation. Atosiban may be preferable to a beta$_2$ agonist because it has fewer side effects. The dihydropyridine calcium-channel blocker nifedipine p. 162 also has fewer side-effects than a beta$_2$ agonist.

The beta$_2$ agonists salbutamol p. 252 and terbutaline sulfate p. 254 are licensed for inhibiting uncomplicated premature labour between 22 and 37 weeks of gestation to permit a delay in delivery of up to 48 hours. Use of high-dose short acting beta$_2$ agonists in obstetric indications has been associated with serious, sometimes fatal cardiovascular events in the mother and fetus, particularly when used for a prolonged period of time. Oral therapy is no longer recommended and parenteral therapy should be restricted to a maximum duration of 48 hours, given under the supervision of a specialist, and with close monitoring.

Indometacin p. 1109, a cyclo-oxygenase inhibitor, also inhibits labour [unlicensed indication] and it can be useful in situations where a beta$_2$ agonist is not appropriate; however, there are concerns about neonatal complications such as transient impairment of renal function and premature closure of ductus arteriosus.

5.1   Induction of labour

> **Other drugs used for Induction of labour** Misoprostol, p. 807

PROSTAGLANDINS AND OXYTOCICS

Dinoprostone

- **INDICATIONS AND DOSE**

PROPESS®

Cervical ripening and induction of labour at term
▸ BY VAGINA
▸ Adult: 1 pessary, insert pessary (in retrieval device) high into posterior fornix and remove when cervical ripening adequate; if oxytocin necessary, remove 30 minutes before oxytocin infusion; remove if cervical ripening inadequate after 24 hours (dose not to be repeated)

PROSTIN E2® VAGINAL GEL

Induction of labour
▸ BY VAGINA
▸ Adult: 1 mg, inserted high into the posterior fornix (avoid administration into the cervical canal), followed by 1–2 mg after 6 hours if required; maximum 3 mg per course

Induction of labour (unfavourable primigravida)
▸ BY VAGINA
▸ Adult: 2 mg, inserted high into the posterior fornix (avoid administration into the cervical canal), followed by 1–2 mg if required, after 6 hours; maximum 4 mg per course

PROSTIN E2® VAGINAL TABLETS

Induction of labour
▸ BY VAGINA
▸ Adult: 3 mg, inserted high into the posterior fornix, followed by 3 mg after 6–8 hours, to be given if labour not established; maximum 6 mg per course

DOSE EQUIVALENCE AND CONVERSION
▸ *Prostin* E2 *Vaginal tablets* and *Vaginal Gel* are not bioequivalent.

- CONTRA-INDICATIONS Active cardiac disease · active pulmonary disease · avoid extra-amniotic route in cervicitis or vaginitis · fetal distress · fetal malpresentation · grand multiparas · history of caesarean section · history of difficult or traumatic delivery · history of major uterine surgery · major cephalopelvic disproportion · multiple pregnancy · placenta praevia or unexplained vaginal bleeding during pregnancy · ruptured membranes · untreated pelvic infection

- CAUTIONS Effect of oxytocin enhanced · history of asthma · history of epilepsy · history of glaucoma and raised intra-ocular pressure · hypertension · risk factors for disseminated intravascular coagulation · uterine rupture · uterine scarring

- SIDE-EFFECTS
▸ **Uncommon** Amniotic cavity infection · febrile disorders · headache · hypotension · pruritus · uterine atony · vaginal burning
▸ **Rare or very rare** Disseminated intravascular coagulation
▸ **Frequency not known** Abdominal pain · diarrhoea · genital oedema · nausea · uterine rupture · vomiting

- HEPATIC IMPAIRMENT Manufacturers advise avoid.

- RENAL IMPAIRMENT Manufacturers advise avoid.

- MONITORING REQUIREMENTS
▸ Monitor for disseminated intravascular coagulation after parturition.
▸ Monitor uterine activity and fetal status (particular care if history of uterine hypertony)
▸ Care needed in monitoring uterine activity when used in sequence following oxytocin.

- PRESCRIBING AND DISPENSING INFORMATION **Important:** Do not confuse dose of *Prostin E2*®**vaginal gel** with that of *Prostin E2*®**vaginal tablets**—not bioequivalent.

- MEDICINAL FORMS
There can be variation in the licensing of different medicines containing the same drug.

Pessary
▸ Prostin E2 (Pfizer Ltd)
  Dinoprostone 3 mg Prostin E2 3mg vaginal tablets |
  8 pessary [PoM] £106.23 (Hospital only)

Vaginal gel
▸ Prostin E2 (Pfizer Ltd)
  Dinoprostone 400 microgram per 1 ml Prostin E2 1mg vaginal gel
  | 2.5 ml [PoM] £13.28 (Hospital only)
  Dinoprostone 800 microgram per 1 ml Prostin E2 2mg vaginal gel
  | 2.5 ml [PoM] £13.28 (Hospital only)

Vaginal device
▸ Propess (Ferring Pharmaceuticals Ltd)
  Dinoprostone 10 mg Propess 10mg vaginal delivery system |
  5 device [PoM] £165.00

Oxytocin

● INDICATIONS AND DOSE

Induction of labour for medical reasons | Stimulation of labour in hypotonic uterine inertia
▸ BY INTRAVENOUS INFUSION
▸ Adult: Initially 0.001–0.004 unit/minute, not to be started for at least 6 hours after administration of vaginal prostaglandin, dose increased at intervals of at least 30 minutes until a maximum of 3–4 contractions occur every 10 minutes (0.01 units/minute is often adequate) up to max. 0.02 units/minute, if regular contractions not established after a total 5 units, stop induction attempt (may be repeated next day starting again at 0.001–0.004 units/minute)

Caesarean section
▸ BY SLOW INTRAVENOUS INJECTION
▸ Adult: 5 units immediately after delivery

Prevention of postpartum haemorrhage after delivery of placenta
▸ BY SLOW INTRAVENOUS INJECTION
▸ Adult: 5 units, if infusion previously used for induction or enhancement of labour, increase rate during third stage and for next few hours
▸ BY INTRAMUSCULAR INJECTION
▸ Adult: 10 units, can be used instead of oxytocin with ergometrine (*Syntometrine*®).

Treatment of postpartum haemorrhage
▸ BY SLOW INTRAVENOUS INJECTION
▸ Adult: 5 units, repeated if necessary

Treatment of severe cases of postpartum haemorrhage (following intravenous injection)
▸ BY INTRAVENOUS INFUSION
▸ Adult: 40 units, given in 500 mL infusion fluid given at a rate sufficient to control uterine atony

Incomplete, inevitable, or missed miscarriage
▸ INITIALLY BY SLOW INTRAVENOUS INJECTION
▸ Adult: 5 units, followed by (by intravenous infusion) 0.02–0.04 unit/minute if required, the rate of infusion can be faster if necessary

● UNLICENSED USE Oxytocin doses in the BNF may differ from those in the product literature. Administration by intramuscular injection is an unlicensed use.

IMPORTANT SAFETY INFORMATION
Prolonged intravenous administration at high doses with large volume of fluid (which is possible in inevitable or missed miscarriage or postpartum haemorrhage) may cause water intoxication with hyponatraemia. To avoid: use electrolyte-containing diluent (i.e. not glucose), increase oxytocin concentration to reduce fluid, restrict fluid intake by mouth; monitor fluid and electrolytes.

● CONTRA-INDICATIONS Any condition where spontaneous labour inadvisable · any condition where vaginal delivery inadvisable · avoid intravenous injection during labour · avoid prolonged administration in oxytocin-resistant uterine inertia · avoid rapid intravenous injection (may transiently reduce blood pressure) · fetal distress (discontinue immediately if this occurs) · hypertonic uterine contractions (discontinue immediately if this occurs) · severe cardiovascular disease · severe pre-eclamptic toxaemia

● CAUTIONS Avoid large infusion volumes and restrict fluid intake by mouth (risk of hyponatraemia and water-intoxication) · enhancement of labour—presence of borderline cephalopelvic disproportion (avoid if significant) · history of lower-uterine segment caesarean section · induction of labour—presence of borderline cephalopelvic disproportion (avoid if significant) · mild

pregnancy-induced cardiac disease · mild pregnancy-induced hypertension · moderate pregnancy-induced cardiac disease · moderate pregnancy-induced hypertension · risk factors for disseminated intravascular coagulation · secondary uterine inertia · women over 35 years

● SIDE-EFFECTS
▸ **Common or very common** Arrhythmias · headache · nausea · vomiting
▸ **Rare or very rare** Dyspnoea · hypotension · rash
▸ **Frequency not known** Angioedema · disseminated intravascular coagulation · electrolyte imbalance · flushing · haemorrhage · myocardial ischaemia · pulmonary oedema · QT interval prolongation · uterine rupture · water intoxication

SIDE-EFFECTS, FURTHER INFORMATION Avoid rapid intravenous injection (may transiently reduce blood pressure).
Uterine hyperstimulation Usually occurs with excessive doses—may cause fetal distress, asphyxia, and death, or may lead to hypertonicity, tetanic contractions, soft-tissue damage or uterine rupture.
Overdose Placental abruption and amniotic fluid embolism reported on overdose.

● MONITORING REQUIREMENTS
▸ Careful monitoring of fetal heart rate and uterine motility essential for dose titration.
▸ Monitor for disseminated intravascular coagulation after parturition.

● DIRECTIONS FOR ADMINISTRATION For *intravenous infusion* (*Syntocinon*®), give continuously in Glucose 5% or Sodium chloride 0.9%. Preferably given *via* a variable-speed infusion pump in a concentration appropriate to the pump; if given by drip infusion for *induction* or *enhancement of labour*, dilute 5 units in 500 mL infusion fluid or for higher doses, 10 units in 500 mL; for *treatment of postpartum uterine haemorrhage* dilute 40 units in 500 mL; if high doses given for prolonged period (e.g. for inevitable or missed abortion or for postpartum haemorrhage), use low volume of an electrolyte-containing infusion fluid (not Glucose 5%) given at higher concentration than for induction or enhancement of labour; close attention to patient's fluid and electrolyte status essential.

● MEDICINAL FORMS
There can be variation in the licensing of different medicines containing the same drug. Forms available from special-order manufacturers include: infusion, solution for infusion

Solution for injection
▸ Oxytocin (Non-proprietary)
   Oxytocin 10 unit per 1 ml Oxytocin 10units/1ml solution for infusion ampoules | 5 ampoule [PoM] £3.00
   Oxytocin 10units/1ml concentrate for solution for infusion ampoules | 5 ampoule [PoM] £4.55 | 10 ampoule [PoM] £9.00
▸ Syntocinon (Novartis Pharmaceuticals UK Ltd)
   Oxytocin 5 unit per 1 ml Syntocinon 5units/1ml solution for injection ampoules | 5 ampoule [PoM] £4.01 (Hospital only)
   Oxytocin 10 unit per 1 ml Syntocinon 10units/1ml solution for injection ampoules | 5 ampoule [PoM] £4.53 (Hospital only)

5.2 Postpartum haemorrhage

Other drugs used for Postpartum haemorrhage Oxytocin, above

PROSTAGLANDINS AND OXYTOCICS

Carbetocin

06-Feb-2018

- **INDICATIONS AND DOSE**

Prevention of uterine atony after caesarean section
- ▸ BY SLOW INTRAVENOUS INJECTION
- ▸ Adult: 100 micrograms for 1 dose, to be given over 1 minute, administer as soon as possible after delivery, preferably before removal of placenta

- **CONTRA-INDICATIONS** Eclampsia · epilepsy · pre-eclampsia
- **CAUTIONS** Asthma · cardiovascular disease (avoid if severe) · hyponatraemia · migraine
- **SIDE-EFFECTS**
- ▸ **Common or very common** Chest pain · chills · dizziness · dyspnoea · feeling hot · flushing · headache · hypotension · nausea · pain · pruritus · taste metallic · tremor · vomiting
- ▸ **Frequency not known** Hyperhidrosis · tachycardia
- **HEPATIC IMPAIRMENT** Manufacturer advises avoid.
- **RENAL IMPAIRMENT** Manufacturer advises avoid.
- **NATIONAL FUNDING/ACCESS DECISIONS**

Scottish Medicines Consortium (SMC) Decisions
The *Scottish Medicines Consortium* has advised (January 2018) that carbetocin (*Pabal®*) is **not** recommended for use within NHS Scotland for the prevention of uterine atony following delivery of the infant by Caesarean section under epidural or spinal anaesthesia as the economic case was not demonstrated.

- **MEDICINAL FORMS**
There can be variation in the licensing of different medicines containing the same drug.
Solution for injection
- ▸ Pabal (Ferring Pharmaceuticals Ltd)
Carbetocin 100 microgram per 1 ml Pabal 100micrograms/1ml solution for injection ampoules | 5 ampoule PoM £88.20 (Hospital only)

Carboprost

- **INDICATIONS AND DOSE**

Postpartum haemorrhage due to uterine atony in patients unresponsive to ergometrine and oxytocin
- ▸ BY DEEP INTRAMUSCULAR INJECTION
- ▸ Adult: 250 micrograms, repeated if necessary, to be given at intervals of not less than 15 minutes. Total dose should not exceed 2 mg (8 doses)

- **CONTRA-INDICATIONS** Cardiac disease · pulmonary disease · untreated pelvic infection
- **CAUTIONS** Excessive dosage may cause uterine rupture · history of anaemia · history of asthma · history of diabetes · history of epilepsy · history of glaucoma · history of hypertension · history of hypotension · history of jaundice · history of raised intra-ocular pressure · uterine scars
- **SIDE-EFFECTS**
- ▸ **Common or very common** Chills · cough · diarrhoea · headache · nausea · uterine disorders · vasodilation · vomiting
- ▸ **Uncommon** Abdominal pain upper · asthma · back pain · breast tenderness · chest discomfort · dizziness · drowsiness · dry mouth · dyspnoea · eye pain · haemorrhage · hiccups · hyperhidrosis · hypertension · increased risk of infection · movement disorders · muscle complaints · paraesthesia · pelvic pain · respiratory disorders · septic shock · sleep disorder · syncope · tachycardia · taste altered · tinnitus · uterine injuries · vertigo · vision blurred

- ▸ **Frequency not known** Anxiety · asthenia · blepharospasm · choking sensation · palpitations · rash · thirst · throat complaints · thyrotoxic crisis
- **HEPATIC IMPAIRMENT** Manufacturer advises avoid.
- **RENAL IMPAIRMENT** Manufacturer advises avoid.

- **MEDICINAL FORMS**
There can be variation in the licensing of different medicines containing the same drug.
Solution for injection
- ▸ Hemabate (Pfizer Ltd)
Carboprost (as Carboprost trometamol) 250 microgram per 1 ml Hemabate 250micrograms/1ml solution for injection ampoules | 10 ampoule PoM £182.01 (Hospital only)

Ergometrine maleate

- **INDICATIONS AND DOSE**

Postpartum haemorrhage caused by uterine atony
- ▸ BY INTRAMUSCULAR INJECTION, OR BY SLOW INTRAVENOUS INJECTION
- ▸ Adult: 250–500 micrograms

- **CONTRA-INDICATIONS** Eclampsia · first stage of labour · induction of labour · second stage of labour · sepsis · severe cardiac disease · severe hypertension · vascular disease
- **CAUTIONS** Acute porphyrias p. 1025 · cardiac disease · hypertension · multiple pregnancy · risk of hypertension associated with intravenous administration
- **INTERACTIONS** → Appendix 1: ergometrine
- **SIDE-EFFECTS** Abdominal pain · arrhythmias · chest pain · coronary vasospasm · dizziness · dyspnoea · headache · hypertension · myocardial infarction · nausea · palpitations · pulmonary oedema · rash · tinnitus · vasoconstriction · vomiting
- **HEPATIC IMPAIRMENT** Manufacturer advises caution in mild or moderate impairment. Manufacturer advises avoid in severe impairment.
- **RENAL IMPAIRMENT** Manufacturer advises caution in mild or moderate impairment. Manufacturer advises avoid in severe impairment.

- **MEDICINAL FORMS**
There can be variation in the licensing of different medicines containing the same drug.
Solution for injection
- ▸ Ergometrine maleate (Non-proprietary)
Ergometrine maleate 500 microgram per 1 ml Ergometrine 500micrograms/1ml solution for injection ampoules | 10 ampoule PoM £12.00-£15.00

Ergometrine with oxytocin

The properties listed below are those particular to the combination only. For the properties of the components please consider, ergometrine maleate above, oxytocin p. 804.

- **INDICATIONS AND DOSE**

Active management of the third stage of labour | Postpartum haemorrhage caused by uterine atony
- ▸ BY INTRAMUSCULAR INJECTION
- ▸ Adult: 1 mL for one dose
- ▸ BY INTRAVENOUS INJECTION
- ▸ Adult: No longer recommended

Bleeding due to incomplete miscarriage or abortion
- ▸ BY INTRAMUSCULAR INJECTION
- ▸ Adult: Adjusted according to response to, the patient's condition and blood loss

- **INTERACTIONS** → Appendix 1: ergometrine

7

Genito-urinary system

- MEDICINAL FORMS
There can be variation in the licensing of different medicines containing the same drug.
Solution for injection
  › Syntometrine (Alliance Pharmaceuticals Ltd)
Ergometrine maleate 500 microgram per 1 ml, Oxytocin 5 unit per 1 ml Syntometrine 500micrograms/1ml solution for injection ampoules | 5 ampoule [PoM] £7.87

5.3 Premature labour

Other drugs used for Premature labour Nifedipine, p. 162 · Salbutamol, p. 252 · Terbutaline sulfate, p. 254

OXYTOCIN RECEPTOR ANTAGONISTS

Atosiban

- INDICATIONS AND DOSE

Uncomplicated premature labour between 24 and 33 weeks of gestation
  › INITIALLY BY INTRAVENOUS INJECTION
  › Adult: Initially 6.75 mg over 1 minute, then (by intravenous infusion) 18 mg/hour for 3 hours, then (by intravenous infusion) reduced to 6 mg/hour for up to 45 hours. Maximum duration of treatment is 48 hours

- CONTRA-INDICATIONS Abruptio placenta · antepartum haemorrhage (requiring immediate delivery) · eclampsia · intra-uterine fetal death · intra-uterine infection · intra-uterine growth restriction with abnormal fetal heart rate · placenta praevia · premature rupture of membranes after 30 weeks' gestation · severe pre-eclampsia
- CAUTIONS Abnormal placental site · intra-uterine growth restriction
- SIDE-EFFECTS
  › **Common or very common** Dizziness · headache · hot flush · hyperglycaemia · hypotension · nausea · tachycardia · vomiting
  › **Uncommon** Fever · insomnia · skin reactions
  › **Rare or very rare** Uterine atony · uterine haemorrhage
  › **Frequency not known** Dyspnoea · pulmonary oedema
- HEPATIC IMPAIRMENT No information available.
- RENAL IMPAIRMENT No information available.
- MONITORING REQUIREMENTS Monitor blood loss after delivery.
- DIRECTIONS FOR ADMINISTRATION For *intravenous infusion* (*Tractocile®* concentrate for intravenous infusion), give continuously *in* Glucose 5% *or* Sodium chloride 0.9%. Withdraw 10 mL infusion fluid from 100-mL bag and replace with 10 mL atosiban concentrate (7.5 mg/mL) to produce a final concentration of 750 micrograms/mL.

- MEDICINAL FORMS
There can be variation in the licensing of different medicines containing the same drug.
Solution for injection
  › Atosiban (Non-proprietary)
Atosiban (as Atosiban acetate) 7.5 mg per 1 ml Atosiban 6.75mg/0.9ml solution for injection vials | 1 vial [PoM] £18.41 (Hospital only)
  › Tractocile (Ferring Pharmaceuticals Ltd)
Atosiban (as Atosiban acetate) 7.5 mg per 1 ml Tractocile 6.75mg/0.9ml solution for injection vials | 1 vial [PoM] £18.41 (Hospital only)
Solution for infusion
  › Atosiban (Non-proprietary)
Atosiban (as Atosiban acetate) 7.5 mg per 1 ml Atosiban 37.5mg/5ml concentrate for solution for infusion vials | 1 vial [PoM] £52.82 (Hospital only) | 1 vial [PoM] £51.99
Atosiban 37.5mg/5ml solution for infusion vials | 1 vial [PoM] £51.09

Atosiban 6.75mg/0.9ml solution for injection ampoules | 1 ampoule [PoM] £17.99
  › Tractocile (Ferring Pharmaceuticals Ltd)
Atosiban (as Atosiban acetate) 7.5 mg per 1 ml Tractocile 37.5mg/5ml solution for infusion vials | 1 vial [PoM] £52.82 (Hospital only)

5.4 Termination of pregnancy

PROGESTERONE RECEPTOR MODULATORS

Mifepristone

- DRUG ACTION Mifepristone, an antiprogestogenic steroid, sensitises the myometrium to prostaglandin-induced contractions and ripens the cervix.

- INDICATIONS AND DOSE

Cervical ripening before mechanical cervical dilatation for termination of pregnancy of up to 84 days gestation (under close medical supervision)
  › BY MOUTH
  › Adult: 200 mg for 1 dose, to be taken 36-48 hours before procedure

Labour induction in fetal death in utero where prostaglandin or oxytocin inappropriate (under close medical supervision)
  › BY MOUTH
  › Adult: 600 mg once daily for 2 days, if labour not started within 72 hours of first dose, another method should be used

Medical termination of intra-uterine pregnancy of up to 49 days gestation (under close medical supervision)
  › BY MOUTH
  › Adult: 600 mg for 1 dose, dose followed 36–48 hours later (unless abortion already complete) by gemeprost 1 mg by vagina *or* misoprostol 400 micrograms by mouth, alternatively 200 mg for 1 dose, dose followed 36–48 hours later (unless abortion already complete) by gemeprost 1 mg by vagina; observe for at least 3 hours (or until bleeding or pain at acceptable level); follow-up visit within 2 weeks to verify complete expulsion and to assess vaginal bleeding

Medical termination of intra-uterine pregnancy of 50–63 days gestation (under close medical supervision)
  › BY MOUTH
  › Adult: 600 mg for 1 dose, alternatively 200 mg for 1 dose, dose followed 36–48 hours later (unless abortion already complete) by gemeprost 1 mg by vagina; observe for at least 3 hours (or until bleeding or pain at acceptable level); follow-up visit within 2 weeks to verify complete expulsion and to assess vaginal bleeding

Termination of pregnancy of 13–24 weeks gestation (in combination with a prostaglandin) (under close medical supervision)
  › BY MOUTH
  › Adult: 600 mg for 1 dose, alternatively 200 mg for 1 dose, dose followed 36–48 hours later by gemeprost 1 mg by vagina every 3 hours up to max. 5 mg *or* misoprostol; if abortion does not occur, 24 hours after start of treatment repeat course of gemeprost 1 mg by vagina up to max. 5 mg; follow-up visit after appropriate interval to assess vaginal bleeding recommended

- CONTRA-INDICATIONS Acute porphyrias p. 1025 · chronic adrenal failure · suspected ectopic pregnancy (use other specific means of termination) · uncontrolled severe asthma

- CAUTIONS Adrenal suppression (may require corticosteroid) · anticoagulant therapy · asthma (avoid if severe and uncontrolled) · existing cardiovascular disease · haemorrhagic disorders · history of endocarditis · prosthetic heart valve · risk factors for cardiovascular disease
- INTERACTIONS → Appendix 1: mifepristone
- SIDE-EFFECTS
- **Common or very common** Abdominal cramps · diarrhoea · infection · nausea · pelvic inflammatory disease · uterine disorders · vaginal haemorrhage (sometimes severe) · vomiting
- **Uncommon** Hypotension
- **Rare or very rare** Angioedema · chills · dizziness · erythema nodosum · fever · headache · hot flush · malaise · skin reactions · toxic epidermal necrolysis · toxic shock syndrome · uterine rupture
- HEPATIC IMPAIRMENT Manufacturer advises avoid.
- RENAL IMPAIRMENT Manufacturer advises avoid.
- MONITORING REQUIREMENTS Careful monitoring of blood pressure and pulse essential for 3 hours after administration of gemeprost pessary (risk of profound hypotension).
- PRESCRIBING AND DISPENSING INFORMATION Supplied to NHS hospitals and premises approved under Abortion Act 1967.
- PATIENT AND CARER ADVICE Patient information leaflet to be provided.

- MEDICINAL FORMS
  There can be variation in the licensing of different medicines containing the same drug.
  Tablet
  CAUTIONARY AND ADVISORY LABELS 10
  ▸ Mifepristone (Non-proprietary)
  Mifepristone 200 mg Mifepristone 200mg tablets | 1 tablet PoM ⓧ (Hospital only)
  ▸ Mifegyne (Nordic Pharma Ltd)
  Mifepristone 200 mg Mifegyne 200mg tablets | 3 tablet PoM £52.66 (Hospital only)

PROSTAGLANDINS AND OXYTOCICS

Gemeprost

- INDICATIONS AND DOSE
  Cervical ripening prior to first trimester surgical abortion
  ▸ BY VAGINA
  ▸ Adult: 1 mg, dose to be inserted into posterior fornix 3 hours before surgery
  Second trimester abortion
  ▸ BY VAGINA
  ▸ Adult: 1 mg every 3 hours for maximum 5 administrations, to be inserted into posterior fornix, second course may begin 24 hours after start of treatment (if treatment fails, pregnancy should be terminated by another method)
  Second trimester intra-uterine death
  ▸ BY VAGINA
  ▸ Adult: 1 mg every 3 hours for maximum 5 administrations only, to be inserted into posterior fornix
  Medical termination of intra-uterine pregnancy of up to 49 days gestation following mifepristone | Medical termination of intra-uterine pregnancy of 50–63 days gestation following mifepristone
  ▸ BY VAGINA
  ▸ Adult: 1 mg

Termination of pregnancy of 13–24 weeks gestation (in combination with a prostaglandin) following mifepristone
▸ BY VAGINA
▸ Adult: 1 mg every 3 hours, if abortion does not occur, 24 hours after start of treatment repeat course of gemeprost 1 mg by vagina up to max. 5 mg; follow-up visit after appropriate interval to assess vaginal bleeding recommended, careful monitoring of blood pressure and pulse essential for 3 hours after administration of gemeprost pessary (risk of profound hypotension); maximum 5 mg per course

- CONTRA-INDICATIONS Placenta praevia · unexplained vaginal bleeding · uterine scarring
- CAUTIONS Cardiovascular insufficiency · cervicitis · obstructive airways disease · raised intra-ocular pressure · vaginitis
- SIDE-EFFECTS Back pain · chest pain · chills · coronary vasospasm · diarrhoea · dizziness · dyspnoea · fever · flushing · headache · hypotension · muscle weakness · myocardial infarction · nausea · palpitations · uterine pain · uterine rupture · vaginal haemorrhage · vomiting
- RENAL IMPAIRMENT Manufacturer advises avoid.
- MONITORING REQUIREMENTS
- ▸ If used in combination with mifepristone, carefully monitor blood pressure and pulse for 3 hours.
- ▸ When used for second trimester intra-uterine death, monitor for coagulopathy during treatment.

- MEDICINAL FORMS
  There can be variation in the licensing of different medicines containing the same drug.
  Pessary
  ▸ Gemeprost (Non-proprietary)
  Gemeprost 1 mg Gemeprost 1mg pessaries | 5 pessary PoM ⓧ

Misoprostol
26-Apr-2018

- DRUG ACTION Misoprostol is a synthetic prostaglandin analogue that acts as a potent uterine stimulant.

- INDICATIONS AND DOSE
  Termination of pregnancy following mifepristone (gestation up to 49 days)
  ▸ BY MOUTH
  ▸ Adult: 400 micrograms for 1 dose, dose to be given 24–48 hours after mifepristone
  Termination of pregnancy following mifepristone (gestation 50 to 63 days)
  ▸ INITIALLY BY VAGINA, OR BY BUCCAL ADMINISTRATION, OR BY SUBLINGUAL ADMINISTRATION
  ▸ Adult: 800 micrograms for 1 dose, dose to be given 24–48 hours after mifepristone, if abortion has not occurred 4 hours after first misoprostol dose a further dose may be given, (by mouth or by vagina) 400 micrograms for 1 dose
  Termination of pregnancy following mifepristone (gestation of 9 to 13 weeks)
  ▸ INITIALLY BY VAGINA
  ▸ Adult: 800 micrograms for 1 dose, dose to be given 36–48 hours after mifepristone, followed by (by vagina or by mouth) 400 micrograms every 3 hours if required for a maximum of 4 doses
  Termination of pregnancy following mifepristone (gestation of 13 to 24 weeks)
  ▸ INITIALLY BY VAGINA
  ▸ Adult: 800 micrograms for 1 dose, dose to be given 36–48 hours after mifepristone, followed by (by vagina or by mouth) 400 micrograms every 3 hours continued →

if required for a maximum of 4 doses, if abortion has not occurred 3 hours after the last dose of misoprostol, a further dose of mifepristone may be given, and misoprostol may be recommenced 12 hours later

MYSODELLE® VAGINAL DELIVERY SYSTEM

Induction of labour (specialist supervision in hospital)

▸ BY VAGINA
▸ Adult: 200 micrograms for 1 dose, to be inserted (in vaginal delivery system) high into posterior fornix; if oxytocin required, remove at least 30 minutes before oxytocin administration, for information on when to remove the delivery system—consult product literature

● UNLICENSED USE Use of misoprostol for termination of pregnancy is an unlicensed use.

> **IMPORTANT SAFETY INFORMATION**
>
> MHRA/CHM ADVICE: MISOPROSTOL VAGINAL DELIVERY SYSTEM (*MYSODELLE®*): REPORTS OF EXCESSIVE UTERINE CONTRACTIONS (TACHYSYSTOLE) UNRESPONSIVE TO TOCOLYTIC TREATMENT (FEBRUARY 2018)
>
> *Mysodelle®* can cause excessive uterine tachysystole that may not respond to tocolytic treatment. Monitor patients closely and remove the vaginal delivery system immediately in cases of excessive or prolonged uterine contractions, at the onset of labour, or if there is clinical concern for mother or baby.
>
> Be prepared to administer tocolytic therapy—if needed, it can be administered immediately after removal of *Mysodelle®*.

● CONTRA-INDICATIONS
MYSODELLE® VAGINAL DELIVERY SYSTEM Before 36 weeks' gestation · chorioamnionitis (unless adequate prior treatment initiated) · fetal malpresentation · placenta praevia · suspicion or evidence of fetal compromise · unexplained vaginal bleeding after 24 weeks gestation · uterine abnormality · uterine scar

● CAUTIONS
▸ When used for termination of pregnancy Cardiovascular disease · risk factors for cardiovascular disease
MYSODELLE® VAGINAL DELIVERY SYSTEM Modified Bishop score greater than 4

● SIDE-EFFECTS
▸ **Common or very common** Constipation · diarrhoea · dizziness · flatulence · gastrointestinal discomfort · headache · nausea · rash · vomiting
▸ **Uncommon** Fever · haemorrhage · menstrual cycle irregularities · postmenopausal haemorrhage · uterine cramps
▸ **Frequency not known** Chills · uterine rupture

● BREAST FEEDING Manufacturer advises avoid—present in milk, and may cause diarrhoea in nursing infants. EvGr Tertiary sources state present in milk but amount probably too small to be harmful; to further reduce risk following termination of pregnancy, consider interrupting breastfeeding for 5 hours after a dose. ◈

● HANDLING AND STORAGE
MYSODELLE® VAGINAL DELIVERY SYSTEM Manufacturer advises store in a freezer (-10 to -25°C); no thawing required prior to use.

● PATIENT AND CARER ADVICE
Driving and skilled tasks Manufacturer advises patients should be cautioned on the effects on driving and performance of skilled tasks—increased risk of dizziness.

● NATIONAL FUNDING/ACCESS DECISIONS
MYSODELLE® VAGINAL DELIVERY SYSTEM
All Wales Medicines Strategy Group (AWMSG) Decisions
AWMSG No. 3627
The *All Wales Medicines Strategy Group* has advised (March 2018) that misoprostol (*Mysodelle®*) is recommended as an option for use within NHS Wales for the induction of labour in women with an unfavourable cervix, from 36 weeks gestation, in whom induction is clinically indicated.

● MEDICINAL FORMS
There can be variation in the licensing of different medicines containing the same drug.

Vaginal delivery system
▸ Mysodelle (Ferring Pharmaceuticals Ltd)
Misoprostol 7 microgram per 1 hour Mysodelle 200micrograms vaginal delivery system | 5 unit PoM £465.00
▸ Misoprostol (Non-proprietary)
Misoprostol 200 microgram Misoprostol 200microgram vaginal tablets | 4 tablet PoM ⓢ (Hospital only)
▸ Topogyne (Nordic Pharma Ltd)
Misoprostol 400 microgram Topogyne 400microgram tablets | 16 tablet PoM £128.00 (Hospital only)

---

6 Vaginal and vulval conditions

Vaginal and vulval conditions

Management

Symptoms are often restricted to the vulva, but infections almost invariably involve the vagina which should also be treated. Applications to the vulva alone are likely to give only symptomatic relief without cure.

Aqueous medicated douches may disturb normal vaginal acidity and bacterial flora.

Topical anaesthetic agents give only symptomatic relief and may cause sensitivity reactions. They are indicated only in cases of pruritus where specific local causes have been excluded.

Systemic drugs are required in the treatment of infections such as gonorrhoea and syphilis.

Vaginal and vulval changes

Topical HRT for vaginal atrophy

A cream containing an oestrogen may be applied on a short-term basis to improve the vaginal epithelium in *menopausal atrophic vaginitis*. It is **important** to bear in mind that topical oestrogens should be used in the **smallest effective** amount to minimise systemic effects. Modified-release vaginal tablets and an impregnated vaginal ring are now also available.

The risk of endometrial hyperplasia and carcinoma is increased when *systemic* oestrogens are administered alone for prolonged periods. The endometrial safety of long-term or repeated use of *topical* vaginal oestrogens is uncertain; treatment should be reviewed at least annually, with special consideration given to any symptoms of endometrial hyperplasia or carcinoma.

Topical oestrogens are also used in postmenopausal women before vaginal surgery for prolapse when there is epithelial atrophy.

Non-hormonal preparations for vaginal atrophy

Several non-hormonal vaginal moisturisers are available and some are prescribable on the NHS (consult Drug Tariff).

Vaginal and vulval infections

Effective specific treatments are available for the common vaginal infections.

Fungal infections

Candidal vulvitis can be treated locally with cream, but is almost invariably associated with vaginal infection which should also be treated. *Vaginal candidiasis* is treated primarily with antifungal pessaries or cream inserted high into the vagina (including during menstruation). Single-dose preparations offer an advantage when compliance is a problem. Local irritation may occur on application of vaginal antifungal products.

    Imidazole drugs (clotrimazole p. 810, econazole nitrate p. 811, fenticonazole nitrate p. 811, and miconazole p. 811) are effective against candida in short courses of 1 to 14 days according to the preparation used; treatment can be repeated if initial course fails to control symptoms or if symptoms recur. Vaginal applications may be supplemented with antifungal cream for vulvitis and to treat other superficial sites of infection.

    Oral treatment of vaginal infection with fluconazole p. 584 or itraconazole p. 586 is also effective.

Vulvovaginal candidiasis in pregnancy

Vulvovaginal candidiasis is common during pregnancy and can be treated with vaginal application of an imidazole (such as clotrimazole), and a topical imidazole cream for vulvitis. Pregnant women need a longer duration of treatment, usually about 7 days, to clear the infection. Oral antifungal treatment should be avoided during pregnancy.

Recurrent vulvovaginal candidiasis

Recurrence of vulvovaginal candidiasis is particularly likely if there are predisposing factors, such as antibacterial therapy, pregnancy, diabetes mellitus, or possibly oral contraceptive use. Reservoirs of infection may also lead to recontamination and should be treated; these include other skin sites such as the digits, nail beds, and umbilicus as well as the gastro-intestinal tract and the bladder. The partner may also be the source of reinfection and, if symptomatic, should be treated with a topical imidazole cream at the same time.

    Treatment against candida may need to be extended for 6 months in recurrent vulvovaginal candidiasis.

Other infections

Trichomonal infections commonly involve the lower urinary tract as well as the genital system and need systemic treatment with metronidazole p. 533 or tinidazole p. 534.

    Bacterial infections with Gram-negative organisms are particularly common in association with gynaecological operations and trauma. Metronidazole is effective against certain Gram-negative organisms, especially *Bacteroides* spp. and can be used prophylactically in gynaecological surgery.

    Clindamycin below cream and metronidazole gel are indicated for bacterial vaginosis.

    Vaginal preparations intended to restore normal acidity may prevent recurrence of vaginal infections and permit the re-establishment of the normal vaginal flora.

    The antiviral drugs aciclovir p. 623, famciclovir p. 625, and valaciclovir p. 625 can be used in the treatment of genital infection due to *herpes simplex virus*, the HSV type 2 being a major cause of genital ulceration; they have a beneficial effect on virus shedding and healing, generally giving relief from pain and other symptoms.

6.1   Vaginal and vulval infections

6.1a   Vaginal and vulval bacterial infections

> **Other drugs used for Vaginal and vulval bacterial infections** Metronidazole, p. 533

ANTIBACTERIALS > LINCOSAMIDES

Clindamycin

- **INDICATIONS AND DOSE**

DALACIN ® 2% CREAM
Bacterial vaginosis
▸ BY VAGINA
▸ Adult: 1 applicatorful daily for 3–7 nights, dose to be administered at night

DOSE EQUIVALENCE AND CONVERSION
▸ 1 applicatorful delivers a 5 g dose of clindamycin 2%.

- **INTERACTIONS** → Appendix 1: clindamycin
- **SIDE-EFFECTS**
▸ **Common or very common** Skin reactions
▸ **Frequency not known** Constipation · diarrhoea (discontinue) · dizziness · gastrointestinal discomfort · headache · increased risk of infection · nausea · vertigo · vomiting · vulvovaginal irritation

SIDE-EFFECTS, FURTHER INFORMATION Clindamycin 2% cream is poorly absorbed into the blood—low risk of systemic effects.

- **CONCEPTION AND CONTRACEPTION**

DALACIN ® 2% CREAM Damages latex condoms and diaphragms.

- **MEDICINAL FORMS**
There can be variation in the licensing of different medicines containing the same drug.

Cream
EXCIPIENTS: May contain Benzyl alcohol, cetostearyl alcohol (including cetyl and stearyl alcohol), polysorbates, propylene glycol
▸ Dalacin (Pfizer Ltd)
  Clindamycin (as Clindamycin phosphate) 20 mg per 1 gram Dalacin 2% cream | 40 gram PoM £10.86 DT = £10.86

ANTISEPTICS AND DISINFECTANTS

Dequalinium chloride   13-Mar-2017

- **DRUG ACTION** Dequalinium chloride is a bactericidal anti-infective which causes bacterial cell death by increasing cell permeability and reducing enzyme activity.

- **INDICATIONS AND DOSE**
Bacterial vaginosis
▸ BY VAGINA
▸ Adult 18–55 years: 10 mg once daily for 6 days, inserted at night

- **CONTRA-INDICATIONS** Vaginal ulceration
- **SIDE-EFFECTS**
▸ **Common or very common** Increased risk of infection · vulvovaginal disorders
▸ **Uncommon** Haemorrhage · headache · nausea
▸ **Frequency not known** Cystitis · fever

- **CONCEPTION AND CONTRACEPTION** Does not affect efficacy of latex condoms; however, manufacturer advises avoid use of non-latex condoms and intravaginal devices—no information available

7

Genito-urinary system

- PREGNANCY Manufacturer advises avoid unless essential—limited information available.
- NATIONAL FUNDING/ACCESS DECISIONS

Scottish Medicines Consortium (SMC) Decisions

The *Scottish Medicines Consortium* has advised (November 2016) that dequalinium chloride (*Fluomizin* ®) is accepted for restricted use within NHS Scotland for treatment of bacterial vaginosis in patients for whom the initial treatment is not effective or well tolerated.

All Wales Medicines Strategy Group (AWMSG) Decisions

The *All Wales Medicines Strategy Group* has advised (November 2016) that dequalinium chloride (*Fluomizin* ®) is recommended as an option for restricted use within NHS Wales for the treatment of bacterial vaginosis only after initial treatment is ineffective or not tolerated, as an alternative option to clindamycin vaginal cream.

- MEDICINAL FORMS

There can be variation in the licensing of different medicines containing the same drug.

Tablet

▸ Fluomizin (KoRa Healthcare)
Dequalinium chloride 10 mg Fluomizin 10mg vaginal tablets | 6 tablet [PoM] £6.95 DT = £6.95

CARBOXYLIC ACIDS

Lactic acid

- INDICATIONS AND DOSE

BALANCE ACTIV RX ® GEL

Prevention of bacterial vaginosis

▸ BY VAGINA
▸ Adult: 5 mL 1–2 times a week, insert the content of 1 tube (5 mL)

RELACTAGEL ® GEL

Prevention of bacterial vaginosis

▸ BY VAGINA
▸ Adult: 5 mL daily for 2–3 nights after menstruation, insert the contents of one tube

Treatment of bacterial vaginosis

▸ BY VAGINA
▸ Adult: 5 mL daily for 7 nights, insert the contents of one tube

- SIDE-EFFECTS Skin irritation
- ALLERGY AND CROSS-SENSITIVITY Contra-indicated in shellfish allergy.
- CONCEPTION AND CONTRACEPTION

RELACTAGEL ® GEL Not recommended if trying to conceive.

- MEDICINAL FORMS

There can be variation in the licensing of different medicines containing the same drug.

Gel

EXCIPIENTS: May contain Propylene glycol

▸ Balance Activ (BBI Healthcare Ltd)
Balance Activ BV vaginal pH correction gel | 7 device £5.25
▸ Relactagel (KoRa Healthcare)
Relactagel vaginal pH correction gel | 7 device £5.25

6.1b Vaginal and vulval fungal infections

Other drugs used for Vaginal and vulval fungal infections
Fluconazole, p. 584 · Itraconazole, p. 586

ANTIFUNGALS ⟩ IMIDAZOLE ANTIFUNGALS

Clotrimazole

- INDICATIONS AND DOSE

Superficial sites of infection in vaginal and vulval candidiasis (dose for 1% or 2% cream)

▸ BY VAGINA USING CREAM
▸ Adult: Apply 2–3 times a day, to be applied to anogenital area

Vaginal candidiasis (dose for 10% intravaginal cream)

▸ BY VAGINA USING VAGINAL CREAM
▸ Adult: 5 g for 1 dose, one applicatorful to be inserted into the vagina at night, dose can be repeated once if necessary

Vaginal candidiasis

▸ BY VAGINA USING PESSARIES
▸ Adult: 200 mg for 3 nights, course can be repeated once if necessary, alternatively 100 mg for 6 nights, course can be repeated once if necessary, alternatively 500 mg for 1 night, dose can be repeated once if necessary

Recurrent vulvovaginal candidiasis

▸ BY VAGINA USING PESSARIES
▸ Adult: 500 mg every week for 6 months, dose to be administered following topical imidazole for 10–14 days

- INTERACTIONS → Appendix 1: antifungals, azoles
- SIDE-EFFECTS Abdominal pain · discomfort · dyspnoea · genital peeling · hypotension · oedema · paraesthesia · pelvic pain · skin reactions · syncope · vaginal haemorrhage
- CONCEPTION AND CONTRACEPTION Cream and pessaries may damage latex condoms and diaphragms.
- PREGNANCY

Dose adjustments Pregnant women need a longer duration of treatment, usually about 7 days, to clear the infection. Oral antifungal treatment should be avoided during pregnancy.

- EXCEPTIONS TO LEGAL CATEGORY Brands for sale to the public include *Canesten* ® Internal Cream.

- MEDICINAL FORMS

There can be variation in the licensing of different medicines containing the same drug.

Pessary

EXCIPIENTS: May contain Benzyl alcohol, cetostearyl alcohol (including cetyl and stearyl alcohol), polysorbates

▸ Clotrimazole (Non-proprietary)
Clotrimazole 500 mg Clotrimazole 500mg pessaries | 1 pessary [P] £3.57 DT = £3.57
▸ Canesten (clotrimazole) (Bayer Plc)
Clotrimazole 100 mg Canesten 100mg pessaries | 6 pessary [P] £3.50 DT = £3.50
Clotrimazole 200 mg Canesten 200mg pessaries | 3 pessary [P] £3.10 DT = £3.10
Clotrimazole 500 mg Canesten 500mg Soft Gel pessaries | 1 pessary [P] £6.99 DT = £3.57
Canesten 500mg pessaries | 1 pessary [P] [Ⓢ] DT = £3.57
Canesten Vaginal 500mg pessaries | 1 pessary [PoM] £2.00 DT = £3.57

Cream

EXCIPIENTS: May contain Benzyl alcohol, cetostearyl alcohol (including cetyl and stearyl alcohol), polysorbates

▸ Clotrimazole (Non-proprietary)
Clotrimazole 10 mg per 1 gram Clotrimazole 1% cream | 20 gram [P] £2.06 DT = £0.72 | 50 gram [P] £5.45 DT = £1.80
▸ Canesten (clotrimazole) (Bayer Plc)
Clotrimazole 10 mg per 1 gram Canesten 1% cream | 20 gram £2.20 DT = £0.72 | 50 gram [P] £3.50 DT = £1.80
Canesten Antifungal 1% cream | 20 gram [P] £1.85 DT = £0.72
Clotrimazole 20 mg per 1 gram Canesten 2% thrush cream | 20 gram [P] £4.76 DT = £4.76
Clotrimazole 100 mg per 1 gram Canesten Internal 10% cream Canesten 10% VC cream | 5 gram [PoM] £4.50 DT = £6.23

Econazole nitrate

- **INDICATIONS AND DOSE**

GYNO-PEVARYL® ONCE

Vaginal and vulval candidiasis
- ▸ BY VAGINA
- ▸ Adult: 1 pessary for 1 dose, pessary to be inserted at night, dose to be repeated once if necessary

GYNO-PEVARYL® CREAM

Vaginal and vulval candidiasis
- ▸ INITIALLY BY VAGINA USING VAGINAL CREAM
- ▸ Adult: 1 applicatorful daily for at least 14 days, dose to be inserted vaginally at night and (to the skin) apply daily for at least 14 days, to be applied to vulva at night, course can be repeated once if necessary

GYNO-PEVARYL® PESSARY

Vaginal and vulval candidiasis
- ▸ BY VAGINA
- ▸ Adult: 1 pessary daily for 3 days, pessary to be inserted at night, course can be repeated once if necessary

- **SIDE-EFFECTS**
- ▸ **Common or very common** Skin reactions
- ▸ **Uncommon** Vaginal burning
- ▸ **Frequency not known** Angioedema
- **CONCEPTION AND CONTRACEPTION** Cream and pessaries damage latex condoms and diaphragms.
- **PREGNANCY** Pregnant women need a longer duration of treatment, usually about 7 days, to clear the infection.

- **MEDICINAL FORMS**
  There can be variation in the licensing of different medicines containing the same drug.

  Pessary
  - ▸ Gyno-Pevaryl (Janssen-Cilag Ltd)
    Econazole nitrate 150 mg Gyno-Pevaryl Once 150mg vaginal pessary | 1 pessary PoM £3.69
    Gyno-Pevaryl 150mg vaginal pessaries | 3 pessary PoM £4.17

  Cream
  EXCIPIENTS: May contain Butylated hydroxyanisole, fragrances
  - ▸ Gyno-Pevaryl (Janssen-Cilag Ltd)
    Econazole nitrate 10 mg per 1 gram Gyno-Pevaryl 1% cream | 15 gram PoM £2.11 | 30 gram PoM £3.78

Fenticonazole nitrate

- **INDICATIONS AND DOSE**

Vaginal and vulva candidiasis
- ▸ BY VAGINA USING CAPSULES
- ▸ Adult: 200 mg daily for 3 days, alternatively 600 mg daily for 1 dose, to be inserted at night
- ▸ BY VAGINA USING CREAM
- ▸ Adult: 1 applicatorful twice daily for 3 days

DOSE EQUIVALENCE AND CONVERSION
- ▸ 1 applicatorful delivers a 5 g dose of fenticonazole 2 %.

- **SIDE-EFFECTS** Paraesthesia
- **CONCEPTION AND CONTRACEPTION** Intravaginal cream and vaginal capsules damage latex condoms and diaphragms.

- **MEDICINAL FORMS**
  There can be variation in the licensing of different medicines containing the same drug.

  Cream
  EXCIPIENTS: May contain Cetostearyl alcohol (including cetyl and stearyl alcohol), propylene glycol, woolfat and related substances (including lanolin)
  - ▸ Gynoxin (Recordati Pharmaceuticals Ltd)
    Fenticonazole nitrate 20 mg per 1 gram Gynoxin 2% vaginal cream | 30 gram PoM £3.74

Capsule
EXCIPIENTS: May contain Hydroxybenzoates (parabens)
- ▸ Gynoxin (Recordati Pharmaceuticals Ltd)
  Fenticonazole nitrate 200 mg Gynoxin 200mg vaginal capsules | 3 capsule PoM £2.42
  Fenticonazole nitrate 600 mg Gynoxin 600mg vaginal capsules | 1 capsule PoM £2.62

Ketoconazole　　　　　　　　　　　　　　　20-Jul-2017

- **INDICATIONS AND DOSE**

Vaginal and vulva candidiasis
- ▸ BY VAGINA USING CREAM
- ▸ Adult: Apply 1–2 times a day, to be applied to the anogenital area

- **INTERACTIONS** → Appendix 1: antifungals, azoles
- **SIDE-EFFECTS**
- ▸ **Common or very common** Skin reactions
- **CONCEPTION AND CONTRACEPTION** Effect on latex condoms and diaphragms not yet known.

- **MEDICINAL FORMS**
  There can be variation in the licensing of different medicines containing the same drug.

  Cream
  EXCIPIENTS: May contain Cetostearyl alcohol (including cetyl and stearyl alcohol), polysorbates, propylene glycol
  - ▸ Nizoral (Janssen-Cilag Ltd)
    Ketoconazole 20 mg per 1 gram Nizoral 2% cream | 30 gram PoM £4.24 DT = £4.24

Miconazole　　　　　　　　　　　　　　　　11-Oct-2017

- **INDICATIONS AND DOSE**

Vaginal and vulval candidiasis
- ▸ BY VAGINA USING CAPSULES
- ▸ Child: 1 capsule daily, ovule to be inserted at night as a single dose, dose can be repeated once if necessary
- ▸ Adult: 1 capsule daily, ovule to be inserted at night as a single dose, dose can be repeated once if necessary
- ▸ BY VAGINA USING CREAM
- ▸ Adult: Apply 1 applicatorful daily for 10 to 14 days, alternatively apply 1 applicatorful twice daily for 7 days, course can be repeated once if necessary

Superficial sites of infection in vaginal and vulval candidiasis | Vulvitis
- ▸ BY VAGINA USING CREAM
- ▸ Adult: Apply twice daily, apply to the anogenital area

- **CAUTIONS** Avoid intravaginal preparations (particularly those that require use of an applicator) in young girls who are not sexually active, unless there is no alternative
- **INTERACTIONS** → Appendix 1: antifungals, azoles
- **SIDE-EFFECTS**
- ▸ **Common or very common** Dysmenorrhoea · skin reactions · vulvovaginal disorders
- ▸ **Frequency not known** Abdominal pain · angioedema · dysuria · headache · nausea · pelvic cramps · urinary tract infection · vaginal haemorrhage
- **CONCEPTION AND CONTRACEPTION** *Gyno-Daktarin®* damages latex condoms and diaphragms.
- **PREGNANCY** Pregnant women need a longer duration of treatment, usually about 7 days, to clear the infection.
- **BREAST FEEDING** Manufacturer advises caution—no information available.

- MEDICINAL FORMS
There can be variation in the licensing of different medicines containing the same drug.

Cream
EXCIPIENTS: May contain Butylated hydroxyanisole
▸ Gyno-Daktarin (Janssen-Cilag Ltd)
Miconazole nitrate 20 mg per 1 gram Gyno-Daktarin 2% vaginal cream | 78 gram PoM £4.33

6.2 Vaginal atrophy

OESTROGENS

Estradiol

- INDICATIONS AND DOSE
ESTRING ®
Postmenopausal urogenital conditions (not suitable for vasomotor symptoms or osteoporosis prophylaxis)
▸ BY VAGINA
▸ Adult: To be inserted into upper third of vagina and worn continuously; replace after 3 months; max. duration of continuous treatment 2 years

VAGIFEM ®
Improve the vaginal epithelium in menopausal atrophic vaginitis
▸ BY VAGINA
▸ Adult: 1 tablet daily for 2 weeks, then reduced to 1 tablet twice weekly

- CONTRA-INDICATIONS Active arterial thromboembolic disease (e.g. angina or myocardial infarction) · active thrombophlebitis · Dubin-Johnson syndrome (or monitor closely) · history of breast cancer · history of recurrent venous thromboembolism (unless already on anticoagulant treatment) · oestrogen-dependent cancer · recent arterial thromboembolic disease (e.g. angina or myocardial infarction) · Rotor syndrome (or monitor closely) · thrombophilic disorder · undiagnosed vaginal bleeding · untreated endometrial hyperplasia · venous thromboembolism

- CAUTIONS Acute porphyrias p. 1025 · diabetes (increased risk of heart disease) · history of breast nodules—closely monitor breast status (risk of breast cancer) · history of endometrial hyperplasia · factors predisposing to thromboembolism · history of fibrocystic disease—closely monitor breast status (risk of breast cancer) · hypophyseal tumours · increased risk of gall-bladder disease · interrupt treatment periodically to assess need for continued treatment · migraine (or migraine-like headaches) · presence of antiphospholipid antibodies (increased risk of thrombotic events) · prolonged exposure to unopposed oestrogens may increase risk of developing endometrial cancer · risk factors for oestrogen-dependent tumours (e.g. breast cancer in first-degree relative) · symptoms of endometriosis may be exacerbated · uterine fibroids may increase in size
CAUTIONS, FURTHER INFORMATION
▸ Risk of breast cancer It is estimated that using *all* types of HRT increases the risk of breast cancer within 1–2 years of initiating treatment. The increased risk is related to the duration of HRT use (but not to the age at which HRT is started) and this excess risk disappears within 5 years of stopping.
  Radiological detection of breast cancer can be made more difficult as mammographic density can increase with HRT use.
▸ Risk of endometrial cancer The increased risk of endometrial cancer depends on the dose and duration of oestrogen-only HRT.

In women with a uterus, the addition of a progestogen cyclically (for at least 10 days per 28-day cycle) reduces the additional risk of endometrial cancer; this additional risk is eliminated if a progestogen is given continuously. However, this should be weighed against the increased risk of breast cancer.
▸ Risk of ovarian cancer Long-term use of combined HRT or oestrogen-only HRT is associated with a small increased risk of ovarian cancer. This excess risk disappears within a few years of stopping.
▸ Risk of venous thromboembolism Women using combined or oestrogen-only HRT are at an increased risk of deep vein thrombosis and of pulmonary embolism especially in the first year of use.
  In *women who have predisposing factors* (such as a personal or family history of deep vein thrombosis or pulmonary embolism, severe varicose veins, obesity, trauma, or prolonged bed-rest) it is prudent to review the need for HRT, as in some cases the risks of HRT may exceed the benefits.
  Travel involving prolonged immobility further increases the risk of deep vein thrombosis.
▸ Risk of stroke Risk of stroke increases with age, therefore older women have a greater absolute risk of stroke. Combined HRT or oestrogen-only HRT slightly increases the risk of stroke.
▸ Risk of coronary heart disease HRT does not prevent coronary heart disease and should not be prescribed for this purpose. There is an increased risk of coronary heart disease in women who start combined HRT more than 10 years after menopause. Although very little information is available on the risk of coronary heart disease in younger women who start HRT close to the menopause, studies suggest a lower relative risk compared with older women.
▸ Other conditions The product literature advises caution in other conditions including hypertension, renal disease, asthma, epilepsy, sickle-cell disease, melanoma, otosclerosis, multiple sclerosis, and systemic lupus erythematosus (but care required if antiphospholipid antibodies present). Evidence for caution in these conditions is unsatisfactory and many women with these conditions may stand to benefit from HRT.

- INTERACTIONS → Appendix 1: hormone replacement therapy

- SIDE-EFFECTS
▸ **Common or very common** Abdominal pain · headaches · nausea · skin reactions · vaginal haemorrhage · vulvovaginal disorders
▸ **Uncommon** Hypertension · vulvovaginal fungal infection · weight increased
▸ **Rare or very rare** Diarrhoea · embolism and thrombosis · endometrial hyperplasia · fluid retention · genital pruritus · increased risk of ischaemic stroke · insomnia · neoplasm malignant · neoplasms · vaginismus
SIDE-EFFECTS, FURTHER INFORMATION Cyclical HRT (where a progestogen is taken for 12–14 days of each 28-day oestrogen treatment cycle) usually results in regular withdrawal bleeding towards the end of the progestogen. Continuous combined HRT commonly produces irregular breakthrough bleeding in the first 4–6 months of treatment. Bleeding beyond 6 months or after a spell of amenorrhoea requires further investigation to exclude serious gynaecological pathology.

- CONCEPTION AND CONTRACEPTION HRT does **not** provide contraception and a woman is considered potentially fertile for 2 years after her last menstrual period if she is under 50 years, and for 1 year if she is over 50 years. A woman who is under 50 years and free of all risk factors for venous and arterial disease can use a low-oestrogen combined oral contraceptive pill to provide both relief of menopausal symptoms and contraception; it is recommended that the oral contraceptive be stopped at 50 years of age since there are more suitable alternatives. If any potentially fertile woman needs HRT, non-hormonal contraceptive measures (such as condoms) are necessary. Measurement of follicle-stimulating hormone can help to determine fertility, but high measurements alone (particularly in women aged under 50 years) do not necessarily preclude the possibility of becoming pregnant. VAGIFEM ® No evidence of damage to latex condoms and diaphragms.

* PREGNANCY Not known to be harmful.
* BREAST FEEDING Avoid; adverse effects on lactation.
* HEPATIC IMPAIRMENT Avoid in active liver disease including disorders of hepatic excretion (e.g. Dubin-Johnson or Rotor syndromes), infective hepatitis (until liver function returns to normal), and liver tumours.
* MONITORING REQUIREMENTS
  ▸ History of breast nodules or fibrocystic disease—closely monitor breast status (risk of breast cancer).
  ▸ The endometrial safety of long-term or repeated use of topical vaginal oestrogens is uncertain; treatment should be reviewed at least annually, with special consideration given to any symptoms of endometrial hyperplasia or carcinoma.
* MEDICINAL FORMS
  There can be variation in the licensing of different medicines containing the same drug. Forms available from special-order manufacturers include: implant

  Pessary
  ▸ Vagifem (Novo Nordisk Ltd)
  Estradiol 10 microgram Vagifem 10microgram vaginal tablets | 24 pessary [PoM] £16.72 DT = £16.72

  Vaginal delivery system
  CAUTIONARY AND ADVISORY LABELS 10
  ▸ Estring (Pfizer Ltd)
  Estradiol (as Estradiol hemihydrate) 7.5 microgram per 24 hour Estring 7.5micrograms/24hours vaginal delivery system | 1 device [PoM] £31.42

Estriol

* **INDICATIONS AND DOSE**

OVESTIN ®

Improve the vaginal epithelium in menopausal atrophic vaginitis (short-term use)
▸ BY VAGINA
▸ Adult: Apply 1 applicatorful daily for 2–3 weeks, then reduced to 1 applicatorful twice weekly, discontinue every 2–3 months for 4 weeks to assess need for further treatment

Vaginal surgery for prolapse when there is epithelial atrophy in postmenopausal women (before surgery)
▸ BY VAGINA
▸ Adult: Apply 1 applicatorful daily for 2 weeks before surgery, resume 2 weeks after surgery

* CONTRA-INDICATIONS Active arterial thromboembolic disease (e.g. angina or myocardial infarction) · active thrombophlebitis · Dubin-Johnson syndrome (or monitor closely) · history of breast cancer · history of recurrent venous thromboembolism (unless already on anticoagulant treatment) · oestrogen-dependent cancer · recent arterial thromboembolic disease (e.g. angina or myocardial infarction) · Rotor syndrome (or monitor closely) · thrombophilic disorder · undiagnosed vaginal bleeding · untreated endometrial hyperplasia · venous thromboembolism
* CAUTIONS Acute porphyrias p. 1025 · diabetes (increased risk of heart disease) · factors predisposing to thromboembolism · history of breast nodules—closely

monitor breast status (risk of breast cancer) · history of endometrial hyperplasia · history of fibrocystic disease—closely monitor breast status (risk of breast cancer) · hypophyseal tumours · increased risk of gall-bladder disease · interrupt treatment periodically to assess need for continued treatment · migraine (or migraine-like headaches) · presence of antiphospholipid antibodies (increased risk of thrombotic events) · prolonged exposure to unopposed oestrogens may increase risk of developing endometrial cancer · risk factors for oestrogen-dependent tumours (e.g. breast cancer in first-degree relative) · symptoms of endometriosis may be exacerbated · uterine fibroids may increase in size

CAUTIONS, FURTHER INFORMATION
▸ Risk of breast cancer It is estimated that using *all* types of HRT increases the risk of breast cancer within 1–2 years of initiating treatment. The increased risk is related to the duration of HRT use (but not to the age at which HRT is started) and this excess risk disappears within 5 years of stopping.
  Radiological detection of breast cancer can be made more difficult as mammographic density can increase with HRT use.
▸ Risk of endometrial cancer The increased risk of endometrial cancer depends on the dose and duration of oestrogen-only HRT.
  In women with a uterus, the addition of a progestogen cyclically (for at least 10 days per 28-day cycle) reduces the additional risk of endometrial cancer; this additional risk is eliminated if a progestogen is given continuously. However, this should be weighed against the increased risk of breast cancer.
▸ Risk of ovarian cancer Long-term use of combined HRT or oestrogen-only HRT is associated with a small increased risk of ovarian cancer. This excess risk disappears within a few years of stopping.
▸ Risk of venous thromboembolism Women using combined or oestrogen-only HRT are at an increased risk of deep vein thrombosis and of pulmonary embolism especially in the first year of use.
  In *women who have predisposing factors* (such as a personal or family history of deep vein thrombosis or pulmonary embolism, severe varicose veins, obesity, trauma, or prolonged bed-rest) it is prudent to review the need for HRT, as in some cases the risks of HRT may exceed the benefits.
  Travel involving prolonged immobility further increases the risk of deep vein thrombosis.
▸ Risk of stroke Risk of stroke increases with age, therefore older women have a greater absolute risk of stroke. Combined HRT or oestrogen-only HRT slightly increases the risk of stroke.
▸ Risk of coronary heart disease HRT does not prevent coronary heart disease and should not be prescribed for this purpose. There is an increased risk of coronary heart disease in women who start combined HRT more than 10 years after menopause. Although very little information is available on the risk of coronary heart disease in younger women who start HRT close to the menopause, studies suggest a lower relative risk compared with older women.
▸ Other conditions The product literature advises caution in other conditions including hypertension, renal disease, asthma, epilepsy, sickle-cell disease, melanoma, otosclerosis, multiple sclerosis, and systemic lupus erythematosus (but care required if antiphospholipid antibodies present). Evidence for caution in these conditions is unsatisfactory and many women with these conditions may stand to benefit from HRT.

* INTERACTIONS → Appendix 1: hormone replacement therapy

- SIDE-EFFECTS Breast abnormalities · cervical mucus increased · dementia · erythema nodosum · gallbladder disorder · headache · increased risk of coronary artery disease · increased risk of ischaemic stroke · increased risk of venous thromboembolism · nausea · neoplasms · skin reactions · vaginal haemorrhage · vaginal spotting · vomiting

  SIDE-EFFECTS, FURTHER INFORMATION Cyclical HRT (where a progestogen is taken for 12–14 days of each 28-day oestrogen treatment cycle) usually results in regular withdrawal bleeding towards the end of the progestogen. Continuous combined HRT commonly produces irregular breakthrough bleeding in the first 4–6 months of treatment. Bleeding beyond 6 months or after a spell of amenorrhoea requires further investigation to exclude serious gynaecological pathology.

- CONCEPTION AND CONTRACEPTION Effect on latex condoms and diaphragms not yet known.

- PREGNANCY Not known to be harmful.

- BREAST FEEDING Avoid; adverse effects on lactation.

- HEPATIC IMPAIRMENT Avoid in active liver disease including disorders of hepatic excretion (e.g. Dubin-Johnson or Rotor syndromes), infective hepatitis (until liver function returns to normal), and liver tumours.

- RENAL IMPAIRMENT Manufacturer advises caution in renal disease. Evidence for caution is unsatisfactory and many women with these conditions may stand to benefit from HRT.

- MONITORING REQUIREMENTS
  ▶ Closely monitor breast status if history of breast nodules or fibrocystic disease (risk of breast cancer).
  ▶ The endometrial safety of long-term or repeated use of topical vaginal oestrogens is uncertain; treatment should be reviewed at least annually, with special consideration given to any symptoms of endometrial hyperplasia or carcinoma.

- MEDICINAL FORMS
  There can be variation in the licensing of different medicines containing the same drug.
  Cream
  EXCIPIENTS: May contain Arachis (peanut) oil, cetostearyl alcohol (including cetyl and stearyl alcohol), polysorbates
  ▶ Ovestin (Aspen Pharma Trading Ltd)
  Estriol 1 mg per 1 gram Ovestin 1mg cream | 15 gram [PoM] £4.45
  DT = £4.45

Chapter 8
Immune system and malignant disease

CONTENTS

Immune system

1 Immune system disorders and transplantation

Immune response

Inflammatory bowel disease

Azathioprine p. 816, ciclosporin p. 818, mercaptopurine p. 887, and methotrexate p. 888 have a role in the treatment of inflammatory bowel disease.

Folic acid p. 993 should be given to reduce the possibility of methotrexate toxicity [unlicensed indication]. Folic acid is usually given weekly on a different day to the methotrexate; alternative regimens may be used in some settings.

Immunosuppressant therapy

Immunosuppressants are used to suppress rejection in organ transplant recipients and to treat a variety of chronic inflammatory and autoimmune diseases. Solid organ transplant patients are maintained on drug regimens, which may include antiproliferative drugs (azathioprine or mycophenolate mofetil p. 826), calcineurin inhibitors (ciclosporin or tacrolimus p. 821), corticosteroids, or sirolimus p. 820. Choice is dependent on the type of organ, time after transplantation, and clinical condition of the patient. Specialist management is required and other immunomodulators may be used to initiate treatment or to treat rejection.

Impaired immune responsiveness

Modification of tissue reactions caused by corticosteroids and other immunosuppressants may result in the rapid *spread of infection*. Corticosteroids may suppress clinical signs of infection and allow diseases such as septicaemia or tuberculosis to reach an advanced stage before being recognised— **important**: normal immunoglobulin administration should be considered as soon as possible after measles exposure, and varicella–zoster immunoglobulin (VZIG) is recommended for individuals who have significant chickenpox (varicella) exposure. Specialist advice should be sought on the use of live vaccines for those being treated with immunosuppressive drugs.

Antiproliferative immunosuppressants

Azathioprine is widely used for transplant recipients and it is also used to treat a number of auto-immune conditions, usually when corticosteroid therapy alone provides inadequate control. It is metabolised to mercaptopurine, and doses should be reduced when allopurinol p. 1086 is given concurrently.

Mycophenolate mofetil is metabolised to mycophenolic acid which has a more selective mode of action than azathioprine.

There is evidence that compared with similar regimens incorporating azathioprine, mycophenolate mofetil reduces the risk of acute rejection episodes; the risk of opportunistic infections (particularly due to tissue-invasive cytomegalovirus) and the occurrence of blood disorders such as leucopenia may be higher.

Cyclophosphamide p. 871 is less commonly prescribed as an immunosuppressant.

Corticosteroids and other immunosuppressants

Prednisolone p. 664 is widely used in oncology. It has a marked antitumour effect in acute lymphoblastic leukaemia, Hodgkin's disease, and the non-Hodgkin lymphomas. It has a role in the palliation of symptomatic end-stage malignant disease when it may enhance appetite and produce a sense of well-being.

The corticosteroids are also powerful immunosuppressants. They are used to prevent organ transplant rejection, and in high dose to treat rejection episodes.

Ciclosporin a calcineurin inhibitor, is a potent immunosuppressant which is virtually non-myelotoxic but markedly nephrotoxic. It has an important role in organ and tissue transplantation, for prevention of graft rejection following bone marrow, kidney, liver, pancreas, heart, lung, and heart-lung transplantation, and for prophylaxis and treatment of graft-versus-host disease.

Tacrolimus is also a calcineurin inhibitor. Although not chemically related to ciclosporin it has a similar mode of action and side-effects, but the incidence of neurotoxicity appears to be greater; cardiomyopathy has also been reported. Disturbance of glucose metabolism also appears to be significant.

Sirolimus is a non-calcineurin inhibiting immunosuppressant licensed for renal transplantation.

Basiliximab p. 825 is used for prophylaxis of acute rejection in allogeneic renal transplantation. It is given with ciclosporin and corticosteroid immunosuppression regimens; its use should be confined to specialist centres.

Belatacept p. 828 is a fusion protein and co-stimulation blocker that prevents T-cell activation; it is licensed for prophylaxis of graft rejection in adults undergoing renal transplantation who are seropositive for the Epstein-Barr virus. It is used with interleukin-2 receptor antagonist induction, in combination with corticosteroids and a mycophenolic acid.

Antimocyte immunoglobulin (rabbit) below is licensed for the prophylaxis of organ rejection in renal and heart allograft recipients and for the treatment of corticosteroid-resistant allograft rejection in renal transplantation. Tolerability is increased by pretreatment with an intravenous corticosteroid and antihistamine; an antipyretic drug such as paracetamol may also be beneficial.

> **Other drugs used for Immune system disorders and transplantation** Chloroquine, p. 604 · Everolimus, p. 950 · Hydroxychloroquine sulfate, p. 1062 · Rituximab, p. 859

IMMUNE SERA AND IMMUNOGLOBULINS >
IMMUNOGLOBULINS

Antithymocyte immunoglobulin (rabbit)

28-Nov-2017

● **INDICATIONS AND DOSE**

Prophylaxis of organ rejection in heart allograft recipients
▸ BY INTRAVENOUS INFUSION
▸ Adult: 1–2.5 mg/kg daily for 3–5 days, to be given over at least 6 hours

Prophylaxis of organ rejection in renal allograft recipients
▸ BY INTRAVENOUS INFUSION
▸ Adult: 1–1.5 mg/kg daily for 3–9 days, to be given over at least 6 hours

Treatment of corticosteroid-resistant allograft rejection in renal transplantation
▸ BY INTRAVENOUS INFUSION
▸ Adult: 1.5 mg/kg daily for 7–14 days, to be given over at least 6 hours

DOSES AT EXTREMES OF BODY-WEIGHT
▸ To avoid excessive dosage in obese patients, calculate dose on the basis of ideal body weight.

● CONTRA-INDICATIONS Infection

● SIDE-EFFECTS
▸ **Common or very common** Chills · diarrhoea · dysphagia · dyspnoea · fever · hypotension · infection · lymphopenia · myalgia · nausea · neoplasm malignant · neoplasms · neutropenia · reactivation of infection · secondary malignancy · sepsis · skin reactions · thrombocytopenia · vomiting
▸ **Uncommon** Cytokine release syndrome · hepatic disorders · hypersensitivity · infusion related reaction

SIDE-EFFECTS, FURTHER INFORMATION Tolerability is increased by pretreatment with an intravenous corticosteroid and antihistamine; an antipyretic drug such as paracetamol may also be beneficial.

● PREGNANCY Manufacturer advises use only if potential benefit outweighs risk—no information available.

● BREAST FEEDING Manufacturer advises avoid—no information available.

● MONITORING REQUIREMENTS Monitor blood count.

● DIRECTIONS FOR ADMINISTRATION For *continuous intravenous infusion* (Thymoglobuline®) in Glucose 5% or Sodium chloride 0.9%; reconstitute each vial with 5 mL water for injections to produce a solution of 5 mg/mL; gently rotate to dissolve. Dilute requisite dose with infusion fluid to a total volume of 50–500 mL (usually 50 mL/vial); begin infusion immediately after dilution;

give through an in-line filter (pore size 0.22 micron); not to be given with unfractionated heparin and hydrocortisone in glucose infusion—precipitation reported.

● NATIONAL FUNDING/ACCESS DECISIONS
NICE decisions
▸ **Immunosuppressive therapy for kidney transplant in adults (October 2017)** NICE TA481
Antithymocyte immunoglobulin (rabbit) is not recommended as an initial treatment to prevent organ rejection in adults having a kidney transplant. Patients whose treatment was started within the NHS before this guidance was published should have the option to continue treatment, without change to their funding arrangements, until they and their NHS clinician consider it appropriate to stop.
www.nice.org.uk/guidance/TA481

● MEDICINAL FORMS
There can be variation in the licensing of different medicines containing the same drug.
Powder and solvent for solution for infusion
▸ Thymoglobulin (Sanofi)
Antithymocyte immunoglobulin (rabbit) 25 mg Thymoglobuline 25mg powder and solvent for solution for infusion vials | 1 vial PoM £158.77 (Hospital only)

IMMUNOSUPPRESSANTS > ANTIMETABOLITES

Azathioprine

21-Mar-2018

● DRUG ACTION Azathioprine is metabolised to mercaptopurine.

● **INDICATIONS AND DOSE**

Severe acute Crohn's disease | Maintenance of remission of Crohn's disease | Maintenance of remission of acute ulcerative colitis
▸ BY MOUTH
▸ Adult: 2–2.5 mg/kg daily, some patients may respond to lower doses

Rheumatoid arthritis that has not responded to other disease-modifying drugs | Severe systemic lupus erythematosus and other connective tissue disorders | Polymyositis in cases of corticosteroid resistance
▸ BY MOUTH
▸ Adult: Initially up to 2.5 mg/kg daily in divided doses, adjusted according to response, rarely more than 3 mg/kg daily; maintenance 1–3 mg/kg daily, consider withdrawal if no improvement within 3 months

Autoimmune conditions
▸ BY MOUTH, OR BY INTRAVENOUS INJECTION, OR BY INTRAVENOUS INFUSION
▸ Adult: 1–3 mg/kg daily, adjusted according to response, consider withdrawal if no improvement within 3 months, oral administration preferable, if not possible then can be given by intravenous injection (intravenous solution very irritant) or by intravenous infusion

Suppression of transplant rejection
▸ BY MOUTH, OR BY INTRAVENOUS INJECTION, OR BY INTRAVENOUS INFUSION
▸ Adult: 1–2.5 mg/kg daily, adjusted according to response, oral administration preferable, if not possible then can be given by intravenous injection (intravenous solution very irritant) or by intravenous infusion

Severe refractory eczema, normal or high TPMT activity
▸ BY MOUTH
▸ Adult: 1–3 mg/kg daily

Severe refractory eczema, intermediate TPMT activity
▸ BY MOUTH
▸ Adult: 0.5–1.5 mg/kg daily

Generalised myasthenia gravis
▸ BY MOUTH, OR BY INTRAVENOUS INJECTION, OR BY
  INTRAVENOUS INFUSION
▸ Adult: Initially 0.5–1 mg/kg daily, then increased to
  2–2.5 mg/kg daily, dose is increased over 3–4 weeks,
  azathioprine is usually started at the same time as the
  corticosteroid and allows a lower maintenance dose of
  the corticosteroid to be used, oral administration
  preferable, if not possible then can be given by
  intravenous injection (intravenous solution very
  irritant) *or* by intravenous infusion

DOSE ADJUSTMENTS DUE TO INTERACTIONS
▸ Manufacturer advises reduce dose to one-quarter of
  the usual dose with concurrent use of allopurinol.

● UNLICENSED USE Azathioprine doses given in BNF for
  suppression of transplant rejection and autoimmune
  conditions may differ from those in product literature.
  Use for severe refractory eczema is unlicensed.

● CONTRA-INDICATIONS
▸ When used for severe refractory eczema Absent thiopurine
  methyltransferase (TPMT) activity · very low thiopurine
  methyltransferase (TPMT) activity

● CAUTIONS Reduce dose in elderly · reduced thiopurine
  methyltransferase activity

● INTERACTIONS → Appendix 1: azathioprine

● SIDE-EFFECTS
GENERAL SIDE-EFFECTS
▸ **Common or very common** Bone marrow depression (dose-
  related) · increased risk of infection · leucopenia ·
  thrombocytopenia
▸ **Uncommon** Anaemia · hepatic disorders · hypersensitivity ·
  pancreatitis
▸ **Rare or very rare** Agranulocytosis · alopecia · bone marrow
  disorders · diarrhoea · gastrointestinal disorders ·
  neoplasms · photosensitivity reaction · pneumonitis ·
  severe cutaneous adverse reactions (SCARs)
▸ **Frequency not known** Nodular regenerative hyperplasia ·
  sinusoidal obstruction syndrome
SPECIFIC SIDE-EFFECTS
▸ With oral use Nausea

SIDE-EFFECTS, FURTHER INFORMATION Side-effects may
require drug withdrawal.
Hypersensitivity reactions Hypersensitivity reactions
(including malaise, dizziness, vomiting, diarrhoea, fever,
rigors, myalgia, arthralgia, rash, hypotension and renal
dysfunction) call for immediate withdrawal.
Neutropenia and thrombocytopenia Neutropenia is
dose-dependent. Management of neutropenia and
thrombocytopenia requires careful monitoring and dose
adjustment.
Nausea Nausea is common early in the course of
treatment and usually resolves after a few weeks without
an alteration in dose. Moderate nausea can be managed by
using divided daily doses, taking doses after food,
prescribing concurrent antiemetics or temporarily
reducing the dose.

● ALLERGY AND CROSS-SENSITIVITY Contra-indicated in
  hypersensitivity to mercaptopurine.

● PREGNANCY Transplant patients immunosuppressed with
  azathioprine should not discontinue it on becoming
  pregnant. However, there have been reports of premature
  birth and low-birth-weight following exposure to
  azathioprine, particularly in combination with
  corticosteroids. Spontaneous abortion has been reported
  following maternal or paternal exposure. Azathioprine is
  teratogenic in *animal* studies. The use of azathioprine

during pregnancy needs to be supervised in specialist
units. Treatment should not generally be initiated during
pregnancy.

● BREAST FEEDING Present in milk in low concentration. No
  evidence of harm in small studies—use if potential benefit
  outweighs risk.

● HEPATIC IMPAIRMENT
Dose adjustments Reduce dose.
Monitoring Monitor liver function.

● RENAL IMPAIRMENT
Dose adjustments Reduce dose.

● PRE-TREATMENT SCREENING
Thiopurine methyltransferase The enzyme thiopurine
methyltransferase (TPMT) metabolises thiopurine drugs
(azathioprine, mercaptopurine, tioguanine); the risk of
myelosuppression is increased in patients with reduced
activity of the enzyme, particularly for the few individuals
in whom TPMT activity is undetectable. Consider
measuring TPMT activity before starting azathioprine,
mercaptopurine, or tioguanine therapy. Patients with
absent TPMT activity should not receive thiopurine drugs;
those with reduced TPMT activity may be treated under
specialist supervision.

● MONITORING REQUIREMENTS
▸ Monitor for toxicity throughout treatment.
▸ Monitor full blood count weekly (more frequently with
  higher doses or if severe hepatic or renal impairment) for
  first 4 weeks (manufacturer advises weekly monitoring for
  8 weeks but evidence of practical value unsatisfactory),
  thereafter reduce frequency of monitoring to at least every
  3 months.
▸ Blood tests and monitoring for signs of myelosuppression
  are essential in long-term treatment.

● DIRECTIONS FOR ADMINISTRATION For *intravenous
  injection*, give over at least 1 minute (followed by 50 mL
  sodium chloride intravenous infusion). For *intravenous
  infusion (Imuran®)*, give intermittently in Glucose 5% *or*
  Sodium Chloride 0.9%. Reconstitute 50 mg with 5–15 mL
  Water for Injections; dilute requisite dose to a volume of
  20–200 mL with infusion fluid. Intravenous injection is
  alkaline and very irritant, intravenous route should
  therefore be used **only** if oral route not feasible.

● PATIENT AND CARER ADVICE
Bone marrow suppression Patients and their carers should be
warned to report immediately any signs or symptoms of
bone marrow suppression e.g. inexplicable bruising or
bleeding, infection.

● MEDICINAL FORMS
There can be variation in the licensing of different medicines
containing the same drug. Forms available from special-order
manufacturers include: capsule, oral suspension, oral solution

Tablet
CAUTIONARY AND ADVISORY LABELS 21
▸ Azathioprine (Non-proprietary)
  Azathioprine 25 mg Azathioprine 25mg tablets | 28 tablet [PoM]
  £8.41 DT = £1.30 | 100 tablet [PoM] £4.64–£33.26
  Azathioprine 50 mg Azathioprine 50mg tablets | 56 tablet [PoM]
  £7.28 DT = £2.20 | 100 tablet [PoM] £3.93–£16.55
▸ Azapress (Ennogen Pharma Ltd)
  Azathioprine 50 mg Azapress 50mg tablets | 56 tablet [PoM] £2.83
  DT = £2.20
▸ Imuran (Aspen Pharma Trading Ltd)
  Azathioprine 25 mg Imuran 25mg tablets | 100 tablet [PoM] £10.99
  Azathioprine 50 mg Imuran 50mg tablets | 100 tablet [PoM] £7.99

Powder for solution for injection
▸ Imuran (Aspen Pharma Trading Ltd)
  Azathioprine 50 mg Imuran 50mg powder for solution for injection
  vials | 1 vial [PoM] £15.38

IMMUNOSUPPRESSANTS › CALCINEURIN INHIBITORS AND RELATED DRUGS

Ciclosporin

(Cyclosporin)

01-Sep-2016

● **DRUG ACTION** Ciclosporin inhibits production and release of lymphokines, thereby suppressing cell-mediated immune response.

● **INDICATIONS AND DOSE**

Severe acute ulcerative colitis refractory to corticosteroid treatment
▶ BY CONTINUOUS INTRAVENOUS INFUSION
▸ Adult: 2 mg/kg, to be given over 24 hours, dose adjusted according to blood-ciclosporin concentration and response

Severe active rheumatoid arthritis when conventional second-line therapy inappropriate or ineffective (administered on expert advice)
▶ BY MOUTH
▸ Adult: Initially 2.5 mg/kg daily in 2 divided doses, increased if necessary up to 4 mg/kg daily after 6 weeks, if dose increases are necessary they should be made gradually, discontinue if response insufficient after 3 months, dose adjusted according to response for maintenance and treatment reviewed after 6 months (continue only if benefits outweigh risks)

Short-term treatment of severe atopic dermatitis where conventional therapy ineffective or inappropriate (administered on expert advice)
▶ BY MOUTH
▸ Adult: Initially 1.25 mg/kg twice daily (max. per dose 2.5 mg/kg twice daily) usual maximum duration of 8 weeks but may be used for longer under specialist supervision, if good initial response not achieved within 2 weeks, increase dose rapidly up to maximum

Short-term treatment of very severe atopic dermatitis where conventional therapy ineffective or inappropriate (administered on expert advice)
▶ BY MOUTH
▸ Adult: 2.5 mg/kg twice daily usual maximum duration of 8 weeks but may be used for longer under specialist supervision

Severe psoriasis where conventional therapy ineffective or inappropriate (administered on expert advice)
▶ BY MOUTH
▸ Adult: Initially 1.25 mg/kg twice daily (max. per dose 2.5 mg/kg twice daily), increased gradually to maximum if no improvement within 1 month, initial dose of 2.5 mg/kg twice daily justified if condition requires rapid improvement; discontinue if inadequate response after 3 months at the optimum dose; max. duration of treatment usually 1 year unless other treatments cannot be used

Organ transplantation (used alone)
▶ BY MOUTH
▸ Adult: 10–15 mg/kg, to be administered 4–12 hours before transplantation, followed by 10–15 mg/kg daily for 1–2 weeks postoperatively, then maintenance 2–6 mg/kg daily, reduce dose gradually to maintenance. Dose should be adjusted according to blood-ciclosporin concentration and renal function; dose is lower if given concomitantly with other immunosuppressant therapy (e.g. corticosteroids); if necessary one-third corresponding oral dose can be given by intravenous infusion over 2–6 hours

Bone-marrow transplantation | Prevention and treatment of graft-versus-host disease
▶ INITIALLY BY INTRAVENOUS INFUSION
▸ Adult: 3–5 mg/kg daily, to be administered over 2–6 hours from day before transplantation to 2 weeks postoperatively, alternatively (by mouth) initially 12.5–15 mg/kg daily, then (by mouth) 12.5 mg/kg daily for 3-6 months and then tailed off (may take up to a year after transplantation)

Nephrotic syndrome
▶ BY MOUTH
▸ Adult: 5 mg/kg daily in 2 divided doses, for maintenance reduce to lowest effective dose according to proteinuria and serum creatinine measurements; discontinue after 3 months if no improvement in glomerulonephritis or glomerulosclerosis (after 6 months in membranous glomerulonephritis)

DOSE ADJUSTMENTS DUE TO INTERACTIONS
▸ With oral use Manufacturer advises increase dose by 50% or switch to intravenous administration with concurrent use of octreotide.

● **UNLICENSED USE** Not licensed for use in severe acute ulcerative colitis refractory to corticosteroid treatment

> **IMPORTANT SAFETY INFORMATION**
> MHRA/CHM ADVICE: CICLOSPORIN MUST BE PRESCRIBED AND DISPENSED BY BRAND NAME (DECEMBER 2009)
> Patients should be stabilised on a particular brand of oral ciclosporin because switching between formulations without close monitoring may lead to clinically important changes in blood-ciclosporin concentration.

● **CONTRA-INDICATIONS** Abnormal baseline renal function (in non-transplant indications) · malignancy (in non-transplant indications) · uncontrolled hypertension (in non-transplant indications) · uncontrolled infections (in non-transplant indications)

● **CAUTIONS** Elderly—monitor renal function · hyperuricaemia · in atopic dermatitis, active herpes simplex infections—allow infection to clear before starting (if they occur during treatment withdraw if severe) · in atopic dermatitis, *Staphylococcus aureus* skin infections—not absolute contra-indication providing controlled (but avoid erythromycin unless no other alternative) · in psoriasis treat, patients with malignant or pre-malignant conditions of skin only after appropriate treatment (and if no other option) · in uveitis, Behcet's syndrome (monitor neurological status) · lymphoproliferative disorders (discontinue treatment) · malignancy

CAUTIONS, FURTHER INFORMATION
▸ Malignancy In psoriasis, exclude malignancies (including those of skin and cervix) before starting (biopsy any lesions not typical of psoriasis) and treat patients with malignant or pre-malignant conditions of skin only after appropriate treatment (and if no other option); discontinue if lymphoproliferative disorder develops.

● **INTERACTIONS** → Appendix 1: ciclosporin

● **SIDE-EFFECTS**
▸ **Common or very common** Appetite decreased · diarrhoea · electrolyte imbalance · fatigue · fever · flushing · gastrointestinal discomfort · gingival hyperplasia · hair changes · headaches · hepatic disorders · hyperglycaemia · hyperlipidaemia · hypertension · hyperuricaemia · leucopenia · muscle complaints · nausea · paraesthesia · peptic ulcer · renal impairment (renal structural changes on long-term administration) · seizure · skin reactions · tremor · vomiting
▸ **Uncommon** Anaemia · encephalopathy · oedema · thrombocytopenia · weight increased

▸ **Rare or very rare** Eye inflammation · gynaecomastia · haemolytic anaemia · idiopathic intracranial hypertension · menstrual disorder · multifocal motor neuropathy · muscle weakness · myopathy · pancreatitis

▸ **Frequency not known** Pain in extremity · thrombotic microangiopathy

● **PREGNANCY** Crosses placenta; manufacturer advises avoid unless potential benefit outweighs risk—toxicity in *animal* studies.

● **BREAST FEEDING** Manufacturer advises avoid—present in milk.

● **HEPATIC IMPAIRMENT**
Dose adjustments Extensively metabolised by the liver—manufacturer advises consider dose adjustment based on bilirubin and liver enzyme levels.

● **RENAL IMPAIRMENT**
Dose adjustments In non-transplant indications, manufacturer advises establishing baseline renal function before initiation of treatment; if baseline function is impaired in non-transplant indications, except nephrotic syndrome—avoid. In nephrotic syndrome, manufacturer advises initial dose should not exceed 2.5 mg/kg daily in patients with baseline renal impairment. *During treatment* for non-transplant indications, manufacturer recommends if eGFR decreases by more than 25% below baseline on more than one measurement, reduce dose by 25–50%. If the eGFR decrease from baseline exceeds 35%, further dose reduction should be considered (even if within normal range); discontinue if reduction not successful within 1 month.

● **MONITORING REQUIREMENTS**

▸ Monitor whole blood ciclosporin concentration (trough level dependent on indication—consult local treatment protocol for details).

▸ Dermatological and physical examination, including blood pressure and renal function measurements required at least twice before starting treatment for psoriasis or atopic dermatitis.

▸ Monitor liver function.

▸ Monitor serum potassium, especially in renal dysfunction (risk of hyperkalaemia).

▸ Monitor serum magnesium.

▸ Measure blood lipids before treatment and after the first month of treatment.

▸ In psoriasis and atopic dermatitis monitor serum creatinine every 2 weeks for first 3 months then every month.

▸ Investigate lymphadenopathy that persists despite improvement in atopic dermatitis.

▸ Monitor kidney function—dose dependent increase in serum creatinine and urea during first few weeks may necessitate dose reduction in transplant patients (exclude rejection if kidney transplant) or discontinuation in non-transplant patients.

▸ Monitor blood pressure—discontinue if hypertension develops that cannot be controlled by antihypertensives.

▸ In long-term management of nephrotic syndrome, perform renal biopsies at yearly intervals.

▸ In rheumatoid arthritis measure serum creatinine at least twice before treatment. During treatment, monitor serum creatinine every 2 weeks for first 3 months, then every month for a further 3 months, then every 4–8 weeks depending on the stability of the disease, concomitant medication, and concomitant diseases (or more frequently if dose increased or concomitant NSAIDs introduced or increased).

▸ Monitor hepatic function if concomitant NSAIDs given.

● **DIRECTIONS FOR ADMINISTRATION**

▸ With oral use Mix solution with orange or apple juice, or other soft drink (to improve taste) immediately before taking (and rinse with more to ensure total dose). Do not

mix with grapefruit juice. Total daily dose should be taken in 2 divided doses.

▸ With intravenous use For *intravenous infusion* (Sandimmun®), give intermittently *or* continously *in* Glucose 5% *or* Sodium Chloride 0.9%; dilute to a concentration of 50 mg in 20–100 mL; give intermittent infusion over 2–6 hours; not to be used with PVC equipment. Observe patient for signs of anaphylaxis for at least 30 minutes after starting infusion and at frequent intervals thereafter.

● **PRESCRIBING AND DISPENSING INFORMATION**
Brand name prescribing Prescribing and dispensing of ciclosporin should be by brand name to avoid inadvertent switching. If it is necessary to switch a patient to a different brand of ciclosporin, the patient should be monitored closely for changes in blood-ciclosporin concentration, serum creatinine, blood pressure, and transplant function (for transplant indications). *Sandimmun*® capsules and oral solution are available direct from Novartis for patients who cannot be transferred to a different oral preparation.

● **PATIENT AND CARER ADVICE** Patients and carers should be counselled on the administration of different formulations of ciclosporin. Manufacturer advises avoid excessive exposure to UV light, including sunlight. In psoriasis and atopic dermatitis, avoid use of UVB or PUVA.

● **MEDICINAL FORMS**
There can be variation in the licensing of different medicines containing the same drug.

Solution for infusion
CAUTIONARY AND ADVISORY LABELS 11
EXCIPIENTS: May contain Alcohol, polyoxyl castor oils

▸ Sandimmun (Novartis Pharmaceuticals UK Ltd)
Ciclosporin 50 mg per 1 ml Sandimmun 250mg/5ml concentrate for solution for infusion ampoules | 10 ampoule PoM £110.05
Sandimmun 50mg/1ml concentrate for solution for infusion ampoules | 10 ampoule PoM £23.23

Oral solution
CAUTIONARY AND ADVISORY LABELS 11
EXCIPIENTS: May contain Alcohol, propylene glycol

▸ Capsorin (Morningside Healthcare Ltd)
Ciclosporin 100 mg per 1 ml Capsorin 100mg/ml oral solution sugar-free | 50 ml PoM £86.96

▸ Neoral (Novartis Pharmaceuticals UK Ltd)
Ciclosporin 100 mg per 1 ml Neoral 100mg/ml oral solution sugar-free | 50 ml PoM £102.30

▸ Sandimmun (Novartis Pharmaceuticals UK Ltd)
Ciclosporin 100 mg per 1 ml Sandimmun 100mg/ml oral solution sugar-free | 50 ml PoM £164.72

Capsule
CAUTIONARY AND ADVISORY LABELS 11
EXCIPIENTS: May contain Ethanol, ethyl lactate, propylene glycol

▸ Ciclosporin (Non-proprietary)
Ciclosporin 25 mg Ciclosporin 25mg capsules | 30 capsule PoM ⬛
DT = £18.37
Ciclosporin 50 mg Ciclosporin 50mg capsules | 30 capsule PoM ⬛
DT = £35.97
Ciclosporin 100 mg Ciclosporin 100mg capsules |
30 capsule PoM ⬛ DT = £68.28

▸ Capimune (Mylan)
Ciclosporin 25 mg Capimune 25mg capsules | 30 capsule PoM
£13.05 DT = £18.37
Ciclosporin 50 mg Capimune 50mg capsules | 30 capsule PoM
£25.50 DT = £35.97
Ciclosporin 100 mg Capimune 100mg capsules | 30 capsule PoM
£48.50 DT = £68.28

▸ Capsorin (Morningside Healthcare Ltd)
Ciclosporin 25 mg Capsorin 25mg capsules | 30 capsule PoM
£11.14 DT = £18.37
Ciclosporin 50 mg Capsorin 50mg capsules | 30 capsule PoM
£21.80 DT = £35.97
Ciclosporin 100 mg Capsorin 100mg capsules | 30 capsule PoM
£41.59 DT = £68.28

Immune system and malignant disease

8

▶ Deximune (Dexcel-Pharma Ltd)

Ciclosporin 25 mg Deximune 25mg capsules | 30 capsule PoM
£13.06 DT = £18.37

Ciclosporin 50 mg Deximune 50mg capsules | 30 capsule PoM
£25.60 DT = £35.97

Ciclosporin 100 mg Deximune 100mg capsules | 30 capsule PoM
£48.90 DT = £68.28

▶ Neoral (Novartis Pharmaceuticals UK Ltd)

Ciclosporin 10 mg Neoral 10mg capsules | 60 capsule PoM £18.25
DT = £18.25

Ciclosporin 25 mg Neoral 25mg capsules | 30 capsule PoM £18.37
DT = £18.37

Ciclosporin 50 mg Neoral 50mg capsules | 30 capsule PoM £35.97
DT = £35.97

Ciclosporin 100 mg Neoral 100mg capsules | 30 capsule PoM
£68.28 DT = £68.28

▶ Sandimmun (Novartis Pharmaceuticals UK Ltd)

Ciclosporin 25 mg Sandimmun 25mg capsules | 30 capsule PoM
£29.58 DT = £18.37

Ciclosporin 50 mg Sandimmun 50mg capsules | 30 capsule PoM
£57.92 DT = £35.97

Ciclosporin 100 mg Sandimmun 100mg capsules | 30 capsule PoM
£109.93 DT = £68.28

▶ Vanquoral (Teva UK Ltd)

Ciclosporin 10 mg Vanquoral 10mg capsules | 60 capsule PoM
£12.75 DT = £18.25

Ciclosporin 25 mg Vanquoral 25mg capsules | 30 capsule PoM
£13.05 DT = £18.37

Ciclosporin 50 mg Vanquoral 50mg capsules | 30 capsule PoM
£25.59 DT = £35.97

Ciclosporin 100 mg Vanquoral 100mg capsule | 30 capsule PoM
£48.89 DT = £68.28

Sirolimus

16-Nov-2017

● **DRUG ACTION** Sirolimus is a non-calcineurin inhibiting immunosuppressant.

● **INDICATIONS AND DOSE**

Prophylaxis of organ rejection in kidney allograft recipients

▶ BY MOUTH

▶ Adult: Initially 6 mg for 1 dose, to be given after surgery once wound has healed, then 2 mg once daily; to be given in combination with ciclosporin and corticosteroid for 2–3 months (sirolimus doses should be given 4 hours after ciclosporin), ciclosporin should then be withdrawn over 4–8 weeks (if not possible, sirolimus should be discontinued and an alternate immunosuppressive regimen used), dose to be adjusted according to whole blood-sirolimus trough concentration

DOSE EQUIVALENCE AND CONVERSION

▶ The 500 microgram tablet is not bioequivalent to the 1 mg and 2 mg tablets. Multiples of 500 microgram tablets should **not** be used as a substitute for other tablet strengths.

● CAUTIONS Hyperlipidaemia · increased susceptibility to infection (especially urinary-tract infection) · increased susceptibility to lymphoma and other malignancies, particularly of the skin (limit exposure to UV light)

● INTERACTIONS → Appendix 1: sirolimus

● SIDE-EFFECTS

▶ **Common or very common** Abdominal pain · anaemia · arthralgia · ascites · constipation · diabetes mellitus · diarrhoea · dyslipidaemia · electrolyte imbalance · embolism and thrombosis · fever · haemolytic uraemic syndrome · haemorrhage · headache · healing impaired · hyperglycaemia · hypertension · increased risk of infection · leucopenia · lymphatic vessel disorders · menstrual cycle irregularities · nausea · neoplasms · neutropenia · oedema · osteonecrosis · ovarian cyst · pain · pancreatitis · pericardial effusion · proteinuria · respiratory disorders ·

sepsis · skin reactions · stomatitis · tachycardia · thrombocytopenia

▶ **Uncommon** Antibiotic associated colitis · focal segmental glomerulosclerosis · hepatic failure · nephrotic syndrome · pancytopenia · post transplant lymphoproliferative disorder

▶ **Frequency not known** Posterior reversible encephalopathy syndrome (PRES)

● CONCEPTION AND CONTRACEPTION Effective contraception must be used during treatment and for 12 weeks after stopping.

● PREGNANCY Avoid unless essential—toxicity in *animal* studies.

● BREAST FEEDING Discontinue breast-feeding.

● HEPATIC IMPAIRMENT Clearance reduced in mild to moderate impairment.
Dose adjustments In severe impairment decrease dose by 50% and monitor whole blood-sirolimus trough concentration every 5–7 days until 3 consecutive measurements have shown stable blood-sirolimus concentration.
Monitoring Monitor whole blood-sirolimus level closely and consult local treatment protocol in hepatic impairment.

● MONITORING REQUIREMENTS

▶ Monitor whole blood-sirolimus trough concentration (Afro-Caribbean patients may require higher doses).

▶ Manufacturer advises pre-dose ('trough') whole blood-sirolimus concentration (using **chromatographic** assay) when used with ciclosporin should be 4–12 micrograms/litre (local treatment protocols may differ); after withdrawal of ciclosporin pre-dose whole blood-sirolimus concentration should be 12–20 micrograms/litre (local treatment protocols may differ).

▶ Close monitoring of whole blood-sirolimus concentration required if concomitant treatment with potent inducers or inhibitors of metabolism and after discontinuing them, or if ciclosporin dose reduced significantly or stopped.

▶ When changing between oral solution and tablets, measurement of whole blood 'trough' sirolimus concentration after 1–2 weeks is recommended.

▶ Therapeutic drug monitoring assays Sirolimus whole-blood concentration is measured using either high performance liquid chromatography (HPLC) or immunoassay. Switching between different immunoassays or between an immunoassay and HPLC can lead to clinically significant differences in results and therefore incorrect dose adjustments. Adjustment to the target therapeutic dose range should be made with knowledge of the assay used and corresponding reference range.

▶ Monitor kidney function when given with ciclosporin; monitor lipids; monitor urine proteins.

● DIRECTIONS FOR ADMINISTRATION Food may affect absorption (take at the same time with respect to food). Sirolimus oral solution should be mixed with at least 60 mL water or orange juice in a glass or plastic container immediately before taking; refill container with at least 120 mL of water or orange juice and drink immediately (to ensure total dose). Do not mix with any other liquids.

● PATIENT AND CARER ADVICE Patient or carers should be given advice on how to administer sirolimus.
Patients should be advised to avoid excessive exposure to UV light.

● NATIONAL FUNDING/ACCESS DECISIONS

NICE decisions

▶ **Immunosuppressive therapy for kidney transplant in adults (October 2017)** NICE TA481
Sirolimus is not recommended as an initial treatment to prevent organ rejection in adults having a kidney transplant. Patients whose treatment was started within

the NHS before this guidance was published should have the option to continue treatment, without change to their funding arrangements, until they and their NHS clinician consider it appropriate to stop.
www.nice.org.uk/guidance/TA481

● MEDICINAL FORMS
There can be variation in the licensing of different medicines containing the same drug.

Oral solution
EXCIPIENTS: May contain Ethanol
▸ Rapamune (Pfizer Ltd)
  Sirolimus 1 mg per 1 ml Rapamune 1mg/ml oral solution sugar-free | 60 ml [PoM] £162.41

Tablet
▸ Rapamune (Pfizer Ltd)
  Sirolimus 500 microgram Rapamune 0.5mg tablets | 30 tablet [PoM] £69.00 DT = £69.00
  Sirolimus 1 mg Rapamune 1mg tablets | 30 tablet [PoM] £86.49 = £86.49
  Sirolimus 2 mg Rapamune 2mg tablets | 30 tablet [PoM] £172.98 DT = £172.98

Tacrolimus
19-Mar-2018

● DRUG ACTION Tacrolimus is a calcineurin inhibitor.

● INDICATIONS AND DOSE

ADOPORT®
Prophylaxis of graft rejection following liver transplantation, starting 12 hours after transplantation
▸ BY MOUTH
▸ Adult: Initially 100–200 micrograms/kg daily in 2 divided doses

Prophylaxis of graft rejection following kidney transplantation, starting within 24 hours of transplantation
▸ BY MOUTH
▸ Adult: Initially 200–300 micrograms/kg daily in 2 divided doses

Prophylaxis of graft rejection following heart transplantation following antibody induction, starting within 5 days of transplantation
▸ BY MOUTH
▸ Adult: Initially 75 micrograms/kg daily in 2 divided doses

Prophylaxis of graft rejection following heart transplantation without antibody induction, starting within 12 hours of transplantation
▸ BY MOUTH
▸ Adult: Initially 75 micrograms/kg daily in 2 divided doses

Allograft rejection resistant to conventional immunosuppressive therapy
▸ BY MOUTH
▸ Adult: Seek specialist advice

ADVAGRAF®
Prophylaxis of graft rejection following liver transplantation, starting 12–18 hours after transplantation
▸ BY MOUTH
▸ Adult: Initially 100–200 micrograms/kg once daily, to be taken in the morning

Prophylaxis of graft rejection following kidney transplantation, starting within 24 hours of transplantation
▸ BY MOUTH
▸ Adult: Initially 200–300 micrograms/kg once daily, to be taken in the morning

Allograft rejection resistant to conventional immunosuppressive therapy
▸ BY MOUTH
▸ Adult: Seek specialist advice

CAPEXION®
Prophylaxis of graft rejection following liver transplantation, starting 12 hours after transplantation
▸ BY MOUTH
▸ Adult: Initially 100–200 micrograms/kg daily in 2 divided doses

Prophylaxis of graft rejection following kidney transplantation, starting within 24 hours of transplantation
▸ BY MOUTH
▸ Adult: Initially 200–300 micrograms/kg daily in 2 divided doses

Prophylaxis of graft rejection following heart transplantation following antibody induction, starting within 5 days of transplantation
▸ BY MOUTH
▸ Adult: Initially 75 micrograms/kg daily in 2 divided doses

Prophylaxis of graft rejection following heart transplantation without antibody induction, starting within 12 hours of transplantation
▸ BY MOUTH
▸ Adult: Initially 75 micrograms/kg daily in 2 divided doses

Allograft rejection resistant to conventional immunosuppressive therapy
▸ BY MOUTH
▸ Adult: Seek specialist advice

ENVARSUS® MODIFIED-RELEASE TABLETS
Prophylaxis of graft rejection following liver transplantation, starting within 24 hours of transplantation
▸ BY MOUTH
▸ Adult: Initially 110–130 micrograms/kg once daily, to be taken in the morning

Prophylaxis of graft rejection following renal transplantation, starting within 24 hours of transplantation
▸ BY MOUTH
▸ Adult: Initially 170 micrograms/kg once daily, to be taken in the morning

Rejection therapy
▸ BY MOUTH
▸ Adult: Seek specialist advice

MODIGRAF®
Prophylaxis of graft rejection following liver transplantation, starting 12 hours after transplantation
▸ BY MOUTH
▸ Adult: Initially 100–200 micrograms/kg daily in 2 divided doses

Prophylaxis of graft rejection following kidney transplantation, starting within 24 hours of transplantation
▸ BY MOUTH
▸ Adult: Initially 200–300 micrograms/kg daily in 2 divided doses

Prophylaxis of graft rejection following heart transplantation following antibody induction, starting within 5 days of transplantation
▸ BY MOUTH
▸ Adult: Initially 75 micrograms/kg daily in 2 divided doses

continued →

Prophylaxis of graft rejection following heart transplantation without antibody induction, starting within 12 hours of transplantation
▸ BY MOUTH
▸ Adult: Initially 75 micrograms/kg daily in 2 divided doses

Rejection therapy
▸ BY MOUTH
▸ Adult: Seek specialist advice

PROGRAF ® CAPSULES

Prophylaxis of graft rejection following liver transplantation, starting 12 hours after transplantation
▸ BY MOUTH
▸ Adult: Initially 100–200 micrograms/kg daily in 2 divided doses

Prophylaxis of graft rejection following kidney transplantation, starting within 24 hours of transplantation
▸ BY MOUTH
▸ Adult: Initially 200–300 micrograms/kg daily in 2 divided doses

Prophylaxis of graft rejection following heart transplantation following antibody induction, starting within 5 days of transplantation
▸ BY MOUTH
▸ Adult: Initially 75 micrograms/kg daily in 2 divided doses

Prophylaxis of graft rejection following heart transplantation without antibody induction, starting within 12 hours of transplantation
▸ BY MOUTH
▸ Adult: Initially 75 micrograms/kg daily in 2 divided doses

Allograft rejection resistant to conventional immunosuppressive therapy
▸ BY MOUTH
▸ Adult: Seek specialist advice

PROGRAF ® INFUSION

Prophylaxis of graft rejection following liver transplantation, starting 12 hours after transplantation when oral route not appropriate
▸ BY INTRAVENOUS INFUSION
▸ Adult: Initially 10–50 micrograms/kg daily for up to 7 days (then transfer to oral therapy), dose to be administered over 24 hours

Prophylaxis of graft rejection following kidney transplantation, starting within 24 hours of transplantation when oral route not appropriate
▸ BY INTRAVENOUS INFUSION
▸ Adult: Initially 50–100 micrograms/kg daily for up to 7 days (then transfer to oral therapy), dose to be administered over 24 hours

Prophylaxis of graft rejection following heart transplantation following antibody induction, starting within 5 days of transplantation
▸ BY INTRAVENOUS INFUSION
▸ Adult: Initially 10–20 micrograms/kg daily for up to 7 days (then transfer to oral therapy), dose to be administered over 24 hours

Prophylaxis of graft rejection following heart transplantation without antibody induction, starting within 12 hours of transplantation
▸ BY INTRAVENOUS INFUSION
▸ Adult: Initially 10–20 micrograms/kg daily for up to 7 days (then transfer to oral therapy), dose to be administered over 24 hours

Allograft rejection resistant to conventional immunosuppressive therapy
▸ BY CONTINUOUS INTRAVENOUS INFUSION
▸ Adult: Seek specialist advice (consult local protocol)

TACNI ®

Prophylaxis of graft rejection following liver transplantation, starting 12 hours after transplantation
▸ BY MOUTH
▸ Adult: Initially 100–200 micrograms/kg daily in 2 divided doses

Prophylaxis of graft rejection following kidney transplantation, starting within 24 hours of transplantation
▸ BY MOUTH
▸ Adult: Initially 200–300 micrograms/kg daily in 2 divided doses

Prophylaxis of graft rejection following heart transplantation following antibody induction, starting within 5 days of transplantation
▸ BY MOUTH
▸ Adult: Initially 75 micrograms/kg daily in 2 divided doses

Prophylaxis of graft rejection following heart transplantation without antibody induction, starting within 12 hours of transplantation
▸ BY MOUTH
▸ Adult: Initially 75 micrograms/kg daily in 2 divided doses

Allograft rejection resistant to conventional immunosuppressive therapy
▸ BY MOUTH
▸ Adult: Seek specialist advice

VIVADEX ®

Prophylaxis of graft rejection following liver transplantation, starting 12 hours after transplantation
▸ BY MOUTH
▸ Adult: Initially 100–200 micrograms/kg daily in 2 divided doses

Prophylaxis of graft rejection following kidney transplantation, starting within 24 hours of transplantation
▸ BY MOUTH
▸ Adult: Initially 200–300 micrograms/kg daily in 2 divided doses

Prophylaxis of graft rejection following heart transplantation following antibody induction, starting within 5 days of transplantation
▸ BY MOUTH
▸ Adult: Initially 75 micrograms/kg daily in 2 divided doses

Prophylaxis of graft rejection following heart transplantation without antibody induction, starting within 12 hours of transplantation
▸ BY MOUTH
▸ Adult: Initially 75 micrograms/kg daily in 2 divided doses

Allograft rejection resistant to conventional immunosuppressive therapy
▸ BY MOUTH
▸ Adult: Seek specialist advice

IMPORTANT SAFETY INFORMATION

MHRA/CHM ADVICE: ORAL TACROLIMUS PRODUCTS: PRESCRIBE AND DISPENSE BY BRAND NAME ONLY, TO MINIMISE THE RISK OF INADVERTENT SWITCHING BETWEEN PRODUCTS, WHICH HAS BEEN ASSOCIATED WITH REPORTS OF TOXICITY AND GRAFT REJECTION (JUNE 2012)

Inadvertent switching between oral tacrolimus products has been associated with reports of toxicity and graft rejection. To ensure maintenance of therapeutic response when a patient is stabilised on a particular brand, oral tacrolimus products should be prescribed and dispensed by brand name only.

- *Adoport*®, *Prograf*®, *Capexion*®, *Tacni*®, and *Vivadex*® are immediate-release capsules that are taken twice daily, once in the morning and once in the evening;
- *Modigraf*® granules are used to prepare an immediate-release oral suspension which is taken twice daily, once in the morning and once in the evening;
- *Advagraf*® is a prolonged-release capsule that is taken once daily in the morning.

Switching between tacrolimus brands requires careful supervision and therapeutic monitoring by an appropriate specialist.

Important: *Envarsus*® is not interchangeable with other oral tacrolimus containing products; the MHRA has advised (June 2012) that oral tacrolimus products should be prescribed and dispensed by brand only.

- **CAUTIONS** Increased risk of infections · lymphoproliferative disorders · malignancies · neurotoxicity · QT-interval prolongation · UV light (avoid excessive exposure to sunlight and sunlamps)
- **INTERACTIONS** → Appendix 1: tacrolimus
- **SIDE-EFFECTS**

GENERAL SIDE-EFFECTS

- **Common or very common** Alopecia · anaemia · anxiety · appetite decreased · arrhythmias · ascites · asthenic conditions · bile duct disorders · confusion · consciousness impaired · constipation · coronary artery disease · cough · depression · diabetes mellitus · diarrhoea · dizziness · dysgraphia · dyslipidaemia · dyspnoea · electrolyte imbalance · embolism and thrombosis · eye disorder · febrile disorders · fluid imbalance · gastrointestinal discomfort · gastrointestinal disorders · gastrointestinal inflammatory disorders · haemorrhage · hallucination · headache · hearing impairment · hepatic disorders · hyperglycaemia · hyperhidrosis · hypertension · hyperuricaemia · hypotension · increased risk of infection · ischaemia · joint disorders · leucocytosis · leucopenia · metabolic acidosis · mood altered · muscle spasms · nasal complaints · nausea · nephropathy · nervous system disorder · oedema · oral disorders · pain · peripheral neuropathy · peripheral vascular disease · primary transplant dysfunction · psychiatric disorder · renal impairment · renal tubular necrosis · respiratory disorders · seizure · sensation abnormal · skin reactions · sleep disorders · temperature sensation altered · thrombocytopenia · tremor · urinary tract disorder · urine abnormal · vision disorders · vomiting · weight changes
- **Uncommon** Asthma · cardiac arrest · cardiomyopathy · cataract · central nervous system haemorrhage · chest discomfort · coagulation disorders · coma · dysmenorrhoea · encephalopathy · feeling abnormal · haemolytic anaemia · heart failure · hypoglycaemia · hypoproteinaemia · influenza like illness · memory loss · multi organ failure · neutropenia · palpitations · pancreatitis · pancytopenia · paralysis · paresis · photosensitivity reaction · psychotic disorder · shock · speech disorder · stroke · ventricular hypertrophy
- **Rare or very rare** Fall · hirsutism · mobility decreased · muscle tone increased · muscle weakness · pancreatic pseudocyst · pericardial effusion · QT interval prolongation · severe cutaneous adverse reactions (SCARs) · sinusoidal obstruction syndrome · thirst · ulcer
- **Frequency not known** Agranulocytosis · malignancy · neoplasms · polyomavirus-associated nephropathy · progressive multifocal leukoencephalopathy · pure red cell aplasia

SPECIFIC SIDE-EFFECTS

- With intravenous use Anaphylactoid reaction (due to excipient) · hypersensitivity

SIDE-EFFECTS, FURTHER INFORMATION Cardiomyopathy has been reported to occur primarily in children with tacrolimus blood trough concentrations much higher than the recommended maximum levels. Patients should be monitored by echocardiography for hypertrophic changes—consider dose reduction or discontinuation if these occur.

- **ALLERGY AND CROSS-SENSITIVITY** Contra-indicated if history of hypersensitivity to macrolides.
- **CONCEPTION AND CONTRACEPTION** Exclude pregnancy before treatment.
- **PREGNANCY** Avoid unless potential benefit outweighs risk—crosses the placenta and risk of premature delivery, intra-uterine growth restriction, and hyperkalaemia.
- **BREAST FEEDING** Avoid—present in breast milk (following systemic administration).
- **HEPATIC IMPAIRMENT**
  Dose adjustments Dose reduction may be necessary in severe impairment.
- **MONITORING REQUIREMENTS**
- After initial dosing, and for maintenance treatment, tacrolimus doses should be adjusted according to whole-blood concentration. Monitor whole blood-tacrolimus trough concentration (especially during episodes of diarrhoea)—consult local treatment protocol for details.
- Monitor blood pressure, ECG (for hypertrophic changes—risk of cardiomyopathy), fasting blood-glucose concentration, haematological and neurological (including visual) and coagulation parameters, electrolytes, hepatic and renal function.
- **DIRECTIONS FOR ADMINISTRATION** For *intravenous infusion* (*Prograf*®); give continuously in Glucose 5% *or* Sodium Chloride 0.9%. Dilute concentrate in infusion fluid to a final concentration of 4–100 micrograms/mL; give over 24 hours. Tacrolimus is incompatible with PVC.
- **PATIENT AND CARER ADVICE** Avoid excessive exposure to UV light including sunlight.
  Driving and skilled tasks May affect performance of skilled tasks (e.g. driving).
- **NATIONAL FUNDING/ACCESS DECISIONS**

NICE decisions

- **Immunosuppressive therapy for kidney transplant in adults (October 2017) NICE TA481**
  Immediate-release tacrolimus, when used as part of an immunosuppressive regimen, is recommended as an initial option to prevent organ rejection in adults having a kidney transplant. Treatment should be started with the least expensive product, but if this is not suitable, an alternative dosage form may be given. Tacrolimus granules for oral suspension (*Modigraf*®) should be used only if the manufacturer provides it at the same price or lower than that agreed with the Commercial Medicines Unit. Patients whose treatment was started within the NHS before this guidance was published should have the option to continue treatment, without change to their funding arrangements, until they and their NHS clinician consider it appropriate to stop.
  www.nice.org.uk/guidance/TA481
- **Immunosuppressive therapy for kidney transplant in adults (October 2017) NICE TA481**
  Prolonged-release tacrolimus is not recommended as an initial treatment to prevent organ rejection in adults having a kidney transplant. Patients whose treatment was started within the NHS before this guidance was published should have the option to continue treatment, without

change to their funding arrangements, until they and their NHS clinician consider it appropriate to stop.
www.nice.org.uk/guidance/TA481

Scottish Medicines Consortium (SMC) Decisions
The *Scottish Medicines Consortium* has advised (December 2010) that tacrolimus granules for suspension (*Modigraf*®) are accepted for restricted use within NHS Scotland in patients for whom tacrolimus is an appropriate choice of immunosuppressive therapy and where small changes (less than 500 micrograms) in dosing increments are required (such as, in paediatric patients) or in seriously ill patients who are unable to swallow tacrolimus capsules.

The *Scottish Medicines Consortium* has advised (April 2015) that tacrolimus (*Envarsus*®) is accepted for use in NHS Scotland for prophylaxis of graft rejection and treatment of rejection resistant to treatment with other immunosuppressive medicinal products in adults.

● MEDICINAL FORMS
There can be variation in the licensing of different medicines containing the same drug.

Modified-release tablet
▸ Envarsus (Chiesi Ltd)
Tacrolimus (as Tacrolimus monohydrate)
750 microgram Envarsus 750microgram modified-release tablets | 30 tablet [PoM] £44.33
Tacrolimus (as Tacrolimus monohydrate) 1 mg Envarsus 1mg modified-release tablets | 30 tablet [PoM] £59.10
Tacrolimus (as Tacrolimus monohydrate) 4 mg Envarsus 4mg modified-release tablets | 30 tablet [PoM] £236.40

Granules
CAUTIONARY AND ADVISORY LABELS 13, 23
▸ Modigraf (Astellas Pharma Ltd)
Tacrolimus (as Tacrolimus monohydrate)
200 microgram Modigraf 0.2mg granules sachets sugar-free | 50 sachet [PoM] £71.30 DT = £71.30
Tacrolimus (as Tacrolimus monohydrate) 1 mg Modigraf 1mg granules sachets sugar-free | 50 sachet [PoM] £356.65 DT = £356.65

Modified-release capsule
CAUTIONARY AND ADVISORY LABELS 23, 25
▸ Advagraf (Astellas Pharma Ltd)
Tacrolimus (as Tacrolimus monohydrate)
500 microgram Advagraf 0.5mg modified-release capsules | 50 capsule [PoM] £35.79
Tacrolimus (as Tacrolimus monohydrate) 1 mg Advagraf 1mg modified-release capsules | 50 capsule [PoM] £71.59 | 100 capsule [PoM] £143.17
Tacrolimus (as Tacrolimus monohydrate) 3 mg Advagraf 3mg modified-release capsules | 50 capsule [PoM] £214.76 DT = £214.76
Tacrolimus (as Tacrolimus monohydrate) 5 mg Advagraf 5mg modified-release capsules | 50 capsule [PoM] £266.92 DT = £266.92

Solution for infusion
EXCIPIENTS: May contain Polyoxyl castor oils
▸ Prograf (Astellas Pharma Ltd)
Tacrolimus 5 mg per 1 ml Prograf 5mg/1ml solution for infusion ampoules | 10 ampoule [PoM] £584.51

Capsule
CAUTIONARY AND ADVISORY LABELS 23
▸ Adoport (Sandoz Ltd)
Tacrolimus 500 microgram Adoport 0.5mg capsules | 50 capsule [PoM] £42.92 DT = £61.88
Tacrolimus 1 mg Adoport 1mg capsules | 50 capsule [PoM] £55.69 DT = £80.28 | 100 capsule [PoM] £111.36
Tacrolimus 5 mg Adoport 5mg capsules | 50 capsule [PoM] £205.74 DT = £296.58
▸ Capexion (Mylan)
Tacrolimus 500 microgram Capexion 0.5mg capsules | 50 capsule [PoM] £52.50 DT = £61.88
▸ Prograf (Astellas Pharma Ltd)
Tacrolimus 500 microgram Prograf 500microgram capsules | 50 capsule [PoM] £61.88 DT = £61.88
Tacrolimus 1 mg Prograf 1mg capsules | 50 capsule [PoM] £80.28 DT = £80.28 | 100 capsule [PoM] £160.54
Tacrolimus 5 mg Prograf 5mg capsules | 50 capsule [PoM] £296.58 DT = £296.58

▸ Tacni (Teva UK Ltd)
Tacrolimus 500 microgram Tacni 0.5mg capsules | 50 capsule [PoM] £50.48 DT = £61.88
Tacrolimus 1 mg Tacni 1mg capsules | 50 capsule [PoM] £65.49 DT = £80.28 | 100 capsule [PoM] £130.99
Tacrolimus 5 mg Tacni 5mg capsules | 50 capsule [PoM] £242.01 DT = £296.58

IMMUNOSUPPRESSANTS › MONOCLONAL ANTIBODIES

Canakinumab

● DRUG ACTION Canakinumab is a recombinant human monoclonal antibody that selectively inhibits interleukin-1 beta receptor binding.

● INDICATIONS AND DOSE
Acute gout in patients whose condition has not responded adequately to treatment with NSAIDs or colchicine, or who are intolerant of them
▸ BY SUBCUTANEOUS INJECTION
▸ Adult: 150 mg for 1 dose, dose may be repeated at least 12 weeks after initial response if symptoms recur, patients who do not respond to initial dose should not be retreated

Treatment of cryopyrin-associated periodic syndromes, including severe forms of familial cold auto-inflammatory syndrome (or familial cold urticaria), Muckle-Wells syndrome, and neonatal-onset multisystem inflammatory disease (also known as chronic infantile neurological cutaneous and articular syndrome)
▸ BY SUBCUTANEOUS INJECTION
▸ Adult: (consult product literature)

● CONTRA-INDICATIONS Active infection · leucopenia · neutropenia

● CAUTIONS History of recurrent infection · latent and active tuberculosis · predisposition to infection
CAUTIONS, FURTHER INFORMATION
▸ Vaccinations Patients should receive all recommended vaccinations (including pneumococcal and inactivated influenza vaccine) before starting treatment; avoid live vaccines unless potential benefit outweighs risk—consult product literature for further information.

● INTERACTIONS → Appendix 1: monoclonal antibodies

● SIDE-EFFECTS
▸ Common or very common Abdominal pain upper · arthralgia · asthenia · dizziness · increased risk of infection · leucopenia · neutropenia · pain · proteinuria · vertigo
▸ Uncommon Gastrooesophageal reflux disease

● CONCEPTION AND CONTRACEPTION Effective contraception required during treatment and for up to 3 months after last dose.

● PREGNANCY Manufacturer advises avoid unless potential benefit outweighs risk.

● BREAST FEEDING Consider if benefit outweighs risk—not known if present in human milk.

● HEPATIC IMPAIRMENT No information available.

● RENAL IMPAIRMENT Limited information available but manufacturer advises no dose adjustment required.

● PRE-TREATMENT SCREENING Patients should be evaluated for latent and active tuberculosis before starting treatment.

● MONITORING REQUIREMENTS
▸ Monitor full blood count including neutrophil count before starting treatment, 1–2 months after starting treatment, and periodically thereafter.
▸ Monitor for signs and symptoms of tuberculosis during and after treatment.

- **MEDICINAL FORMS**
There can be variation in the licensing of different medicines containing the same drug.
Solution for injection
  - Ilaris (Novartis Pharmaceuticals UK Ltd)
  Canakinumab 150 mg per 1 ml Ilaris 150mg/1ml solution for injection vials | 1 vial [PoM] £9,927.80

IMMUNOSUPPRESSANTS > MONOCLONAL ANTIBODIES > ANTI-LYMPHOCYTE

Basiliximab

16-Nov-2017

- **DRUG ACTION** Basiliximab is a monoclonal antibody that acts as an interleukin-2 receptor antagonist and prevents T-lymphocyte proliferation.

- **INDICATIONS AND DOSE**
Prophylaxis of acute rejection in allogeneic renal transplantation used in combination with ciclosporin and corticosteroid-containing immunosuppression regimens (specialist use only)
  - BY INTRAVENOUS INJECTION, OR BY INTRAVENOUS INFUSION
  - Adult: Initially 20 mg, administered within 2 hours before transplant surgery, followed by 20 mg after 4 days, dose to be administered after surgery, withhold second dose if severe hypersensitivity or graft loss occurs

- **CAUTIONS** Off-label use in cardiac transplantation—increased risk of serious cardiac side-effects
- **INTERACTIONS** → Appendix 1: monoclonal antibodies
- **SIDE-EFFECTS** Anaemia · capillary leak syndrome · constipation · cytokine release syndrome · diarrhoea · dyspnoea · electrolyte imbalance · headache · heart failure · hypercholesterolaemia · hypersensitivity · hypertension · hypotension · increased risk of infection · myocardial infarction · nausea · pain · peripheral oedema · post procedural wound complication · pulmonary oedema · respiratory disorders · skin reactions · sneezing · tachycardia · weight increased
- **CONCEPTION AND CONTRACEPTION** Adequate contraception must be used during treatment and for 16 weeks after last dose.
- **PREGNANCY** Manufacturer advises avoid—no information available.
- **BREAST FEEDING** Manufacturer advises avoid—no information available.
- **DIRECTIONS FOR ADMINISTRATION** For *intravenous infusion* (*Simulect*®) give intermittently in Glucose 5% or Sodium chloride 0.9%; reconstitute 10 mg with 2.5 mL water for injections then dilute to at least 25 mL with infusion fluid; reconstitute 20 mg with 5 mL water for injections then dilute to at least 50 mL with infusion fluid; give over 20-30 minutes.
- **NATIONAL FUNDING/ACCESS DECISIONS**
  NICE decisions
  - **Immunosuppressive therapy for kidney transplant in adults (October 2017) NICE TA481**
  Basiliximab, when used as part of an immunosuppressive regimen that includes a calcineurin inhibitor, is recommended as an initial option to prevent organ rejection in adults having a kidney transplant. The use of basiliximab with tacrolimus is outside the terms of the marketing authorisation. If this combination is prescribed, the prescriber should follow relevant professional guidance, taking full responsibility for the decision. Informed consent should be obtained and documented.
      Patients whose treatment was started within the NHS before this guidance was published should have the option to continue treatment, without change to their funding

arrangements, until they and their NHS clinician consider it appropriate to stop.
www.nice.org.uk/guidance/TA481

- **MEDICINAL FORMS**
There can be variation in the licensing of different medicines containing the same drug.
Powder and solvent for solution for injection
  - Simulect (Novartis Pharmaceuticals UK Ltd)
  Basiliximab 10 mg Simulect 10mg powder and solvent for solution for injection vials | 1 vial [PoM] £758.69 (Hospital only)
  Basiliximab 20 mg Simulect 20mg powder and solvent for solution for injection vials | 1 vial [PoM] £842.38 (Hospital only)

Belimumab

24-Oct-2016

- **INDICATIONS AND DOSE**
Adjunctive therapy in patients with active, autoantibody-positive systemic lupus erythematosus with a high degree of disease activity despite standard therapy
  - BY INTRAVENOUS INFUSION
  - Adult: 10 mg/kg every 2 weeks for 3 doses, then 10 mg/kg every 4 weeks, review treatment if no response within 6 months

- **CAUTIONS** Do not initiate until active infections controlled · history or development of malignancy · predisposition to infection
- **INTERACTIONS** → Appendix 1: monoclonal antibodies
- **SIDE-EFFECTS**
  - **Common or very common** Cystitis · depression · diarrhoea · fever · hypersensitivity · increased risk of infection · insomnia · leucopenia · migraine · nausea · pain in extremity
  - **Uncommon** Angioedema · skin reactions
  - **Frequency not known** Progressive multifocal leukoencephalopathy · vomiting
  SIDE-EFFECTS, FURTHER INFORMATION Infusion-related side-effects are reported commonly, including severe or life-threatening hypersensitivity and infusion reactions. Premedication with an antihistamine, with or without an antipyretic may be considered.
- **CONCEPTION AND CONTRACEPTION** Manufacturer advises adequate contraception during treatment and for at least 4 months after last dose.
- **PREGNANCY** Avoid unless essential.
- **BREAST FEEDING** Avoid—present in milk in *animal* studies.
- **RENAL IMPAIRMENT** Caution in severe impairment—no information available.
- **MONITORING REQUIREMENTS** Delay in the onset of acute hypersensitivity reactions has been observed; patients should remain under clinical supervision for several hours following at least the first 2 infusions.
- **DIRECTIONS FOR ADMINISTRATION** For *intravenous infusion* (*Benlysta*®), give intermittently in Sodium chloride 0.9%; reconstitute with water for injections (120 mg in 1.5 mL, 400 mg in 4.8 mL) to produce a solution containing 80 mg/mL; gently swirl vial for 60 seconds, then allow to stand; swirl vial (without shaking) for 60 seconds every 5 minutes until dissolved; dilute requisite dose with infusion fluid to a final volume of 250 mL and give over 1 hour.
- **NATIONAL FUNDING/ACCESS DECISIONS**
  NICE decisions
  - **Belimumab for treating active autoantibody-positive systemic lupus erythematosus (June 2016) NICE TA397**
  Belimumab is recommended as an add-on treatment option in adults with active autoantibody-positive systemic lupus erythematosus, only if all of the following criteria apply:

- there is evidence for serological disease activity (defined as positive anti-double-stranded DNA and low complement) and a Safety of Estrogen in Lupus National Assessment – Systemic Lupus Erythematosus Disease Activity Index (SELENA-SLEDAI) score of greater than or equal to 10 despite standard therapy;
- treatment with belimumab is continued after 24 weeks only if the SELENA-SLEDAI score has improved by 4 points or more;
- the manufacturer provides belimumab with the discount agreed in the patient access scheme; **and**
- under the conditions specified in the NICE managed access agreement documentation.

Patients whose treatment was started before this guidance was published should continue treatment until they and their clinician consider it appropriate to stop.
www.nice.org.uk/TA397

Scottish Medicines Consortium (SMC) Decisions
The *Scottish Medicines Consortium* has advised (May 2017) that belimumab (*Benlysta®*) is accepted for restricted use within NHS Scotland as adjunctive therapy in patients with active, autoantibody-positive systemic lupus erythematosus with a high degree of disease activity despite standard therapy, and who have evidence of serological disease activity and a Safety of Estrogens in Lupus Erythematosus National Assessment–Systemic Lupus Erythematosus Disease Activity Index (SELENA-SLEDAI) score of 10 or greater. This advice is contingent upon the continuing availability of the Patient Access Scheme in NHS Scotland or a list price that is equivalent or lower.

- ● MEDICINAL FORMS
There can be variation in the licensing of different medicines containing the same drug.
Powder for solution for infusion
  - Benlysta (GlaxoSmithKline UK Ltd) ▼
  Belimumab 120 mg Benlysta 120mg powder for concentrate for solution for infusion vials | 1 vial [PoM] £121.50 (Hospital only)
  Belimumab 400 mg Benlysta 400mg powder for concentrate for solution for infusion vials | 1 vial [PoM] £405.00 (Hospital only)

IMMUNOSUPPRESSANTS > PURINE SYNTHESIS INHIBITORS

Mycophenolate mofetil
09-Mar-2018

- ● INDICATIONS AND DOSE
Prophylaxis of acute rejection in renal transplantation (in combination with a corticosteroid and ciclosporin) (under expert supervision)
  - ▸ BY MOUTH
  - ▸ Adult: 1 g twice daily, to be started within 72 hours of transplantation
  - ▸ BY INTRAVENOUS INFUSION
  - ▸ Adult: 1 g twice daily for maximum 14 days, then transfer to oral therapy, to be started within 24 hours of transplantation

Prophylaxis of acute rejection in cardiac transplantation (in combination with ciclosporin and corticosteroids) (under expert supervision)
  - ▸ BY MOUTH
  - ▸ Adult: 1.5 g twice daily, to be started within 5 days of transplantation

Prophylaxis of acute rejection in hepatic transplantation (in combination with ciclosporin and corticosteroids) (under expert supervision)
  - ▸ INITIALLY BY INTRAVENOUS INFUSION
  - ▸ Adult: 1 g twice daily for 4 days, up to a maximum of 14 days, to be started within 24 hours of

transplantation, then (by mouth) 1.5 g twice daily, the dose route should be changed as soon as is tolerated

CEPTAVA ®
Renal transplantation (specialist use only)
  - ▸ BY MOUTH
  - ▸ Adult: 720 mg twice daily, to be started within 72 hours of transplantation

DOSE EQUIVALENCE AND CONVERSION
  - ▸ For *Ceptava®*: mycophenolic acid 720 mg is approximately equivalent to mycophenolate mofetil 1 g but avoid unnecessary switching because of pharmacokinetic differences.

MYFORTIC ®
Renal transplantation (specialist use only)
  - ▸ BY MOUTH
  - ▸ Adult: 720 mg twice daily, to be started within 72 hours of transplantation

DOSE EQUIVALENCE AND CONVERSION
  - ▸ For *Myfortic®*: mycophenolic acid 720 mg is approximately equivalent to mycophenolate mofetil 1 g but avoid unnecessary switching because of pharmacokinetic differences.

> IMPORTANT SAFETY INFORMATION
> MHRA/CHM ADVICE: MYCOPHENOLATE MOFETIL, MYCOPHENOLIC ACID: UPDATED CONTRACEPTION ADVICE FOR MALE PATIENTS (FEBRUARY 2018)
> Available clinical evidence does not indicate an increased risk of malformations or miscarriage in pregnancies where the father was taking mycophenolate medicines, however mycophenolate mofetil and mycophenolic acid are genotoxic and a risk cannot be fully excluded; for further information, see Conception and contraception and Patient and carer advice.

- ● CAUTIONS Active serious gastro-intestinal disease (risk of haemorrhage, ulceration and perforation) · children (higher incidence of side-effects may call for temporary reduction of dose or interruption) · delayed graft function · elderly (increased risk of infection, gastro-intestinal haemorrhage and pulmonary oedema) · increased susceptibility to skin cancer (avoid exposure to strong sunlight) · risk of hypogammaglobulinaemia or bronchiectasis when used in combination with other immunosuppressants

CAUTIONS, FURTHER INFORMATION
  - ▸ Hypogammaglobulinaemia or bronchiectasis Measure serum immunoglobulin levels if recurrent infections develop, and consider bronchiectasis or pulmonary fibrosis if persistent respiratory symptoms such as cough and dyspnoea develop.

- ● INTERACTIONS → Appendix 1: mycophenolate
- ● SIDE-EFFECTS
GENERAL SIDE-EFFECTS
  - ▸ **Common or very common** Acidosis · alopecia · anaemia · appetite decreased · arthralgia · asthenia · bone marrow disorders · chills · constipation · cough · depression · diarrhoea · drowsiness · dyslipidaemia · dyspnoea · electrolyte imbalance · fever · gastrointestinal discomfort · gastrointestinal disorders · gastrointestinal haemorrhage · headache · hyperglycaemia · hypertension · hypotension · increased risk of infection · insomnia · leucocytosis · leucopenia · malaise · nausea · neoplasms · oedema · oral disorders · pain · pancreatitis · paraesthesia · renal impairment · respiratory disorders · seizure · sepsis · skin reactions · tachycardia · thinking abnormal · thrombocytopenia · tremor · vomiting · weight decreased
  - ▸ **Uncommon** Agranulocytosis
  - ▸ **Frequency not known** Endocarditis · hypogammaglobulinaemia · malignancy · meningitis ·

neutropenia · polyomavirus-associated nephropathy · progressive multifocal leukoencephalopathy · pure red cell aplasia

SPECIFIC SIDE-EFFECTS
▸ **Common or very common**
▸ With intravenous use Hepatitis · muscle tone increased
▸ With oral use Anxiety · burping · confusion · dizziness · gout · hepatic disorders · hyperbilirubinaemia · hyperuricaemia · neuromuscular dysfunction · taste altered · vasodilation

SIDE-EFFECTS, FURTHER INFORMATION Cases of pure red cell aplasia have been reported with mycophenolate mofetil; dose reduction or discontinuation should be considered under specialist supervision.

● CONCEPTION AND CONTRACEPTION
Pregnancy prevention The MHRA advises to exclude pregnancy in females of child-bearing potential before treatment—2 pregnancy tests 8–10 days apart are recommended. Women should use at least 1 method of effective contraception before and during treatment, and for 6 weeks after discontinuation—2 methods of effective contraception are preferred. Male patients or their female partner should use effective contraception during treatment and for 90 days after discontinuation.

● PREGNANCY Avoid unless no suitable alternative—congenital malformations and spontaneous abortions reported.

● BREAST FEEDING Manufacturer advises avoid—present in milk in *animal* studies.

● RENAL IMPAIRMENT No data available in cardiac or hepatic transplant patients with renal impairment.

● MONITORING REQUIREMENTS Monitor full blood count every week for 4 weeks then twice a month for 2 months then every month in the first year (consider interrupting treatment if neutropenia develops).

● DIRECTIONS FOR ADMINISTRATION For *intravenous infusion* (*CellCept*®), give intermittently in Glucose 5%; reconstitute each 500−mg vial with 14 mL glucose 5% and dilute the contents of 2 vials in 140 mL infusion fluid; give over 2 hours.

● PATIENT AND CARER ADVICE
Pregnancy prevention advice The MHRA advises that prescribers should ensure that female patients understand the need to comply with the pregnancy prevention advice, and they should be informed to seek immediate medical attention if there is a possibility of pregnancy; male patients planning to conceive children should be informed of the implications of both immunosuppression and the effect of the prescribed medications on the pregnancy. Bone marrow suppression Patients should be warned to report immediately any signs or symptoms of bone marrow suppression e.g. infection or inexplicable bruising or bleeding.

● NATIONAL FUNDING/ACCESS DECISIONS
NICE decisions
▸ **Immunosuppressive therapy for kidney transplant in adults (October 2017) NICE TA481**
Mycophenolate mofetil, when used as part of an immunosuppressive regimen, is recommended as an initial option to prevent organ rejection in adults having a kidney transplant. Treatment should be started with the least expensive product, but if this is not suitable, an alternative dosage form may be given. The use of mycophenolate mofetil with tacrolimus is outside the terms of the marketing authorisation. If this combination is prescribed, the prescriber should follow relevant professional guidance, taking full responsibility for the decision. Informed consent should be obtained and documented.

Patients whose treatment was started within the NHS before this guidance was published should have the option to continue treatment, without change to their funding

arrangements, until they and their NHS clinician consider it appropriate to stop.
www.nice.org.uk/guidance/TA481
▸ **Immunosuppressive therapy for kidney transplant in adults (October 2017) NICE TA481**
Mycophenolate sodium (*Ceptava*®, *Myfortic*®) is not recommended as an initial treatment to prevent organ rejection in adults having a kidney transplant. Patients whose treatment was started within the NHS before this guidance was published should have the option to continue treatment, without change to their funding arrangements, until they and their NHS clinician consider it appropriate to stop.
www.nice.org.uk/guidance/TA481

● MEDICINAL FORMS
There can be variation in the licensing of different medicines containing the same drug. Forms available from special-order manufacturers include: oral suspension

Gastro-resistant tablet
CAUTIONARY AND ADVISORY LABELS 25
▸ Mycophenolate mofetil (Non-proprietary)
Mycophenolic acid (as Mycophenolate sodium)
180 mg Mycophenolic acid 180mg gastro-resistant tablets | 120 tablet PoM £96.72
Mycophenolic acid (as Mycophenolate sodium)
360 mg Mycophenolic acid 360mg gastro-resistant tablets | 120 tablet PoM £193.43
▸ Ceptava (Sandoz Ltd)
Mycophenolic acid (as Mycophenolate sodium) 180 mg Ceptava 180mg gastro-resistant tablets | 120 tablet PoM £77.38
Mycophenolic acid (as Mycophenolate sodium) 360 mg Ceptava 360mg gastro-resistant tablets | 120 tablet PoM £154.75
▸ Myfortic (Novartis Pharmaceuticals UK Ltd)
Mycophenolic acid (as Mycophenolate sodium) 180 mg Myfortic 180mg gastro-resistant tablets | 120 tablet PoM £96.72
Mycophenolic acid (as Mycophenolate sodium) 360 mg Myfortic 360mg gastro-resistant tablets | 120 tablet PoM £193.43

Tablet
▸ Mycophenolate mofetil (Non-proprietary)
Mycophenolate mofetil 500 mg Mycophenolate mofetil 500mg tablets | 50 tablet PoM £42.50 DT = £5.66
▸ CellCept (Roche Products Ltd)
Mycophenolate mofetil 500 mg CellCept 500mg tablets | 50 tablet PoM £82.26 DT = £5.66
▸ Myfenax (Teva UK Ltd)
Mycophenolate mofetil 500 mg Myfenax 500mg tablets | 50 tablet PoM £78.15 DT = £5.66

Oral suspension
EXCIPIENTS: May contain Aspartame
▸ CellCept (Roche Products Ltd)
Mycophenolate mofetil 200 mg per 1 ml CellCept 1g/5ml oral suspension sugar-free | 175 ml PoM £115.16 DT = £115.16

Powder for solution for infusion
▸ Mycophenolate mofetil (Non-proprietary)
Mycophenolate mofetil (as Mycophenolate mofetil hydrochloride) 500 mg Mycophenolate mofetil 500mg powder for concentrate for solution for infusion vials | 4 vial PoM £34.67 (Hospital only)
▸ CellCept (Roche Products Ltd)
Mycophenolate mofetil (as Mycophenolate mofetil hydrochloride) 500 mg CellCept 500mg powder for solution for infusion vials | 4 vial PoM £36.49

Capsule
▸ Mycophenolate mofetil (Non-proprietary)
Mycophenolate mofetil 250 mg Mycophenolate mofetil 250mg capsules | 100 capsule PoM £82.26 DT = £82.26
▸ CellCept (Roche Products Ltd)
Mycophenolate mofetil 250 mg CellCept 250mg capsules | 100 capsule PoM £82.26 DT = £82.26
▸ Myfenax (Teva UK Ltd)
Mycophenolate mofetil 250 mg Myfenax 250mg capsules | 100 capsule PoM £78.15 DT = £82.26

IMMUNOSUPPRESSANTS > T-CELL ACTIVATION INHIBITORS

Belatacept

16-Nov-2017

● **INDICATIONS AND DOSE**

Prophylaxis of graft rejection in adults undergoing renal transplantation who are seropositive for the Epstein-Barr virus

▶ BY INTRAVENOUS INFUSION
  ▶ Adult: (consult product literature)

● CAUTIONS Increased risk of acute graft rejection—with tapering of corticosteroid, particularly in patients with high immunologic risk · increased risk of infection · latent and active tuberculosis · risk factors for post-transplant lymphoproliferative disorder

● INTERACTIONS → Appendix 1: belatacept

● SIDE-EFFECTS

▶ **Common or very common** Acidosis · alopecia · anaemia · angina pectoris · arrhythmias · arterial fibrosis · cataract · chest pain · constipation · cough · Cushing's syndrome · decreased leucocytes · diabetes mellitus · diarrhoea · dizziness · dyslipidaemia · dyspnoea · ear pain · electrolyte imbalance · embolism and thrombosis · eye erythema · fatigue · fever · fluid imbalance · gastrointestinal discomfort · gastrointestinal disorders · haemorrhage · headaches · healing impaired · hearing impairment · heart failure · hepatic disorders · hypercapnia · hyperglycaemia · hypertension · hypoproteinaemia · hypotension · increased risk of infection · intervertebral disc disorder · joint disorders · lethargy · leucocytosis · lymphocele · malaise · muscle complaints · muscle weakness · nausea · neoplasms · nerve disorders · neutropenia · oral disorders · oropharyngeal complaints · osteoarthritis · pain · paraesthesia · peripheral oedema · polyomavirus infections · pulmonary oedema · red blood cell abnormalities · renal disorders · renal tubular necrosis · respiratory disorders · scrotal disorders · sepsis · shock · skin reactions · stroke · sweat changes · syncope · thrombocytopenia · transplant rejection · tremor · urinary disorders · urine abnormalities · vascular disorders · ventricular hypertrophy · vertigo · vesicoureteric reflux · vision disorders · vomiting · weight changes

▶ **Uncommon** Acute coronary syndrome · adrenal insufficiency · agranulocytosis · alkalosis · anxiety · aortic valve disease · appetite decreased · arterial stenosis · atrioventricular block · attention deficit/hyperactivity disorder · bone disorders · bone fracture · breast mass · broken nails · cervical dysplasia · cholelithiasis · cognitive disorder · demyelination · depression · diabetic foot · disease recurrence · dysphonia · encephalopathy · endocarditis · eye inflammation · facial paralysis · facial swelling · feeling hot · fibrosis · flushing · haemolysis · hair changes · hemiparesis · hypercalcaemia · hypogammaglobulinaemia · infertility · inflammation · infusion related reaction · intermittent claudication · intracranial pressure increased · lymphangitis · memory loss · mood altered · nephritis · nephrosclerosis · pancreatitis · penile ulceration · post procedural haematoma · progressive multifocal leukoencephalopathy · pulmonary hypertension · renal tubular atrophy · restless legs · seasonal allergy · seizure · sexual dysfunction · sleep apnoea · sleep disorders · taste altered · tendon rupture · testicular pain · ulcer · vitamin D deficiency · vulvovaginal disorders · wound dehiscence

SIDE-EFFECTS, FURTHER INFORMATION Side effects are reported when used in combination with basiliximab, mycophenolate mofetil and corticosteroids.

● CONCEPTION AND CONTRACEPTION Adequate contraception must be used during treatment and for up to 8 weeks after last dose.

● PREGNANCY Use only if essential.

● BREAST FEEDING Avoid—no information available.

● PRE-TREATMENT SCREENING Patients should be evaluated for latent and active tuberculosis before starting treatment.

● MONITORING REQUIREMENTS Patients should be monitored for signs and symptoms of tuberculosis during and after treatment.

● PATIENT AND CARER ADVICE Patients should be advised to avoid excessive exposure to UV light including sunlight.

● NATIONAL FUNDING/ACCESS DECISIONS

NICE decisions

▶ **Immunosuppressive therapy for kidney transplant in adults (October 2017)** NICE TA481
Belatacept is not recommended as an initial treatment to prevent organ rejection in adults having a kidney transplant. Patients whose treatment was started within the NHS before this guidance was published should have the option to continue treatment, without change to their funding arrangements, until they and their NHS clinician consider it appropriate to stop.
www.nice.org.uk/guidance/TA481

● MEDICINAL FORMS
There can be variation in the licensing of different medicines containing the same drug.

Powder for solution for infusion

▶ Nulojix (Bristol-Myers Squibb Pharmaceuticals Ltd)
Belatacept 250 mg Nulojix 250mg powder for concentrate for solution for infusion vials | 1 vial [PoM] £354.52 (Hospital only) | 2 vial [PoM] £709.04 (Hospital only)

1.1 Multiple sclerosis

Multiple sclerosis

02-Nov-2016

Description of condition

Multiple sclerosis is a chronic, immune-mediated, demyelinating inflammatory condition of the central nervous system, which affects the brain, optic nerves and spinal cord, and leads to progressive severe disability.

Relapsing-remitting multiple sclerosis is the most common pattern of the disease. It is characterised by periods of exacerbation of symptoms (relapses) followed by unpredictable periods of stability (remission). The severity and frequency of relapses varies greatly between patients, but on average occur once or twice per year. This clinical pattern often develops into *secondary-progressive* multiple sclerosis, with progressive disability unrelated to relapses. Most patients develop secondary progressive disease 6–10 years after onset.

Primary-progressive multiple sclerosis follows a gradual course, with the development of symptoms that worsen over time, without relapses and remissions.

Progressive-relapsing multiple sclerosis follows a course of steadily worsening neurological function from onset, in addition to acute relapses.

Disease activity in relapsing-remitting multiple sclerosis

Active disease is defined as at least two clinically significant relapses occurring within the last 2 years. *Highly active* disease is characterised by an unchanged/increased relapse rate or by ongoing severe relapses compared with the previous year, despite treatment with interferon beta p. 830. *Rapidly-evolving severe* relapsing-remitting multiple sclerosis is defined by two or more disabling relapses in 1 year, and one or more gadolinium-enhancing lesions on brain magnetic resonance imaging (MRI) or a significant increase in T2 lesion load compared with a previous MRI.

Aims of treatment

There is no cure for multiple sclerosis. The overall aims of treatment are to modify the course of the disease and manage symptoms, in order to improve quality of life. Treatment is aimed at reducing the frequency and duration of relapses and at preventing or slowing disability.

Drug treatment

Shared decision-making between the patient and their clinicians is particularly important in the treatment of multiple sclerosis, due to the unpredictability of the condition and the lack of evidence of long-term benefit of treatments. [EvGr] A discussion about treatment options, disease activity, risk, and benefit should take place to ensure that treatment choices are right for the patient and their circumstances. [A] The choice of drug also depends on the patient's disability status, individual tolerance, disease severity and disease activity (see *Disease activity in relapsing-remitting multiple sclerosis* above). [EvGr] Treatment should be initiated as early as possible, under the supervision of a specialist. [A]

Note: NHS England (May 2014) has provided guidance on the use of interferon beta, glatiramer acetate p. 832, fingolimod p. 834 and natalizumab p. 837 for the treatment of multiple sclerosis in England, see *Useful resources* below. This Clinical Commissioning Policy outlines the funding arrangements and the criteria for initiating and discontinuing these treatment options. See also *National funding/access decisions*, under individual monographs for teriflunomide p. 839, dimethyl fumarate p. 833 and alemtuzumab p. 837.

Low levels of vitamin D are believed to be a risk factor for developing multiple sclerosis. Patients with diagnosed multiple sclerosis are usually given regular vitamin D after assessment of their serum levels of vitamin D, but there is insufficient evidence to support its use as a treatment for multiple sclerosis. [EvGr] Patients should not be offered vitamin D solely for the purpose of treating multiple sclerosis. [A]

Relapsing-remitting multiple sclerosis

[EvGr] Disease-modifying drugs are the recommended treatment for patients presenting with *active* relapsing-remitting multiple sclerosis. Interferon beta and glatiramer acetate may be the preferred choice for some patients, due to their established safety profile, and the long term clinical experience associated with their use. [A] Peginterferon beta-1a p. 832 requires less frequent administration and is available as an alternative to the non-pegylated interferon beta therapies.

Teriflunomide and dimethyl fumarate are treatment options for patients with *active* disease. [EvGr] They may be preferred due to their oral route of administration. [A] There is insufficient evidence for the use of either drug to treat *highly active* or *rapidly-evolving severe* relapsing-remitting multiple sclerosis.

[EvGr] More active disease may be treated with natalizumab or alemtuzumab. Natalizumab may be preferred due to the complex safety profile associated with alemtuzumab. Natalizumab is only recommended for the treatment of *rapidly-evolving severe* relapsing-remitting multiple sclerosis. Although licensed as a treatment option in all patients with *active* disease, alemtuzumab may be used more frequently in patients for whom other disease-modifying treatments have not been effective, due to the risk of serious side effects associated with its use.

Fingolimod is also taken by the oral route and is the recommended treatment for patients with *highly active* disease. [A] The NHS England Clinical Commissioning Policy (see *Useful resources* below) advises that fingolimod is

a suitable alternative for patients receiving natalizumab who are at high risk of developing progressive multifocal leukoencephalopathy (defined as patients previously exposed to the JC virus or who are receiving immunosuppressants or who have been receiving treatment with natalizumab for more than 2 years).

Secondary progressive multiple sclerosis

Currently, only interferon beta 1b is licensed for use in secondary progressive multiple sclerosis. Interferon beta 1b reduces the risk of relapse and of short-term relapse-related disability, but does not prevent the development of permanent physical disability or retard progression once it is established. Therefore its role in secondary progressive disease is limited.

Primary progressive multiple sclerosis

Currently there are no effective disease-modifying treatments licensed for primary progressive multiple sclerosis. Interferon beta [unlicensed indication] has been used, but there is limited evidence to support its use due to the lack of a significant reduction in disability progression.

Progressive-relapsing multiple sclerosis

There are no specific treatment options for this type of multiple sclerosis. None of the currently licensed disease-modifying drugs are recommended in non-relapsing progressive disease.

Management of symptoms

Other than episodes of neurological dysfunction, chronic symptoms (such as fatigue, spasticity, visual problems, and emotional lability) produce much of the disability in multiple sclerosis. [EvGr] Smoking may increase the progression of disability in multiple sclerosis, and cessation should be encouraged. [A]

Relapses

Suspected relapses should be referred to a specialist for diagnosis and treatment. [EvGr] Corticosteroids are recommended for reducing inflammation and accelerating recovery in acute relapses of relapsing-remitting multiple sclerosis. Oral methylprednisolone p. 663 is recommended as the first-line option. Intravenous methylprednisolone should be considered as an alternative if oral methylprednisolone has failed or is not tolerated or if hospitalisation is required. [A]

Fatigue and impaired mobility

[EvGr] Regular exercise may have beneficial effects on mobility and fatigue in patients with multiple sclerosis, and should be encouraged. Cognitive behavioural techniques for fatigue should also be considered in combination with exercise. Amantadine hydrochloride p. 412 [unlicensed indication] may be used to treat fatigue related to multiple sclerosis. Vitamin B_{12} injections are **not** recommended as a treatment for fatigue in patients with multiple sclerosis. [A] Fampridine p. 830 is licensed for the improvement of walking in patients with multiple sclerosis who have a walking disability. [EvGr] NICE do not consider it to be a cost-effective treatment and do not recommend its use. [A]

Spasticity

Many factors may aggravate spasticity in multiple sclerosis, including constipation, infection, poor mobility aids, pressure ulcers, posture and pain. [EvGr] These causes should be managed appropriately. The first-line options for managing spasticity in multiple sclerosis are baclofen p. 1092 or gabapentin p. 314 [unlicensed indication]. They may be used cautiously in combination if the individual drugs are ineffective or if side effects prevent an increase in the dose of either drug. Tizanidine p. 1094 or dantrolene sodium p. 1307 are second-line options; benzodiazepines may be used as third-line therapy and may also be effective in treating nocturnal spasms. [A] A cannabis extract p. 1092 containing dronabinol and cannabidiol is licensed as an adjunct treatment for moderate-to-severe spasticity associated with multiple sclerosis in patients who have not responded adequately to other skeletal muscle relaxants. EvGr NICE do not consider it to be a cost-effective treatment and do not recommend its use. ⚠

Oscillopsia

EvGr Gabapentin [unlicensed indication] is the first-line treatment for oscillopsia; memantine hydrochloride p. 303 [unlicensed indication] is the second-line option. ⚠

Emotional lability

EvGr Amitriptyline hydrochloride p. 369 [unlicensed indication] may be used to treat emotional lability in patients with multiple sclerosis. ⚠

Useful Resources

Clinical Commissioning Policy: disease modifying therapies for patients with multiple sclerosis. NHS England. May 2014. www.england.nhs.uk/commissioning/wp-content/uploads/sites/12/2013/10/d04-p-b.pdf

Multiple sclerosis in adults: management. National Institute for Health and Care Excellence. Clinical guideline 186. October 2014.
www.nice.org.uk/guidance/cg186

> **Other drugs used for Multiple sclerosis** Cladribine, p. 882

CHOLINERGIC RECEPTOR STIMULATING DRUGS

Fampridine

21-Mar-2017

- **INDICATIONS AND DOSE**
  Improvement of walking disability in multiple sclerosis (specialist use only)
  - ▸ BY MOUTH
  - ▸ Adult: 10 mg every 12 hours, discontinue treatment if no improvement within 2 weeks

- CONTRA-INDICATIONS History of seizures (discontinue treatment if seizures occur)
- CAUTIONS Atrioventricular conduction disorders · predisposition to seizures · sinoatrial conduction disorders · symptomatic cardiac rhythm disorders
- INTERACTIONS → Appendix 1: fampridine
- SIDE-EFFECTS
  - ▸ **Common or very common** Anxiety · asthenia · balance impaired · constipation · dizziness · dyspepsia · dyspnoea · headache · insomnia · laryngeal pain · nausea · pain · palpitations · paraesthesia · tremor · urinary tract infection · vomiting
  - ▸ **Uncommon** Seizure · skin reactions · tachycardia
- PREGNANCY Avoid—toxicity in *animal* studies.
- BREAST FEEDING Avoid—no information available.
- RENAL IMPAIRMENT Avoid if eGFR less than 80 mL/minute/1.73 m^2.
- PRESCRIBING AND DISPENSING INFORMATION Dispense in original container (pack contains a desiccant) and discard any tablets remaining 7 days after opening.
- NATIONAL FUNDING/ACCESS DECISIONS
  Scottish Medicines Consortium (SMC) Decisions
  The *Scottish Medicines Consortium* has advised (November 2016) that fampridine (*Fampyra®*) is **not** recommended for use within NHS Scotland for the improvement of walking in adult patients with multiple sclerosis (MS) with walking disability (EDSS [expanded disability status scale] 4 to 7) as the economic case was not demonstrated.

- MEDICINAL FORMS
  There can be variation in the licensing of different medicines containing the same drug. Forms available from special-order manufacturers include: capsule
  Modified-release tablet
  CAUTIONARY AND ADVISORY LABELS 23, 25
  - ▸ Fampyra (Biogen Idec Ltd)
    Fampridine 10 mg Fampyra 10mg modified-release tablets | 28 tablet PoM £181.00 | 56 tablet PoM £362.00

IMMUNOSTIMULANTS > INTERFERONS

Interferon beta

- **INDICATIONS AND DOSE**
  AVONEX® INJECTION
  For relapsing, remitting multiple sclerosis (characterised by at least two attacks of neurological dysfunction over the previous 2 or 3 years, followed by complete or incomplete recovery) who are able to walk unaided | For a single demyelinating event with an active inflammatory process (if severe enough to require intravenous corticosteroid and patient at high risk of developing multiple sclerosis)
  - ▸ BY INTRAMUSCULAR INJECTION
  - ▸ Adult: (consult product literature)
  AVONEX® VIAL
  For relapsing, remitting multiple sclerosis (characterised by at least two attacks of neurological dysfunction over the previous 2 or 3 years, followed by complete or incomplete recovery) who are able to walk unaided | For a single demyelinating event with an active inflammatory process (if severe enough to require intravenous corticosteroid and patient at high risk of developing multiple sclerosis)
  - ▸ BY INTRAMUSCULAR INJECTION
  - ▸ Adult: (consult product literature)
  BETAFERON® INJECTION
  For relapsing, remitting multiple sclerosis (characterised by at least two attacks of neurological dysfunction over the previous 2 or 3 years, followed by complete or incomplete recovery) who are able to walk unaided | For secondary progressive multiple sclerosis with active disease | For a single demyelinating event with an active inflammatory process (if severe enough to require intravenous corticosteroid and patient at high risk of developing multiple sclerosis)
  - ▸ BY SUBCUTANEOUS INJECTION
  - ▸ Adult: (consult product literature)
  EXTAVIA®
  For relapsing, remitting multiple sclerosis (characterised by at least two attacks of neurological dysfunction over the previous 2 or 3 years, followed by complete or incomplete recovery) who are able to walk unaided | For secondary progressive multiple sclerosis with active disease | For a single demyelinating event with an active inflammatory process (if severe enough to require intravenous corticosteroid and patient at high risk of developing multiple sclerosis)
  - ▸ BY SUBCUTANEOUS INJECTION
  - ▸ Adult: (consult product literature)

REBIF ® CARTRIDGE

For relapsing, remitting multiple sclerosis (characterised by at least two attacks of neurological dysfunction over the previous 2 or 3 years, followed by complete or incomplete recovery) who are able to walk unaided | For a single demyelinating event with an active inflammatory process (if severe enough to require intravenous corticosteroid and patient at high risk of developing multiple sclerosis)

▸ BY SUBCUTANEOUS INJECTION
▸ Adult: (consult product literature)

REBIF ® PRE-FILLED PEN AND SYRINGE

For relapsing, remitting multiple sclerosis (characterised by at least two attacks of neurological dysfunction over the previous 2 or 3 years, followed by complete or incomplete recovery) who are able to walk unaided | For a single demyelinating event with an active inflammatory process (if severe enough to require intravenous corticosteroid and patient at high risk of developing multiple sclerosis)

▸ BY SUBCUTANEOUS INJECTION
▸ Adult: (consult product literature)

● CONTRA-INDICATIONS Decompensated liver disease · severe depressive illness
    CONTRA-INDICATIONS, FURTHER INFORMATION
    Consult product literature for further information on contra-indications.
● CAUTIONS History of cardiac disorders · history of depressive disorders (avoid in severe depression or in those with suicidal ideation) · history of seizures · history of severe myelosupression
    CAUTIONS, FURTHER INFORMATION Consult product literature for further information on cautions.
● INTERACTIONS → Appendix 1: interferons
● SIDE-EFFECTS
    GENERAL SIDE-EFFECTS
▸ **Common or very common** Alopecia · appetite decreased · arrhythmias · arthralgia · asthenia · chills · confusion · depression · diarrhoea · fever · headaches · hypothyroidism · influenza like illness (decreasing over time) · insomnia · malaise · menstrual cycle irregularities · nausea · neuromuscular dysfunction · pain · skin reactions · sweat changes · vasodilation · vomiting · weight changes
▸ **Uncommon** Emotional lability · glomerulosclerosis · hepatic disorders · nephrotic syndrome · seizure · suicidal ideation · thrombocytopenia
▸ **Rare or very rare** Cardiomyopathy · dyspnoea · haemolytic uraemic syndrome · hyperthyroidism · thrombotic microangiopathy
▸ **Frequency not known** Anxiety · chest pain · dizziness · hypersensitivity · muscle weakness · palpitations · pulmonary arterial hypertension
    SPECIFIC SIDE-EFFECTS
▸ **Common or very common**
▸ With intramuscular use Muscle complaints · musculoskeletal stiffness · rhinorrhoea · sensation abnormal
▸ With subcutaneous use Anaemia
▸ **Rare or very rare**
▸ With subcutaneous use Bronchospasm · pancreatitis · thyroid disorder
▸ **Frequency not known**
▸ With intramuscular use Angioedema · arthritis · congestive heart failure · neurological effects · pancytopenia · psychosis · syncope · systemic lupus erythematosus (SLE)
▸ With subcutaneous use Abdominal pain · abscess · capillary leak syndrome · conjunctivitis · constipation · cough aggravated · ear pain · erectile dysfunction · eye disorder · hypertension · increased risk of infection · lupus-like

syndrome · lymphadenopathy · myalgia · paraesthesia · peripheral oedema · urinary disorders · visual impairment

● CONCEPTION AND CONTRACEPTION Effective contraception required during treatment—consult product literature.
● PREGNANCY Avoid unless potential benefit outweighs risk (toxicity in *animal* studies).
● BREAST FEEDING Avoid—no information available.
● HEPATIC IMPAIRMENT Caution in severe hepatic impairment.
● RENAL IMPAIRMENT Caution in severe renal impairment.
● MONITORING REQUIREMENTS
▸ Monitor for signs of hepatic injury—hepatic failure has been reported rarely.
▸ Patients should be monitored for clinical features of thrombotic microangiopathy (TMA), including thrombocytopenia, new onset hypertension, fever, central nervous system symptoms (e.g. confusion and paresis), and impaired renal function. Any signs of TMA should be investigated fully and, if diagnosed, interferon beta should be stopped immediately and treatment for TMA promptly initiated (consult product literature for details).
▸ Patients should also be monitored for signs and symptoms of nephrotic syndrome, including oedema, proteinuria, and impaired renal function—monitor renal function periodically. If nephrotic syndrome develops, treat promptly and consider stopping interferon beta treatment.
● PRESCRIBING AND DISPENSING INFORMATION
    REBIF ® CARTRIDGE Cartridges for use with *RebiSmart* ® auto-injector device.
    BETAFERON ® INJECTION An auto-injector device (*Betaject* ® Light) is available from Bayer Schering.
    EXTAVIA ® An auto-injector device (*ExtaviPro* ® 30G) is supplied as part of the *ExtaviPro* ® 30G kit.
● NATIONAL FUNDING/ACCESS DECISIONS
    NICE decisions
▸ **Interferon beta and glatiramer acetate for multiple sclerosis (January 2002)** NICE TA32
    Interferon beta and glatiramer acetate are **not** recommended for the treatment of multiple sclerosis in the NHS in England and Wales.
        Patients who are currently receiving interferon beta or glatiramer acetate for multiple sclerosis, whether as routine therapy or as part of a clinical trial, should have the option to continue treatment until they and their consultant consider it appropriate to stop, having regard to the established criteria for withdrawal from treatment.
    www.nice.org.uk/TA32
    NHS restrictions
    NHS England Clinical Commissioning Policy NHS England (May 2014) has provided guidance on the use of interferon beta for the treatment of multiple sclerosis in England. An NHS England Clinical Commissioning Policy outlines the funding arrangements and the criteria for initiating and discontinuing this treatment option, see
    www.england.nhs.uk/commissioning/wp-content/uploads/sites/12/2013/10/d04-p-b.pdf.
● MEDICINAL FORMS
    There can be variation in the licensing of different medicines containing the same drug.
    Solution for injection
    EXCIPIENTS: May contain Benzyl alcohol
▸ Avonex (Biogen Idec Ltd)
    Interferon beta-1a 12 mega u per 1 ml Avonex 30micrograms/0.5ml (6million units) solution for injection pre-filled syringes | 4 pre-filled disposable injection [PoM] £654.00 | 12 pre-filled disposable injection [PoM] £1,962.00
    Avonex 30micrograms/0.5ml (6million units) solution for injection pre-filled pen | 4 pre-filled disposable injection [PoM] £654.00 | 12 pre-filled disposable injection [PoM] £1,962.00

▸ Rebif (Merck Serono Ltd)

Interferon beta-1a 12 mega u per 1 ml Rebif 22micrograms/0.5ml (6million units) solution for injection pre-filled syringes | 12 pre-filled disposable injection [PoM] £613.52
Rebif 22micrograms/0.5ml (6million units) solution for injection 1.5ml cartridges | 4 cartridge [PoM] £613.52
Rebif 8.8micrograms/0.2ml (2.4million units) solution for injection pre-filled syringes | 6 pre-filled disposable injection [PoM] ⓢ
Rebif 22micrograms/0.5ml (6million units) solution for injection pre-filled pen | 12 pre-filled disposable injection [PoM] £613.52

Interferon beta-1a 24 mega u per 1 ml Rebif 44micrograms/0.5ml (12million units) solution for injection pre-filled pen | 12 pre-filled disposable injection [PoM] £813.21
Rebif 44micrograms/0.5ml (12million units) solution for injection pre-filled syringes | 12 pre-filled disposable injection [PoM] £813.21
Rebif 44micrograms/0.5ml (12million units) solution for injection 1.5ml cartridges | 4 cartridge [PoM] £813.21

Powder and solvent for solution for injection
▸ Betaferon (Bayer Plc)

Interferon beta-1b 300 microgram Betaferon 300microgram powder and solvent for solution for injection vials | 15 vial [PoM] £596.63 (Hospital only)
▸ Extavia (Novartis Pharmaceuticals UK Ltd)

Interferon beta-1b 300 microgram Extavia 300microgram powder and solvent for solution for injection vials | 15 vial [PoM] £596.63

Peginterferon beta-1a

● DRUG ACTION Peginterferon beta-1a is a polyethylene glycol-conjugated ('pegylated') derivative of interferon beta; pegylation increases the persistence of interferon in the blood.

● INDICATIONS AND DOSE
Treatment of relapsing, remitting multiple sclerosis
▸ BY SUBCUTANEOUS INJECTION
▸ Adult: (consult product literature)

● CONTRA-INDICATIONS Severe depression · suicidal ideation
● CAUTIONS History of cardiac disorders · history of depressive disorders (avoid in severe depression or in those with suicidal ideation) · history of seizures · history of severe myelosupression

CAUTIONS, FURTHER INFORMATION Consult product literature for further information about cautions.

● INTERACTIONS → Appendix 1: peginterferon beta-1a
● SIDE-EFFECTS
▸ **Common or very common** Arthralgia · asthenia · chills · depression · fever · headache · hyperthermia · influenza like illness · myalgia · nausea · pain · skin reactions · vomiting
▸ **Uncommon** Seizure · thrombocytopenia
▸ **Rare or very rare** Glomerulosclerosis · haemolytic uraemic syndrome · nephrotic syndrome · thrombotic microangiopathy
▸ **Frequency not known** Pulmonary arterial hypertension
● CONCEPTION AND CONTRACEPTION Effective contraception required during treatment—consult product literature.
● PREGNANCY Do not initiate during pregnancy. Avoid unless potential benefit outweighs risk.
● BREAST FEEDING Avoid—no information available.
● HEPATIC IMPAIRMENT Caution in severe hepatic impairment.
● RENAL IMPAIRMENT Caution in severe renal impairment.
● MONITORING REQUIREMENTS
▸ Monitor for signs of hepatic injury—hepatic failure has been reported rarely.
▸ Thrombotic microangiopathy Patients should be monitored for clinical features of thrombotic microangiopathy (TMA), including thrombocytopenia, new onset hypertension, fever, central nervous system symptoms (e.g. confusion and paresis), and impaired renal function. Any signs of TMA should be investigated fully and, if diagnosed,

interferon beta should be stopped immediately and treatment for TMA promptly initiated (consult product literature for details).
▸ Nephrotic syndrome Patients should also be monitored for signs and symptoms of nephrotic syndrome, including oedema, proteinuria, and impaired renal function—monitor renal function periodically. If nephrotic syndrome develops, treat promptly and consider stopping interferon beta treatment.

● MEDICINAL FORMS
There can be variation in the licensing of different medicines containing the same drug.
Solution for injection
▸ Plegridy (Biogen Idec Ltd) ▼
Peginterferon beta-1a 126 microgram per 1 ml Plegridy 63micrograms/0.5ml solution for injection pre-filled pen | 1 pre-filled disposable injection [PoM] ⓢ
Peginterferon beta-1a 188 microgram per 1 ml Plegridy 94micrograms/0.5ml solution for injection pre-filled pen | 1 pre-filled disposable injection [PoM] ⓢ
Peginterferon beta-1a 250 microgram per 1 ml Plegridy 125micrograms/0.5ml solution for injection pre-filled pen | 2 pre-filled disposable injection [PoM] £654.00 | 6 pre-filled disposable injection [PoM] £1,962.00

IMMUNOSTIMULANTS ⟩ OTHER

Glatiramer acetate

10-Nov-2017

● DRUG ACTION Glatiramer is an immunomodulating drug comprising synthetic polypeptides.

● INDICATIONS AND DOSE
Multiple sclerosis [relapsing-remitting] (initiated under specialist supervision)
▸ BY SUBCUTANEOUS INJECTION
▸ Adult: 20 mg once daily, alternatively 40 mg 3 times a week, doses to be separated by an interval of at least 48 hours

● CAUTIONS Cardiac disorders
● SIDE-EFFECTS
▸ **Common or very common** Anxiety · appetite decreased · arrhythmias · asthenia · chest pain · chills · constipation · cough · depression · dyspepsia · dysphagia · dyspnoea (may occur within minutes of injection) · ear disorder · eye disorders · fever · gastrointestinal disorders · headaches · hyperhidrosis · hypersensitivity · increased risk of infection · joint disorders · local reaction · lymphadenopathy · nausea · neoplasms · neuromuscular dysfunction · oedema · oral disorders · pain · palpitations · rhinitis seasonal · skin reactions · speech disorder · syncope · taste altered · tremor · urinary disorders · vasodilation · vision disorders · vomiting · weight increased
▸ **Uncommon** Abnormal dreams · abscess · alcohol intolerance · angioedema · apnoea · arthritis · breast engorgement · burping · cataract · choking sensation · cholelithiasis · cognitive disorder · confusion · cyst · dry eye · dysgraphia · dyslexia · erythema nodosum · goitre · gout · haemorrhage · hallucination · hangover · hepatic disorders · hostility · hyperlipidaemia · hyperthyroidism · hypothermia · inflammation · leucocytosis · leucopenia · mood altered · movement disorders · mucous membrane disorder · muscle atrophy · nephrolithiasis · nerve disorders · paralysis · pelvic prolapse · personality disorder · post vaccination syndrome · prostatic disorder · respiratory disorders · seizure · sexual dysfunction · skin nodule · splenomegaly · stupor · suicide attempt · testicular disorder · thrombocytopenia · urinary tract disorder · urine abnormal · varicose veins · vulvovaginal disorder
● PREGNANCY Manufacturer advises avoid—no information available.

- BREAST FEEDING Manufacturer advises caution—no information available.
- RENAL IMPAIRMENT No information available—manufacturer advises caution.
- NATIONAL FUNDING/ACCESS DECISIONS

NICE decisions
▶ **Interferon beta and glatiramer acetate for multiple sclerosis (January 2002)** NICE TA32
Interferon beta and glatiramer acetate are **not** recommended for the treatment of multiple sclerosis in the NHS in England and Wales.

Patients who are currently receiving interferon beta or glatiramer acetate for multiple sclerosis, whether as routine therapy or as part of a clinical trial, should have the option to continue treatment until they and their consultant consider it appropriate to stop, having regard to the established criteria for withdrawal from treatment.
www.nice.org.uk/TA32

NHS restrictions
NHS England Clinical Commissioning Policy NHS England (May 2014) has provided guidance on the use of glatiramer acetate for the treatment of multiple sclerosis in England. An NHS England Clinical Commissioning Policy outlines the funding arrangements and the criteria for initiating and discontinuing this treatment option, see
www.england.nhs.uk/commissioning/wp-content/uploads/sites/12/2013/10/d04-p-b.pdf.

- MEDICINAL FORMS
There can be variation in the licensing of different medicines containing the same drug.
Solution for injection
▶ Brabio (Mylan)
Glatiramer acetate 20 mg per 1 ml Brabio 20mg/1ml solution for injection pre-filled syringes | 28 pre-filled disposable injection PoM £462.56
Glatiramer acetate 40 mg per 1 ml Brabio 40mg/1ml solution for injection pre-filled syringes | 12 pre-filled disposable injection PoM £462.56
▶ Copaxone (Teva UK Ltd)
Glatiramer acetate 20 mg per 1 ml Copaxone 20mg/1ml solution for injection pre-filled syringes | 28 pre-filled disposable injection PoM £513.95
Glatiramer acetate 40 mg per 1 ml Copaxone 40mg/1ml solution for injection pre-filled syringes | 12 pre-filled disposable injection PoM £513.95

IMMUNOSUPPRESSANTS >
IMMUNOMODULATING DRUGS

Dimethyl fumarate
06-Dec-2017

- DRUG ACTION Dimethyl fumarate has immunomodulatory and anti-inflammatory properties.

- INDICATIONS AND DOSE

SKILARENCE ®

Plaque psoriasis [moderate-to-severe] (under expert supervision)
▶ BY MOUTH
▶ Adult: Initially 30 mg once daily for 1 week, dose to be taken in the evening, then increased in steps of 30 mg every week for 3 weeks, then increased in steps of 120 mg every week for 5 weeks, for further information on the dose titration and administration schedule, advice on establishing a maintenance dose, and for dose adjustments due to side-effects, consult product literature; maximum 720 mg per day

TECFIDERA ®
Multiple sclerosis [relapsing-remitting] (initiated by a specialist)
▶ BY MOUTH
▶ Adult: Initially 120 mg twice daily for 7 days, then increased to 240 mg twice daily, for dose adjustments due to side effects—consult product literature

- CONTRA-INDICATIONS

SKILARENCE ® Do not initiate if leucocyte count below 3×10^9/litre · do not initiate if lymphocyte count below 1×10^9/litre · do not initiate if pathological haematological abnormalities identified · severe gastro-intestinal disorders

- CAUTIONS Reduced lymphocyte count

TECFIDERA ® Serious infection (do not initiate until infection resolved; consider suspending treatment if infection develops) · severe active gastro-intestinal disease
SKILARENCE ® Significant infection (consider avoiding initiation until infection resolved and suspending treatment if infection develops)

- INTERACTIONS → Appendix 1: dimethyl fumarate

- SIDE-EFFECTS

▶ **Common or very common** Appetite decreased · asthenia · constipation · decreased leucocytes · diarrhoea · eosinophilia · feeling hot · flatulence · gastrointestinal discomfort · headache · leucocytosis · nausea · paraesthesia · progressive multifocal leukoencephalopathy (PML) · skin reactions · vasodilation · vomiting
▶ **Uncommon** Dizziness · proteinuria
▶ **Rare or very rare** Acute lymphocytic leukaemia · pancytopenia
▶ **Frequency not known** Renal failure

SIDE-EFFECTS, FURTHER INFORMATION Severe prolonged lymphopenia reported, and patients are exposed to a potential risk of PML. Treatment should be stopped immediately if PML is suspected.

- PREGNANCY

TECFIDERA ® Manufacturer advises avoid unless essential and potential benefit outweighs risk—toxicity in *animal* studies.
SKILARENCE ® Manufacturer advises avoid—toxicity in *animal* studies.

- BREAST FEEDING Manufacturer advises avoid.

- HEPATIC IMPAIRMENT

TECFIDERA ® Manufacturer advises caution in severe impairment—no information available.
SKILARENCE ® Manufacturer advises avoid in severe impairment—no information available.

- RENAL IMPAIRMENT

TECFIDERA ® Manufacturer advises caution in severe impairment—no information available.
SKILARENCE ® Manufacturer advises avoid in severe impairment—no information available.

- MONITORING REQUIREMENTS

▶ Manufacturer advises monitor full blood count before treatment initiation then every 3 months thereafter—consult product information for further information.
▶ Manufacturer advises monitor patient closely for features of progressive multifocal leukoencephalopathy (PML) (e.g. signs and symptoms of neurological dysfunction) and other opportunistic infections.
▶ Manufacturer advises monitor renal and hepatic function before treatment initiation and during treatment—consult product literature for further information.
▶ Manufacturer of *Tecfidera* ® advises perform a baseline MRI as a reference and repeat as required during treatment.

- PRESCRIBING AND DISPENSING INFORMATION
SKILARENCE® The manufacturer of *Skilarence*® has provided a *Healthcare Professional Guideline*, which includes important safety information on the risk of serious infections.

- PATIENT AND CARER ADVICE Manufacturer advises patients and their carers should be informed of the possibility of experiencing symptoms of flushing; they should also be advised to report symptoms of infection to their doctor. The MHRA recommends that patients and their carers should be counselled on the risk of progressive multifocal leukoencephalopathy and advised to seek immediate medical attention if symptoms develop.

- NATIONAL FUNDING/ACCESS DECISIONS
TECFIDERA®

NICE decisions

▸ **Dimethyl fumarate (*Tecfidera*®) for treating relapsing-remitting multiple sclerosis (August 2014)** NICE TA320
Dimethyl fumarate (*Tecfidera*®) is recommended for the treatment of active relapsing-remitting multiple sclerosis, only if:
  - the patient does not have highly active or rapidly evolving severe relapsing-remitting multiple sclerosis **and**
  - the manufacturer provides dimethyl fumarate with the discount agreed in the patient access scheme
Patients currently receiving dimethyl fumarate whose disease does not meet the above criteria should be able to continue treatment until they and their clinician consider it appropriate to stop.
www.nice.org.uk/guidance/TA320

Scottish Medicines Consortium (SMC) Decisions
The *Scottish Medicines Consortium* has advised (April 2014) that dimethyl fumarate (*Tecfidera*®) is accepted for use within NHS Scotland for the treatment of patients with relapsing remitting multiple sclerosis. This advice is contingent upon the continuing availability of the Patient Access Scheme in NHS Scotland or a list price that is equivalent or lower.
SKILARENCE®

NICE decisions

▸ **Dimethyl fumarate for treating moderate-to-severe plaque psoriasis (September 2017)** NICE TA475
Dimethyl fumarate is recommended as an option for treating plaque psoriasis in adults, only if the disease:
  - is severe, as defined by a total Psoriasis Area and Severity Index (PASI) of 10 or more and a Dermatology Life Quality Index (DLQI) of more than 10, **and**
  - has not responded to other systemic therapies, including, ciclosporin, methotrexate and PUVA (psoralen and long-wave ultraviolet A radiation), or these options are contra-indicated or not tolerated.
Stop dimethyl fumarate treatment at 16 weeks if the psoriasis has not responded adequately. An adequate response is defined as:
  - a 75% reduction in the PASI score (PASI 75) from when treatment started, **or**
  - a 50% reduction in the PASI score (PASI 50) and a 5-point reduction in DLQI from when treatment started.
Patients whose treatment was started within the NHS before this guidance was published should have the option to continue treatment, without change to their funding arrangements, until they and their NHS clinician consider it appropriate to stop.
www.nice.org.uk/guidance/ta475

Scottish Medicines Consortium (SMC) Decisions
SMC No. 1313/18
The *Scottish Medicines Consortium* has advised (April 2018) that dimethyl fumarate (*Skilarence*®) is accepted for restricted use within NHS Scotland for the treatment of moderate-to-severe plaque psoriasis in adults in need of

systemic medicinal therapy, whom other non-biologic systemic treatments (methotrexate, ciclosporin and acitretin) are not appropriate or have failed and who are considered unsuitable for biologic therapy given their current disease state or personal preference.

- MEDICINAL FORMS
There can be variation in the licensing of different medicines containing the same drug.
Gastro-resistant capsule
CAUTIONARY AND ADVISORY LABELS 21, 25
▸ Tecfidera (Biogen Idec Ltd)
  Dimethyl fumarate 120 mg Tecfidera 120mg gastro-resistant capsules | 14 capsule [PoM] £343.00
  Dimethyl fumarate 240 mg Tecfidera 240mg gastro-resistant capsules | 56 capsule [PoM] £1,373.00
Gastro-resistant tablet
CAUTIONARY AND ADVISORY LABELS 21, 25
▸ Skilarence (Almirall Ltd)
  Dimethyl fumarate 30 mg Skilarence 30mg gastro-resistant tablets | 42 tablet [PoM] £89.04
  Dimethyl fumarate 120 mg Skilarence 120mg gastro-resistant tablets | 90 tablet [PoM] £190.80 | 180 tablet [PoM] £381.60

Fingolimod

17-Jul-2017

- DRUG ACTION Fingolimod is an immunomodulating drug.

- INDICATIONS AND DOSE
Treatment of highly active relapsing-remitting multiple sclerosis in patients who have high disease activity despite treatment with at least one disease modifying therapy or in those with rapidly evolving severe relapsing-remitting multiple sclerosis (initiated under specialist supervision)
▸ BY MOUTH
▸ Adult: 500 micrograms once daily

IMPORTANT SAFETY INFORMATION

MHRA/CHM ADVICE: MULTIPLE SCLEROSIS THERAPIES: SIGNAL OF REBOUND EFFECT AFTER STOPPING OR SWITCHING THERAPY (APRIL 2017)
A signal of rebound syndrome in multiple sclerosis patients whose treatment with fingolimod was stopped or switched to other treatments has been reported in two recently published articles. The MHRA advise to be vigilant for such events and report any suspected adverse effects relating to fingolimod, or other treatments for multiple sclerosis, via the Yellow Card Scheme, while this report is under investigation.

MHRA/CHM ADVICE: FINGOLIMOD—NOT RECOMMENDED FOR PATIENTS AT KNOWN RISK OF CARDIOVASCULAR EVENTS. ADVICE FOR EXTENDED MONITORING FOR THOSE WITH SIGNIFICANT BRADYCARDIA OR HEART BLOCK AFTER THE FIRST DOSE AND FOLLOWING TREATMENT INTERRUPTION (JANUARY 2013)
Fingolimod is known to cause transient bradycardias and heart block after the first dose—see Cautions, Contra-indications and Monitoring for further information.

MHRA/CHM ADVICE: FINGOLIMOD: NEW CONTRA-INDICATIONS IN RELATION TO CARDIAC RISK (DECEMBER 2017)
Fingolimod can cause persistent bradycardia, which can increase the risk of serious cardiac arrhythmias. New contra-indications have been introduced for patients with pre-existing cardiac disorders—see Contra-indications for further information.

MHRA/CHM ADVICE: FINGOLIMOD: UPDATED ADVICE ABOUT RISK OF CANCERS AND SERIOUS INFECTIONS (DECEMBER 2017)
Fingolimod has an immunosuppressive effect and can increase the risk of skin cancers and lymphoma. Following a recent EU review, the MHRA has recommended the following strengthened warnings:
  - re-assess the benefit-risk balance of fingolimod therapy in individual patients, particularly those with

additional risk factors for malignancy—either closely monitor for skin cancers or consider discontinuation on a case-by-case basis
- examine all patients for skin lesions before they start fingolimod and then re-examine at least every 6 to 12 months
- advise patients to protect themselves against UV radiation exposure and seek urgent medical advice if they notice any skin lesions
- refer patients with suspicious lesions to a dermatologist

Fingolimod has also been associated with risk of fatal fungal infections and reports of progressive multifocal leukoencephalopathy (PML)—see Monitoring and Side effects for further information.

- **CONTRA-INDICATIONS** Heart failure in the previous 6 months (New York Heart Association class III/IV) · active malignancies · baseline QTc interval 500 milliseconds or greater · cerebrovascular disease (including transient ischaemic attack) · decompensated heart failure (requiring inpatient treatment) · increased risk for opportunistic infections (including immunosuppression) · myocardial infarction · second-degree Mobitz type II atrioventricular block or third-degree AV block, or sick-sinus syndrome, if the patient does not have a pacemaker · severe active infection · severe cardiac arrhythmias requiring treatment with class Ia or class III anti-arrhythmic drugs · unstable angina

- **CAUTIONS** Check varicella zoster virus status—consult product literature for further information · chronic obstructive pulmonary disease · history of myocardial infarction · history of symptomatic bradycardia or recurrent syncope · patients receiving antiarrhythmic or heart-rate lowering drugs including beta blockers, heart rate-lowering calcium channel blockers (seek advice from cardiologist regarding switching to alternative drugs, or if appropriate monitoring if unable to switch) · pulmonary fibrosis · risk of bradycardia and cardiac rhythm disturbance · risk of macular oedema · severe respiratory disease · severe sleep apnoea · significant QT prolongation (QTc greater than 470 milliseconds in women, or QTc greater than 450 milliseconds in men); if QTc 500 milliseconds or greater—see Contra-indications · sino-atrial heart block · susceptibility to QT-interval prolongation (including electrolyte disturbances) · uncontrolled hypertension

  CAUTIONS, FURTHER INFORMATION
- ▸ Washout period A washout period is recommended when switching treatment from some disease modifying therapies—consult product literature for further information.
- ▸ Bradycardia and cardiac rhythm disturbance Fingolimod may cause transient bradycardia, atrioventricular conduction delays and heart block after the first dose. Fingolimod is not recommended in patients with the cardiovascular risks listed above unless the anticipated benefits outweigh the potential risks, and advice from a cardiologist (including monitoring advice) is sought before initiation.

- **INTERACTIONS** → Appendix 1: fingolimod

- **SIDE-EFFECTS**
- ▸ **Common or very common** Alopecia · asthenia · atrioventricular block · back pain · bradycardia · cough · decreased leucocytes · depression · diarrhoea · dizziness · dyspnoea · headaches · hypertension · increased risk of infection · neoplasms · skin reactions · vision blurred
- ▸ **Uncommon** Macular oedema · nausea · thrombocytopenia
- ▸ **Rare or very rare** Posterior reversible encephalopathy syndrome (PRES)
- ▸ **Frequency not known** Peripheral oedema · progressive multifocal leukoencephalopathy

SIDE-EFFECTS, FURTHER INFORMATION
Basal-cell carcinoma Patients should be advised to seek medical advice if they have any signs of basal-cell carcinoma including skin nodules, patches or open sores that do not heal within weeks.
Progressive multifocal leukoencephalopathy (PML) and other opportunistic infections Patients should be advised to seek medical attention if they have any signs of PML or any other infections. Suspension of treatment should be considered if a patient develops a severe infection, taking into consideration the risk-benefit.

- **CONCEPTION AND CONTRACEPTION** Exclude pregnancy before treatment. Ensure effective contraception during and for at least 2 months after treatment.
- **PREGNANCY** Avoid (toxicity in *animal* studies).
- **BREAST FEEDING** Avoid.
- **HEPATIC IMPAIRMENT** Manufacturer advises caution when initiating treatment in mild-to-moderate impairment; avoid in severe impairment.
- **MONITORING REQUIREMENTS**
- ▸ **All** patients receiving fingolimod should be monitored at treatment initiation, (first dose monitoring—before, during and after dose), and after treatment interruption (see note below); monitoring should include:
- ▸ **Pre-treatment**
  - an ECG and blood pressure measurement before starting
- ▸ **During the first 6 hours of treatment**
  - continuous ECG monitoring for 6 hours
  - blood pressure and heart rate measurement every hour
- ▸ **After 6 hours of treatment**
  - a further ECG and blood pressure measurement
- ▸ If heart rate at the end of the 6 hour period is at its lowest since fingolimod was first administered, monitoring should be extended by at least 2 hours and until heart rate increases.
- ▸ If post-dose bradyarrhythmia-related symptoms occur, appropriate clinical management should be initiated and monitoring should be continued until the symptoms have resolved. If pharmacological intervention is required during the first-dose monitoring, overnight monitoring should follow, and the first-dose monitoring should then be repeated after the second dose.
- ▸ If after 6 hours, the heart rate is less than 45 beats per minute, or the ECG shows new onset second degree, higher grade AV block, or a QTc interval of 500 milliseconds or greater, or if third degree AV block occurs, monitoring should be extended (at least overnight, until side-effect resolution).
- ▸ The occurrence at any time of third degree AV block requires extended monitoring (at least overnight, until side-effect resolution).
- ▸ In case of T-wave inversion, ensure there are no associated signs or symptoms of myocardial ischaemia—if suspected seek advice from a cardiologist.
- ▸ **Note**
- ▸ First dose monitoring as above **should be repeated** in all patients whose treatment is interrupted for:
  - 1 day or more during the first 2 weeks of treatment
  - more than 7 days during weeks 3 and 4 of treatment
  - more than 2 weeks after one month of treatment
- ▸ If the treatment interruption is of shorter duration than the above, treatment should be continued with the next dose as planned.
- ▸ Manufacturer advises eye examination recommended 3–4 months after initiation of treatment (and before initiation of treatment in patients with diabetes or history of uveitis).
- ▸ Manufacturer advises skin examination for skin lesions before starting treatment and then every 6 to 12 months thereafter or as clinically indicated.

8

Immune system and malignant disease

▶ Monitor hepatic transaminases before treatment, then every 3 months for 1 year, then periodically thereafter.
▶ Monitor full blood count before treatment, at 3 months, then at least yearly thereafter and if signs of infection (interrupt treatment if lymphocyte count reduced)—consult product literature.
▶ Monitor for signs and symptoms of haemophagocytic syndrome (including pyrexia, asthenia, hepato-splenomegaly and adenopathy—may be associated with hepatic failure and respiratory distress; also progressive cytopenia, elevated serum-ferritin concentrations, hypertriglyceridaemia, hypofibrinogenaemia, coagulopathy, hepatic cytolysis, hyponatraemia)—initiate treatment immediately.
▶ Manufacturer advises to monitor routine MRI for lesions suggestive of progressive multifocal leukoencephalopathy (PML), particularly in patients considered at increased risk; monitor for signs and symptoms of new neurological dysfunction.

● NATIONAL FUNDING/ACCESS DECISIONS

NICE decisions

▶ Fingolimod for the treatment of highly active relapsing-remitting multiple sclerosis (April 2012) NICE TA254
Fingolimod is recommended as an option for the treatment of highly active relapsing-remitting multiple sclerosis in adults, only if:
• they have an unchanged or increased relapse rate or ongoing severe relapses compared with the previous year despite treatment with interferon beta, **and**
• the manufacturer provides fingolimod with the discount agreed as part of the patient access scheme
Patients currently receiving fingolimod whose disease does not meet the above criteria should be able to continue treatment until they and their clinician consider it appropriate to stop.
www.nice.org.uk/guidance/ta254

Scottish Medicines Consortium (SMC) Decisions
The *Scottish Medicines Consortium* has advised (September 2012) that fingolimod (*Gilenya* ®) is accepted for restricted use within NHS Scotland as single disease modifying therapy in highly active relapsing-remitting multiple sclerosis despite treatment with interferon beta, with an unchanged or increased relapse rate or ongoing severe relapses, as compared to the previous year. This advice is contingent upon the continuing availability of the patient access scheme in NHS Scotland.
The *Scottish Medicines Consortium* has advised (October 2014) that fingolimod (*Gilenya* ®) is accepted for restricted use within NHS Scotland as a single disease modifying therapy in highly active relapsing remitting multiple sclerosis for adults with rapidly evolving severe relapsing remitting multiple sclerosis. This advice is contingent upon the continuing availability of the patient access scheme in NHS Scotland, or a list price that is equivalent or lower.
The *Scottish Medicines Consortium* has advised (April 2015) that fingolimod (*Gilenya* ®) is accepted for use within NHS Scotland as a single disease modifying therapy in highly active relapsing remitting multiple sclerosis for adults with high disease activity despite treatment with at least one disease modifying therapy. This advice is contingent upon the continuing availability of the patient access scheme in NHS Scotland, or a list price that is equivalent or lower.

All Wales Medicines Strategy Group (AWMSG) Decisions
The *All Wales Medicines Strategy Group* has advised (January 2017) that fingolimod (*Gilenya* ®) is recommended as an option for use within NHS Wales as a single disease-modifying therapy in highly active relapsing-remitting multiple sclerosis only in patients with rapidly evolving severe relapsing-remitting multiple sclerosis defined by 2 or more disabling relapses in 1 year and with 1 or more

gadolinium-enhancing lesions on brain magnetic resonance imaging (MRI) or a significant increase in T2 lesion load compared with a previous recent MRI, only if the manufacturer provides fingolimod with the discount agreed as part of the patient access scheme or where the list price is equivalent or lower.

NHS restrictions
NHS England Clinical Commissioning Policy NHS England (May 2014) has provided guidance on the use of fingolimod for the treatment of multiple sclerosis in England. An NHS England Clinical Commissioning Policy outlines the funding arrangements and the criteria for initiating and discontinuing this treatment option, see www.england.nhs.uk/commissioning/wp-content/uploads/sites/12/2013/10/d04-p-b.pdf.

● MEDICINAL FORMS
There can be variation in the licensing of different medicines containing the same drug.
Capsule
▶ Gilenya (Novartis Pharmaceuticals UK Ltd) ▼
Fingolimod (as Fingolimod hydrochloride)
500 microgram Gilenya 0.5mg capsules | 7 capsule [PoM] £367.50 | 28 capsule [PoM] £1,470.00

IMMUNOSUPPRESSANTS > MONOCLONAL ANTIBODIES > ANTI-LYMPHOCYTE

Anti-lymphocyte monoclonal antibodies

● DRUG ACTION The anti-lymphocyte monoclonal antibodies cause lysis of B lymphocytes.

> IMPORTANT SAFETY INFORMATION
> All anti-lymphocyte monoclonal antibodies should be given under the supervision of an experienced specialist, in an environment where full resuscitation facilities are immediately available.

● SIDE-EFFECTS
▶ **Common or very common** Alopecia · anaemia · arthralgia · asthenia · back pain · chills · constipation · cough · cytokine release syndrome · depression · diarrhoea · dyspnoea · fever · flushing · headache · hypersensitivity (discontinue permanently) · hypertension · hypotension · increased risk of infection · infusion related reaction · leucopenia · nausea · neutropenia · pruritus · sweat changes · tachycardia · thrombocytopenia · tumour lysis syndrome · vomiting
▶ **Uncommon** Progressive multifocal leukoencephalopathy
▶ **Rare or very rare** Hepatitis B reactivation
▶ **Frequency not known** Anaphylactic reaction

SIDE-EFFECTS, FURTHER INFORMATION
Infusion-related side-effects In rare cases infusion reactions may be fatal. Infusion-related side-effects occur predominantly during the first infusion. Patients should receive premedication before administration of anti-lymphocyte monoclonal antibodies to reduce these effects - consult product literature for details of individual regimens. The infusion may have to be stopped temporarily and the infusion-related effects treated—consult product literature for appropriate management.
Cytokine release syndrome Fatalities following severe cytokine release syndrome (characterised by severe dyspnoea) and associated with features of tumour lysis syndrome have occurred after infusions of anti-lymphocyte monoclonal antibodies. Patients with a high tumour burden as well as those with pulmonary insufficiency or infiltration are at increased risk and should be monitored very closely (and a slower rate of infusion considered).

- PRE-TREATMENT SCREENING All patients should be screened for hepatitis B before treatment.
- MONITORING REQUIREMENTS Patients should also be monitored for cytopenias—consult product literature for specific recommendations.

▶ 836

Alemtuzumab

- INDICATIONS AND DOSE

Treatment of adults with relapsing-remitting multiple sclerosis with active disease defined by clinical or imaging features
  ▶ BY INTRAVENOUS INFUSION
  ▶ Adult: (consult product literature)

- UNLICENSED USE Although no longer licensed for oncological and transplant indications, alemtuzumab is also available through a patient access programme for these indications.

> IMPORTANT SAFETY INFORMATION
> Alemtuzumab should be given under the care of a specialist with facilities for the management of hypersenstivity and anaphylactic reactions.

- CONTRA-INDICATIONS Human immunodeficiency virus
- CAUTIONS Hepatitis B carriers · hepatitis C carriers · in patients with active infection, a delay in initiation of alemtuzumab treatment should be considered until the infection is fully controlled · not recommended for inactive disease · not recommended for stable disease · patients should receive oral prophylaxis for herpes infection starting on the first day of treatment and continuing for at least a month following each treatment course · patients with previous autoimmune conditions other than multiple sclerosis · pretreatment before administration is required (consult product literature)

  CAUTIONS, FURTHER INFORMATION For full details of cautions, consult product literature.
  ▶ Autoimmune mediated conditions The risk of autoimmune mediated conditions may increase during treatment, including immune thrombocytopenic purpura, thyroid disorders, nephropathies, and cytopenias, and should be monitored for throughout the course of treatment (consult product literature).

- INTERACTIONS → Appendix 1: monoclonal antibodies
- SIDE-EFFECTS
  ▶ Common or very common Abdominal pain · anxiety · autoimmune thyroiditis · goitre · haemorrhage · hyperthyroidism · hypothyroidism · influenza like illness · lymphadenopathy · lymphopenia · malaise · menstrual cycle irregularities · multiple sclerosis exacerbated · muscle complaints · muscle weakness · oropharyngeal pain · pain · palpitations · peripheral oedema · proteinuria · sensation abnormal · skin reactions · stomatitis · tremor · vertigo · vision blurred
  ▶ Uncommon Cervical dysplasia · conjunctivitis · dysphagia · gastrooesophageal reflux disease · hiccups · immune thrombocytopenic purpura · throat complaints · weight decreased
  ▶ Frequency not known Goodpasture's syndrome · nephropathy

- CONCEPTION AND CONTRACEPTION Women of childbearing potential should use effective contraception during and for 4 months after treatment.
- PREGNANCY Manufacturer advises avoid unless potential benefit outweighs risk—toxicity in *animal* studies. Autoimmune thyroid disease during treatment may affect fetus (consult product literature).

- BREAST FEEDING Manufacturer advises avoid during and for 4 months after each treatment course unless potential benefit outweighs risk.
- PRE-TREATMENT SCREENING Screening patients at high risk of hepatitis B or C is recommended before treatment. All patients should be evaluated for active or latent tuberculosis before starting treatment.
- MONITORING REQUIREMENTS HPV screening should be carried out annually in female patients.
- PRESCRIBING AND DISPENSING INFORMATION All patients should receive oral prophylaxis for herpes infection starting on the first day of treatment and continuing for at least a month following each treatment course.
- PATIENT AND CARER ADVICE Patients should be provided with a patient alert card and patient guide.
- NATIONAL FUNDING/ACCESS DECISIONS

  NICE decisions
  ▶ Alemtuzumab for treating relapsing-remitting multiple sclerosis (May 2014) NICE TA312
  Alemtuzumab is recommended as an option, within its marketing authorisation, for treating adults with active relapsing-remitting multiple sclerosis.
  www.nice.org.uk/TA312

- MEDICINAL FORMS
  There can be variation in the licensing of different medicines containing the same drug.
  Solution for infusion
  ▶ Lemtrada (Genzyme Therapeutics Ltd) ▼
    Alemtuzumab 10 mg per 1 ml Lemtrada 12mg/1.2ml concentrate for solution for infusion vials | 1 vial PoM £7,045.00 (Hospital only)
  ▶ MabCampath (Genzyme Therapeutics Ltd)
    Alemtuzumab 30 mg per 1 ml MabCampath 30mg/1ml concentrate for solution for infusion vials | 3 vial PoM £792.34 (Hospital only)

▶ 836

Natalizumab

- DRUG ACTION Natalizumab is a monoclonal antibody that inhibits the migration of leucocytes into the central nervous system, hence reducing inflammation and demyelination.

- INDICATIONS AND DOSE

Highly active relapsing-remitting multiple sclerosis despite treatment with interferon beta or glatiramer acetate, or those patients with rapidly evolving severe relapsing-remitting multiple sclerosis (initiated under specialist supervision)
  ▶ BY INTRAVENOUS INFUSION
  ▶ Adult 18–65 years: 300 mg every 4 weeks, treatment should be discontinued if no response after 6 months

- CONTRA-INDICATIONS Active infection · active malignancies (except cutaneous basal cell carcinoma) · immunosuppression · progressive multifocal leucoencephalopathy
- CAUTIONS
  CAUTIONS, FURTHER INFORMATION
  ▶ Progressive Multifocal Leucoencephalopathy Natalizumab is associated with an increased risk of opportunistic infection and progressive multifocal leucoencephalopathy (PML) caused by JC virus. The risk of developing PML increases with the presence of anti-JCV antibodies, previous use of immunosuppressant therapy, and treatment duration (especially beyond 2 years of treatment); the risk beyond 4 years of treatment is not known. Patients with all three risk factors should only be treated with natalizumab if the benefits of treatment outweigh the risks. Treatment should be suspended until PML has been excluded. If a patient develops an opportunistic infection or PML, natalizumab should be permanently discontinued.
    For information on cautions consult product literature.

8

Immune system and malignant disease

- INTERACTIONS → Appendix 1: monoclonal antibodies
- SIDE-EFFECTS Acute retinal necrosis · basophil count increased · eosinophilia · haemolytic anaemia · hyperbilirubinaemia · JC virus granule cell neuronopathy · liver injury · nucleated red cells

SIDE-EFFECTS, FURTHER INFORMATION

Progressive Multifocal Leukoencephalopathy (PML) If suspected, treatment should be suspended until PML has been excluded. If a patient develops an opportunistic infection or PML, natalizumab should be permanently discontinued.

Liver injury Discontinue treatment if significant liver injury occurs.

Infusion-related reactions Infusion-related reactions including dizziness, nausea, urticaria, chills, vomiting and flushing have been reported either during infusion or within 1 hour after completion of infusion.

- PREGNANCY Avoid unless essential—toxicity in *animal* studies.
- BREAST FEEDING Present in milk in *animal* studies—avoid.
- PRE-TREATMENT SCREENING

Progressive Multifocal Leucoencephalopathy A magnetic resonance image (MRI) scan is recommended before starting treatment with natalizumab.

Testing for serum anti-JCV antibodies before starting treatment or in those with unknown antibody status already receiving natalizumab is recommended and should be repeated every 6 months (consult product literature for full details).

- MONITORING REQUIREMENTS
▸ Monitor liver function.
▸ Progressive Multifocal Leucoencephalopathy A magnetic resonance image (MRI) scan is recommended annually. Patients should be monitored for new or worsening neurological symptoms, and for cognitive and psychiatric signs of PML. All patients should continue to be monitored for signs and symptoms that may be suggestive of PML for approximately 6 months following discontinuation of treatment.
▸ Hypersensitivity reactions Patients should be observed for hypersensitivity reactions, including anaphylaxis, during the infusion and for 1 hour after completion of the infusion.
- DIRECTIONS FOR ADMINISTRATION For *intravenous infusion* (*Tysabri*®), give intermittently in Sodium chloride 0.9%; dilute 300 mg in 100 mL infusion fluid; gently invert to mix, do not shake. Use within 8 hours of dilution and give over 1 hour.
- PATIENT AND CARER ADVICE A patient alert card should be provided.

Hypersensitivity reactions Patients should be told the importance of uninterrupted dosing, particularly in the early months of treatment (intermittent therapy may increase risk of sensitisation).

Progressive Multifocal Leucoencephalopathy Patients should be informed about the risks of PML before starting treatment with natalizumab and again after 2 years; they should be given an alert card which includes information about the symptoms of PML.

Liver toxicity Advise patients to seek immediate medical attention if symptoms such as jaundice or dark urine develop.

- NATIONAL FUNDING/ACCESS DECISIONS

NICE decisions
▸ Natalizumab for the treatment of adults with highly active relapsing-remitting multiple sclerosis (August 2007) NICE TA127

Natalizumab is an option for the treatment only of rapidly evolving severe relapsing-remitting multiple sclerosis (RES). RES is defined by 2 or more disabling relapses in

1 year, and 1 or more gadolinium-enhancing lesions on brain magnetic resonance imaging (MRI) or a significant increase in T2 lesion load compared with a previous MRI. www.nice.org.uk/TA127

Scottish Medicines Consortium (SMC) Decisions

The *Scottish Medicines Consortium* has advised (August 2007) that natalizumab is accepted for restricted use as single disease-modifying therapy in highly active relapsing-remitting multiple sclerosis only in patients with rapidly evolving severe relapsing-remitting multiple sclerosis defined by 2 or more disabling relapses in 1 year and with 1 or more gadolinium-enhancing lesions on brain magnetic resonance imaging (MRI) or a significant increase in T2 lesion load compared with a previous MRI.

NHS restrictions

NHS England Clinical Commissioning Policy NHS England (May 2014) has provided guidance on the use of natalizumab for the treatment of multiple sclerosis in England. An NHS England Clinical Commissioning Policy outlines the funding arrangements and the criteria for initiating and discontinuing this treatment option, see www.england.nhs.uk/commissioning/wp-content/uploads/sites/12/2013/10/d04-p-b.pdf.

- MEDICINAL FORMS
There can be variation in the licensing of different medicines containing the same drug.

Solution for infusion
ELECTROLYTES: May contain Sodium
▸ Tysabri (Biogen Idec Ltd) ▼
  Natalizumab 20 mg per 1 ml Tysabri 300mg/15ml concentrate for solution for infusion vials | 1 vial [PoM] £1,130.00 (Hospital only)

⧉ 836

Ocrelizumab

14-Mar-2018

- INDICATIONS AND DOSE

Multiple sclerosis (specialist use only)
▸ BY INTRAVENOUS INFUSION
▸ Adult: Initially 300 mg, then 300 mg after 2 weeks; maintenance 600 mg every 6 months, the first maintenance dose should be given 6 months after the first initial dose; a minimum interval of 5 months should be maintained between each maintenance dose, for dose interruption, adjustment of infusion rate or discontinuation of treatment due to infusion-related reactions or side-effects—consult product literature

- CONTRA-INDICATIONS Active infection · active malignancies · severely immunocompromised patients
- CAUTIONS Complete required vaccinations at least 6 weeks before treatment initiation · hepatitis B reactivation
- INTERACTIONS → Appendix 1: monoclonal antibodies
- CONCEPTION AND CONTRACEPTION Manufacturer advises women of childbearing potential should use contraception during treatment and for 12 months after the last dose.
- PREGNANCY Manufacturer advises avoid unless potential benefit outweighs risk—limited information available; monitor infants for B-cell depletion.
- BREAST FEEDING Manufacturer advises avoid—present in milk in *animal* studies.
- MONITORING REQUIREMENTS
▸ Manufacturer advises monitor for signs and symptoms of progressive multifocal leucoencephalopathy (PML) (including any new onset or worsening of neurological symptoms)—if PML is suspected, interrupt treatment; discontinue treatment permanently if PML is confirmed.
▸ Manufacturer advises monitor for infusion-related reactions during the infusion and observe patients for 1 hour after completion of the infusion—if severe pulmonary symptoms occur, permanently discontinue treatment.

● PRESCRIBING AND DISPENSING INFORMATION
Manufacturer advises to record the batch number after
each administration.

● HANDLING AND STORAGE Manufacturer advises store in a
refrigerator (2–8°C)—consult product literature for further
information regarding storage conditions after preparation
of the infusion.

● PATIENT AND CARER ADVICE Manufacturer advises
patients and carers should be advised that infusion-related
reactions can occur within 24 hours of infusion.

● MEDICINAL FORMS
There can be variation in the licensing of different medicines
containing the same drug.
Solution for infusion
▸ Ocrevus (Roche Products Ltd) ▼
Ocrelizumab 30 mg per 1 ml Ocrevus 300mg/10ml concentrate for
solution for infusion vials | 1 vial [PoM] Ⓢ

IMMUNOSUPPRESSANTS > PYRIMIDINE
SYNTHESIS INHIBITORS

Teriflunomide

● DRUG ACTION Teriflunomide is a metabolite of
leflunomide which has immunomodulating and anti-
inflammatory properties.

● INDICATIONS AND DOSE
**Treatment of relapsing-remitting multiple sclerosis
(initiated under specialist supervision)**
▸ BY MOUTH
▸ Adult: 14 mg once daily

● CONTRA-INDICATIONS Anaemia · leucopenia · neutropenia
· serious infection · severe hypoproteinaemia · severe
immunodeficiency · significantly impaired bone-marrow
function · thrombocytopenia

● CAUTIONS Adult over 65 years · anaemia · dyspnoea—
assess for interstitial lung disease and consider suspending
treatment · hypoproteinaemia (avoid if severe) · impaired
bone-marrow function (avoid if severe) · latent
tuberculosis · leucopenia · persistent cough—assess for
interstitial lung disease and consider suspending
treatment · severe infection—delay or suspend treatment
until resolved · significant alcohol consumption · signs or
symptoms of serious skin reactions (including ulcerative
stomatitis, Stevens-Johnson syndrome, and toxic
epidermal necrolysis)—discontinue treatment · switching
between other immunomodulating drugs ·
thrombocytopenia

● INTERACTIONS → Appendix 1: teriflunomide

● SIDE-EFFECTS
▸ **Common or very common** Abdominal pain upper · alopecia ·
anaemia · anxiety · arthralgia · cystitis · diarrhoea ·
headache · hypersensitivity · hypertension · increased risk
of infection · menorrhagia · myalgia · nausea · nerve
disorders · neutropenia · oral disorders · pain · palpitations
· sensation abnormal · skin reactions · urinary frequency
increased · vomiting · weight decreased
▸ **Uncommon** Thrombocytopenia
▸ **Frequency not known** Asthenia · hepatitis acute · interstitial
lung disease · nail disorder · pancreatitis · sepsis
SIDE-EFFECTS, FURTHER INFORMATION
Hepatic injury Discontinue treatment if signs or
symptoms of hepatic injury, or if liver enzymes exceed
3 times the upper limit of reference range.
Important: accelerated elimination procedure
recommended following discontinuation due to serious
adverse effects (consult product literature).

● CONCEPTION AND CONTRACEPTION Effective
contraception essential for women of child-bearing

potential during treatment and for up to 2 years after
treatment. In patients undergoing treatment with
teriflunomide that are planning to conceive, the
accelerated elimination procedure should be used prior to
conception. Use of non-oral contraception is
recommended during the accelerated elimination
procedure—consult product literature.

● PREGNANCY Avoid—toxicity in animal studies.

● BREAST FEEDING Present in milk in *animal* studies—
manufacturer advises avoid.

● HEPATIC IMPAIRMENT Avoid in severe impairment.

● MONITORING REQUIREMENTS
▸ Monitor full blood count (including differential white cell
count and platelet count) before treatment and as
clinically indicated during treatment.
▸ Monitor blood pressure before treatment and periodically
thereafter.
▸ Hepatic monitoring Monitor liver function before treatment
and every 2 weeks for first 6 months then every 8 weeks
thereafter or as clinically indicated (pre-existing liver
disease may increase risk). Increase to weekly monitoring
if alanine aminotransferase (ALT) is 2–3 times the upper
limit of reference range; discontinue treatment if signs or
symptoms of hepatic injury, or if liver enzymes exceed
3 times the upper limit of reference range.

● TREATMENT CESSATION
Accelerated elimination procedures To aid drug elimination in
case of serious adverse effect or before conception, stop
treatment and give *either* colestyramine p. 196 *or* charcoal,
activated p. 1326. After the accelerated elimination
procedure a plasma concentration of less than
20 micrograms/litre (measured on 2 occasions at least
14 days apart) and a waiting period of one and a half
months are necessary before conception.

● NATIONAL FUNDING/ACCESS DECISIONS
NICE decisions
▸ Teriflunomide for treating relapsing-remitting multiple
sclerosis (January 2014) NICE TA303
Teriflunomide is recommended for the treatment of adults
with active relapsing-remitting multiple sclerosis
(normally defined as 2 clinically significant relapses in the
previous 2 years), in adults who:
● do not have highly active or rapidly evolving severe
relapsing-remitting multiple sclerosis **and**
● the manufacturer provides teriflunomide with the
discount agreed in the patient access scheme
www.nice.org.uk/TA303
Scottish Medicines Consortium (SMC) Decisions
The *Scottish Medicines Consortium* has advised (February
2014) that the use of teriflunomide (*Aubagio*)® in NHS
Scotland is restricted to use in patients with relapsing-
remitting multiple sclerosis who do not have highly active
disease, and only as an alternative to treatment with
interferon beta or glatiramer acetate.

● MEDICINAL FORMS
There can be variation in the licensing of different medicines
containing the same drug.
Tablet
▸ Aubagio (Genzyme Therapeutics Ltd) ▼
Teriflunomide 14 mg Aubagio 14mg tablets | 28 tablet [PoM]
£1,037.84

8

Immune system and malignant disease

Malignant disease

1 Antibody responsive malignancy

ANTINEOPLASTIC DRUGS > MONOCLONAL ANTIBODIES

Atezolizumab

30-Jan-2018

- **DRUG ACTION** Atezolizumab is a monoclonal antibody, which binds to the programmed death-1 (PD-1) receptor, thereby potentiating an immune response to tumour cells.

- **INDICATIONS AND DOSE**

Urothelial carcinoma (specialist use only) | Non-small cell lung cancer (specialist use only)
  - ▶ BY INTRAVENOUS INFUSION
  - ▶ Adult: 1200 mg every 3 weeks, for dose interruption, adjustment of infusion rate or discontinuation of treatment due to side-effects or infusion-related reactions—consult product literature

- **CAUTIONS** Abnormal thyroid function—manufacturer advises to consider appropriate treatment · patients may need pre-medication to minimise the development of infusion-related reactions—consult product literature

- **INTERACTIONS** → Appendix 1: monoclonal antibodies

- **SIDE-EFFECTS**
  - ▶ **Common or very common** Abdominal pain · appetite decreased · arthralgia · asthenia · chills · colitis · diarrhoea · dysphagia · dyspnoea · electrolyte imbalance · fever · hyperthyroidism · hypotension · hypothyroidism · hypoxia · influenza like illness · musculoskeletal pain · nasal congestion · nausea · pneumonitis · skin reactions · thrombocytopenia · vomiting
  - ▶ **Uncommon** Adrenal insufficiency · diabetes mellitus · Guillain-Barre syndrome · hepatitis · meningitis non-infective · pancreatitis
  - ▶ **Rare or very rare** Encephalitis non-infective · hypophysitis

SIDE-EFFECTS, FURTHER INFORMATION
Immune-related reactions Manufacturer advises most immune-related adverse reactions are reversible and managed by temporarily stopping treatment and administration of a corticosteroid—consult product literature.
Infusion-related reactions Manufacturer advises permanently discontinue treatment in patients with severe infusion reactions.

- **CONCEPTION AND CONTRACEPTION** Manufacturer advises effective contraception in women of childbearing potential, during treatment and for 5 months after stopping treatment. See also *Pregnancy and reproductive function* in Cytotoxic drugs p. 865.

- **PREGNANCY** Manufacturer advises avoid unless essential—no information available. See also *Pregnancy and reproductive function* in Cytotoxic drugs p. 865.

- **BREAST FEEDING** Manufacturer advises avoid—no information available.

- **MONITORING REQUIREMENTS** Manufacturer advises monitor for signs and symptoms of infusion- and immune-related reactions—consult product literature.

- **PRESCRIBING AND DISPENSING INFORMATION** Manufacturer advises to record the brand name and batch number after each administration.

All prescribers should be familiar with the *Physician Information and Management Guidelines* provided by the manufacturer.

- **HANDLING AND STORAGE** Manufacturer advises store in a refrigerator (2–8°C); consult product literature for storage conditions after dilution.

- **PATIENT AND CARER ADVICE** An alert card should be provided.
Missed doses Manufacturer advises if a dose is missed, it should be administered as soon as possible—administration schedule should be adjusted to maintain a 3-week interval between doses.
Driving and skilled tasks Manufacturer advises patients should be counselled on the effects on driving and performance of skilled tasks—increased risk of drowsiness.

- **NATIONAL FUNDING/ACCESS DECISIONS**
NICE decisions
  - ▶ Atezolizumab for untreated locally advanced or metastatic urothelial cancer when cisplatin is unsuitable (December 2017) NICE TA492
Atezolizumab is recommended for use within the Cancer Drugs Fund as an option for untreated locally advanced or metastatic urothelial carcinoma in adults, for whom cisplatin-based chemotherapy is unsuitable, only if the conditions of the managed access agreement for atezolizumab are followed.
Patients whose treatment was started within the NHS before this guidance was published should have the option to continue treatment, without change to their funding arrangements, until they and their NHS clinician consider it appropriate to stop.
www.nice.org.uk/guidance/ta492

  - ▶ Atezolizumab for treating locally advanced or metastatic non-small-cell lung cancer after chemotherapy (May 2018) NICE TA520
Atezolizumab is recommended as an option for treating locally advanced or metastatic non-small-cell lung cancer (NSCLC) in adults who have had chemotherapy (and targeted treatment if they have an EGFR- or ALK-positive tumour), only if:
    - atezolizumab is stopped at 2 years of uninterrupted treatment or earlier if the disease progresses, **and**
    - the manufacturer provides atezolizumab with the discount agreed in the patient access scheme.
Patients whose treatment was started within the NHS before this guidance was published should have the option to continue treatment, without change to their funding arrangements, until they and their NHS clinician consider it appropriate to stop.
www.nice.org.uk/guidance/ta520

Scottish Medicines Consortium (SMC) Decisions
SMC No. 1297/18
The *Scottish Medicines Consortium* has advised (March 2018) that atezolizumab (*Tecentriq®*) is **not** recommended for use within NHS Scotland as monotherapy for the treatment of adults with locally advanced or metastatic urothelial carcinoma after prior platinum-containing chemotherapy, or who are considered cisplatin ineligible as the economic case was not demonstrated.

- **MEDICINAL FORMS**
There can be variation in the licensing of different medicines containing the same drug.
Solution for infusion
  - ▶ Tecentriq (Roche Products Ltd) ▼
Atezolizumab 60 mg per 1 ml Tecentriq 1200mg/20ml concentrate for solution for infusion vials | 1 vial PoM £3,807.69

Avelumab
18-May-2018

- DRUG ACTION Avelumab is a monoclonal antibody, which binds to the programmed death-1 (PD-1) receptor, thereby potentiating an immune response to tumour cells.

● INDICATIONS AND DOSE

Metastatic Merkel cell carcinoma (specialist use only)
▶ BY INTRAVENOUS INFUSION
▶ Adult: 10 mg/kg every 2 weeks, for information on dose delay or interruption due to side-effects and infusion-related reactions—consult product literature

- CAUTIONS Patients should receive pre-medication to minimise the development of adverse reactions (consult product literature)
- INTERACTIONS → Appendix 1: monoclonal antibodies
- SIDE-EFFECTS
▶ **Common or very common** Abdominal pain · anaemia · appetite decreased · arthralgia · asthenia · chills · constipation · cough · diarrhoea · dizziness · dry mouth · dyspnoea · endocrine disorders · fever · headache · hypertension · hypotension · influenza like illness · lymphopenia · myalgia · nausea · nerve disorders · peripheral oedema · pneumonitis · skin reactions · vomiting · weight decreased
▶ **Uncommon** Adrenal insufficiency · diabetes mellitus · eosinophilia · flushing · gastrointestinal disorders · hepatic disorders · hypopituitarism · myositis · nephritis tubulointerstitial · systemic inflammatory response syndrome · thrombocytopenia · uveitis
▶ **Rare or very rare** Myocarditis
SIDE-EFFECTS, FURTHER INFORMATION
Infusion-related reactions For treatment modifications in patients with grade 1 or 2 infusion-related reactions, consult product literature. Manufacturer advises permanently discontinue treatment in patients with grade 3 or 4 infusion-related reaction.
Immune-related reactions Most immune-related adverse reactions are reversible and managed by temporarily stopping treatment and administration of a corticosteroid—consult product literature for further information.
- CONCEPTION AND CONTRACEPTION Manufacturer advises women of child-bearing potential should use effective contraception during treatment and for at least 1 month after stopping treatment.
- PREGNANCY Manufacturer advises avoid unless essential—no information available. See also *Pregnancy and reproductive function* in Cytotoxic drugs p. 865.
- BREAST FEEDING Manufacturer advises avoid during treatment and for at least 1 month after stopping treatment—no information available.
- MONITORING REQUIREMENTS Manufacturer advises monitor for signs and symptoms of infusion- and immune-related reactions.
- DIRECTIONS FOR ADMINISTRATION Manufacturer advises for *intermittent intravenous infusion* (Bavencio®), dilute requisite dose with Sodium Chloride 0.9%; give over 60 minutes via a separate line using a low-protein binding 0.2 micron filter.
- HANDLING AND STORAGE Manufacturer advises store in a refrigerator (2–8 °C)—consult product literature for storage conditions after preparation of the infusion.
- NATIONAL FUNDING/ACCESS DECISIONS
NICE decisions
▶ Avelumab for treating metastatic Merkel cell carcinoma (April 2018) NICE TA517
Avelumab is recommended as an option for treating metastatic Merkel cell carcinoma in adults, only if they

have had 1 or more lines of chemotherapy for metastatic disease.
Avelumab is recommended for use within the Cancer Drugs Fund as an option for treating metastatic Merkel cell carcinoma in adults, only if:
- they have not had chemotherapy for metastatic disease, and
- the conditions in the managed access agreement for avelumab are followed.
Patients whose treatment was started within the NHS before this guidance was published should have the option to continue treatment, without change to their funding arrangements, until they and their NHS clinician consider it appropriate to stop.
www.nice.org.uk/guidance/ta517
Scottish Medicines Consortium (SMC) Decisions
SMC No. 1315/18
The *Scottish Medicines Consortium* has advised (May 2018) that avelumab (Bavencio®) is accepted for use within NHS Scotland as monotherapy for treating adults with metastatic Merkel cell carcinoma.

● MEDICINAL FORMS
There can be variation in the licensing of different medicines containing the same drug.
Solution for infusion
▶ Bavencio (Merck Serono Ltd) ▼
Avelumab 20 mg per 1 ml Bavencio 200mg/10ml concentrate for solution for infusion vials | 1 vial [PoM] £768.00

Bevacizumab
28-Jun-2017

- DRUG ACTION Bevacizumab is a monoclonal antibody that inhibits vascular endothelial growth factor.

● INDICATIONS AND DOSE

Treatment of metastatic colorectal cancer in combination with fluoropyrimidine-based chemotherapy | First-line treatment of metastatic breast cancer in combination with paclitaxel when treatment with other chemotherapy, including taxanes or anthracyclines is not appropriate | First-line treatment of metastatic breast cancer in combination with capecitabine when treatment with other chemotherapy, including taxanes or anthracyclines is not appropriate (patients who have received adjuvant taxane or anthracycline-containing regimens in the previous 12 months should not be treated with bevacizumab in combination with capecitabine) | Advanced or metastatic renal cell carcinoma in combination with interferon alfa-2a | First-line treatment of unresectable advanced, metastatic or recurrent non-small cell lung cancer other than predominantly squamous cell histology (In combination with platinum-based chemotherapy) | First-line treatment of advanced (FIGO stages IIIB, IIIC and IV) epithelial ovarian, fallopian tube, or primary peritoneal cancer (in combination with carboplatin and paclitaxel) | First recurrence of platinum-sensitive epithelial ovarian, fallopian tube, or primary peritoneal cancer in patients who have not been treated previously with bevacizumab or other drugs that target vascular endothelial growth factor (in combination with carboplatin and gemcitabine)
▶ BY INTRAVENOUS INFUSION
▶ Adult: (consult local protocol)

IMPORTANT SAFETY INFORMATION
MHRA/CHM ADVICE: BEVACIZUMAB AND SUNITINIB: RISK OF OSTEONECROSIS OF THE JAW (JANUARY 2011)
Treatment with bevacizumab or sunitinib may be a risk factor for the development of osteonecrosis of the jaw.

8

Immune system and malignant disease

Patients treated with bevacizumab or sunitinib, who have previously received bisphosphonates, or are treated concurrently with bisphosphonates, may be particularly at risk.

Dental examination and appropriate preventive dentistry should be considered before treatment with bevacizumab or sunitinib.

If possible, invasive dental procedures should be avoided in patients treated with bevacizumab or sunitinib who have previously received, or who are currently receiving, intravenous bisphosphonates.

● CAUTIONS Elective surgery (withhold treatment and avoid for at least 28 days after major surgery or until wound fully healed) · history of arterial thromboembolism · history of cardiovascular disease (increased risk of cardiovascular events, especially in the elderly) · history of hypertension (increased risk of proteinuria—discontinue if nephrotic syndrome) · increased risk of fistulas (discontinue permanently if tracheo-oesophageal or grade 4 fistula develops) · increased risk of haemorrhage · increased risk of tumour-associated haemorrhage · intra-abdominal inflammation (risk of gastro-intestinal perforation and gall bladder perforation · uncontrolled hypertension · untreated CNS metastases

● INTERACTIONS → Appendix 1: monoclonal antibodies

● SIDE-EFFECTS

▶ **Common or very common** Abscess · anaemia · appetite decreased · arthralgia · asthenia · congestive heart failure · constipation · cough · decreased leucocytes · dehydration · diarrhoea · drowsiness · dysarthria · dysphonia · dyspnoea · electrolyte imbalance · embolism and thrombosis · eye disorders · fever · fistula · gastrointestinal discomfort · gastrointestinal disorders · haemorrhage · headache · healing impaired · hypersensitivity · hypertension · hypoxia · increased risk of infection · infusion related reaction · mucositis · muscle weakness · myalgia · nausea · neutropenia · ovarian failure · pain · pelvic pain · peripheral neuropathy · proteinuria · rectovaginal fistula · sepsis · skin reactions · stomatitis · stroke · supraventricular tachycardia · syncope · taste altered · thrombocytopenia · vomiting · weight decreased

▶ **Rare or very rare** Encephalopathy · necrotising fasciitis (discontinue and initiate treatment promptly)

▶ **Frequency not known** Chest pain · chills · flushing · gallbladder perforation · hyperglycaemia · hypotension · nasal septum perforation · osteonecrosis · pulmonary hypertension · renal thrombotic microangiopathy

● CONCEPTION AND CONTRACEPTION Effective contraception required during and for at least 6 months after treatment in women.

● PREGNANCY Avoid—toxicity in *animal* studies. See also *Pregnancy and reproductive function* in Cytotoxic drugs p. 865.

● BREAST FEEDING Manufacturer advises avoid breast-feeding during and for at least 6 months after treatment.

● MONITORING REQUIREMENTS

▶ Monitor for necrotising fasciitis (usually secondary to wound healing complications, gastro-intestinal perforation or fistula formation)—discontinue and initiate treatment promptly.

▶ Monitor blood pressure.

▶ Monitor for congestive heart failure.

▶ Monitor for posterior reversible encephalopathy syndrome (presenting as seizures, headache, altered mental status, visual disturbance or cortical blindness, with or without hypertension).

▶ Consider dental check-up before initiating treatment (risk of osteonecrosis of the jaw).

● NATIONAL FUNDING/ACCESS DECISIONS

NICE decisions

▶ **Bevacizumab and cetuximab for the treatment of metastatic colorectal cancer (January 2007)** NICE TA118
Bevacizumab in combination with fluorouracil plus folinic acid, with or without irinotecan, is **not** recommended for the first-line treatment of metastatic colorectal cancer; see also NICE guidance Cetuximab, bevacizumab and panitumumab for the treatment of metastatic colorectal cancer after first-line chemotherapy.
www.nice.org.uk/guidance/TA118

▶ **Bevacizumab in combination with oxaliplatin and either fluorouracil plus folinic acid or capecitabine for the treatment of metastatic colorectal cancer (December 2010)** NICE TA212
Bevacizumab in combination with oxaliplatin and either fluorouracil plus folinic acid or capecitabine is **not** recommended for the treatment of metastatic colorectal cancer.
www.nice.org.uk/guidance/TA212

▶ **Cetuximab, bevacizumab and panitumumab for the treatment of metastatic colorectal cancer after first-line chemotherapy (January 2012)** NICE TA242
Bevacizumab in combination with non-oxaliplatin (fluoropyrimidine-based) chemotherapy is **not** recommended for the treatment of patients with metastatic colorectal cancer that has progressed after first-line chemotherapy; see also NICE guidance Bevacizumab and cetuximab for the treatment of metastatic colorectal cancer (January 2007).
www.nice.org.uk/guidance/TA242

▶ **Bevacizumab (first-line), sorafenib (first and second-line), sunitinib (second-line) and temsirolimus (first-line) for the treatment of advanced and/or metastatic renal cell carcinoma (August 2009)** NICE TA178
Bevacizumab, sorafenib, and temsirolimus are **not** recommended as first-line treatments for people with advanced and/or metastatic renal cell carcinoma. Sorafenib and sunitinib are not recommended as second-line treatments for people with advanced and/or metastatic renal cell carcinoma.
www.nice.org.uk/guidance/TA178

▶ **Bevacizumab in combination with a taxane for the first-line treatment of metastatic breast cancer (February 2011)** NICE TA214
Bevacizumab in combination with a taxane is **not** recommended for the first-line treatment of metastatic breast cancer.
www.nice.org.uk/guidance/TA214

▶ **Bevacizumab in combination with capecitabine for the first-line treatment of metastatic breast cancer (August 2012)** NICE TA263
Bevacizumab in combinations with capecitabine is **not** recommended within its marketing authorisation for the first-line treatment of metastatic breast cancer, that is, when treatment with other chemotherapy options including taxanes or anthracyclines is not considered appropriate, or when taxanes or anthracyclines have been used as part of adjuvant treatment in the previous 12 months.
www.nice.org.uk/guidance/TA263

▶ **Bevacizumab in combination with paclitaxel and carboplatin for the first-line treatment of advanced ovarian cancer (May 2013)** NICE TA284
Bevacizumab in combination with paclitaxel and carboplatin is **not** recommended for the first-line treatment of advanced ovarian cancer (including fallopian tube and primary peritoneal cancer).
www.nice.org.uk/guidance/TA284

▶ **Bevacizumab in combination with gemcitabine and carboplatin for the treatment of the first recurrence of**

platinum-sensitive advanced ovarian cancer (May 2013)
NICE TA285
Bevacizumab in combination with gemcitabine and carboplatin is **not** recommended within its marketing authorisation, that is, for the treatment of the first recurrence of platinum-sensitive advanced ovarian cancer (including fallopian tube and primary peritoneal cancer) that has not been previously treated with bevacizumab or other vascular endothelial growth factor (VEGF) inhibitors or VEGF receptor-targeted agents.
www.nice.org.uk/guidance/TA285

Scottish Medicines Consortium (SMC) Decisions
The *Scottish Medicines Consortium* has advised (May 2012) that bevacizumab (*Avastin*®) is **not** recommended for use within NHS Scotland for the first line treatment of patients with metastatic breast cancer in whom treatment with other chemotherapy options including taxanes or anthracyclines is not considered appropriate.

The *Scottish Medicines Consortium* has advised (September 2015) that bevacizumab (*Avastin*®) is accepted for restricted use within NHS Scotland in combination with paclitaxel for the treatment of adult patients with platinum-resistant recurrent epithelial ovarian, fallopian tube, or primary peritoneal cancer who received no more than two prior chemotherapy regimens and who have not received prior therapy with bevacizumab or other vascular endothelial growth factor (VEGF) inhibitors or VEGF receptor-targeted agents.

The *Scottish Medicines Consortium* has advised (November 2015) that bevacizumab (*Avastin*®) is accepted for restricted use within NHS Scotland in combination with carboplatin and paclitaxel for the first-line treatment of advanced FIGO stage IV epithelial ovarian, fallopian tube, or primary peritoneal cancer.

All Wales Medicines Strategy Group (AWMSG) Decisions
The *All Wales Medicines Strategy Group* has advised (September 2017) that bevacizumab (*Avastin*®) is not recommended for use within NHS Wales in combination with paclitaxel and cisplatin, or alternatively, paclitaxel and topotecan in patients who cannot receive platinum therapy, for the treatment of adults with persistent, recurrent, or metastatic carcinoma of the cervix. The case for cost-effectiveness has not been proven.

● MEDICINAL FORMS
There can be variation in the licensing of different medicines containing the same drug.
Solution for infusion
▸ Avastin (Roche Products Ltd)
Bevacizumab 25 mg per 1 ml Avastin 400mg/16ml solution for infusion vials | 1 vial [PoM] £924.40 (Hospital only)
Avastin 100mg/4ml solution for infusion vials | 1 vial [PoM] £242.66 (Hospital only)

Blinatumomab

20-Jul-2017

● DRUG ACTION The anti-lymphocyte monoclonal antibodies cause lysis of B lymphocytes.

● INDICATIONS AND DOSE
Relapsed or refractory Philadelphia chromosome-negative acute lymphoblastic leukaemia
▸ BY CONTINUOUS INTRAVENOUS INFUSION
▸ Adult (body-weight 45 kg and above): Initially 9 micrograms/24 hours on days 1–7 of first cycle, followed by 28 micrograms/24 hours on days 8–28, first cycle is followed by a 2 week treatment-free interval, then 28 micrograms/24 hours for days 1–28 of second and subsequent cycles—patients who achieve complete remission after 2 treatment cycles may receive up to 3 additional cycles of consolidation treatment, for dose adjustments due to side-effects and infusion-related

reactions or patients with high tumour burden—consult product literature

● CAUTIONS Aphasia · brain injuries (severe) · cerebellar disease · dementia · elderly—limited information available · epilepsy · paresis · Parkinson's disease · patients may need pre-medication to minimise adverse reactions · psychosis · seizure · severe hepatic impairment · severe renal impairment · stroke

CAUTIONS, FURTHER INFORMATION
▸ Pre-medication Manufacturer advises pre-medication with intravenous dexamethasone and an anti-pyretic—consult product literature.
▸ Neurological events There is potentially a higher risk of neurological events in patients with clinically relevant CNS pathology—manufacturer advises caution.

● INTERACTIONS → Appendix 1: monoclonal antibodies

● SIDE-EFFECTS
▸ **Common or very common** Abdominal pain · anaemia · aphasia · appetite decreased · arthralgia · chest pain · chills · cognitive disorder · confusion · constipation · cough · decreased leucocytes · diarrhoea · dizziness · dyspnoea · electrolyte imbalance · encephalopathy · facial swelling · fatigue · fever · flushing · headache · hyperglycaemia · hypersensitivity · hypertension · hypoalbuminaemia · hypotension · immune disorder · increased risk of infection · insomnia · leucocytosis · memory loss · nausea · neutropenia · oedema · pain · paraesthesia · rash · seizure · sepsis · tachycardia · thrombocytopenia · tremor · tumour lysis syndrome · vomiting · wheezing
▸ **Uncommon** Capillary leak syndrome · cranial nerve disorder · pancreatitis

SIDE-EFFECTS, FURTHER INFORMATION
Pancreatitis Life-threatening or fatal cases of pancreatitis have been reported; manufacturer advises monitor for signs and symptoms of pancreatitis during treatment—temporary interruption or discontinuation may be required (consult product literature).
Cytokine release syndrome, infusion-reactions and tumour lysis syndrome Life-threatening (including fatal) cases of cytokine release syndrome and tumour lysis syndrome have been reported in patients taking blinatumomab. Manufacturer advises monitor signs and symptoms of cytokine release syndrome and infusion reactions during treatment; temporary interruption or discontinuation may be required—consult product literature.

● CONCEPTION AND CONTRACEPTION Manufacturer advises effective contraception during treatment and for at least 48 hours after treatment in women of child-bearing potential. See also Pregnancy and reproductive function in Cytotoxic drugs p. 865.

● PREGNANCY Manufacturer advises avoid unless potential benefit outweighs risk—no information available; if exposed during pregnancy, monitor infant for B-cell depletion. See also Pregnancy and reproductive function in Cytotoxic drugs p. 865.

● BREAST FEEDING Manufacturer advises avoid during and for at least 48 hours after treatment—no information available.

● HEPATIC IMPAIRMENT Manufacturer advises caution in severe impairment—no information available.

● RENAL IMPAIRMENT Manufacturer advises caution in severe impairment—no information available.

● MONITORING REQUIREMENTS Manufacturer advises neurological examination prior to the initiation of treatment and continued monitoring during treatment—consult product literature.

- HANDLING AND STORAGE Manufacturer advises store in a refrigerator (2–8°C); consult product literature for storage conditions after reconstitution and dilution.
- PATIENT AND CARER ADVICE A patient alert card should be provided. Educational materials should be provided to patients, carers and healthcare professionals to ensure blinatumomab is used in a safe and effective way, and to prevent the risk of medication errors and neurological events—consult product information.
  Driving and skilled tasks Manufacturer advises patients and carers should be counselled about the effects on driving and performance of skilled tasks—increased risk of confusion, disorientation, co-ordination and balance disorders, seizures and disturbances in consciousness.
- NATIONAL FUNDING/ACCESS DECISIONS
  NICE decisions
  ▶ **Blinatumomab for previously treated Philadelphia-chromosome-negative acute lymphoblastic leukaemia (June 2017)** NICE TA450
  Blinatumomab is recommended within its marketing authorisation as an option for treating Philadelphia-chromosome-negative relapsed or refractory precursor B-cell acute lymphoblastic leukaemia in adults, only if the company provides it with the discount agreed in the patient access scheme.
  www.nice.org.uk/guidance/TA450
- MEDICINAL FORMS
  There can be variation in the licensing of different medicines containing the same drug.
  Powder for solution for infusion
  ▶ Blincyto (Amgen Ltd) ▼
  Blinatumomab 38.5 microgram Blincyto 38.5micrograms powder for concentrate and solution for solution for infusion vials | 1 vial [PoM] £2,017.00

Brentuximab vedotin

19-Jul-2017

- **INDICATIONS AND DOSE**
  Treatment of relapsed or refractory CD-30 positive Hodgkin's disease following autologous stem cell transplant or following at least two prior therapies, when autologous stem cell transplant or multi-agent chemotherapy is not a treatment option | Relapsed or refractory systemic anaplastic large cell lymphoma
  ▶ BY INTRAVENOUS INFUSION
  ▶ Adult: (consult product literature)

- CAUTIONS Elevated BMI—risk of hyperglycaemia · high tumour burden—risk of tumour lysis syndrome · rapidly proliferating tumours—risk of tumour lysis syndrome
- INTERACTIONS → Appendix 1: monoclonal antibodies
- SIDE-EFFECTS
  ▶ **Common or very common** Abdominal pain · alopecia · anaemia · arthralgia · back pain · chills · constipation · cough · diarrhoea · dizziness · dyspnoea · fatigue · fever · hyperglycaemia · increased risk of infection · infusion related reaction · myalgia · nausea · nerve disorders · neutropenia · sepsis · skin reactions · thrombocytopenia · vomiting · weight decreased
  ▶ **Uncommon** Cytomegalovirus infection reactivation · pancreatitis acute · tumour lysis syndrome
  ▶ **Rare or very rare** Severe cutaneous adverse reactions (SCARs)
  ▶ **Frequency not known** Acute respiratory distress syndrome (ARDS) · anaphylactic reaction · disease recurrence · gastrointestinal disorders · gastrointestinal haemorrhage · paraesthesia · progressive multifocal leukoencephalopathy
- CONCEPTION AND CONTRACEPTION Effective contraception required during treatment and for 6 months after treatment in men and women.

- PREGNANCY Avoid unless potential benefit outweighs risk (toxicity in *animal* studies).
- BREAST FEEDING Avoid—no information available.
- MONITORING REQUIREMENTS
  ▶ Monitor for symptoms of progressive multifocal leucoencephalopathy (presenting as new or worsening neurological, cognitive or behavioural signs or symptoms).
  ▶ Monitor for new or worsening abdominal pain—investigate and withhold treatment if acute pancreatitis suspected and discontinue if confirmed (fatal cases reported).
  ▶ Monitor for pulmonary toxicity—treat symptoms promptly.
  ▶ Routinely monitor hepatic function.
  ▶ Monitor for infusion-related (including anaphylactic) reactions.
  ▶ Monitor for signs of peripheral neuropathy—consult product literature for treatment adjustment.
- NATIONAL FUNDING/ACCESS DECISIONS
  NICE decisions
  ▶ **Brentuximab vedotin for treating CD30-positive Hodgkin lymphoma (June 2017)** NICE TA446
  Brentuximab vedotin is recommended as a treatment option for CD30-positive Hodgkin lymphoma in adults, only if:
  • they have relapsed or refractory disease after autologous stem cell transplant, **and**
  • the company provides brentuximab vedotin at the price agreed with NHS England in the commercial access agreement
  Brentuximab vedotin is recommended for use within the Cancer Drugs Fund as a treatment option for CD30-positive Hodgkin lymphoma in adults, only if:
  • they have relapsed or refractory disease after at least 2 previous therapies **and**
  • they cannot have autologous stem cell transplant or multi-agent chemotherapy, **and**
  • the conditions of the managed access agreement are followed
  These recommendations are not intended to affect treatment that was started in the NHS before this guidance was published. Adults having treatment outside these recommendations may continue without change to the funding arrangements in place before this guidance was published, until they and their clinician consider it appropriate to stop.
  www.nice.org.uk/guidance/TA446
  ▶ **Brentuximab vedotin for treating relapsed or refractory systemic anaplastic large cell lymphoma (October 2017)** NICE TA478
  Brentuximab vedotin is recommended as an option for treating relapsed or refractory systemic anaplastic large cell lymphoma in adults, only if:
  • they have an Eastern Cooperative Oncology Group performance status of 0 or 1, **and**
  • the manufacturer provides brentuximab vedotin according to the commercial access agreement with NHS England.
  These recommendations are not intended to affect treatment that was started in the NHS before this guidance was published. Adults having treatment outside these recommendations may continue without change to the funding arrangements in place before this guidance was published, until they and their NHS clinician consider it appropriate to stop.
  www.nice.org.uk/guidance/TA478

● MEDICINAL FORMS
There can be variation in the licensing of different medicines containing the same drug.

Powder for solution for infusion
ELECTROLYTES: May contain Sodium

▸ Adcetris (Takeda UK Ltd) ▼
Brentuximab vedotin 50 mg Adcetris 50mg powder for concentrate for solution for infusion vials | 1 vial [PoM] £2,500.00

Cetuximab

26-Jun-2017

● INDICATIONS AND DOSE

Treatment of wild-type RAS metastatic colorectal cancer in patients with tumours expressing epidermal growth factor receptor, as combination therapy, or as monotherapy if oxaliplatin- and irinotecan-based therapy has failed or if irinotecan is not tolerated | **Treatment of locally advanced squamous cell cancer of the head and neck (in combination with radiotherapy)** | **Treatment of recurrent or metastatic squamous cell cancer of the head and neck (in combination with platinum-based chemotherapy)**

▸ BY INTRAVENOUS INFUSION
▸ Adult (initiated by a specialist): (consult product literature or local protocols)

IMPORTANT SAFETY INFORMATION
MHRA/CHM ADVICE: EPIDERMAL GROWTH FACTOR RECEPTOR (EGFR) INHIBITORS: SERIOUS CASES OF KERATITIS AND ULCERATIVE KERATITIS (MAY 2012)
Keratitis and ulcerative keratitis have been reported following treatment with epidermal growth factor receptor (EGFR) inhibitors for cancer (cetuximab, erlotinib, gefitinib and panitumumab). In rare cases, this has resulted in corneal perforation and blindness. Patients undergoing treatment with EGFR inhibitors who present with acute or worsening signs and symptoms suggestive of keratitis should be referred promptly to an ophthalmology specialist. Treatment should be interrupted or discontinued if ulcerative keratitis is diagnosed.

Patients must receive an antihistamine and a corticosteroid at least one hour before infusion. Resuscitation facilities should be available and treatment should be initiated by a specialist.

● CONTRA-INDICATIONS Combination of cetuximab with oxaliplatin-containing chemotherapy is contra-indicated in patients with metastatic colorectal cancer who have mutant or unknown *RAS* status · *RAS* mutated colorectal tumours (or if *RAS* tumour status unknown)

● CAUTIONS Cardiopulmonary disease · cardiovascular disease · history of keratitis · pulmonary disease—discontinue if interstitial lung disease · risk factors for keratitis · severe dry eye · ulcerative keratitis (including contact lens use)

● INTERACTIONS → Appendix 1: monoclonal antibodies

● SIDE-EFFECTS
▸ **Common or very common** Appetite decreased · cytokine release syndrome · dehydration · diarrhoea · electrolyte imbalance · eye inflammation · fatigue · headache · infusion related reaction · mucositis · nausea · skin eruption · vomiting
▸ **Uncommon** Embolism and thrombosis · interstitial lung disease
▸ **Rare or very rare** Severe cutaneous adverse reactions (SCARs)
▸ **Frequency not known** Meningitis aseptic · superinfection of skin lesions

● CONCEPTION AND CONTRACEPTION Contraceptive advice required, see *Pregnancy and reproductive function* in Cytotoxic drugs p. 865.

● PREGNANCY Use only if potential benefit outweighs risk—no information available. See also *Pregnancy and reproductive function* in Cytotoxic drugs p. 865.

● BREAST FEEDING Avoid breast-feeding during and for 2 months after treatment—no information available.

● PRE-TREATMENT SCREENING Evidence of non-mutated (wild-type) *RAS* status (at exons 2, 3 and 4 of *KRAS* and *NRAS*) is required before cetuximab is initiated for the treatment of metastatic colorectal cancer, and should be determined by an experienced laboratory using a validated test method.

● DIRECTIONS FOR ADMINISTRATION Resuscitation facilities should be available.

● NATIONAL FUNDING/ACCESS DECISIONS

NICE decisions
▸ **Cetuximab for the treatment of locally advanced squamous cell cancer of the head and neck (June 2008)** NICE TA145
Cetuximab in combination with radiotherapy is an option for the treatment of locally advanced squamous cell cancer of the head and neck in patients who have a Karnofsky performance status of 90% or greater and when all forms of platinum-based chemoradiotherapy treatment are contra-indicated.
www.nice.org.uk/guidance/TA145

▸ **Cetuximab, bevacizumab and panitumumab for the treatment of metastatic colorectal cancer after first-line chemotherapy (January 2012)** NICE TA242
Cetuximab monotherapy or combination chemotherapy is **not** recommended for the treatment of patients with metastatic colorectal cancer that has progressed after first-line chemotherapy.
www.nice.org.uk/guidance/TA242

▸ **Cetuximab and panitumumab for previously untreated metastatic colorectal cancer (updated September 2017)** NICE TA439
Cetuximab is recommended, within its marketing authorisation, as an option for previously untreated epidermal growth factor receptor-expressing, RAS wild-type metastatic colorectal cancer in patients in combination with:
● 5-fluorouracil, folinic acid and oxaliplatin (FOLFOX), **or**
● 5-fluorouracil, folinic acid and irinotecan (FOLFIRI).
This advice is contingent upon the manufacturer providing cetuximab with the discount agreed in the commercial access agreement.
www.nice.org.uk/guidance/TA439

▸ **Cetuximab for treating recurrent or metastatic squamous cell cancer of the head and neck (August 2017)** NICE TA473
Cetuximab in combination with platinum-based chemotherapy is recommended as an option for treating recurrent or metastatic squamous cell cancer of the head and neck in patients only:
● if the cancer started in the oral cavity, **and**
● when the company provides the drug in line with the commercial access agreement with NHS England.
Patients currently receiving cetuximab whose disease does not meet the above criteria may continue treatment until they and their clinician consider it appropriate to stop.
www.nice.org.uk/guidance/TA473

● MEDICINAL FORMS
There can be variation in the licensing of different medicines containing the same drug.

Solution for infusion
▸ Erbitux (Merck Serono Ltd)
Cetuximab 5 mg per 1 ml Erbitux 100mg/20ml solution for infusion vials | 1 vial [PoM] £178.10 (Hospital only)
Erbitux 500mg/100ml solution for infusion vials | 1 vial [PoM] £890.50 (Hospital only)

8

Immune system and malignant disease

Immune system and malignant disease

8

Daratumumab

12-Dec-2017

- **DRUG ACTION** Daratumumab is a monoclonal antibody that binds to CD38, a cell-surface protein, resulting in tumour cell death by immune-mediated actions and apoptosis.

- **INDICATIONS AND DOSE**

Treatment of relapsed and refractory multiple myeloma (as monotherapy after failure of a proteasome inhibitor and an immunomodulatory agent) (specialist use only)
  - ▸ BY INTRAVENOUS INFUSION
  - ▸ Adult: 16 mg/kg once weekly for weeks 1 to 8, then 16 mg/kg every 2 weeks for weeks 9 to 24, then 16 mg/kg every 4 weeks for week 25 onwards until disease progression, for dose adjustments due to side-effects and infusion-related reactions—consult product literature

- **CAUTIONS** History of obstructive pulmonary disorder (consider additional post-medication—consult product literature) · patients may need pre-medication to minimise adverse reactions · risk of herpes zoster reactivation (consider antiviral prophylaxis)

  CAUTIONS, FURTHER INFORMATION
  - ▸ Infusion-related reactions Serious infusion-related reactions can occur and daratumumab should only be administered when appropriately trained staff and resuscitation facilities are immediately available; manufacturer advises pre-medication with intravenous corticosteroid, an antihistamine and an anti-pyretic and post-medication with oral corticosteroids—consult product literature. Manufacturer advises patients should be closely monitored for signs of infusion-related reactions during and after administration; in the event of a hypersensitivity reaction, treatment should be stopped immediately and appropriate management initiated.

- **INTERACTIONS** → Appendix 1: monoclonal antibodies

- **SIDE-EFFECTS**
  - ▸ **Common or very common** Anaemia · atrial fibrillation · chills · cough · diarrhoea · dyspnoea · fatigue · fever · headache · hypertension · hypoxia · increased risk of infection · lymphopenia · muscle spasms · nasal congestion · nausea · neutropenia · peripheral neuropathy · peripheral oedema · pulmonary oedema · respiratory disorders · throat irritation · thrombocytopenia · vomiting
  - ▸ **Frequency not known** Allergic rhinitis · chest discomfort · hypotension · pruritus

  SIDE-EFFECTS, FURTHER INFORMATION Manufacturer advises treatment should be immediately interrupted if an infusion-related reaction of any grade or severity occurs—consult product literature for specific management recommendations.

- **CONCEPTION AND CONTRACEPTION** Manufacturer advises effective contraception in women of childbearing potential during treatment and for 3 months after stopping treatment. See also *Pregnancy and reproductive function* in Cytotoxic drugs p. 865.

- **PREGNANCY** Manufacturer advises avoid unless potential benefit outweighs risk—no information available. See also *Pregnancy and reproductive function* in Cytotoxic drugs p. 865.

- **BREAST FEEDING** Manufacturer advises avoid—no information available.

- **EFFECT ON LABORATORY TESTS** Possible positive indirect Coombs test (may affect antibody screening).

- **HANDLING AND STORAGE** Manufacturer advises store in a refrigerator at 2–8°C; consult product literature for storage advice following dilution.

- **NATIONAL FUNDING/ACCESS DECISIONS**

  NICE decisions
  - ▸ **Daratumumab monotherapy for treating relapsed and refractory multiple myeloma (March 2018)** NICE TA510
  Daratumumab monotherapy is recommended for use within the Cancer Drugs Fund as an option for treating relapsed and refractory multiple myeloma in adults whose previous therapy included a proteasome inhibitor and an immunomodulator, and whose disease progressed on the last therapy, only if:
    - they have daratumumab after 3 previous therapies, **and**
    - the conditions in the managed access agreement are followed.
  Patients whose treatment was started within the NHS before this guidance was published should have the option to continue treatment, without change to their funding arrangements, until they and their NHS clinician consider it appropriate to stop.
  www.nice.org.uk/guidance/ta510

  Scottish Medicines Consortium (SMC) Decisions
  SMC No. 1205/17
  The *Scottish Medicines Consortium* has advised (October 2017) that daratumumab (*Darzalex®*) is accepted for restricted use within NHS Scotland as monotherapy for use as a fourth-line treatment option for adults with relapsed and refractory multiple myeloma, only if a proteasome inhibitor and an immunomodulatory agent have been used as prior therapy and disease demonstrated progression on the last therapy. This advice is contingent upon the continuing availability of the patient access scheme in NHS Scotland or a list price that is equivalent or lower.

- **MEDICINAL FORMS**
  There can be variation in the licensing of different medicines containing the same drug.
  Solution for infusion
  EXCIPIENTS: May contain Polysorbates
  ELECTROLYTES: May contain Sodium
  - ▸ Darzalex (Janssen-Cilag Ltd) ▼
  Daratumumab 20 mg per 1 ml Darzalex 400mg/20ml concentrate for solution for infusion vials | 1 vial [PoM] £1,440.00
  Darzalex 100mg/5ml concentrate for solution for infusion vials | 1 vial [PoM] £360.00

Elotuzumab

07-Apr-2017

- **DRUG ACTION** Elotuzumab is a monoclonal antibody that targets the signalling lymphocytic activation molecule family member 7 (SLAMF7) protein, thereby activating natural killer cells and mediating myeloma cell death.

- **INDICATIONS AND DOSE**

Multiple myeloma in patients who have received at least one prior therapy (in combination with lenalidomide and dexamethasone) (specialist use only)
  - ▸ BY INTRAVENOUS INFUSION
  - ▸ Adult: 10 mg/kg every week, on days 1, 8, 15 and 22 of cycles 1 and 2, then 10 mg/kg every 2 weeks, on days 1 and 15 of subsequent cycles

- **CAUTIONS** Pre-medication must be administered to minimise the development of infusion-related reactions—consult product literature · secondary primary malignancies

  CAUTIONS, FURTHER INFORMATION
  - ▸ Secondary primary malignancies Manufacturer advises to monitor for the development of secondary primary malignancy before and during treatment with elotuzumab.

- **INTERACTIONS** → Appendix 1: monoclonal antibodies

- **SIDE-EFFECTS**
  - ▸ **Common or very common** Chest pain · cough · deep vein thrombosis · diarrhoea · fatigue · fever · headache ·

hypersensitivity · increased risk of infection · lymphopenia · mood altered · night sweats · numbness · oropharyngeal pain · weight decreased

SIDE-EFFECTS, FURTHER INFORMATION Side-effects reported when used in combination with lenalidomide and dexamethasone or bortezomib and dexamethamsone. **Infusion-related reactions** Manufacturer advises for mild-to-moderate infusion reactions interrupt treatment or reduce infusion rate, and monitor closely (consult product literature); permanently discontinue therapy in severe infusion reactions.

- CONCEPTION AND CONTRACEPTION Manufacturer advises effective contraception in men and women of childbearing potential; male patients should continue effective contraceptive measures for 180 days after stopping treatment if their partner is pregnant or of childbearing potential. See also *Pregnancy and reproductive function* in Cytotoxic drugs p. 865.

- PREGNANCY Manufacturer advises avoid unless essential—no information available. See also *Pregnancy and reproductive function* in Cytotoxic drugs p. 865.

- HANDLING AND STORAGE Manufacturer advises store in a refrigerator (2–8°C); consult product literature for storage conditions after preparation of the infusion.

- MEDICINAL FORMS
There can be variation in the licensing of different medicines containing the same drug.
Powder for solution for infusion
EXCIPIENTS: May contain Polysorbates, sucrose
▸ Empliciti (Bristol-Myers Squibb Pharmaceuticals Ltd) ▼
Elotuzumab 300 mg Empliciti 300mg powder for concentrate for solution for infusion vials | 1 vial PoM £1,085.00
Elotuzumab 400 mg Empliciti 400mg powder for concentrate for solution for infusion vials | 1 vial PoM £1,446.00

Gemtuzumab ozogamicin   21-May-2018

- DRUG ACTION Gemtuzumab ozogamicin is a monoclonal antibody that binds to CD33-expressing tumour cells to induce cell cycle arrest and apoptotic cell death.

- INDICATIONS AND DOSE

CD33-positive acute myeloid leukaemia (specialist use only)
▸ BY INTRAVENOUS INFUSION
▸ Adult: (consult product literature)

- CAUTIONS Adverse-risk cytogenetics (consider benefits and risks of treatment, consult product literature) · haematopoietic stem cell transplantation (increased risk of hepatotoxicity) · pre-medication recommended to minimise adverse reactions

CAUTIONS, FURTHER INFORMATION
▸ Pre-medication Serious infusion-related reactions can occur and gemtuzumab ozogamicin should only be administered when appropriately trained staff and resuscitation facilities are immediately available; manufacturer advises pre-medication with a corticosteroid, paracetamol and antihistamine 1 hour prior to dosing, and to take appropriate measures to help prevent the development of tumour lysis-related hyperuricaemia—consult product literature.

- SIDE-EFFECTS
▸ **Common or very common** Anaemia · appetite decreased · ascites · chills · constipation · decreased leucocytes · diarrhoea · dyspnoea · fatigue · fever · gastrointestinal discomfort · gastrointestinal disorders · haemorrhage · headache · hepatic disorders · hyperbilirubinaemia · hyperglycaemia · hypertension · hypotension · infection · infusion related reaction (including fatal cases) · multi organ failure · nausea · neutropenia · oedema ·

pancytopenia · sinusoidal obstruction syndrome · skin reactions · stomatitis · tachycardia · thrombocytopenia · tumour lysis syndrome (including fatal cases) · vomiting
▸ **Frequency not known** Interstitial pneumonia

SIDE-EFFECTS, FURTHER INFORMATION Infusion-related reactions (including fatal cases) can occur during the first 24 hours after administration. Manufacturer advises interrupt treatment immediately and treat as clinically indicated (consult product literature); permanent discontinuation should be strongly considered in patients who develop signs and symptoms of anaphylaxis.

- CONCEPTION AND CONTRACEPTION Manufacturer advises women of childbearing potential should use 2 methods of effective contraception during treatment and for at least 7 months after the last dose; male patients should use 2 methods of effective contraception during treatment and for at least 4 months after the last dose if their partner is of childbearing potential. See also Pregnancy and reproductive function in Cytotoxic drugs p. 865.

- PREGNANCY Manufacturer advises avoid unless potential benefit outweighs risk—toxicity in *animal* studies. See also Pregnancy and reproductive function in Cytotoxic drugs p. 865.

- BREAST FEEDING Manufacturer advises avoid during treatment and for at least one month after the last dose—no information available.

- HEPATIC IMPAIRMENT Manufacturer advises caution in moderate-to-severe impairment—increased risk of developing hepatotoxicity; postpone treatment if serum transaminases (ALT or AST) greater than 2.5 times the upper limit of normal or total bilirubin greater than 2 times the upper limit of normal.

- MONITORING REQUIREMENTS
▸ Manufacturer advises monitor complete blood counts prior to each dose as well as signs and symptoms of infection, bleeding and other effects of myelosuppression during treatment; dose interruption or discontinuation of treatment may be required—consult product literature.
▸ Manufacturer advises monitor for signs and symptoms of infusion-related reactions—close clinical monitoring, including pulse, blood pressure and temperature, should be performed during infusion; monitor for signs and symptoms of tumour lysis syndrome.
▸ Manufacturer advises monitor for signs and symptoms of hepatotoxicity (including hepatic veno-occlusive disease); liver tests should be monitored prior to each dose—consult product literature.

- PRESCRIBING AND DISPENSING INFORMATION
Gemtuzumab ozogamicin is a biological medicine. Biological medicines must be prescribed and dispensed by brand name, see *Biological medicines* and *Biosimilar medicines*, under Guidance on prescribing p. 1.

- HANDLING AND STORAGE Manufacturer advises store in a refrigerator (2–8°C) and protect from light—consult product literature for storage conditions after reconstitution and dilution.

- PATIENT AND CARER ADVICE
Driving and skilled tasks Manufacturer advises patients and carers should be counselled on the effects on driving and performance of skilled tasks—increased risk of fatigue and headache.

- MEDICINAL FORMS
There can be variation in the licensing of different medicines containing the same drug.
Powder for solution for infusion
▸ Mylotarg (Pfizer Ltd) ▼
Gemtuzumab ozogamicin 5 mg Mylotarg 5mg powder for concentrate for solution for infusion vials | 1 vial PoM £6,300.00 (Hospital only)

Inotuzumab ozogamicin
11-Oct-2017

- DRUG ACTION Inotuzumab ozogamicin is a monoclonal antibody that binds to CD22-expressing tumour cells to induce cell cycle arrest and apoptotic cell death.

- ● INDICATIONS AND DOSE

Monotherapy for relapsed or refractory CD22-positive B cell precursor acute lymphoblastic leukaemia (under expert supervision)
  - ▸ BY INTRAVENOUS INFUSION
  - ▸ Adult: (consult product literature)

- CONTRA-INDICATIONS Prior confirmed severe or ongoing sinusoidal obstruction syndrome

- CAUTIONS History of, or predisposition to QT-interval prolongation (e.g. electrolyte disturbances, concomitant use of drugs that prolong the QT interval) · patients may need pre-medication to minimise adverse reactions · patients undergoing haematopoetic stem cell transplantation (increased risk of hepatotoxicity)

  CAUTIONS, FURTHER INFORMATION
  - ▸ Pre-medication Manufacturer advises pre-medication with a corticosteroid, antipyretic and antihistamine prior to dosing in all patients and pre-medication to reduce uric acid levels and hydration in patients with a high tumour burden (increased risk of tumour lysis syndrome)—consult product literature.

- INTERACTIONS → Appendix 1: monoclonal antibodies

- SIDE-EFFECTS
  - ▸ Common or very common Anaemia · appetite decreased · ascites · bone marrow disorders · central nervous system haemorrhage · chills · constipation · decreased leucocytes · diarrhoea · fatigue · fever · gastrointestinal discomfort · haemorrhage · headache · hyperbilirubinaemia · hypersensitivity · hyperuricaemia · increased risk of infection · nausea · neutropenia · QT interval prolongation · sepsis · sinusoidal obstruction syndrome · stomatitis · thrombocytopenia · tumour lysis syndrome · vomiting

  SIDE-EFFECTS, FURTHER INFORMATION Manufacturer advises interrupt treatment if an infusion related reaction occurs; depending on the severity, discontinuation of the infusion or administration of steroids and antihistamines should be considered (consult product literature); permanently discontinue treatment in severe or life-threatening infusion reactions.

- CONCEPTION AND CONTRACEPTION Manufacturer advises effective contraception in women of childbearing potential during treatment and for at least 8 months after the last dose; male patients should use effective contraception during treatment and for at least 5 months after the last dose if their partner is of childbearing potential. See also Pregnancy and reproductive function in Cytotoxic drugs p. 865.

- PREGNANCY Manufacturer advises avoid unless potential benefit outweighs risk—toxicity in *animal* studies.

- BREAST FEEDING Manufacturer advises avoid during treatment and for at least two months after the last dose—no information available.

- HEPATIC IMPAIRMENT Manufacturer advises careful pre-treatment evaluation in patients with hepatic impairment; dose interruption or discontinuation may be required if serum bilirubin or AST/ALT levels become raised (limited information available)—consult product literature; avoid in severe impairment.

- PRE-TREATMENT SCREENING Manufacturer advises baseline CD22 positivity of greater than 0% is required prior to initiating treatment.

- MONITORING REQUIREMENTS
  - ▸ Manufacturer advises monitor complete blood counts prior to each dose as well as signs and symptoms of infection, bleeding and other effects of myelosupresion during treatment; dose reduction or interruption or discontinuation of treatment may be required—consult product literature.
  - ▸ Manufacturer advises monitor for signs of infusion related-reactions during and for at least 1 hour after infusion; monitor for signs and symptoms of tumour lysis syndrome.
  - ▸ Manufacturer advises ECG and electrolytes should be monitored prior to the start of treatment and periodically during treatment; monitor for increases in serum amylase and lipase.
  - ▸ Manufacturer advises monitor for signs and symptoms of sinusoidal obstruction syndrome; liver tests should be monitored prior to and following each dose—consult product literature.

- DIRECTIONS FOR ADMINISTRATION Manufacturer advises resuscitation facilities should be available during administration.

- PRESCRIBING AND DISPENSING INFORMATION Inotuzumab ozogamicin is a biological medicine. Biological medicines must be prescribed and dispensed by brand name, see *Biological medicines* and *Biosimilar medicines*, under Guidance on prescribing p. 1; manufacturer advises to record the brand name and batch number after each administration.

- HANDLING AND STORAGE Manufacturer advises store in a refrigerator (2–8°C) and protect from light—consult product literature for storage conditions after reconstitution and dilution.

- PATIENT AND CARER ADVICE
  Driving and skilled tasks Manufacturer advises patients and carers should be counselled on the effects on driving and performance of skilled tasks—increased risk of fatigue.

- MEDICINAL FORMS
  There can be variation in the licensing of different medicines containing the same drug.
  Powder for solution for infusion
  ELECTROLYTES: May contain Sodium
  - ▸ Besponsa (Pfizer Ltd) ▼
    Inotuzumab ozogamicin 1 mg Besponsa 1mg powder for concentrate for solution for infusion vials | 1 vial PoM £8,048.00 (Hospital only)

Ipilimumab
24-May-2018

- DRUG ACTION Ipilimumab is a monoclonal antibody which causes T-cell activation resulting in tumour cell death.

- ● INDICATIONS AND DOSE

Advanced melanoma (specialist use only)
  - ▸ BY INTRAVENOUS INFUSION
  - ▸ Adult: 3 mg/kg every 3 weeks for 4 doses, for dose interruption or discontinuation of treatment due to immune-related side-effects—consult product literature

- CAUTIONS

  CAUTIONS, FURTHER INFORMATION For full details consult product literature.

- INTERACTIONS → Appendix 1: monoclonal antibodies

- SIDE-EFFECTS
  - ▸ Common or very common Alopecia · anaemia · appetite decreased · arthralgia · asthenia · cancer pain · chills · confusion · constipation · cough · dehydration · diarrhoea · dizziness · dyspnoea · electrolyte imbalance · eye discomfort · fever · gastrointestinal discomfort · gastrointestinal disorders · haemorrhage · headache ·

hepatic disorders · hypophysitis · hypopituitarism · hypotension · hypothyroidism · influenza like illness · lethargy · lymphopenia · mucositis · muscle complaints · nausea · nerve disorders · night sweats · oedema · pain · skin reactions · vasodilation · vision disorders · vomiting · weight decreased

▶ **Uncommon**   Adrenal hypofunction · alkalosis · allergic rhinitis · amenorrhoea · arrhythmias · arthritis · brain oedema · depression · dysarthria · eosinophilia · eye inflammation · glomerulonephritis · haemolytic anaemia · hair colour changes · hyperthyroidism · hypogonadism · increased risk of infection · infusion related reaction · libido decreased · meningitis · movement disorders · multi organ failure · muscle weakness · myopathy · nephritis autoimmune · neutropenia · pancreatitis · paraneoplastic syndrome · peripheral ischaemia · polymyalgia rheumatica · psychiatric disorder · pulmonary oedema · renal failure · renal tubular acidosis · respiratory disorders · sepsis · severe cutaneous adverse reactions (SCARs) · syncope · systemic inflammatory response syndrome · thrombocytopenia · tremor · tumour lysis syndrome · vascular disorders · vasculitis

▶ **Rare or very rare**   Myasthenia gravis · proteinuria · thyroiditis

SIDE-EFFECTS, FURTHER INFORMATION   A corticosteroid can be used after starting ipilimumab, to treat immune-related reactions.

● CONCEPTION AND CONTRACEPTION   Use effective contraception.

● PREGNANCY   Manufacturer advises avoid unless potential benefit outweighs risk—toxicity in *animal* studies.

● BREAST FEEDING   Manufacturer advises avoid—present in milk in *animal* studies.

● HEPATIC IMPAIRMENT   Use with caution if plasma-bilirubin concentration greater than 3 times upper limit of normal range *or* if plasma-transaminase concentration 5 times or greater than the upper limit of normal range.

● MONITORING REQUIREMENTS
▶ Manufacturer advises monitor liver function tests and thyroid function prior to initiation of treatment and before each dose.
▶ Manufacturer advises monitor for signs or symptoms of immune-related side-effects and gastrointestinal perforation—consult product literature.

● DIRECTIONS FOR ADMINISTRATION   Manufacturer advises for *intravenous infusion*, give undiluted or dilute to a concentration of 1–4 mg/mL with Glucose 5% *or* Sodium Chloride 0.9%; give over 90 minutes.

● PRESCRIBING AND DISPENSING INFORMATION   Infusion-related side-effects have been reported; premedication with paracetamol and an antihistamine is recommended.

● HANDLING AND STORAGE   Manufacturer advises store in a refrigerator (2–8 °C) and protect from light—consult product literature for further information regarding storage conditions outside refrigerator and after preparation of the infusion.

● NATIONAL FUNDING/ACCESS DECISIONS

NICE decisions
▶ Ipilimumab for previously untreated advanced (unresectable or metastatic) melanoma (July 2014) NICE TA319
Ipilimumab is recommended, within its marketing authorisation, as an option for treating adults with previously untreated advanced (unresectable or metastatic) melanoma, only if the manufacturer provides ipilimumab with the discount agreed in the patient access scheme.
www.nice.org.uk/TA319

▶ Ipilimumab for previously treated advanced (unresectable or metastatic) melanoma (December 2012) NICE TA268
Ipilimumab is recommended as an option for the treatment of advanced (unresectable or metastatic) melanoma in patients who have received prior therapy, only if the manufacturer provides ipilimumab with the discount agreed in the patient access scheme.
www.nice.org.uk/TA268

▶ Nivolumab in combination with ipilimumab for treating advanced melanoma (July 2016) NICE TA400
Nivolumab in combination with ipilimumab is recommended, within its marketing authorisation, as a treatment option for advanced (unresectable or metastatic) melanoma in adults, only if the manufacturer provides ipilimumab with the discount agreed in the patient access scheme.
www.nice.org.uk/TA400

Scottish Medicines Consortium (SMC) Decisions
The *Scottish Medicines Consortium* has advised (March 2013) that ipilimumab (*Yervoy®*) is accepted for restricted use within NHS Scotland for the treatment of advanced (unresectable or metastatic) melanoma in adults who have received prior therapy, only whilst ipilimumab is available at the price agreed in the patient access scheme.

● MEDICINAL FORMS
There can be variation in the licensing of different medicines containing the same drug.
Solution for infusion
ELECTROLYTES: May contain Sodium
▶ Yervoy (Bristol-Myers Squibb Pharmaceuticals Ltd) ▼
  Ipilimumab 5 mg per 1 ml Yervoy 50mg/10ml concentrate for solution for infusion vials | 1 vial [PoM] £3,750.00 (Hospital only)
  Yervoy 200mg/40ml concentrate for solution for infusion vials | 1 vial [PoM] £15,000.00 (Hospital only)

Necitumumab   21-Feb-2017

● DRUG ACTION   Necitumumab is a monoclonal antibody that binds to the epidermal growth factor receptor (EGFR).

● **INDICATIONS AND DOSE**

Locally advanced or metastatic epidermal growth factor receptor expressing squamous non-small-cell lung cancer, in patients who have not received previous chemotherapy (in combination with gemcitabine and cisplatin) (specialist use only)
▶ BY INTRAVENOUS INFUSION
▶ Adult: 800 mg once daily on days 1 and 8 of a 3-week cycle, for up to 6 cycles, patients whose disease has not progressed after combination therapy may continue with necitumumab monotherapy, for dose adjustments due to infusion-related reactions or skin reactions—consult product literature

● CAUTIONS   Cardiorespiratory disorders (no information available) · history of thromboembolic events · patients may need pre-medication to minimise the development of infusion-related and skin reactions (consult product literature) · risk factors for thromboembolic events
CAUTIONS, FURTHER INFORMATION
▶ Thromboembolic events   Manufacturer advises that necitumumab should not be administered to patients with multiple risk factors for thromboembolic events unless the benefits outweigh the risks. Thromboprophylaxis should be considered after assessment of a patient's risk factors.

● INTERACTIONS → Appendix 1: monoclonal antibodies

Immune system and malignant disease

8

● SIDE-EFFECTS
▶ **Common or very common** Conjunctivitis · dysuria · electrolyte imbalance · embolism and thrombosis · fever · haemorrhage · headache · hypomagnesaemia (severe) · increased risk of infection · infusion related reaction · muscle spasms · oral disorders · skin reactions · taste altered · vomiting · weight decreased
▶ **Frequency not known** Cardiac arrest · eyelash trichomegaly

● CONCEPTION AND CONTRACEPTION Manufacturer advises women of child-bearing potential should use effective contraception during and for 3 months after treatment.

● PREGNANCY Manufacturer advises avoid unless potential benefit outweighs risk—limited information available. See also *Pregnancy and reproductive function* in Cytotoxic drugs p. 865.

● BREAST FEEDING Manufacturer advises avoid during treatment and for at least 4 months after the last dose—no information available.

● MONITORING REQUIREMENTS Manufacturer advises monitor patients during and following each infusion for signs of hypersensitivity and infusion-related reactions; monitor electrolytes (including magnesium, potassium and calcium) prior to each infusion and after completion of treatment, until within normal limits—correct any electrolyte disturbance promptly.

● DIRECTIONS FOR ADMINISTRATION Manufacturer advises necitumumab should be given under the supervision of an experienced specialist, in an environment where full resuscitation facilities and resources for the treatment of infusion-related reactions are immediately available.

● HANDLING AND STORAGE Manufacturer advises store in a refrigerator (2–8°C); consult product literature for storage conditions after preparation of the infusion.

● PATIENT AND CARER ADVICE Manufacturer advises patients and their carers should be made aware of the symptoms of thromboembolism and advised to seek medical attention if they experience sudden breathlessness, chest pain, or swelling of a limb.

● NATIONAL FUNDING/ACCESS DECISIONS

NICE decisions
▶ **Necitumumab for untreated advanced or metastatic squamous non-small-cell lung cancer (September 2016) NICE TA411**
Necitumumab, in combination with gemcitabine and cisplatin, is **not** recommended within its marketing authorisation for adults with locally advanced or metastatic epidermal growth factor receptor (EGFR)-expressing squamous non-small-cell lung cancer that has not been treated with chemotherapy.
Patients whose treatment was started within the NHS before this guidance was published should have the option to continue treatment, without change to their funding arrangements, until they and their clinician consider it appropriate to stop.
www.nice.org.uk/TA411

● MEDICINAL FORMS
There can be variation in the licensing of different medicines containing the same drug.
Solution for infusion
ELECTROLYTES: May contain Sodium
▶ Portrazza (Eli Lilly and Company Ltd) ▼
Necitumumab 16 mg per 1 ml Portrazza 800mg/50ml concentrate for solution for infusion vials | 1 vial PoM £1,450.00 (Hospital only)

Nivolumab

17-May-2018

● DRUG ACTION Nivolumab is a human immunoglobulin G4 monoclonal antibody, which binds to the programmed death-1 (PD-1) receptor thereby potentiating an immune response to tumour cells.

● INDICATIONS AND DOSE

Unresectable or metastatic advanced melanoma in combination with ipilimumab (specialist use only)
▶ BY INTRAVENOUS INFUSION
▶ Adult: (consult product literature)

Unresectable or metastatic advanced melanoma (as monotherapy) (specialist use only) | Advanced renal cell carcinoma (as monotherapy) (specialist use only)
▶ BY INTRAVENOUS INFUSION
▶ Adult: 240 mg every 2 weeks, alternatively 480 mg every 4 weeks, consult product literature for information on dose adjustments based on individual patient safety and tolerability

Locally advanced or metastatic non-small cell lung cancer (as monotherapy) (specialist use only) | Locally advanced unresectable or metastatic urothelial carcinoma (as monotherapy) (specialist use only) | Squamous cell cancer of the head and neck (as monotherapy) (specialist use only) | Relapsed or refractory classical Hodgkin lymphoma (as monotherapy) (specialist use only)
▶ BY INTRAVENOUS INFUSION
▶ Adult: 240 mg every 2 weeks, consult product literature for information on dose adjustments based on individual patient safety and tolerability

IMPORTANT SAFETY INFORMATION
MHRA/CHM ADVICE: NIVOLUMAB (*OPDIVO*®): REPORTS OF ORGAN TRANSPLANT REJECTION (JULY 2017)
A European review of worldwide data concluded that nivolumab may increase the risk of rejection in organ transplant recipients. The MHRA recommends considering the benefit of treatment with nivolumab versus the risk of possible organ transplant rejection for each patient.

● CAUTIONS May increase risk of severe graft-versus-host reaction in patients who have had prior haematopoietic stem cell transplant (particularly in those with a prior history) · patients may need pre-medication to minimise the development of infusion-related reactions

● INTERACTIONS → Appendix 1: monoclonal antibodies

● SIDE-EFFECTS
▶ **Common or very common** Abdominal pain · alopecia · anaemia · appetite decreased · arthralgia · constipation · cough · decreased leucocytes · diarrhoea · dizziness · dry mouth · dyspnoea · electrolyte imbalance · fatigue · fever · headache · hyperglycaemia · hypersensitivity · hypertension · hyperthyroidism · hypothyroidism · increased risk of infection · nausea · nerve disorders · neutropenia · oedema · pain · respiratory disorders · skin reactions · stomatitis · thrombocytopenia · vomiting · weight decreased
▶ **Uncommon** Adrenal insufficiency · arrhythmias · arthritis · chest pain · dehydration · dry eye · eosinophilia · eye inflammation · gastrointestinal disorders · hepatic disorders · hypophysitis · hypopituitarism · metabolic acidosis · nephritis tubulointerstitial · pancreatitis · polymyalgia rheumatica · renal failure · thyroiditis · vision blurred
▶ **Rare or very rare** Demyelination · diabetes mellitus · histiocytic necrotising lymphadenitis · myasthenic syndrome · myocarditis · myopathy · severe cutaneous adverse reactions (SCARs) · vasculitis

► **Frequency not known** Solid organ transplant rejection

SIDE-EFFECTS, FURTHER INFORMATION

Immune-related reactions Manufacturer advises that most immune-related adverse reactions improved or resolved with appropriate management, including initiation of corticosteroids and treatment modifications—consult product literature for further information.
Infusion-related reactions Manufacturer advises that patients with mild or moderate infusion reactions may continue treatment with close monitoring and use of pre-medication according to local guidelines; discontinue treatment if severe infusion reactions occur.

● CONCEPTION AND CONTRACEPTION Manufacturer advises effective contraception required during treatment and for at least 5 months after treatment in women of childbearing potential.

● PREGNANCY Manufacturer advises avoid unless potential benefit outweighs risk—toxicity in *animal* studies.

● BREAST FEEDING Manufacturer advises avoid—no information available.

● HEPATIC IMPAIRMENT Manufacturer advises use with caution in moderate to severe impairment—limited information available.

● MONITORING REQUIREMENTS Manufacturer advises monitor for signs and symptoms of infusion- and immune-related reactions, cardiac and pulmonary reactions, and electrolyte disturbances before and periodically during treatment. Patients should be monitored for adverse reactions for at least 5 months after the last dose.

● DIRECTIONS FOR ADMINISTRATION Manufacturer advises for *intermittent intravenous infusion*, give undiluted or dilute to a concentration of not less than 1 mg/mL with Glucose 5% *or* Sodium Chloride 0.9%; give over 30 or 60 minutes (depending on dose—consult product literature) through an in-line filter (pore size 0.2–1.2 micron).

● HANDLING AND STORAGE Manufacturer advises store in a refrigerator (2–8 °C)—consult product literature for storage conditions after preparation of the infusion.

● PATIENT AND CARER ADVICE Patients should be provided with a patient alert card with each prescription.

● NATIONAL FUNDING/ACCESS DECISIONS

NICE decisions

► **Nivolumab for treating advanced (unresectable or metastatic) melanoma (February 2016)** NICE TA384
Nivolumab as monotherapy is recommended, within its marketing authorisation, as a treatment option for advanced (unresectable or metastatic) melanoma in adults.
www.nice.org.uk/guidance/ta384

► **Nivolumab in combination with ipilimumab for treating advanced melanoma (July 2016)** NICE TA400
Nivolumab in combination with ipilimumab is recommended, within its marketing authorisation, as a treatment option for advanced (unresectable or metastatic) melanoma in adults, only if the manufacturer provides ipilimumab with the discount agreed in the patient access scheme.
www.nice.org.uk/guidance/ta400

► **Nivolumab for previously treated advanced renal cell carcinoma (updated November 2017)** NICE TA417
Nivolumab is recommended, within its marketing authorisation, as an option for previously treated advanced renal cell carcinoma in adults, when the manufacturer provides nivolumab in line with the commercial access agreement with NHS England.
www.nice.org.uk/guidance/ta417

► **Nivolumab for treating relapsed or refractory classical Hodgkin lymphoma (updated November 2017)** NICE TA462
Nivolumab is recommended, within its marketing authorisation, as an option for treating relapsed or refractory classical Hodgkin lymphoma in adults after autologous stem cell transplant and treatment with brentuximab vedotin, when the manufacturer provides nivolumab in line with the commercial access agreement with NHS England.
www.nice.org.uk/guidance/ta462

► **Nivolumab for previously treated squamous non-small-cell lung cancer (November 2017)** NICE TA483
Nivolumab is recommended for use within the Cancer Drugs Fund as an option for treating locally advanced or metastatic squamous non-small-cell lung cancer in adults after chemotherapy, only if:
● nivolumab is stopped at 2 years of uninterrupted treatment, or earlier in the event of disease progression, **and**
● the conditions in the managed access agreement are followed.
Patients whose treatment was started within the NHS before this guidance was published should have the option to continue treatment, without change to their funding arrangements, until they and their NHS clinician consider it appropriate to stop.
www.nice.org.uk/guidance/ta483

► **Nivolumab for previously treated non-squamous non-small-cell lung cancer (November 2017)** NICE TA484
Nivolumab is recommended for use within the Cancer Drugs Fund as an option for treating locally advanced or metastatic non-squamous non-small-cell lung cancer in adults after chemotherapy, only if:
● their tumours are PD-L1 positive, **and**
● nivolumab is stopped at 2 years of uninterrupted treatment, or earlier in the event of disease progression, **and**
● the conditions in the managed access agreement are followed.
Patients whose treatment was started within the NHS before this guidance was published should have the option to continue treatment, without change to their funding arrangements, until they and their NHS clinician consider it appropriate to stop.
www.nice.org.uk/guidance/ta484

► **Nivolumab for treating squamous cell carcinoma of the head and neck after platinum-based chemotherapy (November 2017)** NICE TA490
Nivolumab is recommended for use within the Cancer Drugs Fund as an option for treating squamous cell carcinoma of the head and neck in adults whose disease has progressed on platinum-based chemotherapy, only if:
● the disease has progressed within 6 months of having chemotherapy, **and**
● nivolumab is stopped at 2 years of uninterrupted treatment, or earlier in the event of disease progression, **and**
● the conditions in the managed access agreement are followed.
Patients whose treatment was started within the NHS before this guidance was published should have the option to continue treatment, without change to their funding arrangements, until they and their NHS clinician consider it appropriate to stop.
www.nice.org.uk/guidance/ta490

Scottish Medicines Consortium (SMC) Decisions
The *Scottish Medicines Consortium* has advised (July 2016) that nivolumab (*Opdivo* ®) is accepted for use within NHS Scotland for the treatment of locally advanced or metastatic squamous non-small cell lung cancer after prior chemotherapy in adults. This advice is contingent upon

8

the continuing availability of the patient access scheme in NHS Scotland or a list price that is equivalent or lower.

The *Scottish Medicines Consortium* has advised (August 2016) that nivolumab (*Opdivo*®) is accepted for restricted use within NHS Scotland as monotherapy for the treatment of advanced (unresectable or metastatic) melanoma in adults previously untreated with ipilimumab. This advice is contingent upon the continuing availability of the patient access scheme in NHS Scotland or a list price that is equivalent or lower.

The *Scottish Medicines Consortium* has advised (October 2016) that nivolumab (*Opdivo*®) is accepted for restricted use within NHS Scotland for the treatment of locally advanced or metastatic non-squamous non-small cell lung cancer after prior chemotherapy in adults, subject to a two-year clinical stopping rule. This advice is contingent upon the continuing availability of the patient access scheme in NHS Scotland or a list price that is equivalent or lower.

The *Scottish Medicines Consortium* has advised (November 2016) that nivolumab (*Opdivo*®) is accepted for restricted use within NHS Scotland in combination with ipilimumab for the first-line treatment of advanced (unresectable or metastatic) melanoma in adults. This advice is contingent upon the continuing availability of the patient access scheme in NHS Scotland or a list price that is equivalent or lower.

The *Scottish Medicines Consortium* has advised (June 2017) that nivolumab (*Opdivo*®) is accepted for use within NHS Scotland as monotherapy for treating adults with advanced renal cell carcinoma after prior therapy. The advice is contingent upon the continuing availability of the patient access scheme in NHS Scotland or a list price that is equivalent or lower.

The *Scottish Medicines Consortium* has advised (July 2017) that nivolumab (*Opdivo*®) is accepted for use within NHS Scotland for the treatment of patients with relapsed or refractory classical Hodgkin lymphoma after autologous stem cell transplant and treatment with brentuximab vedotin. This advice is contingent upon the continuing availability of the patient access scheme in NHS Scotland or a list price that is equivalent or lower.

The *Scottish Medicines Consortium* has advised (September 2017) that nivolumab (*Opdivo*®) is accepted for restricted use within NHS Scotland as monotherapy, for the treatment of squamous cell cancer of the head and neck in adults progressing on or after platinum-based therapy. Treatment with nivolumab is subject to a two year clinical stopping rule. This advice is contingent upon the continuing availability of the patient access scheme in NHS Scotland or a list price that is equivalent or lower.

The *Scottish Medicines Consortium* has advised that nivolumab (*Opdivo*®) is **not** recommended for use within NHS Scotland as monotherapy for the treatment of locally advanced unresectable or metastatic urothelial carcinoma in adults after failure of prior platinum-containing therapy, as the economic case was not demonstrated.

● MEDICINAL FORMS
There can be variation in the licensing of different medicines containing the same drug.
Solution for infusion
CAUTIONARY AND ADVISORY LABELS 3
ELECTROLYTES: May contain Sodium
▸ Nivolumab (non-proprietary) ▼
 Nivolumab 10 mg per 1 ml
▸ Opdivo (Bristol-Myers Squibb Pharmaceuticals Ltd) ▼
 Nivolumab 10 mg per 1 ml Opdivo 40mg/4ml concentrate for solution for infusion vials | 1 vial [PoM] £439.00 (Hospital only)
 Opdivo 100mg/10ml concentrate for solution for infusion vials | 1 vial [PoM] £1,097.00 (Hospital only)
 Opdivo 240mg/24ml concentrate for solution for infusion vials | 1 vial [PoM] £2,633.00 (Hospital only)

⌐ᴳ 836

Obinutuzumab

17-Jul-2017

● INDICATIONS AND DOSE
Treatment of previously untreated chronic lymphocytic leukaemia in patients for whom full-dose fludarabine-based therapy is unsuitable due to co-morbidities | Treatment of previously untreated advanced follicular lymphoma | Treatment of follicular lymphoma in patients who did not respond or who progressed during or up to six months after treatment with rituximab or a rituximab-containing regimen
▸ BY INTRAVENOUS INFUSION
▸ Adult: (consult product literature or local protocols)

● CONTRA-INDICATIONS
CONTRA-INDICATIONS, FURTHER INFORMATION
For obinutuzumab contra-indications, consult product literature.

● CAUTIONS
CAUTIONS, FURTHER INFORMATION For full details on the cautions of obinutuzumab, consult product literature.
▸ Hepatitis B infection and reactivation Hepatitis B infection and reactivation (including fatal cases) have been reported in patients taking **obinutuzumab**. Patients with positive hepatitis B serology should be referred to a liver specialist for monitoring and initiation of antiviral therapy before treatment initiation; treatment should not be initiated in patients with evidence of current hepatitis B infection until the infection has been adequately treated. Patients should be closely monitored for clinical and laboratory signs of active hepatitis B infection during treatment and for up to a year following the last infusion (consult product literature).

● INTERACTIONS → Appendix 1: monoclonal antibodies
● SIDE-EFFECTS
▸ **Common or very common** Arrhythmias · chest pain · dyspepsia · eczema · eye erythema · gastrointestinal disorders · heart failure · hyperuricaemia · lymph node pain · nasal complaints · pain · squamous cell carcinoma · urinary disorders · weight increased
▸ **Frequency not known** Acute coronary syndrome · angina pectoris · dizziness · viral infection reactivation

● CONCEPTION AND CONTRACEPTION Use effective contraception during and for 18 months after treatment.

● PREGNANCY Avoid unless potential benefit outweighs risk of B-lymphocyte depletion in fetus.

● BREAST FEEDING Avoid breast-feeding during and for 18 months after treatment—present in milk in *animal* studies.

● MONITORING REQUIREMENTS Patients should be closely monitored for clinical and laboratory signs of active hepatitis B infection during treatment and for up to a year following the last infusion (consult product literature).

● PRESCRIBING AND DISPENSING INFORMATION Infusion related side-effects have been reported; Patients should receive premedication with paracetamol, an antihistamine, and a corticosteroid before each dose—consult product literature for details.

● NATIONAL FUNDING/ACCESS DECISIONS
NICE decisions
▸ Obinutuzumab in combination with chlorambucil for untreated chronic lymphocytic leukaemia (June 2015) NICE TA343
Obinutuzumab, in combination with chlorambucil, is an option for untreated chronic lymphocytic leukaemia in patients who have comorbidities that make full-dose fludarabine-based therapy unsuitable for them, only if:
● bendamustine-based therapy is not suitable **and**

• the manufacturer provides obinutuzumab with the discount agreed in the patient access scheme.
Patients currently receiving obinutuzumab that is not recommended according to the above criteria should have the option to continue treatment until they and their clinician consider it appropriate to stop.
www.nice.org.uk/guidance/ta343

▶ **Obinutuzumab with bendamustine for treating follicular lymphoma refractory to rituximab (August 2017)** NICE TA472
Obinutuzumab in combination with bendamustine followed by obinutuzumab maintenance, is recommended for use within the Cancer Drugs Fund as an option for treating adults with follicular lymphoma that did not respond or progressed during or up to six months after treatment with rituximab or a rituximab-containing regimen, only if the conditions in the managed access agreement for obinutuzumab are followed.
www.nice.org.uk/guidance/ta472

▶ **Obinutuzumab for untreated advanced follicular lymphoma (March 2018)** NICE TA513
Obinutuzumab is recommended as an option for untreated advanced follicular lymphoma in adults (that is, first as induction treatment with chemotherapy, then alone as maintenance therapy), only if:

• the person has a Follicular Lymphoma International Prognostic Index (FLIPI) score of 2 or more, **and**
• the manufacturer provides obinutuzumab with the discount agreed in the patient access scheme.

Patients whose treatment was started within the NHS before this guidance was published should have the option to continue treatment, without change to their funding arrangements, until they and their NHS clinician consider it appropriate to stop.
www.nice.org.uk/guidance/ta513

Scottish Medicines Consortium (SMC) Decisions
The *Scottish Medicines Consortium* has advised (March 2017) that obinutuzumab (*Gazyvaro®*) is accepted for use within NHS Scotland in combination with bendamustine followed by obinutuzumab maintenance for the treatment of patients with follicular lymphoma who did not respond or who progressed during or up to six months after treatment with rituximab or a rituximab-containing regimen. This advice is contingent upon the continuing availability of the Patient Access Scheme in NHS Scotland or a list price that is equivalent or lower.

The *Scottish Medicines Consortium* has advised (January 2018) that obinutuzumab (*Gazyvaro®*) is **not** recommended for use within NHS Scotland in combination with chemotherapy followed by obinutuzumab maintenance therapy in patients achieving a response, for the treatment of patients with previously untreated advanced follicular lymphoma, as the economic case was not demonstrated.

● MEDICINAL FORMS
There can be variation in the licensing of different medicines containing the same drug.
Solution for infusion
▶ Gazyvaro (Roche Products Ltd) ▼
  Obinutuzumab 25 mg per 1 ml Gazyvaro 1000mg/40ml concentrate for solution for infusion vials | 1 vial PoM £3,312.00 (Hospital only)

Ofatumumab

● INDICATIONS AND DOSE
Treatment of chronic lymphocytic leukaemia (CLL) in patients refractory to fludarabine and alemtuzumab | Treatment of CLL in patients who have not received prior therapy and who are not eligible for fludarabine based therapy (in combination with chlorambucil or bendamustine)
▶ BY INTRAVENOUS INFUSION
▶ Adult: Premedication must be given 30 minutes to 2 hours before each dose—consult product literature for details

● CONTRA-INDICATIONS
CONTRA-INDICATIONS, FURTHER INFORMATION
For full details on the contra-indications for ofatumumab, consult product literature.

● CAUTIONS History of cardiac disease—monitor closely and discontinue treatment if cardiac arrhythmias occur
CAUTIONS, FURTHER INFORMATION
▶ Hepatitis B infection and reactivation Hepatitis B infection and reactivation (including fatal cases) have been reported in patients taking **ofatumumab**. Patients with positive hepatitis B serology should be referred to a liver specialist for monitoring and initiation of antiviral therapy before treatment initiation; treatment should not be initiated in patients with evidence of current hepatitis B infection until the infection has been adequately treated. Patients should be closely monitored for clinical and laboratory signs of active hepatitis B infection during treatment and for up to a year following the last infusion (consult product literature).
    For full details about the cautions for ofatumumab, consult product literature

● INTERACTIONS → Appendix 1: monoclonal antibodies

● SIDE-EFFECTS
▶ **Common or very common** Bronchospasm · chest discomfort · febrile neutropenia · hypoxia · laryngeal pain · nasal congestion · sepsis · skin reactions
▶ **Uncommon** Agranulocytosis · bradycardia · coagulation disorder · gastrointestinal disorders · lymphopenia · pulmonary oedema · pure red cell aplasia
▶ **Rare or very rare** Hepatitis B
SIDE-EFFECTS, FURTHER INFORMATION Infusion-related side-effects (including cytokine release syndrome) have been reported with ofatumumab; premedication with paracetamol, an antihistamine, and a corticosteroid must be given—consult product literature.

● CONCEPTION AND CONTRACEPTION Use effective contraception during and for 12 months after treatment.

● PREGNANCY Avoid unless potential benefit outweighs risk.

● BREAST FEEDING Discontinue breast-feeding during and for 12 months after treatment—no information available.

● RENAL IMPAIRMENT No information available for creatinine clearance less than 30 mL/minute.

● MONITORING REQUIREMENTS
▶ Monitor electrolytes (including potassium and magnesium) before and during administration and correct if abnormal.
▶ Patients must be monitored closely during each infusion for the onset of infusion reactions.

8

Immune system and malignant disease

● NATIONAL FUNDING/ACCESS DECISIONS

NICE decisions

▶ Ofatumumab for the treatment of chronic lymphocytic leukaemia refractory to fludarabine and alemtuzumab (October 2010) NICE TA202

Ofatumumab is **not** recommended for the treatment of chronic lymphocytic leukaemia that is refractory to fludarabine and alemtuzumab.

Patients currently receiving ofatumumab for this condition should have the option to continue treatment until they and their clinician consider it appropriate to stop.

www.nice.org.uk/TA202

▶ Ofatumumab in combination with chlorambucil or bendamustine for untreated chronic lymphocytic leukaemia (June 2015) NICE TA344

Ofatumumab in combination with chlorambucil is an option for untreated chronic lymphocytic leukaemia only if:

● the person is ineligible for fludarabine-based therapy **and**

● bendamustine is not suitable **and**

● the manufacturer provides ofatumumab with the discount agreed in the patient access scheme.

Patients currently receiving ofatumumab that is not recommended according to the above criteria should have the option to continue treatment until they and their clinician consider it appropriate to stop.

www.nice.org.uk/TA344

Scottish Medicines Consortium (SMC) Decisions

The *Scottish Medicines Consortium* has advised (April 2015) that ofatumumab (*Arzerra*®) is accepted for restricted use within NHS Scotland for the treatment of chronic lymphocytic leukaemia in patients who have not received prior therapy and who are not eligible for fludarabine-based therapy. It is restricted to use in patients who would not be considered for bendamustine therapy and who would receive chlorambucil-based therapy.

● MEDICINAL FORMS

There can be variation in the licensing of different medicines containing the same drug.

Solution for infusion

ELECTROLYTES: May contain Sodium

▶ Arzerra (Novartis Pharmaceuticals UK Ltd)

Ofatumumab 20 mg per 1 ml Arzerra 100mg/5ml concentrate for solution for infusion vials | 3 vial [PoM] £546.00 (Hospital only)
Arzerra 1000mg/50ml concentrate for solution for infusion vials | 1 vial [PoM] £1,820.00 (Hospital only)

Olaratumab

15-Aug-2017

● DRUG ACTION Olaratumab is a monoclonal antibody that binds to platelet-derived growth factor receptor alpha to inhibit tumour growth.

● INDICATIONS AND DOSE

Advanced soft tissue sarcoma (in combination with doxorubicin) in patients that are not amenable to curative treatment with surgery or radiotherapy, and who have not been previously treated with doxorubicin (specialist use only)

▶ BY INTRAVENOUS INFUSION

▶ Adult: 15 mg/kg once daily on days 1 and 8 of a 3-week cycle, for up to 8 cycles, patients whose disease has not progressed after combination therapy may continue with olaratumab monotherapy, for dose adjustments due to side-effects and infusion-related reactions—consult product literature

● CAUTIONS Patients should receive pre-medication to minimise the development of adverse reactions (consult product literature)

● INTERACTIONS → Appendix 1: monoclonal antibodies

● SIDE-EFFECTS

▶ **Common or very common** Arthralgia · diarrhoea · headache · lymphopenia · mucositis · muscle complaints · nausea · neutropenia · pain · vomiting

▶ **Rare or very rare** Flushing

▶ **Frequency not known** Bronchospasm · cardiac arrest · chills · dyspnoea · fever · hypersensitivity · hypotension

SIDE-EFFECTS, FURTHER INFORMATION Side-effects were reported for use of olaratumab in combination with doxorubicin.

Infusion-related rections Infusion related reactions have been reported; for grade 1 or 2 infusion-related reactions, manufacturer advises interrupt treatment and treat as clinically indicated; treatment may be recommenced at a reduced dose once the reaction has resolved and pre-medication should be given prior to subsequent infusions—consult product literature. Permanently discontinue treatment in the event of a grade 3 or 4 infusion-related reaction.

● CONCEPTION AND CONTRACEPTION Manufacturer advises women of child-bearing potential should use effective contraception during and for at least 3 months after stopping treatment.

● PREGNANCY Manufacturer advises avoid unless potential benefit outweighs risk—toxicity in *animal* studies. See also *Pregnancy and reproductive function* in Cytotoxic drugs p. 865.

● BREAST FEEDING Manufacturer advises avoid during and for at least 3 months after stopping treatment—no information available.

● MONITORING REQUIREMENTS

▶ Manufacturer advises monitor for signs and symptoms of infusion-related reactions during the infusion.

▶ Manufacturer advises monitor neutrophil and platelet count prior to each dose and during treatment; monitor coagulation profile in patients with increased risk of bleeding.

● DIRECTIONS FOR ADMINISTRATION Manufacturer advises for *intermittent intravenous infusion* (*Lartruvo*®), dilute requisite dose to a final volume of 250 mL with Sodium Chloride 0.9 %; give over approx. 60 minutes at a rate not exceeding 25 mg/minute. Manufacturer advises resuscitation facilities should be available.

● HANDLING AND STORAGE Manufacturer advises store in a refrigerator (2–8 °C)—consult product literature for storage conditions after preparation of the infusion.

● PATIENT AND CARER ADVICE

Driving and skilled tasks Manufacturer advises patients and carers should be counselled on the effects on driving and performance of skilled tasks—increased risk of fatigue.

● NATIONAL FUNDING/ACCESS DECISIONS

NICE decisions

▶ Olaratumab in combination with doxorubicin for treating advanced soft tissue sarcoma (August 2017) NICE TA465

Olaratumab, in combination with doxorubicin, is recommended for use within the Cancer Drugs Fund as an option for advanced soft tissue sarcoma in adults, only if:

● they have not had any previous systemic chemotherapy for advanced soft tissue sarcoma

● they cannot have curative treatment with surgery or their disease does not respond to radiotherapy

● the conditions in the managed access agreement for olaratumab are followed.

This recommendation is not intended to affect treatment with olaratumab that was started in the NHS before this guidance was published. Patients having treatment outside this recommendation may continue without change to the funding arrangements in place for them

before this guidance was published, until they and their NHS clinician consider it appropriate to stop.
www.nice.org.uk/guidance/TA465

Scottish Medicines Consortium (SMC) Decisions
The *Scottish Medicines Consortium* has advised (November 2017) that olaratumab (*Lartruvo®*), in combination with doxorubicin, is accepted for restricted use within NHS Scotland for the first-line treatment of patients with advanced soft-tissue sarcoma not amenable to curative treatment with surgery or radiotherapy. This advice is contingent upon the continuing availability of the patient access scheme in NHS Scotland or a list price that is equivalent or lower.

● MEDICINAL FORMS
There can be variation in the licensing of different medicines containing the same drug.
Solution for infusion
EXCIPIENTS: May contain Polysorbates
ELECTROLYTES: May contain Sodium
▸ Lartruvo (Eli Lilly and Company Ltd) ▼
Olaratumab 10 mg per 1 ml Lartruvo 500mg/50ml concentrate for solution for infusion vials | 1 vial [PoM] £1,000.00
Lartruvo 190mg/19ml concentrate for solution for infusion vials | 1 vial [PoM] £380.00

Panitumumab
02-Aug-2017

● DRUG ACTION Panitumumab is a monoclonal antibody that binds to the epidermal growth factor receptor (EGFR).

● INDICATIONS AND DOSE

Treatment of non-mutated RAS metastatic colorectal cancer (combination therapy) | Treatment of non-mutated RAS metastatic colorectal cancer (monotherapy after failure of fluoropyrimidine-, oxaliplatin-, and irinotecan-containing chemotherapy regimens)
▸ BY INTRAVENOUS INFUSION
▸ Adult: (consult product literature)

IMPORTANT SAFETY INFORMATION
MHRA/CHM ADVICE: SEVERE SKIN REACTIONS
Severe skin reactions have been reported very commonly in patients treated with panitumumab. Patients receiving panitumumab who have severe skin reactions or develop worsening skin reactions should be monitored for the development of inflammatory or infectious sequelae (including cellulitis, sepsis, and necrotising fasciitis). Appropriate treatment should be promptly initiated and panitumumab withheld or discontinued.

MHRA/CHM ADVICE: EPIDERMAL GROWTH FACTOR RECEPTOR (EGFR) INHIBITORS: SERIOUS CASES OF KERATITIS AND ULCERATIVE KERATITIS (MAY 2012)
Keratitis and ulcerative keratitis have been reported following treatment with epidermal growth factor receptor (EGFR) inhibitors for cancer (cetuximab, erlotinib, gefitinib and panitumumab). In rare cases, this has resulted in corneal perforation and blindness. Patients undergoing treatment with EGFR inhibitors who present with acute or worsening signs and symptoms suggestive of keratitis should be referred promptly to an ophthalmology specialist. Treatment should be interrupted or discontinued if ulcerative keratitis is diagnosed.

● CONTRA-INDICATIONS Interstitial pulmonary disease · the combination of panitumumab with oxaliplatin-containing chemotherapy is contra-indicated in patients with mutant *RAS* metastatic colorectal cancer or for whom *RAS* status is unknown

● CAUTIONS History of keratitis · history of severe dry eye · history of ulcerative keratitis · pulmonary disease—discontinue if interstitial lung disease develops · risk factors for keratitis · risk factors for severe dry eye · risk factors for ulcerative keratitis (including contact lens use)

● INTERACTIONS → Appendix 1: monoclonal antibodies

● SIDE-EFFECTS
▸ **Common or very common** Alopecia · anaemia · anxiety · appetite decreased · asthenia · chest pain · chills · constipation · cough · dehydration · diarrhoea · dizziness · dry eye · dry mouth · dyspnoea · electrolyte imbalance · embolism and thrombosis · eye discomfort · eye disorders · eye inflammation · fever · flushing · gastrointestinal discomfort · gastrooesophageal reflux disease · haemorrhage · hair changes · headache · hyperglycaemia · hyperhidrosis · hypersensitivity (may be delayed) · hypertension · hypotension · increased risk of infection · insomnia · leucopenia · mucositis · nail disorders · nausea · oral disorders · pain · peripheral oedema · skin reactions · skin ulcer · tachycardia · vomiting · weight decreased
▸ **Uncommon** Angioedema · cyanosis · infusion related reaction · nasal dryness · onycholysis · respiratory disorders
▸ **Rare or very rare** Anaphylactic reaction · severe cutaneous adverse reactions (SCARs)

● CONCEPTION AND CONTRACEPTION Manufacturer advises effective contraception during and for 6 months after treatment.

● PREGNANCY Avoid (toxicity in *animal* studies). See also *Pregnancy and reproductive function* in Cytotoxic drugs p. 865.

● BREAST FEEDING Manufacturer advises avoid breastfeeding during and for 2 months after treatment.

● PRE-TREATMENT SCREENING Evidence of non-mutated *RAS* status (at exons 2, 3 and 4 of *KRAS* and *NRAS*) is required before panitumumab treatment is initiated, and should be determined by an experienced laboratory using a validated test method.

● MONITORING REQUIREMENTS
▸ Monitor for hypomagnesaemia.
▸ Monitor for hypocalcaemia.
▸ Monitor for dermatological reactions including Stevens-Johnson syndrome and toxic epidermal necrolysis (consult product literature).

● NATIONAL FUNDING/ACCESS DECISIONS

NICE decisions
▸ **Cetuximab, bevacizumab and panitumumab for the treatment of metastatic colorectal cancer after first-line chemotherapy (January 2012)** NICE TA242
Panitinumab monotherapy is **not** recommended for the treatment of patients with metastatic colorectal cancer that has progressed after first-line chemotherapy.
www.nice.org.uk/guidance/TA242
▸ **Cetuximab and panitumumab for previously untreated metastatic colorectal cancer (updated September 2017)** NICE TA439
Panitumumab is recommended, within its marketing authorisation, as an option for previously untreated RAS wild-type metastatic colorectal cancer in adults in combination with:
● 5-fluorouracil, folinic acid and oxaliplatin (FOLFOX), **or**
● 5-fluorouracil, folinic acid and irinotecan (FOLFIRI).
This advice is contingent upon the manufacturer providing panitumumab with the discount agreed in the patient access scheme.
www.nice.org.uk/guidance/TA439

● MEDICINAL FORMS
There can be variation in the licensing of different medicines containing the same drug.
Solution for infusion
ELECTROLYTES: May contain Sodium
▸ Vectibix (Amgen Ltd)
Panitumumab 20 mg per 1 ml Vectibix 400mg/20ml concentrate for solution for infusion vials | 1 vial [PoM] £1,517.16 (Hospital only)
Vectibix 100mg/5ml concentrate for solution for infusion vials | 1 vial [PoM] £379.29 (Hospital only)

Pembrolizumab
20-Oct-2017

● DRUG ACTION Pembrolizumab is a monoclonal antibody, which binds to the programmed death-1 (PD-1) receptor, thereby potentiating an immune response to tumour cells.

● INDICATIONS AND DOSE

Melanoma (specialist use only) | Locally advanced or metastatic non-small cell lung cancer (following prior chemotherapy) (specialist use only)
▸ BY INTRAVENOUS INFUSION
▸ Adult: 2 mg/kg every 3 weeks, for dose adjustments due to side-effects or infusion-related reactions—consult product literature

Metastatic non-small cell lung cancer (first-line treatment) (specialist use only) | Urothelial carcinoma (specialist use only) | Classical Hodgkin lymphoma (specialist use only)
▸ BY INTRAVENOUS INFUSION
▸ Adult: 200 mg every 3 weeks, for dose adjustments due to side-effects or infusion-related reactions—consult product literature

IMPORTANT SAFETY INFORMATION
MHRA/CHM ADVICE: PEMBROLIZUMAB (*KEYTRUDA*®): REPORTS OF ORGAN TRANSPLANT REJECTION (JULY 2017)
A European review of worldwide data concluded that pembrolizumab may increase the risk of rejection in organ transplant recipients. The MHRA recommends considering the benefit of treatment with pembrolizumab versus the risk of possible organ transplant rejection for each patient.

● CAUTIONS Patients may need pretreatment to minimise the development of adverse reactions (consult product literature)
● INTERACTIONS → Appendix 1: monoclonal antibodies
● SIDE-EFFECTS
▸ **Common or very common** Abdominal pain · anaemia · appetite decreased · arthralgia · arthritis · asthenia · chills · constipation · cough · cytokine release syndrome · diarrhoea · dizziness · dry mouth · dyspnoea · fever · gastrointestinal disorders · headache · hypersensitivity · hyperthyroidism · hypothyroidism · influenza like illness · myositis · nausea · oedema · pain · pneumonitis · severe cutaneous adverse reactions (SCARs) · skin reactions · taste altered · vomiting
▸ **Uncommon** Adrenal insufficiency · alopecia · decreased leucocytes · dry eye · electrolyte imbalance · eosinophilia · epilepsy · hair colour changes · hepatitis · hypertension · hypophysitis · insomnia · lethargy · myocarditis · nephritis · nerve disorders · neutropenia · pancreatitis · tenosynovitis · thrombocytopenia · thyroiditis · type 1 diabetes mellitus · uveitis
▸ **Rare or very rare** Erythema nodosum · haemolytic anaemia · myasthenic syndrome · sarcoidosis
▸ **Frequency not known** Solid organ transplant rejection
SIDE-EFFECTS, FURTHER INFORMATION
Immune-related reactions Most immune-related adverse reactions are reversible and managed by

temporarily stopping treatment and administration of a corticosteroid—consult product literature for further information.
Infusion-related reactions Manufacturer advises to permanently discontinue treatment in patients with severe infusion reactions.

● CONCEPTION AND CONTRACEPTION Manufacturer recommends effective contraception during treatment and for at least 4 months after treatment in women of childbearing potential.

● PREGNANCY Manufacturer advises avoid unless potential benefit outweighs risk—no information available

● BREAST FEEDING Manufacturer advises avoid—no information available.

● MONITORING REQUIREMENTS Manufacturer advises monitor for signs and symptoms of infusion- and immune-related reactions.

● HANDLING AND STORAGE Manufacturer advises store in a refrigerator at 2–8°C.

● PATIENT AND CARER ADVICE Patients should be provided with an alert card and advised to keep it with them at all times.

● NATIONAL FUNDING/ACCESS DECISIONS
NICE decisions
▸ **Pembrolizumab for treating advanced melanoma after disease progression with ipilimumab (updated September 2017)** NICE TA357
Pembrolizumab is recommended as an option for treating advanced (unresectable or metastatic) melanoma in adults only:
● after the disease has progressed with ipilimumab and, for BRAF V600 mutation-positive disease, a BRAF or MEK inhibitor, **and**
● the manufacturer provides pembrolizumab in line with the commercial access agreement with NHS England.
www.nice.org.uk/guidance/ta357
▸ **Pembrolizumab for advanced melanoma not previously treated with ipilimumab (updated September 2017)** NICE TA366
Pembrolizumab is recommended as an option for treating advanced (unresectable or metastatic) melanoma that has not been previously treated with ipilimumab, in adults, only when the manufacturer provides pembrolizumab in line with the commercial access agreement with NHS England.
www.nice.org.uk/guidance/ta366
▸ **Pembrolizumab for treating PD-L1-positive non-small-cell lung cancer after chemotherapy (updated September 2017)** NICE TA428
Pembrolizumab is recommended as an option for treating locally advanced or metastatic PD-L1-positive non-small-cell lung cancer in adults who have had at least one chemotherapy (and targeted treatment if they have an epidermal growth factor receptor (EGFR)- or anaplastic lymphoma kinase (ALK)-positive tumour), only if:
● pembrolizumab is stopped at 2 years of uninterrupted treatment and no documented disease progression, **and**
● the manufacturer provides pembrolizumab in line with the commercial access agreement with NHS England.
Patients whose treatment was started within the NHS before this guidance was published should have the option to continue treatment, without change to their funding arrangements, until they or their clinician consider it appropriate to stop.
www.nice.org.uk/guidance/ta428
▸ **Pembrolizumab for untreated PD-L1-positive metastatic non-small-cell lung cancer (June 2017)** NICE TA447
Pembrolizumab is recommended for use within the Cancer Drugs Fund as an option for untreated PD-L1-positive metastatic non-small-cell lung cancer in adults, only if:

- their tumours express PD-L1 with at least a 50% tumour proportion score and have no epidermal growth factor receptor- or anaplastic lymphoma kinase-positive mutations
- pembrolizumab is stopped at 2 years of uninterrupted treatment and no documented disease progression
- the conditions in the managed access agreement for pembrolizumab are followed.

Patients whose treatment was started within the NHS before this guidance was published should have the option to continue treatment, without change to their funding arrangements, until they and their clinician consider it appropriate to stop.

www.nice.org.uk/guidance/ta447

▶ **Pembrolizumab for treating locally advanced or metastatic urothelial carcinoma after platinum-containing chemotherapy (April 2018)** NICE TA519

Pembrolizumab is recommended for use within the Cancer Drugs Fund as an option for treating locally advanced or metastatic urothelial carcinoma in adults who have had platinum-containing chemotherapy, only if:

- pembrolizumab is stopped at 2 years of uninterrupted treatment or earlier in the event of disease progression, **and**
- the conditions in the managed access agreement for pembrolizumab are followed.

Patients whose treatment was started within the NHS before this guidance was published should have the option to continue treatment, without change to their funding arrangements, until they and their NHS clinician consider it appropriate to stop.

www.nice.org.uk/guidance/ta519

Scottish Medicines Consortium (SMC) Decisions

SMC No. 1086/15

The *Scottish Medicines Consortium* has advised (November 2015) that pembrolizumab (*Keytruda®*) is accepted for use within NHS Scotland as monotherapy for the treatment of advanced (unresectable or metastatic) melanoma in adults previously untreated with ipilimumab. The advice is contingent upon the continuing availability of the patient access scheme in NHS Scotland or a list price that is equivalent or lower.

SMC No. 1087/15

The *Scottish Medicines Consortium* has advised (December 2016) that pembrolizumab (*Keytruda®*) is **not** recommended for use within NHS Scotland as monotherapy for the treatment of advanced (unresectable or metastatic) melanoma in adults previously treated with ipilimumab as the economic case was not demonstrated.

SMC No. 1204/17

The *Scottish Medicines Consortium* has advised (January 2017) that pembrolizumab (*Keytruda®*) is accepted for restricted use within NHS Scotland for the treatment of locally advanced or metastatic non-small cell lung carcinoma (NSCLC) in adults whose tumours express programmed death ligand 1 (PD-L1) and who have received at least one prior chemotherapy regimen, subject to a two-year clinical stopping rule. The advice is contingent upon the continuing availability of pembrolizumab at the price agreed in the patient access scheme in NHS Scotland or a list price that is equivalent or lower.

SMC No. 1239/17

The *Scottish Medicines Consortium* has advised (July 2017) that pembrolizumab (*Keytruda®*) is accepted for restricted use within NHS Scotland as monotherapy for the first-line treatment of metastatic non-small cell lung carcinoma (NSCLC) in adults whose tumours express programmed death ligand 1 (PD-L1) with a ≥50% tumour proportion score with no epidermal growth factor receptor or anaplastic lymphoma kinase positive tumour mutations, subject to a two-year clinical stopping rule. The

advice is contingent upon the continuing availability of the patient access scheme in NHS Scotland or a list price that is equivalent or lower.

SMC No. 1291/18

The *Scottish Medicines Consortium* has advised (February 2018) that pembrolizumab (*Keytruda®*) is accepted for restricted use within NHS Scotland as monotherapy for the treatment of locally advanced or metastatic urothelial carcinoma in adults who have received prior platinum-containing chemotherapy. Treatment with pembrolizumab is subject to a two-year clinical stopping rule. This advice is contingent upon the continuing availability of the patient access scheme in NHS Scotland or a list price that is equivalent or lower.

SMC No. 1296/18

The *Scottish Medicines Consortium* has advised (March 2018) that pembrolizumab (*Keytruda®*) is accepted for restricted use within NHS Scotland as monotherapy for the treatment of adults with relapsed or refractory classical Hodgkin lymphoma who have failed autologous stem cell transplant and brentuximab vedotin, or who are transplant-ineligible and have failed brentuximab vedotin. Treatment with pembrolizumab is subject to a two-year clinical stopping rule. This advice is contingent upon the continuing availability of the patient access scheme in NHS Scotland or a list price that is equivalent or lower.

● MEDICINAL FORMS
There can be variation in the licensing of different medicines containing the same drug.

Solution for infusion
CAUTIONARY AND ADVISORY LABELS 3
▶ Keytruda (Merck Sharp & Dohme Ltd) ▼
     Pembrolizumab 25 mg per 1 ml Keytruda 100mg/4ml concentrate for solution for infusion vials | 1 vial PoM £2,630.00 (Hospital only)

Powder for solution for infusion
CAUTIONARY AND ADVISORY LABELS 3
▶ Keytruda (Merck Sharp & Dohme Ltd) ▼
     Pembrolizumab 50 mg Keytruda 50mg powder for concentrate for solution for infusion vials | 1 vial PoM £1,315.00 (Hospital only)

Pertuzumab
               18-Jul-2017

● DRUG ACTION Pertuzumab is a recombinant humanised monoclonal antibody, and acts by inhibiting human epidermal growth factor receptor 2 protein (HER2) dimerisation.

● INDICATIONS AND DOSE

Treatment of HER2-positive metastatic or locally recurrent unresectable breast cancer in combination with trastuzumab and docetaxel, in patients who have not received previous anti-HER2 therapy or chemotherapy (initiated by a specialist)
▶ BY INTRAVENOUS INFUSION
▶ Adult: (consult product literature)

● CAUTIONS Conditions that could impair left ventricular function · history of congestive heart failure · impaired left ventricular function · prior anthracycline exposure · radiotherapy to the chest area · recent myocardial infarction · serious cardiac arrhythmia · uncontrolled hypertension

● INTERACTIONS → Appendix 1: monoclonal antibodies

● SIDE-EFFECTS
▶ **Common or very common** Alopecia · anaemia · appetite decreased · arthralgia · asthenia · chills · congestive heart failure · constipation · cough · cytokine release syndrome · diarrhoea · dizziness · dyspepsia · dyspnoea · excessive tearing · fever · headache · hypersensitivity · increased risk of infection · infusion related reaction · insomnia · left ventricular dysfunction · leucopenia · mucositis · myalgia · nail disorder · nausea · neutropenia · oedema · pain ·

peripheral neuropathy · respiratory disorders · skin reactions · stomatitis · taste altered · vomiting

SIDE-EFFECTS, FURTHER INFORMATION Side effects mostly described for pertuzumab in combination with trastuzumab and docetaxel.

- CONCEPTION AND CONTRACEPTION Ensure effective contraception during and for six months after treatment in women of childbearing potential.
- PREGNANCY Avoid (toxicity in *animal* studies). Most cytotoxic drugs are teratogenic and should not be administered during pregnancy, especially during the first trimester. Considerable caution is necessary if a pregnant woman presents with cancer requiring chemotherapy, and specialist advice should always be sought.
- BREAST FEEDING Avoid—no information available.
- HEPATIC IMPAIRMENT Caution—no information available.
- RENAL IMPAIRMENT Caution in severe impairment—no information available.
- MONITORING REQUIREMENTS
  ▸ Assess for signs and symptoms of congestive heart failure (including left ventricular ejection fraction) before and during treatment—consult product literature, and withhold treatment if necessary.
  ▸ Monitor for febrile neutropenia.
- DIRECTIONS FOR ADMINISTRATION Resuscitation facilities should be available.
- NATIONAL FUNDING/ACCESS DECISIONS

NICE decisions
▸ **Pertuzumab for the neoadjuvant treatment of HER2-positive breast cancer (December 2016)** NICE TA424
Pertuzumab, in combination with trastuzumab and chemotherapy, is recommended, within its marketing authorisation, as an option for neoadjuvant treatment in adults with human epidermal growth factor receptor 2 (HER2-positive), locally advanced, inflammatory or early-stage breast cancer at high risk of recurrence, only if the manufacturer provides it with the discount agreed in the patient access scheme.
www.nice.org.uk/guidance/ta424
▸ **Pertuzumab with trastuzumab and docetaxel for treating HER2-positive breast cancer (March 2018)** NICE TA509
Pertuzumab, in combination with trastuzumab and docetaxel, is recommended, within its marketing authorisation, for treating HER2-positive metastatic or locally recurrent unresectable breast cancer, in adults who have not had previous anti-HER2 therapy or chemotherapy for their metastatic disease, only if the manufacturer provides pertuzumab within the agreed commercial access arrangement.
www.nice.org.uk/guidance/ta509

Scottish Medicines Consortium (SMC) Decisions
SMC No. 1121/16
The *Scottish Medicines Consortium* has advised (December 2016) that pertuzumab (*Perjeta*®) is **not** recommended for use within NHS Scotland in combination with trastuzumab and chemotherapy for the neoadjuvant treatment of patients with human epidermal growth factor receptor 2 (HER2)-positive, locally advanced, inflammatory, or early stage breast cancer at high risk of recurrence, as the economic case was not demonstrated.
SMC No. 897/13
The *Scottish Medicines Consortium* has advised (June 2017) that pertuzumab (*Perjeta*®) is **not** recommended for use within NHS Scotland for the treatment of HER2-positive metastatic or locally recurrent unresectable breast cancer in combination with trastuzumab and docetaxel, in adults who have not received previous anti-HER2 therapy or chemotherapy as the economic case was not sufficient to gain acceptance.

- MEDICINAL FORMS
There can be variation in the licensing of different medicines containing the same drug.
Solution for infusion
▸ Perjeta (Roche Products Ltd) ▼
  Pertuzumab 30 mg per 1 ml Perjeta 420mg/14ml concentrate for solution for infusion vials | 1 vial (PoM) £2,395.00 (Hospital only)

Ramucirumab

31-May-2016

- DRUG ACTION Ramucirumab is a human monoclonal antibody that binds to the vascular endothelial growth factor receptor-2 (VEGFR-2), inhibiting VEGF-induced angiogenesis.

- INDICATIONS AND DOSE

Treatment of advanced gastric cancer or gastro-oesophageal junction adenocarcinoma, in combination with paclitaxel, in patients with disease progression after prior platinum and fluoropyrimidine chemotherapy
▸ BY INTRAVENOUS INFUSION
▸ Adult: 8 mg/kg on days 1 and 15 of a 28 day cycle, dose to be administered prior to paclitaxel infusion, consult product literature for dose adjustments due to side-effects and infusion-related reactions

Treatment of advanced gastric cancer or gastro-oesophageal junction adenocarcinoma, as monotherapy, in patients with disease progression after prior platinum or fluoropyrimidine chemotherapy, and for whom treatment in combination with paclitaxel is not appropriate
▸ BY INTRAVENOUS INFUSION
▸ Adult: 8 mg/kg every 2 weeks, consult product literature for dose adjustments due to side-effects and infusion-related reactions

Treatment of metastatic colorectal cancer, in combination with FOLFIRI (irinotecan, fluorouracil and folinic acid), in patients with disease progression on, or after, prior therapy with bevacizumab, oxaliplatin and a fluoropyrimidine
▸ BY INTRAVENOUS INFUSION
▸ Adult: 8 mg/kg every 2 weeks, dose to be administered prior to FOLFIRI administration, consult product literature for dose adjustments due to side-effects and infusion-related reactions

Treatment of locally advanced or metastatic non-small cell lung cancer, in combination with docetaxel, in patients with disease progression after platinum-based chemotherapy
▸ BY INTRAVENOUS INFUSION
▸ Adult: 10 mg/kg on day 1 of a 21 day cycle, dose to be administered prior to docetaxel infusion, consult product literature for dose adjustments due to side-effects and infusion-related reactions

- CAUTIONS Elective surgery—discontinue treatment for at least 4 weeks prior to surgery · hypertension—must be controlled before initiation · impaired wound healing—discontinue treatment until wound fully healed · pretreatment is recommended to minimise the development of adverse reactions (consult product literature) · risk of bleeding

- INTERACTIONS → Appendix 1: monoclonal antibodies
- SIDE-EFFECTS
▸ **Common or very common** Asthenia · diarrhoea · electrolyte imbalance · gastrointestinal discomfort · gastrointestinal perforation · haemorrhage · hand and foot syndrome · headache · hepatic pain · hypertension · hypoalbuminaemia · leucopenia · mucositis · neutropenia ·

peripheral oedema · proteinuria · sepsis · stomatitis · thrombocytopenia

▶ **Frequency not known** Arterial thrombosis · back pain · back spasms · cardiac arrest · cerebrovascular insufficiency · chest discomfort · chills · dyspnoea · flushing · hypersensitivity · hypotension · hypoxia · myocardial infarction · paraesthesia · respiratory disorders · supraventricular tachycardia · tremor

SIDE-EFFECTS, FURTHER INFORMATION Infusion-related hypersensitivity reactions have been reported with ramucirumab, particularly during or following the first or second infusion; if the patient experiences a grade 1 or 2 infusion-related reaction, the manufacturer advises to reduce rate of infusion by 50% and give premedication for all subsequent infusions—consult product literature. Manufacturer advises to permanently discontinue treatment in the event of a grade 3 or 4 infusion-related reaction.

● CONCEPTION AND CONTRACEPTION Manufacturer advises effective contraception during treatment and for up to 3 months after treatment in women of childbearing potential.

● PREGNANCY Manufacturer advises avoid unless potential benefit outweighs risk—no information available.

● BREAST FEEDING Manufacturer advises discontinue breast-feeding during treatment and for at least 3 months after treatment—no information available.

● HEPATIC IMPAIRMENT Manufacturer advises caution in severe cirrhosis, cirrhosis with hepatic encephalopathy, cirrhosis with clinically significant ascites, or hepatorenal syndrome—use only if potential benefit outweighs risk of progressive hepatic failure.

● MONITORING REQUIREMENTS Manufacturer advises monitor for signs of infusion-related hypersensitivity reactions; monitor blood pressure prior to each infusion; monitor for development or worsening of proteinuria during treatment—consult product literature; monitor blood counts and coagulation parameters in patients at risk of bleeding.

● DIRECTIONS FOR ADMINISTRATION For *intravenous infusion* (*Cyramza®*), give intermittently in Sodium chloride 0.9%; dilute requisite dose with infusion fluid to final volume of 250 mL and invert gently to mix. Do not exceed a rate of 25 mg/minute, and give over approximately 60 minutes via an infusion pump using a separate infusion line with a protein sparing 0.22 micron filter.

● PRESCRIBING AND DISPENSING INFORMATION For *Cyramza®*, each 10 mL vial contains sodium 17 mg (equivalent to Na⁺ 0.74 mmol).

● NATIONAL FUNDING/ACCESS DECISIONS

NICE decisions

▶ Ramucirumab for treating advanced gastric cancer or gastro-oesophageal junction adenocarcinoma previously treated with chemotherapy (January 2016) NICE TA378
Ramucirumab alone or in combination with paclitaxel is **not** recommended for the treatment of advanced gastric cancer or gastro-oesophageal junction adenocarcinoma previously treated with chemotherapy.
 Patients whose treatment was started before this guidance was published, should have the option to continue treatment until they and their clinician consider it appropriate to stop.
www.nice.org.uk/TA378

▶ Ramucirumab for previously treated locally advanced or metastatic non-small-cell lung cancer (August 2016) NICE TA403
Ramucirumab, in combination with docetaxel, is **not** recommended for treating locally advanced or metastatic non-small-cell lung cancer in patients whose disease has progressed after platinum-based chemotherapy.

Patients whose treatment was started within the NHS before this guidance was published should have the option to continue treatment, without change to their funding arrangements, until they and their clinicians consider it appropriate to stop.
www.nice.org.uk/TA403

● MEDICINAL FORMS
There can be variation in the licensing of different medicines containing the same drug.
Solution for infusion
ELECTROLYTES: May contain Sodium
▶ Cyramza (Eli Lilly and Company Ltd) ▼
 Ramucirumab 10 mg per 1 ml Cyramza 100mg/10ml concentrate for solution for infusion vials | 1 vial PoM £500.00 (Hospital only)
 Cyramza 500mg/50ml concentrate for solution for infusion vials | 1 vial PoM £2,500.00 (Hospital only)

Rituximab

21-Feb-2018

● INDICATIONS AND DOSE

Treatment of severe active rheumatoid arthritis in patients whose condition has not responded adequately to other disease-modifying antirheumatic drugs (including one or more tumour necrosis factor inhibitors) or who are intolerant of them (in combination with methotrexate)
▶ BY INTRAVENOUS INFUSION
▶ Adult: 1 g, then 1 g after 2 weeks, patients should receive premedication before each infusion (consult product literature for details)

Treatment of previously untreated stage III–IV follicular lymphoma (in combination with other chemotherapy) | Maintenance therapy in patients with follicular non-Hodgkin's lymphoma that has responded to induction therapy (in combination with other chemotherapy) | Treatment of diffuse large B-cell non-Hodgkin's lymphoma (in combination with other chemotherapy) | Treatment of chemotherapy-resistant or relapsed stage III–IV follicular non-Hodgkin's lymphoma | Previously untreated or relapsed chronic lymphocytic leukaemia | Induction of remission in patients with severe, active granulomatosis with polyangiitis (Wegener's) and microscopic polyangiitis (in combination with glucocorticoids)
▶ BY INTRAVENOUS INFUSION
▶ Adult: Patients should receive premedication before each dose (consult product literature for details) (consult product literature or local protocols)

● CONTRA-INDICATIONS Severe heart failure (when used to treat granulomatosis with polyangiitis or microscopic polyangiitis) · severe infection · severe, uncontrolled heart disease (when used to treat granulomatosis with polyangiitis or microscopic polyangiitis)
CONTRA-INDICATIONS, FURTHER INFORMATION
For full details on contra-indications, consult product literature.

● CAUTIONS
GENERAL CAUTIONS History of cardiovascular disease; in adults exacerbation of angina, arrhythmia, and heart failure have been reported · patients receiving cardiotoxic chemotherapy; in adults exacerbation of angina, arrhythmia, and heart failure have been reported · transient hypotension occurs frequently during infusion (anti-hypertensives may need to be withheld for 12 hours before infusion)

8

Immune system and malignant disease

SPECIFIC CAUTIONS

▸ **When used for rheumatoid arthritis** Predisposition to infection

CAUTIONS, FURTHER INFORMATION

▸ **Hepatitis B infection and reactivation** Hepatitis B infection and reactivation (including fatal cases) have been reported in patients taking **rituximab**. Patients with positive hepatitis B serology should be referred to a liver specialist for monitoring and initiation of antiviral therapy before treatment initiation; treatment should not be initiated in patients with evidence of current hepatitis B infection until the infection has been adequately treated. Patients should be closely monitored for clinical and laboratory signs of active hepatitis B infection during treatment and for up to a year following the last infusion (consult product literature).

For full details on cautions, consult product literature or local treatment protocol.

● INTERACTIONS → Appendix 1: monoclonal antibodies

● SIDE-EFFECTS

▸ **Common or very common** Angioedema · anxiety · appetite decreased · arrhythmias · bone marrow disorders · bursitis · cancer pain · cardiac disorder · chest pain · conjunctivitis · cough aggravated · dizziness · dysphagia · ear pain · gastrointestinal discomfort · gastrointestinal disorders · hearing impairment · hepatitis B · hypercholesterolaemia · hyperglycaemia · hypocalcaemia · increased risk of infection · insomnia · lacrimation disorder · malaise · migraine · multi organ failure · muscle tone increased · myalgia · myocardial infarction · nerve disorders · neutropenia · oedema · oral disorders · oropharyngeal pain · osteoarthritis · pain · postural hypotension · respiratory disorders · sensation abnormal · sepsis · skin reactions · throat irritation · vasodilation · weight decreased

▸ **Uncommon** Asthma · coagulation disorder · haemolytic anaemia · heart failure · hypoxia · ischaemic heart disease · lymphadenopathy · taste altered

▸ **Rare or very rare** Facial paralysis · hypersensitivity · renal failure · Stevens-Johnson syndrome (discontinue) · toxic epidermal necrolysis (discontinue) · vasculitis · vision disorders

▸ **Frequency not known** Hypogammaglobulinaemia · posterior reversible encephalopathy syndrome (PRES) · psychiatric disorder · seizure

SIDE-EFFECTS, FURTHER INFORMATION Associated with infections, sometimes severe, including tuberculosis, septicaemia, and hepatitis B reactivation.

Progressive multifocal leucoencephalopathy has been reported in association with rituximab; patients should be monitored for cognitive, neurological, or psychiatric signs and symptoms. If progressive multifocal leucoencephalopathy is suspected, suspend treatment until it has been excluded.

● CONCEPTION AND CONTRACEPTION Effective contraception (in both sexes) required during and for 12 months after treatment.

● PREGNANCY Avoid unless potential benefit to mother outweighs risk of B-lymphocyte depletion in fetus.

● BREAST FEEDING Avoid breast-feeding during and for 12 months after treatment.

● MONITORING REQUIREMENTS For full details on monitoring requirements consult product literature.

● DIRECTIONS FOR ADMINISTRATION For *intravenous infusion* (*MabThera®*), give intermittently in Glucose 5% or Sodium chloride 0.9%; dilute to 1-4 mg/mL and gently invert bag to avoid foaming.

● PRESCRIBING AND DISPENSING INFORMATION Rituximab is a biological medicine. Biological medicines must be prescribed and dispensed by brand name, see *Biological medicines* and *Biosimilar medicines*, under Guidance on prescribing p. 1.

● PATIENT AND CARER ADVICE

Alert card Patients treated for granulomatosis with polyangiitis and microscopic polyangiitis or rheumatoid arthritis should be provided with a patient alert card with each infusion.

● NATIONAL FUNDING/ACCESS DECISIONS

NICE decisions

▸ **Rituximab in combination with glucocorticoids for treating anti-neutrophil cytoplasmic antibody-associated vasculitis (March 2014)** NICE TA308

This NICE guidance was issued for rituximab by intravenous infusion. Rituximab, in combination with glucocorticoids, is recommended as an option for inducing remission in adults with anti-neutrophil cytoplasmic antibody [ANCA]-associated vasculitis (severely active granulomatosis with polyangiitis [Wegener's] and microscopic polyangiitis), only if:

• further cyclophosphamide treatment would exceed the maximum cumulative cyclophosphamide dose, **or**
• cyclophosphamide is contra-indicated or not tolerated, **or**
• the patient has not completed their family, and treatment with cyclophosphamide may materially affect their fertility, **or**
• the disease has remained active or progressed despite a course of cyclophosphamide lasting 3–6 months **or**
• the patient has had uroepithelial malignancy.
www.nice.org.uk/TA308

▸ **Adalimumab, etanercept, infliximab, rituximab, and abatacept for the treatment of rheumatoid arthritis after the failure of a TNF inhibitor (August 2010)** NICE TA195

Rituximab, in combination with methotrexate, is an option for the treatment of severe active rheumatoid arthritis in adults who have had an inadequate response to, or are intolerant of, other disease-modifying antirheumatic drugs (DMARDs), including at least 1 tumour necrosis factor (TNF) inhibitor. Repeat courses of rituximab should be given no more frequently than every 6 months, and should only be continued if an adequate response is achieved and maintained.
www.nice.org.uk/TA195

▸ **Rituximab for the first-line treatment of stage III-IV follicular lymphoma (January 2012)** NICE TA243

This NICE guidance was issued for rituximab by intravenous infusion. Rituximab, in combination with:

• cyclophosphamide, vincristine and prednisolone (CVP);
• cyclophosphamide, doxorubicin, vincristine and prednisolone (CHOP);
• mitoxantrone, chlorambucil and prednisolone (MCP);
• cyclophosphamide, doxorubicin, etoposide, prednisolone and interferon-alfa (CHVPi); *or*
• chlorambucil

is recommended as an option for the treatment of symptomatic stage III and IV follicular lymphoma in previously untreated patients.
www.nice.org.uk/TA243

▸ **Rituximab for the treatment of relapsed or refractory stage III or IV follicular non-Hodgkin's lymphoma (February 2008)** NICE TA137

This NICE guidance was issued for rituximab by intravenous infusion. Rituximab, in combination with chemotherapy, is an option for the induction of remission in patients with relapsed stage III or IV follicular non-Hodgkin's lymphoma.

Rituximab monotherapy as maintenance therapy is an option for the treatment of patients with relapsed stage III or IV follicular non-Hodgkin's lymphoma in remission induced with chemotherapy (with or without rituximab).

Rituximab monotherapy is an option for the treatment of patients with relapsed or refractory stage III or IV follicular non-Hodgkin's lymphoma, when all alternative

treatment options have been exhausted (that is, if there is resistance to or intolerance of chemotherapy).
www.nice.org.uk/TA137

▶ **Rituximab for the treatment of relapsed or refractory chronic lymphocytic leukaemia (July 2010) NICE TA193**
This NICE guidance was issued for rituximab by intravenous infusion. Rituximab in combination with fludarabine and cyclophosphamide is recommended as a treatment option for people with relapsed or refractory chronic lymphocytic leukaemia except when the condition:

- is refractory to fludarabine (that is, it has not responded to fludarabine, or has relapsed within 6 months of treatment), **or**
- has previously been treated with rituximab, unless it was in the context of a clinical trial, at a dose lower than the dose currently licensed for chronic lymphocytic leukaemia or with chemotherapy other than fludarabine and cyclophosphamide.

Rituximab in combination with fludarabine and cyclophosphamide is recommended only in the context of research for patients with relapsed or refractory chronic lymphocytic leukaemia that has previously been treated with rituximab, unless rituximab has been given as specified above.
www.nice.org.uk/TA193

▶ **Rituximab for the first-line maintenance treatment of follicular non-Hodgkin's lymphoma (June 2011) NICE TA226**
This NICE guidance was issued for rituximab by intravenous infusion. Rituximab maintenance therapy is recommended as an option for the treatment of people with follicular non-Hodgkins's lymphoma that has responded to first-line induction therapy with rituximab in combination with chemotherapy.
www.nice.org.uk/TA226

▶ **Rituximab for the first-line treatment of chronic lymphocytic leukaemia (July 2009) NICE TA174**
This NICE guidance was issued for rituximab by intravenous infusion. Rituximab, in combination with fludarabine and cyclophosphamide, is recommended as an option for the first-line treatment of chronic lymphocytic leukaemia.
www.nice.org.uk/TA174

▶ **Idelalisib for treating chronic lymphocytic leukaemia (October 2015) NICE TA359**
Rituximab, in combination with idelalisib, is recommended as an option for treatment in adults:

- who have untreated chronic lymphocytic leukaemia **or**
- who have chronic lymphocytic leukaemia when the disease has been treated but has relapsed within 24 months **and**
- if the manufacturer provides idelalisib with the discount agreed in the simple discount agreement.

Patients who are already receiving idelalisib should continue treatment until they or their clinician consider it appropriate to stop.
www.nice.org.uk/guidance/TA359

▶ **Rituximab for aggressive non-Hodgkin's lymphoma (September 2003) NICE TA65**
This NICE guidance was issued for rituximab by intravenous infusion. Rituximab, in combination with cyclophosphamide, doxorubicin, vincristine, and prednisolone, is recommended for first-line treatment of CD20-positive diffuse large-B-cell lymphoma at clinical stage II, III or IV.

The use of rituximab for localised (stage I) disease should be limited to clinical trials.
www.nice.org.uk/TA65

Scottish Medicines Consortium (SMC) Decisions
The *Scottish Medicines Consortium* has advised (August 2013) that Rituximab (*MabThera* ®) is accepted for restricted use within NHS Scotland, in combination with glucocorticoids for the induction of remission in adult patients with severe, active granulomatosis with polyangiitis (Wegener's) and microscopic polyangiitis. It is restricted to use in patients who have relapsed following treatment with cyclophosphamide or who are intolerant to or unable to receive cyclophosphamide.

The *Scottish Medicines Consortium* has advised (June 2014) that subcutaneous rituximab (*MabThera*) ® is accepted for restricted use within NHS Scotland, in accordance with UK licensing, except in the maintenance setting, where use is restricted to patients who have responded to induction therapy with rituximab plus chemotherapy.

● MEDICINAL FORMS
There can be variation in the licensing of different medicines containing the same drug.
Solution for infusion

▶ MabThera (Roche Products Ltd)
Rituximab 10 mg per 1 ml MabThera 100mg/10ml concentrate for solution for infusion vials | 2 vial [PoM] £349.25
MabThera 500mg/50ml concentrate for solution for infusion vials | 1 vial [PoM] £873.15

▶ Rixathon (Sandoz Ltd) ▼
Rituximab 10 mg per 1 ml Rixathon 100mg/10ml concentrate for solution for infusion vials | 2 vial [PoM] £314.33 (Hospital only)
Rixathon 500mg/50ml concentrate for solution for infusion vials | 1 vial [PoM] £785.84 (Hospital only) | 2 vial [PoM] £1,571.67 (Hospital only)

▶ Truxima (Napp Pharmaceuticals Ltd) ▼
Rituximab 10 mg per 1 ml Truxima 100mg/10ml concentrate for solution for infusion vials | 2 vial [PoM] £314.33
Truxima 500mg/50ml concentrate for solution for infusion vials | 1 vial [PoM] £785.84

Siltuximab

● DRUG ACTION Siltuximab is a monoclonal antibody that inhibits interleukin-6 receptor binding.

● INDICATIONS AND DOSE

Treatment of multicentric Castleman's disease (MCD) in patients who are human immunodeficiency virus (HIV) negative and human herpesvirus-8 (HHV-8) negative
▶ BY INTRAVENOUS INFUSION
▶ Adult: 11 mg/kg every 3 weeks

● CAUTIONS Patients at increased risk of gastrointestinal perforation—promptly investigate those presenting with symptoms suggestive of gastrointestinal perforation · severe infection—withhold treatment until resolved · treat infection prior to treatment
CAUTIONS, FURTHER INFORMATION
▶ Hypersensitivity reactions Infusion-related side-effects are reported commonly with siltuximab; resuscitation facilities should be available during treatment.
Consult product literature for further information about siltuximab cautions.

● INTERACTIONS → Appendix 1: monoclonal antibodies

● SIDE-EFFECTS
▶ **Common or very common** Abdominal pain · hypersensitivity · hypertension · hypertriglyceridaemia · increased risk of infection · localised oedema · neutropenia · renal impairment · skin reactions · thrombocytopenia · weight increased

SIDE-EFFECTS, FURTHER INFORMATION Siltuximab therapy should be discontinued permanently in the event of a severe infusion-related reaction, anaphylaxis, a severe allergic reaction, or the occurrence of cytokine-release syndrome. Mild to moderate infusion-related reactions may improve by temporarily reducing the rate or stopping the infusion. When restarting treatment, a reduced infusion rate and the administration of antihistamines, paracetamol, and corticosteroids may be considered. Consider discontinuation of siltuximab if more than 2 doses are delayed due to treatment-related toxicities during the first 48 weeks—for full details consult product literature.

- CONCEPTION AND CONTRACEPTION Women of childbearing potential should use effective contraception during and for 3 months after treatment.
- PREGNANCY Manufacturer advises avoid unless potential benefit outweighs risk.
- BREAST FEEDING Manufacturer advises avoid—no information available.
- HEPATIC IMPAIRMENT Use with caution in hepatic impairment.
- MONITORING REQUIREMENTS
- ▶ Monitor neutrophil and platelet count, and haemoglobin levels prior to each dose of siltuximab treatment for the first 12 months and thereafter prior to every third dosing cycle. Consider delaying treatment if required neutrophil, platelet, and haemoglobin levels not achieved—consult product literature for details.
- ▶ Monitor for infection during treatment.
- DIRECTIONS FOR ADMINISTRATION For *intravenous infusion* (*Sylvant*®), give intermittently *in* Glucose 5%. Allow vials to reach room temperature over approximately 30 minutes, then reconstitute each 100 mg vial with 5.2 mL of water for injection, and each 400 mg vial with 20 mL of water for injection, to produce a 20 mg/mL solution. Gently swirl without shaking to dissolve. Further dilute to 250 mL with glucose 5% and gently mix. Use within 6 hours of dilution and give over 60 minutes using an administration set lined with polyvinyl chloride or polyurethane, through a low-protein binding in-line 0.2 micron filter.

- MEDICINAL FORMS
  There can be variation in the licensing of different medicines containing the same drug.

  Powder for solution for infusion
  ▶ Sylvant (Janssen-Cilag Ltd) ▼
  Siltuximab 100 mg Sylvant 100mg powder for concentrate for solution for infusion vials | 1 vial [PoM] £415.00 (Hospital only)
  Siltuximab 400 mg Sylvant 400mg powder for concentrate for solution for infusion vials | 1 vial [PoM] £1,661.00 (Hospital only)

Trastuzumab

01-May-2018

- INDICATIONS AND DOSE

Treatment of early breast cancer which overexpresses human epidermal growth factor receptor-2 (HER2) (initiated by a specialist) | Treatment of metastatic breast cancer in patients with HER2-positive tumours who have not received chemotherapy for metastatic breast cancer and in whom anthracycline treatment is inappropriate (in combination with paclitaxel or docetaxel) (initiated by a specialist) | Treatment of metastatic breast cancer in postmenopausal patients with hormone-receptor positive HER2-positive tumours not previously treated with trastuzumab (in combination with an aromatase inhibitor) (initiated by a specialist)
- ▶ BY INTRAVENOUS INFUSION, OR BY SUBCUTANEOUS INJECTION
- ▶ Adult: (consult product literature or local protocols)

Monotherapy for metastatic breast cancer in patients with tumours that overexpress HER2 who have received at least 2 chemotherapy regimens including, where appropriate, an anthracycline and a taxane (initiated by a specialist)
- ▶ BY INTRAVENOUS INFUSION, OR BY SUBCUTANEOUS INJECTION
- ▶ Adult: Women with oestrogen-receptor-positive breast cancer should also have received hormonal treatment (consult product literature or local protocols)

Treatment of metastatic gastric cancer in patients with HER2-positive tumours who have not received treatment for metastatic gastric cancer (in combination with capecitabine or fluorouracil and cisplatin) (initiated by a specialist)
- ▶ BY INTRAVENOUS INFUSION
- ▶ Adult: (consult product literature or local protocols)

- CONTRA-INDICATIONS Severe dyspnoea at rest
- CAUTIONS Coronary artery disease · history of hypertension · symptomatic heart failure · uncontrolled arrhythmias
- INTERACTIONS → Appendix 1: monoclonal antibodies
- SIDE-EFFECTS
- ▶ Common or very common Alopecia · anaemia · angioedema · anxiety · appetite decreased · arrhythmias · arthralgia · arthritis · asthenia · asthma · ataxia · breast abnormalities · cardiomyopathy · chest pain · chills · constipation · cough · cystitis · depression · diarrhoea · dizziness · drowsiness · dry eye · dry mouth · dyspnoea · excessive tearing · eye inflammation · fever · gastrointestinal discomfort · haemorrhage · haemorrhoids · headache · heart failure · hepatic disorders · hyperhidrosis · hypersensitivity · hypotension · increased risk of infection · influenza like illness · infusion related reaction (may be delayed) · insomnia · leucopenia · malaise · mucositis · muscle complaints · muscle tone increased · nail disorders · nausea · neutropenia · oedema · oral disorders · pain · palpitations · pancreatitis · paraesthesia · peripheral neuropathy · renal disorder · respiratory disorders · rhinorrhoea · sepsis · skin reactions · taste altered · thinking abnormal · thrombocytopenia · tremor · vasodilation · vomiting · weight decreased
- ▶ Uncommon Deafness · pericardial effusion
- ▶ Rare or very rare Paresis
- ▶ Frequency not known Brain oedema · cancer progression · cardiogenic shock · glomerulonephritis · hyperkalaemia · hypoprothrombinaemia · hypoxia · pericarditis · pulmonary fibrosis (may be delayed) · pulmonary oedema (may be delayed) · renal failure
- CONCEPTION AND CONTRACEPTION Contraceptive advice required, see *Pregnancy and reproductive function* in Cytotoxic drugs p. 865.
- PREGNANCY Manufacturer advises avoid—oligohydramnios reported. See also *Pregnancy and reproductive function* in Cytotoxic drugs p. 865.
- BREAST FEEDING Avoid breast-feeding during treatment and for 7 months afterwards.
- MONITORING REQUIREMENTS
- ▶ Cardiotoxicity Monitor cardiac function before and during treatment—for details of monitoring and managing cardiotoxicity, consult product literature.
- DIRECTIONS FOR ADMINISTRATION Resuscitation facilities should be available during administration of trastuzumab.
- PRESCRIBING AND DISPENSING INFORMATION When prescribing, dispensing or administering, check that this is the correct preparation—trastuzumab is **not** interchangeable with trastuzumab emtansine.

● NATIONAL FUNDING/ACCESS DECISIONS

NICE decisions

▶ **Guidance on the use of trastuzumab for the treatment of advanced breast cancer (March 2002)** NICE TA34

Trastuzumab in combination with paclitaxel is recommended as an option for patients with tumours expressing human epidermal growth factor receptor 2 (HER2) scored at levels of 3+ who have not received chemotherapy for metastatic breast cancer, and in whom anthracycline treatment is inappropriate.

Trastuzumab monotherapy is recommended as an option for patients with tumours expressing HER2 scored at levels of 3+ who have received at least two chemotherapy regimens for metastatic breast cancer. Prior chemotherapy must have included at least an anthracycline and a taxane where these treatments are appropriate. It should also have included hormonal therapy in suitable oestrogen-receptor-positive patients.
www.nice.org.uk/guidance/ta34

▶ **Trastuzumab for the adjuvant treatment of early-stage HER2-positive breast cancer (August 2006)** NICE TA107

Trastuzumab, given at 3-week intervals for 1 year or until disease recurrence (whichever is the shorter period), is recommended as an option for women with early-stage HER2-positive breast cancer following surgery, chemotherapy (neoadjuvant or adjuvant) and radiotherapy (if applicable).
www.nice.org.uk/guidance/ta107

▶ **Lapatinib or trastuzumab in combination with an aromatase inhibitor for the first-line treatment of metastatic hormone-receptor-positive breast cancer that overexpresses HER2 (June 2012)** NICE TA257

Lapatinib or trastuzumab in combination with an aromatase inhibitor is **not** recommended for first-line treatment in postmenopausal women of metastatic hormone-receptor-positive breast cancer that overexpresses human epidermal growth factor receptor 2 (HER2).

Postmenopausal women currently receiving lapatinib or trastuzumab in combination with an aromatase inhibitor for this indication should have the option to continue treatment until they and their clinician consider it appropriate to stop.
www.nice.org.uk/guidance/ta257

▶ **Pertuzumab with trastuzumab and docetaxel for treating HER2-positive breast cancer (March 2018)** NICE TA509

Pertuzumab, in combination with trastuzumab and docetaxel, is recommended, within its marketing authorisation, for treating HER2-positive metastatic or locally recurrent unresectable breast cancer, in adults who have not had previous anti-HER2 therapy or chemotherapy for their metastatic disease, only if the manufacturer provides pertuzumab within the agreed commercial access arrangement.
www.nice.org.uk/guidance/ta509

▶ **Trastuzumab for the treatment of HER2-positive metastatic gastric cancer (November 2010)** NICE TA208

Trastuzumab in combination with cisplatin and capecitabine or fluorouracil is recommended for human epidermal growth factor receptor-2-positive metastatic adenocarcinoma of the stomach or gastro-oesophageal junction in patients who:

● have not received treatment for metastatic disease **and**
● have tumours expressing high levels of HER2 as defined by a positive immunohistochemistry score of 3.
www.nice.org.uk/guidance/ta208

Scottish Medicines Consortium (SMC) Decisions
SMC No. 928/13

The *Scottish Medicines Consortium* has advised (January 2014) that subcutaneous trastuzumab injection (*Herceptin*®) is accepted for restricted use within NHS Scotland for the treatment of adults with HER2 positive

metastatic breast cancer and early breast cancer, when used within licensed indications excluding use in combination with an aromatase inhibitor for the treatment of postmenopausal patients with hormone-receptor positive metastatic breast cancer, not previously treated with trastuzumab.
SMC No. 623/10

The *Scottish Medicines Consortium* has advised (October 2015) that trastuzumab solution for infusion (*Herceptin*®) is accepted for restricted use within NHS Scotland in combination with capecitabine or fluorouracil and cisplatin for the treatment of patients with HER2 positive metastatic adenocarcinoma of the stomach or gastro-oesophageal junction, who have not received prior anti-cancer treatment for their metastatic disease. It is restricted to patients with metastatic gastric cancer whose tumours have HER2 over-expression, as determined by an accurate and validated assay.

● MEDICINAL FORMS
There can be variation in the licensing of different medicines containing the same drug.

Solution for injection
▶ Herceptin (Roche Products Ltd)
Trastuzumab 120 mg per 1 ml Herceptin 600mg/5ml solution for injection vials | 1 vial [PoM] £1,222.20 (Hospital only)

Powder for solution for infusion
▶ Herceptin (Roche Products Ltd)
Trastuzumab 150 mg Herceptin 150mg powder for concentrate for solution for infusion vials | 1 vial [PoM] £407.40
▶ Herzuma (Napp Pharmaceuticals Ltd) ▼
Trastuzumab 150 mg Herzuma 150mg powder for concentrate for solution for infusion vials | 1 vial [PoM] £366.66
▶ Ontruzant (Merck Sharp & Dohme Ltd) ▼
Trastuzumab 150 mg Ontruzant 150mg powder for concentrate for solution for infusion vials | 1 vial [PoM] £366.66

Trastuzumab emtansine   02-Aug-2017

● DRUG ACTION Trastuzumab emtansine is an antibody-drug conjugate that contains trastuzumab covalently linked to DM1, a cytotoxic microtubule inhibitor.

● INDICATIONS AND DOSE

Monotherapy for the treatment of HER2-positive, unresectable, locally advanced or metastatic breast cancer, in adult patients who have previously received trastuzumab and a taxane separately or in combination (initiated by a specialist) | Monotherapy for the treatment of HER2-positive, unresectable, locally advanced or metastatic breast cancer, in adult patients who have developed disease recurrence during or within 6 months of completing adjuvant therapy (initiated by a specialist)
▶ BY INTRAVENOUS INFUSION
▶ Adult: (consult product literature or local protocols)

● CAUTIONS Dyspnoea at rest—increased risk of pulmonary events · history of congestive heart failure · patients over 75 years · peripheral neuropathy (temporarily discontinue treatment—consult product literature) · recent history of myocardial infarction · recent history of unstable angina · risk of left ventricular dysfunction—consult product literature for specific risks with trastuzumab treatment · serious arrhythmias

● INTERACTIONS → Appendix 1: monoclonal antibodies

● SIDE-EFFECTS
▶ Common or very common Alopecia · anaemia · arthralgia · asthenia · chills · conjunctivitis · constipation · cough · diarrhoea · dizziness · dry eye · dry mouth · dyspnoea · excessive tearing · fever · gastrointestinal discomfort · haemorrhage · headache · hypersensitivity · hypertension · hypokalaemia · infusion related reaction · insomnia · left

ventricular dysfunction · leucopenia · memory loss · musculoskeletal pain · myalgia · nail disorder · nausea · neutropenia · peripheral neuropathy · peripheral oedema · skin reactions · stomatitis · taste altered · thrombocytopenia · urinary tract infection · vision blurred · vomiting
▸ **Uncommon** Hepatic disorders · nodular regenerative hyperplasia · pneumonitis
● CONCEPTION AND CONTRACEPTION Effective contraception must be used during and for 6 months after stopping treatment in women and men.
● PREGNANCY Manufacturer advises avoid— oligohydramnios reported with trastuzumab. See also Pregnancy and reproductive function in Cytotoxic drugs p. 865.
● BREAST FEEDING Manufacturer advises avoid breast- feeding during and for 6 months after treatment.
● HEPATIC IMPAIRMENT Consult product literature for initiating treatment and discontinuation in cases of abnormal liver function tests.
  Dose adjustments Consult product literature for dose modification in cases of abnormal liver function tests.
● RENAL IMPAIRMENT No information available— manufacturer advises caution in severe impairment.
● MONITORING REQUIREMENTS
▸ Monitor hepatic function before each dose.
▸ Monitor for signs and symptoms of neurotoxicity.
▸ Monitor closely for infusion-related and hypersensitivity reactions.
▸ Monitor platelet count before each dose and as clinically indicated (consult product literature for treatment modification in thrombocytopenia).
▸ Test cardiac function before treatment and regularly during treatment—delay or discontinue treatment in cases of left ventricular dysfunction.
▸ Monitor for dyspnoea, cough, fatigue and pulmonary infiltrates—discontinue if interstitial lung disease or pneumonitis confirmed (fatal cases reported).
● DIRECTIONS FOR ADMINISTRATION Resuscitation facilities should be available during administration of trastuzumab emtansine.
● PRESCRIBING AND DISPENSING INFORMATION When prescribing, dispensing or administering, check that this is the correct preparation— trastuzumab emtansine and trastuzumab are **not** interchangeable.
● NATIONAL FUNDING/ACCESS DECISIONS
  NICE decisions
▸ **Trastuzumab emtansine for treating HER2-positive advanced breast cancer after trastuzumab and a taxane (updated November 2017)** NICE TA458
  Trastuzumab emtansine is recommended, within its marketing authorisation, as an option for treating human epidermal growth factor receptor 2 (HER2)-positive, unresectable, locally advanced or metastatic breast cancer in adults who previously received trastuzumab and a taxane, separately or in combination. Patients should have either received prior therapy for locally advanced or metastatic disease or developed disease recurrence during or within 6 months of completing adjuvant therapy.
  Trastuzumab emtansine is recommended only if the manufacturer provides it with the discount agreed in the patient access scheme.
  www.nice.org.uk/guidance/TA458
  Scottish Medicines Consortium (SMC) Decisions
  The *Scottish Medicines Consortium* has advised (April 2017) that trastuzumab emtansine (*Kadcyla*®) is accepted for use within NHS Scotland as monotherapy for the treatment of patients with human epidermal growth factor type 2 (HER2)-positive, unresectable locally advanced or metastatic breast cancer who previously received

trastuzumab and a taxane, separately or in combination, and have either received prior therapy for locally advanced or metastatic disease *or* developed disease recurrence during or within six months of completing adjuvant therapy. This advice is contingent upon the continuing availability of the Patient Access Scheme in NHS Scotland or a list price that is equivalent or lower.

● MEDICINAL FORMS
  There can be variation in the licensing of different medicines containing the same drug.
  Powder for solution for infusion
  ▸ Kadcyla (Roche Products Ltd) ▼
  Trastuzumab emtansine 100 mg Kadcyla 100mg powder for concentrate for solution for infusion vials | 1 vial [PoM] £1,641.01
  Trastuzumab emtansine 160 mg Kadcyla 160mg powder for concentrate for solution for infusion vials | 1 vial [PoM] £2,625.62

2   Carcinoid syndrome

ENZYME INHIBITORS

Telotristat ethyl

14-Dec-2017

● DRUG ACTION Telotristat ethyl and its active metabolite inhibit L-tryptophan hydroxylases TPH-1 and TPH-2 which reduces the production of serotonin, thereby alleviating symptoms associated with carcinoid syndrome.

● INDICATIONS AND DOSE
  Carcinoid syndrome diarrhoea (specialist use only)
  ▸ BY MOUTH
  ▸ Adult: 250 mg 3 times a day, review treatment if no response after 12 weeks

● INTERACTIONS → Appendix 1: telotristat ethyl
● SIDE-EFFECTS
▸ **Common or very common** Appetite decreased · constipation · fatigue · fever · flatulence · gastrointestinal discomfort · headache · peripheral oedema
● PREGNANCY Manufacturer advises avoid—toxicity in *animal* studies.
● BREAST FEEDING Manufacturer advises avoid—no information available.
● HEPATIC IMPAIRMENT Manufacturer advises avoid in severe impairment—no information available.
  Dose adjustments Manufacturer advises consider dose reduction to 250 mg twice daily in mild impairment; consider dose reduction to 250 mg once daily in moderate impairment—reduce dose according to tolerability and monitor for adverse effects and worsening of liver function.
● RENAL IMPAIRMENT Manufacturer advises caution in mild-to-moderate impairment; avoid in severe impairment—no information available.
● MONITORING REQUIREMENTS Manufacturer advises monitor liver function at initiation and during treatment as clinically indicated—discontinue if liver injury suspected.
● PATIENT AND CARER ADVICE Manufacturer advises inform patients to report any symptoms of depression or decreased interest.

● MEDICINAL FORMS
  There can be variation in the licensing of different medicines containing the same drug.
  Tablet
  CAUTIONARY AND ADVISORY LABELS 3, 21
  ▸ Xermelo (Ipsen Ltd) ▼
  Telotristat ethyl 250 mg Xermelo 250mg tablets | 90 tablet [PoM] £1,120.00

3 Cytotoxic responsive malignancy

Cytotoxic drugs

Overview

The chemotherapy of cancer is complex and should be confined to specialists in oncology. Cytotoxic drugs have both anti-cancer activity and the potential to damage normal tissue; most cytotoxic drugs are teratogenic. Chemotherapy may be given with a curative intent or it may aim to prolong life or to palliate symptoms. In an increasing number of cases chemotherapy may be combined with radiotherapy or surgery or both as either neoadjuvant treatment (initial chemotherapy aimed at shrinking the primary tumour, thereby rendering local therapy less destructive or more effective) or as adjuvant treatment (which follows definitive treatment of the primary disease, when the risk of subclinical metastatic disease is known to be high). All cytotoxic drugs cause side-effects and a balance has to be struck between likely benefit and acceptable toxicity.

Combinations of cytotoxic drugs, as continuous or pulsed cycles of treatment, are frequently more toxic than single drugs but have the advantage in certain tumours of enhanced response, reduced development of drug resistance and increased survival. However for some tumours, single-agent chemotherapy remains the treatment of choice.

Cytotoxic drugs fall into a number of classes, each with characteristic antitumour activity, sites of action, and toxicity. A knowledge of sites of metabolism and excretion is important because impaired drug handling as a result of disease is not uncommon and may result in enhanced toxicity.

Cytotoxic drug handling guidelines

- Trained personnel should reconstitute cytotoxics
- Reconstitution should be carried out in designated pharmacy areas
- Protective clothing (including gloves, gowns, and masks) should be worn
- The eyes should be protected and means of first aid should be specified
- Pregnant staff should avoid exposure to cytotoxic drugs (all females of child-bearing age should be informed of the reproductive hazard)
- Use local procedures for dealing with spillages and safe disposal of waste material, including syringes, containers, and absorbent material
- Staff exposure to cytotoxic drugs should be monitored

Intrathecal chemotherapy

A Health Service Circular (HSC 2008/001) provides guidance on the introduction of safe practice in NHS Trusts where intrathecal chemotherapy is administered; written local guidance covering all aspects of national guidance should be available. Support for training programmes is also available. Copies, and further information may be obtained from:

Department of Health
PO Box 777
London
SE1 6XH
Fax: 01623 724524

It is also available from the Department of Health website (www.dh.gov.uk).

Safe systems for cytotoxic medicines

NHS cancer networks have been established across the UK to bring together all stakeholders in all sectors of care, to work collaboratively to plan and deliver high quality cancer services for a given population. NHS cancer networks have websites containing information on local chemotherapy services and treatment.

Safe system requirements:

- cytotoxic drugs for the treatment of cancer should be given as part of a wider pathway of care coordinated by a multidisciplinary team
- cytotoxic drugs should be prescribed, dispensed, and administered only in the context of a written protocol or treatment plan
- injectable cytotoxic drugs should only be dispensed if they are prepared for administration
- oral cytotoxic medicines should be dispensed with clear directions for use

Cytotoxic drugs: important safety information

Risk of incorrect dosing of oral anti-cancer medicines

The National Patient Safety Agency has advised (January 2008) that the prescribing and use of oral cytotoxic medicines should be carried out to the same standard as parenteral cytotoxic therapy.

- non-specialists who prescribe or administer on-going oral cytotoxic medication should have access to written protocols and treatment plans, including guidance on the monitoring and treatment of toxicity;
- staff dispensing oral cytotoxic medicines should confirm that the prescribed dose is appropriate for the patient. Patients should have written information that includes details of the intended oral anti-cancer regimen, the treatment plan, and arrangements for monitoring, taken from the original protocol from the initiating hospital. Staff dispensing oral cytotoxic medicines should also have access to this information, and to advice from an experienced cancer pharmacist in the initiating hospital.

Cytotoxic drug doses

Doses of cytotoxic drugs are determined using a variety of different methods including body-surface area or body-weight. Alternatively, doses may be fixed. Doses may be further adjusted following consideration of a patient's neutrophil count, renal and hepatic function, and history of previous adverse effects to the cytotoxic drug. Doses may also differ depending on whether a drug is used alone or in combination.

Because of the complexity of dosage regimens in the treatment of malignant disease, dose statements have been omitted from some of the drug entries in this chapter. However, even where dose statements have been provided, detailed specialist literature, individual hospital chemotherapy protocols, or local cancer networks should be consulted before prescribing, dispensing, or administering cytotoxic drugs.

Prescriptions should **not** be repeated except on the instructions of a specialist.

Cytotoxic drug side-effects

Side-effects common to most cytotoxic drugs are discussed below whilst side-effects characteristic of a particular drug or class of drugs (e.g. neurotoxicity with vinca alkaloids) are mentioned in the appropriate sections. Manufacturers' product literature, hospital-trust protocols, and cancer-network protocols should be consulted for full details of side-effects associated with individual drugs and specific chemotherapy regimes.

Many side-effects of cytotoxic drugs often do not occur at the time of administration, but days or weeks later. It is therefore important that patients and healthcare professionals can identify symptoms that cause concern and can contact an expert for advice. Toxicities should be accurately recorded using a recognised scoring system such as the Common Toxicity Criteria for Adverse Events (CTCAE) developed by the National Cancer Institute.

Extravasation of intravenous drugs

A number of cytotoxic drugs will cause severe local tissue necrosis if leakage into the extravascular compartment occurs. To reduce the risk of extravasation injury it is recommended that cytotoxic drugs are administered by appropriately trained staff. See information on the prevention and management of extravasation injury.

Oral mucositis

A sore mouth is a common complication of cancer chemotherapy; it is most often associated with fluorouracil p. 886, methotrexate p. 888, and the anthracyclines. It is best to prevent the complication. Good oral hygiene (rinsing the mouth frequently and effective brushing of the teeth with a soft brush 2–3 times daily) is probably beneficial. For fluorouracil, sucking ice chips during short infusions of the drug is also helpful.

Once a sore mouth has developed, treatment is much less effective. Saline mouthwashes should be used but there is no good evidence to support the use of antiseptic or anti-inflammatory mouthwashes. In general, mucositis is self-limiting but with poor oral hygiene it can be a focus for blood-borne infection.

Tumour lysis syndrome

Tumour lysis syndrome occurs secondary to spontaneous or treatment-related rapid destruction of malignant cells. Patients at risk of tumour lysis syndrome include those with non-Hodgkin's lymphoma (especially if high grade and bulky disease), Burkitt's lymphoma, acute lymphoblastic leukaemia and acute myeloid leukaemia (particularly if high white blood cell counts or bulky disease), and occasionally those with solid tumours. Pre-existing hyperuricaemia, dehydration, and renal impairment are also predisposing factors. Features include hyperkalaemia, hyperuricaemia (see below), and hyperphosphataemia with hypocalcaemia; renal damage and arrhythmias can follow. Early identification of patients at risk, and initiation of prophylaxis or therapy for tumour lysis syndrome, is essential.

Hyperuricaemia

Hyperuricaemia, which may be present in high-grade lymphoma and leukaemia, can be markedly worsened by chemotherapy and is associated with acute renal failure. Allopurinol p. 1086 should be started 24 hours before treating such tumours and patients should be adequately hydrated. The dose of mercaptopurine p. 887 or azathioprine p. 816 should be reduced if allopurinol needs to be given concomitantly. Febuxostat p. 1087 may also be used and should be started 2 days before cytotoxic therapy is initiated.

Rasburicase p. 917, a recombinant urate oxidase, is licensed for hyperuricaemia in patients with haematological malignancy. It rapidly reduces plasma-uric acid concentration and may be of particular value in preventing complications following treatment of leukaemias or bulky lymphomas.

Bone-marrow suppression

All cytotoxic drugs except vincristine sulfate p. 904 and bleomycin p. 894 cause bone-marrow suppression. This commonly occurs 7 to 10 days after administration, but is delayed for certain drugs, such as carmustine p. 870, lomustine p. 873, and melphalan p. 873. Peripheral blood counts must be checked before each treatment, and doses should be reduced or therapy delayed if bone-marrow has not recovered.

Cytotoxic drugs may be contra-indicated in patients with acute infection; any infection should be treated before, or when starting, cytotoxic drugs.

Fever in a neutropenic patient (neutrophil count less than 1.06×10^9/litre) requires immediate broad-spectrum antibacterial therapy. Appropriate bacteriological investigations should be conducted as soon as possible. Patients taking cytotoxic drugs who have signs or symptoms of infection should be advised to seek prompt medical attention. All patients should initially be investigated and treated under the supervision of the appropriate oncology or haematology specialist.

In selected patients, the duration and the severity of neutropenia can be reduced by the use of recombinant human granulocyte-colony stimulating factors.

Symptomatic anaemia is usually treated with red blood cell transfusions. For guidance on the use of erythropoietins in patients with cancer, see MHRA/CHM advice and NICE guidance.

See advice on the use of live vaccines in individuals with impaired immune response, see Vaccines.

Alopecia

Reversible hair loss is a common complication, although it varies in degree between drugs and individual patients. No pharmacological methods of preventing this are available.

Thromboembolism

Venous thromboembolism can be a complication of cancer itself, but chemotherapy increases the risk.

Cytotoxic drugs: effect on pregnancy and reproductive function

Most cytotoxic drugs are teratogenic and should not be administered during pregnancy, especially during the first trimester. Considerable caution is necessary if a pregnant woman presents with cancer requiring chemotherapy, and specialist advice should always be sought.

Exclude pregnancy before treatment with cytotoxic drugs. Contraceptive advice should be given before cytotoxic therapy begins- women of childbearing age should use effective contraception during and after treatment.

Regimens that do not contain an alkylating drug or procarbazine may have less effect on fertility, but those with an alkylating drug or procarbazine carry the risk of causing permanent male sterility (there is no effect on potency). Pretreatment counselling and consideration of sperm storage may be appropriate. Women are less severely affected, though the span of reproductive life may be shortened by the onset of a premature menopause. No increase in fetal abnormalities or abortion rate has been recorded in patients who remain fertile after cytotoxic chemotherapy.

Cytotoxic drugs: nausea and vomiting

Nausea and vomiting cause considerable distress to many patients who receive chemotherapy and to a lesser extent abdominal radiotherapy, and may lead to refusal of further treatment; prophylaxis of nausea and vomiting is therefore extremely important. Symptoms may be acute (occurring within 24 hours of treatment), delayed (first occurring more than 24 hours after treatment), or anticipatory (occurring prior to subsequent doses). Delayed and anticipatory symptoms are more difficult to control than acute symptoms and require different management.

Patients vary in their susceptibility to drug-induced nausea and vomiting; those affected more often include women, patients under 50 years of age, anxious patients, and those who experience motion sickness. Susceptibility also increases with repeated exposure to the cytotoxic drug.

Drugs may be divided according to their emetogenic potential and some examples are given below, but the symptoms vary according to the dose, to other drugs administered and to the individual's susceptibility to emetogenic stimuli.

Mildly emetogenic treatment—fluorouracil, etoposide p. 898, methotrexate p. 888 (less than 100 mg/m^2, low dose in children), the vinca alkaloids, and abdominal radiotherapy.

Moderately emetogenic treatment—the taxanes, doxorubicin hydrochloride p. 876, intermediate and low doses of cyclophosphamide p. 871, mitoxantrone p. 879, and high doses of methotrexate (0.1– 1.2 g/m²).

Highly emetogenic treatment— cisplatin p. 897, dacarbazine p. 872, and high doses of cyclophosphamide.

Prevention of acute symptoms
For patients at *low risk of emesis*, pretreatment with dexamethasone p. 660 or lorazepam p. 335 may be used.

For patients at *high risk of emesis*, a 5HT3-receptor antagonist, usually given by mouth in combination with dexamethasone and the neurokinin receptor antagonist aprepitant p. 427 is effective.

Prevention of delayed symptoms
For delayed symptoms associated with moderately emetogenic chemotherapy, a combination of dexamethasone and 5HT₃-receptor antagonist is effective; for highly emetogenic chemotherapy, a combination of dexamethasone and aprepitant is effective. Rolapitant p. 428 and metoclopramide hydrochloride p. 426 are also licensed for delayed chemotherapy-induced nausea and vomiting.

Prevention of anticipatory symptoms
Good symptom control is the best way to prevent anticipatory symptoms. Lorazepam can be helpful for its amnesic, sedative, and anxiolytic effects.

Treatment of cytotoxic-induced side-effects
Anthracycline side-effects
Anthracycline-induced cardiotoxicity
The anthracycline cytotoxic drugs are associated with dose-related, cumulative, and potentially life-threatening cardiotoxic side-effects.

Anthracycline extravasation
Local guidelines for the management of extravasation should be followed or specialist advice sought.

See further information on the prevention and management of extravasation injury.

Chemotherapy-induced mucositis and myelosuppression
Folinic acid p. 916 (given as calcium folinate) is used to counteract the folate-antagonist action of methotrexate p. 888 and thus speed recovery from methotrexate-induced mucositis or myelosuppression ('folinic acid rescue').

Folinic acid is also used in the management of methotrexate overdose, together with other measures to maintain fluid and electrolyte balance, and to manage possible renal failure.

Folinic acid does not counteract the antibacterial activity of folate antagonists such as trimethoprim p. 563.

When folinic acid and fluorouracil p. 886 are used together in metastatic colorectal cancer the response-rate improves compared to that with fluorouracil alone.

The calcium salt of levofolinic acid p. 917, a single isomer of folinic acid, is also used for rescue therapy following methotrexate administration, for cases of methotrexate overdose, and for use with fluorouracil for colorectal cancer. The dose of calcium levofolinate is generally half that of calcium folinate.

The disodium salts of folinic acid and levofolinic acid are also used for rescue therapy following methotrexate therapy, and for use with fluorouracil for colorectal cancer.

Urothelial toxicity
Haemorrhagic cystitis is a common manifestation of urothelial toxicity which occurs with the oxazaphosphorines, cyclophosphamide p. 871 and ifosfamide p. 872; it is caused by the metabolite acrolein. Mesna p. 915 reacts specifically with this metabolite in the urinary tract, preventing toxicity. Mesna is used routinely (preferably by mouth) in patients receiving ifosfamide, and in patients receiving

cyclophosphamide by the intravenous route at a high dose (e.g. more than 2 g) or in those who experienced urothelial toxicity when given cyclophosphamide previously.

Anthracyclines and other cytotoxic antibiotics
Drugs in this group are widely used. Many cytotoxic antibiotics act as radiomimetics and simultaneous use of radiotherapy should be **avoided** because it may markedly increased toxicity. Daunorubicin p. 876, doxorubicin hydrochloride p. 876, epirubicin hydrochloride p. 877 and idarubicin hydrochloride p. 878 are anthracycline antibiotics. Mitoxantrone p. 879 is an anthracycline derivative.

Doxorubicin hydrochloride is available as both *conventional* and *liposomal* formulations. The different formulations vary in their licensed indications, pharmacokinetics, dosage and administration, and are not interchangeable. *Conventional* doxorubicin hydrochloride is used to treat the acute leukaemias, Hodgkin's and non-Hodgkin's lymphomas, paediatric malignancies, and some solid tumours including breast cancer.

Epirubicin hydrochloride is structurally related to doxorubicin hydrochloride and clinical trials suggest that it is as effective in the treatment of breast cancer.

Idarubicin hydrochloride has general properties similar to those of doxorubicin hydrochloride; it is mostly used in the treatment of haematological malignancies.

Daunorubicin also has general properties similar to those of doxorubicin hydrochloride.

Mitoxantrone is structurally related to doxorubicin hydrochloride.

Pixantrone p. 879 is licensed as monotherapy for the treatment of refractory or multiply relapsed aggressive non-Hodgkin B-cell lymphomas, although the benefits of using it as a fifth-line or greater chemotherapy in refractory patients has not been established.

Bleomycin p. 894 is given intravenously or intramuscularly to treat metastatic germ cell cancer and, in some regimens, non-Hodgkin's lymphoma.

Dactinomycin is principally used to treat paediatric cancers. Its side-effects are similar to those of doxorubicin, except that cardiac toxicity is not a problem.

Mitomycin p. 895 is given intravenously to treat upper gastrointestinal and breast cancers and by bladder instillation for superficial bladder tumours. It causes delayed bone marrow toxicity and therefore it is usually administered at 6-weekly intervals.

Vinca alkaloids
The vinca alkaloids, vinblastine sulfate p. 904, vincristine sulfate p. 904, and vindesine sulfate p. 905, are used to treat a variety of cancers including leukaemias, lymphomas, and some solid tumours (e.g. breast and lung cancer). Vinorelbine p. 906 is a semi-synthetic vinca alkaloid. See also, role of vinorelbine in the treatment of breast cancer.

Antimetabolites
Antimetabolites are incorporated into new nuclear material or combine irreversibly with cellular enzymes, preventing normal cellular division.

Alkylating drugs
Extensive experience is available with these drugs, which are among the most widely used in cancer chemotherapy. They act by damaging DNA, thus interfering with cell replication.

Cyclophosphamide is used mainly in combination with other agents for treating a wide range of malignancies, including some leukaemias, lymphomas, and solid tumours. It is given by mouth or intravenously; it is inactive until metabolised by the liver.

Ifosfamide is related to cyclophosphamide and is given intravenously.

Melphalan p. 873 is licensed for the treatment of multiple myeloma, polycythaemia vera, childhood neuroblastoma, advanced ovarian adenocarcinoma, and advanced breast cancer. However, in practice, melphalan is rarely used for ovarian adenocarcinoma; it is no longer used for advanced breast cancer. Melphalan is also licensed for regional arterial perfusion in localised malignant melanoma of the extremities and localised soft-tissue sarcoma of the extremities.

Lomustine p. 873 is a lipid-soluble nitrosourea and the drug is given at intervals of 4 to 6 weeks.

Carmustine p. 870 has similar activity to lomustine; it is given to patients with multiple myeloma, non-Hodgkin's lymphomas, and brain tumours. Carmustine implants are licensed for intralesional use in adults for the treatment of recurrent glioblastoma multiforme as an adjunct to surgery. Carmustine implants are also licensed for high-grade malignant glioma as adjunctive treatment to surgery and radiotherapy.

Estramustine phosphate p. 872 is a combination of an oestrogen and chlormethine used predominantly in prostate cancer. It is given by mouth and has both an antimitotic effect and (by reducing testosterone concentration) a hormonal effect.

Mitobronitol is occasionally used to treat chronic myeloid leukaemia; it is available on a named-patient basis from specialist importing companies.

ANTINEOPLASTIC DRUGS > ALKYLATING AGENTS

Bendamustine hydrochloride   31-Jul-2017

● INDICATIONS AND DOSE

Treatment of chronic lymphocytic leukaemia | Treatment of non-Hodgkin's lymphoma | Treatment of multiple myeloma
▶ BY INTRAVENOUS INFUSION
▸ Adult: (consult local protocol)

IMPORTANT SAFETY INFORMATION

MHRA/CHM ADVICE: BENDAMUSTINE (*LEVACT*®): INCREASED MORTALITY OBSERVED IN RECENT CLINICAL STUDIES IN OFF-LABEL USE; MONITOR FOR OPPORTUNISTIC INFECTIONS, HEPATITIS B REACTIVATION (JULY 2017)

Recent clinical trials have shown increased mortality when bendamustine was used in combination treatments outside its approved indications. In addition, a recent European review of post-marketing data has suggested that the risk of opportunistic infections for all patients receiving bendamustine treatment may be greater than previously recognised.

The MHRA recommends monitoring patients for opportunistic infections as well as cardiac, neurological, and respiratory adverse events; known carriers of hepatitis B virus (HBV) should be monitored for signs and symptoms of active HBV infection. Patients should be advised to report promptly new signs of infection; consider discontinuing bendamustine if there are signs of opportunistic infections.

● CONTRA-INDICATIONS Jaundice · low leucocyte count · low platelet count · major surgery less than 30 days before start of treatment · severe bone marrow suppression
● CAUTIONS Cardiac disorders—monitor serum potassium and ECG
● INTERACTIONS → Appendix 1: alkylating agents
● SIDE-EFFECTS
▶ Common or very common Alopecia · amenorrhoea · anaemia · angina pectoris · appetite decreased · arrhythmias · cardiac disorder · chills · constipation · decreased leucocytes · dehydration · diarrhoea · dizziness ·

fatigue · fever · haemorrhage · headache · hepatitis B reactivation · hypersensitivity · hypertension · hypokalaemia · hypotension · increased risk of infection · insomnia · mucositis · nausea · neutropenia · pain · palpitations · respiratory disorders · skin reactions · stomatitis · thrombocytopenia · tumour lysis syndrome · vomiting
▶ **Uncommon** Bone marrow disorders · heart failure · myocardial infarction · neoplasms · pericardial effusion
▶ **Rare or very rare** Anticholinergic syndrome · aphonia · ataxia · circulatory collapse · drowsiness · haemolysis · hyperhidrosis · infertility · multi organ failure · nervous system disorder · paraesthesia · peripheral neuropathy · sepsis · taste altered
▶ **Frequency not known** Hepatic failure · necrosis · renal failure · severe cutaneous adverse reactions (SCARs)

SIDE-EFFECTS, FURTHER INFORMATION
Secondary malignancy Use of bendamustine is associated with an increased incidence of acute leukaemias.

Infections Serious and fatal infections are reported, including opportunistic infections such as Pneumocystis jirovecii pneumonia (PJP), varicella zoster virus (VZV) and cytomegalovirus (CMV)—manufacturer advises monitoring for respiratory signs and symptoms throughout treatment; patients should be advised to report new signs of infection, including fever or respiratory symptoms, promptly. Reactivation of hepatitis B is reported in patients who are chronic carriers of the virus—manufacturer advises monitoring for signs and symptoms of active hepatitis B during treatment and for several months after stopping treatment.

● CONCEPTION AND CONTRACEPTION Effective contraception is required during treatment in men or women, and for 6 months after treatment in men. See also *Pregnancy and reproductive function* in Cytotoxic drugs p. 865.
● PREGNANCY Avoid (teratogenic and mutagenic in *animal* studies). See also *Pregnancy and reproductive function* in Cytotoxic drugs p. 865.
● BREAST FEEDING Discontinue breast-feeding.
● HEPATIC IMPAIRMENT Avoid in severe impairment.
Dose adjustments Consider a 30% dose reduction in moderate impairment.
● RENAL IMPAIRMENT No information available on use in patients with creatinine clearance less than 10 mL/minute.
● NATIONAL FUNDING/ACCESS DECISIONS

NICE decisions
▶ **Bendamustine for the first-line treatment of chronic lymphocytic leukaemia (February 2011)** NICE TA216
Bendamustine is recommended as an option for the first-line treatment of chronic lymphocytic leukaemia (Binet stage B or C) in patients for whom fludarabine combination chemotherapy is not appropriate.
www.nice.org.uk/guidance/TA216
▶ **Obinutuzumab with bendamustine for treating follicular lymphoma refractory to rituximab (August 2017)** NICE TA472
Bendamustine in combination with obinutuzumab followed by obinutuzumab maintenance, is recommended for use within the Cancer Drugs Fund as an option for treating adults with follicular lymphoma that did not respond or progressed during or up to 6 months after treatment with rituximab or a rituximab-containing regimen, only if the conditions in the managed access agreement for obinutuzumab are followed.
www.nice.org.uk/guidance/TA472

Scottish Medicines Consortium (SMC) Decisions
The *Scottish Medicines Consortium* has advised (April 2011) that bendamustine (*Levact*®) is accepted for use within NHS Scotland for first-line treatment of chronic lymphocytic leukaemia (Binet stage B or C) in patients for

whom fludarabine combination chemotherapy is not appropriate.

● MEDICINAL FORMS
There can be variation in the licensing of different medicines containing the same drug.

Powder for solution for infusion
▸ Bendamustine hydrochloride (Non-proprietary)
    Bendamustine hydrochloride 25 mg Bendamustine 25mg powder for concentrate for solution for infusion vials | 1 vial PoM £6.85–£65.98 | 5 vial PoM £312.53–£347.26 (Hospital only) | 20 vial PoM £1,241.14 (Hospital only)
    Bendamustine hydrochloride 100 mg Bendamustine 100mg powder for concentrate for solution for infusion vials | 1 vial PoM £27.77–£262.02 | 5 vial PoM £1,241.14–£1,379.04 (Hospital only)
▸ Levact (Napp Pharmaceuticals Ltd)
    Bendamustine hydrochloride 25 mg Levact 25mg powder for concentrate for solution for infusion vials | 5 vial PoM £347.26 (Hospital only)
    Bendamustine hydrochloride 100 mg Levact 100mg powder for concentrate for solution for infusion vials | 5 vial PoM £1,379.04 (Hospital only)

Busulfan

(Busulphan)

● INDICATIONS AND DOSE
Chronic myeloid leukaemia, induction of remission
▸ BY MOUTH
▸ Adult: 60 micrograms/kg daily (max. per dose 4 mg); maintenance 0.5–2 mg daily
Conditioning treatment before haematopoietic progenitor cell transplantation
▸ BY MOUTH, OR BY INTRAVENOUS INFUSION
▸ Adult: (consult local protocol)
Conditioning treatment before haematopoietic progenitor cell transplantation in patients who are candidates for a reduced-intensity conditioning (RIC) regimen
▸ BY INTRAVENOUS INFUSION
▸ Adult: (consult local protocol)

DOSES AT EXTREMES OF BODY-WEIGHT
▸ Dose may need to be calculated based on body surface area or adjusted ideal body weight in obese patients—consult product literature.

IMPORTANT SAFETY INFORMATION
RISKS OF INCORRECT DOSING OF ORAL ANTI-CANCER MEDICINES
See Cytotoxic drugs p. 865.

● CAUTIONS Avoid in Acute porphyrias p. 1025 · high dose (antiepileptic prophylaxis required) · history of seizures (antiepileptic prophylaxis required) · ineffective once in blast crisis phase · previous progenitor cell transplant (increased risk of hepatic veno-occlusive disease) · previous radiation therapy (increased risk of hepatic veno-occlusive disease) · risk of second malignancy · three or more cycles of chemotherapy (increased risk of hepatic veno-occlusive disease)

● INTERACTIONS → Appendix 1: alkylating agents

● SIDE-EFFECTS
GENERAL SIDE-EFFECTS
▸ **Common or very common** Alopecia · diarrhoea · hepatic disorders · nausea · respiratory disorders · sinusoidal obstruction syndrome · skin reactions · thrombocytopenia · vomiting
▸ **Uncommon** Seizure
▸ **Rare or very rare** Cataract · eye disorders
SPECIFIC SIDE-EFFECTS
▸ **Common or very common**
▸ With intravenous use Anaemia · anxiety · appetite decreased · arrhythmias · arthralgia · ascites · asthenia · asthma ·

cardiomegaly · chest pain · chills · confusion · constipation · cough · depression · dizziness · dyspnoea · dysuria · electrolyte imbalance · embolism and thrombosis · fever · gastrointestinal discomfort · gastrointestinal disorders · haemorrhage · headache · hiccups · hyperglycaemia · hypersensitivity · hypertension · hypoalbuminaemia · hypotension · increased risk of infection · insomnia · mucositis · myalgia · nervous system disorder · neutropenia · oedema · pain · pancytopenia · pericardial effusion · pericarditis · reactivation of infections · renal disorder · renal impairment · stomatitis · vasodilation · weight increased
▸ With oral use Amenorrhoea (may be reversible) · azoospermia · bone marrow disorders · cardiac tamponade · delayed puberty · hyperbilirubinaemia · infertility male · leucopenia · leukaemia · menopausal symptoms · oral disorders · ovarian and fallopian tube disorders · testicular atrophy
▸ **Uncommon**
▸ With intravenous use Capillary leak syndrome · delirium · encephalopathy · hallucination · hypoxia · intracranial haemorrhage
▸ **Rare or very rare**
▸ With oral use Dry mouth · erythema nodosum · gynaecomastia · myasthenia gravis · radiation injury · Sjögren's syndrome
▸ **Frequency not known**
▸ With intravenous use Hypogonadism · ovarian failure · premature menopause · sepsis

SIDE-EFFECTS, FURTHER INFORMATION
Lung toxicity Discontinue if lung toxicity develops.
Secondary malignancy Use of busulfan is associated with an increased incidence of secondary malignancy.

● CONCEPTION AND CONTRACEPTION Manufacturers advise effective contraception during and for 6 months after treatment in men or women. See also *Pregnancy and reproductive function* in Cytotoxic drugs p. 865.

● PREGNANCY Avoid (teratogenic in *animals*). See also *Pregnancy and reproductive function* in Cytotoxic drugs p. 865.

● BREAST FEEDING Discontinue breast-feeding.

● HEPATIC IMPAIRMENT Manufacturer advises caution.
Monitoring In patients with hepatic impairment, manufacturer advises regular liver function tests—consult product literature.

● MONITORING REQUIREMENTS
▸ Monitor cardiac and liver function.
▸ Frequent blood tests are necessary because excessive myelosuppression may result in irreversible bone-marrow aplasia.

● MEDICINAL FORMS
There can be variation in the licensing of different medicines containing the same drug. Forms available from special-order manufacturers include: capsule, oral suspension, oral solution

Tablet
▸ Busulfan (Non-proprietary)
    Busulfan 2 mg Busulfan 2mg tablets | 25 tablet PoM £69.02 DT = £69.02

Solution for infusion
▸ Busilvex (Pierre Fabre Ltd)
    Busulfan 6 mg per 1 ml Busilvex 60mg/10ml concentrate for solution for infusion ampoules | 8 ampoule PoM £1,610.00 (Hospital only)

Carmustine

● **INDICATIONS AND DOSE**

Multiple myeloma | Non-Hodgkin's lymphomas | Brain tumours
▶ BY INTRAVENOUS INFUSION
▶ Adult: (consult product literature)

Recurrent glioblastoma multiforme as an adjunct to surgery | High-grade malignant glioma as adjunctive treatment to surgery and radiotherapy
▶ BY INTRALESIONAL IMPLANTATION
▶ Adult: (consult product literature)

● CAUTIONS Avoid in Acute porphyrias p. 1025
● INTERACTIONS → Appendix 1: alkylating agents
● SIDE-EFFECTS
▶ **Common or very common** Abdominal pain · abscess · alopecia · anaemia · anxiety · asthenia · ataxia · chest pain · coma · confusion · conjunctival oedema · constipation · depression · diabetes mellitus · diarrhoea · dizziness · drowsiness · dysphagia · electrolyte imbalance · embolism and thrombosis · eye pain · faecal incontinence · fever · gait abnormal · haemorrhage · hallucination · headache · healing impaired · hydrocephalus · hyperglycaemia · hypersensitivity · hypertension · hypotension · increased risk of infection · injury · insomnia · intracranial pressure increased · leucocytosis · memory loss · meningitis · nausea · oedema · pain · paralysis · paranoia · peripheral neuropathy · personality disorder · rash · seizures · sensation abnormal · sepsis · speech impairment · stupor · thinking abnormal · thrombocytopenia · tremor · urinary incontinence · vision disorders · vomiting
▶ **Uncommon** Cerebral infarction · intracranial haemorrhage
● CONCEPTION AND CONTRACEPTION Manufacturer advises effective contraception during treatment in men or women. See also *Pregnancy and reproductive function* in Cytotoxic drugs p. 865.
● PREGNANCY Avoid (teratogenic and embryotoxic in *animals*). See also *Pregnancy and reproductive function* in Cytotoxic drugs p. 865.
● BREAST FEEDING Discontinue breast-feeding.
● NATIONAL FUNDING/ACCESS DECISIONS
  NICE decisions
▶ **Carmustine implants and temozolomide for the treatment of newly diagnosed high-grade glioma (June 2007)** NICE TA121
  Carmustine implants are an option for the treatment of newly diagnosed high-grade (Grade 3 or 4) glioma **only** for patients in whom at least 90% of the tumour has been resected. Carmustine implants should only be used within specialist centres.
  www.nice.org.uk/TA121

● MEDICINAL FORMS
  There can be variation in the licensing of different medicines containing the same drug.
  Implant
  ▶ Gliadel (Eisai Ltd)
  Carmustine 7.7 mg Gliadel 7.7mg implant | 8 device PoM £5,203.00 (Hospital only)

Chlorambucil

● **INDICATIONS AND DOSE**

Some lymphomas and chronic leukaemias (used either alone or in combination therapy)
▶ BY MOUTH
▶ Adult: (consult local protocol)

IMPORTANT SAFETY INFORMATION
RISKS OF INCORRECT DOSING OF ORAL ANTI-CANCER MEDICINES
See Cytotoxic drugs p. 865.

● CAUTIONS Children with nephrotic syndrome (increased seizure risk) · history of epilepsy (increased seizure risk)
● INTERACTIONS → Appendix 1: alkylating agents
● SIDE-EFFECTS
▶ **Common or very common** Anaemia · bone marrow disorders · diarrhoea · gastrointestinal disorder · leucopenia · nausea · neoplasms · neutropenia · oral ulceration · seizures · thrombocytopenia · vomiting
▶ **Uncommon** Skin reactions
▶ **Rare or very rare** Cystitis · fever · hepatic disorders · movement disorders · muscle twitching · peripheral neuropathy · respiratory disorders · severe cutaneous adverse reactions (SCARs) · tremor
▶ **Frequency not known** Amenorrhoea · azoospermia
  SIDE-EFFECTS, FURTHER INFORMATION
  Secondary malignancy Use of chlorambucil is associated with an increased incidence of acute leukaemia, particularly with prolonged use.
  Skin reactions Manufacturer advises assessing continued use if rash occurs—has been reported to progress to Stevens-Johnson syndrome and toxic epidermal necrolysis.
● CONCEPTION AND CONTRACEPTION Contraceptive advice required, see *Pregnancy and reproductive function* in Cytotoxic drugs p. 865.
● PREGNANCY Avoid. See also *Pregnancy and reproductive function* in Cytotoxic drugs p. 865.
● BREAST FEEDING Discontinue breast-feeding.
● HEPATIC IMPAIRMENT
  Dose adjustments Manufacturer advises consider dose reduction in severe impairment—limited information available.
● NATIONAL FUNDING/ACCESS DECISIONS
  NICE decisions
▶ **Obinutuzumab in combination with chlorambucil for untreated chronic lymphocytic leukaemia (June 2015)** NICE TA343
  Obinutuzumab, in combination with chlorambucil, is an option for untreated chronic lymphocytic leukaemia in patients who have comorbidities that make full-dose fludarabine-based therapy unsuitable for them, only if:
  ● bendamustine-based therapy is not suitable **and**
  ● the manufacturer provides obinutuzumab with the discount agreed in the patient access scheme.
  Patients currently receiving obinutuzumab that is not recommended according to the above criteria should have the option to continue treatment until they and their clinician consider it appropriate to stop.
  www.nice.org.uk/TA343
▶ **Ofatumumab in combination with chlorambucil or bendamustine for untreated chronic lymphocytic leukaemia (June 2015)** NICE TA344
  Ofatumumab in combination with chlorambucil is an option for untreated chronic lymphocytic leukaemia only if:
  ● the person is ineligible for fludarabine-based therapy **and**
  ● bendamustine is not suitable **and**

- the manufacturer provides ofatumumab with the discount agreed in the patient access scheme.

Patients currently receiving ofatumumab that is not recommended according to the above criteria should have the option to continue treatment until they and their clinician consider it appropriate to stop.

www.nice.org.uk/TA344

- ● MEDICINAL FORMS
There can be variation in the licensing of different medicines containing the same drug.

Tablet
▸ Chlorambucil (Non-proprietary)
  Chlorambucil 2 mg Chlorambucil 2mg tablets | 25 tablet [PoM]
  £42.87 DT = £42.87

Cyclophosphamide

- ● INDICATIONS AND DOSE

Rheumatoid arthritis with severe systemic manifestations
▸ BY MOUTH
▸ Adult: 1–1.5 mg/kg daily

Severe systemic rheumatoid arthritis | Other connective tissue diseases (especially with active vasculitis)
▸ BY INTRAVENOUS INJECTION
▸ Adult: 0.5–1 g every 2 weeks, then reduced to 0.5–1 g every month, frequency adjusted according to clinical response and haematological monitoring. To be given with prophylactic mesna

Used, mainly in combination with other agents for treating a wide range of malignancies, including some leukaemias, lymphomas, and solid tumours
▸ BY MOUTH, OR BY INTRAVENOUS INFUSION
▸ Adult: (consult local protocol)

- ● UNLICENSED USE Not licensed for rheumatoid arthritis with severe systemic manifestations.

> IMPORTANT SAFETY INFORMATION
> RISKS OF INCORRECT DOSING OF ORAL ANTI-CANCER MEDICINES
> See Cytotoxic drugs p. 865.

- ● CONTRA-INDICATIONS Haemorrhagic cystitis
- ● CAUTIONS Avoid in Acute porphyrias p. 1025 · diabetes mellitus · previous or concurrent mediastinal irradiation—risk of cardiotoxicity
- ● INTERACTIONS → Appendix 1: alkylating agents
- ● SIDE-EFFECTS
▸ **Common or very common** Agranulocytosis · alopecia · anaemia · asthenia · bone marrow disorders · cystitis · decreased leucocytes · fever · haemolytic uraemic syndrome · haemorrhage · hepatic disorders · immunosuppression · increased risk of infection · mucosal abnormalities · neutropenia · progressive multifocal leukoencephalopathy · reactivation of infections · sperm abnormalities · thrombocytopenia
▸ **Uncommon** Appetite decreased · embolism and thrombosis · flushing · hypersensitivity · ovarian and fallopian tube disorders · sepsis
▸ **Rare or very rare** Bladder disorders · chest pain · confusion · constipation · diarrhoea · disseminated intravascular coagulation · dizziness · eye inflammation · fluid imbalance · headache · hyponatraemia · menstrual cycle irregularities · nail discolouration · nausea · neoplasms · oral disorders · pancreatitis acute · renal failure · secondary neoplasm · seizure · severe cutaneous adverse reactions (SCARs) · SIADH · skin reactions · visual impairment · vomiting
▸ **Frequency not known** Abdominal pain · altered smell sensation · arrhythmias · arthralgia · ascites · cardiac inflammation · cardiogenic shock · cardiomyopathy · cough · dyspnoea · encephalopathy · excessive tearing · facial swelling · gastrointestinal disorders · hearing impairment · heart failure · hyperhidrosis · hypoxia · infertility · influenza like illness · multi organ failure · muscle complaints · myelopathy · myocardial infarction · nasal complaints · nephropathy · nerve disorders · neuralgia · neurotoxicity · oedema · oropharyngeal pain · palpitations · pericardial effusion · peripheral ischaemia · pulmonary hypertension · pulmonary oedema · QT interval prolongation · radiation injuries · renal tubular disorder · renal tubular necrosis · respiratory disorders · rhabdomyolysis · scleroderma · sensation abnormal · sinusoidal obstruction syndrome · taste altered · testicular atrophy · tremor · tumour lysis syndrome · vasculitis

- ● SIDE-EFFECTS, FURTHER INFORMATION
Haemorrhagic cystitis A urinary metabolite of cyclophosphamide, acrolein, can cause haemorrhagic cystitis; this is a rare but serious complication that may be prevented by increasing fluid intake for 24–48 hours after intravenous injection. When high-dose therapy (e.g. more than 2g intravenously) is used or when the patient is considered to be at high risk of cystitis (e.g. because of pelvic irradiation), mesna can also help prevent cystitis.
Secondary malignancy As with all cytotoxic therapy, treatment with cyclophosphamide is associated with an increased incidence of secondary malignancies.

- ● CONCEPTION AND CONTRACEPTION Manufacturer advises effective contraception during and for at least 3 months after treatment in men or women. See also *Pregnancy and reproductive function* in Cytotoxic drugs p. 865.
- ● PREGNANCY Avoid. See also *Pregnancy and reproductive function* in Cytotoxic drugs p. 865.
- ● BREAST FEEDING Discontinue breast-feeding during and for 36 hours after stopping treatment.
- ● HEPATIC IMPAIRMENT
Dose adjustments Reduce dose—consult local treatment protocol for details.
- ● RENAL IMPAIRMENT
Dose adjustments Reduce dose if serum creatinine concentration greater than 120 micromol/litre.
- ● DIRECTIONS FOR ADMINISTRATION
▸ With intravenous use For *intravenous infusion* (cyclophosphamide injection; *Baxter*) give via drip tubing in Glucose 5% or Sodium chloride 0.9%; reconstitute 500 mg with 25 mL sodium chloride 0.9%; reconstitute 1 g with 50 mL sodium chloride 0.9%.
- ● MEDICINAL FORMS
There can be variation in the licensing of different medicines containing the same drug. Forms available from special-order manufacturers include: tablet, oral suspension, oral solution, solution for injection, solution for infusion

Tablet
CAUTIONARY AND ADVISORY LABELS 25, 27
▸ Cyclophosphamide (Non-proprietary)
  Cyclophosphamide (as Cyclophosphamide monohydrate)
  50 mg Cyclophosphamide 50mg tablets | 100 tablet [PoM] £139.00
  DT = £139.00
▸ Cytoxan (Imported (United States))
  Cyclophosphamide 25 mg Cytoxan 25mg tablets |
  100 tablet [PoM] 🅧

Powder for solution for injection
▸ Cyclophosphamide (Non-proprietary)
  Cyclophosphamide (as Cyclophosphamide monohydrate)
  500 mg Cyclophosphamide 500mg powder for solution for injection vials | 1 vial [PoM] £9.66 (Hospital only) | 1 vial [PoM] £9.66
  Cyclophosphamide (as Cyclophosphamide monohydrate)
  1 gram Cyclophosphamide 1g powder for solution for injection vials | 1 vial [PoM] £17.06 (Hospital only) | 1 vial [PoM] £17.91
  Cyclophosphamide (as Cyclophosphamide monohydrate)
  2 gram Cyclophosphamide 2g powder for solution for injection vials | 1 vial [PoM] £34.12 (Hospital only)

Dacarbazine

- **INDICATIONS AND DOSE**

Metastatic melanoma | Soft-tissue sarcomas (combination therapy) | Hodgkin's disease (combination therapy)
  ▶ BY INTRAVENOUS INFUSION, OR BY INTRAVENOUS INJECTION
  ▶ Adult: (consult local protocol)

- **CAUTIONS** Caution in handling—irritant to tissues
- **INTERACTIONS** → Appendix 1: alkylating agents
- **SIDE-EFFECTS**
  ▶ **Common or very common** Anaemia · appetite decreased · leucopenia · nausea · thrombocytopenia · vomiting
  ▶ **Uncommon** Alopecia · infection · influenza like illness · photosensitivity reaction · skin reactions
  ▶ **Rare or very rare** Agranulocytosis · confusion · diarrhoea · flushing · headache · hepatic disorders · lethargy · pancytopenia · paraesthesia · renal impairment · seizure · visual impairment
- **CONCEPTION AND CONTRACEPTION** Ensure effective contraception during and for at least 6 months after treatment in men or women. See also *Pregnancy and reproductive function* in Cytotoxic drugs p. 865.
- **PREGNANCY** Avoid (carcinogenic and teratogenic in *animal* studies). See also *Pregnancy and reproductive function* in Cytotoxic drugs p. 865.
- **BREAST FEEDING** Discontinue breast-feeding.
- **HEPATIC IMPAIRMENT** Avoid in severe impairment.
  Dose adjustments Dose reduction may be required in combined renal and hepatic impairment.
- **RENAL IMPAIRMENT** Avoid in severe impairment.
  Dose adjustments Dose reduction may be required in combined renal and hepatic impairment.
- **PRESCRIBING AND DISPENSING INFORMATION** Dacarbazine is a component of a commonly used combination for Hodgkin's disease (ABVD—doxorubicin [previously *Adriamycin*®], bleomycin, vinblastine, and dacarbazine).
- **MEDICINAL FORMS**
  There can be variation in the licensing of different medicines containing the same drug.
  Powder for solution for infusion
  ▶ Dacarbazine (Non-proprietary)
    Dacarbazine (as Dacarbazine citrate) 500 mg Dacarbazine 500mg powder for solution for infusion vials | 1 vial [PoM] £37.50
    Dacarbazine (as Dacarbazine citrate) 1 gram Dacarbazine 1g powder for solution for infusion vials | 1 vial [PoM] £70.00
  Powder for solution for injection
  ▶ Dacarbazine (Non-proprietary)
    Dacarbazine (as Dacarbazine citrate) 100 mg Dacarbazine 100mg powder for solution for injection vials | 10 vial [PoM] £90.00
    Dacarbazine (as Dacarbazine citrate) 200 mg Dacarbazine 200mg powder for solution for injection vials | 10 vial [PoM] £160.00

Estramustine phosphate

- **INDICATIONS AND DOSE**

Prostate cancer
  ▶ BY MOUTH
  ▶ Adult: Initially 560–840 mg daily in divided doses; maintenance 140–1400 mg daily in divided doses

> **IMPORTANT SAFETY INFORMATION**
> RISKS OF INCORRECT DOSING OF ORAL ANTI-CANCER MEDICINES
> See Cytotoxic drugs p. 865.

- **CONTRA-INDICATIONS** Peptic ulceration · severe cardiovascular disease · thromboembolic disorders
- **CAUTIONS** Cardiovascular disease · cerebrovascular disease · conditions which might be aggravated by fluid retention

(such as epilepsy or migraine) · congestive heart failure · diabetes · hypercalcaemia · hypertension

- **INTERACTIONS** → Appendix 1: alkylating agents
- **SIDE-EFFECTS**
  ▶ **Common or very common** Anaemia · congestive heart failure · diarrhoea · embolism · fluid retention · gynaecomastia · headache · hepatic function abnormal · lethargy · leucopenia · myocardial infarction · nausea · thrombocytopenia · vomiting
  ▶ **Frequency not known** Allergic dermatitis · angioedema · confusion · depression · erectile dysfunction · hypertension · muscle weakness · myocardial ischaemia
- **CONCEPTION AND CONTRACEPTION** Men should use effective contraceptive methods during treatment. See also *Pregnancy and reproductive function* in Cytotoxic drugs p. 865.
- **HEPATIC IMPAIRMENT** Manufacturer advises caution. Avoid in severe impairment.
  Monitoring In hepatic impairment, manufacturer advises regular liver function tests.
- **RENAL IMPAIRMENT** Manufacturer advises caution.
- **DIRECTIONS FOR ADMINISTRATION** Each dose should be taken not less than 1 hour before or 2 hours after meals and should not be taken with products containing calcium, magnesium or aluminium, including dairy products and antacid medication.
- **PATIENT AND CARER ADVICE** Patients should be given advice on how to administer estramustine capsules.

- **MEDICINAL FORMS**
  There can be variation in the licensing of different medicines containing the same drug.
  Capsule
  CAUTIONARY AND ADVISORY LABELS 5, 23
  ▶ Estracyt (Pfizer Ltd)
    Estramustine phosphate (as Estramustine sodium phosphate) 140 mg Estracyt 140mg capsules | 100 capsule [PoM] £171.28

Ifosfamide

- **INDICATIONS AND DOSE**

Malignant disease
  ▶ BY INTRAVENOUS INFUSION
  ▶ Adult: (consult local protocol)

- **CONTRA-INDICATIONS** Acute infection · urinary-tract infection · urinary-tract obstruction · urothelial damage
- **CAUTIONS** Avoid in Acute porphyrias p. 1025 · diabetes mellitus
- **INTERACTIONS** → Appendix 1: alkylating agents
- **SIDE-EFFECTS**
  ▶ **Common or very common** Alopecia · appetite decreased · bone marrow disorders · haemorrhage · hepatic disorders · infection · leucopenia · nausea · reactivation of infection · renal impairment · thrombocytopenia · vascular disorders · vomiting
  ▶ **Uncommon** Cardiotoxicity · diarrhoea · hypotension · oral disorders
  ▶ **Rare or very rare** Skin reactions
  ▶ **Frequency not known** Abdominal pain · agranulocytosis · amenorrhoea · anaemia · angina pectoris · angioedema · arrhythmias · arthralgia · asterixis · behaviour abnormal · blood disorders · bone disorders · cancer progression · cardiac arrest · cardiomyopathy · chills · conjunctivitis · constipation · cough · delirium · delusions · disseminated intravascular coagulation · dysarthria · dyspnoea · electrolyte imbalance · embolism and thrombosis · encephalopathy · eye irritation · fatigue · fever · flushing · gait abnormal · gastrointestinal disorders · growth retardation · haemolytic anaemia · hearing impairment ·

heart failure · hyperglycaemia · hyperhidrosis · hyperphosphaturia · hypertension · hypoxia · immunosuppression · infertility · malaise · mania · memory loss · metabolic acidosis · movement disorders · mucosal ulceration · multi organ failure · muscle complaints · myocardial infarction · nail disorder · neoplasms · nephritis tubulointerstitial · nephrogenic diabetes insipidus · neurotoxicity · oedema · ovarian and fallopian tube disorders · pain · pancreatitis · panic attack · peripheral neuropathy · polydipsia · premature menopause · psychiatric disorders · pulmonary hypertension · pulmonary oedema · radiation recall reaction · respiratory disorders · rhabdomyolysis · secondary malignancy · sensation abnormal · sepsis · severe cutaneous adverse reactions (SCARs) · SIADH · sinusoidal obstruction syndrome · sperm abnormalities · status epilepticus · tumour lysis syndrome · urinary disorders · vasculitis · vertigo · visual impairment

SIDE-EFFECTS, FURTHER INFORMATION
Urothelial toxicity Mesna is routinely given with ifosfamide to reduce urothelial toxicity.
Secondary malignancy Use of ifosfamide is associated with an increased incidence of acute leukaemia.

● CONCEPTION AND CONTRACEPTION Manufacturer advises adequate contraception during and for at least 6 months after treatment in men or women. See also *Pregnancy and reproductive function* in Cytotoxic drugs p. 865.

● PREGNANCY Avoid (teratogenic and carcinogenic in *animals*). See also *Pregnancy and reproductive function* in Cytotoxic drugs p. 865.

● BREAST FEEDING Discontinue breast-feeding.

● HEPATIC IMPAIRMENT Avoid.

● RENAL IMPAIRMENT Avoid if serum creatinine concentration greater than 120 micromol/litre.

● MONITORING REQUIREMENTS Ensure satisfactory electrolyte balance and renal function before each course (risk of tubular dysfunction, Fanconi's syndrome or diabetes insipidus if renal toxicity not treated promptly).

● MEDICINAL FORMS
There can be variation in the licensing of different medicines containing the same drug.
Powder for solution for injection
▸ Ifosfamide (Non-proprietary)
  Ifosfamide 1 gram Ifosfamide 1g powder for concentrate for solution for injection vials | 1 vial [PoM] £115.79
  Ifosfamide 2 gram Ifosfamide 2g powder for concentrate for solution for injection vials | 1 vial [PoM] £228.09

Lomustine

● DRUG ACTION Lomustine is a lipid-soluble nitrosourea.

● INDICATIONS AND DOSE

Hodgkin's disease resistant to conventional therapy | Malignant melanoma | Certain solid tumours
▸ BY MOUTH
▸ Adult: 120–130 mg/m^2 every 6–8 weeks, dose is for when lomustine is used alone

---
IMPORTANT SAFETY INFORMATION
RISKS OF INCORRECT DOSING OF ORAL ANTI-CANCER MEDICINES
See Cytotoxic drugs p. 865.

● CONTRA-INDICATIONS Coeliac disease

● INTERACTIONS → Appendix 1: alkylating agents

● SIDE-EFFECTS
▸ **Common or very common** Leucopenia
▸ **Frequency not known** Alopecia · anaemia · apathy · appetite decreased · azotaemia · bone marrow failure (delayed) ·

confusion · coordination abnormal · diarrhoea · hepatic disorders · lethargy · nausea · neoplasms · neurological effects · renal disorders · renal impairment · respiratory disorders · speech impairment · stomatitis · thrombocytopenia · vision loss (irreversible) · vomiting

SIDE-EFFECTS, FURTHER INFORMATION Prolonged use of lomustine is associated with an increased incidence of acute leukaemias.

● CONCEPTION AND CONTRACEPTION Manufacturer advises effective contraception during and for at least 6 months after treatment in men or women. See also *Pregnancy and reproductive function* in Cytotoxic drugs p. 865.

● PREGNANCY Avoid. See also *Pregnancy and reproductive function* in Cytotoxic drugs p. 865.

● BREAST FEEDING Discontinue breast-feeding.

● RENAL IMPAIRMENT Avoid in severe impairment.

● PRESCRIBING AND DISPENSING INFORMATION The brand name *CCNU*® has been used for lomustine capsules.

● MEDICINAL FORMS
There can be variation in the licensing of different medicines containing the same drug. Forms available from special-order manufacturers include: capsule
Capsule
▸ Lomustine (Non-proprietary)
  Lomustine 40 mg Lomustine 40mg capsules | 20 capsule [PoM] £780.82
  Lomustine 100 mg CeeNU 100mg capsules | 20 capsule [PoM] [℞]

Melphalan

● INDICATIONS AND DOSE

Multiple myeloma
▸ BY MOUTH
▸ Adult: 150 micrograms/kg daily for 4 days, dose to be repeated every 6 weeks, dose may vary according to regimen
▸ BY INTRAVENOUS INJECTION, OR BY INTRAVENOUS INFUSION
▸ Adult: (consult product literature)

Polycythaemia vera
▸ BY MOUTH
▸ Adult: Initially 6–10 mg daily for 5-7 days, then reduced to 2–4 mg daily until satisfactory response, then reduced to 2–6 mg once weekly

Localised malignant melanoma of the extremities | Localised soft-tissue sarcoma of the extremities
▸ BY REGIONAL ARTERIAL PERFUSION
▸ Adult: (consult local protocol)

IMPORTANT SAFETY INFORMATION
RISKS OF INCORRECT DOSING OF ORAL ANTI-CANCER MEDICINES
See Cytotoxic drugs p. 865.

● INTERACTIONS → Appendix 1: alkylating agents

● SIDE-EFFECTS
GENERAL SIDE-EFFECTS
▸ **Common or very common** Alopecia · anaemia · bone marrow depression (delayed) · diarrhoea · nausea · stomatitis · thrombocytopenia · vomiting
▸ **Rare or very rare** Haemolytic anaemia · hepatic disorders · respiratory disorders · skin reactions
SPECIFIC SIDE-EFFECTS
▸ **Common or very common**
▸ With oral use Leucopenia
▸ With parenteral use Feeling hot · myalgia · myopathy · paraesthesia
▸ **Rare or very rare**
▸ With parenteral use Peripheral vascular disease

Immune system and malignant disease

8

SIDE-EFFECTS, FURTHER INFORMATION Use of melphalan is associated with an increased incidence of acute leukaemias.

● CONCEPTION AND CONTRACEPTION Manufacturer advises adequate contraception during treatment in men or women. See also *Pregnancy and reproductive function* in Cytotoxic drugs p. 865.

● PREGNANCY Avoid. See also *Pregnancy and reproductive function* in Cytotoxic drugs p. 865.

● BREAST FEEDING Discontinue breast-feeding.

● RENAL IMPAIRMENT
Dose adjustments Reduce dose initially (consult product literature).

● MONITORING REQUIREMENTS Monitor full blood count before and throughout treatment.

● MEDICINAL FORMS
There can be variation in the licensing of different medicines containing the same drug.
Powder and solvent for solution for injection
▸ Melphalan (Non-proprietary)
Melphalan (as Melphalan hydrochloride) 50 mg Melphalan 50mg powder and solvent for solution for injection vials | 1 vial PoM £137.37
Tablet
▸ Melphalan (Non-proprietary)
Melphalan 2 mg Melphalan 2mg tablets | 25 tablet PoM £45.38 DT = £45.38

Temozolomide

● DRUG ACTION Temozolomide is structurally related to dacarbazine.

● INDICATIONS AND DOSE
Newly diagnosed glioblastoma multiforme in adults (in combination with radiotherapy) and subsequently as monotherapy | Second-line treatment of malignant glioma in adults
▸ BY MOUTH
▸ Adult: (consult product literature)

IMPORTANT SAFETY INFORMATION
RISKS OF INCORRECT DOSING OF ORAL ANTI-CANCER MEDICINES
See Cytotoxic drugs p. 865.

● CAUTIONS *Pneumocystis jirovecii* pneumonia—consult product literature for monitoring and prophylaxis requirements

● INTERACTIONS → Appendix 1: alkylating agents

● SIDE-EFFECTS
▸ **Common or very common** Alopecia · anxiety · appetite decreased · arthralgia · asthenia · chills · concentration impaired · confusion · constipation · cough · decreased leucocytes · diarrhoea · dizziness · drowsiness · dysphagia · dyspnoea · emotional lability · fever · gastrointestinal discomfort · haemorrhage · headache · hearing impairment · hemiparesis · hyperglycaemia · hypersensitivity · increased risk of infection · insomnia · level of consciousness decreased · malaise · memory loss · movement disorders · muscle weakness · nausea · neutropenia · oedema · oral disorders · pain · peripheral neuropathy · radiation injury · seizures · sensation abnormal · skin reactions · speech impairment · taste altered · thrombocytopenia · tremor · urinary disorders · vision disorders · vomiting · weight changes
▸ **Uncommon** Altered smell sensation · anaemia · behaviour disorder · bone marrow disorders · cognitive impairment · condition aggravated · Cushing's syndrome · depression · diabetes insipidus · ear pain · erectile dysfunction · eye pain · gait abnormal · hallucination · hepatic disorders ·

hyperacusia · hyperbilirubinaemia · hypertension · hypokalaemia · intracranial haemorrhage · myalgia · myopathy · nasal congestion · nervous system disorder · palpitations · photosensitivity reaction · reactivation of infections · thirst · vasodilation
▸ **Rare or very rare** Neoplasms · respiratory disorders · secondary malignancy · severe cutaneous adverse reactions (SCARs)

● CONCEPTION AND CONTRACEPTION Manufacturer advises adequate contraception during treatment. Men should avoid fathering a child during and for at least 6 months after treatment. See also *Pregnancy and reproductive function* in Cytotoxic drugs p. 865.

● PREGNANCY Avoid (teratogenic and embryotoxic in *animal* studies). See also *Pregnancy and reproductive function* in Cytotoxic drugs p. 865.

● BREAST FEEDING Discontinue breast-feeding.

● HEPATIC IMPAIRMENT Use with caution in severe impairment—no information available.

● RENAL IMPAIRMENT Manufacturer advises caution—no information available.

● MONITORING REQUIREMENTS
▸ Monitor liver function before treatment initiation, after each treatment cycle and midway through 42-day treatment cycles—consider the balance of benefits and risks of treatment if results are abnormal at any point (fatal liver injury reported).
▸ Monitor for myelodysplastic syndrome.
▸ Monitor for secondary malignancies.

● NATIONAL FUNDING/ACCESS DECISIONS
NICE decisions
▸ **Temozolomide for the treatment of recurrent malignant glioma (brain cancer) (April 2001)** NICE TA23
Temozolomide may be considered for the treatment of recurrent malignant glioma, which has not responded to first-line chemotherapy.
www.nice.org.uk/guidance/ta23
▸ **Carmustine implants and temozolomide for the treatment of newly diagnosed high-grade glioma (June 2007)** NICE TA121
Temozolomide is an option for the treatment of newly diagnosed glioblastoma multiforme in patients with a WHO performance status of 0 or 1.
www.nice.org.uk/TA121

● MEDICINAL FORMS
There can be variation in the licensing of different medicines containing the same drug. Forms available from special-order manufacturers include: oral suspension
Capsule
CAUTIONARY AND ADVISORY LABELS 23, 25
▸ Temozolomide (Non-proprietary)
Temozolomide 5 mg Temozolomide 5mg capsules | 5 capsule PoM £10.06–£16.00
Temozolomide 20 mg Temozolomide 20mg capsules | 5 capsule PoM £40.23–£65.00
Temozolomide 100 mg Temozolomide 100mg capsules | 5 capsule PoM £201.18–£325.00
Temozolomide 140 mg Temozolomide 140mg capsules | 5 capsule PoM £296.47–£465.00
Temozolomide 180 mg Temozolomide 180mg capsules | 5 capsule PoM £381.18–£586.00
Temozolomide 250 mg Temozolomide 250mg capsules | 5 capsule PoM £529.42–£814.00
▸ Temodal (Merck Sharp & Dohme Ltd)
Temozolomide 5 mg Temodal 5mg capsules | 5 capsule PoM £10.59 (Hospital only)
Temozolomide 20 mg Temodal 20mg capsules | 5 capsule PoM £42.35 (Hospital only)
Temozolomide 100 mg Temodal 100mg capsules | 5 capsule PoM £211.77 (Hospital only)
Temozolomide 140 mg Temodal 140mg capsules | 5 capsule PoM £296.48 (Hospital only)
Temozolomide 180 mg Temodal 180mg capsules | 5 capsule PoM £381.19 (Hospital only)

Temozolomide 250 mg Temodal 250mg capsules | 5 capsule PoM £529.43 (Hospital only)

▸ Temomedac (medac UK)

Temozolomide 5 mg Temomedac 5mg capsules | 5 capsule PoM £16.12

Temozolomide 20 mg Temomedac 20mg capsules | 5 capsule PoM £64.49

Temozolomide 100 mg Temomedac 100mg capsules | 5 capsule PoM £322.43

Temozolomide 140 mg Temomedac 140mg capsules | 5 capsule PoM £451.40

Temozolomide 180 mg Temomedac 180mg capsules | 5 capsule PoM £580.37

Temozolomide 250 mg Temomedac 250mg capsules | 5 capsule PoM £806.08

Thiotepa

● **INDICATIONS AND DOSE**

Conditioning treatment before haematopoietic stem cell transplantation in the treatment of haematological disease or solid tumours, in combination with other chemotherapy

▸ BY INTRAVENOUS INFUSION

▸ Adult: (consult local protocol)

● CAUTIONS Avoid in Acute porphyrias p. 1025

● INTERACTIONS → Appendix 1: alkylating agents

● SIDE-EFFECTS

▸ **Common or very common** Alopecia · amenorrhoea · anaemia · anxiety · appetite decreased · arrhythmias · arthralgia · asthenia · azoospermia · cataract · chills · cognitive disorder · confusion · conjunctivitis · constipation · cough · cystitis · delirium · diarrhoea · dizziness · dysuria · embolism · encephalopathy · fever · gastrointestinal discomfort · gastrointestinal disorders · generalised oedema · graft versus host disease · haemorrhage · headache · hearing impairment · heart failure · hepatic disorders · hyperglycaemia · hypersensitivity · hypertension · hypopituitarism · increased risk of infection · infertility · intracranial aneurysm · intracranial haemorrhage · leucopenia · lymphoedema · menopausal symptoms · movement disorders · mucositis · multi organ failure · myalgia · nausea · neutropenia · pain · pancytopenia · paraesthesia · psychiatric disorder · pulmonary oedema · renal impairment · respiratory disorders · secondary malignancy · seizure · sepsis · sinusoidal obstruction syndrome · skin reactions · stomatitis · thrombocytopenia · toxic shock syndrome · vision blurred · vomiting · weight increased

▸ **Uncommon** Cardiomyopathy · hallucination · hypoxia · myocarditis

▸ **Frequency not known** Severe cutaneous adverse reactions (SCARs)

● CONCEPTION AND CONTRACEPTION Contraceptive advice required, see *Pregnancy and reproductive function* in Cytotoxic drugs p. 865.

● PREGNANCY Avoid (teratogenic and embryotoxic in *animals*). See also *Pregnancy and reproductive function* in Cytotoxic drugs p. 865.

● BREAST FEEDING Discontinue breast-feeding.

● NATIONAL FUNDING/ACCESS DECISIONS

Scottish Medicines Consortium (SMC) Decisions

The *Scottish Medicines Consortium* has advised (June 2012) that thiotepa (*Tepadina* ®) is **not** recommended for use within NHS Scotland in combination with other chemotherapy as conditioning treatment in adults or children with haematological diseases, or solid tumours prior to haematopoietic stem cell transplantation.

● MEDICINAL FORMS

There can be variation in the licensing of different medicines containing the same drug.

Powder for solution for infusion

▸ Tepadina (Adienne Pharma & Biotech)

Thiotepa 15 mg Tepadina 15mg powder for concentrate for solution for infusion vials | 1 vial PoM [℥]

Thiotepa 100 mg Tepadina 100mg powder for concentrate for solution for infusion vials | 1 vial PoM [℥]

Treosulfan

● **INDICATIONS AND DOSE**

Ovarian cancer

▸ BY MOUTH, OR BY INTRAVENOUS INJECTION, OR BY INTRAVENOUS INFUSION, OR BY INTRAPERITONEAL INSTILLATION

▸ Adult: (consult product literature)

IMPORTANT SAFETY INFORMATION

RISKS OF INCORRECT DOSING OF ORAL ANTI-CANCER MEDICINES See Cytotoxic drugs p. 865.

● CAUTIONS Avoid in Acute porphyrias p. 1025

● INTERACTIONS → Appendix 1: alkylating agents

● SIDE-EFFECTS

GENERAL SIDE-EFFECTS

▸ **Common or very common** Alopecia · anaemia · bone marrow disorders · increased risk of infection · leucopenia · nausea · skin reactions · thrombocytopenia · vomiting

▸ **Uncommon** Neoplasms · treatment related secondary malignancy

▸ **Rare or very rare** Addison's disease · cardiomyopathy · cystitis haemorrhagic · hypoglycaemia · influenza like illness · paraesthesia · respiratory disorders · scleroderma · sepsis

SPECIFIC SIDE-EFFECTS

▸ **Uncommon**

▸ With oral use Stomatitis

SIDE-EFFECTS, FURTHER INFORMATION Prolonged use of treosulfan is associated with an increased incidence of acute non-lymphocytic leukaemia.

● CONCEPTION AND CONTRACEPTION Contraceptive advice required, see *Pregnancy and reproductive function* in Cytotoxic drugs p. 865.

● PREGNANCY Avoid. See also *Pregnancy and reproductive function* in Cytotoxic drugs p. 865.

● BREAST FEEDING Discontinue breast-feeding.

● MEDICINAL FORMS

There can be variation in the licensing of different medicines containing the same drug.

Capsule

CAUTIONARY AND ADVISORY LABELS 25

▸ Treosulfan (Non-proprietary)

Treosulfan 250 mg Treosulfan 250mg capsules | 100 capsule PoM £653.20

Powder for solution for injection

▸ Treosulfan (Non-proprietary)

Treosulfan 1 gram Treosulfan 1g powder for solution for injection vials | 5 vial PoM £269.17

Treosulfan 5 gram Treosulfan 5g powder for solution for injection vials | 5 vial PoM £1,040.17

8

Immune system and malignant disease

ANTINEOPLASTIC DRUGS > ANTHRACYCLINES AND RELATED DRUGS

Daunorubicin

● INDICATIONS AND DOSE

Acute myelogenous leukaemia | Acute lymphocytic leukaemia
▶ BY INTRAVENOUS INFUSION
▶ Adult: (consult local protocol)

Advanced AIDS-related Kaposi's sarcoma (liposomal formulation only)
▶ BY INTRAVENOUS INFUSION
▶ Adult: (consult product literature)

● CONTRA-INDICATIONS Myocardial insufficiency · previous treatment with maximum cumulative doses of daunorubicin or other anthracycline · recent myocardial infarction · severe arrhythmia
● CAUTIONS Caution in handling—irritant to tissues
● INTERACTIONS → Appendix 1: anthracyclines
● SIDE-EFFECTS Abdominal pain · alopecia · amenorrhoea · anaemia · arrhythmias · ascites · atrioventricular block · azoospermia · bone marrow disorders · cardiac inflammation · cardiomyopathy · chills · congestive heart failure · cyanosis · death · dehydration · diarrhoea · dyspnoea · extravasation · fever · flushing · gastrointestinal disorders · haemorrhage · hepatomegaly · hyperpyrexia · hyperuricaemia · hypoxia · increased risk of infection · ischaemic heart disease · leucopenia · mucositis · myocardial infarction · nail discolouration · nausea · nephropathy · neutropenia · oedema · pain · paraesthesia · pleural effusion · radiation injuries · shock · skin reactions · soft tissue necrosis · stomatitis · thrombocytopenia · thrombophlebitis · urine red · vascular disorders · vomiting
SIDE-EFFECTS, FURTHER INFORMATION Cardiotoxicity is cumulative and may be irreversible, however responds to treatment if detected early.
● CONCEPTION AND CONTRACEPTION Contraceptive advice required, see *Pregnancy and reproductive function* in Cytotoxic drugs p. 865.
● PREGNANCY Avoid (teratogenic and carcinogenic in *animal* studies). See also *Pregnancy and reproductive function* in Cytotoxic drugs p. 865.
● BREAST FEEDING Discontinue breast-feeding.
● HEPATIC IMPAIRMENT Avoid in severe impairment.
Dose adjustments Reduce dose according to serum bilirubin concentration—consult local protocol for details.
● RENAL IMPAIRMENT Avoid in severe impairment.
Dose adjustments Reduce dose by 25% if serum creatinine 105–265 micromol/litre.
Reduce dose by 50% if serum creatinine greater than 265 micromol/litre.
● MONITORING REQUIREMENTS Cardiac monitoring essential.

● MEDICINAL FORMS
There can be variation in the licensing of different medicines containing the same drug.
Solution for infusion
▶ DaunoXome (Galen Ltd)
Daunorubicin (as Daunorubicin hydrochloride citrate) 2 mg per 1 ml DaunoXome 50mg/25ml concentrate for solution for infusion vials | 1 vial PoM £250.00
Powder for solution for infusion
▶ Daunorubicin (Non-proprietary)
Daunorubicin (as Daunorubicin hydrochloride)
20 mg Daunorubicin 20mg powder for solution for infusion vials | 10 vial PoM £650.00 (Hospital only)

Doxorubicin hydrochloride

04-Oct-2017

● INDICATIONS AND DOSE

Acute leukaemias | Hodgkin's lymphoma | Non-Hodgkin's lymphoma | Some solid tumours including breast cancer | Advanced soft-tissue sarcoma
▶ BY INTRAVENOUS INJECTION
▶ Adult: (consult product literature)

Some papillary bladder tumours (bladder instillation) | Recurrent superficial bladder tumours (bladder instillation) | Transitional cell carcinoma (bladder instillation) | Carcinoma in situ (bladder instillation)
▶ BY INTRAVESICAL INSTILLATION
▶ Adult: (consult product literature)

CAELYX ®

For AIDS-related Kaposi's sarcoma in patients with low CD4 count and extensive mucocutaneous or visceral disease | Advanced ovarian cancer when platinum-based chemotherapy has failed | Progressive multiple myeloma (in combination with bortezomib) in patients who have received at least one prior therapy and who have undergone or are unsuitable for bone-marrow transplantation | Monotherapy for metastatic breast cancer in patients with increased cardiac risk
▶ BY INTRAVENOUS INFUSION
▶ Adult: (consult product literature)

MYOCET ®

For use with cyclophosphamide for metastatic breast cancer
▶ Adult: (consult product literature)

● CONTRA-INDICATIONS Consult product literature
● CAUTIONS Cardiac disease · caution in handling—irritant to tissues · consult product literature · elderly · hypertension · previous myocardial irradiation
● INTERACTIONS → Appendix 1: anthracyclines
● SIDE-EFFECTS
▶ Common or very common Alopecia · anaemia · anxiety · appetite decreased · arrhythmias · arthralgia · asthenia · bone marrow depression · breast pain · cachexia · cardiovascular disorder · chest discomfort · chills · constipation · cough · decreased leucocytes · dehydration · depression · diarrhoea · dizziness · drowsiness · dry mouth · dysphagia · dyspnoea · dysuria · electrolyte imbalance · epistaxis · eye inflammation · fever · gastrointestinal discomfort · gastrointestinal disorders · headache · hyperhidrosis · hypersensitivity · hypertension · hyperthermia · hypotension · increased risk of infection · influenza like illness · infusion related reaction · insomnia · malaise · mucosal abnormalities · muscle complaints · muscle tone increased · muscle weakness · nail disorder · nausea · nerve disorders · neutropenia · oedema · oral disorders · pain · scrotal erythema · sensation abnormal · sepsis · skin reactions · skin ulcer · syncope · taste altered · thrombocytopenia · vasodilation · vision blurred · vomiting · weight decreased
▶ Uncommon Confusion · embolism and thrombosis
▶ Rare or very rare Secondary oral neoplasms · severe cutaneous adverse reactions (SCARs)
▶ Frequency not known Asthma · congestive heart failure · secondary malignancy · throat tightness
SIDE-EFFECTS, FURTHER INFORMATION Extravasation can cause tissue necrosis.
Cardiomyopathy Higher cumulative doses are associated with cardiomyopathy and it is usual to limit total cumulative doses to 450 mg/m^2.
Liposomal formulations Liposomal formulations of doxorubicin may reduce the incidence of cardiotoxicity and lower the potential for local necrosis, but infusion reactions, sometimes severe, may occur. Hand-Foot

syndrome (painful, macular reddening skin eruptions) occurs commonly with liposomal doxorubicin and may be dose limiting. It can occur after 2–3 treatment cycles and may be prevented by cooling hands and feet and avoiding socks, gloves, or tight-fitting footwear. It may also occur with non-liposomal formulations.

Elevated bilirubin concentrations Doxorubicin is largely excreted in the bile and an elevated bilirubin concentration is an indication for reducing the dose.

● CONCEPTION AND CONTRACEPTION Manufacturer advises effective contraception during and for at least 6 months after treatment in men or women.

● PREGNANCY Avoid (teratogenic and toxic in *animal* studies). See also *Pregnancy and reproductive function* in Cytotoxic drugs p. 865.

● BREAST FEEDING Discontinue breast-feeding.

● HEPATIC IMPAIRMENT Avoid in severe impairment.
Dose adjustments Reduce dose according to bilirubin concentration—consult product literature or local treatment protocol for details.

● RENAL IMPAIRMENT Consult product literature in severe impairment.

● MONITORING REQUIREMENTS Patients should be assessed before treatment, by echocardiography. Cardiac monitoring during treatment may assist in determining safe dosage.

● DIRECTIONS FOR ADMINISTRATION *Conventional* doxorubicin is given by injection into a fast-running infusion, commonly at 21-day intervals.

● PRESCRIBING AND DISPENSING INFORMATION Doxorubicin is available as both *conventional* and *liposomal* formulations. The different formulations vary in their licensed indications, pharmacokinetics, dosage and administration, and are not interchangeable.

● NATIONAL FUNDING/ACCESS DECISIONS

NICE decisions

▸ **Topotecan, pegylated liposomal doxorubicin hydrochloride, paclitaxel, trabectedin and gemcitabine for treating recurrent ovarian cancer (April 2016)** NICE TA389
Pegylated liposomal doxorubicin hydrochloride (PLDH) monotherapy or in combination with platinum, is recommended as an option for treating recurrent ovarian cancer.

PLDH, in combination with trabectedin, is **not** recommended for treating the first recurrence of platinum-sensitive ovarian cancer.

Patients currently receiving PLDH in combination with trabectedin should have the option to continue their treatment until they and their clinician consider it appropriate to stop.
www.nice.org.uk/guidance/TA389

▸ **Olaratumab in combination with doxorubicin for treating advanced soft tissue sarcoma (August 2017)** NICE TA465
Doxorubicin, in combination with olaratumab, is recommended for use within the Cancer Drugs Fund as an option for advanced soft tissue sarcoma in patients, only if:

● they have not had any previous systemic chemotherapy for advanced soft tissue sarcoma;

● they cannot have curative treatment with surgery or their disease does not respond to radiotherapy;

● the conditions in the managed access agreement for olaratumab are followed.
www.nice.org.uk/guidance/TA465

● MEDICINAL FORMS
There can be variation in the licensing of different medicines containing the same drug. Forms available from special-order manufacturers include: solution for infusion

Solution for injection
▸ Doxorubicin hydrochloride (Non-proprietary)
Doxorubicin hydrochloride 2 mg per 1 ml Doxorubicin 10mg/5ml solution for injection vials | 1 vial [PoM] £18.54 (Hospital only)
Doxorubicin 50mg/25ml solution for injection Cytosafe vials | 1 vial [PoM] £103.00 (Hospital only)
Doxorubicin 50mg/25ml solution for infusion vials | 1 vial [PoM] £103.00 (Hospital only)
Doxorubicin 10mg/5ml solution for injection Cytosafe vials | 1 vial [PoM] £20.60 (Hospital only)
Doxorubicin 10mg/5ml concentrate for solution for infusion vials | 1 vial [PoM] £19.57
Doxorubicin 10mg/5ml solution for infusion vials | 1 vial [PoM] £20.60 (Hospital only)
Doxorubicin 50mg/25ml solution for injection vials | 1 vial [PoM] £92.70 (Hospital only)
Doxorubicin 50mg/25ml concentrate for solution for infusion vials | 1 vial [PoM] £97.85

Solution for infusion
▸ Doxorubicin hydrochloride (Non-proprietary)
Doxorubicin hydrochloride 2 mg per 1 ml Doxorubicin 200mg/100ml solution for injection Cytosafe vials | 1 vial [PoM] £412.00 (Hospital only)
Doxorubicin 200mg/100ml solution for infusion vials | 1 vial [PoM] £412.00 (Hospital only)
Doxorubicin 200mg/100ml concentrate for solution for infusion vials | 1 vial [PoM] £391.40
▸ Caelyx (Janssen-Cilag Ltd)
Doxorubicin hydrochloride (as Doxorubicin hydrochloride liposomal pegylated) 2 mg per 1 ml Caelyx 50mg/25ml concentrate for solution for infusion vials | 1 vial [PoM] £712.49
Caelyx 20mg/10ml concentrate for solution for infusion vials | 1 vial [PoM] £360.23

Powder for solution for injection
▸ Doxorubin (medac UK)
Doxorubicin hydrochloride 50 mg Doxorubin 50mg powder for solution for injection vials | 10 vial [PoM] £914.00

Powder and solvent for suspension for infusion
ELECTROLYTES: May contain Sodium
▸ Myocet (Teva UK Ltd)
Doxorubicin hydrochloride 50 mg Myocet 50mg powder and solvent for suspension for infusion vials | 2 vial [PoM] £912.26 (Hospital only)

Epirubicin hydrochloride

● INDICATIONS AND DOSE

Treatment of breast cancer | Treatment and prophylaxis of certain forms of superficial bladder cancer
▸ BY INTRAVENOUS INFUSION, OR BY INTRAVESICAL INSTILLATION
▸ Adult: (consult product literature or local protocols)

● CONTRA-INDICATIONS Bladder inflammation or contraction (when used as a bladder instillation) · catheterisation difficulties (when used as a bladder instillation) · haematuria (when used as a bladder instillation) · invasive tumours penetrating the bladder (when used as a bladder instillation) · myocardiopathy · previous treatment with maximum cumulative doses of epirubicin or other anthracycline · recent myocardial infarction · severe arrhythmia · severe myocardial insufficiency · unstable angina · urinary tract infections (when used as a bladder instillation)

● CAUTIONS Caution in handling—irritant to tissues

● INTERACTIONS → Appendix 1: anthracyclines

● SIDE-EFFECTS
GENERAL SIDE-EFFECTS
▸ **Common or very common** Paraesthesia · urinary frequency increased

8

Immune system and malignant disease

SPECIFIC SIDE-EFFECTS
▸ **Common or very common**
▸ With intravesical use Chemical cystitis
▸ With parenteral use Alopecia · anaemia · appetite decreased · bone marrow depression · dehydration · diarrhoea · increased risk of infection · leucopenia · mucositis · nausea · neutropenia · oesophagitis · stomatitis · urine red · vasodilation · vomiting
▸ **Uncommon**
▸ With parenteral use Embolism and thrombosis · thrombocytopenia
▸ **Rare or very rare**
▸ With parenteral use Amenorrhoea · arrhythmias · ascites · asthenia · azoospermia · cardiac conduction disorders · cardiomyopathy · cardiotoxicity · chills · congestive heart failure · dizziness · dyspnoea · fever · hepatomegaly · hyperuricaemia · malaise · neoplasms · oedema · pleural effusion · pulmonary oedema · skin reactions
▸ **Frequency not known**
▸ With intravesical use Cystitis bacterial
▸ With parenteral use Eye inflammation · haemorrhage · hypoxia · nail discolouration · photosensitivity reaction · radiation injuries · sepsis · shock
 SIDE-EFFECTS, FURTHER INFORMATION Manufactuer advises extreme caution with cumulative doses exceeding 900 mg/m^2—risk of congestive heart failure increased.
● CONCEPTION AND CONTRACEPTION Contraceptive advice required, see *Pregnancy and reproductive function* in Cytotoxic drugs p. 865.
● PREGNANCY Avoid (carcinogenic in *animal* studies). See also *Pregnancy and reproductive function* in Cytotoxic drugs p. 865.
● BREAST FEEDING Discontinue breast-feeding.
● HEPATIC IMPAIRMENT Avoid in severe impairment.
 Dose adjustments Reduce dose according to bilirubin concentration—consult local treatment protocol for details.
● RENAL IMPAIRMENT
 Dose adjustments Dose reduction may be necessary in severe impairment.

● MEDICINAL FORMS
 There can be variation in the licensing of different medicines containing the same drug. Forms available from special-order manufacturers include: solution for injection, solution for infusion
 Solution for injection
 ▸ Epirubicin hydrochloride (Non-proprietary)
  Epirubicin hydrochloride 2 mg per 1 ml Epirubicin 50mg/25ml solution for injection vials | 1 vial [PoM] £86.89–£100.88
  Epirubicin 10mg/5ml solution for injection vials | 1 vial [PoM] £17.38–£20.18
 ▸ Pharmorubicin (Pfizer Ltd)
  Epirubicin hydrochloride 2 mg per 1 ml Pharmorubicin 50mg/25ml solution for injection Cytosafe vials | 1 vial [PoM] £106.19 (Hospital only)
  Pharmorubicin 10mg/5ml solution for injection Cytosafe vials | 1 vial [PoM] £21.24 (Hospital only)
 Solution for infusion
 ▸ Epirubicin hydrochloride (Non-proprietary)
  Epirubicin hydrochloride 2 mg per 1 ml Epirubicin 200mg/100ml solution for infusion vials | 1 vial [PoM] £306.20–£366.85
  Epirubicin 100mg/50ml solution for infusion vials | 1 vial [PoM] £201.76
 ▸ Pharmorubicin (Pfizer Ltd)
  Epirubicin hydrochloride 2 mg per 1 ml Pharmorubicin 200mg/100ml solution for infusion Cytosafe vials | 1 vial [PoM] £386.16 (Hospital only)

Idarubicin hydrochloride
04-May-2017

● INDICATIONS AND DOSE
Acute non-lymphocytic leukaemias monotherapy
▸ BY MOUTH
▸ Adult: 30 mg/m^2 daily for 3 days; maximum 400 mg/m^2 per course
Acute non-lymphocytic leukaemia in combination therapy
▸ BY MOUTH
▸ Adult: 15–30 mg/m^2 daily for 3 days; maximum 400 mg/m^2 per course
Advanced breast cancer after failure of first-line chemotherapy (not including anthracyclines)—monotherapy
▸ BY MOUTH
▸ Adult: 45 mg/m^2 for 1 dose, repeat treatment every 3–4 weeks, alternatively 15 mg/m^2 daily for 3 consecutive days, repeat treatment every 3–4 weeks; maximum 400 mg/m^2 per course
Acute leukaemias | Advanced breast cancer after failure of first-line chemotherapy (not including anthracyclines)
▸ BY INTRAVENOUS INJECTION
▸ Adult: (consult product literature)

 IMPORTANT SAFETY INFORMATION
 RISKS OF INCORRECT DOSING OF ORAL ANTI-CANCER MEDICINES
 See Cytotoxic drugs p. 865.

● CONTRA-INDICATIONS Previous treatment with maximum cumulative dose of idarubicin or other anthracycline · recent myocardial infarction · severe arrhythmias · severe myocardial insufficiency
● CAUTIONS Caution in handling—irritant to tissues
● INTERACTIONS → Appendix 1: anthracyclines
● SIDE-EFFECTS
 GENERAL SIDE-EFFECTS
▸ **Common or very common** Alopecia · anaemia · appetite decreased · arrhythmias · cardiomyopathy · chills · congestive heart failure · diarrhoea · embolism and thrombosis · fever · haemorrhage · headache · increased risk of infection · leucopenia · nausea · neutropenia · skin reactions · stomatitis · thrombocytopenia · urine red · vomiting
▸ **Uncommon** Dehydration · gastrointestinal disorders · hyperuricaemia · leukaemia secondary · myocardial infarction · nail discolouration · sepsis · shock · soft tissue necrosis
▸ **Rare or very rare** Cardiac conduction disorders · cardiac inflammation · flushing · intracranial haemorrhage
▸ **Frequency not known** Bone marrow disorders · tumour lysis syndrome
 SPECIFIC SIDE-EFFECTS
▸ **Common or very common**
▸ With intravenous use Abdominal pain · mucosal abnormalities · paraesthesia · radiation injuries
▸ With oral use Gastrointestinal discomfort · mucositis · radiation skin sensitivity
● CONCEPTION AND CONTRACEPTION Contraceptive advice required, see *Pregnancy and reproductive function* in Cytotoxic drugs p. 865.
● PREGNANCY Avoid (teratogenic and toxic in *animal* studies). See also *Pregnancy and reproductive function* in Cytotoxic drugs p. 865.
● BREAST FEEDING Discontinue breast-feeding.
● HEPATIC IMPAIRMENT Avoid in severe impairment.
 Dose adjustments Reduce dose according to serum bilirubin concentration.
● RENAL IMPAIRMENT Avoid in severe impairment.
 Dose adjustments Reduce dose.

- MEDICINAL FORMS
There can be variation in the licensing of different medicines containing the same drug.
Powder for solution for injection
▸ Zavedos (Pfizer Ltd)
  Idarubicin hydrochloride 5 mg Zavedos 5mg powder for solution for injection vials | 1 vial PoM £87.36 (Hospital only)
  Idarubicin hydrochloride 10 mg Zavedos 10mg powder for solution for injection vials | 1 vial PoM £174.72 (Hospital only)
Capsule
CAUTIONARY AND ADVISORY LABELS 25
▸ Zavedos (Pfizer Ltd)
  Idarubicin hydrochloride 5 mg Zavedos 5mg capsules | 1 capsule PoM £41.47
  Idarubicin hydrochloride 10 mg Zavedos 10mg capsules | 1 capsule PoM £69.12

Mitoxantrone

(Mitozantrone)

- INDICATIONS AND DOSE
Metastatic breast cancer | Non-Hodgkin's lymphoma | Adult acute non-lymphocytic leukaemia | Non-resectable primary hepatocellular carcinoma
▸ BY INTRAVENOUS INFUSION
▸ Adult: (consult local protocol)

- CAUTIONS Intrathecal administration not recommended
- INTERACTIONS → Appendix 1: anthracyclines
- SIDE-EFFECTS Abdominal pain · acute leukaemia · alopecia · amenorrhoea · anxiety · appetite decreased · arrhythmia · asthenia · bone marrow depression · confusion · constipation · diarrhoea · drowsiness · dyspnoea · fever · gastrointestinal haemorrhage · heart failure · mucositis · nail discolouration · nail dystrophy · nausea · neurological effects · paraesthesia · scleral discolouration · skin discolouration · stomatitis · thrombocytopenia · urine blue · vomiting

  SIDE-EFFECTS, FURTHER INFORMATION Cardiac examinations are recommended after a cumulative dose of 160mg/m^2.

- CONCEPTION AND CONTRACEPTION Manufacturer advises effective contraception during and for at least 6 months after treatment in men or women.
- PREGNANCY Avoid. See also *Pregnancy and reproductive function* in Cytotoxic drugs p. 865.
- BREAST FEEDING Discontinue breast-feeding.
- HEPATIC IMPAIRMENT Use with caution—consult local treatment protocol.

- MEDICINAL FORMS
There can be variation in the licensing of different medicines containing the same drug.
Solution for infusion
▸ Mitoxantrone (Non-proprietary)
  Mitoxantrone (as Mitoxantrone hydrochloride) 2 mg per 1 ml Mitoxantrone 20mg/10ml concentrate for solution for infusion vials | 1 vial PoM £121.85 (Hospital only) | 1 vial PoM £51.43
▸ Onkotrone (Baxter Healthcare Ltd)
  Mitoxantrone (as Mitoxantrone hydrochloride) 2 mg per 1 ml Onkotrone 20mg/10ml solution for infusion vials | 1 vial PoM £103.57
  Onkotrone 25mg/12.5ml solution for infusion vials | 1 vial PoM £129.48

Pixantrone

- INDICATIONS AND DOSE
Treatment of refractory or multiply relapsed aggressive non-Hodgkin B-cell lymphomas (monotherapy)
▸ BY INTRAVENOUS INFUSION
▸ Adult: (consult product literature)

- CONTRA-INDICATIONS Active severe infection · risk factors for severe infection
- CAUTIONS Active cardiovascular disease · cardiac risk factors · caution in handling—irritant to tissues · concurrent radiotherapy to the mediastinal area · history of cardiovascular disease · previous radiotherapy to the mediastinal area · previous therapy with anthracenediones · previous therapy with anthracyclines
- INTERACTIONS → Appendix 1: anthracyclines
- SIDE-EFFECTS
▸ **Common or very common** Alopecia · anaemia · appetite decreased · arrhythmias · asthenia · blood disorder · bundle branch block · cancer progression · cardiac disorder (during or following treatment) · chest pain · congestive heart failure · constipation · cough · decreased leucocytes · diarrhoea · drowsiness · dry mouth · dyspnoea · electrolyte imbalance · eye inflammation · fever · gastrointestinal discomfort · haemorrhage · headache · hypotension · increased risk of infection · left ventricular dysfunction · mucositis · nail disorder · nausea · neutropenia · oedema · oral disorders · pain · paraesthesia · proteinuria · secondary malignancy · skin reactions · taste altered · thrombocytopenia · urine discolouration · vascular disorders · vomiting
▸ **Uncommon** Anxiety · arthralgia · arthritis · bone marrow failure · chills · dizziness · dry eye · eosinophilia · hyperbilirubinaemia · hyperuricaemia · meningitis · muscle weakness · musculoskeletal stiffness · night sweats · oesophagitis · oliguria · respiratory disorders · rhinorrhoea · septic shock · skin ulcer · sleep disorders · spontaneous penile erection · vertigo · weight decreased
- CONCEPTION AND CONTRACEPTION Ensure effective contraception during and for at least 6 months after treatment in men or women.
- PREGNANCY Manufacturer advises avoid—toxicity in *animal* studies. See also *Pregnancy and reproductive function* in Cytotoxic drugs p. 865.
- BREAST FEEDING Manufacturer advises avoid—no information available.
- HEPATIC IMPAIRMENT No information available—manufacturer advises caution in mild to moderate impairment. Avoid in severe impairment.
- RENAL IMPAIRMENT No information available—manufacturer advises caution.
- MONITORING REQUIREMENTS
▸ Baseline investigations should include a full blood count, assessment of cardiac function measured by left ventricular ejection fraction, and measurement of serum concentrations of total bilirubin and total creatinine.
▸ Full blood count and cardiac function should be monitored throughout treatment.
- PATIENT AND CARER ADVICE
Photosensitivity Photosensitivity is a theoretical risk and patients should be advised to follow sun protection strategies.

8

Immune system and malignant disease

8

Immune system and malignant disease

● NATIONAL FUNDING/ACCESS DECISIONS

NICE decisions

▸ Pixantrone monotherapy for treating multiply relapsed or refractory aggressive non-Hodgkin's B-cell lymphoma (February 2014) NICE TA306

Pixantrone monotherapy is recommended as an option for treating adults with multiply relapsed or refractory aggressive non-Hodgkin's B-cell lymphoma in patients:
- who have previously been treated with rituximab **and**
- who are receiving third- or fourth-line treatment **and**
- if the manufacturer provides pixantrone with the discount agreed in the patient access scheme.
www.nice.org.uk/TA306

● MEDICINAL FORMS

There can be variation in the licensing of different medicines containing the same drug.

Powder for solution for infusion
ELECTROLYTES: May contain Sodium
▸ Pixuvri (Servier Laboratories Ltd) ▼
   Pixantrone (as Pixantrone dimaleate) 29 mg Pixuvri 29mg powder for concentrate for solution for infusion vials | 1 vial [PoM] £553.50

ANTINEOPLASTIC DRUGS > ANTIMETABOLITES

Azacitidine

28-Sep-2016

● DRUG ACTION Azacitidine is a pyrimidine analogue.

● INDICATIONS AND DOSE

Treatment of intermediate-2 and high-risk myelodysplastic syndromes, chronic myelomonocytic leukaemia, and acute myeloid leukaemia, in adults who are not eligible for haemotopoietic stem cell transplantation
▸ BY SUBCUTANEOUS INJECTION
▸ Adult: (consult local protocol)

● CONTRA-INDICATIONS Advanced malignant hepatic tumour

● CAUTIONS History of severe congestive heart failure · unstable cardiac disease (consider cardiopulmonary assessment before and during treatment) · unstable pulmonary disease (consider cardiopulmonary assessment before and during treatment)

● INTERACTIONS → Appendix 1: azacitidine

● SIDE-EFFECTS
▸ Common or very common Alopecia · anaemia · anxiety · appetite decreased · arthralgia · asthenia · bone marrow disorders · chest pain · chills · confusion · constipation · dehydration · diarrhoea · dizziness · drowsiness · dyspnoea · fever · gastrointestinal discomfort · haemorrhage · headache · hypertension · hypokalaemia · hypotension · increased risk of infection · inflammation · insomnia · intracranial haemorrhage · laryngeal pain · leucopenia · malaise · muscle complaints · nausea · neutropenia · pain · renal failure · respiratory disorders · sepsis · skin reactions · stomatitis · syncope · thrombocytopenia · vomiting · weight decreased
▸ Uncommon Hepatic coma · hepatic failure · pyoderma gangrenosum · renal tubular acidosis
▸ Rare or very rare Tumour lysis syndrome

● CONCEPTION AND CONTRACEPTION Manufacturer advises effective contraception during and for 3 months after treatment in men or women.

● PREGNANCY Avoid (toxicity in *animal* studies). See also *Pregnancy and reproductive function* in Cytotoxic drugs p. 865.

● BREAST FEEDING Discontinue breast-feeding.

● HEPATIC IMPAIRMENT Caution in severe impairment.

● RENAL IMPAIRMENT

Dose adjustments Delay next treatment cycle if serum-creatinine or blood urea nitrogen greater than twice baseline value and above the upper level of normal until values return to normal or baseline, and then reduce dose by 50% on the next treatment cycle.

Reduce dose by 50% on the next treatment cycle if serum-bicarbonate concentration less than 20 mmol/litre.

● MONITORING REQUIREMENTS
▸ Monitor liver function tests, serum creatinine, and serum bicarbonate before initiation of treatment and before each treatment cycle.
▸ Monitor full blood count before initiation of treatment, before each treatment cycle, and as clinically indicated.
▸ Monitor for bleeding.

● NATIONAL FUNDING/ACCESS DECISIONS

NICE decisions

▸ Azacitidine for treating acute myeloid leukaemia with more than 30% bone marrow blasts (July 2016) NICE TA399

Azacitidine is **not** recommended, within its marketing authorisation, for treating acute myeloid leukaemia with greater than 30% bone marrow blasts in patients aged 65 years or above who are not eligible for haematopoietic stem cell transplant.

Patients whose treatment was started before this guidance was published should continue treatment until they and their clinician consider it appropriate to stop.
www.nice.org.uk/TA399

▸ Azacitidine for the treatment of myelodysplastic syndromes, chronic myelomonocytic leukaemia and acute myeloid leukaemia (March 2011) NICE TA218

Azacitidine is recommended in adults who are not eligible for haematopoietic stem cell transplantation as an option for the treatment of intermediate-2 and high-risk myelodysplastic syndromes, chronic myelomonocytic leukaemia, or acute myeloid leukaemia.
www.nice.org.uk/TA218

● MEDICINAL FORMS

There can be variation in the licensing of different medicines containing the same drug.

Powder for suspension for injection
▸ Vidaza (Celgene Ltd)
   Azacitidine 100 mg Vidaza 100mg powder for suspension for injection vials | 1 vial [PoM] £321.00

Capecitabine

● DRUG ACTION Capecitabine is metabolised to fluorouracil.

● INDICATIONS AND DOSE

Stage III colon cancer, adjuvant following surgery (monotherapy)
▸ BY MOUTH
▸ Adult: 1.25 g/m^2 twice daily for 14 days, subsequent courses repeated after a 7-day interval, recommended duration of treatment is 6 months, adjust dose according to tolerability—consult product literature

Stage III colon cancer, adjuvant following surgery (combination therapy)
▸ BY MOUTH
▸ Adult: 0.8–1 g/m^2 twice daily for 14 days, subsequent courses repeated after a 7-day interval, recommended duration of treatment is 6 months, adjust dose according to tolerability—consult product literature

Metastatic colorectal cancer (monotherapy)
▸ BY MOUTH
▸ Adult: 1.25 g/m^2 twice daily for 14 days, subsequent courses repeated after a 7-day interval, adjust dose according to tolerability—consult product literature

Metastatic colorectal cancer (combination therapy)
▶ BY MOUTH
▸ Adult: 0.8–1 g/m^2 twice daily for 14 days, subsequent courses repeated after a 7-day interval, adjust dose according to tolerability—consult product literature

Advanced gastric cancer (first-line treatment in combination with a platinum based regimen)
▶ BY MOUTH
▸ Adult: 0.8–1 g/m^2 twice daily for 14 days, subsequent courses repeated after a 7-day interval, alternatively 625 mg/m^2 twice daily given continuously, adjust dose according to tolerability—consult product literature

Locally advanced or metastatic breast cancer (second-line treatment as monotherapy after failure of a taxane and anthracycline regimen or where further anthracycline treatment is not indicated) | Locally advanced or metastatic breast cancer (second-line treatment, in combination with docetaxel, where previous therapy included an anthracycline)
▶ BY MOUTH
▸ Adult: 1.25 g/m^2 twice daily for 14 days, subsequent courses repeated after a 7-day interval, adjust dose according to tolerability—consult product literature

---

IMPORTANT SAFETY INFORMATION
RISKS OF INCORRECT DOSING OF ORAL ANTI-CANCER MEDICINES
See Cytotoxic drugs p. 865.

● CONTRA-INDICATIONS Dihydropyrimidine dehydrogenase deficiency
● CAUTIONS Diabetes mellitus · diarrhoea or dehydration—consult product literature for guidance on dose modification and treatment interruption · electrolyte disturbances · history of angina pectoris · history of arrhythmias · history of significant cardiovascular disease · nervous system disease
● INTERACTIONS → Appendix 1: capecitabine
● SIDE-EFFECTS
▶ Common or very common Alopecia · anaemia · appetite abnormal · asthenia · chest pain · constipation · cough · dehydration · depression · diarrhoea · dizziness · dry mouth · dyspnoea · embolism and thrombosis · eye disorders · eye inflammation · eye irritation · fever · gastrointestinal discomfort · gastrointestinal disorders · haemorrhage · headache · hyperbilirubinaemia · increased risk of infection · insomnia · joint disorders · lethargy · malaise · nail disorder · nausea · neutropenia · oedema · pain · rhinorrhoea · sensation abnormal · skin reactions · stomatitis · taste altered · vomiting · weight decreased
▶ Uncommon Acute coronary syndrome · aphasia · arrhythmias · ascites · asthma · chills · confusion · diabetes mellitus · dysphagia · ear pain · facial swelling · haemolytic anaemia · hepatic disorders · hot flush · hydronephrosis · hypertension · hypertriglyceridaemia · hypokalaemia · hypotension · influenza like illness · ischaemic heart disease · leucopenia · libido decreased · lipoma · malnutrition · memory loss · movement disorders · muscle weakness · musculoskeletal stiffness · palpitations · pancytopenia · panic attack · peripheral coldness · peripheral neuropathy · photosensitivity reaction · pneumothorax · radiation recall reaction · sepsis · skin ulcer · syncope · thrombocytopenia · urinary disorders · vertigo · vision disorders
▶ Rare or very rare Cutaneous lupus erythematosus · encephalopathy · QT interval prolongation · severe cutaneous adverse reactions (SCARs) · vasospasm
▶ Frequency not known Cardiomyopathy · heart failure · sudden death

● CONCEPTION AND CONTRACEPTION Contraceptive advice required, see *Pregnancy and reproductive function* in Cytotoxic drugs p. 865.
● PREGNANCY Avoid (teratogenic in *animal* studies). See also *Pregnancy and reproductive function* in Cytotoxic drugs p. 865.
● BREAST FEEDING Discontinue breast-feeding.
● HEPATIC IMPAIRMENT Manufacturer advises monitor liver function in mild to moderate impairment—consult product literature for guidance on treatment interruption; avoid in severe impairment.
● RENAL IMPAIRMENT Avoid if creatinine clearance less than 30 mL/minute.
Dose adjustments Reduce starting dose of 1.25 g/m^2 to 75% if creatinine clearance 30–50 mL/minute.
● MONITORING REQUIREMENTS
▶ Monitor plasma-calcium concentration.
▶ Monitor for eye disorders (including keratitis and corneal disorders).
▶ Severe skin reactions Monitor for symptoms of severe skin reactions (including Stevens-Johnson syndrome and toxic epidermal necrolysis)—permanently discontinue treatment immediately if symptoms occur.
▶ Hand-foot syndrome Monitor for symptoms of hand-foot syndrome—interrupt treatment if significant syndrome occurs and refer to product literature.
● NATIONAL FUNDING/ACCESS DECISIONS

NICE decisions
▶ **Bevacizumab in combination with capecitabine for the first-line treatment of metastatic breast cancer (August 2012)** NICE TA263
Bevacizumab in combinations with capecitabine is **not** recommended within its marketing authorisation for the first-line treatment of metastatic breast cancer, that is, when treatment with other chemotherapy options including taxanes or anthracyclines is not considered appropriate, or when taxanes or anthracyclines have been used as part of adjuvant treatment in the previous 12 months.
www.nice.org.uk/TA263
▶ **Bevacizumab in combination with oxaliplatin and either fluorouracil plus folinic acid or capecitabine for the treatment of metastatic colorectal cancer (December 2010)** NICE TA212
Bevacizumab in combination with oxaliplatin and either fluorouracil plus folinic acid or capecitabine is **not** recommended for the treatment of metastatic colorectal cancer.
www.nice.org.uk/TA212
▶ **Capecitabine for the treatment of advanced gastric cancer (July 2010)** NICE TA191
Capecitabine in combination with a platinum-based regimen is recommended for the first-line treatment of inoperable advanced gastric cancer.
www.nice.org.uk/TA191
▶ **Capecitabine and tegafur with uracil for metastatic colorectal cancer (May 2003)** NICE TA61
Capecitabine or tegafur with uracil [now discontinued] (in combination with folinic acid) is an option for the first-line treatment of metastatic colorectal cancer.
www.nice.org.uk/TA61
▶ **Capecitabine and oxaliplatin in the adjuvant treatment of stage III (Dukes' C) colon cancer (April 2006)** NICE TA100
Capecitabine alone *or* oxaliplatin combined with fluorouracil and folinic acid are options for adjuvant treatment following surgery for stage III (Dukes' C) colon cancer.
www.nice.org.uk/TA100

8

Immune system and malignant disease

● MEDICINAL FORMS
There can be variation in the licensing of different medicines containing the same drug.

Tablet

CAUTIONARY AND ADVISORY LABELS 21

▸ Capecitabine (Non-proprietary)
Capecitabine 150 mg Capecitabine 150mg tablets | 60 tablet [PoM]
£30.00–£39.00
Capecitabine 300 mg Capecitabine 300mg tablets | 60 tablet [PoM]
£76.04
Capecitabine 500 mg Capecitabine 500mg tablets |
120 tablet [PoM] £225.72–£262.00 | 120 tablet [PoM] £265.55
(Hospital only)

▸ Xeloda (Roche Products Ltd)
Capecitabine 150 mg Xeloda 150mg tablets | 60 tablet [PoM]
£40.02
Capecitabine 500 mg Xeloda 500mg tablets | 120 tablet [PoM]
£265.55

Cladribine

20-Feb-2018

● DRUG ACTION Cladribine is a nucleoside analogue that is cytotoxic particularly to lymphocytes and monocytes, inhibiting both DNA synthesis and repair. Its effect on B- and T-lymphocytes is thought to interrupt the cascade of immune events central to multiple sclerosis.

● INDICATIONS AND DOSE

Hairy cell leukaemia (specialist use only)
▸ BY SUBCUTANEOUS INJECTION, OR BY INTRAVENOUS INFUSION
▸ Adult: (consult product literature or local protocols)

B-cell chronic lymphocytic leukaemia (specialist use only)
▸ BY INTRAVENOUS INFUSION
▸ Adult: (consult product literature or local protocols)

Highly active relapsing-remitting multiple sclerosis (specialist use only)
▸ BY MOUTH
▸ Adult: (consult product literature or local protocols)

IMPORTANT SAFETY INFORMATION

MHRA/CHM ADVICE: CLADRIBINE FOR LEUKAEMIA: REPORTS OF PROGRESSIVE MULTIFOCAL ENCEPHALOPATHY (PML); STOP TREATMENT IF PML SUSPECTED (DECEMBER 2017)

The MHRA is aware of 3 confirmed cases of progressive multifocal encephalopathy (PML) that developed 6 months to several years after cladribine treatment for haematological conditions. An association between cladribine and prolonged lymphopenia has been reported.

PML should be considered in the differential diagnosis for patients with new or worsening neurological signs or symptoms. Patients should be monitored for signs and symptoms of new neurological dysfunction, and advised to seek urgent medical attention if they experience symptoms—stop treatment immediately if PML is suspected and ensure specialist investigation is received.

● CONTRA-INDICATIONS
▸ With oral use Active chronic hepatitis · active chronic tuberculosis · active malignancy · HIV infection · immunocompromised patients

● CAUTIONS
GENERAL CAUTIONS Acute infection · use irradiated blood only (haematology consultation advised)
SPECIFIC CAUTIONS
▸ With intravenous use or subcutaneous use High tumour burden—consult product literature · symptomatic or severe bone marrow depression
▸ With oral use No prior exposure to varicella zoster virus · prior malignancy (consider if potential benefit outweighs risk)

CAUTIONS, FURTHER INFORMATION
▸ Immunosuppressive effect of cladribine
▸ With intravenous use or subcutaneous use Cladribine has potent and prolonged myelosuppressive and immunosuppressive effects. Patients treated with cladribine are more prone to serious bacterial, opportunistic fungal, and viral infections, and prophylactic therapy should be considered in those at risk. Acute infections should be treated before initiating cladribine. To prevent potentially fatal transfusion-related graft-versus-host reaction, only irradiated blood products should be administered. Prescribers should consult specialist literature when using highly immunosuppressive drugs.
▸ Varicella zoster virus
▸ With oral use Manufacturer advises vaccination prior to initiation of therapy in patients who have no history of exposure to varicella zoster virus; delay treatment for 4–6 weeks after vaccination.

● INTERACTIONS → Appendix 1: cladribine

● SIDE-EFFECTS
GENERAL SIDE-EFFECTS
▸ **Common or very common** Increased risk of infection · secondary malignancy · skin reactions
SPECIFIC SIDE-EFFECTS
▸ **Common or very common**
▸ With intravenous use Anaemia · anxiety · appetite decreased · arrhythmias · arthritis · asthenia · chest pain · chills · confusion · conjunctivitis · constipation · cough · diarrhoea · dizziness · dyspnoea · febrile neutropenia · fever · flatulence · gastrointestinal discomfort · haemolytic anaemia · headache · hyperhidrosis · hypersensitivity · insomnia · joint disorders · malaise · muscle weakness · myalgia · myocardial ischaemia · nausea · oedema · pain · renal impairment · respiratory disorders · septic shock · thrombocytopenia · vomiting
▸ With oral use Alopecia · lymphopenia
▸ With subcutaneous use Anaemia · anxiety · appetite decreased · arrhythmias · arthralgia · arthritis · asthenia · bone marrow disorders · chills · constipation · cough · diarrhoea · dizziness · dyspnoea · fever · gastrointestinal disorders · gastrointestinal pain · haemorrhage · headache · hyperhidrosis · hypotension · immunosuppression · insomnia · lymphopenia · malaise · mucositis · myalgia · myocardial ischaemia · nausea · neutropenia · oedema · pain · respiratory disorders · sepsis · thrombocytopenia · vomiting
▸ **Uncommon**
▸ With intravenous use Bone marrow disorders · hypereosinophilia · level of consciousness decreased · nerve disorders · neurotoxicity (with high doses) · paralysis · paraparesis · Stevens-Johnson syndrome · tumour lysis syndrome
▸ With subcutaneous use Ataxia · cachexia · confusion · drowsiness · eye inflammation · haemolytic anaemia · paraesthesia · polyneuropathy
▸ **Rare or very rare**
▸ With intravenous use Heart failure
▸ With subcutaneous use Amyloidosis · cholecystitis · depression · dysphagia · epilepsy · graft versus host disease · heart failure · hepatic failure · hypereosinophilia · pulmonary embolism · renal failure · severe cutaneous adverse reactions (SCARs) · speech disorder · tumour lysis syndrome

● CONCEPTION AND CONTRACEPTION Manufacturer advises effective contraception during treatment and for at least 6 months after the last dose in men and women of childbearing potential.
▸ With oral use Manufacturer advises exclude pregnancy before each treatment course; if using a hormonal

contraceptive, a barrier method should also be used for at least 4 weeks after the last dose of each course.

- PREGNANCY Manufacturer advises avoid—teratogenic in *animal* studies. See also *Pregnancy and reproductive function* in Cytotoxic drugs p. 865.

- BREAST FEEDING
  ▸ With intravenous use or subcutaneous use Manufacturer advises avoid during treatment and for 6 months after the last dose—no information available.
  ▸ With oral use Manufacturer advises avoid during treatment and for 1 week after the last dose—no information available.

- HEPATIC IMPAIRMENT
  ▸ With intravenous use Manufacturer advises caution—limited information available.
  ▸ With subcutaneous use Manufacturer advises caution in mild impairment; avoid in moderate-to-severe impairment.
  ▸ With oral use Manufacturer advises avoid in moderate-to-severe impairment—no information available.

- RENAL IMPAIRMENT
  ▸ With subcutaneous use Manufacturer advises caution in mild impairment; avoid in moderate-to-severe impairment.
  ▸ With oral use Manufacturer advises avoid in moderate-to-severe impairment—no information available.
  ▸ With intravenous use Manufacturer advises caution—limited information available.

- PRE-TREATMENT SCREENING
  ▸ With oral use Manufacturer advises exclude HIV infection, active or latent tuberculosis and active or latent hepatitis before starting each treatment course—delay treatment until infection adequately treated.

- MONITORING REQUIREMENTS
  ▸ Manufacturer advises monitor for malignancy—follow routine cancer screening guidelines.
  ▸ Manufacturer advises monitor for progressive multifocal leucoencephalopathy—perform a baseline MRI.
  ▸ Manufacturer advises monitor for haemolysis in patients who are or who become Coombs' positive.
  ▸ Manufacturer advises haematological monitoring required—consult product literature.
  ▸ With intravenous use or subcutaneous use Renal and hepatic function should be monitored periodically as clinically indicated.

- DIRECTIONS FOR ADMINISTRATION *Litak®* for subcutaneous use only—no dilution required; manufacturer advises patients may self-administer, after appropriate training.
  Leustat® for infusion use only.

- HANDLING AND STORAGE
  LITAK® Manufacturer advises store in a refrigerator (2–8°C).
  LEUSTAT® Manufacturer advises store in a refrigerator (2–8°C).

- PATIENT AND CARER ADVICE
  Driving and skilled tasks ▸ With intravenous use or subcutaneous use Manufacturer advises patients and carers should be counselled on the effects on driving and performance of skilled tasks—increased risk of dizziness and drowsiness.

- NATIONAL FUNDING/ACCESS DECISIONS
  NICE decisions
  ▸ **Cladribine tablets for treating relapsing–remitting multiple sclerosis (December 2017)** NICE TA493
  Cladribine tablets are recommended as an option for treating highly active multiple sclerosis in adults, only if the person has:
  - rapidly evolving severe relapsing–remitting multiple sclerosis, that is, at least 2 relapses in the previous year and at least 1 T1 gadolinium-enhancing lesion at baseline MRI, **or**

- relapsing–remitting multiple sclerosis that has responded inadequately to treatment with disease-modifying therapy, defined as 1 relapse in the previous year and MRI evidence of disease activity.

Patients whose treatment was started within the NHS before this guidance was published should have the option to continue treatment, without change to their funding arrangements, until they and their NHS clinician consider it appropriate to stop.
www.nice.org.uk/guidance/ta493

Scottish Medicines Consortium (SMC) Decisions
The *Scottish Medicines Consortium* has advised (February 2018) that cladribine (*Mavenclad®*) is accepted for restricted use within NHS Scotland for the treatment of adults with:
- rapidly evolving severe relapsing-remitting multiple sclerosis: patients with two or more relapses in the prior year whether on treatment or not, and at least one T1 gadolinium-enhancing lesion, **or**
- sub-optimal therapy relapsing-remitting multiple sclerosis: patients with one or more relapses in the previous year while on disease modifying therapy, and at least one T1 gadolinium-enhancing lesion or nine T2 lesions.

- MEDICINAL FORMS
  There can be variation in the licensing of different medicines containing the same drug.
  Solution for injection
  ▸ Litak (Lipomed GmbH)
  Cladribine 2 mg per 1 ml Litak 10mg/5ml solution for injection vials | 1 vial PoM £165.00 (Hospital only)
  Solution for infusion
  ELECTROLYTES: May contain Sodium
  ▸ Leustat (Janssen-Cilag Ltd)
  Cladribine 1 mg per 1 ml Leustat 10mg/10ml solution for infusion vials | 1 vial PoM £159.70
  Tablet
  ▸ Mavenclad (Merck Serono Ltd)
  Cladribine 10 mg Mavenclad 10mg tablets | 1 tablet PoM £2,047.24 | 4 tablet PoM £8,188.97 | 6 tablet PoM £12,283.46

Clofarabine

- INDICATIONS AND DOSE
  Relapsed or refractory acute lymphoblastic leukaemia in patients who have received at least two previous regimens
  ▸ BY INTRAVENOUS INFUSION
  ▸ Adult 18-20 years: (consult local protocol)

- CAUTIONS Cardiac disease
- INTERACTIONS → Appendix 1: clofarabine
- SIDE-EFFECTS
  ▸ **Common or very common** Alopecia · anxiety · appetite decreased · arthralgia · capillary leak syndrome · chills · cough · dehydration · diarrhoea · dizziness · drowsiness · dyspnoea · fatigue · feeling abnormal · feeling hot · fever · flushing · gastrointestinal discomfort · haemorrhage · headache · hearing impairment · hepatic disorders · hyperbilirubinaemia · hyperhidrosis · hypersensitivity · hypotension · increased risk of infection · irritability · mucositis · multi organ failure · myalgia · nausea · neutropenia · oedema · oral disorders · pain · paraesthesia · pericardial effusion · peripheral neuropathy · psychiatric disorder · renal impairment · respiratory disorders · sepsis · sinusoidal obstruction syndrome · skin reactions · systemic inflammatory response syndrome · tachycardia · tremor · tumour lysis syndrome · vomiting · weight decreased
  ▸ **Frequency not known** Antibiotic associated colitis · gastrointestinal disorders · hyponatraemia · pancreatitis · severe cutaneous adverse reactions (SCARs)

- CONCEPTION AND CONTRACEPTION Contraceptive advice required, see *Pregnancy and reproductive function* in Cytotoxic drugs p. 865.
- PREGNANCY Manufacturer advises avoid (teratogenic in *animal* studies). See also *Pregnancy and reproductive function* in Cytotoxic drugs p. 865.
- BREAST FEEDING Discontinue breast-feeding.
- HEPATIC IMPAIRMENT Manufacturer advises caution in mild to moderate impairment. Avoid in severe impairment.
- RENAL IMPAIRMENT Manufacturer advises caution in mild to moderate impairment. Avoid in severe impairment.

- MEDICINAL FORMS
There can be variation in the licensing of different medicines containing the same drug.
Solution for infusion
ELECTROLYTES: May contain Sodium
▸ Clofarabine (Non-proprietary)
Clofarabine 1 mg per 1 ml Clofarabine 20mg/20ml concentrate for solution for infusion vials | 1 vial [PoM] £1,259.87 (Hospital only)
▸ Evoltra (Sanofi) ▼
Clofarabine 1 mg per 1 ml Evoltra 20mg/20ml concentrate for solution for infusion vials | 1 vial [PoM] £1,326.18 (Hospital only)

Cytarabine

- DRUG ACTION Cytarabine acts by interfering with pyrimidine synthesis.

- **INDICATIONS AND DOSE**
Induction of remission of acute myeloblastic leukaemia
▸ BY INTRAVENOUS INFUSION, OR BY INTRAVENOUS INJECTION, OR BY SUBCUTANEOUS INJECTION
▸ Adult: (consult local protocol)
Lymphomatous meningitis
▸ BY INTRATHECAL INJECTION
▸ Adult: (consult local protocol)

IMPORTANT SAFETY INFORMATION
Not all cytarabine preparations can be given by intrathecal injection—consult product literature.

- INTERACTIONS → Appendix 1: cytarabine
- SIDE-EFFECTS
▸ **Common or very common** Alopecia · anaemia · appetite decreased · consciousness impaired · diarrhoea · dysarthria · dysphagia · eye disorders · eye inflammation · eye stinging · fever · gastrointestinal discomfort · gastrointestinal disorders · haemorrhagic conjunctivitis (consider prophylactic corticosteroid eye drops) · hyperuricaemia · leucopenia · nausea · oral disorders · renal impairment · skin reactions · thrombocytopenia · urinary retention · vasculitis · vision disorders · vomiting
▸ **Uncommon** Arthralgia · dyspnoea · headache · increased risk of infection · myalgia · nerve disorders · pain · paralysis · pericarditis · sepsis · skin ulcer · throat pain
▸ **Rare or very rare** Arrhythmias
▸ **Frequency not known** Acute respiratory distress syndrome (ARDS) · amenorrhoea · ataxia · azoospermia · bone marrow disorders · cardiomyopathy · cerebellar dysfunction · chest pain · coma · confusion · cytarabine syndrome · dizziness · drowsiness · haemorrhage · hepatic disorders · hyperbilirubinaemia · neurotoxicity · neurotoxicity rash · neutropenia · pancreatitis · personality change · pulmonary oedema · reticulocytopenia · rhabdomyolysis · seizure · tremor
- CONCEPTION AND CONTRACEPTION Contraceptive advice required, see *Pregnancy and reproductive function* in Cytotoxic drugs p. 865.

- PREGNANCY Avoid (teratogenic in *animal* studies). See also *Pregnancy and reproductive function* in Cytotoxic drugs p. 865.
- BREAST FEEDING Discontinue breast-feeding.
- HEPATIC IMPAIRMENT
Dose adjustments Reduce dose—consult product literature.
- MONITORING REQUIREMENTS
▸ Haematological monitoring Cytarabine is a potent myelosuppressant and requires careful haematological monitoring.
- NATIONAL FUNDING/ACCESS DECISIONS
DEPOCYTE®
Scottish Medicines Consortium (SMC) Decisions
The *Scottish Medicines Consortium* has advised (July 2007) that liposomal cytarabine suspension (*DepoCyte®*) is not recommended for use within NHS Scotland for the intrathecal treatment of lymphomatous meningitis.

- MEDICINAL FORMS
There can be variation in the licensing of different medicines containing the same drug. Forms available from special-order manufacturers include: solution for injection
Solution for injection
▸ Cytarabine (Non-proprietary)
Cytarabine 20 mg per 1 ml Cytarabine 500mg/25ml solution for injection vials | 1 vial [PoM] £19.50 (Hospital only) | 1 vial [PoM] £19.50
Cytarabine 100mg/5ml solution for injection vials | 5 vial [PoM] £20.48–£30.00 (Hospital only) | 5 vial [PoM] £20.98
Cytarabine 100 mg per 1 ml Cytarabine 500mg/5ml solution for injection vials | 5 vial [PoM] £100.00 (Hospital only) | 5 vial [PoM] £89.78
Cytarabine 100mg/1ml solution for injection vials | 5 vial [PoM] £26.93
Cytarabine 2g/20ml solution for injection vials | 1 vial [PoM] £77.50–£79.00 (Hospital only) | 1 vial [PoM] £73.63–£77.50
Cytarabine 1g/10ml solution for injection vials | 1 vial [PoM] £39.00–£40.00 (Hospital only) | 1 vial [PoM] £37.05–£39.00
Suspension for injection
▸ DepoCyte (Napp Pharmaceuticals Ltd)
Cytarabine 10 mg per 1 ml DepoCyte 50mg/5ml suspension for injection vials | 1 vial [PoM] £1,223.75 (Hospital only)

Decitabine

- DRUG ACTION Decitabine is a pyrimidine analogue.

- **INDICATIONS AND DOSE**
Treatment of newly diagnosed acute myeloid leukaemia in patients over 65 years of age who are not candidates for standard induction chemotherapy
▸ BY INTRAVENOUS INFUSION
▸ Elderly: (consult local protocol)

- CAUTIONS History of severe congestive heart failure · history of unstable cardiac disease
- INTERACTIONS → Appendix 1: decitabine
- SIDE-EFFECTS
▸ **Common or very common** Anaemia · diarrhoea · epistaxis · fever · headache · hypersensitivity · increased risk of infection · leucopenia · nausea · neutropenia · sepsis · stomatitis · thrombocytopenia · vomiting
▸ **Uncommon** Acute febrile neutrophilic dermatosis · pancytopenia
▸ **Frequency not known** Gastrointestinal disorders · interstitial lung disease
- CONCEPTION AND CONTRACEPTION Men must avoid fathering a child during and for 3 months after treatment.
- PREGNANCY Avoid (teratogenic in *animal* studies). See also *Pregnancy and reproductive function* in Cytotoxic drugs p. 865.
- BREAST FEEDING Discontinue breast-feeding.

- HEPATIC IMPAIRMENT Manufacturer advises caution—no information available.
- RENAL IMPAIRMENT Manufacturer advises caution if creatinine clearance less than 30 mL/minute—no information available.

- MEDICINAL FORMS
There can be variation in the licensing of different medicines containing the same drug.
Powder for solution for infusion
ELECTROLYTES: May contain Potassium, sodium
  - Dacogen (Janssen-Cilag Ltd)
  Decitabine 50 mg Dacogen 50mg powder for concentrate for solution for infusion vials | 1 vial [PoM] £970.86

Fludarabine phosphate

- INDICATIONS AND DOSE

Initial treatment of advanced B-cell chronic lymphocytic leukaemia (CLL) or after first line treatment in patients with sufficient bone-marrow reserves
  - BY MOUTH
  - Adult: 40 mg/m^2 for 5 days every 28 days, usually given for 6 cycles
  - BY INTRAVENOUS INJECTION, OR BY INTRAVENOUS INFUSION
  - Adult: (consult product literature)

> IMPORTANT SAFETY INFORMATION
> RISKS OF INCORRECT DOSING OF ORAL ANTI-CANCER MEDICINES
> See Cytotoxic drugs p. 865.

- CONTRA-INDICATIONS Haemolytic anaemia
- CAUTIONS Increased susceptibility to skin cancer · worsening of existing skin cancer
  CAUTIONS, FURTHER INFORMATION
  Co-trimoxazole is used to prevent pneumocystis infection.
  - Immunosuppression Fludarabine has a potent and prolonged immunosuppresive effect. Patients treated with fludarabine are more prone to serious bacterial, opportunistic fungal, and viral infections, and prophylactic therapy is recommended in those at risk. To prevent potentially fatal transfusion-related graft-versus-host reaction, only irradiated blood products should be administered. Prescribers should consult specialist literature when using highly immunosuppressive drugs.
- INTERACTIONS → Appendix 1: fludarabine
- SIDE-EFFECTS
  GENERAL SIDE-EFFECTS
  - Common or very common Anaemia · appetite decreased · asthenia · bone marrow depression (may be cumulative) · chills · cough · diarrhoea · fever · increased risk of infection · malaise · mucositis · nausea · neoplasms · nerve disorders · neutropenia · oedema · stomatitis · thrombocytopenia · vision disorders · vomiting
  - Uncommon Autoimmune disorder · confusion · haemorrhage · respiratory disorders · tumour lysis syndrome
  - Rare or very rare Agitation · arrhythmia · coma · heart failure · seizure · severe cutaneous adverse reactions (SCARs)
  SPECIFIC SIDE-EFFECTS
  - Common or very common
  - With oral use Progressive multifocal leukoencephalopathy · skin reactions · viral infection reactivation
  - With parenteral use Rash
  - Uncommon
  - With oral use Acquired haemophilia · crystalluria · dyspnoea · electrolyte imbalance · haemolytic anaemia · hyperuricaemia · metabolic acidosis · renal failure
  - With parenteral use Pulmonary toxicity

  - Frequency not known
  - With parenteral use Encephalopathy · intracranial haemorrhage
- CONCEPTION AND CONTRACEPTION Manufacturer advises effective contraception during and for at least 6 months after treatment in men or women.
- PREGNANCY Avoid (embryotoxic and teratogenic in *animal* studies). See also *Pregnancy and reproductive function* in Cytotoxic drugs p. 865.
- BREAST FEEDING Discontinue breast-feeding.
- RENAL IMPAIRMENT Avoid if creatinine clearance less than 30 mL/minute.
  Dose adjustments Reduce dose by up to 50% if creatinine clearance 30–70 mL/minute.
- MONITORING REQUIREMENTS
  - Monitor for signs of haemolysis.
  - Monitor for neurological toxicity.
  - Assess creatinine clearance in patients over 65 years before treatment initiation.
- DIRECTIONS FOR ADMINISTRATION Concentrate for intravenous injection or infusion must be diluted before administration (consult product literature).
- NATIONAL FUNDING/ACCESS DECISIONS
  NICE decisions
  - **Fludarabine monotherapy for the first-line treatment of chronic lymphocytic leukaemia (February 2007)** NICE TA119
  Fludarabine monotherapy is **not** recommended for the first-line treatment of chronic lymphocytic leukaemia.
  www.nice.org.uk/TA119
  - **Fludarabine for the treatment of B-cell chronic lymphocytic leukaemia (September 2001)** NICE TA29
  Oral fludarabine is recommended for the second-line treatment of B-cell chronic lymphocytic leukaemia in patients who have either failed, or are intolerant of, first line chemotherapy, and who would otherwise have received combination chemotherapy of either:
    - cyclophosphamide, doxorubicin, vincristine and prednisolone (CHOP)
    - cyclophosphamide, doxorubicin and prednisolone (CAP) **or**
    - cyclophosphamide, vincristine and prednisolone (CVP)
  Intravenous fludarabine should only be used when oral fludarabine is contra-indicated.
  www.nice.org.uk/TA29

  Scottish Medicines Consortium (SMC) Decisions
  The *Scottish Medicines Consortium* has advised (October 2006) that fludarabine is accepted for restricted use for the treatment of B-cell chronic lymphocytic leukaemia (CLL) in patients with sufficient bone marrow reserves. First-line treatment should only be initiated in patients with advanced disease, Rai stages III/IV (Binet stage C), or Rai stages I/II (Binet stage A/B) where the patient has disease-related symptoms or evidence of progressive disease.

- MEDICINAL FORMS
  There can be variation in the licensing of different medicines containing the same drug.
  Solution for injection
  - Fludarabine phosphate (Non-proprietary)
  Fludarabine phosphate 25 mg per 1 ml Fludarabine phosphate 50mg/2ml concentrate for solution for injection vials | 1 vial [PoM] £156.00 (Hospital only) | 1 vial [PoM] £155.00
  Tablet
  - Fludara (Sanofi)
  Fludarabine phosphate 10 mg Fludara 10mg tablets | 15 tablet [PoM] £302.48 (Hospital only) | 20 tablet [PoM] £403.31 (Hospital only)
  Powder for solution for injection
  - Fludarabine phosphate (Non-proprietary)
  Fludarabine phosphate 50 mg Fludarabine phosphate 50mg powder for solution for injection vials | 1 vial [PoM] £155.00 (Hospital only)

▶ Fludara (Sanofi)
Fludarabine phosphate 50 mg Fludara 50mg powder for solution
for injection vials | 5 vial [PoM] £735.34 (Hospital only)

Fluorouracil

● INDICATIONS AND DOSE

**Treatment of some solid tumours including gastro-
intestinal tract cancers and breast cancer | In
combination with folinic acid in advanced colorectal
cancer**

▶ BY INTRAVENOUS INJECTION, OR BY INTRAVENOUS INFUSION,
OR BY INTRA-ARTERIAL INFUSION

▶ Adult: (consult product literature)

● INTERACTIONS → Appendix 1: fluorouracil
● SIDE-EFFECTS
SPECIFIC SIDE-EFFECTS

▶ **Common or very common** Agranulocytosis · alopecia ·
anaemia · anal inflammation · appetite decreased ·
asthenia · bone marrow disorders · diarrhoea ·
gastrointestinal disorders · hand and foot syndrome (long
term use) · ischaemic heart disease · leucopenia · malaise ·
nausea · skin reactions · stomatitis · thrombocytopenia ·
vomiting

▶ **Uncommon** Arrhythmia · cardiomyopathy congestive ·
dizziness · drowsiness · euphoric mood · eye disorders ·
gastrointestinal haemorrhage · headache · hypotension ·
movement disorders · myocardial infarction · nail
discolouration · nail disorders · paronychia ·
photosensitivity reaction · vision disorders

▶ **Rare or very rare** Cardiac arrest · cerebral ischaemia · coma
· confusion · embolism and thrombosis · fever ·
leukoencephalopathy · muscle weakness · peripheral
vascular disease · renal failure · seizure · speech
impairment · sudden cardiac death

▶ **Frequency not known** Peripheral neuropathy

● CONCEPTION AND CONTRACEPTION Contraceptive advice
required, see *Pregnancy and reproductive function* in
Cytotoxic drugs p. 865.

● PREGNANCY Avoid (teratogenic). See also *Pregnancy and
reproductive function* in Cytotoxic drugs p. 865.

● BREAST FEEDING Discontinue breast-feeding.

● HEPATIC IMPAIRMENT Manufacturer advises caution.

● HANDLING AND STORAGE Caution in handling—irritant to
tissues.

● MEDICINAL FORMS
There can be variation in the licensing of different medicines
containing the same drug. Forms available from special-order
manufacturers include: solution for injection

Solution for injection

▶ Fluorouracil (Non-proprietary)
Fluorouracil (as Fluorouracil sodium) 25 mg per 1 ml Fluorouracil
500mg/20ml solution for injection vials | 10 vial [PoM] £64.00
(Hospital only)
Fluorouracil 250mg/10ml solution for injection vials | 5 vial [PoM]
£24.00 (Hospital only)
Fluorouracil (as Fluorouracil sodium) 50 mg per 1 ml Fluorouracil
1g/20ml solution for injection vials | 1 vial [PoM] £12.16–£12.80
Fluorouracil 500mg/10ml solution for injection vials | 1 vial [PoM]
£6.08–£6.40 | 5 vial [PoM] £32.00 (Hospital only)

Solution for infusion

▶ Fluorouracil (Non-proprietary)
Fluorouracil (as Fluorouracil sodium) 25 mg per 1 ml Fluorouracil
2.5g/100ml solution for infusion vials | 1 vial [PoM] £32.00 (Hospital
only) | 1 vial [PoM] £32.00
Fluorouracil (as Fluorouracil sodium) 50 mg per 1 ml Fluorouracil
5g/100ml solution for infusion vials | 1 vial [PoM] £64.00 (Hospital
only) | 1 vial [PoM] £60.80–£64.00
Fluorouracil 2.5g/50ml solution for infusion vials | 1 vial [PoM] £32.00
(Hospital only) | 1 vial [PoM] £30.40–£32.00

Gemcitabine

04-Jul-2017

● INDICATIONS AND DOSE

**First-line treatment for locally advanced or metastatic
non-small cell lung cancer (as monotherapy in elderly
patients and in palliative treatment; otherwise in
combination with cisplatin) | Treatment of locally
advanced or metastatic pancreatic cancer | Treatment of
advanced or metastatic bladder cancer (in combination
with cisplatin) | Treatment of locally advanced or
metastatic epithelial ovarian cancer which has relapsed
after a recurrence-free interval of at least 6 months
following previous platinum-based therapy (in
combination with carboplatin) | Treatment of metastatic
breast cancer which has relapsed after previous
chemotherapy including an anthracycline (in
combination with paclitaxel)**

▶ BY INTRAVENOUS INFUSION

▶ Adult: (consult local protocol)

● INTERACTIONS → Appendix 1: gemcitabine
● SIDE-EFFECTS

▶ **Common or very common** Alopecia · anaemia · appetite
decreased · asthenia · back pain · bone marrow depression ·
chills · constipation · cough · diarrhoea · drowsiness ·
dyspnoea · fever · haematuria · headache · hyperhidrosis ·
influenza like illness · insomnia · leucopenia · myalgia ·
nausea · neutropenia · oedema · oral disorders · proteinuria
· rhinitis · skin reactions · thrombocytopenia · vomiting

▶ **Uncommon** Respiratory disorders

▶ **Rare or very rare** Capillary leak syndrome · hypotension ·
myocardial infarction · posterior reversible
encephalopathy syndrome (PRES) · severe cutaneous
adverse reactions (SCARs) · skin ulcer · thrombocytosis

▶ **Frequency not known** Arrhythmias · colitis ischaemic ·
gangrene · haemolytic uraemic syndrome · heart failure ·
hepatic disorders · pulmonary oedema · radiation injuries ·
renal failure · stroke · vasculitis

SIDE-EFFECTS, FURTHER INFORMATION Gemcitabine
should be discontinued if signs of microangiopathic
haemolytic anaemia occur.

● CONCEPTION AND CONTRACEPTION Manufacturer advises
effective contraception during treatment. Men must avoid
fathering a child during and for 6 months after treatment.

● PREGNANCY Avoid (teratogenic in *animal* studies). See
Pregnancy and reproductive function in Cytotoxic drugs
p. 865.

● BREAST FEEDING Discontinue breast-feeding.

● HEPATIC IMPAIRMENT Manufacturer advises caution.

● RENAL IMPAIRMENT Manufacturer advises caution.

● NATIONAL FUNDING/ACCESS DECISIONS

NICE decisions

▶ Gemcitabine for the treatment of pancreatic cancer (May
2001) NICE TA25
Gemcitabine is an option for first-line chemotherapy for
patients with advanced or metastatic adenocarcinoma of
the pancreas and a Karnofsky score of at least 50
[Karnofsky score is a measure of the ability to perform
ordinary tasks].
Gemcitabine is **not** recommended for patients who can
have potentially curative surgery. There is insufficient
evidence to support its use for second-line treatment of
pancreatic adenocarcinoma.
www.nice.org.uk/guidance/TA25

▶ Gemcitabine for the treatment of metastatic breast cancer
(January 2007) NICE TA116
Gemcitabine, in combination with paclitaxel, is an option
for the treatment of metastatic breast cancer **only** when
docetaxel monotherapy or docetaxel plus capecitabine are
also considered appropriate.
www.nice.org.uk/guidance/TA116

▶ **Bevacizumab in combination with gemcitabine and carboplatin for the treatment of the first recurrence of platinum-sensitive advanced ovarian cancer (May 2013) NICE TA285**

Bevacizumab in combination with gemcitabine and carboplatin is **not** recommended within its marketing authorisation, that is, for the treatment of the first recurrence of platinum-sensitive advanced ovarian cancer (including fallopian tube and primary peritoneal cancer) that has not been previously treated with bevacizumab or other vascular endothelial growth factor (VEGF) inhibitors or VEGF receptor-targeted agents.
www.nice.org.uk/guidance/TA285

▶ **Topotecan, pegylated liposomal doxorubicin hydrochloride, paclitaxel, trabectedin and gemcitabine for treating recurrent ovarian cancer (April 2016) NICE TA389**

Gemcitabine, in combination with carboplatin, is **not** recommended for treating the first recurrence of platinum-sensitive ovarian cancer.

Patients currently receiving gemcitabine in combination with carboplatin should have the option to continue their treatment until they and their clinician consider it appropriate to stop.
www.nice.org.uk/guidance/TA389

▶ **Paclitaxel as albumin-bound nanoparticles with gemcitabine for untreated metastatic pancreatic cancer (September 2017) NICE TA476**

Gemcitabine with paclitaxel as albumin-bound nanoparticles (nab-paclitaxel) is recommended as an option for untreated metastatic adenocarcinoma of the pancreas in adults, only if:
• other combination chemotherapies are unsuitable and they would otherwise have gemcitabine monotherapy, **and**
• the manufacturer provides nab-paclitaxel with the discount agreed in the patient access scheme.

Patients whose treatment with nab-paclitaxel was started before this guidance was published, should have the option to continue treatment until they and their NHS clinician consider it appropriate to stop.
www.nice.org.uk/guidance/TA476

Scottish Medicines Consortium (SMC) Decisions

The *Scottish Medicines Consortium* has advised (December 2006) that gemcitabine (*Gemzar®*) is accepted for restricted use within NHS Scotland for the treatment of metastatic breast cancer, which has relapsed following previous chemotherapy including an anthracycline (unless contra-indicated).

● MEDICINAL FORMS
There can be variation in the licensing of different medicines containing the same drug.

Solution for infusion
▶ Gemcitabine (Non-proprietary)
Gemcitabine (as Gemcitabine hydrochloride)
200 mg Gemcitabine 200mg/5.3ml concentrate for solution for infusion vials | 1 vial PoM £32.00 (Hospital only)
Gemcitabine 200mg/2ml concentrate for solution for infusion vials | 1 vial PoM £6.40
Gemcitabine (as Gemcitabine hydrochloride) 1 gram Gemcitabine 1g/26.3ml concentrate for solution for infusion vials | 1 vial PoM £162.00 (Hospital only)
Gemcitabine 1g/25ml concentrate for solution for infusion vials | 1 vial PoM £13.09
Gemcitabine 1g/10ml concentrate for solution for infusion vials | 1 vial PoM £13.09
Gemcitabine (as Gemcitabine hydrochloride) 2 gram Gemcitabine 2g/50ml concentrate for solution for infusion vials | 1 vial PoM £26.86
Gemcitabine 2g/20ml concentrate for solution for infusion vials | 1 vial PoM £26.86
Gemcitabine 2g/52.6ml concentrate for solution for infusion vials | 1 vial PoM £324.00 (Hospital only)

Gemcitabine (as Gemcitabine hydrochloride) 10 mg per 1 ml Gemcitabine 1.6g/160ml infusion bags | 1 bag PoM £140.00
Gemcitabine 2.2g/220ml infusion bags | 1 bag PoM £200.00
Gemcitabine 2g/200ml infusion bags | 1 bag PoM £180.00
Gemcitabine 1.2g/120ml infusion bags | 1 bag PoM £120.00
Gemcitabine 1.8g/180ml infusion bags | 1 bag PoM £160.00

Powder for solution for infusion
▶ Gemcitabine (Non-proprietary)
Gemcitabine (as Gemcitabine hydrochloride)
200 mg Gemcitabine 200mg powder for solution for infusion vials | 1 vial PoM £32.00–£32.55 (Hospital only) | 1 vial PoM £30.93–£32.00
Gemcitabine (as Gemcitabine hydrochloride) 1 gram Gemcitabine 1g powder for solution for infusion vials | 1 vial PoM £162.00–£162.76 (Hospital only) | 1 vial PoM £154.62–£162.00
Gemcitabine (as Gemcitabine hydrochloride)
1.5 gram Gemcitabine 1.5g powder for solution for infusion vials | 1 vial PoM £231.93
Gemcitabine (as Gemcitabine hydrochloride) 2 gram Gemcitabine 2g powder for solution for infusion vials | 1 vial PoM £324.00 (Hospital only) | 1 vial PoM £324.00
▶ Gemzar (Eli Lilly and Company Ltd)
Gemcitabine (as Gemcitabine hydrochloride) 200 mg Gemzar 200mg powder for solution for infusion vials | 1 vial PoM £32.55 (Hospital only)
Gemcitabine (as Gemcitabine hydrochloride) 1 gram Gemzar 1g powder for solution for infusion vials | 1 vial PoM £162.76 (Hospital only)

Mercaptopurine

(6-Mercaptopurine)

● INDICATIONS AND DOSE

Severe acute Crohn's disease | Maintenance of remission of Crohn's disease | Ulcerative colitis
▶ BY MOUTH
▶ Adult: 1–1.5 mg/kg daily, some patients may respond to lower doses

Acute leukaemias | Chronic myeloid leukaemia
▶ BY MOUTH USING TABLETS
▶ Adult: Initially 2.5 mg/kg daily, adjusted according to response, alternatively initially 50–75 mg/m² daily, adjusted according to response
▶ BY MOUTH USING ORAL SUSPENSION
▶ Adult: Initially 25–75 mg/m² daily, adjusted according to response

DOSE ADJUSTMENTS DUE TO INTERACTIONS
▶ Manufacturer advises reduce dose to one-quarter of the usual dose with concurrent use of allopurinol.

DOSE EQUIVALENCE AND CONVERSION
▶ Mercaptopurine tablets and *Xaluprine®* oral suspension are **not** bioequivalent, haematological monitoring is advised when switching formulations.

● UNLICENSED USE Not licensed for use in severe ulcerative colitis and Crohn's disease.

IMPORTANT SAFETY INFORMATION
SAFE PRACTICE
Mercaptopurine has been confused with mercaptamine; care must be taken to ensure the correct drug is prescribed and dispensed.

RISKS OF INCORRECT DOSING OF ORAL ANTI-CANCER MEDICINES
See Cytotoxic drugs p. 865.

● CONTRA-INDICATIONS Absent thiopurine methyltransferase activity
● CAUTIONS Reduced thiopurine methyltransferase activity
CAUTIONS, FURTHER INFORMATION
▶ Thiopurine methyltransferase The enzyme thiopurine methyltransferase (TPMT) metabolises thiopurine drugs (azathioprine, mercaptopurine, tioguanine); the risk of

8

Immune system and malignant disease

myelosuppression is increased in patients with reduced activity of the enzyme, particularly for the few individuals in whom TPMT activity is undetectable. Patients with absent TPMT activity should not receive thiopurine drugs; those with reduced TPMT activity may be treated under specialist supervision.

- INTERACTIONS → Appendix 1: mercaptopurine
- SIDE-EFFECTS
- ▸ **Common or very common** Anaemia · appetite decreased · bone marrow depression · diarrhoea · hepatic disorders · hepatotoxicity (more common at high doses) · leucopenia · nausea · oral disorders · thrombocytopenia · vomiting
- ▸ **Uncommon** Arthralgia · fever · increased risk of infection · neutropenia · pancreatitis · rash
- ▸ **Rare or very rare** Alopecia · face oedema · intestinal ulcer · neoplasms · oligozoospermia
- ▸ **Frequency not known** Photosensitivity reaction
- CONCEPTION AND CONTRACEPTION Contraceptive advice required, see *Pregnancy and reproductive function* in Cytotoxic drugs p. 865.
- PREGNANCY Avoid (teratogenic). See also *Pregnancy and reproductive function* in Cytotoxic drugs p. 865.
- BREAST FEEDING Discontinue breast-feeding.
- HEPATIC IMPAIRMENT
  Dose adjustments May need dose reduction.
- RENAL IMPAIRMENT
  Dose adjustments Reduce dose.
- PRE-TREATMENT SCREENING Consider measuring thiopurine methyltransferase (TPMT) activity before starting mercaptopurine therapy.
- MONITORING REQUIREMENTS Monitor liver function.
- PRESCRIBING AND DISPENSING INFORMATION Flavours of oral liquid formulations may include raspberry.

- MEDICINAL FORMS
  There can be variation in the licensing of different medicines containing the same drug. Forms available from special-order manufacturers include: tablet, capsule, oral suspension
  Tablet
  - ▸ Mercaptopurine (Non-proprietary)
    Mercaptopurine 50 mg Mercaptopurine 50mg tablets | 25 tablet [PoM] £49.15 DT = £49.15

Methotrexate

17-May-2017

- DRUG ACTION Methotrexate inhibits the enzyme dihydrofolate reductase, essential for the synthesis of purines and pyrimidines.

- INDICATIONS AND DOSE
  Severe Crohn's disease
  - ▸ BY INTRAMUSCULAR INJECTION
  - ▸ Adult: Initially 25 mg once weekly until remission induced; maintenance 15 mg once weekly
  Maintenance of remission of severe Crohn's disease
  - ▸ BY MOUTH
  - ▸ Adult: 10–25 mg once weekly
  Moderate to severe active rheumatoid arthritis
  - ▸ BY MOUTH
  - ▸ Adult: 7.5 mg once weekly, adjusted according to response; maximum 20 mg per week
  Severe active rheumatoid arthritis
  - ▸ BY INTRAMUSCULAR INJECTION, OR BY SUBCUTANEOUS INJECTION
  - ▸ Adult: Initially 7.5 mg once weekly, then increased in steps of 2.5 mg once weekly, adjusted according to response; maximum 25 mg per week

Neoplastic diseases
- ▸ BY MOUTH, OR BY INTRAVENOUS INJECTION, OR BY INTRAVENOUS INFUSION, OR BY INTRA-ARTERIAL INFUSION, OR BY INTRAMUSCULAR INJECTION, OR BY INTRATHECAL INJECTION
- ▸ Adult: (consult product literature)
Severe psoriasis unresponsive to conventional therapy (specialist use only)
- ▸ BY MOUTH, OR BY INTRAMUSCULAR INJECTION, OR BY INTRAVENOUS INJECTION, OR BY SUBCUTANEOUS INJECTION
- ▸ Adult: Initially 2.5–10 mg once weekly, then increased in steps of 2.5–5 mg, adjusted according to response, dose to be adjusted at intervals of at least 1 week; usual dose 7.5–15 mg once weekly, stop treatment if inadequate response after 3 months at the optimum dose; maximum 30 mg per week

- UNLICENSED USE Not licensed for use in severe Crohn's disease.

IMPORTANT SAFETY INFORMATION
Note that the dose is a **weekly** dose. To avoid error with low-dose methotrexate, it is recommended that:
- the patient is carefully advised of the **dose** and **frequency** and the reason for taking methotrexate and any other prescribed medicine (e.g. folic acid);
- only one strength of methotrexate tablet (usually 2.5 mg) is prescribed and dispensed;
- the prescription and the dispensing label clearly show the dose and frequency of methotrexate administration;
- the patient is warned to report immediately the onset of any feature of blood disorders (e.g. sore throat, bruising, and mouth ulcers), liver toxicity (e.g. nausea, vomiting, abdominal discomfort, and dark urine), and respiratory effects (e.g. shortness of breath).

- CONTRA-INDICATIONS Active infection (in non-malignant conditions) · ascites · immunodeficiency syndromes (in non-malignant conditions) · significant pleural effusion
- CAUTIONS Photosensitivity—psoriasis lesions aggravated by UV radiation (skin ulceration reported) · diarrhoea · extreme caution in blood disorders (avoid if severe) · peptic ulceration · risk of accumulation in pleural effusion or ascites— drain before treatment · ulcerative colitis · ulcerative stomatitis
  CAUTIONS, FURTHER INFORMATION
- ▸ Blood count Bone marrow suppression can occur abruptly; factors likely to increase toxicity include advanced age, renal impairment, and concomitant use with another anti-folate drug (e.g. trimethoprim). A clinically significant drop in white cell count or platelet count calls for immediate withdrawal of methotrexate and introduction of supportive therapy.
- ▸ Gastro-intestinal toxicity Withdraw treatment if stomatitis develops—may be first sign of gastro-intestinal toxicity.
- ▸ Liver toxicity Liver cirrhosis reported. Treatment should not be started or should be discontinued if any abnormality of liver function tests or liver biopsy is present or develops during therapy. Abnormalities can return to normal within 2 weeks after which treatment may be recommended if judged appropriate.
- ▸ Pulmonary toxicity Pulmonary toxicity may be a special problem in rheumatoid arthritis (patient to seek medical attention if dyspnoea, cough or fever); monitor for symptoms at each visit—discontinue if pneumonitis suspected.

- INTERACTIONS → Appendix 1: methotrexate

- **SIDE-EFFECTS**
  SPECIFIC SIDE-EFFECTS
▸ **Common or very common**
▹ With intra-arterial and intravenous use Abdominal distress · fever · headache · leucopenia · nausea · oral disorders · vomiting
▹ With intramuscular and subcutaneous use Anaemia · appetite decreased · chest pain · cough · diarrhoea · drowsiness · dyspnoea · fatigue · fever · gastrointestinal discomfort · headache · leucopenia · malaise · nausea · oral disorders · respiratory disorders · skin reactions · throat complaints · thrombocytopenia · vomiting
▹ With intrathecal use Arachnoiditis · fever · headache · nausea · necrotising demyelinating leukoencephalopathy · neurotoxicity · vomiting
▹ With oral use Anaemia · appetite decreased · diarrhoea · drowsiness · fatigue · fever · gastrointestinal discomfort · headache · increased risk of infection · leucopenia · nausea · oral disorders · respiratory disorders · skin reactions · throat ulcer · thrombocytopenia · vomiting
▸ **Uncommon**
▹ With intramuscular use Agranulocytosis · alopecia · arthralgia · bone marrow disorders · confusion · cystitis · depression · diabetes mellitus · drug toxicity · dysuria · gastrointestinal disorders · haemorrhage · healing impaired · hepatic disorders · increased risk of infection · lipoatrophy · local reaction · myalgia · neoplasms · osteoporosis · pain · paraesthesia · photosensitivity reaction · rheumatoid arthritis aggravated · seizure · severe cutaneous adverse reactions (SCARs) · sterile abscess · vasculitis · vertigo · vulvovaginal disorders
▹ With oral use Agranulocytosis · alopecia · arthralgia · bone marrow disorders · chills · confusion · cystitis · depression · diabetes mellitus · dysuria · gastrointestinal disorders · haemorrhage · healing impaired · hepatic disorders · myalgia · neoplasms · nephropathy · osteoporosis · photosensitivity reaction · rheumatoid arthritis aggravated · seizure · severe cutaneous adverse reactions (SCARs) · vasculitis · vertigo · vulvovaginal disorders
▹ With subcutaneous use Agranulocytosis · alopecia · arthralgia · bone marrow disorders · confusion · cystitis · depression · diabetes mellitus · drug toxicity · dysuria · gastrointestinal disorders · haemorrhage · healing impaired · hepatic disorders · increased risk of infection · myalgia · neoplasms · osteoporosis · pain · paraesthesia · photosensitivity reaction · rheumatoid arthritis aggravated · seizure · severe cutaneous adverse reactions (SCARs) · vasculitis · vertigo · vulvovaginal disorders
▸ **Rare or very rare**
▹ With intra-arterial and intravenous use Anaemia · bone marrow depression · gastrointestinal disorders · hepatic disorders · hypogammaglobulinaemia · necrosis · respiratory disorders · skin reactions · thrombocytopenia
▹ With intramuscular and subcutaneous use Apnoea · asthma-like conditions · azotaemia · conjunctivitis · eosinophilia · gynaecomastia · hypotension · immune deficiency · infertility · influenza like illness · insomnia · lymphadenopathy · meningism · meningitis aseptic · menstrual disorder · mood swings · muscle weakness · nail discolouration · neutropenia · oligozoospermia · paralysis · pericardial disorders · pericarditis · proteinuria · reactivation of infection · renal impairment · retinopathy · sepsis · sexual dysfunction · stress fracture · taste altered · telangiectasia · thromboembolism · visual impairment
▹ With oral use Azotaemia · brain oedema · cognitive impairment · conjunctivitis · cough · dyspnoea · eosinophilia · gynaecomastia · hypotension · immune deficiency · infertility · insomnia · lymphadenopathy · meningitis aseptic · menstrual disorder · mood altered · muscle weakness · nail discolouration · neutropenia · oligozoospermia · pain · pancreatitis · paresis · pericardial disorders · pericarditis · proteinuria · psychosis · radiation

injuries · renal impairment · retinopathy · sensation abnormal · sepsis · sexual dysfunction · speech impairment · stress fracture · taste metallic · telangiectasia · tinnitus · visual impairment
▸ **Frequency not known**
▹ With intra-arterial and intravenous use Alopecia · aphasia · appetite decreased · arthralgia · azotaemia · chills · cognitive disorder · conjunctivitis · cystitis · defective oogenesis · diabetes mellitus · diarrhoea · dizziness · drowsiness · embolism and thrombosis · fatigue · haemorrhage · hemiparesis · hypotension · increased risk of infection · infertility · leukoencephalopathy · malaise · menstrual disorder · metabolic change · mood altered · mucositis · myalgia · neoplasms · nephropathy · osteoporosis · pancreatitis · pericardial effusion · pericarditis · photosensitivity reaction · pulmonary oedema · renal failure · seizure · sepsis · severe cutaneous adverse reactions (SCARs) · skin ulcer · sperm abnormalities · sudden death · telangiectasia · tinnitus · vaginal ulceration · vasculitis · vision blurred
▹ With oral use Encephalopathy
▹ With intramuscular and subcutaneous use Leukoencephalopathy

SIDE-EFFECTS, FURTHER INFORMATION Give folic acid to reduce side-effects. Folic acid decreases mucosal and gastrointestinal side-effects of methotrexate and may prevent hepatotoxicity; there is no evidence of a reduction in haematological side-effects.
  Withdraw treatment if ulcerative stomatitis develops—may be first sign of gastro-intestinal toxicity.
  Treatment with folinic acid (as calcium folinate) may be required in acute toxicity.

- **CONCEPTION AND CONTRACEPTION** Effective contraception required during and for at least 3 months after treatment in men or women.

- **PREGNANCY** Avoid (teratogenic; fertility may be reduced during therapy but this may be reversible).

- **BREAST FEEDING** Discontinue breast-feeding—present in milk.

- **HEPATIC IMPAIRMENT** When used for malignancy, avoid in severe hepatic impairment—consult local treatment protocol for details. Avoid with hepatic impairment in non-malignant conditions—dose-related toxicity.

- **RENAL IMPAIRMENT** Risk of nephrotoxicity at high doses. Avoid in severe impairment.
  Dose adjustments Reduce dose.

- **PRE-TREATMENT SCREENING** Exclude pregnancy before treatment.
  Patients should have full blood count and renal and liver function tests before starting treatment.

- **MONITORING REQUIREMENTS**
▸ In view of reports of blood dyscrasias (including fatalities) and liver cirrhosis with low-dose methotrexate patients should:
  - have full blood count and renal and liver function tests repeated every 1–2 weeks until therapy stabilised, thereafter patients should be monitored every 2–3 months.
  - be advised to report all symptoms and signs suggestive of infection, especially sore throat
▸ Local protocols for frequency of monitoring may vary.
▸ Treatment with folinic acid (as calcium folinate) may be required in acute toxicity.

- **PRESCRIBING AND DISPENSING INFORMATION** Folinic acid following methotrexate administration helps to prevent methotrexate-induced mucositis and myelosuppression.
  The licensed routes of administration for parenteral preparations vary—further information can be found in the product literature for the individual preparations.

8

Immune system and malignant disease

• PATIENT AND CARER ADVICE Patients and their carers should be warned to report immediately the onset of any feature of blood disorders (e.g. sore throat, bruising, and mouth ulcers), liver toxicity (e.g. nausea, vomiting, abdominal discomfort and dark urine), and respiratory effects (e.g. shortness of breath).

Patients should be advised to avoid self-medication with over-the-counter aspirin or ibuprofen.

Patients should be counselled on the dose, treatment booklet, and the use of NSAIDs.

Methotrexate treatment booklets Methotrexate treatment booklets should be issued where appropriate.

In **England, Wales**, and **Northern Ireland**, they are available for purchase from:
Gorse Street, Chadderton
Oldham
OL9 9QH
Tel: 0845 610 1112

GP practices can obtain supplies through their Local Area Team stores.

NHS Hospitals can order supplies from www.nhsforms.co.uk or by emailing nhsforms@mmm.com.

In **Scotland**, treatment booklets can be obtained by emailing stockorders.dppas@theapsgroup.com or by fax on 0131 629 9967.

These booklets include advice for adults taking oral methotrexate for inflammatory conditions, and a section for recording results of blood tests and dosage information.

• MEDICINAL FORMS
There can be variation in the licensing of different medicines containing the same drug. Forms available from special-order manufacturers include: oral suspension, oral solution, solution for injection

Tablet
▸ Methotrexate (Non-proprietary)
Methotrexate 2.5 mg Methotrexate 2.5mg tablets | 24 tablet PoM £1.23-£3.75 | 28 tablet PoM £3.82 DT = £1.44 | 100 tablet PoM £5.14-£14.01
Methotrexate 10 mg Methotrexate 10mg tablets | 100 tablet PoM £57.21 DT = £49.33
▸ Maxtrex (Pfizer Ltd)
Methotrexate 2.5 mg Maxtrex 2.5mg tablets | 24 tablet PoM £2.39 | 100 tablet PoM £9.96
Methotrexate 10 mg Maxtrex 10mg tablets | 100 tablet PoM £45.16 DT = £49.33

Solution for injection
▸ Methotrexate (Non-proprietary)
Methotrexate (as Methotrexate sodium) 2.5 mg per 1 ml Methotrexate 5mg/2ml solution for injection vials | 5 vial PoM £36.00 (Hospital only)
Methotrexate (as Methotrexate sodium) 25 mg per 1 ml Methotrexate 1g/40ml solution for injection vials | 1 vial PoM £1,452.55 (Hospital only) | 1 vial PoM £44.57
Methotrexate 500mg/20ml solution for injection vials | 1 vial PoM £48.00-£726.28 (Hospital only) | 1 vial PoM £25.07
Methotrexate 50mg/2ml solution for injection vials | 1 vial PoM £2.62-£72.63 | 5 vial PoM £35.00 (Hospital only)
Methotrexate 200mg/8ml solution for injection vials | 1 vial PoM £10.02
Methotrexate (as Methotrexate sodium) 100 mg per 1 ml Methotrexate 1g/10ml solution for injection vials | 1 vial PoM £85.00 (Hospital only)
▸ Methofill (Accord Healthcare Ltd)
Methotrexate 50 mg per 1 ml Methofill 12.5mg/0.25ml solution for injection pre-filled injector | 1 pre-filled disposable injection PoM £14.85 DT = £16.50
Methofill 22.5mg/0.45ml solution for injection pre-filled injector | 1 pre-filled disposable injection PoM £16.61 DT = £18.45
Methofill 30mg/0.6ml solution for injection pre-filled injector | 1 pre-filled disposable injection PoM £17.06 DT = £18.95
Methofill 27.5mg/0.55ml solution for injection pre-filled injector | 1 pre-filled disposable injection PoM £17.00 DT = £18.89
Methofill 7.5mg/0.15ml solution for injection pre-filled injector | 1 pre-filled disposable injection PoM £13.37 DT = £14.85

Methofill 20mg/0.4ml solution for injection pre-filled injector | 1 pre-filled disposable injection PoM £16.06 DT = £17.84
Methofill 10mg/0.2ml solution for injection pre-filled injector | 1 pre-filled disposable injection PoM £13.76 DT = £15.29
Methofill 15mg/0.3ml solution for injection pre-filled injector | 1 pre-filled disposable injection PoM £14.91 DT = £16.57
Methofill 17.5mg/0.35ml solution for injection pre-filled injector | 1 pre-filled disposable injection PoM £15.75 DT = £17.50
Methofill 25mg/0.5ml solution for injection pre-filled injector | 1 pre-filled disposable injection PoM £16.63 DT = £18.48
▸ Metoject PEN (medac UK)
Methotrexate 50 mg per 1 ml Metoject PEN 30mg/0.6ml solution for injection pre-filled pen | 1 pre-filled disposable injection PoM £16.56 DT = £18.95
Metoject PEN 22.5mg/0.45ml solution for injection pre-filled pen | 1 pre-filled disposable injection PoM £16.11 DT = £18.45
Metoject PEN 12.5mg/0.25ml solution for injection pre-filled pen | 1 pre-filled disposable injection PoM £14.35 DT = £16.50
Metoject PEN 20mg/0.4ml solution for injection pre-filled pen | 1 pre-filled disposable injection PoM £15.56 DT = £17.84
Metoject PEN 17.5mg/0.35ml solution for injection pre-filled pen | 1 pre-filled disposable injection PoM £15.25 DT = £17.50
Metoject PEN 7.5mg/0.15ml solution for injection pre-filled pen | 1 pre-filled disposable injection PoM £12.87 DT = £14.85
Metoject PEN 10mg/0.2ml solution for injection pre-filled pen | 1 pre-filled disposable injection PoM £13.26 DT = £15.29
Metoject PEN 27.5mg/0.55ml solution for injection pre-filled pen | 1 pre-filled disposable injection PoM £16.50 DT = £18.89
Metoject PEN 25mg/0.5ml solution for injection pre-filled pen | 1 pre-filled disposable injection PoM £16.13 DT = £18.48
Metoject PEN 15mg/0.3ml solution for injection pre-filled pen | 1 pre-filled disposable injection PoM £14.41 DT = £16.57
▸ Nordimet (Nordic Pharma Ltd)
Methotrexate 25 mg per 1 ml Nordimet 15mg/0.6ml solution for injection pre-filled pens | 1 pre-filled disposable injection PoM £14.92 DT = £14.92
Nordimet 20mg/0.8ml solution for injection pre-filled pens | 1 pre-filled disposable injection PoM £16.06 DT = £16.06
Nordimet 22.5mg/0.9ml solution for injection pre-filled pens | 1 pre-filled disposable injection PoM £16.61 DT = £16.61
Nordimet 12.5mg/0.5ml solution for injection pre-filled pens | 1 pre-filled disposable injection PoM £14.85 DT = £14.85
Nordimet 10mg/0.4ml solution for injection pre-filled pens | 1 pre-filled disposable injection PoM £13.77 DT = £13.77
Nordimet 17.5mg/0.7ml solution for injection pre-filled pens | 1 pre-filled disposable injection PoM £15.75 DT = £15.75
Nordimet 25mg/1ml solution for injection pre-filled pens | 1 pre-filled disposable injection PoM £16.64 DT = £16.64
Nordimet 7.5mg/0.3ml solution for injection pre-filled pens | 1 pre-filled disposable injection PoM £13.37 DT = £13.37
▸ Zlatal (Nordic Pharma Ltd)
Methotrexate (as Methotrexate sodium) 25 mg per 1 ml Zlatal 17.5mg/0.7ml solution for injection pre-filled syringes | 1 pre-filled disposable injection PoM £15.75 DT = £15.75
Zlatal 10mg/0.4ml solution for injection pre-filled syringes | 1 pre-filled disposable injection PoM £13.77 DT = £13.77
Zlatal 25mg/1ml solution for injection pre-filled syringes | 1 pre-filled disposable injection PoM £16.64 DT = £16.64
Zlatal 20mg/0.8ml solution for injection pre-filled syringes | 1 pre-filled disposable injection PoM £16.06 DT = £16.06
Zlatal 12.5mg/0.5ml solution for injection pre-filled syringes | 1 pre-filled disposable injection PoM £14.85 DT = £14.85
Zlatal 7.5mg/0.3ml solution for injection pre-filled syringes | 1 pre-filled disposable injection PoM £13.37 DT = £13.37
Zlatal 22.5mg/0.9ml solution for injection pre-filled syringes | 1 pre-filled disposable injection PoM £16.61 DT = £16.61
Zlatal 15mg/0.6ml solution for injection pre-filled syringes | 1 pre-filled disposable injection PoM £14.92 DT = £14.92

Solution for infusion
▸ Methotrexate (Non-proprietary)
Methotrexate (as Methotrexate sodium) 25 mg per 1 ml Methotrexate 5g/200ml solution for infusion vials | 1 vial PoM £200.57
Methotrexate (as Methotrexate sodium) 100 mg per 1 ml Methotrexate 5g/50ml solution for infusion vials | 1 vial PoM £400.00 (Hospital only)

Oral solution

▸ Methotrexate (Non-proprietary)
Methotrexate (as Methotrexate sodium) 2 mg per 1 ml Methotrexate 2mg/ml oral solution sugar free sugar-free | 35 ml [PoM] £95.00 DT = £95.00 sugar-free | 65 ml [PoM] £125.00 DT = £125.00

▸ Jylamvo (Intrapharm Laboratories Ltd)
Methotrexate (as Methotrexate sodium) 2 mg per 1 ml Jylamvo 2mg/ml oral solution sugar-free | 60 ml [PoM] £112.50

Nelarabine

● **INDICATIONS AND DOSE**

T-cell acute lymphoblastic leukaemia and T-cell lymphoblastic lymphoma in patients who have relapsed or who are refractory after receiving at least two previous regimens

▸ BY INTRAVENOUS INFUSION
▸ Adult: (consult local protocol)

● CAUTIONS Previous or concurrent craniospinal irradiation (increased risk of neurotoxicity) · previous or concurrent intrathecal chemotherapy (increased risk of neurotoxicity)

● INTERACTIONS → Appendix 1: nelarabine

● SIDE-EFFECTS

▸ **Common or very common** Abdominal pain · anaemia · appetite decreased · arthralgia · asthenia · confusion · constipation · cough · diarrhoea · dizziness · drowsiness · dyspnoea · electrolyte imbalance · fever · gait abnormal · headache · hyperbilirubinaemia · hypotension · increased risk of infection · leucopenia · memory loss · movement disorders · muscle weakness · myalgia · nausea · neutropenia · oedema · pain · peripheral neuropathy · respiratory disorders · seizures · sensation abnormal · stomatitis · taste altered · thrombocytopenia · tremor · tumour lysis syndrome · vision blurred · vomiting

▸ **Rare or very rare** Rhabdomyolysis

▸ **Frequency not known** Progressive multifocal leukoencephalopathy

SIDE-EFFECTS, FURTHER INFORMATION If neurotoxicity occurs, treatment should be discontinued.

● CONCEPTION AND CONTRACEPTION Manufacturer advises effective contraception during and for at least 3 months after treatment in men and women.

● PREGNANCY Avoid (toxicity in *animal* studies). See also *Pregnancy and reproductive function* in Cytotoxic drugs p. 865.

● BREAST FEEDING Discontinue breast-feeding.

● MONITORING REQUIREMENTS

▸ Neurotoxicity Close monitoring for neurological events is strongly recommended—discontinue if neurotoxicty occurs.

● PATIENT AND CARER ADVICE
Driving and skilled tasks Drowsiness may affect performance of skilled tasks (e.g. cycling or driving).

● NATIONAL FUNDING/ACCESS DECISIONS

Scottish Medicines Consortium (SMC) Decisions
The *Scottish Medicines Consortium* has advised (March 2008) that the use of nelarabine (*Atriance®*) within NHS Scotland is restricted to bridging treatment before stem cell transplantation.

● MEDICINAL FORMS
There can be variation in the licensing of different medicines containing the same drug.
Solution for infusion
ELECTROLYTES: May contain Sodium
▸ Atriance (Novartis Pharmaceuticals UK Ltd) ▼
Nelarabine 5 mg per 1 ml Atriance 250mg/50ml solution for infusion vials | 6 vial [PoM] £1,332.00

Pemetrexed

07-Jul-2017

● DRUG ACTION Pemetrexed inhibits thymidylate transferase and other folate-dependent enzymes.

● **INDICATIONS AND DOSE**

Treatment of unresectable malignant pleural mesothelioma which has not previously been treated with chemotherapy (in combination with cisplatin) | First-line treatment of locally advanced or metastatic non-small cell lung cancer other than predominantly squamous cell histology (in combination with cisplatin) | Second-line treatment of locally advanced or metastatic non-small cell lung cancer other than predominantly squamous cell histology (monotherapy) | Maintenance treatment in locally advanced or metastatic non-small cell lung cancer other than predominantly squamous cell histology that has not progressed immediately following platinum-based chemotherapy (monotherapy)

▸ BY INTRAVENOUS INFUSION
▸ Adult: (consult local protocol)

● CAUTIONS Diabetes · history of cardiovascular disease · prophylactic folic acid supplementation required (consult product literature) · prophylactic vitamin B_{12} supplementation required (consult product literature)

● INTERACTIONS → Appendix 1: pemetrexed

● SIDE-EFFECTS

▸ **Common or very common** Appetite decreased · fatigue · mucositis · nausea · neuropathy sensory · oedema · pain · renal disorder · skin reactions · stomatitis · vomiting

● CONCEPTION AND CONTRACEPTION Manufacturer advises effective contraception during treatment. Men must avoid fathering a child during and for 6 months after treatment.

● PREGNANCY Avoid (toxicity in *animal* studies). See also *Pregnancy and reproductive function* in Cytotoxic drugs p. 865.

● BREAST FEEDING Discontinue breast-feeding.

● RENAL IMPAIRMENT Manufacturer advises avoid if creatinine clearance less than 45 mL/minute—no information available.

● NATIONAL FUNDING/ACCESS DECISIONS

NICE decisions

▸ **Pemetrexed for the treatment of non-small cell lung cancer (August 2007)** NICE TA124
Pemetrexed is **not** recommended for the treatment of locally advanced or metastatic non-small cell lung cancer which has previously been treated with chemotherapy.
www.nice.org.uk/TA124

▸ **Pemetrexed for the first-line treatment of non-small cell lung cancer (September 2009)** NICE TA181
Pemetrexed, in combination with cisplatin, is an option for the first-line treatment of locally advanced or metastatic non-small cell lung cancer only if the histology of the tumour has been confirmed as adenocarcinoma or large-cell carcinoma.
www.nice.org.uk/TA181

▸ **Pemetrexed for the maintenance treatment of non-small-cell lung cancer (updated August 2017)** NICE TA190
Pemetrexed is recommended as an option for the maintenance treatment of locally advanced or metastatic non-small cell lung cancer other than predominantly squamous cell histology if disease has not progressed immediately following platinum-based chemotherapy in combination with gemcitabine, paclitaxel or docetaxel.
www.nice.org.uk/guidance/TA190

▸ **Pemetrexed maintenance treatment for non-squamous non-small cell lung cancer after pemetrexed and cisplatin (August 2016)** NICE TA402
Pemetrexed is recommended as an option for the maintenance treatment of locally advanced or metastatic

8

Immune system and malignant disease

non-squamous non-small cell lung cancer in patients when:

- their disease has not progressed immediately after 4 cycles of pemetrexed and cisplatin induction therapy
- their Eastern Cooperative Oncology Group performance status is 0 or 1 at the start of maintenance treatment, **and,**
- the company provides the drug according to the terms of the commercial access agreement as agreed with NHS England.

Patients whose treatment was started within the NHS before this guidance was published should have the option to continue treatment, without change to their funding arrangements, until they and their clinician consider it appropriate to stop.
www.nice.org.uk/TA402

▸ Pemetrexed for the treatment of malignant pleural mesothelioma (January 2008) NICE TA135
Pemetrexed is an option for the treatment of malignant pleural mesothelioma only in patients who have a WHO performance status of 0 or 1 [WHO performance status is a measure of the ability to perform ordinary tasks], who are considered to have advanced disease and for whom surgical resection is considered inappropriate.
www.nice.org.uk/TA135

Scottish Medicines Consortium (SMC) Decisions
The *Scottish Medicines Consortium* has advised (September 2008) that pemetrexed (*Alimta* ®) is accepted for restricted use within NHS Scotland as monotherapy for the second-line treatment of locally advanced or metastatic non-small cell lung cancer other than predominantly squamous cell histology. It is restricted for use in patients with good performance status who would otherwise be eligible for docetaxel treatment.

The *Scottish Medicines Consortium* has advised (February 2010) that pemetrexed (*Alimta* ®) is accepted for restricted use within NHS Scotland in combination with cisplatin for the first-line treatment of locally advanced or metastatic non-small-cell lung cancer other than predominantly squamous cell histology. It is restricted to patients in whom histology has been confirmed as adenocarcinoma or large cell carcinoma.

● MEDICINAL FORMS
There can be variation in the licensing of different medicines containing the same drug.

Solution for infusion
▸ Pemetrexed (Non-proprietary)
Pemetrexed (as Pemetrexed ditrometamol) 25 mg per 1 ml Pemetrexed 100mg/4ml concentrate for solution for infusion vials | 1 vial [PoM] £140.00
Pemetrexed 500mg/20ml concentrate for solution for infusion vials | 1 vial [PoM] £700.00
Pemetrexed 1000mg/40ml concentrate for solution for infusion vials | 1 vial [PoM] £1,400.00

Powder for solution for infusion
ELECTROLYTES: May contain Sodium
▸ Pemetrexed (Non-proprietary)
Pemetrexed (as Pemetrexed disodium) 100 mg Pemetrexed 100mg powder for concentrate for solution for infusion vials | 1 vial [PoM] £160.00–£245.00 (Hospital only)
Pemetrexed (as Pemetrexed disodium) 500 mg Pemetrexed 500mg powder for concentrate for solution for infusion vials | 1 vial [PoM] £800.00–£910.00 (Hospital only)
▸ Alimta (Eli Lilly and Company Ltd)
Pemetrexed (as Pemetrexed disodium) 100 mg Alimta 100mg powder for concentrate for solution for infusion vials | 1 vial [PoM] £160.00 (Hospital only)
Pemetrexed (as Pemetrexed disodium) 500 mg Alimta 500mg powder for concentrate for solution for infusion vials | 1 vial [PoM] £800.00 (Hospital only)

Tegafur with gimeracil and oteracil

● DRUG ACTION Tegafur is a prodrug of fluorouracil. Gimeracil inhibits the degradation of fluorouracil and oteracil decreases the activity of fluorouracil in normal gastrointestinal mucosa.

● INDICATIONS AND DOSE
Treatment of advanced gastric cancer when used in combination with cisplatin
▸ BY MOUTH
▸ Adult: (consult local protocol)

> IMPORTANT SAFETY INFORMATION
> RISKS OF INCORRECT DOSING OF ORAL ANTI-CANCER MEDICINES
> See Cytotoxic drugs p. 865.

● CONTRA-INDICATIONS Dihydropyrimidine dehydrogenase deficiency

● INTERACTIONS → Appendix 1: tegafur

● SIDE-EFFECTS
▸ **Common or very common** Anaemia · appetite abnormal · asthenia · constipation · cough · decreased leucocytes · dehydration · diarrhoea · dizziness · dry mouth · dysphagia · dyspnoea · electrolyte imbalance · embolism and thrombosis · eye disorders · eye inflammation · gastrointestinal discomfort · gastrointestinal disorders · haemorrhage · headache · hearing impairment · hiccups · hyperbilirubinaemia · hypertension · hypoproteinaemia · hypotension · insomnia · nausea · nerve disorders · neutropenia · oral disorders · taste altered · thrombocytopenia · vision disorders · vomiting
▸ **Uncommon** Aerophagia · allergic rhinitis · alopecia · angina pectoris · anxiety · aphasia · arrhythmias · ascites · breast abnormalities · burping · cerebrovascular insufficiency · chills · coagulation disorders · confusion · depression · drowsiness · dysphonia · ear discomfort · encephalopathy · eosinophilia · fever · gout · hallucination · heart failure · hemiparesis · hyperglobulinaemia · hyperglycaemia · hyperlipidaemia · hypertrichosis · hypovolaemic shock · increased leucocytes · increased risk of infection · joint disorders · limb discomfort · loss of consciousness · memory loss · movement disorders · mucositis · muscle complaints · muscle weakness · myocardial infarction · nail disorders · nasal complaints · neoplasm complications · nephrotoxicity · oedema · pain · palpitations · pancytopenia · pericardial effusion · personality disorder · renal impairment · seizure · sensation abnormal · sepsis · sexual dysfunction · skin reactions · smell altered · sweat changes · syncope · throat complaints · thrombocytosis · tremor · urinary frequency increased · vascular disorders · vasodilation · vertigo · weight changes
▸ **Rare or very rare** Acute hepatic failure · chest discomfort · feeling cold · interstitial lung disease · local swelling · malaise · multi organ failure · pancreatitis acute · performance status decreased · photosensitivity reaction · rhabdomyolysis · severe cutaneous adverse reactions (SCARs)

● CONCEPTION AND CONTRACEPTION Manufacturer advises effective contraception during and for up to 6 months after treatment.

● PREGNANCY Avoid. See also *Pregnancy and reproductive function* in Cytotoxic drugs p. 865.

● BREAST FEEDING Discontinue breast-feeding.

● RENAL IMPAIRMENT Manufacturer advises avoid if creatinine clearance less than 30 mL/minute.
Dose adjustments Reduce dose if creatinine clearance 30–50 mL/minute—consult product literature.

● NATIONAL FUNDING/ACCESS DECISIONS

Scottish Medicines Consortium (SMC) Decisions
The *Scottish Medicines Consortium* has advised (August 2012) that tegafur with gimeracil and oteracil (*Teysuno*®) is accepted for restricted use within NHS Scotland for the treatment of advanced gastric cancer, when given in combination with cisplatin, in patients who are unsuitable for an anthracycline, fluorouracil and platinum triplet first-line regimen.

● MEDICINAL FORMS
There can be variation in the licensing of different medicines containing the same drug.

Capsule
CAUTIONARY AND ADVISORY LABELS 23
▶ Teysuno (Nordic Pharma Ltd)
Gimeracil 4.35 mg, Oteracil (as Oteracil potassium) 11.8 mg, Tegafur 15 mg Teysuno 15mg/4.35mg/11.8mg capsules | 126 capsule PoM £279.72
Gimeracil 5.8 mg, Oteracil (as Oteracil potassium) 15.8 mg, Tegafur 20 mg Teysuno 20mg/5.8mg/15.8mg capsules | 84 capsule PoM £248.40

Tioguanine

(Thioguanine)

● INDICATIONS AND DOSE

Acute leukaemia | Chronic myeloid leukaemia
▶ BY MOUTH
▶ Adult: 100–200 mg/m^2 daily, can be given at various stages of treatment in short-term cycles

IMPORTANT SAFETY INFORMATION
RISKS OF INCORRECT DOSING OF ORAL ANTI-CANCER MEDICINES
See Cytotoxic drugs p. 865.

● CONTRA-INDICATIONS Absent thiopurine methyltransferase activity
● CAUTIONS Thiopurine methyltransferase status
CAUTIONS, FURTHER INFORMATION
▶ Thiopurine methyltransferase The enzyme thiopurine methyltransferase (TPMT) metabolises thiopurine drugs (azathioprine, mercaptopurine, tioguanine); the risk of myelosuppression is increased in patients with reduced activity of the enzyme, particularly for the few individuals in whom TPMT activity is undetectable. Patients with absent TPMT activity should not receive thiopurine drugs; those with reduced TPMT activity may be treated under specialist supervision.
▶ Long-term therapy Long-term therapy is no longer recommended because of the high risk of liver toxicity.
● INTERACTIONS → Appendix 1: tioguanine
● SIDE-EFFECTS
▶ **Common or very common** Bone marrow failure · gastrointestinal disorders · hepatic disorders · hyperbilirubinaemia · hyperuricaemia · hyperuricosuria · nodular regenerative hyperplasia · oral disorders · sinusoidal obstruction syndrome · splenomegaly · thrombocytopenia · uric acid nephropathy · weight increased
▶ **Frequency not known** Photosensitivity reaction
● CONCEPTION AND CONTRACEPTION Ensure effective contraception during treatment in men or women.
● PREGNANCY Avoid (teratogenicity reported when men receiving tioguanine have fathered children). See also *Pregnancy and reproductive function* in Cytotoxic drugs p. 865.
● BREAST FEEDING Discontinue breast-feeding.

● HEPATIC IMPAIRMENT
Dose adjustments Reduce dose.
● RENAL IMPAIRMENT
Dose adjustments Reduce dose.
● PRE-TREATMENT SCREENING Consider measuring thiopurine methyltransferase (TPMT) activity before starting tioguanine therapy.
● MONITORING REQUIREMENTS Monitor liver function weekly—discontinue if liver toxicity develops.
● MEDICINAL FORMS
There can be variation in the licensing of different medicines containing the same drug. Forms available from special-order manufacturers include: capsule

Tablet
▶ Tioguanine (Non-proprietary)
Tioguanine 40 mg Tioguanine 40mg tablets | 25 tablet PoM £109.57

Trifluridine with tipiracil
24-Apr-2017

● DRUG ACTION Trifluridine is an antimetabolite that interferes with cancer cell DNA synthesis and inhibits cell proliferation; tipiracil is a TPase inhibitor that boosts trifluridine concentrations.

● INDICATIONS AND DOSE

Metastatic colorectal cancer, in patients previously treated with (or unsuitable for treatment with) available therapies including fluoropyrimidine-, oxaliplatin-, and irinotecan-based chemotherapies, or anti-vascular endothelial growth factor (VEGF) agents, or anti-epidermal growth factor receptor (EGFR) agents (specialist use only)
▶ BY MOUTH
▶ Adult: Initially 35 mg/m^2 twice daily (max. per dose 80 mg), given on days 1 to 5 and days 8 to 12 of each 28-day cycle, consult product literature for further information on dose adjustment

IMPORTANT SAFETY INFORMATION
RISKS OF INCORRECT DOSING OF ORAL ANTI-CANCER MEDICINES
See Cytotoxic drugs p. 865.

● SIDE-EFFECTS
▶ **Common or very common** Alopecia · anaemia · appetite decreased · asthenia · constipation · cough · decreased leucocytes · diarrhoea · dizziness · dyspnoea · fever · flushing · gastrointestinal discomfort · headache · hyperbilirubinaemia · hypoalbuminaemia · increased leucocytes · increased risk of infection · insomnia · malaise · mucositis · nausea · neutropenia · oedema · oral disorders · peripheral neuropathy · skin reactions · taste altered · thrombocytopenia · urine abnormalities · vomiting · weight decreased
▶ **Uncommon** Angina pectoris · anxiety · arrhythmia · ascites · bile duct disorders · cancer pain · cataract · conjunctivitis · cystitis · dehydration · dry eye · dysphonia · ear discomfort · electrolyte imbalance · embolism and thrombosis · erythropenia · feeling of body temperature change · gastrointestinal disorders · gout · haemorrhage · hepatotoxicity · hyperglycaemia · hyperhidrosis · hypertension · hypotension · joint disorders · lethargy · menstrual disorder · muscle complaints · muscle weakness · nail disorder · neurotoxicity · oropharyngeal pain · pain · palpitations · pancreatitis acute · pancytopenia · photosensitivity reaction · pleural effusion · QT interval prolongation · renal failure · rhinorrhoea · sensation abnormal · sensation of pressure · septic shock (including fatal cases) · syncope · urinary disorder · vertigo · vision disorders

8

Immune system and malignant disease

- CONCEPTION AND CONTRACEPTION Manufacturer advises effective contraception in women of child-bearing potential and in men with a partner of child-bearing potential, during treatment and for 6 months after stopping treatment. Manufacturer also advises use of an additional barrier method in women using hormonal contraceptives—effect of trifluridine with tipiracil on hormonal contraception unknown.
- PREGNANCY Manufacturer advises avoid unless essential—reproductive toxicity in *animal* studies.
- BREAST FEEDING Manufacturer advises avoid—present in milk in *animal* studies.
- HEPATIC IMPAIRMENT Manufacturer advises avoid in moderate-to-severe impairment—no information available.
- RENAL IMPAIRMENT Manufacturer advises caution if eGFR 30–59 mL/minute/1.73 m^2—monitor for haematological toxicities; manufacturer advises avoid if eGFR less than 30 mL/minute/ 1.73m^2—no information available.
- MONITORING REQUIREMENTS Manufacturer advises obtain baseline blood cell counts before and during treatment; monitor closely for myelosuppression. Manufacturer also advises monitoring for proteinuria before and during treatment.
- NATIONAL FUNDING/ACCESS DECISIONS

NICE decisions

▶ **Trifluridine with tipiracil for previously treated metastatic colorectal cancer (August 2016)** NICE TA405 Trifluridine with tipiracil is recommended, within its marketing authorisation, as an option for treating metastatic colorectal cancer in adults, only when provided by the manufacturer with the discount agreed in the patient access scheme.
www.nice.org.uk/guidance/TA405

Scottish Medicines Consortium (SMC) Decisions
The *Scottish Medicines Consortium* has advised (February 2017) that trifluridine with tipiracil (*Lonsurf*®) is accepted for use within NHS Scotland for the treatment of adults with metastatic colorectal cancer who have been previously treated with, or are not considered candidates for, available therapies including fluoropyrimidine-, oxaliplatin- and irinotecan-based chemotherapies, anti-vascular endothelial growth factor agents, and anti-epidermal growth factor receptor agents.
 This advice is contingent upon the continuing availability of the Patient Access Scheme in NHS Scotland or a list price that is equivalent or lower.

- MEDICINAL FORMS
There can be variation in the licensing of different medicines containing the same drug.
Tablet
CAUTIONARY AND ADVISORY LABELS 21
▶ Lonsurf (Servier Laboratories Ltd) ▼
 Tipiracil (as Tipiracil hydrochloride) 6.14 mg, Trifluridine 15 mg Lonsurf 15mg/6.14mg tablets | 20 tablet [PoM] £500.00 | 60 tablet [PoM] £1,500.00
 Tipiracil (as Tipiracil hydrochloride) 8.19 mg, Trifluridine 20 mg Lonsurf 20mg/8.19mg tablets | 20 tablet [PoM] £666.67 | 60 tablet [PoM] £2,000.00

Bleomycin

- INDICATIONS AND DOSE

Squamous cell carcinoma | Metastatic germ cell cancer | Non-Hodgkin's lymphoma
▶ BY INTRAMUSCULAR INJECTION, OR BY INTRAVENOUS INJECTION, OR BY INTRAVENOUS INFUSION, OR BY INTRA-ARTERIAL INFUSION, OR BY LOCAL INFILTRATION
▶ Adult: (consult product literature or local protocols)

- CAUTIONS Caution in handling—irritant to tissues
- INTERACTIONS → Appendix 1: bleomycin
- SIDE-EFFECTS
▶ **Common or very common** Alopecia · angular stomatitis · appetite decreased · chills · fever (after administration) · haemorrhage · headache · interstitial pneumonia · leucopenia · malaise · nail discolouration · nail disorder · nausea · pain · pulmonary fibrosis (dose-related) · scleroderma · skin reactions · stomatitis · vomiting · weight decreased
▶ **Uncommon** Diarrhoea · dizziness · hepatocellular injury · oliguria · shock · urinary disorders · vein wall hypertrophy · venous stenosis

SIDE-EFFECTS, FURTHER INFORMATION
Progressive pulmonary fibrosis Progressive pulmonary fibrosis is dose-related, and may occur at lower doses in the elderly. Suspicious chest X-ray changes are an indication to stop therapy with this drug.
Pulmonary toxicity Patients who have received bleomycin may be at risk of developing pulmonary toxicity if exposed to high inspired oxygen concentrations, for example peri-operatively, or during lung function testing.

- CONCEPTION AND CONTRACEPTION Contraceptive advice required, see *Pregnancy and reproductive function* in Cytotoxic drugs p. 865.
- PREGNANCY Avoid (teratogenic and carcinogenic in *animal* studies). See also *Pregnancy and reproductive function* in Cytotoxic drugs p. 865
- BREAST FEEDING Discontinue breast feeding.
- RENAL IMPAIRMENT
Dose adjustments Reduce dose by half if serum creatinine 177–354 micromol/litre; reduce dose further if serum-creatinine greater than 354 micromol/litre.
- PRESCRIBING AND DISPENSING INFORMATION To conform to the European Pharmacopoeia vials previously labelled as containing '15 units' of bleomycin are now labelled as containing 15 000 units. The amount of bleomycin in the vial has not changed.

- MEDICINAL FORMS
There can be variation in the licensing of different medicines containing the same drug.
Powder for solution for injection
▶ Bleo-Kyowa (Kyowa Kirin Ltd)
 Bleomycin (as Bleomycin sulfate) 15000 unit Bleo-Kyowa 15,000unit powder for solution for injection vials | 10 vial [PoM] £190.60

Mitomycin

● **INDICATIONS AND DOSE**

Recurrent superficial bladder tumours (bladder instillation)
▶ BY INTRAVESICAL INSTILLATION
▶ Adult: (consult product literature or local protocols)

Upper gastro-intestinal cancers | Breast cancers
▶ BY INTRAVENOUS INJECTION
▶ Adult: (consult product literature or local protocols)

● **CAUTIONS** Caution in handling—irritant to tissues
● **INTERACTIONS** → Appendix 1: mitomycin
● **SIDE-EFFECTS**
GENERAL SIDE-EFFECTS
▶ **Common or very common** Skin reactions
SPECIFIC SIDE-EFFECTS
▶ **Common or very common**
▶ With intravenous use Bone marrow depression · cough · dyspnoea · glomerulonephropathy · interstitial pneumonia · leucopenia · nausea · nephrotoxicity · renal impairment · thrombocytopenia · vomiting
▶ With intravesical use Bladder irritation · cystitis · haemorrhage · urinary disorders
▶ **Uncommon**
▶ With intravenous use Alopecia · appetite decreased · diarrhoea · fever · mucositis · stomatitis
▶ **Rare or very rare**
▶ With intravenous use Haemolytic anaemia · heart failure · hepatic disorders · infection · pulmonary hypertension · sepsis · sinusoidal obstruction syndrome
▶ **Frequency not known**
▶ With intravenous use Neoplasms

SIDE-EFFECTS, FURTHER INFORMATION Mitomycin is usually administered at 6-weekly intervals because it causes delayed bone-marrow toxicity. Prolonged use may result in a cumulative effect.

● **CONCEPTION AND CONTRACEPTION** Contraceptive advice required, see *Pregnancy and reproductive function* in Cytotoxic drugs p. 865.
● **PREGNANCY** Avoid (teratogenic in *animal* studies). See also *Pregnancy and reproductive function* in Cytotoxic drugs p. 865.
● **BREAST FEEDING** Discontinue breast-feeding.

● **MEDICINAL FORMS**
There can be variation in the licensing of different medicines containing the same drug.
Powder for solution for injection
▶ Mitomycin (Non-proprietary)
Mitomycin 2 mg Mitomycin 2mg powder for solution for injection vials | 10 vial [PoM] £55.89
Mitomycin 10 mg Mitomycin 10mg powder for solution for injection vials | 1 vial [PoM] £20.30
▶ Mitomycin-C (Kyowa Kirin Ltd)
Mitomycin 2 mg Mitomycin-C Kyowa 2mg powder for solution for injection vials | 10 vial [PoM] £58.83
Mitomycin 10 mg Mitomycin-C Kyowa 10mg powder for solution for injection vials | 1 vial [PoM] £21.37
Mitomycin 20 mg Mitomycin-C Kyowa 20mg powder for solution for injection vials | 1 vial [PoM] £39.94
Mitomycin 40 mg Mitomycin-C Kyowa 40mg powder for solution for injection vials | 1 vial [PoM] £79.88

Pentostatin

● **INDICATIONS AND DOSE**

Hairy cell leukaemia (initiated in specialist centres)
▶ BY INTRAVENOUS INJECTION, OR BY INTRAVENOUS INFUSION
▶ Adult: To be given on alternate weeks (consult product literature)

● **INTERACTIONS** → Appendix 1: pentostatin
● **SIDE-EFFECTS**
▶ **Common or very common** Agranulocytosis · alopecia · amenorrhoea · anaemia · angina pectoris · anxiety · appetite decreased · arrhythmias · arthritis · asthenia · asthma · atrioventricular block · blood disorder · bone disorder · bone marrow disorders · breast mass · cardiac arrest · chest pain · chills · confusion · constipation · cough · death · depersonalisation · depression · diarrhoea · dizziness · drowsiness · dry eye · dry mouth · dysarthria · dysphagia · dyspnoea · ear pain · electrolyte imbalance · embolism and thrombosis · emotional lability · eosinophilia · eye disorders · eye inflammation · eye pain · febrile neutropenia · fever · fluid imbalance · flushing · gastrointestinal discomfort · gastrointestinal disorders · gout · graft versus host disease · haemorrhage · hallucination · hangover · headaches · hearing impairment · heart failure · hostility · hyperbilirubinaemia · hyperglycaemia · hyperhidrosis · hypersensitivity · hypertension · hypotension · increased risk of infection · influenza like illness · jaundice · joint disorders · leucopenia · lymphadenopathy · malaise · memory loss · meningism · movement disorders · muscle complaints · nausea · neoplasms · nephrolithiasis · nephropathy · nerve disorders · neurotoxicity (withhold or discontinue) · oedema · oral disorders · pain · paralysis · pericardial effusion · photosensitivity reaction · pulmonary oedema · rash (withhold if severe) · renal impairment · respiratory disorders · retinopathy · seborrhoea · seizures · sensation abnormal · sepsis · sexual dysfunction · skin reactions · sleep disorders · splenomegaly · syncope · taste altered · thinking abnormal · thrombocytopenia · tremor · urinary disorders · urogenital disorder · vascular disorders · vasculitis · vertigo · vision disorders · vomiting · weight changes
▶ **Uncommon** Angioedema · antibiotic associated colitis · cardiomyopathy · cystitis · haemolytic anaemia · mucositis · multi organ failure · myocardial infarction · pure red cell aplasia · transplant failure · tumour lysis syndrome
▶ **Rare or very rare** Dementia · pericarditis · shock · Stevens-Johnson syndrome · systemic inflammatory response syndrome

SIDE-EFFECTS, FURTHER INFORMATION Pentostatin can cause myelosuppression, immunosuppression, and a number of other side-effects that may be severe. Treatment should be withheld in patients who develop a severe rash, and withheld or discontinued in patients showing signs of neurotoxicity.

● **CONCEPTION AND CONTRACEPTION** Manufacturer advises that men should not father children during and for 6 months after treatment.
● **PREGNANCY** Avoid (teratogenic in *animal* studies). See also *Pregnancy and reproductive function* in Cytotoxic drugs p. 865.
● **BREAST FEEDING** Discontinue breast-feeding.
● **HEPATIC IMPAIRMENT** Manufacturer advises caution—limited information available.
● **RENAL IMPAIRMENT** Avoid if creatinine clearance less than 60 mL/minute.

Immune system and malignant disease

8

8

Immune system and malignant disease

- MEDICINAL FORMS
  There can be variation in the licensing of different medicines containing the same drug.
  Powder for solution for injection
  - Nipent (Pfizer Ltd)
    Pentostatin 10 mg Nipent 10mg powder for solution for injection vials | 1 vial [PoM] £734.21 (Hospital only)

ANTINEOPLASTIC DRUGS > PLANT ALKALOIDS

Trabectedin

10-Jun-2016

- INDICATIONS AND DOSE
  Treatment of advanced soft-tissue sarcoma when treatment with anthracyclines and ifosfamide has failed or is contra-indicated | Treatment of relapsed platinum-sensitive ovarian cancer (in combination with pegylated liposomal doxorubicin)
  - BY INTRAVENOUS INFUSION
  - Adult: (consult product literature or local protocols)

- CONTRA-INDICATIONS Elevated creatine phosphokinase (consult product literature)
- INTERACTIONS → Appendix 1: trabectedin
- SIDE-EFFECTS
  - **Common or very common** Alopecia · anaemia · appetite decreased · arthralgia · asthenia · back pain · constipation · cough · dehydration · diarrhoea · dizziness · dyspnoea · fever · flushing · gastrointestinal discomfort · headache · hyperbilirubinaemia · hypersensitivity · hypokalaemia · hypotension · infection · insomnia · leucopenia · mucositis · myalgia · nausea · neutropenia · oedema · paraesthesia · peripheral neuropathy · skin reactions · stomatitis · taste altered · thrombocytopenia · vomiting · weight decreased
  - **Uncommon** Capillary leak syndrome · septic shock
  - **Rare or very rare** Hepatic failure
  - **Frequency not known** Rhabdomyolysis

  SIDE-EFFECTS, FURTHER INFORMATION A corticosteroid, such as dexamethasone by intravenous infusion, must be given 30 minutes before therapy for its antiemetic and hepatoprotective effects (consult product literature).

- CONCEPTION AND CONTRACEPTION Effective contraception recommended during and for at least 3 months after treatment in women and during and for at least 5 months after treatment in men.
- PREGNANCY See *Pregnancy and reproductive function* in Cytotoxic drugs p. 865.
- BREAST FEEDING Manufacturer advises avoid breast-feeding during and for 3 months after treatment.
- HEPATIC IMPAIRMENT Avoid in patients with raised bilirubin.
  Dose adjustments Manufacturer advises caution in impairment—consider dose reduction.
  Monitoring Monitor hepatic function closely in patients with hepatic impairment.
- RENAL IMPAIRMENT Avoid monotherapy if creatinine clearance less than 30 mL/minute. Avoid combination regimens if creatinine clearance less than 60 mL/minute.
- MONITORING REQUIREMENTS
  - Specific haematological, renal and hepatic parameters must be monitored and within certain ranges prior to starting treatment and repeated weekly during the first 2 cycles and at least once between treatments in subsequent cycles—consult product literature for full details.
  - Monitor for signs and symptoms of rhabdomyolysis (including myelotoxicity, severe liver function disorder, renal failure, muscle weakness or pain)—monitor creatine phosphokinase closely and discontinue treatment (consult product literature).

- NATIONAL FUNDING/ACCESS DECISIONS
  NICE decisions
  - **Trabectedin for the treatment of advanced soft tissue sarcoma (February 2010)** NICE TA185
    Trabectedin is an option for advanced soft tissue sarcoma when treatment with anthracyclines and ifosfamide has failed, is inappropriate or is not tolerated. The cost of trabectedin for treatment after the fifth cycle is met by the manufacturer.
    www.nice.org.uk/TA185
  - **Topotecan, pegylated liposomal doxorubicin hydrochloride, paclitaxel, trabectedin and gemcitabine for treating recurrent ovarian cancer (April 2016)** NICE TA389
    Trabectedin in combination with pegylated liposomal doxorubicin hydrochloride (PLDH) is **not** recommended for treating the first recurrence of platinum-sensitive ovarian cancer.
    Patients currently receiving trabectedin in combination with PLDH should have the option to continue their treatment until they or their clinician consider it appropriate to stop.
    www.nice.org.uk/TA389

- MEDICINAL FORMS
  There can be variation in the licensing of different medicines containing the same drug.
  Powder for solution for infusion
  - Yondelis (Pharma Mar, S.A.)
    Trabectedin 250 microgram Yondelis 0.25mg powder for concentrate for solution for infusion vials | 1 vial [PoM] £363.00 (Hospital only)
    Trabectedin 1 mg Yondelis 1mg powder for concentrate for solution for infusion vials | 1 vial [PoM] £1,366.00 (Hospital only)

ANTINEOPLASTIC DRUGS > PLATINUM COMPOUNDS

Carboplatin

10-Jun-2016

- INDICATIONS AND DOSE
  Treatment of advanced ovarian cancer and lung cancer (particularly the small cell type)
  - BY INTRAVENOUS INFUSION
  - Adult: The dose of carboplatin is determined according to renal function rather than body surface area (consult product literature)

- INTERACTIONS → Appendix 1: platinum compounds
- SIDE-EFFECTS
  - **Common or very common** Abdominal pain · alopecia · anaemia · asthenia · cardiovascular disorder · constipation · diarrhoea · haemorrhage · hypersensitivity · increased risk of infection · leucopenia · mucosal abnormalities · musculoskeletal disorder · nausea · neutropenia · ototoxicity · peripheral neuropathy · reflexes decreased · respiratory disorders · sensation abnormal · skin reactions · taste altered · thrombocytopenia · urogenital disorder · vision disorders · vomiting
  - **Rare or very rare** Cardiac discomfort · dyspnoea
  - **Frequency not known** Abdominal cramps · appetite decreased · bone marrow failure · chills · dehydration · embolism · encephalopathy · fever · haemolytic uraemic syndrome · heart failure · hypertension · hyponatraemia · hypotension · malaise · pancreatitis · stomatitis · stroke · treatment related secondary malignancy

- CONCEPTION AND CONTRACEPTION Contraceptive advice required, see *Pregnancy and reproductive function* in Cytotoxic drugs p. 865.
- PREGNANCY Avoid (teratogenic and embryotoxic in *animal* studies). See also *Pregnancy and reproductive function* in Cytotoxic drugs p. 865.
- BREAST FEEDING Discontinue breast-feeding.

- RENAL IMPAIRMENT Avoid if creatinine clearance less than 20 mL/minute.
  Dose adjustments Reduce dose.
  Monitoring Monitor haematological parameters in renal impairment.
  Monitor renal function in renal impairment.
- PRESCRIBING AND DISPENSING INFORMATION Carboplatin can be given in an outpatient setting.
- NATIONAL FUNDING/ACCESS DECISIONS

  NICE decisions
  ▶ Bevacizumab in combination with paclitaxel and carboplatin for the first-line treatment of advanced ovarian cancer (May 2013) NICE TA284
  Bevacizumab in combination with paclitaxel and carboplatin is **not** recommended for the first-line treatment of advanced ovarian cancer (including fallopian tube and primary peritoneal cancer).
  www.nice.org.uk/TA284
  ▶ Bevacizumab in combination with gemcitabine and carboplatin for the treatment of the first recurrence of platinum-sensitive advanced ovarian cancer (May 2013) NICE TA285
  Bevacizumab in combination with gemcitabine and carboplatin is **not** recommended within its marketing authorisation, that is, for the treatment of the first recurrence of platinum-sensitive advanced ovarian cancer (including fallopian tube and primary peritoneal cancer) that has not been previously treated with bevacizumab or other vascular endothelial growth factor (VEGF) inhibitors or VEGF receptor-targeted agents.
  www.nice.org.uk/guidance/ta285

- MEDICINAL FORMS
  There can be variation in the licensing of different medicines containing the same drug.
  Solution for infusion
  ▶ Carboplatin (Non-proprietary)
  Carboplatin 10 mg per 1 ml Carboplatin 50mg/5ml concentrate for solution for infusion vials | 1 vial PoM £22.04 (Hospital only) | 1 vial PoM £20.00–£20.20
  Carboplatin 150mg/15ml concentrate for solution for infusion vials | 1 vial PoM £56.92 (Hospital only) | 1 vial PoM £50.00–£60.59
  Carboplatin 600mg/60ml concentrate for solution for infusion vials | 1 vial PoM £232.64–£260.00
  Carboplatin 600mg/60ml solution for infusion vials | 1 vial PoM £260.00 (Hospital only)
  Carboplatin 450mg/45ml concentrate for solution for infusion vials | 1 vial PoM £168.85 (Hospital only) | 1 vial PoM £160.00–£181.77
  Carboplatin 450mg/45ml solution for infusion vials | 1 vial PoM £197.48 (Hospital only)
  Carboplatin 150mg/15ml solution for infusion vials | 1 vial PoM £65.83 (Hospital only)
  Carboplatin 50mg/5ml solution for infusion vials | 1 vial PoM £22.86 (Hospital only)

Cisplatin

- INDICATIONS AND DOSE
  Treatment of testicular, lung, cervical, bladder, head and neck, and ovarian cancer (alone or in combination)
  ▶ BY INTRAVENOUS INFUSION
  ▶ Adult: (consult product literature)

- CAUTIONS
  CAUTIONS, FURTHER INFORMATION
  ▶ Hydration Cisplatin requires intensive intravenous hydration and treatment may be complicated by severe nausea and vomiting.
- INTERACTIONS → Appendix 1: platinum compounds
- SIDE-EFFECTS
  ▶ Common or very common Anaemia · arrhythmias · bone marrow failure · electrolyte imbalance · fever · leucopenia ·

nephrotoxicity (dose-related and potentially cumulative) · sepsis · thrombocytopenia
▶ Uncommon Anaphylactoid reaction · ototoxicity (dose-related and potentially cumulative) · spermatogenesis abnormal
▶ Rare or very rare Acute leukaemia · cardiac arrest · encephalopathy · myocardial infarction · nerve disorders · seizure · stomatitis
▶ Frequency not known Alopecia · appetite decreased · asthenia · autonomic dysfunction · cardiac disorder · cerebrovascular insufficiency · dehydration · diarrhoea · haemolytic anaemia · hearing impairment · hiccups · hyperuricaemia · infection · Lhermitte's sign · malaise · muscle spasms · myelopathy · nausea · papilloedema · pulmonary embolism · rash · Raynaud's phenomenon · renal impairment · renal tubular disorder · retinal discolouration · SIADH · taste loss · tetany · thrombotic microangiopathy · vision disorders · vomiting
- CONCEPTION AND CONTRACEPTION Manufacturer advises effective contraception during and for at least 6 months after treatment in men or women.
- PREGNANCY Avoid (teratogenic and toxic in *animal* studies. See also *Pregnancy and reproductive function* in Cytotoxic drugs p. 865.
- BREAST FEEDING Discontinue breast-feeding.
- RENAL IMPAIRMENT Avoid if possible—nephrotoxic.
- MONITORING REQUIREMENTS
  ▶ Monitor full blood count.
  ▶ Monitor audiology.
  ▶ Monitor plasma electrolytes.
  ▶ Nephrotoxicity Monitoring of renal function is essential.
- DIRECTIONS FOR ADMINISTRATION Cisplatin is increasingly given in a day care setting.

- MEDICINAL FORMS
  There can be variation in the licensing of different medicines containing the same drug.
  Solution for infusion
  ▶ Cisplatin (Non-proprietary)
  Cisplatin 1 mg per 1 ml Cisplatin 50mg/50ml concentrate for solution for infusion vials | 1 vial PoM £26.70 DT = £26.51 | 1 vial PoM £25.11–£28.11 DT = £26.51 (Hospital only)
  Cisplatin 100mg/100ml solution for infusion vials | 1 vial PoM £50.22 (Hospital only) | 1 vial PoM £50.22
  Cisplatin 10mg/10ml solution for infusion vials | 1 vial PoM £5.90 (Hospital only) | 1 vial PoM £5.90
  Cisplatin 50mg/50ml solution for infusion vials | 1 vial PoM £25.37–£28.11 DT = £26.51 | 1 vial PoM £25.37 DT = £26.51 (Hospital only)
  Cisplatin 10mg/10ml concentrate for solution for infusion vials | 1 vial PoM £5.36
  Cisplatin 100mg/100ml concentrate for solution for infusion vials | 1 vial PoM £50.22–£55.64 (Hospital only) | 1 vial PoM £52.86

Oxaliplatin

- INDICATIONS AND DOSE
  Treatment of metastatic colorectal cancer (in combination with fluorouracil and folinic acid) | Treatment of colon cancer after resection of the primary tumour (adjuvant treatment)
  ▶ BY INTRAVENOUS INFUSION
  ▶ Adult: (consult product literature)

- CONTRA-INDICATIONS Peripheral neuropathy with functional impairment
- INTERACTIONS → Appendix 1: platinum compounds
- SIDE-EFFECTS
  ▶ Common or very common Alopecia · anaemia · appetite decreased · arthralgia · asthenia · chills · conjunctivitis · constipation · cough · decreased leucocytes · dehydration · depression · diarrhoea · dizziness · dyspnoea · electrolyte imbalance · embolism and thrombosis · fever · flushing ·

8

Immune system and malignant disease

8

gastrointestinal discomfort · gastrointestinal disorders · haemorrhage · headache · hiccups · hyperglycaemia · hyperhidrosis · hypersensitivity · hypertension · increased risk of infection · insomnia · meningism · mucositis · nail disorder · nausea · necrosis · nerve disorders · neutropenia · neutropenic sepsis · pain · peripheral neuropathy (dose-limiting) · sensation abnormal · skin reactions · stomatitis · taste altered · thrombocytopenia · urinary disorders · vision disorders · vomiting · weight changes

▶ **Uncommon** Hearing impairment · metabolic acidosis · nervousness

▶ **Rare or very rare** Acute kidney injury · acute tubular necrosis · antibiotic associated colitis · disseminated intravascular coagulation · dysarthria · haemolytic anaemia · hepatic disorders · immuno-allergic thrombocytopenia · nephritis acute interstitial · nodular regenerative hyperplasia · pancreatitis · posterior reversible encephalopathy syndrome (PRES) (with oxaliplatin combination chemotherapy) · respiratory disorders · sinusoidal obstruction syndrome · vision loss (reversible on discontinuation)

▶ **Frequency not known** Autoimmune pancytopenia · chest discomfort · dysphagia · gait abnormal · hypersensitivity vasculitis · movement disorders · muscle complaints · muscle contractions involuntary · QT interval prolongation · rhabdomyolysis · throat complaints

SIDE-EFFECTS, FURTHER INFORMATION Neurotoxicity is dose limiting.

Respiratory symptoms If unexplained respiratory symptoms occur, oxaliplatin should be discontinued until investigations exclude interstitial lung disease and pulmonary fibrosis.

● CONCEPTION AND CONTRACEPTION Effective contraception required during and for 4 months after treatment in women and 6 months after treatment in men.

● PREGNANCY Manufacturer advises avoid—toxicity in *animal* studies. See also *Pregnancy and reproductive function* in Cytotoxic drugs p. 865.

● BREAST FEEDING Discontinue breast-feeding.

● RENAL IMPAIRMENT Avoid if creatinine clearance less than 30 mL/minute.
Dose adjustments Reduce dose in mild to moderate impairment (consult product literature).

● NATIONAL FUNDING/ACCESS DECISIONS

NICE decisions

▶ **Capecitabine and oxaliplatin in the adjuvant treatment of stage III (Dukes' C) colon cancer (April 2006)** NICE TA100
Capecitabine alone *or* oxaliplatin combined with fluorouracil and folinic acid are options for adjuvant treatment following surgery for stage III (Dukes' C) colon cancer.
www.nice.org.uk/TA100

▶ **Irinotecan, oxaliplatin, and raltitrexed for advanced colorectal cancer (August 2005)** NICE TA93
A combination of fluorouracil and folinic acid with either irinotecan or oxaliplatin are options for first-line treatment for advanced colorectal cancer.
Irinotecan alone or fluorouracil and folinic acid with oxaliplatin are options for patients who require further treatment subsequently.
www.nice.org.uk/TA93

● MEDICINAL FORMS
There can be variation in the licensing of different medicines containing the same drug.
Solution for infusion
▶ Oxaliplatin (Non-proprietary)
Oxaliplatin 5 mg per 1 ml Oxaliplatin 100mg/20ml concentrate for solution for infusion vials | 1 vial [PoM] £297.49-£330.00 (Hospital only) | 1 vial [PoM] £295.63-£311.00
Oxaliplatin 50mg/10ml concentrate for solution for infusion vials | 1 vial [PoM] £148.55-£165.00 (Hospital only) | 1 vial [PoM] £147.82-£155.00
Oxaliplatin 200mg/40ml concentrate for solution for infusion vials | 1 vial [PoM] £595.65-£627.00 (Hospital only) | 1 vial [PoM] £591.26

ANTINEOPLASTIC DRUGS > PODOPHYLLOTOXIN DERIVATIVES

Etoposide

● INDICATIONS AND DOSE

Small cell carcinoma of the bronchus, the lymphomas and testicular cancer
▶ BY MOUTH
▶ Adult: 120–240 mg/m^2 daily for 5 days
▶ BY INTRAVENOUS INFUSION
▶ Adult: (consult product literature)

IMPORTANT SAFETY INFORMATION
RISKS OF INCORRECT DOSING OF ORAL ANTI-CANCER MEDICINES
See Cytotoxic drugs p. 865.

● INTERACTIONS → Appendix 1: etoposide

● SIDE-EFFECTS

GENERAL SIDE-EFFECTS
▶ **Common or very common** Abdominal pain · acute leukaemia · alopecia · anaemia · appetite decreased · arrhythmia · asthenia · bone marrow depression · constipation · diarrhoea · dizziness · extravasation · hepatotoxicity · hypertension · leucopenia · malaise · mucositis · myocardial infarction · nausea · neutropenia · skin reactions · thrombocytopenia · vomiting
▶ **Uncommon** Nerve disorders
▶ **Rare or very rare** Dysphagia · neurotoxicity · radiation recall reaction · respiratory disorders · seizure · severe cutaneous adverse reactions (SCARs) · taste altered · vision loss

SPECIFIC SIDE-EFFECTS
▶ **Common or very common**
▶ With intravenous use Anaphylactic reaction · hypotension · infection
▶ With oral use Oesophagitis · stomatitis · transient systolic hypotension
▶ **Uncommon**
▶ With intravenous use Haemorrhage
▶ **Rare or very rare**
▶ With intravenous use Fever
▶ With oral use Drowsiness
▶ **Frequency not known**
▶ With intravenous use Angioedema · infertility · tumour lysis syndrome

● CONCEPTION AND CONTRACEPTION Contraceptive advice required, see *Pregnancy and reproductive function* in Cytotoxic drugs p. 865.

● PREGNANCY Avoid (teratogenic in *animal* studies). See also *Pregnancy and reproductive function* in Cytotoxic drugs p. 865.

● BREAST FEEDING Discontinue breast-feeding.

● HEPATIC IMPAIRMENT Avoid in severe impairment.

● RENAL IMPAIRMENT
Dose adjustments Consider dose reduction—consult local treatment protocol for details.

- **DIRECTIONS FOR ADMINISTRATION** Etoposide may be given orally or by slow intravenous infusion, the oral dose being double the intravenous dose. A preparation containing etoposide phosphate can be given by intravenous injection or infusion. Etoposide is usually given daily for 3–5 days and courses should not be repeated more frequently than at intervals of 21 days.

- **MEDICINAL FORMS**
There can be variation in the licensing of different medicines containing the same drug.

Solution for infusion
  ▸ Etoposide (Non-proprietary)
    Etoposide 20 mg per 1 ml Etoposide 100mg/5ml concentrate for solution for infusion vials | 1 vial [PoM] £11.50 (Hospital only) | 1 vial [PoM] £11.50 | 10 vial [PoM] £115.00
    Etoposide 500mg/25ml concentrate for solution for infusion vials | 1 vial [PoM] £73.85 (Hospital only)

Powder for solution for injection
  ▸ Etopophos (Bristol-Myers Squibb Pharmaceuticals Ltd)
    Etoposide (as Etoposide phosphate) 100 mg Etopophos 100mg powder for solution for injection vials | 10 vial [PoM] £261.68 (Hospital only)

Capsule
CAUTIONARY AND ADVISORY LABELS 23
  ▸ Vepesid (Bristol-Myers Squibb Pharmaceuticals Ltd)
    Etoposide 50 mg Vepesid 50mg capsules | 20 capsule [PoM] £99.82 (Hospital only)
    Etoposide 100 mg Vepesid 100mg capsules | 10 capsule [PoM] £87.23 (Hospital only)

ANTINEOPLASTIC DRUGS > TAXANES

Cabazitaxel   17-Mar-2017

- **INDICATIONS AND DOSE**

Treatment of hormone refractory metastatic prostate cancer in patients who have previously been treated with a docetaxel-containing regimen (in combination with prednisone or prednisolone)
  ▸ BY INTRAVENOUS INFUSION
  ▸ Adult: (consult product literature or local protocols)

- **CAUTIONS** Avoid in Acute porphyrias p. 1025
- **INTERACTIONS** → Appendix 1: taxanes
- **SIDE-EFFECTS**
▸ **Common or very common** Acute kidney injury · alopecia · anaemia · anxiety · appetite decreased · arrhythmias · arthralgia · asthenia · chest pain · chills · confusion · conjunctivitis · constipation · cough · cystitis · deep vein thrombosis · dehydration · diarrhoea · dizziness · dry mouth · dyspnoea · excessive tearing · fever · gastrointestinal discomfort · gastrointestinal disorders · haemorrhage · headache · hydronephrosis · hyperglycaemia · hypersensitivity · hypertension · hypokalaemia · hypotension · increased risk of infection · lethargy · leucopenia · malaise · mucositis · muscle complaints · nausea · nerve disorders · neutropenia · oedema · oropharyngeal pain · pain · pelvic pain · renal colic · renal failure (fatal cases of renal failure reported) · sensation abnormal · sepsis · skin reactions · taste altered · thrombocytopenia · tinnitus · ureteral obstruction · urinary disorders · vasodilation · vertigo · vomiting · weight decreased
▸ **Frequency not known** Respiratory disorders
- **CONCEPTION AND CONTRACEPTION** Ensure effective contraception during treatment (women) and for up to 6 months after treatment (men).
- **PREGNANCY** See also *Pregnancy and reproductive function* in Cytotoxic drugs p. 865.
- **BREAST FEEDING** Discontinue breast-feeding.
- **HEPATIC IMPAIRMENT** Avoid.

- **RENAL IMPAIRMENT** Use with caution if creatinine clearance less than 50 mL/minute.
- **MONITORING REQUIREMENTS** Monitor electrolytes—correct dehydration.
- **DIRECTIONS FOR ADMINISTRATION** Intravenous infusion incompatible with PVC.
- **NATIONAL FUNDING/ACCESS DECISIONS**

NICE decisions
▸ **Cabazitaxel for hormone-relapsed metastatic prostate cancer treated with docetaxel (updated August 2016) NICE TA391**
Cabazitaxel in combination with prednisone or prednisolone is recommended as an option for treating metastatic hormone-relapsed prostate cancer in patients whose disease has progressed during or after docetaxel chemotherapy, only if the following criteria are met:
  - the patient has an eastern cooperative oncology group (ECOG) performance status of 0 or 1
  - the patient has had 225 mg/m^2 or more of docetaxel
  - treatment with cabazitaxel is stopped when the disease progresses or after a maximum of 10 cycles
  - the manufacturer provides cabazitaxel with the discount agreed in the patient access scheme
  - NHS trusts purchase cabazitaxel in accordance with the commercial access agreement, either in vials (at a reduced price to reflect the average cost of waste per patient), or in pre-prepared intravenous infusion bags.
Patients currently receiving cabazitaxel that is not recommended according to the above criteria should have the option to continue treatment until they and their clinician consider it appropriate to stop.
www.nice.org.uk/TA391

Scottish Medicines Consortium (SMC) Decisions
The *Scottish Medicines Consortium* has advised (December 2016) that cabazitaxel (*Jevtana*®) in combination with prednisone or prednisolone is accepted for restricted use within NHS Scotland for the treatment of adult patients with hormone refractory metastatic prostate cancer previously treated with a docetaxel-containing regimen (patients who have received at least 225 mg/m^2 (three cycles) of docetaxel and have an Eastern Cooperative Oncology Group (ECOG) performance status of 0 or 1). This advice is contingent upon the continuing availability of the patient access scheme in NHS Scotland or a list price that is equivalent or lower.

- **MEDICINAL FORMS**
There can be variation in the licensing of different medicines containing the same drug.

Solution for infusion
EXCIPIENTS: May contain Ethanol
  ▸ Jevtana (Sanofi)
    Cabazitaxel 40 mg per 1 ml JEVTANA 60mg/1.5ml concentrate and solvent for solution for infusion vials | 1 vial [PoM] £3,696.00 (Hospital only)

Docetaxel

30-Apr-2018

● INDICATIONS AND DOSE

Adjuvant treatment of operable node-positive and operable node-negative breast cancer (in combination with doxorubicin and cyclophosphamide) | Initial chemotherapy of locally advanced or metastatic breast cancer (with doxorubicin) | Locally advanced or metastatic breast cancer where cytotoxic chemotherapy with an anthracycline or an alkylating drug has failed (monotherapy) | Locally advanced or metastatic breast cancer where cytotoxic chemotherapy with an anthracycline has failed (with capecitabine) | Initial chemotherapy of metastatic breast cancer which overexpresses human epidermal growth factor-2 (with trastuzumab) | Locally advanced or metastatic non-small cell lung cancer where previous chemotherapy has failed | Initial chemotherapy of unresectable, locally advanced or metastatic non-small cell lung cancer (with cisplatin) | Hormone-resistant metastatic prostate cancer (in combination with prednisone or prednisolone) | Initial treatment of metastatic gastric adenocarcinoma, including adenocarcinoma of the gastro-oesophageal junction (with cisplatin and fluorouracil) | Induction treatment of locally advanced squamous cell carcinoma of the head and neck (with cisplatin and fluorouracil)

▶ BY INTRAVENOUS INFUSION

▶ Adult: (consult product literature or local protocols)

● CAUTIONS Avoid in Acute porphyrias p. 1025 · consult product literature

● INTERACTIONS → Appendix 1: taxanes

● SIDE-EFFECTS

▶ **Common or very common** Abdominal pain · alopecia · anaemia · appetite decreased · arrhythmia · arthralgia · asthenia · constipation · diarrhoea · dyspnoea · fluid imbalance · haemorrhage · hypersensitivity · hypertension · hypotension · increased risk of infection · myalgia · nail disorders · nausea · neutropenia · pain · peripheral neuropathy · sepsis · skin reactions · stomatitis · taste altered · thrombocytopenia · vomiting

▶ **Uncommon** Gastrointestinal disorders · heart failure

▶ **Frequency not known** Ascites · bone marrow depression · chest tightness · chills · cutaneous lupus erythematosus · disseminated intravascular coagulation · eye disorders · eye inflammation · fever · hearing impairment · hepatitis · hyponatraemia · loss of consciousness · multi organ failure · myocardial infarction · nail discolouration · neurotoxicity · pericardial effusion · peripheral lymphoedema · peripheral oedema · pulmonary oedema · radiation injuries · renal impairment · respiratory disorders · sclerodermal-like changes · seizure · sensation abnormal · severe cutaneous adverse reactions (SCARs) · vasodilation · venous thromboembolism · vision disorders · weight increased

SIDE-EFFECTS, FURTHER INFORMATION Pretreatment with dexamethasone by mouth is recommended for reducing fluid retention and hypersensitivity reactions.

● CONCEPTION AND CONTRACEPTION Manufacturer advises effective contraception for men and women during treatment, and for at least 6 months after stopping treatment in men.

● PREGNANCY Avoid (toxicity in *animal* studies). See also *Pregnancy and reproductive function* in Cytotoxic drugs p. 865.

● BREAST FEEDING Discontinue breast-feeding.

● HEPATIC IMPAIRMENT Avoid in severe impairment.
Dose adjustments Reduce dose according to liver enzymes (consult product literature).
Monitoring
Monitor liver function in hepatic impairment.

● NATIONAL FUNDING/ACCESS DECISIONS
NICE decisions
▶ **Docetaxel for the treatment of hormone-refractory metastatic prostate cancer** (June 2006) NICE TA101
Docetaxel is an option for hormone-refractory metastatic prostate cancer only if their Karnofsky score is at least 60% [Karnofsky score is a measure of the ability to perform ordinary tasks].
www.nice.org.uk/guidance/ta101

▶ **Docetaxel for the adjuvant treatment of early node-positive breast cancer** (September 2006) NICE TA109
Docetaxel, when given concurrently with doxorubicin and cyclophosphamide (TAC regimen), is recommended as an option for the adjuvant treatment of women with early node-positive breast cancer.
www.nice.org.uk/guidance/ta109

▶ **Pertuzumab with trastuzumab and docetaxel for treating HER2-positive breast cancer** (March 2018) NICE TA509
Pertuzumab, in combination with trastuzumab and docetaxel, is recommended, within its marketing authorisation, for treating HER2-positive metastatic or locally recurrent unresectable breast cancer, in adults who have not had previous anti-HER2 therapy or chemotherapy for their metastatic disease, only if the manufacturer provides pertuzumab within the agreed commercial access arrangement.
www.nice.org.uk/guidance/ta509

Scottish Medicines Consortium (SMC) Decisions
SMC No. 369/07
The *Scottish Medicines Consortium* has advised (May 2007) that docetaxel (*Taxotere®*) in combination with cisplatin and fluorouracil is accepted for restricted use within NHS Scotland for the induction treatment of patients with unresectable locally advanced squamous cell carcinoma of the head and neck.
SMC No. 481/08
The *Scottish Medicines Consortium* has advised (July 2008) that docetaxel (*Taxotere®*) in combination with cisplatin and fluorouracil is accepted for restricted use within NHS Scotland for the induction treatment of patients with resectable locally advanced squamous cell carcinoma of the head and neck.

● MEDICINAL FORMS
There can be variation in the licensing of different medicines containing the same drug.
Solution for infusion
EXCIPIENTS: May contain Ethanol
▶ Docetaxel (Non-proprietary)
Docetaxel 10 mg per 1 ml Docetaxel 80mg/8ml concentrate for solution for infusion vials | 1 vial PoM £534.75 (Hospital only)
Docetaxel 160mg/16ml concentrate for solution for infusion vials | 1 vial PoM £1,069.50 (Hospital only)
Docetaxel 20mg/2ml concentrate for solution for infusion vials | 1 vial PoM £162.75 (Hospital only)
Docetaxel 20 mg per 1 ml Docetaxel 80mg/4ml concentrate for solution for infusion vials | 1 vial PoM £479.06–£530.00
Docetaxel 160mg/8ml concentrate for solution for infusion vials | 1 vial PoM £958.11–£1,000.00
Docetaxel 140mg/7ml concentrate for solution for infusion vials | 1 vial PoM £900.00
Docetaxel 20mg/1ml concentrate for solution for infusion vials | 1 vial PoM £145.80–£160.00
▶ Taxceus (medac UK)
Docetaxel 20 mg per 1 ml Taxceus 80mg/4ml concentrate for solution for infusion vials | 1 vial PoM £508.01
Taxceus 140mg/7ml concentrate for solution for infusion vials | 1 vial PoM £720.10
Taxceus 20mg/1ml concentrate for solution for infusion vials | 1 vial PoM £154.61

Paclitaxel

17-Jul-2017

- DRUG ACTION Paclitaxel is a member of the taxane group of drugs.

- INDICATIONS AND DOSE

Treatment of ovarian cancer (advanced or residual disease following laparotomy) in combination with cisplatin (conventional paclitaxel only) | Treatment of metastatic ovarian cancer where platinum-containing therapy has failed (conventional paclitaxel only) | Treatment of locally advanced or metastatic breast cancer (in combination with other cytotoxics or alone if other cytotoxics have failed or are inappropriate) (conventional paclitaxel only) | Adjuvant treatment of node-positive breast cancer following treatment with anthracycline and cyclophosphamide (conventional paclitaxel only) | Treatment of non-small cell lung cancer (in combination with cisplatin) when surgery or radiotherapy not appropriate (conventional paclitaxel only) | Treatment of advanced AIDS-related Kaposi's sarcoma where liposomal anthracycline therapy has failed (conventional paclitaxel only) | First-line treatment of metastatic adenocarcinoma of the pancreas (in combination with gemcitabine) (conventional paclitaxel only) | Monotherapy of metastatic breast cancer when first-line treatment has failed and standard, anthracycline-containing therapy is not indicated (albumin-bound paclitaxel only) | In combination with gemcitabine for the first-line treatment of metastatic adenocarcinoma of the pancreas (albumin-bound paclitaxel only)
  - BY INTRAVENOUS INFUSION
  - Adult: (consult product literature or local protocols)

- CAUTIONS Avoid in Acute porphyrias p. 1025 · consult product literature · patients aged over 75 years with metastatic adenocarcinoma of the pancreas

- INTERACTIONS → Appendix 1: taxanes

- SIDE-EFFECTS
- **Common or very common** Alopecia · anaemia · anxiety · appetite decreased · arrhythmias · arthralgia · asthenia · bone marrow disorders · chest discomfort · chills · constipation · cough · decreased leucocytes · depression · diarrhoea · dizziness · drowsiness · dry eye · dyspnoea · electrolyte imbalance · excessive tearing · eye inflammation · fever · fluid imbalance · gastrointestinal discomfort · gastrointestinal disorders · haemorrhage · headache · hyperpyrexia · hypertension · increased risk of infection · influenza like illness · insomnia · laryngeal pain · lymphoedema · malaise · movement disorders · mucositis · muscle complaints · nail discolouration · nail disorders · nasal complaints · nausea · nerve disorders · neutropenia · oedema · oral disorders · pain · performance status decreased · respiratory disorders · sensation abnormal · skin reactions · taste altered · thrombocytopenia · vasodilation · vertigo · vision disorders · vomiting · weight changes
- **Uncommon** Allergic rhinitis · breast pain · dry mouth · dysphagia · ear pain · embolism and thrombosis · eye discomfort · facial swelling · gait abnormal · hepatomegaly · hoarseness · hyperglycaemia · hypoalbuminaemia · hypoglycaemia · hypotension · limb discomfort · muscle weakness · neoplasm complications · peripheral coldness · photosensitivity reaction · polydipsia · reflexes abnormal · sepsis · sweat changes · swelling · syncope · tinnitus · tremor · urinary disorders
- **Rare or very rare** Atrioventricular block · cardiac arrest · congestive heart failure · left ventricular dysfunction · radiation injuries · severe cutaneous adverse reactions (SCARs)

- SIDE-EFFECTS, FURTHER INFORMATION Manufacturer advises routine premedication with a corticosteroid, an antihistamine and a histamine H2-receptor antagonist is recommended to prevent severe hypersensitivity reactions; hypersensitivity reactions may occur rarely despite premedication.

- CONCEPTION AND CONTRACEPTION Ensure effective contraception during and for at least 6 months after treatment in men or women.

- PREGNANCY Avoid (toxicity in *animal* studies). See also *Pregnancy and reproductive function* in Cytotoxic drugs p. 865.

- BREAST FEEDING Discontinue breast-feeding.

- HEPATIC IMPAIRMENT Avoid in severe impairment.

- MONITORING REQUIREMENTS
  - Cardiac monitoring should be undertaken, particularly if patients have underlying cardiac disease or previous exposure to anthracyclines.
  - Patients should be monitored for signs and symptoms of pneumonitis and sepsis.

- PRESCRIBING AND DISPENSING INFORMATION Paclitaxel is available as both conventional and albumin-bound formulations. The different formulations vary in their licensed indications, pharmacokinetics, dosage and administration, and are not interchangeable.
  Prescribers should specify the brand to be dispensed.

- NATIONAL FUNDING/ACCESS DECISIONS
  NICE decisions
  - **Paclitaxel for ovarian cancer (January 2003)** NICE TA55
  Either paclitaxel in combination with a platinum compound (cisplatin or carboplatin) *or* a platinum compound alone are alternatives for the first-line treatment of ovarian cancer (usually following surgery).
  www.nice.org.uk/guidance/TA55
  - **Paclitaxel for the adjuvant treatment of early node-positive breast cancer (September 2006)** NICE TA108
  Paclitaxel, within its licensed indication, is **not** recommended for the adjuvant treatment of women with early node-positive breast cancer.
  www.nice.org.uk/guidance/TA108
  - **Bevacizumab in combination with paclitaxel and carboplatin for the first-line treatment of advanced ovarian cancer (May 2013)** NICE TA284
  Bevacizumab in combination with paclitaxel and carboplatin is **not** recommended for the first-line treatment of advanced ovarian cancer (including fallopian tube and primary peritoneal cancer).
  www.nice.org.uk/guidance/TA284
  - **Topotecan, pegylated liposomal doxorubicin hydrochloride, paclitaxel, trabectedin and gemcitabine for treating recurrent ovarian cancer (April 2016)** NICE TA389
  Paclitaxel, in combination with platinum or as monotherapy, is recommended as an option for treating recurrent ovarian cancer.
  www.nice.org.uk/guidance/TA389
  - **Paclitaxel as albumin-bound nanoparticles with gemcitabine for untreated metastatic pancreatic cancer (September 2017)** NICE TA476
  Paclitaxel as albumin-bound nanoparticles (nab-paclitaxel) with gemcitabine is recommended as an option for untreated metastatic adenocarcinoma of the pancreas in adults, only if:
    - other combination chemotherapies are unsuitable and they would otherwise have gemcitabine monotherapy, **and**
    - the manufacturer provides nab-paclitaxel with the discount agreed in the patient access scheme.
  Patients whose treatment with nab-paclitaxel was started before this guidance was published, should have the

8

Immune system and malignant disease

option to continue treatment until they and their NHS clinician consider it appropriate to stop. www.nice.org.uk/guidance/TA476

Scottish Medicines Consortium (SMC) Decisions

The *Scottish Medicines Consortium* has advised (April 2010) that paclitaxel albumin (*Abraxane®*) is accepted for restricted use within NHS Scotland for treatment of metastatic breast cancer in patients who have failed first-line treatment for metastatic disease and for whom standard anthracycline containing therapy is not indicated; use is restricted to patients who would otherwise receive docetaxel or 3-weekly solvent-based paclitaxel as second-line treatment for metastatic breast cancer.

The *Scottish Medicines Consortium* has advised (February 2015) that paclitaxel albumin (*Abraxane®*) is accepted for use within NHS Scotland in combination with gemcitabine for the first-line treatment of adult patients with metastatic adenocarcinoma of the pancreas.

● MEDICINAL FORMS
There can be variation in the licensing of different medicines containing the same drug.

Solution for infusion
EXCIPIENTS: May contain Polyoxyl castor oils
▸ Paclitaxel (Non-proprietary)
  Paclitaxel 6 mg per 1 ml Paclitaxel 150mg/25ml concentrate for solution for infusion vials | 1 vial [PoM] £504.90–£561.00 (Hospital only) | 1 vial [PoM] £300.52
  Paclitaxel 30mg/5ml concentrate for solution for infusion vials | 1 vial [PoM] £112.31–£116.05 (Hospital only) | 1 vial [PoM] £66.85–£105.84
  Paclitaxel 300mg/50ml concentrate for solution for infusion vials | 1 vial [PoM] £1,009.80–£1,122.00 (Hospital only) | 1 vial [PoM] £601.03–£951.63
  Paclitaxel 100mg/16.7ml concentrate for solution for infusion vials | 1 vial [PoM] £336.60–£374.00 (Hospital only) | 1 vial [PoM] £200.35–£326.28

Powder for suspension for infusion
ELECTROLYTES: May contain Sodium
▸ Abraxane (Celgene Ltd)
  Paclitaxel albumin 100 mg Abraxane 100mg powder for suspension for infusion vials | 1 vial [PoM] £246.00 (Hospital only)

ANTINEOPLASTIC DRUGS › TOPOISOMERASE I INHIBITORS

Irinotecan hydrochloride
23-May-2017

● DRUG ACTION Irinotecan inhibits topoisomerase I, an enzyme involved in DNA replication.

● INDICATIONS AND DOSE

Metastatic colorectal cancer in combination with fluorouracil and folinic acid or as monotherapy when treatment containing fluorouracil has failed | Treatment of epidermal growth factor receptor-expressing metastatic colorectal cancer after failure of chemotherapy that has included irinotecan (in combination with cetuximab) | First-line treatment of metastatic carcinoma of the colon or rectum (in combination with fluorouracil, folinic acid and bevacizumab) | First-line treatment of metastatic colorectal carcinoma (in combination with capecitabine with or without bevacizumab)
▸ BY INTRAVENOUS INFUSION
▸ Adult: (consult product literature or local protocols)

Metastatic adenocarcinoma of the pancreas in patients who have progressed following gemcitabine based therapy (in combination with fluorouracil and leucovorin) (specialist use only)
▸ BY INTRAVENOUS INFUSION USING LIPID FORMULATION
▸ Adult: (consult product literature or local protocols)

● CONTRA-INDICATIONS Bowel obstruction · chronic inflammatory bowel disease

● CAUTIONS Raised plasma-bilirubin concentration · risk factors for cardiac disease · risk factors for pulmonary toxicity · underweight patients—increased risk of adverse events

● INTERACTIONS → Appendix 1: irinotecan

● SIDE-EFFECTS
▸ Common or very common Abdominal pain · alopecia · anaemia (dose-limiting) · appetite decreased · asthenia · cholinergic syndrome · constipation · diarrhoea (delayed diarrhoea requires prompt treatment) · febrile neutropenia (dose-limiting) · fever · infection · mucositis · nausea · neutropenia (dose-limiting) · thrombocytopenia (dose-limiting) · vomiting

● CONCEPTION AND CONTRACEPTION For *conventional* formulations, manufacturer advises effective contraception during treatment and for up to 1 month after treatment in women of child-bearing potential, and up to 3 months after treatment in men. For *liposomal* formulations, manufacturer advises effective contraception during treatment and for up to 1 month after treatment in women of child-bearing potential, and up to 4 months after treatment in men.

● PREGNANCY Manufacturer advises avoid unless essential—toxicity in *animal* studies. See also Pregnancy and reproductive function in Cytotoxic drugs p. 865.

● BREAST FEEDING For *conventional* formulations, manufacturer advises avoid. For *liposomal* formulations, manufacturer advises avoid until one month after the last dose—no information available.

● HEPATIC IMPAIRMENT For *conventional* formulations, manufacturer advises monitor liver function at baseline and before each cycle; also monitor complete blood counts weekly if plasma-bilirubin concentration 1.5–3 times the upper limit of normal; avoid if plasma-bilirubin concentration greater than 3 times the upper limit of normal. For *liposomal* formulations, manufacturer advises use with caution; avoid if bilirubin greater than 2 mg/dL or if plasma-transaminase greater than 2.5 times the upper limit of normal (greater than 5 times the upper limit of normal if liver metastasis present)—limited information available.

Dose adjustments For *conventional* formulations, manufacturer advises dose adjustment—consult product literature.

● RENAL IMPAIRMENT For *conventional* formulations, manufacturer advises avoid—no information available. For *liposomal* formulations, manufacturer advises avoid in severe impairment—no information available.

● MONITORING REQUIREMENTS Monitor respiratory function.

● PRESCRIBING AND DISPENSING INFORMATION Irinotecan is available as both *conventional* and *liposomal* formulations. Manufacturers advise that the different formulations vary in their licensed indications, pharmacokinetics, dosage and administration, and are **not** interchangeable.

● NATIONAL FUNDING/ACCESS DECISIONS

NICE decisions
▸ Irinotecan, oxaliplatin, and raltitrexed for advanced colorectal cancer (August 2005) NICE TA93
A combination of fluorouracil and folinic acid with either irinotecan or oxaliplatin are options for first-line treatment for advanced colorectal cancer.

Irinotecan alone or fluorouracil and folinic acid with oxaliplatin are options for patients who require further treatment subsequently.
www.nice.org.uk/TA93

▸ **Pegylated liposomal irinotecan for treating pancreatic cancer after gemcitabine (April 2017)** NICE TA440
Pegylated liposomal irinotecan, in combination with fluorouracil and leucovorin, is **not** recommended for treating metastatic adenocarcinoma of the pancreas in adults whose disease has progressed after gemcitabine-based therapy.

Patients whose treatment was started within the NHS before this guidance was published should have the option to continue treatment, without change to their funding arrangements, until they and their clinician consider it appropriate to stop.
www.nice.org.uk/guidance/TA440

Scottish Medicines Consortium (SMC) Decisions
The *Scottish Medicines Consortium* has advised (March 2017) that liposomal irinotecan (*Onivyde*®) is **not** recommended for use within NHS Scotland for the treatment of metastatic adenocarcinoma of the pancreas, in combination with fluorouracil and leucovorin (folinic acid), in patients who have progressed following gemcitabine based therapy as there was insufficient evidence submitted.

● MEDICINAL FORMS
There can be variation in the licensing of different medicines containing the same drug.
Solution for infusion
ELECTROLYTES: May contain Sodium
▸ Irinotecan hydrochloride (Non-proprietary)
  Irinotecan hydrochloride trihydrate 20 mg per 1 ml Irinotecan 500mg/25ml concentrate for solution for infusion vials | 1 vial [PoM] £601.25–£650.00 (Hospital only) | 1 vial [PoM] £601.25
  Irinotecan 40mg/2ml concentrate for solution for infusion vials | 1 vial [PoM] £49.03–£53.00 (Hospital only) | 1 vial [PoM] £49.03–£50.35
  Irinotecan 300mg/15ml concentrate for solution for infusion vials | 1 vial [PoM] £390.00 (Hospital only) | 1 vial [PoM] £365.84–£390.00
  Irinotecan 100mg/5ml concentrate for solution for infusion vials | 1 vial [PoM] £120.25–£130.00 (Hospital only) | 1 vial [PoM] £120.25–£123.50
▸ Campto (Pfizer Ltd)
  Irinotecan hydrochloride trihydrate 20 mg per 1 ml Campto 100mg/5ml concentrate for solution for infusion vials | 1 vial [PoM] £130.00 (Hospital only)
  Campto 40mg/2ml concentrate for solution for infusion vials | 1 vial [PoM] £53.00 (Hospital only)
  Campto 300mg/15ml concentrate for solution for infusion vials | 1 vial [PoM] £390.00 (Hospital only)
▸ Onivyde (Baxalta UK Ltd)
  Irinotecan hydrochloride trihydrate 5 mg per 1 ml Onivyde 50mg/10ml concentrate for solution for infusion vials | 1 vial [PoM] £615.35 (Hospital only)

Topotecan
10-Jun-2016

● DRUG ACTION Topotecan inhibits topoisomerase I, an enzyme involved in DNA replication.

● INDICATIONS AND DOSE

Metastatic ovarian cancer when first-line or subsequent treatment has failed | Treatment of recurrent carcinoma of the cervix, after radiotherapy, and for patients with stage IVB disease (in combination with cisplatin)
▸ BY INTRAVENOUS INFUSION
  ▸ Adult: (consult product literature or local protocols)

Relapsed small-cell lung cancer when retreatment with the first-line regimen is considered inappropriate
▸ BY INTRAVENOUS INFUSION, OR BY MOUTH
  ▸ Adult: (consult product literature or local protocols)

┌───┐
IMPORTANT SAFETY INFORMATION
RISKS OF INCORRECT DOSING OF ORAL ANTI-CANCER MEDICINES
See Cytotoxic drugs p. 865.
└───┘

● INTERACTIONS → Appendix 1: topotecan
● SIDE-EFFECTS
  GENERAL SIDE-EFFECTS
▸ **Common or very common** Alopecia · anaemia · appetite decreased · asthenia · colitis neutropenic · constipation · diarrhoea · fever · gastrointestinal discomfort · hyperbilirubinaemia · hypersensitivity · infection · leucopenia · malaise · mucositis · nausea · neutropenia · pancytopenia · sepsis · skin reactions · thrombocytopenia · vomiting
▸ **Rare or very rare** Angioedema · interstitial lung disease
▸ **Frequency not known** Bone marrow depression (dose-limiting) · haemorrhage

● CONCEPTION AND CONTRACEPTION Contraceptive advice required, see *Pregnancy and reproductive function* in Cytotoxic drugs p. 865.

● PREGNANCY Avoid (teratogenicity and fetal loss in *animal* studies). See also *Pregnancy and reproductive function* in Cytotoxic drugs p. 865.

● BREAST FEEDING Discontinue breast-feeding.

● HEPATIC IMPAIRMENT Avoid in severe impairment.

● RENAL IMPAIRMENT Avoid infusion if creatinine clearance less than 20 mL/minute. Avoid oral route if creatinine clearance less than 60 mL/minute.
  Dose adjustments Reduce dose.

● NATIONAL FUNDING/ACCESS DECISIONS

NICE decisions
▸ **Topotecan for the treatment of recurrent and stage IVB cervical cancer (October 2009)** NICE TA183
Topotecan in combination with cisplatin is recommended as a treatment option for recurrent or stage IVB cervical cancer in patients who have not previously received cisplatin.
www.nice.org.uk/TA183

▸ **Topotecan for the treatment of relapsed small-cell lung cancer (November 2009)** NICE TA184
Oral topotecan is recommended as an option for treatment in patients with relapsed small-cell lung cancer only if re-treatment with the first-line regimen is not considered appropriate, and the combination of cyclophosphamide, doxorubicin and vincristine is contra-indicated. Intravenous topotecan is not recommended for people with relapsed small-cell lung cancer.
www.nice.org.uk/TA184

▸ **Topotecan, pegylated liposomal doxorubicin hydrochloride, paclitaxel, trabectedin and gemcitabine for treating recurrent ovarian cancer (April 2016)** NICE TA389
Topotecan is **not** recommended for treating first recurrence of platinum-sensitive ovarian cancer, recurrent platinum-resistant ovarian cancer, or platinum-refractory ovarian cancer.

Patients currently receiving topotecan should have the option to continue their treatment until they or their clinician consider it appropriate to stop.
www.nice.org.uk/TA389

Scottish Medicines Consortium (SMC) Decisions
The *Scottish Medicines Consortium* has advised (November 2007) that topotecan (*Hycamtin*®) is accepted for restricted use in combination with cisplatin for treatment of recurrent carcinoma of the cervix after radiotherapy and for stage IVB disease; it is restricted to patients who have not previously received cisplatin treatment.

8

Immune system and malignant disease

- **MEDICINAL FORMS**
There can be variation in the licensing of different medicines containing the same drug.
Solution for infusion
  ▸ Topotecan (Non-proprietary)
Topotecan (as Topotecan hydrochloride) 1 mg per 1 ml Topotecan 4mg/4ml concentrate for solution for infusion vials | 1 vial PoM £261.55 (Hospital only) | 1 vial PoM £290.00 | 5 vial PoM £1,453.10 (Hospital only)
Topotecan 1mg/1ml concentrate for solution for infusion vials | 1 vial PoM £87.88 (Hospital only) | 1 vial PoM £97.00
Powder for solution for infusion
  ▸ Hycamtin (Novartis Pharmaceuticals UK Ltd)
Topotecan (as Topotecan hydrochloride) 1mg Hycamtin 1mg powder for concentrate for solution for infusion vials | 1 vial PoM £97.65
Topotecan (as Topotecan hydrochloride) 4 mg Hycamtin 4mg powder for concentrate for solution for infusion vials | 1 vial PoM £348.76
  ▸ Potactasol (Actavis UK Ltd)
Topotecan (as Topotecan hydrochloride) 1 mg Potactasol 1mg powder for concentrate for solution for infusion vials | 1 vial PoM £97.00 (Hospital only)
Topotecan (as Topotecan hydrochloride) 4 mg Potactasol 4mg powder for concentrate for solution for infusion vials | 1 vial PoM £290.00 (Hospital only)
Capsule
CAUTIONARY AND ADVISORY LABELS 25
  ▸ Hycamtin (Novartis Pharmaceuticals UK Ltd)
Topotecan (as Topotecan hydrochloride)
250 microgram Hycamtin 0.25mg capsules | 10 capsule PoM £75.00
Topotecan (as Topotecan hydrochloride) 1 mg Hycamtin 1mg capsules | 10 capsule PoM £360.00

ANTINEOPLASTIC DRUGS ⟩ VINCA ALKALOIDS

Vinblastine sulfate

- **INDICATIONS AND DOSE**
Variety of cancers including leukaemias, lymphomas, and some solid tumours (e.g. breast and lung cancer)
  ▸ Adult: (consult product literature)

> **IMPORTANT SAFETY INFORMATION**
> Vinblastine is for **intravenous administration only**. Inadvertent intrathecal administration can cause severe neurotoxicity, which is usually fatal.
> The National Patient Safety Agency has advised (August 2008) that adult and teenage patients treated in an adult or adolescent unit should receive their vinca alkaloid dose in a 50 mL minibag. Teenagers and children treated in a child unit may receive their vinca alkaloid dose in a syringe.

- **CONTRA-INDICATIONS**
CONTRA-INDICATIONS, FURTHER INFORMATION
Intrathecal injection **contra-indicated**.
- **CAUTIONS** Caution in handling—irritant to tissues
- **INTERACTIONS** → Appendix 1: vinca alkaloids
- **SIDE-EFFECTS**
  ▸ **Rare or very rare** Hearing impairment · nerve disorders
  ▸ **Frequency not known** Abdominal pain · acute respiratory distress syndrome (ARDS) · alopecia (reversible) · anaemia · appetite decreased · asthenia · balance impaired · cancer pain · constipation · depression · diarrhoea · dizziness · dyspnoea · haemorrhage · headache · hypertension · ileus · increased risk of infection · leucopenia (dose-limiting) · malaise · mediastinal disorder · myalgia · myocardial infarction · nausea · nystagmus · oral blistering · pain · Raynaud's phenomenon · reflexes absent · seizure · sensation abnormal · SIADH · skin reactions · stroke · thrombocytopenia · vertigo · vomiting

- **CONCEPTION AND CONTRACEPTION** Contraceptive advice required, see *Pregnancy and reproductive function* in Cytotoxic drugs p. 865.
- **PREGNANCY** Avoid (limited experience suggests fetal harm; teratogenic in *animal* studies). See also *Pregnancy and reproductive function* in Cytotoxic drugs p. 865.
- **BREAST FEEDING** Discontinue breast-feeding.
- **HEPATIC IMPAIRMENT**
Dose adjustments Dose reduction may be necessary—consult local treatment protocol for details.

- **MEDICINAL FORMS**
There can be variation in the licensing of different medicines containing the same drug.
Solution for injection
  ▸ Vinblastine sulfate (Non-proprietary)
Vinblastine sulfate 1 mg per 1 ml Vinblastine 10mg/10ml solution for injection vials | 5 vial PoM £85.00 (Hospital only)

Vincristine sulfate

- **INDICATIONS AND DOSE**
Variety of cancers including leukaemias, lymphomas, and some solid tumours (e.g. breast and lung cancer)
  ▸ Adult: (consult local protocol)

> **IMPORTANT SAFETY INFORMATION**
> Vincristine injections are for **intravenous administration only**. Inadvertent intrathecal administration can cause severe neurotoxicity, which is usually fatal.
> The National Patient Safety Agency has advised (August 2008) that adult and teenage patients treated in an adult or adolescent unit should receive their vinca alkaloid dose in a 50 mL minibag. Teenagers and children treated in a child unit may receive their vinca alkaloid dose in a syringe.

- **CONTRA-INDICATIONS**
CONTRA-INDICATIONS, FURTHER INFORMATION
Intrathecal injection **contra-indicated**.
- **CAUTIONS** Caution in handling—irritant to tissues · neuromuscular disease
- **INTERACTIONS** → Appendix 1: vinca alkaloids
- **SIDE-EFFECTS**
  ▸ **Rare or very rare** Hypersensitivity · rash · SIADH
  ▸ **Frequency not known** Abdominal cramps · adrenal disorder · alopecia · anaemia · appetite decreased · azotaemia · bladder atony · bronchospasm · connective tissue disorders · constipation · coronary artery disease · dehydration · diarrhoea · dizziness · dyspnoea · eighth cranial nerve damage · eye disorders · fever · gait abnormalities · gastrointestinal disorders · haemolytic anaemia · headache · hearing impairment · hypertension · hyponatraemia · hypotension · infection · leucopenia · movement disorders · muscle atrophy · myalgia · myocardial infarction · nausea · neuromuscular effects (dose-limiting) · neutropenia · oedema · oral disorders · pain · paralysis · paresis · reflexes absent · renal disorder · secondary malignancy · sensation abnormal · sepsis · throat pain · thrombocytopenia · urinary disorders · vertigo · vision loss · vomiting · weight decreased

SIDE-EFFECTS, FURTHER INFORMATION
Bronchospasm Severe bronchospasm following administration is more common when used in combination with mitomycin-C.
Neurotoxicity Sensory and motor neuropathies are common and are cumulative. Manufacturer advises monitoring patients for symptoms of neuropathy, such as hypoesthesia, hyperesthesia, paresthesia, hyporeflexia,

areflexia, neuralgia, jaw pain, decreased vibratory sense, cranial neuropathy, ileus, burning sensation, arthralgia, myalgia, muscle spasm, or weakness, both before and during treatment—requires dose reduction, treatment interruption or treatment discontinuation, depending on severity.

Motor weakness can also occur and dose reduction or discontinuation of therapy may be appropriate if motor weakness increases. Recovery from neurotoxic effects is usually slow but complete.

- CONCEPTION AND CONTRACEPTION Contraceptive advice required, see *Pregnancy and reproductive function* in Cytotoxic drugs p. 865.
- PREGNANCY Avoid (teratogenicity and fetal loss in *animal* studies). See also *Pregnancy and reproductive function* in Cytotoxic drugs p. 865.
- BREAST FEEDING Discontinue breast-feeding.
- HEPATIC IMPAIRMENT
  Dose adjustments Dose reduction may be necessary—consult local treatment protocol for details.

- MEDICINAL FORMS
  There can be variation in the licensing of different medicines containing the same drug.
  Solution for injection
  ▸ Vincristine sulfate (Non-proprietary)
    Vincristine sulfate 1 mg per 1 ml Vincristine 2mg/2ml solution for injection vials | 1 vial [PoM] £26.66 (Hospital only) | 5 vial [PoM] £133.30 (Hospital only)
    Vincristine 1mg/1ml solution for injection vials | 1 vial [PoM] £13.47 (Hospital only) | 5 vial [PoM] £67.35 (Hospital only)
    Vincristine 5mg/5ml solution for injection vials | 5 vial [PoM] £329.50 (Hospital only)

Vindesine sulfate

- **INDICATIONS AND DOSE**
  Variety of cancers including leukaemias, lymphomas, and some solid tumours (e.g. breast and lung cancer)
  ▸ Adult: (consult product literature)

IMPORTANT SAFETY INFORMATION
Vindesine injections are for **intravenous administration only**. Inadvertent intrathecal administration can cause severe neurotoxicity, which is usually fatal.

The National Patient Safety Agency has advised (August 2008) that adult and teenage patients treated in an adult or adolescent unit should receive their vinca alkaloid dose in a 50 mL minibag. Teenagers and children treated in a child unit may receive their vinca alkaloid dose in a syringe.

- CONTRA-INDICATIONS
  CONTRA-INDICATIONS, FURTHER INFORMATION
  Intrathecal injection **contra-indicated**.
- CAUTIONS Caution in handling—irritant to tissues · neuromuscular disease
- INTERACTIONS → Appendix 1: vinca alkaloids
- SIDE-EFFECTS
  ▸ **Common or very common** Alopecia
  ▸ **Frequency not known** Anaemia · appetite decreased · asthenia · balance impaired · cellulitis · chills · constipation · depression · diarrhoea · dizziness · dysphagia · fever · gastrointestinal discomfort · gastrointestinal disorders · granulocytopenia (dose-limiting) · headache · hearing impairment · malaise · nausea · nerve disorders · nystagmus · oral disorders · pain · peroneal nerve palsy · rash maculopapular · reflexes absent · seizure · sensation abnormal · thrombocytopenia · thrombocytosis · vertigo · vision loss · vomiting

SIDE-EFFECTS, FURTHER INFORMATION Neurotoxicity, usually as peripheral or autonomic neuropathy; it occurs less often with vindesine than with vincristine. Patients with neurotoxicity commonly have peripheral paraesthesia, loss of deep tendon reflexes; and ototoxicity has been reported. There have been instances in which neurotoxicity has made it necessary to reduce the dosage or temporarily discontinue use of vindesine.

- CONCEPTION AND CONTRACEPTION Contraceptive advice required, see *Pregnancy and reproductive function* in Cytotoxic drugs p. 865.
- PREGNANCY Avoid (teratogenic in *animal* studies). See also *Pregnancy and reproductive function* in Cytotoxic drugs p. 865.
- BREAST FEEDING Discontinue breast-feeding.
- HEPATIC IMPAIRMENT
  Dose adjustments Dose reduction may be necessary.

- MEDICINAL FORMS
  There can be variation in the licensing of different medicines containing the same drug.
  Powder for solution for injection
  ▸ Eldisine (Thornton & Ross Ltd)
    Vindesine sulfate 5 mg Eldisine 5mg powder for solution for injection vials | 1 vial [PoM] £66.55 (Hospital only)

Vinflunine

- **INDICATIONS AND DOSE**
  Treatment of advanced or metastatic transitional cell carcinoma of the urothelial tract after failure of a platinum-containing regimen (monotherapy)
  ▸ Adult: (consult local protocol)

IMPORTANT SAFETY INFORMATION
Vinflunine injections are for **intravenous administration only**. Inadvertent intrathecal administration can cause severe neurotoxicity, which is usually fatal.

The National Patient Safety Agency has advised (August 2008) that adult and teenage patients treated in an adult or adolescent unit should receive their vinca alkaloid dose in a 50 mL minibag. Teenagers and children treated in a child unit may receive their vinca alkaloid dose in a syringe.

- CONTRA-INDICATIONS
  CONTRA-INDICATIONS, FURTHER INFORMATION
  Intrathecal injection **contra-indicated**.
- CAUTIONS Cardiovascular disease · QT-interval prolongation (avoid hypokalaemia)
- INTERACTIONS → Appendix 1: vinca alkaloids
- SIDE-EFFECTS
  ▸ **Common or very common** Alopecia · anaemia · appetite decreased · arthralgia · asthenia · chest pain · chills · constipation · cough · dehydration · diarrhoea · dizziness · dyspnoea · ear pain · fever · gastrointestinal discomfort · gastrointestinal disorders · headache · hyperhidrosis · hypersensitivity · hypertension · hyponatraemia · hypotension · increased risk of infection · insomnia · leucopenia · muscle weakness · myalgia · nausea · neutropenia · oedema · oral disorders · pain · peripheral neuropathy · skin reactions · swallowing difficulty · syncope · tachycardia · taste altered · thrombocytopenia · venous thrombosis · vomiting · weight changes
  ▸ **Uncommon** Acute respiratory distress syndrome (ARDS) · cancer pain · laryngeal pain · myocardial infarction · myocardial ischaemia · neutropenic sepsis · renal failure · SIADH · tinnitus · vertigo · visual impairment

8

Immune system and malignant disease

▶ **Rare or very rare** Posterior reversible encephalopathy syndrome (PRES)

● CONCEPTION AND CONTRACEPTION Manufacturer advises effective contraception during and for up to 3 months after treatment.

● PREGNANCY Avoid unless essential—teratogenicity and embryotoxicity in *animal* studies. See also *Pregnancy and reproductive function* in Cytotoxic drugs p. 865.

● BREAST FEEDING Discontinue breast-feeding.

● HEPATIC IMPAIRMENT
Dose adjustments Reduce dose—consult product literature.

● RENAL IMPAIRMENT
Dose adjustments Reduce dose if creatinine clearance less than 60 mL/minute—consult product literature.

● NATIONAL FUNDING/ACCESS DECISIONS

NICE decisions
▶ **Vinflunine for the treatment of advanced or metastatic transitional cell carcinoma of the urothelial tract (January 2013) NICE TA272**
Vinflunine is **not** recommended for the treatment of advanced or metastatic transitional cell carcinoma of the urothelial tract that has progressed after treatment with platinum-based chemotherapy.
www.nice.org.uk/TA272

● MEDICINAL FORMS
There can be variation in the licensing of different medicines containing the same drug.
Solution for infusion
▶ Javlor (Pierre Fabre Ltd)
Vinflunine (as Vinflunine ditartrate) 25 mg per 1 ml Javlor 250mg/10ml concentrate for solution for infusion vials | 1 vial POM £1,062.50
Javlor 50mg/2ml concentrate for solution for infusion vials | 1 vial POM £212.50

Vinorelbine

● DRUG ACTION Vinorelbine is a semi-synthetic vinca alkaloid.

● **INDICATIONS AND DOSE**

Advanced breast cancer | Advanced non-small cell lung cancer
▶ BY MOUTH
▶ Adult: 60 mg/m^2 once weekly for 3 weeks, then increased if tolerated to 80 mg/m^2 once weekly (max. per dose 160 mg once weekly)
▶ BY INTRAVENOUS INJECTION, OR BY INTRAVENOUS INFUSION
▶ Adult: (consult product literature)

IMPORTANT SAFETY INFORMATION
Vinorelbine injections are for **intravenous administration only**. Inadvertent intrathecal administration can cause severe neurotoxicity, which is usually fatal.
   The National Patient Safety Agency has advised (August 2008) that adult and teenage patients treated in an adult or adolescent unit should receive their vinca alkaloid dose in a 50 mL minibag. Teenagers and children treated in a child unit may receive their vinca alkaloid dose in a syringe.

RISKS OF INCORRECT DOSING OF ORAL ANTI-CANCER MEDICINES
See Cytotoxic drugs p. 865.

● CONTRA-INDICATIONS
▶ With oral use concurrent radiotherapy if treating the liver · long-term oxygen therapy · previous significant surgical resection of small bowel · previous significant surgical resection of stomach

CONTRA-INDICATIONS, FURTHER INFORMATION
Intrathecal injection **contra-indicated**.

● CAUTIONS Caution in handling—irritant to tissues · ischaemic heart disease

● INTERACTIONS → Appendix 1: vinca alkaloids

● SIDE-EFFECTS

GENERAL SIDE-EFFECTS
▶ **Common or very common** Alopecia · anaemia · appetite decreased · arthralgia · bone marrow depression (dose-limiting) · constipation · diarrhoea · dyspnoea · fever · hypertension · hypotension · increased risk of infection · leucopenia · myalgia · nausea · neutropenia (dose-limiting) · pain · reflexes absent · stomatitis · thrombocytopenia · vomiting
▶ **Uncommon** Flushing · peripheral coldness · respiratory disorders · sepsis
▶ **Rare or very rare** Circulatory collapse · hyponatraemia · myocardial infarction · pancreatitis
▶ **Frequency not known** SIADH

SPECIFIC SIDE-EFFECTS
▶ **Common or very common**
▶ With intravenous use Asthenia · cancer pain · chest pain · muscle weakness in legs · nervous system disorder · vascular disorders
▶ With oral use Abdominal pain · chills · cough · dizziness · dysphagia · dysuria · fatigue · gastrointestinal disorders · headache · insomnia · liver disorder · neuromuscular disorders · sensory disorder · skin eruption · taste altered · urogenital disorder · vision disorder · weight changes
▶ **Uncommon**
▶ With intravenous use Paraesthesia
▶ With oral use Ataxia
▶ **Rare or very rare**
▶ With intravenous use Arrhythmias · ischaemic heart disease · necrosis · palpitations · paralytic ileus · skin reactions
▶ **Frequency not known**
▶ With intravenous use Febrile neutropenia
▶ With oral use Gastrointestinal haemorrhage · hypersensitivity

SIDE-EFFECTS, FURTHER INFORMATION
Bronchospasm Severe bronchospasm following administration of the vinca alkaloids is more common when used in combination with mitomycin-C.
Neurotoxicity Neurotoxicity reported in clinical trials, most commonly as constipation, paresthesia, hypersthesia, and hyporeflexia

● CONCEPTION AND CONTRACEPTION Manufacturer advises effective contraception during and for 3 months after treatment; men must avoid fathering a child during and for at least 3 months after treatment.

● PREGNANCY Avoid unless essential (teratogenicity, and fetal loss in *animal* studies). See also *Pregnancy and reproductive function* in Cytotoxic drugs p. 865.

● BREAST FEEDING Discontinue breast-feeding.

● HEPATIC IMPAIRMENT Avoid *oral* use in severe impairment.
Dose adjustments ▶ With oral use Reduce *oral* dose in moderate impairment.
▶ With injectable use Reduce *intravenous dose* in severe impairment.

MEDICINAL FORMS

There can be variation in the licensing of different medicines containing the same drug.

Solution for infusion

▸ Vinorelbine (Non-proprietary)

Vinorelbine (as Vinorelbine tartrate) 10 mg per 1 ml Vinorelbine 50mg/5ml concentrate for solution for infusion vials | 1 vial PoM £139.00 | 10 vial PoM £1,539.80
Vinorelbine 10mg/1ml concentrate for solution for infusion vials | 1 vial PoM £29.00 | 10 vial PoM £329.50

▸ Navelbine (Pierre Fabre Ltd)

Vinorelbine (as Vinorelbine tartrate) 10 mg per 1 ml Navelbine 10mg/1ml concentrate for solution for infusion vials | 10 vial PoM £297.45 (Hospital only)
Navelbine 50mg/5ml concentrate for solution for infusion vials | 10 vial PoM £1,399.79 (Hospital only)

Capsule

CAUTIONARY AND ADVISORY LABELS 21, 25

▸ Navelbine (Pierre Fabre Ltd)

Vinorelbine (as Vinorelbine tartrate) 20 mg Navelbine 20mg capsules | 1 capsule PoM £43.98 (Hospital only)
Vinorelbine (as Vinorelbine tartrate) 30 mg Navelbine 30mg capsules | 1 capsule PoM £65.98 (Hospital only)
Vinorelbine (as Vinorelbine tartrate) 80 mg Navelbine 80mg capsules | 1 capsule PoM £175.92 (Hospital only)

ANTINEOPLASTIC DRUGS > OTHER

Amsacrine

24-May-2017

● INDICATIONS AND DOSE

Acute leukaemia (refractory to anthracycline chemotherapy used alone or in combination with other chemotherapy agents) (specialist use only)

▸ BY INTRAVENOUS INFUSION
▸ Adult: (consult product literature)

● CAUTIONS Hypokalaemia—increased risk of ventricular fibrillation (correct hypokalaemia before initiating treatment)

● INTERACTIONS → Appendix 1: amsacrine

● SIDE-EFFECTS

▸ **Common or very common** Abdominal pain · alopecia · arrhythmias · bone marrow disorders · cardiotoxicity · congestive heart failure · diarrhoea · dyspnoea · emotional lability · fever · generalised tonic-clonic seizure · haemorrhage · hepatic disorders · hypokalaemia · hypotension · infection · nausea · necrosis · skin reactions · stomatitis · thrombocytopenia · vomiting

▸ **Rare or very rare** Anaemia · cardiomyopathy · confusion · dizziness · granulocytopenia · headache · lethargy · leucopenia · numbness · peripheral neuropathy · proteinuria · renal impairment · visual impairment · weight changes

▸ **Frequency not known** Cardiac arrest · hyperuricaemia

● CONCEPTION AND CONTRACEPTION Manufacturer advises effective contraception during and for 3 months after treatment in women of child-bearing potential, and during and for 6 months after treatment in men.

● PREGNANCY Manufacturer advises avoid—toxicity in *animal* studies. See also *Pregnancy and reproductive function* in Cytotoxic drugs p. 865.

● BREAST FEEDING Manufacturer advises avoid—no information available.

● HEPATIC IMPAIRMENT Manufacturer advises monitor liver function at baseline and during treatment—increased risk of toxicity.

Dose adjustments Manufacturer advises consider dose reduction in hepatic impairment.

● RENAL IMPAIRMENT Manufacturer advises monitor renal function at baseline and during treatment—increased risk of toxicity.

Dose adjustments Manufacturer advises consider dose reduction in renal impairment.

● MONITORING REQUIREMENTS

▸ Manufacturer advises monitor full blood count, liver function and renal function regularly; electrolytes should be re-evaluated prior to each treatment.

▸ Manufacturer advises monitor for cardiotoxicity during treatment.

● MEDICINAL FORMS

There can be variation in the licensing of different medicines containing the same drug.

Solution for infusion

▸ Amsidine (Eurocept International bv)

Amsacrine 50 mg per 1 ml Amsidine 75mg/1.5ml solution for infusion ampoules and diluent | 6 ampoule PoM £1,200.00 (Hospital only)

Arsenic trioxide

● INDICATIONS AND DOSE

Acute promyelocytic leukaemia in patients who have relapsed or failed to respond to previous treatment with a retinoid and chemotherapy

▸ BY INTRAVENOUS INFUSION
▸ Adult: (consult local protocol)

● CAUTIONS Hypokalaemia (correct before treatment) · hypomagnesaemia (correct before treatment) · previous treatment with anthracyclines (increased risk of QT interval prolongation)

● INTERACTIONS → Appendix 1: arsenic trioxide

● SIDE-EFFECTS

▸ **Common or very common** Abdominal pain · alveolar haemorrhage · anaemia · arrhythmias · arthralgia · chest pain · chills · diarrhoea · differentiation syndrome · dizziness · dyspnoea · electrolyte imbalance · fatigue · fever · headache · hyperbilirubinaemia · hyperglycaemia · hypotension · hypoxia · increased risk of infection · ketoacidosis · leucocytosis · myalgia · nausea · neutropenia · oedema · pain · pancytopenia · paraesthesia · pericardial effusion · QT interval prolongation · renal failure · respiratory disorders · seizure · skin reactions · thrombocytopenia · vasculitis · vision blurred · vomiting · weight increased

▸ **Frequency not known** Confusion · decreased leucocytes · fluid imbalance · heart failure · hepatotoxicity · peripheral neuropathy · sepsis

SIDE-EFFECTS, FURTHER INFORMATION Signs and symptoms of differentiation syndrome (leucocyte activation syndrome) include unexplained fever, dyspnoea, weight gain, pulmonary infiltrates, pleural or pericardial effusions, with or without leucocytosis—treat with high dose corticosteroids, consult product literature.

● CONCEPTION AND CONTRACEPTION Manufacturer advises effective contraception during treatment in men and women.

● PREGNANCY Avoid (teratogenic and embryotoxic in *animal* studies). See also *Pregnancy and reproductive function* in Cytotoxic drugs p. 865.

● BREAST FEEDING Discontinue breast-feeding.

● HEPATIC IMPAIRMENT Manufacturer advises caution—limited information available.

● RENAL IMPAIRMENT Manufacturer advises caution—limited information available.

● MONITORING REQUIREMENTS ECG required before and during treatment—consult product literature.

Immune system and malignant disease

8

● MEDICINAL FORMS
There can be variation in the licensing of different medicines containing the same drug.
Solution for infusion
▸ Trisenox (Teva UK Ltd)
  Arsenic trioxide 1 mg per 1 ml Trisenox 10mg/10ml concentrate for solution for infusion ampoules | 10 ampoule [PoM] £2,920.00 (Hospital only)

Asparaginase

18-May-2018

● DRUG ACTION Asparaginase is an enzyme which acts by breaking down L-asparagine to aspartic acid and ammonia, this disrupts protein synthesis of tumour cells.

● INDICATIONS AND DOSE

Acute lymphoblastic leukaemia (in combination with other antineoplastic drugs) (specialist use only)
▸ BY INTRAVENOUS INFUSION
▸ Adult: 5000 units/m^2 every 3 days

● CONTRA-INDICATIONS History of pancreatitis related to asparaginase therapy · history of serious haemorrhage related to asparaginase therapy · history of serious thrombosis related to asparaginase therapy · pancreatitis · pre-existing known coagulopathy

● CAUTIONS Diabetes (may raise blood glucose) · hypersensitivity reactions · hypertriglyceridaemia (severe)—increased risk of acute pancreatitis
CAUTIONS, FURTHER INFORMATION
▸ Hypersensitivity reactions Serious hypersensitivity reactions, including life-threatening anaphylaxis, can occur—asparaginase should only be administered when appropriately trained staff and resuscitation facilities are immediately available; in the event of a hypersensitivity reaction, treatment should be stopped immediately and appropriate management initiated. Manufacturer advises an intracutaneous or small intravenous test dose can be used but is of limited value for predicting which patients will experience an allergic reaction.

● INTERACTIONS → Appendix 1: asparaginase

● SIDE-EFFECTS
▸ **Common or very common** Abdominal pain · agitation · anaemia · angioedema · appetite decreased · arthralgia · back pain · bronchospasm · confusion · depression · diarrhoea · disseminated intravascular coagulation · dizziness · drowsiness · dyspnoea · embolism and thrombosis · fatigue · flushing · haemorrhage · hallucination · hyperglycaemia · hypersensitivity · hypoalbuminaemia · hypoglycaemia · hypotension · increased risk of infection · leucopenia · nausea · neurological effects · oedema · pancreatitis · skin reactions · thrombocytopenia · vomiting · weight decreased
▸ **Uncommon** Headache · hyperammonaemia · hyperuricaemia
▸ **Rare or very rare** Coma · consciousness impaired · diabetic ketoacidosis · hepatic disorders · hyperparathyroidism · hypoparathyroidism · ischaemic stroke · necrotising pancreatitis · pancreatic pseudocyst · posterior reversible encephalopathy syndrome (PRES) · seizure · tremor
SIDE-EFFECTS, FURTHER INFORMATION There have been rare reports of cholestasis, icterus, hepatic cell necrosis and hepatic failure with fatal outcome; manufacturer advises interrupt treatment if these symptoms develop.

● CONCEPTION AND CONTRACEPTION Manufacturer advises effective contraception in men and women of child-bearing potential during treatment and for at least 3 months after last dose; asparaginase may reduce effectiveness of oral contraceptives—additional precautions (e.g. barrier method) are required, see also

Pregnancy and reproductive function in Cytotoxic drugs p. 865.

● PREGNANCY Manufacturer advises avoid unless essential—toxicity in *animal* studies. See also *Pregnancy and reproductive function* in Cytotoxic drugs p. 865.

● BREAST FEEDING Manufacturer advises avoid—no information available.

● HEPATIC IMPAIRMENT Manufacturer advises avoid in severe impairment—no information available.

● MONITORING REQUIREMENTS
▸ Manufacturer advises monitor trough serum asparaginase levels 3 days after administration; consider switching to a different asparaginase preparation if target levels not reached—seek expert advice.
▸ Manufacturer advises monitor bilirubin, hepatic transaminases, and coagulation parameters before and during treatment; in addition, monitor plasma and urinary glucose, amylase, lipase, triglycerides, cholesterol and serum protein levels during treatment.

● HANDLING AND STORAGE Manufacturer advises store in a refrigerator (2–8°C)—consult product literature for storage conditions after reconstitution and dilution.

● PATIENT AND CARER ADVICE
Driving and skilled tasks Manufacturer advises asparaginase has moderate influence on driving and performance of skilled tasks—increased risk of dizziness and somnolence.

● NATIONAL FUNDING/ACCESS DECISIONS
Scottish Medicines Consortium (SMC) Decisions
SMC No. 1319/18
The *Scottish Medicines Consortium* has advised (April 2018) that asparaginase (*Spectrila*®) is accepted for use within NHS Scotland when used as a component of antineoplastic combination therapy for the treatment of acute lymphoblastic leukaemia in paediatric patients from birth to 18 years and adults.

● MEDICINAL FORMS
There can be variation in the licensing of different medicines containing the same drug.
Powder for solution for infusion
▸ Spectrila (medac UK) ▼
  Asparaginase 10000 unit Spectrila 10,000unit powder for concentrate for solution for infusion vials | 1 vial [PoM] £450.00 (Hospital only)

Crisantaspase

16-Mar-2017

● DRUG ACTION Crisantaspase is the enzyme asparaginase produced by *Erwinia chrysanthemi*.

● INDICATIONS AND DOSE

Acute lymphoblastic leukaemia
▸ BY INTRAMUSCULAR INJECTION, OR BY SUBCUTANEOUS INJECTION, OR BY INTRAVENOUS INJECTION
▸ Adult: (consult product literature)

● CONTRA-INDICATIONS History of pancreatitis related to asparaginase therapy

● CAUTIONS Diabetes (may raise blood glucose)

● INTERACTIONS → Appendix 1: crisantaspase

● SIDE-EFFECTS
▸ **Common or very common** Chills · coagulation disorders · confusion · diarrhoea · dizziness · drowsiness · dyspnoea · face oedema · fever · headache · hepatic disorders · hypersensitivity · limb swelling · lip swelling · neurotoxicity · pain · pallor · pancreatitis · seizures · skin reactions · thrombosis
▸ **Uncommon** Hyperglycaemia · hyperlipidaemia · hypoxia · increased risk of infection · respiratory disorders

▶ **Rare or very rare** Arthritis reactive · coma · diabetic ketoacidosis · dysphagia · dysphasia · encephalopathy · haemorrhage · level of consciousness decreased · myalgia · myocardial infarction · necrotising pancreatitis · neutropenia · paresis · sepsis · thrombocytopenia
▶ **Frequency not known** Abdominal pain · flushing · hyperammonaemia · hypertension · hypotension · nausea · pseudocyst · vomiting
● CONCEPTION AND CONTRACEPTION Contraceptive advice required, see *Pregnancy and reproductive function* in Cytotoxic drugs p. 865.
● PREGNANCY Avoid. See also, *Pregnancy and reproductive function* in Cytotoxic drugs p. 865.
● BREAST FEEDING Discontinue breast-feeding.
● DIRECTIONS FOR ADMINISTRATION Facilities for the management of anaphylaxis should be available.

● MEDICINAL FORMS
There can be variation in the licensing of different medicines containing the same drug.
Powder for solution for injection
▶ Erwinase (Jazz Pharmaceuticals UK)
  Crisantaspase 10000 unit Erwinase 10,000unit powder for solution for injection vials | 5 vial [PoM] £3,065.00

Eribulin   01-May-2018

● INDICATIONS AND DOSE

Treatment of locally advanced or metastatic breast cancer when the disease has progressed after treatment with at least 1 chemotherapy regimen for advanced disease
▶ BY INTRAVENOUS INJECTION
▶ Adult: Give on day 1 and day 8 of a 21-day cycle, previous therapy should have included an anthracycline and a taxane in either the adjuvant or metastatic setting unless the patient is unsuitable for these treatments (consult local protocol)

● CONTRA-INDICATIONS Congenital long QT syndrome
● CAUTIONS Bradyarrhythmias (increased susceptibility to QT-interval prolongation) · congestive heart failure (increased susceptibility to QT-interval prolongation) · electrolyte disturbances (increased susceptibility to QT-interval prolongation) · susceptibility to QT-interval prolongation
● INTERACTIONS → Appendix 1: eribulin
● SIDE-EFFECTS
▶ **Common or very common** Alopecia · anaemia · appetite decreased · arthralgia · asthenia · chest pain · chills · conjunctivitis · constipation · cough · decreased leucocytes · dehydration · depression · diarrhoea · dizziness · dry mouth · dyspnoea · dysuria · electrolyte imbalance · embolism and thrombosis · excessive tearing · fever · gastrointestinal discomfort · gastrooesophageal reflux disease · haemorrhage · headache · hot flush · hyperbilirubinaemia · hyperglycaemia · increased risk of infection · influenza like illness · insomnia · lethargy · mucositis · muscle complaints · muscle weakness · nail disorder · nausea · nerve disorders · neurotoxicity · neutropenia · oral disorders · oropharyngeal pain · pain · peripheral oedema · rhinorrhoea · sensation abnormal · skin reactions · sweat changes · tachycardia · taste altered · thrombocytopenia · tinnitus · vertigo · vomiting · weight decreased
▶ **Uncommon** Angioedema · hepatotoxicity · interstitial lung disease · pancreatitis · proteinuria · renal failure · sepsis
▶ **Rare or very rare** Disseminated intravascular coagulation
▶ **Frequency not known** QT interval prolongation · severe cutaneous adverse reactions (SCARs)

● CONCEPTION AND CONTRACEPTION Ensure effective contraception during and for up to 3 months after treatment in men or women.
● PREGNANCY Avoid unless essential (teratogenic in *animal* studies). See also *Pregnancy and reproductive function* in Cytotoxic drugs p. 865.
● BREAST FEEDING Discontinue breast-feeding.
● HEPATIC IMPAIRMENT
Dose adjustments Reduce dose.
● RENAL IMPAIRMENT
Dose adjustments Consider dose reduction if creatinine clearance less than 40 mL/minute.
● MONITORING REQUIREMENTS
▶ Monitor for signs of peripheral neuropathy—severe peripheral neurotoxicity requires treatment delay or dose reduction (consult product literature).
▶ ECG monitoring recommended in patients prescribed concomitant use of drugs that prolong the QT-interval or who are susceptible to QT-interval prolongation.
▶ Monitor electrolytes periodically.
● NATIONAL FUNDING/ACCESS DECISIONS

NICE decisions
▶ Eribulin for treating locally advanced or metastatic breast cancer after 2 or more chemotherapy regimens (December 2016) NICE TA423
Eribulin is recommended for the treatment of locally advanced or metastatic breast cancer, only if:
● the condition has progressed after at least 2 chemotherapy regimens (which may include an anthracycline or a taxane, and capecitabine), **and**
● the manufacturer provides eribulin with the discount agreed in the patient access scheme.
Patients whose treatment was started within the NHS before this guidance was published should continue treatment, without change to their funding arrangements, until they and their NHS clinician consider it appropriate to stop.
www.nice.org.uk/guidance/ta423
▶ Eribulin for treating locally advanced or metastatic breast cancer after 1 chemotherapy regimen (March 2018)
NICE TA515
Eribulin is **not** recommended for treating locally advanced or metastatic breast cancer in adults who have had only 1 chemotherapy regimen.
Patients whose treatment was started within the NHS before this guidance was published should have the option to continue treatment, without change to their funding arrangements, until they and their NHS clinician consider it appropriate to stop.
www.nice.org.uk/guidance/ta515
Scottish Medicines Consortium (SMC) Decisions
SMC No. 1065/15
The *Scottish Medicines Consortium* has advised (March 2016) that eribulin (*Halaven*®) is accepted for restricted use within NHS Scotland for the treatment of patients with locally advanced or metastatic breast cancer that has progressed after at least two prior chemotherapy regimens for advanced disease, which includes capecitabine if indicated. This advice is contingent upon the continuing availability of the patient access scheme in NHS Scotland or a list price that is equivalent or lower.

● MEDICINAL FORMS
There can be variation in the licensing of different medicines containing the same drug.
Solution for injection
EXCIPIENTS: May contain Ethanol
▶ Halaven (Eisai Ltd)
  Eribulin.44 mg per 1 ml Halaven 0.88mg/2ml solution for injection vials | 1 vial [PoM] £361.00 (Hospital only)
  Halaven 1.32mg/3ml solution for injection vials | 1 vial [PoM] £541.50 (Hospital only)

8

Immune system and malignant disease

Hydroxycarbamide

(Hydroxyurea)

22-Mar-2018

INDICATIONS AND DOSE

Polycythaemia vera (specialist use only)
▸ BY MOUTH
  ▸ Adult: Initially 15–20 mg/kg daily, adjusted according to response, for information on dose adjustment based on haematocrit and platelet count—consult product literature; usual dose 500–1000 mg daily, dosage should be based on actual or ideal body weight, whichever is less

Essential thrombocythaemia (specialist use only)
▸ BY MOUTH
  ▸ Adult: Initially 15 mg/kg daily, adjusted according to response, for information on dose adjustment based on platelet count and white cell count—consult product literature, dosage should be based on actual or ideal body weight, whichever is less

Chronic myeloid leukaemia (specialist use only)
▸ BY MOUTH
  ▸ Adult: Initially 40 mg/kg daily, then reduced to 20 mg/kg daily, adjusted according to response, for information on dose adjustment based on white cell count—consult product literature, dosage should be based on actual or ideal body weight, whichever is less

HYDREA ®

Chronic myeloid leukaemia (specialist use only) | Cancer of the cervix (specialist use only)
▸ BY MOUTH
  ▸ Adult: 20–30 mg/kg daily, alternatively 80 mg/kg every 3 days, for information on dose adjustment based on platelet count, white cell count and actual or ideal body weight—consult product literature

SIKLOS ®

Sickle-cell disease [prevention of recurrent vaso-occlusive crises] (initiated by a specialist)
▸ BY MOUTH
  ▸ Adult: Initially 15 mg/kg daily, increased in steps of 2.5–5 mg/kg daily, dose to be increased every 12 weeks according to response; usual dose 15–30 mg/kg daily; maximum 35 mg/kg per day

> **IMPORTANT SAFETY INFORMATION**
> RISKS OF INCORRECT DOSING OF ORAL ANTI-CANCER MEDICINES
> See Cytotoxic drugs p. 865.

- **CAUTIONS** Leg ulcers (review treatment if cutaneous vasculitic ulcerations develop)
- **INTERACTIONS** → Appendix 1: hydroxycarbamide
- **SIDE-EFFECTS**
  ▸ **Common or very common** Alopecia · anaemia · appetite decreased · asthenia · bone marrow failure · chills · constipation · cutaneous vasculitis · dermatomyositis · diarrhoea · disorientation · dizziness · drowsiness · dyspnoea · dysuria · fever · gastrointestinal discomfort · hallucination · headache · hepatic disorders · leucopenia · malaise · melaena · mucositis · nail disorder · nausea · pancreatitis · peripheral neuropathy · pulmonary oedema · respiratory disorders · seizure · skin cancer · skin reactions · skin ulcer · sperm abnormalities · stomatitis · thrombocytopenia · vomiting
  ▸ **Rare or very rare** Gangrene
- **CONCEPTION AND CONTRACEPTION** Manufacturer advises effective contraception before and during treatment.
- **PREGNANCY** Avoid (teratogenic in *animal* studies). See also *Pregnancy and reproductive function* in Cytotoxic drugs p. 865.
- **BREAST FEEDING** Discontinue breast-feeding.
- **HEPATIC IMPAIRMENT** Manufacturer advises caution in mild to moderate impairment. Avoid in severe impairment, unless used for malignant conditions.
- **RENAL IMPAIRMENT** In sickle-cell disease, avoid if eGFR less than 30 mL/minute/1.73 m². Use with caution in malignant disease.
  Dose adjustments In sickle-cell disease, reduce initial dose by 50% if eGFR less than 60 mL/minute/1.73 m².
- **MONITORING REQUIREMENTS**
  ▸ Monitor renal and hepatic function before and during treatment.
  ▸ Monitor full blood count before treatment, and repeatedly throughout use; in sickle-cell disease monitor every 2 weeks for the first 2 months and then every 2 months thereafter (or every 2 weeks if on maximum dose).
  ▸ Patients receiving long-term therapy for malignant disease should be monitored for secondary malignancies.
- **PATIENT AND CARER ADVICE** Patients receiving long-term therapy with hydroxycarbamide should be advised to protect skin from sun exposure.

- **MEDICINAL FORMS**
  There can be variation in the licensing of different medicines containing the same drug. Forms available from special-order manufacturers include: capsule, oral suspension, oral solution
  Tablet
  ▸ Siklos (Nordic Pharma Ltd)
    Hydroxycarbamide 100 mg Siklos 100mg tablets | 60 tablet [PoM] £100.00 DT = £100.00
    Hydroxycarbamide 1 gram Siklos 1000mg tablets | 30 tablet [PoM] £500.00 DT = £500.00
  Capsule
  ▸ Hydroxycarbamide (Non-proprietary)
    Hydroxycarbamide 500 mg Hydroxycarbamide 500mg capsules | 100 capsule [PoM] £86.00 DT = £12.14
  ▸ Droxia (Imported (United States))
    Hydroxycarbamide 300 mg Droxia 300mg capsules | 60 capsule [PoM] ⊠
  ▸ Hydrea (Bristol-Myers Squibb Pharmaceuticals Ltd)
    Hydroxycarbamide 500 mg Hydrea 500mg capsules | 100 capsule [PoM] £10.47 DT = £12.14

Mitotane

- **DRUG ACTION** Mitotane selectively inhibits the activity of the adrenal cortex, necessitating corticosteroid replacement therapy.

INDICATIONS AND DOSE

Symptomatic treatment of advanced or inoperable adrenocortical carcinoma
▸ BY MOUTH
  ▸ Adult: Initially 2–3 g daily in 2–3 divided doses adjusted according to plasma-concentration monitoring, in severe illness initial dose can be increased up to 6 g daily, reduce dose or interrupt treatment if signs of toxicity, discontinue if inadequate response after 3 months

> **IMPORTANT SAFETY INFORMATION**
> RISKS OF INCORRECT DOSING OF ORAL ANTI-CANCER MEDICINES
> See Cytotoxic drugs p. 865.

- **CAUTIONS** Avoid in Acute porphyrias p. 1025 · risk of accumulation in overweight patients
- **INTERACTIONS** → Appendix 1: mitotane
- **SIDE-EFFECTS**
  ▸ **Common or very common** Adrenal insufficiency · anaemia · appetite decreased · asthenia · cognitive impairment · confusion · diarrhoea · dizziness · drowsiness · dyslipidaemia · gastrointestinal discomfort ·

gynaecomastia · headache · hepatic disorders · leucopenia · movement disorders · mucositis · muscle weakness · nausea · paraesthesia · polyneuropathy · rash · thrombocytopenia · vertigo · vomiting

▶ **Frequency not known** Encephalopathy · eye disorders · flushing · fungal infection · generalised pain · growth retardation · haemorrhage · hyperpyrexia · hypersalivation · hypertension · hypothyroidism · hypouricaemia · lens opacity · neuro-psychological retardation · ovarian cyst · postural hypotension · proteinuria · taste altered · thyroid disorder · vision disorders

● CONCEPTION AND CONTRACEPTION Contraceptive advice required, see *Pregnancy and reproductive* function in Cytotoxic drugs p. 865.

● PREGNANCY Manufacturer advises avoid. See also *Pregnancy and reproductive function* in Cytotoxic drugs p. 865.

● BREAST FEEDING Discontinue breast-feeding.

● HEPATIC IMPAIRMENT Manufacturer advises caution in mild to moderate impairment. Avoid in severe impairment.
Monitoring In mild to moderate hepatic impairment, monitoring of plasma-mitotane concentration is recommended.

● RENAL IMPAIRMENT Manufacturer advises caution in mild to moderate impairment. Avoid in severe impairment.
Monitoring In mild to moderate renal impairment, monitoring of plasma-mitotane concentration is recommended.

● MONITORING REQUIREMENTS
▶ Plasma-mitotane concentration for optimum response 14–20 mg/litre.
▶ Monitor plasma-mitotane concentration—consult product literature.

● PRESCRIBING AND DISPENSING INFORMATION
Corticosteroid replacement therapy Corticosteroid replacement therapy is necessary with treatment with mitotane. The dose of glucocorticoid should be increased in case of shock, trauma, or infection.

● PATIENT AND CARER ADVICE Patients should be warned to contact doctor immediately if injury, infection, or illness occurs (because of risk of acute adrenal insufficiency).
Driving and skilled tasks Central nervous system toxicity may affect performance of skilled tasks (e.g. driving).

● MEDICINAL FORMS
There can be variation in the licensing of different medicines containing the same drug.

Tablet
CAUTIONARY AND ADVISORY LABELS 2, 10, 21
▶ Lysodren (HRA Pharma UK Ltd)
Mitotane 500 mg Lysodren 500mg tablets | 100 tablet [PoM]
£590.97

Panobinostat

01-Feb-2017

● DRUG ACTION Panobinostat is a histone deacetylase inhibitor, which promotes cell-cycle arrest and apoptosis of tumour cells via multiple pathways.

● INDICATIONS AND DOSE

Treatment of relapsed or refractory multiple myeloma (in combination with bortezomib and dexamethasone), in patients who have received at least two prior regimens, including bortezomib and an immunomodulatory agent

▶ BY MOUTH
▶ Adult 18–74 years: 20 mg once daily, on days 1, 3, 5, 8, 10 and 12 of a 21-day cycle for 8 cycles. Patients with clinical benefit should continue treatment for 8 additional cycles; total duration 16 cycles (48 weeks),

for doses of dexamethasone and bortezomib, or dose adjustment due to side-effects—consult product literature
▶ Adult 75 years and over: 20 mg once daily, on days 1, 3, 5, 8, 10 and 12 of a 21-day cycle for 8 cycles. Patients with clinical benefit should continue treatment for 8 additional cycles; total duration 16 cycles (48 weeks), alternatively initially 15 mg once daily, on days 1, 3, 5, 8, 10 and 12 of a 21-day cycle for 1 cycle, increased if tolerated to 20 mg once daily, on days 1, 3, 5, 8, 10 and 12 of a 21-day cycle for 7 subsequent cycles, patients with clinical benefit should continue treatment for 8 additional cycles; total duration 16 cycles (48 weeks), lower dose may be used for the first cycle depending on patient's condition and co-morbidities, for doses of dexamethasone and bortezomib, or dose adjustment due to side-effects—consult product literature

DOSE ADJUSTMENTS DUE TO INTERACTIONS
▶ Manufacturer advises reduce dose to 10 mg with concurrent use of potent inhibitors of CYP3A4; if the potent inhibitor of CYP3A4 is to be continued, consider increasing the dose to 15 mg if tolerated.
▶ Manufacturer advises avoid potent inhibitors of CYP3A4 if possible in patients taking a reduced panobinostat dose due to side-effects, or in those with hepatic impairment.

IMPORTANT SAFETY INFORMATION
RISKS OF INCORRECT DOSING OF ORAL ANTI-CANCER MEDICINES
See Cytotoxic drugs p. 865.

● CAUTIONS Coagulation disorders · elderly · QT-interval prolongation · risk factors for QT-interval prolongation
CAUTIONS, FURTHER INFORMATION
▶ Risk factors for QT-interval prolongation Patients at risk of developing QT-interval prolongation include those with long QT syndrome, or uncontrolled or significant cardiac disease.

● INTERACTIONS → Appendix 1: panobinostat

● SIDE-EFFECTS
▶ **Common or very common** Anaemia · antibiotic associated colitis · appetite decreased · arrhythmias · asthenia · cheilitis · chills · cough · decreased leucocytes · diarrhoea · dizziness · dry mouth · dyspnoea · electrolyte imbalance · fever · fluid imbalance · gastrointestinal discomfort · gastrointestinal disorders · haemorrhage · headache · hepatic disorders · hyperbilirubinaemia · hyperglycaemia · hypertension · hyperuricaemia · hypoalbuminaemia · hypotension · hypothyroidism · increased risk of infection · insomnia · intracranial haemorrhage · joint swelling · malaise · nausea · neutropenia · palpitations · pancytopenia · peripheral oedema · QT interval prolongation · renal failure · respiratory disorders · sepsis · skin reactions · syncope · taste altered · thrombocytopenia · tremor · urinary incontinence · vomiting · weight decreased
▶ **Uncommon** Haemorrhagic shock · myocardial infarction

SIDE-EFFECTS, FURTHER INFORMATION Side-effects are reported when used in combination with bortezomib and dexamethasone.
Gastro-intestinal disorders Manufacturer advises that patients are treated with anti-diarrhoeals, or any additional treatment, in accordance with local treatment guidelines at the first sign of abdominal cramping or onset of diarrhoea.

● CONCEPTION AND CONTRACEPTION Manufacturer advises exclude pregnancy before starting treatment in women of child-bearing potential, and ensure highly effective contraception used during treatment and for 3 months after last dose. Women using hormonal contraceptives should also use a barrier method of contraception. Highly effective contraception also required for men and their female partners during treatment and for 6 months after last dose.

- **PREGNANCY** Manufacturer advises avoid unless potential benefit outweighs risk—toxicity in *animal* studies. See also *Pregnancy and reproductive function* in Cytotoxic drugs p. 865.
- **BREAST FEEDING** Manufacturer advises avoid—no information available.
- **HEPATIC IMPAIRMENT** Manufacturer advises frequent monitoring of hepatic function in mild and moderate impairment, particularly during the dose escalation phase; avoid in severe impairment—no information available. **Dose adjustments** Manufacturer advises reduce initial dose to 15 mg during the first treatment cycle in mild impairment—dose may be increased to 20 mg based on patient tolerability; reduce initial dose to 10 mg during the first treatment cycle in moderate impairment—dose may be increased to 15 mg based on patient tolerability.
- **MONITORING REQUIREMENTS**
  ▶ Manufacturer advises monitor full blood count before treatment, then frequently during treatment; reduce dose or interrupt treatment if thrombocytopenia or neutropenia occur—consult product literature.
  ▶ Manufacturer advises monitor ECG before treatment and repeat periodically before each treatment cycle; QTcF should be <480 milliseconds before treatment initiation—consult product literature.
  ▶ Manufacturer advises monitor electrolytes before treatment and periodically as clinically indicated, especially in patients with diarrhoea; monitor thyroid and pituitary function (free T4 and TSH) as clinically indicated; monitor hepatic function before treatment and regularly during treatment as clinically indicated.
  ▶ Manufacturer advises monitor patients over 65 years more frequently, especially for thrombocytopenia and gastro-intestinal toxicity.
- **PATIENT AND CARER ADVICE** Manufacturer advises that patients and their carers should be told to seek medical advice if severe gastro-intestinal toxicity occurs. **Missed doses** Manufacturer advises if a dose is missed, it can be taken up to 12 hours after the specified dose time. **Driving and skilled tasks** Dizziness may affect performance of skilled tasks (e.g. driving).
- **NATIONAL FUNDING/ACCESS DECISIONS**

  NICE decisions
  ▶ **Panobinostat for treating multiple myeloma after at least 2 previous treatments (January 2016)** NICE TA380
  Panobinostat, in combination with bortezomib and dexamethasone, is recommended as an option for treating relapsed or refractory multiple myeloma in patients who have received at least 2 prior regimens including bortezomib and an immunomodulatory agent when the manufacturer provides panobinostat with the discount agreed in the patient access scheme.
  www.nice.org.uk/TA380

- **MEDICINAL FORMS**
  There can be variation in the licensing of different medicines containing the same drug.

  Capsule
  CAUTIONARY AND ADVISORY LABELS 25
  ▶ Farydak (Novartis Pharmaceuticals UK Ltd) ▼
  Panobinostat (as Panobinostat lactate anhydrous)
  10 mg Farydak 10mg capsules | 6 capsule [PoM] £3,492.00
  Panobinostat (as Panobinostat lactate anhydrous) 15 mg Farydak 15mg capsules | 6 capsule [PoM] £3,492.00
  Panobinostat (as Panobinostat lactate anhydrous)
  20 mg Farydak 20mg capsules | 6 capsule [PoM] £4,656.00

Pegaspargase

- **DRUG ACTION** Pegaspargase breaks down the amino acid L-asparagine, thereby interfering with the growth of malignant cells, which are unable to synthesise L-asparagine.

- **INDICATIONS AND DOSE**

  Acute lymphoblastic leukaemia (in combination with other antineoplastic drugs) (specialist use only)
  ▶ BY INTRAMUSCULAR INJECTION, OR BY INTRAVENOUS INFUSION
  ▶ Adult 18–21 years: 2500 units/m^2 every 14 days
  ▶ Adult 22 years and over: 2000 units/m^2 every 14 days

- **CONTRA-INDICATIONS** History of pancreatitis · history of serious haemorrhagic event with previous L-asparaginase therapy · history of serious thrombosis with previous L-asparaginase therapy

- **CAUTIONS** Concomitant use of other hepatotoxic drugs (particularly in pre-existing hepatic impairment)—monitor hepatic function · diabetes (may raise blood glucose) · hypersensitivity reactions · marked decrease of leukocyte count at start of treatment is possible—may be associated with significant rise in serum uric acid and development of uric acid nephropathy

  CAUTIONS, FURTHER INFORMATION
  ▶ Hypersensitivity reactions Serious hypersensitivity reactions, including life-threatening anaphylaxis, can occur—pegaspargase should only be administered when appropriately trained staff and resuscitation facilities are immediately available; manufacturer advises patients should be closely monitored for signs of hypersensitivity during treatment and for an hour after administration. In the event of a hypersensitivity reaction, treatment should be stopped immediately and appropriate management initiated.

- **INTERACTIONS** → Appendix 1: pegaspargase

- **SIDE-EFFECTS**
  ▶ **Common or very common** Abdominal pain · bone marrow depression · diarrhoea · hyperglycaemia · hypersensitivity · hypoxia · pain in extremity · pancreatitis (discontinue if suspected and do not restart if confirmed) · peripheral neuropathy · rash · seizure · stomatitis · syncope · thrombosis (discontinue) · vomiting
  ▶ **Rare or very rare** Acute kidney injury · posterior reversible encephalopathy syndrome (PRES) · tremor
  ▶ **Frequency not known** Confusion · diabetic ketoacidosis · drowsiness · hepatobiliary disorder · hyperammonaemia (monitor if symptoms present) · toxic epidermal necrolysis

  SIDE-EFFECTS, FURTHER INFORMATION There have been rare reports of cholestasis, icterus, hepatic cell necrosis and hepatic failure with fatal outcome in patients receiving pegaspargase.

- **CONCEPTION AND CONTRACEPTION** Manufacturer advises effective contraception in men and women of child-bearing potential during treatment and for at least 6 months after discontinuing treatment; pegaspargase may reduce effectiveness of oral contraceptives—additional precautions (e.g. barrier method) are required, see also *Pregnancy and reproductive function* in Cytotoxic drugs p. 865.

- **PREGNANCY** Manufacturer advises avoid unless essential. See also *Pregnancy and reproductive function* in Cytotoxic drugs p. 865.

- **BREAST FEEDING** Manufacturer advises avoid—no information available.

- **HEPATIC IMPAIRMENT** Manufacturer advises avoid in severe impairment.

- **MONITORING REQUIREMENTS**
  ▶ Manufacturer advises trough serum asparaginase activity levels may be measured before the next administration of

pegaspargase; consider switching to a different asparaginase preparation if target levels not reached—seek expert advice.
▸ Manufacturer advises monitor plasma and urine glucose levels during treatment; monitor coagulation profile at baseline and periodically during and after treatment (particularly with concomitant use of other drugs that inhibit coagulation); monitor serum amylase.

● DIRECTIONS FOR ADMINISTRATION Manufacturer advises *for intramuscular injection*, volumes over 3 mL must be divided between more than one site.

● HANDLING AND STORAGE Manufacturer advises store in a refrigerator between 2–8°C.

● PATIENT AND CARER ADVICE
Pancreatitis Manufacturer advises patients and carers should be told how to recognise signs and symptoms of pancreatitis and advised to seek medical attention if symptoms such as persistent, severe abdominal pain develop.
Driving and skilled tasks Manufacturer advises patients and carers should be counselled on the effects on driving and performance of skilled tasks—increased risk of confusion and somnolence.

● NATIONAL FUNDING/ACCESS DECISIONS
NICE decisions
▸ **Pegaspargase for treating acute lymphoblastic leukaemia (September 2016)** NICE TA408
Pegaspargase, as part of antineoplastic combination therapy, is recommended as an option for treating acute lymphoblastic leukaemia only in patients with untreated newly diagnosed disease.
    Patients whose treatment was started within the NHS before this guidance was published may continue treatment until they and their clinician consider it appropriate to stop.
www.nice.org.uk/guidance/ta408
Scottish Medicines Consortium (SMC) Decisions
The *Scottish Medicines Consortium* has advised (October 2016) that pegaspargase (*Oncaspar*®) is accepted for use within NHS Scotland as a component of antineoplastic combination therapy in acute lymphoblastic leukaemia.

● MEDICINAL FORMS
There can be variation in the licensing of different medicines containing the same drug.
Solution for injection
▸ Oncaspar (Imported (United States)) ▼
Pegaspargase 750 unit per 1 ml Oncaspar 3,750 units/5ml solution for injection vials | 1 vial [PoM] 🚫

Procarbazine

● DRUG ACTION Procarbazine is a mild monoamine-oxidase inhibitor.

● INDICATIONS AND DOSE
Hodgkin's lymphoma
▸ BY MOUTH
▸ Adult: (consult local protocol)

IMPORTANT SAFETY INFORMATION
RISKS OF INCORRECT DOSING OF ORAL ANTI-CANCER MEDICINES
See Cytotoxic drugs p. 865.

● CONTRA-INDICATIONS Pre-existing severe leucopenia · pre-existing severe thrombocytopenia

● CAUTIONS Cardiovascular disease · cerebrovascular disease · epilepsy · phaeochromocytoma · procarbazine is a mild monoamineoxidase inhibitor (dietary restriction is rarely considered necessary)

● INTERACTIONS → Appendix 1: procarbazine

● SIDE-EFFECTS
▸ **Common or very common** Appetite decreased
▸ **Frequency not known** Azoospermia · hepatic disorders · infection · lethargy · leucopenia · nausea · neutropenia · ovarian failure · pneumonitis · skin reactions · thrombocytopenia · vomiting

● CONCEPTION AND CONTRACEPTION Contraceptive advice required, see *Pregnancy and reproductive function* in Cytotoxic drugs p. 865.

● PREGNANCY Avoid (teratogenic in *animal* studies and isolated reports in humans). See also *Pregnancy and reproductive function* in Cytotoxic drugs p. 865.

● BREAST FEEDING Discontinue breast-feeding.

● HEPATIC IMPAIRMENT Caution in mild to moderate impairment. Avoid in severe impairment.

● RENAL IMPAIRMENT Caution in mild to moderate impairment. Avoid in severe impairment.

● MEDICINAL FORMS
There can be variation in the licensing of different medicines containing the same drug.
Capsule
CAUTIONARY AND ADVISORY LABELS 4
▸ Procarbazine (Non-proprietary)
Procarbazine (as Procarbazine hydrochloride)
50 mg Procarbazine 50mg capsules | 50 capsule [PoM] £411.34–£411.35 DT = £411.35

Raltitrexed

● DRUG ACTION Raltitrexed is a thymidylate synthase inhibitor.

● INDICATIONS AND DOSE
Palliation of advanced colorectal cancer when fluorouracil and folinic acid cannot be used
▸ BY INTRAVENOUS INFUSION
▸ Adult: (consult local protocol)

● INTERACTIONS → Appendix 1: raltitrexed

● SIDE-EFFECTS
▸ **Common or very common** Alopecia · anaemia · appetite decreased · arthralgia · asthenia · cellulitis · conjunctivitis · constipation · dehydration · diarrhoea · fever · gastrointestinal discomfort · headache · hyperbilirubinaemia · hyperhidrosis · influenza like illness · leucopenia · malaise · mucositis · muscle cramps · muscle tone increased · nausea · neutropenia · oral disorders · pain · peripheral oedema · sepsis · skin reactions · taste altered · thrombocytopenia · vomiting · weight decreased
▸ **Frequency not known** Gastrointestinal haemorrhage

● CONCEPTION AND CONTRACEPTION Ensure effective contraception during and for at least 6 months after treatment in men or women.

● PREGNANCY See *Pregnancy and reproductive function* in Cytotoxic drugs p. 865.

● BREAST FEEDING Discontinue breast-feeding.

● HEPATIC IMPAIRMENT Caution in mild to moderate impairment. Avoid in severe impairment.

● RENAL IMPAIRMENT Avoid if creatinine clearance less than 25 mL/minute.
Dose adjustments Reduce dose and increase dosing interval if creatinine clearance less than 65 mL/minute (consult product literature).

● NATIONAL FUNDING/ACCESS DECISIONS
NICE decisions
▶ **Irinotecan, oxaliplatin, and raltitrexed for advanced colorectal cancer (August 2005)** NICE TA93
Raltitrexed is **not** recommended for the treatment of advanced colorectal cancer. Its use should be confined to clinical studies.
www.nice.org.uk/TA93

● MEDICINAL FORMS
There can be variation in the licensing of different medicines containing the same drug.
Powder for solution for infusion
▶ Tomudex (Pfizer Ltd)
Raltitrexed 2 mg Tomudex 2mg powder for solution for infusion vials | 1 vial [PoM] £148.75 (Hospital only)

RETINOID AND RELATED DRUGS

Bexarotene

● DRUG ACTION Bexarotene is an agonist at the retinoid X receptor, which is involved in the regulation of cell differentiation and proliferation. Bexarotene can cause regression of cutaneous T-cell lymphoma.

● INDICATIONS AND DOSE
Skin manifestations of cutaneous T-cell lymphoma refractory to previous systemic treatment
▶ BY MOUTH
▶ Adult: Initially 300 mg/m^2 once daily, adjusted according to response, to be taken with a meal

IMPORTANT SAFETY INFORMATION
RISKS OF INCORRECT DOSING OF ORAL ANTI-CANCER MEDICINES
See Cytotoxic drugs p. 865.

● CONTRA-INDICATIONS History of pancreatitis · hypervitaminosis A · uncontrolled hyperlipidaemia · uncontrolled hypothyroidism
● CAUTIONS Avoid in Acute porphyrias p. 1025 · hyperlipidaemia · hypothyroidism
● INTERACTIONS → Appendix 1: retinoids
● SIDE-EFFECTS
▶ **Common or very common** Alopecia · anaemia · appetite decreased · arthralgia · asthenia · chills · constipation · diarrhoea · dizziness · dry eye · dry mouth · dyslipidaemia · eye disorders · gastrointestinal discomfort · gastrointestinal disorders · headaches · hearing impairment · hyperhidrosis · hypersensitivity · hypoproteinaemia · hypothyroidism · increased risk of infection · insomnia · leucopenia · lymphadenopathy · muscle complaints · nausea · oedema · oral disorders · pain · pseudolymphoma · sensation abnormal · skin nodule · skin reactions · skin ulcer · thyroid disorder · vomiting · weight changes
▶ **Uncommon** Albuminuria · anxiety · arrhythmias · ataxia · blood disorder · cataract · coagulation disorder · depression · ear disorder · eosinophilia · eye inflammation · fever · gout · haemorrhage · hair disorder · hepatic failure · hyperbilirubinaemia · hypertension · hyperthyroidism · increased leucocytes · mucous membrane disorder · muscle weakness · nail disorder · neoplasms · nerve disorders · pancreatitis · renal impairment · serous drainage · thrombocytopenia · thrombocytosis · varicose veins · vasodilation · vertigo · vision disorders
▶ **Frequency not known** Burping · chest pain · confusion · cough aggravated · dehydration · drowsiness · dysphagia · dyspnoea · emotional lability · hypercalcaemia · hyperuricaemia · libido decreased · muscle tone increased · pelvic pain · peripheral vascular disease · red blood cell

abnormality · taste altered · thirst · white blood cell abnormalities
● ALLERGY AND CROSS-SENSITIVITY Caution—hypersensitivity to retinoids.
● CONCEPTION AND CONTRACEPTION Manufacturer advises effective contraception during and for at least 1 month after treatment in men and women.
● PREGNANCY Avoid. See also *Pregnancy and reproductive function* in Cytotoxic drugs p. 865.
● BREAST FEEDING Discontinue breast-feeding.
● HEPATIC IMPAIRMENT Avoid.
● NATIONAL FUNDING/ACCESS DECISIONS
Scottish Medicines Consortium (SMC) Decisions
The *Scottish Medicines Consortium* has advised (November 2002) that bexarotene is recommended for restricted use as a second-line treatment for patients with advanced cutaneous T-cell lymphoma.

● MEDICINAL FORMS
There can be variation in the licensing of different medicines containing the same drug.
Capsule
▶ Targretin (Eisai Ltd)
Bexarotene 75 mg Targretin 75mg capsules | 100 capsule [PoM] £937.50

Tretinoin

● INDICATIONS AND DOSE
Induction of remission in acute promyelocytic leukaemia (used in previously untreated patients as well as in those who have relapsed after standard chemotherapy or who are refractory to it)
▶ BY MOUTH
▶ Adult: 45 mg/m^2 daily in 2 divided doses maximum duration of treatment is 90 days, consult product literature for details of concomitant chemotherapy

● CAUTIONS Increased risk of thromboembolism during first month of treatment
● INTERACTIONS → Appendix 1: retinoids
● SIDE-EFFECTS
▶ **Common or very common** Abdominal pain · alopecia · anxiety · appetite decreased · arrhythmia · asthma · bone pain · cheilitis · chest pain · chills · confusion · constipation · depression · diarrhoea · dizziness · dry mouth · flushing · headache · hearing impairment · hyperhidrosis · idiopathic intracranial hypertension · insomnia · intracranial pressure increased · malaise · nasal dryness · nausea · pancreatitis · paraesthesia · respiratory disorders · skin reactions · visual impairment · vomiting
▶ **Frequency not known** Embolism and thrombosis · erythema nodosum · genital ulceration · hepatotoxicity · hypercalcaemia · increased leucocytes · myocardial infarction · myositis · necrotising fasciitis · QT interval prolongation · stroke · thrombocytosis · vasculitis
SIDE-EFFECTS, FURTHER INFORMATION
Retinoic acid syndrome Fever, dyspnoea, acute respiratory distress, pulmonary infiltrates, pleural effusion, hyperleucocytosis, hypotension, oedema, weight gain, hepatic, renal and multi-organ failure requires immediate treatment—consult product literature.
● CONCEPTION AND CONTRACEPTION Effective contraception must be used for at least 1 month before oral treatment, during treatment and for at least 1 month after stopping (oral progestogen-only contraceptives not considered effective).
● PREGNANCY Teratogenic. See *Pregnancy and reproductive function* in Cytotoxic drugs p. 865.
● BREAST FEEDING Avoid (discontinue breast-feeding).

- HEPATIC IMPAIRMENT
  Dose adjustments Reduce dose to 25 mg/m^2.
- RENAL IMPAIRMENT
  Dose adjustments Reduce dose to 25 mg/m^2.
- MONITORING REQUIREMENTS Monitor haematological and coagulation profile, liver function, serum calcium and plasma lipids before and during treatment.
- PRESCRIBING AND DISPENSING INFORMATION Tretinoin is the acid form of vitamin A.

- MEDICINAL FORMS
  There can be variation in the licensing of different medicines containing the same drug.
  Capsule
  CAUTIONARY AND ADVISORY LABELS 21, 25
  ▶ Tretinoin (Non-proprietary)
  Tretinoin 10 mg Tretinoin 10mg capsules | 100 capsule PoM
  £240.00–£256.80 DT = £240.00

3.1 Cytotoxic drug-induced side effects

ANTIDOTES AND CHELATORS 〉 **IRON CHELATORS**

Dexrazoxane

- DRUG ACTION Dexrazoxane is an iron chelator.

- **INDICATIONS AND DOSE**
  CARDIOXANE ®
  Prevention of chronic cumulative cardiotoxicity caused by doxorubicin or epirubicin treatment in advanced or metastatic breast cancer patients who have received a prior cumulative dose of 300 mg/m^2 of doxorubicin or a prior cumulative dose of 540 mg/m^2 of epirubicin when further anthracycline treatment is required
  ▶ BY INTRAVENOUS INFUSION
  ▶ Adult: Administer 10 times the doxorubicin-equivalent dose or 10 times the epirubicin-equivalent dose, dose to be given 30 minutes before anthracycline administration

  SAVENE ®
  Anthracycline extravasation
  ▶ BY INTRAVENOUS INFUSION
  ▶ Adult: Initially 1 g/m^2 daily (max. per dose 2 g) for 2 days, then 500 mg/m^2 for 1 day, first dose to be given as soon as possible and within 6 hours after injury

- CONTRA-INDICATIONS Children
- CAUTIONS Myelosuppression (effects may be additive to those of chemotherapy)
  CARDIOXANE ® Manufacturer advises caution in patients with heart failure—no information available · manufacturer advises caution in patients with myocardial infarction in previous 12 months—no information available · manufacturer advises caution in patients with symptomatic valvular heart disease—no information available · manufacturer advises caution in patients with uncontrolled angina—no information available
- INTERACTIONS → Appendix 1: iron chelators
- SIDE-EFFECTS
  ▶ **Common or very common** Alopecia · anaemia · appetite decreased · asthenia · constipation · cough · diarrhoea · dizziness · drowsiness · dry mouth · dyspnoea · embolism and thrombosis · fever · gastrointestinal discomfort · headache · increased risk of infection · leucopenia · myalgia · nail disorder · nausea · neutropenia · peripheral neuropathy · peripheral oedema · post procedural infection · sensation abnormal · skin reactions · stomatitis · syncope ·

tachycardia · thrombocytopenia · tremor · vaginal haemorrhage · vomiting · weight decreased · wound complications
▶ **Uncommon** Acute myeloid leukaemia · lymphoedema · sepsis · thirst · vertigo
▶ **Frequency not known** Anaphylactic reaction

- CONCEPTION AND CONTRACEPTION Ensure effective contraception during and for at least 3 months after treatment in men and women.
- PREGNANCY Avoid unless essential (toxicity in *animal* studies).
- BREAST FEEDING Discontinue breast-feeding.
- HEPATIC IMPAIRMENT
  CARDIOXANE ® **Dose adjustments** Manufacturer advises that if anthracycline dose is reduced, reduce the *Cardioxane*® dose by a similar ratio.
  SAVENE ® Manufacturer advises avoid—no information available.
- RENAL IMPAIRMENT
  CARDIOXANE ® **Dose adjustments** Manufacturer advises reduce dose by 50% if creatinine clearance less than 40 mL/minute.
  SAVENE ® Manufacturer advises avoid—risk of accumulation.
- MONITORING REQUIREMENTS
  ▶ Monitor full blood count.
  ▶ Monitor for cardiac toxicity.
  ▶ Monitor liver function.
- DIRECTIONS FOR ADMINISTRATION Local coolants such as ice packs should be removed at least 15 minutes before administration.
  CARDIOXANE ® For *intravenous infusion*, give intermittently *in* Compound sodium lactate; reconstitute each vial with 25 mL water for injections and dilute each vial with 25–100 mL infusion fluid; give requisite dose over 15 minutes.
  SAVENE ® For *intravenous infusion*, give intermittently *in* diluent; reconstitute each 500-mg vial with 25 mL of diluent; dilute requisite dose further in remaining diluent and give over 1–2 hours into a large vein in an area other than the one affected.

- MEDICINAL FORMS
  There can be variation in the licensing of different medicines containing the same drug.
  Powder for solution for infusion
  ▶ Cardioxane (Clinigen Healthcare Ltd)
  Dexrazoxane 500 mg Cardioxane 500mg powder for solution for infusion vials | 1 vial PoM £156.57
  Powder and solvent for solution for infusion
  ELECTROLYTES: May contain Potassium, sodium
  ▶ Savene (Clinigen Healthcare Ltd)
  Dexrazoxane 500 mg Savene 500mg powder for concentrate and solvent for solution for infusion vials | 10 vial PoM ⓢ

DETOXIFYING DRUGS 〉 **UROPROTECTIVE DRUGS**

Mesna

- **INDICATIONS AND DOSE**
  Cytotoxic induced urothelial toxicity
  ▶ BY MOUTH, OR BY INTRAVENOUS INJECTION
  ▶ Adult: Dose to be calculated according to oxazaphosphorine (cyclophosphamide or ifosfamide) treatment (consult product literature)

- SIDE-EFFECTS
  ▶ **Common or very common** Appetite decreased · arthralgia · asthenia · chest pain · chills · concentration impaired · conjunctivitis · constipation · cough · dehydration · diarrhoea · dizziness · drowsiness · dry mouth · dyspnoea ·

dysuria · fever · flatulence · flushing · gastrointestinal discomfort · haemorrhage · headache · hyperhidrosis · influenza like illness · laryngeal discomfort · lymphadenopathy · malaise · myalgia · nasal congestion · nausea · oral irritation · pain · palpitations · respiratory disorders · sensation abnormal · skin reactions · sleep disorders · syncope · vision disorders · vomiting
▶ **Frequency not known** Acute kidney injury · angioedema · drug reaction with eosinophilia and systemic symptoms (DRESS) · hypotension · hypoxia · oedema · tachycardia · ulcer · vulvovaginal rash
● ALLERGY AND CROSS-SENSITIVITY Contra-indicated if history of hypersensitivity to thiol-containing compounds.
● PREGNANCY Not known to be harmful. See also *Pregnancy and reproductive function* in Cytotoxic drugs p. 865.
● EFFECT ON LABORATORY TESTS False positive urinary ketones. False positive or false negative urinary erythrocytes.
● DIRECTIONS FOR ADMINISTRATION For oral administration of the injection, contents of ampoule are taken in a flavoured drink such as orange juice or cola which may be stored in a refrigerator for up to 24 hours in a sealed container.

● MEDICINAL FORMS
There can be variation in the licensing of different medicines containing the same drug. Forms available from special-order manufacturers include: oral solution
Solution for injection
▶ Mesna (Non-proprietary)
Mesna 100 mg per 1 ml Mesna 1g/10ml solution for injection ampoules | 15 ampoule [PoM] £441.15
Mesna 400mg/4ml solution for injection ampoules | 5 ampoule [PoM] £18.90 | 15 ampoule [PoM] £201.15
Tablet
▶ Mesna (Non-proprietary)
Mesna 400 mg Mesna 400mg tablets | 10 tablet [PoM] £134.30
Mesna 600 mg Mesna 600mg tablets | 10 tablet [PoM] £190.60

VITAMINS AND TRACE ELEMENTS › FOLATES

Folinic acid

● INDICATIONS AND DOSE
Prevention of methotrexate-induced adverse effects
▶ BY INTRAMUSCULAR INJECTION, OR BY INTRAVENOUS INJECTION, OR BY INTRAVENOUS INFUSION
▶ Adult: 15 mg every 6 hours for 24 hours, to be started usually 12–24 hours after start of methotrexate infusion, dose may be continued by mouth, consult local treatment protocol for further information
Suspected methotrexate overdosage
▶ BY INTRAVENOUS INJECTION, OR BY INTRAVENOUS INFUSION
▶ Adult: Initial dose equal to or exceeding dose of methotrexate, to be given at a maximum rate of 160 mg/minute, consult poisons information centres for advice on continuing management
Adjunct to fluorouracil in colorectal cancer
▶ BY SLOW INTRAVENOUS INJECTION
▶ Adult: (consult product literature)
SODIOFOLIN ®
As an antidote to methotrexate
▶ BY INTRAVENOUS INFUSION, OR BY INTRAVENOUS INJECTION
▶ Adult: (consult product literature)
Adjunct to fluorouracil in colorectal cancer
▶ BY INTRAVENOUS INJECTION, OR BY INTRAVENOUS INFUSION
▶ Adult: (consult product literature)

● CONTRA-INDICATIONS Intrathecal injection
● CAUTIONS Avoid simultaneous administration of methotrexate · **not** indicated for pernicious anaemia or

other megaloblastic anaemias caused by vitamin B$_{12}$ deficiency
● INTERACTIONS → Appendix 1: folates
● SIDE-EFFECTS
GENERAL SIDE-EFFECTS
▶ **Uncommon** Fever
▶ **Rare or very rare** Agitation (with high doses) · depression (with high doses) · epilepsy exacerbated · gastrointestinal disorder (with high doses) · insomnia (with high doses) · urticaria
SPECIFIC SIDE-EFFECTS
▶ **Common or very common**
▶ With intravenous use Bone marrow failure · dehydration · diarrhoea (with high doses) · mucositis · nausea · oral disorders · skin reactions · vomiting
▶ **Rare or very rare**
▶ With intravenous use Sensitisation
▶ **Frequency not known**
▶ With intravenous use Hyperammonaemia
● PREGNANCY Not known to be harmful; benefit outweighs risk.
● BREAST FEEDING Presence in milk unknown but benefit outweighs risk.
● NATIONAL FUNDING/ACCESS DECISIONS
NICE decisions
▶ **Bevacizumab in combination with oxaliplatin and either fluorouracil plus folinic acid or capecitabine for the treatment of metastatic colorectal cancer (December 2010)** NICE TA212 Bevacizumab in combination with oxaliplatin and either fluorouracil plus folinic acid or capecitabine is not recommended for the treatment of metastatic colorectal cancer.
www.nice.org.uk/TA212

● MEDICINAL FORMS
There can be variation in the licensing of different medicines containing the same drug. Forms available from special-order manufacturers include: oral suspension, oral solution
Tablet
▶ Folinic acid (Non-proprietary)
Folinic acid (as Calcium folinate) 15 mg Calcium folinate 15mg tablets | 10 tablet [PoM] £49.00 DT = £46.92
▶ Refolinon (Pfizer Ltd)
Folinic acid (as Calcium folinate) 15 mg Refolinon 15mg tablets | 30 tablet [PoM] £85.74
Solution for injection
▶ Folinic acid (Non-proprietary)
Folinic acid (as Calcium folinate) 7.5 mg per 1 ml Calcium folinate 15mg/2ml solution for injection ampoules | 5 ampoule [PoM] £39.00 DT = £39.00 | 5 ampoule [PoM] £39.00 DT = £39.00 (Hospital only)
Folinic acid (as Calcium folinate) 10 mg per 1 ml Calcium folinate 300mg/30ml solution for injection vials | 1 vial [PoM] £100.00 (Hospital only)
Calcium folinate 50mg/5ml solution for injection vials | 1 vial [PoM] £20.00 (Hospital only)
Calcium folinate 100mg/10ml solution for injection vials | 1 vial [PoM] £37.50 (Hospital only)
Folinic acid (as Disodium folinate) 50 mg per 1 ml Disodium folinate 50mg/1ml solution for injection vials | 1 vial [PoM] £24.70
Disodium folinate 200mg/4ml solution for injection vials | 1 vial [PoM] £80.40
▶ Refolinon (Pfizer Ltd)
Folinic acid (as Calcium folinate) 3 mg per 1 ml Refolinon 30mg/10ml solution for injection ampoules | 5 ampoule [PoM] £23.12 (Hospital only)
▶ Sodiofolin (medac UK)
Folinic acid (as Disodium folinate) 50 mg per 1 ml Sodiofolin 400mg/8ml solution for injection vials | 1 vial [PoM] £126.25 (Hospital only)
Sodiofolin 100mg/2ml solution for injection vials | 1 vial [PoM] £35.09 (Hospital only)

Levofolinic acid

- **DRUG ACTION** Levofolinic acid is an isomer of folinic acid.

- **INDICATIONS AND DOSE**

Prevention of methotrexate-induced adverse effects
▸ BY INTRAMUSCULAR INJECTION, OR BY INTRAVENOUS INJECTION, OR BY INTRAVENOUS INFUSION
▹ Adult: Usual dose 7.5 mg every 6 hours for 10 doses, usually started 12–24 hours after beginning of methotrexate infusion

Suspected methotrexate overdosage
▸ BY INTRAVENOUS INFUSION, OR BY INTRAVENOUS INJECTION
▹ Adult: Initial dose at least 50% of the dose of methotrexate, intravenous infusion to be administered at a maximum rate of 160 mg/minute, consult poisons information centres for advice on continuing management

Adjunct to fluorouracil in colorectal cancer
▸ BY SLOW INTRAVENOUS INJECTION
▹ Adult: (consult product literature)

- **CONTRA-INDICATIONS** Intrathecal injection
- **CAUTIONS** Avoid simultaneous administration of methotrexate is **not** indicated for pernicious anaemia or other megaloblastic anaemias caused by vitamin B$_{12}$ deficiency
- **INTERACTIONS** → Appendix 1: folates
- **SIDE-EFFECTS**
▸ **Common or very common** Dehydration · diarrhoea · mucosal toxicity · nausea · vomiting
▸ **Uncommon** Fever
▸ **Rare or very rare** Agitation (with high doses) · depression (with high doses) · epilepsy exacerbated · gastrointestinal disorder · insomnia (with high doses) · urticaria
- **PREGNANCY** Not known to be harmful; benefit outweighs risk.
- **BREAST FEEDING** Presence in milk unknown but benefit outweighs risk.

- **MEDICINAL FORMS**
There can be variation in the licensing of different medicines containing the same drug.
Solution for injection
▹ Isovorin (Pfizer Ltd)
Levofolinic acid (as Calcium levofolinate) 10 mg per 1 ml Isovorin 175mg/17.5ml solution for injection vials | 1 vial [PoM] £81.33 (Hospital only)
Isovorin 25mg/2.5ml solution for injection vials | 1 vial [PoM] £11.62 (Hospital only)

3.1a Hyperuricaemia associated with cytotoxic drugs

Other drugs used for Hyperuricaemia associated with cytotoxic drugs Allopurinol, p. 1086 · Febuxostat, p. 1087

DETOXIFYING DRUGS > URATE OXIDASES

Rasburicase

- **INDICATIONS AND DOSE**

Prophylaxis and treatment of acute hyperuricaemia, before and during initiation of chemotherapy, in patients with haematological malignancy and high tumour burden at risk of rapid lysis
▸ BY INTRAVENOUS INFUSION
▹ Adult: 200 micrograms/kg once daily for up to 7 days according to plasma-uric acid concentration

- **CONTRA-INDICATIONS** G6PD deficiency
- **CAUTIONS** Atopic allergies
- **SIDE-EFFECTS**
▸ **Common or very common** Diarrhoea · fever · headache · nausea · skin reactions · vomiting
▸ **Uncommon** Bronchospasm · haemolysis · haemolytic anaemia · hypersensitivity · hypotension · methaemoglobinaemia · seizure
▸ **Rare or very rare** Rhinitis
▸ **Frequency not known** Muscle contractions involuntary
- **PREGNANCY** Manufacturer advises avoid—no information available.
- **BREAST FEEDING** Manufacturer advises avoid—no information available.
- **MONITORING REQUIREMENTS** Monitor closely for hypersensitivity.
- **EFFECT ON LABORATORY TESTS** May interfere with test for uric acid—consult product literature.
- **DIRECTIONS FOR ADMINISTRATION** For *intravenous infusion* (*Fasturtec*®), give intermittently in Sodium chloride 0.9%; reconstitute with solvent provided; gently swirl vial without shaking to dissolve; dilute requisite dose to 50 mL with infusion fluid and give over 30 minutes.

- **MEDICINAL FORMS**
There can be variation in the licensing of different medicines containing the same drug.
Powder and solvent for solution for infusion
▹ Fasturtec (Sanofi)
Rasburicase 1.5 mg Fasturtec 1.5mg powder and solvent for solution for infusion vials | 3 vial [PoM] £208.39 (Hospital only)
Rasburicase 7.5 mg Fasturtec 7.5mg powder and solvent for solution for infusion vials | 1 vial [PoM] £347.32 (Hospital only)

4 Hormone responsive malignancy

Breast cancer   01-Jun-2016

Description of condition

Breast cancer is the most common form of malignancy in women. The causes of breast cancer are complex and there are several risk factors. Established risk factors include age, early onset of menstruation, late menopause, greater age at first completed pregnancy, and a family history. The use of oral contraceptives and postmenopausal HRT are also associated with a small excess risk.

Non-invasive breast cancer, also known as ductal carcinoma *in situ*, is when the cancer remains localised in the ducts. However, in most cases, the cancer is invasive at the time of diagnosis, which means that malignant cells are liable to spread beyond the immediate area of the tumour. Invasive breast cancer, where malignant cells spread beyond the ducts, can be defined as early breast cancer (operable, primary, stage I/II), locally advanced disease (inoperable local, stage III) and advanced disease (metastatic, stage IV).

Aims of treatment

Reducing mortality, increasing progression-free and disease-free survival and improving quality of life are the main aims of the available treatments for breast cancer and are dependant on the stage of the disease.

Surgery and radiotherapy aim to remove the tumour mass, while adjuvant drug therapy aims to reduce the risk of recurrence and the risk of developing invasive disease. Advanced breast cancer is not curable and treatment aims to achieve remission, to prolong the disease free survival, to relieve symptoms and improve quality of life.

8

Immune system and malignant disease

Treatment

The course of the disease and the therapeutic approach vary depending on the characteristics of the cancer; factors such as patient age and menopausal status, tumour size and grade, involvement of axillary lymph nodes or skin, and presence of hormone receptors within the tumour may inform the extent and aggressiveness of the disease. The management of patients with breast cancer involves surgery, radiotherapy, drug therapy, or a combination of these.

Early and locally advanced breast cancer

EvGr For operable breast cancer, primary treatment is surgical using breast-conserving surgery or mastectomy, followed by adjuvant therapy to eradicate the micro-metastases that cause relapses. Radiotherapy is recommended after breast conserving surgery, as it reduces local recurrence rates. It is also used after mastectomy if there is a high risk of recurrence.

Drug therapy can be used after surgery (adjuvant therapy) or may be offered before surgery (neoadjuvant therapy) to achieve local tumour downsizing in order to make breast-conserving surgery possible. The choice of adjuvant therapy is determined by the safety and efficacy of the drugs, the oestrogen-receptor status, and the human epidermal growth factor 2 (HER2) status of the primary tumour.

Adjuvant chemotherapy or radiotherapy should be considered for all patients, irrespective of age, and it should be started as soon as clinically possible within 31 days of surgery.

A high-dose anthracycline-based chemotherapy regimen is usually preferred to a low-dose anthracycline-based regimen or to a non-anthracycline-based regimen. Choice of chemotherapy regimen is usually guided by local policy, Clinical Cancer Networks, and funding arrangements.

Adjuvant anthracycline-taxane combination chemotherapy should be considered in patients where the additional benefit outweighs risk. For patients with lymph node-positive breast cancer, docetaxel p. 900 can be added as part of an adjuvant chemotherapy regimen; paclitaxel p. 901 is not recommended.

Following surgery, tamoxifen p. 927, alone or in combination with chemotherapy, can be given to premenopausal women with oestrogen-receptor-positive early invasive breast cancer. If chemotherapy has not been selected, tamoxifen can be used in combination with ovarian ablation or suppression. Tamoxifen is not recommended for non-invasive (ductal carcinoma *in situ*) early breast cancer. Premenopausal women with oestrogen-receptor-positive breast cancer who decline chemotherapy may benefit from treatment with goserelin p. 721 or ovarian ablation.

For postmenopausal women with oestrogen-receptor-positive early invasive breast cancer, not considered to be low risk, an aromatase inhibitor, such as anastrozole p. 928 or letrozole p. 929, is first-line therapy. Tamoxifen is an alternative if an aromatase inhibitor is not tolerated or is contra-indicated. An aromatase inhibitor should be given as initial adjuvant therapy for 5 years, or by switching to an aromatase inhibitor after 2–3 years of tamoxifen for a total of 5 years. Postmenopausal women who have already received tamoxifen for 5 years may be considered for extended therapy (5 years) with letrozole. ⒶED

There is some evidence that in postmenopausal women with early breast cancer, adjuvant bisphosphonate therapy can prevent breast cancer recurrence in the bone and improve survival. EvGr Intravenous zoledronic acid p. 715 [unlicensed indication] or oral sodium clodronate p. 714 [unlicensed indication] are the preferred options in these patients. ⒶED There is no evidence of benefit in premenopausal women.

EvGr Adjuvant trastuzumab p. 862 is recommended as an option in patients with HER2 positive breast cancer following surgery, chemotherapy (neoadjuvant or adjuvant)

and radiotherapy. Trastuzumab should not be given concurrently with anthracycline-containing regimens (because of the risk of congestive heart failure) but it may be given either concurrently with taxane-based regimens or sequentially. ⒶED

Advanced breast cancer

Treatment of advanced breast cancer depends on the patient's drug history, disease severity, and oestrogen receptor and HER2 status.

EvGr For the majority of patients with oestrogen-receptor-positive advanced breast cancer, endocrine therapy is first-line treatment. Aromatase inhibitors, such as anastrozole, letrozole and exemestane p. 928, may be offered to patients with no previous history of endocrine treatment or in those previously treated with tamoxifen.

Tamoxifen should be considered as first-line treatment for pre- and perimenopausal women with oestrogen-receptor-positive breast cancer not previously treated with tamoxifen. Ovarian suppression is used in pre- and perimenopausal women who have had disease progression despite treatment with tamoxifen.

In patients with advanced breast cancer that is imminently life-threatening or with visceral organ involvement, which requires early relief of symptoms, an anthracycline-based chemotherapy regimen is the preferred treatment. If anthracyclines are not suitable, the alternative is docetaxel monotherapy as first-line treatment, vinorelbine p. 906 or capecitabine p. 880 as second-line treatment or, for third-line treatment, whichever of the two drugs was not used second line. Gemcitabine p. 886 in combination with paclitaxel is recommended for the treatment of metastatic breast cancer only when docetaxel monotherapy or docetaxel with capecitabine are also considered appropriate.

Trastuzumab is recommended for the treatment of HER2-positive advanced breast cancer. It is used in combination with paclitaxel in those who have not received chemotherapy for metastatic breast cancer and as monotherapy for patients who have received at least two chemotherapy regimens for metastatic breast cancer (see trastuzumab *National funding/access decisions*). ⒶED

Lapatinib p. 956 in combination with an aromatase inhibitor, fulvestrant p. 926, trastuzumab emtansine p. 863, and toremifene p. 927 are all licensed for use in patients with metastatic breast cancer, however their use is not recommended (see drug monographs for *Indications* and *National funding/access decisions*).

The gonadorelin analogue, goserelin p. 721 is licensed for advanced breast cancer in pre- and perimenopausal women suitable for hormone manipulation. Some progestogen preparations, such as medroxyprogesterone acetate p. 791, norethisterone p. 747, megestrol acetate p. 926 are also licensed for the treatment of breast cancer (see drug monographs).

EvGr The use of bisphosphonates in patients with metastatic breast cancer may reduce pain and prevent skeletal complications of bone metastases. ⒶED

Familial breast cancer

EvGr Chemoprevention should be **offered** to all women who have been identified as **high-risk** of developing breast cancer. For women at **moderate-risk**, chemoprevention should only be **considered**. Other strategies should also be considered to reduce the risk.

Chemoprevention should not be given to patients at high-risk of developing breast cancer who have had a risk-reducing bilateral mastectomy. ⒶED

Treatment options for chemoprevention

EvGr Chemoprevention should only be continued for 5 years.

Tamoxifen p. 927 [unlicensed indication] is recommended for *premenopausal* women who do not have a history or increased risk of thromboembolic disease or endometrial cancer.

In *post-menopausal* women (who do not have severe osteoporosis), anastrozole p. 928 [unlicensed indication] is recommended. Women who have severe osteoporosis, or who do not wish to take anastrozole, can be treated with tamoxifen provided there is no history or risk of thromboembolic disease or endometrial cancer. Alternatively, raloxifene hydrochloride p. 736 is an option [unlicensed indication] in *post-menopausal* women with a uterus who do not wish to take tamoxifen, unless there is a history or increased risk of thromboembolic disease. ⒶＡ

Treatment of menopausal symptoms

EvGr Discontinue hormone replacement therapy (HRT) in women who are diagnosed with breast cancer. Do not offer HRT routinely to women with menopausal symptoms and a history of breast cancer. HRT may, in exceptional cases, be offered to women with severe menopausal symptoms and with whom the associated risks have been discussed. Paroxetine p. 363 or fluoxetine p. 362 [unlicensed indications] may be offered to women with breast cancer for relieving menopausal symptoms, particularly hot flushes, but not to those taking tamoxifen—risk of interactions. Clonidine hydrochloride p. 144, venlafaxine p. 365 [unlicensed indication] and gabapentin p. 314 [unlicensed indication] should only be offered to treat hot flushes in women with breast cancer after they have been fully informed of the significant side effects. ⒶＡ

Breast cancer in men

Breast cancer in men is rare. Although, not fully understood, risk factors may be associated with sex hormone metabolism, including those acquired through liver disease or testicular trauma, environmental risk factors such as industrial exposure to heat, and genetic predisposition. Treatment is similar to that for women involving surgery, radiotherapy, drug therapy, or a combination of these.

Useful Resources

Early and locally advanced breast cancer: Diagnosis and treatment. National Institute for Health and Care Excellence. Clinical guideline CG80. February 2009 (updated July 2014).
www.nice.org.uk/guidance/cg80

Advanced breast cancer (update): Diagnosis and treatment. National Institute for Health and Care Excellence. Clinical guideline CG81. July 2014.
www.nice.org.uk/guidance/cg81

Treatment of primary breast cancer. Scottish Intercollegiate Guidelines Network. Clinical guideline 134. September 2013.
www.sign.ac.uk/sign-134-treatment-of-primary-breast-cancer.html

Familial breast cancer: classification, care and managing breast cancer and related risks in people with a family history of breast cancer. National Institute for Health and Care Excellence. Clinical guideline CG164. June 2013 (updated March 2017).
www.nice.org.uk/guidance/cg164

Prostate Cancer
31-May-2016

Description of condition

Prostate cancer is the most common form of cancer affecting men. The main risk factors are age (most cases being diagnosed in men over 65 years of age), ethnicity (more common in black African-Caribbean men), and a familial component. Prostate cancer is usually slow-growing and asymptomatic at diagnosis, however, the presenting symptoms of advanced disease are usually urinary outflow obstruction, or, pelvic or back pain due to bone metastases. Treatment decisions are guided by baseline prostate specific antigen (PSA) levels, tumour grade (Gleason score), the stage of the tumour, the patient's life expectancy (based on age

and comorbid conditions), treatment morbidity, and patient preference.

Aims of treatment

In early or locally advanced prostate cancer, radical treatment aims to eliminate the malignancy. In metastatic disease, drug therapy is aimed at prolonging survival and reducing symptoms.

Drug treatment

Treatment options for patients with prostate cancer include active monitoring, radical prostatectomy, external beam radiotherapy, and brachytherapy. Hormone therapy (androgen deprivation or anti-androgens) is the primary treatment for metastatic prostate cancer, but is also increasingly being used for patients with locally advanced, non-metastatic disease.

In patients with localised prostate cancer, the choice of treatment is guided by whether the disease is considered low, intermediate, or high risk according to the Gleason score, the serum PSA level, and the tumour stage.

Localised or locally advanced prostate cancer

EvGr In patients with **low-risk localised prostate cancer**, and those at **intermediate risk** who decline radical treatments (prostatectomy or radiotherapy), active monitoring is a suitable option. This involves close monitoring to avoid unnecessary treatment until disease progression occurs (or until the patient requests treatment).

In patients with **intermediate-risk** or **high-risk localised prostate cancer** (when there is a realistic prospect of long-term disease control) and in those with **locally advanced disease**, radical prostatectomy or radical radiotherapy should be offered. Other treatment options include a combination of radical radiotherapy and androgen deprivation therapy, consisting of 6 months of androgen deprivation therapy before, during or after radiotherapy. Pelvic radiotherapy should be considered in those with locally advanced prostate cancer who have a higher than 15% risk of pelvic lymph node involvement and are to receive neoadjuvant hormonal therapy.

Androgen deprivation therapy involves the use of a luteinising hormone-releasing hormone (LHRH) agonist (buserelin p. 720, goserelin p. 721, leuprorelin acetate p. 722, or triptorelin p. 723), or bilateral orchidectomy, which removes the supply of endogenous hormone. Androgen deprivation therapy may be continued for up to 3 years in patients with high-risk localised prostate cancer.

Patients should be informed about the side-effects of treatment, particularly urinary and sexual dysfunction, loss of fertility, radiation-induced enteropathy, and hot flushes. Although there is limited evidence, intermittent therapy may be considered for patients who are having long-term androgen deprivation therapy, to reduce drug toxicity. Tumour flare, due to an initial surge in testosterone concentrations, has been reported in the initial stages of treatment with androgen deprivation therapy and prophylactic anti-androgen therapy (such as cyproterone acetate p. 753) may be added.

Medroxyprogesterone acetate p. 791 [unlicensed indication] can be used, initially for up to 10 weeks, to manage troublesome hot flushes caused by long-term androgen suppression; cyproterone acetate is an alternative if medroxyprogesterone acetate is not effective or not tolerated.

Patients who experience a reduction in libido and loss of sexual function should have access to specialist erectile dysfunction services and be considered for treatment with a phosphodiesterase type-5 inhibitor.

Osteoporosis and fatigue may also be a problem with androgen deprivation therapy. A bisphosphonate can be offered to men who have osteoporosis; denosumab p. 717 is an alternative if bisphosphonates are not appropriate.

8

Immune system and malignant disease

Gynaecomastia can occur with long-term (longer than 6 months) bicalutamide p. 921 treatment. Prophylactic radiotherapy (within the first month of treatment), or weekly tamoxifen p. 927 [unlicensed indication], if radiotherapy is unsuccessful, can be considered. ⚠

Metastatic prostate cancer

EvGr Bilateral orchidectomy should be offered to all patients with **metastatic prostate cancer** as an alternative to continuous LHRH agonist treatment. Anti-androgen monotherapy with bicalutamide [unlicensed indication] can be offered to those who are willing to accept the adverse impact on overall survival and gynaecomastia in the hope of retaining sexual function. However, if satisfactory sexual function is not maintained, stop bicalutamide and start androgen deprivation therapy.

Abiraterone acetate below (in combination with prednisone p. 666 or prednisolone p. 664) and enzalutamide p. 921 are both recommended as options for the treatment of castration-resistant metastatic prostate cancer in patients whose disease has progressed during or after treatment with a docetaxel p. 900-containing chemotherapy regimen.

In patients who develop **hormone-relapsed metastatic tumour**, chemotherapy with docetaxel can be used. It is recommended to stop the treatment with docetaxel after 10 cycles, or if severe adverse events occurred, or if there is evidence of disease progression.

Abiraterone acetate (in combination with prednisone or prednisolone) is also recommended as an option for treating **metastatic hormone-relapsed prostate cancer** in patients who have no or mild symptoms after androgen deprivation therapy has failed, and before chemotherapy is indicated.

In patients with hormone-relapsed prostate cancer, a corticosteroid, such as dexamethasone p. 660, can be offered as third line therapy, after androgen deprivation therapy and anti-androgen therapy. ⚠

Useful Resources

Prostate cancer: diagnosis and management. National Institute for Health and Care Excellence. Clinical guideline 175. January 2014.
www.nice.org.uk/guidance/cg175

> **Other drugs used for Hormone responsive malignancy**
> Ethinylestradiol, p. 742

ANTINEOPLASTIC DRUGS > ANTI-ANDROGENS

Abiraterone acetate

31-May-2016

● **INDICATIONS AND DOSE**

Metastatic castration-resistant prostate cancer in patients whose disease has progressed during or after treatment with a docetaxel-containing chemotherapy regimen (in combination with prednisone or prednisolone) | **Metastatic castration-resistant prostate cancer in patients who are asymptomatic or mildly symptomatic after failure of androgen deprivation therapy in whom chemotherapy is not yet clinically indicated (in combination with prednisone or prednisolone)**

▸ BY MOUTH
▸ Adult: 1 g once daily, for dose of concurrent prednisone or prednisolone—consult product literature

● CAUTIONS Diabetes (increased risk of hyperglycaemia—monitor blood sugar frequently) · history of cardiovascular disease

CAUTIONS, FURTHER INFORMATION

▸ Cardiovascular disease Correct hypertension and hypokalaemia before treatment (if significant risk of congestive heart failure, such as history of cardiac failure, uncontrolled hypertension or cardiac events, consult product literature for management and increased monitoring).

● INTERACTIONS → Appendix 1: abiraterone

● SIDE-EFFECTS
▸ **Common or very common** Angina pectoris · arrhythmias · bone fracture · diarrhoea · dyspepsia · haematuria · heart failure · hepatic disorders · hypertension · hypertriglyceridaemia · hypokalaemia · left ventricular dysfunction · osteoporosis · peripheral oedema · rash · sepsis · urinary tract infection
▸ **Uncommon** Adrenal insufficiency · myopathy
▸ **Rare or very rare** Alveolitis allergic
▸ **Frequency not known** Myocardial infarction · QT interval prolongation

● CONCEPTION AND CONTRACEPTION Men should use condoms if their partner is pregnant, and use condoms in combination with another effective contraceptive method if their partner is of child-bearing potential—toxicity in *animal* studies.

● HEPATIC IMPAIRMENT Use with caution in moderate impairment and only if benefit clearly outweighs risk. Avoid in severe impairment.

● RENAL IMPAIRMENT Use with caution in severe impairment—no information available.

● MONITORING REQUIREMENTS
▸ Monitor blood pressure, serum potassium concentration, and fluid balance before treatment, and at least monthly during treatment—consult product literature for management of hypertension, hypokalaemia and oedema.
▸ Monitor liver function before treatment, then every 2 weeks for the first 3 months of treatment, then monthly thereafter—interrupt treatment if serum alanine aminotransferase or aspartate aminotransferase greater than 5 times the upper limit (consult product literature for details of restarting treatment at a lower dose) and discontinue permanently if 20 times the upper limit.

● NATIONAL FUNDING/ACCESS DECISIONS

NICE decisions
▸ **Abiraterone for castration-resistant metastatic prostate cancer previously treated with a docetaxel-containing regimen (June 2012)** NICE TA259
Abiraterone in combination with prednisone or prednisolone is recommended as an option for the treatment of castration-resistant metastatic prostate cancer only if:
● their disease has progressed on or after one docetaxel-containing chemotherapy regimen, **and**
● the manufacturer provides abiraterone with the discount agreed in the patient access scheme.
Patients currently receiving abiraterone in combination with prednisone or prednisolone whose disease does not meet the first criteria should be able to continue therapy until they and their clinician consider it appropriate to stop.
www.nice.org.uk/TA259

▸ **Abiraterone for treating metastatic hormone-relapsed prostate cancer before chemotherapy is indicated (April 2016)** NICE TA387
Abiraterone, in combination with prednisone or prednisolone, is recommended as an option for treating metastatic hormone-relapsed prostate cancer in patients who have mild or no symptoms after androgen deprivation therapy has failed, and before chemotherapy is indicated. In addition, the manufacturer is required to rebate the cost of abiraterone from the 11th month until the end of treatment for patients who remain on treatment for more than 10 months.
www.nice.org.uk/TA387

Scottish Medicines Consortium (SMC) Decisions

The *Scottish Medicines Consortium* has advised (July 2012) that abiraterone (*Zytiga*®), in combination with prednisone or prednisolone, is accepted for restricted use within NHS Scotland for the treatment of metastatic castration-resistant prostate cancer in patients whose disease has progressed during or after treatment with docetaxel-containing chemotherapy regimen, and have received only one prior chemotherapy regimen.

● MEDICINAL FORMS
There can be variation in the licensing of different medicines containing the same drug.

Tablet
CAUTIONARY AND ADVISORY LABELS 23
▸ Zytiga (Janssen-Cilag Ltd)
  Abiraterone acetate 500 mg Zytiga 500mg tablets |
  56 tablet PoM £2,735.00

Bicalutamide

10-Apr-2017

● INDICATIONS AND DOSE

Locally advanced prostate cancer at high risk of disease progression either alone or as adjuvant treatment to prostatectomy or radiotherapy | Locally advanced, non-metastatic prostate cancer when surgical castration or other medical intervention inappropriate
▸ BY MOUTH
▸ Adult: 150 mg once daily

Advanced prostate cancer, in combination with gonadorelin analogue or surgical castration
▸ BY MOUTH
▸ Adult: 50 mg once daily, to be started at the same time as surgical castration or at least 3 days before gonadorelin therapy

Prostate cancer (metastatic) with the aim of retaining sexual function.
▸ BY MOUTH
▸ Adult: 150 mg once daily

● UNLICENSED USE EvGr Not licensed for use in prostate cancer (metastatic), with the aim of retaining sexual function. ◬

● CAUTIONS Risk of photosensitivity—avoid excessive exposure to UV light and sunlight

● INTERACTIONS → Appendix 1: bicalutamide

● SIDE-EFFECTS
▸ Common or very common Alopecia · anaemia · appetite decreased · asthenia · breast tenderness · chest pain · constipation · depression · dizziness · drowsiness · flatulence · gastrointestinal discomfort · gynaecomastia · haematuria · hair changes · hepatic disorders · hot flush · hypertransaminasaemia · nausea · oedema · sexual dysfunction · skin reactions · weight increased
▸ Uncommon Angioedema · interstitial lung disease
▸ Rare or very rare Photosensitivity reaction
▸ Frequency not known QT interval prolongation

● HEPATIC IMPAIRMENT Increased accumulation possible in moderate to severe impairment—manufacturer advises caution.

● MONITORING REQUIREMENTS Consider periodic liver function tests.

● PATIENT AND CARER ADVICE
Risk of photosensitivity Patients should be advised to consider the use of sunscreen.

● MEDICINAL FORMS
There can be variation in the licensing of different medicines containing the same drug. Forms available from special-order manufacturers include: oral suspension

Tablet
▸ Bicalutamide (Non-proprietary)
  Bicalutamide 50 mg Bicalutamide 50mg tablets | 28 tablet PoM
  £128.00 DT = £2.20
  Bicalutamide 150 mg Bicalutamide 150mg tablets | 28 tablet PoM
  £240.00 DT = £5.72
▸ Casodex (AstraZeneca UK Ltd)
  Bicalutamide 50 mg Casodex 50mg tablets | 28 tablet PoM
  £119.79 DT = £2.20
  Bicalutamide 150 mg Casodex 150mg tablets | 28 tablet PoM
  £240.00 DT = £5.72

Enzalutamide

23-May-2017

● INDICATIONS AND DOSE

Metastatic castration-resistant prostate cancer in patients whose disease has progressed during or after docetaxel therapy
▸ BY MOUTH
▸ Adult: 160 mg once daily, for dose adjustments due to side-effects, consult product literature

DOSE ADJUSTMENTS DUE TO INTERACTIONS
▸ Manufacturer advises if concurrent use of potent inhibitors of CYP2C8 is unavoidable, reduce dose to 80 mg daily.

● CAUTIONS Alcoholism · bradycardia · brain injury · brain metastases · brain tumours · history of QT-interval prolongation · history or risk of seizure · recent cardiovascular disease · risk factors for QT-interval prolongation · stroke · uncontrolled hypertension

● INTERACTIONS → Appendix 1: enzalutamide

● SIDE-EFFECTS
▸ Common or very common Anxiety · asthenia · bone fracture · concentration impaired · fall · gynaecomastia · headache · hot flush · hypertension · memory loss · restless legs · skin reactions
▸ Uncommon Cognitive disorder · leucopenia · neutropenia · seizure · visual hallucinations
▸ Frequency not known Back pain · diarrhoea · muscle complaints · muscle weakness · nausea · oral disorders · posterior reversible encephalopathy syndrome (PRES) · QT interval prolongation · throat oedema · thrombocytopenia · vomiting

● CONCEPTION AND CONTRACEPTION Men should use condoms during treatment and for 3 months after stopping treatment if their partner is pregnant, and use condoms in combination with another effective contraceptive method if their partner is of child-bearing potential—toxicity in *animal* studies.

● HEPATIC IMPAIRMENT Manufacturer advises caution in moderate impairment. Avoid in severe impairment.

● RENAL IMPAIRMENT Caution in severe impairment—no information available.

● NATIONAL FUNDING/ACCESS DECISIONS

NICE decisions
▸ Enzalutamide for treating metastatic hormone-relapsed prostate cancer before chemotherapy is indicated (January 2016) NICE TA377
Enzalutamide is recommended as an option for treating metastatic hormone-relapsed prostate cancer in patients who have mild or no symptoms after androgen deprivation therapy has failed, and before chemotherapy is indicated, **and** only if the manufacturer provides enzalutamide with the discount agreed in the patient access scheme.
www.nice.org.uk/TA377

8

Immune system and malignant disease

8

▶ **Enzalutamide for metastatic hormone relapsed prostate cancer previously treated with a docetaxel containing regimen** (July 2014) NICE TA316

Enzalutamide is recommended, within its marketing authorisation, as an option for treating metastatic hormone-relapsed prostate cancer in adults only if, their disease has progressed during or after docetaxel-containing chemotherapy, **and** the manufacturer provides enzalutamide with the discount agreed in the patient access scheme. This guidance does not cover the use of enzalutamide for metastatic hormone-relapsed prostate cancer previously treated with abiraterone.
www.nice.org.uk/TA316

● MEDICINAL FORMS
There can be variation in the licensing of different medicines containing the same drug.

Capsule
CAUTIONARY AND ADVISORY LABELS 25
▶ Xtandi (Astellas Pharma Ltd)
   Enzalutamide 40 mg Xtandi 40mg capsules | 112 capsule [PoM]
   £2,734.67

Flutamide

● INDICATIONS AND DOSE

Advanced prostate cancer | Metastatic prostate cancer refractory to gonadorelin analogue therapy (monotherapy)
▶ BY MOUTH
▶ Adult: 250 mg 3 times a day

● CAUTIONS Avoid excessive alcohol consumption · avoid in Acute porphyrias p. 1025 · cardiac disease (oedema reported)
● SIDE-EFFECTS
▶ **Common or very common** Appetite abnormal · asthenia · breast abnormalities · diarrhoea · drowsiness · galactorrhoea · gynaecomastia · hepatic function abnormal (sometimes fatal) · hepatitis (sometimes fatal) · insomnia · nausea · vomiting
▶ **Rare or very rare** Alopecia · anxiety · breast neoplasm · cardiovascular disorder · chest pain · constipation · cough · depression · dizziness · dyspnoea · gastrointestinal discomfort · gastrointestinal disorders · hair growth abnormal · headache · herpes zoster · hot flush · hypertension · interstitial pneumonitis · libido decreased · lupus-like syndrome · lymphoedema · malaise · muscle cramps · oedema · photosensitivity reaction · skin reactions · thirst · vision blurred
▶ **Frequency not known** QT interval prolongation
● HEPATIC IMPAIRMENT Use with caution (hepatotoxic).
● MONITORING REQUIREMENTS Liver function tests, monthly for first 4 months, periodically thereafter and at the first sign or symptom of liver disorder (e.g. pruritus, dark urine, persistent anorexia, jaundice, abdominal pain, unexplained influenza-like symptoms).

● MEDICINAL FORMS
There can be variation in the licensing of different medicines containing the same drug.

Tablet
▶ Flutamide (Non-proprietary)
   Flutamide 250 mg Flutamide 250mg tablets | 84 tablet [PoM]
   £106.24 DT = £106.24

OESTROGENS

Diethylstilbestrol

(Stilboestrol)

● INDICATIONS AND DOSE

Breast cancer in postmenopausal women
▶ BY MOUTH
▶ Adult: 10–20 mg daily

Prostate cancer
▶ BY MOUTH
▶ Adult: 1–3 mg daily

● CAUTIONS Cardiovascular disease
● SIDE-EFFECTS Bone pain (in breast cancer) · breast abnormalities · cervical mucus increased · cholelithiasis · contact lens intolerance · depression · erectile dysfunction · erythema nodosum · feminisation · fluid retention · gynaecomastia · headaches · hypercalcaemia (in breast cancer) · hypertension · increased risk of thrombosis · jaundice cholestatic · mood altered · nausea · neoplasms · skin reactions · sodium retention · testicular atrophy · uterine disorders · vomiting · weight changes · withdrawal bleed
● PREGNANCY In first trimester, high doses associated with vaginal carcinoma, urogenital abnormalities, and reduced fertility in female offspring. Increased risk of hypospadias in male offspring.
● HEPATIC IMPAIRMENT Avoid. Avoid in active liver disease including disorders of hepatic excretion (e.g. Dubin-Johnson or Rotor syndromes), infective hepatitis (until liver function returns to normal), and liver tumours.

● MEDICINAL FORMS
There can be variation in the licensing of different medicines containing the same drug.

Tablet
▶ Diethylstilbestrol (Non-proprietary)
   Diethylstilbestrol 1 mg Diethylstilbestrol 1mg tablets | 28 tablet [PoM] £123.00 DT = £120.34
   Diethylstilbestrol 5 mg Diethylstilbestrol 5mg tablets | 28 tablet [PoM] £185.00–£208.00 DT = £208.00

PITUITARY AND HYPOTHALAMIC HORMONES AND ANALOGUES > ANTI-GONADOTROPHIN-RELEASING HORMONES

Degarelix

● INDICATIONS AND DOSE

Advanced hormone-dependent prostate cancer
▶ BY SUBCUTANEOUS INJECTION
▶ Adult: Initially 240 mg, to be administered as 2 injections of 120 mg, then 80 mg every 28 days, dose to be administered into the abdominal region

● CAUTIONS Diabetes · susceptibility to QT-interval prolongation
● SIDE-EFFECTS
▶ **Common or very common** Anaemia · chills · diarrhoea · dizziness · fatigue · fever · gynaecomastia · headache · hot flush · influenza like illness · insomnia · musculoskeletal discomfort · musculoskeletal pain · nausea · sexual dysfunction · skin reactions · sweat changes · testicular disorders · weight changes
▶ **Uncommon** Alopecia · appetite decreased · arrhythmias · bone disorders · breast pain · cognitive impairment · constipation · depression · diabetes mellitus · dry mouth · dyspnoea · gastrointestinal discomfort · genital discomfort · hyperglycaemia · hypertension · hypotension · joint disorders · malaise · muscle spasms · muscle weakness ·

numbness · palpitations · pelvic pain · peripheral oedema ·
QT interval prolongation · renal impairment · urinary
disorders · vision blurred · vomiting
▸ **Rare or very rare** Febrile neutropenia · heart failure ·
myocardial infarction

● **HEPATIC IMPAIRMENT** Manufacturer advises caution in
severe impairment—no information available.

● **RENAL IMPAIRMENT** Manufacturer advises caution in
severe impairment—no information available.

● **MONITORING REQUIREMENTS** Monitor bone density.

● **NATIONAL FUNDING/ACCESS DECISIONS**

NICE decisions

▸ **Degarelix for treating advanced hormone-dependent prostate
cancer (August 2016)** NICE TA404
Degarelix is recommended as an option for treating
advanced hormone-dependent prostate cancer in patients
with spinal metastases, only if at least the same
discounted drug cost which was available to the NHS in
June 2016 is achieved by the commissioner.

Patients whose treatment was started within the NHS
before this guidance was published should have the option
to continue treatment, without change to their funding
arrangements, until they and their clinician consider it
appropriate to stop.
www.nice.org.uk/guidance/TA404

● **MEDICINAL FORMS**
There can be variation in the licensing of different medicines
containing the same drug.

Powder and solvent for solution for injection
▸ Firmagon (Ferring Pharmaceuticals Ltd)
Degarelix (as Degarelix acetate) 80 mg Firmagon 80mg powder
and solvent for solution for injection vials | 1 vial PoM £129.37 DT =
£129.37
Degarelix (as Degarelix acetate) 120 mg Firmagon 120mg powder
and solvent for solution for injection vials | 2 vial PoM £260.00 DT =
£260.00

**PITUITARY AND HYPOTHALAMIC HORMONES
AND ANALOGUES** ›SOMATOSTATIN ANALOGUES

Somatostatin analogues, malignant disease

Overview

Lanreotide below, octreotide p. 924 and pasireotide p. 925
are analogues of the hypothalamic release-inhibiting
hormone somatostatin. Lanreotide and octreotide are
indicated for the relief of symptoms associated with
neuroendocrine (particularly carcinoid) tumours and
acromegaly. Additionally, lanreotide is licensed for the
treatment of thyroid tumours and octreotide is also licensed
for the prevention of complications following pancreatic
surgery. Lanreotide (*Somatuline Autogel*®) is also licensed for
the treatment of unresectable locally advanced or metastatic
gastroenteropancreatic neuroendocrine tumours of midgut,
pancreatic or unknown origin where hindgut sites of origin
have been excluded. Octreotide long-acting depot injection
is licensed for treatment of advanced neuroendocrine
tumours of the midgut, or treatment where primary origin is
not known but non-midgut sites of origin have been
excluded. Octreotide may also be valuable in reducing
vomiting in palliative care and in stopping variceal bleeding
[unlicensed indication]—see also vasopressin p. 655 and
terlipressin acetate p. 90. Pasireotide is licensed for the
treatment of Cushing's disease when surgery has failed or is
inappropriate.

Somatostatin analogues　

● **CAUTIONS** Diabetes mellitus (antidiabetic requirements
may be reduced) · insulinoma (increased depth and
duration of hypoglycaemia may occur—observe patients
and monitor blood glucose levels when initiating
treatment and changing doses) · may cause growth
hormone-secreting pituitary tumour expansion during
treatment (causing serious complications)

● **SIDE-EFFECTS**
▸ **Common or very common** Adrenal insufficiency · alopecia ·
appetite decreased · arrhythmias · arthralgia · asthenia ·
biliary dilatation · cholelithiasis (following long term use) ·
constipation · diabetes mellitus · diarrhoea · dizziness ·
dyspnoea · gallbladder disorders · gastrointestinal
discomfort · gastrointestinal disorders · glucose tolerance
impaired (following long term use) · headache · hepatic
disorders · hyperbilirubinaemia · hyperglycaemia (long
term use) · hypoglycaemia · hypotension · hypothyroidism ·
lethargy · musculoskeletal pain · myalgia · nausea · QT
interval prolongation · skin reactions · thyroid disorder ·
vomiting · weight decreased
▸ **Uncommon** Anaemia · dehydration · hot flush · insomnia
▸ **Frequency not known** Pancreatitis · pancreatitis acute (after
administration)

● **MONITORING REQUIREMENTS**
▸ Monitor for signs of tumour expansion (e.g. visual field
defects).
▸ Ultrasound examination of the gallbladder is
recommended before treatment and at intervals of
6–12 months during treatment.

● **DIRECTIONS FOR ADMINISTRATION** Injection sites should
be rotated.

◤ above

Lanreotide

● **INDICATIONS AND DOSE**

SOMATULINE AUTOGEL®

**Acromegaly (if somatostatin analogue not given
previously)**
▸ BY DEEP SUBCUTANEOUS INJECTION
▸ Adult: Initially 60 mg every 28 days, adjusted according
to response, (consult product literature), for patients
treated previously with somatostatin analogue, consult
product literature for initial dose, dose to be given in
the gluteal region

Neuroendocrine (particularly carcinoid) tumours
▸ BY DEEP SUBCUTANEOUS INJECTION
▸ Adult: Initially 60–120 mg every 28 days, adjusted
according to response, dose to be given in the gluteal
region

**Unresectable locally advanced or metastatic
gastroenteropancreatic neuroendocrine tumours of
midgut, pancreatic or unknown origin where hindgut
sites of origin have been excluded**
▸ BY DEEP SUBCUTANEOUS INJECTION
▸ Adult: 120 mg every 28 days

SOMATULINE LA®

**Acromegaly and neuroendocrine (particularly carcinoid)
tumours**
▸ BY INTRAMUSCULAR INJECTION
▸ Adult: Initially 30 mg every 14 days, increased to 30 mg
every 7–10 days, adjusted according to response

Thyroid tumours
▸ BY INTRAMUSCULAR INJECTION
▸ Adult: Initially 30 mg every 14 days, increased to 30 mg
every 10 days, adjusted according to response

8

Immune system and malignant disease

- CAUTIONS Cardiac disorders (including bradycardia) · patients with carcinoid tumours—exclude the presence of an obstructive intestinal tumour before treatment
- INTERACTIONS → Appendix 1: lanreotide
- PREGNANCY Manufacturer advises use only if potential benefit outweighs risk.
- BREAST FEEDING Manufacturer advises caution—no information available.
- MONITORING REQUIREMENTS Monitor for hypothyroidism when clinically indicated.

- MEDICINAL FORMS
There can be variation in the licensing of different medicines containing the same drug.
Solution for injection
- Somatuline Autogel (Ipsen Ltd)
  Lanreotide (as Lanreotide acetate) 120 mg per 1 ml Somatuline Autogel 60mg/0.5ml solution for injection pre-filled syringes with safety system | 1 pre-filled disposable injection [PoM] £551.00 DT = £551.00
  Lanreotide (as Lanreotide acetate) 180 mg per 1 ml Somatuline Autogel 90mg/0.5ml solution for injection pre-filled syringes with safety system | 1 pre-filled disposable injection [PoM] £736.00 DT = £736.00
  Lanreotide (as Lanreotide acetate) 240 mg per 1 ml Somatuline Autogel 120mg/0.5ml solution for injection pre-filled syringes with safety system | 1 pre-filled disposable injection [PoM] £937.00 DT = £937.00

Powder and solvent for suspension for injection
- Somatuline LA (Ipsen Ltd)
  Lanreotide (as Lanreotide acetate) 30 mg Somatuline LA 30mg powder and solvent for suspension for injection vials | 1 vial [PoM] £323.00

Octreotide

☞ 923

17-Oct-2016

- INDICATIONS AND DOSE
Symptoms associated with carcinoid tumours with features of carcinoid syndrome, VIPomas, glucagonomas
▶ BY SUBCUTANEOUS INJECTION
- Adult: Initially 50 micrograms 1–2 times a day, adjusted according to response; increased to 200 micrograms 3 times a day, higher doses may be required exceptionally; maintenance doses are variable; in carcinoid tumours, discontinue after 1 week if no effect, if rapid response required, initial dose may be given by intravenous injection (with ECG monitoring and after dilution)

Acromegaly, short-term treatment before pituitary surgery or long-term treatment in those inadequately controlled by other treatment or until radiotherapy becomes fully effective
▶ BY SUBCUTANEOUS INJECTION
- Adult: 100–200 micrograms 3 times a day, discontinue if no improvement within 3 months

Prevention of complications following pancreatic surgery
▶ BY SUBCUTANEOUS INJECTION
- Adult: (consult product literature)

Test dose before use of depot preparation
▶ BY SUBCUTANEOUS INJECTION
- Adult: Test dose 50–100 micrograms for 1 dose, test dose should be given if subcutanous octreotide not previously given

Acromegaly | Neuroendocrine (particularly carcinoid) tumour adequately controlled by subcutaneous octreotide
▶ BY DEEP INTRAMUSCULAR INJECTION USING DEPOT INJECTION
- Adult: Initially 20 mg every 4 weeks for 3 months then adjusted according to response, increased if necessary up to 30 mg every 4 weeks, to be administered into the gluteal muscle, for *acromegaly*, start depot 1 day after

the last dose of subcutaneous octreotide, for *neuroendocrine tumours*, continue subcutaneous octreotide for 2 weeks after first dose of depot octreotide

Advanced neuroendocrine tumours of the midgut, or tumours of unknown primary origin where non-midgut sites of origin have been excluded
▶ BY DEEP INTRAMUSCULAR INJECTION USING DEPOT INJECTION
- Adult: 30 mg every 4 weeks

Reduce intestinal secretions in palliative care | Reduce vomiting due to bowel obstruction in palliative care
▶ BY CONTINUOUS SUBCUTANEOUS INFUSION
- Adult: 0.25–0.5 mg/24 hours (max. per dose 0.75 mg/24 hours), occasionally doses higher than the maximum are sometimes required

- INTERACTIONS → Appendix 1: octreotide
- SIDE-EFFECTS
SIDE-EFFECTS, FURTHER INFORMATION Administering non-depot injections of octreotide between meals and at bedtime may reduce gastrointestinal side-effects.
- CONCEPTION AND CONTRACEPTION Effective contraception required during treatment.
- PREGNANCY Possible effect on fetal growth; manufacturer advises use only if potential benefit outweighs risk.
- BREAST FEEDING Manufacturer advises avoid—present in milk in *animal* studies.
- HEPATIC IMPAIRMENT
Dose adjustments Adjustment of maintenance dose of non-depot preparations may be necessary in patients with liver cirrhosis.
- MONITORING REQUIREMENTS
- Monitor thyroid function on long-term therapy.
- Monitor liver function.
- With intravenous use ECG monitoring required with intravenous administration.
- TREATMENT CESSATION Avoid abrupt withdrawal of short-acting subcutaneous octreotide (associated with biliary colic and pancreatitis).
- DIRECTIONS FOR ADMINISTRATION For *intravenous injection* or *intravenous infusion*, dilute with Sodium Chloride 0.9% to a concentration of 10–50%.
- PRESCRIBING AND DISPENSING INFORMATION
Palliative care For further information on the use of octreotide in palliative care, see www.palliativedrugs.com/formulary/en/octreotide.html.

- MEDICINAL FORMS
There can be variation in the licensing of different medicines containing the same drug.
Solution for injection
- Octreotide (Non-proprietary)
  Octreotide (as Octreotide acetate) 50 microgram per 1 ml Octreotide 50micrograms/1ml solution for injection pre-filled syringes | 5 pre-filled disposable injection [PoM] £18.85 DT = £18.85
  Octreotide 50micrograms/1ml solution for injection ampoules | 5 ampoule [PoM] £14.85–£18.60
  Octreotide 50micrograms/1ml solution for injection vials | 5 vial [PoM] £22.00 DT = £22.00
  Octreotide (as Octreotide acetate) 100 microgram per 1 ml Octreotide 100micrograms/1ml solution for injection ampoules | 5 ampoule [PoM] £32.65 DT = £27.97
  Octreotide 100micrograms/1ml solution for injection pre-filled syringes | 5 pre-filled disposable injection [PoM] £30.34–£32.90 DT = £30.34
  Octreotide 100micrograms/1ml solution for injection vials | 5 vial [PoM] £32.65 DT = £32.65
  Octreotide (as Octreotide acetate) 200 microgram per 1 ml Octreotide 1mg/5ml solution for injection vials | 1 vial [PoM] £65.00–£69.66
  Octreotide (as Octreotide acetate) 500 microgram per 1 ml Octreotide 500micrograms/1ml solution for injection vials | 5 vial [PoM] £158.25

Octreotide 500micrograms/1ml solution for injection ampoules |
5 ampoule [PoM] £169.35 DT = £135.47

Octreotide 500micrograms/1ml solution for injection pre-filled
syringes | 5 pre-filled disposable injection [PoM] £154.22–£169.00 DT
= £154.22

‣ Sandostatin (Novartis Pharmaceuticals UK Ltd)

Octreotide (as Octreotide acetate) 50 microgram per
1 ml Sandostatin 50micrograms/1ml solution for injection ampoules
| 5 ampoule [PoM] £14.87

Octreotide (as Octreotide acetate) 100 microgram per
1 ml Sandostatin 100micrograms/1ml solution for injection ampoules
| 5 ampoule [PoM] £27.97 DT = £27.97

Octreotide (as Octreotide acetate) 500 microgram per
1 ml Sandostatin 500micrograms/1ml solution for injection ampoules
| 5 ampoule [PoM] £135.47 DT = £135.47

Powder and solvent for suspension for injection

‣ Sandostatin LAR (Novartis Pharmaceuticals UK Ltd)

Octreotide (as Octreotide acetate) 10 mg Sandostatin LAR 10mg
powder and solvent for suspension for injection vials | 1 vial [PoM]
£549.71 DT = £549.71

Octreotide (as Octreotide acetate) 20 mg Sandostatin LAR 20mg
powder and solvent for suspension for injection vials | 1 vial [PoM]
£799.33 DT = £799.33

Octreotide (as Octreotide acetate) 30 mg Sandostatin LAR 30mg
powder and solvent for suspension for injection vials | 1 vial [PoM]
£998.41 DT = £998.41

F 923

Pasireotide
02-Mar-2018

● **INDICATIONS AND DOSE**

Cushing's disease [when surgery has failed or is
inappropriate]

▸ BY SUBCUTANEOUS INJECTION

▸ Adult: Initially 600 micrograms twice daily for
2 months, then increased if necessary to
900 micrograms twice daily, consider discontinuation if
no response after 2 months of treatment, for dose
adjustment due to side-effects—consult product
literature

▸ BY DEEP INTRAMUSCULAR INJECTION

▸ Adult: Initially 10 mg every 4 weeks, increased if
necessary up to 40 mg every 4 weeks, dose may be
titrated every 2–4 months based on response and
tolerability, consider discontinuation if no clinical
benefit observed, for dose adjustment due to side-
effects—consult product literature

Acromegaly [when surgery has failed or is inappropriate,
and control with another somatostatin analogue is
inadequate]

▸ BY DEEP INTRAMUSCULAR INJECTION

▸ Adult: Initially 40 mg every 4 weeks, increased if
necessary up to 60 mg every 4 weeks, dose may be
increased if levels of growth hormone and/or insulin-
like growth factor-1 are not fully controlled after
3 months of initial dosing, for dose adjustment due to
side-effects—consult product literature

● CAUTIONS Cardiac disorders (including bradycardia) ·
susceptibility to QT-interval prolongation (including
electrolyte disturbances)

● INTERACTIONS → Appendix 1: pasireotide

● PREGNANCY Manufacturer advises avoid—toxicity in
animal studies.

● BREAST FEEDING Manufacturer advises avoid—present in
milk in *animal* studies.

● HEPATIC IMPAIRMENT Manufacturer advises avoid in
severe impairment.

Dose adjustments ▸ With subcutaneous use for Cushing's
disease Manufacturer advises reduce initial dose to
300 micrograms twice daily (max. dose 600 micrograms
twice daily) in moderate impairment.

▸ With intramuscular use for Cushing's disease Manufacturer
advises max. dose 20 mg in moderate impairment.

▸ When used for Acromegaly Manufacturer advises reduce
initial dose to 20 mg (max. dose 40 mg) in moderate
impairment.

● RENAL IMPAIRMENT Manufacturer advises caution in
severe impairment—increased plasma-pasireotide
exposure.

● MONITORING REQUIREMENTS

▸ Manufacturer advises consider monitoring pituitary
function before treatment initiation and periodically
thereafter.

▸ With subcutaneous use Manufacturer advises monitor liver
function before treatment initiation, after 1, 2, 4, 8, and
12 weeks of treatment, and thereafter as clinically
indicated. Manufacturer advises assess glycaemic status
before treatment initiation, weekly for the first
2–3 months of treatment, over the first 2–4 weeks after
any dose increase, periodically thereafter, and 3 months
after treatment is complete—if glycaemic control is poor,
diabetes management and monitoring should be
intensified before and during treatment. Manufacturer
advises monitor ECG and electrolytes before treatment
initiation, after one week of treatment, and periodically
thereafter.

▸ With intramuscular use Manufacturer advises monitor liver
function before treatment initiation, after the first
2–3 weeks of treatment, then monthly for 3 months, and
thereafter as clinically indicated. Manufacturer advises
assess glycaemic status before treatment initiation, weekly
for the first 3 months of treatment, over the first
4–6 weeks after any dose increase, periodically thereafter,
and 3 months after treatment is complete—if glycaemic
control is poor, diabetes management and monitoring
should be intensified before and during treatment.
Manufacturer advises monitor ECG and electrolytes before
treatment initiation, after 3 weeks of treatment, and
periodically thereafter.

● PRESCRIBING AND DISPENSING INFORMATION
Switching between formulations

▸ When used for Cushing's disease There are no clinical data
available on switching between formulations; if a switch is
required, manufacturer advises to maintain an interval of
at least 28 days between the last intramuscular injection
and the first subcutaneous injection—for further
information, consult product literature.

● PATIENT AND CARER ADVICE Manufacturer advises
patients and their carers should be informed of the signs
and symptoms of hypocortisolism (including weakness,
fatigue, anorexia, nausea, vomiting, hypotension,
hyperkalaemia, hyponatraemia, hypoglycaemia).

Driving and skilled tasks Manufacturer advises patients and
carers should be counselled on the effects on driving and
performance of skilled tasks—increased risk of fatigue and
dizziness.

● MEDICINAL FORMS
There can be variation in the licensing of different medicines
containing the same drug.

Solution for injection

▸ Signifor (Novartis Pharmaceuticals UK Ltd)

Pasireotide (as Pasireotide diaspartate) 300 microgram per
1 ml Signifor 0.3mg/1ml solution for injection ampoules |
60 ampoule [PoM] £2,800.00

Pasireotide (as Pasireotide diaspartate) 600 microgram per
1 ml Signifor 0.6mg/1ml solution for injection ampoules |
60 ampoule [PoM] £3,240.00

Pasireotide (as Pasireotide diaspartate) 900 microgram per
1 ml Signifor 0.9mg/1ml solution for injection ampoules |
60 ampoule [PoM] £3,240.00

Powder and solvent for suspension for injection

▸ Signifor (Novartis Pharmaceuticals UK Ltd)

Pasireotide (as Pasireotide pamoate) 20 mg Signifor 20mg
powder and solvent for suspension for injection vials | 1 vial [PoM]
£2,300.00

Pasireotide (as Pasireotide pamoate) 40 mg Signifor 40mg powder and solvent for suspension for injection vials | 1 vial [PoM] £2,300.00

Pasireotide (as Pasireotide pamoate) 60 mg Signifor 60mg powder and solvent for suspension for injection vials | 1 vial [PoM] £2,300.00

PROGESTOGENS

Megestrol acetate

- **INDICATIONS AND DOSE**

Treatment of breast cancer
▶ BY MOUTH
▶ Adult: 160 mg once daily

- **CONTRA-INDICATIONS** Acute porphyrias p. 1025 · breast cancer (unless progestogens are being used in the management of this condition) · genital cancer (unless progestogens are being used in the management of this condition) · history during pregnancy of idiopathic jaundice · history during pregnancy of pemphigoid gestationis · history during pregnancy of severe pruritus · history of liver tumours · severe arterial disease · undiagnosed vaginal bleeding

- **CAUTIONS** Asthma · cardiac dysfunction · conditions that may worsen with fluid retention · diabetes (progestogens can decrease glucose tolerance—monitor patient closely) · epilepsy · history of depression · hypertension · migraine · susceptibility to thromboembolism (particular caution with high dose)

- **SIDE-EFFECTS**
▶ **Common or very common** Adrenal insufficiency · alopecia · appetite increased · asthenia · carpal tunnel syndrome · constipation · Cushing's syndrome · diabetes mellitus · diarrhoea · dyspnoea · embolism and thrombosis · erectile dysfunction · flatulence · glucose tolerance impaired · heart failure · hot flush · hypercalcaemia · hyperglycaemia · hypertension · lethargy · menorrhagia · mood altered · nausea · oedema · pain · skin reactions · tumour flare · urinary frequency increased · vomiting · weight increased

- **PREGNANCY** Avoid. Reversible feminisation of male fetuses reported in *animal* studies. Risk of hypospadias in male fetuses and masculinisation of female fetuses.

- **BREAST FEEDING** Discontinue breast-feeding.

- **HEPATIC IMPAIRMENT** Manufacturer advises caution in severe impairment.

- **MEDICINAL FORMS**
There can be variation in the licensing of different medicines containing the same drug. Forms available from special-order manufacturers include: tablet, capsule, oral suspension

Oral suspension
▶ Megestrol acetate (Non-proprietary)
Megestrol acetate 40 mg per 1 ml Megestrol 200mg/5ml oral suspension | 240 ml [PoM] [S]

Tablet
▶ Megestrol acetate (Non-proprietary)
Megestrol acetate 40 mg Megestrol 40mg tablets | 100 tablet [S]
▶ Megace (Swedish Orphan Biovitrum Ltd)
Megestrol acetate 160 mg Megace 160mg tablets | 30 tablet [PoM] £19.52 DT = £19.52

4.1 Hormone responsive breast cancer

ANTINEOPLASTIC DRUGS › ANTI-OESTROGENS

Fulvestrant

20-Mar-2018

- **INDICATIONS AND DOSE**

Oestrogen-receptor-positive breast cancer
▶ BY DEEP INTRAMUSCULAR INJECTION
▶ Adult: 500 mg every 2 weeks for the first 3 doses, then 500 mg every month, to be administered into the buttock

- **INTERACTIONS** → Appendix 1: fulvestrant

- **SIDE-EFFECTS**
▶ **Common or very common** Appetite decreased · arthralgia · asthenia · diarrhoea · headache · hot flush · hypersensitivity · increased risk of infection · nausea · pain · rash · vaginal haemorrhage · venous thromboembolism · vomiting
▶ **Uncommon** Hepatic disorders · vaginal discharge
▶ **Frequency not known** Myalgia

- **PREGNANCY** Manufacturer advises avoid—increased incidence of fetal abnormalities and death in *animal* studies.

- **BREAST FEEDING** Manufacturer advises avoid—present in milk in *animal* studies.

- **HEPATIC IMPAIRMENT** Manufacturer advises caution in mild to moderate impairment. Avoid in severe impairment.

- **RENAL IMPAIRMENT** Manufacturer advises caution if creatinine clearance less than 30 mL/minute—no information available.

- **DIRECTIONS FOR ADMINISTRATION** 500 mg dose should be administered as one 250-mg injection (slowly over 1–2 minutes) into each buttock.

- **NATIONAL FUNDING/ACCESS DECISIONS**

NICE decisions
▶ **Fulvestrant for untreated locally advanced or metastatic oestrogen-receptor positive breast cancer (January 2018)** NICE TA503
Fulvestrant is **not** recommended, within its marketing authorisation, for treating locally advanced or metastatic oestrogen-receptor positive breast cancer in postmenopausal women who have not had endocrine therapy before.
Patients whose treatment was started within the NHS before this guidance was published should have the option to continue treatment, without change to their funding arrangements, until they and their NHS clinician consider it appropriate to stop.
www.nice.org.uk/guidance/ta503

- **MEDICINAL FORMS**
There can be variation in the licensing of different medicines containing the same drug.
Solution for injection
▶ Faslodex (AstraZeneca UK Ltd)
Fulvestrant 50 mg per 1 ml Faslodex 250mg/5ml solution for injection pre-filled syringes | 2 pre-filled disposable injection [PoM] £522.41

Tamoxifen

07-Sep-2017

- **DRUG ACTION** An anti-oestrogen which induces gonadotrophin release by occupying oestrogen receptors in the hypothalamus, thereby interfering with feedback mechanisms; chorionic gonadotrophin is sometimes used as an adjunct in the treatment of female infertility.

- **INDICATIONS AND DOSE**

Pre- and perimenopausal women with oestrogen-receptor-positive breast cancer not previously treated with tamoxifen
- ▸ BY MOUTH
- ▸ Adult: 20 mg daily

Anovulatory infertility
- ▸ BY MOUTH
- ▸ Adult: Initially 20 mg daily on days 2, 3, 4 and 5 of cycle, if necessary the daily dose may be increased to 40 mg then 80 mg for subsequent courses; if cycles irregular, start initial course on any day, with subsequent course starting 45 days later or on day 2 of cycle if menstruation occurs

Gynaecomastia [prevention in men undergoing long-term bicalutamide treatment, if radiotherapy unsuccessful]
- ▸ BY MOUTH
- ▸ Adult: 20 mg once weekly

Breast cancer [chemoprevention in women at moderate-to-high risk]
- ▸ BY MOUTH
- ▸ Adult: 20 mg daily for 5 years

- **UNLICENSED USE** EvGr Not licensed for prevention of gynaecomastia in men.
  Not licensed for chemoprevention of breast cancer. ◁E▷

- **CONTRA-INDICATIONS** Treatment of infertility contra-indicated if personal or family history of idiopathic venous thromboembolism or genetic predisposition to thromboembolism

- **CAUTIONS** Acute porphyrias p. 1025

- **INTERACTIONS** → Appendix 1: tamoxifen

- **SIDE-EFFECTS**
- ▸ **Common or very common** Alopecia · anaemia · cataract · cerebral ischaemia · constipation · diarrhoea · dizziness · embolism and thrombosis · fatigue · fluid retention · headache · hepatic disorders · hot flush · hypersensitivity · hypertriglyceridaemia · muscle complaints · nausea · neoplasms · retinopathy · sensation abnormal · skin reactions · taste altered · uterine disorders · vaginal haemorrhage · vomiting · vulvovaginal disorders
- ▸ **Uncommon** Hypercalcaemia · interstitial pneumonitis · leucopenia · pancreatitis · thrombocytopenia · vision disorders
- ▸ **Rare or very rare** Agranulocytosis · angioedema · corneal changes · cutaneous lupus erythematosus · cutaneous vasculitis · cystic ovarian swelling · nerve disorders · neutropenia · radiation recall reaction · Stevens-Johnson syndrome · tumour flare
- ▸ **Frequency not known** Amenorrhoea

  SIDE-EFFECTS, FURTHER INFORMATION
  Endometrial changes Increased endometrial changes, including hyperplasia, polyps, cancer, and uterine sarcoma reported; prompt investigation required if abnormal vaginal bleeding including menstrual irregularities, vaginal discharge, and pelvic pain or pressure in those receiving (or who have received) tamoxifen.
  Risk of thromboembolism Tamoxifen can increase the risk of thromboembolism particularly during and immediately after major surgery or periods of immobility (consider interrupting treatment and initiating anticoagulant measures).

- **CONCEPTION AND CONTRACEPTION** Unless being used in the treatment of female infertility, effective contraception must be used during treatment and for 2 months after stopping. Patients being treated for infertility should be warned that there is a risk of multiple pregnancy (*rarely* more than twins).

- **PREGNANCY** Avoid—possible effects on fetal development.

- **BREAST FEEDING** Suppresses lactation. Avoid unless potential benefit outweighs risk.

- **PATIENT AND CARER ADVICE**
  Endometrial changes Patients should be informed of the risk of endometrial cancer and told to report relevant symptoms promptly.
  Thromboembolism Patients should be made aware of the symptoms of thromboembolism and advised to report sudden breathlessness and any pain in the calf of one leg.

- **MEDICINAL FORMS**
  There can be variation in the licensing of different medicines containing the same drug. Forms available from special-order manufacturers include: oral suspension, oral solution

Oral solution
- ▸ Tamoxifen (Non-proprietary)
  Tamoxifen (as Tamoxifen citrate) 2 mg per 1 ml Tamoxifen 10mg/5ml oral solution sugar free sugar-free | 150 ml PoM £29.61
  DT = £29.61

Oral suspension
- ▸ Tamoxifen (Non-proprietary)
  Tamoxifen (as Tamoxifen citrate) 2 mg per 1 ml Tamoxifen 10mg/5ml oral suspension | 150 ml PoM ⊠

Tablet
- ▸ Tamoxifen (Non-proprietary)
  Tamoxifen (as Tamoxifen citrate) 10 mg Tamoxifen 10mg tablets | 30 tablet PoM £47.21 DT = £40.71
  Tamoxifen (as Tamoxifen citrate) 20 mg Tamoxifen 20mg tablets | 30 tablet PoM £13.00 DT = £2.48
  Tamoxifen (as Tamoxifen citrate) 40 mg Tamoxifen 40mg tablets | 30 tablet PoM £54.75 DT = £48.72

Toremifene

- **INDICATIONS AND DOSE**

Hormone-dependent metastatic breast cancer in postmenopausal women
- ▸ BY MOUTH
- ▸ Adult: 60 mg daily

- **CONTRA-INDICATIONS** Bradycardia · electrolyte disturbances (particularly uncorrected hypokalaemia) · endometrial hyperplasia · heart failure with reduced left-ventricular ejection fraction · history of arrhythmias · QT prolongation

- **CAUTIONS** Avoid in Acute porphyrias p. 1025 · history of severe thromboembolic disease

- **INTERACTIONS** → Appendix 1: toremifene

- **SIDE-EFFECTS**
- ▸ **Common or very common** Dizziness · fatigue · hot flush · hyperhidrosis · nausea · oedema · skin reactions · vaginal discharge · vomiting
- ▸ **Uncommon** Appetite decreased · constipation · depression · dyspnoea · headache · insomnia · thromboembolism · uterine disorders · weight increased
- ▸ **Rare or very rare** Alopecia · corneal opacity · endometrial cancer · hepatic disorders · uterine haemorrhage · vertigo
- ▸ **Frequency not known** Anaemia · leucopenia · thrombocytopenia

  SIDE-EFFECTS, FURTHER INFORMATION Increased endometrial changes, including hyperplasia, polyps and cancer reported.

- **PREGNANCY** Avoid.

- **BREAST FEEDING** Avoid.

- **HEPATIC IMPAIRMENT** Elimination decreased in hepatic impairment—avoid if severe.

- **MEDICINAL FORMS**
  There can be variation in the licensing of different medicines containing the same drug.
  Tablet
  ▸ Fareston (Orion Pharma (UK) Ltd)
    Toremifene (as Toremifene citrate) 60 mg Fareston 60mg tablets | 30 tablet [PoM] £29.08

HORMONE ANTAGONISTS AND RELATED AGENTS > AROMATASE INHIBITORS

Anastrozole

- **INDICATIONS AND DOSE**
  Adjuvant treatment of oestrogen-receptor-positive early invasive breast cancer in postmenopausal women | Adjuvant treatment of oestrogen-receptor-positive early breast cancer in postmenopausal women following 2–3 years of tamoxifen therapy | Advanced breast cancer in postmenopausal women which is oestrogen-receptor-positive or responsive to tamoxifen
  ▸ BY MOUTH
  ▸ Adult: 1 mg daily

  Breast cancer [chemoprevention in postmenopausal women at moderate to high risk] (initiated under specialist supervision)
  ▸ BY MOUTH
  ▸ Adult: 1 mg daily for 5 years

- **UNLICENSED USE** [EvGr] Not licensed for chemoprevention of breast cancer. ⚑
- **CONTRA-INDICATIONS** Not for premenopausal women
- **CAUTIONS** Susceptibility to osteoporosis
- **SIDE-EFFECTS**
  ▸ **Common or very common** Alopecia · appetite decreased · arthritis · asthenia · bone pain · carpal tunnel syndrome · diarrhoea · drowsiness · headache · hot flush · hypercholesterolaemia · hypersensitivity · joint disorders · myalgia · nausea · osteoporosis · sensation abnormal · skin reactions · taste altered · vaginal haemorrhage · vomiting · vulvovaginal dryness
  ▸ **Uncommon** Hepatitis · hypercalcaemia · trigger finger
  ▸ **Rare or very rare** Angioedema · Stevens-Johnson syndrome · vasculitis
  ▸ **Frequency not known** Mood altered
- **PREGNANCY** Avoid.
- **BREAST FEEDING** Avoid.
- **HEPATIC IMPAIRMENT** Avoid in moderate to severe impairment.
- **RENAL IMPAIRMENT** Avoid if creatinine clearance less than 20 mL/minute.
- **PRE-TREATMENT SCREENING** Laboratory test for menopause if doubt.
- **MONITORING REQUIREMENTS**
  ▸ Osteoporosis Assess bone mineral density before treatment and at regular intervals.
- **PATIENT AND CARER ADVICE**
  Driving and skilled tasks Asthenia and drowsiness may initially affect ability to drive or operate machinery.
- **NATIONAL FUNDING/ACCESS DECISIONS**
  ARIMIDEX ®
  Scottish Medicines Consortium (SMC) Decisions
  The *Scottish Medicines Consortium* has advised (August 2005 and October 2006) that anastrozole (*Arimidex®*) is accepted for restricted use within NHS Scotland, within the licensed indications, for early breast cancer and early invasive breast cancer.

- **MEDICINAL FORMS**
  There can be variation in the licensing of different medicines containing the same drug.
  Tablet
  ▸ Anastrozole (Non-proprietary)
    Anastrozole 1 mg Anastrozole 1mg tablets | 28 tablet [PoM] £65.13 DT = £6.34
  ▸ Arimidex (AstraZeneca UK Ltd)
    Anastrozole 1 mg Arimidex 1mg tablets | 28 tablet [PoM] £68.56 DT = £6.34

Exemestane

- **INDICATIONS AND DOSE**
  Adjuvant treatment of oestrogen-receptor-positive early breast cancer in postmenopausal women following 2–3 years of tamoxifen therapy | Advanced breast cancer in postmenopausal women in whom anti-oestrogen therapy has failed
  ▸ BY MOUTH
  ▸ Adult: 25 mg daily

- **CONTRA-INDICATIONS** Not indicated for premenopausal women
- **INTERACTIONS** → Appendix 1: exemestane
- **SIDE-EFFECTS**
  ▸ **Common or very common** Alopecia · appetite decreased · arthralgia · asthenia · bone fracture · carpal tunnel syndrome · constipation · depression · diarrhoea · dizziness · gastrointestinal discomfort · headache · hot flush · hyperhidrosis · insomnia · leucopenia · nausea · osteoporosis · pain · paraesthesia · peripheral oedema · skin reactions · thrombocytopenia · vomiting
  ▸ **Rare or very rare** Acute generalised exanthematous pustulosis (AGEP) · drowsiness · hepatic disorders
- **PREGNANCY** Avoid.
- **BREAST FEEDING** Avoid.
- **HEPATIC IMPAIRMENT** Manufacturer advises caution.
- **RENAL IMPAIRMENT** Manufacturer advises caution.
- **NATIONAL FUNDING/ACCESS DECISIONS**
  Scottish Medicines Consortium (SMC) Decisions
  The *Scottish Medicines Consortium* has advised (October 2005) that exemestane (*Aromasin®*) is accepted for restricted use within NHS Scotland as an adjuvant treatment in postmenopausal women with oestrogen-receptor-positive invasive early breast cancer, following 2–3 years of initial adjuvant tamoxifen therapy.

- **MEDICINAL FORMS**
  There can be variation in the licensing of different medicines containing the same drug.
  Tablet
  CAUTIONARY AND ADVISORY LABELS 21
  ▸ Exemestane (Non-proprietary)
    Exemestane 25 mg Exemestane 25mg tablets | 30 tablet [PoM] £88.80 DT = £17.25
  ▸ Aromasin (Pfizer Ltd)
    Exemestane 25 mg Aromasin 25mg tablets | 30 tablet [PoM] £88.80 DT = £17.25

8

Immune system and malignant disease

Letrozole

- **INDICATIONS AND DOSE**

First-line treatment in postmenopausal women with hormone-dependent advanced breast cancer | Adjuvant treatment of oestrogen-receptor-positive invasive early breast cancer in postmenopausal women | Advanced breast cancer in postmenopausal women (naturally or artificially induced menopause) in whom other anti-oestrogen therapy has failed | Extended adjuvant treatment of hormone-dependent invasive breast cancer in postmenopausal women who have received standard adjuvant tamoxifen therapy for 5 years | Neo-adjuvant treatment in postmenopausal women with localised hormone-receptor-positive, human epidermal growth factor-2 negative breast cancer where chemotherapy is not suitable and surgery not yet indicated

- ▸ BY MOUTH
- ▸ Adult: 2.5 mg daily

- **CONTRA-INDICATIONS** Not indicated for premenopausal women
- **CAUTIONS** Susceptibility to osteoporosis
- **SIDE-EFFECTS**
- ▸ **Common or very common** Alopecia · appetite abnormal · arthralgia · asthenia · bone fracture · bone pain · constipation · depression · diarrhoea · dizziness · gastrointestinal discomfort · headache · hot flush · hypercholesterolaemia · hyperhidrosis · hypertension · malaise · myalgia · nausea · oedema · osteoporosis · skin reactions · vaginal haemorrhage · vomiting · weight changes
- ▸ **Uncommon** Anxiety · arthritis · breast pain · cancer pain · carpal tunnel syndrome · cataract · cerebrovascular insufficiency · cough · drowsiness · dry mouth · dysaesthesia · dyspnoea · embolism and thrombosis · eye irritation · fever · insomnia · irritability · ischaemic heart disease · leucopenia · memory loss · mucosal dryness · myocardial infarction · palpitations · stomatitis · tachycardia · taste altered · thirst · urinary frequency increased · urinary tract infection · vision blurred · vulvovaginal disorders
- ▸ **Frequency not known** Angioedema · hepatitis · toxic epidermal necrolysis · trigger finger
- **CONCEPTION AND CONTRACEPTION** Manufacturer advises effective contraception required until postmenopausal status fully established (return of ovarian function reported in postmenopausal women).
- **PREGNANCY** Avoid (isolated cases of birth defects reported).
- **BREAST FEEDING** Manufacturer advises avoid.
- **HEPATIC IMPAIRMENT** Manufacturer advises caution in severe impairment.
- **RENAL IMPAIRMENT** Manufacturer advises caution if creatinine clearance less than 10 mL/minute.
- **MONITORING REQUIREMENTS**
- ▸ Osteoporosis Assess bone mineral density before treatment and at regular intervals.
- **MEDICINAL FORMS**
  There can be variation in the licensing of different medicines containing the same drug.

  Tablet
  - ▸ Letrozole (Non-proprietary)
    Letrozole 2.5 mg Letrozole 2.5mg tablets | 14 tablet [PoM] £49.90
    DT = £0.79 | 28 tablet [PoM] £1.58–£73.24
  - ▸ Femara (Novartis Pharmaceuticals UK Ltd)
    Letrozole 2.5 mg Femara 2.5mg tablets | 30 tablet [PoM] £90.92

5   Immunotherapy responsive malignancy

ANTINEOPLASTIC DRUGS

Talimogene laherparepvec   10-Feb-2017

- **DRUG ACTION** Talimogene laherparepvec is an oncolytic immunotherapy derived from herpes simplex virus type-1 which causes tumour lysis and the release of tumour-derived antigens.

- **INDICATIONS AND DOSE**

Unresectable metastatic melanoma with no bone, brain, or visceral disease
- ▸ BY INTRALESIONAL INJECTION
- ▸ Adult: (consult product literature)

- **CONTRA-INDICATIONS** Severely immunocompromised patients
  CONTRA-INDICATIONS, FURTHER INFORMATION
  Manufacturer advises avoid in patients who are severely immunocompromised, for example, those with severe congenital or acquired cellular and/or humoral immune deficiency—may be at increased risk of disseminated herpetic infection.
- **CAUTIONS** Administration of antivirals (may interfere with effectiveness of *Imlygic®*) · autoimmune disease · immunocompromised patients · multiple myeloma (risk of plasmacytoma at injection site)
  CAUTIONS, FURTHER INFORMATION
- ▸ Immunocompromised patients Manufacturer advises caution in patients who are immunocompromised, for example, those with HIV/AIDS, leukaemia, lymphoma, common variable immunodeficiency, or in those who require chronic high-dose steroids or other immunosuppressive agents—risk of disseminated herpetic infection.
- **SIDE-EFFECTS**
- ▸ **Common or very common** Anaemia · anxiety · arthralgia · chills · confusion · constipation · cough · deep vein thrombosis · dehydration · depression · diarrhoea · dizziness · dyspnoea exertional · ear pain · fatigue · fever · flushing · gastrointestinal discomfort · headache · hypertension · immune-mediated events · increased risk of infection · influenza like illness · insomnia · malaise · myalgia · nausea · neoplasm complications · oropharyngeal pain · pain · peripheral oedema · secretion discharge · skin reactions · tachycardia · vomiting · weight decreased · wound complications
- ▸ **Uncommon** Glomerulonephritis · injection site plasmacytoma · post procedural infection · respiratory disorders · vasculitis
  SIDE-EFFECTS, FURTHER INFORMATION Necrosis or ulceration of tumour tissue may occur, and impaired healing at the injection site has been reported. Manufacturer advises careful wound care and infection precautions; if persistent infection or delayed healing develops, the risks and benefits of continuing treatment should be considered.
- **CONCEPTION AND CONTRACEPTION** Manufacturer advises use of latex condoms.
- **PREGNANCY** Manufacturer advises avoid—no information available.
- **BREAST FEEDING** Manufacturer advises avoid—no information available.
- **DIRECTIONS FOR ADMINISTRATION** Consult product literature for information on injection technique.

- HANDLING AND STORAGE Manufacturer advises caution in handling—risk of accidental exposure; avoid preparation or administration if immunocompromised or pregnant. For further information, see the *Physician's Brochure* provided by the manufacturer. Store and transport frozen at -90°C to -70°C—consult product literature for further information on thawing and storage after thawing.

- PATIENT AND CARER ADVICE Manufacturer advises that patients and carers should be informed about the risks of treatment, advised to avoid touching or scratching injection sites, and to keep these sites covered with occlusive dressings. Close contacts should avoid direct contact with injected lesions or body fluids of treated patients during treatment and for up to 30 days after last treatment—if exposed, clean the affected area and seek medical attention if symptoms of herpetic infection develop; close contacts who are immunocompromised or pregnant should not be exposed to potentially contaminated materials. For further information, see the *Information for Patients and Close Contacts* provided by the manufacturer.

  Provide patient alert card—record batch number for each administration of *Imlygic* ®.

  Driving and skilled tasks Manufacturer advises that patients and their carers should be counselled on the effects on driving and performance of skilled tasks—risk of dizziness and confusion.

- NATIONAL FUNDING/ACCESS DECISIONS

  NICE decisions

  ▸ **Talimogene laherparepvec for treating unresectable metastatic melanoma (September 2016)**
  Talimogene laherparepvec is recommended as an option for treating unresectable, regionally or distantly metastatic (Stage IIIB, IIIC or IVM1a) melanoma that has not spread to bone, brain or other internal organs, only if:
  - treatment with systemically administered immunotherapies is not suitable **and**,
  - the manufacturer provides talimogene laherparepvec with the discount agreed in the patient access scheme.
  Patients whose treatment was started within the NHS before this guidance was published should have the option to continue treatment, without change to their funding arrangements, until they and their clinician consider it appropriate to stop.
  www.nice.org.uk/TA410

- MEDICINAL FORMS
  There can be variation in the licensing of different medicines containing the same drug.

  Solution for injection
  EXCIPIENTS: May contain Sorbitol
  ELECTROLYTES: May contain Sodium
  ▸ Imlygic (Amgen Ltd) ▼
    Talimogene laherparepvec 1 mega u per 1 ml Imlygic 1million plaque forming units/1ml solution for injection vials | 1 vial [PoM] £1,670.00
    Talimogene laherparepvec 100 mega u per 1 ml Imlygic 100million plaque forming units/1ml solution for injection vials | 1 vial [PoM] £1,670.00

IMMUNOSTIMULANTS > INTERFERONS

Interferon alfa

- DRUG ACTION Interferon alfa has shown some antitumour effect in certain lymphomas and solid tumours.

- INDICATIONS AND DOSE
  INTRONA ® PEN

  Chronic myelogenous leukaemia (as monotherapy or in combination with cytarabine) | Hairy cell leukaemia | Follicular lymphoma | Lymph or liver metastases of carcinoid tumour | Chronic hepatitis B | Chronic hepatitis C | Adjunct to surgery in malignant melanoma | Maintenance of remission in multiple myeloma
  ▸ BY SUBCUTANEOUS INJECTION
  ▸ Adult: (consult local protocol)

  INTRONA ® VIALS

  Chronic myelogenous leukaemia (as monotherapy or in combination with cytarabine) | Hairy cell leukaemia | Follicular lymphoma | Lymph or liver metastases of carcinoid tumour | Chronic hepatitis B | Chronic hepatitis C | Adjunct to surgery in malignant melanoma | Maintenance of remission in multiple myeloma
  ▸ BY SUBCUTANEOUS INJECTION, OR BY INTRAVENOUS INFUSION
  ▸ Adult: (consult local protocol)

  ROFERON-A ®

  Chronic myelogenous leukaemia | Hairy cell leukaemia | Chronic hepatitis B | Chronic hepatitis C | Adjunct to surgery in malignant melanoma | AIDS-related Kaposi's sarcoma | Advanced renal cell carcinoma | Progressive cutaneous T-cell lymphoma | Follicular non-Hodgkin's lymphoma
  ▸ BY SUBCUTANEOUS INJECTION
  ▸ Adult: (consult local protocol)

- CONTRA-INDICATIONS
  CONTRA-INDICATIONS, FURTHER INFORMATION
  For contra-indications consult product literature and local treatment protocol.

- CAUTIONS
  CAUTIONS, FURTHER INFORMATION For cautions consult product literature and local treatment protocol.

- INTERACTIONS → Appendix 1: interferons

- SIDE-EFFECTS
  ▸ **Common or very common** Alopecia · anaemia · anxiety · appetite abnormal · arrhythmias · arthralgia · arthritis · asthenia · atrioventricular block · breast pain · chest pain · chills · concentration impaired · confusion · constipation · cough · cyanosis · decreased leucocytes · dehydration · depression · diarrhoea · dizziness · drowsiness · dry mouth · dyspnoea · electrolyte imbalance · eye disorders · eye inflammation · eye pain · fever · flushing · gastrointestinal discomfort · haemorrhage · headaches · hearing impairment · hepatic disorders · hyperhidrosis · hypertension · hyperthyroidism · hyperuricaemia · hypothyroidism · increased risk of infection · influenza like illness · lymphadenopathy · malaise · menstrual cycle irregularities · mood altered · muscle complaints · nasal complaints · nausea · oedema · oral disorders · pain · palpitations · respiratory disorders · sensation abnormal · sexual dysfunction · skin reactions · sleep disorders · taste altered · thirst · thrombocytopenia · tremor · urinary disorders · vaginal disorder · vertigo · vision disorders · vomiting · weight decreased
  ▸ **Uncommon** Behaviour abnormal · hypotension · memory loss · nerve disorders · pericarditis · proteinuria · psychiatric disorders
  ▸ **Rare or very rare** Agranulocytosis · angioedema · aplastic anaemia · autoimmune disorder · cardiac arrest ·

cardiomyopathy · central nervous system haemorrhage · cerebrovascular insufficiency · coma (more common with high doses in the elderly) · congestive heart failure · consciousness impaired · diabetes mellitus · embolism and thrombosis · encephalopathy · gastrointestinal disorders · haemolytic anaemia · hallucination · hyperglycaemia · hyperlipidaemia · hypertriglyceridaemia (sometimes severe) · mucosal dryness · myocardial infarction · myocardial ischaemia · myopathy · nephrotic syndrome · pancreatitis · peripheral ischaemia · psychosis · pulmonary oedema · renal impairment · retinopathy · sarcoidosis · seizure (more common at high doses) · sepsis · severe cutaneous adverse reactions (SCARs) · suicidal tendencies; systemic lupus erythematosus (SLE) · thyroid disorder · ulcerative colitis · vasculitis
▸ **Frequency not known** Hepatitis B reactivation · neutropenia · pericardial effusion · pulmonary arterial hypertension · pure red cell aplasia · transplant rejection
● **CONCEPTION AND CONTRACEPTION** Effective contraception required during treatment—consult product literature.
● **PREGNANCY** Avoid unless potential benefit outweighs risk (toxicity in *animal* studies).
● **BREAST FEEDING** Unlikely to be harmful.
● **HEPATIC IMPAIRMENT** Avoid in severe hepatic impairment. **Monitoring** Close monitoring required in mild to moderate hepatic impairment.
● **RENAL IMPAIRMENT** Avoid in severe renal impairment. **Monitoring** Close monitoring required in mild to moderate renal impairment.
● **MONITORING REQUIREMENTS** Monitoring of lipid concentration is recommended.
● **DIRECTIONS FOR ADMINISTRATION** INTRONA® VIALS *IntronA*® injection vials for subcutaneous injection or intravenous infusion. ROFERON-A® *Roferon-A*® injection for subcutaneous injection.
● **NATIONAL FUNDING/ACCESS DECISIONS**

NICE decisions
▸ **Peginterferon alfa, interferon alfa, and ribavirin for moderate to severe chronic hepatitis C (January 2004 and September 2010)** NICE TA200
Interferon alfa for either monotherapy or combined therapy should be used only if neutropenia and thrombocytopenia are a particular risk. Patients receiving interferon alfa may be switched to peginterferon alfa.
www.nice.org.uk/TA200

● **MEDICINAL FORMS**
There can be variation in the licensing of different medicines containing the same drug.
Solution for injection
EXCIPIENTS: May contain Benzyl alcohol
▸ IntronA (Merck Sharp & Dohme Ltd)
Interferon alfa-2b 10 mega u per 1 ml IntronA 10million units/1ml solution for injection vials | 1 vial PoM ⓢ
IntronA 25million units/2.5ml solution for injection multidose vials | 1 vial PoM £103.94
Interferon alfa-2b 15 mega u per 1 ml IntronA 18million units/1.2ml solution for injection multidose pens | 1 pre-filled disposable injection PoM £74.83
Interferon alfa-2b 25 mega u per 1 ml IntronA 30million units/1.2ml solution for injection multidose pens | 1 pre-filled disposable injection PoM £124.72
Interferon alfa-2b 50 mega u per 1 ml IntronA 60million units/1.2ml solution for injection multidose pens | 1 pre-filled disposable injection PoM £249.45
▸ Roferon-A (Roche Products Ltd)
Interferon alfa-2a 6 mega u per 1 ml Roferon-A 3million units/0.5ml solution for injection pre-filled syringes | 1 pre-filled disposable injection PoM £14.20

Interferon alfa-2a 9 mega u per 1 ml Roferon-A 4.5million units/0.5ml solution for injection pre-filled syringes | 1 pre-filled disposable injection PoM £21.29
Interferon alfa-2a 12 mega u per 1 ml Roferon-A 6million units/0.5ml solution for injection pre-filled syringes | 1 pre-filled disposable injection PoM £28.37
Interferon alfa-2a 18 mega u per 1 ml Roferon-A 9million units/0.5ml solution for injection pre-filled syringes | 1 pre-filled disposable injection PoM £42.57

Interferon gamma-1b

(Immune interferon)

● **INDICATIONS AND DOSE**

To reduce the frequency of serious infection in chronic granulomatous disease
▸ BY SUBCUTANEOUS INJECTION
▸ Adult: 50 micrograms/m^2 3 times a week
To reduce the frequency of serious infection in severe malignant osteopetrosis
▸ BY SUBCUTANEOUS INJECTION
▸ Adult: 50 micrograms/m^2 3 times a week

● **CONTRA-INDICATIONS** Simultaneous administration of foreign proteins including immunological products (such as vaccines)—risk of exaggerated immune response
● **CAUTIONS** Arrhythmias · cardiac disease · congestive heart failure · ischaemia · seizure disorders (including seizures associated with fever)
● **SIDE-EFFECTS**
▸ **Common or very common** Abdominal pain · arthralgia · back pain · chills · depression · diarrhoea · fatigue · fever · headache · nausea · rash · vomiting
▸ **Frequency not known** Atrioventricular block · chest discomfort · confusion · connective tissue disorders · embolism and thrombosis · gait abnormal · gastrointestinal haemorrhage · hallucination · heart failure · hepatic failure · hypertriglyceridaemia · hypoglycaemia · hyponatraemia · hypotension · influenza like illness · myocardial infarction · neutropenia · pancreatitis · parkinsonism · proteinuria · renal failure · respiratory disorders · seizure · syncope · systemic lupus erythematosus (SLE) · tachycardia · thrombocytopenia · transient ischaemic attack
● **CONCEPTION AND CONTRACEPTION** Effective contraception required during treatment—consult product literature.
● **PREGNANCY** Manufacturers recommend avoid unless potential benefit outweighs risk (toxicity in *animal* studies).
● **BREAST FEEDING** Manufacturers advise avoid—no information available.
● **HEPATIC IMPAIRMENT** Manufacturer advises caution in severe impairment—risk of accumulation.
● **RENAL IMPAIRMENT** Manufacturer advises caution in severe impairment—risk of accumulation.
● **MONITORING REQUIREMENTS** Monitor before and during treatment: haematological tests (including full blood count, differential white cell count, and platelet count), blood chemistry tests (including renal and liver function tests) and urinalysis.

● **MEDICINAL FORMS**
There can be variation in the licensing of different medicines containing the same drug.
Solution for injection
▸ Immukin (Horizon Pharma Ireland Ltd)
Interferon gamma-1b (recombinant human) 200 microgram per 1 ml Immukin 100micrograms/0.5ml solution for injection vials | 6 vial PoM £450.00

8

Immune system and malignant disease

IMMUNOSTIMULANTS > INTERLEUKINS

Aldesleukin

- **DRUG ACTION** Aldesleukin produces tumour shrinkage in a small proportion of patients, but it has not been shown to increase survival.

- ● **INDICATIONS AND DOSE**

  Metastatic renal cell carcinoma (specialist use only)
  - ▶ BY SUBCUTANEOUS INJECTION, OR BY INTRAVENOUS INFUSION
  - ▶ Adult: (consult product literature)

- **UNLICENSED USE** Aldesleukin is not licensed for use in patients in whom all three of the following prognostic factors are present: performance status of Eastern Co-operative Oncology Group of 1 or greater, more than one organ with metastatic disease sites, and a period of less than 24 months between initial diagnosis of primary tumour and date of evaluation of treatment.

- **CONTRA-INDICATIONS**

  CONTRA-INDICATIONS, FURTHER INFORMATION Consult product literature for information about aldesleukin contra-indications.

- **CAUTIONS**

  CAUTIONS, FURTHER INFORMATION Consult product literature for information about aldesleukin cautions.

- **SIDE-EFFECTS**
  - ▶ **Common or very common** Acidosis · alopecia · anaemia · anxiety · appetite decreased · arrhythmias · arthralgia · ascites · asthenia · cardiovascular disorders · chest pain · chills · coagulation disorders · confusion · conjunctivitis · constipation · cough · cyanosis · dehydration · depression · diarrhoea · dizziness · drowsiness · dyspepsia · dysphagia · dyspnoea · electrolyte imbalance · eosinophilia · fever · gastrointestinal disorders · haemorrhage · hallucination · headache · heart failure · hepatic disorders · hyperbilirubinaemia · hyperglycaemia · hyperhidrosis · hypertension · hyperthyroidism · hypotension · hypothermia · hypothyroidism · hypoxia · increased risk of infection · insomnia · irritability · ischaemic heart disease · leucopenia · malaise · mucositis · myalgia · nasal congestion · nausea · nerve disorders · oedema · oral disorders · pain · palpitations · paraesthesia · pulmonary oedema · renal impairment · respiratory disorders · sepsis · skin reactions · speech disorder · syncope · taste loss · thrombocytopenia · vascular disorders · vomiting · weight changes
  - ▶ **Uncommon** Angioedema · cardiac arrest · cardiac inflammation · cardiomyopathy · coma · embolism and thrombosis · hypoglycaemia · muscle weakness · myopathy · neutropenia · pancreatitis · paralysis · pericardial disorders · seizure
  - ▶ **Rare or very rare** Agranulocytosis · aplastic anaemia · cholecystitis · Crohn's disease aggravated · diabetes mellitus · haemolytic anaemia · Stevens-Johnson syndrome · ventricular dysfunction
  - ▶ **Frequency not known** Immune complex RPGN · inflammatory arthritis · intracranial haemorrhage · leukoencephalopathy · myocardial infarction · oculo-bulbar myasthenia gravis · psychiatric disorder · stroke · thyroiditis · vasculitis cerebral

- **CONCEPTION AND CONTRACEPTION** Ensure effective contraception during treatment in men and women.

- **PREGNANCY** Use only if potential benefit outweighs risk (toxicity in *animal* studies). See also *Pregnancy and reproductive function* in Cytotoxic drugs p. 865.

- **BREAST FEEDING** Discontinue breast-feeding.

- **DIRECTIONS FOR ADMINISTRATION** Aldesleukin is now rarely given by intravenous infusion because of an increased risk of capillary leak syndrome, which can cause pulmonary oedema and hypotension.

- **MEDICINAL FORMS**
  There can be variation in the licensing of different medicines containing the same drug.
  Powder for solution for injection
  - ▶ Proleukin (Novartis Pharmaceuticals UK Ltd)
    Aldesleukin 18 mega u Proleukin 18million unit powder for solution for injection vials | 1 vial [PoM] £112.00 | 10 vial [PoM] £1,036.00

IMMUNOSTIMULANTS > OTHER

Bacillus Calmette-Guérin

- **DRUG ACTION** Bacillus Calmette-Guérin is a live attenuated strain derived from *Mycobacterium bovis*.

- ● **INDICATIONS AND DOSE**

  Bladder instillation for the treatment of primary or recurrent bladder carcinoma and for the prevention of recurrence following transurethral resection
  - ▶ BY INTRAVESICAL INSTILLATION
  - ▶ Adult: (consult product literature)

- **CONTRA-INDICATIONS** Fever of unknown origin · HIV infection · impaired immune response · severe haematuria · tuberculosis · urinary-tract infection

- **CAUTIONS** Bladder injury (delay administration until mucosal damage healed) · traumatic catheterisation (delay administration until mucosal damage healed) · urethral injury (delay administration until mucosal damage healed)

- **SIDE-EFFECTS**
  - ▶ **Common or very common** Appetite decreased · arthritis · bladder cramps · bladder disorders · cardiovascular event · chills · cystitis · diarrhoea · fatigue · fever · haematuria · hepatic disorders · increased risk of infection · joint disorders · malaise · myalgia · nausea · pain · skin reactions · urinary disorders · vomiting
  - ▶ **Uncommon** Abdominal pain · anaemia · coagulation disorder · constipation · dizziness · genital pain · headache · leucopenia · mucositis · nephrotoxicity · stomatitis · thrombocytopenia · tissue in urine · ulcer · ureteral obstruction
  - ▶ **Frequency not known** Erythema nodosum · eye disorders · eye inflammation · glomerulonephritis · influenza like illness · interstitial lung disease · nephritis · renal abscess · renal failure

- **PREGNANCY** Avoid.

- **BREAST FEEDING** Avoid.

- **PRE-TREATMENT SCREENING** Screen for active tuberculosis (contra-indicated if tuberculosis confirmed).

- **MEDICINAL FORMS**
  There can be variation in the licensing of different medicines containing the same drug.
  Powder for reconstitution for instillation
  - ▶ ImmuCyst (Alliance Pharmaceuticals Ltd)
    Connaught strain Bacillus of Calmette-Guerin 81 mg ImmuCyst 81mg powder for reconstitution for instillation vials | 1 vial [PoM] £118.73 (Hospital only)
  - ▶ OncoTICE (Merck Sharp & Dohme Ltd)
    TICE strain Bacillus of Calmette-Guerin 12.5 mg OncoTICE 12.5mg powder for reconstitution for instillation vials | 1 vial [PoM] £71.61 (Hospital only)

Mifamurtide

- **INDICATIONS AND DOSE**

Treatment of high-grade, resectable, non-metastatic osteosarcoma after complete surgical resection (in combination with chemotherapy)
  ▸ BY INTRAVENOUS INFUSION
    ▸ Adult: Infusion to be given over 1 hour (consult product literature or local protocols)

- **UNLICENSED USE** Not licensed for use in patients over 30 years of age at initial diagnosis.

- **CAUTIONS** Asthma—consider prophylactic bronchodilator therapy · chronic obstructive pulmonary disease—consider prophylactic bronchodilator therapy · history of autoimmune disease · history of collagen disease · history of inflammatory disease

- **INTERACTIONS** → Appendix 1: mifamurtide

- **SIDE-EFFECTS**
  ▸ **Common or very common** Alopecia · anaemia · anxiety · appetite decreased · arthralgia · asthenia · cancer pain · chest discomfort · chills · confusion · constipation · cough · cyanosis · dehydration · depression · diarrhoea · dizziness · drowsiness · dysmenorrhoea · dyspnoea · feeling cold · fever · flushing · gastrointestinal discomfort · haemorrhage · headache · hearing impairment · hepatic pain · hyperhidrosis · hypertension · hypokalaemia · hypotension · hypothermia · increased risk of infection · insomnia · laryngeal pain · leucopenia · malaise · mucositis · muscle complaints · musculoskeletal stiffness · nasal congestion · nausea · neutropenia · oedema · pain · palpitations · respiratory disorders · sensation abnormal · sepsis · skin reactions · tachycardia · thrombocytopenia · tremor · urinary disorders · vascular disorders · vertigo · vision blurred · vomiting · weight decreased

- **CONCEPTION AND CONTRACEPTION** Effective contraception required.

- **PREGNANCY** Avoid.

- **BREAST FEEDING** Avoid—no information available.

- **HEPATIC IMPAIRMENT** Use with caution—no information available.

- **RENAL IMPAIRMENT** Use with caution—no information available.

- **MONITORING REQUIREMENTS**
  ▸ Monitor renal function, hepatic function and clotting parameters.
  ▸ Monitor patients with history of venous thrombosis, vasculitis, or unstable cardiovascular disorders for persistent or worsening symptoms during administration—consult product literature.

- **NATIONAL FUNDING/ACCESS DECISIONS**

NICE decisions
  ▸ Mifamurtide for the treatment of osteosarcoma (October 2011) NICE TA235
  Mifamurtide in combination with postoperative multi-agent chemotherapy is recommended (within its licensed indication), as an option for the treatment of high-grade resectable non-metastatic osteosarcoma after macroscopically complete surgical resection in children, adolescents and young adults and when mifamurtide is made available at a reduced cost to the NHS under the patient access scheme.
  www.nice.org.uk/TA235

- **MEDICINAL FORMS**
  There can be variation in the licensing of different medicines containing the same drug.
  Powder for suspension for infusion
    ▸ Mepact (Takeda UK Ltd)
    Mifamurtide 4 mg Mepact 4mg powder for suspension for infusion vials | 1 vial [PoM] £2,375.00

IMMUNOSUPPRESSANTS ⟩ THALIDOMIDE AND RELATED ANOLOGUES

Lenalidomide

12-Jul-2017

- **DRUG ACTION** Lenalidomide is an immunomodulating drug with anti-neoplastic, anti-angiogenic, and pro-erythropoietic properties.

- **INDICATIONS AND DOSE**

Multiple myeloma (newly diagnosed) in patients not eligible for transplant, given in combination with dexamethasone until disease progression
  ▸ BY MOUTH
    ▸ Adult: 25 mg once daily for 21 consecutive days of repeated 28-day cycles, for doses of dexamethasone, and dose adjustments due to side-effects, consult product literature

Multiple myeloma (newly diagnosed) in patients not eligible for transplant, given in combination with melphalan and prednisone followed by maintenance monotherapy
  ▸ BY MOUTH
    ▸ Adult: 10 mg once daily for 21 consecutive days of repeated 28-day cycles for up to 9 cycles, for doses of melphalan and prednisone, and dose adjustments due to side- effects, consult product literature

Multiple myeloma in patients who have received at least one prior therapy, given in combination with dexamethasone
  ▸ BY MOUTH
    ▸ Adult: 25 mg once daily for 21 consecutive days of repeated 28-day cycles, for doses of dexamethasone, and dose adjustments due to side-effects, consult product literature

Treatment of transfusion-dependent anaemia due to low- or intermediate-1-risk myelodysplastic syndromes (MDS) associated with an isolated deletion 5q cytogenetic abnormality when other treatment options are insufficient or inadequate
  ▸ BY MOUTH
    ▸ Adult: 10 mg once daily for 21 consecutive days of repeated 28-day cycles, for dose adjustments due to side-effects, consult product literature

- **CAUTIONS** High tumour burden—risk of tumour lysis syndrome · patients with risk factors for myocardial infarction
  CAUTIONS, FURTHER INFORMATION
  ▸ Thromboembolism Risk factors for thromboembolism (such as smoking, hypertension, hyperlipidaemia) should be minimised and thromboprophylaxis should be considered in patients with multiple risk factors.
  ▸ Second primary malignancy Patients should be carefully evaluated before and during treatment with lenalidomide using routine cancer screening for occurrence of second primary malignancy and treatment should be instituted as indicated.

- **INTERACTIONS** → Appendix 1: lenalidomide

- **SIDE-EFFECTS**
  ▸ **Common or very common** Anaemia · appetite decreased · arthralgia · asthenia · atrial fibrillation · chills · constipation · cough · decreased leucocytes · dehydration · diarrhoea · dizziness · dry mouth · dyspnoea · electrolyte imbalance · embolism and thrombosis · fall · fever · gastrointestinal discomfort · haemorrhage · headache · heart failure · hyperglycaemia · hypertension · hyperthyroidism · hypotension · hypothyroidism · increased risk of infection · influenza like illness · insomnia · iron overload · lethargy · mood altered · muscle complaints · muscle weakness · myocardial infarction ·

8

Immune system and malignant disease

nausea · neoplasms · neutropenia · night sweats · pain · pancytopenia · paraesthesia · peripheral neuropathy · peripheral oedema · renal failure · rhinorrhoea · sepsis · skin reactions · taste altered · thrombocytopenia · toothache · tumour flare · vertigo · vomiting · weight decreased

▸ **Uncommon** Angioedema

▸ **Rare or very rare** Severe cutaneous adverse reactions (SCARs) · tumour lysis syndrome

▸ **Frequency not known** Acquired haemophilia · gastrointestinal disorders · hepatic disorders · hypersensitivity · hypersensitivity vasculitis · interstitial pneumonitis · pancreatitis · reactivation of infections

SIDE-EFFECTS, FURTHER INFORMATION If rash occurs, treatment should be discontinued and only restarted following appropriate clinical evaluation.

Discontinue permanently if angioedema, exfoliative or bullous rash, or if Stevens-Johnson syndrome or toxic epidermal necrolysis is suspected.

● CONCEPTION AND CONTRACEPTION For women of child-bearing potential, pregnancy must be excluded before starting treatment with lenalidomide (perform pregnancy test on initiation or within 3 days prior to initiation). Women must practise effective contraception at least 1 month before, during, and for at least 1 month after treatment, including during dose interruptions (oral combined hormonal contraceptives and copper-releasing intra-uterine devices not recommended) and men should use condoms during treatment, during dose interruption, and for at least 1 week after stopping if their partner is pregnant or is of childbearing potential and not using effective contraception. Patients, prescribers and pharmacists must comply with pregnancy prevention measures as specified in the manufacturer's Pregnancy Prevention Programme.

● PREGNANCY **Important: teratogenic risk.** Lenalidomide is structurally related to thalidomide and there is a risk of teratogenesis.

● BREAST FEEDING Discontinue breast-feeding—no information available.

● RENAL IMPAIRMENT
Dose adjustments Reduce dose in moderate to severe impairment—consult product literature.

● MONITORING REQUIREMENTS

▸ Monitor full blood count (including differential white cell count, platelet count, haemoglobin, and haematocrit) and liver function before treatment, then every week for the first 8 weeks, then monthly thereafter (reduce dose or interrupt treatment if neutropenia, thrombocytopenia or impaired liver function develop—consult product literature.

▸ Monitor for arterial or venous thromboembolism (if thromboembolic event occurs, discontinue lenalidomide and treat with standard anticoagulation therapy; lenalidomide may be restarted with continued anticoagulation therapy once thromboembolic event resolved—consult product literature).

▸ Monitor thyroid function.

▸ Monitor for signs and symptoms of peripheral neuropathy.

▸ Monitor visual ability regularly (risk of cataract).

▸ Hepatic disorders Liver function should be monitored particularly when there is history of, or concurrent viral liver infection, or when lenalidomide is combined with drugs known to be associated with liver dysfunction (e.g. paracetamol).

● PRESCRIBING AND DISPENSING INFORMATION Patient, prescriber, and supplying pharmacy must comply with a pregnancy prevention programme. Every prescription must be accompanied by a completed Prescription Authorisation Form.

● PATIENT AND CARER ADVICE
Thromboembolism Patients and their carers should be made aware of the symptoms of thromboembolism and advised to report sudden breathlessness, chest pain, or swelling of a limb.

Neutropenia and thrombocytopenia Patients and their carers should be made aware of the symptoms of neutropenia and advised to seek medical advice if symptoms suggestive of neutropenia (such as fever, sore throat) or of thrombocytopenia (such as bleeding) develop.

Conception and contraception Patient counselling is advised for lenalidomide capsules (pregnancy and contraception).

● NATIONAL FUNDING/ACCESS DECISIONS

NICE decisions

▸ **Lenalidomide for treating myelodysplastic syndromes associated with an isolated deletion 5q cytogenetic abnormality (September 2014)** NICE TA322
Lenalidomide is recommended as an option, within its marketing authorisation, for treating transfusion-dependent anaemia caused by low or intermediate-1-risk myelodysplastic syndromes associated with an isolated deletion 5q cytogenetic abnormality when other therapeutic options are insufficient or inadequate, with the following condition:

● the drug cost of lenalidomide (excluding any related costs) for people who remain on treatment for more than 26 cycles (each of 28 days; normally a period of 2 years) will be met by the company.
www.nice.org.uk/guidance/ta322

▸ **Lenalidomide for the treatment of multiple myeloma (updated April 2014)** NICE TA171
Lenalidomide in combination with dexamethasone is an option for the treatment of multiple myeloma in patients who have received two or more prior therapies. The drug cost of lenalidomide will be met by the manufacturer for patients who remain on treatment for more than 26 cycles.
www.nice.org.uk/guidance/ta171

▸ **Ixazomib with lenalidomide and dexamethasone for treating relapsed or refractory multiple myeloma (February 2018)** NICE TA505
Ixazomib, with lenalidomide and dexamethasone, is recommended for use within the Cancer Drugs Fund as an option for treating multiple myeloma in adults only if:

● they have already had 2 or 3 lines of therapy, **and**

● the conditions in the managed access agreement for ixazomib are followed.

Patients whose treatment was started within the NHS before this guidance was published should have the option to continue treatment, without change to their funding arrangements, until they and their NHS clinician consider it appropriate to stop.
www.nice.org.uk/guidance/ta505

Scottish Medicines Consortium (SMC) Decisions
The *Scottish Medicines Consortium* has advised (May 2010) that lenalidomide, in combination with dexamethasone, is accepted for restricted use within NHS Scotland for patients with multiple myeloma who have received at least two prior therapies.

The *Scottish Medicines Consortium* has advised (April 2014) that lenalidomide, in combination with dexamethasone, is accepted for restricted use within NHS Scotland for treatment of multiple myeloma in adults to use at first relapse in those who have received prior therapy with bortezomib and for whom thalidomide has not been tolerated or is contra-indicated.

The *Scottish Medicines Consortium* has advised (December 2015) that lenalidomide is accepted for restricted use within NHS Scotland for patients with previously untreated multiple myeloma who are not eligible for transplant and when thalidomide-containing regimens are unsuitable.

● MEDICINAL FORMS
There can be variation in the licensing of different medicines containing the same drug.

Capsule
CAUTIONARY AND ADVISORY LABELS 25
▸ Revlimid (Celgene Ltd) ▼
Lenalidomide 2.5 mg Revlimid 2.5mg capsules | 21 capsule PoM
£3,426.00
Lenalidomide 5 mg Revlimid 5mg capsules | 21 capsule PoM
£3,570.00
Lenalidomide 7.5 mg Revlimid 7.5mg capsules | 21 capsule PoM
£3,675.00
Lenalidomide 10 mg Revlimid 10mg capsules | 21 capsule PoM
£3,780.00
Lenalidomide 15 mg Revlimid 15mg capsules | 21 capsule PoM
£3,969.00
Lenalidomide 20 mg Revlimid 20mg capsules | 21 capsule PoM
£4,168.50
Lenalidomide 25 mg Revlimid 25mg capsules | 21 capsule PoM
£4,368.00

Pomalidomide

02-Jun-2017

● DRUG ACTION Pomalidomide is structurally related to thalidomide and has immunomodulatory properties and direct anti-myeloma tumoricidal activity.

● INDICATIONS AND DOSE

Treatment of relapsed and refractory multiple myeloma in patients who have received at least two prior treatment regimens, including both lenalidomide and bortezomib, and who have had disease progression during the last treatment (in combination with dexamethasone)
▸ BY MOUTH
▸ Adult: 4 mg once daily for 21 consecutive days of repeated 28–day cycles, for doses of dexamethasone and dose adjustment due to side effects—consult product literature

DOSE ADJUSTMENTS DUE TO INTERACTIONS
▸ Manufacturer advises halve dose with concurrent use of potent inhibitors of CYP1A2 and ciprofloxacin.

IMPORTANT SAFETY INFORMATION
MHRA/CHM ADVICE (MAY 2016): RISK OF HEPATITIS B REACTIVATION
An EU wide review has concluded that pomalidomide can cause hepatitis B reactivation; the MHRA recommends to establish hepatitis B virus status in all patients before initiation of treatment.

● CAUTIONS Cardiac disease · cardiac risk factors · hepatitis B infection · high tumour burden—risk of tumour lysis syndrome · interstitial lung disease—discontinue if suspected · peripheral neuropathy
CAUTIONS, FURTHER INFORMATION
▸ Thromboembolism Risk factors for thromboembolism (such as smoking, hypertension, hyperlipidaemia) should be minimised. Thromboprophylaxis should be considered, particularly in patients with additional risk factors.
▸ Second primary malignancy Patients should be carefully evaluated before and during treatment with pomalidomide using routine cancer screening for occurrence of second primary malignancy and treatment should be instituted as indicated.
▸ Hepatitis B infection The MHRA advises that those with a history of hepatitis B infection should be closely monitored for signs and symptoms of active infection throughout treatment; expert advice should be sought for patients who test positive for active infection.

● INTERACTIONS → Appendix 1: pomalidomide

● SIDE-EFFECTS
▸ **Common or very common** Anaemia · angioedema · appetite decreased · atrial fibrillation · bone pain · confusion · constipation · cough · diarrhoea · dizziness · dyspnoea · electrolyte imbalance · embolism and thrombosis · fatigue · fever · haemorrhage · heart failure · hyperuricaemia · increased risk of infection · interstitial lung disease · intracranial haemorrhage · leucopenia · level of consciousness decreased · muscle spasms · myocardial infarction · nausea · neutropenia · neutropenic sepsis · pancytopenia · pelvic pain · peripheral neuropathy · peripheral oedema · renal failure · skin reactions · thrombocytopenia · tremor · urinary retention · vertigo · vomiting
▸ **Uncommon** Hepatitis · hyperbilirubinaemia · neoplasms · stroke · tumour lysis syndrome
▸ **Frequency not known** Hepatitis B reactivation

● CONCEPTION AND CONTRACEPTION For women of child-bearing potential, pregnancy must be excluded before starting treatment with pomalidomide (perform pregnancy test on initiation or within 3 days prior to initiation). Women must practise effective contraception at least 1 month before, during, and for at least 1 month after treatment, including during dose interruptions (oral combined hormonal contraceptives and copper-releasing intra-uterine devices not recommended) and men should use condoms during treatment, during dose interruption, and for at least 1 week after stopping if their partner is pregnant or is of childbearing potential and not using effective contraception. Patients, prescribers and pharmacists must comply with pregnancy prevention measures as specified in the manufacturer's Pregnancy Prevention Programme.

● PREGNANCY **Important: teratogenic risk**.

● BREAST FEEDING Avoid—present in milk in *animal* studies.

● HEPATIC IMPAIRMENT Manufacturer advises caution—no information available.

● RENAL IMPAIRMENT Manufacturer advises caution—no information available.

● MONITORING REQUIREMENTS
▸ Maufacturer advises monitor full blood count before treatment, then every week for the first 8 weeks, then monthly thereafter (reduce dose or interrupt treatment if neutropenia or thrombocytopenia develop—consult product literature).
▸ Manufacturer advises monitor for arterial or venous thromboembolism.
▸ Manufacturer advises monitor for signs and symptoms of cardiac failure.
▸ Manufacturer advises monitor for acute onset or unexplained worsening of respiratory symptoms.
▸ Manufacturer advises monitor liver function for 6 months after initiation, then as clinically indicated.

● PRESCRIBING AND DISPENSING INFORMATION Patient, prescriber, and supplying pharmacy must comply with a pregnancy prevention programme. Every prescription must be accompanied by a completed Prescription Authorisation Form.

● PATIENT AND CARER ADVICE Patients and their carers should be made aware of the symptoms of thromboembolism and advised to report sudden breathlessness, chest pain, or swelling of a limb.
Patients and their carers should be made aware of the symptoms of neutropenia and advised to seek medical advice if symptoms suggestive of neutropenia (such as fever, sore throat) or of thrombocytopenia (such as bleeding) develop.
Conception and contraception Patient counselling is advised for pomalidomide capsules (pregnancy and contraception).

8

Immune system and malignant disease

● NATIONAL FUNDING/ACCESS DECISIONS

NICE decisions

▶ **Pomalidomide for multiple myeloma previously treated with lenalidomide and bortezomib (January 2017)** NICE TA427
Pomalidomide, in combination with low-dose dexamethasone, is recommended as an option for treating multiple myeloma in adults at third or subsequent relapse (that is, after three previous treatments including both lenalidomide and bortezomib), only when the manufacturer provides pomalidomide with the discount agreed in the patient access scheme. Patients whose treatment was started within the NHS before this guidance was published should have the option to continue treatment, without change to their funding arrangements, until they and their clinician consider it appropriate to stop.
www.nice.org.uk/TA427

● MEDICINAL FORMS
There can be variation in the licensing of different medicines containing the same drug.

Capsule

CAUTIONARY AND ADVISORY LABELS 3, 25
EXCIPIENTS: May contain Propylene glycol
▶ Imnovid (Celgene Ltd) ▼

Pomalidomide 1 mg Imnovid 1mg capsules | 21 capsule [PoM]
£8,884.00

Pomalidomide 2 mg Imnovid 2mg capsules | 21 capsule [PoM]
£8,884.00

Pomalidomide 3 mg Imnovid 3mg capsules | 21 capsule [PoM]
£8,884.00

Pomalidomide 4 mg Imnovid 4mg capsules | 21 capsule [PoM]
£8,884.00

Thalidomide

● DRUG ACTION Thalidomide has immunomodulatory and anti-inflammatory activity.

● INDICATIONS AND DOSE

First-line treatment for untreated multiple myeloma, in patients aged 65 years and over, or for those not eligible for high-dose chemotherapy (for example, patients with significant co-morbidity such as cardiac risk factors) in combination with melphalan and prednisolone

▶ BY MOUTH
▶ Adult 18–75 years: 200 mg once daily for 6–week cycle for a maximum of 12 cycles, dose to be taken at bedtime
▶ Adult 76 years and over: 100 mg once daily for 6–week cycle for a maximum of 12 cycles, dose to be taken at bedtime

● CAUTIONS High tumour burden—risk of tumour lysis syndrome · patients aged 76 years and over—increased risk of serious side-effects

CAUTIONS, FURTHER INFORMATION
▶ Thromboembolism Risk factors for thromboembolism (such as smoking, hypertension, hyperlipidaemia) should be minimised. Thromboprophylaxis is recommended for at least the first 5 months of treatment, especially in patients with additional thrombotic risk factors.
▶ Second primary malignancy Patients should be carefully evaluated before and during treatment with thalidomide using routine cancer screening for occurrence of second primary malignancy and treatment should be instituted as indicated.
▶ Peripheral neuropathy Patients with pre-existing peripheral neuropathy should not be treated with thalidomide unless the potential clinical benefits outweigh the risk.

● INTERACTIONS → Appendix 1: thalidomide

● SIDE-EFFECTS

▶ **Common or very common** Anaemia · arrhythmias · asthenia · confusion · constipation · decreased leucocytes · depression · dizziness · drowsiness · dry mouth · dyspnoea · embolism and thrombosis · fever · heart failure · increased risk of infection · malaise · movement disorders · neutropenia · peripheral neuropathy · peripheral oedema · respiratory disorders · sensation abnormal · skin reactions · thrombocytopenia · tremor · vomiting

▶ **Frequency not known** Atrioventricular block · gastrointestinal disorders · gastrointestinal haemorrhage · hearing impairment · hypothyroidism · liver disorder · menstrual cycle irregularities · myocardial infarction · neoplasms · pancreatitis · pancytopenia · posterior reversible encephalopathy syndrome (PRES) · pulmonary hypertension · reactivation of infections · renal failure · seizure · sexual dysfunction · toxic epidermal necrolysis · tumour lysis syndrome

SIDE-EFFECTS, FURTHER INFORMATION
Rash If rash occurs, treatment should be discontinued and only restarted following appropriate clinical evaluation.
Peripheral neuropathy If symptoms suggestive of peripheral neuropathy develop (such as paraesthesia, abnormal coordination, or weakness) dose reduction, dose interruption, or treatment discontinuation may be necessary—consult product literature.

● CONCEPTION AND CONTRACEPTION For women of child-bearing potential, pregnancy must be excluded before starting treatment with thalidomide (perform pregnancy test on initiation or within 3 days prior to initiation). Women must practise effective contraception at least 1 month before, during, and for at least 1 month after treatment, including during dose interruptions (oral combined hormonal contraceptives and copper-releasing intra-uterine devices not recommended) and men should use condoms during treatment, during dose interruption, and for at least 1 week after stopping if their partner is pregnant or is of childbearing potential and not using effective contraception. Patients, prescribers and pharmacists must comply with pregnancy prevention measures as specified in the manufacturer's Pregnancy Prevention Programme.

● PREGNANCY **Important: teratogenic risk**.

● BREAST FEEDING Avoid—present in milk in *animal* studies.

● HEPATIC IMPAIRMENT Caution in severe impairment—no information available.

● RENAL IMPAIRMENT Caution in severe impairment—no information available.

● MONITORING REQUIREMENTS
▶ Monitor white blood cell count (including differential count) and platelet count (reduce dose or interrupt treatment if neutropenia or thrombocytopenia develop—consult product literature).
▶ Monitor for arterial or venous thromboembolism.
▶ Monitor patients for signs and symptoms of peripheral neuropathy.
▶ Hepatic disorder Liver function should be monitored, particularly when there is history of, or concurrent viral liver infection, or when thalidomide is combined with drugs known to be associated with liver dysfunction (e.g. paracetamol).

● PRESCRIBING AND DISPENSING INFORMATION Patient, prescriber, and supplying pharmacy must comply with a pregnancy prevention programme. Every prescription must be accompanied by a complete Prescription Authorisation Form.

● PATIENT AND CARER ADVICE Patients and their carers should be made aware of the symptoms of thromboembolism and advised to report sudden breathlessness, chest pain, or swelling of a limb.

Patients and their carers should be made aware of the symptoms of neutropenia and advised to seek medical advice if symptoms suggestive of neutropenia (such as fever, sore throat) or of thrombocytopenia (such as bleeding) develop.

Patients and their carers should be advised to seek medical advice if symptoms of peripheral neuropathy such as paraesthesia, abnormal coordination, or weakness develop.

Conception and contraception Patient counselling advised for thalidomide capsules (pregnancy and contraception).

● NATIONAL FUNDING/ACCESS DECISIONS

NICE decisions

▸ **Bortezomib and thalidomide for the first-line treatment of multiple myeloma (July 2011)** NICE TA228
Thalidomide in combination with an alkylating drug and a corticosteroid is recommended as an option for the first-line treatment of multiple myeloma in people for whom high-dose chemotherapy with stem cell transplantation is considered inappropriate.
www.nice.org.uk/TA228

● MEDICINAL FORMS
There can be variation in the licensing of different medicines containing the same drug. Forms available from special-order manufacturers include: tablet, oral suspension, oral solution.

Tablet
▸ Talidex (Alan Pharmaceuticals)
Thalidomide 25 mg Talidex 25mg tablets | 30 tablet £1,075.00

Capsule
CAUTIONARY AND ADVISORY LABELS 2
▸ Thalidomide (Non-proprietary)
Thalidomide 50 mg Thalidomide Celgene 50mg capsules | 28 capsule PoM £298.48

6 Photodynamic therapy responsive malignancy

PHOTOSENSITISERS

Porfimer sodium

● DRUG ACTION Porfimer sodium accumulates in malignant tissue and is activated by laser light to produce a cytotoxic effect.

● INDICATIONS AND DOSE

Photodynamic therapy of non-small cell lung cancer and obstructing oesophageal cancer
▸ BY SLOW INTRAVENOUS INJECTION
▸ Adult: (consult product literature)

● CONTRA-INDICATIONS Acute porphyrias p. 1025 · broncho-oesophageal fistula · tracheo-oesophageal fistula
● SIDE-EFFECTS Alopecia · bone marrow depression · constipation · extravasation · hyperuricaemia · nausea · photosensitivity reaction (sunscreens ineffective) · stomatitis · thromboembolism · tumour lysis syndrome · vomiting
● PREGNANCY Manufacturer advises avoid unless essential.
● BREAST FEEDING No information available—manufacturer advises avoid.
● HEPATIC IMPAIRMENT Avoid in severe impairment.
● PATIENT AND CARER ADVICE
Photosensitivity Avoid exposure of skin and eyes to direct sunlight or bright indoor light for at least 30 days.

● MEDICINAL FORMS
There can be variation in the licensing of different medicines containing the same drug.
Powder for solution for injection
▸ Photofrin (Axcan Pharma Inc, Pinnacle Biologics BV)
Porfimer sodium 15 mg Photofrin 15mg powder for solution for injection vials | 1 vial PoM ⑤ (Hospital only)
Porfimer sodium 75 mg Photofrin 75mg powder for solution for injection vials | 1 vial PoM £1,011.00 (Hospital only)

Temoporfin

● DRUG ACTION Temoporfin accumulates in malignant tissue and is activated by laser light to produce a cytotoxic effect.

● INDICATIONS AND DOSE

Photodynamic therapy of advanced head and neck squamous cell carcinoma refractory to, or unsuitable for, other treatments
▸ BY SLOW INTRAVENOUS INJECTION
▸ Adult: (consult product literature)

● CONTRA-INDICATIONS Acute porphyrias p. 1025 · concomitant photosensitising treatment · diseases exacerbated by light · elective surgery · ophthalmic slit-lamp examination for 30 days after administration
● SIDE-EFFECTS Alopecia · bone marrow depression · constipation · dizziness · dysphagia · haemorrhage · hyperuricaemia · nausea · oedema · pain · photosensitivity reaction (sunscreens ineffective) · skin reactions · stomatitis · thromboembolism · tumour lysis syndrome · vomiting
● CONCEPTION AND CONTRACEPTION Manufacturer advises avoid pregnancy for at least 3 months after treatment.
● PREGNANCY Toxicity in *animal* studies. See also Pregnancy and reproductive function in Cytotoxic drugs p. 865.
● BREAST FEEDING Manufacturer advises avoid breastfeeding for at least 1 month after treatment—no information available.
● PATIENT AND CARER ADVICE
Photosensitivity Avoid exposure of skin and eyes to direct sunlight or bright indoor light for at least 15 days after administration.
Avoid prolonged exposure of injection site arm to direct sunlight for 6 months after administration.
If extravasation occurs protect area from light for at least 3 months.

● MEDICINAL FORMS
There can be variation in the licensing of different medicines containing the same drug.
Solution for injection
▸ Foscan (Biolitec Pharma Ltd)
Temoporfin 1 mg per 1 ml Foscan 3mg/3ml solution for injection vials | 1 vial PoM £1,800.00 (Hospital only)
Foscan 6mg/6ml solution for injection vials | 1 vial PoM £3,400.00 (Hospital only)

7 Targeted therapy responsive malignancy

ANTINEOPLASTIC DRUGS > PROTEASOME INHIBITORS

Bortezomib

14-Apr-2016

● DRUG ACTION Bortezomib is a proteasome inhibitor.

● INDICATIONS AND DOSE
Treatment of multiple myeloma that has progressed despite the use of at least one therapy, and where the patient has already had, or is unable to have, haematopoietic stem cell transplantation (either as monotherapy, or in combination with pegylated liposomal doxorubicin or dexamethasone) | Treatment of previously untreated multiple myeloma in patients who are not eligible for high-dose chemotherapy with haematopoietic stem cell transplantation (in combination with melphalan and prednisolone) | Induction treatment of previously untreated multiple myeloma in patients who are eligible for high-dose chemotherapy with haematopoietic stem cell transplantation (in combination with dexamethasone, or with dexamethasone and thalidomide)
▶ BY INTRAVENOUS INJECTION, OR BY SUBCUTANEOUS INJECTION
▶ Adult: (consult local protocol)

> IMPORTANT SAFETY INFORMATION
> Bortezomib injection is for **intravenous or subcutaneous administration** only. Inadvertent intrathecal administration with fatal outcome has been reported.

● CONTRA-INDICATIONS Acute diffuse infiltrative pulmonary disease · pericardial disease

● CAUTIONS Amyloidosis · cardiovascular disease · consider antiviral prophylaxis for herpes zoster infection · dehydration · diabetes (may affect blood glucose) · history of syncope · pulmonary disease (discontinue if interstitial lung disease develops) · risk factors for seizures · risk of neuropathy—consult product literature

● INTERACTIONS → Appendix 1: bortezomib

● SIDE-EFFECTS
▶ **Common or very common** Anaemia · anxiety · appetite abnormal · arrhythmias · asthenia · chills · constipation · cough · decreased leucocytes · diabetes mellitus · diarrhoea · dizziness · dysphagia · dyspnoea · electrolyte imbalance · encephalopathy · enzyme abnormality · eye inflammation · fever · fluid imbalance · gastrointestinal discomfort · gastrointestinal disorders · haemorrhage · hair disorder · headaches · hearing impairment · heart failure · hepatic disorders · hiccups · hyperbilirubinaemia · hypersensitivity · hypertension · hypotension · increased risk of infection · ischaemic heart disease · lethargy · loss of consciousness · malaise · mood altered · muscle complaints · muscle weakness · nausea · nerve disorders · neuromuscular dysfunction · neutropenia · oedema · oral disorders · oropharyngeal complaints · pain · renal impairment · sensation abnormal · sepsis · skin reactions · sleep disorder · syncope · taste altered · thrombocytopenia · ventricular dysfunction · vertigo · vision disorders · vomiting · weight changes
▶ **Uncommon** Altered smell sensation · angioedema · antibiotic associated colitis · arthritis · azotaemia · cardiac arrest · cardiomyopathy · cardiovascular disorder · cerebrovascular insufficiency · chest discomfort · circulation impaired · circulatory collapse · coagulation

disorders · concentration impaired · confusion · Cushing's syndrome · dry eye · dysphonia · ear discomfort · embolism and thrombosis · eye discomfort · eye disorders · failure to thrive · gait abnormal · gas exchange abnormal · genital pain · haemolytic anaemia · hallucination · hyperthyroidism · increased leucocytes · injury · irritable bowel syndrome · joint disorders · lymphadenopathy · memory loss · movement disorders · mucous membrane disorder · myopathy · neurotoxicity · palpitations · pancreatitis · pancytopenia · pericardial disorders · pericarditis · posterior reversible encephalopathy syndrome (PRES) (discontinue) · proteinuria · psychiatric disorders · psychotic disorder · pulmonary hypertension · pulmonary oedema · reflexes abnormal · respiratory disorders · rhinorrhoea · seizure · sensation of pressure · severe cutaneous adverse reactions (SCARs) · sexual dysfunction · shock · SIADH · skin mass · skin ulcers · speech disorder · sweat changes · temperature sensation altered · thirst change · tremor · tumour lysis syndrome · urinary disorders · urinary tract disorder · vascular disorders · vasculitis · vasodilation
▶ **Rare or very rare** Acidosis · acute coronary syndrome · alcohol intolerance · amyloidosis · apnoea · ascites · atrioventricular block · bladder irritation · blood disorders · bone disorder · bone fracture · brain oedema · breast disorder · cardiac valve disorder · cholelithiasis · CNS haemorrhage · cognitive disorder · coma · coronary artery insufficiency · delirium · drooling · ear disorder · erythromelalgia · fistula · gout · healing impaired · hypothyroidism · inflammation · lymphoedema · macrophage activation · mass · meningitis · metabolic disorder · multi organ failure · musculoskeletal and connective tissue infections and inflammations · nail disorder · neoplasm malignant · neoplasms · nervous system disorder · paralysis · paresis · pelvic pain · perforation · photosensitivity reaction · platelet abnormalities · prostatitis · radiation injury · seborrhoea · sudden death · suicidal ideation · testicular disorders · throat complaints · ulcer · vaginal ulceration · venous insufficiency · vitamin deficiencies
▶ **Frequency not known** Herpes zoster reactivation · JC virus infection · progressive multifocal leukoencephalopathy

● CONCEPTION AND CONTRACEPTION Manufacturer advises effective contraception during and for 3 months after treatment in men or women.

● PREGNANCY Toxicity in *animal* studies. See also *Pregnancy and reproductive function* in Cytotoxic drugs p. 865.

● BREAST FEEDING Discontinue breast-feeding.

● HEPATIC IMPAIRMENT
Dose adjustments Reduce dose in moderate to severe impairment—consult product literature.

● RENAL IMPAIRMENT No information available for creatinine clearance less than 20 mL/minute/1.73 m^2.

● MONITORING REQUIREMENTS
▶ Monitor blood-glucose concentration in patients on oral antidiabetics.
▶ Monitor for symptoms of progressive multifocal leucoencephalopathy (presenting as new or worsening neurological signs or symptoms)—discontinue treatment if diagnosed.
▶ Chest x-ray recommended before treatment to monitor for pulmonary disease—discontinue if interstitial lung disease develops.

● NATIONAL FUNDING/ACCESS DECISIONS
NICE decisions
▶ Bortezomib for previously untreated mantle cell lymphoma (December 2015) NICE TA370
Bortezomib is recommended as an option for the treatment of previously untreated mantle cell lymphoma

in adults for whom haematopoietic stem cell transplantation is unsuitable.
www.nice.org.uk/TA370

▸ **Bortezomib for induction therapy in multiple myeloma before high-dose chemotherapy and autologous stem cell transplantation (April 2014)** NICE TA311
Bortezomib is recommended as an option within its marketing authorisation, in combination with dexamethasone, or with dexamethasone and thalidomide, for the induction treatment of adults with previously untreated multiple myeloma, who are eligible for high-dose chemotherapy with haematopoietic stem cell transplantation.
www.nice.org.uk/TA311

▸ **Bortezomib and thalidomide for the first-line treatment of multiple myeloma (July 2011)** NICE TA228
Bortezomib in combination with an alkylating drug and a corticosteroid is recommended as an option for the first-line treatment of multiple myeloma if:
- high-dose chemotherapy with stem cell transplantation is considered inappropriate **and**
- the person is unable to tolerate or has contra-indications to thalidomide.
www.nice.org.uk/TA228

▸ **Bortezomib monotherapy for relapsed multiple myeloma (October 2007)** NICE TA129
Bortezomib monotherapy is an option for the treatment of progressive multiple myeloma in patients who are at first relapse having received one prior therapy and who have undergone, or are unsuitable for, bone-marrow transplantation, under the following circumstances:
- the response to bortezomib is measured using serum M protein after a maximum of four cycles of treatment, and treatment is continued only in patients who have a reduction in serum M protein of 50% or more (where serum M protein is not measurable, an appropriate alternative biochemical measure of response should be used) **and**
- the manufacturer rebates the full cost of bortezomib if there is an inadequate response (as defined above) after four cycles of treatment.
www.nice.org.uk/TA129

Scottish Medicines Consortium (SMC) Decisions
The *Scottish Medicines Consortium*, has advised (December 2013) that bortezomib (*Velcade®*) is accepted for restricted use within NHS Scotland in combination with dexamethasone and thalidomide for the induction treatment of adults with previously untreated multiple myeloma who are eligible for high-dose chemotherapy with haematopoietic stem cell transplantation.

● MEDICINAL FORMS
There can be variation in the licensing of different medicines containing the same drug.
Powder for solution for injection
▸ Velcade (Janssen-Cilag Ltd)
Bortezomib 3.5 mg Velcade 3.5mg powder for solution for injection vials | 1 vial PoM £762.38 (Hospital only)

Carfilzomib   14-Sep-2017

● DRUG ACTION Carfilzomib is an irreversible selective proteasome inhibitor that disrupts tumour cell turnover and induces apoptosis.

● INDICATIONS AND DOSE
Treatment of multiple myeloma in patients who have received at least one prior therapy (in combination with dexamethasone, or with dexamethasone and lenalidomide) (specialist use only)
▸ BY INTRAVENOUS INFUSION
▸ Adult: (consult product literature or local protocols)

● CAUTIONS Elderly (over 75 years)—higher incidence of adverse effects · ensure adequate hydration · infusion-related reactions · recent history of myocardial infarction · risk of cardiac failure · risk of herpes zoster reactivation · uncontrolled angina · uncontrolled arrhythmias
CAUTIONS, FURTHER INFORMATION
▸ Infusion-related reactions Manufacturer advises premedication with dexamethasone to reduce incidence and severity of infusion-related reactions.
▸ Risk of herpes zoster reactivation Manufacturer advises consider antiviral prophylaxis for herpes zoster infection.

● INTERACTIONS → Appendix 1: carfilzomib

● SIDE-EFFECTS
▸ **Common or very common** Anaemia · anxiety · appetite decreased · arrhythmias · arthralgia · asthenia · cataract · chest pain · chills · constipation · cough · decreased leucocytes · dehydration · diarrhoea · dizziness · dysphonia · dyspnoea · electrolyte imbalance · embolism and thrombosis · fever · flushing · gastrointestinal discomfort · haemorrhage · headache · heart failure · hyperbilirubinaemia · hyperglycaemia · hyperhidrosis · hypertension · hyperuricaemia · hypoalbuminaemia · hypotension · increased risk of infection · infusion related reaction · insomnia · muscle complaints · muscle weakness · nausea · neutropenia · oropharyngeal pain · pain · palpitations · peripheral neuropathy · peripheral oedema · pulmonary hypertension · pulmonary oedema · renal impairment · respiratory disorders · sensation abnormal · sepsis · skin reactions · thrombocytopenia · tinnitus · toothache · vision blurred · vomiting
▸ **Uncommon** Cardiac arrest · gastrointestinal perforation · haemolytic uraemic syndrome · hepatic disorders · intracranial haemorrhage · multi organ failure · myocardial infarction · myocardial ischaemia · pericardial effusion · pericarditis · stroke · tumour lysis syndrome
▸ **Rare or very rare** Posterior reversible encephalopathy syndrome (PRES) · thrombotic microangiopathy

● CONCEPTION AND CONTRACEPTION Manufacturer recommends effective contraception during and for 1 month after treatment in women of childbearing potential; efficacy of oral contraceptives may be reduced, and hormonal contraceptives associated with a risk of thrombosis should be avoided. Male patients should use effective contraception during and for 3 months after treatment if their partner is pregnant or of childbearing potential. See also *Pregnancy and reproductive function* in Cytotoxic drugs p. 865.

● PREGNANCY Manufacturer advises avoid unless potential benefit outweighs risk—toxicity in *animal* studies. See also *Pregnancy and reproductive function* in Cytotoxic drugs p. 865.

● BREAST FEEDING Manufacturer advises avoid during and for at least 2 days after treatment—no information available.

● HEPATIC IMPAIRMENT Manufacturer advises caution in mild-to-moderate impairment (increased incidence of adverse effects), and in severe impairment (no information available).

● RENAL IMPAIRMENT Manufacturer advises caution—increased incidence of adverse effects.

● MONITORING REQUIREMENTS Manufacturer advises monitoring of the following patient parameters: serum potassium concentration at least monthly; signs and symptoms of fluid overload, especially in those at risk of cardiac failure; renal function at treatment initiation and at least monthly during treatment—consider dose modification; hepatic function at treatment initiation and monthly during treatment—consider dose modification; platelet count and blood pressure. Also monitor for signs and symptoms of thrombotic microangiopathy.

8

Immune system and malignant disease

- HANDLING AND STORAGE Manufacturer advises store in a refrigerator at 2–8°C.
- PATIENT AND CARER ADVICE Manufacturer advises that patients and carers are warned to report signs and symptoms of thromboembolism (such as dyspnoea, chest pain, arm or leg swelling or pain).
  Driving and skilled tasks Patients and their carers should be counselled on the effects on driving and skilled tasks—increased risk of dizziness, hypotension and blurred vision.
- NATIONAL FUNDING/ACCESS DECISIONS
  NICE decisions
- ▸ Carfilzomib for previously treated multiple myeloma (July 2017) NICE TA457
  Carfilzomib in combination with dexamethasone is recommended as an option for treating multiple myeloma in adults, only if:
  - they have had only 1 previous therapy, which did not include bortezomib **and**
  - the company provides carfilzomib with the discount agreed in the patient access scheme.
  Patients currently receiving carfilzomib whose disease does not meet the above criteria should have the option to continue their treatment until they and their clinician consider it appropriate to stop.
  www.nice.org.uk/guidance/TA457

  Scottish Medicines Consortium (SMC) Decisions
  The *Scottish Medicines Consortium* has advised (January 2017) that carfilzomib (*Kyprolis*®) in combination with lenalidomide and dexamethasone is **not** recommended for use within NHS Scotland for the treatment of patients with multiple myeloma who have received at least one prior therapy as the economic case was not demonstrated.
  The *Scottish Medicines Consortium* has advised (August 2017) that carfilzomib (*Kyprolis*®) is accepted for use within NHS Scotland, in combination with dexamethasone alone for the treatment of patients with multiple myeloma who have received at least one prior therapy. This advice is contingent upon the continuing availability of the patient access scheme in NHS Scotland or a list price that is equivalent or lower.

- MEDICINAL FORMS
  There can be variation in the licensing of different medicines containing the same drug.
  Powder for solution for infusion
  ELECTROLYTES: May contain Sodium
  ▸ Kyprolis (Amgen Ltd) ▼
  Carfilzomib 10 mg Kyprolis 10mg powder for solution for infusion vials | 1 vial [PoM] £176.00
  Carfilzomib 30 mg Kyprolis 30mg powder for solution for infusion vials | 1 vial [PoM] £528.00
  Carfilzomib 60 mg Kyprolis 60mg powder for solution for infusion vials | 1 vial [PoM] £1,056.00

Ixazomib

21-Mar-2018

- DRUG ACTION Ixazomib is a proteasome inhibitor.

- INDICATIONS AND DOSE
  Multiple myeloma in patients who have received at least one prior therapy, in combination with lenalidomide and dexamethasone (specialist use only)
  ▸ BY MOUTH
  ▸ Adult: 4 mg once weekly on days 1, 8, and 15 of a 28-day treatment cycle, for dose adjustments due to side-effects, consult product literature

  IMPORTANT SAFETY INFORMATION
  RISKS OF INCORRECT DOSING OF ORAL ANTI-CANCER MEDICINES
  See Cytotoxic drugs p. 865.

- CAUTIONS Risk of herpes zoster reactivation
  CAUTIONS, FURTHER INFORMATION
- ▸ Herpes zoster reactivation Manufacturer advises consider concomitant antiviral prophylaxis to decrease the risk of herpes zoster reactivation.
- INTERACTIONS → Appendix 1: ixazomib
- SIDE-EFFECTS
- **Common or very common** Back pain · constipation · diarrhoea · increased risk of infection · nausea · neutropenia · peripheral neuropathy (monitor for symptoms) · peripheral oedema · rash · thrombocytopenia · vomiting
- **Frequency not known** Posterior reversible encephalopathy syndrome (PRES) (discontinue)
- CONCEPTION AND CONTRACEPTION Manufacturer advises effective contraception in women of child-bearing potential and in men with a partner of child-bearing potential, during treatment and for at least 90 days after stopping treatment; additional barrier method recommended in women using hormonal contraceptives.
- PREGNANCY Manufacturer advises avoid—toxicity in *animal* studies. See also *Pregnancy and reproductive function* in Cytotoxic drugs p. 865.
- BREAST FEEDING Manufacturer advises avoid—no information available.
- HEPATIC IMPAIRMENT
  Dose adjustments Manufacturer advises reduce dose to 3 mg in moderate-to-severe impairment.
- RENAL IMPAIRMENT
  Dose adjustments Manufacturer advises reduce dose to 3 mg in severe impairment (creatinine clearance less than 30 mL/min).
- MONITORING REQUIREMENTS Manufacturer advises to monitor hepatic function regularly and adjust dose accordingly—consult product literature.
- PATIENT AND CARER ADVICE
  Missed doses Manufacturer advises if less than 72 hours remain before the next scheduled dose, the missed dose should not be taken and the next dose should be taken at the normal time.
- NATIONAL FUNDING/ACCESS DECISIONS
  NICE decisions
- ▸ Ixazomib with lenalidomide and dexamethasone for treating relapsed or refractory multiple myeloma (February 2018) NICE TA505
  Ixazomib, with lenalidomide and dexamethasone, is recommended for use within the Cancer Drugs Fund as an option for treating multiple myeloma in adults only if:
  - they have already had 2 or 3 lines of therapy, **and**
  - the conditions in the managed access agreement for ixazomib are followed.
  Patients whose treatment was started within the NHS before this guidance was published should have the option to continue treatment, without change to their funding arrangements, until they and their NHS clinician consider it appropriate to stop.
  www.nice.org.uk/guidance/ta505

- MEDICINAL FORMS
  There can be variation in the licensing of different medicines containing the same drug.
  Capsule
  CAUTIONARY AND ADVISORY LABELS 23, 25
  ▸ Ninlaro (Takeda UK Ltd) ▼
  Ixazomib (as Ixazomib citrate) 2.3 mg Ninlaro 2.3mg capsules | 3 capsule [PoM] £6,336.00
  Ixazomib (as Ixazomib citrate) 3 mg Ninlaro 3mg capsules | 3 capsule [PoM] £6,336.00
  Ixazomib (as Ixazomib citrate) 4 mg Ninlaro 4mg capsules | 3 capsule [PoM] £6,336.00

ANTINEOPLASTIC DRUGS > PROTEIN KINASE INHIBITORS

Afatinib

- DRUG ACTION Afatinib is a protein kinase inhibitor.

- **INDICATIONS AND DOSE**

  Treatment of locally advanced or metastatic non-small cell lung cancer with activating epidermal growth factor receptor (EGFR) mutations, in patients who have not previously been treated with EGFR tyrosine kinase inhibitor
  ▸ BY MOUTH
    ▸ Adult: 40 mg once daily; increased if tolerated to up to 50 mg once daily, dose increase may be considered after 3 weeks at initial dose; consult product literature for details on dosing and dose adjustment due to side effects

  > IMPORTANT SAFETY INFORMATION
  > RISKS OF INCORRECT DOSING OF ORAL ANTI-CANCER MEDICINES
  > See Cytotoxic drugs p. 865.

- CAUTIONS Cardiac risk factors · conditions which may affect left ventricular ejection fraction—consider cardiac monitoring, including assessment of left ventricular ejection fraction, at baseline and during treatment · diarrhoea—proactive management recommended (consult product literature) · exposure to sun (protect skin from exposure to sun) · history of keratitis · new pulmonary symptoms (including dyspnoea, cough, fever)—interrupt treatment until interstitial lung disease is excluded · severe dry eyes · signs and symptoms of keratitis— promptly refer to ophthalmologist for assessment · signs and symptoms of skin reaction—treat promptly and interrupt afatinib treatment if severe or if Stevens-Johnson syndrome suspected (consult product literature) · ulcerative keratitis · use of contact lenses · worsening pulmonary symptoms (including dyspnoea, cough, fever)—interrupt treatment until interstitial lung disease is excluded

- INTERACTIONS → Appendix 1: afatinib

- SIDE-EFFECTS
  ▸ **Common or very common** Appetite decreased · cystitis · dehydration · diarrhoea · dry eye · dyspepsia · epistaxis · eye inflammation · fever · hypokalaemia · muscle spasms · nausea · oral disorders · paronychia · renal impairment · rhinorrhoea · skin reactions · taste altered · vomiting · weight decreased
  ▸ **Uncommon** Interstitial lung disease · pancreatitis
  ▸ **Rare or very rare** Severe cutaneous adverse reactions (SCARs)

- CONCEPTION AND CONTRACEPTION Ensure effective contraception during and for at least one month after treatment in women of childbearing potential.

- PREGNANCY Manufacturer advises avoid. See also *Pregnancy and reproductive function* in Cytotoxic drugs p. 865.

- BREAST FEEDING Manufacturer advises avoid—present in milk in *animal* studies.

- HEPATIC IMPAIRMENT Manufacturer advises avoid in severe hepatic impairment.
  Dose adjustments Monitor hepatic function regularly and consult product literature for dose adjustment in worsening liver function.

- RENAL IMPAIRMENT Manufacturer advises avoid in severe renal impairment.

- DIRECTIONS FOR ADMINISTRATION Tablets should be taken whole on an empty stomach. Food should not be

consumed for at least 3 hours before and at least 1 hour after each dose.

Giotrif® tablets may be dispersed in approximately 100 mL of noncarbonated water by stirring occasionally for up to 15 minutes (must not be crushed). The dispersion should be swallowed immediately, and the glass rinsed with the same volume of water which should also be swallowed. The dispersion can also be administered via a gastric tube.

- PATIENT AND CARER ADVICE Patient counselling advised (administration).
  Driving and skilled tasks Ocular adverse reactions may affect performance of skilled tasks e.g. driving.

- NATIONAL FUNDING/ACCESS DECISIONS
  NICE decisions
  ▸ **Afatinib for treating epidermal growth factor receptor mutation-positive locally advanced or metastatic non-small-cell lung cancer (April 2014)** NICE TA310
  Afatinib is recommended as an option, within its marketing authorisation, for treating locally advanced or metastatic non-small-cell lung cancer in adults:
  - whose tumour tests positive for the epidermal growth factor receptor tyrosine kinase (EGFR-TK) mutation, **and**
  - who have not previously had an EGFR-TK inhibitor, **and**
  - if the manufacturer provides afatinib with the discount agreed in the patient access scheme.
  www.nice.org.uk/TA310

- MEDICINAL FORMS
  There can be variation in the licensing of different medicines containing the same drug.

  Tablet
  CAUTIONARY AND ADVISORY LABELS 25
  ▸ Giotrif (Boehringer Ingelheim Ltd) ▼

Afatinib 20 mg Giotrif 20mg tablets	28 tablet POM	£2,023.28
Afatinib 30 mg Giotrif 30mg tablets	28 tablet POM	£2,023.28
Afatinib 40 mg Giotrif 40mg tablets	28 tablet POM	£2,023.28
Afatinib 50 mg Giotrif 50mg tablets	28 tablet POM	£2,023.28

Alectinib

17-Jul-2017

- DRUG ACTION Alectinib is a tyrosine kinase inhibitor.

- **INDICATIONS AND DOSE**

  Anaplastic lymphoma kinase (ALK)-positive advanced non-small cell lung cancer previously treated with crizotinib (specialist use only)
  ▸ BY MOUTH
    ▸ Adult: 600 mg twice daily, for dose adjustments due to side-effects—consult product literature

  > IMPORTANT SAFETY INFORMATION
  > RISKS OF INCORRECT DOSING OF ORAL ANTI-CANCER MEDICINES
  > See Cytotoxic drugs p. 865.

- INTERACTIONS → Appendix 1: alectinib

- SIDE-EFFECTS
  ▸ **Common or very common** Anaemia · arrhythmias · constipation · diarrhoea · eye disorders · eye inflammation · hyperbilirubinaemia · musculoskeletal pain · myalgia · nausea · oedema · photosensitivity reaction · skin reactions · vision disorders · vomiting
  ▸ **Uncommon** Drug-induced liver injury · respiratory disorders

- CONCEPTION AND CONTRACEPTION Manufacturer advises women of child-bearing potential should use effective contraception during and for at least 3 months after stopping treatment.

8

Immune system and malignant disease

- PREGNANCY Manufacturer advises avoid—toxicity in *animal* studies. See also *Pregnancy and reproductive function* in Cytotoxic drugs p. 865.
- BREAST FEEDING Manufacturer advises avoid—no information available.
- HEPATIC IMPAIRMENT Manufacturer advises avoid in moderate-to-severe impairment—no information available.
- MONITORING REQUIREMENTS
  ▶ Manufacturer advises monitor creatine phosphokinase every 2 weeks for the first month and as clinically indicated thereafter in patients reporting symptoms of myalgia.
  ▶ Manufacturer advises monitor heart rate and blood pressure as clinically indicated.
  ▶ Manufacturer advises monitor liver function at baseline then every 2 weeks during the first 3 months and periodically thereafter as clinically indicated.
  ▶ Manufacturer advises monitor for symptoms of interstitial lung disease and pneumonitis.
- PATIENT AND CARER ADVICE
  Photosensitivity Manufacturer advises patients should use a broad spectrum sunscreen and lip balm and be advised to avoid prolonged sun exposure during treatment, and for 7 days after discontinuation.
  Myalgia Manufacturer advises patients advised to report any unexplained muscle pain, tenderness or weakness.
  Vomiting Manufacturer advises if vomiting occurs after taking tablets, no additional dose should be taken on that day and the next dose should be taken at the usual time.
  Missed doses Manufacturer advises if a dose is more than 6 hours late, the missed dose should not be taken and the next dose should be taken at the normal time.
  Driving and skilled tasks Manufacturer advises patients and carers should be counselled on the effects on driving and performance of skilled tasks—increased risk of symptomatic bradycardia and vision disorders.

- MEDICINAL FORMS
  There can be variation in the licensing of different medicines containing the same drug.
  Capsule
  CAUTIONARY AND ADVISORY LABELS 11, 21
  ELECTROLYTES: May contain Sodium
  ▶ Alecensa (Roche Products Ltd) ▼
  Alecensa (as Alectinib hydrochloride) 150 mg Alecensa 150mg capsules | 224 capsule [PoM] £5,032.00

Axitinib

- DRUG ACTION Axitinib is a tyrosine kinase inhibitor.

- INDICATIONS AND DOSE
  Treatment of advanced renal cell carcinoma following failure of previous treatment with sunitinib or a cytokine (aldesleukin or interferon alfa)
  ▶ BY MOUTH
  ▶ Adult: (consult product literature)

  IMPORTANT SAFETY INFORMATION
  RISKS OF INCORRECT DOSING OF ORAL ANTI-CANCER MEDICINES
  See Cytotoxic drugs p. 865.

- CONTRA-INDICATIONS Recent active gastro-intestinal bleeding · untreated brain metastases
- CAUTIONS Hypertension (blood pressure should be well-controlled before starting and monitored during treatment)
- INTERACTIONS → Appendix 1: axitinib

- SIDE-EFFECTS
  ▶ **Common or very common** Alopecia · anaemia · appetite decreased · arthralgia · asthenia · constipation · cough · dehydration · diarrhoea · dizziness · dysphonia · dyspnoea · electrolyte imbalance · embolism and thrombosis · gastrointestinal discomfort · gastrointestinal disorders · haemorrhage · headache · heart failure · hyperbilirubinaemia · hypertension · hyperthyroidism · hypothyroidism · mucositis · myalgia · nausea · oral disorders · oropharyngeal pain · pain in extremity · polycythaemia · proteinuria · renal failure · skin reactions · taste altered · thrombocytopenia · tinnitus · vomiting · weight decreased
  ▶ **Uncommon** Leucopenia · neutropenia · posterior reversible encephalopathy syndrome (PRES)
- CONCEPTION AND CONTRACEPTION Effective contraception required during and for up to 1 week after treatment.
- PREGNANCY Manufacturer advises avoid unless potential benefit outweighs risk (toxicity in *animal* studies). See also *Pregnancy and reproductive function* in Cytotoxic drugs p. 865.
- HEPATIC IMPAIRMENT Avoid in severe impairment—no information available.
  Dose adjustments Reduce starting dose in moderate impairment.
- MONITORING REQUIREMENTS
  ▶ Monitor for thyroid dysfunction.
  ▶ Monitor haemoglobin or haematocrit before and during treatment.
  ▶ Monitor for symptoms of gastro-intestinal perforation.
  ▶ Monitor for symptoms of fistula.
  ▶ Monitor for proteinuria before and during treatment.
  ▶ Monitor liver function before and during treatment.
- NATIONAL FUNDING/ACCESS DECISIONS
  NICE decisions
  ▶ Axitinib for treating advanced renal cell carcinoma after failure of prior systemic treatment (February 2015) NICE TA333
  Axitinib is recommended as an option for treating adults with advanced renal cell carcinoma after failure of treatment with a first-line tyrosine kinase inhibitor or a cytokine, **only** if the company provides axitinib with the discount agreed in the patient access scheme.
  www.nice.org.uk/TA333

- MEDICINAL FORMS
  There can be variation in the licensing of different medicines containing the same drug.
  Tablet
  CAUTIONARY AND ADVISORY LABELS 25
  ▶ Inlyta (Pfizer Ltd)
  Axitinib 1 mg Inlyta 1mg tablets | 56 tablet [PoM] £703.40 (Hospital only)
  Axitinib 3 mg Inlyta 3mg tablets | 56 tablet [PoM] £2,110.20 (Hospital only)
  Axitinib 5 mg Inlyta 5mg tablets | 56 tablet [PoM] £3,517.00 (Hospital only)
  Axitinib 7 mg Inlyta 7mg tablets | 56 tablet [PoM] £4,923.80 (Hospital only)

Bosutinib

17-May-2018

- INDICATIONS AND DOSE
  Previously treated chronic, accelerated and blast phase Philadelphia chromosome-positive chronic myeloid leukaemia (specialist use only)
  ▶ BY MOUTH
  ▶ Adult: 500 mg once daily, consult product literature for dose adjustment due to side-effects, or incomplete

haematologic response by week 8, or incomplete cytogenetic response by week 12

Newly-diagnosed chronic phase Philadelphia chromosome-positive chronic myeloid leukaemia (specialist use only)
▸ BY MOUTH
▸ Adult: 400 mg once daily, consult product literature for dose adjustment due to side-effects, or failure to demonstrate breakpoint cluster region-Abelson (BCR-ABL) transcripts ≤10% by month 3

> **IMPORTANT SAFETY INFORMATION**
>
> RISKS OF INCORRECT DOSING OF ORAL ANTI-CANCER MEDICINES
> See Cytotoxic drugs p. 865.
>
> MHRA/CHM ADVICE (MAY 2016): RISK OF HEPATITIS B VIRUS REACTIVATION WITH BCR-ABL TYROSINE KINASE INHIBITORS
> An EU wide review has concluded that bosutinib can cause hepatitis B reactivation; the MHRA recommends establishing hepatitis B virus status in all patients before initiation of treatment.

● CAUTIONS Cardiac disease · hepatitis B infection · history of pancreatitis—withhold treatment if lipase elevated and abdominal symptoms occur · history of QT prolongation—monitor ECG and correct hypokalaemia and hypomagnesaemia before and during treatment · recent cardiac event—monitor ECG and correct hypokalaemia and hypomagnesaemia before and during treatment · risk factors for QT prolongation—monitor ECG and correct hypokalaemia and hypomagnesaemia before and during treatment · significant gastrointestinal disorder

CAUTIONS, FURTHER INFORMATION
▸ Hepatitis B infection The MHRA advises that patients who are carriers of hepatitis B virus should be closely monitored for signs and symptoms of active infection throughout treatment and for several months after stopping treatment; expert advice should be sought for patients who test positive for hepatitis B virus and in those with active infection.

● INTERACTIONS → Appendix 1: bosutinib

● SIDE-EFFECTS
▸ **Common or very common** Anaemia · appetite decreased · arthralgia · asthenia · chest discomfort · cough · dehydration · diarrhoea · dizziness · dyspnoea · electrolyte imbalance · fever · gastritis · gastrointestinal discomfort · headache · hepatic disorders · hypersensitivity · hypertension · increased risk of infection · leucopenia · long QT syndrome · malaise · myalgia · nausea · neutropenia · oedema · pain · pericardial effusion · QT interval prolongation · renal impairment · respiratory disorders · skin reactions · taste altered · thrombocytopenia · vomiting
▸ **Uncommon** Haemorrhage · pancreatitis acute · pericarditis · pulmonary hypertension · pulmonary oedema · tinnitus · tumour lysis syndrome
▸ **Frequency not known** Severe cutaneous adverse reactions (SCARs)

● CONCEPTION AND CONTRACEPTION Effective contraception required during treatment in women.

● PREGNANCY Avoid—toxicity in *animal* studies. See also *Pregnancy and reproductive function* in Cytotoxic drugs p. 865.

● BREAST FEEDING Manufacturer advises avoid—no information available.

● HEPATIC IMPAIRMENT Caution—no information available.

● RENAL IMPAIRMENT
  Dose adjustments For *chronic, accelerated and blast phase Philadelphia chromosome-positive chronic myeloid leukaemia*, manufacturer advises reduce dose to 400 mg in moderate impairment; reduce dose to 300 mg in severe

impairment; consult product literature for dose adjustment due to side-effects, or incomplete haematological, cytogenetic, or molecular response.

  For *newly-diagnosed chronic phase Philadelphia chromosome-positive chronic myeloid leukaemia*, manufacturer advises reduce dose to 300 mg in moderate impairment; reduce dose to 200 mg in severe impairment; consult product literature for dose adjustment due to side-effects, or incomplete haematological, cytogenetic, or molecular response.

● MONITORING REQUIREMENTS
▸ Manufacturer advises monitor liver function before treatment initiation, then monthly for the first 3 months and thereafter as clinically indicated—consult product literature for management of raised transaminases.
▸ Manufacturer advises monitor full blood count weekly for the first month and then monthly thereafter or as clinically indicated.
▸ Manufacturer advises monitor for signs and symptoms of fluid retention (including pericardial effusion, pleural effusion and pulmonary oedema).

● NATIONAL FUNDING/ACCESS DECISIONS
NICE decisions
▸ **Bosutinib for previously treated chronic myeloid leukaemia (August 2016)** NICE TA401
Bosutinib is recommended as a treatment option, within its marketing authorisation, for chronic, accelerated and blast phase Philadelphia-chromosome-positive CML in adults, when:
● they have previously been treated with 1 or more tyrosine kinase inhibitor, **and**
● imatinib, nilotinib and dasatinib are not appropriate, **and**
● the manufacturer provides bosutinib with the discount agreed in the patient access scheme.
www.nice.org.uk/TA401

● MEDICINAL FORMS
There can be variation in the licensing of different medicines containing the same drug.
Tablet
CAUTIONARY AND ADVISORY LABELS 21
▸ Bosulif (Pfizer Ltd) ▼
  Bosutinib 100 mg Bosulif 100mg tablets | 28 tablet PoM £859.17 (Hospital only)
  Bosutinib 500 mg Bosulif 500mg tablets | 28 tablet PoM £3,436.67 (Hospital only)

Cabozantinib   29-Aug-2017

● DRUG ACTION Cabozantinib is an inhibitor of several protein kinases.

● INDICATIONS AND DOSE
Treatment of progressive, unresectable locally advanced or metastatic medullary thyroid carcinoma (initiated by a specialist)
▸ BY MOUTH USING CAPSULES
▸ Adult: 140 mg once daily, for dose adjustment or treatment interruption due to side-effects, consult product literature (closely monitor for first 8 weeks of therapy)

Advanced renal cell carcinoma following prior vascular endothelial growth factor (VEGF)-targeted therapy (initiated by a specialist)
▸ BY MOUTH USING TABLETS
▸ Adult: 60 mg once daily, for dose adjustment or treatment interruption due to side-effects, consult product literature (closely monitor for first 8 weeks of therapy) continued →

DOSE EQUIVALENCE AND CONVERSION
▶ Cabozantinib tablets and capsules are not bioequivalent—consult product literature when switching formulations.

IMPORTANT SAFETY INFORMATION
RISKS OF INCORRECT DOSING OF ORAL ANTI-CANCER MEDICINES
See Cytotoxic drugs p. 865.

● CONTRA-INDICATIONS Reversible Posterior Leukoencephalopathy Syndrome
● CAUTIONS Hypertension—discontinue treatment if uncontrolled despite medical intervention · palmar-plantar erythrodysaesthesia syndrome—consider treatment interruption if severe and restart at a lower dose when resolved to grade 1 · patients at increased risk of fistulas—consult product literature · patients at increased risk of gastro-intestinal perforation—consult product literature · patients at increased risk of intra-abdominal abscess—consult product literature · patients at risk of haemorrhage (including tumour involvement of the trachea or bronchi)—discontinue if symptoms develop · patients at risk of thromboembolic events including myocardial infarction—discontinue if symptoms develop · risk of osteonecrosis of the jaw · susceptibility to QT-interval prolongation (e.g. cardiac disease, electrolyte disturbances, bradycardia, concomitant use of drugs that prolong the QT interval)—monitor ECG and electrolytes periodically

CAUTIONS, FURTHER INFORMATION
▶ Elective surgery Withhold treatment for at least 28 days before elective surgery and restart only if adequate wound healing—discontinue in patients with wound healing complications requiring medical intervention.
▶ Risk of osteonecrosis of the jaw Discontinue treatment at least 28 days before elective invasive dental procedures—monitor for symptoms before and during treatment and discontinue if osteonecrosis develops.

● INTERACTIONS → Appendix 1: cabozantinib
● SIDE-EFFECTS
▶ Common or very common Abscess · alopecia · anxiety · appetite decreased · arrhythmias · arthralgia · asthenia · chills · cholelithiasis · confusion · constipation · dehydration · depression · diarrhoea · dizziness · dysphagia · dysphonia · dysuria · ear pain · electrolyte imbalance · embolism and thrombosis · fistula · gastrointestinal discomfort · gastrointestinal disorders · haemorrhage · hair changes · headache · healing impaired · hearing impairment · hyperbilirubinaemia · hypertension · hypoalbuminaemia · hypotension · hypothyroidism · increased risk of infection · lymphopenia · mucositis · muscle spasms · nausea · neutropenia · oedema · oral disorders · oropharyngeal pain · osteonecrosis of jaw · pain · pallor · pancreatitis · paraesthesia · peripheral coldness · peripheral neuropathy · proteinuria · skin reactions · taste altered · thrombocytopenia · tremor · vision blurred · vomiting · weight decreased
▶ Uncommon Abnormal dreams · acute kidney injury · amenorrhoea · angina pectoris · ataxia · cataract · concentration impaired · conjunctivitis · cyst · delirium · encephalopathy · loss of consciousness · respiratory disorders · rhabdomyolysis · skin ulcer · speech disorder · telangiectasia · throat oedema · transient ischaemic attack
● CONCEPTION AND CONTRACEPTION Patients and their sexual partners must use effective contraception (in addition to barrier method) during treatment and for at least 4 months after the last dose.
● PREGNANCY Manufacturer advises avoid unless potential benefit outweighs risk—toxicity in *animal* studies. See also

Pregnancy and reproductive function in Cytotoxic drugs p. 865.
● BREAST FEEDING Manufacturer advises discontinue breast-feeding during treatment and for at least 4 months after the last dose.
● HEPATIC IMPAIRMENT Manufacturer advises avoid in severe impairment—no information available.
Dose adjustments For *capsules* manufacturer recommends dose of 60 mg once daily in mild-to-moderate impairment—monitor for adverse events and consult product literature for dose adjustments or dose interruption as needed.
For *tablets* manufacturer recommends dose of 40 mg once daily in mild-to-moderate impairment—monitor for adverse events and consult product literature for dose adjustments or dose interruption as needed.
● RENAL IMPAIRMENT Manufacturer advises caution in renal impairment. Avoid in severe impairment.
● MONITORING REQUIREMENTS Monitor urine protein regularly and discontinue if nephrotic syndrome develops.
● PATIENT AND CARER ADVICE Food should not be consumed for at least 2 hours before and at least 1 hour after each dose.
Driving and skilled tasks Fatigue and weakness may affect performance of skilled tasks e.g. driving.
● NATIONAL FUNDING/ACCESS DECISIONS
NICE decisions
▶ Cabozantinib for previously treated advanced renal cell carcinoma (August 2017) NICE TA463
Cabozantinib (*Cabometyx*®) is recommended, within its marketing authorisation, as an option for treating advanced renal cell carcinoma in adults after vascular endothelial growth factor (VEGF)-targeted therapy, only if the company provides cabozantinib with the discount agreed in the patient access scheme.
www.nice.org.uk/guidance/ta463
▶ Cabozantinib for treating medullary thyroid cancer (March 2018) NICE TA516
Cabozantinib (*Cometriq*®) is recommended, within its marketing authorisation, as an option for treating progressive medullary thyroid cancer in adults with unresectable, locally advanced or metastatic disease, only if the manufacturer provides cabozantinib with the discount agreed in the patient access scheme.
www.nice.org.uk/guidance/ta516
Scottish Medicines Consortium (SMC) Decisions
SMC No. 1234/17
The *Scottish Medicines Consortium* has advised (June 2017) that cabozantinib (*Cabometyx*®) is accepted for use within NHS Scotland for the treatment of advanced renal cell carcinoma in adults following vascular endothelial growth factor (VEGF)-targeted therapy. This advice is contingent upon continuing availability of the patient access scheme or a list price that is equivalent or lower.

● MEDICINAL FORMS
There can be variation in the licensing of different medicines containing the same drug.
Tablet
CAUTIONARY AND ADVISORY LABELS 23, 25
▶ Cabometyx (Ipsen Ltd) ▼
Cabozantinib (as Cabozantinib s-malate) 20 mg Cabometyx 20mg tablets | 30 tablet [PoM] £5,143.00
Cabozantinib (as Cabozantinib s-malate) 40 mg Cabometyx 40mg tablets | 30 tablet [PoM] £5,143.00
Cabozantinib (as Cabozantinib s-malate) 60 mg Cabometyx 60mg tablets | 30 tablet [PoM] £5,143.00
Capsule
CAUTIONARY AND ADVISORY LABELS 23, 25
▶ Cometriq (Ipsen Ltd) ▼
Cabozantinib (as Cabozantinib s-malate) 20 mg Cometriq 20mg capsules | 84 capsule [PoM] £4,800.00

Cabozantinib (as Cabozantinib s-malate) 80 mg Cometriq 80mg
capsules | 7 capsule PoM ⚠️
Cometriq 20mg capsules and Cometriq 80mg capsules |
56 capsule PoM £4,800.00 | 112 capsule PoM £4,800.00

Ceritinib
31-Jul-2017

- **DRUG ACTION** Ceritinib is a tyrosine kinase inhibitor, with
particular activity against anaplastic lymphoma kinase
(ALK).

- **INDICATIONS AND DOSE**

**Anaplastic lymphoma kinase (ALK)-positive advanced
non-small cell lung cancer (specialist use only)**
  - BY MOUTH
    - Adult: 750 mg once daily, dose should be taken at the
    same time every day, temporary dose interruption or
    dose reduction may be required based on tolerability—
    consult product literature; discontinue treatment if
    patient unable to tolerate at least 300 mg daily

DOSE ADJUSTMENTS DUE TO INTERACTIONS
  - Manufacturer advises if concurrent use of potent
  inhibitors of CYP3A4 is unavoidable, reduce the dose
  by one-third (rounded to the nearest multiple of the
  150 mg dosage form).

> IMPORTANT SAFETY INFORMATION
> RISKS OF INCORRECT DOSING OF ORAL ANTI-CANCER MEDICINES
> See Cytotoxic drugs p. 865.

- **CONTRA-INDICATIONS** Congenital long QT syndrome
- **CAUTIONS** Diabetes mellitus · history or susceptibility to
QT-interval prolongation

CAUTIONS, FURTHER INFORMATION
  - QT-interval prolongation QT-interval prolongation has been
  observed in clinical studies, which may lead to an
  increased risk for ventricular tachyarrhythmias (e.g.
  torsade de pointes) or sudden death. Risk factors include
  pre-existing bradycardia, other relevant pre-existing
  cardiac disease or electrolyte disturbances; manufacturer
  advises to monitor ECG and electrolytes periodically.

- **INTERACTIONS** → Appendix 1: ceritinib

- **SIDE-EFFECTS**
- **Common or very common** Anaemia · appetite decreased ·
arrhythmias · asthenia · azotaemia · constipation ·
diarrhoea · dysphagia · gastrointestinal discomfort ·
gastrooesophageal reflux disease · hepatic disorders ·
hyperbilirubinaemia · hyperglycaemia ·
hypophosphataemia · nausea · oesophageal disorder ·
pericardial effusion · pericarditis · QT interval prolongation
· renal impairment · respiratory disorders · skin reactions ·
vision disorders · vitreous floater · vomiting · weight
decreased
- **Uncommon** Pancreatitis

SIDE-EFFECTS, FURTHER INFORMATION
Gastro-intestinal effects Manufacturer advises monitor
for signs of gastro-intestinal toxicity and consider dose
reduction or discontinuation of treatment.
Interstitial lung disease Manufacturer advises monitor
patients who exhibit pulmonary symptoms and consider
dose reduction or discontinuation of treatment.

- **CONCEPTION AND CONTRACEPTION** Manufacturer
recommends effective contraception in women of
childbearing potential during treatment and for up to
3 months after discontinuation of treatment.

- **PREGNANCY** Manufacturer advises avoid unless
essential—no information available. See also *Pregnancy
and reproductive function* in Cytotoxic drugs p. 865.

- **BREAST FEEDING** Manufacturer advises avoid—no
information available.

- **HEPATIC IMPAIRMENT** Manufacturer advises avoid in
moderate to severe impairment—no information available
but extensively metabolised by the liver.

- **RENAL IMPAIRMENT** Manufacturer advises caution in
severe impairment—no information available.

- **MONITORING REQUIREMENTS**
  - Manufacturer advises to monitor fasting blood glucose
  concentration prior to initiation of treatment and
  periodically thereafter. Also monitor for amylase and
  lipase elevations periodically during treatment. Consider
  dose reduction, interruption or discontinuation of
  treatment if outside of normal range.
  - In addition, manufacturer advises measure baseline liver
  function, then monitor every 2 weeks for the first month
  and monthly thereafter; consider discontinuation if severe
  changes in liver function occur—increased risk of
  hepatoxicity. Monitor heart rate and blood pressure
  regularly; consider dose reduction or discontinuation if
  bradycardia is reported—consult product literature.

- **DIRECTIONS FOR ADMINISTRATION** Capsules should be
taken on an empty stomach—no food should be eaten for
2 hours before or after dose.

- **PATIENT AND CARER ADVICE** Patients and carers should be
counselled on the administration of capsules.
Missed doses If a dose is more than 12 hours late, the
missed dose should not be taken and the next dose should
be taken at the normal time.
Driving and skilled tasks Manufacturer advises patients and
their carers should be counselled on the effects on driving
and skilled tasks—increased risk of fatigue and vision
disorders.

- **NATIONAL FUNDING/ACCESS DECISIONS**

NICE decisions
  - **Ceritinib for previously treated anaplastic lymphoma kinase-
  positive non small cell lung cancer (June 2016)** NICE TA395
  Ceritinib is recommended, within its marketing
  authorisation, as an option for treating advanced
  anaplastic lymphoma kinase-positive non-small-cell lung
  cancer in adults previously treated with crizotinib; only if
  the manufacturer provides the discount agreed in the
  patient access scheme.
  www.nice.org.uk/guidance/ta395
  - **Ceritinib for untreated ALK-positive non-small-cell lung cancer
  (January 2018)** NICE TA500
  Ceritinib is recommended, within its marketing
  authorisation, as an option for untreated anaplastic
  lymphoma kinase (ALK)-positive advanced non-small-cell
  lung cancer in adults, only if the manufacturer provides it
  with the discount agreed in the patient access scheme.
  www.nice.org.uk/guidance/ta500

Scottish Medicines Consortium (SMC) Decisions
The *Scottish Medicines Consortium* has advised (December
2015) that ceritinib (*Zykadia®*) is accepted for use within
NHS Scotland for the treatment of adults with anaplastic
lymphoma kinase (ALK)-positive advanced non-small cell
lung cancer (NSCLC) previously treated with crizotinib.
This advice is contingent upon the continuing availability
of the Patient Access Scheme in NHS Scotland or a list
price that is equivalent or lower.

- **MEDICINAL FORMS**
There can be variation in the licensing of different medicines
containing the same drug.

Capsule
CAUTIONARY AND ADVISORY LABELS 25
EXCIPIENTS: May contain Gelatin, propylene glycol
  - Zykadia (Novartis Pharmaceuticals UK Ltd) ▼
  Ceritinib 150 mg Zykadia 150mg capsules | 150 capsule PoM
  £4,923.45

8

Immune system and malignant disease

Cobimetinib

12-Jun-2017

- **DRUG ACTION** Cobimetinib is a mitogen-activated protein kinase (MAPK) inhibitor.

- **INDICATIONS AND DOSE**

Treatment of BRAF V600 mutation-positive unresectable or metastatic melanoma (in combination with vemurafenib) (specialist use only)
  - BY MOUTH
  - Adult: 60 mg once daily for 21 days; subsequent cycles repeated after a 7-day interval, for dose adjustment due to side-effects—consult product literature

---

IMPORTANT SAFETY INFORMATION
RISKS OF INCORRECT DOSING OF ORAL ANTI-CANCER MEDICINES
See Cytotoxic drugs p. 865.

- **CAUTIONS** Left ventricular dysfunction · risk factors for bleeding
- **INTERACTIONS** → Appendix 1: cobimetinib
- **SIDE-EFFECTS**
  - **Common or very common** Anaemia · basal cell carcinoma · chills · dehydration · diarrhoea · electrolyte imbalance · fever · haemorrhage · hyperglycaemia · hypertension · nausea · photosensitivity reaction · pneumonitis · serous retinopathy · skin reactions · vision disorders · vomiting
  - **Uncommon** Rhabdomyolysis
- **CONCEPTION AND CONTRACEPTION** Manufacturer advises use of two effective contraceptive methods during treatment and for at least 3 months after stopping treatment.
- **PREGNANCY** Manufacturer advises avoid unless essential—toxicity in *animal* studies. See also *Pregnancy and reproductive function* in Cytotoxic drugs p. 865.
- **BREAST FEEDING** Manufacturer advises avoid—no information available.
- **HEPATIC IMPAIRMENT** Manufacturer advises caution.
- **RENAL IMPAIRMENT** Manufacturer advises caution in severe impairment—limited information available.
- **MONITORING REQUIREMENTS**
  - Creatine kinase elevation Manufacturer advises baseline creatine kinase and creatinine levels should be measured before starting treatment, and then at monthly intervals during treatment or as clinically indicated—consult product literature if elevated.
  - Left ventricular function Manufacturer advises ejection fraction should be evaluated before initiation of treatment, then after the first month of treatment and at least every 3 months thereafter (or as clinically indicated) until treatment discontinuation.
  - Liver function Manufacturer advises liver function should be evaluated before initiation of treatment and monthly thereafter (or more frequently as clinically indicated).
  - Visual disturbances Manufacturer advises assess for new or worsening visual disturbances at each visit; if symptoms of new or worsening visual disturbances are identified, an ophthalmologic examination is recommended.
- **PATIENT AND CARER ADVICE**
Vomiting Manufacturer advises if vomiting occurs after taking tablets, no additional dose should be taken on that day and the next dose should be taken at the usual time.
Missed doses Manufacturer advises if a dose is more than 12 hours late, the missed dose should not be taken and the next dose should be taken at the normal time.
Driving and skilled tasks Manufacturer advises patients should be counselled on the effects on driving and performance of skilled tasks—increased risk of visual disturbances.

- **NATIONAL FUNDING/ACCESS DECISIONS**
NICE decisions
  - **Cobimetinib in combination with vemurafenib for treating unresectable or metastatic BRAF V600 mutation-positive melanoma (October 2016) NICE TA414**
Cobimetinib in combination with vemurafenib is **not** recommended within its marketing authorisation for treating unresectable or metastatic melanoma with a BRAF V600 mutation.
    Patients currently receiving cobimetinib may continue without change to prior funding arrangements, until they and their clinician consider it appropriate to stop.
www.nice.org.uk/TA414

- **MEDICINAL FORMS**
There can be variation in the licensing of different medicines containing the same drug.
Tablet
  - Cotellic (Roche Products Ltd) ▼
  Cobimetinib (as Cobimetinib hemifumarate) 20 mg Cotellic 20mg tablets | 63 tablet [PoM] £4,275.67

Crizotinib

10-Feb-2017

- **DRUG ACTION** Crizotinib is a tyrosine kinase inhibitor.

- **INDICATIONS AND DOSE**

Treatment of previously treated anaplastic lymphoma kinase (ALK)-positive advanced non-small cell lung cancer | First-line treatment of anaplastic lymphoma kinase (ALK)-positive advanced non-small cell lung cancer
  - BY MOUTH
  - Adult: 250 mg twice daily, consult product literature for information on dose adjustments based on individual patient safety and tolerability

---

IMPORTANT SAFETY INFORMATION
RISKS OF INCORRECT DOSING OF ORAL ANTI-CANCER MEDICINES
See Cytotoxic drugs p. 865.

MHRA/CHM ADVICE (NOVEMBER 2015): RISK OF CARDIAC FAILURE
Severe, sometimes fatal cases of cardiac failure have been reported in patients treated with crizotinib. The MHRA has issued the following advice:
- Monitor all patients for signs and symptoms of heart failure (including dyspnoea, oedema, or rapid weight gain from fluid retention)
- Consider reducing the dose, or interrupting or stopping treatment if symptoms of heart failure occur

---

- **CAUTIONS** History of diverticulitis (risk of gastro-intestinal perforation—discontinue treatment if gastrointestinal perforation occurs) · metastases of gastrointestinal tract (risk of gastro-intestinal perforation—discontinue treatment if gastrointestinal perforation occurs) · patients with susceptibility to QT-prolongation (including bradycardia, history of cardiac disease, concomitant use of drugs that prolong QT interval, and electrolyte disturbances)—periodic renal monitoring required · risk of gastro-intestinal perforation—discontinue treatment if gastrointestinal perforation occurs · vision disorders reported—consider full ophthalmological evaluation if vision disorder worsens or persists

CAUTIONS, FURTHER INFORMATION
- Fatal interstitial lung disease and pneumonitis Fatal interstitial lung disease and pneumonitis reported (monitor patients with pulmonary symptoms, withdraw treatment if suspected, and permanently discontinue treatment if diagnosed).

- **INTERACTIONS** → Appendix 1: crizotinib

- **SIDE-EFFECTS**
▸ **Common or very common** Anaemia · appetite decreased · arrhythmias · constipation · diarrhoea · dizziness · fatigue · gait abnormal · gastrointestinal discomfort · gastrointestinal disorders · heart failure · hepatic function abnormal · hypogonadism · hypophosphataemia · leucopenia · local swelling · movement disorders · muscle atrophy · muscle tone decreased · muscle weakness · nausea · nerve disorders · neuralgia · neurotoxicity · neutropenia · oedema · periorbital oedema · peroneal nerve palsy · pulmonary oedema · QT interval prolongation · renal abscess · renal cyst · respiratory disorders · sensation abnormal · skin reactions · syncope · taste altered · vision disorders · vitreous floater · vomiting
▸ **Uncommon** Gastrointestinal perforation (including fatal cases) · hepatic failure (including fatal cases) · renal impairment
   SIDE-EFFECTS, FURTHER INFORMATION Consider reducing the dose, or interrupting or stopping treatment if symptoms of cardiac failure occur.

- **CONCEPTION AND CONTRACEPTION** Ensure effective contraception during and for at least 90 days after treatment.

- **PREGNANCY** Avoid (toxicity in *animal* studies). See also *Pregnancy and reproductive function* in Cytotoxic drugs p. 865.

- **BREAST FEEDING** Avoid—no information available.

- **HEPATIC IMPAIRMENT** Manufacturer advises caution in mild to moderate impairment. Avoid in severe impairment.

- **RENAL IMPAIRMENT**
   Dose adjustments Reduce dose to 250 mg once daily in severe impairment not requiring peritoneal dialysis or hemodialysis, may be increased to 200 mg twice daily after at least 4 weeks, based on individual assessment of safety and tolerability.

- **MONITORING REQUIREMENTS** Monitor liver function once a week during the first 2 months of treatment, then at least monthly thereafter and as clinically indicated. Monitor ECG and electrolytes (correct if abnormal) in all patients before starting treatment, then periodically and as clinically indicated thereafter. Monitor for signs and symptoms of treatment emergent bradycardia (including syncope, dizziness and hypotension)—monitor blood pressure and heart rate regularly.

- **PATIENT AND CARER ADVICE** Counsel all patients on the early signs and symptoms of gastrointestinal perforation—advice to seek immediate medical attention.
   Driving and skilled tasks Symptomatic bradycardia (including syncope, dizziness and hypotension), vision disorder and fatigue may affect performance of skilled tasks (e.g. driving or operating machinery).

- **NATIONAL FUNDING/ACCESS DECISIONS**
   NICE decisions
▸ **Crizotinib for untreated anaplastic lymphoma kinase-positive advanced non-small-cell lung cancer (September 2016)** NICE TA406
   Crizotinib is recommended, within its marketing authorisation, as an option for untreated anaplastic lymphoma kinase-positive advanced non-small-cell lung cancer in adults, only if the manufacturer provides it with the discount agreed in the patient access scheme.
   www.nice.org.uk/TA406
▸ **Crizotinib for previously treated anaplastic lymphoma kinase-positive advanced non-small-cell lung cancer (December 2016)** NICE TA422
   Crizotinib is recommended, within its marketing authorisation, as an option for previously treated anaplastic lymphoma kinase-positive advanced non-small-cell lung cancer in adults, only if the manufacturer

provides it with the discount agreed in the patient access scheme.
www.nice.org.uk/TA422

- **MEDICINAL FORMS**
There can be variation in the licensing of different medicines containing the same drug.

Capsule
CAUTIONARY AND ADVISORY LABELS 25
▸ Xalkori (Pfizer Ltd) ▼
   Crizotinib 200 mg Xalkori 200mg capsules | 60 capsule [PoM] £4,689.00 (Hospital only)
   Crizotinib 250 mg Xalkori 250mg capsules | 60 capsule [PoM] £4,689.00 (Hospital only)

Dabrafenib

21-Feb-2017

- **DRUG ACTION** Dabrafenib is a BRAF kinase inhibitor, which inhibits BRAF V600 mutation-positive melanoma cell growth.

- **INDICATIONS AND DOSE**

Unresectable or metastatic melanoma with a BRAF V600 mutation (as monotherapy or in combination with trametinib)
▸ BY MOUTH
▸ **Adult:** 150 mg every 12 hours, for dose adjustments due to side-effects, consult product literature

---

IMPORTANT SAFETY INFORMATION
RISKS OF INCORRECT DOSING OF ORAL ANTI-CANCER MEDICINES
See Cytotoxic drugs p. 865.

- **CONTRA-INDICATIONS** BRAF wild-type melanoma

- **CAUTIONS** Elderly (more frequent dose adjustments may be required) · prior or concurrent cancer associated with RAS mutations—risk of secondary or recurrent malignancy

- **INTERACTIONS** → Appendix 1: dabrafenib

- **SIDE-EFFECTS**
▸ **Common or very common** Alopecia · appetite decreased · arthralgia · asthenia · chills · constipation · cough · diarrhoea · fever · headache · hyperglycaemia · hypophosphataemia · influenza like illness · myalgia · nausea · neoplasms · pain in extremity · photosensitivity reaction · skin reactions · vomiting
▸ **Uncommon** Nephritis · pancreatitis · panniculitis · renal impairment · uveitis
   SIDE-EFFECTS, FURTHER INFORMATION Additional side-effects reported when used in combination with trametinib include dizziness, hyperhidrosis, hyponatraemia, hypotension, leucopenia, muscle spasms, myocarditis, neutropenia, night sweats, and thrombocytopenia.

- **CONCEPTION AND CONTRACEPTION** Manufacturer advises women of child-bearing potential should use effective non-hormonal contraception during and for 4 weeks after stopping treatment.

- **PREGNANCY** Manufacturer advises avoid unless potential benefit outweighs risk—toxicity in *animal* studies. See also *Pregnancy and reproductive function* in Cytotoxic drugs p. 865.

- **BREAST FEEDING** Manufacturer advises avoid—no information available.

- **HEPATIC IMPAIRMENT** Manufacturer advises caution in moderate to severe impairment.

- **RENAL IMPAIRMENT** Manufacturer advises caution in severe impairment—no information available.

- **MONITORING REQUIREMENTS** Manufacturer advises assess for cutaneous squamous cell carcinoma and new primary melanoma before treatment, monthly during treatment, and for 6 months after discontinuation or until initiation of alternative treatment; assess and monitor for non-cutaneous secondary or recurrent malignancy before, during, and for 6 months after discontinuation or until initiation of alternative treatment—consult product literature; monitor full blood count as clinically indicated; monitor for ophthalmologic reactions including uveitis, iridocyclitis and iritis; monitor serum creatinine.

- PATIENT AND CARER ADVICE Manufacturer advises patients should be informed to immediately report new skin lesions—risk of cutaneous squamous cell carcinoma and new primary melanoma.
  Missed doses Manufacturer advises if a dose is more than 6 hours late, the missed dose should not be taken and the next dose should be taken at the normal time.
  Driving and skilled tasks Manufacturer advises patients and carers should be counselled on the effects on driving and performance of skilled tasks—increased risk of ocular adverse reactions.

- NATIONAL FUNDING/ACCESS DECISIONS
  NICE decisions
  ▸ **Dabrafenib for treating unresectable or metastatic BRAF V600 mutation-positive melanoma (October 2014)** NICE TA321
  Dabrafenib is recommended, within its marketing authorisation, as an option for treating unresectable or metastatic BRAF V600 mutation-positive melanoma only if the manufacturer provides dabrafenib with the discount agreed in the patient access scheme.
  www.nice.org.uk/TA321

  ▸ **Trametinib in combination with dabrafenib for treating unresectable or metastatic melanoma (June 2016)** NICE TA396
  Trametinib in combination with dabrafenib is recommended within its marketing authorisation, as an option for treating unresectable or metastatic melanoma in adults with a BRAF V600 mutation, only when the company provides trametinib and dabrafenib with the discounts agreed in the patient access schemes.
  www.nice.org.uk/TA396

  Scottish Medicines Consortium (SMC) Decisions
  The *Scottish Medicines Consortium* has advised (February 2015) that dabrafenib (*Tafinlar*®) is accepted for restricted use within NHS Scotland, as monotherapy, for the treatment of unresectable or metastatic BRAFV600 mutation-positive melanoma in patients who have received no prior therapy.

- MEDICINAL FORMS
  There can be variation in the licensing of different medicines containing the same drug.
  Capsule
  CAUTIONARY AND ADVISORY LABELS 3, 23, 25
  ▸ Tafinlar (Novartis Pharmaceuticals UK Ltd) ▼
  Dabrafenib (as Dabrafenib mesilate) 50 mg Tafinlar 50mg capsules | 28 capsule PoM £933.33 (Hospital only)
  Dabrafenib (as Dabrafenib mesilate) 75 mg Tafinlar 75mg capsules | 28 capsule PoM £1,400.00 (Hospital only)

Dasatinib

22-Mar-2017

- DRUG ACTION Dasatinib is a tyrosine kinase inhibitor.

- INDICATIONS AND DOSE
  Chronic phase chronic myeloid leukaemia (consult product literature for details)
  ▸ BY MOUTH
  ▸ Adult: 100 mg once daily, then increased if necessary up to 140 mg once daily

Accelerated and blast phase chronic myeloid leukaemia (consult product literature for details) | Acute lymphoblastic leukaemia (consult product literature for details)
▸ BY MOUTH
▸ Adult: 140 mg once daily, then increased if necessary up to 180 mg once daily

---

IMPORTANT SAFETY INFORMATION

RISKS OF INCORRECT DOSING OF ORAL ANTI-CANCER MEDICINES
See Cytotoxic drugs p. 865.

MHRA/CHM ADVICE (MAY 2016): RISK OF HEPATITIS B VIRUS REACTIVATION WITH BCR-ABL TYROSINE KINASE INHIBITORS
An EU wide review has concluded that dasatinib can cause hepatitis B reactivation; the MHRA recommends establishing hepatitis B virus status in all patients before initiation of treatment.

- CAUTIONS Hepatitis B infection · risk of cardiac dysfunction (monitor closely) · susceptibility to QT-interval prolongation (correct hypokalaemia or hypomagnesaemia before starting treatment)
  CAUTIONS, FURTHER INFORMATION
  ▸ Pulmonary arterial hypertension Patients should be evaluated for signs and symptoms of underlying cardiopulmonary disease before starting treatment; echocardiography should be performed at the start of treatment in patients with symptoms of cardiac disease and considered for patients with risk factors for cardiac or pulmonary disease.
    Treatment should be interrupted or the dose reduced in patients who develop dyspnoea or fatigue, while they are evaluated for common aetiologies (e.g. pleural effusion, pulmonary oedema, anaemia or lung infiltration); pulmonary arterial hypertension should be considered in the absence of these conditions, and if there is no improvement following dose reduction or interruption.
    If pulmonary arterial hypertension is confirmed, dasatinib should be permanently discontinued.
  ▸ Hepatitis B infection The MHRA advises that patients who are carriers of hepatitis B virus should be closely monitored for signs and symptoms of active infection throughout treatment and for several months after stopping treatment; expert advice should be sought for patients who test positive for hepatitis B virus and in those with active infection.

- INTERACTIONS → Appendix 1: dasatinib

- SIDE-EFFECTS
  ▸ **Common or very common** Alopecia · anaemia · appetite abnormal · arrhythmias · arthralgia · asthenia · bone marrow depression · cardiac disorder · cardiomyopathy · chest pain · chills · constipation · cough · depression · diarrhoea · dizziness · drowsiness · dry eye · dyspnoea · eye inflammation · facial swelling · fever · fluid imbalance · flushing · gastrointestinal discomfort · gastrointestinal disorders · genital abnormalities · haemorrhage · headache · hearing impairment · heart failure · hypertension · hyperuricaemia · increased risk of infection · insomnia · milia · mucositis · muscle complaints · muscle weakness · musculoskeletal stiffness · myocardial dysfunction · nausea · nerve disorders · neutropenia · oedema · oral disorders · pain · palpitations · pericardial effusion · perinephric effusion · pulmonary hypertension · pulmonary oedema · respiratory disorders · sepsis · skin reactions · sweat changes · taste altered · thrombocytopenia · vision disorders · vomiting · weight changes
  ▸ **Uncommon** Acute coronary syndrome · anxiety · arthritis · ascites · asthma · cardiac inflammation · cardiomegaly · cerebrovascular insufficiency · cholecystitis · CNS haemorrhage · confusion · dysphagia · embolism and thrombosis · emotional lability · excessive tearing · gynaecomastia · hair disorder · hepatic disorders ·

hypercholesterolaemia · hypoalbuminaemia · hypotension · hypothyroidism · ischaemic heart disease · libido decreased · lymphadenopathy · lymphopenia · malaise · memory loss · menstrual disorder · movement disorders · myopathy · nail disorder · osteonecrosis · pancreatitis · panniculitis · penile disorders · photosensitivity reaction · proteinuria · QT interval prolongation · renal impairment · scrotal oedema · skin ulcer · syncope · tendinitis · testicular swelling · tremor · tumour lysis syndrome · urinary frequency increased · vertigo · vulvovaginal swelling

▸ **Rare or very rare** Cardiac arrest · dementia · diabetes mellitus · facial paralysis · gait abnormal · hypersensitivity vasculitis · hyperthyroidism · pure red cell aplasia · seizure · thyroiditis

▸ **Frequency not known** Hepatitis B reactivation · nephrotic syndrome · Stevens-Johnson syndrome

● CONCEPTION AND CONTRACEPTION Effective contraception required during treatment.

● PREGNANCY Manufacturer advises avoid unless potential benefit outweighs risk—toxicity in *animal* studies. See also *Pregnancy and reproductive function* in Cytotoxic drugs p. 865.

● BREAST FEEDING Discontinue breast-feeding.

● HEPATIC IMPAIRMENT Manufacturer advises caution in hepatic impairment.

● NATIONAL FUNDING/ACCESS DECISIONS

NICE decisions

▸ **Dasatinib, nilotinib and imatinib for untreated chronic myeloid leukaemia (CML) (December 2016)** NICE TA426
Dasatinib is recommended, within its marketing authorisation, as an option for untreated chronic phase Philadelphia-chromosome-positive CML, only if the manufacturer provides it with the discount agreed in the patient access scheme.
www.nice.org.uk/TA426

▸ **Dasatinib, nilotinib and high-dose imatinib for treating imatinib-resistant or intolerant chronic myeloid leukaemia (CML) (December 2016)** NICE TA425
Dasatinib is recommended as an option for treating chronic or accelerated phase Philadelphia-chromosome-positive CML in adults, if they cannot have imatinib, or their disease is imatinib-resistant **and** the manufacturer provides dasatinib with the discount agreed in the patient access scheme.

Patients whose treatment was started within the NHS before this guidance was published should have the option to continue treatment, without change to their funding arrangements, until they and their clinician consider it appropriate to stop.
www.nice.org.uk/TA425

Scottish Medicines Consortium (SMC) Decisions
The *Scottish Medicines Consortium* has advised (September 2016) that dasatinib (*Sprycel®*) is accepted for use within NHS Scotland for the treatment of adults with chronic, accelerated or blast phase chronic myelogenous leukaemia (CML) with resistance or intolerance to prior therapy including imatinib mesilate, only if the manufacturer provides dasatinib with the discount agreed in the patient access scheme in NHS Scotland or a list price that is equivalent or lower.

The *Scottish Medicines Consortium* has advised (September 2016) that dasatinib (*Sprycel®*) is accepted for use within NHS Scotland for the treatment of adults with newly diagnosed Philadelphia chromosome positive (Ph+) chronic myelogenous leukaemia (CML) in the chronic phase, only if the manufacturer provides dasatinib with the discount agreed in the patient access scheme in NHS Scotland or a list price that is equivalent or lower.

● MEDICINAL FORMS
There can be variation in the licensing of different medicines containing the same drug.

Tablet
CAUTIONARY AND ADVISORY LABELS 25
▸ Sprycel (Bristol-Myers Squibb Pharmaceuticals Ltd)
  Dasatinib 20 mg Sprycel 20mg tablets | 60 tablet [PoM] £1,252.48
  Dasatinib 50 mg Sprycel 50mg tablets | 60 tablet [PoM] £2,504.96
  Dasatinib 80 mg Sprycel 80mg tablets | 30 tablet [PoM] £2,504.96
  Dasatinib 100 mg Sprycel 100mg tablets | 30 tablet [PoM] £2,504.96
  Dasatinib 140 mg Sprycel 140mg tablets | 30 tablet [PoM] £2,504.96

Erlotinib
18-Apr-2016

● DRUG ACTION Erlotinib is a tyrosine kinase inhibitor.

● INDICATIONS AND DOSE

Treatment of locally advanced or metastatic non-small cell lung cancer after failure of previous chemotherapy | Monotherapy for maintenance treatment of locally advanced or metastatic non-small cell lung cancer with stable disease after four cycles of platinum-based chemotherapy
▸ BY MOUTH
▸ Adult: 150 mg once daily

Treatment of metastatic pancreatic cancer (in combination with gemcitabine)
▸ BY MOUTH
▸ Adult: 100 mg once daily

DOSE ADJUSTMENTS DUE TO INTERACTIONS
▸ Manufacturer advises if concurrent use of potent inducers of CYP3A4 is unavoidable, increase dose to 300 mg daily, if well tolerated for more than 2 weeks, further increase to 450 mg daily could be considered with close monitoring.

IMPORTANT SAFETY INFORMATION

EPIDERMAL GROWTH FACTOR RECEPTOR (EGFR) INHIBITORS: SERIOUS CASES OF KERATITIS AND ULCERATIVE KERATITIS (MAY 2012)
Keratitis and ulcerative keratitis have been reported following treatment with epidermal growth factor receptor (EGFR) inhibitors for cancer (cetuximab, erlotinib, gefitinib and panitumumab). In rare cases, this has resulted in corneal perforation and blindness. Patients undergoing treatment with EGFR inhibitors who present with acute or worsening signs and symptoms suggestive of keratitis should be referred promptly to an ophthalmology specialist. Treatment should be interrupted or discontinued if ulcerative keratitis is diagnosed.

RISKS OF INCORRECT DOSING OF ORAL ANTI-CANCER MEDICINES
See Cytotoxic drugs p. 865.

● INTERACTIONS → Appendix 1: erlotinib
● SIDE-EFFECTS
▸ **Common or very common** Alopecia · diarrhoea · eye inflammation · haemorrhage · increased risk of infection · renal failure · skin reactions
▸ **Uncommon** Brittle nails · eye disorders · gastrointestinal disorders · hair changes · interstitial lung disease · nephritis · proteinuria
▸ **Rare or very rare** Hepatic failure · severe cutaneous adverse reactions (SCARs)
▸ **Frequency not known** Appetite decreased · chills · cough · depression · dyspnoea · fatigue · fever · gastrointestinal discomfort · headache · nausea · neuropathy sensory · stomatitis · vomiting · weight decreased

- **CONCEPTION AND CONTRACEPTION** Effective contraception required during and for at least 2 weeks after treatment.
- **PREGNANCY** Manufacturer advises avoid—toxicity in *animal* studies. See also *Pregnancy and reproductive function* in Cytotoxic drugs p. 865.
- **BREAST FEEDING** Manufacturer advises avoid- no information available.
- **HEPATIC IMPAIRMENT** Manufacturer advises caution in mild to moderate impairment. Avoid in severe impairment. Monitor liver function in pre-existing liver disease.
- **RENAL IMPAIRMENT** Manufacturer advises avoid in severe impairment.
- **NATIONAL FUNDING/ACCESS DECISIONS**

  NICE decisions
  ▸ Erlotinib monotherapy for maintenance treatment of non-small-cell lung cancer (June 2011) NICE TA227
  Erlotinib monotherapy is **not** recommended for maintenance treatment in patients with locally advanced or metastatic non-small-cell lung cancer who have stable disease after platinum-based first-line chemotherapy.
  www.nice.org.uk/TA227
  ▸ Erlotinib for the first-line treatment of locally advanced or metastatic EGFR-TK mutation-positive non-small-cell lung cancer (June 2012) NICE TA258
  Erlotinib is recommended as an option in patients for the first-line treatment of locally advanced or metastatic non-small-cell lung cancer if:
    • they test positive for the epidermal growth factor tyrosine kinase (EGFR-TK) mutation **and**
    • the manufacturer provides erlotinib at the discounted price agreed under the patient access scheme (as revised in 2012).
  www.nice.org.uk/TA258
  ▸ Erlotinib and gefitinib for treating non-small-cell lung cancer that has progressed after prior chemotherapy (December 2015) NICE TA374
  Erlotinib is recommended as an option for treating locally advanced or metastatic non-small-cell lung cancer that has progressed after non-targeted chemotherapy in patients with tumours of unknown epidermal growth factor receptor tyrosine kinase (EGFR-TK) mutation status, only if all of the following criteria are met:
    • the result of an EGFR-TK mutation diagnostic test is unobtainable because of an inadequate tissue sample or poor-quality DNA,
    • the treating clinician considers that the tumour is very likely to be EGFR-TK mutation-positive,
    • the patient's condition responds to the first 2 cycles of treatment with erlotinib, **and**,
    • the manufacturer provides erlotinib with the discount agreed in the patient access scheme.
  Erlotinib is **not** recommended for treating locally advanced or metastatic non-small-cell lung cancer that has progressed after non-targeted chemotherapy in patients with tumours that are EGFR-TK mutation-negative.
  Patients who are already receiving erlotinib should continue treatment until they and their clinician consider it appropriate to stop.
  www.nice.org.uk/TA374

- **MEDICINAL FORMS**
  There can be variation in the licensing of different medicines containing the same drug.

  Tablet
  CAUTIONARY AND ADVISORY LABELS 23
  ▸ Tarceva (Roche Products Ltd)
  Erlotinib (as Erlotinib hydrochloride) 25 mg Tarceva 25mg tablets | 30 tablet [PoM] £378.33

Erlotinib (as Erlotinib hydrochloride) 100 mg Tarceva 100mg tablets | 30 tablet [PoM] £1,324.14
Erlotinib (as Erlotinib hydrochloride) 150 mg Tarceva 150mg tablets | 30 tablet [PoM] £1,631.53

Everolimus

24-Jul-2017

- **DRUG ACTION** Everolimus is a protein kinase inhibitor.

- **INDICATIONS AND DOSE**

  AFINITOR ®

  Treatment of advanced renal cell carcinoma when the disease has progressed despite treatment with vascular endothelial growth factor-targeted therapy | Treatment of unresectable or metastatic, well- or moderately-differentiated neuroendocrine tumours of pancreatic origin | Treatment of hormone-receptor-positive, human epidermal growth factor-2 (HER-2) negative advanced breast cancer, in combination with exemestane, in postmenopausal women without symptomatic visceral disease after recurrence or progression following a non-steroidal aromatase inhibitor
  ▸ BY MOUTH
  ▸ Adult: 10 mg once daily

  CERTICAN ®

  Liver transplantation
  ▸ BY MOUTH
  ▸ Adult: Initially 1 mg twice daily, to be started approximately 4 weeks after transplantation; maintenance, dose adjusted according to response and whole blood everolimus concentration; dose adjustments can be made every 4–5 days

  Renal transplantation | Heart transplantation
  ▸ BY MOUTH
  ▸ Adult: Initially 750 micrograms twice daily, to be started as soon as possible after transplantation; maintenance, dose adjusted according to response and whole blood everolimus concentration; dose adjustments can be made every 4–5 days

  VOTUBIA ® DISPERSIBLE TABLETS

  Subependymal giant cell astrocytoma associated with tuberous sclerosis complex
  ▸ BY MOUTH USING DISPERSIBLE TABLETS
  ▸ Adult: (consult product literature)

  Adjunctive treatment of refractory partial-onset seizures, with or without secondary generalisation, associated with tuberous sclerosis complex
  ▸ BY MOUTH USING DISPERSIBLE TABLETS
  ▸ Adult: (consult product literature)

  VOTUBIA ® TABLETS

  Subependymal giant cell astrocytoma associated with tuberous sclerosis complex
  ▸ BY MOUTH USING TABLETS
  ▸ Adult: (consult product literature)

  Renal angiomyolipoma associated with tuberous sclerosis complex
  ▸ BY MOUTH USING TABLETS
  ▸ Adult: (consult product literature)

  IMPORTANT SAFETY INFORMATION
  RISKS OF INCORRECT DOSING OF ORAL ANTI-CANCER MEDICINES
  See Cytotoxic drugs p. 865.

- **CAUTIONS** History of bleeding disorders
- **INTERACTIONS** → Appendix 1: everolimus
- **SIDE-EFFECTS**
  ▸ Common or very common Alopecia · anaemia · appetite decreased · arthralgia · asthenia · cough · decreased leucocytes · dehydration · diabetes mellitus · diarrhoea · d

mouth · dyslipidaemia · dysphagia · dyspnoea · electrolyte imbalance · eye inflammation · fever · gastrointestinal discomfort · haemorrhage · headache · hyperglycaemia · hypertension · increased risk of infection · insomnia · menstrual cycle irregularities · mucositis · nail disorders · nausea · neutropenia · oral disorders · peripheral oedema · proteinuria · renal impairment · respiratory disorders · skin reactions · taste altered · thrombocytopenia · vomiting · weight decreased

▸ **Uncommon** Congestive heart failure · embolism and thrombosis · flushing · healing impaired · hepatitis B · musculoskeletal chest pain · pancytopenia · sepsis · urinary frequency increased

▸ **Rare or very rare** Pure red cell aplasia

▸ **Frequency not known** Hepatitis B reactivation

SIDE-EFFECTS, FURTHER INFORMATION Reduce dose or discontinue if severe side-effects occur—consult product literature.

● CONCEPTION AND CONTRACEPTION Effective contraception must be used during and for up to 8 weeks after treatment.

● PREGNANCY Manufacturer advises avoid (toxicity in *animal* studies). See also *Pregnancy and reproductive function* in Cytotoxic drugs p. 865.

● BREAST FEEDING Manufacturer advises avoid.

● HEPATIC IMPAIRMENT Consult product literature.

● MONITORING REQUIREMENTS
▸ For *Votubia*® preparations: manufacturer advises everolimus blood concentration monitoring is required—consult product literature.
▸ For *Certican*®: manufacturer advises pre-dose ('trough') whole blood everolimus concentration should be 3–8 nanograms/mL; monitoring should be performed every 4–5 days (using **chromatographic** assay) after initiation or dose adjustment until 2 consecutive stable concentrations; monitor patients with hepatic impairment taking concomitant strong CYP3A4 inducers and inhibitors when switching formulation, and/or if concomitant ciclosporin dose is reduced.
▸ Monitor blood-glucose concentration, serum-triglycerides and serum-cholesterol before treatment and periodically thereafter.
▸ Monitor renal function before treatment and periodically thereafter.

● DIRECTIONS FOR ADMINISTRATION
VOTUBIA® DISPERSIBLE TABLETS Manufacturer advises tablets must be dispersed in water before administration—consult product literature for details.
VOTUBIA® TABLETS Tablets may be dispersed in approximately 30 mL of water by gently stirring, immediately before drinking. After solution has been swallowed, any residue must be re-dispersed in the same volume of water and swallowed.

● PRESCRIBING AND DISPENSING INFORMATION *Votubia*® is available as both *tablets* and *dispersible tablets*. These formulations vary in their licensed indications and are not interchangeable—consult product literature for information on switching between formulations.

● PATIENT AND CARER ADVICE
Pneumonitis Non-infectious pneumonitis reported. Patients should be advised to seek urgent medical advice if new or worsening respiratory symptoms occur.

● NATIONAL FUNDING/ACCESS DECISIONS
NICE decisions
▸ **Everolimus with exemestane for treating advanced breast cancer after endocrine therapy (December 2016)** NICE TA421
Everolimus, in combination with exemestane, is recommended within its marketing authorisation for treating advanced human epidermal growth factor receptor 2 (HER2)-negative, hormone-receptor-positive

breast cancer in postmenopausal women without symptomatic visceral disease that has recurred or progressed following treatment with a non-steroidal aromatase inhibitor. Everolimus is recommended only if the manufacturer provides it with the discount agreed in the patient access scheme.
www.nice.org.uk/TA421

▸ **Everolimus for advanced renal cell carcinoma after previous treatment (February 2017)** NICE TA432
Everolimus is recommended within its marketing authorisation as an option for treating advanced renal cell carcinoma that has progressed during or after treatment with vascular endothelial growth factor targeted therapy. Everolimus is only recommended if the manufacturer provides it with the discount agreed in the patient access scheme.
www.nice.org.uk/TA432

▸ **Everolimus and sunitinib for treating unresectable or metastatic neuroendocrine tumours in people with progressive disease (June 2017)** NICE TA449
Everolimus and sunitinib are recommended, within their marketing authorisations, as options for treating well- or moderately differentiated unresectable or metastatic neuroendocrine tumours (NETs) of pancreatic origin in adults with progressive disease.

Everolimus is recommended, within its marketing authorisation, as an option for treating well-differentiated (grade 1 or grade 2) non-functional unresectable or metastatic NETs of gastrointestinal or lung origin in adults with progressive disease.

Everolimus is recommended only when the company provides it with the discount agreed in the patient access scheme.
www.nice.org.uk/TA449

AFINITOR®
NICE decisions
▸ **Lenvatinib with everolimus for previously treated advanced renal cell carcinoma (January 2018)** NICE TA498
Lenvatinib plus everolimus is recommended as an option for treating advanced renal cell carcinoma in adults who have had one previous vascular endothelial growth factor (VEGF)-targeted therapy, only if:
● their Eastern Cooperative Oncology Group (ECOG) performance status score is 0 or 1, **and**
● the manufacturer provides lenvatinib with the discount agreed in the patient access scheme.
Patients whose treatment was started within the NHS before this guidance was published should have the option to continue treatment, without change to their funding arrangements, until they and their NHS clinician consider it appropriate to stop.
www.nice.org.uk/guidance/ta498

CERTICAN®
NICE decisions
▸ **Everolimus for preventing organ rejection in liver transplantation (July 2015)** NICE TA348
Everolimus (*Certican*®) is **not** recommended within its marketing authorisation for preventing organ rejection in patients who have undergone a liver transplant. Patients currently receiving everolimus for this indication should have the option to continue treatment until they and their clinician consider it appropriate to stop.
www.nice.org.uk/guidance/TA348

▸ **Immunosuppressive therapy for kidney transplant in adults (October 2017)** NICE TA481
Everolimus is not recommended as an initial treatment to prevent organ rejection in adults having a kidney transplant. Patients whose treatment was started within the NHS before this guidance was published should have the option to continue treatment, without change to their

Immune system and malignant disease

8

funding arrangements, until they and their NHS clinician consider it appropriate to stop.
www.nice.org.uk/guidance/TA481

- MEDICINAL FORMS
  There can be variation in the licensing of different medicines containing the same drug.

Dispersible tablet
CAUTIONARY AND ADVISORY LABELS 13
- Votubia (Novartis Pharmaceuticals UK Ltd)
  Everolimus 2 mg Votubia 2mg dispersible tablets sugar-free | 30 tablet [PoM] £960.00
  Everolimus 3 mg Votubia 3mg dispersible tablets sugar-free | 30 tablet [PoM] £1,440.00
  Everolimus 5 mg Votubia 5mg dispersible tablets sugar-free | 30 tablet [PoM] £2,250.00

Tablet
CAUTIONARY AND ADVISORY LABELS 25
- Afinitor (Novartis Pharmaceuticals UK Ltd)
  Everolimus 2.5 mg Afinitor 2.5mg tablets | 30 tablet [PoM] £1,200.00
  Everolimus 5 mg Afinitor 5mg tablets | 30 tablet [PoM] £2,250.00
  Everolimus 10 mg Afinitor 10mg tablets | 30 tablet [PoM] £2,673.00
- Certican (Novartis Pharmaceuticals UK Ltd)
  Everolimus 250 microgram Certican 0.25mg tablets | 60 tablet [PoM] £148.50
  Everolimus 750 microgram Certican 0.75mg tablets | 60 tablet [PoM] £445.50
- Votubia (Novartis Pharmaceuticals UK Ltd)
  Everolimus 2.5 mg Votubia 2.5mg tablets | 30 tablet [PoM] £1,200.00
  Everolimus 5 mg Votubia 5mg tablets | 30 tablet [PoM] £2,250.00
  Everolimus 10 mg Votubia 10mg tablets | 30 tablet [PoM] £2,970.00

Gefitinib

27-May-2016

- DRUG ACTION Gefitinib is a tyrosine kinase inhibitor.

- INDICATIONS AND DOSE
  Treatment of locally advanced or metastatic non-small cell lung cancer with activating mutations of epidermal growth factor receptor
  - BY MOUTH
  - Adult: 250 mg once daily

IMPORTANT SAFETY INFORMATION
MHRA/CHM ADVICE: EPIDERMAL GROWTH FACTOR RECEPTOR (EGFR) INHIBITORS: SERIOUS CASES OF KERATITIS AND ULCERATIVE KERATITIS (MAY 2012)
Keratitis and ulcerative keratitis have been reported following treatment with epidermal growth factor receptor (EGFR) inhibitors for cancer (cetuximab, erlotinib, gefitinib and panitumumab). In rare cases, this has resulted in corneal perforation and blindness. Patients undergoing treatment with EGFR inhibitors who present with acute or worsening signs and symptoms suggestive of keratitis should be referred promptly to an ophthalmology specialist. Treatment should be interrupted or discontinued if ulcerative keratitis is diagnosed.

RISKS OF INCORRECT DOSING OF ORAL ANTI-CANCER MEDICINES
See Cytotoxic drugs p. 865.

- INTERACTIONS → Appendix 1: gefitinib
- SIDE-EFFECTS
- **Common or very common** Alopecia · angioedema · appetite decreased · asthenia · cystitis · dehydration · diarrhoea · dry eye · dry mouth · eye inflammation · fever · haemorrhage · hypersensitivity · interstitial lung disease · nail disorder · nausea · proteinuria · skin reactions · stomatitis · vomiting
- **Uncommon** Corneal erosion · gastrointestinal perforation · hepatitis · pancreatitis
- **Rare or very rare** Cutaneous vasculitis · severe cutaneous adverse reactions (SCARs)

- CONCEPTION AND CONTRACEPTION Contraceptive advice required, see *Pregnancy and reproductive function* in Cytotoxic drugs p. 865.
- PREGNANCY Manufacturer advises avoid unless essential—toxicity in *animal* studies. See also *Pregnancy and reproductive function* in Cytotoxic drugs p. 865.
- BREAST FEEDING Discontinue breast-feeding.
- HEPATIC IMPAIRMENT Manufacturer advises caution in moderate to severe impairment due to cirrhosis.
- RENAL IMPAIRMENT Manufacturer advises caution if creatinine clearance less than 20 mL/minute.
- MONITORING REQUIREMENTS
  - Monitor for worsening of dyspnoea, cough and fever—discontinue if interstitial lung disease confirmed.
  - Monitor liver function—consider discontinuing if severe changes in liver function occur.
- NATIONAL FUNDING/ACCESS DECISIONS
  NICE decisions
  - **Gefitinib for the first-line treatment of locally advanced or metastatic non-small-cell lung cancer (July 2010)** NICE TA192
    Gefitinib is recommended as an option for the first-line treatment of locally advanced or metastatic non-small-cell lung cancer if the patient tests positive for the epidermal growth factor receptor tyrosine kinase (EGFR-TK) mutation and the manufacturer provides gefitinib at the fixed price agreed under the patient access scheme.
    www.nice.org.uk/TA192
  - **Erlotinib and gefitinib for treating non-small-cell lung cancer that has progressed after prior chemotherapy (December 2015)** NICE TA374
    Gefitinib is **not** recommended for treating locally advanced or metastatic non-small-cell lung cancer that has progressed after non-targeted chemotherapy in patients with tumours that are EGFR-TK mutation-positive.
    Patients who are already receiving treatment should continue treatment until they and their clinician consider it appropriate to stop.
    www.nice.org.uk/TA374

  Scottish Medicines Consortium (SMC) Decisions
  The *Scottish Medicines Consortium* has advised (December 2015) that gefitinib (*Iressa®*) is accepted for restricted use within NHS Scotland for the treatment of adult patients with previously untreated locally advanced or metastatic non-small cell lung cancer (NSCLC) with activating mutations of epidermal growth factor receptor tyrosine kinase (EGFR-TK).

- MEDICINAL FORMS
  There can be variation in the licensing of different medicines containing the same drug.

Tablet
- Iressa (AstraZeneca UK Ltd)
  Gefitinib 250 mg Iressa 250mg tablets | 30 tablet [PoM] £2,167.71

Ibrutinib

19-Sep-2017

- DRUG ACTION Ibrutinib is a tyrosine kinase inhibitor.

- INDICATIONS AND DOSE
  Treatment of relapsed or refractory mantle cell lymphoma
  - BY MOUTH
  - Adult: 560 mg once daily, for dose adjustments due to side effects consult product literature

Treatment of chronic lymphocytic leukaemia, in patients who have received at least one prior therapy, or as first-line treatment in patients with 17p deletion or TP53 mutation who are unsuitable for chemo-immunotherapy | Treatment of Waldenström's macroglobulinaemia, in patients who have received at least one prior therapy, or as first-line treatment in patients who are unsuitable for chemo-immunotherapy

▶ BY MOUTH
▶ Adult: 420 mg once daily, for dose adjustments due to side effects consult product literature

DOSE ADJUSTMENTS DUE TO INTERACTIONS

▶ Manufacturer advises if concurrent use of moderate inhibitors of CYP3A4, amiodarone or ciprofloxacin is unavoidable, reduce dose to 280 mg once daily.
▶ Manufacturer advises if concurrent use of potent inhibitors of CYP3A4 is unavoidable, reduce dose to 140 mg once daily, or withhold ibrutinib for up to 7 days.

IMPORTANT SAFETY INFORMATION

RISKS OF INCORRECT DOSING OF ORAL ANTI-CANCER MEDICINES
See Cytotoxic drugs p. 865.

MHRA/CHM ADVICE: IBRUTINIB (*IMBRUVICA*®): REPORTS OF VENTRICULAR TACHYARRHYTHMIA; RISK OF HEPATITIS B REACTIVATION AND OF OPPORTUNISTIC INFECTIONS (AUGUST 2017)

Cases of ventricular tachyarrhythmia have been reported with the use of ibrutinib. The MHRA advises that ibrutinib should be temporarily discontinued in patients who develop symptoms suggestive of ventricular arrhythmia and to assess benefit-risk before restarting therapy.

Hepatitis B virus status should be established before initiating therapy—for patients with positive hepatitis B serology, consultation with a liver disease expert is recommended before the start of treatment; monitor and manage patients according to local protocols to minimise the risk of hepatitis B virus reactivation. Prophylaxis should be considered for those at an increased risk of opportunistic infections.

● CAUTIONS Family history of congenital short QT syndrome · increased lymphocytes—increased risk of leukostasis, consider withholding treatment temporarily and monitor closely · patients at risk from further shortening of QTc interval · personal history of congenital short QT syndrome · risk of haemorrhagic events—withhold ibrutinib treatment for at least 3 to 7 days before and after surgery depending on risk of bleeding

● INTERACTIONS → Appendix 1: ibrutinib

● SIDE-EFFECTS

▶ **Common or very common** Arrhythmias · arthralgia · broken nails · CNS haemorrhage · constipation · diarrhoea · dizziness · fever · haemorrhage · headache · hypertension · hyperuricaemia · increased leucocytes · increased risk of infection · interstitial lung disease · muscle spasms · musculoskeletal pain · nausea · neoplasms · neutropenia · peripheral oedema · sepsis · skin reactions · stomatitis · thrombocytopenia · tumour lysis syndrome · vision blurred · vomiting

▶ **Uncommon** Angioedema · hepatitis B reactivation · leukostasis syndrome · panniculitis

▶ **Frequency not known** Anaemia · hepatic failure · progressive multifocal leukoencephalopathy · Stevens-Johnson syndrome

● CONCEPTION AND CONTRACEPTION Highly effective contraception (must include a non-hormonal method) required during and for 3 months after stopping treatment.

● PREGNANCY Manufacturer advises avoid—toxicity in *animal* studies. See also *Pregnancy and reproductive function* in Cytotoxic drugs p. 865.

● BREAST FEEDING Manufacturer advises discontinue breastfeeding—no information available.

● HEPATIC IMPAIRMENT Avoid in severe impairment.
Dose adjustments Reduce dose to 280 mg daily in mild impairment and reduce dose to 140 mg daily in moderate impairment—monitor for toxicity and adjust dose if necessary (consult product literature).

● RENAL IMPAIRMENT Use in severe impairment only if benefit outweighs risk and with close monitoring for toxicity.
Monitoring Maintain hydration and monitor serum creatinine periodically in mild to moderate renal impairment.

● MONITORING REQUIREMENTS
▶ Monitor full blood count once a month.
▶ Monitor for atrial fibrillation (increased risk in cardiac risk factors, acute infections and history of atrial fibrillation), monitor all patients periodically and complete ECG if arrhythmic symptoms or dyspnoea develop—consult product literature for treatment options.

● NATIONAL FUNDING/ACCESS DECISIONS

NICE decisions

▶ Ibrutinib for previously treated chronic lymphocytic leukaemia and untreated chronic lymphocytic leukaemia with 17p deletion or TP53 mutation (January 2017) NICE TA429
Ibrutinib alone is recommended within its marketing authorisation as an option for treating chronic lymphocytic leukaemia in adults who have had at least one prior therapy **or** who have a 17p deletion or TP53 mutation, and in whom chemo-immunotherapy is unsuitable, only when the manufacturer provides ibrutinib with the discount agreed in the patient access scheme.
www.nice.org.uk/guidance/ta429

▶ Ibrutinib for treating Waldenstrom's macroglobulinaemia (November 2017) NICE TA491
Ibrutinib is recommended for use in the Cancer Drugs Fund as an option for treating Waldenstrom's macroglobulinaemia in adults who have had at least 1 prior therapy, only if the conditions in the managed access agreement for ibrutinib are followed.
Patients whose treatment was started within the NHS before this guidance was published should have the option to continue treatment, without change to their funding arrangements, until they and their NHS clinician consider it appropriate to stop.
www.nice.org.uk/guidance/ta491

▶ Ibrutinib for treating relapsed or refractory mantle cell lymphoma (January 2018) NICE TA502
Ibrutinib is recommended as an option for treating relapsed or refractory mantle cell lymphoma in adults, only if:
● they have had only one previous line of therapy, **and**
● the manufacturer provides ibrutinib with the discount agreed in the commercial access agreement with NHS England.
Patients whose treatment was started within the NHS before this guidance was published should have the option to continue treatment, without change to their funding arrangements, until they and their NHS clinician consider it appropriate to stop.
www.nice.org.uk/guidance/ta502

Scottish Medicines Consortium (SMC) Decisions
The *Scottish Medicines Consortium* has advised (April 2017) that ibrutinib (*Imbruvica*®) is accepted for restricted use within NHS Scotland for the treatment of relapsed or refractory chronic lymphocytic leukaemia in adults who have received at least one prior therapy and for whom fludarabine-based regimens are inappropriate. This advice

8

Immune system and malignant disease

is contingent upon the continuing availability of the Patient Access Scheme in NHS Scotland or a list price that is equivalent or lower.

- MEDICINAL FORMS
There can be variation in the licensing of different medicines containing the same drug.

Capsule

CAUTIONARY AND ADVISORY LABELS 25
- Imbruvica (Janssen-Cilag Ltd) ▼
Ibrutinib 140 mg Imbruvica 140mg capsules | 90 capsule [PoM] £4,599.00 | 120 capsule [PoM] £6,132.00

Idelalisib
16-Nov-2016
- DRUG ACTION Idelalisib is a protein kinase inhibitor.

- INDICATIONS AND DOSE

Treatment of chronic lymphocytic leukaemia in patients who have received at least one previous therapy, or as first-line treatment in the presence of 17p deletion or TP53 mutation in patients who are not eligible for any other therapies (in combination with rituximab) | Treatment of follicular lymphoma refractory to two lines of treatment (monotherapy)
- BY MOUTH
- Adult: 150 mg twice daily, for dose adjustment due to side effects, consult product literature

> IMPORTANT SAFETY INFORMATION
>
> RISKS OF INCORRECT DOSING OF ORAL ANTI-CANCER MEDICINES
> See Cytotoxic drugs p. 865.
>
> MHRA/CHM ADVICE: IDELALISIB (ZYDELIG®): UPDATED INDICATIONS AND ADVICE ON MINIMISING THE RISK OF INFECTION (SEPTEMBER 2016)
> In light of a recent safety review the indications for idelalisib have been updated. Manufacturer recommendations regarding monitoring for infection and prophylaxis of *Pneumocystis jirovecii* pneumonia have also been updated. Patients should be advised on the risk of serious or fatal infections during treatment, and idelalisib should not be initiated in patients with any evidence of infection.

- CAUTIONS Active hepatitis · diarrhoea—symptomatic management recommended (consult product literature) · pneumonitis—withhold treatment (consult product literature)
- INTERACTIONS → Appendix 1: idelalisib
- SIDE-EFFECTS
- **Common or very common** Colitis · diarrhoea · fever · infection · neutropenia · pneumonitis · rash
- **Rare or very rare** Severe cutaneous adverse reactions (SCARs)
- CONCEPTION AND CONTRACEPTION Highly effective contraception (in addition to barrier method) required during and for one month after treatment.
- PREGNANCY Manufacturer advises avoid (toxicity in *animal* studies). See also *Pregnancy and reproductive function* in Cytotoxic drugs p. 865.
- BREAST FEEDING Manufacturer advises avoid—no information available.
- HEPATIC IMPAIRMENT Manufacturer advises caution in hepatic impairment.
- MONITORING REQUIREMENTS
- Manufacturer advises monitor liver function—consult product literature.
- Manufacturer advises monitor for signs and symptoms of infection, including *cytomegalovirus* infection and respiratory infections; new symptoms should be reported promptly. Neutrophil count should be monitored in all

patients every 2 weeks for the first 6 months of treatment; patients with neutrophil count <1000 per mm³ should be monitored weekly.

- NATIONAL FUNDING/ACCESS DECISIONS
NICE decisions
- **Idelalisib for treating chronic lymphocytic leukaemia (October 2015)** NICE TA359
Idelalisib, in combination with rituximab, is recommended as an option for treatment in adults:
- who have untreated chronic lymphocytic leukaemia **or**
- who have chronic lymphocytic leukaemia when the disease has been treated but has relapsed within 24 months **and**
- if the manufacturer provides idelalisib with the discount agreed in the simple discount agreement.
Patients who are already receiving idelalisib should continue treatment until they and their clinician consider it appropriate to stop.
www.nice.org.uk/guidance/TA359

Scottish Medicines Consortium (SMC) Decisions
The *Scottish Medicines Consortium* has advised (March 2015) that idelalisib (*Zydelig*®) is accepted for restricted use within NHS Scotland, in combination with rituximab, for the treatment of relapsed chronic lymphocytic leukaemia in patients who are unsuitable for chemotherapy and treatment naïve patients with 17p depletion or TP53 mutation who are unsuitable for chemo-immunotherapy, only whilst idelalisib is available at the price agreed in the patient access scheme.

All Wales Medicines Strategy Group (AWMSG) Decisions
The *All Wales Medicines Strategy Group* has advised (April 2017) that idelalisib (*Zydelig*®) is recommended as an option for use within NHS Wales as monotherapy for the treatment of patients with follicular lymphoma, that is refractory to two prior lines of treatment. The recommendation applies only if the approved Wales Patient Access Scheme (WPAS) is used or where the list price is equivalent or lower.

- MEDICINAL FORMS
There can be variation in the licensing of different medicines containing the same drug.

Tablet

CAUTIONARY AND ADVISORY LABELS 25
- Zydelig (Gilead Sciences International Ltd) ▼
Idelalisib 100 mg Zydelig 100mg tablets | 60 tablet [PoM] £3,114.75 (Hospital only)
Idelalisib 150 mg Zydelig 150mg tablets | 60 tablet [PoM] £3,114.75 (Hospital only)

Imatinib
21-Jul-2016
- DRUG ACTION Imatinib is a tyrosine kinase inhibitor.

- INDICATIONS AND DOSE

Treatment of chronic myeloid leukaemia in chronic phase after failure with interferon alfa
- BY MOUTH
- Adult: 400 mg once daily, increased if necessary up to 800 mg daily in 2 divided doses

Treatment of chronic myeloid leukaemia in accelerated phase, or in blast crisis
- BY MOUTH
- Adult: 600 mg once daily, then increased if necessary up to 800 mg daily in 2 divided doses

Treatment of newly diagnosed acute lymphoblastic leukaemia (in combination with other chemotherapy) | Monotherapy for relapsed or refractory acute lymphoblastic leukaemia
- BY MOUTH
- Adult: 600 mg once daily

Treatment of c-kit (CD117)-positive unresectable or metastatic malignant gastro-intestinal stromal tumours (GIST) | Adjuvant treatment following resection of c-kit (CD117)-positive GIST, in patients at significant risk of relapse | Treatment of myelodysplastic/myeloproliferative diseases associated with platelet-derived growth factor receptor gene rearrangement

▶ BY MOUTH
▶ Adult: 400 mg once daily

Treatment of unresectable dermatofibrosarcoma protuberans | Recurrent or metastatic dermatofibrosarcoma protuberans, in patients who cannot have surgery

▶ BY MOUTH
▶ Adult: 800 mg daily in 2 divided doses

Treatment of advanced hypereosinophilic syndrome and chronic eosinophilic leukaemia

▶ BY MOUTH
▶ Adult: 100–400 mg once daily

IMPORTANT SAFETY INFORMATION

RISKS OF INCORRECT DOSING OF ORAL ANTI-CANCER MEDICINES
See Cytotoxic drugs p. 865.

MHRA/CHM ADVICE (MAY 2016): RISK OF HEPATITIS B VIRUS REACTIVATION WITH BCR-ABL TYROSINE KINASE INHIBITORS
An EU wide review has concluded that imatinib can cause hepatitis B reactivation; the MHRA recommends establishing hepatitis B virus status in all patients before initiation of treatment.

● CAUTIONS Cardiac disease · hepatitis B infection · history of renal failure · risk factors for heart failure
  CAUTIONS, FURTHER INFORMATION
▶ Hepatitis B infection The MHRA advises that patients who are carriers of hepatitis B virus should be closely monitored for signs and symptoms of active infection throughout treatment and for several months after stopping treatment; expert advice should be sought for patients who test positive for hepatitis B virus and in those with active infection.

● INTERACTIONS → Appendix 1: imatinib

● SIDE-EFFECTS
▶ Common or very common Alopecia · anaemia · appetite abnormal · asthenia · bone marrow disorders · chills · constipation · cough · diarrhoea · dizziness · dry eye · dry mouth · dyspnoea · excessive tearing · eye inflammation · fever · fluid imbalance · flushing · gastrointestinal discomfort · gastrointestinal disorders · haemorrhage · headaches · insomnia · joint disorders · muscle complaints · nausea · neutropenia · oedema · pain · photosensitivity reaction · sensation abnormal · skin reactions · sweat changes · taste altered · thrombocytopenia · vision blurred · vomiting · weight changes
▶ Uncommon Anxiety · arrhythmias · ascites · breast abnormalities · broken nails · burping · chest pain · CNS haemorrhage · congestive heart failure · depression · drowsiness · dysphagia · electrolyte imbalance · eosinophilia · eye discomfort · gout · gynaecomastia · hearing impairment · hepatic disorders · hyperbilirubinaemia · hyperglycaemia · hypertension · hyperuricaemia · hypotension · increased risk of infection · laryngeal pain · lymphadenopathy · lymphopenia · malaise · memory loss · menstrual cycle irregularities · nerve disorders · oral disorders · palpitations · pancreatitis · peripheral coldness · pulmonary oedema · Raynaud's phenomenon · renal impairment · renal pain · respiratory disorders · restless legs · scrotal oedema · sepsis · sexual dysfunction · syncope · thrombocytosis · tremor · urinary frequency increased · vertigo

▶ Rare or very rare Angina pectoris · angioedema · arthritis · cardiac arrest · cataract · confusion · glaucoma · haemolytic anaemia · haemorrhagic ovarian cyst · hepatic failure (including fatal cases) · hypersensitivity vasculitis · inflammatory bowel disease · intracranial pressure increased · muscle weakness · myocardial infarction · myopathy · nail discolouration · pericardial disorders · pulmonary hypertension · seizure · severe cutaneous adverse reactions (SCARs) · tumour lysis syndrome
▶ Frequency not known Embolism and thrombosis · hepatitis B reactivation · neoplasm complications · osteonecrosis · pericarditis

● CONCEPTION AND CONTRACEPTION Effective contraception required during treatment.

● PREGNANCY Manufacturer advises avoid unless potential benefit outweighs risk. See also *Pregnancy and reproductive function* in Cytotoxic drugs p. 865.

● BREAST FEEDING Discontinue breast-feeding.

● HEPATIC IMPAIRMENT
  Dose adjustments Max. 400 mg daily; reduce dose further if not tolerated.

● RENAL IMPAIRMENT
  Dose adjustments Maximum starting dose 400 mg daily if creatinine clearance less than 60 mL/minute; reduce dose further if not tolerated.

● MONITORING REQUIREMENTS
▶ Monitor for gastrointestinal haemorrhage.
▶ Monitor complete blood counts regularly.
▶ Monitor for fluid retention.
▶ Monitor liver function.
▶ Monitor growth in children (may cause growth retardation).

● DIRECTIONS FOR ADMINISTRATION Tablets may be dispersed in water or apple juice.

● PATIENT AND CARER ADVICE Patients or carers should be given advice on how to administer imatinib tablets.

● NATIONAL FUNDING/ACCESS DECISIONS

NICE decisions
▶ Imatinib for the adjuvant treatment of gastro-intestinal stromal tumours (November 2014) NICE TA326
Imatinib is recommended as an option for adjuvant treatment of adult patients who are at high risk of relapse after surgery for KIT (CD117)-positive gastro-intestinal stromal tumours, as defined by the Miettinen 2006 criteria (based on tumour size, location, and mitotic rate), for up to 3 years.
  Patients currently receiving treatment initiated within the NHS with imatinib that is not recommended for them by NICE in this guidance should be able to continue treatment until they and their NHS clinician consider it appropriate to stop.
www.nice.org.uk/TA326
▶ Imatinib for chronic myeloid leukaemia (updated January 2016) NICE TA70
Imatinib is recommended as an option for patients with Philadelphia-chromosome-positive chronic myeloid leukaemia who initially present in the accelerated phase or with blast crisis. Imatinib is also recommended as an option for patients who present in the chronic phase and then progress to the accelerated phase or blast crisis if they have not received imatinib previously.
www.nice.org.uk/TA70
▶ Imatinib for the treatment of unresectable and/or metastatic gastro-intestinal stromal tumours (October 2004) NICE TA86
Imatinib 400 mg daily is recommended as first-line management of KIT (CD117)-positive unresectable or metastatic, or both, gastro-intestinal stromal tumours. Continued therapy is recommended only if a response to initial treatment [as defined by Southwest Oncology Group criteria available at www.nice.org.uk/TA86] is achieved

8

Immune system and malignant disease

within 12 weeks. Patients who have responded should be assessed at 12-week intervals. Discontinue if tumour ceases to respond.
www.nice.org.uk/TA86

▶ **Imatinib for the treatment of unresectable and/or metastatic gastro-intestinal stromal tumours (November 2010)** NICE TA209
Imatinib 600 mg daily or 800 mg daily is **not** recommended for unresectable or metastatic, or both, gastro-intestinal stromal tumours whose disease has progressed after treatment with imatinib 400 mg daily.
www.nice.org.uk/TA209

▶ **Dasatinib, nilotinib and imatinib for untreated chronic myeloid leukaemia (CML) (December 2016)** NICE TA426
Imatinib is recommended as an option for untreated chronic phase Philadelphia-chromosome-positive CML in adults.
www.nice.org.uk/TA426

▶ **Dasatinib, nilotinib and high-dose imatinib for treating imatinib-resistant or intolerant chronic myeloid leukaemia (CML) (December 2016)** NICE TA425
High-dose imatinib (600 mg in the chronic phase or 800 mg in the accelerated and blast-crisis phases) is **not** recommended for treating Philadelphia-chromosome-positive CML in adults whose disease is imatinib-resistant.
Patients whose treatment was started within the NHS before this guidance was published should have the option to continue treatment, without change to their funding arrangements, until they and their clinician consider it appropriate to stop.
www.nice.org.uk/TA425

Scottish Medicines Consortium (SMC) Decisions
The *Scottish Medicines Consortium* has advised (March 2002) that imatinib (*Glivec*®) should be used for chronic myeloid leukaemia only under specialist supervision in accordance with British Society of Haematology guidelines (November 2001).
The *Scottish Medicines Consortium* has also advised (February 2012) that imatinib (*Glivec*®) is accepted for restricted use within NHS Scotland for the treatment of adult patients who are at significant risk of relapse following resection of a KIT (CD117) positive gastrointestinal stromal tumour (GIST) and who are at high risk of recurrence following complete resection (according to the Armed Forces Institute of Pathology (AFIP) risk criteria).

● MEDICINAL FORMS
There can be variation in the licensing of different medicines containing the same drug.
Tablet
CAUTIONARY AND ADVISORY LABELS 21, 27
▶ Imatinib (Non-proprietary)
Imatinib (as Imatinib mesilate) 100 mg Imatinib 100mg tablets | 30 tablet [PoM] £486.66 | 60 tablet [PoM] £973.32 DT = £405.85
Imatinib (as Imatinib mesilate) 400 mg Imatinib 400mg tablets | 30 tablet [PoM] £1,946.67 DT = £811.72 | 60 tablet [PoM] £3,893.34
▶ Glivec (Novartis Pharmaceuticals UK Ltd) ▼
Imatinib (as Imatinib mesilate) 100 mg Glivec 100mg tablets | 60 tablet [PoM] £973.32 DT = £405.85
Imatinib (as Imatinib mesilate) 400 mg Glivec 400mg tablets | 30 tablet [PoM] £1,946.67 DT = £811.72

Lapatinib

● DRUG ACTION Lapatinib is a tyrosine kinase inhibitor.

● INDICATIONS AND DOSE
Treatment of advanced or metastatic breast cancer in patients with tumours that overexpress human epidermal growth factor receptor-2 (HER2) with hormone-receptor-negative disease who have had previous treatment with trastuzumab in combination with chemotherapy (in combination with trastuzumab)
▶ BY MOUTH
▸ Adult: 1 g once daily
Treatment of advanced or metastatic breast cancer in patients with tumours that overexpress human epidermal growth factor receptor-2 (HER2), for patients who have had previous treatment with an anthracycline, a taxane, and trastuzumab (in combination with capecitabine)
▶ BY MOUTH
▸ Adult: 1.25 g once daily
Treatment of advanced or metastatic breast cancer with tumours that overexpress human epidermal growth factor receptor-2 (HER2), for postmenopausal women with hormone-receptor-positive disease (in combination with an aromatase inhibitor)
▶ BY MOUTH
▸ Adult: 1.5 g once daily

IMPORTANT SAFETY INFORMATION
RISKS OF INCORRECT DOSING OF ORAL ANTI-CANCER MEDICINES
See Cytotoxic drugs p. 865.

● CAUTIONS Diarrhoea—withhold treatment if severe (consult product literature) · low gastric pH (reduced absorption) · susceptibility to QT-interval prolongation (including electrolyte disturbances)
● INTERACTIONS → Appendix 1: lapatinib
● SIDE-EFFECTS
▶ **Common or very common** Alopecia · appetite decreased · arthralgia · asthenia · constipation · cough · dehydration · diarrhoea (treat promptly) · dyspnoea · epistaxis · gastrointestinal discomfort · headache · hepatotoxicity (discontinue permanently if severe) · hot flush · hyperbilirubinaemia · insomnia · mucositis · nail disorder · nausea · pain · paronychia · skin reactions · stomatitis · vomiting
▶ **Uncommon** Respiratory disorders
▶ **Frequency not known** Severe cutaneous adverse reactions (SCARs)
● CONCEPTION AND CONTRACEPTION Contraceptive advice required, see *Pregnancy and reproductive function* in Cytotoxic drugs p. 865.
● PREGNANCY Avoid unless potential benefit outweighs risk—toxicity in *animal* studies. See also Pregnancy and reproductive function in Cytotoxic drugs p. 865.
● BREAST FEEDING Discontinue breast-feeding.
● HEPATIC IMPAIRMENT Caution in moderate to severe impairment—metabolism reduced.
● RENAL IMPAIRMENT Caution in severe impairment—no information available.
● MONITORING REQUIREMENTS
▶ Monitor left ventricular function.
▶ Monitor for pulmonary toxicity.
▶ Monitor liver function before treatment and at monthly intervals.
● DIRECTIONS FOR ADMINISTRATION Always take at the same time in relation to food: either one hour before or one hour after food.

- **PATIENT AND CARER ADVICE** Counselling advised (administration). Patients should be advised to report any unexpected changes in bowel habit.
- **NATIONAL FUNDING/ACCESS DECISIONS**

NICE decisions

▶ Lapatinib or trastuzumab in combination with an aromatase inhibitor for the first-line treatment of metastatic hormone-receptor-positive breast cancer that overexpresses HER2 (June 2012) NICE TA257

Lapatinib or trastuzumab in combination with an aromatase inhibitor is **not** recommended for first-line treatment in postmenopausal women of metastatic hormone-receptor-positive breast cancer that overexpresses human epidermal growth factor receptor 2 (HER2).

Postmenopausal women currently receiving lapatinib or trastuzumab in combination with an aromatase inhibitor for this indication should have the option to continue treatment until they and their clinician consider it appropriate to stop.

www.nice.org.uk/TA257

- **MEDICINAL FORMS**
There can be variation in the licensing of different medicines containing the same drug.

Tablet

▶ Tyverb (Novartis Pharmaceuticals UK Ltd)
  Lapatinib ditosylate monohydrate 250 mg Tyverb 250mg tablets
  | 84 tablet [PoM] £965.16 | 105 tablet [PoM] £1,206.45

Lenvatinib   20-Mar-2018

- **DRUG ACTION** Lenvatinib is a multireceptor tyrosine kinase inhibitor.

- **INDICATIONS AND DOSE**

KISPLYX ®

Advanced renal cell carcinoma following one prior vascular endothelial growth factor-targeted therapy (in combination with everolimus) (specialist use only)

▶ BY MOUTH
▶ Adult: 18 mg once daily, dose should be taken at the same time every day, for dose adjustment due to side-effects—consult product literature

LENVIMA ®

Progressive, locally advanced, or metastatic, differentiated thyroid carcinoma that is refractory to radioactive iodine (specialist use only)

▶ BY MOUTH
▶ Adult: 24 mg once daily, dose should be taken at the same time every day, for dose adjustments due to side-effects—consult product literature

> **IMPORTANT SAFETY INFORMATION**
> RISKS OF INCORRECT DOSING OF ORAL ANTI-CANCER MEDICINES
> See Cytotoxic drugs p. 865.

- **CONTRA-INDICATIONS** Fistulae
- **CAUTIONS** Arterial thromboembolism within the previous 6 months · elderly (75 years and over)—reduced tolerability · hypertension—blood pressure should be well-controlled prior to treatment
- **SIDE-EFFECTS**
▶ **Common or very common** Alopecia · appetite decreased · arthralgia · asthenia · cerebrovascular insufficiency · cholecystitis · constipation · dehydration · diarrhoea · dizziness · dry mouth · dysphonia · electrolyte imbalance · embolism and thrombosis · gastrointestinal discomfort · gastrointestinal disorders · headache · heart failure · hepatic disorders · hypercholesterolaemia · hypertension ·

hypoalbuminaemia · hypotension · hypothyroidism · increased risk of infection · insomnia · lymphopenia · malaise · metrorrhagia · mucositis · myalgia · myocardial infarction · nausea · oral disorders · oropharyngeal pain · pain · peripheral oedema · proteinuria · QT interval prolongation · renal impairment · renal tubular necrosis · skin reactions · taste altered · thrombocytopenia · vomiting · weight decreased

▶ **Uncommon** Pancreatitis · paresis · posterior reversible encephalopathy syndrome (PRES) · splenic infarction
▶ **Frequency not known** Fistula

SIDE-EFFECTS, FURTHER INFORMATION Manufacturer advises gastrointestinal toxicity should be actively managed—dehydration and/or hypovolaemia caused by gastrointestinal toxicity are identified as primary risk factors for renal impairment or failure.

- **CONCEPTION AND CONTRACEPTION** Manufacturer advises women of child-bearing potential should use highly effective contraception during treatment and for 1 month after the last dose, an additional barrier method of contraception should be used in women using oral hormonal contraceptives. See also *Pregnancy and reproductive function* in Cytotoxic drugs p. 865.

- **PREGNANCY** Manufacturer advises avoid unless potential benefit outweighs risk—teratogenic in *animal* studies. See also *Pregnancy and reproductive function* in Cytotoxic drugs p. 865.

- **BREAST FEEDING** Manufacturer advises avoid—present in milk in *animal* studies.

- **HEPATIC IMPAIRMENT**
KISPLYX ® Manufacturer advises use only if potential benefit outweighs risk in severe impairment.
Dose adjustments Manufacturer advises reduce dose to 10 mg once daily in severe impairment; further dose adjustments may be necessary based on individual tolerability—consult product literature.

LENVIMA ® **Dose adjustments** Manufacturer advises reduce dose to 14 mg once daily in severe impairment; further dose adjustments may be necessary based on tolerability—consult product literature.

- **RENAL IMPAIRMENT**
KISPLYX ® Manufacturer advises avoid in end-stage renal disease.
Dose adjustments Manufacturer advises reduce dose to 10 mg once daily in severe impairment; further dose adjustments may be necessary based on individual tolerability—consult product literature.

LENVIMA ® Manufacturer advises avoid in end-stage renal disease.
Dose adjustments Manufacturer advises reduce dose to 14 mg once daily in severe impairment; further dose adjustments may be necessary based on tolerability—consult product literature.

- **MONITORING REQUIREMENTS**
▶ Manufacturer advises monitor blood pressure after 1 week of treatment, then every 2 weeks for the first 2 months, and then monthly thereafter; monitor for signs and symptoms of cardiac decompensation (adjust dose as necessary—consult product literature).
▶ Manufacturer advises monitor liver function before treatment, then every 2 weeks for the first 2 months, and then monthly thereafter; monitor urine protein regularly.
▶ Manufacturer advises monitor ECG and electrolytes before and periodically during treatment (calcium levels should be monitored at least monthly), correct electrolyte abnormalities prior to treatment; monitor thyroid function before and regularly during treatment.

- **DIRECTIONS FOR ADMINISTRATION**
KISPLYX ® Manufacturer advises capsules should be swallowed whole, or alternatively, capsules may be

dissolved in a tablespoon of water or apple juice (do not break or crush capsules), allow to sit for at least 10 minutes for capsule shell to dissolve.

● PATIENT AND CARER ADVICE

Missed doses Manufacturer advises if a dose is more than 12 hours late, the missed dose should not be taken and the next dose should be taken at the normal time.

Driving and skilled tasks Manufacturer advises patients and carers should be counselled on the effects on driving and performance of skilled tasks—increased risk of fatigue and dizziness.

● NATIONAL FUNDING/ACCESS DECISIONS

KISPLYX ®

NICE decisions

▶ Lenvatinib with everolimus for previously treated advanced renal cell carcinoma (January 2018) NICE TA498

Lenvatinib plus everolimus is recommended as an option for treating advanced renal cell carcinoma in adults who have had one previous vascular endothelial growth factor (VEGF)-targeted therapy, only if:

● their Eastern Cooperative Oncology Group (ECOG) performance status score is 0 or 1, **and**

● the manufacturer provides lenvatinib with the discount agreed in the patient access scheme.

Patients whose treatment was started within the NHS before this guidance was published should have the option to continue treatment, without change to their funding arrangements, until they and their NHS clinician consider it appropriate to stop.

www.nice.org.uk/guidance/ta498

LENVIMA ®

Scottish Medicines Consortium (SMC) Decisions

The *Scottish Medicines Consortium* has advised (October 2016) that lenvatinib (*Lenvima* ®) is accepted for use within NHS Scotland for treatment of adults with progressive, locally advanced or metastatic, differentiated (papillary/follicular/Hürthle cell) thyroid carcinoma, refractory to radioactive iodine. This advice is contingent upon the continuing availability of the patient access scheme in NHS Scotland or a list price that is equivalent or lower.

All Wales Medicines Strategy Group (AWMSG) Decisions

The *All Wales Medicines Strategy Group* has advised (October 2017) that lenvatinib (*Lenvima* ®) is recommended as an option for restricted use within NHS Wales for the treatment of adults with progressive, locally advanced or metastatic, differentiated (papillary/follicular/Hürthle cell) thyroid carcinoma, refractory to radioactive iodine. This recommendation applies only in circumstances where the approved Wales Patient Access Scheme (WPAS) is utilised or where the list/contract price is equivalent or lower.

● MEDICINAL FORMS

There can be variation in the licensing of different medicines containing the same drug.

Capsule

CAUTIONARY AND ADVISORY LABELS 25

▶ Kisplyx (Eisai Ltd) ▼

Lenvatinib (as Lenvatinib mesilate) 4 mg Kisplyx 4mg capsules | 30 capsule PoM £1,437.00 (Hospital only)

Lenvatinib (as Lenvatinib mesilate) 10 mg Kisplyx 10mg capsules | 30 capsule PoM £1,437.00 (Hospital only)

▶ Lenvima (Eisai Ltd) ▼

Lenvatinib (as Lenvatinib mesilate) 4 mg Lenvima 4mg capsules | 30 capsule PoM £1,437.00

Lenvatinib (as Lenvatinib mesilate) 10 mg Lenvima 10mg capsules | 30 capsule PoM £1,437.00

Midostaurin

11-May-2018

● DRUG ACTION Midostaurin is an inhibitor of multiple tyrosine kinases.

● INDICATIONS AND DOSE

Acute myeloid leukaemia (specialist use only)

▶ BY MOUTH

▶ Adult: 50 mg twice daily, on days 8–21 of induction and consolidation chemotherapy cycles; for administration following consolidation chemotherapy, and dose adjustment or treatment interruption due to side-effects—consult product literature

Aggressive systemic mastocytosis (specialist use only) | Systemic mastocytosis with associated haematological neoplasm (specialist use only) | Mast cell leukaemia (specialist use only)

▶ BY MOUTH

▶ Adult: 100 mg twice daily, for dose adjustment or treatment interruption due to side-effects—consult product literature

---

IMPORTANT SAFETY INFORMATION

RISKS OF INCORRECT DOSING OF ORAL ANTI-CANCER MEDICINES

See Cytotoxic drugs p. 865.

● CAUTIONS Active severe infection (control before initiation of monotherapy) · elderly (limited experience) · patients at risk of congestive heart failure · risk factors for QT-interval prolongation

● INTERACTIONS → Appendix 1: midostaurin

● SIDE-EFFECTS

▶ **Common or very common** Concentration impaired · constipation · cough · diarrhoea · dizziness · dyspepsia · dyspnoea · fatigue · febrile neutropenia · fever · haemorrhage · headache · hypotension · infection · nausea · oropharyngeal pain · peripheral oedema · respiratory disorders · tremor · vertigo · vomiting · weight increased

▶ **Frequency not known** Congestive heart failure · QT interval prolongation

● CONCEPTION AND CONTRACEPTION Manufacturer advises perform pregnancy test in women of childbearing potential within 7 days prior to treatment initiation; effective contraception must be used during treatment and for at least 4 months after stopping treatment—additional barrier method recommended in women using hormonal contraceptives. See also *Pregnancy and reproductive function* in Cytotoxic drugs p. 865.

● PREGNANCY Manufacturer advises avoid—toxicity in *animal* studies. See also *Pregnancy and reproductive function* in Cytotoxic drugs p. 865.

● BREAST FEEDING Manufacturer advises avoid during treatment and for 4 months after stopping treatment—present in milk in *animal* studies.

● HEPATIC IMPAIRMENT Manufacturer advises caution in severe impairment and monitor for toxicity—no information available.

● RENAL IMPAIRMENT Manufacturer advises caution in severe impairment and monitor for toxicity—limited information available.

● MONITORING REQUIREMENTS

▶ Manufacturer advises monitor white blood cell count regularly, especially at treatment initiation; also monitor for signs and symptoms of infection.

▶ Manufacturer advises assess left ventricular ejection fraction in patients at risk of congestive heart failure at baseline and during treatment as clinically indicated; consider performing ECGs if concomitant use with drugs that can prolong QT-interval.

▸ Manufacturer advises monitor for pulmonary symptoms indicative of interstitial lung disease or pneumonitis.

● MEDICINAL FORMS
There can be variation in the licensing of different medicines containing the same drug.

Capsule
CAUTIONARY AND ADVISORY LABELS 21, 25
EXCIPIENTS: May contain Alcohol
▸ Rydapt (Novartis Pharmaceuticals UK Ltd) ▼
Midostaurin 25 mg Rydapt 25mg capsules | 56 capsule [PoM]
£5,609.94

Nilotinib

10-Apr-2018

● DRUG ACTION Nilotinib is a tyrosine kinase inhibitor.

● INDICATIONS AND DOSE

Newly diagnosed chronic phase Philadelphia chromosome-positive chronic myeloid leukaemia (initiated by a specialist)
▸ BY MOUTH
▸ Adult: 300 mg twice daily, for dose adjustments due to side-effects—consult product literature

Chronic and accelerated phase Philadelphia chromosome-positive chronic myeloid leukaemia resistant or intolerant to previous therapy, including imatinib (initiated by a specialist)
▸ BY MOUTH
▸ Adult: 400 mg twice daily, for dose adjustments due to side-effects—consult product literature

IMPORTANT SAFETY INFORMATION
RISKS OF INCORRECT DOSING OF ORAL ANTI-CANCER MEDICINES
See Cytotoxic drugs p. 865.

MHRA/CHM ADVICE (MAY 2016): RISK OF HEPATITIS B VIRUS REACTIVATION WITH TYROSINE KINASE INHIBITORS
An EU wide review has concluded that nilotinib can cause hepatitis B virus reactivation; the MHRA recommends establishing hepatitis B virus status in all patients before initiation of treatment.

● CAUTIONS Clinically significant bradycardia · congestive heart failure · hepatitis B infection · history of pancreatitis · recent myocardial infarction · susceptibility to QT-interval prolongation (including electrolyte disturbances) · unstable angina
CAUTIONS, FURTHER INFORMATION
▸ Hepatitis B infection The MHRA advises that patients who are carriers of hepatitis B virus should be closely monitored for signs and symptoms of active infection throughout treatment and for several months after stopping treatment; expert advice should be sought for patients who test positive for hepatitis B virus and in those with active infection.

● INTERACTIONS → Appendix 1: nilotinib

● SIDE-EFFECTS
▸ Common or very common Alopecia · anaemia · angina pectoris · anxiety · appetite abnormal · arrhythmias · arthralgia · asthenia · bone marrow disorders · cardiac conduction disorders · chest discomfort · constipation · cough · decreased leucocytes · depression · diabetes mellitus · diarrhoea · dizziness · dry eye · dyslipidaemia · dyspnoea · electrolyte imbalance · eosinophilia · eye discomfort · eye disorders · eye inflammation · fever · flushing · gastrointestinal discomfort · gastrointestinal disorders · headaches · hepatic disorders · hyperbilirubinaemia · hyperglycaemia · hypertension · increased risk of infection · insomnia · muscle complaints · muscle weakness · myocardial infarction · nausea · neoplasms · neutropenia · oedema · pain · palpitations ·

peripheral neuropathy · QT interval prolongation · respiratory disorders · sensation abnormal · skin reactions · sweat changes · taste altered · thrombocytopenia · vertigo · vomiting · weight changes
▸ Uncommon Atherosclerosis · cerebrovascular insufficiency · chills · cyanosis · erectile dysfunction · gout · haemorrhage · heart failure · hyperaemia · malaise · oral disorders · pancreatitis · peripheral vascular disease · temperature sensation altered · vision disorders
▸ Frequency not known Breast abnormalities · chorioretinopathy · diastolic dysfunction · dry mouth · facial swelling · gynaecomastia · hepatitis B reactivation · hyperparathyroidism · hyperuricaemia · hypoglycaemia · lethargy · memory loss · menorrhagia · oropharyngeal pain · pericardial effusion · pericarditis · restless legs · sebaceous hyperplasia · syncope · tremor · urinary disorders · urine discolouration

● CONCEPTION AND CONTRACEPTION Manufacturer advises highly effective contraception in women of childbearing potential during treatment and for up to two weeks after stopping treatment.

● PREGNANCY Manufacturer advises avoid unless potential benefit outweighs risk—toxicity in *animal* studies; see also *Pregnancy and reproductive function* in Cytotoxic drugs p. 865.

● BREAST FEEDING Manufacturer advises avoid—present in milk in *animal* studies.

● HEPATIC IMPAIRMENT Manufacturer advises caution.

● MONITORING REQUIREMENTS
▸ Manufacturer advises monitor lipid profiles before initiating treatment, at 3 and 6 months, and then yearly thereafter; monitor blood glucose before initiating treatment and then periodically during treatment, as clinically indicated.
▸ Manufacturer advises monitor full blood count every 2 weeks for the first 2 months of treatment, then monthly thereafter, or as clinically indicated.
▸ Manufacturer advises perform baseline ECG before treatment and as clinically indicated thereafter; correct any electrolyte disturbances before treatment and monitor periodically during treatment.
▸ Manufacturer advises monitor and actively manage cardiovascular risk factors during treatment.

● DIRECTIONS FOR ADMINISTRATION Manufacturer advises capsules should either be swallowed whole or the contents of each capsule may be dispersed in one teaspoon of apple sauce and taken immediately.

● PRESCRIBING AND DISPENSING INFORMATION All prescribers should be familiar with the *Summary of Key Safety Recommendations for Tasigna ® (nilotinib)* provided by the manufacturer.

● PATIENT AND CARER ADVICE Manufacturer advises patients and carers should seek immediate medical attention if signs or symptoms of cardiovascular events occur.
All patients should be provided with the *Important Information About How to Take Your Medication* leaflet provided by the manufacturer.

● NATIONAL FUNDING/ACCESS DECISIONS

NICE decisions
▸ **Dasatinib, nilotinib and imatinib for untreated chronic myeloid leukaemia (CML) (December 2016)** NICE TA426
Nilotinib is recommended, within its marketing authorisation, as an option for untreated chronic phase Philadelphia-chromosome-positive CML in adults, only if the manufacturer provides it with the discount agreed in the patient access scheme.
www.nice.org.uk/guidance/ta426

8

Immune system and malignant disease

▸ **Dasatinib, nilotinib and high-dose imatinib for treating imatinib-resistant or intolerant chronic myeloid leukaemia (CML) (December 2016)** NICE TA425
Nilotinib is recommended as an option for treating chronic or accelerated phase Philadelphia-chromosome-positive CML in adults, if they cannot have imatinib, or their disease is imatinib-resistant **and** the manufacturer provides nilotinib with the discount agreed in the patient access scheme.
www.nice.org.uk/guidance/ta425

● **MEDICINAL FORMS**
There can be variation in the licensing of different medicines containing the same drug.
Capsule
CAUTIONARY AND ADVISORY LABELS 23, 25, 27
▸ Tasigna (Novartis Pharmaceuticals UK Ltd)
Nilotinib (as Nilotinib hydrochloride monohydrate)
150 mg Tasigna 150mg capsules | 112 capsule PoM £2,432.85
Nilotinib (as Nilotinib hydrochloride monohydrate)
200 mg Tasigna 200mg capsules | 112 capsule PoM £2,432.85

Nintedanib

23-Feb-2016

● **DRUG ACTION** Nintedanib is a tyrosine protein kinase inhibitor.

● **INDICATIONS AND DOSE**
OFEV®

Treatment of idiopathic pulmonary fibrosis
▸ BY MOUTH
▸ Adult: 150 mg twice daily, reduced if not tolerated to 100 mg twice daily, for dose adjustments due to side-effects, consult product literature

VARGATEF®

Treatment of locally advanced, metastatic or locally recurrent non-small cell lung cancer of adenocarcinoma histology after first-line chemotherapy (in combination with docetaxel) (initiated under specialist supervision)
▸ BY MOUTH
▸ Adult: 200 mg twice daily on days 2–21 of a standard 21 day docetaxel cycle, for treatment following discontinuation of docetaxel and for dose adjustments due to side-effects, consult product literature

IMPORTANT SAFETY INFORMATION
FOR *VARGATEF®*—RISKS OF INCORRECT DOSING OF ORAL ANTI-CANCER MEDICINES
See Cytotoxic drugs p. 865.

● **CAUTIONS** History or risk factors for QT prolongation · impaired wound healing · increased risk of bleeding · patients at high risk of cardiovascular disease · previous abdominal surgery · recent history of hollow organ perforation · theoretical increased risk of gastrointestinal perforation · theoretical increased risk of venous thromboembolism

● **INTERACTIONS** → Appendix 1: nintedanib

● **SIDE-EFFECTS**
▸ **Common or very common** Abdominal pain · appetite decreased · diarrhoea · haemorrhage · nausea · vomiting · weight decreased
▸ **Uncommon** Dehydration · hyperbilirubinaemia · hypertension · pancreatitis · thrombocytopenia
▸ **Frequency not known** Drug-induced liver injury

● **ALLERGY AND CROSS-SENSITIVITY** Contra-indicated in patients with peanut or soya hypersensitivity.

● **CONCEPTION AND CONTRACEPTION** Manufacturer advises exclude pregnancy before treatment and ensure effective contraception (in addition to barrier method) during treatment and for at least 3 months after last dose.

● **PREGNANCY** Manufacturer advises avoid—toxicity in *animal* studies.
VARGATEF® See also *Pregnancy and reproductive function* in Cytotoxic drugs p. 865.

● **BREAST FEEDING** Manufacturer advises avoid—present in milk in *animal* studies.

● **HEPATIC IMPAIRMENT** Manufacturer advises avoid in moderate to severe impairment—no information available. **Dose adjustments** Consult product literature for dose adjustment in worsening liver function.

● **RENAL IMPAIRMENT** Manufacturer advises caution in severe impairment—no information available.

● **MONITORING REQUIREMENTS** For *Vargatef®*, monitor full blood count and hepatic function before each treatment cycle and regularly thereafter, monitor prothrombin time and INR if used concomitantly with anticoagulants and monitor for signs and symptoms of cerebral bleeding.

● **PRESCRIBING AND DISPENSING INFORMATION**
VARGATEF® Not to be taken on the same day as docetaxel therapy.

● **NATIONAL FUNDING/ACCESS DECISIONS**
NICE decisions
▸ **Nintedanib for previously treated locally advanced, metastatic, or locally recurrent non-small cell lung cancer (July 2015)** NICE TA347
Nintedanib (*Vargatef®*), in combination with docetaxel is recommended as an option for the treatment of patients with locally advanced, metastatic, or locally recurrent non-small cell lung cancer of adenocarcinoma histology, that has progressed after first-line chemotherapy, only if the manufacturer provides nintedanib with the discount agreed in the patient access scheme.
www.nice.org.uk/TA347
▸ **Nintedanib for treating idiopathic pulmonary fibrosis (January 2016)** NICE TA379
Nintedanib is recommended as an option for treating idiopathic pulmonary fibrosis, only if:
● the patient has a forced vital capacity (FVC) between 50% and 80% of predicted,
● the manufacturer provides nintedanib with the discount agreed in the patient access scheme, **and**,
● treatment is stopped if disease progresses (a confirmed decline in percent predicted FVC of 10% or more) in any 12-month period.
www.nice.org.uk/TA379

Scottish Medicines Consortium (SMC) Decisions
The *Scottish Medicines Consortium* has advised (September 2015) that nintedanib (*Ofev®*) is accepted for restricted use within NHS Scotland for the treatment of idiopathic pulmonary fibrosis in patients with a predicted forced vital capacity less than or equal to 80%.

● **MEDICINAL FORMS**
There can be variation in the licensing of different medicines containing the same drug.
Capsule
CAUTIONARY AND ADVISORY LABELS 25
EXCIPIENTS: May contain Lecithin
▸ Ofev (Boehringer Ingelheim Ltd) ▼
Nintedanib (as Nintedanib esilate) 100 mg Ofev 100mg capsules | 60 capsule PoM £2,151.10 (Hospital only)
Nintedanib (as Nintedanib esilate) 150 mg Ofev 150mg capsules | 60 capsule PoM £2,151.10 (Hospital only)
▸ Vargatef (Boehringer Ingelheim Ltd) ▼
Nintedanib (as Nintedanib esilate) 100 mg Vargatef 100mg capsules | 120 capsule PoM £2,151.10 (Hospital only)
Nintedanib (as Nintedanib esilate) 150 mg Vargatef 150mg capsules | 60 capsule PoM £2,151.10 (Hospital only)

Osimertinib
21-Apr-2017

- DRUG ACTION Osimertinib is a tyrosine kinase inhibitor.

- **INDICATIONS AND DOSE**

Locally advanced or metastatic epidermal growth factor receptor T790M mutation-positive non-small-cell lung cancer (specialist use only)
- BY MOUTH
- Adult: 80 mg once daily, for dose adjustment due to side-effects—consult product literature

> **IMPORTANT SAFETY INFORMATION**
> RISKS OF INCORRECT DOSING OF ORAL ANTI-CANCER MEDICINES
> See Cytotoxic drugs p. 865.

- CONTRA-INDICATIONS Congenital long QT syndrome
- CAUTIONS Elderly (more frequent dose adjustments may be required) · history of interstitial lung disease · radiation pneumonitis requiring steroid treatment · risk factors for QTc interval prolongation
- INTERACTIONS → Appendix 1: osimertinib
- SIDE-EFFECTS
- **Common or very common** Diarrhoea · eyelid pruritus · increased risk of infection · nail discolouration · nail disorders · respiratory disorders · skin reactions · stomatitis
- **Uncommon** Eye disorders · eye inflammation · QT interval prolongation
- CONCEPTION AND CONTRACEPTION Manufacturer advises use of effective, non-hormonal, contraception during and for 2 months after treatment in women, and 4 months after treatment in men.
- PREGNANCY Manufacturer advises avoid unless essential—toxicity in *animal* studies. See also *Pregnancy and reproductive function* in Cytotoxic drugs p. 865.
- BREAST FEEDING Manufacturer advises avoid—may be present in milk based on *animal* studies.
- HEPATIC IMPAIRMENT Manufacturer advises caution in mild impairment. Avoid in moderate and severe impairment—limited information available.
- RENAL IMPAIRMENT Manufacturer advises caution in severe and end-stage impairment—limited information available.
- MONITORING REQUIREMENTS Manufacturer advises monitor ECG and electrolytes periodically in patients with risk factors for QTc interval prolongation; dose adjustment is advised if QTc interval is more than 500 milliseconds on at least 2 separate ECGs—consult product literature.
- DIRECTIONS FOR ADMINISTRATION Manufacturer advises tablet may be dispersed in 50 mL of non-carbonated water, by stirring until dispersed and swallowed immediately (do not crush). The residue must then be re-dispersed in an additional half a glass of water and immediately swallowed. Manufacturer advises if administration via a nasogastric tube is required, the tablet may be dispersed in 15 mL of non-carbonated water, by stirring until dispersed and the residue re-dispersed in an additional 15 mL of water (do not crush). The total 30 mL of liquid should then be administered as per the nasogastric tube manufacturer's instructions with appropriate water flushes; the solution should be administered within 30 minutes of adding the tablets to water.
- PATIENT AND CARER ADVICE
Missed doses Manufacturer advises if a dose is more than 12 hours late, the missed dose should not be taken and the next dose should be taken at the normal time.

- NATIONAL FUNDING/ACCESS DECISIONS
NICE decisions
- Osimertinib for treating locally advanced or metastatic EGFR T790M mutation-positive non-small-cell lung cancer (October 2016) NICE TA416
Osimertinib is recommended as an option, for use within the Cancer Drugs Fund, for treating locally advanced or metastatic epidermal growth factor receptor (EGFR) T790M mutation-positive non-small-cell lung cancer in adults whose disease has progressed only:
 - after first-line treatment with an EGFR tyrosine kinase inhibitor, **and**
 - if the conditions in the managed access agreement for osimertinib are followed.
Patients whose treatment was started within the NHS before this guidance was published should have the option to continue treatment, without change to their funding arrangements, until they and their clinician consider it appropriate to stop.
www.nice.org.uk/TA416

Scottish Medicines Consortium (SMC) Decisions
The *Scottish Medicines Consortium* has advised (February 2017) that osimertinib (*Tagrisso*®) is accepted for restricted use within NHS Scotland for the treatment of adult patients with locally advanced or metastatic epidermal growth factor receptor (EGFR) T790M mutation-positive non-small-cell lung cancer, only in patients who have received previous treatment with an EGFR tyrosine kinase inhibitor. This advice is contingent upon the continuing availability of the patient access scheme in NHS Scotland or a list price that is equivalent or lower.

- MEDICINAL FORMS
There can be variation in the licensing of different medicines containing the same drug.
Tablet
- Tagrisso (AstraZeneca UK Ltd) ▼
Osimertinib (as Osimertinib mesylate) 40 mg Tagrisso 40mg tablets | 30 tablet [PoM] £5,770.00
Osimertinib (as Osimertinib mesylate) 80 mg Tagrisso 80mg tablets | 30 tablet [PoM] £5,770.00

Palbociclib
29-Jan-2018

- DRUG ACTION Palbociclib is a highly selective inhibitor of cyclin-dependent kinases 4 and 6, which leads to disruption of cancer cell proliferation.

- **INDICATIONS AND DOSE**

Locally advanced or metastatic breast cancer (initiated by a specialist)
- BY MOUTH
- Adult: 125 mg once daily for 21 consecutive days of repeated 28 day cycles, for dose adjustments due to side-effects—consult product literature

DOSE ADJUSTMENTS DUE TO INTERACTIONS
- If concomitant use with potent CYP3A4 inhibitors (such as clarithromycin, itraconazole, ketoconazole, lopinavir boosted with ritonavir, posaconazole, saquinavir, or voriconazole) is unavoidable, reduce palbociclib dose to 75 mg once daily. If the CYP3A4 inhibitor is stopped, increase the palbociclib dose (after 3–5 half lives of the inhibitor) to the dose used before starting the CYP3A4 inhibitor.

> **IMPORTANT SAFETY INFORMATION**
> RISKS OF INCORRECT DOSING OF ORAL ANTI-CANCER MEDICINES
> See Cytotoxic drugs p. 865.

- INTERACTIONS → Appendix 1: palbociclib

● SIDE-EFFECTS
▶ **Common or very common** Alopecia · anaemia · appetite decreased · asthenia · diarrhoea · dry eye · epistaxis · excessive tearing · fever · infection · leucopenia · mucositis · nausea · neutropenia · oral disorders · oropharyngeal complaints · skin reactions · taste altered · thrombocytopenia · vision blurred · vomiting

SIDE-EFFECTS, FURTHER INFORMATION Side-effects are reported when used in combination with letrozole or fulvestrant.

● CONCEPTION AND CONTRACEPTION Manufacturer advises effective contraception in women of childbearing potential during treatment and for at least 3 weeks after completing treatment. Male patients should use effective contraception during treatment and for at least 14 weeks after completing treatment if their partner is of childbearing potential. See also Pregnancy and reproductive function in Cytotoxic drugs p. 865.

● PREGNANCY Manufacturer advises avoid—toxicity in *animal* studies. See also Pregnancy and reproductive function in Cytotoxic drugs p. 865.

● BREAST FEEDING Manufacturer advises avoid—no information available.

● HEPATIC IMPAIRMENT Manufacturer advises caution and close monitoring for signs of toxicity in moderate-to-severe impairment.
Dose adjustments Manufacturer advises reduce dose to 75 mg once daily in severe impairment.

● RENAL IMPAIRMENT Manufacturer advises caution and monitor closely for signs of toxicity in moderate-to-severe impairment.

● MONITORING REQUIREMENTS Manufacturer advises monitor full blood count prior to starting therapy, at the start of each cycle, on day 14 of the first 2 cycles and as clinically indicated.

● PATIENT AND CARER ADVICE
Missed doses Manufacturer advises to take palbociclib at the same time each day; if a dose is missed, the missed dose should not be taken and the next dose should be taken at the usual time.

● NATIONAL FUNDING/ACCESS DECISIONS
NICE decisions
▶ **Palbociclib with an aromatase inhibitor for previously untreated, hormone receptor-positive, HER2-negative, locally advanced or metastatic breast cancer (December 2017)**
NICE TA495
Palbociclib, with an aromatase inhibitor, is recommended within its marketing authorisation, as an option for treating hormone receptor-positive, human epidermal growth factor receptor 2-negative, locally advanced or metastatic breast cancer as initial endocrine-based therapy in adults. Palbociclib is recommended only if the manufacturer provides it with the discount agreed in the patient access scheme.
www.nice.org.uk/guidance/ta495

Scottish Medicines Consortium (SMC) Decisions
The *Scottish Medicines Consortium* has advised (December 2017) that palbociclib (*Ibrance®*) is accepted for restricted use within NHS Scotland in combination with an aromatase inhibitor for the first-line treatment of hormone receptor (HR)-positive, human epidermal growth factor receptor 2 (HER2)-negative locally advanced or metastatic breast cancer. This advice is contingent upon the continuing availability of the patient access scheme in NHS Scotland or a list price that is equivalent or lower.

● MEDICINAL FORMS
There can be variation in the licensing of different medicines containing the same drug.
Capsule
CAUTIONARY AND ADVISORY LABELS 1, 21, 25
▶ Ibrance (Pfizer Ltd) ▼
Palbociclib 75 mg Ibrance 75mg capsules | 21 capsule [PoM] £2,950.00 (Hospital only)
Palbociclib 100 mg Ibrance 100mg capsules | 21 capsule [PoM] £2,950.00 (Hospital only)
Palbociclib 125 mg Ibrance 125mg capsules | 21 capsule [PoM] £2,950.00 (Hospital only)

Pazopanib

02-Jun-2017

● DRUG ACTION Pazopanib is a tyrosine kinase inhibitor.

● INDICATIONS AND DOSE
First-line treatment of advanced renal cell carcinoma | Treatment of advanced renal cell carcinoma in patients who have had previous treatment with cytokine therapy
▶ BY MOUTH
▶ Adult: 800 mg daily, adjust dose in steps of 200 mg according to tolerability; maximum 800 mg per day
Treatment of selective subtypes of advanced soft-tissue sarcoma
▶ BY MOUTH
▶ Adult: (consult product literature)
DOSE ADJUSTMENTS DUE TO INTERACTIONS
▶ Manufacturer advises if concurrent use of potent inhibitors of CYP3A4 is unavoidable, reduce dose to 400 mg daily.

IMPORTANT SAFETY INFORMATION
RISKS OF INCORRECT DOSING OF ORAL ANTI-CANCER MEDICINES
See Cytotoxic drugs p. 865.

● CONTRA-INDICATIONS Cerebral haemorrhage · clinically significant gastro-intestinal haemorrhage · haemoptysis in the past 6 months

● CAUTIONS Cardiac disease · increased risk of gastro-intestinal fistulas · increased risk of gastro-intestinal perforation · increased risk of haemorrhage · increased risk of thrombotic microangiopathy—permanently discontinue if symptoms develop · ischaemic stroke · myocardial infarction · risk of thrombotic events · susceptibility to QT-interval prolongation (including electrolyte disturbances) · transient ischaemic attack

CAUTIONS, FURTHER INFORMATION
▶ Elective surgery Discontinue treatment 7 days before elective surgery and restart only if adequate wound healing.
▶ Blood pressure Blood pressure must be controlled before initiating treatment.

● INTERACTIONS → Appendix 1: pazopanib

● SIDE-EFFECTS
▶ **Common or very common** Alopecia · appetite decreased · arthralgia · asthenia · bradycardia · cancer pain · cardiac disorder · chest pain · chills · cough · dehydration · diarrhoea · dizziness · drowsiness · dry mouth · dysphonia · dyspnoea · electrolyte imbalance · gastrointestinal discomfort · gastrointestinal disorders · haemorrhage · hair colour changes · headache · hepatic disorders · hiccups · hyperbilirubinaemia · hyperhidrosis · hypertension · hypoalbuminaemia · hypothyroidism · increased risk of infection · insomnia · left ventricular dysfunction · leucopenia · mucosal abnormalities · muscle complaints · musculoskeletal pain · nail disorder · nausea · neutropenia · oedema · oral disorders · peripheral neuropathy · proteinuria · respiratory disorders · sensation abnormal · skin reactions · taste altered · thrombocytopenia ·

vasodilation · venous thromboembolism · vision blurred · vomiting · weight decreased

▶ **Uncommon** Cerebrovascular insufficiency · eye disorders · haemolytic uraemic syndrome · menstrual cycle irregularities · myocardial infarction · myocardial ischaemia · oropharyngeal pain · pancreatitis · photosensitivity reaction · polycythaemia · QT interval prolongation · rhinorrhoea · skin ulcer · thrombotic microangiopathy

▶ **Rare or very rare** Posterior reversible encephalopathy syndrome (PRES)

● CONCEPTION AND CONTRACEPTION Effective contraception advised during treatment.

● PREGNANCY Avoid unless potential benefit outweighs risk—toxicity in *animal* studies. See also *Pregnancy and reproductive function* in Cytotoxic drugs p. 865.

● BREAST FEEDING Discontinue breast-feeding.

● HEPATIC IMPAIRMENT Use with caution in mild to moderate impairment. Avoid in severe impairment.
Dose adjustments Reduce dose to 200 mg once daily in moderate impairment.

● RENAL IMPAIRMENT Use with caution if creatinine clearance less than 30 mL/minute—no information available.

● MONITORING REQUIREMENTS

▶ Monitor liver function before treatment and at weeks 3, 5, 7, and 9, then at months 3 and 4, and periodically thereafter as clinically indicated—consult product literature if elevated liver enzymes observed.

▶ Monitor blood pressure within 1 week of treatment initiation, then frequently throughout treatment (consider dose reduction or interruption if hypertension uncontrolled despite anti-hypertensive therapy; discontinue if blood pressure persistently elevated despite anti-hypertensive therapy and pazopanib dose reduction—consult product literature).

▶ Monitor for signs or symptoms of congestive heart failure—monitor left ventricular ejection fraction in patients at risk of heart failure before and during treatment.

▶ Monitor for proteinuria.

▶ Monitor thyroid function.

▶ Monitor for signs and symptoms of posterior reversible encephalopathy syndrome (including headache, hypertension, seizure, lethargy, confusion, visual and neurological disturbances)—permanently discontinue treatment if symptoms occur.

● NATIONAL FUNDING/ACCESS DECISIONS

NICE decisions

▶ **Pazopanib for the first-line treatment of advanced renal cell carcinoma (updated August 2013) NICE TA215**
Pazopanib is recommended as a first-line treatment option for people with advanced renal cell carcinoma:

● who have not received prior cytokine therapy and have an Eastern Cooperative Oncology Group performance status of 0 or 1 **and**

● if the manufacturer provides pazopanib at the discounted price agreed under the patient access scheme.

www.nice.org.uk/TA215

Scottish Medicines Consortium (SMC) Decisions
The *Scottish Medicines Consortium* has advised (February 2011) that pazopanib (*Votrient*®) is accepted for restricted use within NHS Scotland for the first-line treatment of advanced renal cell carcinoma and (December 2012) is **not** recommended for use within NHS Scotland for the treatment of selective subtypes of advanced soft tissue sarcoma in patients who have received prior chemotherapy for metastatic disease, or who have progressed within 12 months after neoadjuvant therapy.

● MEDICINAL FORMS
There can be variation in the licensing of different medicines containing the same drug.

Tablet
CAUTIONARY AND ADVISORY LABELS 23, 25

▶ Votrient (Novartis Pharmaceuticals UK Ltd)
Pazopanib (as Pazopanib hydrochloride) 200 mg Votrient 200mg tablets | 30 tablet [PoM] £560.50
Pazopanib (as Pazopanib hydrochloride) 400 mg Votrient 400mg tablets | 30 tablet [PoM] £1,121.00

Ponatinib
19-Jul-2017

● INDICATIONS AND DOSE

Treatment of chronic, accelerated, or blast phase chronic myeloid leukaemia in patients who have the T315I mutation or who have resistance to or intolerance of dasatinib or nilotinib, and for whom subsequent treatment with imatinib is not clinically appropriate | Treatment of Philadelphia chromosome-positive acute lymphoblastic leukaemia in patients who have the T315I mutation or who have resistance to or intolerance of dasatinib or nilotinib, and for whom subsequent treatment with imatinib is not clinically appropriate

▶ BY MOUTH

▶ Adult: 45 mg once daily, for dose adjustments due to side-effects or dose reduction due to risk of vascular occlusive events, consult product literature

DOSE ADJUSTMENTS DUE TO INTERACTIONS

▶ Manufacturer advises consider a reduced initial dose of 30 mg daily with concurrent use of potent inhibitors of CYP3A4.

IMPORTANT SAFETY INFORMATION

MHRA/CHM ADVICE: PONATINIB: RISK OF VASCULAR OCCLUSIVE EVENTS—UPDATED ADVICE ON POSSIBLE DOSE REDUCTION (UPDATED APRIL 2017)
The benefits and risks of ponatinib were reviewed by the European Medicines Agency's Committee on Medicinal Products for Human Use in 2014, which recommended that strengthened warnings should be added to the product information aimed at minimising the risk of blood clots and blockages in the arteries. Additional long-term follow-up data are now available that supports new advice on dose modification to reduce this risk. The MHRA advise that although the recommended starting dose of ponatinib remains unchanged, prescribers should consider reducing the dose for patients with chronic phase chronic myeloid leukaemia (CP-CML) who have achieved a major cytogenetic response while on treatment. The following factors should be taken into account in the individual patient assessment:

● cardiovascular risk;

● side-effects of ponatinib therapy (including cardiovascular and other dose-related toxicity);

● time to cytogenetic response;

● BCR-ABL transcript levels.
The MHRA recommends close monitoring of response, if dose reduction is undertaken.

MHRA/CHM ADVICE (MAY 2016): RISK OF HEPATITIS B VIRUS REACTIVATION WITH BCR-ABL TYROSINE KINASE INHIBITORS
An EU wide review has concluded that ponatinib can cause hepatitis B reactivation; the MHRA recommends establishing hepatitis B virus status in all patients before initiation of treatment.

RISKS OF INCORRECT DOSING OF ORAL ANTI-CANCER MEDICINES
See Cytotoxic drugs p. 865.

● CAUTIONS Alcohol abuse—increased risk of pancreatitis · current severe hypertriglyceridaemia—increased risk of

8

Immune system and malignant disease

pancreatitis · discontinue treatment if a complete haematologic response has not occurred within 3 months · hepatitis B infection · history of myocardial infarction—do not use unless potential benefit outweighs potential risk · history of pancreatitis · history of stroke—do not use unless potential benefit outweighs potential risk · hypertension—medically control during treatment and interrupt treatment if uncontrolled

CAUTIONS, FURTHER INFORMATION
▸ Cardiovascular status Assess cardiovascular status before treatment—manage cardiovascular risk factors before and during treatment.
▸ Hepatitis B infection The MHRA advises that patients who are carriers of hepatitis B virus should be closely monitored for signs and symptoms of active infection throughout treatment and for several months after stopping treatment; expert advice should be sought for patients who test positive for hepatitis B virus and in those with active infection.

● INTERACTIONS → Appendix 1: ponatinib

● SIDE-EFFECTS
▸ **Common or very common** Acute coronary syndrome · alopecia · anaemia · appetite decreased · arrhythmias · arthralgia · asthenia · cerebrovascular insufficiency · chills · constipation · cough · diarrhoea · dizziness · dry eye · dry mouth · dysphonia · dyspnoea · electrolyte imbalance · embolism and thrombosis · erectile dysfunction · eye inflammation · febrile neutropenia · fever · fluid imbalance · gastrointestinal discomfort · gastrooesophageal reflux disease · haemorrhage · headaches · heart failure · hyperglycaemia · hypertension · hypertriglyceridaemia · hyperuricaemia · hypothyroidism · increased risk of infection · influenza like illness · insomnia · ischaemic heart disease · lethargy · mass · muscle complaints · nausea · oedema · pain · pancreatitis · pancytopenia · pericardial effusion · peripheral neuropathy · peripheral vascular disease · pleural effusion · pulmonary hypertension · sensation abnormal · sepsis · skin reactions · stomatitis · sweat changes · vasodilation · vision disorders · vomiting · weight decreased
▸ **Uncommon** Cardiac discomfort · cardiomyopathy ischaemic · coronary vasospasm · hepatic disorders · hepatic failure (including fatal cases) · intracranial haemorrhage · left ventricular dysfunction · renal artery stenosis · splenic infarction · tumour lysis syndrome

● CONCEPTION AND CONTRACEPTION Ensure effective contraception during treatment in men and women; effectiveness of hormonal contraception unknown—alternative or additional methods of contraception should be used.

● PREGNANCY Avoid—toxicity in *animal* studies. See also *Pregnancy and reproductive function* in Cytotoxic drugs p. 865.

● BREAST FEEDING Manufacturer advises discontinue breastfeeding—no information available.

● HEPATIC IMPAIRMENT Manufacturer advises caution in severe impairment.

● RENAL IMPAIRMENT No information available—manufacturer advises caution if creatinine clearance less than 50 mL/minute.

● MONITORING REQUIREMENTS
▸ Manufacturer advises monitor serum lipase every 2 weeks for the first 2 months and periodically thereafter—withhold treatment if lipase elevated and abdominal symptoms occur.
▸ Manufacturer advises a full blood count every 2 weeks for the first 3 months and then monthly thereafter or as clinically indicated.
▸ Manufacturer advises monitor liver function periodically.

▸ Manufacturer advises monitor for vascular occlusion or thromboembolism—interrupt treatment immediately if this occurs.

● NATIONAL FUNDING/ACCESS DECISIONS
NICE decisions
▸ **Ponatinib for treating chronic myeloid leukaemia and acute lymphoblastic leukaemia (June 2017)** NICE TA451
Ponatinib is recommended, within its marketing authorisation, as an option for treating chronic-, accelerated- or blast-phase chronic myeloid leukaemia in adults when:
  ● the disease is resistant to dasatinib or nilotinib **or**
  ● they cannot tolerate dasatinib or nilotinib and for whom subsequent treatment with imatinib is not clinically appropriate **or**
  ● the T315I gene mutation is present.
Ponatinib is recommended, within its marketing authorisation, as an option for treating Philadelphia-chromosome-positive acute lymphoblastic leukaemia in adults when:
  ● the disease is resistant to dasatinib **or**
  ● they cannot tolerate dasatinib and for whom subsequent treatment with imatinib is not clinically appropriate **or**
  ● the T315I gene mutation is present.
Ponatinib is recommended only if the company provides the drug with the discount agreed in the patient access scheme.
www.nice.org.uk/guidance/ta451

● MEDICINAL FORMS
There can be variation in the licensing of different medicines containing the same drug.
Tablet
CAUTIONARY AND ADVISORY LABELS 3, 25
  ▸ Iclusig (Incyte Biosciences UK Ltd) ▼
  Ponatinib (as Ponatinib hydrochloride) 15 mg Iclusig 15mg tablets | 30 tablet [PoM] £2,525.00
  Ponatinib (as Ponatinib hydrochloride) 30 mg Iclusig 30mg tablets | 30 tablet [PoM] £5,050.00
  Ponatinib (as Ponatinib hydrochloride) 45 mg Iclusig 45mg tablets | 30 tablet [PoM] £5,050.00

Regorafenib

21-Dec-2017

● DRUG ACTION Regorafenib is an inhibitor of several protein kinases.

● INDICATIONS AND DOSE
Metastatic colorectal cancer (specialist use only) | Unresectable or metastatic gastrointestinal stromal tumours (specialist use only) | Hepatocellular carcinoma (specialist use only)
▸ BY MOUTH
▸ Adult: 160 mg once daily for 21 consecutive days of repeated 28-day cycles, for dose adjustment due to side effects—consult product literature

IMPORTANT SAFETY INFORMATION
RISKS OF INCORRECT DOSING OF ORAL ANTI-CANCER MEDICINES
See Cytotoxic drugs p. 865.

● CAUTIONS Ensure measures to prevent hand-foot skin reaction · Gilbert's syndrome—risk of hyperbilirubinaemia · history of ischaemic heart disease—monitor for signs and symptoms of myocardial ischaemia and interrupt treatment if signs of ischaemia or infarction develop · hypertension—control blood pressure before treatment initiation and monitor as clinically indicated during treatment (review dose and consider treatment interruption if severe or persistent hypertension develops; discontinue treatment if hypertensive crisis occurs) · may impair wound healing— withhold treatment for major surgical procedures · predisposition to bleeding

● INTERACTIONS → Appendix 1: regorafenib

● SIDE-EFFECTS

▸ **Common or very common** Alopecia · anaemia · appetite decreased · asthenia · diarrhoea · dry mouth · dysphonia · electrolyte imbalance · fever · gastrooesophageal reflux disease · headache · hyperbilirubinaemia · hypertension · hyperuricaemia · hypothyroidism · increased risk of infection · leucopenia · mucositis · musculoskeletal stiffness · nausea · pain · proteinuria · skin reactions · stomatitis · taste altered · thrombocytopenia · tremor · vomiting · weight decreased

▸ **Uncommon** Gastrointestinal fistula (discontinue) · gastrointestinal perforation (including fatal cases, discontinue) · hepatic disorders · myocardial infarction · myocardial ischaemia · nail disorder

▸ **Rare or very rare** Neoplasms · posterior reversible encephalopathy syndrome (PRES) · severe cutaneous adverse reactions (SCARs)

● CONCEPTION AND CONTRACEPTION Women of childbearing potential and men must use effective contraception during treatment and up to 8 weeks after last dose.

● PREGNANCY Manufacturer advises avoid unless potential benefit outweighs risk—toxicity in *animal* studies. See also *Pregnancy and reproductive function* in Cytotoxic drugs p. 865.

● BREAST FEEDING Avoid—present in milk in *animal* studies.

● HEPATIC IMPAIRMENT Manufacturer advises caution in moderate impairment. Avoid in severe impairment.

● RENAL IMPAIRMENT Caution in severe impairment—no information available.

● MONITORING REQUIREMENTS

▸ Monitor blood count and coagulation parameters and consider permanent discontinuation in event of severe bleeding.

▸ Monitor hepatic function before treatment, then at least every two weeks for the first 2 months, then at least monthly thereafter and as clinically indicated—consult product literature if changes in liver function observed.

▸ Monitor for signs and symptoms of posterior reversible encephalopathy syndrome (including seizure, headache, altered mental status, visual disturbances or cortical blindness, with or without hypertension)—discontinue treatment if symptoms occur.

▸ Monitor biochemical, electrolyte and metabolic parameters during treatment; ensure measures to prevent hand-foot skin reaction—consult product literature if signs or symptoms develop.

● DIRECTIONS FOR ADMINISTRATION Tablets should be taken at the same time each day, swallowed whole with water after a light meal that contains less than 30% fat.

● PATIENT AND CARER ADVICE Counselling advised (administration).

● NATIONAL FUNDING/ACCESS DECISIONS

NICE decisions

▸ **Regorafenib for previously treated unresectable or metastatic gastrointestinal stromal tumours (November 2017) NICE TA488**

Regorafenib is recommended as an option for treating unresectable or metastatic gastrointestinal stromal tumours in adults whose disease has progressed on, or who are intolerant to, prior treatment with imatinib and sunitinib, only if:

● their Eastern Cooperative Oncology Group (ECOG) performance status is 0 to 1, **and**

● the manufacturer provides regorafenib with the discount agreed in the patient access scheme.

Patients whose treatment was started within the NHS before this guidance was published should have the option to continue treatment, without change to their funding arrangements, until they and their NHS clinician consider it appropriate to stop.
www.nice.org.uk/guidance/ta488

▸ **Regorafenib for previously treated advanced hepatocellular carcinoma (March 2018) NICE TA514**

Regorafenib is **not** recommended for treating advanced unresectable hepatocellular carcinoma in adults who have had sorafenib.

Patients whose treatment was started within the NHS before this guidance was published should have the option to continue treatment, without change to their funding arrangements, until they and their NHS clinician consider it appropriate to stop.
www.nice.org.uk/guidance/ta514

Scottish Medicines Consortium (SMC) Decisions

SMC No. 1316/18

The *Scottish Medicines Consortium* has advised (May 2018) that regorafenib (*Stivarga*®) is accepted for use within NHS Scotland as monotherapy for the treatment of adults with hepatocellular carcinoma who have been previously treated with sorafenib. This advice is contingent upon the continuing availability of the patient access scheme in NHS Scotland or a list price that is equivalent or lower.

● MEDICINAL FORMS
There can be variation in the licensing of different medicines containing the same drug.

Tablet

CAUTIONARY AND ADVISORY LABELS 21
ELECTROLYTES: May contain Sodium

▸ Stivarga (Bayer Plc) ▼
   Regorafenib 40 mg Stivarga 40mg tablets | 84 tablet PoM
   £3,744.00 (Hospital only)

Ribociclib   29-Jan-2018

● DRUG ACTION Ribociclib is an inhibitor of cyclin-dependent kinases 4 and 6, which are involved in cancer cell proliferation; their inhibition results in prevention of cancer cell growth.

● INDICATIONS AND DOSE

Locally advanced or metastatic breast cancer (specialist use only)

▸ BY MOUTH

▸ Adult: 600 mg once daily for 21 consecutive days of repeated 28 day cycles, to be taken at approximately the same time each day, preferably in the morning, for dose adjustments due to side-effects—consult product literature

DOSE ADJUSTMENTS DUE TO INTERACTIONS

▸ Manufacturer advises if concurrent use of potent inhibitors of CYP3A4 is unavoidable, reduce dose to 400 mg once daily; in those already taking 400 mg once daily, reduce dose to 200 mg once daily.

┌───┐
│ IMPORTANT SAFETY INFORMATION   │
│ RISKS OF INCORRECT DOSING OF ORAL ANTI-CANCER MEDICINES │
│ See Cytotoxic drugs p. 865.   │
└───┘

● CONTRA-INDICATIONS Pre-existing QTc prolongation · risk factors for QTc prolongation (including concomitant use of drugs known to prolong QTc interval)

● INTERACTIONS → Appendix 1: ribociclib

● SIDE-EFFECTS

▸ **Common or very common** Alopecia · anaemia · appetite decreased · asthenia · back pain · constipation · decreased leucocytes · diarrhoea · dry eye · dyspnoea · electrolyte imbalance · epistaxis · excessive tearing · fever · gastrointestinal discomfort · headache · hepatotoxicity · insomnia · nausea · neutropenia · peripheral oedema · QT interval prolongation · skin reactions · stomatitis · syncope · taste altered · thrombocytopenia · urinary tract infection · vomiting · weight decreased

- **ALLERGY AND CROSS-SENSITIVITY** Contra-indicated in patients with hypersensitivity to peanut or soya products.
- **HEPATIC IMPAIRMENT**
Dose adjustments Manufacturer advises reduce starting dose to 400 mg once daily in moderate-to-severe impairment.
- **RENAL IMPAIRMENT** Manufacturer advises use with caution in severe renal impairment—limited information available.
- **MONITORING REQUIREMENTS**
  ▸ Manufacturer advises to perform full blood counts and liver function tests before initiating treatment, every 2 weeks for the first 2 cycles, at the beginning of the subsequent 4 cycles, and then as clinically indicated thereafter.
  ▸ Manufacturer advises to assess ECG before initiating treatment (only initiate treatment in patients with QTcF values <450 milliseconds); ECG should be repeated at approx. day 14 of the first cycle and at the beginning of the second cycle, then as clinically indicated.
  ▸ Manufacturer advises to monitor serum electrolytes (including potassium, calcium, phosphorus and magnesium) before initiating treatment, at the beginning of the first 6 cycles and then as clinically indicated; any abnormality should be corrected before initiating treatment.
- **NATIONAL FUNDING/ACCESS DECISIONS**

NICE decisions
  ▸ Ribociclib with an aromatase inhibitor for previously untreated, hormone receptor-positive, HER2-negative, locally advanced or metastatic breast cancer (December 2017) NICE TA496
Ribociclib, with an aromatase inhibitor, is recommended within its marketing authorisation, as an option for treating hormone receptor-positive, human epidermal growth factor receptor 2-negative, locally advanced or metastatic breast cancer as initial endocrine-based therapy in adults. Ribociclib is recommended only if the manufacturer provides it with the discount agreed in the patient access scheme.
www.nice.org.uk/guidance/ta496

Scottish Medicines Consortium (SMC) Decisions
SMC No. 1295/18
The *Scottish Medicines Consortium* has advised (March 2018) that ribociclib (*Kisqali®*) is accepted for use within NHS Scotland in combination with an aromatase inhibitor, for the treatment of postmenopausal women with hormone receptor (HR)-positive, human epidermal growth factor receptor 2 (HER2)-negative locally advanced or metastatic breast cancer as initial endocrine-based therapy. This advice is contingent upon the continuing availability of the patient access scheme in NHS Scotland or a list price that is equivalent or lower.

- **MEDICINAL FORMS**
There can be variation in the licensing of different medicines containing the same drug.

Tablet
CAUTIONARY AND ADVISORY LABELS 3, 25
  ▸ Kisqali (Novartis Pharmaceuticals UK Ltd) ▼
  Ribociclib (as Ribociclib succinate) 200 mg Kisqali 200mg tablets | 21 tablet [PoM] £983.33 | 42 tablet [PoM] £1,966.67 | 63 tablet [PoM] £2,950.00

Ruxolitinib

02-Jun-2016

- **DRUG ACTION** Ruxolitinib is a selective inhibitor of the Janus-associated tyrosine kinases JAK1 and JAK2.

- **INDICATIONS AND DOSE**

Treatment of disease-related splenomegaly or symptoms in patients with primary myelofibrosis, post-polycythaemia vera myelofibrosis, or post-essential thrombocythaemia myelofibrosis
  ▸ BY MOUTH
  ▸ Adult: (consult product literature or local protocols)

IMPORTANT SAFETY INFORMATION
RISKS OF INCORRECT DOSING OF ORAL ANTI-CANCER MEDICINES
See Cytotoxic drugs p. 865.

- **CAUTIONS** Assess risk of developing infection before treatment—do not initiate until active serious infections are resolved
CAUTIONS, FURTHER INFORMATION
  ▸ Tuberculosis Patients should be evaluated for latent and active tuberculosis before starting treatment and monitored for signs and symptoms of tuberculosis during treatment.
- **INTERACTIONS** → Appendix 1: ruxolitinib
- **SIDE-EFFECTS**
  ▸ Common or very common Anaemia · bruising · constipation · dizziness · dyslipidaemia · flatulence · haemorrhage · headache · hypertension · increased risk of infection · intracranial haemorrhage · neutropenia · sepsis · thrombocytopenia · weight increased
- **CONCEPTION AND CONTRACEPTION** Contraceptive advice required, see *Pregnancy and reproductive function* in Cytotoxic drugs p. 865.
- **PREGNANCY** Avoid—toxicity in *animal* studies.
- **BREAST FEEDING** Avoid—present in milk in *animal* studies.
- **HEPATIC IMPAIRMENT**
Dose adjustments Reduce dose (consult product literature).
- **RENAL IMPAIRMENT**
Dose adjustments Reduce dose in severe impairment (consult product literature).
- **MONITORING REQUIREMENTS**
  ▸ Monitor full blood count (including differential white cell count) before treatment, then every 2–4 weeks until dose stabilised, then as clinically indicated.
  ▸ Monitor for infection during treatment.
  ▸ Monitor for symptoms of progressive multifocal leucoencephalopathy (presenting as new or worsening neurological, cognitive or psychiatric signs or symptoms)—withhold treatment if suspected.
- **NATIONAL FUNDING/ACCESS DECISIONS**

NICE decisions
  ▸ Ruxolitinib for treating disease-related splenomegaly or symptoms in adults with myelofibrosis (March 2016) NICE TA386
Ruxolitinib is recommended as an option for treating disease-related splenomegaly or symptoms in patients with primary myelofibrosis (also known as chronic idiopathic myelofibrosis), post polycythaemia vera myelofibrosis or post essential thrombocythaemia myelofibrosis, only if the patient has intermediate-2 or high-risk disease, **and** if the manufacturer provides ruxolitinib with the discount agreed in the patient access scheme.

Patients currently receiving ruxolitinib whose disease does not meet the above criteria should have the option to continue their treatment until they and their clinician consider it appropriate to stop.
www.nice.org.uk/TA386

- **MEDICINAL FORMS**
There can be variation in the licensing of different medicines containing the same drug.

Tablet
▸ Jakavi (Novartis Pharmaceuticals UK Ltd)
  Ruxolitinib (as Ruxolitinib phosphate) 5 mg Jakavi 5mg tablets | 56 tablet [PoM] £1,428.00
  Ruxolitinib (as Ruxolitinib phosphate) 10 mg Jakavi 10mg tablets | 56 tablet [PoM] £2,856.00
  Ruxolitinib (as Ruxolitinib phosphate) 15 mg Jakavi 15mg tablets | 56 tablet [PoM] £2,856.00
  Ruxolitinib (as Ruxolitinib phosphate) 20 mg Jakavi 20mg tablets | 56 tablet [PoM] £2,856.00

Sorafenib

29-Jun-2017

- **DRUG ACTION** Sorafenib is an inhibitor of multiple kinases.

- **INDICATIONS AND DOSE**

Treatment of advanced renal cell carcinoma when treatment with interferon alfa or interleukin-2 has failed or is unsuitable | Treatment of progressive, locally advanced, or metastatic, differentiated thyroid carcinoma that is refractory to radioactive iodine | Treatment of hepatocellular carcinoma
▸ BY MOUTH
▸ Adult: 400 mg twice daily, for dose adjustments due to side effects, consult product literature

---

IMPORTANT SAFETY INFORMATION
RISKS OF INCORRECT DOSING OF ORAL ANTI-CANCER MEDICINES
See Cytotoxic drugs p. 865.

- **CAUTIONS** Cardiac ischaemia · major surgical procedures · potential risk of bleeding—treat tracheal, bronchial, or oesophageal infiltration with localised therapy before initiating sorafenib in patients with differentiated thyroid carcinoma (DTC) and consider permanent withdrawal of sorafenib in any patient that requires medical intervention for bleeding · susceptibility to QT-interval prolongation

- **INTERACTIONS** → Appendix 1: sorafenib

- **SIDE-EFFECTS**
▸ **Common or very common** Alopecia · anaemia · appetite decreased · arthralgia · asthenia · congestive heart failure · constipation · decreased leucocytes · depression · diarrhoea · dry mouth · dysphagia · dysphonia · electrolyte imbalance · erectile dysfunction · fever · flushing · gastrointestinal discomfort · gastrointestinal disorders · haemorrhage · headache · hypertension · hypothyroidism · increased risk of infection · influenza like illness · intracranial haemorrhage · mucositis · muscle complaints · myocardial infarction · myocardial ischaemia · nausea · neoplasms · neutropenia · oral disorders · pain · peripheral neuropathy · proteinuria · renal failure · rhinorrhoea · skin reactions · taste altered · thrombocytopenia · tinnitus · vomiting · weight decreased
▸ **Uncommon** Cholangitis · cholecystitis · dehydration · encephalopathy · gynaecomastia · hepatic disorders · hyperthyroidism · pancreatitis · radiation injuries · respiratory disorders
▸ **Rare or very rare** Angioedema · hypersensitivity vasculitis · nephrotic syndrome · QT interval prolongation · rhabdomyolysis · severe cutaneous adverse reactions (SCARs)

- **CONCEPTION AND CONTRACEPTION** Contraceptive advice required, see *Pregnancy and reproductive function* in Cytotoxic drugs p. 865.

- **PREGNANCY** Manufacturer advises avoid unless essential—toxicity in *animal* studies. See also *Pregnancy and reproductive function* in Cytotoxic drugs p. 865.

- **BREAST FEEDING** Discontinue breast-feeding.

- **HEPATIC IMPAIRMENT** Manufacturer advises caution in severe impairment—no information available.

- **MONITORING REQUIREMENTS**
▸ Consider periodic monitoring of ECG and electrolytes in patients susceptible to QT-interval prolongation.
▸ Monitor blood pressure regularly and consider permanent discontinuation of sorafenib if resistant to antihypertensive therapy.
▸ Monitor plasma-calcium concentration (increased risk of hypocalcaemia if history of hypoparathyroidism).
▸ Monitor thyroid stimulating hormone in patients with differentiated thyroid carcinoma.

- **NATIONAL FUNDING/ACCESS DECISIONS**

NICE decisions
▸ **Bevacizumab (first-line), sorafenib (first- and second-line), sunitinib (second-line) and temsirolimus (first-line) for the treatment of advanced and/or metastatic renal cell carcinoma (August 2009)** NICE TA178
Bevacizumab, sorafenib, and temsirolimus are **not** recommended as first-line treatments for people with advanced and/or metastatic renal cell carcinoma.
  Sorafenib and sunitinib are not recommended as second-line treatments for people with advanced or metastatic renal cell carcinoma.
www.nice.org.uk/TA178
▸ **Sorafenib for treating advanced hepatocellular carcinoma (September 2017)** NICE TA474
Sorafenib is recommended as an option for treating advanced hepatocellular carcinoma only for patients with Child-Pugh grade A liver impairment, only if the company provides sorafenib within the agreed commercial access arrangement. Patients whose treatment was started within the NHS before this guidance was published should have the option to continue treatment, without change to their funding arrangements, until they and their clinician consider it appropriate to stop.
www.nice.org.uk/guidance/TA474

Scottish Medicines Consortium (SMC) Decisions
The *Scottish Medicines Consortium* has advised (January 2016) that sorafenib (*Nexavar* ®) is accepted for restricted use within NHS Scotland for the treatment of advanced hepatocellular carcinoma in patients where surgical or loco-regional therapies have failed or are unsuitable. This advice is contingent upon the continuing availability of the patient access scheme in NHS Scotland or a list price that is equivalent or lower.

- **MEDICINAL FORMS**
There can be variation in the licensing of different medicines containing the same drug.

Tablet
CAUTIONARY AND ADVISORY LABELS 23
▸ Nexavar (Bayer Plc)
  Sorafenib (as Sorafenib tosylate) 200 mg Nexavar 200mg tablets | 112 tablet [PoM] £3,576.56

Sunitinib

24-Jul-2017

- **DRUG ACTION** Sunitinib is a tyrosine kinase inhibitor.

- **INDICATIONS AND DOSE**

Treatment of unresectable or metastatic malignant gastro-intestinal stromal tumours, after failure of imatinib | Treatment of advanced or metastatic renal cell carcinoma
▸ BY MOUTH
▸ Adult: 50 mg once daily for 4 weeks, followed by a 2-week treatment-free period to complete 6-week cycle, adjusted in steps of 12.5 mg, doses adjusted according to tolerability; usual dose 25–75 mg daily

continued →

8

Immune system and malignant disease

Treatment of unresectable or metastatic pancreatic neuroendocrine tumours

▶ BY MOUTH
▶ Adult: 37.5 mg once daily without treatment-free period; adjusted in steps of 12.5 mg, doses adjusted according to tolerability; maximum 50 mg per day

DOSE ADJUSTMENTS DUE TO INTERACTIONS
▶ Manufacturer advises if concurrent use of potent inducers of CYP3A4 is unavoidable, dose may need to be increased in steps of 12.5 mg to a max. dose of 87.5 mg per day for gastro-intestinal stromal tumours or renal cell carcinoma, or to a max. dose of 62.5 mg per day for pancreatic neuroendocrine tumours.
▶ Manufacturer advises if concurrent use of potent inhibitors of CYP3A4 is unavoidable, dose may need to be decreased to a minimum of 37.5 mg per day for gastrointestinal stromal tumours or renal cell carcinoma, or to a minimum of 25 mg per day for pancreatic neuroendocrine tumours.

IMPORTANT SAFETY INFORMATION

RISK OF OSTEONECROSIS OF THE JAW (JANUARY 2011)
Treatment with sunitinib may be a risk factor for the development of osteonecrosis of the jaw.

Patients treated with sunitinib, who have previously received bisphosphonates, or are treated concurrently with bisphosphonates, may be particularly at risk.

Dental examination and appropriate preventive dentistry should be considered before treatment with sunitinib.

If possible, invasive dental procedures should be avoided in patients treated with sunitinib who have previously received, or who are currently receiving, intravenous bisphosphonates.

RISKS OF INCORRECT DOSING OF ORAL ANTI-CANCER MEDICINES
See Cytotoxic drugs p. 865.

● CAUTIONS Cardiovascular disease—discontinue if congestive heart failure develops · hypertension · increased risk of bleeding · susceptibility to QT-interval prolongation
● INTERACTIONS → Appendix 1: sunitinib
● SIDE-EFFECTS
▶ Common or very common Abscess · alopecia · anaemia · appetite decreased · arthralgia · burping · chest pain · chills · constipation · cough · dehydration · depression · diarrhoea · dizziness · dry mouth · dysphagia · dyspnoea · embolism and thrombosis · excessive tearing · eye inflammation · fatigue · fever · gastrointestinal discomfort · gastrointestinal disorders · haemorrhage · hair colour changes · headache · hypertension · hypoglycaemia · hypothyroidism · increased risk of infection · influenza like illness · insomnia · leucopenia · mucositis · muscle complaints · muscle weakness · myocardial ischaemia · nail disorder · nasal complaints · nausea · neutropenia · oedema · oral disorders · oropharyngeal pain · pain · peripheral neuropathy · proteinuria · renal impairment · respiratory disorders · sensation abnormal · sepsis · skin reactions · taste altered · thrombocytopenia · urine discolouration · vasodilation · vomiting · weight decreased
▶ Uncommon Anal fistula (interrupt treatment) · cardiomyopathy · cerebrovascular insufficiency · cholecystitis · fistula (interrupt treatment) · healing impaired · heart failure · hepatic disorders · hypersensitivity · hyperthyroidism · intracranial haemorrhage · myocardial infarction · osteonecrosis of jaw · pancreatitis · pancytopenia · pericardial effusion · QT interval prolongation · tumour haemorrhage
▶ Rare or very rare Angioedema · myopathy · nephrotic syndrome · posterior reversible encephalopathy syndrome (PRES) · pyoderma gangrenosum · severe cutaneous

adverse reactions (SCARs) · thrombotic microangiopathy · thyroiditis · torsade de pointes · tumour lysis syndrome
● CONCEPTION AND CONTRACEPTION Effective contraception required during treatment.
● PREGNANCY Manufacturer advises avoid unless potential benefit outweighs risk—toxicity in *animal* studies. See also *Pregnancy and reproductive function* in Cytotoxic drugs p. 865.
● BREAST FEEDING Discontinue breast-feeding.
● MONITORING REQUIREMENTS Monitor for thyroid dysfunction.
● NATIONAL FUNDING/ACCESS DECISIONS

NICE decisions
▶ Sunitinib for advanced or metastatic renal cell carcinoma (March 2009) NICE TA169
Sunitinib is recommended as first-line treatment for advanced or metastatic renal cell carcinoma in patients who are suitable for immunotherapy and have an Eastern Cooperative Oncology Group performance status of 0 or 1.
www.nice.org.uk/TA169
▶ Sunitinib for the treatment of gastrointestinal stromal tumours (September 2009) NICE TA179
Sunitinib is recommended as an option for treatment in patients with unresectable or metastatic gastrointestinal tumours if imatinib treatment has failed because of resistance or intolerance, and the cost of sunitinib for the first treatment cycle is met by the manufacturer.
www.nice.org.uk/TA179
▶ Bevacizumab (first-line), sorafenib (first- and second-line), sunitinib (second-line) and temsirolimus (first-line) for the treatment of advanced or metastatic renal cell carcinoma (August 2009) NICE TA178
Sorafenib and sunitinib are not recommended as second-line treatments for people with advanced or metastatic renal cell carcinoma.
www.nice.org.uk/TA178
▶ Everolimus and sunitinib for treating unresectable or metastatic neuroendocrine tumours in people with progessive disease (June 2017) NICE TA449
Everolimus and sunitinib are recommended, within their marketing authorisations, as options for treating well- or moderately differentiated unresectable or metastatic neuroendocrine tumours (NETs) of pancreatic origin in adults with progressive disease.
www.nice.org.uk/guidance/TA449

Scottish Medicines Consortium (SMC) Decisions
The *Scottish Medicines Consortium* has advised (November 2009) that sunitinib (*Sutent*®) is accepted for use within NHS Scotland for the treatment of unresectable and/or metastatic malignant gastrointestinal stromal tumours after failure of imatinib.

The *Scottish Medicines Consortium* has advised (May 2011) that sunitinib (*Sutent*®) is accepted for use within NHS Scotland for the treatment of unresectable or metastatic, well-differentiated pancreatic neuroendocrine tumours with disease progression in adults.

● MEDICINAL FORMS
There can be variation in the licensing of different medicines containing the same drug.

Capsule
CAUTIONARY AND ADVISORY LABELS 14
▶ Sutent (Pfizer Ltd)
Sunitinib (as Sunitinib malate) 12.5 mg Sutent 12.5mg capsules | 28 capsule [PoM] £784.70 (Hospital only)
Sunitinib (as Sunitinib malate) 25 mg Sutent 25mg capsules | 28 capsule [PoM] £1,569.40 (Hospital only)
Sunitinib (as Sunitinib malate) 50 mg Sutent 50mg capsules | 28 capsule [PoM] £3,138.80 (Hospital only)

Temsirolimus

- DRUG ACTION Temsirolimus is a protein kinase inhibitor.

- **INDICATIONS AND DOSE**

First-line treatment of advanced renal cell carcinoma | Treatment of relapsed or refractory mantle cell lymphoma
- ▶ BY INTRAVENOUS INFUSION
- ▶ Adult: (consult product literature or local protocols)

- INTERACTIONS → Appendix 1: temsirolimus

- SIDE-EFFECTS

- ▶ **Common or very common** Abscess · anaemia · anxiety · appetite decreased · arthralgia · asthenia · chest pain · chills · conjunctivitis · constipation · cough · cystitis · decreased leucocytes · dehydration · depression · diabetes mellitus · diarrhoea · dizziness · drowsiness · dyslipidaemia · dysphagia · dyspnoea · electrolyte imbalance · embolism and thrombosis · fever · gastrointestinal discomfort · gastrointestinal disorders · genital oedema · haemorrhage · headache · hypersensitivity · hypertension · increased risk of infection · insomnia · lacrimation disorder · mucositis · myalgia · nail disorder · nausea · neutropenia · oedema · oral disorders · pain · paraesthesia · post procedural infection · renal failure · respiratory disorders · scrotal oedema · sepsis · skin reactions · taste altered · thrombocytopenia · vomiting
- ▶ **Uncommon** Healing impaired · intracranial haemorrhage · pericardial effusion

  SIDE-EFFECTS, FURTHER INFORMATION Hypersensitivity reactions, including some life-threatening and rare fatal reactions, are associated with temsirolimus therapy. Symptoms include flushing, chest pain, dyspnoea, apnoea, hypotension, loss of consciousness, and anaphylaxis. Patients should receive an intravenous dose of antihistamine 30 minutes before starting the temsirolimus infusion. The infusion may have to be stopped temporarily for the treatment of infusion-related effects—consult product literature for appropriate management. If adverse reactions are not managed with dose delays, a dose reduction should be considered—consult product literature.

- CONCEPTION AND CONTRACEPTION Ensure effective contraception during treatment in men and women.

- PREGNANCY Manufacturer advises avoid (toxicity in *animal* studies). See also *Pregnancy and reproductive function* in Cytotoxic drugs p. 865.

- BREAST FEEDING Manufacturer advises discontinue breast-feeding.

- HEPATIC IMPAIRMENT Use with caution. In mantle cell lymphoma, avoid in moderate or severe impairment. **Dose adjustments** In renal cell carcinoma, reduce dose in severe impairment (consult product literature).

- RENAL IMPAIRMENT Manufacturer advises caution in severe impairment—no information available.

- MONITORING REQUIREMENTS
- ▶ Monitor respiratory function.
- ▶ Monitor blood lipids.

- NATIONAL FUNDING/ACCESS DECISIONS

NICE decisions
- ▶ Bevacizumab (first-line), sorafenib (first- and second-line), sunitinib (second-line) and temsirolimus (first-line) for the treatment of advanced or metastatic renal cell carcinoma (August 2009) NICE TA178
  Bevacizumab, sorafenib, and temsirolimus are **not** recommended as first-line treatments for people with advanced or metastatic renal cell carcinoma.
  www.nice.org.uk/TA178

- MEDICINAL FORMS
  There can be variation in the licensing of different medicines containing the same drug.
  Solution for infusion
  EXCIPIENTS: May contain Ethanol, propylene glycol
  ▶ Torisel (Pfizer Ltd)
    Temsirolimus 25 mg per 1 ml Torisel 30mg/1.2ml concentrate for solution for infusion vials and diluent | 1 vial PoM £620.00 (Hospital only)

Tivozanib

26-Apr-2018

- DRUG ACTION Tivozanib is a tyrosine kinase inhibitor.

- **INDICATIONS AND DOSE**

Advanced renal cell carcinoma (specialist use only)
- ▶ BY MOUTH
- ▶ Adult: 1340 micrograms once daily for 21 consecutive days of repeated 28 day cycles, for dose adjustments due to side effects—consult product literature

> IMPORTANT SAFETY INFORMATION
> RISKS OF INCORRECT DOSING OF ORAL ANTI-CANCER MEDICINES
> See Cytotoxic drugs p. 865.

- CAUTIONS History of arterial thromboembolic events · history of bleeding disorders · history of posterior reversible encephalopathy syndrome following tivozanib treatment · history of QT-interval prolongation · history of venous thromboembolic events · major surgical procedures—interrupt treatment · patients aged over 65 years—increased risk of adverse effects · pre-existing cardiac disease · risk factors for arterial thromboembolic events · risk factors for gastro-intestinal fistula · risk factors for gastro-intestinal perforation · risk factors for venous thromboembolic events · risk of bleeding

- INTERACTIONS → Appendix 1: tivozanib

- SIDE-EFFECTS

- ▶ **Common or very common** Alopecia · anaemia · angina pectoris · appetite decreased · arthralgia · asthenia · chills · constipation · cough · diarrhoea · dizziness · dry mouth · dysphagia · dysphonia · dyspnoea · embolism and thrombosis · fever · flushing · gastrointestinal discomfort · gastrointestinal disorders · haemorrhage · headache · hypertension · hypothyroidism · increased risk of infection · insomnia · myalgia · myocardial infarction · nasal complaints · nausea · oral disorders · pain · pancreatitis · peripheral neuropathy · peripheral oedema · proteinuria · skin reactions · tachycardia · taste altered · tinnitus · vertigo · visual impairment · vomiting · weight decreased
- ▶ **Uncommon** Ear congestion · excessive tearing · goitre · hyperhidrosis · hyperthyroidism · memory loss · mucositis · muscle weakness · pulmonary oedema · QT interval prolongation · thrombocytopenia · transient ischaemic attack
- ▶ **Rare or very rare** Posterior reversible encephalopathy syndrome (PRES)

- CONCEPTION AND CONTRACEPTION Manufacturer advises effective contraception in men, women of childbearing potential, and their partners during treatment and for at least one month after the last dose; an additional barrier method of contraception should be used in women using hormonal contraceptives. See also *Pregnancy and reproductive function* in Cytotoxic drugs p. 865.

- PREGNANCY Manufacturer advises avoid—toxicity in *animal* studies. See also *Pregnancy and reproductive function* in Cytotoxic drugs p. 865.

- BREAST FEEDING Manufacturer advises avoid—no information available.

- HEPATIC IMPAIRMENT Manufacturer advises caution in mild-to-moderate impairment—monitor patients for tolerability; avoid in severe impairment.
Dose adjustments Manufacturer advises reduce dose to 1340 micrograms on alternate days in moderate impairment—increased risk of adverse effects due to increased exposure.
- RENAL IMPAIRMENT Manufacturer advises caution in severe impairment—limited information available.
- MONITORING REQUIREMENTS
  - ▶ Manufacturer advises perform liver function tests (including ALT, AST and AP) before and during treatment; monitor for proteinuria before treatment and periodically thereafter.
  - ▶ Manufacturer advises monitor blood pressure before and during treatment; monitor for signs or symptoms of cardiac failure during treatment.
  - ▶ Manufacturer advises perform baseline ECG and monitor electrolytes before treatment and as clinically indicated thereafter.
  - ▶ Manufacturer advises monitor thyroid function before treatment and periodically thereafter.
  - ▶ Manufacturer advises monitor for symptoms of gastro-intestinal perforation or fistula.
- NATIONAL FUNDING/ACCESS DECISIONS
NICE decisions
  - ▶ Tivozanib for treating advanced renal cell carcinoma (March 2018) NICE TA512
Tivozanib is recommended as an option for treating advanced renal cell carcinoma in adults, only if:
    - they have had no previous treatment, **and**
    - the manufacturer provides tivozanib with the discount agreed in the patient access scheme.
Patients whose treatment was started within the NHS before this guidance was published should have the option to continue treatment, without change to their funding arrangements, until they and their NHS clinician consider it appropriate to stop.
www.nice.org.uk/guidance/ta512
- MEDICINAL FORMS
There can be variation in the licensing of different medicines containing the same drug.
Capsule
CAUTIONARY AND ADVISORY LABELS 25
  - ▶ Fotivda (EUSA Pharma Ltd) ▼
Tivozanib (as Tivozanib hydrochloride monohydrate)
1.34 mg Fotivda 1340microgram capsules | 21 capsule [PoM] £2,052.00

Trametinib

04-May-2017

- DRUG ACTION Trametinib is a protein kinase inhibitor.

- INDICATIONS AND DOSE
Unresectable or metastatic melanoma with a BRAF V600 mutation (as monotherapy or in combination with dabrafenib)
  - ▶ BY MOUTH
  - ▶ Adult: 2 mg once daily, when used in combination with dabrafenib, the dose should be taken at the same time each day with *either* the morning or evening dose of dabrafenib, for dose adjustments due to side-effects, consult product literature

IMPORTANT SAFETY INFORMATION
MHRA/CHM ADVICE (MARCH 2016): TRAMETINIB: RISK OF GASTROINTESTINAL PERFORATION AND COLITIS
A review by EU medicines regulators has concluded that trametinib can cause gastrointestinal perforation or colitis.

Trametinib should be used with caution in patients with risk factors for gastrointestinal perforation, such as gastrointestinal metastases, diverticulitis, or use of concomitant medicines that can cause gastrointestinal perforation. Prescribers should be vigilant for signs and symptoms of gastrointestinal perforation and should advise patients to seek urgent medical attention if they develop severe abdominal pain.

RISKS OF INCORRECT DOSING OF ORAL ANTI-CANCER MEDICINES
See Cytotoxic drugs p. 865.

- CONTRA-INDICATIONS History of retinal vein occlusion
- CAUTIONS Concomitant antiplatelet or anticoagulant therapy—increased risk of haemorrhage · conditions that could impair left ventricular function · elderly (more frequent dose adjustments may be required) · impaired left ventricular function · predisposing factors for retinal vein occlusion · risk factors for gastrointestinal perforation
- INTERACTIONS → Appendix 1: trametinib
- SIDE-EFFECTS
  - ▶ **Common or very common** Abdominal pain · alopecia · anaemia · asthenia · bradycardia · constipation · cough · dehydration · diarrhoea · dry mouth · dyspnoea · eye inflammation · fever · haemorrhage · hypersensitivity · hypertension · increased risk of infection · intracranial haemorrhage · left ventricular dysfunction · lymphoedema · mucositis · nausea · oedema · respiratory disorders · skin reactions · stomatitis · vision disorders · vomiting
  - ▶ **Uncommon** Chorioretinopathy · gastrointestinal disorders · heart failure · retinal detachment · retinal occlusion · rhabdomyolysis

SIDE-EFFECTS, FURTHER INFORMATION Additional side-effects reported when used in combination with dabrafenib include dizziness, hyperhidrosis, hyponatraemia, hypotension, leucopenia, muscle spasms, myocarditis, neutropenia, night sweats, and thrombocytopenia.

- CONCEPTION AND CONTRACEPTION Manufacturer advises women of child-bearing potential should use highly effective non-hormonal contraception during, and for 4 months after stopping treatment.
- PREGNANCY Manufacturer advises avoid—toxicity in *animal* studies. See also *Pregnancy and reproductive function* in Cytotoxic drugs p. 865.
- BREAST FEEDING Manufacturer advises avoid—no information available.
- HEPATIC IMPAIRMENT Manufacturer advises caution in moderate to severe impairment—no information available.
- RENAL IMPAIRMENT Manufacturer advises caution in severe impairment—no information available.
- MONITORING REQUIREMENTS Manufacturer advises measure blood pressure at baseline and monitor during treatment; evaluate left ventricular ejection fraction before treatment, after one month of treatment, and then approximately every 3 months thereafter; monitor liver function every 4 weeks for 6 months after treatment initiation, and thereafter as clinically indicated.
- HANDLING AND STORAGE Manufacturer advises store in refrigerator (2–8 °C); once opened, bottle may be stored for 30 days at not more than 30 °C.
- PATIENT AND CARER ADVICE Manufacturer advises patients and their carers should be told to seek immediate medical attention if symptoms of pulmonary embolism or deep vein thrombosis occur; patients and their carers should also be advised to report new visual disturbances.
Missed doses Manufacturer advises if a dose is more than 12 hours late, the missed dose should not be taken and the next dose should be taken at the normal time.
Driving and skilled tasks Manufacturer advises patients and carers should be counselled on the effects on driving and

performance of skilled tasks—risk of dizziness and visual disturbances.

- **NATIONAL FUNDING/ACCESS DECISIONS**
  NICE decisions
  ▸ **Trametinib in combination with dabrafenib for treating unresectable or metastatic melanoma (June 2016)** NICE TA396
  Trametinib in combination with dabrafenib is recommended, within its marketing authorisation, as an option for treating unresectable or metastatic melanoma in adults with a BRAF V600 mutation only when the company provides trametinib and dabrafenib with the discounts agreed in the patient access schemes.
  www.nice.org.uk/TA396

  Scottish Medicines Consortium (SMC) Decisions
  The *Scottish Medicines Consortium* has advised (August 2016) that trametinib (*Mekinist* ®), in combination with dabrafenib, is accepted for restricted use within NHS Scotland for first-line treatment of adult patients with unresectable or metastatic melanoma with a BRAF V600 mutation.

- **MEDICINAL FORMS**
  There can be variation in the licensing of different medicines containing the same drug.
  Tablet
  CAUTIONARY AND ADVISORY LABELS 3, 23, 25
  ▸ Mekinist (Novartis Pharmaceuticals UK Ltd) ▼
    Trametinib 500 microgram Mekinist 0.5mg tablets | 7 tablet PoM £280.00 | 30 tablet PoM £1,200.00
    Trametinib 2 mg Mekinist 2mg tablets | 7 tablet PoM £1,120.00 | 30 tablet PoM £4,800.00

Vandetanib

- **DRUG ACTION** Vandetanib is a tyrosine kinase inhibitor.

- **INDICATIONS AND DOSE**
  Treatment of aggressive and symptomatic medullary thyroid cancer in patients with unresectable locally advanced or metastatic disease
  ▸ BY MOUTH
  ▸ Adult: 300 mg once daily, for dose adjustment due to side effects—consult product literature

---

IMPORTANT SAFETY INFORMATION
RISKS OF INCORRECT DOSING OF ORAL ANTI-CANCER MEDICINES
See Cytotoxic drugs p. 865.

- **CONTRA-INDICATIONS** Congenital long QT syndrome · QT interval greater than 480 milliseconds
- **CAUTIONS** Brain metastases (intracranial haemorrhage reported) · electrolyte disturbances · history of torsades de pointes · hypertension · phototoxicity reactions reported (wear protective clothing and/or sunscreen) · susceptibility to QT-prolongation
- **INTERACTIONS** → Appendix 1: vandetanib
- **SIDE-EFFECTS**
  ▸ **Common or very common** Alopecia · anxiety · appetite decreased · asthenia · cerebral ischaemia · cholelithiasis · constipation · corneal deposits · cystitis · dehydration · depression · diarrhoea · dizziness · dry eye · dry mouth · dysphagia · electrolyte imbalance · eye disorders · eye inflammation · fever · gastrointestinal discomfort · gastrointestinal disorders · glaucoma · haemorrhage · headache · hyperglycaemia · hypertension · hypothyroidism · increased risk of infection · insomnia · lethargy · loss of consciousness · movement disorders · nail disorder · nausea · nephrolithiasis · oedema · pain · photosensitivity reaction · proteinuria · QT interval prolongation · renal impairment · respiratory disorders · sensation abnormal · sepsis · skin reactions · stomatitis ·

taste altered · tremor · urinary disorders · vision disorders · vomiting · weight decreased
  ▸ **Uncommon** Arrhythmias · brain oedema · cardiac arrest · cardiac conduction disorder · cataract · healing impaired · heart failure · malnutrition · pancreatitis · posterior reversible encephalopathy syndrome (PRES) · seizure · Stevens-Johnson syndrome · urine discolouration
- **CONCEPTION AND CONTRACEPTION** Effective contraception required during and for at least 4 months after treatment.
- **PREGNANCY** Manufacturer advises avoid unless potential benefit outweighs risk. Most cytotoxic drugs are teratogenic and should not be administered during pregnancy, especially during the first trimester. Considerable caution is necessary if a pregnant woman presents with cancer requiring chemotherapy, and specialist advice should always be sought.
- **BREAST FEEDING** Avoid—no information available.
- **HEPATIC IMPAIRMENT** Manufacturer advises avoid in severe impairment (serum bilirubin greater than 1.5 times the upper limit of normal).
- **RENAL IMPAIRMENT** Avoid if creatinine clearance less than 30 mL/minute.
  Dose adjustments Reduce dose to 200 mg if creatinine clearance 30–49 mL/minute.
- **MONITORING REQUIREMENTS** Monitor ECG, plasma potassium, calcium, magnesium and thyroid stimulating hormone before treatment, then 1, 3, 6 and 12 weeks after starting treatment and following dose adjustment or interruption, then every 3 months for at least 1 year.
- **DIRECTIONS FOR ADMINISTRATION** Tablets may be dispersed in half a glass of water by stirring until dispersed (approximately 10 minutes), immediately before drinking (do not crush). After solution has been swallowed, any residue must be re-dispersed in the same volume of water and swallowed. The solution can also be administered via nasogastric or gastrostomy tubes.
- **PATIENT AND CARER ADVICE** Patients or carers should be given advice on how to administer vandetanib tablets. Phototoxicity reactions Patients should be advised to wear protective clothing and/or sunscreen.
  Alert card should be provided.

- **MEDICINAL FORMS**
  There can be variation in the licensing of different medicines containing the same drug.
  Tablet
  ▸ Caprelsa (Genzyme Therapeutics Ltd) ▼
    Vandetanib 100 mg Caprelsa 100mg tablets | 30 tablet PoM £2,500.00
    Vandetanib 300 mg Caprelsa 300mg tablets | 30 tablet PoM £5,000.00

Vemurafenib

- **DRUG ACTION** Vemurafenib is a BRAF kinase inhibitor.

- **INDICATIONS AND DOSE**
  Monotherapy for the treatment of BRAF V600 mutation-positive unresectable or metastatic melanoma
  ▸ BY MOUTH
  ▸ Adult: 960 mg twice daily, for dose adjustment due to side effects—consult product literature

---

IMPORTANT SAFETY INFORMATION
DRUG RASH WITH EOSINOPHILIA AND SYSTEMIC SYMPTOMS (DRESS SYNDROME)
DRESS syndrome has been reported in patients taking vemurafenib. DRESS syndrome starts with rash, fever, swollen glands, and increased white cell count, and it

can affect the liver, kidneys and lungs; DRESS can also be fatal.

Patients should be advised to stop taking vemurafenib and consult their doctor immediately if skin rash develops. Treatment with vemurafenib should not be restarted.

MHRA/CHM ADVICE (NOVEMBER 2015): RISK OF POTENTIATION OF RADIATION TOXICITY

Potentiation of radiation toxicity has been reported in patients treated with vemurafenib before, during, or after radiotherapy— use with caution.

RISKS OF INCORRECT DOSING OF ORAL ANTI-CANCER MEDICINES
See Cytotoxic drugs p. 865.

- CONTRA-INDICATIONS Wild-type BRAF malignant melanoma
- CAUTIONS Electrolyte disturbances · prior or concurrent cancer associated with RAS mutation—increased risk of tumour progression · susceptibility to QT-prolongation
- INTERACTIONS → Appendix 1: vemurafenib
- SIDE-EFFECTS
- **Common or very common** 7th nerve paralysis · alopecia · appetite decreased · arthralgia · arthritis · asthenia · connective tissue disorders · constipation · cough · diarrhoea · dizziness · eye inflammation · fever · folliculitis · headache · myalgia · nausea · neoplasms · pain · panniculitis · peripheral oedema · photosensitivity reaction · QT interval prolongation · radiation injuries · skin reactions · taste altered · vomiting · weight decreased
- **Uncommon** Liver injury · neutropenia · pancreatitis · peripheral neuropathy · retinal occlusion · severe cutaneous adverse reactions (SCARs) · vasculitis
- **Rare or very rare** Acute tubular necrosis · nephritis acute interstitial
- **Frequency not known** Acute kidney injury
- CONCEPTION AND CONTRACEPTION Effective contraception required during for at least 6 months after treatment.
- PREGNANCY Manufacturer advises avoid unless potential benefit outweighs risk. See also *Pregnancy and reproductive function* in Cytotoxic drugs p. 865.
- BREAST FEEDING Avoid—no information available.
- HEPATIC IMPAIRMENT
  Monitoring Manufacturer advises more frequent monitoring in moderate to severe hepatic impairment (including monthly ECG monitoring during first 3 months of treatment).
- RENAL IMPAIRMENT Manufacturer advises caution in severe impairment.
- MONITORING REQUIREMENTS
- Monitor ECG and electrolytes before treatment, after one month and following dose adjustment (treatment not recommended if QT interval greater than 500 milliseconds at baseline).
- Monitor liver function before treatment and periodically thereafter.
- Monitor for uveitis, iritis and retinal vein occlusion.
- Monitor for cutaneous and non-cutaneous squamous cell carcinoma and new primary melanoma before, during and for up to 6 months after treatment—consult product literature.
- DIRECTIONS FOR ADMINISTRATION Food may affect absorption (take at the same time with respect to food).
- PATIENT AND CARER ADVICE Counselling advised (administration).
  Drug rash with eosinophilia and systemic symptoms (DRESS syndrome) Patients should be advised to stop taking vemurafenib and consult their doctor immediately if skin rash develops.

- NATIONAL FUNDING/ACCESS DECISIONS
  NICE decisions
- **Vemurafenib for treating locally advanced or metastatic BRAF V600 mutation-positive malignant melanoma (December 2012)** NICE TA269
  Vemurafenib is recommended as an option for the treatment of BRAF V600 mutation-positive unresectable or metastatic melanoma only if the manufacturer provides vemurafenib with the discount agreed in the patient access scheme.
  www.nice.org.uk/TA269

  Scottish Medicines Consortium (SMC) Decisions
  The *Scottish Medicines Consortium* has advised (November 2013) that vemurafenib (*Zelboraf*®) is accepted for restricted use within NHS Scotland as monotherapy for the first-line treatment of BRAF V600 mutation-positive unresectable or metastatic melanoma.

- MEDICINAL FORMS
  There can be variation in the licensing of different medicines containing the same drug.
  Tablet
  CAUTIONARY AND ADVISORY LABELS 25
  - Zelboraf (Roche Products Ltd)
    Vemurafenib 240 mg Zelboraf 240mg tablets | 56 tablet PoM £1,750.00 (Hospital only)

ANTINEOPLASTIC DRUGS > OTHER

Niraparib
06-Feb-2018

- DRUG ACTION Niraparib is an inhibitor of PARP enzymes which are involved in DNA repair. PARP inhibition results in disruption of cellular homoeostasis and cell death.

- INDICATIONS AND DOSE
  Ovarian cancer (initiated by a specialist) | Fallopian tube cancer (initiated by a specialist) | Peritoneal cancer (initiated by a specialist)
  - BY MOUTH
  - Adult: 300 mg once daily, consider initial dose of 200 mg in patients with body-weight less than 58 kg, for dose adjustments due to side-effects—consult product literature

  IMPORTANT SAFETY INFORMATION
  RISKS OF INCORRECT DOSING OF ORAL ANTI-CANCER MEDICINES
  See Cytotoxic drugs p. 865.

- CAUTIONS Pre-existing hypertension (control before treatment initiation)
- SIDE-EFFECTS
- **Common or very common** Anaemia · anxiety · appetite decreased · arthralgia · back pain · conjunctivitis · constipation · cough · depression · diarrhoea · dizziness · dry mouth · dyspnoea · epistaxis · fatigue · gastrointestinal discomfort · headache · hypertension · hypokalaemia · increased risk of infection · insomnia · leucopenia · mucositis · myalgia · nausea · neutropenia · palpitations · peripheral oedema · photosensitivity reaction · rash · stomatitis · tachycardia · taste altered · thrombocytopenia · vomiting
- **Uncommon** Pancytopenia
- **Frequency not known** Neoplasms
- CONCEPTION AND CONTRACEPTION Manufacturer advises effective contraception in women of childbearing potential during treatment and for 1 month after receiving the last dose.
- PREGNANCY Manufacturer advises avoid—limited information available.

- BREAST FEEDING Manufacturer advises avoid during treatment and for 1 month after last dose—no information available.
- HEPATIC IMPAIRMENT Manufacturer advises caution in severe impairment—no information available.
- RENAL IMPAIRMENT Manufacturer advises caution in severe impairment—no information available.
- MONITORING REQUIREMENTS
▶ Manufacturer advises monitor full blood count weekly for the first month of treatment, then monthly for the next 10 months and periodically thereafter.
▶ Manufacturer advises monitor blood pressure monthly for the first year of treatment and periodically thereafter.
- PATIENT AND CARER ADVICE
Driving and skilled tasks Manufacturer advises patients and their carers should be counselled on the effects on driving and skilled tasks—increased risk of dizziness and fatigue.

- MEDICINAL FORMS
There can be variation in the licensing of different medicines containing the same drug.
Capsule
CAUTIONARY AND ADVISORY LABELS 25
▶ Zejula (Tesaro UK Ltd) ▼
Niraparib (as Niraparib tosylate monohydrate) 100 mg Zejula 100mg capsules | 56 capsule [PoM] £4,500.00 (Hospital only) | 84 capsule [PoM] £6,750.00 (Hospital only)

Olaparib
09-Feb-2018
- DRUG ACTION Olaparib is a PARP inhibitor. PARP are enzymes that repair damaged DNA in cancer cells and, in the absence of functional BRCA, inhibition of PARP results in an inability of cancer cells to repair. Therefore inhibition of PARP results in an antineoplastic effect.

- INDICATIONS AND DOSE
Ovarian cancer (initiated by a specialist) | Fallopian tube cancer (initiated by a specialist) | Peritoneal cancer (initiated by a specialist)
▶ BY MOUTH
▶ Adult: 400 mg twice daily; reduced if not tolerated to 200 mg twice daily, then reduced if not tolerated to 100 mg twice daily, take at least 1 hour after food and avoid food for 2 hours after taking, patients should start treatment within 8 weeks of receiving the final dose of their platinum-containing chemotherapy regimen

DOSE ADJUSTMENTS DUE TO INTERACTIONS
▶ Manufacturer advises if concurrent use of moderate inhibitors of CYP3A4 is unavoidable, reduce dose to 200 mg twice daily.
▶ Manufacturer advises if concurrent use of potent inhibitors of CYP3A4 is unavoidable, reduce dose to 150 mg twice daily.

PHARMACOKINETICS
▶ Peak plasma concentrations are typically achieved 1 to 3 hours after dosing; steady-state is achieved within 3 to 4 days.

IMPORTANT SAFETY INFORMATION
RISKS OF INCORRECT DOSING OF ORAL ANTI-CANCER MEDICINES
See Cytotoxic drugs p. 865.

- INTERACTIONS → Appendix 1: olaparib
SIDE-EFFECTS
Common or very common Anaemia · appetite decreased · diarrhoea · dizziness · fatigue · gastrointestinal discomfort · headache · lymphopenia · nausea · neutropenia · skin reactions · stomatitis · taste altered · thrombocytopenia · vomiting

SIDE-EFFECTS, FURTHER INFORMATION
Haematological toxicity Withhold treatment if severe haematological toxicity develops; further analysis recommended if toxicity still present 4 weeks after treatment withdrawal.
Pneumonitis If dyspnoea, cough and fever, or radiological abnormalities develop, withhold treatment and investigate; if pneumonitis confirmed, discontinue.
- CONCEPTION AND CONTRACEPTION Manufacturer advises effective contraception during treatment and for 1 month after receiving the last dose. Consider an additional non-hormonal method of contraception.
- PREGNANCY Manufacturer advises avoid—toxicity in *animal* studies.
- BREAST FEEDING Manufacturer advises avoid during treatment and for 1 month after last dose—no information available.
- HEPATIC IMPAIRMENT Manufacturer advises avoid—no information available.
- RENAL IMPAIRMENT Manufacturer advises avoid in severe impairment unless benefit outweighs potential risk—no information available.
Dose adjustments Manufacturer advises reduce dose to 300 mg twice daily in moderate impairment.
- MONITORING REQUIREMENTS Manufacturer advises monitor full blood count every month for the first 12 months of treatment and periodically thereafter.
- PATIENT AND CARER ADVICE
Missed doses If a dose is missed, the missed dose should not be taken and the next dose should be taken at the usual time.
Driving and skilled tasks Malaise and dizziness may affect performance of skilled tasks e.g. driving or operating machinery.
- NATIONAL FUNDING/ACCESS DECISIONS
NICE decisions
▶ Olaparib for maintenance treatment of relapsed, platinum-sensitive, BRCA mutation-positive ovarian, fallopian tube and peritoneal cancer after response to second-line or subsequent platinum-based chemotherapy (January 2016) NICE TA381
Olaparib is recommended as an option for treating adults with relapsed, platinum sensitive ovarian, fallopian tube or peritoneal cancer who have BRCA1 or BRCA2 mutations and whose disease has responded to platinum based chemotherapy only if:
  • they have had 3 or more courses of platinum-based chemotherapy and;
  • the drug cost of olaparib for people who remain on treatment after 15 months will be met by the company.
www.nice.org.uk/guidance/ta381
Scottish Medicines Consortium (SMC) Decisions
The *Scottish Medicines Consortium* has advised (November 2016) that olaparib (*Lynparza* ®) is accepted for use within NHS Scotland as monotherapy for the maintenance treatment of adults with platinum-sensitive relapsed BRCA-mutated (germline and/or somatic) high grade serous epithelial ovarian, fallopian tube, or primary peritoneal cancer who are in response (complete response or partial response) to platinum-based chemotherapy.

- MEDICINAL FORMS
There can be variation in the licensing of different medicines containing the same drug.
Capsule
▶ Lynparza (AstraZeneca UK Ltd) ▼
Olaparib 50 mg Lynparza 50mg capsules | 448 capsule [PoM] £3,550.00

8

Immune system and malignant disease

Venetoclax

07-Sep-2017

- **DRUG ACTION** Venetoclax is a potent, selective inhibitor of B-cell lymphoma-2 (BCL-2).

- **INDICATIONS AND DOSE**

Chronic lymphocytic leukaemia in the presence of 17p deletion or TP53 mutation when a B-cell receptor pathway inhibitor is unsuitable or ineffective (specialist use only) | Chronic lymphocytic leukaemia in the absence of 17p deletion or TP53 mutation when both chemo-immunotherapy and a B-cell receptor pathway inhibitor has been ineffective (specialist use only)

  ▸ BY MOUTH

  ▸ Adult: Initially 20 mg once daily for 7 days, then increased to 50 mg once daily for 7 days, then increased to 100 mg once daily for 7 days, then increased to 200 mg once daily for 7 days, then maintenance 400 mg once daily, dose to be taken in the morning during dose-titration phase; dose should be taken at the same time every day, for dose adjustment due to side effects—consult product literature

  DOSE ADJUSTMENTS DUE TO INTERACTIONS

  ▸ Avoid concomitant use of potent or moderate CYP3A4 inhibitors during initiation and dose-titration; once stable reduce dose by 75% with concomitant use of potent CYP3A4 inhibitors and by 50% with concomitant use of moderate CYP3A4 inhibitors.

IMPORTANT SAFETY INFORMATION

RISKS OF INCORRECT DOSING OF ORAL ANTI-CANCER MEDICINES
See Cytotoxic drugs p. 865.

- **CAUTIONS** Ensure adequate hydration

- **INTERACTIONS** → Appendix 1: venetoclax

- **SIDE-EFFECTS**

  ▸ **Common or very common** Anaemia · constipation · diarrhoea · electrolyte imbalance · fatigue · hyperuricaemia · increased risk of infection · lymphopenia · nausea · neutropenia · tumour lysis syndrome · vomiting

- **CONCEPTION AND CONTRACEPTION** Manufacturer advises ensure effective, non-hormonal contraception during and for 30 days after treatment in women of child-bearing potential. See also *Pregnancy and reproductive function* in Cytotoxic drugs p. 865.

- **PREGNANCY** Manufacturer advises avoid—toxicity in *animal* studies. See also *Pregnancy and reproductive function* in Cytotoxic drugs p. 865.

- **BREAST FEEDING** Manufacturer advises avoid—no information available.

- **HEPATIC IMPAIRMENT** Manufacturer advises close monitoring during initiation and dose titration in moderate impairment (increased risk of toxicity); avoid in severe impairment—no information available.

- **RENAL IMPAIRMENT** Manufacturer advises close monitoring (increased risk of tumour lysis syndrome); use only if potential benefit outweighs risk in severe impairment—no information available.

- **MONITORING REQUIREMENTS** Manufacturer advises monitor renal function before starting treatment.

- **PATIENT AND CARER ADVICE**
  Hydration Manufacturer advises patients should drink 1.5–2 L of water daily, starting 2 days before and throughout the dose-titration phase; intravenous fluids should be administered for those who cannot maintain an adequate level of oral hydration with consideration of overall risk of tumour lysis syndrome.
  Vomiting Manufacturer advises that if vomiting occurs following dose administration, no additional doses should be taken on that day and the next dose should be taken at the normal time.
  Missed doses Manufacturer advises that if a dose is more than 8 hours late, the missed dose should not be taken and the next dose should be taken at the normal time.

- **NATIONAL FUNDING/ACCESS DECISIONS**

  NICE decisions

  ▸ Venetoclax for treating chronic lymphocytic leukaemia (November 2017) NICE TA487
  Venetoclax is recommended for use within the Cancer Drugs Fund, within its authorisation, as an option for treating chronic lymphocytic leukaemia in adults:

  - with a 17p deletion or TP53 mutation and when a B-cell receptor pathway inhibitor is unsuitable, or whose disease has progressed after a B-cell receptor pathway inhibitor **or**
  - without a 17p deletion or TP53 mutation, and whose disease has progressed after both chemo-immunotherapy and a B-cell receptor pathway inhibitor, **and**
  - only if the conditions in the managed access agreement are followed.

  Patients whose treatment was started within the NHS before this guidance was published should have the option to continue treatment, without change to their funding arrangements, until they and their NHS clinician consider it appropriate to stop.
  www.nice.org.uk/guidance/TA487

  Scottish Medicines Consortium (SMC) Decisions
  The *Scottish Medicines Consortium* has advised (August 2017) that venetoclax (*Venclyxto®*) is accepted for use within NHS Scotland as monotherapy for the treatment of chronic lymphocytic leukaemia:

  - in the presence of 17p deletion or TP53 mutation in patients who are unsuitable for or have failed a B-cell receptor pathway inhibitor; *or*
  - in the absence of 17p deletion or TP53 mutation in patients who have failed both chemoimmunotherapy and a B-cell receptor pathway inhibitor.

  This advice is contingent upon the continuing availability of the patient access scheme in NHS Scotland or a list price that is equivalent or lower.

- **MEDICINAL FORMS**
  There can be variation in the licensing of different medicines containing the same drug.
  Tablet
  CAUTIONARY AND ADVISORY LABELS 21, 25
  ▸ Venclyxto (AbbVie Ltd) ▼
  Venetoclax 10 mg Venclyxto 10mg tablets | 14 tablet [PoM] £59.87
  Venetoclax 50 mg Venclyxto 50mg tablets | 7 tablet [PoM] £149.67
  Venetoclax 100 mg Venclyxto 100mg tablets | 7 tablet [PoM] £299.34 | 14 tablet [PoM] £598.68 | 112 tablet [PoM] £4,789.47

Vismodegib

17-Jan-2018

- **DRUG ACTION** Vismodegib is a hedgehog pathway inhibitor.

- **INDICATIONS AND DOSE**

Symptomatic metastatic basal cell carcinoma | Locally advanced basal cell carcinoma not appropriate for surgery or radiotherapy

  ▸ BY MOUTH

  ▸ Adult: 150 mg once daily

IMPORTANT SAFETY INFORMATION

RISKS OF INCORRECT DOSING OF ORAL ANTI-CANCER MEDICINES
See Cytotoxic drugs p. 865.

- **INTERACTIONS** → Appendix 1: vismodegib

- SIDE-EFFECTS
► **Common or very common** Alopecia · amenorrhoea · appetite decreased · arthralgia · asthenia · constipation · dehydration · diarrhoea · gastrointestinal discomfort · hair growth abnormal · muscle complaints · nausea · pain · skin reactions · taste altered · vomiting · weight decreased
► **Frequency not known** Epiphyses premature fusion
- CONCEPTION AND CONTRACEPTION For women of child-bearing potential, pregnancy must be excluded before initiation of treatment, and monthly during treatment. Women must use two contraceptive methods (including one highly effective method and one barrier method) during treatment and for 24 months after the final dose of vismodegib. Men must use a condom during treatment and for 2 months after the final dose.
- PREGNANCY **Important: teratogenic risk**—may cause severe birth defects and embryo-fetal death.
- BREAST FEEDING Avoid during treatment and for 24 months after final dose.
- HEPATIC IMPAIRMENT No information available—manufacturer advises caution in moderate to severe impairment.
- RENAL IMPAIRMENT No information available—manufacturer advises caution in severe impairment.
- PRESCRIBING AND DISPENSING INFORMATION Prescribers and pharmacists must comply with prescribing and dispensing restrictions as specified in the manufacturer's Pregnancy Prevention Programme, and ensure that the patient fully acknowledges the programme's pregnancy prevention measures—consult product literature for further information.
- PATIENT AND CARER ADVICE
Conception and contraception Counselling on pregnancy and contraception advised. Patients must comply with the manufacturer's pregnancy prevention programme.
- NATIONAL FUNDING/ACCESS DECISIONS
► **NICE decisions**
► **Vismodegib for treating basal cell carcinoma (November 2017)** NICE TA489
Vismodegib is not recommended within its marketing authorisation for treating symptomatic metastatic basal cell carcinoma, or locally advanced basal cell carcinoma that is inappropriate for surgery or radiotherapy, in adults.
   Patients whose treatment was started within the NHS before this guidance was published should have the option to continue treatment, without change to their funding arrangements, until they and their NHS clinician consider it appropriate to stop.
www.nice.org.uk/guidance/TA489

- MEDICINAL FORMS
There can be variation in the licensing of different medicines containing the same drug.
Capsule
CAUTIONARY AND ADVISORY LABELS 25
► Erivedge (Roche Products Ltd) ▼
   Vismodegib 150 mg Erivedge 150mg capsules | 28 capsule PoM
   £6,285.00 (Hospital only)

ANTINEOVASCULARISATION DRUGS ›
VASCULAR ENDOTHELIAL GROWTH FACTOR INHIBITORS

| **Aflibercept** | 06-Dec-2017 |

- DRUG ACTION Aflibercept is a recombinant fusion protein that acts as a soluble decoy receptor and binds to vascular endothelial growth factors A and B (VEGF-A, VEGF-B) and placental growth factor (PlGF). Aflibercept inhibits the activation of VEGF receptors and the proliferation of endothelial cells, thereby inhibiting the growth of new vessels that supply tumours with oxygen and nutrients.

- **INDICATIONS AND DOSE**
In combination with irinotecan, fluorouracil and folinic acid (FOLFIRI) chemotherapy, in metastatic colorectal cancer that is resistant to, or has progressed after, an oxaliplatin-containing regimen
► BY INTRAVENOUS INFUSION
► Adult: (consult local protocol)

- CONTRA-INDICATIONS Moderate or severe congestive heart failure · uncontrolled hypertension
- CAUTIONS Febrile neutropenia · history of cardiovascular disease (may be exacerbated by hypertension) · increased risk of haemorrhage (including fatal events) · increased risk of hypertension · increased risk of thromboembolic events (consult product literature if event occurs) · may impair wound healing—withhold treatment for at least 4 weeks before elective surgery and for at least 4 weeks after major surgery, or until wound fully healed · neutropenic infection · risk of fistula formation (discontinue if fistula develops) · risk of neutropenia · risk of thrombocytopenia
- INTERACTIONS → Appendix 1: aflibercept
- SIDE-EFFECTS
► **Common or very common** Cataract · eye discomfort · eye disorders · eye inflammation · haemorrhage · retinal pigment epithelial tear · vision disorders
► **Uncommon** Lens opacity
- CONCEPTION AND CONTRACEPTION Exclude pregnancy before treatment. Effective contraception required during and for at least 6 months after treatment in men and women. Contraceptive advice should be given to men and women before therapy begins (and should cover the duration of contraception required after therapy has ended).
- PREGNANCY Manufacturer advises avoid—toxicity in *animal* studies. Considerable caution is necessary if a pregnant woman presents with cancer requiring chemotherapy, and specialist advice should always be sought.
- BREAST FEEDING Manufacturer advises avoid—no information available.
- HEPATIC IMPAIRMENT Caution in severe impairment—no information available.
- RENAL IMPAIRMENT Caution in severe impairment— no information available.
- MONITORING REQUIREMENTS
► Monitor blood pressure at initiation and at least fortnightly during treatment (do not initiate treatment if pre-existing hypertension is uncontrolled)—consult product literature if hypertension develops during treatment.
► Monitor for signs of gastro-intestinal perforation (discontinue if perforation develops).
► Monitor full blood count, including differential count and platelets at baseline and before each treatment cycle.

8

Immune system and malignant disease

- Monitor for proteinuria before each treatment administration (consult product literature if symptoms develop).
- Monitor for signs and symptoms of diarrhoea and dehydration, particularly in elderly—consult product literature if severe diarrhoea occurs.
- Monitor for posterior reversible encephalopathy syndrome (presenting as seizures, altered mental status, nausea, vomiting, headache, or visual disturbance).

● NATIONAL FUNDING/ACCESS DECISIONS

NICE decisions
▶ Aflibercept in combination with irinotecan and fluorouracil-based therapy for treating metastatic colorectal cancer that has progressed following prior oxaliplatin-based chemotherapy (March 2014) NICE TA307
Aflibercept in combination with irinotecan and fluorouracil-based therapy is **not** recommended within its marketing authorisation for treating metastatic colorectal cancer that is resistant to or has progressed after an oxaliplatin-containing regimen.
www.nice.org.uk/guidance/TA307

● MEDICINAL FORMS
There can be variation in the licensing of different medicines containing the same drug.
Solution for infusion
▶ Zaltrap (Sanofi)
Aflibercept 25 mg per 1 ml Zaltrap 200mg/8ml concentrate for solution for infusion vials | 1 vial [PoM] £591.30 (Hospital only)
Zaltrap 100mg/4ml concentrate for solution for infusion vials | 1 vial [PoM] £295.65 (Hospital only)

Chapter 9
Blood and nutrition

CONTENTS

Blood and blood-forming organs

1 Anaemias

Anaemias

Anaemia treatment considerations

Before initiating treatment for anaemia it is essential to determine which type is present. Iron salts may be harmful and result in iron overload if given alone to patients with anaemias other than those due to iron deficiency.

Sickle-cell anaemia

Sickle-cell disease is caused by a structural abnormality of haemoglobin resulting in deformed, less flexible red blood cells. Acute complications in the more severe forms include sickle-cell crisis, where infarction of the microvasculature and blood supply to organs results in severe pain. Sickle-cell crisis requires hospitalisation, intravenous fluids, analgesia and treatment of any concurrent infection. Chronic complications include skin ulceration, renal failure, and increased susceptibility to infection. Pneumococcal vaccine, haemophilus influenzae type b vaccine, an annual influenza

vaccine and prophylactic penicillin reduce the risk of infection. Hepatitis B vaccine should be considered if the patient is not immune.

In most forms of sickle-cell disease, varying degrees of haemolytic anaemia are present accompanied by increased erythropoiesis; this may increase folate requirements and folate supplementation may be necessary.

Hydroxycarbamide p. 910 can reduce the frequency of crises and the need for blood transfusions in sickle-cell disease. The beneficial effects of hydroxycarbamide may not become evident for several months.

G6PD deficiency

Glucose 6-phosphate dehydrogenase (G6PD) deficiency is highly prevalent in individuals originating from most parts of Africa, from most parts of Asia, from Oceania, and from Southern Europe; it can also occur, rarely, in any other individuals. G6PD deficiency is more common in males than it is in females.

Individuals with G6PD deficiency are susceptible to developing acute haemolytic anaemia when they take a number of common drugs. They are also susceptible to developing acute haemolytic anaemia when they eat fava beans (broad beans, *Vicia faba*); this is termed *favism* and can be more severe in children or when the fresh fava beans are eaten raw.

When prescribing drugs for patients with G6PD deficiency, the following three points should be kept in mind:

- G6PD deficiency is genetically heterogeneous; susceptibility to the haemolytic risk from drugs varies; thus, a drug found to be safe in some G6PD-deficient individuals may not be equally safe in others;
- manufacturers do not routinely test drugs for their effects in G6PD-deficient individuals;
- the risk and severity of haemolysis is almost always dose-related.

The lists below should be read with these points in mind. Ideally, information about G6PD deficiency should be available before prescribing a drug listed below. However, in the absence of this information, the possibility of haemolysis should be considered, especially if the patient belongs to a group in which G6PD deficiency is common.

A very few G6PD-deficient individuals with chronic non-spherocytic haemolytic anaemia have haemolysis even in the absence of an exogenous trigger. These patients must be regarded as being at high risk of severe exacerbation of haemolysis following administration of any of the drugs listed below.

Drugs with definite risk of haemolysis in most G6PD-deficient individuals

- Dapsone and other sulfones (higher doses for dermatitis herpetiformis more likely to cause problems)
- Methylthioninium chloride
- Niridazole [not on UK market]
- Nitrofurantoin
- Pamaquin [not on UK market]
- Primaquine (30 mg weekly for 8 weeks has been found to be without undue harmful effects in African and Asian people)
- Quinolones (including ciprofloxacin, moxifloxacin, nalidixic acid, norfloxacin, and ofloxacin)
- Rasburicase
- Sulfonamides (including co-trimoxazole; some sulfonamides, e.g. sulfadiazine, have been tested and found not to be haemolytic in many G6PD-deficient individuals)

Drugs with possible risk of haemolysis in some G6PD-deficient individuals

- Aspirin (acceptable up to a dose of at least 1 g daily in most G6PD-deficient individuals)
- Chloroquine (acceptable in acute malaria and malaria chemoprophylaxis)
- Menadione, water-soluble derivatives (e.g. menadiol sodium phosphate)
- Quinidine (acceptable in acute malaria) [not on UK market]
- Quinine (acceptable in acute malaria)
- Sulfonylureas

Naphthalene in mothballs also causes haemolysis in individuals with G6PD deficiency.

Hypoplastic, haemolytic, and renal anaemias

Anabolic steroids, pyridoxine hydrochloride p. 1047, antilymphocyte immunoglobulin, rituximab p. 859 [unlicensed indication], and various corticosteroids are used in hypoplastic and haemolytic anaemias.

Antilymphocyte immunoglobulin given intravenously through a central line over 12–18 hours each day for 5 days produces a response in about 50% of cases of acquired *aplastic anaemia*; the response rate may be increased when ciclosporin p. 818 is given as well. Severe reactions are common in the first 2 days and profound immunosuppression can occur; antilymphocyte immunoglobulin should be given under specialist supervision with appropriate resuscitation facilities. Alternatively, oxymetholone tablets (available from 'special order' manufacturers or specialist importing companies) can be used in aplastic anaemia for 3 to 6 months.

It is unlikely that dietary deprivation of pyridoxine hydrochloride produces clinically relevant haematological effects. However, certain forms of *sideroblastic anaemia* respond to pharmacological doses, possibly reflecting its role as a co-enzyme during haemoglobin synthesis. Pyridoxine hydrochloride is indicated in both *idiopathic acquired* and *hereditary sideroblastic anaemias*. Although complete cures have not been reported, some increase in haemoglobin can occur; the dose required is usually high. *Reversible sideroblastic anaemias* respond to treatment of the underlying cause but in pregnancy, haemolytic anaemias, and alcohol dependence, or during isoniazid p. 576 treatment, pyridoxine hydrochloride is also indicated.

Corticosteroids have an important place in the management of haematological disorders. They include conditions with an *autoimmune haemolytic anaemia*, *immune thrombocytopenias* and *neutropenias*, and *major transfusion reactions*. They are also used in chemotherapy schedules for many types of *lymphoma*, *lymphoid leukaemias*, and *paraproteinaemias*, including *multiple myeloma*.

Erythropoietins

Epoetins (recombinant human erythropoietins) are used to treat the anaemia associated with erythropoietin deficiency in chronic renal failure, to increase the yield of autologous blood in normal individuals and to shorten the period of symptomatic anaemia in patients receiving cytotoxic chemotherapy.

Epoetin beta p. 982 is also used for the prevention of anaemia in preterm neonates of low birth-weight; only unpreserved formulations should be used in neonates because other preparations may contain benzyl alcohol.

Darbepoetin alfa p. 979 is a hyperglycosylated derivative of epoetin; it has a longer half life and can be administered less frequently than epoetin.

Methoxy polyethylene glycol-epoetin beta p. 984 is a continuous erythropoietin receptor activator that is licensed for the treatment of symptomatic anaemia associated with chronic kidney disease. It has a longer duration of action than epoetin.

1.1 Hypoplastic, haemolytic, and renal anaemias

> **Other drugs used for Hypoplastic, haemolytic, and renal anaemias** Eltrombopag, p. 1001

ANABOLIC STEROIDS > ANDROSTAN DERIVATIVES

Oxymetholone

- **INDICATIONS AND DOSE**

Aplastic anaemia
- ▶ BY MOUTH
- ▶ Adult: 1–5 mg/kg daily for 3 to 6 months

- **INTERACTIONS** → Appendix 1: oxymetholone

- **MEDICINAL FORMS**
There can be variation in the licensing of different medicines containing the same drug. Forms available from special-order manufacturers include: oral suspension

Capsule
- ▶ Oxymetholone (Non-proprietary)
  Oxymetholone 50 mg Oxymetholone 50mg capsules |
  50 capsule [PoM] £475.00 [CD4-2]

EPOETINS

Epoetins

> **IMPORTANT SAFETY INFORMATION**
>
> MHRA/CHM ADVICE: RECOMBINANT HUMAN ERYTHROPOIETINS: VERY RARE RISK OF SEVERE CUTANEOUS ADVERSE REACTIONS (UPDATED JANUARY 2018)
>
> The MHRA is aware of very rare cases of severe cutaneous adverse reactions, including Stevens-Johnson syndrome and toxic epidermal necrolysis, in patients treated with erythropoietins; some cases were fatal. More severe cases were recorded with long-acting agents (darbepoetin alfa and methoxy polyethylene glycol-epoetin beta).
>
> Patients and their carers should be advised of the signs and symptoms of severe skin reactions when starting treatment and instructed to stop treatment and seek immediate medical attention if they develop widespread rash and blistering; these rashes often follow fever or flu-like symptoms—discontinue treatment permanently if such reactions occur.
>
> MHRA/CHM ADVICE (DECEMBER 2007) ERYTHROPOIETINS–HAEMOGLOBIN CONCENTRATION
>
> Overcorrection of haemoglobin concentration in patients with chronic kidney disease may increase the risk of death and serious cardiovascular events, and in patients with cancer may increase the risk of thrombosis and related complications:
> - patients should not be treated with erythropoietins for the licensed indications in chronic kidney disease or cancer in patients receiving chemotherapy *unless* symptoms of anaemia are present
> - the haemoglobin concentration should be maintained within the range 10–12 g/100 mL
> - haemoglobin concentrations higher than 12 g/100 mL should be avoided
> - the aim of treatment is to relieve symptoms of anaemia, and in patients with chronic kidney disease to avoid the need for blood transfusion; the haemoglobin concentration should not be increased beyond that which provides adequate control of symptoms of anaemia (in some patients, this may be achieved at concentrations lower than the recommended range)
>
> MHRA/CHM ADVICE (DECEMBER 2007 AND JULY 2008) ERYTHROPOIETINS–TUMOUR PROGRESSION AND SURVIVAL IN PATIENTS WITH CANCER
>
> Clinical trial data show an unexplained excess mortality and increased risk of tumour progression in patients with anaemia associated with cancer who have been treated with erythropoietins. Many of these trials used erythropoietins outside of the licensed indications (i.e. overcorrected haemoglobin concentration or given to patients who have not received chemotherapy):
> - erythropoietins licensed for the treatment of *symptomatic* anaemia associated with cancer, are licensed only for patients who are receiving chemotherapy
> - the decision to use erythropoietins should be based on an assessment of the benefits and risks for individual patients; blood transfusion may be the preferred treatment for anaemia associated with cancer chemotherapy, particularly in those with a good cancer prognosis

● CONTRA-INDICATIONS Patients unable to receive thromboprophylaxis · pure red cell aplasia following erythropoietin therapy · uncontrolled hypertension

● CAUTIONS Aluminium toxicity (can impair the response to erythropoietin) · concurrent infection (can impair the

response to erythropoietin) · correct factors that contribute to the anaemia of chronic renal failure, such as iron or folate deficiency, before treatment. · during dialysis (increase in unfractionated or low molecular weight heparin dose may be needed) · epilepsy · inadequately treated or poorly controlled blood pressure—interrupt treatment if blood pressure uncontrolled · ischaemic vascular disease · malignant disease · other inflammatory disease (can impair the response to erythropoietin) · risk of thrombosis can be increased when used for anaemia before orthopaedic surgery—avoid in cardiovascular disease including recent myocardial infarction or cerebrovascular accident · risk of thrombosis may be increased when used for anaemia in adults receiving cancer chemotherapy · sickle-cell disease (lower target haemoglobin concentration may be appropriate) · sudden stabbing migraine-like pain (warning of a hypertensive crisis) · thrombocytosis (monitor platelet count for first 8 weeks)

● SIDE-EFFECTS
▶ **Common or very common** Arthralgia · embolism and thrombosis · headache · hypertension (dose-dependent) · influenza like illness · skin reactions · stroke
▶ **Uncommon** Hypertensive crisis (in isolated patients with normal or low blood pressure) · respiratory tract congestion · seizure
▶ **Rare or very rare** Thrombocytosis
▶ **Frequency not known** Pure red cell aplasia (more common following subcutaneous administration in patients with chronic renal failure)

SIDE-EFFECTS, FURTHER INFORMATION
Hypertensive crisis In isolated patients with normal or low blood pressure, hypertensive crisis with encephalopathy-like symptoms and generalised tonic-clonic seizures requiring immediate medical attention has occurred with epoetin.
Pure red cell aplasia There have been very rare reports of pure red cell aplasia in patients treated with erythropoietins. In patients who develop a lack of efficacy with erythropoietin therapy and with a diagnosis of pure red cell aplasia, treatment with erythropoietins must be discontinued and testing for erythropoietin antibodies considered. Patients who develop pure red cell aplasia should not be switched to another form of erythropoietin.

● MONITORING REQUIREMENTS
▶ Monitor closely blood pressure, reticulocyte counts, haemoglobin, and electrolytes—interrupt treatment if blood pressure uncontrolled.
▶ Other factors, such as iron or folate deficiency, that contribute to the anaemia of chronic renal failure should be corrected before treatment and monitored during therapy. Supplemental iron may improve the response in resistant patients.

☞ above

Darbepoetin alfa

● INDICATIONS AND DOSE

Symptomatic anaemia associated with chronic renal failure in patients on dialysis
▶ BY SUBCUTANEOUS INJECTION, OR BY INTRAVENOUS INJECTION
▶ Adult: Initially 450 nanograms/kg once weekly, dose to be adjusted according to response by approximately 25% at intervals of at least 4 weeks, maintenance dose to be given once weekly or once every 2 weeks, reduce dose by approximately 25% if rise in haemoglobin concentration exceeds 2 g/100 mL over 4 weeks or if haemoglobin concentration exceeds 12 g/100 mL; if haemoglobin concentration continues to rise, despite dose reduction, suspend treatment until haemoglobin concentration decreases and then restart at continued →

a dose approximately 25% lower than the previous dose, when changing route give same dose then adjust according to weekly or fortnightly haemoglobin measurements, adjust doses not more frequently than every 2 weeks during maintenance treatment

Symptomatic anaemia associated with chronic renal failure in patients not on dialysis
▸ BY SUBCUTANEOUS INJECTION
▸ Adult: Initially 450 nanograms/kg once weekly, alternatively initially 750 nanograms/kg every 2 weeks, dose to be adjusted according to response by approximately 25% at intervals of at least 4 weeks, maintenance dose can be given once weekly, every 2 weeks, or once a month, subcutaneous route preferred in patients not on haemodialysis, reduce dose by approximately 25% if rise in haemoglobin concentration exceeds 2 g/100 mL over 4 weeks or if haemoglobin concentration exceeds 12 g/100 mL; if haemoglobin concentration continues to rise, despite dose reduction, suspend treatment until haemoglobin concentration decreases and then restart at a dose approximately 25% lower than the previous dose, when changing route give same dose then adjust according to weekly or fortnightly haemoglobin measurements, adjust doses not more frequently than every 2 weeks during maintenance treatment

Symptomatic anaemia associated with chronic renal failure in patients not on dialysis
▸ BY INTRAVENOUS INJECTION
▸ Adult: Initially 450 nanograms/kg once weekly, dose to be adjusted according to response by approximately 25% at intervals of at least 4 weeks, maintenance dose given once weekly, subcutaneous route preferred in patients not on haemodialysis, reduce dose by approximately 25% if rise in haemoglobin concentration exceeds 2 g/100 mL over 4 weeks or if haemoglobin concentration exceeds 12 g/100 mL; if haemoglobin concentration continues to rise, despite dose reduction, suspend treatment until haemoglobin concentration decreases and then restart at a dose approximately 25% lower than the previous dose, when changing route give same dose then adjust according to weekly or fortnightly haemoglobin measurements, adjust doses not more frequently than every 2 weeks during maintenance treatment

Symptomatic anaemia in adults with non-myeloid malignancies receiving chemotherapy
▸ BY SUBCUTANEOUS INJECTION
▸ Adult: Initially 6.75 micrograms/kg every 3 weeks, alternatively initially 2.25 micrograms/kg once weekly, if response inadequate after 9 weeks further treatment may not be effective; if adequate response obtained then reduce dose by 25–50%, reduce dose by approximately 25–50% if rise in haemoglobin concentration exceeds 2 g/100 mL over 4 weeks or if haemoglobin concentration exceeds 12 g/100 mL; if haemoglobin concentration continues to rise, despite dose reduction, suspend treatment until haemoglobin concentration decreases and restart at a dose approximately 25% lower than the previous dose. Discontinue approximately 4 weeks after ending chemotherapy

● INTERACTIONS → Appendix 1: darbepoetin alfa
● SIDE-EFFECTS
▸ **Common or very common** Hypersensitivity · oedema
● PREGNANCY No evidence of harm in *animal* studies—manufacturer advises caution.
● BREAST FEEDING Manufacturer advises avoid—no information available.
● HEPATIC IMPAIRMENT Manufacturer advises caution.

● NATIONAL FUNDING/ACCESS DECISIONS
NICE decisions
▸ **Erythropoiesis-stimulating agents (epoetin and darbepoetin) for treating anaemia in people with cancer having chemotherapy (November 2014)** NICE TA323
Erythropoiesis-stimulating agents (epoetin alfa, beta, theta and zeta, and darbepoetin alfa) are recommended, within their marketing authorisations, as options for treating anaemia in people with cancer who are having chemotherapy.
  If different erythropoiesis-stimulating agents are equally suitable, the product with the lowest acquisition cost for the course of treatment should be used.
www.nice.org.uk/TA323

● MEDICINAL FORMS
There can be variation in the licensing of different medicines containing the same drug.
Solution for injection
▸ Aranesp (Amgen Ltd)
Darbepoetin alfa 25 microgram per 1 ml Aranesp 10micrograms/0.4ml solution for injection pre-filled syringes | 4 pre-filled disposable injection PoM £58.72
Darbepoetin alfa 40 microgram per 1 ml Aranesp 20micrograms/0.5ml solution for injection pre-filled syringes | 4 pre-filled disposable injection PoM £117.45
Darbepoetin alfa 100 microgram per 1 ml Aranesp 50micrograms/0.5ml solution for injection pre-filled syringes | 4 pre-filled disposable injection PoM £293.62
Aranesp 40micrograms/0.4ml solution for injection pre-filled syringes | 4 pre-filled disposable injection PoM £234.90
Aranesp 30micrograms/0.3ml solution for injection pre-filled syringes | 4 pre-filled disposable injection PoM £176.17
Darbepoetin alfa 200 microgram per 1 ml Aranesp 100micrograms/0.5ml solution for injection pre-filled syringes | 4 pre-filled disposable injection PoM £587.24
Aranesp 130micrograms/0.65ml solution for injection pre-filled syringes | 4 pre-filled disposable injection PoM £763.42
Aranesp 80micrograms/0.4ml solution for injection pre-filled syringes | 4 pre-filled disposable injection PoM £469.79
Aranesp 60micrograms/0.3ml solution for injection pre-filled syringes | 4 pre-filled disposable injection PoM £352.35
Darbepoetin alfa 500 microgram per 1 ml Aranesp 300micrograms/0.6ml solution for injection pre-filled syringes | 1 pre-filled disposable injection PoM £440.43
Aranesp 500micrograms/1ml solution for injection pre-filled syringes | 1 pre-filled disposable injection PoM £734.05
Aranesp 150micrograms/0.3ml solution for injection pre-filled syringes | 4 pre-filled disposable injection PoM £880.86
▸ Aranesp SureClick (Amgen Ltd)
Darbepoetin alfa 40 microgram per 1 ml Aranesp SureClick 20micrograms/0.5ml solution for injection pre-filled disposable devices | 1 pre-filled disposable injection PoM £29.36
Darbepoetin alfa 100 microgram per 1 ml Aranesp SureClick 40micrograms/0.4ml solution for injection pre-filled disposable devices | 1 pre-filled disposable injection PoM £58.72
Aranesp SureClick 80micrograms/0.4ml solution for injection pre-filled disposable devices | 1 pre-filled disposable injection PoM £117.45
Darbepoetin alfa 200 microgram per 1 ml Aranesp SureClick 60micrograms/0.3ml solution for injection pre-filled disposable devices | 1 pre-filled disposable injection PoM £88.09
Aranesp SureClick 100micrograms/0.5ml solution for injection pre-filled disposable devices | 1 pre-filled disposable injection PoM £146.81
Darbepoetin alfa 500 microgram per 1 ml Aranesp SureClick 150micrograms/0.3ml solution for injection pre-filled disposable devices | 1 pre-filled disposable injection PoM £220.22
Aranesp SureClick 300micrograms/0.6ml solution for injection pre-filled disposable devices | 1 pre-filled disposable injection PoM £440.43
Aranesp SureClick 500micrograms/1ml solution for injection pre-filled disposable devices | 1 pre-filled disposable injection PoM £734.05

◄ 979

Epoetin alfa

● INDICATIONS AND DOSE

BINOCRIT ® PRE-FILLED SYRINGES

Symptomatic anaemia associated with chronic renal failure in patients on haemodialysis

▶ BY INTRAVENOUS INJECTION
▶ Adult: Initially 50 units/kg 3 times a week, adjusted in steps of 25 units/kg 3 times a week, dose adjusted according to response at intervals of at least 4 weeks; maintenance 25–100 units/kg 3 times a week, intravenous injection to be given over 1–5 minutes, reduce dose by approximately 25% if rise in haemoglobin concentration exceeds 2 g/100 mL over 4 weeks or if haemoglobin concentration exceeds 12 g/100 mL; if haemoglobin concentration continues to rise, despite dose reduction, suspend treatment until haemoglobin concentration decreases and then restart at a dose approximately 25% lower than the previous dose

Symptomatic anaemia associated with chronic renal failure in adults on peritoneal dialysis

▶ BY INTRAVENOUS INJECTION
▶ Adult: Initially 50 units/kg twice weekly; maintenance 25–50 units/kg twice weekly, intravenous injection to be given over 1–5 minutes, reduce dose by approximately 25% if rise in haemoglobin concentration exceeds 2 g/100 mL over 4 weeks or if haemoglobin concentration exceeds 12 g/100 mL; if haemoglobin concentration continues to rise, despite dose reduction, suspend treatment until haemoglobin concentration decreases and then restart at a dose approximately 25% lower than the previous dose

Severe symptomatic anaemia of renal origin in adults with renal insufficiency not yet on dialysis

▶ BY INTRAVENOUS INJECTION
▶ Adult: Initially 50 units/kg 3 times a week, increased in steps of 25 units/kg 3 times a week, adjusted according to response, dose to be increased at intervals of at least 4 weeks; maintenance 17–33 units/kg 3 times a week (max. per dose 200 units/kg 3 times a week), intravenous injection to be given over 1–5 minutes, reduce dose by approximately 25% if rise in haemoglobin concentration exceeds 2 g/100 mL over 4 weeks or if haemoglobin concentration exceeds 12 g/100 mL; if haemoglobin concentration continues to rise, despite dose reduction, suspend treatment until haemoglobin concentration decreases and then restart at a dose approximately 25% lower than the previous dose

Symptomatic anaemia in adults receiving cancer chemotherapy

▶ BY SUBCUTANEOUS INJECTION
▶ Adult: Initially 150 units/kg 3 times a week, alternatively initially 450 units/kg once weekly, increased to 300 units/kg 3 times a week, increased if appropriate rise in haemoglobin (or reticulocyte count) not achieved after 4 weeks; discontinue if inadequate response after 4 weeks at higher dose, subcutaneous injection maximum 1 mL per injection site, reduce dose by approximately 25–50% if rise in haemoglobin concentration exceeds 2 g/100 mL over 4 weeks or if haemoglobin concentration exceeds 12 g/100 mL; if haemoglobin concentration continues to rise, despite dose reduction, suspend treatment until haemoglobin concentration decreases and then restart at a dose approximately 25% lower than the previous dose. Discontinue approximately 4 weeks after ending chemotherapy

To increase yield of autologous blood (to avoid homologous blood) in predonation programme in moderate anaemia either when large volume of blood required or when sufficient blood cannot be saved for elective major surgery

▶ BY INTRAVENOUS INJECTION
▶ Adult: 600 units/kg twice weekly for 3 weeks before surgery, consult product literature for details and advice on ensuring high iron stores, intravenous injection to be given over 1–5 minutes

Moderate anaemia (haemoglobin concentration 10–13 g/100 mL) before elective orthopaedic surgery in adults with expected moderate blood loss to reduce exposure to allogeneic blood transfusion or if autologous transfusion unavailable

▶ BY SUBCUTANEOUS INJECTION
▶ Adult: 600 units/kg once weekly for 3 weeks before surgery and on day of surgery, alternatively 300 units/kg daily for 15 days starting 10 days before surgery, consult product literature for details, subcutaneous injection maximum 1 mL per injection site

EPREX ® PRE-FILLED SYRINGES

Symptomatic anaemia associated with chronic renal failure in patients on haemodialysis

▶ BY INTRAVENOUS INJECTION, OR BY SUBCUTANEOUS INJECTION
▶ Adult: Initially 50 units/kg 3 times a week, adjusted in steps of 25 units/kg 3 times a week, dose adjusted according to response at intervals of at least 4 weeks; maintenance 75–300 units/kg once weekly, intravenous route preferred, intravenous injection to be given over 1–5 minutes, subcutaneous injection, maximum 1 mL per injection site, maintenance dose can be given as a single dose or in divided doses, reduce dose by approximately 25% if rise in haemoglobin concentration exceeds 2 g/100 mL over 4 weeks or if haemoglobin concentration exceeds 12 g/100 mL; if haemoglobin concentration continues to rise, despite dose reduction, suspend treatment until haemoglobin concentration decreases and then restart at a dose approximately 25% lower than the previous dose

Symptomatic anaemia associated with chronic renal failure in adults on peritoneal dialysis

▶ BY INTRAVENOUS INJECTION, OR BY SUBCUTANEOUS INJECTION
▶ Adult: Initially 50 units/kg twice weekly; maintenance 25–50 units/kg twice weekly, intravenous route preferred, intravenous injection to be given over 1–5 minutes, subcutaneous injection, maximum 1 mL per injection site, reduce dose by approximately 25% if rise in haemoglobin concentration exceeds 2 g/100 mL over 4 weeks or if haemoglobin concentration exceeds 12 g/100 mL; if haemoglobin concentration continues to rise, despite dose reduction, suspend treatment until haemoglobin concentration decreases and then restart at a dose approximately 25% lower than the previous dose

Severe symptomatic anaemia of renal origin in adults with renal insufficiency not yet on dialysis

▶ BY INTRAVENOUS INJECTION, OR BY SUBCUTANEOUS INJECTION
▶ Adult: Initially 50 units/kg 3 times a week, increased in steps of 25 units/kg 3 times a week, adjusted according to response, dose to be increased at intervals of at least 4 weeks; maintenance 17–33 units/kg 3 times a week (max. per dose 200 units/kg 3 times a week), intravenous route preferred, intravenous injection to be given over 1–5 minutes, subcutaneous injection, maximum 1 mL per injection site, reduce dose by approximately 25% if rise in haemoglobin concentration exceeds 2 g/100 mL over 4 weeks or if haemoglobin concentration exceeds continued →

9

Blood and nutrition

12 g/100 mL; if haemoglobin concentration continues to rise, despite dose reduction, suspend treatment until haemoglobin concentration decreases and then restart at a dose approximately 25% lower than the previous dose

Symptomatic anaemia in adults receiving cancer chemotherapy
▶ BY SUBCUTANEOUS INJECTION
▶ Adult: Initially 150 units/kg 3 times a week, alternatively initially 450 units/kg once weekly, increased to 300 units/kg 3 times a week, increased if appropriate rise in haemoglobin (or reticulocyte count) not achieved after 4 weeks; discontinue if inadequate response after 4 weeks at higher dose, subcutaneous injection maximum 1 mL per injection site, reduce dose by approximately 25–50% if rise in haemoglobin concentration exceeds 2 g/100 mL over 4 weeks or if haemoglobin concentration exceeds 12 g/100 mL; if haemoglobin concentration continues to rise, despite dose reduction, suspend treatment until haemoglobin concentration decreases and then restart at a dose approximately 25% lower than the previous dose. Discontinue approximately 4 weeks after ending chemotherapy

To increase yield of autologous blood (to avoid homologous blood) in predonation programme in moderate anaemia either when large volume of blood required or when sufficient blood cannot be saved for elective major surgery
▶ BY INTRAVENOUS INJECTION
▶ Adult: 600 units/kg twice weekly for 3 weeks before surgery, consult product literature for details and advice on ensuring high iron stores, intravenous injection to be given over 1–5 minutes

Moderate anaemia (haemoglobin concentration 10–13 g/100 mL) before elective orthopaedic surgery in adults with expected moderate blood loss to reduce exposure to allogeneic blood transfusion or if autologous transfusion unavailable
▶ BY SUBCUTANEOUS INJECTION
▶ Adult: 600 units/kg once weekly for 3 weeks before surgery and on day of surgery, alternatively 300 units/kg daily for 15 days starting 10 days before surgery, consult product literature for details, subcutaneous injection maximum 1 mL per injection site

● INTERACTIONS → Appendix 1: epoetin alfa

● SIDE-EFFECTS
▶ **Common or very common** Chills · cough · diarrhoea · fever · myalgia · nausea · pain · peripheral oedema · vomiting
▶ **Uncommon** Hyperkalaemia

● PREGNANCY No evidence of harm. Benefits probably outweigh risk of anaemia and of blood transfusion in pregnancy.

● BREAST FEEDING Unlikely to be present in milk. Minimal effect on infant.

● HEPATIC IMPAIRMENT Manufacturers advise caution in chronic hepatic failure.

● PRESCRIBING AND DISPENSING INFORMATION Epoetin alfa is a biological medicine. Biological medicines must be prescribed and dispensed by brand name, see *Biological medicines* and *Biosimilar medicines*, under Guidance on prescribing p. 1.

● NATIONAL FUNDING/ACCESS DECISIONS
NICE decisions
▶ Erythropoiesis-stimulating agents (epoetin and darbepoetin) for treating anaemia in people with cancer having chemotherapy (November 2014) NICE TA323
Erythropoiesis-stimulating agents (epoetin alfa, beta, theta and zeta, and darbepoetin alfa) are recommended,

within their marketing authorisations, as options for treating anaemia in people with cancer who are having chemotherapy.
If different erythropoiesis-stimulating agents are equally suitable, the product with the lowest acquisition cost for the course of treatment should be used.
www.nice.org.uk/TA323

● MEDICINAL FORMS
There can be variation in the licensing of different medicines containing the same drug.
Solution for injection
▶ Eprex (Janssen-Cilag Ltd)
Epoetin alfa 2000 unit per 1 ml Eprex 1,000units/0.5ml solution for injection pre-filled syringes | 6 pre-filled disposable injection (PoM) £33.18

Epoetin alfa 4000 unit per 1 ml Eprex 2,000units/0.5ml solution for injection pre-filled syringes | 6 pre-filled disposable injection (PoM) £66.37

Epoetin alfa 10000 unit per 1 ml Eprex 6,000units/0.6ml solution for injection pre-filled syringes | 6 pre-filled disposable injection (PoM) £199.11
Eprex 4,000units/0.4ml solution for injection pre-filled syringes | 6 pre-filled disposable injection (PoM) £132.74
Eprex 5,000units/0.5ml solution for injection pre-filled syringes | 6 pre-filled disposable injection (PoM) £165.92
Eprex 3,000units/0.3ml solution for injection pre-filled syringes | 6 pre-filled disposable injection (PoM) £99.55
Eprex 10,000units/1ml solution for injection pre-filled syringes | 6 pre-filled disposable injection (PoM) £331.85
Eprex 8,000units/0.8ml solution for injection pre-filled syringes | 6 pre-filled disposable injection (PoM) £265.48

Epoetin alfa 40000 unit per 1 ml Eprex 20,000units/0.5ml solution for injection pre-filled syringes | 1 pre-filled disposable injection (PoM) £110.62
Eprex 30,000units/0.75ml solution for injection pre-filled syringes | 1 pre-filled disposable injection (PoM) £199.11
Eprex 40,000units/1ml solution for injection pre-filled syringes | 1 pre-filled disposable injection (PoM) £265.48

◀ 979

Epoetin beta

● INDICATIONS AND DOSE

Symptomatic anaemia associated with chronic renal failure
▶ BY SUBCUTANEOUS INJECTION
▶ Adult: Initially 20 units/kg 3 times a week for 4 weeks, increased in steps of 20 units/kg 3 times a week, according to response at intervals of 4 weeks, total weekly dose may be divided into daily doses; maintenance dose, initially reduce dose by half then adjust according to response at intervals of 1–2 weeks, total weekly maintenance dose may be given as a single dose or in 3 or 7 divided doses. Subcutaneous route preferred in patients not on haemodialysis. Reduce dose by approximately 25% if rise in haemoglobin concentration exceeds 2 g/100 mL over 4 weeks or if haemoglobin concentration approaches or exceeds 12 g/100 mL; if haemoglobin concentration continues to rise, despite dose reduction, suspend treatment until haemoglobin concentration decreases and then restart at a dose approximately 25% lower than the previous dose; maximum 720 units/kg per week
▶ BY INTRAVENOUS INJECTION
▶ Adult: Initially 40 units/kg 3 times a week for 4 weeks, then increased to 80 units/kg 3 times a week, then increased in steps of 20 units/kg 3 times a week if required, at intervals of 4 weeks; maintenance dose, initially reduce dose by half then adjust according to response at intervals of 1–2 weeks. Intravenous injection to be administered over 2 minutes. Subcutaneous route preferred in patients not on haemodialysis. Reduce dose by approximately 25% if rise in haemoglobin concentration exceeds 2 g/100 mL

9

Blood and nutrition

over 4 weeks or if haemoglobin concentration approaches or exceeds 12 g/100 mL; if haemoglobin concentration continues to rise, despite dose reduction, suspend treatment until haemoglobin concentration decreases and then restart at a dose approximately 25% lower than the previous dose; maximum 720 units/kg per week

Symptomatic anaemia in adults with non-myeloid malignancies receiving chemotherapy
▸ BY SUBCUTANEOUS INJECTION
▸ Adult: Initially 450 units/kg once weekly for 4 weeks, dose to be given weekly as a single dose or in 3–7 divided doses, increase dose after 4 weeks (if a rise in haemoglobin of at least 1 g/100 mL not achieved), increased to 900 units/kg once weekly, dose to be given weekly as a single dose or in 3–7 divided doses, if adequate response obtained reduce dose by 25–50%, discontinue treatment if haemoglobin concentration does not increase by at least 1 g/100 mL after 8 weeks of therapy (response unlikely). Reduce dose by approximately 25–50% if rise in haemoglobin concentration exceeds 2 g/100 mL over 4 weeks or if haemoglobin concentration exceeds 12 g/100 mL; if haemoglobin concentration continues to rise, despite dose reduction, suspend treatment until haemoglobin concentration decreases and then restart at a dose approximately 25% lower than the previous dose. Discontinue approximately 4 weeks after ending chemotherapy; maximum 60 000 units per week

To increase yield of autologous blood (to avoid homologous blood) in predonation programme in moderate anaemia when blood-conserving procedures are insufficient or unavailable
▸ BY INTRAVENOUS INJECTION, OR BY SUBCUTANEOUS INJECTION
▸ Adult: (consult product literature)

● INTERACTIONS → Appendix 1: epoetin beta
● SIDE-EFFECTS Severe cutaneous adverse reactions (SCARs)
● PREGNANCY No evidence of harm. Benefits probably outweigh risk of anaemia and of blood transfusion in pregnancy.
● BREAST FEEDING Unlikely to be present in milk. Minimal effect on infant.
● HEPATIC IMPAIRMENT Manufacturers advise caution in chronic hepatic failure.
● NATIONAL FUNDING/ACCESS DECISIONS
NICE decisions
▸ Erythropoiesis-stimulating agents (epoetin and darbepoetin) for treating anaemia in people with cancer having chemotherapy (November 2014) NICE TA323
Erythropoiesis-stimulating agents (epoetin alfa, beta, theta and zeta, and darbepoetin alfa) are recommended, within their marketing authorisations, as options for treating anaemia in people with cancer who are having chemotherapy.
   If different erythropoiesis-stimulating agents are equally suitable, the product with the lowest acquisition cost for the course of treatment should be used.
www.nice.org.uk/TA323

● MEDICINAL FORMS
There can be variation in the licensing of different medicines containing the same drug.
Solution for injection
EXCIPIENTS: May contain Phenylalanine
▸ NeoRecormon (Roche Products Ltd)
Epoetin beta 1667 unit per 1 ml NeoRecormon 500units/0.3ml solution for injection pre-filled syringes | 6 pre-filled disposable injection PoM £21.05

Epoetin beta 6667 unit per 1 ml NeoRecormon 2,000units/0.3ml solution for injection pre-filled syringes | 6 pre-filled disposable injection PoM £84.17
Epoetin beta 10000 unit per 1 ml NeoRecormon 3,000units/0.3ml solution for injection pre-filled syringes | 6 pre-filled disposable injection PoM £126.25
Epoetin beta 13333 unit per 1 ml NeoRecormon 4,000units/0.3ml solution for injection pre-filled syringes | 6 pre-filled disposable injection PoM £168.34
Epoetin beta 16667 unit per 1 ml NeoRecormon 10,000units/0.6ml solution for injection pre-filled syringes | 6 pre-filled disposable injection PoM £420.85
NeoRecormon 5,000units/0.3ml solution for injection pre-filled syringes | 6 pre-filled disposable injection PoM £210.42
Epoetin beta 20000 unit per 1 ml NeoRecormon 6,000units/0.3ml solution for injection pre-filled syringes | 6 pre-filled disposable injection PoM £252.50
Epoetin beta 33333 unit per 1 ml NeoRecormon 20,000units/0.6ml solution for injection pre-filled syringes | 6 pre-filled disposable injection PoM £841.71
Epoetin beta 50000 unit per 1 ml NeoRecormon 30,000units/0.6ml solution for injection pre-filled syringes | 4 pre-filled disposable injection PoM £841.71

☞ 979

Epoetin zeta

● INDICATIONS AND DOSE
Symptomatic anaemia associated with chronic renal failure in patients on haemodialysis
▸ BY INTRAVENOUS INJECTION, OR BY SUBCUTANEOUS INJECTION
▸ Adult: Initially 50 units/kg 3 times a week, adjusted according to response, adjusted in steps of 25 units/kg 3 times a week, dose to be adjusted at intervals of at least 4 weeks; maintenance 25–100 units/kg 3 times a week, intravenous injection to be given over 1–5 minutes, if given by subcutaneous injection, a maximum of 1 mL can be given per injection site, avoid increasing haemoglobin concentration at a rate exceeding 2 g/100 mL over 4 weeks

Symptomatic anaemia associated with chronic renal failure in adults on peritoneal dialysis
▸ BY INTRAVENOUS INJECTION, OR BY SUBCUTANEOUS INJECTION
▸ Adult: Initially 50 units/kg twice weekly; maintenance 25–50 units/kg twice weekly, intravenous injection to be given over 1–5 minutes, if given by subcutaneous injection, a maximum of 1 mL can be given per injection site, avoid increasing haemoglobin concentration at a rate exceeding 2 g/100 mL over 4 weeks

Severe symptomatic anaemia of renal origin in adults with renal insufficiency not yet on dialysis
▸ BY INTRAVENOUS INJECTION, OR BY SUBCUTANEOUS INJECTION
▸ Adult: Initially 50 units/kg 3 times a week, adjusted according to response, adjusted in steps of 25 units/kg 3 times a week, dose to be increased at intervals of at least 4 weeks; maintenance 17–33 units/kg 3 times a week (max. per dose 200 units/kg 3 times a week), intravenous injection to be given over 1–5 minutes, if given by subcutaneous injection, a maximum of 1 mL can be given per injection site, avoid increasing haemoglobin concentration at a rate exceeding 2 g/100 mL over 4 weeks

Symptomatic anaemia in adults receiving cancer chemotherapy
▸ BY SUBCUTANEOUS INJECTION
▸ Adult: Initially 150 units/kg 3 times a week, alternatively initially 450 units/kg once weekly, increased to 300 units/kg 3 times a week, only increase dose if appropriate rise in haemoglobin (or reticulocyte count) not achieved after 4 weeks; discontinue if inadequate response after 4 weeks at higher dose, maximum 1 mL per injection site, reduce dose by approximately 25–50% if rise in   continued →

haemoglobin concentration exceeds 2 g/100 mL over 4 weeks or if haemoglobin concentration exceeds 12 g/100 mL; if haemoglobin concentration continues to rise, despite dose reduction, suspend treatment until haemoglobin concentration decreases and then restart at a dose approximately 25% lower than the previous dose. Discontinue approximately 4 weeks after ending chemotherapy

To increase yield of autologous blood (to avoid homologous blood) in predonation programme in moderate anaemia either when large volume of blood required or when sufficient blood cannot be saved for elective major surgery

▸ BY INTRAVENOUS INJECTION

▸ Adult: 600 units/kg twice weekly for 3 weeks before surgery, intravenous injection to be given over 1–5 minutes, consult product literature for details and advice on ensuring high iron stores

Moderate anaemia (haemoglobin concentration 10–13 g/100 mL) before elective orthopaedic surgery in adults with expected moderate blood loss to reduce exposure to allogeneic blood transfusion or if autologous transfusion unavailable

▸ BY SUBCUTANEOUS INJECTION

▸ Adult: 600 units/kg every week for 3 weeks before surgery and on day of surgery, alternatively 300 units/kg daily for 15 days starting 10 days before surgery, maximum 1 mL per injection site, consult product literature for details

● INTERACTIONS → Appendix 1: epoetin zeta

● SIDE-EFFECTS

▸ **Common or very common** Asthenia · dizziness

▸ **Uncommon** Intracranial haemorrhage

▸ **Rare or very rare** Angioedema

▸ **Frequency not known** Aneurysm · cerebrovascular insufficiency · hypertensive encephalopathy · myocardial infarction · myocardial ischaemia

● PREGNANCY No evidence of harm. Benefits probably outweigh risk of anaemia and of blood transfusion in pregnancy.

● BREAST FEEDING Unlikely to be present in milk. Minimal effect on infant.

● HEPATIC IMPAIRMENT Manufacturers advise caution in chronic hepatic failure.

● PRESCRIBING AND DISPENSING INFORMATION Epoetin zeta is a biological medicine. Biological medicines must be prescribed and dispensed by brand name, see *Biological medicines* and *Biosimilar medicines*, under Guidance on prescribing p. 1.

● NATIONAL FUNDING/ACCESS DECISIONS

NICE decisions

▸ **Erythropoiesis-stimulating agents (epoetin and darbepoetin) for treating anaemia in people with cancer having chemotherapy (November 2014)** NICE TA323
Erythropoiesis-stimulating agents (epoetin alfa, beta, theta and zeta, and darbepoetin alfa) are recommended, within their marketing authorisations, as options for treating anaemia in people with cancer who are having chemotherapy.

If different erythropoiesis-stimulating agents are equally suitable, the product with the lowest acquisition cost for the course of treatment should be used.
www.nice.org.uk/TA323

● MEDICINAL FORMS
There can be variation in the licensing of different medicines containing the same drug.

Solution for injection
EXCIPIENTS: May contain Phenylalanine

▸ Retacrit (Pfizer Ltd)
Epoetin zeta 3333 unit per 1 ml Retacrit 2,000units/0.6ml solution for injection pre-filled syringes | 6 pre-filled disposable injection `PoM` £57.70 (Hospital only)
Retacrit 3,000units/0.9ml solution for injection pre-filled syringes | 6 pre-filled disposable injection `PoM` £86.55 (Hospital only)
Retacrit 1,000units/0.3ml solution for injection pre-filled syringes | 6 pre-filled disposable injection `PoM` £28.85 (Hospital only)
Epoetin zeta 10000 unit per 1 ml Retacrit 6,000units/0.6ml solution for injection pre-filled syringes | 6 pre-filled disposable injection `PoM` £173.09 (Hospital only)
Retacrit 10,000units/1ml solution for injection pre-filled syringes | 6 pre-filled disposable injection `PoM` £288.48 (Hospital only)
Retacrit 8,000units/0.8ml solution for injection pre-filled syringes | 6 pre-filled disposable injection `PoM` £230.79 (Hospital only)
Retacrit 4,000units/0.4ml solution for injection pre-filled syringes | 6 pre-filled disposable injection `PoM` £115.40 (Hospital only)
Retacrit 5,000units/0.5ml solution for injection pre-filled syringes | 6 pre-filled disposable injection `PoM` £144.25 (Hospital only)
Epoetin zeta 40000 unit per 1 ml Retacrit 20,000units/0.5ml solution for injection pre-filled syringes | 1 pre-filled disposable injection `PoM` £96.16 (Hospital only)
Retacrit 40,000units/1ml solution for injection pre-filled syringes | 1 pre-filled disposable injection `PoM` £193.32 (Hospital only)
Retacrit 30,000units/0.75ml solution for injection pre-filled syringes | 1 pre-filled disposable injection `PoM` £144.25 (Hospital only)

Methoxy polyethylene glycol-epoetin beta

29-Nov-2017

● INDICATIONS AND DOSE

Symptomatic anaemia associated with chronic kidney disease in patients on dialysis and not currently treated with erythropoietins

▸ BY SUBCUTANEOUS INJECTION, OR BY INTRAVENOUS INJECTION

▸ Adult: Initially 600 nanograms/kg every 2 weeks, subcutaneous route preferred in patients not on haemodialysis, dose to be adjusted according to response at intervals of at least 1 month, maintenance dose of double the previous fortnightly dose may be given once a month if haemoglobin concentration is above 10 g/100 mL, reduce dose by approximately 25% if rate of rise in haemoglobin concentration exceeds 2 g/100 mL in 1 month or if haemoglobin concentration is increasing or approaching 12 g/100 mL; if haemoglobin concentration continues to rise, despite dose reduction, suspend treatment until haemoglobin concentration decreases and then restart at a dose approximately 25% lower than the previous dose, dose may be increased by approximately 25% if the rate of rise in haemoglobin concentration is less than 1 g/100 mL over 1 month; further increases of approximately 25% may be made at monthly intervals until the individual target haemoglobin concentration is obtained

Symptomatic anaemia associated with chronic kidney disease in patients not on dialysis and not currently treated with erythropoietins

▸ INITIALLY BY SUBCUTANEOUS INJECTION

▸ Adult: Initially 1.2 micrograms/kg every month, alternatively (by subcutaneous injection or by intravenous injection) initially 600 nanograms/kg every 2 weeks, subcutaneous route preferred in patients not on haemodialysis, dose to be adjusted according to response at intervals of at least 1 month, patients treated once every 2 weeks may be given a maintenance dose of double the previous fortnightly dose once a month if haemoglobin concentration is above 10 g/100 mL, reduce dose by approximately 25% if rate of rise in haemoglobin concentration exceeds 2 g/100 mL in 1 month or if haemoglobin concentration is increasing or approaching 12 g/100 mL; if haemoglobin concentration continues to rise, despite dose reduction, suspend treatment until haemoglobin concentration decreases and then restart at a dose approximately 25% lower than the previous dose, dose may be increased by approximately 25% if the rate of rise in haemoglobin concentration is less than 1 g/100 mL over 1 month; further increases of approximately 25% may be made at monthly intervals until the individual target haemoglobin concentration is obtained

Symptomatic anaemia associated with chronic kidney disease in patients currently treated with erythropoietins
▶ BY SUBCUTANEOUS INJECTION, OR BY INTRAVENOUS INJECTION
▶ Adult: (consult product literature)

IMPORTANT SAFETY INFORMATION

MHRA/CHM ADVICE: RECOMBINANT HUMAN ERYTHROPOIETINS: VERY RARE RISK OF SEVERE CUTANEOUS ADVERSE REACTIONS (UPDATED JANUARY 2018)

The MHRA is aware of very rare cases of severe cutaneous adverse reactions, including Stevens-Johnson syndrome and toxic epidermal necrolysis, in patients treated with erythropoietins; some cases were fatal. More severe cases were recorded with long-acting agents (darbepoetin alfa and methoxy polyethylene glycol-epoetin beta).

Patients and their carers should be advised of the signs and symptoms of severe skin reactions when starting treatment and instructed to stop treatment and seek immediate medical attention if they develop widespread rash and blistering; these rashes often follow fever or flu-like symptoms—discontinue treatment permanently if such reactions occur.

MHRA/CHM ADVICE (DECEMBER 2007) ERYTHROPOIETINS—HAEMOGLOBIN CONCENTRATION

Overcorrection of haemoglobin concentration in patients with chronic kidney disease may increase the risk of death and serious cardiovascular events, and in patients with cancer may increase the risk of thrombosis and related complications:
• patients should not be treated with erythropoietins for the licensed indications in chronic kidney disease or cancer in patients receiving chemotherapy *unless* symptoms of anaemia are present
• the haemoglobin concentration should be maintained within the range 10–12 g/100 mL
• haemoglobin concentrations higher than 12 g/100 mL should be avoided
• the aim of treatment is to relieve symptoms of anaemia, and in patients with chronic kidney disease to avoid the need for blood transfusion; the haemoglobin concentration should not be increased beyond that which provides adequate control of symptoms of anaemia (in some patients, this may be achieved at concentrations lower than the recommended range)

● CONTRA-INDICATIONS Pure red cell aplasia following erythropoietin therapy · uncontrolled hypertension
● CAUTIONS Bone marrow fibrosis (can impair the response to erythropoietin) · concurrent infection (can impair the response to erythropoietin) · haematological disease (can impair the response to erythropoietin) · haemolysis (can impair the response to erythropoietin) · inflammatory or traumatic episodes (can impair the response to erythropoietin) · malignant disease · occult blood loss (can

impair the response to erythropoietin) · severe aluminium toxicity (can impair the response to erythropoietin)
● SIDE-EFFECTS
▶ Common or very common Hypertension (dose-dependent)
▶ Uncommon Embolism and thrombosis · headache
▶ Rare or very rare Hot flush · hypertensive encephalopathy · rash maculopapular
▶ Frequency not known Pure red cell aplasia (discontinue) · severe cutaneous adverse reactions (SCARs) · thrombocytopenia
● PREGNANCY No evidence of harm in *animal* studies—manufacturer advises caution.
● BREAST FEEDING Manufacturer advises use only if potential benefit outweighs risk—present in milk in *animal* studies.
● RENAL IMPAIRMENT Manufacturer advises caution with escalation of doses in chronic renal failure.
● MONITORING REQUIREMENTS
▶ Manufacturer advises monitor haemoglobin concentration every 2 weeks until stabilised and periodically thereafter—if patient fails to respond, check reticulocyte count, and search for causative factors such as deficiencies of iron, folic acid or vitamin B12, and correct if necessary. Monitor iron status before and during treatment.
▶ Manufacturer advises monitor blood pressure before and during treatment––if inadequately controlled, reduce dose or discontinue treatment.
● PRESCRIBING AND DISPENSING INFORMATION Methoxy polyethylene glycol-epoetin beta is a biological medicine. Biological medicines must be prescribed and dispensed by brand name, see *Biological medicines* and *Biosimilar medicines*, under Guidance on prescribing p. 1.
The manufacturer of *Mircera*® has provided a *Physician's Guide* which includes important safety information to minimise the risk of pure red cell aplasia.

● MEDICINAL FORMS
There can be variation in the licensing of different medicines containing the same drug.
Solution for injection
▶ Mircera (Roche Products Ltd)
Methoxy polyethylene glycol-epoetin beta 100 microgram per 1 ml Mircera 30micrograms/0.3ml solution for injection pre-filled syringes | 1 pre-filled disposable injection PoM £44.05
Methoxy polyethylene glycol-epoetin beta 166.667 microgram per 1 ml Mircera 50micrograms/0.3ml solution for injection pre-filled syringes | 1 pre-filled disposable injection PoM £73.41
Methoxy polyethylene glycol-epoetin beta 250 microgram per 1 ml Mircera 75micrograms/0.3ml solution for injection pre-filled syringes | 1 pre-filled disposable injection PoM £110.11
Methoxy polyethylene glycol-epoetin beta 333.333 microgram per 1 ml Mircera 100micrograms/0.3ml solution for injection pre-filled syringes | 1 pre-filled disposable injection PoM £146.81
Methoxy polyethylene glycol-epoetin beta 400 microgram per 1 ml Mircera 120micrograms/0.3ml solution for injection pre-filled syringes | 1 pre-filled disposable injection PoM £176.18
Methoxy polyethylene glycol-epoetin beta 500 microgram per 1 ml Mircera 150micrograms/0.3ml solution for injection pre-filled syringes | 1 pre-filled disposable injection PoM £220.22
Methoxy polyethylene glycol-epoetin beta 600 microgram per 1 ml Mircera 360micrograms/0.6ml solution for injection pre-filled syringes | 1 pre-filled disposable injection PoM £528.56
Methoxy polyethylene glycol-epoetin beta 666.667 microgram per 1 ml Mircera 200micrograms/0.3ml solution for injection pre-filled syringes | 1 pre-filled disposable injection PoM £293.62
Methoxy polyethylene glycol-epoetin beta 833.333 microgram per 1 ml Mircera 250micrograms/0.3ml solution for injection pre-filled syringes | 1 pre-filled disposable injection PoM £367.03

1.1a Atypical haemolytic uraemic syndrome and paroxysmal nocturnal haemoglobinuria

IMMUNOSUPPRESSANTS ⟩ MONOCLONAL ANTIBODIES

Eculizumab

04-Dec-2017

- **DRUG ACTION** Eculizumab, a recombinant monoclonal antibody, inhibits terminal complement activation at the C5 protein and thereby reduces haemolysis and thrombotic microangiopathy.

- ● **INDICATIONS AND DOSE**

  Reduce haemolysis in paroxysmal nocturnal haemoglobinuria (PNH), in those with a history of blood transfusions (under expert supervision)
  - ▸ BY INTRAVENOUS INFUSION
  - ▸ Adult: Initially 600 mg once weekly for 4 weeks, then increased to 900 mg once weekly for 1 week; maintenance 900 mg every 12–16 days

  Reduce thrombotic microangiopathy in atypical haemolytic uraemic syndrome (aHUS) (specialist use only)
  - ▸ BY INTRAVENOUS INFUSION
  - ▸ Adult: Initially 900 mg once weekly for 4 weeks, then increased to 1.2 g once weekly for 1 week; maintenance 1.2 g every 12–16 days

- ● **CONTRA-INDICATIONS** Patients unvaccinated against *Neisseria meningitidis* · unresolved *Neisseria meningitidis* infection

- ● **CAUTIONS** Active systemic infection

  CAUTIONS, FURTHER INFORMATION
  - ▸ Meningococcal infection Vaccinate against *Neisseria meningitidis* at least 2 weeks before treatment (tetravalent vaccine against serotypes A, C, W135 and Y recommended); revaccinate according to current medical guidelines. Patients receiving eculizumab less than 2 weeks after receiving meningococcal vaccine must be given prophylactic antibiotics until 2 weeks after vaccination. Advise patient to report promptly any signs of meningococcal infection. Other immunisations should also be up to date.

- ● **INTERACTIONS** → Appendix 1: monoclonal antibodies

- ● **SIDE-EFFECTS**
  - ▸ **Common or very common** Alopecia · asthenia · chills · cough · decreased leucocytes · diarrhoea · dizziness · fever · gastrointestinal discomfort · headache · hypertension · increased risk of infection · influenza like illness · joint disorders · muscle complaints · nausea · oropharyngeal pain · pain · skin reactions · sleep disorders · taste altered · tremor · vomiting
  - ▸ **Uncommon** Abscess · anxiety · appetite decreased · chest discomfort · constipation · cystitis · depression · dysuria · haemorrhage · hot flush · hyperhidrosis · hypersensitivity · hypotension · meningitis meningococcal · mood swings · nasal complaints · oedema · palpitations · paraesthesia · sepsis · spontaneous penile erection · throat irritation · tinnitus · vascular disorders · vertigo · vision blurred
  - ▸ **Rare or very rare** Abnormal clotting factor · conjunctival irritation · feeling hot · gastrooesophageal reflux disease · gingival discomfort · Grave's disease · infusion related reaction · jaundice · malignant melanoma · menstrual disorder · syncope · urogenital tract gonococcal infection

- ● **CONCEPTION AND CONTRACEPTION** Manufacturer advises effective contraception during and for 5 months after treatment.

- ● **PREGNANCY** No information available—use only if potential benefit outweighs risk. Human IgG antibodies known to cross placenta.

- ● **BREAST FEEDING** No information available—manufacturer advises avoid breast-feeding during and for 5 months after treatment.

- ● **MONITORING REQUIREMENTS**
  - ▸ Monitor for 1 hour after infusion.
  - ▸ For *paroxysmal nocturnal haemoglobinuria*, monitor for intravascular haemolysis (including serum-lactate dehydrogenase concentration) during treatment and for at least 8 weeks after discontinuation.
  - ▸ For *atypical haemolytic uraemic syndrome*, monitor for thrombotic microangiopathy (measure platelet count, serum-lactate dehydrogenase concentration, and serum creatinine) during treatment and for at least 12 weeks after discontinuation.

- ● **DIRECTIONS FOR ADMINISTRATION** For *intravenous infusion* (*Soliris®*), give intermittently in Glucose 5% or Sodium chloride 0.9%. Dilute requisite dose to a concentration of 5 mg/mL and mix gently; give over 25–45 minutes (infusion time may be increased to 2 hours if infusion-related reactions occur).

- ● **PRESCRIBING AND DISPENSING INFORMATION** Consult product literature for details of supplemental doses with concomitant plasmapheresis, plasma exchange, or plasma infusion.

- ● **PATIENT AND CARER ADVICE** Patient or carers should be advised to report promptly any signs of meningococcal infection.

  A patient information card should be provided.

- ● **NATIONAL FUNDING/ACCESS DECISIONS**

  NICE decisions
  - ▸ **Eculizumab for treating atypical haemolytic uraemic syndrome (January 2015) NICE HST1**
  Eculizumab, within its marketing authorisation, is recommended for funding for treating atypical haemolytic uraemic syndrome, only if all the following arrangements are in place:
    - coordination of eculizumab use through an expert centre, **and**
    - monitoring systems to record the number of people with a diagnosis of atypical haemolytic uraemic syndrome and the number who have eculizumab, and the dose and duration of treatment, **and**
    - a national protocol for starting and stopping eculizumab for clinical reasons, **and**
    - a research programme with robust methods to evaluate when stopping treatment or dose adjustment might occur.

  The long-term budget impact of eculizumab for treating atypical haemolytic uraemic syndrome is uncertain but will be considerable. NHS England and the manufacturer should consider what opportunities might exist to reduce the cost of eculizumab to the NHS.
  www.nice.org.uk/guidance/HST1

- ● **MEDICINAL FORMS**
  There can be variation in the licensing of different medicines containing the same drug.

  Solution for infusion
  ELECTROLYTES: May contain Sodium
  - ▸ Soliris (Alexion Pharma UK Ltd)
    Eculizumab 10 mg per 1 ml Soliris 300mg/30ml concentrate for solution for infusion vials | 1 vial [PoM] £3,150.00 (Hospital only)

1.2 Iron deficiency anaemia

Anaemia, iron deficiency

Iron deficiency, treatment and prophylaxis

Treatment with an iron preparation is justified only in the presence of a demonstrable iron-deficiency state. Before starting treatment, it is important to exclude any serious underlying cause of the anaemia (e.g. gastric erosion, gastrointestinal cancer).

Prophylaxis with an iron preparation may be appropriate in malabsorption, menorrhagia, pregnancy, after subtotal or total gastrectomy, in haemodialysis patients, and in the management of low birth-weight infants such as preterm neonates.

Oral iron

Iron salts should be given by mouth unless there are good reasons for using another route.

Ferrous salts show only marginal differences between one another in efficiency of absorption of iron. Haemoglobin regeneration rate is little affected by the type of salt used provided sufficient iron is given, and in most patients the speed of response is not critical. Choice of preparation is thus usually decided by the incidence of side-effects and cost.

The oral dose of elemental iron for iron-deficiency anaemia should be 100 to 200 mg daily. It is customary to give this as dried ferrous sulfate; for prophylaxis of iron-deficiency anaemia, ferrous sulfate may be effective.

Iron content of different iron salts		
Iron salt/amount		Content of ferrous iron
ferrous fumarate	200 mg	65 mg
ferrous gluconate	300 mg	35 mg
ferrous sulfate	300 mg	60 mg
ferrous sulfate, dried	200 mg	65 mg

Compound preparations

Preparations containing iron and folic acid p. 993 are used during pregnancy in women who are at high risk of developing iron and folic acid deficiency; they should be distinguished from those used for the prevention of neural tube defects in women planning a pregnancy.

It is important to note that the small doses of folic acid contained in these preparations are inadequate for the treatment of megaloblastic anaemias.

Some oral preparations contain ascorbic acid p. 1049 to aid absorption of the iron but the therapeutic advantage of such preparations is minimal and cost may be increased.

There is no justification for the inclusion of other ingredients, such as the **B group of vitamins** (except folic acid for pregnant women).

Modified-release preparations

Modified-release preparations of iron are licensed for once-daily dosage, but have no therapeutic advantage and should not be used. These preparations are formulated to release iron gradually; the low incidence of side-effects may reflect the small amounts of iron available for absorption as the iron is carried past the first part of the duodenum into an area of the gut where absorption may be poor.

Parenteral iron

Iron can be administered parenterally as iron dextran p. 988, iron sucrose p. 989, ferric carboxymaltose p. 988, or iron isomaltoside 1000 p. 988. Parenteral iron is generally reserved for use when oral therapy is unsuccessful because the patient cannot tolerate oral iron, or does not take it

reliably, or if there is continuing blood loss, or in malabsorption. Parenteral iron may also have a role in the management of chemotherapy-induced anaemia, when given with erythropoietins, in specific patient groups (see NICE guidance).

Many patients with chronic renal failure who are receiving haemodialysis (and some who are receiving peritoneal dialysis) also require iron by the intravenous route on a regular basis.

With the exception of patients with severe renal failure receiving haemodialysis, parenteral iron does not produce a faster haemoglobin response than oral iron provided that the oral iron preparation is taken reliably and is absorbed adequately. Depending on the preparation used, parenteral iron is given as a total dose or in divided doses. Further treatment should be guided by monitoring haemoglobin and serum iron concentrations.

MINERALS AND TRACE ELEMENTS ⟩ IRON, INJECTABLE

Iron (injectable)

> **IMPORTANT SAFETY INFORMATION**
>
> MHRA/CHM ADVICE: SERIOUS HYPERSENSITIVITY REACTIONS WITH INTRAVENOUS IRON (AUGUST 2013)
>
> Serious hypersensitivity reactions, including life-threatening and fatal anaphylactic reactions, have been reported in patients receiving intravenous iron. These reactions can occur even when a previous administration has been tolerated (including a negative test dose). Test doses are no longer recommended and caution is needed with every dose of intravenous iron.
>
> Intravenous iron products should only be administered when appropriately trained staff and resuscitation facilities are immediately available; patients should be closely monitored for signs of hypersensitivity during and for at least 30 minutes after every administration. In the event of a hypersensitivity reaction, treatment should be stopped immediately and appropriate management initiated.
>
> The risk of hypersensitivity is increased in patients with known allergies, immune or inflammatory conditions, or those with a history of severe asthma, eczema, or other atopic allergy; in these patients, intravenous iron should only be used if the benefits outweigh the risks.
>
> Intravenous iron should be avoided in the first trimester of pregnancy and used in the second or third trimesters only if the benefit outweighs the potential risks for both mother and fetus.

- **SIDE-EFFECTS**
- ▶ **Common or very common** Dizziness · flushing · headache · hypertension · hypophosphataemia · hypotension · nausea · taste altered
- ▶ **Uncommon** Arrhythmias · arthralgia · bronchospasm · chest pain · chills · constipation · diarrhoea · dyspnoea · fatigue · fever · gastrointestinal discomfort · hyperhidrosis · hypersensitivity · loss of consciousness · muscle complaints · pain · peripheral oedema · sensation abnormal · skin reactions · vascular disorders · vision blurred · vomiting
- ▶ **Rare or very rare** Angioedema · anxiety · circulatory collapse · influenza like illness · malaise · palpitations · psychiatric disorder · seizure · syncope · tremor

SIDE-EFFECTS, FURTHER INFORMATION Anaphylactic reactions can occur with parenteral administration of iron complexes and facilities for cardiopulmonary resuscitation must be available.

Overdose For details on the management of poisoning, see Iron salts, under Emergency treatment of poisoning p. 1319.

Ferric carboxymaltose [F] 987

- **INDICATIONS AND DOSE**

Iron-deficiency anaemia

▶ BY SLOW INTRAVENOUS INJECTION, OR BY INTRAVENOUS INFUSION
▶ Adult: Dose calculated according to body-weight and iron deficit (consult product literature)

- CAUTIONS Allergic disorders · asthma · eczema · hypersensitivity can occur with parenteral iron and facilities for cardiopulmonary resuscitation must be available · infection (discontinue if ongoing bacteraemia) · oral iron should not be given until 5 days after last injection
- INTERACTIONS → Appendix 1: iron (injectable)
- SIDE-EFFECTS
▶ Rare or very rare Face oedema · flatulence · presyncope
- PREGNANCY Avoid in first trimester; crosses the placenta in *animal* studies. May influence skeletal development.
- HEPATIC IMPAIRMENT Use with caution. Avoid in conditions where iron overload increases risk of impairment.
- DIRECTIONS FOR ADMINISTRATION For *intravenous infusion* (*Ferinject*®), give intermittently in Sodium chloride 0.9%, dilute 200–500 mg in up to 100 mL infusion fluid and give over at least 6 minutes; dilute 0.5–1 g in up to 250 mL infusion fluid and give over at least 15 minutes.
- PRESCRIBING AND DISPENSING INFORMATION A ferric carboxymaltose complex containing 5% (50 mg/mL) of iron.

- MEDICINAL FORMS
There can be variation in the licensing of different medicines containing the same drug.
Solution for injection
ELECTROLYTES: May contain Sodium
▶ Ferinject (Vifor Pharma UK Ltd) ▼
Iron (as Ferric carboxymaltose) 50 mg per 1 ml Ferinject 1000mg/20ml solution for injection vials | 1 vial [PoM] £154.23
Ferinject 100mg/2ml solution for injection vials | 5 vial [PoM] £81.18
Ferinject 500mg/10ml solution for injection vials | 5 vial [PoM] £405.88

Iron dextran [F] 987

- **INDICATIONS AND DOSE**

Iron-deficiency anaemia

▶ BY DEEP INTRAMUSCULAR INJECTION
▶ Adult: Intramuscular injection to be administered into the gluteal muscle, doses calculated according to body-weight and iron deficit (consult product literature)
▶ BY SLOW INTRAVENOUS INJECTION, OR BY INTRAVENOUS INFUSION
▶ Adult: Doses calculated according to body-weight and iron deficit (consult product literature)

- CONTRA-INDICATIONS Active rheumatoid arthritis · asthma · eczema · history of allergic disorders · infection
- CAUTIONS Hypersensitivity can occur with parenteral iron and facilities for cardiopulmonary resuscitation must be available · oral iron should not be given until 5 days after last injection
- INTERACTIONS → Appendix 1: iron (injectable)
- SIDE-EFFECTS
▶ Uncommon Feeling hot · muscle cramps

▶ Rare or very rare Deafness (transient) · haemolysis · restlessness
▶ **Frequency not known** Rheumatoid arthritis aggravated
- PREGNANCY Avoid in first trimester.
- HEPATIC IMPAIRMENT Avoid in severe impairment.
- RENAL IMPAIRMENT Avoid in acute renal failure.
- DIRECTIONS FOR ADMINISTRATION
▶ With intravenous use For *intravenous infusion* (*Cosmofer*®), give intermittently in Glucose 5% *or* Sodium chloride 0.9%, dilute 100–200 mg in 100 mL infusion fluid; give 25mg over 15 minutes initially, then give at a rate not exceeding 6.67 mg/minute; *total dose infusion* diluted in 500 mL infusion fluid and given over 4–6 hours (initial dose 25 mg over 15 minutes).
- PRESCRIBING AND DISPENSING INFORMATION A complex of ferric hydroxide with dextran containing 5% (50 mg/mL) of iron.

- MEDICINAL FORMS
There can be variation in the licensing of different medicines containing the same drug.
Solution for injection
▶ CosmoFer (Pharmacosmos UK Ltd) ▼
Iron (as Iron dextran) 50 mg per 1 ml CosmoFer 500mg/10ml solution for injection ampoules | 2 ampoule [PoM] £79.70
CosmoFer 100mg/2ml solution for injection ampoules | 5 ampoule [PoM] £39.85

Iron isomaltoside 1000 [F] 987   21-Mar-2017

- **INDICATIONS AND DOSE**

Iron-deficiency anaemia

▶ BY INTRAVENOUS INJECTION
▶ Adult: (consult product literature)

- CONTRA-INDICATIONS Active rheumatoid arthritis · asthma · eczema · history of allergic disorders
- CAUTIONS Hypersensitivity can occur with parenteral iron and facilities for cardiopulmonary resuscitation must be available · infection (discontinue if ongoing bacteraemia) · oral iron should not be given until 5 days after last injection
- INTERACTIONS → Appendix 1: iron (injectable)
- SIDE-EFFECTS
▶ Uncommon Dermatitis · infection
▶ Rare or very rare Anaphylactic reaction · dysphonia
- PREGNANCY Avoid in first trimester.
- HEPATIC IMPAIRMENT Avoid in decompensated liver disease and hepatitis.
- NATIONAL FUNDING/ACCESS DECISIONS
Scottish Medicines Consortium (SMC) Decisions
The *Scottish Medicines Consortium* has advised (February 2017) that iron (III) isomaltoside 1000 5% (*Diafer*®) is accepted for use within NHS Scotland for the treatment of iron deficiency in adults with chronic kidney disease on dialysis, when oral iron preparations are ineffective or cannot be used. The advice is contingent upon the continuing availability of the patient access scheme in NHS Scotland or a list price that is equivalent or lower.

- MEDICINAL FORMS
There can be variation in the licensing of different medicines containing the same drug.
Solution for injection
▶ Diafer (Pharmacosmos UK Ltd) ▼
Iron isomaltoside 1000 50 mg per 1 ml Diafer 100mg/2ml solution for injection ampoules | 25 ampoule [PoM] £423.75
▶ Monofer (Pharmacosmos UK Ltd) ▼
Iron isomaltoside 1000 100 mg per 1 ml Monofer 500mg/5ml solution for injection vials | 5 vial [PoM] £423.75
Monofer 100mg/1ml solution for injection vials | 5 vial [PoM] £84.75
Monofer 1g/10ml solution for injection vials | 2 vial [PoM] £339.00

Iron sucrose

☞ 987

● INDICATIONS AND DOSE
Iron-deficiency anaemia
▶ BY SLOW INTRAVENOUS INJECTION, OR BY INTRAVENOUS INFUSION
▶ Adult: Doses calculated according to body-weight and iron deficit (consult product literature)

● CONTRA-INDICATIONS Anaphylaxis · asthma · eczema · history of allergic disorders

● CAUTIONS Hypersensitivity reactions can occur with parenteral iron and facilities for cardiopulmonary resuscitation must be available · infection (discontinue if ongoing bacteraemia · oral iron should not be given until 5 days after last injection

● INTERACTIONS → Appendix 1: iron (injectable)

● SIDE-EFFECTS
▶ **Uncommon** Asthenia · pain
▶ **Rare or very rare** Drowsiness · urine discolouration
▶ **Frequency not known** Bradycardia · cold sweat · confusion · level of consciousness decreased

● PREGNANCY Avoid in first trimester.

● HEPATIC IMPAIRMENT Use with caution. Avoid in conditions where iron overload increases risk of impairment.

● DIRECTIONS FOR ADMINISTRATION For *intravenous infusion* (*Venofer*®), give intermittently in Sodium chloride 0.9%, dilute 100 mg in up to 100 mL infusion fluid; give 25 mg over 15 minutes initially, then give at a rate not exceeding 3.33 mg/minute.

● PRESCRIBING AND DISPENSING INFORMATION A complex of ferric hydroxide with sucrose containing 2% (20 mg/mL) of iron.

● MEDICINAL FORMS
There can be variation in the licensing of different medicines containing the same drug.
Solution for injection
▶ Venofer (Vifor Pharma UK Ltd, Imported (United States)) ▼
Iron (as Iron sucrose) 20 mg per 1 ml Venofer 100mg/5ml solution for injection vials | 5 vial [PoM] £43.52
Venofer 50mg/2.5ml solution for injection vials | 5 vial [PoM] [ⓢ]

MINERALS AND TRACE ELEMENTS > IRON, ORAL

Iron (oral)

● SIDE-EFFECTS
▶ **Common or very common** Constipation · diarrhoea · gastrointestinal discomfort · nausea
▶ **Uncommon** Vomiting
▶ **Frequency not known** Appetite decreased · faeces discoloured

SIDE-EFFECTS, FURTHER INFORMATION Iron can be constipating and occasionally lead to faecal impaction. Oral iron, particularly modified-release preparations, can exacerbate diarrhoea in patients with inflammatory bowel disease; care is also needed in patients with intestinal strictures and diverticular disease.
Overdose For details on the management of poisoning, see Iron salts, under Emergency treatment of poisoning p. 1319.
Iron preparations are an important cause of accidental overdose in children and as little as 20mg/kg of elemental iron can lead to symptoms of toxicity.

● MONITORING REQUIREMENTS
▶ Therapeutic response The haemoglobin concentration should rise by about 100–200 mg/100 mL (1–2 g/litre) per day *or* 2 g/100 mL (20 g/litre) over 3–4 weeks. When the haemoglobin is in the normal range, treatment should be continued for a further 3 months to replenish the iron stores. Epithelial tissue changes such as atrophic glossitis and koilonychia are usually improved, but the response is often slow.

● PRESCRIBING AND DISPENSING INFORMATION
▶ In children Express the dose in terms of elemental iron and iron salt and select the most appropriate preparation; specify both the iron salt and formulation on the prescription. The iron content of artificial formula feeds should also be considered. The most common reason for lack of response in children is poor compliance; poor absorption is rare in children.

● PATIENT AND CARER ADVICE Although iron preparations are best absorbed on an empty stomach they can be taken after food to reduce gastro-intestinal side-effects. May discolour stools.

Ferric maltol

☞ above

20-Mar-2017

● INDICATIONS AND DOSE
Treatment of iron-deficiency anaemia in patients with inflammatory bowel disease
▶ BY MOUTH
▶ Adult: 30 mg twice daily continued until iron stores are replenished; usual duration at least 12 weeks

● CONTRA-INDICATIONS Exacerbation of inflammatory bowel disease · haemochromatosis · haemoglobin less than 9.5 g/dL · iron overload syndromes · repeated blood transfusions

● INTERACTIONS → Appendix 1: iron (oral)

● SIDE-EFFECTS
▶ **Common or very common** Flatulence
▶ **Uncommon** Headache · joint stiffness · pain in extremity · skin reactions · small intestinal bacterial overgrowth · thirst

● NATIONAL FUNDING/ACCESS DECISIONS
Scottish Medicines Consortium (SMC) Decisions
The *Scottish Medicines Consortium* has advised (December 2016) that ferric maltol (*Feraccru*®) is **not** recommended for use within NHS Scotland for the treatment of iron deficiency anaemia in adults with inflammatory bowel disease as the economic case was not demonstrated.

● MEDICINAL FORMS
There can be variation in the licensing of different medicines containing the same drug.
Capsule
▶ Feraccru (Shield Therapeutics (UK) Ltd)
Iron (as Ferric maltol) 30 mg Feraccru 30mg capsules | 56 capsule [PoM] £47.60 DT = £47.60

Ferrous fumarate

☞ above

● INDICATIONS AND DOSE
Iron-deficiency anaemia (prophylactic)
▶ BY MOUTH USING TABLETS
▶ Child 12–17 years: 210 mg 1–2 times a day
▶ Adult: 210 mg 1–2 times a day
▶ BY MOUTH USING SYRUP
▶ Child 12–17 years: 140 mg twice daily
▶ Adult: 140 mg twice daily

continued →

9

Blood and nutrition

Iron-deficiency anaemia (therapeutic)
▸ BY MOUTH USING TABLETS
▸ Child 12–17 years: 210 mg 2–3 times a day
▸ Adult: 210 mg 2–3 times a day
▸ BY MOUTH USING SYRUP
▸ Child 12–17 years: 280 mg twice daily
▸ Adult: 280 mg twice daily

FERSADAY ®

Iron-deficiency anaemia (prophylactic)
▸ BY MOUTH
▸ Adult: 322 mg daily

Iron-deficiency anaemia (therapeutic)
▸ BY MOUTH
▸ Adult: 322 mg twice daily

GALFER ® CAPSULES

Iron-deficiency anaemia (prophylactic)
▸ BY MOUTH
▸ Child 12–17 years: 305 mg daily
▸ Adult: 305 mg daily

Iron-deficiency anaemia (therapeutic)
▸ BY MOUTH
▸ Child 12–17 years: 305 mg twice daily
▸ Adult: 305 mg twice daily

GALFER ® SYRUP

Iron-deficiency anaemia (prophylaxis)
▸ BY MOUTH
▸ Child 1 month–11 years: 0.25 mL/kilogram twice daily, the total daily dose may alternatively be given in 3 divided doses, prophylactic iron supplementation may be required in babies of low birth-weight who are solely breast-fed; supplementation is started 4–6 weeks after birth and continued until mixed feeding is established; maximum 20 mL per day
▸ Child 12–17 years: 10 mL once daily
▸ Adult: 10 mL once daily

Iron-deficiency anaemia (therapeutic)
▸ BY MOUTH
▸ Child 1 month–11 years: 0.25 mL/kilogram twice daily, the total daily dose may alternatively be given in 3 divided doses; maximum 20 mL per day
▸ Child 12–17 years: 10 mL 1–2 times a day
▸ Adult: 10 mL 1–2 times a day

● INTERACTIONS → Appendix 1: iron (oral)
● SIDE-EFFECTS Faecal impaction · haemosiderosis
● PRESCRIBING AND DISPENSING INFORMATION Non-proprietary ferrous fumarate tablets may contain 210 mg (68 mg iron), syrup may contain approx. 140 mg (45 mg iron)/5 mL; *Galfer* ® capsules contain ferrous fumarate 305 mg (100 mg iron); *Fersaday* ® tablets contain ferrous fumarate 322 mg (100 mg iron).
● PATIENT AND CARER ADVICE
Medicines for Children leaflet: Ferrous fumarate for iron-deficiency anaemia www.medicinesforchildren.org.uk/ferrous-fumarate-for-iron-deficiency-anaemia

● MEDICINAL FORMS
There can be variation in the licensing of different medicines containing the same drug.
Oral solution
▸ Ferrous fumarate (Non-proprietary)
Ferrous fumarate 28 mg per 1 ml Ferrous fumarate 140mg/5ml oral solution | 200 ml Ⓟ £3.92 DT = £3.92
▸ Galfer (Thornton & Ross Ltd)
Ferrous fumarate 28 mg per 1 ml Galfer 140mg/5ml syrup sugar-free | 300 ml Ⓟ £5.33 DT = £5.33
Tablet
▸ Ferrous fumarate (Non-proprietary)
Ferrous fumarate 210 mg Ferrous fumarate 210mg tablets | 84 tablet Ⓟ £3.50 DT = £3.50 | 84 tablet Ⓧ DT = £3.50

Ferrous fumarate 322 mg Ferrous fumarate 322mg tablets | 28 tablet Ⓟ £1.00 DT = £1.00
Capsule
▸ Galfer (Thornton & Ross Ltd)
Ferrous fumarate 305 mg Galfer 305mg capsules | 100 capsule Ⓟ £2.33 DT = £2.33 | 250 capsule Ⓟ £5.00

Ferrous fumarate with folic acid

The properties listed below are those particular to the combination only. For the properties of the components please consider, ferrous fumarate p. 989, folic acid p. 993.

● INDICATIONS AND DOSE
Iron-deficiency anaemia
▸ BY MOUTH USING CAPSULES
▸ Adult: 1 capsule daily, to be taken before food
▸ BY MOUTH USING TABLETS
▸ Adult: 1 tablet daily

● INTERACTIONS → Appendix 1: folates · iron (oral)
● PRESCRIBING AND DISPENSING INFORMATION *Pregaday* ® contains ferrous fumarate 322 mg (100 mg iron), folic acid 350 micrograms; *Galfer FA* ® contains ferrous fumarate 305 mg (100 mg iron), folic acid 350 micrograms.

● MEDICINAL FORMS
There can be variation in the licensing of different medicines containing the same drug.
Tablet
▸ Pregaday 322mg/350microgram tablets (RPH Pharmaceuticals AB)
Folic acid 350 microgram, Ferrous fumarate 322 mg Pregaday 322mg/350microgram tablets | 28 tablet Ⓟ £1.25 DT = £1.25
Capsule
▸ Galfer FA (Thornton & Ross Ltd)
Folic acid 350 microgram, Ferrous fumarate 305 mg Galfer FA capsules | 100 capsule Ⓟ £3.25 DT = £3.25

🏳 989

Ferrous gluconate

● INDICATIONS AND DOSE
Prophylaxis of iron-deficiency anaemia
▸ BY MOUTH USING TABLETS
▸ Child 6–11 years: 300–900 mg daily
▸ Child 12–17 years: 600 mg daily
▸ Adult: 600 mg daily

Treatment of iron-deficiency anaemia
▸ BY MOUTH USING TABLETS
▸ Child 6–11 years: 300–900 mg daily
▸ Child 12–17 years: 1.2–1.8 g daily in divided doses
▸ Adult: 1.2–1.8 g daily in divided doses

● INTERACTIONS → Appendix 1: iron (oral)
● SIDE-EFFECTS Gastrointestinal disorders
● PRESCRIBING AND DISPENSING INFORMATION Ferrous gluconate 300 mg contains 35 mg iron.
● PATIENT AND CARER ADVICE
Medicines for Children leaflet: Ferrous gluconate for iron-deficiency anaemia www.medicinesforchildren.org.uk/ferrous-gluconate-for-iron-deficiency-anaemia

● MEDICINAL FORMS
There can be variation in the licensing of different medicines containing the same drug.
Tablet
▸ Ferrous gluconate (Non-proprietary)
Ferrous gluconate 300 mg Ferrous gluconate 300mg tablets | 28 tablet Ⓟ £3.35 DT = £0.64 | 1000 tablet Ⓟ £15.00–£119.64

Ferrous sulfate

20-Jul-2017

⚑ 989

● INDICATIONS AND DOSE

Iron-deficiency anaemia (prophylactic)
▸ BY MOUTH USING TABLETS
▸ Child 6–17 years: 200 mg daily
▸ Adult: 200 mg daily

Iron-deficiency anaemia (therapeutic)
▸ BY MOUTH USING TABLETS
▸ Child 6–17 years: 200 mg 2–3 times a day
▸ Adult: 200 mg 2–3 times a day

FEOSPAN ®

Iron-deficiency anaemia
▸ BY MOUTH
▸ Child 1–17 years: 1 capsule daily, capsule can be opened and sprinkled on food
▸ Adult: 1–2 capsules daily, capsule can be opened and sprinkled on food

FERROGRAD ®

Iron-deficiency anaemia (prophylactic and therapeutic)
▸ BY MOUTH
▸ Child 12–17 years: 1 tablet daily
▸ Adult: 1 tablet daily

IRONORM ® DROPS

Iron-deficiency anaemia (prophylactic)
▸ BY MOUTH
▸ Adult: 2.4–4.8 mL daily

Iron-deficiency anaemia (therapeutic)
▸ BY MOUTH
▸ Adult: 4 mL 1–2 times a day

● INTERACTIONS → Appendix 1: iron (oral)

● SIDE-EFFECTS Tooth discolouration

● PRESCRIBING AND DISPENSING INFORMATION
Iron content Ferrous sulfate 200 mg is equivalent to 65 mg iron; *Ironorm* ® drops contain ferrous sulfate 125 mg (equivalent to 25 mg iron)/mL; *Feospan* ® spansules contains ferrous sulfate 150 mg (47 mg iron) (spansule (= capsules m/r)); *Ferrograd* ® tablets contain ferrous sulfate 325 mg (105 mg iron).
▸ With oral use in adults Modified-release preparations of iron are licensed for once-daily dosage, but have no therapeutic advantage and should not be used. These preparations are formulated to release iron gradually; the low incidence of side-effects may reflect the small amounts of iron available for absorption as the iron is carried past the first part of the duodenum into an area of the gut where absorption may be poor.

● PATIENT AND CARER ADVICE
Medicines for Children leaflet: Ferrous sulfate for iron-deficiency anaemia www.medicinesforchildren.org.uk/ferrous-sulfate-iron-deficiency-anaemia

● NATIONAL FUNDING/ACCESS DECISIONS
NHS restrictions *Feospan* ® is not prescribable in NHS primary care.

● LESS SUITABLE FOR PRESCRIBING *Feospan* ® is less suitable for prescribing. *Ferrograd* ® is less suitable for prescribing.

● MEDICINAL FORMS
There can be variation in the licensing of different medicines containing the same drug.
Modified-release tablet
CAUTIONARY AND ADVISORY LABELS 25
▸ Ferrograd (Teofarma)
Ferrous sulfate dried 325 mg Ferrograd 325mg modified-release tablets | 30 tablet ℗ £2.58 DT = £2.58

Tablet
▸ Ferrous sulfate (Non-proprietary)
Ferrous sulfate dried 200 mg Ferrous sulfate 200mg tablets | 28 tablet ℗ £8.15 DT = £0.95 | 60 tablet ℗ £1.78-£3.05 | 100 tablet ℗ £3.39-£10.80 | 1000 tablet ℗ £38.37-£108.00

Modified-release capsule
CAUTIONARY AND ADVISORY LABELS 25
▸ Feospan Spansules (Intrapharm Laboratories Ltd)
Ferrous sulfate dried 150 mg Feospan 150mg Spansules | 30 capsule ℗ £3.95

Oral drops
▸ Ironorm (Wallace Manufacturing Chemists Ltd)
Ferrous sulfate 125 mg per 1 ml Ironorm 125mg/ml oral drops sugar-free | 15 ml ℗ £30.00 DT = £30.00

Ferrous sulfate with ascorbic acid

20-Jul-2017

The properties listed below are those particular to the combination only. For the properties of the components please consider, ferrous sulfate above, ascorbic acid p. 1049.

● INDICATIONS AND DOSE

Iron-deficiency anaemia
▸ BY MOUTH USING MODIFIED-RELEASE TABLETS
▸ Adult: 1 tablet daily, dose to be taken before food

● INTERACTIONS → Appendix 1: ascorbic acid · iron (oral)

● NATIONAL FUNDING/ACCESS DECISIONS
NHS restrictions *Ferrograd C* ® is not prescribable in NHS primary care.

● LESS SUITABLE FOR PRESCRIBING *Ferrograd C* ® is less suitable for prescribing.

● MEDICINAL FORMS
There can be variation in the licensing of different medicines containing the same drug.
Modified-release tablet
CAUTIONARY AND ADVISORY LABELS 25
▸ Ferrograd C (Teofarma)
Ferrous sulfate dried 325 mg, Ascorbic acid (as Sodium ascorbate) 500 mg Ferrograd C modified-release tablets | 30 tablet ℗ £3.20

Ferrous sulfate with folic acid

20-Jul-2017

The properties listed below are those particular to the combination only. For the properties of the components please consider, ferrous sulfate above, folic acid p. 993.

● INDICATIONS AND DOSE

Iron-deficiency anaemia
▸ BY MOUTH USING MODIFIED-RELEASE CAPSULES
▸ Adult: 1 capsule daily
▸ BY MOUTH USING MODIFIED-RELEASE TABLETS
▸ Child 12–17 years: 1 tablet daily, to be taken before food
▸ Adult: 1 tablet daily, to be taken before food

● INTERACTIONS → Appendix 1: folates · iron (oral)

● NATIONAL FUNDING/ACCESS DECISIONS
NHS restrictions *Fefol* ® is not prescribable in NHS primary care.

● LESS SUITABLE FOR PRESCRIBING *Fefol* ® is less suitable for prescribing. *Ferrograd Folic* ® is less suitable for prescribing.

- **MEDICINAL FORMS**
There can be variation in the licensing of different medicines containing the same drug.
Modified-release tablet
CAUTIONARY AND ADVISORY LABELS 25
  ‣ Ferrograd Folic (Teofarma)
  Folic acid 350 microgram, Ferrous sulfate dried 325 mg Ferrograd Folic 325mg/350microgram modified-release tablets | 30 tablet P £2.64 DT = £2.64
Modified-release capsule
CAUTIONARY AND ADVISORY LABELS 25
  ‣ Fefol Spansules (Intrapharm Laboratories Ltd)
  Folic acid 500 microgram, Ferrous sulfate dried 150 mg Fefol Spansules | 30 capsule P £4.25

Polysaccharide-iron complex

F 989
20-Jul-2017

- **INDICATIONS AND DOSE**
Iron-deficiency anaemia (prophylactic)
  ‣ BY MOUTH
  ‣ **Child 1 month–1 year:** 1 drop (approximately 500 micrograms iron) per 450 g body-weight to be to be given 3 times a daily, dose to be administered from dropper bottle, prophylactic iron supplementation may be required in babies of low birth-weight who are solely breast-fed; supplementation is started 4–6 weeks after birth and continued until mixed feeding is established
  ‣ **Child 12–17 years:** 2.5 mL daily
  ‣ **Adult:** 2.5 mL daily
Iron-deficiency anaemia (therapeutic)
  ‣ BY MOUTH
  ‣ **Child 2–5 years:** 2.5 mL daily
  ‣ **Child 6–11 years:** 5 mL daily
  ‣ **Child 12–17 years:** 5 mL 1–2 times a day
  ‣ **Adult:** 5 mL 1–2 times a day
Iron-deficiency anaemia (therapeutic) if required during second and third trimester of pregnancy
  ‣ BY MOUTH
  ‣ **Child 12–17 years:** 5 mL once daily
  ‣ **Adult:** 5 mL once daily

- **INTERACTIONS** → Appendix 1: iron (oral)
- **PATIENT AND CARER ADVICE** Counselling on the use of the dropper advised.
- **NATIONAL FUNDING/ACCESS DECISIONS**
NHS restrictions *Niferex®* elixir is not prescribable in NHS primary care, except for the 30-mL paediatric dropper bottle for prophylaxis and treatment of iron deficiency in infants born prematurely; endorse prescription 'SLS'.

- **MEDICINAL FORMS**
There can be variation in the licensing of different medicines containing the same drug.
Oral solution
  ‣ Niferex (Tillomed Laboratories Ltd)
  Iron (as Polysaccharide-iron complex) 100 mg Niferex 100mg/5ml elixir sugar-free | 30 ml P £2.16 sugar-free | 240 ml P £6.06

Sodium feredetate

F 989

(Sodium ironedetate)

- **INDICATIONS AND DOSE**
Iron-deficiency anaemia (therapeutic)
  ‣ BY MOUTH USING ORAL SOLUTION
  ‣ **Child 1–11 months:** Up to 2.5 mL twice daily, smaller doses to be used initially
  ‣ **Child 1–4 years:** 2.5 mL 3 times a day
  ‣ **Child 5–11 years:** 5 mL 3 times a day
  ‣ **Child 12–17 years:** 5 mL 3 times a day, increased to 10 mL 3 times a day, dose to be increased gradually

  ‣ **Adult:** 5 mL 3 times a day, increased to 10 mL 3 times a day, dose to be increased gradually

- **INTERACTIONS** → Appendix 1: iron (oral)
- **PRESCRIBING AND DISPENSING INFORMATION** *Sytron®* contains 207.5 mg sodium feredetate trihydrate, which is equivalent to 27.5 mg of iron/5 mL.
- **PATIENT AND CARER ADVICE**
Medicines for Children leaflet: Sytron (sodium feredetate) for the treatment of anaemia www.medicinesforchildren.org.uk/sytron-sodium-feredetate-for-treatment-of-anaemia

- **MEDICINAL FORMS**
There can be variation in the licensing of different medicines containing the same drug.
Oral solution
  ‣ Sodium feredetate (Non-proprietary)
  Iron (as Sodium feredetate) 5.5 mg per 1 ml Sodium feredetate 190mg/5ml oral solution sugar free sugar-free | 500 ml PoM £14.95 DT = £14.95
  ‣ Sytron (Forum Health Products Ltd)
  Iron (as Sodium feredetate) 5.5 mg per 1 ml Sytron oral solution sugar-free | 500 ml P £14.95 DT = £14.95

1.3 Megaloblastic anaemia

Anaemia, megaloblastic

Overview

Most megaloblastic anaemias result from a lack of either vitamin B_12 or folate, and it is essential to establish in every case which deficiency is present and the underlying cause. In emergencies, when delay might be dangerous, it is sometimes necessary to administer both substances after the bone marrow test while plasma assay results are awaited. Normally, however, appropriate treatment should not be instituted until the results of tests are available.

One cause of megaloblastic anaemia in the UK is *pernicious anaemia* in which lack of gastric intrinsic factor resulting from an autoimmune gastritis causes malabsorption of vitamin B_12.

Vitamin B_12 is also needed in the treatment of megaloblastosis caused by *prolonged nitrous oxide anaesthesia*, which inactivates the vitamin, and in the rare syndrome of *congenital transcobalamin II deficiency*.

Vitamin B_12 should be given prophylactically after *total gastrectomy* or *total ileal resection* (or after *partial gastrectomy* if a vitamin B_12 absorption test shows vitamin B_12 malabsorption).

Apart from dietary deficiency, all other causes of vitamin B_12 deficiency are attributable to malabsorption. There is little place for the use of low-dose vitamin B_12 orally and none for vitamin B_12 intrinsic factor complexes given by mouth. Vitamin B_12 in larger oral doses [unlicensed] may be effective.

Hydroxocobalamin p. 994 has completely replaced cyanocobalamin p. 993 as the form of vitamin B_12 of choice for therapy; it is retained in the body longer than cyanocobalamin and thus for maintenance therapy can be given at intervals of up to 3 months. Treatment is generally initiated with frequent administration of intramuscular injections to replenish the depleted body stores. Thereafter, maintenance treatment, which is usually for life, can be instituted. There is no evidence that doses larger than those recommended provide any additional benefit in vitamin B_12 neuropathy.

Folic acid p. 993 has few indications for long-term therapy since most causes of folate deficiency are self-limiting or will yield to a short course of treatment. It should not be used in undiagnosed megaloblastic anaemia unless vitamin B_12 is administered concurrently otherwise neuropathy may be precipitated.

In *folate-deficient megaloblastic anaemia* (e.g. because of poor nutrition, pregnancy, or antiepileptic drugs), daily folic acid supplementation for 4 months brings about haematological remission and replenishes body stores.

For prophylaxis in *chronic haemolytic states*, *malabsorption*, or *in renal dialysis*, folic acid is given daily or sometimes weekly, depending on the diet and the rate of haemolysis.

Folic acid is also used for the prevention of methotrexate-induced side-effects in severe Crohn's disease, rheumatic disease, and severe psoriasis.

Folinic acid p. 916 is also effective in the treatment of folate deficient megaloblastic anaemia but it is generally used in association with cytotoxic drugs; it is given as calcium folinate.

There is **no** justification for prescribing multiple ingredient vitamin preparations containing vitamin B$_{12}$ or folic acid.

For the use of folic acid before and during pregnancy, see Neural tube defects (prevention in pregnancy) p. 1057.

VITAMINS AND TRACE ELEMENTS > FOLATES

Folic acid

09-Jun-2016

- ● INDICATIONS AND DOSE

Folate-deficient megaloblastic anaemia
- ▶ BY MOUTH
  - ▸ Child 1-11 months: Initially 500 micrograms/kg once daily (max. per dose 5 mg) for up to 4 months, doses up to 10 mg daily may be required in malabsorption states
  - ▸ Child 1-17 years: 5 mg daily for 4 months (until term in pregnant women), doses up to 15 mg daily may be required in malabsorption states
  - ▸ Adult: 5 mg daily for 4 months (until term in pregnant women), doses up to 15 mg daily may be required in malabsorption states

Prevention of neural tube defects (in those at a low risk of conceiving a child with a neural tube defect see Neural tube defects (prevention in pregnancy) p. 1057)
- ▶ BY MOUTH
  - ▸ Females of childbearing potential: 400 micrograms daily, to be taken before conception and until week 12 of pregnancy

Prevention of neural tube defects (in those in the high-risk group who wish to become pregnant or who are at risk of becoming pregnant see Neural tube defects (prevention in pregnancy) p. 1057)
- ▶ BY MOUTH
  - ▸ Females of childbearing potential: 5 mg daily, to be taken before conception and until week 12 of pregnancy

Prevention of neural tube defects (in those with sickle-cell disease)
- ▶ BY MOUTH
  - ▸ Females of childbearing potential: 5 mg daily, patient should continue taking their normal dose of folic acid 5 mg daily (or increase the dose to 5 mg daily) before conception and continue this throughout pregnancy

Prevention of methotrexate-induced side-effects in rheumatic disease
- ▶ BY MOUTH
  - ▸ Adult: 5 mg once weekly, dose to be taken on a different day to methotrexate dose

Prevention of methotrexate side-effects in severe Crohn's disease | Prevention of methotrexate side-effects in severe psoriasis
- ▶ BY MOUTH
  - ▸ Adult: 5 mg once weekly, dose to be taken on a different day to methotrexate dose

Prophylaxis in chronic haemolytic states
- ▶ BY MOUTH
  - ▸ Adult: 5 mg every 1–7 days, frequency dependent on underlying disease

Prophylaxis of folate deficiency in dialysis
- ▶ BY MOUTH
  - ▸ Child 1 month-11 years: 250 micrograms/kg once daily (max. per dose 10 mg)
  - ▸ Child 12-17 years: 5–10 mg once daily
  - ▸ Adult: 5 mg every 1–7 days

Prophylaxis of folate deficiency in patients receiving parenteral nutrition
- ▶ BY INTRAVENOUS INFUSION
  - ▸ Adult: 15 mg 1–2 times a week, usually given by *intravenous infusion* in the parenteral nutrition solution

- ● UNLICENSED USE Not licensed for prevention of methotrexate-induced side-effects in severe Crohn's disease, rheumatic disease and severe psoriasis.
- ● CAUTIONS Should never be given alone for pernicious anaemia (may precipitate subacute combined degeneration of the spinal cord)
- ● INTERACTIONS → Appendix 1: folates
- ● SIDE-EFFECTS Abdominal distension · appetite decreased · flatulence · nausea · vitamin B12 deficiency exacerbated
- ● PATIENT AND CARER ADVICE
Medicines for Children leaflet: Folic acid for megaloblastic anaemia caused by folate deficiency and haemolytic anaemia
www.medicinesforchildren.org.uk/folic-acid-megaloblastic-anaemia-caused-folate-deficiency-and-haemolytic-anaemia
- ● EXCEPTIONS TO LEGAL CATEGORY
  - ▸ With oral use Can be sold to the public provided daily doses do not exceed 500 micrograms.

- ● MEDICINAL FORMS
There can be variation in the licensing of different medicines containing the same drug. Forms available from special-order manufacturers include: capsule, oral suspension, oral solution, solution for injection

Tablet
- ▸ Folic acid (Non-proprietary)
  Folic acid 400 microgram Folic acid 400microgram tablets | 90 tablet [PoM] [⅀] DT = £2.71
  Folic acid 5 mg Folic acid 5mg tablets | 28 tablet [PoM] £2.00 DT = £0.47 | 1000 tablet [PoM] £16.79–£20.00

Oral solution
- ▸ Folic acid (Non-proprietary)
  Folic acid 500 microgram per 1 ml Folic acid 2.5mg/5ml oral solution sugar free sugar-free | 150 ml [PoM] £9.16 DT = £9.16 sugar-free | 150 ml £9.16 DT = £9.16
  Folic acid 1 mg per 1 ml Folic acid 5mg/5ml oral solution sugar free sugar-free | 150 ml [PoM] £13.74–£23.49 DT = £22.13
- ▸ Lexpec (Rosemont Pharmaceuticals Ltd)
  Folic acid 500 microgram per 1 ml Lexpec Folic Acid 2.5mg/5ml oral solution sugar-free | 150 ml [PoM] £9.16 DT = £9.16

VITAMINS AND TRACE ELEMENTS > VITAMIN B GROUP

Cyanocobalamin

20-Jul-2017

- ● INDICATIONS AND DOSE

Vitamin B$_{12}$ deficiency of dietary origin
- ▶ BY MOUTH
  - ▸ Adult: 50–150 micrograms daily, dose to be taken between meals
- ▶ BY INTRAMUSCULAR INJECTION
  - ▸ Adult: Initially 1 mg every 2–3 days for 11 doses; maintenance 1 mg every month

- ● PRESCRIBING AND DISPENSING INFORMATION The BP directs that when vitamin B$_{12}$ injection is prescribed or demanded hydroxocobalamin injection shall be dispensed or supplied.

Currently available brands of the tablet may not be suitable for vegans.

- **NATIONAL FUNDING/ACCESS DECISIONS**
NHS restrictions *Cyanocobalamin* solution and *Cytamen*® injection are not prescribable in NHS primary care.

- **LESS SUITABLE FOR PRESCRIBING** Cyanocobalamin is less suitable for prescribing.

- **MEDICINAL FORMS**
There can be variation in the licensing of different medicines containing the same drug. Forms available from special-order manufacturers include: tablet

Tablet
▸ Cyanocobalamin (Non-proprietary)
Cyanocobalamin 50 microgram Cyanocobalamin 50microgram tablets | 50 tablet ⓢ DT = £9.79 | 50 tablet Ⓟ £9.84 DT = £9.79
Cyanocobalamin 1 mg Behepan 1mg tablets | 100 tablet PoM ⓢ

Solution for injection
▸ Cytamen (RPH Pharmaceuticals AB)
Cyanocobalamin 1 mg per 1 ml Cytamen 1000micrograms/1ml solution for injection ampoules | 5 ampoule PoM £14.50 DT = £14.50

Oral solution
▸ Cyanocobalamin (Non-proprietary)
Cyanocobalamin 7 microgram per 1 ml Cyanocobalamin 35micrograms/5ml oral solution | 200 ml Ⓟ £8.75

Hydroxocobalamin

20-Jul-2017

- **INDICATIONS AND DOSE**
Prophylaxis of macrocytic anaemias associated with vitamin B$_{12}$ deficiency
▸ BY INTRAMUSCULAR INJECTION
▸ Adult: 1 mg every 2–3 months

Pernicious anaemia and other macrocytic anaemias without neurological involvement
▸ BY INTRAMUSCULAR INJECTION
▸ Adult: Initially 1 mg 3 times a week for 2 weeks, then 1 mg every 3 months

Pernicious anaemia and other macrocytic anaemias with neurological involvement
▸ BY INTRAMUSCULAR INJECTION
▸ Adult: Initially 1 mg once daily on alternate days until no further improvement, then 1 mg every 2 months

Tobacco amblyopia
▸ BY INTRAMUSCULAR INJECTION
▸ Adult: Initially 1 mg daily for 2 weeks, then 1 mg twice weekly until no further improvement, then 1 mg every 1–3 months

Leber's optic atrophy
▸ BY INTRAMUSCULAR INJECTION
▸ Adult: Initially 1 mg daily for 2 weeks, then 1 mg twice weekly until no further improvement, then 1 mg every 1–3 months

CYANOKIT®

Poisoning with cyanides
▸ BY INTRAVENOUS INFUSION
▸ Child (body-weight 5 kg and above): Initially 70 mg/kg (max. per dose 5 g), to be given over 15 minutes, then 70 mg/kg (max. per dose 5 g) if required, this second dose can be given over 15 minutes–2 hours depending on severity of poisoning and patient stability
▸ Adult: Initially 5 g, to be given over 15 minutes, then 5 g if required, this second dose can be given over 15 minutes–2 hours depending on severity of poisoning and patient stability

- **CAUTIONS**
▸ With intramuscular use Should not be given before diagnosis fully established

- **SIDE-EFFECTS**
GENERAL SIDE-EFFECTS Diarrhoea · dizziness · hot flush · skin reactions · urine discolouration
SPECIFIC SIDE-EFFECTS
▸ With intramuscular use Arrhythmia · chills · drug fever · headache · hypokalaemia · malaise · nausea · pain · thrombocytosis · tremor · vomiting
▸ With intravenous use Angioedema · dysphagia · extrasystole · gastrointestinal discomfort · hypersensitivity · memory loss · mucosal discolouration red · peripheral oedema · pleural effusion · rash pustular · red discolouration of plasma · restlessness · swelling · throat complaints

- **BREAST FEEDING** Present in milk but not known to be harmful.

- **EFFECT ON LABORATORY TESTS**
▸ With intravenous use Deep red colour of hydroxocobalamin may interfere with laboratory tests.

- **DIRECTIONS FOR ADMINISTRATION** For *intravenous infusion (Cyanokit)*®, given intermittently *in* Sodium chloride 0.9%, reconstitute 5 g vial with 200 mL Sodium Chloride 0.9%; gently invert vial for at least 1 minute to mix (do not shake).

- **PRESCRIBING AND DISPENSING INFORMATION**
▸ With intramuscular use The BP directs that when vitamin B$_{12}$ injection is prescribed or demanded, hydroxocobalamin injection shall be dispensed or supplied.
Poisoning by cyanides
▸ With intravenous use *Cyanokit*® is the only preparation of hydroxocobalamin that is suitable for use in victims of smoke inhalation who show signs of significant cyanide poisoning.

- **NATIONAL FUNDING/ACCESS DECISIONS**
NHS restrictions *Cobalin-H*® is not prescribable in NHS primary care.
Neo-Cytamen® is not prescribable in NHS primary care.

- **MEDICINAL FORMS**
There can be variation in the licensing of different medicines containing the same drug.

Solution for injection
▸ Hydroxocobalamin (Non-proprietary)
Hydroxocobalamin 1 mg per 1 ml Hydroxocobalamin 1mg/1ml solution for injection ampoules | 5 ampoule PoM £12.49 DT = £6.70
▸ Cobalin (AMCo)
Hydroxocobalamin 1 mg per 1 ml Cobalin-H 1mg/1ml solution for injection ampoules | 5 ampoule PoM £9.50 DT = £6.70
▸ Neo-Cytamen (RPH Pharmaceuticals AB)
Hydroxocobalamin 1 mg per 1 ml Neo-Cytamen 1000micrograms/1ml solution for injection ampoules | 5 ampoule PoM £12.49 DT = £6.70

Powder for solution for infusion
▸ Cyanokit (SERB)
Hydroxocobalamin 5 gram Cyanokit 5g powder for solution for infusion vials | 1 vial PoM £772.00

2   Iron overload

Iron overload

Overview

Severe tissue iron overload can occur in aplastic and other refractory anaemias, mainly as the result of repeated blood transfusions. It is a particular problem in refractory anaemias with hyperplastic bone marrow, especially *thalassaemia major*, where excessive iron absorption from the gut and inappropriate iron therapy can add to the tissue siderosis.

Iron overload associated with haemochromatosis can be treated with repeated venesection. Venesection may also be used for patients who have received multiple transfusions and whose bone marrow has recovered. Where venesection is contra-indicated, the long-term administration of the iron chelating compound desferrioxamine mesilate p. 996 is useful. Desferrioxamine mesilate (up to 2 g per unit of blood) may also be given at the time of blood transfusion, provided that the desferrioxamine mesilate is **not** added to the blood and is **not** given through the same line as the blood (but the two may be given through the same cannula).

Iron excretion induced by desferrioxamine mesilate is enhanced by administration of ascorbic acid (vitamin C) p. 1049 daily by mouth; it should be given separately from food since it also enhances iron absorption. Ascorbic acid should not be given to patients with cardiac dysfunction; in patients with normal cardiac function ascorbic acid should be introduced 1 month after starting desferrioxamine mesilate.

Desferrioxamine mesilate infusion can be used to treat *aluminium overload* in dialysis patients; theoretically 100 mg of desferrioxamine binds with 4.1 mg of aluminium.

ANTIDOTES AND CHELATORS > IRON CHELATORS

Deferasirox
18-Jul-2017

● **DRUG ACTION** Deferasirox is an oral iron chelator.

● **INDICATIONS AND DOSE**

Transfusion-related chronic iron overload in patients with beta thalassaemia major who receive frequent blood transfusions (7 mL/kg/month or more of packed red blood cells) (specialist use only)
▶ BY MOUTH
▶ Adult: Initially 7–21 mg/kg once daily, dose adjusted according to serum-ferritin concentration and amount of transfused blood—consult product literature, then adjusted in steps of 3.5–7 mg/kg every 3–6 months, maintenance dose adjusted according to serum-ferritin concentration; maximum 28 mg/kg per day; Usual maximum 21 mg/kg

Transfusion-related chronic iron overload when desferrioxamine is contra-indicated or inadequate in patients with beta thalassaemia major who receive infrequent blood transfusions (less than 7 mL/kg/month of packed red blood cells) (specialist use only) | **Transfusion-related chronic iron overload when desferrioxamine is contra-indicated or inadequate in patients with other anaemias (specialist use only)**
▶ BY MOUTH
▶ Adult: Initially 7–21 mg/kg once daily, dose adjusted according to serum-ferritin concentration and amount of transfused blood—consult product literature, then adjusted in steps of 3.5–7 mg/kg every 3–6 months, maintenance dose adjusted according to serum-ferritin concentration; maximum 28 mg/kg per day; Usual maximum 21 mg/kg

Chronic iron overload when desferrioxamine is contra-indicated or inadequate in non-transfusion-dependent thalassaemia syndromes (specialist use only)
▶ BY MOUTH
▶ Adult: Initially 7 mg/kg once daily, then adjusted in steps of 3.5–7 mg/kg every 3–6 months, maintenance dose adjusted according to serum-ferritin concentration and liver-iron concentration (consult product literature); maximum 14 mg/kg per day

● CAUTIONS Elderly (increased risk of side-effects) · history of liver cirrhosis · not recommended in conditions which may reduce life expectancy (e.g. high-risk myelodysplastic syndromes) · platelet count less than 50x10⁹/litre · risk of gastro-intestinal ulceration and haemorrhage · unexplained cytopenia—consider treatment interruption

● INTERACTIONS → Appendix 1: iron chelators
● SIDE-EFFECTS
▶ **Common or very common** Constipation · diarrhoea · gastrointestinal discomfort · headache · nausea · skin reactions · urine abnormalities · vomiting
▶ **Uncommon** Anxiety · cataract · cholelithiasis · deafness · dizziness · fatigue · fever · gastrointestinal disorders · gastrointestinal haemorrhage (including fatal cases) · hepatic disorders · laryngeal pain · maculopathy · oedema · renal tubular disorders · sleep disorder
▶ **Rare or very rare** Optic neuritis
▶ **Frequency not known** Acute kidney injury · alopecia · anaemia aggravated · angioedema · hypersensitivity vasculitis · metabolic acidosis · nephritis tubulointerstitial · nephrolithiasis · neutropenia · pancreatitis acute · pancytopenia · renal tubular necrosis · severe cutaneous adverse reactions (SCARs) · thrombocytopenia

● PREGNANCY Manufacturer advises avoid unless essential— toxicity in *animal* studies.

● BREAST FEEDING Manufacturer advises avoid—present in milk in *animal* studies.

● HEPATIC IMPAIRMENT Avoid in severe impairment.
Dose adjustments Use with caution in moderate impairment, reduce dose considerably then gradually increase to max. 50% of normal dose.

● RENAL IMPAIRMENT Manufacturer advises avoid if estimated creatinine clearance less than 60 mL/minute.
Dose adjustments Manufacturer advises reduce dose if creatinine clearance less than 90 mL/minute and serum creatinine increased by more than 33% of baseline measurement on 2 consecutive occasions—consult product literature.

● MONITORING REQUIREMENTS Manufacturer advises monitoring of the following patient parameters: baseline serum creatinine twice and creatinine clearance once before initiation of treatment, weekly in the first month after treatment initiation or modification, then monthly thereafter; proteinuria before treatment initiation then monthly thereafter, and other markers of renal tubular function as needed; liver function before treatment initiation, every 2 weeks during the first month of treatment, then monthly thereafter; eye and ear examinations before treatment and annually during treatment; serum-ferritin concentration monthly.

● DIRECTIONS FOR ADMINISTRATION For *film-coated tablets*, manufacturer advises tablets may be crushed and sprinkled on to soft food (yoghurt or apple sauce), then administered immediately.

● PATIENT AND CARER ADVICE Patient or carers should be given advice on how to administer deferasirox tablets.

● NATIONAL FUNDING/ACCESS DECISIONS
Scottish Medicines Consortium (SMC) Decisions
The *Scottish Medicines Consortium* has advised (June 2017) that deferasirox (*Exjade®*) is accepted for restricted use within NHS Scotland for the treatment of chronic iron overload associated with the treatment of rare acquired or inherited anaemias requiring recurrent blood transfusions. It is not recommended for patients with myelodysplastic syndromes.

Patients with myelodysplastic syndromes, the commonest cause of transfusion-dependent anaemia, were poorly represented in the clinical trial population and the economic case was not demonstrated in this group.

● MEDICINAL FORMS
There can be variation in the licensing of different medicines containing the same drug.

Tablet
CAUTIONARY AND ADVISORY LABELS 25
▸ Exjade (Novartis Pharmaceuticals UK Ltd) ▼
Deferasirox 90 mg Exjade 90mg tablets | 30 tablet PoM £126.00
Deferasirox 180 mg Exjade 180mg tablets | 30 tablet PoM £252.00
Deferasirox 360 mg Exjade 360mg tablets | 30 tablet PoM £504.00

Deferiprone

● DRUG ACTION Deferiprone is an oral iron chelator.

● INDICATIONS AND DOSE
Treatment of iron overload in patients with thalassaemia major in whom desferrioxamine is contra-indicated or is inadequate
▸ BY MOUTH
▸ Adult: 25 mg/kg 3 times a day; maximum 100 mg/kg per day

● CONTRA-INDICATIONS History of agranulocytosis or recurrent neutropenia
● INTERACTIONS → Appendix 1: deferiprone
● SIDE-EFFECTS
▸ **Common or very common** Abdominal pain (reducing dose and increasing gradually may improve tolerance) · agranulocytosis · appetite increased · arthralgia · diarrhoea (reducing dose and increasing gradually may improve tolerance) · fatigue · headache · nausea (reducing dose and increasing gradually may improve tolerance) · neutropenia · urine discolouration · vomiting (reducing dose and increasing gradually may improve tolerance)
▸ **Frequency not known** Skin reactions · zinc deficiency
● CONCEPTION AND CONTRACEPTION Manufacturer advises avoid before intended conception—teratogenic and embryotoxic in *animal* studies. Contraception advised in females of child-bearing potential.
● PREGNANCY Manufacturer advises avoid during pregnancy—teratogenic and embryotoxic in *animal* studies.
● BREAST FEEDING Manufacturer advises avoid—no information available.
● HEPATIC IMPAIRMENT Manufacturer advises monitor liver function—interrupt treatment if persistent elevation in serum alanine aminotransferase.
● RENAL IMPAIRMENT Manufacturer advises caution—no information available.
● MONITORING REQUIREMENTS
▸ Monitor neutrophil count weekly and discontinue treatment if neutropenia develops.
▸ Monitor plasma-zinc concentration.
● PATIENT AND CARER ADVICE
Blood disorders Patients or their carers should be told how to recognise signs of neutropenia and advised to seek immediate medical attention if symptoms such as fever or sore throat develop.

● MEDICINAL FORMS
There can be variation in the licensing of different medicines containing the same drug. Forms available from special-order manufacturers include: capsule, oral suspension, oral solution
Oral solution
CAUTIONARY AND ADVISORY LABELS 14
▸ Ferriprox (Swedish Orphan Biovitrum Ltd)
Deferiprone 100 mg per 1 ml Ferriprox 100mg/ml oral solution sugar-free | 500 ml PoM £152.39 DT = £152.39

Tablet
CAUTIONARY AND ADVISORY LABELS 14
▸ Ferriprox (Swedish Orphan Biovitrum Ltd)
Deferiprone 500 mg Ferriprox 500mg tablets | 100 tablet PoM £152.39 DT = £152.39
Deferiprone 1 gram Ferriprox 1000mg tablets | 50 tablet PoM £175.25 DT = £175.25

Desferrioxamine mesilate
(Deferoxamine Mesilate)

● INDICATIONS AND DOSE
Iron poisoning
▸ BY CONTINUOUS INTRAVENOUS INFUSION
▸ Adult: Initially up to 15 mg/kg/hour, max. 80 mg/kg in 24 hours, dose to be reduced after 4–6 hours, in severe cases, higher doses may be given on advice from the National Poisons Information Service
Aluminium overload in dialysis patients
▸ BY INTRAVENOUS INFUSION
▸ Adult: (consult product literature or local protocols)
Chronic iron overload (low iron overload)
▸ BY SUBCUTANEOUS INFUSION
▸ Adult: The dose should reflect the degree of iron overload
Chronic iron overload (established overload)
▸ BY SUBCUTANEOUS INFUSION
▸ Adult: 20–50 mg/kg daily

● CAUTIONS Aluminium-related encephalopathy (may exacerbate neurological dysfunction)
● INTERACTIONS → Appendix 1: iron chelators
● SIDE-EFFECTS
▸ **Common or very common** Arthralgia · bone disorder · fever · growth retardation · headache · muscle complaints · nausea · skin reactions
▸ **Uncommon** Abdominal pain · asthma · hearing impairment · vomiting
▸ **Rare or very rare** Angioedema · blood disorder · cataract · diarrhoea · dizziness · encephalopathy · eye disorders · hypersensitivity · hypotension (more common when given too rapidly by intravenous injection) · increased risk of infection · nerve disorders · nervous system disorder · paraesthesia · respiratory disorders · shock · tachycardia · thrombocytopenia · vision disorders
▸ **Frequency not known** Acute kidney injury · hypocalcaemia · leucopenia · renal tubular disorder · seizure · urine red
● PREGNANCY Teratogenic in *animal* studies. Manufacturer advises use only if potential benefit outweighs risk.
● BREAST FEEDING Manufacturer advises use only if potential benefit outweighs risk—no information available.
● RENAL IMPAIRMENT Use with caution.
● MONITORING REQUIREMENTS
▸ Eye and ear examinations before treatment and at 3-month intervals during treatment.
▸ Monitor body-weight and height in children at 3-month intervals—risk of growth retardation with excessive doses.
● DIRECTIONS FOR ADMINISTRATION For full details and warnings relating to administration, consult product literature.
For *intravenous infusion* (Desferal®), give continuously or intermittently in Glucose 5% or Sodium chloride 0.9%. Reconstitute with water for injections to a concentration of 100 mg/mL; dilute with infusion fluid.

● **MEDICINAL FORMS**
There can be variation in the licensing of different medicines containing the same drug.

Powder for solution for injection

▸ Desferrioxamine mesilate (Non-proprietary)
Desferrioxamine mesilate 500 mg Desferrioxamine 500mg powder for solution for injection vials | 10 vial PoM £39.90 | 10 vial PoM £50.00 (Hospital only)
Desferrioxamine mesilate 2 gram Desferrioxamine 2g powder for solution for injection vials | 1 vial PoM £20.00 (Hospital only)

▸ Desferal (Novartis Pharmaceuticals UK Ltd)
Desferrioxamine mesilate 500 mg Desferal 500mg powder for solution for injection vials | 10 vial PoM £46.63

3   Neutropenia and stem cell mobilisation

3.1   Neutropenia

Neutropenia

Management

Recombinant human granulocyte-colony stimulating factor (rhG-CSF) stimulates the production of neutrophils and may reduce the duration of chemotherapy-induced neutropenia and thereby reduce the incidence of associated sepsis; there is as yet no evidence that it improves overall survival. Filgrastim below (unglycosylated rhG-CSF) and lenograstim p. 998 (glycosylated rhG-CSF) have similar effects; both have been used in a variety of clinical settings, but they do not have any clear-cut routine indications. In congenital neutropenia filgrastim usually increases the neutrophil count with an appropriate clinical response. Pegfilgrastim p. 999 is a polyethylene glycol-conjugated ('pegylated') derivative of filgrastim; pegylation increases the duration of filgrastim activity. Lipegfilgrastim p. 999 is a polyethylene glycol-conjugated via a glycine linker derivative of filgrastim.
Granulocyte-colony stimulating factors should only be prescribed by those experienced in their use.

IMMUNOSTIMULANTS ⟩ GRANULOCYTE-COLONY STIMULATING FACTORS

Granulocyte-colony stimulating factors

● **DRUG ACTION** Recombinant human granulocyte-colony stimulating factor (rhG-CSF) stimulates the production of neutrophils.

● **CAUTIONS** Malignant myeloid conditions · pre-malignant myeloid conditions · risk of splenomegaly and rupture—spleen size should be monitored · sickle-cell disease

CAUTIONS, FURTHER INFORMATION
▸ Acute respiratory distress syndrome There have been reports of pulmonary infiltrates leading to acute respiratory distress syndrome—patients with a recent history of pulmonary infiltrates or pneumonia may be at higher risk.

● **SIDE-EFFECTS**
▸ **Common or very common** Arthralgia · cutaneous vasculitis · dyspnoea · haemoptysis · headache · hypersensitivity · leucocytosis · pain · spleen abnormalities · thrombocytopenia
▸ **Uncommon** Acute febrile neutrophilic dermatosis · capillary leak syndrome · hypoxia · pulmonary oedema · respiratory disorders · sickle cell anaemia with crisis

SIDE-EFFECTS, FURTHER INFORMATION Treatment should be withdrawn in patients who develop signs of pulmonary infiltration.

● **PREGNANCY** There have been reports of toxicity in *animal* studies and manufacturers advise not to use granulocyte-colony stimulating factors during pregnancy unless the potential benefit outweighs the risk.

● **BREAST FEEDING** There is no evidence for the use of granulocyte-colony stimulating factors during breast-feeding and manufacturers advise avoiding their use.

● **MONITORING REQUIREMENTS**
▸ Full blood counts including differential white cell and platelet counts should be monitored.
▸ Spleen size should be monitored during treatment—risk of splenomegaly and rupture.

◣ above

Filgrastim

(Recombinant human granulocyte-colony stimulating factor; G-CSF)

● **INDICATIONS AND DOSE**

Reduction in duration of neutropenia and incidence of febrile neutropenia in cytotoxic chemotherapy for malignancy (except chronic myeloid leukaemia and myelodysplastic syndromes) (specialist use only)
▸ BY SUBCUTANEOUS INJECTION, OR BY INTRAVENOUS INFUSION
▸ Adult: 5 micrograms/kg daily until neutrophil count in normal range, usually for up to 14 days (up to 38 days in acute myeloid leukaemia), to be started at least 24 hours after cytotoxic chemotherapy. Preferably given by subcutaneous injection; if given by intravenous infusion, administer over 30 minutes

Reduction in duration of neutropenia (and associated sequelae) in myeloablative therapy followed by bone-marrow transplantation (specialist use only)
▸ BY SUBCUTANEOUS INFUSION, OR BY INTRAVENOUS INFUSION
▸ Adult: 10 micrograms/kg daily, to be started at least 24 hours following cytotoxic chemotherapy and within 24 hours of bone-marrow infusion, then adjusted according to neutrophil count— consult product literature, doses administered over 30 minutes or 24 hours via intravenous route and over 24 hours via subcutaneous route

Mobilisation of peripheral blood progenitor cells for autologous infusion, used alone (specialist use only)
▸ BY SUBCUTANEOUS INFUSION, OR BY SUBCUTANEOUS INJECTION
▸ Adult: 10 micrograms/kg daily for 5–7 days, to be administered over 24 hours if given by subcutaneous infusion

Mobilisation of peripheral blood progenitor cells for autologous infusion, used following adjunctive myelosuppressive chemotherapy—to improve yield (specialist use only)
▸ BY SUBCUTANEOUS INJECTION
▸ Adult: 5 micrograms/kg daily until neutrophil count in normal range, to be started the day after completing chemotherapy, for timing of leucopheresis, consult product literature

Mobilisation of peripheral blood progenitor cells in normal donors for allogeneic infusion (specialist use only)
▸ BY SUBCUTANEOUS INJECTION
▸ Adult 18-59 years: 10 micrograms/kg daily for 4–5 days, for timing of leucopheresis, consult product literature

continued →

9

Blood and nutrition

Severe congenital neutropenia and history of severe or recurrent infections (distinguish carefully from other haematological disorders) (specialist use only)
▸ BY SUBCUTANEOUS INJECTION
▸ Adult: Initially 12 micrograms/kg daily, adjusted according to response, can be given in single or divided doses, consult product literature and local protocol

Severe cyclic neutropenia, or idiopathic neutropenia and history of severe or recurrent infections (distinguish carefully from other haematological disorders) (specialist use only)
▸ BY SUBCUTANEOUS INJECTION
▸ Adult: Initially 5 micrograms/kg daily, adjusted according to response, can be given in single or divided doses, consult product literature and local protocol

Persistent neutropenia in HIV infection (specialist use only)
▸ BY SUBCUTANEOUS INJECTION
▸ Adult: Initially 1 microgram/kg daily, subsequent doses increased as necessary until neutrophil count in normal range, then adjusted to maintain neutrophil count in normal range—consult product literature; maximum 4 micrograms/kg per day

● CONTRA-INDICATIONS Severe congenital neutropenia (Kostmann's syndrome) with abnormal cytogenetics
● CAUTIONS Osteoporotic bone disease (monitor bone density if given for more than 6 months) · secondary acute myeloid leukaemia
● SIDE-EFFECTS
▸ Common or very common Anaemia · diarrhoea · dysuria · haemorrhage · hepatomegaly · hyperuricaemia · hypotension · osteoporosis · rash
▸ Uncommon Fluid imbalance · graft versus host disease · peripheral vascular disease · pseudogout · rheumatoid arthritis aggravated · urine abnormalities
● MONITORING REQUIREMENTS Regular morphological and cytogenetic bone-marrow examinations recommended in severe congenital neutropenia (possible risk of myelodysplastic syndromes or leukaemia).
● DIRECTIONS FOR ADMINISTRATION For *intravenous infusion* (*Neupogen®*); (*Nivestim®*); (*Zarzio®*) give continuously or intermittently *in* Glucose 5%; for a filgrastim concentration of less than 1 500 000 units/mL (15 micrograms/mL) albumin solution (human albumin solution) is added to produce a final albumin concentration of 2 mg/mL; should not be diluted to a filgrastim concentration of less than 200 000 units/mL (2 micrograms/mL) and should not be diluted with sodium chloride solution.
● PRESCRIBING AND DISPENSING INFORMATION Filgrastim is a biological medicine. Biological medicines must be prescribed and dispensed by brand name, see *Biological medicines* and *Biosimilar medicines*, under Guidance on prescribing p. 1.
   1 million units of filgrastim solution for injection contains 10 micrograms filgrastim.

● MEDICINAL FORMS
There can be variation in the licensing of different medicines containing the same drug.

Solution for injection
▸ Accofil (Accord Healthcare Ltd) ▼
   Filgrastim 60 mega u per 1 ml Accofil 30million units/0.5ml solution for injection pre-filled syringes | 5 pre-filled disposable injection [PoM] £284.20
   Filgrastim 96 mega u per 1 ml Accofil 48million units/0.5ml solution for injection pre-filled syringes | 5 pre-filled disposable injection [PoM] £455.70
▸ Neupogen (Amgen Ltd)
   Filgrastim 30 mega u per 1 ml Neupogen 30million units/1ml solution for injection vials | 5 vial [PoM] £263.52

▸ Neupogen Singleject (Amgen Ltd)
   Filgrastim 60 mega u per 1 ml Neupogen Singleject 30million units/0.5ml solution for injection pre-filled syringes | 1 pre-filled disposable injection [PoM] £52.70
   Filgrastim 96 mega u per 1 ml Neupogen Singleject 48million units/0.5ml solution for injection pre-filled syringes | 1 pre-filled disposable injection [PoM] £84.06
▸ Nivestim (Pfizer Ltd)
   Filgrastim 60 mega u per 1 ml Nivestim 30million units/0.5ml solution for injection pre-filled syringes | 5 pre-filled disposable injection [PoM] £246.50 (Hospital only)
   Nivestim 12million units/0.2ml solution for injection pre-filled syringes | 5 pre-filled disposable injection [PoM] £153.00 (Hospital only)
   Filgrastim 96 mega u per 1 ml Nivestim 48million units/0.5ml solution for injection pre-filled syringes | 5 pre-filled disposable injection [PoM] £395.25 (Hospital only)
▸ Zarzio (Sandoz Ltd)
   Filgrastim 60 mega u per 1 ml Zarzio 30million units/0.5ml solution for injection pre-filled syringes | 5 pre-filled disposable injection [PoM] £250.75
   Filgrastim 96 mega u per 1 ml Zarzio 48million units/0.5ml solution for injection pre-filled syringes | 5 pre-filled disposable injection [PoM] £399.50

◀ 997

Lenograstim

(Recombinant human granulocyte-colony stimulating factor; rHuG-CSF)

● INDICATIONS AND DOSE

Reduction in the duration of neutropenia and associated complications following bone-marrow transplantation for non-myeloid malignancy (specialist use only) | Reduction in the duration of neutropenia and associated complications following peripheral stem cells transplantation for non-myeloid malignancy (specialist use only)
▸ BY INTRAVENOUS INFUSION, OR BY SUBCUTANEOUS INJECTION
▸ Adult: 150 micrograms/m^2 daily until neutrophil count stable in acceptable range (max. 28 days), to be started the day after transplantation. Intravenous infusion to be given over 30 minutes

Reduction in the duration of neutropenia and associated complications following treatment with cytotoxic chemotherapy associated with a significant incidence of febrile neutropenia (specialist use only)
▸ BY SUBCUTANEOUS INJECTION
▸ Adult: 150 micrograms/m^2 daily until neutrophil count stable in acceptable range (max. 28 days), to be started on the day after completion of chemotherapy

Mobilisation of peripheral blood progenitor cells for harvesting and subsequent infusion, used alone (specialist use only)
▸ BY SUBCUTANEOUS INJECTION
▸ Adult: 10 micrograms/kg daily for 4–6 days (5–6 days in healthy donors)

Mobilisation of peripheral blood progenitor cells, used following adjunctive myelosuppressive chemotherapy (to improve yield) (specialist use only)
▸ BY SUBCUTANEOUS INJECTION
▸ Adult: 150 micrograms/m^2 daily until neutrophil count stable in acceptable range, to be started 1–5 days after completion of chemotherapy, for timing of leucopheresis, consult product literature

● SIDE-EFFECTS
▸ Common or very common Abdominal pain · asthenia · pain
▸ Rare or very rare Erythema nodosum · pyoderma gangrenosum · toxic epidermal necrolysis
● DIRECTIONS FOR ADMINISTRATION For *intravenous infusion* (*Granocyte®*), give intermittently *in* Sodium chloride 0.9%; initially reconstitute with 1 mL water for injection provided (do not shake vigorously) then dilute with up to

50 mL infusion fluid for each vial of *Granocyte*-13 or up to 100 mL infusion fluid for *Granocyte*-34; give over 30 minutes.

● PRESCRIBING AND DISPENSING INFORMATION *Granocyte*® solution for injection contains 105 micrograms of lenograstim per 13.4 mega unit vial and 263 micrograms lenograstim per 33.6 mega unit vial.

● MEDICINAL FORMS
There can be variation in the licensing of different medicines containing the same drug.
Powder and solvent for solution for injection
EXCIPIENTS: May contain Phenylalanine
▸ Granocyte (Chugai Pharma UK Ltd)
  Lenograstim 13.4 mega u Granocyte-13 powder and solvent for solution for injection vials | 1 vial PoM £40.11 | 5 vial PoM £200.55
  Lenograstim 33.6 mega u Granocyte-34 powder and solvent for solution for injection vials | 1 vial PoM £62.54 | 5 vial PoM £312.69

F 997

Lipegfilgrastim

(Glycopegylated recombinant methionyl human granulocyte-colony stimulating factor)

● INDICATIONS AND DOSE
Reduction in duration of neutropenia and incidence of febrile neutropenia in cytotoxic chemotherapy for malignancy (except chronic myeloid leukaemia and myelodysplastic syndromes)
▸ BY SUBCUTANEOUS INJECTION
▸ Adult (specialist use only): 6 mg, for each chemotherapy cycle, given approximately 24 hours after chemotherapy, dose expressed as filgrastim

● CAUTIONS Myelosuppressive chemotherapy

● SIDE-EFFECTS
▸ **Common or very common** Chest pain · hypokalaemia · skin eruption

● MEDICINAL FORMS
There can be variation in the licensing of different medicines containing the same drug.
Solution for injection
▸ Lonquex (Teva UK Ltd) ▼
  Lipegfilgrastim 10 mg per 1 ml Lonquex 6mg/0.6ml solution for injection pre-filled syringes | 1 pre-filled disposable injection PoM £652.06

F 997

Pegfilgrastim

(Pegylated recombinant methionyl human granulocyte-colony stimulating factor)

● INDICATIONS AND DOSE
Reduction in duration of neutropenia and incidence of febrile neutropenia in cytotoxic chemotherapy for malignancy (except chronic myeloid leukaemia and myelodysplastic syndromes) (specialist use only)
▸ BY SUBCUTANEOUS INJECTION
▸ Adult: 6 mg for each chemotherapy cycle, to be given at least 24 hours after chemotherapy, dose is expressed as filgrastim

● CAUTIONS Acute leukaemia · myelosuppressive chemotherapy

● SIDE-EFFECTS
▸ **Common or very common** Myalgia · nausea · pain
▸ **Uncommon** Glomerulonephritis

● MEDICINAL FORMS
There can be variation in the licensing of different medicines containing the same drug.
Solution for injection
▸ Neulasta (Amgen Ltd)
  Filgrastim (as Pegfilgrastim) 10 mg per 1 ml Neulasta 6mg/0.6ml solution for injection pre-filled syringes | 1 pre-filled disposable injection PoM £686.38
  Neulasta 6mg/0.6ml solution for injection pre-filled syringes with Onpro kit | 1 pre-filled disposable injection PoM £686.38 (Hospital only)

3.2 Stem cell mobilisation

IMMUNOSTIMULANTS > CHEMOKINE RECEPTOR ANTAGONISTS

Plerixafor

● DRUG ACTION Plerixafor is a chemokine receptor antagonist.

● INDICATIONS AND DOSE
Mobilise haematopoietic stem cells to peripheral blood for collection and subsequent autologous transplantation in patients with lymphoma or multiple myeloma (specialist use only)
▸ BY SUBCUTANEOUS INJECTION
▸ Adult: 240 micrograms/kg daily usually for 2–4 days (max 7 days), to be administered 6–11 hours before initiation of apheresis, dose to be given following 4 days treatment with a granulocyte-colony stimulating factor

● SIDE-EFFECTS
▸ **Common or very common** Arthralgia · constipation · diarrhoea · dizziness · dry mouth · erythema · fatigue · flatulence · gastrointestinal discomfort · headache · hyperhidrosis · malaise · musculoskeletal pain · nausea · oral hypoaesthesia · sleep disorders · vomiting
▸ **Uncommon** Hypersensitivity

● CONCEPTION AND CONTRACEPTION Use effective contraception during treatment— teratogenic in *animal* studies.

● PREGNANCY Manufacturer advises avoid unless essential— teratogenic in *animal* studies.

● BREAST FEEDING Manufacturer advises avoid—no information available.

● RENAL IMPAIRMENT No information available if creatinine clearance less than 20 mL/minute.
Dose adjustments Reduce dose to 160 micrograms/kg daily if creatinine clearance 20–50 mL/minute.

● MONITORING REQUIREMENTS Monitor platelets and white blood cell count.

● MEDICINAL FORMS
There can be variation in the licensing of different medicines containing the same drug.
Solution for injection
▸ Mozobil (Sanofi)
  Plerixafor 20 mg per 1 ml Mozobil 24mg/1.2ml solution for injection vials | 1 vial PoM £4,882.77

9

Blood and nutrition

4 Platelet disorders

Platelet disorders

Idiopathic thrombocytopenic purpura

Acute idiopathic thrombocytopenic purpura is usually self-limiting in children. In adults, idiopathic thrombocytopenic purpura can be treated with a **corticosteroid**, e.g. prednisolone p. 664, gradually reducing the dose over several weeks. Splenectomy is considered if a satisfactory platelet count is not achieved or if there is a relapse on reducing the dose of corticosteroid or withdrawing it.

Immunoglobulin preparations, are also used in idiopathic thrombocytopenic purpura or where a temporary rapid rise in platelets is needed, as in pregnancy or pre-operatively; they are also used for children often in preference to a corticosteroid. Anti-D (Rh₀) immunoglobulin p. 1254 is effective in raising the platelet count in about 80% of unsplenectomised rhesus-positive individuals; its effects may last longer than normal immunoglobulin p. 1255 for intravenous use, but further doses are usually required.

Other therapy that has been tried in refractory idiopathic thrombocytopenic purpura includes azathioprine p. 816, cyclophosphamide p. 871, vincristine sulfate p. 904, ciclosporin p. 818, and danazol p. 725. Rituximab p. 859 [unlicensed indication] may also be effective and in some cases induces prolonged remission. For patients with chronic severe thrombocytopenia refractory to other therapy, tranexamic acid p. 110 may be given to reduce the severity of haemorrhage.

Eltrombopag p. 1001 and romiplostim p. 1002 are thrombopoietin receptor agonists licensed for the treatment of chronic idiopathic thrombocytopenic purpura in splenectomised patients refractory to other treatments, such as corticosteroids or immunoglobulins, or as a second-line treatment in non-splenectomised patients when surgery is contra-indicated (see also NICE guidance). Eltrombopag is an oral preparation and romiplostim is an injection which is made biosynthetically by recombinant DNA technology; they should both be used under the supervision of a specialist.

Essential thrombocythaemia

Anagrelide below inhibits platelet formation. It is licensed for essential thrombocythaemia in patients at risk of thrombo-haemorrhagic events who have not responded adequately to other drugs or who cannot tolerate other drugs. An at risk patient is defined by one or more of the following features: over 60 years of age, or a platelet count greater than 1000 x 10⁹/L or history of thrombo-haemorrhagic events. Anagrelide should be initiated under specialist supervision.

4.1 Essential thrombocythaemia

> **Other drugs used for Essential thrombocythaemia**
> Hydroxycarbamide, p. 910

Anagrelide

- **INDICATIONS AND DOSE**

Essential thrombocythaemia in patients at risk of thrombo-haemorrhagic events who have not responded adequately to other drugs or who cannot tolerate other drugs (initiated under specialist supervision)

▸ BY MOUTH

- ▸ Adult: Initially 500 micrograms twice daily, dose to be adjusted at weekly intervals according to response, increased in steps of 500 micrograms daily; usual dose 1–3 mg daily in divided doses (max. per dose 2.5 mg); maximum 10 mg per day

- CAUTIONS Cardiovascular disease—assess cardiac function before and regularly during treatment · concomitant use of drugs that prolong QT-interval—assess cardiac function before and regularly during treatment · risk factors for QT-interval prolongation—assess cardiac function before and regularly during treatment

- INTERACTIONS → Appendix 1: anagrelide

- SIDE-EFFECTS

▸ **Common or very common** Anaemia · arrhythmias · asthenia · diarrhoea · dizziness · fluid retention · gastrointestinal discomfort · gastrointestinal disorders · headaches · nausea · palpitations · skin reactions · vomiting

▸ **Uncommon** Alopecia · appetite decreased · arthralgia · chest pain · chills · confusion · congestive heart failure · constipation · depression · dry mouth · dyspnoea · erectile dysfunction · fever · haemorrhage · hypertension · insomnia · malaise · memory loss · myalgia · nervousness · oedema · pain · pancreatitis · pancytopenia · pneumonia · pulmonary hypertension · respiratory disorders · sensation abnormal · syncope · thrombocytopenia · weight changes

▸ **Rare or very rare** Angina pectoris · cardiomegaly · cardiomyopathy · coordination abnormal · drowsiness · dysarthria · influenza like illness · myocardial infarction · nocturia · pericardial effusion · postural hypotension · renal failure · tinnitus · vasodilation · vision disorders

▸ **Frequency not known** Hepatitis · nephritis tubulointerstitial

- CONCEPTION AND CONTRACEPTION Effective contraception required during treatment.

- PREGNANCY Manufacturer advises avoid (toxicity in *animal* studies).

- BREAST FEEDING Manufacturer advises avoid—present in milk in *animal* studies.

- HEPATIC IMPAIRMENT Manufacturer advises caution in mild impairment. Avoid in moderate to severe impairment.

- RENAL IMPAIRMENT Manufacturer advises avoid if eGFR less than 50 mL/minute/1.73 m².

- MONITORING REQUIREMENTS

▸ Monitor full blood count (monitor platelet count every 2 days for 1 week, then weekly until maintenance dose established).

▸ Monitor liver function.

▸ Monitor serum creatinine.

▸ Monitor urea.

▸ Monitor electrolytes (including potassium, magnesium and calcium) before and during treatment.

- PATIENT AND CARER ADVICE

Driving and skilled tasks Dizziness may affect performance of skilled tasks (e.g. cycling, driving).

● MEDICINAL FORMS
There can be variation in the licensing of different medicines containing the same drug.

Capsule

▸ Anagrelide (Non-proprietary)
Anagrelide (as Anagrelide hydrochloride)
500 microgram Anagrelide 500microgram capsules |
100 capsule PoM £280.00–£404.57 DT = £350.70
▸ Xagrid (Shire Pharmaceuticals Ltd) ▼
Anagrelide (as Anagrelide hydrochloride) 500 microgram Xagrid 500microgram capsules | 100 capsule PoM £404.57 DT = £350.70

4.2 Idiopathic thrombocytopenic purpura

ANTIHAEMORRHAGICS ˃ THROMBOPOIETIN RECEPTOR AGONISTS

Eltrombopag   09-Jun-2017

● INDICATIONS AND DOSE

Chronic immune (idiopathic) thrombocytopenic purpura in patients refractory to other treatments (such as corticosteroids or immunoglobulins) (under expert supervision)

▸ BY MOUTH

▸ Adult: Initially 50 mg once daily, dose to be adjusted to achieve a platelet count of 50x10⁹/litre or more—consult product literature for dose adjustments, discontinue if inadequate response after 4 weeks treatment at maximum dose; maximum 75 mg per day

▸ Adult (patients of East Asian origin): Initially 25 mg once daily, dose to be adjusted to achieve a platelet count of 50x10⁹/litre or more—consult product literature for dose adjustments, discontinue if inadequate response after 4 weeks treatment at maximum dose; maximum 75 mg per day.

Treatment of thrombocytopenia associated with chronic hepatitis C infection, where the degree of thrombocytopenia is the main factor preventing the initiation or limiting the ability to maintain optimal interferon-based therapy (under expert supervision)

▸ BY MOUTH

▸ Adult: Initially 25 mg once daily, dose to be adjusted to achieve a platelet count sufficient to initiate antiviral therapy then a platelet count of 50–75x10⁹/litre during antiviral therapy—consult product literature for dose adjustments, discontinue if inadequate response after 2 weeks treatment at maximum dose; maximum 100 mg per day

Acquired severe aplastic anaemia in patients either refractory to or heavily pretreated with prior immunosuppressive therapy and are unsuitable for haematopoietic stem cell transplantation (under expert supervision)

▸ BY MOUTH

▸ Adult: Initially 50 mg once daily, dose to be adjusted to achieve a platelet count of 50x10⁹/litre or more—consult product literature for dose adjustments, discontinue if no haematological response after 16 weeks treatment; maximum 150 mg per day

▸ Adult (patients of East Asian origin): Initially 25 mg once daily, dose to be adjusted to achieve a platelet count of 50x10⁹/litre or more—consult product literature for dose adjustments, discontinue if no haematological response after 16 weeks treatment; maximum 150 mg per day.

● CAUTIONS Patients of East Asian origin · risk factors for thromboembolism

● INTERACTIONS → Appendix 1: eltrombopag

● SIDE-EFFECTS

▸ **Common or very common** Abnormal loss of weight · alopecia · anaemia · anxiety · appetite abnormal · arthralgia · asthenia · chills · concentration impaired · confusion · constipation · cough · depression · diarrhoea · dizziness · dry eye · dry mouth · dysphagia · dyspnoea · fever · gastrointestinal discomfort · gastrointestinal disorders · haemolytic anaemia · hepatic disorders · hyperbilirubinaemia · hyperglycaemia · hypoglycaemia · increased risk of infection · influenza like illness · iron overload · lymphopenia · malaise · memory loss · menorrhagia · muscle complaints · nausea · neutropenia · oedema · oral disorders · pain · palpitations · QT interval prolongation · sensation abnormal · skin reactions · sleep disorders · splenic infarction · sweat changes · syncope · taste altered · urine discolouration · vertigo · vision disorders · vomiting · weight decreased

▸ **Uncommon** Anisocytosis · arrhythmias · balance impaired · cardiovascular disorder · cataract · chest discomfort · cyanosis · drowsiness · ear pain · electrolyte imbalance · embolism and thrombosis · eosinophilia · eye discomfort · eye disorders · eye inflammation · feeling hot · feeling jittery · food poisoning · gout · haemorrhage · headaches · hemiparesis · increased leucocytes · lens opacity · mood altered · muscle weakness · myocardial infarction · nasal complaints · nephritis lupus · nerve disorders · oropharyngeal complaints · rectosigmoid cancer · renal failure · retinal pigment epitheliopathy · sinus disorder · sleep apnoea · speech disorder · sunburn · thrombocytopenia · tremor · urinary disorders · urine abnormalities · vasodilation · wound inflammation

● CONCEPTION AND CONTRACEPTION Ensure effective contraception during treatment.

● PREGNANCY Avoid—toxicity in *animal* studies.

● BREAST FEEDING Manufacturer advises avoid.

● HEPATIC IMPAIRMENT For *thrombocytopenia associated with chronic hepatitis C infection*, manufacturer advises use only if potential benefit outweighs risk in severe impairment and monitor closely—increased risk of hepatic decompensation and thromboembolic events.
Dose adjustments For *idiopathic thrombocytopenic purpura*, manufacturer advises avoid unless potential benefit outweighs risk—reduce initial dose to 25 mg once daily and wait at least 3 weeks before upwards titration of dose.
For *severe aplastic anaemia*, manufacturer advises reduce initial dose to 25 mg once daily and wait at least 2 weeks before upwards titration of dose.
For *thrombocytopenia associated with chronic hepatitis C infection*, manufacturer advises reduce initial dose to 25 mg once daily and wait at least 2 weeks before upwards titration of dose in moderate-to-severe impairment.

● RENAL IMPAIRMENT Use with caution.

● PRE-TREATMENT SCREENING For *severe aplastic anaemia*, manufacturer advises do not initiate if patients have existing cytogenetic abnormalities of chromosome 7.

● MONITORING REQUIREMENTS

▸ Manufacturer advises monitor liver function before treatment, every two weeks when adjusting the dose, and monthly thereafter.

▸ Manufacturer advises regular ophthalmological examinations for cataract formation.

▸ Manufacturer advises peripheral blood smear prior to initiation to establish baseline level of cellular morphologic abnormalities; once stabilised, full blood count with white blood cell count differential should be performed monthly.

▸ For *idiopathic thrombocytopenic purpura*, manufacturer advises monitor full blood count including platelet count and peripheral blood smears every week during treatment until a stable platelet count is reached (50x10⁹/litre or more for at least 4 weeks), then monthly thereafter; monitor platelet count weekly for 4 weeks following treatment discontinuation.

▶ For *severe aplastic anaemia*, manufacturer advises bone marrow examination with aspirations for cytogenetics prior to initiation, at 3 months of treatment and 6 months thereafter.

▶ For *thrombocytopenia associated with chronic hepatitis C infection*, manufacturer advises monitor platelet count every week before and during antiviral treatment until a stable platelet count is reached (50–75x10^9/litre), then monitor full blood count including platelet count and peripheral blood smears monthly thereafter.

● DIRECTIONS FOR ADMINISTRATION Each dose should be taken at least 4 hours before or after any dairy products (or foods containing calcium), indigestion remedies, or medicines containing aluminium, calcium, iron, magnesium, zinc, or selenium to reduce possible interference with absorption.

● PATIENT AND CARER ADVICE Patient counselling is advised on how to administer eltrombopag tablets.

● NATIONAL FUNDING/ACCESS DECISIONS

NICE decisions

▶ Eltrombopag for treating chronic immune (idiopathic) thrombocytopenic purpura (July 2013) NICE TA293
Eltrombopag is recommended for the treatment of chronic immune (idiopathic) thrombocytopenic purpura in splenectomised adults refractory to other treatments, or as a second-line treatment in non-splenectomised adults when surgery is contra-indicated, only if:

● the manufacturer provides eltrombopag at the agreed discount as part of the patient access scheme *and*

● their condition is refractory to standard active treatments and rescue therapies *or*

● they have severe disease and a high risk of bleeding that needs frequent courses of rescue therapies.

Patients currently receiving eltrombopag whose disease does not meet these criteria should have the option to continue treatment until they and their clinician consider it appropriate to stop.
www.nice.org.uk/TA293

Scottish Medicines Consortium (SMC) Decisions

The *Scottish Medicines Consortium* has advised (July 2010) that eltrombopag (*Revolade* $^®$) is accepted for restricted use within NHS Scotland for the treatment of both splenectomised and non-splenectomised patients with severe symptomatic immune (idiopathic) thrombocytopenic purpura or a high risk of bleeding.

● MEDICINAL FORMS
There can be variation in the licensing of different medicines containing the same drug.

Tablet

▶ Revolade (Novartis Pharmaceuticals UK Ltd)
Eltrombopag (as Eltrombopag olamine) 25 mg Revolade 25mg tablets | 28 tablet [PoM] £770.00
Eltrombopag (as Eltrombopag olamine) 50 mg Revolade 50mg tablets | 28 tablet [PoM] £1,540.00
Eltrombopag (as Eltrombopag olamine) 75 mg Revolade 75mg tablets | 28 tablet [PoM] £2,310.00

Romiplostim

● INDICATIONS AND DOSE

Treatment of chronic idiopathic thrombocytopenic purpura in splenectomised patients refractory to other treatments (such as corticosteroids or immunoglobulins) (under expert supervision) | Second-line treatment of chronic idiopathic thrombocytopenic purpura in non-splenectomised patients when surgery is contra-indicated (under expert supervision)

▶ BY SUBCUTANEOUS INJECTION

▶ Adult: Initially 1 microgram/kg once weekly, adjusted in steps of 1 microgram/kg once weekly (max. per dose 10 micrograms/kg once weekly) until a stable platelet count of 50x10^9/litre is reached, discontinue treatment if inadequate response after 4 weeks at maximum dose, consult product literature for dose adjustments

● SIDE-EFFECTS

▶ **Common or very common** Anaemia · angioedema · arthralgia · asthenia · bone marrow disorders · chills · constipation · diarrhoea · dizziness · embolism and thrombosis · fever · flushing · gastrointestinal discomfort · headaches · hypersensitivity · increased risk of infection · influenza like illness · muscle complaints · nausea · pain · palpitations · peripheral oedema · sensation abnormal · skin reactions · sleep disorders

▶ **Uncommon** Alopecia · appetite decreased · chest pain · clonus · cough · dehydration · depression · dry throat · dysphagia · dyspnoea · erythromelalgia · eye disorders · eye pruritus · feeling hot · feeling jittery · gastrooesophageal reflux disease · gout · haemorrhage · hair growth abnormal · hypotension · irritability · leucocytosis · malaise · muscle weakness · myocardial infarction · nasal complaints · neoplasms · oral disorders · papilloedema · peripheral ischaemia · peripheral neuropathy · phlebitis · photosensitivity reaction · pleuritic pain · portal vein thrombosis · skin nodule · splenomegaly · taste altered · thrombocytosis · vertigo · vision disorders · vomiting · weight changes

● PREGNANCY Manufacturer advises use only if essential—toxicity in *animal* studies.

● BREAST FEEDING Manufacturer advises avoid—no information available.

● HEPATIC IMPAIRMENT Avoid in moderate or severe impairment unless potential benefit outweighs risk (e.g. of portal vein thrombosis).

● RENAL IMPAIRMENT Manufacturer advises caution—no information available.

● MONITORING REQUIREMENTS

▶ Monitor full blood count and peripheral blood smears for morphological abnormalities before and during treatment.

▶ Monitor platelet count weekly until platelet count reaches 50x10^9/litre or more for at least 4 weeks without dose adjustment, then monthly thereafter.

● PATIENT AND CARER ADVICE
Driving and skilled tasks Dizziness may affect performance of skilled tasks (e.g. driving).

● NATIONAL FUNDING/ACCESS DECISIONS

NICE decisions

▶ Romiplostim for the treatment of chronic immune (idiopathic) thrombocytopenic purpura (April 2011) NICE TA221
Romiplostim is recommended for the treatment of chronic immune (idiopathic) thrombocytopenic purpura in adults:

● if the manufacturer provides romiplostin at the agreed discount as part of the patient access scheme *and*

● whose condition is refractory to standard active treatments and rescue therapies *or*

- who have severe disease and a high risk of bleeding that needs frequent courses of rescue therapies.
www.nice.org.uk/TA221

Scottish Medicines Consortium (SMC) Decisions

The *Scottish Medicines Consortium* has advised (September 2009) that romiplostim (*Nplate®*) is accepted for restricted use within NHS Scotland for patients with severe symptomatic idiopathic thrombocytopenic purpura or those at high risk of bleeding.

- **MEDICINAL FORMS**
There can be variation in the licensing of different medicines containing the same drug.

Powder and solvent for solution for injection

▸ Nplate (Amgen Ltd)
Romiplostim 250 microgram Nplate 250microgram powder and solvent for solution for injection pre-filled disposable devices | 1 pre-filled disposable injection [PoM] £482.00

Nutrition and metabolic disorders

1   Fluid and electrolyte imbalances

Fluids and electrolytes

Electrolyte replacement therapy

The electrolyte concentrations (intravenous fluid) table and the electrolyte content (gastro-intestinal secretions) table may be helpful in planning replacement electrolyte therapy; faeces, vomit, or aspiration should be saved and analysed where possible if abnormal losses are suspected.

Oral preparations for fluid and electrolyte imbalance

Sodium and potassium salts, may be given by mouth to prevent deficiencies or to treat established deficiencies of mild or moderate degree.

Oral potassium

Compensation for potassium loss is especially necessary:

- in those taking digoxin or anti-arrhythmic drugs, where potassium depletion may induce arrhythmias;
- in patients in whom secondary hyperaldosteronism occurs, e.g. renal artery stenosis, cirrhosis of the liver, the nephrotic syndrome, and severe heart failure;
- in patients with excessive losses of potassium in the faeces, e.g. chronic diarrhoea associated with intestinal malabsorption or laxative abuse.

Measures to compensate for potassium loss may also be required in the elderly since they frequently take inadequate amounts of potassium in the diet (but see **warning** on **renal insufficiency**). Measures may also be required during long-term administration of drugs known to induce potassium loss (e.g. corticosteroids). Potassium supplements are **seldom required** with the small doses of diuretics given to treat hypertension; **potassium-sparing diuretics** (rather than potassium supplements) are recommended for prevention of hypokalaemia due to diuretics such as furosemide p. 226 or the thiazides when these are given to eliminate oedema.

If potassium salts are used for the prevention of hypokalaemia, then doses of potassium chloride daily (in divided doses) by mouth are suitable in patients taking a normal diet. *Smaller doses* must be used if there is *renal insufficiency (common in the elderly)* to reduce the **risk** of **hyperkalaemia**.

Potassium salts cause nausea and vomiting and poor compliance is a major limitation to their effectiveness; when appropriate, potassium-sparing diuretics are preferable.

When there is *established potassium depletion* larger doses may be necessary, the quantity depending on the severity of any continuing potassium loss (monitoring of plasma-potassium concentration and specialist advice would be required). Potassium depletion is frequently associated with chloride depletion and with metabolic alkalosis, and these disorders require correction.

Management of hyperkalaemia

Acute severe hyperkalaemia (plasma-potassium concentration above 6.5 mmol/litre or in the presence of ECG changes) calls for urgent treatment with calcium gluconate 10% p. 1014 by slow intravenous injection, titrated and adjusted to ECG improvement, to temporarily protect against myocardial excitability. An intravenous injection of soluble insulin (5–10 units) p. 696 with 50 mL glucose 50% given over 5–15 minutes, reduces serum-potassium concentration; this is repeated if necessary or a continuous infusion instituted. Salbutamol p. 252 [unlicensed indication], by nebulisation or slow intravenous injection may also reduce plasma-potassium concentration; it should be used with caution in patients with cardiovascular disease. The correction of causal or compounding acidosis with sodium bicarbonate infusion p. 1006 should be considered (**important**: preparations of sodium bicarbonate and calcium salts should not be administered in the same line—risk of precipitation). Drugs exacerbating hyperkalaemia should be reviewed and stopped as appropriate; occasionally haemodialysis is needed.

Ion-exchange resins may be used to remove excess potassium in *mild hyperkalaemia* or in *moderate hyperkalaemia* when there are no ECG changes.

Oral sodium and water

Sodium chloride p. 1008 is indicated in states of sodium depletion and usually needs to be given intravenously. In chronic conditions associated with mild or moderate degrees of sodium depletion, e.g. in salt-losing bowel or renal disease, oral supplements of sodium chloride or sodium bicarbonate, according to the acid-base status of the patient, may be sufficient.

Oral rehydration therapy (ORT)

As a worldwide problem *diarrhoea* is by far the most important indication for fluid and electrolyte replacement. Intestinal absorption of sodium and water is enhanced by glucose (and other carbohydrates). Replacement of fluid and electrolytes lost through diarrhoea can therefore be achieved by giving solutions containing sodium, potassium, and glucose or another carbohydrate such as rice starch.

Oral rehydration solutions should:

- enhance the absorption of water and electrolytes;
- replace the electrolyte deficit adequately and safely;
- contain an alkalinising agent to counter acidosis;
- be slightly hypo-osmolar (about 250 mmol/litre) to prevent the possible induction of osmotic diarrhoea;
- be simple to use in hospital and at home;
- be palatable and acceptable, especially to children;
- be readily available.

It is the policy of the World Health Organization (WHO) to promote a single oral rehydration solution but to use it flexibly (e.g. by giving extra water between drinks of oral rehydration solution to moderately dehydrated infants).

The WHO oral rehydration salts formulation contains sodium chloride 2.6 g, potassium chloride 1.5 g, sodium citrate 2.9 g, anhydrous glucose 13.5 g. It is dissolved in sufficient water to produce 1 litre (providing Na^+ 75 mmol, K^+ 20 mmol, Cl^- 65 mmol, citrate 10 mmol, glucose 75 mmol/litre). This formulation is recommended by the

WHO and the United Nations Children's fund, but it is not commonly used in the UK.

Oral rehydration solutions used in the UK are lower in sodium (50–60 mmol/litre) than the WHO formulation since, in general, patients suffer less severe sodium loss.

Rehydration should be rapid over 3 to 4 hours (except in hypernatraemic dehydration in which case rehydration should occur more slowly over 12 hours). The patient should be reassessed after initial rehydration and if still dehydrated rapid fluid replacement should continue.

Once rehydration is complete further dehydration is prevented by encouraging the patient to drink normal volumes of an appropriate fluid and by replacing continuing losses with an oral rehydration solution; in infants, breast-feeding or formula feeds should be offered between oral rehydration drinks.

Oral bicarbonate

Sodium bicarbonate is given by mouth for *chronic acidotic states* such as uraemic acidosis or renal tubular acidosis. The dose for correction of metabolic acidosis is not predictable and the response must be assessed. For severe *metabolic acidosis*, sodium bicarbonate can be given intravenously.

Sodium bicarbonate may also be used to increase the pH of the urine; it is also used in dyspepsia.

Sodium supplements may increase blood pressure or cause fluid retention and pulmonary oedema in those at risk; hypokalaemia may be exacerbated.

Where *hyperchloraemic acidosis* is associated with potassium deficiency, as in some renal tubular and gastrointestinal disorders it may be appropriate to give oral **potassium bicarbonate**, although acute or severe deficiency should be managed by intravenous therapy.

Parenteral preparations for fluid and electrolyte imbalance

Electrolytes and water

Solutions of electrolytes are given intravenously, to meet normal fluid and electrolyte requirements or to replenish substantial deficits or continuing losses, when the patient is nauseated or vomiting and is unable to take adequate amounts by mouth. When intravenous administration is not possible, fluid (as sodium chloride 0.9% p. 1008 or glucose 5% p. 1009) can also be given by subcutaneous infusion (hypodermoclysis).

The nature and severity of the electrolyte imbalance must be assessed from the history and clinical and biochemical investigations. Sodium, potassium, chloride, magnesium, phosphate, and water depletion can occur singly and in combination with or without disturbances of acid-base balance.

Isotonic solutions may be infused safely into a peripheral vein. Solutions more concentrated than plasma, e.g. 20% glucose, are best given through an indwelling catheter positioned in a large vein.

Intravenous sodium

Sodium chloride in isotonic solution provides the most important extracellular ions in near physiological concentrations and is indicated in *sodium depletion*, which can arise from such conditions as gastro-enteritis, diabetic ketoacidosis, ileus, and ascites. In a severe deficit of 4 to 8 litres, 2 to 3 litres of isotonic sodium chloride may be given over 2 to 3 hours; thereafter the infusion can usually be at a slower rate.

Chronic hyponatraemia arising from inappropriate secretion of antidiuretic hormone should ideally be corrected by fluid restriction. However, if sodium chloride is required for acute or chronic hyponatraemia, regardless of the cause, the deficit should be corrected slowly to avoid the risk of osmotic demyelination syndrome and the rise in plasma-sodium concentration should not exceed 10 mmol/litre in 24 hours. In severe hyponatraemia, sodium chloride 1.8% may be used cautiously.

Compound sodium lactate (Hartmann's solution) can be used instead of isotonic sodium chloride solution during or after surgery, or in the initial management of the injured or wounded; it may reduce the risk of hyperchloraemic acidosis.

Sodium chloride with glucose solutions p. 1009 are indicated when there is combined *water and sodium depletion*. A 1:1 mixture of isotonic sodium chloride and 5% glucose allows some of the water (free of sodium) to enter body cells which suffer most from dehydration while the sodium salt with a volume of water determined by the normal plasma Na^+ remains extracellular.

Combined sodium, potassium, chloride, and water depletion may occur, for example, with severe diarrhoea or persistent vomiting; replacement is carried out with sodium chloride intravenous infusion 0.9% and glucose intravenous infusion 5% with potassium as appropriate.

Intravenous glucose

Glucose solutions (5%) are used mainly to replace water deficit. Average water requirements in a healthy adult are 1.5 to 2.5 litres daily and this is needed to balance unavoidable losses of water through the skin and lungs and to provide sufficient for urinary excretion. Water depletion (dehydration) tends to occur when these losses are not matched by a comparable intake, as may occur in coma or dysphagia or in the elderly or apathetic who may not drink enough water on their own initiative.

Excessive loss of water without loss of electrolytes is uncommon, occurring in fevers, hyperthyroidism, and in uncommon water-losing renal states such as diabetes insipidus or hypercalcaemia. The volume of glucose solution needed to replace deficits varies with the severity of the disorder, but usually lies within the range of 2 to 6 litres.

Glucose solutions are also used to correct and prevent hypoglycaemia and to provide a source of energy in those too ill to be fed adequately by mouth; glucose solutions are a key component of parenteral nutrition.

Glucose solutions are given in regimens with calcium and insulin for the emergency management of *hyperkalaemia*. They are also given, after correction of hyperglycaemia, during treatment of diabetic ketoacidosis, when they must be accompanied by continuing insulin infusion.

Intravenous potassium

Potassium chloride with sodium chloride intravenous infusion p. 1008 is the initial treatment for the correction of *severe hypokalaemia* and when sufficient potassium cannot be taken by mouth.

Repeated measurement of plasma-potassium concentration is necessary to determine whether further infusions are required and to avoid the development of hyperkalaemia, which is especially likely in renal impairment.

Initial potassium replacement therapy should **not** involve glucose infusions, because glucose may cause a further decrease in the plasma-potassium concentration.

Bicarbonate and lactate

Sodium bicarbonate p. 1006 is used to control severe *metabolic acidosis* (pH<7.1) particularly that caused by loss of bicarbonate (as in renal tubular acidosis or from excessive gastro-intestinal losses). Mild metabolic acidosis associated with volume depletion should first be managed by appropriate fluid replacement because acidosis usually resolves as tissue and renal perfusion are restored. In more severe metabolic acidosis or when the acidosis remains unresponsive to correction of anoxia or hypovolaemia, sodium bicarbonate (1.26%) can be infused over 3–4 hours with plasma-pH and electrolyte monitoring. In severe shock, for example in cardiac arrest, metabolic acidosis can develop without sodium or volume depletion; in these circumstances sodium bicarbonate is best given as a small volume of hypertonic solution, such as 50 mL of 8.4% solution intravenously.

Fluids and electrolytes

Electrolyte concentrations—intravenous fluids

Intravenous infusion	Millimoles per litre				
	Na$^+$	K$^+$	HCO$_3^-$	Cl$^-$	Ca^{2+}
Normal plasma values	142	4.5	26	103	2.5
Sodium Chloride 0.9%	150	-	-	150	-
Compound Sodium Lactate (Hartmann's)	131	5	29	111	2
Sodium Chloride 0.18% and Glucose 4% (Adults only)	30	-	-	30	-
Sodium Chloride 0.45% and Glucose 5% (Children only)	75	-	-	75	-
Potassium Chloride 0.15% and Glucose 5% (Children only)	-	20	-	20	-
Potassium Chloride 0.15% and Sodium Chloride 0.9% (Children only)	150	20	-	170	-
Potassium Chloride 0.3% and Glucose 5%	-	40	-	40	-
Potassium Chloride 0.3% and Sodium Chloride 0.9%	150	40	-	190	-
To correct metabolic acidosis					
Sodium Bicarbonate 1.26%	150	-	150	-	-
Sodium Bicarbonate 8.4% for cardiac arrest	1000	-	1000	-	-
Sodium Lactate (m/6)	167	-	167	-	-

Electrolyte content—gastro-intestinal secretions

Type of fluid	Millimoles per litre				
	H$^+$	Na$^+$	K$^+$	HCO$_3^-$	Cl$^-$
Gastric	40–60	20–80	5–20	-	100–150
Biliary	-	120–140	5–15	30–50	80–120
Pancreatic	-	120–140	5–15	70–110	40–80
Small bowel	-	120–140	5–15	20–40	90–130

Sodium lactate intravenous infusion is no longer used in metabolic acidosis because of the risk of producing lactic acidosis, particularly in seriously ill patients with poor tissue perfusion or impaired hepatic function.

For *chronic acidotic states*, sodium bicarbonate can be given by mouth.

Plasma and plasma substitutes

Plasma and plasma substitutes ('colloids') contain large molecules that do not readily leave the intravascular space where they exert osmotic pressure to maintain circulatory volume. Compared to fluids containing electrolytes such as sodium chloride and glucose ('crystalloids'), a smaller volume of colloid is required to produce the same expansion of blood volume, thereby shifting salt and water from the extravascular space. If resuscitation requires a volume of fluid that exceeds the maximum dose of the colloid then crystalloids can be given; packed red cells may also be required.

Albumin solution p. 1015, prepared from whole blood, contain soluble proteins and electrolytes but no clotting factors, blood group antibodies, or plasma cholinesterases; they may be given without regard to the recipient's blood group.

Albumin is usually used after the acute phase of illness, to correct a plasma-volume deficit; hypoalbuminaemia itself is not an appropriate indication. The use of albumin solution in acute plasma or blood loss may be wasteful; plasma substitutes are more appropriate. Concentrated albumin solution (20%) can be used under specialist supervision in patients with an intravascular fluid deficit and oedema because of interstitial fluid overload, to restore intravascular plasma volume with less exacerbation of the salt and water

overload than isotonic solutions. Concentrated albumin solution p. 1015 may also be used to obtain a diuresis in hypoalbuminaemic patients (e.g. in hepatic cirrhosis).

Recent evidence does not support the previous view that the use of albumin increases mortality.

Plasma substitutes

Dextran, gelatin p. 1016, and the hydroxyethyl starch, tetrastarch, are macromolecular substances which are metabolised slowly. Dextran and gelatin may be used at the outset to expand and maintain blood volume in shock arising from conditions such as burns or septicaemia; they may also be used as an immediate short-term measure to treat haemorrhage until blood is available. Dextran and gelatin are rarely needed when shock is due to sodium and water depletion because, in these circumstances, the shock responds to water and electrolyte repletion.

Hydroxyethyl starches should only be used for the treatment of hypovolaemia due to acute blood loss when crystalloids alone are not sufficient; they should be used at the lowest effective dose for the first 24 hours of fluid resuscitation.

Plasma substitutes should **not** be used to maintain plasma volume in conditions such as burns or peritonitis where there is loss of plasma protein, water, and electrolytes over periods of several days or weeks. In these situations, plasma or plasma protein fractions containing large amounts of albumin should be given.

Large volumes of *some* plasma substitutes can increase the risk of bleeding through depletion of coagulation factors.

9

Blood and nutrition

Blood and nutrition

9

BICARBONATE

Sodium bicarbonate

● INDICATIONS AND DOSE

Alkalinisation of urine | Relief of discomfort in mild urinary-tract infections
▸ BY MOUTH
▸ **Adult:** 3 g every 2 hours until urinary pH exceeds 7, to be dissolved in water

Maintenance of alkaline urine
▸ BY MOUTH
▸ **Adult:** 5–10 g daily, to be dissolved in water

Chronic acidotic states such as uraemic acidosis or renal tubular acidosis
▸ BY MOUTH
▸ **Adult:** 4.8 g daily, (57 mmol each of Na$^+$ and HCO$_3^-$), higher doses may be required and should be adjusted according to response

Severe metabolic acidosis
▸ BY SLOW INTRAVENOUS INJECTION, OR BY INTRAVENOUS INFUSION
▸ **Adult:** Administer an amount appropriate to the body base deficit, to be given by slow intravenous injection of a strong solution (up to 8.4%), or by continuous intravenous infusion of a weaker solution (usually 1.26%)

● CONTRA-INDICATIONS
▸ With oral use Salt restricted diet

● CAUTIONS Avoid prolonged use in urinary conditions · cardiac disease · elderly · patients on sodium-restricted diet · respiratory acidosis

● INTERACTIONS → Appendix 1: sodium bicarbonate

● SIDE-EFFECTS
▸ With intravenous use Skin exfoliation · soft tissue necrosis · ulcer
▸ With oral use Abdominal cramps · burping · flatulence · hypokalaemia · metabolic alkalosis

● PREGNANCY
▸ With oral use Use with caution in urinary conditions.

● HEPATIC IMPAIRMENT In patients with fluid retention, avoid large amounts of sodium.

● RENAL IMPAIRMENT
▸ With oral use Avoid (except for specialised role in some forms of renal disease).

● MONITORING REQUIREMENTS
▸ With intravenous use Plasma-pH and electrolytes should be monitored.

● DIRECTIONS FOR ADMINISTRATION
▸ With intravenous use For *slow intravenous injection* use a small volume of hypertonic solution (such as 50 mL of 8.4%). For *continuous intravenous infusion* a weaker solution of 1.26% solution can be infused over 3–4 hours.
▸ With oral use Sodium bicarbonate may affect the stability or absorption of other drugs if administered at the same time. If possible, allow 1–2 hours before administering other drugs orally.

● PRESCRIBING AND DISPENSING INFORMATION
▸ With oral use *Sodium bicarbonate* 500*mg* capsules contain approximately 6 mmol each of Na$^+$ and HCO$_3^-$; *Sodium bicarbonate* 600*mg* capsules contain approximately 7 mmol each of Na$^+$ and HCO$_3^-$. Oral solutions of sodium bicarbonate are required occasionally; these are available from 'special-order' manufacturers or specialist importing companies; the strength of sodium bicarbonate should be stated on the prescription.
▸ With intravenous use Usual strength Sodium bicarbonate 1.26% (12.6 g, 150 mmol each of Na$^+$ and HCO$_3^-$/litre), various other strengths available.

● PATIENT AND CARER ADVICE Patients or carers should be given advice on the administration of sodium bicarbonate oral medicines.

● MEDICINAL FORMS
There can be variation in the licensing of different medicines containing the same drug. Forms available from special-order manufacturers include: capsule, oral suspension, oral solution, solution for injection

Tablet
▸ Sodium bicarbonate (Non-proprietary)
 Sodium bicarbonate 600 mg Sodium bicarbonate 600mg tablets | 100 tablet £125.50 DT = £26.77 | 100 tablet GSL £29.75 DT = £26.77

Solution for injection
▸ Sodium bicarbonate (Non-proprietary)
 Sodium bicarbonate 84 mg per 1 ml Sodium bicarbonate 8.4% (1mmol/ml) solution for injection 10ml ampoules | 10 ampoule PoM £81.27–£89.40
 Sodium bicarbonate 8.4% (1mmol/ml) solution for injection 250ml bottles | 10 bottle PoM £62.04
 Sodium bicarbonate 8.4% (1mmol/ml) solution for injection 100ml bottles | 10 bottle PoM £65.34 DT = £65.34

Oral solution
▸ Thamicarb (Thame Laboratories Ltd)
 Sodium bicarbonate 84 mg per 1 ml Thamicarb 84mg/1ml oral solution sugar-free | 100 ml P £39.80 DT = £39.80 sugar-free | 500 ml P £199.20 DT = £199.20

Capsule
▸ Sodium bicarbonate (Non-proprietary)
 Sodium bicarbonate 500 mg Sodium bicarbonate 500mg capsules | 56 capsule P £17.56 DT = £1.55 | 100 capsule £2.89

Infusion
▸ Sodium bicarbonate (Non-proprietary)
 Sodium bicarbonate 12.6 mg per 1 ml Polyfusor BC sodium bicarbonate 1.26% infusion 500ml bottles | 1 bottle PoM £10.87
 Sodium bicarbonate 14 mg per 1 ml Polyfusor BD sodium bicarbonate 1.4% infusion 500ml bottles | 1 bottle PoM £10.87
 Sodium bicarbonate 27.4 mg per 1 ml Polyfusor V sodium bicarbonate 2.74% infusion 500ml bottles | 1 bottle PoM £10.87
 Sodium bicarbonate 42 mg per 1 ml Polyfusor BE sodium bicarbonate 4.2% infusion 500ml bottles | 1 bottle PoM £10.87
 Sodium bicarbonate 84 mg per 1 ml Polyfusor B sodium bicarbonate 8.4% infusion 200ml bottles | 1 bottle PoM £10.87

ELECTROLYTES AND MINERALS ❭ POTASSIUM

Potassium chloride with calcium chloride and sodium chloride and sodium lactate

(Sodium Lactate Intravenous Infusion, Compound; Compound, Hartmann's Solution for Injection; Ringer-Lactate Solution for Injection)

The properties listed below are those particular to the combination only. For the properties of the components please consider, potassium chloride p. 1025, sodium chloride p. 1008, calcium chloride p. 1014.

● INDICATIONS AND DOSE

For prophylaxis, and replacement therapy, requiring the use of sodium chloride and lactate, with minimal amounts of calcium and potassium
▸ BY INTRAVENOUS INFUSION
▸ **Adult:** (consult product literature)

● INTERACTIONS → Appendix 1: calcium salts · potassium chloride

● PRESCRIBING AND DISPENSING INFORMATION Compound sodium lactate intravenous infusion contains Na$^+$ 131 mmol, K$^+$ 5 mmol, Ca^{2+} 2 mmol, HCO$_3^-$ (as lactate) 29 mmol, Cl$^-$ 111 mmol/litre.

• MEDICINAL FORMS
There can be variation in the licensing of different medicines containing the same drug.

Infusion

▸ Potassium chloride with calcium chloride and sodium chloride and sodium lactate (Non-proprietary)
Calcium chloride 270 microgram per 1 ml, Potassium chloride 400 microgram per 1 ml, Sodium lactate 3.17 mg per 1 ml, Sodium chloride 6 mg per 1 ml Sodium lactate compound infusion 1litre Macoflex N bags | 1 bag PoM ⛄
Sodium lactate compound infusion 1litre bags | 1 bag PoM ⛄

Potassium chloride with calcium chloride dihydrate and sodium chloride

(Ringer's solution)

The properties listed below are those particular to the combination only. For the properties of the components please consider, potassium chloride p. 1025, sodium chloride p. 1008.

● INDICATIONS AND DOSE

Electrolyte imbalance
▸ BY INTRAVENOUS INFUSION
▸ Adult: Dosed according to the deficit or daily maintenance requirements (consult product literature)

● INTERACTIONS → Appendix 1: potassium chloride

● PRESCRIBING AND DISPENSING INFORMATION Ringer's solution for injection provides the following ions (in mmol/litre), Ca^{2+} 2.2, K^+ 4, Na^+ 147, Cl^- 156.

● MEDICINAL FORMS
There can be variation in the licensing of different medicines containing the same drug.

Infusion

▸ Potassium chloride with calcium chloride dihydrate and sodium chloride (Non-proprietary)
Potassium chloride 300 microgram per 1 ml, Calcium chloride 320 microgram per 1 ml, Sodium chloride 8.6 mg per 1 ml Polyfusor C ringers infusion 500ml bottles | 1 bottle PoM £3.25
Steriflex No.9 ringers infusion 1litre bags | 1 bag PoM £2.22
Steriflex No.9 ringers infusion 500ml bags | 1 bag PoM £1.96

Potassium chloride with glucose

The properties listed below are those particular to the combination only. For the properties of the components please consider, potassium chloride p. 1025, glucose p. 1009.

● INDICATIONS AND DOSE

Electrolyte imbalance
▸ BY INTRAVENOUS INFUSION
▸ Adult: Dosed according to the deficit or daily maintenance requirements

● INTERACTIONS → Appendix 1: glucose · potassium chloride

● PRESCRIBING AND DISPENSING INFORMATION Potassium chloride 0.3% contains 40 mmol each of K^+ and Cl^-/litre or 0.15% contains 20 mmol each of K^+ and Cl^-/litre with 5% of anhydrous glucose.

● MEDICINAL FORMS
There can be variation in the licensing of different medicines containing the same drug. Forms available from special-order manufacturers include: infusion, solution for infusion

Infusion

▸ Potassium chloride with glucose (Non-proprietary)
Potassium chloride 3 mg per 1 ml, Glucose anhydrous 50 mg per 1 ml Potassium chloride 0.3% (potassium 20mmol/500ml) / glucose 5% infusion 500ml bags | 1 bag PoM £1.67

Potassium chloride 0.3% (potassium 40mmol/1litre) / Glucose 5% infusion 1litre bags | 1 bag PoM £3.11
Potassium chloride 2 mg per 1 ml, Glucose anhydrous 50 mg per 1 ml Steriflex No.29 potassium chloride 0.2% (potassium 27mmol/1litre) / glucose 5% infusion 1litre bags | 1 bag PoM £2.20
Steriflex No.29 potassium chloride 0.2% (potassium 13.3mmol/500ml) / glucose 5% infusion 500ml bags | 1 bag PoM £1.67
Potassium chloride 1.5 mg per 1 ml, Glucose anhydrous 50 mg per 1 ml Steriflex No.13 potassium chloride 0.15% (potassium 10mmol/500ml) / glucose 5% infusion 500ml bags | 1 bag PoM £1.67
Potassium chloride 0.15% (potassium 20mmol/1litre) / glucose 5% infusion 1litre bags | 1 bag PoM £1.07–£2.20
Potassium chloride 0.15% (potassium 20mmol/1litre) / Glucose 5% infusion 1litre bags | 1 bag PoM ⛄

Potassium chloride with glucose and sodium chloride

The properties listed below are those particular to the combination only. For the properties of the components please consider, potassium chloride p. 1025, glucose p. 1009, sodium chloride p. 1008.

● INDICATIONS AND DOSE

Electrolyte imbalance
▸ BY INTRAVENOUS INFUSION
▸ Adult: Dosed according to the deficit or daily maintenance requirements

● INTERACTIONS → Appendix 1: glucose · potassium chloride

● PRESCRIBING AND DISPENSING INFORMATION
Concentration of potassium chloride to be specified by the prescriber (usually K^+ 10–40 mmol/litre).

● MEDICINAL FORMS
There can be variation in the licensing of different medicines containing the same drug. Forms available from special-order manufacturers include: infusion, solution for infusion

Infusion

▸ Potassium chloride with glucose and sodium chloride (Non-proprietary)
Sodium chloride 1.8 mg per 1 ml, Potassium chloride 3 mg per 1 ml, Glucose anhydrous 40 mg per 1 ml Potassium chloride 0.3% (potassium 20mmol/500ml) / Glucose 4% / Sodium chloride 0.18% infusion 500ml bags | 1 bag PoM ⛄
Potassium chloride 0.3% (potassium 40mmol/1litre) / Glucose 4% / Sodium chloride 0.18% infusion 1litre bags | 1 bag PoM ⛄
Potassium chloride 1.5 mg per 1 ml, Sodium chloride 1.8 mg per 1 ml, Glucose anhydrous 40 mg per 1 ml Potassium chloride 0.15% (potassium 20mmol/1litre) / Glucose 4% / Sodium chloride 0.18% infusion 1litre bags | 1 bag PoM ⛄
Potassium chloride 0.15% (potassium 10mmol/500ml) / Glucose 4% / Sodium chloride 0.18% infusion 500ml bags | 1 bag PoM ⛄
Sodium chloride 1.8 mg per 1 ml, Potassium chloride 2 mg per 1 ml, Glucose anhydrous 40 mg per 1 ml Steriflex No.30 potassium chloride 0.2% (potassium 13.3mmol/500ml) / glucose 4% / sodium chloride 0.18% infusion 500ml bags | 1 bag PoM £1.67
Steriflex No.30 potassium chloride 0.2% (potassium 27mmol/1litre) / glucose 4% / sodium chloride 0.18% infusion 1litre bags | 1 bag PoM £2.20
Potassium chloride 1.5 mg per 1 ml, Sodium chloride 4.5 mg per 1 ml, Glucose anhydrous 50 mg per 1 ml Intraven potassium chloride 0.15% (potassium 10mmol/500ml) / glucose 5% / sodium chloride 0.45% infusion 500ml bags | 1 bag PoM £3.12

9 Blood and nutrition

9

Blood and nutrition

Potassium chloride with potassium bicarbonate

The properties listed below are those particular to the combination only. For the properties of the components please consider, potassium chloride p. 1025.

● INDICATIONS AND DOSE

Potassium depletion

▸ BY MOUTH

▸ Adult: Dosed according to the deficit or daily maintenance requirements (consult product literature)

● INTERACTIONS → Appendix 1: potassium chloride

● PRESCRIBING AND DISPENSING INFORMATION Each *Sando-K*® tablet contains potassium 470 mg (12 mmol of K⁺) and chloride 285mg (8 mmol of Cl⁻).

● MEDICINAL FORMS
There can be variation in the licensing of different medicines containing the same drug.
Effervescent tablet
CAUTIONARY AND ADVISORY LABELS 13, 21
▸ Sando-K (HK Pharma Ltd)
Potassium bicarbonate 400 mg, Potassium chloride 600 mg Sando-K effervescent tablets | 100 tablet P £9.95 DT = £9.95

Potassium chloride with sodium chloride

The properties listed below are those particular to the combination only. For the properties of the components please consider, potassium chloride p. 1025, sodium chloride below.

● INDICATIONS AND DOSE

Electrolyte imbalance

▸ BY INTRAVENOUS INFUSION

▸ Adult: Depending on the deficit or the daily maintenance requirements (consult product literature)

● INTERACTIONS → Appendix 1: potassium chloride

● PRESCRIBING AND DISPENSING INFORMATION Potassium chloride 0.15% with sodium chloride 0.9% contains K⁺ 20 mmol, Na⁺ 150 mmol, and Cl⁻ 170 mmol/litre or potassium chloride 0.3% with sodium chloride 0.9% contains K⁺ 40 mmol, Na⁺ 150 mmol, and Cl⁻ 190 mmol/litre.

● MEDICINAL FORMS
There can be variation in the licensing of different medicines containing the same drug. Forms available from special-order manufacturers include: infusion, solution for infusion
Infusion
▸ Potassium chloride with sodium chloride (Non-proprietary)
Potassium chloride 3 mg per 1 ml, Sodium chloride 9 mg per 1 ml Potassium chloride 0.3% (potassium 20mmol/500ml) / Sodium chloride 0.9% infusion 500ml bags | 1 bag PoM £1.67-£2.46
Potassium chloride 0.3% (potassium 40mmol/1litre) / Sodium chloride 0.9% infusion 1litre bags | 1 bag PoM ⓢ
Potassium chloride 1.5 mg per 1 ml, Sodium chloride 9 mg per 1 ml Potassium chloride 0.15% (potassium 10mmol/500ml) / Sodium chloride 0.9% infusion 500ml bags | 1 bag PoM ⓢ
Potassium chloride 0.15% (potassium 20mmol/1litre) / Sodium chloride 0.9% infusion 1litre bags | 1 bag PoM ⓢ
Potassium chloride 2 mg per 1 ml, Sodium chloride 9 mg per 1 ml Steriflex No.28 potassium chloride 0.2% (potassium 13.3mmol/500ml) / sodium chloride 0.9% infusion 500ml bags | 1 bag PoM £1.67
Steriflex No.28 potassium chloride 0.2% (potassium 27mmol/1litre) / sodium chloride 0.9% infusion 1litre bags | 1 bag PoM £2.20

ELECTROLYTES AND MINERALS › SODIUM CHLORIDE

Sodium chloride

● INDICATIONS AND DOSE

Prophylaxis of sodium chloride deficiency

▸ BY MOUTH

▸ Adult: 4–8 tablets daily, to be taken with water, up to maximum 20 tablets daily in severe depletion

Chronic renal salt wasting

▸ BY MOUTH

▸ Adult: Up to 20 tablets daily, to be taken with appropriate fluid intake

Management of diabetic ketoacidosis (to restore circulating volume if systolic blood pressure is below 90 mmHg and adjusted for age, sex, and medication as appropriate)

▸ BY INTRAVENOUS INFUSION

▸ Adult: 500 mL, sodium chloride 0.9% to be given over 10–15 minutes, repeat if blood pressure remains below 90 mmHg and seek senior medical advice, when blood pressure is over 90 mmHg, sodium chloride 0.9% should be given by intravenous infusion at a rate that replaces deficit and provides maintenance, management regimen also includes administration of potassium chloride, soluble insulin, long acting insulin analogues and glucose 10% solution

Diluent for instillation of drugs to the bladder

▸ BY INTRAVESICAL INSTILLATION

▸ Adult: (consult product literature)

● CAUTIONS

▸ With intravenous use Avoid excessive administration · cardiac failure · dilutional hyponatraemia especially in the elderly · hypertension · peripheral oedema · pulmonary oedema · restrict intake in impaired renal function · toxaemia of pregnancy

● SIDE-EFFECTS

▸ With intravenous use Chills · fever · hypervolaemia · hypotension · local reaction · localised pain · paraesthesia · skin reactions · tremor · vascular disorders · venous thrombosis

▸ With oral use Abdominal cramps · acidosis hyperchloraemic · diarrhoea · generalised oedema · hypertension · hypotension · irritability · muscle complaints · nausea · vomiting

● MONITORING REQUIREMENTS

▸ With intravenous use The jugular venous pressure should be assessed, the bases of the lungs should be examined for crepitations, and in elderly or seriously ill patients it is often helpful to monitor the right atrial (central) venous pressure.

● PRESCRIBING AND DISPENSING INFORMATION

▸ With intravenous use Sodium chloride 0.9% intravenous infusion contains Na⁺ and Cl⁻ each 150 mmol/litre. The term 'normal saline' should not be used to describe sodium chloride intravenous infusion 0.9%; the term 'physiological saline' is acceptable but it is preferable to give the composition (i.e. sodium chloride intravenous infusion 0.9%).

▸ With oral use Each *Slow Sodium*® tablet contains approximately 10 mmol each of Na⁺ and Cl⁻; EvGr tablets can be crushed before administration ⓔ.

- MEDICINAL FORMS
There can be variation in the licensing of different medicines containing the same drug. Forms available from special-order manufacturers include: capsule, solution for injection, infusion, solution for infusion

Modified-release tablet
CAUTIONARY AND ADVISORY LABELS 25
▸ Slow Sodium (HK Pharma Ltd)
Sodium chloride 600 mg Slow Sodium 600mg tablets | 100 tablet [GSL] £9.20 DT = £9.20

Solution for injection
▸ Sodium chloride (Non-proprietary)
Sodium chloride 9 mg per 1 ml Sodium chloride 0.9% solution for injection 5ml Sure-Amp ampoules | 20 ampoule [PoM] £7.15
Sodium chloride 0.9% solution for injection 50ml vials | 25 vial [PoM] £85.00–£85.25
Sodium chloride 0.9% solution for injection 10ml ampoules | 10 ampoule [PoM] £2.96–£3.26 DT = £2.96 | 50 ampoule [PoM] £14.75
Sodium chloride 0.9% solution for injection 20ml Mini-Plasco ampoules | 20 ampoule [PoM] £18.93
Sodium chloride 0.9% solution for injection 5ml Mini-Plasco ampoules | 20 ampoule [PoM] £8.96
Sodium chloride 0.9% solution for injection 2ml Sure-Amp ampoules | 20 ampoule [PoM] £7.15
Sodium chloride 0.9% solution for injection 20ml ampoules | 20 ampoule [PoM] £15.75
Sodium chloride 0.9% solution for injection 2ml ampoules | 10 ampoule [PoM] £2.07–£2.57 DT = £2.07
Sodium chloride 0.9% solution for injection 5ml ampoules | 10 ampoule [PoM] £2.11–£2.32 DT = £2.11 | 50 ampoule [PoM] £10.50
Sodium chloride 0.9% solution for injection 10ml Sure-Amp ampoules | 20 ampoule [PoM] £8.15
Sodium chloride 0.9% solution for injection 10ml Mini-Plasco ampoules | 20 ampoule [PoM] £10.21
Sodium chloride 300 mg per 1 ml Sodium chloride 30% solution for injection 10ml ampoules | 10 ampoule [PoM] £70.43 DT = £70.43
▸ Drytec saline (GE Healthcare Biosciences)
Sodium chloride 9 mg per 1 ml Drytec saline eluent 5ml vials | 20 vial [PoM] [℞] (Hospital only)
Drytec saline eluent 10ml vials | 20 vial [PoM] [℞] (Hospital only)
Drytec saline eluent 20ml vials | 20 vial [PoM] [℞] (Hospital only)

Solution for infusion
▸ Sodium chloride (Non-proprietary)
Sodium chloride 300 mg per 1 ml Sodium chloride 30% concentrate for solution for infusion 100ml vials | 10 vial [PoM] £50.60
Sodium chloride 30% concentrate for solution for infusion 50ml vials | 1 vial [PoM] £13.30 | 10 vial [PoM] £50.60
Sodium chloride 30% concentrate for solution for infusion 10ml ampoules | 10 ampoule [PoM] £70.40

Intravesical solution
▸ Sodium chloride (Non-proprietary)
Sodium chloride 9 mg per 1 ml Sodium chloride 0.9% intravesical solution 50ml bags | 1 bag [P] £5.00

Infusion
▸ Sodium chloride (Non-proprietary)
Sodium chloride 1.8 mg per 1 ml Polyfusor O sodium chloride 0.18% infusion 500ml bottles | 1 bottle [PoM] £3.79
Sodium chloride 4.5 mg per 1 ml Sodium chloride 0.45% infusion 500ml bags | 1 bag [PoM] [℞]
Sodium chloride 0.45% infusion 500ml bottles | 1 bottle [PoM] £3.79
Sodium chloride 9 mg per 1 ml Sodium chloride 0.9% infusion 100ml bags | 1 bag [PoM] £0.55
Sodium chloride 0.9% infusion 250ml bags | 1 bag [PoM] [℞]
Sodium chloride 0.9% infusion 1litre bags | 1 bag [PoM] [℞]
Sodium chloride 0.9% infusion 500ml bags | 1 bag [PoM] [℞]
Sodium chloride 0.9% infusion 50ml bags | 1 bag [PoM] [℞]
Sodium chloride 0.9% infusion 2litre bags | 1 bag [PoM] £3.01
Sodium chloride 0.9% infusion 100ml polyethylene bottles | 1 bottle [PoM] £0.55 | 20 bottle [PoM] £11.00
Polyfusor S sodium chloride 0.9% infusion 500ml bottles | 1 bottle [PoM] £2.57
Sodium chloride 0.9% infusion 1litre bottles | 1 bottle [PoM] £3.42
Sodium chloride 18 mg per 1 ml Polyfusor SC sodium chloride 1.8% infusion 500ml bottles | 1 bottle [PoM] £3.79
Sodium chloride 27 mg per 1 ml Polyfusor SD sodium chloride 2.7% infusion 500ml bottles | 1 bottle [PoM] £3.79
Sodium chloride 50 mg per 1 ml Polyfusor SE sodium chloride 5% infusion 500ml bottles | 1 bottle [PoM] £3.79

Combinations available: *Potassium chloride with calcium chloride and sodium chloride and sodium lactate*, p. 1006 ·

Potassium chloride with calcium chloride dihydrate and sodium chloride, p. 1007 · *Potassium chloride with glucose and sodium chloride*, p. 1007 · *Potassium chloride with sodium chloride*, p. 1008

Sodium chloride with glucose

The properties listed below are those particular to the combination only. For the properties of the components please consider, sodium chloride p. 1008, glucose below.

- INDICATIONS AND DOSE
Combined water and sodium depletion
▸ BY INTRAVENOUS INFUSION
▸ Adult: (consult product literature)

- INTERACTIONS → Appendix 1: glucose
- MONITORING REQUIREMENTS Maintenance fluid should accurately reflect daily requirements and close monitoring is required to avoid fluid and electrolyte imbalance.

- MEDICINAL FORMS
There can be variation in the licensing of different medicines containing the same drug. Forms available from special-order manufacturers include: solution for infusion

Infusion
▸ Sodium chloride with glucose (Non-proprietary)
Sodium chloride 4.5 mg per 1 ml, Glucose anhydrous 25 mg per 1 ml Sodium chloride 0.45% / Glucose 2.5% infusion 500ml bags | 1 bag [PoM] [℞]
Sodium chloride 1.8 mg per 1 ml, Glucose anhydrous 40 mg per 1 ml Sodium chloride 0.18% / Glucose 4% infusion 500ml bags | 1 bag [PoM] [℞]
Sodium chloride 0.18% / Glucose 4% infusion 1litre bags | 1 bag [PoM] [℞]
Sodium chloride 9 mg per 1 ml, Glucose 50 mg per 1 ml Sodium chloride 0.9% / Glucose 5% infusion 500ml bags | 1 bag [PoM] £2.19
Glucose 5% / sodium chloride 0.9% infusion 1litre bags | 1 bag [PoM] £2.10
Sodium chloride 4.5 mg per 1 ml, Glucose anhydrous 50 mg per 1 ml Sodium chloride 0.45% / Glucose 5% infusion 500ml bags | 1 bag [PoM] [℞]
Sodium chloride 1.8 mg per 1 ml, Glucose anhydrous 100 mg per 1 ml Steriflex No.19 glucose 10% / sodium chloride 0.18% infusion 500ml bags | 1 bag [PoM] £2.23

NUTRIENTS > SUGARS

Glucose

(Dextrose Monohydrate)

- INDICATIONS AND DOSE
Establish presence of gestational diabetes
▸ BY MOUTH
▸ Adult: Test dose 75 g, anhydrous glucose to be given to the fasting patient and blood-glucose concentrations measured at intervals, to be given with 200–300 mL fluid

Oral glucose tolerance test
▸ BY MOUTH
▸ Adult: Test dose 75 g, anhydrous glucose to be given to the fasting patient and blood-glucose concentrations measured at intervals, to be given with 200–300 mL fluid

Hypoglycaemia
▸ BY INTRAVENOUS INFUSION
▸ Child: 500 mg/kg, to be administered as Glucose 10% intravenous infusion into a large vein through a large-gauge needle; care is required since this concentration is irritant especially if extravasation occurs
▸ Adult: 10 g, to be administered as Glucose 20% intravenous infusion into a large vein continued →

through a large-gauge needle; care is required since this concentration is irritant especially if extravasation occurs

Energy source
▸ BY INTRAVENOUS INFUSION
▸ Adult: 1–3 litres daily, solution concentration of 20–50% to be administered

Water replacement
▸ BY INTRAVENOUS INFUSION
▸ Adult: The volume of glucose solution needed to replace deficits may vary (consult product literature)

Persistent cyanosis (in combination with propranolol) when blood glucose less than 3 mmol/litre (followed by morphine)
▸ BY INTRAVENOUS INFUSION
▸ Child: 200 mg/kg, to be administered as Glucose 10% intravenous infusion over 10 minutes

Management of diabetic ketoacidosis
▸ BY INTRAVENOUS INFUSION
▸ Child: Glucose 5% or 10% should be added to replacement fluid once blood-glucose concentration falls below 14 mmol/litre
▸ Adult: Glucose 10% should be given once blood-glucose concentration falls below 14 mmol/litre, to be administered into a large vein through a large-gauge needle at a rate of 125 mL/hour, in addition to the sodium chloride 0.9% infusion

DOSE EQUIVALENCE AND CONVERSION
▸ 75 g anhydrous glucose is equivalent to Glucose BP 82.5 g.

● CAUTIONS Do not give alone except when there is no significant loss of electrolytes · prolonged administration of glucose solutions without electrolytes can lead to hyponatraemia and other electrolyte disturbances

● INTERACTIONS → Appendix 1: glucose

● SIDE-EFFECTS Chills · electrolyte imbalance · fever · fluid imbalance · hypersensitivity · local reaction · localised pain · polyuria · rash · venous thrombosis

● DIRECTIONS FOR ADMINISTRATION
▸ With intravenous use in children Injections containing more than 10% glucose can be irritant and should be given into a central venous line; however, solutions containing up to 12.5% can be administered for a short period into a peripheral line.

● PRESCRIBING AND DISPENSING INFORMATION Glucose BP is the monohydrate but Glucose Intravenous Infusion BP is a sterile solution of anhydrous glucose or glucose monohydrate, potency being expressed in terms of anhydrous glucose.

● EXCEPTIONS TO LEGAL CATEGORY
▸ With intravenous use Prescription only medicine restriction does not apply to 50% solution where administration is for saving life in emergency.

● MEDICINAL FORMS
There can be variation in the licensing of different medicines containing the same drug. Forms available from special-order manufacturers include: oral solution, solution for injection, solution for infusion

Solution for infusion
▸ Glucose (Non-proprietary)
Glucose anhydrous 200 mg per 1 ml Glucose 20% solution for infusion 100ml vials | 1 vial [PoM] £5.00
Glucose anhydrous 500 mg per 1 ml Glucose 50% solution for infusion 20ml ampoules | 10 ampoule [PoM] £12.00 DT = £12.00
Glucose 50% solution for infusion 50ml vials | 25 vial [PoM] £50.00–£50.25

Oral solution
▸ Rapilose OGTT (Galen Ltd)
Glucose 250 mg per 1 ml Rapilose OGTT solution | 300 ml £3.48

Oral gel
▸ Dextrogel (Neoceuticals Ltd)
Glucose 400 mg per 1 gram Dextrogel 40% gel | 75 gram £7.16 DT = £7.16 | 80 gram £6.84
▸ GlucoBoost (Ennogen Healthcare Ltd)
Glucose 400 mg per 1 gram GlucoBoost 40% gel | 75 gram £5.72 DT = £7.16 | 80 gram £6.11
▸ GlucoGel (BBI Healthcare Ltd)
Glucose 400 mg per 1 gram GlucoGel 40% gel original | 75 gram [GSL] £7.16 DT = £7.16 | 80 gram [GSL] £6.84
▸ Rapilose (Galen Ltd)
Glucose 400 mg per 1 gram Rapilose 40% gel | 75 gram £5.49 DT = £7.16

Infusion
▸ Glucose (Non-proprietary)
Glucose anhydrous 50 mg per 1 ml Glucose 5% infusion 1litre bags | 1 bag [PoM] [⧄]
Glucose 5% infusion 500ml bags | 1 bag [PoM] [⧄]
Glucose 5% infusion 100ml bags | 1 bag [PoM] [⧄]
Glucose 5% infusion 50ml bags | 1 bag [PoM] [⧄]
Glucose 5% infusion 250ml bags | 1 bag [PoM] [⧄]
Glucose anhydrous 100 mg per 1 ml Glucose 10% infusion 1litre bags | 1 bag [PoM] [⧄]
Glucose 10% infusion 500ml bags | 1 bag [PoM] [⧄]
Glucose anhydrous 200 mg per 1 ml Steriflex No.31 glucose 20% infusion 500ml bags | 1 bag [PoM] £2.64
Glucose (as Glucose monohydrate) 300 mg per 1 ml Glucose 30% infusion 500ml polyethylene bottles | 10 bottle [PoM] £40.21
Glucose anhydrous 400 mg per 1 ml Steriflex No.33 glucose 40% infusion 500ml bags | 1 bag [PoM] £2.81
Glucose anhydrous 500 mg per 1 ml Steriflex No.34 glucose 50% infusion 500ml bags | 1 bag [PoM] £3.11
Glucose 50% infusion 500ml polyethylene bottles | 1 bottle [PoM] £5.10
Glucose anhydrous 700 mg per 1 ml Glucose 70% concentrate for solution for infusion 500ml Viaflex bags | 1 bag [PoM] [⧄]

Combinations available: *Potassium chloride with glucose,* p. 1007 · *Potassium chloride with glucose and sodium chloride,* p. 1007 · *Sodium chloride with glucose,* p. 1009

ORAL REHYDRATION SALTS

Disodium hydrogen citrate with glucose, potassium chloride and sodium chloride

(Formulated as oral rehydration salts)

● INDICATIONS AND DOSE
Fluid and electrolyte loss in diarrhoea
▸ BY MOUTH
▸ Child 1–11 months: 1–1½ times usual feed volume to be given
▸ Child 1–11 years: 200 mL, to be given after every loose motion
▸ Child 12–17 years: 200–400 mL, to be given after every loose motion, dose according to fluid loss
▸ Adult: 200–400 mL, to be given after every loose motion, dose according to fluid loss

● DIRECTIONS FOR ADMINISTRATION Reconstitute 1 sachet with 200mL of water (freshly boiled and cooled for infants); 5 sachets reconstituted with 1 litre of water provide Na⁺ 60 mmol, K⁺ 20 mmol, Cl⁻ 60 mmol, citrate 10 mmol, and glucose 90 mmol.

● PRESCRIBING AND DISPENSING INFORMATION Flavours of oral powder formulations may include black currant, citrus, or natural.

● PATIENT AND CARER ADVICE After reconstitution any unused solution should be discarded no later than 1 hour after preparation unless stored in a refrigerator when it may be kept for up to 24 hours.
Medicines for Children leaflet: Oral rehydration salts
www.medicinesforchildren.org.uk/oral-rehydration-salts

- **MEDICINAL FORMS**
  There can be variation in the licensing of different medicines containing the same drug.

Powder
- Dioralyte (Sanofi)
  Potassium chloride 300 mg, Sodium chloride 470 mg, Disodium hydrogen citrate 530 mg, Glucose 3.56 gram Dioralyte oral powder sachets citrus | 20 sachet P £6.72
  Dioralyte oral powder sachets plain | 20 sachet P £6.72
  Dioralyte oral powder sachets blackcurrant | 20 sachet P £6.72

Potassium chloride with rice powder, sodium chloride and sodium citrate

(Formulated as oral rehydration salts)

- **INDICATIONS AND DOSE**

  Fluid and electrolyte loss in diarrhoea
  - BY MOUTH
  - Adult: 200–400 mL, to be given after every loose motion, dose according to fluid loss

- **DIRECTIONS FOR ADMINISTRATION** Reconstitute 1 sachet with 200 mL of water (freshly boiled and cooled for infants); 5 sachets when reconstituted with 1 litre of water provide Na⁺ 60 mmol, K⁺ 20 mmol, Cl⁻ 50 mmol and citrate 10 mmol.

- **PRESCRIBING AND DISPENSING INFORMATION** Flavours of oral powder formulations may include apricot, black currant, or raspberry.

- **PATIENT AND CARER ADVICE** Patients and carers should be advised how to reconstitute *Dioralyte* ® Relief oral powder. After reconstitution any unused solution should be discarded no later than 1 hour after preparation unless stored in a refrigerator when it may be kept for up to 24 hours.

- **MEDICINAL FORMS**
  There can be variation in the licensing of different medicines containing the same drug.

Powder
  EXCIPIENTS: May contain Aspartame
- Dioralyte Relief (Sanofi)
  Potassium chloride 300 mg, Sodium chloride 350 mg, Sodium citrate 580 mg, Rice powder pre-cooked 6 gram Dioralyte Relief oral powder sachets blackcurrant sugar-free | 20 sachet P £7.13

1.1 Calcium imbalance

Calcium

Calcium supplements
Calcium supplements are usually only required where dietary calcium intake is deficient. This dietary requirement varies with age and is relatively greater in childhood, pregnancy, and lactation, due to an increased demand, and in old age, due to impaired absorption. In osteoporosis, a calcium intake which is double the recommended amount reduces the rate of bone loss. If the actual dietary intake is less than the recommended amount, a supplement of as much as 40 mmol is appropriate.

In severe acute hypocalcaemia or hypocalcaemic tetany, an initial slow intravenous injection of calcium gluconate injection 10% p. 1014 should be given, with plasma-calcium and ECG monitoring (risk of arrhythmias if given too rapidly), and either repeated as required or, if only temporary improvement, followed by a continuous intravenous infusion to prevent recurrence. Calcium chloride injection p. 1014 is also available, but is more irritant; care should be taken to prevent extravasation. Oral supplements of calcium and vitamin D may also be required in persistent hypocalcaemia. Concurrent hypomagnesaemia should be corrected with magnesium sulfate p. 1019.

See the role of calcium gluconate in temporarily reducing the toxic effects of hyperkalaemia.

Severe hypercalcaemia
Severe hypercalcaemia calls for urgent treatment before detailed investigation of the cause. Dehydration should be corrected first with intravenous infusion of sodium chloride **0.9%** p. 1008. Drugs (such as thiazides and vitamin D compounds) which promote hypercalcaemia, should be discontinued and dietary calcium should be restricted.

If *severe hypercalcaemia persists* drugs which inhibit mobilisation of calcium from the skeleton may be required. The **bisphosphonates** are useful and pamidronate disodium p. 712 is probably the most effective.

Corticosteroids are widely given, but may only be useful where hypercalcaemia is due to sarcoidosis or vitamin D intoxication; they often take several days to achieve the desired effect.

Calcitonin (salmon) p. 716 can be used for the treatment of hypercalcaemia associated with malignancy; it is rarely effective where bisphosphonates have failed to reduce serum calcium adequately.

After treatment of severe hypercalcaemia the underlying cause must be established. *Further treatment* is governed by the same principles as for initial therapy. Salt and water depletion and drugs promoting hypercalcaemia should be avoided; oral administration of a bisphosphonate may be useful.

Hyperparathyroidism
Paricalcitol p. 1055 is licensed for the prevention and treatment of secondary hyperparathyroidism associated with chronic renal failure.

Parathyroidectomy may be indicated for hyperparathyroidism.

Hypercalciuria
Hypercalciuria should be investigated for an underlying cause, which should be treated. Where a cause is not identified (idiopathic hypercalciuria), the condition is managed by increasing fluid intake and giving bendroflumethiazide p. 165. Reducing dietary calcium intake may be beneficial but severe restriction of calcium intake has not proved beneficial and may even be harmful.

1.1a Hypercalcaemia and hypercalciuria

CALCIUM REGULATING DRUGS › BONE RESORPTION INHIBITORS

Cinacalcet

- **DRUG ACTION** Cinacalcet reduces parathyroid hormone which leads to a decrease in serum calcium concentrations.

- **INDICATIONS AND DOSE**

  Secondary hyperparathyroidism in patients with end-stage renal disease on dialysis
  - BY MOUTH
  - Adult: Initially 30 mg once daily, dose to be adjusted every 2–4 weeks; maximum 180 mg per day continued →

9

Blood and nutrition

Treatment of hypercalcaemia in parathyroid carcinoma | Primary hyperparathyroidism in patients where parathyroidectomy is inappropriate

▸ BY MOUTH
▸ Adult: Initially 30 mg twice daily (max. per dose 90 mg 4 times a day), dose to be adjusted every 2–4 weeks according to response

● CAUTIONS Treatment should not be initiated in patients with hypocalcaemia
● INTERACTIONS → Appendix 1: cinacalcet
● SIDE-EFFECTS
▸ Common or very common Appetite decreased · asthenia · back pain · constipation · cough · diarrhoea · dizziness · dyspnoea · electrolyte imbalance · gastrointestinal discomfort · headache · hypersensitivity · hypotension · muscle complaints · nausea · paraesthesia · rash · seizure · upper respiratory tract infection · vomiting
▸ Frequency not known Heart failure aggravated · osteodystrophy · QT interval prolongation · tetany · ventricular arrhythmia
● PREGNANCY Manufacturer advises use only if potential benefit outweighs risk—no information available.
● BREAST FEEDING Manufacturer advises avoid—present in milk in *animal* studies.
● HEPATIC IMPAIRMENT Manufacturer advises caution in moderate to severe impairment.
 Monitoring Monitor closely in hepatic impairment especially when increasing dose.
● MONITORING REQUIREMENTS
▸ Measure serum-calcium concentration before initiation of treatment and within 1 week after starting treatment or adjusting dose, then monthly for secondary hyperparathyroidism, and every 2–3 months for primary hyperparathyroidism and parathyroid carcinoma.
▸ In secondary hyperparathyroidism measure parathyroid hormone concentration 1–4 weeks after starting treatment or adjusting dose, then every 1–3 months.
● NATIONAL FUNDING/ACCESS DECISIONS
 NICE decisions
▸ **Cinacalcet for the treatment of secondary hyperparathyroidism in patients with end-stage renal disease on maintenance dialysis therapy (January 2007)** NICE TA117
 Cinacalcet is not recommended for the routine treatment of secondary hyperparathyroidism in patients with end-stage renal disease on maintenance dialysis therapy.
 Cinacalcet is recommended for the treatment of refractory secondary hyperparathyroidism in patients with end-stage renal disease (including those with calciphylaxis) **only** in those:
 • who have 'very uncontrolled' plasma concentration of intact parathyroid hormone (defined as greater than 85 picomol/litre) refractory to standard therapy, and a normal or high adjusted serum calcium concentration, **and**
 • in whom surgical parathyroidectomy is contra-indicated, in that the risks of surgery outweigh the benefits.
 Response to treatment should be monitored regularly and treatment should be continued only if a reduction in the plasma concentration of intact parathyroid hormone of 30% or greater is seen within 4 months of treatment.
 www.nice.org.uk/TA117

● MEDICINAL FORMS
 There can be variation in the licensing of different medicines containing the same drug.
 Tablet
 CAUTIONARY AND ADVISORY LABELS 21
 ▸ Mimpara (Amgen Ltd)
  Cinacalcet (as Cinacalcet hydrochloride) 30 mg Mimpara 30mg tablets | 28 tablet [PoM] £125.75 DT = £125.75

Cinacalcet (as Cinacalcet hydrochloride) 60 mg Mimpara 60mg tablets | 28 tablet [PoM] £231.97 DT = £231.97
Cinacalcet (as Cinacalcet hydrochloride) 90 mg Mimpara 90mg tablets | 28 tablet [PoM] £347.96 DT = £347.96

Etelcalcetide
26-Jul-2017

● DRUG ACTION Etelcalcetide reduces parathyroid hormone secretion, which leads to a decrease in serum calcium concentrations.

● INDICATIONS AND DOSE
 Secondary hyperparathyroidism in patients with chronic kidney disease on haemodialysis
 ▸ BY INTRAVENOUS INJECTION
 ▸ Adult: Initially 5 mg 3 times a week, then increased in steps of 2.5–5 mg if required, dose to be increased at intervals of at least 4 weeks; usual maintenance 2.5–15 mg 3 times a week, max. dose 15 mg 3 times a week; consult product literature for information on missed doses, and for dose adjustment due to parathyroid hormone levels or serum-calcium concentrations

● CAUTIONS Conditions that may worsen with hypocalcaemia · hypocalcaemia (do not initiate if serum-calcium concentration is less than the lower limit of normal range) · switching from cinacalcet (do not initiate until 7 days after the last dose of cinacalcet)
 CAUTIONS, FURTHER INFORMATION
▸ Conditions that may worsen with hypocalcaemia Manufacturer advises caution with use in patients with conditions that may worsen with hypocalcaemia, including predisposition to QT-interval prolongation, history of seizures, and history of congestive heart failure—serum-calcium concentration should be closely monitored.
● INTERACTIONS → Appendix 1: etelcalcetide
● SIDE-EFFECTS
▸ Common or very common Diarrhoea · electrolyte imbalance · headache · heart failure aggravated · hypotension · muscle complaints · nausea · paraesthesia · QT interval prolongation · vomiting
 SIDE-EFFECTS, FURTHER INFORMATION Manufacturer advises if formation of anti-etelcalcetide antibodies with a clinically significant effect is suspected, contact manufacturer to discuss antibody testing.
● PREGNANCY Manufacturer advises avoid—limited information available.
● BREAST FEEDING Manufacturer advises avoid—present in milk in *animal* studies.
● MONITORING REQUIREMENTS Manufacturer advises monitor parathyroid hormone level 4 weeks after treatment initiation or dose adjustment and approximately every 1–3 months during maintenance treatment; monitor serum-calcium concentration before treatment initiation, within 1 week of initiation or dose adjustment, and then approximately every 4 weeks during maintenance treatment.
● HANDLING AND STORAGE Manufacturer advises store in a refrigerator (2–8°C)—consult product literature for further information regarding storage outside refrigerator.
● PATIENT AND CARER ADVICE Manufacturer advises patients and their carers should be told to seek medical advice if symptoms of hypocalcaemia occur.
● NATIONAL FUNDING/ACCESS DECISIONS
 NICE decisions
▸ **Etelcalcetide for treating secondary hyperparathyroidism (June 2017)** NICE TA448
 Etelcalcetide is recommended as an option for treating secondary hyperparathyroidism in patients with chronic

kidney disease on haemodialysis, only if treatment with a calcimimetic is indicated but cinacalcet is not suitable, and the manufacturer provides etelcalcetide with the discount agreed in the patient access scheme.

Patients whose treatment was started within the NHS before this guidance was published should have the option to continue treatment, without change to their funding arrangements, until they and their clinician consider it appropriate to stop.
www.nice.org.uk/guidance/TA448

Scottish Medicines Consortium (SMC) Decisions
The *Scottish Medicines Consortium* has advised (September 2017) that etelcalcetide (*Parsabiv*®) is not recommended for use within NHS Scotland for the treatment of secondary hyperparathyroidism in patients with chronic kidney disease on haemodialysis as the economic case was not demonstrated.

● MEDICINAL FORMS There can be variation in the licensing of different medicines containing the same drug.
Solution for injection
  ▸ Parsabiv (Amgen Ltd) ▼
    Etelcalcetide (as Etelcalcetide hydrochloride) 5 mg per 1 ml Parsabiv 2.5mg/0.5ml solution for injection vials | 6 vial PoM £136.87
    Parsabiv 10mg/2ml solution for injection vials | 6 vial PoM £327.84
    Parsabiv 5mg/1ml solution for injection vials | 6 vial PoM £163.92

1.1b Hypocalcaemia

ELECTROLYTES AND MINERALS > CALCIUM

Calcium salts

● CONTRA-INDICATIONS Conditions associated with hypercalcaemia (e.g. some forms of malignant disease) · conditions associated with hypercalciuria (e.g. some forms of malignant disease)
● CAUTIONS History of nephrolithiasis · sarcoidosis
● SIDE-EFFECTS
  ▸ **Uncommon** Constipation · diarrhoea · hypercalcaemia · nausea
● RENAL IMPAIRMENT Use with caution.

⌐ above

Calcium carbonate

● INDICATIONS AND DOSE
Phosphate binding in renal failure and hyper-phosphataemia
  ▸ BY MOUTH
  ▸ Adult: (consult product literature)
Calcium deficiency
  ▸ BY MOUTH
  ▸ Adult: (consult product literature)

● INTERACTIONS → Appendix 1: calcium salts
● SIDE-EFFECTS
  ▸ **Uncommon** Hypercalciuria
  ▸ **Rare or very rare** Flatulence · gastrointestinal discomfort · milk-alkali syndrome · skin reactions
● PRESCRIBING AND DISPENSING INFORMATION *Adcal*® contains calcium carbonate 1.5 g (calcium 600 mg or Ca²⁺ 15 mmol); *Calcichew*® contains calcium carbonate 1.25 g (calcium 500 mg or Ca²⁺ 12.5 mmol); *Calcichew Forte*® contains calcium carbonate 2.5 g (calcium 1 g or Ca²⁺ 25 mmol); *Cacit*® contains calcium carbonate 1.25 g, providing calcium citrate when dispersed in water (calcium 500 mg or Ca²⁺ 12.5 mmol); consult product literature for details of other available products.

Flavours of chewable tablet formulations may include orange or fruit flavour.

● MEDICINAL FORMS There can be variation in the licensing of different medicines containing the same drug. Forms available from special-order manufacturers include: tablet, capsule, oral suspension
Tablet
CAUTIONARY AND ADVISORY LABELS 25
  ▸ Calcium carbonate (Non-proprietary)
    Calcium carbonate 1.25 gram Calcium carbonate 1.25g tablets | 100 tablet Ⓢ
Effervescent tablet
CAUTIONARY AND ADVISORY LABELS 13
  ▸ Cacit (Warner Chilcott UK Ltd)
    Calcium carbonate 1.25 gram Cacit 500mg effervescent tablets sugar-free | 76 tablet P £11.81 DT = £11.81
Chewable tablet
CAUTIONARY AND ADVISORY LABELS 24
EXCIPIENTS: May contain Aspartame
  ▸ Calcium carbonate (Non-proprietary)
    Calcium carbonate 1.25 gram Calcium carbonate 1.25g chewable tablets sugar free sugar-free | 100 tablet £12.50 DT = £9.33
  ▸ Adcal (Kyowa Kirin Ltd)
    Calcium carbonate 1.5 gram Adcal 1500mg chewable tablets sugar-free | 100 tablet P £8.70 DT = £8.70
  ▸ Calcichew (Takeda UK Ltd)
    Calcium carbonate 1.25 gram Calcichew 500mg chewable tablets sugar-free | 100 tablet P £9.33 DT = £9.33
    Calcium carbonate 2.5 gram Calcichew Forte chewable tablets sugar-free | 60 tablet P £13.16 DT = £13.16
  ▸ Remegel (SSL International Plc)
    Calcium carbonate 800 mg Remegel 800mg chewable tablets mint | 24 tablet GSL £2.58
  ▸ Rennie (Bayer Plc)
    Calcium carbonate 500 mg Rennie Orange 500mg chewable tablets | 24 tablet GSL £1.50 | 48 tablet GSL £2.57 DT = £2.57
  ▸ Setlers Antacid (Thornton & Ross Ltd)
    Calcium carbonate 500 mg Setlers Antacid spearmint chewable tablets | 36 tablet GSL £1.40
    Setlers Antacid peppermint chewable tablets | 36 tablet GSL £1.40
  ▸ TUMS (GlaxoSmithKline Consumer Healthcare)
    Calcium carbonate 500 mg Tums Assorted Fruit Antacid tablets | 36 tablet GSL £1.33 | 75 tablet GSL £2.14

Calcium carbonate with calcium lactate gluconate

The properties listed below are those particular to the combination only. For the properties of the components please consider, calcium carbonate above.

● INDICATIONS AND DOSE
Calcium deficiency
  ▸ BY MOUTH
  ▸ Adult: Dose according to requirements

● INTERACTIONS → Appendix 1: calcium salts
● PRESCRIBING AND DISPENSING INFORMATION Each *Sandocal*® tablet contains 1 g calcium (Ca²⁺ 25 mmol); flavours of soluble tablet formulations may include orange.

● MEDICINAL FORMS There can be variation in the licensing of different medicines containing the same drug.
Effervescent tablet
CAUTIONARY AND ADVISORY LABELS 13
EXCIPIENTS: May contain Aspartame
  ▸ Sandocal (GlaxoSmithKline Consumer Healthcare)
    Calcium carbonate 1.75 gram, Calcium lactate gluconate 2.263 gram Sandocal 1000 effervescent tablets sugar-free | 30 tablet P £11.65 DT = £11.65

Calcium chloride

⚐ 1013

- **INDICATIONS AND DOSE**

Severe acute hypocalcaemia or hypocalcaemic tetany
- ▶ BY INTRAVENOUS INJECTION
- ▶ Adult: Dose according to requirements

- **CAUTIONS** Avoid in respiratory acidosis · avoid in respiratory failure
- **INTERACTIONS** → Appendix 1: calcium salts
- **SIDE-EFFECTS** Soft tissue calcification · taste unpleasant · vasodilation
- **DIRECTIONS FOR ADMINISTRATION** Care should be taken to avoid extravasation.
- **PRESCRIBING AND DISPENSING INFORMATION** Non-proprietary *Calcium chloride dihydrate* 7.35%(calcium 20 mg or Ca^{2+} 500 micromol/mL); *Calcium chloride dihydrate* 10%(calcium 27.3 mg or Ca^{2+} 680 micromol/mL); *Calcium chloride dihydrate* 14.7%(calcium 40.1 mg or Ca^{2+} 1000 micromol/mL).

- **MEDICINAL FORMS**
There can be variation in the licensing of different medicines containing the same drug. Forms available from special-order manufacturers include: solution for infusion
Solution for injection
- ▶ Calcium chloride (Non-proprietary)
Calcium chloride dihydrate 73.5 mg per 1 ml Calcium chloride 7.35% solution for injection 10ml ampoules | 10 ampoule [PoM] £66.38
Calcium chloride dihydrate 100 mg per 1 ml Calcium chloride 10% solution for injection 10ml pre-filled syringes | 1 pre-filled disposable injection [PoM] £9.42 DT = £9.42
Calcium chloride dihydrate 147 mg per 1 ml Calcium chloride 14.7% solution for injection 5ml ampoules | 10 ampoule [PoM] £109.98
Calcium chloride 14.7% solution for injection 10ml ampoules | 10 ampoule [PoM] £77.95 DT = £77.95

Calcium gluconate

⚐ 1013

- **INDICATIONS AND DOSE**

Severe acute hypocalcaemia or hypocalcaemic tetany
- ▶ INITIALLY BY SLOW INTRAVENOUS INJECTION
- ▶ Adult: Initially 10–20 mL, calcium gluconate injection 10% (providing approximately 2.25–4.5 mmol of calcium) should be administered with plasma-calcium and ECG monitoring, and either repeated as required or, if only temporary improvement, followed by a continuous intravenous infusion to prevent recurrence, alternatively (by continuous intravenous infusion), initially 50 mL/hour, adjusted according to response, infusion to be administered using 100 mL of calcium gluconate 10% diluted in 1 litre of glucose 5% or sodium chloride 0.9%

Acute severe hyperkalaemia (plasma-potassium concentration above 6.5 mmol/litre or in the presence of ECG changes)
- ▶ BY SLOW INTRAVENOUS INJECTION
- ▶ Adult: 10–20 mL, calcium gluconate 10% should be administered, dose titrated and adjusted to ECG improvement

Calcium deficiency | Mild asymptomatic hypocalcaemia
- ▶ BY MOUTH
- ▶ Adult: Dose according to requirements

DOSE EQUIVALENCE AND CONVERSION
- ▶ 0.11 mmol/kg is equivalent to 0.5 mL/kg of calcium gluconate 10%.

> **IMPORTANT SAFETY INFORMATION**
> The MHRA has advised that repeated or prolonged administration of calcium gluconate injection packaged in 10 mL glass containers is contra-indicated in children under 18 years and in patients with renal impairment owing to the risk of aluminium accumulation; in these patients the use of calcium gluconate injection packaged in plastic containers is recommended.

- **INTERACTIONS** → Appendix 1: calcium salts
- **SIDE-EFFECTS**
GENERAL SIDE-EFFECTS Arrhythmias
SPECIFIC SIDE-EFFECTS
- ▶ With intravenous use Circulatory collapse · feeling hot · hyperhidrosis · hypotension · vasodilation · vomiting
- ▶ With oral use Gastrointestinal disorder
- **MONITORING REQUIREMENTS**
- ▶ With intravenous use Plasma-calcium and ECG monitoring required for administration by slow intravenous injection (risk of arrhythmias if given too rapidly).
- **DIRECTIONS FOR ADMINISTRATION**
- ▶ With intravenous use For continuous intravenous infusion, dilute 100 mL of calcium gluconate 10% in 1 litre of glucose 5% or sodium chloride 0.9% and give at an initial rate of 50 mL/hour adjusted according to response. Avoid bicarbonates, phosphates, or sulfates.
- **PRESCRIBING AND DISPENSING INFORMATION** Calcium gluconate 1 g contains calcium 89 mg or Ca^{2+} 2.23 mmol.

- **MEDICINAL FORMS**
There can be variation in the licensing of different medicines containing the same drug. Forms available from special-order manufacturers include: tablet, capsule, oral suspension, oral solution, solution for injection, solution for infusion
Solution for injection
- ▶ Calcium gluconate (Non-proprietary)
Calcium gluconate 100 mg per 1 ml Calcium gluconate 10% solution for injection 10ml ampoules | 10 ampoule [PoM] £7.50–£12.50 DT = £12.50 | 20 ampoule [PoM] £30.00
Effervescent tablet
CAUTIONARY AND ADVISORY LABELS 13
ELECTROLYTES: May contain Sodium
- ▶ Calcium gluconate (Non-proprietary)
Calcium gluconate 1 gram Calcium gluconate 1g effervescent tablets | 28 tablet [GSL] £15.68 DT = £15.68

Calcium lactate

⚐ 1013

- **INDICATIONS AND DOSE**

Calcium deficiency
- ▶ BY MOUTH
- ▶ Adult: Dose according to requirements

- **INTERACTIONS** → Appendix 1: calcium salts

- **MEDICINAL FORMS**
There can be variation in the licensing of different medicines containing the same drug.
Tablet
- ▶ Calcium lactate (Non-proprietary)
Calcium lactate 300 mg Calcium lactate 300mg tablets | 84 tablet [N] DT = £4.57 | 84 tablet [GSL] £4.57 DT = £4.57

⬛ 1013

Calcium phosphate

- **INDICATIONS AND DOSE**

Indications listed in combination monographs (available in the UK only in combination with other drugs)
  - ▸ BY MOUTH
  - ▸ Adult: Doses listed in combination monographs

- **INTERACTIONS** → Appendix 1: calcium salts
- **SIDE-EFFECTS** Epigastric pain · gastrointestinal disorder · hypercalciuria

- **MEDICINAL FORMS**
  No licensed medicines listed.

PARATHYROID HORMONES AND ANALOGUES

Parathyroid hormone   21-Nov-2017

(Human recombinant parathyroid hormone)

- **DRUG ACTION** Parathyroid hormone is produced by recombinant DNA technology; endogenous parathyroid hormone is involved in modulating serum calcium and phosphate levels, regulating renal calcium and phosphate excretion, activating vitamin D, and maintaining normal bone turnover.

- **INDICATIONS AND DOSE**

Chronic hypoparathyroidism (specialist use only)
  - ▸ BY SUBCUTANEOUS INJECTION
  - ▸ Adult: (consult product literature)

- **CONTRA-INDICATIONS** Bone metastases · current or previous radiation therapy to skeleton · increased risk factors for osteosarcoma (including Paget's disease or hereditary disorders) · pseudohypoparathyroidism · skeletal malignancy · unexplained raised levels of bone-specific alkaline phosphatase

- **CAUTIONS** Concomitant use of cardiac glycosides (hypercalcaemia may predispose to digitalis toxicity)—monitor cardiac glycoside levels and check for signs and symptoms of digitalis toxicity · concomitant use of drugs that affect calcium levels · young adults with open epiphyses—increased risk of osteosarcoma

- **INTERACTIONS** → Appendix 1: parathyroid hormone
- **SIDE-EFFECTS**
  - ▸ **Common or very common** Electrolyte imbalance · fatigue · pain in extremity

  SIDE-EFFECTS, FURTHER INFORMATION Hypercalcaemia is more likely during initial dose titration; if severe hypercalcaemia develops, hydrate and consider suspending treatment (including calcium supplement and active vitamin D).

- **PREGNANCY** Manufacturer advises use only if potential benefit outweighs risk—no information available.

- **BREAST FEEDING** Manufacturer advises avoid—present in milk in *animal* studies.

- **HEPATIC IMPAIRMENT** Manufacturer advises caution in severe impairment—no information available.

- **RENAL IMPAIRMENT** Manufacturer advises caution in severe impairment—no information available.

- **PRE-TREATMENT SCREENING** Manufacturer advises confirm sufficient 25-hydroxyvitamin D stores and normal serum magnesium before treatment.

- **MONITORING REQUIREMENTS**
  - ▸ Manufacturer advises monitor serum calcium and assess for signs and symptoms of hypocalcaemia and hypercalcaemia—adjust active vitamin D and calcium supplement as necessary; consult product literature.

- ▸ Manufacturer advises periodic monitoring of the response of serum calcium to treatment (response may decrease over time—if 25-hydroxyvitamin D is low, supplementation may restore serum calcium response).

- **TREATMENT CESSATION** Abrupt interruption or discontinuation can result in severe hypocalcaemia—manufacturer advises to monitor serum calcium and adjust calcium supplement and active vitamin D treatment.

- **PRESCRIBING AND DISPENSING INFORMATION** Manufacturer advises record the brand name and batch number after each administration.

- **HANDLING AND STORAGE** Manufacturer advises store in a refrigerator (2–8 °C); reconstituted solution may be stored for up to 14 days in a refrigerator, and up to 3 days outside of a refrigerator (below 25 °C), during the 14-day use period.

- **PATIENT AND CARER ADVICE** Patients may self-administer *Natpar®*, after appropriate training in subcutaneous injection technique.
  Missed doses | Manufacturer advises missed doses should be administered as soon as possible, and additional treatment with calcium and/or active vitamin D must be taken, based on symptoms of hypocalcaemia.

- **MEDICINAL FORMS**
  There can be variation in the licensing of different medicines containing the same drug.

  Powder and solvent for solution for injection
  ELECTROLYTES: May contain Sodium
  - ▸ Natpar (Shire Pharmaceuticals Ltd) ▼
    Parathyroid hormone 25 microgram Natpar 25micrograms/dose powder and solvent for solution for injection cartridges | 2 cartridge [PoM] £4,880.00
    Parathyroid hormone 50 microgram Natpar 50micrograms/dose powder and solvent for solution for injection cartridges | 2 cartridge [PoM] £4,880.00
    Parathyroid hormone 75 microgram Natpar 75micrograms/dose powder and solvent for solution for injection cartridges | 2 cartridge [PoM] £4,880.00
    Parathyroid hormone 100 microgram Natpar 100micrograms/dose powder and solvent for solution for injection cartridges | 2 cartridge [PoM] £4,880.00

1.2   Low blood volume

BLOOD AND RELATED PRODUCTS > PLASMA PRODUCTS

Albumin solution

(Human Albumin Solution)

- **INDICATIONS AND DOSE**

Acute or sub-acute loss of plasma volume e.g. in burns, pancreatitis, trauma, and complications of surgery (with isotonic solutions) | Plasma exchange (with isotonic solutions) | Severe hypoalbuminaemia associated with low plasma volume and generalised oedema where salt and water restriction with plasma volume expansion are required (with concentrated solutions 20%) | Paracentesis of large volume ascites associated with portal hypertension (with concentrated solutions 20%)
  - ▸ BY INTRAVENOUS INFUSION
  - ▸ Adult: (consult product literature)

- **CONTRA-INDICATIONS** Cardiac failure · severe anaemia
- **CAUTIONS** Correct dehydration when administering concentrated solution · history of cardiac disease (administer slowly to avoid rapid rise in blood pressure and cardiac failure, and monitor cardiovascular and respiratory function) · history of circulatory disease (administer slowly to avoid rapid rise in blood pressure and cardiac failure,

and monitor cardiovascular and respiratory function) · increased capillary permeability

- SIDE-EFFECTS
- ▸ **Rare or very rare** Fever · flushing · nausea · shock · urticaria
- MONITORING REQUIREMENTS Plasma and plasma substitutes are often used in very ill patients whose condition is unstable. Therefore, close monitoring is required and fluid and electrolyte therapy should be adjusted according to the patient's condition at all times.
- PRESCRIBING AND DISPENSING INFORMATION A solution containing protein derived from plasma, serum, or normal placentas; at least 95% of the protein is albumin. The solution may be isotonic (containing 3.5–5% protein) or concentrated (containing 15–25% protein).

- MEDICINAL FORMS
  There can be variation in the licensing of different medicines containing the same drug.
  Infusion
  ▸ Flexbumin (Baxalta UK Ltd)
  Albumin solution human 200 gram per 1 litre Flexbumin 20% infusion 100ml bags | 1 bag [PoM] 🛇
  Flexbumin 20% infusion 50ml bags | 1 bag [PoM] 🛇
  Solution for infusion
  ▸ Albumin solution (Non-proprietary)
  Albumin solution human 200 mg per 1 ml Albunorm 20% solution for infusion 50ml bottles | 1 bottle [PoM] £24.00
  ▸ Albunorm (Octapharma Ltd)
  Albumin solution human 50 mg per 1 ml Albunorm 5% solution for infusion 250ml bottles | 1 bottle [PoM] £30.00
  Albunorm 5% solution for infusion 100ml bottles | 1 bottle [PoM] £12.00
  Albunorm 5% solution for infusion 500ml bottles | 1 bottle [PoM] £60.00
  Albumin solution human 200 mg per 1 ml Albunorm 20% solution for infusion 100ml bottles | 1 bottle [PoM] £48.00
  ▸ Alburex (CSL Behring UK Ltd)
  Albumin solution human 50 mg per 1 ml Alburex 5% solution for infusion 500ml vials | 1 vial [PoM] £50.00
  Albumin solution human 200 mg per 1 ml Alburex 20% solution for infusion 100ml vials | 1 vial [PoM] £40.00
  ▸ Biotest (Biotest (UK) Ltd)
  Albumin solution human 50 mg per 1 ml Human Albumin Biotest 5% solution for infusion 250ml vials | 1 vial [PoM] 🛇
  Albumin solution human 200 mg per 1 ml Human Albumin Biotest 20% solution for infusion 50ml vials | 1 vial [PoM] 🛇
  Human Albumin Biotest 20% solution for infusion 100ml vials | 1 vial [PoM] 🛇
  ▸ Grifols (Grifols UK Ltd)
  Albumin solution human 50 mg per 1 ml Human albumin Grifols 5% solution for infusion 500ml bottles | 1 bottle [PoM] £49.50
  Human albumin Grifols 5% solution for infusion 250ml bottles | 1 bottle [PoM] £24.75
  Human albumin Grifols 5% solution for infusion 100ml bottles | 1 bottle [PoM] £9.90
  ▸ Zenalb (Bio Products Laboratory Ltd)
  Albumin solution human 45 mg per 1 ml Zenalb 4.5% solution for infusion 250ml bottles | 1 bottle [PoM] £27.51
  Zenalb 4.5% solution for infusion 500ml bottles | 1 bottle [PoM] £55.02
  Albumin solution human 200 mg per 1 ml Zenalb 20% solution for infusion 100ml bottles | 1 bottle [PoM] £54.00
  Zenalb 20% solution for infusion 50ml bottles | 1 bottle [PoM] £27.00

PLASMA SUBSTITUTES

Dextran 70 with sodium chloride

- ● INDICATIONS AND DOSE
  Initial treatment of hypovolaemia with hypotension induced by traumatic injury
  ▸ BY INTRAVENOUS INFUSION
  ▸ **Adult:** 250 mL, to be given over 2–5 minutes using *RescueFlow®*, followed immediately by administration of isotonic fluids.

- CAUTIONS Cardiac disease · hyperosmolality · severe hypoglycaemia · severe liver disease
- SIDE-EFFECTS Anaphylactic reaction
- PREGNANCY Avoid—reports of anaphylaxis in mother causing fetal anoxia, neurological damage and death.
- HEPATIC IMPAIRMENT Use with caution in severe impairment.
- RENAL IMPAIRMENT Use with caution.
- MONITORING REQUIREMENTS
- ▸ Where possible, monitor central venous pressure.
- ▸ Urine output should be monitored. Care should be taken to avoid haematocrit concentration from falling below 25–30% and the patient should be monitored for hypersensitivity reactions.
- ▸ Plasma and plasma substitutes are often used in very ill patients whose condition is unstable. Therefore, close monitoring is required and fluid and electrolyte therapy should be adjusted according to the patient's condition at all times.
- EFFECT ON LABORATORY TESTS Can interfere with some laboratory tests—dextran may interfere with blood group cross-matching or biochemical measurements, and these should be carried out before infusion is begun.
- PRESCRIBING AND DISPENSING INFORMATION Dextran 70 is dextran with an average molecular weight of about '70 000'.

- MEDICINAL FORMS
  There can be variation in the licensing of different medicines containing the same drug.
  Infusion
  ▸ RescueFlow (Waymade Healthcare Plc)
  Dextran 70 60 mg per 1 ml, Sodium chloride 75 mg per 1 ml RescueFlow 6% infusion 250ml bags | 6 bag [PoM] 🛇

Gelatin

- ● INDICATIONS AND DOSE
  Low blood volume in hypovolaemic shock, burns and cardiopulmonary bypass
  ▸ BY INTRAVENOUS INFUSION
  ▸ **Adult:** Initially 500–1000 mL, use 3.5–4% solution

- CAUTIONS Cardiac disease · severe liver disease
- SIDE-EFFECTS
- ▸ **Rare or very rare** Chills · dyspnoea · fever · hyperhidrosis · hypersensitivity · hypertension · hypotension · hypoxia · tachycardia · tremor · urticaria · wheezing
- PREGNANCY Manufacturer of *Geloplasma®* advises avoid at the end of pregnancy.
- HEPATIC IMPAIRMENT Use with caution in severe impairment.
- RENAL IMPAIRMENT Use with caution in renal impairment.
- MONITORING REQUIREMENTS
- ▸ Urine output should be monitored. Care should be taken to avoid haematocrit concentration from falling below 25–30% and the patient should be monitored for hypersensitivity reactions.
- ▸ Plasma and plasma substitutes are often used in very ill patients whose condition is unstable. Therefore, close monitoring is required and fluid and electrolyte therapy should be adjusted according to the patient's condition at all times.
- PRESCRIBING AND DISPENSING INFORMATION The gelatin is partially degraded.
  Gelaspan® contains succinylated gelatin (modified fluid gelatin, average molecular weight 26 500) 40 g, Na^+ 151 mmol, K^+ 4 mmol, Mg^{2+} 1 mmol, Cl^- 103 mmol, Ca^{2+} 1 mmol, acetate 24 mmol/litre; *Gelofusine®* contains

succinylated gelatin (modified fluid gelatin, average molecular weight 30 000) 40 g (4%), Na$^+$ 154 mmol, Cl$^-$ 124 mmol/litre; *Geloplasma*® contains partially hydrolysed and succinylated gelatin (modified liquid gelatin) (as anhydrous gelatin) 30 g (3%), Na$^+$ 150 mmol, K$^+$ 5 mmol, Mg^{2+} 1.5 mmol, Cl$^-$ 100 mmol, lactate 30 mmol/litre; *Isoplex*® contains succinylated gelatin (modified fluid gelatin, average molecular weight 30 000) 40g (4%), Na$^+$ 145 mmol, K$^+$ 4 mmol, Mg^{2+} 0.9 mmol, Cl$^-$ 105 mmol, lactate 25mmol/litre; *Volplex*® contains succinylated gelatin (modified fluid gelatin, average molecular weight 30 000) 40 g (4%), Na$^+$ 154 mmol, Cl$^-$ 125 mmol/litre.

● MEDICINAL FORMS
There can be variation in the licensing of different medicines containing the same drug.

Infusion
▸ Gelaspan (B.Braun Medical Ltd)
Gelatin 40 mg per 1 ml Gelaspan 4% infusion 500ml Ecobags | 1 bag PoM £5.95 (Hospital only)
▸ Gelofusine (B.Braun Medical Ltd)
Gelatin 40 mg per 1 ml Gelofusine 4% infusion 1litre Ecobags | 1 bag PoM £9.31
Gelofusine 4% infusion 500ml Ecobags | 1 bag PoM £4.97
▸ Geloplasma (Fresenius Kabi Ltd)
Gelatin 30 mg per 1 ml Geloplasma 3% infusion 500ml Freeflex bags | 20 bag PoM [℞]
▸ Isoplex (Kent Pharmaceuticals Ltd)
Gelatin 40 mg per 1 ml Isoplex 4% infusion 500ml bags | 10 bag PoM £75.00 (Hospital only)
▸ Volplex (Kent Pharmaceuticals Ltd)
Gelatin 40 mg per 1 ml Volplex 4% infusion 500ml bags | 10 bag PoM £47.00 (Hospital only)

Tetrastarch

● INDICATIONS AND DOSE

VOLULYTE® INFUSION

Treatment of hypovolaemia due to acute blood loss when crystalloids alone are not sufficient
▸ BY INTRAVENOUS INFUSION
▸ Adult: Initially 10–20 mL, then increased to up to 30 mL/kilogram daily for a maximum duration of treatment of 24 hours, the initial dose must be given slowly and with careful monitoring of the patient to allow any anaphylactic reaction to be detected as early as possible

VOLUVEN® INFUSION

Treatment of hypovolaemia due to acute blood loss when crystalloids alone are not sufficient
▸ BY INTRAVENOUS INFUSION
▸ Adult: Initially 10–20 mL, then increased to up to 30 mL/kilogram daily for maximum duration of treatment of 24 hours, the initial dose must be given slowly and with careful monitoring of the patient to allow any anaphylactic reaction to be detected as early as possible

● CONTRA-INDICATIONS Burns · cerebral haemorrhage · critically ill patients · dehydration · hyperhydration · intracranial haemorrhage · pulmonary oedema · sepsis · severe coagulopathy

● CAUTIONS Cardiac disease · care should be taken to avoid haematocrit concentration from falling below 25-30% · children · renal impairment · severe liver disease · surgery · trauma

● SIDE-EFFECTS
▸ Rare or very rare Hypersensitivity
▸ Frequency not known Pruritus

● HEPATIC IMPAIRMENT Avoid in severe impairment.

● RENAL IMPAIRMENT Avoid.

● MONITORING REQUIREMENTS
▸ Plasma and plasma substitutes are often used in very ill patients whose condition is unstable. Therefore, close monitoring is required and fluid and electrolyte therapy should be adjusted according to the patient's condition at all times. Treatment with hydroxyethyl starches should be guided by continuous haemodynamic monitoring so that the infusion is stopped as soon as appropriate haemodynamic goals have been achieved.
▸ Monitor renal function.
▸ Monitor for hypersensitivity reactions.
▸ Urine output should be monitored.

● PRESCRIBING AND DISPENSING INFORMATION
Hydroxyethyl starch is composed of more than 90% of amylopectin that has been etherified with hydroxyethyl groups; the term tetrastarch reflects the degree of etherification. Hydroxyethyl starches should only be used for the treatment of hypovolaemia due to acute blood loss when crystalloids alone are not sufficient; they should be used at the lowest effective dose for the first 24 hours of fluid resuscitation.
Volulyte® contains hydroxyethyl starch 6% (average molecular weight 130 000) in sodium chloride intravenous infusion 0.6%, containing Na$^+$ 137 mmol, K$^+$ 4 mmol, Mg^{2+} 1.5 mmol, Cl$^-$ 110 mmol, acetate 34 mmol/litre.

● MEDICINAL FORMS
There can be variation in the licensing of different medicines containing the same drug.

Infusion
▸ Volulyte (Fresenius Kabi Ltd) ▼
Magnesium chloride hexahydrate 300 mg per 1 litre, Potassium chloride 300 mg per 1 litre, Sodium acetate trihydrate 4.63 gram per 1 litre, Sodium chloride 6.02 gram per 1 litre, Tetrastarch 60 gram per 1 litre Volulyte 6% infusion 500ml Freeflex bags | 15 bag PoM £229.62
▸ Voluven (Fresenius Kabi Ltd) ▼
Tetrastarch 60 mg per 1 gram Voluven 6% infusion 500ml Freeflex bags | 1 bag PoM £10.63
Tetrastarch 100 mg per 1 ml Voluven 10% infusion 500ml Freeflex bags | 20 bag PoM [℞]

1.3 Magnesium imbalance

Magnesium

Magnesium is an essential constituent of many enzyme systems, particularly those involved in energy generation; the largest stores are in the skeleton.

Magnesium salts are not well absorbed from the gastrointestinal tract, which explains the use of magnesium sulfate as an osmotic laxative.

Magnesium is excreted mainly by the kidneys and is therefore retained in renal failure, but significant *hypermagnesaemia* (causing muscle weakness and arrhythmias) is rare.

Hypomagnesaemia
Since magnesium is secreted in large amounts in the gastro-intestinal fluid, excessive losses in diarrhoea, stoma or fistula are the most common causes of *hypomagnesaemia*; deficiency may also occur in alcoholism or as a result of treatment with certain drugs. Hypomagnesaemia often causes secondary hypocalcaemia, and also hypokalaemia and hyponatraemia.

Symptomatic *hypomagnesaemia* is associated with a deficit of 0.5–1 mmol/kg; up to 160 mmol Mg^{2+} over up to 5 days may be required to replace the deficit (allowing for urinary losses). Magnesium is given initially by intravenous infusion or by intramuscular injection of magnesium sulfate; the intramuscular injection is painful. Plasma magnesium concentration should be measured to determine the rate and

9

Blood and nutrition

duration of infusion and the dose should be reduced in renal impairment. To prevent *recurrence of the deficit*, magnesium may be given by mouth, but there is limited evidence of benefit. Magnesium aspartate powder for oral solution below is available as a licensed preparation and, magnesium glycerophosphate tablets and liquid [unlicensed] below are available from 'special-order' manufacturers or specialist importing companies.

Arrhythmias

Magnesium sulfate injection has also been recommended for the emergency treatment of *serious arrhythmias*, especially in the presence of hypokalaemia (when hypomagnesaemia may also be present) and when salvos of rapid ventricular tachycardia show the characteristic twisting wave front known as *torsade de pointes*.

Myocardial infarction

Limited evidence that magnesium sulfate prevents arrhythmias and reperfusion injury in patients with suspected myocardial infarction has not been confirmed by large studies. Routine use of magnesium sulfate for this purpose is not recommended.

Eclampsia and pre-eclampsia

Magnesium sulfate injection is the drug of choice for the treatment of seizures and the prevention of recurrent seizures in women with *eclampsia*. Regimens may vary between hospitals. Calcium gluconate injection is used for the management of magnesium toxicity.

Magnesium sulfate injection is also of benefit in women with *pre-eclampsia* in whom there is concern about developing eclampsia. The patient should be monitored carefully.

1.3a Hypomagnesaemia

ELECTROLYTES AND MINERALS > MAGNESIUM

Magnesium aspartate

- ● INDICATIONS AND DOSE
  Treatment and prevention of magnesium deficiency
  ▶ BY MOUTH
  ▸ Adult: 10–20 mmol daily, taken as 1–2 sachets of *Magnaspartate*® powder.

- ● CONTRA-INDICATIONS Disorders of cardiac conduction
- ● INTERACTIONS → Appendix 1: magnesium
- ● SIDE-EFFECTS
  ▶ **Uncommon** Diarrhoea · faeces soft
  ▶ **Rare or very rare** Fatigue · hypermagnesaemia
  ▶ **Frequency not known** Gastrointestinal irritation

  SIDE-EFFECTS, FURTHER INFORMATION Side-effects generally occur at higher doses; if side-effects (such as diarrhoea) occur, consider interrupting treatment and restarting at a reduced dose.

  Overdose Symptoms of hypermagnesaemia may include nausea, vomiting, flushing of the skin, thirst, hypotension due to peripheral vasodilatation, drowsiness, confusion, loss of tendon reflexes and respiratory depression due to neuromuscular blockade, slurred speech, double vision, muscle weakness, bradycardia, cardiac arrhythmias, coma, and cardiac arrest.

- ● RENAL IMPAIRMENT Avoid in severe impairment (eGFR less than 30 mL/minute/1.73^2).

- ● DIRECTIONS FOR ADMINISTRATION Dissolve sachet contents in 50–200 mL water, tea or orange juice and take immediately.

- ● PRESCRIBING AND DISPENSING INFORMATION *Magnaspartate*® contains magnesium aspartate 6.5 g (10 mmol Mg^{2+})/sachet.

- ● PATIENT AND CARER ADVICE Patients and carers should be given advice on how to administer magnesium aspartate powder.

- ● MEDICINAL FORMS
  There can be variation in the licensing of different medicines containing the same drug.
  Powder
  EXCIPIENTS: May contain Sucrose
  ▸ Magnaspartate (KoRa Healthcare)
    Magnesium (as Magnesium aspartate) 243 mg Magnaspartate 243mg (magnesium 10mmol) oral powder sachets | 10 sachet [PoM] £8.95 DT = £8.95

Magnesium glycerophosphate

24-Oct-2017

- ● INDICATIONS AND DOSE
  Prevent recurrence of magnesium deficit
  ▶ BY MOUTH
  ▸ Adult: 24 mmol daily in divided doses, dose expressed as Mg^{2+}

  DOSE EQUIVALENCE AND CONVERSION
  ▸ Magnesium glycerophosphate 1 g is approximately equivalent to Mg^{2+} 4 mmol *or* magnesium 97 mg.

  NEOMAG® CHEWABLE TABLETS
  Hypomagnesaemia
  ▶ BY MOUTH
  ▸ Adult: Initially 1–2 tablets 3 times a day, dose to be adjusted according to the serum total magnesium level

  DOSE EQUIVALENCE AND CONVERSION
  ▸ Each *Neomag*® chewable tablet contains Mg^{2+} 4 mmol *or* magnesium 97 mg.

- ● UNLICENSED USE Preparations other than *Neomag*® are not licensed for use.

- ● INTERACTIONS → Appendix 1: magnesium

- ● SIDE-EFFECTS Diarrhoea · hypermagnesaemia

- ● RENAL IMPAIRMENT Increased risk of toxicity.
  Dose adjustments Avoid or reduce dose.
  NEOMAG® CHEWABLE TABLETS Manufacturer advises avoid in severe impairment.

- ● MONITORING REQUIREMENTS Manufacturer advises to monitor serum magnesium levels every 3–6 months.

- ● DIRECTIONS FOR ADMINISTRATION
  NEOMAG® CHEWABLE TABLETS Manufacturer advises that tablets may be broken into quarters and chewed or swallowed with water.

- ● NATIONAL FUNDING/ACCESS DECISIONS
  NEOMAG® CHEWABLE TABLETS

  Scottish Medicines Consortium (SMC) Decisions
  The *Scottish Medicines Consortium* has advised (September 2017) that magnesium glycerophosphate (*Neomag*®) is accepted for use within NHS Scotland as an oral magnesium supplement for the treatment of patients with chronic magnesium loss, hypomagnesaemia or drug-induced hypomagnesaemia.

- ● MEDICINAL FORMS
  There can be variation in the licensing of different medicines containing the same drug. Forms available from special-order manufacturers include: tablet, capsule, oral suspension, oral solution, powder
  Oral solution
  ▸ LiquaMag GP (Fontus Health Ltd)
    Magnesium (as Magnesium glycerophosphate) 24.25 mg per 1 ml LiquaMag GP (magnesium 121.25mg/5ml (5mmol/5ml)) oral solution sugar-free | 200 ml £49.99

▸ MagnaPhos (TriOn Pharma Ltd)
**Magnesium (as Magnesium glycerophosphate) 19.44 mg per
1 ml** MagnaPhos 97.2mg/5ml (4mmol/5ml) oral solution | 200 ml
£37.87 DT = £133.68
**Magnesium (as Magnesium glycerophosphate) 24.25 mg per
1 ml** MagnaPhos 121.25mg/5ml (5mmol/5ml) oral solution | 200 ml
£37.87 DT = £37.87

Chewable tablet
EXCIPIENTS: May contain Aspartame
▸ MagnaPhate (Arjun Products Ltd)
**Magnesium (as Magnesium glycerophosphate)
97.2 mg** MagnaPhate (magnesium 97.2mg (4mmol)) chewable tablets
sugar-free | 50 tablet £22.64 DT = £22.77
▸ MagnaPhos (TriOn Pharma Ltd)
**Magnesium (as Magnesium glycerophosphate)
97.2 mg** MagnaPhos 97.2mg (4mmol) chewable tablets sugar-free |
50 tablet £17.89 DT = £22.77
▸ Neomag (Neoceuticals Ltd)
Magnesium (as Magnesium glycerophosphate) 97.2 mg Neomag
(magnesium 97mg (4mmol)) chewable tablets sugar-free |
50 tablet PoM £22.77 DT = £22.77

Capsule
▸ MagnaPhos (TriOn Pharma Ltd)
**Magnesium (as Magnesium glycerophosphate)
48.6 mg** MagnaPhos 48.6mg (2mmol) capsules | 50 capsule £35.87
**Magnesium (as Magnesium glycerophosphate)
97.2 mg** MagnaPhos 97.2mg (4mmol) capsules | 50 capsule £37.87

Magnesium sulfate

● **INDICATIONS AND DOSE**
**Severe acute asthma | Continuing respiratory
deterioration in anaphylaxis**
▸ BY INTRAVENOUS INFUSION
▸ Child 2-17 years: 40 mg/kg (max. per dose 2 g), to be
given over 20 minutes
▸ Adult: 1.2–2 g, to be given over 20 minutes

Prevention of seizures in pre-eclampsia
▸ INITIALLY BY INTRAVENOUS INJECTION
▸ Adult: Initially 4 g, to be given over 5–15 minutes,
followed by (by intravenous infusion) 1 gram/hour for
24 hours, if seizure occurs, additional dose of 2 g by
intravenous injection to be administered

**Treatment of seizures and prevention of seizure
recurrence in eclampsia**
▸ INITIALLY BY INTRAVENOUS INJECTION
▸ Adult: Initially 4 g, to be given over 5–15 minutes,
followed by (by intravenous infusion) 1 gram/hour for
24 hours after seizure or delivery (whichever is later), if
seizure recurs, increase the infusion rate to
1.5–2 g/hour or give an additional dose of 2 g by
intravenous injection

Hypomagnesaemia
▸ BY INTRAVENOUS INFUSION, OR BY INTRAMUSCULAR INJECTION
▸ Adult: Up to 40 g, given over a period of up to 5 days,
dose given depends on the amount required to replace
the deficit (allowing for urinary losses)

**Hypomagnesaemia maintenance (e.g. in intravenous
nutrition)**
▸ BY INTRAVENOUS INFUSION, OR BY INTRAMUSCULAR INJECTION
▸ Adult: 2.5–5 g daily, usual dose 3 g daily

Emergency treatment of serious arrhythmias
▸ BY INTRAVENOUS INJECTION
▸ Adult: 2 g, to be given over 10-15 minutes, dose may be
repeated once if necessary

Rapid bowel evacuation (acts in 2–4 hours)
▸ BY MOUTH
▸ Adult: 5–10 g, dose to be mixed in a glass of water,
taken preferably before breakfast

DOSE EQUIVALENCE AND CONVERSION
▸ Magnesium sulfate heptahydrate 1 g equivalent to
Mg^{2+} approx. 4 mmol.

● UNLICENSED USE Unlicensed indication in severe acute
asthma and continuing respiratory deterioration in
anaphylaxis.
● CONTRA-INDICATIONS
▸ With oral use In rapid bowel evacuation—acute gastro-
intestinal conditions
● CAUTIONS
▸ With oral use In rapid bowel evacuation—elderly and
debilitated patients
● INTERACTIONS → Appendix 1: magnesium
● SIDE-EFFECTS
▸ Rare or very rare
▸ With oral use Paralytic ileus
▸ Frequency not known
▸ With intravenous use Electrolyte imbalance
▸ With oral use Diarrhoea · gastrointestinal discomfort ·
hypermagnesaemia
● PREGNANCY
▸ When used for Hypomagnesaemia or Arrhythmias or Prevention of
seizures in pre-eclampsia or Treatment of seizures and prevention
of seizure recurrence in eclampsia or Severe acute asthma or
Continuing respiratory deterioration in anaphylaxis Not known
to be harmful for short-term intravenous administration in
eclampsia. Sufficient amount may cross the placenta in
mothers treated with high doses, causing hypotonia and
respiratory depression in newborns.
● HEPATIC IMPAIRMENT Avoid in hepatic coma if risk of
renal failure.
● RENAL IMPAIRMENT Increased risk of toxicity.
Dose adjustments Avoid or reduce dose.
● MONITORING REQUIREMENTS Monitor blood pressure,
respiratory rate, urinary output and for signs of
overdosage (loss of patellar reflexes, weakness, nausea,
sensation of warmth, flushing, drowsiness, double vision,
and slurred speech).
● DIRECTIONS FOR ADMINISTRATION
▸ With intravenous use In severe hypomagnesaemia
administer initially via controlled infusion device
(preferably syringe pump).
For *intravenous injection*, in arrhythmias,
hypomagnesaemia, eclampsia, and pre-eclampsia, give
continuously in Glucose 5% or Sodium chloride 0.9%.
Concentration of magnesium sulfate heptahydrate should
not exceed 20% (200 mg/mL or 0.8 mmol/mL Mg^{2+}); dilute
1 part of magnesium sulfate injection 50% with at least
1.5 parts of water for injections. Max. rate 150 mg/minute
(0.6 mmol/minute Mg^{2+}).
● PRESCRIBING AND DISPENSING INFORMATION
▸ With intramuscular use or intravenous use The BP directs that
the label states the strength as the % w/v of magnesium
sulfate heptahydrate and as the approximate
concentration of magnesium ions (Mg^{2+}) in mmol/mL.
Magnesium Sulfate Injection BP is a sterile solution of
Magnesium Sulfate Heptahydrate.
● EXCEPTIONS TO LEGAL CATEGORY
▸ With oral use Magnesium sulfate is on sale to the public as
Epsom Salts.

● MEDICINAL FORMS
There can be variation in the licensing of different medicines
containing the same drug. Forms available from special-order
manufacturers include: solution for injection, infusion,
solution for infusion
Solution for injection
▸ Magnesium sulfate (Non-proprietary)
Magnesium sulfate heptahydrate 500 mg per 1 ml Magnesium
sulfate 50% (magnesium 2mmol/ml) solution for injection 10ml
ampoules | 10 ampoule PoM £21.70–£21.71 DT = £21.63
Magnesium sulfate 50% (magnesium 2mmol/ml) solution for injection
20ml vials | 10 vial PoM £49.20

Magnesium sulfate 50% (magnesium 2mmol/ml) solution for injection 5ml ampoules | 10 ampoule [PoM] £37.80–£61.26
Magnesium sulfate 50% (magnesium 2mmol/ml) solution for injection 2ml ampoules | 10 ampoule [PoM] £17.30–£17.35 DT = £17.35

Solution for infusion
▸ Magnesium sulfate (Non-proprietary)
Magnesium sulfate heptahydrate 100 mg per 1 ml Magnesium sulfate 10% (magnesium 0.4mmol/ml) solution for injection 10ml ampoules | 10 ampoule [PoM] £66.26 DT = £66.26
Magnesium sulfate heptahydrate 500 mg per 1 ml Magnesium sulfate 50% (magnesium 2mmol/ml) solution for infusion 50ml vials | 10 vial [PoM] £73.00

Powder
▸ Magnesium sulfate (Non-proprietary)
Magnesium sulfate dried 1 mg per 1 mg Magnesium sulfate powder | 300 gram [GSL] £2.09 | 500 gram [GSL] £3.20 DT = £3.20 | 2000 gram [GSL] £5.60 | 5000 gram [GSL] £11.49
▸ Brands may include Epsom salts

1.4 Phosphate imbalance

Phosphorus

Phosphate supplements

Oral phosphate supplements p. 1023 may be required in addition to vitamin D in a small minority of patients with hypophosphataemic vitamin D-resistant rickets.

Phosphate infusion is occasionally needed in alcohol dependence or in phosphate deficiency arising from use of parenteral nutrition deficient in phosphate supplements; phosphate depletion also occurs in severe diabetic ketoacidosis.

For phosphate requirements in total parenteral nutrition regimens, see Intravenous nutrition p. 1038.

Phosphate-binding agents

Calcium-containing preparations are used as phosphate-binding agents in the management of hyperphosphataemia complicating renal failure. Aluminium-containing preparations are rarely used as phosphate binding agents and can cause aluminium accumulation.

Sevelamer p. 1022 is licensed for the treatment of hyperphosphataemia in patients on haemodialysis or peritoneal dialysis. Sevelamer carbonate is also licensed for the treatment of patients with chronic kidney disease not on dialysis who have a serum-phosphate concentration of 1.78 mmol/litre or more.

Lanthanum p. 1021 is licensed for the control of hyperphosphataemia in patients with chronic renal failure on haemodialysis or continuous ambulatory peritoneal dialysis (CAPD), and in patients with chronic kidney disease not on dialysis who have a serum-phosphate concentration of 1.78 mmol/litre or more that cannot be controlled by a low-phosphate diet.

Sucroferric oxyhydroxide p. 1022 is licensed for the control of hyperphosphataemia in patients with chronic kidney disease on haemodialysis or peritoneal dialysis. It is used as part of a multiple therapeutic approach to control the development of renal bone disease; this could include the concomitant use of a calcium supplement, a vitamin D analogue or calcimimetics.

1.4a Hyperphosphataemia

ELECTROLYTES AND MINERALS ⟩ ALUMINIUM

Aluminium hydroxide

● **INDICATIONS AND DOSE**

Hyperphosphataemia in renal failure
▸ **BY MOUTH USING CAPSULES**
▸ Adult: 4–20 capsules daily in divided doses, to be taken with meals

Antacid
▸ **BY MOUTH USING CAPSULES**
▸ Adult: 475 mg 5 times a day, last dose to be taken at bedtime

● **CONTRA-INDICATIONS** Hypophosphataemia
● **INTERACTIONS** → Appendix 1: antacids
● **SIDE-EFFECTS** Constipation
● **HEPATIC IMPAIRMENT** Avoid; can cause constipation which can precipitate coma.
● **RENAL IMPAIRMENT** There is a risk of accumulation and aluminium toxicity with antacids containing aluminium salts. Absorption of aluminium from aluminium salts is increased by citrates, which are contained in many effervescent preparations (such as effervescent analgesics).

● **MEDICINAL FORMS**
There can be variation in the licensing of different medicines containing the same drug.
Capsule
▸ Alu-Cap (Meda Pharmaceuticals Ltd)
Aluminium hydroxide 475 mg Alu-Cap 475mg capsules | 120 capsule [P] £13.71 DT = £13.71

ELECTROLYTES AND MINERALS ⟩ CALCIUM

⚑ 1013

Calcium acetate

● **INDICATIONS AND DOSE**

PHOSEX ® TABLETS

Hyperphosphataemia
▸ **BY MOUTH**
▸ Adult: Initially 1 tablet 3 times a day, to be taken with meals, dose to be adjusted according to serum-phosphate concentration, usual dose 4–6 tablets daily in divided doses, (1 or 2 tablets with each meal); maximum 12 tablets per day

RENACET ® TABLETS

Hyperphosphataemia
▸ **BY MOUTH**
▸ Adult: 475–950 mg, to be taken with breakfast and with snacks, 0.95–2.85 g, to be taken with main meals and 0.95–1.9 g, to be taken with supper, dose to be adjusted according to serum-phosphate concentration; maximum 6.65 g per day

● **INTERACTIONS** → Appendix 1: calcium salts
● **SIDE-EFFECTS**
▸ **Uncommon** Vomiting
● **DIRECTIONS FOR ADMINISTRATION**
PHOSEX ® TABLETS *Phosex*® tablets are taken with meals. Tablets can be broken to aid swallowing, but not chewed (bitter taste).
RENACET ® TABLETS Manufacturer advises that other drugs should be taken 1 to 2 hours before or after *Renacet*®

to reduce the possible interference with absorption of other drugs. *Renacet*® tablets are taken with meals.
- PRESCRIBING AND DISPENSING INFORMATION *Renacet*® tablets contain calcium acetate 475 mg (equivalent to calcium 120.25 mg or Ca^{2+} 3 mmol); *Phosex*® tablets contain calcium acetate 1 g (equivalent to calcium 250 mg or Ca^{2+} 6.2 mmol).
- PATIENT AND CARER ADVICE
  PHOSEX® TABLETS Patients or carers should be given advice on how to administer *Phosex*® tablets.
  RENACET® TABLETS Patients or carers should be given advice on how to administer *Renacet*® tablets.
- MEDICINAL FORMS
  There can be variation in the licensing of different medicines containing the same drug. Forms available from special-order manufacturers include: tablet

Tablet
CAUTIONARY AND ADVISORY LABELS 25
▸ Phosex (Pharmacosmos UK Ltd)
  Calcium acetate 1 gram Phosex 1g tablets | 180 tablet [PoM] £19.79
  DT = £19.79
▸ Renacet (Stanningley Pharma Ltd)
  Calcium acetate 475 mg Renacet 475mg tablets | 200 tablet [PoM]
  £9.71 DT = £9.71
  Calcium acetate 950 mg Renacet 950mg tablets | 200 tablet [PoM]
  £18.45 DT = £18.45

Combinations available: *Calcium acetate with magnesium carbonate,* below

PHOSPHATE BINDERS

Calcium acetate with magnesium carbonate

The properties listed below are those particular to the combination only. For the properties of the components please consider, calcium acetate p. 1020, magnesium carbonate p. 70.

- INDICATIONS AND DOSE
  Hyperphosphataemia
  ▸ BY MOUTH
  ▸ Adult: Initially 1 tablet 3 times a day, adjusted according to serum-phosphate concentration, to be taken with food; usual dose 3–10 tablets daily; maximum 12 tablets per day

- CONTRA-INDICATIONS Hypercalcaemia · hypermagnesaemia · myasthenia gravis · third-degree AV block
- INTERACTIONS → Appendix 1: antacids · calcium salts
- DIRECTIONS FOR ADMINISTRATION Manufacturer advises that other drugs should be taken at least 2 hours before or 3 hours after calcium acetate with magnesium carbonate to reduce possible interference with absorption of other drugs.
- PATIENT AND CARER ADVICE Patients or carers should be given advice on how to administer calcium acetate with magnesium carbonate tablets.

- MEDICINAL FORMS
  There can be variation in the licensing of different medicines containing the same drug.

Tablet
CAUTIONARY AND ADVISORY LABELS 25
▸ Rephoren (Vifor Fresenius Medical Care Renal Pharma UK Ltd)
  Magnesium carbonate heavy 235 mg, Calcium acetate 435 mg Osvaren 435mg/235mg tablets | 180 tablet [PoM] £24.00

Lanthanum

- INDICATIONS AND DOSE
  Hyperphosphataemia in patients with chronic renal failure on haemodialysis or continuous ambulatory peritoneal dialysis (CAPD) | Hyperphosphataemia in patients with chronic kidney disease not on dialysis who have a serum-phosphate concentration of 1.78 mmol/litre or more that cannot be controlled by a low-phosphate diet
  ▸ BY MOUTH
  ▸ Adult: 1.5–3 g daily in divided doses, dose to be adjusted according to serum-phosphate concentration every 2–3 weeks, to be taken with or immediately after meals

- CAUTIONS Acute peptic ulcer · bowel obstruction · Crohn's disease · ulcerative colitis
- INTERACTIONS → Appendix 1: lanthanum
- SIDE-EFFECTS
  ▸ Common or very common Constipation · diarrhoea · electrolyte imbalance · gastrointestinal discomfort · gastrointestinal disorders · headache · nausea · vomiting
  ▸ Uncommon Alopecia · appetite abnormal · arthralgia · asthenia · burping · chest pain · dizziness · dry mouth · eosinophilia · hyperglycaemia · hyperhidrosis · hyperparathyroidism · increased risk of infection · irritable bowel syndrome · malaise · myalgia · oral disorders · osteoporosis · pain · peripheral oedema · taste altered · thirst · vertigo · weight decreased
- PREGNANCY Manufacturer advises avoid—toxicity in *animal* studies.
- BREAST FEEDING Manufacturer advises caution—no information available.
- HEPATIC IMPAIRMENT Lanthanum excreted in bile—possible accumulation in obstructive jaundice.
- DIRECTIONS FOR ADMINISTRATION Tablets are to be chewed. Each sachet of powder to be mixed with soft food and consumed within 15 minutes.
- PATIENT AND CARER ADVICE Patient and carers should be given advice on how to administer lanthanum tablets and powder.
- NATIONAL FUNDING/ACCESS DECISIONS
  Scottish Medicines Consortium (SMC) Decisions
  The *Scottish Medicines Consortium* has advised (March 2007) that lanthanum (*Fosrenol*®) is accepted for restricted use within NHS Scotland for the control of hyperphosphataemia in patients with chronic renal failure on haemodialysis or continuous ambulatory peritoneal dialysis, as a second-line agent, where a non-aluminium, non-calcium phosphate binder is required.

- MEDICINAL FORMS
  There can be variation in the licensing of different medicines containing the same drug.
  Powder
  CAUTIONARY AND ADVISORY LABELS 21
  ▸ Fosrenol (Shire Pharmaceuticals Ltd)
    Lanthanum (as Lanthanum carbonate) 750 mg Fosrenol 750mg oral powder sachets | 90 sachet [PoM] £182.60 DT = £182.60
    Lanthanum (as Lanthanum carbonate) 1 gram Fosrenol 1000mg oral powder sachets | 90 sachet [PoM] £193.59 DT = £193.59
  Chewable tablet
  CAUTIONARY AND ADVISORY LABELS 21
  ▸ Fosrenol (Shire Pharmaceuticals Ltd)
    Lanthanum (as Lanthanum carbonate) 500 mg Fosrenol 500mg chewable tablets | 90 tablet [PoM] £124.06 DT = £124.06
    Lanthanum (as Lanthanum carbonate) 750 mg Fosrenol 750mg chewable tablets | 90 tablet [PoM] £182.60 DT = £182.60
    Lanthanum (as Lanthanum carbonate) 1 gram Fosrenol 1000mg chewable tablets | 90 tablet [PoM] £193.59 DT = £193.59

9

Blood and nutrition

Sevelamer

19-Mar-2018

● **INDICATIONS AND DOSE**

RENAGEL ®

Hyperphosphataemia in patients on haemodialysis or peritoneal dialysis

▸ BY MOUTH

▸ Adult: Initially 2.4–4.8 g daily in 3 divided doses, dose to be given with meals and adjusted according to serum-phosphate concentration; usual dose 2.4–12 g daily in 3 divided doses

RENVELA ® 2.4G ORAL POWDER SACHETS

Hyperphosphataemia in patients on haemodialysis or peritoneal dialysis | Hyperphosphataemia in patients with chronic kidney disease not on dialysis who have a serum-phosphate concentration of 1.78 mmol/litre or more

▸ BY MOUTH

▸ Adult: Initially 2.4–4.8 g daily in 3 divided doses, dose to be taken with meals and adjusted according to serum-phosphate concentration every 2–4 weeks—consult product literature; usual dose 6 g daily in 3 divided doses

RENVELA ® 800MG TABLETS

Hyperphosphataemia in patients on haemodialysis or peritoneal dialysis | Hyperphosphataemia in patients with chronic kidney disease not on dialysis who have a serum-phosphate concentration of 1.78 mmol/litre or more

▸ BY MOUTH

▸ Adult: Initially 2.4–4.8 g daily in 3 divided doses, dose to be taken with meals and adjusted according to serum-phosphate concentration every 2–4 weeks; usual dose 6 g daily in 3 divided doses

● CONTRA-INDICATIONS Bowel obstruction

● CAUTIONS Gastro-intestinal disorders

● SIDE-EFFECTS

▸ **Common or very common** Constipation · diarrhoea · gastrointestinal discomfort · gastrointestinal disorders · nausea · vomiting

▸ **Frequency not known** Skin reactions

● PREGNANCY Manufacturer advises use only if potential benefit outweighs risk.

● BREAST FEEDING

RENVELA ® 2.4G ORAL POWDER SACHETS Unlikely to be present in milk (however, manufacturer advises avoid).

RENVELA ® 800MG TABLETS Unlikely to be present in milk (however, manufacturer advises avoid).

RENAGEL ® Manufacturer advises use only if potential benefit outweighs risk.

● DIRECTIONS FOR ADMINISTRATION

RENVELA ® 2.4G ORAL POWDER SACHETS Manufacturer advises each sachet should be dispersed in 60 mL water, or mixed with a small amount of cool food (100 g), prior to administration and discarded if unused after 30 minutes.

● PATIENT AND CARER ADVICE

RENVELA ® 2.4G ORAL POWDER SACHETS Patients and carers should be advised on how to administer powder for oral suspension.

● NATIONAL FUNDING/ACCESS DECISIONS

RENVELA ® 2.4G ORAL POWDER SACHETS

Scottish Medicines Consortium (SMC) Decisions

The *Scottish Medicines Consortium* has advised (April 2011) that sevelamer carbonate (*Renvela ®*) is accepted for restricted use within NHS Scotland for the second-line management of hyperphosphataemia in adults receiving haemodialysis.

RENVELA ® 800MG TABLETS

Scottish Medicines Consortium (SMC) Decisions

The *Scottish Medicines Consortium* has advised (April 2011) that sevelamer carbonate (*Renvela ®*) is accepted for restricted use within NHS Scotland for the second-line management of hyperphosphataemia in adults receiving haemodialysis.

● MEDICINAL FORMS

There can be variation in the licensing of different medicines containing the same drug.

Powder

CAUTIONARY AND ADVISORY LABELS 13

▸ Renvela (Sanofi)

Sevelamer carbonate 2.4 gram Renvela 2.4g oral powder sachets sugar-free | 60 sachet [PoM] £167.04 DT = £167.04

Tablet

CAUTIONARY AND ADVISORY LABELS 25

EXCIPIENTS: May contain Propylene glycol

▸ Renagel (Sanofi)

Sevelamer 800 mg Renagel 800mg tablets | 180 tablet [PoM] £167.04 DT = £30.52

▸ Renvela (Sanofi)

Sevelamer 800 mg Renvela 800mg tablets | 180 tablet [PoM] £167.04 DT = £30.52

Sucroferric oxyhydroxide

16-Feb-2016

● **INDICATIONS AND DOSE**

Hyperphosphataemia in patients with chronic kidney disease on haemodialysis or peritoneal dialysis

▸ BY MOUTH

▸ Adult: Initially 1.5 g daily in 3 divided doses, dose to be taken with meals, then adjusted in steps of 500 mg every 2–4 weeks, dose adjusted according to serum-phosphate concentration; maintenance 1.5–2 g daily in divided doses; maximum 3 g per day

● CONTRA-INDICATIONS Haemochromatosis · iron accumulation disorders

● CAUTIONS Gastric disorders · hepatic disorders · major gastrointestinal surgery · peritonitis in the last 3 months

● SIDE-EFFECTS

▸ **Common or very common** Constipation · diarrhoea · gastrointestinal discomfort · gastrointestinal disorders · nausea · oral disorders · product taste abnormal · vomiting

▸ **Uncommon** Dysphagia · dyspnoea · electrolyte imbalance · fatigue · headache · skin reactions

SIDE-EFFECTS, FURTHER INFORMATION Discoloured faeces may mask the visual signs of gastrointestinal bleeding.

● PREGNANCY Manufacturer advises use only if potential benefit outweighs risk—no information available.

● BREAST FEEDING Manufacturer advises avoid—no information available.

● DIRECTIONS FOR ADMINISTRATION *Velphoro ®* tablets must be chewed or crushed, not swallowed whole.

● PATIENT AND CARER ADVICE Patients or carers should be counselled on administration of sucroferric oxyhydroxide tablets and advised that this medication can cause discoloured black stools.

● MEDICINAL FORMS

There can be variation in the licensing of different medicines containing the same drug.

Chewable tablet

▸ Velphoro (Vifor Fresenius Medical Care Renal Pharma UK Ltd) ▼

Iron (as Sucroferric oxyhydroxide) 500 mg Velphoro 500mg chewable tablets | 90 tablet [PoM] £179.00

1.4b Hypophosphataemia

ELECTROLYTES AND MINERALS > PHOSPHATES

Phosphate

- **INDICATIONS AND DOSE**

Treatment of moderate to severe hypophosphatemia
- ▸ BY INTRAVENOUS INFUSION
- ▸ Adult: (consult product literature)

Established hypophosphataemia (with monobasic potassium phosphate)
- ▸ BY INTRAVENOUS INFUSION
- ▸ Adult: 9 mmol every 12 hours, increased if necessary up to 0.5 mmol/kg (max. per dose 50 mmol), increased dose to be used in critically ill patients; dose to be infused over 6–12 hours, according to severity

Vitamin D-resistant hypophosphataemic osteomalacia
- ▸ BY MOUTH USING EFFERVESCENT TABLETS
- ▸ Adult: 4–6 tablets daily, using *Phosphate Sandoz®*.

- **SIDE-EFFECTS**
  GENERAL SIDE-EFFECTS
- ▸ **Common or very common** Diarrhoea
- ▸ **Frequency not known** Nausea
  SPECIFIC SIDE-EFFECTS
- ▸ With intravenous use Acute kidney injury · hypocalcaemia · hypotension · metastatic calcification · oedema
- ▸ With oral use Abdominal distress
  SIDE-EFFECTS, FURTHER INFORMATION Diarrhoea is a common side-effect and should prompt a reduction in dosage.

- **RENAL IMPAIRMENT**
  Dose adjustments Reduce dose.
  Monitoring Monitor closely in renal impairment.

- **MONITORING REQUIREMENTS** It is essential to monitor closely plasma concentrations of calcium, phosphate, potassium, and other electrolytes—excessive doses of phosphates may cause hypocalcaemia and metastatic calcification.

- **PRESCRIBING AND DISPENSING INFORMATION** *Phosphate Sandoz®* contains sodium dihydrogen phosphate anhydrous (anhydrous sodium acid phosphate) 1.936 g, sodium bicarbonate 350 mg, potassium bicarbonate 315 mg, equivalent to phosphorus 500 mg (phosphate 16.1 mmol), sodium 468.8 mg (Na⁺ 20.4 mmol), potassium 123 mg (K⁺ 3.1 mmol); *Polyfusor NA®* contains Na⁺ 162 mmol/litre, K⁺ 19 mmol/litre, PO_4^{3-} 100 mmol/litre; non-proprietary *potassium dihydrogen phosphate injection* (potassium acid phosphate) 13.6% may contain 1 mmol/mL phosphate, 1 mmol/mL potassium.

- **MEDICINAL FORMS**
  There can be variation in the licensing of different medicines containing the same drug. Forms available from special-order manufacturers include: infusion, solution for infusion

Effervescent tablet
CAUTIONARY AND ADVISORY LABELS 13
- ▸ Phosphate Sandoz (HK Pharma Ltd)
  Sodium dihydrogen phosphate anhydrous 1.936 gram Phosphate Sandoz effervescent tablets | 100 tablet P £19.39

Solution for infusion
- ▸ Phosphate (Non-proprietary)
  Potassium dihydrogen phosphate 136 mg per 1 ml Potassium dihydrogen phosphate 13.6% (potassium 10mmol/10ml) solution for infusion 10ml ampoules | 10 ampoule PoM £80.25–£92.69 DT = £92.69

Infusion
- ▸ Phosphate (Non-proprietary)
  Potassium dihydrogen phosphate 1.295 gram per 1 litre, Disodium hydrogen phosphate anhydrous 5.75 gram per 1 litre Polyfusor NA phosphates infusion 500ml bottles | 1 bottle PoM £5.15

1.5 Potassium imbalance

1.5a Hyperkalaemia

> **Other drugs used for Hyperkalaemia** Calcium gluconate, p. 1014

ANTIDOTES AND CHELATORS > CATION EXCHANGE RESINS

Calcium polystyrene sulfonate

- **INDICATIONS AND DOSE**

Hyperkalaemia associated with anuria or severe oliguria, and in dialysis patients
- ▸ BY MOUTH
- ▸ Adult: 15 g 3–4 times a day
- ▸ BY RECTUM
- ▸ Adult: 30 g, retained for 9 hours followed by irrigation to remove resin from colon

- **CONTRA-INDICATIONS** Hyperparathyroidism · metastatic carcinoma · multiple myeloma · obstructive bowel disease · sarcoidosis
- **INTERACTIONS** → Appendix 1: polystyrene sulfonate
- **SIDE-EFFECTS** Appetite decreased · constipation (discontinue—avoid magnesium-containing laxatives) · diarrhoea · electrolyte imbalance · epigastric discomfort · gastrointestinal disorders · gastrointestinal necrosis (in combination with sorbitol) · hypercalcaemia (in dialysed patients and occasionally in those with renal impairment) · increased risk of infection · nausea · vomiting
- **PREGNANCY** Manufacturers advise use only if potential benefit outweighs risk—no information available.
- **BREAST FEEDING** Manufacturers advise use only if potential benefit outweighs risk—no information available.
- **MONITORING REQUIREMENTS** Monitor for electrolyte disturbances (stop if plasma-potassium concentration below 5 mmol/litre).
- **DIRECTIONS FOR ADMINISTRATION**
- ▸ With rectal use Mix each 30 g of resin with 150 mL of water or 10% glucose.

- **MEDICINAL FORMS**
  There can be variation in the licensing of different medicines containing the same drug. Forms available from special-order manufacturers include: enema

Powder
CAUTIONARY AND ADVISORY LABELS 13, 21 (Sorbisterit® powder only)
EXCIPIENTS: May contain Sucrose
- ▸ Calcium Resonium (Sanofi)
  Calcium polystyrene sulfonate 999.34 mg per 1 gram Calcium Resonium powder sugar-free | 300 gram P £82.16

Patiromer calcium

15-Oct-2017

- DRUG ACTION Patiromer is a non-absorbed cation-exchange polymer that acts as a potassium binder in the gastro-intestinal tract.

- INDICATIONS AND DOSE

Hyperkalaemia

▶ BY MOUTH
▶ Adult: Initially 8.4 g once daily; adjusted in steps of 8.4 g as required, dose adjustments should be made at intervals of at least one week; maximum 25.2 g per day

PHARMACOKINETICS
▶ Onset of action 4–7 hours.

- CAUTIONS Risk factors for hypercalcaemia (calcium partially released from counterion complex) · severe gastro-intestinal disorders (ischaemia, necrosis, and intestinal perforation reported with other potassium binders)

- INTERACTIONS → Appendix 1: patiromer

- SIDE-EFFECTS
▶ **Common or very common** Abdominal pain · constipation · diarrhoea · flatulence · hypomagnesaemia
▶ **Uncommon** Nausea · vomiting

- PREGNANCY Manufacturer advises avoid—no information available.

- BREAST FEEDING Manufacturer advises avoid—no information available (although no effects on the infant are anticipated).

- MONITORING REQUIREMENTS Manufacturer advises monitor for electrolyte disturbances, particularly plasma-potassium (as clinically indicated) and plasma-magnesium (continue to monitor for at least 1 month after initiation of treatment).

- DIRECTIONS FOR ADMINISTRATION Manufacturer advises *Veltassa*® should be mixed with approx. 40 mL of water, then stirred and mixed with a further approx. 40 mL of water; the powder will not dissolve. More water may be added as needed. The mixture should be taken within 1 hour of preparation. Apple juice or cranberry juice may be used instead of water, other liquids should be avoided as they may contain high amounts of potassium.

- HANDLING AND STORAGE Store in a refrigerator (2–8°C) prior to dispensing; once dispensed, patient may store below 25°C for up to 6 months.

- MEDICINAL FORMS
There can be variation in the licensing of different medicines containing the same drug.
Powder
CAUTIONARY AND ADVISORY LABELS 13, 21
▶ Veltassa (Vifor Pharma UK Ltd) ▼
Patiromer calcium (as Patiromer sorbitex calcium)
8.4 gram Veltassa 8.4g oral powder sachets | 30 sachet [PoM] £300.00
Patiromer calcium (as Patiromer sorbitex calcium)
16.8 gram Veltassa 16.8g oral powder sachets | 30 sachet [PoM] £300.00

Sodium polystyrene sulfonate

- INDICATIONS AND DOSE

Hyperkalaemia associated with anuria or severe oliguria, and in dialysis patients

▶ BY MOUTH
▶ Adult: 15 g 3–4 times a day
▶ BY RECTUM
▶ Adult: 30 g, retain for 9 hours followed by irrigation to remove resin from colon

- CONTRA-INDICATIONS Obstructive bowel disease

- CAUTIONS Congestive heart failure · hypertension · oedema

- INTERACTIONS → Appendix 1: polystyrene sulfonate

- SIDE-EFFECTS Appetite decreased · bezoar · constipation (discontinue—avoid magnesium-containing laxatives) · diarrhoea · electrolyte imbalance · epigastric discomfort · gastrointestinal disorders · increased risk of infection · nausea · necrosis (in combination with sorbitol) · vomiting

- PREGNANCY Manufacturers advise use only if potential benefit outweighs risk—no information available.

- BREAST FEEDING Manufacturers advise use only if potential benefit outweighs risk—no information available.

- RENAL IMPAIRMENT Use with caution.

- MONITORING REQUIREMENTS Monitor for electrolyte disturbances (stop if plasma-potassium concentration below 5 mmol/litre).

- DIRECTIONS FOR ADMINISTRATION
▶ With rectal use Mix each 30 g of resin with 150 mL of water or 10% glucose.
▶ With oral use Administer dose (powder) in a small amount of water or honey—do not give with fruit juice or squash, which have a high potassium content.

- MEDICINAL FORMS
There can be variation in the licensing of different medicines containing the same drug. Forms available from special-order manufacturers include: oral suspension
Powder
CAUTIONARY AND ADVISORY LABELS 13
▶ Resonium A (Sanofi)
Sodium polystyrene sulfonate 999.34 mg per 1 gram Resonium A powder sugar-free | 454 gram [P] £81.11

1.5b Hypokalaemia

ELECTROLYTES AND MINERALS > POTASSIUM

Potassium bicarbonate with potassium acid tartrate

- INDICATIONS AND DOSE

Hyperchloraemic acidosis associated with potassium deficiency (as in some renal tubular and gastro-intestinal disorders)

▶ BY MOUTH
▶ Adult: (consult product literature)

- CONTRA-INDICATIONS Hypochloraemia · plasma-potassium concentration above 5 mmol/litre

- CAUTIONS Cardiac disease · elderly

- SIDE-EFFECTS Abdominal pain · diarrhoea · flatulence · nausea · vomiting

- RENAL IMPAIRMENT Avoid in severe impairment.
Monitoring Close monitoring required in renal impairment—high risk of hyperkalaemia.

- DIRECTIONS FOR ADMINISTRATION To be dissolved in water before administration.

- PRESCRIBING AND DISPENSING INFORMATION These tablets do not contain chloride.

• MEDICINAL FORMS
There can be variation in the licensing of different medicines containing the same drug.
Effervescent tablet
CAUTIONARY AND ADVISORY LABELS 13, 21
▸ Potassium bicarbonate with potassium acid tartrate (Non-proprietary)
Potassium acid tartrate 300 mg, Potassium bicarbonate 500 mg Potassium (potassium 6.5mmol) effervescent tablets BPC 1968 | 56 tablet GSL £77.77–£93.33 DT = £88.15

Potassium chloride

• INDICATIONS AND DOSE
Prevention of hypokalaemia (patients with normal diet)
▸ BY MOUTH
▸ Adult: 2–4 g daily in divided doses
Electrolyte imbalance
▸ BY INTRAVENOUS INFUSION
▸ Adult: Dose dependent on deficit or the daily maintenance requirements

> **IMPORTANT SAFETY INFORMATION**
> SAFE PRACTICE
> Potassium overdose can be fatal. Ready-mixed infusion solutions containing potassium should be used. Exceptionally, if potassium chloride concentrate is used for preparing an infusion, the infusion solution should be **thoroughly mixed**. Local policies on avoiding inadvertent use of potassium chloride concentrate should be followed.

• CONTRA-INDICATIONS Plasma-potassium concentration above 5 mmol/litre
• CAUTIONS
▸ With intravenous use seek specialist advice in very severe potassium depletion or difficult cases
▸ With oral use Cardiac disease · elderly · hiatus hernia (*with modified-release preparations*) · history of peptic ulcer (*with modified-release preparations*) · intestinal stricture (*with modified-release preparations*)
• INTERACTIONS → Appendix 1: potassium chloride
• SIDE-EFFECTS
GENERAL SIDE-EFFECTS Hyperkalaemia
SPECIFIC SIDE-EFFECTS
▸ With oral use Abdominal cramps · diarrhoea · gastrointestinal disorders · nausea · vomiting
• RENAL IMPAIRMENT Avoid in severe impairment.
Dose adjustments Smaller doses must be used in the prevention of hypokalaemia, to reduce the risk of hyperkalaemia.
Monitoring Close monitoring required in renal impairment—high risk of hyperkalaemia.
• MONITORING REQUIREMENTS
▸ Regular monitoring of plasma-potassium concentration is essential in those taking potassium supplements.
▸ With intravenous use ECG monitoring should be performed in difficult cases.
• DIRECTIONS FOR ADMINISTRATION
▸ With oral use Potassium salts are preferably given as a liquid (or effervescent) preparation, rather than modified-release tablets; they should be given as the chloride (the use of effervescent potassium tablets BPC 1968 should be restricted to *hyperchloraemic* states).
▸ With intravenous use Potassium chloride concentrate must be diluted with **not less** than 50 times its volume of sodium chloride intravenous infusion 0.9% or other suitable diluent and **mixed well**. Ready-mixed infusion solutions should be used where possible; alternatively,

potassium chloride concentrate as ampoules containing 1.5 g (K^+ 20 mmol) in 10 mL, is **thoroughly mixed** with 500 mL of sodium chloride 0.9% intravenous infusion and given slowly over 2 to 3 hours with specialist advice and ECG monitoring in difficult cases. For *peripheral intravenous infusion*, the concentration of potassium should not usually exceed 40 mmol/L. Higher concentrations of potassium chloride may be given in very severe depletion, but require specialist advice.
• PRESCRIBING AND DISPENSING INFORMATION Kay-Cee-L ® contains 1 mmol/mL each of K^+ and Cl^-.
Potassium Tablets Do not confuse Effervescent Potassium Tablets BPC 1968 with effervescent potassium chloride tablets. Effervescent Potassium Tablets BPC 1968 do not contain chloride ions and their use should be restricted to hyperchloraemic states.
• PATIENT AND CARER ADVICE Patient or carers should be given advice on how to administer potassium chloride modified-release tablets.
Salt substitutes A number of salt substitutes which contain significant amounts of potassium chloride are readily available as health food products (e.g. *LoSalt* ® and *Ruthmol* ®). These should not be used by patients with renal failure as potassium intoxication may result.
• LESS SUITABLE FOR PRESCRIBING Modified-release tablets are less suitable for prescribing. Modified-release preparations should be avoided unless effervescent tablets or liquid preparations inappropriate.

• MEDICINAL FORMS
There can be variation in the licensing of different medicines containing the same drug. Forms available from special-order manufacturers include: modified-release tablet, oral solution, solution for injection, infusion, solution for infusion
Modified-release tablet
CAUTIONARY AND ADVISORY LABELS 25, 27
▸ Potassium chloride (Non-proprietary)
Potassium chloride 600 mg Kaleorid LP 600mg tablets | 30 tablet PoM ⓢ
Duro-K 600mg tablets | 100 tablet PoM ⓢ
Solution for infusion
▸ Potassium chloride (Non-proprietary)
Potassium chloride 150 mg per 1 ml Potassium chloride 15% (potassium 20mmol/10ml) solution for infusion 10ml ampoules | 10 ampoule PoM £5.00 | 20 ampoule PoM £6.50–£10.70
Potassium chloride 15% (potassium 20mmol/10ml) solution for infusion 10ml Mini-Plasco ampoules | 20 ampoule PoM £10.70
Potassium chloride 200 mg per 1 ml Potassium chloride 20% (potassium 13.3mmol/5ml) solution for infusion 5ml ampoules | 10 ampoule PoM £3.84–£4.00
Potassium chloride 20% (potassium 27mmol/10ml) solution for infusion 10ml ampoules | 10 ampoule PoM £121.25
Oral solution
CAUTIONARY AND ADVISORY LABELS 21
▸ Kay-Cee-L (Geistlich Sons Ltd)
Potassium chloride 75 mg per 1 ml Kay-Cee-L syrup sugar-free | 500 ml Ⓟ £8.43

2 Metabolic disorders
2.1 Acute porphyrias

Acute porphyrias   01-Oct-2017

Overview

The acute porphyrias (acute intermittent porphyria, variegate porphyria, hereditary coproporphyria, and 5-aminolaevulinic acid dehydratase deficiency porphyria) are hereditary disorders of haem biosynthesis; they have a prevalence of about 1 in 75 000 of the population.

Great care must be taken when prescribing for patients with acute porphyria, since certain drugs can induce acute porphyric crises. Since acute porphyrias are hereditary, relatives of affected individuals should be screened and advised about the potential danger of certain drugs.

EvGr Where there is no safe alternative, drug treatment for serious or life-threatening conditions should not be withheld from patients with acute porphyria. Where possible, the clinical situation should be discussed with a porphyria specialist for advice on how to proceed and monitor the patient. In the UK clinical advice can be obtained from the National Acute Porphyria Service or from the UK Porphyria Medicines Information Service (UKPMIS)—see details below. Ⓔ

Haem arginate p. 1027 is administered by short intravenous infusion as haem replacement in moderate, severe, or unremitting acute porphyria crises.

In the United Kingdom the National Acute Porphyria Service (NAPS) provides clinical support and treatment with haem arginate from two centres (University Hospital of Wales and King's College Hospital). To access the service telephone (029) 2074 7747 and ask for the Acute Porphyria Service.

Drugs unsafe for use in acute porphyrias

EvGr The following list contains drugs on the UK market that have been classified as 'unsafe' in porphyria because they have been shown to be porphyrinogenic in animals or in vitro, or have been associated with acute attacks in patients. Absence of a drug from the following lists does not necessarily imply that the drug is safe. For many drugs no information about porphyria is available. Ⓔ

An up-to-date list of drugs considered safe in acute porphyrias is available from the UKPMIS, see *Useful resources* below.

Further information may be obtained from: porphyria.eu/ and also from:
The UK Porphyria Medicines Information Service (UKPMIS)
University Hospital of Wales
CF14 4XW
Cardiff
(029) 2074 2979/3877
Quite modest changes in chemical structure can lead to changes in porphyrinogenicity but where possible general statements have been made about groups of drugs; these should be checked first.

Unsafe Drug Groups (check first)

- Anabolic steroids
- Antidepressants, MAOIs (contact UKPMIS for advice)
- Antidepressants, Tricyclic and related (contact UKPMIS for advice)
- Barbiturates (includes primidone and thiopental)
- Contraceptives, hormonal (for detailed advice contact UKPMIS or a porphyria specialist)
- Hormone replacement therapy (for detailed advice contact UKPMIS or a porphyria specialist)
- Imidazole antifungals (applies to oral and intravenous use; topical antifungals are thought to be safe due to low systemic exposure)
- Non-nucleoside reverse transcriptase inhibitors (contact UKPMIS for advice)
- Progestogens (for detailed advice contact UKPMIS or a porphyria specialist)
- Protease inhibitors (contact UKPMIS for advice)
- Sulfonamides (includes co-trimoxazole and sulfasalazine)
- Sulfonylureas (glipizide and glimepiride are thought to be safe)
- Taxanes (contact UKPMIS for advice)
- Triazole antifungals (applies to oral and intravenous use; topical antifungals are thought to be safe due to low systemic exposure)

Unsafe Drugs (check groups above first)

- Aceclofenac
- Alcohol
- Amiodarone
- Aprepitant
- Artemether with lumefantrine
- Bexarotene
- Bosentan
- Busulfan
- Carbamazepine
- Chloral hydrate (although evidence of hazard is uncertain, manufacturer advises avoid)
- Chloramphenicol
- Chloroform (small amounts in medicines probably safe)
- Clemastine
- Clindamycin
- Cocaine
- Danazol
- Dapsone
- Diltiazem
- Disopyramide
- Disulfiram
- Ergometrine
- Ergotamine
- Erythromycin
- Etamsylate
- Ethosuximide
- Etomidate
- Flutamide
- Fosaprepitant
- Fosphenytoin
- Griseofulvin
- Hydralazine
- Ifosfamide
- Indapamide
- Isometheptene mucate
- Isoniazid (safety uncertain, contact UKPMIS for advice)
- Ketamine
- Mefenamic acid (safety uncertain, contact UKPMIS for advice)
- Meprobamate
- Methyldopa
- Metolazone
- Metyrapone
- Mifepristone
- Minoxidil (safety uncertain, contact UKPMIS for advice)
- Mitotane
- Nalidixic acid
- Nitrazepam
- Nitrofurantoin
- Orphenadrine
- Oxcarbazepine
- Oxybutynin
- Pentazocine
- Pentoxifylline
- Pergolide
- Phenoxybenzamine
- Phenytoin
- Pivmecillinam
- Pizotifen
- Porfimer
- Raloxifene
- Rifabutin (safety uncertain, contact UKPMIS for advice)
- Rifampicin
- Riluzole
- Risperidone
- Spironolactone
- Sulfinpyrazone
- Tamoxifen
- Temoporfin
- Thiotepa
- Tiagabine

- Tibolone
- Topiramate
- Toremifene
- Trimethoprim
- Valproate
- Verapamil
- Xipamide

Useful Resources

Acute porphyrias safe list. UK Porphyria Medicines Information Service. 2017.
www.wmic.wales.nhs.uk/specialist-services/drugs-in-porphyria

BLOOD AND RELATED PRODUCTS 〉 HAEM DERIVATIVES

Haem arginate

(Human hemin)

- **INDICATIONS AND DOSE**

Acute porphyrias | Acute intermittent porphyria | Porphyria variegata | Hereditary coproporphyria
- ▸ BY INTRAVENOUS INFUSION
- ▸ Adult: Initially 3 mg/kg once daily for 4 days, if response inadequate, repeat 4-day course with close biochemical monitoring; maximum 250 mg per day

- **SIDE-EFFECTS**
- ▸ **Rare or very rare** Fever
- ▸ **Frequency not known** Headache · skin discolouration · venous thrombosis
- **PREGNANCY** Manufacturer advises avoid unless essential.
- **BREAST FEEDING** Manufacturer advises avoid unless essential—no information available.
- **DIRECTIONS FOR ADMINISTRATION** For *intravenous infusion* (*Normosang*®), give intermittently in Sodium chloride 0.9%; dilute requisite dose in 100 mL infusion fluid in glass bottle and give over at least 30 minutes through a filter *via* large antebrachial or central vein; administer within 1 hour after dilution.
- **MEDICINAL FORMS**
There can be variation in the licensing of different medicines containing the same drug.
Solution for infusion
- ▸ Normosang (Orphan Europe (UK) Ltd)
Haem arginate 25 mg per 1 ml Normosang 250mg/10ml solution for infusion ampoules | 4 ampoule [PoM] £1,737.00

2.2 Carnitine deficiency

AMINO ACIDS AND DERIVATIVES

Levocarnitine

(Carnitine)

- **INDICATIONS AND DOSE**

Primary carnitine deficiency due to inborn errors of metabolism
- ▸ BY MOUTH
- ▸ Adult: Up to 200 mg/kg daily in 2–4 divided doses; maximum 3 g per day
- ▸ BY SLOW INTRAVENOUS INJECTION
- ▸ Adult: Up to 100 mg/kg daily in 2–4 divided doses, to be administered over 2–3 minutes

Secondary carnitine deficiency in haemodialysis patients
- ▸ INITIALLY BY SLOW INTRAVENOUS INJECTION
- ▸ Adult: 20 mg/kg, to be administered over 2–3 minutes, after each dialysis session, dosage adjusted according to plasma-carnitine concentration, then (by mouth) maintenance 1 g daily, administered if benefit is gained from first intravenous course

- **CAUTIONS** Diabetes mellitus
- **SIDE-EFFECTS**
- ▸ **Rare or very rare** Abdominal cramps · diarrhoea · nausea · skin odour abnormal · vomiting

SIDE-EFFECTS, FURTHER INFORMATION Side-effects may be dose-related—monitor tolerance during first week and after any dose increase.
- **PREGNANCY** Appropriate to use; no evidence of teratogenicity in *animal* studies.
- **RENAL IMPAIRMENT** Accumulation of metabolites may occur with chronic oral administration in severe impairment.
- **MONITORING REQUIREMENTS**
- ▸ Monitoring of free and acyl carnitine in blood and urine recommended.
- **MEDICINAL FORMS**
There can be variation in the licensing of different medicines containing the same drug. Forms available from special-order manufacturers include: capsule
Solution for injection
- ▸ Carnitor (Logixx Pharma Solutions Ltd)
L-Carnitine 200 mg per 1 ml Carnitor 1g/5ml solution for injection ampoules | 5 ampoule [PoM] £59.50
Oral solution
- ▸ Levocarnitine (Non-proprietary)
L-Carnitine 300 mg per 1 ml Levocarnitine 1.5g/5ml (30%) oral solution paediatric | 20 ml [PoM] £71.40 DT = £71.40 | 40 ml [PoM] £69.80
- ▸ Carnitor (Logixx Pharma Solutions Ltd)
L-Carnitine 100 mg per 1 ml Carnitor oral single dose 1g solution sugar-free | 10 unit dose [PoM] £35.00
Chewable tablet
- ▸ Carnitor (Logixx Pharma Solutions Ltd)
L-Carnitine 1 gram Carnitor 1g chewable tablets | 10 tablet [PoM] £35.00

2.3 Cystinosis

2.3a Nephropathic cystinosis

AMINO ACIDS AND DERIVATIVES

Mercaptamine

21-Nov-2017

(Cysteamine)

- **INDICATIONS AND DOSE**

Nephropathic cystinosis (specialist use only)
- ▸ BY MOUTH
- ▸ Adult (body-weight 50 kg and above): Initially one-sixth to one-quarter of the expected maintenance dose, increased gradually over 4–6 weeks to avoid intolerance, maintenance 2 g daily in 4 divided doses

Corneal cystine crystal deposits in patients with cystinosis (specialist use only)
- ▸ TO THE EYE
- ▸ Adult: Apply 1 drop 4 times a day, to be applied to both eyes (minimum 4 hours between doses); dose may be reduced according to response (minimum daily dose 1 drop in each eye)

continued →

9

Blood and nutrition

DOSE EQUIVALENCE AND CONVERSION
‣ With oral use
‣ 1.3 g/m^2 is approximately equivalent to 50 mg/kg.

IMPORTANT SAFETY INFORMATION
SAFE PRACTICE
Mercaptamine has been confused with mercaptopurine; care must be taken to ensure the correct drug is prescribed and dispensed.

● CAUTIONS
‣ When used by eye Contact lens wearers
‣ With oral use Dose of phosphate supplement may need to be adjusted if transferring from phosphocysteamine to mercaptamine
● SIDE-EFFECTS
‣ Common or very common
‣ When used by eye Dry eye · eye discomfort · eye erythema · excessive tearing · vision blurred
‣ With oral use Appetite decreased · asthenia · breath odour · diarrhoea · drowsiness · encephalopathy · fever · gastroenteritis · gastrointestinal discomfort · headache · nausea · skin reactions · vomiting
‣ Uncommon
‣ With oral use Compression fracture · gastrointestinal ulcer · hair colour changes · hallucination · joint hyperextension · leg pain · leucopenia · musculoskeletal disorders · nephrotic syndrome · nervousness · osteopenia · seizure
‣ Frequency not known
‣ With oral use Depression · intracranial pressure increased · papilloedema
● ALLERGY AND CROSS-SENSITIVITY Contra-indicated if history of hypersensitivity to penicillamine.
● PREGNANCY
‣ With oral use Manufacturer advises avoid—teratogenic and toxic in *animal* studies.
● BREAST FEEDING
‣ With oral use Manufacturer advises avoid—no information available.
● MONITORING REQUIREMENTS
‣ With oral use Leucocyte-cystine concentration and haematological monitoring required—consult product literature.
● PRESCRIBING AND DISPENSING INFORMATION
Mercaptamine has a very unpleasant taste and smell, which can affect compliance.
● HANDLING AND STORAGE
‣ When used by eye Manufacturer advises store in a refrigerator (2–8°C)—after opening store at room temperature up to 25°C for up to 7 days; protect from light.
● NATIONAL FUNDING/ACCESS DECISIONS
Scottish Medicines Consortium (SMC) Decisions
‣ With oral use The *Scottish Medicines Consortium* has advised (November 2017) that mercaptamine (*Procysbi*®) is **not** recommended for use within NHS Scotland for the treatment of proven nephropathic cystinosis.

● MEDICINAL FORMS
There can be variation in the licensing of different medicines containing the same drug. Forms available from special-order manufacturers include: eye drops
Gastro-resistant capsule
‣ Procysbi (Chiesi Ltd)
Mercaptamine (as Mercaptamine bitartrate) 25 mg Procysbi 25mg gastro-resistant capsules | 60 capsule [PoM] £335.97
Mercaptamine (as Mercaptamine bitartrate) 75 mg Procysbi 75mg gastro-resistant capsules | 250 capsule [PoM] £4,199.65

Eye drops
EXCIPIENTS: May contain Benzalkonium chloride, disodium edetate
‣ Cystadrops (Orphan Europe (UK) Ltd)
Mercaptamine (as Mercaptamine hydrochloride) 3.8 mg per 1 ml Cystadrops 3.8mg/ml eye drops | 5 ml [PoM] £865.00
Capsule
CAUTIONARY AND ADVISORY LABELS 21
‣ Cystagon (Orphan Europe (UK) Ltd)
Mercaptamine (as Mercaptamine bitartrate) 50 mg Cystagon 50mg capsules | 100 capsule [PoM] £70.00
Mercaptamine (as Mercaptamine bitartrate) 150 mg Cystagon 150mg capsules | 100 capsule [PoM] £190.00

2.4 Fabry's disease

ENZYMES

Agalsidase alfa

● DRUG ACTION Agalsidase alfa, an enzyme produced by recombinant DNA technology are licensed for long-term enzyme replacement therapy in Fabry's disease (a lysosomal storage disorder caused by deficiency of alpha-galactosidase A).

● INDICATIONS AND DOSE
Fabry's disease (specialist use only)
‣ BY INTRAVENOUS INFUSION
‣ Adult: 200 micrograms/kg every 2 weeks

● INTERACTIONS → Appendix 1: agalsidase

● SIDE-EFFECTS
‣ Common or very common Arrhythmias · asthenia · chest discomfort · chills · cough · diarrhoea · dizziness · dyspnoea · excessive tearing · fever · flushing · gastrointestinal discomfort · headache · hearing impairment · hoarseness · hypersomnia · hypertension · increased risk of infection · influenza like illness · joint disorders · malaise · musculoskeletal discomfort · myalgia · nausea · pain · palpitations · peripheral oedema · peripheral swelling · rhinorrhoea · sensation abnormal · skin reactions · taste altered · temperature sensation altered · throat complaints · tremor · vomiting
‣ Uncommon Altered smell sensation · angioedema · hypersensitivity · sensation of pressure
‣ Frequency not known Heart failure · hyperhidrosis · hypotension · myocardial ischaemia
SIDE-EFFECTS, FURTHER INFORMATION Infusion-related reactions; manage by interrupting the infusion, or minimise by pre-treatment with an antihistamine or corticosteroid—consult product literature.

● PREGNANCY Use with caution.
● BREAST FEEDING Use with caution—no information available.
● DIRECTIONS FOR ADMINISTRATION Administration for *intravenous infusion*, give intermittently *in* sodium chloride 0.9%; dilute requisite dose with 100 mL infusion fluid and give over 40 minutes using an in-line filter; use within 3 hours of dilution.

● MEDICINAL FORMS
There can be variation in the licensing of different medicines containing the same drug.
Solution for infusion
‣ Replagal (Shire Pharmaceuticals Ltd)
Agalsidase alfa 1 mg per 1 ml Replagal 3.5mg/3.5ml solution for infusion vials | 1 vial [PoM] £1,049.94

Agalsidase beta

- **DRUG ACTION** Agalsidase beta, an enzyme produced by recombinant DNA technology are licensed for long-term enzyme replacement therapy in Fabry's disease (a lysosomal storage disorder caused by deficiency of alpha-galactosidase A).

● **INDICATIONS AND DOSE**

Fabry's disease (specialist use only)
▶ BY INTRAVENOUS INFUSION
▶ Adult: 1 mg/kg every 2 weeks

● **INTERACTIONS** → Appendix 1: agalsidase

● **SIDE-EFFECTS**
▶ **Common or very common** Angioedema · arrhythmias · arthralgia · asthenia · chest discomfort · chills · cough · diarrhoea · dizziness · drowsiness · dyspnoea · eye disorders · fever · gastrointestinal discomfort · headache · hypertension · hyperthermia · hypotension · increased risk of infection · muscle complaints · musculoskeletal stiffness · nasal complaints · nausea · oedema · oral hypoaesthesia · pain · pallor · palpitations · respiratory disorders · sensation abnormal · skin reactions · syncope · temperature sensation altered · throat complaints · tinnitus · vasodilation · vertigo · vomiting
▶ **Uncommon** Dysphagia · ear discomfort · eye pruritus · influenza like illness · malaise · peripheral coldness · tremor
▶ **Frequency not known** Anaphylactoid reaction · hypersensitivity vasculitis · hypoxia
  SIDE-EFFECTS, FURTHER INFORMATION Infusion-related reactions; manage by slowing the infusion rate, or minimise by pre-treatment with an antihistamine, antipyretic, or corticosteroid—consult product literature.

● **PREGNANCY** Use with caution.

● **BREAST FEEDING** Use with caution—no information available.

● **DIRECTIONS FOR ADMINISTRATION** For *intravenous infusion*, given intermittently *in* Sodium chloride 0.9%, reconstitute initially with Water for Injections (5 mg in 1.1 mL, 35 mg in 7.2 mL) to produce a solution containing 5 mg/mL. Dilute with Sodium Chloride 0.9% (for doses less than 35 mg dilute with at least 50 mL; doses 35–70 mg dilute with at least 100 mL; doses 70–100 mg dilute with at least 250 mL; doses greater than 100 mg dilute with 500 mL) and give through an in-line low protein-binding 0.2 micron filter at an initial rate of no more than 15 mg/hour; for subsequent infusions, infusion rate may be increased gradually once tolerance has been established.

● **MEDICINAL FORMS**
There can be variation in the licensing of different medicines containing the same drug.

Powder for solution for infusion
▶ Fabrazyme (Genzyme Therapeutics Ltd)
  Agalsidase beta 5 mg Fabrazyme 5mg powder for solution for infusion vials | 1 vial PoM £315.08
  Agalsidase beta 35 mg Fabrazyme 35mg powder for solution for infusion vials | 1 vial PoM £2,196.59

ENZYME STABILISERS

Migalastat

24-Nov-2017

- **DRUG ACTION** Migalastat is a pharmacological chaperone that binds to the active sites of certain mutant forms of alpha-galactosidase A, thereby stabilising these mutant forms in the endoplasmic reticulum, and facilitating normal trafficking to lysosomes.

● **INDICATIONS AND DOSE**

Fabry's disease (specialist use only)
▶ BY MOUTH
▶ Adult: 123 mg once daily on alternate days, take at the same time of day, at least 2 hours before or after food

● **SIDE-EFFECTS**
▶ **Common or very common** Constipation · defaecation urgency · depression · diarrhoea · dizziness · dry mouth · dyspnoea · epistaxis · fatigue · gastrointestinal discomfort · headache · muscle complaints · nausea · pain in extremity · palpitations · proteinuria · sensation abnormal · skin reactions · torticollis · vertigo

● **PREGNANCY** Manufacturer advises avoid—toxicity in *animal* studies.

● **BREAST FEEDING** Manufacturer advises avoid—present in milk in *animal* studies.

● **RENAL IMPAIRMENT** Manufacturer advises avoid if eGFR less than 30 mL/minute/1.73 m^2.

● **MONITORING REQUIREMENTS** Manufacturer advises monitor renal function, echocardiographic parameters and biochemical markers every 6 months.

● **PATIENT AND CARER ADVICE**
Missed doses Manufacturer advises if a dose is missed entirely for the day, the missed dose should not be taken and the next dose should be taken on the normal day and at the normal time (not to be taken on 2 consecutive days).

● **NATIONAL FUNDING/ACCESS DECISIONS**
NICE decisions
▶ **Migalastat for treating Fabry disease (February 2017)**
NICE HST4
Migalastat is recommended, within its marketing authorisation, as an option for treating Fabry disease in people over 16 years of age with an amenable mutation, only if migalastat is provided with the discount agreed in the patient access scheme, and only if enzyme replacement therapy would otherwise be offered.
www.nice.org.uk/guidance/hst4
Scottish Medicines Consortium (SMC) Decisions
The *Scottish Medicines Consortium* (November 2016) has advised that migalastat (*Galafold®*) is accepted for restricted use within NHS Scotland for long-term treatment of adults and adolescents aged 16 years and older with a confirmed diagnosis of Fabry disease (α-galactosidase A deficiency) and who have an amenable mutation—consult SMC advice for full details of restriction.

● **MEDICINAL FORMS**
There can be variation in the licensing of different medicines containing the same drug.

Capsule
▶ Galafold (Amicus Therapeutics UK Ltd) ▼
  Migalastat (as Migalastat hydrochloride) 123 mg Galafold 123mg capsules | 14 capsule PoM £16,153.85

2.5 Gaucher's disease

Other drugs used for Gaucher's disease Miglustat, p. 1034

ENZYME INHIBITORS > GLUCOSYLCERAMIDE SYNTHASE INHIBITORS

Eliglustat

04-Dec-2017

- **DRUG ACTION** Eliglustat is an inhibitor of glucosylceramide synthase.

● INDICATIONS AND DOSE

Type 1 Gaucher disease (CYP2D6 poor metabolisers) (under expert supervision)
  - ‣ BY MOUTH
  - ‣ Adult: 84 mg once daily

Type 1 Gaucher disease (CYP2D6 intermediate or extensive metabolisers) (under expert supervision)
  - ‣ BY MOUTH
  - ‣ Adult: 84 mg twice daily

- **CONTRA-INDICATIONS** Cardiac disease (no information available) · concurrent use of Class IA and Class III antiarrhythmics · long QT syndrome (no information available)
- **INTERACTIONS** → Appendix 1: eliglustat
- **SIDE-EFFECTS**
  - ‣ **Common or very common** Arthralgia · constipation · dyspepsia · fatigue · gastrointestinal disorders · nausea · palpitations
  - ‣ **Frequency not known** Syncope
- **PREGNANCY** Manufacturer advises avoid—limited information available.
- **BREAST FEEDING** Manufacturer advises avoid—present in milk in *animal* studies.
- **PRE-TREATMENT SCREENING** Manufacturer advises CYP2D6 metaboliser status should be determined before initiation of treatment.
- **MONITORING REQUIREMENTS**
  - ‣ For treatment-naive patients showing less than 20% spleen volume reduction after 9 months of treatment, manufacturer advises monitor for further improvement or consider an alternative treatment.
  - ‣ For patients with stable disease who have switched from enzyme replacement therapy, manufacturer advises monitor for disease progression—consider reinstitution of enzyme replacement therapy or an alternative treatment if response sub-optimal.
- **PRESCRIBING AND DISPENSING INFORMATION** The manufacturer of *Cerdelga*® has provided a *Prescriber Guide*, which includes a prescriber checklist.
- **PATIENT AND CARER ADVICE** A patient alert card should be provided.
- **NATIONAL FUNDING/ACCESS DECISIONS**

  NICE decisions
  - ‣ **Eliglustat for treating type 1 Gaucher disease (June 2017)** NICE HST5
  Eliglustat is recommended within its marketing authorisation for treating type 1 Gaucher disease, that is, for long-term treatment in adults who are cytochrome P450 2D6 poor, intermediate or extensive metabolisers. Eliglustat is only recommended when the manufacturer provides it with the discount agreed in the patient access scheme.
  www.nice.org.uk/guidance/hst5

Scottish Medicines Consortium (SMC) Decisions
The *Scottish Medicines Consortium* has advised (December 2017) that eliglustat (*Cerdelga*®) is accepted for use within NHS Scotland for the long-term treatment of adult patients with type 1 Gaucher disease who are CYP2D6 poor metabolisers, intermediate metabolisers or extensive metabolisers. This advice is contingent upon the continuing availability of the patient access scheme in NHS Scotland or a list price that is equivalent to or lower.

- **MEDICINAL FORMS** There can be variation in the licensing of different medicines containing the same drug.
  Capsule
  CAUTIONARY AND ADVISORY LABELS 10
  - ‣ Cerdelga (Sanofi) ▼
    Eliglustat (as Eliglustat tartrate) 84.4 mg Cerdelga 84mg capsules | 56 capsule [PoM] £19,164.96

ENZYMES

Imiglucerase

- **DRUG ACTION** Imiglucerase is an enzyme produced by recombinant DNA technology that is administered as enzyme replacement therapy for non-neurological manifestations of type I or type III Gaucher's disease, a familial disorder affecting principally the liver, spleen, bone marrow, and lymph nodes.

● INDICATIONS AND DOSE

Non-neurological manifestations of type I Gaucher's disease (specialist use only) | Non-neurological manifestations of type III Gaucher's disease (specialist use only)
  - ‣ BY INTRAVENOUS INFUSION
  - ‣ Adult: Initially 60 units/kg every 2 weeks; maintenance, adjusted according to response, doses as low as 15 units/kg once every 2 weeks may improve haematological parameters and organomegaly

- **SIDE-EFFECTS**
  - ‣ **Common or very common** Angioedema · cough · dyspnoea · hypersensitivity · skin reactions
  - ‣ **Uncommon** Abdominal cramps · arthralgia · back pain · chest discomfort · chills · cyanosis · diarrhoea · dizziness · fatigue · fever · flushing · headache · hypotension · nausea · paraesthesia · tachycardia · vomiting
- **PREGNANCY** Manufacturer advises use with caution—limited information available.
- **BREAST FEEDING** No information available.
- **MONITORING REQUIREMENTS**
  - ‣ Monitor for immunoglobulin G (IgG) antibodies to imiglucerase.
  - ‣ When stabilised, monitor all parameters and response to treatment at intervals of 6–12 months.
- **DIRECTIONS FOR ADMINISTRATION** For *intravenous infusion* (*Cerezyme*®), give intermittently in Sodium chloride 0.9%; initially reconstitute with water for injections (200 units in 5.1 mL, 400 units in 10.2 mL) to give 40 units/mL solution; dilute requisite dose with infusion fluid to a final volume of 100–200 mL and give initial dose at a rate not exceeding 0.5 units/kg/minute, subsequent doses to be given at a rate not exceeding 1 unit/kg/minute; administer within 3 hours after reconstitution.

- **MEDICINAL FORMS** There can be variation in the licensing of different medicines containing the same drug.
  Powder for solution for infusion
  ELECTROLYTES: May contain Sodium
  - ‣ Cerezyme (Genzyme Therapeutics Ltd)
    Imiglucerase 400 unit Cerezyme 400unit powder for solution for infusion vials | 1 vial [PoM] £1,071.29

Velaglucerase alfa

- **DRUG ACTION** Velaglucerase alfa is an enzyme produced by recombinant DNA technology that is administered as enzyme replacement therapy for the treatment of type I Gaucher's disease.

- **INDICATIONS AND DOSE**

Type I Gaucher's disease (specialist use only)
▸ BY INTRAVENOUS INFUSION
▸ Adult: Initially 60 units/kg every 2 weeks; adjusted according to response to 15–60 units/kg every 2 weeks

- **SIDE-EFFECTS**
▸ **Common or very common** Arthralgia · asthenia · chest discomfort · dizziness · dyspnoea · fever · flushing · gastrointestinal discomfort · headache · hypersensitivity · hypertension · hypotension · infusion related reaction · nausea · pain · skin reactions · tachycardia

SIDE-EFFECTS, FURTHER INFORMATION Infusion-related reactions are very common; manage by slowing the infusion rate, or interrupting the infusion, or minimise by pre-treatment with an antihistamine, antipyretic, or corticosteroid—consult product literature.

- **PREGNANCY** Manufacturer advises use with caution—limited information available.

- **BREAST FEEDING** Manufacturer advises use with caution—no information available.

- **MONITORING REQUIREMENTS** Monitor immunoglobulin G (IgG) antibody concentration in severe infusion-related reactions or if there is a lack or loss of effect with velaglucerase alfa.

- **DIRECTIONS FOR ADMINISTRATION** For *intravenous infusion* (*VPRIV®*), give intermittently *in* Sodium chloride 0.9%; reconstitute each 400-unit vial with 4.3 mL water for injections to produce a 100 units/mL solution; dilute requisite dose in 100 mL infusion fluid; give over 60 minutes through a 0.22 micron filter; start infusion within 24 hours of reconstitution.

- **MEDICINAL FORMS**
There can be variation in the licensing of different medicines containing the same drug.
Powder for solution for infusion
ELECTROLYTES: May contain Sodium
▸ VPRIV (Shire Pharmaceuticals Ltd)
Velaglucerase alfa 400 unit VPRIV 400units powder for solution for infusion vials | 1 vial [PoM] £1,410.20

2.6 Homocystinuria

METHYL DONORS

Betaine

- **INDICATIONS AND DOSE**

Adjunctive treatment of homocystinuria involving deficiencies or defects in cystathionine beta-synthase, 5,10-methylene-tetrahydrofolate reductase, or cobalamin cofactor metabolism (specialist use only)
▸ BY MOUTH
▸ Adult: 3 g twice daily (max. per dose 10 g), adjusted according to response; maximum 20 g per day

- **SIDE-EFFECTS**
▸ **Uncommon** Abdominal discomfort · agitation · alopecia · appetite decreased · brain oedema · diarrhoea · glossitis · irritability · nausea · skin reactions · urinary incontinence · vomiting

- **PREGNANCY** Manufacturer advises avoid unless essential—limited information available.

- **BREAST FEEDING** Manufacturer advises caution—no information available.

- **MONITORING REQUIREMENTS** Monitor plasma-methionine concentration before and during treatment—interrupt treatment if symptoms of cerebral oedema occur.

- **DIRECTIONS FOR ADMINISTRATION** Powder should be mixed with water, juice, milk, formula, or food until completely dissolved and taken immediately; measuring spoons are provided to measure 1 g, 150 mg, and 100 mg of *Cystadane®* powder.

- **PRESCRIBING AND DISPENSING INFORMATION** Betaine should be used in conjunction with dietary restrictions and may be given with supplements of Vitamin B12, pyridoxine, and folate under specialist advice.

- **NATIONAL FUNDING/ACCESS DECISIONS**

Scottish Medicines Consortium (SMC) Decisions
The *Scottish Medicines Consortium* has advised (July 2010) that betaine anhydrous (Cystadane ®) is accepted for restricted use within NHS Scotland for the adjunctive treatment of homocystinuria involving deficiencies or defects in cystathionine beta-synthase, 5,10-methylene-tetrahydrofolate reductase, or cobalamin cofactor metabolism in patients who are not responsive to pyridoxine treatment.

- **MEDICINAL FORMS**
There can be variation in the licensing of different medicines containing the same drug. Forms available from special-order manufacturers include: tablet, oral solution
Powder
▸ Cystadane (Orphan Europe (UK) Ltd)
Betaine 1 gram per 1 gram Cystadane oral powder | 180 gram [PoM] £347.00

2.7 Hypophosphatasia

ENZYMES

Asfotase alfa

04-Dec-2017

- **DRUG ACTION** Asfotase alfa is a human recombinant tissue-nonspecific alkaline phosphatase that promotes mineralisation of the skeleton.

- **INDICATIONS AND DOSE**

Paediatric-onset hypophosphatasia (initiated by a specialist)
▸ BY SUBCUTANEOUS INJECTION
▸ Adult: 2 mg/kg 3 times a week, alternatively 1 mg/kg 6 times a week, dosing frequency depends on body-weight—consult product literature for further information

- **CAUTIONS** Hypersensitivity reactions

CAUTIONS, FURTHER INFORMATION
▸ Hypersensitivity reactions Reactions, including signs and symptoms consistent with anaphylaxis, have occurred within minutes of administration and can occur in patients on treatment for more than one year; if these reactions occur, manufacturer advises immediate discontinuation of treatment and initiation of appropriate medical treatment. For information on re-administration, consult product literature.

- **SIDE-EFFECTS**
▸ **Common or very common** Bruising tendency · chills · cutis laxa · fever · headache · hypersensitivity · irritability · lipohypertrophy · myalgia · nausea · oral hypoaesthesia · pain · skin reactions · vasodilation

SIDE-EFFECTS, FURTHER INFORMATION Injection-site reactions including hypertrophy, induration, skin discolouration, and cellulitis may occur, particularly in patients receiving treatment 6 times a week. Manufacturer advises rotation of injection sites to manage these reactions; interrupt treatment if severe reactions occur and administer appropriate medical therapy.

- PREGNANCY Manufacturer advises avoid—no information available.
- BREAST FEEDING Manufacturer advises avoid—no information available.
- MONITORING REQUIREMENTS
- ▶ Manufacturer advises monitor serum parathyroid hormone and calcium concentrations—supplements of calcium and oral vitamin D may be required.
- ▶ Manufacturer advises periodic ophthalmological examination and renal ultrasounds.
- DIRECTIONS FOR ADMINISTRATION Manufacturer advises max. 1 mL per injection site; administer multiple injections if more than 1 mL is required—consult product literature.
- HANDLING AND STORAGE Manufacturer advises store in a refrigerator (2–8 °C).
- PATIENT AND CARER ADVICE
Injection guides The manufacturer has produced injection guides for patients and carers to support training given by health care professionals.
- NATIONAL FUNDING/ACCESS DECISIONS
NICE decisions
- ▶ Asfotase alfa for treating paediatric-onset hypophosphatasia (August 2017) NICE HST6
Asfotase alfa is recommended as an option for treating paediatric-onset hypophosphatasia only:
  - for people who meet the criteria for treatment within the managed access arrangement (see section 4.18 of the guidance), **and**
  - for the duration of this arrangement and in line with the other conditions it specifies, **and**
  - when the manufacturer provides asfotase alfa with the confidential commercial terms agreed with NHS England.
  Patients whose treatment was started within the NHS before this guidance was published should have the option to continue treatment, without change to their funding arrangements, until they and their NHS clinician consider it appropriate to stop.
  www.nice.org.uk/guidance/HST6

- MEDICINAL FORMS
There can be variation in the licensing of different medicines containing the same drug.
Solution for injection
- ▶ Strensiq (Alexion Pharma UK Ltd) ▼
Asfotase alfa 40 mg per 1 ml Strensiq 18mg/0.45ml solution for injection vials | 12 vial [PoM] £12,700.80 (Hospital only)
Strensiq 28mg/0.7ml solution for injection vials | 12 vial [PoM] £19,756.80 (Hospital only)
Strensiq 40mg/1ml solution for injection vials | 12 vial [PoM] £28,224.00 (Hospital only)
Asfotase alfa 100 mg per 1 ml Strensiq 80mg/0.8ml solution for injection vials | 12 vial [PoM] £56,448.00 (Hospital only)

2.8 Mucopolysaccharidosis

ENZYMES

Elosulfase alfa

04-Dec-2017

- DRUG ACTION Elosulfase alfa is an enzyme produced by recombinant DNA technology that provides replacement therapy in conditions caused by N-acetylgalactosamine-6-sulfatase (GALNS) deficiency.

- INDICATIONS AND DOSE
Mucopolysaccharidosis IVA (specialist use only)
▶ BY INTRAVENOUS INFUSION
  ▶ Adult: 2 mg/kg once weekly

- CAUTIONS Elderly—no information available · infusion-related reactions
CAUTIONS, FURTHER INFORMATION
▶ Infusion-related reactions Infusion-related reactions can occur; manufacturer advises these may be minimised by pre-treatment with an antihistamine and antipyretic, given 30-60 minutes before treatment. If reaction is severe, stop infusion and start appropriate treatment. Caution and close monitoring is advised during re-administration following a severe reaction.

- SIDE-EFFECTS
▶ **Common or very common** Abdominal pain · chills · diarrhoea · dizziness · dyspnoea · fever · headache · hypersensitivity · infusion related reaction · myalgia · nausea · oropharyngeal pain · vomiting

- PREGNANCY Manufacturer advises avoid unless essential—limited information available.

- BREAST FEEDING Manufacturer advises use only if potential benefit outweighs risk—present in milk in *animal* studies.

- DIRECTIONS FOR ADMINISTRATION For *intravenous infusion* (*Vimizim*®), give intermittently *in* Sodium chloride 0.9%; body-weight under 25 kg, dilute requisite dose to final volume of 100 mL infusion fluid and mix gently, give over 4 hours through in-line filter (0.2 micron) initially at a rate of 3 mL/hour, then increase to a rate of 6 mL/hour after 15 minutes, then increase gradually if tolerated every 15 minutes by 6 mL/hour to max. 36 mL/hour; body-weight 25 kg or over, dilute requisite dose to final volume of 250 mL and mix gently, give over 4 hours through in-line filter (0.2 micron) initially at a rate of 6 mL/hour, then increase to a rate of 12 mL/hour after 15 minutes, then increase gradually if tolerated every 15 minutes by 12 mL/hour to max. 72 mL/hour.

- HANDLING AND STORAGE Manufacturer advises store in a refrigerator at 2–8°C. After dilution use immediately or, if necessary, store at 2-8°C for max. 24 hours, followed by up to 24 hours at 23–27°C.

- PATIENT AND CARER ADVICE
Driving and skilled tasks Manufacturer advises patients and carers should be counselled about the effects on driving and performance of skilled tasks—increased risk of dizziness.

- NATIONAL FUNDING/ACCESS DECISIONS
NICE decisions
▶ Elosulfase alfa for treating mucopolysaccharidosis type IVa (December 2015) NICE HST2
Elosulfase alfa, within its marketing authorisation, is recommended for funding for treating mucopolysaccharidosis type IVa (MPS IVa) according to the conditions in the managed access agreement for elosulfase alfa.
www.nice.org.uk/guidance/HST2

● MEDICINAL FORMS
There can be variation in the licensing of different medicines containing the same drug.

Solution for infusion
EXCIPIENTS: May contain Polysorbates, sorbitol
ELECTROLYTES: May contain Sodium
▸ Vimizim (BioMarin Europe Ltd) ▼
  Elosulfase alfa 1 mg per 1 ml Vimizim 5mg/5ml concentrate for solution for infusion vials | 1 vial PoM £750.00

Galsulfase

● DRUG ACTION Galsulfase is a recombinant form of human N-acetylgalactosamine-4-sulfatase.

● INDICATIONS AND DOSE

Mucopolysaccharidosis VI (specialist use only)
▸ BY INTRAVENOUS INFUSION
▸ Adult: 1 mg/kg once weekly

● CAUTIONS Acute febrile illness (consider delaying treatment) · acute respiratory illness (consider delaying treatment) · infusion-related reactions can occur · respiratory disease

● SIDE-EFFECTS Abdominal pain · apnoea · chest pain · chills · conjunctivitis · corneal opacity · dyspnoea · ear pain · face oedema · hypertension · increased risk of infection · malaise · nasal congestion · reflexes absent · umbilical hernia

SIDE-EFFECTS, FURTHER INFORMATION Infusion-related reactions often occur, they can be managed by slowing the infusion rate or interrupting the infusion, and can be minimised by pre-treatment with an antihistamine and an antipyretic. Recurrent infusion-related reactions may require pre-treatment with a corticosteroid—consult product literature for details.

● PREGNANCY Manufacturer advises avoid unless essential.

● BREAST FEEDING Manufacturer advises avoid—no information available.

● DIRECTIONS FOR ADMINISTRATION For *intravenous infusion* (*Naglazyme*®), give intermittently *in* Sodium chloride 0.9%; dilute requisite dose with infusion fluid to final volume of 250 mL and mix gently; infuse through a 0.2 micron in-line filter; give approx. 2.5% of the total volume over 1 hour, then infuse remaining volume over next 3 hours; if body-weight under 20 kg and at risk of fluid overload, dilute requisite dose in 100 mL infusion fluid and give over at least 4 hours.

● MEDICINAL FORMS
There can be variation in the licensing of different medicines containing the same drug.

Solution for infusion
▸ Naglazyme (BioMarin Europe Ltd) ▼
  Galsulfase 1 mg per 1 ml Naglazyme 5mg/5ml solution for infusion vials | 1 vial PoM £982.00

Idursulfase

● DRUG ACTION Idursulfase is an enzyme produced by recombinant DNA technology licensed for long-term replacement therapy in mucopolysaccharidosis II (Hunter syndrome), a lysosomal storage disorder caused by deficiency of iduronate-2-sulfatase.

● INDICATIONS AND DOSE

Mucopolysaccharidosis II (specialist use only)
▸ BY INTRAVENOUS INFUSION
▸ Adult: 500 micrograms/kg once weekly

● CAUTIONS Acute febrile respiratory illness (consider delaying treatment) · infusion-related reactions can occur · severe respiratory disease

● SIDE-EFFECTS
▸ Common or very common Arrhythmias · arthralgia · chest pain · cough · cyanosis · diarrhoea · dizziness · dyspnoea · fever · flushing · gastrointestinal discomfort · headache · hypertension · hypotension · hypoxia · nausea · oedema · respiratory disorders · skin reactions · tongue swelling · tremor · vomiting
▸ Frequency not known Hypersensitivity

SIDE-EFFECTS, FURTHER INFORMATION Infusion-related reactions often occur, they can be managed by slowing the infusion rate or interrupting the infusion, and can be minimised by pre-treatment with an antihistamine and an antipyretic. Recurrent infusion-related reactions may require pre-treatment with a corticosteroid—consult product literature for details.

● CONCEPTION AND CONTRACEPTION Contra-indicated in women of child-bearing potential.

● PREGNANCY Manufacturer advises avoid.

● BREAST FEEDING Manufacturer advises avoid—present in milk in *animal* studies.

● DIRECTIONS FOR ADMINISTRATION For *intravenous infusion* (*Elaprase*®), give intermittently *in* Sodium chloride 0.9%; dilute requisite dose in 100 mL infusion fluid and mix gently (do not shake); give over 3 hours (gradually reduced to 1 hour if no infusion-related reactions).

● MEDICINAL FORMS
There can be variation in the licensing of different medicines containing the same drug.

Solution for infusion
▸ Elaprase (Shire Pharmaceuticals Ltd) ▼
  Idursulfase 2 mg per 1 ml Elaprase 6mg/3ml concentrate for solution for infusion vials | 1 vial PoM £1,985.00

Laronidase

● DRUG ACTION Laronidase is an enzyme produced by recombinant DNA technology licensed for long-term replacement therapy in the treatment of non-neurological manifestations of mucopolysaccharidosis I, a lysosomal storage disorder caused by deficiency of alpha-L-iduronidase.

● INDICATIONS AND DOSE

Non-neurological manifestations of mucopolysaccharidosis I (specialist use only)
▸ BY INTRAVENOUS INFUSION
▸ Adult: 100 units/kg once weekly

● CAUTIONS Infusion-related reactions can occur

● INTERACTIONS → Appendix 1: laronidase

● SIDE-EFFECTS
▸ Common or very common Abdominal pain · alopecia · anaphylactic reaction · angioedema · chills · cough · diarrhoea · dizziness · dyspnoea · fatigue · fever · flushing · headache · hypotension · influenza like illness · joint disorders · nausea · pain · pallor · paraesthesia · peripheral coldness · respiratory disorders · restlessness · skin reactions · sweat changes · tachycardia · temperature sensation altered · vomiting
▸ Frequency not known Cyanosis · hypoxia · oedema

SIDE-EFFECTS, FURTHER INFORMATION Infusion-related reactions often occur, they can be managed by slowing the infusion rate or interrupting the infusion, and can be minimised by pre-treatment with an antihistamine and an antipyretic. Recurrent infusion-related reactions may require pre-treatment with a corticosteroid—consult product literature for details.

9

Blood and nutrition

- **PREGNANCY** Manufacturer advises avoid unless essential—no information available.
- **BREAST FEEDING** Manufacturer advises avoid—no information available.
- **MONITORING REQUIREMENTS** Monitor immunoglobulin G (IgG) antibody concentration.
- **DIRECTIONS FOR ADMINISTRATION** For *intravenous infusion* (*Aldurazyme®*), give intermittently in Sodium chloride 0.9%; body-weight under 20 kg, use 100 mL infusion fluid; body-weight over 20 kg use 250 mL infusion fluid; withdraw volume of infusion fluid equivalent to volume of laronidase concentrate being added; give through in-line filter (0.22 micron) initially at a rate of 2 units/kg/hour then increase gradually every 15 minutes to max. 43 units/kg/hour.

- **MEDICINAL FORMS**
There can be variation in the licensing of different medicines containing the same drug.
Solution for infusion
ELECTROLYTES: May contain Sodium
▸ Aldurazyme (Genzyme Therapeutics Ltd)
Laronidase 100 unit per 1 ml Aldurazyme 500units/5ml solution for infusion vials | 1 vial PoM £444.70

2.9 Niemann-Pick type C disease

ENZYME INHIBITORS ⟩ GLUCOSYLCERAMIDE SYNTHASE INHIBITORS

Miglustat

- **DRUG ACTION** Miglustat is an inhibitor of glucosylceramide synthase.

- **INDICATIONS AND DOSE**
Mild to moderate type I Gaucher's disease for whom enzyme replacement therapy is unsuitable (under expert supervision)
▸ BY MOUTH
▸ Adult: 100 mg 3 times a day, reduced if not tolerated to 100 mg 1–2 times a day
Treatment of progressive neurological manifestations of Niemann-Pick type C disease (under expert supervision)
▸ BY MOUTH
▸ Adult: 200 mg 3 times a day

- **SIDE-EFFECTS**
▸ **Common or very common** Appetite decreased · asthenia · chills · constipation · depression · diarrhoea · dizziness · flatulence · gastrointestinal discomfort · headache · insomnia · libido decreased · malaise · muscle spasms · muscle weakness · nausea · peripheral neuropathy · sensation abnormal · thrombocytopenia · tremor · vomiting · weight decreased

- **CONCEPTION AND CONTRACEPTION** Effective contraception must be used during treatment. Men should avoid fathering a child during and for 3 months after treatment.
- **PREGNANCY** Manufacturer advises avoid—toxicity in *animal* studies.
- **BREAST FEEDING** Manufacturer advises avoid—no information available.
- **HEPATIC IMPAIRMENT** No information available—manufacturer advises caution.
- **RENAL IMPAIRMENT** Avoid if eGFR less than 30 mL/minute/1.73 m².
Dose adjustments For Gaucher's disease initially 100 mg twice daily if eGFR 50–70 mL/minute/1.73 m². Initially 100 mg once daily if eGFR 30–50 mL/minute/1.73 m².

For Niemann-Pick type C disease, initially 200 mg twice daily if eGFR 50–70 mL/minute/1.73 m². Initially 100 mg twice daily if eGFR 30–50 mL/minute/1.73 m²

- **MONITORING REQUIREMENTS**
▸ Monitor cognitive and neurological function.
▸ Monitor growth and platelet count in Niemann-Pick type C disease.

- **MEDICINAL FORMS**
There can be variation in the licensing of different medicines containing the same drug.
Capsule
▸ Zavesca (Actelion Pharmaceuticals UK Ltd)
Miglustat 100 mg Zavesca 100mg capsules | 84 capsule PoM £3,934.17 (Hospital only)

2.10 Pompe disease

ENZYMES

Alglucosidase alfa

- **DRUG ACTION** Alglucosidase alfa is an enzyme produced by recombinant DNA technology licensed for long-term replacement therapy in Pompe disease, a lysosomal storage disorder caused by deficiency of acid alpha-glucosidase.

- **INDICATIONS AND DOSE**
Pompe disease (specialist use only)
▸ BY INTRAVENOUS INFUSION
▸ Adult: 20 mg/kg every 2 weeks

- **CAUTIONS** Cardiac dysfunction · infusion-related reactions—consult product literature · respiratory dysfunction

- **SIDE-EFFECTS**
▸ **Common or very common** Anxiety · arrhythmias · chest discomfort · chills · cough · cyanosis · diarrhoea · dizziness · fatigue · feeling hot · fever · flushing · hyperhidrosis · hypersensitivity · hypertension · irritability · local swelling · muscle complaints · nausea · oedema · pallor · paraesthesia · respiratory disorders · skin reactions · throat complaints · tremor · vomiting
▸ **Frequency not known** Abdominal pain · angioedema · apnoea · arthralgia · cardiac arrest · dyspnoea · excessive tearing · eye inflammation · headache · hypotension · nephrotic syndrome · peripheral coldness · proteinuria · vasoconstriction
SIDE-EFFECTS, FURTHER INFORMATION Infusion-related reactions are very common, calling for use of antihistamine, antipyretic, or corticosteroid; consult product literature for details.
- **PREGNANCY** Toxicity in *animal* studies, but treatment should not be withheld.
- **BREAST FEEDING** Manufacturer advises avoid—no information available.
- **MONITORING REQUIREMENTS**
▸ Monitor closely if cardiac dysfunction.
▸ Monitor closely if respiratory dysfunction.
▸ Monitor immunoglobulin G (IgG) antibody concentration.
- **DIRECTIONS FOR ADMINISTRATION** For *intravenous infusion* (*Myozyme®*), give intermittently *in* Sodium chloride 0.9%; reconstitute 50 mg with 10.3 mL water for injections to produce 5 mg/mL solution; gently rotate vial without shaking; dilute requisite dose with infusion fluid to give a final concentration of 0.5–4 mg/mL; give through a low protein-binding in-line filter (0.2 micron) at an initial rate of 1 mg/kg/hour increased by 2 mg/kg/hour every 30 minutes to max. 7 mg/kg/hour.

- MEDICINAL FORMS
There can be variation in the licensing of different medicines containing the same drug.
Powder for solution for infusion
▸ Myozyme (Genzyme Therapeutics Ltd)
 Alglucosidase alfa 50 mg Myozyme 50mg powder for concentrate for solution for infusion vials | 1 vial [PoM] £356.06 (Hospital only)

2.11 Tyrosinaemia type I

ENZYME INHIBITORS ›
4-HYDROXYPHENYLPYRUVATE DIOXYGENASE INHIBITORS

Nitisinone

(NTBC)

- INDICATIONS AND DOSE
Hereditary tyrosinaemia type I (in combination with dietary restriction of tyrosine and phenylalanine) (specialist use only)
▸ BY MOUTH
▸ Adult: Initially 500 micrograms/kg twice daily, adjusted according to response; maximum 2 mg/kg per day

- INTERACTIONS → Appendix 1: nitisinone
- SIDE-EFFECTS
▸ **Common or very common** Corneal opacity · eye inflammation · eye pain · granulocytopenia · leucopenia · photophobia · thrombocytopenia
▸ **Uncommon** Leucocytosis · skin reactions
- PREGNANCY Manufacturer advises avoid unless potential benefit outweighs risk—toxicity in *animal* studies.
- BREAST FEEDING Manufacturer advises avoid—adverse effects in *animal* studies.
- PRE-TREATMENT SCREENING Slit-lamp examination of eyes recommended before treatment.
- MONITORING REQUIREMENTS
▸ Monitor liver function regularly.
▸ Monitor platelet and white blood cell count every 6 months.
- DIRECTIONS FOR ADMINISTRATION Capsules can be opened and the contents suspended in a small amount of water or formula diet and taken immediately.

- MEDICINAL FORMS
There can be variation in the licensing of different medicines containing the same drug.
Oral suspension
▸ Orfadin (Swedish Orphan Biovitrum Ltd)
 Nitisinone 4 mg per 1 ml Orfadin 4mg/1ml oral suspension sugar-free | 90 ml [PoM] £1,692.00 DT = £1,692.00
Capsule
▸ Nitisinone (Non-proprietary)
 Nitisinone 2 mg Nitisinone 2mg capsules | 60 capsule [PoM] £423.00
 Nitisinone 5 mg Nitisinone 5mg capsules | 60 capsule [PoM] £845.25
 Nitisinone 10 mg Nitisinone 10mg capsules | 60 capsule [PoM] £1,546.50
▸ Orfadin (Swedish Orphan Biovitrum Ltd)
 Nitisinone 2 mg Orfadin 2mg capsules | 60 capsule [PoM] £564.00
 Nitisinone 5 mg Orfadin 5mg capsules | 60 capsule [PoM] £1,127.00
 Nitisinone 10 mg Orfadin 10mg capsules | 60 capsule [PoM] £2,062.00
 Nitisinone 20 mg Orfadin 20mg capsules | 60 capsule [PoM] £4,512.00

2.12 Urea cycle disorders

AMINO ACIDS AND DERIVATIVES

Carglumic acid

- INDICATIONS AND DOSE
Hyperammonaemia due to N-acetylglutamate synthase deficiency (under expert supervision)
▸ BY MOUTH
▸ Adult: Initially 50–125 mg/kg twice daily, to be taken immediately before food, dose adjusted according to plasma–ammonia concentration; maintenance 5–50 mg/kg twice daily, the total daily dose may alternatively be given in 3–4 divided doses
Hyperammonaemia due to organic acidaemia (under expert supervision)
▸ BY MOUTH
▸ Adult: Initially 50–125 mg/kg twice daily, to be taken immediately before food, dose adjusted according to plasma-ammonia concentration, the total daily dose may alternatively be given in 3–4 divided doses

> **IMPORTANT SAFETY INFORMATION**
> EMERGENCY MANAGEMENT OF UREA CYCLE DISORDERS
> For further information on the emergency management of urea cycle disorders consult the British Inherited Metabolic Disease Group (BIMDG) website at www.bimdg.org.uk.

- SIDE-EFFECTS
▸ **Common or very common** Hyperhidrosis
▸ **Uncommon** Bradycardia · diarrhoea · fever · vomiting
▸ **Frequency not known** Rash
- PREGNANCY Manufacturer advises avoid unless essential—no information available.
- BREAST FEEDING Manufacturer advises avoid—present in milk in *animal* studies.
- DIRECTIONS FOR ADMINISTRATION Dispersible tablets must be dispersed in at least 5–10 mL of water and taken orally immediately, or administered via a nasogastric tube.

- MEDICINAL FORMS
There can be variation in the licensing of different medicines containing the same drug.
Dispersible tablet
CAUTIONARY AND ADVISORY LABELS 13
▸ Carbaglu (Orphan Europe (UK) Ltd)
 Carglumic acid 200 mg Carbaglu 200mg dispersible tablets sugar-free | 5 tablet [PoM] £299.00 sugar-free | 15 tablet [PoM] £897.00 sugar-free | 60 tablet [PoM] £3,499.00
▸ Ucedane (Lucane Pharma Ltd)
 Carglumic acid 200 mg Ucedane 200mg dispersible tablets sugar-free | 60 tablet [PoM] £3,300.00

DRUGS FOR METABOLIC DISORDERS ›
AMMONIA LOWERING DRUGS

Glycerol phenylbutyrate

14-May-2018

- DRUG ACTION Glycerol phenylbutyrate is a nitrogen-binding agent that provides an alternative vehicle for waste nitrogen excretion.
- INDICATIONS AND DOSE
Urea cycle disorders (specialist use only)
▸ BY MOUTH, OR BY GASTROSTOMY TUBE, OR BY NASOGASTRIC TUBE
▸ Adult (body surface area up to 1.3 m²): Initially 9.4 g/m² daily in divided doses, usual maintenance continued →

9

Blood and nutrition

5.3–12.4 g/m^2 daily in divided doses, with meals, each dose should be rounded up to the nearest 0.5 mL. For dose adjustments based on individual requirements—consult product literature
- ▸ Adult (body surface area 1.3 m^2 and above): Initially 8 g/m^2 daily in divided doses, usual maintenance 5.3–12.4 g/m^2 daily in divided doses, with meals, each dose should be rounded up to the nearest 0.5 mL. For dose adjustments based on individual requirements—consult product literature

DOSE EQUIVALENCE AND CONVERSION
- ▸ 1 mL of liquid contains 1.1 g of glycerol phenylbutyrate.
- ▸ For patients switching from sodium phenylbutyrate—consult product literature.

IMPORTANT SAFETY INFORMATION
EMERGENCY MANAGEMENT OF UREA CYCLE DISORDERS
For further information on the emergency management of urea cycle disorders consult the British Inherited Metabolic Disease Group (BIMDG) website at www.bimdg.org.uk.

- CONTRA-INDICATIONS Treatment of acute hyperammonaemia
- CAUTIONS Elderly—limited information available · intestinal malabsorption · pancreatic insufficiency
- INTERACTIONS → Appendix 1: glycerol phenylbutyrate
- SIDE-EFFECTS
- ▸ **Common or very common** Constipation · diarrhoea · dizziness · fatigue · gastrointestinal discomfort · gastrointestinal disorders · headache · menstrual disorder · nausea · oral disorders · peripheral oedema · skin reactions · tremor · vomiting
- ▸ **Uncommon** Akathisia · alopecia · biliary colic · bladder pain · confusion · depressed mood · drowsiness · epistaxis · hot flush · hyperhidrosis · hypoalbuminaemia · hypokalaemia · hypothyroidism · joint swelling · muscle spasms · pain · paraesthesia · plantar fasciitis · speech disorder · taste altered · ventricular arrhythmia · weight change
- PREGNANCY Manufacturer advises avoid unless essential—toxicity in *animal* studies.
- BREAST FEEDING Manufacturer advises avoid—no information available.
- HEPATIC IMPAIRMENT Manufacturer advises use with caution—use lowest possible dose.
- RENAL IMPAIRMENT Manufacturer advises use with caution in severe impairment—no information available.
- DIRECTIONS FOR ADMINISTRATION Manufacturer advises may be added to a small amount of apple sauce, ketchup, or squash and used within 2 hours. For administration advice via nasogastric or gastrostomy tube—consult product literature.
- HANDLING AND STORAGE Manufacturer advises discard contents of bottle 14 days after opening.
- PATIENT AND CARER ADVICE
  Driving and skilled tasks Manufacturer advises patients and carers should be counselled on the effects on driving and performance of skilled tasks—increased risk of dizziness.

- MEDICINAL FORMS
There can be variation in the licensing of different medicines containing the same drug.
Liquid
- ▸ Ravicti (Swedish Orphan Biovitrum Ltd) ▼
  Glycerol phenylbutyrate 1.1 gram per 1 ml Ravicti 1.1g/ml oral liquid | 25 ml [PoM] £161.00

Sodium phenylbutyrate

- INDICATIONS AND DOSE
Long-term treatment of urea cycle disorders (as adjunctive therapy in all patients with neonatal-onset disease and in those with late-onset disease who have a history of hyperammonaemic encephalopathy) (under expert supervision)
- ▸ BY MOUTH
- ▸ Adult: 9.9–13 g/m^2 daily in divided doses, with meals; maximum 20 g per day

IMPORTANT SAFETY INFORMATION
EMERGENCY MANAGEMENT OF UREA CYCLE DISORDERS
For further information on the emergency management of urea cycle disorders consult the British Inherited Metabolic Disease Group (BIMDG) website at www.bimdg.org.uk.

- CAUTIONS Congestive heart failure (preparations contain significant amounts of sodium)
- INTERACTIONS → Appendix 1: sodium phenylbutyrate
- SIDE-EFFECTS
- ▸ **Common or very common** Abdominal pain · anaemia · appetite decreased · constipation · depression · headache · irritability · leucocytosis · leucopenia · menstrual cycle irregularities · metabolic acidosis · metabolic alkalosis · nausea · oedema · renal tubular acidosis · skin reactions · syncope · taste altered · thrombocytopenia · thrombocytosis · vomiting · weight increased
- ▸ **Uncommon** Anorectal haemorrhage · aplastic anaemia · arrhythmia · gastrointestinal disorders · pancreatitis
- CONCEPTION AND CONTRACEPTION Manufacturer advises adequate contraception during administration in women of child-bearing potential.
- PREGNANCY Avoid—toxicity in *animal* studies.
- BREAST FEEDING Manufacturer advises avoid—no information available.
- HEPATIC IMPAIRMENT Manufacturer advises use with caution.
- RENAL IMPAIRMENT Manufacturer advises use with caution (preparations contain significant amounts of sodium).
- DIRECTIONS FOR ADMINISTRATION Granules should be mixed with food before taking. *Pheburane*® granules must not be administered by nasogastric or gastrostromy tubes.

- MEDICINAL FORMS
There can be variation in the licensing of different medicines containing the same drug. Forms available from special-order manufacturers include: capsule, oral suspension, oral solution, solution for infusion
Granules
- ▸ Ammonaps (Swedish Orphan Biovitrum Ltd)
  Sodium phenylbutyrate 940 mg per 1 gram Ammonaps 940mg/g granules sugar-free | 266 gram [PoM] £860.00
- ▸ Pheburane (Lucane Pharma Ltd)
  Sodium phenylbutyrate 483 mg per 1 gram Pheburane 483mg/g granules | 174 gram [PoM] £331.00
Tablet
- ▸ Ammonaps (Swedish Orphan Biovitrum Ltd)
  Sodium phenylbutyrate 500 mg Ammonaps 500mg tablets | 250 tablet [PoM] £493.00

2.13 Wilson's disease

> **Other drugs used for Wilson's disease** Penicillamine, p. 1063

ANTIDOTES AND CHELATORS > COPPER ABSORPTION INHIBITORS

Zinc acetate

- DRUG ACTION Zinc prevents the absorption of copper in Wilson's disease.

- ● INDICATIONS AND DOSE

Wilson's disease (initiated under specialist supervision)
▶ BY MOUTH
▷ Adult: 50 mg 3 times a day (max. per dose 50 mg 5 times a day), adjusted according to response
DOSE EQUIVALENCE AND CONVERSION
▷ Doses expressed as elemental zinc.
PHARMACOKINETICS
▷ Symptomatic Wilson's disease patients should be treated initially with a chelating agent because zinc has a slow onset of action. When transferring from chelating treatment to zinc maintenance therapy, chelating treatment should be co-administered for 2–3 weeks until zinc produces its maximal effect.

- ● CAUTIONS Portal hypertension (risk of hepatic decompensation when switching from chelating agent)
- ● INTERACTIONS → Appendix 1: zinc
- ● SIDE-EFFECTS
▶ **Common or very common** Epigastric discomfort (usually transient)
▶ **Uncommon** Leucopenia · sideroblastic anaemia
  SIDE-EFFECTS, FURTHER INFORMATION Transient gastric irritation may be reduced if first dose is taken mid-morning or with a little protein.
- ● PREGNANCY
Dose adjustments Reduce dose to 25 mg 3 times daily adjusted according to plasma-copper concentration and urinary copper excretion.
- ● BREAST FEEDING Manufacturer advises avoid; present in milk—may cause zinc-induced copper deficiency in infant.
- ● MONITORING REQUIREMENTS Monitor full blood count and serum cholesterol.

- ● MEDICINAL FORMS
There can be variation in the licensing of different medicines containing the same drug.
Capsule
CAUTIONARY AND ADVISORY LABELS 23
▷ Wilzin (Orphan Europe (UK) Ltd)
  Zinc (as Zinc acetate) 25 mg Wilzin 25mg capsules | 250 capsule [PoM] £132.00
  Zinc (as Zinc acetate) 50 mg Wilzin 50mg capsules | 250 capsule [PoM] £242.00

ANTIDOTES AND CHELATORS > COPPER CHELATORS

Trientine dihydrochloride

- ● INDICATIONS AND DOSE
Wilson's disease in patients intolerant of penicillamine
▶ BY MOUTH
▷ Adult: 1.2–2.4 g daily in 2–4 divided doses, adjusted according to response, to be taken before food

- ● INTERACTIONS → Appendix 1: trientine
- ● SIDE-EFFECTS
▶ **Rare or very rare** Anaemia
▶ **Frequency not known** Gastrointestinal disorders · nausea · neurological deterioration in Wilson's Disease · rash
- ● PREGNANCY Teratogenic in *animal* studies—use only if benefit outweighs risk.
Monitoring Monitor maternal and neonatal serum-copper concentrations.
- ● PRESCRIBING AND DISPENSING INFORMATION Trientine is **not** an alternative to penicillamine for rheumatoid arthritis or cystinuria. Penicillamine-induced systemic lupus erythematosus may not resolve on transfer to trientine.

- ● MEDICINAL FORMS
There can be variation in the licensing of different medicines containing the same drug.
Capsule
CAUTIONARY AND ADVISORY LABELS 6, 22
▷ Trientine dihydrochloride (Non-proprietary)
  Trientine dihydrochloride 250 mg Metalite 250mg capsules | 100 capsule [PoM] [X]
  Trientine dihydrochloride 300 mg Trientine dihydrochloride 300mg capsules | 100 capsule [PoM] £3,090.00 DT = £3,090.00

3   Mineral and trace elements deficiencies

3.1 Selenium deficiency

Selenium

Selenium deficiency can occur as a result of inadequate diet or prolonged parenteral nutrition. A selenium supplement should not be given unless there is good evidence of deficiency.

VITAMINS AND TRACE ELEMENTS

Selenium

- ● INDICATIONS AND DOSE
Selenium deficiency
▶ BY MOUTH, OR BY INTRAMUSCULAR INJECTION, OR BY INTRAVENOUS INJECTION
▷ Adult: 100–500 micrograms daily

- ● INTERACTIONS → Appendix 1: selenium

- ● MEDICINAL FORMS
There can be variation in the licensing of different medicines containing the same drug.
Tablet
▷ SelenoPrecise (Pharma Nord (UK) Ltd)
  Selenium (as L-Selenomethionine) 100 microgram SelenoPrecise 100microgram tablets | 60 tablet £4.02
  L-Selenomethionine 200 microgram SelenoPrecise 200microgram tablets | 60 tablet £4.41 | 150 tablet £8.01

9

Blood and nutrition

Solution for injection

▸ Selenase (Baxter Healthcare Ltd)
Selenium (as Sodium selenite) 50 microgram per 1 ml Selenase 100micrograms/2ml solution for injection ampoules | 10 ampoule [PoM] 🅢
Selenase 500micrograms/10ml solution for injection vials | 10 vial [PoM] 🅢

Solution for infusion

▸ Selenium (Non-proprietary)
Selenium (as Sodium selenite) 10 microgram per 1 ml Selenium 100micrograms/10ml solution for infusion vials | 10 vial [PoM] 🅢

Oral solution

▸ Selenase (Baxter Healthcare Ltd)
Selenium (as Sodium selenite) 50 microgram per 1 ml Selenase 100micrograms/2ml oral solution 2ml unit dose ampoules | 20 unit dose [P] 🅢
Selenase 500micrograms/10ml oral solution unit dose vials | 10 unit dose [P] 🅢

Capsule

▸ Selenium (Non-proprietary)
L-Selenomethionine 200 microgram Selenium 200microgram capsules | 30 capsule £3.20 | 60 capsule £5.79

3.2 Zinc deficiency

Zinc

Zinc supplements should not be given unless there is good evidence of deficiency (hypoproteinaemia spuriously lowers plasma-zinc concentration) or in zinc-losing conditions. Zinc deficiency can occur as a result of inadequate diet or malabsorption; excessive loss of zinc can occur in trauma, burns, and protein-losing conditions. A zinc supplement is given until clinical improvement occurs, but it may need to be continued in severe malabsorption, metabolic disorders, or in zinc-losing states.

Zinc is used in the treatment of Wilson's disease and acrodermatitis enteropathica, a rare inherited abnormality of zinc absorption.

Parenteral nutrition regimens usually include trace amounts of zinc. If necessary, further zinc can be added to intravenous feeding regimens.

ELECTROLYTES AND MINERALS ❭ ZINC

Zinc sulfate

● **INDICATIONS AND DOSE**

Zinc deficiency or supplementation in zinc-losing conditions

▸ BY MOUTH USING EFFERVESCENT TABLETS

▸ Child (body-weight up to 10 kg): 22.5 mg daily, dose to be adjusted as necessary, to be dissolved in water and taken after food, dose expressed as elemental zinc

▸ Child (body-weight 10–30 kg): 22.5 mg 1–3 times a day, dose to be adjusted as necessary, to be dissolved in water and taken after food, dose expressed as elemental zinc

▸ Child (body-weight 31 kg and above): 45 mg 1–3 times a day, dose to be adjusted as necessary, to be dissolved in water and taken after food, dose expressed as elemental zinc

▸ Adult (body-weight 31 kg and above): 45 mg 1–3 times a day, dose to be adjusted as necessary, to be dissolved in water and taken after food, dose expressed as elemental zinc

Additional elemental zinc for intravenous nutrition

▸ BY INTRAVENOUS INJECTION

▸ Adult: 6.5 mg daily (Zn^{2+} 100 micromol)

● UNLICENSED USE *Solvazinc*® is not licensed for use in acrodermatitis enteropathica.

● INTERACTIONS → Appendix 1: zinc

● SIDE-EFFECTS Diarrhoea · gastritis · gastrointestinal discomfort · nausea · vomiting

● PREGNANCY Crosses placenta; risk theoretically minimal, but no information available.

● BREAST FEEDING Present in milk; risk theoretically minimal, but no information available.

● RENAL IMPAIRMENT Accumulation may occur in acute renal failure.

● PRESCRIBING AND DISPENSING INFORMATION Each *Solvazinc*® tablet contains zinc sulfate monohydrate 125 mg (45 mg zinc).

● MEDICINAL FORMS
There can be variation in the licensing of different medicines containing the same drug.

Effervescent tablet
CAUTIONARY AND ADVISORY LABELS 13, 21
▸ Solvazinc (Galen Ltd)
Zinc sulfate monohydrate 125 mg Solvazinc 125mg effervescent tablets sugar-free | 90 tablet [P] £17.20 DT = £17.20

4 Nutrition (intravenous)

Intravenous nutrition

Overview

When adequate feeding through the alimentary tract is not possible, nutrients may be given by intravenous infusion. This may be in addition to ordinary oral or tube feeding— **supplemental parenteral nutrition**, or may be the sole source of nutrition— **total parenteral nutrition** (TPN). Indications for this method include preparation of undernourished patients for surgery, chemotherapy, or radiation therapy; severe or prolonged disorders of the gastro-intestinal tract; major surgery, trauma, or burns; prolonged coma or refusal to eat; and some patients with renal or hepatic failure. The composition of proprietary preparations available is given under Proprietary Infusion Fluids for Parenteral Feeding p. 1039.

Parenteral nutrition requires the use of a solution containing amino acids, glucose, fat, electrolytes, trace elements, and vitamins. This is now commonly provided by the pharmacy in the form of a 3-litre bag. A single dose of vitamin B_{12}, as hydroxocobalamin p. 994, is given by intramuscular injection; regular vitamin B_{12} injections are not usually required unless total parenteral nutrition continues for many months. Folic acid p. 993 is given in a dose of 15 mg once or twice each week, usually in the nutrition solution. Other vitamins are usually given daily; they are generally introduced in the parenteral nutrition solution. Alternatively, if the patient is able to take small amounts by mouth, vitamins may be given orally.

The nutrition solution is infused through a central venous catheter inserted under full surgical precautions. Alternatively, infusion through a peripheral vein may be used for supplementary as well as total parenteral nutrition for periods of up to a month, depending on the availability of peripheral veins; factors prolonging cannula life and preventing thrombophlebitis include the use of soft polyurethane paediatric cannulas and use of feeds of low osmolality and neutral pH. Only nutritional fluids should be given by the dedicated intravenous line.

Before starting, the patient should be well oxygenated with a near normal circulating blood volume and attention should be given to renal function and acid-base status. Appropriate biochemical tests should have been carried out beforehand and serious deficits corrected. Nutritional and electrolyte status must be monitored throughout treatment.

Proprietary Infusion Fluids for Parenteral Feeding

Preparation	Nitrogen g/litre	1,2 Energy kJ/litre	Electrolytes mmol/litre					Other components/litre
			K⁺	Mg²⁺	Na⁺	Acet⁻	Cl⁻	

Preparation	Nitrogen g/litre	1,2 Energy kJ/litre	K⁺	Mg²⁺	Na⁺	Acet⁻	Cl⁻	Other components/litre
Aminoven 25 (Fresenius Kabi Ltd) Net price 500 ml = £19.72	25.7	–	–	–	–	–	–	
Clinimix N9G20E (Baxter Healthcare Ltd) Net price (dual compartment bag of amino acids with electrolytes 1000 mL and glucose 20% with calcium 1000 mL) 2 litre: no price available	4.6	1680	30.0	2.5	35.0	50.0	40.0	Ca²⁺ 2.3 mmol, phosphate 15 mmol, anhydrous glucose 100 g
Clinimix N14G30E (Baxter Healthcare Ltd) Net price (dual compartment bag of amino acids with electrolytes 1000 mL and glucose 30% with calcium 1000 mL) 2 litre: no price available	7.0	2520	30.0	2.5	35.0	70.0	40.0	Ca²⁺ 2.3 mmol, phosphate 15 mmol, anhydrous glucose 150 g
ClinOleic 20% (Baxter Healthcare Ltd) Net price 100 ml: no price available; Net price 250 ml: no price available; Net price 500 ml: no price available	–	8360	–	–	–	–	–	purified olive and soya oil 200 g, glycerol 22.5 g, egg phosphatides 12 g
Hyperamine 30 (B.Braun Medical Ltd) Net price 500 ml: no price available	30.0	–	–	–	5.0	–	–	
Intralipid 10% (Fresenius Kabi Ltd) Net price 100 ml = £4.12; Net price 500 ml = £9.01	–	4600	–	–	–	–	–	soya oil 100 g, glycerol 22 g, purified egg phospholipids 12 g, phosphate 15 mmol
Intralipid 20% (Fresenius Kabi Ltd) Net price 100 ml = £6.21; Net price 250 ml = £10.16; Net price 500 ml = £13.52	–	8400	–	–	–	–	–	soya oil 200 g, glycerol 22 g, purified egg phospholipids 12 g, phosphate 15 mmol
Intralipid 30% (Fresenius Kabi Ltd) Net price 333 ml: no price available	–	12600	–	–	–	–	–	soya oil 300 g, glycerol 16.7 g, purified egg phospholipids 12 g, phosphate 15 mmol
Kabiven (Fresenius Kabi Ltd) Net price (triple compartment bag of amino acids and electrolytes 300 mL, 450 mL, 600 mL, or 750 mL; glucose 526 mL, 790 mL, 1053 mL, or 1316 mL; lipid emulsion 200 mL, 300 mL, 400 mL, or 500 mL) 1.026 litre: no price available; Net price 1.54 litre = £44.09; Net price 2.053 litre = £57.42; Net price 2.566 litre = £59.92	5.3	3275	23.0	4.0	31.0	38.0	45.0	Ca²⁺ 2 mmol, phosphate 9.7 mmol, anhydrous glucose 97 g, soya oil 39 g
Kabiven peripheral (Fresenius Kabi Ltd) Net price (triple compartment bag of amino acids and electrolytes 300 mL, 400 mL, or 500 mL; glucose 885 mL, 1180 mL, or 1475 mL; lipid emulsion 255 mL, 340 mL, or 425 mL) 1.44 litre = £30.77; Net price 1.92 litre = £44.09; Net price 2.4 litre = £55.72	3.75	2625	17.0	2.8	22.0	27.0	33.0	Ca²⁺ 1.4 mmol, phosphate 7.5 mmol, anhydrous glucose 67.5 g, soya oil 35.4 g
Lipidem (B.Braun Medical Ltd) Net price 100 ml = £19.11; Net price 250 ml = £31.85; Net price 500 ml = £40.34	–	7900	–	–	–	–	–	omega-3-acid triglycerides 20 g, soya oil 80 g, medium chain triglycerides 100 g
Lipofundin MCT/LCT 10% (B.Braun Medical Ltd) Net price 100 ml: no price available; Net price 500 ml = £13.69	–	4430	–	–	–	–	–	soya oil 50 g, medium-chain triglycerides 50 g
Lipofundin MCT/LCT 20% (B.Braun Medical Ltd) Net price 100 ml = £13.28; Net price 250 ml: no price available; Net price 500 ml = £20.36	–	8000	–	–	–	–	–	soya oil 100 g, medium-chain triglycerides 100 g

1 1000 kcal = 4200kJ; 1000 kJ = 238.8 kcal. All entries are Prescription-only medicines.

2 Excludes protein- or amino acid-derived energy

9

Blood and nutrition

Blood and nutrition

9

Preparation	Nitrogen g/litre	[1,2]Energy kJ/litre	Electrolytes mmol/litre					Other components/litre
			K⁺	Mg²⁺	Na⁺	Acet⁻	Cl⁻	
Nutriflex basal (B.Braun Medical Ltd) Net price (dual compartment bag of amino acids 400 mL or 800 mL; glucose 600 mL or 1200 mL) 1 litre: no price available; Net price 2 litre = £29.20	4.6	2095	30.0	5.7	49.9	35.0	50.0	Ca²⁺ 3.6 mmol, acid phosphate 12.8 mmol, anhydrous glucose 125 g
Nutriflex peri (B.Braun Medical Ltd) Net price (dual compartment bag of amino acids 400 mL or 800 mL; glucose 600 mL or 1200 mL) 1 litre: no price available; Net price 2 litre = £30.47	5.7	1340	15.0	4.0	27.0	19.5	31.6	Ca²⁺ 2.5 mmol, acid phosphate 5.7 mmol, anhydrous glucose 80 g
Nutriflex plus (B.Braun Medical Ltd) Net price (dual compartment bag of amino acids 400 mL or 800 mL; glucose 600 mL or 1200 mL) 1 litre: no price available; Net price 2 litre = £33.02	6.8	2510	25.0	5.7	37.2	22.9	35.5	Ca²⁺ 3.6 mmol, acid phosphate 20 mmol, anhydrous glucose 150 g
Nutriflex special (B.Braun Medical Ltd) Net price (dual compartment bag of amino acids 500 mL or 750 mL; glucose 500 mL or 750 mL) 1 litre: no price available; Net price 1.5 litre = £27.60	10.0	4020	25.7	5.0	40.5	22.0	49.5	Ca²⁺ 4.1 mmol, acid phosphate 14.7 mmol, anhydrous glucose 240 g
NuTRIflex Lipid peri (B.Braun Medical Ltd) Net price (triple compartment bag of amino acids 500 mL, 750 mL or 1000 mL; glucose 500 mL, 750 mL or 1000 mL; lipid emulsion 20% 250 mL, 375 mL or 500 mL) 1.25 litre = £42.83; Net price 1.875 litre = £54.37; Net price 2.5 litre = £64.22	4.56	2664	24.0	2.4	40.0	32.0	38.4	Ca²⁺ 2.4 mmol, Zn²⁺ 24 micromol, phosphate 6 mmol, anhydrous glucose 64 g, soya oil 20 g, medium-chain triglycerides 20 g
NuTRIflex Lipid plus (B.Braun Medical Ltd) Net price (triple compartment bag of amino acids 500 mL, 750 mL or 1000 mL; glucose 500 mL, 750 mL or 1000 mL; lipid emulsion 20% 250 mL, 375 mL or 500 mL) 1.25 litre = £46.56; Net price 1.875 litre = £59.46; Net price 2.5 litre = £68.39	5.44	3600	28.0	3.2	40.0	36.0	36.0	Ca²⁺ 3.2 mmol, Zn²⁺ 24 micromol, phosphate 12 mmol, anhydrous glucose 120 g, soya oil 20 g, medium-chain triglycerides 20 g
NuTRIflex Lipid plus without Electrolytes (B.Braun Medical Ltd) Net price (triple compartment bag of amino acids 500 mL, 750 mL or 1000 mL; glucose 500 mL, 750 mL or 1000 mL; lipid emulsion 20% 250 mL, 375 mL or 500 mL) 1.25 litre = £46.56; Net price 1.875 litre = £59.45; Net price 2.5 litre = £84.64	5.44	3600	-	-	-	-	-	anhydrous glucose 120 g, soya oil 20 g, medium-chain triglycerides 20 g
NuTRIflex Lipid special (B.Braun Medical Ltd) Net price (triple compartment bag of amino acids 500 mL, 750 mL or 1000 mL; glucose 500 mL, 750 mL or 1000 mL; lipid emulsion 20% 250 mL, 375 mL or 500 mL) 1.25 litre = £56.95; Net price 1.875 litre = £74.62; Net price 2.5 litre: no price available	8.0	4004	37.6	4.24	53.6	48.0	48.0	Ca²⁺ 4.24 mmol, Zn²⁺ 32 micromol, phosphate 16 mmol, anhydrous glucose 144 g, soya oil 20 g, medium-chain triglycerides 20 g
NuTRIflex Lipid special without Electrolytes (B.Braun Medical Ltd) Net price (triple compartment bag of amino acids 500 mL, 750 mL or 1000 mL; glucose 500 mL, 750 mL or 1000 mL; lipid emulsion 20% 250 mL, 375 mL or 500 mL) 1.25 litre = £56.95; Net price 1.875 litre = £74.62	8.0	4004	-	-	-	-	-	anhydrous glucose 144 g, soya oil 20 g, medium-chain triglycerides 20 g

1 1000 kcal = 4200kJ; 1000 kJ = 238.8 kcal. All entries are Prescription-only medicines.
2 Excludes protein- or amino acid-derived energy

Preparation	Nitrogen g/litre	1,2 Energy kJ/litre	Electrolytes mmol/litre					Other components/litre
			K⁺	Mg²⁺	Na⁺	Acet⁻	Cl⁻	
NuTRIflex Omega plus (B.Braun Medical Ltd) Net price (triple compartment bag of amino acids 500 mL, 750 mL or 1000 mL; glucose 500 mL, 750 mL or 1000 mL; lipid emulsion 250 mL, 375 mL or 500 mL) 1.25 litre = £47.43; Net price 1.875 litre = £60.57; Net price 2.5 litre = £69.66	5.4	3600	28.0	3.2	40.0	36.0	36.0	Ca^{2+} 3.2 mmol, Zn^{2+} 24 micromol, phosphate 12 mmol, anhydrous glucose 120 g, refined soya oil 16 g, medium-chain triglycerides 20 g, omega-3-acid triglycerides 4 g
NuTRIflex Omega special (B.Braun Medical Ltd) Net price (triple compartment bag of amino acids 250 mL, 500 mL, 750 mL or 1000 mL; glucose 250 mL, 500 mL, 750 mL or 1000 mL; lipid emulsion 125 mL, 250 mL, 375 mL or 500 mL) 625 ml = £43.62; Net price 1.25 litre = £58.01; Net price 1.875 litre = £76.01; Net price 2.5 litre = £89.71	8.0	4004	37.6	4.24	53.6	48.0	48.0	Ca^{2+} 4.24 mmol, Zn^{2+} 30 micromol, phosphate 16 mmol, anhydrous glucose 144 g, refined soya oil 16 g, medium-chain triglycerides 20 g, omega-3-acid triglycerides 4 g
OliClinomel N4-550E (Baxter Healthcare Ltd) Net price (triple compartment bag of amino acids with electrolytes 1000 mL; glucose 20% 1000 mL; lipid emulsion 10% 500 mL) 2.5 litre: no price available	3.6	2184	16.0	2.2	21.0	30.0	33.0	Ca^{2+} 2 mmol, phosphate 8.5 mmol, refined olive and soya oil 20 g, anhydrous glucose 80 g
OliClinomel N4-720E (Baxter Healthcare Ltd) Net price (triple compartment bag of amino acids with electrolytes 1000 mL; glucose 20% 1000 mL; lipid emulsion 20% 500 mL) 2.5 litre: no price available	3.64	3024	24.0	2.0	28.0	40.0	40.0	Ca^{2+} 1.8 mmol, phosphate 8 mmol, refined olive and soya oil 40 g, anhydrous glucose 80 g
OliClinomel N5-800E (Baxter Healthcare Ltd) Net price (triple compartment bag of amino acids with electrolytes 800 mL or 1000 mL; glucose 25% 800 mL or 1000 mL; lipid emulsion 20% 400 mL or 500 mL) 2 litre: no price available; Net price 2.5 litre: no price available	4.6	3360	24.0	2.2	32.0	49.0	44.0	Ca^{2+} 2 mmol, phosphate 10 mmol, refined olive and soya oil 40 g, anhydrous glucose 100 g
OliClinomel N6-900E (Baxter Healthcare Ltd) Net price (triple compartment bag of amino acids with electrolytes 800 mL or 1000 mL; glucose 30% 800 mL or 1000 mL; lipid emulsion 20% 400 mL or 500 mL) 2 litre: no price available; Net price 2.5 litre: no price available	5.6	3696	24.0	2.2	32.0	53.0	46.0	Ca^{2+} 2 mmol, phosphate 10 mmol, refined olive and soya oil 40 g, anhydrous glucose 120 g
OliClinomel N7-1000 (Baxter Healthcare Ltd) Net price (triple compartment bag of amino acids 600 mL; glucose 40% 600 mL; lipid emulsion 20% 300 mL) 1.5 litre: no price available	6.6	4368	–	–	–	37.0	16.0	phosphate 3 mmol, refined olive and soya oil 40 g, anhydrous glucose 160 g
OliClinomel N7-1000E (Baxter Healthcare Ltd) Net price (triple compartment bag of amino acids with electrolytes 800 mL; glucose 40% 800 mL; lipid emulsion 20% 400 mL) 2 litre: no price available	6.6	4368	24.0	2.2	32.0	57.0	48.0	Ca^{2+} 2 mmol, phosphate 10 mmol, refined olive and soya oil 40 g, anhydrous glucose 160 g
OliClinomel N8-800 (Baxter Healthcare Ltd) Net price (triple compartment bag of amino acids 800 mL; glucose 31.25% 800 mL; lipid emulsion 15% 400 mL) 2 litre: no price available	8.25	3360	–	–	–	42.5	20.0	phosphate 2.25 mmol, refined olive and soya oil 30 g, anhydrous glucose 125 g

1 1000 kcal = 4200kJ; 1000 kJ = 238.8 kcal. All entries are Prescription-only medicines.

2 Excludes protein- or amino acid-derived energy

9

Blood and nutrition

Preparation	Nitrogen g/litre	[1,2]Energy kJ/litre	Electrolytes mmol/litre						Other components/litre
			K^+	Mg^{2+}	Na^+	$Acet^-$	Cl^-		
Omegaven (Fresenius Kabi Ltd) Net price 100 ml: no price available	–	4700	–	–	–	–	–		highly refined fish oil 100 g, glycerol 25 g, egg phosphatide 12 g
Plasma-Lyte 148 (water) (Baxter Healthcare Ltd) Net price 1 litre: no price available	–	–	5.0	1.5	140.0	27.0	98.0	gluconate 23 mmol
Plasma-Lyte 148 (dextrose 5%) (Baxter Healthcare Ltd) Net price 1 litre: no price available	–	840	5.0	1.5	140.0	27.0	98.0	gluconate 23 mmol, anhydrous glucose 50 g
Plasma-Lyte M (dextrose 5%) (Baxter Healthcare Ltd) Net price 1 litre: no price available	–	840	16.0	1.5	40.0	12.0	40.0	Ca^{2+} 2.5 mmol, lactate 12 mmol, anhydrous glucose 50 g
SMOFlipid (Fresenius Kabi Ltd) Net price 500 ml = £174.30	–	8400	–	–	–	–	–	fish oil 30 g, olive oil 50 g, soya oil 60 g, medium-chain triglycerides 60 g
Synthamin 9 (Baxter Healthcare Ltd) Net price 500 ml: no price available; Net price 1 litre: no price available	9.1	–	60.0	5.0	70.0	100.0	70.0	acid phosphate 30 mmol
Synthamin 9 EF (electrolyte-free) (Baxter Healthcare Ltd) Net price 500 ml: no price available; Net price 1 litre: no price available	9.1	–	–	–	–	44.0	22.0	
Synthamin 14 (Baxter Healthcare Ltd) Net price 500 ml: no price available; Net price 1 litre: no price available; Net price 3 litre: no price available	14.0	–	60.0	5.0	70.0	140.0	70.0	acid phosphate 30 mmol
Synthamin 14 EF (electrolyte-free) (Baxter Healthcare Ltd) Net price 500 ml: no price available; Net price 1 litre: no price available	14.0	–	–	–	–	68.0	34.0	
Synthamin 17 (Baxter Healthcare Ltd) Net price 500 ml: no price available; Net price 1 litre: no price available	16.5	–	60.0	5.0	70.0	150.0	70.0	acid phosphate 30 mmol
Synthamin 17 EF (electrolyte-free) (Baxter Healthcare Ltd) Net price 500 ml: no price available; Net price 3 litre: no price available	16.5	–	–	–	–	82.0	40.0	
Vamin 9 Glucose (Fresenius Kabi Ltd) Net price 100 ml: no price available; Net price 500 ml: no price available; Net price 1 litre: no price available	9.4	1700	20.0	1.5	50.0	–	50.0	Ca^{2+} 2.5 mmol, anhydrous glucose 100 g
Vamin 14 (Fresenius Kabi Ltd) Net price 500 ml: no price available; Net price 1 litre = £16.02	13.5	–	50.0	8.0	100.0	135.0	100.0	Ca^{2+} 5 mmol, SO_4^{2-} 8 mmol
Vamin 14 (electrolyte-free) (Fresenius Kabi Ltd) Net price 500 ml = £9.48; Net price 1 litre = £16.02	13.5	–	–	–	–	90.0	–	
Vamin 18 (electrolyte-free) (Fresenius Kabi Ltd) Net price 500 ml = £11.99; Net price 1 litre = £23.38	18.0	–	–	–	–	110.0	–	

1 1000 kcal = 4200 kJ; 1000 kJ = 238.8 kcal. All entries are Prescription-only medicines.
2 Excludes protein- or amino acid-derived energy

Complications of long-term parenteral nutrition include gall bladder sludging, gall stones, cholestasis and abnormal liver function tests. For details of the prevention and management of parenteral nutrition complications, specialist literature should be consulted.

Protein is given as mixtures of essential and non-essential synthetic L-amino acids. Ideally, all essential amino acids should be included with a wide variety of nonessential ones to provide sufficient nitrogen together with electrolytes. Solutions vary in their composition of amino acids; they often contain an energy source (usually glucose p. 1009) and electrolytes.

Energy is provided in a ratio of 0.6 to 1.1 megajoules (150–250 kcals) per gram of protein nitrogen. Energy requirements must be met if amino acids are to be utilised for tissue maintenance. A mixture of carbohydrate and fat energy sources (usually 30–50% as fat) gives better utilisation of amino acids than glucose alone.

Glucose is the preferred source of carbohydrate, but if more than 180 g is given per day frequent monitoring of blood glucose is required, and insulin may be necessary. Glucose in various strengths from 10 to 50% must be infused through a central venous catheter to avoid thrombosis.

In parenteral nutrition regimens, it is necessary to provide adequate **phosphate** in order to allow phosphorylation of glucose and to prevent hypophosphataemia; between 20 and 30 mmol of phosphate is required daily.

Fructose and sorbitol have been used in an attempt to avoid the problem of hyperosmolar hyperglycaemic non-ketotic acidosis but other metabolic problems may occur, as with xylitol and ethanol which are now rarely used.

Fat emulsions have the advantages of a high energy to fluid volume ratio, neutral pH, and iso-osmolarity with plasma, and provide essential fatty acids. Several days of adaptation may be required to attain maximal utilisation. Reactions include occasional febrile episodes (usually only with 20% emulsions) and rare anaphylactic responses. Interference with biochemical measurements such as those for blood gases and calcium may occur if samples are taken before fat has been cleared. Daily checks are necessary to ensure complete clearance from the plasma in conditions where fat metabolism may be disturbed. **Additives should not be mixed with fat emulsions unless compatibility is known.**

Administration

Because of the complex requirements relating to parenteral nutrition full details relating to administration have been omitted. In all cases *product literature and other specialist literature should be consulted.*

NUTRIENTS > PARENTERAL NUTRITION

Parenteral nutrition supplements

● **INDICATIONS AND DOSE**

Supplement in intravenous nutrition

▶ BY INTRAVENOUS INFUSION, OR BY SLOW INTRAVENOUS INJECTION

▸ Adult: (consult product literature)

DIPEPTIVEN 20G/100ML CONCENTRATE FOR SOLUTION FOR INFUSION BOTTLES

Amino acid supplement for hypercatabolic or hypermetabolic states

▶ BY INTRAVENOUS INFUSION

▸ Adult: 300–400 mg/kg daily, dose not to exceed 20% of total amino acid intake

● DIRECTIONS FOR ADMINISTRATION Because of the complex requirements relating to parenteral nutrition, full details relating to administration have been omitted. In all cases *specialist pharmacy advice, product literature, and other*

specialist literature should be consulted. Compatibility with the infusion solution must be ascertained before adding supplementary preparations. **Additives should not be mixed with fat emulsions unless compatibility is known.**

CERNEVIT SOLUTION FOR INJECTION VIALS AND DILUENT Dissolve in 5 mL water for injections.

ADDITRACE SOLUTION FOR INFUSION 10ML AMPOULES For addition to *Vamin*® solutions and glucose intravenous infusions.

DIPEPTIVEN 20G/100ML CONCENTRATE FOR SOLUTION FOR INFUSION BOTTLES For addition to infusion solutions containing amino acids.

ADDIPHOS® VIALS For addition to *Vamin*® solutions and glucose intravenous infusions.

DECAN CONCENTRATE FOR SOLUTION FOR INFUSION 40ML BOTTLES For addition to infusion solutions.

TRACUTIL® AMPOULES For addition to infusion solutions.

SOLIVITO N POWDER FOR SOLUTION FOR INFUSION VIALS Dissolve in water for injections or glucose intravenous infusion for adding to glucose intravenous infusion or *Intralipid*®; dissolve in *Vitlipid N*® or *Intralipid*® for adding to *Intralipid*® only.

VITLIPID N ADULT EMULSION FOR INJECTION 10ML AMPOULES For addition to *Intralipid*®.

● PRESCRIBING AND DISPENSING INFORMATION

CERNEVIT SOLUTION FOR INJECTION VIALS AND DILUENT *Cernevit*® solution contains *dl*-alpha tocopherol 11.2 units, ascorbic acid 125 mg, biotin 69 micrograms, colecalciferol 220 units, cyanocobalamin 6 micrograms, folic acid 414 micrograms, glycine 250 mg, nicotinamide 46 mg, pantothenic acid (as dexpanthenol) 17.25 mg, pyridoxine hydrochloride 5.5 mg, retinol (as palmitate) 3500 units, riboflavin (as dihydrated sodium phosphate) 4.14 mg, thiamine (as cocarboxylase tetrahydrate) 3.51 mg.

ADDITRACE SOLUTION FOR INFUSION 10ML AMPOULES For patients over 40 kg. *Additrace*® solution contains traces of Fe^{3+}, Zn^{2+}, Mn^{2+}, Cu^{2+}, Cr^{3+}, Se^{4+}, Mo^{6+}, F^-, I^-.

DIPEPTIVEN 20G/100ML CONCENTRATE FOR SOLUTION FOR INFUSION BOTTLES *Dipeptiven*® solution contains N(2)-L-alanyl-L-glutamine 200 mg/mL (providing L-alanine 82 mg, L-glutamine 134.6 mg).

ADDIPHOS® VIALS *Addiphos*® sterile solution contains phosphate 40 mmol, K^+ 30 mmol, Na^+ 30 mmol/20 mL.

DECAN CONCENTRATE FOR SOLUTION FOR INFUSION 40ML BOTTLES For patients over 40 kg. *Decan*® solution contains trace elements Fe^{2+}, Zn^{2+}, Cu^{2+}, Mn^{2+}, F^-, Co^{2+}, I^-, Se^{4+}, Mo^{6+}, Cr^{3+}.

TRACUTIL® AMPOULES *Tracutil*® solution contains trace elements Fe^{2+}, Zn^{2+}, Mn^{2+}, Cu^{2+}, Cr^{3+}, Se^{4+}, Mo^{6+}, I^-, F^-.

SOLIVITO N POWDER FOR SOLUTION FOR INFUSION VIALS *Solivito N*® powder for reconstitution contains biotin 60 micrograms, cyanocobalamin 5 micrograms, folic acid 400 micrograms, glycine 300 mg, nicotinamide 40 mg, pyridoxine hydrochloride 4.9 mg, riboflavin sodium phosphate 4.9 mg, sodium ascorbate 113 mg, sodium pantothenate 16.5 mg, thiamine mononitrate 3.1 mg.

VITLIPID N ADULT EMULSION FOR INJECTION 10ML AMPOULES *Vitlipid N*® adult emulsion contains vitamin A 330 units, ergocalciferol 20 units, *dl*-alpha tocopherol 1 unit, phytomenadione 15 micrograms/mL.

For adults and children over 11 years.

9

Blood and nutrition

● MEDICINAL FORMS
There can be variation in the licensing of different medicines containing the same drug. Forms available from special-order manufacturers include: solution for infusion

Solution for injection

▸ Cernevit (Baxter Healthcare Ltd)
Cyanocobalamin 6 microgram, Biotin 69 microgram, Folic acid 414 microgram, Thiamine 3.51 mg, Riboflavin (as Riboflavin sodium phosphate) 4.14 mg, Pyridoxine (as Pyridoxine hydrochloride) 4.53 mg, Pantothenic acid (as Dexpanthenol) 17.25 mg, Nicotinamide 46 mg, Ascorbic acid 125 mg, Alpha tocopherol 11.2 unit, Colecalciferol 220 unit, Retinol 3500 unit Cernevit solution for injection vials and diluent | 10 vial PoM ⚖

Solution for infusion

▸ Parenteral nutrition supplements (Non-proprietary)
Sodium glycerophosphate 216 mg per 1 ml Sodium glycerophosphate 4.32g/20ml concentrate for solution for infusion vials | 1 vial PoM £5.33

▸ Additrace (Fresenius Kabi Ltd)
Sodium molybdate 4.85 microgram per 1 ml, Chromic chloride 5.33 microgram per 1 ml, Sodium selenite 10.5 microgram per 1 ml, Potassium iodide 16.6 microgram per 1 ml, Manganese chloride 99 microgram per 1 ml, Sodium fluoride 210 microgram per 1 ml, Copper chloride 340 microgram per 1 ml, Ferric chloride 544 microgram per 1 ml, Zinc chloride 1.36 mg per 1 ml Additrace solution for infusion 10ml ampoules | 1 ampoule PoM £1.96

▸ Dipeptiven (Fresenius Kabi Ltd)
N(2)-L-alanyl-L-glutamine 200 mg per 1 ml Dipeptiven 20g/100ml concentrate for solution for infusion bottles | 1 bottle PoM £25.93
Dipeptiven 10g/50ml concentrate for solution for infusion bottles | 1 bottle PoM £13.94

▸ Tracutil (B.Braun Melsungen AG)
Sodium molybdate dihydrate 2.42 microgram per 1 ml, Chromic chloride 5.3 microgram per 1 ml, Sodium selenite pentahydrate 7.89 microgram per 1 ml, Potassium iodide 16.6 microgram per 1 ml, Sodium fluoride 126 microgram per 1 ml, Manganese chloride 197.9 microgram per 1 ml, Copper chloride 204.6 microgram per 1 ml, Zinc chloride 681.5 microgram per 1 ml, Ferrous chloride 695.8 microgram per 1 ml Tracutil concentrate for solution for infusion 10ml ampoules | 5 ampoule PoM £7.96

Powder for solution for infusion

▸ Solivito N (Fresenius Kabi Ltd)
Cyanocobalamin 5 microgram, Biotin 60 microgram, Folic acid 400 microgram, Thiamine nitrate 3.1 mg, Pyridoxine hydrochloride 4.9 mg, Riboflavin sodium phosphate 4.9 mg, Sodium pantothenate 16.5 mg, Nicotinamide 40 mg, Sodium ascorbate 113 mg Solivito N powder for solution for infusion vials | 1 vial PoM £1.97

Emulsion for injection

▸ Vitlipid N Adult (Fresenius Kabi Ltd)
Ergocalciferol 500 nanogram per 1 ml, Phytomenadione 15 microgram per 1 ml, Retinol palmitate 99 microgram per 1 ml, Alpha tocopherol 910 microgram per 1 ml Vitlipid N Adult emulsion for injection 10ml ampoules | 1 ampoule PoM £1.97

5   Nutrition (oral)

Enteral nutrition

Overview

The body's reserves of protein rapidly become exhausted in severely ill patients, especially during chronic illness or in those with severe burns, extensive trauma, pancreatitis, or intestinal fistula. Much can be achieved by frequent meals and by persuading the patient to take supplementary snacks of ordinary food between the meals.

However, extra calories, protein, other nutrients, and vitamins are often best given by supplementing ordinary meals with enteral sip or tube feeds.

When patients cannot feed normally, for example, patients with severe facial injury, oesophageal obstruction, or coma, a

nutritionally complete diet of enteral feeds must be given. The advice of a dietitian should be sought to determine the protein and total energy requirement of the patient and the form and relative contribution of carbohydrate and fat to the energy requirements.

Most enteral feeds contain protein derived from cows' milk or soya. Elemental feeds containing protein hydrolysates or free amino acids can be used for patients who have diminished ability to break down protein, for example in inflammatory bowel disease or pancreatic insufficiency.

Even when nutritionally complete feeds are given, water and electrolyte balance should be monitored. Haematological and biochemical parameters should also be monitored, particularly in clinically unstable patients. Extra minerals (e.g. magnesium and zinc) may be needed in patients where gastro-intestinal secretions are being lost. Additional vitamins may also be needed.

Enteral nutrition in children

Children have special requirements and in most situations liquid feeds prepared for adults are totally unsuitable—the advice of a paediatric dietitian should be sought.

5.1   Special diets

Nutrition in special diets

Overview

These are preparations that have been modified to eliminate a particular constituent from a food or that are nutrient mixtures formulated as food substitutes for patients who either cannot tolerate or cannot metabolise certain common constituents of food. In certain clinical conditions, some food preparations are regarded as drugs and can be prescribed within the NHS if they have been approved by the Advisory Committee on Borderline Substances (ACBS).

Coeliac disease

Coeliac disease is caused by an abnormal immune response to gluten. For management and further information, see Coeliac disease p. 35.

Phenylketonuria

Phenylketonuria (hyperphenylalaninaemia, PKU), which results from the inability to metabolise **phenylalanine**, is managed by restricting dietary intake of **phenylalanine** to a small amount sufficient for tissue building and repair.

Sapropterin dihydrochloride p. 1045, a synthetic form of tetrahydrobiopterin, is licensed as an adjunct to dietary restriction of **phenylalanine** in the management of patients with *phenylketonuria* and *tetrahydrobiopterin deficiency*.

Aspartame (used as a sweetener in some foods and medicines) contributes to the **phenylalanine** intake and may affect control of *phenylketonuria*. Where the presence of **aspartame** is specified in the product literature this is indicated in the BNF against the preparation; the patient should be informed of this.

5.1a Phenylketonuria

DRUGS FOR METABOLIC DISORDERS >
TETRAHYDROBIOPTERIN AND DERIVATIVES

Sapropterin dihydrochloride

- ● **INDICATIONS AND DOSE**

  Phenylketonuria (adjunct to dietary restriction of phenylalanine) (specialist use only)
  - ▸ BY MOUTH
  - ▹ Adult: Initially 10 mg/kg once daily, adjusted according to response; usual dose 5–20 mg/kg once daily, dose to be taken preferably in the morning

  Tetrahydrobiopterin deficiency (adjunct to dietary restriction of phenylalanine) (specialist use only)
  - ▸ BY MOUTH
  - ▹ Adult: Initially 2–5 mg/kg once daily, adjusted according to response, dose to be taken preferably in the morning, the total daily dose may alternatively be given in 2–3 divided doses; maximum 20 mg/kg per day

- ● CAUTIONS History of convulsions
- ● INTERACTIONS → Appendix 1: sapropterin
- ● SIDE-EFFECTS
  - ▸ Common or very common Abdominal pain · cough · diarrhoea · headache · laryngeal pain · nasal congestion · vomiting
  - ▸ Frequency not known Hypersensitivity
- ● PREGNANCY Manufacturer advises caution—consider only if strict dietary management inadequate.
- ● BREAST FEEDING Manufacturer advises avoid—no information available.
- ● HEPATIC IMPAIRMENT Manufacturer advises caution—no information available.
- ● RENAL IMPAIRMENT Manufacturer advises caution—no information available.
- ● MONITORING REQUIREMENTS
  - ▸ Monitor blood-phenylalanine concentration before and after first week of treatment—if unsatisfactory response increase dose at weekly intervals to max. dose and monitor blood-phenylalanine concentration weekly; discontinue treatment if unsatisfactory response after 1 month.
  - ▸ Monitor blood-phenylalanine and tyrosine concentrations 1–2 weeks after dose adjustment and during treatment.
- ● DIRECTIONS FOR ADMINISTRATION Tablets should be dissolved in water and taken within 20 minutes.
- ● PRESCRIBING AND DISPENSING INFORMATION Sapropterin is a synthetic form of tetrahydrobiopterin.
- ● PATIENT AND CARER ADVICE Patient or carers should be given advice on how to administer sapropterin dihydrochloride dispersible tablets.

- ● MEDICINAL FORMS
  There can be variation in the licensing of different medicines containing the same drug.
  Soluble tablet
  CAUTIONARY AND ADVISORY LABELS 13, 21
  - ▸ Kuvan (BioMarin Europe Ltd)
  Sapropterin dihydrochloride 100 mg Kuvan 100mg soluble tablets sugar-free | 30 tablet [PoM] £597.22

6   Vitamin deficiency

Vitamins

Overview

Vitamins are used for the prevention and treatment of specific deficiency states or where the diet is known to be inadequate; they may be prescribed in the NHS to prevent or treat deficiency but not as dietary supplements.

Their use as general 'pick-me-ups' is of unproven value and, in the case of preparations containing vitamin A or D, may actually be harmful if patients take more than the prescribed dose. The 'fad' for mega-vitamin therapy with water-soluble vitamins, such as ascorbic acid p. 1049 and pyridoxine hydrochloride p. 1047, is unscientific and can be harmful.

Dietary reference values for vitamins are available in the Department of Health publication:

Dietary Reference Values for Food Energy and Nutrients for the United Kingdom: Report of the Panel on Dietary Reference Values of the Committee on Medical Aspects of Food Policy. *Report on Health and Social Subjects* 41. London: HMSO, 1991.

Dental patients

It is unjustifiable to treat stomatitis or glossitis with mixtures of vitamin preparations; this delays diagnosis and correct treatment.

Most patients who develop a nutritional deficiency despite an adequate intake of vitamins have malabsorption and if this is suspected the patient should be referred to a medical practitioner.

Vitamin A

Deficiency of vitamin A (retinol) p. 1047 is associated with ocular defects (particularly xerophthalmia) and an increased susceptibility to infections, but deficiency is rare in the UK (even in disorders of fat absorption).

Vitamin B group

Deficiency of the B vitamins, other than vitamin B_{12}, is rare in the UK and is usually treated by preparations containing thiamine (B_1) p. 1048, riboflavin (B_2), and nicotinamide p. 1237, which is used in preference to nicotinic acid p. 199, as it does not cause vasodilatation. Other members (or substances traditionally classified as members) of the vitamin B complex such as aminobenzoic acid, biotin, choline, inositol nicotinate p. 232, and pantothenic acid or panthenol may be included in vitamin B preparations but there is no evidence of their value.

The severe deficiency states Wernicke's encephalopathy and Korsakoff's psychosis, especially as seen in chronic alcoholism, are best treated initially by the parenteral administration of B vitamins (*Pabrinex*®), followed by oral administration of thiamine in the longer term. Anaphylaxis has been reported with parenteral B vitamins.

As with other vitamins of the B group, pyridoxine hydrochloride (B_6) deficiency is rare, but it may occur during isoniazid p. 576 therapy or penicillamine p. 1063 treatment in Wilson's disease and is characterised by peripheral neuritis. High doses of pyridoxine hydrochloride are given in some metabolic disorders, such as hyperoxaluria, and it is also used in sideroblastic anaemia. There is evidence to suggest that pyridoxine hydrochloride may provide some benefit in premenstrual syndrome. It has been tried for a wide variety of other disorders, but there is little sound evidence to support the claims of efficacy.

Nicotinic acid inhibits the synthesis of cholesterol and triglyceride. Folic acid p. 993 and vitamin B_{12} are used in the treatment of megaloblastic anaemia. Folinic acid p. 916

9

Blood and nutrition

(available as calcium folinate) is used in association with cytotoxic therapy.

Vitamin C

Vitamin C (ascorbic acid) therapy is essential in scurvy, but less florid manifestations of vitamin C deficiency are commonly found, especially in the elderly.

Severe scurvy causes gingival swelling and bleeding margins as well as petechiae on the skin. This is, however, exceedingly rare and a patient with these signs is more likely to have leukaemia. Investigation should not be delayed by a trial period of vitamin treatment.

Claims that vitamin C ameliorates colds or promotes wound healing have not been proven.

Vitamin D

The term Vitamin D is used for a range of compounds which possess the property of preventing or curing rickets. They include ergocalciferol (calciferol, vitamin D_2) p. 1054, colecalciferol (vitamin D_3) p. 1051, dihydrotachysterol p. 1054, alfacalcidol (1α-hydroxycholecalciferol) p. 1050, and calcitriol (1,25-dihydroxycholecalciferol) p. 1050.

Simple vitamin D deficiency can be prevented by taking an oral supplement of ergocalciferol (calciferol, vitamin D_2) or colecalciferol (vitamin D_3) daily. Vitamin D deficiency can occur in people whose exposure to sunlight is limited and in those whose diet is deficient in vitamin D. In these individuals, ergocalciferol or colecalciferol daily by mouth may be given to treat vitamin D deficiency; higher doses may be necessary for *severe* deficiency. Patients who do not respond should be referred to a specialist.

Preparations containing colecalciferol with calcium carbonate p. 1053 are available for the management of combined calcium and vitamin D deficiency, or for those at high risk of deficiency.

Vitamin D deficiency caused by *intestinal malabsorption* or *chronic liver disease* usually requires vitamin D in pharmacological doses.

Vitamin D requires hydroxylation by the kidney to its active form, therefore the hydroxylated derivatives alfacalcidol or calcitriol should be prescribed if patients with *severe renal impairment* require vitamin D therapy. Calcitriol is also licensed for the management of postmenopausal osteoporosis.

Paricalcitol p. 1055, a synthetic vitamin D analogue, is licensed for the prevention and treatment of secondary hyperparathyroidism associated with chronic renal failure.

Vitamin E

The daily requirement of vitamin E (tocopherol) has not been well defined but is probably 3 to 15 mg daily. There is little evidence that oral supplements of vitamin E are essential in adults, even where there is fat malabsorption secondary to cholestasis. In young children with congenital cholestasis, abnormally low vitamin E concentrations may be found in association with neuromuscular abnormalities, which usually respond only to the parenteral administration of vitamin E.

Vitamin E has been tried for various other conditions but there is little scientific evidence of its value.

Vitamin K

Vitamin K is necessary for the production of blood clotting factors and proteins necessary for the normal calcification of bone.

Because vitamin K is fat soluble, patients with fat malabsorption, especially in biliary obstruction or hepatic disease, may become deficient. Menadiol sodium phosphate p. 1056 is a water-soluble synthetic vitamin K derivative that can be given orally to prevent vitamin K deficiency in malabsorption syndromes.

Oral coumarin anticoagulants act by interfering with vitamin K metabolism in the hepatic cells and their effects can be antagonised by giving vitamin K.

Other compounds

Potassium aminobenzoate p. 1047 has been used in the treatment of various disorders associated with excessive fibrosis such as scleroderma and Peyronie's disease. In Peyronie's disease there is some evidence to support efficacy in reducing progression when given early in the disease; however, there is no evidence for reversal of the condition. The therapeutic value of potassium aminobenzoate p. 1047 in scleroderma is doubtful.

VITAMINS AND TRACE ELEMENTS ⟩
MULTIVITAMINS

Vitamins A and D

- ● **INDICATIONS AND DOSE**
Prevention of vitamin A and D deficiency
▶ BY MOUTH
▸ Child: 1 capsule daily, 1 capsule contains 4000 units vitamin A and 400 units (10 micrograms) vitamin D
▸ Adult: (consult product literature)

- ● **UNLICENSED USE** Not licensed in children under 6 months of age.

- ● **SIDE-EFFECTS**
Overdose
Excessive ingestion Prolonged excessive ingestion of vitamins A and D can lead to hypervitaminosis.

- ● **PRESCRIBING AND DISPENSING INFORMATION** This drug contains vitamin D; consult individual vitamin D monographs.

- ● **MEDICINAL FORMS**
There can be variation in the licensing of different medicines containing the same drug.
Capsule
▸ Vitamins a and d (Non-proprietary)
Vitamin D 400 unit, Vitamin A 4000 unit Vitamins A and D capsules BPC 1973 | 28 capsule £2.81 | 28 capsule GSL £2.81 | 84 capsule £6.75–£8.42 DT = £8.42

Vitamins A, C and D

The properties listed below are those particular to the combination only. For the properties of the components please consider, vitamin A p. 1047, ascorbic acid p. 1049.

- ● **INDICATIONS AND DOSE**
Prevention of vitamin deficiency
▶ BY MOUTH
▸ Child 1 month–4 years: 5 drops daily, 5 drops contain vitamin A approx. 700 units, vitamin D approx. 300 units (7.5 micrograms), ascorbic acid approx. 20 mg

- ● **INTERACTIONS** → Appendix 1: ascorbic acid · vitamin A

- ● **PRESCRIBING AND DISPENSING INFORMATION** This drug contains vitamin D; consult individual vitamin D monographs.
Available free of charge to children under 4 years in families on the Healthy Start Scheme, or alternatively may be available direct to the public—further information for healthcare professionals can be accessed at www.healthystart.nhs.uk. Beneficiaries can contact their midwife or health visitor for further information on where to obtain supplies.
Healthy Start Vitamins for women (containing ascorbic acid, vitamin D, and folic acid) are also available free of charge to women on the Healthy Start Scheme during

pregnancy and until their baby is one year old, or alternatively may be available direct to the public—further information for healthcare professionals can be accessed at www.healthystart.nhs.uk. Beneficiaries can contact their midwife or health visitor for further information on where to obtain supplies.

- **MEDICINAL FORMS**
There can be variation in the licensing of different medicines containing the same drug.

Oral drops
▸ Healthy Start Children's Vitamin (Secretary of State for Health)
  Vitamin A and D3 concentrate.55 mg per 1 ml, Sodium ascorbate 18.58 mg per 1 ml, Ascorbic acid 150 mg per 1 ml, Vitamin D 2000 iu per 1 ml, Vitamin A 5000 iu per 1 ml Healthy Start Children's Vitamin drops | 10 ml 🅂

VITAMINS AND TRACE ELEMENTS 〉 VITAMIN A

Vitamin A

(Retinol)

- **INDICATIONS AND DOSE**

Vitamin A deficiency
▸ BY MOUTH
  ▸ Child 1–11 months: 5000 units daily, to be taken with or after food, higher doses may be used initially for treatment of severe deficiency
  ▸ Child 1–17 years: 10 000 units daily, to be taken with or after food, higher doses may be used initially for treatment of severe deficiency

- **UNLICENSED USE** Preparations containing only vitamin A are not licensed.

- **INTERACTIONS** → Appendix 1: vitamin A

- **SIDE-EFFECTS**
Overdose Massive overdose can cause rough skin, dry hair, an enlarged liver, and a raised erythrocyte sedimentation rate and raised serum calcium and serum alkaline phosphatase concentrations.

- **PREGNANCY** Excessive doses may be teratogenic. In view of evidence suggesting that high levels of vitamin A may cause birth defects, women who are (or may become) pregnant are advised not to take vitamin A supplements (including tablets and fish liver oil drops), except on the advice of a doctor or an antenatal clinic; nor should they eat liver or products such as liver paté or liver sausage.

- **BREAST FEEDING** Theoretical risk of toxicity in infants of mothers taking large doses.

- **MONITORING REQUIREMENTS** Treatment is sometimes initiated with very high doses of vitamin A and the child should be monitored closely; very high doses are associated with acute toxicity.

- **MEDICINAL FORMS**
There can be variation in the licensing of different medicines containing the same drug. Forms available from special-order manufacturers include: oral drops, solution for injection

Oral drops
▸ Arovit (Imported (Italy))
  Vitamin A 150000 unit per 1 ml Arovit 150,000units/ml drops | 7.5 ml PoM 🅂

Combinations available: *Vitamins A, C and D,* p. 1046

VITAMINS AND TRACE ELEMENTS 〉 VITAMIN B GROUP

Potassium aminobenzoate

- **INDICATIONS AND DOSE**

Peyronie's disease | Scleroderma
▸ BY MOUTH
  ▸ Adult: 12 g daily in divided doses, to be taken after food

- **SIDE-EFFECTS** Hepatitis · hypoglycaemia

- **MEDICINAL FORMS**
There can be variation in the licensing of different medicines containing the same drug.

Powder
CAUTIONARY AND ADVISORY LABELS 13, 21
▸ Potaba (Cheplapharm Arzneimittel GmbH)
  Potassium aminobenzoate 3 gram Potaba 3g sachets | 40 sachet P £34.31

Capsule
CAUTIONARY AND ADVISORY LABELS 21
▸ Potaba (Cheplapharm Arzneimittel GmbH)
  Potassium aminobenzoate 500 mg Potaba 500mg capsules | 240 capsule P £44.75

Pyridoxine hydrochloride

(Vitamin B_6)

- **INDICATIONS AND DOSE**

Deficiency states
▸ BY MOUTH
  ▸ Adult: 20–50 mg 1–3 times a day

Isoniazid-induced neuropathy (prophylaxis)
▸ BY MOUTH
  ▸ Adult: 10–20 mg daily

Isoniazid-induced neuropathy (treatment)
▸ BY MOUTH
  ▸ Adult: 50 mg 3 times a day

Idiopathic sideroblastic anaemia
▸ BY MOUTH
  ▸ Adult: 100–400 mg daily in divided doses

Prevention of penicillamine-induced neuropathy in Wilson's disease
▸ BY MOUTH
  ▸ Adult: 20 mg daily

Premenstrual syndrome
▸ BY MOUTH
  ▸ Adult: 50–100 mg daily

- **UNLICENSED USE** Not licensed for prophylaxis of penicillamine-induced neuropathy in Wilson's disease. Not licensed for treatment of premenstrual syndrome.

┌───┐
IMPORTANT SAFETY INFORMATION
Prolonged use of pyridoxine in a dose of 10 mg daily is considered safe but the long-term use of pyridoxine in a dose of 200 mg or more daily has been associated with neuropathy. The safety of long-term pyridoxine supplementation with doses above 10 mg daily has not been established.
└───┘

- **SIDE-EFFECTS** Peripheral neuritis
Overdose Overdosage induces toxic effects.

9

Blood and nutrition

● MEDICINAL FORMS
There can be variation in the licensing of different medicines containing the same drug. Forms available from special-order manufacturers include: capsule, oral suspension, oral solution

Tablet
▸ Pyridoxine hydrochloride (Non-proprietary)
  Pyridoxine hydrochloride 10 mg Pyridoxine 10mg tablets | 28 tablet PoM £16.95 DT = £12.95
  Pyridoxine hydrochloride 20 mg Pyridoxine 20mg tablets | 500 tablet GSL 🔄
  Pyridoxine hydrochloride 50 mg Pyridoxine 50mg tablets | 28 tablet P 🔄 DT = £12.00

Capsule
▸ Pyridoxine hydrochloride (Non-proprietary)
  Pyridoxine hydrochloride 100 mg G & G Vitamin B6 100mg capsules | 120 capsule £6.00
  Solgar Vitamin B6 100mg capsules | 100 capsule 🔄

Thiamine

(Vitamin B₁)

● INDICATIONS AND DOSE

Mild deficiency
▸ BY MOUTH
▸ Adult: 25–100 mg daily

Severe deficiency
▸ BY MOUTH
▸ Adult: 200–300 mg daily in divided doses

IMPORTANT SAFETY INFORMATION
MHRA/CHM ADVICE (SEPTEMBER 2007)
Although potentially serious allergic adverse reactions may rarely occur during, or shortly after, parenteral administration, the CHM has recommended that:
● This should not preclude the use of parenteral thiamine in patients where this route of administration is required, particularly in patients at risk of Wernicke-Korsakoff syndrome where treatment with thiamine is essential;
● Intravenous administration should be by infusion over 30 minutes;
● Facilities for treating anaphylaxis (including resuscitation facilities) should be available when parenteral thiamine is administered.

● CAUTIONS Anaphylaxis may occasionally follow injection
● BREAST FEEDING Severely thiamine-deficient mothers should avoid breast-feeding as toxic methyl-glyoxal present in milk.

● MEDICINAL FORMS
There can be variation in the licensing of different medicines containing the same drug. Forms available from special-order manufacturers include: oral suspension, oral solution

Modified-release tablet
▸ Thiamine (Non-proprietary)
  Thiamine hydrochloride 100 mg Vitamin B1 100mg modified-release tablets | 90 tablet £4.46

Tablet
▸ Thiamine (Non-proprietary)
  Thiamine hydrochloride 25 mg Vitamin B1 25mg tablets | 100 tablet P 🔄
  Thiamine hydrochloride 50 mg Thiamine 50mg tablets | 28 tablet P £1.32-£1.80 | 100 tablet 🔄 DT = £4.72 | 100 tablet P £6.72 DT = £4.72
  Thiamine hydrochloride 100 mg Thiamine 100mg tablets | 28 tablet P £1.91-£6.72 | 100 tablet P £11.55 DT = £6.83 | 100 tablet 🔄 DT = £6.83
▸ Benerva (Teofarma)
  Thiamine hydrochloride 50 mg Benerva 50mg tablets | 100 tablet P £4.00 DT = £4.72
  Thiamine hydrochloride 100 mg Benerva 100mg tablets | 100 tablet P £6.29 DT = £6.83

▸ Tyvera (Auden McKenzie (Pharma Division) Ltd)
  Thiamine hydrochloride 100 mg Tyvera 100mg tablets | 100 tablet P £6.99 DT = £6.83

Vitamin B complex

20-Jul-2017

● INDICATIONS AND DOSE

Treatment of deficiency
▸ BY MOUTH USING TABLETS
▸ Adult: 1–2 tablets 3 times a day, this dose is for vitamin B compound **strong** tablets

Prophylaxis of deficiency
▸ BY MOUTH USING TABLETS
▸ Adult: 1–2 tablets daily, this dose is for vitamin B compound tablets

● LESS SUITABLE FOR PRESCRIBING Vitamin B compound tablets and vitamin B compound strong tablets are less suitable for prescribing.

● MEDICINAL FORMS
There can be variation in the licensing of different medicines containing the same drug.

Tablet
▸ Vitamin b complex (Non-proprietary)
  Riboflavin 1 mg, Thiamine hydrochloride 1 mg, Nicotinamide 15 mg Vitamin B compound tablets | 28 tablet 🔄 DT = £26.63
  Pyridoxine hydrochloride 2 mg, Riboflavin 2 mg, Thiamine hydrochloride 5 mg, Nicotinamide 20 mg Vitamin B compound strong tablets | 28 tablet P 🔄 DT = £5.64

Vitamin B substances with ascorbic acid

The properties listed below are those particular to the combination only. For the properties of the components please consider, thiamine above, ascorbic acid p. 1049.

● INDICATIONS AND DOSE

Parenteral vitamins B and C for rapid correction of severe depletion or malabsorption (e.g. in alcoholism, after acute infections, postoperatively, or in psychiatric states) | Maintenance of vitamins B and C in chronic intermittent haemodialysis
▸ BY INTRAVENOUS INFUSION
▸ Adult: See MHRA/CHM advice in thiamine above monograph (consult product literature).

Treatment of Wernicke's encephalopathy
▸ INITIALLY BY INTRAVENOUS INFUSION
▸ Adult: 2–3 pairs 3 times a day for 2 days, discontinue if no response, continue treatment if symptoms respond after 2 days; (by intravenous infusion or by deep intramuscular injection) 1 pair once daily for 5 days or for as long as improvement continues, give deep intramuscular injection into the gluteal muscle

Prophylaxis of Wernicke's encephalopathy in alcohol dependence
▸ BY INTRAVENOUS INFUSION, OR BY DEEP INTRAMUSCULAR INJECTION
▸ Adult: 1 pair once daily for at least 3–5 days, give deep intramuscular injection into the gluteal muscle

Psychosis following narcosis or electroconvulsive therapy | Toxicity from acute infections
▸ BY INTRAVENOUS INFUSION, OR BY DEEP INTRAMUSCULAR INJECTION
▸ Adult: 1 pair twice daily for up to 7 days, give deep intramuscular injection into the gluteal muscle

Haemodialysis
▸ BY INTRAVENOUS INFUSION
▸ Adult: 1 pair every 2 weeks

- UNLICENSED USE *Pabrinex*® doses in BNF may differ from those in product literature.
- INTERACTIONS → Appendix 1: ascorbic acid
- DIRECTIONS FOR ADMINISTRATION Give (*Pabrinex*® I/V High Potency) intermittently *or* via drip tubing *in* Glucose 5% *or* Sodium chloride 0.9%. Ampoules contents should be mixed, diluted, and administered without delay; give over 30 minutes.
- PRESCRIBING AND DISPENSING INFORMATION Some formulations of *Pabrinex*® may contain benzyl alcohol (avoid in neonates). *Pabrinex*® I/M High Potency injection is for intramuscular use only. *Pabrinex*® I/V High Potency injection is for intravenous use only.
- MEDICINAL FORMS
  There can be variation in the licensing of different medicines containing the same drug.
  Solution for injection
  EXCIPIENTS: May contain Benzyl alcohol
  ▸ Pabrinex Intramuscular High Potency (Kyowa Kirin Ltd)
  Pabrinex Intramuscular High Potency solution for injection 5ml and 2ml ampoules | 20 ampoule [PoM] £22.53 DT = £22.53
  ▸ Pabrinex Intravenous High Potency (Kyowa Kirin Ltd)
  Pabrinex Intravenous High Potency solution for injection 5ml and 5ml ampoules | 12 ampoule [PoM] £16.23 | 20 ampoule [PoM] £22.53 DT = £22.53

Vitamins with minerals and trace elements

- INDICATIONS AND DOSE
  FORCEVAL® CAPSULES
  Vitamin and mineral deficiency and as adjunct in synthetic diets
  ▸ BY MOUTH
  ▸ Adult: 1 capsule daily, one hour after a meal
  KETOVITE® LIQUID
  Prevention of vitamin deficiency in disorders of carbohydrate or amino-acid metabolism | Adjunct in restricted, specialised, or synthetic diets
  ▸ BY MOUTH
  ▸ Adult: 5 mL daily, use with *Ketovite*® Tablets for complete vitamin supplementation.
  KETOVITE® TABLETS
  Prevention of vitamin deficiency in disorders of carbohydrate or amino-acid metabolism | Adjunct in restricted, specialised, or synthetic diets
  ▸ BY MOUTH
  ▸ Adult: 1 tablet 3 times a day, use with *Ketovite*® Liquid for complete vitamin supplementation.

- PRESCRIBING AND DISPENSING INFORMATION To avoid potential toxicity, the content of all vitamin preparations, particularly vitamin A, should be considered when used together with other supplements.
- PATIENT AND CARER ADVICE
  KETOVITE® LIQUID *Ketovite*® liquid may be mixed with milk, cereal, or fruit juice.
  KETOVITE® TABLETS Tablets may be crushed immediately before use.
- MEDICINAL FORMS
  There can be variation in the licensing of different medicines containing the same drug.
  Oral emulsion
  ▸ Ketovite (Essential Pharmaceuticals Ltd)
  Cyanocobalamin 2.5 microgram per 1 ml, Choline chloride 30 mg per 1 ml, Ergocalciferol 80 unit per 1 ml, Vitamin A 500 unit per 1 ml Ketovite liquid sugar-free | 150 ml [P] £19.10

Tablet
▸ Ketovite (Essential Pharmaceuticals Ltd)
Biotin 170 microgram, Folic acid 250 microgram, Pyridoxine hydrochloride 330 microgram, Acetomenaphthone 500 microgram, Riboflavin 1 mg, Thiamine hydrochloride 1 mg, Calcium pantothenate 1.16 mg, Nicotinamide 3.3 mg, Alpha tocopheryl acetate 5 mg, Ascorbic acid 16.6 mg, Inositol 50 mg Ketovite tablets | 100 tablet [PoM] £9.21
Capsule
▸ Forceval (Alliance Pharmaceuticals Ltd)
Cyanocobalamin 3 microgram, Selenium 50 microgram, Biotin 100 microgram, Iodine 140 microgram, Chromium 200 microgram, Molybdenum 250 microgram, Folic acid 400 microgram, Pyridoxine 2 mg, Manganese 3 mg, Pantothenic acid 4 mg, Potassium 4 mg, Tocopheryl acetate 10 mg, Iron 12 mg, Zinc 15 mg, Nicotinamide 18 mg, Magnesium 30 mg, Ascorbic acid 60 mg, Phosphorus 77 mg, Calcium 100 mg, Ergocalciferol 400 unit, Vitamin A 2500 unit Forceval capsules | 15 capsule [P] £4.86 | 30 capsule [P] £8.48 | 90 capsule [P] £25.44

VITAMINS AND TRACE ELEMENTS > VITAMIN C

Ascorbic acid
(Vitamin C)

- INDICATIONS AND DOSE
  Prevention of scurvy
  ▸ BY MOUTH
  ▸ Adult: 25–75 mg daily
  Treatment of scurvy
  ▸ BY MOUTH
  ▸ Adult: Not less than 250 mg daily in divided doses

- CAUTIONS
  CAUTIONS, FURTHER INFORMATION
  ▸ Iron overload Ascorbic acid should not be given to patients with cardiac dysfunction.
    In patients with normal cardiac function ascorbic acid should be introduced 1 month after starting desferrioxamine.
- INTERACTIONS → Appendix 1: ascorbic acid
- PRESCRIBING AND DISPENSING INFORMATION It is rarely necessary to prescribe more than 100 mg daily except early in the treatment of scurvy.

- MEDICINAL FORMS
  There can be variation in the licensing of different medicines containing the same drug. Forms available from special-order manufacturers include: tablet, oral suspension, oral solution
  Tablet
  EXCIPIENTS: May contain Aspartame
  ▸ Ascorbic acid (Non-proprietary)
  Ascorbic acid 50 mg Ascorbic acid 50mg tablets | 28 tablet [GSL] £15.05 DT = £15.05
  Ascorbic acid 100 mg Ascorbic acid 100mg tablets | 28 tablet [GSL] £14.30 DT = £14.30
  Ascorbic acid 200 mg Ascorbic acid 200mg tablets | 28 tablet [GSL] £19.86 DT = £19.86
  Ascorbic acid 250 mg Ascorbic acid 250mg tablets | 1000 tablet [PoM] [S]
  Ascorbic acid 500 mg Ascorbic acid 500mg tablets | 28 tablet [GSL] £26.87 DT = £26.87
  Chewable tablet
  CAUTIONARY AND ADVISORY LABELS 24
  EXCIPIENTS: May contain Aspartame
  ▸ Ascur (Ennogen Healthcare Ltd)
  Ascorbic acid 100 mg Ascur 100mg chewable tablets | 30 tablet £3.95
  Ascorbic acid (as Sodium ascorbate) 500 mg Ascur 500mg chewable tablets sugar-free | 30 tablet £2.99

Combinations available: *Vitamin B substances with ascorbic acid*, p. 1048 · *Vitamins A, C and D*, p. 1046

9

Blood and nutrition

Blood and nutrition

9

Vitamin D and analogues (systemic)

- CONTRA-INDICATIONS Hypercalcaemia · metastatic calcification
- SIDE-EFFECTS
- ▶ Common or very common Abdominal pain · headache · hypercalcaemia · hypercalciuria · nausea · skin reactions
- ▶ Uncommon Appetite decreased · constipation · thirst · vomiting

SIDE-EFFECTS, FURTHER INFORMATION
Overdose Symptoms of overdosage include anorexia, lassitude, nausea and vomiting, diarrhoea, constipation, weight loss, polyuria, sweating, headache, thirst, vertigo, and raised concentrations of calcium and phosphate in plasma and urine.

- PREGNANCY High doses teratogenic in *animals* but therapeutic doses unlikely to be harmful.
- BREAST FEEDING Caution with high doses; may cause hypercalcaemia in infant—monitor serum-calcium concentration.
- MONITORING REQUIREMENTS **Important**: all patients receiving pharmacological doses of vitamin D should have their plasma-calcium concentration checked at intervals (initially once or twice weekly) and whenever nausea or vomiting occur.

Alfacalcidol

(1α-Hydroxycholecalciferol)

- INDICATIONS AND DOSE
Patients with severe renal impairment requiring vitamin D therapy
- ▶ BY MOUTH, OR BY INTRAVENOUS INJECTION
- ▶ Adult: Initially 1 microgram daily, dose to be adjusted to avoid hypercalcaemia; maintenance 0.25–1 microgram daily
- ▶ Elderly: Initially 500 nanograms daily, dose adjusted to avoid hypercalcaemia; maintenance 0.25–1 microgram daily

Hypophosphataemic rickets | Persistent hypocalcaemia due to hypoparathyroidism or pseudohypoparathyroidism
- ▶ BY MOUTH, OR BY INTRAVENOUS INJECTION
- ▶ Child 1 month–11 years: 25–50 nanograms/kg once daily, dose to be adjusted as necessary; maximum 1 microgram per day
- ▶ Child 12–17 years: 1 microgram once daily, dose to be adjusted as necessary

Prevention of vitamin D deficiency in renal or cholestatic liver disease
- ▶ BY MOUTH, OR BY INTRAVENOUS INJECTION
- ▶ Child 1 month–11 years (body-weight up to 20 kg): 15–30 nanograms/kg once daily (max. per dose 500 nanograms)
- ▶ Child 1 month–11 years (body-weight 20 kg and above): 250–500 nanograms once daily, dose to be adjusted as necessary
- ▶ Child 12–17 years: 250–500 nanograms once daily, dose to be adjusted as necessary

DOSE EQUIVALENCE AND CONVERSION
- ▶ One drop of alfacalcidol 2 microgram/mL oral drops contains approximately 100 nanograms alfacalcidol.

- CAUTIONS Nephrolithiasis · take care to ensure correct dose in infants
- INTERACTIONS → Appendix 1: vitamin D substances
- SIDE-EFFECTS
- ▶ Common or very common Abdominal discomfort · hyperphosphataemia
- ▶ Uncommon Asthenia · diarrhoea · malaise · myalgia · urolithiases
- ▶ Rare or very rare Dizziness
- ▶ Frequency not known Confusion · renal impairment
- RENAL IMPAIRMENT
Monitoring Monitor plasma-calcium concentration in renal impairment.
- MONITORING REQUIREMENTS Monitor plasma-calcium concentration in patients receiving high doses.
- DIRECTIONS FOR ADMINISTRATION
- ▶ With intravenous use For injection, shake ampoule for at least 5 seconds before use, and give over 30 seconds.

- MEDICINAL FORMS
There can be variation in the licensing of different medicines containing the same drug. Forms available from special-order manufacturers include: oral suspension, oral solution
Solution for injection
EXCIPIENTS: May contain Alcohol, propylene glycol
- ▶ One-Alpha (LEO Pharma)
Alfacalcidol 2 microgram per 1 ml One-Alpha 2micrograms/1ml solution for injection ampoules | 10 ampoule [PoM] £41.13
One-Alpha 1micrograms/0.5ml solution for injection ampoules | 10 ampoule [PoM] £21.57
Oral drops
EXCIPIENTS: May contain Alcohol
- ▶ One-Alpha (LEO Pharma)
Alfacalcidol 2 microgram per 1 ml One-Alpha 2micrograms/ml oral drops sugar-free | 10 ml [PoM] £21.30 DT = £21.30
Capsule
EXCIPIENTS: May contain Sesame oil
- ▶ Alfacalcidol (Non-proprietary)
Alfacalcidol 250 nanogram Alfacalcidol 250nanogram capsules | 30 capsule [PoM] £5.00 DT = £4.82
Alfacalcidol 500 nanogram Alfacalcidol 500nanogram capsules | 30 capsule [PoM] £10.00 DT = £9.68
Alfacalcidol 1 microgram Alfacalcidol 1microgram capsules | 30 capsule [PoM] £14.00 DT = £13.49 | 30 capsule [⊠] DT = £13.49
- ▶ One-Alpha (LEO Pharma)
Alfacalcidol 250 nanogram One-Alpha 250nanogram capsules | 30 capsule [PoM] £3.37 DT = £4.82
Alfacalcidol 500 nanogram One-Alpha 0.5microgram capsules | 30 capsule [PoM] £6.27 DT = £9.68
Alfacalcidol 1 microgram One-Alpha 1microgram capsules | 30 capsule [PoM] £8.75 DT = £13.49

Calcitriol

(1,25-Dihydroxycholecalciferol)

- INDICATIONS AND DOSE
Renal osteodystrophy
- ▶ BY MOUTH
- ▶ Adult: Initially 250 nanograms daily, adjusted in steps of 250 nanograms every 2–4 weeks if required; usual dose 0.5–1 microgram daily

Renal osteodystrophy (in patients with normal or only slightly reduced plasma-calcium concentration)
- ▶ BY MOUTH
- ▶ Adult: Initially 250 nanograms once daily on alternate days, adjusted in steps of 250 nanograms every 2–4 weeks if required; usual dose 0.5–1 microgram daily

Established postmenopausal osteoporosis
▸ BY MOUTH
▸ Adult: 250 nanograms twice daily, plasma-calcium concentration and creatinine to be monitored (consult product literature)

● INTERACTIONS → Appendix 1: vitamin D substances
● SIDE-EFFECTS
▸ **Common or very common** Urinary tract infection
▸ **Frequency not known** Abdominal pain upper · apathy · arrhythmia · dehydration · drowsiness · fever · growth retardation · muscle weakness · paralytic ileus · polydipsia · psychiatric disorder · sensory disorder · urinary disorders · weight decreased
● HEPATIC IMPAIRMENT Manufacturer advises avoid—no information available.
● RENAL IMPAIRMENT Manufacturer advises avoid—no information available.
Monitoring Monitor plasma-calcium concentration in renal impairment.
● MONITORING REQUIREMENTS
▸ Monitor plasma calcium, phosphate, and creatinine during dosage titration.
▸ Monitor plasma-calcium concentration in patients receiving high doses.
● DIRECTIONS FOR ADMINISTRATION Contents of capsule may be administered by oral syringe.

● MEDICINAL FORMS
There can be variation in the licensing of different medicines containing the same drug. Forms available from special-order manufacturers include: oral suspension, oral solution
Capsule
▸ Calcitriol (Non-proprietary)
Calcitriol 250 nanogram Calcitriol 250nanogram capsules | 30 capsule PoM £5.41-£18.04 | 100 capsule PoM ⊠ DT = £18.04
Calcitriol 500 nanogram Calcitriol 500nanogram capsules | 30 capsule PoM £9.68-£32.25 | 100 capsule PoM ⊠ DT = £32.25
▸ Rocaltrol (Roche Products Ltd)
Calcitriol 250 nanogram Rocaltrol 250nanogram capsules | 100 capsule PoM £18.04 DT = £18.04
Calcitriol 500 nanogram Rocaltrol 500nanogram capsules | 100 capsule PoM £32.25 DT = £32.25

⚑ 1050

Colecalciferol

(Cholecalciferol; Vitamin D₃)

● INDICATIONS AND DOSE
Prevention of vitamin D deficiency
▸ BY MOUTH
▸ Adult: 400 units daily
Treatment of vitamin D deficiency
▸ BY MOUTH
▸ Adult: 800 units daily, higher doses may be necessary for severe deficiency

● INTERACTIONS → Appendix 1: vitamin D substances
● SIDE-EFFECTS Laryngeal oedema
● RENAL IMPAIRMENT
Monitoring Monitor plasma-calcium concentration in renal impairment.
● MONITORING REQUIREMENTS Monitor plasma-calcium concentration in patients receiving high doses.
● DIRECTIONS FOR ADMINISTRATION
INVITA D3 ® ORAL SOLUTION May be mixed with a small amount of cold or lukewarm food immediately before administration.

● MEDICINAL FORMS
There can be variation in the licensing of different medicines containing the same drug. Forms available from special-order manufacturers include: tablet, capsule, oral suspension, oral solution, oral drops
Tablet
▸ Colecalciferol (Non-proprietary)
Colecalciferol 400 unit Colecalciferol 400unit tablets | 60 tablet £15.50
Colecalciferol 800 unit Colecalciferol 800unit tablets | 30 tablet PoM £3.60 DT = £3.60
Colecalciferol 5000 unit D3 5,000unit tablets | 60 tablet £5.00
Colecalciferol 10000 unit Colecalciferol 10,000unit tablets | 30 tablet £36.00
Colecalciferol 20000 unit Colecalciferol 20,000unit tablets | 20 tablet £36.00
▸ Aciferol D3 (Rhodes Pharma Ltd)
Colecalciferol 400 unit Aciferol D3 400unit tablets | 90 tablet £9.99
Colecalciferol 2200 unit Aciferol D3 2,200unit tablets | 90 tablet £25.99
Colecalciferol 3000 unit Aciferol D3 3,000unit tablets | 60 tablet £14.99
Colecalciferol 5000 unit Aciferol D3 5,000unit tablets | 60 tablet £19.99
Colecalciferol 10000 unit Aciferol D3 10,000unit tablets | 30 tablet £13.99
Colecalciferol 20000 unit Aciferol D3 20,000unit tablets | 30 tablet £18.99
▸ Cubicole D3 (Cubic Pharmaceuticals Ltd)
Colecalciferol 400 unit Cubicole D3 400unit tablets | 30 tablet £5.95
▸ Desunin (Meda Pharmaceuticals Ltd)
Colecalciferol 800 unit Desunin 800unit tablets | 30 tablet PoM £3.60 DT = £3.60 | 90 tablet PoM £10.17
Colecalciferol 4000 unit Desunin 4,000unit tablets | 70 tablet PoM £15.90 DT = £15.90
▸ E-D3 (Ennogen Healthcare Ltd)
Colecalciferol 400 unit E-D3 400unit tablets | 30 tablet £78.50
Colecalciferol 10000 unit E-D3 10,000unit tablets | 30 tablet £95.00
Colecalciferol 20000 unit E-D3 20,000unit tablets | 30 tablet £95.90
▸ Iso D3 (Nutri Advanced Ltd)
Colecalciferol 2000 unit Iso D3 2,000unit tablets | 90 tablet £16.72
▸ Stexerol-D3 (Kyowa Kirin Ltd)
Colecalciferol 1000 unit Stexerol-D3 1,000unit tablets | 28 tablet PoM £2.95 DT = £2.95
Colecalciferol 25000 unit Stexerol-D3 25,000unit tablets | 12 tablet PoM £17.00 DT = £17.00
▸ SunVit D3 (SunVit-D3 Ltd)
Colecalciferol 400 unit SunVit-D3 400unit tablets | 28 tablet £2.55
Colecalciferol 2000 unit SunVit-D3 2,000unit tablets | 28 tablet £3.99
Colecalciferol 3000 unit SunVit-D3 3,000unit tablets | 28 tablet £5.49
Colecalciferol 5000 unit SunVit-D3 5,000unit tablets | 28 tablet £4.99
Colecalciferol 10000 unit SunVit-D3 10,000unit tablets | 28 tablet £6.99
Colecalciferol 20000 unit SunVit-D3 20,000unit tablets | 28 tablet £4.40
Colecalciferol 50000 unit SunVit-D3 50,000unit tablets | 15 tablet £19.99
Oral drops
▸ Colecalciferol (Non-proprietary)
Colecalciferol 1000 unit per 1 ml D3 Drops 1000 oral drops sugar-free | 30 ml £6.12
Colecalciferol 20000 unit per 1 ml Vigantol 20,000units/ml oral drops | 10 ml ⊠
▸ E-D3 (Ennogen Healthcare Ltd)
Colecalciferol 2000 unit per 1 ml E-D3 2,000units/ml oral drops sugar-free | 20 ml ⊠
▸ Fultium-D3 (Internis Pharmaceuticals Ltd)
Colecalciferol 2740 unit per 1 ml Fultium-D3 2,740units/ml oral drops sugar-free | 25 ml PoM £10.70 DT = £10.70
▸ InVita D3 (Consilient Health Ltd)
Colecalciferol 2400 unit per 1 ml InVita D3 2,400units/ml oral drops sugar-free | 10 ml PoM £3.60

9

Blood and nutrition

▸ Pro D3 (Synergy Biologics Ltd)
Colecalciferol 2000 unit per 1 ml Pro D3 2,000units/ml liquid drops sugar-free | 20 ml £9.80

▸ Sapvit-D3 (Stirling Anglian Pharmaceuticals Ltd)
Colecalciferol 14400 unit per 1 ml Sapvit-D3 14,400units/ml oral drops sugar-free | 12.5 ml PoM £8.95

▸ SunVit D3 (SunVit-D3 Ltd)
Colecalciferol 2000 unit per 1 ml SunVit-D3 2,000units/ml oral drops sugar-free | 20 ml £6.20

▸ Thorens (Galen Ltd)
Colecalciferol 10000 unit per 1 ml Thorens 10,000units/ml oral drops sugar-free | 10 ml PoM £5.85 DT = £5.85

Oral solution

CAUTIONARY AND ADVISORY LABELS 21

▸ Colecalciferol (Non-proprietary)
Colecalciferol 3000 unit per 1 ml Colecalciferol 3,000units/ml oral solution | 100 ml £144.00 DT = £144.00
Colecalciferol 10000 unit per 1 ml ZymaD 10,000units/ml oral solution | 10 ml PoM ⓧ

▸ Aciferol D3 (Rhodes Pharma Ltd)
Colecalciferol 2000 unit per 1 ml Aciferol D3 2,000units/ml liquid | 100 ml £18.00

▸ InVita D3 (Consilient Health Ltd)
Colecalciferol 25000 unit per 1 ml InVita D3 25,000units/1ml oral solution sugar-free | 3 ampoule PoM £4.45 DT = £4.45
Colecalciferol 50000 unit per 1 ml InVita D3 50,000units/1ml oral solution sugar-free | 3 ampoule PoM £6.25 DT = £6.25

▸ Pro D3 (Synergy Biologics Ltd)
Colecalciferol 2000 unit per 1 ml Pro D3 2,000units/ml liquid | 50 ml £16.80 | 100 ml £22.50

▸ SunVit D3 (SunVit-D3 Ltd)
Colecalciferol 2000 unit per 1 ml SunVit-D3 10,000units/5ml oral solution sugar-free | 50 ml £8.90
SunVit-D3 2,000units/ml oral solution sugar-free | 50 ml £8.90

▸ Thorens (Galen Ltd)
Colecalciferol 10000 unit per 1 ml Thorens 25,000units/2.5ml oral solution sugar-free | 2.5 ml PoM £1.55 DT = £1.55 sugar-free | 10 ml PoM £5.85 DT = £5.85

Chewable tablet

▸ EveryDay-D (Vega Nutritionals Ltd)
Colecalciferol 400 unit EveryDay-D 400unit chewable tablets | 100 tablet £3.22 | 500 tablet £14.60

▸ Urgent-D (Vega Nutritionals Ltd)
Colecalciferol 2000 unit Urgent-D 2,000unit chewable tablets | 60 tablet £4.31

Capsule

CAUTIONARY AND ADVISORY LABELS 25

▸ Colecalciferol (Non-proprietary)
Colecalciferol 400 unit Colecalciferol 400unit capsules | 30 capsule ⓧ
Colecalciferol 600 unit Colecalciferol 600unit capsules | 30 capsule ⓧ
Colecalciferol 2200 unit Colecalciferol 2,200unit capsules | 30 capsule ⓧ
Colecalciferol 2500 unit FSC High Strength Vitamin D3 2,500unit capsules | 60 capsule £1.95
Colecalciferol 2,500unit capsules | 30 capsule ⓧ
Colecalciferol 3000 unit Colecalciferol 3,000unit capsules | 30 capsule ⓧ
Colecalciferol 5000 unit Colecalciferol 5,000unit capsules | 30 capsule ⓧ
Colecalciferol 10000 unit Colecalciferol 10,000unit capsules | 30 capsule ⓧ
Colecalciferol 20000 unit Colecalciferol 20,000unit capsules | 20 capsule £2.62–£22.72 | 20 capsule PoM £37.99 | 30 capsule £35.99 DT = £29.00 | 30 capsule PoM £29.00 DT = £29.00
Colecalciferol 30000 unit Colecalciferol 30,000unit capsules | 10 capsule
Colecalciferol 50000 unit Colecalciferol 50,000unit capsules | 10 capsule £36.00

▸ Aciferol D3 (Rhodes Pharma Ltd)
Colecalciferol 30000 unit Aciferol D3 30,000unit capsules | 10 capsule £19.99

▸ Aviticol (Colonis Pharma Ltd)
Colecalciferol 1000 unit Aviticol 1,000unit capsules | 30 capsule PoM £3.16 DT = £3.16
Colecalciferol 20000 unit Aviticol 20,000unit capsules | 30 capsule PoM £20.25 DT = £29.00

▸ Bio-Vitamin D3 (Pharma Nord (UK) Ltd)
Colecalciferol 5000 unit Bio-Vitamin D3 5,000unit capsules | 40 capsule £5.51

▸ Cubicole D3 (Cubic Pharmaceuticals Ltd)
Colecalciferol 400 unit Cubicole D3 400unit capsules | 30 capsule £3.95
Colecalciferol 600 unit Cubicole D3 600unit capsules | 30 capsule £6.95
Colecalciferol 2200 unit Cubicole D3 2,200unit capsules | 30 capsule £9.95
Colecalciferol 3000 unit Cubicole D3 3,000unit capsules | 30 capsule £11.95
Colecalciferol 10000 unit Cubicole D3 10,000unit capsules | 30 capsule £12.95

▸ D-Max (Nutraconcepts Ltd)
Colecalciferol 400 unit D-Max 400unit capsules | 30 capsule £3.95
Colecalciferol 5000 unit D-Max 5,000unit capsules | 30 capsule £4.85
Colecalciferol 10000 unit D-Max 10,000unit capsules | 30 capsule £6.89

▸ E-D3 (Ennogen Healthcare Ltd)
Colecalciferol 400 unit E-D3 400unit capsules | 30 capsule £78.50
Colecalciferol 600 unit E-D3 600unit capsules | 30 capsule £82.10
Colecalciferol 2200 unit E-D3 2,200unit capsules | 30 capsule £86.20
Colecalciferol 2500 unit E-D3 2,500unit capsules | 30 capsule £86.20
Colecalciferol 3000 unit E-D3 3,000unit capsules | 30 capsule £88.60
Colecalciferol 5000 unit E-D3 5,000unit capsules | 30 capsule £94.00
Colecalciferol 10000 unit E-D3 10,000unit capsules | 30 capsule £95.00
Colecalciferol 30000 unit E-D3 30,000unit capsules | 10 capsule £94.40

▸ Fultium daily D3 (Internis Pharmaceuticals Ltd)
Colecalciferol 400 unit Fultium daily D3 400unit capsules | 30 capsule £2.58 | 60 capsule £4.84 | 90 capsule £7.09

▸ Fultium-D3 (Internis Pharmaceuticals Ltd)
Colecalciferol 800 unit Fultium-D3 800unit capsules | 30 capsule PoM £3.60 DT = £3.60 | 90 capsule PoM £8.85
Colecalciferol 3200 unit Fultium-D3 3,200unit capsules | 30 capsule PoM £13.32 DT = £13.32 | 90 capsule PoM £39.96
Colecalciferol 20000 unit Fultium-D3 20,000unit capsules | 15 capsule PoM £17.04 DT = £17.04 | 30 capsule PoM £29.00 DT = £29.00

▸ InVita D3 (Consilient Health Ltd)
Colecalciferol 800 unit InVita D3 800unit capsules | 28 capsule PoM £2.50
Colecalciferol 5600 unit InVita D3 5,600unit capsules | 4 capsule PoM £2.50 DT = £2.50
Colecalciferol 25000 unit InVita D3 25,000unit capsules | 3 capsule PoM £3.95 DT = £3.95
Colecalciferol 50000 unit InVita D3 50,000unit capsules | 3 capsule PoM £4.95 DT = £4.95

▸ Plenachol (Auden McKenzie (Pharma Division) Ltd)
Colecalciferol 20000 unit Plenachol 20,000unit capsules | 10 capsule PoM £9.00
Colecalciferol 40000 unit Plenachol 40,000unit capsules | 10 capsule PoM £15.00 DT = £15.00

▸ Pro D3 (Synergy Biologics Ltd)
Colecalciferol 400 unit Pro D3 400unit capsules | 30 capsule £4.99
Colecalciferol 2500 unit Pro D3 2,500unit capsules | 30 capsule £9.99
Colecalciferol 10000 unit Pro D3 10,000unit capsules | 30 capsule £14.99
Colecalciferol 30000 unit Pro D3 30,000unit capsules | 10 capsule £24.99

▸ Strivit-D3 (Strides Arcolab International Ltd)
Colecalciferol 800 unit Strivit-D3 800unit capsules | 30 capsule PoM £2.34 DT = £3.60

▸ SunVit D3 (SunVit-D3 Ltd)
Colecalciferol 400 unit SunVit-D3 400unit capsules | 28 capsule £2.30 DT = £1.85
Colecalciferol 2200 unit SunVit-D3 2,200unit capsules | 28 capsule £4.99
Colecalciferol 2500 unit SunVit-D3 2,500unit capsules | 28 capsule £5.49
Colecalciferol 10000 unit SunVit-D3 10,000unit capsules | 28 capsule £6.99

Orodispersible tablet

▸ Colecalciferol (Non-proprietary)
  Colecalciferol 2000 unit D3 Lemon Melts 2,000unit tablets sugar-free | 120 tablet £4.88

Colecalciferol with calcium carbonate

The properties listed below are those particular to the combination only. For the properties of the components please consider, colecalciferol p. 1051, calcium carbonate p. 1013.

- **INDICATIONS AND DOSE**
  ### Prevention and treatment of vitamin D and calcium deficiency
  ▸ BY MOUTH
  ▸ Adult: Dosed according to the deficit or daily maintenance requirements (consult product literature)

- **INTERACTIONS** → Appendix 1: calcium salts · vitamin D substances

- **PRESCRIBING AND DISPENSING INFORMATION** *Accrete D*3 ® contains calcium carbonate 1.5 g (calcium 600 mg or Ca²⁺ 15 mmol), colecalciferol 10 micrograms (400 units); *Adcal-D3* ® tablets contain calcium carbonate 1.5 g (calcium 600 mg or Ca²⁺ 15 mmol), colecalciferol 10 micrograms (400 units); *Cacit* ® *D3* contains calcium carbonate 1.25 g (calcium 500 mg or Ca²⁺ 12.5 mmol), colecalciferol 11 micrograms (440 units)/sachet; *Calceos* ® contains calcium carbonate 1.25 g (calcium 500 mg or Ca²⁺ 12.5 mmol), colecalciferol 10 micrograms (400 units); *Calcichew-D3* ® tablets contain calcium carbonate 1.25 g (calcium 500 mg or Ca²⁺ 12.5 mmol), colecalciferol 5 micrograms (200 units); *Calcichew-D3* ® *Forte* tablets contain calcium carbonate 1.25 g (calcium 500 mg or Ca²⁺ 12.5 mmol), colecalciferol 10 micrograms (400 units); *Calcichew-D3* ® 500 mg/400 unit caplets contain calcium carbonate (calcium 500 mg or Ca²⁺ 12.5 mmol), colecalciferol 10 micrograms (400 units); *Kalcipos-D* ® contains calcium carbonate (calcium 500 mg or Ca²⁺ 12.5 mmol), colecalciferol 20 micrograms (800 units); *Natecal D3* ® contains calcium carbonate 1.5 g (calcium 600 mg or Ca²⁺ 15 mmol), colecalciferol 10 micrograms (400 units); consult product literature for details of other available products.
  Flavours of chewable and soluble forms may include orange, lemon, aniseed, peppermint, molasses, or tutti-frutti.

- **MEDICINAL FORMS**
  There can be variation in the licensing of different medicines containing the same drug.

Effervescent granules
CAUTIONARY AND ADVISORY LABELS 13
▸ Colecalciferol with calcium carbonate (Non-proprietary)
  Calcium carbonate 2.5 gram, Colecalciferol 880 unit Colecalciferol 880unit / Calcium carbonate 2.5g effervescent granules sachets | 24 sachet PoM ⊠
▸ Cacit D3 (Teva UK Ltd)
  Calcium carbonate 1.25 gram, Colecalciferol 440 unit Cacit D3 effervescent granules sachets | 30 sachet P £4.06 DT = £4.06

Effervescent tablet
CAUTIONARY AND ADVISORY LABELS 13
▸ Adcal-D3 (Kyowa Kirin Ltd)
  Calcium carbonate 1.5 gram, Colecalciferol 400 unit Adcal-D3 Dissolve 1500mg/400unit effervescent tablets | 56 tablet P £5.99 DT = £5.99

Tablet
EXCIPIENTS: May contain Propylene glycol
▸ Accrete D3 (Internis Pharmaceuticals Ltd)
  Calcium carbonate 1.5 gram, Colecalciferol 400 unit Accrete D3 tablets | 60 tablet P £2.95 DT = £2.95

▸ Adcal-D3 (Kyowa Kirin Ltd)
  Calcium carbonate 750 mg, Colecalciferol 200 unit Adcal-D3 750mg/200unit caplets | 112 tablet P £2.95 DT = £2.95
▸ Calcichew D3 (Takeda UK Ltd)
  Calcium carbonate 1.25 gram, Colecalciferol 400 unit Calcichew D3 500mg/400unit caplets | 100 tablet P £7.43 DT = £7.43
▸ Kalcipos-D (Meda Pharmaceuticals Ltd)
  Calcium carbonate 1.25 gram, Colecalciferol 800 unit Kalcipos-D 500mg/800unit tablets | 30 tablet PoM £4.21 DT = £4.21

Chewable tablet
CAUTIONARY AND ADVISORY LABELS 24
EXCIPIENTS: May contain Aspartame
▸ Colecalciferol with calcium carbonate (Non-proprietary)
  Calcium carbonate 1.5 gram, Colecalciferol 400 unit Colecalciferol 400unit / Calcium carbonate 1.5g chewable tablets | 56 tablet P £3.65 DT = £3.65 | 60 tablet P £3.91
▸ Accrete D3 One a Day (Sandoz Ltd)
  Calcium carbonate 2.5 gram, Colecalciferol 880 unit Accrete D3 One a Day 1000mg/880unit chewable tablets | 30 tablet P £2.95 DT = £2.95
▸ Adcal-D3 (Kyowa Kirin Ltd)
  Calcium carbonate 1.5 gram, Colecalciferol 400 unit Adcal-D3 Lemon chewable tablets | 56 tablet P £3.65 DT = £3.65 | 112 tablet P £7.49
  Adcal-D3 chewable tablets tutti frutti | 56 tablet P £3.65 DT = £3.65 | 112 tablet P £7.49
▸ Calceos (Galen Ltd)
  Calcium carbonate 1.25 gram, Colecalciferol 400 unit Calceos 500mg/400unit chewable tablets | 60 tablet P £3.88 DT = £4.24
▸ Calci-D (Consilient Health Ltd)
  Calcium carbonate 2.5 gram, Colecalciferol 1000 iu Calci-D 1000mg/1,000unit chewable tablets | 28 tablet PoM £2.25 DT = £2.25
▸ Calcichew D3 (Takeda UK Ltd)
  Calcium carbonate 2.5 gram, Colecalciferol 800 iu Calcichew D3 1000mg/800unit Once Daily chewable tablets | 30 tablet P £6.75 DT = £6.75
  Calcium carbonate 1.25 gram, Colecalciferol 200 unit Calcichew D3 chewable tablets | 100 tablet P £7.68 DT = £7.68
▸ Calcichew D3 Forte (Takeda UK Ltd)
  Calcium carbonate 1.25 gram, Colecalciferol 400 unit Calcichew D3 Forte chewable tablets | 60 tablet P £4.24 DT = £4.24 | 100 tablet P £7.08
▸ Evacal D3 (Teva UK Ltd)
  Calcium carbonate 1.5 gram, Colecalciferol 400 unit Evacal D3 1500mg/400unit chewable tablets | 56 tablet P £2.75 DT = £3.65 | 112 tablet P £5.50
▸ Kalcipos-D (Meda Pharmaceuticals Ltd)
  Calcium carbonate 1.25 gram, Colecalciferol 800 unit Kalcipos-D 500mg/800unit chewable tablets | 30 tablet PoM £4.21 DT = £4.21
▸ Natecal (Chiesi Ltd)
  Calcium carbonate 1.5 gram, Colecalciferol 400 unit Natecal D3 600mg/400unit chewable tablets | 60 tablet P £3.63
▸ TheiCal-D3 (Stirling Anglian Pharmaceuticals Ltd)
  Calcium carbonate 2.5 gram, Colecalciferol 880 unit TheiCal-D3 1000mg/880unit chewable tablets | 30 tablet P £2.95 DT = £2.95

Colecalciferol with calcium phosphate

The properties listed below are those particular to the combination only. For the properties of the components please consider, colecalciferol p. 1051, calcium phosphate p. 1015.

- **INDICATIONS AND DOSE**
  ### Calcium and vitamin D deficiency
  ▸ BY MOUTH
  ▸ Adult: (consult product literature)

- **INTERACTIONS** → Appendix 1: calcium salts · vitamin D substances

9

Blood and nutrition

● MEDICINAL FORMS
There can be variation in the licensing of different medicines
containing the same drug.
Powder
CAUTIONARY AND ADVISORY LABELS 13, 21
▶ Calfovit D3 (A. Menarini Farmaceutica Internazionale SRL)
  Calcium phosphate 3.1 gram, Colecalciferol 800 unit Calfovit D3
  oral powder sachets | 30 sachet Ⓟ £4.32 DT = £4.32

☛ 1050

Dihydrotachysterol

● INDICATIONS AND DOSE
**Acute, chronic, and latent forms of hypocalcaemic tetany
due to hypoparathyroidism**
▶ BY MOUTH
▶ Adult: (consult product literature)

● INTERACTIONS → Appendix 1: vitamin D substances

● SIDE-EFFECTS Abdominal cramps · apathy · dehydration ·
hypertension · paralysis · renal failure · stupor · urinary
disorders · vertigo

● RENAL IMPAIRMENT
Monitoring Monitor plasma-calcium concentration in
renal impairment.

● MONITORING REQUIREMENTS Monitor plasma-calcium
concentration in patients receiving high doses.

● MEDICINAL FORMS
There can be variation in the licensing of different medicines
containing the same drug.
Oral solution
EXCIPIENTS: May contain Arachis (peanut) oil
▶ AT10 (Intrapharm Laboratories Ltd)
  Dihydrotachysterol 250 microgram per 1 ml AT10
  250micrograms/ml oral solution sugar-free | 15 ml Ⓟ £22.87

☛ 1050

Ergocalciferol

(Calciferol; Vitamin D$_2$)

● INDICATIONS AND DOSE
**Vitamin D deficiency caused by intestinal malabsorption
or chronic liver disease**
▶ BY MOUTH
▶ Adult: Up to 40 000 units daily
**Hypocalcaemia of hypoparathyroidism to achieve
normocalcaemia**
▶ BY MOUTH
▶ Adult: Up to 100 000 units daily
Prevention of vitamin D deficiency
▶ BY MOUTH
▶ Adult: 400 units daily
Treatment of vitamin D deficiency
▶ BY MOUTH
▶ Adult: 800 units daily, higher doses may be necessary
for severe deficiency

● INTERACTIONS → Appendix 1: vitamin D substances

● RENAL IMPAIRMENT
Monitoring Monitor plasma-calcium concentration in
renal impairment.

● MONITORING REQUIREMENTS Monitor plasma-calcium
concentration in patients receiving high doses.

● PRESCRIBING AND DISPENSING INFORMATION The BP
directs that when calciferol is prescribed or demanded,
colecalciferol or ergocalciferol should be dispensed or
supplied.
    When the strength of the tablets ordered or prescribed is
not clear, the intention of the prescriber with respect to
the strength (expressed in micrograms or milligrams per
tablet) should be ascertained.

● MEDICINAL FORMS
There can be variation in the licensing of different medicines
containing the same drug. Forms available from special-order
manufacturers include: tablet, capsule, oral suspension, oral
solution
Tablet
▶ Ergocalciferol (Non-proprietary)
  Ergocalciferol 12.5 microgram Ergocalciferol 12.5microgram tablets
  | 30 tablet Ⓢ
  Ergo-D2 12.5microgram tablets | 30 tablet Ⓢ
▶ Ergoral (Cubic Pharmaceuticals Ltd)
  Ergocalciferol 125 microgram Ergoral D2 5,000unit tablets |
  30 tablet £14.95
  Ergocalciferol 250 microgram Ergoral D2 10,000unit tablets |
  30 tablet £19.95
Oral solution
▶ Eciferol (Rhodes Pharma Ltd)
  Ergocalciferol 3000 unit per 1 ml Eciferol D2 3,000units/ml liquid
  | 60 ml £55.00 DT = £89.20
Capsule
▶ Ergocalciferol (Non-proprietary)
  Ergocalciferol 1.25 mg Ergocalciferol 1.25mg capsules |
  30 capsule PoM Ⓢ
▶ Eciferol (Rhodes Pharma Ltd)
  Ergocalciferol 1.25 mg Eciferol D2 50,000unit capsules | 10 capsule
  £29.99
▶ Ergoral (Cubic Pharmaceuticals Ltd)
  Ergocalciferol 1.25 mg Ergoral D2 50,000unit capsules | 10 capsule
  £19.95

Ergocalciferol with calcium lactate and calcium phosphate

(Calcium and vitamin D)

The properties listed below are those particular to the
combination only. For the properties of the components
please consider, ergocalciferol above, calcium lactate
p. 1014.

● INDICATIONS AND DOSE
**Prevention of calcium and vitamin D deficiency |
Treatment of calcium and vitamin D deficiency**
▶ BY MOUTH
▶ Adult: (consult product literature)

● INTERACTIONS → Appendix 1: calcium salts · vitamin D
substances

● SIDE-EFFECTS Hypercalcaemia

● DIRECTIONS FOR ADMINISTRATION Tablets may be crushed
before administration, or may be chewed.

● PRESCRIBING AND DISPENSING INFORMATION Each tablet
contains calcium lactate 300 mg, calcium phosphate
150 mg (calcium 97 mg or Ca^{2+} 2.4 mmol), ergocalciferol
10 micrograms (400 units).

● PATIENT AND CARER ADVICE Patient or carers should be
given advice on how to administer calcium and
ergocalciferol tablets.

● MEDICINAL FORMS
There can be variation in the licensing of different medicines
containing the same drug.
Tablet
▶ Ergocalciferol with calcium lactate and calcium phosphate (Non-
  proprietary)
  **Ergocalciferol 10 microgram, Calcium phosphate 150 mg, Calcium
  lactate 300 mg** Calcium and Ergocalciferol tablets | 28 tablet Ⓟ
  £22.38 DT = £21.28 | 28 tablet Ⓢ DT = £21.28

☞ 1050

Paricalcitol

- **INDICATIONS AND DOSE**

For prevention and treatment of secondary hyperparathyroidism associated with chronic renal failure

▸ BY MOUTH
▸ Adult: (consult product literature)

For prevention and treatment of secondary hyperparathyroidism associated with chronic renal failure in patients on haemodialysis

▸ Adult: To be administered via haemodialysis access (consult product literature)

- **INTERACTIONS** → Appendix 1: vitamin D substances
- **SIDE-EFFECTS**

GENERAL SIDE-EFFECTS
▸ **Common or very common** Electrolyte imbalance · hypoparathyroidism · taste altered
▸ **Uncommon** Asthenia · diarrhoea · dizziness · dry mouth · malaise · muscle complaints · pain
▸ **Frequency not known** Angioedema · laryngeal oedema

SPECIFIC SIDE-EFFECTS
▸ **Uncommon**
▸▸ With oral use Acne · breast tenderness · gastrointestinal discomfort · gastrooesophageal reflux disease · palpitations · peripheral oedema · pneumonia
▸▸ With parenteral use Alopecia · anaemia · anxiety · arrhythmias · asthma · breast cancer · breast pain · bullous dermatitis · cardiac arrest · cerebrovascular insufficiency · chest pain · coma · condition aggravated · confusion · conjunctivitis · cough · delirium · depersonalisation · dyspepsia · dysphagia · dyspnoea · ear disorder · erectile dysfunction · fever · gait abnormal · gastrointestinal disorders · glaucoma · haemorrhage · hirsutism · hyperhidrosis · hyperparathyroidism · hypertension · hypotension · increased risk of infection · insomnia · joint disorders · leucopenia · lymphadenopathy · myoclonus · oedema · pulmonary oedema · sensation abnormal · sepsis · syncope · weight decreased

- **PREGNANCY** Toxicity in *animal* studies—manufacturer advises avoid unless potential benefit outweighs risk.
- **BREAST FEEDING** Manufacturer advises caution—no information available.
- **MONITORING REQUIREMENTS**
▸ Monitor plasma calcium and phosphate during dose titration and at least monthly when stabilised.
▸ Monitor parathyroid hormone concentration.

- **MEDICINAL FORMS**
There can be variation in the licensing of different medicines containing the same drug.

Solution for injection
EXCIPIENTS: May contain Propylene glycol
▸ Zemplar (AbbVie Ltd)
Paricalcitol 5 microgram per 1 ml Zemplar 5micrograms/1ml solution for injection vials | 5 vial [PoM] £62.00 (Hospital only)

Capsule
▸ Zemplar (AbbVie Ltd)
Paricalcitol 1 microgram Zemplar 1microgram capsules | 28 capsule [PoM] £69.44
Paricalcitol 2 microgram Zemplar 2microgram capsules | 28 capsule [PoM] £138.88

VITAMINS AND TRACE ELEMENTS > VITAMIN E

Alpha tocopherol

(Tocopherol)

- **INDICATIONS AND DOSE**

Vitamin E deficiency because of malabsorption in congenital or hereditary chronic cholestasis

▸ BY MOUTH USING ORAL SOLUTION
▸ Child: 17 mg/kg daily, dose to be adjusted as necessary

- **CAUTIONS** Predisposition to thrombosis
- **INTERACTIONS** → Appendix 1: vitamin E substances
- **SIDE-EFFECTS**
▸ **Common or very common** Diarrhoea
▸ **Uncommon** Alopecia · asthenia · headache · skin reactions
▸ **Frequency not known** Abdominal pain

- **PREGNANCY** Manufacturer advises caution, no evidence of harm in *animal* studies.
- **BREAST FEEDING** Manufacturer advises use only if potential benefit outweighs risk—no information available.
- **HEPATIC IMPAIRMENT** Manufacturer advises caution—no information available.
Monitoring Manufacturer advises monitor closely in hepatic impairment.
- **RENAL IMPAIRMENT** Manufacturer advises caution. Risk of renal toxicity due to polyethylene glycol content.
Monitoring Manufacturer advises monitor closely in renal impairment.
- **PRESCRIBING AND DISPENSING INFORMATION**
Tocofersolan is a water-soluble form of D-alpha tocopherol.

- **MEDICINAL FORMS**
There can be variation in the licensing of different medicines containing the same drug.
Oral solution
▸ Vedrop (Orphan Europe (UK) Ltd) ▼
D-alpha tocopherol (as Tocofersolan) 50 mg per 1 ml Vedrop 50mg/ml oral solution sugar-free | 20 ml [PoM] £54.55 sugar-free | 60 ml [PoM] £163.65

Alpha tocopheryl acetate

(Tocopherol)

- **INDICATIONS AND DOSE**

Vitamin E deficiency
▸ BY MOUTH
▸ Child: 2–10 mg/kg daily, increased if necessary up to 20 mg/kg daily

Malabsorption in cystic fibrosis
▸ BY MOUTH
▸ Child 1–11 months: 50 mg once daily, dose to be adjusted as necessary, to be taken with food and pancreatic enzymes
▸ Child 1–11 years: 100 mg once daily, dose to be adjusted as necessary, to be taken with food and pancreatic enzymes
▸ Child 12–17 years: 100–200 mg once daily, dose to be adjusted as necessary, to be taken with food and pancreatic enzymes
▸ Adult: 100–200 mg once daily, dose to be adjusted as necessary, to be taken with food and pancreatic enzymes

continued →

9

Blood and nutrition

Vitamin E deficiency in cholestasis and severe liver disease

▶ BY MOUTH
▶ Child 1 month–11 years: Initially 100 mg daily, adjusted according to response, increased if necessary up to 200 mg/kg daily
▶ Child 12–17 years: Initially 200 mg daily, adjusted according to response, increased if necessary up to 200 mg/kg daily

Malabsorption in abetalipoproteinaemia

▶ BY MOUTH
▶ Adult: 50–100 mg/kg once daily

● CAUTIONS Predisposition to thrombosis
● INTERACTIONS → Appendix 1: vitamin E substances
● SIDE-EFFECTS Abdominal pain (more common at high doses) · bleeding tendency · diarrhoea (more common at high doses) · increased risk of thrombosis
● PREGNANCY No evidence of safety of high doses.
● BREAST FEEDING Excreted in milk; minimal risk, although caution with large doses.
● MONITORING REQUIREMENTS Increased bleeding tendency in vitamin-K deficient patients or those taking anticoagulants (prothrombin time and INR should be monitored).

● MEDICINAL FORMS
There can be variation in the licensing of different medicines containing the same drug. Forms available from special-order manufacturers include: chewable tablet

Oral suspension
EXCIPIENTS: May contain Sucrose
▶ Alpha tocopheryl acetate (Non-proprietary)
   Alpha tocopheryl acetate 100 mg per 1 ml Alpha tocopheryl acetate 500mg/5ml oral suspension | 100 ml GSL £67.97 DT = £67.97

Chewable tablet
▶ Alpha tocopheryl acetate (Non-proprietary)
   Alpha tocopheryl acetate 100 mg Alpha tocopheryl acetate 100mg chewable tablets | 30 tablet Ⓟ
▶ E-Tabs (Ennogen Healthcare Ltd)
   Alpha tocopheryl acetate 100 mg E-Tabs 100mg chewable tablets | 30 tablet £87.30
▶ Ephynal (Imported (Italy))
   Alpha tocopheryl acetate 100 mg Ephynal 100mg chewable tablets | 30 tablet Ⓟ

Capsule
▶ E-Caps (Ennogen Healthcare Ltd)
   Alpha tocopherol 75 unit E-Caps 75unit capsules | 100 capsule £109.50
   Alpha tocopherol 100 unit E-Caps 100unit capsules | 30 capsule £84.40
   Alpha tocopherol 200 unit E-Caps 200unit capsules | 30 capsule £89.50
   Alpha tocopherol 400 unit E-Caps 400unit capsules | 30 capsule £128.50
   Alpha tocopherol 1000 unit E-Caps 1,000unit capsules | 30 capsule £130.20
▶ Vita-E (Typharm Ltd)
   Alpha tocopherol 75 unit Vita-E 75unit capsules | 100 capsule £4.35
   Alpha tocopherol 200 unit Vita-E 200unit capsules | 30 capsule £3.35 | 100 capsule £10.34
   Alpha tocopherol 400 unit Vita-E 400unit capsules | 30 capsule £5.04 | 100 capsule £16.44

VITAMINS AND TRACE ELEMENTS > VITAMIN K

Menadiol sodium phosphate

● INDICATIONS AND DOSE

Prevention of Vitamin K deficiency in malabsorption syndromes

▶ BY MOUTH
▶ Adult: 10–40 mg daily, dose to be adjusted as necessary

● CAUTIONS G6PD deficiency (risk of haemolysis) · vitamin E deficiency (risk of haemolysis)
● SIDE-EFFECTS Haemolysis
● PREGNANCY Avoid in late pregnancy and labour unless benefit outweighs risk of neonatal haemolytic anaemia, hyperbilirubinaemia, and kernicterus in neonate.

● MEDICINAL FORMS
Forms available from special-order manufacturers include: tablet, oral suspension, oral solution

Phytomenadione

(Vitamin K₁)

● INDICATIONS AND DOSE

Major bleeding in patients on warfarin (in combination with dried prothrombin complex or fresh frozen plasma)

▶ BY SLOW INTRAVENOUS INJECTION
▶ Adult: 5 mg for 1 dose, stop warfarin treatment

INR > 8.0 with minor bleeding in patients on warfarin

▶ BY SLOW INTRAVENOUS INJECTION
▶ Adult: 1–3 mg, stop warfarin treatment, dose may be repeated if INR still too high after 24 hours, restart warfarin treatment when INR <5

INR > 8.0 with no bleeding in patients on warfarin

▶ BY MOUTH
▶ Adult: 1–5 mg, intravenous preparation to be used orally, stop warfarin treatment, repeat dose if INR still too high after 24 hours, restart warfarin treatment when INR <5

INR 5.0–8.0 with minor bleeding in patients on warfarin

▶ BY SLOW INTRAVENOUS INJECTION
▶ Adult: 1–3 mg, stop warfarin treatment, restart warfarin treatment when INR <5

Reversal of anticoagulation prior to elective surgery (after warfarin stopped)

▶ BY MOUTH
▶ Adult: 1–5 mg, intravenous preparation to be used orally, dose to be given the day before surgery if INR ≥1.5

Reversal of anticoagulation prior to emergency surgery (when surgery can be delayed 6–12 hours)

▶ BY INTRAVENOUS INJECTION
▶ Adult: 5 mg as a single dose, if surgery cannot be delayed, dried prothrombin complex can be given in addition to phytomenadione and the INR checked before surgery

● UNLICENSED USE Oral use of intravenous preparations is unlicensed.
● CAUTIONS Intravenous injections should be given very slowly—risk of vascular collapse
   KONAKION ® MM Reduce dose in elderly
● PREGNANCY Use if potential benefit outweighs risk.
● BREAST FEEDING Present in milk.
● HEPATIC IMPAIRMENT
   KONAKION ® MM Caution—glycocholic acid may displace bilirubin.
● DIRECTIONS FOR ADMINISTRATION
   KONAKION ® MM PAEDIATRIC Konakion ® MM Paediatric may be administered by mouth or by intramuscular injection or by intravenous injection. For intramuscular injection, may be diluted with Glucose 5% if necessary.
   KONAKION ® MM Konakion ® MM may be administered by slow intravenous injection or by intravenous infusion in glucose 5%; not for intramuscular injection. For intravenous infusion (Konakion ® MM), give intermittently

in Glucose 5%; dilute with 55 mL; may be injected into lower part of infusion apparatus.

● MEDICINAL FORMS
There can be variation in the licensing of different medicines containing the same drug. Forms available from special-order manufacturers include: tablet, capsule, oral suspension, oral solution

Solution for injection
EXCIPIENTS: May contain Glycocholic acid, lecithin
▸ Konakion MM (Roche Products Ltd)
   Phytomenadione 10 mg per 1 ml Konakion MM Paediatric 2mg/0.2ml solution for injection ampoules | 5 ampoule [PoM] £4.71
   Konakion MM 10mg/1ml solution for injection ampoules | 10 ampoule [PoM] £3.78 DT = £3.78

6.1   Neural tube defects (prevention in pregnancy)

Neural tube defects (prevention in pregnancy)
01-Aug-2017

Description of condition
Neural tube defects represent a group of congenital defects, caused by incomplete closure of the neural tube within 28 days of conception. The most common forms are anencephaly, spina bifida and encephalocele.

The main risk factors are maternal folate deficiency, maternal vitamin B_{12} deficiency, previous history of having an infant with a neural tube defect, smoking, diabetes, obesity, and use of antiepileptic drugs.

Prevention in pregnancy
[EvGr] Pregnant women or women who wish to become pregnant should be advised to take supplementation with folic acid p. 993 before conception and until week 12 of pregnancy.

A higher daily dose (see folic acid) is recommended for women at a high risk of conceiving a child with a neural tube defect, including women who have previously had an infant with a neural tube defect, who are receiving antiepileptic medication (see Epilepsy p. 304), or who have diabetes or sickle-cell disease. Ⓐ

Useful Resources
Antenatal care for uncomplicated pregnancies. National Institute for Health and Care Excellence. Clinical guideline 62. March 2008 (Updated March 2016).
www.nice.org.uk/guidance/cg62

Fertility problems: assessment and treatment. National Institute for Health and Care Excellence. Clinical guideline 156. June 2015.
www.nice.org.uk/guidance/cg156

Chapter 10
Musculoskeletal system

CONTENTS

1   Arthritis

Arthritis

Rheumatoid arthritis and other inflammatory disorders

A non-steroidal anti-inflammatory drug (NSAID) is indicated for pain and stiffness resulting from inflammatory rheumatic disease; analgesics such as paracetamol p. 438 or codeine phosphate p. 448 can also be used.

Drugs are also used to influence the rheumatic disease process itself. For *rheumatoid arthritis* these disease-modifying antirheumatic drugs (DMARDs) include methotrexate p. 888, cytokine modulators, azathioprine p. 816, ciclosporin p. 818, cyclophosphamide p. 871, leflunomide p. 1063, penicillamine p. 1063, gold, antimalarials (chloroquine p. 604 and hydroxychloroquine sulfate p. 1062), and sulfasalazine p. 42. Corticosteroids also have a significant role in the management of rheumatoid arthritis.

Drugs which may affect the disease process in *psoriatic arthritis* include sulfasalazine, gold, azathioprine, methotrexate, leflunomide, and cytokine modulators.

Osteoarthritis and soft-tissue disorders

For pain relief in osteoarthritis and soft-tissue disorders, paracetamol should be used first and may need to be taken regularly. A topical NSAID or topical capsaicin 0.025% p. 476 should also be considered, particularly in knee or hand osteoarthritis. An oral NSAID can be substituted for, or used in addition to, paracetamol. If further pain relief is required in osteoarthritis, then the addition of an opioid analgesic may be considered, but with a substantial risk of adverse effects; however, an opioid analgesic should be considered before a NSAID in patients taking low-dose aspirin.

Intra-articular corticosteroid injections may produce temporary benefit in osteoarthritis, especially if associated with soft-tissue inflammation.

Non-drug measures, such as weight reduction and exercise, should also be encouraged.

Glucosamine p. 1061 and rubefacients are not recommended for the treatment of osteoarthritis.

Hyaluronic acid and its derivatives are available for osteoarthritis of the knee, but are not recommended. Sodium hyaluronate (*Durolane*®, *Euflexxa*®, *Fermathron*®, *Orthovisc*®, *Ostenil*®, *Ostenil Plus*®, *RenehaVis*®, *Suplasyn*®, *Synocrom*®, *Synopsis*®) or hylan G-F 20 (*Synvisc*®) is injected intra-articularly to supplement natural hyaluronic acid in the synovial fluid. These injections may reduce pain over 1–6 months, but are associated with a short-term increase in knee inflammation. Sodium hyaluronate (*SportVis*®) is also licensed for the relief of pain and optimisation of recovery following ankle sprain, and for the relief of chronic pain and disability associated with tennis elbow.

Spondyloarthritis

01-Sep-2017

Description of condition

Spondyloarthritis refers to a group of inflammatory musculoskeletal conditions with shared features which affect both axial and peripheral joints. Most people with these conditions have either axial spondyloarthritis (which includes ankylosing spondylitis and non-radiographic axial spondyloarthritis) or psoriatic arthritis. Axial spondyloarthritis primarily affects the spine, in particular the sacroiliac joint.

Psoriatic arthritis may present in several forms, including involvement of small joints (in the hands and feet), large joints (particularly in the knees), or combinations of both. Psoriatic arthritis may also involve the axial joints, finger and toe joints, and inflammation of the connective tissue between tendon/ligament and bone.

Less common subgroups are enteropathic spondyloarthritis, which is associated with inflammatory bowel disease (Crohn's disease p. 36 and Ulcerative colitis p. 37), and reactive arthritis (a form of peripheral arthritis), which can occur following gastro-intestinal or genito-urinary infections.

Aims of treatment

The aims of treatment are to relieve symptoms, slow the progression of the condition, and improve quality of life.

Non-drug treatment

EvGr Patients who have difficulties with everyday activities should be referred to a specialist therapist (such as a physiotherapist, occupational therapist, hand therapist, orthotist or podiatrist). Hydrotherapy can be considered as an adjunctive therapy to manage pain and maintain or improve function for people with axial spondyloarthritis. ⟨A⟩

Drug treatment

Axial spondyloarthritis

EvGr For pain associated with axial spondyloarthritis, start one of the Non-steroidal anti-inflammatory drugs p. 1094 (NSAIDs) at the lowest effective dose. Clinical assessment, monitoring of risk factors, and the use of gastroprotective treatment should be considered. If an NSAID taken at the maximum tolerated dose for 2–4 weeks does not provide adequate pain relief, consider switching to a different NSAID.

A tumour necrosis factor (TNF) alpha inhibitor (or biological DMARD) such as adalimumab p. 1073, certolizumab pegol p. 1076, etanercept p. 1078, golimumab p. 1080, or infliximab p. 1082 is recommended as an option for treating severe active **ankylosing spondylitis** in patients whose disease has responded inadequately to, or who are intolerant of, NSAIDs.

Secukinumab p. 1066 is recommended as an option for treating active ankylosing spondylitis in patients who have responded inadequately to NSAIDs or TNF-alpha inhibitors (see *National funding/access decisions* under secukinumab p. 1066).

Adalimumab p. 1073, certolizumab pegol p. 1076 and etanercept p. 1078 are also recommended as options for treating severe **non-radiographic axial spondyloarthritis** in patients whose disease has responded inadequately to, or who are intolerant of, NSAIDs.

The choice of treatment should depend on patient preference and extra-articular involvement. The response to treatment should be assessed after 12 weeks and should only be continued if there is clear evidence of response.

Treatment with another TNF-alpha inhibitor is recommended in those who cannot tolerate, or whose disease has not responded to, treatment with the first TNF-alpha inhibitor, or in those whose disease has stopped responding after an initial response. ⟨A⟩

Psoriatic arthritis and other peripheral spondyloarthritides

EvGr Monotherapy with local corticosteroid injections should be considered for non-progressive **monoarthritis** (see Corticosteroids, inflammatory disorders p. 1118).

Standard DMARDs, such as methotrexate p. 888, leflunomide p. 1063 or sulfasalazine p. 42, can be used for patients with peripheral **polyarthritis**, **oligoarthritis**, or persistent or progressive **monoarthritis** associated with peripheral spondyloarthritis.

Standard DMARDs, such as methotrexate p. 888 or leflunomide p. 1063 can also be used for patients with **psoriatic arthritis**.

The choice of DMARD will depend on numerous factors such as the patient's circumstances (such as pregnancy planning and alcohol consumption), comorbidities (such as uveitis, psoriasis and inflammatory bowel disease), and potential side-effects.

If a standard DMARD taken at the maximum tolerated dose for at least 3 months does not provide adequate relief from symptoms, a switch to, or the addition of, another standard DMARD can be considered.

An NSAID can be used as an adjunct to standard DMARDs or biological DMARDs to manage symptoms. If NSAIDs do not provide adequate relief from symptoms, consider corticosteroid injections or short-term oral corticosteroid therapy as an adjunct to standard DMARDs or biological DMARDs to manage symptoms.

If extra-articular disease is adequately controlled by an existing standard DMARD but peripheral spondyloarthritis is not, consider adding another standard DMARD. ⟨A⟩

Further options for psoriatic arthritis

EvGr The targeted DMARD apremilast p. 1084, used alone or in combination with standard DMARDs, is recommended for the treatment of active and progressive psoriatic arthritis if the patient has peripheral arthritis with 3 or more tender joints and 3 or more swollen joints, and the psoriatic arthritis has not responded to at least 2 standard DMARDs given alone or in combination.

The biological DMARDs etanercept p. 1078, infliximab p. 1082, golimumab p. 1080 and adalimumab p. 1073 (TNF-alpha inhibitors) are recommended for the treatment of active and progressive psoriatic arthritis if the patients has

peripheral arthritis with 3 or more tender joints and 3 or more swollen joints, and the psoriatic arthritis has not responded to at least 2 standard DMARDs given alone or in combination.

Ustekinumab p. 1069, alone or in combination with methotrexate, is recommended for treating active psoriatic arthritis when treatment with TNF-alpha inhibitors is contra-indicated but would otherwise be considered or the patient has had treatment with one or more TNF-alpha inhibitors. The response to treatment should be assessed at 24 weeks and should only be continued if there is clear evidence of response. ⟨A⟩

Reactive arthritis

EvGr After treating the initial infection, do not offer long-term (4 weeks or longer) treatment with an antibacterial solely to manage reactive arthritis caused by a gastro-intestinal or genito-urinary infection. ⟨A⟩

Useful Resources

Spondyloarthritis in over 16s: diagnosis and management. National Institute for Health and Care Excellence. Clinical Guideline NG65. February 2017.
www.nice.org.uk/guidance/ng65

Rheumatic disease, suppressing drugs

Overview

Certain drugs such as those affecting the immune response can suppress the disease process in *rheumatoid arthritis* and *psoriatic arthritis*; gold, penicillamine p. 1063, hydroxychloroquine sulfate p. 1062, chloroquine p. 604, and sulfasalazine p. 42 can also suppress the disease process in *rheumatoid arthritis* while sulfasalazine and possibly gold can suppress the disease process in *psoriatic arthritis*. Unlike NSAIDs, which are used only for symptom control, disease-modifying anti-rheumatic drugs (DMARDs) can affect the progression of disease but may require 2–6 months of treatment for a full therapeutic response. Response to DMARDs may allow the NSAID dose to be reduced or withdrawn. All patients with suspected inflammatory joint disease should be referred to a specialist as soon as possible to confirm diagnosis and evaluate disease activity; early initiation of DMARDs is recommended to control the signs and symptoms, and to limit joint damage.

Choice

The choice of a disease-modifying antirheumatic drug should take into account co-morbidity and patient preference. Methotrexate p. 888, sulfasalazine, intramuscular gold, and penicillamine are similar in efficacy. However, methotrexate or sulfasalazine may be better tolerated.

A combination of **DMARDs** (including methotrexate and at least one other DMARD) and a short-term **corticosteroid**, should be given to patients with newly diagnosed active rheumatoid arthritis, ideally within 3 months of the onset of persistent symptoms. If the use of particular DMARDs is contra-indicated and combination therapy is not possible, monotherapy with a suitable DMARD should be given and the dose rapidly increased until clinically effective. In patients with established and stable rheumatoid arthritis, cautiously reduce drug doses to the lowest that are clinically effective. Response to drug treatment often produces a reduction in requirements of both corticosteroids and other drugs.

Gold and penicillamine are effective in *palindromic rheumatism*. *Systemic* and *discoid lupus erythematosus* are sometimes treated with chloroquine or hydroxychloroquine sulfate.

If a disease-modifying anti-rheumatic drug does not lead to an objective benefit within 6 months, it should be replaced by a different one.

Gold

Gold can be given as sodium aurothiomalate p. 1064 for active progressive rheumatoid arthritis; it must be given by deep intramuscular injection and the area gently massaged. A test dose must be given followed by doses at weekly intervals until there is definite evidence of remission. In patients who do respond, the interval between injections is then gradually increased to 4 weeks and treatment is continued for up to 5 years after complete remission. If relapse occurs the dosage frequency may be immediately increased and only once control has been obtained again should the dosage frequency be decreased; if no response is seen within 2 months, alternative treatment should be sought. It is important to avoid complete relapse since second courses of gold are not usually effective.

Penicillamine

Penicillamine has a similar action to gold. More patients are able to continue treatment than with gold but side-effects are common.

Patients should be warned not to expect improvement for at least 6 to 12 weeks after treatment is initiated. Penicillamine should be discontinued if there is no improvement within 1 year.

Sulfasalazine

Sulfasalazine has a beneficial effect in suppressing the inflammatory activity of rheumatoid arthritis. Sulfasalazine may also be used by specialists, in the management of psoriatic arthritis affecting peripheral joints [unlicensed indication]. Haematological abnormalities occur usually in the first 3 to 6 months of treatment and are reversible on cessation of treatment.

Antimalarials

The antimalarial hydroxychloroquine sulfate is used to treat rheumatoid arthritis of moderate inflammatory activity; chloroquine is also licensed for treating inflammatory disorders but is used much less frequently and is generally reserved for use if other drugs have failed.

Chloroquine and hydroxychloroquine sulfate are effective for mild systemic lupus erythematosus, particularly involving the skin and joints. These drugs should not be used for psoriatic arthritis. Chloroquine and hydroxychloroquine sulfate are better tolerated than gold or penicillamine. Retinopathy rarely occurs provided that the recommended doses are not exceeded; in the elderly it is difficult to distinguish drug-induced retinopathy from changes of ageing.

Mepacrine hydrochloride p. 498 is sometimes used in discoid lupus erythematosus [unlicensed].

Drugs affecting the immune response

Methotrexate is a disease-modifying antirheumatic drug suitable for moderate to severe rheumatoid arthritis. Azathioprine p. 816, ciclosporin p. 818, cyclophosphamide p. 871, leflunomide p. 1063, and the **cytokine modulators** are considered more toxic and they are used in cases that have not responded to other disease-modifying drugs.

Methotrexate is usually given by mouth once a week, adjusted according to response. In patients who experience mucosal or gastro-intestinal side-effects with methotrexate, folic acid p. 993 given every week [unlicensed indication], on a different day from the methotrexate, may help to reduce the frequency of such side-effects.

Leflunomide acts on the immune system as a disease-modifying antirheumatic drug. Its therapeutic effect starts after 4–6 weeks and improvement may continue for a further

4–6 months. Leflunomide, which is similar in efficacy to sulfasalazine and methotrexate, may be chosen when these drugs cannot be used.

Ciclosporin is licensed for severe active rheumatoid arthritis when conventional second-line therapy is inappropriate or ineffective. There is some evidence that ciclosporin may retard the rate of erosive progression and improve symptom control in those who respond only partially to methotrexate.

Cyclophosphamide may be used for rheumatoid arthritis with severe systemic manifestations [unlicensed indication]; it is toxic and regular blood counts (including platelet counts) should be carried out. Cyclophosphamide can also be given for *severe systemic rheumatoid arthritis* and for other connective tissue diseases (especially with active vasculitis).

Drugs that affect the immune response are also used in the management of severe cases of *systemic lupus erythematosus* and other connective tissue disorders. They are often given in conjunction with corticosteroids for patients with severe or progressive renal disease. They may be used in cases of *polymyositis* that are resistant to corticosteroids. They are used for their corticosteroid-sparing effect in patients whose corticosteroid requirements are excessive. Azathioprine is usually used.

In the specialist management of psoriatic arthritis affecting peripheral joints, leflunomide, methotrexate, or azathioprine [unlicensed indication] may be used.

Juvenile idiopathic arthritis

Many children with *juvenile idiopathic arthritis* (juvenile chronic arthritis) do not require disease-modifying antirheumatic drugs. Methotrexate is effective; sulfasalazine is an alternative [unlicensed indication] but it should be avoided in *systemic-onset juvenile idiopathic arthritis*. Gold and penicillamine are no longer used. Cytokine modulators have a role in *juvenile idiopathic arthritis*.

Cytokine modulators

Cytokine modulators should be used under specialist supervision.

Adalimumab p. 1073, certolizumab pegol p. 1076, etanercept p. 1078, golimumab p. 1080, and infliximab p. 1082 inhibit the activity of tumour necrosis factor alpha (TNF-α).

Adalimumab is licensed for moderate to severe active *rheumatoid arthritis* when response to other disease modifying antirheumatic drugs (including methotrexate p. 888) has been inadequate; it is also licensed for severe, active, and progressive disease in adults not previously treated with methotrexate. In the treatment of rheumatoid arthritis, adalimumab should be used in combination with methotrexate, but it can be given alone if methotrexate is inappropriate. Adalimumab is also licensed for the treatment of active and progressive *psoriatic arthritis* and severe active *ankylosing spondylitis* that have not responded adequately to other disease-modifying antirheumatic drugs. It is also licensed for the treatment of severe axial spondyloarthritis without radiographic evidence of ankylosing spondylitis but with objective signs of inflammation, in patients who have had an inadequate response to, or are intolerant of NSAIDs. Adalimumab also has a role in inflammatory bowel disease and plaque psoriasis.

Certolizumab pegol is licensed for use in patients with moderate to severe active *rheumatoid arthritis* when response to disease-modifying antirheumatic drugs (including methotrexate) has been inadequate. Certolizumab pegol can be used in combination with methotrexate, or as a monotherapy if methotrexate is not tolerated or is contra-indicated. Certolizumab pegol is also licensed for the treatment of severe active *ankylosing spondylitis* in patients who have had an inadequate response to, or are intolerant of NSAIDs. It is also licensed for the treatment of severe active axial *spondyloarthritis*, without radiographic evidence of ankylosing spondylitis but with objective signs of inflammation, in patients who have had an inadequate response to, or are intolerant of NSAIDs.

Etanercept is licensed for the treatment of moderate to severe active *rheumatoid arthritis* either alone or in combination with methotrexate when the response to other disease-modifying antirheumatic drugs is inadequate and in severe, active and progressive *rheumatoid arthritis* in patients not previously treated with methotrexate. It is also licensed for the treatment of active and progressive *psoriatic arthritis* inadequately responsive to other disease-modifying antirheumatic drugs, and for severe *ankylosing spondylitis* inadequately responsive to conventional therapy. Etanercept also has a role in plaque psoriasis.

Golimumab is licensed in combination with methotrexate for the treatment of moderate to severe active *rheumatoid arthritis* when response to disease-modifying antirheumatic drug (DMARD) therapy (including methotrexate has been inadequate; it is also licensed in combination with methotrexate for patients with severe, active, and progressive rheumatoid arthritis not previously treated with methotrexate. Golimumab is also licensed for the treatment of active and progressive *psoriatic arthritis*, as monotherapy or in combination with methotrexate, when response to DMARD therapy has been inadequate; it is also licensed for the treatment of severe active *ankylosing spondylitis* when there is an inadequate response to conventional treatment.

Infliximab is licensed for the treatment of active *rheumatoid arthritis* in combination with methotrexate when the response to other disease-modifying antirheumatic drugs, including methotrexate, is inadequate; it is also licensed in combination with methotrexate for patients not previously treated with methotrexate or other DMARDs who have severe, active, and progressive rheumatoid arthritis. Infliximab is also licensed for the treatment of *ankylosing spondylitis*, in patients with severe axial symptoms who have not responded adequately to conventional therapy, and in combination with methotrexate (or alone if methotrexate is not tolerated or is contra-indicated) for the treatment of active and progressive *psoriatic arthritis* which has not responded adequately to disease-modifying antirheumatic drugs.

Rituximab p. 859 is licensed in combination with methotrexate for the treatment of severe active *rheumatoid arthritis* in patients whose condition has not responded adequately to other disease-modifying antirheumatic drugs (including one or more tumour necrosis factor inhibitors) or who are intolerant of them. Rituximab has a role in malignant disease.

Abatacept p. 1073 prevents the full activation of T-lymphocytes. It is licensed for moderate to severe active *rheumatoid arthritis* in combination with methotrexate, in patients unresponsive to other disease-modifying antirheumatic drugs (including methotrexate or a tumour necrosis factor (TNF) inhibitor). Abatacept is not recommended for use in combination with TNF inhibitors.

Anakinra p. 1065 inhibits the activity of interleukin-1. Anakinra (in combination with methotrexate) is licensed for the treatment of *rheumatoid arthritis* which has not responded to methotrexate alone. Anakinra is not recommended for the treatment of rheumatoid arthritis except when used in a controlled long-term clinical study. Patients who are already receiving anakinra for rheumatoid arthritis should continue treatment until they and their specialist consider it appropriate to stop.

Baricitinib p. 1071 and tofacitinib p. 1072 are licensed alone or in combination with methotrexate for the treatment of moderate to severe active *rheumatoid arthritis* in patients who have had an inadequate response to, or who are intolerant to, one or more disease-modifying antirheumatic drugs.

Belimumab p. 825 inhibits the activity of B-lymphocyte stimulator. Belimumab is licensed as adjunctive therapy in patients with active, autoantibody-positive systemic lupus erythematosus with a high degree of disease activity despite standard therapy.

Sarilumab p. 1065 is a recombinant human monoclonal antibody that specifically binds to interleukin-6 receptors and blocks the activity of pro-inflammatory cytokines; it is licensed alone or in combination with methotrexate for the treatment of moderate to severe active rheumatoid arthritis in patients who have had an inadequate response to, or are intolerant to one or more disease-modifying anti-rheumatic drugs.

Secukinumab p. 1066 inhibits the activity of interleukin-17A. Secukinumab is licensed for the treatment of active *psoriatic arthritis*, in combination with methotrexate or alone, which has not responded adequately to disease-modifying antirheumatic drugs; it is also licensed for the treatment of *ankylosing spondylitis*, in patients who have not responded adequately to conventional therapy. Secukinumab also has a role in plaque psoriasis.

Tocilizumab p. 1068 antagonises the actions of interleukin-6. Tocilizumab is licensed for use in patients with moderate to severe active *rheumatoid arthritis* when response to at least one disease-modifying antirheumatic drug or tumour necrosis factor inhibitor has been inadequate, or in those who are intolerant of these drugs. Tocilizumab can be used in combination with methotrexate, or as monotherapy if methotrexate is not tolerated or is contra-indicated.

Ustekinumab p. 1069 inhibits the activity of interleukins 12 and 23. It is licensed for the treatment of active *psoriatic arthritis* (in combination with methotrexate or alone) in patients who have had an inadequate response to one or more disease-modifying antirheumatic drugs.

> **Other drugs used for Arthritis** Aceclofenac, p. 1096 · Acemetacin, p. 1097 · Celecoxib, p. 1097 · Dexibuprofen, p. 1098 · Diclofenac potassium, p. 1100 · Diclofenac sodium, p. 1101 · Etodolac, p. 1103 · Etoricoxib, p. 1104 · Fenoprofen, p. 1105 · Flurbiprofen, p. 1106 · Ibuprofen, p. 1106 · Indometacin, p. 1109 · Ixekizumab, p. 1224 · Ketoprofen, p. 1110 · Mefenamic acid, p. 1111 · Meloxicam, p. 1112 · Nabumetone, p. 1113 · Naproxen, p. 1113 · Piroxicam, p. 1115 · Prednisone, p. 666 · Sulindac, p. 1116 · Tenoxicam, p. 1117 · Tiaprofenic acid, p. 1117

CHONDROPROTECTIVE DRUGS

Glucosamine

● DRUG ACTION Glucosamine is a natural substance found in mucopolysaccharides, mucoproteins, and chitin.

● INDICATIONS AND DOSE

ALATERIS®

Symptomatic relief of mild to moderate osteoarthritis of the knee
▶ BY MOUTH
▶ Adult: 1250 mg once daily, review treatment if no benefit after 2–3 months

DOLENIO®

Symptomatic relief of mild to moderate osteoarthritis of the knee
▶ BY MOUTH
▶ Adult: 1500 mg once daily, review treatment if no benefit after 2–3 months continued →

GLUSARTEL ®

Symptomatic relief of mild to moderate osteoarthritis of the knee
▶ BY MOUTH
▶ Adult: 1500 mg once daily, dose to be dissolved in at least 250 mL of water, review treatment if no benefit after 2–3 months

● CAUTIONS Asthma · impaired glucose tolerance · predisposition to cardiovascular disease
● INTERACTIONS → Appendix 1: glucosamine
● SIDE-EFFECTS
▶ Common or very common Constipation · diarrhoea · fatigue · gastrointestinal discomfort · headache · nausea
▶ Uncommon Flushing · skin reactions
▶ Rare or very rare Jaundice
▶ Frequency not known Angioedema · asthma · diabetes mellitus · dizziness · hypercholesterolaemia · oedema · vomiting
● ALLERGY AND CROSS-SENSITIVITY Contra-indicated if patient has a shellfish allergy.
● PREGNANCY Manufacturers advise avoid—no information available.
● BREAST FEEDING Manufacturers advise avoid—no information available.
● MONITORING REQUIREMENTS
▶ Monitor blood-glucose concentration before treatment and periodically thereafter in patients with impaired glucose tolerance.
▶ Monitor cholesterol in patients with predisposition to cardiovascular disease.
● NATIONAL FUNDING/ACCESS DECISIONS
Scottish Medicines Consortium (SMC) Decisions
The *Scottish Medicines Consortium* has advised (May 2008) that glucosamine (*Alateris*®) and (July 2011) glucosamine (*Glusartel*®) are **not** recommended for use within NHS Scotland for the symptomatic relief of mild to moderate osteoarthritis of the knee.
● LESS SUITABLE FOR PRESCRIBING Less suitable for prescribing—the mechanism of action is not understood and there is limited evidence to show it is effective.

● MEDICINAL FORMS
There can be variation in the licensing of different medicines containing the same drug.
Tablet
ELECTROLYTES: May contain Sodium
▶ Dolenio (Alissa Healthcare Research Ltd)
Dolenio 1500mg tablets | 30 tablet [PoM] £18.20 DT = £18.20

DISEASE-MODIFYING ANTI-RHEUMATIC DRUGS

Hydroxychloroquine sulfate

● INDICATIONS AND DOSE
Active rheumatoid arthritis (administered on expert advice) | Systemic and discoid lupus erythematosus (administered on expert advice) | Dermatological conditions caused or aggravated by sunlight (administered on expert advice)
▶ BY MOUTH
▶ Adult: 200–400 mg daily, daily maximum dose to be based on ideal body-weight; maximum 6.5 mg/kg per day

● CAUTIONS Acute porphyrias p. 1025 · diabetes (may lower blood glucose) · elderly · G6PD deficiency · may aggravate myasthenia gravis · may exacerbate psoriasis · neurological disorders (especially in those with a history of epilepsy) · severe gastro-intestinal disorders

CAUTIONS, FURTHER INFORMATION
▶ Screening for ocular toxicity A review group convened by the Royal College of Ophthalmologists has updated guidelines for screening to prevent ocular toxicity on long-term treatment with chloroquine and hydroxychloroquine (*Hydroxychloroquine and Ocular Toxicity: Recommendations on Screening* 2009). The following recommendations relate to hydroxychloroquine, which is only rarely associated with toxicity.
Before treatment:
● Assess renal and liver function (adjust dose if impaired)
● Ask patient about visual impairment (not corrected by glasses). If impairment or eye disease present, assessment by an optometrist is advised and any abnormality should be referred to an ophthalmologist
● Record near visual acuity of each eye (with glasses where appropriate) using a standard reading chart
● Initiate hydroxychloroquine treatment if no abnormality detected (at a dose not exceeding hydroxychloroquine sulfate 6.5 mg/kg daily)
During treatment:
● Ask patient about visual symptoms and monitor visual acuity annually using the standard reading chart
● Refer to ophthalmologist if visual acuity changes or if vision blurred and warn patient to seek prescribing doctor's advice about stopping treatment
● If long-term treatment is required (more than 5 years), individual arrangement should be agreed with the local ophthalmologist
● INTERACTIONS → Appendix 1: hydroxychloroquine
● SIDE-EFFECTS
▶ Common or very common Abdominal pain · appetite decreased · diarrhoea · emotional lability · headache · nausea · skin reactions · vision disorders · vomiting
▶ Uncommon Alopecia · corneal oedema · dizziness · eye disorders · hair colour changes · hearing impairment · nervousness · neuromuscular dysfunction · retinopathy · seizure · vertigo
▶ Frequency not known Acute hepatic failure · agranulocytosis · anaemia · angioedema · bone marrow disorders · bronchospasm · cardiac conduction disorders · cardiomyopathy · hypoglycaemia · leucopenia · movement disorders · muscle weakness · myopathy · photosensitivity reaction · psychosis · reflexes absent · severe cutaneous adverse reactions (SCARs) · thrombocytopenia · tremor · ventricular hypertrophy
Overdose Hydroxychloroquine is very toxic in overdosage; overdosage is extremely hazardous and difficult to treat. Urgent advice from the National Poisons Information Service is essential. Life-threatening features include arrhythmias (which can have a very rapid onset) and convulsions (which can be intractable).
● PREGNANCY It is not necessary to withdraw an antimalarial drug during pregnancy if the rheumatic disease is well controlled; however, the manufacturer of hydroxychloroquine advises avoiding use.
● BREAST FEEDING Avoid—risk of toxicity in infant.
● HEPATIC IMPAIRMENT Caution in moderate to severe hepatic impairment.
● RENAL IMPAIRMENT Manufacturer advises caution.
Monitoring Monitor plasma-hydroxychloroquine concentration in severe renal impairment.
● MONITORING REQUIREMENTS Manufacturers recommend regular ophthalmological examination but the evidence of practical value is unsatisfactory (see advice of the Royal College of Ophthalmologists).
● PRESCRIBING AND DISPENSING INFORMATION To avoid excessive dosage in obese patients, the dose of hydroxychloroquine should be calculated on the basis of ideal body-weight.

- MEDICINAL FORMS
  There can be variation in the licensing of different medicines
  containing the same drug. Forms available from special-order
  manufacturers include: oral suspension, oral solution

Tablet
CAUTIONARY AND ADVISORY LABELS 21
- Hydroxychloroquine sulfate (Non-proprietary)
  Hydroxychloroquine sulfate 200 mg Hydroxychloroquine 200mg
  tablets | 60 tablet PoM £32.49 DT = £5.83
- Quinoric (Bristol Laboratories Ltd)
  Hydroxychloroquine sulfate 200 mg Quinoric 200mg tablets |
  60 tablet PoM £4.75 DT = £5.83

Leflunomide

- **INDICATIONS AND DOSE**

Moderate to severe active rheumatoid arthritis (specialist use only)
- BY MOUTH
  - Adult: Initially 100 mg once daily for 3 days, then
    reduced to 10–20 mg once daily

Active psoriatic arthritis (specialist use only)
- BY MOUTH
  - Adult: Initially 100 mg once daily for 3 days, then
    reduced to 20 mg once daily

- CONTRA-INDICATIONS Serious infection · severe
  hypoproteinaemia · severe immunodeficiency
- CAUTIONS Anaemia (avoid if significant and due to causes
  other than rheumatoid arthritis) · history of tuberculosis ·
  impaired bone-marrow function (avoid if significant and
  due to causes other than rheumatoid arthritis) · leucopenia
  (avoid if significant and due to causes other than
  rheumatoid arthritis) · thrombocytopenia (avoid if
  significant and due to causes other than rheumatoid
  arthritis)
- INTERACTIONS → Appendix 1: leflunomide
- SIDE-EFFECTS
- **Common or very common** Abdominal pain · accelerated hair
  loss · appetite decreased · asthenia · diarrhoea · dizziness ·
  gastrointestinal disorders · headache · leucopenia · nausea ·
  oral disorders · paraesthesia · peripheral neuropathy · skin
  reactions · tendon disorders · vomiting · weight decreased
- **Uncommon** Anaemia · anxiety · electrolyte imbalance ·
  hyperlipidaemia · taste altered · thrombocytopenia
- **Rare or very rare** Agranulocytosis · eosinophilia · hepatic
  disorders · infection · pancreatitis · pancytopenia ·
  respiratory disorders · sepsis · severe cutaneous adverse
  reactions (SCARs) · vasculitis
- **Frequency not known** Cutaneous lupus erythematosus ·
  hypouricaemia · pulmonary hypertension · renal failure
  SIDE-EFFECTS, FURTHER INFORMATION Discontinue
  treatment and institute washout procedure in case of
  serious side-effect (consult product literature).
  Hepatotoxicity Potentially life-threatening
  hepatotoxicity reported usually in the first 6 months.
  Discontinue treatment (and institute washout procedure—
  consult product literature) or reduce dose according to
  liver-function abnormality; if liver-function abnormality
  persists after dose reduction, discontinue treatment and
  institute washout procedure.
- CONCEPTION AND CONTRACEPTION Effective
  contraception **essential** during treatment and for at least
  2 years after treatment in women and at least 3 months
  after treatment in men (plasma concentration monitoring
  required; waiting time before conception may be reduced
  with washout procedure—consult product literature). The
  concentration of the active metabolite after washout
  should be less than 20 micrograms/litre (measured on 2
  occasions 14 days apart) in men or women before
  conception—consult product literature.

- PREGNANCY Avoid—active metabolite teratogenic in
  animal studies.
- BREAST FEEDING Present in milk in *animal* studies—
  manufacturer advises avoid.
- HEPATIC IMPAIRMENT Avoid—active metabolite may
  accumulate.
- RENAL IMPAIRMENT Manufacturer advises avoid in
  moderate or severe impairment—no information available.
- PRE-TREATMENT SCREENING Exclude pregnancy before
  treatment.
- MONITORING REQUIREMENTS
- Monitor full blood count (including differential white cell
  count and platelet count) before treatment and every
  2 weeks for 6 months then every 8 weeks.
- Monitor liver function before treatment and every 2 weeks
  for first 6 months then every 8 weeks.
- Monitor blood pressure.
- TREATMENT CESSATION
  Washout Procedure The active metabolite persists for a long
  period; to aid drug elimination in case of serious adverse
  effect, or before starting another disease-modifying
  antirheumatic drug, or before conception, stop treatment
  and give *either* colestyramine p. 196 *or* charcoal, activated
  p. 1326. Procedure may be repeated as necessary.

- MEDICINAL FORMS
  There can be variation in the licensing of different medicines
  containing the same drug.
Tablet
CAUTIONARY AND ADVISORY LABELS 4
- Leflunomide (Non-proprietary)
  Leflunomide 10 mg Leflunomide 10mg tablets | 30 tablet PoM
  £46.00 DT = £7.08
  Leflunomide 15 mg Leflunomide 15mg tablets | 30 tablet PoM
  £46.00 DT = £46.00
  Leflunomide 20 mg Leflunomide 20mg tablets | 30 tablet PoM
  £61.36 DT = £7.43
- Arava (Sanofi)
  Leflunomide 10 mg Arava 10mg tablets | 30 tablet PoM £51.13 DT
  = £7.08
  Leflunomide 20 mg Arava 20mg tablets | 30 tablet PoM £61.36 DT
  = £7.43
  Leflunomide 100 mg Arava 100mg tablets | 3 tablet PoM £30.67

Penicillamine

- DRUG ACTION Penicillamine aids the elimination of copper
  ions in Wilson's disease (hepatolenticular degeneration).

- **INDICATIONS AND DOSE**

Severe active rheumatoid arthritis (administered on expert advice)
- BY MOUTH
  - Adult: Initially 125–250 mg daily for 1 month, then
    increased in steps of 125–250 mg, at intervals of not
    less than 4 weeks; maintenance 500–750 mg daily in
    divided doses, then reduced in steps of 125–250 mg
    every 12 weeks, dose reduction attempted only if
    remission sustained for 6 months; maximum 1.5 g per
    day
  - Elderly: Initially up to 125 mg daily for 1 month, then
    increased in steps of up to 125 mg, at intervals of at
    least 4 weeks; maximum 1 g per day

Wilson's disease
- BY MOUTH
  - Adult: 1.5–2 g daily in divided doses, adjusted
    according to response, to be taken before food;
    maintenance 0.75–1 g daily, a dose of 2 g daily should
    not be continued for more than one year; maximum 2 g
    per day
  - Elderly: 20 mg/kg daily in divided doses, adjusted
    according to response

continued →

Autoimmune hepatitis (used rarely; after disease controlled with corticosteroids)
▸ BY MOUTH
▸ Adult: Initially 500 mg daily in divided doses, to be increased slowly over 3 months; maintenance 1.25 g daily

Cystinuria, therapeutic
▸ BY MOUTH
▸ Adult: 1–3 g daily in divided doses, to be adjusted to maintain urinary cystine below 200 mg/litre, to be taken before food

Cystinuria, prophylactic
▸ BY MOUTH
▸ Adult: 0.5–1 g daily, maintain urinary cystine below 300 mg/litre and adequate fluid intake (at least 3 litres daily), to be taken at bedtime
▸ Elderly: Minimum dose to maintain urinary cystine below 200 mg/litre is recommended

● CONTRA-INDICATIONS Lupus erythematosus
● CAUTIONS Neurological involvement in Wilson's disease
● INTERACTIONS → Appendix 1: penicillamine
● SIDE-EFFECTS
▸ **Common or very common** Proteinuria · thrombocytopenia
▸ **Rare or very rare** Alopecia · breast enlargement (males and females) · connective tissue disorders · haematuria (discontinue immediately if cause unknown) · hypersensitivity · oral disorders · skin reactions
▸ **Frequency not known** Agranulocytosis · aplastic anaemia · appetite decreased · fever · glomerulonephritis · Goodpasture's syndrome · haemolytic anaemia · increased risk of infection · jaundice cholestatic · leucopenia · lupus-like syndrome · myasthenia gravis · nausea · nephrotic syndrome · neurological deterioration in Wilson's Disease · neutropenia · pancreatitis · polymyositis · pulmonary haemorrhage · rash (consider dose reduction) · respiratory disorders · Stevens-Johnson syndrome · taste loss (mineral supplements not recommended) · vomiting · yellow nail syndrome

SIDE-EFFECTS, FURTHER INFORMATION Proteinuria occurs in up to 30% of patients—can be a sign of immune-mediated nephropathy. Discontinue immediately if nephrotoxicity occurs.

Nausea and rash more common early in treatment if full dose used from initiation. Delayed rash can occur after months or years of treatment—manufacturer advises reduce dose.

● ALLERGY AND CROSS-SENSITIVITY Patients who are hypersensitive to penicillin may react rarely to penicillamine.
● PREGNANCY Fetal abnormalities reported rarely; avoid if possible.
● BREAST FEEDING Manufacturer advises avoid unless potential benefit outweighs risk—no information available.
● RENAL IMPAIRMENT
Dose adjustments Reduce dose and monitor renal function or avoid (consult product literature).
● MONITORING REQUIREMENTS
▸ Consider withdrawal if platelet count falls below 120 000/mm^3 or white blood cells below 2500/mm^3 or if 3 successive falls within reference range (can restart at reduced dose when counts return to within reference range but permanent withdrawal necessary if recurrence of leucopenia or thrombocytopenia).
▸ Blood counts, including platelets, and urine examinations should be carried out before starting treatment and then every 1 or 2 weeks for the first 2 months then every 4 weeks to detect blood disorders and proteinuria (they

should also be carried out in the week after any dose increase).
▸ A reduction in platelet count calls for discontinuation with subsequent re-introduction at a lower dosage and then, if possible, gradual increase.
▸ Longer intervals may be adequate in cystinuria and Wilson's disease.
● PATIENT AND CARER ADVICE Counselling on the symptoms of blood disorders is advised. Warn patient and carers to tell doctor immediately if sore throat, fever, infection, non-specific illness, unexplained bleeding and bruising, purpura, mouth ulcers, or rashes develop.

● MEDICINAL FORMS
There can be variation in the licensing of different medicines containing the same drug. Forms available from special-order manufacturers include: oral solution
Tablet
CAUTIONARY AND ADVISORY LABELS 6, 22
▸ Penicillamine (Non-proprietary)
Penicillamine 125 mg Penicillamine 125mg tablets | 56 tablet [PoM] £45.00 DT = £45.00
Penicillamine 250 mg Penicillamine 250mg tablets | 56 tablet [PoM] £88.77 DT = £88.77

Sodium aurothiomalate

● INDICATIONS AND DOSE
Active progressive rheumatoid arthritis (administered on expert advice)
▸ BY DEEP INTRAMUSCULAR INJECTION
▸ Adult: Test dose 10 mg, followed by 50 mg once weekly until there is definite evidence of remission, then reduced to 50 mg every 4 weeks continued for up to 5 years after complete remission, dose to be reduced gradually. Benefit is not expected until 300–500 mg has been given; it should be discontinued if there is no remission after 1 g has been given

Relapse in patients who have previously received sodium aurothiomalate therapy for active progressive rheumatoid arthritis (administered on expert advice)
▸ BY DEEP INTRAMUSCULAR INJECTION
▸ Adult: 50 mg once weekly until control has been obtained again, then reduced to 50 mg every 4 weeks continued for up to 5 years after complete remission, if no response is seen within 2 months, alternative treatment should be sought

● CONTRA-INDICATIONS Exfoliative dermatitis · history of blood disorders · history of bone marrow aplasia · necrotising enterocolitis · pulmonary fibrosis · systemic lupus erythematosus
● CAUTIONS Colitis · eczema · elderly · history of urticaria
CAUTIONS, FURTHER INFORMATION Sodium aurothiomalate should be discontinued in the presence of blood disorders, gastro-intestinal bleeding (associated with ulcerative enterocolitis), or unexplained proteinuria (associated with immune complex nephritis) which is repeatedly above 300 mg/litre.
● INTERACTIONS → Appendix 1: sodium aurothiomalate
● SIDE-EFFECTS Abdominal pain · agranulocytosis · albuminuria · alopecia · asthenia · blood disorder · bone marrow disorders · circulatory collapse · dry cough · dyspnoea · encephalopathy · enterocolitis · eosinophilia · flushing · hepatic disorders · hypersensitivity · hypotension · leucopenia · nephrotic syndrome · nerve disorders · neutropenia · palpitations · respiratory disorders · shock · skin reactions · tachycardia · thrombocytopenia

SIDE-EFFECTS, FURTHER INFORMATION Rashes with pruritus often occur after 2 to 6 months of treatment and may necessitate discontinuation.

- PREGNANCY Manufacturer advises avoid but limited data suggests usually not necessary to withdraw if condition well controlled.
  Dose adjustments Consider reducing dose and frequency.
- BREAST FEEDING Manufacturer advises avoid—present in milk; theoretical possibility of rashes and idiosyncratic reactions.
- HEPATIC IMPAIRMENT Caution in mild to moderate impairment. Avoid in severe impairment.
- RENAL IMPAIRMENT Caution in mild to moderate impairment. Avoid in severe impairment.
- MONITORING REQUIREMENTS
  ► Urine tests and full blood counts (including total and differential white cell and platelet counts) must be performed before starting treatment and before each intramuscular injection.
  ► Monitor for pulmonary fibrosis with annual chest X-ray.
- PATIENT AND CARER ADVICE Patients should be advised to seek prompt medical attention if diarrhoea, sore throat, fever, infection, non-specific illness, unexplained bleeding and bruising, purpura, mouth ulcers, metallic taste, rash, breathlessness, or cough develop.

- MEDICINAL FORMS
  There can be variation in the licensing of different medicines containing the same drug.
  Solution for injection
  CAUTIONARY AND ADVISORY LABELS 11
  ► Myocrisin (Sanofi)
  Sodium aurothiomalate 20 mg per 1 ml Myocrisin 10mg/0.5ml solution for injection ampoules | 10 ampoule [PoM] £45.55
  Sodium aurothiomalate 100 mg per 1 ml Myocrisin 50mg/0.5ml solution for injection ampoules | 10 ampoule [PoM] £134.80

IMMUNOSUPPRESSANTS › INTERLEUKIN INHIBITORS

Anakinra

- INDICATIONS AND DOSE
  Treatment of rheumatoid arthritis (in combination with methotrexate) which has not responded to methotrexate alone
  ► BY SUBCUTANEOUS INJECTION
  ► Adult: 100 mg once daily

- CONTRA-INDICATIONS Neutropenia
- CAUTIONS History of asthma (risk of serious infection) · predisposition to infection
- INTERACTIONS → Appendix 1: anakinra
- SIDE-EFFECTS
  ► **Common or very common** Headache · infection · neutropenia · thrombocytopenia
  ► **Uncommon** Skin reactions
  ► **Frequency not known** Hepatitis
  SIDE-EFFECTS, FURTHER INFORMATION Neutropenia reported commonly—discontinue if neutropenia develops.
- CONCEPTION AND CONTRACEPTION Effective contraception must be used during treatment.
- PREGNANCY Manufacturer advises avoid.
- BREAST FEEDING Manufacturer advises avoid—no information available.
- RENAL IMPAIRMENT Caution if eGFR 30–50 mL/minute/1.73 m². Avoid if eGFR less than 30 mL/minute/1.73 m².
- MONITORING REQUIREMENTS Monitor neutrophil count before treatment, then every month for 6 months, then every 3 months.

- PATIENT AND CARER ADVICE
  Blood disorders Patients should be instructed to seek medical advice if symptoms suggestive of neutropenia (such as fever, sore throat, bruising or, bleeding) develop.
- NATIONAL FUNDING/ACCESS DECISIONS
  Scottish Medicines Consortium (SMC) Decisions
  The *Scottish Medicines Consortium* has advised (July 2002) that anakinra is **not** recommended for the treatment of rheumatoid arthritis within NHS Scotland.

- MEDICINAL FORMS
  There can be variation in the licensing of different medicines containing the same drug.
  Solution for injection
  ► Kineret (Swedish Orphan Biovitrum Ltd)
  Anakinra 150 mg per 1 ml Kineret 100mg/0.67ml solution for injection pre-filled syringes | 28 pre-filled disposable injection [PoM] £734.44

Sarilumab

30-Nov-2017

- DRUG ACTION Sarilumab is a recombinant human monoclonal antibody that specifically binds to interleukin-6 receptors and blocks the activity of pro-inflammatory cytokines.

- INDICATIONS AND DOSE
  Moderate-to-severe active rheumatoid arthritis in patients who have had an inadequate response to, or are intolerant to one or more disease-modifying anti-rheumatic drugs (as monotherapy or in combination with methotrexate) (specialist use only)
  ► BY SUBCUTANEOUS INJECTION
  ► Adult: 200 mg every 2 weeks, for dose adjustments due to neutropenia, thrombocytopenia, or liver enzyme elevations—consult product literature

- CONTRA-INDICATIONS Do not initiate if absolute neutrophil count less than 2×10^9/litre · do not initiate if platelet count less than 150×10^3/microlitre · do not initiate if serum transaminases (ALT or AST) greater than 1.5 times the upper limit of normal · severe active infection
- CAUTIONS Chronic or recurrent infection · elderly (increased risk of infection) · history of diverticulitis · history of intestinal ulceration · history of serious or opportunistic infection · predisposition to infection
  CAUTIONS, FURTHER INFORMATION
  ► Infection Manufacturer advises caution in patients who have been exposed to tuberculosis, or who have lived in or travelled to areas of endemic tuberculosis or mycoses. Patients with latent tuberculosis should complete anti-tuberculosis therapy before initiation of sarilumab; consider anti-tuberculosis therapy before initiation of sarilumab in patients with a past history of latent or active tuberculosis in whom an adequate course of treatment cannot be confirmed, and for those with a negative test for latent tuberculosis but have risk factors for tuberculosis—consultation with a tuberculosis specialist may be appropriate.
    Manufacturer advises patients should be brought up-to-date with current immunisation schedule before initiating treatment.
- INTERACTIONS → Appendix 1: monoclonal antibodies
- SIDE-EFFECTS
  ► **Common or very common** Dyslipidaemia · increased risk of infection · neutropenia · thrombocytopenia
  ► **Frequency not known** Hypersensitivity · skin reactions
- CONCEPTION AND CONTRACEPTION Manufacturer advises effective contraception in women of childbearing potential during treatment and for up to 3 months after treatment.

- PREGNANCY Manufacturer advises avoid unless essential—limited information available.
- BREAST FEEDING Manufacturer advises avoid—no information available.
- HEPATIC IMPAIRMENT Manufacturer advises avoid in active hepatic disease or hepatic impairment—no information available.
- PRE-TREATMENT SCREENING Manufacturer advises that patients should be evaluated for tuberculosis before treatment.
- MONITORING REQUIREMENTS
  ▶ Manufacturer advises monitor for signs and symptoms of infection; monitor neutrophil count 4 to 8 weeks after treatment initiation and according to clinical judgement thereafter—discontinue if absolute neutrophil count less than 0.5×10^9/litre.
  ▶ Manufacturer advises monitor platelet count 4 to 8 weeks after treatment initiation and according to clinical judgement thereafter—discontinue if platelet count less than 50×10^3/microlitre.
  ▶ Manufacturer advises monitor hepatic transaminases (ALT and AST) 4 to 8 weeks after treatment initiation and every 3 months thereafter, and consider other liver function tests if clinically indicated—discontinue if ALT is greater than 5 times the upper limit of normal.
  ▶ Manufacturer advises monitor lipid profile approximately 4 to 8 weeks after treatment initiation and approximately every 6 months thereafter—hyperlipidaemia should be managed according to clinical guidelines.
- DIRECTIONS FOR ADMINISTRATION Manufacturer advises to avoid injecting into areas of the skin that are tender, damaged, or have bruises or scars; patients may self-administer *Kevzara®*, after appropriate training in subcutaneous injection technique.
- PRESCRIBING AND DISPENSING INFORMATION Sarilumab is a biological medicine. Biological medicines must be prescribed and dispensed by brand name, see *Biological medicines* and *Biosimilar medicines*, under Guidance on prescribing p. 1; manufacturer advises to record the brand name and batch number after each administration.
- HANDLING AND STORAGE Manufacturer advises store in a refrigerator (2–8°C) and protect from light—consult product literature for further information regarding storage outside refrigerator.
- PATIENT AND CARER ADVICE Manufacturer advises patients should be advised to seek immediate medical attention if symptoms of a hypersensitivity reaction occur. Self-administration Manufacturer advises patients and their carers should be given training in subcutaneous injection technique if appropriate.

  An alert card should be provided.

  Missed doses Manufacturer advises if a dose is more than 3 days late, the missed dose should not be taken and the next dose should be taken at the normal time.
- NATIONAL FUNDING/ACCESS DECISIONS

  NICE decisions
  ▶ Sarilumab for moderate-to-severe rheumatoid arthritis (November 2017) NICE TA485

  Sarilumab, with methotrexate, is recommended as an option for treating active rheumatoid arthritis in adults whose disease has responded inadequately to intensive therapy with a combination of conventional disease-modifying antirheumatic drugs (DMARDs), only if:
- disease is severe (a disease activity score [DAS28] of more than 5.1), **and**
- the manufacturer provides sarilumab with the discount agreed in the patient access scheme.

  Sarilumab, with methotrexate, is recommended as an option for treating active rheumatoid arthritis in adults whose disease has responded inadequately to or who

cannot have other DMARDs, including at least 1 biological DMARD, only if:
- disease is severe (a DAS28 of more than 5.1), **and**
- they cannot have rituximab, **and**
- the manufacturer provides sarilumab with the discount agreed in the patient access scheme.

Sarilumab can be used as monotherapy for people who cannot take methotrexate because it is contra-indicated or because of intolerance, when the above criteria are met.

  Sarilumab, with methotrexate, is recommended as an option for treating active rheumatoid arthritis in adults whose disease has responded inadequately to rituximab and at least 1 biological DMARD, only if:
- disease is severe (a DAS28 of more than 5.1), **and**
- the manufacturer provides sarilumab with the discount agreed in the patient access scheme.

Continue treatment only if there is a moderate response measured using European League Against Rheumatism (EULAR) criteria at 6 months after starting therapy. After an initial response within 6 months, withdraw treatment if at least 1 moderate EULAR response is not maintained.

  Patients whose treatment was started within the NHS before this guidance was published should have the option to continue treatment, without change to their funding arrangements, until they and their NHS clinician consider it appropriate to stop.
www.nice.org.uk/guidance/ta485

Scottish Medicines Consortium (SMC) Decisions
SMC No. 1314/18

The *Scottish Medicines Consortium* has advised (April 2018) that sarilumab (*Kevzara®*) is accepted for restricted use within NHS Scotland for treatment of severely active rheumatoid arthritis (a disease activity score [DAS28] greater than 5.1) that has not responded to intensive therapy with a combination of conventional disease-modifying anti-rheumatic drugs (DMARDs). In patients with severe disease inadequately controlled by a TNF antagonist, it may be used in patients ineligible to receive rituximab. This advice is contingent upon the continuing availability of the patient access scheme in NHS Scotland or a list price that is equivalent or lower.

- MEDICINAL FORMS
There can be variation in the licensing of different medicines containing the same drug.

Solution for injection
CAUTIONARY AND ADVISORY LABELS 10
▶ Kevzara (Sanofi) ▼
  Sarilumab 131.6 mg per 1 ml Kevzara 150mg/1.14ml solution for injection pre-filled syringes | 2 pre-filled disposable injection [PoM] £912.25
  Kevzara 150mg/1.14ml solution for injection pre-filled pen | 2 pre-filled disposable injection [PoM] £912.25
  Sarilumab 175 mg per 1 ml Kevzara 200mg/1.14ml solution for injection pre-filled syringes | 2 pre-filled disposable injection [PoM] £912.25
  Kevzara 200mg/1.14ml solution for injection pre-filled pen | 2 pre-filled disposable injection [PoM] £912.25

Secukinumab

15-Aug-2017

- DRUG ACTION Secukinumab is a recombinant human monoclonal antibody that selectively binds to cytokine interleukin-17A (IL-17A) and inhibits the release of proinflammatory cytokines and chemokines.

- INDICATIONS AND DOSE
Psoriatic arthritis | Ankylosing spondylitis
▶ BY SUBCUTANEOUS INJECTION
  ▶ Adult: 150 mg every week for 5 doses, then maintenance 150 mg every month, review treatment if no response within 16 weeks of initial dose

Psoriatic arthritis with concomitant moderate to severe plaque psoriasis or if inadequate response to anti-TNFα treatment | Plaque psoriasis
‣ BY SUBCUTANEOUS INJECTION
  ‣ Adult: 300 mg every week for 5 doses, then maintenance 300 mg every month, review treatment if no response within 16 weeks of initial dose

● CONTRA-INDICATIONS Severe active infection
● CAUTIONS Chronic infection · Crohn's disease (monitor for exacerbations) · history of recurrent infection · predisposition to infection (discontinue if new serious infection develops)
  CAUTIONS, FURTHER INFORMATION
‣ Tuberculosis Manufacturer advises that patients with latent tuberculosis should complete anti-tuberculosis therapy before starting secukinumab.
● INTERACTIONS → Appendix 1: monoclonal antibodies
● SIDE-EFFECTS
  ‣ Common or very common Diarrhoea · increased risk of infection · rhinorrhoea
  ‣ Uncommon Conjunctivitis · neutropenia (usually mild and reversible) · urticaria
● CONCEPTION AND CONTRACEPTION Manufacturer advises that women of childbearing potential should use effective contraception during treatment and for at least 20 weeks after stopping treatment.
● PREGNANCY Manufacturer advises avoid—no information available.
● BREAST FEEDING Manufacturer advises avoid during treatment and for up to 20 weeks after discontinuing treatment—no information available.
● DIRECTIONS FOR ADMINISTRATION Manufacturer advises to take the syringe or pen out of the refrigerator 20 minutes before administration and to avoid injecting into areas of the skin that show psoriasis. Patients may self-administer *Cosentyx*® pre-filled pen.
● PATIENT AND CARER ADVICE
  Self-administration Patients and their carers should be given training in subcutaneous injection technique.
  Infection Patients and their carers should be advised to seek immediate medical attention if symptoms of infection develop during treatment with secukinumab.
● NATIONAL FUNDING/ACCESS DECISIONS
  NICE decisions
  ‣ Secukinumab for treating moderate to severe plaque psoriasis (July 2015) NICE TA350
  Secukinumab is recommended as an option for the treatment of moderate to severe plaque psoriasis in adults if:
  ● the disease has failed to respond to standard systemic treatments (including ciclosporin, methotrexate, and PUVA), or when standard treatments are contra-indicated or not tolerated; *and*
  ● the manufacturer provides secukinumab with the discount agreed in the patient access scheme
  Secukinumab should be withdrawn in patients whose psoriasis has not responded adequately within 12 weeks of initial dose; further treatment cycles are not recommended.
    Patients whose treatment with secukinumab was started before this guidance was published, but does not meet these criteria, should have the option to continue treatment until they and their clinician consider it appropriate to stop.
  www.nice.org.uk/TA350

‣ Secukinumab for active ankylosing spondylitis after treatment with non-steroidal anti-inflammatory drugs or TNF-alpha inhibitors (September 2016) NICE TA407
Secukinumab is recommended, within its marketing authorisation, as an option for treating active ankylosing spondylitis in adults who have responded inadequately to conventional therapy (non-steroidal anti-inflammatory drugs or TNF-alpha inhibitors) only if the manufacturer provides secukinumab with the discount agreed in the patient access scheme.
  Assess response to secukinumab after 16 weeks of treatment and continue only if there is clear evidence of response, defined as a reduction in the Bath Ankylosing Spondylitis Disease Activity Index (BASDAI) score to 50% of the pre-treatment value or by 2 or more units **and** a reduction in the spinal pain visual analogue scale (VAS) by 2 cm or more.
www.nice.org.uk/TA407

‣ Certolizumab pegol and secukinumab for treating active psoriatic arthritis after inadequate response to DMARDs (May 2017) NICE TA445
Secukinumab alone, or in combination with methotrexate, is recommended as an option for treating active psoriatic arthritis in adults only if:
  ● it is used as described in the NICE technology appraisal guidance on etanercept, infliximab and adalimumab for the treatment of psoriatic arthritis (TA199 recommendations 1.1 and 1.2) or,
  ● the person has had a tumour necrosis factor (TNF)-alpha inhibitor but their disease has not responded within the first 12 weeks or has stopped responding after 12 weeks or,
  ● TNF-alpha inhibitors are contra-indicated but would otherwise be considered.
Secukinumab is only recommended if the manufacturer provides it as agreed in the patient access scheme.
  Assess the response to secukinumab after 16 weeks of treatment. Treatment should only be continued if there is clear evidence of response, defined as an improvement in at least 2 of the 4 Psoriatic Arthritis Response Criteria (PsARC), 1 of which must be joint tenderness or swelling score, with no worsening in any of the 4 criteria. People whose disease has a Psoriasis Area and Severity Index (PASI) 75 response but whose PsARC response does not justify continuing treatment should be assessed by a dermatologist.
  Patients whose treatment was started within the NHS before this guidance was published should have the option to continue treatment, without change to their funding arrangements, until they and their clinician consider it appropriate to stop.
www.nice.org.uk/guidance/TA445

Scottish Medicines Consortium (SMC) Decisions
The *Scottish Medicines Consortium* has advised (June 2015) that secukinumab *(Cosentyx*®) is accepted for restricted use within NHS Scotland for the treatment of moderate to severe plaque psoriasis in adults who have failed to respond to standard systemic therapies (including ciclosporin, methotrexate and phototherapy), or when standard treatments cannot be used because of intolerance or contra-indications.

● MEDICINAL FORMS
There can be variation in the licensing of different medicines containing the same drug.
Solution for injection
‣ Cosentyx (Novartis Pharmaceuticals UK Ltd) ▼
  Secukinumab 150 mg per 1 ml Cosentyx 150mg/1ml solution for injection pre-filled pens | 2 pre-filled disposable injection PoM £1,218.78
  Cosentyx 150mg/1ml solution for injection pre-filled syringes | 2 pre-filled disposable injection PoM ⊠

10

Musculoskeletal system

Tocilizumab

24-May-2018

● INDICATIONS AND DOSE

Rheumatoid arthritis [severe, active and progressive, not previously treated with methotrexate] | Rheumatoid arthritis [moderate-to-severe, in combination with methotrexate or alone if methotrexate inappropriate, when response to at least one disease-modifying antirheumatic drug or tumour necrosis factor inhibitor has been inadequate, or in those who are intolerant of these drugs]

▸ BY INTRAVENOUS INFUSION
▸ Adult: 8 mg/kg every 4 weeks (max. per dose 800 mg), for dose adjustments in patients with liver enzyme abnormalities, or low absolute neutrophil or platelet count—consult product literature
▸ BY SUBCUTANEOUS INJECTION
▸ Adult: 162 mg once weekly, administer to abdomen, thigh or upper arm, for dose adjustments in patients with liver enzyme abnormalities, or low absolute neutrophil or platelet count—consult product literature

Giant cell arteritis [in combination with a tapering course of glucocorticoid or alone following discontinuation of glucocorticoid]

▸ BY SUBCUTANEOUS INJECTION
▸ Adult: 162 mg once weekly, administer to abdomen, thigh or upper arm, for dose adjustments in patients with liver enzyme abnormalities, or low absolute neutrophil or platelet count—consult product literature, not to be used alone for acute relapses; review need for treatment beyond 52 weeks

● CONTRA-INDICATIONS Do not initiate if absolute neutrophil count less than 2×10^9/litre · severe active infection

● CAUTIONS History of diverticulitis · history of intestinal ulceration · history of recurrent or chronic infection (interrupt treatment if serious infection occurs) · low absolute neutrophil count · low platelet count · predisposition to infection (interrupt treatment if serious infection occurs)

CAUTIONS, FURTHER INFORMATION
▸ Tuberculosis Patients with latent tuberculosis should be treated with standard therapy before starting tocilizumab.

● INTERACTIONS → Appendix 1: monoclonal antibodies

● SIDE-EFFECTS
▸ **Common or very common** Abdominal pain · conjunctivitis · cough · dizziness · dyslipidaemia · dyspnoea · gastrointestinal disorders · headache · hypersensitivity · hypertension · increased risk of infection · leucopenia · neutropenia · oral disorders · peripheral oedema · skin reactions · weight increased
▸ **Uncommon** Hypothyroidism · nephrolithiasis
▸ **Frequency not known** Infusion related reaction · interstitial lung disease · pancytopenia · Stevens-Johnson syndrome

SIDE-EFFECTS, FURTHER INFORMATION Discontinue if absolute neutrophil count less than 0.5×10^9/litre or platelet count less than 50×10^3/microlitre).

● CONCEPTION AND CONTRACEPTION Effective contraception required during and for 3 months after treatment.

● PREGNANCY Manufacturer advises avoid unless essential—toxicity in *animal* studies.

● BREAST FEEDING Manufacturer advises avoid—no information available.

● HEPATIC IMPAIRMENT Manufacturer advises caution—consult product literature.

● RENAL IMPAIRMENT
▸ With intravenous use Manufacturer advises monitor renal function closely in moderate-to-severe impairment—no information available.
▸ With subcutaneous use Manufacturer advises monitor renal function closely in severe impairment—no information available.

● PRE-TREATMENT SCREENING
Tuberculosis Patients should be evaluated for tuberculosis before treatment.

● MONITORING REQUIREMENTS
▸ Manufacturer advises monitor lipid profile 4–8 weeks after starting treatment and then as indicated.
▸ Manufacturer advises monitor for demyelinating disorders.
▸ Manufacturer advises monitor hepatic transaminases every 4–8 weeks for first 6 months of treatment, then every 12 weeks thereafter.
▸ Manufacturer advises monitor neutrophil and platelet count 4–8 weeks after starting treatment and then as indicated.

● DIRECTIONS FOR ADMINISTRATION
▸ With intravenous use For *intravenous infusion*, manufacturer advises give intermittently in Sodium chloride 0.9%; dilute requisite dose to a volume of 100 mL with infusion fluid and give over 1 hour.
▸ With subcutaneous use For *subcutaneous injection*, manufacturer advises rotate injection site and avoid skin that is tender, damaged or scarred. Patients may self-administer RoActemra ®, after appropriate training in subcutaneous injection technique.

● PRESCRIBING AND DISPENSING INFORMATION
Manufacturer advises to record the brand name and batch number after each administration.

● HANDLING AND STORAGE Manufacturer advises protect from light and store in a refrigerator (2–8 °C)—consult product literature for further information regarding storage conditions outside refrigerator and after preparation of the infusion.

● PATIENT AND CARER ADVICE Manufacturer advises patients and their carers should be advised to seek immediate medical attention if symptoms of infection occur, or if symptoms of diverticular perforation such as abdominal pain, haemorrhage, or fever accompanying change in bowel habits occur.
An alert card should be provided.
Driving and skilled tasks Manufacturer advises patients should be counselled on the effects on driving and performance of skilled tasks—increased risk of dizziness.

● NATIONAL FUNDING/ACCESS DECISIONS

NICE decisions
▸ **Adalimumab, etanercept, infliximab, certolizumab pegol, golimumab, tocilizumab and abatacept for rheumatoid arthritis not previously treated with DMARDs or after conventional DMARDs only have failed (January 2016)** NICE TA375
Tocilizumab, in combination with methotrexate, is recommended as an option for treating rheumatoid arthritis, only if **all** the following criteria are met:
● disease is severe, that is, a disease activity score (DAS28) greater than 5.1,
● disease has not responded to intensive therapy with a combination of conventional disease-modifying antirheumatic drugs (DMARDs), and
● the manufacturers provide tocilizumab as agreed in the patient access schemes.
Tocilizumab can be used as monotherapy in patients who cannot take methotrexate because it is contra-indicated or because of intolerance, when the criteria above are met.
Continue treatment only if there is a moderate response measured using European League Against Rheumatism

(EULAR) criteria at 6 months after starting therapy. After initial response within 6 months, withdraw treatment if a moderate EULAR response is not maintained.

Patients currently receiving tocilizumab whose disease does not meet the above criteria should have the option to continue their treatment until they and their NHS clinician consider it appropriate to stop.
www.nice.org.uk/guidance/ta375

▸ **Tocilizumab for the treatment of rheumatoid arthritis (updated January 2016)** NICE TA247
Tocilizumab, in combination with methotrexate, is recommended as an option for the treatment of rheumatoid arthritis in adults if:
- the disease has responded inadequately to DMARDs and a TNF inhibitor and the patient cannot receive rituximab because of contra-indications or intolerance, **and** tocilizumab is used as described for TNF inhibitor treatments (specifically the recommendations on disease activity) in the NICE guidance Adalimumab, etanercept, infliximab, rituximab and abatacept for the treatment of rheumatoid arthritis after the failure of a TNF inhibitor (August 2010), *or*
- the disease has responded inadequately to one or more TNF inhibitor treatments and to rituximab
- **and** the manufacturer provides tocilizumab with the discount agreed as part of the patient access scheme.
Patients currently receiving tocilizumab for the treatment of rheumatoid arthritis who do not meet these criteria should have the option to continue treatment until they and their clinicians consider it appropriate to stop.
www.nice.org.uk/guidance/ta247

▸ **Tocilizumab for treating giant cell arteritis (April 2018)** NICE TA518
Tocilizumab, when used with a tapering course of glucocorticoids (and when used alone after glucocorticoids), is recommended as an option for treating giant cell arteritis in adults, only if:
- they have relapsing or refractory disease,
- they have not already had tocilizumab,
- tocilizumab is stopped after 1 year of uninterrupted treatment at most, **and**
- the manufacturer provides it with the discount agreed in the patient access scheme.
Patients whose treatment was started within the NHS before this guidance was published should have the option to continue treatment, without change to their funding arrangements, until they and their NHS clinician consider it appropriate to stop.
www.nice.org.uk/guidance/ta518

● **MEDICINAL FORMS**
There can be variation in the licensing of different medicines containing the same drug.

Solution for injection
▸ RoActemra (Roche Products Ltd)
Tocilizumab 180 mg per 1 ml RoActemra 162mg/0.9ml solution for injection pre-filled syringes | 4 pre-filled disposable injection PoM £913.12 (Hospital only)
RoActemra 162mg/0.9ml solution for injection pre-filled pen | 4 pre-filled disposable injection PoM £913.12

Solution for infusion
ELECTROLYTES: May contain Sodium
▸ RoActemra (Roche Products Ltd)
Tocilizumab 20 mg per 1 ml RoActemra 400mg/20ml concentrate for solution for infusion vials | 1 vial PoM £512.00 (Hospital only)
RoActemra 200mg/10ml concentrate for solution for infusion vials | 1 vial PoM £256.00 (Hospital only)
RoActemra 80mg/4ml concentrate for solution for infusion vials | 1 vial PoM £102.40 (Hospital only)

Ustekinumab
03-Oct-2017

● **INDICATIONS AND DOSE**
Moderate-to-severe plaque psoriasis that has not responded for other systemic treatments or photochemotherapy, or when these treatments cannot be used because of intolerance or contra-indications (specialist use only)
▸ BY SUBCUTANEOUS INJECTION
▸ Adult (body-weight up to 100 kg): Initially 45 mg, then 45 mg after 4 weeks, then 45 mg every 12 weeks, consider discontinuation if no response within 28 weeks
▸ Adult (body-weight 100 kg and above): Initially 90 mg, then 90 mg after 4 weeks, then 90 mg every 12 weeks, consider discontinuation if no response within 28 weeks

Active psoriatic arthritis (in combination with methotrexate or alone) in patients who have had an inadequate response to one or more disease-modifying antirheumatic drugs (specialist use only)
▸ BY SUBCUTANEOUS INJECTION
▸ Adult: Initially 45 mg, then 45 mg after 4 weeks, then 45 mg every 12 weeks, consider discontinuation if no response within 28 weeks, higher doses of 90 mg may be used in patients with body-weight over 100 kg

Moderate to severe active Crohn's disease in patients who have had an inadequate response with, lost response to, are intolerant to, or have contra-indications to either conventional therapy or a tumour necrosis factor alpha inhibitor (specialist use only)
▸ INITIALLY BY INTRAVENOUS INFUSION
▸ Adult (body-weight up to 56 kg): 260 mg, then (by subcutaneous injection) 90 mg after 8 weeks, then (by subcutaneous injection) 90 mg every 12 weeks, if response is inadequate 8 weeks after first subcutaneous dose, or if treatment is interrupted or response is lost, dosing frequency may be increased—consult product literature; review treatment if no response within 16 weeks of initial dose or increase in dosing frequency
▸ Adult (body-weight 56–85 kg): 390 mg, then (by subcutaneous injection) 90 mg after 8 weeks, then (by subcutaneous injection) 90 mg every 12 weeks, if response is inadequate 8 weeks after first subcutaneous dose, or if treatment is interrupted or response is lost, dosing frequency may be increased—consult product literature; review treatment if no response within 16 weeks of initial dose or increase in dosing frequency
▸ Adult (body-weight 86 kg and above): 520 mg, then (by subcutaneous injection) 90 mg after 8 weeks, then (by subcutaneous injection) 90 mg every 12 weeks, if response is inadequate 8 weeks after first subcutaneous dose, or if treatment is interrupted or response is lost, dosing frequency may be increased—consult product literature; review treatment if no response within 16 weeks of initial dose or increase in dosing frequency

● **CONTRA-INDICATIONS** Active infection
● **CAUTIONS** Development of malignancy · elderly · history of malignancy · predisposition to infection · start appropriate treatment if widespread erythema and skin exfoliation develop, and stop ustekinumab treatment if exfoliative dermatitis suspected

CAUTIONS, FURTHER INFORMATION
▸ Tuberculosis Active tuberculosis should be treated with standard treatment for at least 2 months before starting ustekinumab. Patients who have previously received adequate treatment for tuberculosis can start ustekinumab but should be monitored every 3 months for possible recurrence. In patients without active tuberculosis but who were previously not treated adequately,

10

Musculoskeletal system

chemoprophylaxis should ideally be completed before starting ustekinumab. In patients at high risk of tuberculosis who cannot be assessed by tuberculin skin test, chemoprophylaxis can be given concurrently with ustekinumab.

● INTERACTIONS → Appendix 1: monoclonal antibodies

● SIDE-EFFECTS

▶ **Common or very common** Arthralgia · asthenia · back pain · diarrhoea · dizziness · headache · increased risk of infection · myalgia · nausea · oropharyngeal pain · skin reactions · vomiting

▶ **Uncommon** Depression · facial paralysis · hypersensitivity (may be delayed) · nasal congestion

● CONCEPTION AND CONTRACEPTION Manufacturer advises effective contraception during treatment and for 15 weeks after stopping treatment.

● PREGNANCY Avoid.

● BREAST FEEDING Manufacturer advises avoid—present in milk in *animal* studies.

● PRE-TREATMENT SCREENING
Tuberculosis Patients should be evaluated for tuberculosis before treatment.

● MONITORING REQUIREMENTS
▶ Monitor for non-melanoma skin cancer, especially in patients with a history of PUVA treatment or prolonged immunosuppressant therapy, or those over 60 years of age.
▶ Monitor for signs and symptoms of exfoliative dermatitis or erythrodermic psoriasis.

● DIRECTIONS FOR ADMINISTRATION Manufacturer advises for *intravenous infusion* (Stelara®), give intermittently in Sodium Chloride 0.9%; dilute requisite dose with infusion fluid to final volume of 250 mL and give over at least 1 hour through an in-line low-protein binding filter (pore size 0.2 micron); use within 4 hours of dilution.

● PATIENT AND CARER ADVICE
Exfoliative dermatitis Patients should be advised to seek prompt medical attention if symptoms suggestive of exfoliative dermatitis or erythrodermic psoriasis (such as increased redness and shedding of skin over a larger area of the body) develop.
Tuberculosis Patients should be advised to seek medical attention if symptoms suggestive of tuberculosis (e.g. persistent cough, weight loss, and fever) develop.

● NATIONAL FUNDING/ACCESS DECISIONS
NICE decisions
▶ **Ustekinumab for the treatment of adults with moderate to severe psoriasis (updated March 2017)** NICE TA180
Ustekinumab is recommended as a treatment option for adults with plaque psoriasis only if:
● the disease is severe, defined by a total Psoriasis Area Severity Index (PASI) score of 10 or more and a Dermatology Life Quality Index (DLQI) score of 10 or more, **and**
● the psoriasis has not responded to standard systemic therapies (e.g. ciclosporin, methotrexate and psoralen and long-wave ultraviolet radiation), or patients are intolerant to or have a contra-indication to these treatments.
Ustekinumab treatment should be stopped 16 weeks after starting treatment if the psoriasis has not shown a 75% reduction in the PASI score from when treatment started, or a 50% reduction in the PASI score and a 5-point reduction in the DLQI score from when treatment started.
www.nice.org.uk/guidance/TA180

▶ **Ustekinumab for treating active psoriatic arthritis (updated March 2017)** NICE TA340
Ustekinumab is recommended as an option, alone or in combination with methotrexate, for treating active psoriatic arthritis in adults only when:

● treatment with tumour necrosis factor (TNF) alpha inhibitors is contra-indicated but would otherwise be considered, *or*
● the patient has had treatment with 1 or more TNF-alpha inhibitors.
Ustekinumab should be stopped at 24 weeks, if the psoriatic arthritis has not shown adequate response using the Psoriatic Arthritis Response Criteria (PsARC).
Patients currently receiving ustekinumab who do not meet the above criteria and whose treatment was started within the NHS before this guidance was published, should have the option to continue treatment until they and their clinician consider it appropriate to stop.
www.nice.org.uk/guidance/TA340

▶ **Ustekinumab for moderately to severely active Crohn's disease after previous treatment (July 2017)** NICE TA456
Ustekinumab is recommended as an option for treating moderately to severely active Crohn's disease in adults who have had an inadequate response with, lost response to, or were intolerant to either conventional therapy or a TNF-alpha inhibitor or have medical contra-indications to such therapies.
Ustekinumab should be given until treatment failure (including the need for surgery) or until 12 months after the start of treatment, whichever is shorter.
www.nice.org.uk/guidance/TA456

Scottish Medicines Consortium (SMC) Decisions
The *Scottish Medicines Consortium* has advised (February 2014) that ustekinumab (*Stelara®*) is accepted for restricted use within NHS Scotland either alone or in combination with methotrexate, for the treatment of active psoriatic arthritis in adults who have responded inadequately to previous therapy with a non-biological disease-modifying anti-rheumatic drug, and failed on, or are unsuitable for, treatment with a TNF inhibitor.
The *Scottish Medicines Consortium* has advised (July 2017) that ustekinumab (*Stelara®*) is accepted for use within NHS Scotland for the treatment of adults with moderately to severely active Crohn's disease who have had an inadequate response with, lost response to, or were intolerant to either conventional therapy or a tumour necrosis factor-alpha antagonist or have medical contra-indications to such therapies. This advice is contingent upon the continuing availability of the patient access scheme in NHS Scotland or a list price that is equivalent or lower.

● MEDICINAL FORMS
There can be variation in the licensing of different medicines containing the same drug.
Solution for injection
CAUTIONARY AND ADVISORY LABELS 10
▶ Stelara (Janssen-Cilag Ltd)
Ustekinumab 90 mg per 1 ml Stelara 90mg/1ml solution for injection pre-filled syringes | 1 pre-filled disposable injection [PoM] £2,147.00
Stelara 45mg/0.5ml solution for injection vials | 1 vial [PoM] £2,147.00
Stelara 45mg/0.5ml solution for injection pre-filled syringes | 1 pre-filled disposable injection [PoM] £2,147.00
Solution for infusion
CAUTIONARY AND ADVISORY LABELS 10
▶ Stelara (Janssen-Cilag Ltd)
Ustekinumab 5 mg per 1 ml Stelara 130mg/26ml concentrate for solution for infusion vials | 1 vial [PoM] £2,147.00

IMMUNOSUPPRESSANTS > PROTEIN KINASE INHIBITORS

Baricitinib

28-Sep-2017

- **DRUG ACTION** Baricitinib selectively and reversibly inhibits the Janus-associated tyrosine kinases JAK1 and JAK2.

- **INDICATIONS AND DOSE**

  Moderate-to-severe active rheumatoid arthritis in patients who have had an inadequate response to, or are intolerant to, one or more disease-modifying anti-rheumatic drugs (as monotherapy or in combination with methotrexate) (initiated by a specialist)
  - ▸ BY MOUTH
  - ▸ Adult 18-74 years: 4 mg once daily, for dose adjustments due to side-effects or dose reduction due to history of infection or sustained control of disease activity, consult product literature
  - ▸ Adult 75 years and over: 2 mg once daily, for dose adjustments due to side-effects, consult product literature

- **CONTRA-INDICATIONS** Absolute lymphocyte count less than 0.5×10^9 cells/litre (do not initiate) · absolute neutrophil count less than 1×10^9 cells/litre (do not initiate) · active tuberculosis · haemoglobin less than 8 g/dL (do not initiate)

- **CAUTIONS** Active, chronic or recurrent infection (interrupt treatment if no response to standard therapy) · risk of viral reactivation (consult product literature)

  CAUTIONS, FURTHER INFORMATION
  - ▸ Tuberculosis Manufacturer advises consider anti-tuberculosis therapy prior to initiation of baricitinib in patients with previously untreated latent tuberculosis.

- **INTERACTIONS** → Appendix 1: baricitinib

- **SIDE-EFFECTS**
- **Common or very common** Dyslipidaemia · herpes zoster (interrupt treatment) · increased risk of infection · nausea · oropharyngeal pain · thrombocytosis
- ▸ **Uncommon** Acne · neutropenia · weight increased

- **CONCEPTION AND CONTRACEPTION** Manufacturer advises effective contraception during and for at least 1 week after treatment in women of child-bearing potential.

- **PREGNANCY** Manufacturer advises avoid—toxicity in *animal* studies.

- **BREAST FEEDING** Manufacturer advises avoid—present in milk in *animal* studies.

- **HEPATIC IMPAIRMENT** Manufacturer advises avoid in severe impairment—no information available.

- **RENAL IMPAIRMENT** Manufacturer advises avoid if creatinine clearance less than 30 mL/minute.
  Dose adjustments Manufacturer advises reduce dose to 2 mg once daily if creatinine clearance 30–60 mL/minute.

- **PRE-TREATMENT SCREENING** Manufacturer advises patients should be evaluated for tuberculosis and viral hepatitis before treatment.

- **MONITORING REQUIREMENTS**
  - ▸ Manufacturer advises monitor patients with hepatitis B surface antibody and hepatitis B core antibody, without hepatitis B surface antigen, for expression of hepatitis B virus (HBV) DNA—if HBV DNA detected, consult liver specialist for advice.
  - ▸ Manufacturer advises monitor lipid profile 12 weeks after treatment initiation—hyperlipidaemia should be managed according to international clinical guidelines; monitor hepatic transaminases routinely—interrupt treatment if drug-induced liver injury suspected.
  - ▸ Manufacturer advises monitor for haematological abnormalities; interrupt treatment if absolute neutrophil count less than 1×10^9 cells/litre, absolute lymphocyte count less than 0.5×10^9 cells/litre, or haemoglobin less than 8 g/dL—treatment may be restarted when levels return above these values.

- **NATIONAL FUNDING/ACCESS DECISIONS**

  NICE decisions
  - ▸ **Baricitinib for moderate to severe rheumatoid arthritis (August 2017)** NICE TA466
  Baricitinib, with methotrexate, is recommended as an option for treating active rheumatoid arthritis in patients whose disease has responded inadequately to intensive therapy with a combination of conventional disease-modifying antirheumatic drugs (DMARDs), only if:
  - disease is severe (a disease activity score [DAS28] of more than 5.1), **and**
  - the company provides baricitinib with the discount agreed in the patient access scheme (PAS).

  Baricitinib, with methotrexate, is recommended as an option for treating active rheumatoid arthritis in patients whose disease has responded inadequately to or who cannot have other DMARDs, including at least one biological DMARD, only if:
  - disease is severe (a DAS28 of more than 5.1), **and**
  - they cannot have rituximab, **and**
  - the company provides baricitinib with the discount agreed in the PAS.

  Baricitinib can be used as monotherapy for people who cannot take methotrexate because it is contra-indicated or because of intolerance, when the above two sets of criteria are met.

  Continue treatment only if there is a moderate response measured using European League Against Rheumatism (EULAR) criteria at 6 months after starting therapy. After an initial response within 6 months, withdraw treatment if at least a moderate EULAR response is not maintained.

  Patients currently receiving baricitinib whose disease does not meet the above criteria should be able to continue treatment until they and their clinician consider it appropriate to stop.

  www.nice.org.uk/guidance/TA466

  Scottish Medicines Consortium (SMC) Decisions
  The *Scottish Medicines Consortium* has advised (September 2017) that baricitinib (*Olumiant®*) is accepted for restricted use within NHS Scotland for the treatment of active rheumatoid arthritis only if the following criteria are met:
  - disease is severe, that is, a disease activity score (DAS28) greater than 5.1, **and**
  - disease has not responded to intensive therapy with a combination of conventional disease-modifying anti-rheumatic drugs, **or**
  - disease inadequately controlled by a tumour necrosis factor antagonist and patients are ineligible to receive rituximab.

  This advice is contingent upon the continuing availability of the patient access scheme in NHS Scotland or a list price that is equivalent of lower.

- **MEDICINAL FORMS**
  There can be variation in the licensing of different medicines containing the same drug.
  Tablet
  - ▸ Olumiant (Eli Lilly and Company Ltd) ▼
    Baricitinib 2 mg Olumiant 2mg tablets | 28 tablet [PoM] £805.56
    Baricitinib 4 mg Olumiant 4mg tablets | 28 tablet [PoM] £805.56 | 84 tablet [PoM] £2,416.68

10

Musculoskeletal system

Tofacitinib

30-Nov-2017

- **DRUG ACTION** Tofacitinib selectively inhibits the Janus-associated tyrosine kinases JAK1 and JAK3.

- **INDICATIONS AND DOSE**

Moderate-to-severe active rheumatoid arthritis in patients who have had an inadequate response to, or are intolerant to one or more disease-modifying anti-rheumatic drugs (as monotherapy or in combination with methotrexate) (specialist use only)
  - ▸ BY MOUTH
  - ▸ Adult: 5 mg twice daily, for dose adjustments due to side-effects—consult product literature

  DOSE ADJUSTMENTS DUE TO INTERACTIONS
  - ▸ Manufacturer advises reduce dose to 5 mg once daily with concurrent use of potent CYP3A4 inhibitors or drugs which are both moderate CYP3A4 and potent CYP2C19 inhibitors.

- **CONTRA-INDICATIONS** Absolute lymphocyte count less than 750 cells/mm³ (do not initiate) · absolute neutrophil count less than 1000 cells/mm³ (do not initiate) · active infection including localised infection · active tuberculosis · haemoglobin less than 9 g/dL (do not initiate)

- **CAUTIONS** Active, chronic or recurrent infection · elderly · predisposition to infection · previous or current malignancy · raised serum transaminases (particularly in combination with potentially hepatotoxic drugs) · risk of gastrointestinal perforation (new onset abdominal signs and symptoms should be evaluated promptly) · risk of viral reactivation (consult product literature)

  CAUTIONS, FURTHER INFORMATION Manufacturer advises patients should receive all recommended vaccinations before starting treatment (consider prophylactic varicella zoster vaccination); live vaccines should be given at least 2 weeks, but preferably 4 weeks before treatment initiation—consult product literature.
  - ▸ Tuberculosis Manufacturer advises consider anti-tuberculosis therapy prior to initiation of tofacitinib in patients with previously untreated latent tuberculosis.

- **INTERACTIONS** → Appendix 1: tofacitinib

- **SIDE-EFFECTS**
  - ▸ **Common or very common** Anaemia · cough · decreased leucocytes · diarrhoea · dyslipidaemia · dyspnoea · fatigue · fever · gastritis · gastrointestinal discomfort · headache · hypertension · increased risk of infection · insomnia · joint disorders · musculoskeletal pain · nausea · peripheral oedema · skin reactions · vomiting · weight increased
  - ▸ **Uncommon** Dehydration · hepatic steatosis · ligament sprain · muscle strain · neutropenia · non-melanoma skin cancer · paraesthesia · sepsis · sinus congestion · tendinitis
  - ▸ **Rare or very rare** Meningitis cryptococcal

- **CONCEPTION AND CONTRACEPTION** Manufacturer advises effective contraception during and for at least 4 weeks after treatment in women of child-bearing potential.

- **PREGNANCY** Manufacturer advises avoid—toxicity in *animal* studies.

- **BREAST FEEDING** Manufacturer advises avoid—present in milk in *animal* studies.

- **HEPATIC IMPAIRMENT** Manufacturer advises avoid in severe impairment.
  Dose adjustments Manufacturer advises reduce dose to 5 mg once daily in moderate impairment.

- **RENAL IMPAIRMENT**
  Dose adjustments Manufacturer advises reduce dose to 5 mg once daily in severe impairment.

- **PRE-TREATMENT SCREENING** Manufacturer advises patients should be evaluated for tuberculosis and viral hepatitis before treatment.

- **MONITORING REQUIREMENTS**
  - ▸ Manufacturer advises monitor for signs and symptoms of infection during and after treatment.
  - ▸ Manufacturer advises periodic skin examination in patients at increased risk for skin cancer.
  - ▸ Manufacturer advises monitor liver function routinely; monitor lipid profile 8 weeks after treatment initiation.
  - ▸ Manufacturer advises monitor lymphocytes at baseline and every 3 months thereafter; neutrophils and haemoglobin should be monitored at baseline, after 4 to 8 weeks of treatment and every 3 months thereafter.

- **DIRECTIONS FOR ADMINISTRATION** Manufacturer advises tablets may be crushed and taken with water.

- **NATIONAL FUNDING/ACCESS DECISIONS**

NICE decisions
- ▸ **Tofacitinib for moderate-to-severe rheumatoid arthritis (October 2017)** NICE TA480
Tofacitinib, with methotrexate, is recommended as an option for treating active rheumatoid arthritis in adults whose disease has responded inadequately to intensive therapy with a combination of conventional disease-modifying antirheumatic drugs (DMARDs), only if:
  - disease is severe (a disease activity score [DAS28] of more than 5.1), **and**
  - the manufacturer provides tofacitinib with the discount agreed in the patient access scheme.
Tofacitinib, with methotrexate, is recommended as an option for treating active rheumatoid arthritis in adults whose disease has responded inadequately to, or who cannot have, other DMARDs, including at least 1 biological DMARD, only if:
  - disease is severe (a DAS28 of more than 5.1), **and**
  - they cannot have rituximab, **and**
  - the manufacturer provides tofacitinib with the discount agreed in the patient access scheme.
Tofacitinib can be used as monotherapy for adults who cannot take methotrexate because it is contra-indicated or because of intolerance, when the above criteria are met.

  Continue treatment only if there is a moderate response measured using European League Against Rheumatism (EULAR) criteria at 6 months after starting therapy. After an initial response within 6 months, withdraw treatment if at least a moderate EULAR response is not maintained.

  Patients whose treatment was started within the NHS before this guidance was published should have the option to continue treatment, without change to their funding arrangements, until they and their NHS clinician consider it appropriate to stop.
  www.nice.org.uk/guidance/ta480

Scottish Medicines Consortium (SMC) Decisions
The *Scottish Medicines Consortium* has advised (February 2018) that tofacitinib citrate (*Xeljanz®*) is accepted for restricted use within NHS Scotland in combination with methotrexate in adults with severe active rheumatoid arthritis (a disease activity score [DAS28] greater than 5.1) that has not responded to intensive therapy with a combination of conventional disease-modifying anti-rheumatic drugs (DMARDs). In patients with severe disease inadequately controlled by a tumour necrosis factor (TNF) antagonist it may be used in patients ineligible to receive rituximab.

  This advice is contingent upon the continuing availability of the patient access scheme in NHS Scotland or a list price that is equivalent to or lower.

- **MEDICINAL FORMS**
There can be variation in the licensing of different medicines containing the same drug.
Tablet
  - ▸ Xeljanz (Pfizer Ltd) ▼
    Tofacitinib 5 mg Xeljanz 5mg tablets | 56 tablet [PoM] £690.03 (Hospital only)

IMMUNOSUPPRESSANTS > T-CELL ACTIVATION
INHIBITORS

Abatacept

01-Dec-2017

● **INDICATIONS AND DOSE**

Moderate-to-severe active rheumatoid arthritis (specialist use only) | Active psoriatic arthritis (specialist use only)

▸ BY INTRAVENOUS INFUSION

▸ Adult (body-weight up to 60 kg): 500 mg every 2 weeks for 3 doses, then 500 mg every 4 weeks, review treatment if no response within 6 months

▸ Adult (body-weight 60-100 kg): 750 mg every 2 weeks for 3 doses, then 750 mg every 4 weeks, review treatment if no response within 6 months

▸ Adult (body-weight 101 kg and above): 1 g every 2 weeks for 3 doses, then 1 g every 4 weeks, review treatment if no response within 6 months

Moderate-to-severe active rheumatoid arthritis (specialist use only) | Active psoriatic arthritis (specialist use only)

▸ BY SUBCUTANEOUS INJECTION

▸ Adult: 125 mg once weekly, review treatment if no response within 6 months, subcutaneous dosing may be initiated with or without an intravenous loading dose—consult product literature

● **CONTRA-INDICATIONS** Severe infection

● **CAUTIONS** Do not initiate until active infections are controlled · elderly (increased risk of side-effects) · predisposition to infection (screen for latent tuberculosis and viral hepatitis) · progressive multifocal leucoencephalopathy (discontinue treatment if neurological symptoms present)

● **INTERACTIONS** → Appendix 1: abatacept

● **SIDE-EFFECTS**

▸ **Common or very common** Asthenia · cough · diarrhoea · dizziness · gastrointestinal discomfort · headaches · hypertension · increased risk of infection · nausea · oral ulceration · skin reactions · vomiting

▸ **Uncommon** Alopecia · anxiety · arrhythmias · arthralgia · bruising tendency · conjunctivitis · depression · dry eye · dyspnoea · gastritis · hyperhidrosis · hypotension · influenza like illness · leucopenia · menstrual cycle irregularities · musculoskeletal and connective tissue infections and inflammations · pain in extremity · palpitations · paraesthesia · respiratory disorders · sepsis · sleep disorders · throat tightness · thrombocytopenia · vasculitis · vasodilation · vertigo · visual acuity decreased · weight increased

▸ **Rare or very rare** Pelvic inflammatory disease · respiratory malignancy

● **CONCEPTION AND CONTRACEPTION** Effective contraception required during treatment and for 14 weeks after last dose.

● **PREGNANCY** Manufacturer advises avoid unless essential.

● **BREAST FEEDING** Present in milk in *animal* studies—manufacturer advises avoid breast-feeding during treatment and for 14 weeks after last dose.

● **DIRECTIONS FOR ADMINISTRATION** For *intravenous infusion*, given intermittently *in* Sodium chloride 0.9%; reconstitute each vial with 10 mL water for injections using the silicone-free syringe provided; dilute requisite dose in Sodium Chloride 0.9% to 100 mL (using the same silicone-free syringe); give over 30 minutes through a low protein-binding filter (pore size 0.2–1.2 micron).

● **NATIONAL FUNDING/ACCESS DECISIONS**

NICE decisions

▸ **Adalimumab, etanercept, infliximab, rituximab, and abatacept for the treatment of rheumatoid arthritis after the failure of a TNF inhibitor (August 2010)** NICE TA195

Abatacept, in combination with methotrexate, is an option for the treatment of severe active rheumatoid arthritis in adults who have had an inadequate response to, or have an intolerance of, other disease-modifying antirheumatic drugs (DMARDs) including at least 1 tumour necrosis factor (TNF) inhibitor, and who cannot use rituximab because of contra-indications or intolerance. Treatment should be continued only if there is adequate response. Patients should be monitored at least every 6 months.
www.nice.org.uk/TA195

▸ **Adalimumab, etanercept, infliximab, certolizumab pegol, golimumab, tocilizumab and abatacept for rheumatoid arthritis not previously treated with DMARDs or after conventional DMARDs only have failed (January 2016)** NICE TA375

Abatacept, in combination with methotrexate, is recommended as an option for treating rheumatoid arthritis, only if **all** the following criteria are met:

● disease is severe, that is, a disease activity score (DAS28) greater than 5.1,

● disease has not responded to intensive therapy with a combination of conventional disease-modifying antirheumatic drugs (DMARDs),

● the manufacturers provides abatacept as agreed in the patient access schemes.

Continue treatment only if there is a moderate response measured using European League Against Rheumatism (EULAR) criteria at 6 months after starting therapy. After initial response within 6 months, withdraw treatment if a moderate EULAR response is not maintained.

Patients currently receiving abatacept whose disease does not meet the above criteria should have the option to continue their treatment until they and their clinician consider it appropriate to stop.
www.nice.org.uk/TA375

● **MEDICINAL FORMS**
There can be variation in the licensing of different medicines containing the same drug.

Solution for injection

▸ Orencia (Bristol-Myers Squibb Pharmaceuticals Ltd)
Abatacept 125 mg per 1 ml Orencia 125mg/1ml solution for injection pre-filled syringes | 4 pre-filled disposable injection PoM £1,209.60 (Hospital only)

▸ Orencia ClickJect (Bristol-Myers Squibb Pharmaceuticals Ltd)
Abatacept 125 mg per 1 ml Orencia ClickJect 125mg/1ml solution for injection pre-filled pen | 4 pre-filled disposable injection PoM £1,209.60

Powder for solution for infusion

ELECTROLYTES: May contain Sodium

▸ Orencia (Bristol-Myers Squibb Pharmaceuticals Ltd)
Abatacept 250 mg Orencia 250mg powder for concentrate for solution for infusion vials | 1 vial PoM £302.40 (Hospital only)

IMMUNOSUPPRESSANTS > TUMOR NECROSIS
FACTOR ALPHA (TNF-α) INHIBITORS

Adalimumab

21-Feb-2018

● **INDICATIONS AND DOSE**

Plaque psoriasis (initiated by a specialist)

▸ BY SUBCUTANEOUS INJECTION

▸ Adult: Initially 80 mg, then 40 mg every 2 weeks, to be started 1 week after initial dose, review treatment if no response within 16 weeks—consult product literature

continued →

10

Musculoskeletal system

Rheumatoid arthritis (initiated by a specialist)
▸ BY SUBCUTANEOUS INJECTION
▸ Adult: 40 mg every 2 weeks, then increased if necessary to 40 mg once weekly, dose to be increased only in patients receiving adalimumab alone, review treatment if no response within 12 weeks

Psoriatic arthritis (initiated by a specialist) | Ankylosing spondylitis (initiated by a specialist) | Axial spondyloarthritis (initiated by a specialist)
▸ BY SUBCUTANEOUS INJECTION
▸ Adult: 40 mg every 2 weeks, review treatment if no response within 12 weeks

Crohn's disease (initiated by a specialist)
▸ BY SUBCUTANEOUS INJECTION
▸ Adult: Initially 80 mg, then 40 mg after 2 weeks; maintenance 40 mg every 2 weeks, increased if necessary to 40 mg once weekly, maximum 40 mg administered at a single site, review treatment if no response within 12 weeks of initial dose

Crohn's disease (accelerated regimen) (initiated by a specialist)
▸ BY SUBCUTANEOUS INJECTION
▸ Adult: Initially 160 mg, dose can alternatively be given as divided injections over 2 days, then 80 mg after 2 weeks; maintenance 40 mg every 2 weeks, increased if necessary to 40 mg once weekly, maximum 40 mg administered at a single site, review treatment if no response within 12 weeks of initial dose

Ulcerative colitis (initiated by a specialist)
▸ BY SUBCUTANEOUS INJECTION
▸ Adult: Initially 160 mg, dose can alternatively be given as divided injections over 2 days, then 80 mg after 2 weeks; maintenance 40 mg every 2 weeks, increased if necessary to 40 mg once weekly, maximum 40 mg administered at a single site, review treatment if no response within 8 weeks of initial dose

Hidradenitis suppurativa (initiated by a specialist)
▸ BY SUBCUTANEOUS INJECTION
▸ Adult: Initially 160 mg, given as either four 40 mg injections in one day or as two 40 mg injections per day for 2 consecutive days, followed by 80 mg after 2 weeks, given as two 40 mg injections in one day, then 40 mg after 2 weeks; maintenance 40 mg once weekly, review treatment if no response within 12 weeks; if treatment interrupted—consult product literature

Uveitis (initiated by a specialist)
▸ BY SUBCUTANEOUS INJECTION
▸ Adult: Initially 80 mg, given as two 40 mg injections in one day, then 40 mg after 1 week; maintenance 40 mg every 2 weeks

● CONTRA-INDICATIONS Moderate or severe heart failure · severe infection
● CAUTIONS Demyelinating disorders (risk of exacerbation) · development of malignancy · do not initiate until active infections are controlled (discontinue if new serious infection develops) · hepatitis B virus—monitor for active infection · history of malignancy · mild heart failure (discontinue if symptoms develop or worsen) · predisposition to infection
   CAUTIONS, FURTHER INFORMATION
▸ Tuberculosis Active tuberculosis should be treated with standard treatment for at least 2 months before starting adalimumab. Patients who have previously received adequate treatment for tuberculosis can start adalimumab but should be monitored every 3 months for possible recurrence. In patients without active tuberculosis but who were previously not treated adequately, chemoprophylaxis should ideally be completed before starting adalimumab. In patients at high risk of tuberculosis who cannot be assessed by tuberculin skin test, chemoprophylaxis can be given concurrently with adalimumab.

● INTERACTIONS → Appendix 1: monoclonal antibodies
● SIDE-EFFECTS
▸ **Common or very common** Agranulocytosis · alopecia · anaemia · anxiety · arrhythmias · arterial occlusion · asthma · broken nails · chest pain · coagulation disorder · connective tissue disorders · cough · dehydration · depression · dyspnoea · electrolyte imbalance · embolism and thrombosis · eye inflammation · fever · flushing · gastrointestinal discomfort · gastrointestinal disorders · haemorrhage · headaches · healing impaired · hyperglycaemia · hypersensitivity · hypertension · increased risk of infection · insomnia · leucocytosis · leucopenia · mood altered · muscle spasms · musculoskeletal pain · nausea · neoplasms · nerve disorders · neutropenia · oedema · renal impairment · seasonal allergy · sensation abnormal · sepsis · skin reactions · sweat changes · thrombocytopenia · vasculitis · vertigo · vision disorders · vomiting
▸ **Uncommon** Aortic aneurysm · congestive heart failure · demyelinating disorders · dysphagia · erectile dysfunction · gallbladder disorders · hearing impairment · hepatic disorders · inflammation · lupus erythematosus · meningitis viral · myocardial infarction · nocturia · pancreatitis · respiratory disorders · rhabdomyolysis · sarcoidosis · solid organ neoplasm · stroke · tremor
▸ **Rare or very rare** Cardiac arrest · pancytopenia · Stevens-Johnson syndrome
   SIDE-EFFECTS, FURTHER INFORMATION Associated with infections, sometimes severe, including tuberculosis, septicaemia, and hepatitis B reactivation.
● CONCEPTION AND CONTRACEPTION Manufacturer advises effective contraception required during treatment and for at least 5 months after last dose.
● PREGNANCY Avoid.
● BREAST FEEDING Avoid; manufacturer advises avoid for at least 5 months after last dose.
● PRE-TREATMENT SCREENING
   Tuberculosis Patients should be evaluated for tuberculosis before treatment.
● MONITORING REQUIREMENTS
▸ Manufacturer advises monitor for infection before, during, and for 4 months after treatment.
▸ Manufacturer advises monitor for non-melanoma skin cancer before and during treatment, especially in patients with a history of PUVA treatment for psoriasis or extensive immunosuppressant therapy.
▸ For uveitis, manufacturer advises patients should be assessed for pre-existing or developing central demyelinating disorders before and at regular intervals during treatment.
● PRESCRIBING AND DISPENSING INFORMATION
   Adalimumab is a biological medicine. Biological medicines must be prescribed and dispensed by brand name, see Biological medicines and Biosimilar medicines, under Guidance on prescribing p. 1.
● PATIENT AND CARER ADVICE When used to treat hidradenitis suppurativa, patients and their carers should be advised to use a daily topical antiseptic wash on lesions during treatment with adalimumab.
   An alert card should be provided.
   Tuberculosis Patients and their carers should be advised to seek medical attention if symptoms suggestive of tuberculosis (e.g. persistent cough, weight loss, and fever) develop.
   Blood disorders Patients and their carers should be advised to seek medical attention if symptoms suggestive of blood disorders (such as fever, sore throat, bruising, or bleeding) develop.

● NATIONAL FUNDING/ACCESS DECISIONS

NICE decisions

▶ **Adalimumab for plaque psoriasis in adults (June 2008)**
NICE TA146

Adalimumab is recommended for the treatment of severe plaque psoriasis which has failed to respond to standard systemic treatments (including ciclosporin and methotrexate) and photochemotherapy, or when standard treatments cannot be used because of intolerance or contra-indications. Adalimumab should be withdrawn if the response is not adequate after 16 weeks.
www.nice.org.uk/guidance/ta146

▶ **Infliximab and adalimumab for Crohn's disease (May 2010)**
NICE TA187

Adalimumab is recommended for the treatment of severe active Crohn's disease that has not responded to conventional therapy (including corticosteroids and other drugs affecting the immune response) or when conventional therapy cannot be used because of intolerance or contra-indications.

Adalimumab should be given as a planned course of treatment for 12 months or until treatment failure, whichever is shorter. Treatment should be continued beyond 12 months only if there is evidence of active disease—in these cases the need for treatment should be reviewed at least annually. If the disease relapses after stopping treatment, adalimumab can be restarted.
www.nice.org.uk/guidance/ta187

▶ **Infliximab, adalimumab and golimumab for treating moderately to severely active ulcerative colitis after the failure of conventional therapy (February 2015)** NICE TA329

Adalimumab is an option for treating moderately to severely active ulcerative colitis in adults whose disease has responded inadequately to conventional therapy including corticosteroids and mercaptopurine or azathioprine, or in adults who are intolerant to or have contra-indications for conventional therapies.

The choice of treatment should be made on an individual basis and if more than one treatment is suitable, the least expensive should be chosen.

Adalimumab should be given as a planned course of treatment until treatment fails (including the need for surgery) or until 12 months after starting treatment, whichever is shorter. Treatment should be continued only if there is clear evidence of a response. Patients who continue treatment should be reassessed at least every 12 months to determine whether ongoing treatment is still clinically appropriate.
www.nice.org.uk/guidance/ta329

▶ **Etanercept, infliximab, and adalimumab for the treatment of psoriatic arthritis (August 2010)** NICE TA199

Adalimumab is recommended for the treatment of active and progressive psoriatic arthritis in adults who have peripheral arthritis with at least 3 tender joints and at least 3 swollen joints, and who have not responded adequately to at least 2 standard disease-modifying antirheumatic drugs (used alone or in combination).

Adalimumab should be discontinued if there is an inadequate response at 12 weeks.
www.nice.org.uk/guidance/ta199

▶ **Adalimumab, etanercept, infliximab, rituximab, and abatacept for the treatment of rheumatoid arthritis after the failure of a TNF inhibitor (August 2010)** NICE TA195

Adalimumab, in combination with methotrexate, is an option for the treatment of severe active rheumatoid arthritis in adults who have had an inadequate response to, or have an intolerance of, other DMARDs including at least 1 TNF inhibitor, and who cannot use rituximab because of contra-indications or intolerance. In patients who cannot use methotrexate because of intolerance or contra-indications, adalimumab can be given as monotherapy. Treatment should be continued only if there

is adequate response. Patients should be monitored at least every 6 months.
www.nice.org.uk/guidance/ta195

▶ **Adalimumab, etanercept, infliximab, certolizumab pegol, golimumab, tocilizumab and abatacept for rheumatoid arthritis not previously treated with DMARDs or after conventional DMARDs only have failed (January 2016)**
NICE TA375

Adalimumab, in combination with methotrexate, is recommended as an option for treating rheumatoid arthritis, only if the following criteria are met:
● disease is severe, that is, a disease activity score (DAS28) greater than 5.1, **and**,
● disease has not responded to intensive therapy with a combination of conventional disease-modifying antirheumatic drugs (DMARDs).

Adalimumab can be used as monotherapy in patients who cannot take methotrexate because it is contra-indicated or because of intolerance, when the criteria above are met.

Continue treatment only if there is a moderate response measured using European League Against Rheumatism (EULAR) criteria at 6 months after starting therapy. After initial response within 6 months, withdraw treatment if a moderate EULAR response is not maintained.

Patients currently receiving adalimumab whose disease does not meet the above criteria should have the option to continue their treatment until they and their clinician consider it appropriate to stop.
www.nice.org.uk/guidance/ta375

▶ **TNF-alpha inhibitors for ankylosing spondylitis and non-radiographic axial spondyloarthritis (February 2016)**
NICE TA383

Adalimumab, certolizumab pegol, etanercept, golimumab and infliximab are recommended as options for treating severe active ankylosing spondylitis in patients whose disease has responded inadequately to, or who are intolerant of, non-steroidal anti-inflammatory drugs (NSAIDs).

Adalimumab, certolizumab pegol and etanercept are also recommended as options for treating severe non-radiographic axial spondyloarthritis in patients whose disease has responded inadequately to, or who are intolerant of, NSAIDs.

The response to treatment should be assessed 12 weeks after the start of treatment and should only be continued if there is clear evidence of response.

Treatment with another tumour necrosis factor (TNF) -alpha inhibitor is recommended in those who cannot tolerate, or whose disease has not responded to, treatment with the first TNF-alpha inhibitor, or in those whose disease has stopped responding after an initial response.
www.nice.org.uk/guidance/ta383

▶ **Adalimumab for treating moderate-to-severe hidradenitis suppurativa (June 2016)** NICE TA392

Adalimumab is recommended, within its marketing authorisation, as an option for treating active moderate-to-severe hidradenitis suppurativa in adults whose disease has not responded to conventional systemic therapy. The drug is recommended only if the manufacturer provides it at the price agreed in the patient access scheme. Response should be assessed after 12 weeks of treatment, and the drug continued only if there is clear evidence of response, defined as a reduction of 25% or more in the total abscess and inflammatory nodule count and no increase in abscesses and draining fistulas.
www.nice.org.uk/guidance/ta392

▶ **Adalimumab and dexamethasone for treating non-infectious uveitis (July 2017)** NICE TA460

Adalimumab is recommended as an option for treating non-infectious uveitis in the posterior segment of the eye in adults with inadequate response to corticosteroids, only if there is:

10

Musculoskeletal system

- active disease (that is, current inflammation in the eye), **and**
- inadequate response or intolerance to immunosuppressants, **and**
- systemic disease or both eyes are affected (or one eye is affected if the second eye has poor visual acuity), **and**
- worsening vision with a high risk of blindness (for example, risk of blindness that is similar to that seen in people with macular oedema).

Stop adalimumab for non-infectious uveitis in the posterior segment of the eye in adults with inadequate response to corticosteroids if there is one of the following:
- new active inflammatory chorioretinal or inflammatory retinal vascular lesions, or both, **or**
- a two-step increase in vitreous haze or anterior chamber cell grade, **or**
- worsening of best corrected visual acuity by three or more lines or 15 letters.

Patients currently receiving adalimumab whose disease does not meet the above criteria should be able to continue treatment until they and their clinician consider it appropriate to stop.

www.nice.org.uk/guidance/ta460

Scottish Medicines Consortium (SMC) Decisions

The *Scottish Medicines Consortium* issued similar advice for plaque psoriasis to NICE TA146 in May 2008.

- **MEDICINAL FORMS**
  There can be variation in the licensing of different medicines containing the same drug.
  Solution for injection
  CAUTIONARY AND ADVISORY LABELS 10
  ▸ Humira (AbbVie Ltd)
  Adalimumab 50 mg per 1 ml Humira 40mg/0.8ml solution for injection vials | 2 vial [PoM] £704.28
  Adalimumab 100 mg per 1 ml Humira 40mg/0.4ml solution for injection pre-filled pen | 2 pre-filled disposable injection [PoM] £704.28 DT = £704.28
  Humira 20mg/0.2ml solution for injection pre-filled syringes | 2 pre-filled disposable injection [PoM] £352.14
  Humira 40mg/0.4ml solution for injection pre-filled syringes | 2 pre-filled disposable injection [PoM] £704.28 DT = £704.28

Certolizumab pegol

07-Aug-2017

- **INDICATIONS AND DOSE**

  Moderate to severe active rheumatoid arthritis when response to disease-modifying antirheumatic drugs (including methotrexate) has been inadequate (as monotherapy or in combination with methotrexate) | Severe, active and progressive rheumatoid arthritis in patients not previously treated with methotrexate or other disease-modifying antirheumatic drugs (in combination with methotrexate) | Active psoriatic arthritis when response to disease-modifying antirheumatic drugs has been inadequate (as monotherapy or in combination with methotrexate)
  ▸ BY SUBCUTANEOUS INJECTION
  ▸ Adult: Loading dose 400 mg every 2 weeks for 3 doses, then maintenance 200 mg every 2 weeks, once clinical response is confirmed, an alternative maintenance dosing of 400 mg every 4 weeks can be considered, review treatment if no response within 12 weeks

Treatment of severe active ankylosing spondylitis in patients who have had an inadequate response to, or are intolerant of NSAIDs | Treatment of severe active axial spondyloarthritis, without radiographic evidence of ankylosing spondylitis but with objective signs of inflammation, in patients who have had an inadequate response to, or are intolerant of NSAIDs
▸ BY SUBCUTANEOUS INJECTION
▸ Adult: Loading dose 400 mg every 2 weeks for 3 doses, then maintenance 200 mg every 2 weeks, alternatively maintenance 400 mg every 4 weeks, review treatment if no response within 12 weeks

- **CONTRA-INDICATIONS** Moderate to severe heart failure · severe active infection

- **CAUTIONS** Demyelinating CNS disorders (risk of exacerbation) · do not initiate until active infections are controlled (discontinue if new serious infection develops and until infection controlled) · hepatitis B virus (monitor for active infection) · history or development of malignancy · mild heart failure (discontinue if symptoms develop or worsen) · predisposition to infection
  CAUTIONS, FURTHER INFORMATION
  ▸ Tuberculosis Active tuberculosis should be treated with standard treatment for at least 2 months before starting certolizumab pegol. Patients who have previously received adequate treatment for tuberculosis can start certolizumab pegol but should be monitored every 3 months for possible recurrence. In patients without active tuberculosis but who were previously not treated adequately, chemoprophylaxis should ideally be completed before starting certolizumab pegol. In patients at high risk of tuberculosis who cannot be assessed by tuberculin skin test, chemoprophylaxis can be given concurrently with certolizumab pegol.

- **INTERACTIONS** → Appendix 1: monoclonal antibodies

- **SIDE-EFFECTS**
  ▸ **Common or very common** Abscess · asthenia · decreased leucocytes · eosinophilic disorders · fever · headaches · hepatic disorders · hypertension · increased risk of infection · nausea · neoplasms · neutropenia · pain · sensory disorder · skin reactions
  ▸ **Uncommon** Alopecia · anaemia · anxiety · appetite disorder · arrhythmias · ascites · asthma · breast disorder · cardiomyopathy · chills · coronary artery disease · cough · cyst · dizziness · dyslipidaemia · electrolyte imbalance · embolism and thrombosis · eye inflammation · flushing · gastrointestinal discomfort · gastrointestinal disorders · haemorrhage · healing impaired · heart failure · hypercoagulation · influenza like illness · lacrimation disorder · lymphadenopathy · menstrual cycle irregularities · mood disorder · muscle disorder · nail disorder · nerve disorders · oedema · oral disorders · oropharyngeal dryness · palpitations · photosensitivity reaction · renal impairment · respiratory disorders · sepsis · skin ulcer · solid organ neoplasm · sweat changes · syncope · systemic lupus erythematosus (SLE) · temperature perception abnormal · thrombocytopenia · thrombocytosis · tinnitus · tremor · urinary tract disorder · vasculitides · vertigo · vision disorders · weight change
  ▸ **Rare or very rare** Atherosclerosis · atrioventricular block · cholelithiasis · cognitive impairment · delirium · fistula · haemosiderosis · hair texture abnormal · movement disorders · nephritis · nephropathy · odynophagia · pancytopenia · panniculitis · pericarditis · polycythaemia · Raynaud's phenomenon · sarcoidosis · seizure · serum sickness · sexual dysfunction · splenomegaly · stroke · suicide attempt · telangiectasia · thyroid disorder
  ▸ **Frequency not known** Multiple sclerosis

SIDE-EFFECTS, FURTHER INFORMATION Associated with infections, sometimes severe, including tuberculosis, septicaemia, and hepatitis B reactivation.

● CONCEPTION AND CONTRACEPTION Manufacturer advises adequate contraception during treatment and for at least 5 months after last dose.

● PREGNANCY Avoid.

● BREAST FEEDING Manufacturer advises use only if potential benefit outweighs risk—no information available.

● PRE-TREATMENT SCREENING
Tuberculosis Patients should be evaluated for tuberculosis before treatment.

● MONITORING REQUIREMENTS Monitor for infection before, during, and for 5 months after treatment.

● PATIENT AND CARER ADVICE An alert card should be provided.
Blood disorders Patients should be advised to seek medical attention if symptoms suggestive of blood disorders (such as fever, sore throat, bruising, or bleeding) develop.
Tuberculosis Patients should be advised to seek medical attention if symptoms suggestive of tuberculosis (e.g persistent cough, weight loss and fever) develop.

● NATIONAL FUNDING/ACCESS DECISIONS
NICE decisions
▸ **Adalimumab, etanercept, infliximab, certolizumab pegol, golimumab, tocilizumab and abatacept for rheumatoid arthritis not previously treated with DMARDs or after conventional DMARDs only have failed (January 2016)** NICE TA375
Certolizumab pegol, in combination with methotrexate, is recommended as an option for treating rheumatoid arthritis, only if the following criteria are met:
● disease is severe, that is, a disease activity score (DAS28) greater than 5.1,
● disease has not responded to intensive therapy with a combination of conventional disease-modifying antirheumatic drugs (DMARDs),
● the manufacturers provide certolizumab pegol as agreed in the patient access schemes.
Certolizumab pegol can be used as monotherapy in patients who cannot take methotrexate because it is contra-indicated or because of intolerance, when the criteria above are met.
   Continue treatment only if there is a moderate response measured using European League Against Rheumatism (EULAR) criteria at 6 months after starting therapy. After initial response within 6 months, withdraw treatment if a moderate EULAR response is not maintained.
   Patients currently receiving certolizumab pegol within the NHS whose disease does not meet the above criteria should have the option to continue their treatment until they and their clinician consider it appropriate to stop. www.nice.org.uk/TA375

▸ **TNF-alpha inhibitors for ankylosing spondylitis and non-radiographic axial spondyloarthritis (February 2016)** NICE TA383
Adalimumab, certolizumab pegol, etanercept, golimumab and infliximab are recommended as options for treating severe active ankylosing spondylitis in adult patients whose disease has responded inadequately to, or who are intolerant of, non-steroidal anti-inflammatory drugs.
   Adalimumab, certolizumab pegol and etanercept are also recommended as options for treating severe non-radiographic axial spondyloarthritis in patients whose disease has responded inadequately to, or who are intolerant of, non-steroidal anti-inflammatory drugs (NSAIDs).
   The response to treatment should be assessed 12 weeks after the start of treatment. Treatment should only be continued if there is clear evidence of response.

Treatment with another tumour necrosis factor (TNF)-alpha inhibitor is recommended in those who cannot tolerate, or whose disease has not responded to, treatment with the first TNF-alpha inhibitor, or in those whose disease has stopped responding after an initial response. www.nice.org.uk/TA383

▸ **Certolizumab pegol for treating rheumatoid arthritis after inadequate response to a TNF-alpha inhibitor (October 2016)** NICE TA415
Certolizumab pegol, in combination with methotrexate, or as monotherapy, is recommended as an option for treating active rheumatoid arthritis in adults who have had an inadequate response to, or who cannot tolerate, other disease-modifying antirheumatic drugs (DMARDs) including at least 1 tumour necrosis factor-alpha (TNF-alpha) inhibitor, only if the following criteria are met:
● disease activity is severe **and**
● rituximab is contra-indicated or not tolerated, or if monotherapy, rituximab cannot be given because methotrexate is contra-indicated or not tolerated **and**
● the manufacturers provide certolizumab pegol as agreed in the patient access scheme.
Continue treatment only if there is at least a moderate response measured using European League Against Rheumatism (EULAR) criteria at 6 months after starting therapy. After initial response within 6 months, withdraw treatment if at least a moderate EULAR response is not maintained.
   Patients whose treatment was started within the NHS before this guidance was published should have the option to continue treatment, without change to their funding arrangements, until they and their clinician consider it appropriate to stop. www.nice.org.uk/TA415

▸ **Certolizumab pegol and secukinumab for treating active psoriatic arthritis after inadequate response to DMARDs (May 2017)** NICE TA445
Certolizumab pegol alone, or in combination with methotrexate, is recommended as an option for treating active psoriatic arthritis in adults only if:
● it is used as described in the NICE technology appraisal guidance on etanercept, infliximab and adalimumab for the treatment of psoriatic arthritis (TA199 recommendations 1.1 and 1.2) or,
● the person has had a tumour necrosis factor (TNF)-alpha inhibitor but their disease has stopped responding after the first 12 weeks.
Certolizumab pegol is only recommended if the manufacturer provides it as agreed in the patient access scheme.
   Assess the response to treatment after 12 weeks. Treatment should only be continued if there is clear evidence of response, defined as an improvement in at least 2 of the 4 Psoriatic Arthritis Response Criteria (PsARC), 1 of which must be joint tenderness or swelling score, with no worsening in any of the 4 criteria. People whose disease has a Psoriasis Area and Severity Index (PASI) 75 response but whose PsARC response does not justify continuing treatment should be assessed by a dermatologist.
   Patients whose treatment was started within the NHS before this guidance was published should have the option to continue treatment, without change to their funding arrangements, until they and their clinician consider it appropriate to stop. www.nice.org.uk/guidance/TA445

Scottish Medicines Consortium (SMC) Decisions
The *Scottish Medicines Consortium* has advised (July 2014) that certolizumab pegol is accepted for restricted use within NHS Scotland, in combination with methotrexate, for the treatment of active psoriatic arthritis in patients

whose disease has not responded to adequate trials of at least two standard disease-modifying antirheumatic drugs (DMARDs), administered either individually or in combination.

- MEDICINAL FORMS
There can be variation in the licensing of different medicines containing the same drug.
Solution for injection
CAUTIONARY AND ADVISORY LABELS 10
▸ Cimzia (UCB Pharma Ltd)
Certolizumab pegol 200 mg per 1 ml Cimzia 200mg/1ml solution for injection pre-filled pen | 2 pre-filled disposable injection [PoM] £715.00
Cimzia 200mg/1ml solution for injection pre-filled syringes | 2 syringe [PoM] £715.00

Etanercept

14-Sep-2017

- INDICATIONS AND DOSE
BENEPALI ® SOLUTION FOR INJECTION
Moderate-to-severe active rheumatoid arthritis (alone or in combination with methotrexate) when the response to other disease-modifying antirheumatic drugs is inadequate | Severe, active and progressive rheumatoid arthritis not previously treated with methotrexate | Active and progressive psoriatic arthritis when the response to other disease-modifying antirheumatic drugs is inadequate | Severe active ankylosing spondylitis when the response to conventional therapy is inadequate | Severe, non-radiographic axial spondyloarthritis when the response to non-steroidal anti-inflammatory drugs is inadequate
▸ BY SUBCUTANEOUS INJECTION
▸ Adult: 50 mg once weekly, review treatment if no response within 12 weeks of initial dose
Moderate-to-severe plaque psoriasis when the response to other systemic therapies or psoralen and ultraviolet-A light (PUVA) is inadequate, or when these therapies cannot be used because of intolerance or contra-indications
▸ BY SUBCUTANEOUS INJECTION
▸ Adult: 50 mg once weekly, alternatively 50 mg twice weekly for up to 12 weeks, followed by 50 mg once weekly if required continue treatment for up to 24 weeks—continuous therapy beyond 24 weeks may be appropriate in some patients (consult product literature), discontinue if no response after 12 weeks

ENBREL ® POWDER AND SOLVENT FOR SOLUTION FOR INJECTION
Moderate-to-severe active rheumatoid arthritis (alone or in combination with methotrexate) when the response to other disease-modifying antirheumatic drugs is inadequate | Severe, active and progressive rheumatoid arthritis not previously treated with methotrexate | Active and progressive psoriatic arthritis when the response to other disease-modifying antirheumatic drugs is inadequate | Severe active ankylosing spondylitis when the response to conventional therapy is inadequate | Severe, non-radiographic axial spondyloarthritis when the response to non-steroidal anti-inflammatory drugs is inadequate
▸ BY SUBCUTANEOUS INJECTION
▸ Adult: 25 mg twice weekly, alternatively 50 mg once weekly, review treatment if no response within 12 weeks of initial dose

Moderate-to-severe plaque psoriasis when the response to other systemic therapies or psoralen and ultraviolet-A light (PUVA) is inadequate, or when these therapies cannot be used because of intolerance or contra-indications
▸ BY SUBCUTANEOUS INJECTION
▸ Adult: 25 mg twice weekly, alternatively 50 mg once weekly, alternatively 50 mg twice weekly for up to 12 weeks, followed by 25 mg twice weekly, alternatively 50 mg once weekly if required continue treatment for up to 24 weeks—continuous therapy beyond 24 weeks may be appropriate in some patients (consult product literature), discontinue if no response after 12 weeks

ENBREL ® SOLUTION FOR INJECTION
Moderate-to-severe active rheumatoid arthritis (alone or in combination with methotrexate) when the response to other disease-modifying antirheumatic drugs is inadequate | Severe, active and progressive rheumatoid arthritis not previously treated with methotrexate | Active and progressive psoriatic arthritis when the response to other disease-modifying antirheumatic drugs is inadequate | Severe active ankylosing spondylitis when the response to conventional therapy is inadequate | Severe, non-radiographic axial spondyloarthritis when the response to non-steroidal anti-inflammatory drugs is inadequate
▸ BY SUBCUTANEOUS INJECTION
▸ Adult: 25 mg twice weekly, alternatively 50 mg once weekly, review treatment if no response within 12 weeks of initial dose

Moderate-to-severe plaque psoriasis when the response to other systemic therapies or psoralen and ultraviolet-A light (PUVA) is inadequate, or when these therapies cannot be used because of intolerance or contra-indications
▸ BY SUBCUTANEOUS INJECTION
▸ Adult: 25 mg twice weekly, alternatively 50 mg once weekly, alternatively 50 mg twice weekly for up to 12 weeks, followed by 25 mg twice weekly, alternatively 50 mg once weekly if required continue treatment for up to 24 weeks—continuous therapy beyond 24 weeks may be appropriate in some patients (consult product literature), discontinue if no response after 12 weeks

- CONTRA-INDICATIONS Active infection
- CAUTIONS Development of malignancy · diabetes mellitus · heart failure (risk of exacerbation) · hepatitis B virus—monitor for active infection · hepatitis C infection (monitor for worsening infection) · history of blood disorders · history of malignancy · history or increased risk of demyelinating disorders · predisposition to infection (avoid if predisposition to septicaemia) · significant exposure to herpes zoster virus—interrupt treatment and consider varicella–zoster immunoglobulin
CAUTIONS, FURTHER INFORMATION
▸ Tuberculosis Active tuberculosis should be treated with standard treatment for at least 2 months before starting etanercept. Patients who have previously received adequate treatment for tuberculosis can start etanercept but should be monitored every 3 months for possible recurrence. In patients without active tuberculosis but who were previously not treated adequately, chemoprophylaxis should ideally be completed before starting etanercept. In patients at high risk of tuberculosis who cannot be assessed by tuberculin skin test, chemoprophylaxis can be given concurrently with etanercept.
- INTERACTIONS → Appendix 1: etanercept

- SIDE-EFFECTS
▸ **Common or very common** Cystitis · fever · hypersensitivity · increased risk of infection (frequency not known in children) · pain · skin reactions · swelling
▸ **Uncommon** Abscess · bursitis · cholecystitis · diarrhoea · endocarditis · eye inflammation · gastritis · hepatic disorders · myositis · neoplasms · respiratory disorders · sepsis (frequency not known in children) · skin ulcers · thrombocytopenia · vasculitis
▸ **Rare or very rare** Anaemia · bone marrow disorders · congestive heart failure · cutaneous lupus erythematosus · demyelination · leucopenia · lupus-like syndrome · nerve disorders · neutropenia · sarcoidosis · seizure · severe cutaneous adverse reactions (SCARs) · transverse myelitis
▸ **Frequency not known** Dermatomyositis exacerbated · hepatitis B reactivation

SIDE-EFFECTS, FURTHER INFORMATION Associated with infections, sometimes severe, including tuberculosis, septicaemia, and hepatitis B reactivation.

● CONCEPTION AND CONTRACEPTION Manufacturer advises effective contraception required during treatment and for 3 weeks after last dose.
● PREGNANCY Avoid—limited information available.
● BREAST FEEDING Manufacturer advises avoid—present in milk in *animal* studies.
● HEPATIC IMPAIRMENT Use with caution in moderate to severe alcoholic hepatitis.
● PRE-TREATMENT SCREENING
Tuberculosis Patients should be evaluated for tuberculosis before treatment.
● MONITORING REQUIREMENTS Monitor for skin cancer before and during treatment, particularly in those at risk (including patients with psoriasis or a history of PUVA treatment).
● PRESCRIBING AND DISPENSING INFORMATION Etanercept is a biological medicine. Biological medicines must be prescribed and dispensed by brand name, see *Biological medicines* and *Biosimilar medicines*, under Guidance on prescribing p. 1.
● PATIENT AND CARER ADVICE An alert card should be provided.
Blood disorders Patients and their carers should be advised to seek medical attention if symptoms suggestive of blood disorders (such as fever, sore throat, bruising, or bleeding) develop.
Tuberculosis Patients and their carers should be advised to seek medical attention if symptoms suggestive of tuberculosis (e.g. persistent cough, weight loss, and fever) develop.
● NATIONAL FUNDING/ACCESS DECISIONS

NICE decisions

▸ **Etanercept and efalizumab for plaque psoriasis (July 2006)** NICE TA103
Etanercept is recommended for severe plaque psoriasis which has failed to respond to standard systemic treatments (including ciclosporin and methotrexate) and to photochemotherapy, or when standard treatments cannot be used because of intolerance or contra-indications. Etanercept should be withdrawn if the response is not adequate after 12 weeks.
www.nice.org.uk/TA103

▸ **Adalimumab, etanercept, infliximab, rituximab, and abatacept for the treatment of rheumatoid arthritis after the failure of a TNF inhibitor (August 2010)** NICE TA195
Etanercept, in combination with methotrexate, is an option for the treatment of severe active rheumatoid arthritis in adults who have had an inadequate response to, or have an intolerance of, other DMARDs including at least 1 TNF inhibitor, and who cannot use rituximab because of contra-indications or intolerance. In patients

who cannot use methotrexate because of intolerance or contra-indications, etanercept can be given as monotherapy. Treatment should be continued only if there is adequate response. Patients should be monitored at least every 6 months.
www.nice.org.uk/TA195

▸ **Etanercept, infliximab, and adalimumab for the treatment of psoriatic arthritis (August 2010)** NICE TA199
Etanercept is recommended for the treatment of active and progressive psoriatic arthritis in adults who have peripheral arthritis with at least 3 tender joints and at least 3 swollen joints, and who have not responded adequately to at least 2 standard disease-modifying antirheumatic drugs (used alone or in combination).
Etanercept should be discontinued if there is an inadequate response at 12 weeks.
www.nice.org.uk/TA199

▸ **Adalimumab, etanercept, infliximab, certolizumab pegol, golimumab, tocilizumab and abatacept for rheumatoid arthritis not previously treated with DMARDs or after conventional DMARDs only have failed (January 2016)** NICE TA375
Etanercept, in combination with methotrexate, is recommended as an option for treating rheumatoid arthritis, only if the following criteria are met:
● disease is severe, that is, a disease activity score (DAS28) greater than 5.1, **and**
● disease has not responded to intensive therapy with a combination of conventional disease-modifying antirheumatic drugs (DMARDs)
Etanercept can be used as monotherapy in patients who cannot take methotrexate because it is contra-indicated or because of intolerance, when the criteria above are met.
Continue treatment only if there is a moderate response measured using European League Against Rheumatism (EULAR) criteria at 6 months after starting therapy. After initial response within 6 months, withdraw treatment if a moderate EULAR response is not maintained.
Patients currently receiving etanercept whose disease does not meet the above criteria should have the option to continue their treatment until they and their clinician consider it appropriate to stop.
www.nice.org.uk/TA375

▸ **TNF-alpha inhibitors for ankylosing spondylitis and non-radiographic axial spondyloarthritis (February 2016)** NICE TA383
Etanercept is recommended as an option for treating severe active ankylosing spondylitis in patients whose disease has responded inadequately to, or who are intolerant of, non-steroidal anti-inflammatory drugs (NSAIDs).
Etanercept is also recommended as an option for treating severe non-radiographic axial spondyloarthritis in patients whose disease has responded inadequately to, or who are intolerant of, NSAIDs.
The response to treatment should be assessed 12 weeks after the start of treatment and should only be continued if there is clear evidence of response.
Treatment with another tumour necrosis factor (TNF)-alpha inhibitor is recommended in those who cannot tolerate, or whose disease has not responded to, treatment with the first TNF-alpha inhibitor, or in those whose disease has stopped responding after an initial response.
www.nice.org.uk/TA383

● MEDICINAL FORMS
There can be variation in the licensing of different medicines containing the same drug.
Solution for injection
CAUTIONARY AND ADVISORY LABELS 10
▸ Benepali (Biogen Idec Ltd) ▼
Etanercept 50 mg per 1 ml Benepali 50mg/1ml solution for injection pre-filled syringes | 4 pre-filled disposable injection [PoM] £656.00

Benepali 50mg/1ml solution for injection pre-filled pen | 4 pre-filled disposable injection [PoM] £656.00

▸ Enbrel (Pfizer Ltd)
Etanercept 50 mg per 1 ml Enbrel 50mg/1ml solution for injection pre-filled syringes | 4 pre-filled disposable injection [PoM] £715.00 (Hospital only)
Enbrel 25mg/0.5ml solution for injection pre-filled syringes | 4 pre-filled disposable injection [PoM] £357.50 (Hospital only)

▸ Enbrel MyClic (Pfizer Ltd)
Etanercept 50 mg per 1 ml Enbrel 50mg/1ml solution for injection pre-filled MyClic pen | 4 pre-filled disposable injection [PoM] £715.00 (Hospital only)
Enbrel 25mg/0.5ml solution for injection pre-filled MyClic pen | 4 pre-filled disposable injection [PoM] £357.50 (Hospital only)

Powder and solvent for solution for injection
CAUTIONARY AND ADVISORY LABELS 10
EXCIPIENTS: May contain Benzyl alcohol

▸ Enbrel (Pfizer Ltd)
Etanercept 10 mg Enbrel Paediatric 10mg powder and solvent for solution for injection vials | 4 vial [PoM] £143.00 (Hospital only)
Etanercept 25 mg Enbrel 25mg powder and solvent for solution for injection vials | 4 vial [PoM] £357.50 (Hospital only)

Golimumab

01-Mar-2018

● INDICATIONS AND DOSE
Ulcerative colitis (initiated by a specialist)
▸ BY SUBCUTANEOUS INJECTION
▸ Adult (body-weight up to 80 kg): Initially 200 mg, then 100 mg after 2 weeks; maintenance 50 mg every 4 weeks, review treatment if no response after 4 doses
▸ Adult (body-weight 80 kg and above): Initially 200 mg, then 100 mg after 2 weeks; maintenance 100 mg every 4 weeks, review treatment if no response after 4 doses

Rheumatoid arthritis (initiated by a specialist) | Psoriatic arthritis (initiated by a specialist) | Ankylosing spondylitis (initiated by a specialist) | Non-radiographic axial spondyloarthritis (initiated by a specialist)
▸ BY SUBCUTANEOUS INJECTION
▸ Adult (body-weight up to 100 kg): 50 mg once a month, on the same date each month, review treatment if no response after 3–4 doses
▸ Adult (body-weight 100 kg and above): Initially 50 mg once a month for 3–4 doses, on the same date each month, dose may be increased if inadequate response, increased to 100 mg once a month, review treatment if inadequate response to this higher dose after 3–4 doses

● CONTRA-INDICATIONS Moderate or severe heart failure · severe active infection

● CAUTIONS Active infection (do not initiate until active infections are controlled; discontinue if new serious infection develops until infection controlled) · demyelinating disorders (risk of exacerbation) · hepatitis B virus—monitor for active infection · history or development of malignancy · mild heart failure (discontinue if symptoms develop or worsen) · predisposition to infection · risk factors for dysplasia or carcinoma of the colon—screen for dysplasia regularly

CAUTIONS, FURTHER INFORMATION
▸ Tuberculosis Active tuberculosis should be treated with standard treatment for at least 2 months before starting golimumab. Patients who have previously received adequate treatment for tuberculosis can start golimumab but should be monitored every 3 months for possible recurrence. In patients without active tuberculosis but who were previously not treated adequately, chemoprophylaxis should ideally be completed before starting golimumab. In patients at high risk of tuberculosis who cannot be assessed by tuberculin skin test, chemoprophylaxis can be given concurrently with golimumab. Patients who have tested negative for latent

tuberculosis, and those who are receiving or who have completed treatment for latent tuberculosis, should be monitored closely for symptoms of active infection.

● INTERACTIONS → Appendix 1: monoclonal antibodies

● SIDE-EFFECTS
▸ **Common or very common** Abscess · alopecia · anaemia · asthenia · asthma · bone fracture · chest discomfort · depression · dizziness · fever · gastrointestinal discomfort · gastrointestinal disorders · gastrointestinal inflammatory disorders · headache · hypersensitivity · hypertension · increased risk of infection · insomnia · nausea · paraesthesia · respiratory disorders · skin reactions · stomatitis
▸ **Uncommon** Arrhythmia · balance impaired · bone marrow disorders · breast disorder · cholelithiasis · constipation · eye inflammation · eye irritation · flushing · goitre · hyperthyroidism · hypothyroidism · leucopenia · liver disorder · menstrual disorder · myocardial ischaemia · neoplasms · sepsis · thrombocytopenia · thrombosis · thyroid disorder · vision disorders
▸ **Rare or very rare** Bladder disorder · congestive heart failure · demyelination · healing impaired · hepatitis B reactivation · lupus-like syndrome · Raynaud's phenomenon · renal disorder · sarcoidosis · taste altered · vasculitis

SIDE-EFFECTS, FURTHER INFORMATION Associated with infections, sometimes severe, including tuberculosis, septicaemia, and hepatitis B reactivation.

● CONCEPTION AND CONTRACEPTION Manufacturer advises adequate contraception during treatment and for at least 6 months after last dose.

● PREGNANCY Use only if essential.

● BREAST FEEDING Manufacturer advises avoid during and for at least 6 months after treatment—present in milk in *animal* studies.

● HEPATIC IMPAIRMENT Manufacturer advises caution—no information available.

● PRE-TREATMENT SCREENING
Tuberculosis Patients should be evaluated for tuberculosis before treatment.

● MONITORING REQUIREMENTS Monitor for infection before, during, and for 5 months after treatment.

● DIRECTIONS FOR ADMINISTRATION For doses requiring multiple injections, each injection should be administered at a different site.
Missed dose If dose administered more than 2 weeks late, subsequent doses should be administered on the new monthly due date.

● PATIENT AND CARER ADVICE An alert card should be provided.
Tuberculosis All patients and their carers should be advised to seek medical attention if symptoms suggestive of tuberculosis (e.g. persistent cough, weight loss, and fever) develop.
Blood disorders Patients and their carers should be advised to seek medical attention if symptoms suggestive of blood disorders (such as fever, sore throat, bruising, or bleeding) develop.

● NATIONAL FUNDING/ACCESS DECISIONS
NICE decisions
▸ **Golimumab for the treatment of psoriatic arthritis (April 2011)** NICE TA220
Golimumab is an option for the treatment of active and progressive psoriatic arthritis in adults only if:
● golimumab is used as described in the NICE guidance (August 2010) for other tumour necrosis factor (TNF) inhibitors, **and**
● the manufacturer provides the 100 mg dose of golimumab at the same price as the 50 mg dose.
www.nice.org.uk/guidance/ta220

▸ **Adalimumab, etanercept, infliximab, certolizumab pegol, golimumab, tocilizumab and abatacept for rheumatoid arthritis not previously treated with DMARDs or after conventional DMARDs only have failed (January 2016)** NICE TA375
Golimumab, in combination with methotrexate, is recommended as an option for treating rheumatoid arthritis, only if **all** the following criteria are met:
● disease is severe, that is, a disease activity score (DAS28) greater than 5.1,
● disease has not responded to intensive therapy with a combination of conventional disease-modifying antirheumatic drugs (DMARDs),
● the manufacturers provides golimumab as agreed in the patient access schemes.
Continue treatment only if there is a moderate response measured using European League Against Rheumatism (EULAR) criteria at 6 months after starting therapy. After initial response within 6 months, withdraw treatment if a moderate EULAR response is not maintained.

Patients currently receiving treatment with golimumab whose disease does not meet the above criteria should have the option to continue their treatment until they and their NHS clinician consider it appropriate to stop.
www.nice.org.uk/guidance/ta375

▸ **Golimumab for the treatment of rheumatoid arthritis after the failure of previous disease-modifying antirheumatic drugs (June 2011)** NICE TA225
Golimumab, in combination with methotrexate, is an option for the treatment of rheumatoid arthritis in patients who have had an inadequate response to DMARDs, including a TNF inhibitor, if golimumab is used as described in the NICE technology appraisal guidance 195 (August 2010) for other TNF inhibitors, **and** the manufacturer provides the 100 mg dose of golimumab at the same price as the 50 mg dose.
www.nice.org.uk/guidance/ta225

▸ **TNF-alpha inhibitors for ankylosing spondylitis and non-radiographic axial spondyloarthritis (February 2016)** NICE TA383
Adalimumab, certolizumab pegol, etanercept, golimumab and infliximab are recommended as options for treating severe active ankylosing spondylitis in patients whose disease has responded inadequately to, or who are intolerant of, non-steroidal anti-inflammatory drugs (NSAIDs).

The response to treatment should be assessed 12 weeks after the start of treatment. Treatment should only be continued if there is clear evidence of response.

Treatment with another tumour necrosis factor (TNF)-alpha inhibitor is recommended in those who cannot tolerate, or whose disease has not responded to, treatment with the first TNF-alpha inhibitor, or in those whose disease has stopped responding after an initial response.
www.nice.org.uk/guidance/ta383

▸ **Golimumab for treating non-radiographic axial spondyloarthritis (January 2018)** NICE TA497
Golimumab is recommended, within its marketing authorisation, as an option for treating severe non-radiographic axial spondyloarthritis in adults whose disease has responded inadequately to, or who cannot tolerate, nonsteroidal anti-inflammatory drugs.

If patients and their clinicians consider golimumab to be one of a range of suitable treatments, including adalimumab, etanercept and certolizumab pegol, the least expensive (taking into account administration costs and patient access schemes) should be chosen.

Assess the response to golimumab 12 weeks after the start of treatment. Continue treatment only if there is clear evidence of response, defined as:

● a reduction in the Bath Ankylosing Spondylitis Disease Activity Index (BASDAI) score to 50% of the pre-treatment value or by 2 or more units, **and**
● a reduction in the spinal pain visual analogue scale (VAS) score by 2 cm or more.
www.nice.org.uk/guidance/ta497

▸ **Infliximab, adalimumab and golimumab for treating moderately-to-severely active ulcerative colitis after the failure of conventional therapy (February 2015)** NICE TA329
Golimumab is an option for treating moderately-to-severely active ulcerative colitis in adults whose disease has responded inadequately to conventional therapy including corticosteroids and mercaptopurine or azathioprine, or in adults who are intolerant to or have contra-indications for conventional therapies.

Golimumab is recommended only if the manufacturer provides the 100 mg dose of golimumab at the same cost as the 50 mg dose, as agreed in the patient access scheme.

The choice of treatment should be made on an individual basis and if more than one treatment is suitable, the least expensive should be chosen.

Golimumab should be given as a planned course of treatment until treatment fails (including the need for surgery) or until 12 months after starting treatment, whichever is shorter. Treatment should be continued only if there is clear evidence of a response. Patients who continue treatment should be reassessed at least every 12 months to determine whether ongoing treatment is still clinically appropriate.
www.nice.org.uk/guidance/ta329

Scottish Medicines Consortium (SMC) Decisions
The *Scottish Medicines Consortium* has advised (July 2012) that golimumab (*Simponi*®) is accepted for restricted use within NHS Scotland at a dose of 50 mg, alone or in combination with methotrexate, for the treatment of active and progressive psoriatic arthritis in adults whose disease has not responded to adequate trials of at least two standard DMARDs, administered either individually or in combination.

The *Scottish Medicines Consortium* has advised (February 2016) that golimumab (*Simponi*®) is accepted for use within NHS Scotland for the treatment of adults with severe, active non-radiographic axial spondyloarthritis with objective signs of inflammation as indicated by elevated C-reactive protein (CRP) and/or magnetic resonance imaging (MRI) evidence, who have had an inadequate response to, or are intolerant to non-steroidal anti-inflammatory drugs (NSAIDs). This advice is contingent upon the continuing availability of the patient access scheme in NHS Scotland or a list price that is equivalent or lower.

● MEDICINAL FORMS
There can be variation in the licensing of different medicines containing the same drug.
Solution for injection
CAUTIONARY AND ADVISORY LABELS 10
▸ Simponi (Merck Sharp & Dohme Ltd)
Golimumab 100 mg per 1 ml Simponi 50mg/0.5ml solution for injection pre-filled disposable devices | 1 pre-filled disposable injection PoM £762.97
Simponi 50mg/0.5ml solution for injection pre-filled syringes | 1 pre-filled disposable injection PoM £762.97
Simponi 100mg/1ml solution for injection pre-filled pen | 1 pre-filled disposable injection PoM £1,525.94

10

Musculoskeletal system

Infliximab

31-May-2016

● **INDICATIONS AND DOSE**

Severe active Crohn's disease
▸ BY INTRAVENOUS INFUSION
▸ Adult: Initially 5 mg/kg, then 5 mg/kg after 2 weeks, then 5 mg/kg after 4 weeks, if condition has responded, then maintenance 5 mg/kg every 8 weeks

Fistulating Crohn's disease
▸ BY INTRAVENOUS INFUSION
▸ Adult: Initially 5 mg/kg, then 5 mg/kg after 2 weeks, followed by 5 mg/kg after 4 weeks, if condition has responded consult product literature for guidance on further doses

Severe active ulcerative colitis
▸ BY INTRAVENOUS INFUSION
▸ Adult: Initially 5 mg/kg, then 5 mg/kg after 2 weeks, followed by 5 mg/kg after 4 weeks, then 5 mg/kg every 8 weeks, discontinue if no response 14 weeks after initial dose

Rheumatoid arthritis (in combination with methotrexate)
▸ BY INTRAVENOUS INFUSION
▸ Adult: Initially 3 mg/kg, then 3 mg/kg after 2 weeks, followed by 3 mg/kg after 4 weeks, then 3 mg/kg every 8 weeks, dose to be increased only if response is inadequate after 12 weeks of initial treatment; increased in steps of 1.5 mg/kg every 8 weeks, increased if necessary up to 7.5 mg/kg every 8 weeks, alternatively increased if necessary to 3 mg/kg every 4 weeks, discontinue if no response by 12 weeks of initial infusion or after dose adjustment

Ankylosing spondylitis
▸ BY INTRAVENOUS INFUSION
▸ Adult: 5 mg/kg, then 5 mg/kg after 2 weeks, followed by 5 mg/kg after 4 weeks, then 5 mg/kg every 6–8 weeks, discontinue if no response by 6 weeks of initial infusion

Psoriatic arthritis (in combination with methotrexate)
▸ BY INTRAVENOUS INFUSION
▸ Adult: 5 mg/kg, then 5 mg/kg after 2 weeks, followed by 5 mg/kg after 4 weeks, followed by 5 mg/kg every 8 weeks

Plaque psoriasis
▸ BY INTRAVENOUS INFUSION
▸ Adult: 5 mg/kg, then 5 mg/kg after 2 weeks, followed by 5 mg/kg after 4 weeks, then 5 mg/kg every 8 weeks, discontinue if no response within 14 weeks of initial infusion

> **IMPORTANT SAFETY INFORMATION**
> Adequate resuscitation facilities must be available when infliximab is used.

● CONTRA-INDICATIONS Moderate or severe heart failure · severe infections
● CAUTIONS Demyelinating disorders (risk of exacerbation) · dermatomyositis · development of malignancy · hepatitis B virus—monitor for active infection · history of colon carcinoma (in inflammatory bowel disease) · history of dysplasia (in inflammatory bowel disease) · history of malignancy · history of prolonged immunosuppressant or PUVA treatment in patients with psoriasis · mild heart failure (discontinue if symptoms develop or worsen) · predisposition to infection (discontinue if new serious infection develops) · risk of delayed hypersensitivity reactions if drug-free interval exceeds 16 weeks (re-administration after interval exceeding 16 weeks not recommended)

CAUTIONS, FURTHER INFORMATION
▸ Tuberculosis Manufacturer advises to evaluate patients for active and latent tuberculosis before treatment. Active tuberculosis should be treated with standard treatment for at least 2 months before starting infliximab. If latent tuberculosis is diagnosed, treatment should be started before commencing treatment with infliximab. Patients who have previously received adequate treatment for tuberculosis can start infliximab but should be monitored every 3 months for possible recurrence. In patients without active tuberculosis but who were previously not treated adequately, chemoprophylaxis should ideally be completed before starting infliximab. In patients at high risk of tuberculosis who cannot be assessed by tuberculin skin test, chemoprophylaxis can be given concurrently with infliximab. Patients should be advised to seek medical attention if symptoms suggestive of tuberculosis develop (e.g. persistent cough, weight loss and fever).
▸ Hypersensitivity reactions Hypersensitivity reactions (including fever, chest pain, hypotension, hypertension, dyspnoea, transient visual loss, pruritus, urticaria, serum sickness-like reactions, angioedema, anaphylaxis) reported during or within 1–2 hours after infusion (risk greatest during first or second infusion or in patients who discontinue other immunosuppressants). Manufacturer advises prophylactic antipyretics, antihistamines, or hydrocortisone may be administered.

● INTERACTIONS → Appendix 1: monoclonal antibodies
● SIDE-EFFECTS
▸ **Common or very common** Abscess · alopecia · anaemia · arrhythmias · arthralgia · chest pain · chills · constipation · decreased leucocytes · depression · diarrhoea · dizziness · dyspnoea · eye inflammation · fatigue · fever · gastrointestinal discomfort · gastrointestinal disorders · haemorrhage · headache · hepatic disorders · hyperhidrosis · hypertension · hypotension · increased risk of infection · infusion related reaction · insomnia · lymphadenopathy · myalgia · nausea · neutropenia · oedema · pain · palpitations · respiratory disorders · sensation abnormal · sepsis · skin reactions · vasodilation · vertigo
▸ **Uncommon** Anxiety · cheilitis · cholecystitis · confusion · drowsiness · healing impaired · heart failure · hypersensitivity · lupus-like syndrome · lymphocytosis · memory loss · neoplasms · nerve disorders · pancreatitis · peripheral ischaemia · pulmonary oedema · seborrhoea · seizure · syncope · thrombocytopenia
▸ **Rare or very rare** Agranulocytosis · circulatory collapse · cyanosis · demyelinating disorders · granuloma · haemolytic anaemia · hepatitis B reactivation · meningitis · pancytopenia · pericardial effusion · sarcoidosis · severe cutaneous adverse reactions (SCARs) · transverse myelitis · vasculitis · vasospasm
▸ **Frequency not known** Dermatomyositis exacerbated · hepatosplenic T-cell lymphoma (increased risk in inflammatory bowel disease) · myocardial infarction · myocardial ischaemia · vision loss

● CONCEPTION AND CONTRACEPTION Manufacturer advises adequate contraception during and for at least 6 months after last dose.
● PREGNANCY Use only if essential.
● BREAST FEEDING Amount probably too small to be harmful.
● PRE-TREATMENT SCREENING
Tuberculosis Patients should be evaluated for tuberculosis before treatment.
● MONITORING REQUIREMENTS
▸ Monitor for infection before, during, and for 6 months after treatment.
▸ All patients should be observed carefully for 1–2 hours after infusion and resuscitation equipment should be

available for immediate use (risk of hypersensitivity reactions).
▸ Monitor for symptoms of delayed hypersensitivity if re-administered after a prolonged period.
▸ Manufacturer advises periodic skin examination for non-melanoma skin cancer, particularly in patients with risk factors.

● DIRECTIONS FOR ADMINISTRATION For *intravenous infusion* (*Remicade*®), give intermittently *in* Sodium chloride 0.9%; reconstitute each 100-mg vial with 10 mL water for injections using a 21-gauge or smaller needle; gently swirl vial without shaking to dissolve; allow to stand for 5 minutes; dilute requisite dose with infusion fluid to a final volume of 250 mL and give through a low protein-binding filter (1.2 micron or less) over at least 2 hours (adults over 18 years who have tolerated 3 initial 2-hour infusions may be given subsequent infusions of up to 6 mg/kg over at least 1 hour); start infusion within 3 hours of reconstitution.

● PRESCRIBING AND DISPENSING INFORMATION Infliximab is a biological medicine. Biological medicines must be prescribed and dispensed by brand name, see *Biological medicines* and *Biosimilar medicines*, under Guidance on prescribing p. 1.

● PATIENT AND CARER ADVICE An alert card should be provided.
Tuberculosis Patients and carers should be advised to seek medical attention if symptoms suggestive of tuberculosis (e.g. persistent cough, weight loss, and fever) develop.
Blood disorders Patients and carers should be advised to seek medical attention if symptoms suggestive of blood disorders (such as fever, sore throat, bruising, or bleeding) develop.
Hypersensitivity reactions Patients and carers should be advised to keep Alert card with them at all times and seek medical advice if symptoms of delayed hypersensitivity develop.

● NATIONAL FUNDING/ACCESS DECISIONS

NICE decisions
▸ **Infliximab for plaque psoriasis in adults (January 2008)** NICE TA134
Infliximab is recommended for the treatment of very severe plaque psoriasis which has failed to respond to standard systemic treatments (including ciclosporin and methotrexate) or to photochemotherapy, or when standard treatments cannot be used because of intolerance or contra-indications. Infliximab should be withdrawn if the response is not adequate after 10 weeks.
www.nice.org.uk/TA134

▸ **Infliximab for acute exacerbations of ulcerative colitis (December 2008)** NICE TA163
Infliximab is recommended as an option for the treatment of acute exacerbations of severe ulcerative colitis when treatment with ciclosporin is contra-indicated or inappropriate.
www.nice.org.uk/TA163

▸ **Infliximab and adalimumab for Crohn's disease (May 2010)** NICE TA187
Infliximab is recommended for the treatment of severe active Crohn's disease that has not responded to conventional therapy (including corticosteroids and other drugs affecting the immune response) or when conventional therapy cannot be used because of intolerance or contra-indications; infliximab can also be used in a similar way in children over 6 years of age. In adults over 18 years of age, infliximab is recommended for the treatment of fistulating Crohn's disease that has not responded to conventional therapy (including antibacterials, drainage, and other drugs affecting the immune response) or when conventional therapy cannot be used because of intolerance or contra-indications.

Infliximab should be given as a planned course of treatment for 12 months or until treatment failure, whichever is shorter. Treatment should be continued beyond 12 months only if there is evidence of active disease—in these cases the need for treatment should be reviewed at least annually. If the disease relapses after stopping treatment, infliximab can be restarted.
www.nice.org.uk/TA187

▸ **Adalimumab, etanercept, infliximab, rituximab, and abatacept for the treatment of rheumatoid arthritis after the failure of a TNF inhibitor (August 2010)** NICE TA195
Infliximab, in combination with methotrexate, is an option for the treatment of severe active rheumatoid arthritis in adults who have had an inadequate response to, or have an intolerance of, other DMARDs including at least 1 TNF inhibitor, and who cannot use rituximab because of contra-indications or intolerance. Treatment should be continued only if there is adequate response. Patients should be monitored at least every 6 months.
www.nice.org.uk/TA195

▸ **Etanercept, infliximab, and adalimumab for the treatment of psoriatic arthritis (August 2010)** NICE TA199
Infliximab is recommended for the treatment of active and progressive psoriatic arthritis in adults who have peripheral arthritis with at least 3 tender joints and at least 3 swollen joints, and who have not responded adequately to at least 2 standard disease-modifying antirheumatic drugs (used alone or in combination).
Infliximab should be discontinued if there is an inadequate response at 12 weeks.
www.nice.org.uk/TA199

▸ **Infliximab, adalimumab and golimumab for treating moderately to severely active ulcerative colitis after the failure of conventional therapy (February 2015)** NICE TA329
Infliximab is an option for treating moderately to severely active ulcerative colitis in adults whose disease has responded inadequately to conventional therapy including corticosteroids and mercaptopurine or azathioprine, or in adults who are intolerant to or have contra-indications for conventional therapies.
The choice of treatment should be made on an individual basis and if more than one treatment is suitable, the least expensive should be chosen.
Infliximab should be given as a planned course of treatment until treatment fails (including the need for surgery) or until 12 months after starting treatment, whichever is shorter. Treatment should be continued only if there is clear evidence of a response. Patients who continue treatment should be reassessed at least every 12 months to determine whether ongoing treatment is still clinically appropriate.
www.nice.org.uk/TA329

▸ **Adalimumab, etanercept, infliximab, certolizumab pegol, golimumab, tocilizumab and abatacept for rheumatoid arthritis not previously treated with DMARDs or after conventional DMARDs only have failed (January 2016)** NICE TA375
Infliximab, in combination with methotrexate, is recommended as an option for treating rheumatoid arthritis, only if the following criteria are met:
● disease is severe, that is, a disease activity score (DAS28) greater than 5.1, **and,**
● disease has not responded to intensive therapy with a combination of conventional disease-modifying antirheumatic drugs (DMARDs).
Continue treatment only if there is a moderate response measured using European League Against Rheumatism (EULAR) criteria at 6 months after starting therapy. After initial response within 6 months, withdraw treatment if a moderate EULAR response is not maintained.
Patients currently receiving infliximab whose disease does not meet the above criteria should have the option to

continue their treatment until they and their clinician consider it appropriate to stop.
www.nice.org.uk/TA375

▶ **TNF-alpha inhibitors for ankylosing spondylitis and non-radiographic axial spondyloarthritis (February 2016)** NICE TA383

Adalimumab, certolizumab pegol, etanercept, golimumab and infliximab are recommended as options for treating severe active ankylosing spondylitis in patients whose disease has responded inadequately to, or who are intolerant of, non-steroidal anti-inflammatory drugs (NSAIDs). Infliximab is recommended only if treatment is started with the least expensive infliximab product. Patients currently receiving infliximab should continue treatment with the same infliximab product until they and their clinician considers it appropriate to stop.

The response to treatment should be assessed 12 weeks after the start of treatment and should only be continued if there is clear evidence of response.

Treatment with another tumour necrosis factor (TNF)-alpha inhibitor is recommended in those who cannot tolerate, or whose disease has not responded to, treatment with the first TNF-alpha inhibitor, or in those whose disease has stopped responding after an initial response.
www.nice.org.uk/TA383

● MEDICINAL FORMS
There can be variation in the licensing of different medicines containing the same drug.

Powder for solution for infusion
CAUTIONARY AND ADVISORY LABELS 10
▶ Flixabi (Biogen Idec Ltd) ▼
Infliximab 100 mg Flixabi 100mg powder for concentrate for solution for infusion vials | 1 vial [PoM] £377.00 (Hospital only)
▶ Inflectra (Pfizer Ltd) ▼
Infliximab 100 mg Inflectra 100mg powder for concentrate for solution for infusion vials | 1 vial [PoM] £377.66 (Hospital only)
▶ Remicade (Merck Sharp & Dohme Ltd)
Infliximab 100 mg Remicade 100mg powder for concentrate for solution for infusion vials | 1 vial [PoM] £419.62 (Hospital only)
▶ Remsima (Napp Pharmaceuticals Ltd) ▼
Infliximab 100 mg Remsima 100mg powder for concentrate for solution for infusion vials | 1 vial [PoM] £377.66 (Hospital only)

PHOSPHODIESTERASE TYPE-4 INHIBITORS

Apremilast
13-Apr-2017

● DRUG ACTION Apremilast inhibits the activity of phosphodiesterase type-4 (PDE4) which results in suppression of pro-inflammatory mediator synthesis and promotes anti-inflammatory mediators.

● INDICATIONS AND DOSE

Active psoriatic arthritis (in combination with disease-modifying antirheumatic drugs or alone) in patients who have had an inadequate response or who have been intolerant to a prior disease-modifying antirheumatic drug therapy | Moderate to severe chronic plaque psoriasis that has not responded to standard systemic treatments or photochemotherapy, or when these treatments cannot be used because of intolerance or contra-indications
▶ BY MOUTH
▶ Adult: Initially 10 mg daily on day 1, then 10 mg twice daily on day 2, then 10 mg in the morning and 20 mg in the evening on day 3, then 20 mg twice daily on day 4, then 20 mg in the morning and 30 mg in the evening on day 5, then maintenance 30 mg twice daily, doses should be taken approximately 12 hours apart; review treatment if no response within 24 weeks of initiation

● CAUTIONS Concomitant use of drugs likely to cause psychiatric symptoms · history of psychiatric illness · low body-weight—consider discontinuation if weight loss is unexplained or clinically significant

● INTERACTIONS → Appendix 1: apremilast

● SIDE-EFFECTS
▶ **Common or very common** Appetite decreased · back pain · cough · depression · diarrhoea · fatigue · gastrointestinal discomfort · gastrointestinal disorders · headaches · increased risk of infection · insomnia · nausea · vomiting
▶ **Uncommon** Gastrointestinal haemorrhage · rash · suicidal tendencies · weight decreased

● CONCEPTION AND CONTRACEPTION Exclude pregnancy before treatment and ensure effective contraception during treatment.

● PREGNANCY Avoid—teratogenic in *animal* studies.

● BREAST FEEDING Manufacturer advises avoid—present in milk in *animal* studies.

● RENAL IMPAIRMENT
Dose adjustments Reduce dose if eGFR less than 30 mL/minute/1.73 m^2; consult product literature for initial dose titration.

● MONITORING REQUIREMENTS
▶ Manufacturer advises monitor body-weight regularly in patients underweight at the start of treatment.
▶ Manufacturer advises monitor for psychiatric symptoms (including depression, suicidal ideation and behaviour)—discontinue treatment if new or worsening psychiatric symptoms are identified.

● PATIENT AND CARER ADVICE Manufacturer advises patients and carers should be instructed to notify the prescriber of any changes in behaviour or mood, and of any suicidal ideation.

● NATIONAL FUNDING/ACCESS DECISIONS
NICE decisions
▶ **Apremilast for treating active psoriatic arthritis (February 2017)** NICE TA433
Apremilast, alone or in combination with disease-modifying antirheumatic drugs (DMARDs), is recommended as an option for treating active psoriatic arthritis in adults only if:
● they have peripheral arthritis with 3 or more tender joints and 3 or more swollen joints **and**
● their disease has not responded to adequate trials of at least 2 standard DMARDs, given either alone or in combination **and**
● the manufacturer provides apremilast with the discount agreed in the patient access scheme.
Patients whose treatment was started within the NHS before this guidance was published should have the option to continue treatment, without change to their funding arrangements, until they and their clinician consider it appropriate to stop.
www.nice.org.uk/TA433
▶ **Apremilast for treating moderate to severe plaque psoriasis (November 2016)** NICE TA419
Apremilast is recommended as an option for treating chronic plaque psoriasis in patients whose disease has not responded to other systemic therapies, including

ciclosporin, methotrexate and PUVA, or when these treatments are contra-indicated or not tolerated, only if:
- the disease is severe, as defined by a total Psoriasis Area Severity Index (PASI) of 10 or more and a Dermatology Life Quality Index (DLQI) of more than 10 **and**
- treatment is stopped if the psoriasis has not responded adequately at 16 weeks (defined as a 75% reduction in the PASI score (PASI 75) from when treatment started or a 50% reduction in the PASI score (PASI 50) and a 5-point reduction in DLQI from start of treatment), **and**
- the manufacturer provides apremilast with the discount agreed in the patient access scheme.

Patients whose treatment was started within the NHS before this guidance was published should have the option to continue treatment, without change to their funding arrangements, until they and their clinician consider it appropriate to stop.
www.nice.org.uk/TA419

Scottish Medicines Consortium (SMC) Decisions
The *Scottish Medicines Consortium* has advised (June 2015) that apremilast (*Otezla* ®) is accepted for restricted use within NHS Scotland for the treatment of active psoriatic arthritis in patients who have had an inadequate response with at least two prior Disease Modifying Antirheumatic Drug (DMARD) therapies or who are intolerant to such therapies.

● MEDICINAL FORMS
There can be variation in the licensing of different medicines containing the same drug.

Tablet
CAUTIONARY AND ADVISORY LABELS 25
▸ Otezla (Celgene Ltd) ▼
  Apremilast 10 mg Otezla 10mg tablets | 4 tablet PoM Ⓢ
  Apremilast 20 mg Otezla 20mg tablets | 4 tablet PoM Ⓢ
  Apremilast 30 mg Otezla 30mg tablets | 56 tablet PoM £550.00

2   Hyperuricaemia and gout

Gout

Overview
It is important to distinguish drugs used for the treatment of acute attacks of gout from those used in the long-term control of the disease. The latter exacerbate and prolong the acute manifestations if started during an attack. The management of gout in adolescents requires specialist supervision.

Acute attacks of gout
Acute attacks of gout are usually treated with high doses of NSAIDs such as diclofenac sodium p. 1101, diclofenac potassium p. 1100, etoricoxib p. 1104, indometacin p. 1109, ketoprofen p. 1110, naproxen p. 1113 or sulindac p. 1116. Colchicine below is an alternative in patients in whom NSAIDs are contra-indicated. Aspirin p. 121 is *not* indicated in gout. Allopurinol p. 1086, febuxostat p. 1087, and uricosurics are not effective in treating an acute attack and may prolong it indefinitely if started during the acute episode.

The use of colchicine is limited by the development of toxicity at higher doses, but it is of value in patients with heart failure since, unlike NSAIDs, it does not induce fluid retention; moreover, it can be given to patients receiving anticoagulants.

Oral or parenteral corticosteroids are an effective alternative in those who cannot tolerate NSAIDs or who are resistant to other treatments. Intra-articular injection of a corticosteroid can be used in acute monoarticular

gout [unlicensed indication]. A corticosteroid by intramuscular injection can be effective in podagra.

Canakinumab p. 824, a recombinant monoclonal antibody, can be used for the symptomatic treatment of frequent gouty arthritis attacks (at least 3 in the previous 12 months). It is licensed for use in patients whose condition has not responded adequately to treatment with NSAIDs or colchicine, or who are intolerant of them.

Long-term control of gout
Frequent recurrence of acute attacks of gout, the presence of tophi, or signs of chronic gouty arthritis may call for the initiation of long-term ('interval') treatment. For long-term control of gout the formation of uric acid from purines may be reduced with the xanthine-oxidase inhibitors allopurinol or febuxostat alternatively the uricosuric drug sulfinpyrazone p. 1086 may be used to increase the excretion of uric acid in the urine. Treatment should be continued indefinitely to prevent attacks of gout by correcting the hyperuricaemia. These drugs should never be started during an acute attack; they are usually started 1–2 weeks after the attack has settled. The initiation of treatment may precipitate an acute attack, and therefore an anti-inflammatory analgesic or colchicine should be used as a prophylactic and continued for at least one month after the hyperuricaemia has been corrected. However, if an acute attack develops during treatment, then the treatment should continue at the same dosage and the acute attack treated in its own right.

Allopurinol is widely used and is especially useful in patients with renal impairment or urate stones when uricosuric drugs cannot be used; it is *not* indicated for the treatment of asymptomatic hyperuricaemia. It can cause rashes.

Febuxostat is licensed for the treatment of chronic hyperuricaemia where urate deposition has already occurred; it is *not* indicated for patients in whom the rate of urate formation is greatly increased, such as in malignant disease or in Lesch-Nyhan syndrome.

Sulfinpyrazone can be used instead of allopurinol or in conjunction with it in cases that are resistant to treatment.

Benzbromarone (available from 'special-order' manufacturers or specialist importing companies) is a uricosuric drug that can be used in patients with mild renal impairment.

Crystallisation of urate in the urine can occur with the uricosuric drugs and it is important to ensure an adequate urine output especially in the first few weeks of treatment. As an additional precaution the urine may be rendered alkaline.

Aspirin and other salicylates antagonise the uricosuric drugs; they do not antagonise allopurinol but are nevertheless *not* indicated in gout.

ALKALOIDS ⟩ PLANT ALKALOIDS

Colchicine

● INDICATIONS AND DOSE

Acute gout
▸ BY MOUTH
▸ Adult: 500 micrograms 2–4 times a day until symptoms relieved, maximum 6 mg per course, do not repeat course within 3 days

Short-term prophylaxis during initial therapy with allopurinol and uricosuric drugs
▸ BY MOUTH
▸ Adult: 500 micrograms twice daily

continued →

10

Musculoskeletal system

Prophylaxis of familial Mediterranean fever (recurrent polyserositis)
▶ BY MOUTH
▶ Adult: 0.5–2 mg once daily
DOSE ADJUSTMENTS DUE TO INTERACTIONS
▶ Manufacturer advises reduce dose by half with concurrent use of moderate inhibitors of CYP3A4.
▶ Manufacturer advises reduce dose by 75% (to one quarter of usual dose) with concurrent use of potent inhibitors of CYP3A4 or P-glycoprotein inhibitors; avoid concurrent use in patients with hepatic or renal impairment.

● UNLICENSED USE BNF doses may differ from those in the product literature. Use of colchicine for prophylaxis of familial Mediterranean fever (recurrent polyserositis) is an unlicensed indication.
● CONTRA-INDICATIONS Blood disorders
● CAUTIONS Cardiac disease · elderly · gastro-intestinal disease
● INTERACTIONS → Appendix 1: colchicine
● SIDE-EFFECTS
▶ Common or very common Abdominal pain · diarrhoea · nausea · vomiting
▶ Frequency not known Agranulocytosis · alopecia · bone marrow disorders · gastrointestinal haemorrhage · kidney injury · liver injury · menstrual cycle irregularities · myopathy · nerve disorders · rash · sperm abnormalities · thrombocytopenia
● PREGNANCY Avoid—teratogenicity in *animal* studies.
● BREAST FEEDING Present in milk but no adverse effects reported. Manufacturers advise caution.
● HEPATIC IMPAIRMENT Use with caution.
● RENAL IMPAIRMENT Avoid if eGFR less than 10 mL/minute/1.73 m².
Dose adjustments Reduce dose or increase dosage interval if eGFR 10–50 mL/minute/1.73 m².

● MEDICINAL FORMS
There can be variation in the licensing of different medicines containing the same drug.
Tablet
▶ Colchicine (Non-proprietary)
Colchicine **500 microgram** Colchicine 500microgram tablets | 100 tablet PoM £21.95 DT = £12.12

URICOSURICS

Sulfinpyrazone

(Sulphinpyrazone)

● INDICATIONS AND DOSE
Gout prophylaxis | Hyperuricaemia
▶ BY MOUTH
▶ Adult: Initially 100–200 mg daily, dose to be taken with food (or milk); increased to 600–800 mg daily over 2–3 weeks, 800 mg daily is rarely given; continue until serum uric acid concentration normal then reduce dose for maintenance (maintenance dose may be as low as 200 mg daily)

● CONTRA-INDICATIONS Acute gout attack · Acute porphyrias p. 1025 · history of blood disorders · peptic ulceration
● CAUTIONS Cardiac disease (may cause salt and water retention) · ensure adequate fluid intake (about 2–3 litres daily) and render urine alkaline during initial treatment
● INTERACTIONS → Appendix 1: sulfinpyrazone
● SIDE-EFFECTS Abdominal distress · acute kidney injury · agranulocytosis · allergic dermatitis · aplastic anaemia ·

fluid retention · gastrointestinal haemorrhage · gastrointestinal ulcer · hepatic disorders · leucopenia · sodium retention · thrombocytopenia
● ALLERGY AND CROSS-SENSITIVITY Avoid in hypersensitivity to aspirin, salicylates, NSAIDs.
● PREGNANCY Manufacturer advises caution—no information available.
● BREAST FEEDING No information available.
● HEPATIC IMPAIRMENT Avoid in severe impairment.
● RENAL IMPAIRMENT Avoid in severe impairment.
Dose adjustments Reduce dose.
● MONITORING REQUIREMENTS Regular blood counts before treatment and at regular intervals during treatment.
● MEDICINAL FORMS
There can be variation in the licensing of different medicines containing the same drug. Forms available from special-order manufacturers include: tablet

XANTHINE OXIDASE INHIBITORS

Allopurinol

● INDICATIONS AND DOSE
Prophylaxis of gout and of uric acid and calcium oxalate renal stones | Prophylaxis of hyperuricaemia associated with cancer chemotherapy
▶ BY MOUTH
▶ Adult: Initially 100 mg daily, for maintenance adjust dose according to plasma or urinary uric acid concentration, dose to be taken preferably after food
Prophylaxis of gout and of uric acid and calcium oxalate renal stones (usual maintenance in mild conditions) | Prophylaxis of hyperuricaemia associated with cancer chemotherapy (usual maintenance in mild conditions)
▶ BY MOUTH
▶ Adult: 100–200 mg daily, dose to be taken preferably after food
Prophylaxis of gout and of uric acid and calcium oxalate renal stones (usual maintenance in moderately severe conditions) | Prophylaxis of hyperuricaemia associated with cancer chemotherapy (usual maintenance in moderately severe conditions)
▶ BY MOUTH
▶ Adult: 300–600 mg daily in divided doses (max. per dose 300 mg), dose to be taken preferably after food
Prophylaxis of gout and of uric acid and calcium oxalate renal stones (usual maintenance in severe conditions) | Prophylaxis of hyperuricaemia associated with cancer chemotherapy (usual maintenance in severe conditions)
▶ BY MOUTH
▶ Adult: 700–900 mg daily in divided doses (max. per dose 300 mg), dose to be taken preferably after food

● CONTRA-INDICATIONS Not a treatment for acute gout but continue if attack develops when already receiving allopurinol, and treat attack separately
● CAUTIONS Ensure adequate fluid intake (2–3 litres/day) · for hyperuricaemia associated with cancer therapy, allopurinol treatment should be started before cancer therapy
CAUTIONS, FURTHER INFORMATION Administer prophylactic NSAID (*not* aspirin or salicylates) or colchicine until at least 1 month after hyperuricaemia corrected (usually for first 3 months) to avoid precipitating an acute attack.
● INTERACTIONS → Appendix 1: allopurinol

● SIDE-EFFECTS
▶ **Common or very common** Rash (discontinue therapy; if rash mild re-introduce cautiously but discontinue immediately if recurrence)
▶ **Uncommon** Hypersensitivity · nausea · vomiting
▶ **Rare or very rare** Agranulocytosis · alopecia · angina pectoris · angioedema · angioimmunoblastic T-cell lymphoma · aplastic anaemia · asthenia · ataxia · boil · bradycardia · cataract · coma · depression · diabetes mellitus · drowsiness · erectile dysfunction · fever · gastrointestinal disorders · gynaecomastia · haemorrhage · hair colour changes · headache · hepatic disorders · hyperlipidaemia · hypertension · infertility male · maculopathy · malaise · oedema · paraesthesia · paralysis · peripheral neuropathy · severe cutaneous adverse reactions (SCARs) · skin reactions · stomatitis · taste altered · thrombocytopenia · vertigo · visual impairment
● PREGNANCY Toxicity not reported. Manufacturer advises use only if no safer alternative and disease carries risk for mother or child.
● BREAST FEEDING Present in milk—not known to be harmful.
● HEPATIC IMPAIRMENT
Dose adjustments Reduce dose.
● RENAL IMPAIRMENT
Dose adjustments Max. 100 mg daily, increased only if response inadequate; in severe impairment, reduce daily dose below 100 mg, or increase dose interval; if facilities available, adjust dose to maintain plasma-oxipurinol concentration below 100 micromol/litre.

● MEDICINAL FORMS
There can be variation in the licensing of different medicines containing the same drug. Forms available from special-order manufacturers include: oral suspension, oral solution, mouthwash
Tablet
CAUTIONARY AND ADVISORY LABELS 8, 21, 27
▶ Allopurinol (Non-proprietary)
  Allopurinol 100 mg Allopurinol 100mg tablets | 28 tablet [PoM] £8.15 DT = £0.38
  Allopurinol 300 mg Allopurinol 300mg tablets | 28 tablet [PoM] £5.85 DT = £0.89
▶ Uricto (Ennogen Pharma Ltd)
  Allopurinol 100 mg Uricto 100mg tablets | 28 tablet [PoM] £1.25 DT = £0.38
  Allopurinol 300 mg Uricto 300mg tablets | 28 tablet [PoM] £0.94 DT = £0.89
▶ Zyloric (Aspen Pharma Trading Ltd)
  Allopurinol 100 mg Zyloric 100mg tablets | 100 tablet [PoM] £10.19
  Allopurinol 300 mg Zyloric 300mg tablets | 28 tablet [PoM] £7.31 DT = £0.89

Febuxostat

28-Sep-2016

● INDICATIONS AND DOSE
Treatment of chronic hyperuricaemia in gout
▶ BY MOUTH
▶ Adult: Initially 80 mg once daily, if after 2–4 weeks of initial dose, serum uric acid greater than 6 mg/100 mL then increase dose; increased if necessary to 120 mg once daily

Prophylaxis and treatment of acute hyperuricaemia with initial chemotherapy for haematologic malignancies
▶ BY MOUTH
▶ Adult: 120 mg once daily, to be started 2 days before start of cytotoxic therapy and continued for 7–9 days, according to chemotherapy duration

┌──┐
│ IMPORTANT SAFETY INFORMATION
│ MHRA/CHM ADVICE: SERIOUS HYPERSENSITIVITY REACTIONS
│ (JUNE 2012)
│ There have been rare but serious reports of hypersensitivity reactions, including Stevens-Johnson syndrome and acute anaphylactic shock with febuxostat. Patients should be advised of the signs and symptoms of severe hypersensitivity; febuxostat must be stopped immediately if these occur (early withdrawal is associated with a better prognosis), and must not be restarted in patients who have ever developed a hypersensitivity reaction to febuxostat. Most cases occur during the first month of treatment; a prior history of hypersensitivity to allopurinol and/or renal disease may indicate potential hypersensitivity to febuxostat.
└──┘

● CONTRA-INDICATIONS Not a treatment for acute gout but continue if attack develops when already receiving febuxostat, and treat attack separately
● CAUTIONS Congestive heart failure · ischaemic heart disease · thyroid disorders · transplant recipients
  CAUTIONS, FURTHER INFORMATION Administer prophylactic NSAID (*not* aspirin or salicylates) or colchicine for at least 6 months after starting febuxostat to avoid precipitating an acute attack.
● INTERACTIONS → Appendix 1: febuxostat
● SIDE-EFFECTS
▶ **Common or very common** Diarrhoea · gout aggravated · headache · hepatic disorders · nausea · oedema · skin reactions
▶ **Uncommon** Altered smell sensation · appetite abnormal · arrhythmias · arthritis · bundle branch block · chest discomfort · cholelithiasis · constipation · cough · diabetes mellitus · dizziness · drowsiness · dry mouth · dyspnoea · fatigue · gastrointestinal discomfort · gastrointestinal disorders · haemorrhage · hemiparesis · hyperlipidaemia · hypertension · increased risk of infection · insomnia · joint disorders · muscle complaints · muscle weakness · musculoskeletal pain · nephrolithiasis · palpitations · proteinuria · renal failure · sensation abnormal · sexual dysfunction · taste altered · urinary disorders · vasodilation · vomiting · weight changes
▶ **Rare or very rare** Alopecia · angioedema · hyperhidrosis · hypersensitivity · musculoskeletal stiffness · nephritis tubulointerstitial · nervousness · oral ulceration · pancreatitis · pancytopenia · rhabdomyolysis · severe cutaneous adverse reactions (SCARs) · thirst · thrombocytopenia · tinnitus · vision blurred
● PREGNANCY Manufacturer advises avoid—limited information available.
● BREAST FEEDING Manufacturer advises avoid—present in milk in *animal* studies.
● HEPATIC IMPAIRMENT
Dose adjustments Max. 80 mg daily in mild impairment.
  No dose information available in moderate or severe impairment.
● RENAL IMPAIRMENT Use with caution if eGFR less than 30 mL/minute/1.73 m^2—no information available.
● PRE-TREATMENT SCREENING Monitor liver function tests before treatment as indicated.
● MONITORING REQUIREMENTS Monitor liver function tests periodically during treatment as indicated.
● NATIONAL FUNDING/ACCESS DECISIONS
NICE decisions
▶ **Febuxostat for the management of hyperuricaemia in patients with gout (December 2008)** NICE TA164
Febuxostat is recommended as an option for the management of chronic hyperuricaemia in gout only for patients who are intolerant of allopurinol or for whom allopurinol is contra-indicated.

10

Musculoskeletal system

For the purposes of this guidance, intolerance of allopurinol is defined as adverse effects that are sufficiently severe to warrant discontinuation, or to prevent full dose escalation for optimal effectiveness. www.nice.org.uk/TA164

Scottish Medicines Consortium (SMC) Decisions

The *Scottish Medicines Consortium* issued similar advice to NICE guidance: Febuxostat for the management of hyperuricaemia in patients with gout (December 2008), in August 2010.

The *Scottish Medicines Consortium* has advised (June 2016) that febuxostat (*Adenuric*®) is accepted for restricted use within NHS Scotland for the prevention and treatment of hyperuricaemia in patients undergoing chemotherapy for haematological malignancies at intermediate to high risk of tumour lysis syndrome, only when allopurinol is not tolerated or contra-indicated.

● MEDICINAL FORMS
There can be variation in the licensing of different medicines containing the same drug.

Tablet

▸ Adenuric (A. Menarini Farmaceutica Internazionale SRL)
Febuxostat 80 mg Adenuric 80mg tablets | 28 tablet [PoM] £24.36 DT = £24.36
Febuxostat 120 mg Adenuric 120mg tablets | 28 tablet [PoM] £24.36 DT = £24.36

3 Neuromuscular disorders

Neuromuscular disorders

Drugs that enhance neuromuscular transmission

Anticholinesterases are used as first-line treatment in *ocular myasthenia gravis* and as an adjunct to immunosuppressant therapy for *generalised myasthenia gravis*.

Corticosteroids are used when anticholinesterases do not control symptoms completely. A second-line immunosuppressant such as azathioprine p. 816 is frequently used to reduce the dose of corticosteroid.

Plasmapheresis or infusion of intravenous immunoglobulin [unlicensed indication] may induce temporary remission in severe relapses, particularly where bulbar or respiratory function is compromised or before thymectomy.

Anticholinesterases

Anticholinesterase drugs enhance neuromuscular transmission in voluntary and involuntary muscle in myasthenia gravis. Excessive dosage of these drugs can impair neuromuscular transmission and precipitate cholinergic crises by causing a depolarising block. This may be difficult to distinguish from a worsening myasthenic state.

Muscarinic side-effects of anticholinesterases include increased sweating, increased salivary and gastric secretions, increased gastro-intestinal and uterine motility, and bradycardia. These parasympathomimetic effects are antagonised by atropine sulfate p. 1131.

Neostigmine p. 1090 produces a therapeutic effect for up to 4 hours. Its pronounced muscarinic action is a disadvantage, and simultaneous administration of an antimuscarinic drug such as atropine sulfate or propantheline bromide p. 85 may be required to prevent colic, excessive salivation, or diarrhoea. In severe disease neostigmine can be given every 2 hours. The maximum that most patients can tolerate is 180 mg daily.

Pyridostigmine bromide p. 1091 is less powerful and slower in action than neostigmine but it has a longer duration of action. It is preferable to neostigmine because of its smoother action and the need for less frequent dosage. It

is particularly preferred in patients whose muscles are weak on waking. It has a comparatively mild gastrointestinal effect but an antimuscarinic drug may still be required.

Neostigmine is also used to reverse the actions of the non-depolarising neuromuscular blocking drugs.

Immunosuppressant therapy

Corticosteroids are established as treatment for myasthenia gravis; although they are commonly given on alternate days there is little evidence of benefit over daily administration. Corticosteroid treatment is usually initiated under in-patient supervision and all patients should receive osteoporosis prophylaxis.

In *generalised myasthenia gravis* prednisolone p. 664 is given. About 10% of patients experience a transient but very serious worsening of symptoms in the first 2–3 weeks, especially if the corticosteroid is started at a high dose. Smaller doses of corticosteroid are usually required in *ocular myasthenia*. Once clinical remission has occurred (usually after 2–6 months), the dose of prednisolone should be reduced slowly to the minimum effective dose.

In generalised myasthenia gravis azathioprine is usually started at the same time as the corticosteroid and it allows a lower maintenance dose of the corticosteroid to be used. Ciclosporin p. 818, methotrexate p. 888, or mycophenolate mofetil p. 826 can be used in patients unresponsive or intolerant to other treatments [unlicensed indications].

Acetylcholine-release enhancers

Amifampridine p. 1091 is licensed for the symptomatic treatment of Lambert-Eaton myasthenic syndrome (LEMS), a rare disorder of neuromuscular transmission.

Fampridine p. 830 is licensed for the improvement of walking in patients with Multiple sclerosis p. 828 who have a walking disability.

Skeletal muscle relaxants

The drugs described are used for the relief of chronic muscle spasm or spasticity associated with Multiple sclerosis p. 828 or other neurological damage; they are not indicated for spasm associated with minor injuries. Baclofen, diazepam, and tizanidine act principally on the central nervous system. Dantrolene has a peripheral site of action; cannabis extract has both a central and a peripheral action. Skeletal muscle relaxants differ in action from the muscle relaxants used in anaesthesia, which block transmission at the neuromuscular junction.

The underlying cause of spasticity should be treated and any aggravating factors (e.g. pressure sores, infection) remedied. Skeletal muscle relaxants are effective in most forms of spasticity except the rare alpha variety. The major disadvantage of treatment with these drugs is that reduction in muscle tone can cause a loss of splinting action of the spastic leg and trunk muscles and sometimes lead to an increase in disability.

Baclofen p. 1092 inhibits transmission at spinal level and also depresses the central nervous system. The dose should be increased slowly to avoid the major side-effects of sedation and muscular hypotonia (other adverse events are uncommon).

A cannabis extract p. 1092 containing dronabinol (delta-9-tetrahydrocannabinol) and cannabidiol is licensed as an adjunct treatment for moderate to severe spasticity associated with Multiple sclerosis p. 828 in patients who have not responded adequately to other skeletal muscle relaxants. The dose should be titrated over 2 weeks; response to treatment should be reviewed after 4 weeks and treatment stopped if an adequate response is not achieved.

Dantrolene sodium p. 1307 acts directly on skeletal muscle and produces fewer central adverse effects making it a drug of choice. The dose should be increased slowly.

Diazepam p. 340 can also be used. Sedation and occasionally extensor hypotonus are disadvantages. Other benzodiazepines also have muscle-relaxant properties.

Muscle-relaxant doses of benzodiazepines are similar to anxiolytic doses.

Tizanidine p. 1094 is an alpha$_2$-adrenoceptor agonist indicated for spasticity associated with Multiple sclerosis p. 828 or spinal cord injury.

Other muscle relaxants
The clinical efficacy of methocarbamol p. 1093 and meprobamate p. 343 as muscle relaxants are **not** well established, although they have been included in compound analgesic preparations.

NEUROPROTECTIVE DRUGS

Riluzole

● INDICATIONS AND DOSE

To extend life in patients with amyotrophic lateral sclerosis, initiated by specialist experienced in the management of motor neurone disease
▸ BY MOUTH
▸ Adult: 50 mg twice daily

● CONTRA-INDICATIONS Acute porphyrias p. 1025
● CAUTIONS History of abnormal hepatic function (consult product literature for details) · interstitial lung disease
CAUTIONS, FURTHER INFORMATION
▸ Interstitial lung disease Perform chest radiography if symptoms such as dry cough or dyspnoea develop; discontinue if interstitial lung disease is diagnosed.
● INTERACTIONS → Appendix 1: riluzole
● SIDE-EFFECTS
▸ **Common or very common** Abdominal pain · asthenia · diarrhoea · dizziness · drowsiness · headache · nausea · oral paraesthesia · pain · tachycardia · vomiting
▸ **Uncommon** Anaemia · angioedema · interstitial lung disease · pancreatitis
▸ **Frequency not known** Hepatitis · neutropenia
SIDE-EFFECTS, FURTHER INFORMATION White blood cell counts should be determined in febrile illness; neutropenia requires discontinuation of riluzole.
● PREGNANCY Avoid—no information available.
● BREAST FEEDING Avoid—no information available.
● HEPATIC IMPAIRMENT Avoid.
● RENAL IMPAIRMENT Avoid—no information available.
● PATIENT AND CARER ADVICE
Blood disorders Patients or their carers should be told how to recognise signs of neutropenia and advised to seek immediate medical attention if symptoms such as fever occur.
Driving and skilled tasks Dizziness or vertigo may affect performance of skilled tasks (e.g. driving).
● NATIONAL FUNDING/ACCESS DECISIONS
NICE decisions
▸ Riluzole for motor neurone disease (January 2001) NICE TA20
Riluzole is recommended for treating the amyotrophic lateral sclerosis (ALS) form of motor neurone disease (MND). Treatment should be initiated by a specialist in MND but it can then be supervised under a shared-care arrangement involving the general practitioner.
www.nice.org.uk/TA20

● MEDICINAL FORMS
There can be variation in the licensing of different medicines containing the same drug. Forms available from special-order manufacturers include: oral suspension, oral solution, powder
Oral suspension
▸ Teglutik (Martindale Pharmaceuticals Ltd)
Riluzole 5 mg per 1 ml Teglutik 5mg/1ml oral suspension sugar-free | 300 ml [PoM] £100.00 DT = £100.00

Tablet
▸ Riluzole (Non-proprietary)
Riluzole 50 mg Riluzole 50mg tablets | 56 tablet [PoM] £320.00 DT = £15.89
▸ Rilutek (Sanofi)
Riluzole 50 mg Rilutek 50mg tablets | 56 tablet [PoM] £320.33 DT = £15.89

3.1 Muscular dystrophy

DRUGS FOR NEUROMUSCULAR DISORDERS

Ataluren
24-May-2017

● DRUG ACTION Ataluren restores the synthesis of dystrophin by allowing ribosomes to read through premature stop codons that cause incomplete dystrophin synthesis in nonsense mutation Duchenne muscular dystrophy.

● INDICATIONS AND DOSE

Duchenne muscular dystrophy resulting from a nonsense mutation in the dystrophin gene, in ambulatory patients (initiated by a specialist)
▸ BY MOUTH
▸ Adult: (consult product literature)

● INTERACTIONS → Appendix 1: ataluren
● SIDE-EFFECTS
▸ **Common or very common** Appetite decreased · constipation · cough · enuresis · fever · flatulence · gastrointestinal discomfort · haemorrhage · headache · hypertension · hypertriglyceridaemia · nausea · pain · rash erythematous · vomiting · weight decreased
● PREGNANCY Manufacturer advises avoid—toxicity in *animal* studies.
● BREAST FEEDING Manufacturer advises discontinue breastfeeding—present in milk in *animal* studies.
● HEPATIC IMPAIRMENT Manufacturer advises close monitoring—safety and efficacy not established.
● RENAL IMPAIRMENT Manufacturer advises close monitoring—safety and efficacy not established.
● MONITORING REQUIREMENTS Manufacturer advises monitor renal function at least every 6–12 months, and cholesterol and triglyceride concentrations at least annually.
● DIRECTIONS FOR ADMINISTRATION Manufacturer advises the contents of each sachet should be mixed with at least 30 mL of liquid (water, milk, fruit juice), or 3 tablespoons of semi-solid food (yoghurt or apple sauce).
● PATIENT AND CARER ADVICE Manufacturer advises patients should maintain adequate hydration during treatment.
Missed doses Manufacturer advises if a morning or midday dose is more than 3 hours late, or an evening dose is more than 6 hours late, the missed dose should not be taken and the next dose should be taken at the normal time.
● NATIONAL FUNDING/ACCESS DECISIONS
NICE decisions
▸ Ataluren for treating Duchenne muscular dystrophy with a nonsense mutation in the dystrophin gene (July 2016) NICE HST3
Ataluren, within its marketing authorisation, is recommended for treating Duchenne muscular dystrophy resulting from a nonsense mutation in the dystrophin gene in people aged 5 years and older who can walk, only when:
● the manufacturer provides ataluren with the discount agreed in the patient access scheme, **and**

10

Musculoskeletal system

- the conditions under which ataluren is made available are set out in the managed access agreement between the manufacturer and NHS England, which should include the conditions set out in sections 5.12–5.15 and 5.23 of the guidance.

Patients whose treatment was started within the NHS before this guidance was published should have the option to continue treatment, without change to their funding arrangements, until they and their NHS clinician consider it appropriate to stop.
www.nice.org.uk/guidance/HST3

Scottish Medicines Consortium (SMC) Decisions
The *Scottish Medicines Consortium* has advised (April 2016) that ataluren (*Translarna*®) is **not** recommended for use within NHS Scotland for the treatment of Duchenne muscular dystrophy resulting from a nonsense mutation in the dystrophin gene, in ambulatory patients aged 5 years and older as the economic case was not demonstrated.

All Wales Medicines Strategy Group (AWMSG) Decisions
The *All Wales Medicines Strategy Group* has advised (August 2016) that the NICE HST advice for ataluren (*Translarna*®) should be implemented within NHS Wales.

● MEDICINAL FORMS
There can be variation in the licensing of different medicines containing the same drug.
Granules
▸ Translarna (PTC Therapeutics Ltd) ▼
  Ataluren 125 mg Translarna 125mg granules for oral suspension sachets | 30 sachet [PoM] £2,532.00
  Ataluren 250 mg Translarna 250mg granules for oral suspension sachets | 30 sachet [PoM] £5,064.00
  Ataluren 1 gram Translarna 1,000mg granules for oral suspension sachets | 30 sachet [PoM] £20,256.00

Nusinersen

18-May-2018

● DRUG ACTION Nusinersen is an antisense oligonucleotide that increases the production of survival motor neurone (SMN) protein, thereby helping to compensate for the defect in the SMN1 gene found in 5q spinal muscular atrophy.

● INDICATIONS AND DOSE
5q spinal muscular atrophy (initiated by a specialist)
▸ BY INTRATHECAL INJECTION
▸ Adult: Initially 12 mg for 4 doses, on days 0, 14, 28 and 63, then 12 mg every 4 months, for advice on missed doses—consult product literature

● CAUTIONS Risk factors for renal toxicity—monitor urine protein (preferably using a first morning urine specimen) · risk factors for thrombocytopenia and coagulation disorders—monitor platelet and coagulation profile before treatment

● PREGNANCY Manufacturer advises avoid—no information available.

● BREAST FEEDING Manufacturer advises avoid—no information available.

● RENAL IMPAIRMENT Manufacturer advises close monitoring—safety and efficacy not established.

● HANDLING AND STORAGE Manufacturer advises store in a refrigerator (2–8 °C); may be stored (in the original carton, protected from light) at or below 30 °C, for up to 14 days.

● MEDICINAL FORMS
There can be variation in the licensing of different medicines containing the same drug.
Solution for injection
▸ Spinraza (Biogen Idec Ltd) ▼
  Nusinersen (as Nusinersen sodium) 2.4 mg per 1 ml Spinraza 12mg/5ml solution for injection vials | 1 vial [PoM] £75,000.00

3.2 Myasthenia gravis and Lambert-Eaton myasthenic syndrome

ANTICHOLINESTERASES

Anticholinesterases

● DRUG ACTION They prolong the action of acetylcholine by inhibiting the action of the enzyme acetylcholinesterase.

● CONTRA-INDICATIONS Intestinal obstruction · urinary obstruction

● CAUTIONS Arrhythmias · asthma (extreme caution) · atropine or other antidote to muscarinic effects may be necessary (particularly when neostigmine is given by injection) but not given routinely because it may mask signs of overdosage · bradycardia · epilepsy · hyperthyroidism · hypotension · parkinsonism · peptic ulceration · recent myocardial infarction · vagotonia

● SIDE-EFFECTS Abdominal cramps · diarrhoea · excessive tearing · gastrointestinal disorders · hypersalivation · muscle complaints · nausea · rash · vomiting

Overdose Signs of overdosage include bronchoconstriction, increased bronchial secretions, lacrimation, excessive sweating, involuntary defaecation, involuntary micturition, miosis, nystagmus, bradycardia, heart block, arrhythmias, hypotension, agitation, excessive dreaming, and weakness eventually leading to fasciculation and paralysis.

● PREGNANCY Manufacturer advises use only if potential benefit outweighs risk.

● BREAST FEEDING Amount probably too small to be harmful.

⚑ above

Neostigmine

(Neostigmine methylsulfate)

● INDICATIONS AND DOSE
Treatment of myasthenia gravis
▸ BY MOUTH
▸ Adult: Initially 15–30 mg, dose repeated at suitable intervals throughout the day, total daily dose 75–300 mg, the maximum that most patients can tolerate is 180 mg daily
▸ BY SUBCUTANEOUS INJECTION, OR BY INTRAMUSCULAR INJECTION
▸ Adult: 1–2.5 mg, dose repeated at suitable intervals throughout the day (usual total daily dose 5–20 mg)

Reversal of non-depolarising (competitive) neuromuscular blockade
▸ BY INTRAVENOUS INJECTION
▸ Adult: 2.5 mg (max. per dose 5 mg), repeated if necessary after or with glycopyrronium or atropine, to be given over 1 minute

● CAUTIONS Glycopyrronium or atropine should also be given when reversing neuromuscular blockade

● INTERACTIONS → Appendix 1: neostigmine

● RENAL IMPAIRMENT
Dose adjustments May need dose reduction.

- **MEDICINAL FORMS**
  There can be variation in the licensing of different medicines containing the same drug. Forms available from special-order manufacturers include: oral solution
  Solution for injection
  ▸ Neostigmine (Non-proprietary)
    Neostigmine metilsulfate 2.5 mg per 1 ml Neostigmine 2.5mg/1ml solution for injection ampoules | 10 ampoule [PoM] £5.45 DT = £5.45
  Tablet
  ▸ Neostigmine (Non-proprietary)
    Neostigmine bromide 15 mg Neostigmine 15mg tablets | 140 tablet [PoM] £120.52 DT = £120.52

◀ 1090

Pyridostigmine bromide

- **DRUG ACTION** Pyridostigmine bromide has weaker muscarinic action than neostigmine.

- **INDICATIONS AND DOSE**
  Myasthenia gravis
  ▸ INITIALLY BY MOUTH
  ▸ Adult: 30–120 mg, doses to be given at suitable intervals throughout day; (by mouth) usual dose 0.3–1.2 g daily in divided doses, it is inadvisable to exceed a total daily dose of 450 mg in order to avoid acetylcholine receptor down-regulation; patients requiring doses exceeding 450 mg daily will usually require input from a specialised neuromuscular service. Immunosuppressant therapy is usually considered if the dose of pyridostigmine exceeds 360 mg daily

- **INTERACTIONS** → Appendix 1: pyridostigmine
- **RENAL IMPAIRMENT**
  Dose adjustments Reduce dose; excreted by kidney.

- **MEDICINAL FORMS**
  There can be variation in the licensing of different medicines containing the same drug. Forms available from special-order manufacturers include: oral suspension, oral solution
  Tablet
  ▸ Pyridostigmine bromide (Non-proprietary)
    Pyridostigmine bromide 60 mg Pyridostigmine bromide 60mg tablets | 200 tablet [PoM] £45.48 DT = £44.02
  ▸ Mestinon (Meda Pharmaceuticals Ltd)
    Pyridostigmine bromide 60 mg Mestinon 60mg tablets | 200 tablet [PoM] £45.57 DT = £44.02

CHOLINERGIC RECEPTOR STIMULATING DRUGS

Amifampridine

- **INDICATIONS AND DOSE**
  Symptomatic treatment of Lambert-Eaton myasthenic syndrome (specialist use only)
  ▸ BY MOUTH
  ▸ Adult: Initially 15 mg daily in 3 divided doses, then increased in steps of 5 mg every 4–5 days, increased to up to 60 mg daily in 3–4 divided doses (max. per dose 20 mg); maximum 60 mg per day

- **CONTRA-INDICATIONS** Congenital QT syndromes · epilepsy · uncontrolled asthma
- **CAUTIONS** Non-paraneoplastic form of Lambert- Eaton myasthenic syndrome
- **INTERACTIONS** → Appendix 1: amifampridine
- **SIDE-EFFECTS** Anxiety · arrhythmia · asthenia · asthma · bronchial secretion increased · cough · dizziness · drowsiness · gastrointestinal disorder · headache · movement disorders · palpitations · paraesthesia · Raynaud's phenomenon · seizure · sleep disorder · vision blurred

- **CONCEPTION AND CONTRACEPTION** Ensure effective contraception during treatment in men and women.
- **PREGNANCY** Manufacturer advises avoid.
- **BREAST FEEDING** Manufacturer advises avoid—no information available.
- **HEPATIC IMPAIRMENT** Use with caution.
  Dose adjustments In mild impairment reduce initial dose to 10 mg daily in divided doses, increased in steps of 5 mg every 7 days.
      In moderate or severe impairment reduce initial dose to 5 mg daily in divided doses, increased in steps of 5 mg every 7 days.
- **RENAL IMPAIRMENT** Use with caution.
  Dose adjustments In mild impairment reduce initial dose to 10 mg daily in divided doses, increased in steps of 5 mg every 7 days.
      In moderate or severe impairment reduce initial dose to 5 mg daily in divided doses, increased in steps of 5 mg every 7 days.
- **MONITORING REQUIREMENTS** Clinical and ECG monitoring required at treatment initiation and yearly thereafter.
- **NATIONAL FUNDING/ACCESS DECISIONS**
  Scottish Medicines Consortium (SMC) Decisions
  The *Scottish Medicines Consortium* has advised (July 2012) that amifampridine phosphate (*Firdapse®*) is not recommended for use within NHS Scotland for the symptomatic treatment of Lambert-Eaton myasthenic syndrome (LEMS).

- **MEDICINAL FORMS**
  There can be variation in the licensing of different medicines containing the same drug. Forms available from special-order manufacturers include: tablet
  Tablet
  CAUTIONARY AND ADVISORY LABELS 3, 21
  ▸ Firdapse (BioMarin Europe Ltd) ▼
    Amifampridine (as Amifampridine phosphate) 10 mg Firdapse 10mg tablets | 100 tablet [PoM] £1,815.00

3.3 Nocturnal leg cramps

Nocturnal leg cramps

Quinine salts

Quinine salts p. 608, such as quinine sulfate are effective in reducing the frequency of nocturnal leg cramps by about 25% in ambulatory patients; however, because of potential toxicity, quinine is not recommended for routine treatment and should not be used unless cramps cause regular disruption to sleep. Quinine should only be considered when cramps are very painful or frequent; when other treatable causes of cramp have been excluded; and when non-pharmacological treatments have not worked (e.g. passive stretching exercises). It may take up to 4 weeks for improvement to become apparent; if there is benefit, quinine treatment can be continued. Treatment should be interrupted at intervals of approximately 3 months to assess the need for further quinine treatment. In patients taking quinine long term, a trial discontinuation may be considered. Quinine is toxic in overdosage and accidental fatalities have occurred.

3.4 Spasticity

Other drugs used for Spasticity Dantrolene sodium, p. 1307
· Diazepam, p. 340

CANNABINOIDS

Cannabis extract

- **INDICATIONS AND DOSE**

Adjunct in moderate to severe spasticity in multiple sclerosis (specialist use only)
▶ BY BUCCAL ADMINISTRATION
▶ Adult: (consult product literature)

- CONTRA-INDICATIONS Family history of psychosis · history of other severe psychiatric disorder · personal history of psychosis
- CAUTIONS History of epilepsy · significant cardiovascular disease
- INTERACTIONS → Appendix 1: cannabis extract
- SIDE-EFFECTS
▶ **Common or very common** Appetite abnormal · balance impaired · concentration impaired · constipation · depression · diarrhoea · disorientation · dizziness · drowsiness · dry mouth · dysarthria · euphoric mood · feeling drunk · malaise · memory loss · nausea · oral disorders · perception altered · taste altered · vertigo · vision blurred · vomiting
▶ **Uncommon** Abdominal pain upper · delusions · hallucinations · hypertension · palpitations · paranoia · pharyngitis · suicidal ideation · syncope · tachycardia · throat irritation

- CONCEPTION AND CONTRACEPTION Manufacturer recommends effective contraception during and for 3 months after treatment in men and women.
- PREGNANCY Manufacturer advises use only if potential benefit outweighs risks.
- BREAST FEEDING Avoid—present in milk.
- HEPATIC IMPAIRMENT
Monitoring Manufacturer advises more frequent monitoring in significant hepatic impairment—possible risk of prolonged or enhanced effect.
- RENAL IMPAIRMENT
Monitoring Manufacturer advises more frequent monitoring in significant renal impairment—possible risk of prolonged or enhanced effect.
- MONITORING REQUIREMENTS Monitor oral mucosa—interrupt treatment if lesions or persistent soreness.
- PATIENT AND CARER ADVICE
Driving and skilled tasks For information on 2015 legislation regarding driving whilst taking certain controlled drugs, including cannabis, see Drugs and driving under Guidance on prescribing p. 1.

- MEDICINAL FORMS
There can be variation in the licensing of different medicines containing the same drug.
Spray
EXCIPIENTS: May contain Propylene glycol
▶ Sativex (Bayer Plc)
Cannabidiol 2.5 mg per 1 dose, Dronabinol 2.7 mg per 1 dose Sativex oromucosal spray | 270 dose [PoM] £375.00 [CD4-1]

MUSCLE RELAXANTS > CENTRALLY ACTING

Baclofen

21-Nov-2016

- **INDICATIONS AND DOSE**

Pain of muscle spasm in palliative care
▶ BY MOUTH
▶ Adult: 5–10 mg 3 times a day
Hiccup due to gastric distension (in palliative care)
▶ BY MOUTH
▶ Adult: 5 mg twice daily
Chronic severe spasticity resulting from disorders such as multiple sclerosis or traumatic partial section of spinal cord
▶ BY MOUTH
▶ Adult: Initially 5 mg 3 times a day, gradually increased; maintenance up to 60 mg daily in divided doses, review treatment if no benefit within 6 weeks of achieving maximum dose; maximum 100 mg per day
Severe chronic spasticity unresponsive to oral antispastic drugs (or where side-effects of oral therapy unacceptable) or as alternative to ablative neurosurgical procedures (specialist use only)
▶ BY INTRATHECAL INJECTION
▶ Adult: Test dose 25–50 micrograms, to be given over at least 1 minute via catheter or lumbar puncture, then increased in steps of 25 micrograms (max. per dose 100 micrograms), not given more often than every 24 hours to determine appropriate dose, then *dose-titration phase*, most often using infusion pump (implanted into chest wall or abdominal wall tissues) to establish maintenance dose (ranging from 12 micrograms to 2 mg daily for spasticity of spinal origin or 22 micrograms to 1.4 mg daily for spasticity of cerebral origin) retaining some spasticity to avoid sensation of paralysis

> **IMPORTANT SAFETY INFORMATION**
> Consult product literature for details on test dose and titration—important to monitor patients closely in appropriately equipped and staffed environment during screening and immediately after pump implantation. Resuscitation equipment must be available for immediate use. Treatment with continuous pump-administered intrathecal baclofen should be initiated within 3 months of a satisfactory response to intrathecal baclofen testing.

- CONTRA-INDICATIONS
▶ With intrathecal use Local infection · systemic infection
▶ With oral use Avoid oral route in active peptic ulceration
- CAUTIONS
GENERAL CAUTIONS Cerebrovascular disease · diabetes · elderly · epilepsy · history of peptic ulcer · hypertonic bladder sphincter · Parkinson's disease · psychiatric illness · respiratory impairment
SPECIFIC CAUTIONS
▶ With intrathecal use Coagulation disorders · malnutrition (increased risk of post-surgical complications) · previous spinal fusion procedure
- INTERACTIONS → Appendix 1: baclofen
- SIDE-EFFECTS
GENERAL SIDE-EFFECTS
▶ **Common or very common** Asthenia · confusion · constipation · depression · diarrhoea · dizziness · drowsiness · dry mouth · euphoric mood · hallucination · headache · hyperhidrosis · hypotension · nausea · paraesthesia · respiratory disorders · sexual dysfunction · skin reactions · sleep disorders · urinary disorders · vision disorders · vomiting

▶ **Uncommon** Bradycardia · hypothermia · taste altered
▶ **Rare or very rare** Withdrawal syndrome
  SPECIFIC SIDE-EFFECTS
▶ **Common or very common**
 ▸ With intrathecal use Anxiety · appetite decreased · chills · dyspnoea · fever · hypersalivation · neuromuscular dysfunction · oedema · pain · pneumonia · seizure
 ▸ With oral use Gastrointestinal disorder · muscle weakness · myalgia
▶ **Uncommon**
 ▸ With intrathecal use Alopecia · deep vein thrombosis · dehydration · flushing · hypertension · ileus · memory loss · pallor · paranoia · suicidal tendencies
▶ **Rare or very rare**
 ▸ With oral use Abdominal pain · hepatic function abnormal
▶ **Frequency not known**
 ▸ With intrathecal use Scoliosis

● PREGNANCY Manufacturer advises use only if potential benefit outweighs risk (toxicity in *animal* studies).

● BREAST FEEDING Present in milk—amount probably too small to be harmful.

● HEPATIC IMPAIRMENT
● With oral use Manufacturer advises use with caution.

● RENAL IMPAIRMENT Excreted by the kidney.
  Dose adjustments ▸ With oral use Risk of toxicity—use smaller doses (e.g. 5 mg daily by mouth) and if necessary increase dosage interval; if eGFR less than 15 mL/minute/1.73 m^2 manufacturer advises use by mouth only if potential benefit outweighs risk.

● TREATMENT CESSATION Avoid abrupt withdrawal (risk of hyperactive state, may exacerbate spasticity, and precipitate autonomic dysfunction including hyperthermia, psychiatric reactions and convulsions; to minimise risk, discontinue by gradual dose reduction over at least 1–2 weeks (longer if symptoms occur)).

● PRESCRIBING AND DISPENSING INFORMATION Flavours of oral liquid formulations may include raspberry.
  Palliative care For further information on the use of baclofen in palliative care, see www.palliativedrugs.com/formulary/en/baclofen.html.

● PATIENT AND CARER ADVICE
  Driving and skilled tasks Drowsiness may affect performance of skilled tasks (e.g. driving); effects of alcohol enhanced.

● MEDICINAL FORMS
  There can be variation in the licensing of different medicines containing the same drug. Forms available from special-order manufacturers include: oral suspension, oral solution, solution for injection

Tablet
CAUTIONARY AND ADVISORY LABELS 2, 8, 21
EXCIPIENTS: May contain Gluten
 ▸ Baclofen (Non-proprietary)
  Baclofen 10 mg Baclofen 10mg tablets | 84 tablet PoM £9.99 DT = £1.07
 ▸ Lioresal (Novartis Pharmaceuticals UK Ltd)
  Baclofen 10 mg Lioresal 10mg tablets | 100 tablet PoM £14.86

Solution for injection
 ▸ Baclofen (Non-proprietary)
  Baclofen 50 microgram per 1 ml Baclofen 50micrograms/1ml solution for injection ampoules | 10 ampoule PoM £25.00–£27.60
 ▸ Lioresal (Novartis Pharmaceuticals UK Ltd)
  Baclofen 50 microgram per 1 ml Lioresal Intrathecal 50micrograms/1ml solution for injection ampoules | 1 ampoule PoM £3.16

Solution for infusion
 ▸ Baclofen (Non-proprietary)
  Baclofen 500 microgram per 1 ml Baclofen 10mg/20ml solution for infusion ampoules | 1 ampoule PoM £50.00–£57.00
  Baclofen 2 mg per 1 ml Baclofen 40mg/20ml solution for infusion ampoules | 1 ampoule PoM £228.00–£250.00

Baclofen 10mg/5ml solution for infusion ampoules | 10 ampoule PoM £500.00–£570.00
 ▸ Lioresal (Novartis Pharmaceuticals UK Ltd)
  Baclofen 500 microgram per 1 ml Lioresal Intrathecal 10mg/20ml solution for infusion ampoules | 1 ampoule PoM £70.01
  Baclofen 2 mg per 1 ml Lioresal Intrathecal 10mg/5ml solution for infusion ampoules | 1 ampoule PoM £70.01

Oral solution
CAUTIONARY AND ADVISORY LABELS 2, 8, 21
 ▸ Baclofen (Non-proprietary)
  Baclofen 1 mg per 1 ml Baclofen 5mg/5ml oral solution sugar free sugar-free | 300 ml PoM £13.45 DT = £2.71
 ▸ Lioresal (Novartis Pharmaceuticals UK Ltd)
  Baclofen 1 mg per 1 ml Lioresal 5mg/5ml liquid sugar-free | 300 ml PoM £10.31 DT = £2.71
 ▸ Lyflex (Chemidex Pharma Ltd)
  Baclofen 1 mg per 1 ml Lyflex 5mg/5ml oral solution sugar-free | 300 ml PoM £7.95 DT = £2.71

Methocarbamol

● **INDICATIONS AND DOSE**
Short-term symptomatic relief of muscle spasm
▶ BY MOUTH
 ▸ **Adult:** 1.5 g 4 times a day; reduced to 750 mg 3 times a day if required
 ▸ **Elderly:** Up to 750 mg 4 times a day, dose may be sufficient

● CONTRA-INDICATIONS Brain damage · coma · epilepsy · myasthenia gravis · pre-coma

● INTERACTIONS → Appendix 1: methocarbamol

● SIDE-EFFECTS Angioedema · anxiety · bradycardia · confusion · conjunctivitis · dizziness · drowsiness · dyspepsia · fever · flushing · headache · hepatic disorders · hypotension · insomnia · leucopenia · memory loss · nasal congestion · nausea · seizures · skin reactions · syncope · taste metallic · vertigo · vision disorders · vomiting

● PREGNANCY Manufacturer advises avoid unless potential benefit outweighs risk.

● BREAST FEEDING Present in milk in *animal studies*— manufacturer advises caution.

● HEPATIC IMPAIRMENT Manufacturer advises caution; half-life may be prolonged.

● RENAL IMPAIRMENT Manufacturer advises caution.

● PATIENT AND CARER ADVICE
  Driving and skilled tasks Drowsiness may affect performance of skilled tasks (e.g. driving); effects of alcohol enhanced.

● LESS SUITABLE FOR PRESCRIBING Less suitable for prescribing.

● MEDICINAL FORMS
  There can be variation in the licensing of different medicines containing the same drug. Forms available from special-order manufacturers include: oral suspension

Tablet
CAUTIONARY AND ADVISORY LABELS 2
 ▸ Methocarbamol (Non-proprietary)
  Methocarbamol 750 mg Methocarbamol 750mg tablets | 100 tablet PoM £12.78 DT = £12.72
 ▸ Robaxin (Almirall Ltd)
  Methocarbamol 750 mg Robaxin 750 tablets | 100 tablet PoM £12.65 DT = £12.72

Musculoskeletal system

Tizanidine

● **INDICATIONS AND DOSE**

Spasticity associated with multiple sclerosis or spinal cord injury or disease

▸ BY MOUTH

▸ Adult: Initially 2 mg daily, then increased in steps of 2 mg daily in divided doses, increased at intervals of at least 3–4 days and adjust according to response; usual dose up to 24 mg daily in 3–4 divided doses; maximum 36 mg per day

● CAUTIONS Elderly

● INTERACTIONS → Appendix 1: tizanidine

● SIDE-EFFECTS

▸ **Common or very common** Arrhythmias · dizziness · drowsiness · dry mouth · fatigue · hypotension · rebound hypertension

▸ **Rare or very rare** Gastrointestinal disorder · hallucination · hepatic disorders · muscle weakness · nausea · sleep disorders

▸ **Frequency not known** Abdominal pain · accommodation disorder · anxiety · appetite decreased · confusion · headache · QT interval prolongation · skin reactions · vomiting · withdrawal syndrome

SIDE-EFFECTS, FURTHER INFORMATION Treatment should be discontinued if liver enzymes are persistently raised—consult product literature.

● PREGNANCY Avoid (toxicity in *animal* studies).

● BREAST FEEDING Avoid (present in milk in *animal* studies).

● HEPATIC IMPAIRMENT Avoid in severe impairment; use in moderate impairment only if potential benefit outweighs risk.

● RENAL IMPAIRMENT Manufacturer advises caution.

● MONITORING REQUIREMENTS Monitor liver function monthly for first 4 months and in those who develop unexplained nausea, anorexia or fatigue.

● TREATMENT CESSATION Avoid abrupt withdrawal (risk of rebound hypertension and tachycardia); to minimise risk, discontinue gradually and monitor blood pressure.

● PATIENT AND CARER ADVICE

Driving and skilled tasks Drowsiness may affect performance of skilled tasks (e.g. driving); effects of alcohol enhanced.

● MEDICINAL FORMS

There can be variation in the licensing of different medicines containing the same drug. Forms available from special-order manufacturers include: oral suspension, oral solution

Tablet

CAUTIONARY AND ADVISORY LABELS 2, 8

▸ Tizanidine (Non-proprietary)

Tizanidine (as Tizanidine hydrochloride) 2 mg Tizanidine 2mg tablets | 120 tablet [PoM] £28.89 DT = £3.45

Tizanidine (as Tizanidine hydrochloride) 4 mg Tizanidine 4mg tablets | 120 tablet [PoM] £40.07 DT = £39.56

---

4 Pain and inflammation in musculoskeletal disorders

Non-steroidal anti-inflammatory drugs

05-Jun-2017

Therapeutic effects

In *single doses* non-steroidal anti-inflammatory drugs (NSAIDs) have analgesic activity comparable to that of paracetamol p. 438, but paracetamol is preferred, particularly in the elderly.

In regular *full dosage* NSAIDs have both a lasting analgesic and an anti-inflammatory effect which makes them particularly useful for the treatment of continuous or regular pain associated with inflammation. Therefore, although paracetamol often gives adequate pain control in osteoarthritis, NSAIDs are more appropriate than paracetamol or the opioid analgesics in the *inflammatory arthritides* (e.g. rheumatoid arthritis) and in some cases of *advanced osteoarthritis*. NSAIDs can also be of benefit in the less well defined conditions of *back pain* and *soft-tissue disorders*.

Choice

Differences in anti-inflammatory activity between NSAIDs are small, but there is considerable variation in individual response and tolerance to these drugs. About 60% of patients will respond to any NSAID; of the others, those who do not respond to one may well respond to another. Pain relief starts soon after taking the first dose and a full analgesic effect should normally be obtained within a week, whereas an anti-inflammatory effect may not be achieved (or may not be clinically assessable) for up to 3 weeks. If appropriate responses are not obtained within these times, another NSAID should be tried.

NSAIDs reduce the production of prostaglandins by inhibiting the enzyme cyclo-oxygenase. They vary in their selectivity for inhibiting different types of cyclo-oxygenase; selective inhibition of cyclo-oxygenase-2 is associated with less gastro-intestinal intolerance. Several other factors also influence susceptibility to gastrointestinal effects, and a NSAID should be chosen on the basis of the incidence of gastro-intestinal and other side-effects.

Ibuprofen p. 1106 is a propionic acid derivative with anti-inflammatory, analgesic, and antipyretic properties. It has fewer side-effects than other non-selective NSAIDs but its anti-inflammatory properties are weaker. It is unsuitable for conditions where inflammation is prominent, such as acute gout. Dexibuprofen p. 1098 is the active enantiomer of ibuprofen. It has similar properties to ibuprofen and is licensed for the relief of mild to moderate pain and inflammation.

Other propionic acid derivatives:

Naproxen p. 1113 is one of the first choices because it combines good efficacy with a low incidence of side-effects (but more than ibuprofen).

Fenoprofen p. 1105 is as effective as naproxen, and flurbiprofen p. 1106 may be slightly more effective. Both are associated with slightly more gastro-intestinal side-effects than ibuprofen.

Ketoprofen p. 1110 has anti-inflammatory properties similar to ibuprofen and has more side-effects. Dexketoprofen p. 1099, an isomer of ketoprofen, has been introduced for the short-term relief of mild to moderate pain.

Tiaprofenic acid p. 1117 is as effective as naproxen; it has more side-effects than ibuprofen.

Drugs with properties similar to those of propionic acid derivatives:

Diclofenac sodium p. 1101 and aceclofenac p. 1096 are similar in efficacy to naproxen.

Etodolac p. 1103 is comparable in efficacy to naproxen; it is licensed for symptomatic relief of osteoarthritis and rheumatoid arthritis.

Indometacin p. 1109 has an action equal to or superior to that of naproxen, but with a high incidence of side-effects including headache, dizziness, and gastro-intestinal disturbances.

Mefenamic acid p. 1111 has minor anti-inflammatory properties. It has occasionally been associated with diarrhoea and haemolytic anaemia which require discontinuation of treatment.

Meloxicam p. 1112 is licensed for the short-term relief of pain in osteoarthritis and for long-term treatment of rheumatoid arthritis and ankylosing spondylitis.

Nabumetone p. 1113 is comparable in effect to naproxen.

Phenylbutazone is licensed for ankylosing spondylitis, but is not recommended because it is associated with serious side-effects, in particular haematological reactions; it should be used only by a specialist in severe cases where other treatments have been found unsuitable.

Piroxicam p. 1115 is as effective as naproxen and has a long duration of action which permits once-daily administration. However, it has more gastro-intestinal side-effects than most other NSAIDs, and is associated with more frequent serious skin reactions.

Sulindac p. 1116 is similar in tolerance to naproxen.

Tenoxicam p. 1117 is similar in activity and tolerance to naproxen. Its long duration of action allows once-daily administration.

Tolfenamic acid p. 469 is licensed for the treatment of migraine.

Ketorolac trometamol p. 1144 and the selective inhibitor of cyclo-oxygenase-2, parecoxib p. 1303, are licensed for the short-term management of postoperative pain.

The selective inhibitors of cyclo-oxygenase-2, etoricoxib p. 1104 and celecoxib p. 1097, are as effective as non-selective NSAIDs such as diclofenac sodium and naproxen. Although selective inhibitors can cause serious gastro-intestinal events, available evidence appears to indicate that the risk of serious upper gastro-intestinal events is lower with selective inhibitors compared to non-selective NSAIDs; this advantage may be lost in patients who require concomitant low-dose aspirin.

Celecoxib and etoricoxib are licensed for the relief of pain in osteoarthritis, rheumatoid arthritis, and ankylosing spondylitis; etoricoxib is also licensed for the relief of pain from acute gout.

Aspirin p. 121 has been used in high doses to treat rheumatoid arthritis, but other NSAIDs are now preferred.

Dental and orofacial pain

Most mild to moderate dental pain and inflammation is effectively relieved by NSAIDs. Those used for dental pain include ibuprofen, diclofenac sodium, and diclofenac potassium p. 1100.

Asthma

Any degree of worsening of asthma may be related to the ingestion of NSAIDs, either prescribed or (in the case of ibuprofen **and** others) purchased over the counter.

NSAIDs and cardiovascular events

All NSAID use (including cyclo-oxygenase-2 selective inhibitors) can, to varying degrees, be associated with a small increased risk of thrombotic events (e.g. myocardial infarction and stroke) independent of baseline cardiovascular risk factors or duration of NSAID use; however, the greatest risk may be in those receiving high doses long term.

Cyclo-oxygenase-2 selective inhibitors, diclofenac (150 mg daily) and ibuprofen (2.4 g daily) are associated with an increased risk of thrombotic events. Although there are limited data regarding the thrombotic effects of aceclofenac, treatment advice has been updated in line with diclofenac, based on aceclofenac's structural similarity to diclofenac and its metabolism to diclofenac. The increased risk for diclofenac is similar to that of licensed doses of etoricoxib. Naproxen (1 g daily) is associated with a lower thrombotic risk, and low doses of ibuprofen (1.2 g daily or less) have not been associated with an increased risk of myocardial infarction.

The lowest effective dose of NSAID should be prescribed for the shortest period of time to control symptoms and the need for long-term treatment should be reviewed periodically.

NSAIDs and gastro-intestinal events

All NSAIDs are associated with serious gastro-intestinal toxicity; the risk is higher in the elderly. Evidence on the relative safety of non-selective NSAIDs indicates differences in the risks of serious upper gastro-intestinal side-effects—piroxicam p. 1115, ketoprofen p. 1110, and ketorolac trometamol p. 1144 are associated with the highest risk; indometacin p. 1109, diclofenac, and naproxen p. 1113 are associated with intermediate risk, and ibuprofen p. 1106 with the lowest risk (although high doses of ibuprofen have been associated with intermediate risk). Selective inhibitors of cyclo-oxygenase-2 are associated with a *lower risk* of serious upper gastro-intestinal side-effects than non-selective NSAIDs.

Recommendations are that NSAIDs associated with a low risk e.g. ibuprofen are *generally preferred*, to start at the *lowest recommended dose* **and** not to use more than one oral NSAID at a time.

The combination of a NSAID **and** low-dose aspirin can increase the risk of gastro-intestinal side-effects; this combination should be used only if absolutely necessary **and** the patient should be monitored closely.

While it is preferable to avoid NSAIDs in patients with active or previous gastro-intestinal ulceration or bleeding, and to withdraw them if gastro-intestinal lesions develop, nevertheless patients with serious rheumatic diseases (e.g. rheumatoid arthritis) are usually dependent on NSAIDs for effective relief of pain and stiffness.

Patients at risk of gastro-intestinal ulceration (including the elderly), who need NSAID treatment should receive gastroprotective treatment.

Systemic as well as local effects of NSAIDs contribute to gastro–intestinal damage; taking oral formulations with milk or food, or using enteric-coated formulations, or changing the route of administration may only partially reduce symptoms such as dyspepsia.

NSAIDs and alcohol

Alcohol increases the risk of gastro-intestinal haemorrhage associated with NSAIDs. Specialist sources recommend that concurrent use need not be avoided with moderate alcohol intake, but greater caution is warranted in those who drink more than the recommended daily limits.

Some cases of acute kidney injury have been attributed to use of NSAIDs and acute excessive alcohol consumption.

Low back pain and sciatica
08-Mar-2017

Description of condition

Low back pain is pain in the lumbosacral area of the back. It can be described as *non-specific, mechanical, musculoskeletal* or *simple* (if it is not associated with serious or potentially serious causes). Episodes of back pain do not usually last long, with rapid improvements in pain and disability seen within a few weeks to months.

Sciatica (*radicular pain* or *radiculopathy*) is neuropathic leg pain secondary to compressive lumbosacral nerve root pathology.

Non-drug treatment

EvGr Exercise programmes, manual therapy, and psychological therapies should be considered for managing low back pain with or without sciatica.

Spinal decompression may be considered in patients with sciatica when pain and function has not improved with non-surgical treatment (including drug treatment). ⟨A⟩

Drug treatment

EvGr An oral NSAID (see Non-steroidal anti-inflammatory drugs p. 1094) should be considered for managing acute low back pain, taking into consideration the gastro-intestinal, cardio-renal and hepatic risks associated with NSAIDs; as well as the need for continued monitoring, and the possible need for gastroprotective treatment (see *NSAID-associated ulcers* under Peptic ulceration p. 71).

A weak opioid, either alone or with paracetamol p. 438, can be used to manage acute low back pain only if an NSAID is contra-indicated, not tolerated or ineffective (see *Opioid analgesics* under Analgesics p. 436). Paracetamol alone is ineffective for managing low back pain. Ⓐ

EvGr Benzodiazepines are sometimes used to manage acute low back pain (particularly in loss of lordosis); however evidence to support their use is very weak. Ⓔ

EvGr In patients with chronic low back pain who have had an inadequate response to non-drug treatment, NSAIDs should be considered as first-line therapy. Opioids should be the last treatment option considered and should be considered only in patients for whom other therapies have failed and only if the potential benefits outweigh the risks for individual patients. If indicated, opioids should only be prescribed for a limited period of time. Long term opioid therapy should be avoided.

Selective serotonin re-uptake inhibitors (SSRIs), serotonin and noradrenaline re-uptake inhibitors (SNRIs), tricyclic antidepressants, and antiepileptic drugs should **not** be offered for managing low back pain.

When non-surgical treatment is ineffective in patients with moderate and severe localised back pain arising from structures supplied by the medial branch nerve, radiofrequency denervation can be considered. Ⓐ

Sciatica

Patients with sciatica may require specific treatment for Neuropathic pain p. 475.

EvGr Patients with acute and severe sciatica may benefit from treatment with epidural injections of local anaesthetic and/or corticosteroid. Ⓐ

Useful Resources

Low back pain and sciatica. National Institute for Health and Care Excellence. Clinical guideline NG59. November 2016. www.nice.org.uk/guidance/ng59

ANALGESICS ⟩ NON-STEROIDAL ANTI-INFLAMMATORY DRUGS

| Aceclofenac

01-Jun-2016

- ● INDICATIONS AND DOSE

Pain and inflammation in rheumatoid arthritis, osteoarthritis and ankylosing spondylitis
  ▶ BY MOUTH
  ▶ Adult: 100 mg twice daily

- ● CONTRA-INDICATIONS Active gastro-intestinal bleeding · active gastro-intestinal ulceration · cerebrovascular disease · history of gastro-intestinal bleeding related to previous NSAID therapy · history of gastro-intestinal perforation related to previous NSAID therapy · history of recurrent gastro-intestinal haemorrhage (two or more distinct episodes) · history of recurrent gastro-intestinal ulceration (two or more distinct episodes) · ischaemic heart disease · mild heart failure · peripheral arterial disease · severe heart failure

- ● CAUTIONS Allergic disorders · avoid in Acute porphyrias p. 1025 · cardiac impairment (NSAIDs may impair renal function) · coagulation defects · connective-tissue disorders · Crohn's disease (may be exacerbated) · elderly (risk of serious side-effects and fatalities) · history of

cardiac failure · hypertension · left ventricular dysfunction · oedema · risk factors for cardiovascular events · ulcerative colitis (may be exacerbated)

- ● INTERACTIONS → Appendix 1: NSAIDs

- ● SIDE-EFFECTS
  ▶ **Common or very common** Diarrhoea · dizziness · gastrointestinal discomfort · nausea
  ▶ **Uncommon** Constipation · gastrointestinal disorders · oral disorders · skin reactions · vomiting
  ▶ **Rare or very rare** Anaemia · angiooedema · bone marrow disorders · depression · drowsiness · dyspnoea · fatigue · haemolytic anaemia · haemorrhage · headache · heart failure · hepatic disorders · hyperkalaemia · hypersensitivity · hypertension · inflammatory bowel disease · leg cramps · nephrotic syndrome · neutropenia · oedema · palpitations · pancreatitis · paraesthesia · renal failure (more common in patients with pre-existing renal impairment) · respiratory disorders · severe cutaneous adverse reactions (SCARs) · sleep disorders · taste altered · thrombocytopenia · tinnitus · tremor · vasculitis · vasodilation · vertigo · visual impairment · weight increased
  ▶ **Frequency not known** Acute coronary syndrome · agranulocytosis · asthma · confusion · hallucination · increased risk of arterial thromboembolism · increased risk of ischaemic stroke · malaise · meningitis aseptic (patients with connective-tissue disorders such as systemic lupus erythematosus may be especially susceptible) · nephritis tubulointerstitial · optic neuritis · photosensitivity reaction · platelet aggregation inhibition · respiratory tract reaction
  SIDE-EFFECTS, FURTHER INFORMATION For information about cardiovascular and gastrointestinal side-effects, and a possible exacerbation of symptoms in asthma, see Non-steroidal anti-inflammatory drugs p. 1094.

- ● ALLERGY AND CROSS-SENSITIVITY Contra-indicated in patients with a history of hypersensitivity to aspirin or any other NSAID—which includes those in whom attacks of asthma, angiooedema, urticaria or rhinitis have been precipitated by aspirin or any other NSAID.

- ● CONCEPTION AND CONTRACEPTION Caution—long-term use of some NSAIDs is associated with reduced female fertility, which is reversible on stopping treatment.

- ● PREGNANCY Most manufacturers advise avoiding the use of NSAIDs during pregnancy or avoiding them unless the potential benefit outweighs the risk. NSAIDs should be avoided during the third trimester because use is associated with a risk of closure of fetal ductus arteriosus *in utero* and possibly persistent pulmonary hypertension of the newborn. In addition, the onset of labour may be delayed and its duration may be increased.

- ● BREAST FEEDING Use with caution during breast-feeding. Manufacturer advises avoid.

- ● HEPATIC IMPAIRMENT Use with caution; there is an increased risk of gastro-intestinal bleeding and fluid retention. Avoid in severe liver disease.
  Dose adjustments Initially 100 mg daily.

- ● RENAL IMPAIRMENT Avoid if possible or use with caution; avoid in moderate to severe impairment.
  Dose adjustments The lowest effective dose should be used for the shortest possible duration.
  Monitoring In renal impairment monitor renal function; sodium and water retention may occur and renal function may deteriorate, possibly leading to renal failure.

● MEDICINAL FORMS
There can be variation in the licensing of different medicines
containing the same drug.

Tablet
CAUTIONARY AND ADVISORY LABELS 21
▸ Aceclofenac (Non-proprietary)
  Aceclofenac 100 mg Aceclofenac 100mg tablets | 60 tablet PoM
  £11.50 DT = £9.63
▸ Preservex (Almirall Ltd)
  Aceclofenac 100 mg Preservex 100mg tablets | 60 tablet PoM
  £9.63 DT = £9.63

Acemetacin

● DRUG ACTION Glycolic acid ester of indometacin.

● INDICATIONS AND DOSE
**Pain and inflammation in rheumatic disease | Pain and
inflammation in other musculoskeletal disorders |
Postoperative analgesia**
▸ BY MOUTH
▸ Adult: 120 mg daily in divided doses, then increased if
  necessary to 180 mg daily in divided doses, dose to be
  taken with food

● CONTRA-INDICATIONS Active gastro-intestinal bleeding ·
active gastro-intestinal ulceration · history of gastrointestinal bleeding related to previous NSAID therapy ·
history of gastro-intestinal perforation related to previous
NSAID therapy · history of recurrent gastro-intestinal
haemorrhage (two or more distinct episodes) · history of
recurrent gastro-intestinal ulceration (two or more
distinct episodes) · severe heart failure

● CAUTIONS Allergic disorders · cardiac impairment (NSAIDs
may impair renal function) · cerebrovascular disease ·
coagulation defects · connective-tissue disorders · Crohn's
disease (may be exacerbated) · elderly (risk of serious side-
effects and fatalities) · epilepsy · heart failure · ischaemic
heart disease · parkinsonism · peripheral arterial disease ·
psychiatric disturbances · risk factors for cardiovascular
events · ulcerative colitis (may be exacerbated) ·
uncontrolled hypertension

● INTERACTIONS → Appendix 1: NSAIDs

● SIDE-EFFECTS
▸ **Common or very common** Anxiety · appetite decreased ·
central nervous system disorders · diarrhoea · dizziness ·
drowsiness · fatigue · gastrointestinal discomfort ·
gastrointestinal disorders · haemorrhage · headache ·
hypersensitivity · malaise · nausea · skin reactions ·
vomiting
▸ **Uncommon** Alopecia · eye discolouration · hepatic
disorders · oedema
▸ **Rare or very rare** Acute kidney injury (more common in
patients with pre-existing renal impairment) ·
agranulocytosis · anaemia · angioedema · asthma · bone
marrow disorders · coma · confusion · constipation ·
depression · enanthema · eyelid oedema · haemolytic
anaemia · hallucination · hearing impairment ·
hyperglycaemia · hyperhidrosis · hyperkalaemia ·
hypersensitivity vasculitis · hypertension · inflammatory
bowel disease · irritability · kidney injury (more common in
patients with pre-existing renal impairment) · leucopenia ·
loss of consciousness · memory loss · meningitis aseptic
(patients with connective-tissue disorders such as
systemic lupus erythematosus may be especially
susceptible) · muscle weakness · nephritis
tubulointerstitial · nephrotic syndrome · oral disorders ·
pancreatitis · photosensitivity reaction · psychiatric
disorders · psychosis · renal papillary necrosis · respiratory
disorders · seizure · severe cutaneous adverse reactions
(SCARs) · shock · sleep disorders · tachycardia · taste

altered · thrombocytopenia · tremor · urinary disorder ·
urine abnormalities
▸ **Frequency not known** Circulatory collapse · dyspnoea ·
fertility decreased female · heart failure · increased risk of
arterial thromboembolism · increased risk of infection ·
increased risk of ischaemic stroke · increased risk of
myocardial infarction · optic neuritis · paraesthesia ·
respiratory tract reaction

SIDE-EFFECTS, FURTHER INFORMATION For information
about cardiovascular and gastrointestinal side-effects, and
a possible exacerbation of symptoms in asthma, see Non-
steroidal anti-inflammatory drugs p. 1094.

● ALLERGY AND CROSS-SENSITIVITY Contra-indicated in
patients with a history of hypersensitivity to aspirin or any
other NSAID—which includes those in whom attacks of
asthma, angioedema, urticaria or rhinitis have been
precipitated by aspirin or any other NSAID.

● CONCEPTION AND CONTRACEPTION Caution—long-term
use of some NSAIDs is associated with reduced female
fertility, which is reversible on stopping treatment.

● PREGNANCY Most manufacturers advise avoiding the use
of NSAIDs during pregnancy or avoiding them unless the
potential benefit outweighs the risk. NSAIDs should be
avoided during the third trimester because use is
associated with a risk of closure of fetal ductus arteriosus
in utero and possibly persistent pulmonary hypertension of
the newborn. In addition, the onset of labour may be
delayed and its duration may be increased.

● BREAST FEEDING Use with caution during breast-feeding.
Manufacturer advises avoid.

● HEPATIC IMPAIRMENT Use with caution; there is an
increased risk of gastro-intestinal bleeding and fluid
retention. Avoid in severe liver disease.

● RENAL IMPAIRMENT Avoid if possible or use with caution.
Dose adjustments The lowest effective dose should be used
for the shortest possible duration.
Monitoring In renal impairment monitor renal function;
sodium and water retention may occur and renal function
may deteriorate, possibly leading to renal failure.

● MONITORING REQUIREMENTS During prolonged therapy
ophthalmic and blood examinations particularly advisable.

● PATIENT AND CARER ADVICE
Driving and skilled tasks Dizziness may affect performance
of skilled tasks (e.g. driving).

● MEDICINAL FORMS
No licensed medicines listed.

Celecoxib
02-Jun-2017

● INDICATIONS AND DOSE
Pain and inflammation in osteoarthritis
▸ BY MOUTH
▸ Adult: 200 mg daily in 1–2 divided doses, then
  increased if necessary up to 200 mg twice daily,
  discontinue if no improvement after 2 weeks on
  maximum dose

Pain and inflammation in rheumatoid arthritis
▸ BY MOUTH
▸ Adult: 100 mg twice daily, then increased if necessary
  to 200 mg twice daily, discontinue if no improvement
  after 2 weeks on maximum dose

Ankylosing spondylitis
▸ BY MOUTH
▸ Adult: 200 mg daily in 1–2 divided doses, then
  increased if necessary up to 400 mg daily in 1–2 divided
  doses, discontinue if no improvement after 2 weeks on
  maximum dose   continued →

10

Musculoskeletal system

DOSE ADJUSTMENTS DUE TO INTERACTIONS
▶ Manufacturer advises reduce dose by half with concurrent use of fluconazole.

● CONTRA-INDICATIONS Active gastro-intestinal bleeding · active gastro-intestinal ulceration · cerebrovascular disease · inflammatory bowel disease · ischaemic heart disease · mild to severe heart failure · peripheral arterial disease

● CAUTIONS Allergic disorders · cardiac impairment (NSAIDs may impair renal function) · coagulation defects · connective-tissue disorders · Crohn's disease (may be exacerbated) · elderly (risk of serious side-effects and fatalities) · history of cardiac failure · hypertension · left ventricular dysfunction · oedema · risk factors for cardiovascular events · ulcerative colitis (may be exacerbated)

● INTERACTIONS → Appendix 1: NSAIDs

● SIDE-EFFECTS
▶ **Common or very common** Angina pectoris · benign prostatic hyperplasia · cough · diarrhoea · dizziness · dysphagia · dyspnoea · fluid retention · gastrointestinal discomfort · gastrointestinal disorders · headache · hypersensitivity · hypertension · increased risk of infection · influenza like illness · injury · insomnia · irritable bowel syndrome · joint disorders · muscle tone increased · myocardial infarction · nausea · nephrolithiasis · oedema · skin reactions · vomiting · weight increased
▶ **Uncommon** Anaemia · anxiety · arrhythmias · breast tenderness · burping · cerebral infarction · chest pain · conjunctivitis · constipation · depression · drowsiness · dysphonia · electrolyte imbalance · embolism and thrombosis · fatigue · haemorrhage · hearing impairment · heart failure · hepatic disorders · lipoma · lower limb fracture · muscle complaints · nocturia · oral disorders · palpitations · paraesthesia · respiratory disorders · vision blurred · vitreous floater
▶ **Rare or very rare** Acute kidney injury (more common in patients with pre-existing renal impairment) · alopecia · angioedema · anosmia · ataxia · confusion · flushing · hallucination · intracranial haemorrhage · leucopenia · meningitis aseptic · menstrual disorder · myositis · nephritis tubulointerstitial · nephropathy · pancreatitis · pancytopenia · photosensitivity reaction · seizures · severe cutaneous adverse reactions (SCARs) · taste altered · thrombocytopenia · vasculitis
▶ **Frequency not known** Infertility

SIDE-EFFECTS, FURTHER INFORMATION For information about cardiovascular and gastrointestinal side-effects, and a possible exacerbation of symptoms in asthma, see Non-steroidal anti-inflammatory drugs p. 1094.

● ALLERGY AND CROSS-SENSITIVITY Contra-indicated in patients with a history of hypersensitivity to aspirin or any other NSAID—which includes those in whom attacks of asthma, angioedema, urticaria or rhinitis have been precipitated by aspirin or any other NSAID.
    Contra-indicated in patients with sulfonamide sensitivity.

● CONCEPTION AND CONTRACEPTION Caution—long-term use of some NSAIDs is associated with reduced female fertility, which is reversible on stopping treatment.

● PREGNANCY Avoid (teratogenic in *animal* studies).

● BREAST FEEDING Avoid—present in milk in *animal* studies.

● HEPATIC IMPAIRMENT Use with caution; there is an increased risk of gastro-intestinal bleeding and fluid retention. Avoid in severe liver disease.
Dose adjustments Halve initial dose in moderate impairment.

● RENAL IMPAIRMENT Avoid if possible or use with caution. Avoid if eGFR less than 30 mL/minute/1.73 m².

Dose adjustments The lowest effective dose should be used for the shortest possible duration.
Monitoring In renal impairment monitor renal function; sodium and water retention may occur and renal function may deteriorate, possibly leading to renal failure.

● MONITORING REQUIREMENTS Monitor blood pressure before and during treatment.

● MEDICINAL FORMS
There can be variation in the licensing of different medicines containing the same drug.
Capsule
▶ Celecoxib (Non-proprietary)
    Celecoxib 100 mg Celecoxib 100mg capsules | 60 capsule [PoM]
    £21.55 DT = £1.95
    Celecoxib 200 mg Celecoxib 200mg capsules | 30 capsule [PoM]
    £21.55 DT = £1.69
▶ Celebrex (Pfizer Ltd)
    Celecoxib 100 mg Celebrex 100mg capsules | 60 capsule [PoM]
    £21.55 DT = £1.95
    Celecoxib 200 mg Celebrex 200mg capsules | 30 capsule [PoM]
    £21.55 DT = £1.69

Dexibuprofen

21-May-2018

● **INDICATIONS AND DOSE**
Osteoarthritis
▶ BY MOUTH
▶ Adult: 600–900 mg daily in up to 3 divided doses; increased if necessary up to 1200 mg daily (max. per dose 400 mg)

Dysmenorrhoea
▶ BY MOUTH
▶ Adult: 600–900 mg daily in up to 3 divided doses (max. per dose 400 mg)

Mild-to-moderate pain
▶ BY MOUTH
▶ Adult: 600 mg daily in up to 3 divided doses; increased if necessary up to 1200 mg daily (max. per dose 400 mg), higher dose for short-term use for acute pain

● CONTRA-INDICATIONS Active gastro-intestinal bleeding · active gastro-intestinal ulceration · history of gastro-intestinal bleeding related to previous NSAID therapy · history of gastro-intestinal perforation related to previous NSAID therapy · history of recurrent gastro-intestinal haemorrhage (two or more distinct episodes) · history of recurrent gastro-intestinal ulceration (two or more distinct episodes) · severe heart failure

● CAUTIONS Allergic disorders · cardiac impairment (NSAIDs may impair renal function) · cerebrovascular disease · coagulation defects · congestive heart failure · connective-tissue disorders · Crohn's disease (may be exacerbated) · elderly (risk of serious side-effects and fatalities) · ischaemic heart disease · peripheral arterial disease · risk factors for cardiovascular events · ulcerative colitis (may be exacerbated) · uncontrolled hypertension

CAUTIONS, FURTHER INFORMATION
▶ High-dose dexibuprofen A small increase in cardiovascular risk, similar to the risk associated with cyclo-oxygenase-2 inhibitors and diclofenac, has been reported with high-dose dexibuprofen (≥ 1.2 g daily); use should be avoided in patients with established ischaemic heart disease, peripheral arterial disease, cerebrovascular disease, congestive heart failure (New York Heart Association classification II-III), and uncontrolled hypertension.

● INTERACTIONS → Appendix 1: NSAIDs

● SIDE-EFFECTS
▶ **Common or very common** Diarrhoea · dizziness · drowsiness · fatigue · gastrointestinal discomfort · headache · nausea · skin reactions · vertigo · vomiting

▸ **Uncommon** Angioedema · anxiety · gastrointestinal disorders · haemorrhage · hearing impairment · increased risk of infection · insomnia · oral disorders · respiratory disorders · vasculitis · vision disorders

▸ **Rare or very rare** Agranulocytosis · alopecia · asthma · blood disorder · bone marrow disorders · confusion · constipation · depression · fever · granulocytopenia · haemolytic anaemia · hepatic disorders · hypersensitivity · hypotension · inflammatory bowel disease · irritability · leucopenia · meningitis aseptic (patients with connective-tissue disorders such as systemic lupus erythematosus may be especially susceptible) · nephritis tubulointerstitial · nephrotic syndrome · photosensitivity reaction · psychotic disorder · renal failure (more common in patients with pre-existing renal impairment) · severe cutaneous adverse reactions (SCARs) · shock · tachycardia · thrombocytopenia

▸ **Frequency not known** Fluid retention · generalised oedema · glomerulonephritis · increased risk of arterial thromboembolism · renal impairment · renal papillary necrosis

SIDE-EFFECTS, FURTHER INFORMATION For information about cardiovascular and gastrointestinal side-effects, and a possible exacerbation of symptoms in asthma, see Non-steroidal anti-inflammatory drugs p. 1094.

● ALLERGY AND CROSS-SENSITIVITY Contra-indicated in patients with a history of hypersensitivity to aspirin or any other NSAID—which includes those in whom attacks of asthma, angioedema, urticaria or rhinitis have been precipitated by aspirin or any other NSAID.

● CONCEPTION AND CONTRACEPTION Caution—long-term use of some NSAIDs is associated with reduced female fertility, which is reversible on stopping treatment.

● PREGNANCY Avoid unless the potential benefit outweighs the risk. Avoid during the third trimester (risk of closure of fetal ductus arteriosus *in utero* and possibly persistent pulmonary hypertension of the newborn); onset of labour may be delayed and duration may be increased.

● BREAST FEEDING Use with caution during breast-feeding. Present in milk—but risk to infant minimal.

● HEPATIC IMPAIRMENT Manufacturer advises close monitoring in mild-to-moderate impairment; avoid in severe impairment.
Dose adjustments Manufacturer advises reduce initial dose in mild-to-moderate impairment.

● RENAL IMPAIRMENT Avoid if possible or use with caution. Avoid if eGFR less than 30 mL/minute/1.73 m^2.
Dose adjustments Reduce initial dose.
The lowest effective dose should be used for the shortest possible duration.
Monitoring Monitor renal function; sodium and water retention may occur and renal function may deteriorate, possibly leading to renal failure.

● MEDICINAL FORMS
There can be variation in the licensing of different medicines containing the same drug.
Tablet
CAUTIONARY AND ADVISORY LABELS 21
▸ Seractil (Gebro Pharma GmbH)
Dexibuprofen 300 mg Seractil 300mg tablets | 60 tablet [PoM] £9.47

Dexketoprofen   23-Apr-2018

● INDICATIONS AND DOSE
Short-term treatment of mild to moderate pain including dysmenorrhoea
▸ BY MOUTH
▸ Adult: 12.5 mg every 4–6 hours, alternatively 25 mg every 8 hours; maximum 75 mg per day

▸ Elderly: 12.5 mg every 4–6 hours, alternatively 25 mg every 8 hours, initial max. 50 mg; maximum 75 mg daily

● CONTRA-INDICATIONS Active bleeding or bleeding disorders · active or recurrent gastro-intestinal haemorrhage · active or recurrent gastro-intestinal ulcer · chronic dyspepsia · Crohn's disease · history of NSAID-associated gastro-intestinal bleeding or perforation · known photoallergic or phototoxic reactions during treatment with ketoprofen or fibrates · severe dehydration · severe heart failure · ulcerative colitis · varicella infection

● CAUTIONS Allergic disorders · asthma · cerebrovascular disease · coagulation defects · congenital disorder of porphyrin metabolism · congestive heart failure · dehydration · elderly (risk of serious side-effects and fatalities) · following major surgery · haematopoietic disorders · history of cardiac disease (NSAIDs may cause fluid retention and oedema) · history of gastro-intestinal disease · history of gastro-intestinal toxicity · ischaemic heart disease · mixed connective-tissue disorders · peripheral arterial disease · risk factors for cardiovascular events · systemic lupus erythematosus · uncontrolled hypertension

● INTERACTIONS → Appendix 1: NSAIDs

● SIDE-EFFECTS
▸ **Common or very common** Diarrhoea · gastrointestinal discomfort · nausea · vomiting

▸ **Uncommon** Anxiety · asthenia · chills · constipation · dizziness · drowsiness · dry mouth · flushing · gastrointestinal disorders · headache · insomnia · malaise · pain · palpitations · skin reactions · vertigo

▸ **Rare or very rare** Angioedema · appetite decreased · dyspnoea · haemorrhage · hepatic disorders · hyperhidrosis · hypersensitivity · hypertension · hypotension · menstrual disorder · nephritis · nephrotic syndrome · neutropenia · oedema · pancreatitis · paraesthesia · photosensitivity reaction · polyuria · prostatic disorder · respiratory disorders · severe cutaneous adverse reactions (SCARs) · syncope · tachycardia · thrombocytopenia · tinnitus · vision blurred

▸ **Frequency not known** Acute kidney injury (more common in patients with pre-existing renal impairment) · agranulocytosis · anaemia · aplastic anaemia · haemolytic anaemia · inflammatory bowel disease · meningitis aseptic · oral ulceration · platelet aggregation inhibition · renal papillary necrosis

SIDE-EFFECTS, FURTHER INFORMATION For information about cardiovascular and gastrointestinal side-effects, and a possible exacerbation of symptoms in asthma, see Non-steroidal anti-inflammatory drugs p. 1094.

● ALLERGY AND CROSS-SENSITIVITY Contra-indicated in patients with a history of hypersensitivity to aspirin or any other NSAID—which includes those in whom attacks of asthma, angioedema, urticaria or rhinitis have been precipitated by aspirin or any other NSAID.

● CONCEPTION AND CONTRACEPTION Caution—long-term use of some NSAIDs is associated with reduced female fertility, which is reversible on stopping treatment.

● PREGNANCY Avoid unless the potential benefit outweighs the risk. Avoid during the third trimester (risk of closure of fetal ductus arteriosus *in utero* and possibly persistent pulmonary hypertension of the newborn); onset of labour may be delayed and duration may be increased.

● BREAST FEEDING Use with caution during breast-feeding. Manufacturer advises avoid—no information available.

● HEPATIC IMPAIRMENT Use with caution; there is an increased risk of gastro-intestinal bleeding and fluid retention. Avoid in severe liver disease.
Dose adjustments Reduce initial dose to max. 50 mg daily in mild to moderate impairment.

10

Musculoskeletal system

● RENAL IMPAIRMENT Avoid if possible or use with caution. Avoid in moderate to severe impairment.
Dose adjustments Reduce initial dose to 50 mg daily. The lowest effective dose should be used for the shortest possible duration.
Monitoring In renal impairment monitor renal function; sodium and water retention may occur and renal function may deteriorate, possibly leading to renal failure.

● MEDICINAL FORMS
There can be variation in the licensing of different medicines containing the same drug.
Tablet
CAUTIONARY AND ADVISORY LABELS 22
▸ Keral (A. Menarini Farmaceutica Internazionale SRL)
Dexketoprofen (as Dexketoprofen trometamol) 25 mg Keral 25mg tablets | 20 tablet [PoM] £3.67 | 50 tablet [PoM] £9.18 DT = £9.18

Combinations available: *Tramadol with dexketoprofen,* p. 466

Diclofenac potassium

● INDICATIONS AND DOSE

Pain and inflammation in rheumatic disease and other musculoskeletal disorders
▸ BY MOUTH
▸ Child 14–17 years: 75–100 mg daily in 2–3 divided doses
▸ Adult: 75–150 mg daily in 2–3 divided doses

Acute gout
▸ BY MOUTH
▸ Adult: 75–150 mg daily in 2–3 divided doses

Postoperative pain
▸ BY MOUTH
▸ Child 9–13 years (body-weight 35 kg and above): Up to 2 mg/kg daily in 3 divided doses; maximum 100 mg per day
▸ Child 14–17 years: 75–100 mg daily in 2–3 divided doses
▸ Adult: 75–150 mg daily in 2–3 divided doses

Migraine
▸ BY MOUTH
▸ Adult: 50 mg, to be given at onset of migraine, then 50 mg after 2 hours if required, then 50 mg after 4–6 hours; maximum 200 mg per day

Fever in ear, nose, or throat infection
▸ BY MOUTH
▸ Child 9–17 years (body-weight 35 kg and above): Up to 2 mg/kg daily in 3 divided doses; maximum 100 mg per day

● UNLICENSED USE *Voltarol® Rapid* not licensed for use in children under 14 years or in fever.

● CONTRA-INDICATIONS Active gastro-intestinal bleeding · active gastro-intestinal ulceration · cerebrovascular disease · history of gastro-intestinal bleeding related to previous NSAID therapy · history of gastro-intestinal perforation related to previous NSAID therapy · history of recurrent gastro-intestinal haemorrhage (two or more distinct episodes) · history of recurrent gastro-intestinal ulceration (two or more distinct episodes) · ischaemic heart disease · mild to severe heart failure · peripheral arterial disease

● CAUTIONS Allergic disorders · cardiac impairment (NSAIDs may impair renal function) · coagulation defects · connective-tissue disorders · Crohn's disease (may be exacerbated) · elderly (risk of serious side-effects and fatalities) · history of cardiac failure · hypertension · left ventricular dysfunction · oedema · risk factors for cardiovascular events · ulcerative colitis (may be exacerbated)

● INTERACTIONS → Appendix 1: NSAIDs

● SIDE-EFFECTS
▸ **Common or very common** Appetite decreased · diarrhoea · dizziness · gastrointestinal discomfort · gastrointestinal disorders · headache · nausea · skin reactions · vertigo · vomiting
▸ **Uncommon** Chest pain · heart failure · myocardial infarction · palpitations
▸ **Rare or very rare** Acute kidney injury · agranulocytosis · alopecia · anaemia · angioedema · anxiety · aplastic anaemia · asthma · confusion · constipation · depression · drowsiness · dyspnoea · erectile dysfunction · fatigue · haemolytic anaemia · haemorrhage · hearing impairment · hepatic disorders · hypersensitivity · hypertension · hypotension · inflammatory bowel disease · irritability · leucopenia · memory loss · meningitis aseptic (patients with connective-tissue disorders such as systemic lupus erythematosus may be especially susceptible) · nephritis tubulointerstitial · nephrotic syndrome · oedema · oral disorders · pancreatitis · photosensitivity reaction · pneumonitis · proteinuria · psychotic disorder · renal papillary necrosis · seizure · sensation abnormal · severe cutaneous adverse reactions (SCARs) · shock · sleep disorders · stroke · taste altered · thrombocytopenia · tremor · vasculitis · vision disorders
▸ **Frequency not known** Hallucination · malaise · optic neuritis

● ALLERGY AND CROSS-SENSITIVITY Contra-indicated in patients with a history of hypersensitivity to aspirin or any other NSAID—which includes those in whom attacks of asthma, angioedema, urticaria or rhinitis have been precipitated by aspirin or any other NSAID.

● CONCEPTION AND CONTRACEPTION Caution—long-term use of some NSAIDs is associated with reduced female fertility, which is reversible on stopping treatment.

● PREGNANCY Avoid unless the potential benefit outweighs the risk. Avoid during the third trimester (risk of closure of fetal ductus arteriosus *in utero* and possibly persistent pulmonary hypertension of the newborn); onset of labour may be delayed and duration may be increased.

● BREAST FEEDING Use with caution during breast-feeding. Amount in milk too small to be harmful.

● HEPATIC IMPAIRMENT Use with caution; there is an increased risk of gastro-intestinal bleeding and fluid retention. Avoid in severe liver disease.

● RENAL IMPAIRMENT Avoid if possible or use with caution. Avoid in severe impairment.
Dose adjustments The lowest effective dose should be used for the shortest possible duration.
Monitoring In renal impairment monitor renal function; sodium and water retention may occur and renal function may deteriorate, possibly leading to renal failure.

● PATIENT AND CARER ADVICE
Medicines for Children leaflet: Diclofenac for pain and inflammation www.medicinesforchildren.org.uk/diclofenac-for-pain-and-inflammation

● MEDICINAL FORMS
There can be variation in the licensing of different medicines containing the same drug.
Tablet
CAUTIONARY AND ADVISORY LABELS 21
▸ Diclofenac potassium (Non-proprietary)
Diclofenac potassium 25 mg Diclofenac potassium 25mg tablets | 28 tablet [PoM] £3.87 DT = £3.87
Diclofenac potassium 50 mg Diclofenac potassium 50mg tablets | 28 tablet [PoM] £6.18–£7.41
▸ Voltarol Rapid (Novartis Pharmaceuticals UK Ltd)
Diclofenac potassium 50 mg Voltarol Rapid 50mg tablets | 30 tablet [PoM] £7.94 DT = £7.94

Diclofenac sodium

● INDICATIONS AND DOSE

Pain and inflammation in musculoskeletal disorders | Acute gout

▸ BY MOUTH USING IMMEDIATE-RELEASE MEDICINES
▸ Adult: 75–150 mg daily in 2–3 divided doses
▸ BY RECTUM
▸ Adult: 75–150 mg daily in divided doses

Pain and inflammation in rheumatic disease including juvenile idiopathic arthritis

▸ BY MOUTH USING IMMEDIATE-RELEASE MEDICINES
▸ Adult: 75–150 mg daily in 2–3 divided doses
▸ BY RECTUM
▸ Adult: 75–150 mg daily in divided doses

Postoperative pain

▸ BY MOUTH USING IMMEDIATE-RELEASE MEDICINES
▸ Adult: 75–150 mg daily in 2–3 divided doses
▸ BY RECTUM
▸ Adult: 75–150 mg daily in divided doses

DICLOMAX RETARD ®

Pain and inflammation in rheumatic disease (including juvenile idiopathic arthritis) and other musculoskeletal disorders | Acute gout | Postoperative pain

▸ BY MOUTH
▸ Adult: 1 capsule once daily

DICLOMAX SR ®

Pain and inflammation in rheumatic disease (including juvenile idiopathic arthritis) and other musculoskeletal disorders | Acute gout | Postoperative pain

▸ BY MOUTH
▸ Adult: 1 capsule 1–2 times a day, alternatively 2 capsules once daily

MOTIFENE ®

Pain and inflammation in rheumatic disease (including juvenile idiopathic arthritis) and other musculoskeletal disorders | Acute gout | Postoperative pain

▸ BY MOUTH
▸ Adult: 1 capsule 1–2 times a day

VOLTAROL ® 75MG SR TABLETS

Pain and inflammation in rheumatic disease (including juvenile idiopathic arthritis) and other musculoskeletal disorders | Acute gout | Postoperative pain

▸ BY MOUTH
▸ Adult: 1 tablet 1–2 times a day

VOLTAROL ® EMULGEL

Relief of pain in musculoskeletal conditions | Adjunctive treatment in knee or hand osteoarthritis

▸ TO THE SKIN
▸ Adult: Apply 3–4 times a day, therapy should be reviewed after 14 days (or after 28 days for osteoarthritis)

VOLTAROL ® RETARD

Pain and inflammation in rheumatic disease (including juvenile idiopathic arthritis) and other musculoskeletal disorders | Acute gout | Postoperative pain

▸ BY MOUTH
▸ Adult: 1 tablet once daily

VOLTAROL ® SOLUTION FOR INJECTION

Postoperative pain

▸ BY DEEP INTRAMUSCULAR INJECTION
▸ Adult: 75 mg 1–2 times a day for maximum 2 days, twice daily administration in severe cases, to be injected into the gluteal muscle

Acute exacerbations of pain

▸ BY DEEP INTRAMUSCULAR INJECTION
▸ Adult: 75 mg 1–2 times a day for maximum 2 days, twice daily administration in severe cases, to be injected into the gluteal muscle

Ureteric colic

▸ BY DEEP INTRAMUSCULAR INJECTION
▸ Adult: 75 mg, then 75 mg after 30 minutes if required

Acute postoperative pain (in hospital setting)

▸ BY INTRAVENOUS INFUSION
▸ Adult: 75 mg, then 75 mg after 4–6 hours if required for maximum 2 days; maximum 150 mg per day

Prevention of postoperative pain (in hospital setting)

▸ BY INTRAVENOUS INFUSION
▸ Adult: Initially 25–50 mg, to be given after surgery over 15–60 minutes, then 5 mg/hour for maximum 2 days; maximum 150 mg per day

● CONTRA-INDICATIONS
▸ With intravenous use Dehydration · history of asthma · history of confirmed or suspected cerebrovascular bleeding · history of haemorrhagic diathesis · hypovolaemia · operations with high risk of haemorrhage
▸ With systemic use Active gastro-intestinal bleeding · active gastro-intestinal ulceration · avoid suppositories in proctitis · cerebrovascular disease · history of gastro-intestinal bleeding related to previous NSAID therapy · history of gastro-intestinal perforation related to previous NSAID therapy · history of recurrent gastro-intestinal haemorrhage (two or more distinct episodes) · history of recurrent gastro-intestinal ulceration (two or more distinct episodes) · ischaemic heart disease · mild to severe heart failure · peripheral arterial disease

● CAUTIONS
▸ With systemic use Allergic disorders · cardiac impairment (NSAIDs may impair renal function) · coagulation defects · connective-tissue disorders · Crohn's disease (may be exacerbated) · elderly (risk of serious side-effects and fatalities) · history of cardiac failure · hypertension · left ventricular dysfunction · oedema · risk factors for cardiovascular events · ulcerative colitis (may be exacerbated)
▸ With topical use Avoid contact with eyes · avoid contact with inflamed or broken skin · avoid contact with mucous membranes · not for use with occlusive dressings · topical application of large amounts can result in systemic effects, including hypersensitivity and asthma (renal disease has also been reported)

● INTERACTIONS → Appendix 1: NSAIDs

● SIDE-EFFECTS

SPECIFIC SIDE-EFFECTS
▸ **Common or very common**
▸ With systemic use Appetite decreased · diarrhoea · dizziness · gastrointestinal discomfort · gastrointestinal disorders · headache · nausea · oedema · rash (discontinue) · skin reactions · vertigo · vomiting
▸ **Uncommon**
▸ With systemic use Chest pain · heart failure · myocardial infarction · palpitations
▸ **Rare or very rare**
▸ With systemic use Acute kidney injury · agranulocytosis · alopecia · anaemia · angioedema · anxiety · aplastic anaemia · asthma · confusion · constipation · Crohn's disease · depression · disorientation · drowsiness · dyspnoea · erectile dysfunction · haemolytic anaemia · haemorrhage · hearing impairment · hepatic disorders · hypersensitivity · hypertension · hypotension · irritability · leucopenia · memory loss · meningitis aseptic (patients with connective-tissue disorders such as systemic lupus erythematosus may be especially susceptible) · nephritis tubulointerstitial · nephrotic syndrome · oral disorders ·

10

Musculoskeletal system

pancreatitis · paraesthesia · photosensitivity reaction · pneumonitis · proteinuria · psychotic disorder · renal papillary necrosis · seizure · sensation abnormal · severe cutaneous adverse reactions (SCARs) · shock · sleep disorders · stroke · taste altered · thrombocytopenia · tremor · vasculitis · vision disorders
‣ **Frequency not known**
‣ With systemic use Fertility decreased female · fluid retention · hallucination · malaise · optic neuritis · platelet aggregation inhibition
‣ With topical use Hair colour changes
SIDE-EFFECTS, FURTHER INFORMATION For information about cardiovascular and gastrointestinal side-effects, and a possible exacerbation of symptoms in asthma, see Non-steroidal anti-inflammatory drugs p. 1094.
‣ With topical use Topical application of large amounts of diclofenac can result in systemic effects.
● ALLERGY AND CROSS-SENSITIVITY Contra-indicated in patients with a history of hypersensitivity to aspirin or any other NSAID—which includes those in whom attacks of asthma, angioedema, urticaria or rhinitis have been precipitated by aspirin or any other NSAID.
● CONCEPTION AND CONTRACEPTION
‣ With systemic use Caution—long-term use of some NSAIDs is associated with reduced female fertility, which is reversible on stopping treatment.
● PREGNANCY
‣ With systemic use Avoid unless the potential benefit outweighs the risk. Avoid during the third trimester (risk of closure of fetal ductus arteriosus *in utero* and possibly persistent pulmonary hypertension of the newborn); onset of labour may be delayed and duration may be increased.
‣ With topical use Patient packs for topical preparations carry a warning to avoid during pregnancy.
● BREAST FEEDING
‣ With systemic use Use with caution during breast-feeding. Amount in milk too small to be harmful.
‣ With topical use Patient packs for topical preparations carry a warning to avoid during breast-feeding.
● HEPATIC IMPAIRMENT
‣ With systemic use Use with caution; there is an increased risk of gastro-intestinal bleeding and fluid retention. Avoid in severe liver disease.
● RENAL IMPAIRMENT
‣ With systemic use Avoid if possible or use with caution. Avoid in severe impairment.
‣ With intravenous use Avoid intravenous use if serum creatinine greater than 160 micromol/litre. Contra-indicated in moderate or severe renal impairment.
Dose adjustments ‣ With systemic use The lowest effective dose should be used for the shortest possible duration.
Monitoring ‣ With systemic use In renal impairment monitor renal function; sodium and water retention may occur and renal function may deteriorate, possibly leading to renal failure.
● DIRECTIONS FOR ADMINISTRATION
‣ With intravenous use For *intravenous infusion* (*Voltarol*®), give continuously or intermittently in Glucose 5% or Sodium chloride 0.9%. Dilute 75 mg with 100–500 mL infusion fluid (previously buffered with 0.5 mL sodium bicarbonate 8.4% solution *or* with 1 mL sodium bicarbonate 4.2% solution). For intermittent infusion give 25–50 mg over 15–60 minutes or 75 mg over 30–120 minutes. For continuous infusion give at a rate of 5 mg/hour.
‣ With topical use For topical preparations, apply with gentle massage only.
● PRESCRIBING AND DISPENSING INFORMATION *Voltarol*® dispersible tablets are more suitable for **short-term** use in acute conditions for which treatment required for no more than 3 months (no information on use beyond 3 months).

● PROFESSION SPECIFIC INFORMATION
Dental practitioners' formulary
Diclofenac Sodium Tablets may be prescribed.

● MEDICINAL FORMS
There can be variation in the licensing of different medicines containing the same drug. Forms available from special-order manufacturers include: dispersible tablet, oral suspension, oral solution

Gastro-resistant tablet
CAUTIONARY AND ADVISORY LABELS 5, 25
‣ Diclofenac sodium (Non-proprietary)
 Diclofenac sodium 25 mg Diclofenac sodium 25mg gastro-resistant tablets | 28 tablet PoM £5.49-£8.99 DT = £2.02 | 84 tablet PoM £1.50-£26.97
 Diclofenac sodium 50 mg Diclofenac sodium 50mg gastro-resistant tablets | 28 tablet PoM £4.97 DT = £2.25 | 84 tablet PoM £3.00-£15.00
‣ Dicloflex (Dexcel-Pharma Ltd)
 Diclofenac sodium 25 mg Dicloflex 25mg gastro-resistant tablets | 84 tablet PoM £4.42
 Diclofenac sodium 50 mg Dicloflex 50mg gastro-resistant tablets | 28 tablet PoM £2.75 DT = £2.25 (Hospital only) | 84 tablet PoM £8.05
‣ Fenactol (Discovery Pharmaceuticals)
 Diclofenac sodium 50 mg Fenactol 50mg gastro-resistant tablets | 100 tablet PoM £3.70

Suppository
‣ Diclofenac sodium (Non-proprietary)
 Diclofenac sodium 100 mg Diclofenac 100mg suppositories | 10 suppository PoM £3.64 DT = £3.64
‣ Econac (AMCo)
 Diclofenac sodium 100 mg Econac 100mg suppositories | 10 suppository PoM £3.04 DT = £3.64
‣ Voltarol (Novartis Pharmaceuticals UK Ltd)
 Diclofenac sodium 12.5 mg Voltarol 12.5mg suppositories | 10 suppository PoM £0.70 DT = £0.70
 Diclofenac sodium 25 mg Voltarol 25mg suppositories | 10 suppository PoM £1.24 DT = £1.24
 Diclofenac sodium 50 mg Voltarol 50mg suppositories | 10 suppository PoM £2.04 DT = £2.04
 Diclofenac sodium 100 mg Voltarol 100mg suppositories | 10 suppository PoM £3.64 DT = £3.64

Solution for injection
EXCIPIENTS: May contain Benzyl alcohol, propylene glycol
‣ Voltarol (Novartis Pharmaceuticals UK Ltd)
 Diclofenac sodium 25 mg per 1 ml Voltarol 75mg/3ml solution for injection ampoules | 10 ampoule PoM £9.91 DT = £9.91

Modified-release capsule
CAUTIONARY AND ADVISORY LABELS 21(does not apply to Motifene® 75 mg), 25
EXCIPIENTS: May contain Propylene glycol
‣ Diclomax Retard (Galen Ltd)
 Diclofenac sodium 100 mg Diclomax Retard 100mg capsules | 28 capsule PoM £8.20 DT = £8.20
‣ Diclomax SR (Galen Ltd)
 Diclofenac sodium 75 mg Diclomax SR 75mg capsules | 56 capsule PoM £11.40 DT = £11.40
‣ Motifene (Daiichi Sankyo UK Ltd)
 Diclofenac sodium 75 mg Motifene 75mg modified-release capsules | 56 capsule PoM £8.00 DT = £8.00

Gel
‣ Voltarol Emulgel (GlaxoSmithKline Consumer Healthcare)
 Diclofenac diethylammonium 11.6 mg per 1 gram Voltarol 1.16% Emulgel | 100 gram PoM £5.63 DT = £5.63

Diclofenac sodium with misoprostol

The properties listed below are those particular to the combination only. For the properties of the components please consider, diclofenac sodium p. 1101, misoprostol p. 77.

● **INDICATIONS AND DOSE**

ARTHROTEC® 50/200

Prophylaxis against NSAID-induced gastroduodenal ulceration in patients requiring diclofenac for rheumatoid arthritis or osteoarthritis
▸ Adult: 1 tablet 2–3 times a day, take with food

ARTHROTEC® 75/200

Prophylaxis against NSAID-induced gastroduodenal ulceration in patients requiring diclofenac for rheumatoid arthritis or osteoarthritis
▸ BY MOUTH
▸ Adult: 1 tablet twice daily, take with food

MISOFEN® 50/200

Prophylaxis against NSAID-induced gastroduodenal ulceration in patients requiring diclofenac for rheumatoid arthritis or osteoarthritis
▸ BY MOUTH
▸ Adult: 1 tablet 2–3 times a day, take with food

MISOFEN® 75/200

Prophylaxis against NSAID-induced gastroduodenal ulceration in patients requiring diclofenac for rheumatoid arthritis or osteoarthritis
▸ BY MOUTH
▸ Adult: 1 tablet twice daily, take with food

● **UNLICENSED USE** The BNF recommends a higher starting dose of misoprostol for prophylaxis against NSAID-induced gastroduodenal ulceration than that provided by the combination preparations of diclofenac and misoprostol.

● **INTERACTIONS** → Appendix 1: NSAIDs

● **MEDICINAL FORMS**
There can be variation in the licensing of different medicines containing the same drug.
Gastro-resistant tablet
CAUTIONARY AND ADVISORY LABELS 21, 25
▸ Arthrotec (Pfizer Ltd)
  Misoprostol 200 microgram, Diclofenac sodium 50 mg Arthrotec 50 gastro-resistant tablets | 60 tablet [PoM] £11.98 DT = £11.98
  Misoprostol 200 microgram, Diclofenac sodium 75 mg Arthrotec 75 gastro-resistant tablets | 60 tablet [PoM] £15.83 DT = £15.83
▸ Misofen (Morningside Healthcare Ltd)
  Misoprostol 200 microgram, Diclofenac sodium 50 mg Misofen 50mg/200microgram gastro-resistant tablets | 60 tablet [PoM] £11.98 DT = £11.98
  Misoprostol 200 microgram, Diclofenac sodium 75 mg Misofen 75mg/200microgram gastro-resistant tablets | 60 tablet [PoM] £15.83 DT = £15.83

Etodolac

● **INDICATIONS AND DOSE**

Pain and inflammation in rheumatoid arthritis and osteoarthritis
▸ BY MOUTH USING IMMEDIATE-RELEASE MEDICINES
▸ Adult: 300–600 mg daily in 1–2 divided doses
▸ BY MOUTH USING MODIFIED-RELEASE MEDICINES
▸ Adult: 600 mg daily

● **CONTRA-INDICATIONS** Active gastro-intestinal bleeding · active gastro-intestinal ulceration · history of gastro-intestinal bleeding related to previous NSAID therapy · history of gastro-intestinal perforation related to previous

NSAID therapy · history of recurrent gastro-intestinal haemorrhage (two or more distinct episodes) · history of recurrent gastro-intestinal ulceration (two or more distinct episodes) · severe heart failure

● **CAUTIONS** Allergic disorders · cardiac impairment (NSAIDs may impair renal function) · cerebrovascular disease · coagulation defects · connective-tissue disorders · Crohn's disease (may be exacerbated) · elderly (risk of serious side-effects and fatalities) · heart failure · ischaemic heart disease · peripheral arterial disease · risk factors for cardiovascular events · ulcerative colitis (may be exacerbated) · uncontrolled hypertension

● **INTERACTIONS** → Appendix 1: NSAIDs

● **SIDE-EFFECTS** Agranulocytosis · angioedema · aplastic anaemia · asthenia · asthma · bilirubinuria · bronchospasm · chills · confusion · constipation · Crohn's disease aggravated · depression · diarrhoea · dizziness · drowsiness · dyspnoea · fever · gastrointestinal discomfort · gastrointestinal disorders · haemolytic anaemia · haemorrhage · hallucination · headache · heart failure · hepatic disorders · hypersensitivity · hypertension · insomnia · malaise · meningitis aseptic (patients with connective-tissue disorders such as systemic lupus erythematosus may be especially susceptible) · nausea · nephritic syndrome · nephritis tubulointerstitial · nephrotoxicity · nervousness · neutropenia · oedema · optic neuritis · oral ulceration · palpitations · pancreatitis · paraesthesia · photosensitivity reaction · renal failure (more common in patients with pre-existing renal impairment) · severe cutaneous adverse reactions (SCARs) · skin reactions · thrombocytopenia · tinnitus · tremor · urinary disorders · vasculitis · vertigo · visual impairment · vomiting

SIDE-EFFECTS, FURTHER INFORMATION For information about cardiovascular and gastrointestinal side-effects, and a possible exacerbation of symptoms in asthma, see Non-steroidal anti-inflammatory drugs p. 1094.

● **ALLERGY AND CROSS-SENSITIVITY** Contra-indicated in patients with a history of hypersensitivity to aspirin or any other NSAID—which includes those in whom attacks of asthma, angioedema, urticaria or rhinitis have been precipitated by aspirin or any other NSAID.

● **CONCEPTION AND CONTRACEPTION** Caution—long-term use of some NSAIDs is associated with reduced female fertility, which is reversible on stopping treatment.

● **PREGNANCY** Avoid unless the potential benefit outweighs the risk. Avoid during the third trimester (risk of closure of fetal ductus arteriosus *in utero* and possibly persistent pulmonary hypertension of the newborn); onset of labour may be delayed and duration may be increased.

● **BREAST FEEDING** Use with caution during breast-feeding. Manufacturer advises avoid.

● **HEPATIC IMPAIRMENT** Use with caution; there is an increased risk of gastro-intestinal bleeding and fluid retention. Avoid in severe liver disease.

● **RENAL IMPAIRMENT** Avoid if possible or use with caution. Avoid in severe impairment.
Dose adjustments The lowest effective dose should be used for the shortest possible duration.
Monitoring In renal impairment monitor renal function; sodium and water retention may occur and renal function may deteriorate, possibly leading to renal failure.

● **MEDICINAL FORMS**
There can be variation in the licensing of different medicines containing the same drug.
Modified-release tablet
CAUTIONARY AND ADVISORY LABELS 25
▸ Etodolac (Non-proprietary)
  Etodolac 600 mg Etodolac 600mg modified-release tablets | 30 tablet [PoM] £21.40 DT = £15.50

▸ Etolyn (Mylan)
Etodolac 600 mg Etolyn 600mg modified-release tablets |
30 tablet [PoM] £12.40 DT = £15.50
▸ Etopan XL (Sun Pharmaceuticals UK Ltd)
Etodolac 600 mg Etopan XL 600mg tablets | 30 tablet [PoM] £14.60
DT = £15.50
▸ Lodine SR (Almirall Ltd)
Etodolac 600 mg Lodine SR 600mg tablets | 30 tablet [PoM] £15.50
DT = £15.50

Capsule
▸ Eccoxolac (Meda Pharmaceuticals Ltd)
Etodolac 300 mg Eccoxolac 300mg capsules | 60 capsule [PoM]
£8.14 DT = £8.14

Etoricoxib
23-Nov-2016

● **INDICATIONS AND DOSE**

Pain and inflammation in osteoarthritis
▸ BY MOUTH
▸ Child 16–17 years: 30 mg once daily, increased if
necessary to 60 mg once daily
▸ Adult: 30 mg once daily, increased if necessary to
60 mg once daily

**Pain and inflammation in rheumatoid arthritis |
Ankylosing spondylitis**
▸ BY MOUTH
▸ Child 16–17 years: 60 mg once daily, increased if
necessary to 90 mg once daily
▸ Adult: 60 mg once daily, increased if necessary to
90 mg once daily

Acute gout
▸ BY MOUTH
▸ Child 16–17 years: 120 mg once daily for maximum
8 days
▸ Adult: 120 mg once daily for maximum 8 days

● CONTRA-INDICATIONS Active gastro-intestinal bleeding ·
active gastro-intestinal ulceration · cerebrovascular
disease · inflammatory bowel disease · ischaemic heart
disease · mild to severe heart failure · peripheral arterial
disease · uncontrolled hypertension (persistently above
140/90 mmHg)

● CAUTIONS Allergic disorders · cardiac impairment (NSAIDs
may impair renal function) · coagulation defects ·
connective-tissue disorders · Crohn's disease (may be
exacerbated) · dehydration · elderly (risk of serious side-
effects and fatalities) · history of cardiac failure ·
hypertension · left ventricular dysfunction · oedema · risk
factors for cardiovascular events · ulcerative colitis (may be
exacerbated)

● INTERACTIONS → Appendix 1: NSAIDs

● SIDE-EFFECTS

▸ **Common or very common** Arrhythmias · asthenia ·
bronchospasm · constipation · diarrhoea · dizziness · fluid
retention · gastrointestinal discomfort · gastrointestinal
disorders · headache · hypertension · increased risk of
infection · influenza like illness · nausea · oedema · oral
ulceration · palpitations · skin reactions · vomiting
▸ **Uncommon** Alertness decreased · anaemia · angina pectoris
· anxiety · appetite abnormal · cerebrovascular
insufficiency · chest pain · congestive heart failure ·
conjunctivitis · cough · depression · drowsiness · dry mouth
· dyspnoea · flushing · haemorrhage · hallucination ·
hyperkalaemia · hypersensitivity · insomnia · irritable
bowel syndrome · leucopenia · myocardial infarction ·
pancreatitis · proteinuria · renal failure (more common in
patients with pre-existing renal impairment) · sensation
abnormal · taste altered · thrombocytopenia · tinnitus ·
vasculitis · vertigo · vision blurred · weight increased

▸ **Rare or very rare** Angioedema · confusion · hepatic
disorders · muscle complaints · severe cutaneous adverse
reactions (SCARs) · shock
▸ **Frequency not known** Nephritis tubulointerstitial ·
nephropathy

SIDE-EFFECTS, FURTHER INFORMATION For information
about cardiovascular and gastrointestinal side-effects, and
a possible exacerbation of symptoms in asthma, see Non-
steroidal anti-inflammatory drugs p. 1094.

● ALLERGY AND CROSS-SENSITIVITY Contra-indicated in
patients with a history of hypersensitivity to aspirin or any
other NSAID—which includes those in whom attacks of
asthma, angioedema, urticaria or rhinitis have been
precipitated by aspirin or any other NSAID.

● CONCEPTION AND CONTRACEPTION Caution—long-term
use of some NSAIDs is associated with reduced female
fertility, which is reversible on stopping treatment.

● PREGNANCY Manufacturer advises avoid (teratogenic in
animal studies). Avoid during the third trimester (risk of
closure of fetal ductus arteriosus *in utero* and possibly
persistent pulmonary hypertension of the newborn); onset
of labour may be delayed and duration may be increased.

● BREAST FEEDING Use with caution during breast-feeding.
Manufacturer advises avoid—present in milk in *animal*
studies.

● HEPATIC IMPAIRMENT Use with caution; there is an
increased risk of gastro-intestinal bleeding and fluid
retention. Avoid in severe liver disease.
Dose adjustments Max. 60 mg daily in mild impairment.
Max. 60 mg on alternate days or 30 mg once daily in
moderate impairment.

● RENAL IMPAIRMENT Avoid if possible or use with caution.
▸ In adults Avoid if eGFR less than 30 mL/minute/1.73 m^2.
▸ In children Avoid if estimated glomerular filtration rate less
than 30 mL/minute/1.73 m^2.
Dose adjustments The lowest effective dose should be used
for the shortest possible duration.
Monitoring In renal impairment monitor renal function;
sodium and water retention may occur and renal function
may deteriorate, possibly leading to renal failure.

● MONITORING REQUIREMENTS Monitor blood pressure
before treatment, 2 weeks after initiation and periodically
during treatment.

● MEDICINAL FORMS
There can be variation in the licensing of different medicines
containing the same drug.
Tablet
▸ Etoricoxib (Non-proprietary)
Etoricoxib 30 mg Etoricoxib 30mg tablets | 28 tablet [PoM] £2.80–
£13.99 DT = £13.99
Etoricoxib 60 mg Etoricoxib 60mg tablets | 28 tablet [PoM] £3.01–
£20.11 DT = £3.01
Etoricoxib 90 mg Etoricoxib 90mg tablets | 28 tablet [PoM] £3.64–
£22.96 DT = £3.64
Etoricoxib 120 mg Etoricoxib 120mg tablets | 7 tablet [PoM] £1.80–
£5.73 | 28 tablet [PoM] £7.23–£24.11 DT = £24.11
▸ Arcoxia (Grunenthal Ltd)
Etoricoxib 30 mg Arcoxia 30mg tablets | 28 tablet [PoM] £13.99 DT
= £13.99
Etoricoxib 60 mg Arcoxia 60mg tablets | 28 tablet [PoM] £20.11 DT
= £3.01
Etoricoxib 90 mg Arcoxia 90mg tablets | 5 tablet [PoM] £4.10 |
28 tablet [PoM] £22.96 DT = £3.64
Etoricoxib 120 mg Arcoxia 120mg tablets | 7 tablet [PoM] £6.03 |
28 tablet [PoM] £24.11 DT = £24.11

Felbinac

- **DRUG ACTION** Felbinac is an active metabolite of the NSAID fenbufen.

- **INDICATIONS AND DOSE**

Relief of pain in musculoskeletal conditions | Treatment in knee or hand osteoarthritis (adjunct)
  ▶ TO THE SKIN
  ▶ Adult: Apply 2–4 times a day, therapy should be reviewed after 14 days; maximum 25 g per day

- **CONTRA-INDICATIONS** Active gastro-intestinal bleeding · active gastro-intestinal ulceration · history of gastro-intestinal bleeding related to previous NSAID therapy · history of gastro-intestinal haemorrhage (two or more distinct episodes) · history of gastro-intestinal perforation related to previous NSAID therapy · history of recurrent gastro-intestinal ulceration (two or more distinct episodes) · severe heart failure

- **CAUTIONS** Allergic disorders · avoid contact with eyes · avoid contact with inflamed or broken skin · avoid contact with mucous membranes · cardiac impairment (NSAIDs may impair renal function) · cerebrovascular disease · coagulation defects · connective-tissue disorders · Crohn's disease (may be exacerbated) · elderly (risk of serious side-effects and fatalities) · heart failure · ischaemic heart disease · not for use with occlusive dressings · peripheral arterial disease · risk factors for cardiovascular events · topical application of large amounts can result in systemic effects, including hypersensitivity and asthma (renal disease has also been reported) · ulcerative colitis (may be exacerbated) · uncontrolled hypertension

- **INTERACTIONS** → Appendix 1: NSAIDs

- **SIDE-EFFECTS** Bronchospasm · gastrointestinal disorder · hypersensitivity · paraesthesia · photosensitivity reaction · skin reactions

  SIDE-EFFECTS, FURTHER INFORMATION For information about cardiovascular and gastrointestinal side-effects, and a possible exacerbation of symptoms in asthma, see Non-steroidal anti-inflammatory drugs p. 1094.

- **ALLERGY AND CROSS-SENSITIVITY** Contra-indicated in patients with a history of hypersensitivity to aspirin or any other NSAID—which includes those in whom attacks of asthma, angioedema, urticaria or rhinitis have been precipitated by aspirin or any other NSAID.

- **CONCEPTION AND CONTRACEPTION** Caution—long-term use of some NSAIDs is associated with reduced female fertility, which is reversible on stopping treatment.

- **PREGNANCY** Patient packs for topical preparations carry a warning to avoid during pregnancy.

- **BREAST FEEDING** Patient packs for topical preparations carry a warning to avoid during breast-feeding.

- **HEPATIC IMPAIRMENT** Use with caution; there is an increased risk of gastro-intestinal bleeding and fluid retention. Avoid in severe liver disease.

- **RENAL IMPAIRMENT** Avoid if possible or use with caution. Deterioration in renal function has also been reported after topical use.
  Dose adjustments The lowest effective dose should be used for the shortest possible duration.
  Monitoring In renal impairment monitor renal function; sodium and water retention may occur and renal function may deteriorate, possibly leading to renal failure.

- **DIRECTIONS FOR ADMINISTRATION** For topical preparations, apply with gentle massage only.

- **PRESCRIBING AND DISPENSING INFORMATION** Caution—topical preparations not generally suitable for children.

- **PATIENT AND CARER ADVICE** For topical preparations patients and carers should be advised to wash hands immediately after use.

Photosensitivity Patients should be advised against excessive exposure to sunlight of area treated in order to avoid possibility of photosensitivity.

- **MEDICINAL FORMS**
There can be variation in the licensing of different medicines containing the same drug.
Gel
  ▶ Traxam (AMCo)
  Felbinac 30 mg per 1 gram Traxam 3% gel | 100 gram [PoM] £8.03
  DT = £8.03
  Traxam Pain Relief 3% gel | 7.5 gram [P] £1.24 | 30 gram [P] £2.26
  DT = £2.26
Foam
  CAUTIONARY AND ADVISORY LABELS 15
  EXCIPIENTS: May contain Cetostearyl alcohol (including cetyl and stearyl alcohol)
  ▶ Traxam (AMCo)
  Felbinac 31.7 mg per 1 gram Traxam 3.17% foam | 100 gram [PoM] £8.41 DT = £8.41

Fenoprofen

- **INDICATIONS AND DOSE**

Pain and inflammation in rheumatic disease and other musculoskeletal disease | Mild to moderate pain
  ▶ BY MOUTH
  ▶ Adult: 300–600 mg 3–4 times a day; maximum 3 g per day

- **CONTRA-INDICATIONS** Active gastro-intestinal bleeding · active gastro-intestinal ulceration · history of gastro-intestinal bleeding related to previous NSAID therapy · history of gastro-intestinal perforation related to previous NSAID therapy · history of recurrent gastro-intestinal haemorrhage (two or more distinct episodes) · history of recurrent gastro-intestinal ulceration (two or more distinct episodes) · severe heart failure

- **CAUTIONS** Allergic disorders · cardiac impairment (NSAIDs may impair renal function) · cerebrovascular disease · coagulation defects · connective-tissue disorders · Crohn's disease (may be exacerbated) · elderly (risk of serious side-effects and fatalities) · heart failure · ischaemic heart disease · peripheral arterial disease · risk factors for cardiovascular events · ulcerative colitis (may be exacerbated) · uncontrolled hypertension

- **INTERACTIONS** → Appendix 1: NSAIDs

- **SIDE-EFFECTS** Agranulocytosis · alopecia · angioedema · aplastic anaemia · arrhythmias · arthralgia · asthma · azotaemia · breast pain · bronchospasm · confusion · constipation · Crohn's disease · cystitis · depression · diarrhoea · dizziness · drowsiness · dry mouth · dyspnoea · dysuria · fatigue · fertility decreased female · fever · gastrointestinal discomfort · gastrointestinal disorders · haemolytic anaemia · haemorrhage · hallucination · headache · hearing impairment · heart failure · hepatic disorders · hyperhidrosis · hypersensitivity · hypertension · increased risk of infection · lymphadenopathy · malaise · meningitis aseptic (patients with connective-tissue disorders such as systemic lupus erythematosus may be especially susceptible) · nausea · nephritis tubulointerstitial · nephropathy · nervousness · neutropenia · optic neuritis · oral disorders · palpitations · pancreatitis · paraesthesia · personality change · photosensitivity reaction · platelet aggregation inhibition · pulmonary oedema · renal failure (more common in patients with pre-existing renal impairment) · renal impairment · renal papillary necrosis · severe cutaneous adverse reactions (SCARs) · skin reactions · taste metallic · thrombocytopenia · vertigo · vision disorders · vomiting

  SIDE-EFFECTS, FURTHER INFORMATION For information about cardiovascular and gastrointestinal side-effects, and

10

Musculoskeletal system

a possible exacerbation of symptoms in asthma, see Non-steroidal anti-inflammatory drugs p. 1094.

- ALLERGY AND CROSS-SENSITIVITY Contra-indicated in patients with a history of hypersensitivity to aspirin or any other NSAID—which includes those in whom attacks of asthma, angioedema, urticaria or rhinitis have been precipitated by aspirin or any other NSAID.
- CONCEPTION AND CONTRACEPTION Caution—long-term use of some NSAIDs is associated with reduced female fertility, which is reversible on stopping treatment.
- PREGNANCY Avoid unless the potential benefit outweighs the risk. Avoid during the third trimester (risk of closure of fetal ductus arteriosus *in utero* and possibly persistent pulmonary hypertension of the newborn); onset of labour may be delayed and duration may be increased.
- BREAST FEEDING Use with caution during breast-feeding. Amount too small to be harmful.
- HEPATIC IMPAIRMENT Use with caution; there is an increased risk of gastro-intestinal bleeding and fluid retention. Avoid in severe liver disease.
- RENAL IMPAIRMENT Avoid if possible or use with caution.
  Dose adjustments The lowest effective dose should be used for the shortest possible duration.
  Monitoring In renal impairment monitor renal function; sodium and water retention may occur and renal function may deteriorate, possibly leading to renal failure.

- MEDICINAL FORMS
  No licensed medicines listed.

Flurbiprofen

- INDICATIONS AND DOSE
Pain and inflammation in rheumatic disease and other musculoskeletal disorders | Migraine | Postoperative analgesia | Mild to moderate pain
  ▸ BY MOUTH
  ▸ Child 12-17 years: 150–200 mg daily in 2–4 divided doses, then increased to 300 mg daily, dose to be increased only in acute conditions
  ▸ Adult: 150–200 mg daily in 2–4 divided doses, then increased to 300 mg daily, dose to be increased only in acute conditions

Dysmenorrhoea
  ▸ BY MOUTH
  ▸ Child 12-17 years: Initially 100 mg, then 50–100 mg every 4–6 hours; maximum 300 mg per day
  ▸ Adult: Initially 100 mg, then 50–100 mg every 4–6 hours; maximum 300 mg per day

- CONTRA-INDICATIONS Active gastro-intestinal bleeding · active gastro-intestinal ulceration · history of gastro-intestinal bleeding related to previous NSAID therapy · history of gastro-intestinal perforation related to previous NSAID therapy · history of recurrent gastro-intestinal haemorrhage (two or more distinct episodes) · history of recurrent gastro-intestinal ulceration (two or more distinct episodes) · severe heart failure
- CAUTIONS Allergic disorders · cardiac impairment (NSAIDs may impair renal function) · cerebrovascular disease · coagulation defects · connective-tissue disorders · Crohn's disease (may be exacerbated) · elderly (risk of serious side-effects and fatalities) · heart failure · ischaemic heart disease · peripheral arterial disease · risk factors for cardiovascular events · ulcerative colitis (may be exacerbated) · uncontrolled hypertension
- INTERACTIONS → Appendix 1: NSAIDs
- SIDE-EFFECTS
  ▸ Common or very common Haemorrhage
  ▸ Frequency not known Agranulocytosis · angioedema · aplastic anaemia · asthma · bronchospasm · confusion ·

constipation · Crohn's disease · depression · diarrhoea · dizziness · drowsiness · dyspnoea · fatigue · fertility decreased female · gastrointestinal discomfort · gastrointestinal disorders · haemolytic anaemia · hallucination · headache · heart failure · hepatic disorders · hypersensitivity · hypertension · malaise · meningitis aseptic (patients with connective-tissue disorders such as systemic lupus erythematosus may be especially susceptible) · nausea · nephritis tubulointerstitial · nephropathy · neutropenia · oedema · optic neuritis · oral ulceration · pancreatitis · paraesthesia · photosensitivity reaction · platelet aggregation inhibition · renal failure (more common in patients with pre-existing renal impairment) · respiratory tract reaction · severe cutaneous adverse reactions (SCARs) · skin reactions · stroke · thrombocytopenia · tinnitus · vertigo · visual impairment · vomiting

SIDE-EFFECTS, FURTHER INFORMATION For information about cardiovascular and gastrointestinal side-effects, and a possible exacerbation of symptoms in asthma, see Non-steroidal anti-inflammatory drugs p. 1094.

- ALLERGY AND CROSS-SENSITIVITY Contra-indicated in patients with a history of hypersensitivity to aspirin or any other NSAID—which includes those in whom attacks of asthma, angioedema, urticaria or rhinitis have been precipitated by aspirin or any other NSAID.
- CONCEPTION AND CONTRACEPTION Caution—long-term use of some NSAIDs is associated with reduced female fertility, which is reversible on stopping treatment.
- PREGNANCY Avoid unless the potential benefit outweighs the risk. Avoid during the third trimester (risk of closure of fetal ductus arteriosus *in utero* and possibly persistent pulmonary hypertension of the newborn); onset of labour may be delayed and duration may be increased.
- BREAST FEEDING Use with caution during breast-feeding. Small amount present in milk—manufacturer advises avoid.
- HEPATIC IMPAIRMENT Use with caution; there is an increased risk of gastro-intestinal bleeding and fluid retention. Avoid in severe liver disease.
- RENAL IMPAIRMENT Avoid if possible or use with caution. Avoid in severe impairment.
  Dose adjustments The lowest effective dose should be used for the shortest possible duration.
  Monitoring In renal impairment monitor renal function; sodium and water retention may occur and renal function may deteriorate, possibly leading to renal failure.

- MEDICINAL FORMS
  There can be variation in the licensing of different medicines containing the same drug.
  Tablet
  CAUTIONARY AND ADVISORY LABELS 21
  ▸ Flurbiprofen (Non-proprietary)
  Flurbiprofen 50 mg Flurbiprofen 50mg tablets | 100 tablet [PoM] £21.30–£35.97 DT = £35.97
  Flurbiprofen 100 mg Flurbiprofen 100mg tablets | 100 tablet [PoM] £64.34 DT = £64.34

Ibuprofen

- INDICATIONS AND DOSE
Pain and inflammation in rheumatic disease and other musculoskeletal disorders | Mild to moderate pain including dysmenorrhoea | Postoperative analgesia | Migraine | Dental pain
  ▸ BY MOUTH USING IMMEDIATE-RELEASE MEDICINES
  ▸ Adult: Initially 300–400 mg 3–4 times a day; increased if necessary up to 600 mg 4 times a day; maintenance 200–400 mg 3 times a day, may be adequate

▸ BY MOUTH USING MODIFIED-RELEASE MEDICINES
▸ Adult: 1.6 g once daily, dose to be taken in the early evening, increased if necessary to 2.4 g daily in 2 divided doses, dose to be increased only in severe cases

Mild to moderate pain | Pain and inflammation of soft-tissue injuries | Pyrexia with discomfort
▸ BY MOUTH USING IMMEDIATE-RELEASE MEDICINES
▸ Child 3–5 months: 50 mg 3 times a day, maximum daily dose to be given in 3–4 divided doses; maximum 30 mg/kg per day
▸ Child 6–11 months: 50 mg 3–4 times a day, maximum daily dose to be given in 3–4 divided doses; maximum 30 mg/kg per day
▸ Child 1–3 years: 100 mg 3 times a day, maximum daily dose to be given in 3–4 divided doses; maximum 30 mg/kg per day
▸ Child 4–6 years: 150 mg 3 times a day, maximum daily dose to be given in 3–4 divided doses; maximum 30 mg/kg per day
▸ Child 7–9 years: 200 mg 3 times a day, maximum daily dose to be given in 3–4 divided doses; maximum 30 mg/kg per day; maximum 2.4 g per day
▸ Child 10–11 years: 300 mg 3 times a day, maximum daily dose to be given in 3–4 divided doses; maximum 30 mg/kg per day; maximum 2.4 g per day
▸ Child 12–17 years: Initially 300–400 mg 3–4 times a day; increased if necessary up to 600 mg 4 times a day; maintenance 200–400 mg 3 times a day, may be adequate

Pain and inflammation
▸ BY MOUTH USING MODIFIED-RELEASE MEDICINES
▸ Child 12–17 years: 1.6 g once daily, dose preferably taken in the early evening, increased to 2.4 g daily in 2 divided doses, dose to be increased only in severe cases

Pain and inflammation in rheumatic disease including juvenile idiopathic arthritis
▸ BY MOUTH USING IMMEDIATE-RELEASE MEDICINES
▸ Child 3 months–17 years: 30–40 mg/kg daily in 3–4 divided doses; maximum 2.4 g per day

Pain and inflammation in systemic juvenile idiopathic arthritis
▸ BY MOUTH USING IMMEDIATE-RELEASE MEDICINES
▸ Child 3 months–17 years: Up to 60 mg/kg daily in 4–6 divided doses; maximum 2.4 g per day

Post-immunisation pyrexia in infants (on doctor's advice only)
▸ BY MOUTH USING IMMEDIATE-RELEASE MEDICINES
▸ Child 2–3 months: 50 mg for 1 dose, followed by 50 mg after 6 hours if required

Pain relief in musculoskeletal conditions | Treatment in knee or hand osteoarthritis (adjunct)
▸ TO THE SKIN
▸ Adult: Apply up to 3 times a day, ibuprofen gel 5% gel to be administered

FENBID ® FORTE
Pain relief in musculoskeletal conditions | Treatment in knee or hand osteoarthritis (adjunct)
▸ TO THE SKIN
▸ Adult: Apply up to 4 times a day, therapy should be reviewed after 14 days

IBUGEL ® FORTE
Pain relief in musculoskeletal conditions | Treatment in knee or hand osteoarthritis (adjunct)
▸ TO THE SKIN
▸ Adult: Apply up to 3 times a day

● UNLICENSED USE Not licensed for use in children under 3 months or body-weight under 5 kg. Maximum dose for systemic juvenile idiopathic arthritis is unlicensed.
● CONTRA-INDICATIONS
▸ With systemic use Active gastro-intestinal bleeding · active gastro-intestinal ulceration · history of gastro-intestinal bleeding related to previous NSAID therapy · history of gastro-intestinal perforation related to previous NSAID therapy · history of recurrent gastro-intestinal haemorrhage (two or more distinct episodes) · history of recurrent gastro-intestinal ulceration (two or more distinct episodes) · severe heart failure
● CAUTIONS
▸ With systemic use Allergic disorders (in adults) · cardiac impairment (NSAIDs may impair renal function) · cerebrovascular disease · coagulation defects · connective-tissue disorders · Crohn's disease (may be exacerbated) · elderly (risk of serious side-effects and fatalities) · heart failure · ischaemic heart disease · peripheral arterial disease · risk factors for cardiovascular events · risk factors for cardiovascular events · ulcerative colitis (may be exacerbated) · uncontrolled hypertension
▸ With topical use Avoid contact with eyes · avoid contact with inflamed or broken skin · avoid contact with mucous membranes · not for use with occlusive dressings · topical application of large amounts can result in systemic effects, including hypersensitivity and asthma (renal disease has also been reported)

CAUTIONS, FURTHER INFORMATION
▸ High-dose ibuprofen A small increase in cardiovascular risk, similar to the risk associated with cyclo-oxygenase-2 inhibitors and diclofenac, has been reported with high-dose ibuprofen ($\geq$ 2.4 g daily); use should be avoided in patients with established ischaemic heart disease, peripheral arterial disease, cerebrovascular disease, congestive heart failure (New York Heart Association classification II-III), and uncontrolled hypertension.
● INTERACTIONS → Appendix 1: NSAIDs
● SIDE-EFFECTS
▸ Common or very common
▸ With intravenous use Fluid retention · gastrointestinal disorders · haemorrhage · intraventricular haemorrhage · neutropenia · periventricular leukomalacia · renal impairment · thrombocytopenia
▸ Uncommon
▸ With oral use Gastrointestinal discomfort · headache · hypersensitivity · nausea · rash (discontinue) · skin reactions
▸ Rare or very rare
▸ With oral use Acute kidney injury · agranulocytosis · anaemia · angioedema · constipation · diarrhoea · dyspnoea · fatigue · fever · gastrointestinal disorders · haemorrhage · hypotension · influenza like illness · leucopenia · liver disorder · meningitis aseptic (patients with connective-tissue disorders such as systemic lupus erythematosus may be especially susceptible) · oedema · oral disorders · pancytopenia · renal papillary necrosis · respiratory disorders · severe cutaneous adverse reactions (SCARs) · shock · tachycardia · throat pain · thrombocytopenia · vomiting
▸ Frequency not known
▸ With oral use Asthma · Crohn's disease · fertility decreased female · fluid retention · heart failure · hypertension · increased risk of arterial thromboembolism · renal failure (more common in patients with pre-existing renal impairment) · respiratory tract reaction
▸ With topical use Angioedema · asthma · bronchospasm · dyspnoea · gastrointestinal discomfort · hypersensitivity · rash (discontinue) · renal impairment · skin reactions · toxic epidermal necrolysis

SIDE-EFFECTS, FURTHER INFORMATION For information about cardiovascular and gastrointestinal side-effects, and a possible exacerbation of symptoms in asthma, see Non-steroidal anti-inflammatory drugs p. 1094.

With topical use Topical application of large amounts can result in systemic effects, including hypersensitivity and asthma (renal disease has also been reported).

Overdose Overdosage with ibuprofen may cause nausea, vomiting, epigastric pain, and tinnitus, but more serious toxicity is very uncommon. Charcoal, activated followed by symptomatic measures are indicated if more than 100mg/kg has been ingested within the preceding hour.

For details on the management of poisoning, see Emergency treatment of poisoning p. 1319.

● ALLERGY AND CROSS-SENSITIVITY Contra-indicated in patients with a history of hypersensitivity to aspirin or any other NSAID—which includes those in whom attacks of asthma, angioedema, urticaria or rhinitis have been precipitated by aspirin or any other NSAID.

● CONCEPTION AND CONTRACEPTION Caution—long-term use of some NSAIDs is associated with reduced female fertility, which is reversible on stopping treatment.

● PREGNANCY
▸ With systemic use Avoid unless the potential benefit outweighs the risk. Avoid during the third trimester (risk of closure of fetal ductus arteriosus *in utero* and possibly persistent pulmonary hypertension of the newborn); onset of labour may be delayed and duration may be increased.
▸ With topical use Patient packs for topical preparations carry a warning to avoid during pregnancy.

● BREAST FEEDING
▸ With oral use Use with caution during breast-feeding. Amount too small to be harmful but some manufacturers advise avoid.
▸ With topical use Patient packs for topical preparations carry a warning to avoid during breast-feeding.

● HEPATIC IMPAIRMENT
▸ With oral use Use with caution; there is an increased risk of gastro-intestinal bleeding and fluid retention. Avoid in severe liver disease.

● RENAL IMPAIRMENT
▸ With oral use Avoid if possible or use with caution. Avoid in severe impairment.
▸ With topical use Deterioration in renal function has also been reported after topical use.
Dose adjustments ▸ With systemic use The lowest effective dose should be used for the shortest possible duration.
Monitoring ▸ With systemic use In renal impairment monitor renal function; sodium and water retention may occur and renal function may deteriorate, possibly leading to renal failure.

● DIRECTIONS FOR ADMINISTRATION For topical preparations, apply with gentle massage only.

● PRESCRIBING AND DISPENSING INFORMATION Flavours of syrup may include orange.

● PATIENT AND CARER ADVICE
Medicines for Children leaflet: Ibuprofen for pain and inflammation www.medicinesforchildren.org.uk/ibuprofen-for-pain-and-inflammation
▸ With topical use For topical preparations, patients and their carers should be advised to wash hands immediately after use.
Photosensitivity For topical preparations, patients or their carers should be advised against excessive exposure to sunlight of area treated in order to avoid possibility of photosensitivity.

● PROFESSION SPECIFIC INFORMATION
Dental practitioners' formulary
Ibuprofen Oral Suspension Sugar-free may be prescribed. Ibuprofen Tablets may be prescribed.

● EXCEPTIONS TO LEGAL CATEGORY Smaller pack sizes of gel preparations may be available on sale to the public. Oral preparations can be sold to the public in certain circumstances.

● MEDICINAL FORMS
There can be variation in the licensing of different medicines containing the same drug. Forms available from special-order manufacturers include: oral suspension

Effervescent granules
CAUTIONARY AND ADVISORY LABELS 13, 21
ELECTROLYTES: May contain Sodium
▸ Brufen (Mylan)
Ibuprofen 600 mg Brufen 600mg effervescent granules sachets | 20 sachet [PoM] £6.80 DT = £6.80

Modified-release tablet
CAUTIONARY AND ADVISORY LABELS 25, 27
▸ Brufen Retard (Mylan)
Ibuprofen 800 mg Brufen Retard 800mg tablets | 56 tablet [PoM] £7.74 DT = £7.74

Foam
▸ Ibumousse (Dermal Laboratories Ltd)
Ibuprofen 50 mg per 1 gram Ibumousse 5% | 125 gram [P] £5.85

Tablet
CAUTIONARY AND ADVISORY LABELS 21
▸ Ibuprofen (Non-proprietary)
Ibuprofen 200 mg Ibuprofen 200mg tablets | 16 tablet [P] £0.25 | 24 tablet [P] £0.91 DT = £0.66 | 48 tablet [P] £0.80-£1.47 | 84 tablet [P] £3.29 DT = £2.31 | 96 tablet [P] £1.69
Ibuprofen 200mg caplets | 16 tablet [P] £0.25 | 24 tablet [℞] DT = £0.66
Ibuprofen 400 mg Ibuprofen 400mg tablets film coated | 250 tablet [PoM] £10.54
Ibuprofen 600 mg Ibuprofen 600mg tablets | 84 tablet [PoM] £6.95 DT = £3.60
Ibuprofen 600mg tablets film coated | 84 tablet [PoM] £3.60 DT = £3.60
▸ Brufen (Mylan)
Ibuprofen 400 mg Brufen 400mg tablets | 60 tablet [PoM] £4.90
Ibuprofen 600 mg Brufen 600mg tablets | 60 tablet [PoM] £7.34
▸ Ibucalm (Aspar Pharmaceuticals Ltd)
Ibuprofen 200 mg Ibucalm 200mg tablets | 24 tablet [P] £0.77 DT = £0.66 | 48 tablet [P] £1.43 | 96 tablet [P] £2.43
▸ Nurofen (Reckitt Benckiser Healthcare (UK) Ltd)
Ibuprofen 200 mg Nurofen 200mg caplets | 24 tablet [P] £2.49 DT = £0.66
Nurofen 200mg tablets | 24 tablet [P] £2.38 DT = £0.66 | 48 tablet [P] £4.36 | 96 tablet [P] £7.20
Ibuprofen (as Ibuprofen lysine) 400 mg Nurofen Maximum Strength Migraine Pain 684mg caplets | 12 tablet [P] £3.49

Oral suspension
CAUTIONARY AND ADVISORY LABELS 21
▸ Ibuprofen (Non-proprietary)
Ibuprofen 20 mg per 1 ml Ibuprofen 100mg/5ml oral suspension sugar free | 500 ml [PoM] £6.45
▸ Brufen (Mylan)
Ibuprofen 20 mg per 1 ml Brufen 100mg/5ml syrup | 500 ml [PoM] £8.88 DT = £8.88

Modified-release capsule
▸ Nurofen Back Pain SR (Reckitt Benckiser Healthcare (UK) Ltd)
Ibuprofen 300 mg Nurofen Back Pain SR 300mg capsules | 24 capsule [P] £4.20 DT = £4.20

Chewable capsule
▸ Nurofen (Reckitt Benckiser Healthcare (UK) Ltd)
Ibuprofen 100 mg Nurofen for Children 100mg chewable capsules | 12 capsule [P] £3.23

Gel
EXCIPIENTS: May contain Benzyl alcohol
▸ Ibuprofen (Non-proprietary)
Ibuprofen 50 mg per 1 gram Mentholatum Ibuprofen 5% gel | 100 gram [P] £5.01 DT = £1.74
Ibuprofen 5% gel | 30 gram [P] £1.35 | 50 gram [P] £1.01 DT = £0.87 | 100 gram [P] £2.01 DT = £1.74
▸ Fenbid (AMCo)
Ibuprofen 100 mg per 1 gram Fenbid Forte 10% gel | 100 gram [PoM] £4.00 DT = £5.79

▸ Ibugel (Dermal Laboratories Ltd)
Ibuprofen 50 mg per 1 gram Ibugel 5% gel | 100 gram ℗ £4.87 DT = £1.74
▸ Ibuleve (Dendron Ltd)
Ibuprofen 50 mg per 1 gram Ibuleve 5% gel | 30 gram ℗ £2.64 | 50 gram ℗ £3.70 DT = £0.87 | 100 gram ℗ £6.80 DT = £1.74
▸ Phorpain (AMCo)
Ibuprofen 50 mg per 1 gram Phorpain 5% gel | 100 gram ℗ £0.89 DT = £1.74

Capsule
▸ Ibuprofen (Non-proprietary)
Ibuprofen 200 mg Ibuprofen 200mg capsules | 30 capsule ℗ 🅂 DT = £4.39
Ibuprofen 400 mg Ibuprofen 400mg capsules | 20 capsule ℗ 🅂 DT = £5.82
▸ Flarin (infirst Healthcare Ltd)
Ibuprofen 200 mg Flarin 200mg capsules | 30 capsule ℗ £6.85 DT = £4.39
▸ Nurofen Express (Reckitt Benckiser Healthcare (UK) Ltd)
Ibuprofen 200 mg Nurofen Express 200mg liquid capsules | 30 capsule ℗ £4.39 DT = £4.39
Ibuprofen 400 mg Nurofen Express 400mg liquid capsules | 10 capsule ℗ £3.55 | 20 capsule ℗ £5.82 DT = £5.82

Orodispersible tablet
▸ Ibuprofen (Non-proprietary)
Ibuprofen 200 mg Ibuprofen 200mg orodispersible tablets | 12 tablet GSL 🅂 DT = £2.19
▸ Brands may include Nurofen Meltlets

Indometacin
(Indomethacin)

● **INDICATIONS AND DOSE**

Pain and moderate to severe inflammation in rheumatic disease and other musculoskeletal disorders
▸ BY MOUTH USING IMMEDIATE-RELEASE MEDICINES
▸ Adult: 50–200 mg daily in divided doses
▸ BY RECTUM
▸ Adult: 100 mg twice daily if required, dose to be administered at night and in the morning, combined oral and rectal treatment, maximum total daily dose 150–200 mg
▸ BY MOUTH USING MODIFIED-RELEASE MEDICINES
▸ Adult: 75 mg 1–2 times a day

Acute gout
▸ BY MOUTH USING IMMEDIATE-RELEASE MEDICINES
▸ Adult: 150–200 mg daily in divided doses
▸ BY RECTUM
▸ Adult: 100 mg twice daily if required, dose to be administered at night and in the morning, combined oral and rectal treatment, maximum total daily dose 150–200 mg
▸ BY MOUTH USING MODIFIED-RELEASE MEDICINES
▸ Adult: 75 mg 1–2 times a day

Dysmenorrhoea
▸ BY MOUTH USING IMMEDIATE-RELEASE MEDICINES
▸ Adult: Up to 75 mg daily
▸ BY RECTUM
▸ Adult: 100 mg twice daily if required, dose to be administered at night and in the morning, combined oral and rectal treatment, maximum total daily dose 150–200 mg
▸ BY MOUTH USING MODIFIED-RELEASE MEDICINES
▸ Adult: 75 mg daily

● **CONTRA-INDICATIONS** Active gastro-intestinal bleeding · active gastro-intestinal ulceration · history of gastro-intestinal bleeding related to previous NSAID therapy · history of gastro-intestinal perforation related to previous NSAID therapy · history of recurrent gastro-intestinal haemorrhage (two or more distinct episodes) · history of recurrent gastro-intestinal ulceration (two or more distinct episodes) · severe heart failure

● **CAUTIONS**
GENERAL CAUTIONS Heart failure
SPECIFIC CAUTIONS Allergic disorders · cardiac impairment (NSAIDs may impair renal function) · cerebrovascular disease · coagulation defects · connective-tissue disorders · Crohn's disease (may be exacerbated) · elderly (risk of serious side-effects and fatalities) · epilepsy · ischaemic heart disease · parkinsonism · peripheral arterial disease · psychiatric disturbances · risk factors for cardiovascular events · ulcerative colitis (may be exacerbated) · uncontrolled hypertension
▸ With rectal use Avoid rectal administration in haemorrhoids · avoid rectal administration in proctitis

● **INTERACTIONS** → Appendix 1: NSAIDs

● **SIDE-EFFECTS**
GENERAL SIDE-EFFECTS
Agranulocytosis · alopecia · anaphylactic reaction · angioedema · anxiety · appetite decreased · arrhythmias · asthma · blood disorder · bone marrow disorders · breast abnormalities · chest pain · coma · confusion · congestive heart failure · constipation · corneal deposits · depression · diarrhoea · disseminated intravascular coagulation · dizziness · drowsiness · dysarthria · erythema nodosum · eye disorder · eye pain · fatigue · fluid retention · flushing · gastrointestinal discomfort · gastrointestinal disorders · gynaecomastia · haemolytic anaemia · haemorrhage · hallucination · headache · hearing impairment · hepatic disorders · hyperglycaemia · hyperhidrosis · hyperkalaemia · hypotension · inflammatory bowel disease · insomnia · leucopenia · movement disorders · muscle weakness · nausea · nephritis tubulointerstitial · nephrotic syndrome · oedema · oral disorders · palpitations · pancreatitis · paraesthesia · peripheral neuropathy · photosensitivity reaction · platelet aggregation inhibition · psychiatric disorders · renal failure (more common in patients with pre-existing renal impairment) · respiratory disorders · seizures · severe cutaneous adverse reactions (SCARs) · skin reactions · syncope · thrombocytopenia · urine abnormalities · vasculitis · vertigo · vision disorders · vomiting

SPECIFIC SIDE-EFFECTS
▸ With oral use Anaemia · dyspnoea · eosinophilia · malaise · pulmonary oedema · sigmoid lesion perforation
SIDE-EFFECTS, FURTHER INFORMATION For information about cardiovascular and gastrointestinal side-effects, and a possible exacerbation of symptoms in asthma, see Non-steroidal anti-inflammatory drugs p. 1094.

● **ALLERGY AND CROSS-SENSITIVITY** Contra-indicated in patients with a history of hypersensitivity to aspirin or any other NSAID—which includes those in whom attacks of asthma, angioedema, urticaria or rhinitis have been precipitated by aspirin or any other NSAID.

● **CONCEPTION AND CONTRACEPTION** Caution—long-term use of some NSAIDs is associated with reduced female fertility, which is reversible on stopping treatment.

● **PREGNANCY** Avoid unless the potential benefit outweighs the risk. Avoid during the third trimester (risk of closure of fetal ductus arteriosus *in utero* and possibly persistent pulmonary hypertension of the newborn); onset of labour may be delayed and duration may be increased.

● **BREAST FEEDING** Amount probably too small to be harmful—manufacturers advise avoid. Use with caution during breast-feeding.

● **HEPATIC IMPAIRMENT** Use with caution; there is an increased risk of gastro-intestinal bleeding and fluid retention. Avoid in severe liver disease.

● **RENAL IMPAIRMENT** Avoid if possible or use with caution. Avoid in severe impairment.
Dose adjustments The lowest effective dose should be used for the shortest possible duration.

Monitoring In renal impairment monitor renal function; sodium and water retention may occur and renal function may deteriorate, possibly leading to renal failure.

● MONITORING REQUIREMENTS During prolonged therapy ophthalmic and blood examinations particularly advisable.

● PATIENT AND CARER ADVICE
Driving and skilled tasks Dizziness may affect performance of skilled tasks (e.g. driving).

● MEDICINAL FORMS
There can be variation in the licensing of different medicines containing the same drug. Forms available from special-order manufacturers include: oral suspension, oral solution
Suppository
▸ Indometacin (Non-proprietary)
Indometacin 100 mg Indometacin 100mg suppositories |
10 suppository [PoM] [⚠] DT = £17.61
▸ Indocid (Aspen Pharma Trading Ltd)
Indometacin 100 mg Indocid 100mg suppositories |
10 suppository [PoM] £17.61 DT = £17.61
Modified-release capsule
CAUTIONARY AND ADVISORY LABELS 21, 25
▸ Indometacin (Non-proprietary)
Indometacin 75 mg Indometacin 75mg modified-release capsules |
100 capsule [PoM] [⚠] DT = £8.65
▸ Berlind Retard (Tillomed Laboratories Ltd)
Indometacin 75 mg Berlind 75 Retard capsules | 100 capsule [PoM]
£8.65 DT = £8.65
Capsule
CAUTIONARY AND ADVISORY LABELS 21
▸ Indometacin (Non-proprietary)
Indometacin 25 mg Indometacin 25mg capsules | 28 capsule [PoM]
£5.00 DT = £0.83
Indometacin 50 mg Indometacin 50mg capsules | 28 capsule [PoM]
£7.50 DT = £1.24

Ketoprofen

15-May-2018

● INDICATIONS AND DOSE
Pain and mild inflammation in rheumatic disease and musculoskeletal conditions | Dysmenorrhoea | Acute gout
▸ BY MOUTH
▸ Adult: 100–200 mg once daily
Relief of pain in rheumatic disease and musculoskeletal conditions
▸ TO THE SKIN
▸ Adult: Apply 2–4 times a day for up to 7 days, ketoprofen 2.5% gel to be administered; maximum 15 g per day

POWERGEL ®
Relief of pain in musculoskeletal conditions | Adjunctive treatment in knee or hand osteoarthritis
▸ TO THE SKIN
▸ Adult: Apply 2–3 times a day for up to max. 10 days

● CONTRA-INDICATIONS
▸ With systemic use Active gastro-intestinal bleeding · active gastro-intestinal ulceration · history of gastro-intestinal bleeding · history of gastro-intestinal perforation · history of gastro-intestinal ulceration · severe heart failure

● CAUTIONS
▸ With systemic use Allergic disorders · cardiac impairment (NSAIDs may impair renal function) · cerebrovascular disease · coagulation defects · connective-tissue disorders · Crohn's disease (may be exacerbated) · elderly (risk of serious side-effects and fatalities) · heart failure · ischaemic heart disease · peripheral arterial disease · risk factors for cardiovascular events · ulcerative colitis (may be exacerbated) · uncontrolled hypertension
▸ With topical use Avoid contact with eyes · avoid contact with inflamed or broken skin · avoid contact with mucous membranes · not for use with occlusive dressings · topical

application of large amounts can result in systemic effects, including hypersensitivity and asthma (renal disease has also been reported)

● INTERACTIONS → Appendix 1: NSAIDs

● SIDE-EFFECTS
GENERAL SIDE-EFFECTS
▸ **Uncommon** Diarrhoea
▸ **Rare or very rare** Hypersensitivity · photosensitivity reaction
▸ **Frequency not known** Angioedema
SPECIFIC SIDE-EFFECTS
▸ **Common or very common**
▹ With oral use Gastrointestinal discomfort · nausea · vomiting
▸ **Uncommon**
▹ With oral use Constipation · dizziness · drowsiness · fatigue · gastrointestinal disorders · headache · oedema · rash (discontinue) · skin reactions
▹ With topical use Increased risk of infection · paraesthesia · skin reactions
▸ **Rare or very rare**
▹ With oral use Asthma · haemorrhagic anaemia · hepatic disorders · pancreatitis · paraesthesia · shock · stomatitis · tinnitus · vision disorders · weight increased
▹ With topical use Renal impairment
▸ **Frequency not known**
▹ With oral use Acute kidney injury (more common in patients with pre-existing renal impairment) · agranulocytosis · alopecia · bone marrow failure · bronchospasm · confusion · Crohn's disease aggravated · depression · dyspnoea · fertility decreased female · haemorrhage · hallucination · heart failure · hypertension · increased risk of arterial thromboembolism · increased risk of ischaemic stroke · increased risk of myocardial infarction · malaise · meningitis aseptic (patients with connective-tissue disorders such as systemic lupus erythematosus may be especially susceptible) · mood altered · nephritic syndrome · nephritis tubulointerstitial · neutropenia · optic neuritis · rhinitis · seizure · severe cutaneous adverse reactions (SCARs) · taste altered · thrombocytopenia · vasodilation · vertigo
▹ With topical use Eosinophilia · eyelid oedema · fever · gastrointestinal haemorrhage · lip swelling · peptic ulcer · vasculitis · wound complications
SIDE-EFFECTS, FURTHER INFORMATION For information about cardiovascular and gastrointestinal side-effects, and a possible exacerbation of symptoms in asthma, see Non-steroidal anti-inflammatory drugs p. 1094.
▹ With topical use Topical application of large amounts can result in systemic effects, including hypersensitivity and asthma (renal disease has also been reported).

● ALLERGY AND CROSS-SENSITIVITY Contra-indicated in patients with a history of hypersensitivity to aspirin or any other NSAID—which includes those in whom attacks of asthma, angioedema, urticaria or rhinitis have been precipitated by aspirin or any other NSAID.

● CONCEPTION AND CONTRACEPTION
▸ With systemic use Caution—long-term use of some NSAIDs is associated with reduced female fertility, which is reversible on stopping treatment.

● PREGNANCY
▸ With systemic use Avoid unless the potential benefit outweighs the risk. Avoid during the third trimester (risk of closure of fetal ductus arteriosus *in utero* and possibly persistent pulmonary hypertension of the newborn); onset of labour may be delayed and duration may be increased.
▸ With topical use Patient packs for topical preparations carry a warning to avoid during pregnancy.

- **BREAST FEEDING**
- With systemic use   Use with caution during breast-feeding. Amount probably too small to be harmful but manufacturers advise avoid.
- With topical use   Patient packs for topical preparations carry a warning to avoid during breast-feeding.

- **HEPATIC IMPAIRMENT**
- With systemic use   Use with caution; there is an increased risk of gastro-intestinal bleeding and fluid retention. Should be avoided in severe liver disease.

- **RENAL IMPAIRMENT**
- With systemic use   Avoid if possible or use with caution. Avoid in severe impairment.
- With topical use   Deterioration in renal function has also been reported after topical use.
  Dose adjustments ‣ With systemic use   The lowest effective dose should be used for the shortest possible duration.
  Monitoring ‣ With systemic use   In renal impairment monitor renal function; sodium and water retention may occur and renal function may deteriorate, possibly leading to renal failure.

- **DIRECTIONS FOR ADMINISTRATION** For topical preparations apply with gentle massage only.

- **PRESCRIBING AND DISPENSING INFORMATION** Flavours of oral liquid formulations may include strawberry.

- **PATIENT AND CARER ADVICE** For topical preparations, patients and their carers should be advised to wash hands immediately after use.
  Photosensitivity
- With topical use   Patients should be advised against excessive exposure to sunlight of area treated in order to avoid possibility of photosensitivity. Patients should be advised not to expose area treated to sunbeds or sunlight (even on a bright but cloudy day) during, and for two weeks after stopping treatment; treated areas should be protected with clothing.

- **EXCEPTIONS TO LEGAL CATEGORY** Smaller pack sizes of gel preparations may be available on sale to the public.

- **MEDICINAL FORMS**
  There can be variation in the licensing of different medicines containing the same drug. Forms available from special-order manufacturers include: gel

Modified-release capsule
CAUTIONARY AND ADVISORY LABELS 21, 25
‣ Ketoprofen (Non-proprietary)
  Ketoprofen 200 mg Ketoprofen 200mg modified-release capsules | 28 capsule [PoM] [🟢] DT = £23.85
‣ Larafen CR (Ennogen Pharma Ltd)
  Ketoprofen 200 mg Larafen CR 200mg capsules | 28 capsule [PoM] £19.08 DT = £23.85
‣ Oruvail (Sanofi)
  Ketoprofen 100 mg Oruvail 100 modified-release capsules | 56 capsule [PoM] £23.93 DT = £23.93
  Ketoprofen 200 mg Oruvail 200 modified-release capsules | 28 capsule [PoM] £23.85 DT = £23.85
‣ Tiloket CR (Tillomed Laboratories Ltd)
  Ketoprofen 100 mg Tiloket CR 100mg capsules | 56 capsule [PoM] £10.70 DT = £23.93
  Ketoprofen 200 mg Tiloket CR 200mg capsules | 28 capsule [PoM] £10.70 DT = £23.85
‣ Valket Retard (Tillomed Laboratories Ltd)
  Ketoprofen 200 mg Valket 200 Retard capsules | 28 capsule [PoM] £10.70 DT = £23.85

Gel
CAUTIONARY AND ADVISORY LABELS 11
EXCIPIENTS: May contain Ethanol, fragrances
‣ Ketoprofen (Non-proprietary)
  Ketoprofen 25 mg per 1 gram Ketoprofen 2.5% gel | 50 gram [PoM] £1.19 DT = £1.19 | 100 gram [PoM] £2.38 DT = £2.38
‣ Oruvail (Sanofi)
  Ketoprofen 25 mg per 1 gram Oruvail 2.5% gel | 100 gram [PoM] £6.84 DT = £2.38

‣ Powergel (A. Menarini Farmaceutica Internazionale SRL)
  Ketoprofen 25 mg per 1 gram Powergel 2.5% gel | 50 gram [PoM] £3.06 DT = £1.19 | 100 gram [PoM] £5.89 DT = £2.38
‣ Tiloket (Tillomed Laboratories Ltd)
  Ketoprofen 25 mg per 1 gram Tiloket 2.5% gel | 50 gram [PoM] £3.00 DT = £1.19 | 100 gram [PoM] £6.00 DT = £2.38

Mefenamic acid   05-Oct-2016

- **INDICATIONS AND DOSE**

Pain and inflammation in rheumatoid arthritis and osteoarthritis | Postoperative pain | Mild to moderate pain
‣ BY MOUTH
‣ Adult: 500 mg 3 times a day

Acute pain including dysmenorrhoea | Menorrhagia
‣ BY MOUTH
‣ Child 12–17 years: 500 mg 3 times a day
‣ Adult: 500 mg 3 times a day

- **CONTRA-INDICATIONS** Active gastro-intestinal bleeding · active gastro-intestinal ulceration · history of gastro-intestinal bleeding related to previous NSAID therapy · history of gastro-intestinal perforation related to previous NSAID therapy · history of recurrent gastro-intestinal haemorrhage (two or more distinct episodes) · history of recurrent gastro-intestinal ulceration (two or more distinct episodes) · inflammatory bowel disease · severe heart failure

- **CAUTIONS** Acute porphyrias p. 1025 · allergic disorders · cardiac impairment (NSAIDs may impair renal function) · cerebrovascular disease · coagulation defects · connective-tissue disorders · Crohn's disease (may be exacerbated) · elderly (risk of serious side-effects and fatalities) · epilepsy · heart failure · ischaemic heart disease · peripheral arterial disease · risk factors for cardiovascular events · ulcerative colitis (may be exacerbated) · uncontrolled hypertension

- **INTERACTIONS** → Appendix 1: NSAIDs

- **SIDE-EFFECTS** Agranulocytosis · anaemia · angioedema · appetite decreased · asthma · bone marrow disorders · confusion · constipation · Crohn's disease · depression · diarrhoea (discontinue) · disseminated intravascular coagulation · dizziness · drowsiness · dyspnoea · dysuria · ear pain · eosinophilia · eye irritation · fatigue · fertility decreased female · gastrointestinal discomfort · gastrointestinal disorders · glomerulonephritis · glucose tolerance impaired · haemolytic anaemia · haemorrhage · hallucination · headache · heart failure · hepatic disorders · hyperhidrosis · hypersensitivity · hypertension · hyponatraemia · hypotension · insomnia · leucopenia · malaise · meningitis aseptic (patients with connective-tissue disorders such as systemic lupus erythematosus may be especially susceptible) · multi organ failure · nausea · nephritis acute interstitial · nephrotic syndrome · nervousness · neutropenia · oedema · optic neuritis · oral ulceration · palpitations · pancreatitis · paraesthesia · photosensitivity reaction · proteinuria · rash (discontinue) · renal failure (more common in patients with pre-existing renal impairment) · renal failure non-oliguric · renal papillary necrosis · respiratory disorders · seizure · sepsis · severe cutaneous adverse reactions (SCARs) · skin reactions · thrombocytopenia · tinnitus · vertigo · vision disorders · vomiting

SIDE-EFFECTS, FURTHER INFORMATION For information about cardiovascular and gastrointestinal side-effects, and a possible exacerbation of symptoms in asthma, see Non-steroidal anti-inflammatory drugs p. 1094.

Overdose   Mefenamic acid has important consequences in overdosage because it can cause convulsions, which if prolonged or recurrent, require treatment.

10

Musculoskeletal system

For details on the management of poisoning, see Emergency treatment of poisoning , in particular, Convulsions p. 1319.

- ALLERGY AND CROSS-SENSITIVITY Contra-indicated in patients with a history of hypersensitivity to aspirin or any other NSAID—which includes those in whom attacks of asthma, angioedema, urticaria or rhinitis have been precipitated by aspirin or any other NSAID.

- CONCEPTION AND CONTRACEPTION Caution—long-term use of some NSAIDs is associated with reduced female fertility, which is reversible on stopping treatment.

- PREGNANCY Avoid unless the potential benefit outweighs the risk. Avoid during the third trimester (risk of closure of fetal ductus arteriosus *in utero* and possibly persistent pulmonary hypertension of the newborn); onset of labour may be delayed and duration may be increased.

- BREAST FEEDING Use with caution during breast-feeding. Amount too small to be harmful but manufacturer advises avoid.

- HEPATIC IMPAIRMENT Use with caution; there is an increased risk of gastro-intestinal bleeding and fluid retention. Avoid in severe liver disease.

- RENAL IMPAIRMENT Avoid if possible or use with caution. Avoid in severe impairment.
  Dose adjustments The lowest effective dose should be used for the shortest possible duration.
  Monitoring In renal impairment monitor renal function; sodium and water retention may occur and renal function may deteriorate, possibly leading to renal failure.

- MEDICINAL FORMS
There can be variation in the licensing of different medicines containing the same drug. Forms available from special-order manufacturers include: oral suspension

Oral suspension
CAUTIONARY AND ADVISORY LABELS 21
EXCIPIENTS: May contain Ethanol
▸ Mefenamic acid (Non-proprietary)
  Mefenamic acid 10 mg per 1 ml Mefenamic acid 50mg/5ml oral suspension | 125 ml PoM £179.00 DT = £179.00

Tablet
CAUTIONARY AND ADVISORY LABELS 21
▸ Mefenamic acid (Non-proprietary)
  Mefenamic acid 500 mg Mefenamic acid 500mg tablets | 28 tablet PoM £60.00 DT = £42.50 | 84 tablet PoM £108.00–£170.00
▸ Ponstan (Chemidex Pharma Ltd)
  Mefenamic acid 500 mg Ponstan Forte 500mg tablets | 100 tablet PoM £15.72

Capsule
CAUTIONARY AND ADVISORY LABELS 21
▸ Mefenamic acid (Non-proprietary)
  Mefenamic acid 250 mg Mefenamic acid 250mg capsules | 100 capsule PoM £60.10 DT = £18.66
▸ Ponstan (Chemidex Pharma Ltd)
  Mefenamic acid 250 mg Ponstan 250mg capsules | 100 capsule PoM £8.17 DT = £18.66

Meloxicam

- INDICATIONS AND DOSE
Exacerbation of osteoarthritis (short-term)
▸ BY MOUTH
▹ Child 16–17 years: 7.5 mg once daily, then increased if necessary up to 15 mg once daily
▹ Adult: 7.5 mg once daily, then increased if necessary up to 15 mg once daily

Pain and inflammation in rheumatic disease | Ankylosing spondylitis
▸ BY MOUTH
▹ Child 16–17 years: 15 mg once daily, then reduced to 7.5 mg once daily if required
▹ Adult: 15 mg once daily, then reduced to 7.5 mg once daily if required
▹ Elderly: 7.5 mg once daily

Relief of pain and inflammation in juvenile idiopathic arthritis and other musculoskeletal disorders in children intolerant to other NSAIDs
▸ BY MOUTH
▹ Child 12–17 years (body-weight up to 50 kg): 7.5 mg once daily
▹ Child 12–17 years (body-weight 50 kg and above): 15 mg once daily

- UNLICENSED USE Not licensed for use in children under 16 years.

- CONTRA-INDICATIONS Active gastro-intestinal bleeding · active gastro-intestinal ulceration · history of gastro-intestinal bleeding related to previous NSAID therapy · history of gastro-intestinal perforation related to previous NSAID therapy · history of recurrent gastro-intestinal haemorrhage (two or more distinct episodes) · history of recurrent gastro-intestinal ulceration (two or more distinct episodes) · severe heart failure

- CAUTIONS Allergic disorders · cardiac impairment (NSAIDs may impair renal function) · cerebrovascular disease · coagulation defects · connective-tissue disorders · Crohn's disease (may be exacerbated) · elderly (risk of serious side-effects and fatalities) · heart failure · ischaemic heart disease · peripheral arterial disease · risk factors for cardiovascular events · ulcerative colitis (may be exacerbated) · uncontrolled hypertension

- INTERACTIONS → Appendix 1: NSAIDs

- SIDE-EFFECTS
▸ **Common or very common** Constipation · diarrhoea · gastrointestinal discomfort · gastrointestinal disorders · headache · nausea · vomiting
▸ **Uncommon** Anaemia · angioedema · burping · dizziness · drowsiness · electrolyte imbalance · fluid retention · flushing · haemorrhage · hepatic disorders · hypersensitivity · oedema · skin reactions · stomatitis · vertigo
▸ **Rare or very rare** Acute kidney injury · asthma · conjunctivitis · leucopenia · mood altered · nightmare · palpitations · severe cutaneous adverse reactions (SCARs) · thrombocytopenia · tinnitus · vision disorders
▸ **Frequency not known** Agranulocytosis · confusion · fertility decreased female · heart failure · increased risk of arterial thromboembolism · nephritis tubulointerstitial · nephrotic syndrome · photosensitivity reaction · renal necrosis
SIDE-EFFECTS, FURTHER INFORMATION For information about cardiovascular and gastrointestinal side-effects, and a possible exacerbation of symptoms in asthma, see Non-steroidal anti-inflammatory drugs p. 1094.

- ALLERGY AND CROSS-SENSITIVITY Contra-indicated in patients with a history of hypersensitivity to aspirin or any other NSAID—which includes those in whom attacks of asthma, angioedema, urticaria or rhinitis have been precipitated by aspirin or any other NSAID.

- CONCEPTION AND CONTRACEPTION Caution—long-term use of some NSAIDs is associated with reduced female fertility, which is reversible on stopping treatment.

- PREGNANCY Avoid unless the potential benefit outweighs the risk. Avoid during the third trimester (risk of closure of fetal ductus arteriosus *in utero* and possibly persistent pulmonary hypertension of the newborn); onset of labour may be delayed and duration may be increased.

- BREAST FEEDING Use with caution during breast-feeding. Present in milk in *animal* studies—manufacturer advises avoid.
- HEPATIC IMPAIRMENT Use with caution; there is an increased risk of gastro-intestinal bleeding and fluid retention. Avoid in severe liver disease.
- RENAL IMPAIRMENT Avoid if possible or use with caution.
  - In adults Avoid if eGFR less than 25 mL/minute/1.73 m².
  - In children Avoid if estimated glomerular filtration rate less than 25 mL/minute/1.73 m².

  Dose adjustments The lowest effective dose should be used for the shortest possible duration.

  Monitoring In renal impairment monitor renal function; sodium and water retention may occur and renal function may deteriorate, possibly leading to renal failure.

- MEDICINAL FORMS
  There can be variation in the licensing of different medicines containing the same drug. Forms available from special-order manufacturers include: oral suspension

  Orodispersible tablet
  - Meloxicam (Non-proprietary)
    Meloxicam 7.5 mg Meloxicam 7.5mg orodispersible tablets sugar free sugar-free | 30 tablet [PoM] £15.50
    Meloxicam 15 mg Meloxicam 15mg orodispersible tablets sugar free sugar-free | 30 tablet [PoM] £15.50

  Tablet
  CAUTIONARY AND ADVISORY LABELS 21
  - Meloxicam (Non-proprietary)
    Meloxicam 7.5 mg Meloxicam 7.5mg tablets | 30 tablet [PoM] £4.00
    DT = £0.87
    Meloxicam 15 mg Meloxicam 15mg tablets | 30 tablet [PoM] £4.00
    DT = £0.91

Nabumetone

- INDICATIONS AND DOSE

Pain and inflammation in osteoarthritis and rheumatoid arthritis
- BY MOUTH
  - Adult: 1 g once daily, dose to be taken at night
  - Elderly: 0.5–1 g daily

Pain and inflammation in osteoarthritis and rheumatoid arthritis (severe and persistent symptoms)
- BY MOUTH
  - Adult: 0.5–1 g, dose to be taken in the morning and 1 g, dose to be taken at night
  - Elderly: 0.5–1 g daily

- CONTRA-INDICATIONS Active gastro-intestinal bleeding · active gastro-intestinal ulceration · history of gastro-intestinal bleeding related to previous NSAID therapy · history of gastro-intestinal perforation related to previous NSAID therapy · history of recurrent gastro-intestinal haemorrhage (two or more distinct episodes) · history of recurrent gastro-intestinal ulceration (two or more distinct episodes) · severe heart failure
- CAUTIONS Allergic disorders · cardiac impairment (NSAIDs may impair renal function) · cerebrovascular disease · coagulation defects · connective-tissue disorders · Crohn's disease (may be exacerbated) · elderly (risk of serious side-effects and fatalities) · heart failure · ischaemic heart disease · peripheral arterial disease · risk factors for cardiovascular events · ulcerative colitis (may be exacerbated) · uncontrolled hypertension
- INTERACTIONS → Appendix 1: NSAIDs
- SIDE-EFFECTS
- Common or very common Constipation · diarrhoea · ear disorder · gastrointestinal discomfort · gastrointestinal disorders · nausea · oedema · skin reactions · tinnitus
- Uncommon Anxiety · asthenia · confusion · dizziness · drowsiness · dry mouth · dyspnoea · eye disorder ·

haemorrhage · headache · hyperhidrosis · insomnia · myopathy · oral disorders · paraesthesia · photosensitivity reaction · respiratory disorders · urinary tract disorder · visual impairment · vomiting
- Rare or very rare Alopecia · angioedema · hepatic disorders · hypersensitivity · menorrhagia · nephrotic syndrome · pancreatitis · renal failure (more common in patients with pre-existing renal impairment) · severe cutaneous adverse reactions (SCARs) · thrombocytopenia
- Frequency not known Agranulocytosis · aplastic anaemia · asthma · Crohn's disease aggravated · depression · fertility decreased female · haemolytic anaemia · hallucination · heart failure · hypertension · increased risk of arterial thromboembolism · leucopenia · malaise · meningitis aseptic (patients with connective-tissue disorders such as systemic lupus erythematosus may be especially susceptible) · nephritis tubulointerstitial · neutropenia · optic neuritis · vertigo
  SIDE-EFFECTS, FURTHER INFORMATION For information about cardiovascular and gastrointestinal side-effects, and a possible exacerbation of symptoms in asthma, see Non-steroidal anti-inflammatory drugs p. 1094.

- ALLERGY AND CROSS-SENSITIVITY Contra-indicated in patients with a history of hypersensitivity to aspirin or any other NSAID—which includes those in whom attacks of asthma, angioedema, urticaria or rhinitis have been precipitated by aspirin or any other NSAID.
- CONCEPTION AND CONTRACEPTION Caution—long-term use of some NSAIDs is associated with reduced female fertility, which is reversible on stopping treatment.
- PREGNANCY Avoid unless the potential benefit outweighs the risk. Avoid during the third trimester (risk of closure of fetal ductus arteriosus *in utero* and possibly persistent pulmonary hypertension of the newborn); onset of labour may be delayed and duration may be increased.
- BREAST FEEDING Use with caution during breast-feeding. Manufacturer advises avoid.
- HEPATIC IMPAIRMENT Use with caution; there is an increased risk of gastro-intestinal bleeding and fluid retention. Avoid in severe liver disease.
- RENAL IMPAIRMENT Avoided if possible or use with caution. Avoid in severe impairment.
  Dose adjustments The lowest effective dose should be used for the shortest possible duration.
  Monitoring In renal impairment monitor renal function; sodium and water retention may occur and renal function may deteriorate, possibly leading to renal failure.

- MEDICINAL FORMS
  There can be variation in the licensing of different medicines containing the same drug.
  Tablet
  CAUTIONARY AND ADVISORY LABELS 21
  - Nabumetone (Non-proprietary)
    Nabumetone 500 mg Nabumetone 500mg tablets | 56 tablet [PoM] £20.00 DT = £6.82
  - Relifex (Meda Pharmaceuticals Ltd)
    Nabumetone 500 mg Relifex 500mg tablets | 60 tablet [PoM] £6.18

Naproxen

- INDICATIONS AND DOSE

Pain and inflammation in rheumatic disease
- BY MOUTH
  - Adult: 0.5–1 g daily in 1–2 divided doses

Pain and inflammation in musculoskeletal disorders | Dysmenorrhoea
- BY MOUTH
  - Adult: Initially 500 mg, then 250 mg every 6–8 hours as required, maximum dose after the first day 1.25 g daily

  continued →

10

Musculoskeletal system

Acute gout

▶ BY MOUTH

▶ Adult: Initially 750 mg, then 250 mg every 8 hours until attack has passed

● CONTRA-INDICATIONS Active gastro-intestinal bleeding · active gastro-intestinal ulceration · history of gastro-intestinal bleeding related to previous NSAID therapy · history of gastro-intestinal perforation related to previous NSAID therapy · history of recurrent gastro-intestinal haemorrhage (two or more distinct episodes) · history of recurrent gastro-intestinal ulceration (two or more distinct episodes) · severe heart failure

● CAUTIONS Allergic disorders · cardiac impairment (NSAIDs may impair renal function) · cerebrovascular disease · coagulation defects · connective-tissue disorders · Crohn's disease (may be exacerbated) · elderly (risk of serious side-effects and fatalities) · heart failure · ischaemic heart disease · peripheral arterial disease · risk factors for cardiovascular events · ulcerative colitis (may be exacerbated) · uncontrolled hypertension

● INTERACTIONS → Appendix 1: NSAIDs

● SIDE-EFFECTS Agranulocytosis · alopecia · angioedema · aplastic anaemia · asthma · cognitive impairment · concentration impaired · confusion · constipation · corneal opacity · depression · diarrhoea · dizziness · drowsiness · dyspnoea · erythema nodosum · fatigue · gastrointestinal discomfort · gastrointestinal disorders · glomerulonephritis · haemolytic anaemia · haemorrhage · hallucination · headache · hearing impairment · heart failure · hepatic disorders · hyperhidrosis · hyperkalaemia · hypersensitivity · hypertension · increased risk of arterial thromboembolism · infertility female · inflammatory bowel disease · malaise · meningitis aseptic (patients with connective-tissue disorders such as systemic lupus erythematosus may be especially susceptible) · muscle weakness · myalgia · nausea · nephritis tubulointerstitial · nephropathy · neutropenia · oedema · optic neuritis · oral disorders · palpitations · pancreatitis · papillitis · papilloedema · paraesthesia · photosensitivity reaction · platelet aggregation inhibition · pulmonary oedema · rash pustular · renal failure (more common in patients with pre-existing renal impairment) · renal papillary necrosis · respiratory disorders · seizure · severe cutaneous adverse reactions (SCARs) · skin reactions · sleep disorders · thirst · thrombocytopenia · vasculitis · vertigo · visual impairment · vomiting

SIDE-EFFECTS, FURTHER INFORMATION For information about cardiovascular and gastrointestinal side-effects, and a possible exacerbation of symptoms in asthma, see Non-steroidal anti-inflammatory drugs p. 1094.

● ALLERGY AND CROSS-SENSITIVITY Contra-indicated in patients with a history of hypersensitivity to aspirin or any other NSAID—which includes those in whom attacks of asthma, angioedema, urticaria or rhinitis have been precipitated by aspirin or any other NSAID.

● CONCEPTION AND CONTRACEPTION Caution—long-term use of some NSAIDs is associated with reduced female fertility, which is reversible on stopping treatment.

● PREGNANCY Avoid unless the potential benefit outweighs the risk. Avoid during the third trimester (risk of closure of fetal ductus arteriosus *in utero* and possibly persistent pulmonary hypertension of the newborn); onset of labour may be delayed and duration may be increased.

● BREAST FEEDING Use with caution during breast-feeding. Amount too small to be harmful but manufacturer advises avoid.

● HEPATIC IMPAIRMENT Use with caution; there is an increased risk of gastro-intestinal bleeding and fluid retention. Avoid in severe liver disease.

● RENAL IMPAIRMENT Avoid if possible or use with caution. Avoid if eGFR less than 30 mL/minute/1.73 m^2.
Dose adjustments The lowest effective dose should be used for the shortest possible duration.
Monitoring In renal impairment monitor renal function; sodium and water retention may occur and renal function may deteriorate, possibly leading to renal failure.

● EXCEPTIONS TO LEGAL CATEGORY Can be sold to the public for the treatment of primary dysmenorrhoea in women aged 15–50 years subject to max. single dose of 500 mg, max. daily dose of 750 mg for max. 3 days, and a max. pack size of 9 × 250 mg tablets.

● MEDICINAL FORMS
There can be variation in the licensing of different medicines containing the same drug. Forms available from special-order manufacturers include: oral suspension

Gastro-resistant tablet
CAUTIONARY AND ADVISORY LABELS 5, 25
▶ Naproxen (Non-proprietary)
Naproxen 250 mg Naproxen 250mg gastro-resistant tablets | 56 tablet P℥M £7.00 DT = £2.19
Naproxen 375 mg Naproxen 375mg gastro-resistant tablets | 56 tablet P℥M £26.82 DT = £26.82
Naproxen 500 mg Naproxen 500mg gastro-resistant tablets | 56 tablet P℥M £7.34 DT = £4.89
▶ Feminax Ultra (Bayer Plc)
Naproxen 250 mg Feminax Ultra 250mg gastro-resistant tablets | 9 tablet P £3.04
▶ Naprosyn EC (Atnahs Pharma UK Ltd)
Naproxen 250 mg Naprosyn EC 250mg tablets | 56 tablet P℥M £4.29 DT = £2.19
Naproxen 375 mg Naprosyn EC 375mg tablets | 56 tablet P℥M £6.42 DT = £26.82
Naproxen 500 mg Naprosyn EC 500mg tablets | 56 tablet P℥M £8.56 DT = £4.89

Tablet
CAUTIONARY AND ADVISORY LABELS 21
▶ Naproxen (Non-proprietary)
Naproxen 250 mg Naproxen 250mg tablets | 28 tablet P℥M £2.10 DT = £0.70 | 56 tablet P℥M £2.33
Naproxen 500 mg Naproxen 500mg tablets | 28 tablet P℥M £4.27 DT = £1.13 | 56 tablet P℥M £3.99
▶ Naprosyn (Atnahs Pharma UK Ltd)
Naproxen 250 mg Naprosyn 250mg tablets | 56 tablet P℥M £4.29
Naproxen 500 mg Naprosyn 500mg tablets | 56 tablet P℥M £8.56

Oral suspension
▶ Naproxen (Non-proprietary)
Naproxen 25 mg per 1 ml Naproxen 25mg/ml oral suspension sugar free sugar-free | 100 ml P℥M £110.00 DT = £119.00
Naproxen 125mg/5ml oral suspension sugar free sugar-free | 100 ml P℥M £110.00-£128.00 DT = £119.00
Naproxen 50 mg per 1 ml Naproxen 50mg/ml oral suspension | 100 ml P℥M £45.00-£75.00 DT = £75.00

Effervescent tablet
▶ Stirlescent (Stirling Anglian Pharmaceuticals Ltd)
Naproxen 250 mg Stirlescent 250mg effervescent tablets sugar-free | 20 tablet P℥M £52.72 DT = £52.72

Naproxen with esomeprazole

The properties listed below are those particular to the combination only. For the properties of the components please consider, naproxen p. 1113, esomeprazole p. 78.

● INDICATIONS AND DOSE

Patients requiring naproxen for osteoarthritis, rheumatoid arthritis, or ankylosing spondylitis, who are at risk of NSAID-associated duodenal or gastric ulcer and when treatment with lower doses of naproxen or other NSAIDs ineffective

▶ BY MOUTH
▶ Adult: 500/20 mg twice daily, dose expressed as *x*/*y* mg naproxen/esomeprazole

- INTERACTIONS → Appendix 1: NSAIDs · proton pump inhibitors
- PRESCRIBING AND DISPENSING INFORMATION Naproxen component is gastro-resistant.

- MEDICINAL FORMS
There can be variation in the licensing of different medicines containing the same drug.
Modified-release tablet
CAUTIONARY AND ADVISORY LABELS 22, 25
  ▸ Vimovo (AstraZeneca UK Ltd)
  Esomeprazole (as Esomeprazole magnesium trihydrate) 20 mg, Naproxen 500 mg Vimovo 500mg/20mg modified-release tablets | 60 tablet [PoM] £14.95 DT = £14.95

Piroxicam

- INDICATIONS AND DOSE
Rheumatoid arthritis (initiated by a specialist) | Osteoarthritis (initiated by a specialist) | Ankylosing spondylitis (initiated by a specialist)
  ▸ BY MOUTH
  ▸ Adult: Up to 20 mg once daily
Pain relief in musculoskeletal conditions | Treatment in knee or hand osteoarthritis (adjunct)
  ▸ TO THE SKIN
  ▸ Adult: Apply 3–4 times a day, 0.5% gel to be applied; review treatment after 4 weeks

> IMPORTANT SAFETY INFORMATION
> CHMP ADVICE—PIROXICAM (JUNE 2007)
> The CHMP has recommended restrictions on the use of piroxicam because of the increased risk of gastro-intestinal side effects and serious skin reactions. The CHMP has advised that:
> - piroxicam should be initiated only by physicians experienced in treating inflammatory or degenerative rheumatic diseases
> - piroxicam should not be used as first-line treatment
> - in adults, use of piroxicam should be limited to the symptomatic relief of osteoarthritis, rheumatoid arthritis, and ankylosing spondylitis
> - piroxicam dose should not exceed 20 mg daily
> - piroxicam should no longer be used for the treatment of acute painful and inflammatory conditions
> - treatment should be reviewed 2 weeks after initiating piroxicam, and periodically thereafter
> - concomitant administration of a gastro-protective agent should be considered.
> Topical preparations containing piroxicam are not affected by these restrictions.

- CONTRA-INDICATIONS
  ▸ With systemic use Active gastro-intestinal bleeding · active gastro-intestinal ulceration · history of gastro-intestinal bleeding · history of gastro-intestinal perforation · history of gastro-intestinal ulceration · inflammatory bowel disease · severe heart failure
- CAUTIONS
  ▸ With systemic use Allergic disorders · cardiac impairment (NSAIDs may impair renal function) · cerebrovascular disease · coagulation defects · connective-tissue disorders · Crohn's disease (may be exacerbated) · elderly (risk of serious side-effects and fatalities) · heart failure · ischaemic heart disease · peripheral arterial disease · risk factors for cardiovascular events · ulcerative colitis (may be exacerbated) · uncontrolled hypertension
  ▸ With topical use Avoid contact with eyes · avoid contact with inflamed or broken skin · avoid contact with mucous membranes · not for use with occlusive dressings · topical application of large amounts can result in systemic effects,

including hypersensitivity and asthma (renal disease has also been reported)
- INTERACTIONS → Appendix 1: NSAIDs
- SIDE-EFFECTS
  GENERAL SIDE-EFFECTS
  ▸ **Common or very common** Gastrointestinal discomfort · gastrointestinal disorders · nausea · skin reactions
  ▸ **Rare or very rare** Severe cutaneous adverse reactions (SCARs)
  ▸ **Frequency not known** Bronchospasm · dyspnoea · photosensitivity reaction
  SPECIFIC SIDE-EFFECTS
  ▸ **Common or very common**
  ▸ With oral use Anaemia · appetite decreased · constipation · diarrhoea · dizziness · drowsiness · eosinophilia · headache · hearing impairment · hyperglycaemia · leucopenia · oedema · rash (discontinue) · thrombocytopenia · vertigo · vomiting · weight changes
  ▸ **Uncommon**
  ▸ With oral use Hypoglycaemia · palpitations · stomatitis · vision blurred
  ▸ **Rare or very rare**
  ▸ With oral use Nephritis tubulointerstitial · nephrotic syndrome · renal failure · renal papillary necrosis
  ▸ **Frequency not known**
  ▸ With oral use Alopecia · angioedema · aplastic anaemia · confusion · depression · embolism and thrombosis · eye irritation · eye swelling · fertility decreased female · fluid retention · haemolytic anaemia · haemorrhage · hallucination · heart failure · hepatic disorders · hypersensitivity · hypertension · malaise · mood altered · nervousness · onycholysis · pancreatitis · paraesthesia · sleep disorders · vasculitis
  SIDE-EFFECTS, FURTHER INFORMATION For information about cardiovascular and gastrointestinal side-effects, and a possible exacerbation of symptoms in asthma, see Non-steroidal anti-inflammatory drugs p. 1094.
  ▸ With topical use Topical application of large amounts can result in systemic effects.
- ALLERGY AND CROSS-SENSITIVITY Contra-indicated in patients with a history of hypersensitivity to aspirin or any other NSAID—which includes those in whom attacks of asthma, angioedema, urticaria or rhinitis have been precipitated by aspirin or any other NSAID.
- CONCEPTION AND CONTRACEPTION
  ▸ With systemic use Caution—long-term use of some NSAIDs is associated with reduced female fertility, which is reversible on stopping treatment.
- PREGNANCY
  ▸ With systemic use Avoid unless the potential benefit outweighs the risk. Avoid during the third trimester (risk of closure of fetal ductus arteriosus *in utero* and possibly persistent pulmonary hypertension of the newborn); onset of labour may be delayed and duration may be increased.
  ▸ With topical use Patient packs for topical preparations carry a warning to avoid during pregnancy.
- BREAST FEEDING
  ▸ With systemic use Use with caution during breast-feeding. Amount too small to be harmful.
  ▸ With topical use Patient packs for topical preparations carry a warning to avoid during breast-feeding.
- HEPATIC IMPAIRMENT
  ▸ With systemic use Use with caution; there is an increased risk of gastro-intestinal bleeding and fluid retention. Avoid in severe liver disease.
- RENAL IMPAIRMENT
  ▸ With systemic use Avoid if possible or use with caution.
  ▸ With topical use Deterioration in renal function has also been reported after topical use.

10

Musculoskeletal system

Dose adjustments ▸ With systemic use The lowest effective dose should be used for the shortest possible duration.
Monitoring ▸ With systemic use In renal impairment monitor renal function; sodium and water retention may occur and renal function may deteriorate, possibly leading to renal failure.

● DIRECTIONS FOR ADMINISTRATION Piroxicam orodispersible tablets can be taken by placing on the tongue and allowing to dissolve or by swallowing.
▸ With topical use For topical preparations apply with gentle massage only.

● PRESCRIBING AND DISPENSING INFORMATION Caution—topical preparations not generally suitable for children.

● PATIENT AND CARER ADVICE For topical preparations, patients and their carers should be advised to wash hands immediately after use.
Photosensitivity
▸ With topical use Patients should be advised against excessive exposure to sunlight of area treated in order to avoid possibility of photosensitivity.

● LESS SUITABLE FOR PRESCRIBING
▸ With oral use Piroxicam is less suitable for prescribing.

● MEDICINAL FORMS
There can be variation in the licensing of different medicines containing the same drug.
Orodispersible tablet
CAUTIONARY AND ADVISORY LABELS 10, 21
EXCIPIENTS: May contain Aspartame
▸ Feldene Melt (Pfizer Ltd)
Piroxicam 20 mg Feldene Melt 20mg tablets sugar-free | 30 tablet [PoM] £10.53 DT = £10.53
Gel
EXCIPIENTS: May contain Benzyl alcohol, propylene glycol
▸ Piroxicam (Non-proprietary)
Piroxicam 5 mg per 1 gram Piroxicam 0.5% gel | 60 gram [PoM] £3.50 DT = £2.54 | 100 gram [PoM] £4.80 | 112 gram [PoM] £7.25 DT = £4.74
▸ Feldene (Pfizer Ltd)
Piroxicam 5 mg per 1 gram Feldene 0.5% gel | 60 gram [PoM] £6.00 DT = £2.54 | 112 gram [PoM] £9.41 DT = £4.74
Capsule
CAUTIONARY AND ADVISORY LABELS 21
▸ Piroxicam (Non-proprietary)
Piroxicam 10 mg Piroxicam 10mg capsules | 56 capsule [PoM] £16.82 DT = £4.93
Piroxicam 20 mg Piroxicam 20mg capsules | 28 capsule [PoM] £5.76 DT = £4.51
▸ Feldene (Pfizer Ltd)
Piroxicam 10 mg Feldene 10mg capsules | 30 capsule [PoM] £3.86
Piroxicam 20 mg Feldene 20 capsules | 30 capsule [PoM] £7.71

Sulindac

● INDICATIONS AND DOSE

Pain and inflammation in rheumatic disease and other musculoskeletal disorders | Acute gout
▸ BY MOUTH
▸ Adult: 200 mg twice daily for maximum duration 7–10 days in peri-articular disorders, dose may be reduced according to response; acute gout should respond within 7 days; maximum 400 mg per day

● CONTRA-INDICATIONS Active gastro-intestinal bleeding · active gastro-intestinal ulceration · history of gastro-intestinal bleeding related to previous NSAID therapy · history of gastro-intestinal perforation related to previous NSAID therapy · history of recurrent gastro-intestinal haemorrhage (two or more distinct episodes) · history of recurrent gastro-intestinal ulceration (two or more distinct episodes) · severe heart failure

● CAUTIONS Allergic disorders · cardiac impairment (NSAIDs may impair renal function) · cerebrovascular disease ·

coagulation defects · connective-tissue disorders · Crohn's disease (may be exacerbated) · elderly (risk of serious side-effects and fatalities) · ensure adequate hydration · heart failure · history of renal stones · ischaemic heart disease · peripheral arterial disease · risk factors for cardiovascular events · ulcerative colitis (may be exacerbated) · uncontrolled hypertension

● INTERACTIONS → Appendix 1: NSAIDs

● SIDE-EFFECTS Acute psychosis · agranulocytosis · alopecia · angioedema · appetite decreased · arrhythmia · asthenia · asthma · bone marrow disorders · cholecystitis · confusion · constipation · Crohn's disease aggravated · depression · diarrhoea · dizziness · drowsiness · dyspnoea · dysuria · eye disorder · fever · gastrointestinal discomfort · gastrointestinal disorders · gynaecomastia · haemolytic anaemia · haemorrhage · hallucination · headache · hearing impairment · heart failure · hepatic disorders · hyperglycaemia · hyperhidrosis · hyperkalaemia · hypersensitivity · hypersensitivity vasculitis · hypertension · increased risk of arterial thromboembolism · increased risk of infection · insomnia · leucopenia · malaise · meningitis aseptic (patients with connective-tissue disorders such as systemic lupus erythematosus may be especially susceptible) · mucosal abnormalities · muscle weakness · nausea · nephritis tubulointerstitial · nephrotic syndrome · nerve disorders · nervousness · neutropenia · oedema · oral disorders · palpitations · pancreatitis · paraesthesia · photosensitivity reaction · psychiatric disorder · renal impairment · respiratory disorders · seizure · severe cutaneous adverse reactions (SCARs) · skin reactions · syncope · taste altered · thrombocytopenia · urine abnormalities · urine discolouration · vertigo · vision disorders · vomiting

SIDE-EFFECTS, FURTHER INFORMATION For information about cardiovascular and gastrointestinal side-effects, and a possible exacerbation of symptoms in asthma, see Non-steroidal anti-inflammatory drugs p. 1094.

● ALLERGY AND CROSS-SENSITIVITY Contra-indicated in patients with a history of hypersensitivity to aspirin or any other NSAID—which includes those in whom attacks of asthma, angioedema, urticaria or rhinitis have been precipitated by aspirin or any other NSAID.

● CONCEPTION AND CONTRACEPTION Caution—long-term use of some NSAIDs is associated with reduced female fertility, which is reversible on stopping treatment.

● PREGNANCY Avoid unless the potential benefit outweighs the risk. Avoid during the third trimester (risk of closure of fetal ductus arteriosus *in utero* and possibly persistent pulmonary hypertension of the newborn); onset of labour may be delayed and duration may be increased.

● BREAST FEEDING Use with caution during breast-feeding.

● HEPATIC IMPAIRMENT Use with caution; there is an increased risk of gastro-intestinal bleeding and fluid retention. Avoid in severe liver disease.

● RENAL IMPAIRMENT Avoid if possible or use with caution. Avoid in severe impairment.
Dose adjustments The lowest effective dose should be used for the shortest possible duration.
Monitoring In renal impairment monitor renal function; sodium and water retention may occur and renal function may deteriorate, possibly leading to renal failure.

● MEDICINAL FORMS
There can be variation in the licensing of different medicines containing the same drug.
Tablet
CAUTIONARY AND ADVISORY LABELS 21
▸ Sulindac (Non-proprietary)
Sulindac 100 mg Sulindac 100mg tablets | 56 tablet [PoM] £48.00 DT = £29.78
Sulindac 200 mg Sulindac 200mg tablets | 56 tablet [PoM] £96.00 DT = £38.29

Tenoxicam

● **INDICATIONS AND DOSE**

Pain and inflammation in rheumatic disease

▶ BY MOUTH
▶ Adult: 20 mg once daily
▶ BY INTRAVENOUS INJECTION, OR BY INTRAMUSCULAR INJECTION
▶ Adult: 20 mg once daily as initial treatment for 1–2 days if oral administration not possible

Pain and inflammation in acute musculoskeletal disorders

▶ BY MOUTH
▶ Adult: 20 mg once daily for 7 days; maximum duration of treatment 14 days (including treatment by intravenous or intramuscular injection)
▶ BY INTRAVENOUS INJECTION, OR BY INTRAMUSCULAR INJECTION
▶ Adult: 20 mg once daily as initial treatment for 1–2 days if oral administration not possible

● CONTRA-INDICATIONS Active gastro-intestinal bleeding · active gastro-intestinal ulceration · history of gastro-intestinal bleeding related to previous NSAID therapy · history of gastro-intestinal perforation related to previous NSAID therapy · history of recurrent gastro-intestinal haemorrhage (two or more distinct episodes) · history of recurrent gastro-intestinal ulceration (two or more distinct episodes) · severe heart failure

● CAUTIONS Allergic disorders · cardiac impairment (NSAIDs may impair renal function) · cerebrovascular disease · coagulation defects · connective-tissue disorders · Crohn's disease (may be exacerbated) · elderly (risk of serious side-effects and fatalities) · heart failure · ischaemic heart disease · peripheral arterial disease · risk factors for cardiovascular events · ulcerative colitis (may be exacerbated) · uncontrolled hypertension

● INTERACTIONS → Appendix 1: NSAIDs

● SIDE-EFFECTS

GENERAL SIDE-EFFECTS

▶ **Common or very common** Constipation · Crohn's disease aggravated · diarrhoea · gastrointestinal discomfort · gastrointestinal disorders · haemorrhage · headache · nausea · vomiting
▶ **Uncommon** Fatigue · oedema · skin reactions
▶ **Rare or very rare** Asthma · bronchospasm · depression · dyspnoea · hyperglycaemia · nervousness · palpitations · pancreatitis · severe cutaneous adverse reactions (SCARs) · sleep disorders · vertigo · weight changes
▶ **Frequency not known** Agranulocytosis · alopecia · anaemia · angioedema · aplastic anaemia · confusion · eosinophilia · fertility decreased female · haemolytic anaemia · hallucination · heart failure · hepatic disorders · hypersensitivity · hypertension · leucopenia · malaise · nail disorder · nephritis tubulointerstitial · nephropathy · paraesthesia · photosensitivity reaction · platelet aggregation inhibition · purpura non-thrombocytopenic · renal failure (more common in patients with pre-existing renal impairment) · thrombocytopenia · tinnitus · vasculitis · vision disorders

SPECIFIC SIDE-EFFECTS

▶ **Common or very common**
▶ With oral use Dizziness · dry mouth · oral disorders
▶ **Rare or very rare**
▶ With oral use Embolism and thrombosis · metabolic disorder
▶ **Frequency not known**
▶ With oral use Drowsiness · eye irritation · eye swelling
▶ With parenteral use Appetite decreased · increased risk of arterial thromboembolism · increased risk of ischaemic stroke · increased risk of myocardial infarction · meningitis aseptic (patients with connective-tissue disorders such as

systemic lupus erythematosus may be especially susceptible) · neutropenia · oral ulceration

SIDE-EFFECTS, FURTHER INFORMATION For information about cardiovascular and gastrointestinal side-effects, and a possible exacerbation of symptoms in asthma, see Non-steroidal anti-inflammatory drugs p. 1094.

● ALLERGY AND CROSS-SENSITIVITY Contra-indicated in patients with a history of hypersensitivity to aspirin or any other NSAID—which includes those in whom attacks of asthma, angioedema, urticaria or rhinitis have been precipitated by aspirin or any other NSAID.

● CONCEPTION AND CONTRACEPTION Caution—long-term use of some NSAIDs is associated with reduced female fertility, which is reversible on stopping treatment.

● PREGNANCY Avoid unless the potential benefit outweighs the risk. Avoid during the third trimester (risk of closure of fetal ductus arteriosus *in utero* and possibly persistent pulmonary hypertension of the newborn); onset of labour may be delayed and duration may be increased.

● BREAST FEEDING Use with caution during breast-feeding. Present in milk in *animal* studies.

● HEPATIC IMPAIRMENT Use with caution; there is an increased risk of gastro-intestinal bleeding and fluid retention. Avoid in severe liver disease.

● RENAL IMPAIRMENT Avoid if possible or use with caution. Avoid in severe impairment.
Dose adjustments The lowest effective dose should be used for the shortest possible duration.
Monitoring In renal impairment monitor renal function; sodium and water retention may occur and renal function may deteriorate, possibly leading to renal failure.

● MEDICINAL FORMS
There can be variation in the licensing of different medicines containing the same drug.
Powder and solvent for solution for injection
▶ Tenoxicam (Non-proprietary)
   Tenoxicam 20 mg Tenoxicam 20mg powder and solvent for solution for injection vials | 1 vial PoM £3.98
Tablet
CAUTIONARY AND ADVISORY LABELS 21
▶ Tenoxicam (Non-proprietary)
   Tenoxicam 20 mg Tenoxicam 20mg tablets | 28 tablet PoM [S]
▶ Mobiflex (Meda Pharmaceuticals Ltd)
   Tenoxicam 20 mg Mobiflex 20mg tablets | 30 tablet PoM £13.42
   DT = £13.42

Tiaprofenic acid

● **INDICATIONS AND DOSE**

Pain and inflammation in rheumatic disease and other musculoskeletal disorders

▶ BY MOUTH
▶ Adult: 300 mg twice daily

IMPORTANT SAFETY INFORMATION
CSM ADVICE
Following reports of **severe cystitis** the CSM has recommended that tiaprofenic acid should not be given to patients with urinary-tract disorders and should be stopped if urinary symptoms develop.
   Patients should be advised to stop taking tiaprofenic acid and to report to their doctor promptly if they develop urinary-tract symptoms (such as increased frequency, nocturia, urgency, pain on urinating, or blood in urine).

● CONTRA-INDICATIONS Active bladder disease (or symptoms) · active gastro-intestinal bleeding · active gastro-intestinal ulceration · active prostate disease (or

10

Musculoskeletal system

symptoms) · history of gastro-intestinal bleeding related to previous NSAID therapy · history of gastro-intestinal perforation related to previous NSAID therapy · history of recurrent gastro-intestinal haemorrhage (two or more distinct episodes) · history of recurrent gastro-intestinal ulceration (two or more distinct episodes) · history of recurrent urinary-tract disorders (if urinary symptoms develop discontinue immediately and perform urine tests and culture) · severe heart failure

● CAUTIONS Allergic disorders · cardiac impairment (NSAIDs may impair renal function) · cerebrovascular disease · coagulation defects · connective-tissue disorders · Crohn's disease (may be exacerbated) · elderly (risk of serious side-effects and fatalities) · heart failure · ischaemic heart disease · peripheral arterial disease · risk factors for cardiovascular events · ulcerative colitis (may be exacerbated) · uncontrolled hypertension

● INTERACTIONS → Appendix 1: NSAIDs

● SIDE-EFFECTS Agranulocytosis · alopecia · anaemia · angioedema · aplastic anaemia · appetite decreased · asthma · bladder pain · bronchospasm · confusion · constipation · Crohn's disease aggravated · cystitis · depression · diarrhoea · dizziness · drowsiness · dyspnoea · fatigue · fertility decreased female · fluid retention · gastrointestinal discomfort · gastrointestinal disorders · haemolytic anaemia · haemorrhage · hallucination · headache · heart failure · hepatic disorders · hypersensitivity · hypertension · increased risk of arterial thromboembolism · malaise · meningitis aseptic (patients with connective-tissue disorders such as systemic lupus erythematosus may be especially susceptible) · nausea · nephritis tubulointerstitial · nephropathy · neutropenia · oedema · optic neuritis · oral ulceration · pancreatitis · paraesthesia · photosensitivity reaction · renal failure (more common in patients with pre-existing renal impairment) · severe cutaneous adverse reactions (SCARs) · skin reactions · sodium retention · thrombocytopenia · tinnitus · urinary disorders · urinary tract inflammation · vertigo · visual impairment · vomiting

SIDE-EFFECTS, FURTHER INFORMATION For information about cardiovascular and gastrointestinal side-effects, and a possible exacerbation of symptoms in asthma, see Non-steroidal anti-inflammatory drugs p. 1094.

● ALLERGY AND CROSS-SENSITIVITY Contra-indicated in patients with a history of hypersensitivity to aspirin or any other NSAID—which includes those in whom attacks of asthma, angioedema, urticaria or rhinitis have been precipitated by aspirin or any other NSAID.

● CONCEPTION AND CONTRACEPTION Caution—long-term use of some NSAIDs is associated with reduced female fertility, which is reversible on stopping treatment.

● PREGNANCY Avoid unless the potential benefit outweighs the risk. Avoid during the third trimester (risk of closure of fetal ductus arteriosus *in utero* and possibly persistent pulmonary hypertension of the newborn); onset of labour may be delayed and duration may be increased.

● BREAST FEEDING Use with caution during breast-feeding. Amount too small to be harmful.

● HEPATIC IMPAIRMENT Use with caution; there is an increased risk of gastro-intestinal bleeding and fluid retention. Avoid in severe liver disease.
Dose adjustments Reduce dose in mild or moderate impairment.

● RENAL IMPAIRMENT Avoid if possible or use with caution. Avoid in severe impairment.
Dose adjustments Reduce dose in mild or moderate impairment. The lowest effective dose should be used for the shortest possible duration.

Monitoring In renal impairment monitor renal function; sodium and water retention may occur and renal function may deteriorate, possibly leading to renal failure.

● MEDICINAL FORMS
There can be variation in the licensing of different medicines containing the same drug.
Tablet
CAUTIONARY AND ADVISORY LABELS 21
▶ Surgam (Sanofi)
   Tiaprofenic acid 300 mg Surgam 300mg tablets | 56 tablet [PoM] £14.95 DT = £14.95

5 Soft tissue and joint disorders

5.1 Local inflammation of joints and soft tissue

> **Other drugs used for Local inflammation of joints and soft tissue** Betamethasone, p. 660

CORTICOSTEROIDS

Corticosteroids, inflammatory disorders

Systemic corticosteroids

Short-term treatment with corticosteroids can help to rapidly improve symptoms of rheumatoid arthritis. Long-term treatment in rheumatoid arthritis should be considered only after evaluating the risks and all other treatment options have been considered. Corticosteroids can induce osteoporosis, and prophylaxis should be considered on long-term treatment.

In severe, possibly life-threatening, situations a high initial dose of corticosteroid is given to induce remission and the dose is then reduced gradually and discontinued altogether. Relapse may occur as the dose of corticosteroid is reduced, particularly if the reduction is too rapid. The tendency is therefore to increase the maintenance dose and consequently the patient becomes dependent on corticosteroids. For this reason pulse doses of corticosteroids (e.g. methylprednisolone p. 663 up to 1 g intravenously on 3 consecutive days) are used to suppress highly active inflammatory disease while longer-term treatment with a disease-modifying drug is commenced.

Prednisolone p. 664 may reduce the rate of joint destruction in moderate to severe *rheumatoid arthritis* of less than 2 years' duration. The reduction in joint destruction must be distinguished from mere symptomatic improvement (which lasts only 6 to 12 months at this dose) and care should be taken to avoid increasing the dose above 7.5 mg daily. Evidence supports maintenance of this anti-erosive dose for 2–4 years only after which treatment should be tapered off to reduce long-term adverse effects.

A modified-release preparation of prednisone p. 666 is available for the treatment of moderate to severe rheumatoid arthritis.

Polymyalgia rheumatica and *giant cell (temporal) arteritis* are always treated with corticosteroids. Relapse is common if therapy is stopped prematurely. Many patients require treatment for at least 2 years and in some patients it may be necessary to continue long-term low-dose corticosteroid treatment.

Polyarteritis nodosa and *polymyositis* are usually treated with corticosteroids.

Systemic lupus erythematosus is treated with corticosteroids when necessary using a similar dosage regimen to that for polyarteritis nodosa and polymyositis. Patients with pleurisy, pericarditis, or other systemic manifestations will respond to corticosteroids. It may then be possible to reduce the dosage; alternate-day treatment is sometimes adequate, and the drug may be gradually withdrawn. In some mild cases corticosteroid treatment may be stopped after a few months. Many mild cases of systemic lupus erythematosus do not require corticosteroid treatment. Alternative treatment with anti-inflammatory analgesics, and possibly chloroquine p. 604 or hydroxychloroquine sulfate p. 1062, should be considered.

Ankylosing spondylitis should not be treated with long-term corticosteroids; rarely, pulse doses may be needed and may be useful in extremely active disease that does not respond to conventional treatment.

Local corticosteroid injections

Corticosteroids are injected locally for an anti-inflammatory effect. In inflammatory conditions of the joints, particularly in rheumatoid arthritis, they are given by *intra-articular injection* to relieve pain, increase mobility, and reduce deformity in one or a few joints; they can also provide symptomatic relief while waiting for DMARDs to take effect. Full aseptic precautions are essential; infected areas should be avoided. Occasionally an acute inflammatory reaction develops after an intra-articular or soft-tissue injection of a corticosteroid. This may be a reaction to the microcrystalline suspension of the corticosteroid used, but must be distinguished from sepsis introduced into the injection site.

Smaller amounts of corticosteroids may also be injected directly into soft tissues for the relief of inflammation in conditions such as *tennis* or *golfer's elbow* or *compression neuropathies*. In *tendinitis*, injections should be made into the tendon sheath and not directly into the tendon (due to the absence of a true tendon sheath and a high risk of rupture, the Achilles tendon should not be injected).

Hydrocortisone acetate below or one of the synthetic analogues is generally used for local injection. Intra-articular corticosteroid injections can cause flushing and may affect the hyaline cartilage. Each joint should not usually be treated more than 4 times in one year.

Corticosteroid injections are also injected into soft tissues for the treatment of skin lesions.

F 658

Dexamethasone
21-Dec-2017

● **INDICATIONS AND DOSE**

Local inflammation of joints
▸ BY INTRA-ARTICULAR INJECTION
▸ Adult: 0.3–3.3 mg, where appropriate, dose may be repeated at intervals of 3–21 days according to response, dose given according to size—consult product literature

Local inflammation of soft tissues
▸ BY LOCAL INFILTRATION
▸ Adult: 1.7–5 mg, dose given according to size—consult product literature, where appropriate may be repeated at intervals of 3–21 days, use the 3.3 mg/mL injection preparation for this dose

● **INTERACTIONS** → Appendix 1: corticosteroids
● **PREGNANCY** Dexamethasone readily crosses the placenta.
● **PRESCRIBING AND DISPENSING INFORMATION**
▸ With systemic use Dexamethasone 3.8 mg/mL Injection has replaced Dexamethasone 4 mg/mL Injection. All dosage recommendations for intravenous, intramuscular, intrarticular use or local infiltration; are given in units of dexamethasone base.

● **MEDICINAL FORMS**
There can be variation in the licensing of different medicines containing the same drug.
Solution for injection
CAUTIONARY AND ADVISORY LABELS 10
▸ Dexamethasone (Non-proprietary)
Dexamethasone (as Dexamethasone sodium phosphate) 3.3 mg per 1 ml Dexamethasone 6.6mg/2ml solution for injection vials | 5 vial PoM £24.00 DT = £24.00
Dexamethasone 6.6mg/2ml solution for injection ampoules | 5 ampoule PoM £11.00 DT = £11.00 | 10 ampoule PoM £22.00
Dexamethasone 3.3mg/1ml solution for injection ampoules | 5 ampoule PoM £12.00 | 10 ampoule PoM £12.00–£19.67 DT = £19.67
Dexamethasone (as Dexamethasone sodium phosphate) 3.8 mg per 1 ml Dexamethasone 3.8mg/1ml solution for injection vials | 10 vial PoM £19.99–£20.01 DT = £20.00

F 658

Hydrocortisone
21-Dec-2017

● **INDICATIONS AND DOSE**

HYDROCORTISTAB ®

Local inflammation of joints and soft-tissues
▸ BY INTRA-ARTICULAR INJECTION
▸ Adult: 5–50 mg, select dose according to size of patient and joint; where appropriate dose may be repeated at intervals of 21 days. Not more than 3 joints should be treated on any one day, for details consult product literature

● **INTERACTIONS** → Appendix 1: corticosteroids
● **SIDE-EFFECTS** Bruising · increased risk of infection · malaise · myocardial rupture (following recent myocardial infarction)

● **MEDICINAL FORMS**
There can be variation in the licensing of different medicines containing the same drug.
Suspension for injection
▸ Hydrocortistab (AMCo)
Hydrocortisone acetate 25 mg per 1 ml Hydrocortistab 25mg/1ml suspension for injection ampoules | 10 ampoule PoM £68.72 DT = £68.72

F 658

Methylprednisolone
03-Nov-2017

● **INDICATIONS AND DOSE**

DEPO-MEDRONE ®

Local inflammation of joints and soft tissues
▸ BY INTRA-ARTICULAR INJECTION
▸ Adult: 4–80 mg, select dose according to size; where appropriate dose may be repeated at intervals of 7–35 days, for details consult product literature

● **INTERACTIONS** → Appendix 1: corticosteroids
● **PATIENT AND CARER ADVICE** Patient counselling is advised for methylprednisolone tablets and injections (steroid card).

● **MEDICINAL FORMS**
There can be variation in the licensing of different medicines containing the same drug.
Suspension for injection
CAUTIONARY AND ADVISORY LABELS 10
▸ Depo-Medrone (Pfizer Ltd)
Methylprednisolone acetate 40 mg per 1 ml Depo-Medrone 40mg/1ml suspension for injection vials | 1 vial PoM £3.44 DT = £3.44 | 10 vial PoM £34.04
Depo-Medrone 80mg/2ml suspension for injection vials | 1 vial PoM £6.18 DT = £6.18 | 10 vial PoM £61.39
Depo-Medrone 120mg/3ml suspension for injection vials | 1 vial PoM £8.96 DT = £8.96 | 10 vial PoM £88.81

Methylprednisolone with lidocaine

The properties listed below are those particular to the combination only. For the properties of the components please consider, methylprednisolone p. 1119, lidocaine hydrochloride p. 1312.

- ● **INDICATIONS AND DOSE**

Local inflammation of joints
- ▶ BY INTRA-ARTICULAR INJECTION
- ▶ Adult: 4–80 mg, dose adjusted according to size; where appropriate may be repeated at intervals of 7–35 days, for details consult product literature

- ● INTERACTIONS → Appendix 1: antiarrhythmics · corticosteroids

- ● MEDICINAL FORMS
There can be variation in the licensing of different medicines containing the same drug.
Suspension for injection
- ▶ Depo-Medrone with Lidocaine (Pfizer Ltd)
Lidocaine hydrochloride 10 mg per 1 ml, Methylprednisolone acetate 40 mg per 1 ml Depo-Medrone with Lidocaine suspension for injection 2ml vials | 1 vial [PoM] £7.06 DT = £7.06 | 10 vial [PoM] £70.13
Depo-Medrone with Lidocaine suspension for injection 1ml vials | 1 vial [PoM] £3.94 DT = £3.94 | 10 vial [PoM] £38.88

Prednisolone

21-Dec-2017

- ● **INDICATIONS AND DOSE**
DELTASTAB ®

Local inflammation of joints
- ▶ BY INTRA-ARTICULAR INJECTION
- ▶ Adult: 5–25 mg, dose according to size; not more than 3 joints should be treated on any one day; where appropriate may be repeated when relapse occurs, for details consult product literature

> **IMPORTANT SAFETY INFORMATION**
> SAFE PRACTICE
> Prednisolone has been confused with propranolol; care must be taken to ensure the correct drug is prescribed and dispensed.

- ● INTERACTIONS → Appendix 1: corticosteroids
- ● SIDE-EFFECTS Abdominal pain · bruising · diarrhoea · dizziness · exophthalmos · hiccups · Kaposi's sarcoma · malaise · myocardial rupture (following recent myocardial infarction) · vomiting
- ● PREGNANCY As it crosses the placenta 88% of prednisolone is inactivated.
- ● BREAST FEEDING Prednisolone appears in small amounts in breast milk but maternal doses of up to 40 mg daily are unlikely to cause systemic effects in the infant.

- ● MEDICINAL FORMS
There can be variation in the licensing of different medicines containing the same drug.
Suspension for injection
- ▶ Deltastab (AMCo)
Prednisolone acetate 25 mg per 1 ml Deltastab 25mg/1ml suspension for injection ampoules | 10 ampoule [PoM] £68.72

Triamcinolone acetonide

21-Dec-2017

- ● **INDICATIONS AND DOSE**
ADCORTYL ® INTRA-ARTICULAR/INTRADERMAL

Local inflammation of joints and soft tissues
- ▶ BY INTRA-ARTICULAR INJECTION
- ▶ Adult: 2.5–15 mg, adjusted according to size (for larger doses use Kenalog ®). Where appropriate dose may be repeated when relapse occurs, for details consult product literature.
- ▶ BY INTRADERMAL INJECTION
- ▶ Adult: 2–3 mg, max. 5 mg at any one site (total max. 30 mg). Where appropriate may be repeated at intervals of 1–2 weeks, for details consult product literature

KENALOG ® VIALS

Local inflammation of joints and soft tissues
- ▶ BY INTRA-ARTICULAR INJECTION
- ▶ Adult: 5–40 mg (max. per dose 80 mg), for further details consult product literature, select dose according to size. For doses below 5 mg use Adcortyl ® Intra-articular/Intradermal injection, where appropriate dose may be repeated when relapse occurs.

- ● INTERACTIONS → Appendix 1: corticosteroids

- ● MEDICINAL FORMS
There can be variation in the licensing of different medicines containing the same drug.
Suspension for injection
CAUTIONARY AND ADVISORY LABELS 10
EXCIPIENTS: May contain Benzyl alcohol
- ▶ Adcortyl Intra-articular / Intradermal (Bristol-Myers Squibb Pharmaceuticals Ltd)
Triamcinolone acetonide 10 mg per 1 ml Adcortyl Intra-articular / Intradermal 50mg/5ml suspension for injection vials | 1 vial [PoM] £3.63
Adcortyl Intra-articular / Intradermal 10mg/1ml suspension for injection ampoules | 5 ampoule [PoM] £4.47 DT = £4.47
- ▶ Kenalog (Bristol-Myers Squibb Pharmaceuticals Ltd)
Triamcinolone acetonide 40 mg per 1 ml Kenalog Intra-articular / Intramuscular 40mg/1ml suspension for injection vials | 5 vial [PoM] £7.45 DT = £7.45

Triamcinolone hexacetonide

21-Dec-2017

- ● **INDICATIONS AND DOSE**

Local inflammation of joints and soft-tissues (for details, consult product literature)
- ▶ BY INTRA-ARTICULAR INJECTION
- ▶ Adult: 2–20 mg, adjusted according to size of joint, no more than 2 joints should be treated on any one day, where appropriate, may be repeated at intervals of 3–4 weeks
- ▶ BY PERI-ARTICULAR INJECTION
- ▶ Adult: 10–20 mg, adjusted according to size of joint, no more than 2 joints should be treated on any one day

- ● CONTRA-INDICATIONS Consult product literature
- ● CAUTIONS Consult product literature
- ● INTERACTIONS → Appendix 1: corticosteroids
- ● SIDE-EFFECTS Protein catabolism · skin fragility
- ● PRESCRIBING AND DISPENSING INFORMATION Various strengths available from 'special order' manufacturers or specialist importing companies.

- MEDICINAL FORMS
There can be variation in the licensing of different medicines containing the same drug.
Suspension for injection
EXCIPIENTS: May contain Benzyl alcohol
▸ Triamcinolone hexacetonide (Non-proprietary)
Triamcinolone hexacetonide 20 mg per 1 ml Triamcinolone hexacetonide 20mg/1ml suspension for injection ampoules | 10 ampoule [PoM] £120.00

5.2 Soft tissue disorders

Soft-tissue disorders

Extravasation

Local guidelines for the management of extravasation should be followed where they exist or specialist advice sought.

Extravasation injury follows leakage of drugs or intravenous fluids from the veins or inadvertent administration into the subcutaneous or subdermal tissue. It must be dealt with **promptly** to prevent tissue necrosis.

Acidic or alkaline preparations and those with an osmolarity greater than that of plasma can cause extravasation injury; excipients including alcohol and polyethylene glycol have also been implicated. Cytotoxic drugs commonly cause extravasation injury. In addition, certain patients such as the very young and the elderly are at increased risk. Those receiving anticoagulants are more likely to lose blood into surrounding tissues if extravasation occurs, while those receiving sedatives or analgesics may not notice the early signs or symptoms of extravasation.

Extravasation prevention

Precautions should be taken to avoid extravasation; ideally, drugs likely to cause extravasation injury should be given through a central line and patients receiving repeated doses of hazardous drugs peripherally should have the cannula resited at regular intervals. Attention should be paid to the manufacturers' recommendations for administration. Placing a glyceryl trinitrate patch p. 217 distal to the cannula may improve the patency of the vessel in patients with small veins or in those whose veins are prone to collapse.

Patients should be asked to report any pain or burning at the site of injection immediately.

Extravasation management

If extravasation is suspected the infusion should be stopped immediately but the cannula should not be removed until after an attempt has been made to aspirate the area (through the cannula) in order to remove as much of the drug as possible. Aspiration is sometimes possible if the extravasation presents with a raised bleb or blister at the injection site and is surrounded by hardened tissue, but it is often unsuccessful if the tissue is soft or soggy.

Corticosteroids are usually given to treat inflammation, although there is little evidence to support their use in extravasation. Hydrocortisone or dexamethasone p. 1119 can be given either locally by subcutaneous injection or intravenously at a site distant from the injury.

Antihistamines and **analgesics** may be required for symptom relief.

The management of extravasation beyond these measures is not well standardised and calls for specialist advice. Treatment depends on the nature of the offending substance; one approach is to localise and neutralise the substance whereas another is to spread and dilute it.

The first method may be appropriate following extravasation of vesicant drugs and involves administration of an antidote (if available) and the application of cold compresses 3–4 times a day (consult specialist literature for details of specific antidotes). Spreading and diluting the offending substance involves infiltrating the area with physiological saline, applying warm compresses, elevating the affected limb, and administering hyaluronidase p. 1122. A saline flush-out technique (involving flushing the subcutaneous tissue with physiological saline) may be effective but requires specialist advice. Hyaluronidase should not be administered following extravasation of vesicant drugs (unless it is either specifically indicated or used in the saline flush-out technique). Dexrazoxane p. 915 is licensed for the treatment of anthracycline-induced extravasation.

Enzymes used in soft-tissue disorders

Collagenase

Collagenase below are proteolytic enzymes that are derived from the fermentation of *Clostridium histolyticum* and have the ability to break down collagen. A preparation containing a mixture of two collagenases is licensed for the treatment of Dupuytren's contracture; the preparation should be injected into a palpable cord with a contracture of a metacarpophalangeal joint or proximal interphalangeal joint.

Hyaluronidase

Hyaluronidase is used to render the tissues more readily permeable to injected fluids, e.g. for introduction of fluids by subcutaneous infusion (termed hypodermoclysis).

Rubefacients

Rubefacients act by counter-irritation. Pain, whether superficial or deep-seated, is relieved by any method that itself produces irritation of the skin. Topical rubefacient preparations may contain nicotinate and salicylate compounds, essential oils, capsicum, and camphor. The evidence available does not support the use of topical rubefacients in acute or chronic musculoskeletal pain.

Topical NSAIDs

The use of a NSAID by mouth is effective for relieving musculoskeletal pain. **Topical NSAIDs** (e.g. felbinac p. 1105, ibuprofen p. 1106, ketoprofen p. 1110, and piroxicam p. 1115 may provide some relief of pain in musculoskeletal conditions; they can be considered as an adjunctive treatment in knee or hand osteoarthritis.

Capsaicin

A preparation containing capsaicin 0.025% p. 476 can be considered as an adjunct in hand or knee osteoarthritis.It may need to be used for 1–2 weeks before pain is relieved.

A capsaicin 0.075% cream is licensed for the symptomatic relief of postherpetic neuralgia after lesions have healed, and for the relief of painful diabetic neuropathy.

A self-adhesive patch containing capsaicin 8% is licensed for the treatment of peripheral neuropathic pain in non-diabetic patients.

ENGYMES

Collagenase   20-Sep-2017

- INDICATIONS AND DOSE
Dupuytren's contracture in patients with a palpable cord
▸ BY INTRALESIONAL INJECTION
▸ Adult: 580 micrograms, then 580 micrograms every 4 weeks if required, inject into palpable cord, maximum 3 injections per cord, maximum 8 injections in total and only one cord may be treated at a time

- CONTRA-INDICATIONS Avoid injecting into other structures containing collagen (e.g. tendons, nerves, and blood vessels)—risk of tendon rupture or ligament damage
- CAUTIONS Coagulation disorders · use of anticoagulants

- SIDE-EFFECTS
- ▶ **Common or very common** Axillary mass · dizziness · headache · hyperhidrosis · inflammation · joint disorders · lymphatic abnormalities · muscle complaints · nausea · pain · peripheral oedema · sensation abnormal · skin reactions
- ▶ **Uncommon** Abdominal pain upper · anxiety · breast abnormalities · disorientation · dyspnoea · eyelid oedema · facial swelling · fatigue · feeling hot · fever · haematoma · hypersensitivity · hypotension · influenza like illness · insomnia · irritability · ligament injury · limb discomfort · limb injury · local swelling · lymphangitis · malaise · monoplegia · muscle weakness · musculoskeletal discomfort · syncope · tendon disorders · thrombocytopenia · tremor · vomiting · wound complications
- PREGNANCY Manufacturer advises avoid.
- BREAST FEEDING Systemic absorption by mother negligible.
- DIRECTIONS FOR ADMINISTRATION Reconstitution and injected volumes vary with site of injection—consult product literature.
- NATIONAL FUNDING/ACCESS DECISIONS

NICE decisions
- ▶ **Collagenase clostridium histolyticum for treating Dupuytren's contracture (July 2017)** NICE TA459
For people not taking part in the ongoing clinical trial (HTA-15/102/04), collagenase clostridium histolyticum (CCH) is recommended as an option for treating Dupuytren's contracture with a palpable cord in patients only if the following apply:
  - There is evidence of moderate disease (functional problems and metacarpophalangeal joint contracture of 30° to 60° and proximal interphalangeal joint contracture of less than 30° or first web contracture) plus up to 2 affected joints, **and**
  - Percutaneous needle fasciotomy is not considered appropriate, but limited fasciectomy is considered appropriate by the treating hand surgeon, **and**
  - The choice of treatment (CCH or limited fasciectomy) is made on an individual basis after discussion between the responsible hand surgeon and the patient about the risks and benefits of the treatments available, **and**
  - One injection is given per treatment session by a hand surgeon in an outpatient setting.

Patients currently receiving CCH whose disease does not meet the above criteria should be able to continue treatment until they and their clinician consider it appropriate to stop.
www.nice.org.uk/TA459

- MEDICINAL FORMS
There can be variation in the licensing of different medicines containing the same drug.
Powder and solvent for solution for injection
- ▶ Xiapex (Swedish Orphan Biovitrum Ltd)
Collagenase clostridium histolyticum **900 microgram** Xiapex 0.9mg powder and solvent for solution for injection vials | 1 vial [PoM] £572.00

Hyaluronidase

- INDICATIONS AND DOSE

Enhance permeation of subcutaneous or intramuscular injections
- ▶ BY SUBCUTANEOUS INJECTION, OR BY INTRAMUSCULAR INJECTION
- ▶ Adult: 1500 units, to be dissolved directly into the solution to be injected (ensure compatibility)

Enhance permeation of local anaesthetics
- ▶ BY LOCAL INFILTRATION
- ▶ Adult: 1500 units, to be mixed with the local anaesthetic solution

Enhance permeation of ophthalmic local anaesthetic
- ▶ TO THE EYE
- ▶ Adult: 15 units/mL, to be mixed with the local anaesthetic solution

Hypodermoclysis
- ▶ BY SUBCUTANEOUS INJECTION
- ▶ Adult: 1500 units, to be dissolved in 1 mL water for injections or 0.9% sodium chloride injection, administered before start of 500–1000 mL infusion fluid

Extravasation
- ▶ BY LOCAL INFILTRATION
- ▶ Adult: 1500 units, to be dissolved in 1 mL water for injections or 0.9% sodium chloride and infiltrated into affected area as soon as possible after extravasation

Haematoma
- ▶ BY LOCAL INFILTRATION
- ▶ Adult: 1500 units, to be dissolved in 1 mL water for injections or 0.9% sodium chloride and infiltrated into affected area

- CONTRA-INDICATIONS Avoid sites where infection is present · avoid sites where malignancy is present · do not apply direct to cornea · not for anaesthesia in unexplained premature labour · not for intravenous administration · not to be used to enhance the absorption and dispersion of dopamine and/or alpha-adrenoceptor agonists · not to be used to reduce swelling of bites · not to be used to reduce swelling of stings
- CAUTIONS Elderly (control speed and total volume and avoid overhydration especially in renal impairment)
- SIDE-EFFECTS Oedema · periorbital oedema

- MEDICINAL FORMS
There can be variation in the licensing of different medicines containing the same drug.
Powder for solution for injection
- ▶ Hyaluronidase (Non-proprietary)
Hyaluronidase **1500 unit** Hyaluronidase 1,500unit powder for solution for injection ampoules | 10 ampoule [PoM] £136.55

Chapter 11
Eye

CONTENTS

Eye

Eye treatment: drug administration

Drugs are most commonly administered to the eye by topical application as eye drops or eye ointments. When a higher drug concentration is required within the eye, a local injection may be necessary.

Eye-drop dispenser devices are available to aid the instillation of eye drops from plastic bottles and some are prescribable on the NHS (consult Drug Tariff—see Appliances and Reagents). Product-specific devices may be supplied by manufacturers—consult individual manufacturers for information. They are particularly useful for the elderly, visually impaired, arthritic, or otherwise physically limited patients.

Eye drops and eye ointments

Eye drops are generally instilled into the pocket formed by gently pulling down the lower eyelid and keeping the eye closed for as long as possible after application; one drop is all that is needed. Instillation of more than one drop should be discouraged because it may increase systemic side-effects. A small amount of eye ointment is applied similarly; the ointment melts rapidly and blinking helps to spread it.

When two different eye-drop preparations are used at the same time of day, dilution and overflow may occur when one immediately follows the other. The patient should therefore leave an interval of at least 5 minutes between the two; the interval should be extended when eye drops with a prolonged contact time, such as gels and suspensions, are used. Eye ointment should be applied after drops.

Systemic effects may arise from absorption of drugs into the general circulation from conjunctival vessels or from the nasal mucosa where the excess preparation has drained down through the tear ducts. The extent of systemic absorption following ocular administration is highly variable; nasal drainage of drugs is associated with eye drops much more often than with eye ointments. Pressure on the lacrimal punctum for at least a minute after applying eye drops reduces nasolacrimal drainage and therefore decreases systemic absorption from the nasal mucosa.

After using eye drops or eye ointments, patients should be warned not to drive or perform other skilled tasks until vision is clear.

Also see warnings relating to eye drops and contact lenses.

Eye lotions

These are solutions for the irrigation of the conjunctival sac. They act mechanically to flush out irritants or foreign bodies as a first-aid treatment. Sterile sodium chloride 0.9% solution p. 1134 is usually used. Clean water will suffice in an emergency.

Other preparations administered to the eye

Subconjunctival injection may be used to administer anti-infective drugs, mydriatics, or corticosteroids for conditions not responding to topical therapy; intracameral and intravitreal routes can also be used to administer certain drugs, for example antibacterials. These injections should only be used under specialist supervision.

Drugs such as antimicrobials and corticosteroids may be administered systemically to treat susceptible eye conditions.

Ophthalmic Specials

Certain eye drops, e.g. amphotericin p. 583, ceftazidime p. 519, cefuroxime p. 1137, colistimethate sodium p. 546, desferrioxamine mesilate p. 996, dexamethasone p. 1127, gentamicin p. 1136, and vancomycin p. 525 can be prepared aseptically from material supplied for injection.

The Royal College of Ophthalmologists and the UK Ophthalmic Pharmacy Group have produced the Ophthalmic Specials Guidance to help prescribers and pharmacists manage and restrict the use of unlicensed eye preparations. 'Specials' should only be prescribed in situations where a licensed product is not suitable for a patient's needs. The Ophthalmic Specials Guidance can be accessed on the Royal College of Ophthalmologists website (www.rcophth.ac.uk). The guidance will be reviewed every six months to ensure the most accurate and up-to-date information is available.

Preservatives and sensitisers

Information on preservatives and substances identified as skin sensitisers is provided under Excipients statements in preparation entries. Very rarely, cases of corneal calcification have been reported with the use of phosphate-containing eye drops in patients with significantly damaged corneas—consult product literature for further information.

Eye preparations: control of microbial contamination

Preparations for the eye should be sterile when issued. Care should be taken to avoid contamination of the contents during use.

Eye drops in multiple-application containers for *domiciliary use* should not be used for more than 4 weeks after first opening (unless otherwise stated by the manufacturer).

Multiple application eye drops for use in *hospital wards* are normally discarded 1 week after first opening—local practice may vary. Individual containers should be provided for each patient. A separate container should be supplied for each eye only if there are special concerns about contamination. Containers used before an eye operation should be discarded at the time of the operation and fresh containers supplied postoperatively. A fresh supply should also be provided upon discharge from hospital; in specialist ophthalmology units, it may be acceptable to issue containers that have been dispensed to the patient on the day of discharge.

In *out-patient departments* single-application containers should be used; if multiple-application containers are used, they should be discarded after single patient use within one clinical session.

In *eye surgery* single-application containers should be used if possible; if a multiple-application container is used, it should be discarded after single use. Preparations used during intra-ocular procedures and others that may penetrate into the anterior chamber must be isotonic and without preservatives and buffered if necessary to a neutral pH. Specially formulated fluids should be used for intra-ocular surgery; intravenous infusion preparations are not usually suitable for this purpose (Hartmann's solution may be used in some ocular surgery). For all surgical procedures, a previously unopened container is used for each patient.

Contact lenses

For cosmetic reasons many people prefer to wear contact lenses rather than spectacles; contact lenses are also sometimes required for medical indications. Visual defects are corrected by either rigid ('hard' or gas permeable) lenses or soft (hydrogel or silicone hydrogel—in adults only) lenses; soft lenses are the most popular type, because they are initially the most comfortable, but they may not give the best vision. Lenses should usually be worn for a specified number of hours each day and removed for sleeping. The risk of infectious and non-infectious keratitis is increased by extended continuous contact lens wear, which is not recommended, except when medically indicated.

Contact lenses require meticulous care. Poor compliance with directions for use, and with daily cleaning and disinfection, can result in complications including ulcerative keratitis or conjunctivitis. One-day disposable lenses, which are worn only once and therefore require no disinfection or cleaning, are becoming increasingly popular.

Acanthamoeba keratitis, a painful and sight-threatening condition, is associated with ineffective lens cleaning and disinfection, the use of contaminated lens cases, or tap water coming into contact with the lenses. The condition is especially associated with the use of soft lenses (including frequently replaced lenses) and should be treated by specialists.

Contact lenses and drug treatment

Special care is required in prescribing eye preparations for contact lens users. Some drugs and preservatives in eye preparations can accumulate in hydrogel lenses and may induce toxic and adverse reactions. Therefore, unless medically indicated, the lenses should be removed before instillation of the eye preparation and not worn during the period of treatment. Alternatively, unpreserved drops can be used. Eye drops may, however, be instilled while patients are wearing rigid corneal contact lenses. Ointment preparations should never be used in conjunction with contact lens wear; oily eye drops should also be avoided.

Many drugs given systemically can also have adverse effects on contact lens wear. These include oral contraceptives (particularly those with a higher oestrogen content), drugs which reduce blink rate (e.g. anxiolytics, hypnotics, antihistamines, and muscle relaxants), drugs which reduce lacrimation (e.g. antihistamines, antimuscarinics, phenothiazines and related drugs, some beta-blockers, diuretics, and tricyclic antidepressants), and drugs which increase lacrimation (including ephedrine hydrochloride p. 271 and hydralazine hydrochloride p. 180). Other drugs that may affect contact lens wear are isotretinoin p. 1234 (can cause conjunctival inflammation), aspirin p. 121 (salicylic acid appears in tears and can be absorbed by contact lenses—leading to irritation), and rifampicin p. 571 and sulfasalazine p. 42 (can discolour lenses).

1 Allergic and inflammatory eye conditions

Eye, allergy and inflammation

Corticosteroids

Corticosteroids administered locally to the eye or given by mouth are effective for treating anterior segment inflammation, including that which results from surgery.

Topical corticosteroids are applied frequently for the first 24–48 hours; once inflammation is controlled, the frequency of application is reduced. They should normally only be used under expert supervision; three main dangers are associated with their use:

- a 'red eye', when the diagnosis is unconfirmed, may be due to herpes simplex virus, and a corticosteroid may aggravate the condition, leading to corneal ulceration, with possible damage to vision and even loss of the eye. Bacterial, fungal, and amoebic infections pose a similar hazard;
- 'steroid glaucoma' can follow the use of corticosteroid eye preparations in susceptible individuals;
- a 'steroid cataract' can follow prolonged use.

Combination products containing a corticosteroid with an anti-infective drug are sometimes used after ocular surgery to reduce inflammation and prevent infection; use of combination products is otherwise rarely justified.

Systemic corticosteroids may be useful for ocular conditions. The risk of producing a 'steroid cataract' increases with the dose and duration of corticosteroid use.

Intravitreal corticosteroids

An intravitreal implant containing dexamethasone p. 1127 (*Ozurdex®*) is licensed for the treatment of adults with macular oedema following either branch retinal vein occlusion or central retinal vein occlusion; it is also licensed for the treatment of adult patients with inflammation of the posterior segment of the eye presenting as non-infectious uveitis.

An intravitreal implant containing fluocinolone acetonide p. 1157 (*Iluvien®*) is licensed for the treatment of visual impairment associated with chronic diabetic macular oedema which is insufficiently responsive to available therapies. It should be administered by specialists experienced in the use of intravitreal injections.

Eye care, other anti-inflammatory preparations

Other preparations used for the topical treatment of inflammation and allergic conjunctivitis include antihistamines, lodoxamide p. 1126, and sodium cromoglicate p. 1126.

Eye drops containing antihistamines, such as **antazoline** (with xylometazoline hydrochloride p. 1125 as *Otrivine-Antistin®*), azelastine hydrochloride p. 1125, epinastine hydrochloride p. 1125, ketotifen p. 1125, and olopatadine p. 1126, can be used for allergic conjunctivitis.

Sodium cromoglicate (sodium cromoglycate) and nedocromil sodium eye drops p. 1126 can be useful for vernal keratoconjunctivitis and other allergic forms of conjunctivitis.

Lodoxamide eye drops are used for allergic conjunctival conditions including seasonal allergic conjunctivitis.

Diclofenac sodium eye drops p. 1144 are also licensed for seasonal allergic conjunctivitis.

Non-steroidal anti-inflammatory eye drops are used for the prophylaxis and treatment of inflammation of the eye following surgery or laser treatment.

Ciclosporin p. 1130 is licensed for severe keratitis in patients with dry eye disease, which has not improved despite treatment with tear substitutes.

Cenegermin p. 1130 is licensed for moderate to severe neurotrophic keratitis.

1.1 Allergic conjunctivitis

ANTIHISTAMINES

Antazoline with xylometazoline

- **INDICATIONS AND DOSE**
Allergic conjunctivitis
▸ TO THE EYE
▹ Child 12–17 years: Apply 2–3 times a day for maximum 7 days
▹ Adult: Apply 2–3 times a day for maximum 7 days

- CAUTIONS Angle-closure glaucoma · cardiovascular disease · diabetes mellitus · hypertension · hyperthyroidism · phaeochromocytoma · urinary retention

- INTERACTIONS → Appendix 1: antihistamines, sedating · sympathomimetics, vasoconstrictor

- SIDE-EFFECTS Drowsiness · eye irritation · headache · hyperhidrosis · hypertension · mydriasis · nausea · palpitations · vascular disorders · vision blurred

  SIDE-EFFECTS, FURTHER INFORMATION Absorption of antazoline and xylometazoline may result in systemic side-effects.

- MEDICINAL FORMS
There can be variation in the licensing of different medicines containing the same drug.
Eye drops
EXCIPIENTS: May contain Benzalkonium chloride, disodium edetate
▹ Otrivine Antistin (Thea Pharmaceuticals Ltd)
Xylometazoline hydrochloride 500 microgram per 1 ml, Antazoline sulfate 5 mg per 1 ml Otrivine Antistin 0.5%/0.05% eye drops | 10 ml $\boxed{P}$ £3.35 DT = £3.35

Azelastine hydrochloride

- **INDICATIONS AND DOSE**
Seasonal allergic conjunctivitis
▸ TO THE EYE
▹ Child 4–17 years: Apply twice daily, increased if necessary to 4 times a day
▹ Adult: Apply twice daily, increased if necessary to 4 times a day
Perennial conjunctivitis
▸ TO THE EYE
▹ Child 12–17 years: Apply twice daily; increased if necessary to 4 times a day, maximum duration of treatment 6 weeks
▹ Adult: Apply twice daily; increased if necessary to 4 times a day, maximum duration of treatment 6 weeks

- INTERACTIONS → Appendix 1: antihistamines, non-sedating

- SIDE-EFFECTS
▸ **Common or very common** Eye irritation
▸ **Uncommon** Taste bitter

- MEDICINAL FORMS
There can be variation in the licensing of different medicines containing the same drug.
Eye drops
EXCIPIENTS: May contain Benzalkonium chloride, disodium edetate
▹ Optilast (Meda Pharmaceuticals Ltd)
Azelastine hydrochloride 500 microgram per 1 ml Optilast 0.05% eye drops | 8 ml $\boxed{PoM}$ £6.40 DT = £6.40

Epinastine hydrochloride

- **INDICATIONS AND DOSE**
Seasonal allergic conjunctivitis
▸ TO THE EYE
▹ Child 12–17 years: Apply twice daily for maximum 8 weeks
▹ Adult: Apply twice daily for maximum 8 weeks

- SIDE-EFFECTS
▸ **Common or very common** Eye discomfort
▸ **Uncommon** Dry eye · eye disorders · headache · nasal irritation · rhinitis · taste altered · visual impairment

- MEDICINAL FORMS
There can be variation in the licensing of different medicines containing the same drug.
Eye drops
EXCIPIENTS: May contain Benzalkonium chloride, disodium edetate
▹ Relestat (Allergan Ltd)
Epinastine hydrochloride 500 microgram per 1 ml Relestat 500micrograms/ml eye drops | 5 ml $\boxed{PoM}$ £9.90 DT = £9.90

Ketotifen

- **INDICATIONS AND DOSE**
Seasonal allergic conjunctivitis
▸ TO THE EYE
▹ Child 3–17 years: Apply twice daily
▹ Adult: Apply twice daily

- INTERACTIONS → Appendix 1: antihistamines, sedating

- SIDE-EFFECTS
▸ **Common or very common** Eye discomfort · eye disorders · eye inflammation
▸ **Uncommon** Conjunctival haemorrhage · drowsiness · dry eye · dry mouth · headache · skin reactions · vision disorders
▸ **Frequency not known** Asthma exacerbated · facial swelling · oedema

- MEDICINAL FORMS
There can be variation in the licensing of different medicines containing the same drug.
Eye drops
EXCIPIENTS: May contain Benzalkonium chloride
▹ Ketofall (Scope Ophthalmics Ltd)
Ketotifen (as Ketotifen hydrogen fumarate) 250 microgram per 1 ml Ketofall 0.25mg/ml eye drops 0.4ml unit dose | 30 unit dose $\boxed{PoM}$ £6.95
▹ Zaditen (Thea Pharmaceuticals Ltd)
Ketotifen (as Ketotifen fumarate) 250 microgram per 1 ml Zaditen 250micrograms/ml eye drops | 5 ml $\boxed{PoM}$ £7.80 DT = £7.80

Olopatadine

- INDICATIONS AND DOSE

Seasonal allergic conjunctivitis

▸ TO THE EYE
  ‣ Child 3–17 years: Apply twice daily for maximum 4 months
  ‣ Adult: Apply twice daily for maximum 4 months

- SIDE-EFFECTS
▸ **Common or very common** Asthenia · dry eye · eye discomfort · headache · nasal dryness · taste altered
▸ **Uncommon** Dizziness · eye disorders · eye inflammation · increased risk of infection · numbness · skin reactions · vision disorders
▸ **Frequency not known** Drowsiness · dyspnoea · malaise · nausea · vomiting

- MEDICINAL FORMS
  There can be variation in the licensing of different medicines containing the same drug.
  Eye drops
  EXCIPIENTS: May contain Benzalkonium chloride
  ‣ Opatanol (Novartis Pharmaceuticals UK Ltd)
    Olopatadine (as Olopatadine hydrochloride) 1 mg per 1 ml Opatanol 1mg/ml eye drops | 5 ml [PoM] £4.68 DT = £4.68

MAST-CELL STABILISERS

Lodoxamide

- INDICATIONS AND DOSE

Allergic conjunctivitis

▸ TO THE EYE
  ‣ Child 4–17 years: Apply 4 times a day, improvement of symptoms may sometimes require treatment for up to 4 weeks
  ‣ Adult: Apply 4 times a day, improvement of symptoms may sometimes require treatment for up to 4 weeks

- SIDE-EFFECTS
▸ **Common or very common** Dry eye · eye discomfort · eye disorders · vision disorders
▸ **Uncommon** Corneal deposits · dizziness · eye inflammation · headache · nausea
▸ **Rare or very rare** Nasal complaints · rash · taste altered

- EXCEPTIONS TO LEGAL CATEGORY Lodoxamide 0.1% eye drops can be sold to the public for treatment of allergic conjunctivitis in adults and children over 4 years.

- MEDICINAL FORMS
  There can be variation in the licensing of different medicines containing the same drug.
  Eye drops
  EXCIPIENTS: May contain Benzalkonium chloride, disodium edetate
  ‣ Alomide (Novartis Pharmaceuticals UK Ltd)
    Lodoxamide (as Lodoxamide trometamol) 1 mg per 1 ml Alomide 0.1% eye drops | 10 ml [PoM] £5.21 DT = £5.21

Nedocromil sodium

- INDICATIONS AND DOSE

Seasonal and perennial conjunctivitis

▸ TO THE EYE
  ‣ Child 6–17 years: Apply twice daily, increased if necessary to 4 times a day, max.12 weeks duration of treatment for seasonal allergic conjunctivitis
  ‣ Adult: Apply twice daily, increased if necessary to 4 times a day, max.12 weeks duration of treatment for seasonal allergic conjunctivitis

Seasonal keratoconjunctivitis

▸ TO THE EYE
  ‣ Child 6–17 years: Apply 4 times a day
  ‣ Adult: Apply 4 times a day

- SIDE-EFFECTS
▸ **Common or very common** Eye discomfort · eye strain · taste altered

- MEDICINAL FORMS
  No licensed medicines listed.

Sodium cromoglicate

(Sodium cromoglycate)

- INDICATIONS AND DOSE

Allergic conjunctivitis | Seasonal keratoconjunctivitis

▸ TO THE EYE
  ‣ Child: Apply 4 times a day
  ‣ Adult: Apply 4 times a day

- SIDE-EFFECTS Eye stinging

- EXCEPTIONS TO LEGAL CATEGORY Sodium cromoglicate 2% eye drops can be sold to the public (in max. pack size of 10 mL) for treatment of acute seasonal and perennial allergic conjunctivitis.

- MEDICINAL FORMS
  There can be variation in the licensing of different medicines containing the same drug. Forms available from special-order manufacturers include: eye drops
  Eye drops
  ‣ Sodium cromoglicate (Non-proprietary)
    Sodium cromoglicate 20 mg per 1 ml Sodium cromoglicate 2% eye drops | 13.5 ml [PoM] £11.25 DT = £9.87
  ‣ Opticrom (Sanofi)
    Sodium cromoglicate 20 mg per 1 ml Opticrom Aqueous 2% eye drops | 13.5 ml [PoM] £8.03 DT = £9.87
  ‣ Vividrin (Bausch & Lomb UK Ltd)
    Sodium cromoglicate 20 mg per 1 ml Vividrin 2% eye drops | 13.5 ml [PoM] £10.95 DT = £9.87

1.2   Inflammatory eye conditions

Other drugs used for Inflammatory eye conditions
Adalimumab, p. 1073

ANALGESICS › NON-STEROIDAL ANTI-INFLAMMATORY DRUGS

Nepafenac

06-Jun-2017

- INDICATIONS AND DOSE

Prophylaxis and treatment of postoperative pain and inflammation associated with cataract surgery | Reduction in the risk of postoperative macular oedema associated with cataract surgery in diabetic patients

▸ TO THE EYE
  ‣ Adult: (consult product literature)

- CAUTIONS Avoid sunlight · corneal epithelial breakdown (if evidence of, then discontinue immediately)
- INTERACTIONS → Appendix 1: NSAIDs
- SIDE-EFFECTS
▸ **Uncommon** Eye discomfort · eye disorders · eye inflammation
▸ **Rare or very rare** Allergic dermatitis · corneal deposits · dizziness · dry eye · headache · nausea

▶ **Frequency not known** Cutis laxa · vision disorders · vomiting

● NATIONAL FUNDING/ACCESS DECISIONS

Scottish Medicines Consortium (SMC) Decisions
The *Scottish Medicines Consortium* has advised (May 2017) that nepafenac (*Nevanac*®) 3 mg/mL eye drops are accepted for use within NHS Scotland for the reduction in risk of postoperative macular oedema associated with cataract surgery in diabetic patients.

● MEDICINAL FORMS
There can be variation in the licensing of different medicines containing the same drug.

Eye drops
EXCIPIENTS: May contain Benzalkonium chloride, disodium edetate
▶ Nevanac (Novartis Pharmaceuticals UK Ltd)
Nepafenac 1 mg per 1 ml Nevanac 1mg/ml eye drops | 5 ml PoM
£14.92 DT = £14.92
Nepafenac 3 mg per 1 ml Nevanac 3mg/ml eye drops | 3 ml PoM
£14.92 DT = £14.92

CORTICOSTEROIDS

Betamethasone

21-Dec-2017

● INDICATIONS AND DOSE

Local treatment of inflammation (short-term)
▶ TO THE EYE USING EYE DROP
▶ Child: Apply every 1–2 hours until controlled then reduce frequency
▶ Adult: Apply every 1–2 hours until controlled then reduce frequency
▶ TO THE EYE USING EYE OINTMENT
▶ Child: Apply 2–4 times a day, alternatively apply at night when used in combination with eye drops
▶ Adult: Apply 2–4 times a day, alternatively apply at night when used in combination with eye drops

> IMPORTANT SAFETY INFORMATION
> MHRA/CHM ADVICE: CORTICOSTEROIDS: RARE RISK OF CENTRAL SEROUS CHORIORETINOPATHY WITH LOCAL AS WELL AS SYSTEMIC ADMINISTRATION (AUGUST 2017)
> See *Corticosteroids, general use* p. 656.

● INTERACTIONS → Appendix 1: corticosteroids
● SIDE-EFFECTS Vision disorders

● MEDICINAL FORMS
There can be variation in the licensing of different medicines containing the same drug.
Ear/eye/nose drops solution
EXCIPIENTS: May contain Benzalkonium chloride, disodium edetate
▶ Betnesol (RPH Pharmaceuticals AB)
Betamethasone sodium phosphate 1 mg per 1 ml Betnesol 0.1% eye/ear/nose drops | 10 ml PoM £2.32 DT = £2.32
▶ Vistamethasone (Martindale Pharmaceuticals Ltd)
Betamethasone sodium phosphate 1 mg per 1 ml Vistamethasone 0.1% ear/eye/nose drops | 5 ml PoM £1.02 | 10 ml PoM £1.16 DT = £2.32
Eye ointment
▶ Betamethasone (Non-proprietary)
Betamethasone sodium phosphate 1 mg per 1 gram Betamethasone 0.1% eye ointment | 3 gram PoM £3.48 DT = £1.41
▶ Betnesol (Focus Pharmaceuticals Ltd)
Betamethasone sodium phosphate 1 mg per 1 gram Betnesol 0.1% eye ointment | 3 gram PoM £1.41 DT = £1.41

Combinations available: *Betamethasone with neomycin,* p. 1129

Dexamethasone

21-Dec-2017

● INDICATIONS AND DOSE

Local treatment of inflammation (short-term)
▶ TO THE EYE USING EYE DROP
▶ Child: Apply 4–6 times a day
▶ Adult: Apply every 30–60 minutes until controlled, then reduced to 4–6 times a day

Short term local treatment of inflammation (severe conditions)
▶ TO THE EYE USING EYE DROP
▶ Child: Apply every 30–60 minutes until controlled, reduce frequency when control achieved

Macular oedema following either branch retinal vein occlusion or central retinal vein occlusion (specialist use only) | Visual impairment due to diabetic macular oedema in adults who are pseudophakic, or who are insufficiently responsive to, or unsuitable for non-corticosteroid therapy (specialist use only) | For the treatment of inflammation of the posterior segment of the eye presenting as non-infectious uveitis (specialist use only)
▶ BY INTRAVITREAL INJECTION
▶ Adult: 700 micrograms, to be administered into the affected eye, concurrent administration to both eyes not recommended. For further information on pre-treatment, administration and repeat dosing, consult product literature

● UNLICENSED USE *Maxidex*® not licensed for use in children under 2 years. *Dropodex*® not licensed for use in children.

> IMPORTANT SAFETY INFORMATION
> MHRA/CHM ADVICE: CORTICOSTEROIDS: RARE RISK OF CENTRAL SEROUS CHORIORETINOPATHY WITH LOCAL AS WELL AS SYSTEMIC ADMINISTRATION (AUGUST 2017)
> See *Corticosteroids, general use* p. 656.

● CONTRA-INDICATIONS
▶ With intravitreal use Active ocular herpes simplex · active or suspected ocular infection · active or suspected periocular infection · rupture of the posterior lens capsule in patients with aphakia, iris or transscleral fixated intra-ocular lens or anterior chamber intra-ocular lens · uncontrolled advanced glaucoma

● CAUTIONS
▶ With intravitreal use history of ocular viral infection (including herpes simplex) · posterior capsule tear or iris defect (risk of implant migration into the anterior chamber which may cause corneal oedema and, in persistent severe cases, the need for corneal transplantation) · retinal vein occlusion with significant retinal ischaemia

● INTERACTIONS → Appendix 1: corticosteroids

● SIDE-EFFECTS
▶ **Common or very common** Eye discomfort
▶ **Uncommon**
▶ When used by eye (topical) Photophobia · taste altered
▶ With intravitreal use Retinitis necrotising

● PREGNANCY Dexamethasone readily crosses the placenta.
▶ With intravitreal use Manufacturer advises avoid unless potential benefit outweighs risk—no information available.

● BREAST FEEDING
▶ With intravitreal use Manufacturer advises avoid unless potential benefit outweighs risk—no information available.

● MONITORING REQUIREMENTS
▶ With intravitreal use Monitor intra-ocular pressure and for signs of ocular infection. In patients with posterior capsule

11

Eye

tear or iris defect monitor for implant migration to allow for; early diagnosis and management.

- PRESCRIBING AND DISPENSING INFORMATION Although multi-dose dexamethasone eye drops commonly contain preservatives, preservative-free unit dose vials may be available.

- NATIONAL FUNDING/ACCESS DECISIONS

NICE decisions

▶ **Dexamethasone intravitreal implant for the treatment of macular oedema secondary to retinal vein occlusion (July 2011)** NICE TA229
Dexamethasone intravitreal implant is recommended as an option for the treatment of macular oedema following central retinal vein occlusion. Dexamethasone intravitreal implant is also recommended as an option for the treatment of macular oedema following branch retinal vein occlusion when:

- treatment with laser photocoagulation has not been beneficial, *or*
- treatment with laser photocoagulation is not considered suitable because of the extent of macular haemorrhage.
www.nice.org.uk/TA229

▶ **Dexamethasone intravitreal implant for treating diabetic macular oedema (July 2015)** NICE TA349
Dexamethasone intravitreal implant is recommended as an option for treating diabetic macular oedema only if:

- the implant is to be used in an eye with an intraocular (pseudophakic) lens **and**
- the diabetic macular oedema does not respond to non-corticosteroid treatment, or such treatment is unsuitable.
www.nice.org.uk/TA349

▶ **Adalimumab and dexamethasone for treating non-infectious uveitis (July 2017)** NICE TA460
Dexamethasone intravitreal implant is recommended as an option for treating non-infectious uveitis in the posterior segment of the eye in patients, only if there is:

- active disease (that is, current inflammation in the eye), **and**
- worsening vision with a risk of blindness.
Patients currently receiving dexamethasone whose disease does not meet the above criteria should be able to continue treatment until they and their clinician consider it appropriate to stop.
www.nice.org.uk/TA460

Scottish Medicines Consortium (SMC) Decisions
The *Scottish Medicines Consortium* has advised (June 2012) that dexamethasone intravitreal implant (*Ozurdex*®) is accepted for restricted use within NHS Scotland for the treatment of patients with macular oedema following central retinal vein occlusion, and in patients with branch retinal vein occlusion who are not clinically suitable for laser treatment, including patients with dense macular haemorrhage, or patients who have received and failed on previous laser treatment.

- MEDICINAL FORMS
There can be variation in the licensing of different medicines containing the same drug. Forms available from special-order manufacturers include: eye drops
Eye drops
EXCIPIENTS: May contain Benzalkonium chloride, disodium edetate, polysorbates
▶ Dexamethasone (Non-proprietary)
Dexamethasone sodium phosphate 1 mg per 1 ml Minims dexamethasone 0.1% eye drops 0.5ml unit dose | 20 unit dose PoM £11.46 DT = £11.46
▶ Dexafree (Thea Pharmaceuticals Ltd)
Dexamethasone sodium phosphate 1 mg per 1 ml Dexafree 1mg/1ml eye drops 0.4ml unit dose | 30 unit dose PoM £9.70
▶ Dropodex (Rayner Pharmaceuticals Ltd)
Dexamethasone sodium phosphate 1 mg per 1 ml Dropodex 0.1% eye drops 0.4ml unit dose | 20 unit dose PoM £10.48 DT = £10.48

▶ Maxidex (Novartis Pharmaceuticals UK Ltd)
Dexamethasone 1 mg per 1 ml Maxidex 0.1% eye drops | 5 ml PoM £1.42 DT = £1.42 | 10 ml PoM £2.80 DT = £2.80

Implant
▶ Ozurdex (Allergan Ltd)
Dexamethasone 700 microgram Ozurdex 700microgram intravitreal implant in applicator | 1 device PoM £870.00 (Hospital only)

Combinations available: *Dexamethasone with framycetin sulfate and gramicidin*, p. 1129 · *Dexamethasone with hypromellose, neomycin and polymyxin B sulfate*, p. 1129 · *Dexamethasone with tobramycin*, p. 1130

Fluorometholone
21-Dec-2017

- **INDICATIONS AND DOSE**

Local treatment of inflammation (short term)
▶ TO THE EYE
▶ Child 2-17 years: Apply every 1 hour for 24–48 hours, then reduced to 2–4 times a day
▶ Adult: Apply every 1 hour for 24–48 hours, then reduced to 2–4 times a day

- UNLICENSED USE Not licensed for use in children under 2 years.

> **IMPORTANT SAFETY INFORMATION**
> MHRA/CHM ADVICE: CORTICOSTEROIDS: RARE RISK OF CENTRAL SEROUS CHORIORETINOPATHY WITH LOCAL AS WELL AS SYSTEMIC ADMINISTRATION (AUGUST 2017)
> See *Corticosteroids, general use* p. 656.

- SIDE-EFFECTS Cataract · eye discomfort · eye disorders · eye infection · eye inflammation · rash · taste altered · vision disorders

- MEDICINAL FORMS
There can be variation in the licensing of different medicines containing the same drug.
Eye drops
EXCIPIENTS: May contain Benzalkonium chloride, disodium edetate, polysorbates
▶ FML Liquifilm (Allergan Ltd)
Fluorometholone 1 mg per 1 ml FML Liquifilm 0.1% ophthalmic suspension | 5 ml PoM £1.71 DT = £1.71 | 10 ml PoM £2.95 DT = £2.95

Prednisolone
21-Dec-2017

- **INDICATIONS AND DOSE**

Local treatment of inflammation (short-term)
▶ TO THE EYE
▶ Child: Apply every 1–2 hours until controlled then reduce frequency
▶ Adult: Apply every 1–2 hours until controlled then reduce frequency

- UNLICENSED USE *Pred Forte*® not licensed for use in children (age range not specified by manufacturer).

> **IMPORTANT SAFETY INFORMATION**
> SAFE PRACTICE
> Prednisolone has been confused with propranolol; care must be taken to ensure the correct drug is prescribed and dispensed.
> MHRA/CHM ADVICE: CORTICOSTEROIDS: RARE RISK OF CENTRAL SEROUS CHORIORETINOPATHY WITH LOCAL AS WELL AS SYSTEMIC ADMINISTRATION (AUGUST 2017)
> See *Corticosteroids, general use* p. 656.

- INTERACTIONS → Appendix 1: corticosteroids

- SIDE-EFFECTS Eye discomfort · increased risk of infection · taste altered · visual impairment
- PRESCRIBING AND DISPENSING INFORMATION Although multi-dose prednisolone eye drops commonly contain preservatives, preservative-free unit dose vials may be available.
- MEDICINAL FORMS
There can be variation in the licensing of different medicines containing the same drug. Forms available from special-order manufacturers include:eye drops

Eye drops
EXCIPIENTS: May contain Benzalkonium chloride, disodium edetate, polysorbates
  ▸ Prednisolone (Non-proprietary)
  Prednisolone sodium phosphate 5 mg per 1 ml Minims prednisolone sodium phosphate 0.5% eye drops 0.5ml unit dose | 20 unit dose [PoM] £12.25 DT = £12.25
  ▸ Pred Forte (Allergan Ltd)
  Prednisolone acetate 10 mg per 1 ml Pred Forte 1% eye drops | 5 ml [PoM] £1.82 DT = £1.82 | 10 ml [PoM] £3.66 DT = £3.66

Ear/eye drops solution
EXCIPIENTS: May contain Benzalkonium chloride, disodium edetate
  ▸ Predsol (RPH Pharmaceuticals AB)
  Prednisolone sodium phosphate 5 mg per 1 ml Predsol 0.5% ear/eye drops | 10 ml [PoM] £2.00 DT = £2.00

Rimexolone
21-Dec-2017

- INDICATIONS AND DOSE

Local treatment of postoperative inflammation (short term use)
  ▸ TO THE EYE
  ▸ Adult: Apply 4 times a day for 2 weeks, treatment to begin 24 hours after surgery

Local treatment of steroid-responsive inflammation (short term use)
  ▸ TO THE EYE
  ▸ Adult: Apply in at least 4 times a day divided doses for up to 4 weeks

Uveitis (short term use)
  ▸ TO THE EYE
  ▸ Adult: Apply every 1 hour during the day time for week 1, then apply every 2 hours for week 2, then apply 4 times a day for week 3, then apply twice daily for the first 4 days of week 4, then apply once daily for the remaining 3 days of week 4

IMPORTANT SAFETY INFORMATION

MHRA/CHM ADVICE: CORTICOSTEROIDS: RARE RISK OF CENTRAL SEROUS CHORIORETINOPATHY WITH LOCAL AS WELL AS SYSTEMIC ADMINISTRATION (AUGUST 2017)
See *Corticosteroids, general use* p. 656.

- SIDE-EFFECTS
  ▸ Common or very common Eye discomfort · vision disorders
  ▸ Uncommon Dry eye · eye disorders · eye inflammation · headache · taste altered
  ▸ Frequency not known Increased risk of eye infections · optic nerve damage

- MEDICINAL FORMS
No licensed medicines listed.

CORTICOSTEROIDS > CORTICOSTEROID COMBINATIONS WITH ANTI-INFECTIVES

Betamethasone with neomycin

The properties listed below are those particular to the combination only. For the properties of the components please consider, betamethasone p. 1127.

- INDICATIONS AND DOSE

Local treatment of eye inflammation and bacterial infection (short-term)
  ▸ TO THE EYE USING EYE DROP
  ▸ Adult: Apply up to 6 times a day

- LESS SUITABLE FOR PRESCRIBING Betamethasone with neomycin eye-drops are less suitable for prescribing.

- MEDICINAL FORMS
There can be variation in the licensing of different medicines containing the same drug.

Ear/eye/nose drops solution
EXCIPIENTS: May contain Benzalkonium chloride, disodium edetate
  ▸ Betnesol-N (RPH Pharmaceuticals AB)
  Betamethasone (as Betamethasone sodium phosphate) 1 mg per 1 ml, Neomycin sulfate 5 mg per 1 ml Betnesol-N ear/eye/nose drops | 10 ml [PoM] £2.39 DT = £2.39

Dexamethasone with framycetin sulfate and gramicidin
21-Dec-2017

The properties listed below are those particular to the combination only. For the properties of the components please consider, dexamethasone p. 1127, framycetin sulfate p. 1160.

- INDICATIONS AND DOSE

Local treatment of inflammation (short-term)
  ▸ TO THE EYE
  ▸ Child: Apply 4–6 times a day, may be administered every 30–60 minutes in severe conditions until controlled, then reduce frequency
  ▸ Adult: Apply 4–6 times a day, may be administered every 30–60 minutes in severe conditions until controlled, then reduce frequency

- LESS SUITABLE FOR PRESCRIBING *Sofradex®* is less suitable for prescribing.

- MEDICINAL FORMS
There can be variation in the licensing of different medicines containing the same drug.

Ear/eye drops solution
EXCIPIENTS: May contain Polysorbates
  ▸ Sofradex (Sanofi)
  Gramicidin 50 microgram per 1 ml, Dexamethasone (as Dexamethasone sodium metasulfobenzoate) 500 microgram per 1 ml, Framycetin sulfate 5 mg per 1 ml Sofradex ear/eye drops | 8 ml [PoM] £7.50

Dexamethasone with hypromellose, neomycin and polymyxin B sulfate

The properties listed below are those particular to the combination only. For the properties of the components please consider, dexamethasone p. 1127.

- INDICATIONS AND DOSE

Local treatment of inflammation (short-term)
  ▸ TO THE EYE USING EYE DROP
  ▸ Adult: Apply every 30–60 minutes until controlled, then reduced to 4–6 times a day

continued →

Local treatment of inflammation (short-term)
▶ TO THE EYE USING EYE OINTMENT
▶ Adult: Apply 3–4 times a day, alternatively, apply at night when used with eye drops

● LESS SUITABLE FOR PRESCRIBING Dexamethasone with neomycin and polymixin B sulfate is less suitable for prescribing.

● MEDICINAL FORMS
There can be variation in the licensing of different medicines containing the same drug.
Eye ointment
EXCIPIENTS: May contain Hydroxybenzoates (parabens), woolfat and related substances (including lanolin).
▶ Maxitrol (Novartis Pharmaceuticals UK Ltd)
Dexamethasone 1 mg per 1 gram, Neomycin (as Neomycin sulfate) 3500 unit per 1 gram, Polymyxin B sulfate 6000 unit per 1 gram Maxitrol eye ointment | 3.5 gram PoM £1.44
Eye drops
EXCIPIENTS: May contain Benzalkonium chloride, polysorbates
▶ Maxitrol (Novartis Pharmaceuticals UK Ltd)
Dexamethasone 1 mg per 1 ml, Hypromellose 5 mg per 1 ml, Neomycin (as Neomycin sulfate) 3500 unit per 1 ml, Polymyxin B sulfate 6000 unit per 1 ml Maxitrol eye drops | 5 ml PoM £1.68

Dexamethasone with tobramycin

The properties listed below are those particular to the combination only. For the properties of the components please consider, dexamethasone p. 1127, tobramycin p. 1137.

● INDICATIONS AND DOSE
Local treatment of inflammation (short-term)
▶ TO THE EYE
▶ Adult: (consult product literature)

● LESS SUITABLE FOR PRESCRIBING Dexamethasone with tobramycin eye-drops are less suitable for prescribing.

● MEDICINAL FORMS
There can be variation in the licensing of different medicines containing the same drug.
Eye drops
EXCIPIENTS: May contain Benzalkonium chloride, disodium edetate
▶ Tobradex (Novartis Pharmaceuticals UK Ltd)
Dexamethasone 1 mg per 1 ml, Tobramycin 3 mg per 1 ml Tobradex 3mg/ml / 1mg/ml eye drops | 5 ml PoM £5.37 DT = £5.37

IMMUNOSUPPRESSANTS > CALCINEURIN INHIBITORS AND RELATED DRUGS

Ciclosporin

01-Sep-2016

(Cyclosporin)

● DRUG ACTION Ciclosporin inhibits production and release of lymphokines, thereby suppressing cell-mediated immune response.

● INDICATIONS AND DOSE
Severe keratitis in dry eye disease that has not responded to treatment with tear substitutes (initiated by a specialist)
▶ TO THE EYE
▶ Adult: Apply 1 drop once daily, to be applied to the affected eye(s) at bedtime, review treatment at least every 6 months

● CONTRA-INDICATIONS Active or suspected ocular or peri-ocular infection

● CAUTIONS Glaucoma—limited information available · history of ocular herpes—no information available

● INTERACTIONS → Appendix 1: ciclosporin

● SIDE-EFFECTS
▶ Common or very common Eye discomfort · eye disorders · eye inflammation · vision blurred
▶ Uncommon Eye deposit · ophthalmic herpes zoster

● CONCEPTION AND CONTRACEPTION Manufacturer recommends effective contraception during treatment in women of child-bearing potential.

● PREGNANCY Manufacturer advises avoid unless potential benefit outweighs risk—no information available.

● BREAST FEEDING Manufacturer advises avoid—limited information.

● DIRECTIONS FOR ADMINISTRATION Keep eyes closed for 2 minutes after using *Ikervis*® eye drops, to increase local drug action and reduce systemic absorption.

● NATIONAL FUNDING/ACCESS DECISIONS
NICE decisions
▶ Ciclosporin for treating dry eye disease that has not improved despite treatment with artificial tears (December 2015)
NICE TA369
Ciclosporin (*Ikervis*®) is recommended as an option for treating dry eye disease that has not improved despite treatment with tear substitutes.
www.nice.org.uk/TA369

● MEDICINAL FORMS
There can be variation in the licensing of different medicines containing the same drug. Forms available from special-order manufacturers include: eye drops, eye ointment
Eye drops
▶ Ikervis (Santen UK Ltd)
Ciclosporin 1 mg per 1 ml Ikervis 0.1% eye drops 0.3ml unit dose | 30 unit dose PoM £72.00 DT = £72.00

NERVE GROWTH FACTORS

Cenegermin

13-Dec-2017

● DRUG ACTION Cenegermin is a recombinant form of human nerve growth factor which allows restoration of corneal integrity; endogenous human nerve growth factor is involved in the differentiation and maintenance of neurons.

● INDICATIONS AND DOSE
Moderate or severe neurotrophic keratitis (specialist use only)
▶ TO THE EYE
▶ Adult: Apply 1 drop 6 times a day, to be applied every 2 hours, starting in the morning and completing within 12 hours; treatment should be continued for 8 weeks

● CONTRA-INDICATIONS Eye infection—resolve before initiating treatment (if an infection occurs during treatment, cenegermin should be suspended until infection resolution) · patients requiring immediate corneal surgery (assess for risk of corneal melting or impending perforation before initiating treatment)

● CAUTIONS Ocular cancer—manufacturer recommends monitor for cancer progression before and after treatment

● SIDE-EFFECTS
▶ Common or very common Eye disorders · eye inflammation · eye pain · headache · photophobia
▶ Uncommon Corneal abscess

● PREGNANCY Manufacturer advises avoid—no information available.

● BREAST FEEDING Manufacturer advises avoid—no information available.

● DIRECTIONS FOR ADMINISTRATION Manufacturer advises that other topical ophthalmic preparations should be administered at least 15 minutes before or after use.

- HANDLING AND STORAGE For information on storage of cenegermin, consult product literature.
- PATIENT AND CARER ADVICE Manufacturer advises patients and carers should be counselled on how to administer cenegermin eye drops.

- MEDICINAL FORMS
There can be variation in the licensing of different medicines containing the same drug.
  Eye drops
  ‣ Oxervate (Dompe UK Ltd) ▼
  Cenegermin 20 microgram per 1 ml Oxervate 20micrograms/ml eye drops preservative free | 1 ml [PoM] [Ṡ] (Hospital only)

1.2a Anterior uveitis

ANTIMUSCARINICS

Antimuscarinics (eye) ⬤

- CAUTIONS Children under 3 months owing to the possible association between cycloplegia and the development of amblyopia · darkly pigmented iris is more resistant to pupillary dilatation and caution should be exercised to avoid overdosage · mydriasis can precipitate acute angle-closure glaucoma (usually in those aged over 60 years and hypermetropic (long-sighted), who are predisposed to the condition because of a shallow anterior chamber) · mydriasis can precipitate acute angle-closure glaucoma (usually in those who are predisposed to the condition because of a shallow anterior chamber) (in children) · neonates at increased risk of systemic toxicity
- SIDE-EFFECTS Arrhythmias · conjunctivitis (on prolonged administration) · dry mouth · dry skin · eye oedema (on prolonged administration) · flushing · hyperaemia (on prolonged administration) · gastrointestinal disorders · urinary disorders
- PATIENT AND CARER ADVICE Patients may not be able to undertake skilled tasks until vision clears after mydriasis.

🖝 above

Atropine sulfate

- INDICATIONS AND DOSE
Cycloplegia
▸ TO THE EYE USING EYE DROP
  ‣ Adult: (consult product literature)
Anterior uveitis
▸ TO THE EYE USING EYE DROP
  ‣ Adult: (consult product literature)

- INTERACTIONS → Appendix 1: atropine
- SIDE-EFFECTS
  SIDE-EFFECTS, FURTHER INFORMATION Systemic side-effects can occur.
- PRESCRIBING AND DISPENSING INFORMATION Although multi-dose atropine sulphate eye drops commonly contain preservatives, preservative-free unit dose vials may be available.

- MEDICINAL FORMS
There can be variation in the licensing of different medicines containing the same drug. Forms available from special-order manufacturers include: eye drops, eye ointment
  Eye drops
  ‣ Atropine sulfate (Non-proprietary)
  Atropine sulfate 10 mg per 1 ml Atropine 1% eye drops | 10 ml [PoM] £132.25 DT = £132.25
  ‣ Atropine sulfate (Bausch & Lomb UK Ltd)
  Atropine sulfate 10 mg per 1 ml Minims atropine sulfate 1% eye drops 0.5ml unit dose | 20 unit dose [PoM] £15.10 DT = £15.10

Cyclopentolate hydrochloride

- INDICATIONS AND DOSE
Cycloplegia
▸ TO THE EYE
  ‣ Child 3 months–11 years: Apply 1 drop, 30–60 minutes before examination, using 1% eye drops
  ‣ Child 12–17 years: Apply 1 drop, 30–60 minutes before examination, using 0.5% eye drops
Uveitis
▸ TO THE EYE
  ‣ Child 3 months–17 years: Apply 1 drop 2–4 times a day, using 0.5% eye drops (1% for deeply pigmented eyes)
Anterior uveitis | Cycloplegia
▸ TO THE EYE
  ‣ Adult: (consult product literature)

- INTERACTIONS → Appendix 1: cyclopentolate
- SIDE-EFFECTS Mydriasis · photophobia
  SIDE-EFFECTS, FURTHER INFORMATION Systemic side-effects can occur, particularly in children and the elderly.
- PRESCRIBING AND DISPENSING INFORMATION Although multi-dose cyclopentolate eye drops commonly contain preservatives, preservative-free unit dose vials may be available.

- MEDICINAL FORMS
There can be variation in the licensing of different medicines containing the same drug.
  Eye drops
  EXCIPIENTS: May contain Benzalkonium chloride
  ‣ Cyclopentolate hydrochloride (Bausch & Lomb UK Ltd)
  Cyclopentolate hydrochloride 5 mg per 1 ml Minims cyclopentolate hydrochloride 0.5% eye drops 0.5ml unit dose | 20 unit dose [PoM] £11.41 DT = £11.41
  Cyclopentolate hydrochloride 10 mg per 1 ml Minims cyclopentolate hydrochloride 1% eye drops 0.5ml unit dose | 20 unit dose [PoM] £11.68 DT = £11.68
  ‣ Mydrilate (Intrapharm Laboratories Ltd)
  Cyclopentolate hydrochloride 5 mg per 1 ml Mydrilate 0.5% solution | 5 ml [PoM] £8.08 DT = £8.08
  Cyclopentolate hydrochloride 10 mg per 1 ml Mydrilate 1% solution | 5 ml [PoM] £8.08 DT = £8.08

🖝 above

Homatropine hydrobromide

- INDICATIONS AND DOSE
Anterior uveitis
▸ TO THE EYE
  ‣ Adult: (consult product literature)

- INTERACTIONS → Appendix 1: homatropine

- MEDICINAL FORMS
Forms available from special-order manufacturers include: eye drops

2 Dry eye conditions

Dry eye

Tear deficiency, ocular lubricants, and astringents

Chronic soreness of the eyes associated with reduced or abnormal tear secretion (e.g. in Sjögren's syndrome) often responds to tear replacement therapy or pilocarpine p. 1149 given by mouth in adults. The severity of the condition and patient preference will often guide the choice of preparation.

Hypromellose p. 1133 is the traditional choice of treatment for tear deficiency. It may need to be instilled

11

Eye

frequently (e.g. hourly) for adequate relief. Ocular surface mucin is often abnormal in tear deficiency and the combination of hypromellose with a mucolytic such as acetylcysteine below can be helpful.

The ability of **carbomers** to cling to the eye surface may help reduce frequency of application to 4 times daily.

Polyvinyl alcohol p. 1134 increases the persistence of the tear film and is useful when the ocular surface mucin is reduced.

Sodium hyaluronate eye drops p. 1135, with or without trehalose, are also used in the management of tear deficiency.

Sodium chloride 0.9% drops p. 1134 are sometimes useful in tear deficiency, and can be used as 'comfort drops' by contact lens wearers, and to facilitate lens removal. They are also used to irrigate the eye. Special presentations of sodium chloride 0.9% and other irrigation solutions are used routinely for intra-ocular surgery. Sodium chloride 5% eye drops are used for the short-term treatment of corneal oedema in adults.

Eye ointments containing a paraffin can be used to lubricate the eye surface, especially in cases of recurrent corneal epithelial erosion. They may cause temporary visual disturbance and are best suited for application before sleep. Ointments should not be used during contact lens wear.

OCULAR LUBRICANTS

Acetylcysteine

07-Feb-2017

- ● **INDICATIONS AND DOSE**

Tear deficiency | **Impaired or abnormal mucus production**
- ▸ TO THE EYE
- ▸ Adult: Apply 3–4 times a day

- ● MEDICINAL FORMS
There can be variation in the licensing of different medicines containing the same drug. Forms available from special-order manufacturers include: eye drops

Eye drops
EXCIPIENTS: May contain Benzalkonium chloride, disodium edetate
- ▸ Ilube (Rayner Pharmaceuticals Ltd)
Acetylcysteine 50 mg per 1 ml Ilube 5% eye drops | 10 ml £16.90 DT = £16.90 PoM

Carbomers

(Polyacrylic acid)

- ● **INDICATIONS AND DOSE**

Dry eyes including keratoconjunctivitis sicca, unstable tear film
- ▸ TO THE EYE
- ▸ Child: Apply 3–4 times a day or when required
- ▸ Adult: Apply 3–4 times a day or when required

- ● UNLICENSED USE Some preparations not licensed for use in children.

- ● PRESCRIBING AND DISPENSING INFORMATION Synthetic high molecular weight polymers of acrylic acid cross-linked with either allyl ethers of sucrose or allyl ethers of pentaerithrityl.

- ● MEDICINAL FORMS
There can be variation in the licensing of different medicines containing the same drug.

Eye gel
EXCIPIENTS: May contain Benzalkonium chloride, cetrimide, disodium edetate
- ▸ Blephagel (Thea Pharmaceuticals Ltd)
Carbomer 3.5 mg per 1 gram Blephagel 0.35% eye gel | 40 gram £6.66
Carbomer 3.6 mg per 1 gram Blephagel 0.36% eye gel preservative free | 30 gram £7.53
- ▸ Liquivisc (Thea Pharmaceuticals Ltd)
Carbomer 974P 2.5 mg per 1 gram Liquivisc 0.25% eye gel | 10 gram P £4.50 DT = £4.50

Eye drops
- ▸ Carbomers (Non-proprietary)
Carbomer 980 2 mg per 1 gram EyeGel 0.2% eye gel | 10 gram £2.80 DT = £2.80
Carbomer '980' 0.2% eye drops | 10 gram P £2.80 DT = £2.80
Carbomer 0.2% eye gel | 10 gram £2.80 DT = £2.80
- ▸ Artelac Nighttime (Bausch & Lomb UK Ltd)
Carbomer 980 2 mg per 1 gram Artelac Nighttime 0.2% eye gel | 10 gram £2.96 DT = £2.80
- ▸ Clinitas Carbomer (Altacor Ltd)
Carbomer 980 2 mg per 1 gram Clinitas Carbomer 0.2% eye gel | 10 gram £1.49 DT = £2.80
- ▸ GelTears (Bausch & Lomb UK Ltd)
Carbomer 980 2 mg per 1 gram GelTears 0.2% gel | 10 gram P £2.80 DT = £2.80
- ▸ Lumecare Long Lasting (Medicom Healthcare Ltd)
Carbomer 980 2 mg per 1 gram Lumecare Carbomer 0.2% eye gel | 10 gram £1.51 DT = £2.80
- ▸ Viscotears (Bausch & Lomb UK Ltd)
Carbomer 980 2 mg per 1 gram Viscotears 2mg/g liquid gel | 10 gram P £1.59 DT = £2.80
Viscotears 2mg/g eye gel 0.6ml unit dose | 30 unit dose P £5.42 DT = £5.42
- ▸ Xailin (Visufarma UK Ltd)
Carbomer 980 2 mg per 1 gram Xailin 0.2% eye gel | 10 gram £3.28 DT = £2.80

Carmellose sodium

- ● **INDICATIONS AND DOSE**

Dry eye conditions
- ▸ TO THE EYE
- ▸ Child: Apply as required
- ▸ Adult: Apply as required

- ● PRESCRIBING AND DISPENSING INFORMATION Some preparations are contained units which are resealable and may be used for up to 12 hours.

- ● MEDICINAL FORMS
There can be variation in the licensing of different medicines containing the same drug.

Eye drops
- ▸ Carmellose sodium (Non-proprietary)
Carmellose 0.5% eye drops | 10 ml £7.49
Carmellose 1% eye drops 0.4ml unit dose preservative free | 30 unit dose PoM ⓢ DT = £3.00 | 30 unit dose £3.00 DT = £3.00 | 30 unit dose P ⓢ DT = £3.00
Carmellose sodium 5 mg per 1 ml Carmellose 0.5% eye drops 0.4ml unit dose preservative free | 30 unit dose P ⓢ = £4.80 | 30 unit dose £5.75 DT = £4.80
- ▸ Carmellose (Moorfields Pharmaceuticals, Medicom Healthcare Ltd)
PF Drops Carmellose 0.5% eye drops preservative free | 10 ml £7.49
PF Drops Carmellose 1% eye drops preservative free | 10 ml £7.49
Lumecare Advance Carmellose 0.5% eye drops | 10 ml £5.99
- ▸ Carmize (Aspire Pharma Ltd)
Carmize 1% eye drops | 10 ml £8.49
Carmize 1% eye drops 0.4ml unit dose preservative free | 30 unit dose £3.00 DT = £3.00 | 60 unit dose £6.00
Carmize 0.5% eye drops | 10 ml £7.49
Carmellose sodium 5 mg per 1 ml Carmize 0.5% eye drops 0.4ml unit dose preservative free | 30 unit dose £5.75 DT = £4.80 | 90 unit dose £15.53

▸ Cellusan (Farmigea S.p.A.)
Cellusan 1% eye drops preservative free | 10 ml £4.80
Cellusan 1% eye drops 0.4ml unit dose preservative free | 30 unit dose £3.00 DT = £3.00
Cellusan Light 0.5% eye drops preservative free | 10 ml £4.80
Carmellose sodium 5 mg per 1 ml Cellusan Light 0.5% eye drops 0.4ml unit dose preservative free | 30 unit dose £5.75 DT = £4.80

▸ Celluvisc (Allergan Ltd)
Celluvisc 1% eye drops 0.4ml unit dose | 30 unit dose ℗ £3.00 DT = £3.00 | 60 unit dose ℗ £10.99
Carmellose sodium 5 mg per 1 ml Celluvisc 0.5% eye drops 0.4ml unit dose | 30 unit dose ℗ £4.80 DT = £4.80 | 90 unit dose ℗ £15.53

▸ Lumecare (Carmellose) (Medicom Healthcare Ltd)
Carmellose sodium 5 mg per 1 ml Lumecare Singles Carmellose 0.5% eye drops 0.4ml unit dose | 30 unit dose £4.60 DT = £4.80

▸ Optho-Lique (Essential-Healthcare Ltd)
Optho-Lique 0.5% eye drops | 10 ml £3.73
Optho-Lique Forte 1% eye drops | 10 ml £3.97

▸ Optive (Allergan Ltd)
Optive 0.5% eye drops | 10 ml £7.49

▸ Optive Plus (Allergan Ltd)
Optive Plus 0.5% eye drops | 10 ml £7.49

✗ Xailin Fresh (Visufarma UK Ltd)
Carmellose sodium 5 mg per 1 ml Xailin Fresh 0.5% eye drops 0.4ml unit dose | 30 unit dose £3.87 DT = £4.80

Hydroxyethylcellulose

● **INDICATIONS AND DOSE**

Tear deficiency
▸ TO THE EYE
▸ Child: Apply as required
▸ Adult: Apply as required

● **PRESCRIBING AND DISPENSING INFORMATION** Although multi-dose hydroxyethylcellulose eye drops commonly contain preservatives, preservative-free unit dose vials may be available.

● **MEDICINAL FORMS**
There can be variation in the licensing of different medicines containing the same drug.
Eye drops
▸ Artificial tears (Bausch & Lomb UK Ltd)
Hydroxyethylcellulose 4.4 mg per 1 ml Minims artificial tears 0.44% eye drops 0.5ml unit dose | 20 unit dose ℗ £9.33

Hydroxypropyl guar with polyethylene glycol and propylene glycol

(Formulated as an ocular lubricant)

● **INDICATIONS AND DOSE**

Dry eye conditions
▸ TO THE EYE
▸ Child: Apply as required
▸ Adult: Apply as required

● **MEDICINAL FORMS**
No licensed medicines listed.

Hypromellose

● **INDICATIONS AND DOSE**

Tear deficiency
▸ TO THE EYE
▸ Child: Apply as required
▸ Adult: Apply as required

● **PRESCRIBING AND DISPENSING INFORMATION** Although multi-dose hypromellose eye drops commonly contain preservatives, preservative-free unit dose vials may be available.

● **MEDICINAL FORMS**
There can be variation in the licensing of different medicines containing the same drug. Forms available from special-order manufacturers include: eye drops
Eye drops
EXCIPIENTS: May contain Benzalkonium chloride, cetrimide, disodium edetate
▸ Hypromellose (Non-proprietary)
Hypromellose 3 mg per 1 ml Hypromellose 0.3% eye drops preservative free | 10 ml £5.75
Hypromellose 0.3% eye drops | 10 ml £0.99–£1.50 DT = £1.06 | 10 ml ℗ £1.06 DT = £1.06
Hypromellose 5 mg per 1 ml Hypromellose 0.5% eye drops | 10 ml £0.81 DT = £0.81

▸ Artelac (Bausch & Lomb UK Ltd)
Hypromellose 3.2 mg per 1 ml Artelac Single Dose Unit 0.32% eye drops 0.5ml unit dose | 30 unit dose ℗ £16.95 | 60 unit dose ℗ £32.85
Artelac 0.32% eye drops | 10 ml ℗ £4.99 DT = £4.99

▸ Brolene Cool (Sanofi)
Hypromellose 3 mg per 1 ml Brolene Cool Eyes 0.3% eye drops | 10 ml GSL £2.38 DT = £1.06

▸ Hydromoor (Moorfields Pharmaceuticals)
Hydromoor 0.3% eye drops 0.4ml unit dose preservative free | 30 unit dose £5.75

▸ Hypromellose (Moorfields Pharmaceuticals)
Hypromellose 3 mg per 1 ml PF Drops Hypromellose 0.3% eye drops preservative free | 10 ml £5.75

▸ Hypromol (Ennogen Healthcare Ltd)
Hypromellose 3 mg per 1 ml Hypromol 0.3% eye drops preservative free | 10 ml £4.55

▸ Isopto Plain (Novartis Pharmaceuticals UK Ltd)
Hypromellose 5 mg per 1 ml Isopto Plain 0.5% eye drops | 10 ml ℗ £0.81 DT = £0.81

▸ Lumecare (Hypromellose) (Medicom Healthcare Ltd)
Hypromellose 3 mg per 1 ml Lumecare Hypromellose 0.3% eye drops | 10 ml £1.67 DT = £1.06

▸ Lumecare Tear Drops (Medicom Healthcare Ltd)
Hypromellose 3 mg per 1 ml Lumecare Tear Drops 0.3% eye drops | 10 ml £0.79 DT = £1.06

▸ Mandanol (Hydroxypropyl methylcellulose) (M & A Pharmachem Ltd)
Hypromellose 3 mg per 1 ml Mandanol eye drops | 10 ml £1.33 DT = £1.06

▸ Ocu-Lube (Sai-Meds Ltd)
Hypromellose 3 mg per 1 ml Ocu-Lube 0.3% eye drops preservative free | 10 ml £5.75

▸ SoftDrops (Farmigea S.p.A.)
Hypromellose 3 mg per 1 ml SoftDrops 0.3% eye drops | 10 ml £1.67 DT = £1.06

▸ Tear-Lac (Scope Ophthalmics Ltd)
Hypromellose 3 mg per 1 ml Tear-Lac Hypromellose 0.3% eye drops preservative free | 10 ml £5.80

▸ Vizulize Hypromellose (East Midlands Pharma Ltd)
Hypromellose 3 mg per 1 ml Vizulize Hypromellose 0.3% eye drops | 10 ml £1.25 DT = £1.06

▸ Xailin Hydrate (Visufarma UK Ltd)
Hypromellose 3 mg per 1 ml Xailin Hydrate 0.3% eye drops preservative free | 10 ml £4.64

11

Eye

Hypromellose with dextran 70

The properties listed below are those particular to the combination only. For the properties of the components please consider, hypromellose p. 1133.

- ● INDICATIONS AND DOSE
Tear deficiency
▸ TO THE EYE
▸ Adult: Apply as required

- ● MEDICINAL FORMS
There can be variation in the licensing of different medicines containing the same drug.
Eye drops
EXCIPIENTS: May contain Benzalkonium chloride, disodium edetate
▸ Tears Naturale (Novartis Pharmaceuticals UK Ltd)
Dextran 70 1 mg per 1 ml, Hypromellose 3 mg per 1 ml Tears Naturale eye drops | 15 ml P £1.89 DT = £1.89
Tears Naturale eye drops 0.4ml unit dose | 28 unit dose P £13.26 DT = £13.26

Liquid paraffin with white soft paraffin and wool alcohols

- ● INDICATIONS AND DOSE
Dry eye conditions
▸ TO THE EYE
▸ Child: Apply as required, best suited for application before sleep
▸ Adult: Apply as required, best suited for application before sleep

- ● PATIENT AND CARER ADVICE May cause temporary visual disturbance. Should not be used during contact lens wear.

- ● MEDICINAL FORMS
There can be variation in the licensing of different medicines containing the same drug.
Eye ointment
▸ Lacri-Lube (Allergan Ltd)
Wool alcohols 2 mg per 1 gram, Liquid paraffin 425 mg per 1 gram, White soft paraffin 573 mg per 1 gram Lacri-lube eye ointment | 3.5 gram P £3.01 | 5 gram P £3.98

Paraffin, yellow, soft

- ● INDICATIONS AND DOSE
Eye surface lubrication
▸ TO THE EYE
▸ Child: Apply every 2 hours as required
▸ Adult: Apply every 2 hours as required

- ● PATIENT AND CARER ADVICE Ophthalmic preparations may cause temporary visual disturbance. Should not be used during contact lens wear.

- ● MEDICINAL FORMS
There can be variation in the licensing of different medicines containing the same drug.
Eye ointment
▸ Paraffin, yellow, soft (Non-proprietary)
Liquid paraffin 100 mg per 1 gram, Wool fat 100 mg per 1 gram, Yellow soft paraffin 800 mg per 1 gram Simple eye ointment | 4 gram P £18.62 DT = £18.46

Polyvinyl alcohol

- ● INDICATIONS AND DOSE
Tear deficiency
▸ TO THE EYE
▸ Child: Apply as required
▸ Adult: Apply as required

- ● PRESCRIBING AND DISPENSING INFORMATION Although multi-dose polyvinyl alcohol eye drops commonly contain preservatives, preservative-free unit dose vials may be available.

- ● MEDICINAL FORMS
There can be variation in the licensing of different medicines containing the same drug. Forms available from special-order manufacturers include: eye drops
Eye drops
EXCIPIENTS: May contain Benzalkonium chloride, disodium edetate
▸ Liquifilm Tears (Allergan Ltd)
Polyvinyl alcohol 14 mg per 1 ml Liquifilm Tears 1.4% eye drops | 15 ml £1.93
Liquifilm Tears 1.4% eye drops 0.4ml unit dose preservative free | 30 unit dose £5.35
▸ Refresh Ophthalmic (Allergan Ltd)
Polyvinyl alcohol 14 mg per 1 ml Refresh Ophthalmic 1.4% eye drops 0.4ml unit dose | 30 unit dose £2.25
▸ Sno Tears (Bausch & Lomb UK Ltd)
Polyvinyl alcohol 14 mg per 1 ml Sno Tears 1.4% eye drops | 10 ml £1.06

Retinol palmitate with white soft paraffin and light liquid paraffin and liquid paraffin and wool fat

(Formulated as an ocular lubricant)

- ● INDICATIONS AND DOSE
Dry eye conditions
▸ TO THE EYE
▸ Adult: (consult product literature)

- ● MEDICINAL FORMS
There can be variation in the licensing of different medicines containing the same drug.
Eye ointment
▸ VitA-POS (Scope Ophthalmics Ltd)
VitA-POS eye ointment preservative free | 5 gram £2.75

Sodium chloride

- ● INDICATIONS AND DOSE
Tear deficiency | Ocular lubricants and astringents | Irrigation, including first-aid removal of harmful substances | Intra-ocular or topical irrigation during surgical procedures
▸ TO THE EYE
▸ Child: Apply as required, use 0.9% eye preparations
▸ Adult: Apply as required, use 0.9% eye preparations
Corneal oedema
▸ TO THE EYE
▸ Adult: Use 5% eye preparations (consult product literature)

- ● PRESCRIBING AND DISPENSING INFORMATION Although multi-dose sodium chloride eye drops commonly contain preservatives, preservative-free unit dose vials may be available.

MEDICINAL FORMS

There can be variation in the licensing of different medicines containing the same drug. Forms available from special-order manufacturers include: eye drops, eye ointment

Eye drops

▸ Sodium chloride (Non-proprietary)
Sodium chloride 50 mg per 1 ml Sodium chloride 5% eye drops | 10 ml £25.25

▸ Hypersal (Ennogen Healthcare Ltd)
Sodium chloride 50 mg per 1 ml Hypersal 5% eye drops | 10 ml £25.25

▸ ODM5 (Kestrel Ophthalmics Ltd)
Sodium chloride 50 mg per 1 ml ODM5 5% eye drops preservative free | 10 ml £24.00 DT = £0.00

▸ Saline (Bausch & Lomb UK Ltd)
Sodium chloride 9 mg per 1 ml Minims saline 0.9% eye drops 0.5ml unit dose | 20 unit dose [P] £7.43 DT = £7.43

▸ Sodium chloride (Essential Pharmaceuticals Ltd, Moorfields Pharmaceuticals)
Sodium chloride 50 mg per 1 ml NaCl 5% eye drops 0.45ml unit dose preservative free | 20 unit dose £19.70
PF Drops Sodium Chloride 5% eye drops preservative free | 10 ml £25.20 DT = £0.00

Eye ointment

▸ Sodium chloride (Non-proprietary)
Sodium chloride 50 mg per 1 ml Sodium chloride 5% eye ointment preservative free | 5 gram £22.50

Sodium hyaluronate

INDICATIONS AND DOSE

Dry eye conditions

▸ TO THE EYE
▸ Adult: Apply as required

PRESCRIBING AND DISPENSING INFORMATION Some preparations are contained in units which are resealable and may be used for up to 12 hours.

Although multi-dose sodium hyaluronate eye drops commonly contain preservatives, preservative-free unit dose vials may be available.

MEDICINAL FORMS

There can be variation in the licensing of different medicines containing the same drug.

Eye drops

▸ Artelac Rebalance (Bausch & Lomb UK Ltd)
Artelac Rebalance 0.15% eye drops | 10 ml £4.00

▸ Artelac Splash (Bausch & Lomb UK Ltd)
Artelac Splash 0.2% eye drops 0.5ml unit dose | 30 unit dose £7.00 | 60 unit dose £11.20

▸ Blink Intensive (AMO UK Ltd)
Blink Intensive Tears 0.2% eye drops 0.4ml unit dose | 20 unit dose £2.97
Blink Intensive Tears 0.2% eye drops | 10 ml £2.97

▸ Clinitas (Altacor Ltd)
Clinitas Multi 0.4% eye drops preservative free | 10 ml £6.99
Clinitas 0.4% eye drops 0.5ml unit dose | 30 unit dose £5.70

▸ Evolve HA (Medicom Healthcare Ltd)
Evolve HA 0.2% eye drops preservative free | 10 ml £5.99

▸ Hy-Opti (Alissa Healthcare Research Ltd)
Hy-Opti 0.1% eye drops preservative free | 10 ml £8.50
Hy-Opti 0.2% eye drops preservative free | 10 ml £9.50

▸ Hyabak (Thea Pharmaceuticals Ltd)
Hyabak 0.15% eye drops preservative free | 10 ml £7.99

▸ Hycosan (Scope Ophthalmics Ltd)
Hycosan Extra 0.2% eye drops | 7.5 ml 🖫
Hycosan 0.1% eye drops | 7.5 ml 🖫

▸ HydraMed (Farmigea S.p.A.)
HydraMed 0.2% eye drops preservative free | 10 ml £5.60
HydraMed 0.2% eye drops 0.5ml unit dose preservative free | 30 unit dose £5.60

▸ Hylo-Comod (Scope Ophthalmics Ltd)
Hylo-Tear 0.1% eye drops preservative free | 10 ml £8.50
Hylo-Forte 0.2% eye drops preservative free | 10 ml £9.50

▸ Hylo-fresh (Scope Ophthalmics Ltd)
Hylo-Fresh 0.03% eye drops preservative free | 10 ml £4.95

▸ Lubristil (Moorfields Pharmaceuticals)
Lubristil 0.15% eye drops 0.3ml unit dose preservative free | 20 unit dose £4.99

▸ Ocusan (Agepha Pharma s.r.o.)
Ocusan 0.2% eye drops 0.5ml unit dose | 20 unit dose £5.41

▸ Optive Fusion (Allergan Ltd)
Optive Fusion 0.1% eye drops | 10 ml £7.49

▸ Oxyal (Bausch & Lomb Ltd)
Oxyal 0.15% eye drops | 10 ml £4.15

▸ Vismed (TRB Chemidica (UK) Ltd)
Vismed Gel Multi 0.3% eye drops preservative free | 10 ml £8.01
Vismed Multi 0.18% eye drops preservative free | 10 ml £6.87
Vismed 0.18% eye drops 0.3ml unit dose preservative free | 20 unit dose £5.14

▸ Vizulize (East Midlands Pharma Ltd)
Vizulize 0.1% eye drops | 10 ml £1.71

▸ Xailin HA (Visufarma UK Ltd)
Xailin HA 0.2% eye drops | 10 ml £7.19
Xailin HA 0.2% eye drops preservative free | 10 ml £7.19

Eye gel

▸ Lubristil (Moorfields Pharmaceuticals)
Lubristil 0.15% eye gel 0.4ml unit dose preservative free | 20 unit dose £6.49

▸ Vismed (TRB Chemidica (UK) Ltd)
Vismed Gel 0.3% eye gel 0.45ml unit dose preservative free | 20 unit dose £6.03

Sodium hyaluronate and trehalose

21-Nov-2017

INDICATIONS AND DOSE

Dry eye conditions

▸ TO THE EYE
▸ Adult: Apply 1 drop 4–6 times a day

PRESCRIBING AND DISPENSING INFORMATION Sodium hyaluronate and trehalose preparations do not contain preservatives; multi-dose preparation can be used for up to 3 months.

MEDICINAL FORMS

There can be variation in the licensing of different medicines containing the same drug.

Eye drops

▸ Thealoz Duo (Thea Pharmaceuticals Ltd)
Thealoz Duo eye drops preservative free | 10 ml £8.99
Thealoz Duo UD eye drops 0.4ml unit dose preservative free | 30 unit dose £6.99

Soybean oil

INDICATIONS AND DOSE

Dry eye conditions

▸ TO THE EYE
▸ Child: Apply up to 4 times a day
▸ Adult: Apply up to 4 times a day

MEDICINAL FORMS

There can be variation in the licensing of different medicines containing the same drug.

Eye drops

▸ Emustil (Moorfields Pharmaceuticals)
Emustil eye drops 0.3ml unit dose preservative free | 20 unit dose £6.22

11

Eye

3   Eye infections

Eye, infections

Eye infections

Most acute superficial eye infections can be treated topically. Blepharitis and conjunctivitis are often caused by staphylococci; keratitis and endophthalmitis may be bacterial, viral, or fungal.

Bacterial *blepharitis* is treated by application of an antibacterial eye ointment to the conjunctival sac or to the lid margins. Systemic treatment may occasionally be required and is usually undertaken after culturing organisms from the lid margin and determining their antimicrobial sensitivity; antibiotics such as the tetracyclines given for 3 months or longer may be appropriate.

Most cases of acute bacterial conjunctivitis are self limiting; where treatment is appropriate, antibacterial eye drops or an eye ointment are used. A poor response might indicate viral or allergic conjunctivitis.

Corneal ulcer and *keratitis* require specialist treatment and may call for hospital admission for intensive therapy.

Endophthalmitis is a medical emergency which also calls for specialist management and requires intravitreal administration of antimicrobials; concomitant systemic treatment is required in some cases. Surgical intervention, such as vitrectomy, is sometimes indicated.

Antibacterials for eye infections

Bacterial eye infections are generally treated topically with eye drops and eye ointments. Systemic administration is sometimes appropriate in blepharitis.

Chloramphenicol p. 1139 has a broad spectrum of activity and is the drug of choice for *superficial eye infections*. Chloramphenicol eye drops are well tolerated and the recommendation that chloramphenicol eye drops should be avoided because of an increased risk of aplastic anaemia is not well founded.

Other antibacterials with a broad spectrum of activity include the quinolones, ciprofloxacin p. 1137, levofloxacin p. 1138, moxifloxacin p. 1138, and ofloxacin p. 1138; the aminoglycosides, gentamicin below and tobramycin p. 1137 are also active against a wide variety of bacteria. Gentamicin, tobramycin, quinolones (except moxifloxacin), and **polymyxin B** are effective for infections caused by *Pseudomonas aeruginosa*.

Ciprofloxacin eye drops are licensed for corneal ulcers; intensive application (especially in the first 2 days) is required throughout the day and night.

Azithromycin eye drops p. 1137 are licensed for trachomatous conjunctivitis caused by *Chlamydia trachomatis* and for purulent bacterial conjunctivitis. *Trachoma* which results from chronic infection with *Chlamydia trachomatis* can be treated with azithromycin by mouth [unlicensed indication].

Fusidic acid is useful for staphylococcal infections. Propamidine isetionate p. 1139 is of little value in bacterial infections but is used by specialists to treat the rare, but potentially sight-threatening, condition of *acanthamoeba keratitis* [unlicensed indication].

Cefuroxime p. 1137 can be administered by intracameral injection for the prophylaxis of endophthalmitis following cataract surgery.

With corticosteroids

Many antibacterial preparations also incorporate a corticosteroid but such mixtures should **not** be used unless a patient is under close specialist supervision. In particular they should not be prescribed for undiagnosed 'red eye'

which is sometimes caused by the herpes simplex virus and may be difficult to diagnose.

Administration

Frequency of application depends on the severity of the infection and the potential for irreversible ocular damage; antibacterial eye preparations are usually administered as follows:

- *Eye drops*, apply 1 drop at least every 2 hours then reduce frequency as infection is controlled and continue for 48 hours after healing.
- *Eye ointment*, apply *either* at night (if eye drops used during the day) *or* 3–4 times daily (if eye ointment used alone).

Antifungals for eye infections

Fungal infections of the cornea are rare but can occur after agricultural injuries, especially in hot and humid climates. Orbital mycosis is rarer, and when it occurs it is usually because of direct spread of infection from the paranasal sinuses. Increasing age, debility, or immunosuppression can encourage fungal proliferation. The spread of infection through blood occasionally produces metastatic endophthalmitis.

Many different fungi are capable of producing ocular infection; they can be identified by appropriate laboratory procedures.

Antifungal preparations for the eye are not generally available. Treatment will normally be carried out at specialist centres, but requests for information about supplies of preparations not available commercially should be addressed to the Strategic Health Authority (or equivalent), or to the nearest hospital ophthalmology unit, or to Moorfields Eye Hospital, 162 City Road, London EC1V 2PD (tel. (020) 7253 3411) or www.moorfields.nhs.uk.

Antivirals for eye infections

Herpes simplex infections producing, for example, dendritic corneal ulcers can be treated with aciclovir p. 1140 or ganciclovir p. 1140. Aciclovir eye ointment is used in combination with systemic treatment for ophthalmic zoster.

Slow-release ocular implants containing ganciclovir (available on a named-patient basis from specialist importing companies) may be inserted surgically to treat immediate sight-threatening CMV retinitis. Local treatments do not protect against systemic infection or infection in the other eye. See systemic treatment of CMV retinitis.

3.1   Bacterial eye infection

ANTIBACTERIALS > AMINOGLYCOSIDES

Gentamicin

11-Dec-2017

- **● INDICATIONS AND DOSE**

Bacterial eye infections
- ▶ TO THE EYE
  - ▶ Child: Apply 1 drop at least every 2 hours in severe infection, reduce frequency as infection is controlled and continue for 48 hours after healing, frequency of eye drops depends on the severity of the infection and the potential for irreversible ocular damage; for less severe infection 3–4 times daily is generally sufficient
  - ▶ Adult: Apply 1 drop at least every 2 hours, reduce frequency as infection is controlled and continue for 48 hours after healing, frequency of eye drops depends on the severity of the infection and the potential for irreversible ocular damage; for less severe infection 3–4 times daily is generally sufficient

- **● INTERACTIONS** → Appendix 1: aminoglycosides

- PRESCRIBING AND DISPENSING INFORMATION Eye drops may be sourced as a manufactured special or from specialist importing companies.

- MEDICINAL FORMS
There can be variation in the licensing of different medicines containing the same drug. Forms available from special-order manufacturers include: eye drops
Ear/eye drops solution
EXCIPIENTS: May contain Benzalkonium chloride
▸ Gentamicin (Non-proprietary)
  Gentamicin (as Gentamicin sulfate) 3 mg per 1 ml Gentamicin 0.3% ear/eye drops | 10 ml [PoM] £2.63 DT = £2.47

Tobramycin
22-Nov-2016

- INDICATIONS AND DOSE
Local treatment of infections
▸ TO THE EYE
▸ Child 1-17 years: Apply twice daily for 6–8 days
▸ Adult: Apply twice daily for 6–8 days
Local treatment of infections (severe infection)
▸ TO THE EYE
▸ Child 1-17 years: Apply 4 times a day for first day, then apply twice daily for 5–7 days
▸ Adult: Apply 4 times a day for first day, then apply twice daily for 5–7 days

- INTERACTIONS → Appendix 1: aminoglycosides

- MEDICINAL FORMS
No licensed medicines listed.

ANTIBACTERIALS > CEPHALOSPORINS, SECOND-GENERATION

▸ 515

Cefuroxime

- INDICATIONS AND DOSE
APROKAM ® INTRACAMERAL INJECTION
Prophylaxis of endophthalmitis after cataract surgery
▸ BY INTRACAMERAL INJECTION
▸ Adult: 1 mg, dose to be injected into the anterior chamber of the eye at the end of cataract surgery

- CAUTIONS
APROKAM ® INTRACAMERAL INJECTION Combined operations with cataract surgery · complicated cataracts · reduced corneal endothelial cells (less than 2000) · severe risk of infection · severe thyroid disease

- INTERACTIONS → Appendix 1: cephalosporins
- PREGNANCY Not known to be harmful.
- BREAST FEEDING Present in milk in low concentration, but appropriate to use.
- NATIONAL FUNDING/ACCESS DECISIONS
APROKAM ® INTRACAMERAL INJECTION
Scottish Medicines Consortium (SMC) Decisions
The *Scottish Medicines Consortium* has advised (December 2016) that cefuroxime (*Aprokam ®*) is accepted for use within NHS Scotland for antibiotic prophylaxis of postoperative endophthalmitis after cataract surgery.
All Wales Medicines Strategy Group (AWMSG) Decisions
The *All Wales Medicines Strategy Group* has advised (August 2017) that cefuroxime (*Aprokam ®*) is recommended as an option for use within NHS Wales for the antibiotic prophylaxis of postoperative endophthalmitis after cataract surgery.

- MEDICINAL FORMS
There can be variation in the licensing of different medicines containing the same drug.
Powder for solution for injection
▸ Aprokam (Thea Pharmaceuticals Ltd)
  Cefuroxime sodium 50 mg Aprokam 50mg powder for solution for injection vials | 10 vial [PoM] £49.95

ANTIBACTERIALS > MACROLIDES

Azithromycin

- INDICATIONS AND DOSE
Trachomatous conjunctivitis caused by *Chlamydia trachomatis* | Purulent bacterial conjunctivitis
▸ TO THE EYE
▸ Child: Apply twice daily for 3 days, review if no improvement after 3 days of treatment
▸ Adult: Apply twice daily for 3 days, review if no improvement after 3 days of treatment

- INTERACTIONS → Appendix 1: macrolides

- SIDE-EFFECTS
▸ **Common or very common** Eye discomfort · vision blurred
▸ **Uncommon** Angioedema · eye allergy

- MEDICINAL FORMS
There can be variation in the licensing of different medicines containing the same drug.
Eye drops
▸ Azyter (Thea Pharmaceuticals Ltd)
  Azithromycin dihydrate 15 mg per 1 gram Azyter 15mg/g eye drops 0.25g unit dose | 6 unit dose [PoM] £6.99 DT = £6.99

ANTIBACTERIALS > QUINOLONES

Ciprofloxacin
26-Apr-2018

- INDICATIONS AND DOSE
Superficial bacterial eye infection
▸ TO THE EYE USING EYE DROP
▸ Child: Apply 4 times a day for maximum duration of treatment 21 days
▸ Adult: Apply 4 times a day for maximum duration of treatment 21 days
▸ TO THE EYE USING EYE OINTMENT
▸ Child 1-17 years: Apply 1.25 centimetres 3 times a day for 2 days, then apply 1.25 centimetres twice daily for 5 days
▸ Adult: Apply 1.25 centimetres 3 times a day for 2 days, then apply 1.25 centimetres twice daily for 5 days
Superficial bacterial eye infection (severe infection)
▸ TO THE EYE USING EYE DROP
▸ Child: Apply every 2 hours during waking hours for 2 days, then apply 4 times a day for maximum duration of treatment 21 days
▸ Adult: Apply every 2 hours during waking hours for 2 days, then apply 4 times a day for maximum duration of treatment 21 days
Corneal ulcer
▸ TO THE EYE USING EYE DROP
▸ Child: Apply every 15 minutes for 6 hours, then apply every 30 minutes for the remainder of day 1, then apply every 1 hour on day 2, then apply every 4 hours on days 3–14, maximum duration of treatment 21 days, to be administered throughout the day and night
▸ Adult: Apply every 15 minutes for 6 hours, then apply every 30 minutes for the remainder of day 1, then apply every 1 hour on day 2, then apply every 4 hours on days 3–14, maximum duration of treatment 21 days, to be administered throughout the day and night   continued →

11

Eye

▶ TO THE EYE USING EYE OINTMENT
- ▶ **Child 1–17 years:** Apply 1.25 centimetres every 1–2 hours for 2 days, then apply 1.25 centimetres every 4 hours for the next 12 days, to be administered throughout the day and night
- ▶ **Adult:** Apply 1.25 centimetres every 1–2 hours for 2 days, then apply 1.25 centimetres every 4 hours for the next 12 days, to be administered throughout the day and night

- ● UNLICENSED USE Eye ointment not licensed for use in children under 1 year.
- ● INTERACTIONS → Appendix 1: quinolones
- ● SIDE-EFFECTS
- ▶ **Common or very common** Corneal deposits (reversible after completion of treatment)
- ▶ **Uncommon** Eye disorders · eye inflammation · eyelid crusting · vision disorders
- ▶ **Rare or very rare** Dermatitis · ear pain · increased risk of infection · paranasal sinus hypersecretion
- ▶ **Frequency not known** Tendon disorder
- ● PREGNANCY Manufacturer advises use only if potential benefit outweighs risk.
- ● BREAST FEEDING Manufacturer advises caution.

- ● MEDICINAL FORMS
There can be variation in the licensing of different medicines containing the same drug. Forms available from special-order manufacturers include: eye drops
  Eye drops
  EXCIPIENTS: May contain Benzalkonium chloride
  - ▶ Ciloxan (Novartis Pharmaceuticals UK Ltd)
  Ciprofloxacin (as Ciprofloxacin hydrochloride) 3 mg per 1 ml Ciloxan 0.3% eye drops | 5 ml [PoM] £4.70 DT = £4.70

Levofloxacin

13-Jul-2017

- ● **INDICATIONS AND DOSE**
Local treatment of eye infections
- ▶ TO THE EYE
- ▶ **Child 1–17 years:** Apply every 2 hours for first 2 days, to be applied maximum 8 times a day, then apply 4 times a day for 3 days
- ▶ **Adult:** Apply every 2 hours for first 2 days, to be applied maximum 8 times a day, then apply 4 times a day for 3 days

- ● INTERACTIONS → Appendix 1: quinolones
- ● SIDE-EFFECTS
- ▶ **Common or very common** Eye discomfort
- ▶ **Uncommon** Eye disorders · rhinitis
- ▶ **Rare or very rare** Laryngeal oedema
- ● PREGNANCY Manufacturer advises use only if potential benefit outweighs risk.
- ● BREAST FEEDING Manufacturer advises use only if potential benefit outweighs risk.
- ● PRESCRIBING AND DISPENSING INFORMATION Although multi-dose levofloxacin eye drops commonly contain preservatives, preservative-free unit dose vials may be available.

- ● MEDICINAL FORMS
There can be variation in the licensing of different medicines containing the same drug.
  Eye drops
  EXCIPIENTS: May contain Benzalkonium chloride
  - ▶ Levofloxacin (Non-proprietary)
  Levofloxacin (as Levofloxacin hemihydrate) 5 mg per 1 ml Levofloxacin 5mg/ml eye drops | 5 ml [PoM] £6.95 DT = £6.95

- ▶ Oftaquix (Santen UK Ltd)
  Levofloxacin (as Levofloxacin hemihydrate) 5 mg per 1 ml Oftaquix 5mg/ml eye drops 0.3ml unit dose | 30 unit dose [PoM] £17.95 DT = £17.95
  Oftaquix 5mg/ml eye drops | 5 ml [PoM] £6.95 DT = £6.95

Moxifloxacin

- ● **INDICATIONS AND DOSE**
Local treatment of infections
- ▶ TO THE EYE
- ▶ **Child:** Apply 3 times a day continue treatment for 2–3 days after infection improves; review if no improvement within 5 days
- ▶ **Adult:** Apply 3 times a day continue treatment for 2–3 days after infection improves; review if no improvement within 5 days

- ● INTERACTIONS → Appendix 1: quinolones
- ● SIDE-EFFECTS
- ▶ **Uncommon** Conjunctival haemorrhage · eye inflammation · palpitations · sensation abnormal
- ▶ **Rare or very rare** Eye disorders · laryngeal pain · nasal discomfort · visual acuity decreased
- ▶ **Frequency not known** Abnormal sensation in eye · corneal deposits · erythema

- ● MEDICINAL FORMS
There can be variation in the licensing of different medicines containing the same drug.
  Eye drops
  - ▶ Moxivig (Novartis Pharmaceuticals UK Ltd)
  Moxifloxacin (as Moxifloxacin hydrochloride) 5 mg per 1 ml Moxivig 0.5% eye drops | 5 ml [PoM] £9.80 DT = £9.80

Ofloxacin

- ● **INDICATIONS AND DOSE**
Local treatment of infections
- ▶ TO THE EYE
- ▶ **Child 1–17 years:** Apply every 2–4 hours for the first 2 days, then reduced to 4 times a day for maximum 10 days treatment
- ▶ **Adult:** Apply every 2–4 hours for the first 2 days, then reduced to 4 times a day for maximum 10 days treatment

- ● CAUTIONS Corneal ulcer (risk of corneal perforation) · epithelial defect (risk of corneal perforation)
- ● INTERACTIONS → Appendix 1: quinolones
- ● SIDE-EFFECTS Eye discomfort · eye inflammation · face oedema · oropharyngeal swelling · tongue swelling
- ● PREGNANCY Manufacturer advises use only if benefit outweighs risk (systemic quinolones have caused arthropathy in *animal* studies).
- ● BREAST FEEDING Manufacturer advises avoid.

- ● MEDICINAL FORMS
There can be variation in the licensing of different medicines containing the same drug.
  Eye drops
  EXCIPIENTS: May contain Benzalkonium chloride
  - ▶ Exocin (Allergan Ltd)
  Ofloxacin 3 mg per 1 ml Exocin 0.3% eye drops | 5 ml [PoM] £2.17 DT = £2.17

Chloramphenicol

- **DRUG ACTION** Chloramphenicol is a potent broad-spectrum antibiotic.

- **INDICATIONS AND DOSE**
Superficial eye infections
▶ TO THE EYE USING EYE DROP
▸ Child: Apply 1 drop every 2 hours then reduce frequency as infection is controlled and continue for 48 hours after healing, frequency dependent on the severity of the infection. For less severe infection 3–4 times daily is generally sufficient
▸ Adult: Apply 1 drop every 2 hours then reduce frequency as infection is controlled and continue for 48 hours after healing, frequency dependent on the severity of the infection. For less severe infection 3–4 times daily is generally sufficient
▶ TO THE EYE USING EYE OINTMENT
▸ Child: Apply daily, to be applied at night (if eye drops used during the day), alternatively apply 3–4 times a day, if ointment used alone
▸ Adult: Apply daily, to be applied at night (if eye drops used during the day), alternatively apply 3–4 times a day, if ointment used alone

- **INTERACTIONS** → Appendix 1: chloramphenicol
- **SIDE-EFFECTS** Angioedema · bone marrow disorders · eye stinging · fever · paraesthesia · skin reactions
- **PREGNANCY** Avoid unless essential—no information on *topical* use but risk of 'neonatal grey-baby syndrome' with *oral* use in third trimester.
- **BREAST FEEDING** Avoid unless essential— *theoretical* risk of bone-marrow toxicity.
- **PRESCRIBING AND DISPENSING INFORMATION** Although multi-dose chloramphenicol eye drops commonly contain preservatives, preservative-free unit dose vials may be available.
- **PATIENT AND CARER ADVICE**
Medicines for Children leaflet: Chloramphenicol for eye infections www.medicinesforchildren.org.uk/chloramphenicol-eye-infections-0
- **EXCEPTIONS TO LEGAL CATEGORY** Chloramphenicol 0.5% eye drops (in max. pack size 10 mL) and 1% eye ointment (in max. pack size 4 g) can be sold to the public for treatment of acute bacterial conjunctivitis in adults and children over 2 years; max. duration of treatment 5 days.

- **MEDICINAL FORMS**
There can be variation in the licensing of different medicines containing the same drug.
Eye drops
EXCIPIENTS: May contain Phenylmercuric acetate
▸ Chloramphenicol (Non-proprietary)
Chloramphenicol 5 mg per 1 ml Minims chloramphenicol 0.5% eye drops 0.5ml unit dose | 20 unit dose [PoM] £11.43 DT = £11.43
Chloramphenicol 0.5% eye drops | 10 ml [PoM] £2.20 DT = £1.14
▸ Chloromycetin (AMCo)
Chloramphenicol 5 mg per 1 ml Chloromycetin Redidrops 0.5% | 10 ml [PoM] £0.90 DT = £1.14
▸ Eykappo (Aspire Pharma Ltd)
Chloramphenicol 5 mg per 1 ml Eykappo 5mg/ml eye drops | 10 ml [PoM] £10.12 DT = £10.12
Eye ointment
▸ Chloramphenicol (Non-proprietary)
Chloramphenicol 10 mg per 1 gram Chloramphenicol 1% eye ointment | 4 gram [PoM] £1.89 DT = £1.89

Fusidic acid

16-Jun-2017

- **DRUG ACTION** Fusidic acid and its salts are narrow-spectrum antibiotics used for staphylococcal infections.

- **INDICATIONS AND DOSE**
Staphylococcal eye infections
▶ TO THE EYE
▸ Child: Apply twice daily
▸ Adult: Apply twice daily

- **INTERACTIONS** → Appendix 1: fusidic acid

- **MEDICINAL FORMS**
There can be variation in the licensing of different medicines containing the same drug.
Modified-release drops
EXCIPIENTS: May contain Benzalkonium chloride, disodium edetate
▸ Fusidic acid (Non-proprietary)
Fusidic acid 10 mg per 1 gram Fusidic acid 1% modified-release eye drops | 5 gram [PoM] £29.06 DT = £29.06

Propamidine isetionate

- **INDICATIONS AND DOSE**
***Acanthamoeba keratitis* infections (specialist use only)** |
Local treatment of eye infections
▶ TO THE EYE USING EYE OINTMENT
▸ Adult: Apply 1–2 times a day
▶ TO THE EYE USING EYE DROP
▸ Adult: Apply up to 4 times a day

- **UNLICENSED USE** Not licensed for *acanthamoeba keratitis* infections.
- **SIDE-EFFECTS** Eye discomfort · vision blurred
- **PREGNANCY** Manufacturer advises avoid unless essential—no information available.
- **BREAST FEEDING** Manufacturer advises avoid unless essential—no information available.

- **MEDICINAL FORMS**
There can be variation in the licensing of different medicines containing the same drug.
Eye ointment
▸ Golden Eye (dibromopropamidine) (Cambridge Healthcare Supplies Ltd)
Dibromopropamidine isetionate 1.5 mg per 1 gram Golden Eye 0.15% ointment | 5 gram [P] £3.98 DT = £3.98
Eye drops
EXCIPIENTS: May contain Benzalkonium chloride
▸ Brolene (Propamidine) (Sanofi)
Propamidine isetionate 1 mg per 1 ml Brolene 0.1% eye drops | 10 ml [P] £2.80
▸ Golden Eye (propamidine) (Cambridge Healthcare Supplies Ltd)
Propamidine isetionate 1 mg per 1 ml Golden Eye 0.1% drops | 10 ml [P] £3.62

11

Eye

3.2 Viral eye infection
3.2a Ophthalmic herpes simplex

ANTIVIRALS > NUCLEOSIDE ANALOGUES

Aciclovir
(Acyclovir)

- **INDICATIONS AND DOSE**
Herpes simplex infection (local treatment)
  ▶ TO THE EYE USING EYE OINTMENT
  ▶ **Child:** Apply 1 centimetre 5 times a day continue for at least 3 days after complete healing
  ▶ **Adult:** Apply 1 centimetre 5 times a day continue for at least 3 days after complete healing

- **INTERACTIONS** → Appendix 1: aciclovir
- **SIDE-EFFECTS**
  ▶ **Common or very common** Eye inflammation · eye pain
- **PATIENT AND CARER ADVICE**
Medicines for Children leaflet: Aciclovir eye ointment for herpes simplex infections www.medicinesforchildren.org.uk/aciclovir-eye-ointment-for-herpes-simplex-infection

- **MEDICINAL FORMS**
There can be variation in the licensing of different medicines containing the same drug.
Eye ointment
  ▶ Zovirax (GlaxoSmithKline UK Ltd)
  Aciclovir 30 mg per 1 gram Zovirax 3% ophthalmic ointment | 4.5 gram [PoM] £9.34 DT = £9.34

Ganciclovir

31-May-2018

- **INDICATIONS AND DOSE**
Acute herpetic keratitis
  ▶ TO THE EYE
  ▶ **Adult:** Apply 5 times a day until healing complete, then apply 3 times a day for a further 7 days, treatment does not usually exceed 21 days

- **INTERACTIONS** → Appendix 1: ganciclovir
- **SIDE-EFFECTS**
  ▶ **Common or very common** Eye stinging · punctate keratitis
- **ALLERGY AND CROSS-SENSITIVITY** Contra-indicated in patients hypersensitive to valganciclovir, aciclovir, or valaciclovir.
- **CONCEPTION AND CONTRACEPTION** As teratogenicity and impaired fertility observed in animal studies with *oral* and *intravenous* ganciclovir, manufacturer advises women of childbearing potential should use effective contraception during treatment; men with partners of childbearing potential should be advised to use barrier contraception during and for at least 90 days after treatment.
- **PREGNANCY** Manufacturer advises avoid unless no suitable alternative—limited information available.
- **BREAST FEEDING** Manufacturer advises avoid unless no suitable alternative—limited information available.

- **MEDICINAL FORMS**
There can be variation in the licensing of different medicines containing the same drug.
Eye gel
EXCIPIENTS: May contain Benzalkonium chloride
  ▶ Virgan (Thea Pharmaceuticals Ltd)
  Ganciclovir 1.5 mg per 1 gram Virgan 0.15% eye gel | 5 gram [PoM] £19.99 DT = £19.99

4 Eye procedures

Mydriatics and cycloplegics

Overview

Antimuscarinics dilate the pupil and paralyse the ciliary muscle; they vary in potency and duration of action.

Short-acting, relatively weak mydriatics, such as tropicamide 0.5% below (action lasts for 4–6 hours), facilitate the examination of the fundus of the eye. Longer-acting options include cyclopentolate hydrochloride 1% p. 1131 (action up to 24 hours) or atropine sulfate p. 1131 (action up to 7 days).

Phenylephrine hydrochloride p. 1141 is used for mydriasis in diagnostic or therapeutic procedures; mydriasis occurs within 60–90 minutes and lasts up to 5–7 hours.

Mydriatics and cycloplegics are used in the treatment of anterior uveitis, usually as an adjunct to corticosteroids. Atropine sulfate is used in anterior uveitis mainly to prevent posterior synechiae and to relieve ciliary spasm; cyclopentolate hydrochloride or homatropine hydrobromide p. 1131 (action up to 3 days) can also be used and may be preferred because they have a shorter duration of action.

> **Other drugs used for Eye procedures** Apraclonidine, p. 1153

ANTIMUSCARINICS

ᴳ 1131

Tropicamide

- **INDICATIONS AND DOSE**
Funduscopy
  ▶ TO THE EYE
  ▶ **Child:** 0.5% eye drops to be applied 20 minutes before examination
  ▶ **Adult:** (consult product literature)

- **INTERACTIONS** → Appendix 1: tropicamide
- **PRESCRIBING AND DISPENSING INFORMATION** Although multi-dose tropicamide eye drops commonly contain preservatives, preservative-free unit dose vials may be available.

- **MEDICINAL FORMS**
There can be variation in the licensing of different medicines containing the same drug.
Eye drops
EXCIPIENTS: May contain Benzalkonium chloride, edetic acid (edta)
  ▶ Mydriacyl (Novartis Pharmaceuticals UK Ltd)
  Tropicamide 10 mg per 1 ml Mydriacyl 1% eye drops | 5 ml [PoM] £1.60
  ▶ Tropicamide (Bausch & Lomb UK Ltd)
  Tropicamide 5 mg per 1 ml Minims tropicamide 0.5% eye drops 0.5ml unit dose | 20 unit dose [PoM] £11.18
  Tropicamide 10 mg per 1 ml Minims tropicamide 1% eye drops 0.5ml unit dose | 20 unit dose [PoM] £11.31

Combinations available: *Phenylephrine with tropicamide,* p. 1142 · *Tropicamide with phenylephrine and lidocaine,* p. 1142

ANTISEPTICS AND DISINFECTANTS > IODINE PRODUCTS

Povidone-iodine

- **INDICATIONS AND DOSE**

Cutaneous peri-ocular and conjunctival antisepsis before ocular surgery
- ▸ TO THE EYE
- ▸ Adult: Apply, leave for 2 minutes, then irrigate thoroughly with sodium chloride 0.9%

- **CONTRA-INDICATIONS** Concomitant use of ocular antimicrobial drugs · concomitant use of ocular formulations containing mercury-based preservatives · preterm neonates
- **SIDE-EFFECTS**
- ▸ **Rare or very rare** Eye erythema · punctate keratitis
- ▸ **Frequency not known** Cytotoxicity · eye discolouration
- **BREAST FEEDING** Avoid regular or excessive use.
- **PRESCRIBING AND DISPENSING INFORMATION** Although multi-dose povidone iodine eye drops commonly contain preservatives, preservative-free unit dose vials may be available.

- **MEDICINAL FORMS**
There can be variation in the licensing of different medicines containing the same drug. Forms available from special-order manufacturers include: eye drops, eye lotion
Eye drops
- ▸ Povidone-iodine (Bausch & Lomb UK Ltd)
Povidone-Iodine 50 mg per 1 ml Minims povidone iodine 5% eye drops 0.4ml unit dose | 20 unit dose PoM £16.00

DIAGNOSTIC AGENTS > DYES

Fluorescein sodium

- **INDICATIONS AND DOSE**

Detection of lesions and foreign bodies
- ▸ TO THE EYE USING EYE DROP
- ▸ Adult: Use sufficient amount to stain damaged areas

- **PRESCRIBING AND DISPENSING INFORMATION** Although multi-dose fluorescein eye drops commonly contain preservatives, preservative-free unit dose vials may be available.

- **MEDICINAL FORMS**
There can be variation in the licensing of different medicines containing the same drug.
Eye drops
- ▸ Fluorescein sodium (Bausch & Lomb UK Ltd)
Fluorescein sodium 10 mg per 1 ml Minims fluorescein sodium 1% eye drops 0.5ml unit dose | 20 unit dose P £9.25
Fluorescein sodium 20 mg per 1 ml Minims fluorescein sodium 2% eye drops 0.5ml unit dose | 20 unit dose P £9.25

MIOTICS > PARASYMPATHOMIMETICS

Acetylcholine chloride

- **INDICATIONS AND DOSE**

Cataract surgery | Penetrating keratoplasty | Iridectomy | Anterior segment surgery requiring rapid complete miosis
- ▸ TO THE EYE
- ▸ Adult: (consult product literature)

- **CAUTIONS** Asthma · gastro-intestinal spasm · heart failure · hyperthyroidism · parkinsonism · peptic ulcer · urinary-tract obstruction

- **SIDE-EFFECTS** Bradycardia · corneal decompensation · corneal oedema · dyspnoea · flushing · hyperhidrosis · hypotension
- **PREGNANCY** Avoid unless potential benefit outweighs risk—no information available.
- **BREAST FEEDING** Avoid unless potential benefit outweighs risk—no information available.

- **MEDICINAL FORMS**
There can be variation in the licensing of different medicines containing the same drug.
Irrigation
- ▸ Miochol-E (Bausch & Lomb UK Ltd)
Acetylcholine chloride 20 mg Miochol-E 20mg powder and solvent for solution for intraocular irrigation vials | 1 vial PoM £7.28
- ▸ Miphtel (Farmigea S.p.A.)
Acetylcholine chloride 20 mg Miphtel 20mg powder and solvent for solution for intraocular irrigation ampoules | 6 ampoule PoM £43.68 (Hospital only)

SYMPATHOMIMETICS > VASOCONSTRICTOR

Phenylephrine hydrochloride

- **INDICATIONS AND DOSE**

Mydriasis
- ▸ TO THE EYE
- ▸ Child: Apply 1 drop, to be administered before procedure, a drop of proxymetacaine topical anaesthetic may be applied to the eye a few minutes before using phenylephrine to prevent stinging
- ▸ Adult: Apply 1 drop, to be administered before procedure, then apply 1 drop after 60 minutes if required, a drop of topical anaesthetic may be applied to the eye a few minutes before using phenylephrine to prevent stinging

- **CONTRA-INDICATIONS** 10% strength eye drops in children · 10% strength eye drops in elderly · aneurysms · cardiovascular disease · hypertension · thyrotoxicosis
- **CAUTIONS** Asthma · cerebral arteriosclerosis (in adults) · corneal epithelial damage · darkly pigmented iris is more resistant to pupillary dilatation and caution should be exercised to avoid overdosage · diabetes (avoid eye drops in long standing diabetes) · mydriasis can precipitate acute angle-closure glaucoma in a few patients, usually over 60 years and hypermetropic (long-sighted), who are pre-disposed to the condition because of a shallow anterior chamber · mydriasis can precipitate acute angle-closure glaucoma in the very few children who are predisposed to the condition because of a shallow anterior chamber · ocular hyperaemia · susceptibility to angle-closure glaucoma
- **INTERACTIONS** → Appendix 1: sympathomimetics, vasoconstrictor
- **SIDE-EFFECTS** Arrhythmias · conjunctivitis allergic · eye discomfort · hypertension · myocardial infarction (usually after use of 10% strength in patients with pre-existing cardiovascular disease) · palpitations · periorbital pallor (in children) · vision disorders
- **PREGNANCY** Use only if potential benefit outweighs risk.
- **BREAST FEEDING** Use only if potential benefit outweighs risk—no information available.
- **PRESCRIBING AND DISPENSING INFORMATION** Although multi-dose phenylephrine eye drops commonly contain preservatives, preservative-free unit dose vials may be available.
- **PATIENT AND CARER ADVICE**
Driving and skilled tasks Patients should be warned not to undertake skilled tasks (e.g. driving) until vision clears after mydriasis.

11

Eye

- **MEDICINAL FORMS**
  There can be variation in the licensing of different medicines containing the same drug. Forms available from special-order manufacturers include: eye drops

  Eye drops
  EXCIPIENTS: May contain Disodium edetate, sodium metabisulfite
  ▸ Phenylephrine hydrochloride (Bausch & Lomb UK Ltd)
    Phenylephrine hydrochloride 25 mg per 1 ml Minims phenylephrine hydrochloride 2.5% eye drops 0.5ml unit dose | 20 unit dose P £11.87
    Phenylephrine hydrochloride 100 mg per 1 ml Minims phenylephrine hydrochloride 10% eye drops 0.5ml unit dose | 20 unit dose P £11.87

Phenylephrine with tropicamide

The properties listed below are those particular to the combination only. For the properties of the components please consider, phenylephrine hydrochloride p. 1141, tropicamide p. 1140.

- **INDICATIONS AND DOSE**

  Pre-operative mydriasis | Diagnostic procedures when monotherapy insufficient
  ▸ TO THE EYE
  ▸ Adult: One insert to be applied into the lower conjunctival sac up to max. 2 hours before procedure; remove insert within 30 minutes of satisfactory mydriasis, and within 2 hours of application

- **INTERACTIONS** → Appendix 1: sympathomimetics, vasoconstrictor · tropicamide

- **DIRECTIONS FOR ADMINISTRATION** Patients with severe dry eyes may require a drop of saline to improve insert tolerance.

- **MEDICINAL FORMS**
  There can be variation in the licensing of different medicines containing the same drug.

  Ophthalmic insert
  ▸ Mydriasert (Thea Pharmaceuticals Ltd)
    Tropicamide.28 mg, Phenylephrine hydrochloride 5.4 mg Mydriasert 5.4mg/0.28mg ophthalmic inserts | 20 insert PoM £84.00

Tropicamide with phenylephrine and lidocaine

17-Aug-2017

- **INDICATIONS AND DOSE**

  Mydriasis and intraocular anaesthesia during cataract surgery
  ▸ BY INTRACAMERAL INJECTION
  ▸ Adult: 0.2 mL for 1 dose, to be injected slowly at the start of the surgical procedure

  DOSE EQUIVALENCE AND CONVERSION
  ▸ Each 0.2 mL dose of *Mydrane*® solution for injection contains 0.04 mg of tropicamide, 0.62 mg of phenylephrine hydrochloride and 2 mg of lidocaine hydrochloride.

- **CONTRA-INDICATIONS** Cataract surgery combined with vitrectomy · history of acute, narrow-angle glaucoma · shallow anterior chamber

- **CAUTIONS** Conditions where systemic exposure to phenylephrine or lidocaine could be harmful (consult product literature) · risk of floppy iris syndrome (consult product literature)

- **INTERACTIONS** → Appendix 1: antiarrhythmics · sympathomimetics, vasoconstrictor · tropicamide

- **SIDE-EFFECTS**
  ▸ **Uncommon** Headache · hyperaemia · hypertension · keratitis

- **ALLERGY AND CROSS-SENSITIVITY** Contra-indicated in patients with known hypersensitivity to amide-type anaesthetics or atropine derivatives.

- **PREGNANCY** Manufacturer advises avoid (systemic uptake after administration cannot be excluded)—insufficient data available for phenylephrine and tropicamide in pregnancy; lidocaine crosses the placenta but is not known to be harmful in *animal* studies.

- **BREAST FEEDING** Manufacturer advises avoid—no data available for phenylephrine or tropicamide; lidocaine present in milk in small amount.

- **PRE-TREATMENT SCREENING** Manufacturer advises patients must have demonstrated, at a previous visit, a satisfactory pupil dilation with topical mydriatic treatment.

- **PATIENT AND CARER ADVICE**
  Driving and skilled tasks Manufacturer advises patients should be counselled about the effects on driving and skilled tasks.

- **MEDICINAL FORMS**
  There can be variation in the licensing of different medicines containing the same drug.

  Solution for injection
  EXCIPIENTS: May contain Disodium edetate
  ▸ Mydrane (Thea Pharmaceuticals Ltd)
    Tropicamide 200 microgram per 1 ml, Phenylephrine hydrochloride 3.1 mg per 1 ml, Lidocaine hydrochloride 10 mg per 1 ml Mydrane 0.2mg/ml / 3.1mg/ml / 10mg/ml solution for injection 0.6ml ampoules | 20 ampoule PoM £119.95

4.1 Post-operative pain and inflammation

Eye, surgical and peri-operative drug use

Ocular peri-operative drugs

Drugs used to prepare the eye for surgery, drugs that are injected into the anterior chamber at the time of surgery, and those used after eye surgery, are included here.

Cefuroxime p. 1137, administered by intra-ocular injection into the anterior chamber of the eye (intracameral use), is used for the prophylaxis of endophthalmitis after cataract surgery.

Non-steroidal anti-inflammatory eye drops such as diclofenac sodium p. 1144, flurbiprofen p. 1144, ketorolac trometamol p. 1144, and nepafenac p. 1126, are used for the prophylaxis and treatment of inflammation, pain, and other symptoms associated with ocular surgery or laser treatment of the eye. Bromfenac p. 1143 is used for the treatment of postoperative inflammation following cataract surgery. Diclofenac sodium and flurbiprofen are also used to prevent miosis during ocular surgery.

Apraclonidine p. 1153, an alpha₂-adrenoreceptor agonist, reduces intra-ocular pressure possibly by reducing the production of aqueous humour. It is used to control increases in intra-ocular pressure associated with ocular surgery and as short-term treatment to reduce intraocular pressure prior to surgery.

Acetylcholine chloride p. 1141, administered into the anterior chamber of the eye during surgery, rapidly produces miosis which lasts approximately 20 minutes. If prolonged miosis is required, it can be applied again.

Intra-ocular sodium hyaluronate p. 1135 and balanced salt solution are used during surgical procedures on the eye.

Povidone-iodine p. 1141 is used for peri-ocular and conjunctival antisepsis before ocular surgery to support postoperative infection control.

Ocular local anaesthetics

Oxybuprocaine hydrochloride below and tetracaine below are widely used topical local anaesthetics. Proxymetacaine hydrochloride below causes less initial stinging and is useful for children. Oxybuprocaine hydrochloride or a combined preparation of lidocaine hydrochloride and fluorescein sodium p. 1143 is used for tonometry. Tetracaine produces a more profound anaesthesia and is suitable for use before minor surgical procedures, such as the removal of corneal sutures. It has a temporary disruptive effect on the corneal epithelium. Lidocaine hydrochloride p. 1312, with or without adrenaline/epinephrine p. 1313, is injected into the eyelids for minor surgery. Local anaesthetics should never be used for the management of ocular symptoms.

ANAESTHETICS, LOCAL

Fluorescein with lidocaine

● **INDICATIONS AND DOSE**

Local anaesthesia
▶ TO THE EYE
▶ Adult: Apply as required

● PRESCRIBING AND DISPENSING INFORMATION Although multi-dose lidocaine and fluorescein eye drops commonly contain preservatives, preservative-free unit dose vials may be available.

● MEDICINAL FORMS There can be variation in the licensing of different medicines containing the same drug.
Eye drops
▶ Lidocaine and Fluorescein (Bausch & Lomb UK Ltd)
Fluorescein sodium 2.5 mg per 1 ml, Lidocaine hydrochloride 40 mg per 1 ml Minims lidocaine and fluorescein eye drops 0.5ml unit dose | 20 unit dose PoM £11.69

Oxybuprocaine hydrochloride

(Benoxinate hydrochloride)

● **INDICATIONS AND DOSE**

Local anaesthetic
▶ TO THE EYE
▶ Adult: Apply as required

● CONTRA-INDICATIONS Avoid in preterm neonates
● INTERACTIONS → Appendix 1: anaesthetics, local
● PRESCRIBING AND DISPENSING INFORMATION Although multi-dose oxybuprocaine eye drops commonly contain preservatives, preservative-free unit dose vials may be available.

● MEDICINAL FORMS There can be variation in the licensing of different medicines containing the same drug.
Eye drops
▶ Oxybuprocaine hydrochloride (Bausch & Lomb UK Ltd)
Oxybuprocaine hydrochloride 4 mg per 1 ml Minims oxybuprocaine hydrochloride 0.4% eye drops 0.5ml unit dose | 20 unit dose PoM £10.56

Proxymetacaine hydrochloride

● **INDICATIONS AND DOSE**

Local anaesthetic
▶ TO THE EYE
▶ Adult: Apply as required

● CONTRA-INDICATIONS Avoid in preterm neonates
● INTERACTIONS → Appendix 1: anaesthetics, local
● PRESCRIBING AND DISPENSING INFORMATION Although multi-dose proxymetacaine eye drops commonly contain preservatives, preservative-free unit dose vials may be available.

● MEDICINAL FORMS There can be variation in the licensing of different medicines containing the same drug.
Eye drops
▶ Proxymetacaine (Bausch & Lomb UK Ltd)
Proxymetacaine hydrochloride 5 mg per 1 ml Minims proxymetacaine 0.5% eye drops 0.5ml unit dose | 20 unit dose PoM £12.12

Tetracaine

(Amethocaine)

● **INDICATIONS AND DOSE**

Local anaesthetic
▶ TO THE EYE
▶ Adult: Apply as required

● INTERACTIONS → Appendix 1: anaesthetics, local
● PRESCRIBING AND DISPENSING INFORMATION Although multi-dose tetracaine eye drops commonly contain preservatives, preservative-free unit dose vials may be available.

● MEDICINAL FORMS There can be variation in the licensing of different medicines containing the same drug.
Eye drops
▶ Tetracaine (Non-proprietary)
Tetracaine hydrochloride 5 mg per 1 ml Minims tetracaine hydrochloride 0.5% eye drops 0.5ml unit dose | 20 unit dose PoM £10.57 DT = £10.57
Tetracaine hydrochloride 10 mg per 1 ml Minims tetracaine hydrochloride 1% eye drops 0.5ml unit dose | 20 unit dose PoM £10.57 DT = £10.57

ANALGESICS › NON-STEROIDAL ANTI-INFLAMMATORY DRUGS

Bromfenac

● **INDICATIONS AND DOSE**

Postoperative inflammation following cataract surgery
▶ TO THE EYE
▶ Adult: (consult product literature)

● INTERACTIONS → Appendix 1: NSAIDs

● MEDICINAL FORMS There can be variation in the licensing of different medicines containing the same drug.
Eye drops
EXCIPIENTS: May contain Benzalkonium chloride, disodium edetate, sulfites
▶ Yellox (Bausch & Lomb UK Ltd)
Bromfenac (as Bromfenac sodium sesquihydrate) 900 microgram per 1 ml Yellox 900micrograms/ml eye drops | 5 ml PoM £8.50 DT = £8.50

11

Eye

Diclofenac sodium

- **INDICATIONS AND DOSE**

Inhibition of intra-operative miosis during cataract surgery (but does not possess intrinsic mydriatic properties) | Postoperative inflammation in cataract surgery, strabismus surgery or argon laser trabeculoplasty | Pain in corneal epithelial defects after photorefractive keratectomy, radial keratotomy or accidental trauma | Seasonal allergic conjunctivitis
  - ▸ TO THE EYE
  - ▸ Adult: (consult product literature)

- **INTERACTIONS** → Appendix 1: NSAIDs
- **ALLERGY AND CROSS-SENSITIVITY** Contra-indicated in patients with a history of hypersensitivity to aspirin or any other NSAID—which includes those in whom attacks of asthma, angioedema, urticaria or rhinitis have been precipitated by aspirin or any other NSAID.
- **PRESCRIBING AND DISPENSING INFORMATION** Although multi-dose diclofenac sodium eye drops commonly contain preservatives, preservative-free unit dose vials may be available.

- **MEDICINAL FORMS**
  There can be variation in the licensing of different medicines containing the same drug.
  Eye drops
  EXCIPIENTS: May contain Benzalkonium chloride, disodium edetate, propylene glycol
  - ▸ Voltarol Ophtha (Thea Pharmaceuticals Ltd)
    Diclofenac sodium 1 mg per 1 ml Voltarol Ophtha 0.1% eye drops 0.3ml unit dose | 5 unit dose [PoM] £4.00 DT = £4.00 | 40 unit dose [PoM] £32.00 DT = £32.00
  - ▸ Voltarol Ophtha Multidose (Thea Pharmaceuticals Ltd)
    Diclofenac sodium 1 mg per 1 ml Voltarol Ophtha Multidose 0.1% eye drops | 5 ml [PoM] £6.68 DT = £6.68

Flurbiprofen

- **INDICATIONS AND DOSE**

Inhibition of intra-operative miosis (but does not possess intrinsic mydriatic properties) | Control of anterior segment inflammation following postoperative and post-laser trabeculoplasty when corticosteroids contra-indicated
  - ▸ TO THE EYE
  - ▸ Adult: (consult product literature)

- **INTERACTIONS** → Appendix 1: NSAIDs
- **ALLERGY AND CROSS-SENSITIVITY** Contra-indicated in patients with a history of hypersensitivity to aspirin or any other NSAID—which includes those in whom attacks of asthma, angioedema, urticaria or rhinitis have been precipitated by aspirin or any other NSAID.

- **MEDICINAL FORMS**
  There can be variation in the licensing of different medicines containing the same drug.
  Eye drops
  - ▸ Ocufen (Allergan Ltd)
    Flurbiprofen sodium 300 microgram per 1 ml Ocufen 0.03% eye drops 0.4ml unit dose | 40 unit dose [PoM] £37.15

Ketorolac trometamol

- **INDICATIONS AND DOSE**

Prophylaxis and reduction of inflammation and associated symptoms following ocular surgery
  - ▸ TO THE EYE
  - ▸ Adult: (consult product literature)

- **INTERACTIONS** → Appendix 1: NSAIDs
- **ALLERGY AND CROSS-SENSITIVITY** Contra-indicated in patients with a history of hypersensitivity to aspirin or any other NSAID—which includes those in whom attacks of asthma, angioedema, urticaria or rhinitis have been precipitated by aspirin or any other NSAID.

- **MEDICINAL FORMS**
  There can be variation in the licensing of different medicines containing the same drug.
  Eye drops
  EXCIPIENTS: May contain Benzalkonium chloride, disodium edetate
  - ▸ Ketorolac trometamol (Non-proprietary)
    Ketorolac trometamol 5 mg per 1 ml Ketorolac 0.5% eye drops | 5 ml [PoM] £2.85-£3.00 DT = £3.00
  - ▸ Acular (Allergan Ltd)
    Ketorolac trometamol 5 mg per 1 ml Acular 0.5% eye drops | 5 ml [PoM] £3.00 DT = £3.00

CORTICOSTEROIDS

Loteprednol etabonate

21-Dec-2017

- **INDICATIONS AND DOSE**

Treatment of post-operative inflammation following ocular surgery
  - ▸ TO THE EYE
  - ▸ Adult: Apply 4 times a day for maximum duration of treatment of 14 days, to be started 24 hours after surgery

---

IMPORTANT SAFETY INFORMATION

MHRA/CHM ADVICE: CORTICOSTEROIDS: RARE RISK OF CENTRAL SEROUS CHORIORETINOPATHY WITH LOCAL AS WELL AS SYSTEMIC ADMINISTRATION (AUGUST 2017)

See *Corticosteroids, general use* p. 656.

- **SIDE-EFFECTS**
  - ▸ **Common or very common** Dry eye · eye discomfort · eye disorders · headaches
  - ▸ **Uncommon** Conjunctival oedema · vision disorders
  - ▸ **Rare or very rare** Breast neoplasm · face oedema · muscle twitching · taste altered

- **MEDICINAL FORMS**
  There can be variation in the licensing of different medicines containing the same drug.
  Eye drops
  EXCIPIENTS: May contain Benzalkonium chloride, disodium edetate
  - ▸ Lotemax (Bausch & Lomb UK Ltd)
    Loteprednol etabonate 5 mg per 1 ml Lotemax 0.5% eye drops | 5 ml [PoM] £5.50 DT = £5.50

5 Glaucoma and ocular hypertension

Glaucoma

Overview

Glaucoma describes a group of disorders characterised by a loss of visual field associated with cupping of the optic disc and optic nerve damage. While glaucoma is generally associated with raised intra-ocular pressure, it can occur when the intra-ocular pressure is within the normal range.

The most common form of glaucoma is primary open-angle glaucoma (chronic open-angle glaucoma), where drainage of the aqueous humour through the trabecular meshwork is restricted. The condition is often asymptomatic, but the patient may present with significant loss of visual-field. Patients with ocular hypertension are at high risk of developing primary open-angle glaucoma.

Drugs that reduce intra-ocular pressure by different mechanisms are available for managing ocular hypertension and glaucoma. A topical beta-blocker or a prostaglandin analogue is usually the drug of first choice for the treatment of ocular hypertension. A prostaglandin analogue should be used to manage patients with early or moderate primary open-angle glaucoma. After checking compliance and eye drop instillation technique, it may be necessary to combine these drugs or add others, such as sympathomimetics, carbonic anhydrase inhibitors, or miotics to control intra-ocular pressure.

Acute angle-closure glaucoma

Acute angle-closure glaucoma occurs when the outflow of aqueous humour from the eye is obstructed by bowing of the iris against the trabecular meshwork; it is a medical emergency that requires urgent reduction of intra-ocular pressure to prevent loss of vision. Patients with acute angle-closure glaucoma should be referred immediately to specialist ophthalmology assessment and treatment.

Standard antiglaucoma therapy is used if supplementary treatment is required after iridotomy, iridectomy, laser treatment, or drainage surgery in either primary open-angle or acute angle-closure glaucoma.

Beta-blockers for glaucoma

Topical application of a beta-blocker to the eye reduces intra-ocular pressure effectively in *primary open-angle glaucoma*, probably by reducing the rate of production of aqueous humour. Administration by mouth also reduces intra-ocular pressure but this route is not used since side-effects may be troublesome.

Beta-blockers used as eye drops include betaxolol below, levobunolol hydrochloride p. 1146, and timolol maleate p. 1146.

Prostaglandin analogues and prostamides for glaucoma

The prostaglandin analogues latanoprost p. 1150, tafluprost p. 1151 and travoprost, and the synthetic prostamide, bimatoprost, increase uveoscleral outflow and subsequently reduce intra-ocular pressure. They are used to reduce intra-ocular pressure in ocular hypertension or open-angle glaucoma.

Sympathomimetics for glaucoma

Brimonidine tartrate, a selective alpha$_2$-adrenoceptor agonist, is thought to lower intra-ocular pressure by reducing aqueous humour formation and increasing uveoscleral outflow. It is licensed for the reduction of intra-ocular pressure in open-angle glaucoma or ocular hypertension in patients for whom beta-blockers are inappropriate; it may also be used as adjunctive therapy when intra-ocular pressure is inadequately controlled by other anti-glaucoma therapy.

Apraclonidine p. 1153 is another alpha$_2$- adrenoceptor agonist that lowers intra-ocular pressure by reducing aqueous humour formation. Eye drops containing apraclonidine 0.5% are used short-term to delay laser treatment or surgery in patients with glaucoma not adequately controlled by another drug; eye drops containing 1% are used for control of intra-ocular pressure after anterior segment laser surgery. Apraclonidine may not provide additional benefit in patients already using two drugs that suppress the production of aqueous humour.

Carbonic anhydrase inhibitors and systemic drugs for glaucoma

The **carbonic anhydrase inhibitors**, acetazolamide p. 1147, brinzolamide p. 1147, and dorzolamide p. 1148, reduce intra-

ocular pressure by reducing aqueous humour production. Systemic use of acetazolamide also produces weak diuresis.

Acetazolamide is given by mouth or by intravenous injection (intramuscular injections are painful because of the alkaline pH of the solution). It is used as an adjunct to other treatment for reducing intra-ocular pressure. Acetazolamide is not generally recommended for long-term use.

Dorzolamide and brinzolamide are topical carbonic anhydrase inhibitors. They are licensed for use in patients resistant to beta-blockers or those in whom beta-blockers are contra-indicated. They are used alone or as an adjunct to a topical beta-blocker. Brinzolamide can also be used as an adjunct to a prostaglandin analogue or the alpha2-adrenoceptor agonist, brimonidine tartrate p. 1153. Systemic absorption can rarely cause sulfonamide-like side-effects and may require discontinuation if severe.

The **osmotic diuretics**, intravenous hypertonic mannitol p. 228 or glycerol by mouth are useful short-term ocular hypotensive drugs.

Miotics for glaucoma

Miotics act by opening the inefficient drainage channels in the trabecular meshwork.

Pilocarpine p. 1149, a miotic, is not commonly used for the treatment of primary open-angle glaucoma because side-effects are poorly tolerated. It is used mainly in the treatment of primary angle-closure glaucoma and in some secondary glaucomas.

BETA-ADRENOCEPTOR BLOCKERS

Betaxolol

● **INDICATIONS AND DOSE**

Primary open-angle glaucoma

▶ TO THE EYE
▶ **Adult:** Apply twice daily

● CONTRA-INDICATIONS Also consider contra-indications listed for systemically administered beta blockers · bradycardia · heart block

● CAUTIONS Patients with corneal disease
 CAUTIONS, FURTHER INFORMATION Systemic absorption can follow topical application to the eyes; consider cautions listed for systemically administered beta blockers.

● INTERACTIONS → Appendix 1: beta blockers, selective

● SIDE-EFFECTS
▶ **Common or very common** Eye discomfort · eye disorders · vision disorders
▶ **Uncommon** Dry eye · eye inflammation · rhinitis
▶ **Rare or very rare** Cataract · rhinorrhoea · skin reactions
▶ **Frequency not known** Angioedema · hypersensitivity
 SIDE-EFFECTS, FURTHER INFORMATION Systemic absorption can follow topical application to the eyes; consider side effects listed for systemically administered beta blockers.

● PRESCRIBING AND DISPENSING INFORMATION Although multi-dose bextaxolol eye drops commonly contain preservatives, preservative-free unit dose vials may be available.

● MEDICINAL FORMS
 There can be variation in the licensing of different medicines containing the same drug.
 Eye drops
 EXCIPIENTS: May contain Benzalkonium chloride, disodium edetate
▶ Betaxolol (Non-proprietary)
  Betaxolol (as Betaxolol hydrochloride) 5 mg per 1 ml Betaxolol 0.5% eye drops | 5 ml [PoM] [🚫] DT = £1.90
▶ Betoptic (Novartis Pharmaceuticals UK Ltd)
  Betaxolol (as Betaxolol hydrochloride) 2.5 mg per 1 ml Betoptic 0.25% suspension eye drops | 5 ml [PoM] £2.66 DT = £2.66

11

Eye

Betoptic 0.25% eye drops suspension 0.25ml unit dose | 50 unit dose [PoM] £13.77 DT = £13.77
Betaxolol (as Betaxolol hydrochloride) 5 mg per 1 ml Betoptic 0.5% eye drops | 5 ml [PoM] £1.90 DT = £1.90

Levobunolol hydrochloride

● **INDICATIONS AND DOSE**

Primary open-angle glaucoma
▸ TO THE EYE
▸ Adult: Apply 1–2 times a day

● CONTRA-INDICATIONS Also consider contra-indications listed for systemically administered beta blockers · bradycardia · heart block
● CAUTIONS Patients with corneal disease
CAUTIONS, FURTHER INFORMATION Systemic absorption can follow topical application to the eyes; consider cautions listed for systemically administered beta blockers.
● INTERACTIONS → Appendix 1: beta blockers, non-selective
● SIDE-EFFECTS
▸ **Common or very common** Eye discomfort · eye inflammation
▸ **Frequency not known** Dry eye · eye disorders · vision blurred
SIDE-EFFECTS, FURTHER INFORMATION Systemic absorption can follow topical application to the eyes; consider side effects listed for systemically administered beta blockers.
● PRESCRIBING AND DISPENSING INFORMATION Although multi-dose (Levobunolol) eye drops commonly contain preservatives, preservative-free unit dose vials may be available.

● MEDICINAL FORMS
There can be variation in the licensing of different medicines containing the same drug.
Eye drops
EXCIPIENTS: May contain Benzalkonium chloride, disodium edetate, sodium metabisulfite
▸ Betagan (Allergan Ltd)
Levobunolol hydrochloride 5 mg per 1 ml Betagan 0.5% eye drops | 5 ml [PoM] £1.85 DT = £1.85
Betagan Unit Dose 0.5% eye drops 0.4ml unit dose | 30 unit dose [PoM] £9.98

Timolol maleate

● **INDICATIONS AND DOSE**

Reduction of intra-ocular pressure in primary open-angle glaucoma
▸ TO THE EYE
▸ Adult: Apply twice daily
TIMOPTOL-LA ®

Reduction of intra-ocular pressure in primary open-angle glaucoma
▸ TO THE EYE
▸ Adult: Apply once daily
TIOPEX ®

Reduction of intra-ocular pressure in primary open-angle glaucoma
▸ TO THE EYE
▸ Adult: Apply once daily, to be applied in the morning

● CONTRA-INDICATIONS Also consider contra-indications listed for systemically administered beta blockers · bradycardia · heart block
● CAUTIONS Consider also cautions listed for systemically administered beta blockers · patients with corneal disease
● INTERACTIONS → Appendix 1: beta blockers, non-selective

● SIDE-EFFECTS
▸ **Common or very common** Eye discomfort · eye disorders · eye inflammation · vision disorders
▸ **Rare or very rare** Angioedema
SIDE-EFFECTS, FURTHER INFORMATION Systemic absorption can follow topical application to the eyes; consider side effects listed for systemically administered beta blockers.
● BREAST FEEDING Manufacturer advises avoidance.
● PRESCRIBING AND DISPENSING INFORMATION Although multi-dose timolol eye drops commonly contain preservatives, preservative-free unit dose vials may be available.
● NATIONAL FUNDING/ACCESS DECISIONS
TIOPEX ®
Scottish Medicines Consortium (SMC) Decisions
▸ When used by eye The *Scottish Medicines Consortium* has advised (February 2014) that timolol gel eye drops (*Tiopex*®) are accepted for restricted use within NHS Scotland for the reduction of elevated intraocular pressure in patients with ocular hypertension or chronic open angle glaucoma who have proven sensitivity to preservatives.

● MEDICINAL FORMS
There can be variation in the licensing of different medicines containing the same drug.
Eye gel
EXCIPIENTS: May contain Benzododecinium bromide
▸ Timoptol-LA (Santen UK Ltd)
Timolol (as Timolol maleate) 2.5 mg per 1 ml Timoptol-LA 0.25% ophthalmic gel-forming solution | 2.5 ml [PoM] £3.12 DT = £3.12
Timolol (as Timolol maleate) 5 mg per 1 ml Timoptol-LA 0.5% ophthalmic gel-forming solution | 2.5 ml [PoM] £3.12 DT = £3.12
Eye drops
EXCIPIENTS: May contain Benzalkonium chloride
▸ Timolol maleate (Non-proprietary)
Timolol (as Timolol maleate) 2.5 mg per 1 ml Timolol 0.25% eye drops | 5 ml [PoM] £0.78 DT = £0.78
Timolol (as Timolol maleate) 5 mg per 1 ml Timolol 0.5% eye drops | 5 ml [PoM] £0.80 DT = £0.80
▸ Eysano (Aspire Pharma Ltd)
Timolol (as Timolol maleate) 2.5 mg per 1 ml Eysano 2.5mg/ml eye drops | 5 ml [PoM] £8.45 DT = £8.45
Timolol (as Timolol maleate) 5 mg per 1 ml Eysano 5mg/ml eye drops | 5 ml [PoM] £9.65 DT = £9.65
▸ Timoptol (Santen UK Ltd)
Timolol (as Timolol maleate) 2.5 mg per 1 ml Timoptol 0.25% eye drops | 5 ml [PoM] £3.12 DT = £0.78
Timolol (as Timolol maleate) 5 mg per 1 ml Timoptol 0.5% eye drops | 5 ml [PoM] £3.12 DT = £0.80
Timoptol Unit Dose 0.5% ophthalmic solution 0.2ml unit dose | 30 unit dose [PoM] £9.65 DT = £9.65
▸ Tiopex (Thea Pharmaceuticals Ltd)
Timolol (as Timolol maleate) 1 mg per 1 gram Tiopex 1mg/g eye gel 0.4g unit dose | 30 unit dose [PoM] £7.49 DT = £7.49

Combinations available: *Bimatoprost with timolol*, p. 1150 · *Brimonidine with timolol*, p. 1154 · *Brinzolamide with timolol*, p. 1148 · *Dorzolamide with timolol*, p. 1149 · *Latanoprost with timolol*, p. 1151 · *Tafluprost with timolol*, p. 1152 · *Travoprost with timolol*, p. 1152

CARBONIC ANHYDRASE INHIBITORS

Acetazolamide

● **INDICATIONS AND DOSE**

Reduction of intra-ocular pressure in open-angle glaucoma | Reduction of intra-ocular pressure in secondary glaucoma | Reduction of intra-ocular pressure perioperatively in angle-closure glaucoma

▸ BY MOUTH USING IMMEDIATE-RELEASE MEDICINES, OR BY INTRAVENOUS INJECTION, OR BY INTRAMUSCULAR INJECTION

▸ Adult: 0.25–1 g daily in divided doses, intramuscular injection preferably avoided because of alkalinity

Glaucoma

▸ BY MOUTH USING MODIFIED-RELEASE MEDICINES

▸ Adult: 250–500 mg daily

Epilepsy

▸ BY MOUTH USING IMMEDIATE-RELEASE MEDICINES, OR BY INTRAVENOUS INJECTION, OR BY INTRAMUSCULAR INJECTION

▸ Adult: 0.25–1 g daily in divided doses, intramuscular injection preferably avoided because of alkalinity

● CONTRA-INDICATIONS Adrenocortical insufficiency · hyperchloraemic acidosis · hypokalaemia · hyponatraemia · long-term administration in chronic angle-closure glaucoma

● CAUTIONS Avoid extravasation at injection site (risk of necrosis) · diabetes mellitus · elderly · impaired alveolar ventilation (risk of acidosis) · not generally recommended for long-term use · pulmonary obstruction (risk of acidosis) · renal calculi

● INTERACTIONS → Appendix 1: acetazolamide

● SIDE-EFFECTS

GENERAL SIDE-EFFECTS

▸ **Common or very common** Haemorrhage · metabolic acidosis · nephrolithiasis · sensation abnormal

▸ **Uncommon** Bone marrow disorders · depression · dizziness · electrolyte imbalance · hearing impairment · hepatic disorders · leucopenia · nausea · renal colic · renal impairment · renal lesions · severe cutaneous adverse reactions (SCARs) · skin reactions · thrombocytopenia · urinary tract discomfort · urine abnormalities · vomiting

▸ **Rare or very rare** Anaphylactic reaction · appetite changes · confusion · diarrhoea · fatigue · fever · flushing · headache · irritability · libido decreased · paralysis · photosensitivity reaction · seizure

▸ **Frequency not known** Agranulocytosis · drowsiness · myopia · polyuria · taste altered · thirst

SPECIFIC SIDE-EFFECTS

▸ **Uncommon**

▸ With oral use Osteomalacia

▸ **Rare or very rare**

▸ With oral use Ataxia · hyperglycaemia · hypoglycaemia · renal tubular necrosis

▸ **Frequency not known**

▸ With oral use Agitation

SIDE-EFFECTS, FURTHER INFORMATION Acetazolamide is a sulfonamide derivative; blood disorders, rashes, and other sulfonamide-related side-effects occur occasionally—patients should be told to report any unusual skin rash.

If electrolyte disturbances and metabolic acidosis occur, these can be corrected by administering bicarbonate.

● ALLERGY AND CROSS-SENSITIVITY Contra-indicated if history of sulfonamide hypersensitivity.

● PREGNANCY Manufacturer advises avoid, especially in first trimester (toxicity in *animal* studies).

● BREAST FEEDING Amount too small to be harmful.

● HEPATIC IMPAIRMENT Manufacturer advises avoid.

● RENAL IMPAIRMENT Avoid—risk of metabolic acidosis.

● MONITORING REQUIREMENTS Monitor blood count and plasma electrolyte concentrations with prolonged use.

● MEDICINAL FORMS
There can be variation in the licensing of different medicines containing the same drug. Forms available from special-order manufacturers include: oral suspension, oral solution

Tablet

CAUTIONARY AND ADVISORY LABELS 3

▸ Acetazolamide (Non-proprietary)
Acetazolamide 250 mg Acetazolamide 250mg tablets | 112 tablet PoM £75.36 DT = £16.86

Powder for solution for injection

▸ Diamox (AMCo)
Acetazolamide 500 mg Diamox Sodium Parenteral 500mg powder for solution for injection vials | 1 vial PoM £17.71

Modified-release capsule

CAUTIONARY AND ADVISORY LABELS 3, 25

▸ Diamox SR (AMCo)
Acetazolamide 250 mg Diamox SR 250mg capsules | 30 capsule PoM £16.66 DT = £16.66

▸ Eytazox (Teva UK Ltd)
Acetazolamide 250 mg Eytazox 250mg modified-release capsules | 30 capsule PoM £16.60 DT = £16.66

Brinzolamide

● **INDICATIONS AND DOSE**

Reduction of intra-ocular pressure in ocular hypertension and open-angle glaucoma either as adjunct to beta-blockers or prostaglandin analogues or used alone in patients unresponsive to beta-blockers or if beta-blockers contra-indicated

▸ TO THE EYE

▸ Adult: Apply twice daily, then increased if necessary up to 3 times a day

● CONTRA-INDICATIONS Hyperchloraemic acidosis

● CAUTIONS Renal tubular immaturity or abnormality · systemic absorption follows topical application

● INTERACTIONS → Appendix 1: brinzolamide

● SIDE-EFFECTS

▸ **Common or very common** Eye discomfort · eye disorders · taste altered · vision disorders

▸ **Uncommon** Arrhythmias · asthenia · cardio-respiratory distress · chest discomfort · cough · depression · diarrhoea · dizziness · dry eye · dry mouth · dyspnoea · epistaxis · eye deposit · eye inflammation · feeling abnormal · foreign body in eye · gastrointestinal discomfort · gastrointestinal disorders · headache · increased risk of infection · memory loss · motor dysfunction · muscle complaints · nasal complaints · nausea · nervousness · oral disorders · oropharyngeal pain · pain · palpitations · renal pain · scleral discolouration · sensation abnormal · sexual dysfunction · skin reactions · sleep disorders · throat complaints · vomiting

▸ **Rare or very rare** Alopecia · angina pectoris · drowsiness · irritability · optic nerve disorder · respiratory disorders · tinnitus

▸ **Frequency not known** Appetite decreased · arthralgia · asthma · hypertension · malaise · peripheral oedema · tremor · urinary frequency increased · vertigo

SIDE-EFFECTS, FURTHER INFORMATION Systemic absorption can rarely cause sulfonamide-like side-effects and may require discontinuation if severe.

● ALLERGY AND CROSS-SENSITIVITY Contra-indicated if history of sulfonamide hypersensitivity.

● PREGNANCY Avoid—toxicity in *animal* studies.

● BREAST FEEDING Use only if benefit outweighs risk.

● HEPATIC IMPAIRMENT Manufacturer advises avoid.

11

Eye

- RENAL IMPAIRMENT Avoid if eGFR less than 30 mL/minute/1.73 m².

- MEDICINAL FORMS
  There can be variation in the licensing of different medicines containing the same drug.
  Eye drops
  EXCIPIENTS: May contain Benzalkonium chloride, disodium edetate
  ▸ Brinzolamide (Non-proprietary)
  Brinzolamide 10 mg per 1 ml Brinzolamide 10mg/ml eye drops | 5 ml [PoM] £6.92 DT = £1.89
  ▸ Azopt (Novartis Pharmaceuticals UK Ltd)
  Brinzolamide 10 mg per 1 ml Azopt 10mg/ml eye drops | 5 ml [PoM] £6.92 DT = £1.89

Brinzolamide with brimonidine   27-Sep-2016

The properties listed below are those particular to the combination only. For the properties of the components please consider, brinzolamide p. 1147, brimonidine tartrate p. 1153.

- INDICATIONS AND DOSE
  Raised intra-ocular pressure in open-angle glaucoma and in ocular hypertension when monotherapy is inadequate
  ▸ TO THE EYE
  ▸ Adult: Apply 1 drop twice daily

- INTERACTIONS → Appendix 1: brimonidine · brinzolamide

- MEDICINAL FORMS
  There can be variation in the licensing of different medicines containing the same drug.
  Eye drops
  CAUTIONARY AND ADVISORY LABELS 3
  EXCIPIENTS: May contain Benzalkonium chloride, propylene glycol
  ▸ Simbrinza (Novartis Pharmaceuticals UK Ltd)
  Brimonidine tartrate 2 mg per 1 ml, Brinzolamide 10 mg per 1 ml Simbrinza 10mg/ml / 2mg/ml eye drops | 5 ml [PoM] £9.23 DT = £9.23

Brinzolamide with timolol

The properties listed below are those particular to the combination only. For the properties of the components please consider, brinzolamide p. 1147, timolol maleate p. 1146.

- INDICATIONS AND DOSE
  Raised intra-ocular pressure in open-angle glaucoma or ocular hypertension when beta-blocker alone not adequate
  ▸ TO THE EYE
  ▸ Adult: Apply twice daily

- INTERACTIONS → Appendix 1: beta blockers, non-selective · brinzolamide

- MEDICINAL FORMS
  There can be variation in the licensing of different medicines containing the same drug.
  Eye drops
  EXCIPIENTS: May contain Benzalkonium chloride, disodium edetate
  ▸ Azarga (Novartis Pharmaceuticals UK Ltd)
  Timolol (as Timolol maleate) 5 mg per 1 ml, Brinzolamide 10 mg per 1 ml Azarga 10mg/ml / 5mg/ml eye drops | 5 ml [PoM] £11.05 DT = £11.05

Dorzolamide

- INDICATIONS AND DOSE
  Raised intra-ocular pressure in ocular hypertension used alone in patients unresponsive to beta-blockers or if beta-blockers contra-indicated | Open-angle glaucoma used alone in patients unresponsive to beta-blockers or if beta-blockers contra-indicated | Pseudo-exfoliative glaucoma used alone in patients unresponsive to beta-blockers or if beta-blockers contra-indicated
  ▸ TO THE EYE
  ▸ Adult: Apply 3 times a day

  Raised intra-ocular pressure in ocular hypertension as adjunct to beta-blocker | Open-angle glaucoma as adjunct to beta-blocker | Pseudo-exfoliative glaucoma as adjunct to beta-blocker
  ▸ TO THE EYE
  ▸ Adult: Apply twice daily

- CONTRA-INDICATIONS Hyperchloraemic acidosis
- CAUTIONS Chronic corneal defects · history of intra-ocular surgery · history of renal calculi · low endothelial cell count · systemic absorption follows topical application
- INTERACTIONS → Appendix 1: dorzolamide
- SIDE-EFFECTS
  ▸ Common or very common Asthenia · eye discomfort · eye disorders · eye inflammation · headache · nausea · paraesthesia · taste bitter · vision disorders
  ▸ Rare or very rare Angioedema · bronchospasm · dizziness · dry mouth · dyspnoea · epistaxis · local reaction · pain · severe cutaneous adverse reactions (SCARs) · skin reactions · throat irritation · urolithiasis
  SIDE-EFFECTS, FURTHER INFORMATION Systemic absorption can cause sulfonamide-like side-effects and may require discontinuation if severe.
- ALLERGY AND CROSS-SENSITIVITY Contra-indicated if history of sulfonamide hypersensitivity.
- PREGNANCY Manufacturer advises avoid—toxicity in *animal* studies.
- BREAST FEEDING Manufacturer advises avoid—no information available.
- HEPATIC IMPAIRMENT Manufacturer advises caution— no information available.
- RENAL IMPAIRMENT Avoid if eGFR less than 30 mL/minute/1.73 m².
- PRESCRIBING AND DISPENSING INFORMATION Although multi-dose dorzolamide eye drops commonly contain preservatives, preservative-free unit dose vials may be available.

- MEDICINAL FORMS
  There can be variation in the licensing of different medicines containing the same drug.
  Eye drops
  EXCIPIENTS: May contain Benzalkonium chloride
  ▸ Dorzolamide (Non-proprietary)
  Dorzolamide (as Dorzolamide hydrochloride) 20 mg per 1 ml Dorzolamide 20mg/ml eye drops | 5 ml [PoM] £5.69 DT = £1.55
  ▸ Eydelto (Aspire Pharma Ltd)
  Dorzolamide (as Dorzolamide hydrochloride) 20 mg per 1 ml Eydelto 20mg/ml eye drops | 5 ml [PoM] £12.09 DT = £12.09
  ▸ Trusopt (Santen UK Ltd)
  Dorzolamide (as Dorzolamide hydrochloride) 20 mg per 1 ml Trusopt 20mg/ml eye drops 0.2ml unit dose preservative free | 60 unit dose [PoM] £24.18 DT = £24.18
  Trusopt 20mg/ml eye drops | 5 ml [PoM] £6.33 DT = £1.55

Dorzolamide with timolol

The properties listed below are those particular to the combination only. For the properties of the components please consider, dorzolamide p. 1148, timolol maleate p. 1146.

- **INDICATIONS AND DOSE**
  Raised intra-ocular pressure in ocular hypertension when beta-blockers alone not adequate | Raised intra-ocular pressure in open-angle glaucoma when beta-blockers alone not adequate | Raised intra-ocular pressure in pseudo-exfoliative glaucoma when beta-blockers alone not adequate
  ▶ TO THE EYE
  ▶ Adult: Apply twice daily

- INTERACTIONS → Appendix 1: beta blockers, non-selective · dorzolamide

- **PRESCRIBING AND DISPENSING INFORMATION** Although multi-dose dorzolamide with timolol eye drops commonly contain preservatives, preservative-free unit dose vials may be available.

- MEDICINAL FORMS
  There can be variation in the licensing of different medicines containing the same drug.
  Eye drops
  EXCIPIENTS: May contain Benzalkonium chloride
  ▶ Dorzolamide with timolol (Non-proprietary)
  Timolol (as Timolol maleate) 5 mg per 1 ml, Dorzolamide (as Dorzolamide hydrochloride) 20 mg per 1 ml Dorzolamide 20mg/ml / Timolol 5mg/ml eye drops 0.2ml unit dose preservative free | 60 unit dose ⟨PoM⟩ £25.99–£28.59 DT = £28.59
  Dorzolamide 20mg/ml / Timolol 5mg/ml eye drops | 5 ml ⟨PoM⟩ £27.16 DT = £1.50
  ▶ Cosopt (Santen UK Ltd)
  Timolol (as Timolol maleate) 5 mg per 1 ml, Dorzolamide (as Dorzolamide hydrochloride) 20 mg per 1 ml Cosopt 20mg/ml / 5mg/ml eye drops 0.2ml unit dose preservative free | 60 unit dose ⟨PoM⟩ £28.59 DT = £28.59
  Cosopt 20mg/ml / 5mg/ml eye drops | 5 ml ⟨PoM⟩ £10.05 DT = £1.50
  ▶ Eylamdo (Aspire Pharma Ltd)
  Timolol (as Timolol maleate) 5 mg per 1 ml, Dorzolamide (as Dorzolamide hydrochloride) 20 mg per 1 ml Eylamdo 20mg/ml / 5mg/ml eye drops | 5 ml ⟨PoM⟩ £14.29 DT = £14.29

MIOTICS › PARASYMPATHOMIMETICS

Pilocarpine

- DRUG ACTION Pilocarpine acts by opening the inefficient drainage channels in the trabecular meshwork.

- **INDICATIONS AND DOSE**
  Primary angle-closure glaucoma | Some secondary glaucomas
  ▶ TO THE EYE
  ▶ Adult: Apply up to 4 times a day

- CONTRA-INDICATIONS Acute inflammatory disease of the anterior segment · acute iritis · anterior uveitis · conditions where pupillary constriction is undesirable · some forms of secondary glaucoma (where pupillary constriction is undesirable)

- CAUTIONS A darkly pigmented iris may require a higher concentration of the miotic or more frequent administration and care should be taken to avoid overdosage · asthma · cardiac disease · care in conjunctival damage · care in corneal damage · epilepsy · gastro-intestinal spasm · hypertension · hyperthyroidism · hypotension · marked vasomotor instability · Parkinson's disease · peptic ulceration · retinal detachment has occurred in susceptible individuals and those with retinal disease · urinary-tract obstruction

- INTERACTIONS → Appendix 1: pilocarpine
- SIDE-EFFECTS
  ▶ **Common or very common** Diarrhoea · headache · hyperhidrosis · hypersalivation · nausea · skin reactions · vision disorders · vomiting
  ▶ **Frequency not known** Bradycardia · bronchospasm · conjunctival vascular congestion · eye disorder (long term use) · hypotension · pain · paraesthesia · pulmonary oedema · sensitisation · vitreous haemorrhage

- PREGNANCY Avoid unless the potential benefit outweighs risk—limited information available.

- BREAST FEEDING Avoid unless the potential benefit outweighs risk—no information available.

- PRE-TREATMENT SCREENING Fundus examination is advised before starting treatment with a miotic (retinal detachment has occurred).

- MONITORING REQUIREMENTS Intra-ocular pressure and visual fields should be monitored in those with chronic simple glaucoma and those receiving long-term treatment with a miotic.

- PRESCRIBING AND DISPENSING INFORMATION Although multi-dose pilocarpine eye drops commonly contain preservatives, preservative-free unit dose vials may be available.

- PATIENT AND CARER ADVICE
  Driving and skilled tasks Blurred vision may affect performance of skilled tasks (e.g. driving) particularly at night or in reduced lighting.

- MEDICINAL FORMS
  There can be variation in the licensing of different medicines containing the same drug. Forms available from special-order manufacturers include: oral solution, eye drops
  Eye drops
  EXCIPIENTS: May contain Benzalkonium chloride
  ▶ Pilocarpine (Non-proprietary)
  Pilocarpine hydrochloride 10 mg per 1 ml Pilocarpine hydrochloride 1% eye drops | 10 ml ⟨PoM⟩ £20.78 DT = £19.95
  Pilocarpine hydrochloride 20 mg per 1 ml Pilocarpine hydrochloride 2% eye drops | 10 ml ⟨PoM⟩ £21.52 DT = £19.88
  Pilocarpine hydrochloride 40 mg per 1 ml Pilocarpine hydrochloride 4% eye drops | 10 ml ⟨PoM⟩ £27.20 DT = £23.14
  ▶ Pilocarpine nitrate (Bausch & Lomb UK Ltd)
  Pilocarpine nitrate 20 mg per 1 ml Minims pilocarpine nitrate 2% eye drops 0.5ml unit dose | 20 unit dose ⟨PoM⟩ £12.47

PROSTAGLANDIN ANALOGUES AND PROSTAMIDES

Bimatoprost

- **INDICATIONS AND DOSE**
  Raised intra-ocular pressure in open-angle glaucoma | Ocular hypertension
  ▶ TO THE EYE
  ▶ Adult: Apply once daily, to be administered preferably in the evening

- CAUTIONS Angle-closure glaucoma (no experience of use) · aphakia · asthma · chronic obstructive pulmonary disease · compromised respiratory function · congenital glaucoma (no experience of use) · contact lens wearers · history of significant ocular viral infections · inflammatory ocular conditions (no experience of use) · narrow-angle glaucoma (no experience of use) · neovascular glaucoma (no experience of use) · predisposition to bradycardia · predisposition to hypotension · pseudophakia with torn posterior lens capsule or anterior chamber lenses · risk factors for cystoid macular oedema · risk factors for iritis · risk factors for uveitis

11

Eye

- SIDE-EFFECTS
  - **Common or very common** Dry eye · eye discolouration · eye discomfort · eye disorders · eye inflammation · headache · hypertension · hypertrichosis · skin reactions · vision disorders
  - **Uncommon** Asthenia · dizziness · madarosis · nausea · retinal haemorrhage
  - **Frequency not known** Asthma · bradycardia · dyspnoea · hypotension · reactivation of infection
- PREGNANCY Manufacturer advises use only if potential benefit outweighs risk.
- BREAST FEEDING Manufacturer advises avoid—present in milk in *animal* studies.
- HEPATIC IMPAIRMENT Use with caution in moderate to severe impairment—no information available.
- RENAL IMPAIRMENT Use with caution—no information available.
- PRESCRIBING AND DISPENSING INFORMATION Although multi-dose bimatoprost eye drops commonly contain preservatives, preservative-free unit dose vials may be available.
- PATIENT AND CARER ADVICE
  Changes to eye colour Before initiating treatment, patients should be warned of a possible change in eye colour as an increase in the brown pigment in the iris can occur, which may be permanent; particular care is required in those with mixed coloured irides and those receiving treatment to one eye only. Changes in eyelashes and vellus hair can also occur, and patients should also be advised to avoid repeated contact of the eye drop solution with skin as this can lead to hair growth or skin pigmentation.
- NATIONAL FUNDING/ACCESS DECISIONS
  LUMIGAN ®
  Scottish Medicines Consortium (SMC) Decisions
  The *Scottish Medicines Consortium* has advised (March 2013) that bimatoprost 300 micrograms/mL preservative-free eye drops (*Lumigan*® single-dose eye drops) are accepted for restricted use within NHS Scotland for the reduction of elevated intra-ocular pressure in chronic open-angle glaucoma and ocular hypertension (as monotherapy or as adjunctive therapy to beta-blockers) in adults who have proven sensitivity to benzalkonium chloride.

- MEDICINAL FORMS
  There can be variation in the licensing of different medicines containing the same drug.
  Eye drops
  EXCIPIENTS: May contain Benzalkonium chloride
  - Bimatoprost (Non-proprietary)
    Bimatoprost 300 microgram per 1 ml Bimatoprost 300micrograms/ml eye drops | 3 ml PoM £10.30 DT = £10.30
  - Eyreida (Aspire Pharma Ltd)
    Bimatoprost 300 microgram per 1 ml Eyreida 0.3mg/ml eye drops | 3 ml PoM £11.71
  - Lumigan (Allergan Ltd)
    Bimatoprost 100 microgram per 1 ml Lumigan 100micrograms/ml eye drops | 3 ml PoM £11.71 DT = £11.71 | 9 ml PoM £35.13
    Bimatoprost 300 microgram per 1 ml Lumigan 300micrograms/ml eye drops 0.4ml unit dose | 30 unit dose PoM £13.75 DT = £13.75
  - Sturiban (Actavis UK Ltd)
    Bimatoprost 300 microgram per 1 ml Sturiban 0.3mg/ml eye drops | 3 ml PoM £9.27 DT = £10.30 | 9 ml PoM £27.81

Bimatoprost with timolol

The properties listed below are those particular to the combination only. For the properties of the components please consider, bimatoprost p. 1149, timolol maleate p. 1146.

- INDICATIONS AND DOSE
  Raised intra-ocular pressure in patients with open-angle glaucoma or ocular hypertension when beta-blocker or prostaglandin analogue alone not adequate
  - TO THE EYE
  - Adult: Apply once daily
- INTERACTIONS → Appendix 1: beta blockers, non-selective
- NATIONAL FUNDING/ACCESS DECISIONS
  GANFORT ® SINGLE USE
  Scottish Medicines Consortium (SMC) Decisions
  The Scottish Medicines Consortium has advised (October 2013) that *Ganfort*® unit dose eye drops are accepted for restricted use within NHS Scotland for the reduction of intra-ocular pressure in patients with open-angle glaucoma or ocular hypertension insufficiently responsive to topical beta-blockers or prostaglandin analogues who have proven sensitivity to preservatives.

- MEDICINAL FORMS
  There can be variation in the licensing of different medicines containing the same drug.
  Eye drops
  EXCIPIENTS: May contain Benzalkonium chloride
  - Ganfort (Allergan Ltd)
    Bimatoprost 300 microgram per 1 ml, Timolol (as Timolol maleate) 5 mg per 1 ml Ganfort 0.3mg/ml / 5mg/ml eye drops | 3 ml PoM £14.16 DT = £14.16 | 9 ml PoM £38.15
    Ganfort 0.3mg/ml / 5mg/ml eye drops 0.4ml unit dose | 30 unit dose PoM £17.94 DT = £17.94

Latanoprost

- INDICATIONS AND DOSE
  Raised intra-ocular pressure in open-angle glaucoma | Ocular hypertension
  - TO THE EYE
  - Adult: Apply once daily, to be administered preferably in the evening

> IMPORTANT SAFETY INFORMATION
> MHRA/CHM ADVICE: LATANOPROST (*XALATAN*®): INCREASED REPORTING OF EYE IRRITATION SINCE REFORMULATION (JULY 2015)
> Following reformulation of *Xalatan*®, to allow for long-term storage at room temperature, there has been an increase in the number of reports of eye irritation from across the EU. Patients should be advised to tell their health professional promptly (within a week) if they experience eye irritation (e.g. excessive watering) severe enough to make them consider stopping treatment. Review treatment and prescribe a different formulation if necessary.

- CONTRA-INDICATIONS Active herpes simplex keratitis · history of recurrent herpetic keratitis associated with prostaglandin analogues
- CAUTIONS Angle-closure glaucoma (no experience of use) · aphakia · asthma · chronic obstructive pulmonary disease · compromised respiratory function · congenital glaucoma (no experience of use) · contact lens wearers · do not use within 5 minutes of thiomersal-containing preparations · history of significant ocular viral infections · inflammatory ocular conditions (no experience of use) · narrow-angle glaucoma (no experience of use) · neovascular glaucoma

(no experience of use) · peri-operative period of cataract surgery · pseudophakia with torn posterior lens capsule or anterior chamber lenses · risk factors for cystoid macular oedema · risk factors for iritis · risk factors for uveitis

● SIDE-EFFECTS
▶ **Common or very common** Eye discolouration · eye discomfort · eye disorders · eye inflammation · vision disorders
▶ **Uncommon** Dry eye · rash
▶ **Rare or very rare** Asthma · chest pain · dyspnoea · unstable angina
▶ **Frequency not known** Arthralgia · dizziness · headache · myalgia · ophthalmic herpes simplex · palpitations

● PREGNANCY Manufacturer advises avoid.

● BREAST FEEDING May be present in milk—manufacturer advises avoid.

● PRESCRIBING AND DISPENSING INFORMATION Although multi-dose latanoprost eye drops commonly contain preservatives, preservative-free unit dose vials may be available.

● PATIENT AND CARER ADVICE
Changes in eye colour Before initiating treatment, patients should be warned of a possible change in eye colour as an increase in the brown pigment in the iris can occur, which may be permanent; particular care is required in those with mixed coloured irides and those receiving treatment to one eye only. Changes in eyelashes and vellus hair can also occur, and patients should also be advised to avoid repeated contact of the eye drop solution with skin as this can lead to hair growth or skin pigmentation.

● NATIONAL FUNDING/ACCESS DECISIONS
MONOPOST ®
Scottish Medicines Consortium (SMC) Decisions
The *Scottish Medicines Consortium* has advised (June 2013) that *Monopost* ® is accepted for restricted use within NHS Scotland for the reduction of elevated intra-ocular pressure in patients with open-angle glaucoma and ocular hypertension who have proven sensitivity to benzalkonium chloride.

● MEDICINAL FORMS
There can be variation in the licensing of different medicines containing the same drug.
Eye drops
EXCIPIENTS: May contain Benzalkonium chloride
▶ Latanoprost (Non-proprietary)
  Latanoprost 50 microgram per 1 ml Latanoprost 50micrograms/ml eye drops | 2.5 ml [PoM] £12.48 DT = £1.53
▶ Medizol (Medicom Healthcare Ltd)
  Latanoprost 50 microgram per 1 ml Medizol 0.005% eye drops | 2.5 ml [PoM] £1.40 DT = £1.53
▶ Monopost (Thea Pharmaceuticals Ltd)
  Latanoprost 50 microgram per 1 ml Monopost 50micrograms/ml eye drops 0.2ml unit dose | 30 unit dose [PoM] £8.49 DT = £8.49 | 90 unit dose [PoM] £25.47 DT = £25.47
▶ Xalatan (Pfizer Ltd)
  Latanoprost 50 microgram per 1 ml Xalatan 50micrograms/ml eye drops | 2.5 ml [PoM] £12.48 DT = £1.53

Latanoprost with timolol

The properties listed below are those particular to the combination only. For the properties of the components please consider, latanoprost p. 1150, timolol maleate p. 1146.

● **INDICATIONS AND DOSE**
Raised intra-ocular pressure in patients with open-angle glaucoma and ocular hypertension when beta-blocker or prostaglandin analogue alone not adequate
▶ TO THE EYE
▶ Adult: Apply once daily

● INTERACTIONS → Appendix 1: beta blockers, non-selective

● MEDICINAL FORMS
There can be variation in the licensing of different medicines containing the same drug.
Eye drops
EXCIPIENTS: May contain Benzalkonium chloride
▶ Latanoprost with timolol (Non-proprietary)
  Latanoprost 50 microgram per 1 ml, Timolol (as Timolol maleate) 5 mg per 1 ml Latanoprost 50micrograms/ml / Timolol 5mg/ml eye drops | 2.5 ml [PoM] £14.32 DT = £2.44
▶ Xalacom (Pfizer Ltd)
  Latanoprost 50 microgram per 1 ml, Timolol (as Timolol maleate) 5 mg per 1 ml Xalacom eye drops | 2.5 ml [PoM] £14.32 DT = £2.44

Tafluprost

● **INDICATIONS AND DOSE**
Raised intra-ocular pressure in open-angle glaucoma | Ocular hypertension
▶ TO THE EYE
▶ Adult: Apply once daily, to be administered preferably in the evening

● CAUTIONS Angle-closure glaucoma (no experience of use) · aphakia · asthma · chronic obstructive pulmonary disease · compromised respiratory function · congenital glaucoma (no experience of use) · contact lens wearers · history of significant ocular viral infections · inflammatory ocular conditions (no experience of use) · narrow-angle glaucoma (no experience of use) · neovascular glaucoma (no experience of use) · pseudophakia with torn posterior lens capsule or anterior chamber lenses · risk factors for cystoid macular oedema · risk factors for iritis · risk factors for uveitis

● SIDE-EFFECTS
▶ **Common or very common** Dry eye · eye discolouration · eye discomfort · eye disorders · eye inflammation · headache · vision disorders
▶ **Uncommon** Hypertrichosis
▶ **Frequency not known** Asthma exacerbated · dyspnoea

● PREGNANCY Manufacturer advises avoid unless potential benefit outweighs risk—toxicity in *animal* studies.

● BREAST FEEDING Manufacturer advises avoid—present in milk in *animal* studies.

● HEPATIC IMPAIRMENT Use with caution—no information available.

● RENAL IMPAIRMENT Use with caution—no information available.

● PRESCRIBING AND DISPENSING INFORMATION Although multi-dose tafluprost eye drops commonly contain preservatives, preservative-free unit dose vials may be available.

● PATIENT AND CARER ADVICE
Changes to eye colour Before initiating treatment, patients should be warned of a possible change in eye colour as an increase in the brown pigment in the iris can occur, which may be permanent; particular care is required in those with mixed coloured irides and those receiving treatment to one eye only. Changes in eyelashes and vellus hair can also occur, and patients should also be advised to avoid repeated contact of the eye drop solution with skin as this can lead to hair growth or skin pigmentation.

● MEDICINAL FORMS
There can be variation in the licensing of different medicines containing the same drug.
Eye drops
EXCIPIENTS: May contain Disodium edetate
▶ Saflutan (Santen UK Ltd)
  Tafluprost 15 microgram per 1 ml Saflutan 15micrograms/ml eye drops 0.3ml unit dose | 30 unit dose [PoM] £12.20 DT = £12.20

11

Eye

Tafluprost with timolol

30-Mar-2016

The properties listed below are those particular to the combination only. For the properties of the components please consider, tafluprost p. 1151, timolol maleate p. 1146.

- **INDICATIONS AND DOSE**

Raised intra-ocular pressure in open-angle glaucoma and ocular hypertension when beta-blocker or prostaglandin analogue alone not adequate
  - ▸ TO THE EYE
  - ▸ Adult: Apply 1 drop once daily

- **INTERACTIONS** → Appendix 1: beta blockers, non-selective
- **PATIENT AND CARER ADVICE**
  Driving and skilled tasks Blurred vision may affect performance of skilled tasks (e.g. driving or operating machinery).
- **NATIONAL FUNDING/ACCESS DECISIONS**
  Scottish Medicines Consortium (SMC) Decisions
  The *Scottish Medicines Consortium* has advised (September 2015) that *Taptiqom®* (tafluprost with timolol) is accepted for restricted use within NHS Scotland, within the licensed indications, in patients who have proven sensitivity to preservatives.

- **MEDICINAL FORMS**
  There can be variation in the licensing of different medicines containing the same drug.

  Eye drops
  EXCIPIENTS: May contain Disodium edetate
  - ▸ Taptiqom (Santen UK Ltd)
    Tafluprost 15 microgram per 1 ml, Timolol (as Timolol maleate) 5 mg per 1 ml Taptiqom 15micrograms/ml / 5mg/ml eye drops 0.3ml unit dose | 30 unit dose [PoM] £14.50

Travoprost

- **INDICATIONS AND DOSE**

Raised intra-ocular pressure in open-angle glaucoma | Ocular hypertension
  - ▸ TO THE EYE
  - ▸ Adult: Apply once daily, to be administered preferably in the evening

- **CAUTIONS** History of significant ocular viral infections · angle-closure glaucoma (no experience of use) · aphakia · asthma · chronic obstructive pulmonary disease · compromised respiratory function · congenital glaucoma (no experience of use) · contact lens wearers · inflammatory ocular conditions (no experience of use) · narrow-angle glaucoma (no experience of use) · neovascular glaucoma (no experience of use) · pseudophakia with torn posterior lens capsule or anterior chamber lenses · risk factors for cystoid macular oedema · risk factors for iritis · risk factors for uveitis

- **SIDE-EFFECTS**
  - ▸ **Common or very common** Dry eye · eye discolouration · eye discomfort · eye disorders
  - ▸ **Uncommon** Cataract · cough · eye inflammation · hair changes · headache · nasal complaints · palpitations · seasonal allergy · skin reactions · throat irritation · vision disorders
  - ▸ **Rare or very rare** Allergic rhinitis · arthralgia · asthenia · asthma · constipation · dizziness · dry mouth · dysphonia · dyspnoea · gastrointestinal disorders · hypertension · hypotension · madarosis · musculoskeletal pain · ophthalmic herpes simplex · oropharyngeal pain · respiratory disorder · taste altered
  - ▸ **Frequency not known** Abdominal pain · anxiety · arrhythmias · chest pain · depression · diarrhoea · epistaxis

· insomnia · nausea · tinnitus · urinary disorders · vertigo · vomiting

- **PREGNANCY** Manufacturer advises avoid unless potential benefit outweighs risk—toxicity in *animal* studies.
- **BREAST FEEDING** Present in milk in *animal* studies; manufacturer advises avoid.
- **PATIENT AND CARER ADVICE**
  Changes to eye colour Before initiating treatment, patients should be warned of a possible change in eye colour as an increase in the brown pigment in the iris can occur, which may be permanent; particular care is required in those with mixed coloured irides and those receiving treatment to one eye only. Changes in eyelashes and vellus hair can also occur, and patients should also be advised to avoid repeated contact of the eye drop solution with skin as this can lead to hair growth or skin pigmentation.

- **MEDICINAL FORMS**
  There can be variation in the licensing of different medicines containing the same drug.

  Eye drops
  EXCIPIENTS: May contain Propylene glycol
  - ▸ Travoprost (Non-proprietary)
    Travoprost 40 microgram per 1 ml Travoprost 40micrograms/ml eye drops | 2.5 ml [PoM] £7.27–£10.95 DT = £7.27
  - ▸ Bondulc (Actavis UK Ltd)
    Travoprost 40 microgram per 1 ml Bondulc 40micrograms/ml eye drops | 2.5 ml [PoM] £10.94 DT = £7.27
  - ▸ Travatan (Novartis Pharmaceuticals UK Ltd)
    Travoprost 40 microgram per 1 ml Travatan 40micrograms/ml eye drops | 2.5 ml [PoM] £10.95 DT = £7.27

Travoprost with timolol

The properties listed below are those particular to the combination only. For the properties of the components please consider, travoprost above, timolol maleate p. 1146.

- **INDICATIONS AND DOSE**

Raised intra-ocular pressure in patients with open-angle glaucoma or ocular hypertension when beta-blocker or prostaglandin analogue alone not adequate
  - ▸ TO THE EYE
  - ▸ Adult: Apply once daily

- **INTERACTIONS** → Appendix 1: beta blockers, non-selective

- **MEDICINAL FORMS**
  There can be variation in the licensing of different medicines containing the same drug.

  Eye drops
  EXCIPIENTS: May contain Propylene glycol
  - ▸ Travoprost with timolol (Non-proprietary)
    Travoprost 40 microgram per 1 ml, Timolol (as Timolol maleate) 5 mg per 1 ml Travoprost 40micrograms/ml / Timolol 5mg/ml eye drops | 2.5 ml [PoM] £13.95 DT = £13.95
  - ▸ DuoTrav (Novartis Pharmaceuticals UK Ltd)
    Travoprost 40 microgram per 1 ml, Timolol (as Timolol maleate) 5 mg per 1 ml DuoTrav 40micrograms/ml / 5mg/ml eye drops | 2.5 ml [PoM] £13.95 DT = £13.95 | 7.5 ml [PoM] £39.68

SYMPATHOMIMETICS > ALPHA₂-ADRENOCEPTOR AGONISTS

Apraclonidine

- **DRUG ACTION** Apraclonidine is an alpha₂-adrenoceptor agonist that lowers intra-ocular pressure by reducing aqueous humour formation. It is a derivative of clonidine.

- **INDICATIONS AND DOSE**

  Control or prevention of postoperative elevation of intra-ocular pressure after anterior segment laser surgery
  - TO THE EYE
  - Adult: Apply 1 drop, 1 hour before laser procedure, then 1 drop, immediately after completion of procedure, 1% eye drops to be administered

  Short-term adjunctive treatment of chronic glaucoma in patients not adequately controlled by another drug
  - TO THE EYE
  - Adult: Apply 1 drop 3 times a day usually for maximum 1 month, 0.5% eye drops to be administered, may not provide additional benefit if patient already using two drugs that suppress the production of aqueous humour

- **CONTRA-INDICATIONS** History of severe or unstable and uncontrolled cardiovascular disease

- **CAUTIONS** Cerebrovascular disease · depression · heart failure · history of angina · hypertension · loss of effect may occur over time · Parkinson's syndrome · Raynaud's syndrome · recent myocardial infarction · reduction in vision in end-stage glaucoma (suspend treatment) · severe coronary insufficiency · thromboangiitis obliterans · vasovagal attack

- **INTERACTIONS** → Appendix 1: apraclonidine

- **SIDE-EFFECTS**
  - **Common or very common** Eye disorders
  - **Uncommon** Bradycardia · conjunctival haemorrhage · diarrhoea · dry eye · eye discomfort · eye inflammation · gastrointestinal discomfort · irritability · libido decreased · nasal dryness · palpitations · postural hypotension · sensation abnormal · sleep disorders · syncope · vision disorders · vomiting
  - **Rare or very rare** Chest pain · dry mouth · fatigue · headache · hyperhidrosis · pain in extremity · pruritus · taste altered · temperature sensation altered

    SIDE-EFFECTS, FURTHER INFORMATION Since systemic absorption may follow topical application, see clonidine hydrochloride p. 144.
    Ocular intolerance Manufacturer advises withdrawal if eye pruritus, ocular hyperaemia, increased lacrimation, or oedema of the eyelids and conjunctiva occur.

- **PREGNANCY** Manufacturer advises avoid—no information available.

- **BREAST FEEDING** Manufacturer advises avoid—no information available.

- **HEPATIC IMPAIRMENT** Manufacturer advises caution.

- **RENAL IMPAIRMENT** Use with caution in chronic renal failure.

- **MONITORING REQUIREMENTS**
  - Monitor intra-ocular pressure and visual fields.
  - Monitor for excessive reduction in intra-ocular pressure following peri-operative use.

- **PATIENT AND CARER ADVICE**
  Driving and skilled tasks Drowsiness may affect performance of skilled tasks (e.g. driving).

- **MEDICINAL FORMS**
  There can be variation in the licensing of different medicines containing the same drug.
  Eye drops
  EXCIPIENTS: May contain Benzalkonium chloride
  - Iopidine (Novartis Pharmaceuticals UK Ltd)
    Apraclonidine (as Apraclonidine hydrochloride) 5 mg per 1 ml Iopidine 5mg/ml eye drops | 5 ml [PoM] £10.88 DT = £10.88
    Apraclonidine (as Apraclonidine hydrochloride) 10 mg per 1 ml Iopidine 1% eye drops 0.25ml unit dose | 24 unit dose [PoM] £77.85 DT = £77.85

Brimonidine tartrate

12-Jul-2017

- **DRUG ACTION** Brimonidine, an alpha₂-adrenoceptor agonist, is thought to lower intra-ocular pressure by reducing aqueous humour formation and increasing uveoscleral outflow.

- **INDICATIONS AND DOSE**

  Raised intra-ocular pressure in open-angle glaucoma in patients for whom beta-blockers are inappropriate | Ocular hypertension in patients for whom beta-blockers are inappropriate | Adjunctive therapy when intra-ocular pressure is inadequately controlled by other antiglaucoma therapy
  - TO THE EYE
  - Adult: Apply twice daily

- **CAUTIONS** Cerebral insufficiency · coronary insufficiency · depression · postural hypotension · Raynaud's syndrome · severe cardiovascular disease · thromboangitis obliterans

- **INTERACTIONS** → Appendix 1: brimonidine

- **SIDE-EFFECTS**
  - **Common or very common** Asthenia · dizziness · drowsiness · dry eye · dry mouth · eye discomfort · eye disorders · eye inflammation · gastrointestinal disorder · headache · hypersensitivity · respiratory disorders · sensation of foreign body · skin reactions · taste altered · vascular disorders · vision disorders
  - **Uncommon** Arrhythmias · nasal dryness · palpitations
  - **Rare or very rare** Dyspnoea · hypertension · hypotension · insomnia · syncope
  - **Frequency not known** Face oedema · vasodilation

- **PREGNANCY** Manufacturer advises use only if benefit outweighs risk—limited information available.

- **BREAST FEEDING** Manufacturer advises avoid—no information available.

- **HEPATIC IMPAIRMENT** Manufacturer advises use with caution.

- **RENAL IMPAIRMENT** Manufacturer advises use with caution.

- **PATIENT AND CARER ADVICE**
  Driving and skilled tasks Drowsiness may affect performance of skilled tasks (e.g. driving).

- **MEDICINAL FORMS**
  There can be variation in the licensing of different medicines containing the same drug.
  Eye drops
  EXCIPIENTS: May contain Benzalkonium chloride
  - Brimonidine tartrate (Non-proprietary)
    Brimonidine tartrate 2 mg per 1 ml Brimonidine 0.2% eye drops | 5 ml [PoM] £6.85 DT = £1.13
  - Alphagan (Allergan Ltd)
    Brimonidine tartrate 2 mg per 1 ml Alphagan 0.2% eye drops | 5 ml [PoM] £6.85 DT = £1.13
  - Brymont (Blumont Pharma Ltd)
    Brimonidine tartrate 2 mg per 1 ml Brymont 2mg/ml eye drops | 5 ml [PoM] £2.27 DT = £1.13

  Combinations available: *Brinzolamide with brimonidine,* p. 1148

11

Eye

Brimonidine with timolol

The properties listed below are those particular to the combination only. For the properties of the components please consider, brimonidine tartrate p. 1153, timolol maleate p. 1146.

- ● INDICATIONS AND DOSE

Raised intra-ocular pressure in open-angle glaucoma and for ocular hypertension when beta-blocker alone not adequate
  - ▸ TO THE EYE
  - ▸ Adult: Apply twice daily

- ● INTERACTIONS → Appendix 1: beta blockers, non-selective · brimonidine

- ● MEDICINAL FORMS
  There can be variation in the licensing of different medicines containing the same drug.

  Eye drops
  EXCIPIENTS: May contain Benzalkonium chloride
  - ▸ Combigan (Allergan Ltd)
    Brimonidine tartrate 2 mg per 1 ml, Timolol (as Timolol maleate) 5 mg per 1 ml Combigan eye drops | 5 ml [PoM] £10.00 DT = £10.00 | 15 ml [PoM] £27.00

6 Retinal disorders
6.1 Macular degeneration

Subfoveal choroidal neovascularisation

Treatment

Aflibercept p. 1154, pegaptanib sodium and ranibizumab p. 1155 are vascular endothelial growth factor inhibitors licensed for the treatment of neovascular (wet) age-related macular degeneration. Aflibercept is also licensed for the treatment of macular oedema secondary to central retinal vein occlusion, and diabetic macular oedema; ranibizumab is also licensed for the treatment of visual impairment due to diabetic macular oedema, macular oedema secondary to branch or central retinal vein occlusion, and choroidal neovascularisation secondary to pathologic myopia. Ranibizumab can be administered concomitantly with laser photocoagulation for the treatment of diabetic macular oedema and for macular oedema secondary to branch retinal vein occlusion.

ANTINEOVASCULARISATION DRUGS ›
VASCULAR ENDOTHELIAL GROWTH FACTOR INHIBITORS

Aflibercept

06-Dec-2017

- ● DRUG ACTION Aflibercept is a recombinant fusion protein that acts as a soluble decoy receptor and binds to vascular endothelial growth factors A and B (VEGF-A, VEGF-B) and placental growth factor (PlGF). Aflibercept inhibits the activation of VEGF receptors and the proliferation of endothelial cells, thereby inhibiting the growth of new vessels.

- ● INDICATIONS AND DOSE

Neovascular (wet) age-related macular degeneration (specialist use only)
  - ▸ BY INTRAVITREAL INJECTION
  - ▸ Adult: Initially 2 mg once a month for 3 months, then 2 mg every 2 months, review treatment frequency after 12 months

Macular oedema secondary to retinal vein occlusion (specialist use only)
  - ▸ BY INTRAVITREAL INJECTION
  - ▸ Adult: Initially 2 mg once a month until maximum visual acuity is achieved or there are no signs of disease activity (discontinue treatment if no improvement in visual and anatomic outcomes)

Diabetic macular oedema (specialist use only)
  - ▸ BY INTRAVITREAL INJECTION
  - ▸ Adult: Initially 2 mg once a month for 5 months, then maintenance 2 mg every 2 months, review treatment frequency after 12 months (discontinue treatment if no improvement in visual and anatomic outcomes)

Myopic choroidal neovascularisation (specialist use only)
  - ▸ BY INTRAVITREAL INJECTION
  - ▸ Adult: 2 mg for 1 dose, if visual or anatomic outcomes indicate that disease persists, additional doses may be administered; the interval between 2 doses should be greater than 1 month

- ● CONTRA-INDICATIONS Clinical signs of irreversible ischaemic visual function loss · ocular or periocular infection · severe intra-ocular inflammation

- ● CAUTIONS Active systemic infection · diabetic patients with uncontrolled hypertension · discontinue treatment if stage 3 or 4 macular holes develop—consult product literature for full details · discontinue treatment in the event of a retinal break—consult product literature for full details · discontinue treatment in the event of rhegmatogenous retinal detachment—consult product literature for full details · patients at risk of retinal pigment epithelial tear · poorly controlled glaucoma · recent history of myocardial infarction · recent history of stroke · recent history of transient ischaemic attack

  CAUTIONS, FURTHER INFORMATION Aflibercept is given by intravitreal injection by specialists experienced in the management of this condition. There is a potential risk of arterial thromboembolic events and non-ocular haemorrhage following the intravitreal injection of vascular endothelial growth factor inhibitors. Endophthalmitis can occur after intravitreal injections—patients should be advised to report any signs of infection immediately.

- ● INTERACTIONS → Appendix 1: aflibercept

- ● SIDE-EFFECTS
  - ▸ **Common or very common** Cataract · eye discomfort · eye disorders · eye inflammation · haemorrhage · retinal pigment epithelial tear · vision disorders
  - ▸ **Uncommon** Lens opacity

- ● CONCEPTION AND CONTRACEPTION Manufacturer recommends women use effective contraception during and for at least 3 months after treatment.

- ● PREGNANCY Manufacturer advises avoid unless potential benefit outweighs risk.

- ● BREAST FEEDING Manufacturer advises avoid—no information available.

- ● MONITORING REQUIREMENTS Monitor intra-ocular pressure following injection.

- ● DIRECTIONS FOR ADMINISTRATION For further information on administration, consult product literature.

- ● NATIONAL FUNDING/ACCESS DECISIONS

  NICE decisions
  - ▸ **Aflibercept solution for injection for treating wet age-related macular degeneration (July 2013)** NICE TA294
    Aflibercept solution for injection is recommended as an option for treating wet age-related macular degeneration only if:
    - ● it is used in accordance with the recommendations for ranibizumab in NICE TA 155 **and**

- the manufacturer provides aflibercept solution for injection with the discount agreed in the patient access scheme

www.nice.org.uk/guidance/TA294

▸ **Aflibercept for treating visual impairment caused by macular oedema secondary to central retinal vein occlusion** (February 2014) NICE TA305

Aflibercept solution for injection is recommended as an option for treating visual impairment caused by macular oedema secondary to central retinal vein occlusion only if the manufacturer provides aflibercept solution for injection with the discount agreed in the patient access scheme.

www.nice.org.uk/guidance/TA305

▸ **Aflibercept for treating diabetic macular oedema** (July 2015) NICE TA346

Aflibercept solution for injection is recommended as an option for treating visual impairment caused by diabetic macular oedema only if:

- the eye has a central retinal thickness of 400 micrometres or more at the start of treatment **and**
- the manufacturer provides aflibercept with the discount agreed in the patient access scheme.

www.nice.org.uk/guidance/TA346

▸ **Aflibercept for treating visual impairment caused by macular oedema after branch retinal vein occlusion** (September 2016) NICE TA409

Aflibercept is recommended, within its marketing authorisation, as an option for treating visual impairment in adults caused by macular oedema after branch retinal vein occlusion, only if the manufacturer provides aflibercept with the discount agreed in the patient access scheme.

www.nice.org.uk/guidance/TA409

▸ **Aflibercept for treating choroidal neovascularisation** (November 2017) NICE TA486

Aflibercept is recommended, within its marketing authorisation, as an option for treating visual impairment because of myopic choroidal neovascularisation in adults, only if the manufacturer provides aflibercept with the discount agreed in the patient access scheme.

If patients and their clinicians consider both aflibercept and ranibizumab to be suitable treatments, the least costly should be used, taking into account anticipated administration costs, dosage and price per dose.

www.nice.org.uk/guidance/TA486

Scottish Medicines Consortium (SMC) Decisions
The *Scottish Medicines Consortium* has advised (October 2016) that aflibercept (*Eylea* ®) is accepted for use within NHS Scotland in adults for the treatment of visual impairment due to myopic choroidal neovascularisation. This advice is contingent upon the continuing availability of the patient access scheme in NHS Scotland or a list price that is equivalent or lower.

- MEDICINAL FORMS
There can be variation in the licensing of different medicines containing the same drug.
Solution for injection
▸ Eylea (Bayer Plc)
   Aflibercet 40 mg per 1 ml Eylea 2nm/50 microlitres solution for injection | 1 vial [PoM] £816.00

Ranibizumab

- INDICATIONS AND DOSE

Neovascular (wet) age-related macular degeneration (specialist use only)
▸ BY INTRAVITREAL INJECTION
▸ Adult: 500 micrograms once a month, to be administered into the affected eye, monitor visual acuity monthly, continue treatment until visual acuity is stable for 3 consecutive months, thereafter monitor visual acuity monthly, if necessary subsequent doses may be given at least 1 month apart

Diabetic macular oedema | Macular oedema secondary to retinal vein occlusion (specialist use only)
▸ BY INTRAVITREAL INJECTION
▸ Adult: Initially 500 micrograms once a month, to be administered into the affected eye, monitor visual acuity monthly, continue treatment until visual acuity is stable for 3 consecutive months (discontinue treatment if no improvement in visual acuity after initial 3 injections), thereafter monitor visual acuity monthly, if necessary subsequent doses may be given at least 1 month apart

Choroidal neovascularisation secondary to pathologic myopia (specialist use only)
▸ BY INTRAVITREAL INJECTION
▸ Adult: Initially 500 micrograms, to be administered as a single injection into the affected eye, monitor for disease activity monthly for first 2 months, then at least every 3 months thereafter during the first year, then as required, if necessary subsequent doses may be given at least 1 month apart

Concomitant treatment of diabetic macular oedema, or macular oedema secondary to branch retinal vein occlusion, with laser photocoagulation (specialist use only)
▸ BY INTRAVITREAL INJECTION
▸ Adult: 500 micrograms, to be administered at least 30 minutes after laser photocoagulation

- CONTRA-INDICATIONS Ocular or periocular infection · severe intra-ocular inflammation · signs of irreversible ischaemic visual function loss in patients with retinal vein occlusion

- CAUTIONS Active systemic infection · diabetic macular oedema due to type 1 diabetes (limited information available) · diabetic patients with HbA$_{1c}$ over 12% · history of stroke · history of transient ischaemic attack · patients at risk of retinal pigment epithelial tear · previous intravitreal injections · proliferative diabetic retinopathy · retinal detachment or macular hole (discontinue treatment if rhegmatogenous retinal detachment or stage 3 or 4 macular holes develop) · uncontrolled hypertension

   CAUTIONS, FURTHER INFORMATION Ranibizumab is given by intravitreal injection by specialists. There is a potential risk of arterial thromboembolic events and non-ocular haemorrhage following the intravitreal injection of vascular endothelial growth factor inhibitors. Endophthalmitis can occur after intravitreal injections—patients should be advised to report any signs of infection immediately.

- INTERACTIONS → Appendix 1: ranibizumab

- SIDE-EFFECTS
▸ **Common or very common** Anaemia · anxiety · arthralgia · cataract · cough · dry eye · eye discomfort · eye disorders · eye inflammation · haemorrhage · headache · hypersensitivity · increased risk of infection · lens opacity · nausea · retinal pigment epithelial tear · vision disorders
▸ **Uncommon** Corneal deposits
▸ **Frequency not known** Arterial thromboembolism

11

Eye

- CONCEPTION AND CONTRACEPTION Manufacturer recommends women use effective contraception during and for at least 3 months after treatment.
- PREGNANCY Manufacturer advises avoid unless potential benefit outweighs risk.
- BREAST FEEDING Manufacturer advises avoid—no information available.
- MONITORING REQUIREMENTS
▶ Monitor intra-ocular pressure, perfusion of the optic nerve head, and for signs of ocular infection following injection.
▶ Monitor visual acuity, see individual indications and dose for frequency.
- DIRECTIONS FOR ADMINISTRATION For further information on administration, consult product literature.
- NATIONAL FUNDING/ACCESS DECISIONS

NICE decisions
▶ **Ranibizumab for treating choroidal neovascularisation associated with pathological myopia (November 2013)** NICE TA298
Ranibizumab is recommended as an option for treating visual impairment due to choroidal neovascularisation secondary to pathological myopia when the manufacturer provides ranibizumab with the discount agreed in the patient access scheme.
www.nice.org.uk/TA298
▶ **Ranibizumab for the treatment of visual impairment caused by macular oedema secondary to retinal vein occlusion (May 2013)** NICE TA283
Ranibizumab is recommended as an option for treating visual impairment caused by macular oedema:
 - following central retinal vein occlusion **or**
 - following branch retinal vein occlusion only if treatment with laser photocoagulation has not been beneficial, or when laser photocoagulation is not suitable because of the extent of macular haemorrhage **and**
 - only if the manufacturer provides ranibizumab with the discount agreed in the patient access scheme revised in the context of NICE technology appraisal guidance 274.
www.nice.org.uk/TA283
▶ **Ranibizumab for the treatment of diabetic macular oedema (February 2013)** NICE TA274
Ranibizumab is recommended as an option for the treatment of visual impairment due to diabetic macular oedema only if:
 - the eye has a central retinal thickness of 400 micrometres or more at the start of treatment **and**
 - the manufacturer provides ranibizumab with the discount agreed in the patient access scheme (as revised in 2012).
Patients currently receiving ranibizumab for treating visual impairment due to diabetic macular oedema whose disease does not meet the criteria should be able to continue treatment until they and their clinician consider it appropriate to stop.
www.nice.org.uk/TA274
▶ **Ranibizumab and pegaptanib for the treatment of age-related macular degeneration (updated May 2012)** NICE TA155
Ranibizumab is recommended for the treatment of wet age-related macular degeneration if all of the following apply:
 - the best corrected visual acuity is between 6/12 and 6/96;
 - there is no permanent structural damage to the central fovea;
 - the lesion size is less than or equal to 12 disc areas in greatest linear dimension;
 - there is evidence of recent disease progression;
 - the manufacturer provides ranibizumab with the discount agreed in the patient access scheme (as revised in 2012).

Ranibizumab should only be continued in patients who maintain adequate response to therapy.
www.nice.org.uk/TA155

Scottish Medicines Consortium (SMC) Decisions
The *Scottish Medicines Consortium* has advised (May 2007) that ranibizumab (*Lucentis*®) is accepted for use within NHS Scotland for the treatment of neovascular (wet) age-related macular degeneration.

The *Scottish Medicines Consortium* has advised (October 2011 and April 2013) that ranibizumab (*Lucentis*®) is accepted for use within NHS Scotland for the treatment of macular oedema secondary to branch or central retinal vein occlusion, and (November 2012) for restricted use for the treatment of visual impairment due to diabetic macular oedema in adults with best corrected visual acuity 75 Early Treatment Diabetic Retinopathy Study letters or less at baseline, and (October 2013) for the treatment of visual impairment due to choroidal neovascularisation secondary to pathologic myopia in adults; SMC advice is contingent upon the continuing availability of ranibizumab at the price agreed in the patient access scheme.

- MEDICINAL FORMS
There can be variation in the licensing of different medicines containing the same drug.

Solution for injection
▶ Lucentis (Novartis Pharmaceuticals UK Ltd)
Ranibizumab 10 mg per 1 ml Lucentis 2.3mg/0.23ml solution for injection vials | 1 vial [PoM] £551.00 (Hospital only)
Lucentis 1.65mg/0.165ml solution for injection pre-filled syringes | 1 pre-filled disposable injection [PoM] £551.00

PHOTOSENSITISERS

Verteporfin

- DRUG ACTION Following intravenous infusion, verteporfin is activated by local irradiation using non-thermal red light to produce cytotoxic derivatives.

- INDICATIONS AND DOSE

Photodynamic treatment of age-related macular degeneration associated with predominantly classic subfoveal choroidal neovascularisation or with pathological myopia (specialist use only)
▶ BY INTRAVENOUS INFUSION
▶ Adult: 6 mg/m², dose to be given over 10 minutes

- CONTRA-INDICATIONS Acute porphyrias p. 1025
- CAUTIONS Avoid extravasation · biliary obstruction · photosensitivity
- INTERACTIONS → Appendix 1: verteporfin
- SIDE-EFFECTS
▶ **Common or very common** Asthenia · dizziness · dyspnoea · headache · hypercholesterolaemia · hypersensitivity · infusion related reaction · nausea · photosensitivity reaction · syncope · vision disorders
▶ **Uncommon** Eye inflammation · fever · haemorrhage · hyperaesthesia · hypertension · pain · retinal detachment · skin reactions
▶ **Rare or very rare** Malaise · retinal ischaemia
▶ **Frequency not known** Myocardial infarction · retinal pigment epithelial tear
- PREGNANCY Manufacturer advises use only if potential benefit outweighs risk (teratogenic in *animal* studies).
- BREAST FEEDING No information available—manufacturer advises avoid breast-feeding for 48 hours after administration.
- HEPATIC IMPAIRMENT Use with caution in moderate hepatic impairment. Avoid in severe hepatic impairment.

- DIRECTIONS FOR ADMINISTRATION For information on administration and light activation, consult product literature.

  For *intravenous infusion* (*Visudyne*®), give intermittently in Glucose 5%; reconstitute each 15 mg with 7 ml water for injections to produce a 2 mg/ml solution then dilute requisite dose with infusion fluid to a final volume of 30 mL and give over 10 minutes; protect infusion from light and administer within 4 hours of reconstitution. Incompatible with sodium chloride infusion.

- PATIENT AND CARER ADVICE Photosensitivity—avoid exposure of unprotected skin and eyes to bright light during infusion and for 48 hours afterwards.

- NATIONAL FUNDING/ACCESS DECISIONS

  NICE decisions

  ▶ Verteporfin photodynamic therapy for wet age-related macular degeneration (September 2003) NICE TA68
  Photodynamic therapy is recommended for wet age-related macular degeneration with a confirmed diagnosis of classic (no occult) subfoveal choroidal neovascularisation and best-corrected visual acuity of 6/60 or better.

  Photodynamic therapy is **not** recommended for wet age-related macular degeneration with predominantly classic but partly occult subfoveal choroidal neovascularisation *except* in clinical studies.
  www.nice.org.uk/TA68

- MEDICINAL FORMS
  There can be variation in the licensing of different medicines containing the same drug.

  Powder for solution for infusion
  EXCIPIENTS: May contain Butylated hydroxytoluene
  ▶ Visudyne (Novartis Pharmaceuticals UK Ltd)
  Verteporfin 15 mg Visudyne 15mg powder for solution for infusion vials | 1 vial PoM £850.00 (Hospital only)

6.2 Macular oedema

Other drugs used for Macular oedema Aflibercept, p. 1154
· Dexamethasone, p. 1127 · Ranibizumab, p. 1155

CORTICOSTEROIDS

Fluocinolone acetonide   21-Dec-2017

- ● INDICATIONS AND DOSE

  Treatment of visual impairment associated with chronic diabetic macular oedema which is insufficiently responsive to available therapies (specialist use only)
  ▶ BY INTRAVITREAL INJECTION
  ▸ Adult: 190 micrograms, to be administered into the affected eye

  IMPORTANT SAFETY INFORMATION
  MHRA/CHM ADVICE: CORTICOSTEROIDS: RARE RISK OF CENTRAL SEROUS CHORIORETINOPATHY WITH LOCAL AS WELL AS SYSTEMIC ADMINISTRATION (AUGUST 2017)
  See *Corticosteroids, general use* p. 656.

- CONTRA-INDICATIONS Active or suspected ocular infection · active or suspected peri-ocular infection · pre-existing glaucoma
- CAUTIONS Raised baseline intra-ocular pressure
- INTERACTIONS → Appendix 1: fluocinolone
- SIDE-EFFECTS
  ▶ **Common or very common** Cataract · eye discomfort · glaucoma · haemorrhage · vision blurred
  ▶ **Uncommon** Eye disorders · headache

- ▶ **Frequency not known** Thromboembolism
- PREGNANCY Manufacturer advises avoid unless potential benefit outweighs risk—no information available.
- BREAST FEEDING Manufacturer advises avoid unless essential.
- MONITORING REQUIREMENTS
  ▶ Monitor for raised intra-ocular pressure (particularly if raised at baseline), retinal detachment, endophthalmitis, vitreous haemorrhage or detachment within 2–7 days following the procedure.
  ▶ Monitor intra-ocular pressure at least every 3 months thereafter (for approximately 36 months).
- DIRECTIONS FOR ADMINISTRATION Concurrent administration to both eyes not recommended. For further information on administration and repeat dosing, consult product literature.
- NATIONAL FUNDING/ACCESS DECISIONS

  NICE decisions

  ▶ Fluocinolone acetonide intravitreal implant for treating chronic diabetic macular oedema after an inadequate response to prior therapy (November 2013) NICE TA301
  Fluocinolone acetonide intravitreal implant is recommended as an option for treating chronic diabetic macular oedema that is insufficiently responsive to available therapies only if:
  ● the implant is to be used in an eye with an intra-ocular (pseudophakic lens) **and**
  ● the manufacturer provides fluocinolone acetonide intravitreal implant with the discount agreed in the patient access scheme.
  www.nice.org.uk/TA301

  Scottish Medicines Consortium (SMC) Decisions
  The *Scottish Medicines Consortium* has advised (February 2014) that fluocinolone acetonide intravitreal implant (*Iluvien*®) is recommended for restricted use within NHS Scotland for the treatment of vision impairment associated with chronic diabetic macular oedema, considered insufficiently responsive to available therapies, only in patients in whom the affected eye is pseudophakic (has an artificial lens after cataract surgery), **and** retreatment would take place only if the patient had previously responded to treatment with fluocinolone acetonide and subsequently best corrected visual acuity had deteriorated to less than 20/32.

- MEDICINAL FORMS
  There can be variation in the licensing of different medicines containing the same drug.

  Implant
  ▶ Iluvien (Alimera Sciences Ltd)
  Fluocinolone acetonide 190 microgram ILUVIEN 190microgram intravitreal implant in applicator | 1 device PoM £5,500.00

6.3 Optic neuropathy

DRUGS FOR METABOLIC DISORDERS ›
ANTIOXIDANTS

Idebenone   31-May-2017

- DRUG ACTION Idebenone is a nootropic and antioxidant that is thought to act by restoring cellular ATP generation, thereby reactivating retinal ganglion cells.

- ● INDICATIONS AND DOSE

  Leber's Hereditary Optic Neuropathy (initiated by a specialist)
  ▶ BY MOUTH
  ▸ Adult: 300 mg 3 times a day

- SIDE-EFFECTS
  - **Common or very common** Cough · diarrhoea · increased risk of infection · pain
  - **Frequency not known** Agranulocytosis · anaemia · anxiety · appetite decreased · azotaemia · delirium · dizziness · dyspepsia · hallucination · headache · hepatitis · leucopenia · malaise · movement disorders · nausea · neutropenia · poriomania · seizure · skin reactions · stupor · thrombocytopenia · urine discolouration · vomiting

  SIDE-EFFECTS, FURTHER INFORMATION The metabolites of idebenone may cause red-brown discolouration of the urine. This effect is harmless, but the manufacturer advises caution as this may mask colour changes due to other causes (e.g. renal or blood disorders).

- PREGNANCY Manufacturer advises avoid unless potential benefit outweighs risk—no information available.

- BREAST FEEDING Manufacturer advises avoid—present in milk in *animal* studies.

- HEPATIC IMPAIRMENT Manufacturer advises use with caution—no information available.

- RENAL IMPAIRMENT Manufacturer advises use with caution—no information available.

- NATIONAL FUNDING/ACCESS DECISIONS

  Scottish Medicines Consortium (SMC) Decisions
  The *Scottish Medicines Consortium* has advised (May 2017) that idebenone (*Raxone®*) is accepted for restricted use within NHS Scotland for the treatment of visual impairment in patients with Leber's Hereditary Optic Neuropathy (LHON) who are not yet blind i.e. they do not meet the UK criteria to be registered as severely sight impaired. This advice is contingent upon the continuing availability of the Patient Access Scheme in NHS Scotland or a list price that is equivalent or lower.

- MEDICINAL FORMS
  There can be variation in the licensing of different medicines containing the same drug. Forms available from special-order manufacturers include: tablet

  Tablet
  CAUTIONARY AND ADVISORY LABELS 14, 21
  - Raxone (Santhera (UK) Ltd) ▼
    Idebenone 150 mg Raxone 150mg tablets | 180 tablet [PoM]
    £6,364.00

6.4 Vitreomacular traction

RECOMBINANT PROTEOLYTIC ENZYMES

Ocriplasmin

- INDICATIONS AND DOSE

  Treatment of vitreomacular traction, including when associated with a macular hole of diameter less than or equal to 400 microns (specialist use only)
  - BY INTRAVITREAL INJECTION
  - **Adult:** 125 micrograms for 1 dose, to be administered into the affected eye, concurrent administration to both eyes is not recommended

- CONTRA-INDICATIONS Active or suspected ocular or periocular infection · aphakia · exudative age-related macular degeneration · high myopia · history of rhegmatogenous retinal detachment · ischaemic retinopathies · large diameter macular hole (> 400 microns) · lens zonule instability · proliferative diabetic retinopathy · recent intra-ocular injection (including laser therapy) · recent ocular surgery · retinal vein occlusions · vitreous haemorrhage

- CAUTIONS History of uveitis (including severe active inflammation) · non-proliferative diabetic retinopathy · significant eye trauma

- SIDE-EFFECTS
  - **Common or very common** Dry eye · eye discomfort · eye disorders · eye inflammation · haemorrhage · retinal pigment epitheliopathy · vision disorders

- PREGNANCY Manufacturer advises use only if potential benefit outweighs risk—no information available.

- BREAST FEEDING Manufacturer advises use only if potential benefit outweighs risk—no information available.

- MONITORING REQUIREMENTS Monitor intra-ocular pressure, visual acuity, and for signs of intra-ocular inflammation or infection following injection.

- DIRECTIONS FOR ADMINISTRATION For further information on administration, consult product literature.

- NATIONAL FUNDING/ACCESS DECISIONS
  NICE decisions
  - **Ocriplasmin for treating vitreomacular traction (October 2013)** NICE TA297
    Ocriplasmin is recommended as an option for treating vitreomacular traction in adults, only if:
    - an epiretinal membrane is not present **and**
    - they have a stage II full-thickness macular hole with a diameter of 400 microns or less **and/or**
    - they have severe symptoms.
    www.nice.org.uk/TA297

  Scottish Medicines Consortium (SMC) Decisions
  The *Scottish Medicines Consortium* has advised (July 2014) that ocriplasmin (*Jetrea®*) is accepted for restricted use within NHS Scotland for the treatment of patients with vitreomacular traction plus macular hole, regardless of whether they have epiretinal membrane formation, and in patients with vitreomacular traction alone (no epiretinal membrane and no macular hole).

- MEDICINAL FORMS
  There can be variation in the licensing of different medicines containing the same drug.
  Solution for injection
  - Jetrea (Alcon Laboratories (UK) Ltd)
    Ocriplasmin 2.5 mg per 1 ml Jetrea 0.5mg/0.2ml concentrate for solution for injection vials | 1 vial [PoM] £2,500.00

Chapter 12
Ear, nose and oropharynx

Ear

Ear

Otitis externa

Otitis externa is an inflammatory reaction of the meatal skin. It is important to exclude an underlying chronic otitis media before treatment is commenced. Many cases recover after thorough cleansing of the external ear canal by suction or dry mopping. A frequent problem in resistant cases is the difficulty in applying lotions and ointments satisfactorily to the relatively inaccessible affected skin. The most effective method is to introduce a ribbon gauze dressing or sponge wick soaked with **corticosteroid** ear drops or with an astringent such as aluminium acetate solution p. 1164. When this is not practical, the ear should be gently cleansed with a probe covered in cotton wool and the patient encouraged to lie with the affected ear uppermost for ten minutes after the canal has been filled with a liberal quantity of the appropriate solution.

If infection is present, a topical anti-infective which is not used systemically (such as neomycin sulfate p. 1161 or **clioquinol**) may be used, but for only about a week as excessive use may result in fungal infections; these may be difficult to treat and require expert advice. Sensitivity to the anti-infective or solvent may occur and resistance to antibacterials is a possibility with prolonged use. Aluminium acetate ear drops are also effective against bacterial infection and inflammation of the ear. Chloramphenicol p. 1161 may be used but the ear drops contain propylene glycol and cause hypersensitivity reactions in about 10% of patients. Solutions containing an anti-infective and a corticosteroid are used for treating cases where infection is present with inflammation and eczema.

In view of reports of ototoxicity, manufacturers contra-indicate treatment with topical **aminoglycosides** or **polymyxins** in patients with a perforated tympanic membrane (eardrum) or patent grommet. However, some specialists do use these drops cautiously in the presence of a perforation or patent grommet in patients with chronic suppurative otitis media and when other measures have failed for otitis externa; treatment should be considered only **by specialists** in the following circumstances:

- drops should only be used in the presence of obvious infection;
- treatment should be for no longer than 2 weeks;

- patients should be counselled on the risk of ototoxicity and given justification for the use of these topical antibiotics;
- baseline audiometry should be performed, if possible, before treatment is commenced.

Clinical expertise and judgement should be used to assess the risk of treatment versus the benefit to the patient in such circumstances.

A solution of **acetic acid** 2% acts as an antifungal and antibacterial in the external ear canal. It may be used to treat mild otitis externa but in severe cases an antiinflammatory preparation with or without an anti-infective drug is required. A proprietary preparation containing acetic acid 2% (*EarCalm*® spray) is on sale to the public.

For severe pain associated with otitis externa, a simple analgesic, such as paracetamol p. 438 or ibuprofen p. 1106, can be used. A systemic antibacterial can be used if there is spreading cellulitis or if the patient is systemically unwell. When a resistant staphylococcal infection (a boil) is present in the external auditory meatus, flucloxacillin p. 544 is the drug of choice; ciprofloxacin p. 548 (or an aminoglycoside) may be needed in pseudomonal infections which may occur if the patient has diabetes or is immunocompromised.

The skin of the pinna adjacent to the ear canal is often affected by eczema. A topical corticosteroid cream or ointment is then required, but prolonged use should be avoided.

Otitis media

Acute otitis media

Acute otitis media is the commonest cause of severe aural pain in small children. Many infections, especially those accompanying coryza, are caused by viruses. Most uncomplicated cases resolve without antibacterial treatment and a **simple analgesic**, such as paracetamol, may be sufficient. In children without systemic features, a **systemic antibacterial** may be started after 72 hours if there is no improvement, or earlier if there is deterioration, if the patient is systemically unwell, if the patient is at high risk of serious complications (e.g. in immunosuppression, cystic fibrosis), if mastoiditis is present, or in children under 2 years of age with bilateral otitis media. Perforation of the tympanic membrane in patients with *acute otitis media* usually heals spontaneously without treatment; if there is no improvement, e.g. pain or discharge persists, systemic antibacterial can be given. Topical treatment of acute otitis media is ineffective and there is no place for drops containing a local anaesthetic.

Otitis media with effusion

Otitis media with effusion (glue ear) occurs in about 10% of children and in 90% of children with cleft palates. Systemic antibacterials are not usually required. If glue ear persists for more than a month or two, the child should be referred for assessment and follow up because of the risk of long-term hearing impairment which can delay language development. Untreated or resistant glue ear may be responsible for some types of *chronic otitis media*.

Chronic otitis media

Opportunistic organisms are often present in the debris, keratin, and necrotic bone of the middle ear and mastoid in patients with chronic otitis media. The mainstay of treatment is thorough cleansing with aural microsuction which may completely resolve long-standing infection. Local cleansing of the meatal and middle ear may be followed by treatment with a sponge wick or ribbon gauze dressing soaked with corticosteroid ear drops or with an astringent such as aluminium acetate solution; this is particularly beneficial for discharging ears or infections of the mastoid cavity. An antibacterial ear ointment may also be used. Acute exacerbations of chronic infection may also require systemic treatment with amoxicillin p. 539 (or erythromycin p. 530 if penicillin-allergic); treatment is adjusted according to the results of sensitivity testing.

In view of reports of ototoxicity, manufacturers contraindicate topical treatment with ototoxic antibacterials in the presence of a tympanic perforation or patent grommet. Ciprofloxacin p. 1137 or ofloxacin eye drops p. 1138 used in the ear [unlicensed use] or ear drops p. 1161 [both unlicensed; available from 'special-order' manufacturers or specialist importing companies] are an effective alternative to such ototoxic ear drops for chronic otitis media in patients with perforation of the tympanic membrane.

However, some specialists do use ear drops containing **aminoglycosides** or **polymyxins** [unlicensed indications] cautiously in patients with chronic suppurative otitis media and a perforation of the tympanic membrane, if the otitis media has failed to settle with systemic antibacterials; treatment should be considered only **by specialists** in the following circumstances:

- drops should only be used in the presence of obvious infection;
- treatment should be for no longer than 2 weeks;
- patients should be counselled on the risk of ototoxicity and given justification for the use of these topical antibiotics;
- baseline audiometry should be performed, if possible, before treatment is commenced.

Clinical expertise and judgement should be used to assess the risk of treatment versus the benefit to the patient in such circumstances. It is considered that the pus in the middle ear associated with otitis media also carries a risk of ototoxicity.

Removal of ear wax

Ear wax (cerumen) is a normal bodily secretion which provides a protective film on the meatal skin and need only be removed if it causes hearing loss or interferes with a proper view of the ear drum.

Ear wax can be softened using simple remedies such as **olive oil** ear drops or **almond oil** ear drops; sodium bicarbonate ear drops p. 1164 are also effective, but may cause dryness of the ear canal. If the wax is hard and impacted, the drops can be used twice daily for several days and this may reduce the need for mechanical removal of the wax. The patient should lie with the affected ear uppermost for 5 to 10 minutes after a generous amount of the softening remedy has been introduced into the ear. Some proprietary preparations containing organic solvents can irritate the meatal skin, and in most cases the simple remedies indicated above are just as effective and less likely to cause irritation.

Docusate sodium p. 1164 or urea hydrogen peroxide p. 1165 are ingredients in a number of proprietary preparations for softening ear wax.

If necessary, wax may be removed by irrigation with water (warmed to body temperature). Ear irrigation is generally best avoided in young children, in patients unable to co-operate with the procedure, in those with otitis media in the last six weeks, in otitis externa, in patients with cleft palate, a history of ear drum perforation, or previous ear surgery. A person who has hearing in one ear only should not have that ear irrigated because even a very slight risk of damage is unacceptable in this situation.

1   Otitis externa

ANTIBACTERIALS › AMINOGLYCOSIDES

Framycetin sulfate

- **INDICATIONS AND DOSE**

Bacterial infection in otitis externa
▶ TO THE EAR
▸ Adult: (consult product literature)

- **CONTRA-INDICATIONS** Perforated tympanic membrane
- **CAUTIONS** Avoid prolonged use
- **SIDE-EFFECTS** Local reaction

- **MEDICINAL FORMS**
No licensed medicines listed.

Combinations available: *Dexamethasone with framycetin sulfate and gramicidin*, p. 1129

Gentamicin   11-Dec-2017

- **INDICATIONS AND DOSE**

Bacterial infection in otitis externa
▶ TO THE EAR
▸ Child: Apply 2–3 drops 4–5 times a day, (including a dose at bedtime)
▸ Adult: Apply 2–3 drops 4–5 times a day, (including a dose at bedtime)

- **CONTRA-INDICATIONS** Patent grommet (although may be used by specialists, see Ear p. 1159) · perforated tympanic membrane (although may be used by specialists, see Ear p. 1159)
- **CAUTIONS** Avoid prolonged use
- **SIDE-EFFECTS** Dermatitis

- **MEDICINAL FORMS**
There can be variation in the licensing of different medicines containing the same drug.
Ear/eye drops solution
EXCIPIENTS: May contain Benzalkonium chloride
▸ Gentamicin (Non-proprietary)
Gentamicin (as Gentamicin sulfate) 3 mg per 1 ml Gentamicin 0.3% ear/eye drops | 10 ml [PoM] £2.63 DT = £2.47

Gentamicin with hydrocortisone
21-Dec-2017

- **INDICATIONS AND DOSE**

Eczematous inflammation in otitis externa
▶ TO THE EAR
▸ Child: Apply 2–4 drops 4–5 times a day, (including a dose at bedtime)

▸ Adult: Apply 2–4 drops 4–5 times a day, (including a dose at bedtime)

> IMPORTANT SAFETY INFORMATION
> MHRA/CHM ADVICE: CORTICOSTEROIDS: RARE RISK OF CENTRAL SEROUS CHORIORETINOPATHY WITH LOCAL AS WELL AS SYSTEMIC ADMINISTRATION (AUGUST 2017)
> See Corticosteroids, general use p. 656.

- CONTRA-INDICATIONS Patent grommet (although may be used by specialists, see Ear p. 1159) · perforated tympanic membrane (although may be used by specialists, see Ear p. 1159)
- CAUTIONS Avoid prolonged use
- SIDE-EFFECTS Local reaction
- PATIENT AND CARER ADVICE
  Medicines for Children leaflet: Gentamicin and hydrocortisone ear drops for inflammatory ear infections
  www.medicinesforchildren.org.uk/gentamicin-and-hydrocortisone-ear-drops-inflammatory-ear-infections

- MEDICINAL FORMS
  There can be variation in the licensing of different medicines containing the same drug.
  Ear drops
  EXCIPIENTS: May contain Benzalkonium chloride, disodium edetate
  ▸ Gentamicin with hydrocortisone (Non-proprietary)
    Gentamicin (as Gentamicin sulfate) 3 mg per 1 ml, Hydrocortisone acetate 10 mg per 1 ml Gentamicin 0.3% / Hydrocortisone acetate 1% ear drops | 10 ml [PoM] £26.19 DT = £26.19

Neomycin sulfate

- ● INDICATIONS AND DOSE
  Bacterial infection in otitis externa
  ▸ TO THE EAR
  ▸ Child: (consult product literature)
  ▸ Adult: (consult product literature)

- CONTRA-INDICATIONS Patent grommet (although may be used by specialists, see Ear p. 1159) · perforated tympanic membrane (although may be used by specialists, see Ear p. 1159)
- CAUTIONS Avoid prolonged use
- SIDE-EFFECTS Local reaction

- MEDICINAL FORMS
  No licensed medicines listed.

  Combinations available: *Betamethasone with neomycin,* p. 1129 · *Dexamethasone with glacial acetic acid and neomycin sulfate,* p. 1163 · *Hydrocortisone with neomycin and polymyxin B sulfate,* p. 1164

ANTIBACTERIALS > QUINOLONES

Ciprofloxacin   26-Apr-2018

- ● INDICATIONS AND DOSE
  Acute otitis externa
  ▸ TO THE EAR
  ▸ Child 1–17 years: Apply 0.25 mL twice daily for 7 days, each 0.25 mL dose contains 0.5 mg ciprofloxacin
  ▸ Adult: Apply 0.25 mL twice daily for 7 days, each 0.25 mL dose contains 0.5 mg ciprofloxacin

- CAUTIONS Known (or at risk of) perforated tympanic membrane
- SIDE-EFFECTS
  ▸ **Uncommon** Dermatitis · ear pruritus

- HANDLING AND STORAGE Manufacturer advises discard any ampoules remaining 8 days after opening the pouch.
- PATIENT AND CARER ADVICE
  Medicines for Children leaflet: Ciprofloxacin ear drops for ear infections www.medicinesforchildren.org.uk/ciprofloxacin-ear-drops-ear-infections-0
- NATIONAL FUNDING/ACCESS DECISIONS
  Scottish Medicines Consortium (SMC) Decisions
  SMC No. 1320/18
  The *Scottish Medicines Consortium* has advised (April 2018) that ciprofloxacin ear drops (*Cetraxal®*) are recommended for use within NHS Scotland for treatment of acute otitis externa in adults and children over 1 year with an intact tympanic membrane, caused by ciprofloxacin susceptible microorganisms when off-label or unlicensed ciprofloxacin formulations would otherwise be used.

- MEDICINAL FORMS
  There can be variation in the licensing of different medicines containing the same drug. Forms available from special-order manufacturers include: ear drops
  Ear drops
  ▸ Cetraxal (Aspire Pharma Ltd)
    Ciprofloxacin (as Ciprofloxacin hydrochloride) 2 mg per 1 ml Cetraxal 2mg/ml ear drops 0.25ml unit dose | 15 unit dose [PoM] £6.01

  Combinations available: *Dexamethasone with ciprofloxacin,* p. 1163

ANTIBACTERIALS > OTHER

Chloramphenicol

- DRUG ACTION Chloramphenicol is a potent broad-spectrum antibiotic.

- ● INDICATIONS AND DOSE
  Bacterial infection in otitis externa
  ▸ TO THE EAR
  ▸ Child: Apply 2–3 drops 2–3 times a day
  ▸ Adult: Apply 2–3 drops 2–3 times a day

- CAUTIONS Avoid prolonged use
- SIDE-EFFECTS Blood disorder · bone marrow depression
- PATIENT AND CARER ADVICE
  Medicines for Children leaflet: Chloramphenicol ear drops for ear infections (otitis externa) www.medicinesforchildren.org.uk/chloramphenicol-ear-drops-ear-infections-otitis-externa-0
- LESS SUITABLE FOR PRESCRIBING Chloramphenicol ear drops are less suitable for prescribing.

- MEDICINAL FORMS
  There can be variation in the licensing of different medicines containing the same drug.
  Ear drops
  EXCIPIENTS: May contain Propylene glycol
  ▸ Chloramphenicol (Non-proprietary)
    Chloramphenicol 50 mg per 1 ml Chloramphenicol 5% ear drops | 10 ml [PoM] £63.69 DT = £63.69
    Chloramphenicol 100 mg per 1 ml Chloramphenicol 10% ear drops | 10 ml [PoM] £87.84 DT = £87.84

ANTIFUNGALS > IMIDAZOLE ANTIFUNGALS

Clotrimazole

- ● INDICATIONS AND DOSE
  Fungal infection in otitis externa
  ▸ TO THE EAR
  ▸ Child: Apply 2–3 times a day continue for at least 14 days after disappearance of infection
  ▸ Adult: Apply 2–3 times a day continue for at least 14 days after disappearance of infection

12

Ear, nose and oropharynx

- SIDE-EFFECTS Local reaction

- MEDICINAL FORMS
There can be variation in the licensing of different medicines containing the same drug.
Liquid
▸ Canesten (clotrimazole) (Bayer Plc)
  Clotrimazole 10 mg per 1 ml Canesten 1% solution | 20 ml [P] £2.30 DT = £2.30

CORTICOSTEROIDS

Betamethasone

21-Dec-2017

- **INDICATIONS AND DOSE**
BETNESOL ®

Eczematous inflammation in otitis externa
▸ TO THE EAR
▸ Adult: Apply 2–3 drops every 2–3 hours, reduce frequency when relief obtained

VISTAMETHASONE ®

Eczematous inflammation in otitis externa
▸ TO THE EAR
▸ Adult: Apply 2–3 drops every 3–4 hours, reduce frequency when relief obtained

---

IMPORTANT SAFETY INFORMATION

MHRA/CHM ADVICE: CORTICOSTEROIDS: RARE RISK OF CENTRAL SEROUS CHORIORETINOPATHY WITH LOCAL AS WELL AS SYSTEMIC ADMINISTRATION (AUGUST 2017)
See *Corticosteroids, general use* p. 656.

- CONTRA-INDICATIONS Avoid alone in the presence of untreated infection (combine with suitable anti-infective)
- CAUTIONS Avoid prolonged use
- SIDE-EFFECTS Local reaction

- MEDICINAL FORMS
There can be variation in the licensing of different medicines containing the same drug.
Ear/eye/nose drops solution
EXCIPIENTS: May contain Benzalkonium chloride, disodium edetate
▸ Betnesol (RPH Pharmaceuticals AB)
  Betamethasone sodium phosphate 1 mg per 1 ml Betnesol 0.1% eye/ear/nose drops | 10 ml [PoM] £2.32 DT = £2.32
▸ Vistamethasone (Martindale Pharmaceuticals Ltd)
  Betamethasone sodium phosphate 1 mg per 1 ml Vistamethasone 0.1% ear/eye/nose drops | 5 ml [PoM] £1.02 | 10 ml [PoM] £1.16 DT = £2.32

Combinations available: *Betamethasone with neomycin,* p. 1129

Flumetasone pivalate with clioquinol

21-Dec-2017

- **INDICATIONS AND DOSE**

Eczematous inflammation in otitis externa | Mild bacterial or fungal infections in otitis externa
▸ TO THE EAR
▸ Child 2-17 years: 2–3 drops twice daily for 7–10 days, to be instilled into the ear
▸ Adult: 2–3 drops twice daily for 7–10 days, to be instilled into the ear

---

IMPORTANT SAFETY INFORMATION

MHRA/CHM ADVICE: CORTICOSTEROIDS: RARE RISK OF CENTRAL SEROUS CHORIORETINOPATHY WITH LOCAL AS WELL AS SYSTEMIC ADMINISTRATION (AUGUST 2017)
See *Corticosteroids, general use* p. 656.

- CONTRA-INDICATIONS Iodine sensitivity
- CAUTIONS Avoid prolonged use · manufacturer advises avoid in perforated tympanic membrane (but used by specialists for short periods)
- SIDE-EFFECTS Paraesthesia · skin reactions
- PATIENT AND CARER ADVICE Clioquinol stains skin and clothing

- MEDICINAL FORMS
There can be variation in the licensing of different medicines containing the same drug.
Ear drops
▸ Flumetasone pivalate with clioquinol (Non-proprietary)
  Flumetasone pivalate 200 microgram per 1 ml, Clioquinol 10 mg per 1 ml Flumetasone 0.02% / Clioquinol 1% ear drops | 7.5 ml [PoM] £11.34 DT = £11.34 | 10 ml [PoM] £15.13 DT = £15.13

Prednisolone

21-Dec-2017

- **INDICATIONS AND DOSE**

Eczematous inflammation in otitis externa
▸ TO THE EAR
▸ Child: Apply 2–3 drops every 2–3 hours, frequency to be reduced when relief obtained
▸ Adult: Apply 2–3 drops every 2–3 hours, frequency to be reduced when relief obtained

---

IMPORTANT SAFETY INFORMATION

SAFE PRACTICE
Prednisolone has been confused with propranolol; care must be taken to ensure the correct drug is prescribed and dispensed.

MHRA/CHM ADVICE: CORTICOSTEROIDS: RARE RISK OF CENTRAL SEROUS CHORIORETINOPATHY WITH LOCAL AS WELL AS SYSTEMIC ADMINISTRATION (AUGUST 2017)
See *Corticosteroids, general use* p. 656.

- CONTRA-INDICATIONS Avoid alone in the presence of untreated infection (combine with suitable anti-infective)
- CAUTIONS Avoid prolonged use
- SIDE-EFFECTS Local reaction

- MEDICINAL FORMS
There can be variation in the licensing of different medicines containing the same drug.
Ear/eye drops solution
EXCIPIENTS: May contain Benzalkonium chloride, disodium edetate
▸ Predsol (RPH Pharmaceuticals AB)
  Prednisolone sodium phosphate 5 mg per 1 ml Predsol 0.5% ear/eye drops | 10 ml [PoM] £2.00 DT = £2.00

CORTICOSTEROIDS › CORTICOSTEROID COMBINATIONS WITH ANTI-INFECTIVES

Betamethasone with neomycin

The properties listed below are those particular to the combination only. For the properties of the components please consider, betamethasone above.

- **INDICATIONS AND DOSE**

Eczematous inflammation in otitis externa
▸ TO THE EAR USING EAR DROPS
▸ Child: Apply 2–3 drops 3–4 times a day
▸ Adult: Apply 2–3 drops 3–4 times a day

- CONTRA-INDICATIONS Patent grommet (although may be used by specialists, see Ear p. 1159) · perforated tympanic membrane (although may be used by specialists, see Ear p. 1159)
- CAUTIONS Avoid prolonged use

- **MEDICINAL FORMS**
There can be variation in the licensing of different medicines containing the same drug.
Ear/eye/nose drops solution
EXCIPIENTS: May contain Benzalkonium chloride, disodium edetate
▸ Betnesol-N (RPH Pharmaceuticals AB)
  Betamethasone (as Betamethasone sodium phosphate) 1 mg per 1 ml, Neomycin sulfate 5 mg per 1 ml Betnesol-N ear/eye/nose drops | 10 ml PoM £2.39 DT = £2.39

Dexamethasone with ciprofloxacin

21-Dec-2017

The properties listed below are those particular to the combination only. For the properties of the components please consider, ciprofloxacin p. 1161.

- **INDICATIONS AND DOSE**
Acute otitis media in patients with tympanostomy tubes
▸ TO THE EAR
▸ Adult: Apply 4 drops twice daily for 7 days
Acute otitis externa
▸ TO THE EAR
▸ Adult: Apply 4 drops twice daily for 7 days

> **IMPORTANT SAFETY INFORMATION**
> MHRA/CHM ADVICE: CORTICOSTEROIDS: RARE RISK OF CENTRAL SEROUS CHORIORETINOPATHY WITH LOCAL AS WELL AS SYSTEMIC ADMINISTRATION (AUGUST 2017)
> See *Corticosteroids, general use* p. 656.

- **CONTRA-INDICATIONS** Fungal ear infections · viral ear infections
- **CAUTIONS** Avoid prolonged use
- **PREGNANCY** Manufacturer advises use only if potential benefit outweighs risk—no information available.
- **BREAST FEEDING** Manufacturer advises caution—no information available.
- **PATIENT AND CARER ADVICE** Manufacturer advises counselling on administration.
- **NATIONAL FUNDING/ACCESS DECISIONS**
Scottish Medicines Consortium (SMC) Decisions
The *Scottish Medicines Consortium* has advised (July 2017) that dexamethasone with ciprofloxacin (*Cilodex®*) is accepted for restricted use within NHS Scotland for the treatment of acute otitis media in patients with tympanostomy tubes (AOMT).

- **MEDICINAL FORMS**
There can be variation in the licensing of different medicines containing the same drug.
Ear drops
EXCIPIENTS: May contain Benzalkonium chloride, disodium edetate
▸ Cilodex (Novartis Pharmaceuticals UK Ltd)
  Dexamethasone 1 mg per 1 ml, Ciprofloxacin (as Ciprofloxacin hydrochloride) 3 mg per 1 ml Cilodex ear drops | 5 ml PoM £6.12 DT = £6.12

Dexamethasone with framycetin sulfate and gramicidin

21-Dec-2017

The properties listed below are those particular to the combination only. For the properties of the components please consider, framycetin sulfate p. 1160.

- **INDICATIONS AND DOSE**
Eczematous inflammation in otitis externa
▸ TO THE EAR
▸ Child: 2–3 drops 3–4 times a day

▸ Adult: 2–3 drops 3–4 times a day

> **IMPORTANT SAFETY INFORMATION**
> MHRA/CHM ADVICE: CORTICOSTEROIDS: RARE RISK OF CENTRAL SEROUS CHORIORETINOPATHY WITH LOCAL AS WELL AS SYSTEMIC ADMINISTRATION (AUGUST 2017)
> See *Corticosteroids, general use* p. 656.

- **SIDE-EFFECTS** Dermatitis
- **LESS SUITABLE FOR PRESCRIBING** *Sofradex®* is less suitable for prescribing.
- **MEDICINAL FORMS**
There can be variation in the licensing of different medicines containing the same drug.
Ear/Eye drops
EXCIPIENTS: May contain polysorbates
▸ Sofradex ear/eye drops (Sanofi)
  Gramicidin 50 microgram per 1 ml, Framycetin sulfate 5 mg per 1 ml, Dexamethasone 500 microgram per 1 ml Sofradex ear/eye drops | 8 ml PoM £7.50

Dexamethasone with glacial acetic acid and neomycin sulfate

21-Dec-2017

The properties listed below are those particular to the combination only. For the properties of the components please consider, neomycin sulfate p. 1161.

- **INDICATIONS AND DOSE**
Eczematous inflammation in otitis externa
▸ TO THE EAR
▸ Child 2–17 years: Apply 1 spray 3 times a day
▸ Adult: Apply 1 spray 3 times a day

> **IMPORTANT SAFETY INFORMATION**
> MHRA/CHM ADVICE: CORTICOSTEROIDS: RARE RISK OF CENTRAL SEROUS CHORIORETINOPATHY WITH LOCAL AS WELL AS SYSTEMIC ADMINISTRATION (AUGUST 2017)
> See *Corticosteroids, general use* p. 656.

- **CONTRA-INDICATIONS** Patent grommet (although may be used by specialists, see Ear p. 1159) · perforated tympanic membrane (although may be used by specialists, see Ear p. 1159)
- **CAUTIONS** Avoid prolonged use
- **SIDE-EFFECTS** Paraesthesia · skin reactions

- **MEDICINAL FORMS**
There can be variation in the licensing of different medicines containing the same drug.
Spray
EXCIPIENTS: May contain Hydroxybenzoates (parabens)
▸ Otomize (Teva UK Ltd)
  Dexamethasone 1 mg per 1 gram, Neomycin sulfate 5 mg per 1 gram, Acetic acid glacial 20 mg per 1 gram Otomize ear spray | 5 ml PoM £3.27

12

Ear, nose and oropharynx

Hydrocortisone with neomycin and polymyxin B sulfate

21-Dec-2017

The properties listed below are those particular to the combination only. For the properties of the components please consider, neomycin sulfate p. 1161.

- ● INDICATIONS AND DOSE

Bacterial infection in otitis externa
- ▶ TO THE EAR
- ▶ Child 3-17 years: Apply 3 drops 3–4 times a day for 7 days (review treatment if there is no clinical improvement)
- ▶ Adult: Apply 3 drops 3–4 times a day for 7 days (review treatment if there is no clinical improvement)

> IMPORTANT SAFETY INFORMATION
>
> MHRA/CHM ADVICE: CORTICOSTEROIDS: RARE RISK OF CENTRAL SEROUS CHORIORETINOPATHY WITH LOCAL AS WELL AS SYSTEMIC ADMINISTRATION (AUGUST 2017)
> See *Corticosteroids, general use* p. 656.

- ● SIDE-EFFECTS
- ▶ **Rare or very rare** Headache · paraesthesia · skin reactions · telangiectasia
- ● RENAL IMPAIRMENT Manufacturer advises avoid prolonged, unsupervised use.
  Dose adjustments Manufacturer advises reduce dose.

- ● MEDICINAL FORMS
  There can be variation in the licensing of different medicines containing the same drug.
  Ear drops
  EXCIPIENTS: May contain Cetostearyl alcohol (including cetyl and stearyl alcohol), hydroxybenzoates (parabens), polysorbates
  - ▶ Otosporin (Phoenix Labs Ltd)
    Hydrocortisone 10 mg per 1 ml, Neomycin sulfate 3400 unit per 1 ml, Polymyxin B sulfate 10000 unit per 1 ml Otosporin ear drops | 10 ml PoM £7.45

DERMATOLOGICAL DRUGS > ASTRINGENTS

Aluminium acetate

- ● INDICATIONS AND DOSE

Inflammation in otitis externa
- ▶ TO THE EAR
- ▶ Adult: To be inserted into meatus or apply on a ribbon gauze dressing or sponge wick which should be kept saturated with the ear drops

- ● DIRECTIONS FOR ADMINISTRATION For ear drops 8%—dilute 8 parts aluminium acetate ear drops (13%) with 5 parts purified water. Must be freshly prepared.

- ● MEDICINAL FORMS
  Forms available from special-order manufacturers include: ear drops

2   Removal of earwax

BICARBONATE

Sodium bicarbonate

- ● INDICATIONS AND DOSE

Removal of earwax (with 5% ear drop solution)
- ▶ TO THE EAR
- ▶ Child: (consult product literature)
- ▶ Adult: (consult product literature)

- ● SIDE-EFFECTS Dry ear
- ● MEDICINAL FORMS
  There can be variation in the licensing of different medicines containing the same drug.
  Ear drops
  - ▶ Sodium bicarbonate (Non-proprietary)
    Sodium bicarbonate 50 mg per 1 ml Sodium bicarbonate 5% ear drops | 10 ml £1.23-£1.25

SOFTENING DRUGS

Almond oil

- ● INDICATIONS AND DOSE

Removal of earwax
- ▶ TO THE EAR
- ▶ Child: Allow drops to warm to room temperature before use (consult product literature)
- ▶ Adult: Allow drops to warm to room temperature before use (consult product literature)

- ● DIRECTIONS FOR ADMINISTRATION The patient should lie with the affected ear uppermost for 5 to 10 minutes after a generous amount of the softening remedy has been introduced into the ear.

- ● MEDICINAL FORMS
  There can be variation in the licensing of different medicines containing the same drug.
  Liquid
  - ▶ Almond oil (Non-proprietary)
    Almond oil 1 ml per 1 ml Almond oil liquid | 50 ml £0.95 DT = £0.95 | 70 ml £0.85 | 200 ml £2.68 | 500 ml £11.90

Arachis oil with chlorobutanol

- ● INDICATIONS AND DOSE

Removal of earwax
- ▶ TO THE EAR
- ▶ Adult: (consult product literature)

- ● SIDE-EFFECTS Skin reactions
- ● LESS SUITABLE FOR PRESCRIBING Arachis (peanut) oil with chlorobutanol ear drops are less suitable for prescribing.

- ● MEDICINAL FORMS
  There can be variation in the licensing of different medicines containing the same drug.
  Ear drops
  - ▶ Cerumol (Thornton & Ross Ltd)
    Chlorobutanol 50 mg per 1 ml, Arachis oil 573 mg per 1 ml Cerumol ear drops | 11 ml P £2.05

Docusate sodium

20-Apr-2016

(Dioctyl sodium sulphosuccinate)

- ● INDICATIONS AND DOSE

Removal of ear wax
- ▶ TO THE EAR
- ▶ Adult: (consult product literature)

- ● LESS SUITABLE FOR PRESCRIBING Ear drops less suitable for prescribing.

- MEDICINAL FORMS
There can be variation in the licensing of different medicines containing the same drug.

Ear drops
EXCIPIENTS: May contain Propylene glycol
- ▸ Molcer (Wallace Manufacturing Chemists Ltd)
  Docusate sodium 50 mg per 1 ml Molcer ear drops | 15 ml P
  £5.60
- ▸ Waxsol (Meda Pharmaceuticals Ltd)
  Docusate sodium 5 mg per 1 ml Waxsol ear drops | 10 ml P £1.95
  DT = £1.95

Olive oil

- INDICATIONS AND DOSE
Removal of earwax
- ▸ TO THE EAR
- ▸ Child: Apply twice daily for several days (if wax is hard and impacted)
- ▸ Adult: Apply twice daily for several days (if wax is hard and impacted)

- DIRECTIONS FOR ADMINISTRATION The patient should lie with the affected ear uppermost for 5 to 10 minutes after a generous amount of the softening remedy has been introduced into the ear. Allow ear drops to warm to room temperature before use.

- MEDICINAL FORMS
There can be variation in the licensing of different medicines containing the same drug.

Spray
- ▸ Earol (HL Healthcare Ltd)
  Earol olive oil ear spray | 10 ml ⓢ

Ear drops
- ▸ Olive oil (Non-proprietary)
  Olive oil ear drops | 10 ml £1.35–£1.42
- ▸ Arjun (Arjun Products Ltd)
  Arjun ear drops | 10 ml £1.26
- ▸ Cerumol (olive oil) (Thornton & Ross Ltd)
  Cerumol olive oil ear drops | 10 ml ⓢ
- ▸ KliarVax (Essential-Healthcare Ltd)
  KliarVax ear drops | 10 ml £0.97
- ▸ Oleax (JR Biomedical Ltd)
  Oleax ear drops | 15 ml £1.40
- ▸ Olive oil (Thornton & Ross Ltd)
  Care olive oil ear drops | 10 ml £1.42
- ▸ St George's (St Georges Medical Ltd)
  Olive oil ear drops | 10 ml £1.40 | 20 ml £2.70

Urea hydrogen peroxide

- INDICATIONS AND DOSE
Softening and removal of earwax
- ▸ TO THE EAR
- ▸ Adult: (consult product literature)

- PATIENT AND CARER ADVICE The patient should lie with the affected ear uppermost for 5 to 10 minutes after a generous amount of the softening remedy has been introduced into the ear.

- LESS SUITABLE FOR PRESCRIBING Urea-hydrogen peroxide ear drops are less suitable for prescribing.

- MEDICINAL FORMS
There can be variation in the licensing of different medicines containing the same drug.

Ear drops
- ▸ Exterol (Dermal Laboratories Ltd)
  Urea hydrogen peroxide 50 mg per 1 gram Exterol 5% ear drops |
  8 ml P £1.75 DT = £2.89
- ▸ Otex (Dendron Ltd)
  Urea hydrogen peroxide 50 mg per 1 gram Otex 5% ear drops |
  8 ml P £2.89 DT = £2.89

Nose

Nose

31-Oct-2017

Rhinitis

Rhinitis is often self-limiting. There are few indications for nasal sprays and drops except in allergic rhinitis and perennial rhinitis. Many nasal preparations contain sympathomimetic drugs which may damage the nasal cilia. Sodium chloride 0.9% solution p. 1008 may be used as a douche or 'sniff' following endonasal surgery.

Drugs used in nasal allergy

Mild allergic rhinitis is controlled by **antihistamines** (see under Antihistamines, allergen immunotherapy and allergic emergencies p. 276) or topical **nasal corticosteroids**; systemic nasal decongestants are of doubtful value. Topical nasal decongestants can be used for a short period to relieve congestion and allow penetration of a topical nasal corticosteroid.

More persistent symptoms and nasal congestion can be relieved by topical nasal **corticosteroids**; sodium cromoglicate p. 1173 is an alternative, but may be less effective. The topical antihistamine azelastine hydrochloride p. 1169 is useful for controlling breakthrough symptoms in allergic rhinitis. Topical antihistamines are considered less effective than topical corticosteroids but probably more effective than cromoglicate. In seasonal allergic rhinitis (e.g. hay fever), treatment should begin 2 to 3 weeks before the season commences and may have to be continued for several months; continuous treatment may be required for years in perennial rhinitis.

Montelukast p. 268 is less effective than topical nasal corticosteroids; montelukast can be used in patients with seasonal allergic rhinitis and concomitant asthma.

Sometimes allergic rhinitis is accompanied by vasomotor rhinitis. In this situation, the addition of topical nasal ipratropium bromide can reduce watery rhinorrhoea.

Very disabling symptoms occasionally justify the use of **systemic corticosteroids** for short periods, for example, in students taking important examinations. They may also be used at the beginning of a course of treatment with a corticosteroid spray to relieve severe mucosal oedema and allow the spray to penetrate the nasal cavity.

Corticosteroids

Corticosteroid nasal preparations should be avoided in the presence of untreated nasal infections, after nasal surgery (until healing has occurred), and in pulmonary tuberculosis. Patients transferred from systemic corticosteroids may experience exacerbation of some symptoms. Systemic absorption may follow nasal administration particularly if high doses are used or if treatment is prolonged; for cautions and side-effects of systemic corticosteroids. The risk of systemic effects may be greater with nasal drops than with nasal sprays; drops are administered incorrectly more often than sprays. The height of children receiving prolonged treatment with nasal corticosteroids should be monitored; if growth is slowed, referral to a paediatrician should be considered.

Nasal polyps

Short-term use of corticosteroid nasal drops helps to shrink nasal polyps; to be effective, the drops must be administered with the patient in the 'head down' position. A short course of a systemic corticosteroid may be required initially to shrink large polyps. A corticosteroid nasal spray can be used to maintain the reduction in swelling and also for the initial treatment of small polyps.

Pregnancy

If a pregnant woman cannot tolerate the symptoms of allergic rhinitis, treatment with nasal beclometasone dipropionate p. 1170, budesonide p. 1171, fluticasone p. 1171, or sodium cromoglicate p. 1173 may be considered.

Topical nasal decongestants

The nasal mucosa is sensitive to changes in atmospheric temperature and humidity and these alone may cause slight nasal congestion. The nose and nasal sinuses produce a litre of mucus in 24 hours and much of this finds its way silently into the stomach via the nasopharynx. Slight changes in the nasal airway, accompanied by an awareness of mucus passing along the nasopharynx causes some patients to be inaccurately diagnosed as suffering from chronic sinusitis. These symptoms are particularly noticeable in the later stages of the common cold. Sodium chloride 0.9% given as nasal drops or spray may relieve nasal congestion by helping to liquefy mucous secretions.

Inhalation of **warm moist air** may be useful in the treatment of symptoms of acute infective conditions. The addition of volatile substances such as menthol and eucalyptus may encourage the use of warm moist air (see under Aromatic inhalations, cough preparations and systemic nasal decongestants p. 294).

Symptoms of nasal congestion associated with vasomotor rhinitis and the common cold can be relieved by the short-term use (usually not longer than 7 days) of decongestant nasal drops and sprays. These all contain sympathomimetic drugs which exert their effect by vasoconstriction of the mucosal blood vessels which in turn reduces oedema of the nasal mucosa. They are of limited value because they can give rise to a rebound congestion (rhinitis medicamentosa) on withdrawal, due to a secondary vasodilatation with a subsequent temporary increase in nasal congestion. This in turn tempts the further use of the decongestant, leading to a vicious cycle of events. Ephedrine hydrochloride nasal drops below is the safest sympathomimetic preparation and can give relief for several hours. The more potent sympathomimetic drugs oxymetazoline and xylometazoline hydrochloride p. 1167 are more likely to cause a rebound effect.

Non-allergic watery rhinorrhoea often responds well to treatment with the antimuscarinic ipratropium bromide p. 1169.

Nasal preparations for infection

There is **no** evidence that topical anti-infective nasal preparations have any therapeutic value in rhinitis; see elimination of nasal staphylococci.

Nasal staphylococci

Elimination of organisms such as staphylococci from the nasal vestibule can be achieved by the use of a cream containing **chlorhexidine** and **neomycin** (*Naseptin®*), but re-colonisation frequently occurs. Coagulase-positive staphylococci are present in the noses of 40% of the population.

A nasal ointment containing mupirocin p. 1168 is also available; it should probably be held in reserve for resistant infections. In hospitals or in care establishments, mupirocin nasal ointment should be reserved for the eradication (in both patients and staff) of nasal carriage of meticillin-resistant *Staphylococcus aureus* (MRSA). A sample should be taken 2 days after treatment to confirm eradication. The course may be repeated if the sample is positive (and the throat is not colonised). To avoid the development of resistance, the treatment course should not exceed 7 days and the course should not be repeated on more than one occasion. If the MRSA strain is mupirocin-resistant or does not respond after 2 courses, consider alternative products such as chlorhexidine and neomycin cream.

1 Nasal congestion

SYMPATHOMIMETICS › VASOCONSTRICTOR

Ephedrine hydrochloride

● **INDICATIONS AND DOSE**

Nasal congestion | Sinusitis affecting the maxillary antrum
▶ BY INTRANASAL ADMINISTRATION
▶ Child 12–17 years: Apply 1–2 drops up to 4 times a day as required for a maximum of 7 days, to be instilled into each nostril, administer ephedrine 0.5% nasal drops
▶ Adult: Apply 1–2 drops up to 4 times a day as required for a maximum of 7 days, to be instilled into each nostril

IMPORTANT SAFETY INFORMATION
CHM/MHRA ADVICE
The CHM/MHRA has stated that non-prescription cough and cold medicines containing ephedrine can be considered for up to 5 days' treatment in children aged 6–12 years after basic principles of best care have been tried; these medicines should not be used in children under 6 years of age.

● CAUTIONS Avoid excessive or prolonged use · cardiovascular disease (in children) · diabetes mellitus · elderly · hypertension · hyperthyroidism · ischaemic heart disease (in adults) · prostatic hypertrophy (risk of acute urinary retention) (in adults)
● INTERACTIONS → Appendix 1: sympathomimetics, vasoconstrictor
● SIDE-EFFECTS
▶ **Common or very common** Anxiety · headache · insomnia · nausea
▶ **Frequency not known** Appetite decreased · arrhythmia · circulation impaired · dermatitis · dizziness · drug dependence · drug tolerance · dry mouth · dyspnoea · hallucination · hyperglycaemia · hyperhidrosis · hypersalivation · hypertension · hypokalaemia · hypotension · irritability · muscle weakness · mydriasis · pain · palpitations · paranoia · piloerection · rebound congestion · syncope · thirst · tremor · urinary disorders · vasoconstriction · vasodilation · vomiting
● PREGNANCY Manufacturer advises avoid.
● BREAST FEEDING Present in milk; manufacturer advises avoid—irritability and disturbed sleep reported.
● PRESCRIBING AND DISPENSING INFORMATION For nasal drops, the BP directs that if no strength is specified 0.5% drops should be supplied.
● PROFESSION SPECIFIC INFORMATION
Dental practitioners' formulary
Ephedrine nasal drops may be prescribed.
● EXCEPTIONS TO LEGAL CATEGORY Ephedrine nasal drops can be sold to the public provided no more than 180 mg of ephedrine base (or salts) are supplied at one time, and pseudoephedrine salts are not supplied at the same time; for conditions that apply to supplies made at the request of a patient, see *Medicines, Ethics and Practice*, London, Pharmaceutical Press (always consult latest edition).
● MEDICINAL FORMS
There can be variation in the licensing of different medicines containing the same drug.
Nasal drops
▶ Ephedrine hydrochloride (Non-proprietary)
Ephedrine hydrochloride 5 mg per 1 ml Ephedrine 0.5% nasal drops | 10 ml P £1.90–£1.94 DT = £1.90
Ephedrine hydrochloride 10 mg per 1 ml Ephedrine 1% nasal drops | 10 ml P £1.94–£2.01 DT = £1.94

Pseudoephedrine hydrochloride

- **INDICATIONS AND DOSE**

Congestion of mucous membranes of upper respiratory tract

- ▸ BY MOUTH
- ▸ Child 6–11 years: 30 mg 3–4 times a day
- ▸ Child 12–17 years: 60 mg 3–4 times a day
- ▸ Adult: 60 mg 3–4 times a day

IMPORTANT SAFETY INFORMATION

MHRA/CHM ADVICE (MARCH 2008 AND FEBRUARY 2009): OVER-THE-COUNTER COUGH AND COLD MEDICINES FOR CHILDREN
Children under 6 years should not be given over-the-counter cough and cold medicines containing pseudoephedrine.

- CAUTIONS Diabetes · heart disease · hypertension · hyperthyroidism · ischaemic heart disease (in adults) · prostatic hypertrophy (in adults) · raised intra-ocular pressure (in children) · susceptibility to angle-closure glaucoma (in adults)
- INTERACTIONS → Appendix 1: sympathomimetics, vasoconstrictor
- SIDE-EFFECTS Angle closure glaucoma · anxiety · arrhythmias · circulation impaired · dry mouth · hallucination · headache · hypertension · irritability · nausea · palpitations · psychotic disorder · skin reactions · sleep disorders · tremor · urinary retention · vomiting
- PREGNANCY Defective closure of the abdominal wall (gastroschisis) reported very rarely in newborns after first trimester exposure.
- BREAST FEEDING May suppress lactation; avoid if lactation not well established or if milk production insufficient.
- HEPATIC IMPAIRMENT Manufacturer advises use with caution in severe impairment.
- RENAL IMPAIRMENT Use with caution in mild to moderate renal impairment. Manufacturer advises avoid in severe renal impairment.
- LESS SUITABLE FOR PRESCRIBING Pseudoephedrine hydrochloride is less suitable for prescribing.
- EXCEPTIONS TO LEGAL CATEGORY *Galpseud®* and *Sudafed®* can be sold to the public provided no more than 720 mg of pseudoephedrine salts are supplied, and ephedrine base (or salts) are not supplied at the same time; for details see *Medicines, Ethics and Practice*, London, Pharmaceutical Press (always consult latest edition).

- MEDICINAL FORMS
There can be variation in the licensing of different medicines containing the same drug.

Oral solution
EXCIPIENTS: May contain Alcohol
- ▸ Pseudoephedrine hydrochloride (Non-proprietary)
Pseudoephedrine hydrochloride 6 mg per 1 ml Care Decongestant 30mg/5ml oral liquid sugar-free | 100 ml [P] £1.67 DT = £1.67
- ▸ Galpseud (Thornton & Ross Ltd)
Pseudoephedrine hydrochloride 6 mg per 1 ml Galpseud 30mg/5ml linctus sugar-free | 2000 ml [PoM] £14.00
- ▸ Sudafed Non-Drowsy Decongestant (pseudoephedrine) (McNeil Products Ltd)
Pseudoephedrine hydrochloride 6 mg per 1 ml Sudafed Decongestant 30mg/5ml liquid | 100 ml [P] £2.22

Tablet
- ▸ Pseudoephedrine hydrochloride (Non-proprietary)
Pseudoephedrine hydrochloride 60 mg Care Decongestant 60mg tablets | 12 tablet [P] £1.29
- ▸ Galpseud (Thornton & Ross Ltd)
Pseudoephedrine hydrochloride 60 mg Galpseud 60mg tablets | 24 tablet [PoM] £2.25 | 100 tablet [PoM] £5.42 DT = £5.42

- ▸ Sudafed Non-Drowsy Decongestant (pseudoephedrine) (McNeil Products Ltd)
Pseudoephedrine hydrochloride 60 mg Sudafed Decongestant 60mg tablets | 12 tablet [P] £2.43

Xylometazoline hydrochloride

- **DRUG ACTION** Xylometazoline is a sympathomimetic.

- **INDICATIONS AND DOSE**

Nasal congestion
- ▸ BY INTRANASAL ADMINISTRATION USING NASAL DROPS
- ▸ Child 6–11 years: 1–2 drops 1–2 times a day as required for maximum duration of 5 days, 0.05% solution to be administered into each nostril
- ▸ Child 12–17 years: 2–3 drops 2–3 times a day as required for maximum duration of 7 days, 0.1% solution to be administered into each nostril
- ▸ Adult: 2–3 drops 2–3 times a day as required for maximum duration of 7 days, 0.1% solution to be administered into each nostril
- ▸ BY INTRANASAL ADMINISTRATION USING NASAL SPRAY
- ▸ Child 12–17 years: 1 spray 1–3 times a day as required for maximum duration of 7 days, to be administered into each nostril
- ▸ Adult: 1 spray 1–3 times a day as required for maximum duration of 7 days, to be administered into each nostril

---

IMPORTANT SAFETY INFORMATION
The CHM/MHRA has stated that non-prescription cough and cold medicines containing oxymetazoline or xylometazoline can be considered for up to 5 days' treatment in children aged 6–12 years after basic principles of best care have been tried; these medicines should not be used in children under 6 years of age.

- CAUTIONS Angle-closure glaucoma · avoid excessive or prolonged use · cardiovascular disease (in children) · diabetes mellitus · elderly · hypertension · hyperthyroidism · ischaemic heart disease (in adults) · prostatic hypertrophy (risk of acute retention)(in adults) · rebound congestion
CAUTIONS, FURTHER INFORMATION
- ▸ Rebound congestion Sympathomimetic drugs are of limited value in the treatment of nasal congestion because they can, following prolonged use (more than 7 days), give rise to a rebound congestion (rhinitis medicamentosa) on withdrawal, due to a secondary vasodilatation with a subsequent temporary increase in nasal congestion. This in turn tempts the further use of the decongestant, leading to a vicious cycle of events.
- INTERACTIONS → Appendix 1: sympathomimetics, vasoconstrictor
- SIDE-EFFECTS Cardiovascular effects · headache · hypersensitivity · nasal dryness · nausea · paraesthesia · visual impairment
SIDE-EFFECTS, FURTHER INFORMATION Use of decongestants in infants and children under 6 years has been associated with agitated psychosis, ataxia, hallucinations, and even death—avoid.
- PREGNANCY Manufacturer advises avoid.
- BREAST FEEDING Manufacturer advises caution—no information available.

12

Ear, nose and oropharynx

- MEDICINAL FORMS
There can be variation in the licensing of different medicines containing the same drug.

Spray

▶ Otrivine (GlaxoSmithKline Consumer Healthcare)
Xylometazoline hydrochloride 1 mg per 1 ml Otrivine Congestion Relief 0.1% nasal spray | 10 ml GSL £3.05 DT = £2.18
Otrivine Adult Measured Dose Sinusitis spray | 10 ml GSL £2.62 DT = £2.18
Otrivine Allergy Relief 0.1% nasal spray | 10 ml GSL £2.62 DT = £2.18
Otrivine Adult nasal spray | 10 ml GSL £2.18 DT = £2.18
Otrivine Adult Metered Dose 0.1% nasal spray | 10 ml GSL £2.62 DT = £2.18

▶ Sudafed Congestion Relief (McNeil Products Ltd)
Xylometazoline hydrochloride 1 mg per 1 ml Sudafed Congestion Relief 0.1% nasal spray | 10 ml GSL £3.46 DT = £2.18

▶ Sudafed Mucus Relief (McNeil Products Ltd)
Xylometazoline hydrochloride 1 mg per 1 ml Sudafed Mucus Relief 0.1% nasal spray | 15 ml GSL £2.76

▶ Sudafed Non-Drowsy Decongestant (xylometazoline) (McNeil Products Ltd)
Xylometazoline hydrochloride 1 mg per 1 ml Sudafed Blocked Nose 0.1% spray | 15 ml GSL £2.76

Nasal drops

▶ Otrivine (GlaxoSmithKline Consumer Healthcare)
Xylometazoline hydrochloride 500 microgram per 1 ml Otrivine Child nasal drops | 10 ml P £1.91 DT = £1.91
Xylometazoline hydrochloride 1 mg per 1 ml Otrivine Adult 0.1% nasal drops | 10 ml GSL £2.18 DT = £2.18

2   Nasal infection

Sinusitis (acute)

31-Oct-2017

Description of condition

Sinusitis is an inflammation of the mucosal lining of the paranasal sinuses. Acute sinusitis (rhinosinusitis) is a self-limiting condition usually triggered by a viral upper-respiratory tract infection such as the 'common cold'. Occasionally, acute sinusitis may become complicated by a bacterial infection (see *Antibacterial therapy for acute sinusitis* in Nose infections, antibacterial therapy p. 506).

Patients with acute sinusitis usually present with symptoms of nasal blockage or congestion, nasal discharge, dental or facial pain or pressure, and reduction or loss of the sense of smell.

Symptoms usually improve within 2 to 3 weeks without requiring treatment.

Rarely, acute sinusitis may lead to orbital, intracranial or skeletal complications (e.g. periorbital cellulitis, symptoms or signs of meningitis).

Aims of treatment

Treatment is aimed at managing symptoms including pain, fever, and nasal congestion as well as treatment of bacterial infection if present.

Treatment

EvGr Patients presenting with symptoms for around 10 *days or less*, should be given advice about the usual duration of acute sinusitis, self-care of pain or fever with paracetamol p. 438 or ibuprofen p. 1106, and when to seek medical help. Patients should be reassured that antibiotics are usually not required. Some patients may try nasal saline or nasal decongestants, however there is limited evidence to show they help to relieve nasal congestion.

Patients presenting with symptoms for around 10 *days or more* with no improvement could be considered for treatment with a high-dose nasal corticosteroid, such as mometasone furoate p. 1172 [unlicensed use] or fluticasone p. 1171 [unlicensed use] for 14 days. Supply of a back-up

antibiotic prescription could be considered and used if symptoms do not improve within 7 days, or if they worsen rapidly or significantly.

If the patient is systemically very unwell, has signs and symptoms of a more serious illness or condition, or is at high-risk of complications, an immediate antibiotic should be given. Ⓐ (see *Antibacterial therapy for acute sinusitis* in Nose infections, antibacterial therapy p. 506).

EvGr Patients presenting with symptoms of acute sinusitis associated with a severe systemic infection or with orbital or intracranial complications should be referred to hospital. Ⓐ

Useful Resources

Sinusitis (acute): antimicrobial prescribing. National Institute for Health and Care Excellence. NICE guideline 79. October 2017.
www.nice.org.uk/guidance/ng79

ANTIBACTERIALS › AMINOGLYCOSIDES

Chlorhexidine with neomycin

- INDICATIONS AND DOSE

Eradication of nasal carriage of staphylococci
▶ BY INTRANASAL ADMINISTRATION
▶ Child: Apply 4 times a day for 10 days
▶ Adult: Apply 4 times a day for 10 days

Preventing nasal carriage of staphylococci
▶ BY INTRANASAL ADMINISTRATION
▶ Child: Apply twice daily
▶ Adult: Apply twice daily

- MEDICINAL FORMS
There can be variation in the licensing of different medicines containing the same drug.

Cream
EXCIPIENTS: May contain Arachis (peanut) oil, cetostearyl alcohol (including cetyl and stearyl alcohol)

▶ Naseptin (Alliance Pharmaceuticals Ltd)
Chlorhexidine hydrochloride 1 mg per 1 gram, Neomycin sulfate 5 mg per 1 gram Naseptin nasal cream | 15 gram PoM £2.03 DT = £2.24

ANTIBACTERIALS › OTHER

Mupirocin

- INDICATIONS AND DOSE

BACTROBAN NASAL ®

For eradication of nasal carriage of staphylococci, including meticillin-resistant *Staphylococcus aureus* (MRSA)
▶ BY INTRANASAL ADMINISTRATION
▶ Child: Apply 2–3 times a day for 5 days; a sample should be taken 2 days after treatment to confirm eradication. Course may be repeated once if sample positive (and throat not colonised), dose to be applied to the inner surface of each nostril
▶ Adult: Apply 2–3 times a day for 5 days; a sample should be taken 2 days after treatment to confirm eradication. Course may be repeated once if sample positive (and throat not colonised), dose to be applied to the inner surface of each nostril

- SIDE-EFFECTS
- Common or very common Skin reactions
▶ Uncommon Nasal mucosal disorder
- PREGNANCY Manufacturer advises avoid unless potential benefit outweighs risk—no information available.
- BREAST FEEDING No information available.

- RENAL IMPAIRMENT Manufacturer advises caution when mupirocin ointment used in moderate or severe impairment because it contains macrogols (polyethylene glycol).

- MEDICINAL FORMS
There can be variation in the licensing of different medicines containing the same drug.
Nasal ointment
  ► Bactroban (GlaxoSmithKline UK Ltd)
  Mupirocin (as Mupirocin calcium) 20 mg per 1 gram Bactroban 2% nasal ointment | 3 gram [PoM] £4.24 DT = £4.24

CORTICOSTEROIDS > CORTICOSTEROID COMBINATIONS WITH ANTI-INFECTIVES

Betamethasone with neomycin

The properties listed below are those particular to the combination only. For the properties of the components please consider, betamethasone p. 1170,

- INDICATIONS AND DOSE
Nasal infection
  ► BY INTRANASAL ADMINISTRATION USING NASAL DROPS
  ► Child: Apply 2–3 drops 2–3 times a day, to be applied into each nostril
  ► Adult: Apply 2–3 drops 2–3 times a day, to be applied into each nostril

- INTERACTIONS → Appendix 1: corticosteroids · neomycin
- LESS SUITABLE FOR PRESCRIBING Betamethasone with neomycin nasal-drops are less suitable for prescribing; there is no evidence that topical anti-infective nasal preparations have any therapeutic value in rhinitis or sinusitis.

- MEDICINAL FORMS
There can be variation in the licensing of different medicines containing the same drug.
Ear/eye/nose drops solution
EXCIPIENTS: May contain Benzalkonium chloride, disodium edetate
  ► Betnesol-N (RPH Pharmaceuticals AB)
  Betamethasone (as Betamethasone sodium phosphate) 1 mg per 1 ml, Neomycin sulfate 5 mg per 1 ml Betnesol-N ear/eye/nose drops | 10 ml [PoM] £2.39 DT = £2.39

3 Nasal inflammation, nasal polyps and rhinitis

Other drugs used for Nasal inflammation, nasal polyps and rhinitis Desloratadine, p. 279 · Fexofenadine hydrochloride, p. 280 · Ketotifen, p. 285 · Rupatadine, p. 282

ANTIHISTAMINES > NON-SEDATING

Azelastine hydrochloride

- INDICATIONS AND DOSE
Allergic rhinitis
  ► BY INTRANASAL ADMINISTRATION
  ► Child 6–17 years: 1 spray twice daily, to be administered into each nostril
  ► Adult: 1 spray twice daily, to be administered into each nostril
  DOSE EQUIVALENCE AND CONVERSION
  ► 1 spray equivalent to 140 micrograms.

- INTERACTIONS → Appendix 1: antihistamines, non-sedating

- SIDE-EFFECTS
  ► Common or very common Taste bitter
  ► Uncommon Nasal irritation

- MEDICINAL FORMS
There can be variation in the licensing of different medicines containing the same drug.
Spray
  ► Rhinolast (Meda Pharmaceuticals Ltd)
  Azelastine hydrochloride 140 microgram per 1 actuation Rhinolast 140micrograms/dose nasal spray | 22 ml [PoM] £10.50 DT = £10.50

Combinations available: *Fluticasone with azelastine*, p. 1172

ANTIMUSCARINICS

Ipratropium bromide   22-Jan-2018

- INDICATIONS AND DOSE
Rhinorrhoea associated with allergic and non-allergic rhinitis
  ► BY INTRANASAL ADMINISTRATION
  ► Child 12–17 years: 2 sprays 2–3 times a day, dose to be sprayed into each nostril
  ► Adult: 2 sprays 2–3 times a day, dose to be sprayed into each nostril
  DOSE EQUIVALENCE AND CONVERSION
  ► 1 metered spray of nasal spray = 21 micrograms.

- CAUTIONS Avoid spraying near eyes · bladder outflow obstruction · cystic fibrosis · prostatic hyperplasia (in adults) · susceptibility to angle-closure glaucoma
- INTERACTIONS → Appendix 1: ipratropium
- SIDE-EFFECTS
  ► Common or very common Gastrointestinal motility disorder · nasal complaints · throat complaints
  ► Uncommon Corneal oedema · eye disorders · eye pain · respiratory disorders · vision disorders
- ALLERGY AND CROSS-SENSITIVITY Contra-indicated in patients with hypersensitivity to atropine or its derivatives.
- PREGNANCY Manufacturer advises only use if potential benefit outweighs the risk.
- BREAST FEEDING No information available—manufacturer advises only use if potential benefit outweighs risk.
- PATIENT AND CARER ADVICE Patients or carers should be counselled on appropriate administration technique and warned against accidental contact with the eye (due to risk of ocular complications).
  Driving and skilled tasks Manufacturer advises patients and carers should be counselled on the effects on driving and performance of skilled tasks—increased risk of dizziness and vision disorders.

- MEDICINAL FORMS
There can be variation in the licensing of different medicines containing the same drug.
Spray
EXCIPIENTS: May contain Benzalkonium chloride, disodium edetate
  ► Rinatec (Boehringer Ingelheim Ltd)
  Ipratropium bromide 21 microgram per 1 dose Rinatec 21micrograms/dose nasal spray | 180 dose [PoM] £6.54 DT = £6.54

12

Ear, nose and oropharynx

CORTICOSTEROIDS

Corticosteroids (intranasal)

IMPORTANT SAFETY INFORMATION

MHRA/CHM ADVICE: CORTICOSTEROIDS: RARE RISK OF CENTRAL SEROUS CHORIORETINOPATHY WITH LOCAL AS WELL AS SYSTEMIC ADMINISTRATION (AUGUST 2017)

Central serous chorioretinopathy is a retinal disorder that has been linked to the systemic use of corticosteroids. Recently, it has also been reported after local administration of corticosteroids via inhaled and intranasal, epidural, intra-articular, topical dermal, and periocular routes. The MHRA recommends that patients should be advised to report any blurred vision or other visual disturbances with corticosteroid treatment given by any route; consider referral to an ophthalmologist for evaluation of possible causes if a patient presents with vision problems.

- CAUTIONS Avoid after nasal surgery (until healing has occurred) · avoid in pulmonary tuberculosis · avoid in the presence of untreated nasal infections · patients transferred from systemic corticosteroids may experience exacerbation of some symptoms

  CAUTIONS, FURTHER INFORMATION
  - Systemic absorption Systemic absorption may follow nasal administration particularly if high doses are used or if treatment is prolonged; therefore also consider the cautions and side-effects of systemic corticosteroids. The risk of systemic effects may be greater with nasal drops than with nasal sprays; drops are administered incorrectly more often than sprays.

- SIDE-EFFECTS
  - **Common or very common** Altered smell sensation · amenorrhoea · anxiety · behaviour abnormal · cognitive impairment · Cushing's syndrome · dyspepsia · electrolyte imbalance · epistaxis · hair changes · headache · healing impaired · hypertension · increased risk of infection · mood altered · nasal complaints · nausea · osteoporosis · skin reactions · sleep disorder · taste altered · throat irritation · voice alteration
  - **Uncommon** Adrenal suppression · cataract · diabetic control impaired · glaucoma · osteonecrosis · pancreatitis · peptic ulcer · psychotic disorder · thromboembolism · vision blurred
  - **Rare or very rare** Bronchospasm paradoxical · nasal septum perforation (more common following nasal surgery) · telangiectasia
  - **Frequency not known** Growth retardation (uncommon in children) · local reaction · pneumonia (in patients with COPD)

  SIDE-EFFECTS, FURTHER INFORMATION Systemic absorption may follow nasal administration particularly if high doses are used or if treatment is prolonged. Therefore also consider the side-effects of systemic corticosteroids.

- MONITORING REQUIREMENTS The height of children receiving prolonged treatment with nasal corticosteroids should be monitored; if growth is slowed, referral to a paediatrician should be considered.

Beclometasone dipropionate

04-Jan-2016

(Beclomethasone dipropionate)

- INDICATIONS AND DOSE

Prophylaxis and treatment of allergic and vasomotor rhinitis
- BY INTRANASAL ADMINISTRATION
  - Child 6–17 years: 100 micrograms twice daily, dose to be administered into each nostril, reduced to 50 micrograms twice daily, dose to be administered into each nostril, dose to be reduced when symptoms controlled; maximum 400 micrograms per day
  - Adult: 100 micrograms twice daily, dose to be administered into each nostril, reduced to 50 micrograms twice daily, dose to be administered into each nostril, dose to be reduced when symptoms controlled; maximum 400 micrograms per day

- INTERACTIONS → Appendix 1: corticosteroids
- EXCEPTIONS TO LEGAL CATEGORY Preparations of beclometasone dipropionate can be sold to the public for nasal administration as a nasal spray if supplied for the prevention and treatment of allergic rhinitis in adults over 18 years subject to max. single dose of 100 micrograms per nostril, max. daily dose of 200 micrograms per nostril for max. 3 months, and a pack size of 20 mg.

- MEDICINAL FORMS
There can be variation in the licensing of different medicines containing the same drug.

Spray

EXCIPIENTS: May contain Benzalkonium chloride, polysorbates
- Beclometasone dipropionate (Non-proprietary)
  Beclometasone dipropionate 50 microgram per 1 dose Beclometasone 50micrograms/dose nasal spray | 200 dose [PoM] [🔔] DT = £2.55 | 200 dose [P] £2.55 DT = £2.55
- Beconase (GlaxoSmithKline UK Ltd, Omega Pharma Ltd)
  Beclometasone dipropionate 50 microgram per 1 dose Beconase Aqueous 50micrograms/dose nasal spray | 200 dose [PoM] £2.63 DT = £2.55
  Beconase Hayfever 50micrograms/dose nasal spray | 180 dose [P] £7.11
  Beconase Hayfever Relief for Adults 50micrograms/dose nasal spray | 100 dose [GSL] £5.16
- Nasobec (Teva UK Ltd)
  Beclometasone dipropionate 50 microgram per 1 dose Nasobec Aqueous 50micrograms/dose nasal spray | 200 dose [PoM] £3.06 DT = £2.55
  Nasobec Hayfever 50micrograms/dose nasal spray | 180 dose [P] £5.78
- Pollenase (beclometasone) (E M Pharma)
  Beclometasone dipropionate 50 microgram per 1 dose Pollenase Hayfever Relief for Adults 50micrograms/dose nasal spray | 100 dose [GSL] £3.49
  Pollenase Hayfever 50micrograms/dose nasal spray | 200 dose [P] £4.97 DT = £2.55

Betamethasone

21-Dec-2017

- INDICATIONS AND DOSE

BETNESOL ®

Non-infected inflammatory conditions of nose
- BY INTRANASAL ADMINISTRATION
  - Adult: Apply 2–3 drops 2–3 times a day, dose to be applied into each nostril

VISTAMETHASONE ®

Non-infected inflammatory conditions of nose
- BY INTRANASAL ADMINISTRATION
  - Adult: Apply 2–3 drops twice daily, dose to be applied into each nostril

- INTERACTIONS → Appendix 1: corticosteroids

- **MEDICINAL FORMS**
There can be variation in the licensing of different medicines containing the same drug.

Ear/eye/nose drops solution
EXCIPIENTS: May contain Benzalkonium chloride, disodium edetate
▸ Betnesol (RPH Pharmaceuticals AB)
Betamethasone sodium phosphate 1 mg per 1 ml Betnesol 0.1% eye/ear/nose drops | 10 ml [PoM] £2.32 DT = £2.32
▸ Vistamethasone (Martindale Pharmaceuticals Ltd)
Betamethasone sodium phosphate 1 mg per 1 ml Vistamethasone 0.1% ear/eye/nose drops | 5 ml [PoM] £1.02 | 10 ml [PoM] £1.16 DT = £2.32

⎯⎯⎯⎯⎯⎯⎯⎯⎯⎯⎯⎯⎯⎯⎯ ⚑ 1170

Budesonide
21-Dec-2017

- **DRUG ACTION** Budesonide is a glucocorticoid, which exerts significant local anti-inflammatory effects.

- **INDICATIONS AND DOSE**

Allergic rhinitis | Nasal polyps
▸ BY INTRANASAL ADMINISTRATION
▹ Child 6–17 years: 128 micrograms once daily, dose to be administered into each nostril in the morning, alternatively 64 micrograms twice daily, dose to be administered to each nostril, reduce dose when control achieved
▹ Adult: 128 micrograms once daily, dose to be administered into each nostril in the morning, alternatively 64 micrograms twice daily, dose to be administered to each nostril, reduce dose when control achieved

Prophylaxis and treatment of allergic and vasomotor rhinitis
▸ BY INTRANASAL ADMINISTRATION
▹ Child 12–17 years: Initially 200 micrograms once daily, dose to be administered into each nostril in the morning, alternatively initially 100 micrograms twice daily, dose to be administered to each nostril; reduced to 100 micrograms once daily, dose to be administered into each nostril, dose can be reduced when control achieved
▹ Adult: Initially 200 micrograms once daily, dose to be administered into each nostril in the morning, alternatively initially 100 micrograms twice daily, dose to be administered to each nostril; reduced to 100 micrograms once daily, dose to be administered into each nostril, dose can be reduced when control achieved

Nasal polyps
▸ BY INTRANASAL ADMINISTRATION
▹ Child 12–17 years: 100 micrograms twice daily for up to 3 months, dose to be administered into each nostril
▹ Adult: 100 micrograms twice daily for up to 3 months, dose to be administered into each nostril

RHINOCORT AQUA ®

Rhinitis
▸ BY INTRANASAL ADMINISTRATION
▹ Adult: 128 micrograms once daily, dose to be administered into each nostril in the morning, alternatively 64 micrograms twice daily, dose to be administered into each nostril; reduced to 64 micrograms once daily when control achieved. Use for maximum 3 months, doses to be administered into each nostril

Nasal polyps
▸ BY INTRANASAL ADMINISTRATION
▹ Adult: 64 micrograms twice daily for up to 3 months, dose to be administered into each nostril

- **UNLICENSED USE** *Rhinocort Aqua* ® is not licensed for use in children.

- **INTERACTIONS** → Appendix 1: corticosteroids
- **EXCEPTIONS TO LEGAL CATEGORY** Preparations of budesonide can be sold to the public for nasal administration as a nasal spray if supplied for the prevention and treatment of seasonal allergic rhinitis in adults over 18 years subject to max. single dose of 200 micrograms per nostril, max. daily dose of 200 micrograms per nostril for max. period of 3 months, and a pack size of 10 mg.

- **MEDICINAL FORMS**
There can be variation in the licensing of different medicines containing the same drug.

Spray
EXCIPIENTS: May contain Disodium edetate, polysorbates, potassium sorbate
▸ Budesonide (Non-proprietary)
Budesonide 64 microgram per 1 dose Budesonide 64micrograms/dose nasal spray | 120 dose [PoM] £4.77 DT = £4.77
▸ Budesonide (Import)
Budesonide 100 microgram per 1 dose Budeflam Aquanase 100micrograms/dose nasal spray | 150 dose [PoM] ⓈⒽ Aircort 100micrograms/dose nasal spray | 200 dose [PoM] ⓈⒽ
▸ Rhinocort (Johnson & Johnson Ltd)
Budesonide 64 microgram per 1 dose Rhinocort Aqua 64 nasal spray | 120 dose [PoM] £3.77 DT = £4.77

⎯⎯⎯⎯⎯⎯⎯⎯⎯⎯⎯⎯⎯⎯⎯ ⚑ 1170

Fluticasone
21-Dec-2017

- **INDICATIONS AND DOSE**

Prophylaxis and treatment of allergic rhinitis and perennial rhinitis
▸ BY INTRANASAL ADMINISTRATION USING NASAL SPRAY
▹ Child 4–11 years: 50 micrograms once daily, to be administered into each nostril preferably in the morning, increased if necessary to 50 micrograms twice daily
▹ Child 12–17 years: 100 micrograms once daily, to be administered into each nostril preferably in the morning, increased if necessary to 100 micrograms twice daily; reduced to 50 micrograms once daily, dose to be administered into each nostril, dose to be reduced when control achieved
▹ Adult: 100 micrograms once daily, to be administered into each nostril preferably in the morning, increased if necessary to 100 micrograms twice daily; reduced to 50 micrograms once daily, dose to be administered into each nostril, dose to be reduced when control achieved

Nasal polyps
▸ BY INTRANASAL ADMINISTRATION USING NASAL DROPS
▹ Child 16–17 years: 200 micrograms 1–2 times a day, to be administered into each nostril, alternative treatment should be considered if no improvement after 4–6 weeks, (200 micrograms is equivalent to approximately 6 drops)
▹ Adult: 200 micrograms 1–2 times a day, to be administered into each nostril, alternative treatment should be considered if no improvement after 4–6 weeks, (200 micrograms is equivalent to approximately 6 drops)

AVAMYS ® SPRAY

Prophylaxis and treatment of allergic rhinitis
▸ BY INTRANASAL ADMINISTRATION
▹ Child 6–11 years: 27.5 micrograms once daily, dose to be sprayed into each nostril, then increased if necessary to 55 micrograms once daily, dose to be sprayed into each nostril, reduced to 27.5 micrograms once daily, to be sprayed into each nostril, dose to be reduced once control achieved; use minimum effective dose
▹ Child 12–17 years: 55 micrograms once daily, dose to be sprayed into each nostril, reduced to continued →

12

Ear, nose and oropharynx

27.5 micrograms once daily, to be sprayed into each nostril, dose to be reduced once control achieved; use minimum effective dose

▸ Adult: 55 micrograms once daily, dose to be sprayed into each nostril, reduced to 27.5 micrograms once daily, to be sprayed into each nostril, dose to be reduced once control achieved; use minimum effective dose

DOSE EQUIVALENCE AND CONVERSION

▸ For *Avamys*® spray: 1 spray equivalent to 27.5 micrograms.

● INTERACTIONS → Appendix 1: corticosteroids

● SIDE-EFFECTS

SIDE-EFFECTS, FURTHER INFORMATION Nasal ulceration occurs commonly with nasal preparations containing fluticasone furoate.

● EXCEPTIONS TO LEGAL CATEGORY Preparations of fluticasone propionate can be sold to the public for nasal administration (other than by pressurised nasal spray) if supplied for the prevention and treatment of allergic rhinitis in adults over 18 years, subject to max. single dose of 100 micrograms per nostril, max. daily dose of 200 micrograms per nostril for max. 3 months, and a pack size of 3 mg.

● MEDICINAL FORMS
There can be variation in the licensing of different medicines containing the same drug.

Spray
EXCIPIENTS: May contain Benzalkonium chloride, disodium edetate, polysorbates

▸ Fluticasone (Non-proprietary)
Fluticasone propionate 50 microgram per 1 dose Fluticasone propionate 50micrograms/dose nasal spray | 150 dose [PoM] 🛇 DT = £11.01

▸ Avamys (GlaxoSmithKline UK Ltd)
Fluticasone furoate 27.5 microgram per 1 dose Avamys 27.5micrograms/dose nasal spray | 120 dose [PoM] £6.44 DT = £6.44

▸ Flixonase (GlaxoSmithKline Consumer Healthcare, GlaxoSmithKline UK Ltd)
Fluticasone propionate 50 microgram per 1 dose Flixonase 50micrograms/dose aqueous nasal spray | 150 dose [PoM] £11.01 DT = £11.01

▸ Nasofan (Teva UK Ltd)
Fluticasone propionate 50 microgram per 1 dose Nasofan 50micrograms/dose aqueous nasal spray | 150 dose [PoM] £8.04 DT = £11.01

▸ Pirinase Hayfever (GlaxoSmithKline Consumer Healthcare)
Fluticasone propionate 50 microgram per 1 dose Pirinase Hayfever Relief for Adults 0.05% nasal spray | 60 dose [GSL] £5.05

Nasal drops
EXCIPIENTS: May contain Polysorbates

▸ Flixonase (GlaxoSmithKline UK Ltd)
Fluticasone propionate 400 microgram Flixonase Nasule 400microgram/unit dose nasal drops | 28 unit dose [PoM] £12.99 DT = £12.99

Fluticasone with azelastine

The properties listed below are those particular to the combination only. For the properties of the components please consider, fluticasone p. 1171, azelastine hydrochloride p. 1169.

● INDICATIONS AND DOSE

Moderate to severe seasonal and perennial allergic rhinitis, if monotherapy with antihistamine or corticosteroid is inadequate

▸ BY INTRANASAL ADMINISTRATION

▸ Child 12–17 years: 1 spray twice daily, dose to be administered into each nostril

▸ Adult: 1 spray twice daily, dose to be administered into each nostril

● INTERACTIONS → Appendix 1: antihistamines, non-sedating · corticosteroids

● MEDICINAL FORMS
There can be variation in the licensing of different medicines containing the same drug.

Spray
EXCIPIENTS: May contain Benzalkonium chloride, polysorbates

▸ Fluticasone with azelastine (Non-proprietary)
Fluticasone propionate 50 microgram per 1 actuation, Azelastine hydrochloride 137 microgram per 1 actuation Fluticasone propionate 50micrograms/dose / Azelastine 137micrograms/dose nasal spray | 120 dose [PoM] 🛇 DT = £14.80

▸ Dymista (Meda Pharmaceuticals Ltd)
Fluticasone propionate 50 microgram per 1 actuation, Azelastine hydrochloride 137 microgram per 1 actuation Dymista 137micrograms/dose / 50micrograms/dose nasal spray | 120 dose [PoM] £14.80 DT = £14.80

Mometasone furoate

⚑ 1170

21-Dec-2017

● INDICATIONS AND DOSE

Prophylaxis and treatment of allergic rhinitis

▸ BY INTRANASAL ADMINISTRATION

▸ Child 6–11 years: 50 micrograms daily, dose to be sprayed into each nostril

▸ Child 12–17 years: 100 micrograms daily, increased if necessary up to 200 micrograms daily, dose to be sprayed into each nostril; reduced to 50 micrograms daily, dose to be reduced when control achieved, dose to be sprayed into each nostril

▸ Adult: 100 micrograms daily, increased if necessary up to 200 micrograms daily, dose to be sprayed into each nostril; reduced to 50 micrograms daily, dose to be reduced when control achieved, dose to be sprayed into each nostril

Nasal polyps

▸ BY INTRANASAL ADMINISTRATION

▸ Adult: Initially 100 micrograms daily for 5–6 weeks, dose to be sprayed into each nostril, then increased if necessary to 100 micrograms twice daily, dose to be sprayed into each nostril, consider alternative treatment if no improvement after further 5–6 weeks, reduce to the lowest effective dose when control achieved

● INTERACTIONS → Appendix 1: corticosteroids

● SIDE-EFFECTS

SIDE-EFFECTS, FURTHER INFORMATION Nasal ulceration occurs commonly with preparations containing mometasone furoate.

● MEDICINAL FORMS
There can be variation in the licensing of different medicines containing the same drug.

Spray
EXCIPIENTS: May contain Benzalkonium chloride, polysorbates

▸ Mometasone furoate (Non-proprietary)
Mometasone furoate 50 microgram per 1 dose Mometasone 50micrograms/dose nasal spray | 140 dose [PoM] £7.30 DT = £1.70

▸ Nasonex (Merck Sharp & Dohme Ltd)
Mometasone furoate 50 microgram per 1 dose Nasonex 50micrograms/dose nasal spray | 140 dose [PoM] £7.68 DT = £1.70

Triamcinolone acetonide

⚑ 1170

21-Dec-2017

● INDICATIONS AND DOSE

Prophylaxis and treatment of allergic rhinitis

▸ BY INTRANASAL ADMINISTRATION

▸ Child 6–11 years: 55 micrograms once daily, dose to be sprayed into each nostril, increased if necessary to 110 micrograms once daily, dose to be sprayed into each nostril; reduced to 55 micrograms once daily, dose to be sprayed into each nostril, reduce dose when control achieved; maximum duration of treatment 3 months

- Child 12-17 years: 110 micrograms once daily, dose to be sprayed into each nostril, reduced to 55 micrograms once daily, dose to be sprayed into each nostril, reduce dose when control achieved
- Adult: 110 micrograms once daily, dose to be sprayed into each nostril, reduced to 55 micrograms once daily, dose to be sprayed into each nostril, reduce dose when control achieved

- INTERACTIONS → Appendix 1: corticosteroids

- EXCEPTIONS TO LEGAL CATEGORY Preparations of triamcinolone acetonide can be sold to the public for nasal administration as a non-pressurised nasal spray if supplied for the symptomatic treatment of seasonal allergic rhinitis in adults over 18 years, subject to maximum daily dose of 110 micrograms per nostril for maximum 3 months, and a pack size of 3.575 mg.

- MEDICINAL FORMS
There can be variation in the licensing of different medicines containing the same drug.

Spray
EXCIPIENTS: May contain Benzalkonium chloride, disodium edetate, polysorbates

▸ Nasacort (Sanofi)
Triamcinolone acetonide 55 microgram per 1 dose Nasacort 55micrograms/dose nasal spray | 120 dose [PoM] £7.39 DT = £7.39

MAST-CELL STABILISERS

Sodium cromoglicate

(Sodium cromoglycate)

- INDICATIONS AND DOSE
Prophylaxis of allergic rhinitis
▸ BY INTRANASAL ADMINISTRATION
▸ Child: 1 spray 2–4 times a day, to be administered into each nostril
▸ Adult: 1 spray 2–4 times a day, to be administered into each nostril

- UNLICENSED USE Licensed for use in children (age range not specified by manufacturers).

- MEDICINAL FORMS
No licensed medicines listed.

Oropharynx

1 Dry mouth

Treatment of dry mouth

Overview

Dry mouth (xerostomia) may be caused by drugs with antimuscarinic (anticholinergic) side-effects (e.g. antispasmodics, tricyclic antidepressants, and some antipsychotics), by diuretics, by irradiation of the head and neck region or by damage to or disease of the salivary glands. Patients with a persistently dry mouth may develop a burning or scalded sensation and have poor oral hygiene; they may develop increased dental caries, periodontal disease, intolerance of dentures, and oral infections (particularly candidiasis). Dry mouth may be relieved in many patients by simple measures such as frequent sips of cool drinks or sucking pieces of ice or sugar-free fruit

pastilles. Sugar-free chewing gum stimulates salivation in patients with residual salivary function.

Artificial saliva can provide useful relief of dry mouth. A properly balanced artificial saliva should be of a neutral pH and contain electrolytes (including fluoride) to correspond approximately to the composition of saliva. The acidic pH of some artificial saliva products may be inappropriate. Of the proprietary preparations, *Aquoral®*, *Biotène Oralbalance®* gel or *Xerotin®* can be used for any condition giving rise to a dry mouth. *BioXtra®*, *Glandosane®*, *Saliva Orthana®*, and *Saliveze®*, have ACBS approval for dry mouth associated only with radiotherapy or sicca syndrome. *Salivix®* pastilles, which act locally as salivary stimulants, are also available for any condition leading to a dry mouth and SST tablets may be prescribed for dry mouth in patients with salivary gland impairment (and patent salivary ducts).

Pilocarpine tablets p. 1174 are licensed for the treatment of xerostomia following irradiation for head and neck cancer and for dry mouth and dry eyes (xerophthalmia) in Sjögren's syndrome. They are effective only in patients who have some residual salivary gland function, and therefore should be withdrawn if there is no response.

LUBRICANTS

Artificial saliva products

- ARTIFICIAL SALIVA PRODUCTS
AS SALIVA ORTHANA® LOZENGES
Mucin 65 mg, xylitol 59 mg, in a sorbitol basis, pH neutral

- INDICATIONS AND DOSE
Dry mouth as a result of having (or having undergone) radiotherapy (ACBS) | Dry mouth as a result of sicca syndrome (ACBS)
▸ BY MOUTH
▸ Adult: 1 lozenge as required, allow to dissolve slowly in the mouth

- PRESCRIBING AND DISPENSING INFORMATION *AS Saliva Orthana®* lozenges do not contain fluoride.

AS Saliva Orthana lozenges (A S Pharma Ltd)
30 lozenge(ACBS) • NHS indicative price = £3.50 • Drug Tariff (Part VIIIA Category C) price = £3.50

AS SALIVA ORTHANA® SPRAY
Gastric mucin (porcine) 3.5%, xylitol 2%, sodium fluoride 4.2 mg/litre, with preservatives and flavouring agents, pH neutral

- INDICATIONS AND DOSE
Symptomatic treatment of dry mouth
▸ BY MOUTH
▸ Adult: Apply 2–3 sprays as required, spray onto oral and pharyngeal mucosa

- PROFESSION SPECIFIC INFORMATION
Dental practitioners' formulary
AS Saliva Orthana® Oral Spray may be prescribed.

BIOXTRA® GEL
Lactoperoxidase, lactoferrin, lysozyme, whey colostrum, xylitol and other ingredients.

- INDICATIONS AND DOSE
Dry mouth as a result of having (or having undergone) radiotherapy | Dry mouth as a result of sicca syndrome
▸ BY MOUTH
▸ Adult: Apply as required, apply to oral mucosa

- PROFESSION SPECIFIC INFORMATION
Dental practitioners' formulary
BioXtra® Gel may be prescribed.

BioXtra Dry Mouth oral gel (R.I.S. Products Ltd)
40 ml • NHS indicative price = £3.94 • Drug Tariff (Part IXa)

BIOTENE ORALBALANCE®
Lactoperoxidase, lactoferrin, lysozyme, glucose oxidase, xylitol in a gel basis

● **INDICATIONS AND DOSE**

Symptomatic treatment of dry mouth
▶ BY MOUTH
▸ Adult: Apply as required, apply to gums and tongue

● **PATIENT AND CARER ADVICE** Avoid use with toothpastes containing detergents (including foaming agents).

● **PROFESSION SPECIFIC INFORMATION**

Dental practitioners' formulary
Biotene Oralbalance® Saliva Replacement Gel may be prescribed as Artificial Saliva Gel.

Biotene Oralbalance dry mouth saliva replacement gel
(GlaxoSmithKline Consumer Healthcare) Glucose oxidase 12000 unit, Lactoferrin 12 mg, Lactoperoxidase 12000 unit, Muramidase 12 mg 50 gram • NHS indicative price = £4.46 • Drug Tariff (Part IXa)

GLANDOSANE®
Carmellose sodium 500 mg, sorbitol 1.5 g, potassium chloride 60 mg, sodium chloride 42.2 mg, magnesium chloride 2.6 mg, calcium chloride 7.3 mg, and dipotassium hydrogen phosphate 17.1 mg/50 g, pH 5.75.

● **INDICATIONS AND DOSE**

Dry mouth as a result of having (or having undergone) radiotherapy (ACBS) | Dry mouth as a result of sicca syndrome (ACBS)
▶ BY MOUTH
▸ Adult: Apply as required, spray onto oral and pharyngeal mucosa

● **PROFESSION SPECIFIC INFORMATION**

Dental practitioners' formulary
Glandosane® Aerosol Spray may be prescribed.

Glandosane synthetic saliva spray lemon (Fresenius Kabi Ltd)
50 ml • NHS indicative price = £5.68

Glandosane synthetic saliva spray natural (Fresenius Kabi Ltd)
50 ml • NHS indicative price = £5.68

Glandosane synthetic saliva spray peppermint (Fresenius Kabi Ltd)
50 ml • NHS indicative price = £5.68

ORALIEVE GEL

● **INDICATIONS AND DOSE**

Symptomatic treatment of dry mouth
▶ BY MOUTH
▸ Adult: Apply as required, particularly at night, to oral mucosa

● **PRESCRIBING AND DISPENSING INFORMATION** Contains traces of milk protein and egg white protein.

SST®
Sugar-free, citric acid, malic acid and other ingredients in a sorbitol base.

● **INDICATIONS AND DOSE**

Symptomatic treatment of dry mouth in patients with impaired salivary gland function and patent salivary ducts
▶ BY MOUTH
▸ Adult: 1 tablet as required, allow tablet to dissolve slowly in the mouth

● **PROFESSION SPECIFIC INFORMATION**

Dental practitioners' formulary
May be prescribed as Saliva Stimulating Tablets.

SST saliva stimulating tablets (Sinclair IS Pharma Plc)
100 tablet • NHS indicative price = £4.86 • Drug Tariff (Part IXa)

SALIVEZE®
Carmellose sodium (sodium carboxymethylcellulose), calcium chloride, magnesium chloride, potassium chloride, sodium chloride, and dibasic sodium phosphate, pH neutral

● **INDICATIONS AND DOSE**

Dry mouth as a result of having (or having undergone) radiotherapy (ACBS) | Dry mouth as a result of sicca syndrome (ACBS)
▶ BY MOUTH
▸ Adult: Apply 1 spray as required, spray onto oral mucosa

● **PROFESSION SPECIFIC INFORMATION**

Dental practitioners' formulary
Saliveze® Oral Spray may be prescribed.

Saliveze mouth spray (Wyvern Medical Ltd)
50 ml(ACBS) • NHS indicative price = £3.50

SALIVIX®
Sugar-free, reddish-amber, acacia, malic acid and other ingredients.

● **INDICATIONS AND DOSE**

Symptomatic treatment of dry mouth
▶ BY MOUTH USING PASTILLES
▸ Adult: 1 unit as required, suck pastille

● **PROFESSION SPECIFIC INFORMATION**

Dental practitioners' formulary
Salivix® Pastilles may be prescribed as Artificial Saliva Pastilles.

Salivix pastilles (Galen Ltd)
50 pastille • NHS indicative price = £3.55 • Drug Tariff (Part IXa)

XEROTIN®
Sugar-free, water, sorbitol, carmellose (carboxymethylcellulose), potassium chloride, sodium chloride, potassium phosphate, magnesium chloride, calcium chloride and other ingredients, pH neutral.

● **INDICATIONS AND DOSE**

Symptomatic treatment of dry mouth
▶ BY MOUTH
▸ Adult: 1 spray as required

● **PROFESSION SPECIFIC INFORMATION**

Dental practitioners' formulary
Xerotin® Oral Spray may be prescribed as Artificial Saliva Oral Spray.

Xerotin spray (SpePharm UK Ltd)
100 ml • NHS indicative price = £6.86 • Drug Tariff (Part IXa)

PARASYMPATHOMIMETICS

Pilocarpine

● **INDICATIONS AND DOSE**

Xerostomia following irradiation for head and neck cancer
▶ BY MOUTH
▸ Adult: 5 mg 3 times a day for 4 weeks, then increased if tolerated to up to 30 mg daily in divided doses if required, dose to be taken with or immediately after meals (last dose always with evening meal), maximum therapeutic effect normally within 4–8 weeks; discontinue if no improvement after 2–3 months

Dry mouth and dry eyes in Sjögren's syndrome
▶ BY MOUTH
▸ Adult: 5 mg 4 times a day; increased if tolerated to up to 30 mg daily in divided doses if required, dose to be taken with meals and at bedtime, discontinue if no improvement after 2–3 months

- CONTRA-INDICATIONS Acute iritis · chronic obstructive pulmonary disease (increased bronchial secretions and increased airways resistance) · uncontrolled asthma (increased bronchial secretions and increased airways resistance) · uncontrolled cardiorenal disease

- CAUTIONS Asthma (avoid if uncontrolled) · biliary-tract disease · cardiovascular disease (avoid if uncontrolled) · cholelithiasis · chronic obstructive pulmonary disease (avoid if uncontrolled) · cognitive disturbances · maintain adequate fluid intake to avoid dehydration associated with excessive sweating · peptic ulceration · psychiatric disturbances · risk of increased renal colic · risk of increased urethral smooth muscle tone · susceptibility to angle-closure glaucoma

- INTERACTIONS → Appendix 1: pilocarpine

- SIDE-EFFECTS
  ▸ **Common or very common** Asthenia · conjunctivitis · constipation · diarrhoea · dizziness · excessive tearing · eye pain · flushing · gastrointestinal discomfort · headache · hyperhidrosis · hypersalivation · hypersensitivity · hypertension · increased risk of infection · nausea · palpitations · skin reactions · urinary disorders · vision disorders · vomiting
  ▸ **Uncommon** Gastrointestinal disorders
  ▸ **Frequency not known** Affective disorder · agitation · arrhythmias · atrioventricular block · chills · confusion · hallucination · hypotension · memory loss · psychiatric disorder · respiratory distress · shock · tremor

- PREGNANCY Avoid—smooth muscle stimulant; toxicity in *animal* studies.

- BREAST FEEDING Manufacturer advises avoid—present in milk in *animal* studies.

- HEPATIC IMPAIRMENT **Dose adjustments** Reduce initial oral dose in moderate or severe cirrhosis.

- RENAL IMPAIRMENT Manufacturer advises caution with tablets.

- PATIENT AND CARER ADVICE
  Driving and skilled tasks Blurred vision may affect performance of skilled tasks (e.g. driving) particularly at night or in reduced lighting.

- MEDICINAL FORMS
  There can be variation in the licensing of different medicines containing the same drug. Forms available from special-order manufacturers include: oral solution
  Tablet
  CAUTIONARY AND ADVISORY LABELS 21, 27
  ▸ Salagen (Merus Labs Luxco S.a R.L.)
  Pilocarpine hydrochloride 5 mg Salagen 5mg tablets
  84 tablet PoM £41.14 DT = £41.14

2 Oral hygiene

Mouthwashes and other preparations for oropharyngeal use

Lozenges and sprays

There is no convincing evidence that antiseptic lozenges and sprays have a beneficial action and they sometimes irritate and cause sore tongue and sore lips. Some of these preparations also contain local anaesthetics which relieve pain but may cause sensitisation.

Mouthwashes, gargles, and dentifrices

Superficial infections of the mouth are often helped by warm mouthwashes which have a mechanical cleansing effect and cause some local hyperaemia. However, to be effective, they must be used frequently and vigorously. A warm saline

mouthwash is ideal and can be prepared either by dissolving half a teaspoonful of salt in a glassful of warm water or by diluting compound sodium chloride mouthwash p. 1177 with an equal volume of warm water.

Mouthwashes containing an oxidising agent, such as hydrogen peroxide p. 1176, may be useful in the treatment of acute ulcerative gingivitis (Vincent's infection) since the organisms involved are anaerobes. It also has a mechanical cleansing effect arising from frothing when in contact with oral debris.

Chlorhexidine below is an effective antiseptic which has the advantage of inhibiting plaque formation on the teeth. It does not, however, completely control plaque deposition and is not a substitute for effective toothbrushing. Moreover, chlorhexidine preparations do not penetrate significantly into stagnation areas and are therefore of little value in the control of dental caries or of periodontal disease once pocketing has developed.

Chlorhexidine mouthwash is used in the treatment of denture stomatitis. It is also used in the prevention of oral candidiasis in immunocompromised patients. Chlorhexidine mouthwash reduces the incidence of alveolar osteitis following tooth extraction. Chlorhexidine mouthwash should not be used for the prevention of endocarditis in patients undergoing dental procedures.

Chlorhexidine can be used as a mouthwash, spray or gel for secondary infection in mucosal ulceration and for controlling gingivitis, as an adjunct to other oral hygiene measures. These preparations may also be used instead of toothbrushing where there is a painful periodontal condition (e.g. primary herpetic stomatitis) or if the patient has a haemorrhagic disorder, or is disabled.

Chlorhexidine preparations are of little value in the control of acute necrotising ulcerative gingivitis. With prolonged use, chlorhexidine causes reversible brown staining of teeth and tongue. Chlorhexidine may be incompatible with some ingredients in toothpaste, causing an unpleasant taste in the mouth; rinse the mouth thoroughly with water between using toothpaste and chlorhexidine-containing products.

There is no convincing evidence that gargles are effective in adults.

ANTISEPTICS AND DISINFECTANTS

Chlorhexidine

- INDICATIONS AND DOSE
  Oral hygiene and plaque inhibition | Oral candidiasis | Gingivitis | Management of aphthous ulcers
  ▸ BY MOUTH USING MOUTHWASH
  ▸ Child: Rinse or gargle 10 mL twice daily (rinse or gargle for about 1 minute)
  ▸ Adult: Rinse or gargle 10 mL twice daily (rinse or gargle for about 1 minute)

  Denture stomatitis
  ▸ MOUTHWASH
  ▸ Adult: Cleanse and soak dentures in mouthwash solution for 15 minutes twice daily

  Oral hygiene and plaque inhibition and gingivitis
  ▸ BY MOUTH USING DENTAL GEL
  ▸ Child: Apply 1–2 times a day, to be brushed on the teeth
  ▸ Adult: Apply 1–2 times a day, to be brushed on the teeth

  Oral candidiasis | Management of aphthous ulcers
  ▸ BY MOUTH USING DENTAL GEL
  ▸ Child: Apply 1–2 times a day, to affected areas
  ▸ Adult: Apply 1–2 times a day, to affected areas

continued →

12

Ear, nose and oropharynx

Oral hygiene and plaque inhibition | Oral candidiasis | Gingivitis | Management of aphthous ulcers
▶ BY MOUTH USING OROMUCOSAL SPRAY
▶ Child: Apply up to 12 sprays twice daily as required, to be applied tooth, gingival, or ulcer surfaces
▶ Adult: Apply up to 12 sprays twice daily as required, to be applied tooth, gingival, or ulcer surfaces

Bladder irrigation and catheter patency solutions
▶ BY INTRAVESICAL INSTILLATION
▶ Adult: (consult product literature)

● UNLICENSED USE *Corsodyl*® not licensed for use in children under 12 years (unless on the advice of a healthcare professional).
● SIDE-EFFECTS
● **Common or very common** Dry mouth · hypersensitivity · oral disorders · taste altered
   SIDE-EFFECTS, FURTHER INFORMATION If desquamation occurs with mucosal irritation, discontinue treatment.
● PATIENT AND CARER ADVICE Chlorhexidine gluconate may be incompatible with some ingredients in toothpaste; rinse the mouth thoroughly with water between using toothpaste and chlorhexidine-containing product.
● PROFESSION SPECIFIC INFORMATION
   Dental practitioners' formulary *Corsodyl*® dental gel may be prescribed as Chlorhexidine Gluconate Gel; *Corsodyl*® mouthwash may be prescribed as Chlorhexidine Mouthwash; *Corsodyl*® oral spray may be prescribed as Chlorhexidine Oral Spray.
● MEDICINAL FORMS
   There can be variation in the licensing of different medicines containing the same drug.
   Dental gel
   ▶ Corsodyl (GlaxoSmithKline Consumer Healthcare)
      Chlorhexidine gluconate 10 mg per 1 gram Corsodyl 1% dental gel sugar-free | 50 gram [P] £1.56 DT = £1.56
   Mouthwash
   ▶ Chlorhexidine (Non-proprietary)
      Chlorhexidine gluconate 2 mg per 1 ml Chlorhexidine gluconate 0.2% mouthwash aniseed | 300 ml [GSL] £2.09 DT = £4.09
      Chlorhexidine gluconate 0.2% mouthwash natural | 300 ml [GSL] £4.02 DT = £4.09
      Chlorhexidine gluconate 0.2% mouthwash plain | 300 ml [GSL] £4.09 DT = £4.09
      Chlorhexidine gluconate 0.2% mouthwash peppermint | 300 ml [GSL] £4.09 DT = £4.09
      Chlorhexidine gluconate 0.2% mouthwash original | 300 ml [GSL] £4.18 DT = £4.09
      Chlorhexidine gluconate 0.2% mouthwash alcohol free | 300 ml [GSL] [⬧] DT = £4.09
   ▶ Corsodyl (GlaxoSmithKline Consumer Healthcare)
      Chlorhexidine gluconate 2 mg per 1 ml Corsodyl 0.2% mouthwash aniseed | 300 ml [GSL] £2.44 DT = £4.09
      Corsodyl Mint 0.2% mouthwash | 300 ml [GSL] £2.44 DT = £4.09 | 600 ml [GSL] £4.50
      Corsodyl 0.2% mouthwash alcohol free | 300 ml [GSL] £3.06 DT = £4.09
   ▶ Curasept (Curaprox (UK) Ltd)
      Chlorhexidine gluconate 2 mg per 1 ml Curasept 0.2% oral rinse | 200 ml [⬧]
   Irrigation
   ▶ Chlorhexidine (Non-proprietary)
      Chlorhexidine acetate 200 microgram per 1 ml Chlorhexidine acetate 0.02% catheter maintenance solution | 100 ml [P] [⬧]
   ▶ Uro-Tainer (chlorhexidine) (B.Braun Medical Ltd)
      Chlorhexidine acetate 200 microgram per 1 ml Uro-Tainer chlorhexidine 1:5000 catheter maintenance solution | 100 ml [P] £2.70
   Irrigation solution
   ▶ Chlorhexidine (Non-proprietary)
      Chlorhexidine acetate 200 microgram per 1 ml Chlorhexidine acetate 0.02% irrigation solution 1litre bottles | 1 bottle [P] [⬧]
      Chlorhexidine acetate 500 microgram per 1 ml Chlorhexidine acetate 0.05% irrigation solution 1litre bottles | 1 bottle [P] [⬧]

Hexetidine

● INDICATIONS AND DOSE
Oral hygiene
▶ BY MOUTH USING MOUTHWASH
▶ Child 6–17 years: Rinse or gargle 15 mL 2–3 times a day, to be used undiluted
▶ Adult: Rinse or gargle 15 mL 2–3 times a day, to be used undiluted

● SIDE-EFFECTS
▶ **Rare or very rare** Anaesthesia · taste altered
▶ **Frequency not known** Cough · dry mouth · dysphagia · dyspnoea · nausea · salivary gland enlargement · vomiting

● MEDICINAL FORMS
   There can be variation in the licensing of different medicines containing the same drug.
   Mouthwash
   ▶ Oraldene (McNeil Products Ltd)
      Hexetidine 1 mg per 1 ml Oraldene 0.1% mouthwash peppermint sugar-free | 200 ml [GSL] £2.92

Hydrogen peroxide

● DRUG ACTION Hydrogen peroxide is an oxidising agent.

● INDICATIONS AND DOSE
Oral hygiene (with hydrogen peroxide 6%)
▶ BY MOUTH USING MOUTHWASH
▶ Child: Rinse or gargle 15 mL 2–3 times a day for 2–3 minutes, to be diluted in half a tumblerful of warm water
▶ Adult: Rinse or gargle 15 mL 2–3 times a day for 2–3 minutes, to be diluted in half a tumblerful of warm water
PEROXYL®
Oral hygiene
▶ BY MOUTH USING MOUTHWASH
▶ Child 6–17 years: Rinse or gargle 10 mL 3 times a day for about 1 minute, for maximum 7 days, to be used after meals and at bedtime
▶ Adult: Rinse or gargle 10 mL up to 4 times a day for about 1 minute, to be used after meals and at bedtime

● SIDE-EFFECTS Tongue papilla hypertrophy
● PRESCRIBING AND DISPENSING INFORMATION When prepared extemporaneously, the BP states Hydrogen Peroxide Mouthwash, BP consists of hydrogen peroxide 6% solution (= approx. 20 volume) BP.
● HANDLING AND STORAGE Hydrogen peroxide bleaches fabric.
● PROFESSION SPECIFIC INFORMATION
   Dental practitioners' formulary Hydrogen Peroxide Mouthwash may be prescribed.
● MEDICINAL FORMS
   There can be variation in the licensing of different medicines containing the same drug.
   Mouthwash
   ▶ Peroxyl (Colgate-Palmolive (UK) Ltd)
      Hydrogen peroxide 15 mg per 1 ml Peroxyl 1.5% mouthwash sugar-free | 300 ml [GSL] £2.94 DT = £2.94

Sodium bicarbonate with sodium chloride

● INDICATIONS AND DOSE
Oral hygiene
▶ BY MOUTH USING MOUTHWASH
▶ Adult: (consult product literature)

● DIRECTIONS FOR ADMINISTRATION For mouthwash, extemporaneous preparations should be prepared according to the following formula: sodium chloride 1.5 g, sodium bicarbonate 1 g, concentrated peppermint emulsion 2.5 mL, double-strength chloroform water 50 mL, water to 100 mL. To be diluted with an equal volume of warm water prior to administration.

- **PRESCRIBING AND DISPENSING INFORMATION** Flavours of mouthwash may include peppermint.
- **PROFESSION SPECIFIC INFORMATION**

Dental practitioners' formulary Compound sodium chloride mouthwash may be prescribed.

- **MEDICINAL FORMS**
Forms available from special-order manufacturers include: mouthwash

Sodium chloride

- **INDICATIONS AND DOSE**

Oral hygiene
- ▶ BY MOUTH USING MOUTHWASH
- ▹ Child: Rinse or gargle as required
- ▹ Adult: Rinse or gargle as required

- **DIRECTIONS FOR ADMINISTRATION** Extemporaneous mouthwash preparations should be prepared according to the following formula: sodium chloride 1.5 g, sodium bicarbonate 1 g, concentrated peppermint emulsion 2.5 mL, double-strength chloroform water 50 mL, water to 100 mL. To be diluted with an equal volume of warm water.
- **PRESCRIBING AND DISPENSING INFORMATION** No mouthwash preparations available—when prepared extemporaneously, the BP states Sodium Chloride Mouthwash, Compound, BP consists of sodium bicarbonate 1%, sodium chloride 1.5% in a suitable vehicle with peppermint flavour.
- ▹ In children The RCPCH and NPPG recommend that, when a liquid special of sodium chloride is required, the following strength is used: 5 mmol/mL.
- **PROFESSION SPECIFIC INFORMATION**

Dental practitioners' formulary Compound Sodium Chloride Mouthwash may be prescribed.

- **MEDICINAL FORMS**
No licensed medicines listed.

2.1 Dental caries

Fluoride

Availability of adequate fluoride confers significant resistance to dental caries. It is now considered that the topical action of fluoride on enamel and plaque is more important than the systemic effect.

When the fluoride content of drinking water is less than 700 micrograms per litre (0.7 parts per million), daily administration of fluoride tablets or drops provides suitable supplementation. Systemic fluoride supplements should not be prescribed without reference to the fluoride content of the local water supply. Infants need not receive fluoride supplements until the age of 6 months.

Dentifrices which incorporate sodium fluoride or monofluorophosphate are also a convenient source of fluoride.

Individuals who are either particularly caries prone or medically compromised may be given additional protection by use of fluoride rinses or by application of fluoride gels. Rinses may be used daily or weekly; daily use of a less concentrated rinse is more effective than weekly use of a more concentrated one. High-strength gels must be applied regularly under professional supervision; extreme caution is

necessary to prevent children from swallowing any excess. Less concentrated gels are available for home use. Varnishes are also available and are particularly valuable for young or disabled children since they adhere to the teeth and set in the presence of moisture.

VITAMINS AND TRACE ELEMENTS

Sodium fluoride

- **INDICATIONS AND DOSE**

Prophylaxis of dental caries for water content less than 300micrograms/litre (0.3 parts per million) of fluoride ion
- ▶ BY MOUTH USING TABLETS
- ▹ Child 6 months-2 years: 250 micrograms daily, doses expressed as fluoride ion (F⁻)
- ▹ Child 3-5 years: 500 micrograms daily, doses expressed as fluoride ion (F⁻)
- ▹ Child 6-17 years: 1 mg daily, doses expressed as fluoride ion (F⁻)
- ▹ Adult: 1 mg daily, doses expressed as fluoride ion (F⁻)

Prophylaxis of dental caries for water content between 300 and 700micrograms/litre (0.3-0.7 parts per million) of fluoride ion
- ▶ BY MOUTH USING TABLETS
- ▹ Child 3-5 years: 250 micrograms daily, doses expressed as fluoride ion (F⁻)
- ▹ Child 6-17 years: 500 micrograms daily, doses expressed as fluoride ion (F⁻)
- ▹ Adult: 500 micrograms daily, doses expressed as fluoride ion (F⁻)

Prophylaxis of dental caries for water content above 700micrograms/litre (0.7 parts per million) of fluoride ion
- ▹ Child 6 months-17 years: Supplements not advised
- ▹ Adult: Supplements not advised

Prophylaxis of dental caries for individuals who are caries prone or medically compromised
- ▶ BY MOUTH USING MOUTHWASH
- ▹ Adult: Rinse or gargle 10 mL daily

DOSE EQUIVALENCE AND CONVERSION
- ▹ Sodium fluoride 2.2 mg provides approx. 1 mg fluoride ion.
- ▹ These doses reflect the recommendations of the British Dental Association, the British Society of Paediatric Dentistry and the British Association for the Study of Community Dentistry (*Br Dent J* 1997; **182**: 6–7).

COLGATE DURAPHAT ® 2800PPM FLUORIDE TOOTHPASTE
Prophylaxis of dental caries
- ▶ BY MOUTH USING PASTE
- ▹ Child 10-17 years: Apply 1 centimetre twice daily, to be applied using a toothbrush
- ▹ Adult: Apply 1 centimetre twice daily, to be applied using a toothbrush

COLGATE DURAPHAT ® 5000PPM FLUORIDE TOOTHPASTE
Prophylaxis of dental caries
- ▶ BY MOUTH USING PASTE
- ▹ Child 16-17 years: Apply 2 centimetres 3 times a day, to be applied after meals using a toothbrush
- ▹ Adult: Apply 2 centimetres 3 times a day, to be applied after meals using a toothbrush

EN-DE-KAY ® FLUORINSE
Prophylaxis of dental carries for individuals who are caries prone or medically compromised
- ▶ BY MOUTH USING MOUTHWASH
- ▹ Adult: 5 drops daily, dilute 5 drops to 10 mL of water, alternatively 20 drops once weekly, dilute 20 drops to 10 mL

- CONTRA-INDICATIONS Not for areas where drinking water is fluoridated
- SIDE-EFFECTS Dental fluorosis
- DIRECTIONS FOR ADMINISTRATION
  - ▶ With oral use Tablets should be sucked or dissolved in the mouth and taken preferably in the evening.
  - ▶ With oral (topical) use For mouthwash, rinse mouth for 1 minute and then spit out.

  COLGATE DURAPHAT ® 5000PPM FLUORIDE
  TOOTHPASTE Brush teeth for 3 minutes before spitting out.

  COLGATE DURAPHAT ® 2800PPM FLUORIDE
  TOOTHPASTE Brush teeth for 1 minute before spitting out.
- PRESCRIBING AND DISPENSING INFORMATION Flavours of oral tablet formulations may include orange.
- PATIENT AND CARER ADVICE
  Mouthwash Avoid eating, drinking, or rinsing mouth for 15 minutes after use.

  COLGATE DURAPHAT ® 5000PPM FLUORIDE
  TOOTHPASTE Patients or carers should be given advice on how to administer Sodium fluoride toothpaste.

  COLGATE DURAPHAT ® 2800PPM FLUORIDE
  TOOTHPASTE Patients or carers should be given advice on how to administer sodium fluoride toothpaste.
  Avoid drinking or rinsing mouth for 30 minutes after use.
- PROFESSION SPECIFIC INFORMATION
  Dental practitioners' formulary
  Tablets may be prescribed as Sodium Fluoride Tablets.
  Oral drops may be prescribed as Sodium Fluoride Oral Drops.
  Mouthwashes may be prescribed as Sodium Fluoride Mouthwash 0.05% or Sodium Fluoride Mouthwash 2%.
  COLGATE DURAPHAT ® 5000PPM FLUORIDE
  TOOTHPASTE May be prescribed as Sodium Fluoride Toothpaste 1.1%.
  COLGATE DURAPHAT ® 2800PPM FLUORIDE
  TOOTHPASTE May be prescribed as Sodium Fluoride Toothpaste 0.619%.
  Dental information
  Fluoride mouthwash, oral drops, tablets and toothpaste are prescribable on form FP10D (GP14 in Scotland, WP10D in Wales).
  There are also arrangements for health authorities to supply fluoride tablets in the course of pre-school dental schemes, and they may also be supplied in school dental schemes.
  Fluoride gels are not prescribable on form FP10D (GP14 in Scotland, WP10D in Wales).
- MEDICINAL FORMS
  There can be variation in the licensing of different medicines containing the same drug.
  Tablet
  ▶ Sodium fluoride (Manx Healthcare Ltd)
  Sodium fluoride 1.1 mg Endekay Fluotabs 3-6 Years 1.1mg tablets | 200 tablet P £2.38 DT = £2.38
  Sodium fluoride 2.2 mg Endekay Fluotabs 6+ Years 2.2mg tablets | 200 tablet P £2.38 DT = £2.38
  Paste
  ▶ Sodium fluoride (Non-proprietary)
  Fluoride (as Sodium fluoride) 2.8 mg per 1 gram Sodium fluoride 0.619% dental paste sugar free sugar-free | 75 ml PoM £3.26 DT = £3.26
  Fluoride (as Sodium fluoride) 5 mg per 1 gram Sodium fluoride 1.1% dental paste sugar free sugar-free | 51 gram PoM £6.50 DT = £6.50
  ▶ Colgate Duraphat (Colgate-Palmolive (UK) Ltd)
  Fluoride (as Sodium fluoride) 2.8 mg per 1 gram Colgate Duraphat 2800ppm fluoride toothpaste sugar-free | 75 ml PoM £3.26 DT = £3.26

Fluoride (as Sodium fluoride) 5 mg per 1 gram Colgate Duraphat 5000ppm fluoride toothpaste sugar-free | 51 gram PoM £6.50 DT = £6.50
Oral drops
▶ Endekay (Manx Healthcare Ltd)
Sodium fluoride 3.7 mg per 1 ml Endekay Fluodrops 0.37% drops paediatric sugar-free | 60 ml P £2.38 DT = £2.38
Mouthwash
▶ Sodium fluoride (Non-proprietary)
Sodium fluoride 500 microgram per 1 ml Sodium fluoride 0.05% mouthwash sugar free sugar-free | 250 ml GSL ⓢ DT = £1.51
▶ Colgate FluoriGard (Colgate-Palmolive (UK) Ltd)
Sodium fluoride 500 microgram per 1 ml Colgate FluoriGard 0.05% daily dental rinse alcohol free sugar-free | 400 ml £2.99
Colgate FluoriGard 0.05% daily dental rinse sugar-free | 400 ml GSL £2.99
▶ Endekay (Manx Healthcare Ltd)
Sodium fluoride 500 microgram per 1 ml Endekay 0.05% daily fluoride mouthrinse sugar-free | 250 ml GSL £1.51 DT = £1.51 sugar-free | 500 ml GSL £2.45
Sodium fluoride 20 mg per 1 ml Endekay Fluorinse 2% mouthwash sugar-free | 100 ml PoM £4.97

---

3 Oral ulceration and inflammation

Oral ulceration and inflammation

Ulceration and inflammation

Ulceration of the oral mucosa may be caused by trauma (physical or chemical), recurrent aphthae, infections, carcinoma, dermatological disorders, nutritional deficiencies, gastro-intestinal disease, haematopoietic disorders, and drug therapy (see also *Chemotherapy induced mucositis and myelosuppression* under Cytotoxic drugs p. 865). It is important to establish the diagnosis in each case as the majority of these lesions require specific management in addition to local treatment. Local treatment aims to protect the ulcerated area, to relieve pain, to reduce inflammation, or to control secondary infection. Patients with an unexplained mouth ulcer of more than 3 weeks' duration require urgent referral to hospital to exclude oral cancer.

Simple mouthwashes

A **saline** mouthwash may relieve the pain of traumatic ulceration. The mouthwash is made up with warm water and used at frequent intervals until the discomfort and swelling subsides.

Antiseptic mouthwashes

Secondary bacterial infection may be a feature of any mucosal ulceration; it can increase discomfort and delay healing. Use of a chlorhexidine mouthwash p. 1175 is often beneficial and may accelerate healing of recurrent aphthae.

Corticosteroids

Topical corticosteroid therapy may be used for some forms of oral ulceration. In the case of aphthous ulcers it is most effective if applied in the 'prodromal' phase.
Thrush or other types of candidiasis are recognised complications of corticosteroid treatment.
Hydrocortisone **oromucosal tablets** p. 1181 are allowed to dissolve next to an ulcer and are useful in recurrent aphthae and erosive lichenoid lesions.
Beclometasone dipropionate inhaler p. 1180 sprayed on the oral mucosa is used to manage oral ulceration [unlicensed indication]. Alternatively, betamethasone soluble tablets p. 1180 dissolved in water can be used as a mouthwash to treat oral ulceration [unlicensed indication].

Systemic corticosteroid therapy (see under Corticosteroids, inflammatory disorders p. 1118), is reserved for severe conditions such as pemphigus vulgaris.

Local analgesics
Local analgesics have a limited role in the management of oral ulceration. When applied topically their action is of a relatively short duration so that analgesia cannot be maintained continuously throughout the day. The main indication for a topical local analgesic is to relieve the pain of otherwise intractable oral ulceration particularly when it is due to major aphthae. For this purpose lidocaine hydrochloride 5% ointment below or lozenges containing a local anaesthetic are applied to the ulcer. Lidocaine hydrochloride 10% solution as spray can be applied thinly to the ulcer [unlicensed indication] using a cotton bud. When local anaesthetics are used in the mouth care must be taken not to produce anaesthesia of the pharynx before meals as this might lead to choking.

Preparations on sale to the public: many mouth ulcer preparations, throat lozenges, and throat sprays on sale to the public contain a local anaesthetic. To identify the active ingredients in such preparations, consult the product literature of the manufacturer— the correct proprietary name should be ascertained as many products have very similar names but different active ingredients.

Benzydamine hydrochloride p. 1180 and flurbiprofen p. 1180 are non-steroidal anti-inflammatory drugs (NSAIDs). Benzydamine hydrochloride mouthwash or spray may be useful in reducing the discomfort associated with a variety of ulcerative conditions. It has also been found to be effective in reducing the discomfort of tonsillectomy and post-irradiation mucositis. Some patients find the full-strength mouthwash causes some stinging and, for them, it should be diluted with an equal volume of water. Flurbiprofen lozenges are licensed for the relief of sore throat.

Choline salicylate p. 1181 is a derivative of salicylic acid and has some analgesic action. The dental gel may provide relief for recurrent aphthae, but excessive application or confinement under a denture irritates the mucosa and can itself cause ulceration.

Other preparations
Doxycycline p. 1182 rinsed in the mouth may be of value for recurrent aphthous ulceration.

Periodontitis
Low-dose doxycycline (*Periostat*®) is licensed as an adjunct to scaling and root planing for the treatment of periodontitis; a low dose of doxycycline reduces collagenase activity without inhibiting bacteria associated with periodontitis.

For anti-infectives used in the treatment of destructive (refractory) forms of periodontal disease, see under Oropharyngeal infections, antibacterial therapy p. 1182. See also Mouthwashes and other preparations for oropharyngeal use p. 1175 for mouthwashes used for oral hygiene and plaque inhibition.

ANAESTHETICS, LOCAL

Lidocaine hydrochloride
(Lignocaine hydrochloride)

● **INDICATIONS AND DOSE**
Dental practice
▶ BY BUCCAL ADMINISTRATION USING OINTMENT
▸ Adult: Rub gently into dry gum
Relief of pain in oral lesions
▶ TO THE LESION USING OINTMENT
▸ Adult: Apply as required, rub sparingly and gently on affected areas

XYLOCAINE®
Bronchoscopy | Laryngoscopy | Oesophagoscopy | Endotracheal intubation
▶ TO MUCOUS MEMBRANES
▸ Adult: Up to 20 doses
Dental practice
▶ TO MUCOUS MEMBRANES
▸ Adult: 1–5 doses
Maxillary sinus puncture
▶ TO MUCOUS MEMBRANES
▸ Adult: 3 doses
Relief of pain in oral lesions
▶ TO THE LESION
▸ Adult: Apply thinly to the ulcer using a cotton bud

● UNLICENSED USE Spray not licensed for the relief of pain in oral lesions.
● CAUTIONS Avoid anaesthesia of the pharynx before meals—risk of choking · can damage plastic cuffs of endotracheal tubes
● INTERACTIONS → Appendix 1: antiarrhythmics
● ALLERGY AND CROSS-SENSITIVITY
▶ Hypersensitivity and cross-sensitivity Hypersensitivity reactions occur mainly with the ester-type local anaesthetics, such as tetracaine; reactions are less frequent with the amide types, such as articaine, bupivacaine, levobupivacaine, lidocaine, mepivacaine, prilocaine, and ropivacaine. Cross-sensitivity reactions may be avoided by using the alternative chemical type.
● PREGNANCY Crosses the placenta but not known to be harmful in *animal* studies—use if benefit outweighs risk. When used as a local anaesthetic, large doses can cause fetal bradycardia; if given during delivery can also cause neonatal respiratory depression, hypotonia, or bradycardia after paracervical or epidural block.
● BREAST FEEDING Present in milk but amount too small to be harmful.
● HEPATIC IMPAIRMENT Caution—increased risk of side-effects.
● RENAL IMPAIRMENT Possible accumulation of lidocaine and active metabolite; caution in severe impairment.
● PROFESSION SPECIFIC INFORMATION
Dental practitioners' formulary
Lidocaine ointment 5% may be prescribed.
Spray may be prescribed as Lidocaine Spray 10%.
XYLOCAINE® May be prescribed as lidocaine spray 10%.
● NATIONAL FUNDING/ACCESS DECISIONS
VERSATIS®
Scottish Medicines Consortium (SMC) Decisions
The *Scottish Medicines Consortium* has advised (July 2008) that *Versatis*® is accepted for restricted use within NHS Scotland for the treatment of postherpetic neuralgia in patients who are intolerant of first-line systemic therapies or when they have been ineffective.

● MEDICINAL FORMS
There can be variation in the licensing of different medicines containing the same drug.
Ointment
▶ Lidocaine hydrochloride (Non-proprietary)
  Lidocaine hydrochloride **50 mg per 1 gram** Lidocaine 5% ointment | 15 gram ℗ £6.50 DT = £6.18

ANALGESICS > NON-STEROIDAL ANTI-INFLAMMATORY DRUGS

Benzydamine hydrochloride

- **INDICATIONS AND DOSE**

Painful inflammatory conditions of oropharynx
- ▸ TO THE LESION USING MOUTHWASH
  - ▸ Child 13-17 years: Rinse or gargle 15 mL every 1.5-3 hours as required usually for not more than 7 days, dilute with an equal volume of water if stinging occurs
  - ▸ Adult: Rinse or gargle 15 mL every 1.5-3 hours as required usually for not more than 7 days, dilute with an equal volume of water if stinging occurs
- ▸ TO THE LESION USING OROMUCOSAL SPRAY
  - ▸ Child 1 month-5 years (body-weight 4-7 kg): 1 spray every 1.5-3 hours, to be administered onto the affected area
  - ▸ Child 1 month-5 years (body-weight 8-11 kg): 2 sprays every 1.5-3 hours, to be administered onto the affected area
  - ▸ Child 1 month-5 years (body-weight 12-15 kg): 3 sprays every 1.5-3 hours, to be administered onto the affected area
  - ▸ Child 1 month-5 years (body-weight 16 kg and above): 4 sprays every 1.5-3 hours, to be administered onto the affected area
  - ▸ Child 6-11 years: 4 sprays every 1.5-3 hours, to be administered onto affected area
  - ▸ Child 12-17 years: 4-8 sprays every 1.5-3 hours, to be administered onto affected area
  - ▸ Adult: 4-8 sprays every 1.5-3 hours, to be administered onto affected area

- **INTERACTIONS** → Appendix 1: NSAIDs
- **SIDE-EFFECTS**
- ▸ **Uncommon** Oral disorders
- ▸ **Rare or very rare** Photosensitivity reaction · respiratory disorders · skin reactions
- ▸ **Frequency not known** Angioedema
- **PROFESSION SPECIFIC INFORMATION**

Dental practitioners' formulary
Benzydamine Oromucosal Spray 0.15% may be prescribed. Benzydamine mouthwash may be prescribed as Benzydamine Mouthwash 0.15%.

- **MEDICINAL FORMS**
There can be variation in the licensing of different medicines containing the same drug.
Spray
  - ▸ Benzydamine hydrochloride (Non-proprietary)
    Benzydamine hydrochloride 1.5 mg per 1 ml Benzydamine 0.15% oromucosal spray sugar free sugar-free | 30 ml P £4.24 DT = £4.21
  - ▸ Difflam (Meda Pharmaceuticals Ltd)
    Benzydamine hydrochloride 1.5 mg per 1 ml Difflam 0.15% spray sugar-free | 30 ml P £4.24 DT = £4.21
Mouthwash
  - ▸ Benzydamine hydrochloride (Non-proprietary)
    Benzydamine hydrochloride 1.5 mg per 1 ml Benzydamine 0.15% mouthwash sugar free sugar-free | 300 ml P £6.53 DT = £6.53
  - ▸ Difflam (Meda Pharmaceuticals Ltd)
    Benzydamine hydrochloride 1.5 mg per 1 ml Difflam Oral Rinse 0.15% solution sugar-free | 300 ml P £6.50 DT = £6.53
    Difflam 0.15% Sore Throat Rinse sugar-free | 200 ml P £4.64

Flurbiprofen

- **INDICATIONS AND DOSE**

Relief of sore throat
- ▸ BY MOUTH USING LOZENGES
  - ▸ Child 12-17 years: 1 lozenge every 3-6 hours for maximum 3 days, allow lozenge to dissolve slowly in the mouth; maximum 5 lozenges per day
  - ▸ Adult: 1 lozenge every 3-6 hours for maximum 3 days, allow lozenge to dissolve slowly in the mouth; maximum 5 lozenges per day

- **INTERACTIONS** → Appendix 1: NSAIDs
- **SIDE-EFFECTS**
- ▸ **Common or very common** Haemorrhage
- **ALLERGY AND CROSS-SENSITIVITY** Contra-indicated in patients with a history of hypersensitivity to aspirin or any other NSAID—which includes those in whom attacks of asthma, angioedema, urticaria or rhinitis have been precipitated by aspirin or any other NSAID.

- **MEDICINAL FORMS**
There can be variation in the licensing of different medicines containing the same drug.
Lozenge
  - ▸ Strefen (Reckitt Benckiser Healthcare (UK) Ltd)
    Flurbiprofen 8.75 mg Strefen 8.75mg lozenges | 16 lozenge P £2.58 DT = £2.58

CORTICOSTEROIDS

Beclometasone dipropionate   04-Jan-2016

(Beclomethasone dipropionate)

- **INDICATIONS AND DOSE**

Management of oral ulceration
- ▸ TO THE LESION
  - ▸ Adult: 50-100 micrograms twice daily, administered using an inhaler device

- **UNLICENSED USE** Use of inhaler unlicensed in oral ulceration.

> **IMPORTANT SAFETY INFORMATION**
>
> MHRA/CHM ADVICE: CORTICOSTEROIDS: RARE RISK OF CENTRAL SEROUS CHORIORETINOPATHY WITH LOCAL AS WELL AS SYSTEMIC ADMINISTRATION (AUGUST 2017)
> See *Corticosteroids, general use* p. 656.

- **INTERACTIONS** → Appendix 1: corticosteroids
- **MEDICINAL FORMS**
For preparations see inhaled beclometasone, p. 257.

Betamethasone   21-Dec-2017

- **INDICATIONS AND DOSE**

Oral ulceration
- ▸ TO THE LESION USING SOLUBLE TABLETS
  - ▸ Child 12-17 years: 500 micrograms 4 times a day, to be dissolved in 20 mL water and rinsed around the mouth; not to be swallowed
  - ▸ Adult: 500 micrograms 4 times a day, to be dissolved in 20 mL water and rinsed around the mouth; not to be swallowed

- UNLICENSED USE Betamethasone soluble tablets not licensed for use as mouthwash or in oral ulceration.

> **IMPORTANT SAFETY INFORMATION**
> MHRA/CHM ADVICE: CORTICOSTEROIDS: RARE RISK OF CENTRAL SEROUS CHORIORETINOPATHY WITH LOCAL AS WELL AS SYSTEMIC ADMINISTRATION (AUGUST 2017)
> See *Corticosteroids, general use* p. 656.

- CONTRA-INDICATIONS Untreated local infection
- INTERACTIONS → Appendix 1: corticosteroids
- PATIENT AND CARER ADVICE Patient counselling is advised for betamethasone soluble tablets (administration).
- PROFESSION SPECIFIC INFORMATION

  Dental practitioners' formulary Betamethasone Soluble Tablets 500 micrograms may be prescribed for oral ulceration.

- MEDICINAL FORMS
  There can be variation in the licensing of different medicines containing the same drug.
  Soluble tablet
  CAUTIONARY AND ADVISORY LABELS 10, 13, 21 (not for use as mouthwash for oral ulceration)
  ▶ Betamethasone (Non-proprietary)
  Betamethasone (as Betamethasone sodium phosphate)
  500 microgram Betamethasone 500microgram soluble tablets sugar free sugar-free | 100 tablet [PoM] £51.12 DT = £51.12

Hydrocortisone   21-Dec-2017

- **INDICATIONS AND DOSE**
  Oral and perioral lesions
  ▶ TO THE LESION USING BUCCAL TABLET
  ▶ Child 1 month–11 years: Only on medical advice
  ▶ Child 12–17 years: 1 lozenge 4 times a day, allowed to dissolve slowly in the mouth in contact with the ulcer
  ▶ Adult: 1 lozenge 4 times a day, allowed to dissolve slowly in the mouth in contact with the ulcer

- UNLICENSED USE *Hydrocortisone mucoadhesive buccal tablets* licensed for use in children (under 12 years—on medical advice only).

> **IMPORTANT SAFETY INFORMATION**
> MHRA/CHM ADVICE: CORTICOSTEROIDS: RARE RISK OF CENTRAL SEROUS CHORIORETINOPATHY WITH LOCAL AS WELL AS SYSTEMIC ADMINISTRATION (AUGUST 2017)
> See *Corticosteroids, general use* p. 656.

- CONTRA-INDICATIONS Untreated local infection
- INTERACTIONS → Appendix 1: corticosteroids
- PROFESSION SPECIFIC INFORMATION
  Dental practitioners' formulary Mucoadhesive buccal tablets may be prescribed as Hydrocortisone Oromucosal Tablets.

- MEDICINAL FORMS
  There can be variation in the licensing of different medicines containing the same drug.
  Muco-adhesive buccal tablet
  ▶ Hydrocortisone (Non-proprietary)
  Hydrocortisone (as Hydrocortisone sodium succinate)
  2.5 mg Hydrocortisone 2.5mg muco-adhesive buccal tablets sugar free sugar-free | 20 tablet [P] £8.30 DT = £7.70

SALICYLIC ACID AND DERIVATIVES

Choline salicylate

- **INDICATIONS AND DOSE**
  Mild oral and perioral lesions
  ▶ TO THE LESION
  ▶ Child 16–17 years: Apply 0.5 inch, apply with gentle massage, not more often than every 3 hours
  ▶ Adult: Apply 0.5 inch, apply with gentle massage, not more often than every 3 hours

- CONTRA-INDICATIONS Children under 16 years
  CONTRA-INDICATIONS, FURTHER INFORMATION
  ▶ Reye's syndrome The CHM has advised that topical oral pain relief products containing salicylate salts should not be used in children under 16 years, as a cautionary measure due to the theoretical risk of Reye's syndrome.

- CAUTIONS Frequent application, especially in children, may give rise to salicylate poisoning · not to be applied to dentures—leave at least 30 minutes before re-insertion of dentures (in adults)

- INTERACTIONS → Appendix 1: choline salicylate

- SIDE-EFFECTS Bronchospasm

- PRESCRIBING AND DISPENSING INFORMATION When prepared extemporaneously, the BP states Choline Salicylate Dental Gel, BP consists of choline salicylate 8.7% in a flavoured gel basis.

- PROFESSION SPECIFIC INFORMATION
  Dental practitioners' formulary
  Choline Salicylate Dental Gel may be prescribed.

- MEDICINAL FORMS
  There can be variation in the licensing of different medicines containing the same drug.
  Oromucosal gel
  ▶ Bonjela (Reckitt Benckiser Healthcare (UK) Ltd)
  Choline salicylate 87 mg per 1 gram Bonjela Cool Mint gel sugar-free | 15 gram [GSL] £3.55 DT = £2.58
  Bonjela Original gel sugar-free | 15 gram [GSL] £2.58 DT = £2.58

Salicylic acid with rhubarb extract

- **INDICATIONS AND DOSE**
  Mild oral and perioral lesions
  ▶ TO THE LESION
  ▶ Child 16–17 years: Apply 3–4 times a day maximum duration 7 days
  ▶ Adult: Apply 3–4 times a day maximum duration 7 days

- CONTRA-INDICATIONS Children under 16 years
  CONTRA-INDICATIONS, FURTHER INFORMATION
  ▶ Reye's syndrome The CHM has advised that topical oral pain relief products containing salicylate salts should not be used in children under 16 years, as a cautionary measure due to the theoretical risk of Reye's syndrome.

- CAUTIONS Frequent application, especially in children, may give rise to salicylate poisoning · not to be applied to dentures—leave at least 30 minutes before re-insertion of dentures (in adults)

- SIDE-EFFECTS
  ▶ **Common or very common** Paraesthesia · oral disorders

- PATIENT AND CARER ADVICE May cause temporary discolouration of teeth and oral mucosa.

12

Ear, nose and oropharynx

- MEDICINAL FORMS
There can be variation in the licensing of different medicines containing the same drug.
Paint
EXCIPIENTS: May contain Ethanol
▸ Pyralvex (Meda Pharmaceuticals Ltd)
Salicylic acid 10 mg per 1 ml, Rhubarb extract 50 mg per 1 ml Pyralvex solution | 10 ml P £3.25

4 Oropharyngeal bacterial infections

Oropharyngeal infections, antibacterial therapy

Pericoronitis

Antibacterial required only in presence of systemic features of infection, or of trismus, or persistent swelling despite local treatment.
- Metronidazole p. 533, or *alternatively*, amoxicillin p. 539
▸ *Suggested duration of treatment* 3 days or until symptoms resolve.

Gingivitis (acute necrotising ulcerative)

Antibacterial required only if systemic features of infection.
- Metronidazole, or *alternatively*, amoxicillin
▸ *Suggested duration of treatment* 3 days or until symptoms resolve.

Abscess (periapical or periodontal)

Antibacterial required only in severe disease with cellulitis or if systemic features of infection.
- Amoxicillin, or *alternatively*, metronidazole
▸ *Suggested duration of treatment* 5 days.

Periodontitis

Antibacterial used as an adjunct to debridement in severe disease or disease unresponsive to local treatment alone.
- Metronidazole, or *alternatively in adults and children over 12 years*, doxycycline p. 555

Throat infections

Most throat infections are caused by viruses and many do not require antibacterial therapy. Consider antibacterial, if history of valvular heart disease, if marked systemic upset, if peritonsillar cellulitis or abscess, or if at increased risk from acute infection (e.g. in immunosuppression, cystic fibrosis); prescribe antibacterial for beta-haemolytic streptococcal pharyngitis.
- Phenoxymethylpenicillin p. 538
▸ In severe infection, initial parenteral therapy with benzylpenicillin sodium p. 537, then oral therapy with phenoxymethylpenicillin *or* amoxicillin (*or* ampicillin p. 540). **Avoid** amoxicillin if possibility of glandular fever.
▸ *Suggested duration of treatment* 10 days.
▸ *If penicillin-allergic*, clarithromycin p. 529 (*or* azithromycin p. 528 *or* erythromycin p. 530)
▸ *Suggested duration of treatment* 10 days

ANTIBACTERIALS ⟩ TETRACYCLINES AND RELATED DRUGS

▸ 554

| Doxycycline

- INDICATIONS AND DOSE
Treatment of recurrent aphthous ulceration
▸ BY MOUTH USING SOLUBLE TABLETS
▸ Child 12–17 years: 100 mg 4 times a day usually for 3 days, dispersible tablet can be stirred into a small amount of water then rinsed around the mouth for 2–3 minutes, it should preferably not be swallowed
▸ Adult: 100 mg 4 times a day usually for 3 days, dispersible tablet can be stirred into a small amount of water then rinsed around the mouth for 2–3 minutes, it should preferably not be swallowed

- UNLICENSED USE Not licensed for severe recurrent aphthous ulceration. Not licensed for use in children under 12 years.
- CAUTIONS Alcohol dependence
- INTERACTIONS → Appendix 1: tetracyclines
- SIDE-EFFECTS
▸ **Common or very common** Dyspnoea · hypotension · peripheral oedema · serum sickness · skin reactions · tachycardia
▸ **Uncommon** Gastritis · gastrointestinal discomfort
▸ **Rare or very rare** Antibiotic associated colitis · arthralgia · flushing · hepatic function abnormal · myalgia · photoonycholysis · severe cutaneous adverse reactions (SCARs) · tinnitus · vision disorders
- RENAL IMPAIRMENT Use with caution (avoid excessive doses).
- PATIENT AND CARER ADVICE Counselling on administration advised.
Photosensitivity Patients should be advised to avoid exposure to sunlight or sun lamps.
- PROFESSION SPECIFIC INFORMATION
Dental practitioners' formulary
Dispersible tablets may be prescribed as Dispersible Doxycycline Tablets.

- MEDICINAL FORMS
There can be variation in the licensing of different medicines containing the same drug.
Dispersible tablet
CAUTIONARY AND ADVISORY LABELS 6, 9, 11, 13
▸ Vibramycin-D (Pfizer Ltd)
Doxycycline (as Doxycycline monohydrate) 100 mg Vibramycin-D 100mg dispersible tablets sugar-free | 8 tablet PoM £4.91 DT = £4.91

5 Oropharyngeal fungal infections

Oropharyngeal fungal infections

Overview

Fungal infections of the mouth are usually caused by *Candida* spp. (candidiasis or candidosis). Different types of oropharyngeal candidiasis are managed as follows:

Thrush

Acute pseudomembranous candidiasis (thrush), is usually an acute infection but it may persist for months in patients receiving inhaled corticosteroids, cytotoxics or broad-spectrum antibacterials. Thrush also occurs in patients with serious systemic disease associated with reduced immunity such as leukaemia, other malignancies, and HIV infection.

Any predisposing condition should be managed appropriately. When thrush is associated with corticosteroid inhalers, rinsing the mouth with water (or cleaning a child's teeth) immediately after using the inhaler may avoid the problem. Treatment with nystatin p. 1184 or miconazole below may be needed. Fluconazole p. 584 is effective for unresponsive infections or if a topical antifungal drug cannot be used or if the patient has dry mouth. Topical therapy may not be adequate in immunocompromised patients and an oral triazole antifungal is preferred.

Acute erythematous candidiasis

Acute erythematous (atrophic) candidiasis is a relatively uncommon condition associated with corticosteroid and broad-spectrum antibacterial use and with HIV disease. It is usually treated with fluconazole.

Denture stomatitis

Patients with denture stomatitis (chronic atrophic candidiasis), should cleanse their dentures thoroughly and leave them out as often as possible during the treatment period. To prevent recurrence of the problem, dentures should not normally be worn at night. New dentures may be required if these measures fail despite good compliance.

Miconazole oral gel can be applied to the fitting surface of the denture before insertion (for short periods only). Denture stomatitis is not always associated with candidiasis and other factors such as mechanical or chemical irritation, bacterial infection, or rarely allergy to the dental base material, may be the cause.

Chronic hyperplastic candidiasis

Chronic hyperplastic candidiasis (candidal leucoplakia) carries an increased risk of malignancy; biopsy is essential—this type of candidiasis may be associated with varying degrees of dysplasia, with oral cancer present in a high proportion of cases. Chronic hyperplastic candidiasis is treated with a systemic antifungal such as fluconazole to eliminate candidal overlay. Patients should avoid the use of tobacco.

Angular cheilitis

Angular cheilitis (angular stomatitis) is characterised by soreness, erythema and fissuring at the angles of the mouth. It is commonly associated with denture stomatitis but may represent a nutritional deficiency or it may be related to orofacial granulomatosis or HIV infection. Both yeasts (*Candida* spp.) and bacteria (*Staphylococcus aureus* and beta-haemolytic streptococci) are commonly involved as interacting, infective factors. A reduction in facial height related to ageing and tooth loss with maceration in the deep occlusive folds that may subsequently arise, predisposes to such infection. While the underlying cause is being identified and treated, it is often helpful to apply miconazole cream p. 1199 or fusidic acid ointment p. 561; if the angular cheilitis is unresponsive to treatment, hydrocortisone with miconazole cream or ointment p. 1218 can be used.

Immunocompromised patients

See advice on prevention of fungal infections in *Immunocompromised patients* under Antifungals, systemic use p. 580.

Drugs used in oropharyngeal candidiasis

Nystatin is not absorbed from the gastro-intestinal tract and is applied locally (as a suspension) to the mouth for treating local fungal infections. Miconazole is applied locally (as an oral gel) in the mouth but it is absorbed to the extent that potential interactions need to be considered. Miconazole also has some activity against Gram-positive bacteria including streptococci and staphylococci. Fluconazole is given by mouth for infections that do not respond to topical therapy or when topical therapy cannot be used. It is reliably absorbed and effective. Itraconazole p. 586 can be used for fluconazole-resistant infections.

If candidal infection fails to respond to 1 to 2 weeks of treatment with antifungal drugs the patient should be sent for investigation to eliminate the possibility of underlying disease. Persistent infection may also be caused by reinfection from the genito-urinary or gastro-intestinal tract. Infection can be eliminated from these sources by appropriate anticandidal therapy; the patient's partner may also require treatment to prevent reinfection.

Antiseptic mouthwashes are used in the prevention of oral candidiasis in immunocompromised patients and in the treatment of denture stomatitis.

ANTIFUNGALS > IMIDAZOLE ANTIFUNGALS

Miconazole
11-Oct-2017

- **INDICATIONS AND DOSE**

Oral candidiasis
▶ BY MOUTH USING ORAL GEL
- Child 2-17 years: 2.5 mL 4 times a day treatment should be continued for at least 7 days after lesions have healed or symptoms have cleared, to be administered after meals, retain near oral lesions before swallowing (dental prostheses and orthodontic appliances should be removed at night and brushed with gel)
- Adult: 2.5 mL 4 times a day treatment should be continued for at least 7 days after lesions have healed or symptoms have cleared, to be administered after meals, retain near oral lesions before swallowing (dental prostheses and orthodontic appliances should be removed at night and brushed with gel)

Intestinal candidiasis
▶ BY MOUTH USING ORAL GEL
- Child 4 months-17 years: 5 mg/kg 4 times a day (max. per dose 250 mg) treatment should be continued for at least 7 days after lesions have healed or symptoms have cleared
- Adult: 5 mg/kg 4 times a day (max. per dose 250 mg) treatment should be continued for at least 7 days after lesions have healed or symptoms have cleared

- **UNLICENSED USE** Not licensed for use in children under 4 months of age or during first 5–6 months of life of an infant born pre-term.
- **CONTRA-INDICATIONS** Infants with impaired swallowing reflex
- **CAUTIONS** Avoid in Acute porphyrias p. 1025
- **INTERACTIONS** → Appendix 1: antifungals, azoles
- **SIDE-EFFECTS**
▶ **Common or very common** Dry mouth · nausea · oral disorders · regurgitation · skin reactions
▶ **Uncommon** Taste altered
▶ **Frequency not known** Angioedema · choking (in children) · diarrhoea · hepatitis · severe cutaneous adverse reactions (SCARs)
- **PREGNANCY** Manufacturer advises avoid if possible—toxicity at high doses in *animal* studies.
- **BREAST FEEDING** Manufacturer advises caution—no information available.
- **HEPATIC IMPAIRMENT** Avoid.
- **DIRECTIONS FOR ADMINISTRATION** Oral gel should be held in mouth, after food.
- **PRESCRIBING AND DISPENSING INFORMATION** Flavours of oral gel may include orange.
- **PATIENT AND CARER ADVICE** Patients or carers should be given advice on how to administer miconazole oromucosal gel.
- **PROFESSION SPECIFIC INFORMATION**
Dental practitioners' formulary Miconazole Oromucosal Gel may be prescribed.

- EXCEPTIONS TO LEGAL CATEGORY 15-g tube of oral gel can be sold to the public.

- MEDICINAL FORMS
There can be variation in the licensing of different medicines containing the same drug.
Oromucosal gel
CAUTIONARY AND ADVISORY LABELS 9
▸ Daktarin (McNeil Products Ltd, Janssen-Cilag Ltd)
Miconazole 20 mg per 1 gram Daktarin 20mg/g oromucosal gel sugar-free | 80 gram [PoM] £4.38 DT = £4.38

ANTIFUNGALS > POLYENE ANTIFUNGALS

Nystatin   08-Feb-2017

- INDICATIONS AND DOSE
Oral candidiasis
▸ BY MOUTH
▸ Child: 100 000 units 4 times a day usually for 7 days, and continued for 48 hours after lesions have resolved
▸ Adult: 100 000 units 4 times a day usually for 7 days, and continued for 48 hours after lesions have resolved

- CAUTIONS Contact with eyes and mucous membranes should be avoided

- SIDE-EFFECTS Abdominal distress · angioedema · diarrhoea · face oedema · nausea · sensitisation · skin reactions · Stevens-Johnson syndrome · vomiting

- PATIENT AND CARER ADVICE Counselling advised with oral suspension (use of pipette, hold in mouth, after food).
Medicines for Children leaflet: Nystatin for Candida infection www.medicinesforchildren.org.uk/nystatin-for-candida-infection

- PROFESSION SPECIFIC INFORMATION
Dental practitioners' formulary
Nystatin Oral Suspension may be prescribed.

- MEDICINAL FORMS
There can be variation in the licensing of different medicines containing the same drug.
Oral suspension
CAUTIONARY AND ADVISORY LABELS 9
EXCIPIENTS: May contain Ethanol
▸ Nystatin (Non-proprietary)
Nystatin 100000 unit per 1 ml Nystatin 100,000units/ml oral suspension | 30 ml [PoM] £2.22 DT = £2.22

6   Oropharyngeal viral infections

Oropharyngeal viral infections

Management

Viral infections are the most common cause of a sore throat. They do not benefit from anti-infective treatment.

The management of primary herpetic gingivostomatitis is a soft diet, adequate fluid intake, and analgesics as required, including local use of benzydamine hydrochloride p. 1180. The use of chlorhexidine mouthwash p. 1175 will control plaque accumulation if toothbrushing is painful and will also help to control secondary infection in general.

In the case of severe herpetic stomatitis, a systemic antiviral such as aciclovir p. 623 is required. Valaciclovir p. 625 and famciclovir p. 625 are suitable alternatives for oral lesions associated with herpes zoster. Aciclovir and valaciclovir are also used for the prevention of frequently recurring herpes simplex lesions of the mouth, particularly when implicated in the initiation of erythema multiforme.

Chapter 13
Skin

13

Skin

Skin conditions, management

Vehicles

The British Association of Dermatologists list of preferred unlicensed dermatological preparations (specials) is available at www.bad.org.uk/specials.

Both vehicle and active ingredients are important in the treatment of skin conditions; the vehicle alone may have more than a mere placebo effect. The vehicle affects the degree of hydration of the skin, has a mild anti-inflammatory effect, and aids the penetration of active drug.

Applications are usually viscous solutions, emulsions, or suspensions for application to the skin (including the scalp) or nails.

Collodions are painted on the skin and allowed to dry to leave a flexible film over the site of application.

Creams are emulsions of oil and water and are generally well absorbed into the skin. They may contain an antimicrobial preservative unless the active ingredient or basis is intrinsically bactericidal and fungicidal. Generally, creams are cosmetically more acceptable than ointments because they are less greasy and easier to apply.

Gels consist of active ingredients in suitable hydrophilic or hydrophobic bases; they generally have a high water content. Gels are particularly suitable for application to the face and scalp.

Lotions have a cooling effect and may be preferred to ointments or creams for application over a hairy area. Lotions in alcoholic basis can sting if used on broken skin. *Shake lotions* (such as calamine lotion) contain insoluble powders which leave a deposit on the skin surface.

Ointments are greasy preparations which are normally anhydrous and insoluble in water, and are more occlusive than creams. They are particularly suitable for chronic, dry lesions. The most commonly used ointment bases consist of soft paraffin or a combination of soft, liquid, and hard paraffin. Some ointment bases have both *hydrophilic and lipophilic* properties; they may have occlusive properties on the skin surface, encourage hydration, and also be miscible with water; they often have a mild anti-inflammatory effect. *Water-soluble ointments* contain macrogols which are freely soluble in water and are therefore readily washed off; they have a limited but useful role where ready removal is desirable.

Pastes are stiff preparations containing a high proportion of finely powdered solids such as zinc oxide and starch suspended in an ointment. They are used for circumscribed lesions such as those which occur in lichen simplex, chronic eczema, or psoriasis. They are less occlusive than ointments and can be used to protect inflamed, lichenified, or excoriated skin.

Dusting powders are used only rarely. They reduce friction between opposing skin surfaces. Dusting powders should not be applied to moist areas because they can cake and abrade the skin. Talc is a lubricant but it does not absorb moisture; it can cause respiratory irritation. Starch is less lubricant but absorbs water.

Dilution

The BP directs that creams and ointments should **not** normally be diluted but that should dilution be necessary care should be taken, in particular, to prevent microbial contamination. The appropriate diluent should be used and heating should be avoided during mixing; excessive dilution may affect the stability of some creams. Diluted creams should normally be used within 2 weeks of preparation.

Suitable quantities for prescribing

Suitable quantities of dermatological preparations to be prescribed for specific areas of the body		
Area of body	Creams and Ointments	Lotions
Face	15–30 g	100 ml
Both hands	25–50 g	200 ml
Scalp	50–100 g	200 ml
Both arms or both legs	100–200 g	200 ml
Trunk	400 g	500 ml
Groins and genitalia	15–25 g	100 ml

These amounts are usually suitable for an adult for twice daily application for 1 week. The recommendations **do not apply** to corticosteroid preparations. For suitable quantities of corticosteroid preparations, see relevant table.

Excipients and sensitisation

Excipients in topical products rarely cause problems. If a patch test indicates allergy to an excipient, products containing the substance should be avoided. The following excipients in topical preparations are associated, rarely, with sensitisation; the presence of these excipients is indicated in the entries for topical products.

- Beeswax
- Benzyl alcohol
- Butylated hydroxyanisole
- Butylated hydroxytoluene
- Cetostearyl alcohol (including cetyl and stearyl alcohol)
- Chlorocresol
- Edetic acid (EDTA)
- Ethylenediamine
- Fragrances
- Hydroxybenzoates (parabens)
- Imidurea
- Isopropyl palmitate
- N-(3-Chloroallyl)hexaminium chloride (quaternium 15)
- Polysorbates
- Propylene glycol
- Sodium metabisulfite
- Sorbic acid
- Wool fat and related substances including lanolin (purified versions of wool fat have reduced the problem)

1 Dry and scaling skin disorders

Emollient and barrier preparations

Borderline substances

The preparations marked 'ACBS' are regarded as drugs when prescribed in accordance with the advice of the Advisory Committee on Borderline Substances for the clinical conditions listed. Prescriptions issued in accordance with this advice and endorsed 'ACBS' will normally not be investigated.

Emollients

Emollients soothe, smooth and hydrate the skin and are indicated for all dry or scaling disorders. Their effects are short lived and they should be applied frequently even after improvement occurs. They are useful in dry and eczematous disorders, and to a lesser extent in psoriasis. The choice of an appropriate emollient will depend on the severity of the condition, patient preference, and the site of application. Some ingredients rarely cause sensitisation and this should be suspected if an eczematous reaction occurs. The use of aqueous cream as a leave-on emollient may increase the risk of skin reactions, particularly in eczema.

Preparations such as **aqueous cream** and **emulsifying ointment** can be used as soap substitutes for hand washing and in the bath; the preparation is rubbed on the skin before rinsing off completely. The addition of a bath oil may also be helpful.

Urea is occasionally used with other topical agents such as corticosteroids to enhance penetration of the skin.

Emollient bath and shower preparations

Emollient bath additives should be added to bath water; hydration can be improved by soaking in the bath for 10–20 minutes. Some bath emollients can be applied to wet skin undiluted and rinsed off. In dry skin conditions soap should be avoided.

The quantities of bath additives recommended for adults are suitable for an adult-size bath. Proportionately less should be used for a child-size bath or a washbasin; recommended bath additive quantities for children reflect this.

MHRA/CHM update (April 2016): Fire risk with paraffin-based skin emollients on dressings and clothing

When patients are being treated with a paraffin-based emollient product that is covered by a dressing or clothing, there is a danger that smoking or using a naked flame could cause dressings or clothing to catch fire.

Patients should be advised not to smoke, use naked flames (or be near people who are smoking or using naked flames), or go near anything that may cause a fire while emollients are in contact with their medical dressings or clothing. Patients' clothing and bedding should be changed regularly—preferably daily—because emollients soak into fabric and can become a fire hazard.

Barrier preparations

Barrier preparations often contain water-repellent substances such as dimeticone p. 1202 or other silicones. They are used on the skin around stomas, bedsores, and pressure areas in the elderly where the skin is intact. Where the skin has broken down, barrier preparations have a limited role in protecting adjacent skin. Barrier preparations are not a substitute for adequate nursing care.

Nappy rash

The first line of treatment is to ensure that nappies are changed frequently and that tightly fitting water-proof pants are avoided. The rash may clear when left exposed to the air and a barrier preparation, applied with each nappy change, can be helpful. A mild corticosteroid such as hydrocortisone 0.5% or 1% p. 1213 can be used if inflammation is causing discomfort, but it should be avoided in neonates. The barrier preparation should be applied after the corticosteroid preparation to prevent further damage. Preparations containing hydrocortisone should be applied for no more than a week; the hydrocortisone should be discontinued as soon as the inflammation subsides. The occlusive effect of nappies and waterproof pants may increase absorption of corticosteroids. If the rash is associated with candidal infection, a topical antifungal such as clotrimazole cream p. 1197 can be used. Topical antibacterial preparations can be used if bacterial infection is present; treatment with an oral antibacterial may occasionally be required in severe or recurrent infection. Hydrocortisone may be used in combination with antimicrobial preparations if there is considerable inflammation, erosion, and infection.

DERMATOLOGICAL DRUGS > BARRIER PREPARATIONS

Barrier creams and ointments

- **INDICATIONS AND DOSE**

For use as a barrier preparation
  ▸ TO THE SKIN
  ▸ Child: (consult product literature)
  ▸ Adult: (consult product literature)

- MEDICINAL FORMS
  There can be variation in the licensing of different medicines containing the same drug.

Ointment
  EXCIPIENTS: May contain Woolfat and related substances (including lanolin)

  ▸ Barrier creams and ointments (Non-proprietary)
  Cetostearyl alcohol 20 mg per 1 gram, Zinc oxide 75 mg per 1 gram, Beeswax white 100 mg per 1 gram, Arachis oil 305 mg per 1 gram, Castor oil 500 mg per 1 gram Zinc and Castor oil ointment | 100 gram GSL £1.46 | 500 gram GSL £4.99–£5.38 DT = £5.38
  Zinc and Castor oil cream | 100 gram GSL £1.46
  ▸ Brands may include Metanium

Spray

CAUTIONARY AND ADVISORY LABELS 15

EXCIPIENTS: May contain Cetostearyl alcohol (including cetyl and stearyl alcohol), hydroxybenzoates (parabens), woolfat and related substances (including lanolin)

▸ Sprilon (J M Loveridge Ltd)

Dimeticone 10.4 mg per 1 gram, Zinc oxide 125 mg per 1 gram Sprilon aerosol spray | 115 gram GSL £8.90 DT = £8.90

Cream

EXCIPIENTS: May contain Beeswax, butylated hydroxyanisole, butylated hydroxytoluene, cetostearyl alcohol (including cetyl and stearyl alcohol), chlorocresol, fragrances, hydroxybenzoates (parabens), propylene glycol, woolfat and related substances (including lanolin)

▸ Conotrane (LEO Pharma)

Benzalkonium chloride 1 mg per 1 gram, Dimeticone 220 mg per 1 gram Conotrane cream | 100 gram GSL £0.88 DT = £0.88 | 500 gram GSL £3.51

▸ Drapolene (Supra Enterprises Ltd)

Benzalkonium chloride 100 microgram per 1 gram, Cetrimide 2 mg per 1 gram Drapolene cream | 100 gram GSL £1.76 | 200 gram GSL £2.86 | 350 gram GSL £4.28

▸ Siopel (Derma UK Ltd)

Cetrimide 3 mg per 1 gram, Dimeticone 1000 100 mg per 1 gram Siopel cream | 50 gram GSL £4.65

▸ Sudocrem (Teva UK Ltd)

Benzyl cinnamate 1.5 mg per 1 gram, Benzyl alcohol 3.9 mg per 1 gram, Benzyl benzoate 10.1 mg per 1 gram, Wool fat hydrous 40 mg per 1 gram, Zinc oxide 152.5 mg per 1 gram Sudocrem antiseptic healing cream | 30 gram GSL £1.45 | 60 gram GSL £1.45 | 125 gram GSL £2.15 | 250 gram GSL £3.67 | 400 gram GSL £5.25

DERMATOLOGICAL DRUGS › EMOLLIENTS

Emollient bath and shower products, antimicrobial-containing

31-Aug-2016

● **INDICATIONS AND DOSE**

DERMOL ® 200 SHOWER EMOLLIENT

Dry and pruritic skin conditions including eczema and dermatitis

▸ TO THE SKIN

▸ Child: To be applied to the skin or used as a soap substitute

▸ Adult: To be applied to the skin or used as a soap substitute

DERMOL ® 600 BATH EMOLLIENT

Dry and pruritic skin conditions including eczema and dermatitis

▸ TO THE SKIN

▸ Child 1–23 months: 5–15 mL/bath, not to be used undiluted

▸ Child 2–17 years: 15–30 mL/bath, not to be used undiluted

▸ Adult: Up to 30 mL/bath, not to be used undiluted

DERMOL ® WASH EMULSION

Dry and pruritic skin conditions including eczema and dermatitis

▸ TO THE SKIN

▸ Child: To be applied to the skin or used as a soap substitute

▸ Adult: To be applied to the skin or used as a soap substitute

EMULSIDERM ®

Dry skin conditions including eczema and ichthyosis

▸ TO THE SKIN

▸ Child 1–23 months: 5–10 mL/bath, alternatively, to be rubbed into dry skin until absorbed

▸ Child 2–17 years: 7–30 mL/bath, alternatively, to be rubbed into dry skin until absorbed

▸ Adult: 7–30 mL/bath, alternatively, to be rubbed into dry skin until absorbed

OILATUM ® PLUS

Topical treatment of eczema, including eczema at risk from infection

▸ TO THE SKIN

▸ Child 6–11 months: 1 mL/bath, not to be used undiluted

▸ Child 1–17 years: 1–2 capfuls/bath, not to be used undiluted

▸ Adult: 1–2 capfuls/bath, not to be used undiluted

IMPORTANT SAFETY INFORMATION

These preparations make skin and surfaces slippery—particular care is needed when bathing.

MHRA/CHM UPDATE (APRIL 2016): FIRE RISK WITH PARAFFIN-BASED SKIN EMOLLIENTS ON DRESSINGS OR CLOTHING

See Emollient and barrier preparations p. 1186.

● DIRECTIONS FOR ADMINISTRATION Emollient bath additives should be added to bath water; hydration can be improved by soaking in the bath for 10–20 minutes. Some bath emollients can be applied to wet skin undiluted and rinsed off. Emollient preparations contained in tubs should be removed with a clean spoon or spatula to reduce bacterial contamination of the emollient. Emollients should be applied in the direction of hair growth to reduce the risk of folliculitis.

● PRESCRIBING AND DISPENSING INFORMATION Preparations containing an antibacterial should be avoided unless infection is present or is a frequent complication.

● MEDICINAL FORMS There can be variation in the licensing of different medicines containing the same drug.

Bath additive

CAUTIONARY AND ADVISORY LABELS 15

EXCIPIENTS: May contain Acetylated lanolin alcohols, isopropyl palmitate, polysorbates

▸ Dermol 600 (Dermal Laboratories Ltd)

Benzalkonium chloride 5 mg per 1 gram, Isopropyl myristate 250 mg per 1 gram, Liquid paraffin 250 mg per 1 gram Dermol 600 bath emollient | 600 ml P £7.55

▸ Emulsiderm (Dermal Laboratories Ltd)

Benzalkonium chloride 5 mg per 1 gram, Isopropyl myristate 250 mg per 1 gram, Liquid paraffin 250 mg per 1 gram Emulsiderm emollient | 300 ml P £3.85 | 1000 ml P £12.00

▸ Oilatum Plus (GlaxoSmithKline Consumer Healthcare)

Triclosan 20 mg per 1 gram, Benzalkonium chloride 60 mg per 1 gram, Liquid paraffin light 525 mg per 1 gram Oilatum Plus bath additive | 500 ml GSL £7.22

Liquid

CAUTIONARY AND ADVISORY LABELS 15

EXCIPIENTS: May contain Cetostearyl alcohol (including cetyl and stearyl alcohol)

▸ Dermol 200 (Dermal Laboratories Ltd)

Benzalkonium chloride 1 mg per 1 gram, Chlorhexidine hydrochloride 1 mg per 1 gram, Isopropyl myristate 25 mg per 1 gram, Liquid paraffin 25 mg per 1 gram Dermol 200 shower emollient | 200 ml P £3.55

▸ Dermol Wash (Dermal Laboratories Ltd)

Benzalkonium chloride 1 mg per 1 gram, Chlorhexidine hydrochloride 1 mg per 1 gram, Isopropyl myristate 25 mg per 1 gram, Liquid paraffin 25 mg per 1 gram Dermol Wash cutaneous emulsion | 200 ml P £3.55

13

Skin

Emollient bath and shower products, colloidal oatmeal-containing

● **INDICATIONS AND DOSE**

Endogenous and exogenous eczema | Xeroderma | Ichthyosis

▸ TO THE SKIN
▸ Child 2-17 years: 20–30 mL/bath, alternatively apply to wet skin and rinse
▸ Adult: 20–30 mL/bath, alternatively apply to wet skin and rinse

Pruritus of the elderly associated with dry skin

▸ TO THE SKIN
▸ Elderly: 20–30 mL/bath, alternatively apply to wet skin and rinse

IMPORTANT SAFETY INFORMATION
These preparations make skin and surfaces slippery—particular care is needed when bathing.

● DIRECTIONS FOR ADMINISTRATION Emollient bath additives should be added to bath water; hydration can be improved by soaking in the bath for 10–20 minutes. Some bath emollients can be applied to wet skin undiluted and rinsed off. Emollient preparations contained in tubs should be removed with a clean spoon or spatula to reduce bacterial contamination of the emollient. Emollients should be applied in the direction of hair growth to reduce the risk of folliculitis.

● MEDICINAL FORMS
No licensed medicines listed.

Emollient bath and shower products, paraffin-containing

15-Aug-2016

● **INDICATIONS AND DOSE**

AQUAMAX ® WASH

Dry skin conditions
▸ TO THE SKIN
▸ Child: To be applied to wet or dry skin and rinse
▸ Adult: To be applied to wet or dry skin and rinse

CETRABEN ® BATH

Dry skin conditions, including eczema
▸ TO THE SKIN
▸ Child 1 month-11 years: 0.5–1 capful/bath, alternatively, to be applied to wet skin and rinse
▸ Child 12-17 years: 1–2 capfuls/bath, alternatively, to be applied to wet skin and rinse
▸ Adult: 1–2 capfuls/bath, alternatively, to be applied to wet skin and rinse

DERMALO ®

Dermatitis | Dry skin conditions, including ichthyosis
▸ TO THE SKIN
▸ Child 1 month-11 years: 5–10 mL/bath, alternatively, to be applied to wet skin and rinse
▸ Child 12-17 years: 15–20 mL/bath, alternatively, to be applied to wet skin and rinse
▸ Adult: 15–20 mL/bath, alternatively, to be applied to wet skin and rinse

Pruritus of the elderly
▸ TO THE SKIN
▸ Elderly: 15–20 mL/bath, alternatively, to be applied to wet skin and rinse

DOUBLEBASE ® EMOLLIENT BATH ADDITIVE

Dry skin conditions including dermatitis and ichthyosis
▸ TO THE SKIN
▸ Child 1 month-11 years: 5–10 mL/bath
▸ Child 12-17 years: 15–20 mL/bath
▸ Adult: 15–20 mL/bath

Pruritus of the elderly
▸ TO THE SKIN
▸ Elderly: 15–20 mL/bath

DOUBLEBASE ® EMOLLIENT SHOWER GEL

Dry, chapped, or itchy skin conditions
▸ TO THE SKIN
▸ Child: To be applied to wet or dry skin and rinse, or apply to dry skin after showering
▸ Adult: To be applied to wet or dry skin and rinse, or apply to dry skin after showering

E45 ® BATH OIL

Endogenous and exogenous eczema, xeroderma, and ichthyosis
▸ TO THE SKIN
▸ Child 1 month-11 years: 5–10 mL/bath, alternatively, to be applied to wet skin and rinse
▸ Child 12-17 years: 15 mL/bath, alternatively, to be applied to wet skin and rinse
▸ Adult: 15 mL/bath, alternatively, to be applied to wet skin and rinse

Pruritus of the elderly associated with dry skin
▸ TO THE SKIN
▸ Elderly: 15 mL/bath, alternatively, to be applied to wet skin and rinse

E45 ® WASH CREAM

Endogenous and exogenous eczema, xeroderma, and ichthyosis
▸ TO THE SKIN
▸ Child: To be used as a soap substitute
▸ Adult: To be used as a soap substitute

Pruritus of the elderly associated with dry skin
▸ TO THE SKIN
▸ Elderly: To be used as a soap substitute

HYDROMOL ® BATH AND SHOWER EMOLLIENT

Dry skin conditions | Eczema | Ichthyosis
▸ TO THE SKIN
▸ Child 1 month-11 years: 0.5–2 capfuls/bath, alternatively apply to wet skin and rinse
▸ Child 12-17 years: 1–3 capfuls/bath, alternatively apply to wet skin and rinse
▸ Adult: 1–3 capfuls/bath, alternatively apply to wet skin and rinse

Pruritus of the elderly
▸ TO THE SKIN
▸ Elderly: 1–3 capfuls/bath, alternatively apply to wet skin and rinse

LPL 63.4 ®

Dry skin conditions
▸ TO THE SKIN
▸ Child 1 month-11 years: 0.5–2 capfuls/bath, alternatively, to be applied to wet skin and rinse
▸ Child 12-17 years: 1–3 capfuls/bath, alternatively, to be applied to wet skin and rinse
▸ Adult: 1–3 capfuls/bath, alternatively, to be applied to wet skin and rinse

OILATUM ® EMOLLIENT BATH ADDITIVE

Dry skin conditions including dermatitis and ichthyosis
▸ TO THE SKIN
▸ Child 1 month-11 years: Apply 0.5–2 capfuls/bath, alternatively, to be applied to wet skin and rinse

- Child 12–17 years: 1–3 capfuls/bath, alternatively, to be applied to wet skin and rinse
- Adult: 1–3 capfuls/bath, alternatively, to be applied to wet skin and rinse

Pruritus of the elderly

▶ TO THE SKIN
- Elderly: 1–3 capfuls/bath, alternatively, to be applied to wet skin and rinse

OILATUM ® JUNIOR BATH ADDITIVE

Dry skin conditions including dermatitis and ichthyosis

▶ TO THE SKIN
- Child 1 month–11 years: 0.5–2 capfuls/bath, alternatively, apply to wet skin and rinse
- Child 12–17 years: 1–3 capfuls/bath, alternatively, apply to wet skin and rinse
- Adult: 1–3 capfuls/bath, alternatively, apply to wet skin and rinse

Pruritus of the elderly

▶ TO THE SKIN
- Elderly: 1–3 capfuls/bath, alternatively, apply to wet skin and rinse

QV ® BATH OIL

Dry skin conditions including eczema, psoriasis, ichthyosis, and pruritus

▶ TO THE SKIN
- Child 1–11 months: 5 mL/bath, alternatively, to be applied to wet skin and rinse
- Child 1–17 years: 10 mL/bath, alternatively, to be applied to wet skin and rinse
- Adult: 10 mL/bath, alternatively, to be applied to wet skin and rinse

QV ® GENTLE WASH

Dry skin conditions including eczema, psoriasis, ichthyosis, and pruritus

▶ TO THE SKIN
- Child: To be used as a soap substitute
- Adult: To be used as a soap substitute

ZEROLATUM ®

Dry skin conditions | Dermatitis | Ichthyosis

▶ TO THE SKIN
- Child 1 month–11 years: 5–10 mL/bath
- Child 12–17 years: 15–20 mL/bath
- Adult: 15–20 mL/bath

Pruritus of the elderly

▶ TO THE SKIN
- Elderly: 15–20 mL/bath

IMPORTANT SAFETY INFORMATION

These preparations make the skin and surfaces slippery—particular care is needed when bathing.

MHRA/CHM UPDATE (APRIL 2016): FIRE RISK WITH PARAFFIN-BASED SKIN EMOLLIENTS ON DRESSINGS OR CLOTHING
See Emollient and barrier preparations p. 1186.

● DIRECTIONS FOR ADMINISTRATION Emollient bath additives should be added to bath water; hydration can be improved by soaking in the bath for 10–20 minutes. Some bath emollients can be applied to wet skin undiluted and rinsed off. Emollient preparations contained in tubs should be removed with a clean spoon or spatula to reduce bacterial contamination of the emollient. Emollients should be applied in the direction of hair growth to reduce the risk of folliculitis.

● MEDICINAL FORMS
There can be variation in the licensing of different medicines containing the same drug.

Bath additive

CAUTIONARY AND ADVISORY LABELS 15
EXCIPIENTS: May contain Acetylated lanolin alcohols, cetostearyl alcohol (including cetyl and stearyl alcohol), fragrances, isopropyl palmitate

▶ Cetraben (Thornton & Ross Ltd)
Liquid paraffin light 828 mg per 1 gram Cetraben emollient 82.8% bath additive | 500 ml GSL £5.75
▶ Dermalo (Dermal Laboratories Ltd)
Acetylated wool alcohols 50 mg per 1 gram, Liquid paraffin 650 mg per 1 gram Dermalo bath emollient | 500 ml GSL £3.44
▶ Doublebase (Dermal Laboratories Ltd)
Liquid paraffin 650 mg per 1 gram Doublebase emollient bath additive | 500 ml GSL £5.45
▶ Hydromol (Alliance Pharmaceuticals Ltd)
Isopropyl myristate 130 mg per 1 ml, Liquid paraffin light 378 mg per 1 ml Hydromol Bath & Shower emollient | 350 ml £3.91 | 500 ml £4.46 | 1000 ml £8.87
▶ LPL (Huxley Europe Ltd)
Liquid paraffin light 634 mg per 1 ml LPL 63.4 bath additive and emollient | 500 ml £3.10 DT = £4.71
▶ Oilatum (GlaxoSmithKline Consumer Healthcare)
Liquid paraffin light 634 mg per 1 ml Oilatum Bath Formula | 150 ml GSL £2.95 DT = £2.95 | 300 ml GSL £5.02 DT = £5.02
▶ Oilatum junior (GlaxoSmithKline Consumer Healthcare)
Liquid paraffin light 634 mg per 1 ml Oilatum Junior bath additive | 150 ml GSL £2.95 DT = £2.95 | 250 ml GSL £4.44 DT = £2.75 | 300 ml GSL £5.02 DT = £5.02 | 600 ml GSL £6.67 DT = £6.67
▶ QV (Crawford Healthcare Ltd)
Liquid paraffin light 850.9 mg per 1 gram QV 85.09% bath oil | 250 ml £2.93 | 500 ml £4.79
▶ Zerolatum (Thornton & Ross Ltd)
Acetylated wool alcohols 50 mg per 1 gram, Liquid paraffin 650 mg per 1 gram Zerolatum Emollient bath additive | 500 ml £4.79

Gel

CAUTIONARY AND ADVISORY LABELS 15
EXCIPIENTS: May contain Cetostearyl alcohol (including cetyl and stearyl alcohol)

▶ Doublebase (Dermal Laboratories Ltd)
Isopropyl myristate 150 mg per 1 gram, Liquid paraffin 150 mg per 1 gram Doublebase emollient shower gel | 200 gram P £5.21

Form unstated

CAUTIONARY AND ADVISORY LABELS 15
▶ E45 emollient bath (Forum Health Products Ltd)
E45 emollient bath oil | 250 ml(ACBS) £3.30 | 500 ml(ACBS) £5.29

Products without form

CAUTIONARY AND ADVISORY LABELS 15
EXCIPIENTS: May contain Hydroxybenzoates (parabens)
▶ QV Gentle (Crawford Healthcare Ltd)
QV Gentle wash | 250 ml £3.19 | 500 ml £5.32

Wash

CAUTIONARY AND ADVISORY LABELS 15
EXCIPIENTS: May contain Cetostearyl alcohol (including cetyl and stearyl alcohol), polysorbates
▶ Aquamax (Intrapharm Laboratories Ltd)
Aquamax wash | 250 gram £2.99
▶ E45 emollient wash (Forum Health Products Ltd)
E45 emollient wash cream | 250 ml(ACBS) £3.30

Emollient bath and shower products, soya-bean oil-containing

● INDICATIONS AND DOSE

BALNEUM ® BATH OIL

Dry skin conditions including those associated with dermatitis and eczema

▶ TO THE SKIN
- Child 1–23 months: 5–15 mL/bath, not to be used undiluted

continued →

13

Skin

► Child 2-17 years: 20–60 mL/bath, not to be used undiluted
► Adult: 20–60 mL/bath, not to be used undiluted

BALNEUM ® PLUS BATH OIL

Dry skin conditions including those associated with dermatitis and eczema where pruritus also experienced
► TO THE SKIN
► Child 1-23 months: 5 mL/bath, alternatively, to be applied to wet skin and rinse
► Child 2-17 years: 10–20 mL/bath, alternatively, to be applied to wet skin and rinse
► Adult: 20 mL/bath, alternatively, to be applied to wet skin and rinse

ZERONEUM ®

Dry skin conditions including eczema
► TO THE SKIN
► Child 1 month–11 years: 5 mL/bath
► Child 12-17 years: 20 mL/bath
► Adult: 20 mL/bath

> **IMPORTANT SAFETY INFORMATION**
> These preparations make skin and surfaces slippery—particular care is needed when bathing.

● DIRECTIONS FOR ADMINISTRATION Emollient bath additives should be added to bath water; hydration can be improved by soaking in the bath for 10–20 minutes. Some bath emollients can be applied to wet skin undiluted and rinsed off. Emollient preparations contained in tubs should be removed with a clean spoon or spatula to reduce bacterial contamination of the emollient. Emollients should be applied in the direction of hair growth to reduce the risk of folliculitis.

● MEDICINAL FORMS
There can be variation in the licensing of different medicines containing the same drug.
Bath additive
EXCIPIENTS: May contain Butylated hydroxytoluene, fragrances, propylene glycol
► Balneum (Almirall Ltd)
Lauromacrogols 150 mg per 1 gram, Soya oil 829.5 mg per 1 gram Balneum Plus bath oil | 500 ml [GSL] £6.66
Soya oil 847.5 mg per 1 gram Balneum 84.75% bath oil | 500 ml [GSL] £5.38 DT = £5.38 | 1000 ml [GSL] £10.39 DT = £10.39
► Zeroneum (Thornton & Ross Ltd)
Soya oil 833.5 mg per 1 gram Zeroneum 83.35% bath additive | 500 ml £4.48

Emollient bath and shower products, tar-containing

17-Aug-2016

● INDICATIONS AND DOSE

POLYTAR EMOLLIENT ®

Psoriasis, eczema, atopic and pruritic dermatoses
► TO THE SKIN
► Adult: 2–4 capfuls/bath, add 15–30 mL to an adult-size bath; soak for 20 minutes

PSORIDERM ® EMULSION

Psoriasis
► TO THE SKIN
► Adult: Up to 30 mL/bath, use 30mL in adult-size bath, soak for 5 minutes

> **IMPORTANT SAFETY INFORMATION**
> These preparations make skin and surfaces slippery—particular care is needed when bathing.

● DIRECTIONS FOR ADMINISTRATION Emollient bath additives should be added to bath water; hydration can be

improved by soaking in the bath for 10–20 minutes. Some bath emollients can be applied to wet skin undiluted and rinsed off. Emollient preparations contained in tubs should be removed with a clean spoon or spatula to reduce bacterial contamination of the emollient. Emollients should be applied in the direction of hair growth to reduce the risk of folliculitis.

● MEDICINAL FORMS
There can be variation in the licensing of different medicines containing the same drug.
Bath additive
EXCIPIENTS: May contain Isopropyl palmitate, polysorbates
► Psoriderm (Dermal Laboratories Ltd)
Coal tar distilled 400 mg per 1 ml Psoriderm Emulsion 40% bath additive | 200 ml [P] £2.74

Emollient creams and ointments, antimicrobial-containing

17-Aug-2016

● INDICATIONS AND DOSE
Dry and pruritic skin conditions including eczema and dermatitis
► TO THE SKIN
► Child: To be applied to the skin or used as a soap substitute
► Adult: To be applied to the skin or used as a soap substitute

> **IMPORTANT SAFETY INFORMATION**
> These preparations make skin and surfaces slippery—particular care is needed when bathing.
>
> MHRA/CHM UPDATE (APRIL 2016): FIRE RISK WITH PARAFFIN-BASED SKIN EMOLLIENTS ON DRESSINGS OR CLOTHING
> See Emollient and barrier preparations p. 1186.

● DIRECTIONS FOR ADMINISTRATION Emollients should be applied immediately after washing or bathing to maximise the effect of skin hydration. Emollient preparations contained in tubs should be removed with a clean spoon or spatula to reduce bacterial contamination of the emollient. Emollients should be applied in the direction of hair growth to reduce the risk of folliculitis.

● PRESCRIBING AND DISPENSING INFORMATION
Preparations containing an antibacterial should be avoided unless infection is present or is a frequent complication.

● MEDICINAL FORMS
There can be variation in the licensing of different medicines containing the same drug.
Cream
CAUTIONARY AND ADVISORY LABELS 15
EXCIPIENTS: May contain Cetostearyl alcohol (including cetyl and stearyl alcohol)
► Dermol (Dermal Laboratories Ltd)
Benzalkonium chloride 1 mg per 1 gram, Chlorhexidine hydrochloride 1 mg per 1 gram, Isopropyl myristate 100 mg per 1 gram, Liquid paraffin 100 mg per 1 gram Dermol cream | 100 gram [P] £2.86 | 500 gram [P] £6.63
► Hibitane Obstetric (Derma UK Ltd)
Chlorhexidine gluconate 10 mg per 1 gram Hibitane Obstetric 1% cream | 250 ml [GSL] £16.95

Liquid

CAUTIONARY AND ADVISORY LABELS 15
EXCIPIENTS: May contain Cetostearyl alcohol (including cetyl and stearyl alcohol)
‣ Dermol 500 (Dermal Laboratories Ltd)
Benzalkonium chloride 1 mg per 1 gram, Chlorhexidine hydrochloride 1 mg per 1 gram, Isopropyl myristate 25 mg per 1 gram, Liquid paraffin 25 mg per 1 gram Dermol 500 lotion | 500 ml P £6.04

Emollient creams and ointments, colloidal oatmeal-containing   01-Jun-2018

● **INDICATIONS AND DOSE**

Endogenous and exogenous eczema | Xeroderma | Ichthyosis
▸ TO THE SKIN
▸ Child: (consult product literature)
▸ Adult: (consult product literature)

Senile pruritus (pruritus of the elderly) associated with dry skin
▸ TO THE SKIN
▸ Elderly: (consult product literature)

> **IMPORTANT SAFETY INFORMATION**
> MHRA/CHM UPDATE (APRIL 2016): FIRE RISK WITH PARAFFIN-BASED SKIN EMOLLIENTS ON DRESSINGS OR CLOTHING
> See Emollient and barrier preparations p. 1186.

● **DIRECTIONS FOR ADMINISTRATION** Emollients should be applied immediately after washing or bathing to maximise the effect of skin hydration. Emollient preparations contained in tubs should be removed with a clean spoon or spatula to reduce bacterial contamination of the emollient. Emollients should be applied in the direction of hair growth to reduce the risk of folliculitis.

● **MEDICINAL FORMS**
There can be variation in the licensing of different medicines containing the same drug.

Cream and Lotion

CAUTIONARY AND ADVISORY LABELS 15
EXCIPIENTS: May contain Benzyl alcohol, cetostearyl alcohol (including cetyl and stearyl alcohol), isopropyl palmitate
‣ Aveeno (Johnson & Johnson Ltd)
Aveeno lotion | 500 ml(ACBS) £6.66
Aveeno cream | 100 ml(ACBS) £3.97 | 300 ml(ACBS) £6.80 | 500 ml (ACBS) £7.19

Emollient creams and ointments, paraffin-containing   31-Aug-2016

● **INDICATIONS AND DOSE**

Dry skin conditions | Eczema | Psoriasis | Ichthyosis | Pruritus
▸ TO THE SKIN
▸ Child: (consult product literature)
▸ Adult: (consult product literature)

> **IMPORTANT SAFETY INFORMATION**
> MHRA/CHM UPDATE (APRIL 2016): FIRE RISK WITH PARAFFIN-BASED SKIN EMOLLIENTS ON DRESSINGS OR CLOTHING
> See Emollient and barrier preparations p. 1186.

● **DIRECTIONS FOR ADMINISTRATION** Emollients should be applied immediately after washing or bathing to maximise the effect of skin hydration. Emollient preparations contained in tubs should be removed with a clean spoon or spatula to reduce bacterial contamination of the emollient.

Emollients should be applied in the direction of hair growth to reduce the risk of folliculitis.

● **MEDICINAL FORMS**
There can be variation in the licensing of different medicines containing the same drug.

Spray

CAUTIONARY AND ADVISORY LABELS 15
‣ Dermamist (Alliance Pharmaceuticals Ltd)
White soft paraffin 100 mg per 1 gram Dermamist 10% spray | 250 ml P £5.97 DT = £5.97
‣ Emollin (C D Medical Ltd)
Emollin aerosol spray | 150 ml £4.00 | 240 ml £6.39

Gel

CAUTIONARY AND ADVISORY LABELS 15
‣ AproDerm (isopropyl myristate / liquid paraffin) (Fontus Health Ltd)
Isopropyl myristate 150 mg per 1 gram, Liquid paraffin 150 mg per 1 gram AproDerm gel | 100 gram £1.99 DT = £2.65 | 500 gram £3.99 DT = £5.83
‣ Doublebase (Dermal Laboratories Ltd)
Isopropyl myristate 150 mg per 1 gram, Liquid paraffin 150 mg per 1 gram Doublebase Dayleve gel | 100 gram P £2.65 DT = £2.65 | 500 gram P £6.29 DT = £5.83
Doublebase gel | 100 gram P £2.65 DT = £2.65 | 500 gram P £5.83 DT = £5.83 | 1000 gram P £10.98
Doublebase emollient wash gel | 200 gram P £5.21
Doublebase emollient shower gel | 200 gram P £5.21
‣ Exmabase (Ascot Laboratories Ltd)
Isopropyl myristate 150 mg per 1 gram, Liquid paraffin 150 mg per 1 gram Exmabase gel | 500 gram £2.85 DT = £5.83
‣ HypoBase (Aspire Pharma Ltd)
Isopropyl myristate 150 mg per 1 gram, Liquid paraffin 150 mg per 1 gram HypoBase gel | 500 gram £5.83 DT = £5.83
‣ MyriBase (Penlan Healthcare Ltd)
Isopropyl myristate 150 mg per 1 gram, Liquid paraffin 150 mg per 1 gram MyriBase gel | 100 gram £2.12 DT = £2.65 | 500 gram £4.66 DT = £5.83
‣ Zerodouble (Thornton & Ross Ltd)
Isopropyl myristate 150 mg per 1 gram, Liquid paraffin 150 mg per 1 gram Zerodouble gel | 100 gram £2.25 DT = £2.65 | 475 gram £4.71 | 500 gram £4.90 DT = £5.83
‣ Isomol (Dermato Logical Ltd)
Isopropyl myristate 150 mg per 1 gram, Liquid paraffin 150 mg per 1 gram isomol gel | 100 gram £1.99 DT = £2.65 | 500 gram £2.92 DT = £5.83

Cream

CAUTIONARY AND ADVISORY LABELS 15
EXCIPIENTS: May contain Benzyl alcohol, cetostearyl alcohol (including cetyl and stearyl alcohol), chlorocresol, disodium edetate, fragrances, hydroxybenzoates (parabens), polysorbates, propylene glycol, sorbic acid, lanolin
‣ Aquamol (Thornton & Ross Ltd)
Aquamol cream | 50 gram £1.22 | 500 gram £6.40
‣ Cetraben (Thornton & Ross Ltd)
Liquid paraffin light 105 mg per 1 gram, White soft paraffin 132 mg per 1 gram Cetraben cream | 50 gram £1.40 | 150 gram £3.98 | 500 gram £5.99 | 1050 gram £11.62
‣ Diprobase (Bayer Plc)
Diprobase cream | 50 gram GSL £1.28 | 500 gram GSL £6.32
‣ E45 (Forum Health Products Ltd)
Wool fat 10 mg per 1 gram, Liquid paraffin light 126 mg per 1 gram, White soft paraffin 145 mg per 1 gram E45 cream | 50 gram GSL £1.61 | 125 gram GSL £2.90 | 350 gram GSL £5.49 | 500 gram GSL £5.99
‣ Enopen (Ennogen Healthcare Ltd)
Liquid paraffin light 105 mg per 1 gram, White soft paraffin 132 mg per 1 gram Enopen cream | 50 gram £1.40 | 150 gram £3.98 | 500 gram £5.99 | 1050 gram £11.62
‣ Epaderm (Molnlycke Health Care Ltd)
Epaderm cream | 50 gram £1.70 | 150 gram £3.58 | 500 gram £6.95
‣ ExCetra (Dermato Logical Ltd)
Liquid paraffin light 105 mg per 1 gram, White soft paraffin 132 mg per 1 gram ExCetra cream | 100 gram £1.75 | 500 gram £2.95
‣ ExmaQS (Ascot Laboratories Ltd)
Liquid paraffin light 60 mg per 1 gram, White soft paraffin 150 mg per 1 gram ExmaQS cream | 500 gram £2.95

13

Skin

‣ Exmaben (Ascot Laboratories Ltd)
Liquid paraffin light 105 mg per 1 gram, White soft paraffin 132 mg per 1 gram Exmaben cream | 500 gram £4.25
‣ Exmalatum (Ascot Laboratories Ltd)
Liquid paraffin light 60 mg per 1 gram, White soft paraffin 150 mg per 1 gram Exmalatum cream | 500 gram £4.45
‣ Lipobase (LEO Pharma)
Lipobase cream | 50 gram P £1.46
‣ Oilatum (GlaxoSmithKline Consumer Healthcare)
Liquid paraffin light 60 mg per 1 gram, White soft paraffin 150 mg per 1 gram Oilatum cream | 150 gram GSL £3.06 DT = £3.06 | 500 ml GSL £5.28 DT = £5.28
‣ Oilatum junior (GlaxoSmithKline Consumer Healthcare)
Liquid paraffin light 60 mg per 1 gram, White soft paraffin 150 mg per 1 gram Oilatum Junior cream | 150 gram GSL £3.06 DT = £3.06 | 350 ml GSL £4.65 DT = £4.65 | 500 ml GSL £5.28 DT = £5.28
‣ Soffen (Vitame Ltd)
Liquid paraffin light 105 mg per 1 gram, White soft paraffin 132 mg per 1 gram Soffen cream | 500 gram £4.79
‣ Unguentum M (Almirall Ltd)
Unguentum M cream | 100 gram GSL £2.78 | 500 gram GSL £8.48
‣ ZeroAQS (Thornton & Ross Ltd)
ZeroAQS emollient cream | 500 gram £3.29
‣ Zerobase (Thornton & Ross Ltd)
Liquid paraffin 110 mg per 1 gram Zerobase 11% cream | 50 gram £1.04 | 500 gram £5.26
‣ Zerocream (Thornton & Ross Ltd)
Liquid paraffin 126 mg per 1 gram, White soft paraffin 145 mg per 1 gram Zerocream | 50 gram £1.17 | 500 gram £4.08
‣ Zeroguent (Thornton & Ross Ltd)
White soft paraffin 40 mg per 1 gram, Soya oil 50 mg per 1 gram, Liquid paraffin light 80 mg per 1 gram Zeroguent cream | 100 gram £2.33 | 500 gram £6.99

Ointment

CAUTIONARY AND ADVISORY LABELS 15
EXCIPIENTS: May contain Cetostearyl alcohol (including cetyl and stearyl alcohol), polysorbates

‣ Emollient creams and ointments, paraffin-containing (Non-proprietary)
Liquid paraffin 200 mg per 1 gram, Emulsifying wax 300 mg per 1 gram, White soft paraffin 500 mg per 1 gram Emulsifying ointment | 500 gram GSL £3.83 DT = £3.83 | 500 gram ⊠ DT = £3.83 | 500 gram PoM ⊠ DT = £3.83
Liquid paraffin 500 mg per 1 gram, White soft paraffin 500 mg per 1 gram White soft paraffin 50% / Liquid paraffin 50% ointment | 250 gram £1.87–£1.92 | 500 gram £4.32 DT = £4.57 | 500 gram P £4.57 DT = £4.57
White soft paraffin 1 mg per 1 mg White soft paraffin solid | 500 gram GSL £4.33 DT = £3.23 | 4500 gram GSL £19.17–£29.07
Yellow soft paraffin 1 mg per 1 mg Yellow soft paraffin solid | 15 gram GSL £1.16–£1.21 | 500 gram GSL £18.40 DT = £18.40 | 4500 gram GSL £19.02
‣ Diprobase (Bayer Plc)
Liquid paraffin 50 mg per 1 gram, White soft paraffin 950 mg per 1 gram Diprobase ointment | 50 gram GSL £1.28 DT = £1.28 | 500 gram GSL £5.99 DT = £5.99
‣ Emelpin (Vitame Ltd)
Emulsifying wax 300 mg per 1 gram, Yellow soft paraffin 300 mg per 1 gram Emelpin ointment | 125 gram £3.08 | 500 gram £5.22
‣ Epaderm (Molnlycke Health Care Ltd)
Emulsifying wax 300 mg per 1 gram, Yellow soft paraffin 300 mg per 1 gram Epaderm ointment | 125 gram £3.85 | 500 gram £6.53 | 1000 gram £12.12
‣ Fifty:50 (Ennogen Healthcare Ltd)
Liquid paraffin 500 mg per 1 gram, White soft paraffin 500 mg per 1 gram Fifty:50 ointment | 250 gram £1.83 | 500 gram £3.66 DT = £4.57
‣ Hydromol (Alliance Pharmaceuticals Ltd)
Emulsifying wax 300 mg per 1 gram, Yellow soft paraffin 300 mg per 1 gram Hydromol ointment | 125 gram £2.92 | 500 gram £4.96 | 1000 gram £8.20
‣ KreaMoint (Essential-Healthcare Ltd)
Liquid paraffin 500 mg per 1 gram, White soft paraffin 500 mg per 1 gram KreaMoint 50:50 ointment | 500 gram £3.17 DT = £4.57
‣ Thirty:30 (Ennogen Healthcare Ltd)
Emulsifying wax 300 mg per 1 gram, Yellow soft paraffin 300 mg per 1 gram Thirty:30 ointment | 125 gram £3.81 | 250 gram £4.29 | 500 gram £6.47

‣ Vaseline (Unilever UK Home & Personal Care)
White soft paraffin 1 mg per 1 mg Vaseline Pure Petroleum jelly | 50 ml GSL ⊠

Liquid

CAUTIONARY AND ADVISORY LABELS 15
EXCIPIENTS: May contain Benzyl alcohol, cetostearyl alcohol (including cetyl and stearyl alcohol), hydroxybenzoates (parabens), isopropyl palmitate

‣ E45 (Forum Health Products Ltd)
E45 lotion | 200 ml £2.45 | 500 ml £4.59
‣ QV (Crawford Healthcare Ltd)
White soft paraffin 50 mg per 1 gram QV 5% skin lotion | 250 ml £3.19 | 500 ml £5.32

Emollients, urea-containing

● DRUG ACTION Urea is a keratin softener and hydrating agent used in the treatment of dry, scaling conditions (including ichthyosis) and may be useful in elderly patients.

● INDICATIONS AND DOSE

AQUADRATE ®

Dry, scaling, and itching skin
▸ TO THE SKIN
▸ Child: Apply twice daily, to be applied thinly
▸ Adult: Apply twice daily, to be applied thinly

BALNEUM ® CREAM

Dry skin conditions
▸ TO THE SKIN
▸ Child: Apply twice daily
▸ Adult: Apply twice daily

BALNEUM ® PLUS CREAM

Dry, scaling, and itching skin
▸ TO THE SKIN
▸ Child: Apply twice daily
▸ Adult: Apply twice daily

CALMURID ®

Dry, scaling, and itching skin
▸ TO THE SKIN
▸ Child: Apply twice daily, apply a thick layer for 3–5 minutes, massage into area, and remove excess. Can be diluted with aqueous cream (life of diluted cream is 14 days). Half-strength cream can be used for 1 week if stinging occurs
▸ Adult: Apply twice daily, apply a thick layer for 3–5 minutes, massage into area, and remove excess. Can be diluted with aqueous cream (life of diluted cream is 14 days). Half-strength cream can be used for 1 week if stinging occurs

DERMATONICS ONCE HEEL BALM ®

Dry skin on soles of feet
▸ TO THE SKIN
▸ Child 12–17 years: Apply once daily
▸ Adult: Apply once daily

E45 ® ITCH RELIEF CREAM

Dry, scaling, and itching skin
▸ TO THE SKIN
▸ Child: Apply twice daily
▸ Adult: Apply twice daily

EUCERIN ® INTENSIVE CREAM

Dry skin conditions including eczema, ichthyosis, xeroderma, and hyperkeratosis
▸ TO THE SKIN
▸ Child: Apply twice daily, to be applied thinly and rubbed into area
▸ Adult: Apply twice daily, to be applied thinly and rubbed into area

EUCERIN® INTENSIVE LOTION

Dry skin conditions including eczema, ichthyosis, xeroderma, and hyperkeratosis

▸ TO THE SKIN
▸ Child: Apply twice daily, to be applied sparingly and rubbed into area
▸ Adult: Apply twice daily, to be applied sparingly and rubbed into area

FLEXITOL®

Dry skin on soles of feet and heels

▸ TO THE SKIN
▸ Child 12–17 years: Apply 1–2 times a day
▸ Adult: Apply 1–2 times a day

HYDROMOL® INTENSIVE

Dry, scaling, and itching skin

▸ TO THE SKIN
▸ Child: Apply twice daily, to be applied thinly
▸ Adult: Apply twice daily, to be applied thinly

IMUDERM® EMOLLIENT

Dry skin conditions including eczema, psoriasis or dermatitis

▸ TO THE SKIN
▸ Adult: Apply to skin or use as a soap substitute

NUTRAPLUS®

Dry, scaling, and itching skin

▸ TO THE SKIN
▸ Child: Apply 2–3 times a day
▸ Adult: Apply 2–3 times a day

● DIRECTIONS FOR ADMINISTRATION Emollients should be applied immediately after washing or bathing to maximise the effect of skin hydration. Emollient preparations contained in tubs should be removed with a clean spoon or spatula to reduce bacterial contamination of the emollient. Emollients should be applied in the direction of hair growth to reduce the risk of folliculitis.

● MEDICINAL FORMS
There can be variation in the licensing of different medicines containing the same drug.

Cream
EXCIPIENTS: May contain Benzyl alcohol, cetostearyl alcohol (including cetyl and stearyl alcohol), hydroxybenzoates (parabens), isopropyl palmitate, polysorbates, propylene glycol, woolfat and related substances (including lanolin)
▸ Aquadrate (Alliance Pharmaceuticals Ltd)
  Urea 100 mg per 1 gram Aquadrate 10% cream | 30 gram £1.64 | 100 gram £4.37
▸ Balneum (Almirall Ltd)
  Balneum cream | 50 gram £2.85 | 500 gram £9.97
▸ Balneum Plus (Almirall Ltd)
  Lauromacrogols 30 mg per 1 gram, Urea 50 mg per 1 gram Balneum Plus cream | 100 gram GSL £3.29 DT = £4.28 | 500 gram GSL £14.99 DT = £14.99
▸ Calmurid (Galderma (UK) Ltd)
  Lactic acid 50 mg per 1 gram, Urea 100 mg per 1 gram Calmurid cream | 100 gram P £5.75 DT = £5.75 | 500 gram P £33.40 DT = £33.40
▸ E45 Itch Relief (Forum Health Products Ltd)
  Lauromacrogols 30 mg per 1 gram, Urea 50 mg per 1 gram E45 Itch Relief cream | 50 gram GSL £2.81 DT = £2.81 | 100 gram GSL £4.28 DT = £4.28 | 500 gram GSL £14.99 DT = £14.99
▸ Eucerin Intensive (Beiersdorf UK Ltd)
  Urea 100 mg per 1 gram Eucerin Intensive 10% cream | 100 ml GSL £7.59
▸ Hydromol Intensive (Alliance Pharmaceuticals Ltd)
  Urea 100 mg per 1 gram Hydromol Intensive 10% cream | 30 gram £1.65 | 100 gram £4.41
▸ Nutraplus (Galderma (UK) Ltd)
  Urea 100 mg per 1 gram Nutraplus 10% cream | 100 gram P £4.37

Liquid
EXCIPIENTS: May contain Benzyl alcohol, isopropyl palmitate
▸ Eucerin Intensive (Beiersdorf UK Ltd)
  Urea 100 mg per 1 gram Eucerin Intensive 10% lotion | 250 ml GSL £7.93 DT = £7.93

Balm
EXCIPIENTS: May contain Beeswax, benzyl alcohol, cetostearyl alcohol (including cetyl and stearyl alcohol), fragrances, lanolin
▸ Emollients, urea-containing (Non-proprietary)
  imuDERM emollient | 500 gram £6.55
▸ Dermatonics Once (Dermatonics Ltd)
  Dermatonics Once Heel Balm | 75 ml £3.60 | 200 ml £8.50
▸ Flexitol (Thornton & Ross Ltd)
  Flexitol 25% Urea Heel Balm | 40 gram £2.75 | 75 gram £3.80 | 200 gram £9.40 | 500 gram £14.75

2 Infections of the skin

Skin infections

Antibacterial preparations for the skin

Cellulitis, a rapidly spreading deeply seated inflammation of the skin and subcutaneous tissue, requires systemic antibacterial treatment. Lower leg infections or infections spreading around wounds are almost always cellulitis. *Erysipelas*, a superficial infection with clearly defined edges (and often affecting the face), is also treated with a systemic antibacterial.

In the community, acute *impetigo* on small areas of the skin may be treated by short-term topical application of fusidic acid p. 561; mupirocin p. 1197 should be used only to treat meticillin-resistant *Staphylococcus aureus*. If the impetigo is extensive or longstanding, an oral antibacterial such as flucloxacillin p. 544 (or clarithromycin p. 529 in penicillin allergy) should be used. Mild antiseptics can be used to soften crusts.

Although many antibacterial drugs are available in topical preparations, some are potentially hazardous and frequently their use is not necessary if adequate hygienic measures can be taken. Moreover, not all skin conditions that are oozing, crusted, or characterised by pustules are actually infected. Topical antibacterials should be **avoided** on *leg ulcers* unless used in short courses for defined infections; treatment of bacterial colonisation is generally inappropriate.

To minimise the development of resistant organisms it is advisable to limit the choice of antibacterials applied topically to those not used systemically. Unfortunately some of these, for example neomycin sulfate p. 1195, may cause sensitisation, and there is cross-sensitivity with other aminoglycoside antibiotics, such as gentamicin p. 510. If *large areas of skin* are being treated, ototoxicity may also be a hazard with aminoglycoside antibiotics (and also with polymyxins p. 1196), particularly in children, in the elderly, and in those with renal impairment. *Resistant organisms* are more common in hospitals, and whenever possible swabs should be taken for bacteriological examination before beginning treatment.

Mupirocin is not related to any other antibacterial in use; it is effective for skin infections, particularly those due to Gram-positive organisms but it is not indicated for pseudomonal infection. Although *Staphylococcus aureus* strains with low-level resistance to mupirocin are emerging, it is generally useful in infections resistant to other antibacterials. To avoid the development of resistance, mupirocin or fusidic acid should not be used for longer than 10 days and local microbiology advice should be sought before using it in hospital. In the presence of mupirocin-resistant MRSA infection, a topical antiseptic such as povidone-iodine p. 1241, chlorhexidine p. 1241, or alcohol can be used; their use should be discussed with the local microbiologist.

13

Skin

Retapamulin p. 1197 can be used for impetigo and other superficial bacterial skin infections caused by *Staphylococcus aureus* and *Streptococcus pyogenes* that are resistant to first-line topical antibacterials. However, it is not effective against MRSA.

Tedizolid p. 563 is licensed for the treatment of acute bacterial skin and skin structure infections.

Silver sulfadiazine p. 1196 is used in the treatment of infected burns.

Antibacterial preparations also used systemically

Fusidic acid is a narrow-spectrum antibacterial used for staphylococcal infections. Fusidic acid has a role in the treatment of impetigo.

An ointment containing fusidic acid is used in the fissures of angular cheilitis when associated with staphylococcal infection. See Oropharyngeal fungal infections p. 1182 for further information on angular cheilitis.

Metronidazole p. 1196 is used topically for rosacea and to reduce the odour associated with anaerobic infections; oral metronidazole is used to treat wounds infected with anaerobic bacteria.

Antifungal preparations for the skin

Most localised fungal infections are treated with topical preparations. To prevent relapse, local antifungal treatment should be continued for 1–2 weeks after the disappearance of all signs of infection. Systemic therapy is necessary for scalp infection or if the skin infection is widespread, disseminated, or intractable; although topical therapy may be used to treat some nail infections, systemic therapy is more effective. Skin scrapings should be examined if systemic therapy is being considered or where there is doubt about the diagnosis.

Dermatophytoses

Ringworm infection can affect the scalp (tinea capitis), body (tinea corporis), groin (tinea cruris), hand (tinea manuum), foot (tinea pedis, athlete's foot), or nail (tinea unguium). Scalp infection requires systemic treatment; additional application of a topical antifungal, during the early stages of treatment, may reduce the risk of transmission. A topical antifungal can also be used to treat asymptomatic carriers of scalp ringworm. Most other local ringworm infections can be treated adequately with topical antifungal preparations (including shampoos). The imidazole antifungals clotrimazole p. 1197, econazole nitrate p. 1198, ketoconazole p. 1198, and miconazole p. 1199 are all effective. Terbinafine cream p. 1200 is also effective but it is more expensive. Other topical antifungals include griseofulvin p. 1200 and the **undecenoates**. **Compound benzoic acid ointment** (Whitfield's ointment) has been used for ringworm infections but it is cosmetically less acceptable than proprietary preparations. Topical preparations for athlete's foot containing **tolnaftate** are on sale to the public.

Antifungal dusting powders are of little therapeutic value in the treatment of fungal skin infections and may cause skin irritation; they may have some role in preventing re-infection.

Antifungal treatment may not be necessary in asymptomatic patients with tinea infection of the nails. If treatment is necessary, a systemic antifungal is more effective than topical therapy. However, topical application of amorolfine p. 1199 or tioconazole p. 1199 may be useful for treating early onychomycosis when involvement is limited to mild distal disease, or for superficial white onychomycosis, or where there are contra-indications to systemic therapy.

Pityriasis versicolor

Pityriasis (tinea) versicolor can be treated with ketoconazole shampoo. Alternatively, **selenium sulfide** shampoo [unlicensed indication] can be used as a lotion (diluting with

a small amount of water can reduce irritation) and left on the affected area for 10 minutes before rinsing off; it should be applied once daily for 7 days, and the course repeated if necessary.

Topical imidazole antifungals such as clotrimazole, econazole nitrate, ketoconazole, and miconazole, or topical terbinafine are alternatives, but large quantities may be required.

If topical therapy fails, or if the infection is widespread, pityriasis versicolor is treated systemically with a triazole antifungal. Relapse is common, especially in the immunocompromised.

Candidiasis

Candidal skin infections can be treated with a topical imidazole antifungal, such as clotrimazole, econazole nitrate, ketoconazole, or miconazole; topical terbinafine is an alternative. Topical application of nystatin p. 1184 is also effective for candidiasis but it is ineffective against dermatophytosis. Refractory candidiasis requires systemic treatment generally with a triazole such as fluconazole p. 584; systemic treatment with terbinafine is **not appropriate** for refractory candidiasis.

Angular cheilitis

Miconazole cream is used in the fissures of angular cheilitis when associated with *Candida*.

Compound topical preparations

Combination of an imidazole and a mild corticosteroid (such as hydrocortisone 1% p. 1214) may be of value in the treatment of eczematous intertrigo and, in the first few days only, of a severely inflamed patch of ringworm.

Combination of a mild corticosteroid with either an imidazole or nystatin may be of use in the treatment of intertrigo associated with candida.

Antiviral preparations for the skin

Aciclovir cream p. 1203 is licensed for the treatment of initial and recurrent labial and genital *herpes simplex infections*; treatment should begin as early as possible. Systemic treatment is necessary for buccal or vaginal infections and for *herpes zoster* (shingles).

Herpes labialis

Aciclovir cream can be used for the treatment of initial and recurrent labial herpes simplex infections (cold sores). It is best applied at the earliest possible stage, usually when prodromal changes of sensation are felt in the lip and before vesicles appear.

Penciclovir cream is also licensed for the treatment of herpes labialis; it needs to be applied more frequently than aciclovir cream.

Systemic treatment is necessary if cold sores recur frequently or for infections in the mouth.

Parasiticidal preparations for the skin

Suitable quantities of parasiticidal preparations

Area of body	Skin creams	Lotions	Cream rinses
Scalp (head lice)		50–100 mL	50–100 mL
Body (scabies)	30–60 g	100 mL	
Body (crab lice)	30–60 g	100 mL	

These amounts are usually suitable for an adult for single application.

Scabies

Permethrin p. 1203 is used for the treatment of *scabies* (*Sarcoptes scabiei*); malathion p. 1202 can be used if permethrin is inappropriate.

Benzyl benzoate p. 1202 is an irritant and should be avoided in children; it is less effective than malathion and permethrin.

Ivermectin p. 593 (available on a named patient basis from 'special-order' manufacturers or specialist importing companies) by mouth has been used, in combination with topical drugs, for the treatment of hyperkeratotic (crusted or 'Norwegian') scabies that does not respond to topical treatment alone; further doses may be required.

Application
Although acaricides have traditionally been applied after a hot bath, this is **not** necessary and there is even evidence that a hot bath may increase absorption into the blood, removing them from their site of action on the skin.

All members of the affected household should be treated simultaneously. Treatment should be applied to the whole body including the scalp, neck, face, and ears. Particular attention should be paid to the webs of the fingers and toes and lotion brushed under the ends of nails. It is now recommended that malathion and permethrin should be applied twice, one week apart; in the case of benzyl benzoate in adults, up to 3 applications on consecutive days may be needed. It is important to warn users to reapply treatment to the hands if they are washed. Patients with hyperkeratotic scabies may require 2 or 3 applications of acaricide on consecutive days to ensure that enough penetrates the skin crusts to kill all the mites.

Itching
The *itch* and *eczema* of scabies persists for some weeks after the infestation has been eliminated and treatment for pruritus and eczema may be required. Application of crotamiton p. 1230 can be used to control itching after treatment with more effective acaricides. A topical corticosteroid may help to reduce itch and inflammation after scabies has been treated successfully; however, persistent symptoms suggest that scabies eradication was not successful. Oral administration of a **sedating antihistamine** at night may also be useful.

Head lice
Dimeticone p. 1202 is effective against head lice (*Pediculus humanus capitis*). It coats head lice and interferes with water balance in lice by preventing the excretion of water; it is less active against eggs and treatment should be repeated after 7 days. Malathion, an organophosphorus insecticide, is an alternative, but resistance has been reported. Benzyl benzoate is licensed for the treatment of head lice but it is less effective than other drugs and not recommended for use in children. Permethrin is active against head lice but the formulation and licensed methods of application of the current products make them unsuitable for the treatment of head lice.

Head lice infestation (pediculosis) should be treated using lotion or liquid formulations only if live lice are present. Shampoos are diluted too much in use to be effective. A contact time of 8–12 hours or overnight treatment is recommended for lotions and liquids; a 2-hour treatment is not sufficient to kill eggs.

In general, a course of treatment for head lice should be 2 applications of product 7 days apart to kill lice emerging from any eggs that survive the first application. All affected household members should be treated simultaneously.

MHRA/CHM advice: Head lice eradication products: risk of serious burns if treated hair is exposed to open flames or other sources of ignition (March 2018)
Some products for the eradication of head lice infestations are combustible/flammable when on the hair and can ignite and cause serious harm in the presence of an open flame or other source of ignition such as when lighting cigarettes.

Patients and carers should be advised on the safe and correct use of head lice eradication treatments and if appropriate, should be advised that they should not smoke

around treated hair and that it should be kept away from open flames or other sources of ignition, including in the morning after overnight application until hair is washed.

Wet combing methods
Head lice can be mechanically removed by combing wet hair meticulously with a plastic detection comb (probably for at least 30 minutes each time) over the whole scalp at 4-day intervals for a minimum of 2 weeks, and continued until no lice are found on 3 consecutive sessions; hair conditioner or vegetable oil can be used to facilitate the process.

Several devices for the removal of head lice such as combs and topical solutions, are available and some are prescribable on the NHS.

The Drug Tariffs can be accessed online at:
- National Health Service Drug Tariff for England and Wales: www.ppa.org.uk/ppa/edt_intro.htm
- Health and Personal Social Services for Northern Ireland Drug Tariff: www.hscbusiness.hscni.net/services/2034.htm
- Scottish Drug Tariff: www.isdscotland.org/Health-topics/Prescribing-and-Medicines/Scottish-Drug-Tariff/

Crab lice
Permethrin and malathion are used to eliminate *crab lice* (*Pthirus pubis*). An aqueous preparation should be applied, allowed to dry naturally and washed off after 12 hours; a second treatment is needed after 7 days to kill lice emerging from surviving eggs. All surfaces of the body should be treated, including the scalp, neck, and face (paying particular attention to the eyebrows and other facial hair). A different insecticide should be used if a course of treatment fails.

2.1 Bacterial skin infections

ANTIBACTERIALS › AMINOGLYCOSIDES

Neomycin sulfate

- **INDICATIONS AND DOSE**
Bacterial skin infections
▶ TO THE SKIN
▶ **Child:** Apply up to 3 times a day, for short-term use only
▶ **Adult:** Apply up to 3 times a day, for short-term use only

- **UNLICENSED USE**
▶ In children *Neomycin Cream BPC*—no information available.
- **CONTRA-INDICATIONS** Neonates
- **CAUTIONS** If large areas of skin are being treated ototoxicity may be a hazard, particularly in children, the elderly, and in those with renal impairment.
- **INTERACTIONS** → Appendix 1: neomycin
- **SIDE-EFFECTS** Sensitisation (cross sensitivity with other aminoglycosides may occur)
- **RENAL IMPAIRMENT** Ototoxicity may be a hazard if large areas of skin are treated.
- **LESS SUITABLE FOR PRESCRIBING** Neomycin sulfate cream is less suitable for prescribing.

- **MEDICINAL FORMS**
Forms available from special-order manufacturers include: cream

13

Skin

ANTIBACTERIALS > NITROIMIDAZOLE DERIVATIVES

Metronidazole

- **DRUG ACTION** Metronidazole is an antimicrobial drug with high activity against anaerobic bacteria and protozoa.

- **INDICATIONS AND DOSE**

ACEA ®

Acute inflammatory exacerbation of rosacea
- TO THE SKIN
- Adult: Apply twice daily for 8 weeks, to be applied thinly

ANABACT ®

Malodorous fungating tumours and malodorous gravitational and decubitus ulcers
- TO THE SKIN
- Adult: Apply 1–2 times a day, to be applied to clean wound and covered with non-adherent dressing

METROGEL ®

Acute inflammatory exacerbation of rosacea
- TO THE SKIN
- Adult: Apply twice daily for 8–9 weeks, to be applied thinly

Malodorous fungating tumours
- TO THE SKIN
- Adult: Apply 1–2 times a day, to be applied to clean wound and covered with non-adherent dressing

METROSA ®

Acute exacerbation of rosacea
- TO THE SKIN
- Adult: Apply twice daily for up to 8 weeks, to be applied thinly

ROSICED ®

Inflammatory papules and pustules of rosacea
- TO THE SKIN
- Adult: Apply twice daily for 6 weeks (longer if necessary)

ROZEX ® **CREAM**

Inflammatory papules, pustules and erythema of rosacea
- TO THE SKIN
- Adult: Apply twice daily for 3–4 months

ROZEX ® **GEL**

Inflammatory papules, pustules and erythema of rosacea
- TO THE SKIN
- Adult: Apply twice daily for 3–4 months

ZYOMET ®

Acute inflammatory exacerbation of rosacea
- TO THE SKIN
- Adult: Apply twice daily for 8–9 weeks, to be applied thinly

- **CAUTIONS** Avoid exposure to strong sunlight or UV light
- **INTERACTIONS** → Appendix 1: metronidazole

- **MEDICINAL FORMS**
There can be variation in the licensing of different medicines containing the same drug. Forms available from special-order manufacturers include: cream, gel

Gel

EXCIPIENTS: May contain Benzyl alcohol, disodium edetate, hydroxybenzoates (parabens), propylene glycol
- Acea (Ferndale Pharmaceuticals Ltd)
Metronidazole 7.5 mg per 1 gram Acea 0.75% gel | 40 gram [PoM] £9.95 DT = £22.63
- Anabact (Cambridge Healthcare Supplies Ltd)
Metronidazole 7.5 mg per 1 gram Anabact 0.75% gel | 15 gram [PoM] £4.47 DT = £4.47 | 30 gram [PoM] £7.89 | 40 gram [PoM] £15.89 DT = £22.63

- Metrogel (Galderma (UK) Ltd)
Metronidazole 7.5 mg per 1 gram Metrogel 0.75% gel | 40 gram [PoM] £22.63 DT = £22.63
- Metrosa (M & A Pharmachem Ltd)
Metronidazole 7.5 mg per 1 gram Metrosa 0.75% gel | 30 gram [PoM] £12.00 | 40 gram [PoM] £19.90 DT = £22.63
- Rozex (Galderma (UK) Ltd)
Metronidazole 7.5 mg per 1 gram Rozex 0.75% gel | 30 gram [PoM] £6.60 | 40 gram [PoM] £9.88 DT = £22.63
- Zyomet (AMCo)
Metronidazole 7.5 mg per 1 gram Zyomet 0.75% gel | 30 gram [PoM] £12.00

Cream

EXCIPIENTS: May contain Benzyl alcohol, isopropyl palmitate, propylene glycol
- Rosiced (Pierre Fabre Dermo-Cosmetique)
Metronidazole 7.5 mg per 1 gram Rosiced 0.75% cream | 30 gram [PoM] £6.60 DT = £6.60
- Rozex (Galderma (UK) Ltd)
Metronidazole 7.5 mg per 1 gram Rozex 0.75% cream | 30 gram [PoM] £6.60 DT = £6.60 | 40 gram [PoM] £9.88 DT = £9.88

ANTIBACTERIALS > POLYMYXINS

Polymyxins

- **INDICATIONS AND DOSE**

Bacterial skin infections
- TO THE SKIN
- Adult: Apply twice daily, may be applied more frequently if required

- **CAUTIONS** If large areas of skin are being treated nephrotoxicity and neurotoxicity may be a hazard, particularly in children, in the elderly, and in those with renal impairment.
- **INTERACTIONS** → Appendix 1: polymyxins
- **SIDE-EFFECTS** Sensitisation

- **MEDICINAL FORMS**
No licensed medicines listed.

ANTIBACTERIALS > SULFONAMIDES

Silver sulfadiazine

- **INDICATIONS AND DOSE**

Prophylaxis and treatment of infection in burn wounds
- TO THE SKIN
- Child: Apply daily, may be applied more frequently if very exudative
- Adult: Apply daily, may be applied more frequently if very exudative

For conservative management of finger-tip injuries
- TO THE SKIN
- Child: Apply every 2–3 days, consult product literature for details
- Adult: Apply every 2–3 days, consult product literature for details

Adjunct to prophylaxis of infection in skin graft donor sites and extensive abrasions
- TO THE SKIN
- Adult: (consult product literature)

Adjunct to short-term treatment of infection in pressure sores
- TO THE SKIN
- Adult: Apply once daily or on alternate days

As an adjunct to short-term treatment of infection in leg ulcers
- TO THE SKIN
- Adult: Apply once daily or on alternate days, not recommended if ulcer is very exudative

- UNLICENSED USE
▸ In children No age range specified by manufacturer.
- CONTRA-INDICATIONS Not recommended for neonates
- CAUTIONS G6PD deficiency
   CAUTIONS, FURTHER INFORMATION
▸ Large areas Plasma-sulfadiazine concentrations may
   approach therapeutic levels with *side-effects* and
   interactions as for sulfonamides if large areas of skin are
   treated.
- INTERACTIONS → Appendix 1: silver sulfadiazine
- SIDE-EFFECTS
▸ **Common or very common** Leucopenia · skin reactions
▸ **Rare or very rare** Argyria (following treatment of large
   areas of skin or long term use) · renal failure
   SIDE-EFFECTS, FURTHER INFORMATION Leucopenia
   developing 2–3 days after starting treatment of burns
   patients is reported usually to be self-limiting and silver
   sulfadiazine need not usually be discontinued provided
   blood counts are monitored carefully to ensure return to
   normality within a few days.
- ALLERGY AND CROSS-SENSITIVITY Contra-indicated in
   patients with sensitivity to sulfonamides.
- PREGNANCY Risk of neonatal haemolysis and
   methaemoglobinaemia in third trimester.
- BREAST FEEDING Small risk of kernicterus in jaundiced
   infants and of haemolysis in G6PD-deficient infants.
- HEPATIC IMPAIRMENT Manufacturer advises caution if
   significant impairment.
- RENAL IMPAIRMENT Manufacturer advises caution if
   significant impairment.
- MONITORING REQUIREMENTS Monitor for leucopenia.
- DIRECTIONS FOR ADMINISTRATION Apply with sterile
   applicator.
- MEDICINAL FORMS
   There can be variation in the licensing of different medicines
   containing the same drug.
   Cream
   EXCIPIENTS: May contain Cetostearyl alcohol (including cetyl and
   stearyl alcohol), polysorbates, propylene glycol
   ▸ Flamazine (Smith & Nephew Healthcare Ltd)
      Sulfadiazine silver 10 mg per 1 gram Flamazine 1% cream |
      20 gram [PoM] £2.91 | 50 gram [PoM] £3.85 DT = £3.85 |
      250 gram [PoM] £10.32 DT = £10.32 | 500 gram [PoM] £18.27 DT =
      £18.27

ANTIBACTERIALS > OTHER

Mupirocin

- INDICATIONS AND DOSE
   **Bacterial skin infections, particularly those caused by
   Gram-positive organisms (except pseudomonal
   infection)**
   ▸ TO THE SKIN
   ▸ Child: Apply up to 3 times a day for up to 10 days
   ▸ Adult: Apply up to 3 times a day for up to 10 days

- UNLICENSED USE Mupirocin ointment licensed for use in
   children (age range not specified by manufacturer).
   Bactroban® cream not recommended for use in children
   under 1 year.
- SIDE-EFFECTS
▸ **Common or very common** Skin reactions
- PREGNANCY Manufacturer advises avoid unless potential
   benefit outweighs risk—no information available.
- BREAST FEEDING No information available.
- RENAL IMPAIRMENT Manufacturer advises caution when
   mupirocin ointment used in moderate or severe

impairment because it contains macrogols (polyethylene
glycol).

- MEDICINAL FORMS
   There can be variation in the licensing of different medicines
   containing the same drug.
   Ointment
   ▸ Mupirocin (Non-proprietary)
      Mupirocin 20 mg per 1 gram Mupirocin 2% ointment |
      15 gram [PoM] £12.50 DT = £5.26
   ▸ Bactroban (GlaxoSmithKline UK Ltd)
      Mupirocin 20 mg per 1 gram Bactroban 2% ointment |
      15 gram [PoM] £5.26 DT = £5.26
   Cream
   EXCIPIENTS: May contain Benzyl alcohol, cetostearyl alcohol (including
   cetyl and stearyl alcohol)
   ▸ Bactroban (GlaxoSmithKline UK Ltd)
      Mupirocin (as Mupirocin calcium) 20 mg per 1 gram Bactroban
      2% cream | 15 gram [PoM] £5.26 DT = £5.26

Retapamulin

- INDICATIONS AND DOSE
   **Superficial bacterial skin infection caused by
   Staphylococcus aureus and *Streptococcus pyogenes* (if
   resistant to first line topical antibacterials)**
   ▸ TO THE SKIN
   ▸ Child 9 months-17 years: Apply twice daily for 5 days, to
      be applied thinly, maximum area of skin treated 2% of
      body surface area, review treatment if no response
      within 2–3 days
   ▸ Adult: Apply twice daily for 5 days, to be applied thinly,
      maximum area of skin treated 100 cm^2 or lesion length
      10 cm, review treatment if no response within 2–3 days

- CONTRA-INDICATIONS Contact with eyes · contact with
   mucous membranes
- SIDE-EFFECTS
▸ **Uncommon** Contact dermatitis
- NATIONAL FUNDING/ACCESS DECISIONS
   Scottish Medicines Consortium (SMC) Decisions
   The *Scottish Medicines Consortium* has advised (March
   2008) that retapamulin (*Altargo*®) is **not** recommended for
   use within NHS Scotland for the treatment of superficial
   skin infections.

- MEDICINAL FORMS
   No licensed medicines listed.

2.2 Fungal skin infections

ANTIFUNGALS > IMIDAZOLE ANTIFUNGALS

Clotrimazole

- INDICATIONS AND DOSE
   Fungal skin infections
   ▸ TO THE SKIN
   ▸ Child: Apply 2–3 times a day
   ▸ Adult: Apply 2–3 times a day

- CAUTIONS Contact with eyes and mucous membranes
   should be avoided
- INTERACTIONS → Appendix 1: antifungals, azoles
- SIDE-EFFECTS Oedema · pain · paraesthesia · skin reactions
- PREGNANCY Minimal absorption from skin; not known to
   be harmful.
- PRESCRIBING AND DISPENSING INFORMATION Spray may
   be useful for application of clotrimazole to large or hairy
   areas of the skin.

13

Skin

● MEDICINAL FORMS
There can be variation in the licensing of different medicines containing the same drug.

Cream
EXCIPIENTS: May contain Benzyl alcohol, cetostearyl alcohol (including cetyl and stearyl alcohol), polysorbates
▸ Clotrimazole (Non-proprietary)
Clotrimazole 10 mg per 1 gram Clotrimazole 1% cream |
20 gram P £2.06 DT = £0.72 | 50 gram P £5.45 DT = £1.80
▸ Canesten (clotrimazole) (Bayer Plc)
Clotrimazole 10 mg per 1 gram Canesten 1% cream | 20 gram P
£2.20 DT = £0.72 | 50 gram P £3.50 DT = £1.80
Canesten Antifungal 1% cream | 20 gram P £1.85 DT = £0.72
Canesten Dual Action 1% cream | 15 gram GSL £2.14 |
30 gram GSL £2.76
Clotrimazole 20 mg per 1 gram Canesten 2% thrush cream |
20 gram P £4.76 DT = £4.76
Clotrimazole 100 mg per 1 gram Canesten Internal 10% cream |
5 gram P £6.23 DT = £6.23
Canesten 10% VC cream | 5 gram PoM £4.50 DT = £6.23

Liquid
▸ Canesten (clotrimazole) (Bayer Plc)
Clotrimazole 10 mg per 1 ml Canesten 1% solution | 20 ml P
£2.30 DT = £2.30

Spray
CAUTIONARY AND ADVISORY LABELS 15
EXCIPIENTS: May contain propylene glycol
▸ Canesten (clotrimazole) (Bayer Plc)
Clotrimazole 10 mg per 1 ml Canesten, Dermatological 1% spray |
40 ml P £4.72 DT = £4.72

Combinations available: *Hydrocortisone with clotrimazole,*
p. 1217

Econazole nitrate

● INDICATIONS AND DOSE
Fungal skin infections
▸ TO THE SKIN
▸ Child: Apply twice daily
▸ Adult: Apply twice daily
Fungal nail infections
▸ BY TRANSUNGUAL APPLICATION
▸ Child: Apply once daily, applied under occlusive dressing
▸ Adult: Apply once daily, applied under occlusive dressing

● CAUTIONS Avoid contact with eyes and mucous membranes
● SIDE-EFFECTS
▸ Common or very common Pain · skin reactions
▸ Uncommon Swelling
▸ Frequency not known Angioedema
SIDE-EFFECTS, FURTHER INFORMATION Treatment should be discontinued if side-effects are severe.
● PREGNANCY Minimal absorption from skin; not known to be harmful.

● MEDICINAL FORMS
There can be variation in the licensing of different medicines containing the same drug.

Cream
EXCIPIENTS: May contain Butylated hydroxyanisole, fragrances
▸ Pevaryl (Janssen-Cilag Ltd)
Econazole nitrate 10 mg per 1 gram Pevaryl 1% cream |
30 gram P £3.71

Ketoconazole

20-Jul-2017

● INDICATIONS AND DOSE
Tinea pedis
▸ TO THE SKIN USING CREAM
▸ Adult: Apply twice daily
Fungal skin infection (not Tinea pedis)
▸ TO THE SKIN USING CREAM
▸ Adult: Apply 1–2 times a day
Treatment of seborrhoeic dermatitis and dandruff
▸ TO THE SKIN USING SHAMPOO
▸ Child 12–17 years: Apply twice weekly for 2–4 weeks, leave preparation on for 3–5 minutes before rinsing
▸ Adult: Apply twice weekly for 2–4 weeks, leave preparation on for 3–5 minutes before rinsing
Prophylaxis of seborrhoeic dermatitis and dandruff
▸ TO THE SKIN USING SHAMPOO
▸ Child 12–17 years: Apply every 1–2 weeks, leave preparation on for 3–5 minutes before rinsing
▸ Adult: Apply every 1–2 weeks, leave preparation on for 3–5 minutes before rinsing
Treatment of pityriasis versicolor
▸ TO THE SKIN USING SHAMPOO
▸ Child 12–17 years: Apply once daily for maximum 5 days, leave preparation on for 3–5 minutes before rinsing
▸ Adult: Apply once daily for maximum 5 days, leave preparation on for 3–5 minutes before rinsing
Prophylaxis of pityriasis versicolor
▸ TO THE SKIN USING SHAMPOO
▸ Child 12–17 years: Apply once daily for up to 3 days before sun exposure, leave preparation on for 3–5 minutes before rinsing
▸ Adult: Apply once daily for up to 3 days before sun exposure, leave preparation on for 3–5 minutes before rinsing

● CONTRA-INDICATIONS Acute porphyrias p. 1025
● CAUTIONS Avoid contact with eyes · avoid contact with mucous membranes
● INTERACTIONS → Appendix 1: antifungals, azoles
● SIDE-EFFECTS
▸ Common or very common Skin reactions
▸ Uncommon Excessive tearing · folliculitis · hair changes
● NATIONAL FUNDING/ACCESS DECISIONS
NHS restrictions *Nizoral*® cream is not prescribable in NHS primary care except for the treatment of seborrhoeic dermatitis and pityriasis versicolor; endorse prescription 'SLS'.
● EXCEPTIONS TO LEGAL CATEGORY A 15-g tube is available for sale to the public for the treatment of tinea pedis, tinea cruris, and candidal intertrigo.
Can be sold to the public for the prevention and treatment of dandruff and seborrhoeic dermatitis of the scalp as a shampoo formulation containing ketoconazole maximum 2%, in a pack containing maximum 120 mL and labelled to show a maximum frequency of application of once every 3 days.

● MEDICINAL FORMS
There can be variation in the licensing of different medicines containing the same drug.

Cream
EXCIPIENTS: May contain Cetostearyl alcohol (including cetyl and stearyl alcohol), polysorbates, propylene glycol
▸ Nizoral (Janssen-Cilag Ltd)
Ketoconazole 20 mg per 1 gram Nizoral 2% cream | 30 gram PoM
£4.24 DT = £4.24

Shampoo
EXCIPIENTS: May contain Imidurea
▸ Ketoconazole (Non-proprietary)
Ketoconazole 20 mg per 1 gram Ketoconazole 2% shampoo |
120 ml PoM £3.60 DT = £3.14

▸ Dandrazol (Transdermal Ltd)
Ketoconazole 20 mg per 1 gram Dandrazol 2% shampoo |
120 ml `PoM` £3.39 DT = £3.14
▸ Nizoral (Janssen-Cilag Ltd, McNeil Products Ltd)
Ketoconazole 20 mg per 1 gram Nizoral 2% shampoo |
120 ml `PoM` £3.59 DT = £3.14

Miconazole
11-Oct-2017

● **INDICATIONS AND DOSE**
Fungal skin infections
▸ TO THE SKIN
▸ **Child:** Apply twice daily continuing for 10 days after
lesions have healed
▸ **Adult:** Apply twice daily continuing for 10 days after
lesions have healed

Fungal nail infections
▸ TO THE SKIN
▸ **Child:** Apply 1–2 times a day
▸ **Adult:** Apply 1–2 times a day

● **UNLICENSED USE** Licensed for use in children (age range
not specified by manufacturer).

● **CAUTIONS** Avoid in Acute porphyrias p. 1025 · contact with
eyes and mucous membranes should be avoided

● **INTERACTIONS** → Appendix 1: antifungals, azoles

● **SIDE-EFFECTS**
▸ **Common or very common** Skin reactions
▸ **Frequency not known** Angioedema

● **PREGNANCY** Absorbed from the skin in small amounts;
manufacturer advises caution.

● **BREAST FEEDING** Manufacturer advises caution—no
information available.

● **PROFESSION SPECIFIC INFORMATION**
Dental practitioners' formulary
Miconazole cream may be prescribed.

● **NATIONAL FUNDING/ACCESS DECISIONS**
NHS restrictions Miconazole nitrate 2% powder is not
prescribable in NHS primary care.

● **MEDICINAL FORMS**
There can be variation in the licensing of different medicines
containing the same drug.
Cream
EXCIPIENTS: May contain Butylated hydroxyanisole
▸ Daktarin (McNeil Products Ltd, Janssen-Cilag Ltd)
Miconazole nitrate 20 mg per 1 gram Daktarin 2% cream |
15 gram `P` £2.51 | 30 gram `P` £1.82 DT = £1.82
Powder
▸ Daktarin (McNeil Products Ltd)
Miconazole nitrate 20 mg per 1 gram Daktarin 2% powder |
20 gram `P` £2.95 DT = £2.78

Tioconazole

● **INDICATIONS AND DOSE**
Fungal nail infection
▸ BY TRANSUNGUAL APPLICATION
▸ **Child:** Apply twice daily usually for up to 6 months
(may be extended to 12 months), apply to nails and
surrounding skin
▸ **Adult:** Apply twice daily usually for up to 6 months
(may be extended to 12 months), apply to nails and
surrounding skin

● **UNLICENSED USE** Licensed for use in children (age range
not specified by manufacturer).

● **CAUTIONS** Contact with eyes and mucous membranes
should be avoided · use with caution if child likely to suck
affected digits

● **SIDE-EFFECTS**
▸ **Common or very common** Peripheral oedema
▸ **Uncommon** Skin reactions
▸ **Frequency not known** Nail disorder · pain · paraesthesia ·
periorbital oedema
● **PREGNANCY** Manufacturer advises avoid.

● **MEDICINAL FORMS**
There can be variation in the licensing of different medicines
containing the same drug.
Paint
▸ Tioconazole (Non-proprietary)
Tioconazole 283 mg per 1 ml Tioconazole 283mg/ml medicated nail
lacquer | 12 ml `PoM` £27.38–£28.74 DT = £28.74
▸ Trosyl (Pfizer Ltd)
Tioconazole 283 mg per 1 ml Trosyl 283mg/ml nail solution |
12 ml `PoM` £27.38 DT = £28.74

ANTIFUNGALS > OTHER

Amorolfine

● **INDICATIONS AND DOSE**
Fungal nail infections
▸ BY TRANSUNGUAL APPLICATION
▸ **Child 12–17 years:** Apply 1–2 times a week for 6 months
to treat finger nails and for toe nails 9–12 months
(review at intervals of 3 months), apply to infected
nails after filing and cleansing, allow to dry for
approximately 3 minutes
▸ **Adult:** Apply 1–2 times a week for 6 months to treat
finger nails and for toe nails 9–12 months (review at
intervals of 3 months), apply to infected nails after
filing and cleansing, allow to dry for approximately
3 minutes

● **CAUTIONS** Avoid contact with ears · avoid contact with
eyes and mucous membranes · use with caution in child
likely to suck affected digits

● **SIDE-EFFECTS**
▸ **Rare or very rare** Nail discolouration · skin reactions

● **PATIENT AND CARER ADVICE** Avoid nail varnish or artificial
nails during treatment.

● **EXCEPTIONS TO LEGAL CATEGORY**
▸ In adults Amorolfine nail lacquer can be sold to the public
if supplied for the treatment of mild cases of distal and
lateral subungual onychomycoses caused by
dermatophytes, yeasts and moulds; subject to treatment of
max. 2 nails, max. strength of nail lacquer amorolfine 5%
and a pack size of 3 mL.

● **MEDICINAL FORMS**
There can be variation in the licensing of different medicines
containing the same drug.
Medicated nail lacquer
CAUTIONARY AND ADVISORY LABELS 10
▸ Amorolfine (Non-proprietary)
**Amorolfine (as Amorolfine hydrochloride) 50 mg per
1 ml** Amorolfine 5% medicated nail lacquer | 5 ml `PoM` £16.21 DT =
£6.14
▸ Loceryl (Galderma (UK) Ltd)
Amorolfine (as Amorolfine hydrochloride) 50 mg per 1 ml Loceryl
5% medicated nail lacquer | 2.5 ml `PoM` £7.26 | 5 ml `PoM` £9.08 DT
= £6.14
▸ Omicur (Morningside Healthcare Ltd)
Amorolfine (as Amorolfine hydrochloride) 50 mg per 1 ml Omicur
5% medicated nail lacquer | 2.5 ml `PoM` £9.09 | 5 ml `PoM` £9.09 DT
= £6.14

13

Skin

Griseofulvin

● **INDICATIONS AND DOSE**

Tinea pedis
▶ TO THE SKIN
▶ Adult: Apply 400 micrograms once daily, apply to an area approximately 13 cm^2; increased if necessary to 1.2 mg once daily for maximum treatment duration of 4 weeks, allow each spray to dry between application

● **CAUTIONS** Avoid contact with eyes and mucous membranes

● **INTERACTIONS** → Appendix 1: griseofulvin

● **SIDE-EFFECTS** Paraesthesia · skin irritation · stinging

● **PREGNANCY** Manufacturer advises avoid unless potential benefit outweighs risk.

● **BREAST FEEDING** Manufacturer advises avoid unless potential benefit outweighs risk.

● **MEDICINAL FORMS**
There can be variation in the licensing of different medicines containing the same drug.

Spray
CAUTIONARY AND ADVISORY LABELS 15
EXCIPIENTS: May contain Benzyl alcohol
▶ Grisol AF (Transdermal Ltd)
   Griseofulvin 10 mg per 1 gram Grisol AF 1% spray | 20 ml [P] £4.00

Terbinafine

23-Apr-2018

● **INDICATIONS AND DOSE**

Tinea pedis
▶ TO THE SKIN USING CREAM
▶ Adult: Apply 1–2 times a day for up to 1 week, to be applied thinly
▶ BY MOUTH USING TABLETS
▶ Adult: 250 mg once daily for 2-6 weeks

Tinea corporis
▶ TO THE SKIN USING CREAM
▶ Adult: Apply 1–2 times a day for up to 1–2 weeks, to be applied thinly, review treatment after 2 weeks
▶ BY MOUTH USING TABLETS
▶ Adult: 250 mg once daily for 4 weeks

Tinea cruris
▶ TO THE SKIN USING CREAM
▶ Adult: Apply 1–2 times a day for up to 1–2 weeks, to be applied thinly, review treatment after 2 weeks
▶ BY MOUTH USING TABLETS
▶ Adult: 250 mg once daily for 2-4 weeks

Dermatophyte infections of the nails
▶ BY MOUTH USING TABLETS
▶ Adult: 250 mg once daily for 6 weeks-3 months (occasionally longer in toenail infections)

Cutaneous candidiasis | Pityriasis versicolor
▶ TO THE SKIN USING CREAM
▶ Adult: Apply 1–2 times a day for 2 weeks, to be applied thinly, review treatment after 2 weeks

● **CAUTIONS**
▶ With oral use Autoimmune disease (risk of lupus-erythematosus-like effect) · psoriasis (risk of exacerbation)
▶ With topical use Contact with eyes and mucous membranes should be avoided

● **INTERACTIONS** → Appendix 1: terbinafine

● **SIDE-EFFECTS**
GENERAL SIDE-EFFECTS
▶ Common or very common Skin reactions

SPECIFIC SIDE-EFFECTS
▶ **Common or very common**
▶ With oral use Appetite decreased · arthralgia · diarrhoea · gastrointestinal discomfort · gastrointestinal disorder · headache · myalgia · nausea
▶ **Uncommon**
▶ With oral use Taste altered · weight decreased
▶ **Rare or very rare**
▶ With oral use Agranulocytosis · alopecia · cutaneous lupus erythematosus · dizziness · hepatic disorders · malaise · neutropenia · photosensitivity reaction · sensation abnormal · severe cutaneous adverse reactions (SCARs) · systemic lupus erythematosus (SLE) · thrombocytopenia · vertigo
▶ **Frequency not known**
▶ With oral use Anaemia · anxiety · depressive symptom · fatigue · fever · hearing impairment · influenza like illness · pancreatitis · pancytopenia · rhabdomyolysis · serum sickness-like reaction · smell altered · vasculitis · vision disorders

SIDE-EFFECTS, FURTHER INFORMATION
Liver toxicity With oral use; discontinue treatment if liver toxicity develops (including jaundice, cholestasis and hepatitis).
Serious skin reactions With oral use; discontinue treatment in progressive skin rash (including Stevens-Johnson syndrome and toxic epidermal necrolysis).

● **PREGNANCY**
▶ With topical use Manufacturer advises use only if potential benefit outweighs risk— *animal* studies suggest no adverse effects.
▶ With oral use Manufacturer advises use only if potential benefit outweighs risk—no information available.

● **BREAST FEEDING**
▶ With topical use Manufacturer advises avoid—present in milk. Less than 5% of the dose is absorbed after topical application of terbinafine; avoid application to mother's chest.
▶ With oral use Avoid—present in milk.

● **HEPATIC IMPAIRMENT**
▶ With oral use Manufacturer advises avoid—elimination reduced.

● **RENAL IMPAIRMENT**
Dose adjustments ▶ With oral use Use half normal dose if eGFR less than 50 mL/minute/1.73 m^2 and no suitable alternative available.

● **MONITORING REQUIREMENTS**
▶ With oral use Monitor hepatic function before treatment and then periodically after 4–6 weeks of treatment—discontinue if abnormalities in liver function tests.

● **PATIENT AND CARER ADVICE**
▶ With oral use Manufacturer advises that patients should immediately report any signs or symptoms suggestive of liver dysfunction such as pruritus, unexplained persistent nausea, decreased appetite, anorexia, jaundice, vomiting, fatigue, right upper abdominal pain, dark urine, or pale stools. Patients with these symptoms should discontinue taking terbinafine and the patient's liver function should be immediately evaluated.

● **EXCEPTIONS TO LEGAL CATEGORY** Preparations of terbinafine hydrochloride (maximum 1%) can be sold to the public for use in those over 16 years for external use for the treatment of tinea pedis as a cream in a pack containing maximum 15 g, or for the treatment of tinea pedis and cruris as a cream in a pack containing maximum 15 g, or for the treatment of tinea pedis, cruris, and corporis as a spray in a pack containing maximum 30 mL spray or as a gel in a pack containing maximum 30 g gel.

- **MEDICINAL FORMS**
There can be variation in the licensing of different medicines
containing the same drug.
Tablet
CAUTIONARY AND ADVISORY LABELS 9
▸ Terbinafine (Non-proprietary)
Terbinafine (as Terbinafine hydrochloride) 250 mg Terbinafine
250mg tablets | 14 tablet PoM £18.11 DT = £8.46 | 28 tablet PoM
£5.00–£34.93
▸ Lamisil (Novartis Pharmaceuticals UK Ltd)
Terbinafine (as Terbinafine hydrochloride) 250 mg Lamisil 250mg
tablets | 14 tablet PoM £21.30 DT = £8.46 | 28 tablet PoM £41.09
Cream
EXCIPIENTS: May contain Benzyl alcohol, cetostearyl alcohol (including
cetyl and stearyl alcohol), polysorbates
▸ Terbinafine (Non-proprietary)
Terbinafine hydrochloride 10 mg per 1 gram Terbinafine 1% cream
| 7.5 gram PoM £1.06 | 15 gram PoM £3.17 DT = £0.98 |
30 gram PoM £6.33 DT = £1.96
▸ Lamisil (GlaxoSmithKline Consumer Healthcare)
Terbinafine hydrochloride 10 mg per 1 gram Lamisil 1% cream |
30 gram PoM £8.76 DT = £1.96

ANTISEPTICS AND DISINFECTANTS ›
UNDECENOATES

Undecenoic acid with zinc undecenoate

- **INDICATIONS AND DOSE**
Treatment of athletes foot
▸ TO THE SKIN
▸ Child: Apply twice daily, continue use for 7 days after
lesions have healed
▸ Adult: Apply twice daily, continue use for 7 days after
lesions have healed
Prevention of athletes foot
▸ TO THE SKIN
▸ Child: Apply once daily
▸ Adult: Apply once daily

- **UNLICENSED USE** *Mycota*® licensed for use in children (age
range not specified by manufacturer).
- **CAUTIONS** Avoid broken skin · contact with eyes should be
avoided · contact with mucous membranes should be
avoided
- **SIDE-EFFECTS**
▸ **Rare or very rare** Skin irritation
SIDE-EFFECTS, FURTHER INFORMATION Treatment should
be discontinued if irritation is severe.

- **MEDICINAL FORMS**
There can be variation in the licensing of different medicines
containing the same drug.
Cream
EXCIPIENTS: May contain Cetostearyl alcohol (including cetyl and
stearyl alcohol), fragrances
▸ Mycota (zinc undecenoate / undecenoic acid) (Thornton & Ross
Ltd)
**Undecenoic acid 50 mg per 1 gram, Zinc undecenoate 200 mg per
1 gram** Mycota cream | 25 gram GSL £2.01
Powder
EXCIPIENTS: May contain Fragrances
▸ Mycota (zinc undecenoate / undecenoic acid) (Thornton & Ross
Ltd)
**Undecenoic acid 20 mg per 1 gram, Zinc undecenoate 200 mg per
1 gram** Mycota powder | 70 gram GSL £3.04

ANTISEPTICS AND DISINFECTANTS › OTHER

Chlorhexidine with nystatin

- **INDICATIONS AND DOSE**
Skin infections due to *Candida* spp.
▸ TO THE SKIN
▸ Child: Apply 2–3 times a day, continuing for 7 days
after lesions have healed
▸ Adult: Apply 2–3 times a day, continuing for 7 days
after lesions have healed

- **UNLICENSED USE** Licensed for use in children (age range
not specified by manufacturer).
- **CAUTIONS** Avoid contact with eyes and mucous
membranes
- **SIDE-EFFECTS** Hypersensitivity · skin reactions
SIDE-EFFECTS, FURTHER INFORMATION Treatment should
be discontinued if side-effects are severe.

- **MEDICINAL FORMS**
There can be variation in the licensing of different medicines
containing the same drug.
Cream
EXCIPIENTS: May contain Benzyl alcohol, cetostearyl alcohol (including
cetyl and stearyl alcohol), polysorbates
▸ Chlorhexidine with nystatin (Non-proprietary)
**Chlorhexidine hydrochloride 10 mg per 1 gram, Nystatin
100000 unit per 1 gram** Nystatin 100,000units/g / Chlorhexidine
hydrochloride 1% cream | 30 gram PoM £4.99 DT = £4.99

BENZOATES

Benzoic acid with salicylic acid

- **INDICATIONS AND DOSE**
Ringworm (tinea)
▸ TO THE SKIN
▸ Child: Apply twice daily
▸ Adult: Apply twice daily

- **UNLICENSED USE** Licensed for use in children (age range
not specified by manufacturer).
- **CAUTIONS** Avoid broken or inflamed skin · avoid contact
with eyes · avoid contact with mucous membranes
CAUTIONS, FURTHER INFORMATION
▸ **Salicylate toxicity** Salicylate toxicity may occur particularly
if applied on large areas of skin.
- **SIDE-EFFECTS** Hypersensitivity · skin burning sensation
(mild) · skin reactions
SIDE-EFFECTS, FURTHER INFORMATION Treatment should
be discontinued if side effects are severe.
- **PRESCRIBING AND DISPENSING INFORMATION** Benzoic
Acid Ointment, Compound, BP has also been referred to as
Whitfield's ointment.

- **MEDICINAL FORMS**
Forms available from special-order manufacturers include:
cream, ointment

SALICYLIC ACID AND DERIVATIVES

Boric acid with salicylic acid and tannic acid

- **INDICATIONS AND DOSE**
Fungal nail infection, particularly tinea
▸ BY TRANSUNGUAL APPLICATION
▸ Child 5–17 years: Apply twice daily, and after washing
▸ Adult: Apply twice daily, and after washing

- CAUTIONS Avoid broken or inflamed skin · contact with eyes and mucous membranes should be avoided · use with caution in children likely to suck affected digits

  CAUTIONS, FURTHER INFORMATION
  ▸ Salicylate toxicity Salicylate toxicity can occur particularly if applied on large areas of skin.
- SIDE-EFFECTS Stinging
- PREGNANCY Avoid.

- MEDICINAL FORMS
  No licensed medicines listed.

2.3 Parasitic skin infections

Other drugs used for Parasitic skin infections Ivermectin, p. 593

PARASITICIDES

Benzyl benzoate

- INDICATIONS AND DOSE
  Scabies
  ▸ TO THE SKIN
  ▸ Adult: Apply over the whole body; repeat without bathing on the following day and wash off 24 hours later; a third application may be required in some cases

- CAUTIONS Avoid contact with eyes and mucous membranes · children (not recommended) · do not use on broken or secondarily infected skin
- SIDE-EFFECTS Skin burning sensation (especially on genitalia and excoriations) · skin reactions
- BREAST FEEDING Suspend feeding until product has been washed off.
- PRESCRIBING AND DISPENSING INFORMATION When prepared extemporaneously, the BP states Benzyl Benzoate Application, BP consists of benzyl benzoate 25% in an emulsion basis.
  Some manufacturers recommend application to the body but to exclude the head and neck. However, application should be extended to the scalp, neck, face, and ears. Note—dilution to reduce irritant effect also reduces efficacy.
- LESS SUITABLE FOR PRESCRIBING Benzyl benzoate is less suitable for prescribing.

- MEDICINAL FORMS
  Forms available from special-order manufacturers include: liquid

Dimeticone

06-Apr-2018

- INDICATIONS AND DOSE
  Head lice
  ▸ TO THE SKIN
  ▸ Child: Apply once weekly for 2 doses, rub into dry hair and scalp, allow to dry naturally, shampoo after minimum 8 hours (or overnight)
  ▸ Adult: Apply once weekly for 2 doses, rub into dry hair and scalp, allow to dry naturally, shampoo after minimum 8 hours (or overnight)

- UNLICENSED USE Not licensed for use in children under 6 months except under medical supervision.

> IMPORTANT SAFETY INFORMATION
> MHRA/CHM ADVICE: HEAD LICE ERADICATION PRODUCTS: RISK OF SERIOUS BURNS IF TREATED HAIR IS EXPOSED TO OPEN FLAMES OR OTHER SOURCES OF IGNITION (MARCH 2018)
> See Skin infections p. 1193.

- CAUTIONS Avoid contact with eyes · children under 6 months, medical supervision required
- SIDE-EFFECTS Alopecia · dyspnoea · eye irritation · hypersensitivity · scalp changes · skin reactions

- MEDICINAL FORMS
  There can be variation in the licensing of different medicines containing the same drug.
  Liquid
  ▸ Hedrin (Thornton & Ross Ltd)
    Dimeticone 40 mg per 1 gram Hedrin 4% lotion | 50 ml | ℗ £3.28 DT = £3.28 | 150 ml | ℗ £7.62 DT = £7.62
  ▸ Lyclear (dimeticone) (Omega Pharma Ltd)
    Dimeticone 40 mg per 1 gram Lyclear lotion | 100 ml | 🔲
  Cutaneous spray solution
  ▸ Hedrin (Thornton & Ross Ltd)
    Dimeticone 40 mg per 1 gram Hedrin 4% spray | 120 ml | GSL £7.85

Malathion

06-Apr-2018

- INDICATIONS AND DOSE
  Head lice
  ▸ TO THE SKIN
  ▸ Child: Apply once weekly for 2 doses, rub preparation into dry hair and scalp, allow to dry naturally, remove by washing after 12 hours
  ▸ Adult: Apply once weekly for 2 doses, rub preparation into dry hair and scalp, allow to dry naturally, remove by washing after 12 hours
  Crab lice
  ▸ TO THE SKIN
  ▸ Child: Apply once weekly for 2 doses, apply preparation over whole body, allow to dry naturally, wash off after 12 hours or overnight
  ▸ Adult: Apply once weekly for 2 doses, apply preparation over whole body, allow to dry naturally, wash off after 12 hours or overnight
  Scabies
  ▸ TO THE SKIN
  ▸ Child: Apply once weekly for 2 doses, apply preparation over whole body, and wash off after 24 hours, if hands are washed with soap within 24 hours, they should be retreated
  ▸ Adult: Apply once weekly for 2 doses, apply preparation over whole body, and wash off after 24 hours, if hands are washed with soap within 24 hours, they should be retreated

- UNLICENSED USE Not licensed for use in children under 6 months except under medical supervision.

> IMPORTANT SAFETY INFORMATION
> MHRA/CHM ADVICE: HEAD LICE ERADICATION PRODUCTS: RISK OF SERIOUS BURNS IF TREATED HAIR IS EXPOSED TO OPEN FLAMES OR OTHER SOURCES OF IGNITION (MARCH 2018)
> See Skin infections p. 1193.

- CAUTIONS Alcoholic lotions **not** recommended for head lice in children with severe eczema or asthma, or for scabies or crab lice · avoid contact with eyes · children under 6 months, medical supervision required · do not use lotion more than once a week for 3 consecutive weeks · do not use on broken or secondarily infected skin

13

Skin

- SIDE-EFFECTS Angioedema · eye swelling · hypersensitivity · skin reactions
- PRESCRIBING AND DISPENSING INFORMATION For scabies, manufacturer recommends application to the body but not necessarily to the head and neck. However, application should be extended to the scalp, neck, face, and ears.

- MEDICINAL FORMS
There can be variation in the licensing of different medicines containing the same drug.

Liquid

EXCIPIENTS: May contain Cetostearyl alcohol (including cetyl and stearyl alcohol), fragrances, hydroxybenzoates (parabens)

- Derbac-M (G.R. Lane Health Products Ltd)
  Malathion 5 mg per 1 gram Derbac-M 0.5% liquid | 50 ml P £3.89 DT = £3.89 | 200 ml P £9.09 DT = £9.09

Permethrin

12-Apr-2018

- INDICATIONS AND DOSE

Scabies
- TO THE SKIN
- Child: Apply once weekly for 2 doses, apply 5% preparation over whole body including face, neck, scalp and ears then wash off after 8–12 hours. If hands are washed with soap within 8 hours of application, they should be treated again with cream
- Adult: Apply once weekly for 2 doses, apply 5% preparation over whole body including face, neck, scalp and ears then wash off after 8–12 hours. If hands are washed with soap within 8 hours of application, they should be treated again with cream

Crab lice
- TO THE SKIN
- Adult: Apply once weekly for 2 doses, apply 5% cream over whole body, allow to dry naturally and wash off after 12 hours or after leaving on overnight

Head lice
- TO THE SKIN
- Adult: Not recommended; no information given

- UNLICENSED USE *Dermal Cream* (scabies), not licensed for use in children under 2 months; not licensed for treatment of crab lice in children under 18 years. *Creme Rinse* (head lice) not licensed for use in children under 6 months except under medical supervision.

> **IMPORTANT SAFETY INFORMATION**
> MHRA/CHM ADVICE: HEAD LICE ERADICATION PRODUCTS: RISK OF SERIOUS BURNS IF TREATED HAIR IS EXPOSED TO OPEN FLAMES OR OTHER SOURCES OF IGNITION (MARCH 2018)
> See Skin infections p. 1193.

- CAUTIONS Avoid contact with eyes · children aged 2 months–2 years, medical supervision required for dermal cream (scabies) · children under 6 months, medical supervision required for cream rinse (head lice) · do not use on broken or secondarily infected skin
- SIDE-EFFECTS Scalp irritation · skin reactions
- PRESCRIBING AND DISPENSING INFORMATION Manufacturer recommends application to the body but to exclude head and neck. However, application should be extended to the scalp, neck, face, and ears.
  Larger patients may require up to two 30-g packs for adequate treatment.
- LESS SUITABLE FOR PRESCRIBING Lyclear ® Creme Rinse is less suitable for prescribing.

- MEDICINAL FORMS
There can be variation in the licensing of different medicines containing the same drug.

Cream

CAUTIONARY AND ADVISORY LABELS 10 (Dermal cream only)
EXCIPIENTS: May contain Butylated hydroxytoluene, woolfat and related substances (including lanolin)
- Permethrin (Non-proprietary)
  Permethrin 50 mg per 1 gram Permethrin 5% cream | 30 gram P £7.46 DT = £7.46
- Lyclear (Omega Pharma Ltd)
  Permethrin 50 mg per 1 gram Lyclear 5% dermal cream | 30 gram P £5.71 DT = £7.46

Liquid

EXCIPIENTS: May contain Cetostearyl alcohol (including cetyl and stearyl alcohol)
- Lyclear (Omega Pharma Ltd)
  Permethrin 10 mg per 1 gram Lyclear 1% creme rinse | 59 ml P £4.20 DT = £4.20 | 118 ml P £6.79 DT = £6.79

2.4 Viral skin infections

ANTIVIRALS ⟩ NUCLEOSIDE ANALOGUES

Aciclovir
(Acyclovir)

- INDICATIONS AND DOSE

Herpes simplex infection (local treatment)
- TO THE SKIN
- Child: Apply 5 times a day for 5–10 days, to be applied to lesions approximately every 4 hours, starting at first sign of attack
- Adult: Apply 5 times a day for 5–10 days, to be applied to lesions approximately every 4 hours, starting at first sign of attack

- UNLICENSED USE Cream licensed for use in children (age range not specified by manufacturer).
- CAUTIONS Avoid cream coming in to contact with eyes and mucous membranes
- INTERACTIONS → Appendix 1: aciclovir
- SIDE-EFFECTS
- **Uncommon** Skin reactions
- PREGNANCY Limited absorption from topical aciclovir preparations.
- PATIENT AND CARER ADVICE
  Medicines for Children leaflet: Aciclovir cream for herpes www.medicinesforchildren.org.uk/aciclovir-cream-for-herpes
- PROFESSION SPECIFIC ADVICE
  Dental practitioners' formulary
  Aciclovir Cream may be prescribed.
- EXCEPTIONS TO LEGAL CATEGORY A 2-g tube and a pump pack are on sale to the public for the treatment of cold sores.

- MEDICINAL FORMS
There can be variation in the licensing of different medicines containing the same drug.

Cream

EXCIPIENTS: May contain Cetostearyl alcohol (including cetyl and stearyl alcohol), propylene glycol
- Aciclovir (Non-proprietary)
  Aciclovir 50 mg per 1 gram Aciclovir 5% cream | 2 gram PoM £1.09 DT = £1.09 | 10 gram PoM £5.45 DT = £5.45
- Zovirax (GlaxoSmithKline UK Ltd, GlaxoSmithKline Consumer Healthcare)
  Aciclovir 50 mg per 1 gram Zovirax 5% cream | 2 gram PoM £4.63 DT = £1.09 | 10 gram PoM £13.96 DT = £5.45

13

Skin

3 Inflammatory skin conditions

3.1 Eczema and psoriasis

Eczema

Types and management

Eczema (dermatitis) has several causes, which may influence treatment. The main types of eczema are irritant, allergic contact, atopic, venous and discoid; different types may co-exist. Lichenification, due to scratching and rubbing, may complicate any chronic eczema. *Atopic eczema* is the most common type and it usually involves dry skin as well as infection and lichenification.

Management of eczema involves the removal or treatment of contributory factors including occupational and domestic irritants. Known or suspected contact allergens should be avoided. Rarely, ingredients in topical medicinal products may sensitise the skin; the BNF lists active ingredients together with excipients that have been associated with skin sensitisation.

Skin dryness and the consequent irritant eczema requires **emollients** applied regularly (at least twice daily) and liberally to the affected area; this can be supplemented with bath or shower emollients. The use of emollients should continue even if the eczema improves or if other treatment is being used.

Topical corticosteroids are also required in the management of eczema; the potency of the corticosteroid should be appropriate to the severity and site of the condition. Mild corticosteroids are generally used on the face and on flexures; potent corticosteroids are generally required for use on adults with discoid or lichenified eczema or with eczema on the scalp, limbs, and trunk. Treatment should be reviewed regularly, especially if a potent corticosteroid is required. In patients with frequent flares (2–3 per month), a topical corticosteroid can be applied on 2 consecutive days each week to prevent further flares.

Bandages (including those containing ichthammol with zinc oxide p. 1218) are sometimes applied over topical corticosteroids or emollients to treat eczema of the limbs. Dry-wrap dressings can be used to provide a physical barrier to help prevent scratching and improve retention of emollients. See *Wound management products and elasticated garments* for details of elasticated viscose stockinette tubular bandages and garments, and silk clothing.

See Eczema and psoriasis, drugs affecting the immune response p. 1206 for the role of topical pimecrolimus p. 1221 and tacrolimus p. 1222 in atopic eczema.

Infection

Bacterial infection (commonly with *Staphylococcus aureus* and occasionally with *Streptococcus pyogenes*) can exacerbate eczema and requires treatment with topical or systemic **antibacterial drugs**. Antibacterial drugs should be used in short courses (typically 1 week) to reduce the risk of drug resistance or skin sensitisation. Associated eczema is treated simultaneously with a topical corticosteroid which can be combined with a topical antimicrobial.

Eczema involving widespread or recurrent infection requires the use of a systemic antibacterial that is active against the infecting organism. Products that combine an antiseptic with an emollient application and with a bath emollient can also be used; antiseptic shampoos can be used on the scalp.

Intertriginous eczema commonly involves candida and bacteria; it is best treated with a mild or moderately potent topical corticosteroid and a suitable antimicrobial drug.

Widespread herpes simplex infection may complicate atopic eczema and treatment with a systemic antiviral drug is indicated.

Management of other features of eczema

Lichenification, which results from repeated scratching is treated initially with a potent corticosteroid. Bandages containing **ichthammol** paste p. 1218 (to reduce pruritus) and other substances such as **zinc oxide** can be applied over the corticosteroid or emollient. **Coal tar** and ichthammol can be useful in some cases of *chronic eczema*.

A *non-sedating* **antihistamine** may be of some value in relieving severe itching or urticaria associated with eczema. A *sedating* antihistamine can be used if itching causes sleep disturbance.

Exudative ('weeping') eczema requires a potent corticosteroid initially; infection may also be present and require specific treatment. Potassium permanganate solution (1 in 10,000) p. 1240 can be used in exudating eczema for its antiseptic and astringent effects; treatment should be stopped when exudation stops.

Severe refractory eczema

Severe refractory eczema is best managed under specialist supervision; it may require phototherapy or drugs that act on the immune system. Alitretinoin p. 1226 is licensed for the treatment of severe chronic hand eczema refractory to potent topical corticosteroids; patients with hyperkeratotic features are more likely to respond to alitretinoin than those with pompholyx.

Seborrhoeic dermatitis

Seborrhoeic dermatitis (seborrhoeic eczema) is associated with species of the yeast *Malassezia* and affects the scalp, paranasal areas, and eyebrows. Shampoos active against the yeast (including those containing ketoconazole p. 1198 or coal tar p. 1219) and combinations of mild corticosteroids with suitable antimicrobials are used.

Psoriasis

Management

Psoriasis is characterised by epidermal thickening and scaling. It commonly affects extensor surfaces and the scalp.

Occasionally, psoriasis is provoked or exacerbated by drugs such as lithium, chloroquine and hydroxychloroquine, beta-blockers, non-steroidal anti-inflammatory drugs, and ACE inhibitors. Psoriasis may not be seen until the drug has been taken for weeks or months.

Emollients, in addition to their effects on dryness, scaling and cracking, may have an anti-proliferative effect in psoriasis, and may be the only treatment necessary for mild psoriasis. They are particularly useful in *inflammatory psoriasis* and in *plaque psoriasis of palms and soles*, in which irritant factors can perpetuate the condition. Emollients are useful adjuncts to other more specific treatment.

More specific topical treatment for *chronic stable plaque psoriasis* on extensor surfaces of trunk and limbs involves the use of **vitamin D analogues**, coal tar p. 1219, dithranol p. 1219, and the retinoid tazarotene p. 1227. However, they can irritate the skin and they are not suitable for the more inflammatory forms of psoriasis; their use should be suspended during an inflammatory phase of psoriasis. The efficacy and the irritancy of each substance varies between patients. If a substance irritates significantly, it should be stopped or the concentration reduced; if it is tolerated, its effects should be assessed after 4 to 6 weeks and treatment continued if it is effective.

Scalp psoriasis is usually scaly, and the scale may be thick and adherent; this will require softening with an emollient cream, ointment, or oil. A tar-based shampoo is first-line treatment for scalp psoriasis; a keratolytic, such as salicylic acid, should also be used if there is significant scaling, to allow other treatments to work.

Some preparations prescribed for psoriasis affecting the scalp, combine salicylic acid with coal tar or sulfur. The product should be applied generously, and an adequate quantity should be prescribed. It should be left on for at least an hour, often more conveniently overnight, before washing off. The use of scalp preparations containing a potent corticosteroid or a vitamin D analogue, either alone or in combination, can also be helpful.

Facial, flexural and genital psoriasis can be managed with short-term use of a mild or moderate potency topical corticosteroid (a mild potency topical corticosteroid is preferred for the initial treatment of facial psoriasis). Calcitriol p. 1228 or tacalcitol p. 1228 can be used for longer-term treatment, or if the response to mild or moderate potency topical corticosteroids is inadequate; calcipotriol p. 1227 is more likely to cause irritation. Low strength tar preparations can also be used. Pimecrolimus p. 1221 or tacrolimus p. 1222 by topical application [unlicensed indication] can be used short-term, under specialist supervision, in patients whose condition has not responded adequately to other treatments, or who are intolerant of them.

Widespread *unstable psoriasis* of erythrodermic or generalised pustular type requires urgent specialist assessment. Initial topical treatment should be limited to using emollients frequently and generously; emollients should be prescribed in quantities of 1 kg or more. More localised acute or subacute *inflammatory psoriasis* with hot, spreading or itchy lesions, should be treated topically with emollients or with a corticosteroid of moderate potency.

Calcipotriol and tacalcitol are analogues of vitamin D that affect cell division and differentiation. Calcitriol is an active form of vitamin D. Vitamin D and its analogues are used first-line for the long-term treatment of plaque psoriasis; they do not smell or stain and they may be more acceptable than tar or dithranol products. Of the vitamin D analogues, tacalcitol and calcitriol are less likely to irritate.

Coal tar has anti-inflammatory properties that are useful in chronic plaque psoriasis; it also has antiscaling properties. Crude coal tar (coal tar, BP) is the most effective form, typically in a concentration of 1 to 10% in a soft paraffin base, but few outpatients tolerate the smell and mess. Cleaner extracts of coal tar included in proprietary preparations, are more practicable for home use but they are less effective and improvement takes longer. Contact of coal tar products with normal skin is not normally harmful and they can be used for widespread small lesions; however, irritation, contact allergy, and sterile folliculitis can occur. The milder tar extracts can be used on the face and flexures. Tar baths and tar shampoos are also helpful.

Dithranol is effective for chronic plaque psoriasis. Its major disadvantages are irritation (for which individual susceptibility varies) and staining of skin and of clothing. Dithranol is not generally suitable for widespread small lesions nor should it be used in the flexures or on the face. Proprietary preparations are more suitable for home use; they are usually washed off after 5 to 60 minutes ('short contact'). Specialist nurses may apply intensive treatment with dithranol paste which is covered by stockinette dressings and usually retained overnight. Dithranol should be discontinued if even a low concentration causes acute inflammation; continued use can result in the psoriasis becoming unstable.

Tazarotene, a retinoid, has a similar efficacy to vitamin D and its analogues, but is associated with a greater incidence of irritation. Although irritation is common, it is minimised by applying tazarotene sparingly to the plaques and avoiding normal skin; application to the face and in flexures should also be avoided. Tazarotene does not stain and is odourless.

A topical **corticosteroid** is not generally suitable for long-term use or as the sole treatment of extensive chronic plaque psoriasis; any early improvement is not usually maintained and there is a risk of the condition deteriorating or of precipitating an unstable form of psoriasis (e.g. erythrodermic psoriasis or generalised pustular psoriasis) on withdrawal. Topical use of potent corticosteroids on widespread psoriasis can also lead to systemic as well as local side-effects. However, topical corticosteroids used short-term may be appropriate to treat psoriasis in specific sites such as the face or flexures (with a mild or moderate corticosteroid), and psoriasis of the scalp, palms, and soles (with a potent corticosteroid). Very potent corticosteroids should only be used under specialist supervision.

Combining the use of a corticosteroid with another specific topical treatment may be beneficial in chronic plaque psoriasis; the drugs may be used separately at different times of the day or used together in a single formulation. *Eczema* co-existing with psoriasis may be treated with a corticosteroid, or coal tar, or both.

Phototherapy

Phototherapy is available in specialist centres under the supervision of a dermatologist. **Ultraviolet B** (UVB) radiation is usually effective for *chronic stable psoriasis* and for *guttate psoriasis*. It may be considered for patients with moderately severe psoriasis in whom topical treatment has failed, but it may irritate inflammatory psoriasis.

Photochemotherapy combining long-wave ultraviolet A radiation with a psoralen (PUVA) is available in specialist centres under the supervision of a dermatologist. The psoralen, which enhances the effect of irradiation, is administered either by mouth or topically. PUVA is effective in most forms of psoriasis, including *localised palmoplantar pustular psoriasis*. Early adverse effects include phototoxicity and pruritus. Higher cumulative doses exaggerate skin ageing, increase the risk of dysplastic and neoplastic skin lesions, especially squamous cancer, and pose a theoretical risk of cataracts.

Phototherapy combined with coal tar, dithranol, tazarotene, topical vitamin D or vitamin D analogues, or oral acitretin, allows reduction of the cumulative dose of phototherapy required to treat psoriasis.

Systemic treatment

Systemic treatment is required for severe, resistant, unstable or complicated forms of psoriasis, and it should be initiated only under specialist supervision. Systemic drugs for psoriasis include acitretin and drugs that affect the immune response (such as ciclosporin p. 818 and methotrexate p. 888).

Systemic corticosteroids should be used only rarely in psoriasis because rebound deterioration may occur on reducing the dose.

Acitretin p. 1225, a metabolite of etretinate, is a retinoid (vitamin A derivative); it is prescribed by specialists. The main indication for acitretin is *psoriasis*, but it is also used in disorders of keratinisation such as severe *Darier's disease* (keratosis follicularis), and some forms of *ichthyosis*. Although a minority of cases of psoriasis respond well to acitretin alone, it is only moderately effective in many cases and it is combined with other treatments. A therapeutic effect occurs after 2 to 4 weeks and the maximum benefit after 4 months. Consideration should be given to stopping acitretin if the response is inadequate after 4 months at the optimum dose. The manufacturers of acitretin do not recommend continuous treatment for longer than 6 months. However, some patients may benefit from longer treatment, provided that the lowest effective dose is used, patients are monitored carefully for adverse effects, and the need for treatment is reviewed regularly.

Apart from teratogenicity, which remains a risk for 3 years after stopping, acitretin is the least toxic systemic treatment for psoriasis; in women with a potential for child-bearing,

13

Skin

the possibility of pregnancy must be excluded before treatment and effective contraception used during treatment and for at least 3 years afterwards (oral progestogen-only contraceptives not considered effective).

Topical treatment

The vitamin D and analogues, calcipotriol p. 1227, calcitriol p. 1228, and tacalcitol p. 1228 are used for the management of plaque psoriasis. They should be avoided by those with calcium metabolism disorders, and used with caution in generalised pustular or erythrodermic exfoliative psoriasis (enhanced risk of hypercalcaemia).

Eczema and psoriasis, drugs affecting the immune response

Overview

Drugs affecting the immune response are used for eczema or psoriasis. Systemic drugs acting on the immune system are used under specialist supervision.

Pimecrolimus p. 1221 by topical application is licensed for *mild to moderate atopic eczema*. Tacrolimus p. 1222 is licensed for topical use in *moderate to severe atopic eczema*. Both are drugs whose long-term safety is still being evaluated and they should not usually be considered first-line treatments unless there is a specific reason to avoid or reduce the use of topical corticosteroids. Treatment of atopic eczema with topical pimecrolimus or topical tacrolimus should be initiated only by prescribers experienced in managing the condition. Topical tacrolimus and pimecrolimus have a role in the treatment of psoriasis.

A short course of a systemic corticosteroid can be given for eczema flares that have not improved despite appropriate topical treatment.

Ciclosporin p. 818 by mouth can be used for *severe psoriasis* and for *severe eczema*. Azathioprine p. 816 or mycophenolate mofetil p. 826 are used for severe refractory eczema [unlicensed indication]. Dupilumab p. 1223 is licensed for the treatment of moderate to severe atopic eczema in patients requiring systemic therapy. Dimethyl fumarate p. 833 is licensed for the treatment of moderate to severe plaque psoriasis.

Methotrexate p. 888 can be used for *severe psoriasis*, the dose being adjusted according to severity of the condition and haematological and biochemical measurements. Folic acid p. 993 should be given to reduce the possibility of side-effects associated with methotrexate. Folic acid can be given once weekly [unlicensed indication], on a different day from the methotrexate; alternative regimens of folic acid may be used in some settings.

Etanercept p. 1078, adalimumab p. 1073, and infliximab p. 1082 inhibit the activity of tumour necrosis factor (TNFα). They are used for *severe plaque psoriasis* either refractory to at least 2 standard systemic treatments and photochemotherapy, or when standard treatments cannot be used because of intolerance or contra-indications; while either etanercept or adalimumab is considered to be the first choice in stable disease, infliximab or adalimumab may be useful when rapid disease control is required. Secukinumab p. 1066 and ixekizumab p. 1224 inhibit the activity of interleukin-17A, brodalumab p. 1222 inhibits the activity of interleukin-17RA and guselkumab p. 1224 inhibits the activity of interleukin-23. They are used for *moderate to severe plaque psoriasis* in patients who are candidates for systemic therapy. Secukinumab is also licensed for psoriatic arthritis and ankylosing spondylitis. Ustekinumab p. 1069 (a monoclonal antibody that inhibits interleukins 12 and 23) can be used for *severe plaque psoriasis* that has not responded to at least 2 standard systemic treatments and photochemotherapy, or when these treatments cannot be used because of intolerance or contra-indications.

Adalimumab is also licensed for the treatment of active moderate to severe hidradenitis suppurativa (acne inversa) in patients who have had inadequate response to conventional systemic therapy. Adalimumab, etanercept, infliximab, ixekizumab and ustekinumab are also licensed for psoriatic arthritis.

> **Other drugs used for Eczema and psoriasis** Apremilast, p. 1084

CORTICOSTEROIDS

Topical corticosteroids

Overview

Topical corticosteroids are used for the treatment of inflammatory conditions of the skin (other than those arising from an infection), in particular eczema, contact dermatitis, insect stings, and eczema of scabies. Corticosteroids suppress the inflammatory reaction during use; they are not curative and on discontinuation a rebound exacerbation of the condition may occur. They are generally used to relieve symptoms and suppress signs of the disorder when other measures such as emollients are ineffective.

Topical corticosteroids are not recommended in the routine treatment of urticaria; treatment should only be initiated and supervised by a specialist. They should not be used indiscriminately in pruritus (where they will only benefit if inflammation is causing the itch) and are **not** recommended for acne vulgaris.

Systemic or very potent topical corticosteroids should be avoided or given only under specialist supervision in *psoriasis* because, although they may suppress the psoriasis in the short term, relapse or vigorous rebound occurs on withdrawal (sometimes precipitating severe pustular psoriasis). See the role of topical corticosteroids in the treatment of psoriasis.

In general, the most potent topical corticosteroids should be reserved for recalcitrant dermatoses such as *chronic discoid lupus erythematosus, lichen simplex chronicus, hypertrophic lichen planus,* and *palmoplantar pustulosis.* Potent corticosteroids should generally be avoided on the face and skin flexures, but specialists occasionally prescribe them for use on these areas in certain circumstances.

When topical treatment has failed, intralesional corticosteroid injections may be used. These are more effective than the very potent topical corticosteroid preparations and should be reserved for severe cases where there are localised lesions such as *keloid scars, hypertrophic lichen planus,* or *localised alopecia areata.*

Perioral lesions

Hydrocortisone cream 1% p. 1213 can be used for up to 7 days to treat uninfected inflammatory lesions on the lips. Hydrocortisone with miconazole cream or ointment p. 1218 is useful where infection by susceptible organisms and inflammation co-exist, particularly for initial treatment (up to 7 days) e.g. in angular cheilitis. Organisms susceptible to miconazole include *Candida* spp. and many Gram-positive bacteria including streptococci and staphylococci.

Choice of formulation

Water-miscible corticosteroid *creams* are suitable for moist or weeping lesions whereas *ointments* are generally chosen for dry, lichenified or scaly lesions or where a more occlusive effect is required. *Lotions* may be useful when minimal application to a large or hair-bearing area is required or for the treatment of exudative lesions. *Occlusive polythene* or *hydrocolloid dressings* increase absorption, but also increase the risk of side-effects; they are therefore used only under supervision on a short-term basis for areas of very thick skin (such as the palms and soles). The inclusion of urea or salicylic acid also increases the penetration of the corticosteroid.

In the BNF publications topical corticosteroids for the skin are categorised as 'mild', 'moderately potent', 'potent' or 'very potent'; the **least potent** preparation which is effective should be chosen but dilution should be avoided whenever possible.

Absorption through the skin

Mild and *moderately potent* topical corticosteroids are associated with few side-effects but care is required in the use of *potent* and *very potent* corticosteroids. Absorption through the skin can rarely cause adrenal suppression and even Cushing's syndrome, depending on the area of the body being treated and the duration of treatment. Absorption is greatest where the skin is thin or raw, and from intertriginous areas; it is increased by occlusion.

Suitable quantities of corticosteroid preparations to be prescribed for specific areas of the body	
Area of body	Creams and Ointments
Face and neck	15 to 30 g
Both hands	15 to 30 g
Scalp	15 to 30 g
Both arms	30 to 60g
Both legs	100 g
Trunk	100 g
Groins and genitalia	15 to 30 g

These amounts are usually suitable for an adult for a single daily application for 2 weeks

Compound preparations

The advantages of including other substances (such as antibacterials or antifungals) with corticosteroids in topical preparations are uncertain, but some combinations may have a place where inflammatory skin conditions are associated with bacterial or fungal infection, such as infected eczema. In these cases the antimicrobial drug should be chosen according to the sensitivity of the infecting organism and used regularly for a short period (typically twice daily for 1 week). Longer use increases the likelihood of resistance and of sensitisation.

The keratolytic effect of salicylic acid p. 1250 facilitates the absorption of topical corticosteroids; however, excessive and prolonged use of topical preparations containing salicylic acid may cause salicylism.

Topical corticosteroid preparation potencies

Potency of a topical corticosteroid preparation is a result of the formulation as well as the corticosteroid. Therefore, proprietary names are shown.

Mild

- Hydrocortisone 0.1–2.5%
- Dioderm
- Mildison
- Synalar 1 in 10 dilution

Mild with antimicrobials

- Canesten HC
- Daktacort
- Econacort
- Fucidin H
- Nystaform-HC
- Terra-Cortril
- Timodine

Moderate

- Betnovate-RD

- Eumovate
- Haelan
- Modrasone
- Synalar 1 in 4 Dilution
- Ultralanum Plain

Moderate with antimicrobials

- Trimovate

Moderate with urea:

- Alphaderm

Potent

- Beclometasone dipropionate 0.025%
- Betamethasone valerate 0.1%
- Betacap
- Betesil
- Bettamousse
- Betnovate
- Cutivate
- Diprosone
- Elocon
- Hydrocortisone butyrate
- Locoid
- Locoid Crelo
- Metosyn
- Mometasone furoate 0.1%
- Nerisone
- Synalar

Potent with antimicrobials

- Aureocort
- Betamethasone and clioquinol
- Betamethasone and neomycin
- Fucibet
- Lotriderm
- Synalar C
- Synalar N

Potent with salicylic acid

- Diprosalic

Very potent

- Clarelux
- Dermovate
- Etrivex
- Nerisone Forte

Very potent with antimicrobials

- Clobetasol with neomycin and nystatin

Use in children

Children, especially infants, are particularly susceptible to side-effects. However, concern about the safety of topical corticosteroids in children should not result in the child being undertreated. The aim is to control the condition as well as possible; inadequate treatment will perpetuate the condition. A mild corticosteroid such as hydrocortisone 0.5% or 1% is useful for treating nappy rash and hydrocortisone 1% for atopic eczema in childhood. A moderately potent or potent corticosteroid may be appropriate for severe atopic eczema on the limbs, for 1–2 weeks only, switching to a less potent preparation as the condition improves. In an acute flare-up of atopic eczema, it may be appropriate to use more potent formulations of topical corticosteroids for a short period to regain control of the condition. A very potent corticosteroid should be initiated under the supervision of a specialist. Carers of young children should be advised that treatment should **not** necessarily be reserved to 'treat only the worst areas' and they may need to be advised that patient information leaflets may contain inappropriate advice for the patient's condition.

Corticosteroids (topical)

IMPORTANT SAFETY INFORMATION

MHRA/CHM ADVICE: CORTICOSTEROIDS: RARE RISK OF CENTRAL SEROUS CHORIORETINOPATHY WITH LOCAL AS WELL AS SYSTEMIC ADMINISTRATION (AUGUST 2017)

Central serous chorioretinopathy is a retinal disorder that has been linked to the systemic use of corticosteroids. Recently, it has also been reported after local administration of corticosteroids via inhaled and intranasal, epidural, intra-articular, topical dermal, and periocular routes. The MHRA recommends that patients should be advised to report any blurred vision or other visual disturbances with corticosteroid treatment given by any route; consider referral to an ophthalmologist for evaluation of possible causes if a patient presents with vision problems.

- **CONTRA-INDICATIONS** Acne · perioral dermatitis · potent corticosteroids in widespread plaque psoriasis · rosacea (in adults) · untreated bacterial, fungal or viral skin lesions
- **CAUTIONS** Avoid prolonged use (particularly on the face) · cautions applicable to systemic corticosteroids may also apply if absorption occurs following topical and local use · dermatoses of infancy, including nappy rash (extreme caution required—treatment should be limited to 5–7 days) · infection · keep away from eyes · use potent or very potent topical corticosteroids under specialist supervision (in children) · use potent or very potent topical corticosteroids under specialist supervision in psoriasis (can result in rebound relapse, development of generalised pustular psoriasis, and local and systemic toxicity) (in adults)
- **SIDE-EFFECTS**
- ▸ **Uncommon** Adrenal suppression · skin reactions · telangiectasia
- ▸ **Rare or very rare** Hypertrichosis · skin depigmentation (may be reversible)
- ▸ **Frequency not known** Local reaction · vasodilation

  SIDE-EFFECTS, FURTHER INFORMATION Side-effects applicable to systemic corticosteroids may also apply if absorption occurs following topical and local use. In order to minimise the side-effects of a topical corticosteroid, it is important to apply it thinly to affected areas only, no more frequently than twice daily, and to use the least potent formulation which is fully effective.
- **DIRECTIONS FOR ADMINISTRATION** Topical corticosteroid preparations should be applied no more frequently than twice daily; once daily is often sufficient. Topical corticosteroids should be spread thinly on the skin but in sufficient quantity to cover the affected areas. The length of cream or ointment expelled from a tube may be used to specify the quantity to be applied to a given area of skin. This length can be measured in terms of a *fingertip unit* (the distance from the tip of the adult index finger to the first crease). One fingertip unit (approximately 500 mg from a tube with a standard 5 mm diameter nozzle) is sufficient to cover an area that is twice that of the flat adult handprint (palm and fingers). Mixing topical preparations on the skin should be avoided where possible; several minutes should elapse between application of different preparations.
- ▸ In children 'Wet-wrap bandaging' increases absorption into the skin, but should be initiated only by a dermatologist and application supervised by a healthcare professional trained in the technique.
- **PRESCRIBING AND DISPENSING INFORMATION** The potency of each topical corticosteroid should be included on the label with the directions for use. The label should be attached to the container (for example, the tube) rather than the outer packaging.

- **PATIENT AND CARER ADVICE** Patients or carers should be given advice on how to administer corticosteroid creams and ointments. If a patient is using topical corticosteroids of different potencies, the patient should be told when to use each corticosteroid. Patients and their carers should be reassured that side effects such as skin thinning and systemic effects rarely occur when topical corticosteroids are used appropriately.

⚑ above

Alclometasone dipropionate
21-Dec-2017

- **INDICATIONS AND DOSE**

Inflammatory skin disorders such as eczemas
- ▸ TO THE SKIN
- ▸ **Child:** Apply 1–2 times a day, to be applied thinly
- ▸ **Adult:** Apply 1–2 times a day, to be applied thinly
POTENCY
- ▸ Alclometasone dipropionate cream 0.05%: moderate

- **UNLICENSED USE** Licensed for use in children (age range not specified by manufacturer).
- **PATIENT AND CARER ADVICE** Patients or carers should be counselled on the application of alclometasone dipropionate cream.

- **MEDICINAL FORMS**
There can be variation in the licensing of different medicines containing the same drug.
Cream
CAUTIONARY AND ADVISORY LABELS 28
EXCIPIENTS: May contain Cetostearyl alcohol (including cetyl and stearyl alcohol), chlorocresol, propylene glycol
- ▸ Alclometasone dipropionate (Non-proprietary)
  Alclometasone dipropionate 500 microgram per 1 gram Boots Derma Care Eczema & Dermatitis Flare-Up 0.05% cream | 15 gram Ⓟ Ⓢ

⚑ above

Beclometasone dipropionate
04-Jan-2016
(Beclomethasone dipropionate)

- **INDICATIONS AND DOSE**

Severe inflammatory skin disorders such as eczemas unresponsive to less potent corticosteroids | Psoriasis
- ▸ TO THE SKIN
- ▸ **Child:** Apply 1–2 times a day, to be applied thinly
- ▸ **Adult:** Apply 1–2 times a day, to be applied thinly
POTENCY
- ▸ Beclometasone dipropionate cream and ointment 0.025%: potent.

- **UNLICENSED USE** Not licensed for use in children under 1 year.
- **INTERACTIONS** → Appendix 1: corticosteroids

- **MEDICINAL FORMS**
There can be variation in the licensing of different medicines containing the same drug. Forms available from special-order manufacturers include: cream, ointment
Cream
CAUTIONARY AND ADVISORY LABELS 28
- ▸ Beclometasone dipropionate (Non-proprietary)
  Beclometasone dipropionate 250 microgram per 1 gram Beclometasone 0.025% cream | 30 gram ⓅoM £68.00 DT = £68.00
Ointment
CAUTIONARY AND ADVISORY LABELS 28
- ▸ Beclometasone dipropionate (Non-proprietary)
  Beclometasone dipropionate 250 microgram per 1 gram Beclometasone 0.025% ointment | 30 gram ⓅoM £68.00 DT = £68.00

Betamethasone

☞ 1208

21-Dec-2017

● **INDICATIONS AND DOSE**

Severe inflammatory skin disorders such as eczemas unresponsive to less potent corticosteroids | Psoriasis

▸ TO THE SKIN

▸ Child: Apply 1–2 times a day, to be applied thinly

▸ Adult: Apply 1–2 times a day, to be applied thinly

POTENCY

▸ Betamethasone valerate 0.025% cream and ointment: moderate. Betamethasone valerate 0.1% cream, lotion, ointment, and scalp application: potent. Betamethasone valerate 0.12% foam: potent. Betamethasone dipropionate 0.05% cream, lotion, and ointment: potent.

● UNLICENSED USE *Betacap®*, *Betnovate®* and *Betnovate-RD®* are not licensed for use in children under 1 year. *Bettamousse®* is not licensed for use in children under 6 years.

● CAUTIONS Use of more than 100 g per week of 0.1% preparation likely to cause adrenal suppression

● INTERACTIONS → Appendix 1: corticosteroids

● PATIENT AND CARER ADVICE Patient counselling is advised for betamethasone cream, ointment, scalp application and foam (application).

● MEDICINAL FORMS
There can be variation in the licensing of different medicines containing the same drug. Forms available from special-order manufacturers include: cream, ointment

Foam
CAUTIONARY AND ADVISORY LABELS 15, 28
EXCIPIENTS: May contain Cetostearyl alcohol (including cetyl and stearyl alcohol), polysorbates, propylene glycol
▸ Bettamousse (RPH Pharmaceuticals AB)
Betamethasone (as Betamethasone valerate) 1 mg per 1 gram Bettamousse 0.1% cutaneous foam | 100 gram PoM £9.75 DT = £9.75

Cream
CAUTIONARY AND ADVISORY LABELS 28
EXCIPIENTS: May contain Cetostearyl alcohol (including cetyl and stearyl alcohol), chlorocresol
▸ Betamethasone (Non-proprietary)
Betamethasone (as Betamethasone valerate) 1 mg per 1 gram Betamethasone valerate 0.1% cream | 15 gram PoM £3.00 | 30 gram PoM £5.99 DT = £2.57 | 100 gram PoM £11.99 DT = £8.57
▸ Audavate (Auden McKenzie (Pharma Division) Ltd)
Betamethasone (as Betamethasone valerate) 250 microgram per 1 gram Audavate RD 0.025% cream | 100 gram PoM £2.52 DT = £3.15
▸ Betnovate (GlaxoSmithKline UK Ltd)
Betamethasone (as Betamethasone valerate) 250 microgram per 1 gram Betnovate RD 0.025% cream | 100 gram PoM £3.15 DT = £3.15
Betamethasone (as Betamethasone valerate) 1 mg per 1 gram Betnovate 0.1% cream | 30 gram PoM £1.43 DT = £2.57 | 100 gram PoM £4.05 DT = £8.57
▸ Diprosone (Merck Sharp & Dohme Ltd)
Betamethasone (as Betamethasone dipropionate) 500 microgram per 1 gram Diprosone 0.05% cream | 30 gram PoM £2.16 DT = £2.16 | 100 gram PoM £6.12 DT = £6.12

Ointment
CAUTIONARY AND ADVISORY LABELS 28
▸ Betamethasone (Non-proprietary)
Betamethasone (as Betamethasone valerate) 1 mg per 1 gram Betamethasone valerate 0.1% ointment | 30 gram PoM £5.55 DT = £1.61 | 100 gram PoM £14.99 DT = £5.37
▸ Audavate (Auden McKenzie (Pharma Division) Ltd)
Betamethasone (as Betamethasone valerate) 250 microgram per 1 gram Audavate RD 0.025% ointment | 100 gram PoM £2.52 DT = £3.15

Betamethasone (as Betamethasone valerate) 1 mg per 1 gram Audavate 0.1% ointment | 30 gram PoM £1.14 DT = £1.61 | 100 gram PoM £3.24 DT = £5.37
▸ Betnovate (GlaxoSmithKline UK Ltd)
Betamethasone (as Betamethasone valerate) 250 microgram per 1 gram Betnovate RD 0.025% ointment | 100 gram PoM £3.15 DT = £3.15
Betamethasone (as Betamethasone valerate) 1 mg per 1 gram Betnovate 0.1% ointment | 30 gram PoM £1.43 DT = £1.61 | 100 gram PoM £4.05 DT = £5.37
▸ Diprosone (Merck Sharp & Dohme Ltd)
Betamethasone (as Betamethasone dipropionate) 500 microgram per 1 gram Diprosone 0.05% ointment | 30 gram PoM £2.16 DT = £2.16 | 100 gram PoM £6.12 DT = £6.12

Liquid
CAUTIONARY AND ADVISORY LABELS 15(scalp lotion only), 28
EXCIPIENTS: May contain Cetostearyl alcohol (including cetyl and stearyl alcohol), hydroxybenzoates (parabens)
▸ Betacap (Dermal Laboratories Ltd)
Betamethasone (as Betamethasone valerate) 1 mg per 1 gram Betacap 0.1% scalp application | 100 ml PoM £3.75 DT = £3.75
▸ Betnovate (GlaxoSmithKline UK Ltd)
Betamethasone (as Betamethasone valerate) 1 mg per 1 gram Betnovate 0.1% scalp application | 100 ml PoM £4.99 DT = £3.75
Betnovate 0.1% lotion | 100 ml PoM £4.58 DT = £4.58
▸ Diprosone (Merck Sharp & Dohme Ltd)
Betamethasone (as Betamethasone dipropionate) 500 microgram per 1 ml Diprosone 0.05% lotion | 30 ml PoM £2.73 DT = £2.73 | 100 ml PoM £7.80 DT = £7.80

Combinations available: *Betamethasone with clioquinol*, p. 1214 · *Betamethasone with clotrimazole*, p. 1214 · *Betamethasone with fusidic acid*, p. 1215 · *Betamethasone with neomycin*, p. 1215 · *Betamethasone with salicylic acid*, p. 1215

Calcipotriol with betamethasone

30-May-2017

The properties listed below are those particular to the combination only. For the properties of the components please consider, calcipotriol p. 1227, betamethasone above.

● **INDICATIONS AND DOSE**

DOVOBET® GEL

Scalp psoriasis

▸ TO THE SKIN

▸ Adult: Apply 1–4 g once daily usual duration of therapy 4 weeks; if necessary, treatment may be continued beyond 4 weeks or repeated, on the advice of a specialist, shampoo off after leaving on scalp overnight or during day, when different preparations containing calcipotriol used together, maximum total calcipotriol 5 mg in any one week

Mild to moderate plaque psoriasis

▸ TO THE SKIN

▸ Adult: Apply once daily for 8 weeks; if necessary, treatment may be continued beyond 8 weeks or repeated, on the advice of a specialist, apply to maximum 30% of body surface, when different preparations containing calcipotriol used together, max. total calcipotriol 5 mg in any one week; maximum 15 g per day

DOVOBET® OINTMENT

Stable plaque psoriasis

▸ TO THE SKIN

▸ Adult: Apply once daily for 4 weeks; if necessary, treatment may be continued beyond 4 weeks or repeated, on the advice of a specialist, apply to a maximum 30% of body surface, when different preparations containing calcipotriol used continued →

13

Skin

together, max. total calcipotriol 5 mg in any one week; maximum 15 g per day

ENSTILAR ®

Psoriasis

▶ TO THE SKIN

▶ Adult: Apply once daily to be applied to the affected area for up to 4 weeks—consult product literature for further information; maximum 15 g per day

● CONTRA-INDICATIONS

ENSTILAR ® Erythrodermic psoriasis · pustular psoriasis

● INTERACTIONS → Appendix 1: corticosteroids · vitamin D substances

● NATIONAL FUNDING/ACCESS DECISIONS

ENSTILAR ®

Scottish Medicines Consortium (SMC) Decisions

The *Scottish Medicines Consortium* has advised (September 2016) that calcipotriol with betamethasone (*Enstilar*®) is accepted for use within NHS Scotland for the treatment of psoriasis vulgaris.

● MEDICINAL FORMS

There can be variation in the licensing of different medicines containing the same drug.

Ointment

CAUTIONARY AND ADVISORY LABELS 28

EXCIPIENTS: May contain Butylated hydroxytoluene

▶ Dovobet (LEO Pharma)

Calcipotriol (as Calcipotriol hydrate) 50 microgram per 1 gram, Betamethasone (as Betamethasone dipropionate) 500 microgram per 1 gram Dovobet ointment | 30 gram PoM £19.84 DT = £19.84 | 60 gram PoM £39.68 | 120 gram PoM £73.86

Foam

▶ Enstilar (LEO Pharma)

Calcipotriol (as Calcipotriol monohydrate) 50 microgram per 1 gram, Betamethasone (as Betamethasone dipropionate) 500 microgram per 1 gram Enstilar 50micrograms/g / 0.5 mg/g cutaneous foam | 60 gram | 120 gram PoM £79.36 | Enstilar 50micrograms/g £39.68 DT = £39.68 |

Gel

CAUTIONARY AND ADVISORY LABELS 28

EXCIPIENTS: May contain Butylated hydroxytoluene

▶ Dovobet (LEO Pharma)

Calcipotriol (as Calcipotriol monohydrate) 50 microgram per 1 gram, Betamethasone (as Betamethasone dipropionate) 500 microgram per 1 gram Dovobet gel | 60 gram PoM £37.21 DT = £37.21 | 120 gram PoM £69.11

📰 1208

Clobetasol propionate

21-Dec-2017

● INDICATIONS AND DOSE

Short-term treatment only of severe resistant inflammatory skin disorders such as recalcitrant eczemas unresponsive to less potent corticosteroids | Psoriasis

▶ TO THE SKIN

▶ Child 1-17 years: Apply 1–2 times a day for up to 4 weeks, to be applied thinly

▶ Adult: Apply 1–2 times a day for up to 4 weeks, to be applied thinly, maximum 50 g of 0.05% preparation per week

POTENCY

▶ Clobetasol propionate 0.05% cream, foam, ointment, scalp application, and shampoo: very potent.

ETRIVEX ®

Moderate scalp psoriasis

▶ TO THE SKIN

▶ Adult: Apply once daily maximum duration of treatment 4 weeks, to be applied thinly then rinsed off after 15 minutes; frequency of application should be reduced after clinical improvement

● UNLICENSED USE *Dermovate*® not licensed for use in children under 1 year.

● PATIENT AND CARER ADVICE Patients or carers should be given advice on how to administer clobetasol propionate foam, liquid (scalp application), cream, ointment and shampoo.

Scalp application Patients or carers should be advised to apply foam directly to scalp lesions (foam begins to subside immediately on contact with skin).

● MEDICINAL FORMS

There can be variation in the licensing of different medicines containing the same drug. Forms available from special-order manufacturers include: cream, ointment

Foam

CAUTIONARY AND ADVISORY LABELS 15, 28

EXCIPIENTS: May contain Cetostearyl alcohol (including cetyl and stearyl alcohol), polysorbates, propylene glycol

▶ Clarelux (Pierre Fabre Dermo-Cosmetique)

Clobetasol propionate 500 microgram per 1 gram Clarelux 500micrograms/g foam | 100 gram PoM £11.06 DT = £11.06

Shampoo

CAUTIONARY AND ADVISORY LABELS 28

▶ Etrivex (Galderma (UK) Ltd)

Clobetasol propionate 500 microgram per 1 gram Etrivex 500micrograms/g shampoo | 125 ml PoM £9.15 DT = £9.15

Cream

CAUTIONARY AND ADVISORY LABELS 28

EXCIPIENTS: May contain Beeswax, cetostearyl alcohol (including cetyl and stearyl alcohol), chlorocresol, propylene glycol

▶ Clobetasol propionate (Non-proprietary)

Clobetasol propionate 500 microgram per 1 gram Clobetasol 0.05% cream | 30 gram PoM 🅢 DT = £2.69 | 100 gram PoM 🅢 DT = £7.90

▶ ClobaDerm (Auden McKenzie (Pharma Division) Ltd)

Clobetasol propionate 500 microgram per 1 gram ClobaDerm 0.05% cream | 30 gram PoM £2.15 DT = £2.69 | 100 gram PoM £6.32 = £7.90

▶ Dermovate (GlaxoSmithKline UK Ltd)

Clobetasol propionate 500 microgram per 1 gram Dermovate 0.05% cream | 30 gram PoM £2.69 DT = £2.69 | 100 gram PoM £7.90 DT = £7.90

Ointment

CAUTIONARY AND ADVISORY LABELS 28

EXCIPIENTS: May contain Propylene glycol

▶ Clobetasol propionate (Non-proprietary)

Clobetasol propionate 500 microgram per 1 gram Clobetasol 0.05% ointment | 30 gram PoM 🅢 DT = £2.69 | 100 gram PoM 🅢 DT = £7.90

▶ ClobaDerm (Auden McKenzie (Pharma Division) Ltd)

Clobetasol propionate 500 microgram per 1 gram ClobaDerm 0.05% ointment | 30 gram PoM £2.15 DT = £7.90 | 100 gram PoM £6.32 DT = £7.90

▶ Dermovate (GlaxoSmithKline UK Ltd)

Clobetasol propionate 500 microgram per 1 gram Dermovate 0.05% ointment | 30 gram PoM £2.69 DT = £2.69 | 100 gram PoM £7.90 DT = £7.90

Liquid

CAUTIONARY AND ADVISORY LABELS 15, 28

▶ Dermovate (GlaxoSmithKline UK Ltd)

Clobetasol propionate 500 microgram per 1 gram Dermovate 0.05% scalp application | 30 ml PoM £3.07 DT = £3.07 | 100 ml PoM £10.42 DT = £10.42

Combinations available: *Clobetasol propionate with neomycin sulfate and nystatin*, p. 1216

📰 1208

Clobetasone butyrate

21-Dec-2017

● INDICATIONS AND DOSE

Eczemas and dermatitis of all types | Maintenance between courses of more potent corticosteroids

▶ TO THE SKIN

▶ Child: Apply 1–2 times a day, to be applied thinly

▶ Adult: Apply 1–2 times a day, to be applied thinly

POTENCY
▸ Clobetasone butyrate 0.05% cream and ointment:
moderate.

● UNLICENSED USE Licensed for use in children (age range
not specified by manufacturer).

● PATIENT AND CARER ADVICE Patients or carers should be
advised on the application of clobetasone butyrate
containing preparations.

● EXCEPTIONS TO LEGAL CATEGORY Cream can be sold to the
public for short-term symptomatic treatment and control
of patches of eczema and dermatitis (but not seborrhoeic
dermatitis) in adults and children over 12 years provided
pack does not contain more than 15 g.

● MEDICINAL FORMS
There can be variation in the licensing of different medicines
containing the same drug. Forms available from special-order
manufacturers include: cream, ointment

Ointment
CAUTIONARY AND ADVISORY LABELS 28
▸ Clobavate (Teva UK Ltd)
 Clobetasone butyrate 500 microgram per 1 gram Clobavate
 0.05% ointment | 30 gram PoM £1.49 DT = £1.86 | 100 gram PoM
 £4.35 DT = £5.44
▸ Eumovate (GlaxoSmithKline UK Ltd)
 Clobetasone butyrate 500 microgram per 1 gram Eumovate
 0.05% ointment | 30 gram PoM £1.86 DT = £1.86 | 100 gram PoM
 £5.44 DT = £5.44

Cream
CAUTIONARY AND ADVISORY LABELS 28
EXCIPIENTS: May contain Cetostearyl alcohol (including cetyl and
stearyl alcohol), chlorocresol
▸ Eumovate (GlaxoSmithKline Consumer Healthcare, GlaxoSmithKline
 UK Ltd)
 Clobetasone butyrate 500 microgram per 1 gram Eumovate
 0.05% cream | 30 gram PoM £1.86 DT = £1.86 | 100 gram PoM
 £5.44 DT = £5.44

Combinations available: *Clobetasone butyrate with nystatin
and oxytetracycline*, p. 1216

Ϝ 1208

Diflucortolone valerate   21-Dec-2017

● INDICATIONS AND DOSE
**Severe inflammatory skin disorders such as eczemas
unresponsive to less potent corticosteroids (using 0.3%
diflucortolone valerate) | Short-term treatment of severe
exacerbations (using 0.3% diflucortolone valerate) |
Psoriasis (using 0.3% diflucortolone valerate)**
▸ TO THE SKIN
▸ Child 4-17 years: Apply 1–2 times a day for up to
 2 weeks, reducing strength as condition responds, to be
 applied thinly; maximum 60 g per week
▸ Adult: Apply 1–2 times a day for up to 2 weeks,
 reducing strength as condition responds, to be applied
 thinly; maximum 60 g per week

**Severe inflammatory skin disorders such as eczemas
unresponsive to less potent corticosteroids (using 0.1%
diflucortolone valerate) | Psoriasis (using 0.1%
diflucortolone valerate)**
▸ TO THE SKIN
▸ Child: Apply 1–2 times a day for up to 4 weeks, to be
 applied thinly
▸ Adult: Apply 1–2 times a day for up to 4 weeks, to be
 applied thinly
POTENCY
▸ Diflucortolone valerate 0.1% cream and ointment:
potent.
▸ Diflucortolone valerate 0.3% cream and ointment: very
potent.

● UNLICENSED USE *Nerisone*® licensed for use in children
(age range not specified by manufacturer); *Nerisone Forte*®
not licensed for use in children under 4 years.

● SIDE-EFFECTS Pustular psoriasis

● PRESCRIBING AND DISPENSING INFORMATION Patients or
carers should be advised on application of diflucortolone
valerate containing preparations.

● MEDICINAL FORMS
There can be variation in the licensing of different medicines
containing the same drug.

Ointment
CAUTIONARY AND ADVISORY LABELS 28
▸ Nerisone (Meadow Laboratories Ltd)
 Diflucortolone valerate 1 mg per 1 gram Nerisone 0.1% ointment |
 30 gram PoM £3.98
 Diflucortolone valerate 3 mg per 1 gram Nerisone Forte 0.3%
 ointment | 15 gram PoM £4.70

Cream
CAUTIONARY AND ADVISORY LABELS 28
EXCIPIENTS: May contain Beeswax, cetostearyl alcohol (including cetyl
and stearyl alcohol), disodium edetate, hydroxybenzoates (parabens)
▸ Nerisone (Meadow Laboratories Ltd)
 Diflucortolone valerate 1 mg per 1 gram Nerisone 0.1% cream |
 30 gram PoM £3.98
 Nerisone 0.1% oily cream | 30 gram PoM £4.95 DT = £4.95
 Diflucortolone valerate 3 mg per 1 gram Nerisone Forte 0.3% oily
 cream | 15 gram PoM £4.70 DT = £4.70

Ϝ 1208

Fludroxycortide   21-Dec-2017

(Flurandrenolone)

● INDICATIONS AND DOSE
Inflammatory skin disorders such as eczemas
▸ TO THE SKIN
▸ Child: Apply 1–2 times a day, to be applied thinly
▸ Adult: Apply 1–2 times a day, to be applied thinly
POTENCY
▸ Fludroxycortide 0.0125% cream and ointment: moderate

HAELAN® TAPE
**Chronic localised recalcitrant dermatoses (but not acute
or weeping)**
▸ TO THE SKIN
▸ Child: Cut tape to fit lesion, apply to clean, dry skin
 shorn of hair, usually for 12 hours daily
▸ Adult: Cut tape to fit lesion, apply to clean, dry skin
 shorn of hair, usually for 12 hours daily

● UNLICENSED USE Licensed for use in children (age range
not specified by manufacturer).

● PATIENT AND CARER ADVICE Patients or carers should be
counselled on application of fludroxycortide cream and
ointment.

● MEDICINAL FORMS
There can be variation in the licensing of different medicines
containing the same drug.

Ointment
CAUTIONARY AND ADVISORY LABELS 28
EXCIPIENTS: May contain Beeswax, cetostearyl alcohol (including cetyl
and stearyl alcohol), polysorbates
▸ Fludroxycortide (Non-proprietary)
 Fludroxycortide 125 microgram per 1 gram Fludroxycortide
 0.0125% ointment | 60 gram PoM £5.99

Cream
CAUTIONARY AND ADVISORY LABELS 28
EXCIPIENTS: May contain Cetostearyl alcohol (including cetyl and
stearyl alcohol), propylene glycol
▸ Fludroxycortide (Non-proprietary)
 Fludroxycortide 125 microgram per 1 gram Fludroxycortide
 0.0125% cream | 60 gram PoM £5.99

13

Skin

Impregnated dressing

▸ Fludroxycortide (Non-proprietary)

Fludroxycortide 4 microgram per 1 square cm Fludroxycortide 4micrograms/square cm tape 7.5cm | 20 cm PoM £12.49–£13.67 DT = £13.67

Fluocinolone acetonide

F 1208

21-Dec-2017

● INDICATIONS AND DOSE

Severe inflammatory skin disorders such as eczemas | Psoriasis

▸ TO THE SKIN

▸ **Child 1-17 years:** Apply 1–2 times a day, to be applied thinly, reduce strength as condition responds

▸ **Adult:** Apply 1–2 times a day, to be applied thinly, reduce strength as condition responds

POTENCY

▸ Fluocinolone acetonide 0.025% cream, gel, and ointment: potent.

▸ Fluocinolone acetonide 0.00625% cream and ointment: moderate.

▸ Fluocinolone acetonide 0.0025% cream: mild.

● SIDE-EFFECTS Pustular psoriasis

● PRESCRIBING AND DISPENSING INFORMATION Gel is useful for application to the scalp and other hairy areas.

● PATIENT AND CARER ADVICE Patient counselling is advised for fluocinolone acetonide cream, gel and ointment (application).

● MEDICINAL FORMS
There can be variation in the licensing of different medicines containing the same drug.

Ointment

CAUTIONARY AND ADVISORY LABELS 28

EXCIPIENTS: May contain Propylene glycol, woolfat and related substances (including lanolin)

▸ Synalar (Reig Jofre UK Ltd)

Fluocinolone acetonide 62.5 microgram per 1 gram Synalar 1 in 4 Dilution 0.00625% ointment | 50 gram PoM £4.84 DT = £4.84

Fluocinolone acetonide 250 microgram per 1 gram Synalar 0.025% ointment | 30 gram PoM £4.14 DT = £4.14 | 100 gram PoM £11.75 DT = £11.75

Cream

CAUTIONARY AND ADVISORY LABELS 28

EXCIPIENTS: May contain Benzyl alcohol, cetostearyl alcohol (including cetyl and stearyl alcohol), polysorbates, propylene glycol

▸ Synalar (Reig Jofre UK Ltd)

Fluocinolone acetonide 25 microgram per 1 gram Synalar 1 in 10 Dilution 0.0025% cream | 50 gram PoM £4.58 DT = £4.58

Fluocinolone acetonide 62.5 microgram per 1 gram Synalar 1 in 4 Dilution 0.00625% cream | 50 gram PoM £4.84 DT = £4.84

Fluocinolone acetonide 250 microgram per 1 gram Synalar 0.025% cream | 30 gram PoM £4.14 DT = £4.14 | 100 gram PoM £11.75 DT = £11.75

Gel

CAUTIONARY AND ADVISORY LABELS 28

EXCIPIENTS: May contain Hydroxybenzoates (parabens), propylene glycol

▸ Synalar (Reig Jofre UK Ltd)

Fluocinolone acetonide 250 microgram per 1 gram Synalar 0.025% gel | 30 gram PoM £5.56 DT = £5.56 | 60 gram PoM £10.02 DT = £10.02

Combinations available: *Fluocinolone acetonide with clioquinol*, p. 1216 · *Fluocinolone acetonide with neomycin*, p. 1216

Fluocinonide

F 1208

21-Dec-2017

● INDICATIONS AND DOSE

Severe inflammatory skin disorders such as eczemas unresponsive to less potent corticosteroids | Psoriasis

▸ TO THE SKIN

▸ **Child:** Apply 1–2 times a day, to be applied thinly

▸ **Adult:** Apply 1–2 times a day, to be applied thinly

POTENCY

▸ Fluocinonide 0.05% cream and ointment: potent.

● UNLICENSED USE Not licensed for use in children under 1 year.

● SIDE-EFFECTS Pustular psoriasis

● PATIENT AND CARER ADVICE Patients or carers should be advised on the application of fluocinonide preparations.

● MEDICINAL FORMS
There can be variation in the licensing of different medicines containing the same drug. Forms available from special-order manufacturers include: ointment

Ointment

CAUTIONARY AND ADVISORY LABELS 28

EXCIPIENTS: May contain Propylene glycol, woolfat and related substances (including lanolin)

▸ Metosyn (Reig Jofre UK Ltd)

Fluocinonide 500 microgram per 1 gram Metosyn 0.05% ointment | 25 gram PoM £3.50 DT = £3.50 | 100 gram PoM £13.15 DT = £13.15

Cream

CAUTIONARY AND ADVISORY LABELS 28

EXCIPIENTS: May contain Propylene glycol

▸ Metosyn FAPG (Reig Jofre UK Ltd)

Fluocinonide 500 microgram per 1 gram Metosyn FAPG 0.05% cream | 25 gram PoM £3.96 DT = £3.96 | 100 gram PoM £13.34 DT = £13.34

Fluticasone

F 1208

21-Dec-2017

● INDICATIONS AND DOSE

Severe inflammatory skin disorders such as dermatitis and eczemas unresponsive to less potent corticosteroids | Psoriasis

▸ TO THE SKIN

▸ **Child 3 months-17 years:** Apply 1–2 times a day, to be applied thinly

▸ **Adult:** Apply 1–2 times a day, to be applied thinly

POTENCY

▸ Fluticasone cream 0.05%: potent.

▸ Fluticasone ointment 0.005%: potent.

● INTERACTIONS → Appendix 1: corticosteroids

● PATIENT AND CARER ADVICE Patients or carers should be given advice on application of fluticasone creams and ointments.

● MEDICINAL FORMS
There can be variation in the licensing of different medicines containing the same drug.

Cream

CAUTIONARY AND ADVISORY LABELS 28

EXCIPIENTS: May contain Cetostearyl alcohol (including cetyl and stearyl alcohol), imidurea, propylene glycol

▸ Cutivate (GlaxoSmithKline UK Ltd)

Fluticasone propionate 500 microgram per 1 gram Cutivate 0.05% cream | 15 gram PoM £2.27 DT = £2.27 | 30 gram PoM £4.24 DT = £4.24

Ointment

CAUTIONARY AND ADVISORY LABELS 28

EXCIPIENTS: May contain Propylene glycol

▸ Cutivate (GlaxoSmithKline UK Ltd)

Fluticasone propionate 50 microgram per 1 gram Cutivate 0.005% ointment | 15 gram [PoM] £2.27 DT = £2.27 | 30 gram [PoM] £4.24 DT = £4.24

⚑ 1208

Hydrocortisone

21-Dec-2017

● **INDICATIONS AND DOSE**

Mild inflammatory skin disorders such as eczemas

▸ TO THE SKIN

▸ Child: Apply 1–2 times a day, to be applied thinly

▸ Adult: Apply 1–2 times a day, to be applied thinly

Nappy rash

▸ TO THE SKIN

▸ Child: Apply 1–2 times a day for no longer than 1 week, discontinued as soon as the inflammation subsides

POTENCY

▸ Hydrocortisone cream and ointment 0.5 to 2.5%: mild

● **INTERACTIONS** → Appendix 1: corticosteroids

● **PRESCRIBING AND DISPENSING INFORMATION** When hydrocortisone cream or ointment is prescribed and no strength is stated, the 1% strength should be supplied. Although *Dioderm®* contains only 0.1% hydrocortisone, the formulation is designed to provide a clinical activity comparable to that of Hydrocortisone Cream 1% BP.

● **PATIENT AND CARER ADVICE** Patient counselling is advised for hydrocortisone cream and ointment (application).

● **PROFESSION SPECIFIC INFORMATION**

Dental practitioners' formulary

Hydrocortisone Cream 1% 15 g may be prescribed.

● **EXCEPTIONS TO LEGAL CATEGORY**

Over-the-counter hydrocortisone preparations

Skin creams and ointments containing hydrocortisone (alone or with other ingredients) can be sold to the public for the treatment of allergic contact dermatitis, irritant dermatitis, insect bite reactions and mild to moderate eczema in patients over 10 years, to be applied sparingly over the affected area 1–2 times daily for max. 1 week. Over-the-counter hydrocortisone preparations should not be sold without medical advice for children under 10 years or for pregnant women; they should **not** be sold for application to the face, anogenital region, broken or infected skin (including cold sores, acne, and athlete's foot).

● **MEDICINAL FORMS**

There can be variation in the licensing of different medicines containing the same drug. Forms available from special-order manufacturers include: cream, ointment

Cream

CAUTIONARY AND ADVISORY LABELS 28

EXCIPIENTS: May contain Benzyl alcohol, cetostearyl alcohol (including cetyl and stearyl alcohol), hydroxybenzoates (parabens), propylene glycol

▸ Hydrocortisone (Non-proprietary)

Hydrocortisone 5 mg per 1 gram Hydrocortisone 0.5% cream | 15 gram [PoM] £3.00 DT = £0.79 | 30 gram [PoM] £2.18–£4.90

Hydrocortisone 10 mg per 1 gram Hydrocortisone 1% cream | 15 gram [PoM] £10.50 DT = £0.71 | 15 gram [P] £1.64 DT = £0.71 | 30 gram [PoM] £23.83 DT = £1.42 | 50 gram [PoM] £36.12 DT = £2.37

Hydrocortisone 25 mg per 1 gram Hydrocortisone 2.5% cream | 15 gram [PoM] £44.00 DT = £4.98 | 30 gram [PoM] £12.00–£88.00

▸ Dioderm (Dermal Laboratories Ltd)

Hydrocortisone 1 mg per 1 gram Dioderm 0.1% cream | 30 gram [PoM] £2.39 DT = £2.39

▸ Mildison Lipocream (LEO Pharma)

Hydrocortisone 10 mg per 1 gram Mildison Lipocream 1% cream | 30 gram [PoM] £1.71 DT = £1.42

Ointment

CAUTIONARY AND ADVISORY LABELS 28

▸ Hydrocortisone (Non-proprietary)

Hydrocortisone 5 mg per 1 gram Hydrocortisone 0.5% ointment | 15 gram [PoM] £5.67 DT = £5.67 | 30 gram [PoM] £12.00

Hydrocortisone 10 mg per 1 gram Hydrocortisone 1% ointment | 15 gram [PoM] £10.50 DT = £0.70 | 30 gram [PoM] £23.83 DT = £1.40 | 50 gram [PoM] £36.12 DT = £2.33

Hydrocortisone 25 mg per 1 gram Hydrocortisone 2.5% ointment | 15 gram [PoM] £44.00 DT = £25.08 | 30 gram [PoM] £50.16–£88.00

Combinations available: *Hydrocortisone with benzalkonium chloride, dimeticone and nystatin*, p. 1217 · *Hydrocortisone with chlorhexidine hydrochloride and nystatin*, p. 1217 · *Hydrocortisone with clotrimazole*, p. 1217 · *Hydrocortisone with fusidic acid*, p. 1217 · *Hydrocortisone with miconazole*, p. 1218 · *Hydrocortisone with oxytetracycline*, p. 1218

⚑ 1208

Hydrocortisone butyrate

21-Dec-2017

● **INDICATIONS AND DOSE**

Severe inflammatory skin disorders such as eczemas unresponsive to less potent corticosteroids | Psoriasis

▸ TO THE SKIN

▸ Child 1-17 years: Apply 1–2 times a day, to be applied thinly

▸ Adult: Apply 1–2 times a day, to be applied thinly

POTENCY

▸ Hydrocortisone butyrate 0.1% cream, liquid, and ointment: potent

● **PATIENT AND CARER ADVICE** Patients or carers should be given advice on how to administer hydrocortisone butyrate lotion, cream, ointment and scalp lotion.

Medicines for Children leaflet: Hydrocortisone (topical) for eczema www.medicinesforchildren.org.uk/hydrocortisone-topical-for-eczema

● **MEDICINAL FORMS**

There can be variation in the licensing of different medicines containing the same drug. Forms available from special-order manufacturers include: ointment

Ointment

CAUTIONARY AND ADVISORY LABELS 28

▸ Locoid (LEO Pharma)

Hydrocortisone butyrate 1 mg per 1 gram Locoid 0.1% ointment | 30 gram [PoM] £1.60 DT = £1.60 | 100 gram [PoM] £4.93 DT = £4.93

Cream

CAUTIONARY AND ADVISORY LABELS 28

EXCIPIENTS: May contain Benzyl alcohol, cetostearyl alcohol (including cetyl and stearyl alcohol), hydroxybenzoates (parabens), 28

▸ Locoid (LEO Pharma)

Hydrocortisone butyrate 1 mg per 1 gram Locoid 0.1% cream | 30 gram [PoM] £1.60 DT = £1.60 | 100 gram [PoM] £4.93 DT = £4.93

▸ Locoid Lipocream (LEO Pharma)

Hydrocortisone butyrate 1 mg per 1 gram Locoid 0.1% Lipocream | 30 gram [PoM] £1.69 DT = £1.60 | 100 gram [PoM] £5.17 DT = £4.93

Liquid

CAUTIONARY AND ADVISORY LABELS 15(excluding Locoid Crelo topical emulsion), 28

EXCIPIENTS: May contain Butylated hydroxytoluene, cetostearyl alcohol (including cetyl and stearyl alcohol), hydroxybenzoates (parabens), propylene glycol

▸ Locoid (LEO Pharma)

Hydrocortisone butyrate 1 mg per 1 ml Locoid 0.1% scalp lotion | 100 ml [PoM] £6.83 DT = £6.83

▸ Locoid Crelo (LEO Pharma)

Hydrocortisone butyrate 1 mg per 1 gram Locoid Crelo 0.1% topical emulsion | 100 gram [PoM] £5.91

13

Skin

Hydrocortisone with urea

The properties listed below are those particular to the combination only. For the properties of the components please consider, hydrocortisone p. 1213.

- **INDICATIONS AND DOSE**

Mild inflammatory skin disorders such as eczemas
▸ TO THE SKIN
- Child: To be applied thinly (consult product literature)
- Adult: To be applied thinly (consult product literature)
POTENCY
▸ Hydrocortisone 1% with urea cream: moderate

- **INTERACTIONS** → Appendix 1: corticosteroids
- **PATIENT AND CARER ADVICE** Patients or carers should be advised on application of hydrocortisone with urea cream.

- **MEDICINAL FORMS**
There can be variation in the licensing of different medicines containing the same drug.
Cream
CAUTIONARY AND ADVISORY LABELS 28
▸ Alphaderm (Alliance Pharmaceuticals Ltd)
Hydrocortisone 10 mg per 1 gram, Urea 100 mg per 1 gram Alphaderm 1%/10% cream | 30 gram [PoM] £2.38 DT = £2.38 | 100 gram [PoM] £7.03 DT = £7.03

Mometasone furoate

📕 1208

21-Dec-2017

- **INDICATIONS AND DOSE**

Severe inflammatory skin disorders such as eczemas unresponsive to less potent corticosteroids | Psoriasis
▸ TO THE SKIN
- Child 2-17 years: Apply once daily, to be applied thinly (to scalp in case of lotion)
- Adult: Apply once daily, to be applied thinly (to scalp in case of lotion)
POTENCY
▸ Mometasone furoate 0.1% cream, ointment, and scalp lotion: potent.

- **INTERACTIONS** → Appendix 1: corticosteroids
- **PATIENT AND CARER ADVICE** Patients and carers should be advised on the application of topical mometasone.

- **MEDICINAL FORMS**
There can be variation in the licensing of different medicines containing the same drug. Forms available from special-order manufacturers include: ointment
Cream
CAUTIONARY AND ADVISORY LABELS 28
EXCIPIENTS: May contain Beeswax
▸ Mometasone furoate (Non-proprietary)
Mometasone furoate 1 mg per 1 gram Mometasone 0.1% cream | 30 gram [PoM] £4.36 DT = £1.53 | 100 gram [PoM] £12.58 DT = £5.10
▸ Elocon (Merck Sharp & Dohme Ltd)
Mometasone furoate 1 mg per 1 gram Elocon 0.1% cream | 30 gram [PoM] £4.80 DT = £1.53 | 100 gram [PoM] £15.10 DT = £5.10
Ointment
CAUTIONARY AND ADVISORY LABELS 28
EXCIPIENTS: May contain Beeswax, propylene glycol
▸ Mometasone furoate (Non-proprietary)
Mometasone furoate 1 mg per 1 gram Mometasone 0.1% ointment | 15 gram [PoM] £4.32 | 30 gram [PoM] £4.45 DT = £1.57 | 50 gram [PoM] £12.44 | 100 gram [PoM] £12.82 DT = £5.23
▸ Elocon (Merck Sharp & Dohme Ltd)
Mometasone furoate 1 mg per 1 gram Elocon 0.1% ointment | 30 gram [PoM] £4.32 DT = £1.57 | 100 gram [PoM] £12.44 DT = £5.23
Liquid
CAUTIONARY AND ADVISORY LABELS 28
EXCIPIENTS: May contain Propylene glycol
▸ Elocon (Merck Sharp & Dohme Ltd)
Mometasone furoate 1 mg per 1 gram Elocon 0.1% scalp lotion | 30 ml [PoM] £4.36 DT = £4.36

CORTICOSTEROIDS ❭ CORTICOSTEROID COMBINATIONS WITH ANTI-INFECTIVES

Betamethasone with clioquinol

18-Nov-2015

The properties listed below are those particular to the combination only. For the properties of the components please consider, betamethasone p. 1209.

- **INDICATIONS AND DOSE**

Severe inflammatory skin disorders such as eczemas unresponsive to less potent corticosteroids | Psoriasis
▸ TO THE SKIN
- Child: (consult product literature)
- Adult: (consult product literature)
POTENCY
▸ Betamethasone (as valerate) 0.1% with clioquinol cream and ointment: potent.

- **UNLICENSED USE** Betamethasone and clioquinol preparations is not licensed for use in children under 1 year.
- **PATIENT AND CARER ADVICE** Stains clothing. Patients or carers should be counselled on application of betamethasone with clioquinol preparations.

- **MEDICINAL FORMS**
There can be variation in the licensing of different medicines containing the same drug.
Ointment
CAUTIONARY AND ADVISORY LABELS 28
▸ Betamethasone with clioquinol (Non-proprietary)
Betamethasone (as Betamethasone valerate) 1 mg per 1 gram, Clioquinol 30 mg per 1 gram Betamethasone valerate 0.1% / Clioquinol 3% ointment | 30 gram [PoM] £38.88 DT = £38.88
Cream
CAUTIONARY AND ADVISORY LABELS 28
EXCIPIENTS: May contain Cetostearyl alcohol (including cetyl and stearyl alcohol), chlorocresol
▸ Betamethasone with clioquinol (Non-proprietary)
Betamethasone (as Betamethasone valerate) 1 mg per 1 gram, Clioquinol 30 mg per 1 gram Betamethasone valerate 0.1% / Clioquinol 3% cream | 30 gram [PoM] £38.88 DT = £38.88

Betamethasone with clotrimazole

The properties listed below are those particular to the combination only. For the properties of the components please consider, betamethasone p. 1209, clotrimazole p. 1197.

- **INDICATIONS AND DOSE**

Severe inflammatory skin disorders such as eczemas unresponsive to less potent corticosteroids | Psoriasis
▸ TO THE SKIN
- Child: (consult product literature)
- Adult: (consult product literature)
POTENCY
▸ Betamethasone dipropionate 0.064% (=betamethasone 0.5%) with clotrimazole cream: potent.

- **UNLICENSED USE** *Lotriderm*® not licensed for use in children under 12 years.
- **PATIENT AND CARER ADVICE** Patients or carers should be given advice on how to administer betamethasone with clotrimazole cream.

● MEDICINAL FORMS
There can be variation in the licensing of different medicines containing the same drug.

Cream
CAUTIONARY AND ADVISORY LABELS 28
EXCIPIENTS: May contain Benzyl alcohol, cetostearyl alcohol (including cetyl and stearyl alcohol), propylene glycol
  ▸ Lotriderm (Merck Sharp & Dohme Ltd)
    Betamethasone dipropionate 640 microgram per 1 gram, Clotrimazole 10 mg per 1 gram Lotriderm cream | 30 gram PoM £6.34 DT = £6.34

Betamethasone with fusidic acid

The properties listed below are those particular to the combination only. For the properties of the components please consider, betamethasone p. 1209, fusidic acid p. 561.

● INDICATIONS AND DOSE

Severe inflammatory skin disorders such as eczemas unresponsive to less potent corticosteroids | Psoriasis
  ▸ TO THE SKIN
  ▸ Child: (consult product literature)
  ▸ Adult: (consult product literature)

POTENCY
  ▸ Betamethasone (as valerate) 0.1% with fusidic acid cream: potent.

● UNLICENSED USE *Fucibet® Lipid Cream* is not licensed for use in children under 6 years.

● PATIENT AND CARER ADVICE Patients or carers should be counselled on application of betamethasone with fusidic acid preparations.

● MEDICINAL FORMS
There can be variation in the licensing of different medicines containing the same drug.

Cream
CAUTIONARY AND ADVISORY LABELS 28
EXCIPIENTS: May contain Cetostearyl alcohol (including cetyl and stearyl alcohol), chlorocresol, hydroxybenzoates (parabens)
  ▸ Betamethasone with fusidic acid (Non-proprietary)
    Betamethasone (as Betamethasone valerate) 1 mg per 1 gram, Fusidic acid 20 mg per 1 gram Betamethasone valerate 0.1% / Fusidic acid 2% cream | 30 gram PoM £6.38 DT = £6.38 | 60 gram PoM £12.76 DT = £12.76
  ▸ Fucibet (LEO Pharma)
    Betamethasone (as Betamethasone valerate) 1 mg per 1 gram, Fusidic acid 20 mg per 1 gram Fucibet cream | 30 gram PoM £6.38 DT = £6.38 | 60 gram PoM £12.76 DT = £12.76
    Fucibet Lipid cream | 30 gram PoM £6.74 DT = £6.38
  ▸ Xemacort (Mylan)
    Betamethasone (as Betamethasone valerate) 1 mg per 1 gram, Fusidic acid 20 mg per 1 gram Xemacort cream | 30 gram PoM £6.05 DT = £6.38 | 60 gram PoM £12.45 DT = £12.76

Betamethasone with neomycin

The properties listed below are those particular to the combination only. For the properties of the components please consider, betamethasone p. 1209, neomycin sulfate p. 1195.

● INDICATIONS AND DOSE

Severe inflammatory skin disorders such as eczemas unresponsive to less potent corticosteroids | Psoriasis
  ▸ TO THE SKIN USING OINTMENT, OR TO THE SKIN USING CREAM
  ▸ Child 2–17 years: Apply 1–2 times a day, to be applied thinly
  ▸ Adult: Apply 1–2 times a day, to be applied thinly
POTENCY
  ▸ Betamethasone (as valerate) 0.1% with neomycin cream and ointment: potent.

● PATIENT AND CARER ADVICE Patient counselling is advised for betamethasone with neomycin cream and ointment (application).

● MEDICINAL FORMS
There can be variation in the licensing of different medicines containing the same drug.

Ointment
CAUTIONARY AND ADVISORY LABELS 28
  ▸ Betamethasone with neomycin (Non-proprietary)
    Betamethasone (as Betamethasone valerate) 1 mg per 1 gram, Neomycin sulfate 5 mg per 1 gram Betamethasone valerate 0.1% / Neomycin 0.5% ointment | 30 gram PoM £38.88 DT = £31.36 | 100 gram PoM £97.00 DT = £104.52

Cream
CAUTIONARY AND ADVISORY LABELS 28
EXCIPIENTS: May contain Cetostearyl alcohol (including cetyl and stearyl alcohol), chlorocresol
  ▸ Betamethasone with neomycin (Non-proprietary)
    Betamethasone (as Betamethasone valerate) 1 mg per 1 gram, Neomycin sulfate 5 mg per 1 gram Betamethasone valerate 0.1% / Neomycin 0.5% cream | 30 gram PoM £38.88 DT = £31.36 | 100 gram PoM £97.00 DT = £104.52

Betamethasone with salicylic acid

The properties listed below are those particular to the combination only. For the properties of the components please consider, betamethasone p. 1209, salicylic acid p. 1250.

● INDICATIONS AND DOSE
DIPROSALIC® OINTMENT

Severe inflammatory skin disorders such as eczemas unresponsive to less potent corticosteroids | Psoriasis
  ▸ TO THE SKIN
  ▸ Child: Apply 1–2 times a day, max. 60 g per week
  ▸ Adult: Apply 1–2 times a day, max. 60 g per week
POTENCY
  ▸ For *Diprosalic*® ointment: betamethasone (as dipropionate) 0.05% with salicylic acid 3%: potent.

DIPROSALIC® SCALP APPLICATION

Severe inflammatory skin disorders such as eczemas unresponsive to less potent corticosteroids | Psoriasis
  ▸ TO THE SKIN
  ▸ Child: Apply 1–2 times a day, apply a few drops
  ▸ Adult: Apply 1–2 times a day, apply a few drops
POTENCY
  ▸ For *Diprosalic*® scalp application: betamethasone (as dipropionate) 0.05% with salicylic acid 2%: potent.

● PATIENT AND CARER ADVICE
DIPROSALIC® OINTMENT Patients or carers should be counselled on application of betamethasone and salicylic acid preparations.
DIPROSALIC® SCALP APPLICATION Patients or carers should be counselled on application of betamethasone and salicylic acid scalp application.

● MEDICINAL FORMS
There can be variation in the licensing of different medicines containing the same drug. Forms available from special-order manufacturers include: ointment

Ointment
CAUTIONARY AND ADVISORY LABELS 28
  ▸ Diprosalic (Merck Sharp & Dohme Ltd)
    Betamethasone (as Betamethasone dipropionate) 500 microgram per 1 gram, Salicylic acid 30 mg per 1 gram Diprosalic 0.05%/3% ointment | 30 gram PoM £3.18 DT = £3.18 | 100 gram PoM £9.14 DT = £9.14

13

Skin

Liquid

CAUTIONARY AND ADVISORY LABELS 28

EXCIPIENTS: May contain Disodium edetate

▶ Diprosalic (Merck Sharp & Dohme Ltd)

Betamethasone (as Betamethasone dipropionate) **500 microgram per 1 ml, Salicylic acid 20 mg per 1 ml** Diprosalic 0.05%/2% scalp application | 100 ml [PoM] £10.10 DT = £10.10

Clobetasol propionate with neomycin sulfate and nystatin

The properties listed below are those particular to the combination only. For the properties of the components please consider, clobetasol propionate p. 1210, neomycin sulfate p. 1195.

● INDICATIONS AND DOSE

Short-term treatment only of severe resistant inflammatory skin disorders such as recalcitrant eczemas associated with infection and unresponsive to less potent corticosteroids | Psoriasis associated with infection

▶ TO THE SKIN

▶ Adult: (consult product literature)

POTENCY

▶ Clobetasol propionate 0.05% with neomycin sulfate and nystatin cream and ointment: very potent.

● PATIENT AND CARER ADVICE Patients or carers should be advised on application of clobetasol propionate, neomycin sulfate and nystatin containing preparations.

● MEDICINAL FORMS There can be variation in the licensing of different medicines containing the same drug.

Ointment

CAUTIONARY AND ADVISORY LABELS 28

▶ Clobetasol propionate with neomycin sulfate and nystatin (Non-proprietary)

Clobetasol propionate **500 microgram per 1 gram, Neomycin sulfate 5 mg per 1 gram, Nystatin 100000 unit per 1 gram** Clobetasol 500microgram / Neomycin 5mg / Nystatin 100,000units/g ointment | 30 gram [PoM] £87.00 DT = £87.00

Cream

CAUTIONARY AND ADVISORY LABELS 28

▶ Clobetasol propionate with neomycin sulfate and nystatin (Non-proprietary)

Clobetasol propionate **500 microgram per 1 gram, Neomycin sulfate 5 mg per 1 gram, Nystatin 100000 unit per 1 gram** Clobetasol 500microgram / Neomycin 5mg / Nystatin 100,000units/g cream | 30 gram [PoM] £87.00 DT = £87.00

Clobetasone butyrate with nystatin and oxytetracycline

The properties listed below are those particular to the combination only. For the properties of the components please consider, clobetasone butyrate p. 1210, oxytetracycline p. 557.

● INDICATIONS AND DOSE

Steroid-responsive dermatoses where candidal or bacterial infection is present

▶ TO THE SKIN

▶ Adult: (consult product literature)

POTENCY

▶ Clobetasone butyrate 0.05% with nystatin and oxytetracycline cream: moderate.

● PATIENT AND CARER ADVICE Stains clothing.

● MEDICINAL FORMS Forms available from special-order manufacturers include: cream

Fluocinolone acetonide with clioquinol

The properties listed below are those particular to the combination only. For the properties of the components please consider, fluocinolone acetonide p. 1212.

● INDICATIONS AND DOSE

Inflammatory skin disorders such as eczemas associated with infection | Psoriasis associated with infection

▶ TO THE SKIN

▶ Adult: Apply 1–2 times a day, to be applied thinly, reducing strength as condition responds

POTENCY

▶ Clioquinol 3% with fluocinolone acetonide 0.025% cream and ointment: potent

● PATIENT AND CARER ADVICE Patient counselling is advised for clioquinol with fluocinolone acetonide cream and ointment (application). Ointment stains clothing.

● MEDICINAL FORMS There can be variation in the licensing of different medicines containing the same drug.

Ointment

CAUTIONARY AND ADVISORY LABELS 28

EXCIPIENTS: May contain Propylene glycol, woolfat and related substances (including lanolin)

▶ Synalar C (Reig Jofre UK Ltd)

Fluocinolone acetonide **250 microgram per 1 gram, Clioquinol 30 mg per 1 gram** Synalar C ointment | 15 gram [PoM] £2.66

Cream

CAUTIONARY AND ADVISORY LABELS 28

EXCIPIENTS: May contain Cetostearyl alcohol (including cetyl and stearyl alcohol), disodium edetate, hydroxybenzoates (parabens), polysorbates, propylene glycol

▶ Synalar C (Reig Jofre UK Ltd)

Fluocinolone acetonide **250 microgram per 1 gram, Clioquinol 30 mg per 1 gram** Synalar C cream | 15 gram [PoM] £2.66

Fluocinolone acetonide with neomycin

The properties listed below are those particular to the combination only. For the properties of the components please consider, fluocinolone acetonide p. 1212, neomycin sulfate p. 1195.

● INDICATIONS AND DOSE

Inflammatory skin disorders such as eczemas associated with infection | Psoriasis associated with infection

▶ TO THE SKIN

▶ Child 1-17 years: Apply 1–2 times a day, to be applied thinly, reducing strength as condition responds

▶ Adult: Apply 1–2 times a day, to be applied thinly, reducing strength as condition responds

POTENCY

▶ Fluocinolone acetonide 0.025% with neomycin 0.5% cream and ointment: potent.

● PATIENT AND CARER ADVICE Patients or carers should be counselled on the application of fluocinolone acetonide with neomycin preparations.

● MEDICINAL FORMS There can be variation in the licensing of different medicines containing the same drug.

Ointment

CAUTIONARY AND ADVISORY LABELS 28

EXCIPIENTS: May contain Propylene glycol, woolfat and related substances (including lanolin)

▸ Synalar N (Reig Jofre UK Ltd)
Fluocinolone acetonide 250 microgram per 1 gram, Neomycin sulfate 5 mg per 1 gram Synalar N ointment | 30 gram [PoM] £4.36

Cream
CAUTIONARY AND ADVISORY LABELS 28
EXCIPIENTS: May contain Cetostearyl alcohol (including cetyl and stearyl alcohol), hydroxybenzoates (parabens), polysorbates, propylene glycol

▸ Synalar N (Reig Jofre UK Ltd)
Fluocinolone acetonide 250 microgram per 1 gram, Neomycin sulfate 5 mg per 1 gram Synalar N cream | 30 gram [PoM] £4.36

Hydrocortisone with benzalkonium chloride, dimeticone and nystatin

15-Mar-2016

The properties listed below are those particular to the combination only. For the properties of the components please consider, hydrocortisone p. 1213, dimeticone p. 1202.

● **INDICATIONS AND DOSE**

Mild inflammatory skin disorders such as eczemas associated with infection
▸ TO THE SKIN
▸ Child: Apply 3 times a day until lesion has healed, to be applied thinly
▸ Adult: Apply 3 times a day until lesion has healed, to be applied thinly

POTENCY
▸ Benzalkonium with dimeticone, hydrocortisone acetate 0.5%, and nystatin cream: mild.

● **PATIENT AND CARER ADVICE** Patients or carers should be advised on application of benzalkonium with dimeticone and hydrocortisone and nystatin preparations.

● **MEDICINAL FORMS**
There can be variation in the licensing of different medicines containing the same drug.
Cream
CAUTIONARY AND ADVISORY LABELS 28
EXCIPIENTS: May contain Butylated hydroxyanisole, cetostearyl alcohol (including cetyl and stearyl alcohol), hydroxybenzoates (parabens), sodium metabisulfite, sorbic acid
▸ Timodine (Alliance Pharmaceuticals Ltd)
Benzalkonium chloride 1 mg per 1 gram, Hydrocortisone 5 mg per 1 gram, Dimeticone 350 100 mg per 1 gram, Nystatin 100000 unit per 1 gram Timodine cream | 30 gram [PoM] £3.37

Hydrocortisone with chlorhexidine hydrochloride and nystatin

The properties listed below are those particular to the combination only. For the properties of the components please consider, hydrocortisone p. 1213, chlorhexidine p. 1241.

● **INDICATIONS AND DOSE**

Mild inflammatory skin disorders such as eczemas
▸ TO THE SKIN
▸ Child: To be applied thinly (consult product literature)
▸ Adult: To be applied thinly (consult product literature)

POTENCY
▸ Hydrocortisone 0.5% with chlorhexidine hydrochloride 1% and nystatin cream: mild
▸ Hydrocortisone 1% with chlorhexidine hydrochloride 1% and nystatin ointment: mild

● **PATIENT AND CARER ADVICE** Patients or carers should be given advice on application of chlorhexidine hydrochloride with hydrocortisone and nystatin preparations.

● **MEDICINAL FORMS**
There can be variation in the licensing of different medicines containing the same drug.
Ointment
CAUTIONARY AND ADVISORY LABELS 28
▸ Hydrocortisone with chlorhexidine hydrochloride and nystatin (Non-proprietary)
Chlorhexidine acetate 10 mg per 1 gram, Hydrocortisone 10 mg per 1 gram, Nystatin 100000 unit per 1 gram Nystatin 100,000units/g / Chlorhexidine acetate 1% / Hydrocortisone 1% ointment | 30 gram [PoM] £5.29 DT = £5.29

Cream
CAUTIONARY AND ADVISORY LABELS 28
EXCIPIENTS: May contain Benzyl alcohol, cetostearyl alcohol (including cetyl and stearyl alcohol), polysorbates
▸ Hydrocortisone with chlorhexidine hydrochloride and nystatin (Non-proprietary)
Hydrocortisone 5 mg per 1 gram, Chlorhexidine hydrochloride 10 mg per 1 gram, Nystatin 100000 unit per 1 gram Nystatin 100,000units/g / Chlorhexidine hydrochloride 1% / Hydrocortisone 0.5% cream | 30 gram [PoM] £5.29 DT = £5.29

Hydrocortisone with clotrimazole

The properties listed below are those particular to the combination only. For the properties of the components please consider, hydrocortisone p. 1213, clotrimazole p. 1197.

● **INDICATIONS AND DOSE**

Mild inflammatory skin disorders such as eczemas (associated with fungal infection)
▸ TO THE SKIN
▸ Child: (consult product literature)
▸ Adult: (consult product literature)

POTENCY
▸ Clotrimazole with hydrocortisone 1% cream: mild

● **PATIENT AND CARER ADVICE** Patients or carers should be given advice on how to administer clotrimazole with hydrocortisone cream.

● **EXCEPTIONS TO LEGAL CATEGORY** A 15-g tube is on sale to the public for the treatment of athlete's foot and fungal infection of skin folds with associated inflammation in patients 10 years and over.

● **MEDICINAL FORMS**
There can be variation in the licensing of different medicines containing the same drug.
Cream
CAUTIONARY AND ADVISORY LABELS 28
EXCIPIENTS: May contain Benzyl alcohol, cetostearyl alcohol (including cetyl and stearyl alcohol)
▸ Canesten HC (Bayer Plc)
Clotrimazole 10 mg per 1 gram, Hydrocortisone 10 mg per 1 gram Canesten HC cream | 30 gram [PoM] £2.42 DT = £2.42

Hydrocortisone with fusidic acid

The properties listed below are those particular to the combination only. For the properties of the components please consider, hydrocortisone p. 1213, fusidic acid p. 561.

● **INDICATIONS AND DOSE**

Mild inflammatory skin disorders such as eczemas
▸ TO THE SKIN
▸ Child: To be applied thinly (consult product literature)
▸ Adult: To be applied thinly (consult product literature)

POTENCY
▸ Hydrocortisone with fusidic acid cream: mild

13

Skin

- **PATIENT AND CARER ADVICE** Patients or carers should be advised on application of hydrocortisone with fusidic acid preparations.

- **MEDICINAL FORMS**
There can be variation in the licensing of different medicines containing the same drug.

Cream

CAUTIONARY AND ADVISORY LABELS 28

EXCIPIENTS: May contain Butylated hydroxyanisole, cetostearyl alcohol (including cetyl and stearyl alcohol), polysorbates, potassium sorbate

▸ **Fucidin H** (Fusidic acid / Hydrocortisone) (LEO Pharma)
Hydrocortisone acetate 10 mg per 1 gram, Fusidic acid 20 mg per 1 gram Fucidin H cream | 30 gram [PoM] £6.02 DT = £6.02 | 60 gram [PoM] £12.05 DT = £12.05

Hydrocortisone with miconazole

The properties listed below are those particular to the combination only. For the properties of the components please consider, hydrocortisone p. 1213, miconazole p. 1199.

- **INDICATIONS AND DOSE**

Mild inflammatory skin disorders such as eczemas associated with infections
▸ TO THE SKIN
▸ Adult: (consult product literature)

POTENCY
▸ Hydrocortisone 1% with miconazole cream and ointment: mild

- **PATIENT AND CARER ADVICE** Patients or carers should be advised on application of hydrocortisone with miconazole preparations.

- **PROFESSION SPECIFIC INFORMATION**

Dental practitioners' formulary
May be prescribed as Miconazole and Hydrocortisone Cream or Ointment for max. 7 days.

- **EXCEPTIONS TO LEGAL CATEGORY** A 15-g tube of hydrocortisone with miconazole cream is on sale to the public for the treatment of athlete's foot and candidal intertrigo.

- **MEDICINAL FORMS**
There can be variation in the licensing of different medicines containing the same drug.

Ointment

CAUTIONARY AND ADVISORY LABELS 28

▸ **Daktacort** (Janssen-Cilag Ltd)
Hydrocortisone 10 mg per 1 gram, Miconazole nitrate 20 mg per 1 gram Daktacort ointment | 30 gram [PoM] £2.50 DT = £2.50

Cream

CAUTIONARY AND ADVISORY LABELS 28

EXCIPIENTS: May contain Butylated hydroxyanisole, disodium edetate

▸ **Daktacort** (McNeil Products Ltd, Janssen-Cilag Ltd)
Hydrocortisone 10 mg per 1 gram, Miconazole nitrate 20 mg per 1 gram Daktacort 2%/1% cream | 30 gram [PoM] £2.49 DT = £2.49

Hydrocortisone with oxytetracycline

The properties listed below are those particular to the combination only. For the properties of the components please consider, hydrocortisone p. 1213, oxytetracycline p. 557.

- **INDICATIONS AND DOSE**

Mild inflammatory skin disorders such as eczemas
▸ TO THE SKIN
▸ Child 12–17 years: (consult product literature)
▸ Adult: (consult product literature)

POTENCY
▸ Hydrocortisone 1% with oxytetracycline ointment: mild.

- **CONTRA-INDICATIONS** Children under 12 years

- **PREGNANCY** Tetracyclines should not be given to pregnant women. Effects on skeletal development have been documented when tetracyclines have been used in the first trimester in animal studies. Administration during the second or third trimester may cause discoloration of the child's teeth.

- **BREAST FEEDING** Tetracyclines should not be given to women who are breast-feeding (although absorption and therefore discoloration of teeth in the infant is probably usually prevented by chelation with calcium in milk).

- **PATIENT AND CARER ADVICE** Patients should be given advice on the application of hydrocortisone with oxytetracycline ointment.

- **MEDICINAL FORMS**
There can be variation in the licensing of different medicines containing the same drug.

Ointment

CAUTIONARY AND ADVISORY LABELS 28

▸ **Terra-Cortil** (Intrapharm Laboratories Ltd)
Hydrocortisone 10 mg per 1 gram, Oxytetracycline (as Oxytetracycline hydrochloride) 30 mg per 1 gram Terra-Cortil ointment | 30 gram [PoM] £5.01 DT = £5.01

DERMATOLOGICAL DRUGS ❯ ANTI-INFECTIVES

Ichthammol

- **INDICATIONS AND DOSE**

Chronic lichenified eczema
▸ TO THE SKIN
▸ Child 1–17 years: Apply 1–3 times a day
▸ Adult: Apply 1–3 times a day

- **UNLICENSED USE**
▸ In children No information available.

- **SIDE-EFFECTS** Skin irritation

- **MEDICINAL FORMS**
There can be variation in the licensing of different medicines containing the same drug. Forms available from special-order manufacturers include: ointment, paste

Liquid
▸ Ichthammol (Non-proprietary)
Ichthammol 1 mg per 1 mg Ichthammol liquid | 100 gram [GSL] £11.42 DT = £11.42 | 500 gram [GSL] £34.27

Ichthammol with zinc oxide

The properties listed below are those particular to the combination only. For the properties of the components please consider, ichthammol above.

- **INDICATIONS AND DOSE**

Chronic lichenified eczema
▸ TO THE SKIN
▸ Adult: (consult product literature)

- **MEDICINAL FORMS**
There can be variation in the licensing of different medicines containing the same drug. Forms available from special-order manufacturers include: cream, ointment

Impregnated dressing
▸ Ichthopaste (Evolan Pharma AB)
Ichthopaste bandage 7.5cm × 6m | 1 bandage £3.75

DERMATOLOGICAL DRUGS > ANTRACEN DERIVATIVES

Dithranol

(Anthralin)

- **INDICATIONS AND DOSE**

Subacute and chronic psoriasis

▶ TO THE SKIN
- Adult: (consult product literature)

DITHROCREAM ®

Subacute and chronic psoriasis

▶ TO THE SKIN
- Adult: For application to skin or scalp, 0.1–0.5% cream suitable for overnight treatment, 1–2% cream for maximum 1 hour (consult product literature)

MICANOL ®

Subacute and chronic psoriasis

▶ TO THE SKIN
- Adult: Apply once daily, for application to skin or scalp, to be applied for up to 30 minutes, apply 1% cream, if necessary 3% cream can be used under medical supervision

- **CONTRA-INDICATIONS** Acute and pustular psoriasis · hypersensitivity
- **CAUTIONS** Avoid sensitive areas of skin · avoid use near eyes
- **SIDE-EFFECTS** Skin reactions
- **PREGNANCY** No adverse effects reported.
- **BREAST FEEDING** No adverse effects reported.
- **DIRECTIONS FOR ADMINISTRATION** When applying dithranol, hands should be protected by gloves or they should be washed thoroughly afterwards. Dithranol should be applied to chronic extensor plaques only, carefully avoiding normal skin.

  MICANOL ® At the end of contact time, use plenty of lukewarm (not hot) water to rinse off cream; soap may be used after the cream has been rinsed off; use shampoo before applying cream to scalp and if necessary after cream has been rinsed off.

- **PRESCRIBING AND DISPENSING INFORMATION** Treatment should be started with a low concentration such as dithranol 0.1%, and the strength increased gradually every few days up to 3%, according to tolerance.
- **PATIENT AND CARER ADVICE** Dithranol can stain the skin, hair and fabrics.
- **EXCEPTIONS TO LEGAL CATEGORY** Prescription only medicine if dithranol content more than 1%, otherwise may be sold to the public.

- **MEDICINAL FORMS**
  There can be variation in the licensing of different medicines containing the same drug. Forms available from special-order manufacturers include: ointment

  Cream
  CAUTIONARY AND ADVISORY LABELS 28
  EXCIPIENTS: May contain Cetostearyl alcohol (including cetyl and stearyl alcohol), chlorocresol
  ▶ Dithrocream (Dermal Laboratories Ltd)
    Dithranol 1 mg per 1 gram Dithrocream 0.1% cream | 50 gram Ⓟ £3.77
    Dithranol 2.5 mg per 1 gram Dithrocream 0.25% cream | 50 gram Ⓟ £4.04
    Dithranol 5 mg per 1 gram Dithrocream 0.5% cream | 50 gram Ⓟ £4.66
    Dithranol 10 mg per 1 gram Dithrocream HP 1% cream | 50 gram Ⓟ £5.42

Dithranol 20 mg per 1 gram Dithrocream 2% cream | 50 gram PoM £6.79

Combinations available: *Coal tar with dithranol and salicylic acid,* p. 1220

Dithranol with salicylic acid and zinc oxide

The properties listed below are those particular to the combination only. For the properties of the components please consider, dithranol above, salicylic acid p. 1250.

- **INDICATIONS AND DOSE**

Subacute and chronic psoriasis

▶ TO THE SKIN
- Adult: (consult local protocol)

- **MEDICINAL FORMS**
  Forms available from special-order manufacturers include: ointment, paste

DERMATOLOGICAL DRUGS > TARS

Coal tar

- **INDICATIONS AND DOSE**

Psoriasis | Chronic atopic eczema

▶ TO THE SKIN USING PASTE
- Child: Apply 1–3 times a day, start application with low-strength preparations
- Adult: Apply 1–3 times a day, start application with low-strength preparations

▶ TO THE SKIN
- Child: 100 mL/bath, to be added to an adult sized bath; add proportionally less for a child's bath. Use Coal Tar Solution BP
- Adult: 100 mL/bath, to be added to an adult sized bath. Use Coal Tar Solution BP

ALPHOSYL 2 IN 1 ® SHAMPOO

Psoriasis | Seborrhoeic dermatitis | Scaling | Itching

▶ TO THE SKIN
- Adult: Apply every 2–3 days

Dandruff

▶ TO THE SKIN
- Adult: Apply 1–2 times a week as required

EXOREX ® LOTION

Psoriasis

▶ TO THE SKIN
- Adult: Apply 2–3 times a day, to be applied to skin or scalp; in elderly, lotion can be diluted with a few drops of water before applying

- **CONTRA-INDICATIONS** Avoid broken or inflamed skin · avoid eye area · avoid genital area · avoid mucosal areas · avoid rectal area · infection · sore, acute, or pustular psoriasis
- **CAUTIONS** Application to face · application to skin flexures
- **SIDE-EFFECTS** Photosensitivity reaction · skin reactions
- **PRESCRIBING AND DISPENSING INFORMATION** Coal Tar Solution BP contains coal tar 20%, Strong Coal Tar Solution BP contains coal tar 40%.
- **HANDLING AND STORAGE** Use suitable chemical protection gloves for extemporaneous preparation. May stain skin, hair and fabric.
- **PATIENT AND CARER ADVICE** May stain skin, hair and fabric.

13

Skin

- **MEDICINAL FORMS**
There can be variation in the licensing of different medicines containing the same drug. Forms available from special-order manufacturers include: cream, ointment, paste
Bath additive
▸ Psoriderm (Dermal Laboratories Ltd)
  Coal tar distilled 400 mg per 1 ml Psoriderm Emulsion 40% bath additive | 200 ml P £2.74
Cutaneous emulsion
EXCIPIENTS: May contain Hydroxybenzoates (parabens)
▸ Exorex (Teva UK Ltd)
  Coal tar solution 50 mg per 1 gram Exorex lotion | 100 ml GSL
  £8.11 DT = £8.11 | 250 ml GSL £16.24 DT = £16.24
Shampoo
EXCIPIENTS: May contain Fragrances, hydroxybenzoates (parabens)
▸ Coal tar (Non-proprietary)
  Coal tar extract 20 mg per 1 gram Coal tar extract 2% shampoo |
  125 ml GSL ⬚ DT = £3.90 | 250 ml GSL ⬚ DT = £5.86
▸ Brands may include Alphosyl 2 in 1, Neutrogena T/Gel Therapeutic, Polytar Scalp

Coal tar with calamine

31-Aug-2016

The properties listed below are those particular to the combination only. For the properties of the components please consider, coal tar p. 1219.

- **INDICATIONS AND DOSE**
Psoriasis | Chronic atopic eczema (occasionally)
▸ TO THE SKIN
▸ Adult: Apply 1–2 times a day

IMPORTANT SAFETY INFORMATION

MHRA/CHM UPDATE (APRIL 2016): FIRE RISK WITH PARAFFIN-BASED SKIN EMOLLIENTS ON DRESSINGS OR CLOTHING
See Emollient and barrier preparations p. 1186.

- **PRESCRIBING AND DISPENSING INFORMATION** When prepared extemporaneously, the BP states Calamine and Coal Tar Ointment BP, consists of calamine 12.5 g, strong coal tar solution 2.5 g, zinc oxide 12.5 g, hydrous wool fat 25 g, white soft paraffin 47.5 g.

- **MEDICINAL FORMS**
No licensed medicines listed.

Coal tar with coconut oil and salicylic acid

The properties listed below are those particular to the combination only. For the properties of the components please consider, coal tar p. 1219, salicylic acid p. 1250.

- **INDICATIONS AND DOSE**
Scaly scalp disorders | Psoriasis | Seborrhoeic dermatitis | Dandruff | Cradle cap
▸ TO THE SKIN USING SHAMPOO
▸ Child: Apply daily as required
▸ Adult: Apply daily as required

- **MEDICINAL FORMS**
There can be variation in the licensing of different medicines containing the same drug.
Shampoo
▸ Capasal (Dermal Laboratories Ltd)
  Salicylic acid 5 mg per 1 gram, Coal tar distilled 10 mg per 1 gram, Coconut oil 10 mg per 1 gram Capasal Therapeutic shampoo |
  250 ml P £4.69

Coal tar with dithranol and salicylic acid

The properties listed below are those particular to the combination only. For the properties of the components please consider, coal tar p. 1219, dithranol p. 1219, salicylic acid p. 1250.

- **INDICATIONS AND DOSE**
Subacute and chronic psoriasis
▸ TO THE SKIN
▸ Child: Apply up to twice daily
▸ Adult: Apply up to twice daily

- **UNLICENSED USE** *Psorin*® is licensed for use in children (age range not specified by manufacturer).

- **MEDICINAL FORMS**
Forms available from special-order manufacturers include: ointment

Coal tar with lecithin

The properties listed below are those particular to the combination only. For the properties of the components please consider, coal tar p. 1219.

- **INDICATIONS AND DOSE**
PSORIDERM® CREAM
Psoriasis
▸ TO THE SKIN
▸ Child: Apply 1–2 times a day, cream to be applied to the skin or scalp
▸ Adult: Apply 1–2 times a day, cream to be applied to the skin or scalp
PSORIDERM® SCALP LOTION
Scalp psoriasis
▸ TO THE SKIN
▸ Child: Apply as required
▸ Adult: Apply as required

- **MEDICINAL FORMS**
There can be variation in the licensing of different medicines containing the same drug.
Cream
EXCIPIENTS: May contain Isopropyl palmitate, propylene glycol
▸ Psoriderm (Dermal Laboratories Ltd)
  Lecithin 4 mg per 1 gram, Coal tar distilled 60 mg per 1 gram Psoriderm cream | 225 ml P £9.42
Shampoo
EXCIPIENTS: May contain Disodium edetate
▸ Psoriderm (Dermal Laboratories Ltd)
  Lecithin 3 mg per 1 ml, Coal tar distilled 25 mg per 1 ml Psoriderm scalp lotion | 250 ml P £4.74

Coal tar with salicylic acid

26-Aug-2016

The properties listed below are those particular to the combination only. For the properties of the components please consider, coal tar p. 1219, salicylic acid p. 1250.

- **INDICATIONS AND DOSE**
Psoriasis | Chronic atopic eczema
▸ TO THE SKIN USING OINTMENT
▸ Adult: Apply 1–2 times a day

IMPORTANT SAFETY INFORMATION

MHRA/CHM UPDATE (APRIL 2016): FIRE RISK WITH PARAFFIN-BASED SKIN EMOLLIENTS ON DRESSINGS OR CLOTHING
See Emollient and barrier preparations p. 1186.

- PRESCRIBING AND DISPENSING INFORMATION When prepared extemporaneously, the BP states Coal Tar and Salicylic Acid Ointment, BP consists of coal tar 2 g, salicylic acid 2 g, emulsifying wax 11.4 g, white soft paraffin 19 g, coconut oil 54 g, polysorbate '80' 4 g, liquid paraffin 7.6 g.

- MEDICINAL FORMS
  Forms available from special-order manufacturers include: ointment

Coal tar with salicylic acid and precipitated sulfur

The properties listed below are those particular to the combination only. For the properties of the components please consider, coal tar p. 1219, salicylic acid p. 1250.

- **INDICATIONS AND DOSE**

COCOIS® OINTMENT

Scaly scalp disorders including psoriasis, eczema, seborrhoeic dermatitis and dandruff
▸ INITIALLY TO THE SKIN USING SCALP OINTMENT
▸ Child 6-11 years: Medical supervision required
▸ Child 12-17 years: Apply once weekly as required, alternatively (to the skin) apply daily for the first 3-7 days (if severe), shampoo off after 1 hour
▸ Adult: Apply once weekly as required, alternatively (to the skin) apply daily for the first 3-7 days (if severe), shampoo off after 1 hour

SEBCO® OINTMENT

Scaly scalp disorders including psoriasis, eczema, seborrhoeic dermatitis and dandruff
▸ TO THE SKIN USING SCALP OINTMENT
▸ Child 6-11 years: Medical supervision required
▸ Child 12-17 years: Apply as required, alternatively apply daily for the first 3-7 days (if severe), shampoo off after 1 hour
▸ Adult: Apply as required, alternatively apply daily for the first 3-7 days (if severe), shampoo off after 1 hour

- MEDICINAL FORMS
  There can be variation in the licensing of different medicines containing the same drug.
  Ointment
  EXCIPIENTS: May contain Cetostearyl alcohol (including cetyl and stearyl alcohol)
  ▸ Cocois (RPH Pharmaceuticals AB)
  Salicylic acid 20 mg per 1 gram, Sulfur precipitated 40 mg per 1 gram, Coal tar solution 120 mg per 1 gram Cocois ointment | 40 gram GSL £6.22 | 100 gram GSL £11.69
  ▸ Sebco (Derma UK Ltd)
  Salicylic acid 20 mg per 1 gram, Sulfur precipitated 40 mg per 1 gram, Coal tar solution 120 mg per 1 gram Sebco ointment | 40 gram GSL £6.20 | 100 gram GSL £11.67

Coal tar with zinc oxide

26-Aug-2016

The properties listed below are those particular to the combination only. For the properties of the components please consider, coal tar p. 1219.

- **INDICATIONS AND DOSE**

Psoriasis | Chronic atopic eczema
▸ TO THE SKIN
▸ Child: Apply 1-2 times a day

▸ Adult: Apply 1-2 times a day

> **IMPORTANT SAFETY INFORMATION**
> MHRA/CHM UPDATE (APRIL 2016): FIRE RISK WITH PARAFFIN-BASED SKIN EMOLLIENTS ON DRESSINGS OR CLOTHING
> See Emollient and barrier preparations p. 1186.

- PRESCRIBING AND DISPENSING INFORMATION No preparations available—when prepared extemporaneously, the BP states Zinc and Coal Tar Paste, BP consists of zinc oxide 6%, coal tar 6%, emulsifying wax 5%, starch 38%, yellow soft paraffin 45%.

- MEDICINAL FORMS
  Forms available from special-order manufacturers include: ointment, paste

IMMUNOSUPPRESSANTS ⟩ CALCINEURIN INHIBITORS AND RELATED DRUGS

Pimecrolimus

- **INDICATIONS AND DOSE**

Short-term treatment of mild to moderate atopic eczema (including flares) when topical corticosteroids cannot be used (initiated by a specialist)
▸ TO THE SKIN
▸ Adult: Apply twice daily until symptoms resolve (stop treatment if eczema worsens or no response after 6 weeks)

Short-term treatment of facial, flexural, or genital psoriasis in patients unresponsive to, or intolerant of other topical therapy (initiated by a specialist)
▸ TO THE SKIN
▸ Adult: Apply twice daily until symptoms resolve (maximum duration of treatment 4 weeks)

- UNLICENSED USE Pimecrolimus is not licensed for short-term treatment of facial, flexural, or genital psoriasis in patients unresponsive to, or intolerant of other topical therapy.

- CONTRA-INDICATIONS Application to malignant or potentially malignant skin lesions · application under occlusion · congenital epidermal barrier defects · contact with eyes · contact with mucous membranes · generalised erythroderma · immunodeficiency · infection at treatment site

- CAUTIONS Alcohol consumption (risk of facial flushing and skin irritation) · avoid other topical treatments except emollients at treatment site · UV light (avoid excessive exposure to sunlight and sunlamps)

- INTERACTIONS → Appendix 1: pimecrolimus

- SIDE-EFFECTS
▸ **Common or very common** Increased risk of infection
▸ **Rare or very rare** Skin discolouration
▸ **Frequency not known** Skin papilloma

- PREGNANCY Manufacturer advises avoid; toxicity in *animal* studies following systemic administration.

- BREAST FEEDING Manufacturer advises caution; ensure infant does not come in contact with treated areas.

- NATIONAL FUNDING/ACCESS DECISIONS
  NICE decisions
▸ Tacrolimus and pimecrolimus for atopic eczema (August 2004) NICE TA82
  Topical pimecrolimus is an option for atopic eczema not controlled by maximal topical corticosteroid treatment or if there is a risk of important corticosteroid side-effects (particularly skin atrophy).
  Topical pimecrolimus is recommended for moderate atopic eczema on the face and neck of children aged

13

Skin

2–16 years. Pimecrolimus should be used within its licensed indications.
www.nice.org.uk/TA82

● MEDICINAL FORMS
There can be variation in the licensing of different medicines containing the same drug.
Cream
CAUTIONARY AND ADVISORY LABELS 4, 11, 28
EXCIPIENTS: May contain Benzyl alcohol, cetostearyl alcohol (including cetyl and stearyl alcohol), propylene glycol
▸ Elidel (Meda Pharmaceuticals Ltd)
  Pimecrolimus 10 mg per 1 gram Elidel 1% cream | 30 gram [PoM]
  £19.69 DT = £19.69 | 60 gram [PoM] £37.41 DT = £37.41 |
  100 gram [PoM] £59.07 DT = £59.07

Tacrolimus

19-Mar-2018

● DRUG ACTION Tacrolimus is a calcineurin inhibitor.

● **INDICATIONS AND DOSE**

Short-term treatment of moderate to severe atopic eczema (including flares) in patients unresponsive to, or intolerant of conventional therapy (initiated by a specialist)
▸ TO THE SKIN
▸ Adult: Apply twice daily until lesion clears (consider other treatment if eczema worsens or no improvement after 2 weeks), initially 0.1% ointment to be applied thinly, reduce frequency to once daily or strength of ointment to 0.03% if condition allows

Prevention of flares in patients with moderate to severe atopic eczema and 4 or more flares a year who have responded to initial treatment with topical tacrolimus (initiated by a specialist)
▸ TO THE SKIN
▸ Adult: Apply twice weekly, 0.1% ointment to be applied thinly, with an interval of 2–3 days between applications, use short-term treatment regimen during an acute flare; review need for preventative therapy after 1 year

Short-term treatment of facial, flexural, or genital psoriasis in patients unresponsive to, or intolerant of other topical therapy (initiated under specialist supervision)
▸ TO THE SKIN
▸ Adult: Apply twice daily until symptoms resolve, 0.1% ointment to be applied thinly, reduce to once daily or switch to 0.03% ointment if condition allows, maximum duration of treatment 4 weeks

● UNLICENSED USE Short-term treatment of facial, flexural, or genital psoriasis is unlicensed.

● CONTRA-INDICATIONS Application to malignant or potentially malignant skin lesions · application under occlusion · avoid contact with eyes · avoid contact with mucous membranes · congenital epidermal barrier defects · generalised erythroderma · immunodeficiency · infection at treatment site

● CAUTIONS UV light (avoid excessive exposure to sunlight and sunlamps)

● INTERACTIONS → Appendix 1: tacrolimus

● SIDE-EFFECTS
▸ **Common or very common** Alcohol intolerance · increased risk of infection · sensation abnormal · skin reactions
▸ **Uncommon** Lymphadenopathy
▸ **Frequency not known** Malignancy · neoplasms

● ALLERGY AND CROSS-SENSITIVITY Contra-indicated if history of hypersensitivity to macrolides.

● PREGNANCY Manufacturer advises avoid unless essential; toxicity in *animal* studies following systemic administration.

● BREAST FEEDING Avoid—present in breast milk (following systemic administration).

● PATIENT AND CARER ADVICE Avoid excessive exposure to UV light including sunlight.

● NATIONAL FUNDING/ACCESS DECISIONS
NICE decisions
▸ Tacrolimus and pimecrolimus for atopic eczema (August 2004) NICE TA82
Topical tacrolimus is an option for atopic eczema not controlled by maximal topical corticosteroid treatment or if there is a risk of important corticosteroid side-effects (particularly skin atrophy).
  Topical tacrolimus is recommended as an option for the second-line treatment for moderate to severe atopic eczema in adults and children over 2 years. Tacrolimus should be used within its licensed indications.
www.nice.org.uk/guidance/TA82
Scottish Medicines Consortium (SMC) Decisions
The *Scottish Medicines Consortium* has advised (April 2010) that tacrolimus 0.1% ointment (*Protopic®*) is accepted for restricted use within NHS Scotland for the prevention of flares in patients aged 16 years and over with moderate-to-severe atopic eczema in accordance with the licensed indications; initiation of treatment is restricted to doctors (including general practitioners) with a specialist interest and experience in treating atopic eczema with immunomodulatory therapy.

● MEDICINAL FORMS
There can be variation in the licensing of different medicines containing the same drug.
Ointment
CAUTIONARY AND ADVISORY LABELS 4, 11, 28
EXCIPIENTS: May contain Beeswax
▸ Protopic (LEO Pharma)
  Tacrolimus (as Tacrolimus monohydrate) 300 microgram per 1 gram Protopic 0.03% ointment | 30 gram [PoM] £23.33 DT = £23.33 | 60 gram [PoM] £42.55 DT = £42.55
  Tacrolimus (as Tacrolimus monohydrate) 1 mg per 1 gram Protopic 0.1% ointment | 30 gram [PoM] £25.92 DT = £25.92 | 60 gram [PoM] £47.28 DT = £47.28

IMMUNOSUPPRESSANTS › INTERLEUKIN INHIBITORS

Brodalumab

22-Jan-2018

● DRUG ACTION Brodalumab is a recombinant human monoclonal antibody that binds with high affinity to interleukin-17RA and blocks the activity of pro-inflammatory cytokines.

● **INDICATIONS AND DOSE**

Moderate-to-severe plaque psoriasis (under expert supervision)
▸ BY SUBCUTANEOUS INJECTION
▸ Adult: 210 mg every week for 3 doses, followed by 210 mg every 2 weeks, consider discontinuing treatment if no response after 16 weeks

● CONTRA-INDICATIONS Active Crohn's disease · clinically significant active infection

● CAUTIONS Chronic infection · history of Crohn's disease (monitor for exacerbations) · history of depressive disorders (discontinue if new or worsening symptoms develop) · history of recurrent infection · history of suicidal ideation or behaviour (discontinue if new or worsening symptoms develop)
CAUTIONS, FURTHER INFORMATION
▸ Infection Manufacturer advises to consider anti-tuberculosis therapy for patients with latent tuberculosis before starting treatment with brodalumab.

Manufacturer advises patients should be brought up-to-date with current immunisation schedule before initiating treatment.

- INTERACTIONS → Appendix 1: monoclonal antibodies
- SIDE-EFFECTS
  ▸ **Common or very common** Arthralgia · diarrhoea · fatigue · headache · increased risk of infection · myalgia · nausea · oropharyngeal pain
  ▸ **Uncommon** Conjunctivitis
  ▸ **Frequency not known** Meningitis cryptococcal · suicidal tendencies
- CONCEPTION AND CONTRACEPTION Manufacturer advises that women of childbearing potential should use effective contraception during treatment and for at least 12 weeks after stopping treatment.
- PREGNANCY Manufacturer advises avoid—limited information available.
- BREAST FEEDING Manufacturer advises avoid—no information available.
- DIRECTIONS FOR ADMINISTRATION Manufacturer advises to take the syringe out of the refrigerator at least 30 minutes before administration, and to avoid injecting into areas of the skin that are tender, bruised, or affected by psoriasis. Patients may self-administer *Kyntheum®*, after appropriate training in subcutaneous injection technique.
- PRESCRIBING AND DISPENSING INFORMATION Brodalumab is a biological medicine. Biological medicines must be prescribed and dispensed by brand name, see *Biological medicines* and *Biosimilar medicines*, under Guidance on prescribing p. 1; manufacturer advises to record the brand name and batch number after each administration.
- HANDLING AND STORAGE Manufacturer advises store in a refrigerator (2–8°C) and protect from light—consult product literature for further information regarding storage outside refrigerator.
- PATIENT AND CARER ADVICE Manufacturer advises patients and their carers should be given training in subcutaneous injection technique. Manufacturer advises patients and their carers should seek medical advice if new or worsening symptoms of depression, suicidal ideation, or behaviour occur; they should also be advised to report signs and symptoms of infection.
- NATIONAL FUNDING/ACCESS DECISIONS

NICE decisions
▸ **Brodalumab for treating moderate to severe plaque psoriasis (March 2018)** NICE TA511
Brodalumab is recommended as an option for treating plaque psoriasis in adults, only if:
- the disease is severe, as defined by a total Psoriasis Area and Severity Index (PASI) of 10 or more and a Dermatology Life Quality Index (DLQI) of more than 10, **and**
- the disease has not responded to other systemic therapies, including ciclosporin, methotrexate and PUVA (psoralen and long-wave ultraviolet A radiation), or these options are contra-indicated or not tolerated, **and**
- the manufacturer provides the drug with the discount agreed in the patient access scheme.
Stop brodalumab at 12 weeks if the psoriasis has not responded adequately, defined as:
- a 75% reduction in the PASI score (PASI 75) from when treatment started, **or**
- a 50% reduction in the PASI score (PASI 50) and a 5-point reduction in DLQI from when treatment started.
Patients whose treatment was started within the NHS before this guidance was published should have the option to continue treatment, without change to their funding

arrangements, until they and their NHS clinician consider it appropriate to stop.
www.nice.org.uk/guidance/ta511

Scottish Medicines Consortium (SMC) Decisions
SMC No. 1283/17
The *Scottish Medicines Consortium* has advised (updated May 2018) that brodalumab (*Kyntheum®*) is accepted for restricted use within NHS Scotland for the treatment of moderate-to-severe plaque psoriasis in adults who have failed to respond to standard systemic therapies (including ciclosporin, methotrexate and phototherapy), are intolerant to, or have a contra-indication to these treatments. This advice is contingent upon the continuing availability of the patient access scheme in NHS Scotland or a list price that is equivalent or lower.

- MEDICINAL FORMS
There can be variation in the licensing of different medicines containing the same drug.
Solution for injection
▸ Kyntheum (LEO Pharma) ▼
Brodalumab 140 mg per 1 ml Kyntheum 210mg/1.5ml solution for injection pre-filled syringes | 2 pre-filled disposable injection [PoM] £1,280.00

Dupilumab   15-Jan-2018

- DRUG ACTION Dupilumab is a recombinant human monoclonal antibody that inhibits interleukin-4 and interleukin-13 signaling; these cytokines are involved in atopic eczema.

- INDICATIONS AND DOSE

Moderate-to-severe atopic eczema (specialist use only)
▸ BY SUBCUTANEOUS INJECTION
▸ Adult: Initially 600 mg, followed by 300 mg every 2 weeks, the initial dose should be administered as two consecutive 300 mg injections at different injection sites, review treatment if no response after 16 weeks

- CAUTIONS Asthma—consult product literature · helminth infection

CAUTIONS, FURTHER INFORMATION
▸ Helminth infection Dupilumab may influence the immune response to helminth infections. Resolve pre-existing infection before initiating treatment; suspend treatment if resistant infection develops during therapy.

- INTERACTIONS → Appendix 1: monoclonal antibodies
- SIDE-EFFECTS
  ▸ **Common or very common** Eosinophilia · eye inflammation · eye pruritus · headache · oral herpes
  ▸ **Rare or very rare** Serum sickness-like reaction
  SIDE-EFFECTS, FURTHER INFORMATION Side-effects reported with or without concomitant corticosteroids.
- PREGNANCY Manufacturer advises use only if potential benefit outweighs risk—limited information available.
- BREAST FEEDING Manufacturer advises avoid—no information available.
- DIRECTIONS FOR ADMINISTRATION Manufacturer advises to inject into the thigh or abdomen (except for the 5 cm around the navel), or upper arm (if not self-administered); rotate injection site and avoid skin that is tender, damaged or scarred. Patients may self-administer *Dupixent®* after appropriate training in preparation and administration.
- PRESCRIBING AND DISPENSING INFORMATION Manufacturer advises to record the brand name and batch number after each administration.
- HANDLING AND STORAGE Manufacturer advises store in a refrigerator (2–8°C); pre-filled syringes may be kept at room temperature (max. 25°C) for max. 14 days.

13

Skin

● MEDICINAL FORMS
There can be variation in the licensing of different medicines
containing the same drug.

Solution for injection
▸ Dupixent (Sanofi) ▼
Dupilumab 150 mg per 1 ml Dupixent 300mg/2ml solution for
injection pre-filled syringes | 2 pre-filled disposable injection PoM
£1,264.89

Guselkumab
26-Feb-2018

● DRUG ACTION Guselkumab is a recombinant human
monoclonal antibody that binds selectively to interleukin-
23 and blocks the activity of pro-inflammatory cytokines.

● INDICATIONS AND DOSE

Moderate-to-severe plaque psoriasis (specialist use only)
▸ BY SUBCUTANEOUS INJECTION
▸ Adult: Initially 100 mg, then 100 mg after 4 weeks, then
maintenance 100 mg every 8 weeks, consider
discontinuation if no response after 16 weeks

● CONTRA-INDICATIONS Clinically significant active
infection

● CAUTIONS Risk of infection
CAUTIONS, FURTHER INFORMATION
▸ Risk of infection Manufacturer advises consider anti-
tuberculosis therapy before initiation of guselkumab in
patients with a past history of latent or active tuberculosis
in whom an adequate course of treatment cannot be
confirmed.
     Manufacturer advises consider completion of
appropriate immunisations according to current
guidelines before initiating treatment (consult product
literature for appropriate interval between vaccination and
administration of guselkumab).

● INTERACTIONS → Appendix 1: monoclonal antibodies

● SIDE-EFFECTS
▸ **Common or very common** Arthralgia · diarrhoea · headache ·
increased risk of infection · urticaria

● CONCEPTION AND CONTRACEPTION Manufacturer advises
effective contraception in women of childbearing potential
during treatment and for at least 12 weeks after treatment.

● PREGNANCY Manufacturer advises avoid—no information
available.

● BREAST FEEDING Manufacturer advises avoid during
treatment and for up to 12 weeks after discontinuing
treatment—no information available.

● PRE-TREATMENT SCREENING Manufacturer advises that
patients should be evaluated for tuberculosis infection
before treatment.

● MONITORING REQUIREMENTS Manufacturer advises
monitor for signs and symptoms of active tuberculosis
during and after treatment.

● DIRECTIONS FOR ADMINISTRATION Manufacturer advises
to avoid injecting into areas of the skin that show
psoriasis. Patients may self-administer *Tremfya*®, after
appropriate training in subcutaneous injection technique.

● PRESCRIBING AND DISPENSING INFORMATION
Manufacturer advises to record the brand name and batch
number after each administration.

● HANDLING AND STORAGE Manufacturer advises store in a
refrigerator (2–8°C) and protect from light.

● PATIENT AND CARER ADVICE Manufacturer advises
patients and their carers should be advised to seek medical
attention if signs or symptoms of infection occur (monitor
closely and suspend treatment if infection is clinically
significant or unresponsive to treatment).

Self-administration Manufacturer advises patients may self-
administer following training in subcutaneous injection
technique.

● MEDICINAL FORMS
There can be variation in the licensing of different medicines
containing the same drug.

Solution for injection
▸ Tremfya (Janssen-Cilag Ltd) ▼
Guselkumab 100 mg per 1 ml Tremfya 100mg/1ml solution for
injection pre-filled syringes | 1 pre-filled disposable injection PoM
£2,250.00

Ixekizumab
26-Jun-2017

● DRUG ACTION Ixekizumab is a human monoclonal
antibody that binds to interleukin-17A and inhibits the
release of pro-inflammatory cytokines and chemokines.

● INDICATIONS AND DOSE

**Moderate-to-severe plaque psoriasis (under expert
supervision) | Psoriatic arthritis with concomitant
moderate-to-severe plaque psoriasis (under expert
supervision)**
▸ BY SUBCUTANEOUS INJECTION
▸ Adult: Initially 160 mg for 1 dose, followed by 80 mg
after 2 weeks, then 80 mg every 2 weeks for 5 further
doses (at weeks 4, 6, 8, 10 and 12), then maintenance
80 mg every 4 weeks, consider discontinuation of
treatment if no response after 16–20 weeks

Psoriatic arthritis (under expert supervision)
▸ BY SUBCUTANEOUS INJECTION
▸ Adult: Initially 160 mg for 1 dose, then maintenance
80 mg every 4 weeks, consider discontinuation of
treatment if no response after 16–20 weeks

● CONTRA-INDICATIONS Active infections (including active
tuberculosis)

● CAUTIONS Chronic infection—monitor carefully and
discontinue if serious, unresponsive infection develops ·
Crohn's disease · ulcerative colitis
CAUTIONS, FURTHER INFORMATION
▸ Severe hypersensitivity reactions Severe hypersensitivity
reactions have been reported—discontinue treatment
immediately if symptoms occur.
▸ Latent tuberculosis Manufacturer advises that patients with
latent tuberculosis should complete anti-tuberculosis
therapy before starting ixekizumab.
▸ Inflammatory bowel disease Manufacturer advises to monitor
closely for exacerbation.

● INTERACTIONS → Appendix 1: monoclonal antibodies

● SIDE-EFFECTS
▸ **Common or very common** Increased risk of infection ·
nausea · oropharyngeal pain
▸ **Uncommon** Conjunctivitis · neutropenia · skin reactions ·
thrombocytopenia
▸ **Frequency not known** Angioedema · dyspnoea ·
hypersensitivity (occasionally late-onset) · inflammatory
bowel disease

● CONCEPTION AND CONTRACEPTION Manufacturer advises
effective contraception during treatment and for at least
10 weeks after treatment in women of childbearing
potential.

● PREGNANCY Manufacturer advises avoid—limited
information available.

● BREAST FEEDING Manufacturer advises avoid—present in
milk in *animal* studies.

● DIRECTIONS FOR ADMINISTRATION Manufacturer advises
to avoid injecting into areas of the skin that show
psoriasis; injection sites may be alternated. Patients may

self-administer *Taltz*®, after appropriate training in subcutaneous injection technique.

- HANDLING AND STORAGE Manufacturer advises store in a refrigerator (2–8°C).
- PATIENT AND CARER ADVICE
Self-administration If appropriate, patients and their carers should be given training in subcutaneous injection technique.
- NATIONAL FUNDING/ACCESS DECISIONS
NICE decisions
▶ **Ixekizumab for treating moderate to severe plaque psoriasis (April 2017)** NICE TA442
Ixekizumab is recommended as an option for treating plaque psoriasis only if:

- the disease is severe, defined by a total Psoriasis Area and Severity Index (PASI) of 10 or more and a Dermatology Life Quality Index (DLQI) of 10 or more;
- the disease has not responded to standard systemic therapies (e.g. ciclosporin, methotrexate and PUVA) or these treatments are contra-indicated or not tolerated, **and**
- the manufacturer provides ixekizumab with the discount agreed in the patient access scheme

Ixekizumab should be discontinued if there is an inadequate response at 12 weeks.

Patients currently receiving ixekizumab, whose disease does not meet the above criteria, should have the option to continue treatment until they and their clinician consider it appropriate to stop.
www.nice.org.uk/guidance/TA442

Scottish Medicines Consortium (SMC) Decisions
The *Scottish Medicines Consortium* has advised (April 2017) that ixekizumab (*Taltz*®) is accepted for restricted use within NHS Scotland for the treatment of moderate-to-severe plaque psoriasis only in patients who have failed to respond to standard systemic therapies (including ciclosporin, methotrexate and phototherapy), are intolerant to, or have a contra-indication to these treatments. This advice is contingent upon the continuing availability of the patient access scheme in NHS Scotland, or a list price that is equivalent or lower.

- MEDICINAL FORMS
There can be variation in the licensing of different medicines containing the same drug.
Solution for injection
EXCIPIENTS: May contain Polysorbates
▶ Taltz (Eli Lilly and Company Ltd) ▼
Ixekizumab 80 mg per 1 ml Taltz 80mg/1ml solution for injection pre-filled syringes | 1 pre-filled disposable injection [PoM] £1,125.00 (Hospital only)
Taltz 80mg/1ml solution for injection pre-filled pen | 1 pre-filled disposable injection [PoM] £1,125.00 (Hospital only)

RETINOID AND RELATED DRUGS

Acitretin

- DRUG ACTION Acitretin is a metabolite of etretinate.

- INDICATIONS AND DOSE
Severe extensive psoriasis resistant to other forms of therapy (under expert supervision) | Palmoplantar pustular psoriasis (under expert supervision) | Severe congenital ichthyosis (under expert supervision)
▶ BY MOUTH
▶ Adult: Initially 25–30 mg daily for 2–4 weeks, then adjusted according to response to 25–50 mg daily, increased to up to 75 mg daily, dose only increased to 75 mg daily for short periods in psoriasis

Severe Darier's disease (keratosis follicularis) (under expert supervision)
▶ BY MOUTH
▶ Adult: Initially 10 mg daily for 2–4 weeks, then adjusted according to response to 25–50 mg daily

- CONTRA-INDICATIONS Hyperlipidaemia
- CAUTIONS Avoid excessive exposure to sunlight and unsupervised use of sunlamps · diabetes (can alter glucose tolerance—initial frequent blood glucose checks) · do not donate blood during and for 2 years after stopping therapy (teratogenic risk) · in children use only in exceptional circumstances and monitor growth parameters and bone development (premature epiphyseal closure reported) · investigate atypical musculoskeletal symptoms
- INTERACTIONS → Appendix 1: retinoids
- SIDE-EFFECTS
▶ **Common or very common** Abdominal pain · arthralgia · brittle nails · conjunctivitis · diarrhoea · dry mouth · gastrointestinal disorder · haemorrhage · hair texture abnormal · headache · increased risk of infection · mucosal abnormalities · myalgia · nausea · oral disorders · peripheral oedema · skin reactions · thirst · vomiting · xerophthalmia
▶ **Uncommon** Dizziness · hepatic disorders · photosensitivity reaction · vision disorders
▶ **Rare or very rare** Bone pain · exostosis · idiopathic intracranial hypertension · peripheral neuropathy
▶ **Frequency not known** Angioedema · capillary leak syndrome · drowsiness · dysphonia · flushing · glucose tolerance impaired · granuloma · hearing impairment · hyperhidrosis · malaise · pyogenic granuloma · retinoic acid syndrome · taste altered

SIDE-EFFECTS, FURTHER INFORMATION
Exostosis Skeletal hyperostosis and extra-osseous calcification reported following long-term treatment with etretinate (of which acitretin is a metabolite) and premature epiphyseal closure in children.
Benign intracranial hypertension Discontinue if severe headache, nausea, vomiting, or visual disturbances occur.

- CONCEPTION AND CONTRACEPTION Effective contraception must be used.
Pregnancy prevention In females of child-bearing potential (including those with a history of infertility), exclude pregnancy up to 3 days before treatment, every month during treatment, and every 1–3 months for 3 years after stopping treatment. Treatment should be started on day 2 or 3 of menstrual cycle. Females of child-bearing age must practise effective contraception for at least 1 month before starting treatment, during treatment, and for at least 3 years after stopping treatment. Females should be advised to use at least 1 method of contraception, but ideally they should use 2 methods of contraception. Oral progestogen-only contraceptives are not considered effective. Barrier methods should not be used alone but can be used in conjunction with other contraceptive methods. Females should be advised to seek medical attention immediately if they become pregnant during treatment or within 3 years of stopping treatment. They should also be advised to avoid alcohol during treatment and for 2 months after stopping treatment.
- PREGNANCY Avoid—teratogenic.
- BREAST FEEDING Avoid.
- HEPATIC IMPAIRMENT Avoid in severe impairment—risk of further impairment.
- RENAL IMPAIRMENT Avoid in severe impairment; increased risk of toxicity.
- MONITORING REQUIREMENTS
▶ Monitor serum-triglyceride and serum-cholesterol concentrations before treatment, 1 month after starting, then every 3 months.

13

Skin

▶ Check liver function at start, then every 2–4 weeks for first 2 months and then every 3 months.

● PRESCRIBING AND DISPENSING INFORMATION
Prescribing for women of child-bearing potential Each prescription for acitretin should be limited to a supply of up to 30 days' treatment and dispensed within 7 days of the date stated on the prescription.

● PATIENT AND CARER ADVICE Females of child-bearing potential must be advised on pregnancy prevention.
A patient information leaflet should be provided.

● MEDICINAL FORMS
There can be variation in the licensing of different medicines containing the same drug. Forms available from special-order manufacturers include: oral suspension, oral solution

Capsule

CAUTIONARY AND ADVISORY LABELS 10, 11, 21
▶ Acitretin (Non-proprietary)
Acitretin 10 mg Acitretin 10mg capsules | 60 capsule [PoM] £23.80 DT = £23.80
Acitretin 25 mg Acitretin 25mg capsules | 60 capsule [PoM] £55.24 DT = £55.24
▶ Neotigason (Teva UK Ltd)
Acitretin 10 mg Neotigason 10mg capsules | 60 capsule [PoM] £17.30 DT = £23.80
Acitretin 25 mg Neotigason 25mg capsules | 60 capsule [PoM] £43.00 DT = £55.24

Alitretinoin

● INDICATIONS AND DOSE
Severe chronic hand eczema refractory to potent topical corticosteroids
▶ BY MOUTH
▶ Adult (prescribed by or under supervision of a consultant dermatologist): 30 mg once daily; reduced if not tolerated to 10 mg once daily for 12–24 weeks total duration of treatment, discontinue if no response after 12 weeks, course may be repeated in those who relapse

Severe chronic hand eczema refractory to potent topical corticosteroids in patients with diabetes, history of hyperlipidaemia, or risk factors for cardiovascular disease
▶ BY MOUTH
▶ Adult (prescribed by or under supervision of a consultant dermatologist): Initially 10 mg once daily, increased if necessary up to 30 mg once daily for 12–24 weeks total duration of treatment, discontinue if no response after 12 weeks, course may be repeated in those who relapse

DOSE ADJUSTMENTS DUE TO INTERACTIONS
▶ Manufacturer advises reduce dose to 10 mg once daily with concurrent use of potent inhibitors of CYP3A4, CYP2C8 and moderate inhibitors of CYP2C9.

● CONTRA-INDICATIONS Hypervitaminosis A · uncontrolled hyperlipidaemia · uncontrolled hypothyroidism

● CAUTIONS Avoid blood donation during treatment and for at least 1 month after stopping treatment · dry eye syndrome · history of depression

● INTERACTIONS → Appendix 1: retinoids

● SIDE-EFFECTS
▶ **Common or very common** Alopecia · anaemia · conjunctivitis · depression · dizziness · dry eye · dry mouth · eye irritation · fatigue · flushing · headache · hypercholesterolaemia · hypertension · hypertriglyceridaemia (risk of pancreatitis if triglycerides above 9mmol/litre) · joint disorders · myalgia · nausea · oral disorders · skin reactions · tinnitus · vomiting
▶ **Uncommon** Bone disorders · cataract · dyspepsia · epistaxis · vision disorders
▶ **Rare or very rare** Idiopathic intracranial hypertension · nail disorder · photosensitivity reaction · vasculitis

▶ **Frequency not known** Inflammatory bowel disease · mood altered · peripheral oedema · suicidal ideation
SIDE-EFFECTS, FURTHER INFORMATION
Dry eyes Dry eyes may respond to lubricating eye ointment or tear replacement therapy.
Benign intracranial hypertension Discontinue treatment if headache, nausea, vomiting, papilloedema, or visual disturbances occur.

● CONCEPTION AND CONTRACEPTION Effective contraception must be used.
Pregnancy prevention In women of child-bearing potential, exclude pregnancy 1 month before treatment, up to 3 days before treatment, every month during treatment (unless there are compelling reasons to indicate that there is no risk of pregnancy), and 5 weeks after stopping treatment—perform pregnancy test in the first 3 days of the menstrual cycle.
Women must practise effective contraception for at least 1 month before starting treatment, during treatment, and for at least 1 month after stopping treatment. Women should be advised to use at least 1 method of contraception but ideally they should use 2 methods of contraception. Oral progestogen-only contraceptives are not considered effective. Barrier methods should not be used alone but can be used in conjunction with other contraceptive methods.
Women should be advised to discontinue treatment and to seek prompt medical attention if they become pregnant during treatment or within 1 month of stopping treatment.

● PREGNANCY Avoid—teratogenic.

● BREAST FEEDING Manufacturer advises avoid.

● HEPATIC IMPAIRMENT Manufacturer advises avoid—no information available.

● RENAL IMPAIRMENT Manufacturer advises avoid in severe impairment—no information available.

● MONITORING REQUIREMENTS Monitor serum lipids (more frequently in those with diabetes, history of hyperlipidaemia, or risk factors for cardiovascular disease)—discontinue if uncontrolled hyperlipidaemia.

● PRESCRIBING AND DISPENSING INFORMATION
Prescribing for women of child-bearing potential Each prescription for alitretinoin should be limited to a supply of up to 30 days' treatment and dispensed within 7 days of the date stated on the prescription.
Alitretinoin is **teratogenic** and must **not** be given to women of child-bearing potential unless they practise effective contraception and then only after detailed assessment and explanation by the physician.

● PATIENT AND CARER ADVICE A patient information leaflet should be provided.
Conception and contraception Women of child-bearing potential must be counselled on pregnancy prevention.

● NATIONAL FUNDING/ACCESS DECISIONS
NICE decisions
▶ **Alitretinoin for the treatment of severe chronic hand eczema in adults (August 2009) NICE TA177**
Alitretinoin is recommended for the treatment of severe chronic hand eczema that has not responded to potent topical corticosteroids. Treatment should be stopped as soon as an adequate response has been achieved (hands clear or almost clear), or if the eczema remains severe after 12 weeks, or if an adequate response has not been achieved by 24 weeks.
www.nice.org.uk/TA177

- **MEDICINAL FORMS**
There can be variation in the licensing of different medicines containing the same drug.

Capsule

CAUTIONARY AND ADVISORY LABELS 10, 11, 21
▸ Toctino (Stiefel Laboratories (UK) Ltd)
Alitretinoin 10 mg Toctino 10mg capsules | 30 capsule [PoM]
£411.43
Alitretinoin 30 mg Toctino 30mg capsules | 30 capsule [PoM]
£411.43

| Tazarotene

- **INDICATIONS AND DOSE**

Mild to moderate plaque psoriasis affecting up to 10% of skin area

▸ TO THE SKIN
▸ Adult: Apply once daily usually for up to 12 weeks, apply in the evening

- **CAUTIONS** Avoid contact with eczematous skin · avoid contact with eyes · avoid contact with face · avoid contact with hair-covered scalp · avoid contact with inflamed skin · avoid contact with intertriginous areas
- **INTERACTIONS** → Appendix 1: retinoids
- **SIDE-EFFECTS**
▸ **Common or very common** Paraesthesia · skin reactions · stinging
SIDE-EFFECTS, FURTHER INFORMATION Local irritation is more common with higher concentration and may require treatment interruption.
- **CONCEPTION AND CONTRACEPTION** Effective contraception required (oral progestogen-only contraceptives not considered effective).
- **PREGNANCY** Avoid.
- **BREAST FEEDING** Manufacturer advises avoid—present in milk in *animal* studies.
- **PATIENT AND CARER ADVICE** Avoid excessive exposure to UV light (including sunlight, solariums, PUVA or UVB treatment). Do not apply emollients or cosmetics within 1 hour of application. Wash hands immediately after use.
- **MEDICINAL FORMS**
There can be variation in the licensing of different medicines containing the same drug.

Gel

EXCIPIENTS: May contain Benzyl alcohol, butylated hydroxyanisole, butylated hydroxytoluene, disodium edetate, polysorbates
▸ Zorac (Allergan Ltd)
Tazarotene 500 microgram per 1 gram Zorac 0.05% gel | 30 gram [PoM] £14.09 DT = £14.09
Tazarotene 1 mg per 1 gram Zorac 0.1% gel | 30 gram [PoM] £14.80 DT = £14.80

SALICYLIC ACID AND DERIVATIVES

| Salicylic acid with zinc oxide

- **INDICATIONS AND DOSE**

Hyperkeratotic skin disorders

▸ TO THE SKIN
▸ Adult: Apply twice daily

- **CAUTIONS** Avoid broken skin · avoid inflamed skin
CAUTIONS, FURTHER INFORMATION
▸ **Salicylate toxicity** Salicylate toxicity may occur particularly if applied on large areas of skin or neonatal skin.
- **SIDE-EFFECTS** Skin reactions
- **PRESCRIBING AND DISPENSING INFORMATION** Zinc and Salicylic Acid Paste BP is also referred to as Lassar's Paste. When prepared extemporaneously, the BP states Zinc and

Salicylic Acid Paste, BP (Lassar's Paste) consists of zinc oxide 24%, salicylic acid 2%, starch 24%, white soft paraffin 50%.

- **MEDICINAL FORMS**
Forms available from special-order manufacturers include: paste

VITAMINS AND TRACE ELEMENTS > VITAMIN D AND ANALOGUES

| Calcipotriol

- **INDICATIONS AND DOSE**

Plaque psoriasis

▸ TO THE SKIN USING OINTMENT
▸ Adult: Apply 1–2 times a day, when preparations are used together maximum total calcipotriol 5 mg in any one week (e.g. scalp solution 60 mL with ointment 30 g or scalp solution 30 mL with ointment 60 g); maximum 100 g per week

Scalp psoriasis

▸ TO THE SKIN USING SCALP LOTION
▸ Adult: Apply twice daily, when preparations are used together maximum total calcipotriol 5 mg in any one week (e.g. scalp solution 60 mL with ointment 30 g or scalp solution 30 mL with ointment 60 g); maximum 60 mL per week

- **CONTRA-INDICATIONS** Calcium metabolism disorders
- **CAUTIONS** Avoid excessive exposure to sunlight and sunlamps · avoid use on face · erythrodermic exfoliative psoriasis (enhanced risk of hypercalcaemia) · generalised pustular psoriasis (enhanced risk of hypercalcaemia)
- **INTERACTIONS** → Appendix 1: vitamin D substances
- **SIDE-EFFECTS**
▸ **Common or very common** Skin reactions
▸ **Uncommon** Increased risk of infection
▸ **Rare or very rare** Hypercalcaemia · hypercalciuria · photosensitivity reaction
- **PREGNANCY** Manufacturers advise avoid unless essential.
- **BREAST FEEDING** No information available.
- **PATIENT AND CARER ADVICE**

Advice on application Patient information leaflet for *Dovonex®* ointment advises liberal application. However, patients should be advised of maximum recommended weekly dose.

Hands should be washed thoroughly after application to avoid inadvertent transfer to other body areas.

- **MEDICINAL FORMS**
There can be variation in the licensing of different medicines containing the same drug. Forms available from special-order manufacturers include: ointment

Ointment

EXCIPIENTS: May contain Disodium edetate, propylene glycol
▸ Calcipotriol (Non-proprietary)
Calcipotriol 50 microgram per 1 gram Calcipotriol 50micrograms/g ointment | 30 gram [PoM] £5.78 DT = £5.78 | 60 gram [PoM] £11.56–£13.86 | 120 gram [PoM] £23.12–£27.72
▸ Dovonex (LEO Pharma)
Calcipotriol 50 microgram per 1 gram Dovonex 50micrograms/g ointment | 30 gram [PoM] £5.78 DT = £5.78 | 60 gram [PoM] £11.56

Liquid

▸ Calcipotriol (Non-proprietary)
Calcipotriol (as Calcipotriol hydrate) 50 microgram per 1 ml Calcipotriol 50micrograms/ml scalp solution | 60 ml [PoM] £56.94 DT = £56.94 | 120 ml [PoM] £113.88 DT = £113.88

Combinations available: *Calcipotriol with betamethasone,* p. 1209

13

Skin

Calcitriol

(1,25-Dihydroxycholecalciferol)

● **INDICATIONS AND DOSE**
Mild to moderate plaque psoriasis
▶ TO THE SKIN
▶ Adult: Apply twice daily, not more than 35% of body surface to be treated daily; maximum 30 g per day

● CONTRA-INDICATIONS Do not apply under occlusion · patients with calcium metabolism disorders
● CAUTIONS Erythrodermic exfoliative psoriasis (enhanced risk of hypercalcaemia) · generalised pustular psoriasis (enhanced risk of hypercalcaemia)
● INTERACTIONS → Appendix 1: vitamin D substances
● SIDE-EFFECTS
▶ **Common or very common** Skin reactions
● PREGNANCY Manufacturer advises use in restricted amounts only if clearly necessary.
Monitoring Monitor urine- and serum-calcium concentration in pregnancy.
● BREAST FEEDING Manufacturer advises avoid.
● HEPATIC IMPAIRMENT Manufacturer advises avoid—no information available.
● RENAL IMPAIRMENT Manufacturer advises avoid—no information available.
● HANDLING AND STORAGE Hands should be washed thoroughly after application to avoid inadvertent transfer to other body areas.

● MEDICINAL FORMS
There can be variation in the licensing of different medicines containing the same drug.
Ointment
▶ Silkis (Galderma (UK) Ltd)
Calcitriol 3 microgram per 1 gram Silkis ointment | 100 gram [PoM] £18.06 DT = £18.06

Tacalcitol

● **INDICATIONS AND DOSE**
Plaque psoriasis
▶ TO THE SKIN
▶ Adult: Apply once daily, preferably at bedtime, maximum 10 g ointment or 10 mL lotion daily, when lotion and ointment used together, maximum total tacalcitol 280 micrograms in any one week (e.g. lotion 30 mL with ointment 40 g)

● CONTRA-INDICATIONS Calcium metabolism disorders
● CAUTIONS Avoid eyes · erythrodermic exfoliative psoriasis (enhanced risk of hypercalcaemia) · generalised pustular psoriasis (enhanced risk of hypercalcaemia) · if used in conjunction with UV treatment
CAUTIONS, FURTHER INFORMATION
▶ UV treatment If tacalcitol is used in conjunction with UV treatment, UV radiation should be given in the morning and tacalcitol applied at bedtime.
● INTERACTIONS → Appendix 1: vitamin D substances
● SIDE-EFFECTS
▶ **Uncommon** Skin reactions
▶ **Frequency not known** Hypercalcaemia
● PREGNANCY Manufacturer advises avoid unless no safer alternative—no information available.
● BREAST FEEDING Manufacturer advises avoid application to breast area; no information available on presence in milk.

● MONITORING REQUIREMENTS Monitor serum calcium if risk of hypercalcaemia.
● PATIENT AND CARER ADVICE Hands should be washed thoroughly after application to avoid inadvertent transfer to other body areas.

● MEDICINAL FORMS
There can be variation in the licensing of different medicines containing the same drug.
Ointment
▶ Curatoderm (Almirall Ltd)
Tacalcitol (as Tacalcitol monohydrate) 4 microgram per 1 gram Curatoderm 4micrograms/g ointment | 30 gram [PoM] £13.40 DT = £13.40 | 100 gram [PoM] £30.86 DT = £30.86
Liquid
EXCIPIENTS: May contain Disodium edetate, propylene glycol
▶ Curatoderm (Almirall Ltd)
Tacalcitol (as Tacalcitol monohydrate) 4 microgram per 1 gram Curatoderm 4micrograms/g lotion | 30 ml [PoM] £12.73

4   Perspiration
4.1   Hyperhidrosis

Hyperhidrosis

16-May-2017

Overview

Aluminium chloride hexahydrate p. 1229 is a potent antiperspirant used in the treatment of hyperhidrosis. Aluminium salts are also incorporated in preparations used for minor fungal skin infections associated with hyperhidrosis.

Limited evidence suggests that oxybutynin hydrochloride p. 760 [unlicensed indication] can be used to treat hyperhidrosis in patients whose symptoms are not adequately managed through lifestyle modifications and antiperspirants.

In more severe cases specialists use glycopyrronium bromide below as a 0.05% solution in the iontophoretic treatment of hyperhidrosis of plantar and palmar areas. *Botox*® contains botulinum toxin type A complex p. 403 and is licensed for use intradermally for severe hyperhidrosis of the axillae unresponsive to topical antiperspirant or other antihidrotic treatment.

ANTIMUSCARINICS

Glycopyrronium bromide

F 759

13-Sep-2017

(Glycopyrrolate)

● **INDICATIONS AND DOSE**
Iontophoretic treatment of hyperhidrosis
▶ TO THE SKIN
▶ Adult: Only 1 site to be treated at a time, maximum 2 sites treated in any 24 hours, treatment not to be repeated within 7 days (consult product literature)

● CONTRA-INDICATIONS Infections affecting the treatment site
CONTRA-INDICATIONS, FURTHER INFORMATION Contra-indications applicable to systemic use should be considered; however, glycopyrronium is poorly absorbed and systemic effects unlikely with topical use.
● CAUTIONS Cautions applicable to systemic use should be considered; however, glycopyrronium is poorly absorbed and systemic effects unlikely with topical use.
● SIDE-EFFECTS Abdominal discomfort · eating disorder · pain · paraesthesia · urinary disorder

SIDE-EFFECTS, FURTHER INFORMATION The possibility of systemic side-effects should be considered; however, glycopyrronium is poorly absorbed and systemic effects are unlikely with topical use.

● MEDICINAL FORMS
There can be variation in the licensing of different medicines containing the same drug.
Powder for solution for iontophoresis
▸ Glycopyrronium bromide (Non-proprietary)
Glycopyrronium bromide 1 mg per 1 mg Glycopyrronium bromide powder for solution for iontophoresis | 3 gram PoM £327.00

DERMATOLOGICAL DRUGS 〉 ASTRINGENTS

Aluminium chloride hexahydrate

● INDICATIONS AND DOSE
Hyperhidrosis affecting axillae, hands or feet
▸ TO THE SKIN
▸ Adult: Apply once daily, apply liquid formulation at night to dry skin, wash off the following morning, reduce frequency as condition improves—do not bathe immediately before use

Hyperhidrosis | Bromidrosis | Intertrigo | Prevention of tinea pedis and related conditions
▸ TO THE SKIN
▸ Adult: Apply powder to dry skin

● CAUTIONS Avoid contact with eyes · avoid contact with mucous membranes · avoid use on broken or irritated skin · do not shave axillae or use depilatories within 12 hours of application
● SIDE-EFFECTS Skin reactions
● PATIENT AND CARER ADVICE Avoid contact with clothing.
● EXCEPTIONS TO LEGAL CATEGORY A 30 mL pack of aluminium chloride hexahydrate 20% is on sale to the public.

● MEDICINAL FORMS
There can be variation in the licensing of different medicines containing the same drug.
Liquid
CAUTIONARY AND ADVISORY LABELS 15
▸ Aluminium chloride hexahydrate (Non-proprietary)
Aluminium chloride 200 mg per 1 ml Aluminium chloride 20% solution | 60 ml P ⊠ DT = £2.51
▸ Anhydrol (Dermal Laboratories Ltd)
Aluminium chloride 200 mg per 1 ml Anhydrol Forte 20% solution | 60 ml P £2.51 DT = £2.51
▸ Driclor (GlaxoSmithKline Consumer Healthcare)
Aluminium chloride 200 mg per 1 ml Driclor 20% solution | 75 ml P £3.01 DT = £3.01

5 Pruritus

Topical local antipruritics

Overview

Pruritus may be caused by systemic disease (such as obstructive jaundice, endocrine disease, chronic renal disease, iron deficiency, and certain malignant diseases), skin disease (e.g. psoriasis, eczema, urticaria, and scabies), drug hypersensitivity, or as a side-effect of opioid analgesics. Where possible, the underlying causes should be treated. An emollient may be of value where the pruritus is associated with dry skin. Pruritus that occurs in otherwise healthy elderly people can also be treated with an emollient. Levomenthol cream p. 1230 can be used to relieve pruritus; it

exerts a cooling effect on the skin. Local antipruritics have a role in the treatment of pruritus in palliative care.

Preparations containing crotamiton p. 1230 are sometimes used but are of uncertain value. Preparations containing calamine are often ineffective.

A topical preparation containing doxepin 5% p. 1230 is licensed for the relief of pruritus in eczema; it can cause drowsiness and there may be a risk of sensitisation.

Pruritus is common in biliary obstruction, especially in primary biliary cirrhosis and drug-induced cholestasis. Oral administration of colestyramine p. 196 is the treatment of choice.

Topical antihistamines and local anaesthetics are only marginally effective and occasionally cause hypersensitivity. For *insect stings* and *insect bites*, a short course of a topical corticosteroid is appropriate. Short-term treatment with a **sedating antihistamine** may help in insect stings and in intractable pruritus where sedation is desirable. Calamine preparations are of little value for the treatment of insect stings or bites.

Topical local anaesthetics are indicated for the relief of local pain. Preparations may be absorbed, especially through mucosal surfaces, therefore excessive application should be avoided and they should preferably not be used for more than 3 days; not generally suitable for young children and are less suitable for prescribing.

Topical antihistamines should be avoided in eczema and are not recommended for longer than 3 days. They are less suitable for prescribing.

> **Other drugs used for Pruritus** Alimemazine tartrate, p. 282 · Cetirizine hydrochloride, p. 279 · Chlorphenamine maleate, p. 283 · Coal tar with calamine, p. 1220 · Hydroxyzine hydrochloride, p. 284 · Levocetirizine hydrochloride, p. 280

ANTIPRURITICS

Calamine with zinc oxide   31-Aug-2016

● INDICATIONS AND DOSE
Pruritus
▸ TO THE SKIN
▸ Child: (consult product literature)
▸ Adult: (consult product literature)

IMPORTANT SAFETY INFORMATION
MHRA/CHM UPDATE (APRIL 2016): FIRE RISK WITH PARAFFIN-BASED SKIN EMOLLIENTS ON DRESSINGS OR CLOTHING
See Emollient and barrier preparations p. 1186.

● CONTRA-INDICATIONS Avoid application of preparations containing zinc oxide prior to x-ray (zinc oxide may affect outcome of x-ray)
● LESS SUITABLE FOR PRESCRIBING Less suitable for prescribing.

● MEDICINAL FORMS
There can be variation in the licensing of different medicines containing the same drug.
Cream
CAUTIONARY AND ADVISORY LABELS 15
▸ Calamine with zinc oxide (Non-proprietary)
Phenoxyethanol 5 mg per 1 gram, Zinc oxide 30 mg per 1 gram, Calamine 40 mg per 1 gram, Cetomacrogol emulsifying wax 50 mg per 1 gram, Liquid paraffin 200 mg per 1 gram Aqueous calamine cream | 100 gram GSL £1.43 DT = £1.43
▸ Cala Soothe (Ennogen Healthcare Ltd)
Phenoxyethanol 5 mg per 1 gram, Zinc oxide 30 mg per 1 gram, Calamine 40 mg per 1 gram, Cetomacrogol emulsifying wax 50 mg per 1 gram, Self-emulsifying glyceryl monostearate 50 mg

13

Skin

per 1 gram, Liquid paraffin 200 mg per 1 gram Cala Soothe cream | 100 ml £18.80

Liquid

▸ Calamine with zinc oxide (Non-proprietary)
Phenol liquefied 5 mg per 1 ml, Sodium citrate 5 mg per 1 ml, Bentonite 30 mg per 1 ml, Glycerol 50 mg per 1 ml, Zinc oxide 50 mg per 1 ml, Calamine 150 mg per 1 ml Calamine lotion | 200 ml GSL £0.94–£1.09 DT = £1.09

▸ Cala Soothe (Ennogen Healthcare Ltd)
Phenol liquefied 5 mg per 1 ml, Sodium citrate 5 mg per 1 ml, Bentonite 30 mg per 1 ml, Glycerol 50 mg per 1 ml, Zinc oxide 50 mg per 1 ml, Calamine 150 mg per 1 ml Cala Soothe lotion | 200 ml £19.50 DT = £1.09

Crotamiton

● INDICATIONS AND DOSE

Pruritus (including pruritus after scabies)

▸ TO THE SKIN
▸ Child 1 month–2 years (on doctor's advice only): Apply once daily
▸ Child 3–17 years: Apply 2–3 times a day
▸ Adult: Apply 2–3 times a day

● CONTRA-INDICATIONS Acute exudative dermatoses

● CAUTIONS Avoid use in buccal mucosa · avoid use near eyes · avoid use on broken skin · avoid use on very inflamed skin · use on doctor's advice for children under 3 years

● PREGNANCY Manufacturer advises avoid, especially during the first trimester—no information available.

● BREAST FEEDING No information available; avoid application to nipple area.

● MEDICINAL FORMS
There can be variation in the licensing of different medicines containing the same drug.

Cream
EXCIPIENTS: May contain Beeswax, cetostearyl alcohol (including cetyl and stearyl alcohol), fragrances, hydroxybenzoates (parabens)

▸ Eurax (GlaxoSmithKline Consumer Healthcare)
Crotamiton 100 mg per 1 gram Eurax 10% cream | 30 gram GSL £2.50 DT = £2.50 | 100 gram GSL £4.35 DT = £4.35

Doxepin

● INDICATIONS AND DOSE

Pruritus in eczema

▸ TO THE SKIN
▸ Child 12–17 years: Apply up to 3 g 3–4 times a day, apply thinly; coverage should be less than 10% of body surface area; maximum 12 g per day
▸ Adult: Apply up to 3 g 3–4 times a day, apply thinly; coverage should be less than 10% of body surface area; maximum 12 g per day

● CAUTIONS Avoid application to large areas · cardiac arrhythmias · mania · severe heart disease · susceptibility to angle-closure glaucoma · urinary retention

● INTERACTIONS → Appendix 1: tricyclic antidepressants

● SIDE-EFFECTS Constipation · diarrhoea · dizziness · drowsiness · dry eye · dry mouth · dyspepsia · fever · headache · nausea · paraesthesia · skin reactions · suicidal tendencies · taste altered · urinary retention · vision blurred · vomiting

● PREGNANCY Manufacturer advises use only if potential benefit outweighs risk.

● BREAST FEEDING Manufacturer advises use only if potential benefit outweighs risk.

● HEPATIC IMPAIRMENT Manufacturer advises caution in severe liver disease.

● PATIENT AND CARER ADVICE A patient information leaflet should be provided.
Driving and skilled tasks Drowsiness may affect performance of skilled tasks (e.g. driving). Effects of alcohol enhanced.

● MEDICINAL FORMS
There can be variation in the licensing of different medicines containing the same drug.

Cream
CAUTIONARY AND ADVISORY LABELS 2, 10
EXCIPIENTS: May contain Benzyl alcohol

▸ Xepin (Cambridge Healthcare Supplies Ltd)
Doxepin hydrochloride 50 mg per 1 gram Xepin 5% cream | 30 gram PoM £11.70

MENTHOL AND DERIVATIVES

Levomenthol

● INDICATIONS AND DOSE

Pruritus

▸ TO THE SKIN
▸ Adult: Apply 1–2 times a day

● MEDICINAL FORMS
There can be variation in the licensing of different medicines containing the same drug. Forms available from special-order manufacturers include: cream

Cream

▸ AquaSoothe (Ennogen Healthcare Ltd)
Menthol 10 mg per 1 gram AquaSoothe 1% cream | 100 gram £3.70 DT = £3.97 | 500 gram £15.43 DT = £16.59
Menthol 20 mg per 1 gram AquaSoothe 2% cream | 50 gram £1.86 | 500 gram £15.43 DT = £16.97

▸ Arjun (Arjun Products Ltd)
Menthol 5 mg per 1 gram Arjun 0.5% cream | 500 gram £15.30 DT = £16.07
Menthol 10 mg per 1 gram Arjun 1% cream | 100 gram £3.25 DT = £3.97 | 500 gram £15.30 DT = £16.59
Menthol 20 mg per 1 gram Arjun 2% cream | 500 gram £15.30 DT = £16.97

▸ Dermacool (Pern Consumer Products Ltd)
Menthol 5 mg per 1 gram Dermacool 0.5% cream | 100 gram £3.85 | 500 gram £16.07 DT = £16.07
Menthol 10 mg per 1 gram Dermacool 1% cream | 100 gram £3.97 DT = £3.97 | 250 gram £8.99 | 500 gram £16.59 DT = £16.59
Menthol 20 mg per 1 gram Dermacool 2% cream | 100 gram £4.07 | 500 gram £16.97 DT = £16.97
Menthol 50 mg per 1 gram Dermacool 5% cream | 100 gram £4.69 | 500 gram £17.48

▸ Menthoderm (Derma UK Ltd)
Menthol 5 mg per 1 gram Menthoderm 0.5% cream | 100 gram £3.12 | 500 gram £14.59–£15.07 DT = £16.07
Menthol 10 mg per 1 gram Menthoderm 1% cream | 100 gram £3.20 DT = £3.97 | 500 gram £14.79–£15.59 DT = £16.59
Menthol 20 mg per 1 gram Menthoderm 2% cream | 100 gram £3.85 | 500 gram £14.99–£15.97 DT = £16.97

6 Rosacea and acne

Rosacea and Acne

Acne

Treatment of acne should be commenced early to prevent scarring. Patients should be counselled that an improvement may not be seen for at least a couple of months. The choice of treatment depends on whether the acne is predominantly inflammatory or comedonal and its severity.

Mild to moderate acne is generally treated with topical preparations. Systemic treatment with oral antibacterials is generally used for *moderate to severe acne* or where topical preparations are not tolerated or are ineffective or where application to the site is difficult. Another oral preparation used for acne is the hormone treatment co-cyprindiol p. 1232 (cyproterone acetate with ethinylestradiol); it is for women only.

Severe acne, acne unresponsive to prolonged courses of oral antibacterials, scarring, or acne associated with psychological problems calls for early referral to a consultant dermatologist who may prescribe isotretinoin p. 1234 for administration by mouth.

Acne: topical preparations

In mild to moderate acne, comedones and inflamed lesions respond well to benzoyl peroxide p. 1233 or to a topical retinoid. Alternatively, topical application of an antibacterial such as erythromycin p. 530 or clindamycin p. 1232 may be effective for inflammatory acne. If topical preparations prove inadequate, oral preparations may be needed.

Benzoyl peroxide and azelaic acid

Benzoyl peroxide is effective in mild to moderate acne. Both comedones and inflamed lesions respond well to benzoyl peroxide. The lower concentrations seem to be as effective as higher concentrations in reducing inflammation. It is usual to start with a lower strength and to increase the concentration of benzoyl peroxide gradually. Adverse effects include local skin irritation, particularly when therapy is initiated, but the scaling and redness often subside with treatment continued at a reduced frequency of application. If the acne does not respond after 2 months then use of a topical antibacterial should be considered.

Azelaic acid p. 1233 has antimicrobial and anticomedonal properties. It may be an alternative to benzoyl peroxide or to a topical retinoid for treating mild to moderate comedonal acne, particularly of the face. Some patients prefer azelaic acid because it is less likely to cause local irritation than benzoyl peroxide.

Topical antibacterials for acne

For many patients with mild to moderate inflammatory acne, topical antibacterials may be no more effective than topical benzoyl peroxide or tretinoin p. 914. Topical antibacterials are probably best reserved for patients who wish to avoid oral antibacterials or who cannot tolerate them. Topical preparations of erythromycin and clindamycin are effective for inflammatory acne. Topical antibacterials can produce mild irritation of the skin, and on rare occasions cause sensitisation; gastro-intestinal disturbances have been reported with topical clindamycin.

Antibacterial resistance of *Propionibacterium acnes* is increasing; there is cross-resistance between erythromycin and clindamycin. To avoid development of resistance:

- when possible use non-antibiotic antimicrobials (such as benzoyl peroxide or azelaic acid);
- avoid concomitant treatment with different oral and topical antibacterials;
- if a particular antibacterial is effective, use it for repeat courses if needed (short intervening courses of benzoyl peroxide or azelaic acid may eliminate any resistant propionibacteria);
- do not continue treatment for longer than necessary (however, treatment with a topical preparation should be continued for at least 6 months).

Some manufacturers of topical antibacterial preparations for acne advise that preparations containing alcohol are not suitable for use with benzoyl peroxide.

Topical retinoids and related preparations for acne

Topical tretinoin, its isomer isotretinoin, and adapalene p. 1234 (a retinoid-like drug), are useful for treating comedones and inflammatory lesions in mild to moderate acne. Several months of treatment may be needed to achieve an optimal response and the treatment should be continued

until no new lesions develop. Isotretinoin is given by mouth in severe acne.

Other topical preparations for acne

Preparations containing aluminium oxide are not considered beneficial in acne.

A topical preparation of nicotinamide p. 1237 is available for inflammatory acne.

Acne: oral preparations

Systemic antibacterial treatment is useful for inflammatory acne if topical treatment is not adequately effective or if it is inappropriate. Anticomedonal treatment (e.g. with topical benzoyl peroxide) may also be required.

Either oxytetracycline p. 557 or tetracycline p. 557 is usually given for acne. If there is no improvement after the first 3 months another oral antibacterial should be used. Maximum improvement usually occurs after 4 to 6 months but in more severe cases treatment may need to be continued for 2 years or longer.

Doxycycline p. 555 and lymecycline p. 556 are alternatives to tetracycline.

Although minocycline p. 556 is as effective as other tetracyclines for acne, it is associated with a greater risk of lupus erythematosus-like syndrome. Minocycline sometimes causes irreversible pigmentation; it is given in a once or twice daily dose.

Erythromycin in a twice daily dose is an alternative for the management of acne but *propionibacteria* strains resistant to erythromycin are becoming widespread and this may explain poor response.

Trimethoprim p. 563 may be used for acne resistant to other antibacterials [unlicensed indication]. Prolonged treatment with trimethoprim may depress haematopoiesis; it should generally be initiated by specialists.

Concomitant use of different topical and systemic antibacterials is undesirable owing to the increased likelihood of the development of bacterial resistance.

Hormone treatment for acne

Co-cyprindiol (cyproterone acetate with ethinylestradiol) contains an anti-androgen. It is licensed for use in women with moderate to severe acne that has not responded to topical therapy or oral antibacterials, and for moderately severe hirsutism. Although it is an effective hormonal contraceptive, it should not be used solely for contraception.

Improvement of acne with co-cyprindiol probably occurs because of decreased sebum secretion which is under androgen control. Some women with moderately severe hirsutism may also benefit because hair growth is also androgen-dependent.

Oral retinoid for acne

The retinoid isotretinoin reduces sebum secretion. It is used for the systemic treatment of nodulo-cystic and conglobate acne, severe acne, scarring, acne which has not responded to an adequate course of a systemic antibacterial, or acne which is associated with psychological problems. It is also useful in women who develop acne in the third or fourth decades of life, since late onset acne is frequently unresponsive to antibacterials.

Isotretinoin is a toxic drug that should be prescribed **only** by, or under the supervision of, a consultant dermatologist. It is given for at least 16 weeks; repeat courses are not normally required.

Side-effects of isotretinoin include severe dryness of the skin and mucous membranes, nose bleeds, and joint pains. The drug is **teratogenic** and must **not** be given to women of child-bearing age unless they practise effective contraception (oral progestogen-only contraceptives not considered effective) and then only after detailed assessment and explanation by the physician. Women must also be registered with a pregnancy prevention programme.

13

Skin

13

Skin

Although a causal link between isotretinoin p. 1234 use and psychiatric changes (including suicidal ideation) has not been established, the possibility should be considered before initiating treatment; if psychiatric changes occur during treatment, isotretinoin should be stopped, the prescriber informed, and specialist psychiatric advice should be sought.

Rosacea

Rosacea is not comedonal (but may exist with acne which may be comedonal). Brimonidine tartrate p. 1237 is licensed for the treatment of facial erythema in rosacea. The pustules and papules of rosacea respond to topical azelaic acid p. 1233, topical ivermectin p. 1237 or to topical metronidazole p. 1196. Alternatively oral administration of oxytetracycline p. 557 or tetracycline p. 557, or erythromycin p. 530, can be used; courses usually last 6–12 weeks and are repeated intermittently. Doxycycline p. 555 can be used [unlicensed indication] if oxytetracycline or tetracycline is inappropriate (e.g. in renal impairment). A modified-release preparation of doxycycline is licensed in low daily doses for the treatment of facial rosacea. Isotretinoin is occasionally given in refractory cases [unlicensed indication]. Camouflagers may be required for the redness.

6.1 Acne

ANTI-ANDROGENS

Co-cyprindiol

02-Mar-2017

● **INDICATIONS AND DOSE**

Moderate to severe acne in females of child-bearing age refractory to topical therapy or oral antibacterials | Moderately severe hirsutism

▶ BY MOUTH
▶ Females of childbearing potential: 1 tablet daily for 21 days, to be started on day 1 of menstrual cycle; subsequent courses repeated after a 7-day interval (during which withdrawal bleeding occurs), time to symptom remission, at least 3 months; review need for treatment regularly

● CONTRA-INDICATIONS Acute porphyrias p. 1025 · gallstones · heart disease associated with pulmonary hypertension or risk of embolus · history during pregnancy of cholestatic jaundice · history during pregnancy of chorea · history during pregnancy of pemphigoid gestationis · history during pregnancy of pruritus · history of breast cancer but can be used after 5 years if no evidence of disease and non-hormonal methods unacceptable · history of haemolytic uraemic syndrome · migraine with aura · personal history of venous or arterial thrombosis · presence or history of liver tumours · sclerosing treatment for varicose veins · severe or multiple risk factors for arterial disease or for venous thromboembolism · systemic lupus erythematosus with (or unknown) antiphospholipid antibodies · transient cerebral ischaemic attacks without headaches · undiagnosed vaginal bleeding

● CAUTIONS Active trophoblastic disease (until return to normal of urine- and plasma-gonadotrophin concentration)—seek specialist advice · arterial disease · gene mutations associated with breast cancer (e.g. BRCA 1) · history of severe depression especially if induced by hormonal contraceptive · hyperprolactinaemia—seek specialist advice · inflammatory bowel disease including Crohn's disease · migraine · personal or family history of hypertriglyceridaemia (increased risk of pancreatitis) · risk factors for venous thromboembolism · sickle-cell disease · undiagnosed breast mass

CAUTIONS, FURTHER INFORMATION
▶ Venous thromboembolism There is an increased risk of venous thromboembolism in women taking co-cyprindiol, particularly during the first year of use. The incidence of venous thromboembolism is 1.5–2 times higher in women using co-cyprindiol than in women using combined oral contraceptives containing levonorgestrel, but the risk may be similar to that associated with use of combined oral contraceptives containing third generation progestogens (desogestrel and gestodene) or drospirenone. Women requiring co-cyprindiol may have an inherently increased risk of cardiovascular disease.

● INTERACTIONS → Appendix 1: combined hormonal contraceptives

● SIDE-EFFECTS
▶ Rare or very rare Cholelithiasis · photosensitivity reactions · systemic lupus erythematosus (SLE)
▶ Frequency not known Abdominal cramps · amenorrhoea (on discontinuation) · breast abnormalities · cervical erosion · chorea · contact lens intolerance · depression · fluid retention · headache · hepatic impairment · hepatic neoplasm · hypertension · irritability · leg cramps · libido disorder · lipid metabolism change · melasma · menstrual disorder · nausea · thrombosis (more common when factor V Leiden present or in blood groups A, B, and AB) · vulvovaginal disorders · visual impairment · vomiting

● PREGNANCY Avoid—risk of feminisation of male fetus with cyproterone.

● BREAST FEEDING Manufacturer advises avoid; possibility of anti-androgen effects in neonate with cyproterone.

● HEPATIC IMPAIRMENT Manufacturer advises avoid in severe impairment (until liver function returns to normal.)

● PRESCRIBING AND DISPENSING INFORMATION A mixture of cyproterone acetate and ethinylestradiol in the mass proportions 2000 parts to 35 parts, respectively.

● MEDICINAL FORMS
There can be variation in the licensing of different medicines containing the same drug.
Tablet
▶ Co-cyprindiol (Non-proprietary)
Ethinylestradiol 35 microgram, Cyproterone acetate 2 mg Co-cyprindiol 2000microgram/35microgram tablets | 63 tablet [PoM] £5.70 DT = £5.70
▶ Clairette (Stragen UK Ltd)
Ethinylestradiol 35 microgram, Cyproterone acetate 2 mg Clairette 2000/35 tablets | 63 tablet [PoM] £5.13 DT = £5.70
▶ Dianette (Bayer Plc)
Ethinylestradiol 35 microgram, Cyproterone acetate 2 mg Dianette tablets | 63 tablet [PoM] £7.71 DT = £5.70
▶ Teragezza (Morningside Healthcare Ltd)
Ethinylestradiol 35 microgram, Cyproterone acetate 2 mg Teragezza 2000microgram/35microgram tablets | 63 tablet [PoM] £11.10 DT = £5.70

ANTIBACTERIALS ⟩ LINCOSAMIDES

Clindamycin

● **INDICATIONS AND DOSE**

DALACIN T ® LOTION
Acne vulgaris
▶ TO THE SKIN
▶ Child: Apply twice daily, to be applied thinly
▶ Adult: Apply twice daily, to be applied thinly

DALACIN T ® SOLUTION
Acne vulgaris
▶ TO THE SKIN
▶ Child: Apply twice daily, to be applied thinly
▶ Adult: Apply twice daily, to be applied thinly

ZINDACLIN ® GEL

Acne vulgaris
▶ TO THE SKIN
▸ Child 12-17 years: Apply once daily, to be applied thinly
▸ Adult: Apply once daily, to be applied thinly

● INTERACTIONS → Appendix 1: clindamycin

● MEDICINAL FORMS
There can be variation in the licensing of different medicines containing the same drug.
Gel
EXCIPIENTS: May contain Propylene glycol
▸ Zindaclin (Crawford Healthcare Ltd)
Clindamycin (as Clindamycin phosphate) 10 mg per 1 gram Zindaclin 1% gel | 30 gram [PoM] £8.66 DT = £8.66
Liquid
EXCIPIENTS: May contain Cetostearyl alcohol (including cetyl and stearyl alcohol), hydroxybenzoates (parabens), propylene glycol
▸ Dalacin T (Pfizer Ltd)
Clindamycin (as Clindamycin phosphate) 10 mg per 1 ml Dalacin T 1% topical lotion | 30 ml [PoM] £5.08 DT = £5.08 | 60 ml [PoM] £10.16
Dalacin T 1% topical solution | 30 ml [PoM] £4.34 DT = £4.34 | 50 ml [PoM] £7.23

Combinations available: *Benzoyl peroxide with clindamycin,* below · *Tretinoin with clindamycin,* p. 1236

ANTIBACTERIALS > MACROLIDES

Erythromycin with zinc acetate

● INDICATIONS AND DOSE
Acne vulgaris
▶ TO THE SKIN
▸ Child: Apply twice daily
▸ Adult: Apply twice daily

● CAUTIONS Some manufacturers advise preparations containing alcohol are not suitable for use with benzoyl peroxide

● MEDICINAL FORMS
There can be variation in the licensing of different medicines containing the same drug.
Liquid
▸ Zineryt (LEO Pharma)
Zinc acetate 12 mg per 1 ml, Erythromycin 40 mg per 1 ml Zineryt lotion | 30 ml [PoM] £9.25 DT = £9.25 | 90 ml [PoM] £20.02 DT = £20.02

ANTISEPTICS AND DISINFECTANTS > PEROXIDES

Benzoyl peroxide

● INDICATIONS AND DOSE
Acne vulgaris
▶ TO THE SKIN
▸ Child 12-17 years: Apply 1-2 times a day, preferably apply after washing with soap and water, start treatment with lower-strength preparations
▸ Adult: Apply 1-2 times a day, preferably apply after washing with soap and water, start treatment with lower-strength preparations

● CAUTIONS Avoid contact with broken skin · avoid contact with eyes · avoid contact with mouth · avoid contact with mucous membranes · avoid excessive exposure to sunlight

● SIDE-EFFECTS
▶ **Common or very common** Skin reactions
▶ **Frequency not known** Facial swelling
SIDE-EFFECTS, FURTHER INFORMATION Reduce frequency or suspend use until skin irritation subsides and re-introduce at reduced frequency.

● PATIENT AND CARER ADVICE May bleach fabrics and hair.

● MEDICINAL FORMS
There can be variation in the licensing of different medicines containing the same drug.
Cream
EXCIPIENTS: May contain Cetostearyl alcohol (including cetyl and stearyl alcohol), fragrances, isopropyl palmitate, propylene glycol
▸ Brevoxyl (GlaxoSmithKline Consumer Healthcare)
Benzoyl peroxide 40 mg per 1 gram Brevoxyl 4% cream | 50 gram [P] £4.13 DT = £4.13
Gel
EXCIPIENTS: May contain Fragrances, propylene glycol
▸ Acnecide (Galderma (UK) Ltd)
Benzoyl peroxide 50 mg per 1 gram Acnecide 5% gel | 30 gram [P] £5.44 DT = £5.44 | 60 gram [P] £10.68 DT = £10.68
Acnecide Wash 5% gel | 50 gram [P] £5.44 DT = £5.44

Combinations available: *Adapalene with benzoyl peroxide,* p. 1234

13

Skin

Benzoyl peroxide with clindamycin

The properties listed below are those particular to the combination only. For the properties of the components please consider, benzoyl peroxide above, clindamycin p. 1232.

● INDICATIONS AND DOSE
Acne vulgaris
▶ TO THE SKIN
▸ Child 12-17 years: Apply once daily, dose to be applied in the evening
▸ Adult: Apply once daily, dose to be applied in the evening

● INTERACTIONS → Appendix 1: clindamycin

● MEDICINAL FORMS
There can be variation in the licensing of different medicines containing the same drug.
Gel
EXCIPIENTS: May contain Disodium edetate
▸ Duac (Stiefel Laboratories (UK) Ltd)
Clindamycin (as Clindamycin phosphate) 10 mg per 1 gram, Benzoyl peroxide 30 mg per 1 gram Duac Once Daily gel (3% and 1%) | 30 gram [PoM] £13.14 DT = £13.14 | 60 gram [PoM] £26.28
Clindamycin (as Clindamycin phosphate) 10 mg per 1 gram, Benzoyl peroxide 50 mg per 1 gram Duac Once Daily gel (5% and 1%) | 30 gram [PoM] £13.14 DT = £13.14 | 60 gram [PoM] £26.28 DT = £26.28

DERMATOLOGICAL DRUGS > ANTICOMEDONALS

Azelaic acid

● INDICATIONS AND DOSE
FINACEA ®
Facial acne vulgaris
▶ TO THE SKIN
▸ Child 12-17 years: Apply twice daily, discontinue if no improvement after 1 month
▸ Adult: Apply twice daily, discontinue if no improvement after 1 month
Papulopustular rosacea
▶ TO THE SKIN
▸ Adult: Apply twice daily, discontinue if no improvement after 2 months
SKINOREN ®
Acne vulgaris
▶ TO THE SKIN
▸ Child 12-17 years: Apply twice daily
▸ Adult: Apply twice daily　　　　　　　　continued →

Acne vulgaris in patients with sensitive skin
- ▶ TO THE SKIN
  - ▶ Child 12-17 years: Apply once daily for 1 week, then apply twice daily
  - ▶ Adult: Apply once daily for 1 week, then apply twice daily

- ● CAUTIONS Avoid contact with eyes · avoid contact with mouth · avoid contact with mucous membranes
- ● SIDE-EFFECTS
  - ▶ **Common or very common** Application site irritation (reduce frequency or discontinue temporarily)
  - ▶ **Uncommon** Skin reactions
  - ▶ **Rare or very rare** Asthma exacerbated · cheilitis
  - ▶ **Frequency not known** Angioedema · eye swelling

- ● MEDICINAL FORMS
  There can be variation in the licensing of different medicines containing the same drug.
  Cream
  EXCIPIENTS: May contain Propylene glycol
  - ▶ Skinoren (Bayer Plc)
    Azelaic acid 200 mg per 1 gram Skinoren 20% cream | 30 gram PoM £4.49 DT = £4.49
  Gel
  EXCIPIENTS: May contain Disodium edetate, polysorbates, propylene glycol
  - ▶ Finacea (Bayer Plc)
    Azelaic acid 150 mg per 1 gram Finacea 15% gel | 30 gram PoM £7.48 DT = £7.48

RETINOID AND RELATED DRUGS

Adapalene

- ● INDICATIONS AND DOSE
  Mild to moderate acne vulgaris
  - ▶ TO THE SKIN
    - ▶ Child 12-17 years: Apply once daily, apply thinly in the evening
    - ▶ Adult: Apply once daily, apply thinly in the evening

- ● CAUTIONS Avoid accumulation in angles of the nose · avoid contact with eyes, nostrils, mouth and mucous membranes, eczematous, broken or sunburned skin · avoid exposure to UV light (including sunlight, solariums) · avoid in severe acne involving large areas · caution in sensitive areas such as the neck
- ● INTERACTIONS → Appendix 1: retinoids
- ● CONCEPTION AND CONTRACEPTION Females of child-bearing age must use effective contraception (oral progestogen-only contraceptives not considered effective).
- ● PREGNANCY Avoid.
- ● BREAST FEEDING Amount of drug in milk probably too small to be harmful; ensure infant does not come in contact with treated areas.
- ● PATIENT AND CARER ADVICE If sun exposure is unavoidable, an appropriate sunscreen or protective clothing should be used.

- ● MEDICINAL FORMS
  There can be variation in the licensing of different medicines containing the same drug.
  Cream
  CAUTIONARY AND ADVISORY LABELS 11
  EXCIPIENTS: May contain Disodium edetate, hydroxybenzoates (parabens)
  - ▶ Adapalene (Non-proprietary)
    Adapalene 1 mg per 1 gram Adapalene 0.1% cream | 45 gram PoM £16.43 DT = £16.43

- ▶ Differin (Galderma (UK) Ltd)
  Adapalene 1 mg per 1 gram Differin 0.1% cream | 45 gram PoM £16.43 DT = £16.43
Gel
CAUTIONARY AND ADVISORY LABELS 11
EXCIPIENTS: May contain Disodium edetate, hydroxybenzoates (parabens), propylene glycol
- ▶ Adapalene (Non-proprietary)
  Adapalene 1 mg per 1 gram Adapalene 0.1% gel | 45 gram PoM £16.43 DT = £16.43
- ▶ Differin (Galderma (UK) Ltd)
  Adapalene 1 mg per 1 gram Differin 0.1% gel | 45 gram PoM £16.43 DT = £16.43

Adapalene with benzoyl peroxide

The properties listed below are those particular to the combination only. For the properties of the components please consider, adapalene above, benzoyl peroxide p. 1233.

- ● INDICATIONS AND DOSE
  Acne vulgaris
  - ▶ TO THE SKIN
    - ▶ Child 9-17 years: Apply once daily, to be applied thinly in the evening
    - ▶ Adult: Apply once daily, to be applied thinly in the evening

- ● INTERACTIONS → Appendix 1: retinoids
- ● CONCEPTION AND CONTRACEPTION Females of child-bearing age must use effective contraception (oral progestogen-only contraceptives not considered effective).
- ● PATIENT AND CARER ADVICE Gel may bleach clothing and hair.
- ● NATIONAL FUNDING/ACCESS DECISIONS
  Scottish Medicines Consortium (SMC) Decisions
  The *Scottish Medicines Consortium* has advised (March 2014) that *Epiduo*® should be restricted for use in mild to moderate facial acne when monotherapy with benzoyl peroxide or adapalene is inappropriate.

- ● MEDICINAL FORMS
  There can be variation in the licensing of different medicines containing the same drug.
  Gel
  CAUTIONARY AND ADVISORY LABELS 11
  EXCIPIENTS: May contain Disodium edetate, polysorbates, propylene glycol
  - ▶ Epiduo (Galderma (UK) Ltd)
    Adapalene 1 mg per 1 gram, Benzoyl peroxide 25 mg per 1 gram Epiduo 0.1%/2.5% gel | 45 gram PoM £19.53 DT = £19.53

Isotretinoin

03-Nov-2017

- ● INDICATIONS AND DOSE
  Topical treatment of mild to moderate acne
  - ▶ TO THE SKIN
    - ▶ Adult: Apply 1-2 times a day, to be applied thinly

  Severe acne (under expert supervision) | Acne which is associated with psychological problems (under expert supervision) | Acne which has not responded to an adequate course of a systemic antibacterial (under expert supervision) | Acne with scarring (under expert supervision) | Systemic treatment of nodulo-cystic and conglobate acne (under expert supervision)
  - ▶ BY MOUTH
    - ▶ Adult: Initially 500 micrograms/kg daily in 1-2 divided doses, increased if necessary to 1 mg/kg daily for 16-24 weeks, repeat treatment course after a period of

at least 8 weeks if relapse after first course; maximum 150 mg/kg per course

---

IMPORTANT SAFETY INFORMATION

MHRA/CHM ADVICE: ISOTRETINOIN (*ROACCUTANE*®): RARE REPORTS OF ERECTILE DYSFUNCTION AND DECREASED LIBIDO (OCTOBER 2017)

An EU-wide review has concluded that on rare occasions, oral isotretinoin, indicated for severe acne, may cause sexual side-effects, including erectile dysfunction and decreased libido.

● CONTRA-INDICATIONS
▸ With oral use Hyperlipidaemia · hypervitaminosis A
▸ With topical use Perioral dermatitis · rosacea

● CAUTIONS
▸ With oral use Avoid blood donation during treatment and for at least 1 month after treatment · diabetes · dry eye syndrome (associated with risk of keratitis) · history of depression · monitor for depression
▸ With topical use Allow peeling (resulting from other irritant treatments) to subside before using a topical retinoid · alternating a preparation that causes peeling with a topical retinoid may give rise to contact dermatitis (reduce frequency of retinoid application) · avoid accumulation in angles of the nose · avoid contact with eyes, nostrils, mouth and mucous membranes, eczematous, broken or sunburned skin · avoid exposure to UV light (including sunlight, solariums) · avoid in severe acne involving large areas · avoid use of topical retinoids with abrasive cleaners, comedogenic or astringent cosmetics · caution in sensitive areas such as the neck · personal or familial history of skin cancer

● INTERACTIONS → Appendix 1: retinoids

● SIDE-EFFECTS

GENERAL SIDE-EFFECTS
▸ **Common or very common** Skin reactions
▸ **Rare or very rare** Photosensitivity reaction

SPECIFIC SIDE-EFFECTS
▸ **Common or very common**
▸ With oral use Alopecia · anaemia · arthralgia · back pain · cheilitis · dry eye · eye discomfort · eye inflammation · haemorrhage · headache · increased risk of infection · myalgia · nasal dryness · neutropenia · proteinuria · skin fragility (trauma may cause blistering) · thrombocytopenia · thrombocytosis
▸ **Rare or very rare**
▸ With oral use Anxiety · arthritis · behaviour abnormal · bone disorders · bronchospasm · cataract · corneal opacity · depression · diabetes mellitus · dizziness · drowsiness · dry throat · gastrointestinal disorders · glomerulonephritis · hair changes · hearing impairment · hepatitis · hoarseness · hyperhidrosis · hyperuricaemia · idiopathic intracranial hypertension · inflammatory bowel disease · lymphadenopathy · malaise · mood altered · nail dystrophy · nausea · pancreatitis · psychotic disorder · pyogenic granuloma · seizure · suicidal tendencies · tendinitis · vasculitis · vision disorders
▸ **Frequency not known**
▸ With oral use Rhabdomyolysis · severe cutaneous adverse reactions (SCARs)

SIDE-EFFECTS, FURTHER INFORMATION Risk of pancreatitis if triglycerides above 9 mmol/litre—discontinue if uncontrolled hypertriglyceridaemia or pancreatitis.

Discontinue treatment if skin peeling severe or haemorrhagic diarrhoea develops.

Visual disturbances require expert referral and possible withdrawal.

Psychiatric side-effects could require expert referral.

● CONCEPTION AND CONTRACEPTION
Pregnancy prevention
▸ With oral use Effective contraception must be used. In women of child-bearing potential, exclude pregnancy up to 3 days before treatment (start treatment on day 2 or 3 of menstrual cycle), every month during treatment (unless there are compelling reasons to indicate that there is no risk of pregnancy), and 5 weeks after stopping treatment— perform pregnancy test in the first 3 days of the menstrual cycle. Women must practise effective contraception for at least 1 month before starting treatment, during treatment, and for at least 1 month after stopping treatment. Women should be advised to use at least 1 method of contraception, but ideally they should use 2 methods of contraception. Oral progestogen-only contraceptives are not considered effective. Barrier methods should not be used alone, but can be used in conjunction with other contraceptive methods. Each prescription for isotretinoin should be limited to a supply of up to 30 days' treatment and dispensed within 7 days of the date stated on the prescription; repeat prescriptions or faxed prescriptions are not acceptable. Women should be advised to discontinue treatment and to seek prompt medical attention if they become pregnant during treatment or within 1 month of stopping treatment.
▸ With topical use Females of child-bearing age must use effective contraception (oral progestogen-only contraceptives not considered effective).

● PREGNANCY Contra-indicated in pregnancy (teratogenic).

● BREAST FEEDING Avoid.

● HEPATIC IMPAIRMENT
▸ With oral use Avoid—further impairment may occur.

● RENAL IMPAIRMENT
Dose adjustments ▸ With oral use In severe impairment, reduce initial dose (e.g. 10 mg daily) and increase gradually up to 1 mg/kg daily as tolerated.

● MONITORING REQUIREMENTS
▸ With oral use Measure hepatic function and serum lipids before treatment, 1 month after starting and then every 3 months (reduce dose or discontinue if transaminase or serum lipids persistently raised).

● PRESCRIBING AND DISPENSING INFORMATION Isotretinoin is an isomer of tretinoin.

● PATIENT AND CARER ADVICE
▸ With oral use Warn patient to avoid wax epilation (risk of epidermal stripping), dermabrasion, and laser skin treatments (risk of scarring) during treatment and for at least 6 months after stopping; patient should avoid exposure to UV light (including sunlight) and use sunscreen and emollient (including lip balm) preparations from the start of treatment.

Patients and carers should be told how to recognise signs and symptoms of psychiatric disorders such as depression, anxiety, and rarely suicidal thoughts.
▸ With topical use Patients should be warned that some redness and skin peeling can occur initially but settles with time. If undue irritation occurs, the frequency of application should be reduced or treatment suspended until the reaction subsides; if irritation persists, discontinue treatment. Several months of treatment may be needed to achieve an optimal response and the treatment should be continued until no new lesions develop. If sun exposure is unavoidable, an appropriate sunscreen or protective clothing should be used.

13

Skin

- MEDICINAL FORMS
  There can be variation in the licensing of different medicines containing the same drug.

  Capsule

  CAUTIONARY AND ADVISORY LABELS 10, 11, 21
  ▸ Isotretinoin (Non-proprietary)
    Isotretinoin 5 mg Isotretinoin 5mg capsules | 30 capsule PoM
    £10.10–£10.15 | 56 capsule PoM £14.78 DT = £14.78
    Isotretinoin 10 mg Isotretinoin 10mg capsules | 30 capsule PoM
    £14.54 DT = £14.54
    Isotretinoin 20 mg Isotretinoin 20mg capsules | 30 capsule PoM
    £20.00 DT = £16.66 | 56 capsule PoM £31.01–£37.85
    Isotretinoin 40 mg Isotretinoin 40mg capsules | 30 capsule PoM
    £38.98 DT = £38.98
  ▸ Roaccutane (Roche Products Ltd)
    Isotretinoin 10 mg Roaccutane 10mg capsules | 30 capsule PoM
    £14.54 DT = £14.54
    Isotretinoin 20 mg Roaccutane 20mg capsules | 30 capsule PoM
    £20.02 DT = £16.66

Isotretinoin with erythromycin

The properties listed below are those particular to the combination only. For the properties of the components please consider, isotretinoin p. 1234, erythromycin p. 530.

- ● INDICATIONS AND DOSE

  Topical treatment of mild to moderate acne
  ▸ TO THE SKIN
  ▸ Adult: (consult product literature)

- ● INTERACTIONS → Appendix 1: macrolides · retinoids

- ● MEDICINAL FORMS
  There can be variation in the licensing of different medicines containing the same drug.

  Gel

  CAUTIONARY AND ADVISORY LABELS 11
  EXCIPIENTS: May contain Butylated hydroxytoluene
  ▸ Isotrexin (Stiefel Laboratories (UK) Ltd)
    Isotretinoin 500 microgram per 1 gram, Erythromycin 20 mg per 1 gram Isotrexin gel | 30 gram PoM £7.47 DT = £7.47

Tretinoin with clindamycin

The properties listed below are those particular to the combination only. For the properties of the components please consider, tretinoin p. 914, clindamycin p. 1232.

- ● INDICATIONS AND DOSE

  Facial acne
  ▸ TO THE SKIN
  ▸ Child 12–17 years: Apply daily, (to be applied thinly at bedtime)
  ▸ Adult: Apply daily, (to be applied thinly at bedtime)

- ● CONTRA-INDICATIONS Perioral dermatitis · personal or familial history of skin cancer · rosacea
- ● CAUTIONS Allow peeling (resulting from other irritant treatments) to subside before using a topical retinoid · alternating a preparation that causes peeling with a topical retinoid may give rise to contact dermatitis (reduce frequency of retinoid application) · avoid accumulation in angles of the nose · avoid contact with eyes, nostrils, mouth and mucous membranes, eczematous, broken or sunburned skin · avoid exposure to UV light (including sunlight, solariums) · avoid in severe acne involving large areas · avoid use of topical retinoids with abrasive cleaners, comedogenic or astringent cosmetics · caution in sensitive areas such as the neck
- ● INTERACTIONS → Appendix 1: clindamycin · retinoids
- ● SIDE-EFFECTS Dry skin (discontinue if severe) · eye irritation · oedema · photosensitivity reaction · skin pigmentation change (transient) · skin reactions

- ● CONCEPTION AND CONTRACEPTION Females of child-bearing age must use effective contraception (oral progestogen-only contraceptives not considered effective).
- ● PREGNANCY Contra-indicated in pregnancy.
- ● BREAST FEEDING Amount of drug in milk after topical application probably too small to be harmful; ensure infant does not come in contact with treated areas.
- ● PATIENT AND CARER ADVICE If sun exposure is unavoidable, an appropriate sunscreen or protective clothing should be used.
  Patients and carers should be warned that some redness and skin peeling can occur initially but settles with time. If undue irritation occurs, the frequency of application should be reduced or treatment suspended until the reaction subsides; if irritation persists, discontinue treatment. Several months of treatment may be needed to achieve an optimal response and the treatment should be continued until no new lesions develop.

- ● MEDICINAL FORMS
  There can be variation in the licensing of different medicines containing the same drug.

  Gel

  CAUTIONARY AND ADVISORY LABELS 11
  EXCIPIENTS: May contain Butylated hydroxytoluene, hydroxybenzoates (parabens), polysorbates
  ▸ Treclin (Meda Pharmaceuticals Ltd)
    Tretinoin 250 microgram per 1 gram, Clindamycin (as Clindamycin phosphate) 10 mg per 1 gram Treclin 1%/0.025% gel
    | 30 gram PoM £11.94

Tretinoin with erythromycin

The properties listed below are those particular to the combination only. For the properties of the components please consider, tretinoin p. 914, erythromycin p. 530.

- ● INDICATIONS AND DOSE

  Acne
  ▸ TO THE SKIN
  ▸ Child: Apply 1–2 times a day, apply thinly
  ▸ Adult: Apply 1–2 times a day, apply thinly

- ● CONTRA-INDICATIONS Perioral dermatitis · personal or familial history of skin cancer · rosacea
- ● CAUTIONS Allow peeling (resulting from other irritant treatments) to subside before using a topical retinoid · alternating a preparation that causes peeling with a topical retinoid may give rise to contact dermatitis (reduce frequency of retinoid application) · avoid accumulation in angles of the nose · avoid contact with eyes, nostrils, mouth and mucous membranes, eczematous, broken or sunburned skin · avoid exposure to UV light (including sunlight, solariums) · avoid in severe acne involving large areas · avoid use of topical retinoids with abrasive cleaners, comedogenic or astringent cosmetics · caution in sensitive areas such as the neck
- ● INTERACTIONS → Appendix 1: macrolides · retinoids
- ● SIDE-EFFECTS Dry skin (discontinue if severe) · eye irritation · oedema · photosensitivity reaction · skin pigmentation change (transient) · skin reactions
- ● CONCEPTION AND CONTRACEPTION Females of child-bearing age must use effective contraception (oral progestogen-only contraceptives not considered effective).
- ● PREGNANCY Contra-indicated in pregnancy.
- ● BREAST FEEDING Amount of drug in milk after topical application probably too small to be harmful; ensure infant does not come in contact with treated areas.

- **PATIENT AND CARER ADVICE** Patients and carers should be warned that some redness and skin peeling can occur initially but settles with time. If undue irritation occurs, the frequency of application should be reduced or treatment suspended until the reaction subsides; if irritation persists, discontinue treatment. Several months of treatment may be needed to achieve an optimal response and the treatment should be continued until no new lesions develop. If sun exposure is unavoidable, an appropriate sunscreen or protective clothing should be used.

- **MEDICINAL FORMS** There can be variation in the licensing of different medicines containing the same drug.

Liquid
CAUTIONARY AND ADVISORY LABELS 11
▸ Aknemycin Plus (Almirall Ltd)
   Tretinoin 250 microgram per 1 gram, Erythromycin 40 mg per 1 gram Aknemycin Plus solution | 25 ml P̲o̲M̲ £7.05 DT = £7.05

VITAMINS AND TRACE ELEMENTS ⟩ VITAMIN B GROUP

Nicotinamide

- **INDICATIONS AND DOSE**

Inflammatory acne vulgaris
▸ TO THE SKIN
▸ **Adult:** Apply twice daily, reduced to once daily or on alternate days, dose reduced if irritation occurs

- **CAUTIONS** Avoid contact with eyes · avoid contact with mucous membranes (including nose and mouth) · reduce frequency of application if excessive dryness, irritation or peeling

- **SIDE-EFFECTS** Paraesthesia · skin reactions

- **MEDICINAL FORMS** There can be variation in the licensing of different medicines containing the same drug.

Gel
▸ Freederm (Dendron Ltd)
   Nicotinamide 40 mg per 1 gram Freederm Treatment 4% gel | 25 gram P̲ £5.56
▸ Nicam (Dermal Laboratories Ltd)
   Nicotinamide 40 mg per 1 gram Nicam 4% gel | 60 gram P̲ £7.10

6.2 Rosacea

Other drugs used for Rosacea Azelaic acid, p. 1233

ANTHELMINTICS

Ivermectin   17-May-2017

- **INDICATIONS AND DOSE**

Papulopustular rosacea
▸ TO THE SKIN
▸ **Adult:** Apply daily for up to 4 months, the treatment course may be repeated; discontinue if no improvement after 3 months

- **INTERACTIONS** → Appendix 1: ivermectin
- **SIDE-EFFECTS**
▸ **Common or very common** Skin reactions
- **PREGNANCY** Manufacturer advises avoid—limited information but toxicity following *oral* use in *animal* studies.
- **BREAST FEEDING** Manufacturer advises avoid—limited information but present in milk following *oral* use.

- **HEPATIC IMPAIRMENT** Manufacturer advises use with caution in severe impairment—no information available.
- **DIRECTIONS FOR ADMINISTRATION** Manufacturer advises apply thinly to the face only, avoiding contact with eyes, lips and mucosa.
- **PATIENT AND CARER ADVICE** Wash hands immediately after use.
- **NATIONAL FUNDING/ACCESS DECISIONS**

Scottish Medicines Consortium (SMC) Decisions
The *Scottish Medicines Consortium* has advised (December 2015) that ivermectin (*Soolantra®*) is accepted for restricted use within NHS Scotland for the treatment of moderate-to-severe inflammatory lesions of rosacea (papulopustular) where a topical treatment is considered appropriate.

All Wales Medicines Strategy Group (AWMSG) Decisions
The All Wales Medicines Strategy Group has advised (April 2016) that ivermectin (*Soolantra®*) is recommended as an option for use within NHS Wales for the topical treatment of inflammatory lesions of rosacea (papulopustular) in adult patients.

- **MEDICINAL FORMS** There can be variation in the licensing of different medicines containing the same drug.

Cream
CAUTIONARY AND ADVISORY LABELS 28
EXCIPIENTS: May contain Cetostearyl alcohol (including cetyl and stearyl alcohol), disodium edetate, isopropyl palmitate, propylene glycol
▸ Soolantra (Galderma (UK) Ltd)
   Ivermectin 10 mg per 1 gram Soolantra 10mg/g cream | 30 gram P̲o̲M̲ £18.29

SYMPATHOMIMETICS ⟩ ALPHA₂-ADRENOCEPTOR AGONISTS

Brimonidine tartrate   12-Jul-2017

- **DRUG ACTION** Brimonidine, an alpha$_2$-adrenoceptor agonist, is used to reduce erythema in rosacea by cutaneous vasoconstriction.

- **INDICATIONS AND DOSE**

Facial erythema in rosacea
▸ TO THE SKIN
▸ **Adult:** Apply once daily until erythema subsides, apply thinly, divide dose over forehead, chin, nose, and cheeks, max. 1 g of gel per day

DOSE EQUIVALENCE AND CONVERSION
▸ 1 g of gel contains 5 mg of brimonidine tartrate (equivalent to 3.3 mg of brimonidine).

IMPORTANT SAFETY INFORMATION
MHRA/CHM ADVICE: BRIMONIDINE GEL (*MIRVASO®*): RISK OF SYSTEMIC CARDIOVASCULAR EFFECTS (JUNE 2017)
Systemic cardiovascular effects including bradycardia, hypotension, and dizziness have been reported after application of brimonidine gel. To minimise the possibility of systemic absorption, it is important to avoid application to irritated or damaged skin, including after laser therapy.
MHRA/CHM ADVICE: BRIMONIDINE GEL (*MIRVASO®*): RISK OF EXACERBATION OF ROSACEA (NOVEMBER 2016)
Symptom exacerbation has been reported very commonly in patients treated with brimonidine gel. Treatment should be initiated with a small amount of gel (less than the maximum dose) for at least 1 week, then increased gradually, based on tolerability and response. Patients should be counselled on the importance of not exceeding the maximum daily dose, and advised to stop treatment and seek medical advice if symptoms worsen during treatment.

13

Skin

13

Skin

- CAUTIONS Cerebral insufficiency · coronary insufficiency · depression · postural hypotension · Raynaud's syndrome · severe cardiovascular disease · thromboangitis obliterans
- INTERACTIONS → Appendix 1: brimonidine
- SIDE-EFFECTS
- ▶ **Common or very common** Dizziness · dry mouth · flushing · headache · skin reactions
- ▶ **Uncommon** Angioedema · eyelid oedema · feeling hot · nasal congestion · paraesthesia · peripheral coldness
- ▶ **Rare or very rare** Bradycardia · hypotension
- PREGNANCY Manufacturer advises avoid—limited information available.
- BREAST FEEDING Manufacturer advises avoid—no information available.
- HEPATIC IMPAIRMENT Manufacturer advises use with caution.
- RENAL IMPAIRMENT Manufacturer advises use with caution.
- DIRECTIONS FOR ADMINISTRATION Avoid contact with eyes, mouth, and mucous membranes; avoid use on irritated or damaged skin or open wounds; apply other topical preparations (including cosmetics) only after brimonidine gel has dried on skin.
- PATIENT AND CARER ADVICE Patients should be advised on administration of gel.
  Driving and skilled tasks Drowsiness may affect performance of skilled tasks (e.g. driving).
- NATIONAL FUNDING/ACCESS DECISIONS
  Scottish Medicines Consortium (SMC) Decisions
  The *Scottish Medicines Consortium* has advised (December 2014) that brimonidine (*Mirvaso®*) is accepted for restricted use within NHS Scotland for the symptomatic treatment of moderate to severe persistent facial erythema associated with rosacea in adult patients.

- MEDICINAL FORMS
  There can be variation in the licensing of different medicines containing the same drug.
  Gel
  CAUTIONARY AND ADVISORY LABELS 28
  EXCIPIENTS: May contain Hydroxybenzoates (parabens), propylene glycol
  ▶ Mirvaso (Galderma (UK) Ltd)
  Brimonidine (as Brimonidine tartrate) 3 mg per 1 gram Mirvaso 3mg/g gel | 30 gram [PoM] £33.69 DT = £33.69

7   Scalp and hair conditions

Scalp and hair conditions

Overview

Dandruff is considered to be a mild form of seborrhoeic dermatitis. Shampoos containing antimicrobial agents such as **pyrithione zinc** (which are widely available) and selenium p. 1239 may have beneficial effects. Shampoos containing **tar** extracts may be useful and they are also used in *psoriasis*. Ketoconazole shampoo p. 1198 should be considered for more persistent or severe dandruff or for seborrhoeic dermatitis of the scalp.

Corticosteroid gels and lotions can also be used.

Shampoos containing coal tar with salicylic acid p. 1220 may also be useful. A cream or an ointment containing coal tar with salicylic acid is very helpful in Psoriasis p. 1204 that affects the scalp. Patients who do not respond to these treatments may need to be referred to exclude the possibility of other skin conditions.

Cradle cap in infants may be treated with **coconut oil** or **olive oil** applications followed by shampooing.

Hirsutism

Hirsutism may result from hormonal disorders or as a side-effect of drugs such as minoxidil p. 1239, corticosteroids, anabolic steroids, androgens, danazol p. 725, and progestogens.

Weight loss can reduce hirsutism in obese women.

Women should be advised about local methods of hair removal, and in the mildest cases this may be all that is required.

Eflornithine p. 1239 an antiprotozoal drug, inhibits the enzyme ornithine decarboxylase in hair follicles. Topical eflornithine can be used as an adjunct to laser therapy for facial hirsutism in women.

Co-cyprindiol p. 1232 may be effective for moderately severe hirsutism. Metformin hydrochloride p. 678 is an alternative in women with polycystic ovary syndrome [unlicensed indication]. Systemic treatment is required for 6–12 months before benefit is seen.

Androgenetic alopecia

Finasteride p. 769 is licensed for the treatment of androgenetic alopecia in men. Continuous use for 3–6 months is required before benefit is seen, and effects are reversed 6–12 months after treatment is discontinued.

Topical application of minoxidil may stimulate limited hair growth in a small proportion of adults but only for as long as it is used.

> **Other drugs used for Scalp and hair conditions** Coal tar, p. 1219 · Coal tar with lecithin, p. 1220 · Coal tar with salicylic acid and precipitated sulfur, p. 1221

ANTISEPTICS AND DISINFECTANTS ›
UNDECENOATES

Cetrimide with undecenoic acid

- **INDICATIONS AND DOSE**

Scalp psoriasis | Seborrhoeic dermatitis | Dandruff
- ▶ TO THE SKIN
- ▶ **Child:** Apply 3 times a week for 1 week, then apply twice weekly
- ▶ **Adult:** Apply 3 times a week for 1 week, then apply twice weekly

- MEDICINAL FORMS
  There can be variation in the licensing of different medicines containing the same drug.
  Shampoo
  ▶ Ceanel (Alliance Pharmaceuticals Ltd)
  Undecenoic acid 10 mg per 1 ml, Phenylethyl alcohol 75 mg per 1 ml, Cetrimide 100 mg per 1 ml Ceanel Concentrate shampoo | 150 ml [P] £3.40 | 500 ml [P] £9.80

ANTISEPTICS AND DISINFECTANTS › OTHER

Benzalkonium chloride

- **INDICATIONS AND DOSE**

Seborrhoeic scalp conditions associated with dandruff and scaling
- ▶ TO THE SKIN
- ▶ **Child:** Apply as required
- ▶ **Adult:** Apply as required

- **MEDICINAL FORMS**
There can be variation in the licensing of different medicines containing the same drug.
Shampoo
▸ Dermax (Dermal Laboratories Ltd)
Benzalkonium chloride 5 mg per 1 ml Dermax Therapeutic 0.5% shampoo | 250 ml Ⓟ £5.69

VITAMINS AND TRACE ELEMENTS

Selenium

- **INDICATIONS AND DOSE**

Seborrhoeic dermatitis | Dandruff
▸ TO THE SKIN USING SHAMPOO
▸ Child 5–17 years: Apply twice weekly for 2 weeks, then apply once weekly for 2 weeks, then apply as required
▸ Adult: Apply twice weekly for 2 weeks, then apply once weekly for 2 weeks, then apply as required

Pityriasis versicolor
▸ TO THE SKIN USING SHAMPOO
▸ Adult: Apply once daily for 7 days, apply to the affected area and leave on for 10 minutes before rinsing off. The course may be repeated if necessary. Diluting with a small amount of water prior to application can reduce irritation

- **UNLICENSED USE** The use of selenium sulfide shampoo as a lotion for the treatment of pityriasis (tinea) versicolor is an unlicensed indication.
- **INTERACTIONS** → Appendix 1: selenium
- **PATIENT AND CARER ADVICE** Avoid using 48 hours before or after applying hair colouring, straightening or waving preparations.

- **MEDICINAL FORMS**
There can be variation in the licensing of different medicines containing the same drug.
Shampoo
EXCIPIENTS: May contain Fragrances
▸ Selsun (Chattem (U.K.) Ltd)
Selenium sulfide 25 mg per 1 ml Selsun 2.5% shampoo | 50 ml Ⓟ £1.61 DT = £1.61 | 100 ml Ⓟ £2.15 DT = £2.15 | 150 ml Ⓟ £3.06 DT = £3.06

7.1 Alopecia

Other drugs used for Alopecia Finasteride, p. 769

VASODILATORS

Minoxidil

- **INDICATIONS AND DOSE**

REGAINE® FOR MEN EXTRA STRENGTH FOAM
Androgenetic alopecia
▸ TO THE SKIN
▸ Adult: Apply 0.5 capful twice daily, to be applied to the affected areas of scalp; discontinue if no improvement after 16 weeks

REGAINE® FOR MEN EXTRA STRENGTH SOLUTION
Androgenetic alopecia
▸ TO THE SKIN
▸ Adult: Apply 1 mL twice daily, to be applied to the affected areas of scalp; discontinue if no improvement after 1 year

REGAINE® FOR WOMEN REGULAR STRENGTH
Androgenetic alopecia
▸ TO THE SKIN
▸ Adult: Apply 1 mL twice daily, to be applied to the affected areas of scalp; discontinue if no improvement after 1 year

- **CONTRA-INDICATIONS** Phaeochromocytoma
- **CAUTIONS** Avoid contact with broken, infected, shaved, or inflamed skin · avoid contact with eyes · avoid contact with mouth · avoid contact with mucous membranes · avoid inhalation of spray mist · avoid occlusive dressings
CAUTIONS, FURTHER INFORMATION When used topically systemic effects unlikely; only about 1–2% absorbed (greater absorption may occur with use on inflamed skin).
- **INTERACTIONS** → Appendix 1: minoxidil
- **SIDE-EFFECTS**
▸ **Common or very common** Hair changes
▸ **Uncommon** Hypotension
SIDE-EFFECTS, FURTHER INFORMATION When used topically systemic effects unlikely; only about 1–2% absorbed (greater absorption may occur with use on inflamed skin).
- **PREGNANCY** Avoid—possible toxicity including reduced placental perfusion. Neonatal hirsutism reported.
- **BREAST FEEDING** Present in milk but not known to be harmful.
- **PATIENT AND CARER ADVICE** Ensure hair and scalp dry before application. Patients and their carers should be advised to wash hands after application of liquid or foam.

- **MEDICINAL FORMS**
There can be variation in the licensing of different medicines containing the same drug.
Liquid
CAUTIONARY AND ADVISORY LABELS 15
EXCIPIENTS: May contain Propylene glycol
▸ Regaine (McNeil Products Ltd)
Minoxidil 20 mg per 1 ml Regaine for Women Regular Strength 2% solution | 60 ml GSL £15.43
Minoxidil 50 mg per 1 ml Regaine for Men Extra Strength 5% solution | 60 ml GSL £21.63 | 180 ml Ⓟ £43.28
Foam
CAUTIONARY AND ADVISORY LABELS 15
EXCIPIENTS: May contain Butylated hydroxytoluene, cetostearyl alcohol (including cetyl and stearyl alcohol), polysorbates
▸ Regaine (McNeil Products Ltd)
Minoxidil 50 mg per 1 gram Regaine for Men Extra Strength 5% scalp foam | 60 gram GSL £23.33 | 180 gram GSL £50.01

7.2 Hirsutism

Other drugs used for Hirsutism Co-cyprindiol, p. 1232

ANTIPROTOZOALS

Eflornithine

- **DRUG ACTION** An antiprotozoal drug that inhibits the enzyme ornithine decarboxylase in hair follicles.

- **INDICATIONS AND DOSE**

Adjunct to laser therapy for facial hirsutism in women
▸ TO THE SKIN
▸ Adult: Apply twice daily, to be applied thinly, discontinue use if no improvement after 4 months of treatment

13

Skin

- SIDE-EFFECTS
- ▶ **Common or very common** Alopecia · increased risk of infection · paraesthesia · skin reactions
- ▶ **Uncommon** Face oedema · flushing · hair changes · oral disorders · skin haemorrhage
- ▶ **Rare or very rare** Skin neoplasm
- PREGNANCY Toxicity in *animal* studies—manufacturer advises avoid.
- BREAST FEEDING Manufacturer advises avoid—no information available.
- PATIENT AND CARER ADVICE Medicines must be rubbed in thoroughly. Cosmetics may be applied over treated area 5 minutes after eflornithine, do not wash treated area for 4 hours after application.
- NATIONAL FUNDING/ACCESS DECISIONS

  Scottish Medicines Consortium (SMC) Decisions
  The *Scottish Medicines Consortium* has advised (September 2005) that eflornithine for facial hirsutism be restricted for use in women in whom alternative drug treatment cannot be used.

- MEDICINAL FORMS
  There can be variation in the licensing of different medicines containing the same drug.

  Cream
  EXCIPIENTS: May contain Cetostearyl alcohol (including cetyl and stearyl alcohol), hydroxybenzoates (parabens)
  ▶ Vaniqa (Almirall Ltd)
  Eflornithine (as Eflornithine monohydrate chloride) 115 mg per 1 gram Vaniqa 11.5% cream | 60 gram [PoM] £56.87 DT = £56.87

8 Skin cleansers, antiseptics and desloughing agents

Skin cleansers, antiseptics and desloughing agents

Skin cleansers and antiseptics

Soap or detergent is used with water to cleanse intact skin; emollient preparations such as aqueous cream or emulsifying ointment can be used in place of soap or detergent for cleansing dry skin.

An antiseptic is used for skin that is infected or that is susceptible to recurrent infection. Detergent preparations containing chlorhexidine p. 1241 or povidone-iodine p. 1241, which should be thoroughly rinsed off, are used. Emollients may also contain antiseptics.

Antiseptics such as chlorhexidine or povidone-iodine are used on intact skin before surgical procedures; their antiseptic effect is enhanced by an alcoholic solvent. Antiseptic solutions containing cetrimide can be used if a detergent effect is also required.

Hydrogen peroxide p. 1243, an oxidising agent, can be used in solutions of up to 6% for skin disinfection, such as cleansing and deodorising wounds and ulcers. Hydrogen peroxide is also available as a cream for superficial bacterial skin infections.

For irrigating ulcers or wounds, lukewarm sterile sodium chloride 0.9% solution is used, but tap water is often appropriate.

Potassium permanganate below solution 1 in 10000, a mild antiseptic with astringent properties, can be used for exudative eczematous areas; treatment should be stopped when the skin becomes dry.

Desloughing agents

Alginate, hydrogel and hydrocolloid dressings are effective at wound debridement. Sterile larvae (maggots) (available

from BioMonde) are also used for managing sloughing wounds and are prescribable on the NHS.

Desloughing solutions and creams are of little clinical value. Substances applied to an open area are easily absorbed and perilesional skin is easily sensitised. Gravitational dermatitis may be complicated by superimposed contact sensitivity to substances such as neomycin sulfate p. 1195 or lanolin.

ANTISEPTICS AND DISINFECTANTS

Potassium permanganate

- INDICATIONS AND DOSE

  Cleansing and deodorising suppurating eczematous reactions and wounds
  ▶ TO THE SKIN
  ▶ Adult: For wet dressings or baths, use approximately 0.01% (1 in 10 000) solution

- CAUTIONS Irritant to mucous membranes
- DIRECTIONS FOR ADMINISTRATION Potassium permanganate 0.1% solution to be diluted 1 in 10 to provide a 0.01% (1 in 10 000) solution. With potassium permanganate tablets for solution, 1 tablet dissolved in 4 litres of water provides a 0.01% (1 in 10 000) solution.
- PATIENT AND CARER ADVICE Can stain clothing, skin and nails (especially with prolonged use).

- MEDICINAL FORMS
  There can be variation in the licensing of different medicines containing the same drug. Forms available from special-order manufacturers include: liquid

  Tablet for cutaneous solution
  ▶ Potassium permanganate (Non-proprietary)
  Potassium permanganate 400 mg Potassium permanganate 400mg tablets for cutaneous solution | 30 tablet [S] DT = £19.25
  EN-Potab 400mg tablets for cutaneous solution | 30 tablet [S] DT = £19.25
  ▶ Permitabs (Alliance Pharmaceuticals Ltd)
  Potassium permanganate 400 mg Permitabs 400mg tablets for cutaneous solution | 30 tablet £19.25 DT = £19.25

ANTISEPTICS AND DISINFECTANTS > ALCOHOL DISINFECTANTS

Alcohol

(Industrial methylated spirit)

- INDICATIONS AND DOSE

  Skin preparation before injection
  ▶ TO THE SKIN
  ▶ Child: Apply as required
  ▶ Adult: Apply as required

- CONTRA-INDICATIONS Neonates
- CAUTIONS Avoid broken skin · flammable · patients have suffered severe burns when diathermy has been preceded by application of alcoholic skin disinfectants
- SIDE-EFFECTS

  Overdose
  Features of acute alcohol intoxication include ataxia, dysarthria, nystagmus, and drowsiness, which may progress to coma, with hypotension and acidosis.

  For details on the management of poisoning, see Alcohol, under Emergency treatment of poisoning p. 1319.

- PRESCRIBING AND DISPENSING INFORMATION Industrial methylated spirits defined by the BP as a mixture of 19 volumes of ethyl alcohol of an appropriate strength with 1 volume of approved wood naphtha.

- **MEDICINAL FORMS**
  There can be variation in the licensing of different medicines containing the same drug.

  Liquid
  ▸ Alcohol (Non-proprietary)
    Industrial methylated spirit 70% | 600 ml £6.30–£7.01
    Wood naphtha 50 ml per 1 litre, Ethanol 950 ml per 1 litre Industrial methylated spirit 95% | 600 ml £5.04 | 1000 ml £4.46

ANTISEPTICS AND DISINFECTANTS ⟩ IODINE PRODUCTS

Povidone-iodine

- **INDICATIONS AND DOSE**

  Skin disinfection
  ▸ TO THE SKIN
  ▸ Child: (consult product literature)
  ▸ Adult: (consult product literature)

  BETADINE ® DRY POWDER SPRAY

  Skin disinfection, particularly minor wounds and infections
  ▸ TO THE SKIN
  ▸ Adult: Not for use in serous cavities (consult product literature)

  SAVLON ® DRY

  Skin disinfection of minor wounds
  ▸ TO THE SKIN
  ▸ Adult: (consult product literature)

  VIDENE ® SOLUTION

  Skin disinfection
  ▸ TO THE SKIN
  ▸ Child: Apply undiluted in pre-operative skin disinfection and general antisepsis
  ▸ Adult: Apply undiluted in pre-operative skin disinfection and general antisepsis

  VIDENE ® SURGICAL SCRUB ®

  Skin disinfection
  ▸ TO THE SKIN
  ▸ Child: Use as a pre-operative scrub for hand and skin disinfection
  ▸ Adult: Use as a pre-operative scrub for hand and skin disinfection

  VIDENE ® TINCTURE

  Skin disinfection
  ▸ TO THE SKIN
  ▸ Adult: Apply undiluted in pre-operative skin disinfection

- **CONTRA-INDICATIONS** Avoid regular use in patients with thyroid disorders (in adults) · concomitant use of lithium · corrected gestational age under 32 weeks · infants body-weight under 1.5 kg · regular use in neonates
- **CAUTIONS** Broken skin · large open wounds
  CAUTIONS, FURTHER INFORMATION
  ▸ Large open wounds The application of povidone–iodine to large wounds or severe burns may produce systemic adverse effects such as metabolic acidosis, hypernatraemia and impairment of renal function.
  VIDENE ® TINCTURE Procedures involving hot wire cautery and diathermy
- **SIDE-EFFECTS**
- Rare or very rare Sensitivity
- **PREGNANCY** Sufficient iodine may be absorbed to affect the fetal thyroid in the second and third trimester.
- **BREAST FEEDING** Avoid regular or excessive use.

- **RENAL IMPAIRMENT** Avoid regular application to inflamed or broken skin or mucosa.
- **EFFECT ON LABORATORY TESTS** May interfere with thyroid function tests.
- **MEDICINAL FORMS**
  There can be variation in the licensing of different medicines containing the same drug. Forms available from special-order manufacturers include: liquid

  Spray
  ▸ Betadine (Aspire Pharma Ltd)
    Povidone-Iodine 25 mg per 1 gram Betadine 2.5% dry powder spray | 100 ml GSL £9.95 DT = £9.95

  Liquid
  CAUTIONARY AND ADVISORY LABELS 15 (Only for use with alcoholic solutions)
  ▸ Videne (Ecolab Healthcare Division)
    Povidone-Iodine 75 mg per 1 ml Videne 7.5% surgical scrub solution | 500 ml P £7.67
    Povidone-Iodine 100 mg per 1 ml Videne 10% antiseptic solution | 500 ml GSL £7.67
    Videne 10% alcoholic tincture | 500 ml P £7.67

ANTISEPTICS AND DISINFECTANTS ⟩ OTHER

Chlorhexidine

- **INDICATIONS AND DOSE**

  CEPTON ® LOTION

  For skin disinfection in acne
  ▸ TO THE SKIN
  ▸ Child: (consult product literature)
  ▸ Adult: (consult product literature)

  CEPTON ® SKIN WASH

  For use as skin wash in acne
  ▸ TO THE SKIN
  ▸ Child: (consult product literature)
  ▸ Adult: (consult product literature)

  HIBITANE ® PLUS 5% CONCENTRATE SOLUTION

  General and pre-operative skin disinfection
  ▸ TO THE SKIN
  ▸ Child: (consult product literature)

  HIBISCRUB ®

  Pre-operative hand and skin disinfection | General hand and skin disinfection
  ▸ TO THE SKIN
  ▸ Child: Use as alternative to soap (consult product literature)
  ▸ Adult: Use as alternative to soap (consult product literature)

  HIBITANE OBSTETRIC ®

  For use in obstetrics and gynaecology as an antiseptic and lubricant
  ▸ TO THE SKIN
  ▸ Adult: To be applied to skin around vulva and perineum and to hands of midwife or doctor

  HIBI ® LIQUID HAND RUB+

  Hand and skin disinfection
  ▸ TO THE SKIN
  ▸ Child: To be used undiluted (consult product literature)
  ▸ Adult: To be used undiluted (consult product literature)

  HYDREX ® SOLUTION

  For pre-operative skin disinfection
  ▸ TO THE SKIN
  ▸ Child: (consult product literature)
  ▸ Adult: (consult product literature)

continued →

13

Skin

HYDREX ® SURGICAL SCRUB

For pre-operative hand and skin disinfection | General hand disinfection
▶ TO THE SKIN
▶ Child: (consult product literature)
▶ Adult: (consult product literature)

UNISEPT ®

For cleansing and disinfecting wounds and burns and swabbing in obstetrics
▶ TO THE SKIN
▶ Child: (consult product literature)
▶ Adult: (consult product literature)

● CONTRA-INDICATIONS Alcoholic solutions not suitable before diathermy · not for use in body cavities
● CAUTIONS Avoid contact with brain · avoid contact with eyes · avoid contact with meninges · avoid contact with middle ear
● SIDE-EFFECTS Skin reactions
● DIRECTIONS FOR ADMINISTRATION
HIBITANE ® PLUS 5% CONCENTRATE SOLUTION For pre-operative skin preparation, dilute 1 in 10 (0.5%) with alcohol 70%. For general skin disinfection, dilute 1 in 100 (0.05%) with water. Alcoholic solutions not suitable for use before diathermy or on neonatal skin.

● MEDICINAL FORMS
There can be variation in the licensing of different medicines containing the same drug. Forms available from special-order manufacturers include: liquid, irrigation solution
Cream
CAUTIONARY AND ADVISORY LABELS 15 (For ethanolic solutions (e.g. ChloraPrep ® and Hydrex ® only)
EXCIPIENTS: May contain Fragrances
▶ Cepton (Boston Healthcare Ltd)
Chlorhexidine gluconate 10 mg per 1 ml Cepton 1% medicated skin wash | 150 ml GSL £33.34
▶ HiBiTane Plus (Molnlycke Health Care Ltd)
Chlorhexidine gluconate 50 mg per 1 ml HiBiTane Plus 5% concentrate solution | 5000 ml GSL £14.50 DT = £14.50
▶ Hibi (Molnlycke Health Care Ltd)
Chlorhexidine gluconate 5 mg per 1 ml HiBi Liquid Hand Rub+ 0.5% solution | 500 ml GSL £5.25 DT = £5.25
▶ Hibiscrub (Molnlycke Health Care Ltd)
Chlorhexidine gluconate 40 mg per 1 ml HiBiScrub 4% solution | 250 ml GSL £4.25 DT = £4.25 | 500 ml GSL £5.25 DT = £5.25 | 5000 ml GSL £24.00 DT = £24.00
▶ Hydrex (Ecolab Healthcare Division)
Chlorhexidine gluconate 5 mg per 1 ml Hydrex pink chlorhexidine gluconate 0.5% solution | 600 ml GSL £4.72 DT = £4.72 Hydrex clear chlorhexidine gluconate 0.5% solution | 600 ml GSL £4.72 DT = £4.72
Chlorhexidine gluconate 40 mg per 1 ml Hydrex 4% Surgical Scrub | 250 ml GSL £4.30 DT = £4.25 | 500 ml GSL £4.77 DT = £5.25 | 5000 ml GSL £39.75 DT = £24.00
▶ Sterets Unisept (Molnlycke Health Care Ltd)
Chlorhexidine gluconate 500 microgram per 1 ml Sterets Unisept 0.05% solution 25ml sachets | 25 sachet P £5.54 Sterets Unisept 0.05% solution 100ml sachets | 10 sachet P £6.83

Cream
▶ Hibitane Obstetric (Derma UK Ltd)
Chlorhexidine gluconate 10 mg per 1 gram Hibitane Obstetric 1% cream | 250 ml GSL £16.95
Liquid

Chlorhexidine gluconate with isopropyl alcohol

The properties listed below are those particular to the combination only. For the properties of the components please consider, chlorhexidine p. 1241.

● INDICATIONS AND DOSE
Skin disinfection before invasive procedures
▶ TO THE SKIN
▶ Child 2 months-17 years: (consult product literature)
▶ Adult: (consult product literature)

● MEDICINAL FORMS
There can be variation in the licensing of different medicines containing the same drug. Forms available from special-order manufacturers include: liquid
Liquid
CAUTIONARY AND ADVISORY LABELS 15
▶ ChloraPrep (CareFusion U.K. Ltd)
Chlorhexidine gluconate 20 mg per 1 ml, Isopropyl alcohol 700 ml per 1 litre ChloraPrep with Tint solution 10.5ml applicators | 25 applicator GSL £76.65
ChloraPrep with Tint solution 26ml applicators | 25 applicator GSL £170.75
ChloraPrep solution 3ml applicators | 25 applicator GSL £21.25
ChloraPrep solution 1.5ml applicators | 20 applicator GSL £11.00
ChloraPrep with Tint solution 3ml applicators | 25 applicator GSL £22.31
ChloraPrep solution 0.67ml applicators | 200 applicator GSL £60.00
ChloraPrep solution 10.5ml applicators | 25 applicator GSL £73.00
ChloraPrep solution 26ml applicators | 25 applicator GSL £162.50

Chlorhexidine with cetrimide

The properties listed below are those particular to the combination only. For the properties of the components please consider, chlorhexidine p. 1241.

● INDICATIONS AND DOSE
Skin disinfection such as wound cleansing and obstetrics
▶ TO THE SKIN
▶ Child: To be used undiluted
▶ Adult: To be used undiluted

● MEDICINAL FORMS
There can be variation in the licensing of different medicines containing the same drug.
Cream
▶ Chlorhexidine with cetrimide (Non-proprietary)
Chlorhexidine gluconate 1 mg per 1 gram, Cetrimide 5 mg per 1 gram Savlon antiseptic cream | 15 gram GSL £0.90 | 30 gram GSL £1.19 | 60 gram GSL £1.91 | 100 gram GSL £2.78
Irrigation solution
▶ Chlorhexidine with cetrimide (Non-proprietary)
Chlorhexidine acetate 150 microgram per 1 ml, Cetrimide 1.5 mg per 1 ml Chlorhexidine acetate 0.015% / Cetrimide 0.15% irrigation solution 1litre bottles | 1 bottle P 🚫
Liquid
▶ Sterets Tisept (Molnlycke Health Care Ltd)
Chlorhexidine gluconate 150 microgram per 1 ml, Cetrimide 1.5 mg per 1 ml Sterets Tisept solution 25ml sachets | 25 sachet P £5.33
Sterets Tisept solution 100ml sachets | 10 sachet P £6.85

Diethyl phthalate with methyl salicylate

● INDICATIONS AND DOSE

Skin preparation before injection

▶ TO THE SKIN
▶ Adult: Apply to the area to be disinfected

● MEDICINAL FORMS
There can be variation in the licensing of different medicines containing the same drug.

Liquid
CAUTIONARY AND ADVISORY LABELS 15
▶ Diethyl phthalate with methyl salicylate (Non-proprietary)
  Methyl salicylate 5 ml per 1 litre, Diethyl phthalate 20 ml per 1 litre, Castor oil 25 ml per 1 litre, Industrial methylated spirit 950 ml per 1 litre Surgical spirit | 200 ml GSL £1.17 DT = £1.17 | 1000 ml GSL £3.62

Hydrogen peroxide

● DRUG ACTION Hydrogen peroxide is an oxidising agent.

● INDICATIONS AND DOSE

For skin disinfection, particularly cleansing and deodorising wounds and ulcers

▶ TO THE SKIN
▶ Adult: Use 3% and 6% solutions (consult product literature)

CRYSTACIDE®

Superficial bacterial skin infection

▶ TO THE SKIN
▶ Child: Apply 2–3 times a day for up to 3 weeks
▶ Adult: Apply 2–3 times a day for up to 3 weeks

● UNLICENSED USE Licensed for use in children (age range not specified by manufacturer).

● CONTRA-INDICATIONS Closed body cavities (in adults) · deep wounds (in adults) · large wounds (in adults) · use as disinfection agent for surgical instruments (in adults) · use as enema (in adults) · use during surgery (in adults)

● CAUTIONS Avoid on eyes · avoid on healthy skin · incompatible with products containing iodine or potassium permanganate

● PRESCRIBING AND DISPENSING INFORMATION The BP directs that when hydrogen peroxide is prescribed, hydrogen peroxide solution 6% (20 vols) should be dispensed.
  Strong solutions of hydrogen peroxide which contain 27% (90 vols) and 30% (100 vols) are only for the preparation of weaker solutions.

● HANDLING AND STORAGE Hydrogen peroxide bleaches fabric.

● MEDICINAL FORMS
There can be variation in the licensing of different medicines containing the same drug. Forms available from special-order manufacturers include: liquid

Cream
EXCIPIENTS: May contain Edetic acid (edta), propylene glycol
▶ Crystacide (Reig Jofre UK Ltd)
  Hydrogen peroxide 10 mg per 1 gram Crystacide 1% cream | 25 gram P £8.07 DT = £8.07 | 40 gram P £11.62

Liquid
▶ Hydrogen peroxide (Non-proprietary)
  Hydrogen peroxide 60 mg per 1 ml Hydrogen peroxide 6% solution | 200 ml GSL £0.67 | 500 ml GSL £2.57 | 2000 ml GSL £7.81
  Hydrogen peroxide 90 mg per 1 ml Hydrogen peroxide 9% solution | 200 ml GSL £0.69–£0.72
  Hydrogen peroxide 30 ml per 1 litre Hydrogen peroxide 3% solution | 200 ml GSL £0.63

Proflavine

● INDICATIONS AND DOSE

Infected wounds | Infected burns

▶ TO THE SKIN
▶ Adult: (consult product literature)

● PATIENT AND CARER ADVICE Stains clothing.

● MEDICINAL FORMS
Forms available from special-order manufacturers include: liquid

Irrigation solutions

● IRRIGATION SOLUTIONS

Flowfusor sodium chloride 0.9% irrigation solution 120ml bottles (Fresenius Kabi Ltd) **Sodium chloride 9 mg per 1 ml** | 1 bottle · NHS indicative price = £1.71 · Drug Tariff (Part IXa)

Irriclens sodium chloride 0.9% irrigation solution aerosol spray (ConvaTec Ltd) **Sodium chloride 9 mg per 1 ml** | 240 ml · NHS indicative price = £3.57 · Drug Tariff (Part IXa)

Normasol sodium chloride 0.9% irrigation solution 100ml sachets (Molnlycke Health Care Ltd) **Sodium chloride 9 mg per 1 ml** | 10 unit dose · NHS indicative price = £7.97 · Drug Tariff (Part IXa)

Normasol sodium chloride 0.9% irrigation solution 25ml sachets (Molnlycke Health Care Ltd) **Sodium chloride 9 mg per 1 ml** | 25 unit dose · NHS indicative price = £6.46 · Drug Tariff (Part IXa)

Sodium chloride 0.9% irrigation solution 20ml Clinipod unit dose (Mayors Healthcare Ltd) **Sodium chloride 9 mg per 1 ml** | 25 unit dose · NHS indicative price = £4.80 · Drug Tariff (Part IXa)

Sodium chloride 0.9% irrigation solution 20ml ISO-POD unit dose (St Georges Medical Ltd) **Sodium chloride 9 mg per 1 ml** | 25 unit dose · NHS indicative price = £4.95 · Drug Tariff (Part IXa)

Sodium chloride 0.9% irrigation solution 20ml Irripod unit dose (C D Medical Ltd) **Sodium chloride 9 mg per 1 ml** | 25 unit dose · NHS indicative price = £5.84 · Drug Tariff (Part IXa)

Sodium chloride 0.9% irrigation solution 20ml Sal-e Pods unit dose (Ennogen Healthcare Ltd) **Sodium chloride 9 mg per 1 ml** | 25 unit dose · NHS indicative price = £4.80 · Drug Tariff (Part IXa)

Sodium chloride 0.9% irrigation solution 20ml Salipod unit dose (Sai-Meds Ltd) **Sodium chloride 9 mg per 1 ml** | 25 unit dose · NHS indicative price = £4.99 · Drug Tariff (Part IXa)

Sodium chloride 0.9% irrigation solution 20ml Steripod unit dose (Molnlycke Health Care Ltd) **Sodium chloride 9 mg per 1 ml** | 25 unit dose · NHS indicative price = £7.96 · Drug Tariff (Part IXa)

Sodium chloride 0.9% irrigation solution 20ml Sterowash unit dose (Steroplast Healthcare Ltd) **Sodium chloride 9 mg per 1 ml** | 25 unit dose · NHS indicative price = £5.40 · Drug Tariff (Part IXa)

Sodium chloride 0.9% irrigation solution 20ml unit dose (Alissa Healthcare Research Ltd) **Sodium chloride 9 mg per 1 ml** | 25 unit dose · NHS indicative price = £7.36 · Drug Tariff (Part IXa)

Sodium chloride 0.9% irrigation solution 20ml unit dose (Crest Medical Ltd) **Sodium chloride 9 mg per 1 ml** | 25 unit dose · NHS indicative price = £4.99 · Drug Tariff (Part IXa)

Sodium chloride 0.9% irrigation solution 20ml unit dose (Mylan) **Sodium chloride 9 mg per 1 ml** | 25 unit dose · NHS indicative price = £5.50 · Drug Tariff (Part IXa)

Stericlens sodium chloride 0.9% irrigation solution aerosol spray (C D Medical Ltd) **Sodium chloride 9 mg per 1 ml** | 100 ml · NHS indicative price = £2.07 · Drug Tariff (Part IXa) | 240 ml · NHS indicative price = £3.15 · Drug Tariff (Part IXa)

13

Skin

8.1 Minor cuts and abrasions

Minor cuts and abrasions

Management

Many preparations traditionally used to manage minor burns, and abrasions have fallen out of favour. Preparations containing camphor and sulfonamides should be avoided. Preparations such as magnesium sulfate paste are now rarely used to treat carbuncles and boils as these are best treated with antibiotics.

Cetrimide is used to treat minor cuts and abrasions and proflavine p. 1243 may be used to treat infected wounds or burns, but its use has now been largely superseded by other antiseptics or suitable antibacterials. The effervescent effect of hydrogen peroxide p. 1243 is used to clean minor cuts and abrasions.

Flexible collodion (see castor oil with collodion and colophony below) may be used to seal minor cuts and wounds that have partially healed; skin tissue adhesives are used similarly, and also for additional suture support.

ANTISEPTICS AND DISINFECTANTS > OTHER

Glycerol with magnesium sulfate and phenol

- **INDICATIONS AND DOSE**
  Treat carbuncles and boils
  ▸ TO THE SKIN
  ▸ Adult: To be applied under dressing

- **DIRECTIONS FOR ADMINISTRATION** Paste should be stirred before use.

- **MEDICINAL FORMS**
  There can be variation in the licensing of different medicines containing the same drug.
  Paste
  ▸ Glycerol with magnesium sulfate and phenol (Non-proprietary)
  Phenol 5 mg per 1 gram, Magnesium sulfate dried 450 mg per 1 gram, Glycerol 550 mg per 1 gram Magnesium sulfate paste | 25 gram GSL £0.76-£1.24 | 50 gram GSL £0.91-£2.48 DT = £2.48

DERMATOLOGICAL DRUGS > COLLODIONS

Castor oil with collodion and colophony

- **INDICATIONS AND DOSE**
  Used to seal minor cuts and wounds that have partially healed
  ▸ TO THE SKIN
  ▸ Child: (consult product literature)
  ▸ Adult: (consult product literature)

- **ALLERGY AND CROSS-SENSITIVITY** Contra-indicated if patient has an allergy to colophony in elastic adhesive plasters and tape.

- **MEDICINAL FORMS**
  There can be variation in the licensing of different medicines containing the same drug.
  Flexible collodion
  ▸ Castor oil with collodion and colophony (Non-proprietary)
  Castor oil 25 mg per 1 ml, Colophony 25 mg per 1 ml, Collodion methylated 950 microlitre per 1 ml Flexible collodion methylated | 100 ml £13.54-£13.81 | 500 ml £27.79

Skin adhesives

- SKIN ADHESIVES
  Derma+Flex skin adhesive (Chemence Ltd)
  0.5 ml · NHS indicative price = £5.36 · Drug Tariff (Part IXa)
  Dermabond ProPen skin adhesive (Ethicon Ltd)
  0.5 ml · NHS indicative price = £19.46 · Drug Tariff (Part IXa)
  Histoacryl L skin adhesive (B.Braun Medical Ltd)
  0.5 ml · NHS indicative price = £6.72 · Drug Tariff (Part IXa)
  Histoacryl skin adhesive (B.Braun Medical Ltd)
  0.5 ml · NHS indicative price = £6.50 · Drug Tariff (Part IXa)
  Indermil skin adhesive (Covidien (UK) Commercial Ltd)
  0.5 gram · NHS indicative price = £6.50 · Drug Tariff (Part IXa)
  LiquiBand flow control tissue adhesive (Advanced Medical Solutions Ltd)
  0.5 gram · NHS indicative price = £5.50 · Drug Tariff (Part IXa)
  LiquiBand tissue adhesive (Advanced Medical Solutions Ltd)
  0.5 gram · NHS indicative price = £5.50 · Drug Tariff (Part IXa)

9 Skin disfigurement

Camouflagers

Overview

Disfigurement of the skin can be very distressing to patients and may have a marked psychological effect. In skilled hands, or with experience, camouflage cosmetics can be very effective in concealing scars and birthmarks. The depigmented patches in vitiligo are also very disfiguring and camouflage creams are of great cosmetic value.

Opaque cover foundation or cream is used to mask skin pigment abnormalities; careful application using a combination of dark- and light-coloured cover creams set with powder helps to minimise the appearance of skin deformities.

Borderline substances

The preparations marked 'ACBS' can be prescribed on the NHS for postoperative scars and other deformities and as adjunctive therapy in the relief of emotional disturbances due to disfiguring skin disease, such as vitiligo.

Camouflages

- CAMOUFLAGES
  Covermark classic foundation (Derma UK Ltd)
  15 ml (ACBS) · NHS indicative price = £11.86
  Covermark finishing powder (Derma UK Ltd)
  25 gram (ACBS) · NHS indicative price = £11.86
  Covermark removing cream (Derma UK Ltd)
  200 ml · No NHS indicative price available
  Dermablend Dermasmooth Corrective Foundation (Vichy)
  30 ml · No NHS indicative price available
  Dermacolor Creme Effectiv (Kryolan UK Ltd)
  50 ml · NHS indicative price = £5.73
  Dermacolor body camouflage (Kryolan UK Ltd)
  50 ml · NHS indicative price = £8.94
  Dermacolor camouflage creme (Kryolan UK Ltd)
  30 gram · NHS indicative price = £11.00
  Dermacolor cleansing cream (Kryolan UK Ltd)
  75 gram · No NHS indicative price available
  Dermacolor fixing powder (Kryolan UK Ltd)
  60 gram (ACBS) · NHS indicative price = £9.85
  Keromask finishing powder (Bellava Ltd)
  20 gram (ACBS) · NHS indicative price = £6.07

Keromask masking cream (Bellava Ltd)
15 ml (ACBS) · NHS indicative price = £6.07

Veil cleansing cream (Thomas Blake Cosmetic Creams Ltd)
50 gram · NHS indicative price = £2.45 100 gram · NHS indicative price = £3.90

Veil cover cream (Thomas Blake Cosmetic Creams Ltd)
19 gram (ACBS) · NHS indicative price = £22.42 44 gram (ACBS) · NHS indicative price = £33.35 70 gram (ACBS) · NHS indicative price = £42.10

Veil finishing powder (Thomas Blake Cosmetic Creams Ltd)
35 gram (ACBS) · NHS indicative price = £24.58

10 Sun protection and photodamage

Sunscreen

Sunscreen preparations

Solar ultraviolet irradiation can be harmful to the skin. It is responsible for disorders such as *polymorphic light eruption, solar urticaria,* and it provokes the various *cutaneous porphyrias.* It also provokes (or at least aggravates) skin lesions of *lupus erythematosus* and may aggravate *rosacea* and some other *dermatoses.* Certain drugs, such as demeclocycline, phenothiazines, or amiodarone, can cause photosensitivity. All these conditions (as well as *sunburn*) may occur after relatively short periods of exposure to the sun. Solar ultraviolet irradiation may provoke attacks of recurrent herpes labialis (but it is not known whether the effect of sunlight exposure is local or systemic).

The effects of exposure over longer periods include *ageing changes* and more importantly the initiation of *skin cancer.*

Solar ultraviolet radiation is approximately 200–400 nm in wavelength. The medium wavelengths (290–320 nm, known as UVB) cause *sunburn.* The long wavelengths (320–400 nm, known as UVA) are responsible for many *photosensitivity reactions* and *photodermatoses.* Both UVA and UVB contribute to long-term *photodamage* and to the changes responsible for *skin cancer* and ageing.

Sunscreen preparations contain substances that protect the skin against UVA and UVB radiation, but they are no substitute for covering the skin and avoiding sunlight. The sun protection factor (SPF, usually indicated in the preparation title) provides guidance on the degree of protection offered against UVB; it indicates the multiples of protection provided against burning, compared with unprotected skin; for example, an SPF of 8 should enable a person to remain 8 times longer in the sun without burning. However, in practice, users do not apply sufficient sunscreen product and the protection is lower than that found in experimental studies.

Some manufacturers use a star rating system to indicate the protection against UVA relative to protection against UVB for sunscreen products. However, the usefulness of the star rating system remains controversial. The EU Commission (September 2006) has recommended that the UVA protection factor for a sunscreen should be at least one-third of the sun protection factor (SPF); products that achieve this requirement will be labelled with a UVA logo alongside the SPF classification. Preparations that also contain reflective substances, such as titanium dioxide, provide the most effective protection against UVA.

Sunscreen preparations may rarely cause allergic reactions.

For optimum photoprotection, sunscreen preparations should be applied **thickly** and **frequently** (approximately 2 hourly). In photodermatoses, they should be used from spring to autumn. As maximum protection from sunlight is desirable, preparations with the highest SPF should be prescribed.

Ingredient nomenclature in sunscreen preparations

rINN	INCI
amiloxate	isoamyl *p*-methoxycinnamate
avobenzone	butyl methoxydibenzoylmethane
bemotrizinol	bis-ethylhexyloxyphenol methoxyphenyl triazine
bisoctrizole	methylene bis-benzotriazolyl tetramethylbutylphenol
ecamsule	terephthalylidene dicamphor sulfonic acid
ensulizole	phenylbenzimidazole sulfonic acid
enzacamene	4-methylbenzylidene camphor
octinoxate	octyl (*or* ethylhexyl) methoxycinnamate
octocrilene	octocrylene
oxybenzone	benzophenone-3

The European Commission Cosmetic Products Regulation (EC) 1223/2009 requires the use of INCI (International Nomenclature of Cosmetic Ingredients) for cosmetics and sunscreens. This table includes the rINN and the INCI synonym for the active ingredients of sunscreen preparations in the BNF

Borderline substances

Anthelios® XL SPF 50+ Melt-in cream; *Sunsense*® Ultra; *Uvistat*® Lipscreen SPF 50; and *Uvistat*® Suncream SPF 30 and 50 (see *Borderline substances*) are regarded as drugs when prescribed for skin protection against ultraviolet radiation in abnormal cutaneous photosensitivity resulting from genetic disorders or photodermatoses, including vitiligo and those resulting from radiotherapy; chronic or recurrent herpes simplex labialis. Preparations with SPF less than 30 should not normally be prescribed

Photodamage

Overview

Patients should be advised to use a high-SPF sunscreen and to minimise exposure of the skin to direct sunlight or sun lamps.

Topical treatments can be used for actinic keratosis. An emollient may be sufficient for mild lesions. Diclofenac sodium gel p. 1246 is suitable for the treatment of superficial lesions in mild disease. Fluorouracil cream p. 1246 is effective against most types of non-hypertrophic actinic keratosis; a solution containing fluorouracil with salicylic acid p. 1246 is available for the treatment of low or moderately thick hyperkeratotic actinic keratosis. Imiquimod p. 1249 is used for lesions on the face and scalp when cryotherapy or other topical treatments cannot be used. Fluorouracil and imiquimod produce a more marked inflammatory reaction than diclofenac sodium but lesions resolve faster. A short course of ingenol mebutate p. 1247 is licensed for the treatment of non-hypertrophic actinic keratosis; response to treatment can usually be assessed 8 weeks after the course. Photodynamic therapy in combination with methyl-5-aminolevulinate cream (Metvix®, available from Galderma) or 5-aminolaevulinic acid gel (Ameluz®, available from Spirit Healthcare) is used in specialist centres for treating superficial and confluent, non-hypertrophic actinic keratosis when other treatments are inadequate or unsuitable; it is particularly suitable for multiple lesions, for periorbital lesions, or for lesions located at sites of poor healing.

13

Skin

Imiquimod or topical fluorouracil is used for treating superficial basal cell carcinomas. Photodynamic therapy in combination with methyl-5-aminolevulinate cream is used in specialist centres for treating superficial, nodular basal cell carcinomas when other treatments are unsuitable.

ANALGESICS > NON-STEROIDAL ANTI-INFLAMMATORY DRUGS

Diclofenac sodium

- **INDICATIONS AND DOSE**

SOLARAZE ®

Actinic keratosis
▸ TO THE SKIN
▸ Adult: Apply twice daily for 60–90 days, to be applied thinly; maximum 8 g per day

- CAUTIONS Avoid contact with eyes · avoid contact with inflamed or broken skin · avoid contact with mucous membranes · not for use with occlusive dressings · topical application of large amounts can result in systemic effects, including hypersensitivity and asthma (renal disease has also been reported)
- INTERACTIONS → Appendix 1: NSAIDs
- SIDE-EFFECTS
▸ **Common or very common** Conjunctivitis · muscle tone increased · oedema · rash (discontinue) · sensation abnormal · skin reactions
▸ **Uncommon** Abdominal pain · alopecia · diarrhoea · eye pain · haemorrhage · lacrimation disorder · nausea · seborrhoea
▸ **Rare or very rare** Asthma · hypersensitivity · photosensitivity reaction · rash pustular · renal failure
▸ **Frequency not known** Hair colour changes

SIDE-EFFECTS, FURTHER INFORMATION Topical application of large amounts of diclofenac can result in systemic effects.
- ALLERGY AND CROSS-SENSITIVITY Contra-indicated in patients with a history of hypersensitivity to aspirin or any other NSAID—which includes those in whom attacks of asthma, angioedema, urticaria or rhinitis have been precipitated by aspirin or any other NSAID.
- PREGNANCY Patient packs for topical preparations carry a warning to avoid during pregnancy.
- BREAST FEEDING Patient packs for topical preparations carry a warning to avoid during breast-feeding.
- DIRECTIONS FOR ADMINISTRATION For topical preparations, apply with gentle massage only.
- PATIENT AND CARER ADVICE For topical preparations, patients and their carers should be advised to wash hands immediately after use.
Photosensitivity Patients should be advised against excessive exposure to sunlight of area treated in order to avoid possibility of photosensitivity.
- EXCEPTIONS TO LEGAL CATEGORY Various pack sizes of gel preparations may be available on sale to the public.

- MEDICINAL FORMS
There can be variation in the licensing of different medicines containing the same drug.
Gel
EXCIPIENTS: May contain Benzyl alcohol, fragrances, propylene glycol
▸ Solaraze (Almirall Ltd)
Diclofenac sodium 30 mg per 1 gram Solaraze 3% gel | 50 gram [PoM] £38.30 DT = £38.30 | 100 gram [PoM] £76.60

ANTINEOPLASTIC DRUGS > ANTIMETABOLITES

Fluorouracil

- **INDICATIONS AND DOSE**

Superficial malignant and pre-malignant skin lesions
▸ TO THE SKIN USING CREAM
▸ Adult: Apply 1–2 times a day for 3–4 weeks (usual duration of initial therapy), apply thinly to the affected area, maximum area of skin 500 cm^2 (e.g. 23 cm × 23 cm) treated at one time, alternative regimens may be used in some settings

- CAUTIONS Avoid contact with eyes and mucous membranes · do not apply to bleeding lesions
- INTERACTIONS → Appendix 1: fluorouracil
- SIDE-EFFECTS
▸ **Common or very common** Alopecia · diarrhoea · nausea · skin reactions · stomatitis · thrombocytopenia · vomiting
▸ **Uncommon** Dizziness · headache
▸ **Rare or very rare** Abdominal pain · chills · fever · haemorrhagic diarrhoea · leucocytosis · mucositis · neutropenia · pancytopenia · skin irritation (use a topical corticosteroid for severe discomfort associated with inflammatory reactions) · skin ulcer
▸ **Frequency not known** Conjunctival irritation · excessive tearing · keratitis · taste altered
- CONCEPTION AND CONTRACEPTION Contraceptive advice required, see *Pregnancy and reproductive function* in Cytotoxic drugs p. 865.
- PREGNANCY Manufacturers advise avoid (teratogenic).
- BREAST FEEDING Manufacturers advise avoid.
- HANDLING AND STORAGE Caution in handling—irritant to tissues.

- MEDICINAL FORMS
There can be variation in the licensing of different medicines containing the same drug.
Cream
EXCIPIENTS: May contain Cetostearyl alcohol (including cetyl and stearyl alcohol), hydroxybenzoates (parabens), polysorbates, propylene glycol
▸ Efudix (Meda Pharmaceuticals Ltd)
Fluorouracil 50 mg per 1 gram Efudix 5% cream | 40 gram [PoM] £32.90 DT = £32.90

Fluorouracil with salicylic acid

The properties listed below are those particular to the combination only. For the properties of the components please consider, fluorouracil above, salicylic acid p. 1250.

- **INDICATIONS AND DOSE**

Low or moderately thick hyperkeratotic actinic keratosis
▸ TO THE SKIN
▸ Adult: Apply once daily for up to 12 weeks, reduced to 3 times a week if severe side effects occur and until side-effects improve, to be applied to the affected area, if treating area with thin epidermis, reduce frequency of application and monitor response more often; maximum area of skin treated at one time, 25 cm^2 (e.g. 5 cm × 5 cm)

- INTERACTIONS → Appendix 1: fluorouracil

- MEDICINAL FORMS
There can be variation in the licensing of different medicines containing the same drug.
Cutaneous solution
CAUTIONARY AND ADVISORY LABELS 15
▸ Actikerall (Almirall Ltd)
Fluorouracil 5 mg/g, Salicylic acid 100 mg/g Actikerall 5mg/g / 100mg/g cutaneous solution | 25 ml [PoM] £38.30

PROTEIN KINASE C ACTIVATORS

Ingenol mebutate

● **INDICATIONS AND DOSE**

Actinic keratosis on face and scalp
▶ TO THE SKIN
▶ Adult: Apply once daily for 3 days, use the 150 microgram/g gel

Actinic keratosis on trunk and extremities
▶ TO THE SKIN
▶ Adult: Apply once daily for 2 days, use the 500 microgram/g gel

● CAUTIONS Avoid contact with broken skin · avoid contact with eyes · avoid contact with inside of ears · avoid contact with inside of nostrils · avoid contact with lips · avoid occlusive dressings on treated area

● SIDE-EFFECTS
▶ **Common or very common** Headache · infection · local reaction · oedema · pain · skin reactions
▶ **Uncommon** Paraesthesia · skin ulcer

● PREGNANCY Not absorbed from skin, but manufacturer advises avoid.

● BREAST FEEDING Not absorbed from skin; ensure infant does not come in contact with treated area for 6 hours after application.

● DIRECTIONS FOR ADMINISTRATION One tube covers skin area of 25 cm². Allow gel to dry on treatment area for 15 minutes. Avoid washing or touching the treated area for 6 hours after application; after this time, area may be washed with mild soap and water. Avoid use immediately after shower or less than 2 hours before bedtime.

● MEDICINAL FORMS
There can be variation in the licensing of different medicines containing the same drug.
Gel
CAUTIONARY AND ADVISORY LABELS 15
EXCIPIENTS: May contain Benzyl alcohol
▶ Picato (LEO Pharma)
Ingenol mebutate 150 microgram per 1 gram Picato 150micrograms/g gel | 1.41 gram [PoM] £65.00
Ingenol mebutate 500 microgram per 1 gram Picato 500micrograms/g gel | 0.94 gram [PoM] £65.00

11 Superficial soft-tissue injuries and superficial thrombophlebitis

Topical circulatory preparations

Overview

These preparations are used to improve circulation in conditions such as bruising, superficial thrombophlebitis, chilblains and varicose veins but are of little value. Chilblains are best managed by avoidance of exposure to cold; neither systemic nor topical vasodilator therapy is established as being effective.

HEPARINOIDS

Heparinoid

● **INDICATIONS AND DOSE**

Superficial thrombophlebitis | Bruising | Haematoma
▶ TO THE SKIN
▶ Adult: Apply up to 4 times a day

● CONTRA-INDICATIONS Should not be used on large areas of skin, broken or sensitive skin, or mucous membranes

● LESS SUITABLE FOR PRESCRIBING Hirudoid ® is less suitable for prescribing.

● MEDICINAL FORMS
There can be variation in the licensing of different medicines containing the same drug.
Cream
EXCIPIENTS: May contain Cetostearyl alcohol (including cetyl and stearyl alcohol), hydroxybenzoates (parabens)
▶ Hirudoid (Thornton & Ross Ltd)
Heparinoid 3 mg per 1 gram Hirudoid 0.3% cream | 50 gram [P] £3.99 DT = £3.99
Gel
EXCIPIENTS: May contain Fragrances, propylene glycol
▶ Hirudoid (Thornton & Ross Ltd)
Heparinoid 3 mg per 1 gram Hirudoid 0.3% gel | 50 gram [P] £3.99 DT = £3.99

12 Warts and calluses

Warts and calluses

Overview

Warts (verrucas) are caused by a human papillomavirus, which most frequently affects the hands, feet (plantar warts), and the anogenital region; treatment usually relies on local tissue destruction. Warts may regress on their own and treatment is required only if the warts are painful, unsightly, persistent, or cause distress.

Preparations of salicylic acid p. 1250, formaldehyde p. 1249, glutaraldehyde p. 1249 or silver nitrate p. 1249 are available for purchase by the public; they are suitable for the removal of warts on hands and feet. Salicylic acid is a useful keratolytic which may be considered first-line; it is also suitable for the removal of corns and calluses. Preparations of salicylic acid in a collodion basis are available but some patients may develop an allergy to colophony in the formulation; collodion should be avoided in children allergic to elastic adhesive plaster. Cryotherapy causes pain, swelling, and blistering, and may be no more effective than topical salicylic acid in the treatment of warts.

Anogenital warts

The treatment of anogenital warts (condylomata acuminata) should be accompanied by screening for other sexually transmitted infections. Podophyllotoxin p. 1248 (the major active ingredient of podophyllum) may be used for soft, non-keratinised external anogenital warts. Patients with a limited number of external warts or keratinised lesions may be better treated with cryotherapy or other forms of physical ablation.

Imiquimod cream p. 1249 is licensed for the treatment of external anogenital warts; it may be used for both keratinised and non-keratinised lesions. It is also licensed for the treatment of superficial basal cell carcinoma and actinic keratosis. Camellia sinensis ointment p. 1248 is licensed for the treatment of external anogenital warts.

Inosine pranobex p. 622 is licensed for adjunctive treatment of genital warts but it has been superseded by more effective drugs.

ANTINEOPLASTIC DRUGS > PLANT ALKALOIDS

Camellia sinensis

03-May-2017

- **DRUG ACTION** Camellia sinensis is an extract from green tea leaves. The exact mechanism of action is not known; non-clinical studies have shown inhibition of the growth of activated keratinocytes, and anti-oxidative effects at the site of application.

- **INDICATIONS AND DOSE**

Warts (external genital and perianal) in immunocompetent patients

- ▸ TO THE LESION
  - ▸ **Adult:** Apply up to 250 mg 3 times a day until complete clearance of warts (maximum 16 weeks), do not exceed treatment period even if new warts develop; maximum 750 mg per day

DOSE EQUIVALENCE AND CONVERSION
- ▸ 250 mg is equivalent to 0.5 cm of ointment.

- **CAUTIONS** Avoid broken skin · avoid contact with eyes · avoid contact with lips · avoid contact with mouth · avoid contact with nostrils · avoid inflamed skin · uncircumcised males (risk of phimosis) · vulvar region

- **SIDE-EFFECTS**
  - ▸ **Uncommon** Balanoposthitis · increased risk of infection · lymphatic abnormalities · necrosis · painful sexual intercourse · phimosis · skin reactions · urinary disorders
  - ▸ **Frequency not known** Urinary tract stenosis · vaginal discharge

- **CONCEPTION AND CONTRACEPTION** Manufacturer advises *Catephen* ® may weaken condoms and vaginal diaphragms—alternative methods of contraception should be considered.

- **PREGNANCY** Manufacturer advises avoid—toxicity in *animal* studies.

- **BREAST FEEDING** Manufacturer advises risk to infant cannot be excluded—no information available.

- **HEPATIC IMPAIRMENT** Manufacturer advises avoid in severe impairment—no information available.

- **DIRECTIONS FOR ADMINISTRATION** Manufacturer advises apply to each wart, ensuring a thin layer is left on the wart. It is not necessary to wash off the ointment from the area before next application.

- **PATIENT AND CARER ADVICE** Manufacturer advises the ointment should be washed off before sexual activity. Manufacturer advises female patients using tampons should insert tampon before applying the ointment.

- **NATIONAL FUNDING/ACCESS DECISIONS**

Scottish Medicines Consortium (SMC) Decisions
The *Scottish Medicines Consortium* has advised (April 2016) that camellia sinensis (green tea) leaf extract (*Catephen* ®) is accepted for restricted use within NHS Scotland for the treatment of external genital and perianal warts in patients not suitable for podophyllotoxin or who have not responded to treatment with podophyllotoxin.

All Wales Medicines Strategy Group (AWMSG) Decisions
The *All Wales Medicines Strategy Group* has advised (October 2016) that green tea leaf extract (camellia sinensis), (*Catephen* ®), is recommended for restricted use within NHS Wales for the treatment of external genital and perianal warts in patients not suitable for podophyllotoxin or who have not responded to treatment with podophyllotoxin.

- **MEDICINAL FORMS**
There can be variation in the licensing of different medicines containing the same drug.
Ointment
- ▸ Catephen (KoRa Healthcare)
  Camellia sinensis extract 100 mg per 1 gram Catephen 10% ointment | 15 gram [PoM] £39.00

Podophyllotoxin

- **INDICATIONS AND DOSE**

CONDYLINE ®

Condylomata acuminata affecting the penis or the female external genitalia
- ▸ TO THE LESION
  - ▸ **Adult:** Apply twice daily for 3 consecutive days, treatment may be repeated at weekly intervals if necessary for a total of five 3-day treatment courses, direct medical supervision for lesions in the female and for lesions greater than 4 cm^2 in the male, maximum 50 single applications ('loops') per session (consult product literature)

WARTICON ® CREAM

Condylomata acuminata affecting the penis or the female external genitalia
- ▸ TO THE LESION
  - ▸ **Adult:** Apply twice daily for 3 consecutive days, treatment may be repeated at weekly intervals if necessary for a total of four 3-day treatment courses, direct medical supervision for lesions greater than 4 cm^2

WARTICON ® LIQUID

Condylomata acuminata affecting the penis or the female external genitalia
- ▸ TO THE LESION
  - ▸ **Adult:** Apply twice daily for 3 consecutive days, treatment may be repeated at weekly intervals if necessary for a total of four 3-day treatment courses, direct medical supervision for lesions greater than 4 cm^2, maximum 50 single applications ('loops') per session (consult product literature)

- **CAUTIONS** Avoid normal skin · avoid open wounds · keep away from face · very irritant to eyes

- **SIDE-EFFECTS** Balanoposthitis · skin irritation

- **PREGNANCY** Avoid.

- **BREAST FEEDING** Avoid.

- **MEDICINAL FORMS**
There can be variation in the licensing of different medicines containing the same drug.
Cream
EXCIPIENTS: May contain Butylated hydroxyanisole, cetostearyl alcohol (including cetyl and stearyl alcohol), hydroxybenzoates (parabens), sorbic acid
- ▸ Warticon (Stiefel Laboratories (UK) Ltd)
  Podophyllotoxin 1.5 mg per 1 gram Warticon 0.15% cream | 5 gram [PoM] £17.83 DT = £17.83
Liquid
CAUTIONARY AND ADVISORY LABELS 15
- ▸ Condyline (Takeda UK Ltd)
  Podophyllotoxin 5 mg per 1 ml Condyline 0.5% solution | 3.5 ml [PoM] £14.49 DT = £14.49
- ▸ Warticon (Stiefel Laboratories (UK) Ltd)
  Podophyllotoxin 5 mg per 1 ml Warticon 0.5% solution | 3 ml [PoM] £14.86 DT = £14.86

ANTISEPTICS AND DISINFECTANTS >
ALDEHYDES AND DERIVATIVES

Formaldehyde

- **INDICATIONS AND DOSE**

Warts, particularly plantar warts
▸ TO THE LESION
▸ Child: Apply twice daily
▸ Adult: Apply twice daily

- **UNLICENSED USE** Licensed for use in children (age range not specified by manufacturer).
- **CAUTIONS** Impaired peripheral circulation · not suitable for application to anogenital region · not suitable for application to face · not suitable for application to large areas · patients with diabetes at risk of neuropathic ulcers · protect surrounding skin and avoid broken skin · significant peripheral neuropathy
- **SIDE-EFFECTS** Asthma · cough · dysphagia · eye irritation · increased risk of infection · laryngospasm · skin reactions

- **MEDICINAL FORMS**
There can be variation in the licensing of different medicines containing the same drug. Forms available from special-order manufacturers include: liquid
Liquid
▸ Formaldehyde (Non-proprietary)
  Formaldehyde 40 mg per 1 ml Formaldehyde (Buffered) 4% solution | 100 ml £3.90 DT = £3.90
  Formaldehyde 350 mg per 1 gram Formaldehyde solution | 500 ml £5.90 DT = £5.90 | 2000 ml £16.98

Glutaraldehyde

- **INDICATIONS AND DOSE**

Warts, particularly plantar warts
▸ TO THE LESION
▸ Child: Apply twice daily
▸ Adult: Apply twice daily

- **UNLICENSED USE** Licensed for use in children (age range not specified by manufacturer).
- **CAUTIONS** Not for application to anogenital areas · not for application to face · not for application to mucosa · protect surrounding skin
- **SIDE-EFFECTS**
▸ **Rare or very rare** Severe cutaneous adverse reactions (SCARs)
▸ **Frequency not known** Rash · skin irritation (discontinue if severe)

- **MEDICINAL FORMS**
There can be variation in the licensing of different medicines containing the same drug.
Paint
▸ Glutarol (Dermal Laboratories Ltd)
  Glutaraldehyde 100 mg per 1 ml Glutarol 10% cutaneous solution | 10 ml [P] £2.07 DT = £2.07

ANTISEPTICS AND DISINFECTANTS > OTHER

Silver nitrate

- **INDICATIONS AND DOSE**

Common warts
▸ TO THE LESION
▸ Child: Apply every 24 hours for up to 3 applications, apply moistened caustic pencil tip for 1–2 minutes. Instructions in proprietary packs generally incorporate

advice to remove dead skin before use by gentle filing and to cover with adhesive dressing after application
▸ Adult: Apply every 24 hours for up to 3 applications, apply moistened caustic pencil tip for 1–2 minutes. Instructions in proprietary packs generally incorporate advice to remove dead skin before use by gentle filing and to cover with adhesive dressing after application

Verrucas
▸ TO THE LESION
▸ Child: Apply every 24 hours for up to 6 applications, apply moistened caustic pencil tip for 1–2 minutes. Instructions in proprietary packs generally incorporate advice to remove dead skin before use by gentle filing and to cover with adhesive dressing after application
▸ Adult: Apply every 24 hours for up to 6 applications, apply moistened caustic pencil tip for 1–2 minutes. Instructions in proprietary packs generally incorporate advice to remove dead skin before use by gentle filing and to cover with adhesive dressing after application

Umbilical granulomas
▸ TO THE SKIN
▸ Child: Apply moistened caustic pencil tip (usually containing silver nitrate 40%) for 1–2 minutes, protect surrounding skin with soft paraffin
▸ Adult: Apply moistened caustic pencil tip (usually containing silver nitrate 40%) for 1–2 minutes, protect surrounding skin with soft paraffin

- **UNLICENSED USE**
▸ In children No age range specified by manufacturer.
- **CAUTIONS** Avoid broken skin · not suitable for application to ano-genital region · not suitable for application to face · not suitable for application to large areas · protect surrounding skin
- **SIDE-EFFECTS**
▸ **Rare or very rare** Argyria · methaemoglobinaemia
- **PATIENT AND CARER ADVICE** Patients should be advised that silver nitrate may stain fabric.

- **MEDICINAL FORMS**
There can be variation in the licensing of different medicines containing the same drug.
Stick
▸ Avoca (Bray Group Ltd)
  Silver nitrate 400 mg per 1 gram Avoca 40% silver nitrate pencils | 1 applicator [P] £1.13
  Silver nitrate 750 mg per 1 gram Avoca 75% silver nitrate applicators | 100 applicator [P] £47.82
  Avoca 75% silver nitrate applicators with thick handles | 50 applicator [P] £47.19
  Silver nitrate 950 mg per 1 gram Avoca 95% silver nitrate applicators | 100 applicator [P] £51.17
  Avoca 95% silver nitrate pencils | 1 applicator [P] £2.56 DT = £3.00
  Avoca wart and verruca treatment set | 1 applicator [P] £3.00 DT = £3.00

ANTIVIRALS > IMMUNE RESPONSE MODIFIERS

Imiquimod

- **INDICATIONS AND DOSE**

ALDARA ®

Warts (external genital and perianal)
▸ TO THE LESION
▸ Adult: Apply 3 times a week until lesions resolve (maximum 16 weeks), to be applied thinly at night

Superficial basal cell carcinoma
▸ TO THE LESION
▸ Adult: Apply daily for 5 nights of each week for 6 weeks, to be applied to lesion and 1 cm beyond it, assess response 12 weeks after completing treatment

continued →

13

Skin

Actinic keratosis

▸ TO THE LESION

▸ **Adult:** Apply 3 times a week for 4 weeks, to be applied to lesion at night, assess response after a 4 week treatment-free interval; repeat 4-week course if lesions persist, maximum 2 courses

ZYCLARA ®

Actinic keratosis

▸ TO THE SKIN

▸ **Adult:** Apply once daily for 2 weeks, to be applied at bedtime to lesion on face or balding scalp, repeat course after a 2-week treatment-free interval, assess response 8 weeks after second course; maximum 2 sachets per day

● CAUTIONS Autoimmune disease · avoid broken skin · avoid contact with eyes · avoid contact with lips · avoid contact with nostrils · avoid open wounds · immunosuppressed patients · not suitable for internal genital warts · uncircumcised males (risk of phimosis or stricture of foreskin)

● SIDE-EFFECTS

▸ **Common or very common** Appetite decreased · arthralgia · asthenia · headaches · increased risk of infection · lymphadenopathy · myalgia · nausea · pain

▸ **Uncommon** Anorectal disorder · chills · conjunctival irritation · depression · diarrhoea · dizziness · drowsiness · dry mouth · dysuria · erectile dysfunction · eyelid oedema · face oedema · fever · flushing · gastrointestinal discomfort · genital pain · hyperhidrosis · inflammation · influenza like illness · insomnia · irritability · laryngeal pain · malaise · nasal congestion · painful sexual intercourse · paraesthesia · penis disorder · skin reactions · skin ulcer · tinnitus · uterovaginal prolapse · vomiting · vulvovaginal disorders

▸ **Rare or very rare** Autoimmune disorder exacerbated

▸ **Frequency not known** Alopecia · cutaneous lupus erythematosus · severe cutaneous adverse reactions (SCARs)

● CONCEPTION AND CONTRACEPTION May damage latex condoms and diaphragms.

● PREGNANCY No evidence of teratogenicity or toxicity in *animal* studies; manufacturer advises caution.

● BREAST FEEDING No information available.

● DIRECTIONS FOR ADMINISTRATION

ZYCLARA ® ▸ **Important** Should be rubbed in and allowed to stay on the treated area for 8 hours, then washed off with mild soap and water.

ALDARA ® ▸ **Important** Should be rubbed in and allowed to stay on the treated area for 6–10 hours for warts or for 8 hours for basal cell carcinoma and actinic keratosis, then washed off with mild soap and water (uncircumcised males treating warts under foreskin should wash the area daily). The cream should be washed off before sexual contact.

● PATIENT AND CARER ADVICE A patient information leaflet should be provided.

● MEDICINAL FORMS
There can be variation in the licensing of different medicines containing the same drug.

Cream

CAUTIONARY AND ADVISORY LABELS 10
EXCIPIENTS: May contain Benzyl alcohol, cetostearyl alcohol (including cetyl and stearyl alcohol), hydroxybenzoates (parabens), polysorbates

▸ Aldara (Meda Pharmaceuticals Ltd)
Imiquimod 50 mg per 1 gram Aldara 5% cream 250mg sachets | 12 sachet PoM £48.60 DT = £48.60

▸ Zyclara (Meda Pharmaceuticals Ltd)
Imiquimod 37.5 mg per 1 gram Zyclara 3.75% cream 250mg sachets | 28 sachet PoM £113.00 DT = £113.00

SALICYLIC ACID AND DERIVATIVES

Salicylic acid

● INDICATIONS AND DOSE

OCCLUSAL ®

Common and plantar warts

▸ TO THE LESION

▸ **Child:** Apply daily, treatment may need to be continued for up to 3 months

▸ **Adult:** Apply daily, treatment may need to be continued for up to 3 months

VERRUGON ®

For plantar warts

▸ TO THE LESION

▸ **Child:** Apply daily, treatment may need to be continued for up to 3 months

▸ **Adult:** Apply daily, treatment may need to be continued for up to 3 months

● UNLICENSED USE Not licensed for use in children under 2 years.

● CAUTIONS Avoid broken skin · impaired peripheral circulation · not suitable for application to anogenital region · not suitable for application to face · not suitable for application to large areas · patients with diabetes at risk of neuropathic ulcers · significant peripheral neuropathy

● SIDE-EFFECTS Skin irritation

● PATIENT AND CARER ADVICE Advise patient to apply carefully to wart and to protect surrounding skin (e.g. with soft paraffin or specially designed plaster); rub wart surface gently with file or pumice stone once weekly.

● MEDICINAL FORMS
There can be variation in the licensing of different medicines containing the same drug. Forms available from special-order manufacturers include: liquid, ointment

Ointment

▸ Verrugon (Optima Consumer Health Ltd)
Salicylic acid 500 mg per 1 gram Verrugon complete 50% ointment | 6 gram P £4.44 DT = £4.44

Liquid

CAUTIONARY AND ADVISORY LABELS 15

▸ Occlusal (Alliance Pharmaceuticals Ltd)
Salicylic acid 260 mg per 1 ml Occlusal 26% solution | 10 ml P £3.56 DT = £3.56

Salicylic acid with lactic acid

The properties listed below are those particular to the combination only. For the properties of the components please consider, salicylic acid above.

● INDICATIONS AND DOSE

CUPLEX ®

Plantar and mosaic warts | Corns | Calluses

▸ TO THE LESION

▸ **Adult:** Apply once daily, treatment may need to be continued for up to 3 months

DUOFILM ®

Plantar and mosaic warts

▸ TO THE LESION

▸ **Adult:** Apply daily, treatment may need to be continued for up to 3 months

SALACTOL ®

Warts, particularly plantar warts | Verrucas | Corns | Calluses
▶ TO THE LESION
▶ Adult: Apply daily, treatment may need to be continued for up to 3 months

SALATAC ®

Warts | Verrucas | Corns | Calluses
▶ TO THE LESION
▶ Adult: Apply daily, treatment may need to be continued for up to 3 months

● PRESCRIBING AND DISPENSING INFORMATION
Preparations of salicylic acid in a collodion basis (Cuplex ® and Salactol ®) are available but some patients may develop an allergy to colophony in the formulation.

● MEDICINAL FORMS
There can be variation in the licensing of different medicines containing the same drug.

Paint
CAUTIONARY AND ADVISORY LABELS 15
▶ Duofilm (GlaxoSmithKline UK Ltd)
  Lactic acid 150 mg per 1 gram, Salicylic acid 167 mg per 1 gram Duofilm paint | 15 ml P £2.25 DT = £2.25
▶ Salactol (Dermal Laboratories Ltd)
  Lactic acid 167 mg per 1 gram, Salicylic acid 167 mg per 1 gram Salactol paint | 10 ml P £1.71 DT = £1.71

Gel
CAUTIONARY AND ADVISORY LABELS 15
▶ Cuplex (Crawford Healthcare Ltd)
  Lactic acid 40 mg per 1 gram, Salicylic acid 110 mg per 1 gram Cuplex Verruca gel | 5 gram GSL £2.88 DT = £2.88
▶ Salatac (Dermal Laboratories Ltd)
  Lactic acid 40 mg per 1 gram, Salicylic acid 120 mg per 1 gram Salatac gel | 8 gram P £2.98 DT = £2.98

Chapter 14
Vaccines

CONTENTS

1   Immunoglobulin therapy

IMMUNE SERA AND IMMUNOGLOBULINS >
IMMUNOGLOBULINS

Immunoglobulins

04-Oct-2017

Passive immunity

Immunity with immediate protection against certain infective organisms can be obtained by injecting preparations made from the plasma of immune individuals with adequate levels of antibody to the disease for which protection is sought. The duration of this passive immunity varies according to the dose and the type of immunoglobulin. Passive immunity may last only a few weeks; when necessary, passive immunisation can be repeated. Antibodies of human origin are usually termed immunoglobulins. The term antiserum is applied to material prepared in animals. Because of serum sickness and other allergic-type reactions that may follow injections of antisera, this therapy has been replaced wherever possible by the use of immunoglobulins. Reactions are theoretically possible after injection of human immunoglobulins but reports of such reactions are very rare.

Two types of human immunoglobulin preparation are available, normal immunoglobulin p. 1255 and **disease-specific immunoglobulins**.

Human immunoglobulin is a sterile preparation of concentrated antibodies (immune globulins) recovered from pooled human plasma or serum obtained from outside the UK, tested and found non-reactive for hepatitis B surface antigen and for antibodies against hepatitis C virus and human immunodeficiency virus (types 1 and 2). A global shortage of human immunoglobulin and the rapidly increasing range of clinical indications for treatment with immunoglobulins has resulted in the need for a Demand Management programme in the UK, for further information consult www.ivig.nhs.uk and *Clinical Guidelines for Immunoglobulin Use*, www.gov.uk/dh.

Further information on the use of immunoglobulins is included in Public Health England's *Immunoglobulin Handbook* www.gov.uk/phe, and in the Department of Health's publication, *Immunisation against Infectious Disease*, www.gov.uk/dh.

Availability

Normal immunoglobulin for intramuscular administration is available from some regional Public Health laboratories for protection of contacts and the control of outbreaks of hepatitis A, measles, and rubella only. For other indications, subcutaneous or intravenous normal immunoglobulin should be purchased from the manufacturer.

Disease-specific immunoglobulins are available from some regional Public Health laboratories, with the exception of tetanus immunoglobulin p. 1257 which is available from

BPL, hospital pharmacies, or blood transfusion departments. Rabies immunoglobulin p. 1257 is available from the Specialist and Reference Microbiology Division, Public Health England, Colindale. Hepatitis B immunoglobulin p. 1255 required by transplant centres should be obtained commercially.

In Scotland all immunoglobulins are available from the *Scottish National Blood Transfusion Service* (SNBTS).

In Wales all immunoglobulins are available from the *Welsh Blood Service* (WBS).

In Northern Ireland all immunoglobulins are available from the *Northern Ireland Blood Transfusion Service* (NIBTS).

Normal immunoglobulin

Human normal immunoglobulin ('HNIG') is prepared from pools of at least 1000 donations of human plasma; it contains immunoglobulin G (IgG) and antibodies to hepatitis A, measles, mumps, rubella, varicella, and other viruses that are currently prevalent in the general population.

Uses

Normal immunoglobulin (containing 10%–18% protein) is administered by *intramuscular injection* for the protection of susceptible contacts against **hepatitis A** virus (infectious hepatitis), **measles** and, to a lesser extent, **rubella**. Injection of immunoglobulin produces immediate protection lasting several weeks.

Normal immunoglobulin (containing 3%–12% protein) for *intravenous administration* is used as *replacement therapy* for patients with congenital agammaglobulinaemia and hypogammaglobulinaemia, and for the short-term treatment of idiopathic thrombocytopenic purpura and Kawasaki disease; it is also used for the prophylaxis of infection following bone-marrow transplantation and in children with symptomatic HIV infection who have recurrent bacterial infections. Normal immunoglobulin for replacement therapy may also be given intramuscularly or subcutaneously, but intravenous formulations are normally preferred. Intravenous immunoglobulin is also used in the treatment of Guillain-Barré syndrome as an alternative to plasma exchange.

For guidance on the use of intravenous normal immunoglobulin and alternative therapies for certain conditions, consult *Clinical Guidelines for Immunoglobulin Use* (www.gov.uk/dh).

Hepatitis A

Hepatitis A vaccine p. 1279 is recommended for individuals at risk of infection including those visiting areas where the disease is highly endemic (all countries excluding Northern and Western Europe, North America, Japan, Australia, and New Zealand). In unimmunised individuals, transmission of hepatitis A is reduced by good hygiene. Intramuscular normal immunoglobulin is no longer recommended for prophylaxis in travellers.

Public Health England recommends the use of normal immunoglobulin in addition to hepatitis A vaccine for prevention of infection in close contacts (of confirmed cases of hepatitis A) who are 60 years of age or over, have chronic liver disease (including chronic hepatitis B or C infection), or HIV infection (with a CD4 count < 200 cells per microlitre), or who are immunosuppressed; normal immunoglobulin should be given as soon as possible, preferably within 14 days of exposure to the primary case. However, normal immunoglobulin can still be given to contacts with chronic liver disease up to 28 days after exposure to the primary case. Hepatitis A vaccine can be given at the same time, but it should be given at a separate injection site.

Measles

Intravenous or subcutaneous normal immunoglobulin may be given to prevent or attenuate an attack of measles in individuals who do not have adequate immunity. Patients with compromised immunity who have come into contact with measles should receive intravenous or subcutaneous normal immunoglobulin as soon as possible after exposure. It is most effective if given within 72 hours but can be effective if given within 6 days.

Subcutaneous or intramuscular normal immunoglobulin should also be considered for the following individuals if they have been in contact with a confirmed case of measles or with a person associated with a local outbreak:

- non-immune pregnant women
- infants under 9 months

Further advice should be sought from the Centre for Infections, Public Health England (tel. (020) 8200 6868).

Individuals with normal immunity who are not in the above categories and who have not been fully immunised against measles, can be given measles, mumps and rubella vaccine, live p. 1284 for prophylaxis following exposure to measles.

Rubella

Intramuscular immunoglobulin after exposure to rubella does **not** prevent infection in non-immune contacts and is **not** recommended for protection of pregnant women exposed to rubella. It may, however, reduce the likelihood of a clinical attack which may possibly reduce the risk to the fetus. Risk of intra-uterine transmission is greatest in the first 11 weeks of pregnancy, between 16 and 20 weeks there is minimal risk of deafness only, after 20 weeks there is no increased risk. Intramuscular normal immunoglobulin should be used only if termination of pregnancy would be unacceptable to the pregnant woman—it should be given as soon as possible after exposure. Serological follow-up of recipients is essential to determine if the woman has become infected despite receiving immunoglobulin.

For routine prophylaxis against Rubella, see measles, mumps and rubella vaccine, live p. 1284.

Disease-specific immunoglobulins

Specific immunoglobulins are prepared by pooling the plasma of selected human donors with high levels of the specific antibody required. For further information, see *Immunoglobulin Handbook* (www.gov.uk/phe).

There are no specific immunoglobulins for hepatitis A, measles, or rubella— normal immunoglobulin p. 1255 is used in certain circumstances. There is no specific immunoglobulin for mumps; neither normal immunoglobulin nor measles, mumps and rubella vaccine, live is effective as post-exposure prophylaxis.

Hepatitis B immunoglobulin

Disease-specific hepatitis B immunoglobulin p. 1255 ('HBIG') is available for use in association with hepatitis B vaccine p. 1280 for the prevention of infection in laboratory and other personnel who have been accidentally inoculated with hepatitis B virus, and in infants born to mothers who have become infected with this virus in pregnancy or who are high-risk carriers. Hepatitis B immunoglobulin will not inhibit the antibody response when given at the same time as hepatitis B vaccine but should be given at different sites.

An intravenous and subcutaneous preparation of hepatitis B immunoglobulin is licensed for the prevention of hepatitis B recurrence in HBV-DNA negative patients who have undergone liver transplantation for liver failure caused by the virus.

Rabies immunoglobulin

Following exposure of an unimmunised individual to an animal in or from a country where the risk of rabies is high the site of the bite should be washed with soapy water and specific rabies immunoglobulin p. 1257 of human origin administered. All of the dose should be injected around the site of the wound; if this is difficult or the wound has completely healed it can be given in the anterolateral thigh (remote from the site used for vaccination).

Rabies vaccine p. 1285 should also be given intramuscularly at a different site (for details see rabies vaccine). If there is delay in giving the rabies immunoglobulin, it should be given within 7 days of starting the course of rabies vaccine.

Tetanus immunoglobulin

For the management of tetanus-prone wounds, tetanus immunoglobulin p. 1257 should be used in addition to wound cleansing and, where appropriate, antibacterial prophylaxis and a tetanus-containing vaccine. Tetanus immunoglobulin, together with metronidazole p. 533 and wound cleansing, should also be used for the treatment of established cases of tetanus.

Varicella-zoster immunoglobulin

Varicella-zoster immunoglobulin p. 1257 (VZIG) is recommended for individuals who are at increased risk of severe varicella (neonates, pregnant women and immunosuppressed individuals with varicella-zoster virus immunoglobulin G antibody less than 150 mIU/mL) *and* who have no antibodies to varicella–zoster virus *and* who have significant exposure to chickenpox (varicella) or shingles (herpes zoster) during the infectious period.

Immunosuppressed patients receiving regular intravenous immunoglobulin replacement therapy only require varicella-zoster immunoglobulin if the most recent dose was administered more than 3 weeks before exposure.

Immunosuppressed patients on long term aciclovir p. 623 or valaciclovir p. 625 prophylaxis will require a temporary increase in their dose following exposure; for patients within 12 months of a stem cell transplant, varicella-zoster immunoglobulin should also be considered.

Important: for full details consult *Guidance for issuing varicella-zoster immunoglobulin (VZIG)* and *Immunisation against infectious disease* from Public Health England (www.gov.uk).

Anti-D (Rh₀) immunoglobulin

Anti-D (Rh$_0$) immunoglobulin p. 1254 is prepared from plasma taken from rhesus-negative donors who have been immunised against the anti-D-antigen. Anti-D (Rh$_0$) immunoglobulin is used to prevent a rhesus-negative mother from forming antibodies to fetal rhesus-positive cells which may pass into the maternal circulation. The objective is to protect any subsequent child from the hazard of haemolytic disease of the newborn.

Anti-D (Rh$_0$) immunoglobulin should be administered to the mother following any sensitising episode (e.g. abortion, miscarriage and birth); it should be injected within 72 hours of the episode but even if a longer period has elapsed it may still give protection and should be administered. Anti-D (Rh$_0$) immunoglobulin is also given when significant feto-maternal haemorrhage occurs in rhesus-negative women during delivery. The dose of anti-D (Rh$_0$) immunoglobulin is determined according to the level of exposure to rhesus-positive blood.

Use of routine *antenatal* anti-D prophylaxis should be given irrespective of previous anti-D prophylaxis for a

14

Vaccines

sensitising event early in the same pregnancy. Similarly, *postpartum* anti-D prophylaxis should be given irrespective of previous routine antenatal anti-D prophylaxis or antenatal anti-D prophylaxis for a sensitising event in the same pregnancy.

Anti-D (Rh₀) immunoglobulin is also given to women of child-bearing potential after the inadvertent transfusion of rhesus-incompatible blood components and is used for the treatment of idiopathic thrombocytopenia purpura.

MMR vaccine
Measles, mumps and rubella vaccine, live may be given in the postpartum period with anti-D (Rh₀) immunoglobulin injection provided that separate syringes are used and the products are administered into different limbs. If blood is transfused, the antibody response to the vaccine may be inhibited—measure rubella antibodies after 6–8 weeks and revaccinate if necessary.

Anti-D (Rh₀) immunoglobulin

● INDICATIONS AND DOSE
To rhesus-negative woman for prevention of Rh₀(D) sensitisation, following birth of rhesus-positive infant
▸ BY DEEP INTRAMUSCULAR INJECTION
▸ Females of childbearing potential: 500 units, dose to be administered immediately or within 72 hours; for transplacental bleed of over 4 mL fetal red cells, extra 100–125 units per mL fetal red cells, subcutaneous route used for patients with bleeding disorders

To rhesus-negative woman for prevention of Rh₀(D) sensitisation, following any potentially sensitising episode (e.g. stillbirth, abortion, amniocentesis) up to 20 weeks' gestation
▸ BY DEEP INTRAMUSCULAR INJECTION
▸ Females of childbearing potential: 250 units per episode, dose to be administered immediately or within 72 hours, subcutaneous route used for patients with bleeding disorders

To rhesus-negative woman for prevention of Rh₀(D) sensitisation, following any potentially sensitising episode (e.g. stillbirth, abortion, amniocentesis) after 20 weeks' gestation
▸ BY DEEP INTRAMUSCULAR INJECTION
▸ Females of childbearing potential: 500 units per episode, dose to be administered immediately or within 72 hours, subcutaneous route used for patients with bleeding disorders

To rhesus-negative woman for prevention of Rh₀(D) sensitisation, antenatal prophylaxis
▸ BY DEEP INTRAMUSCULAR INJECTION
▸ Females of childbearing potential: 500 units, dose to be given at weeks 28 and 34 of pregnancy, if infant rhesus-positive, a further dose is still needed immediately or within 72 hours of delivery, subcutaneous route used for patients with bleeding disorders

To rhesus-negative woman for prevention of Rh₀(D) sensitisation, antenatal prophylaxis (alternative NICE recommendation)
▸ BY DEEP INTRAMUSCULAR INJECTION
▸ Females of childbearing potential: 1000–1650 units, dose to be given at weeks 28 and 34 of pregnancy, alternatively 1500 units for 1 dose, dose to be given between 28 and 30 weeks gestation

To rhesus-negative woman for prevention of Rh₀(D) sensitisation, following Rh₀(D) incompatible blood transfusion
▸ BY DEEP INTRAMUSCULAR INJECTION
▸ Females of childbearing potential: 100–125 units per mL of transfused rhesus-positive red cells, subcutaneous route used for patients with bleeding disorders

RHOPHYLAC ®
To rhesus-negative woman for prevention of Rh₀(D) sensitisation, following birth of rhesus-positive infant
▸ BY INTRAMUSCULAR INJECTION, OR BY INTRAVENOUS INJECTION
▸ Females of childbearing potential: 1000–1500 units, dose to administered immediately or within 72 hours; for large transplacental bleed, extra 100 units per mL fetal red cells (preferably by intravenous injection), intravenous route recommended for patients with bleeding disorders

To rhesus-negative woman for prevention of Rh₀(D) sensitisation, following any potentially sensitising episode (e.g. abortion, amniocentesis, chorionic villous sampling) up to 12 weeks' gestation
▸ BY INTRAMUSCULAR INJECTION, OR BY INTRAVENOUS INJECTION
▸ Females of childbearing potential: 1000 units per episode, dose to be administered immediately or within 72 hours, intravenous route recommended for patients with bleeding disorders, higher doses may be required after 12 weeks gestation

To rhesus-negative woman for prevention of Rh₀(D) sensitisation, antenatal prophylaxis
▸ BY INTRAMUSCULAR INJECTION, OR BY INTRAVENOUS INJECTION
▸ Females of childbearing potential: 1500 units, dose to be given between weeks 28–30 of pregnancy; if infant rhesus-positive, a further dose is still needed immediately or within 72 hours of delivery, intravenous route recommended for patients with bleeding disorders

To rhesus-negative woman for prevention of Rh₀(D) sensitisation, following Rh₀(D) incompatible blood transfusion
▸ BY INTRAVENOUS INJECTION
▸ Females of childbearing potential: 50 units per mL of transfused rhesus-positive blood, alternatively 100 units per of mL of erythrocyte concentrate, intravenous route recommended for patients with bleeding disorders

● CONTRA-INDICATIONS Treatment of idiopathic thrombocytopenia purpura in rhesus negative patients · treatment of idiopathic thrombocytopenia purpura in splenectomised patients

● CAUTIONS Immunoglobulin A deficiency · possible interference with live virus vaccines
CAUTIONS, FURTHER INFORMATION
▸ MMR vaccine MMR vaccine may be given in the postpartum period with anti-D (Rh₀) immunoglobulin injection provided that separate syringes are used and the products are administered into different limbs. If blood is transfused, the antibody response to the vaccine may be inhibited—measure rubella antibodies after 6–8 weeks and revaccinate if necessary.

● SIDE-EFFECTS
▸ **Uncommon** Chills · fever · headache · malaise · skin reactions
▸ **Rare or very rare** Arthralgia · dyspnoea · hypersensitivity · hypotension · nausea · tachycardia · vomiting
▸ **Frequency not known** Intravascular haemolysis

- HANDLING AND STORAGE Care must be taken to store all immunological products under the conditions recommended in the product literature, otherwise the preparation may become ineffective. **Refrigerated storage** is usually necessary; many immunoglobulins need to be stored at 2–8°C and not allowed to freeze. Immunoglobulins should be protected from light. Opened multidose vials must be used within the period recommended in the product literature.

- NATIONAL FUNDING/ACCESS DECISIONS

NICE decisions

▸ **Routine antenatal anti-D prophylaxis for rhesus-negative women (August 2008)** NICE TA156
Routine antenatal anti-D prophylaxis should be offered to all non-sensitised pregnant women who are rhesus negative.
www.nice.org.uk/TA156

- MEDICINAL FORMS
There can be variation in the licensing of different medicines containing the same drug.

Solution for injection

▸ D-Gam (Bio Products Laboratory Ltd)
Anti-D (Rh$_0$) immunoglobulin 500 unit D-Gam Anti-D immunoglobulin 500unit solution for injection vials | 1 vial [PoM] £33.75
Anti-D (Rh$_0$) immunoglobulin 1500 unit D-Gam Anti-D immunoglobulin 1,500unit solution for injection vials | 1 vial [PoM] £58.00

▸ Rhophylac (CSL Behring UK Ltd)
Anti-D (Rh$_0$) immunoglobulin 750 unit per 1 ml Rhophylac 1,500units/2ml solution for injection pre-filled syringes | 1 pre-filled disposable injection [PoM] £46.50

Hepatitis B immunoglobulin

- INDICATIONS AND DOSE

Prophylaxis against hepatitis B infection
▸ BY INTRAMUSCULAR INJECTION
▸ Adult: 500 units, dose to be administered as soon as possible after exposure; ideally within 12–48 hours, but no later than 7 days after exposure

Prophylaxis against hepatitis B infection, after exposure to hepatitis B virus-contaminated material
▸ BY INTRAVENOUS INFUSION
▸ Adult: Dose to be administered as soon as possible after exposure, but no later than 72 hours (consult product literature)

Prevention of hepatitis B in haemodialysed patients
▸ BY INTRAVENOUS INFUSION
▸ Adult: (consult product literature)

Prophylaxis against re-infection of transplanted liver
▸ BY INTRAVENOUS INFUSION
▸ Adult: (consult product literature)

Prevention of hepatitis B re-infection more than 6 months after liver transplantation in stable HBV-DNA negative patients
▸ BY SUBCUTANEOUS INJECTION
▸ Adult (body-weight up to 75 kg): 500 units once weekly, increased if necessary up to 1000 units once weekly, dose to be started 2–3 weeks after last dose of intravenous hepatitis B immunoglobulin
▸ Adult (body-weight 75 kg and above): 1000 units once weekly, dose to be started 2–3 weeks after last dose of intravenous hepatitis B immunoglobulin

- CAUTIONS IgA deficiency · interference with live virus vaccines

- SIDE-EFFECTS
- **Uncommon** Abdominal pain upper · headache
▸ **Rare or very rare** Cardiac discomfort · fatigue · hypersensitivity · hypertension · hypotension · muscle

spasms · nasopharyngitis · oropharyngeal pain · palpitations · skin reactions

- PRESCRIBING AND DISPENSING INFORMATION Vials containing 200 units or 500 units (for intramuscular injection), available from selected Public Health England and NHS laboratories (except for Transplant Centres), also available from BPL.

- HANDLING AND STORAGE Care must be taken to store all immunological products under the conditions recommended in the product literature, otherwise the preparation may become ineffective. **Refrigerated storage** is usually necessary; many immunoglobulins need to be stored at 2–8°C and not allowed to freeze. Immunoglobulins should be protected from light. Opened multidose vials must be used within the period recommended in the product literature.

- MEDICINAL FORMS
There can be variation in the licensing of different medicines containing the same drug.

Solution for injection

▸ Hepatitis B immunoglobulin (Non-proprietary)
Hepatitis B immunoglobulin human 200 unit Hepatitis B immunoglobulin human 200unit solution for injection vials | 1 vial [PoM] £150.00
Hepatitis B immunoglobulin human 500 unit Hepatitis B immunoglobulin human 500unit solution for injection vials | 1 vial [PoM] £300.00

▸ Zutectra (Biotest (UK) Ltd)
Zutectra 500units/1ml solution for injection pre-filled syringes | 5 syringe [PoM] £1,500.00

Solution for infusion

▸ Hepatect CP (Biotest (UK) Ltd)
Hepatitis B immunoglobulin human 50 unit per 1 ml Hepatect CP 100units/2ml solution for infusion vials | 1 vial [PoM] £55.00
Hepatect CP 2000units/40ml solution for infusion vials | 1 vial [PoM] £1,100.00
Hepatect CP 500units/10ml solution for infusion vials | 1 vial [PoM] £275.00
Hepatect CP 5000units/100ml solution for infusion vials | 1 vial [PoM] £2,750.00

▸ Omri-Hep-B (Imported (Israel))
Hepatitis B immunoglobulin human 50 unit per 1 ml Omri-Hep-B 5000units/100ml solution for infusion vials | 1 vial [PoM] 🚫

Normal immunoglobulin

- INDICATIONS AND DOSE

To control outbreaks of hepatitis A
▸ BY DEEP INTRAMUSCULAR INJECTION
▸ Adult: 500 mg

Rubella in pregnancy, prevention of clinical attack
▸ BY DEEP INTRAMUSCULAR INJECTION
▸ Females of childbearing potential: 750 mg

Antibody deficiency syndromes
▸ BY SUBCUTANEOUS INFUSION
▸ Adult: (consult product literature)

SUBGAM ®

Hepatitis A prophylaxis in outbreaks
▸ BY INTRAMUSCULAR INJECTION
▸ Adult: 750 mg

- UNLICENSED USE
SUBGAM ® *Subgam* ® is not licensed for prophylactic use, but due to difficulty in obtaining suitable immunoglobulin products, Public Health England recommends intramuscular use for prophylaxis against Hepatitis A or rubella.

- CONTRA-INDICATIONS Patients with selective IgA deficiency who have known antibody against IgA

PRIVIGEN ® Hyperprolinaemia (contains L-proline)
FLEBOGAMMA ® DIF Hereditary fructose intolerance
(contains sorbitol)
HIZENTRA ® Hyperprolinaemia (contains L-proline)
GAMMAPLEX ® Hereditary fructose intolerance (contains
sorbitol)

● CAUTIONS Agammaglobulinaemia with or without IgA
deficiency · hypogammaglobulinaemia with or without IgA
deficiency · interference with live virus vaccines

CAUTIONS, FURTHER INFORMATION

▸ Interference with live virus vaccines Normal immunoglobulin
may **interfere with the immune response to live virus
vaccines** which should therefore only be given **at least
3 weeks before or 3 months after** an injection of normal
immunoglobulin (this does not apply to yellow fever
vaccine since normal immunoglobulin does not contain
antibody to this virus).

OCTAGAM ® Falsely elevated results with blood glucose
testing systems (contains maltose)

● SIDE-EFFECTS

GENERAL SIDE-EFFECTS

▸ **Common or very common** Dizziness · fatigue ·
gastrointestinal discomfort · headache · hypotension ·
myalgia · nausea · pain · skin reactions
▸ **Uncommon** Paraesthesia

SPECIFIC SIDE-EFFECTS

▸ **Common or very common**
▸ With intramuscular use Chills
▸ With subcutaneous use Diarrhoea · drowsiness
▸ **Uncommon**
▸ With intramuscular use Feeling hot
▸ **Rare or very rare**
▸ With intramuscular use Arthralgia · musculoskeletal stiffness
· peripheral coldness · tremor
▸ **Frequency not known**
▸ With intramuscular use Chest discomfort · dyspnoea · facial
swelling · fever · flushing · hyperhidrosis · hypertension ·
malaise · oral paraesthesia · pallor · tachycardia · vomiting

SIDE-EFFECTS, FURTHER INFORMATION Adverse reactions
are more likely to occur in patients receiving normal
immunoglobulin for the first time, or following a
prolonged period between treatments, or when a different
brand of normal immunoglobulin is administered.

● MONITORING REQUIREMENTS Monitor for acute renal
failure; consider discontinuation if renal function
deteriorates. Intravenous preparations with added sucrose
have been associated with cases of renal dysfunction and
acute renal failure.

● DIRECTIONS FOR ADMINISTRATION
Preparations for subcutaneous use May be administered by
intramuscular injection if subcutaneous route not
possible; intramuscular route **not** for patients with
thrombocytopenia or other bleeding disorders.

GAMUNEX ® Use Glucose 5% intravenous infusion if
dilution prior to infusion is required.

KIOVIG ® Use Glucose 5% intravenous infusion if dilution
prior to infusion is required.

● PRESCRIBING AND DISPENSING INFORMATION Antibody
titres can vary widely between normal immunoglobulin
preparations from different manufacturers—formulations
are **not interchangeable**; patients should be maintained
on the same formulation throughout long-term treatment
to avoid adverse effects.

▸ With intramuscular use Available from the Centre for
Infections and other regional Public Health England
offices (for contacts and control of outbreaks only).

● HANDLING AND STORAGE Care must be taken to store all
immunological products under the conditions
recommended in the product literature, otherwise the

preparation may become ineffective. **Refrigerated
storage** is usually necessary; many immunoglobulins need
to be stored at 2–8°C and not allowed to freeze.
Immunoglobulins should be protected from light. Opened
multidose vials must be used within the period
recommended in the product literature.

● MEDICINAL FORMS
There can be variation in the licensing of different medicines
containing the same drug.

Solution for injection
ELECTROLYTES: May contain Sodium
▸ Hizentra (CSL Behring UK Ltd)
Normal immunoglobulin human 200 mg per 1 ml Hizentra 1g/5ml
solution for injection pre-filled syringes | 1 pre-filled disposable
injection PoM £54.00
Hizentra 2g/10ml solution for injection pre-filled syringes | 1 pre-
filled disposable injection PoM £108.00
▸ Subgam (Bio Products Laboratory Ltd)
Normal immunoglobulin human 150 mg per 1 ml Subgam
750mg/5ml solution for injection vials | 1 vial PoM £37.50
Subgam 1.5g/10ml solution for injection vials | 1 vial PoM £75.00

Solution for infusion
EXCIPIENTS: May contain Glucose, maltose, sorbitol, sucrose
▸ Normal immunoglobulin (non-proprietary) ▼
Normal immunoglobulin human 100 mg per 1 ml Panzyga
10g/100ml solution for infusion bottles | 1 bottle PoM £586.50
(Hospital only)
Normal immunoglobulin human 5g/50ml solution for infusion vials |
1 vial PoM 🛇
Normal immunoglobulin human 2.5g/25ml solution for infusion vials
| 1 vial PoM 🛇
Normal immunoglobulin human 20g/200ml solution for infusion vials
| 1 vial PoM 🛇
Normal immunoglobulin human 10g/100ml solution for infusion vials
| 1 vial PoM 🛇
Normal immunoglobulin human 30g/300ml solution for infusion vials
| 1 vial PoM 🛇
▸ Flebogammadif (Grifols UK Ltd)
Normal immunoglobulin human 50 mg per 1 ml Flebogamma DIF
10g/200ml solution for infusion vials | 1 vial PoM £510.00
Flebogamma DIF 2.5g/50ml solution for infusion vials | 1 vial PoM
£127.50
Flebogamma DIF 5g/100ml solution for infusion vials | 1 vial PoM
£255.00
Flebogamma DIF 500mg/10ml solution for infusion vials | 1 vial PoM
£30.00
Flebogamma DIF 20g/400ml solution for infusion vials | 1 vial PoM
£1,020.00
▸ Gammaplex (Bio Products Laboratory Ltd)
Normal immunoglobulin human 50 mg per 1 ml Gammaplex
10g/200ml solution for infusion vials | 1 vial PoM £418.00 (Hospital
only)
Gammaplex 5g/100ml solution for infusion vials | 1 vial PoM
£209.00 (Hospital only)
Gammaplex 20g/400ml solution for infusion vials | 1 vial PoM
£836.00 (Hospital only)
▸ Gamunex (Grifols UK Ltd)
Normal immunoglobulin human 100 mg per 1 ml Gamunex 10%
1g/10ml solution for infusion vials | 1 vial PoM £42.50
Gamunex 10% 10g/100ml solution for infusion vials | 1 vial PoM
£425.00
Gamunex 10% 20g/200ml solution for infusion vials | 1 vial PoM
£850.00
Gamunex 10% 5g/50ml solution for infusion vials | 1 vial PoM
£212.50
▸ Hizentra (CSL Behring UK Ltd)
Normal immunoglobulin human 200 mg per 1 ml Hizentra
2g/10ml solution for infusion vials | 1 vial PoM £108.00
Hizentra 1g/5ml solution for infusion vials | 1 vial PoM £54.00
Hizentra 4g/20ml solution for infusion vials | 1 vial PoM £216.00
▸ Kiovig (Baxalta UK Ltd)
Normal immunoglobulin human 100 mg per 1 ml Kiovig 5g/50ml
solution for infusion vials | 1 vial PoM £245.00
Kiovig 20g/200ml solution for infusion vials | 1 vial PoM £980.00
Kiovig 10g/100ml solution for infusion vials | 1 vial PoM £490.00
Kiovig 30g/300ml solution for infusion vials | 1 vial PoM £1,470.00
Kiovig 2.5g/25ml solution for infusion vials | 1 vial PoM £122.50
Kiovig 1g/10ml solution for infusion vials | 1 vial PoM £49.00

▸ Octagam (Octapharma Ltd)
Normal immunoglobulin human 50 mg per 1 ml Octagam 5%
10g/200ml solution for infusion bottles | 1 bottle [PoM] £480.00
(Hospital only)
Octagam 5% 5g/100ml solution for infusion bottles | 1 bottle [PoM]
£240.00 (Hospital only)
Octagam 5% 2.5g/50ml solution for infusion bottles | 1 bottle [PoM]
£120.00 (Hospital only)
Normal immunoglobulin human 100 mg per 1 ml Octagam 10%
10g/100ml solution for infusion bottles | 1 bottle [PoM] £690.00
(Hospital only)
Octagam 10% 20g/200ml solution for infusion bottles | 1 bottle [PoM]
£1,380.00 (Hospital only)
Octagam 10% 5g/50ml solution for infusion bottles | 1 bottle [PoM]
£345.00 (Hospital only)
Octagam 10% 2g/20ml solution for infusion vials | 1 vial [PoM]
£138.00 (Hospital only)

▸ Privigen (CSL Behring UK Ltd)
Normal immunoglobulin human 100 mg per 1 ml Privigen
5g/50ml solution for infusion vials | 1 vial [PoM] £270.00
Privigen 20g/200ml solution for infusion vials | 1 vial [PoM] £1,080.00
Privigen 10g/100ml solution for infusion vials | 1 vial [PoM] £540.00
Privigen 2.5g/25ml solution for infusion vials | 1 vial [PoM] £135.00

Rabies immunoglobulin

● **INDICATIONS AND DOSE**

Post-exposure prophylaxis against rabies infection
▸ BY LOCAL INFILTRATION, OR BY INTRAMUSCULAR INJECTION
▸ Child: 20 units/kg, dose administered by infiltration in
  and around the cleansed wound; if the wound not
  visible or healed or if infiltration of whole volume not
  possible, give remainder by intramuscular injection
  into anterolateral thigh (remote from vaccination site)
▸ Adult: 20 units/kg, dose administered by infiltration in
  and around the cleansed wound; if the wound not
  visible or healed or if infiltration of whole volume not
  possible, give remainder by intramuscular injection
  into anterolateral thigh (remote from vaccination site)

● CAUTIONS IgA deficiency · interference with live virus
  vaccines
● SIDE-EFFECTS
▸ **Rare or very rare** Arthralgia · chills · fatigue · fever ·
  headache · hypersensitivity · hypotension · influenza like
  illness · malaise · nausea · skin reactions · tachycardia ·
  vomiting
● PRESCRIBING AND DISPENSING INFORMATION The potency
  of individual batches of rabies immunoglobulin from the
  manufacturer may vary; potency may also be described
  differently by different manufacturers. It is therefore
  critical to know the potency of the batch to be used and
  the weight of the patient in order to calculate the specific
  volume required to provide the necessary dose.
      Available from Specialist and Reference Microbiology
  Division, Public Health England (also from BPL).
● HANDLING AND STORAGE Care must be taken to store all
  immunological products under the conditions
  recommended in the product literature, otherwise the
  preparation may become ineffective. **Refrigerated
  storage** is usually necessary; many immunoglobulins need
  to be stored at 2–8°C and not allowed to freeze.
  Immunoglobulins should be protected from light. Opened
  multidose vials must be used within the period
  recommended in the product literature.

● MEDICINAL FORMS
There can be variation in the licensing of different medicines
containing the same drug.
Solution for injection
▸ Rabies immunoglobulin (Non-proprietary)
  Rabies immunoglobulin human 500 unit Rabies immunoglobulin
  human 500unit solution for injection vials | 1 vial [PoM] £600.00

Tetanus immunoglobulin

● **INDICATIONS AND DOSE**

Post-exposure prophylaxis
▸ BY INTRAMUSCULAR INJECTION
▸ Child: Initially 250 units, then increased to 500 units,
  dose is only increased if more than 24 hours have
  elapsed or there is risk of heavy contamination or
  following burns
▸ Adult: Initially 250 units, then increased to 500 units,
  dose is only increased if more than 24 hours have
  elapsed or there is risk of heavy contamination or
  following burns

Treatment of tetanus infection
▸ BY INTRAMUSCULAR INJECTION
▸ Child: 150 units/kg, dose may be given over multiple
  sites
▸ Adult: 150 units/kg, dose may be given over multiple
  sites

● CAUTIONS IgA deficiency · interference with live virus
  vaccines
● SIDE-EFFECTS
▸ **Rare or very rare** Anaphylactic reaction · hypotension
▸ **Frequency not known** Arthralgia · chest pain · dizziness ·
  dyspnoea · face oedema · oral disorders · tremor
● HANDLING AND STORAGE Care must be taken to store all
  immunological products under the conditions
  recommended in the product literature, otherwise the
  preparation may become ineffective. **Refrigerated
  storage** is usually necessary; many immunoglobulins need
  to be stored at 2–8°C and not allowed to freeze.
  Immunoglobulins should be protected from light. Opened
  multidose vials must be used within the period
  recommended in the product literature.

● MEDICINAL FORMS
There can be variation in the licensing of different medicines
containing the same drug.
Solution for injection
▸ Tetanus immunoglobulin (Non-proprietary)
  Tetanus immunoglobulin human 250 unit Tetanus immunoglobulin
  human 250unit solution for injection vials | 1 vial [PoM] £125.00

Varicella-zoster immunoglobulin

(Antivaricella-zoster Immunoglobulin)

● **INDICATIONS AND DOSE**

Prophylaxis against varicella infection
▸ BY DEEP INTRAMUSCULAR INJECTION
▸ Adult: 1 g, to be administered as soon as possible—not
  later than 10 days after exposure, second dose to be
  given if further exposure occurs more than 3 weeks
  after first dose, no evidence that effective in severe
  disease

● CAUTIONS IgA deficiency · interference with live virus
  vaccines
● SIDE-EFFECTS Arthralgia · chills · fever · headache ·
  hypersensitivity · hypotension · malaise · nausea · skin
  reactions · tachycardia · vomiting
● DIRECTIONS FOR ADMINISTRATION Normal
  immunoglobulin for intravenous use may be used in those
  unable to receive intramuscular injections.
● PRESCRIBING AND DISPENSING INFORMATION Available
  from selected Public Health England and NHS laboratories
  (also from BPL).
● HANDLING AND STORAGE Care must be taken to store all
  immunological products under the conditions
  recommended in the product literature, otherwise the

14

Vaccines

preparation may become ineffective. **Refrigerated storage** is usually necessary; many immunoglobulins need to be stored at 2–8°C and not allowed to freeze. Immunoglobulins should be protected from light. Opened multidose vials must be used within the period recommended in the product literature.

- MEDICINAL FORMS
There can be variation in the licensing of different medicines containing the same drug.
Solution for injection
▶ Varicella-Zoster (Bio Products Laboratory Ltd)
Varicella-Zoster immunoglobulin human 250 mg Varicella-Zoster immunoglobulin human 250mg solution for injection vials | 1 vial PoM £450.00

2 Post-exposure prophylaxis

IMMUNE SERA AND IMMUNOGLOBULINS ⟩ ANTITOXINS

Bezlotoxumab

18-Aug-2017

- DRUG ACTION Bezlotoxumab is a human monoclonal antitoxin antibody; it binds to *Clostridium difficile* toxin B and neutralises its activity, preventing recurrence of *Clostridium difficile* infection.

- INDICATIONS AND DOSE
Prevention of recurrence of *Clostridium difficile* infection in patients at high risk of reinfection
▶ BY INTRAVENOUS INFUSION
▶ Adult: 10 mg/kg for 1 dose, to be administered during the course of antibacterial therapy for *Clostridium difficile* infection

- SIDE-EFFECTS
▶ **Common or very common** Dizziness · dyspnoea · fatigue · fever · headache · hypertension · infusion related reaction · nausea
- PREGNANCY Manufacturer advises avoid unless essential—limited information available.
- BREAST-FEEDING Manufacturer advises avoid—no information available.
- DIRECTIONS FOR ADMINISTRATION Manufacturer advises for *intravenous infusion* (Zinplava®), give intermittently in Glucose 5% or Sodium Chloride 0.9%; dilute requisite dose to a concentration of 1–10 mg/mL with infusion fluid; give over 60 minutes via a central venous catheter or peripheral catheter using a low-protein binding filter (0.2–0.5 micron).
- HANDLING AND STORAGE Manufacturer advises store in a refrigerator (2–8°C)—consult product literature for further information regarding storage conditions outside refrigerator and after preparation of the infusion.

- MEDICINAL FORMS
There can be variation in the licensing of different medicines containing the same drug.
Solution for infusion
EXCIPIENTS: May contain Polysorbates
ELECTROLYTES: May contain Sodium
▶ Zinplava (Merck Sharp & Dohme Ltd) ▼
Bezlotoxumab 25 mg per 1 ml Zinplava 1g/40ml concentrate for solution for infusion vials | 1 vial PoM £2,470.00

Botulism antitoxin

- DRUG ACTION A preparation containing the specific antitoxic globulins that have the power of neutralising the toxins formed by types A, B, and E of *Clostridium botulinum*.

- INDICATIONS AND DOSE
Post exposure prophylaxis of botulism
▶ BY INTRAMUSCULAR INJECTION
▶ Adult: (consult product literature)

- SIDE-EFFECTS Hypersensitivity
SIDE-EFFECTS, FURTHER INFORMATION It is essential to read the contra-indications, warnings, and details of sensitivity tests on the package insert. Prior to treatment checks should be made regarding previous administration of any antitoxin and history of any allergic condition, e.g. asthma, hay fever, etc.
- PRE-TREATMENT SCREENING All patients should be tested for sensitivity (diluting the antitoxin if history of allergy).
- PRESCRIBING AND DISPENSING INFORMATION Available from local designated centres, for details see TOXBASE (requires registration) www.toxbase.org. For supplies outside working hours apply to other designated centres or to the Public Health England Colindale duty doctor (Tel (020) 8200 6868). For major incidents, obtain supplies from the local blood bank.
The BP title Botulinum Antitoxin is not used because the preparation currently in use may have a different specification.

- MEDICINAL FORMS
No licensed medicines listed.

Diphtheria antitoxin
(Dip/Ser)

- INDICATIONS AND DOSE
Passive immunisation in suspected cases of diphtheria
▶ BY INTRAVENOUS INFUSION
▶ Adult: Dose should be given without waiting for bacteriological confirmation (consult product literature)

- CAUTIONS
CAUTIONS, FURTHER INFORMATION
▶ Hypersensitivity Hypersensitivity is common after administration; resuscitation facilities should be available. Diphtheria antitoxin is no longer used for prophylaxis because of the risk of hypersensitivity; unimmunised contacts should be promptly investigated and given antibacterial prophylaxis and vaccine.
- SIDE-EFFECTS
▶ **Common or very common** Hypersensitivity
- PRE-TREATMENT SCREENING Diphtheria antitoxin is derived from horse serum and reactions are common; tests for hypersensitivity should be carried out before use.
- PRESCRIBING AND DISPENSING INFORMATION Available from Centre for Infections (Tel (020) 8200 6868) or in Northern Ireland from Public Health Laboratory, Belfast City Hospital (Tel (028) 9032 9241).

- MEDICINAL FORMS
There can be variation in the licensing of different medicines containing the same drug.
Solution for injection
▶ Diphtheria antitoxin (Non-proprietary)
Diphtheria antitoxin 1000 unit per 1 ml Antidiphtheria serum 10,000units/10ml solution for injection ampoules | 1 ampoule PoM ⓧ

3 Tuberculosis diagnostic test

DIAGNOSTIC AGENTS

| Tuberculin purified protein derivative

(Tuberculin PPD)

- **INDICATIONS AND DOSE**

Mantoux test
▸ BY INTRADERMAL INJECTION
- Child: 2 units for one dose
- Adult: 2 units for one dose

Mantoux test (if first test is negative and a further test is considered appropriate)
▸ BY INTRADERMAL INJECTION
- Child: 10 units for 1 dose
- Adult: 10 units for 1 dose

DOSE EQUIVALENCE AND CONVERSION
▸ 2 units is equivalent to 0.1 mL of 20 units/mL strength.
▸ 10 units is equivalent to 0.1 mL of 100 units/mL strength.

- **CAUTIONS**
CAUTIONS, FURTHER INFORMATION
▸ Mantoux test Response to tuberculin may be suppressed by viral infection, sarcoidosis, corticosteroid therapy, or immunosuppression due to disease or treatment and the MMR vaccine. If a tuberculin skin test has already been initiated, then the MMR should be delayed until the skin test has been read unless protection against measles is required urgently. If a child has had a recent MMR, and requires a tuberculin test, then a 4 week interval should be observed. Apart from tuberculin and MMR, all other live vaccines can be administered at any time before or after tuberculin.

- **PRESCRIBING AND DISPENSING INFORMATION** Available from ImmForm (SSI brand).
The strength of tuberculin PPD in currently available products may be different to the strengths of products used previously for the Mantoux test; care is required to select the correct strength.

- **MEDICINAL FORMS**
There can be variation in the licensing of different medicines containing the same drug. Forms available from special-order manufacturers include: solution for injection

Solution for injection
▸ Tuberculin purified protein derivative (Non-proprietary)
Tuberculin purified protein derivative 20 tuberculin unit per 1 ml Tuberculin PPD RT 23 SSI 20 tuberculin units/ml solution for injection 1.5ml vials | 1 vial 🔒
Tuberculin purified protein derivative 100 tuberculin unit per 1 ml Tuberculin PPD RT 23 SSI 100 tuberculin units/ml solution for injection 1.5ml vials | 1 vial 🔒

4 Vaccination

Vaccines

16-Aug-2017

Active immunity

Active immunity can be acquired by natural disease or by vaccination. **Vaccines** stimulate production of antibodies and other components of the immune mechanism; they consist of either:

- a *live attenuated* form of a virus (e.g. measles, mumps and rubella vaccine) or bacteria (e.g. BCG vaccine), or
- *inactivated* preparations of the virus (e.g. influenza vaccine) or bacteria, or
- *detoxified exotoxins* produced by a micro-organism (e.g. tetanus vaccine), or
- *extracts of* a micro-organism, which may be derived from the organism (e.g. pneumococcal vaccine) or produced by recombinant DNA technology (e.g. hepatitis B vaccine).

Live attenuated vaccines usually produce a durable immunity, but not always as long-lasting as that resulting from natural infection.

Inactivated vaccines may require a primary series of injections of vaccine to produce an adequate antibody response, and in most cases booster (reinforcing) injections are required; the duration of immunity varies from months to many years. Some inactivated vaccines are adsorbed onto an adjuvant (such as aluminium hydroxide) to enhance the antibody response.

Advice reflects that in the handbook *Immunisation against Infectious Disease* (2013), which in turn reflects the guidance of the Joint Committee on Vaccination and Immunisation (JCVI).

Chapters from the handbook (including updates since 2013) are available at www.gov.uk/government/collections/immunisation-against-infectious-disease-the-green-book

The advice also incorporates changes announced by the Chief Medical Officer and Health Department Updates.

Immunisation schedule

Vaccines for the childhood immunisation schedule should be obtained from **local health organisations** or from **ImmForm** (www.immform.dh.gov.uk)—not to be prescribed on FP10 (HS21 in Northern Ireland; GP10 in Scotland; WP10 in Wales).

For the most up to date immunisation schedule consult 'The complete routine immunisation schedule', available at www.gov.uk

Preterm birth

Babies born preterm should receive all routine immunisations based on their actual date of birth. The risk of apnoea following vaccination is increased in preterm babies, particularly in those born at or before 28 weeks gestational age. If babies at risk of apnoea are in hospital at the time of their first immunisation, they should be monitored for 48–72 hours after immunisation. If a baby develops apnoea, bradycardia, or desaturation after the first immunisation, the second immunisation should also be given in hospital with similar monitoring. Seroconversion may be unreliable in babies born earlier than 28 weeks' gestation or in babies treated with corticosteroids for chronic lung disease; consideration should be given to testing for antibodies against *Haemophilus influenzae* type b, meningococcal C, and hepatitis B after primary immunisation.

Vaccines and HIV infection

HIV-positive individuals with or without symptoms can receive the following live vaccines:

- MMR (but avoid if immunity significantly impaired; use of normal immunoglobulin should be considered after exposure to measles), varicella-zoster vaccine against chickenpox (but avoid if immunity significantly impaired—consult product literature; varicella–zoster immunoglobulin should be considered after exposure to chickenpox or herpes zoster), rotavirus;

and the following inactivated vaccines:

- anthrax, cholera (oral), diphtheria, haemophilus influenzae type b, hepatitis A, hepatitis B, human papillomavirus, influenza (injection), meningococcal, pertussis, pneumococcal, poliomyelitis, rabies, tetanus, tick-borne encephalitis, typhoid (injection).

Routine immunisation schedule

When to immunise	Vaccine given and dose schedule (for details of dose, see under individual vaccines)
Neonates at risk only	▸ Bacillus Calmette-Guérin vaccine p. 1273 (at birth, see *BCG vaccine*, below) ▸ Hepatitis B vaccine p. 1280 (at birth, see *Hepatitis B* vaccine, below)
2 months	▸ Diphtheria with tetanus, pertussis, hepatitis B, poliomyelitis and haemophilus influenzae type b vaccine p. 1273 (*Infanrix hexa*®). First dose ▸ Meningococcal group B vaccine (rDNA, component, adsorbed) p. 1275 First dose ▸ Pneumococcal polysaccharide conjugate vaccine (adsorbed) p. 1277 First dose ▸ Rotavirus vaccine p. 1286 First dose
3 months	▸ Diphtheria with tetanus, pertussis, hepatitis B, poliomyelitis and haemophilus influenzae type b vaccine p. 1273 (*Infanrix hexa*®). Second dose ▸ Rotavirus vaccine p. 1286 Second dose
4 months	▸ Diphtheria with tetanus, pertussis, hepatitis B, poliomyelitis and haemophilus influenzae type b vaccine p. 1273 (*Infanrix hexa*®). Third dose ▸ Meningococcal group B vaccine (rDNA, component, adsorbed) p. 1275 Second dose ▸ Pneumococcal polysaccharide conjugate vaccine (adsorbed) p. 1277 Second dose
12-13 months	▸ Measles, mumps and rubella vaccine, live p. 1284 First dose ▸ Meningococcal group B vaccine (rDNA, component, adsorbed) p. 1275 Single booster dose ▸ Pneumococcal polysaccharide conjugate vaccine (adsorbed) p. 1277 Single booster dose ▸ Haemophilus influenzae type b with meningococcal group C vaccine p. 1275 Single booster dose
2-8 years (including children in school years 1, 2, 3 and 4)	▸ Influenza vaccine p. 1282 Each year from September. **Note:** Flu nasal spray is recommended (*Fluenz Tetra*®). If contra-indicated and child is in clinical risk group, use inactivated flu vaccine
Between 3 years and 4 months, and 5 years	▸ Diphtheria with pertussis, poliomyelitis vaccine and tetanus p. 1272 Single booster dose. **Note:** Preferably allow interval of at least 3 years after completing primary course ▸ Measles, mumps and rubella vaccine, live p. 1284 Second dose
11-14 years (females only). First dose of HPV vaccine will be offered to females aged 12-13 years of age in England, Wales, and Northern Ireland, and 11-13 years of age in Scotland.	▸ Human papillomavirus vaccines p. 1282 2 doses; second dose 6-24 months after first dose. If a 3-dose course of HPV vaccine has been started under the 2013/2014 programme, where possible, the course should be completed (2 doses less than 6 months apart does not provide long-term protection).The two human papillomavirus vaccines are not interchangeable and, ideally, one vaccine product should be used for the entire course. However, since 2012, only *Gardasil*® is offered as part of the national immunisation programme; for those females who started the schedule with *Cervarix*® under the national immunisation programme, but did not complete the vaccination course, the course can be completed with *Gardasil*®.
13-15 years	▸ Meningococcal groups A with C and W135 and Y vaccine p. 1276 Single booster dose
13-18 years	▸ Diphtheria with poliomyelitis and tetanus vaccine p. 1273 Single booster dose. **Note:** Can be given at the same time as the dose of meningococcal group A with C and W135 and Y vaccine at 13-15 years of age.
During adult life, women of child-bearing age susceptible to rubella	▸ Measles, mumps and rubella vaccine, live p. 1284 Women of child-bearing age who have not received 2 doses of a rubella-containing vaccine or who do not have a positive antibody test for rubella should be offered rubella immunisation (using the MMR vaccine)—exclude pregnancy before immunisation.
Pregnant women	▸ Acellular pertussis-containing vaccine administered as diphtheria with pertussis, poliomyelitis vaccine and tetanus p. 1272 (*Boostrix-IPV*®) 1 dose from the 16th week of pregnancy, preferably after the fetal anomaly scan (weeks 18–20) ▸ Influenza vaccine p. 1282 (inactivated), Single dose administered from September, regardless of the stage of pregnancy
Under 25 years, those entering university who are at risk of meningococcal disease	▸ Meningococcal groups A with C and W135 and Y vaccine p. 1276 Single dose. **Note:** Should be offered to those aged under 25 years entering university who have not received the meningococcal groups A with C and W135 and Y vaccine p. 1276 over the age of 10 years
During adult life, if not previously immunised	▸ Diphtheria with poliomyelitis and tetanus vaccine p. 1273
65 years	▸ Pneumococcal polysaccharide vaccine p. 1277
From 65 years	▸ Influenza vaccine p. 1282 Each year from September
70 years	▸ Varicella-zoster vaccine p. 1287 Single dose

HIV-positive individuals should **not** receive:
- BCG, influenza nasal spray (unless stable HIV infection and receiving antiretroviral therapy), typhoid (oral), yellow fever (if yellow fever risk is unavoidable, specialist advice should be sought)

The above advice differs from that for other immunocompromised patients; *Immunisation Guidelines for HIV-infected Adults* issued by *British HIV Association* (BHIVA)

are available at www.bhiva.org and, *Immunisation of HIV-infected Children* issued by *Children's HIV Association* (CHIVA) are available at www.chiva.org.uk

Vaccines and asplenia
The following vaccines are recommended for asplenic patients, those with splenic dysfunction or complement disorders, depending on the age at which their condition is diagnosed:

- Haemophilus influenzae type b with meningococcal group C vaccine p. 1275;
- Influenza vaccine p. 1282;
- Meningococcal groups A with C and W135 and Y vaccine p. 1276 and meningococcal group B vaccine (rDNA, component, adsorbed) p. 1275;
- pneumococcal polysaccharide vaccine.

Children first diagnosed under 1 year of age should be vaccinated according to the Immunisation Schedule. Additionally, one dose of meningococcal groups A with C and W135 and Y vaccine should be given during infancy followed by a second dose at least one month apart. Two months following the routine 12 month booster vaccines, give a dose of meningococcal groups A with C and W135 and Y vaccine and an additional dose of 13-valent pneumococcal polysaccharide vaccine. An additional dose of haemophilus influenzae type b with meningococcal group C vaccine and 23-valent pneumococcal polysaccharide vaccine should be given after the second birthday. The influenza vaccine should be administered annually in children aged 6 months or older.

Children first diagnosed between 1 and 2 years of age should be vaccinated according to the Immunisation Schedule, including the 12 month boosters. Two months after the routine 12 month booster vaccines, give a dose of meningococcal groups A with C and W135 and Y vaccine and an additional dose of 13-valent pneumococcal polysaccharide vaccine. An additional dose of haemophilus influenzae type b with meningococcal group C vaccine and 23-valent pneumococcal polysaccharide vaccine should be given after the second birthday. The influenza vaccine should be administered annually.

Children first diagnosed over 2 years of age should be vaccinated according to the Immunisation schedule, including the 12 month boosters. The child should receive one additional booster dose of haemophilus influenzae type b with meningococcal group C vaccine along with the 23-valent pneumococcal polysaccharide vaccine, followed by one dose of meningococcal groups A with C and W135 and Y vaccine after 2 months. The influenza vaccine should be administered annually.

Vaccines and antisera availability

Anthrax vaccine p. 1273 and yellow fever vaccine, live p. 1287, botulism antitoxin p. 1258, diphtheria antitoxin p. 1258, and snake and spider venom antitoxins are available from local designated holding centres.

For antivenom, see Poisoning, emergency treatment p. 1319.

Enquiries for vaccines not available commercially can also be made to:

Vaccines and Countermeasures Response Department
Public Health England
Wellington House
133–155 Waterloo Road
London
SE1 8UG
vaccinesupply@phe.gov.uk

In Scotland information about availability of vaccines can be obtained from a Specialist in Pharmaceutical Public Health.

In Wales enquiries for vaccines not available commercially should be directed to:

Welsh Medicines Information Centre
University Hospital of Wales
Cardiff
CF14 4XW
(029) 2074 2979

In Northern Ireland:
Pharmacy and Medicines Management Centre
Northern Health and Social Care Trust
Beech House
Antrim Hospital Site
Bush Road
Antrim
BT41 2RL
rphps.admin@northerntrust.hscni.net

For further details of availability, see under individual vaccines.

Anthrax vaccine

Anthrax vaccine is made from antigens from *B. anthracis*. Anthrax immunisation is indicated for individuals who handle infected animals, for those exposed to imported infected animal products, and for laboratory staff who work with *B. anthracis*. A 4-dose regimen is used for primary immunisation; booster doses should be given annually to workers at continued risk of exposure to anthrax.

In the event of possible contact with *B. anthracis*, post-exposure immunisation may be indicated, in addition to antimicrobial prophylaxis. Advice on the use of anthrax vaccine for post-exposure prophylaxis must be obtained from Public Health England Colindale (tel. 020 8200 4400).

BCG vaccine

Bacillus Calmette-Guérin vaccine p. 1273 should be given intradermally by operators skilled in the technique.

The expected reaction to successful Bacillus Calmette-Guérin vaccine is induration at the site of injection followed by a local lesion which starts as a papule 2 or more weeks after vaccination; the lesion may ulcerate then subside over several weeks or months, leaving a small, flat scar. A dry dressing may be used if the ulcer discharges, but air should **not** be excluded.

BCG is recommended for the following groups if BCG immunisation has not previously been carried out and they are negative for tuberculoprotein hypersensitivity:

- neonates with a family history of tuberculosis in the last 5 years;
- all neonates and infants (0–12 months) born in areas where the incidence of tuberculosis is greater than 40 per 100 000;
- neonates, infants, and children under 16 years with a parent or grandparent born in a country with an incidence of tuberculosis greater than 40 per 100 000;
- new immigrants aged under 16 years who were born in, or lived for more than 3 months in a country with an incidence of tuberculosis greater than 40 per 100 000;
- new immigrants aged 16–35 years from Sub-Saharan Africa or a country with an incidence of tuberculosis greater than 500 per 100 000;
- contacts aged under 36 years of those with active respiratory tuberculosis (for healthcare or laboratory workers who have had contact with clinical materials or patients with tuberculosis, age limit does not apply);
- healthcare workers and laboratory staff (irrespective of age) who are likely to have contact with patients, clinical materials, or derived isolates; other individuals under 35 years (there is inadequate evidence of protection by BCG vaccine in adults aged over 35 years; however, vaccination is recommended for healthcare workers irrespective of age because of the increased risk to them or their patients) at occupational risk including veterinary and other staff who handle animal species susceptible to tuberculosis, and staff working directly with prisoners, in care homes for the elderly, or in hostels or facilities for the homeless or refugees;
- individuals under 16 years intending to live with local people for more than 3 months in a country with an incidence of tuberculosis greater than 40 per 100 000.

14

Vaccines

List of countries or primary care trusts where the incidence of tuberculosis is greater than 40 cases per 100 000 is available at www.gov.uk/phe.

Bladder instillations of BCG are licensed for the management of bladder carcinoma.

See also Tuberculosis p. 567 for advice on chemoprophylaxis; for the treatment of infection following vaccination, seek expert advice.

Tuberculosis Diagnostic Agents

The *Mantoux test* is recommended for tuberculin skin testing, but no licensed preparation is currently available. Guidance for healthcare professionals is available at www.dh.gov.uk/immunisation.

In the Mantoux test, the diagnostic dose is administered by intradermal injection of tuberculin purified protein derivative (PPD) p. 1259.

The *Heaf test* (involving the use of multiple-puncture apparatus) is no longer available.

Two interferon gamma release assay (IGRA) tests are also available as an aid in the diagnosis of tuberculosis infection: *QuantiFERON® TB Gold* and *T-SPOT®. TB*. Both tests measure T-cell mediated immune response to synthetic antigens. For further information on the use of interferon gamma release assay tests for tuberculosis, see www.gov.uk/phe.

Botulism antitoxin

A polyvalent botulism antitoxin p. 1258 is available for the post-exposure prophylaxis of botulism and for the treatment of persons thought to be suffering from botulism. It specifically neutralises the toxins produced by *Clostridium botulinum* types A, B, and E. It is not effective against infantile botulism as the toxin (type A) is seldom, if ever, found in the blood in this type of infection.

Cholera vaccine

Cholera vaccine (oral) p. 1274 contains inactivated Inaba (including El-Tor biotype) and Ogawa strains of *Vibrio cholerae*, serotype O1 together with recombinant B-subunit of the cholera toxin produced in Inaba strains of *V.cholerae*, serotype O1.

Oral cholera vaccine is licensed for travellers to endemic or epidemic areas on the basis of current recommendations. Immunisation should be completed at least 1 week before potential exposure. However, there is no requirement for cholera vaccination for international travel.

Injectable cholera vaccine provides unreliable protection and is no longer available in the UK.

Diphtheria vaccine

Diphtheria-containing vaccines are prepared from the toxin of *Corynebacterium diphtheriae* and adsorption on aluminium hydroxide or aluminium phosphate improves antigenicity. The vaccine stimulates the production of the protective antibody. The quantity of diphtheria toxoid in a preparation determines whether the vaccine is defined as 'high dose' or 'low dose'. Vaccines containing the higher dose of diphtheria toxoid are used for primary immunisation of children under 10 years of age. Vaccines containing the lower dose of diphtheria toxoid are used for primary immunisation in adults and children over 10 years. Single-antigen diphtheria vaccine is not available and adsorbed diphtheria vaccine is given as a combination product containing other vaccines.

For primary immunisation *of children aged between 2 months and 10 years*, vaccination is recommended usually in the form of 3 doses (separated by 1-month intervals) of diphtheria with tetanus, pertussis, hepatitis B, poliomyelitis and haemophilus influenzae type b vaccine p. 1273 (*Infanrix hexa®*) (see Immunisation schedule). In unimmunised individuals aged *over 10 years* the primary course comprises

of 3 doses of **adsorbed diphtheria** [low dose], **tetanus and poliomyelitis (inactivated) vaccine**.

A booster dose should be given 3 years after the primary course (this interval can be reduced to a minimum of 1 year if the primary course was delayed). Children *under 10 years* should receive *either* **adsorbed diphtheria, tetanus, pertussis (acellular, component) and poliomyelitis (inactivated) vaccine** *or* **adsorbed diphtheria** [low dose], **tetanus, pertussis (acellular, component) and poliomyelitis (inactivated) vaccine** . Individuals aged *over* 10 *years* should receive **adsorbed diphtheria** [low dose], **tetanus, and poliomyelitis (inactivated) vaccine**.

A second booster dose, of adsorbed diphtheria [low dose], tetanus and poliomyelitis (inactivated) vaccine, should be given 10 years after the previous booster dose (this interval can be reduced to a minimum of 5 years if previous doses were delayed).

Diphtheria-containing vaccines for children over 10 years and adults

A **low dose** of diphtheria toxoid is sufficient to recall immunity in individuals previously immunised against diphtheria but whose immunity may have diminished with time; it is insufficient to cause serious reactions in an individual who is already immune. Preparations containing low dose diphtheria should be used for adults and children *over* 10 *years*, for both primary immunisation and booster doses.

Travel

Those intending to travel to areas with a risk of diphtheria infection should be fully immunised according to the UK schedule. If more than 10 years have lapsed since completion of the UK schedule, a dose of **adsorbed diphtheria** [low dose], **tetanus and poliomyelitis (inactivated) vaccine** should be administered.

Contacts

Staff in contact with diphtheria patients or with potentially pathogenic clinical specimens or working directly with *C. diphtheriae* or *C. ulcerans* should receive a booster dose if fully immunised (with 5 doses of diphtheria-containing vaccine given at appropriate intervals); further doses should be given at 10-year intervals if risk persists. Individuals at risk who are not fully immunised should complete the primary course; a booster dose should be given after 5 years and then at 10-year intervals. **Adsorbed diphtheria** [low dose], **tetanus and poliomyelitis (inactivated) vaccine** is used for this purpose; immunity should be checked by antibody testing at least 3 months after completion of immunisation.

Advice on the management of cases, carriers, contacts and outbreaks must be sought from health protection units. The immunisation history of infected individuals and their contacts should be determined; those who have been incompletely immunised should complete their immunisation and fully immunised individuals should receive a reinforcing dose. See advice on antibacterial treatment to prevent a secondary case of diphtheria in a non-immune individual.

Haemophilus influenzae type b conjugate vaccine

Haemophilus influenzae type b (Hib) vaccine is made from capsular polysaccharide; it is conjugated with a protein such as tetanus toxoid to increase immunogenicity, especially in young children. *Haemophilus influenzae type b vaccine* immunisation is given in combination with diphtheria, tetanus, pertussis, hepatitis B and poliomyelitis vaccine (*Infanrix hexa®*), as a component of the primary course of childhood immunisation (see Immunisation schedule). For infants under 1 year, the course consists of 3 doses of a vaccine containing *Haemophilus influenzae* type b component with an interval of 1 month between doses. A booster dose of haemophilus influenzae type b vaccine (combined with meningococcal group C conjugate vaccine) should be given at 12–13 months of age.

Children 1–10 years who have not been immunised against *Haemophilus influenzae* type b need to receive only 1 dose of Haemophilus influenzae type b vaccine (combined with meningococcal group C conjugate vaccine). However, if a primary course of immunisation has not been completed, children born before August 2017 should be given 3 doses of the combined vaccine they were started on. The risk of infection falls sharply in older children and the vaccine is not normally required for children over 10 years.

Haemophilus influenzae type b vaccine may be given to those over 10 years who are considered to be at increased risk of invasive *H. influenzae* type b disease (such as those with sickle-cell disease or complement deficiency, or those receiving treatment for malignancy).

Invasive *Haemophilus influenzae* type b disease
After recovery from infection, unimmunised and partially immunised index cases under 10 years of age should complete their age-specific course of immunisation. Previously vaccinated cases under 10 years of age should be given an additional dose of haemophilus influenzae type b vaccine (combined with meningococcal group C conjugate vaccine) if Hib antibody concentrations are low or if it is not possible to measure antibody concentrations. Index cases of any age with asplenia or splenic dysfunction should complete their immunisation according to the recommendations below; fully vaccinated cases with asplenia or splenic dysfunction should be given an additional dose of haemophilus influenzae type b vaccine (combined with meningococcal group C conjugate vaccine) if they received their previous dose over 1 year ago.

See also use of rifampicin p. 571 in the prevention of secondary cases of *Haemophilus influenzae* type b disease.

Hepatitis A vaccine
Hepatitis A vaccine p. 1279 is prepared from formaldehyde-inactivated hepatitis A virus grown in human diploid cells. Immunisation is recommended for:
- laboratory staff who work directly with the virus;
- staff and residents of homes for those with severe learning difficulties;
- workers at risk of exposure to untreated sewage;
- individuals who work with primates;
- patients with haemophilia or other conditions treated with plasma-derived clotting factors;
- patients with severe liver disease;
- travellers to high-risk areas;
- individuals who are at risk due to their sexual behaviour;
- parenteral drug abusers.

Immunisation should be considered for:
- patients with chronic liver disease including chronic hepatitis B or chronic hepatitis C;
- prevention of secondary cases in close contacts of confirmed cases of hepatitis A, within 14 days of exposure to the primary case (within 8 weeks of exposure to the primary case where there is more than 1 contact in the household).

A booster dose is usually given 6–12 months after the initial dose. A second booster dose can be given 20 years after the previous booster dose to those who continue to be at risk. Specialist advice should be sought on re-immunisation of immunocompromised individuals.

For rapid protection against hepatitis A after exposure or during an outbreak, in adults a single dose of a monovalent vaccine is recommended; for children under 16 years, a single dose of the combined vaccine Ambirix® can also be used.

Public Health England recommends the use of intramuscular normal immunoglobulin p. 1255 in addition to hepatitis A vaccine for prevention of infection in close contacts (of confirmed cases of hepatitis A) who are 60 years of age or over, have chronic liver disease, or HIV infection, or who are immunosuppressed. For further guidance, see Immunoglobulins p. 1252.

Post-exposure prophylaxis is not required for healthy children under 1 year of age, so long as all those involved in nappy changing are vaccinated against hepatitis A. However, children 2–12 months of age can be given a dose of hepatitis A vaccine if it is not possible to vaccinate their carers, or if the child becomes a source of infection to others [unlicensed use]; in these cases, if the child goes on to require long-term protection against hepatitis A after the first birthday, the full course of 2 doses should be given.

Hepatitis B vaccine
Hepatitis B vaccine p. 1280 contains inactivated hepatitis B virus surface antigen (HBsAg) adsorbed onto an adjuvant. It is made biosynthetically using recombinant DNA technology.

From August 2017, vaccination against hepatitis B is recommended as part of the **routine immunisation schedule**. Primary immunisation (see *Routine immunisation schedule*) requires 3 doses, administered at intervals of 1 month from the age of 2 months, to be given as part of the combined diphtheria with tetanus, pertussis, hepatitis B, poliomyelitis and haemophilus influenzae type b vaccine p. 1273 (*Infanrix hexa®*).

As part of the **selective neonatal immunisation programme**, vaccination is recommended for neonates whose mothers have had acute hepatitis B during pregnancy *or* are positive for hepatitis B surface antigen (regardless of e-antigen markers). Hepatitis B vaccination is started immediately after birth with a dose of the monovalent hepatitis B vaccine (no later than 24 hours after delivery), followed by a second dose at 4 weeks; the routine immunisation combination vaccine (*Infanrix hexa®*) at weeks 8, 12 and 16; and a further dose of the monovalent hepatitis B vaccine at one year of age.

Neonates born to highly infectious mothers should also receive hepatitis B immunoglobulin p. 1255 at the same time as the first dose of monovalent hepatitis B vaccine, but administered at a different site—more detailed guidance is given in the handbook *Immunisation against Infectious Disease* (www.gov.uk/government/publications/hepatitis-b-the-green-book-chapter-18).

Following **significant exposure to hepatitis B** (e.g. through needle-stick injury or unprotected sex) and for **pre-exposure prophylaxis in high-risk groups**, an 'accelerated schedule' using the single, monovalent hepatitis B vaccine is recommended immediately, with the second dose given 1 month after the initial dose, and the third dose given 2 months after the initial dose. For those at continued high risk following exposure, a fourth dose should be given 12 months after the first dose. More detailed guidance is given in the handbook *Immunisation against Infectious Disease*.

Specific hepatitis B immunoglobulin can also be indicated for use with the vaccine in those accidentally inoculated and in neonates at special risk of infection. If hepatitis B immunoglobulin is indicated, it should be given as soon as possible, ideally at the same time or within 24 hours of the first dose of vaccine, but not after seven days have elapsed since exposure. See also *Hepatitis B immunoglobulin* in Immunoglobulins p. 1252.

In the UK, groups at high-risk of hepatitis B include:
- parenteral drug misusers, their sexual partners, and household contacts; other drug misusers who are likely to 'progress' to injecting;
- individuals who change sexual partners frequently;
- close family contacts of a case or individual with chronic hepatitis B infection;

14 Vaccines

- individuals with haemophilia, those receiving regular blood transfusions or blood products, and carers responsible for the administration of such products;
- patients with chronic renal failure including those on haemodialysis. Haemodialysis patients should be monitored for antibodies annually and re-immunised if necessary. Home carers (of dialysis patients) should be vaccinated;
- individuals with chronic liver disease;
- healthcare personnel (including trainees) who have direct contact with blood or blood-stained body fluids or with patients' tissues;
- laboratory staff who handle material that may contain the virus;
- other occupational risk groups such as morticians and embalmers;
- staff and patients of day-care or residential accommodation for those with severe learning difficulties;
- staff and inmates of custodial institutions;
- those travelling to areas of high or intermediate prevalence who are at increased risk or who plan to remain there for lengthy periods;
- families adopting children from countries with a high or intermediate prevalence of hepatitis B;
- foster carers and their families.

Following a primary course of immunisation, most people do not require a reinforcing dose of a hepatitis B-containing vaccine. A single booster dose should be offered to healthcare workers approximately five years after primary immunisation, to patients on renal dialysis with anti-HBs levels below 10mlU/mL, and at the time of a subsequent significant exposure.

Immunisation does not eliminate the need for commonsense precautions for avoiding the risk of infection from known carriers by the routes of infection which have been clearly established, consult *Guidance for Clinical Health Care Workers: Protection against Infection with Blood-borne Viruses* (available at www.dh.gov.uk). Accidental inoculation of hepatitis B virus-infected blood into a wound, incision, needle-prick, or abrasion may lead to infection, whereas it is unlikely that indirect exposure to a carrier will do so.

A combined hepatitis A and B vaccine p. 1278 is also available.

Human papillomavirus vaccine

Human papillomavirus vaccine is available as a bivalent vaccine (*Cervarix®*) or a quadrivalent vaccine (*Gardasil®*). Since 2012, only *Gardasil®* is offered as part of the national immunisation programme. *Cervarix®* is licensed for use in females for the prevention of cervical cancer and other pre-cancerous lesions caused by human papillomavirus types 16 and 18. *Gardasil* is licensed for use in females for the prevention of cervical and anal cancers, genital warts and pre-cancerous genital (cervical, vulvar, and vaginal) and anal lesions caused by human papillomavirus types 6, 11, 16, and 18. The vaccines may also provide limited protection against disease caused by other types of human papillomavirus. The two vaccines are not interchangeable and one vaccine product should be used for an entire course.

Human papillomavirus vaccine will be most effective if given before sexual activity starts. From September 2014, a 2-dose schedule is recommended, as long as the first dose is received before the age of 15 years. The first dose is given to females aged 11 to 14 years, and the second dose is given 6–24 months after the first dose (for the purposes of planning the national immunisation programme, it is appropriate to give the second dose 12 months after the first—see Immunisation schedule). If the course is interrupted, it should be resumed (using the same vaccine) but not repeated, even if more than 24 months have elapsed since the first dose or if the girl is then aged 15 years or more.

Females receiving their first dose aged 15 years or older require a 3-dose schedule (see *Cervarix®* and *Gardasil®*), with the second and third doses given 1 and 4–6 months after the first dose; all 3 doses should be given within a 12-month period. If the course is interrupted, it should be resumed (using the same vaccine) but not repeated, allowing the appropriate interval between the remaining doses.

If a 3-dose course of vaccination had been started before September 2014 in a female aged under 15 years, then where possible this should be completed; the interrupted course should be resumed (using the same vaccine) but not repeated, allowing the appropriate interval between the remaining doses.

Under the national programme in England, females remain eligible to receive the human papillomavirus vaccine up to the age of 18 years if they did not receive the vaccine when scheduled. Where appropriate, immunisation with human papillomavirus vaccine should be offered to females coming into the UK as they may not have been offered protection in their country of origin. The duration of protection has not been established, but current studies suggest that protection is maintained for at least 6 years after completion of the primary course.

As the vaccines do not protect against all strains of human papillomavirus, routine cervical screening should continue.

Influenza vaccine

While most viruses are antigenically stable, the influenza viruses A and B (especially A) are constantly altering their antigenic structure as indicated by changes in the haemagglutinins (H) and neuraminidases (N) on the surface of the viruses. It is essential that influenza vaccine p. 1282 in use contain the H and N components of the prevalent strain or strains as recommended each year by the World Health Organization.

Immunisation is recommended *for persons at high risk*, and to reduce transmission of infection. Annual immunisation is strongly recommended for individuals aged over 6 months with the following conditions:

- chronic respiratory disease (includes asthma treated with continuous or repeated use of inhaled or systemic corticosteroids or asthma with previous exacerbations requiring hospital admission);
- chronic heart disease;
- chronic liver disease;
- chronic renal disease at stage 3, 4 or 5;
- chronic neurological disease;
- complement disorders;
- diabetes mellitus;
- immunosuppression because of disease (including asplenia or splenic dysfunction) or treatment (including prolonged systemic corticosteroid treatment [for over 1 month at dose equivalents of prednisolone: *adult and child over 20 kg*, 20 mg or more daily; *child under 20 kg*, 1 mg/kg or more daily] and chemotherapy);
- HIV infection (regardless of immune status);
- morbid obesity (BMI of 40 kg/m^2 and above).

Seasonal influenza vaccine (inactivated) is also recommended for all pregnant women, for all persons aged over 65 years, for residents of nursing or residential homes for the elderly and other long-stay facilities, and for carers of persons whose welfare may be at risk if the carer falls ill. Influenza immunisation should also be considered for household contacts of immunocompromised individuals.

As part of winter planning, NHS employers should offer vaccination to health and social care workers who are directly involved in patient care.

Unless contra-indicated, the live influenza vaccine, administered as a nasal spray (*Fluenz Tetra®*), is preferred in children aged 2–17 years because it provides a higher level of protection than the inactivated influenza vaccine. In the 2017/2018 national influenza immunisation programme, seasonal influenza vaccine will also be offered to all children aged 2–8 years on 31 August 2017 (including those in school years 1, 2, 3 and 4) and to all primary school-aged children in former primary school pilot areas.

Information on pandemic influenza, avian influenza and swine influenza may be found at www.dh.gov.uk/pandemicflu and at www.gov.uk/phe.

Japanese encephalitis vaccine

Japanese encephalitis vaccine p. 1283 is indicated for travellers to areas in Asia and the Far East where infection is endemic and for laboratory staff at risk of exposure to the virus. The primary immunisation course of 2 doses should be completed at least one week before potential exposure to Japanese encephalitis virus.

Up-to-date information on the risk of Japanese encephalitis in specific countries can be obtained from the National Travel Health Network and Centre (www.nathnac. org).

Measles, Mumps and Rubella vaccine

Measles vaccine has been replaced by a combined live measles, mumps and rubella vaccine, live p. 1284 (MMR vaccine).

Measles, mumps and rubella vaccine, live aims to eliminate measles, mumps, and rubella (German measles) and congenital rubella syndrome. Every child should receive two doses of measles, mumps and rubella vaccine, live p. 1284 by entry to primary school, unless there is a valid contra-indication. Measles, mumps and rubella vaccine, live should be given irrespective of previous measles, mumps, or rubella infection or vaccination.

The first dose of measles, mumps and rubella vaccine, live is given to children aged 12–13 months. A second dose is given before starting school at 3 years and 4 months–5 years of age (see Immunisation Schedule).

Children presenting for pre-school booster who have not received the first dose of measles, mumps and rubella vaccine, live should be given a dose of measles, mumps and rubella vaccine, live followed 3 months later by a second dose.

At school-leaving age or at entry into further education, measles, mumps and rubella vaccine, live immunisation should be offered to individuals of both sexes who have not received 2 doses during childhood. In those who have received only a single dose of measles, mumps and rubella vaccine, live in childhood, a second dose is recommended to achieve full protection. If 2 doses of measles, mumps and rubella vaccine, live are required, the second dose should be given one month after the initial dose. The decision on whether to vaccinate adults should take into consideration their vaccination history, the likelihood of the individual remaining susceptible, and the future risk of exposure and disease.

Measles, mumps and rubella vaccine, live should be used to protect against rubella in *seronegative women of child-bearing age* (see Immunisation Schedule); unimmunised healthcare workers who might put pregnant women and other vulnerable groups at risk of rubella or measles should be vaccinated. Measles, mumps and rubella vaccine, live may also be offered to previously *unimmunised and seronegative post-partum women* (see measles, mumps and rubella vaccine, live)—vaccination a few days after delivery is important because about 60% of congenital abnormalities from rubella infection occur in babies of women who have borne more than one child. Immigrants arriving after the age of school immunisation are particularly likely to require immunisation.

Contacts

Measles, mumps and rubella vaccine, live may also be used in the control of outbreaks of measles and should be offered to susceptible children aged over 6 months who are contacts of a case, within 3 days of exposure to infection. Children immunised before 12 months of age should still receive two doses of measles, mumps and rubella vaccine, live at the recommended ages. If one dose of measles, mumps and rubella vaccine, live has already been given to a child, then the second dose may be brought forward to at least one month after the first, to ensure complete protection. If the child is under 18 months of age and the second dose is given within 3 months of the first, then the routine dose before starting school at 3 years and 4 months–5 years should still be given. Children aged under 9 months for whom avoidance of measles infection is particularly important (such as those with history of recent severe illness) can be given normal immunoglobulin after exposure to measles; routine measles, mumps and rubella vaccine, live immunisation should then be given after at least 3 months at the appropriate age.

Measles, mumps and rubella vaccine, live is **not suitable** for prophylaxis following exposure to mumps or rubella since the antibody response to the mumps and rubella components is too slow for effective prophylaxis.

Children and adults with impaired immune response should not receive live vaccines (see advice on HIV). If they have been exposed to measles infection they should be given normal immunoglobulin.

Travel

Unimmunised travellers, including children over 6 months, to areas where measles is endemic or epidemic should receive measles, mumps and rubella vaccine, live. Children immunised before 12 months of age should still receive two doses of measles, mumps and rubella vaccine, live at the recommended ages. If one dose of measles, mumps and rubella vaccine, live has already been given to a child, then the second dose should be brought forward to at least one month after the first, to ensure complete protection. If the child is under 18 months of age and the second dose is given within 3 months of the first, then the routine dose before starting school at 3 years and 4 months–5 years should still be given.

Meningococcal vaccines

Almost all childhood meningococcal disease in the UK is caused by *Neisseria meningitidis* serogroups B and C. **Meningococcal group C conjugate vaccine** protects only against infection by serogroup C and **Meningococcal group B vaccine** protects only against infection by serogroup B. The risk of meningococcal disease declines with age—immunisation is not generally recommended after the age of 25 years.

Tetravalent meningococcal vaccines that cover serogroups A, C, W135, and Y are available. Although the duration of protection has not been established, the **meningococcal groups A, C, W135, and Y conjugate vaccine** is likely to provide longer-lasting protection than the unconjugated meningococcal polysaccharide vaccine. The antibody response to serogroup C in unconjugated meningococcal polysaccharide vaccines in young children may be suboptimal [not currently available in the UK].

A **meningococcal group B vaccine**, Bexsero®, is licensed in the UK against infection caused by *Neisseria meningitidis* serogroup B and is recommended in the Immunisation Schedule. Bexsero® contains 3 recombinant *Neisseria meningitidis* serogroup B proteins and the outer membrane vesicles from the NZ 98/254 strain, in order to achieve broad protection against *Neisseria meningitidis* serogroup B; the proteins are adsorbed onto an aluminium compound to stimulate an enhanced immune response.

Childhood immunisation

Meningococcal group C conjugate vaccine provides long-term protection against infection by serogroup C of *Neisseria meningitidis*. Immunisation consists of 1 dose given at 12 months of age (as the haemophilus influenzae type b with meningococcal group C vaccine p. 1275) and a second dose given at 13–15 years of age (as the meningococcal groups A with C and W135 and Y vaccine p. 1276) (see Immunisation Schedule).

Meningococcal group B vaccine provides protection against infection by serogroup B of *Neisseria meningitidis*. Immunisation consists of 1 dose given at 2 months of age, a second dose at 4 months of age, and a booster dose at 12 months of age (see *Immunisation Schedule* above).

Unimmunised children aged under 12 months should be given 1 dose of meningococcal group B vaccine (rDNA, component, adsorbed) p. 1275 followed by a second dose of meningococcal group B vaccine (rDNA, component, adsorbed) two months later. They should then be vaccinated according to the Immunisation Schedule (ensuring at least a two month interval between doses of meningococcal group B vaccines). Unimmunised children aged 12–23 months should be given 2 doses of meningococcal group B vaccine (rDNA, component, adsorbed) separated by an interval of two months if they have received less than 2 doses in the first year of life. Unimmunised children aged 2–9 years should be given a single dose of meningococcal group C vaccine (as the haemophilus influenzae type b with meningococcal group C vaccine) followed by a booster dose of meningococcal groups A with C and W135 and Y vaccine at 13–15 years of age.

From 2015, unimmunised individuals aged 10–25 years, including those aged under 25 years who are attending university for the first time, should be given a single dose of meningococcal groups A with C and W135 and Y vaccine p. 1276; a booster dose is not required.

Patients under 25 years of age with confirmed serogroup C disease, who have previously been immunised with meningococcal group C vaccine, should be offered meningococcal group C conjugate vaccine before discharge from hospital.

Travel

Individuals travelling to countries of risk should be immunised with meningococcal groups A, C, W135, and Y conjugate vaccine, even if they have previously received meningococcal group C conjugate vaccine. If an individual has recently received meningococcal group C conjugate vaccine, an interval of at least 4 weeks should be allowed before administration of the tetravalent (meningococcal groups A, C, W135, and Y) vaccine.

Vaccination is particularly important for those living or working with local people or visiting an area of risk during outbreaks.

Immunisation recommendations and requirements for visa entry for individual countries should be checked before travelling, particularly to countries in Sub-Saharan Africa, Asia, and the Indian sub-continent where epidemics of meningococcal outbreaks and infection are reported. Country-by-country information is available from the National Travel Health Network and Centre (www.nathnac. org).

Proof of vaccination with the tetravalent meningococcal groups A with C and W135 and Y vaccine is required for those travelling to Saudi Arabia during the Hajj and Umrah pilgrimages (where outbreaks of the W135 strain have occurred).

Contacts

For advice on the immunisation of *laboratory workers and close contacts* of cases of meningococcal disease in the UK and on the role of the vaccine in the control of *local outbreaks*, consult Guidance for Public Health Management of Meningococcal Disease in the UK at www.gov.uk/phe. Also see for antibacterial prophylaxis for prevention of secondary cases of meningococcal meningitis.

The need for immunisation of laboratory staff who work directly with *Neisseria meningitidis* should be considered.

Pertussis vaccine

Pertussis vaccine is given as a combination preparation containing other vaccines. Acellular vaccines are derived from highly purified components of *Bordetella pertussis*. Primary immunisation against pertussis (whooping cough) requires 3 doses of an acellular pertussis-containing vaccine (see Immunisation schedule), given at intervals of 1 month from the age of 2 months.

All children up to the age of 10 years should receive primary immunisation with a combination vaccine of diphtheria with tetanus, pertussis, hepatitis B, poliomyelitis and haemophilus influenzae type b vaccine p. 1273 (*Infanrix hexa*®).

A booster dose of an acellular pertussis-containing vaccine should ideally be given 3 years after the primary course, although, the interval can be reduced to 1 year if the primary course was delayed. Children aged 1–10 years who have not received a *pertussis-containing* vaccine as part of their primary immunisation should be offered 1 dose of a suitable pertussis-containing vaccine; after an interval of at least 1 year, a booster dose of a suitable pertussis-containing vaccine should be given. Immunisation against pertussis is not routinely recommended in individuals over 10 years of age.

Vaccination of pregnant women against pertussis

In response to the pertussis outbreak, the UK health departments introduced a temporary programme (October 2012) to vaccinate pregnant women against pertussis, and this programme will continue until further notice. The aim of the programme is to boost the levels of pertussis–specific antibodies that are transferred through the placenta, from the mother to the fetus, so that the newborn is protected before routine immunisation begins at 2 months of age.

Pregnant women should be offered a single dose of acellular pertussis-containing vaccine (as adsorbed diphtheria [low dose], tetanus, pertussis (acellular, component) and poliomyelitis (inactivated) vaccine; *Boostrix-IPV*®) between 16 and 32 weeks of pregnancy. Public Health England has advised (2016) that the vaccine is probably best offered after the fetal anomaly scan at around 18–20 weeks. Pregnant women should be offered a single dose of acellular pertussis-containing vaccine up to the onset of labour if they missed the opportunity for vaccination at 16–32 weeks of pregnancy. A single dose of acellular pertussis-containing vaccine may also be offered to new mothers, who have never previously been vaccinated against pertussis, until the child receives the first vaccination.

While this programme is in place, women who become pregnant again should be offered vaccination during each pregnancy to maximise transplacental transfer of antibody.

Contacts

Vaccination against pertussis should be considered for close contacts of cases with pertussis who have been offered antibacterial prophylaxis. Unimmunised or partially immunised contacts under 10 years of age should complete their vaccination against pertussis. A booster dose of an acellular pertussis-containing vaccine is recommended for contacts aged over 10 years who have not received a pertussis-containing vaccine in the last 5 years and who have not received adsorbed diphtheria [low dose], tetanus, and poliomyelitis (inactivated) vaccine in the last month.

Side-effects

Local reactions do not contra-indicate further doses.

The vaccine should not be withheld from children with a history of a preceding dose of:

- fever, irrespective of severity;
- persistent crying or screaming for more than 3 hours;
- severe local reaction, irrespective of extent.

Pneumococcal vaccine

The pneumococcal polysaccharide conjugate vaccine (adsorbed) p. 1277 and the pneumococcal polysaccharide vaccine p. 1277 protect against infection with *Streptococcus pneumoniae* (pneumococcus). Both vaccines contain polysaccharide from capsular pneumococci. The pneumococcal polysaccharide vaccine contains purified polysaccharide from **23 capsular types** of pneumococci, whereas the pneumococcal polysaccharide conjugate vaccine (adsorbed) contains polysaccharide from either **10 capsular types** (*Synflorix*®) or **13 capsular types** (*Prevenar* 13®), and the polysaccharide is conjugated to protein.

Prevenar 13®, is the 13-valent pneumococcal polysaccharide conjugate vaccine (adsorbed) used in the childhood immunisation schedule. The recommended schedule consists of 3 doses: the first at 2 months of age, the second at 4 months of age, and the third at 12–13 months of age (see *Immunisation Schedule*).

The 23-valent pneumococcal polysaccharide vaccine is recommended for individuals at increased risk of pneumococcal infection as follows:

- age over 65 years or in at-risk groups aged 2 years or over;
- asplenia or splenic dysfunction (including homozygous sickle cell disease and coeliac disease which could lead to splenic dysfunction);
- chronic respiratory disease (includes severe asthma treated with continuous or frequent use of a systemic corticosteroid);
- chronic heart disease;
- chronic renal disease;
- chronic liver disease;
- chronic neurological conditions;
- complement disorders;
- diabetes mellitus requiring insulin or oral hypoglycaemic drugs;
- immune deficiency because of disease (e.g. HIV infection) or treatment (including prolonged systemic corticosteroid treatment for over 1 month at dose equivalents of prednisolone: *adult and child over 20 kg*, 20 mg or more daily; *child under 20 kg*, 1 mg/kg or more daily);
- presence of cochlear implant;
- conditions where leakage of cerebrospinal fluid may occur;
- child under 5 years with a history of invasive pneumococcal disease;
- at risk of occupational exposure to metal fume (e.g. welders).

Where possible, the vaccine should be given at least 2 weeks before splenectomy, cochlear implant surgery, chemotherapy, or radiotherapy; patients should be given advice about increased risk of pneumococcal infection. If it is not practical to vaccinate at least 2 weeks before splenectomy, chemotherapy, or radiotherapy, the vaccine should be given at least 2 weeks after the splenectomy or, where possible, at least 3 months after completion of chemotherapy or radiotherapy. Prophylactic antibacterial therapy against pneumococcal infection should not be stopped after immunisation. A patient card and information leaflet for patients with asplenia are available from the Department of Health or in Scotland from the Scottish Government, Health Protection Division (Tel (0131) 244 2879).

Choice of vaccine

Children under 2 years at increased risk of pneumococcal infection (see list) should receive the 13-valent pneumococcal polysaccharide conjugate vaccine (adsorbed) p. 1277 at the recommended ages, followed by a single dose of the 23-valent pneumococcal polysaccharide vaccine p. 1277 after their second birthday. Children at increased risk of pneumococcal infection presenting late for vaccination should receive 2 doses (separated by at least 1 month) of the 13-valent pneumococcal polysaccharide conjugate vaccine

(adsorbed) before the age of 12 months, and a third dose at 12–13 months. Children over 12 months and under 5 years (who have not been vaccinated or not completed the primary course) should receive a single dose of the 13-valent pneumococcal polysaccharide conjugate vaccine (adsorbed) (2 doses separated by an interval of 2 months in the immunocompromised or those with asplenia or splenic dysfunction). All children under 5 years at increased risk of pneumococcal infection should receive a single dose of the 23-valent pneumococcal polysaccharide vaccine after their second birthday and at least 2 months after the final dose of the 13-valent pneumococcal polysaccharide conjugate vaccine (adsorbed).

Children over 5 years and adults who are at increased risk of pneumococcal disease should receive a single dose of the 23-valent pneumococcal polysaccharide vaccine.

Revaccination

In individuals with higher concentrations of antibodies to pneumococcal polysaccharides, revaccination with the 23-valent pneumococcal polysaccharide vaccine more commonly produces adverse reactions. Revaccination is therefore not recommended, except every 5 years in individuals in whom the antibody concentration is likely to decline rapidly (e.g. asplenia, splenic dysfunction and nephrotic syndrome). If there is doubt, the need for revaccination should be discussed with a haematologist, immunologist, or microbiologist.

Poliomyelitis vaccine

Two types of poliomyelitis vaccines (containing strains of poliovirus types 1, 2, and 3) are available, inactivated poliomyelitis vaccine (for injection) and live (oral) poliomyelitis vaccine. **Inactivated** poliomyelitis vaccines, only available in combined preparation, is recommended for routine immunisation.

A course of primary immunisation consists of 3 doses of a combined preparation containing inactivated poliomyelitis vaccines, starting at 2 months of age with intervals of 1 month between doses (see Immunisation schedule). A course of 3 doses should also be given to all unimmunised adults; no adult should remain unimmunised against poliomyelitis.

Two booster doses of a preparation containing inactivated poliomyelitis vaccines are recommended, the first before school entry and the second before leaving school (see Immunisation schedule). Further booster doses are only necessary for adults at special risk, such as travellers to endemic areas, or laboratory staff likely to be exposed to the viruses, or healthcare workers in possible contact with cases; booster doses should be given to such individuals every 10 years.

Live (oral) poliomyelitis vaccine is no longer available for routine use; its use may be considered during large outbreaks, but advice should be sought from Public Health England. The live (oral) vaccine poses a very rare risk of vaccine-associated paralytic polio because the attenuated strain of the virus can revert to a virulent form. For this reason the live (oral) vaccine must **not** be used for immunosuppressed individuals or their household contacts. The use of inactivated poliomyelitis vaccines removes the risk of vaccine-associated paralytic polio altogether.

Travel

Unimmunised travellers to areas with a high incidence of poliomyelitis should receive a full 3-dose course of a preparation containing inactivated poliomyelitis vaccines. Those who have not been vaccinated in the last 10 years should receive a booster dose of **adsorbed diphtheria [low dose], tetanus and poliomyelitis (inactivated) vaccine**. Information about countries with a high incidence of poliomyelitis can be obtained from www.travax.nhs.uk or from the National Travel Health Network and Centre (www.nathnac.org).

14
Vaccines

14

Vaccines

Rabies vaccine

Rabies vaccine p. 1285 contains inactivated rabies virus cultivated in either human diploid cells or purified chick embryo cells; vaccines are used for pre- and post-exposure prophylaxis.

Pre-exposure prophylaxis

Immunisation should be offered to those at high risk of exposure to rabies— laboratory staff who handle the rabies virus, those working in quarantine stations, animal handlers, veterinary surgeons and field workers who are likely to be bitten by infected wild animals, certain port officials, and bat handlers. Transmission of rabies by humans has not been recorded but it is advised that those caring for patients with the disease should be vaccinated.

Immunisation against rabies is also recommended where there is limited access to prompt medical care for those living in areas where rabies is enzootic, for those travelling to such areas for longer than 1 month, and for those on shorter visits who may be exposed to unusual risk.

Immunisation against rabies is indicated during pregnancy if there is substantial risk of exposure to rabies and rapid access to post-exposure prophylaxis is likely to be limited.

Up-to-date country-by-country information on the incidence of rabies can be obtained from the National Travel Health Network and Centre (www.nathnac.org) and, in Scotland, from Health Protection Scotland (www.hps.scot.nhs.uk).

Immunisation against rabies requires 3 doses of rabies vaccine, with further booster doses for those who remain at frequent risk. To ensure continued protection in persons at high risk (e.g. laboratory workers), the concentration of antirabies antibodies in plasma is used to determine the intervals between doses.

Post-exposure management

Following potential exposure to rabies, the wound or site of exposure (e.g. mucous membrane) should be cleansed under running water and washed for several minutes with soapy water as soon as possible after exposure. Disinfectant and a simple dressing can be applied, but suturing should be delayed because it may increase the risk of introducing rabies virus into the nerves.

Post-exposure prophylaxis against rabies depends on the level of risk in the country, the nature of exposure, and the individual's immunity. In each case, expert risk assessment and advice on appropriate management should be obtained from the local Public Health England Centre or Public Health England's Virus Reference Department, Colindale (tel. (020) 8200 4400) or the PHE Colindale Duty Doctor (tel. (020) 8200 6868), in Wales from the Public Health Wales local Health Protection Team or Public Health Wales Virus Reference Laboratory (tel. (029) 2074 7747), in Scotland from the local on-call infectious diseases consultant, and in Northern Ireland from the Public Health Agency Duty Room (tel (028) 9055 3997/(028) 9063 2662) or the Regional Virology Service (tel. (028) 9024 0503).

There are no specific contra-indications to the use of rabies vaccine p. 1285 for post-exposure prophylaxis and its use should be considered whenever a patient has been attacked by an animal in a country where rabies is enzootic, even if there is no direct evidence of rabies in the attacking animal. Because of the potential consequences of untreated rabies exposure and because rabies vaccination has not been associated with fetal abnormalities, pregnancy is not considered a contra-indication to post-exposure prophylaxis.

For post-exposure prophylaxis of *fully immunised* individuals (who have previously received pre-exposure or post-exposure prophylaxis with cell-derived rabies vaccine), 2 doses of cell-derived vaccine are likely to be sufficient; the first dose is given on day 0 and the second dose is given

between day 3–7. Rabies immunoglobulin p. 1257 is not necessary in such cases.

Post-exposure treatment for *unimmunised individuals* (or those whose prophylaxis is possibly incomplete) comprises 5 doses of rabies vaccine given over 1 month (on days 0, 3, 7, 14, and the fifth dose is given between day 28–30); also, depending on the level of risk (determined by factors such as the nature of the bite and the country where it was sustained), rabies immunoglobulin is given to unimmunised individuals on day 0 or within 7 days of starting the course of rabies vaccine. The immunisation course can be discontinued if it is proved that the individual was not at risk.

Rotavirus vaccine

Rotavirus vaccine p. 1286 is a live, oral vaccine that protects young children against gastro-enteritis caused by rotavirus infection. The recommended schedule consists of 2 doses, the first at 2 months of age, and the second at 3 months of age (see Immunisation schedule). The first dose of rotavirus vaccine must be given between 6–15 weeks of age and the second dose should be given after an interval of at least 4 weeks; the vaccine should not be started in children 15 weeks of age or older. Ideally, the full course should be completed before 16 weeks of age to provide protection before the main burden of disease, and to avoid a temporal association between vaccination and intussusception; the course must be completed before 24 weeks of age.

The rotavirus vaccine virus is excreted in the stool and may be transmitted to close contacts; however, vaccination of those with *immunosuppressed* close contacts may protect the contacts from wild-type rotavirus disease and outweigh any risk from transmission of vaccine virus. Carers of a recently vaccinated baby should be advised of the need to wash their hands after changing the baby's nappies.

Smallpox vaccine

Limited supplies of **smallpox vaccine** are held at the Specialist and Reference Microbiology Division, Public Health England Colindale (Tel. (020) 8200 4400) for the exclusive use of workers in laboratories where pox viruses (such as vaccinia) are handled.

If a wider use of the vaccine is being considered, *Guidelines for smallpox response and management in the post-eradication era* should be consulted at www.gov.uk/phe.

Tetanus vaccine

Tetanus vaccine contains a cell-free purified toxin of *Clostridium tetani* adsorbed on aluminium hydroxide or aluminium phosphate to improve antigenicity.

Primary immunisation for children under 10 years consists of 3 doses of a combined preparation containing adsorbed tetanus vaccine, with an interval of 1 month between doses (see *Routine immunisation schedule*). Following routine childhood vaccination, 2 booster doses of a preparation containing adsorbed tetanus vaccine are recommended, the first before school entry and the second before leaving school.

The recommended schedule of tetanus vaccination not only gives protection against tetanus in childhood but also gives the basic immunity for subsequent booster doses. In most circumstances, a total of 5 doses of tetanus vaccine is considered sufficient for long term protection.

For primary immunisation of adults and children over 10 years previously unimmunised against tetanus, 3 doses of **adsorbed diphtheria [low dose], tetanus and poliomyelitis (inactivated) vaccine** are given with an interval of 1 month between doses (see *Diphtheria-containing vaccines for children over 10 years and adults*).

When an individual presents for a booster dose but has been vaccinated following a tetanus-prone wound, the vaccine preparation administered at the time of injury should be determined. If this is not possible, the booster should still be given to ensure adequate protection against all antigens in the booster vaccine.

Very rarely, tetanus has developed after abdominal surgery; patients awaiting elective surgery should be asked about tetanus immunisation and immunised if necessary.

Parenteral drug abuse is also associated with tetanus; those abusing drugs by injection should be vaccinated if unimmunised—booster doses should be given if there is any doubt about their immunisation status.

All laboratory staff should be offered a primary course if unimmunised.

Wounds

Wounds are considered to be tetanus-prone if they are sustained more than 6 hours before surgical treatment or at any interval after injury and are puncture-type (particularly if contaminated with soil or manure) *or* show much devitalised tissue *or* are septic *or* are compound fractures *or* contain foreign bodies. All wounds should receive thorough cleansing.

- For *clean wounds*: fully immunised individuals (those who have received a total of 5 doses of a tetanus-containing vaccine at appropriate intervals) and those whose primary immunisation is complete (with boosters up to date), do not require tetanus vaccine; individuals whose primary immunisation is incomplete or whose boosters are not up to date require a reinforcing dose of a tetanus-containing vaccine (followed by further doses as required to complete the schedule); non-immunised individuals (or those whose immunisation status is not known or who have been fully immunised but are now immunocompromised) should be given a dose of the appropriate tetanus-containing vaccine immediately (followed by completion of the full course of the vaccine if records confirm the need)
- For *tetanus-prone wounds*: management is as for clean wounds with the addition of a dose of tetanus immunoglobulin given at a different site; in fully immunised individuals and those whose primary immunisation is complete (with boosters up to date) the immunoglobulin is needed only if the risk of infection is especially high (e.g. contamination with manure). Antibacterial prophylaxis (with benzylpenicillin, co-amoxiclav, or metronidazole) may also be required for tetanus-prone wounds.

Tick-borne encephalitis vaccine

Tick-borne encephalitis vaccine, inactivated p. 1286 contains inactivated tick-borne encephalitis virus cultivated in chick embryo cells. It is recommended for immunisation of those working in, or visiting, high-risk areas (see International Travel). Those working, walking or camping in warm forested areas of Central and Eastern Europe, Scandinavia, Northern and Eastern China, and some parts of Japan, particularly from April to November when ticks are most prevalent, are at greatest risk of tick-borne encephalitis. For full protection, 3 doses of the vaccine are required; booster doses are required every 3–5 years for those still at risk. Ideally, immunisation should be completed at least one month before travel.

Typhoid vaccine

Typhoid vaccine p. 1277 is available as Vi capsular polysaccharide (from *Salmonella typhi*) vaccine for injection and as live attenuated *Salmonella typhi* for oral use. Typhoid immunisation is advised for:

- travellers to areas where typhoid is endemic, especially if staying with or visiting local people;
- travellers to endemic areas where frequent or prolonged exposure to poor sanitation and poor food hygiene is likely
- laboratory personnel who, in the course of their work, may be exposed to *Salmonella typhi*.

Typhoid vaccination is not a substitute for scrupulous personal hygiene.

Capsular **polysaccharide** typhoid vaccine is usually given by *intramuscular injection*. Children under 2 years may respond suboptimally to the vaccine, but children aged between 1–2 years should be immunised if the risk of typhoid fever is considered high (immunisation is not recommended for infants under 12 months). Revaccination is needed every 3 years on continued exposure.

Oral typhoid vaccine is a **live attenuated** vaccine contained in an enteric-coated capsule. One capsule taken on alternate days for a total of 3 doses, provides protection 7–10 days after the last dose. Protection may persist for up to 3 years in those constantly (or repeatedly) exposed to *Salmonella typhi*, but those who only occasionally travel to endemic areas require further courses at intervals of 1 year.

Varicella-zoster vaccine

The live varicella-zoster vaccine p. 1287, *Varilrix®* and *Varivax®*, are licensed for immunisation against varicella (chickenpox) in seronegative individuals. They are not recommended for routine use in children, but can be given to seronegative healthy children over 1 year who come into close contact with individuals at high risk of severe varicella infections. The Department of Health recommends these vaccines for seronegative healthcare workers who come into direct contact with patients. Those with a history of chickenpox or shingles can be considered immune, but healthcare workers with a negative or uncertain history should be tested.

Rarely, the varicella-zoster vaccine virus has been transmitted from the vaccinated individual to close contacts. Therefore, contact with the following should be avoided if a vaccine-related cutaneous rash develops within 4–6 weeks of the first or second dose:

- varicella-susceptible pregnant women;
- individuals at high risk of severe varicella, including those with immunodeficiency or those receiving immunosuppressive therapy;

Healthcare workers who develop a generalised papular or vesicular rash on vaccination should avoid contact with patients until the lesions have crusted. Those who develop a localised rash after vaccination should cover the lesions and be allowed to continue working unless in contact with patients at high risk of severe varicella.

National shingles immunisation programme

The aim of the national shingles immunisation programme is to lower the incidence and severity of shingles in older people using the high potency, live varicella-zoster vaccine, *Zostavax®*. It is recommended that vaccination is routinely offered to people aged 70 years. A catch-up programme has also been rolled out (since 2013) in those aged 70-79 years, as this age group is likely to have the greatest benefit from vaccination.

In the 2016–2017 immunisation programme, varicella-zoster vaccine is recommended in adults who were 70 **or** 78 years of age on 1st September 2016. Patients who were eligible for vaccination in the first 3 years of the programme but have not been vaccinated against *herpes zoster* remain eligible until their 80th birthday; this includes patients who were aged 71–73 or 79 on 1st September 2016. Patients who have reached 80 years are no longer eligible for vaccination. A single dose of *Zostavax®* is likely to give protection for at least 7 years, but the need for, or timing of, a booster dose has not been established. Although *Zostavax®* is not recommended for the treatment of shingles or post-herpetic neuralgia, it can be given to those with a previous history of shingles; ideally the vaccine should be delayed until systemic antiviral treatment has been completed.

Varicella-zoster immunoglobulin p. 1257 is used to protect susceptible individuals at increased risk of severe varicella infection (*see* Immunoglobulins p. 1252).

14

Vaccines

Yellow fever vaccine

Yellow fever vaccine, live p. 1287 is indicated for those travelling or living in areas where infection is endemic and for laboratory staff who handle the virus or who handle clinical material from suspected cases. Infants under 6 months of age should not be vaccinated because there is a small risk of encephalitis; infants aged 6–9 months should be vaccinated only if the risk of yellow fever is high and unavoidable (seek expert advice). The immunity which probably lasts for life is officially accepted for 10 years starting from 10 days after primary immunisation and for a further 10 years immediately after revaccination.

Vaccines for travel

Immunisation for travel

See advice on Malaria, treatment p. 602.

No special immunisation is required for travellers to the United States, Europe, Australia, or New Zealand, although all travellers should have immunity to tetanus and poliomyelitis (and childhood immunisations should be up to date); Tick-borne encephalitis vaccine is recommended for immunisation of those working in, or visiting, high-risk areas. Certain special precautions are required in non-European areas surrounding the Mediterranean, in Africa, the Middle East, Asia, and South America.

Travellers to areas that have a high incidence of **poliomyelitis** or **tuberculosis** should be immunised with the appropriate vaccine; in the case of poliomyelitis previously immunised travellers may be given a booster dose of a preparation containing inactivated poliomyelitis vaccine. BCG immunisation is recommended for travellers aged under 16 years proposing to stay for longer than 3 months (or in close contact with the local population) in countries with an incidence of tuberculosis greater than 40 per 100 000 (list of countries where the incidence of tuberculosis is greater than 40 cases per 100 000 is available from www.gov.uk/phe); it should preferably be given 3 months or more before departure.

Yellow fever immunisation is recommended for travel to the endemic zones of Africa and South America. Many countries require an International Certificate of Vaccination from individuals arriving from, or who have been travelling through, endemic areas; other countries require a certificate from all entering travellers (consult the Department of Health handbook, *Health Information for Overseas Travel*, www.dh.gov.uk).

Immunisation against **meningococcal meningitis** is recommended for a number of areas of the world.

Protection against **hepatitis A** is recommended for travellers to high-risk areas outside Northern and Western Europe, North America, Japan, Australia and New Zealand. Hepatitis A vaccine is recommended and it is likely to be effective even if given shortly before departure; Public Health England recommends travellers can be vaccinated with hepatitis A vaccine up to the day of travel, and no longer recommends the use of normal immunoglobulin for travel prophylaxis. Special care must also be taken with food hygiene.

Hepatitis B vaccine is recommended for those travelling to areas of high or intermediate prevalence who intend to seek employment as healthcare workers or who plan to remain there for lengthy periods and who may therefore be at increased risk of acquiring infection as the result of medical or dental procedures carried out in those countries. Short-term tourists or business travellers are not generally at increased risk of infection but may put themselves at risk by their sexual behaviour when abroad.

Prophylactic immunisation against **rabies** is recommended for travellers to enzootic areas on long

journeys or to areas out of reach of immediate medical attention.

Travellers who have not had a **tetanus** booster in the last 10 years and are visiting areas where medical attention may not be accessible should receive a booster dose of adsorbed diphtheria [low dose], tetanus and poliomyelitis (inactivated) vaccine, even if they have received 5 doses of a tetanus-containing vaccine previously.

Typhoid vaccine is indicated for travellers to countries where typhoid is endemic, but the vaccine is no substitute for personal precautions.

There is no requirement for cholera vaccination as a condition for entry into any country, but **oral cholera vaccine** should be considered for backpackers and those travelling to situations where the risk is greatest (e.g. refugee camps). Regardless of vaccination, travellers to areas where cholera is endemic should take special care with food hygiene.

Advice on **diphtheria**, on **Japanese encephalitis**, and on **tick-borne encephalitis** is included in *Health Information for Overseas Travel*.

Food hygiene

In areas where sanitation is poor, good food hygiene is important to help prevent hepatitis A, typhoid, cholera, and other diarrhoeal diseases (including travellers' diarrhoea). Food should be freshly prepared and hot, and uncooked vegetables (including green salads) should be avoided; only fruits which can be peeled should be eaten. Only suitable bottled water, or tap water that has been boiled or treated with sterilising tablets, should be used for drinking.

Information on health advice for travellers

Health professionals and travellers can find the latest information on immunisation requirements and precautions for avoiding disease while travelling from: www.nathnac.org.

The handbook, *Health Information for Overseas Travel* (2010), which draws together essential information *for healthcare professionals* regarding health advice for travellers, can also be obtained from this website.

Immunisation requirements change from time to time, and information on the current requirements for any particular country may be obtained from the embassy or legation of the appropriate country or from:

National Travel Health Network and Centre
UCLH NHS Foundation Trust
3rd Floor Central
250 Euston Road
London
NW1 2PG
Tel: 0845 602 6712
(Monday and Friday: 9–11 a.m. and 1–2 p.m., Tuesday to Thursday: 9–11 a.m. and 1–3:30 p.m. For healthcare professionals only)
www.travelhealthpro.org.uk/

Travel Medicine Team
Health Protection Scotland
Meridian Court
5 Cadogan Street
Glasgow
G2 6QE
Tel: (0141) 300 1130
(2–4 p.m. Monday to Wednesday, 9:30–11:30 a.m. Friday; for registered TRAVAX users only)
www.travax.nhs.uk

(TRAVAX is free for NHS Scotland users (registration required); subscription fee may be payable for users outside NHS Scotland)

Welsh Assembly Government
Tel (029) 2082 5397
(9 a.m.–5:30 p.m. weekdays)

Department of Health, Social Services and Public Safety
Castle Buildings
Stormont
Belfast
BT4 3SQ
Tel: (028) 9052 2118
(9 a.m.–5 p.m. weekdays)
www.dhsspsni.gov.uk

VACCINES

Vaccines ⊙

> **IMPORTANT SAFETY INFORMATION**
> MHRA/CHM ADVICE (UPDATED NOVEMBER 2017)
> Following reports of death in neonates who received a live attenuated vaccine after exposure to a tumor necrosis factor alpha (TNF-a) inhibitor in utero, the MHRA has issued the following advice:
> * any infant who has been exposed to immunosuppressive treatment from the mother either in utero during pregnancy or via breastfeeding should have any live attenuated vaccination deferred for as long as a postnatal influence on the immune status of the infant remains possible;
> * in the case of infants who have been exposed to TNF-a inhibitors and other immunosuppressive biological medicines in utero, PHE advise that any live attenuated vaccination (e.g. BCG vaccine) should be deferred until the infant is age 6 months;
> * PHE advise if there is any doubt as to whether an infant due to receive a live attenuated vaccine may be immunosuppressed due to the mother's therapy, including exposure through breast-feeding, specialist advice should be sought.

● CONTRA-INDICATIONS
  CONTRA-INDICATIONS, FURTHER INFORMATION
▸ Impaired immune response Severely immunosuppressed patients should not be given live vaccines (including those with severe primary immunodeficiency).
● CAUTIONS Acute illness · minor illnesses
  CAUTIONS, FURTHER INFORMATION Vaccination may be postponed if the individual is suffering from an acute illness; however, it is not necessary to postpone immunisation in patients with minor illnesses without fever or systemic upset.
▸ Impaired immune response and drugs affecting immune response Immune response to vaccines may be reduced in immunosuppressed patients and there is also a risk of generalised infection with live vaccines.
  Specialist advice should be sought for those being treated with high doses of corticosteroids (dose equivalents of prednisolone: **adults**, at least 40 mg daily for more than 1 week; **children**, 2 mg/kg (or more than 40 mg) daily for at least 1 week or 1 mg/kg daily for 1 month), or other immunosuppressive drugs, and those being treated for malignant conditions with chemotherapy or generalised radiotherapy. Live vaccines should be postponed until at least 3 months after stopping high-dose systemic corticosteroids and at least 6 months after stopping other immunosuppressive drugs or generalised radiotherapy (at least 12 months after discontinuing immunosuppressants following bone-marrow transplantation).
  The Royal College of Paediatrics and Child Health has produced a statement, *Immunisation of the Immunocompromised Child* (2002)(available at www.rcpch. ac.uk).
▸ Predisposition to neurological problems When there is a personal or family history of *febrile* convulsions, there is an

increased risk of these occurring during fever from any cause including immunisation, but this is not a contra-indication to immunisation. In children who have had a seizure associated with fever without neurological deterioration, immunisation is *recommended*; advice on the *management of fever* (see Post-immunisation Pyrexia in Infants) should be given before immunisation. When a child has had a convulsion not associated with fever, and the neurological condition is not deteriorating, immunisation is *recommended*.
  Children with stable neurological disorders (e.g. spina bifida, congenital brain abnormality, and peri-natal hypoxic-ischaemic encephalopathy) should be immunised according to the recommended schedule.
  When there is a *still evolving neurological problem*, including poorly controlled epilepsy, immunisation should be deferred and the child referred to a specialist. Immunisation is recommended if a cause for the neurological disorder is identified. If a cause is not identified, immunisation should be deferred until the condition is stable.
● SIDE-EFFECTS
▸ **Common or very common** Appetite decreased · arthralgia · diarrhoea · dizziness · fatigue · fever · headache · irritability · lymphadenopathy (uncommon in children) · malaise · myalgia · nausea · skin reactions · vomiting
▸ **Uncommon** Hypersensitivity
● ALLERGY AND CROSS-SENSITIVITY Contra-indicated in patients with a confirmed anaphylactic reaction to a preceding dose of a vaccine containing the same antigens or vaccine component (such as antibacterials in viral vaccines).
● PREGNANCY Live vaccines should not be administered routinely to pregnant women because of the theoretical risk of fetal infection but where there is a significant risk of exposure to disease, the need for vaccination usually outweighs any possible risk to the fetus. Termination of pregnancy following inadvertent immunisation is not recommended. There is no evidence of risk from vaccinating pregnant women with inactivated viral or bacterial vaccines or toxoids.
● BREAST FEEDING Although there is a theoretical risk of live vaccine being present in breast milk, vaccination is not contra-indicated for women who are breast-feeding when there is significant risk of exposure to disease. There is no evidence of risk from vaccinating women who are breast-feeding, with inactivated viral or bacterial vaccines or toxoids.
● DIRECTIONS FOR ADMINISTRATION If alcohol or disinfectant is used for cleansing the skin it should be allowed to evaporate before vaccination to prevent possible inactivation of live vaccines.
  When 2 or more live vaccines are required (and are not available as a combined preparation), they can be administered at any time before or after each other at different sites, preferably in a different limb; if more than one injection is to be given in the same limb, they should be administered at least 2.5 cm apart. See also Bacillus Calmette-Guérin vaccine p. 1273, and Cautions, further information in measles, mumps and rubella vaccine, live p. 1284.
  Vaccines should not be given intravenously. Most vaccines are given by the intramuscular route, although some are given by either the intradermal, deep subcutaneous, or oral route. The intramuscular route should not be used in patients with **bleeding disorders** such as haemophilia or thrombocytopenia, vaccines usually given by the intramuscular route should be given by deep subcutaneous injection instead.

14

Vaccines

The Department of Health has advised *against the use of jet guns* for vaccination owing to the risk of transmitting blood borne infections, such as HIV.

Particular attention must be paid to instructions on the use of diluents. Vaccines which are liquid suspensions or are reconstituted before use should be adequately mixed to ensure uniformity of the material to be injected.

- HANDLING AND STORAGE Care must be taken to store all vaccines under the conditions recommended in the product literature, otherwise the preparation may become ineffective. **Refrigerated storage** is usually necessary; many vaccines need to be stored at 2–8°C and not allowed to freeze. Vaccines should be protected from light. Reconstituted vaccines and opened multidose vials must be used within the period recommended in the product literature. Unused vaccines should be disposed of by incineration at a registered disposal contractor.

VACCINES > BACTERIAL AND VIRAL VACCINES, COMBINED

F 1271

Diphtheria with haemophilus influenzae type b vaccine, pertussis, poliomyelitis and tetanus

- ● INDICATIONS AND DOSE
Primary immunisation
- ▶ BY INTRAMUSCULAR INJECTION
- ▶ Child 2 months–9 years: 0.5 mL every month for 3 doses

- ● UNLICENSED USE *Infanrix-IPV+ Hib®* not licensed for use in children over 36 months; *Pediacel®* not licensed in children over 4 years. However, the Department of Health recommends that these be used for children up to 10 years.
- ● SIDE-EFFECTS
- ▶ **Common or very common** Crying abnormal · drowsiness · restlessness
- ▶ **Uncommon** Cough · extensive swelling of vaccinated limb · increased risk of infection · rhinorrhoea
- ▶ **Frequency not known** Anaphylactoid reaction · angioedema · apnoea · hypotonic-hyporesponsiveness episode · seizure
SIDE-EFFECTS, FURTHER INFORMATION The incidence of local and systemic reactions is lower with acellular pertussis vaccines than with whole-cell pertussis vaccines used previously.

Compared with primary vaccination, injection site reactions are more common with booster doses of vaccines containing acellular pertussis. Public Health England has advised (2016) that the vaccine should not be withheld from children with a history to a preceding dose of: fever, irrespective of severity; hypotonic-hyporesonsive episodes; persistent crying or screaming for more than 3 hours; severe local reaction, irrespective of extent.
- ● PRESCRIBING AND DISPENSING INFORMATION Available as part of childhood schedule from health organisations or ImmForm.

- ● MEDICINAL FORMS
There can be variation in the licensing of different medicines containing the same drug.
Powder and suspension for suspension for injection
- ▶ Infanrix-IPV + Hib (GlaxoSmithKline UK Ltd)
Infanrix-IPV + Hib vaccine powder and suspension for suspension for injection 0.5ml pre-filled syringes | 1 pre-filled disposable injection PoM £27.86

F 1271

Diphtheria with pertussis, poliomyelitis vaccine and tetanus

- ● INDICATIONS AND DOSE
First booster dose
- ▶ BY INTRAMUSCULAR INJECTION
- ▶ Child 3–9 years: 0.5 mL, to be given 3 years after primary immunisation
Vaccination of pregnant women against pertussis (using low dose vaccines)
- ▶ BY INTRAMUSCULAR INJECTION
- ▶ Females of childbearing potential: 0.5 mL for 1 dose

- ● SIDE-EFFECTS
- ▶ **Common or very common** Abdominal pain (uncommon in children)
- ▶ **Uncommon** Apathy (in children) · asthma · chills · drowsiness (very common in children) · dry throat (in children) · extensive swelling of vaccinated limb · common in children) · oral herpes · pain · paraesthesia · sleep disorder (in children)
- ▶ **Frequency not known** Anaphylactoid reaction · angioedema · asthenia · hypotonic-hyporesponsiveness episode · seizure
SIDE-EFFECTS, FURTHER INFORMATION The incidence of local and systemic reactions is lower with acellular pertussis vaccines than with whole-cell pertussis vaccines used previously.

Compared with primary vaccination, injection site reactions are more common with booster doses of vaccines containing acellular pertussis. Public Health England has advised (2016) that the vaccine should not be withheld from children with a history to a preceding dose of: fever, irrespective of severity; hypotonic-hyporesonsive episodes; persistent crying or screaming for more than 3 hours; severe local reaction, irrespective of extent.
- ● PREGNANCY Contra-indicated in pregnant women with a history of encephalopathy of unknown origin within 7 days of previous immunisation with a pertussis-containing vaccine. Contra-indicated in pregnant women with a history of transient thrombocytopenia or neurological complications following previous immunisation against diphtheria or tetanus.
- ● PRESCRIBING AND DISPENSING INFORMATION Pregnant women should be vaccinated using low dose vaccines (brands may include *Boostrix-IPV®* or *Repevax®*).

Available as part of childhood immunisation schedule from health organisations or ImmForm.

Available for vaccination of pregnant women from ImmForm.

- ● MEDICINAL FORMS
There can be variation in the licensing of different medicines containing the same drug.
Suspension for injection
EXCIPIENTS: May contain Neomycin, polymyxin b, streptomycin
- ▶ Boostrix-IPV (GlaxoSmithKline UK Ltd)
Boostrix-IPV suspension for injection 0.5ml pre-filled syringes | 1 pre-filled disposable injection PoM £22.74
- ▶ Repevax (Sanofi Pasteur)
Repevax vaccine suspension for injection 0.5ml pre-filled syringes | 1 pre-filled disposable injection PoM £20.00

Diphtheria with poliomyelitis and tetanus vaccine

● **INDICATIONS AND DOSE**

Primary immunisation

▸ BY INTRAMUSCULAR INJECTION
▸ Child 10-17 years: 0.5 mL every month for 3 doses
▸ Adult: 0.5 mL every month for 3 doses

Booster doses

▸ BY INTRAMUSCULAR INJECTION
▸ Child 10-17 years: 0.5 mL for 1 dose, first booster dose—
should be given 3 years after primary course (this
interval can be reduced to a minimum of 1 year if the
primary course was delayed), then 0.5 mL for 1 dose,
second booster dose—should be given 10 years after
first booster dose (this interval can be reduced to a
minimum of 5 years if previous doses were delayed),
second booster dose may also be used as first booster
dose in those over 10 years who have received only
3 previous doses of a diphtheria-containing vaccine
▸ Adult: 0.5 mL for 1 dose, first booster dose—should be
given 3 years after primary course (this interval can be
reduced to a minimum of 1 year if the primary course
was delayed), then 0.5 mL for 1 dose, second booster
dose—should be given 10 years after first booster dose
(this interval can be reduced to a minimum of 5 years if
previous doses were delayed), second booster dose may
also be used as first booster dose in those over 10 years
who have received only 3 previous doses of a
diphtheria-containing vaccine

● **SIDE-EFFECTS**

▸ **Common or very common** Vertigo
▸ **Frequency not known** Abdominal pain · asthenia · chills ·
face oedema · influenza like illness · nerve disorders · pallor
· seizure · shock · syncope · vaccination reactions

● PRESCRIBING AND DISPENSING INFORMATION Available as
part of childhood schedule from health organisations or
ImmForm.

● MEDICINAL FORMS
There can be variation in the licensing of different medicines
containing the same drug.
Suspension for injection
EXCIPIENTS: May contain Neomycin, polymyxin b, streptomycin
▸ Revaxis (Sanofi Pasteur)
Revaxis vaccine suspension for injection 0.5ml pre-filled syringes |
1 pre-filled disposable injection [PoM] £7.80 DT = £7.80

Diphtheria with tetanus, pertussis, hepatitis B, poliomyelitis and haemophilus influenzae type b vaccine

12-Oct-2017

● **INDICATIONS AND DOSE**

Primary immunisation (first dose)

▸ BY DEEP INTRAMUSCULAR INJECTION
▸ Child 2 months: 0.5 mL for 1 dose

Primary immunisation (second dose)

▸ BY DEEP INTRAMUSCULAR INJECTION
▸ Child 3 months: 0.5 mL for 1 dose, preferably administer
at a different injection site to that of first dose

Primary immunisation (third dose)

▸ BY DEEP INTRAMUSCULAR INJECTION
▸ Child 4 months: 0.5 mL for 1 dose, preferably administer
at a different injection site to that of second dose

● **SIDE-EFFECTS**

▸ **Common or very common** Anxiety · crying abnormal
▸ **Uncommon** Cough · drowsiness · extensive swelling of
vaccinated limb · increased risk of infection
▸ **Rare or very rare** Anaphylactoid reaction · angioedema ·
apnoea · dermatitis · hypotonic-hyporesponsiveness
episode · seizure · swelling · thrombocytopenia

● PRESCRIBING AND DISPENSING INFORMATION Available as
part of childhood schedule from health organisations or
ImmForm.

● MEDICINAL FORMS
There can be variation in the licensing of different medicines
containing the same drug.
Powder and suspension for suspension for injection
EXCIPIENTS: May contain Neomycin, polymyxin b
▸ Infanrix Hexa (GlaxoSmithKline UK Ltd)
Infanrix Hexa vaccine powder and suspension for suspension for
injection 0.5ml pre-filled syringes | 1 pre-filled disposable
injection [PoM] [S]

VACCINES > BACTERIAL VACCINES

Anthrax vaccine

● **INDICATIONS AND DOSE**

Pre-exposure immunisation against anthrax | Post-exposure immunisation

▸ BY INTRAMUSCULAR INJECTION
▸ Adult: Initially 1 dose every 3 weeks for 3 doses,
followed by 1 dose after 6 months, to be administered
in the deltoid region, 1 dose is equivalent to 0.5 mL

Booster

▸ BY INTRAMUSCULAR INJECTION
▸ Adult: 1 dose every 12 months, to be administered in
deltoid region, 1 dose is equivalent to 0.5 mL

● **SIDE-EFFECTS**

▸ **Common or very common** Febrile disorders · influenza like
illness
▸ **Rare or very rare** Angioedema · asthenia · hyperhidrosis ·
paraesthesia
▸ **Frequency not known** Bronchospasm · circulatory collapse ·
hypotension

● PRESCRIBING AND DISPENSING INFORMATION Available
from Public Health England's Centre for Emergency
Preparedness and Response (Porton Down).

● MEDICINAL FORMS
There can be variation in the licensing of different medicines
containing the same drug.
Suspension for injection
EXCIPIENTS: May contain Thiomersal
▸ Anthrax vaccine (Non-proprietary)
Anthrax vaccine (alum precipitated sterile filtrate) suspension for
injection 0.5ml ampoules | 5 ampoule [PoM] [S]

Bacillus Calmette-Guérin vaccine

(BCG Vaccine)

● DRUG ACTION BCG (Bacillus Calmette-Guérin) is a live
attenuated strain derived from *Mycobacterium bovis* which
stimulates the development of immunity to *M.
tuberculosis*.

● **INDICATIONS AND DOSE**

Immunisation against tuberculosis

▸ BY INTRADERMAL INJECTION
▸ Child 1-11 months: 0.05 mL, to be injected at insertion of
deltoid muscle onto humerus (keloid formation more
likely with sites higher on arm); tip of shoulder should
be **avoided**

continued →

14

Vaccines

► Child 1-17 years: 0.1 mL, to be injected at insertion of deltoid muscle onto humerus (keloid formation more likely with sites higher on arm); tip of shoulder should be **avoided**

► Adult: 0.1 mL, to be injected at insertion of deltoid muscle onto humerus (keloid formation more likely with sites higher on arm); tip of shoulder should be **avoided**

● CONTRA-INDICATIONS Generalised septic skin conditions

CONTRA-INDICATIONS, FURTHER INFORMATION A lesion-free site should be used to administer BCG vaccine to patients with eczema.

● CAUTIONS

CAUTIONS, FURTHER INFORMATION BCG vaccine can be given simultaneously with another live vaccine, but if they are not given at the same time an interval of 4 weeks should normally be allowed. When BCG is given to infants, there is no need to delay routine primary immunisations. No further vaccination should be given in the arm used for BCG vaccination for at least 3 months because of the risk of regional lymphadenitis.

● INTERACTIONS → Appendix 1: live vaccines

● SIDE-EFFECTS

► **Rare or very rare** Increased risk of infection · osteitis

● PRE-TREATMENT SCREENING Apart from children under 6 years, any person being considered for BCG immunisation must first be given a skin test for hypersensitivity to tuberculoprotein (see tuberculin purified protein derivative p. 1259). A skin test is not necessary for a child under 6 years provided that the child has not stayed for longer than 3 months in a country with an incidence of tuberculosis greater than 40 per 100 000, the child has not had contact with a person with tuberculosis, and there is no family history of tuberculosis within the last 5 years.

● DIRECTIONS FOR ADMINISTRATION Intradermal injection technique Skin is stretched between thumb and forefinger and needle (size 25G or 26G) inserted (bevel upwards) for about 3 mm into superficial layers of dermis (almost parallel with surface). Needle should be short with short bevel (can usually be seen through epidermis during insertion). Tense raised blanched bleb showing tips of hair follicles is sign of correct injection; 7 mm bleb ≡ 0.1 mL injection, 3 mm bleb ≡ 0.05 mL injection; if considerable resistance not felt, needle too deep and should be removed and reinserted before giving more vaccine.

● PRESCRIBING AND DISPENSING INFORMATION Available from health organisations or direct from ImmForm www.immform.dh.gov.uk (SSI brand, multidose vial with diluent).

● MEDICINAL FORMS
There can be variation in the licensing of different medicines containing the same drug.
Powder and solvent for suspension for injection
► Bacillus calmette-guérin vaccine (Non-proprietary)
Bacillus Calmette-Guerin vaccine powder and solvent for suspension for injection vials | 10 vial [PoM] Ⓢ

⚑ 1271

Cholera vaccine

● INDICATIONS AND DOSE

Immunisation against cholera (for travellers to endemic or epidemic areas on the basis of current recommendations)
► BY MOUTH
► Child 2-5 years: 1 dose every 1–6 weeks for 3 doses, if more than 6 weeks have elapsed between doses, the

primary course should be restarted, immunisation should be completed at least one week before potential exposure

► Child 6-17 years: 1 dose every 1–6 weeks for 2 doses, if more than 6 weeks have elapsed between doses, the primary course should be restarted, immunisation should be completed at least one week before potential exposure

► Adult: 1 dose every 1–6 weeks for 2 doses, if more than 6 weeks have elapsed between doses, the primary course should be restarted, immunisation should be completed at least one week before potential exposure

Booster
► BY MOUTH
► Child 2-5 years: A single booster dose can be given within 6 months after primary course, if more than 6 months have elapsed since the last vaccination, the primary course should be repeated

► Child 6-17 years: A single booster dose can be given within 2 years after primary course, if more than 2 years have elapsed since the last vaccination, the primary course should be repeated

► Adult: A single booster dose can be given within 2 years after primary course, if more than 2 years have elapsed since the last vaccination, the primary course should be repeated

● CONTRA-INDICATIONS Acute gastro-intestinal illness

● INTERACTIONS → Appendix 1: cholera vaccine

● SIDE-EFFECTS

► **Uncommon** Gastrointestinal discomfort · gastrointestinal disorders

► **Rare or very rare** Chills · cough · dehydration · drowsiness · hyperhidrosis · increased risk of infection · insomnia · pulmonary reaction · syncope · taste altered · throat pain

► **Frequency not known** Angioedema · asthenia · dyspnoea · hypertension · influenza like illness · lymphadenitis · pain · paraesthesia · sputum increased

● DIRECTIONS FOR ADMINISTRATION

► In children Dissolve effervescent sodium bicarbonate granules in a glassful of water or chlorinated water (approximately 150 mL). For children over 6 years, add vaccine suspension to make one dose. For child 2–5 years, discard half (approximately 75 mL) of the solution, then add vaccine suspension to make one dose. Drink within 2 hours. Food, drink, and other oral medicines should be avoided for 1 hour before and after vaccination.

► In adults Dissolve effervescent sodium bicarbonate granules in a glassful of water or chlorinated water (approximately 150 mL). Add vaccine suspension to make one dose. Drink within 2 hours. Food, drink, and other oral medicines should be avoided for 1 hour before and after vaccination.

● PATIENT AND CARER ADVICE Counselling on administration advised. Immunisation with cholera vaccine does not provide complete protection and all travellers to a country where cholera exists should be warned that scrupulous attention to food, water, and personal hygiene is **essential**.

● MEDICINAL FORMS
There can be variation in the licensing of different medicines containing the same drug.
Oral suspension
► Dukoral (Valneva UK Ltd)
Dukoral cholera vaccine oral suspension | 2 dose [PoM] £26.35 DT = £26.35

Haemophilus influenzae type b with meningococcal group C vaccine

F 1271

- **INDICATIONS AND DOSE**

Booster dose (for infants who have received primary immunisation with a vaccine containing *Haemophilus influenzae* type b component) and primary immunisation against *Neisseria meningitidis*
- ▶ BY INTRAMUSCULAR INJECTION
- ▹ Child 12–13 months: 0.5 mL for 1 dose

Immunisation against *Neisseria meningitidis* in an unimmunised patient
- ▶ BY INTRAMUSCULAR INJECTION
- ▹ Child 1–9 years: 0.5 mL for 1 dose

Booster dose (for children who have not been immunised against *Haemophilus influenza* type b) | Booster dose after recovery from *Haemophilus influenzae* type b disease (for index cases previously vaccinated, with low Hib antibody concentration or if it is not possible to measure antibody concentration)
- ▶ BY INTRAMUSCULAR INJECTION
- ▹ Child 1–9 years: 0.5 mL for 1 dose

Booster dose after recovery from *Haemophilus influenzae* type b disease (for fully vaccinated index cases with asplenia or splenic dysfunction, if previous dose received over 1 year ago)
- ▶ BY INTRAMUSCULAR INJECTION
- ▹ Child 1–17 years: 0.5 mL for 1 dose
- ▹ Adult: 0.5 mL for 1 dose

Booster dose (for patients diagnosed with asplenia, splenic dysfunction or complement deficiency at under 2 years of age)
- ▶ BY INTRAMUSCULAR INJECTION
- ▹ Child 2–17 years: 0.5 mL for 1 dose, this booster dose should be given after the second birthday, this is the second dose of haemophilus influenzae type b vaccine combined with meningococcal group C conjugate vaccine (the first dose is given during the routine immunisation schedule)

Booster dose (for patients diagnosed with asplenia, splenic dysfunction or complement deficiency at over 2 years of age)
- ▶ BY INTRAMUSCULAR INJECTION
- ▹ Child 2–17 years: 0.5 mL for 1 dose, this booster dose should be followed 2 months later by one dose of meningococcal A, C, W135, and Y conjugate vaccine (in patients from 11 years of age, this interval can be reduced to one month)
- ▹ Adult: 0.5 mL for 1 dose, this booster dose should be followed 1 month later by one dose of meningococcal A, C, W135, and Y conjugate vaccine

- **UNLICENSED USE** Not licensed for use in patients over 2 years.
- **SIDE-EFFECTS**
- ▶ **Common or very common** Drowsiness
- ▶ **Uncommon** Crying
- ▶ **Rare or very rare** Abdominal pain · insomnia
- ▶ **Frequency not known** Anaphylactoid reaction · febrile seizure · meningism (but no evidence that vaccine causes meningococcal C meningitis) · muscle tone decreased
- **PRESCRIBING AND DISPENSING INFORMATION** Available as part of the childhood immunisation schedule from ImmForm.

- **MEDICINAL FORMS**
There can be variation in the licensing of different medicines containing the same drug.
Powder and solvent for solution for injection
- ▶ Menitorix (GlaxoSmithKline UK Ltd)
Menitorix vaccine powder and solvent for solution for injection 0.5ml vials | 1 vial [PoM] £37.76

Meningococcal group B vaccine (rDNA, component, adsorbed)

F 1271

19-Oct-2017

- **INDICATIONS AND DOSE**

BEXSERO®

Immunisation against *Neisseria meningitidis*, primary immunisation
- ▶ BY DEEP INTRAMUSCULAR INJECTION
- ▹ Child 2 months: 0.5 mL for 1 dose, injected preferably into deltoid region (or anterolateral thigh in infants), for information about the use of paracetamol for prophylaxis of post-immunisation pyrexia, see paracetamol p. 438.
- ▹ Child 4 months: 0.5 mL for 1 dose, injected preferably into deltoid region (or anterolateral thigh in infants), for information about the use of paracetamol for prophylaxis of post-immunisation pyrexia, see paracetamol p. 438.

Immunisation against *Neisseria meningitidis*, primary immunisation booster dose
- ▶ BY DEEP INTRAMUSCULAR INJECTION
- ▹ Child 12–23 months: 0.5 mL for 1 dose, injected preferably into deltoid region (or anterolateral thigh in infants)

Immunisation against *Neisseria meningitidis*, primary immunisation (in unimmunised patients)
- ▶ BY DEEP INTRAMUSCULAR INJECTION
- ▹ Child 6–11 months: 0.5 mL for 2 doses, separated by an interval of at least 2 months; booster dose of 0.5 mL given between 1–2 years of age and at least 2 months after completion of primary immunisation, injected preferably into deltoid region (or anterolateral thigh in infants)
- ▹ Child 12–23 months: 0.5 mL for 2 doses, separated by an interval of at least 2 months; booster dose of 0.5 mL given 12–24 months after completion of primary immunisation, injected preferably into deltoid region (or anterolateral thigh in infants)
- ▹ Child 2–10 years: 0.5 mL for 2 doses, separated by an interval of at least 2 months. Injected preferably into deltoid region (or anterolateral thigh in infants)
- ▹ Child 11–17 years: 0.5 mL for 2 doses, separated by an interval of at least 1 month. Injected preferably into deltoid region
- ▹ Adult: 0.5 mL for 2 doses, separated by an interval of at least 1 month. Injected preferably into deltoid region

TRUMENBA®

Immunisation against *Neisseria meningitidis*, primary immunisation
- ▶ BY INTRAMUSCULAR INJECTION
- ▹ Child 10–17 years: 0.5 mL for 2 doses, separated by an interval of 6 months, alternatively 0.5 mL for 2 doses, separated by an interval of at least 1 month, followed by 0.5 mL as a third dose, given at least 4 months after the second dose, injected preferably into deltoid region, a booster dose should be considered for individuals at continued risk—consult product literature
- ▹ Adult: 0.5 mL for 2 doses, separated by an interval of 6 months, alternatively 0.5 mL for 2 doses, separated by an interval of at least 1 month, followed continued →

14

Vaccines

by 0.5 mL as a third dose, given at least 4 months after the second dose, injected preferably into deltoid region, a booster dose should be considered for individuals at continued risk—consult product literature

- SIDE-EFFECTS
▶ **Common or very common** Crying abnormal (in children) · drowsiness (in children) · eating disorder (in children)
▶ **Uncommon** Eczema (in children) · seizures (in children) · vascular disorders (in children)
▶ **Frequency not known** Extensive swelling of vaccinated limb · hypotonic-hyporesponsiveness episode (in children)

- MEDICINAL FORMS
There can be variation in the licensing of different medicines containing the same drug.
Suspension for injection
EXCIPIENTS: May contain Kanamycin
▶ Bexsero (GlaxoSmithKline UK Ltd) ▼
Bexsero vaccine suspension for injection 0.5ml pre-filled syringes | 1 pre-filled disposable injection [PoM] £75.00
▶ Trumenba (Pfizer Ltd) ▼
Trumenba vaccine suspension for injection 0.5ml pre-filled syringes | 1 pre-filled disposable injection [PoM] £75.00

Meningococcal group C vaccine F 1271

- INDICATIONS AND DOSE
Patients with confirmed serogroup C disease (who have previously been immunised)
▶ BY INTRAMUSCULAR INJECTION
▷ Child 1-17 years: 0.5 mL for 1 dose, dose to be given before discharge from hospital
▷ Adult 18-24 years: 0.5 mL for 1 dose, dose to be given before discharge from hospital

- SIDE-EFFECTS
▶ **Common or very common** Anxiety (in children) · cough (in children) · crying (in children) · drowsiness (in children) · gastrointestinal discomfort (in children) · hyperhidrosis (in children) · increased risk of infection (in children)
▶ **Uncommon** Chills · eyelid oedema (in children) · flushing (in children) · influenza like illness (rare in children) · joint stiffness (in children)
▶ **Rare or very rare** Circulatory collapse (in children)
▶ **Frequency not known** Angioedema · apnoea · asthenia (uncommon in children) · dyspnoea · hypotonic-hyporesponsiveness episode · immune thrombocytopenic purpura · meningism (but no evidence that vaccine causes meningococcal C meningitis) · musculoskeletal stiffness (uncommon in children) · nasal congestion (uncommon in children) · oedema (uncommon in children) · pain (very common in children) · respiratory disorders (uncommon in children) · seizures (uncommon in children) · sensation abnormal (uncommon in children) · sleep disorders (very common in children) · Stevens-Johnson syndrome · syncope (uncommon in children)

- PRESCRIBING AND DISPENSING INFORMATION Available as part of childhood immunisation schedule from www.immform.dh.gov.uk.

- MEDICINAL FORMS
There can be variation in the licensing of different medicines containing the same drug.
Suspension for injection
▶ NeisVac-C (Pfizer Ltd)
NeisVac-C vaccine suspension for injection 0.5ml pre-filled syringes | 10 pre-filled disposable injection [PoM] £187.50

Meningococcal groups A with C and W135 and Y vaccine F 1271

- INDICATIONS AND DOSE
MENVEO ®
Primary immunisation against *Neisseria meningitidis*
▶ BY INTRAMUSCULAR INJECTION
▷ Child 13-15 years: 0.5 mL for 1 dose, dose preferably injected into deltoid region
Immunisation against *Neisseria meningitidis* in an unimmunised patient
▶ BY INTRAMUSCULAR INJECTION
▷ Child 10-17 years: 0.5 mL for 1 dose, booster dose is not required
▷ Adult 18-24 years: 0.5 mL for 1 dose, booster dose is not required
Immunisation against *Neisseria meningitidis* in those at risk of exposure to prevent invasive disease
▶ BY INTRAMUSCULAR INJECTION
▷ Child 3-11 months: 0.5 mL every month for 2 doses, dose preferably injected into deltoid region
▷ Child 1-17 years: 0.5 mL for 1 dose, dose preferably injected into deltoid region
▷ Adult: 0.5 mL for 1 dose, dose preferably injected into deltoid region
Patients attending university for the first time (who have not received the routine meningococcal A, C, W135, and Y conjugate vaccine over the age of 10 years)
▶ BY INTRAMUSCULAR INJECTION
▷ Adult 18-24 years: 0.5 mL for 1 dose
NIMENRIX ®
Primary immunisation against *Neisseria meningitidis*
▶ BY INTRAMUSCULAR INJECTION
▷ Child 13-15 years: 0.5 mL for 1 dose, to be injected preferably into deltoid region
Immunisation against *Neisseria meningitidis* in an unimmunised patient
▶ BY INTRAMUSCULAR INJECTION
▷ Child 10-17 years: 0.5 mL for 1 dose, booster dose is not required
▷ Adult 18-24 years: 0.5 mL for 1 dose, booster dose is not required
Immunisation against *Neisseria meningitidis* in those at risk of exposure
▶ BY INTRAMUSCULAR INJECTION
▷ Child 1-17 years: 0.5 mL for 1 dose, to be injected preferably into deltoid region (or anterolateral thigh in child 12–23 months), then 0.5 mL after 1 year if required for 1 dose, second dose should be considered in those who continue to be at risk of *Neisseria meningitidis* serogroup A infection
▷ Adult: 0.5 mL for 1 dose, to be injected preferably into deltoid region, then 0.5 mL after 1 year if required for 1 dose, second dose should be considered in those who continue to be at risk of *Neisseria meningitidis* serogroup A infection
Patients attending university for the first time (who have not received the routine meningococcal A, C, W135, and Y conjugate vaccine over the age of 10 years)
▶ BY INTRAMUSCULAR INJECTION
▷ Adult 18-24 years: 0.5 mL for 1 dose

- UNLICENSED USE
MENVEO ® *Menveo*® is not licensed for use in children under 2 years.
- SIDE-EFFECTS
▶ **Common or very common** Drowsiness

▸ **Uncommon** Crying · insomnia · numbness · pain in extremity
▸ **Frequency not known** Extensive swelling of vaccinated limb

● MEDICINAL FORMS
There can be variation in the licensing of different medicines containing the same drug.
Powder and solvent for solution for injection
▸ Menveo (GlaxoSmithKline UK Ltd)
Menveo vaccine powder and solvent for solution for injection 0.5ml vials | 1 vial PoM £30.00
▸ Nimenrix (Pfizer Ltd)
Nimenrix vaccine powder and solvent for solution for injection 0.5ml pre-filled syringes | 1 pre-filled disposable injection PoM £30.00

F 1271

Pneumococcal polysaccharide conjugate vaccine (adsorbed)

● INDICATIONS AND DOSE
PREVENAR 13 ®
Primary immunisation against pneumococcal infection (first dose)
▸ BY INTRAMUSCULAR INJECTION
▸ Child 2 months: 0.5 mL for 1 dose, anterolateral thigh is preferred site of injection in infants
Primary immunisation against pneumococcal infection (second dose)
▸ BY INTRAMUSCULAR INJECTION
▸ Child 4 months: 0.5 mL for 1 dose, anterolateral thigh is preferred site of injection in infants
Primary immunisation against pneumococcal infection (booster dose)
▸ BY INTRAMUSCULAR INJECTION
▸ Child 12-13 months: 0.5 mL for 1 dose, anterolateral thigh is preferred site of injection in infants
Immunisation against pneumococcal infection (in patients who have not been vaccinated or not completed the primary course)
▸ BY INTRAMUSCULAR INJECTION
▸ Child 12 months-4 years: 0.5 mL for 1 dose, deltoid muscle is preferred site of injection in young children; anterolateral thigh is preferred site in infants
Immunisation against pneumococcal infection, in immunocompromised or asplenic patients or patients with splenic dysfunction (who have not been vaccinated or not completed the primary course)
▸ BY INTRAMUSCULAR INJECTION
▸ Child 12 months-4 years: 0.5 mL every 2 months for 2 doses, deltoid muscle is preferred site of injection in young children; anterolateral thigh is preferred site in infants

SYNFLORIX ®
Immunisation against pneumococcal infection
▸ BY INTRAMUSCULAR INJECTION
▸ Child 6 weeks-4 years: Deltoid muscle is preferred site of injection in young children; anterolateral thigh is preferred site in infants (consult product literature)

● UNLICENSED USE
PREVENAR 13 ® The dose in BNF publications may differ from that in product literature.
● CONTRA-INDICATIONS Concomitant use of high potency varicella-zoster vaccine (*Zostavax*®) with pneumococcal polysaccharide vaccine (in adults)
● SIDE-EFFECTS
▸ **Common or very common** Drowsiness
▸ **Uncommon** Apnoea · crying abnormal · extensive swelling of vaccinated limb

▸ **Rare or very rare** Angioedema · hypotonic-hyporesponsiveness episode · Kawasaki disease · seizure
● PRESCRIBING AND DISPENSING INFORMATION
PREVENAR 13 ® Available as part of childhood immunisation schedule from ImmForm www.immform.dh.gov.uk.

● MEDICINAL FORMS
There can be variation in the licensing of different medicines containing the same drug.
Suspension for injection
▸ Prevenar (Pfizer Ltd)
Prevenar 13 vaccine suspension for injection 0.5ml pre-filled syringes | 1 pre-filled disposable injection PoM £49.10 | 10 pre-filled disposable injection PoM £491.00
▸ Synflorix (GlaxoSmithKline UK Ltd)
Synflorix vaccine suspension for injection 0.5ml pre-filled syringes | 1 pre-filled disposable injection PoM £27.60

F 1271

Pneumococcal polysaccharide vaccine

● INDICATIONS AND DOSE
Immunisation against pneumococcal infection
▸ BY INTRAMUSCULAR INJECTION, OR BY SUBCUTANEOUS INJECTION
▸ Child 2-17 years: 0.5 mL for 1 dose
▸ Adult: 0.5 mL for 1 dose
Immunisation in patients at increased risk of pneumococcal disease
▸ BY INTRAMUSCULAR INJECTION, OR BY SUBCUTANEOUS INJECTION
▸ Child 2-4 years: 0.5 mL for 1 dose, dose should be administered after the second birthday or at least 2 months after the final dose of the 13-valent pneumococcal polysaccharide conjugate vaccine (adsorbed)
▸ Child 5-17 years: 0.5 mL for 1 dose
▸ Adult: 0.5 mL for 1 dose

● SIDE-EFFECTS Angioedema · arthritis · asthenia · chills · febrile seizure · haemolytic anaemia · hypersensitivity · leucocytosis · lymphadenitis · nerve disorders · paraesthesia · peripheral oedema · thrombocytopenia

● MEDICINAL FORMS
There can be variation in the licensing of different medicines containing the same drug.
Solution for injection
▸ Pneumococcal polysaccharide vaccine (Non-proprietary)
Pneumococcal polysaccharide vaccine solution for injection 0.5ml vials | 1 vial PoM £8.32

F 1271

Typhoid vaccine

● INDICATIONS AND DOSE
Immunisation against typhoid fever in children at high risk of typhoid fever
▸ BY INTRAMUSCULAR INJECTION
▸ Child 12-23 months: 0.5 mL for 1 dose, dose should be given at least 2 weeks before potential exposure to typhoid infection, response may be suboptimal
Immunisation against typhoid fever
▸ BY INTRAMUSCULAR INJECTION
▸ Child 2-17 years: 0.5 mL for 1 dose, dose should be given at least 2 weeks before potential exposure to typhoid infection
▸ Adult: 0.5 mL for 1 dose, dose should be given at least 2 weeks before potential exposure to typhoid infection

continued →

14

Vaccines

▸ BY MOUTH
  ▹ Child 6-17 years: 1 capsule every 2 days for 3 doses (on days 1, 3, and 5)
  ▹ Adult: 1 capsule every 2 days for 3 doses (on days 1, 3, and 5)

● UNLICENSED USE Not licensed for use in children under 2 years.
● CONTRA-INDICATIONS
  ▸ With oral use Acute gastro-intestinal illness
● INTERACTIONS → Appendix 1: live vaccines
● SIDE-EFFECTS
  ▸ Common or very common
  ▹ With oral use Gastrointestinal discomfort · influenza like illness
  ▸ Rare or very rare
  ▹ With oral use Asthenia · back pain · chills · flatulence · paraesthesia
  ▸ Frequency not known
  ▹ With parenteral use Abdominal pain · asthma · serum sickness · shock · syncope
● DIRECTIONS FOR ADMINISTRATION Capsule should be taken one hour before a meal. Swallow as soon as possible after placing in mouth with a cold or lukewarm drink.
● HANDLING AND STORAGE It is important to store capsules in a refrigerator.
● PATIENT AND CARER ADVICE Patients or carers should be given advice on how to administer and store typhoid vaccine capsules.

● MEDICINAL FORMS
  There can be variation in the licensing of different medicines containing the same drug.
  Solution for injection
  ▸ Typhim Vi (Sanofi Pasteur)
    Salmonella typhi Vi capsular polysaccharide 50 microgram per 1 ml Typhim Vi 25micrograms/0.5ml vaccine solution for injection pre-filled syringes | 1 pre-filled disposable injection [PoM] £11.16 DT = £11.16 | 10 pre-filled disposable injection [PoM] £93.00 DT = £93.00
  Gastro-resistant capsule
  CAUTIONARY AND ADVISORY LABELS 25
  ▸ Vivotif (PaxVax Ltd)
    Vivotif vaccine gastro-resistant capsules | 3 capsule [PoM] £14.77

  Combinations available: *Hepatitis A with typhoid vaccine*, p. 1280

VACCINES > VIRAL VACCINES

Hepatitis A and B vaccine

The properties listed below are those particular to the combination only. For the properties of the components please consider, hepatitis A vaccine p. 1279, hepatitis B vaccine p. 1280.

● INDICATIONS AND DOSE
AMBIRIX ®
Immunisation against hepatitis A and hepatitis B infection (primary course)
▸ BY INTRAMUSCULAR INJECTION
  ▹ Child 1-15 years: Initially 1 mL for 1 dose, then 1 mL after 6–12 months for 1 dose, the deltoid region is the preferred site of injection in older children; anterolateral thigh is the preferred site in infants; not to be injected into the buttock (vaccine efficacy reduced), subcutaneous route used for patients with bleeding disorders (but immune response may be reduced)

TWINRIX ® ADULT
Immunisation against hepatitis A and hepatitis B infection (primary course)
▸ BY INTRAMUSCULAR INJECTION
  ▹ Child 16-17 years: Initially 1 mL every month for 2 doses, then 1 mL after 5 months for 1 dose, the deltoid region is the preferred site of injection; not to be injected into the buttock (vaccine efficacy reduced), subcutaneous route used for patients with bleeding disorders (but immune response may be reduced)
  ▹ Adult: Initially 1 mL every month for 2 doses, then 1 mL after 5 months for 1 dose, the deltoid region is the preferred site of injection; not to be injected into the buttock (vaccine efficacy reduced), subcutaneous route used for patients with bleeding disorders (but immune response may be reduced)

Immunisation against hepatitis A and hepatitis B infection—accelerated schedule for travellers departing within 1 month
▸ BY INTRAMUSCULAR INJECTION
  ▹ Child 16-17 years: Initially 1 mL for 1 dose, then 1 mL after 7 days for 1 dose, then 1 mL after 14 days for 1 dose, then 1 mL for 1 dose given 12 months after the first dose, the deltoid region is the preferred site of injection; not to be injected into the buttock (vaccine efficacy reduced), subcutaneous route used for patients with bleeding disorders (but immune response may be reduced)
  ▹ Adult: Initially 1 mL for 1 dose, then 1 mL after 7 days for 1 dose, then 1 mL after 14 days for 1 dose, then 1 mL for 1 dose given 12 months after the first dose, the deltoid region is the preferred site of injection; not to be injected into the buttock (vaccine efficacy reduced), subcutaneous route used for patients with bleeding disorders (but immune response may be reduced)

TWINRIX ® PAEDIATRIC
Immunisation against hepatitis A and hepatitis B infection (primary course)
▸ BY INTRAMUSCULAR INJECTION
  ▹ Child 1-15 years: Initially 0.5 mL every month for 2 doses, then 0.5 mL after 5 months for 1 dose, the deltoid region is the preferred site of injection in older children; anterolateral thigh is the preferred site in infants; not to be injected into the buttock (vaccine efficacy reduced), subcutaneous route used for patients with bleeding disorders (but immune response may be reduced)

> IMPORTANT SAFETY INFORMATION
> *Ambirix* ® and *Twinrix* ® are not recommended for post-exposure prophylaxis following percutaneous (needle-stick), ocular, or mucous membrane exposure to hepatitis B virus.

● PRESCRIBING AND DISPENSING INFORMATION
TWINRIX ® PAEDIATRIC Primary course should be completed with *Twinrix* ® (single component vaccines given at appropriate intervals may be used for booster dose).
TWINRIX ® ADULT Primary course should be completed with *Twinrix* ® (single component vaccines given at appropriate intervals may be used for booster dose).
AMBIRIX ® Primary course should be completed with *Ambirix* ® (single component vaccines given at appropriate intervals may be used for booster dose).

● MEDICINAL FORMS
There can be variation in the licensing of different medicines containing the same drug.

Suspension for injection
EXCIPIENTS: May contain Neomycin
▸ Ambirix (GlaxoSmithKline UK Ltd)
Ambirix vaccine suspension for injection 1ml pre-filled syringes | 1 pre-filled disposable injection PoM £31.18 DT = £31.18
▸ Twinrix (GlaxoSmithKline UK Ltd)
Twinrix Paediatric vaccine suspension for injection 0.5ml pre-filled syringes | 1 pre-filled disposable injection PoM £20.79
Twinrix Adult vaccine suspension for injection 1ml pre-filled syringes | 1 pre-filled disposable injection PoM £33.31 DT = £31.18 | 10 pre-filled disposable injection PoM £333.13

🞿 1271

Hepatitis A vaccine

● INDICATIONS AND DOSE

AVAXIM®

Immunisation against hepatitis A infection
▸ BY INTRAMUSCULAR INJECTION
▸ Child 16–17 years: Initially 0.5 mL for 1 dose, then 0.5 mL after 6–12 months, dose given as booster; booster dose may be delayed by up to 3 years if not given after recommended interval following primary dose, the deltoid region is the preferred site of injection. The subcutaneous route may be used for patients with bleeding disorders; not to be injected into the buttock (vaccine efficacy reduced)
▸ Adult: Initially 0.5 mL for 1 dose, then 0.5 mL after 6–12 months, dose given as booster; booster dose may be delayed by up to 3 years if not given after recommended interval following primary dose, the deltoid region is the preferred site of injection. The subcutaneous route may be used for patients with bleeding disorders; not to be injected into the buttock (vaccine efficacy reduced)

HAVRIX MONODOSE®

Immunisation against hepatitis A infection
▸ BY INTRAMUSCULAR INJECTION
▸ Child 1–15 years: Initially 0.5 mL for 1 dose, then 0.5 mL after 6–12 months, dose given as booster; booster dose may be delayed by up to 3 years if not given after recommended interval following primary dose, the deltoid region is the preferred site of injection. The subcutaneous route may be used for patients with bleeding disorders
▸ Child 16–17 years: Initially 1 mL for 1 dose, then 1 mL after 6–12 months, dose given as booster; booster dose may be delayed by up to 3 years if not given after recommended interval following primary dose, the deltoid region is the preferred site of injection. The subcutaneous route may be used for patients with bleeding disorders
▸ Adult: Initially 1 mL for 1 dose, then 1 mL after 6–12 months, dose given as booster; booster dose may be delayed by up to 3 years if not given after recommended interval following primary dose, the deltoid region is the preferred site of injection. The subcutaneous route may be used for patients with bleeding disorders

VAQTA® ADULT

Immunisation against hepatitis A infection
▸ BY INTRAMUSCULAR INJECTION
▸ Adult: Initially 1 mL for 1 dose, then 1 mL after 6–18 months, dose given as booster, the deltoid region is the preferred site of injection. The subcutaneous route may be used for patients with bleeding disorders (but immune response may be delayed)

VAQTA® PAEDIATRIC

Immunisation against hepatitis A infection
▸ BY INTRAMUSCULAR INJECTION
▸ Child 1–17 years: Initially 0.5 mL for 1 dose, then 0.5 mL after 6–18 months, dose given as booster, the deltoid region is the preferred site of injection. The subcutaneous route may be used for patients with bleeding disorders (but immune response may be reduced)

● SIDE-EFFECTS
▸ **Common or very common** Asthenia (uncommon in children) · pain (uncommon in children)
▸ **Uncommon** Anxiety (in children) · chills (in adults) · cough · crying (in children) · ear pain (rare in children) · gastrointestinal discomfort · gastrointestinal disorders (rare in children) · increased risk of infection (in adults) · influenza like illness (rare in children) · muscle weakness (in adults) · musculoskeletal stiffness (rare in children) · nasal complaints · paraesthesia (rare in children) · respiratory disorders (rare in children) · sensation of tightness (rare in children) · temperature sensation altered (rare in children) · vasodilation (rare in children)
▸ **Rare or very rare** Allergic rhinitis (in children) · apathy (in adults) · asthma (in children) · ataxia (in children) · burping (in children) · chest pain · constipation (in children) · dehydration (in children) · drowsiness (uncommon in children) · dry mouth (in adults) · eye discomfort · gait abnormal (in children) · infantile spitting up (in children) · menstrual disorder (in adults) · migraine (in adults) · muscle complaints (in adults) · oral ulceration (in adults) · oropharyngeal pain (in children) · photophobia (in adults) · screaming (in children) · sleep disorders (uncommon in children) · sweat changes · synovitis (in children) · throat oedema (in adults) · tremor (in adults) · vertigo (in adults) · watering eye (in adults)
▸ **Frequency not known** Guillain-Barre syndrome · thrombocytopenia

● MEDICINAL FORMS
There can be variation in the licensing of different medicines containing the same drug.

Suspension for injection
EXCIPIENTS: May contain Neomycin
▸ Avaxim (Sanofi Pasteur)
Avaxim vaccine suspension for injection 0.5ml pre-filled syringes | 1 pre-filled disposable injection PoM £21.72 | 10 pre-filled disposable injection PoM £181.00
▸ Havrix (GlaxoSmithKline UK Ltd)
Havrix Monodose vaccine suspension for injection 1ml pre-filled syringes | 1 pre-filled disposable injection PoM £22.14 | 10 pre-filled disposable injection PoM £221.43
Havrix Junior Monodose vaccine suspension for injection 0.5ml pre-filled syringes | 1 pre-filled disposable injection PoM £16.77 | 10 pre-filled disposable injection PoM £167.68
▸ VAQTA (Merck Sharp & Dohme Ltd)
VAQTA Adult vaccine suspension for injection 1ml pre-filled syringes | 1 pre-filled disposable injection PoM £18.10
VAQTA Paediatric vaccine suspension for injection 0.5ml pre-filled syringes | 1 pre-filled disposable injection PoM £14.74

14

Vaccines

Hepatitis A with typhoid vaccine

The properties listed below are those particular to the combination only. For the properties of the components please consider, hepatitis A vaccine p. 1279, typhoid vaccine p. 1277.

● **INDICATIONS AND DOSE**

HEPATYRIX ®

Immunisation against hepatitis A and typhoid infection (primary course)
▶ BY INTRAMUSCULAR INJECTION
▶ Child 15-17 years: 1 mL for 1 dose, the deltoid region is the preferred site of injection; not to be injected into the buttock (vaccine efficacy reduced). The subcutaneous route may be used for patients with bleeding disorders, booster dose given using single component vaccines
▶ Adult: 1 mL for 1 dose, the deltoid region is the preferred site of injection; not to be injected into the buttock (vaccine efficacy reduced). The subcutaneous route may be used for patients with bleeding disorders, booster dose given using single component vaccines

VIATIM ®

Immunisation against hepatitis A and typhoid infection (primary course)
▶ BY INTRAMUSCULAR INJECTION
▶ Child 16-17 years: 1 mL for 1 dose, the deltoid region is the preferred site of injection; not to be injected into the buttock (vaccine efficacy reduced). The subcutaneous route may be used for patients with bleeding disorders, booster dose given using single component vaccines
▶ Adult: 1 mL for 1 dose, the deltoid region is the preferred site of injection; not to be injected into the buttock (vaccine efficacy reduced). The subcutaneous route may be used for patients with bleeding disorders, booster dose given using single component vaccines

● **MEDICINAL FORMS**
There can be variation in the licensing of different medicines containing the same drug.
Suspension for injection
EXCIPIENTS: May contain Neomycin
▶ ViATIM (Sanofi Pasteur)
ViATIM vaccine suspension for injection 1ml pre-filled syringes | 1 pre-filled disposable injection [PoM] £35.76

�F 1271

Hepatitis B vaccine

● **INDICATIONS AND DOSE**

ENGERIX B ®

Immunisation against hepatitis B infection
▶ BY INTRAMUSCULAR INJECTION
▶ Child 1 month-15 years: 10 micrograms for 1 dose, then 10 micrograms after 1 month for 1 dose, followed by 10 micrograms after 5 months for 1 dose, deltoid muscle is preferred site of injection in older children; anterolateral thigh is preferred site in infants and young children; not to be injected into the buttock (vaccine efficacy reduced)
▶ Child 16-17 years: 20 micrograms for 1 dose, then 20 micrograms after 1 month for 1 dose, followed by 20 micrograms after 5 months for 1 dose, deltoid muscle is preferred site of injection; not to be injected into the buttock (vaccine efficacy reduced)
▶ Adult: 20 micrograms for 1 dose, then 20 micrograms after 1 month for 1 dose, followed by 20 micrograms after 5 months for 1 dose, deltoid muscle is preferred

site of injection; not to be injected into the buttock (vaccine efficacy reduced)

Immunisation against hepatitis B infection (accelerated schedule)
▶ BY INTRAMUSCULAR INJECTION
▶ Neonate: 10 micrograms every month for 3 doses, followed by 10 micrograms after 10 months for 1 dose, anterolateral thigh is preferred site in neonates; not to be injected into the buttock (vaccine efficacy reduced), this dose should not be given to neonates born to hepatitis B surface antigen positive mother.

▶ Child 1 month-15 years: 10 micrograms every month for 3 doses, followed by 10 micrograms after 10 months for 1 dose, deltoid muscle is preferred site of injection in older children; anterolateral thigh is preferred site in infants and young children; not to be injected into the buttock (vaccine efficacy reduced)
▶ Child 16-17 years: 20 micrograms every month for 3 doses, followed by 20 micrograms after 10 months for 1 dose, deltoid muscle is preferred site of injection; not to be injected into the buttock (vaccine efficacy reduced)
▶ Adult: 20 micrograms every month for 3 doses, followed by 20 micrograms after 10 months for 1 dose, deltoid muscle is preferred site of injection; not to be injected into the buttock (vaccine efficacy reduced)

Immunisation against hepatitis B infection, alternative accelerated schedule
▶ BY INTRAMUSCULAR INJECTION
▶ Child 11-15 years: 20 micrograms for 1 dose, followed by 20 micrograms after 6 months, this schedule is not suitable if high risk of infection between doses or if compliance with second dose uncertain, deltoid muscle is preferred site of injection; not to be injected into the buttock (vaccine efficacy reduced)

Immunisation against hepatitis B infection (accelerated schedule in exceptional cases, e.g. for travellers departing within 1 month)
▶ BY INTRAMUSCULAR INJECTION
▶ Adult: 20 micrograms for 1 dose, then 20 micrograms after 7 days for 1 dose, followed by 20 micrograms after 14 days for 1 dose, followed by 20 micrograms for 1 dose, to be given 12 months after the first dose, deltoid muscle is preferred site of injection; not to be injected into the buttock (vaccine efficacy reduced)

Immunisation against hepatitis B infection (in renal insufficiency, including haemodialysis patients)
▶ BY INTRAMUSCULAR INJECTION
▶ Child 1 month-15 years: 10 micrograms every month for 2 doses, followed by 10 micrograms after 5 months for 1 dose, immunisation schedule and booster doses may need to be adjusted in those with low antibody concentration, deltoid muscle is preferred site of injection in older children; anterolateral thigh is preferred site in infants and young children; not to be injected into the buttock (vaccine efficacy reduced)
▶ Child 16-17 years: 40 micrograms every month for 3 doses, followed by 40 micrograms after 4 months for 1 dose, immunisation schedule and booster doses may need to be adjusted in those with low antibody concentration, deltoid muscle is preferred site of injection; not to be injected into the buttock (vaccine efficacy reduced)
▶ Adult: 40 micrograms every month for 3 doses, followed by 40 micrograms after 4 months for 1 dose, immunisation schedule and booster doses may need to be adjusted in those with low antibody concentration, deltoid muscle is preferred site of injection; not to be injected into the buttock (vaccine efficacy reduced)

Immunisation against hepatitis B infection (in renal insufficiency, including haemodialysis patients (accelerated schedule))

▶ BY INTRAMUSCULAR INJECTION

▶ Child 1 month–15 years: 10 micrograms every month for 3 doses, followed by 10 micrograms after 10 months for 1 dose, immunisation schedule and booster doses may need to be adjusted in those with low antibody concentration, deltoid muscle is preferred site of injection in older children; anterolateral thigh is preferred site in infants and young children; not to be injected into the buttock (vaccine efficacy reduced)

FENDRIX ®

Immunisation against hepatitis B infection in renal insufficiency (including pre-haemodialysis and haemodialysis patients)

▶ BY INTRAMUSCULAR INJECTION

▶ Child 15–17 years: 20 micrograms every month for 3 doses, followed by 20 micrograms after 4 months for 1 dose, immunisation schedule and booster doses may need to be adjusted in those with low antibody concentration, deltoid muscle is preferred site of injection; not to be injected into the buttock (vaccine efficacy reduced)

▶ Adult: 20 micrograms every month for 3 doses, followed by 20 micrograms after 4 months for 1 dose, immunisation schedule and booster doses may need to be adjusted in those with low antibody concentration, deltoid muscle is preferred site of injection; not to be injected into the buttock (vaccine efficacy reduced)

HBVAXPRO ®

Immunisation against hepatitis B infection

▶ BY INTRAMUSCULAR INJECTION

▶ Neonate: 5 micrograms for 1 dose, followed by 5 micrograms after 1 month for 1 dose, then 5 micrograms after 5 months for 1 dose, booster doses may be required in immunocompromised patients with low antibody concentration, anterolateral thigh is preferred site in neonates; not to be injected into the buttock (vaccine efficacy reduced), dose not to be used for neonate born to hepatitis B surface antigen positive mother.

▶ Child 1 month–15 years: 5 micrograms for 1 dose, followed by 5 micrograms after 1 month for 1 dose, then 5 micrograms after 5 months for 1 dose, booster doses may be required in immunocompromised patients with low antibody concentration, deltoid muscle is preferred site of injection in adults and older children; anterolateral thigh is preferred site in infants; not to be injected into the buttock (vaccine efficacy reduced)

▶ Child 16–17 years: 10 micrograms for 1 dose, followed by 10 micrograms after 1 month for 1 dose, followed by 10 micrograms after 5 months for 1 dose, booster doses may be required in immunocompromised patients with low antibody concentration, deltoid muscle is preferred site of injection in adults and older children; not to be injected into the buttock (vaccine efficacy reduced)

▶ Adult: 10 micrograms for 1 dose, followed by 10 micrograms after 1 month for 1 dose, followed by 10 micrograms after 5 months for 1 dose, booster doses may be required in immunocompromised patients with low antibody concentration, deltoid muscle is preferred site of injection in adults and older children; not to be injected into the buttock (vaccine efficacy reduced)

Immunisation against hepatitis B infection (accelerated schedule)

▶ BY INTRAMUSCULAR INJECTION

▶ Neonate: 5 micrograms every month for 3 doses, followed by 5 micrograms after 10 months for 1 dose, booster doses may be required in immunocompromised patients with low antibody concentration, anterolateral thigh is preferred site in neonates; not to be injected into the buttock (vaccine efficacy reduced), dose not to be used for neonate born to hepatitis B surface antigen positive mother.

▶ Child 1 month–15 years: 5 micrograms every month for 3 doses, followed by 5 micrograms after 10 months for 1 dose, booster doses may be required in immunocompromised patients with low antibody concentration, deltoid muscle is preferred site of injection in older children; anterolateral thigh is preferred site in infants; not to be injected into the buttock (vaccine efficacy reduced)

▶ Child 16–17 years: 10 micrograms every month for 3 doses, followed by 10 micrograms after 10 months for 1 dose, booster doses may be required in immunocompromised patients with low antibody concentration, deltoid muscle is preferred site of injection in older children; not to be injected into the buttock (vaccine efficacy reduced)

▶ Adult: 10 micrograms every month for 3 doses, followed by 10 micrograms after 10 months for 1 dose, booster doses may be required in immunocompromised patients with low antibody concentration, deltoid muscle is preferred site of injection; not to be injected into the buttock (vaccine efficacy reduced)

Neonate born to hepatitis B surface antigen-positive mother

▶ BY INTRAMUSCULAR INJECTION

▶ Neonate: 5 micrograms every month for 3 doses, first dose given at birth with hepatitis B immunoglobulin injection (separate site), followed by 5 micrograms after 10 months for 1 dose, anterolateral thigh is preferred site in neonates; not to be injected into the buttock (vaccine efficacy reduced).

Chronic haemodialysis patients

▶ BY INTRAMUSCULAR INJECTION

▶ Child 16–17 years: 40 micrograms every month for 2 doses, followed by 40 micrograms after 5 months for 1 dose, booster doses may be required in those with low antibody concentration, deltoid muscle is preferred site of injection in older children; not to be injected into the buttock (vaccine efficacy reduced)

▶ Adult: 40 micrograms every month for 2 doses, followed by 40 micrograms after 5 months for 1 dose, booster doses may be required in those with low antibody concentration, deltoid muscle is preferred site of injection; not to be injected into the buttock (vaccine efficacy reduced)

● SIDE-EFFECTS

▶ **Common or very common** Drowsiness · gastrointestinal disorder

▶ **Uncommon** Influenza like illness

▶ **Rare or very rare** Sensation abnormal

▶ **Frequency not known** Anaphylactoid reaction · angioedema · apnoea · arthritis · encephalitis · encephalopathy · hypotension · meningitis · multiple sclerosis · muscle weakness · nerve disorders · paralysis · seizure · thrombocytopenia · vasculitis

14

Vaccines

14

Vaccines

● MEDICINAL FORMS

There can be variation in the licensing of different medicines containing the same drug.

Suspension for injection

EXCIPIENTS: May contain Thiomersal

▸ Engerix B (GlaxoSmithKline UK Ltd)

Hepatitis B virus surface antigen 20 microgram per 1 ml Engerix B 10micrograms/0.5ml vaccine suspension for injection pre-filled syringes | 1 pre-filled disposable injection PoM £9.67

Engerix B 20micrograms/1ml vaccine suspension for injection pre-filled syringes | 1 pre-filled disposable injection PoM £12.99 | 10 pre-filled disposable injection PoM £129.92

▸ Fendrix (GlaxoSmithKline UK Ltd)

Hepatitis B virus surface antigen 40 microgram per 1 ml Fendrix 20micrograms/0.5ml vaccine suspension for injection pre-filled syringes | 1 pre-filled disposable injection PoM £38.10

▸ HBVAXPRO (Merck Sharp & Dohme Ltd)

Hepatitis B virus surface antigen 10 microgram per 1 ml HBVAXPRO 10micrograms/1ml vaccine suspension for injection pre-filled syringes | 1 pre-filled disposable injection PoM £12.20

HBVAXPRO 5micrograms/0.5ml vaccine suspension for injection pre-filled syringes | 1 pre-filled disposable injection PoM £8.95

Hepatitis B virus surface antigen 40 microgram per 1 ml HBvaxPRO 40micrograms/1ml vaccine suspension for injection vials | 1 vial PoM £27.60

F 1271

Human papillomavirus vaccines

02-Mar-2017

● INDICATIONS AND DOSE

CERVARIX ®

Prevention of premalignant genital lesions and cervical cancer

▸ BY INTRAMUSCULAR INJECTION

▸ **Child 9–14 years (female):** 0.5 mL for 1 dose, followed by 0.5 mL after 5–7 months for 1 dose, if second dose administered earlier than 5 months after the first, a third dose should be administered, dose to be administered into deltoid region, if the course is interrupted, it should be resumed (using the same vaccine) but not repeated, even if more than 24 months have elapsed since the first dose or if the girl is then aged 15 years or more.

▸ **Child 15–17 years (female):** 0.5 mL for 1 dose, followed by 0.5 mL after 1–2.5 months for 1 dose, then 0.5 mL after 5–12 months from the first dose for 1 dose, dose to be administered into deltoid region, if the course is interrupted, it should be resumed (using the same vaccine) but not repeated, allowing the appropriate interval between the remaining doses.

▸ **Adult (female):** 0.5 mL for 1 dose, followed by 0.5 mL after 1–2.5 months for 1 dose, then 0.5 mL after 5–12 months from the first dose for 1 dose, dose to be administered into deltoid region, if the course is interrupted, it should be resumed (using the same vaccine) but not repeated, allowing the appropriate interval between the remaining doses.

GARDASIL ®

Prevention of premalignant genital (cervical, vulvar and vaginal) and anal lesions, cervical and anal cancers, and genital warts

▸ BY INTRAMUSCULAR INJECTION

▸ **Child 9–14 years (female):** 0.5 mL for 1 dose, followed by 0.5 mL after 6 months for 1 dose, if the second dose is administered earlier than 6 months after the first dose, a third dose should be administered preferably into deltoid region or higher anterolateral thigh, if the course is interrupted, it should be resumed (using the same vaccine) but not repeated, even if more than 24 months have elapsed since the first dose or if the girl is then aged 15 years or more.

▸ **Child 15–17 years (female):** 0.5 mL for 1 dose, followed by 0.5 mL for 1 dose, second dose to be given at least 1 month after the first dose, then 0.5 mL for 1 dose, third dose to be given at least 3 months after the second dose, schedule should be completed within 12 months of the first dose, dose to be administered preferably into deltoid region or higher anterolateral thigh, if the course is interrupted, it should be resumed (using the same vaccine) but not repeated, allowing the appropriate interval between the remaining doses.

▸ **Adult (female):** 0.5 mL for 1 dose, followed by 0.5 mL for 1 dose, second dose to be given at least 1 month after the first dose, then 0.5 mL for 1 dose, third dose to be given at least 3 months after the second dose, schedule should be completed within 12 months of the first dose, dose to be administered preferably into deltoid region or higher anterolateral thigh, if the course is interrupted, it should be resumed (using the same vaccine) but not repeated, allowing the appropriate interval between the remaining doses.

Prevention of premalignant genital (cervical, vulvar, and vaginal) and anal lesions, cervical and anal cancers, and genital warts (alternative schedule)

▸ BY INTRAMUSCULAR INJECTION

▸ **Child 9–14 years (female):** 0.5 mL for 1 dose, followed by 0.5 mL for 1 dose, second dose to be given at least 1 month after the first dose, then 0.5 mL for 1 dose, third dose to be given at least 3 months after the second dose, schedule should be completed within 12 months of the first dose, dose to be administered preferably into deltoid region or higher anterolateral thigh, if the course is interrupted, it should be resumed (using the same vaccine) but not repeated, allowing the appropriate interval between the remaining doses.

● UNLICENSED USE

GARDASIL ® Two dose schedule not licensed for use in girls aged 14 years.

● SIDE-EFFECTS

▸ **Common or very common** Pain in extremity

▸ **Rare or very rare** Bronchospasm

▸ **Frequency not known** Acute disseminated encephalomyelitis · anaphylactoid reaction · asthenia · chills · Guillain-Barre syndrome · immune thrombocytopenic purpura · syncope

● PREGNANCY Not known to be harmful, but vaccination should be postponed until completion of pregnancy.

● PRESCRIBING AND DISPENSING INFORMATION To avoid confusion, prescribers should specify the brand to be dispensed.

● MEDICINAL FORMS

There can be variation in the licensing of different medicines containing the same drug.

Suspension for injection

▸ Cervarix (GlaxoSmithKline UK Ltd)

Cervarix vaccine suspension for injection 0.5ml pre-filled syringes | 1 pre-filled disposable injection PoM £80.50

▸ Gardasil (Merck Sharp & Dohme Ltd)

Gardasil vaccine suspension for injection 0.5ml pre-filled syringes | 1 pre-filled disposable injection PoM £86.50

F 1271

Influenza vaccine

● INDICATIONS AND DOSE

Annual immunisation against seasonal influenza

▸ BY INTRAMUSCULAR INJECTION

▸ **Child 6 months–17 years:** 0.5 mL for 1 dose

▸ **Adult:** 0.5 mL for 1 dose

▸ BY INTRADERMAL INJECTION
▸ Adult 18–59 years: 9 micrograms for 1 dose, dose to be injected into deltoid region
▸ Adult 60 years and over: 15 micrograms for 1 dose, dose to be injected into deltoid region
▸ BY INTRANASAL ADMINISTRATION
▸ Child 2–17 years: 0.1 mL for 1 dose, dose to be administered into each nostril

Annual immunisation against seasonal influenza (for children who have not received seasonal influenza vaccine previously)
▸ BY INTRAMUSCULAR INJECTION
▸ Child 6 months–9 years: 0.5 mL for 1 dose, followed by 0.5 mL for 1 dose, after at least 4 weeks
▸ BY INTRANASAL ADMINISTRATION
▸ Child 2–9 years: 0.1 mL for 1 dose, followed by 0.1 mL for 1 dose, after at least 4 weeks. 0.1 mL dose to be administered to each nostril

● UNLICENSED USE Some products containing inactivated influenza vaccine (surface antigen) are not licensed for use in children under 4 years—check product literature.
OPTAFLU ® Not licensed for use in children and adolescents under 18 years.
FLUVIRIN ® Not licensed for use in children under 4 years.
● CONTRA-INDICATIONS Preparations marketed by Pfizer, or CSL Biotherapies in child under 5 years— increased risk of febrile convulsions
FLUENZ TETRA ® Active wheezing · concomitant use with antiviral therapy for influenza · severe asthma
CONTRA-INDICATIONS, FURTHER INFORMATION
▸ Concomitant use with antiviral therapy for influenza Avoid influenza antiviral agents for at least 2 weeks after immunisation; avoid immunisation for at least 48 hours after stopping the influenza antiviral agent.
ENZIRA ® Child under 5 years—increased risk of febrile convulsions
● CAUTIONS Increased risk of fever in child 5–9 years with preparations marketed by Pfizer or CSL Biotherapies—use alternative influenza vaccine if available
ENZIRA ® Child 5–9 years (increased risk of fever)—use alternative influenza vaccine if available
● INTERACTIONS → Appendix 1: live vaccines
● SIDE-EFFECTS
▸ Common or very common
▸ With intradermal or intramuscular use Chills · hyperhidrosis · pain
▸ With intranasal use Nasal complaints
▸ Uncommon
▸ With intranasal use Epistaxis · face oedema
▸ Rare or very rare
▸ With intradermal or intramuscular use Nerve disorders · paraesthesia
▸ Frequency not known
▸ With intradermal or intramuscular use Angioedema · encephalomyelitis · febrile seizure · nervous system disorder · shock · thrombocytopenia · vasculitis
▸ With intramuscular use Extensive swelling of vaccinated limb · presyncope · syncope
▸ With intranasal use Guillain-Barre syndrome
● ALLERGY AND CROSS-SENSITIVITY Individuals with a history of egg allergy can be immunised with either an egg free influenza vaccine, if available, or an influenza vaccine with an ovalbumin content less than 120 nanograms/mL (facilities should be available to treat anaphylaxis). Vaccines with an ovalbumin content more than 120 nanograms/mL or where content is not stated should not be used in individuals with egg allergy. If an influenza vaccine containing ovalbumin is being considered in those with a history of anaphylaxis to egg or egg allergy with

uncontrolled asthma, these individuals should be referred to a specialist in hospital.
● PREGNANCY Inactivated vaccines not known to be harmful.
FLUENZ TETRA ® Avoid in pregnancy.
● BREAST FEEDING Inactivated vaccines not known to be harmful.
FLUENZ TETRA ® Avoid in breast-feeding.
● PRESCRIBING AND DISPENSING INFORMATION
FLUARIX TETRA ® Ovalbumin content less than 100 nanograms/mL.
● PATIENT AND CARER ADVICE
FLUENZ TETRA ® Avoid close contact with severely immunocompromised patients for 1–2 weeks after vaccination.

● MEDICINAL FORMS
There can be variation in the licensing of different medicines containing the same drug.

Spray
EXCIPIENTS: May contain Gelatin, gentamicin
▸ Fluenz Tetra (AstraZeneca UK Ltd) ▼
Fluenz Tetra vaccine nasal suspension 0.2ml unit dose | 10 unit dose PoM £180.00

Suspension for injection
EXCIPIENTS: May contain Gentamicin, kanamycin, neomycin penicillins, polymyxin b
▸ Influenza vaccine (Non-proprietary)
Influenza vaccine (split virion, inactivated) suspension for injection 0.5ml pre-filled syringes | 1 pre-filled disposable injection PoM £5.22–£6.59 | 10 pre-filled disposable injection PoM £52.20–£65.90
Quadrivalent vaccine (split virion, inactivated) suspension for injection 0.5ml pre-filled syringes | 1 pre-filled disposable injection PoM £8.00 | 10 pre-filled disposable injection PoM £80.00
▸ Agrippal (Seqirus Vaccines Ltd)
Agrippal vaccine suspension for injection 0.5ml pre-filled syringes | 1 pre-filled disposable injection PoM £6.59 | 10 pre-filled disposable injection PoM £65.90
▸ Enzira (Pfizer Ltd)
Enzira vaccine suspension for injection 0.5ml pre-filled syringes | 1 pre-filled disposable injection PoM £5.25 | 10 pre-filled disposable injection PoM £52.50
▸ Fluarix Tetra (GlaxoSmithKline UK Ltd) ▼
Fluarix Tetra vaccine suspension for injection 0.5ml pre-filled syringes | 1 pre-filled disposable injection PoM £9.94 | 10 pre-filled disposable injection PoM £99.40
▸ Imuvac (Mylan)
Imuvac vaccine suspension for injection 0.5ml pre-filled syringes | 1 pre-filled disposable injection PoM £6.59 | 10 pre-filled disposable injection PoM £65.90
▸ Influvac Sub-unit (Mylan)
Influvac Sub-unit vaccine suspension for injection 0.5ml pre-filled syringes | 1 pre-filled disposable injection PoM £5.22 | 10 pre-filled disposable injection PoM £52.20

F 1271

Japanese encephalitis vaccine

● INDICATIONS AND DOSE
Immunisation against Japanese encephalitis
▸ BY INTRAMUSCULAR INJECTION
▸ Child 2 months–2 years: 0.25 mL every 28 days for 2 doses, anterolateral thigh is preferred site of injection in infants, the subcutaneous route may be used for patients with bleeding disorders
▸ Child 3–17 years: 0.5 mL every 28 days for 2 doses, deltoid muscle is preferred site in older children; anterolateral thigh is preferred in infants, the subcutaneous route may be used for patients with bleeding disorders
▸ Adult: 0.5 mL every 28 days for 2 doses, deltoid muscle is preferred site of injection, the subcutaneous route may be used for patients with bleeding disorders

continued →

14

Vaccines

Booster dose
▸ BY INTRAMUSCULAR INJECTION
▸ Adult: 0.5 mL after 1–2 years, deltoid muscle is preferred site of injection, the subcutaneous route may be used for patients with bleeding disorders, for those at continued risk, the booster dose should be given 1 year after completing the primary course

● SIDE-EFFECTS
▸ **Common or very common** Influenza like illness (frequency not known in children)
▸ **Uncommon** Abdominal pain (frequency not known in children) · asthenia (in adults) · chills (in adults) · hyperhidrosis (in adults) · migraine (in adults) · musculoskeletal stiffness (in adults) · vertigo (in adults)
▸ **Rare or very rare** Dyspnoea (in adults) · eyelid oedema (in adults) · neuritis (in adults) · pain in extremity (in adults) · palpitations (in adults) · paraesthesia (in adults) · peripheral oedema (in adults) · tachycardia (in adults) · taste altered (in adults) · thrombocytopenia (in adults)
▸ **Frequency not known** Cough (in children)

● PREGNANCY Although manufacturer advises avoid because of limited information, miscarriage has been associated with Japanese encephalitis virus infection acquired during the first 2 trimesters of pregnancy.

● MEDICINAL FORMS
There can be variation in the licensing of different medicines containing the same drug.

Solution for injection
▸ Japanese encephalitis vaccine (Non-proprietary)
Japanese encephalitis GCVC vaccine solution for injection 1ml vials | 1 vial 💊
Japanese encephalitis GCVC vaccine solution for injection 20ml vials | 1 vial 💊
Japanese encephalitis GCVC vaccine solution for injection 10ml vials | 1 vial 💊

Suspension for injection
▸ Ixiaro (Valneva UK Ltd)
Ixiaro vaccine suspension for injection 0.5ml pre-filled syringes | 1 pre-filled disposable injection [PoM] £59.50

⟨F⟩ 1271

Measles, mumps and rubella vaccine, live

● INDICATIONS AND DOSE
Primary immunisation against measles, mumps, and rubella (first dose)
▸ BY INTRAMUSCULAR INJECTION, OR BY DEEP SUBCUTANEOUS INJECTION
▸ Child 12–13 months: 0.5 mL for 1 dose
Primary immunisation against measles, mumps, and rubella (second dose)
▸ BY INTRAMUSCULAR INJECTION, OR BY DEEP SUBCUTANEOUS INJECTION
▸ Child 40 months–5 years: 0.5 mL for 1 dose
Rubella immunisation (in seronegative women, susceptible to rubella and in unimmunised, seronegative women, post-partum)
▸ BY INTRAMUSCULAR INJECTION, OR BY DEEP SUBCUTANEOUS INJECTION
▸ Females of childbearing potential: (consult product literature or local protocols)

Children presenting for pre-school booster, who have not received the primary immunisation (first dose) | Immunisation for patients at school-leaving age or at entry into further education, who have not completed the primary immunisation course | Control of measles outbreak | Immunisation for patients travelling to areas where measles is endemic or epidemic, who have not completed the primary immunisation
▸ BY INTRAMUSCULAR INJECTION, OR BY DEEP SUBCUTANEOUS INJECTION
▸ Child 6 months–17 years: (consult product literature or local protocols)
▸ Adult: (consult product literature or local protocols)

● UNLICENSED USE Not licensed for use in children under 9 months.

> IMPORTANT SAFETY INFORMATION
> MMR VACCINATION AND BOWEL DISEASE OR AUTISM
> Reviews undertaken on behalf of the CSM, the Medical Research Council, and the Cochrane Collaboration, have not found any evidence of a link between MMR vaccination and bowel disease or autism. The Chief Medical Officers have advised that the MMR vaccine is the safest and best way to protect children against measles, mumps, and rubella. Information (including fact sheets and a list of references) may be obtained from www.dh.gov.uk/immunisation.

● CAUTIONS Antibody response to measles component may be reduced after immunoglobulin administration or blood transfusion–leave an interval of at least 3 months before MMR immunisation
CAUTIONS, FURTHER INFORMATION
▸ Administration with other vaccines MMR vaccine should not be administered on the same day as yellow fever vaccine; there should be a 4-week minimum interval between the vaccines. When protection is rapidly required, the vaccines can be given at any interval and an additional dose of MMR may be considered.
   MMR and varicella-zoster vaccine can be given on the same day or separated by a 4-week minimum interval. When protection is rapidly required, the vaccines can be given at any interval and an additional dose of the vaccine given second may be considered.

● INTERACTIONS → Appendix 1: live vaccines

● SIDE-EFFECTS
▸ **Uncommon** Increased risk of infection · rhinorrhoea
▸ **Frequency not known** Anaphylactoid reaction · angioedema · arthritis · ataxia · cough · encephalopathy · eye inflammation · meningitis aseptic · nerve deafness · nerve disorders · oculomotor nerve paralysis · oedema · panniculitis · papillitis · paraesthesia · regional lymphadenopathy · respiratory disorders · seizures · Stevens-Johnson syndrome · subacute sclerosing panencephalitis · syncope · throat pain · thrombocytopenia · vasculitis

SIDE-EFFECTS, FURTHER INFORMATION Malaise, fever, or a rash can occur after the first dose of MMR vaccine–most commonly about a week after vaccination and lasting about 2 to 3 days. Febrile seizures occur rarely 6 to 11 days after MMR vaccination (the incidence is lower than that following measles infection).
Idiopathic thrombocytopenic purpura Idiopathic thrombocytopenic purpura has occurred rarely following MMR vaccination, usually within 6 weeks of the first dose. The risk of idiopathic thrombocytopenic purpura after MMR vaccine is much less than the risk after infection with wild measles or rubella virus. Children who develop idiopathic thrombocytopenic purpura within 6 weeks of the first dose of MMR should undergo serological testing

before the second dose is due; if the results suggest incomplete immunity against measles, mumps or rubella then a second dose of MMR is recommended. Samples should be sent to the Virus Reference Laboratory of the Health Protection Agency.

Frequency of side effects Adverse reactions are considerably less frequent after the second dose of MMR vaccine than after the first.

- ● ALLERGY AND CROSS-SENSITIVITY MMR vaccine can be given safely even when the child has had an anaphylactic reaction to food containing egg. Dislike of eggs, refusal to eat egg, or confirmed anaphylactic reactions to egg-containing food is not a contra-indication to MMR vaccination. Children with a confirmed anaphylactic reaction to the MMR vaccine should be assessed by a specialist.

- ● CONCEPTION AND CONTRACEPTION Exclude pregnancy before immunisation. Avoid pregnancy for at least 1 month after vaccination.

- ● PRESCRIBING AND DISPENSING INFORMATION Available as part of childhood immunisation schedule from health organisations or ImmForm www.immform.dh.gov.uk.

- ● MEDICINAL FORMS
  There can be variation in the licensing of different medicines containing the same drug.

Powder and solvent for suspension for injection
EXCIPIENTS: May contain Gelatin, neomycin
- ▸ M-M-RVAXPRO (Merck Sharp & Dohme Ltd)
  M-M-RVAXPRO vaccine powder and solvent for suspension for injection 0.5ml pre-filled syringes | 1 pre-filled disposable injection [PoM] £11.00

Powder and solvent for solution for injection
EXCIPIENTS: May contain Neomycin
- ▸ Priorix (GlaxoSmithKline UK Ltd)
  Priorix vaccine powder and solvent for solution for injection 0.5ml pre-filled syringes | 1 pre-filled disposable injection [PoM] £7.64

◀ 1271

Rabies vaccine

- ● INDICATIONS AND DOSE

Pre-exposure prophylaxis
- ▸ BY INTRAMUSCULAR INJECTION
- ▸ Child: 1 mL for 2 doses (on days 0 and 7), followed by 1 mL for 1 dose (on day 28), to be administered in deltoid region or anterolateral thigh in infants, for those at continuous risk, measure plasma-concentration of antirabies antibodies every 6 months and give a booster dose if the titre is less than 0.5 units/mL, final dose may be given from day 21, if insufficient time before travel
- ▸ Adult: 1 mL for 2 doses (on days 0 and 7), followed by 1 mL for 1 dose (on day 28), to be administered in deltoid region, for those at continuous risk, measure plasma-concentration of antirabies antibodies every 6 months and give a booster dose if the titre is less than 0.5 units/mL, final dose may be given from day 21, if insufficient time before travel

Pre-exposure prophylaxis booster dose (for patients at frequent risk of exposure)
- ▸ BY INTRAMUSCULAR INJECTION
- ▸ Child: 1 mL after 1 year for 1 dose, to be given 1 year after primary course is completed, then 1 mL every 3–5 years, to be administered in deltoid region or anterolateral thigh in infants, the frequency of booster doses may alternatively be determined according to plasma-concentration of antirabies antibodies
- ▸ Adult: 1 mL for 1 dose, to be given 1 year after primary course is completed, then 1 mL every 3–5 years, to be administered in deltoid region, the frequency of booster doses may alternatively be determined

according to plasma-concentration of antirabies antibodies

Pre-exposure prophylaxis booster dose (for patients at infrequent risk of exposure)
- ▸ BY INTRAMUSCULAR INJECTION
- ▸ Child: 1 mL for 1 dose, to be given 10 years after primary course is completed, administered in deltoid region or anterolateral thigh in infants
- ▸ Adult: 1 mL for 1 dose, to be given 10 years after primary course is completed, administered in deltoid region

Post-exposure prophylaxis of fully immunised individuals (who have previously received pre-exposure or post-exposure prophylaxis with cell-derived rabies vaccine)
- ▸ BY INTRAMUSCULAR INJECTION
- ▸ Child (administered on expert advice): 1 mL for 1 dose, followed by 1 mL after 3–7 days for 1 dose, to be administered in deltoid region or anterolateral thigh in infants, rabies immunoglobulin is not necessary
- ▸ Adult (administered on expert advice): 1 mL for 1 dose, followed by 1 mL after 3–7 days for 1 dose, to be administered in deltoid region, rabies immunoglobulin is not necessary

Post-exposure treatment for unimmunised individuals (or those whose prophylaxis is possibly incomplete)
- ▸ BY INTRAMUSCULAR INJECTION
- ▸ Child (administered on expert advice): 1 mL 5 times a month for 1 month, doses should be given on days 0, 3, 7, 14, and the fifth dose is given between day 28–30, to be administered in deltoid region or anterolateral thigh in infants, depending on the level of risk (determined by factors such as the nature of the bite and the country where it was sustained), rabies immunoglobulin is given to unimmunised individuals on day 0 or within 7 days of starting the course of rabies vaccine, the immunisation course can be discontinued if it is proved that the individual was not at risk
- ▸ Adult (administered on expert advice): 1 mL 5 times a month for 1 month, doses should be given on days 0, 3, 7, 14, and the fifth dose is given between day 28–30, to be administered in deltoid region, depending on the level of risk (determined by factors such as the nature of the bite and the country where it was sustained), rabies immunoglobulin is given to unimmunised individuals on day 0 or within 7 days of starting the course of rabies vaccine, the immunisation course can be discontinued if it is proved that the individual was not at risk

- ● INTERACTIONS → Appendix 1: rabies vaccine

- ● SIDE-EFFECTS
- ▸ **Common or very common** Asthenia · gastrointestinal discomfort
- ▸ **Rare or very rare** Anaphylactic shock · angioedema · chills · encephalitis · Guillain-Barre syndrome · hyperhidrosis · paraesthesia · presyncope · syncope · vertigo

- ● PREGNANCY Because of the potential consequences of untreated rabies exposure and because rabies vaccination has not been associated with fetal abnormalities, pregnancy is not considered a contra-indication to post-exposure prophylaxis. Immunisation against rabies is indicated during pregnancy if there is substantial risk of exposure to rabies and rapid access to post-exposure prophylaxis is likely to be limited.

14

Vaccines

● **MEDICINAL FORMS**
There can be variation in the licensing of different medicines containing the same drug.
Powder and solvent for suspension for injection
EXCIPIENTS: May contain Neomycin
▸ Rabies vaccine (Non-proprietary)
Verorab powder and solvent for suspension for injection 0.5ml vials | 1 vial [PoM] Ⓢ
Rabies vaccine powder and solvent for suspension for injection 1ml vials | 1 vial [PoM] £40.84
Powder and solvent for solution for injection
EXCIPIENTS: May contain Neomycin
▸ Rabipur (GlaxoSmithKline UK Ltd)
Rabipur vaccine powder and solvent for solution for injection 1ml vials | 1 vial [PoM] £34.56
Rabipur vaccine powder and solvent for solution for injection 1ml pre-filled syringes | 1 pre-filled disposable injection [PoM] £34.56

⚑ 1271

Rotavirus vaccine

11-Dec-2017

● **DRUG ACTION** Rotavirus vaccine is a live, oral vaccine that protects young children against gastro-enteritis caused by rotavirus infection.

● **INDICATIONS AND DOSE**
Immunisation against gastro-enteritis caused by rotavirus
▸ BY MOUTH
▸ Child 6–23 weeks: 1.5 mL for 2 doses separated by an interval of at least 4 weeks, first dose must be given between 6–14 weeks of age; course should be completed before 24 weeks of age (preferably before 16 weeks)

> **IMPORTANT SAFETY INFORMATION**
> PUBLIC HEALTH ENGLAND: UPDATE TO GREEN BOOK (OCTOBER 2017)
> Public Health England advises that immunisation with live vaccines should be delayed until 6 months of age in children born to mothers who received immunosuppressive biological therapy during pregnancy. In practice, this means that children born to mothers who were on immunosuppressive biological therapy during pregnancy will not be eligible to receive rotavirus vaccine.

● **CONTRA-INDICATIONS** History of intussusception · predisposition to intussusception · severe combined immunosuppression
CONTRA-INDICATIONS, FURTHER INFORMATION
▸ Immunosuppression With the exception of severe combined immunodeficiency (and children born to mothers who received immunosuppressive biological therapy during pregnancy, see *Important safety information*), rotavirus vaccine is not contra-indicated in immunosuppressed patients—benefit from vaccination is likely to outweigh the risk, if there is any doubt, seek specialist advice.

● **CAUTIONS** Diarrhoea (postpone vaccination) · immunosuppressed close contacts · vomiting (postpone vaccination)
CAUTIONS, FURTHER INFORMATION The rotavirus vaccine virus is excreted in the stool and may be transmitted to close contacts; however, vaccination of those with immunosuppressed close contacts may protect the contacts from wild-type rotavirus disease and outweigh any risk from transmission of vaccine virus.

● **INTERACTIONS** → Appendix 1: live vaccines

● **SIDE-EFFECTS**
▸ **Uncommon** Abdominal pain · dermatitis · gastrointestinal disorders
▸ **Frequency not known** Apnoea · gastroenteritis · haematochezia

● **PATIENT AND CARER ADVICE** The rotavirus vaccine virus is excreted in the stool and may be transmitted to close contacts; carers of a recently vaccinated baby should be advised of the need to wash their hands after changing the baby's nappies.

● **MEDICINAL FORMS**
There can be variation in the licensing of different medicines containing the same drug.
Oral suspension
▸ Rotarix (GlaxoSmithKline UK Ltd)
Rotarix vaccine live oral suspension 1.5ml pre-filled syringes | 1 unit dose [PoM] £34.76
Rotarix vaccine live oral suspension 1.5ml tube | 1 tube [PoM] £34.76

⚑ 1271

Tick-borne encephalitis vaccine, inactivated

● **INDICATIONS AND DOSE**
Initial immunisation against tick-borne encephalitis
▸ BY INTRAMUSCULAR INJECTION
▸ Child 1–15 years: 0.25 mL for 1 dose, followed by 0.25 mL after 1–3 months for 1 dose, then 0.25 mL after further 5–12 months for 1 dose, to achieve more rapid protection, second dose may be given 14 days after first dose, dose to be administered in deltoid region or anterolateral thigh in infants, in immunocompromised patients (including those receiving immunosuppressants), antibody concentration may be measured 4 weeks after second dose and dose repeated if protective levels not achieved
▸ Child 16–17 years: 0.5 mL for 1 dose, followed by 0.5 mL after 1–3 months for 1 dose, then 0.5 mL after further 5–12 months for 1 dose, to achieve more rapid protection, second dose may be given 14 days after first dose, dose to be administered in deltoid region, in immunocompromised patients (including those receiving immunosuppressants), antibody concentration may be measured 4 weeks after second dose and dose repeated if protective levels not achieved
▸ Adult: 0.5 mL for 1 dose, followed by 0.5 mL after 1–3 months for 1 dose, then 0.5 mL after further 5–12 months for 1 dose, to achieve more rapid protection, second dose may be given 14 days after first dose, dose to be administered in deltoid region, in immunocompromised patients (including those receiving immunosuppressants), antibody concentration may be measured 4 weeks after second dose and dose repeated if protective levels not achieved
▸ Elderly: 0.5 mL for 1 dose, followed by 0.5 mL after 1–3 months for 1 dose, then 0.5 mL after further 5–12 months for 1 dose, to achieve more rapid protection, second dose may be given 14 days after first dose, dose to be administered in deltoid region, antibody concentration may be measured 4 weeks after second dose and dose repeated if protective levels not achieved

Immunisation against tick-borne encephalitis, booster doses
▸ BY INTRAMUSCULAR INJECTION
▸ Child 1–17 years: First dose to be given within 3 years after initial course completed and then every 3–5 years, dose to be administered in deltoid region or anterolateral thigh in infants (consult product literature)
▸ Adult: First dose to be given within 3 years after initial course completed and then every 3–5 years, dose to be administered in deltoid region (consult product literature)

● SIDE-EFFECTS
▶ **Common or very common** Restlessness (in children) · sleep disorder (in children)
▶ **Rare or very rare** Asthenia · autoimmune disorder (in adults) · chills (uncommon in children) · demyelination (in adults) · drowsiness (in adults) · dyspnoea · eye pain · gait abnormal · gastrointestinal discomfort (uncommon in children) · hyperhidrosis · increased risk of infection · influenza like illness · joint swelling (in adults) · meningism · meningitis aseptic (in adults) · motor dysfunction · musculoskeletal stiffness · nerve disorders · oedema · pain · seizures · sensory disorder · tachycardia (in adults) · tinnitus · vertigo · vision disorders

● ALLERGY AND CROSS-SENSITIVITY Individuals with evidence of previous anaphylactic reaction to egg should not be given tick-borne encephalitis vaccine.

● MEDICINAL FORMS
There can be variation in the licensing of different medicines containing the same drug.
Suspension for injection
EXCIPIENTS: May contain Gentamicin, neomycin
▶ TicoVac (Pfizer Ltd)
TicoVac Junior vaccine suspension for injection 0.25ml pre-filled syringes | 1 pre-filled disposable injection [PoM] £28.00
TicoVac vaccine suspension for injection 0.5ml pre-filled syringes | 1 pre-filled disposable injection [PoM] £32.00

⬛ 1271

Varicella-zoster vaccine

● INDICATIONS AND DOSE
VARILRIX ®
Prevention of varicella infection (chickenpox)
▶ BY SUBCUTANEOUS INJECTION
▶ Child 1–17 years: 0.5 mL every 4–6 weeks for 2 doses, to be administered into the deltoid region or anterolateral thigh
▶ Adult: 0.5 mL every 4–6 weeks for 2 doses, to be administered into the deltoid region or anterolateral thigh

VARIVAX ®
Prevention of varicella infection (chickenpox)
▶ BY SUBCUTANEOUS INJECTION, OR BY INTRAMUSCULAR INJECTION
▶ Child 1–12 years: 0.5 mL for 2 doses, interval of at least 4 weeks between each dose, to be administered into the deltoid region (or higher anterolateral thigh in young children)
▶ Child 13–17 years: 0.5 mL every 4–8 weeks for 2 doses, to be administered preferably into the deltoid region
▶ Adult: 0.5 mL every 4–8 weeks for 2 doses, to be administered preferably into the deltoid region

Prevention of varicella infection (chickenpox) in children with asymptomatic HIV infection
▶ BY SUBCUTANEOUS INJECTION, OR BY INTRAMUSCULAR INJECTION
▶ Child 1–12 years: 0.5 mL every 12 weeks for 2 doses, to be administered into the deltoid region (or higher anterolateral thigh in young children)

ZOSTAVAX ®
Prevention of herpes zoster (shingles)
▶ BY SUBCUTANEOUS INJECTION
▶ Adult 70–79 years: 0.65 mL for 1 dose, to be administered preferably into the deltoid region

● CAUTIONS Post-vaccination close contact with susceptible individuals
CAUTIONS, FURTHER INFORMATION Rarely, the varicella–zoster vaccine virus has been transmitted from the vaccinated individual to close contacts. Therefore, contact with the following should be avoided if a vaccine-related

cutaneous rash develops within 4–6 weeks of the first or second dose:
● varicella-susceptible pregnant women;
● individuals at high risk of severe varicella, including those with immunodeficiency or those receiving immunosuppressive therapy.
Healthcare workers who develop a generalised papular or vesicular rash on vaccination should avoid contact with patients until the lesions have crusted. Those who develop a localised rash after vaccination should cover the lesions and be allowed to continue working unless in contact with patients at high risk of severe varicella.
▶ Administration with MMR vaccine Varicella–zoster and MMR vaccines can be given on the same day or separated by a 4-week minimum interval. When protection is rapidly required, the vaccines can be given at any interval and an additional dose of the vaccine given second may be considered.

● INTERACTIONS → Appendix 1: live vaccines

● SIDE-EFFECTS
▶ **Uncommon** Cough · drowsiness · increased risk of infection
▶ **Rare or very rare** Abdominal pain · conjunctivitis · Kawasaki disease · seizure · stroke · thrombocytopenia · vasculitis

● CONCEPTION AND CONTRACEPTION Avoid pregnancy for 3 months after vaccination.

● PRESCRIBING AND DISPENSING INFORMATION
ZOSTAVAX ® Advice in the BNF may differ from that in product literature.

● MEDICINAL FORMS
There can be variation in the licensing of different medicines containing the same drug.
Powder and solvent for suspension for injection
EXCIPIENTS: May contain Gelatin, neomycin
▶ Varivax (Merck Sharp & Dohme Ltd)
Varivax vaccine powder and solvent for suspension for injection 0.5ml vials | 1 vial [PoM] £30.28
▶ Zostavax (Merck Sharp & Dohme Ltd)
Zostavax vaccine powder and solvent for suspension for injection 0.65ml pre-filled syringes | 1 pre-filled disposable injection [PoM] £99.96
Powder and solvent for solution for injection
EXCIPIENTS: May contain Neomycin
▶ Varilrix (GlaxoSmithKline UK Ltd)
Varilrix vaccine powder and solvent for solution for injection 0.5ml vials | 1 vial [PoM] £27.31

⬛ 1271

Yellow fever vaccine, live

● INDICATIONS AND DOSE
Immunisation against yellow fever
▶ BY DEEP SUBCUTANEOUS INJECTION
▶ Child 6–8 months (administered on expert advice): Infants under 9 months should be vaccinated only if the risk of yellow fever is high and unavoidable (consult product literature or local protocols)
▶ Child 9 months–17 years: 0.5 mL for 1 dose
▶ Adult: 0.5 mL for 1 dose

● CONTRA-INDICATIONS Children under 6 months · history of thymus dysfunction

● CAUTIONS Individuals over 60 years—greater risk of vaccine-associated adverse effects (in adults)
CAUTIONS, FURTHER INFORMATION
▶ Administration with MMR vaccine Yellow fever and MMR vaccines should not be administered on the same day; there should be a 4-week minimum interval between the vaccines. When protection is rapidly required, the vaccines can be given at any interval and an additional dose of MMR may be considered.

● INTERACTIONS → Appendix 1: live vaccines

14

Vaccines

- SIDE-EFFECTS
- ► **Common or very common** Asthenia · crying (in children) · drowsiness (in children)
- ► **Uncommon** Abdominal pain
- ► **Rare or very rare** Rhinitis · yellow fever vaccine-associated neurotropic disease · yellow fever vaccine-associated viscerotropic disease
- ► **Frequency not known** Anaphylactoid reaction · angioedema · influenza like illness · paraesthesia

  SIDE-EFFECTS, FURTHER INFORMATION Very rare vaccine-associated adverse effects may occur, such as viscerotropic disease (yellow-fever vaccine-associated viscerotropic disease, YEL-AVD), a syndrome which may include metabolic acidosis, muscle and liver cirrhosis, and multi-organ failure. Neurological disorders (yellow fever vaccine-associated neurotropic disease, YEL-AND) such as encephalitis have also been reported. These very rare adverse effects usually occur after the first dose of yellow fever vaccine in those with no previous immunity.

- ● ALLERGY AND CROSS-SENSITIVITY Yellow fever vaccine should only be considered under the guidance of a specialist in individuals with evidence of previous anaphylactic reaction to egg.

- ● PREGNANCY Live yellow fever vaccine should not be given during pregnancy because there is a theoretical risk of fetal infection. Pregnant women should be advised not to travel to areas at high risk of yellow fever. If exposure cannot be avoided during pregnancy, then the vaccine should be given if the risk from disease in the mother outweighs the risk to the fetus from vaccination.

- ● BREAST FEEDING Avoid; seek specialist advice if exposure to virus cannot be avoided.

- ● MEDICINAL FORMS
  There can be variation in the licensing of different medicines containing the same drug.

  Powder and solvent for suspension for injection
  ► Stamaril (Sanofi Pasteur)
    Stamaril vaccine powder and solvent for suspension for injection 0.5ml vials | 1 vial PoM £33.10

Chapter 15
Anaesthesia

CONTENTS

General anaesthesia

Anaesthesia (general)

Overview

Several different types of drug are given together during general anaesthesia. Anaesthesia is induced with either a volatile drug given by inhalation or with an intravenously administered drug; anaesthesia is maintained with an intravenous or inhalational anaesthetic. Analgesics, usually short-acting opioids, are also used. The use of neuromuscular blocking drugs necessitates intermittent positive-pressure ventilation. Following surgery, anticholinesterases can be given to reverse the effects of neuromuscular blocking drugs; specific antagonists can be used to reverse central and respiratory depression caused by some drugs used in surgery. A local topical anaesthetic can be used to reduce pain at the injection site.

Individual requirements vary considerably and the recommended doses are only a guide. Smaller doses are indicated in ill, shocked, or debilitated patients and in significant hepatic impairment, while robust individuals may require larger doses. The required dose of induction agent may be less if the patient has been premedicated with a sedative agent or if an opioid analgesic has been used.

Intravenous anaesthetics

Intravenous anaesthetics may be used either to induce anaesthesia or for maintenance of anaesthesia throughout surgery. Intravenous anaesthetics nearly all produce their effect in one arm-brain circulation time. Extreme care is required in surgery of the mouth, pharynx, or larynx where the airway may be difficult to maintain (e.g. in the presence of a tumour in the pharynx or larynx).

To facilitate tracheal intubation, induction is usually followed by a neuromuscular blocking drug or a short-acting opioid.

The doses of all intravenous anaesthetic drugs should be titrated to effect (except when using 'rapid sequence induction'); lower doses may be required in premedicated patients.

Total intravenous anaesthesia

This is a technique in which major surgery is carried out with all drugs given intravenously. Respiration can be spontaneous, or controlled with oxygen-enriched air. Neuromuscular blocking drugs can be used to provide relaxation and prevent reflex muscle movements. The main problem to be overcome is the assessment of depth of anaesthesia. Target Controlled Infusion (TCI) systems can be used to titrate intravenous anaesthetic infusions to predicted plasma-drug concentrations in ventilated adult patients.

Drugs used for intravenous anaesthesia

Propofol p. 1291, the most widely used intravenous anaesthetic, can be used for induction or maintenance of anaesthesia in adults and children, but it is not commonly used in neonates. Propofol is associated with rapid recovery and less hangover effect than other intravenous anaesthetics. Propofol can also be used for sedation during diagnostic procedures and sedation in adults in intensive care.

Thiopental sodium p. 335 is a barbiturate that is used for induction of anaesthesia, but has no analgesic properties. Induction is generally smooth and rapid, but dose-related cardiovascular and respiratory depression can occur. Awakening from a moderate dose of thiopental sodium is rapid because the drug redistributes into other tissues, particularly fat. However, metabolism is slow and sedative effects can persist for 24 hours. Repeated doses have a cumulative effect and recovery is much slower.

Etomidate p. 1291 is an intravenous agent associated with rapid recovery without a hangover effect. Etomidate causes less hypotension than thiopental sodium and propofol during induction. It produces a high incidence of extraneous muscle movements, which can be minimised by an opioid analgesic or a short-acting benzodiazepine given just before induction.

Ketamine p. 1305 is used rarely. Ketamine causes less hypotension than thiopental sodium and propofol during induction. It is used mainly for paediatric anaesthesia, particularly when repeated administration is required (such as for serial burns dressings); recovery is relatively slow and there is a high incidence of extraneous muscle movements. The main disadvantage of ketamine is the high incidence of hallucinations, nightmares, and other transient psychotic effects; these can be reduced by a benzodiazepine such as diazepam p. 340 or midazolam p. 336.

Inhalational anaesthetics

Inhalational anaesthetics include gases and volatile liquids. *Gaseous anaesthetics* require suitable equipment for storage and administration. *Volatile liquid anaesthetics* are administered using calibrated vaporisers, using air, oxygen, or nitrous oxide-oxygen mixtures as the carrier gas. To prevent hypoxia, the inspired gas mixture should contain a minimum of 25% oxygen at all times. Higher concentrations of oxygen (greater than 30%) are usually required during inhalational anaesthesia when nitrous oxide p. 1293 is being administered.

Volatile liquid anaesthetics

Volatile liquid anaesthetics can be used for induction and maintenance of anaesthesia, and following induction with an intravenous anaesthetic.

Isoflurane p. 1293 is a volatile liquid anaesthetic. Heart rhythm is generally stable during isoflurane anaesthesia, but heart-rate can rise, particularly in younger patients. Systemic arterial pressure and cardiac output can fall, owing to a decrease in systemic vascular resistance. Muscle relaxation occurs and the effects of muscle relaxant drugs are potentiated. Isoflurane is the preferred inhalational anaesthetic for use in obstetrics.

Desflurane p. 1293 is a rapid acting volatile liquid anaesthetic; it is reported to have about one-fifth the potency of isoflurane. Emergence and recovery from anaesthesia are particularly rapid because of its low solubility. Desflurane is not recommended for induction of anaesthesia as it is irritant to the upper respiratory tract.

Sevoflurane p. 1294 is a rapid acting volatile liquid anaesthetic and is more potent than desflurane. Emergence and recovery are particularly rapid, but slower than desflurane. Sevoflurane is non-irritant and is therefore often used for inhalational induction of anaesthesia; it has little effect on heart rhythm compared with other volatile liquid anaesthetics.

Nitrous oxide

Nitrous oxide is used for maintenance of anaesthesia and, in sub-anaesthetic concentrations, for analgesia. For *anaesthesia*, nitrous oxide is commonly used in a concentration of 50 to 66% in oxygen as part of a balanced technique in association with other inhalational or intravenous agents. Nitrous oxide is unsatisfactory as a sole anaesthetic owing to lack of potency, but is useful as part of a combination of drugs since it allows a significant reduction in dosage.

For analgesia (without loss of consciousness), a mixture of nitrous oxide and oxygen containing 50% of each gas (Entonox®, Equanox®) is used. Self-administration using a demand valve is popular in obstetric practice, for changing painful dressings, as an aid to postoperative physiotherapy, and in emergency ambulances.

Nitrous oxide may have a deleterious effect if used in patients with an air-containing closed space since nitrous oxide diffuses into such a space with a resulting increase in pressure. This effect may be dangerous in conditions such as pneumothorax, which may enlarge to compromise respiration, or in the presence of intracranial air after head injury, entrapped air following recent underwater dive, or recent intra-ocular gas injection.

Malignant hyperthermia

Malignant hyperthermia is a rare but potentially lethal complication of anaesthesia. It is characterised by a rapid rise in temperature, increased muscle rigidity, tachycardia, and acidosis. The most common triggers of malignant hyperthermia are the volatile anaesthetics. Suxamethonium chloride p. 1297 has also been implicated, but malignant hyperthermia is more likely if it is given following a volatile anaesthetic. Volatile anaesthetics and suxamethonium chloride should be avoided during anaesthesia in patients at high risk of malignant hyperthermia.

Dantrolene sodium p. 1307 is used in the treatment of malignant hyperthermia.

Sedation, anaesthesia, and resuscitation in dental practice

Overview

Sedation for dental procedures should be limited to conscious sedation. Diazepam p. 340 and temazepam p. 481 are effective anxiolytics for dental treatment in adults.

For details of sedation, anaesthesia, and resuscitation in dental practice see *A Conscious Decision: A review of the use of general anaesthesia and conscious sedation in primary dental care* ; report by a group chaired by the Chief Medical Officer and Chief Dental Officer, July 2000 and associated documents. Further details can also be found in *Standards for Conscious Sedation in the Provision of Dental Care*; report of an Intercollegiate Advisory Committee for Sedation in Dentistry, 2015 https://www.rcseng.ac.uk/-/media/files/rcs/library-and-publications/non-journal-publications/dental-sedation-report.pdf.

Surgery and long-term medication

Overview

The risk of losing disease control on stopping long-term medication before surgery is often greater than the risk posed by continuing it during surgery. It is vital that the anaesthetist knows about **all** drugs that a patient is (or has been) taking.

Patients with adrenal atrophy resulting from long-term corticosteroid use may suffer a precipitous fall in blood pressure unless corticosteroid cover is provided during anaesthesia and in the immediate postoperative period. Anaesthetists must therefore know whether a patient is, or has been, receiving corticosteroids (including high-dose inhaled corticosteroids).

Other drugs that should normally not be stopped before surgery include antiepileptics, antiparkinsonian drugs, antipsychotics, anxiolytics, bronchodilators, cardiovascular drugs (but see potassium-sparing diuretics, angiotensin-converting enzyme inhibitors, and angiotensin-II receptor antagonists), glaucoma drugs, immunosuppressants, drugs of dependence, and thyroid or antithyroid drugs. Expert advice is required for patients receiving antivirals for HIV infection. See general advice on surgery in diabetic patients in Diabetes, surgery and medical illness p. 675.

Patients taking antiplatelet medication or an oral anticoagulant present an increased risk for surgery. In these circumstances, the anaesthetist and surgeon should assess the relative risks and decide jointly whether the antiplatelet or the anticoagulant drug should be stopped or replaced with heparin (unfractionated) p. 132 or low molecular weight heparin therapy.

Drugs that should be stopped before surgery include combined oral contraceptives, see Contraceptives, hormonal p. 772; for advice on hormone replacement therapy, see Sex hormones p. 734. MAOIs can have important interactions with some drugs used during surgery, such as pethidine hydrochloride p. 463. Tricyclic antidepressants need not be stopped, but there may be an increased risk of arrhythmias and hypotension (and dangerous interactions with vasopressor drugs); therefore, the anaesthetist should be informed if they are not stopped. Lithium should be stopped 24 hours before major surgery but the normal dose can be continued for minor surgery (with careful monitoring of fluids and electrolytes). Potassium-sparing diuretics may need to be withheld on the morning of surgery because hyperkalaemia may develop if renal perfusion is impaired or if there is tissue damage. Angiotensin-converting enzyme (ACE) inhibitors and angiotensin-II receptor antagonists can be associated with severe hypotension after induction of anaesthesia; these drugs may need to be discontinued 24 hours before surgery. Herbal medicines may be associated with adverse effects when given with anaesthetic drugs and consideration should be given to stopping them before surgery.

ANAESTHETICS, GENERAL > INTRAVENOUS ANAESTHETICS

Etomidate

● **INDICATIONS AND DOSE**
Induction of anaesthesia
▶ BY SLOW INTRAVENOUS INJECTION
▶ Adult: 150–300 micrograms/kg (max. per dose 60 mg), to be administered over 30-60 seconds (60 seconds in patients in whom hypotension might be hazardous)
▶ Elderly: 150–200 micrograms/kg (max. per dose 60 mg), to be administered over 30-60 seconds (60 seconds in patients in whom hypotension might be hazardous)

IMPORTANT SAFETY INFORMATION
Etomidate should only be administered by, or under the direct supervision of, personnel experienced in its use, with adequate training in anaesthesia and airway management, and when resuscitation equipment is available.

● CAUTIONS Acute circulatory failure (shock) · adrenal insufficiency · Avoid in Acute porphyrias p. 1025 · cardiovascular disease · elderly · fixed cardiac output · hypovolaemia
CAUTIONS, FURTHER INFORMATION
▶ Adrenal insufficiency Etomidate suppresses adrenocortical function, particularly during continuous administration, and it should not be used for maintenance of anaesthesia. It should be used with caution in patients with underlying adrenal insufficiency, for example, those with sepsis.
● INTERACTIONS → Appendix 1: etomidate
● SIDE-EFFECTS
▶ **Common or very common** Apnoea · hypotension · movement disorders · nausea · respiratory disorders · skin reactions · vascular disorders · vomiting
▶ **Uncommon** Arrhythmias · cough · hiccups · hypersalivation · hypertension · muscle rigidity · neuromuscular dysfunction · nystagmus
▶ **Frequency not known** Adrenal insufficiency · atrioventricular block · cardiac arrest · embolism and thrombosis · seizures · shock · Stevens-Johnson syndrome · trismus
SIDE-EFFECTS, FURTHER INFORMATION
Pain on injection Can be reduced by injecting into a larger vein or by giving an opioid analgesic just before induction.
Extraneous muscle movements Extraneous muscle movements can be minimised by an opioid analgesic or a short-acting benzodiazepine given just before induction.
● PREGNANCY May depress neonatal respiration if used during delivery.
● BREAST FEEDING Breast-feeding can be resumed as soon as mother has recovered sufficiently from anaesthesia.
● HEPATIC IMPAIRMENT
Dose adjustments Reduce dose in liver cirrhosis.
● DIRECTIONS FOR ADMINISTRATION To be administered over 30–60 seconds (60 seconds in patients in whom hypotension might be hazardous).
● PATIENT AND CARER ADVICE
Driving and skilled tasks Patients given sedatives and analgesics during minor outpatient procedures should be

very carefully warned about the risk of driving or undertaking skilled tasks afterwards. For a short general anaesthetic the risk extends to **at least 24 hours** after administration. Responsible persons should be available to take patients home. The dangers of taking **alcohol** should also be emphasised.

● MEDICINAL FORMS
There can be variation in the licensing of different medicines containing the same drug.
Solution for injection
EXCIPIENTS: May contain Propylene glycol
▶ Hypnomidate (Piramal Critical Care Ltd)
  Etomidate 2 mg per 1 ml Hypnomidate 20mg/10ml solution for injection ampoules | 5 ampoule PoM £6.90
Emulsion for injection
▶ Etomidate-Lipuro (B.Braun Medical Ltd)
  Etomidate 2 mg per 1 ml Etomidate-Lipuro 20mg/10ml emulsion for injection ampoules | 10 ampoule PoM £16.09

Propofol

● **INDICATIONS AND DOSE**
Induction of anaesthesia using 0.5% or 1% injection
▶ BY SLOW INTRAVENOUS INJECTION, OR BY INTRAVENOUS INFUSION
▶ Adult 18–54 years: Usual dose 1.5–2.5 mg/kg, to be administered at a rate of 20–40 mg every 10 seconds until response, for debilitated patients use dose for 55 years and over
▶ Adult 55 years and over: Usual dose 1–1.5 mg/kg, to be administered at a rate of 20 mg every 10 seconds until response
Induction of anaesthesia using 2% injection
▶ BY INTRAVENOUS INFUSION
▶ Adult 18–54 years: Usual dose 1.5–2.5 mg/kg, to be administered at a rate of 20–40 mg every 10 seconds until response. For debilitated patients use dose for 55 years and over
▶ Adult 55 years and over: Usual dose 1–1.5 mg/kg, to be administered at a rate of 20 mg every 10 seconds until response
Maintenance of anaesthesia using 1% injection
▶ INITIALLY BY INTRAVENOUS INFUSION
▶ Adult: Usual dose 4–12 mg/kg/hour, alternatively (by slow intravenous injection) 25–50 mg, dose may be repeated according to response, for debilitated patients use dose for elderly
▶ Elderly: Usual dose 3–6 mg/kg/hour, alternatively (by slow intravenous injection) 25–50 mg, dose may be repeated according to response
Maintenance of anaesthesia using 2% injection
▶ BY INTRAVENOUS INFUSION
▶ Adult: Usual dose 4–12 mg/kg/hour, for debilitated patients use dose for elderly
▶ Elderly: Usual dose 3–6 mg/kg/hour
Sedation of ventilated patients in intensive care using 1% or 2% injection
▶ BY CONTINUOUS INTRAVENOUS INFUSION
▶ Adult: Usual dose 0.3–4 mg/kg/hour, adjusted according to response
Induction of sedation for surgical and diagnostic procedures using 0.5% or 1% injection
▶ BY SLOW INTRAVENOUS INJECTION
▶ Adult: Initially 0.5–1 mg/kg, to be administered over 1–5 minutes, dose and rate of administration adjusted according to desired level of sedation and response

continued →

15

Anaesthesia

Anaesthesia

15

Maintenance of sedation for surgical and diagnostic procedures using 0.5% injection

▸ INITIALLY BY INTRAVENOUS INFUSION
▸ Adult: Initially 1.5–4.5 mg/kg/hour, dose and rate of administration adjusted according to desired level of sedation and response, followed by (by slow intravenous injection) 10–20 mg, (if rapid increase in sedation required), patients over 55 years or debilitated may require lower initial dose and rate of administration

Maintenance of sedation for surgical and diagnostic procedures using 1% injection

▸ INITIALLY BY INTRAVENOUS INFUSION
▸ Adult: Initially 1.5–4.5 mg/kg/hour, dose and rate of administration adjusted according to desired level of sedation and response, followed by (by slow intravenous injection) 10–20 mg, (if rapid increase in sedation required), patients over 55 years or debilitated may require lower initial dose and rate of administration

Maintenance of sedation for surgical and diagnostic procedures using 2% injection

▸ INITIALLY BY INTRAVENOUS INFUSION
▸ Adult: Initially 1.5–4.5 mg/kg/hour, dose and rate of administration adjusted according to desired level of sedation and response, followed by (by slow intravenous injection) 10–20 mg, using 0.5% or 1% injection (if rapid increase in sedation required), patients over 55 years or debilitated may require lower initial dose and rate of administration

> **IMPORTANT SAFETY INFORMATION**
> Propofol should only be administered by, or under the direct supervision of, personnel experienced in its use, with adequate training in anaesthesia and airway management, and when resuscitation equipment is available.

- CAUTIONS Acute circulatory failure (shock) · cardiac impairment · cardiovascular disease · elderly · epilepsy · fixed cardiac output · hypotension · hypovolaemia · raised intracranial pressure · respiratory impairment
- INTERACTIONS → Appendix 1: propofol
- SIDE-EFFECTS
▸ **Common or very common** Apnoea · arrhythmias · headache · hypotension · nausea · vomiting
▸ **Uncommon** Thrombosis
▸ **Rare or very rare** Epileptiform seizure (may be delayed) · pancreatitis · post procedural complications · pulmonary oedema · sexual disinhibition · urine discolouration
▸ **Frequency not known** Drug use disorders · dyskinesia · euphoric mood · heart failure · hepatomegaly · hyperkalaemia · hyperlipidaemia · metabolic acidosis · renal failure · respiratory depression · rhabdomyolysis

SIDE-EFFECTS, FURTHER INFORMATION
Bradycardia Bradycardia may be profound and may be treated with intravenous administration of an antimuscarinic drug.
Pain on injection Pain on injection can be reduced by intravenous lidocaine.
Propofol infusion syndrome Prolonged infusion of propofol doses exceeding 4mg/kg/hour may result in potentially fatal effects, including metabolic acidosis, arrhythmias, cardiac failure, rhabdomyolysis, hyperlipidaemia, hyperkalaemia, hepatomegaly, and renal failure.

- PREGNANCY May depress neonatal respiration if used during delivery.
Dose adjustments Max. dose for maintenance of anaesthesia 6 mg/kg/hour.

- BREAST FEEDING Breast-feeding can be resumed as soon as mother has recovered sufficiently from anaesthesia.
- HEPATIC IMPAIRMENT Use with caution.
- RENAL IMPAIRMENT Use with caution.
- MONITORING REQUIREMENTS Monitor blood-lipid concentration if risk of fat overload or if sedation longer than 3 days.
- DIRECTIONS FOR ADMINISTRATION Shake before use; microbiological filter not recommended; may be administered via a Y-piece close to injection site co-administered with Glucose 5% or Sodium chloride 0.9%. 0.5% **emulsion** for injection or intermittent infusion; may be administered undiluted, or diluted with Glucose 5% or Sodium chloride 0.9%; dilute to a concentration not less than 1 mg/mL. 1% **emulsion** for injection or infusion; may be administered undiluted, or diluted with Glucose 5% (*Diprivan*®) or (*Propofol-Lipuro*®) or Sodium chloride 0.9% (*Propofol-Lipuro*® only); dilute to a concentration not less than 2 mg/mL; use within 6 hours of preparation. 2% **emulsion** for infusion; do not dilute.
- PATIENT AND CARER ADVICE
Driving and skilled tasks Patients given sedatives and analgesics during minor outpatient procedures should be very carefully warned about the risk of driving or undertaking skilled tasks afterwards. For a short general anaesthetic the risk extends to **at least 24 hours** after administration. Responsible persons should be available to take patients home. The dangers of taking **alcohol** should also be emphasised.

- MEDICINAL FORMS
There can be variation in the licensing of different medicines containing the same drug.
Emulsion for infusion
▸ Propofol (Non-proprietary)
Propofol 10 mg per 1 ml Propofol 500mg/50ml emulsion for infusion vials | 1 vial PoM £3.00 (Hospital only)
Propofol-Lipuro 1% emulsion for infusion 50ml vials | 10 vial PoM £97.56 (Hospital only)
Propofol 1g/100ml emulsion for infusion vials | 1 vial PoM £4.00 (Hospital only)
Propofol 20 mg per 1 ml Propofol 1g/50ml emulsion for infusion vials | 1 vial PoM £3.50 (Hospital only)
▸ Diprivan (Aspen Pharma Trading Ltd)
Propofol 10 mg per 1 ml Diprivan 1% emulsion for infusion 50ml pre-filled syringes | 1 pre-filled disposable injection PoM £10.68
Propofol 20 mg per 1 ml Diprivan 2% emulsion for infusion 50ml pre-filled syringes | 1 pre-filled disposable injection PoM £15.16
Emulsion for injection
▸ Propofol (Non-proprietary)
Propofol 10 mg per 1 ml Propofol 200mg/20ml emulsion for injection vials | 5 vial PoM £4.00 (Hospital only)
▸ Diprivan (Aspen Pharma Trading Ltd)
Propofol 10 mg per 1 ml Diprivan 1% emulsion for injection 20ml ampoules | 5 ampoule PoM £15.36 (Hospital only)
▸ Propofol-Lipuro (B.Braun Melsungen AG)
Propofol 5 mg per 1 ml Propofol-Lipuro 0.5% emulsion for injection 20ml ampoules | 5 ampoule PoM £15.15

ANAESTHETICS, GENERAL ⟩ VOLATILE LIQUID ANAESTHETICS

Volatile halogenated anaesthetics

> **IMPORTANT SAFETY INFORMATION**
> Should only be administered by, or under the direct supervision of, personnel experienced in their use, with adequate training in anaesthesia and airway management, and when resuscitation equipment is available.

- CONTRA-INDICATIONS Susceptibility to malignant hyperthermia
- CAUTIONS Can trigger malignant hyperthermia · raised intracranial pressure (can increase cerebrospinal pressure)
- SIDE-EFFECTS
  - **Common or very common** Agitation · apnoea · arrhythmias · chills · coagulation disorder · conjunctivitis · cough · dizziness · drowsiness · fever · headache · hepatic disorders · hypersalivation · hypertension · hypotension · nausea · respiratory disorders · temperature regulation disorders · vomiting
  - **Uncommon** Asthma · atrioventricular block · confusion · hypoxia · muscle complaints · myocardial infarction · myocardial ischaemia · vasodilation
  - **Frequency not known** Abdominal pain · asthenia · breath holding · carboxyhaemoglobinaemia · cardiac arrest · chest discomfort · cognitive impairment · delirium · dyspnoea · dystonia · electrolyte imbalance · haemorrhage · heart failure · ileus · intracranial pressure increased · malaise · metabolic acidosis · mood altered (that can last several days) · myoglobinuria · nephritis tubulointerstitial · oedema · pancreatitis · QT interval prolongation · rhabdomyolysis · seizure · shock · skin reactions · ventricular dysfunction · visual acuity decreased
- ALLERGY AND CROSS-SENSITIVITY Can cause hepatotoxicity in those sensitised to halogenated anaesthetics.
- DIRECTIONS FOR ADMINISTRATION Volatile liquid anaesthetics are administered using calibrated vaporisers, using air, oxygen, or nitrous oxide-oxygen mixtures as the carrier gas. To prevent hypoxia, the inspired gas mixture should contain a minimum of 25% oxygen at all times.
- PATIENT AND CARER ADVICE
  Driving and skilled tasks Patients given sedatives and analgesics during minor outpatient procedures should be very carefully warned about the risks of driving or undertaking skilled tasks afterwards. For a short general anaesthetic, the risk extends to **at least 24 hours** after administration. Responsible persons should be available to take patients home. The dangers of taking **alcohol** should also be emphasised.

F 1292

Desflurane

- INDICATIONS AND DOSE
Induction of anaesthesia (but not recommended)
  - BY INHALATION
  - Adult: 4–11 %, to be inhaled through specifically calibrated vaporiser
Maintenance of anaesthesia (in nitrous oxide–oxygen)
  - BY INHALATION
  - Adult: 2–6 %, to be inhaled through a specifically calibrated vaporiser
Maintenance of anaesthesia (in oxygen or oxygen-enriched air)
  - BY INHALATION
  - Adult: 2.5–8.5 %, to be inhaled through a specifically calibrated vaporiser

- INTERACTIONS → Appendix 1: volatile halogenated anaesthetics
- PREGNANCY May depress neonatal respiration if used during delivery.
- BREAST FEEDING Breast-feeding can be resumed as soon as mother has recovered sufficiently from anaesthesia.

- MEDICINAL FORMS
There can be variation in the licensing of different medicines containing the same drug.
Inhalation vapour
  - Desflurane (Non-proprietary)
  Desflurane 1 ml per 1 ml Desflurane volatile liquid | 240 ml PoM � (Hospital only)

F 1292

Isoflurane

- INDICATIONS AND DOSE
Induction of anaesthesia (in oxygen or nitrous oxide-oxygen)
  - BY INHALATION
  - Adult: Initially 0.5 %, increased to 3 %, adjusted according to response, administered using specifically calibrated vaporiser
Maintenance of anaesthesia (in nitrous oxide–oxygen)
  - BY INHALATION
  - Adult: 1–2.5 %, to be administered using specifically calibrated vaporiser; an additional 0.5–1% may be required when given with oxygen alone
Maintenance of anaesthesia in caesarean section (in nitrous oxide–oxygen)
  - BY INHALATION
  - Adult: 0.5–0.75 %, to be administered using specifically calibrated vaporiser

- INTERACTIONS → Appendix 1: volatile halogenated anaesthetics
- PREGNANCY May depress neonatal respiration if used during delivery.
- BREAST FEEDING Breast-feeding can be resumed as soon as mother has recovered sufficiently from anaesthesia.

- MEDICINAL FORMS
There can be variation in the licensing of different medicines containing the same drug.
Inhalation vapour
  - Isoflurane (Non-proprietary)
  Isoflurane 1 ml per 1 ml Isoflurane inhalation vapour | 250 ml PoM £35.29 (Hospital only)
  Isoflurane volatile liquid | 250 ml P £47.50 (Hospital only)
  - AErrane (Baxter Healthcare Ltd)
  Isoflurane 1 ml per 1 ml AErrane volatile liquid | 250 ml P � (Hospital only)

Nitrous oxide

- INDICATIONS AND DOSE
Maintenance of anaesthesia in conjunction with other anaesthetic agents
  - BY INHALATION
  - Adult: 50–66 %, to be administered using suitable anaesthetic apparatus in oxygen
Analgesia
  - BY INHALATION
  - Adult: Up to 50 %, to be administered using suitable anaesthetic apparatus in oxygen, adjusted according to the patient's needs

---

IMPORTANT SAFETY INFORMATION
Nitrous oxide should only be administered by, or under the direct supervision of, personnel experienced in its use, with adequate training in anaesthesia and airway management, and when resuscitation equipment is available.

15

Anaesthesia

- CAUTIONS Entrapped air following recent underwater dive · pneumothorax · presence of intracranial air after head injury · recent intra-ocular gas injection

  CAUTIONS, FURTHER INFORMATION Nitrous oxide may have a deleterious effect if used in patients with an air-containing closed space since nitrous oxide diffuses into such a space with a resulting increase in pressure. This effect may be dangerous in conditions such as pneumothorax, which may enlarge to compromise respiration, or in the presence of intracranial air after head injury, entrapped air following recent underwater dive, or recent intra-ocular gas injection.

- INTERACTIONS → Appendix 1: nitrous oxide

- SIDE-EFFECTS Abdominal distension · addiction · agranulocytosis · disorientation · dizziness · euphoric mood · megaloblastic anaemia · middle ear damage · myeloneuropathy · nausea · paraesthesia · sedation · subacute combined cord degeneration · tympanic membrane perforation · vomiting

  SIDE-EFFECTS, FURTHER INFORMATION Exposure of patients to nitrous oxide for prolonged periods, either by continuous or by intermittent administration, may result in megaloblastic anaemia owing to interference with the action of vitamin B_{12}; neurological toxic effects can occur without preceding overt haematological changes. Depression of white cell formation may also occur.

- PREGNANCY May depress neonatal respiration if used during delivery.

- BREAST FEEDING Breast-feeding can be resumed as soon as mother has recovered sufficiently from anaesthesia.

- MONITORING REQUIREMENTS
  - Assessment of plasma-vitamin B_{12} concentration should be considered in those at risk of deficiency, including the elderly, those who have a poor, vegetarian, or vegan diet, and those with a history of anaemia.
  - Nitrous oxide should **not** be given continuously for longer than 24 hours or more frequently than every 4 days without close supervision and haematological monitoring.

- DIRECTIONS FOR ADMINISTRATION For analgesia (without loss of consciousness), a mixture of nitrous oxide and oxygen containing 50% of each gas (Entonox®, Equanox®) is used.

- HANDLING AND STORAGE Exposure of theatre staff to nitrous oxide should be minimised (risk of serious side-effects).

- MEDICINAL FORMS
  There can be variation in the licensing of different medicines containing the same drug.
  Inhalation gas
  - Nitrous oxide (Non-proprietary)
    Nitrous oxide 1 ml per 1 ml Nitrous oxide cylinders size E | 1800 litre (P) (N)
    Medical Nitrous Oxide cylinders size D | 900 litre (P) (N)
    Medical Nitrous Oxide cylinders size G | 9000 litre (P) (N)
    Nitrous oxide cylinders size F | 3600 litre (P) (N)
    Nitrous oxide cylinders size J | 18000 litre (P) (N)
    Nitrous oxide cylinders size G | 9000 litre (P) (N)
    Nitrous oxide cylinders size C | 450 litre (P) (N)
    Medical Nitrous Oxide cylinders size F | 3600 litre (P) (N)
    Nitrous oxide cylinders size D | 900 litre (P) (N)
    Medical Nitrous Oxide cylinders size E | 1800 litre (P) (N)

Sevoflurane

F 1292

- INDICATIONS AND DOSE

  Induction of anaesthesia (in oxygen or nitrous oxide–oxygen)
  - BY INHALATION
  - Adult: Initially 0.5–1 %, then increased to up to 8 %, increased gradually, according to response, to be administered using specifically calibrated vaporiser

  Maintenance of anaesthesia (in oxygen or nitrous oxide–oxygen)
  - BY INHALATION
  - Adult: 0.5–3 %, adjusted according to response, to be administered using specifically calibrated vaporiser

- CAUTIONS Susceptibility to QT-interval prolongation

- INTERACTIONS → Appendix 1: volatile halogenated anaesthetics

- PREGNANCY May depress neonatal respiration if used during delivery.

- BREAST FEEDING Breast-feeding can be resumed as soon as mother has recovered sufficiently from anaesthesia.

- RENAL IMPAIRMENT Use with caution.

- MEDICINAL FORMS
  There can be variation in the licensing of different medicines containing the same drug.
  Inhalation vapour
  - Sevoflurane (Non-proprietary)
    Sevoflurane 1 ml per 1 ml Sevoflurane volatile liquid | 250 ml (PoM)
    £123.00 (Hospital only)

1   Anaesthesia adjuvants

Pre-medication and peri-operative drugs

Drugs that affect gastric pH

Regurgitation and aspiration of gastric contents (Mendelson's syndrome) can be an important complication of general anaesthesia, particularly in obstetrics and during emergency surgery, and requires prophylaxis against acid aspiration. Prophylaxis is also needed in those with gastro-oesophageal reflux disease and in circumstances where gastric emptying may be delayed.

A **H_2-receptor antagonist** can be used before surgery to increase the pH and reduce the volume of gastric fluid. It does not affect the pH of fluid already in the stomach and this limits its value in emergency procedures; an oral H_2-receptor antagonist can be given 1–2 hours before the procedure. Antacids are frequently used to neutralise the acidity of the fluid already in the stomach; 'clear' (non-particulate) antacids such as sodium citrate p. 770 are preferred.

Antimuscarinic drugs

Antimuscarinic drugs are used (less commonly nowadays) as premedicants to dry bronchial and salivary secretions which are increased by intubation, upper airway surgery, or some inhalational anaesthetics. They are also used before or with neostigmine p. 1090 to prevent bradycardia, excessive salivation, and other muscarinic actions of neostigmine. They also prevent bradycardia and hypotension associated with drugs such as propofol p. 1291 and suxamethonium chloride p. 1297.

Atropine sulfate p. 1295 is now rarely used for premedication but still has an emergency role in the treatment of vagotonic side-effects. Atropine sulfate may have a role in acute arrhythmias after myocardial infarction.

Hyoscine hydrobromide p. 433 reduces secretions and also provides a degree of amnesia, sedation, and anti-emesis. Unlike atropine sulfate it may produce bradycardia rather than tachycardia.

Glycopyrronium bromide p. 1296 reduces salivary secretions. When given intravenously it produces less tachycardia than atropine sulfate. It is widely used with neostigmine for reversal of non-depolarising neuromuscular blocking drugs.

Phenothiazines do not effectively reduce secretions when used alone.

Sedative drugs

Fear and anxiety before a procedure (including the night before) can be minimised by using a sedative drug, usually a **benzodiazepine**. Premedication may also augment the action of anaesthetics and provide some degree of pre-operative amnesia. The choice of drug depends on the individual, the nature of the procedure, the anaesthetic to be used, and other prevailing circumstances such as outpatients, obstetrics, and availability of recovery facilities. The choice also varies between elective and emergency procedures.

Premedicants can be given the night before major surgery; a further, smaller dose may be required before surgery. Alternatively, the first dose may be given on the day of the procedure.

Benzodiazepines

Benzodiazepines possess useful properties for premedication including relief of anxiety, sedation, and amnesia; short-acting benzodiazepines taken by mouth are the most common premedicants. Benzodiazepines are also used in intensive care units for sedation, particularly in those receiving assisted ventilation. Flumazenil p. 1328 is used to antagonise the effects of benzodiazepines.

Diazepam p. 340 is used to produce mild sedation with amnesia. It is a long-acting drug with active metabolites and a second period of drowsiness can occur several hours after its administration. Peri-operative use of diazepam in children is not recommended; its effect and timing of response are unreliable and paradoxical effects may occur.

Diazepam is relatively insoluble in water and preparations formulated in organic solvents are painful on intravenous injection and give rise to a high incidence of venous thrombosis (which may not be noticed for several days after the injection). Intramuscular injection of diazepam is painful and absorption is erratic. An emulsion formulated for intravenous injection is less irritant and reduces the risk of venous thrombosis; it is not suitable for intramuscular injection.

Temazepam p. 481 is given by mouth for premedication and has a shorter duration of action and a more rapid onset than oral diazepam; anxiolytic and sedative effects last about 90 minutes although there may be residual drowsiness.

Lorazepam p. 335 produces more prolonged sedation than temazepam and it has marked amnesic effects.

Midazolam p. 336 is a water-soluble benzodiazepine that is often used in preference to intravenous diazepam; recovery is faster than from diazepam, but may be significantly longer in the elderly, in patients with a low cardiac output, or after repeated dosing. Midazolam is associated with profound sedation when high doses are given intravenously or when it is used with certain other drugs.

Other drugs for sedation

Dexmedetomidine p. 1306 and clonidine hydrochloride p. 144 are alpha$_2$-adrenergic agonists with sedative properties. Dexmedetomidine is licensed for the sedation of patients receiving intensive care who need to remain responsive to verbal stimulation. Clonidine hydrochloride

[unlicensed indication] can be used by mouth or by intravenous injection as a sedative agent when adequate sedation cannot be achieved with standard treatment.

Antagonists for central and respiratory depression

Respiratory depression is a major concern with opioid analgesics and it may be treated by artificial ventilation or be reversed by naloxone hydrochloride p. 1329. Naloxone hydrochloride will immediately reverse opioid-induced respiratory depression but the dose may have to be repeated because of the short duration of action of naloxone hydrochloride; however, naloxone hydrochloride will also antagonise the analgesic effect.

Flumazenil is a benzodiazepine antagonist for the reversal of the central sedative effects of benzodiazepines after anaesthetic and similar procedures. Flumazenil has a shorter half-life and duration of action than diazepam or midazolam so patients may become resedated.

Doxapram hydrochloride p. 297 is a central and respiratory stimulant but is of limited value in anaesthesia.

ANTIMUSCARINICS

F 759

| Atropine sulfate

- **INDICATIONS AND DOSE**

Bradycardia due to acute massive overdosage of beta-blockers

▶ BY INTRAVENOUS INJECTION
- Child: 40 micrograms/kg (max. per dose 3 mg)
- Adult: 3 mg

Treatment of poisoning by organophosphorus insecticide or nerve agent (in combination with pralidoxime chloride)

▶ BY INTRAVENOUS INJECTION
- Child: 20 micrograms/kg every 5–10 minutes (max. per dose 2 mg) until the skin becomes flushed and dry, the pupils dilate, and bradycardia is abolished, frequency of administration dependent on the severity of poisoning
- Adult: 2 mg every 5–10 minutes until the skin becomes flushed and dry, the pupils dilate, and bradycardia is abolished, frequency of administration dependent on the severity of poisoning

Symptomatic relief of gastro-intestinal disorders characterised by smooth muscle spasm

▶ BY MOUTH
- Adult: 0.6–1.2 mg daily, dose to be taken at night

Premedication

▶ BY INTRAVENOUS INJECTION
- Child 12-17 years: 300–600 micrograms, to be administered immediately before induction of anaesthesia
- Adult: 300–600 micrograms, to be administered immediately before induction of anaesthesia
▶ BY SUBCUTANEOUS INJECTION, OR BY INTRAMUSCULAR INJECTION
- Child 12-17 years: 300–600 micrograms, to be administered 30–60 minutes before induction of anaesthesia
- Adult: 300–600 micrograms, to be administered 30–60 minutes before induction of anaesthesia

Intra-operative bradycardia

▶ BY INTRAVENOUS INJECTION
- Child 12-17 years: 300–600 micrograms, larger doses may be used in emergencies
- Adult: 300–600 micrograms, larger doses may be used in emergencies

continued →

Control of muscarinic side-effects of neostigmine in reversal of competitive neuromuscular block
▶ BY INTRAVENOUS INJECTION
- Child 12–17 years: 0.6–1.2 mg
- Adult: 0.6–1.2 mg

Excessive bradycardia associated with beta-blocker use
▶ BY INTRAVENOUS INJECTION
- Adult: 0.6–2.4 mg in divided doses (max. per dose 600 micrograms)

Bradycardia following myocardial infarction (particularly if complicated by hypotension)
▶ BY INTRAVENOUS INJECTION
- Adult: 500 micrograms every 3–5 minutes; maximum 3 mg per course

> **IMPORTANT SAFETY INFORMATION**
> Antimuscarinic drugs used for premedication to general anaesthesia should only be administered by, or under the direct supervision of, personnel experienced in their use.

● INTERACTIONS → Appendix 1: atropine
● SIDE-EFFECTS
▶ Common or very common
▶ With intravenous use Anhidrosis · anxiety · bronchial secretion decreased · dysphagia · gastrointestinal disorders · hallucination · hyperthermia · movement disorders · speech disorder · taste loss · thirst · urticaria · visual impairment
▶ Rare or very rare
▶ With intravenous use Angina pectoris · arrhythmias · hypertensive crisis · seizure
▶ Frequency not known
▶ With intravenous use Insomnia
▶ With oral use Angle closure glaucoma · bronchial secretion altered · chest pain · dysphagia · fever · increased gastric reflux · thirst
● PREGNANCY Not known to be harmful; manufacturer advises caution.
● BREAST FEEDING May suppress lactation; small amount present in milk—manufacturer advises caution.
● MONITORING REQUIREMENTS
▶ Control of muscarinic side-effects of neostigmine in reversal of competitive neuromuscular block Since atropine has a shorter duration of action than neostigmine, late unopposed bradycardia may result; close monitoring of the patient is necessary.
● LESS SUITABLE FOR PRESCRIBING Atropine tablets less suitable for prescribing. Any clinical benefit as a gastro-intestinal antispasmodic is outweighed by atropinic side-effects.
● EXCEPTIONS TO LEGAL CATEGORY Prescription only medicine restriction does not apply where administration is for saving life in emergency.

● MEDICINAL FORMS
There can be variation in the licensing of different medicines containing the same drug. Forms available from special-order manufacturers include: oral suspension, oral solution, solution for injection, solution for infusion
Tablet
▶ Atropine sulfate (Non-proprietary)
Atropine sulfate 600 microgram Atropine 600microgram tablets | 28 tablet [PoM] £52.92 DT = £52.92
Solution for injection
▶ Atropine sulfate (Non-proprietary)
Atropine sulfate 100 microgram per 1 ml Atropine 500micrograms/5ml solution for injection pre-filled syringes | 1 pre-filled disposable injection [PoM] £13.00 | 10 pre-filled disposable injection [PoM] £130.00
Atropine sulfate 200 microgram per 1 ml Atropine 1mg/5ml solution for injection pre-filled syringes | 1 pre-filled disposable

injection [PoM] £7.08–£13.00 | 10 pre-filled disposable injection [PoM] £130.00
Atropine sulfate 300 microgram per 1 ml Atropine 3mg/10ml solution for injection pre-filled syringes | 1 pre-filled disposable injection [PoM] £7.08–£13.00 DT = £7.11 | 10 pre-filled disposable injection [PoM] £130.00
Atropine sulfate 400 microgram per 1 ml Atropine 400micrograms/1ml solution for injection ampoules | 10 ampoule [PoM] £90.30 DT = £90.30
Atropine sulfate 600 microgram per 1 ml Atropine 600micrograms/1ml solution for injection ampoules | 10 ampoule [PoM] £11.71 DT = £11.71
Atropine 600micrograms/1ml solution for injection pre-filled syringes | 1 pre-filled disposable injection [PoM] £7.08
Atropine sulfate 1 mg per 1 ml Atropine 1mg/1ml solution for injection ampoules | 10 ampoule [PoM] £83.61 DT = £83.61

▶ F 759

Glycopyrronium bromide
13-Sep-2017

(Glycopyrrolate)

● INDICATIONS AND DOSE
Premedication at induction
▶ BY INTRAMUSCULAR INJECTION, OR BY INTRAVENOUS INJECTION
- Adult: 200–400 micrograms, alternatively 4–5 micrograms/kg (max. per dose 400 micrograms)
Intra-operative bradycardia
▶ BY INTRAVENOUS INJECTION
- Adult: 200–400 micrograms, alternatively 4–5 micrograms/kg (max. per dose 400 micrograms), repeated if necessary
Control of muscarinic side-effects of neostigmine in reversal of non-depolarising neuromuscular block
▶ BY INTRAVENOUS INJECTION
- Adult: 10–15 micrograms/kg, alternatively, 200 micrograms per 1 mg of neostigmine to be administered
Bowel colic in palliative care | Excessive respiratory secretions in palliative care
▶ BY SUBCUTANEOUS INJECTION
- Adult: 200 micrograms every 4 hours and when required, hourly use is occasionally necessary, particularly in excessive respiratory secretions
▶ BY SUBCUTANEOUS INFUSION
- Adult: 0.6–1.2 mg/24 hours

> **IMPORTANT SAFETY INFORMATION**
> Antimuscarinic drugs used for premedication to general anaesthesia should only be administered by, or under the direct supervision of, personnel experienced in their use.

● INTERACTIONS → Appendix 1: glycopyrronium
● SIDE-EFFECTS Angle closure glaucoma · anhidrosis · bradycardia · bronchial secretion decreased · mydriasis · photophobia · urinary urgency
● PRESCRIBING AND DISPENSING INFORMATION
Palliative care For further information on the use of glycopyrronium bromide in palliative care, see www.palliativedrugs.com/formulary/en/glycopyrronium.html.

● MEDICINAL FORMS
There can be variation in the licensing of different medicines containing the same drug.
Solution for injection
▶ Glycopyrronium bromide (Non-proprietary)
Glycopyrronium bromide 200 microgram per 1 ml Glycopyrronium bromide 200micrograms/1ml solution for injection ampoules | 10 ampoule [PoM] £5.72–£14.00 DT = £12.22
Glycopyrronium bromide 600micrograms/3ml solution for injection ampoules | 3 ampoule [PoM] £8.00 | 10 ampoule [PoM] £9.61–£13.97

1.1 Neuromuscular blockade

Neuromuscular blockade

Neuromuscular blocking drugs

Neuromuscular blocking drugs used in anaesthesia are also known as **muscle relaxants**. By specific blockade of the neuromuscular junction they enable light anaesthesia to be used with adequate relaxation of the muscles of the abdomen and diaphragm. They also relax the vocal cords and allow the passage of a tracheal tube. Their action differs from the muscle relaxants used in musculoskeletal disorders that act on the spinal cord or brain.

Patients who have received a neuromuscular blocking drug should **always** have their respiration assisted or controlled until the drug has been inactivated or antagonised. They should also receive sufficient concomitant inhalational or intravenous anaesthetic or sedative drugs to prevent awareness.

Non-depolarising neuromuscular blocking drugs

Non-depolarising neuromuscular blocking drugs (also known as competitive muscle relaxants) compete with acetylcholine for receptor sites at the neuromuscular junction and their action can be reversed with anticholinesterases such as neostigmine p. 1090. Non-depolarising neuromuscular blocking drugs can be divided into the **aminosteroid** group, comprising pancuronium bromide p. 1299, rocuronium bromide p. 1300, and vecuronium bromide p. 1300, and the **benzylisoquinolinium** group, comprising atracurium besilate p. 1298, cisatracurium p. 1299, and mivacurium p. 1299.

Non-depolarising neuromuscular blocking drugs have a slower onset of action than suxamethonium chloride below. These drugs can be classified by their duration of action as short-acting (15–30 minutes), intermediate-acting (30–40 minutes), and long-acting (60–120 minutes), although duration of action is dose-dependent. Drugs with a shorter or intermediate duration of action, such as atracurium besilate and vecuronium bromide, are more widely used than those with a longer duration of action, such as pancuronium bromide.

Non-depolarising neuromuscular blocking drugs have no sedative or analgesic effects and are not considered to trigger malignant hyperthermia.

For patients receiving intensive care and who require tracheal intubation and mechanical ventilation, a non-depolarising neuromuscular blocking drug is chosen according to its onset of effect, duration of action, and side-effects. Rocuronium bromide, with a rapid onset of effect, may facilitate intubation. Atracurium besilate or cisatracurium may be suitable for long-term neuromuscular blockade since their duration of action is not dependent on elimination by the liver or the kidneys.

Atracurium besilate, a mixture of 10 isomers, is a benzylisoquinolinium neuromuscular blocking drug with an intermediate duration of action. It undergoes non-enzymatic metabolism which is independent of liver and kidney function, thus allowing its use in patients with hepatic or renal impairment. Cardiovascular effects are associated with significant histamine release; histamine release can be minimised by administering slowly or in divided doses over at least 1 minute.

Cisatracurium is a single isomer of atracurium besilate. It is more potent and has a slightly longer duration of action than atracurium besilate and provides greater cardiovascular stability because cisatracurium lacks histamine-releasing effects.

Mivacurium, a benzylisoquinolinium neuromuscular blocking drug, has a short duration of action. It is metabolised by plasma cholinesterase and muscle paralysis is prolonged in individuals deficient in this enzyme. It is not associated with vagolytic activity or ganglionic blockade although histamine release can occur, particularly with rapid injection.

Pancuronium bromide, an aminosteroid neuromuscular blocking drug, has a long duration of action and is often used in patients receiving long-term mechanical ventilation in intensive care units. It lacks a histamine-releasing effect, but vagolytic and sympathomimetic effects can cause tachycardia and hypertension.

Rocuronium bromide exerts an effect within 2 minutes and has the most rapid onset of any of the non-depolarising neuromuscular blocking drugs. It is an aminosteroid neuromuscular blocking drug with an intermediate duration of action. It is reported to have minimal cardiovascular effects; high doses produce mild vagolytic activity.

Vecuronium bromide, an aminosteroid neuromuscular blocking drug, has an intermediate duration of action. It does not generally produce histamine release and lacks cardiovascular effects.

Depolarising neuromuscular blocking drugs

Suxamethonium chloride has the most rapid onset of action of any of the neuromuscular blocking drugs and is ideal if fast onset and brief duration of action are required, e.g. with tracheal intubation. Unlike the non-depolarising neuromuscular blocking drugs, its action cannot be reversed and recovery is spontaneous; anticholinesterases such as neostigmine potentiate the neuromuscular block.

Suxamethonium chloride should be given after anaesthetic induction because paralysis is usually preceded by painful muscle fasciculations. While tachycardia occurs with single use, bradycardia may occur with repeated doses in adults and with the first dose in children. Premedication with atropine reduces bradycardia as well as the excessive salivation associated with suxamethonium chloride use.

Prolonged paralysis may occur in **dual block**, which occurs with high or repeated doses of suxamethonium chloride and is caused by the development of a non-depolarising block following the initial depolarising block. Individuals with myasthenia gravis are resistant to suxamethonium chloride but can develop dual block resulting in delayed recovery. Prolonged paralysis may also occur in those with low or atypical plasma cholinesterase. Assisted ventilation should be continued until muscle function is restored.

NEUROMUSCULAR BLOCKING DRUGS ›
DEPOLARISING

Suxamethonium chloride

(Succinylcholine chloride)

- DRUG ACTION Suxamethonium acts by mimicking acetylcholine at the neuromuscular junction but hydrolysis is much slower than for acetylcholine; depolarisation is therefore prolonged, resulting in neuromuscular blockade.

- INDICATIONS AND DOSE

Neuromuscular blockade (short duration) during surgery and intubation
▸ BY INTRAVENOUS INJECTION
▸ Adult: 1–1.5 mg/kg

15

Anaesthesia

- UNLICENSED USE Doses of suxamethonium in BNF may differ from those in product literature.

> IMPORTANT SAFETY INFORMATION
> Should only be administered by, or under the direct supervision of, personnel experienced in its use.

- CONTRA-INDICATIONS Duchenne muscular dystrophy · family history of malignant hyperthermia · hyperkalaemia · low plasma-cholinesterase activity (including severe liver disease) · major trauma · neurological disease involving acute wasting of major muscle · personal or family history of congenital myotonic disease · prolonged immobilisation (risk of hyperkalaemia) · severe burns
- CAUTIONS Cardiac disease · neuromuscular disease · raised intra-ocular pressure (avoid in penetrating eye injury) · respiratory disease · severe sepsis (risk of hyperkalaemia)
- INTERACTIONS → Appendix 1: suxamethonium
- SIDE-EFFECTS
  ‣ **Common or very common** Arrhythmias · bradycardia (may occur with repeated doses) · flushing · muscle contractions involuntary · myoglobinaemia · myoglobinuria · rash
  ‣ **Rare or very rare** Apnoea · cardiac arrest · hypersensitivity · malignant hyperthermia · respiratory disorders · trismus
  SIDE-EFFECTS, FURTHER INFORMATION Premedication with atropine reduces bradycardia associated with suxamethonium use.
- ALLERGY AND CROSS-SENSITIVITY Allergic cross-reactivity between neuromuscular blocking drugs has been reported; caution is advised in cases of hypersensitivity to these drugs.
- PREGNANCY Mildly prolonged maternal neuromuscular blockade may occur.
- BREAST FEEDING Unlikely to be present in breast milk in significant amounts (ionised at physiological pH). Breast-feeding may be resumed once the mother recovered from neuromuscular block.
- HEPATIC IMPAIRMENT Prolonged apnoea may occur in severe liver disease because of reduced hepatic synthesis of pseudocholinesterase.

- MEDICINAL FORMS
  There can be variation in the licensing of different medicines containing the same drug. Forms available from special-order manufacturers include: solution for injection
  Solution for injection
  ‣ Suxamethonium chloride (Non-proprietary)
    Suxamethonium chloride 50 mg per 1 ml Suxamethonium chloride 100mg/2ml solution for injection ampoules | 10 ampoule [PoM] £28.80–£50.00
  ‣ Anectine (Aspen Pharma Trading Ltd)
    Suxamethonium chloride 50 mg per 1 ml Anectine 100mg/2ml solution for injection ampoules | 5 ampoule [PoM] £3.57

NEUROMUSCULAR BLOCKING DRUGS >
NON-DEPOLARISING

Non-depolarising neuromuscular blocking drugs

> IMPORTANT SAFETY INFORMATION
> Non-depolarising neuromuscular blocking drugs should only be administered by, or under direct supervision of, personnel experienced in their use, with adequate training in anaesthesia and airway management.

- CAUTIONS Burns (resistance can develop, increased doses may be required) · cardiovascular disease (reduce rate of administration) · electrolyte disturbances (response unpredictable) · fluid disturbances (response unpredictable) · hypothermia (activity prolonged, lower doses required) · myasthenia gravis (activity prolonged, lower doses required) · neuromuscular disorders (response unpredictable)
- SIDE-EFFECTS
  ‣ **Common or very common** Flushing · hypotension
  ‣ **Uncommon** Bronchospasm · hypersensitivity · skin reactions · tachycardia
  ‣ **Rare or very rare** Circulatory collapse · muscle weakness · myopathy (after prolonged use in intensive care) · shock
- ALLERGY AND CROSS-SENSITIVITY Allergic cross-reactivity between neuromuscular blocking drugs has been reported; caution is advised in cases of hypersensitivity to these drugs.
- PREGNANCY Non-depolarising neuromuscular blocking drugs are highly ionised at physiological pH and are therefore unlikely to cross the placenta in significant amounts.
- BREAST FEEDING Non-depolarising neuromuscular blocking drugs are ionised at physiological pH and are unlikely to be present in milk in significant amounts. Breast-feeding may be resumed once the mother has recovered from neuromuscular block.

‣ above

Atracurium besilate
(Atracurium besylate)

- INDICATIONS AND DOSE
  Neuromuscular blockade (short to intermediate duration) for surgery and intubation
  ‣ INITIALLY BY INTRAVENOUS INJECTION
  ‣ Adult: Initially 300–600 micrograms/kg, then (by intravenous injection) 100–200 micrograms/kg as required, alternatively (by intravenous injection) initially 300–600 micrograms/kg, followed by (by intravenous infusion) 300–600 micrograms/kg/hour
  Neuromuscular blockade during intensive care
  ‣ INITIALLY BY INTRAVENOUS INJECTION
  ‣ Adult: Initially 300–600 micrograms/kg, initial dose is optional, then (by intravenous infusion) 270–1770 micrograms/kg/hour; (by intravenous infusion) usual dose 650–780 micrograms/kg/hour
  DOSES AT EXTREMES OF BODY-WEIGHT
  ‣ To avoid excessive dosage in obese patients, dose should be calculated on the basis of ideal body-weight.

- INTERACTIONS → Appendix 1: neuromuscular blocking drugs, non-depolarising
- SIDE-EFFECTS
  ‣ **Rare or very rare** Cardiac arrest
  ‣ **Frequency not known** Seizure
  SIDE-EFFECTS, FURTHER INFORMATION Hypotension, skin flushing, and bronchospasm is associated with histamine release. Manufacturer advises minimising effects of histamine release by administering over 1 minute in patients with cardiovascular disease or sensitivity to hypotension.
- DIRECTIONS FOR ADMINISTRATION For *intravenous infusion* (*Tracrium*®; Atracurium besilate injection, Hospira; Atracurium injection/infusion, Genus), give continuously in Glucose 5% or Sodium Chloride 0.9%; stability varies with diluent; dilute requisite dose with infusion fluid to a concentration of 0.5–5 mg/mL.

- **MEDICINAL FORMS**
There can be variation in the licensing of different medicines containing the same drug.
Solution for injection
  ▸ Atracurium besilate (Non-proprietary)
    Atracurium besilate 10 mg per 1 ml Atracurium besilate 250mg/25ml solution for injection vials | 1 vial [PoM] £16.50 (Hospital only)
    Atracurium besilate 25mg/2.5ml solution for injection ampoules | 5 ampoule [PoM] £9.25 (Hospital only) | 5 ampoule [PoM] £9.25
    Atracurium besilate 50mg/5ml solution for injection ampoules | 5 ampoule [PoM] £17.50 (Hospital only) | 5 ampoule [PoM] £17.50
  ▸ Tracrium (Aspen Pharma Trading Ltd)
    Atracurium besilate 10 mg per 1 ml Tracrium 250mg/25ml solution for injection vials | 2 vial [PoM] £25.81
    Tracrium 25mg/2.5ml solution for injection ampoules | 5 ampoule [PoM] £8.28
    Tracrium 50mg/5ml solution for injection ampoules | 5 ampoule [PoM] £15.02

⚑ 1298

Cisatracurium

- **INDICATIONS AND DOSE**
Neuromuscular blockade (intermediate duration) during surgery and intubation
  ▸ INITIALLY BY INTRAVENOUS INJECTION
  ▸ Adult: Initially 150 micrograms/kg, then (by intravenous injection) maintenance 30 micrograms/kg every 20 minutes, alternatively (by intravenous infusion) initially 180 micrograms/kg/hour, then (by intravenous infusion) maintenance 60–120 micrograms/kg/hour, maintenance dose administered after stabilisation

Neuromuscular blockade (intermediate duration) during intensive care
  ▸ INITIALLY BY INTRAVENOUS INJECTION
  ▸ Adult: Initially 150 micrograms/kg, initial dose is optional, then (by intravenous infusion) 180 micrograms/kg/hour, adjusted according to response; (by intravenous infusion) usual dose 30–600 micrograms/kg/hour

DOSES AT EXTREMES OF BODY-WEIGHT
  ▸ To avoid excessive dosage in obese patients, dose should be calculated on the basis of ideal body-weight.

- **INTERACTIONS** → Appendix 1: neuromuscular blocking drugs, non-depolarising
- **SIDE-EFFECTS**
  ▸ Common or very common Bradycardia
- **DIRECTIONS FOR ADMINISTRATION** For *intravenous infusion* (Nimbex®, Nimbex Forte®), give continuously in Glucose 5% or Sodium Chloride 0.9%; solutions of 2 mg/mL and 5 mg/mL may be infused undiluted; alternatively dilute with infusion fluid to a concentration of 0.1–2 mg/mL.

- **MEDICINAL FORMS**
There can be variation in the licensing of different medicines containing the same drug.
Solution for injection
  ▸ Cisatracurium (Non-proprietary)
    Cisatracurium (as Cisatracurium besilate) 2 mg per 1 ml Cisatracurium besilate 20mg/10ml solution for injection ampoules | 5 ampoule [PoM] £32.09
    Cisatracurium besilate 20mg/10ml solution for injection vials | 5 vial [PoM] £37.75 (Hospital only)
    Cisatracurium (as Cisatracurium besilate) 5 mg per 1 ml Cisatracurium besilate 150mg/30ml solution for injection vials | 1 vial [PoM] £45.00 (Hospital only) | 5 ampoule [PoM] £26.43-£29.54
  ▸ Nimbex (Aspen Pharma Trading Ltd)
    Cisatracurium (as Cisatracurium besilate) 2 mg per 1 ml Nimbex 20mg/10ml solution for injection ampoules | 5 ampoule [PoM] £37.75
    Cisatracurium (as Cisatracurium besilate) 5 mg per 1 ml Nimbex Forte 150mg/30ml solution for injection vials | 1 vial [PoM] £31.09

⚑ 1298

Mivacurium

- **INDICATIONS AND DOSE**
Neuromuscular blockade (short duration) during surgery and intubation
  ▸ INITIALLY BY INTRAVENOUS INJECTION
  ▸ Adult: 70–250 micrograms/kg; (by intravenous injection) maintenance 100 micrograms/kg every 15 minutes, alternatively (by intravenous infusion) maintenance 8–10 micrograms/kg/minute, (by intravenous infusion) adjusted in steps of 1 microgram/kg/minute every 3 minutes if required; (by intravenous infusion) usual dose 6–7 micrograms/kg/minute

DOSES AT EXTREMES OF BODY-WEIGHT
  ▸ To avoid excessive dosage in obese patients, dose should be calculated on the basis of ideal bodyweight.

- **CAUTIONS** Burns (low plasma cholinesterase activity; dose titration required) · elderly
- **INTERACTIONS** → Appendix 1: neuromuscular blocking drugs, non-depolarising
- **SIDE-EFFECTS**
  ▸ Uncommon Erythema
- **HEPATIC IMPAIRMENT**
  Dose adjustments Reduce dose in severe impairment.
- **RENAL IMPAIRMENT**
  Dose adjustments Clinical effect prolonged in renal failure—reduce dose according to response.
- **DIRECTIONS FOR ADMINISTRATION** For *intravenous infusion*, give continuously in Glucose 5% or Sodium chloride 0.9%. Dilute to a concentration of 500 micrograms/mL; may also be given undiluted. Doses up to 150 micrograms/kg may be given over 5–15 seconds, higher doses should be given over 30 seconds. In asthma, cardiovascular disease or in those sensitive to reduced arterial blood pressure, give over 60 seconds.

- **MEDICINAL FORMS**
There can be variation in the licensing of different medicines containing the same drug.
Solution for injection
  ▸ Mivacron (Aspen Pharma Trading Ltd)
    Mivacurium (as Mivacurium chloride) 2 mg per 1 ml Mivacron 10mg/5ml solution for injection ampoules | 5 ampoule [PoM] £13.95
    Mivacron 20mg/10ml solution for injection ampoules | 5 ampoule [PoM] £22.57

⚑ 1298

Pancuronium bromide

- **INDICATIONS AND DOSE**
Neuromuscular blockade (long duration) during surgery and intubation
  ▸ BY INTRAVENOUS INJECTION
  ▸ Adult: Initially 100 micrograms/kg, then 20 micrograms/kg as required

Neuromuscular blockade (long duration) during intensive care
  ▸ BY INTRAVENOUS INJECTION
  ▸ Adult: Initially 100 micrograms/kg, initial dose is optional, then 60 micrograms/kg every 60–90 minutes

DOSES AT EXTREMES OF BODY-WEIGHT
  ▸ To avoid excessive dosage in obese patients, dose should be calculated on the basis of ideal bodyweight.

- **INTERACTIONS** → Appendix 1: neuromuscular blocking drugs, non-depolarising
- **SIDE-EFFECTS** Apnoea · arrhythmia · hypersalivation · increased cardiac output · miosis

15

Anaesthesia

SIDE-EFFECTS, FURTHER INFORMATION Pancuronium lacks histamine-releasing effect, but vagolytic and sympathomimetic effects can cause tachycardia.

● HEPATIC IMPAIRMENT Possibly slower onset, higher dose requirement, and prolonged recovery time.

● RENAL IMPAIRMENT Use with caution; prolonged duration of block.

● MEDICINAL FORMS
There can be variation in the licensing of different medicines containing the same drug.
Solution for injection
▸ Pancuronium bromide (Non-proprietary)
Pancuronium bromide 2 mg per 1 ml Pancuronium bromide 4mg/2ml solution for injection ampoules | 10 ampoule [PoM] £50.00 (Hospital only)

◤ 1298

Rocuronium bromide

● INDICATIONS AND DOSE
Neuromuscular blockade (intermediate duration) during surgery and intubation
▸ INITIALLY BY INTRAVENOUS INJECTION
▸ Adult: Initially 600 micrograms/kg; (by intravenous injection) maintenance 150 micrograms/kg, alternatively (by intravenous infusion) maintenance 300–600 micrograms/kg/hour, adjusted according to response
▸ Elderly: Initially 600 micrograms/kg; (by intravenous injection) maintenance 75–100 micrograms/kg, alternatively (by intravenous infusion) maintenance up to 400 micrograms/kg/hour, adjusted according to response

Neuromuscular blockade (intermediate duration) during intensive care
▸ INITIALLY BY INTRAVENOUS INJECTION
▸ Adult: Initially 600 micrograms/kg, initial dose is optional; (by intravenous infusion) maintenance 300–600 micrograms/kg/hour for first hour, then (by intravenous infusion), adjusted according to response

DOSES AT EXTREMES OF BODY-WEIGHT
▸ To avoid excessive dosage in obese patients, dose should be calculated on the basis of ideal bodyweight.

● INTERACTIONS → Appendix 1: neuromuscular blocking drugs, non-depolarising

● SIDE-EFFECTS
▸ **Rare or very rare** Angioedema · face oedema · hypersensitivity · malignant hyperthermia · paralysis · rash erythematous

● HEPATIC IMPAIRMENT
Dose adjustments Reduce dose.

● RENAL IMPAIRMENT
Dose adjustments Reduce maintenance dose; prolonged paralysis.

● DIRECTIONS FOR ADMINISTRATION For *continuous intravenous infusion* or via drip tubing, may be diluted with Glucose 5% or Sodium Chloride 0.9%.

● MEDICINAL FORMS
There can be variation in the licensing of different medicines containing the same drug.
Solution for injection
▸ Rocuronium bromide (Non-proprietary)
Rocuronium bromide 10 mg per 1 ml Rocuronium bromide 50mg/5ml solution for injection ampoules | 10 ampoule [PoM] £24.00
Rocuronium bromide 50mg/5ml solution for injection vials | 10 vial [PoM] £28.00-£30.00
Rocuronium bromide 100mg/10ml solution for injection vials | 10 vial [PoM] £57.00-£57.90

▸ Esmeron (Merck Sharp & Dohme Ltd)
Rocuronium bromide 10 mg per 1 ml Esmeron 50mg/5ml solution for injection vials | 10 vial [PoM] £28.92 (Hospital only)
Esmeron 100mg/10ml solution for injection vials | 10 vial [PoM] £57.85 (Hospital only)

◤ 1298

Vecuronium bromide

● INDICATIONS AND DOSE
Neuromuscular blockade (intermediate duration) during surgery and intubation
▸ INITIALLY BY INTRAVENOUS INJECTION
▸ Adult: 80–100 micrograms/kg; (by intravenous injection) maintenance 20–30 micrograms/kg, adjusted according to response, max. 100 micrograms/kg in caesarian section, alternatively (by intravenous infusion) maintenance 0.8–1.4 micrograms/kg/minute, adjusted according to response

DOSES AT EXTREMES OF BODY-WEIGHT
▸ To avoid excessive dosage in obese patients, dose should be calculated on the basis of ideal bodyweight.

● INTERACTIONS → Appendix 1: neuromuscular blocking drugs, non-depolarising

● SIDE-EFFECTS
▸ **Rare or very rare** Angioedema · face oedema · hypersensitivity · paralysis · rash erythematous

● HEPATIC IMPAIRMENT Use with caution in significant impairment.

● RENAL IMPAIRMENT Use with caution.

● DIRECTIONS FOR ADMINISTRATION Reconstitute each vial with 5 mL Water for Injections to give 2 mg/mL solution; *alternatively* reconstitute with up to 10 mL Glucose 5% *or* Sodium Chloride 0.9% *or* Water for Injections—unsuitable for further dilution if not reconstituted with Water for Injections. For *continuous intravenous infusion*, dilute reconstituted solution to a concentration up to 40 micrograms/mL with Glucose 5% or Sodium Chloride 0.9%; reconstituted solution can also be given via drip tubing.

● MEDICINAL FORMS
No licensed medicines listed.

1.2 Neuromuscular blockade reversal

Neuromuscular blockade reversal

Neuromuscular blockade reversal

Anticholinesterases
Anticholinesterases reverse the effects of the non-depolarising (competitive) neuromuscular blocking drugs such as pancuronium bromide but they prolong the action of the depolarising neuromuscular blocking drug suxamethonium chloride.

Neostigmine is used specifically for reversal of non-depolarising (competitive) blockade. It acts within one minute of intravenous injection and its effects last for 20 to 30 minutes; a second dose may then be necessary. Glycopyrronium bromide p. 1296 or alternatively atropine sulfate p. 1295, given before or with neostigmine, prevent bradycardia, excessive salivation, and other muscarinic effects of neostigmine.

Other drugs for reversal of neuromuscular blockade
Sugammadex p. 1301 is a modified gamma cyclodextrin that can be used for rapid reversal of neuromuscular blockade induced by rocuronium bromide or vecuronium bromide. In

practice, sugammadex is used mainly for rapid reversal of neuromuscular blockade in an emergency.

ANTICHOLINESTERASES

Neostigmine with glycopyrronium bromide

The properties listed below are those particular to the combination only. For the properties of the components please consider, neostigmine p. 1090, glycopyrronium bromide p. 246.

● INDICATIONS AND DOSE

Reversal of non-depolarising neuromuscular blockade

▸ BY INTRAVENOUS INJECTION
▸ Adult: 1–2 mL, repeated if necessary, alternatively 0.02 mL/kilogram, repeated if necessary; maximum 2 mL per course

● INTERACTIONS → Appendix 1: glycopyrronium · neostigmine

● DIRECTIONS FOR ADMINISTRATION For *intravenous injection*, give over 10–30 seconds.

● MEDICINAL FORMS
There can be variation in the licensing of different medicines containing the same drug.
Solution for injection
▸ Neostigmine with glycopyrronium bromide (Non-proprietary)
Glycopyrronium bromide 500 microgram per 1 mL, Neostigmine metilsulfate 2.5 mg per 1 mL Neostigmine 2.5mg/1ml / Glycopyrronium bromide 500micrograms/1ml solution for injection ampoules | 10 ampoule PoM £11.50

ANTIDOTES AND CHELATORS

Sugammadex

● INDICATIONS AND DOSE

Routine reversal of neuromuscular blockade induced by rocuronium or vecuronium

▸ BY INTRAVENOUS INJECTION
▸ Adult: Initially 2–4 mg/kg, then 4 mg/kg if required, administered if recurrence of neuromuscular blockade occurs; consult product literature for further details

Immediate reversal of neuromuscular blockade induced by rocuronium

▸ BY INTRAVENOUS INJECTION
▸ Adult: 16 mg/kg (consult product literature)

IMPORTANT SAFETY INFORMATION
Should only be administered by, or under the direct supervision of, personnel experienced in its use.

● CAUTIONS Cardiovascular disease (recovery may be delayed) · elderly (recovery may be delayed) · pre-existing coagulation disorders · recurrence of neuromuscular blockade— monitor respiratory function until fully recovered · use of anticoagulants (unrelated to surgery) · wait 24 hours before re-administering rocuronium · wait 24 hours before re-administering vecuronium

● INTERACTIONS → Appendix 1: sugammadex

● SIDE-EFFECTS
▸ Common or very common Abdominal pain · arrhythmias · cough · dizziness · headache · nausea · skin reactions · taste altered · vomiting
▸ Uncommon Hypersensitivity
▸ Frequency not known Bronchospasm

● PREGNANCY Use with caution—no information available.

● RENAL IMPAIRMENT Avoid if eGFR less than 30 mL/minute/1.73 m^2.

● NATIONAL FUNDING/ACCESS DECISIONS
Scottish Medicines Consortium (SMC) Decisions
The *Scottish Medicines Consortium*, has advised (February 2013) that sugammadex (*Bridion*®) is accepted for restricted use within NHS Scotland for the routine reversal of neuromuscular blockade in high-risk patients only, or where prompt reversal of neuromuscular block is required.

● MEDICINAL FORMS
There can be variation in the licensing of different medicines containing the same drug.
Solution for injection
ELECTROLYTES: May contain Sodium
▸ Bridion (Merck Sharp & Dohme Ltd)
Sugammadex (as Sugammadex sodium) 100 mg per 1 mL Bridion 500mg/5ml solution for injection vials | 10 vial PoM £1,491.00 (Hospital only)
Bridion 200mg/2ml solution for injection vials | 10 vial PoM £596.40 (Hospital only)

1.3 Peri-operative analgesia

Peri-operative analgesia

Non-opioid analgesics

Since non-steroidal anti-inflammatory drugs (NSAIDs) do not depress respiration, do not impair gastro-intestinal motility, and do not cause dependence, they may be useful alternatives or adjuncts to opioids for the relief of postoperative pain. NSAIDs may be inadequate for the relief of severe pain. Acemetacin p. 1097, diclofenac sodium p. 1101, diclofenac potassium p. 1100, flurbiprofen p. 1106, ibuprofen p. 1106, ketoprofen p. 1110, paracetamol p. 438, parecoxib p. 1303, and ketorolac trometamol p. 1144 are licensed for postoperative use. Diclofenac and paracetamol can be given by injection as well as by mouth. Diclofenac sodium can be given by intravenous infusion for the treatment or prevention of postoperative pain. Intramuscular injections of diclofenac sodium and ketoprofen are rarely used; they are given deep into the gluteal muscle to minimise pain and tissue damage. Ketorolac trometamol is less irritant on intramuscular injection but pain has been reported; it can also be given by intravenous injection.

Suppositories of diclofenac sodium and ketoprofen may be effective alternatives to the parenteral use of these drugs.

Opioid analgesics

Opioid analgesics are now rarely used as premedicants; they are more likely to be administered at induction. Pre-operative use of opioid analgesics is generally limited to those patients who require control of existing pain. See general notes on opioid analgesics and their use in postoperative pain.

See the management of opioid-induced respiratory depression in Pre-medication and peri-operative drugs p. 1294.

Intra-operative analgesia

Opioid analgesics given in small doses before or with induction reduce the dose requirement of some drugs used during anaesthesia.

Alfentanil p. 1304, fentanyl p. 451, and remifentanil p. 1304 are particularly useful because they act within 1–2 minutes and have short durations of action. The initial doses of alfentanil or fentanyl are followed either by successive intravenous injections or by an intravenous infusion; prolonged infusions increase the duration of effect. Repeated intra-operative doses of alfentanil or fentanyl should be given with care since the resulting respiratory depression can persist postoperatively and occasionally it may become apparent for the first time postoperatively when monitoring of the patient might be less intensive. Alfentanil, fentanyl, and remifentanil can cause muscle rigidity, particularly of the chest wall or jaw; this can be managed by the use of neuromuscular blocking drugs.

In contrast to other opioids which are metabolised in the liver, remifentanil undergoes rapid metabolism by nonspecific blood and tissue esterases; its short duration of action allows prolonged administration at high dosage, without accumulation, and with little risk of residual postoperative respiratory depression. Remifentanil should not be given by intravenous injection intraoperatively, but it is well suited to continuous infusion; a supplementary analgesic is given before stopping the infusion of remifentanil.

ANAESTHETICS, LOCAL

Bupivacaine with fentanyl

The properties listed below are those particular to the combination only. For the properties of the components please consider, bupivacaine hydrochloride p. 1309, fentanyl p. 451.

- **INDICATIONS AND DOSE**

  During labour (once epidural block established)
  ▸ BY CONTINUOUS LUMBAR EPIDURAL INFUSION
  ▸ Adult: 10–18.75 mg/hour, dose of bupivacaine to be administered, maximum 400 mg bupivacaine in 24 hours and 16–30 micrograms/hour, dose of fentanyl to be administered, maximum 720 micrograms fentanyl in 24 hours

  Postoperative pain (once epidural block established)
  ▸ BY CONTINUOUS EPIDURAL INFUSION
  ▸ Adult: 4–18.75 mg/hour, dose of bupivacaine to be administered, maximum 400 mg bupivacaine in 24 hours and 8–30 micrograms/hour, dose of fentanyl to be administered, maximum 720 micrograms fentanyl in 24 hours, to be administered by thoracic, upper abdominal or lower abdominal epidural infusion

- **INTERACTIONS** → Appendix 1: anaesthetics, local · opioids

- **MEDICINAL FORMS**
  There can be variation in the licensing of different medicines containing the same drug. Forms available from special-order manufacturers include: infusion, solution for infusion

  Solution for infusion
  ▸ Bufyl (AMCo)
  Fentanyl 2 microgram per 1 ml, Bupivacaine hydrochloride 1 mg per 1 ml Bufyl 1mg/ml and 2micrograms/ml 500ml infusion bags | 10 bag [PoM] £92.00 (Hospital only) [CD2]
  Bufyl 1mg/ml and 2micrograms/ml 250ml infusion bags | 20 bag [PoM] £170.00 (Hospital only) [CD2]
  Fentanyl (as Fentanyl citrate) 2 microgram per 1 ml, Bupivacaine hydrochloride 1.25 mg per 1 ml Bufyl 1.25mg/ml and 2micrograms/ml 250ml infusion bags | 20 bag [PoM] £181.00 (Hospital only) [CD2]
  Bufyl 1.25mg/ml and 2micrograms/ml 500ml infusion bags | 10 bag [PoM] £92.00 (Hospital only) [CD2]

ANALGESICS › NON-STEROIDAL ANTI-INFLAMMATORY DRUGS

Ketorolac trometamol

- **INDICATIONS AND DOSE**

  Short-term management of moderate to severe acute postoperative pain only
  ▸ BY INTRAMUSCULAR INJECTION, OR BY INTRAVENOUS INJECTION
  ▸ Adult (body-weight up to 50 kg): Initially 10 mg, then 10–30 mg every 4–6 hours as required for maximum duration of treatment 2 days, frequency may be increased to up to every 2 hours during initial postoperative period; maximum 60 mg per day
  ▸ Adult (body-weight 50 kg and above): Initially 10 mg, then 10–30 mg every 4–6 hours as required for maximum duration of treatment 2 days, frequency may be increased to up to every 2 hours during initial postoperative period; maximum 90 mg per day
  ▸ Elderly: Initially 10 mg, then 10–30 mg every 4–6 hours as required for maximum duration of treatment 2 days, frequency may be increased to up to every 2 hours during initial postoperative period; maximum 60 mg per day

- **CONTRA-INDICATIONS** Active or history of gastro-intestinal bleeding · active or history of gastro-intestinal ulceration · coagulation disorders · complete or partial syndrome of nasal polyps · confirmed or suspected cerebrovascular bleeding · dehydration · following operations with high risk of haemorrhage or incomplete haemostasis · haemorrhagic diatheses · history of gastro-intestinal perforation · hypovolaemia · severe heart failure

- **CAUTIONS** Allergic disorders · cardiac impairment (NSAIDs may impair renal function) · cerebrovascular disease · coagulation defects · connective-tissue disorders · Crohn's disease (may be exacerbated) · elderly (risk of serious side-effects and fatalities) · heart failure · ischaemic heart disease · peripheral arterial disease · risk factors for cardiovascular events · ulcerative colitis (may be exacerbated) · uncontrolled hypertension

- **INTERACTIONS** → Appendix 1: NSAIDs

- **SIDE-EFFECTS** Agranulocytosis · angioedema · anxiety · aplastic anaemia · appetite decreased · asthenia · asthma · azotaemia · bradycardia · burping · chest pain · concentration impaired · confusion · constipation · Crohn's disease aggravated · depression · diarrhoea · dizziness · drowsiness · dry mouth · dyspnoea · electrolyte imbalance · embolism and thrombosis · euphoric mood · fever · flank pain · fluid retention · flushing · gastrointestinal discomfort · gastrointestinal disorders · haemolytic anaemia · haemorrhage · hallucination · headache · hearing impairment · heart failure · hepatic disorders · hyperhidrosis · hyperkinesia · hypersensitivity · hypertension · hypotension · infertility female · malaise · meningitis aseptic (patients with connective-tissue disorders such as systemic lupus erythematosus may be especially susceptible) · musculoskeletal disorder · myalgia · myocardial infarction · nausea · nephritis tubulointerstitial · nephropathy · neutropenia · oedema · optic neuritis · oral disorders · pallor · palpitations · pancreatitis · paraesthesia · perforation · photosensitivity reaction · platelet aggregation inhibition · psychotic disorder · pulmonary oedema · renal impairment · respiratory disorders · seizure · severe cutaneous adverse reactions (SCARs) · skin reactions · sleep disorders · stroke · taste altered · thinking abnormal · thirst · thrombocytopenia · ulcer · urinary disorders · vertigo · visual impairment · vomiting · weight increased · wound haemorrhage

SIDE-EFFECTS, FURTHER INFORMATION For information about cardiovascular and gastrointestinal side-effects, and a possible exacerbation of symptoms in asthma, see Non-steroidal anti-inflammatory drugs p. 1094.

● ALLERGY AND CROSS-SENSITIVITY Contra-indicated in patients with a history of hypersensitivity to aspirin or any other NSAID—which includes those in whom attacks of asthma, angioedema, urticaria or rhinitis have been precipitated by aspirin or any other NSAID.

● CONCEPTION AND CONTRACEPTION Caution—long-term use of some NSAIDs is associated with reduced female fertility, which is reversible on stopping treatment.

● PREGNANCY Avoid unless the potential benefit outweighs the risk. Avoid during the third trimester (risk of closure of fetal ductus arteriosus *in utero* and possibly persistent pulmonary hypertension of the newborn); onset of labour may be delayed and duration may be increased.

● BREAST FEEDING Amount too small to be harmful.

● HEPATIC IMPAIRMENT Use with caution; there is an increased risk of gastro-intestinal bleeding and fluid retention. Avoid in severe liver disease.

● RENAL IMPAIRMENT Avoid if possible or use with caution. Avoid if serum creatinine greater than 160 micromol/litre.
Dose adjustments The lowest effective dose should be used for the shortest possible duration. Max. 60 mg daily by intramuscular injection or intravenous injection.
Monitoring In renal impairment monitor renal function; sodium and water retention may occur and renal function may deteriorate, possibly leading to renal failure.

● DIRECTIONS FOR ADMINISTRATION For *intravenous injection*, give over at least 15 seconds.

● MEDICINAL FORMS
There can be variation in the licensing of different medicines containing the same drug.
Solution for injection
▸ Ketorolac trometamol (Non-proprietary)
Ketorolac trometamol 30 mg per 1 ml Ketorolac 30mg/1ml solution for injection ampoules | 5 ampoule PoM £4.00 (Hospital only) | 5 ampoule PoM £4.00 | 6 ampoule PoM £6.56
▸ Toradol (Atnahs Pharma UK Ltd)
Ketorolac trometamol 30 mg per 1 ml Toradol 30mg/1ml solution for injection ampoules | 5 ampoule PoM £5.36

Parecoxib

● DRUG ACTION Parecoxib is a selective inhibitor of cyclo-oxygenase-2.

● INDICATIONS AND DOSE
Short-term management of acute postoperative pain
▸ BY DEEP INTRAMUSCULAR INJECTION, OR BY INTRAVENOUS INJECTION
▸ Adult: Initially 40 mg, then 20–40 mg every 6–12 hours as required for up to 3 days; maximum 80 mg per day
▸ Elderly (body-weight up to 50 kg): Initially 20 mg; maximum 40 mg per day

● CONTRA-INDICATIONS Active gastro-intestinal bleeding · active gastro-intestinal ulceration · cerebrovascular disease · inflammatory bowel disease · ischaemic heart disease · mild to severe heart failure · peripheral arterial disease

● CAUTIONS Allergic disorders · cardiac impairment (NSAIDs may impair renal function) · coagulation defects · connective-tissue disorders · Crohn's disease (may be exacerbated) · dehydration · elderly (risk of serious side-effects and fatalities) · following coronary artery bypass graft surgery · history of cardiac failure · hypertension · left ventricular dysfunction · oedema · risk factors for cardiovascular events · ulcerative colitis (may be exacerbated)

● INTERACTIONS → Appendix 1: NSAIDs
● SIDE-EFFECTS
▸ **Common or very common** Agitation · back pain · constipation · dizziness · gastrointestinal discomfort · gastrointestinal disorders · hyperhidrosis · hypertension · hypokalaemia · hypotension · increased risk of infection · insomnia · nausea · numbness · peripheral oedema · post procedural complications · renal impairment · respiratory disorders · skin reactions · vomiting
▸ **Uncommon** Appetite decreased · arrhythmias · arthralgia · asthenia · cerebrovascular insufficiency · dry mouth · ear pain · embolism and thrombosis · hyperglycaemia · myocardial infarction · thrombocytopenia
▸ **Rare or very rare** Hypersensitivity · pancreatitis · perioral swelling
▸ **Frequency not known** Angioedema · cardiovascular event · circulatory collapse · congestive heart failure · dyspnoea · hepatitis · renal failure (more common in patients with pre-existing renal impairment) · severe cutaneous adverse reactions (SCARs)

SIDE-EFFECTS, FURTHER INFORMATION For information about cardiovascular and gastrointestinal side-effects, and a possible exacerbation of symptoms in asthma, see Non-steroidal anti-inflammatory drugs p. 1094.

● ALLERGY AND CROSS-SENSITIVITY Contra-indicated in patients with a history of hypersensitivity to aspirin or any other NSAID—which includes those in whom attacks of asthma, angioedema, urticaria or rhinitis have been precipitated by aspirin or any other NSAID. Contra-indicated in patients with a history of allergic drug reactions including sulfonamide hypersensitivity.

● CONCEPTION AND CONTRACEPTION Caution—long-term use of some NSAIDs is associated with reduced female fertility, which is reversible on stopping treatment.

● PREGNANCY Avoid unless the potential benefit outweighs the risk. Avoid during the third trimester (risk of closure of fetal ductus arteriosus *in utero* and possibly persistent pulmonary hypertension of the newborn); onset of labour may be delayed and duration may be increased.

● BREAST FEEDING Avoid—present in milk.

● HEPATIC IMPAIRMENT Use with caution; there is an increased risk of gastro-intestinal bleeding and fluid retention. Avoid in severe liver disease.
Dose adjustments Halve dose in moderate impairment (max. 40 mg daily).

● RENAL IMPAIRMENT Avoid if possible or use with caution.
Dose adjustments The lowest effective dose should be used for the shortest possible duration.
Monitoring In renal impairment monitor renal function; sodium and water retention may occur and renal function may deteriorate, possibly leading to renal failure.

● NATIONAL FUNDING/ACCESS DECISIONS
Scottish Medicines Consortium (SMC) Decisions
The *Scottish Medicines Consortium* has advised (January 2003) that parecoxib is **not** recommended for use within NHS Scotland.

● MEDICINAL FORMS
There can be variation in the licensing of different medicines containing the same drug.
Powder and solvent for solution for injection
▸ Dynastat (Pfizer Ltd)
Parecoxib (as Parecoxib sodium) 40 mg Dynastat 40mg powder and solvent for solution for injection vials | 5 vial PoM £28.34
Powder for solution for injection
▸ Dynastat (Pfizer Ltd)
Parecoxib (as Parecoxib sodium) 40 mg Dynastat 40mg powder for solution for injection vials | 10 vial PoM £49.60

15

Anaesthesia

ANALGESICS > OPIOIDS

F 441

Alfentanil

● INDICATIONS AND DOSE

Spontaneous respiration: analgesia and enhancement of anaesthesia for short procedures
▸ BY INTRAVENOUS INJECTION
▸ Adult: Initially up to 500 micrograms, dose to be administered over 30 seconds; supplemental doses 250 micrograms

Assisted ventilation: analgesia and enhancement of anaesthesia for short procedures
▸ BY INTRAVENOUS INJECTION
▸ Adult: Initially 30–50 micrograms/kg, supplemental doses 15 micrograms/kg

Assisted ventilation: analgesia and enhancement of anaesthesia during maintenance of anaesthesia for longer procedures
▸ BY INTRAVENOUS INFUSION
▸ Adult: Initially 50–100 micrograms/kg, dose to be administered over 10 minutes or as a bolus, followed by maintenance 30–60 micrograms/kg/hour

Assisted ventilation: analgesia and suppression of respiratory activity during intensive care for up to 4 days
▸ BY INTRAVENOUS INFUSION
▸ Adult: Initially 2 mg/hour, adjusted according to response; usual dose 0.5–10 mg/hour, alternatively initially 5 mg in divided doses, to be administered over 10 minutes; dose used for more rapid initial control, reduce rate of administration if hypotension or bradycardia occur; additional doses of 0.5–1 mg may be given by intravenous injection during short painful procedures

DOSES AT EXTREMES OF BODY-WEIGHT
▸ To avoid excessive dosage in obese patients, dose should be calculated on the basis of ideal body-weight.

● CAUTIONS
CAUTIONS, FURTHER INFORMATION
▸ Repeated intra-operative doses Repeated intra-operative doses of alfentanil should be given with care since the resulting respiratory depression can persist postoperatively and occasionally it may become apparent for the first time postoperatively when monitoring of the patient might be less intensive.

● INTERACTIONS → Appendix 1: opioids

● SIDE-EFFECTS
▸ **Common or very common** Apnoea · chills · fatigue · hypertension · movement disorders · muscle rigidity
▸ **Uncommon** Arrhythmia · coma · hiccups · hypercapnia · pain · post procedural complications · respiratory disorders · skin reactions
▸ **Rare or very rare** Agitation · crying · epistaxis · vascular pain
▸ **Frequency not known** Cardiac arrest · cough · disorientation · fever · loss of consciousness · seizure

SIDE-EFFECTS, FURTHER INFORMATION Alfentanil can cause muscle rigidity, particularly of the chest wall or jaw; this can be managed by the use of neuromuscular blocking drugs.

● BREAST FEEDING Present in milk—withhold breast-feeding for 24 hours.

● RENAL IMPAIRMENT Avoid use or reduce dose; opioid effects increased and prolonged and increased cerebral sensitivity occurs.

● DIRECTIONS FOR ADMINISTRATION 5 mg/mL injection to be diluted before use. For *continuous or intermittent*

intravenous infusion dilute in Glucose 5% *or* Sodium Chloride 0.9%.

● MEDICINAL FORMS
There can be variation in the licensing of different medicines containing the same drug. Forms available from special-order manufacturers include: solution for injection
Solution for injection
▸ Alfentanil (Non-proprietary)
Alfentanil (as Alfentanil hydrochloride) 500 microgram per 1 ml Alfentanil 1mg/2ml solution for injection ampoules | 10 ampoule PoM £5.95 CD2
Alfentanil 25mg/50ml solution for injection vials | 1 vial PoM £14.90 CD2
Alfentanil 5mg/10ml solution for injection ampoules | 5 ampoule PoM £13.90 CD2
Alfentanil (as Alfentanil hydrochloride) 5 mg per 1 ml Alfentanil 5mg/1ml solution for injection ampoules | 10 ampoule PoM £21.95 DT = £23.19 CD2
▸ Rapifen (Piramal Critical Care Ltd)
Alfentanil (as Alfentanil hydrochloride) 500 microgram per 1 ml Rapifen 5mg/10ml solution for injection ampoules | 5 ampoule PoM £14.50 CD2
Rapifen 1mg/2ml solution for injection ampoules | 10 ampoule PoM £6.34 CD2
Alfentanil (as Alfentanil hydrochloride) 5 mg per 1 ml Rapifen Intensive Care 5mg/1ml solution for injection ampoules | 10 ampoule PoM £23.19 DT = £23.19 (Hospital only) CD2

Papaveretum with hyoscine hydrobromide

The properties listed below are those particular to the combination only. For the properties of the components please consider, papaveretum p. 462, hyoscine hydrobromide p. 433.

● INDICATIONS AND DOSE
Premedication
▸ BY SUBCUTANEOUS INJECTION, OR BY INTRAMUSCULAR INJECTION
▸ Adult: 0.5–1 mL

● INTERACTIONS → Appendix 1: hyoscine · opioids
● LESS SUITABLE FOR PRESCRIBING Hyoscine hydrobromide with papaveretum is less suitable for prescribing.

● MEDICINAL FORMS
No licensed medicines listed.

F 441

Remifentanil

● INDICATIONS AND DOSE
Analgesia and enhancement of anaesthesia at induction (initial bolus injection)
▸ BY INTRAVENOUS INJECTION
▸ Adult: Initially 0.25–1 microgram/kg, dose to be administered over at least 30 seconds, if patient is to be intubated more than 8 minutes after start of intravenous infusion, initial bolus intravenous injection dose is not necessary

Analgesia and enhancement of anaesthesia at induction with or without initial bolus dose
▸ BY INTRAVENOUS INFUSION
▸ Adult: 30–60 micrograms/kg/hour, if patient is to be intubated more than 8 minutes after start of intravenous infusion, initial bolus intravenous injection dose is not necessary

Assisted ventilation: analgesia and enhancement of anaesthesia during maintenance of anaesthesia (initial bolus injection)
▸ BY INTRAVENOUS INJECTION
▸ Adult: Initially 0.25–1 microgram/kg, dose to be administered over at least 30 seconds

Assisted ventilation: analgesia and enhancement of anaesthesia during maintenance of anaesthesia with or without initial bolus dose
▸ BY INTRAVENOUS INFUSION
▸ Adult: 3–120 micrograms/kg/hour, dose to be administered according to anaesthetic technique and adjusted according to response, in light anaesthesia additional doses can be given *by intravenous injection* every 2–5 minutes during the intravenous infusion

Spontaneous respiration: analgesia and enhancement of anaesthesia during maintenance of anaesthesia
▸ BY INTRAVENOUS INFUSION
▸ Adult: Initially 2.4 micrograms/kg/hour, adjusted according to response; usual dose 1.5–6 micrograms/kg/hour

Assisted ventilation: analgesia and sedation in intensive-care patients (for max 3 days)
▸ BY INTRAVENOUS INFUSION
▸ Adult: Initially 6–9 micrograms/kg/hour, then adjusted in steps of 1.5 micrograms/kg/hour, allow at least 5 minutes between dose adjustments; usual dose 0.36–44.4 micrograms/kg/hour, if an infusion rate of 12 micrograms/kg/hour does not produce adequate sedation add another sedative (consult product literature for details)

Assisted ventilation: additional analgesia during stimulating or painful procedures in intensive-care patients
▸ BY INTRAVENOUS INFUSION
▸ Adult: Usual dose 15–45 micrograms/kg/hour, maintain infusion rate of at least 6 micrograms/kg/hour for at least 5 minutes before procedure and adjust every 2–5 minutes according to requirements

Cardiac surgery
▸ Adult: (consult product literature)
DOSES AT EXTREMES OF BODY-WEIGHT
▸ To avoid excessive dosage in obese patients, dose should be calculated on the basis of ideal body-weight.

● UNLICENSED USE Remifentanil doses in BNF may differ from those in product literature.

● CONTRA-INDICATIONS Analgesia in conscious patients

● INTERACTIONS → Appendix 1: opioids

● SIDE-EFFECTS
▸ **Common or very common** Apnoea · muscle rigidity · post procedural complications
▸ **Uncommon** Hypoxia
▸ **Rare or very rare** Cardiac arrest
▸ **Frequency not known** Agitation · atrioventricular block · hypertension · seizure

SIDE-EFFECTS, FURTHER INFORMATION In contrast to other opioids which are metabolised in the liver, remifentanil undergoes rapid metabolism by plasma esterases; it has short duration of action which is independent of dose and duration of infusion.
Muscle rigidity Remifentanil can cause muscle rigidity that can be managed by the use of neuromuscular blocking drugs.

● PREGNANCY No information available.

● BREAST FEEDING Avoid breast-feeding for 24 hours after administration—present in milk in *animal* studies.

● RENAL IMPAIRMENT
Dose adjustments No dose adjustment necessary in renal impairment.

● DIRECTIONS FOR ADMINISTRATION
▸ With intravenous use For *intravenous infusion* (*Ultiva*®), give continuously in Glucose 5% or Sodium Chloride 0.9% or Water for Injections; reconstitute with infusion fluid to a concentration of 1 mg/mL then dilute further to a concentration of 20–250 micrograms/mL (50 micrograms/mL recommended for general anaesthesia, 20–50 micrograms/mL recommended when used with target controlled infusion (TCI) device).

● PRESCRIBING AND DISPENSING INFORMATION
Remifentanil should not be given by intravenous injection intra-operatively, but it is well suited to continuous infusion; a supplementary analgesic is given before stopping the infusion of remifentanil.

● MEDICINAL FORMS
There can be variation in the licensing of different medicines containing the same drug.
Powder for solution for injection
▸ Remifentanil (Non-proprietary)
 Remifentanil (as Remifentanil hydrochloride) 1 mg Remifentanil 1mg powder for concentrate for solution for injection vials | 5 vial [PoM] £25.60 (Hospital only) [CD2]
 Remifentanil (as Remifentanil hydrochloride) 2 mg Remifentanil 2mg powder for concentrate for solution for injection vials | 5 vial [PoM] £51.13 (Hospital only) [CD2]
 Remifentanil (as Remifentanil hydrochloride) 5 mg Remifentanil 5mg powder for concentrate for solution for injection vials | 5 vial [PoM] £127.90 (Hospital only) [CD2]
▸ Ultiva (Aspen Pharma Trading Ltd)
 Remifentanil (as Remifentanyl hydrochloride) 1 mg Ultiva 1mg powder for solution for injection vials | 5 vial [PoM] £25.58 (Hospital only) [CD2]
 Remifentanil (as Remifentanyl hydrochloride) 2 mg Ultiva 2mg powder for solution for injection vials | 5 vial [PoM] £51.15 (Hospital only) [CD2]
 Remifentanil (as Remifentanyl hydrochloride) 5 mg Ultiva 5mg powder for solution for injection vials | 5 vial [PoM] £127.88 (Hospital only) [CD2]

1.4 Peri-operative sedation

Conscious sedation for clinical procedures

Overview
Sedation of patients during diagnostic and therapeutic procedures is used to reduce fear and anxiety, to control pain, and to minimise excessive movement. The choice of sedative drug will depend upon the intended procedure; some procedures are safer and more successful under anaesthesia. The patient should be *monitored carefully*; monitoring should begin as soon as the sedative is given or when the patient becomes drowsy, and should be continued until the patient wakes up.

ANAESTHETICS, GENERAL > NMDA RECEPTOR ANTAGONISTS

Ketamine

● INDICATIONS AND DOSE
Induction and maintenance of anaesthesia for short procedures
▸ BY INTRAMUSCULAR INJECTION
▸ Adult: Initially 6.5–13 mg/kg, adjusted according to response, a dose of 10 mg/kg usually produces 12–25 minutes of surgical anaesthesia continued →

15

Anaesthesia

► BY INTRAVENOUS INJECTION
► Adult: Initially 1–4.5 mg/kg, adjusted according to response, to be administered over at least 60 seconds, a dose of 2 mg/kg usually produces 5–10 minutes of surgical anaesthesia

Diagnostic manoeuvres and procedures not involving intense pain
► BY INTRAMUSCULAR INJECTION
► Adult: Initially 4 mg/kg

Induction and maintenance of anaesthesia for long procedures
► BY INTRAVENOUS INFUSION
► Adult: Initially 0.5–2 mg/kg, using an infusion solution containing 1 mg/ml; maintenance 10–45 micrograms/kg/minute, adjusted according to response

---

IMPORTANT SAFETY INFORMATION
Ketamine should only be administered by, or under the direct supervision of, personnel experienced in its use, with adequate training in anaesthesia and airway management, and when resuscitation equipment is available.

● CONTRA-INDICATIONS Acute porphyrias p. 1025 · eclampsia · head trauma · hypertension · pre-eclampsia · raised intracranial pressure · severe cardiac disease · stroke
● CAUTIONS Acute circulatory failure (shock) · cardiovascular disease · dehydration · elderly · fixed cardiac output · hallucinations · head injury · hypertension · hypovolaemia · increased cerebrospinal fluid pressure · intracranial mass lesions · nightmares · predisposition to seizures · psychotic disorders · raised intra-ocular pressure · respiratory tract infection · thyroid dysfunction
● INTERACTIONS → Appendix 1: ketamine
● SIDE-EFFECTS
► **Common or very common** Anxiety · behaviour abnormal · confusion · diplopia · hallucination · muscle tone increased · nausea · nystagmus · skin reactions · sleep disorders · tonic clonic movements · vomiting
► **Uncommon** Appetite decreased · arrhythmias · hypotension · respiratory disorders
► **Rare or very rare** Apnoea · cystitis · cystitis haemorrhagic · delirium · dysphoria · flashback · hypersalivation
► **Frequency not known** Drug-induced liver injury
SIDE-EFFECTS, FURTHER INFORMATION Incidence of hallucinations can be reduced by premedication with a benzodiazepine (such as midazolam).
● PREGNANCY May depress neonatal respiration if used during delivery.
● BREAST FEEDING Avoid for at least 12 hours after last dose.
● HEPATIC IMPAIRMENT
Dose adjustments Consider dose reduction.
● DIRECTIONS FOR ADMINISTRATION For *continuous intravenous infusion*, dilute to a concentration of 1 mg/mL with Glucose 5% *or* Sodium Chloride 0.9%; use microdrip infusion for maintenance of anaesthesia. For *intravenous injection*, dilute 100 mg/mL strength to a concentration of not more than 50 mg/mL with Glucose 5% *or* Sodium Chloride 0.9% *or* Water for Injections.
● PATIENT AND CARER ADVICE
Driving and skilled tasks Patients given sedatives and analgesics during minor outpatient procedures should be very carefully warned about the risk of driving or undertaking skilled tasks afterwards. For a short general anaesthetic the risk extends to **at least 24 hours** after administration. Responsible persons should be available to take patients home. The dangers of taking **alcohol** should also be emphasised.

For information on 2015 legislation regarding driving whilst taking certain controlled drugs, including ketamine, see *Drugs and driving* under Guidance on prescribing p. 1.

● MEDICINAL FORMS
There can be variation in the licensing of different medicines containing the same drug. Forms available from special-order manufacturers include: solution for injection
Solution for injection
► Ketamine (Non-proprietary)
  Ketamine (as Ketamine hydrochloride) 50 mg per 1 ml Ketamine 500mg/10ml solution for injection vials | 10 vial [PoM] £70.00 [CD2]
  Ketamin 100mg/2ml solution for injection ampoules | 10 ampoule [PoM] [℥] [CD2]
► Ketalar (Pfizer Ltd)
  Ketamine (as Ketamine hydrochloride) 10 mg per 1 ml Ketalar 200mg/20ml solution for injection vials | 1 vial [PoM] £5.06 (Hospital only) [CD2]
  Ketamine (as Ketamine hydrochloride) 50 mg per 1 ml Ketalar 500mg/10ml solution for injection vials | 1 vial [PoM] £8.77 (Hospital only) [CD2]

HYPNOTICS, SEDATIVES AND ANXIOLYTICS >
NON-BENZODIAZEPINE HYPNOTICS AND SEDATIVES

Dexmedetomidine

● INDICATIONS AND DOSE
Maintenance of sedation during intensive care
► BY INTRAVENOUS INFUSION
► Adult: 0.7 microgram/kg/hour, adjusted according to response; usual dose 0.2–1.4 micrograms/kg/hour

---

IMPORTANT SAFETY INFORMATION
Dexmedetomidine should only be administered by, or under the direct supervision of, personnel experienced in its use, with adequate training in anaesthesia and airway management.

● CONTRA-INDICATIONS Acute cerebrovascular disorders · second- or third-degree AV block (unless pacemaker fitted) · uncontrolled hypotension
● CAUTIONS Abrupt withdrawal after prolonged use · bradycardia · ischaemic heart disease · malignant hyperthermia · severe cerebrovascular disease (especially at higher doses) · severe neurological disorders · spinal cord injury
● INTERACTIONS → Appendix 1: dexmedetomidine
● SIDE-EFFECTS
► **Common or very common** Agitation · arrhythmias · dry mouth · hyperglycaemia · hypertension · hyperthermia · hypoglycaemia · hypotension · myocardial infarction · myocardial ischaemia · nausea · respiratory depression · vomiting
► **Uncommon** Abdominal distension · apnoea · atrioventricular block · drug ineffective · dyspnoea · hallucination · hypoalbuminaemia · metabolic acidosis · thirst
● PREGNANCY Manufacturer advises avoid unless potential benefit outweighs risk—toxicity in *animal* studies.
● BREAST FEEDING Manufacturer advises avoid unless potential benefit outweighs risk—present in milk in *animal* studies.
● HEPATIC IMPAIRMENT Manufacturer advises caution.
Dose adjustments Dose reduction may be required.
● MONITORING REQUIREMENTS
► Monitor cardiac function.
► Monitor respiratory function in non-intubated patients.
● DIRECTIONS FOR ADMINISTRATION To be diluted before use. For *intravenous infusion* given continuously in Glucose

5% or Sodium chloride 0.9%, dilute to a concentration of 4 micrograms/mL.

- **MEDICINAL FORMS**
  There can be variation in the licensing of different medicines containing the same drug.
  Solution for infusion
  ▸ Dexdor (Orion Pharma (UK) Ltd)
    Dexmedetomidine (as Dexmedetomidine hydrochloride)
    100 microgram per 1 ml Dexdor 1mg/10ml concentrate for solution for infusion vials | 4 vial PoM £313.20 (Hospital only)
    Dexdor 400micrograms/4ml concentrate for solution for infusion vials | 4 vial PoM £125.28 (Hospital only)
    Dexdor 200micrograms/2ml concentrate for solution for infusion ampoules | 5 ampoule PoM £78.30 (Hospital only) | 25 ampoule PoM £391.50 (Hospital only)

2   Malignant hyperthermia

MUSCLE RELAXANTS > DIRECTLY ACTING

Dantrolene sodium

- **DRUG ACTION** Acts on skeletal muscle cells by interfering with calcium efflux, thereby stopping the contractile process.

  - **INDICATIONS AND DOSE**
  Malignant hyperthermia
  ▸ BY RAPID INTRAVENOUS INJECTION
  ▸ Adult: Initially 2–3 mg/kg, then 1 mg/kg, repeated if necessary; maximum 10 mg/kg per course
  Chronic severe spasticity of voluntary muscle
  ▸ BY MOUTH
  ▸ Adult: Initially 25 mg daily, then increased to up to 100 mg 4 times a day, dose increased at weekly intervals; usual dose 75 mg 3 times a day

  > **IMPORTANT SAFETY INFORMATION**
  > Should only be administered by, or under the direct supervision of, personnel experienced in the use of dantrolene when used for malignant hyperthermia.

- **CONTRA-INDICATIONS**
  ▸ With oral use Acute muscle spasm · avoid when spasticity is useful, for example, locomotion
- **CAUTIONS**
  ▸ With intravenous use Avoid extravasation (risk of tissue necrosis)
  ▸ With oral use Females (hepatotoxicity) · history of liver disorders (hepatotoxicity) · if doses greater than 400 mg daily (hepatotoxicity) · impaired cardiac function · impaired pulmonary function · patients over 30 years (hepatotoxicity) · therapeutic effect may take a few weeks to develop— discontinue if no response within 6–8 weeks
- **INTERACTIONS** → Appendix 1: dantrolene
- **SIDE-EFFECTS**
  GENERAL SIDE-EFFECTS
  ▸ **Common or very common** Abdominal pain · hepatic disorders · nausea · respiratory disorders · skin reactions · speech disorder · vomiting
  ▸ **Uncommon** Crystalluria · hyperhidrosis
  ▸ **Frequency not known** Arrhythmias · dizziness · drowsiness
  SPECIFIC SIDE-EFFECTS
  ▸ **Common or very common**
  ▸ With oral use Appetite decreased · chills · confusion · depression · eosinophilia · fever · headache · insomnia · nervousness · pericarditis · visual impairment
  ▸ **Uncommon**
  ▸ With oral use Constipation · dysphagia · haemorrhage · heart failure aggravated · urinary disorders

▸ **Frequency not known**
▸ With intravenous use Gastrointestinal haemorrhage · heart failure · pulmonary oedema · seizure
▸ With oral use Asthenia · diarrhoea · dyspnoea · hypertension · malaise
- **PREGNANCY**
  ▸ With intravenous use Use only if potential benefit outweighs risk.
  ▸ With oral use Avoid use in chronic spasticity—embryotoxic in *animal* studies.
- **BREAST FEEDING**
  ▸ With intravenous use Present in milk—use only if potential benefit outweighs risk.
  ▸ With oral use Present in milk—manufacturer advises avoid use in chronic spasticity.
- **HEPATIC IMPAIRMENT** Avoid—may cause severe liver damage (injection may be used in an emergency for malignant hyperthermia).
- **MONITORING REQUIREMENTS**
  ▸ With oral use Test liver function before and at intervals during therapy.
- **PATIENT AND CARER ADVICE**
  Hepatotoxicity ▸ With oral use Patients should be told how to recognise signs of liver disorder and advised to seek prompt medical attention if symptoms such as anorexia, nausea, vomiting, fatigue, abdominal pain, dark urine, or pruritus develop.
  Driving and skilled tasks ▸ With oral use Drowsiness may affect performance of skilled tasks (e.g. driving); effects of alcohol enhanced.
- **MEDICINAL FORMS**
  There can be variation in the licensing of different medicines containing the same drug. Forms available from special-order manufacturers include: oral suspension, oral solution
  Powder for solution for injection
  ▸ Dantrium (Norgine Pharmaceuticals Ltd)
    Dantrolene sodium 20 mg Dantrium Intravenous 20mg powder for solution for injection vials | 12 vial PoM £612.00 (Hospital only) | 36 vial PoM £1,836.00 (Hospital only)
  Capsule
  CAUTIONARY AND ADVISORY LABELS 2
  ▸ Dantrium (Norgine Pharmaceuticals Ltd)
    Dantrolene sodium 25 mg Dantrium 25mg capsules | 100 capsule PoM £16.87 DT = £16.87
    Dantrolene sodium 100 mg Dantrium 100mg capsules | 100 capsule PoM £43.07 DT = £43.07

Local anaesthesia

Anaesthesia (local)

Local anaesthetic drugs

The use of local anaesthetics by injection or by application to mucous membranes to produce local analgesia is discussed in this section.

Local anaesthetic drugs act by causing a reversible block to conduction along nerve fibres. They vary widely in their potency, toxicity, duration of action, stability, solubility in water, and ability to penetrate mucous membranes. These factors determine their application, e.g. topical (surface), infiltration, peripheral nerve block, intravenous regional anaesthesia (Bier's block), plexus, epidural (extradural), or spinal (intrathecal or subarachnoid) block. Local anaesthetics may also be used for postoperative pain relief, thereby reducing the need for analgesics such as opioids.

Bupivacaine hydrochloride p. 1309 has a longer duration of action than other local anaesthetics. It has a slow onset of action, taking up to 30 minutes for full effect. It is often used in lumbar epidural blockade and is particularly suitable for continuous epidural analgesia in labour, or for postoperative pain relief. It is the principal drug used for spinal anaesthesia. Hyperbaric solutions containing glucose may be used for spinal block.

Levobupivacaine p. 1311, an isomer of bupivacaine, has anaesthetic and analgesic properties similar to bupivacaine hydrochloride, but is thought to have fewer adverse effects.

Lidocaine hydrochloride p. 1312 is effectively absorbed from mucous membranes and is a useful surface anaesthetic in concentrations up to 10%. Except for surface anaesthesia and dental anaesthesia, solutions should **not** usually exceed 1% in strength. The duration of the block (with adrenaline/epinephrine p. 221) is about 90 minutes.

Prilocaine hydrochloride p. 1316 is a local anaesthetic of low toxicity which is similar to lidocaine hydrochloride. A hyperbaric solution of prilocaine hydrochloride (containing glucose) may be used for spinal anaesthesia.

Ropivacaine hydrochloride p. 1317 is an amide-type local anaesthetic agent similar to bupivacaine hydrochloride. It is less cardiotoxic than bupivacaine hydrochloride, but also less potent.

Tetracaine p. 1318, a para-aminobenzoic acid ester, is an effective local anaesthetic for topical application; a 4% gel is indicated for anaesthesia before venepuncture or venous cannulation. It is rapidly absorbed from mucous membranes and should **never** be applied to inflamed, traumatised, or highly vascular surfaces. It should never be used to provide anaesthesia for bronchoscopy or cystoscopy because lidocaine hydrochloride is a safer alternative.

Administration by injection

The dose of local anaesthetic depends on the injection site and the procedure used. In determining the safe dosage, it is important to take account of the rate of absorption and excretion, and of the potency. The patient's age, weight, physique, and clinical condition, and the vascularity of the administration site and the duration of administration, must also be considered.

Uptake of local anaesthetics into the systemic circulation determines their duration of action and produces toxicity.

NHS Improvement has advised (September 2016) that, prior to administration, all injectable medicines must be drawn directly from their original ampoule or container into a syringe and should **never** be decanted into gallipots or open containers. This is to avoid the risk of medicines being confused with other substances, e.g. skin disinfectants, and to reduce the risk of contamination.

Great care must be taken to avoid accidental intravascular injection; local anaesthetic injections should be given slowly in order to detect inadvertent intravascular administration. When prolonged analgesia is required, a long-acting local anaesthetic is preferred to minimise the likelihood of cumulative systemic toxicity. Local anaesthesia around the oral cavity may impair swallowing and therefore increases the risk of aspiration.

Epidural anaesthesia is commonly used during surgery, often combined with general anaesthesia, because of its protective effect against the stress response of surgery. It is often used when good postoperative pain relief is essential.

Vasoconstrictors in combination with local anaesthetics

Local anaesthetics cause dilatation of blood vessels. The addition of a vasoconstrictor such as adrenaline/epinephrine to the local anaesthetic preparation diminishes local blood flow, slowing the rate of absorption and thereby prolonging the anaesthetic effect. Great care should be taken to avoid inadvertent intravenous administration of a preparation containing adrenaline/epinephrine, and it is **not** advisable to give adrenaline/epinephrine with a local anaesthetic injection in digits or appendages because of the risk of ischaemic necrosis.

Adrenaline/epinephrine must be used in a low concentration when administered with a local anaesthetic. Care must also be taken to calculate a safe maximum dose of local anaesthetic when using combination products.

In patients with severe hypertension or unstable cardiac rhythm, the use of adrenaline/epinephrine with a local anaesthetic may be hazardous. For these patients an anaesthetic without adrenaline/epinephrine should be used.

Dental anaesthesia

Lidocaine hydrochloride is widely used in dental procedures; it is most often used in combination with adrenaline/epinephrine. Lidocaine hydrochloride 2% combined with adrenaline/epinephrine 1 in 80 000 (12.5 micrograms/mL) is a safe and effective preparation; there is no justification for using higher concentrations of adrenaline/epinephrine.

The amide-type local anaesthetics **articaine** and mepivacaine hydrochloride p. 1315 are also used in dentistry; they are available in cartridges suitable for dental use. Mepivacaine hydrochloride is available with or without adrenaline/epinephrine and articaine is available with adrenaline.

In patients with severe hypertension or unstable cardiac rhythm, mepivacaine hydrochloride without adrenaline/epinephrine may be used. Alternatively, prilocaine hydrochloride with or without felypressin can be used but there is no evidence that it is any safer. Felypressin can cause coronary vasoconstriction when used at high doses; limit dose in patients with coronary artery disease.

Toxicity induced by local anaesthesia

For management of toxicity see Severe local anaesthetic-induced cardiovascular toxicity below.

Severe local anaesthetic-induced cardiovascular toxicity

Overview

After injection of a bolus of local anaesthetic, toxicity may develop at any time in the following hour. In the event of signs of toxicity during injection, the administration of the local anaesthetic must be stopped immediately.

Cardiovascular status must be assessed and cardiopulmonary resuscitation procedures must be followed.

In the event of local anaesthetic-induced cardiac arrest, standard cardiopulmonary resuscitation should be initiated immediately. Lidocaine must not be used as anti-arrhythmic therapy.

If the patient does not respond rapidly to standard procedures, 20% lipid emulsion such as *Intralipid*® [unlicensed indication] should be given intravenously at an initial bolus dose of 1.5 mL/kg over 1 minute, followed by an infusion of 15 mL/kg/hour. After 5 minutes, if cardiovascular stability has not been restored or circulation deteriorates, give a maximum of two further bolus doses of 1.5 mL/kg over 1 minute, 5 minutes apart, and increase the infusion rate to 30 mL/kg/hour. Continue infusion until cardiovascular stability and adequate circulation are restored or maximum cumulative dose of 12 mL/kg is given.

Standard cardiopulmonary resuscitation must be maintained throughout lipid emulsion treatment.

Propofol is not a suitable alternative to lipid emulsion.

Further advice on ongoing treatment should be obtained from the National Poisons Information Service.

Detailed treatment algorithms and accompanying notes are available at www.toxbase.org or can be found in the Association of Anaesthetists of Great Britain and Ireland safety guideline, Management of Severe Local Anaesthetic Toxicity and Management of Severe Local Anaesthetic Toxicity – Accompanying notes.

ANAESTHETICS, LOCAL

Adrenaline with articaine hydrochloride

(Carticaine hydrochloride with epinephrine)

● INDICATIONS AND DOSE

Infiltration anaesthesia in dentistry

▶ BY REGIONAL ADMINISTRATION

▶ Adult: Consult expert dental sources

DOSES AT EXTREMES OF BODY-WEIGHT

▶ To avoid excessive dosage in obese patients, dose should be calculated on the basis of ideal body-weight.

IMPORTANT SAFETY INFORMATION

Should only be administered by, or under the direct supervision of, personnel experienced in their use, with adequate training in anaesthesia and airway management, and should not be administered parenterally unless adequate resuscitation equipment is available.

Adrenaline/epinephrine must be used in a low concentration when administered with a local anaesthetic. The total dose of adrenaline should not exceed 500 micrograms and it is essential not to exceed a concentration of 1 in 200 000 (5 micrograms/mL) if more than 50 mL of the mixture is to be injected.

● CONTRA-INDICATIONS Application to damaged skin · application to the middle ear (may cause ototoxicity) · complete heart block · injection into infected tissues · injection into inflamed tissues · preparations containing preservatives should not be used for caudal, epidural, or spinal block, or for intravenous regional anaesthesia (Bier's block)

CONTRA-INDICATIONS, FURTHER INFORMATION

▶ Injection site Local anaesthetics should not be injected into inflamed or infected tissues nor should they be applied to damaged skin. Increased absorption into the blood increases the possibility of systemic side-effects, and the local anaesthetic effect may also be reduced by altered local pH.

● CAUTIONS Arrhythmias · arteriosclerosis · cardiovascular disease · cerebrovascular disease · cor pulmonale · debilitated patients (consider dose reduction) · diabetes mellitus · elderly (consider dose reduction) · epilepsy · hypercalcaemia · hyperreflexia · hypertension · hyperthyroidism · hypokalaemia · hypovolaemia · impaired cardiac conduction · impaired respiratory function · ischaemic heart disease · myasthenia gravis · obstructive cardiomyopathy · occlusive vascular disease · organic brain damage · phaeochromocytoma · prostate disorders · psychoneurosis · severe angina · shock · susceptibility to angle-closure glaucoma

CAUTIONS, FURTHER INFORMATION

▶ Use of vasoconstrictors In patients with severe hypertension or unstable cardiac rhythm, the use of adrenaline with a local anaesthetic may be hazardous. For these patients an anaesthetic without adrenaline should be used.

● INTERACTIONS → Appendix 1: articaine · sympathomimetics, vasoconstrictor

● SIDE-EFFECTS Face oedema · gingivitis · headache · nausea · sensation abnormal

SIDE-EFFECTS, FURTHER INFORMATION Toxic effects after administration of local anaesthetics are a result of excessively high plasma concentrations; severe toxicity usually results from inadvertent intravascular injection. The toxicity mainly involves the central nervous and cardiovascular systems. The onset of toxicity can be

unpredictable and delayed. Monitor as per local protocol for at least 30 minutes after administration.

● ALLERGY AND CROSS-SENSITIVITY

▶ Hypersensitivity and cross-sensitivity Hypersensitivity reactions occur mainly with the ester-type local anaesthetics, such as tetracaine; reactions are less frequent with the amide types, such as articaine, bupivacaine, levobupivacaine, lidocaine, mepivacaine, prilocaine, and ropivacaine. Cross-sensitivity reactions may be avoided by using the alternative chemical type.

● PREGNANCY Use only if potential benefit outweighs risk—no information available.

● BREAST FEEDING Avoid breast-feeding for 48 hours after administration.

● HEPATIC IMPAIRMENT Use with caution; increased risk of side-effects in severe impairment.

● RENAL IMPAIRMENT Manufacturers advise use with caution in severe impairment.

● MONITORING REQUIREMENTS Consider monitoring blood pressure and ECG (advised with systemic adrenaline/epinephrine).

● MEDICINAL FORMS
There can be variation in the licensing of different medicines containing the same drug.

Solution for injection
EXCIPIENTS: May contain Sulfites

▶ Septanest (Septodont Ltd)
Adrenaline (as Adrenaline acid tartrate) 10 microgram per 1 ml, Articaine hydrochloride 40 mg per 1 ml Septanest 1 in 100,000 solution for injection cartridges | 50 cartridge [PoM] £24.95
Adrenaline (as Adrenaline acid tartrate) 5 microgram per 1 ml, Articaine hydrochloride 40 mg per 1 ml Septanest 1 in 200,000 solution for injection cartridges | 50 cartridge [PoM] £24.95

Bupivacaine hydrochloride

● INDICATIONS AND DOSE

Surgical anaesthesia, lumbar epidural block

▶ BY REGIONAL ADMINISTRATION

▶ Adult: 75–150 mg, dose administered using a 5 mg/mL (0.5%) solution

Surgical anaesthesia, field block

▶ BY REGIONAL ADMINISTRATION

▶ Adult: Up to 150 mg, dose administered using a 2.5 mg/mL (0.25%) or 5 mg/mL (0.5%) solution

Surgical anaesthesia, thoracic epidural block

▶ BY THORACIC EPIDURAL

▶ Adult: 12.5–50 mg, dose administered using a 2.5 mg/mL (0.25%) or 5 mg/mL (0.5%) solution

Surgical anaesthesia, caudal epidural block

▶ BY REGIONAL ADMINISTRATION

▶ Adult: 50–150 mg, dose administered using a 2.5 mg/mL (0.25%) or 5 mg/mL (0.5%) solution

Surgical anaesthesia, major nerve block

▶ BY REGIONAL ADMINISTRATION

▶ Adult: 50–175 mg, dose administered using a 5 mg/mL (0.5%) solution

Acute pain, intra-articular block

▶ BY INTRA-ARTICULAR INJECTION

▶ Adult: Up to 100 mg, dose administered using a 2.5 mg/mL (0.25%) solution; when co-administered with bupivacaine by another route, total max. 150 mg

Acute pain, thoracic epidural block

▶ BY CONTINUOUS EPIDURAL INFUSION

▶ Adult: 6.3–18.8 mg/hour, dose administered using a 1.25 mg/mL (0.125%) or 2.5 mg/mL (0.25%) solution; maximum 400 mg per day

continued →

15

Anaesthesia

Acute pain, labour
▸ BY CONTINUOUS EPIDURAL INFUSION
▸ Adult: 6.25–12.5 mg/hour, dose administered using a 1.25 mg/mL (0.125%) solution; maximum 400 mg per day

Acute pain, lumbar epidural block
▸ INITIALLY BY LUMBAR EPIDURAL
▸ Adult: 15–37.5 mg, then (by lumbar epidural) 15–37.5 mg, repeated when required at intervals of at least 30 minutes, dose administered by intermittent injection using a 2.5 mg/mL (0.25%) solution, alternatively (by continuous epidural infusion) 12.5–18.8 mg/hour, dose administered using a 1.25 mg/mL (0.125%) or 2.5 mg/mL (0.25%) solution; maximum 400 mg per day

Acute pain, field block
▸ BY REGIONAL ADMINISTRATION
▸ Adult: Up to 150 mg, dose administered using a 2.5 mg/mL (0.25%) solution

MARCAIN HEAVY ®

Intrathecal anaesthesia for surgery
▸ BY INTRATHECAL INJECTION
▸ Adult: 10–20 mg

DOSES AT EXTREMES OF BODY-WEIGHT
▸ To avoid excessive dosage in obese patients, dose should be calculated on the basis of ideal body-weight.

> **IMPORTANT SAFETY INFORMATION**
> The licensed doses stated may not be appropriate in some settings and expert advice should be sought.
>   Should only be administered by, or under the direct supervision of, personnel experienced in their use, with adequate training in anaesthesia and airway management, and should not be administered parenterally unless adequate resuscitation equipment is available.

● CONTRA-INDICATIONS Application to the middle ear (can cause ototoxicity) · avoid injection into infected tissues · avoid injection into inflamed tissues · complete heart block · preparations containing preservatives should not be used for caudal, epidural, or spinal block, or for intravenous regional anaesthesia (Bier's block) · should not be applied to damaged skin

CONTRA-INDICATIONS, FURTHER INFORMATION
▸ Injection site Local anaesthetics should not be injected into inflamed or infected tissues nor should they be applied to damaged skin. Increased absorption into the blood increases the possibility of systemic side-effects, and the local anaesthetic effect may also be reduced by altered local pH.

● CAUTIONS Cardiovascular disease · cerebral atheroma · debilitated patients (consider dose reduction) · elderly (consider dose reduction) · epilepsy · hypertension · hypotension · hypovolaemia · impaired cardiac conduction · impaired respiratory function · myasthenia gravis · myocardial depression may be more severe and more resistant to treatment · shock

● INTERACTIONS → Appendix 1: anaesthetics, local

● SIDE-EFFECTS
▸ **Common or very common** Arrhythmias · dizziness · hypertension · hypotension · nausea · paraesthesia · urinary retention · vomiting
▸ **Uncommon** Neurotoxicity
▸ **Rare or very rare** Arachnoiditis · cardiac arrest · diplopia · nerve disorders · paraplegia · paresis · respiratory depression

SIDE-EFFECTS, FURTHER INFORMATION Toxic effects after administration of local anaesthetics are a result of

excessively high plasma concentrations; severe toxicity usually results from inadvertent intravascular injection. The systemic toxicity of local anaesthetics mainly involves the central nervous and cardiovascular systems. The onset of toxicity can be unpredictable and delayed. Monitor as per local protocol for at least 30 minutes after administration.

● ALLERGY AND CROSS-SENSITIVITY
▸ Hypersensitivity and cross-sensitivity Hypersensitivity reactions occur mainly with the ester-type local anaesthetics, such as tetracaine; reactions are less frequent with the amide types, such as articaine, bupivacaine, levobupivacaine, lidocaine, mepivacaine, prilocaine, and ropivacaine. Cross-sensitivity reactions may be avoided by using the alternative chemical type.

● PREGNANCY Large doses during delivery can cause neonatal respiratory depression, hypotonia, and bradycardia after epidural block.
  Dose adjustments Use lower doses for intrathecal use during late pregnancy.

● BREAST FEEDING Amount too small to be harmful.

● HEPATIC IMPAIRMENT Use with caution in severe impairment.

● RENAL IMPAIRMENT Use with caution in severe impairment.

● MEDICINAL FORMS
There can be variation in the licensing of different medicines containing the same drug. Forms available from special-order manufacturers include: solution for injection, infusion, solution for infusion

Solution for injection
▸ Bupivacaine hydrochloride (Non-proprietary)
  Bupivacaine hydrochloride 2.5 mg per 1 ml Bupivacaine 25mg/10ml (0.25%) solution for injection vials | 10 vial ⓢ
  Bupivacaine 0.25% solution for injection 10ml Sure-Amp ampoules | 20 ampoule [PoM] £17.50
  Bupivacaine hydrochloride 5 mg per 1 ml Bupivacaine 0.5% solution for injection 10ml Sure-Amp ampoules | 20 ampoule [PoM] £18.30
  Bupivacaine 100mg/20ml (0.5%) solution for injection vials | 10 vial [PoM] ⓢ
  Bupivacaine 50mg/10ml (0.5%) solution for injection ampoules | 10 ampoule [PoM] £17.58
  Bupivacaine hydrochloride anhydrous 40 mg per 1 ml Bupivacain Sintetica 40mg/ml (4%) solution for injection ampoules | 10 ampoule [PoM] ⓢ
▸ Marcain (Aspen Pharma Trading Ltd)
  Bupivacaine hydrochloride 2.5 mg per 1 ml Marcain 0.25% solution for injection 10ml Polyamp Steripack ampoules | 5 ampoule [PoM] £7.92
  Bupivacaine hydrochloride 5 mg per 1 ml Marcain 0.5% solution for injection 10ml Polyamp Steripack ampoules | 5 ampoule [PoM] £9.25

Infusion
▸ Bupivacaine hydrochloride (Non-proprietary)
  Bupivacaine hydrochloride 1 mg per 1 ml Bupivacaine 100mg/100ml (0.1%) infusion bags | 20 bag [PoM] ⓢ
  Bupivacaine 250mg/250ml (0.1%) infusion bags | 20 bag [PoM] £211.72
  Bupivacaine hydrochloride 1.25 mg per 1 ml Bupivacaine 312.5mg/250ml (0.125%) infusion bags | 20 bag [PoM] £216.06

Bupivacaine with adrenaline

The properties listed below are those particular to the combination only. For the properties of the components please consider, bupivacaine hydrochloride p. 1309, adrenaline/epinephrine p. 221.

● **INDICATIONS AND DOSE**

Surgical anaesthesia

▸ BY LUMBAR EPIDURAL, OR BY LOCAL INFILTRATION, OR BY CAUDAL EPIDURAL
▸ Adult: (consult product literature)

Acute pain management

▸ BY LUMBAR EPIDURAL, OR BY LOCAL INFILTRATION
▸ Adult: (consult product literature)

IMPORTANT SAFETY INFORMATION
Adrenaline/epinephrine must be used in a low concentration when administered with a local anaesthetic. The total dose of adrenaline should not exceed 500 micrograms and it is essential not to exceed a concentration of 1 in 200 000 (5 micrograms/mL) if more than 50 mL of the mixture is to be injected.

● **CAUTIONS**
CAUTIONS, FURTHER INFORMATION In patients with severe hypertension or unstable cardiac rhythm, the use of adrenaline with a local anaesthetic may be hazardous. For these patients an anaesthetic without adrenaline should be used.

● **INTERACTIONS** → Appendix 1: anaesthetics, local · sympathomimetics, vasoconstrictor

● **MEDICINAL FORMS**
There can be variation in the licensing of different medicines containing the same drug.

Solution for injection
▸ Bupivacaine with adrenaline (Non-proprietary)
  Adrenaline (as Adrenaline acid tartrate) 5 microgram per 1 ml, Bupivacaine hydrochloride 2.5 mg per 1 ml Bupivacaine 25mg/10ml (0.25%) / Adrenaline (base) 50micrograms/10ml (1 in 200,000) solution for injection ampoules | 10 ampoule [PoM] £40.00
  Adrenaline (as Adrenaline acid tartrate) 5 microgram per 1 ml, Bupivacaine hydrochloride 5 mg per 1 ml Bupivacaine 50mg/10ml (0.5%) / Adrenaline (base) 50micrograms/10ml (1 in 200,000) solution for injection ampoules | 10 ampoule [PoM] £45.00

Levobupivacaine

● **INDICATIONS AND DOSE**

Acute postoperative pain

▸ BY CONTINUOUS EPIDURAL INFUSION
▸ Adult: 12.5–18.75 mg/hour, dose administered using a 1.25 mg/mL (0.125%) or 2.5 mg/mL (0.25%) solution; maximum 400 mg per day

Acute labour pain

▸ BY LUMBAR EPIDURAL
▸ Adult: 15–25 mg, repeated at intervals of at least 15 minutes, dose administered using a 2.5 mg/mL (0.25%) solution; maximum 400 mg per day
▸ BY CONTINUOUS EPIDURAL INFUSION
▸ Adult: 5–12.5 mg/hour, dose administered using a 1.25 mg/mL (0.125%) solution; maximum 400 mg per day

Surgical anaesthesia, peripheral nerve block

▸ BY REGIONAL ADMINISTRATION
▸ Adult: 2.5–150 mg, dose administered using a 2.5 mg/mL (0.25%) or 5 mg/mL (0.5%) solution

Surgical anaesthesia, peribulbar nerve block

▸ BY REGIONAL ADMINISTRATION
▸ Adult: 37.5–112.5 mg, dose administered using a 7.5 mg/mL (0.75%) solution

Surgical anaesthesia for caesarean section

▸ BY LUMBAR EPIDURAL
▸ Adult: 75–150 mg, to be given over 15–20 minutes, dose administered using a 5 mg/mL (0.5%) solution

Surgical anaesthesia

▸ BY LUMBAR EPIDURAL
▸ Adult: 50–150 mg, to be given over 5 minutes, dose administered using a 5 mg/mL (0.5%) or 7.5 mg/mL (0.75%) solution
▸ BY INTRATHECAL INJECTION
▸ Adult: 15 mg, dose administered using a 5 mg/mL (0.5%) solution
▸ BY LOCAL INFILTRATION
▸ Adult: 2.5–150 mg, dose administered using a 2.5 mg/mL (0.25%) solution

DOSES AT EXTREMES OF BODY-WEIGHT
▸ To avoid excessive dosage in obese patients, dose should be calculated on the basis of ideal body-weight.

IMPORTANT SAFETY INFORMATION
The licensed doses stated may not be appropriate in some settings and expert advice should be sought.
  Should only be administered by, or under the direct supervision of, personnel experienced in their use, with adequate training in anaesthesia and airway management, and should not be administered parenterally unless adequate resuscitation equipment is available.

● **CONTRA-INDICATIONS** Application to the middle ear (can cause ototoxicity) · avoid injection into infected tissues · avoid injection into inflamed tissues · complete heart block · preparations containing preservatives should not be used for caudal, epidural, or spinal block, or for intravenous regional anaesthesia (Bier's block) · should not be applied to damaged skin

CONTRA-INDICATIONS, FURTHER INFORMATION
▸ Injection site Local anaesthetics should not be injected into inflamed or infected tissues nor should they be applied to damaged skin. Increased absorption into the blood increases the possibility of systemic side-effects, and the local anaesthetic effect may also be reduced by altered local pH.

● **CAUTIONS** Cardiovascular disease · debilitated patients (consider dose reduction) · elderly (consider dose reduction) · epilepsy · hypovolaemia · impaired cardiac conduction · impaired respiratory function · myasthenia gravis · shock

● **INTERACTIONS** → Appendix 1: anaesthetics, local

● **SIDE-EFFECTS**
▸ Common or very common Anaemia · back pain · dizziness · fever · headache · hypotension · nausea · vomiting
▸ Frequency not known Angioedema · apnoea · arrhythmias · asthenia · atrioventricular block · bladder disorder · cardiac arrest · drowsiness · eye disorders · faecal incontinence · flushing · loss of consciousness · muscle twitching · muscle weakness · nerve disorders · neurological injury · oral hypoaesthesia · paralysis · priapism · respiratory disorders · seizure · sensation abnormal · skin reactions · sneezing · sweat changes · syncope · vision blurred

SIDE-EFFECTS, FURTHER INFORMATION The systemic toxicity of local anaesthetics mainly involves the central nervous and cardiovascular systems. Systemic toxicity can occur due to inadvertent intravascular injection. The onset of toxicity can be unpredictable and delayed. Monitor as

15

Anaesthesia

per local protocol for at least 30 minutes after administration.

• **ALLERGY AND CROSS-SENSITIVITY**
▸ Hypersensitivity and cross-sensitivity Hypersensitivity reactions occur mainly with the ester-type local anaesthetics, such as tetracaine; reactions are less frequent with the amide types, such as articaine, bupivacaine, levobupivacaine, lidocaine, mepivacaine, prilocaine, and ropivacaine. Cross-sensitivity reactions may be avoided by using the alternative chemical type.

• **PREGNANCY** Large doses during delivery can cause neonatal respiratory depression, hypotonia, and bradycardia after epidural block. Avoid if possible in the first trimester—toxicity in *animal* studies. May cause fetal distress syndrome. Do not use for paracervical block in obstetrics. Do not use 7.5 mg/mL strength in obstetrics.

• **BREAST FEEDING** Amount too small to be harmful.

• **HEPATIC IMPAIRMENT** Use with caution.

• **DIRECTIONS FOR ADMINISTRATION** For 1.25 mg/mL concentration dilute standard solutions with sodium chloride 0.9%.

• **PRESCRIBING AND DISPENSING INFORMATION** Levobupivacaine is an isomer of bupivacaine.

• **MEDICINAL FORMS**
There can be variation in the licensing of different medicines containing the same drug.

Solution for injection
▸ Chirocaine (AbbVie Ltd)
Levobupivacaine (as Levobupivacaine hydrochloride) 2.5 mg per 1 ml Chirocaine 25mg/10ml solution for injection ampoules | 10 ampoule [PoM] £14.11 (Hospital only)
Levobupivacaine (as Levobupivacaine hydrochloride) 5 mg per 1 ml Chirocaine 50mg/10ml solution for injection ampoules | 10 ampoule [PoM] £16.15 (Hospital only)
Levobupivacaine (as Levobupivacaine hydrochloride) 7.5 mg per 1 ml Chirocaine 75mg/10ml solution for injection ampoules | 10 ampoule [PoM] £24.23 (Hospital only)

Infusion
▸ Chirocaine (AbbVie Ltd)
Levobupivacaine (as Levobupivacaine hydrochloride) 1.25 mg per 1 ml Chirocaine 125mg/100ml infusion bags | 24 bag [PoM] £174.22
Chirocaine 250mg/200ml infusion bags | 12 bag [PoM] [S]

Lidocaine hydrochloride
(Lignocaine hydrochloride)

• **INDICATIONS AND DOSE**
Infiltration anaesthesia
▸ BY LOCAL INFILTRATION
▸ Adult: Dose to be given according to patient's weight and nature of procedure; max. 200 mg, maximum dose 500 mg if given in solutions containing adrenaline

DOSES AT EXTREMES OF BODY-WEIGHT
▸ When used by local infiltration To avoid excessive dosage in obese patients, weight-based doses for non-emergency indications may need to be calculated on the basis of ideal body-weight.

Intravenous regional anaesthesia and nerve block
▸ BY REGIONAL ADMINISTRATION
▸ Adult: Seek expert advice

Pain relief (in anal fissures, haemorrhoids, pruritus ani, pruritus vulvae, herpes zoster, or herpes labialis) | Lubricant in cystoscopy | Lubricant in proctoscopy
▸ TO THE SKIN USING OINTMENT
▸ Adult: Apply 1–2 mL as required, avoid long-term use

Sore nipples from breast-feeding
▸ TO THE SKIN USING OINTMENT
▸ Adult: Apply using gauze and wash off immediately before next feed

LMX 4 ®
Anaesthesia before venous cannulation or venepuncture
▸ TO THE SKIN
▸ Child 1-2 months: Apply up to 1 g, apply thick layer to small area (2.5 cm × 2.5 cm) of non-irritated skin at least 30 minutes before procedure; may be applied under an occlusive dressing; max. application time 60 minutes, remove cream with gauze and perform procedure after approximately 5 minutes
▸ Child 3-11 months: Apply up to 1 g, apply thick layer to small area (2.5 cm × 2.5 cm) of non-irritated skin at least 30 minutes before procedure; may be applied under an occlusive dressing; max. application time 4 hours, remove cream with gauze and perform procedure after approximately 5 minutes
▸ Child 1-17 years: Apply 1–2.5 g, apply thick layer to small area (2.5 cm × 2.5 cm) of non-irritated skin at least 30 minutes before procedure; may be applied under an occlusive dressing; max. application time 5 hours, remove cream with gauze and perform procedure after approximately 5 minutes
▸ Adult: Apply 1–2.5 g, apply thick layer to small area (2.5 cm × 2.5 cm) of non-irritated skin at least 30 minutes before procedure; may be applied under an occlusive dressing; max. application time 5 hours, remove cream with gauze and perform procedure after approximately 5 minutes

VERSATIS ®
Postherpetic neuralgia
▸ TO THE SKIN
▸ Adult: Apply once daily for up to 12 hours, followed by a 12-hour plaster-free period; discontinue if no response after 4 weeks, to be applied to intact, dry, non-hairy, non-irritated skin, up to 3 plasters may be used to cover large areas; plasters may be cut

XYLOCAINE ®
During delivery in obstetrics
▸ TO THE SKIN
▸ Adult: Up to 20 doses

IMPORTANT SAFETY INFORMATION
▸ When used by local infiltration
The licensed doses stated may not be appropriate in some settings and expert advice should be sought. Should only be administered by, or under the direct supervision of, personnel experienced in their use, with adequate training in anaesthesia and airway management, and should not be administered parenterally unless adequate resuscitation equipment is available.

• **CONTRA-INDICATIONS**
▸ When used by regional administration All grades of atrioventricular block · application to the middle ear (can cause ototoxicity) · avoid injection into infected tissues · avoid injection into inflamed tissues · preparations containing preservatives should not be used for caudal, epidural, or spinal block, or for intravenous regional anaesthesia (Bier's block) · severe myocardial depression · should not be applied to damaged skin · sino-atrial disorders

CONTRA-INDICATIONS, FURTHER INFORMATION
▸ When used by regional administration Local anaesthetics should not be injected into inflamed or infected tissues nor should they be applied to damaged skin. Increased absorption into the blood increases the possibility of systemic side-effects, and the local anaesthetic effect may also be reduced by altered local pH.

- CAUTIONS
▸ When used by regional administration Acute porphyrias p. 1025 (consider infusion with glucose for its anti-porphyrinogenic effects) · children (consider dose reduction) · congestive cardiac failure (consider lower dose) · debilitated patients (consider dose reduction) · elderly (consider dose reduction) · epilepsy · hypovolaemia · impaired cardiac conduction · impaired respiratory function · myasthenia gravis · post cardiac surgery (consider lower dose) · shock

- INTERACTIONS → Appendix 1: antiarrhythmics

- SIDE-EFFECTS
▸ With parenteral use Anxiety · arrhythmias · atrioventricular block · cardiac arrest · circulatory collapse · confusion · dizziness · drowsiness · euphoric mood · headache · hypotension (may lead to cardiac arrest) · loss of consciousness · methaemoglobinaemia · muscle twitching · myocardial contractility decreased · nausea · neurological effects · nystagmus · pain · psychosis · respiratory disorders · seizure · sensation abnormal · temperature sensation altered · tinnitus · tremor · vision blurred · vomiting

SIDE-EFFECTS, FURTHER INFORMATION
Toxic effects The systemic toxicity of local anaesthetics mainly involves the central nervous and cardiovascular systems.
Methaemoglobinaemia Methylthioninium chloride is licensed for the acute symptomatic treatment of drug-induced methaemoglobinaemia.

- ALLERGY AND CROSS-SENSITIVITY
▸ Hypersensitivity and cross-sensitivity Hypersensitivity reactions occur mainly with the ester-type local anaesthetics, such as tetracaine; reactions are less frequent with the amide types, such as articaine, bupivacaine, levobupivacaine, lidocaine, mepivacaine, prilocaine, and ropivacaine. Cross-sensitivity reactions may be avoided by using the alternative chemical type.

- PREGNANCY Crosses the placenta but not known to be harmful in *animal* studies—use if benefit outweighs risk. When used as a local anaesthetic, large doses can cause fetal bradycardia; if given during delivery can also cause neonatal respiratory depression, hypotonia, or bradycardia after paracervical or epidural block.

- BREAST FEEDING Present in milk but amount too small to be harmful.

- HEPATIC IMPAIRMENT Caution—increased risk of side-effects.

- RENAL IMPAIRMENT Possible accumulation of lidocaine and active metabolite; caution in severe impairment.

- MONITORING REQUIREMENTS
▸ With systemic use Monitor ECG and have resuscitation facilities available.

- NATIONAL FUNDING/ACCESS DECISIONS

VERSATIS ®

Scottish Medicines Consortium (SMC) Decisions
The *Scottish Medicines Consortium* has advised (July 2008) that *Versatis*® is accepted for restricted use within NHS Scotland for the treatment of postherpetic neuralgia in patients who are intolerant of first-line systemic therapies or when they have been ineffective.

- MEDICINAL FORMS
There can be variation in the licensing of different medicines containing the same drug. Forms available from special-order manufacturers include: solution for injection, liquid, ointment

Solution for injection
▸ Lidocaine hydrochloride (Non-proprietary)
Lidocaine hydrochloride 5 mg per 1 ml Lidocaine 50mg/10ml (0.5%) solution for injection ampoules | 10 ampoule PoM £7.00
Lidocaine hydrochloride 10 mg per 1 ml Lidocaine 100mg/10ml (1%) solution for injection Mini-Plasco ampoules | 20 ampoule PoM £11.21

Lidocaine 100mg/10ml (1%) solution for injection ampoules | 10 ampoule PoM £4.40 DT = £4.40
Lidocaine 100mg/10ml (1%) solution for injection Sure-Amp ampoules | 20 ampoule PoM £8.80
Lidocaine 200mg/20ml (1%) solution for injection vials | 10 vial PoM £19.00
Lidocaine 200mg/20ml (1%) solution for injection ampoules | 10 ampoule PoM £7.00–£9.63 DT = £9.63
Lidocaine 50mg/5ml (1%) solution for injection ampoules | 10 ampoule PoM £2.59–£3.10 DT = £2.59
Lidocaine 20mg/2ml (1%) solution for injection ampoules | 10 ampoule PoM £3.50 DT = £2.20
Lidocaine 50mg/5ml (1%) solution for injection Sure-Amp ampoules | 20 ampoule PoM £6.00
Lidocaine hydrochloride 20 mg per 1 ml Lidocaine 100mg/5ml (2%) solution for injection ampoules | 10 ampoule PoM £2.70–£3.80 DT = £2.70
Lidocaine 400mg/20ml (2%) solution for injection vials | 10 vial PoM £19.50
Lidocaine 200mg/10ml (2%) solution for injection Mini-Plasco ampoules | 20 ampoule PoM £14.95
Lidocaine 40mg/2ml (2%) solution for injection ampoules | 10 ampoule PoM £4.00 DT = £2.37
Lidocaine 100mg/5ml (2%) solution for injection Sure-Amp ampoules | 20 ampoule PoM £6.00
Lidocaine 400mg/20ml (2%) solution for injection ampoules | 10 ampoule PoM £8.00–£9.90 DT = £9.90

Medicated plaster
EXCIPIENTS: May contain Hydroxybenzoates (parabens), propylene glycol
▸ Versatis (Grunenthal Ltd)
Lidocaine 50 mg per 1 gram Versatis 700mg medicated plasters | 30 plaster PoM £72.40 DT = £72.40

Cream
EXCIPIENTS: May contain Benzyl alcohol, propylene glycol
▸ LMX 4 (Ferndale Pharmaceuticals Ltd)
Lidocaine 40 mg per 1 gram LMX 4 cream | 5 gram P £2.98 DT = £2.98 | 30 gram P £14.90 DT = £14.90

Ointment
▸ Lidocaine hydrochloride (Non-proprietary)
Lidocaine hydrochloride 50 mg per 1 gram Lidocaine 5% ointment | 15 gram P £6.50 DT = £6.18

Spray
▸ Xylocaine (Aspen Pharma Trading Ltd)
Lidocaine 10 mg per 1 actuation Xylocaine 10mg/dose spray sugar-free | 50 ml P £6.29 DT = £6.29

Lidocaine with adrenaline

The properties listed below are those particular to the combination only. For the properties of the components please consider, lidocaine hydrochloride p. 1312, adrenaline/epinephrine p. 221.

- INDICATIONS AND DOSE

Local anaesthesia
▸ BY LOCAL INFILTRATION
▸ Adult: Dosed according to the type of nerve block required (consult product literature)

IMPORTANT SAFETY INFORMATION
Adrenaline/epinephrine must be used in a low concentration when administered with a local anaesthetic. The total dose of adrenaline should not exceed 500 micrograms and it is essential not to exceed a concentration of 1 in 200 000 (5 micrograms/mL) if more than 50 mL of the mixture is to be injected.

- INTERACTIONS → Appendix 1: antiarrhythmics · sympathomimetics, vasoconstrictor
- PROFESSION SPECIFIC INFORMATION

Dental information
A variety of lidocaine injections with adrenaline is available in dental cartridges.
Consult expert dental sources for specific advice in relation to dose of lidocaine for dental anaesthesia.

15

Anaesthesia

- MEDICINAL FORMS
There can be variation in the licensing of different medicines containing the same drug. Forms available from special-order manufacturers include: solution for injection

Solution for injection
EXCIPIENTS: May contain Sulfites

▸ Lignospan Special (Septodont Ltd)
Adrenaline (as Adrenaline acid tartrate) 12.5 microgram per 1 ml, Lidocaine hydrochloride 20 mg per 1 ml Lignospan Special 2% injection 2.2ml cartridges | 50 cartridges [PoM] £21.95
Lignospan Special 2% injection 1.8ml cartridges | 50 cartridge [PoM] £21.95

▸ Rexocaine (Henry Schein Ltd)
Adrenaline (as Adrenaline acid tartrate) 12.5 microgram per 1 ml, Lidocaine hydrochloride 20 mg per 1 ml Rexocaine 2% injection 2.2ml cartridges | 50 cartridge [PoM] £23.29

▸ Xylocaine with Adrenaline (Aspen Pharma Trading Ltd)
Adrenaline (as Adrenaline acid tartrate) 5 microgram per 1 ml, Lidocaine hydrochloride 10 mg per 1 ml Xylocaine 1% with Adrenaline 100micrograms/20ml (1 in 200,000) solution for injection vials | 5 vial [PoM] £9.66 DT = £9.66
Adrenaline (as Adrenaline acid tartrate) 5 microgram per 1 ml, Lidocaine hydrochloride 20 mg per 1 ml Xylocaine 2% with Adrenaline 100micrograms/20ml (1 in 200,000) solution for injection vials | 5 vial [PoM] £8.85 DT = £8.85

Lidocaine with cetrimide
27-Apr-2018

The properties listed below are those particular to the combination only. For the properties of the components please consider, lidocaine hydrochloride p. 1312.

- INDICATIONS AND DOSE
Anaesthesia and disinfection in dental practice
▸ TO MUCOUS MEMBRANES USING OROMUCOSAL SPRAY
▸ Adult: 10–20 mg, no more than 30 mg should be applied to the same quadrant of the buccal cavity—consult product literature, dose expressed as lidocaine
Anaesthesia in dental practice
▸ TO MUCOUS MEMBRANES USING DENTAL GEL
▸ Adult: Apply 100–500 mg, use cotton pellet for application to dried mucosa, dose expressed as weight of gel
DOSE EQUIVALENCE AND CONVERSION
▸ 1 metered dose of *Xylonor*® spray is equivalent to 10 mg of lidocaine.
▸ 2 millimetres of *Xylonor*® gel is approximately equivalent to 100 mg of gel (approximately equivalent to 5 mg of lidocaine).

- CAUTIONS Sepsis (risk of rapid systemic absorption) · traumatised mucosa (risk of rapid systemic absorption)
- INTERACTIONS → Appendix 1: antiarrhythmics
- MEDICINAL FORMS
There can be variation in the licensing of different medicines containing the same drug.
Oromucosal gel
▸ Xylonor (Septodont Ltd)
Cetrimide 1.5 mg per 1 gram, Lidocaine 50 mg per 1 gram Xylonor 5% gel sugar-free | 15 gram [PoM] £4.00
Spray
▸ Xylonor (Septodont Ltd)
Cetrimide 100 microgram per 1 gram, Lidocaine 10 mg per 1 gram Xylonor 10% spray sugar-free | 36 gram [PoM] £20.15

Lidocaine with phenylephrine

The properties listed below are those particular to the combination only. For the properties of the components please consider, lidocaine hydrochloride p. 1312, phenylephrine hydrochloride p. 188.

- INDICATIONS AND DOSE
Anaesthesia before nasal surgery, endoscopy, laryngoscopy, or removal of foreign bodies from the nose
▸ BY INTRANASAL ADMINISTRATION
▸ Adult: Up to 8 sprays

- INTERACTIONS → Appendix 1: antiarrhythmics · sympathomimetics, vasoconstrictor

- MEDICINAL FORMS
There can be variation in the licensing of different medicines containing the same drug.
Spray
▸ Lidocaine with phenylephrine (Non-proprietary)
Phenylephrine hydrochloride 5 mg per 1 ml, Lidocaine hydrochloride 50 mg per 1 ml Lidocaine 5% / Phenylephrine 0.5% nasal spray | 2.5 ml [PoM] £12.90 DT = £12.90

Lidocaine with prilocaine
14-Jun-2017

The properties listed below are those particular to the combination only. For the properties of the components please consider, lidocaine hydrochloride p. 1312, prilocaine hydrochloride p. 1316.

- INDICATIONS AND DOSE
Anaesthesia before minor skin procedures including venepuncture
▸ TO THE SKIN
▸ Child 1-2 months: Apply up to 1 g for maximum 1 hour before procedure, to be applied under occlusive dressing, shorter application time of 15–30 minutes is recommended for children with atopic dermatitis (30 minutes before removal of mollusca); maximum 1 dose per day
▸ Child 3-11 months: Apply up to 2 g for maximum 1 hour before procedure, to be applied under occlusive dressing, shorter application time of 15–30 minutes is recommended for children with atopic dermatitis (30 minutes before removal of mollusca); maximum 2 doses per day
▸ Child 1-11 years: Apply 1–5 hours before procedure, a thick layer should be applied under occlusive dressing, shorter application time of 15–30 minutes is recommended for children with atopic dermatitis (30 minutes before removal of mollusca); maximum 2 doses per day
▸ Child 12-17 years: Apply 1–5 hours before procedure (2–5 hours before procedures on large areas e.g. split skin grafting), a thick layer should be applied under occlusive dressing, shorter application time of 15–30 minutes is recommended for children with atopic dermatitis (30 minutes before removal of mollusca)
▸ Adult: Apply 1–5 hours before procedure (2–5 hours before procedures on large areas e.g. split skin grafting), a thick layer should be applied under occlusive dressing
Anaesthesia on genital skin before injection of local anaesthetics
▸ TO THE SKIN
▸ Adult: Apply under occlusive dressing for 15 minutes (males) or 60 minutes (females) before procedure

Anaesthesia before surgical treatment of lesions on genital mucosa
▶ TO THE SKIN
▶ Adult: Apply up to 10 g, to be applied 5–10 minutes before procedure

Anaesthesia before cervical curettage
▶ TO THE SKIN
▶ Adult: Apply 10 g in lateral vaginal fornices for 10 minutes

Anaesthesia before mechanical cleansing or debridement of leg ulcer
▶ TO THE SKIN
▶ Adult: Apply up to 10 g for 30–60 minutes, to be applied under occlusive dressing

● CONTRA-INDICATIONS Use in child less than 37 weeks corrected gestational age
● INTERACTIONS → Appendix 1: anaesthetics, local · antiarrhythmics
● PATIENT AND CARER ADVICE
Medicines for Children leaflet: EMLA cream for local anaesthesia www.medicinesforchildren.org.uk/emla-cream-for-local-anaesthesia

● MEDICINAL FORMS
There can be variation in the licensing of different medicines containing the same drug.
Cream
▶ Lidocaine with prilocaine (Non-proprietary)
Lidocaine 25 mg per 1 gram, Prilocaine 25 mg per 1 gram Lidocaine 2.5% / Prilocaine 2.5% cream | 5 gram P ▦
▶ Denela (Teva UK Ltd)
Lidocaine 25 mg per 1 gram, Prilocaine 25 mg per 1 gram Denela 5% cream | 5 gram P £2.84-£3.29 | 25 gram P £12.99 | 30 gram P £14.75 DT = £12.30
▶ Emla (Aspen Pharma Trading Ltd)
Lidocaine 25 mg per 1 gram, Prilocaine 25 mg per 1 gram Emla 5% cream | 5 gram P £2.25-£2.99 | 25 gram P £11.70 | 30 gram P £12.30 DT = £12.30
▶ Nulbia (Glenmark Pharmaceuticals Europe Ltd)
Lidocaine 25 mg per 1 gram, Prilocaine 25 mg per 1 gram Nulbia 5% cream | 5 gram P £1.58 | 25 gram P £7.88 | 30 gram P £8.61 DT = £12.30

Mepivacaine hydrochloride

● **INDICATIONS AND DOSE**
Infiltration anaesthesia and nerve block in dentistry
▶ Child 3-17 years: Consult expert dental sources
▶ Adult: Consult expert dental sources
DOSES AT EXTREMES OF BODY-WEIGHT
▶ To avoid excessive dosage in obese patients, dose should be calculated on the basis of ideal body-weight.

IMPORTANT SAFETY INFORMATION
Should only be administered by, or under the direct supervision of, personnel experienced in their use, with adequate training in anaesthesia and airway management, and should not be administered parenterally unless adequate resuscitation equipment is available.

● CONTRA-INDICATIONS Application to the middle ear (can cause ototoxicity) · avoid injection into infected tissues · avoid injection into inflamed tissues · complete heart block · preparations containing preservatives should not be used for caudal, epidural, or spinal block, or for intravenous regional anaesthesia (Bier's block) · should not be applied to damaged skin

CONTRA-INDICATIONS, FURTHER INFORMATION
▶ Injection site Local anaesthetics should not be injected into inflamed or infected tissues nor should they be applied to damaged skin. Increased absorption into the blood increases the possibility of systemic side-effects, and the local anaesthetic effect may also be reduced by altered local pH.
● CAUTIONS Cardiovascular disease · children (consider dose reduction) · debilitated patients (consider dose reduction) · elderly (consider dose reduction) · epilepsy · hypovolaemia · impaired cardiac conduction · impaired respiratory function · myasthenia gravis · shock
● INTERACTIONS → Appendix 1: anaesthetics, local
● SIDE-EFFECTS
▶ **Common or very common** Arrhythmias · dizziness · hypertension · hypotension · nausea · paraesthesia · vomiting
▶ **Uncommon** Neurotoxicity
▶ **Rare or very rare** Arachnoiditis · cardiac arrest · diplopia · nerve disorders · respiratory depression
SIDE-EFFECTS, FURTHER INFORMATION Toxic effects after administration of local anaesthetics are a result of excessively high plasma concentrations; severe toxicity usually results from inadvertent intravascular injection or too rapid injection. The systemic toxicity of local anaesthetics mainly involves the central nervous and cardiovascular systems. The onset of toxicity can be unpredictable and delayed. Monitor as per local protocol for at least 30 minutes after administration.
● ALLERGY AND CROSS-SENSITIVITY
▶ Hypersensitivity and cross-sensitivity Hypersensitivity reactions occur mainly with the ester-type local anaesthetics, such as tetracaine; reactions are less frequent with the amide types, such as articaine, bupivacaine, levobupivacaine, lidocaine, mepivacaine, prilocaine, and ropivacaine. Cross-sensitivity reactions may be avoided by using the alternative chemical type.
● PREGNANCY Use with caution in early pregnancy.
● BREAST FEEDING Use with caution.
● HEPATIC IMPAIRMENT Use with caution; increased risk of side-effects in severe impairment.
● RENAL IMPAIRMENT Use with caution; increased risk of side-effects.

● MEDICINAL FORMS
There can be variation in the licensing of different medicines containing the same drug.
Solution for injection
▶ Scandonest plain (Septodont Ltd)
Mepivacaine hydrochloride 30 mg per 1 ml Scandonest plain 3% solution for injection 2.2ml cartridges | 50 cartridge PoM £21.95

Mepivacaine with adrenaline

The properties listed below are those particular to the combination only. For the properties of the components please consider, mepivacaine hydrochloride above, adrenaline/epinephrine p. 221.

● **INDICATIONS AND DOSE**
Infiltration anaesthesia and nerve block in dentistry
▶ BY LOCAL INFILTRATION
▶ Adult: (consult product literature)

IMPORTANT SAFETY INFORMATION
Adrenaline/epinephrine must be used in a low concentration when administered with a local anaesthetic. The total dose of adrenaline should not exceed 500 micrograms and it is essential not to exceed a

concentration of 1 in 200 000 (5 micrograms/mL) if more than 50 mL of the mixture is to be injected.

- INTERACTIONS → Appendix 1: anaesthetics, local · sympathomimetics, vasoconstrictor

- MEDICINAL FORMS
There can be variation in the licensing of different medicines containing the same drug.
Solution for injection
EXCIPIENTS: May contain Sulfites
▸ Scandonest special (Septodont Ltd)
Adrenaline 10 microgram per 1 ml, Mepivacaine hydrochloride 20 mg per 1 ml Scandonest special 2% solution for injection 2.2ml cartridges | 50 cartridge [PoM] £21.95

Prilocaine hydrochloride

- INDICATIONS AND DOSE
DOSES AT EXTREMES OF BODY-WEIGHT
To avoid excessive dosage in obese patients, dose should be calculated on the basis of ideal body-weight.
CITANEST 1% ®
Infiltration anaesthesia | Nerve block
▸ BY REGIONAL ADMINISTRATION
▸ Adult: 100–200 mg/minute, alternatively may be given in incremental doses; dose adjusted according to site of administration and response, and in elderly and debilitated patients (smaller doses may be required); maximum 400 mg per course
PRILOTEKAL ®
Spinal anaesthesia
▸ BY INTRATHECAL INJECTION
▸ Adult: Usual dose 40–60 mg (max. per dose 80 mg); dose may need to be reduced in elderly or debilitated patients, or in late pregnancy

---

IMPORTANT SAFETY INFORMATION
Should only be administered by, or under the direct supervision of, personnel experienced in their use, with adequate training in anaesthesia and airway management, and should not be administered parenterally unless adequate resuscitation equipment is available.

- CONTRA-INDICATIONS Acquired methaemoglobinaemia · anaemia · application to the middle ear (can cause ototoxicity) · avoid injection into infected tissues · avoid injection into inflamed tissues · complete heart block · congenital methaemoglobinaemia · preparations containing preservatives should not be used for caudal, epidural, or spinal block, or for intravenous regional anaesthesia (Bier's block) · should not be applied to damaged skin
CONTRA-INDICATIONS, FURTHER INFORMATION
▸ Injection site Local anaesthetics should not be injected into inflamed or infected tissues nor should they be applied to damaged skin. Increased absorption into the blood increases the possibility of systemic side-effects, and the local anaesthetic effect may also be reduced by altered local pH.
- CAUTIONS Cardiovascular disease · debilitated patients (consider dose reduction) · elderly (consider dose reduction) · epilepsy · hypovolaemia · impaired cardiac conduction · impaired respiratory function · myasthenia gravis · severe or untreated hypertension · shock
- INTERACTIONS → Appendix 1: anaesthetics, local

- SIDE-EFFECTS
▸ **Common or very common** Arrhythmias · dizziness · hypertension · hypotension · nausea · paraesthesia · vomiting
▸ **Uncommon** Neurotoxicity
▸ **Rare or very rare** Cardiac arrest · methaemoglobinaemia · nerve disorders
▸ **Frequency not known** Diplopia · respiratory depression
SIDE-EFFECTS, FURTHER INFORMATION
Toxic effects Toxic effects after administration of local anaesthetics are a result of excessively high plasma concentrations; severe toxicity usually results from inadvertent intravascular injection or too rapid injection. The systemic toxicity of local anaesthetics mainly involves the central nervous and cardiovascular systems. The onset of toxicity can be unpredictable and delayed. Monitor as per local protocol for at least 30 minutes after administration.
Methaemoglobinaemia Methaemoglobinaemia can be treated with an intravenous injection of methylthioninium chloride.

- ALLERGY AND CROSS-SENSITIVITY
▸ Hypersensitivity and cross-sensitivity Hypersensitivity reactions occur mainly with the ester-type local anaesthetics, such as tetracaine; reactions are less frequent with the amide types, such as articaine, bupivacaine, levobupivacaine, lidocaine, mepivacaine, prilocaine, and ropivacaine. Cross-sensitivity reactions may be avoided by using the alternative chemical type.
- PREGNANCY Large doses during delivery can cause neonatal respiratory depression, hypotonia, and bradycardia after epidural block. Avoid paracervical or pudendal block in obstetrics (neonatal methaemoglobinaemia reported).
Dose adjustments Use lower doses for intrathecal use during late pregnancy.
- BREAST FEEDING Present in milk but not known to be harmful.
- HEPATIC IMPAIRMENT Use with caution.
Dose adjustments Lower doses may be required for intrathecal anaesthesia.
- RENAL IMPAIRMENT Use with caution.
Dose adjustments Lower doses may be required for intrathecal anaesthesia.
- NATIONAL FUNDING/ACCESS DECISIONS
PRILOTEKAL ®
Scottish Medicines Consortium (SMC) Decisions
▸ With intrathecal use The *Scottish Medicines Consortium* has advised (December 2010) that prilocaine 2% hyperbaric solution for injection (*Prilotekal*®) is accepted for restricted use within NHS Scotland for use in spinal anaesthesia in ambulatory surgery settings.

- MEDICINAL FORMS
There can be variation in the licensing of different medicines containing the same drug.
Solution for injection
▸ Citanest (Aspen Pharma Trading Ltd)
Prilocaine hydrochloride 10 mg per 1 ml Citanest 1% solution for injection 50ml vials | 1 vial [PoM] £5.06
▸ Prilotekal (Sintetica SA Pharmaceuticals)
Prilocaine hydrochloride 20 mg per 1 ml Prilotekal 100mg/5ml solution for injection ampoules | 10 ampoule [PoM] [X]

Prilocaine with felypressin

The properties listed below are those particular to the combination only. For the properties of the components please consider, prilocaine hydrochloride p. 1316.

- **● INDICATIONS AND DOSE**

Dental anaesthesia
▸ BY REGIONAL ADMINISTRATION
▸ Adult: Consult expert dental sources for specific advice

- **● INTERACTIONS** → Appendix 1: anaesthetics, local
- **● SIDE-EFFECTS** Bradycardia · cardiac arrest · dizziness · drowsiness · hypotension · loss of consciousness · methaemoglobinaemia · myocardial contractility decreased · nervousness · respiratory arrest · seizure · tremor · vision blurred

- **● MEDICINAL FORMS**
There can be variation in the licensing of different medicines containing the same drug.
Solution for injection
▸ Citanest with Octapressin (Dentsply Ltd)
Prilocaine hydrochloride 30 mg per 1 ml, Felypressin.03 unit per 1 ml Citanest 3% with Octapressin Dental 0.066units/2.2ml solution for injection self aspirating cartridges | 50 cartridge [PoM] Ⓢ

Ropivacaine hydrochloride

- **● INDICATIONS AND DOSE**

Acute pain, peripheral nerve block
▸ BY REGIONAL ADMINISTRATION
▸ Adult: 10–20 mg/hour, dose administered as a continuous infusion or by intermittent injection using a 2 mg/mL (0.2%) solution

Acute pain, field block
▸ BY REGIONAL ADMINISTRATION
▸ Adult: 2–200 mg, dose administered using a 2 mg/mL (0.2%) solution

Acute pain, lumbar epidural block
▸ BY LUMBAR EPIDURAL
▸ Adult: 20–40 mg, followed by 20–30 mg at least every 30 minutes, dose administered using a 2 mg/mL (0.2%) solution

Acute labour pain
▸ BY CONTINUOUS EPIDURAL INFUSION
▸ Adult: 12–20 mg/hour, dose administered using a 2 mg/mL (0.2%) solution

Acute postoperative pain
▸ BY CONTINUOUS EPIDURAL INFUSION
▸ Adult: Up to 28 mg/hour, dose administered using a 2 mg/mL (0.2%) solution

Postoperative pain, thoracic epidural block
▸ BY CONTINUOUS EPIDURAL INFUSION
▸ Adult: 12–28 mg/hour, dose administered using a 2 mg/mL (0.2%) solution

Surgical anaesthesia, field block
▸ BY REGIONAL ADMINISTRATION
▸ Adult: 7.5–225 mg, dose administered using a 7.5 mg/mL (0.75%) solution

Surgical anaesthesia, major nerve block (brachial plexus block)
▸ BY REGIONAL ADMINISTRATION
▸ Adult: 225–300 mg, dose administered using a 7.5 mg/mL (0.75%) solution

Surgical anaesthesia, thoracic epidural block (to establish block for postoperative pain)
▸ BY THORACIC EPIDURAL
▸ Adult: 38–113 mg, dose administered using a 7.5 mg/mL (0.75%) solution

Surgical anaesthesia for caesarean section
▸ BY LUMBAR EPIDURAL
▸ Adult: 113–150 mg, to be administered in incremental doses using a 7.5 mg/mL (0.75%) solution

Surgical anaesthesia, lumbar epidural block
▸ BY LUMBAR EPIDURAL
▸ Adult: 113–200 mg, dose administered using a 7.5 mg/mL (0.75%) or 10 mg/mL (1%) solution

DOSES AT EXTREMES OF BODY-WEIGHT
▸ To avoid excessive dosage in obese patients, dose may need to be calculated on the basis of ideal bodyweight.

> **IMPORTANT SAFETY INFORMATION**
> Should only be administered by, or under the direct supervision of, personnel experienced in their use, with adequate training in anaesthesia and airway management, and should not be administered parenterally unless adequate resuscitation equipment is available.

- **● CONTRA-INDICATIONS** Application to the middle ear (can cause ototoxicity) · avoid injection into infected tissues · avoid injection into inflamed tissues · complete heart block · preparations containing preservatives should not be used for caudal, epidural, or spinal block, or for intravenous regional anaesthesia (Bier's block) · should not be applied to damaged skin
CONTRA-INDICATIONS, FURTHER INFORMATION
▸ Injection site Local anaesthetics should not be injected into inflamed or infected tissues nor should they be applied to damaged skin. Increased absorption into the blood increases the possibility of systemic side-effects, and the local anaesthetic effect may also be reduced by altered local pH.

- **● CAUTIONS** Acute porphyrias p. 1025 · cardiovascular disease · debilitated patients (consider dose reduction) · elderly (consider dose reduction) · epilepsy · hypovolaemia · impaired cardiac conduction · impaired respiratory function · myasthenia gravis · shock

- **● INTERACTIONS** → Appendix 1: anaesthetics, local

- **● SIDE-EFFECTS**
▸ **Common or very common** Arrhythmias · back pain · chills · dizziness · headache · hypertension · hypotension · nausea · sensation abnormal · urinary retention · vomiting
▸ **Uncommon** Anxiety · dyspnoea · hypothermia · neurotoxicity · syncope
▸ **Rare or very rare** Cardiac arrest
▸ **Frequency not known** Dyskinesia
SIDE-EFFECTS, FURTHER INFORMATION Toxic effects after administration of local anaesthetics are a result of excessively high plasma concentrations; severe toxicity usually results from inadvertent intravascular injection. The systemic toxicity of local anaesthetics mainly involves the central nervous and cardiovascular systems. The onset of toxicity can be unpredictable and delayed. Monitor as per local protocol for at least 30 minutes after administration.

- **● ALLERGY AND CROSS-SENSITIVITY**
▸ Hypersensitivity and cross-sensitivity Hypersensitivity reactions occur mainly with the ester-type local anaesthetics, such as tetracaine; reactions are less frequent with the amide types, such as articaine, bupivacaine, levobupivacaine, lidocaine, mepivacaine, prilocaine, and ropivacaine. Cross-sensitivity reactions may be avoided by using the alternative chemical type.

- **● PREGNANCY** Not known to be harmful. Do not use for paracervical block in obstetrics.

- **● BREAST FEEDING** Not known to be harmful.

15

Anaesthesia

- **HEPATIC IMPAIRMENT** Use with caution in severe impairment.
- **RENAL IMPAIRMENT** Caution in severe impairment. Increased risk of systemic toxicity in chronic renal failure.

- **MEDICINAL FORMS**
There can be variation in the licensing of different medicines containing the same drug.
Solution for injection
ELECTROLYTES: May contain Sodium
▸ Ropivacaine hydrochloride (Non-proprietary)
Ropivacaine hydrochloride 2 mg per 1 ml Ropivacaine 20mg/10ml solution for injection ampoules | 10 ampoule [PoM] £16.50 (Hospital only)
Ropivacaine hydrochloride 7.5 mg per 1 ml Ropivacaine 75mg/10ml solution for injection ampoules | 10 ampoule [PoM] £25.00 (Hospital only)
Ropivacaine hydrochloride 10 mg per 1 ml Ropivacaine 100mg/10ml solution for injection ampoules | 10 ampoule [PoM] £30.00 (Hospital only)
▸ Naropin (Aspen Pharma Trading Ltd)
Ropivacaine hydrochloride 2 mg per 1 ml Naropin 20mg/10ml solution for injection ampoules | 5 ampoule [PoM] £12.79
Ropivacaine hydrochloride 7.5 mg per 1 ml Naropin 75mg/10ml solution for injection ampoules | 5 ampoule [PoM] £15.90
Ropivacaine hydrochloride 10 mg per 1 ml Naropin 100mg/10ml solution for injection ampoules | 5 ampoule [PoM] £19.22
Infusion
ELECTROLYTES: May contain Sodium
▸ Ropivacaine hydrochloride (Non-proprietary)
Ropivacaine hydrochloride 2 mg per 1 ml Ropivacaine 400mg/200ml infusion bags | 10 bag [PoM] £137.00 (Hospital only)
▸ Naropin (Aspen Pharma Trading Ltd)
Ropivacaine hydrochloride 2 mg per 1 ml Naropin 400mg/200ml infusion Polybags | 5 bag [PoM] £86.70

Tetracaine
(Amethocaine)

- **INDICATIONS AND DOSE**
Anaesthesia before venepuncture or venous cannulation
▸ TO THE SKIN
▸ Child 1 month–4 years: Apply contents of up to 1 tube (applied at separate sites at a single time or appropriate proportion) to site of venepuncture or venous cannulation and cover with occlusive dressing; remove gel and dressing after 30 minutes for venepuncture and after 45 minutes for venous cannulation
▸ Child 5–17 years: Apply contents of up to 5 tubes (applied at separate sites at a single time or appropriate proportion) to site of venepuncture or venous cannulation and cover with occlusive dressing; remove gel and dressing after 30 minutes for venepuncture and after 45 minutes for venous cannulation
▸ Adult: Apply contents of up to 5 tubes (applied at separate sites at a single time or appropriate proportion) to site of venepuncture or venous cannulation and cover with occlusive dressing; remove gel and dressing after 30 minutes for venepuncture and after 45 minutes for venous cannulation

- **CONTRA-INDICATIONS** Should not be applied to damaged skin
- **INTERACTIONS** → Appendix 1: anaesthetics, local
- **SIDE-EFFECTS** Oedema · skin reactions
SIDE-EFFECTS, FURTHER INFORMATION The systemic toxicity of local anaesthetics mainly involves the central nervous system; systemic side effects unlikely as minimal absorption following topical application.
- **ALLERGY AND CROSS-SENSITIVITY**
▸ Hypersensitivity and cross-sensitivity Hypersensitivity reactions occur mainly with the ester-type local anaesthetics, such as tetracaine; reactions are less

frequent with the amide types, such as articaine, bupivacaine, levobupivacaine, lidocaine, mepivacaine, prilocaine, and ropivacaine. Cross-sensitivity reactions may be avoided by using the alternative chemical type.
- **BREAST FEEDING** Not known to be harmful.
- **PATIENT AND CARER ADVICE**
Medicines for Children leaflet: Tetracaine gel for local anaesthesia www.medicinesforchildren.org.uk/tetracaine-gel-for-local-anaesthesia

- **MEDICINAL FORMS**
There can be variation in the licensing of different medicines containing the same drug.
Gel
EXCIPIENTS: May contain Hydroxybenzoates (parabens)
▸ Ametop (Alliance Pharmaceuticals Ltd)
Tetracaine 40 mg per 1 gram Ametop 4% gel | 1.5 gram [P] £1.08

Chapter 16
Emergency treatment of poisoning

CONTENTS

Poisoning, emergency treatment

Overview

These notes provide only an overview of the treatment of poisoning, and it is strongly recommended that either **TOXBASE** or the **UK National Poisons Information Service** be consulted when there is doubt about the degree of risk or about management.

Hospital admission

Patients who have features of poisoning should generally be admitted to hospital. Patients who have taken poisons with delayed action should also be admitted, even if they appear well. Delayed-action poisons include aspirin p. 121, iron, paracetamol p. 438, tricyclic antidepressants, and co-phenotrope (diphenoxylate with atropine, *Lomotil*®) p. 66; the effects of modified-release preparations are also delayed. A note of all relevant information, including what treatment has been given, should accompany the patient to hospital.

Further information

TOXBASE, the primary clinical toxicology database of the National Poisons Information Service, is available on the internet to registered users at www.toxbase.org (a backup site is available at www.toxbasebackup.org if the main site cannot be accessed). It provides information about routine diagnosis, treatment, and management of patients exposed to drugs, household products, and industrial and agricultural chemicals.

Specialist information and advice on the treatment of poisoning is available day and night from the **UK National Poisons Information Service** on the following number: Tel: 0344 892 0111.

Advice on laboratory analytical services can be obtained from TOXBASE or from the National Poisons Information Service. Help with identifying capsules or tablets may be available from a regional medicines information centre or from the National Poisons Information Service (out of hours).

General care

It is often impossible to establish with certainty the identity of the poison and the size of the dose. This is not usually important because only a few poisons (such as opioids, paracetamol, and iron) have specific antidotes; few patients require active removal of the poison. In most patients, treatment is directed at managing symptoms as they arise. Nevertheless, knowledge of the type and timing of poisoning can help in anticipating the course of events. All relevant information should be sought from the poisoned individual and from carers or parents. However, such information

should be interpreted with care because it may not be complete or entirely reliable. Sometimes symptoms arise from other illnesses and patients should be assessed carefully. Accidents may involve domestic and industrial products (the contents of which are not generally known). The **National Poisons Information Service** should be consulted when there is doubt about any aspect of suspected poisoning.

Respiration

Respiration is often impaired in unconscious patients. An obstructed airway requires immediate attention. In the absence of trauma, the airway should be opened with simple measures such as chin lift or jaw thrust. An oropharyngeal or nasopharyngeal airway may be useful in patients with reduced consciousness to prevent obstruction, provided ventilation is adequate. Intubation and ventilation should be considered in patients whose airway cannot be protected or who have respiratory acidosis because of inadequate ventilation; such patients should be monitored in a critical care area.

Most poisons that impair consciousness also depress respiration. Assisted ventilation (either mouth-to-mouth or using a bag-valve-mask device) may be needed. Oxygen is not a substitute for adequate ventilation, although it should be given in the highest concentration possible in poisoning with carbon monoxide and irritant gases.

Blood pressure

Hypotension is common in severe poisoning with central nervous system depressants. A systolic blood pressure of less than 70 mmHg may lead to irreversible brain damage or renal tubular necrosis. Hypotension should be corrected initially by raising the foot of the bed and administration of an infusion of either sodium chloride p. 1008 or a colloid. Vasoconstrictor sympathomimetics are rarely required and their use may be discussed with the National Poisons Information Service.

Fluid depletion without hypotension is common after prolonged coma and after aspirin poisoning due to vomiting, sweating, and hyperpnoea.

Hypertension, often transient, occurs less frequently than hypotension in poisoning; it may be associated with sympathomimetic drugs such as amfetamines, phencyclidine, and cocaine.

Heart

Cardiac conduction defects and arrhythmias can occur in acute poisoning, notably with tricyclic antidepressants, some antipsychotics, and some antihistamines. Arrhythmias often respond to correction of underlying hypoxia, acidosis,

16

Emergency treatment of poisoning

or other biochemical abnormalities, but ventricular arrhythmias that cause serious hypotension require treatment. If the QT interval is prolonged, specialist advice should be sought because the use of some anti-arrhythmic drugs may be inappropriate. Supraventricular arrhythmias are seldom life-threatening and drug treatment is best withheld until the patient reaches hospital.

Body temperature

Hypothermia may develop in patients of any age who have been deeply unconscious for some hours, particularly following overdose with barbiturates or phenothiazines. It may be missed unless core temperature is measured using a low-reading rectal thermometer or by some other means. Hypothermia should be managed by prevention of further heat loss and appropriate re-warming as clinically indicated.

Hyperthermia can develop in patients taking CNS stimulants; children and the elderly are also at risk when taking therapeutic doses of drugs with antimuscarinic properties. Hyperthermia is initially managed by removing all unnecessary clothing and using a fan. Sponging with **tepid** water will promote evaporation. Advice should be sought from the National Poisons Information Service on the management of severe hyperthermia resulting from conditions such as the serotonin syndrome.

Both hypothermia and hyperthermia require **urgent** hospitalisation for assessment and supportive treatment.

Convulsions during poisoning

Single short-lived convulsions (lasting less than 5 minutes) do not require treatment. If convulsions are protracted or recur frequently, lorazepam p. 335 or diazepam (preferably as emulsion) p. 340 should be given by slow intravenous injection into a large vein. Benzodiazepines should not be given by the intramuscular route for convulsions. If the intravenous route is not readily available, midazolam oromucosal solution p. 336 [unlicensed use in adults and children under 3 months] can be given by the buccal route or diazepam can be administered as a rectal solution.

Methaemoglobinaemia

Drug- or chemical-induced methaemoglobinaemia should be treated with methylthioninium chloride p. 1331 if the methaemoglobin concentration is 30% or higher, or if symptoms of tissue hypoxia are present despite oxygen therapy. Methylthioninium chloride reduces the ferric iron of methaemoglobin back to the ferrous iron of haemoglobin; in high doses, methylthioninium chloride can itself cause methaemoglobinaemia.

Poison removal and elimination

Prevention of absorption

Given by mouth, charcoal, activated p. 1326 can bind many poisons in the gastro-intestinal system, thereby reducing their absorption. The **sooner** it is given the **more effective** it is, but it may still be effective up to 1 hour after ingestion of the poison—longer in the case of modified-release preparations or of drugs with antimuscarinic (anticholinergic) properties. It is particularly useful for the prevention of absorption of poisons that are toxic in small amounts, such as antidepressants.

Active elimination techniques

Repeated doses of charcoal, activated by mouth *enhance the elimination* of some drugs after they have been absorbed; repeated doses are given after overdosage with:

- Carbamazepine
- Dapsone
- Phenobarbital
- Quinine
- Theophylline

If vomiting occurs after dosing it should be treated (e.g. with an antiemetic drug) since it may reduce the efficacy of

charcoal treatment. In cases of intolerance, the dose may be reduced and the frequency increased but this may compromise efficacy.

Charcoal, activated should **not** be used for poisoning with petroleum distillates, corrosive substances, alcohols, malathion, cyanides and metal salts including iron and lithium salts.

Other techniques intended to enhance the elimination of poisons after absorption are only practicable in hospital and are only suitable for a small number of severely poisoned patients. Moreover, they only apply to a limited number of poisons. Examples include:

- haemodialysis for ethylene glycol, lithium, methanol, phenobarbital, salicylates, and sodium valproate;
- alkalinisation of the urine for salicylates.

Removal from the gastro-intestinal tract

Gastric lavage is rarely required; for substances that cannot be removed effectively by other means (e.g. iron), it should be considered only if a life-threatening amount has been ingested within the previous hour. It should be carried out only if the airway can be protected adequately. Gastric lavage is contra-indicated if a corrosive substance or a petroleum distillate has been ingested, but it may occasionally be considered in patients who have ingested drugs that are not adsorbed by charcoal, such as iron or lithium. Induction of *emesis* (e.g. with ipecacuanha) is **not** recommended because there is no evidence that it affects absorption and it may increase the risk of aspiration.

Whole bowel irrigation (by means of a bowel cleansing preparation) has been used in poisoning with certain modified-release or enteric-coated formulations, in severe poisoning with iron and lithium salts, and if illicit drugs are carried in the gastro-intestinal tract ('body-packing'). However, it is not clear that the procedure improves outcome and advice should be sought from the National Poisons Information Service.

Alcohol, acute intoxication

Acute intoxication with alcohol (ethanol) is common in adults but also occurs in children. The features include ataxia, dysarthria, nystagmus, and drowsiness, which may progress to coma, with hypotension and acidosis. Aspiration of vomit is a special hazard and hypoglycaemia may occur in children and some adults. Patients are managed supportively, with particular attention to maintaining a clear airway and measures to reduce the risk of aspiration of gastric contents. The blood glucose is measured and glucose given if indicated.

Aspirin poisoning

The main features of salicylate poisoning are hyperventilation, tinnitus, deafness, vasodilatation, and sweating. Coma is uncommon but indicates very severe poisoning. The associated acid-base disturbances are complex.

Treatment must be in hospital, where plasma salicylate, pH, and electrolytes can be measured; absorption of aspirin may be slow and the plasma-salicylate concentration may continue to rise for several hours, requiring repeated measurement. Plasma-salicylate concentration may not correlate with clinical severity in the young and the elderly, and clinical and biochemical assessment is necessary. Generally, the clinical severity of poisoning is less below a plasma-salicylate concentration of 500 mg/litre (3.6 mmol/litre), unless there is evidence of metabolic acidosis. Activated charcoal can be given within 1 hour of ingesting more than 125 mg/kg of aspirin. Fluid losses should be replaced and intravenous sodium bicarbonate may be given (ensuring plasma-potassium concentration is within the reference range) to enhance urinary salicylate excretion (optimum urinary pH 7.5–8.5).

Paracetamol overdose treatment graph

Patients whose plasma-paracetamol concentrations are on or above the **treatment line** should be treated with acetylcysteine by intravenous infusion.

The prognostic accuracy after 15 hours is uncertain, but a plasma-paracetamol concentration on or above the treatment line should be regarded as carrying a serious risk of liver damage.

Graph reproduced courtesy of Medicines and Healthcare products Regulatory Agency

Plasma-potassium concentration should be corrected before giving sodium bicarbonate as hypokalaemia may complicate alkalinisation of the urine.

Haemodialysis is the treatment of choice for severe salicylate poisoning and should be considered when the plasma-salicylate concentration exceeds 700 mg/litre (5.1 mmol/litre) or in the presence of severe metabolic acidosis.

Opioid poisoning

Opioids (narcotic analgesics) cause coma, respiratory depression, and pinpoint pupils. The specific antidote naloxone hydrochloride p. 1329 is indicated if there is coma or bradypnoea. Since naloxone has a shorter duration of action than many opioids, close monitoring and repeated injections are necessary according to the respiratory rate and depth of coma. When repeated administration of naloxone is required, it can be given by continuous intravenous infusion instead and the rate of infusion adjusted according to vital signs. The effects of some opioids, such as buprenorphine, are only partially reversed by naloxone.
Dextropropoxyphene and methadone have very long durations of action; patients may need to be monitored for long periods following large overdoses.

Naloxone reverses the opioid effects of dextropropoxyphene. The long duration of action of dextropropoxyphene calls for prolonged monitoring and further doses of naloxone may be required.
Norpropoxyphene, a metabolite of dextropropoxyphene, also has cardiotoxic effects which may require treatment

with sodium bicarbonate p. 1006 or magnesium sulfate p. 1019, or both. Arrhythmias may occur for up to 12 hours.

Paracetamol poisoning

In cases of **intravenous paracetamol poisoning** contact the National Poisons Information Service for advice on risk assessment and management.

Toxic doses of paracetamol p. 438 may cause severe hepatocellular necrosis and, much less frequently, renal tubular necrosis. Nausea and vomiting, the only early features of poisoning, usually settle within 24 hours. Persistence beyond this time, often associated with the onset of right subcostal pain and tenderness, usually indicates development of hepatic necrosis. Liver damage is maximal 3–4 days after paracetamol overdose and may lead to encephalopathy, haemorrhage, hypoglycaemia, cerebral oedema, and death. Therefore, despite a lack of significant early symptoms, patients who have taken an overdose of paracetamol should be transferred to hospital urgently.

To avoid underestimating the potentially toxic paracetamol dose ingested by obese patients who weigh more than 110 kg, use a body-weight of 110 kg (rather than their actual body-weight) when calculating the total dose of paracetamol ingested (in mg/kg).

Acetylcysteine p. 1330 protects the liver if infused up to, and possibly beyond, 24 hours of ingesting paracetamol. It is most effective if given within 8 hours of ingestion, after which effectiveness declines. Very rarely, giving acetylcysteine by mouth [unlicensed route] is an alternative if intravenous access is not possible—contact the National Poisons Information Service for advice.

Neonates less than 45 weeks corrected gestational age may be more susceptible to paracetamol-induced liver toxicity, therefore, treatment with acetylcysteine should be considered in all paracetamol overdoses, and advice should be sought from the National Poisons Information Service.

Acute overdose

Hepatotoxicity may occur after a single ingestion of more than 150 mg/kg paracetamol taken in less than 1 hour. Rarely, hepatotoxicity may develop with single ingestions as low as 75 mg/kg of paracetamol taken in less than 1 hour. Patients who have ingested 75 mg/kg or more of paracetamol in less than 1 hour should be referred to hospital. Administration of charcoal, activated p. 1326 should be considered if paracetamol in excess of 150 mg/kg is thought to have been ingested within the previous hour.

Patients at risk of liver damage and, therefore, requiring acetylcysteine, can be identified from a single measurement of the plasma-paracetamol concentration, related to the time from ingestion, provided this time interval is not less than 4 hours; earlier samples may be misleading. The concentration is plotted on a paracetamol treatment graph, with a reference line ('treatment line') joining plots of 100 mg/litre (0.66 mmol/litre) at 4 hours and 3.13 mg/litre (0.02 mmol/litre) at 24 hours. Acetylcysteine treatment should commence immediately in patients:

- whose plasma-paracetamol concentration falls on or above the *treatment line* on the paracetamol treatment graph;
- who present 8–24 hours after taking an acute overdose of more than 150 mg/kg of paracetamol, even if the plasma-paracetamol concentration is not yet available; acetylcysteine can be discontinued if the plasma-paracetamol concentration is later reported to be below the *treatment line* on the paracetamol treatment graph, provided that the patient is asymptomatic and liver function tests, serum creatinine and INR are normal.

The prognostic accuracy of a plasma-paracetamol concentration taken after 15 hours is uncertain, but a concentration on or above the *treatment line* on the paracetamol treatment graph should be regarded as carrying a serious risk of liver damage. If more than 15 hours have elapsed since ingestion, or there is doubt about appropriate management, advice should be sought from the National Poisons Information Service.

'Staggered' overdose, uncertain time of overdose, or therapeutic excess

A 'staggered' overdose involves ingestion of a potentially toxic dose of paracetamol over more than one hour, with the possible intention of causing self-harm. Therapeutic excess is the inadvertent ingestion of a potentially toxic dose of paracetamol during its clinical use. The paracetamol treatment graph is unreliable if a 'staggered' overdose is taken, if there is uncertainty about the time of the overdose, or if there is therapeutic excess. In these cases, patients who have taken more than 150 mg/kg of paracetamol in any 24-hour period are at risk of toxicity and should be commenced on acetylcysteine immediately, unless it is more than 24 hours since the last ingestion, the patient is asymptomatic, the plasma-paracetamol concentration is undetectable, and liver function tests, serum creatinine and INR are normal.

Rarely, toxicity can occur with paracetamol doses between 75–150 mg/kg in any 24-hour period; clinical judgement of the individual case is necessary to determine whether to treat those who have ingested this amount of paracetamol. For small adults, this may be within the licensed dose, but ingestion of a licensed dose of paracetamol is not considered an overdose.

Although there is some evidence suggesting that factors such as the use of liver enzyme-inducing drugs (e.g.

carbamazepine p. 309, efavirenz p. 632, nevirapine p. 633, phenobarbital p. 331, phenytoin p. 321, primidone p. 332, rifabutin p. 564, rifampicin p. 571, St John's wort), chronic alcoholism, and starvation may increase the risk of hepatotoxicity, the CHM has advised that these should no longer be used in the assessment of paracetamol toxicity.

Significant toxicity is unlikely if, 24 hours or longer after the last paracetamol ingestion, the patient is asymptomatic, the plasma-paracetamol concentration is undetectable, and liver function tests, serum creatinine and INR are normal. Patients with clinical features of hepatic injury such as jaundice or hepatic tenderness should be treated urgently with acetylcysteine. If there is uncertainty about a patient's risk of toxicity after paracetamol overdose, treatment with acetylcysteine should be commenced. Advice should be sought from the National Poisons Information Service whenever necessary.

Acetylcysteine dose and administration

For paracetamol overdosage, acetylcysteine is given in a total dose that is divided into 3 consecutive intravenous infusions over a total of 21 hours. The tables below include the dose of acetylcysteine, for adults and children of body-weight 40 kg and over, in terms of the volume of acetylcysteine Concentrate for Intravenous Infusion required for each of the 3 infusions. The requisite dose of acetylcysteine is added to glucose Intravenous Infusion 5% p. 1009.

First infusion	
Body-weight	Volume of Acetylcysteine Concentrate for Intravenous Infusion 200 mg/mL required to prepare first infusion
40-49 kg	34 mL
50-59 kg	42 mL
60-69 kg	49 mL
70-79 kg	57 mL
80-89 kg	64 mL
90-99 kg	72 mL
100-109 kg	79 mL
≥110 kg	83 mL (max. dose)

First infusion (based on an acetylcysteine dose of approx. 150 mg/kg)—add requisite volume of Acetylcysteine Concentrate for Intravenous Infusion to 200 mL Glucose Intravenous Infusion 5%; infuse over 1 hour.

Second infusion	
Body-weight	Volume of Acetylcysteine Concentrate for Intravenous Infusion 200 mg/mL required to prepare second infusion
40-49 kg	12 mL
50-59 kg	14 mL
60-69 kg	17 mL
70-79 kg	19 mL
80-89 kg	22 mL
90-99 kg	24 mL
100-109 kg	27 mL
≥110 kg	28 mL (max. dose)

Second infusion (based on an acetylcysteine dose of approx. 50 mg/kg; start immediately after completion of first infusion)—add requisite volume of Acetylcysteine Concentrate for Intravenous Infusion to 500 mL Glucose Intravenous Infusion 5%; infuse over 4 hours.

Third infusion

Body-weight	Volume of Acetylcysteine Concentrate for Intravenous Infusion 200 mg/mL required to prepare third infusion
40-49 kg	23 mL
50-59 kg	28 mL
60-69 kg	33 mL
70-79 kg	38 mL
80-89 kg	43 mL
90-99 kg	48 mL
100-109 kg	53 mL
≥110 kg	55 mL (max. dose)

Third infusion (based on an acetylcysteine dose of approx. 100 mg/kg; start immediately after completion of second infusion)—add requisite volume of Acetylcysteine Concentrate for Intravenous Infusion to 1 litre Glucose Intravenous Infusion 5%; infuse over 16 hours.

Antidepressant poisoning

Tricyclic and related antidepressants

Tricyclic and related antidepressants cause dry mouth, coma of varying degree, hypotension, hypothermia, hyperreflexia, extensor plantar responses, convulsions, respiratory failure, cardiac conduction defects, and arrhythmias. Dilated pupils and urinary retention also occur. Metabolic acidosis may complicate severe poisoning; delirium with confusion, agitation, and visual and auditory hallucinations are common during recovery.

Assessment in hospital is strongly advised in case of poisoning by tricyclic and related antidepressants but symptomatic treatment can be given before transfer. Supportive measures to ensure a clear airway and adequate ventilation during transfer are mandatory. Intravenous lorazepam or intravenous diazepam (preferably in emulsion form) may be required to treat convulsions. Activated charcoal given within 1 hour of the overdose reduces absorption of the drug. Although arrhythmias are worrying, some will respond to correction of hypoxia and acidosis. The use of anti-arrhythmic drugs is best avoided, but intravenous infusion of sodium bicarbonate can arrest arrhythmias or prevent them in those with an extended QRS duration. Diazepam given by mouth is usually adequate to sedate delirious patients but large doses may be required.

Selective serotonin re-uptake inhibitors (SSRIs)

Symptoms of poisoning by selective serotonin re-uptake inhibitors include nausea, vomiting, agitation, tremor, nystagmus, drowsiness, and sinus tachycardia; convulsions may occur. Rarely, severe poisoning results in the serotonin syndrome, with marked neuropsychiatric effects, neuromuscular hyperactivity, and autonomic instability; hyperthermia, rhabdomyolysis, renal failure, and coagulopathies may develop.

Management of SSRI poisoning is supportive. Activated charcoal given within 1 hour of the overdose reduces absorption of the drug. Convulsions can be treated with lorazepam, diazepam, or midazolam oromucosal solution [unlicensed use in adults and children under 3 months] (see *Convulsions*). Contact the National Poisons Information Service for the management of hyperthermia or the serotonin syndrome.

Antimalarial poisoning

Overdosage with quinine, chloroquine, or hydroxychloroquine is extremely hazardous and difficult to treat. Urgent advice from the National Poisons Information Service is essential. Life-threatening features include arrhythmias (which can have a very rapid onset) and convulsions (which can be intractable).

Antipsychotic poisoning

Phenothiazines and related drugs

Phenothiazines cause less depression of consciousness and respiration than other sedatives. Hypotension, hypothermia, sinus tachycardia, and arrhythmias may complicate poisoning. Dystonic reactions can occur with therapeutic doses (particularly with prochlorperazine and trifluoperazine), and convulsions may occur in severe cases. Arrhythmias may respond to correction of hypoxia, acidosis, and other biochemical abnormalities, but specialist advice should be sought if arrhythmias result from a prolonged QT interval; the use of some anti-arrhythmic drugs can worsen such arrhythmias. Dystonic reactions are rapidly abolished by injection of drugs such as procyclidine hydrochloride p. 406 or diazepam (emulsion preferred) p. 340.

Second-generation antipsychotic drugs

Features of poisoning by second-generation antipsychotic drugs include drowsiness, convulsions, extrapyramidal symptoms, hypotension, and ECG abnormalities (including prolongation of the QT interval). Management is supportive. Charcoal, activated p. 1326 can be given within 1 hour of ingesting a significant quantity of a second-generation antipsychotic drug.

Benzodiazepine poisoning

Benzodiazepines taken alone cause drowsiness, ataxia, dysarthria, nystagmus, and occasionally respiratory depression, and coma. Charcoal, activated can be given within 1 hour of ingesting a significant quantity of benzodiazepine, provided the patient is awake and the airway is protected. Benzodiazepines potentiate the effects of other central nervous system depressants taken concomitantly. Use of the benzodiazepine antagonist flumazenil p. 1328 [unlicensed indication] can be hazardous, particularly in mixed overdoses involving tricyclic antidepressants or in benzodiazepine-dependent patients. Flumazenil may prevent the need for ventilation, particularly in patients with severe respiratory disorders; it should be used on expert advice only and not as a diagnostic test in patients with a reduced level of consciousness.

Beta blockers poisoning

Therapeutic overdosages with beta-blockers may cause lightheadedness, dizziness, and possibly syncope as a result of bradycardia and hypotension; heart failure may be precipitated or exacerbated. These complications are most likely in patients with conduction system disorders or impaired myocardial function. Bradycardia is the most common arrhythmia caused by beta-blockers, but sotalol may induce ventricular tachyarrhythmias (sometimes of the torsade de pointes type). The effects of massive overdosage can vary from one beta-blocker to another; propranolol overdosage in particular may cause coma and convulsions.

Acute massive overdosage must be managed in hospital and expert advice should be obtained. Maintenance of a clear airway and adequate ventilation is mandatory. An intravenous injection of atropine sulfate p. 1131 is required to treat bradycardia. Cardiogenic shock unresponsive to atropine sulfate is probably best treated with an intravenous injection of glucagon p. 707 [unlicensed] in glucose 5% (with precautions to protect the airway in case of vomiting) followed by an intravenous infusion. If glucagon is not available, intravenous isoprenaline (available from 'special-order' manufacturers or specialist importing companies) is an alternative. A cardiac pacemaker can be used to increase the heart rate.

Calcium-channel blockers poisoning

Features of calcium-channel blocker poisoning include nausea, vomiting, dizziness, agitation, confusion, and coma in severe poisoning. Metabolic acidosis and hyperglycaemia may occur. Verapamil and diltiazem have a profound cardiac depressant effect causing hypotension and arrhythmias, including complete heart block and asystole. The dihydropyridine calcium-channel blockers cause severe hypotension secondary to profound peripheral vasodilatation.

Charcoal, activated should be considered if the patient presents within 1 hour of overdosage with a calcium-channel blocker; repeated doses of activated charcoal are considered if a modified-release preparation is involved. In patients with significant features of poisoning, calcium chloride p. 1014 or calcium gluconate p. 1014 is given by injection; atropine sulfate is given to correct symptomatic bradycardia. In severe cases, an insulin and glucose infusion may be required in the management of hypotension and myocardial failure. For the management of hypotension, the choice of inotropic sympathomimetic depends on whether hypotension is secondary to vasodilatation or to myocardial depression—advice should be sought from the National Poisons Information Service.

Iron salts poisoning

Iron poisoning in childhood is usually accidental. The symptoms are nausea, vomiting, abdominal pain, diarrhoea, haematemesis, and rectal bleeding. Hypotension and hepatocellular necrosis can occur later. Coma, shock, and metabolic acidosis indicate severe poisoning.

Advice should be sought from the National Poisons Information Service if a significant quantity of iron has been ingested within the previous hour.

Mortality is reduced by intensive and specific therapy with desferrioxamine mesilate p. 996, which chelates iron. The serum-iron concentration is measured as an emergency and intravenous desferrioxamine mesilate given to chelate absorbed iron in excess of the expected iron binding capacity. In severe toxicity intravenous desferrioxamine mesilate should be given immediately without waiting for the result of the serum-iron measurement.

Lithium poisoning

Most cases of lithium intoxication occur as a complication of long-term therapy and are caused by reduced excretion of the drug because of a variety of factors including dehydration, deterioration of renal function, infections, and co-administration of diuretics or NSAIDs (or other drugs that interact). Acute deliberate overdoses may also occur with delayed onset of symptoms (12 hours or more) owing to slow entry of lithium into the tissues and continuing absorption from modified-release formulations.

The early clinical features are non-specific and may include apathy and restlessness which could be confused with mental changes arising from the patient's depressive illness. Vomiting, diarrhoea, ataxia, weakness, dysarthria, muscle twitching, and tremor may follow. Severe poisoning is associated with convulsions, coma, renal failure, electrolyte imbalance, dehydration, and hypotension.

Therapeutic serum-lithium concentrations are within the range of 0.4–1 mmol/litre; concentrations in excess of 2 mmol/litre are usually associated with serious toxicity and such cases may need treatment with haemodialysis if neurological symptoms or renal failure are present. In acute overdose much higher serum-lithium concentrations may be present without features of toxicity and all that is usually necessary is to take measures to increase urine output (e.g. by increasing fluid intake but avoiding diuretics). Otherwise, treatment is supportive with special regard to electrolyte balance, renal function, and control of convulsions. Gastric lavage may be considered if it can be performed within 1 hour of ingesting significant quantities of lithium. Whole-bowel irrigation should be considered for significant ingestion, but advice should be sought from the National Poisons Information Service.

Stimulant-drug poisoning

Amfetamines cause wakefulness, excessive activity, paranoia, hallucinations, and hypertension followed by exhaustion, convulsions, hyperthermia, and coma. The early stages can be controlled by diazepam p. 340 or lorazepam p. 335; advice should be sought from the National Poisons Information Service on the management of hypertension. Later, tepid sponging, anticonvulsants, and artificial respiration may be needed.

Cocaine

Cocaine stimulates the central nervous system, causing agitation, dilated pupils, tachycardia, hypertension, hallucinations, hyperthermia, hypertonia, and hyperreflexia; cardiac effects include chest pain, myocardial infarction, and arrhythmias.

Initial treatment of cocaine poisoning involves intravenous administration of diazepam to control agitation and cooling measures for hyperthermia (see Body temperature); hypertension and cardiac effects require specific treatment and expert advice should be sought.

Ecstasy

Ecstasy (methylenedioxymethamfetamine, MDMA) may cause severe reactions, even at doses that were previously tolerated. The most serious effects are delirium, coma, convulsions, ventricular arrhythmias, hyperthermia, rhabdomyolysis, acute renal failure, acute hepatitis, disseminated intravascular coagulation, adult respiratory distress syndrome, hyperreflexia, hypotension and intracerebral haemorrhage; hyponatraemia has also been associated with ecstasy use.

Treatment of methylenedioxymethamfetamine poisoning is supportive, with diazepam to control severe agitation or persistent convulsions and close monitoring including ECG. Self-induced water intoxication should be considered in patients with ecstasy poisoning.

'Liquid ecstasy' is a term used for sodium oxybate (gamma-hydroxybutyrate, GHB), which is a sedative.

Theophylline poisoning

Theophylline and related drugs are often prescribed as modified-release formulations and toxicity can therefore be delayed. They cause vomiting (which may be severe and intractable), agitation, restlessness, dilated pupils, sinus tachycardia, and hyperglycaemia. More serious effects are haematemesis, convulsions, and supraventricular and ventricular arrhythmias. Severe hypokalaemia may develop rapidly.

Repeated doses of activated charcoal can be used to eliminate theophylline even if more than 1 hour has elapsed after ingestion and especially if a modified-release preparation has been taken (see also under Active Elimination Techniques). Ondansetron p. 430 may be effective for severe vomiting that is resistant to other antiemetics [unlicensed indication]. Hypokalaemia is corrected by intravenous infusion of potassium chloride p. 1025 and may be so severe as to require 60 mmol/hour (high doses require ECG monitoring). Convulsions should be controlled by intravenous administration of lorazepam or diazepam (see Convulsions). Sedation with diazepam may be necessary in agitated patients.

Provided the patient does not suffer from asthma, a short-acting beta-blocker can be administered intravenously to reverse severe tachycardia, hypokalaemia, and hyperglycaemia.

Cyanide poisoning

Oxygen should be administered to patients with cyanide poisoning. The choice of antidote depends on the severity of poisoning, certainty of diagnosis, and the cause. Dicobalt edetate p. 1327 is the antidote of choice when there is a strong clinical suspicion of severe cyanide poisoning, but it should **not** be used as a precautionary measure. Dicobalt edetate itself is toxic, associated with anaphylactoid reactions, and is potentially fatal if administered in the absence of cyanide poisoning. A regimen of sodium nitrite p. 1327 followed by sodium thiosulfate p. 1327 is an alternative if dicobalt edetate is not available.

Hydroxocobalamin (*Cyanokit*®—no other preparation of hydroxocobalamin is suitable) p. 994 can be considered for use in victims of smoke inhalation who show signs of significant cyanide poisoning.

Ethylene glycol and methanol poisoning

Fomepizole (available from 'special-order' manufacturers or specialist importing companies) is the treatment of choice for ethylene glycol and methanol (methyl alcohol) poisoning. If necessary, **ethanol** (by mouth or by intravenous infusion) can be used, but with caution. Advice on the treatment of ethylene glycol and methanol poisoning should be obtained from the National Poisons Information Service. It is important to start antidote treatment promptly in cases of suspected poisoning with these agents.

Heavy metal poisoning

Heavy metal antidotes include succimer (DMSA) [unlicensed], unithiol (DMPS) [unlicensed], sodium calcium edetate [unlicensed], and dimercaprol. Dimercaprol in the management of heavy metal poisoning has been superseded by other chelating agents. In all cases of heavy metal poisoning, the advice of the National Poisons Information Service should be sought.

Noxious gases poisoning

Carbon monoxide

Carbon monoxide poisoning is usually due to inhalation of smoke, car exhaust, or fumes caused by blocked flues or incomplete combustion of fuel gases in confined spaces.

Immediate treatment of carbon monoxide poisoning is essential. The person should be moved to fresh air, the airway cleared, and high-flow **oxygen** 100% administered through a tight-fitting mask with an inflated face seal. Artificial respiration should be given as necessary and continued until adequate spontaneous breathing starts, or stopped only after persistent and efficient treatment of cardiac arrest has failed. The patient should be admitted to hospital because complications may arise after a delay of hours or days. Cerebral oedema may occur in severe poisoning and is treated with an intravenous infusion of mannitol p. 228. Referral for hyperbaric oxygen treatment should be discussed with the National Poisons Information Service if the patient is pregnant or in cases of severe poisoning, such as if the patient is or has been unconscious, or has psychiatric or neurological features other than a headache, or has myocardial ischaemia or an arrhythmia, or has a blood carboxyhaemoglobin concentration of more than 20%.

Sulfur dioxide, chlorine, phosgene, and ammonia

All of these gases can cause upper respiratory tract and conjunctival irritation. Pulmonary oedema, with severe breathlessness and cyanosis may develop suddenly up to 36 hours after exposure. Death may occur. Patients are kept under observation and those who develop pulmonary oedema are given oxygen. Assisted ventilation may be necessary in the most serious cases.

CS Spray poisoning

CS spray, which is used for riot control, irritates the eyes (hence 'tear gas') and the respiratory tract; symptoms normally settle spontaneously within 15 minutes. If symptoms persist, the patient should be removed to a well-ventilated area, and the exposed skin washed with soap and water after removal of contaminated clothing. Contact lenses should be removed and rigid ones washed (soft ones should be discarded). Eye symptoms should be treated by irrigating the eyes with physiological saline (or water if saline is not available) and advice sought from an ophthalmologist. Patients with features of severe poisoning, particularly respiratory complications, should be admitted to hospital for symptomatic treatment.

Nerve agent poisoning

Treatment of nerve agent poisoning is similar to organophosphorus insecticide poisoning, but advice must be sought from the National Poisons Information Service. The risk of cross-contamination is significant; adequate decontamination and protective clothing for healthcare personnel are essential. In emergencies involving the release of nerve agents, kits ('NAAS pods') containing pralidoxime chloride p. 1327 can be obtained through the Ambulance Service from the National Blood Service (or the Welsh Blood Service in South Wales or designated hospital pharmacies in Northern Ireland and Scotland—see TOXBASE for list of designated centres).

Pesticide poisoning

Organophosphorus insecticides

Organophosphorus insecticides are usually supplied as powders or dissolved in organic solvents. All are absorbed through the bronchi and intact skin as well as through the gut and inhibit cholinesterase activity, thereby prolonging and intensifying the effects of acetylcholine. Toxicity between different compounds varies considerably, and onset may be delayed after skin exposure.

Anxiety, restlessness, dizziness, headache, miosis, nausea, hypersalivation, vomiting, abdominal colic, diarrhoea, bradycardia, and sweating are common features of organophosphorus poisoning. Muscle weakness and fasciculation may develop and progress to generalised flaccid paralysis, including the ocular and respiratory muscles. Convulsions, coma, pulmonary oedema with copious bronchial secretions, hypoxia, and arrhythmias occur in severe cases. Hyperglycaemia and glycosuria without ketonuria may also be present.

Further absorption of the organophosphorus insecticide should be prevented by moving the patient to fresh air, removing soiled clothing, and washing contaminated skin. In severe poisoning it is vital to ensure a clear airway, frequent removal of bronchial secretions, and adequate ventilation and oxygenation; gastric lavage may be considered provided that the airway is protected. Atropine sulfate p. 1295 will reverse the muscarinic effects of acetylcholine and is given by intravenous injection until the skin becomes flushed and dry, the pupils dilate, and bradycardia is abolished.

Pralidoxime chloride, a cholinesterase reactivator, is used as an adjunct to atropine sulfate in moderate or severe poisoning. It improves muscle tone within 30 minutes of administration. Pralidoxime chloride is continued until the patient has not required atropine sulfate for 12 hours. Pralidoxime chloride can be obtained from designated centres, the names of which are held by the National Poisons Information Service.

Snake bites and animal stings

Snake bites

Envenoming from snake bite is uncommon in the UK. Many exotic snakes are kept, some illegally, but the only indigenous venomous snake is the adder (*Vipera berus*). The bite may cause local and systemic effects. Local effects include pain, swelling, bruising, and tender enlargement of regional lymph nodes. Systemic effects include early anaphylactic symptoms (transient hypotension with syncope, angioedema, urticaria, abdominal colic, diarrhoea, and vomiting), with later persistent or recurrent hypotension, ECG abnormalities, spontaneous systemic bleeding, coagulopathy, adult respiratory distress syndrome, and acute renal failure. Fatal envenoming is rare but the potential for severe envenoming must not be underestimated.

Early anaphylactic symptoms should be treated with **adrenaline/epinephrine p. 221**. Indications for european viper snake venom antiserum treatment p. 1331 include *systemic envenoming*, especially hypotension, ECG abnormalities, vomiting, haemostatic abnormalities, and marked local envenoming such that after bites on the hand or foot, swelling extends beyond the wrist or ankle within 4 hours of the bite. For those patients who present with clinical features of *severe envenoming* (e.g. shock, ECG abnormalities, or local swelling that has advanced from the foot to above the knee or from the hand to above the elbow within 2 hours of the bite), a higher initial dose of the european viper snake venom antiserum is recommended; if symptoms of *systemic envenoming* persist contact the National Poisons Information Service. Adrenaline/epinephrine injection must be immediately to hand for treatment of anaphylactic reactions to the european viper snake venom antiserum.

European viper snake venom antiserum is available for bites by certain foreign snakes and spiders, stings by scorpions and fish. For information on identification, management, and for supply in an emergency, telephone the National Poisons Information Service. Whenever possible the TOXBASE entry should be read, and relevant information collected, before telephoning the National Poisons Information Service.

Insect stings

Stings from ants, wasps, hornets, and bees cause local pain and swelling but seldom cause severe direct toxicity unless many stings are inflicted at the same time. If the sting is in the mouth or on the tongue local swelling may threaten the upper airway. The stings from these insects are usually treated by cleaning the area with a topical antiseptic. Bee stings should be removed as quickly as possible. Anaphylactic reactions require immediate treatment with intramuscular **adrenaline/epinephrine**; self-administered intramuscular adrenaline/epinephrine (e.g. *EpiPen*®) is the best first-aid treatment for patients with severe hypersensitivity. An inhaled bronchodilator should be used for asthmatic reactions, see also the management of anaphylaxis. A short course of an **oral antihistamine** or a **topical corticosteroid** may help to reduce inflammation and relieve itching. A vaccine containing extracts of bee and wasp venom can be used to reduce the risk of anaphylaxis and systemic reactions in patients with systemic hypersensitivity to bee or wasp stings.

Marine stings

The severe pain of weeverfish (*Trachinus vipera*) and Portuguese man-o'-war stings can be relieved by immersing the stung area immediately in uncomfortably hot, but not scalding, water (not more than 45°C). People stung by jellyfish and Portuguese man-o'-war around the UK coast should be removed from the sea as soon as possible. Adherent tentacles should be lifted off carefully (wearing gloves or using tweezers) or washed off with seawater. Alcoholic solutions, including suntan lotions, should **not** be applied because they can cause further discharge of stinging hairs. Ice packs can be used to reduce pain.

Other poisons

Consult either the National Poisons Information Service day and night or TOXBASE.

The **National Poisons Information Service** (Tel: 0344 892 0111) will provide specialist advice on all aspects of poisoning day and night.

1 Active elimination from the gastro-intestinal tract

ANTIDOTES AND CHELATORS › INTESTINAL ADSORBENTS

Charcoal, activated

● INDICATIONS AND DOSE

Reduction of absorption of poisons in the gastro-intestinal system
▸ BY MOUTH

▸ Neonate: 1 g/kg.

▸ Child 1 month–11 years: 1 g/kg (max. per dose 50 g)
▸ Child 12–17 years: 50 g
▸ Adult: 50 g

Active elimination of poisons
▸ BY MOUTH

▸ Neonate: 1 g/kg every 4 hours, dose may be reduced and the frequency increased if not tolerated, reduced dose may compromise efficacy

▸ Child 1 month–11 years: 1 g/kg every 4 hours (max. per dose 50 g), dose may be reduced and the frequency increased if not tolerated, reduced dose may compromise efficacy
▸ Child 12–17 years: Initially 50 g, then 50 g every 4 hours, reduced if not tolerated to 25 g every 2 hours, alternatively 12.5 g every 1 hour, reduced dose may compromise efficacy
▸ Adult: Initially 50 g, then 50 g every 4 hours, reduced if not tolerated to 25 g every 2 hours, alternatively 12.5 g every 1 hour, reduced dose may compromise efficacy

Accelerated elimination of teriflunomide
▸ BY MOUTH USING GRANULES
▸ Adult: 50 g every 12 hours for 11 days

Accelerated elimination of leflunomide (washout procedure)
▸ BY MOUTH USING GRANULES
▸ Adult: 50 g 4 times a day for 11 days

● UNLICENSED USE
▸ In adults Activated charcoal doses in BNF may differ from those in product literature.

● CAUTIONS Comatose patient (risk of aspiration—ensure airway is protected) · drowsy patient (risk of aspiration—ensure airway protected) · reduced gastrointestinal motility (risk of obstruction)

● SIDE-EFFECTS Bezoar · constipation · diarrhoea · gastrointestinal disorders

● DIRECTIONS FOR ADMINISTRATION Suspension or reconstituted powder may be mixed with soft drinks (e.g. caffeine-free diet cola) or fruit juices to mask the taste.

- MEDICINAL FORMS
There can be variation in the licensing of different medicines containing the same drug.
Oral suspension
▸ Charcodote (Teva UK Ltd)
Activated charcoal 200 mg per 1 ml Charcodote 200mg/ml oral suspension sugar-free | 250 ml ℗ £11.88
Granules
▸ Carbomix (Kent Pharmaceuticals Ltd)
Activated charcoal 813 mg per 1 gram Carbomix 81.3% granules sugar-free | 50 gram ℗ £11.90

2 Chemical toxicity

2.1 Cyanide toxicity

ANTIDOTES AND CHELATORS

Dicobalt edetate

- INDICATIONS AND DOSE
Severe poisoning with cyanides
▸ BY INTRAVENOUS INJECTION
▸ Child: Consult the National Poisons Information Service
▸ Adult: 300 mg, to be given over 1 minute (or 5 minutes if condition less serious), dose to be followed immediately by 50 mL of glucose intravenous infusion 50%; if response inadequate a second dose of both may be given, but risk of cobalt toxicity

- CAUTIONS Owing to toxicity to be used only for definite cyanide poisoning when patient tending to lose, or has lost, consciousness

- SIDE-EFFECTS Reflex tachycardia · vomiting

- EXCEPTIONS TO LEGAL CATEGORY Prescription only medicine restriction does not apply where administration is for saving life in emergency.

- MEDICINAL FORMS
There can be variation in the licensing of different medicines containing the same drug.
Solution for injection
▸ Dicobalt edetate (Non-proprietary)
Dicobalt edetate 15 mg per 1 ml Dicobalt edetate 300mg/20ml solution for injection ampoules | 6 ampoule [PoM] £117.20

Sodium nitrite   16-Mar-2018

- INDICATIONS AND DOSE
Poisoning with cyanides (used in conjunction with sodium thiosulfate)
▸ BY INTRAVENOUS INJECTION
▸ Child: Consult the National Poisons Information Service
▸ Adult: 300 mg

- SIDE-EFFECTS Arrhythmias · dizziness · headache · hypotension · palpitations

- EXCEPTIONS TO LEGAL CATEGORY Prescription only medicine restriction does not apply where administration is for saving life in emergency.

- MEDICINAL FORMS
There can be variation in the licensing of different medicines containing the same drug.
Solution for injection
▸ Sodium nitrite (Non-proprietary)
Sodium nitrite 30 mg per 1 ml Sodium nitrite 300mg/10ml solution for injection vials | 1 vial [PoM] [☒]

Sodium thiosulfate   16-Mar-2018

- INDICATIONS AND DOSE
Poisoning with cyanides
▸ BY INTRAVENOUS INJECTION
▸ Child: Consult the National Poisons Information Service
▸ Adult: 12.5 g, to be given over 10 minutes, dose may be repeated in severe cyanide poisoning

DOSE EQUIVALENCE AND CONVERSION
▸ 12.5 g equates to 50 mL of a 25% solution *or* 25 mL of a 50% solution.

- EXCEPTIONS TO LEGAL CATEGORY Prescription only medicine restriction does not apply where administration is for saving life in emergency.

- MEDICINAL FORMS
There can be variation in the licensing of different medicines containing the same drug. Forms available from special-order manufacturers include: solution for injection
Solution for injection
▸ Sodium thiosulfate (Non-proprietary)
Sodium thiosulfate 250 mg per 1 ml Sodium thiosulfate 12.5g/50ml solution for injection vials | 1 vial [PoM] [☒]

2.2 Organophosphorus toxicity

Other drugs used for Organophosphorus toxicity Atropine sulfate, p. 1295

ANTIDOTES AND CHELATORS

Pralidoxime chloride

- INDICATIONS AND DOSE
Adjunct to atropine in the treatment of poisoning by organophosphorus insecticide or nerve agent
▸ BY INTRAVENOUS INFUSION
▸ Child: Initially 30 mg/kg, to be given over 20 minutes, followed by 8 mg/kg/hour; maximum 12 g per day
▸ Adult: Initially 30 mg/kg, to be given over 20 minutes, followed by 8 mg/kg/hour; maximum 12 g per day

- UNLICENSED USE Pralidoxime chloride doses may differ from those in product literature. Licensed for use in children (age range not specified by manufacturer).

- CONTRA-INDICATIONS Poisoning with carbamates · poisoning with organophosphorus compounds without anticholinesterase activity

- CAUTIONS Myasthenia gravis

- SIDE-EFFECTS Dizziness · drowsiness · headache · hyperventilation · muscle weakness · nausea · tachycardia · visual impairment

- RENAL IMPAIRMENT Use with caution.

- DIRECTIONS FOR ADMINISTRATION The loading dose may be administered by intravenous injection (diluted to a concentration of 50 mg/mL with water for injections) over at least 5 minutes if pulmonary oedema is present or if it is not practical to administer an intravenous infusion.
▸ In children For *intravenous infusion*, reconstitute each vial with 20 mL Water for Injections, then dilute to a concentration of 10–20 mg/mL with Sodium Chloride 0.9%.

- PRESCRIBING AND DISPENSING INFORMATION Available from designated centres for organophosphorus insecticide poisoning or from the National Blood Service (or Welsh Ambulance Services for Mid West and South East Wales)—see TOXBASE for list of designated centres.

16

Emergency treatment of poisoning

- **EXCEPTIONS TO LEGAL CATEGORY** Prescription only medicine restriction does not apply where administration is for saving life in emergency.

- **MEDICINAL FORMS**
There can be variation in the licensing of different medicines containing the same drug.
  Powder for solution for injection
  ▸ Protopam (imported (United States))
  Pralidoxime chloride 1 gram Protopam Chloride 1g powder for solution for injection vials | 6 vial PoM ⓧ

3　Drug toxicity

3.1　Benzodiazepine toxicity

ANTIDOTES AND CHELATORS ⟩
BENZODIAZEPINE ANTAGONISTS

Flumazenil

- **INDICATIONS AND DOSE**
Reversal of sedative effects of benzodiazepines in anaesthesia and clinical procedures
  ▸ **BY INTRAVENOUS INJECTION**
  ▸ Adult:　200 micrograms, dose to be administered over 15 seconds, then 100 micrograms every 1 minute if required; usual dose 300–600 micrograms; maximum 1 mg per course

Reversal of sedative effects of benzodiazepines in intensive care
  ▸ **BY INTRAVENOUS INJECTION**
  ▸ Adult:　300 micrograms, dose to be administered over 15 seconds, then 100 micrograms every 1 minute if required; maximum 2 mg per course

Reversal of sedative effects of benzodiazepines in intensive care (if drowsiness recurs after injection)
  ▸ **INITIALLY BY INTRAVENOUS INFUSION**
  ▸ Adult:　100–400 micrograms/hour, adjusted according to response, alternatively (by intravenous injection) 300 micrograms, adjusted according to response

> **IMPORTANT SAFETY INFORMATION**
> Flumazenil should only be administered by, or under the direct supervision of, personnel experienced in its use.

- **CONTRA-INDICATIONS** Life-threatening condition (e.g. raised intracranial pressure, status epilepticus) controlled by benzodiazepines

- **CAUTIONS** Avoid rapid injection following major surgery · avoid rapid injection in high-risk or anxious patients · benzodiazepine dependence (may precipitate withdrawal symptoms) · elderly · ensure neuromuscular blockade cleared before giving · head injury (rapid reversal of benzodiazepine sedation may cause convulsions) · history of panic disorders (risk of recurrence) · prolonged benzodiazepine therapy for epilepsy (risk of convulsions) · short-acting (repeat doses may be necessary— benzodiazepine effects may persist for at least 24 hours)

- **SIDE-EFFECTS**
  ▸ **Common or very common** Anxiety · diplopia · dry mouth · eye disorders · flushing · headache · hiccups · hyperhidrosis · hyperventilation · hypotension · insomnia · nausea · palpitations · paraesthesia · speech disorder · tremor · vertigo · vomiting
  ▸ **Uncommon** Abnormal hearing · arrhythmias · chest pain · chills · cough · dyspnoea · nasal congestion · seizure (more common in patients with epilepsy)
  ▸ **Frequency not known** Withdrawal syndrome

- **PREGNANCY** Not known to be harmful.
- **BREAST FEEDING** Avoid breast-feeding for 24 hours.
- **HEPATIC IMPAIRMENT** **Dose adjustments** Carefully titrate dose.
- **DIRECTIONS FOR ADMINISTRATION** For *continuous intravenous infusion*, dilute with Glucose 5% or Sodium Chloride 0.9%.

- **MEDICINAL FORMS**
There can be variation in the licensing of different medicines containing the same drug.
  Solution for injection
  ▸ Flumazenil (Non-proprietary)
  Flumazenil 100 microgram per 1 ml Flumazenil 500micrograms/5ml solution for injection ampoules | 5 ampoule PoM £65.50–£70.00

3.2　Digoxin toxicity

ANTIDOTES AND CHELATORS ⟩ ANTIBODIES

Digoxin-specific antibody

- **INDICATIONS AND DOSE**
Treatment of known or strongly suspected life-threatening digoxin toxicity associated with ventricular arrhythmias or bradyarrhythmias unresponsive to atropine and when measures beyond the withdrawal of digoxin and correction of any electrolyte abnormalities are considered necessary
  ▸ **BY INTRAVENOUS INFUSION**
  ▸ Child:　Serious cases of digoxin toxicity should be discussed with the National Poisons Information Service (consult product literature)
  ▸ Adult:　Serious cases of digoxin toxicity should be discussed with the National Poisons Information Service (consult product literature)

- **DIRECTIONS FOR ADMINISTRATION**
  ▸ In adults For *intravenous infusion* (*DigiFab*®), given intermittently in Sodium chloride 0.9%. Reconstitute with water for injections (4 mL/vial), then dilute with infusion fluid and give over 30 minutes.

- **MEDICINAL FORMS**
There can be variation in the licensing of different medicines containing the same drug.
  Powder for solution for infusion
  ▸ DigiFab (BTG International Ltd)
  Digoxin-specific antibody fragments 40 mg DigiFab 40mg powder for solution for infusion vials | 1 vial PoM £750.00 (Hospital only)

3.3　Heparin toxicity

ANTIDOTES AND CHELATORS

Protamine sulfate

- **INDICATIONS AND DOSE**
Overdosage with intravenous injection of unfractionated heparin
  ▸ **BY INTRAVENOUS INJECTION**
  ▸ Adult:　Dose to be administered at a rate not exceeding 5 mg/minute, 1 mg neutralises 80–100 units heparin when given within 15 minutes; if longer than 15 minute since heparin, less protamine required (consult product literature for details) as heparin rapidly excreted; maximum 50 mg

Overdosage with intravenous infusion of unfractionated heparin

▶ BY INTRAVENOUS INJECTION

▶ Adult: 25–50 mg, to be administered once heparin infusion stopped at a rate not exceeding 5 mg/minute

Overdosage with subcutaneous injection of unfractionated heparin

▶ INITIALLY BY INTRAVENOUS INJECTION

▶ Adult: Initially 25–50 mg, to be administered at a rate not exceeding 5 mg/minute, 1 mg neutralises 100 units heparin, then (by intravenous infusion), any remaining dose to be administered over 8–16 hours; maximum 50 mg per course

Overdosage with subcutaneous injection of low molecular weight heparin

▶ BY INTRAVENOUS INJECTION, OR BY CONTINUOUS INTRAVENOUS INFUSION

▶ Adult: Dose to be administered by intermittent intravenous injection at a rate not exceeding 5 mg/minute, 1 mg neutralises approx. 100 units low molecular weight heparin (consult product literature of low molecular weight heparin for details); maximum 50 mg

● CAUTIONS Excessive doses can have an anticoagulant effect

● SIDE-EFFECTS
▶ **Rare or very rare** Hypertension · pulmonary oedema non-cardiogenic
▶ **Frequency not known** Acute pulmonary vasoconstriction · back pain · bradycardia · circulatory collapse · dyspnoea · fatigue · feeling hot · flushing · nausea · pulmonary hypertension · vomiting

● ALLERGY AND CROSS-SENSITIVITY Caution if increased risk of allergic reaction to protamine (includes previous treatment with protamine or protamine insulin, allergy to fish, men who are infertile or who have had a vasectomy and who may have antibodies to protamine).

● MONITORING REQUIREMENTS Monitor activated partial thromboplastin time or other appropriate blood clotting parameters.

● PRESCRIBING AND DISPENSING INFORMATION The long half-life of low molecular weight heparins should be taken into consideration when determining the dose of protamine sulfate; the effects of low molecular weight heparins can persist for up to 24 hours after administration.

● MEDICINAL FORMS
There can be variation in the licensing of different medicines containing the same drug.
Solution for injection
▶ Protamine sulfate (Non-proprietary)
  Protamine sulfate 10 mg per 1 ml Protamine sulfate 100mg/10ml solution for injection ampoules | 5 ampoule [PoM] S
  Protamine sulfate 50mg/5ml solution for injection ampoules | 10 ampoule [PoM] £49.55

3.4 Opioid toxicity

OPIOID RECEPTOR ANTAGONISTS

| Naloxone hydrochloride

● INDICATIONS AND DOSE
Overdosage with opioids
▶ BY INTRAVENOUS INJECTION
▶ Child 1 month–11 years: Initially 100 micrograms/kg (max. per dose 2 mg), if no response, repeat at intervals of 1 minute to a max. of 2 mg, then review diagnosis;

further doses may be required if respiratory function deteriorates, doses can be given by subcutaneous or intramuscular routes but only if intravenous route is not feasible; intravenous administration has more rapid onset of action
▶ Child 12-17 years: Initially 400 micrograms, then 800 micrograms for up to 2 doses at 1 minute intervals if no response to preceding dose, then increased to 2 mg for 1 dose if still no response (4 mg dose may be required in seriously poisoned patients), then review diagnosis; further doses may be required if respiratory function deteriorates, doses can be given by subcutaneous or intramuscular routes but only if intravenous route is not feasible; intravenous administration has more rapid onset of action
▶ Adult: Initially 400 micrograms, then 800 micrograms for up to 2 doses at 1 minute intervals if no response to preceding dose, then increased to 2 mg for 1 dose if still no response (4 mg dose may be required in seriously poisoned patients), then review diagnosis; further doses may be required if respiratory function deteriorates, doses can be given by subcutaneous or intramuscular routes but only if intravenous route is not feasible; intravenous administration has more rapid onset of action

▶ BY CONTINUOUS INTRAVENOUS INFUSION
▶ Child: Using an infusion pump, adjust rate according to response (initially, rate may be set at 60% of the initial resuscitative intravenous injection dose per hour). The initial resuscitative *intravenous injection* dose is that which maintained satisfactory ventilation for at least 15 minutes
▶ Adult: Using an infusion pump, adjust rate according to response (initially, rate may be set at 60% of the initial resuscitative intravenous injection dose per hour). The initial resuscitative *intravenous injection* dose is that which maintained satisfactory ventilation for at least 15 minutes

Overdosage with opioids in a non-medical setting
▶ BY INTRAMUSCULAR INJECTION
▶ Adult: 400 micrograms every 2–3 minutes, each dose given in subsequent resuscitation cycles if patient not breathing normally, continue until consciousness regained, breathing normally, medical assistance available, or contents of syringe used up; to be injected into deltoid region or anterolateral thigh

Reversal of postoperative respiratory depression
▶ INITIALLY BY INTRAVENOUS INJECTION
▶ Child 1 month-11 years: 1 microgram/kg, repeated every 2–3 minutes if required
▶ Child 12-17 years: Initially 100–200 micrograms, alternatively (by intravenous injection) initially 1.5–3 micrograms/kg, if response inadequate, give subsequent doses, (by intravenous injection) 100 micrograms every 2 minutes, alternatively (by intramuscular injection) 100 micrograms every 1–2 hours
▶ Adult: Initially 100–200 micrograms, alternatively (by intravenous injection) initially 1.5–3 micrograms/kg, if response inadequate, give subsequent doses, (by intravenous injection) 100 micrograms every 2 minutes, alternatively (by intramuscular injection) 100 micrograms every 1–2 hours

PHARMACOKINETICS
▶ Naloxone has a short duration of action; repeated doses or infusion may be necessary to reverse effects of opioids with longer duration of action.

16

Emergency treatment of poisoning

- UNLICENSED USE Naloxone doses in BNF may differ from those in product literature.

> IMPORTANT SAFETY INFORMATION
> SAFE PRACTICE
> Doses used in acute opioid overdosage may not be appropriate for the management of opioid-induced respiratory depression and sedation in those receiving palliative care and in chronic opioid use.

- CAUTIONS Cardiovascular disease or those receiving cardiotoxic drugs (serious adverse cardiovascular effects reported) · maternal physical dependence on opioids (may precipitate withdrawal in newborn) · pain · physical dependence on opioids (precipitates withdrawal)
  CAUTIONS, FURTHER INFORMATION
- Titration of dose In postoperative use, the dose should be titrated for each patient in order to obtain sufficient respiratory response; however, naloxone antagonises analgesia.
- SIDE-EFFECTS
- Common or very common Arrhythmias · dizziness · headache · hypertension · hypotension · nausea · vomiting
- Uncommon Diarrhoea · dry mouth · hyperhidrosis · hyperventilation · pain · tremor
- Rare or very rare Anxiety · cardiac arrest · erythema multiforme · pulmonary oedema · seizure
- Frequency not known Analgesia reversed · asthenia · chills · death · dyspnoea · fever · irritability · nasal complaints · piloerection · withdrawal syndrome · yawning
- PREGNANCY Use only if potential benefit outweighs risk.
- BREAST FEEDING Not orally bioavailable.
- DIRECTIONS FOR ADMINISTRATION
- With intravenous use in children For *continuous intravenous infusion*, dilute to a concentration of up to 200 micrograms/mL with Glucose 5% or Sodium Chloride 0.9%.
- With intravenous use in adults For *intravenous infusion* (*Minijet*® Naloxone Hydrochloride), give continuously in Glucose 5% or Sodium Chloide 0.9%. Dilute to a concentration of up to 200 micrograms/mL and administer via an infusion pump.

- MEDICINAL FORMS
  There can be variation in the licensing of different medicines containing the same drug.
  Solution for injection
  - Naloxone hydrochloride (Non-proprietary)
    Naloxone hydrochloride 20 microgram per 1 ml Naloxone 40micrograms/2ml solution for injection ampoules | 10 ampoule [PoM] £55.00
    Naloxone hydrochloride 400 microgram per 1 ml Naloxone 400micrograms/1ml solution for injection ampoules | 10 ampoule [PoM] £41.00–£53.70
    Naloxone hydrochloride 1 mg per 1 ml Naloxone 2mg/2ml solution for injection pre-filled syringes | 1 pre-filled disposable injection [PoM] £16.80

3.5 Paracetamol toxicity

ANTIDOTES AND CHELATORS

Acetylcysteine

03-Apr-2018

- INDICATIONS AND DOSE
  Paracetamol overdosage
  - BY INTRAVENOUS INFUSION
  - Child (body-weight up to 20 kg): Initially 150 mg/kg over 1 hour, dose to be administered in 3 mL/kg glucose 5%, followed by 50 mg/kg over 4 hours, dose to be administered in 7 mL/kg glucose 5%, then 100 mg/kg

over 16 hours, dose to be administered in 14 mL/kg glucose 5%
  - Child (body-weight 20–39 kg): Initially 150 mg/kg over 1 hour, dose to be administered in 100 mL glucose 5%, followed by 50 mg/kg over 4 hours, dose to be administered in 250 mL glucose 5%, then 100 mg/kg over 16 hours, dose to be administered in 500 mL glucose 5%
  - Child (body-weight 40 kg and above): 150 mg/kg over 1 hour, dose to be administered in 200 mL Glucose Intravenous Infusion 5%, then 50 mg/kg over 4 hours, to be started immediately after completion of first infusion, dose to be administered in 500 mL Glucose Intravenous Infusion 5%, then 100 mg/kg over 16 hours, to be started immediately after completion of second infusion, dose to be administered in 1 litre Glucose Intravenous Infusion 5%
  - Adult (body-weight 40 kg and above): 150 mg/kg over 1 hour, dose to be administered in 200 mL Glucose Intravenous Infusion 5%, then 50 mg/kg over 4 hours, to be started immediately after completion of first infusion, dose to be administered in 500 mL Glucose Intravenous Infusion 5%, then 100 mg/kg over 16 hours, to be started immediately after completion of second infusion, dose to be administered in 1 litre Glucose Intravenous Infusion 5%

DOSES AT EXTREMES OF BODY-WEIGHT
- To avoid excessive dosage in obese patients, a ceiling weight of 110 kg should be used when calculating the dose for paracetamol overdosage.

> IMPORTANT SAFETY INFORMATION
> MHRA/CHM ADVICE: INTRAVENOUS ACETYLCYSTEINE FOR PARACETAMOL OVERDOSE: REMINDER OF AUTHORISED DOSE REGIMEN; POSSIBLE NEED FOR CONTINUED TREATMENT (JANUARY 2017)
> The authorised dose regimen for acetylcysteine in paracetamol overdose is 3 consecutive intravenous infusions given over a total of 21 hours.
>   Continued treatment (given at the dose and rate as used in the third infusion) may be necessary depending on the clinical evaluation of the individual patient.

- CAUTIONS Asthma (see Side-effects for management of asthma but do not delay acetylcysteine treatment) · atopy · may slightly increase INR · may slightly increase prothrombin time
- SIDE-EFFECTS Acidosis · anaphylactoid reaction · angioedema · anxiety · arrhythmias · cardiac arrest · chest discomfort · cough · cyanosis · eye pain · eye swelling · generalised seizure · hyperhidrosis · hypertension · hypotension · joint disorders · malaise · nausea · pain facial · respiratory disorders · skin reactions · syncope · thrombocytopenia · vasodilation · vision blurred · vomiting
  SIDE-EFFECTS, FURTHER INFORMATION Anaphylactoid reactions can be managed by suspending treatment and initiating appropriate management. Treatment may then be restarted at lower rate.

- DIRECTIONS FOR ADMINISTRATION
- In children Glucose 5% is preferred fluid; Sodium Chloride 0.9% is an alternative if Glucose 5% unsuitable.
- In adults For *intravenous infusion* (*Parvolex*®), give continuously in Glucose 5% or Sodium chloride 0.9%. Glucose Intravenous Infusion 5% is the preferred fluid; Sodium Chloride Intravenous Infusion 0.9% is an alternative if Glucose Intravenous Infusion 5% is unsuitable.

- MEDICINAL FORMS
There can be variation in the licensing of different medicines containing the same drug.
Solution for infusion
ELECTROLYTES: May contain Sodium
▸ Acetylcysteine (Non-proprietary)
  Acetylcysteine 200 mg per 1 ml Acetylcysteine 2g/10ml solution for infusion ampoules | 10 ampoule [PoM] £21.26-£24.99 DT = £21.26
▸ Parvolex (Phoenix Labs Ltd)
  Acetylcysteine 200 mg per 1 ml Parvolex 2g/10ml concentrate for solution for infusion ampoules | 10 ampoule [PoM] £22.50 DT = £21.26

4 Methaemoglobinaemia

ANTIDOTES AND CHELATORS

Methylthioninium chloride

(Methylene blue)

- INDICATIONS AND DOSE
Drug- or chemical-induced methaemoglobinaemia
▸ BY SLOW INTRAVENOUS INJECTION
▸ Child 3 months–17 years: Initially 1–2 mg/kg, then 1–2 mg/kg after 30–60 minutes if required, to be given over 5 minutes, seek advice from National Poisons Information Service if further repeat doses are required; maximum 7 mg/kg per course
▸ Adult: Initially 1–2 mg/kg, then 1–2 mg/kg after 30–60 minutes if required, to be given over 5 minutes, seek advice from National Poisons Information Service if further repeat doses are required; maximum 7 mg/kg per course
Aniline- or dapsone-induced methaemoglobinaemia
▸ BY SLOW INTRAVENOUS INJECTION
▸ Child 3 months–17 years: Initially 1–2 mg/kg, then 1–2 mg/kg after 30–60 minutes if required, to be given over 5 minutes, seek advice from National Poisons Information Service if further repeat doses are required; maximum 4 mg/kg per course
▸ Adult: Initially 1–2 mg/kg, then 1–2 mg/kg after 30–60 minutes if required, to be given over 5 minutes, seek advice from National Poisons Information Service if further repeat doses are required; maximum 4 mg/kg per course

- CAUTIONS Chlorate poisoning (reduces efficacy of methylthioninium) · G6PD deficiency (seek advice from National Poisons Information Service) · methaemoglobinaemia due to treatment of cyanide poisoning with sodium nitrite (seek advice from National Poisons Information Service) · pulse oximetry may give false estimation of oxygen saturation
- INTERACTIONS → Appendix 1: methylthioninium chloride
- SIDE-EFFECTS
▸ **Common or very common** Abdominal pain · anxiety · chest pain · dizziness · headache · hyperhidrosis · nausea · pain in extremity · paraesthesia · skin reactions · taste altered · urine discolouration · vomiting
▸ **Frequency not known** Aphasia · arrhythmias · confusion · faeces discoloured · fever · haemolytic anaemia · hyperbilirubinaemia (in infants) · hypertension · hypotension · mydriasis · tremor
- PREGNANCY No information available, but risk to fetus of untreated methaemoglobinaemia likely to be significantly higher than risk of treatment.
- BREAST FEEDING Manufacturer advises avoid breastfeeding for up to 6 days after administration—no information available.

- RENAL IMPAIRMENT **Dose adjustments** Use with caution in severe impairment; dose reduction may be required.
- DIRECTIONS FOR ADMINISTRATION
▸ In children For *intravenous injection*, may be diluted with Glucose 5% to minimise injection-site pain; not compatible with Sodium Chloride 0.9%.
- MEDICINAL FORMS
There can be variation in the licensing of different medicines containing the same drug. Forms available from special-order manufacturers include: solution for injection
Solution for injection
▸ Methylthioninium chloride (Non-proprietary)
  Methylthioninium chloride 5 mg per 1 ml Methylthioninium chloride Proveblue 50mg/10ml solution for injection ampoules | 5 ampoule [PoM] £196.89

5 Snake bites

IMMUNE SERA AND IMMUNOGLOBULINS ›
ANTITOXINS

European viper snake venom antiserum

- INDICATIONS AND DOSE
Systemic envenoming from snake bites | Marked local envenoming
▸ BY INTRAVENOUS INJECTION, OR BY INTRAVENOUS INFUSION
▸ Child: Initially 10 mL for 1 dose, then 10 mL after 1–2 hours if required, the second dose should only be given if symptoms of systemic envenoming persist after the first dose, if symptoms of systemic envenoming persist contact the National Poisons Information Service
▸ Adult: Initially 10 mL for 1 dose, then 10 mL after 1–2 hours if required, the second dose should only be given if symptoms of systemic envenoming persist after the first dose, if symptoms of systemic envenoming persist contact the National Poisons Information Service
Severe systemic envenoming from snake bites in patients presenting with clinical features
▸ BY INTRAVENOUS INJECTION, OR BY INTRAVENOUS INFUSION
▸ Child: Initially 20 mL for 1 dose, if symptoms of systemic envenoming persist contact the National Poisons Information Service
▸ Adult: Initially 20 mL for 1 dose, if symptoms of systemic envenoming persist contact the National Poisons Information Service

- DIRECTIONS FOR ADMINISTRATION By *intravenous injection* given over 10–15 minutes or by *intravenous infusion* over 30 minutes after diluting in sodium chloride 0.9% (use 5 mL diluent/kg body-weight).
- PRESCRIBING AND DISPENSING INFORMATION To order, email immform@dh.gsi.gov.uk.
- MEDICINAL FORMS
There can be variation in the licensing of different medicines containing the same drug.
Solution for injection
▸ European viper snake venom antiserum (Non-proprietary)
  European viper snake venom antiserum 100 mg per 1 ml Viper venom antiserum, European (equine) 1g/10ml solution for injection vials | 1 vial [PoM] [℞]

16

Emergency treatment of poisoning

Appendix 1
Interactions

Changes have been made to the interactions content in BNF publications. For more information, see www.bnf.org/new-bnf-interactions/.

Two or more drugs given at the same time can exert their effects independently or they can interact. Interactions may be beneficial and exploited therapeutically; this type of interaction is not within the scope of this appendix. Many interactions are harmless, and even those that are potentially harmful can often be managed, allowing the drugs to be used safely together. Nevertheless, adverse drug interactions should be reported to the Medicines and Healthcare products Regulatory Agency (MHRA), through the Yellow Card Scheme (see Adverse reactions to drugs p. 12), as for other adverse drug reactions.

Potentially harmful drug interactions may occur in only a small number of patients, but the true incidence is often hard to establish. Furthermore the severity of a harmful interaction is likely to vary from one patient to another. Patients at increased risk from drug interactions include the elderly and those with impaired renal or hepatic function.

Interactions can result in the potentiation or antagonism of one drug by another, or result in another effect, such as renal impairment. Drug interactions may develop either through pharmacokinetic or pharmacodynamic mechanisms.

Pharmacodynamic interactions

These are interactions between drugs which have similar or antagonistic pharmacological effects or side-effects. They might be due to competition at receptor sites, or occur between drugs acting on the same physiological system. They are usually predictable from a knowledge of the pharmacology of the interacting drugs; in general, those demonstrated with one drug are likely to occur with related drugs.

Pharmacokinetic interactions

These occur when one drug alters the absorption, distribution, metabolism, or excretion of another, thus increasing or decreasing the amount of drug available to produce its pharmacological effects. Pharmacokinetic interactions occurring with one drug do not necessarily occur uniformly across a group of related drugs.

Affecting absorption The rate of absorption and the total amount absorbed can both be altered by drug interactions. Delayed absorption is rarely of clinical importance unless a rapid effect is required (e.g. when giving an analgesic). Reduction in the total amount absorbed, however, can result in ineffective therapy.

Affecting distribution *Due to changes in protein binding*: To a variable extent most drugs are loosely bound to plasma proteins. Protein-binding sites are non-specific and one drug can displace another thereby increasing the proportion free to diffuse from plasma to its site of action. This only produces a detectable increase in effect if it is an extensively bound drug (more than 90%) that is not widely distributed throughout the body. Even so displacement rarely produces

more than transient potentiation because this increased concentration of free drug will usually be eliminated.

Displacement from protein binding plays a part in the potentiation of warfarin by sulfonamides but these interactions become clinically relevant mainly because warfarin metabolism is also inhibited.

Induction or inhibition of drug transporter proteins: Drug transporter proteins, such as P-glycoprotein, actively transport drugs across biological membranes. Transporters can be induced or inhibited, resulting in changes in the concentrations of drugs that are substrates for the transporter. For example, rifampicin induces P-glycoprotein, particularly in the gut wall, resulting in decreased plasma concentrations of digoxin, a P-glycoprotein substrate.

Affecting metabolism Many drugs are metabolised in the liver. Drugs are either metabolised by phase I reactions (oxidation, reduction, or hydrolysis) or by phase II reactions (e.g. glucuronidation).

Phase I reactions are mainly carried out by the cytochrome P450 family of isoenzymes, of which CYP3A4 is the most important isoenzyme involved in the metabolism of drugs. Induction of cytochrome P450 isoenzymes by one drug can increase the rate of metabolism of another, resulting in lower plasma concentrations and a reduced effect. On withdrawal of the inducing drug, plasma concentrations increase and toxicity can occur.

Conversely when one drug inhibits cytochrome P450 isoenzymes, it can decrease the metabolism of another, leading to higher plasma concentrations, resulting in an increased effect with a risk of toxicity.

Isoenzymes of the hepatic cytochrome P450 system interact with a wide range of drugs. With knowledge of which isoenzymes are involved in a drug's metabolism, it is possible to predict whether certain pharmacokinetic interactions will occur. For example, carbamazepine is a potent inducer of CYP3A4, ketoconazole is potent inhibitor of CYP3A4, and midazolam is a substrate of CYP3A4. Carbamazepine reduces midazolam concentrations, and it is therefore likely that other drugs that are potent inducers of CYP3A4 will interact similarly with midazolam. Ketoconazole, however, increases midazolam concentrations, and it can be predicted that other drugs that are potent inhibitors of CYP3A4 will interact similarly.

Less is known about the enzymes involved in phase II reactions. These include UDP-glucuronyltransferases which, for example, might be induced by rifampicin, resulting in decreased metabolism of mycophenolate (a substrate for this enzyme) to its active form, mycophenolic acid.

Affecting renal excretion Drugs are eliminated through the kidney both by glomerular filtration and by active tubular secretion. Competition occurs between those which share active transport mechanisms in the proximal tubule. For example, salicylates and some other NSAIDs delay the excretion of methotrexate; serious methotrexate toxicity is possible. Changes in urinary pH can also affect the reabsorption of a small number of drugs, including methenamine.

Relative importance of interactions

Levels of severity: Most interactions have been assigned a severity; this describes the likely effect of an unmanaged interaction on the patient.

Severe—the result may be a life-threatening event or have a permanent detrimental effect.

Moderate—the result could cause considerable distress or partially incapacitate a patient; they are unlikely to be life-threatening or result in long-term effects.

Mild—the result is unlikely to cause concern or incapacitate the majority of patients.

Unknown—used for those interactions that are predicted, but there is insufficient evidence to hazard a guess at the outcome.

Levels of evidence: Most interactions have been assigned a rating to indicate the weight of evidence behind the interaction.

Study—for interactions where the information is based on formal study including those for other drugs with same mechanism (e.g. known inducers, inhibitors, or substrates of cytochrome P450 isoenzymes or P-glycoprotein).

Anecdotal—interactions based on either a single case report or a limited number of case reports.

Theoretical—interactions that are predicted based on sound theoretical considerations. The information may have been derived from *in vitro* studies or based on the way other members in the same class act.

Action messages: Each interaction describes the effect that occurs, and the action to be taken, either based on manufacturer's advice from the relevant Summary of Product Characteristics or advice from a relevant authority (e.g. MHRA). An action message is only included where the combination is to be avoided, where a dose adjustment is required, or where specific administration requirements (e.g timing of doses) are recommended. **Pharmacodynamic interactions**, with the exception of interactions with drugs that may prolong the QT interval, do not have an action message included as these will depend on individual patient circumstances.

Appendix 1 structure

❶ Drugs

Drugs are listed alphabetically. If a drug is a member of a drug class, all interactions for that drug will be listed under the drug class entry; in this case the drug entry provides direction to the relevant drug class where its interactions can be found.

Within a drug or drug class entry, interactions are listed alphabetically by the interacting drug or drug class. The interactions describe the effect that occurs, and the action to be taken, either based on manufacturer's advice from the relevant Summary of Product Characteristics or advice from a relevant authority (e.g. MHRA). An action message is only included where the combination is to be avoided, where a dose adjustment is required, or where specific administration requirements (e.g. timing of doses) are recommended. If two drugs have a pharmacodynamic effect in addition to a pharmacokinetic interaction, a cross-reference to the relevant pharmacodynamic effect table is included at the end of the pharmacokinetic message.

❷ Drug classes

The drugs that are members of a drug class are listed underneath the drug class entry in a blue box. Interactions for the class are then listed alphabetically by the interacting drug or drug class. If the interaction only applies to certain drugs in the class, these drugs will be shown in brackets after the drug class name.

❸ Supplementary information

If a drug has additional important information to be considered, this is shown in a blue box underneath the drug or drug class entry. This information might be food and lifestyle advice (including smoking and alcohol consumption), relate to the pharmacology of the drug or applicability of interactions to certain routes of administration, or it might be advice about separating administration times.

❹ Pharmacodynamic effects

Tables at the beginning of Appendix 1 cover pharmacodynamic effects. If a drug is included in one or more of these tables, this will be indicated at the top of the

---

❶ **Drug entry**
  ▸ Details of interaction between **drug entry** and another drug or drug class. Action statement. [Severity] Evidence
  ▸ Details of interaction between **drug entry** and another drug or drug class. Action statement. [Severity] Evidence
    → Also see TABLE 1

Drug entry → see Drug class entry

❷ **Drug class entry**

  Drug A · Drug B · Drug C · Drug D

  ▸ Details of interaction between **drug class entry** and another drug or drug class. Action statement. [Severity] Evidence

❸ **Drug entry or Drug class entry**

  Supplementary information

❹ **Drug entry or Drug class entry** → see TABLE 1

  TABLE 1
  Name of pharmacodynamic effect
  Explanation of the effect

  | Drug | Drug | Drug |
  | Drug | Drug | Drug |

---

list of interactions for the drug or drug class. In addition to the list of interactions for a drug or drug class, these tables should always be consulted.

Each table describes the relevant pharmacodynamic effect and lists those drugs that are commonly associated with the effect. Concurrent use of two or more drugs from the same table is expected to increase the risk of the pharmacodynamic effect occurring. Please note these tables are not exhaustive.

TABLE 1
Drugs that cause hepatotoxicity

The following is a list of some drugs that cause hepatotoxicity (note that this list is not exhaustive). Concurrent use of two or more drugs from the list might increase this risk.

alcohol (beverage)	dantrolene	itraconazole	minocycline	tetracycline
alectinib	demeclocycline	leflunomide	oxytetracycline	tigecycline
asparaginase	didanosine	lenalidomide	paracetamol	trabectedin
atorvastatin	doxycycline	lomitapide	pegaspargase	valproate
carbamazepine	flucloxacillin	lymecycline	pravastatin	vincristine
clavulanic acid	fluconazole	mercaptopurine	rosuvastatin	
crisantaspase	fluvastatin	methotrexate	simvastatin	
dactinomycin	isoniazid	micafungin	sulfasalazine	

TABLE 2
Drugs that cause nephrotoxicity

The following is a list of some drugs that cause nephrotoxicity (note that this list is not exhaustive). Concurrent use of two or more drugs from the list might increase this risk.

aceclofenac	ceftaroline	etodolac	methotrexate	telavancin
acemetacin	ceftazidime	etoricoxib	nabumetone	tenofovir disoproxil
aciclovir	ceftobiprole	fenoprofen	naproxen	tenoxicam
amikacin	ceftolozane	flurbiprofen	neomycin	tiaprofenic acid
amphotericin	ceftriaxone	foscarnet	oxaliplatin	tobramycin
bacitracin	cefuroxime	ganciclovir	parecoxib	tolfenamic acid
capreomycin	celecoxib	gentamicin	pemetrexed	trimethoprim
carboplatin	ciclosporin	ibuprofen	penicillamine	valaciclovir
cefaclor	cisplatin	ifosfamide	pentamidine	valganciclovir
cefadroxil	colistimethate (particularly	indometacin	piroxicam	vancomycin
cefalexin	intravenous)	ketoprofen	polymyxins	zidovudine
cefixime	dexibuprofen	ketorolac	streptomycin	zoledronic acid
cefotaxime	dexketoprofen	mefenamic acid	sulindac	
cefradine	diclofenac	meloxicam	tacrolimus	

TABLE 3
Drugs with anticoagulant effects

The following is a list of drugs that have anticoagulant effects. Concurrent use of two or more drugs from this list might increase the risk of bleeding; concurrent use of drugs with antiplatelet effects (see table of drugs with antiplatelet effects) might also increase this risk.

acenocoumarol	dabigatran	fondaparinux	phenindione	urokinase
alteplase	dalteparin	glucose	rivaroxaban	warfarin
apixaban	danaparoid	heparin (unfractionated)	streptokinase	
argatroban	edoxaban	nicotinic acid	tenecteplase	
bivalirudin	enoxaparin	omega-3-acid ethyl esters	tinzaparin	

TABLE 4
Drugs with antiplatelet effects

The following is a list of drugs that have antiplatelet effects (note that this list is not exhaustive). Concurrent use of two or more drugs from this list might increase the risk of bleeding; concurrent use of drugs with anticoagulant effects (see table of drugs with anticoagulant effects) might also increase this risk.

abciximab	dapoxetine	etoricoxib	mefenamic acid	sulindac
aceclofenac	dasatinib	fenoprofen	meloxicam	tenoxicam
acemetacin	dexibuprofen	fluoxetine	nabumetone	tiaprofenic acid
anagrelide	dexketoprofen	flurbiprofen	naproxen	ticagrelor
aspirin	diclofenac	fluvoxamine	parecoxib	tirofiban
bevacizumab	dipyridamole	ibrutinib	paroxetine	tolfenamic acid
cangrelor	duloxetine	ibuprofen	piroxicam	trastuzumab
celecoxib	epoprostenol	iloprost	prasugrel	trastuzumab emtansine
cilostazol	eptifibatide	indometacin	regorafenib	venlafaxine
citalopram	escitalopram	ketoprofen	sertraline	vortioxetine
clopidogrel	etodolac	ketorolac	sulfinpyrazone	

TABLE 5
Drugs that cause thromboembolism

The following is a list of some drugs that cause thromboembolism (note that this list is not exhaustive). Concurrent use of two or more drugs from the list might increase this risk.

bleomycin	epoetin zeta	pentostatin	toremifene	vinflunine
cyclophosphamide	fluorouracil	pomalidomide	tranexamic acid	vinorelbine
darbepoetin alfa	fulvestrant	raloxifene	tretinoin	
doxorubicin	lenalidomide	tamoxifen	vinblastine	
epoetin alfa	methotrexate	thalidomide	vincristine	
epoetin beta	mitomycin	tibolone	vindesine	

TABLE 6
Drugs that cause bradycardia
The following is a list of drugs that cause bradycardia (note that this list is not exhaustive). Concurrent use of two or more drugs from the list might increase this risk.

acebutolol	carvedilol	fentanyl	nadolol	rivastigmine
alectinib	celiprolol	fingolimod	nebivolol	selegiline
alfentanil	cisatracurium	flecainide	neostigmine	sotalol
amiodarone	clonidine	galantamine	oxprenolol	sufentanil
apraclonidine	crizotinib	ivabradine	pasireotide	thalidomide
atenolol	digoxin	labetalol	pindolol	timolol
betaxolol	diltiazem	levobunolol	propranolol	tizanidine
bisoprolol	donepezil	methadone	pyridostigmine	verapamil
brimonidine	esmolol	metoprolol	remifentanil	

TABLE 7
Drugs that cause first dose hypotension
The following is a list of some drugs that can cause first-dose hypotension (note that this list is not exhaustive). Concurrent use of two or more drugs from the list might increase this risk.

alfuzosin	eprosartan	isosorbide dinitrate	prazosin	trandolapril
azilsartan	fosinopril	isosorbide mononitrate	quinapril	valsartan
candesartan	glyceryl trinitrate	lisinopril	ramipril	
captopril	imidapril	losartan	tamsulosin	
doxazosin	indoramin	olmesartan	telmisartan	
enalapril	irbesartan	perindopril	terazosin	

TABLE 8
Drugs that cause hypotension
The following is a list of some drugs that cause hypotension (note that this list is not exhaustive). Concurrent use of two or more drugs from the list might increase this risk.

acebutolol	chlorpromazine	haloperidol	moxisylyte	riociguat
alcohol (beverage)	chlortalidone	hydralazine	moxonidine	risperidone
alfuzosin	clevidipine	hydrochlorothiazide	nadolol	ropinirole
aliskiren	clomipramine	hydroflumethiazide	nebivolol	rotigotine
alprostadil	clonidine	imidapril	nicardipine	sacubitril
amantadine	clopamide	imipramine	nicorandil	sapropterin
amitriptyline	clozapine	indapamide	nifedipine	selegiline
amlodipine	cyclopenthiazide	indoramin	nimodipine	sevoflurane
apomorphine	dapagliflozin	irbesartan	nitrous oxide	sildenafil
apraclonidine	desflurane	isocarboxazid	nortriptyline	sodium nitroprusside
aripiprazole	diazoxide	isoflurane	olanzapine	sodium oxybate
asenapine	diltiazem	isosorbide dinitrate	olmesartan	sotalol
atenolol	dipyridamole	isosorbide mononitrate	oxprenolol	spironolactone
avanafil	dosulepin	ketamine	paliperidone	sulpiride
azilsartan	doxazosin	labetalol	pergolide	tadalafil
baclofen	doxepin	lacidipine	pericyazine	tamsulosin
bendroflumethiazide	droperidol	lercanidipine	perindopril	telmisartan
benperidol	empagliflozin	levobunolol	perphenazine	terazosin
betaxolol	enalapril	levodopa	phenelzine	thiopental
bisoprolol	eplerenone	levomepromazine	pimozide	timolol
bortezomib	eprosartan	lisinopril	pindolol	tizanidine
brimonidine	esmolol	lofepramine	pramipexole	torasemide
bromocriptine	etomidate	lofexidine	prazosin	trandolapril
bumetanide	felodipine	losartan	prochlorperazine	tranylcypromine
cabergoline	flupentixol	loxapine	promazine	trifluoperazine
canagliflozin	fluphenazine	lurasidone	propofol	trimipramine
candesartan	fosinopril	methoxyflurane	propranolol	valsartan
captopril	furosemide	methyldopa	quetiapine	vardenafil
carvedilol	glyceryl trinitrate	metolazone	quinagolide	verapamil
celiprolol	guanethidine	metoprolol	quinapril	xipamide
chlorothiazide	guanfacine	minoxidil	ramipril	zuclopenthixol

TABLE 9
Drugs that prolong the QT interval

The following is a list of some drugs that prolong the QT-interval (note that this list is not exhaustive). In general, manufacturers advise that the use of two or more drugs that are associated with QT prolongation should be avoided. Increasing age, female sex, cardiac disease, and some metabolic disturbances (notably hypokalaemia) predispose to QT prolongation—concurrent use of drugs that reduce serum potassium might further increase this risk (see table of drugs that reduce serum potassium).

Drugs that are not known to prolong the QT interval but are predicted (by the manufacturer) to increase the risk of QT prolongation include: domperidone, fingolimod, granisetron, ivabradine, mefloquine, mizolastine, palonosetron, and intravenous pentamidine. Most manufacturers advise avoiding concurrent use with drugs that prolong the QT interval.

amifampridine	clarithromycin	fluphenazine	panobinostat	telavancin
amiodarone	clomipramine	haloperidol	pasireotide	tetrabenazine
amisulpride	crizotinib	hydroxyzine	pazopanib	tizanidine
anagrelide	dasatinib	inotuzumab ozogamicin	pimozide	tolterodine
apomorphine	delamanid	lapatinib	quinine	toremifene
arsenic trioxide	disopyramide	levomepromazine	ranolazine	vandetanib
artemether	dronedarone	lithium	ribociclib	vardenafil
artenimol	droperidol	lofexidine	risperidone	vemurafenib
bedaquiline	efavirenz	methadone	saquinavir	venlafaxine
bosutinib	eribulin	moxifloxacin	sildenafil	vinflunine
cabozantinib	erythromycin	nilotinib	sorafenib	voriconazole
ceritinib	escitalopram	ondansetron	sotalol	zuclopenthixol
chlorpromazine	flecainide	osimertinib	sulpiride	
citalopram	fluconazole	paliperidone	sunitinib	

TABLE 10
Drugs with antimuscarinic effects

The following is a list of some drugs that have antimuscarinic effects (note that this list is not exhaustive). Concurrent use of two or more drugs from this list might increase the risk of these effects occurring.

aclidinium	cyclopentolate	haloperidol	orphenadrine	tiotropium
amantadine	cyproheptadine	homatropine	oxybutynin	tolterodine
amitriptyline	darifenacin	hydroxyzine	perphenazine	trifluoperazine
atropine	dicycloverine	hyoscine	pimozide	trihexyphenidyl
baclofen	dimenhydrinate	imipramine	prochlorperazine	trimipramine
chlorphenamine	disopyramide	ipratropium	procyclidine	tropicamide
chlorpromazine	dosulepin	levomepromazine	promethazine	trospium
clemastine	doxepin	lofepramine	propafenone	umeclidinium
clomipramine	fesoterodine	loxapine	propantheline	
clozapine	flavoxate	nefopam	propiverine	
cyclizine	glycopyrronium	nortriptyline	solifenacin	

TABLE 11
Drugs with CNS depressant effects

The following is a list of some drugs with CNS depressant effects (note that this list is not exhaustive). Concurrent use of two or more drugs from this list might increase the risk of CNS depressant effects, such as drowsiness, which might affect the ability to perform skilled tasks (see 'Drugs and Driving' in Guidance on Prescribing p. 1).

agomelatine	clomethiazole	isoflurane	moxonidine	quetiapine
alcohol (beverage)	clonazepam	ketamine	nabilone	remifentanil
alfentanil	clonidine	ketotifen	nitrazepam	risperidone
alimemazine	clozapine	lamotrigine	nitrous oxide	ropivacaine
alprazolam	codeine	levetiracetam	olanzapine	sevoflurane
amisulpride	cyclizine	levomepromazine	oxazepam	sodium oxybate
apraclonidine	cyproheptadine	lidocaine	oxycodone	sufentanil
aripiprazole	desflurane	lofexidine	paliperidone	sulpiride
articaine	dexmedetomidine	loprazolam	papaveretum	tapentadol
asenapine	diamorphine	lorazepam	pentazocine	temazepam
baclofen	diazepam	lormetazepam	perampanel	tetracaine
benperidol	dihydrocodeine	loxapine	pericyazine	thalidomide
brimonidine	dipipanone	lurasidone	perphenazine	thiopental
buclizine	droperidol	melatonin	pethidine	tizanidine
bupivacaine	etomidate	mepivacaine	phenobarbital	tramadol
buprenorphine	fentanyl	meprobamate	pimozide	trazodone
cannabis extract	flupentixol	meptazinol	pizotifen	trifluoperazine
chloral hydrate	fluphenazine	methadone	pregabalin	venlafaxine
chlordiazepoxide	flurazepam	methocarbamol	prilocaine	zaleplon
chlorphenamine	gabapentin	methoxyflurane	primidone	zolpidem
chlorpromazine	guanfacine	mianserin	prochlorperazine	zopiclone
cinnarizine	haloperidol	midazolam	promazine	zuclopenthixol
clemastine	hydromorphone	mirtazapine	promethazine	
clobazam	hydroxyzine	morphine	propofol	

TABLE 12
Drugs that cause peripheral neuropathy

The following is a list of some drugs that cause peripheral neuropathy (note that this list is not exhaustive). Concurrent use of two or more drugs from the list might increase this risk.

amiodarone	didanosine	isoniazid	phenytoin	vindesine
bortezomib	disulfiram	lamivudine	stavudine	vinflunine
brentuximab vedotin	docetaxel	metronidazole	thalidomide	vinorelbine
cabazitaxel	eribulin	nitrofurantoin	vinblastine	
cisplatin	fosphenytoin	paclitaxel	vincristine	

TABLE 13
Drugs that cause serotonin syndrome

The following is a list of some drugs that cause serotonin syndrome (note that this list is not exhaustive). See 'Serotonin Syndrome' and 'Monoamine-Oxidase Inhibitors' under Antidepressant drugs p. 355 for more information and for specific advice on avoiding monoamine-oxidase inhibitors during and after administration of other serotonergic drugs.

almotriptan	fentanyl	methadone	pethidine	tapentadol
bupropion	fluoxetine	methylthioninium chloride	phenelzine	tramadol
buspirone	fluvoxamine	mianserin	procarbazine	tranylcypromine
citalopram	frovatriptan	mirtazapine	rasagiline	trazodone
clomipramine	granisetron	moclobemide	rizatriptan	tryptophan
dapoxetine	imipramine	naratriptan	safinamide	venlafaxine
dexamfetamine	isocarboxazid	ondansetron	selegiline	vortioxetine
duloxetine	linezolid	palonosetron	sertraline	zolmitriptan
eletriptan	lisdexamfetamine	paroxetine	St John's Wort	
escitalopram	lithium	pentazocine	sumatriptan	

TABLE 14
Antidiabetic drugs

The following is a list of antidiabetic drugs (note that this list is not exhaustive). Concurrent use of two or more drugs from the list might increase the risk of hypoglycaemia.

acarbose	dulaglutide	glimepiride	lixisenatide	saxagliptin
albiglutide	empagliflozin	glipizide	metformin	sitagliptin
alogliptin	exenatide	insulins	nateglinide	tolbutamide
canagliflozin	glibenclamide	linagliptin	pioglitazone	vildagliptin
dapagliflozin	gliclazide	liraglutide	repaglinide	

TABLE 15
Drugs that cause myelosuppression

The following is a list of some drugs that cause myelosuppression (note that this list is not exhaustive). Concurrent use of two or more drugs from the list might increase this risk.

afatinib	carmustine	everolimus	nilotinib	rituximab
aflibercept	ceritinib	fludarabine	nivolumab	ruxolitinib
alemtuzumab	cetuximab	fluorouracil	obinutuzumab	siltuximab
amsacrine	chlorambucil	ganciclovir	ofatumumab	sorafenib
anakinra	cisplatin	gefitinib	olanzapine	sulfadiazine
arsenic trioxide	cladribine	gemcitabine	olaparib	sulfasalazine
asparaginase	clofarabine	hydroxycarbamide	olsalazine	sunitinib
axitinib	clozapine	ibrutinib	oxaliplatin	temozolomide
azacitidine	co-trimoxazole	idarubicin	paclitaxel	temsirolimus
azathioprine	crisantaspase	idelalisib	panitumumab	thalidomide
balsalazide	crizotinib	ifosfamide	panobinostat	thiotepa
belimumab	cyclophosphamide	imatinib	pazopanib	tioguanine
bendamustine	cytarabine	interferon alfa	pegaspargase	topotecan
bevacizumab	dabrafenib	interferon beta	peginterferon alfa	trabectedin
bleomycin	dacarbazine	irinotecan	peginterferon beta-1a	trastuzumab emtansine
blinatumomab	dactinomycin	leflunomide	pemetrexed	treosulfan
bortezomib	dasatinib	lenalidomide	pentamidine	valganciclovir
bosutinib	daunorubicin	linezolid	pentostatin	vinblastine
brentuximab vedotin	decitabine	lomustine	pixantrone	vincristine
busulfan	deferiprone	melphalan	pomalidomide	vindesine
cabazitaxel	docetaxel	mercaptopurine	primaquine	vinflunine
cabozantinib	doxorubicin	methotrexate	procarbazine	vinorelbine
canakinumab	epirubicin	mitomycin	propylthiouracil	vismodegib
capecitabine	eribulin	mitotane	pyrimethamine	zidovudine
carbimazole	estramustine	mitoxantrone	raltitrexed	
carboplatin	ethosuximide	mycophenolate	ramucirumab	
carfilzomib	etoposide	nelarabine	regorafenib	

TABLE 16
Drugs that increase serum potassium

The following is a list of some drugs that increase serum potassium concentrations (note that this list is not exhaustive). Concurrent use of two or more drugs from this list might increase the risk of hyperkalaemia (hyperkalaemia is particularly notable when ACE inhibitors or angiotensin-II receptor antagonists are given with spironolactone or eplerenone).

aceclofenac	dexketoprofen	fenoprofen	meloxicam	sulindac
acemetacin	diclofenac	flurbiprofen	nabumetone	tacrolimus
aliskiren	drospirenone	heparin (unfractionated)	naproxen	telmisartan
amiloride	enalapril	ibuprofen	olmesartan	tenoxicam
azilsartan	enoxaparin	imidapril	parecoxib	tiaprofenic acid
candesartan	eplerenone	indometacin	perindopril	tinzaparin
captopril	epoetin alfa	irbesartan	piroxicam	tolfenamic acid
celecoxib	epoetin beta	ketoprofen	potassium canrenoate	tolvaptan
ciclosporin	epoetin zeta	ketorolac	potassium chloride	trandolapril
dalteparin	eprosartan	lisinopril	quinapril	triamterene
darbepoetin alfa	etodolac	losartan	ramipril	trimethoprim
dexibuprofen	etoricoxib	mefenamic acid	spironolactone	valsartan

TABLE 17
Drugs that reduce serum potassium

The following is a list of some drugs that reduce serum potassium concentrations (note that this list is not exhaustive and that other drugs can cause hypokalaemia in overdose). Concurrent use of two or more drugs from this list might increase the risk of hypokalaemia. Hypokalaemia can increase the risk of torsade de pointes, which might be additive with the effects of drugs that prolong the QT interval (see table of drugs that prolong the QT interval).

aminophylline	bumetanide	fludrocortisone	indapamide	salmeterol
amphotericin	chlorothiazide	formoterol	methylprednisolone	terbutaline
bambuterol	chlortalidone	furosemide	metolazone	theophylline
beclometasone	clopamide	hydrochlorothiazide	olodaterol	torasemide
bendroflumethiazide	cyclopenthiazide	hydrocortisone	prednisolone	triamcinolone
betamethasone	deflazacort	hydroflumethiazide	prednisone	vilanterol
budesonide	dexamethasone	indacaterol	salbutamol	xipamide

TABLE 18
Drugs that cause hyponatraemia

The following is a list of some drugs that reduce sodium concentrations (note that this list is not exhaustive). Concurrent use of two or more drugs from this list might increase the risk of hyponatraemia.

aceclofenac	clopamide	etodolac	indometacin	sertraline
acemetacin	cyclopenthiazide	etoricoxib	ketoprofen	sodium picosulfate
amiloride	dapoxetine	fenoprofen	ketorolac	spironolactone
amitriptyline	desmopressin	fluoxetine	mefenamic acid	sulindac
bendroflumethiazide	dexibuprofen	flurbiprofen	meloxicam	tenoxicam
bumetanide	dexketoprofen	fluvoxamine	metolazone	tiaprofenic acid
carbamazepine	diclofenac	furosemide	nabumetone	tolfenamic acid
celecoxib	dosulepin	hydrochlorothiazide	naproxen	torasemide
chlorothiazide	doxepin	hydroflumethiazide	nortriptyline	triamterene
chlortalidone	duloxetine	ibuprofen	parecoxib	trimethoprim
citalopram	eplerenone	imipramine	paroxetine	trimipramine
clomipramine	escitalopram	indapamide	piroxicam	xipamide

TABLE 19
Drugs that cause ototoxicity

The following is a list of some drugs that cause ototoxicity (note that this list is not exhaustive). Concurrent use of two or more drugs from the list might increase this risk.

amikacin	cisplatin	oxaliplatin	torasemide	vindesine
bumetanide	furosemide	streptomycin	vancomycin	vinflunine
capreomycin	gentamicin	telavancin	vinblastine	vinorelbine
carboplatin	neomycin	tobramycin	vincristine	

TABLE 20
Drugs with neuromuscular blocking effects

The following is a list of some drugs with neuromuscular blocking effects (note that this list is not exhaustive). Concurrent use of two or more drugs from the list might increase this risk.

amikacin	cisatracurium	neomycin	pyridostigmine	tobramycin
atracurium	colistimethate	neostigmine	rocuronium	vecuronium
botulinum toxin type A	gentamicin	pancuronium	streptomycin	
botulinum toxin type B	mivacurium	polymyxins	suxamethonium	

List of drug interactions

The following is an alphabetical list of drugs and their interactions; to avoid excessive cross-referencing each drug or group is listed twice: in the alphabetical list and also against the drug or group with which it interacts.

Abacavir
▸ Antiepileptics (carbamazepine, fosphenytoin, phenobarbital, phenytoin, primidone) are predicted to decrease the exposure to **abacavir**. Moderate Theoretical
▸ HIV-protease inhibitors (tipranavir) slightly decrease the exposure to **abacavir**. Avoid. Severe Study

Abatacept
▸ Live vaccines are predicted to increase the risk of generalised infection (possibly life-threatening) when given with **abatacept**. Public Health England advises avoid (refer to Green Book). Severe Theoretical

Abciximab → see TABLE 4 p. 1334 (antiplatelet effects)

Abiraterone

GENERAL INFORMATION Caution with concurrent chemotherapy—safety and efficacy not established.

▸ Antiepileptics (carbamazepine, fosphenytoin, phenobarbital, phenytoin, primidone) are predicted to decrease the exposure to **abiraterone**. Avoid. Severe Theoretical
▸ Antifungals, azoles (itraconazole, ketoconazole, voriconazole) are predicted to increase the exposure to **abiraterone**. Severe Theoretical
▸ **Abiraterone** is predicted to increase the exposure to beta blockers, selective (metoprolol). Moderate Study
▸ Cobicistat is predicted to increase the exposure to **abiraterone**. Severe Theoretical
▸ **Abiraterone** is predicted to increase the exposure to eliglustat. Avoid or adjust dose—consult product literature. Severe Study
▸ Enzalutamide is predicted to decrease the exposure to **abiraterone**. Avoid. Severe Theoretical
▸ HIV-protease inhibitors are predicted to increase the exposure to **abiraterone**. Severe Theoretical
▸ Idelalisib is predicted to increase the exposure to **abiraterone**. Severe Theoretical
▸ Macrolides (clarithromycin) are predicted to increase the exposure to **abiraterone**. Severe Theoretical
▸ Mitotane is predicted to decrease the exposure to **abiraterone**. Avoid. Severe Theoretical
▸ **Abiraterone** is predicted to increase the exposure to pitolisant. Use with caution and adjust dose. Moderate Study
▸ Rifampicin is predicted to decrease the exposure to **abiraterone**. Avoid. Severe Theoretical
▸ **Abiraterone** potentially increases the exposure to venlafaxine. Severe Theoretical

Acarbose → see TABLE 14 p. 1337 (antidiabetic drugs)
▸ **Acarbose** decreases the concentration of digoxin. Moderate Study
▸ Pancreatin is predicted to decrease the effects of **acarbose**. Avoid. Moderate Theoretical

ACE inhibitors → see TABLE 7 p. 1335 (first-dose hypotension), TABLE 8 p. 1335 (hypotension), TABLE 16 p. 1338 (increased serum potassium)

captopril · enalapril · fosinopril · imidapril · lisinopril · perindopril · quinapril · ramipril · trandolapril

▸ **ACE inhibitors** increase the risk of renal impairment when given with aliskiren. Use with caution or avoid aliskiren in selected patients, p. 179. Severe Study → Also see TABLE 8 p. 1335 → Also see TABLE 16 p. 1338
▸ **ACE inhibitors** are predicted to increase the risk of hypersensitivity and haematological reactions when given with allopurinol. Severe Anecdotal
▸ **ACE inhibitors** are predicted to increase the risk of anaemia and/or leucopenia when given with azathioprine. Severe Anecdotal
▸ **ACE inhibitors** are predicted to decrease the efficacy of icatibant and icatibant is predicted to decrease the efficacy of **ACE inhibitors**. Avoid. Moderate Theoretical
▸ **ACE inhibitors** are predicted to increase the concentration of lithium. Monitor and adjust dose. Severe Anecdotal

▸ **ACE inhibitors** are predicted to increase the risk of hypersensitivity when given with sodium aurothiomalate. Severe Anecdotal
▸ Quinapril (tablet) decreases the absorption of oral tetracyclines (tetracycline). Avoid. Moderate Study

Acebutolol → see beta blockers, selective
Aceclofenac → see NSAIDs
Acemetacin → see NSAIDs
Acenocoumarol → see coumarins
Acetazolamide
▸ **Acetazolamide** potentially increases the risk of toxicity when given with antiepileptics (valproate). Severe Study
▸ **Acetazolamide** potentially increases the risk of overheating and dehydration when given with antiepileptics (zonisamide). Avoid in children. Severe Theoretical
▸ **Acetazolamide** increases the risk of severe toxic reaction when given with aspirin (high-dose). Severe Study
▸ **Acetazolamide** alters the concentration of lithium. Severe Anecdotal
▸ **Acetazolamide** is predicted to decrease the efficacy of methenamine. Avoid. Moderate Theoretical
▸ **Acetazolamide** increases the urinary excretion of methotrexate. Moderate Study

Aciclovir → see TABLE 2 p. 1334 (nephrotoxicity)

ROUTE-SPECIFIC INFORMATION Since systemic absorption can follow topical application, the possibility of interactions should be borne in mind.

▸ **Aciclovir** increases the exposure to aminophylline. Monitor and adjust dose. Severe Anecdotal
▸ Mycophenolate is predicted to increase the risk of haematological toxicity when given with **aciclovir**. Moderate Theoretical
▸ **Aciclovir** is predicted to increase the exposure to theophylline. Monitor and adjust dose. Severe Theoretical

Acitretin → see retinoids
Aclidinium → see TABLE 10 p. 1336 (antimuscarinics)
Acrivastine → see antihistamines, non-sedating
Adalimumab → see monoclonal antibodies
Adapalene → see retinoids
Adefovir
▸ Ataluren increases the exposure to **adefovir**. Moderate Study
Adenosine → see antiarrhythmics
Adrenaline/epinephrine → see sympathomimetics, vasoconstrictor
Afatinib → see TABLE 15 p. 1337 (myelosuppression)
▸ Antiarrhythmics (amiodarone, dronedarone) are predicted to increase the exposure to **afatinib**. Separate administration by 12 hours. Moderate Study
▸ Antiepileptics (carbamazepine) are predicted to decrease the exposure to **afatinib**. Moderate Study
▸ Antifungals, azoles (itraconazole, ketoconazole) are predicted to increase the exposure to **afatinib**. Separate administration by 12 hours. Moderate Study
▸ Calcium channel blockers (verapamil) are predicted to increase the exposure to **afatinib**. Separate administration by 12 hours. Moderate Study
▸ Ciclosporin is predicted to increase the exposure to **afatinib**. Separate administration by 12 hours. Moderate Study
▸ HIV-protease inhibitors (lopinavir, ritonavir, saquinavir) are predicted to increase the exposure to **afatinib**. Separate administration by 12 hours. Moderate Study
▸ Lapatinib is predicted to increase the exposure to **afatinib**. Separate administration by 12 hours. Moderate Study
▸ Macrolides are predicted to increase the exposure to **afatinib**. Separate administration by 12 hours. Moderate Study
▸ Ranolazine is predicted to increase the exposure to **afatinib**. Separate administration by 12 hours. Moderate Study
▸ Rifampicin is predicted to decrease the exposure to **afatinib**. Moderate Study
▸ St John's Wort is predicted to decrease the exposure to **afatinib**. Moderate Study
▸ Vemurafenib is predicted to increase the exposure to **afatinib**. Separate administration by 12 hours. Moderate Study

Aflibercept → see TABLE 15 p. 1337 (myelosuppression)

Agalsidase

▸ Aminoglycosides are predicted to decrease the effects of **agalsidase**. Avoid. Moderate Theoretical
▸ Antiarrhythmics (amiodarone) are predicted to decrease the effects of **agalsidase**. Avoid. Moderate Theoretical
▸ Antimalarials (chloroquine) are predicted to decrease the effects of **agalsidase**. Avoid. Moderate Theoretical
▸ Hydroxychloroquine is predicted to decrease the effects of **agalsidase**. Moderate Theoretical

Agomelatine → see TABLE 11 p. 1336 (CNS depressant effects)

> ▸ Dose adjustment might be necessary if smoking started or stopped during treatment.
> ▸ Caution with concomitant use of drugs associated with hepatic injury.

▸ Antiepileptics (fosphenytoin, phenytoin) are predicted to decrease the exposure to **agomelatine**. Moderate Theoretical
▸ Combined hormonal contraceptives are predicted to increase the exposure to **agomelatine**. Moderate Study
▸ HIV-protease inhibitors (ritonavir) are predicted to decrease the exposure to **agomelatine**. Moderate Theoretical
▸ Leflunomide is predicted to decrease the exposure to **agomelatine**. Moderate Theoretical
▸ Quinolones (ciprofloxacin) are predicted to increase the exposure to **agomelatine**. Moderate Study
▸ Rifampicin is predicted to decrease the exposure to **agomelatine**. Moderate Theoretical
▸ SSRIs (fluvoxamine) very markedly increase the exposure to **agomelatine**. Avoid. Severe Study
▸ Teriflunomide is predicted to decrease the exposure to **agomelatine**. Moderate Theoretical

Albendazole

▸ Antiepileptics (carbamazepine, fosphenytoin, phenobarbital, phenytoin, primidone) decrease the concentration of **albendazole**. Moderate Study
▸ H$_2$ receptor antagonists (cimetidine) decrease the clearance of **albendazole**. Moderate Study
▸ HIV-protease inhibitors (ritonavir) decrease the exposure to **albendazole**. Moderate Study
▸ **Albendazole** slightly decreases the exposure to levamisole and levamisole moderately decreases the exposure to **albendazole**. Moderate Study

Albiglutide → see TABLE 14 p. 1337 (antidiabetic drugs)

Alcohol (beverage) → see TABLE 1 p. 1334 (hepatotoxicity), TABLE 8 p. 1335 (hypotension), TABLE 11 p. 1336 (CNS depressant effects)

▸ **Alcohol (beverage)** potentially increases the risk of visual disturbances when given with antiepileptics (retigabine). Moderate Study
▸ **Alcohol (beverage)** potentially causes a disulfiram-like reaction when given with antifungals, azoles (ketoconazole). Avoid. Moderate Anecdotal
▸ **Alcohol (beverage)** causes serious, potentially fatal, CNS depression when given with clomethiazole. Avoid. Severe Study → Also see TABLE 11 p. 1336
▸ **Alcohol (beverage)** (in those who drink heavily) potentially decreases the anticoagulant effect of coumarins. Severe Study
▸ **Alcohol (beverage)** (excessive consumption) potentially increases the risk of gastrointestinal side-effects when given with dimethyl fumarate. Avoid. Moderate Theoretical
▸ **Alcohol (beverage)** causes an extremely unpleasant systemic reaction when given with disulfiram. Avoid for at least 24 hours before and up to 14 days after stopping treatment. Severe Study
▸ **Alcohol (beverage)** potentially causes a disulfiram-like reaction when given with griseofulvin. Moderate Anecdotal
▸ **Alcohol (beverage)** potentially causes a disulfiram-like reaction when given with levamisole. Moderate Study
▸ **Alcohol (beverage)** (excessive consumption) potentially increases the risk of lactic acidosis when given with metformin. Avoid excessive alcohol consumption. Moderate Theoretical
▸ **Alcohol (beverage)** potentially causes a disulfiram-like reaction when given with metronidazole. Avoid for at least 48 hours stopping treatment. Moderate Study

▸ **Alcohol (beverage)** causes rapid release of opioids (hydromorphone, morphine) (from extended-release preparations). Avoid. Severe Study → Also see TABLE 11 p. 1336
▸ **Alcohol (beverage)** (in those who drink heavily) causes severe liver damage when given with paracetamol. Severe Study → Also see TABLE 1 p. 1334
▸ **Alcohol (beverage)** increases the risk of facial flushing and skin irritation when given with topical pimecrolimus. Moderate Study
▸ **Alcohol (beverage)** potentially causes a disulfiram-like reaction when given with procarbazine. Moderate Anecdotal
▸ **Alcohol (beverage)** potentially increases the concentration of retinoids (acitretin). Avoid and for 2 months after stopping acitretin. Moderate Study
▸ **Alcohol (beverage)** increases the risk of facial flushing and skin irritation when given with topical tacrolimus. Moderate Study
▸ **Alcohol (beverage)** potentially causes a disulfiram-like reaction when given with tinidazole. Avoid for 72 hours stopping treatment. Moderate Theoretical

Aldosterone antagonists → see TABLE 18 p. 1338 (hyponatraemia), TABLE 8 p. 1335 (hypotension), TABLE 16 p. 1338 (increased serum potassium)

eplerenone · spironolactone

▸ Antiarrhythmics (amiodarone) are predicted to increase the exposure to **eplerenone**. Adjust **eplerenone** dose, p. 190. Severe Theoretical
▸ Antiarrhythmics (dronedarone) are predicted to increase the exposure to **eplerenone**. Adjust **eplerenone** dose, p. 190. Severe Study
▸ Antiepileptics (carbamazepine, fosphenytoin, phenobarbital, phenytoin, primidone) are predicted to decrease the exposure to **eplerenone**. Avoid. Moderate Theoretical → Also see TABLE 18 p. 1338
▸ Antifungals, azoles (fluconazole, isavuconazole, posaconazole) are predicted to increase the exposure to **eplerenone**. Adjust **eplerenone** dose, p. 190. Severe Study
▸ Antifungals, azoles (itraconazole, ketoconazole, voriconazole) are predicted to markedly increase the exposure to **eplerenone**. Avoid. Severe Study
▸ Aprepitant is predicted to increase the exposure to **eplerenone**. Adjust **eplerenone** dose, p. 190. Severe Study
▸ Calcium channel blockers (diltiazem, verapamil) are predicted to increase the exposure to **eplerenone**. Adjust **eplerenone** dose, p. 190. Severe Study → Also see TABLE 8 p. 1335
▸ Cobicistat is predicted to markedly increase the exposure to **eplerenone**. Avoid. Severe Study
▸ Crizotinib is predicted to increase the exposure to **eplerenone**. Adjust **eplerenone** dose, p. 190. Severe Study
▸ **Eplerenone** very slightly increases the exposure to digoxin. Mild Study
▸ **Spironolactone** increases the concentration of digoxin. Monitor and adjust dose. Moderate Study
▸ Enzalutamide is predicted to decrease the exposure to **eplerenone**. Avoid. Moderate Theoretical
▸ HIV-protease inhibitors are predicted to markedly increase the exposure to **eplerenone**. Avoid. Severe Study
▸ Idelalisib is predicted to markedly increase the exposure to **eplerenone**. Avoid. Severe Study
▸ Imatinib is predicted to increase the exposure to **eplerenone**. Adjust **eplerenone** dose, p. 190. Severe Study
▸ **Eplerenone** potentially increases the concentration of lithium. Avoid. Moderate Theoretical
▸ **Spironolactone** potentially increases the concentration of lithium. Moderate Study
▸ Macrolides (clarithromycin) are predicted to markedly increase the exposure to **eplerenone**. Avoid. Severe Study
▸ Macrolides (erythromycin) are predicted to increase the exposure to **eplerenone**. Adjust **eplerenone** dose, p. 190. Severe Study
▸ Mitotane is predicted to decrease the exposure to **eplerenone**. Avoid. Moderate Theoretical
▸ **Spironolactone** is predicted to decrease the effects of mitotane. Avoid. Severe Anecdotal
▸ Netupitant is predicted to increase the exposure to **eplerenone**. Adjust **eplerenone** dose, p. 190. Severe Study

▶ Nilotinib is predicted to increase the exposure to eplerenone. Adjust eplerenone dose, p. 190. [Severe] Study
▶ Rifampicin is predicted to decrease the exposure to eplerenone. Avoid. [Moderate] Theoretical
▶ St John's Wort is predicted to slightly decrease the exposure to eplerenone. Avoid. [Moderate] Study

Alectinib → see TABLE 6 p. 1335 (bradycardia), TABLE 1 p. 1334 (hepatotoxicity)

Alemtuzumab → see monoclonal antibodies

Alendronic acid → see bisphosphonates

Alfacalcidol → see vitamin D substances

Alfentanil → see opioids

Alfuzosin → see alpha blockers

Alimemazine → see antihistamines, sedating

Aliskiren → see TABLE 8 p. 1335 (hypotension), TABLE 16 p. 1338 (increased serum potassium)

FOOD AND LIFESTYLE Avoid apple juice and orange juice as they greatly decrease aliskiren concentrations and plasma renin activity.

▶ ACE inhibitors increase the risk of renal impairment when given with aliskiren. Use with caution or avoid aliskiren in selected patients, p. 179. [Severe] Study → Also see TABLE 8 p. 1335 → Also see TABLE 16 p. 1338
▶ Angiotensin-II receptor antagonists increase the risk of renal impairment when given with aliskiren. Use with caution or avoid aliskiren in selected patients, p. 179. [Severe] Study → Also see TABLE 8 p. 1335 → Also see TABLE 16 p. 1338
▶ Antiarrhythmics (amiodarone, dronedarone) are predicted to increase the exposure to aliskiren. [Severe] Study
▶ Antiepileptics (carbamazepine) decrease the exposure to aliskiren. [Moderate] Theoretical
▶ Antifungals, azoles (itraconazole) markedly increase the exposure to aliskiren. Avoid. [Severe] Study
▶ Antifungals, azoles (ketoconazole) moderately increase the exposure to aliskiren. [Moderate] Study
▶ Calcium channel blockers (verapamil) moderately increase the exposure to aliskiren. [Moderate] Study → Also see TABLE 8 p. 1335
▶ Ceritinib is predicted to increase the exposure to aliskiren. [Moderate] Theoretical
▶ Ciclosporin markedly increases the exposure to aliskiren. Avoid. [Severe] Study → Also see TABLE 16 p. 1338
▶ Eliglustat is predicted to increase the exposure to aliskiren. Adjust dose. [Moderate] Study
▶ Grapefruit juice moderately decreases the exposure to aliskiren. Avoid. [Severe] Study
▶ HIV-protease inhibitors (ritonavir, saquinavir) are predicted to increase the exposure to aliskiren. [Moderate] Theoretical
▶ Lapatinib is predicted to increase the exposure to aliskiren. [Moderate] Theoretical
▶ Aliskiren slightly decreases the exposure to loop diuretics (furosemide). [Moderate] Study → Also see TABLE 8 p. 1335
▶ Macrolides (azithromycin) are predicted to increase the exposure to aliskiren. [Moderate] Theoretical
▶ Macrolides (clarithromycin, erythromycin) are predicted to increase the exposure to aliskiren. [Moderate] Study
▶ Mirabegron is predicted to increase the exposure to aliskiren. [Mild] Theoretical
▶ Ranolazine is predicted to increase the exposure to aliskiren. [Moderate] Theoretical
▶ Rifampicin decreases the exposure to aliskiren. [Moderate] Study
▶ St John's Wort decreases the exposure to aliskiren. [Moderate] Study
▶ Statins (atorvastatin) slightly to moderately increase the exposure to aliskiren. [Moderate] Study
▶ Velpatasvir is predicted to increase the exposure to aliskiren. [Severe] Theoretical
▶ Vemurafenib is predicted to increase the exposure to aliskiren. Use with caution and adjust dose. [Moderate] Theoretical

Alitretinoin → see retinoids

Alkylating agents → see TABLE 15 p. 1337 (myelosuppression), TABLE 2 p. 1334 (nephrotoxicity), TABLE 5 p. 1334 (thromboembolism)

bendamustine · busulfan · carmustine · chlorambucil · cyclophosphamide · dacarbazine · estramustine · ifosfamide · lomustine · melphalan · temozolomide · thiotepa · treosulfan

▶ Antacids are predicted to decrease the absorption of estramustine. Avoid. [Moderate] Study
▶ Antifungals, azoles (isavuconazole) are predicted to increase the exposure to cyclophosphamide. [Moderate] Study
▶ Antifungals, azoles (itraconazole) increase the risk of busulfan toxicity when given with busulfan. Monitor and adjust dose. [Moderate] Study
▶ Antifungals, azoles (miconazole) are predicted to increase the concentration of busulfan. Use with caution and adjust dose. [Moderate] Theoretical
▶ Oral calcium salts decrease the absorption of estramustine. [Severe] Study
▶ Live vaccines are predicted to increase the risk of generalised infection (possibly life-threatening) when given with alkylating agents. Public Health England advises avoid (refer to Green Book). [Severe] Theoretical
▶ Metronidazole increases the risk of toxicity when given with busulfan. [Severe] Study
▶ Paracetamol is predicted to decrease the clearance of busulfan. [Moderate] Theoretical
▶ Cyclophosphamide (high-dose) increases the risk of toxicity when given with pentostatin. Avoid. [Severe] Anecdotal → Also see TABLE 15 p. 1337 → Also see TABLE 5 p. 1334
▶ Rolapitant is predicted to increase the exposure to bendamustine. Avoid or monitor. [Moderate] Study
▶ Cyclophosphamide increases the risk of prolonged neuromuscular blockade when given with suxamethonium. [Moderate] Study

Allopurinol
▶ ACE inhibitors are predicted to increase the risk of hypersensitivity and haematological reactions when given with allopurinol. [Severe] Anecdotal
▶ Allopurinol potentially increases the risk of haematological toxicity when given with azathioprine. Adjust azathioprine dose, p. 816. [Severe] Study
▶ Allopurinol is predicted to decrease the effects of capecitabine. Avoid. [Severe] Study
▶ Allopurinol moderately increases the exposure to didanosine. Avoid. [Severe] Study
▶ Allopurinol potentially increases the risk of haematological toxicity when given with mercaptopurine. Adjust mercaptopurine dose, p. 887. [Severe] Study
▶ Allopurinol increases the risk of skin rash when given with penicillins (amoxicillin, ampicillin). [Moderate] Study
▶ Allopurinol is predicted to increase the risk of hyperuricaemia when given with pyrazinamide. [Moderate] Theoretical
▶ Thiazide diuretics are predicted to increase the risk of hypersensitivity reactions when given with allopurinol. [Severe] Theoretical

Almotriptan → see TABLE 13 p. 1337 (serotonin syndrome)
▶ Antifungals, azoles (itraconazole, ketoconazole, voriconazole) increase the exposure to almotriptan. [Moderate] Study
▶ Cobicistat increases the exposure to almotriptan. [Mild] Study
▶ Almotriptan is predicted to increase the risk of vasoconstriction when given with ergotamine. Ergotamine should be taken at least 24 hours before or 6 hours after almotriptan. [Severe] Theoretical
▶ HIV-protease inhibitors increase the exposure to almotriptan. [Mild] Study
▶ Idelalisib increases the exposure to almotriptan. [Mild] Study
▶ Macrolides (clarithromycin) increase the exposure to almotriptan. [Mild] Study

Alogliptin → see TABLE 14 p. 1337 (antidiabetic drugs)

Alpha blockers → see TABLE 7 p. 1335 (first-dose hypotension), TABLE 8 p. 1335 (hypotension)

alfuzosin · doxazosin · indoramin · prazosin · tamsulosin · terazosin

▶ Antiarrhythmics (dronedarone) are predicted to increase the exposure to tamsulosin. [Moderate] Theoretical
▶ Antifungals, azoles (fluconazole, isavuconazole, posaconazole) are predicted to increase the exposure to tamsulosin. [Moderate] Theoretical
▶ Antifungals, azoles (itraconazole, ketoconazole, voriconazole) are predicted to increase the exposure to doxazosin. [Moderate] Study

A1

Interactions | Appendix 1

Alpha blockers (continued)

▸ Antifungals, azoles (itraconazole, ketoconazole, voriconazole) are predicted to moderately increase the exposure to alpha blockers **(alfuzosin, tamsulosin).** Use with caution or avoid. Moderate Study

▸ Aprepitant is predicted to increase the exposure to **tamsulosin.** Moderate Theoretical

▸ Calcium channel blockers (diltiazem, verapamil) are predicted to increase the exposure to **tamsulosin.** Moderate Theoretical → Also see TABLE 8 p. 1335

▸ Cobicistat is predicted to moderately increase the exposure to alpha blockers **(alfuzosin, tamsulosin).** Use with caution or avoid. Moderate Study

▸ Cobicistat is predicted to increase the exposure to **doxazosin.** Moderate Study

▸ Crizotinib is predicted to increase the exposure to **tamsulosin.** Moderate Theoretical

▸ HIV-protease inhibitors are predicted to moderately increase the exposure to alpha blockers **(alfuzosin, tamsulosin).** Use with caution or avoid. Moderate Study

▸ HIV-protease inhibitors are predicted to increase the exposure to **doxazosin.** Moderate Study

▸ Idelalisib is predicted to moderately increase the exposure to alpha blockers **(alfuzosin, tamsulosin).** Use with caution or avoid. Moderate Study

▸ Idelalisib is predicted to increase the exposure to **doxazosin.** Moderate Study

▸ Imatinib is predicted to increase the exposure to **tamsulosin.** Moderate Theoretical

▸ Macrolides (clarithromycin) are predicted to increase the exposure to **doxazosin.** Moderate Study

▸ Macrolides (erythromycin) are predicted to increase the exposure to **tamsulosin.** Moderate Theoretical

▸ Macrolides (clarithromycin) are predicted to moderately increase the exposure to alpha blockers **(alfuzosin, tamsulosin).** Use with caution or avoid. Moderate Study

▸ Monoamine-oxidase A and B inhibitors, irreversible are predicted to increase the effects of **indoramin.** Avoid. Severe Theoretical → Also see TABLE 8 p. 1335

▸ Netupitant is predicted to increase the exposure to **tamsulosin.** Moderate Theoretical

▸ Nilotinib is predicted to increase the exposure to **tamsulosin.** Moderate Theoretical

▸ **Alpha blockers** cause significant hypotensive effects when given with phosphodiesterase type-5 inhibitors. Patient should be stabilised on first drug then second drug should be added at the lowest recommended dose. Severe Study → Also see TABLE 8 p. 1335

▸ Ribociclib (high-dose) is predicted to increase the exposure to **alfuzosin.** Avoid. Moderate Theoretical

Alpha tocopherol → see vitamin E substances

Alpha tocopheryl acetate → see vitamin E substances

Alprazolam → see TABLE 11 p. 1336 (CNS depressant effects)

▸ Antiarrhythmics (dronedarone) are predicted to increase the exposure to **alprazolam.** Severe Study

▸ Antiepileptics (carbamazepine, fosphenytoin, phenobarbital, phenytoin, primidone) are predicted to decrease the exposure to **alprazolam.** Adjust dose. Moderate Theoretical → Also see TABLE 11 p. 1336

▸ Antifungals, azoles (fluconazole, isavuconazole, posaconazole) are predicted to increase the exposure to **alprazolam.** Severe Study

▸ Antifungals, azoles (itraconazole, ketoconazole, voriconazole) moderately increase the exposure to **alprazolam.** Avoid. Moderate Study

▸ Antifungals, azoles (miconazole) are predicted to increase the exposure to **alprazolam.** Use with caution and adjust dose. Moderate Theoretical

▸ Aprepitant is predicted to increase the exposure to **alprazolam.** Severe Study

▸ Calcium channel blockers (diltiazem, verapamil) are predicted to increase the exposure to **alprazolam.** Severe Study

▸ Cobicistat moderately increases the exposure to **alprazolam.** Avoid. Moderate Study

▸ Crizotinib is predicted to increase the exposure to **alprazolam.** Severe Study

▸ Enzalutamide is predicted to decrease the exposure to **alprazolam.** Adjust dose. Moderate Theoretical

▸ HIV-protease inhibitors moderately increase the exposure to **alprazolam.** Avoid. Moderate Study

▸ Idelalisib moderately increases the exposure to **alprazolam.** Avoid. Moderate Study

▸ Imatinib is predicted to increase the exposure to **alprazolam.** Severe Study

▸ **Alprazolam** is predicted to increase the exposure to **lomitapide.** Separate administration by 12 hours. Moderate Theoretical

▸ Macrolides (clarithromycin) moderately increase the exposure to **alprazolam.** Avoid. Moderate Study

▸ Macrolides (erythromycin) are predicted to increase the exposure to **alprazolam.** Severe Study

▸ Mitotane is predicted to decrease the exposure to **alprazolam.** Adjust dose. Moderate Theoretical

▸ Monoclonal antibodies (tocilizumab) are predicted to decrease the exposure to **alprazolam.** Monitor and adjust dose. Moderate Theoretical

▸ Netupitant is predicted to increase the exposure to **alprazolam.** Severe Study

▸ Nilotinib is predicted to increase the exposure to **alprazolam.** Severe Study

▸ Rifampicin is predicted to decrease the exposure to **alprazolam.** Adjust dose. Moderate Theoretical

▸ SSRIs (fluvoxamine) moderately increase the exposure to **alprazolam.** Adjust dose. Moderate Study

▸ St John's Wort moderately decreases the exposure to **alprazolam.** Moderate Study

Alprostadil → see TABLE 8 p. 1335 (hypotension)

Alteplase → see TABLE 3 p. 1334 (anticoagulant effects)

Aluminium hydroxide → see antacids

Amantadine → see dopamine receptor agonists

Ambrisentan

▸ Ciclosporin moderately increases the exposure to **ambrisentan.** Adjust **ambrisentan** dose, p. 184. Moderate Study

▸ Rifampicin transiently increases the exposure to **ambrisentan.** Moderate Study

Amfetamines → see TABLE 13 p. 1337 (serotonin syndrome)

dexamfetamine · lisdexamfetamine

▸ **Amfetamines** are predicted to decrease the effects of apraclonidine. Avoid. Severe Theoretical

▸ **Amfetamines** are predicted to increase the risk of side-effects when given with atomoxetine. Severe Theoretical

▸ **Dexamfetamine** decreases the effects of guanethidine. Severe Study

▸ HIV-protease inhibitors (ritonavir, tipranavir) are predicted to increase the exposure to **amfetamines.** Severe Theoretical

▸ Moclobemide is predicted to increase the risk of a hypertensive crisis when given with **amfetamines.** Avoid. Severe Theoretical → Also see TABLE 13 p. 1337

▸ Monoamine-oxidase A and B inhibitors, irreversible are predicted to increase the risk of a hypertensive crisis when given with **amfetamines.** Avoid and for 14 days after stopping the MAOI. Severe Anecdotal → Also see TABLE 13 p. 1337

▸ Monoamine-oxidase B inhibitors (rasagiline, selegiline) are predicted to increase the risk of severe hypertension when given with **amfetamines.** Avoid. Severe Theoretical → Also see TABLE 13 p. 1337

▸ Monoamine-oxidase B inhibitors (safinamide) are predicted to increase the risk of severe hypertension when given with **amfetamines.** Severe Theoretical → Also see TABLE 13 p. 1337

▸ Nabilone is predicted to increase the risk of cardiovascular side-effects when given with **amfetamines.** Severe Theoretical

▸ Phenothiazines are predicted to decrease the effects of **amfetamines.** Moderate Study

▸ **Amfetamines** are predicted to decrease the effects of phenothiazines (chlorpromazine). Moderate Study

▸ SSRIs (fluoxetine, paroxetine) are predicted to increase the exposure to **amfetamines.** Severe Theoretical → Also see TABLE 13 p. 1337

Amifampridine → see TABLE 9 p. 1336 (QT-interval prolongation)

Amikacin → see aminoglycosides

Amiloride → see potassium-sparing diuretics
Aminoglycosides → see TABLE 2 p. 1334 (nephrotoxicity), TABLE 19 p. 1338 (ototoxicity), TABLE 20 p. 1338 (neuromuscular blocking effects)

amikacin · gentamicin · streptomycin · tobramycin

► **Aminoglycosides** are predicted to decrease the effects of agalsidase. Avoid. Moderate Theoretical
► Antifungals, azoles (miconazole) potentially decrease the exposure to **tobramycin**. Moderate Anecdotal
► Ataluren is predicted to increase the risk of nephrotoxicity when given with intravenous **aminoglycosides**. Avoid. Severe Study
► **Aminoglycosides** increase the risk of hypocalcaemia when given with bisphosphonates. Moderate Anecdotal → Also see TABLE 2 p. 1334
► **Aminoglycosides** potentially increase the concentration of digoxin. Monitor and adjust dose. Mild Study
► Loop diuretics increase the risk of nephrotoxicity when given with **aminoglycosides**. Avoid. Moderate Study → Also see TABLE 19 p. 1338
► **Aminoglycosides** are predicted to decrease the effects of neostigmine. Moderate Theoretical → Also see TABLE 20 p. 1338
► **Aminoglycosides** are predicted to decrease the effects of pyridostigmine. Moderate Theoretical → Also see TABLE 20 p. 1338

Aminophylline → see TABLE 17 p. 1338 (reduced serum potassium)

FOOD AND LIFESTYLE Smoking can increase aminophylline clearance and increased doses of aminophylline are therefore required; dose adjustments are likely to be necessary if smoking started or stopped during treatment.

► Aciclovir increases the exposure to **aminophylline**. Monitor and adjust dose. Severe Anecdotal
► **Aminophylline** is predicted to decrease the efficacy of antiarrhythmics (adenosine). Separate administration by 24 hours. Mild Theoretical
► Antiepileptics (fosphenytoin) are predicted to decrease the exposure to **aminophylline**. Adjust dose. Moderate Study
► Antiepileptics (phenobarbital) are predicted to decrease the exposure to **aminophylline**. Adjust dose. Moderate Theoretical
► Antiepileptics (phenytoin) decrease the exposure to **aminophylline**. Adjust dose. Moderate Study
► Antiepileptics (primidone) are predicted to increase the clearance of **aminophylline**. Adjust dose. Moderate Theoretical
► Antiepileptics (stiripentol) are predicted to increase the exposure to **aminophylline**. Avoid. Moderate Theoretical
► Beta blockers, non-selective are predicted to increase the risk of bronchospasm when given with **aminophylline**. Avoid. Severe Theoretical
► Beta blockers, selective are predicted to increase the risk of bronchospasm when given with **aminophylline**. Avoid. Severe Theoretical
► Combined hormonal contraceptives are predicted to increase the exposure to **aminophylline**. Adjust dose. Moderate Theoretical
► **Aminophylline** increases the risk of agitation when given with doxapram. Moderate Study
► H$_2$ receptor antagonists (cimetidine) increase the concentration of **aminophylline**. Adjust dose. Severe Study
► HIV-protease inhibitors (ritonavir) decrease the exposure to aminophylline. Adjust dose. Moderate Study
► Interferons are predicted to slightly increase the exposure to **aminophylline**. Adjust dose. Moderate Theoretical
► Iron chelators (deferasirox) are predicted to increase the exposure to **aminophylline**. Avoid. Moderate Theoretical
► Isoniazid is predicted to affect the clearance of **aminophylline**. Severe Theoretical
► Leflunomide decreases the exposure to **aminophylline**. Adjust dose. Moderate Study
► **Aminophylline** is predicted to decrease the concentration of lithium. Moderate Theoretical
► Macrolides (azithromycin) are predicted to increase the exposure to **aminophylline**. Moderate Theoretical
► Macrolides (clarithromycin) are predicted to increase the exposure to **aminophylline**. Adjust dose. Moderate Theoretical
► **Aminophylline** is predicted to decrease the exposure to macrolides (erythromycin). Adjust dose. Severe Study

► Methotrexate is predicted to decrease the clearance of **aminophylline**. Moderate Theoretical
► Monoclonal antibodies (blinatumomab) are predicted to transiently increase the exposure to **aminophylline**. Monitor and adjust dose. Moderate Theoretical
► Monoclonal antibodies (sarilumab) potentially affect the exposure to **aminophylline**. Monitor and adjust dose. Moderate Theoretical
► Monoclonal antibodies (tocilizumab) are predicted to decrease the exposure to **aminophylline**. Monitor and adjust dose. Moderate Theoretical
► Pentoxifylline is predicted to increase the concentration of **aminophylline**. Use with caution or avoid. Severe Theoretical
► Quinolones (ciprofloxacin, norfloxacin) are predicted to increase the exposure to **aminophylline**. Adjust dose. Moderate Theoretical
► Rifampicin decreases the exposure to **aminophylline**. Adjust dose. Moderate Study
► **Aminophylline** is predicted to slightly increase the exposure to roflumilast. Avoid. Moderate Theoretical
► SSRIs (fluvoxamine) moderately to markedly increase the exposure to **aminophylline**. Avoid. Severe Study
► St John's Wort is predicted to decrease the concentration of **aminophylline**. Severe Theoretical
► Sympathomimetics, vasoconstrictor (ephedrine) increase the risk of side-effects when given with **aminophylline**. Avoid in children. Moderate Study
► Teriflunomide decreases the exposure to **aminophylline**. Adjust dose. Moderate Study
► Valaciclovir is predicted to increase the exposure to **aminophylline**. Severe Anecdotal

Aminosalicylic acid
► **Aminosalicylic acid** is predicted to increase the risk of methaemoglobinaemia when given with topical anaesthetics, local (prilocaine). Use with caution or avoid. Severe Theoretical
► **Aminosalicylic acid** is predicted to increase the risk of methaemoglobinaemia when given with dapsone. Severe Theoretical

Amiodarone → see antiarrhythmics
Amisulpride → see TABLE 9 p. 1336 (QT-interval prolongation), TABLE 11 p. 1336 (CNS depressant effects)
► **Amisulpride** is predicted to decrease the effects of dopamine receptor agonists. Avoid. Moderate Theoretical → Also see TABLE 9 p. 1336
► **Amisulpride** is predicted to decrease the effects of levodopa. Avoid. Severe Theoretical

Amitriptyline → see tricyclic antidepressants
Amlodipine → see calcium channel blockers
Amoxicillin → see penicillins
Amphotericin → see TABLE 2 p. 1334 (nephrotoxicity), TABLE 17 p. 1338 (reduced serum potassium)
► **Amphotericin** increases the risk of toxicity when given with flucytosine. Severe Study
► Micafungin slightly increases the exposure to **amphotericin**. Avoid or monitor toxicity. Moderate Study
► Sodium stibogluconate increases the risk of cardiovascular side-effects when given with **amphotericin**. Separate administration by 14 days. Severe Study

Ampicillin → see penicillins
Amsacrine → see TABLE 15 p. 1337 (myelosuppression)
► Live vaccines are predicted to increase the risk of generalised infection (possibly life-threatening) when given with **amsacrine**. Public Health England advises avoid (refer to Green Book). Severe Theoretical

Anaesthetics, local → see TABLE 11 p. 1336 (CNS depressant effects)

bupivacaine · levobupivacaine · mepivacaine · oxyprocaine · prilocaine · proxymetacaine · ropivacaine · tetracaine

► Aminosalicylic acid is predicted to increase the risk of methaemoglobinaemia when given with topical **prilocaine**. Use with caution or avoid. Severe Theoretical
► **Anaesthetics, local** are predicted to increase the risk of cardiodepression when given with antiarrhythmics. Severe Theoretical → Also see TABLE 11 p. 1336
► Antiepileptics (fosphenytoin, phenobarbital, phenytoin, primidone) are predicted to increase the risk of

Anaesthetics, local (continued)

methaemoglobinaemia when given with topical **prilocaine**. Use with caution or avoid. Severe Theoretical → Also see TABLE 11 p. 1336

▶ Antiepileptics (phenytoin) are predicted to decrease the exposure to **ropivacaine**. Moderate Theoretical

▶ Antimalarials (chloroquine, primaquine) are predicted to increase the risk of methaemoglobinaemia when given with topical **prilocaine**. Use with caution or avoid. Severe Theoretical

▶ Dapsone is predicted to increase the risk of methaemoglobinaemia when given with topical **prilocaine**. Use with caution or avoid. Severe Theoretical

▶ HIV-protease inhibitors (ritonavir) are predicted to decrease the exposure to **ropivacaine**. Moderate Theoretical

▶ Leflunomide is predicted to decrease the exposure to **ropivacaine**. Moderate Theoretical

▶ Metoclopramide is predicted to increase the risk of methaemoglobinaemia when given with topical **prilocaine**. Avoid. Severe Theoretical

▶ Nitrates are predicted to increase the risk of methaemoglobinaemia when given with topical **prilocaine**. Avoid. Severe Theoretical

▶ Nitrofurantoin is predicted to increase the risk of methaemoglobinaemia when given with topical **prilocaine**. Use with caution or avoid. Severe Theoretical

▶ Paracetamol is predicted to increase the risk of methaemoglobinaemia when given with topical **prilocaine**. Use with caution or avoid. Severe Theoretical

▶ Rifampicin is predicted to decrease the exposure to **ropivacaine**. Moderate Theoretical

▶ Sodium nitroprusside is predicted to increase the risk of methaemoglobinaemia when given with topical **prilocaine**. Use with caution or avoid. Severe Theoretical

▶ SSRIs (fluvoxamine) decrease the clearance of **ropivacaine**. Avoid prolonged use. Moderate Study

▶ Sulfonamides potentially increase the risk of methaemoglobinaemia when given with topical **prilocaine**. Use with caution or avoid. Severe Anecdotal

▶ Teriflunomide is predicted to decrease the exposure to **ropivacaine**. Moderate Theoretical

Anagrelide → see TABLE 9 p. 1336 (QT-interval prolongation), TABLE 4 p. 1334 (antiplatelet effects)

▶ Combined hormonal contraceptives are predicted to increase the exposure to **anagrelide**. Moderate Theoretical

▶ Quinolones (ciprofloxacin) are predicted to increase the exposure to **anagrelide**. Moderate Theoretical

▶ SSRIs (fluvoxamine) are predicted to increase the exposure to **anagrelide**. Moderate Theoretical → Also see TABLE 4 p. 1334

Anakinra → see TABLE 15 p. 1337 (myelosuppression)

▶ Live vaccines are predicted to increase the risk of generalised infection (possibly life-threatening) when given with **anakinra**. Public Health England advises avoid (refer to Green Book). Severe Theoretical

Angiotensin-II receptor antagonists → see TABLE 7 p. 1335 (first-dose hypotension), TABLE 8 p. 1335 (hypotension), TABLE 16 p. 1338 (increased serum potassium)

azilsartan · candesartan · eprosartan · irbesartan · losartan · olmesartan · telmisartan · valsartan

▶ Angiotensin-II receptor antagonists increase the risk of renal impairment when given with aliskiren. Use with caution or avoid **aliskiren** in selected patients, p. 179. Severe Study → Also see TABLE 8 p. 1335 → Also see TABLE 16 p. 1338

▶ Angiotensin-II receptor antagonists potentially increase the concentration of lithium. Monitor concentration and adjust dose. Severe Anecdotal

Antacids

aluminium hydroxide · magnesium carbonate · magnesium trisilicate

SEPARATION OF ADMINISTRATION Antacids should preferably not be taken at the same time as other drugs since they might impair absorption. Antacids might damage enteric coatings designed to prevent dissolution in the stomach.

▶ Antacids are predicted to decrease the absorption of alkylating agents (estramustine). Avoid. Moderate Study

▶ Antacids decrease the absorption of antiepileptics (gabapentin). Gabapentin should be taken 2 hours after **antacids**. Moderate Study

▶ Antacids decrease the absorption of antifungals, azoles (itraconazole) (capsule). **Antacids** should be taken 1 hour before or 2 hours after **itraconazole**. Moderate Study

▶ Antacids decrease the absorption of antifungals, azoles (ketoconazole). Separate administration by at least 2 hours. Moderate Study

▶ Antacids decrease the absorption of antihistamines, non-sedating (fexofenadine). Separate administration by 2 hours. Mild Study

▶ Antacids decrease the absorption of antimalarials (chloroquine). Separate administration by at least 4 hours. Moderate Study

▶ Antacids are predicted to decrease the absorption of antimalarials (proguanil). Separate administration by at least 2 hours. Moderate Study

▶ Antacids decrease the absorption of aspirin (high-dose). Moderate Study

▶ Antacids decrease the absorption of bisphosphonates (alendronic acid). Alendronic acid should be taken at least 30 minutes before **antacids**. Moderate Study

▶ Antacids are predicted to decrease the absorption of bisphosphonates (ibandronic acid). Avoid **antacids** for at least 6 hours before or 1 hour after **ibandronic acid**. Moderate Theoretical

▶ Antacids decrease the absorption of bisphosphonates (risedronate). Separate administration by at least 2 hours. Moderate Study

▶ Antacids decrease the absorption of bisphosphonates (sodium clodronate). Avoid **antacids** for 2 hours before or 1 hour after **sodium clodronate**. Moderate Study

▶ Antacids are predicted to decrease the absorption of bosutinib. Bosutinib should be taken at least 12 hours before **antacids**. Moderate Theoretical

▶ Antacids are predicted to decrease the absorption of ceritinib. Separate administration by 2 hours. Moderate Theoretical

▶ Oral **aluminium hydroxide** decreases the absorption of chenodeoxycholic acid. Moderate Study

▶ Antacids are predicted to decrease the absorption of cholic acid. Separate administration by 5 hours. Mild Theoretical

▶ Antacids are predicted to decrease the absorption of corticosteroids (deflazacort). Separate administration by 2 hours. Moderate Theoretical

▶ Antacids decrease the absorption of corticosteroids (dexamethasone). Moderate Study

▶ Antacids decrease the absorption of dasatinib. Separate administration by at least 2 hours. Moderate Study

▶ **Aluminium hydroxide** is predicted to decrease the absorption of deferiprone. Avoid. Moderate Theoretical

▶ Antacids decrease the absorption of digoxin. Separate administration by 2 hours. Mild Study

▶ Antacids are predicted to decrease the absorption of dipyridamole (immediate release tablets). Moderate Theoretical

▶ Antacids moderately decrease the exposure to dolutegravir. Dolutegravir should be taken 2 hours before or 6 hours after **antacids**. Moderate Study

▶ Antacids are predicted to decrease the absorption of eltrombopag. Eltrombopag should be taken 2 hours before or 4 hours after **antacids**. Severe Study

▶ Antacids moderately decrease the exposure to elvitegravir. Separate administration by at least 4 hours. Moderate Study

▶ **Aluminium hydroxide** increases the risk of blocked enteral or nasogastric tubes when given with enteral feeds. Moderate Study

▶ Antacids are predicted to decrease the absorption of erlotinib. **Antacids** should be taken 4 hours before or 2 hours after **erlotinib**. Moderate Theoretical

▶ Antacids slightly to moderately decrease the exposure to fibrates (gemfibrozil). Moderate Study

▶ Antacids are predicted to slightly decrease the exposure to gefitinib. Moderate Theoretical

▸ **Antacids** are predicted to decrease the absorption of HIV-protease inhibitors (atazanavir). **Atazanavir should be taken 2 hours before or 1 hour after antacids.** Severe Theoretical

▸ **Antacids** are predicted to decrease the absorption of HIV-protease inhibitors (tipranavir). Separate administration by 2 hours. Moderate Study

▸ **Antacids** decrease the absorption of hydroxychloroquine. Separate administration by at least 4 hours. Moderate Study

▸ **Antacids** decrease the absorption of iron (oral). **Iron (oral)** should be taken 1 hour before or 2 hours after **antacids**. Moderate Study

▸ **Aluminium hydroxide** is predicted to decrease the exposure to iron chelators (deferasirox). Avoid. Moderate Theoretical

▸ **Antacids** are predicted to decrease the absorption of lapatinib. Avoid. Moderate Theoretical

▸ **Antacids** are predicted to decrease the exposure to ledipasvir. Separate administration by 4 hours. Moderate Theoretical

▸ **Antacids** decrease the exposure to mycophenolate. Moderate Study

▸ **Antacids** are predicted to decrease the absorption of nilotinib. Separate administration by at least 2 hours. Moderate Theoretical

▸ **Magnesium trisilicate** decreases the absorption of nitrofurantoin. Moderate Study

▸ **Antacids** are predicted to decrease the absorption of pazopanib. **Pazopanib should be taken 1 hour before or 2 hours after antacids,** p. 962. Moderate Theoretical

▸ **Antacids** decrease the absorption of penicillamine. Separate administration by 2 hours. Mild Study

▸ **Antacids** decrease the absorption of phenothiazines. Moderate Anecdotal

▸ **Antacids** increase the risk of metabolic alkalosis when given with polystyrene sulfonate. Severe Anecdotal

▸ **Antacids** decrease the absorption of quinolones. **Quinolones** should be taken 2 hours before or 4 hours after **antacids**. Moderate Study

▸ **Antacids** slightly decrease the exposure to raltegravir. Avoid. Moderate Study

▸ **Antacids** decrease the absorption of rifampicin. **Rifampicin** should be taken 1 hour before **antacids**. Moderate Study

▸ **Antacids** are predicted to decrease the exposure to rilpivirine. **Antacids should be taken 2 hours before or 4 hours after rilpivirine.** Severe Theoretical

▸ **Antacids** slightly decrease the exposure to riociguat. **Antacids** should be taken 2 hours before or 1 hour after **riociguat**. Mild Study

▸ **Antacids** moderately decrease the absorption of statins (rosuvastatin). Separate administration by 2 hours. Moderate Study

▸ **Antacids** decrease the absorption of sulpiride. Separate administration by 2 hours. Moderate Study

▸ **Antacids** decrease the absorption of tetracyclines. Separate administration by 2 to 3 hours. Moderate Study

▸ **Antacids** are predicted to decrease the absorption of thyroid hormones (levothyroxine). Separate administration by at least 4 hours. Moderate Anecdotal

▸ **Antacids** are predicted to decrease the absorption of ursodeoxycholic acid. Separate administration by 2 hours. Moderate Theoretical

▸ **Antacids** are predicted to decrease the concentration of velpatasvir. Separate administration by 4 hours. Moderate Theoretical

Antazoline → see antihistamines, sedating

Anthracyclines → see TABLE 15 p. 1337 (myelosuppression), TABLE 5 p. 1334 (thromboembolism)

daunorubicin · doxorubicin · epirubicin · idarubicin · mitoxantrone · pixantrone

GENERAL INFORMATION Caution is necessary with concurrent use of cardiotoxic drugs, or drugs that reduce cardiac contractility.

▸ **Calcium channel blockers** (verapamil) moderately increase the exposure to **doxorubicin**. Moderate Study

▸ **Ciclosporin** increases the concentration of anthracyclines (**daunorubicin, doxorubicin, epirubicin, idarubicin, mitoxantrone**). Severe Study

▸ **H₂ receptor antagonists** (cimetidine) slightly increase the exposure to **epirubicin**. Avoid. Moderate Study

▸ **Live vaccines** are predicted to increase the risk of generalised infection (possibly life-threatening) when given with **anthracyclines**. Public Health England advises avoid (refer to Green Book). Severe Theoretical

▸ **Anthracyclines** are predicted to increase the risk of cardiotoxicity when given with monoclonal antibodies (trastuzumab, trastuzumab emtansine). Avoid. Severe Theoretical → Also see TABLE 15 p. 1337

▸ **Rolapitant** is predicted to increase the exposure to anthracyclines (**doxorubicin, mitoxantrone**). Avoid or monitor. Moderate Study

Antiarrhythmics → see TABLE 6 p. 1335 (bradycardia), TABLE 12 p. 1337 (peripheral neuropathy), TABLE 9 p. 1336 (QT-interval prolongation), TABLE 11 p. 1336 (CNS depressant effects), TABLE 10 p. 1336 (antimuscarinics)

adenosine · amiodarone · disopyramide · dronedarone · flecainide · lidocaine · propafenone

▸ Amiodarone has a long half-life; there is potential for drug interactions to occur for several weeks (or even months) after treatment with it has been stopped.

▸ Since systemic absorption can follow topical application of **lidocaine**, the possibility of interactions should be borne in mind.

▸ **Antiarrhythmics** (**amiodarone, dronedarone**) are predicted to increase the exposure to afatinib. Separate administration by 12 hours. Moderate Study

▸ **Amiodarone** is predicted to decrease the effects of agalsidase. Avoid. Moderate Theoretical

▸ **Amiodarone** is predicted to increase the exposure to aldosterone antagonists (eplerenone). Adjust **eplerenone** dose, p. 190. Severe Theoretical

▸ **Dronedarone** is predicted to increase the exposure to aldosterone antagonists (eplerenone). Adjust **eplerenone** dose, p. 190. Severe Study

▸ **Antiarrhythmics** (**amiodarone, dronedarone**) are predicted to increase the exposure to aliskiren. Severe Study

▸ **Dronedarone** is predicted to increase the exposure to alpha blockers (tamsulosin). Moderate Theoretical

▸ **Dronedarone** is predicted to increase the exposure to alprazolam. Severe Study

▸ **Aminophylline** is predicted to decrease the efficacy of **adenosine**. Separate administration by 24 hours. Mild Theoretical

▸ **Anaesthetics, local** are predicted to increase the risk of cardiodepression when given with **antiarrhythmics**. Severe Theoretical → Also see TABLE 11 p. 1336

▸ **Antiarrhythmics** (**propafenone**) are predicted to increase the risk of cardiodepression when given with antiarrhythmics (**amiodarone**). Monitor and adjust dose. Severe Theoretical

▸ **Antiarrhythmics** (**amiodarone**) increase the concentration of antiarrhythmics (**flecainide**). Adjust **flecainide** dose and monitor side effects. Severe Study → Also see TABLE 6 p. 1335 → Also see TABLE 9 p. 1336

▸ **Antiarrhythmics** (**propafenone**) are predicted to increase the risk of cardiodepression when given with antiarrhythmics (**lidocaine**). Moderate Study

▸ **Antiarrhythmics** (**dronedarone**) are predicted to increase the exposure to antiarrhythmics (**propafenone**). Monitor and adjust dose. Moderate Study

▸ **Amiodarone** increases the risk of bradycardia when given with anticholinesterases, centrally acting. Moderate Anecdotal → Also see TABLE 6 p. 1335

▸ **Antiepileptics** (carbamazepine, fosphenytoin, phenobarbital, phenytoin, primidone) are predicted to decrease the efficacy of **propafenone**. Moderate Study

▸ **Antiepileptics** (fosphenytoin, phenytoin) are predicted to decrease the exposure to **lidocaine**. Severe Anecdotal

▸ **Antiepileptics** (carbamazepine, fosphenytoin, phenobarbital, phenytoin, primidone) are predicted to decrease the exposure

A1

Interactions | Appendix 1

Antiarrhythmics (continued)

to antiarrhythmics **(disopyramide, dronedarone)**. Avoid. Severe Study

▸ **Amiodarone** is predicted to slightly increase the concentration of antiepileptics **(fosphenytoin, phenytoin)**. Monitor and adjust dose. Severe Study → Also see TABLE 12 p. 1337

▸ Antifungals, azoles **(fluconazole)** are predicted to increase the exposure to **dronedarone**. Severe Theoretical → Also see TABLE 9 p. 1336

▸ Antifungals, azoles **(fluconazole, isavuconazole, posaconazole)** are predicted to increase the exposure to **propafenone**. Monitor and adjust dose. Moderate Study

▸ Antifungals, azoles **(itraconazole, ketoconazole, voriconazole)** are predicted to increase the exposure to **disopyramide**. Avoid. Severe Theoretical → Also see TABLE 9 p. 1336

▸ Antifungals, azoles **(itraconazole, ketoconazole, voriconazole)** very markedly increase the exposure to **dronedarone**. Avoid. Severe Study → Also see TABLE 9 p. 1336

▸ Antifungals, azoles **(itraconazole, ketoconazole, voriconazole)** are predicted to increase the exposure to **propafenone**. Monitor and adjust dose. Severe Study

▸ Antifungals, azoles **(miconazole)** are predicted to increase the exposure to **disopyramide**. Use with caution and adjust dose. Severe Theoretical

▸ Antifungals, azoles **(posaconazole)** are predicted to increase the exposure to antiarrhythmics **(disopyramide, dronedarone)**. Avoid. Severe Theoretical

▸ **Dronedarone** is predicted to increase the exposure to antihistamines, non-sedating **(fexofenadine, mizolastine)**. Severe Theoretical

▸ **Dronedarone** is predicted to increase the exposure to antihistamines, non-sedating **(rupatadine)**. Avoid. Moderate Study

▸ **Dronedarone** is predicted to increase the concentration of antimalarials **(piperaquine)**. Severe Theoretical

▸ **Dronedarone** is predicted to increase the exposure to apixaban. Moderate Theoretical

▸ Aprepitant increases the exposure to **dronedarone**. Severe Theoretical

▸ Aprepitant is predicted to increase the exposure to **propafenone**. Monitor and adjust dose. Moderate Study

▸ **Dronedarone** is predicted to increase the exposure to axitinib. Moderate Theoretical

▸ **Dronedarone** is predicted to increase the exposure to bedaquiline. Avoid prolonged use. Mild Theoretical → Also see TABLE 9 p. 1336

▸ Antiarrhythmics **(amiodarone, disopyramide, dronedarone, flecainide, lidocaine)** are predicted to increase the risk of cardiovascular side-effects when given with beta blockers, non-selective. Use with caution or avoid. Severe Study → Also see TABLE 6 p. 1335 → Also see TABLE 9 p. 1336

▸ **Propafenone** is predicted to increase the risk of cardiovascular side-effects when given with beta blockers, non-selective **(labetalol, levobunolol, nadolol, oxprenolol, pindolol, sotalol)**. Use with caution or avoid. Severe Study

▸ **Propafenone** increases the risk of cardiovascular side-effects when given with beta blockers, non-selective **(propranolol)**. Use with caution or avoid. Severe Study

▸ **Propafenone** is predicted to increase the exposure to beta blockers, non-selective **(timolol)** and beta blockers, non-selective **(timolol)** are predicted to increase the risk of cardiodepression when given with **propafenone**. Severe Anecdotal

▸ Antiarrhythmics **(amiodarone, disopyramide, dronedarone, flecainide, lidocaine)** are predicted to increase the risk of cardiovascular side-effects when given with beta blockers, selective. Use with caution or avoid. Severe Study → Also see TABLE 6 p. 1335

▸ **Propafenone** is predicted to increase the risk of cardiovascular side-effects when given with beta blockers, selective **(acebutolol, atenolol, betaxolol, bisoprolol, celiprolol, esmolol)**. Use with caution or avoid. Severe Study

▸ **Propafenone** is predicted to increase the exposure to beta blockers, selective **(metoprolol)**. Moderate Study

▸ **Propafenone** is predicted to increase the exposure to beta blockers, selective **(nebivolol)** and beta blockers, selective **(nebivolol)** are predicted to increase the risk of

cardiodepression when given with **propafenone**. Avoid. Severe Theoretical

▸ Bosentan is predicted to decrease the exposure to **dronedarone**. Severe Theoretical

▸ **Dronedarone** is predicted to increase the exposure to bosutinib. Avoid or adjust dose. Severe Theoretical → Also see TABLE 9 p. 1336

▸ **Dronedarone** is predicted to increase the exposure to buspirone. Use with caution and adjust dose. Moderate Study

▸ **Dronedarone** is predicted to increase the exposure to cabozantinib. Moderate Theoretical → Also see TABLE 9 p. 1336

▸ Caffeine citrate decreases the efficacy of **adenosine**. Separate administration by 24 hours. Mild Study

▸ Calcium channel blockers **(diltiazem, verapamil)** increase the exposure to **dronedarone** and **dronedarone** increases the exposure to calcium channel blockers **(diltiazem, verapamil)**. Moderate Study

▸ Calcium channel blockers **(diltiazem, verapamil)** are predicted to increase the exposure to **propafenone**. Monitor and adjust dose. Moderate Study

▸ Calcium channel blockers **(verapamil)** increase the risk of cardiodepression when given with **flecainide**. Severe Anecdotal → Also see TABLE 6 p. 1335

▸ **Dronedarone** is predicted to increase the exposure to calcium channel blockers **(amlodipine, felodipine, lacidipine, lercanidipine, nicardipine, nifedipine, nimodipine)**. Monitor and adjust dose. Moderate Study

▸ **Amiodarone** is predicted to increase the risk of cardiodepression when given with calcium channel blockers **(diltiazem, verapamil)**. Avoid. Severe Theoretical → Also see TABLE 6 p. 1335

▸ **Disopyramide** is predicted to increase the risk of cardiodepression when given with calcium channel blockers **(verapamil)**. Severe Theoretical

▸ Antiarrhythmics **(amiodarone, dronedarone)** are predicted to increase the exposure to ceritinib. Moderate Theoretical → Also see TABLE 9 p. 1336

▸ **Amiodarone** increases the concentration of ciclosporin. Monitor concentration and adjust dose. Severe Study

▸ **Dronedarone** increases the concentration of ciclosporin. Severe Study

▸ Ciclosporin increases the exposure to **dronedarone**. Avoid. Severe Theoretical

▸ Cobicistat very markedly increases the exposure to **dronedarone**. Avoid. Severe Study

▸ Cobicistat is predicted to increase the exposure to **propafenone**. Monitor and adjust dose. Severe Study

▸ **Dronedarone** is predicted to increase the exposure to cobimetinib. Severe Theoretical

▸ **Dronedarone** is predicted to increase the exposure to colchicine. Adjust **colchicine** dose with moderate inhibitors of CYP3A4, p. 1085. Severe Study

▸ **Dronedarone** is predicted to increase the exposure to corticosteroids **(methylprednisolone)**. Monitor and adjust dose. Moderate Study

▸ **Amiodarone** increases the anticoagulant effect of coumarins. Severe Study

▸ **Propafenone** increases the anticoagulant effect of coumarins. Monitor INR and adjust dose. Moderate Study

▸ Crizotinib is predicted to increase the exposure to **propafenone**. Monitor and adjust dose. Moderate Study

▸ **Amiodarone** increases the exposure to dabigatran. Adjust **dabigatran** dose, p. 135. Moderate Study

▸ **Dronedarone** slightly increases the exposure to dabigatran. Avoid. Severe Study

▸ Daclatasvir is predicted to increase the risk of severe bradycardia or heart block when given with **amiodarone**. Refer to specialist literature. Severe Anecdotal

▸ **Dronedarone** is predicted to slightly increase the exposure to darifenacin. Moderate Study

▸ Darifenacin is predicted to increase the concentration of **flecainide**. Moderate Theoretical

▸ **Dronedarone** is predicted to increase the exposure to dasatinib. Severe Study → Also see TABLE 9 p. 1336

▸ Antiarrhythmics **(amiodarone, dronedarone)** are predicted to moderately increase the exposure to digoxin. Monitor and adjust **digoxin** dose, p. 109. [Severe] Study → Also see TABLE 6 p. 1335

▸ Propafenone increases the concentration of digoxin. Monitor and adjust dose. [Severe] Study

▸ Dipyridamole increases the exposure to **adenosine**. Avoid or adjust dose. [Severe] Study

▸ Dronedarone increases the risk of QT-prolongation when given with domperidone. [Severe] Study

▸ Dronedarone is predicted to increase the exposure to dopamine receptor agonists (bromocriptine). [Severe] Theoretical

▸ Dronedarone is predicted to increase the concentration of dopamine receptor agonists (cabergoline). [Severe] Anecdotal

▸ Dronedarone is predicted to moderately increase the exposure to dutasteride. [Severe] Study

▸ Amiodarone slightly increases the exposure to edoxaban. [Severe] Study

▸ Dronedarone slightly increases the exposure to edoxaban. Adjust **edoxaban** dose, p. 125. [Severe] Study

▸ Efavirenz is predicted to decrease the exposure to dronedarone. [Severe] Theoretical → Also see TABLE 9 p. 1336

▸ Antiarrhythmics **(dronedarone, propafenone)** are predicted to increase the exposure to eliglustat. Avoid or adjust dose—consult product literature. [Severe] Study

▸ Enzalutamide is predicted to decrease the exposure to antiarrhythmics **(disopyramide, dronedarone)**. Avoid. [Severe] Study

▸ Enzalutamide is predicted to decrease the efficacy of **propafenone**. [Moderate] Study

▸ Dronedarone is predicted to increase the risk of ergotism when given with ergometrine. [Severe] Theoretical

▸ Dronedarone is predicted to increase the risk of ergotism when given with ergotamine. [Severe] Theoretical

▸ Antiarrhythmics **(amiodarone, dronedarone)** are predicted to increase the exposure to erlotinib. [Moderate] Theoretical

▸ Dronedarone is predicted to increase the concentration of everolimus. Avoid or adjust dose. [Moderate] Study

▸ Dronedarone is predicted to increase the exposure to fesoterodine. Adjust **fesoterodine** dose with moderate inhibitors of CYP3A4 in hepatic and renal impairment, p. 759. [Mild] Study

▸ Antiarrhythmics **(amiodarone, dronedarone)** are predicted to increase the exposure to fidaxomicin. Avoid. [Moderate] Study

▸ Dronedarone is predicted to increase the exposure to gefitinib. [Moderate] Theoretical

▸ Dronedarone potentially increases the exposure to glecaprevir. [Moderate] Theoretical

▸ Grapefruit juice increases the exposure to **amiodarone**. Avoid. [Moderate] Study

▸ Grapefruit juice moderately increases the exposure to **dronedarone**. Avoid. [Severe] Study

▸ Grapefruit juice increases the exposure to **propafenone**. Monitor and adjust dose. [Moderate] Study

▸ Dronedarone is predicted to increase the concentration of guanfacine. Adjust **guanfacine** dose, p. 349. [Moderate] Theoretical

▸ H_2 receptor antagonists (cimetidine) increase the exposure to **amiodarone**. [Moderate] Study

▸ H_2 receptor antagonists (cimetidine) slightly increase the exposure to **flecainide**. Monitor and adjust dose. [Mild] Study

▸ H_2 receptor antagonists (cimetidine) increase the exposure to **lidocaine**. Monitor and adjust dose. [Moderate] Study

▸ H_2 receptor antagonists (cimetidine) are predicted to increase the exposure to **propafenone**. Monitor and adjust dose. [Moderate] Theoretical

▸ HIV-protease inhibitors are predicted to increase the exposure to **amiodarone**. Avoid. [Severe] Theoretical → Also see TABLE 9 p. 1336

▸ HIV-protease inhibitors are predicted to increase the exposure to **disopyramide**. [Severe] Theoretical → Also see TABLE 9 p. 1336

▸ HIV-protease inhibitors very markedly increase the exposure to **dronedarone**. Avoid. [Severe] Study → Also see TABLE 9 p. 1336

▸ HIV-protease inhibitors are predicted to increase the exposure to **lidocaine**. Avoid. [Severe] Study

▸ HIV-protease inhibitors are predicted to increase the exposure to **propafenone**. Monitor and adjust dose. [Severe] Study

▸ Amiodarone is predicted to increase the exposure to ibrutinib. Adjust **ibrutinib** dose, p. 952. [Severe] Theoretical

▸ Dronedarone is predicted to increase the exposure to ibrutinib. Adjust **ibrutinib** dose with moderate inhibitors of CYP3A4, p. 952. [Severe] Study

▸ Idelalisib is predicted to increase the exposure to **amiodarone**. Avoid. [Moderate] Theoretical

▸ Idelalisib very markedly increases the exposure to **dronedarone**. Avoid. [Severe] Study

▸ Idelalisib is predicted to increase the exposure to **propafenone**. Monitor and adjust dose. [Severe] Study

▸ Imatinib is predicted to increase the exposure to **dronedarone**. [Severe] Theoretical

▸ Imatinib is predicted to increase the exposure to **propafenone**. Monitor and adjust dose. [Moderate] Study

▸ Dronedarone is predicted to increase the exposure to ivabradine. Adjust **ivabradine** dose, p. 210. [Severe] Theoretical

▸ Dronedarone is predicted to increase the exposure to ivacaftor. Adjust **ivacaftor** dose with moderate inhibitors of CYP3A4, p. 292. [Severe] Study

▸ Dronedarone is predicted to increase the exposure to lapatinib. [Moderate] Study → Also see TABLE 9 p. 1336

▸ Ledipasvir increases the risk of severe bradycardia or heart block when given with **amiodarone**. Refer to specialist literature. [Severe] Anecdotal

▸ Amiodarone is predicted to increase the exposure to lomitapide. Separate administration by 12 hours. [Moderate] Theoretical

▸ Dronedarone is predicted to increase the exposure to lomitapide. Avoid. [Moderate] Theoretical

▸ Dronedarone is predicted to increase the exposure to loperamide. [Severe] Theoretical

▸ Dronedarone is predicted to increase the exposure to lurasidone. [Moderate] Study

▸ Macrolides (clarithromycin) very markedly increase the exposure to **dronedarone**. Avoid. [Severe] Study → Also see TABLE 9 p. 1336

▸ Macrolides (clarithromycin) are predicted to increase the exposure to **propafenone**. Monitor and adjust dose. [Severe] Study

▸ Macrolides (clarithromycin, erythromycin) are predicted to increase the exposure to **lidocaine**. [Moderate] Theoretical

▸ Macrolides (erythromycin) are predicted to moderately increase the exposure to **dronedarone**. Avoid. [Severe] Theoretical → Also see TABLE 9 p. 1336

▸ Macrolides (erythromycin) are predicted to increase the exposure to **propafenone**. Monitor and adjust dose. [Moderate] Study

▸ Dronedarone is predicted to increase the exposure to midazolam. Monitor side effects and adjust dose. [Severe] Study

▸ Dronedarone is predicted to increase the exposure to midostaurin. [Moderate] Theoretical

▸ Mitotane is predicted to decrease the exposure to antiarrhythmics **(disopyramide, dronedarone)**. Avoid. [Severe] Study

▸ Mitotane is predicted to decrease the efficacy of **propafenone**. [Moderate] Study

▸ Dronedarone increases the risk of neutropenia when given with monoclonal antibodies (brentuximab vedotin). Monitor and adjust dose. [Severe] Theoretical

▸ Dronedarone is predicted to increase the exposure to naloxegol. Adjust **naloxegol** dose and monitor side effects, p. 64. [Moderate] Study

▸ Netupitant is predicted to increase the exposure to **propafenone**. Monitor and adjust dose. [Moderate] Study

▸ Nevirapine is predicted to decrease the exposure to dronedarone. [Severe] Theoretical

▸ Nilotinib is predicted to increase the exposure to **propafenone**. Monitor and adjust dose. [Moderate] Study

▸ Antiarrhythmics **(amiodarone, dronedarone)** are predicted to increase the exposure to nintedanib. [Moderate] Study

▸ NSAIDs (celecoxib) are predicted to increase the exposure to antiarrhythmics **(flecainide, propafenone)**. Monitor and adjust dose. [Moderate] Theoretical

Antiarrhythmics (continued)

▸ **Dronedarone** is predicted to increase the exposure to olaparib. Avoid moderate inhibitors of CYP3A4 or adjust **olaparib** dose, p. 973. Moderate Theoretical

▸ **Dronedarone** is predicted to increase the exposure to opioids (alfentanil, buprenorphine, fentanyl, oxycodone). Monitor and adjust dose. Moderate Study

▸ **Amiodarone** is predicted to increase the concentration of opioids (fentanyl). Moderate Theoretical → Also see TABLE 6 p. 1335

▸ **Dronedarone** is predicted to increase the exposure to opioids (methadone, sufentanil). Moderate Theoretical → Also see TABLE 9 p. 1336

▸ **Dronedarone** is predicted to increase the exposure to oxybutynin. Mild Theoretical

▸ Antiarrhythmics **(amiodarone, dronedarone)** are predicted to increase the exposure to panobinostat. Adjust dose. Moderate Theoretical → Also see TABLE 9 p. 1336

▸ **Dronedarone** is predicted to increase the exposure to pazopanib. Moderate Theoretical → Also see TABLE 9 p. 1336

▸ **Propafenone** is predicted to increase the anticoagulant effect of phenindione. Monitor and adjust dose. Moderate Theoretical

▸ **Dronedarone** is predicted to increase the exposure to phosphodiesterase type-5 inhibitors (avanafil). Adjust **avanafil** dose, p. 794. Moderate Theoretical

▸ **Dronedarone** is predicted to increase the exposure to phosphodiesterase type-5 inhibitors (sildenafil). Monitor or adjust **sildenafil** dose with moderate inhibitors of CYP3A4, p. 794. Moderate Study → Also see TABLE 9 p. 1336

▸ **Dronedarone** is predicted to increase the exposure to phosphodiesterase type-5 inhibitors (tadalafil). Severe Theoretical

▸ **Dronedarone** is predicted to increase the exposure to phosphodiesterase type-5 inhibitors (vardenafil). Adjust dose. Severe Theoretical → Also see TABLE 9 p. 1336

▸ **Dronedarone** potentially increases the exposure to pibrentasvir. Moderate Theoretical

▸ **Dronedarone** is predicted to increase the exposure to pimozide. Avoid. Severe Theoretical → Also see TABLE 9 p. 1336

▸ **Propafenone** is predicted to increase the exposure to pitolisant. Use with caution and adjust dose. Moderate Study

▸ **Dronedarone** is predicted to increase the exposure to quetiapine. Avoid. Moderate Study

▸ Quinolones (ciprofloxacin) slightly increase the exposure to lidocaine. Mild Study

▸ **Dronedarone** is predicted to increase the exposure to ranolazine. Severe Study → Also see TABLE 9 p. 1336

▸ **Amiodarone** is predicted to increase the exposure to retinoids (alitretinoin). Adjust **alitretinoin** dose, p. 1226. Moderate Theoretical

▸ Ribociclib (high-dose) is predicted to increase the exposure to **amiodarone**. Avoid. Moderate Theoretical → Also see TABLE 9 p. 1336

▸ **Dronedarone** is predicted to increase the exposure to ribociclib. Moderate Study → Also see TABLE 9 p. 1336

▸ Rifampicin is predicted to decrease the exposure to antiarrhythmics **(disopyramide, dronedarone)**. Avoid. Severe Study

▸ Rifampicin is predicted to decrease the efficacy of **propafenone**. Moderate Study

▸ **Dronedarone** is predicted to increase the exposure to rivaroxaban. Avoid. Moderate Theoretical

▸ Rolapitant is predicted to increase the exposure to **propafenone**. Severe Study

▸ **Dronedarone** is predicted to increase the exposure to ruxolitinib. Moderate Theoretical

▸ **Dronedarone** is predicted to increase the exposure to saxagliptin. Mild Study

▸ Simeprevir is predicted to increase the concentration of **amiodarone**. Refer to specialist literature. Severe Anecdotal

▸ **Dronedarone** is predicted to increase the exposure to simeprevir. Avoid. Severe Study

▸ **Amiodarone** is predicted to increase the concentration of sirolimus. Severe Anecdotal

▸ **Dronedarone** increases the concentration of sirolimus. Monitor and adjust dose. Moderate Study

▸ Sofosbuvir is predicted to increase the risk of severe bradycardia or heart block when given with **amiodarone**. Refer to specialist literature. Severe Anecdotal

▸ SSRIs (fluvoxamine) are predicted to increase the exposure to **propafenone**. Monitor and adjust dose. Moderate Study

▸ **Dronedarone** is predicted to increase the exposure to SSRIs (citalopram, escitalopram, fluoxetine, fluvoxamine, paroxetine, sertraline). Severe Theoretical → Also see TABLE 9 p. 1336

▸ **Dronedarone** is predicted to increase the exposure to SSRIs (dapoxetine). Adjust **dapoxetine** dose with moderate inhibitors of CYP3A4, p. 801. Moderate Theoretical

▸ St John's Wort is predicted to decrease the exposure to **dronedarone**. Avoid. Severe Theoretical

▸ **Amiodarone** is predicted to increase the risk of rhabdomyolysis when given with statins (atorvastatin). Monitor and adjust dose. Moderate Theoretical

▸ **Dronedarone** is predicted to increase the exposure to statins (atorvastatin). Monitor and adjust dose. Severe Study

▸ **Amiodarone** is predicted to increase the exposure to statins (fluvastatin). Severe Theoretical

▸ **Dronedarone** slightly increases the exposure to statins (rosuvastatin). Adjust dose. Severe Study

▸ **Amiodarone** increases the risk of rhabdomyolysis when given with statins (simvastatin). Adjust **simvastatin** dose, p. 203. Severe Study

▸ **Dronedarone** is predicted to increase the exposure to statins (simvastatin). Use with caution and adjust **simvastatin** dose, p. 203. Severe Study

▸ **Amiodarone** is predicted to increase the exposure to sulfonylureas. Use with caution and adjust dose. Moderate Study

▸ **Dronedarone** is predicted to increase the exposure to sunitinib. Moderate Theoretical → Also see TABLE 9 p. 1336

▸ **Lidocaine** is predicted to increase the effects of suxamethonium. Moderate Study

▸ **Amiodarone** is predicted to increase the concentration of tacrolimus. Severe Anecdotal

▸ **Dronedarone** is predicted to increase the concentration of tacrolimus. Severe Study

▸ **Dronedarone** is predicted to increase the exposure to taxanes (cabazitaxel). Moderate Theoretical

▸ **Dronedarone** is predicted to increase the exposure to taxanes (paclitaxel). Severe Theoretical

▸ **Dronedarone** is predicted to increase the concentration of temsirolimus. Moderate Theoretical

▸ Theophylline decreases the efficacy of **adenosine**. Separate administration by 24 hours. Mild Study

▸ **Amiodarone** is predicted to increase the risk of thyroid dysfunction when given with thyroid hormones. Avoid. Moderate Study

▸ **Amiodarone** is predicted to increase the exposure to ticagrelor. Use with caution or avoid. Severe Study

▸ **Dronedarone** is predicted to increase the exposure to tofacitinib. Moderate Study

▸ **Dronedarone** is predicted to increase the exposure to tolterodine. Mild Theoretical → Also see TABLE 9 p. 1336

▸ **Dronedarone** is predicted to increase the exposure to tolvaptan. Adjust dose. Moderate Study

▸ Antiarrhythmics **(amiodarone, dronedarone)** are predicted to increase the exposure to topotecan. Severe Study

▸ Antiarrhythmics **(amiodarone, dronedarone)** are predicted to increase the concentration of trametinib. Moderate Theoretical

▸ **Dronedarone** is predicted to increase the exposure to trazodone. Moderate Theoretical

▸ **Dronedarone** is predicted to increase the exposure to tricyclic antidepressants. Avoid. Severe Theoretical → Also see TABLE 9 p. 1336

▸ **Propafenone** is predicted to increase the concentration of tricyclic antidepressants. Moderate Theoretical → Also see TABLE 10 p. 1336

▸ **Dronedarone** is predicted to increase the exposure to ulipristal. Avoid if used for uterine fibroids. Moderate Study

▸ **Amiodarone** is predicted to increase the concentration of velpatasvir. Avoid or monitor. Moderate Theoretical

- **Amiodarone** is predicted to increase the exposure to venetoclax. Avoid or monitor for toxicity. Severe Theoretical
- **Dronedarone** is predicted to increase the exposure to venetoclax. Avoid moderate inhibitors of CYP3A4 or adjust **venetoclax** dose, p. 974. Severe Study
- **Dronedarone** is predicted to increase the exposure to vinca alkaloids. Severe Theoretical → Also see TABLE 9 p. 1336
- **Dronedarone** is predicted to increase the exposure to zopiclone. Adjust dose. Moderate Study

Anticholinesterases, centrally acting → see TABLE 6 p. 1335 (bradycardia)

donepezil · galantamine · rivastigmine

- Antiarrhythmics (amiodarone) increase the risk of bradycardia when given with **anticholinesterases, centrally acting**. Moderate Anecdotal → Also see TABLE 6 p. 1335
- Antiepileptics (carbamazepine, fosphenytoin, phenobarbital, phenytoin, primidone) are predicted to decrease the exposure to **donepezil**. Mild Study
- Antifungals, azoles (itraconazole, ketoconazole, voriconazole) are predicted to increase the exposure to **galantamine**. Monitor and adjust dose. Moderate Study
- **Anticholinesterases, centrally acting** are predicted to increase the risk of bradycardia when given with beta blockers, non-selective. Moderate Anecdotal → Also see TABLE 6 p. 1335
- **Anticholinesterases, centrally acting** are predicted to increase the risk of bradycardia when given with beta blockers, selective. Moderate Anecdotal → Also see TABLE 6 p. 1335
- **Bupropion** is predicted to increase the exposure to galantamine. Monitor and adjust dose. Moderate Study
- Calcium channel blockers (diltiazem, verapamil) increase the risk of bradycardia when given with **anticholinesterases, centrally acting**. Moderate Anecdotal → Also see TABLE 6 p. 1335
- **Cinacalcet** is predicted to increase the exposure to galantamine. Monitor and adjust dose. Moderate Study
- **Cobicistat** is predicted to increase the exposure to galantamine. Monitor and adjust dose. Moderate Study
- **Enzalutamide** is predicted to decrease the exposure to donepezil. Mild Study
- HIV-protease inhibitors are predicted to increase the exposure to galantamine. Monitor and adjust dose. Moderate Study
- **Idelalisib** is predicted to increase the exposure to **galantamine**. Monitor and adjust dose. Moderate Study
- Macrolides (clarithromycin) are predicted to increase the exposure to **galantamine**. Monitor and adjust dose. Moderate Study
- **Mitotane** is predicted to decrease the exposure to **donepezil**. Mild Study
- **Anticholinesterases, centrally acting** are predicted to increase the effects of neuromuscular blocking drugs, non-depolarising. Moderate Theoretical → Also see TABLE 6 p. 1335
- **Rifampicin** is predicted to decrease the exposure to **donepezil**. Mild Study
- SSRIs (fluoxetine, paroxetine) are predicted to increase the exposure to **galantamine**. Monitor and adjust dose. Moderate Study
- **Anticholinesterases, centrally acting** increase the effects of suxamethonium. Moderate Theoretical
- **Terbinafine** is predicted to increase the exposure to galantamine. Monitor and adjust dose. Moderate Study

Antiepileptics → see TABLE 1 p. 1334 (hepatotoxicity), TABLE 18 p. 1338 (hyponatraemia), TABLE 15 p. 1337 (myelosuppression), TABLE 12 p. 1337 (peripheral neuropathy), TABLE 11 p. 1336 (CNS depressant effects)

brivaracetam · carbamazepine · eslicarbazepine · ethosuximide · fosphenytoin · gabapentin · lacosamide · lamotrigine · levetiracetam · oxcarbazepine · paraldehyde · perampanel · phenobarbital · phenytoin · pregabalin · primidone · retigabine · rufinamide · stiripentol · tiagabine · topiramate · valproate · vigabatrin · zonisamide

FOOD AND LIFESTYLE Avoid milk or dairy products, carbonated drinks, and fruit juices at the same time as stiripentol.

- Antiepileptics (carbamazepine, fosphenytoin, phenobarbital, phenytoin, primidone) are predicted to decrease the exposure to abacavir. Moderate Theoretical
- Antiepileptics (carbamazepine, fosphenytoin, phenobarbital, phenytoin, primidone) are predicted to decrease the exposure to abiraterone. Avoid. Severe Theoretical
- **Acetazolamide** potentially increases the risk of toxicity when given with valproate. Severe Study
- **Acetazolamide** potentially increases the risk of overheating and dehydration when given with zonisamide. Avoid in children. Severe Theoretical
- **Carbamazepine** is predicted to decrease the exposure to afatinib. Moderate Study
- Antiepileptics (fosphenytoin, phenytoin) are predicted to decrease the exposure to agomelatine. Moderate Theoretical
- Antiepileptics (carbamazepine, fosphenytoin, phenobarbital, phenytoin, primidone) decrease the concentration of albendazole. Moderate Study
- Alcohol (beverage) potentially increases the risk of visual disturbances when given with retigabine. Moderate Study
- Antiepileptics (carbamazepine, fosphenytoin, phenobarbital, phenytoin, primidone) are predicted to decrease the exposure to aldosterone antagonists (eplerenone). Avoid. Moderate Theoretical → Also see TABLE 18 p. 1338
- **Carbamazepine** decreases the exposure to aliskiren. Moderate Study
- Antiepileptics (carbamazepine, fosphenytoin, phenobarbital, phenytoin, primidone) are predicted to decrease the exposure to alprazolam. Adjust dose. Moderate Theoretical → Also see TABLE 11 p. 1336
- **Fosphenytoin** is predicted to decrease the exposure to aminophylline. Adjust dose. Moderate Study
- **Phenobarbital** is predicted to decrease the exposure to aminophylline. Adjust dose. Moderate Theoretical
- **Phenytoin** decreases the exposure to aminophylline. Adjust dose. Moderate Study
- **Primidone** is predicted to increase the clearance of aminophylline. Adjust dose. Moderate Theoretical
- **Stiripentol** is predicted to increase the exposure to aminophylline. Avoid. Moderate Theoretical
- Antiepileptics (fosphenytoin, phenobarbital, phenytoin, primidone) are predicted to increase the risk of methaemoglobinaemia when given with topical anaesthetics, local (prilocaine). Use with caution or avoid. Severe Theoretical → Also see TABLE 11 p. 1336
- **Phenytoin** is predicted to decrease the exposure to anaesthetics, local (ropivacaine). Moderate Theoretical
- **Antacids** decrease the absorption of gabapentin. Gabapentin should be taken 2 hours after antacids. Moderate Study
- Antiepileptics (carbamazepine, fosphenytoin, phenobarbital, phenytoin, primidone) are predicted to decrease the exposure to antiarrhythmics (disopyramide, dronedarone). Avoid. Severe Study
- Antiarrhythmics (amiodarone) are predicted to slightly increase the concentration of antiepileptics (fosphenytoin, phenytoin). Monitor and adjust dose. Severe Study → Also see TABLE 12 p. 1337
- Antiepileptics (fosphenytoin, phenytoin) are predicted to decrease the exposure to antiarrhythmics (lidocaine). Severe Anecdotal
- Antiepileptics (carbamazepine, fosphenytoin, phenobarbital, phenytoin, primidone) are predicted to decrease the efficacy of antiarrhythmics (propafenone). Moderate Study
- Antiepileptics (carbamazepine, fosphenytoin, phenobarbital, phenytoin, primidone) are predicted to decrease the exposure to anticholinesterases, centrally acting (donepezil). Mild Study
- Antiepileptics (carbamazepine) decrease the concentration of antiepileptics (brivaracetam). Moderate Study
- Antiepileptics (fosphenytoin, phenytoin) decrease the concentration of antiepileptics (brivaracetam). Moderate Study
- Antiepileptics (lamotrigine) potentially increase the concentration of antiepileptics (carbamazepine) and antiepileptics (carbamazepine) decrease the concentration of antiepileptics (lamotrigine). Adjust lamotrigine dose and monitor carbamazepine concentration, p. 316, p. 309. Moderate Study

Antiepileptics (continued)

▶ Antiepileptics **(phenobarbital)** affect the concentration of antiepileptics **(carbamazepine)** and antiepileptics **(carbamazepine)** increase the concentration of antiepileptics **(phenobarbital)**. Adjust dose. Moderate Study

▶ Antiepileptics **(topiramate)** increase the risk of carbamazepine toxicity when given with antiepileptics **(carbamazepine)**. Moderate Study

▶ Antiepileptics **(stiripentol)** increase the concentration of antiepileptics **(carbamazepine, phenobarbital)**. Avoid in Dravet syndrome. Severe Study

▶ Antiepileptics **(carbamazepine)** slightly decrease the exposure to antiepileptics **(eslicarbazepine, oxcarbazepine)**. Monitor and adjust dose. Moderate Study

▶ Antiepileptics **(oxcarbazepine)** are predicted to increase the concentration of antiepileptics **(fosphenytoin)**. Monitor concentration and adjust dose. Moderate Study

▶ Antiepileptics **(stiripentol)** are predicted to increase the concentration of antiepileptics **(fosphenytoin)**. Severe Study

▶ Antiepileptics **(carbamazepine)** affect the concentration of antiepileptics **(fosphenytoin, phenytoin)** and antiepileptics **(fosphenytoin, phenytoin)** decrease the concentration of antiepileptics **(carbamazepine)**. Monitor and adjust dose. Severe Study

▶ Antiepileptics **(eslicarbazepine)** increase the exposure to antiepileptics **(fosphenytoin, phenytoin)** and antiepileptics **(fosphenytoin, phenytoin)** decrease the exposure to antiepileptics **(eslicarbazepine)**. Monitor and adjust dose. Moderate Study

▶ Antiepileptics **(valproate)** affect the concentration of antiepileptics **(fosphenytoin, phenytoin)** and antiepileptics **(fosphenytoin, phenytoin)** decrease the concentration of antiepileptics **(valproate)**. Severe Study

▶ Antiepileptics **(vigabatrin)** decrease the concentration of antiepileptics **(fosphenytoin, phenytoin)**. Mild Study

▶ Antiepileptics **(fosphenytoin)** decrease the concentration of antiepileptics **(lamotrigine)**. Monitor and adjust **lamotrigine** dose, p. 316. Moderate Study

▶ Antiepileptics **(phenobarbital, phenytoin, primidone)** decrease the concentration of antiepileptics **(lamotrigine)**. Monitor and adjust **lamotrigine** dose, p. 316. Moderate Study → Also see **TABLE 11** p. 1336

▶ Antiepileptics **(valproate)** increase the exposure to antiepileptics **(lamotrigine)**. Adjust **lamotrigine** dose and monitor rash, p. 316. Severe Study

▶ Antiepileptics **(lamotrigine)** are predicted to increase the concentration of antiepileptics **(oxcarbazepine)** and antiepileptics **(oxcarbazepine)** are predicted to decrease the concentration of antiepileptics **(lamotrigine)**. Monitor side effects and adjust dose. Moderate Study

▶ Antiepileptics **(carbamazepine, fosphenytoin)** are predicted to decrease the exposure to antiepileptics **(perampanel)**. Monitor and adjust dose. Moderate Study

▶ Antiepileptics **(oxcarbazepine)** decrease the concentration of antiepileptics **(perampanel)** and antiepileptics **(perampanel)** increase the concentration of antiepileptics **(oxcarbazepine)**. Monitor and adjust dose. Moderate Study

▶ Antiepileptics **(phenobarbital, phenytoin, primidone)** are predicted to decrease the exposure to antiepileptics **(perampanel)**. Monitor and adjust dose. Moderate Study → Also see **TABLE 11** p. 1336

▶ Antiepileptics **(phenytoin)** increase the concentration of antiepileptics **(phenobarbital)** and antiepileptics **(phenobarbital)** affect the concentration of antiepileptics **(phenytoin)**. Moderate Study

▶ Antiepileptics **(fosphenytoin)** increase the concentration of antiepileptics **(phenobarbital, primidone)** and antiepileptics **(phenobarbital, primidone)** affect the concentration of antiepileptics **(fosphenytoin)**. Moderate Study

▶ Antiepileptics **(oxcarbazepine)** are predicted to increase the concentration of antiepileptics **(phenytoin)**. Monitor concentration and adjust dose. Moderate Study

▶ Antiepileptics **(stiripentol)** are predicted to increase the concentration of antiepileptics **(phenytoin)**. Avoid in Dravet syndrome. Severe Study

▶ Antiepileptics **(carbamazepine)** potentially decrease the concentration of antiepileptics **(primidone)** and antiepileptics **(primidone)** potentially decrease the concentration of antiepileptics **(carbamazepine)**. Adjust dose. Moderate Anecdotal

▶ Antiepileptics **(phenytoin)** increase the concentration of antiepileptics **(primidone)** and antiepileptics **(primidone)** affect the concentration of antiepileptics **(phenytoin)**. Moderate Study

▶ Antiepileptics **(stiripentol)** are predicted to increase the concentration of antiepileptics **(primidone)**. Severe Theoretical

▶ Antiepileptics **(valproate)** affect the concentration of antiepileptics **(primidone)**. Monitor and adjust dose. Severe Study

▶ Antiepileptics **(carbamazepine)** slightly increase the clearance of antiepileptics **(retigabine)**. Moderate Study

▶ Antiepileptics **(fosphenytoin, phenytoin)** are predicted to slightly increase the clearance of antiepileptics **(retigabine)**. Moderate Study

▶ Antiepileptics **(valproate)** increase the exposure to antiepileptics **(rufinamide)**. Adjust rufinamide dose, p. 324. Moderate Study

▶ Antiepileptics **(carbamazepine, fosphenytoin, phenobarbital, phenytoin, primidone)** are predicted to decrease the exposure to antiepileptics **(tiagabine)**. Monitor and adjust **tiagabine** dose, p. 327. Moderate Study

▶ Antiepileptics **(fosphenytoin, phenytoin)** decrease the concentration of antiepileptics **(topiramate)** and antiepileptics **(topiramate)** increase the concentration of antiepileptics **(fosphenytoin, phenytoin)**. Monitor and adjust dose. Moderate Study

▶ Antiepileptics **(phenobarbital, primidone)** are predicted to decrease the concentration of antiepileptics **(topiramate)**. Mild Study

▶ Antiepileptics **(phenobarbital)** decrease the concentration of antiepileptics **(valproate)** and antiepileptics **(valproate)** increase the concentration of antiepileptics **(phenobarbital)**. Monitor and adjust dose. Moderate Study

▶ Antiepileptics **(topiramate)** increase the risk of toxicity when given with antiepileptics **(valproate)**. Severe Study

▶ Antiepileptics **(carbamazepine)** slightly to moderately decrease the concentration of antiepileptics **(zonisamide)** and antiepileptics **(zonisamide)** affect the concentration of antiepileptics **(carbamazepine)**. Monitor and adjust dose. Moderate Study

▶ Antiepileptics **(fosphenytoin, phenytoin)** slightly to moderately decrease the concentration of antiepileptics **(zonisamide)**. Monitor and adjust dose. Moderate Study

▶ Antiepileptics **(phenobarbital, primidone)** are predicted to decrease the concentration of antiepileptics **(zonisamide)**. Monitor and adjust dose. Moderate Study

▶ Antiepileptics **(topiramate)** potentially increase the risk of overheating and dehydration when given with antiepileptics **(zonisamide)**. Avoid in children. Severe Theoretical

▶ Antifungals, azoles (itraconazole, ketoconazole, voriconazole) are predicted to very slightly increase the exposure to **perampanel**. Mild Study

▶ Antifungals, azoles (miconazole) increase the risk of carbamazepine toxicity when given with **carbamazepine**. Monitor and adjust dose. Severe Anecdotal

▶ Antifungals, azoles (miconazole) increase the risk of phenytoin toxicity when given with **fosphenytoin**. Monitor and adjust dose. Severe Anecdotal

▶ Antifungals, azoles (miconazole) increase the risk of phenytoin toxicity when given with **phenytoin**. Monitor and adjust dose. Severe Anecdotal

▶ **Carbamazepine** is predicted to decrease the efficacy of antifungals, azoles (fluconazole) and antifungals, azoles (fluconazole) increase the concentration of **carbamazepine**. Avoid or monitor **carbamazepine** concentration and adjust dose accordingly, p. 309. Severe Theoretical → Also see **TABLE 1** p. 1334

▶ Antifungals, azoles (fluconazole) increase the concentration of antiepileptics **(fosphenytoin, phenytoin)**. Monitor concentration and adjust dose. Moderate Study

▶ Antiepileptics **(carbamazepine, fosphenytoin, phenobarbital, phenytoin, primidone)** are predicted to decrease the exposure to antifungals, azoles (isavuconazole). Avoid. Severe Study

- **Fosphenytoin** very markedly decreases the exposure to antifungals, azoles (itraconazole). Avoid and for 14 days after stopping **fosphenytoin**, p. 313. Moderate Study
- **Phenobarbital** decreases the concentration of antifungals, azoles (itraconazole). Avoid and for 14 days after stopping **phenobarbital**, p. 331. Moderate Study
- **Phenytoin** very markedly decreases the exposure to antifungals, azoles (itraconazole). Avoid and for 14 days after stopping **phenytoin**, p. 321. Moderate Study
- **Primidone** is predicted to decrease the concentration of antifungals, azoles (itraconazole). Moderate Theoretical
- **Carbamazepine** is predicted to decrease the efficacy of antifungals, azoles (itraconazole, voriconazole) and antifungals, azoles (itraconazole, voriconazole) increase the concentration of **carbamazepine**. Avoid or adjust dose. Moderate Theoretical → Also see TABLE 1 p. 1334
- **Carbamazepine** is predicted to decrease the efficacy of antifungals, azoles (ketoconazole) and antifungals, azoles (ketoconazole) slightly increase the concentration of **carbamazepine**. Avoid or monitor **carbamazepine** concentration and adjust dose accordingly, p. 309. Moderate Study
- **Phenobarbital** is predicted to decrease the concentration of antifungals, azoles (ketoconazole). Avoid. Moderate Study
- Antiepileptics **(fosphenytoin, phenytoin)** decrease the exposure to antifungals, azoles (ketoconazole). Avoid. Moderate Study
- **Primidone** is predicted to decrease the concentration of antifungals, azoles (ketoconazole, posaconazole). Avoid. Moderate Study
- **Carbamazepine** is predicted to decrease the efficacy of antifungals, azoles (posaconazole) and antifungals, azoles (posaconazole) increase the concentration of **carbamazepine**. Avoid. Moderate Theoretical
- **Phenobarbital** is predicted to decrease the concentration of antifungals, azoles (posaconazole). Avoid. Moderate Study
- Antiepileptics **(fosphenytoin, phenytoin)** are predicted to decrease the exposure to antifungals, azoles (posaconazole). Avoid. Moderate Study
- **Fosphenytoin** decreases the exposure to antifungals, azoles (voriconazole) and antifungals, azoles (voriconazole) increase the exposure to **fosphenytoin**. Avoid or adjust **voriconazole** dose and monitor phenytoin concentration, p. 588. Moderate Study
- **Phenytoin** decreases the exposure to antifungals, azoles (voriconazole) and antifungals, azoles (voriconazole) increase the exposure to **phenytoin**. Avoid or adjust **voriconazole** dose and monitor **phenytoin** concentration, p. 588, p. 321. Moderate Study
- Antiepileptics **(phenobarbital, primidone)** are predicted to decrease the concentration of antifungals, azoles (voriconazole). Avoid. Moderate Theoretical
- Antihistamines, sedating (hydroxyzine) potentially increase the risk of overheating and dehydration when given with zonisamide. Avoid in children. Severe Theoretical
- Antiepileptics **(carbamazepine, fosphenytoin, phenobarbital, phenytoin, primidone)** are predicted to decrease the exposure to antimalarials (artemether) (with lumefantrine). Avoid. Severe Study
- Antimalarials (pyrimethamine) increase the risk of haematological toxicity when given with antiepileptics **(fosphenytoin, phenytoin)**. Severe Study
- Antimalarials (pyrimethamine) are predicted to increase the risk of haematological toxicity when given with antiepileptics **(phenobarbital, primidone)**. Severe Theoretical
- Antiepileptics **(carbamazepine, fosphenytoin, phenobarbital, phenytoin, primidone)** are predicted to decrease the concentration of antimalarials (piperaquine). Avoid. Moderate Theoretical
- Antiepileptics **(carbamazepine, phenobarbital, primidone)** potentially increase the risk of toxicity when given with antimalarials (quinine). Unknown Study
- Antiepileptics **(carbamazepine, fosphenytoin, phenobarbital, phenytoin, primidone)** are predicted to moderately decrease the exposure to apixaban. Use with caution or avoid. Severe Study

- Antiepileptics **(carbamazepine, fosphenytoin, phenobarbital, phenytoin, primidone)** moderately decrease the exposure to apremilast. Avoid. Severe Study
- Antiepileptics **(carbamazepine, fosphenytoin, phenobarbital, phenytoin, primidone)** are predicted to markedly decrease the exposure to aprepitant. Avoid. Moderate Study
- Antiepileptics **(carbamazepine, fosphenytoin, phenobarbital, phenytoin, primidone)** are predicted to moderately decrease the exposure to aripiprazole. Adjust **aripiprazole** dose, p. 391. Moderate Study → Also see TABLE 11 p. 1336
- Antiepileptics **(carbamazepine, fosphenytoin, phenobarbital, phenytoin, primidone)** are predicted to decrease the exposure to axitinib. Avoid or adjust dose. Moderate Study
- Antiepileptics **(carbamazepine, fosphenytoin, phenobarbital, phenytoin, primidone)** are predicted to decrease the exposure to bazedoxifene. Moderate Theoretical
- Antiepileptics **(carbamazepine, fosphenytoin, phenobarbital, phenytoin, primidone)** decrease the exposure to bedaquiline. Avoid. Severe Study
- Antiepileptics **(phenobarbital, primidone)** are predicted to decrease the exposure to beta blockers, non-selective (carvedilol, labetalol). Moderate Theoretical
- Antiepileptics **(phenobarbital, primidone)** are predicted to decrease the exposure to beta blockers, non-selective (propranolol). Moderate Study
- Antiepileptics **(phenobarbital, primidone)** are predicted to decrease the exposure to beta blockers, selective (acebutolol, bisoprolol, metoprolol, nebivolol). Moderate Study
- Antiepileptics **(carbamazepine, fosphenytoin, phenobarbital, phenytoin, primidone)** slightly decrease the exposure to bortezomib. Avoid. Severe Study → Also see TABLE 12 p. 1337
- Antiepileptics **(carbamazepine, fosphenytoin, phenobarbital, phenytoin, primidone)** affect the exposure to bosentan. Avoid. Severe Study
- Antiepileptics **(carbamazepine, fosphenytoin, phenobarbital, phenytoin, primidone)** are predicted to very markedly decrease the exposure to bosutinib. Severe Study
- Antiepileptics **(carbamazepine, fosphenytoin, phenobarbital, phenytoin, primidone)** are predicted to markedly decrease the exposure to bupropion. Severe Study
- **Valproate** increases the exposure to bupropion. Severe Study
- Antiepileptics **(carbamazepine, fosphenytoin, phenobarbital, phenytoin, primidone)** are predicted to decrease the exposure to buspirone. Use with caution and adjust dose. Severe Study
- Antiepileptics **(carbamazepine, fosphenytoin, phenobarbital, phenytoin, primidone)** moderately decrease the exposure to cabozantinib. Avoid. Moderate Study
- Antiepileptics **(fosphenytoin, phenytoin)** are predicted to moderately increase the clearance of caffeine citrate. Monitor and adjust dose. Moderate Study
- Calcium channel blockers (diltiazem) increase the concentration of **carbamazepine** and **carbamazepine** is predicted to decrease the exposure to calcium channel blockers (diltiazem). Monitor concentration and adjust dose. Severe Anecdotal
- Calcium channel blockers (verapamil) increase the concentration of **carbamazepine** and **carbamazepine** is predicted to decrease the exposure to calcium channel blockers (verapamil). Severe Anecdotal
- Antiepileptics **(carbamazepine, fosphenytoin, phenobarbital, phenytoin, primidone)** are predicted to decrease the exposure to calcium channel blockers (amlodipine, felodipine, lacidipine, lercanidipine, nicardipine, nifedipine, nimodipine). Monitor and adjust dose. Moderate Study
- Antiepileptics **(phenobarbital, primidone)** are predicted to decrease the exposure to calcium channel blockers (diltiazem, verapamil). Severe Study
- Calcium channel blockers (diltiazem, verapamil) potentially increase the concentration of antiepileptics **(fosphenytoin, phenytoin)** and antiepileptics **(fosphenytoin, phenytoin)** are predicted to decrease the exposure to calcium channel blockers (diltiazem, verapamil). Severe Study
- Antiepileptics **(carbamazepine, fosphenytoin, phenobarbital, phenytoin, primidone)** are predicted to decrease the exposure to cannabis extract. Avoid. Severe Theoretical → Also see TABLE 11 p. 1336

Antiepileptics (continued)

▶ Capecitabine increases the concentration of antiepileptics (**fosphenytoin, phenytoin**). [Severe] Anecdotal

▶ Carbapenems decrease the concentration of **valproate**. Avoid. [Severe] Anecdotal

▶ Antiepileptics (**carbamazepine, fosphenytoin, phenytoin**) are predicted to decrease the concentration of caspofungin. Adjust **caspofungin** dose, p. 582. [Moderate] Theoretical

▶ Antiepileptics (**carbamazepine, fosphenytoin, phenobarbital, phenytoin, primidone**) are predicted to decrease the exposure to ceritinib. Avoid. [Severe] Study

▶ Antiepileptics (**phenobarbital, primidone**) are predicted to affect the efficacy of chenodeoxycholic acid. Monitor and adjust dose. [Moderate] Theoretical

▶ Antiepileptics (**phenobarbital, primidone**) decrease the concentration of chloramphenicol. [Moderate] Study

▶ Intravenous chloramphenicol increases the concentration of antiepileptics (**fosphenytoin, phenytoin**) and antiepileptics (**fosphenytoin, phenytoin**) affect the concentration of intravenous chloramphenicol. Monitor concentration and adjust dose. [Severe] Study

▶ Chlordiazepoxide affects the concentration of antiepileptics (**fosphenytoin, phenytoin**). [Severe] Study

▶ **Phenobarbital** decreases the effects of cholic acid. Avoid. [Moderate] Study

▶ Antiepileptics (**carbamazepine, fosphenytoin, phenobarbital, phenytoin, primidone**) decrease the concentration of ciclosporin. [Severe] Study

▶ **Oxcarbazepine** decreases the concentration of ciclosporin. [Severe] Anecdotal

▶ Antiepileptics (**carbamazepine, fosphenytoin, phenobarbital, phenytoin, primidone**) are predicted to alter the effects of cilostazol. [Moderate] Theoretical

▶ Antiepileptics (**carbamazepine, fosphenytoin, phenobarbital, phenytoin, primidone**) are predicted to decrease the exposure to cinacalcet. Monitor and adjust dose. [Moderate] Study

▶ **Carbamazepine** is predicted to increase the risk of haematological toxicity when given with oral cladribine. [Moderate] Theoretical

▶ Clobazam potentially affects the concentration of antiepileptics (**fosphenytoin, phenytoin**). [Severe] Anecdotal

▶ **Stiripentol** increases the concentration of clobazam. [Severe] Study

▶ Antiepileptics (**carbamazepine, fosphenytoin, phenobarbital, phenytoin, primidone**) decrease the exposure to clomethiazole. Monitor and adjust dose. [Moderate] Study → Also see **TABLE 11** p. 1336

▶ Clonazepam potentially affects the concentration of antiepileptics (**fosphenytoin, phenytoin**). [Severe] Anecdotal

▶ Antiepileptics (**fosphenytoin, phenobarbital, phenytoin, primidone**) are predicted to decrease the exposure to clozapine. [Moderate] Anecdotal → Also see **TABLE 11** p. 1336

▶ **Carbamazepine** is predicted to increase the risk of myelosuppression when given with clozapine. Avoid. [Severe] Anecdotal

▶ Antiepileptics (**carbamazepine, fosphenytoin, phenobarbital, phenytoin, primidone**) are predicted to decrease the exposure to cobicistat. Avoid. [Severe] Theoretical

▶ **Oxcarbazepine** is predicted to decrease the concentration of cobicistat. [Severe] Theoretical

▶ Cobicistat is predicted to very slightly increase the exposure to perampanel. [Mild] Study

▶ Antiepileptics (**carbamazepine, fosphenytoin, phenobarbital, phenytoin, primidone**) are predicted to decrease the exposure to cobimetinib. Avoid. [Severe] Theoretical

▶ Antiepileptics (**carbamazepine, eslicarbazepine, fosphenytoin, oxcarbazepine, perampanel, phenobarbital, phenytoin, primidone, rufinamide, topiramate**) are predicted to decrease the efficacy of combined hormonal contraceptives. For FSRH guidance, see Contraceptives, interactions p. 775. [Severe] Study

▶ Combined hormonal contraceptives alter the exposure to lamotrigine. Adjust dose. [Moderate] Study

▶ Antiepileptics (**carbamazepine, fosphenytoin, phenobarbital, phenytoin, primidone**) are predicted to decrease the exposure to corticosteroids (budesonide, deflazacort, dexamethasone, fludrocortisone, hydrocortisone, methylprednisolone, prednisolone, prednisone, triamcinolone). Monitor and adjust dose. [Moderate] Study

▶ Antiepileptics (**carbamazepine, fosphenytoin, phenobarbital, phenytoin, primidone**) are predicted to decrease the exposure to corticosteroids (fluticasone). [Unknown] Theoretical

▶ Antiepileptics (**fosphenytoin, phenytoin**) are predicted to alter the anticoagulant effect of coumarins. [Moderate] Anecdotal

▶ Antiepileptics (**phenobarbital, primidone**) decrease the anticoagulant effect of coumarins. Monitor INR and adjust dose. [Moderate] Study

▶ **Carbamazepine** decreases the effects of coumarins. Monitor and adjust dose. [Severe] Study

▶ Antiepileptics (**carbamazepine, fosphenytoin, phenobarbital, phenytoin, primidone**) are predicted to markedly decrease the exposure to crizotinib. Avoid. [Severe] Study

▶ **Carbamazepine** is predicted to decrease the exposure to dabigatran. Avoid. [Severe] Study

▶ Antiepileptics (**carbamazepine, fosphenytoin, phenobarbital, phenytoin, primidone**) are predicted to decrease the exposure to dabrafenib. Avoid. [Moderate] Theoretical

▶ Antiepileptics (**carbamazepine, fosphenytoin, phenobarbital, phenytoin, primidone**) are predicted to moderately decrease the exposure to daclatasvir. Avoid. [Severe] Study

▶ **Oxcarbazepine** is predicted to decrease the exposure to daclatasvir. Avoid. [Severe] Theoretical

▶ Danazol moderately increases the concentration of **carbamazepine**. Monitor and adjust dose. [Severe] Study

▶ Antiepileptics (**fosphenytoin, phenobarbital, phenytoin, primidone**) are predicted to increase the risk of methaemoglobinaemia when given with dapsone. [Severe] Theoretical

▶ Antiepileptics (**carbamazepine, fosphenytoin, phenobarbital, phenytoin, primidone**) are predicted to decrease the exposure to darifenacin. [Moderate] Theoretical

▶ Antiepileptics (**carbamazepine, fosphenytoin, phenobarbital, phenytoin, primidone**) are predicted to decrease the exposure to dasabuvir. Avoid. [Severe] Theoretical

▶ Antiepileptics (**carbamazepine, fosphenytoin, phenobarbital, phenytoin, primidone**) are predicted to markedly decrease the exposure to dasatinib. Avoid. [Severe] Study

▶ Antiepileptics (**carbamazepine, fosphenytoin, phenobarbital, phenytoin, primidone**) are predicted to slightly decrease the exposure to delamanid. Avoid. [Moderate] Study

▶ **Lamotrigine** is predicted to increase the risk of hyponatraemia when given with desmopressin. [Severe] Theoretical

▶ Antiepileptics (**carbamazepine, eslicarbazepine, fosphenytoin, oxcarbazepine, perampanel, phenobarbital, phenytoin, primidone, rufinamide, topiramate**) are predicted to decrease the efficacy of desogestrel. For FSRH guidance, see Contraceptives, interactions p. 775. [Severe] Theoretical

▶ Desogestrel is predicted to increase the exposure to lamotrigine. [Moderate] Study

▶ Diazepam potentially affects the concentration of antiepileptics (**fosphenytoin, phenytoin**). Monitor concentration and adjust dose. [Severe] Study

▶ Diazoxide decreases the concentration of antiepileptics (**fosphenytoin, phenytoin**) and antiepileptics (**fosphenytoin, phenytoin**) are predicted to decrease the effects of diazoxide. Monitor concentration and adjust dose. [Moderate] Anecdotal

▶ Antiepileptics (**fosphenytoin, phenytoin**) are predicted to decrease the concentration of digoxin. [Moderate] Anecdotal

▶ Disulfiram increases the concentration of antiepileptics (**fosphenytoin, phenytoin**). Monitor concentration and adjust dose. [Severe] Study → Also see **TABLE 12** p. 1337

▶ Antiepileptics (**carbamazepine, fosphenytoin, phenobarbital, phenytoin, primidone**) decrease the exposure to dolutegravir. Adjust dose. [Severe] Study

▶ **Oxcarbazepine** is predicted to decrease the exposure to dolutegravir. Adjust dose. [Severe] Theoretical

▶ **Phenytoin** is predicted to decrease the exposure to duloxetine. [Moderate] Theoretical

▶ **Carbamazepine** is predicted to decrease the exposure to edoxaban. [Moderate] Study

▸ Antiepileptics **(fosphenytoin, phenytoin)** slightly decrease the exposure to efavirenz and efavirenz affects the concentration of antiepileptics **(fosphenytoin, phenytoin)**. Severe Study

▸ Carbamazepine slightly decreases the exposure to efavirenz and efavirenz slightly decreases the exposure to **carbamazepine**. Severe Study

▸ **Phenobarbital** is predicted to decrease the exposure to efavirenz and efavirenz affects the concentration of **phenobarbital**. Severe Theoretical

▸ Efavirenz is predicted to affect the efficacy of **primidone** and **primidone** is predicted to slightly decrease the exposure to efavirenz. Severe Theoretical

▸ Antiepileptics **(carbamazepine, fosphenytoin, phenobarbital, phenytoin, primidone)** are predicted to decrease the exposure to elbasvir. Avoid. Severe Study

▸ Antiepileptics **(carbamazepine, fosphenytoin, phenobarbital, phenytoin, primidone)** are predicted to decrease the exposure to eliglustat. Avoid. Severe Study

▸ Antiepileptics **(carbamazepine, fosphenytoin, phenobarbital, phenytoin, primidone)** are predicted to decrease the concentration of elvitegravir. Avoid. Severe Theoretical

▸ Enteral feeds decrease the absorption of **phenytoin**. Severe Study

▸ Enzalutamide is predicted to slightly decrease the exposure to **brivaracetam**. Moderate Theoretical

▸ Enzalutamide is predicted to decrease the exposure to **perampanel**. Monitor and adjust dose. Moderate Study

▸ Antiepileptics **(carbamazepine, fosphenytoin, phenobarbital, phenytoin, primidone)** are predicted to decrease the effects of ergotamine. Moderate Theoretical

▸ Antiepileptics **(carbamazepine, fosphenytoin, phenobarbital, phenytoin, primidone)** are predicted to decrease the exposure to erlotinib. Avoid or adjust **erlotinib** dose, p. 949. Severe Study

▸ Antiepileptics **(carbamazepine, eslicarbazepine, fosphenytoin, oxcarbazepine, perampanel, phenobarbital, phenytoin, primidone, rufinamide, topiramate)** are predicted to decrease the efficacy of etonogestrel. For FSRH guidance, see Contraceptives, interactions p. 775. Severe Theoretical

▸ Antiepileptics **(carbamazepine, fosphenytoin, phenobarbital, phenytoin, primidone)** are predicted to decrease the efficacy of etoposide. Moderate Study

▸ Antiepileptics **(carbamazepine, fosphenytoin, phenobarbital, phenytoin, primidone)** are predicted to decrease the exposure to etravirine. Avoid. Severe Theoretical

▸ Antiepileptics **(carbamazepine, fosphenytoin, phenobarbital, phenytoin, primidone)** are predicted to decrease the concentration of everolimus. Avoid or adjust dose. Severe Study

▸ Antiepileptics **(carbamazepine, fosphenytoin, phenobarbital, phenytoin, primidone)** moderately decrease the exposure to exemestane. Moderate Study

▸ Antiepileptics **(carbamazepine, fosphenytoin, phenobarbital, phenytoin, primidone)** are predicted to decrease the exposure to fesoterodine. Avoid. Moderate Study

▸ Antiepileptics **(carbamazepine, fosphenytoin, phenobarbital, phenytoin, primidone)** are predicted to decrease the exposure to fingolimod. Moderate Study

▸ Fluorouracil increases the concentration of antiepileptics **(fosphenytoin, phenytoin)**. Monitor concentration and adjust dose. Severe Anecdotal

▸ Folates are predicted to decrease the concentration of antiepileptics **(fosphenytoin, phenobarbital, phenytoin, primidone)**. Monitor concentration and adjust dose. Severe Study

▸ Antiepileptics **(carbamazepine, fosphenytoin, phenobarbital, phenytoin, primidone)** are predicted to decrease the exposure to fosaprepitant. Avoid. Moderate Theoretical

▸ Antiepileptics **(carbamazepine, fosphenytoin, phenobarbital, phenytoin, primidone)** are predicted to decrease the exposure to gefitinib. Avoid. Severe Study

▸ Antiepileptics **(carbamazepine, fosphenytoin, phenobarbital, phenytoin, primidone)** are predicted to moderately decrease the exposure to glecaprevir. Avoid. Severe Study

▸ Antiepileptics **(eslicarbazepine, oxcarbazepine)** potentially decrease the exposure to glecaprevir. Avoid. Severe Theoretical

▸ **Valproate** potentially opposes the effects of glycerol phenylbutyrate. Moderate Theoretical

▸ Grapefruit juice slightly increases the exposure to **carbamazepine**. Monitor and adjust dose. Moderate Study

▸ Antiepileptics **(carbamazepine, fosphenytoin, phenobarbital, phenytoin, primidone)** are predicted to decrease the exposure to grazoprevir. Avoid. Severe Study

▸ Antiepileptics **(phenobarbital, primidone)** decrease the effects of griseofulvin. Moderate Study

▸ Antiepileptics **(carbamazepine, fosphenytoin, phenobarbital, phenytoin, primidone)** are predicted to decrease the concentration of guanfacine. Adjust **guanfacine** dose, p. 349. Moderate Study → Also see TABLE 11 p. 1336

▸ **Oxcarbazepine** is predicted to decrease the concentration of guanfacine. Monitor and adjust **guanfacine** dose, p. 349. Moderate Theoretical

▸ Guanfacine increases the concentration of **valproate**. Monitor and adjust dose. Moderate Study

▸ H₂ receptor antagonists (cimetidine) transiently increase the concentration of **carbamazepine**. Monitor concentration and adjust dose. Moderate Study

▸ H₂ receptor antagonists (cimetidine) increase the concentration of antiepileptics **(fosphenytoin, phenytoin)**. Monitor concentration and adjust dose. Severe Study

▸ Antiepileptics **(carbamazepine, fosphenytoin, phenobarbital, phenytoin, primidone)** decrease the concentration of haloperidol. Adjust dose. Moderate Study → Also see TABLE 11 p. 1336

▸ Haloperidol potentially increases the risk of overheating and dehydration when given with **zonisamide**. Avoid in children. Severe Theoretical

▸ HIV-protease inhibitors (ritonavir) slightly decrease the exposure to **lamotrigine**. Severe Study

▸ HIV-protease inhibitors are predicted to affect the exposure to antiepileptics **(fosphenytoin, phenytoin)** and antiepileptics **(fosphenytoin, phenytoin)** decrease the concentration of HIV-protease inhibitors. Severe Study

▸ HIV-protease inhibitors are predicted to affect the concentration of antiepileptics **(phenobarbital, primidone)** and antiepileptics **(phenobarbital, primidone)** are predicted to decrease the concentration of HIV-protease inhibitors. Severe Theoretical

▸ HIV-protease inhibitors are predicted to increase the exposure to **carbamazepine** and **carbamazepine** is predicted to decrease the exposure to HIV-protease inhibitors. Monitor and adjust dose. Severe Theoretical

▸ HIV-protease inhibitors are predicted to very slightly increase the exposure to **perampanel**. Mild Study

▸ HIV-protease inhibitors (ritonavir) are predicted to decrease the concentration of **valproate**. Severe Anecdotal

▸ Antiepileptics **(carbamazepine, eslicarbazepine, fosphenytoin, oxcarbazepine, perampanel, phenobarbital, phenytoin, primidone, rufinamide, topiramate)** are predicted to decrease the effects of hormone replacement therapy. Moderate Anecdotal

▸ Hormone replacement therapy is predicted to alter the exposure to **lamotrigine**. Moderate Theoretical

▸ Antiepileptics **(carbamazepine, fosphenytoin, phenobarbital, phenytoin, primidone)** are predicted to decrease the exposure to ibrutinib. Avoid or adjust **ibrutinib** dose, p. 952. Severe Study

▸ Antiepileptics **(carbamazepine, fosphenytoin, phenobarbital, phenytoin, primidone)** are predicted to decrease the exposure to idelalisib. Avoid. Severe Study

▸ Idelalisib is predicted to very slightly increase the exposure to **perampanel**. Mild Study

▸ Antiepileptics **(carbamazepine, fosphenytoin, phenobarbital, phenytoin, primidone)** are predicted to decrease the exposure to imatinib. Avoid. Moderate Study

▸ **Oxcarbazepine** decreases the exposure to imatinib. Avoid. Moderate Study

▸ Antiepileptics **(carbamazepine, fosphenytoin, phenobarbital, phenytoin, primidone)** are predicted to decrease the exposure to irinotecan. Avoid. Severe Study

▸ Antiepileptics **(carbamazepine, fosphenytoin, phenobarbital, phenytoin, primidone)** are predicted to decrease the exposure

Antiepileptics (continued)

‣ to iron chelators (deferasirox). Monitor serum ferritin and adjust dose. Moderate Theoretical

‣ Isoniazid increases the concentration of antiepileptics **(fosphenytoin, phenytoin)**. Moderate Study → Also see TABLE 12 p. 1337

‣ Isoniazid markedly increases the concentration of **carbamazepine** and **carbamazepine** increases the risk of hepatotoxicity when given with isoniazid. Monitor concentration and adjust dose. Severe Study → Also see TABLE 1 p. 1334

‣ Antiepileptics **(carbamazepine, fosphenytoin, phenobarbital, phenytoin, primidone)** are predicted to decrease the exposure to ivabradine. Adjust dose. Moderate Theoretical

‣ Antiepileptics **(carbamazepine, fosphenytoin, phenobarbital, phenytoin, primidone)** are predicted to moderately to markedly decrease the exposure to ivacaftor. Avoid. Severe Study

‣ Antiepileptics **(carbamazepine, fosphenytoin, phenobarbital, phenytoin, primidone)** are predicted to decrease the exposure to ixazomib. Avoid. Severe Study

‣ Antiepileptics **(carbamazepine, fosphenytoin, phenobarbital, phenytoin, primidone)** are predicted to decrease the exposure to lapatinib. Avoid. Severe Study

‣ **Carbamazepine** is predicted to decrease the exposure to ledipasvir. Avoid. Severe Theoretical

‣ Antiepileptics **(fosphenytoin, phenytoin)** decrease the effects of levodopa. Moderate Study

‣ Antiepileptics **(carbamazepine, eslicarbazepine, fosphenytoin, oxcarbazepine, perampanel, phenobarbital, phenytoin, primidone, rufinamide, topiramate)** are predicted to decrease the efficacy of levonorgestrel. For FSRH guidance, see Contraceptives, interactions p. 775. Severe Theoretical

‣ Antiepileptics **(carbamazepine, fosphenytoin, phenobarbital, phenytoin, primidone)** are predicted to decrease the exposure to linagliptin. Moderate Study

‣ Antiepileptics **(carbamazepine, oxcarbazepine)** are predicted to increase the risk of neurotoxicity when given with lithium. Severe Anecdotal

‣ Antiepileptics **(carbamazepine, fosphenytoin, phenobarbital, phenytoin, primidone)** are predicted to decrease the exposure to lomitapide. Monitor and adjust dose. Moderate Theoretical → Also see TABLE 1 p. 1334

‣ Antiepileptics **(fosphenytoin, phenytoin)** decrease the effects of loop diuretics (furosemide). Moderate Study

‣ Lumacaftor is predicted to decrease the exposure to antiepileptics **(carbamazepine, fosphenytoin, phenobarbital, phenytoin, primidone)**. Avoid. Severe Theoretical

‣ Antiepileptics **(carbamazepine, fosphenytoin, phenobarbital, phenytoin, primidone)** are predicted to decrease the exposure to lurasidone. Avoid. Moderate Study → Also see TABLE 11 p. 1336

‣ Antiepileptics **(carbamazepine, fosphenytoin, phenobarbital, phenytoin, primidone)** are predicted to decrease the exposure to macitentan. Avoid. Severe Study

‣ Macrolides (clarithromycin) slightly increase the concentration of **carbamazepine**. Monitor concentration and adjust dose. Severe Study

‣ Macrolides (clarithromycin) are predicted to very slightly increase the exposure to **perampanel**. Mild Study

‣ Macrolides (erythromycin) markedly increase the concentration of **carbamazepine**. Monitor concentration and adjust dose. Severe Study

‣ Antiepileptics **(carbamazepine, fosphenytoin, phenobarbital, phenytoin, primidone)** are predicted to decrease the exposure to maraviroc. Adjust dose. Severe Study

‣ **Phenytoin** is predicted to decrease the exposure to melatonin. Moderate Theoretical

‣ **Levetiracetam** decreases the clearance of methotrexate. Severe Anecdotal

‣ Antiepileptics **(phenobarbital, primidone)** are predicted to decrease the exposure to metronidazole. Moderate Study

‣ Antiepileptics **(fosphenytoin, phenobarbital, phenytoin, primidone)** are predicted to decrease the effects of metyrapone. Avoid. Moderate Study

‣ Antiepileptics **(phenobarbital, primidone)** are predicted to decrease the exposure to mianserin. Moderate Study → Also see TABLE 11 p. 1336

‣ **Carbamazepine** markedly decreases the exposure to mianserin. Adjust dose. Moderate Study

‣ Antiepileptics **(carbamazepine, fosphenytoin, phenobarbital, phenytoin, primidone)** are predicted to decrease the exposure to midazolam. Monitor and adjust dose. Moderate Study → Also see TABLE 11 p. 1336

‣ Antiepileptics **(carbamazepine, fosphenytoin, phenobarbital, phenytoin, primidone)** are predicted to decrease the exposure to midostaurin. Avoid. Severe Study

‣ Antiepileptics **(carbamazepine, fosphenytoin, phenobarbital, phenytoin, primidone)** are predicted to decrease the exposure to mirtazapine. Adjust dose. Moderate Study → Also see TABLE 11 p. 1336

‣ Mitotane is predicted to decrease the exposure to **perampanel**. Monitor and adjust dose. Moderate Study

‣ Antiepileptics **(carbamazepine, phenobarbital, primidone)** are predicted to decrease the exposure to modafinil. Mild Theoretical

‣ Antiepileptics **(fosphenytoin, phenytoin)** are predicted to decrease the exposure to modafinil and modafinil is predicted to increase the concentration of antiepileptics **(fosphenytoin, phenytoin)**. Monitor concentration and adjust dose. Moderate Theoretical

‣ Antiepileptics **(phenobarbital, primidone)** are predicted to increase the effects of monoamine-oxidase A and B inhibitors, irreversible. Severe Theoretical

‣ **Carbamazepine** is predicted to increase the risk of severe toxic reaction when given with monoamine-oxidase A and B inhibitors, irreversible. Avoid and for 14 days after stopping the MAOI. Severe Theoretical

‣ **Carbamazepine** is predicted to decrease the effects of monoclonal antibodies (brentuximab vedotin). Severe Theoretical

‣ Monoclonal antibodies (tocilizumab) are predicted to decrease the exposure to antiepileptics **(fosphenytoin, phenytoin)**. Monitor and adjust dose. Moderate Theoretical

‣ Antiepileptics **(carbamazepine, fosphenytoin, phenobarbital, phenytoin, primidone)** are predicted to decrease the exposure to montelukast. Mild Study

‣ Antiepileptics **(carbamazepine, fosphenytoin, phenobarbital, phenytoin, primidone)** are predicted to markedly decrease the exposure to naloxegol. Avoid. Moderate Study

‣ Antiepileptics **(carbamazepine, fosphenytoin, phenobarbital, phenytoin, primidone)** are predicted to slightly decrease the exposure to nateglinide. Mild Study

‣ Antiepileptics **(carbamazepine, fosphenytoin, phenobarbital, phenytoin, primidone)** are predicted to decrease the exposure to netupitant. Avoid. Severe Study

‣ **Carbamazepine** is predicted to decrease the effects of (but acute use increases the effects of) neuromuscular blocking drugs, non-depolarising (atracurium, cisatracurium, pancuronium, rocuronium, vecuronium). Monitor and adjust dose. Moderate Study

‣ Antiepileptics **(fosphenytoin, phenytoin)** decrease the effects of (but acute use increases the effects of) neuromuscular blocking drugs, non-depolarising (atracurium, cisatracurium, pancuronium, rocuronium, vecuronium). Moderate Study

‣ Nevirapine is predicted to decrease the concentration of antiepileptics **(carbamazepine, fosphenytoin, phenobarbital, phenytoin, primidone)** and antiepileptics **(carbamazepine, fosphenytoin, phenobarbital, phenytoin, primidone)** are predicted to decrease the concentration of nevirapine. Severe Study

‣ Antiepileptics **(carbamazepine, fosphenytoin, phenobarbital, phenytoin, primidone)** are predicted to moderately decrease the exposure to nilotinib. Avoid. Severe Study

‣ **Carbamazepine** is predicted to decrease the exposure to nintedanib. Moderate Study

‣ Antiepileptics **(carbamazepine, fosphenytoin, phenobarbital, phenytoin, primidone)** are predicted to decrease the exposure to nitisinone. Adjust dose. Moderate Theoretical

‣ Antiepileptics **(carbamazepine, eslicarbazepine, fosphenytoin, oxcarbazepine, perampanel, phenobarbital, phenytoin,** primidone, rufinamide, topiramate) are predicted to decrease the efficacy of norethisterone. For FSRH guidance, see Contraceptives, interactions p. 775. Severe Anecdotal

▸ **Carbamazepine** potentially decreases the exposure to olanzapine. Monitor and adjust dose. Moderate Study

▸ **Phenytoin** is predicted to decrease the exposure to olanzapine. Monitor and adjust dose. Moderate Study

▸ Antiepileptics (carbamazepine, fosphenytoin, phenobarbital, phenytoin, primidone) are predicted to decrease the exposure to olaparib. Avoid. Moderate Theoretical

▸ **Carbamazepine** is predicted to decrease the exposure to ombitasvir. Avoid. Severe Theoretical

▸ Antiepileptics (carbamazepine, fosphenytoin, phenobarbital, phenytoin, primidone) are predicted to decrease the exposure to ondansetron. Moderate Study

▸ Antiepileptics (carbamazepine, fosphenytoin, phenobarbital, phenytoin, primidone) are predicted to decrease the exposure to opioids (alfentanil, fentanyl). Moderate Study → Also see TABLE 11 p. 1336

▸ Antiepileptics (carbamazepine, fosphenytoin, phenobarbital, phenytoin, primidone) are predicted to decrease the exposure to opioids (buprenorphine). Monitor and adjust dose. Moderate Theoretical → Also see TABLE 11 p. 1336

▸ Antiepileptics (carbamazepine, fosphenytoin, phenobarbital, phenytoin, primidone) decrease the exposure to opioids (methadone). Monitor and adjust dose. Severe Study → Also see TABLE 11 p. 1336

▸ Antiepileptics (carbamazepine, fosphenytoin, phenobarbital, phenytoin, primidone) are predicted to decrease the exposure to opioids (oxycodone). Monitor and adjust dose. Moderate Study → Also see TABLE 11 p. 1336

▸ **Carbamazepine** decreases the concentration of opioids (tramadol). Adjust dose. Severe Study

▸ Antiepileptics (carbamazepine, fosphenytoin, phenobarbital, phenytoin, primidone) are predicted to moderately decrease the exposure to osimertinib. Avoid. Moderate Study

▸ Oxybutynin potentially increases the risk of overheating and dehydration when given with **zonisamide**. Avoid in children. Severe Theoretical

▸ Antiepileptics (carbamazepine, fosphenytoin, phenobarbital, phenytoin, primidone) are predicted to decrease the exposure to palbociclib. Avoid. Severe Study

▸ Antiepileptics (carbamazepine, fosphenytoin, phenobarbital, phenytoin, primidone) are predicted to decrease the exposure to paliperidone. Monitor and adjust dose. Severe Study → Also see TABLE 11 p. 1336

▸ **Valproate** slightly increases the exposure to paliperidone. Adjust dose. Moderate Study

▸ Antiepileptics (carbamazepine, fosphenytoin, phenobarbital, phenytoin, primidone) are predicted to decrease the exposure to panobinostat. Avoid. Moderate Theoretical

▸ Antiepileptics (carbamazepine, fosphenytoin, phenobarbital, phenytoin, primidone) decrease the exposure to paracetamol. Moderate Study → Also see TABLE 1 p. 1334

▸ Antiepileptics (carbamazepine, fosphenytoin, phenobarbital, phenytoin, primidone) are predicted to decrease the exposure to paritaprevir (with ritonavir and ombitasvir). Avoid. Severe Study

▸ Antiepileptics (carbamazepine, fosphenytoin, phenobarbital, phenytoin, primidone) are predicted to decrease the exposure to pazopanib. Avoid. Severe Theoretical

▸ **Valproate** increases the risk of side-effects when given with penicillins (pivmecillinam). Avoid. Severe Anecdotal

▸ Phenothiazines (chlorpromazine) decrease the concentration of antiepileptics (phenobarbital, primidone) and antiepileptics (phenobarbital, primidone) decrease the concentration of phenothiazines (chlorpromazine). Moderate Study → Also see TABLE 11 p. 1336

▸ Antiepileptics (carbamazepine, fosphenytoin, phenobarbital, phenytoin, primidone) are predicted to decrease the exposure to phosphodiesterase type-5 inhibitors (avanafil, tadalafil). Avoid. Severe Study

▸ Antiepileptics (carbamazepine, fosphenytoin, phenobarbital, phenytoin, primidone) are predicted to decrease the exposure

to phosphodiesterase type-5 inhibitors (sildenafil, vardenafil). Moderate Theoretical

▸ Antiepileptics (carbamazepine, fosphenytoin, phenobarbital, phenytoin, primidone) are predicted to moderately to markedly decrease the exposure to pibrentasvir. Avoid. Severe Study

▸ Antiepileptics (eslicarbazepine, oxcarbazepine) potentially decrease the exposure to pibrentasvir. Avoid. Severe Theoretical

▸ Antiepileptics (fosphenytoin, phenytoin) are predicted to decrease the exposure to pirfenidone. Moderate Theoretical

▸ Antiepileptics (carbamazepine, fosphenytoin, phenobarbital, phenytoin, primidone) are predicted to moderately decrease the exposure to pitolisant. Moderate Study

▸ Antiepileptics (carbamazepine, fosphenytoin, phenobarbital, phenytoin, primidone) are predicted to decrease the exposure to ponatinib. Avoid. Moderate Theoretical

▸ Antiepileptics (carbamazepine, fosphenytoin, phenobarbital, phenytoin, primidone) are predicted to markedly decrease the exposure to praziquantel. Avoid. Moderate Study

▸ Antiepileptics (carbamazepine, phenobarbital, phenytoin, primidone) are predicted to increase the risk of hypersensitivity reactions when given with procarbazine. Severe Anecdotal

▸ **Fosphenytoin** is predicted to increase the risk of hypersensitivity when given with procarbazine. Severe Anecdotal

▸ **Valproate** potentially increases the concentration of propofol. Adjust dose. Severe Theoretical

▸ Antiepileptics (carbamazepine, fosphenytoin, phenobarbital, phenytoin, primidone) are predicted to decrease the exposure to quetiapine. Moderate Study → Also see TABLE 11 p. 1336

▸ **Valproate** potentially increases the risk of neutropenia when given with quetiapine. Moderate Study

▸ Quinolones (ciprofloxacin) affect the concentration of antiepileptics (fosphenytoin, phenytoin). Monitor concentration and adjust dose. Severe Study

▸ Antiepileptics (fosphenytoin, phenobarbital, phenytoin, primidone) are predicted to affect the exposure to raltegravir. Use with caution or avoid. Moderate Theoretical

▸ **Carbamazepine** is predicted to affect the exposure to raltegravir. Moderate Theoretical

▸ Antiepileptics (carbamazepine, fosphenytoin, phenobarbital, phenytoin, primidone) are predicted to decrease the exposure to ranolazine. Avoid. Severe Study

▸ Antiepileptics (carbamazepine, fosphenytoin, phenobarbital, phenytoin, primidone) are predicted to decrease the exposure to reboxetine. Moderate Anecdotal

▸ Antiepileptics (carbamazepine, fosphenytoin, phenobarbital, phenytoin, primidone) are predicted to decrease the exposure to regorafenib. Avoid. Moderate Study

▸ Antiepileptics (carbamazepine, fosphenytoin, phenobarbital, phenytoin, primidone) are predicted to decrease the exposure to repaglinide. Monitor blood glucose and adjust dose. Moderate Study

▸ Antiepileptics (carbamazepine, fosphenytoin, phenobarbital, phenytoin, primidone) are predicted to markedly decrease the exposure to ribociclib. Avoid. Severe Study

▸ Antiepileptics (phenobarbital, primidone) are predicted to decrease the exposure to rifampicin and rifampicin is predicted to decrease the exposure to antiepileptics (phenobarbital, primidone). Use with caution and adjust dose. Moderate Study

▸ Rifampicin decreases the concentration of antiepileptics (fosphenytoin, phenytoin). Use with caution and adjust dose. Moderate Study

▸ Rifampicin slightly decreases the exposure to **brivaracetam**. Adjust dose. Moderate Study

▸ Rifampicin markedly increases the clearance of **lamotrigine**. Adjust **lamotrigine** dose, p. 316. Moderate Study

▸ Rifampicin is predicted to decrease the exposure to **perampanel**. Monitor and adjust dose. Moderate Study

▸ Antiepileptics (carbamazepine, fosphenytoin, phenobarbital, phenytoin, primidone) markedly decrease the exposure to rilpivirine. Avoid. Severe Study

▸ **Oxcarbazepine** is predicted to decrease the concentration of rilpivirine. Avoid. Severe Theoretical

Antiepileptics (continued)

▶ Antiepileptics **(carbamazepine, fosphenytoin, phenobarbital, phenytoin, primidone)** are predicted to decrease the exposure to risperidone. Adjust dose. Moderate Study → Also see TABLE 11 p. 1336

▶ Antiepileptics **(carbamazepine, fosphenytoin, phenobarbital, phenytoin, primidone)** are predicted to moderately decrease the exposure to rivaroxaban. Avoid unless patient can be monitored for signs of thrombosis. Severe Study

▶ Antiepileptics **(carbamazepine, fosphenytoin, phenobarbital, phenytoin, primidone)** are predicted to decrease the exposure to roflumilast. Avoid. Moderate Study

▶ Antiepileptics **(carbamazepine, fosphenytoin, phenobarbital, phenytoin, primidone)** are predicted to markedly decrease the exposure to rolapitant. Avoid. Severe Study

▶ Antiepileptics **(carbamazepine, fosphenytoin, phenobarbital, phenytoin, primidone)** are predicted to decrease the exposure to ruxolitinib. Monitor and adjust dose. Moderate Study

▶ Antiepileptics **(carbamazepine, fosphenytoin, phenobarbital, phenytoin, primidone)** are predicted to moderately decrease the exposure to saxagliptin. Moderate Study

▶ Antiepileptics **(carbamazepine, fosphenytoin, phenytoin)** are predicted to decrease the exposure to the active metabolite of selexipag. Adjust dose. Moderate Study

▶ Valproate is predicted to increase the exposure to selexipag. Unknown Theoretical

▶ Antiepileptics **(carbamazepine, fosphenytoin, phenobarbital, phenytoin, primidone)** are predicted to decrease the exposure to simeprevir. Avoid. Severe Study

▶ **Oxcarbazepine** is predicted to decrease the exposure to simeprevir. Avoid. Severe Theoretical

▶ Antiepileptics **(carbamazepine, fosphenytoin, phenobarbital, phenytoin, primidone)** are predicted to decrease the concentration of sirolimus. Avoid. Severe Study

▶ **Valproate** increases the exposure to sodium oxybate. Adjust **sodium oxybate** dose, p. 484. Moderate Study

▶ **Valproate** potentially decreases the effects of sodium phenylbutyrate. Moderate Anecdotal

▶ Antiepileptics **(fosphenytoin, oxcarbazepine, phenobarbital, phenytoin, primidone)** are predicted to decrease the exposure to sofosbuvir. Avoid. Severe Theoretical

▶ **Carbamazepine** is predicted to decrease the exposure to sofosbuvir. Avoid. Severe Study

▶ Antiepileptics **(carbamazepine, fosphenytoin, phenobarbital, phenytoin, primidone)** are predicted to decrease the exposure to solifenacin. Moderate Theoretical

▶ Antiepileptics **(carbamazepine, fosphenytoin, phenobarbital, phenytoin, primidone)** are predicted to decrease the exposure to sorafenib. Moderate Theoretical

▶ SSRIs (fluoxetine, fluvoxamine) are predicted to increase the concentration of antiepileptics **(fosphenytoin, phenytoin)**. Monitor and adjust dose. Severe Anecdotal

▶ SSRIs (sertraline) potentially increase the risk of toxicity when given with antiepileptics **(fosphenytoin, phenytoin)**. Monitor concentration and adjust dose. Severe Anecdotal

▶ Antiepileptics **(fosphenytoin, phenytoin)** decrease the concentration of SSRIs (paroxetine). Moderate Study

▶ St John's Wort is predicted to decrease the concentration of antiepileptics **(fosphenytoin, phenobarbital, phenytoin, primidone)**. Avoid. Severe Theoretical

▶ St John's Wort is predicted to decrease the exposure to brivaracetam. Moderate Theoretical

▶ St John's Wort is predicted to decrease the concentration of **carbamazepine**. Monitor and adjust dose. Moderate Theoretical

▶ St John's Wort is predicted to decrease the exposure to **perampanel**. Monitor and adjust dose. Moderate Theoretical

▶ St John's Wort is predicted to decrease the exposure to **tiagabine**. Avoid. Mild Theoretical

▶ Antiepileptics **(carbamazepine, eslicarbazepine)** are predicted to decrease the exposure to statins (atorvastatin). Monitor and adjust dose. Moderate Theoretical → Also see TABLE 1 p. 1334

▶ Antiepileptics **(fosphenytoin, phenytoin)** potentially decrease the exposure to statins (atorvastatin, simvastatin). Moderate Anecdotal

▶ **Carbamazepine** moderately decreases the exposure to statins (simvastatin). Monitor and adjust dose. Severe Study → Also see TABLE 1 p. 1334

▶ **Eslicarbazepine** moderately decreases the exposure to statins (simvastatin). Monitor and adjust dose. Moderate Study

▶ Sulfinpyrazone increases the concentration of antiepileptics **(fosphenytoin, phenytoin)**. Moderate Study

▶ Sulfonamides (sulfadiazine) are predicted to increase the concentration of **fosphenytoin**. Monitor and adjust dose. Moderate Study

▶ Sulfonamides (sulfadiazine) increase the concentration of **phenytoin**. Monitor and adjust dose. Moderate Study

▶ Antiepileptics **(carbamazepine, fosphenytoin, phenobarbital, phenytoin, primidone)** are predicted to decrease the exposure to sunitinib. Avoid or adjust **sunitinib** dose, p. 967. Moderate Study

▶ Antiepileptics **(fosphenytoin, phenytoin)** increase the effects of suxamethonium. Moderate Study

▶ **Carbamazepine** increases the risk of prolonged neuromuscular blockade when given with suxamethonium. Moderate Study

▶ Antiepileptics **(carbamazepine, fosphenytoin, phenobarbital, phenytoin, primidone)** decrease the concentration of tacrolimus. Monitor and adjust dose. Severe Study

▶ Antiepileptics **(carbamazepine, fosphenytoin, phenobarbital, phenytoin, primidone)** are predicted to decrease the exposure to taxanes (cabazitaxel, paclitaxel). Avoid. Severe Study → Also see TABLE 12 p. 1337

▶ Antiepileptics **(carbamazepine, fosphenytoin, phenobarbital, phenytoin, primidone)** are predicted to decrease the exposure to taxanes (docetaxel). Severe Theoretical → Also see TABLE 12 p. 1337

▶ Tegafur potentially increases the concentration of antiepileptics **(fosphenytoin, phenytoin)**. Monitor concentration and adjust dose. Severe Anecdotal

▶ Antiepileptics **(carbamazepine, fosphenytoin, phenobarbital, phenytoin, primidone)** are predicted to decrease the concentration of temsirolimus. Avoid. Severe Study

▶ Antiepileptics **(carbamazepine, fosphenytoin, oxcarbazepine, phenobarbital, phenytoin, primidone)** are predicted to decrease the exposure to tenofovir alafenamide. Avoid. Moderate Theoretical

▶ Antiepileptics **(carbamazepine, fosphenytoin, phenobarbital, phenytoin, primidone)** decrease the exposure to tetracyclines (doxycycline). Monitor and adjust dose. Moderate Study → Also see TABLE 1 p. 1334

▶ Antiepileptics **(fosphenytoin, phenytoin)** are predicted to decrease the exposure to theophylline. Adjust dose. Moderate Study

▶ Antiepileptics **(phenobarbital, primidone)** are predicted to increase the clearance of theophylline. Adjust dose. Moderate Theoretical

▶ **Carbamazepine** potentially increases the clearance of theophylline and theophylline decreases the exposure to **carbamazepine**. Adjust dose. Moderate Anecdotal

▶ **Stiripentol** is predicted to increase the exposure to theophylline. Avoid. Moderate Theoretical

▶ Antiepileptics **(carbamazepine, fosphenytoin, phenytoin)** are predicted to increase the risk of hypothyroidism when given with thyroid hormones. Moderate Study

▶ Antiepileptics **(phenobarbital, primidone)** are predicted to decrease the effects of thyroid hormones. Moderate Theoretical

▶ Antiepileptics **(carbamazepine, fosphenytoin, phenobarbital, phenytoin, primidone)** are predicted to markedly decrease the exposure to ticagrelor. Avoid. Severe Study

▶ Antiepileptics **(carbamazepine, fosphenytoin, phenobarbital, phenytoin, primidone)** are predicted to decrease the exposure to tivozanib. Severe Study

▶ Antiepileptics **(fosphenytoin, phenytoin)** moderately decrease the exposure to tizanidine. Mild Study

▶ Antiepileptics **(carbamazepine, fosphenytoin, phenobarbital, phenytoin, primidone)** are predicted to decrease the exposure to tofacitinib. Avoid. Severe Study

▶ Antiepileptics **(carbamazepine, fosphenytoin, phenobarbital, phenytoin, primidone)** are predicted to decrease the exposure to tolvaptan. Avoid. Severe Study

▶ Antiepileptics **(fosphenytoin, phenytoin)** increase the clearance of topotecan. Moderate Study

▶ Antiepileptics **(carbamazepine, fosphenytoin, phenobarbital, phenytoin, primidone)** are predicted to decrease the exposure to toremifene. Adjust dose. Moderate Study

▶ Antiepileptics **(carbamazepine, fosphenytoin, phenobarbital, phenytoin, primidone)** are predicted to decrease the exposure to trabectedin. Avoid. Severe Theoretical → Also see TABLE 1 p. 1334

▶ **Carbamazepine** decreases the concentration of trazodone. Adjust dose. Moderate Anecdotal

▶ Antiepileptics **(phenobarbital, primidone)** are predicted to decrease the exposure to tricyclic antidepressants. Moderate Study

▶ **Carbamazepine** decreases the exposure to tricyclic antidepressants. Adjust dose. Moderate Study → Also see TABLE 18 p. 1338

▶ Tricyclic antidepressants (clomipramine, imipramine) potentially increase the risk of overheating and dehydration when given with zonisamide. Avoid in children. Severe Theoretical

▶ Trimethoprim increases the concentration of antiepileptics **(fosphenytoin, phenytoin)**. Moderate Study

▶ Antiepileptics **(carbamazepine, eslicarbazepine, fosphenytoin, oxcarbazepine, perampanel, phenobarbital, phenytoin, primidone, rufinamide, topiramate)** decrease the efficacy of ulipristal. For FSRH guidance, see Contraceptives, interactions p. 775. Severe Anecdotal

▶ Antiepileptics **(carbamazepine, fosphenytoin, phenobarbital, phenytoin, primidone)** are predicted to decrease the exposure to vandetanib. Avoid. Moderate Study

▶ Antiepileptics **(carbamazepine, fosphenytoin, phenobarbital, phenytoin, primidone)** are predicted to moderately decrease the exposure to velpatasvir. Avoid. Severe Study

▶ **Oxcarbazepine** is predicted to decrease the exposure to velpatasvir. Avoid. Severe Theoretical

▶ Antiepileptics **(carbamazepine, fosphenytoin, phenobarbital, phenytoin, primidone)** are predicted to decrease the exposure to vemurafenib. Avoid. Severe Theoretical

▶ Antiepileptics **(carbamazepine, fosphenytoin, phenobarbital, phenytoin, primidone)** are predicted to decrease the exposure to venetoclax. Avoid. Severe Study

▶ Antiepileptics **(carbamazepine, fosphenytoin, phenobarbital, phenytoin, primidone)** are predicted to decrease the exposure to vinca alkaloids (vinblastine, vincristine, vindesine). Severe Theoretical → Also see TABLE 1 p. 1334 → Also see TABLE 12 p. 1337

▶ Antiepileptics **(carbamazepine, fosphenytoin, phenobarbital, phenytoin, primidone)** are predicted to decrease the exposure to vinca alkaloids (vinflunine). Avoid. Severe Theoretical → Also see TABLE 12 p. 1337

▶ Antiepileptics **(carbamazepine, fosphenytoin, phenobarbital, phenytoin, primidone)** are predicted to decrease the exposure to vinca alkaloids (vinorelbine). Use with caution or avoid. Severe Theoretical → Also see TABLE 12 p. 1337

▶ Antiepileptics **(carbamazepine, fosphenytoin, phenobarbital, phenytoin, primidone)** are predicted to decrease the exposure to vismodegib. Avoid. Moderate Theoretical

▶ Antiepileptics **(fosphenytoin, phenytoin)** decrease the effects of vitamin D substances. Moderate Study

▶ Antiepileptics **(phenobarbital, primidone)** are predicted to decrease the effects of vitamin D substances. Moderate Theoretical

▶ **Carbamazepine** is predicted to decrease the effects of vitamin D substances. Moderate Study

▶ Antiepileptics **(phenobarbital, primidone)** potentially increase the risk of nephrotoxicity when given with volatile halogenated anaesthetics (methoxyflurane). Avoid. Severe Theoretical → Also see TABLE 11 p. 1336

▶ Antiepileptics **(carbamazepine, fosphenytoin, phenobarbital, phenytoin, primidone)** are predicted to decrease the exposure to vortioxetine. Monitor and adjust dose. Moderate Study

▶ Antiepileptics **(carbamazepine, fosphenytoin, phenobarbital, phenytoin, primidone)** are predicted to decrease the concentration of voxilaprevir. Avoid. Severe Study

▶ **Oxcarbazepine** is predicted to decrease the concentration of voxilaprevir. Avoid. Severe Theoretical

▶ **Valproate** slightly increases the exposure to zidovudine. Moderate Study

▶ **Carbamazepine** moderately decreases the exposure to zolpidem. Moderate Study

▶ Antiepileptics **(carbamazepine, fosphenytoin, phenobarbital, phenytoin, primidone)** are predicted to decrease the exposure to zopiclone. Adjust dose. Moderate Study → Also see TABLE 11 p. 1336

Antifungals, azoles → see TABLE 1 p. 1334 (hepatotoxicity), TABLE 9 p. 1336 (QT-interval prolongation)

clotrimazole · fluconazole · isavuconazole · itraconazole · ketoconazole · miconazole · posaconazole · voriconazole

▶ In general, **fluconazole** interactions relate to multiple-dose treatment.

▶ The use of carbonated drinks, such as cola, improves **itraconazole, ketoconazole,** and **posaconazole** bioavailability.

▶ Since systemic absorption can follow topical application, the possibility of interactions with topical **ketoconazole** should be borne in mind.

▶ Interactions of **miconazole** apply to the oral gel formulation, as a sufficient quantity can be absorbed to cause systemic effects. Systemic absorption from intravaginal and topical formulations might also occur.

▶ Antifungals, azoles **(itraconazole, ketoconazole, voriconazole)** are predicted to increase the exposure to abiraterone. Severe Theoretical

▶ Antifungals, azoles **(itraconazole, ketoconazole)** are predicted to increase the exposure to afatinib. Separate administration by 12 hours. Moderate Study

▶ Alcohol (beverage) potentially causes a disulfiram-like reaction when given with **ketoconazole.** Avoid. Moderate Anecdotal

▶ Antifungals, azoles **(fluconazole, isavuconazole, posaconazole)** are predicted to increase the exposure to aldosterone antagonists (eplerenone). Adjust **eplerenone** dose, p. 190. Severe Study

▶ Antifungals, azoles **(itraconazole, ketoconazole, voriconazole)** are predicted to markedly increase the exposure to aldosterone antagonists (eplerenone). Avoid. Severe Study

▶ **Itraconazole** markedly increases the exposure to aliskiren. Avoid. Severe Study

▶ **Ketoconazole** moderately increases the exposure to aliskiren. Moderate Study

▶ **Itraconazole** increases the risk of busulfan toxicity when given with alkylating agents (busulfan). Monitor and adjust dose. Moderate Study

▶ **Miconazole** is predicted to increase the concentration of alkylating agents (busulfan). Use with caution and adjust dose. Moderate Theoretical

▶ **Isavuconazole** is predicted to increase the exposure to alkylating agents (cyclophosphamide). Moderate Study

▶ Antifungals, azoles **(itraconazole, ketoconazole, voriconazole)** increase the exposure to almotriptan. Mild Study

▶ Antifungals, azoles **(itraconazole, ketoconazole, voriconazole)** are predicted to moderately increase the exposure to alpha blockers (alfuzosin, tamsulosin). Use with caution or avoid. Moderate Study

▶ Antifungals, azoles **(itraconazole, ketoconazole, voriconazole)** are predicted to increase the exposure to alpha blockers (doxazosin). Moderate Study

▶ Antifungals, azoles **(fluconazole, isavuconazole, posaconazole)** are predicted to increase the exposure to alpha blockers (tamsulosin). Moderate Theoretical

▶ Antifungals, azoles **(fluconazole, isavuconazole, posaconazole)** are predicted to increase the exposure to alprazolam. Severe Study

▶ Antifungals, azoles **(itraconazole, ketoconazole, voriconazole)** moderately increase the exposure to alprazolam. Avoid. Moderate Study

▶ **Miconazole** is predicted to increase the exposure to alprazolam. Use with caution and adjust dose. Moderate Theoretical

Antifungals, azoles (continued)

▸ **Miconazole** potentially decreases the exposure to aminoglycosides (tobramycin). [Moderate] Anecdotal
▸ Antacids decrease the absorption of **itraconazole** (capsule). Antacids should be taken 1 hour before or 2 hours after **itraconazole**. [Moderate] Study
▸ Antacids decrease the absorption of **ketoconazole**. Separate administration by at least 2 hours. [Moderate] Study
▸ **Miconazole** is predicted to increase the exposure to antiarrhythmics (disopyramide). Use with caution and adjust dose. [Severe] Theoretical
▸ Antifungals, azoles **(itraconazole, ketoconazole, voriconazole)** are predicted to increase the exposure to antiarrhythmics (disopyramide). Avoid. [Severe] Theoretical → Also see TABLE 9 p. 1336
▸ **Posaconazole** is predicted to increase the exposure to antiarrhythmics (disopyramide, dronedarone). Avoid. [Severe] Theoretical
▸ **Fluconazole** is predicted to increase the exposure to antiarrhythmics (dronedarone). [Severe] Theoretical → Also see TABLE 9 p. 1336
▸ Antifungals, azoles **(itraconazole, ketoconazole, voriconazole)** very markedly increase the exposure to antiarrhythmics (dronedarone). Avoid. [Severe] Study → Also see TABLE 9 p. 1336
▸ Antifungals, azoles **(fluconazole, isavuconazole, posaconazole)** are predicted to increase the exposure to antiarrhythmics (propafenone). Monitor and adjust dose. [Moderate] Study
▸ Antifungals, azoles **(itraconazole, ketoconazole, voriconazole)** are predicted to increase the exposure to antiarrhythmics (propafenone). Monitor and adjust dose. [Severe] Study
▸ Antifungals, azoles **(itraconazole, ketoconazole, voriconazole)** are predicted to increase the exposure to anticholinesterases, centrally acting (galantamine). Monitor and adjust dose. [Moderate] Study
▸ Antiepileptics (carbamazepine) are predicted to decrease the efficacy of **fluconazole** and **fluconazole** increases the concentration of antiepileptics (carbamazepine). Avoid or monitor carbamazepine concentration and adjust dose accordingly. [Severe] Theoretical → Also see TABLE 1 p. 1334
▸ Antiepileptics (carbamazepine) are predicted to decrease the efficacy of **ketoconazole** and **ketoconazole** slightly increases the concentration of antiepileptics (carbamazepine). Avoid or monitor carbamazepine concentration and adjust dose accordingly. [Moderate] Study
▸ Antiepileptics (carbamazepine) are predicted to decrease the efficacy of **posaconazole** and **posaconazole** increases the concentration of antiepileptics (carbamazepine). Avoid. [Moderate] Theoretical
▸ Antiepileptics (carbamazepine, fosphenytoin, phenobarbital, phenytoin, primidone) are predicted to decrease the exposure to **isavuconazole**. Avoid. [Severe] Study
▸ Antiepileptics (fosphenytoin) very markedly decrease the exposure to **itraconazole**. Avoid and for 14 days after stopping **fosphenytoin**. [Moderate] Study
▸ Antiepileptics (fosphenytoin) decrease the exposure to **voriconazole** and **voriconazole** increases the exposure to antiepileptics (fosphenytoin). Avoid or adjust **voriconazole** dose, p. 588 and monitor phenytoin concentration. [Moderate] Study
▸ Antiepileptics (fosphenytoin, phenytoin) decrease the exposure to **ketoconazole**. Avoid. [Moderate] Study
▸ Antiepileptics (fosphenytoin, phenytoin) are predicted to decrease the exposure to **posaconazole**. Avoid. [Moderate] Study
▸ Antiepileptics (phenobarbital) decrease the concentration of **itraconazole**. Avoid and for 14 days after stopping **phenobarbital**. [Moderate] Study
▸ Antiepileptics (phenobarbital) are predicted to decrease the concentration of **ketoconazole**. Avoid. [Moderate] Study
▸ Antiepileptics (phenobarbital) are predicted to decrease the concentration of **posaconazole**. Avoid. [Moderate] Study
▸ Antiepileptics (phenobarbital, primidone) are predicted to decrease the concentration of **voriconazole**. Avoid. [Moderate] Theoretical
▸ Antiepileptics (phenytoin) very markedly decrease the exposure to **itraconazole**. Avoid and for 14 days after stopping **phenytoin**. [Moderate] Study

▸ Antiepileptics (phenytoin) decrease the exposure to **voriconazole** and **voriconazole** increases the exposure to antiepileptics (phenytoin). Avoid or adjust **voriconazole** dose, p. 588 and monitor **phenytoin** concentration. [Moderate] Study
▸ Antiepileptics (primidone) are predicted to decrease the concentration of **itraconazole**. [Moderate] Theoretical
▸ **Miconazole** increases the risk of carbamazepine toxicity when given with antiepileptics (carbamazepine). Monitor and adjust dose. [Severe] Anecdotal
▸ **Miconazole** increases the risk of phenytoin toxicity when given with antiepileptics (fosphenytoin). Monitor and adjust dose. [Severe] Anecdotal
▸ **Fluconazole** increases the concentration of antiepileptics (fosphenytoin, phenytoin). Monitor concentration and adjust dose. [Moderate] Study
▸ Antiepileptics (carbamazepine) are predicted to decrease the efficacy of antifungals, azoles **(itraconazole, voriconazole)** and antifungals, azoles **(itraconazole, voriconazole)** increase the concentration of antiepileptics (carbamazepine). Avoid or adjust dose. [Moderate] Theoretical → Also see TABLE 1 p. 1334
▸ Antiepileptics (primidone) are predicted to decrease the concentration of antifungals, azoles **(ketoconazole, posaconazole)**. Avoid. [Moderate] Study
▸ Antifungals, azoles **(itraconazole, ketoconazole, voriconazole)** are predicted to very slightly increase the exposure to antiepileptics (perampanel). [Mild] Study
▸ **Miconazole** increases the risk of phenytoin toxicity when given with antiepileptics (phenytoin). Monitor and adjust dose. [Severe] Anecdotal
▸ Antifungals, azoles **(fluconazole)** are predicted to increase the exposure to antifungals, azoles **(isavuconazole)**. [Severe] Theoretical
▸ Antifungals, azoles **(itraconazole, ketoconazole, voriconazole)** are predicted to increase the exposure to antifungals, azoles **(isavuconazole)**. Avoid or monitor side effects. [Severe] Study
▸ Antifungals, azoles **(posaconazole)** are predicted to increase the exposure to antifungals, azoles **(isavuconazole)**. [Moderate] Theoretical
▸ **Miconazole** is predicted to increase the exposure to antihistamines, non-sedating (mizolastine). Avoid. [Moderate] Theoretical
▸ Antifungals, azoles **(fluconazole, isavuconazole, posaconazole)** are predicted to increase the exposure to antihistamines, non-sedating (mizolastine). [Severe] Theoretical
▸ Antifungals, azoles **(itraconazole, ketoconazole, voriconazole)** are predicted to increase the exposure to antihistamines, non-sedating (mizolastine). Avoid. [Severe] Study
▸ Antifungals, azoles **(fluconazole, isavuconazole, itraconazole, ketoconazole, posaconazole, voriconazole)** are predicted to increase the exposure to antihistamines, non-sedating (rupatadine). Avoid. [Moderate] Study
▸ **Ketoconazole** increases the exposure to antimalarials (mefloquine). [Moderate] Study
▸ Antifungals, azoles **(fluconazole, itraconazole, posaconazole, voriconazole)** are predicted to increase the exposure to antimalarials (mefloquine). [Moderate] Theoretical
▸ Antifungals, azoles **(fluconazole, isavuconazole, itraconazole, ketoconazole, posaconazole, voriconazole)** are predicted to increase the concentration of antimalarials (piperaquine). [Severe] Theoretical
▸ **Itraconazole** is predicted to increase the exposure to apixaban. Avoid. [Severe] Theoretical
▸ **Ketoconazole** slightly to moderately increases the exposure to apixaban. Avoid. [Severe] Study
▸ Antifungals, azoles **(itraconazole, ketoconazole, voriconazole)** are predicted to markedly increase the exposure to aprepitant. [Moderate] Study
▸ Aprepitant is predicted to increase the exposure to **isavuconazole**. [Moderate] Theoretical
▸ Antifungals, azoles **(itraconazole, ketoconazole, voriconazole)** are predicted to slightly increase the exposure to aripiprazole. Adjust aripiprazole dose, p. 391. [Moderate] Study
▸ Antifungals, azoles **(fluconazole, isavuconazole, posaconazole)** are predicted to increase the exposure to axitinib. [Moderate] Theoretical

▸ Antifungals, azoles **(itraconazole, ketoconazole, voriconazole)** are predicted to increase the exposure to axitinib. Avoid or adjust dose. [Moderate] Study

▸ Antifungals, azoles **(fluconazole, isavuconazole, posaconazole)** are predicted to increase the exposure to bedaquiline. Avoid prolonged use. [Mild] Theoretical → Also see TABLE 9 p. 1336

▸ Antifungals, azoles **(itraconazole, ketoconazole, voriconazole)** are predicted to increase the exposure to bedaquiline. Avoid prolonged use. [Mild] Study → Also see TABLE 9 p. 1336

▸ Antifungals, azoles **(itraconazole, ketoconazole)** are predicted to increase the exposure to beta blockers, non-selective **(nadolol)**. [Moderate] Study

▸ Antifungals, azoles **(itraconazole, ketoconazole, voriconazole)** are predicted to increase the exposure to beta$_2$ agonists **(salmeterol)**. Avoid. [Severe] Study

▸ Antifungals, azoles **(itraconazole, ketoconazole, voriconazole)** slightly increase the exposure to bortezomib. [Moderate] Study

▸ **Fluconazole** is predicted to increase the exposure to bosentan. Avoid. [Severe] Study

▸ **Bosentan** is predicted to decrease the exposure to **isavuconazole**. Avoid. [Severe] Theoretical

▸ **Itraconazole** is predicted to increase the exposure to bosentan. [Moderate] Theoretical

▸ **Ketoconazole** moderately increases the exposure to bosentan. [Moderate] Study

▸ **Voriconazole** is predicted to increase the exposure to bosentan. Avoid. [Severe] Theoretical

▸ Antifungals, azoles **(fluconazole, isavuconazole, posaconazole)** are predicted to increase the exposure to bosutinib. Avoid or adjust dose. [Severe] Theoretical → Also see TABLE 9 p. 1336

▸ Antifungals, azoles **(itraconazole, ketoconazole, voriconazole)** are predicted to markedly increase the exposure to bosutinib. Avoid or adjust dose. [Severe] Study → Also see TABLE 9 p. 1336

▸ **Isavuconazole** slightly increases the exposure to bupropion. Adjust dose. [Moderate] Study

▸ Antifungals, azoles **(fluconazole, isavuconazole, posaconazole)** are predicted to increase the exposure to buspirone. Use with caution and adjust dose. [Moderate] Study

▸ Antifungals, azoles **(itraconazole, ketoconazole, voriconazole)** are predicted to increase the exposure to buspirone. Adjust **buspirone** dose, p. 338. [Severe] Study

▸ **Miconazole** is predicted to increase the concentration of buspirone. Use with caution and adjust dose. [Moderate] Theoretical

▸ Antifungals, azoles **(fluconazole, isavuconazole, posaconazole)** are predicted to increase the exposure to cabozantinib. [Moderate] Theoretical → Also see TABLE 9 p. 1336

▸ Antifungals, azoles **(itraconazole, ketoconazole, voriconazole)** slightly increase the exposure to cabozantinib. [Moderate] Study → Also see TABLE 9 p. 1336

▸ Calcium channel blockers **(diltiazem, verapamil)** are predicted to increase the exposure to **isavuconazole**. [Moderate] Theoretical

▸ **Miconazole** is predicted to increase the exposure to calcium channel blockers **(amlodipine, clevidipine, felodipine, lacidipine, lercanidipine, nicardipine, nifedipine, nimodipine, verapamil)**. Use with caution and adjust dose. [Moderate] Theoretical

▸ Antifungals, azoles **(fluconazole, isavuconazole, posaconazole)** are predicted to increase the exposure to calcium channel blockers **(amlodipine, felodipine, lacidipine, lercanidipine, nicardipine, nifedipine, nimodipine)**. Monitor and adjust dose. [Moderate] Study

▸ Antifungals, azoles **(itraconazole, ketoconazole, voriconazole)** are predicted to increase the exposure to calcium channel blockers **(amlodipine, felodipine, lacidipine, nicardipine, nifedipine, nimodipine)**. Monitor and adjust dose. [Moderate] Study

▸ **Fluconazole** (high-dose) is predicted to increase the exposure to calcium channel blockers **(diltiazem, verapamil)**. [Moderate] Theoretical

▸ **Posaconazole** is predicted to increase the exposure to calcium channel blockers **(diltiazem, verapamil)**. [Moderate] Theoretical

▸ Antifungals, azoles **(itraconazole, ketoconazole, voriconazole)** are predicted to increase the exposure to calcium channel blockers **(diltiazem, verapamil)**. [Severe] Study

▸ Antifungals, azoles **(itraconazole, ketoconazole, voriconazole)** are predicted to markedly increase the exposure to calcium channel blockers **(lercanidipine)**. Avoid. [Severe] Study

▸ Antifungals, azoles **(itraconazole, ketoconazole, voriconazole)** are predicted to increase the exposure to cannabis extract. Use with caution and adjust dose. [Moderate] Theoretical

▸ Antifungals, azoles **(fluconazole, isavuconazole, posaconazole)** are predicted to increase the exposure to ceritinib. [Moderate] Theoretical → Also see TABLE 9 p. 1336

▸ Antifungals, azoles **(itraconazole, ketoconazole, voriconazole)** are predicted to increase the exposure to ceritinib. Avoid or adjust **ceritinib** dose, p. 945. [Severe] Study → Also see TABLE 9 p. 1336

▸ Antifungals, azoles **(fluconazole, isavuconazole, itraconazole, ketoconazole, posaconazole, voriconazole)** increase the concentration of ciclosporin. [Severe] Study

▸ **Miconazole** increases the concentration of ciclosporin. Monitor and adjust dose. [Severe] Anecdotal

▸ Antifungals, azoles **(itraconazole, ketoconazole, voriconazole)** are predicted to moderately increase the exposure to cilostazol. Adjust **cilostazol** dose, p. 231. [Moderate] Study

▸ **Fluconazole** is predicted to increase the exposure to cilostazol. Adjust **cilostazol** dose, p. 231. [Moderate] Theoretical

▸ **Miconazole** is predicted to increase the exposure to cilostazol. Use with caution and adjust dose. [Moderate] Theoretical

▸ Antifungals, azoles **(itraconazole, ketoconazole, voriconazole)** are predicted to moderately increase the exposure to cinacalcet. Adjust dose. [Moderate] Study

▸ Antifungals, azoles **(fluconazole, voriconazole)** potentially increase the exposure to clobazam. Adjust dose. [Moderate] Theoretical

▸ **Fluconazole** is predicted to decrease the efficacy of clopidogrel. Avoid. [Severe] Theoretical

▸ **Voriconazole** is predicted to decrease the efficacy of clopidogrel. Avoid. [Moderate] Study

▸ **Cobicistat** is predicted to increase the exposure to antifungals, azoles **(fluconazole, posaconazole)**. [Moderate] Theoretical

▸ **Cobicistat** is predicted to increase the exposure to antifungals, azoles **(itraconazole, ketoconazole)**. Adjust dose. [Moderate] Theoretical

▸ **Cobicistat** is predicted to increase the exposure to **isavuconazole**. Avoid or monitor side effects. [Severe] Study

▸ **Cobicistat** is predicted to affect the exposure to **voriconazole**. Avoid. [Moderate] Theoretical

▸ Antifungals, azoles **(fluconazole, isavuconazole, miconazole, posaconazole)** are predicted to increase the exposure to cobimetinib. [Severe] Theoretical

▸ Antifungals, azoles **(itraconazole, ketoconazole, voriconazole)** are predicted to markedly increase the exposure to cobimetinib. Avoid or monitor for toxicity. [Severe] Study

▸ Antifungals, azoles **(fluconazole, isavuconazole, posaconazole)** are predicted to increase the exposure to colchicine. Adjust **colchicine** dose with moderate inhibitors of CYP3A4, p. 1085. [Severe] Study

▸ Antifungals, azoles **(itraconazole, ketoconazole, voriconazole)** are predicted to increase the exposure to colchicine. Avoid potent inhibitors of CYP3A4 or adjust **colchicine** dose, p. 1085. [Severe] Study

▸ Corticosteroids **(prednisone)** potentially decrease the exposure to **isavuconazole**. Use with caution or avoid. [Moderate] Theoretical

▸ Antifungals, azoles **(itraconazole, ketoconazole, voriconazole)** are predicted to increase the exposure to corticosteroids **(beclometasone)** (risk with beclometasone is likely to be lower than with other corticosteroids). [Moderate] Theoretical

▸ Antifungals, azoles **(itraconazole, ketoconazole, voriconazole)** are predicted to increase the exposure to corticosteroids **(betamethasone, budesonide, ciclesonide, deflazacort, dexamethasone, fludrocortisone, fluticasone, hydrocortisone, methylprednisolone, mometasone, prednisolone, prednisone, triamcinolone)**. Avoid or monitor side effects. [Severe] Study

▸ **Miconazole** is predicted to increase the concentration of corticosteroids **(methylprednisolone)**. Monitor and adjust dose. [Moderate] Theoretical

Antifungals, azoles (continued)

▶ Antifungals, azoles **(fluconazole, isavuconazole, posaconazole)** are predicted to increase the exposure to corticosteroids (methylprednisolone). Monitor and adjust dose. Moderate Study

▶ **Fluconazole** increases the anticoagulant effect of coumarins. Monitor INR and adjust dose. Severe Study

▶ **Itraconazole** potentially increases the anticoagulant effect of coumarins. Severe Anecdotal

▶ **Ketoconazole** potentially increases the anticoagulant effect of coumarins **(warfarin)**. Monitor INR and adjust dose. Severe Anecdotal

▶ **Miconazole** greatly increases the anticoagulant effect of coumarins. MHRA advises avoid unless INR can be monitored closely; monitor for signs of bleeding. Severe Study

▶ **Voriconazole** increases the anticoagulant effect of coumarins. Monitor INR and adjust dose. Moderate Study

▶ Antifungals, azoles **(itraconazole, ketoconazole, voriconazole)** are predicted to moderately increase the exposure to crizotinib. Avoid. Moderate Study → Also see TABLE 9 p. 1336

▶ Antifungals, azoles **(itraconazole, ketoconazole)** are predicted to increase the exposure to dabigatran. Avoid. Severe Study

▶ **Isavuconazole** is predicted to increase the exposure to dabigatran. Monitor and adjust dose. Moderate Study

▶ Antifungals, azoles **(itraconazole, ketoconazole, voriconazole)** are predicted to increase the exposure to dabrafenib. Use with caution or avoid. Moderate Study

▶ Antifungals, azoles **(itraconazole, ketoconazole, voriconazole)** are predicted to moderately increase the exposure to daclatasvir. Adjust **daclatasvir** dose, p. 614. Moderate Study

▶ Antifungals, azoles **(fluconazole, isavuconazole, posaconazole)** are predicted to slightly increase the exposure to darifenacin. Moderate Study

▶ Antifungals, azoles **(itraconazole, ketoconazole, voriconazole)** are predicted to markedly to very markedly increase the exposure to darifenacin. Avoid. Severe Study

▶ Antifungals, azoles **(fluconazole, isavuconazole, posaconazole)** are predicted to increase the exposure to dasatinib. Severe Study → Also see TABLE 9 p. 1336

▶ Antifungals, azoles **(itraconazole, ketoconazole, voriconazole)** are predicted to markedly increase the exposure to dasatinib. Avoid. Severe Study → Also see TABLE 9 p. 1336

▶ Antifungals, azoles **(itraconazole, ketoconazole, voriconazole)** very slightly increase the exposure to delamanid. Severe Study → Also see TABLE 9 p. 1336

▶ Antifungals, azoles **(fluconazole, voriconazole)** moderately increase the exposure to diazepam. Monitor and adjust dose. Moderate Study

▶ Didanosine (buffered) decreases the exposure to antifungals, azoles **(itraconazole, ketoconazole)**. Separate administration by 2 hours. Severe Study → Also see TABLE 1 p. 1334

▶ **Isavuconazole** slightly increases the exposure to digoxin. Monitor and adjust dose. Moderate Study

▶ **Itraconazole** is predicted to markedly increase the concentration of digoxin. Monitor and adjust dose. Severe Study

▶ **Ketoconazole** is predicted to markedly increase the concentration of digoxin. Severe Study

▶ **Posaconazole** is predicted to increase the concentration of digoxin. Severe Study

▶ Antifungals, azoles **(fluconazole, isavuconazole, itraconazole, ketoconazole, posaconazole, voriconazole)** increase the risk of QT-prolongation when given with domperidone. Avoid. Severe Study

▶ Antifungals, azoles **(fluconazole, isavuconazole, posaconazole)** are predicted to increase the exposure to dopamine receptor agonists (bromocriptine). Severe Theoretical

▶ Antifungals, azoles **(itraconazole, ketoconazole, voriconazole)** increase the exposure to dopamine receptor agonists (bromocriptine). Severe Study

▶ Antifungals, azoles **(fluconazole, isavuconazole, itraconazole, ketoconazole, posaconazole, voriconazole)** are predicted to increase the concentration of dopamine receptor agonists (cabergoline). Moderate Anecdotal

▶ **Ketoconazole** moderately increases the exposure to drospirenone. Severe Study

▶ Antifungals, azoles **(fluconazole, isavuconazole, posaconazole)** are predicted to moderately increase the exposure to dutasteride. Mild Study

▶ Antifungals, azoles **(itraconazole, ketoconazole, voriconazole)** are predicted to increase the exposure to dutasteride. Monitor side effects and adjust dose. Moderate Theoretical

▶ **Itraconazole** is predicted to slightly increase the exposure to edoxaban. Severe Theoretical

▶ **Ketoconazole** slightly increases the exposure to edoxaban. Adjust **edoxaban** dose, p. 125. Severe Study

▶ **Efavirenz** is predicted to decrease the exposure to isavuconazole. Avoid. Severe Theoretical

▶ **Efavirenz** slightly decreases the exposure to itraconazole. Avoid and for 14 days after stopping **efavirenz**. Moderate Study

▶ **Efavirenz** moderately decreases the exposure to ketoconazole. Severe Study

▶ **Efavirenz** slightly decreases the exposure to posaconazole. Severe Study

▶ **Efavirenz** moderately decreases the exposure to voriconazole and **voriconazole** slightly increases the exposure to efavirenz. Adjust dose. Severe Study → Also see TABLE 9 p. 1336

▶ Antifungals, azoles **(itraconazole, ketoconazole, voriconazole)** slightly to moderately increase the exposure to elbasvir. Avoid. Moderate Study

▶ Antifungals, azoles **(itraconazole, ketoconazole, voriconazole)** are predicted to markedly increase the exposure to eletriptan. Avoid. Severe Study

▶ Antifungals, azoles **(fluconazole, isavuconazole, itraconazole, ketoconazole, posaconazole, voriconazole)** are predicted to increase the exposure to eliglustat. Avoid or adjust dose— consult product literature. Severe Study

▶ **Enzalutamide** is predicted to decrease the exposure to isavuconazole. Avoid. Severe Study

▶ Antifungals, azoles **(fluconazole, isavuconazole, posaconazole)** are predicted to increase the risk of ergotism when given with ergometrine. Severe Theoretical

▶ Antifungals, azoles **(itraconazole, ketoconazole, voriconazole)** are predicted to increase the risk of ergotism when given with ergometrine. Avoid. Severe Theoretical

▶ **Miconazole** is predicted to increase the exposure to ergometrine. Avoid. Moderate Theoretical

▶ Antifungals, azoles **(fluconazole, isavuconazole, posaconazole)** are predicted to increase the risk of ergotism when given with ergotamine. Severe Theoretical

▶ Antifungals, azoles **(itraconazole, ketoconazole, voriconazole)** are predicted to increase the risk of ergotism when given with ergotamine. Avoid. Severe Theoretical

▶ **Miconazole** is predicted to increase the exposure to ergotamine. Avoid. Moderate Theoretical

▶ Antifungals, azoles **(fluconazole, isavuconazole, posaconazole)** are predicted to increase the exposure to erlotinib. Moderate Theoretical

▶ Antifungals, azoles **(itraconazole, ketoconazole, voriconazole)** are predicted to slightly increase the exposure to erlotinib. Use with caution and adjust dose. Moderate Study

▶ Antifungals, azoles **(fluconazole, isavuconazole, posaconazole)** are predicted to increase the concentration of everolimus. Avoid or adjust dose. Moderate Study

▶ Antifungals, azoles **(itraconazole, ketoconazole, voriconazole)** are predicted to increase the concentration of everolimus. Avoid. Severe Study

▶ Antifungals, azoles **(fluconazole, isavuconazole, posaconazole)** are predicted to increase the exposure to fesoterodine. Adjust **fesoterodine** dose with moderate inhibitors of CYP3A4 in hepatic and renal impairment, p. 759. Mild Study

▶ Antifungals, azoles **(itraconazole, ketoconazole, voriconazole)** are predicted to moderately increase the exposure to fesoterodine. Adjust **fesoterodine** dose with potent inhibitors of CYP3A4; avoid in hepatic and renal impairment, p. 759. Severe Study

▶ Antifungals, azoles **(itraconazole, ketoconazole)** are predicted to increase the exposure to fidaxomicin. Avoid. Moderate Study

▶ Antifungals, azoles **(itraconazole, ketoconazole, voriconazole)** are predicted to increase the exposure to fosaprepitant. Moderate Theoretical

- Antifungals, azoles **(fluconazole, isavuconazole, posaconazole)** are predicted to increase the exposure to gefitinib. Moderate Theoretical
- Antifungals, azoles **(itraconazole, ketoconazole, voriconazole)** are predicted to increase the exposure to gefitinib. Moderate Study
- Antifungals, azoles **(itraconazole, ketoconazole)** potentially increase the exposure to glecaprevir. Moderate Theoretical
- Antifungals, azoles **(itraconazole, ketoconazole, voriconazole)** are predicted to moderately to markedly increase the exposure to grazoprevir. Avoid. Severe Study
- Antifungals, azoles **(fluconazole, isavuconazole, posaconazole)** are predicted to increase the concentration of guanfacine. Adjust **guanfacine** dose, p. 349. Moderate Theoretical
- Antifungals, azoles **(itraconazole, ketoconazole, voriconazole)** are predicted to increase the exposure to guanfacine. Adjust **guanfacine** dose, p. 349. Moderate Study
- H$_2$ receptor antagonists are predicted to decrease the absorption of **itraconazole**. Administer **itraconazole** capsules with an acidic beverage. Moderate Study
- H$_2$ receptor antagonists are predicted to decrease the absorption of **ketoconazole**. Administer **ketoconazole** with an acidic beverage. Moderate Study
- H$_2$ receptor antagonists are predicted to decrease the exposure to **posaconazole**. Avoid use of posaconazole oral suspension. Moderate Study
- **Itraconazole** increases the concentration of haloperidol. Moderate Study
- **Fluconazole** slightly increases the exposure to HIV-protease inhibitors (tipranavir). Avoid or adjust dose. Moderate Study
- HIV-protease inhibitors are predicted to increase the exposure to **isavuconazole**. Avoid or monitor side effects. Severe Study
- HIV-protease inhibitors are predicted to increase the exposure to **itraconazole**. Use with caution and adjust dose. Severe Study
- HIV-protease inhibitors are predicted to increase the exposure to **ketoconazole**. Use with caution and adjust dose. Moderate Study
- **Miconazole** is predicted to increase the concentration of HIV-protease inhibitors. Use with caution and adjust dose. Moderate Theoretical
- **Posaconazole** is predicted to increase the exposure to HIV-protease inhibitors. Moderate Study
- HIV-protease inhibitors are predicted to affect the exposure to **voriconazole** and **voriconazole** potentially affects the exposure to HIV-protease inhibitors. Severe Study → Also see TABLE 9 p. 1336
- Antifungals, azoles **(fluconazole, isavuconazole, posaconazole)** are predicted to increase the exposure to ibrutinib. Adjust **ibrutinib** dose with moderate inhibitors of CYP3A4, p. 952. Severe Study
- Antifungals, azoles **(itraconazole, ketoconazole, voriconazole)** are predicted to very markedly increase the exposure to ibrutinib. Avoid potent inhibitors of CYP3A4 or adjust **ibrutinib** dose, p. 952. Severe Study
- Idelalisib is predicted to increase the exposure to **isavuconazole**. Avoid or monitor side effects. Severe Study
- Antifungals, azoles **(fluconazole, posaconazole)** are predicted to increase the exposure to imatinib. Moderate Theoretical
- Antifungals, azoles **(itraconazole, ketoconazole, voriconazole)** are predicted to increase the exposure to imatinib. Moderate Study
- Imatinib is predicted to decrease the exposure to **isavuconazole**. Moderate Theoretical
- Antifungals, azoles **(itraconazole, ketoconazole, voriconazole)** are predicted to increase the risk of toxicity when given with irinotecan. Avoid. Moderate Study
- Antifungals, azoles **(fluconazole, isavuconazole, posaconazole)** are predicted to increase the exposure to ivabradine. Adjust **ivabradine** dose, p. 210. Severe Theoretical
- Antifungals, azoles **(itraconazole, ketoconazole, voriconazole)** are predicted to increase the exposure to ivabradine. Avoid. Severe Study
- Antifungals, azoles **(fluconazole, isavuconazole, posaconazole)** are predicted to increase the exposure to ivacaftor. Adjust **ivacaftor** dose with moderate inhibitors of CYP3A4, p. 292. Severe Study
- Antifungals, azoles **(itraconazole, ketoconazole, voriconazole)** are predicted to increase the exposure to ivacaftor. Adjust

ivacaftor, p. 292 or **lumacaftor with ivacaftor** p. 293 dose with potent inhibitors of CYP3A4. Severe Study
- Lanthanum is predicted to decrease the absorption of **ketoconazole**. Separate administration by at least 2 hours. Moderate Theoretical
- Antifungals, azoles **(fluconazole, isavuconazole, posaconazole)** are predicted to increase the exposure to lapatinib. Moderate Study → Also see TABLE 9 p. 1336
- Antifungals, azoles **(itraconazole, ketoconazole, voriconazole)** are predicted to increase the exposure to lapatinib. Avoid. Moderate Study → Also see TABLE 9 p. 1336
- Antifungals, azoles **(fluconazole, isavuconazole, posaconazole)** are predicted to increase the exposure to lomitapide. Avoid. Moderate Theoretical → Also see TABLE 1 p. 1334
- Antifungals, azoles **(itraconazole, ketoconazole, voriconazole)** are predicted to markedly increase the exposure to lomitapide. Avoid. Severe Study → Also see TABLE 1 p. 1334
- **Clotrimazole** is predicted to increase the exposure to lomitapide. Separate administration by 12 hours. Moderate Theoretical
- Lumacaftor is predicted to decrease the exposure to antifungals, azoles **(itraconazole, ketoconazole, posaconazole, voriconazole)**. Avoid or monitor efficacy. Moderate Theoretical
- Lumacaftor is predicted to decrease the exposure to **fluconazole**. Adjust dose. Mild Theoretical
- Antifungals, azoles **(fluconazole, isavuconazole, posaconazole)** are predicted to increase the exposure to lurasidone. Moderate Study
- Antifungals, azoles **(itraconazole, ketoconazole, voriconazole)** are predicted to increase the exposure to lurasidone. Avoid. Severe Study
- Antifungals, azoles **(itraconazole, ketoconazole, voriconazole)** are predicted to increase the exposure to macitentan. Moderate Study
- Macrolides (clarithromycin) are predicted to increase the exposure to **isavuconazole**. Avoid or monitor side effects. Severe Study
- Macrolides (erythromycin) are predicted to increase the exposure to **isavuconazole**. Moderate Theoretical
- Antifungals, azoles **(itraconazole, ketoconazole, voriconazole)** are predicted to markedly increase the exposure to maraviroc. Adjust dose. Severe Study
- Metoclopramide potentially decreases the absorption of **posaconazole** (oral suspension). Moderate Study
- Antifungals, azoles **(fluconazole, isavuconazole, posaconazole)** are predicted to increase the exposure to midazolam. Monitor side effects and adjust dose. Severe Study
- Antifungals, azoles **(itraconazole, ketoconazole, voriconazole)** are predicted to markedly to very markedly increase the exposure to midazolam. Avoid or adjust dose. Severe Study
- **Miconazole** is predicted to increase the exposure to intravenous midazolam. Use with caution and adjust dose. Moderate Theoretical
- **Miconazole** is predicted to increase the exposure to oral midazolam. Avoid. Moderate Theoretical
- Antifungals, azoles **(fluconazole, isavuconazole, posaconazole)** are predicted to increase the exposure to midostaurin. Moderate Theoretical
- Antifungals, azoles **(itraconazole, ketoconazole, voriconazole)** are predicted to very markedly increase the exposure to midostaurin. Avoid or monitor for toxicity. Severe Study
- Antifungals, azoles **(itraconazole, ketoconazole, voriconazole)** are predicted to increase the exposure to mirabegron. Adjust **mirabegron** dose in hepatic and renal impairment, p. 763. Moderate Study
- Antifungals, azoles **(itraconazole, ketoconazole, voriconazole)** are predicted to increase the exposure to mirtazapine. Moderate Study
- Mitotane is predicted to decrease the exposure to **isavuconazole**. Avoid. Severe Study
- Antifungals, azoles **(itraconazole, ketoconazole, voriconazole)** are predicted to increase the exposure to modafinil. Mild Theoretical
- Antifungals, azoles **(itraconazole, ketoconazole)** increase the risk of neutropenia when given with monoclonal antibodies (brentuximab vedotin). Monitor and adjust dose. Severe Study

Antifungals, azoles (continued)

▶ Antifungals, azoles **(itraconazole, ketoconazole, voriconazole)** are predicted to increase the exposure to monoclonal antibodies (trastuzumab emtansine). Avoid. Severe Theoretical
▶ **Isavuconazole** increases the exposure to mycophenolate. Moderate Study
▶ Antifungals, azoles **(fluconazole, isavuconazole, posaconazole)** are predicted to increase the exposure to naloxegol. Adjust **naloxegol** dose and monitor side effects, p. 64. Moderate Study
▶ Antifungals, azoles **(itraconazole, ketoconazole, voriconazole)** are predicted to markedly increase the exposure to naloxegol. Avoid. Severe Study
▶ Antifungals, azoles **(itraconazole, ketoconazole, voriconazole)** are predicted to increase the exposure to netupitant. Moderate Study
▶ **Netupitant** is predicted to decrease the exposure to **isavuconazole**. Moderate Theoretical
▶ **Fluconazole** slightly to moderately increases the exposure to nevirapine. Moderate Study
▶ **Nevirapine** is predicted to decrease the exposure to **isavuconazole**. Avoid. Severe Theoretical
▶ **Nevirapine** moderately decreases the exposure to **itraconazole**. Avoid and for 14 days after stopping **nevirapine**. Moderate Study
▶ **Nevirapine** moderately decreases the exposure to **ketoconazole**. Avoid. Severe Study
▶ **Nevirapine** is predicted to decrease the exposure to **voriconazole** and **voriconazole** increases the exposure to nevirapine. Monitor and adjust dose. Severe Theoretical
▶ Antifungals, azoles **(fluconazole, posaconazole)** are predicted to increase the exposure to nilotinib. Moderate Theoretical → Also see TABLE 9 p. 1336
▶ Antifungals, azoles **(itraconazole, ketoconazole, voriconazole)** are predicted to moderately increase the exposure to nilotinib. Avoid. Severe Study → Also see TABLE 9 p. 1336
▶ Antifungals, azoles **(itraconazole, ketoconazole, voriconazole)** are predicted to increase the exposure to nintedanib. Moderate Study
▶ Antifungals, azoles **(itraconazole, ketoconazole, voriconazole)** are predicted to increase the exposure to nitisinone. Adjust dose. Moderate Theoretical
▶ **Fluconazole** moderately increases the exposure to NSAIDs (celecoxib). Adjust **celecoxib** dose, p. 1097. Moderate Study
▶ **Voriconazole** slightly increases the exposure to NSAIDs (diclofenac). Monitor and adjust dose. Moderate Study
▶ **Voriconazole** moderately increases the exposure to NSAIDs (ibuprofen). Adjust dose. Moderate Study
▶ **Fluconazole** increases the exposure to NSAIDs (parecoxib). Monitor and adjust dose. Moderate Study
▶ Antifungals, azoles **(fluconazole, isavuconazole, posaconazole)** are predicted to increase the exposure to olaparib. Avoid moderate inhibitors of CYP3A4 or adjust **olaparib** dose, p. 973. Moderate Theoretical
▶ Antifungals, azoles **(itraconazole, ketoconazole, voriconazole)** are predicted to increase the exposure to olaparib. Avoid potent inhibitors of CYP3A4 or adjust **olaparib** dose, p. 973. Moderate Study
▶ **Miconazole** is predicted to increase the exposure to opioids (alfentanil). Use with caution and adjust dose. Moderate Theoretical
▶ Antifungals, azoles **(fluconazole, isavuconazole, posaconazole)** are predicted to increase the exposure to opioids (alfentanil, buprenorphine, fentanyl, oxycodone). Monitor and adjust dose. Moderate Study
▶ Antifungals, azoles **(itraconazole, ketoconazole, voriconazole)** are predicted to increase the exposure to opioids (alfentanil, buprenorphine, fentanyl, oxycodone, sufentanil). Monitor and adjust dose. Severe Study
▶ Antifungals, azoles **(itraconazole, ketoconazole, voriconazole)** are predicted to increase the exposure to opioids (methadone). Adjust dose. Severe Theoretical → Also see TABLE 9 p. 1336
▶ Antifungals, azoles **(fluconazole, isavuconazole, posaconazole)** are predicted to increase the exposure to opioids (methadone, sufentanil). Moderate Theoretical → Also see TABLE 9 p. 1336
▶ Antifungals, azoles **(fluconazole, isavuconazole, posaconazole)** are predicted to increase the exposure to oxybutynin. Mild Theoretical

▶ Antifungals, azoles **(itraconazole, ketoconazole, voriconazole)** are predicted to increase the exposure to oxybutynin. Mild Study
▶ Antifungals, azoles **(itraconazole, ketoconazole, voriconazole)** are predicted to increase the exposure to palbociclib. Avoid or adjust **palbociclib** dose, p. 961. Severe Study
▶ Antifungals, azoles **(itraconazole, ketoconazole, voriconazole)** are predicted to increase the exposure to panobinostat. Adjust **panobinostat** dose; in hepatic impairment avoid, p. 911. Moderate Study → Also see TABLE 9 p. 1336
▶ **Posaconazole** is predicted to increase the exposure to panobinostat. Adjust dose. Moderate Theoretical
▶ Antifungals, azoles **(itraconazole, ketoconazole, voriconazole)** are predicted to increase the exposure to paritaprevir (with ritonavir and ombitasvir). Avoid. Severe Theoretical
▶ **Posaconazole** is predicted to increase the exposure to paritaprevir (with ritonavir and ombitasvir) and paritaprevir (with ritonavir and ombitasvir) is predicted to increase the exposure to **posaconazole**. Avoid. Severe Theoretical
▶ Antifungals, azoles **(fluconazole, isavuconazole, posaconazole)** are predicted to increase the exposure to pazopanib. Moderate Theoretical → Also see TABLE 9 p. 1336
▶ Antifungals, azoles **(itraconazole, ketoconazole, voriconazole)** are predicted to increase the exposure to pazopanib. Avoid or adjust **pazopanib** dose, p. 962. Moderate Study → Also see TABLE 9 p. 1336
▶ **Miconazole** greatly increases the anticoagulant effect of phenindione. Severe Theoretical
▶ Antifungals, azoles **(fluconazole, isavuconazole, posaconazole)** are predicted to increase the exposure to phosphodiesterase type-5 inhibitors (avanafil). Adjust **avanafil** dose, p. 794. Moderate Theoretical
▶ Antifungals, azoles **(itraconazole, ketoconazole, voriconazole)** are predicted to increase the exposure to phosphodiesterase type-5 inhibitors (avanafil, vardenafil). Avoid. Severe Study → Also see TABLE 9 p. 1336
▶ **Miconazole** is predicted to increase the exposure to phosphodiesterase type-5 inhibitors (sildenafil). Use with caution and adjust dose. Severe Theoretical
▶ Antifungals, azoles **(fluconazole, isavuconazole, posaconazole)** are predicted to increase the exposure to phosphodiesterase type-5 inhibitors (sildenafil). Monitor or adjust **sildenafil** dose with moderate inhibitors of CYP3A4, p. 794. Moderate Study → Also see TABLE 9 p. 1336
▶ Antifungals, azoles **(itraconazole, ketoconazole, voriconazole)** are predicted to increase the exposure to phosphodiesterase type-5 inhibitors (sildenafil). Avoid potent inhibitors of CYP3A4 or adjust **sildenafil** dose, p. 794. Severe Study → Also see TABLE 9 p. 1336
▶ Antifungals, azoles **(fluconazole, isavuconazole, posaconazole)** are predicted to increase the exposure to phosphodiesterase type-5 inhibitors (tadalafil). Severe Theoretical
▶ Antifungals, azoles **(itraconazole, ketoconazole, voriconazole)** are predicted to increase the exposure to phosphodiesterase type-5 inhibitors (tadalafil). Use with caution or avoid. Severe Study
▶ Antifungals, azoles **(fluconazole, isavuconazole, posaconazole)** are predicted to increase the exposure to phosphodiesterase type-5 inhibitors (vardenafil). Adjust dose. Severe Theoretical → Also see TABLE 9 p. 1336
▶ Antifungals, azoles **(itraconazole, ketoconazole, voriconazole)** potentially increase the exposure to pibrentasvir. Moderate Theoretical
▶ Antifungals, azoles **(fluconazole, isavuconazole, posaconazole)** are predicted to increase the exposure to pimozide. Avoid. Severe Theoretical → Also see TABLE 9 p. 1336
▶ Antifungals, azoles **(itraconazole, ketoconazole, voriconazole)** are predicted to increase the exposure to pimozide. Avoid. Severe Study → Also see TABLE 9 p. 1336
▶ **Miconazole** is predicted to increase the exposure to pimozide. Avoid. Moderate Theoretical
▶ **Pioglitazone** potentially decreases the exposure to **isavuconazole**. Use with caution or avoid. Moderate Theoretical
▶ Antifungals, azoles **(itraconazole, ketoconazole, voriconazole)** are predicted to slightly increase the exposure to ponatinib. Monitor and adjust **ponatinib** dose, p. 963. Moderate Study

- Antifungals, azoles **(itraconazole, ketoconazole, voriconazole)** are predicted to moderately increase the exposure to praziquantel. Mild Study
- Proton pump inhibitors decrease the absorption of **itraconazole**. Administer **itraconazole** capsules with an acidic beverage. Moderate Study
- Proton pump inhibitors decrease the absorption of **ketoconazole**. Administer **ketoconazole** with an acidic beverage. Moderate Study
- Proton pump inhibitors decrease the absorption of **posaconazole** (oral suspension). Avoid. Moderate Study
- **Voriconazole** increases the exposure to proton pump inhibitors (esomeprazole, omeprazole). Adjust dose. Moderate Study
- Antifungals, azoles **(fluconazole, isavuconazole, posaconazole)** are predicted to increase the exposure to quetiapine. Avoid. Moderate Study
- Antifungals, azoles **(itraconazole, ketoconazole, voriconazole)** are predicted to increase the exposure to quetiapine. Avoid. Severe Study
- Antifungals, azoles **(fluconazole, isavuconazole, posaconazole)** are predicted to increase the exposure to ranolazine. Severe Study → Also see TABLE 9 p. 1336
- Antifungals, azoles **(itraconazole, ketoconazole, voriconazole)** are predicted to increase the exposure to ranolazine. Avoid. Severe Study → Also see TABLE 9 p. 1336
- Antifungals, azoles **(itraconazole, ketoconazole, voriconazole)** are predicted to increase the exposure to reboxetine. Avoid. Moderate Study
- **Miconazole** is predicted to increase the concentration of reboxetine. Use with caution and adjust dose. Moderate Theoretical
- Antifungals, azoles **(itraconazole, ketoconazole, voriconazole)** are predicted to increase the exposure to regorafenib. Avoid. Moderate Study
- Antifungals, azoles **(itraconazole, ketoconazole, voriconazole)** are predicted to increase the exposure to repaglinide. Moderate Study
- Antifungals, azoles **(fluconazole, itraconazole, ketoconazole, miconazole, voriconazole)** are predicted to increase the exposure to retinoids (alitretinoin). Adjust **alitretinoin** dose, p. 1226. Moderate Theoretical
- Antifungals, azoles **(fluconazole, ketoconazole, voriconazole)** are predicted to increase the risk of tretinoin toxicity when given with retinoids (tretinoin). Moderate Study
- Antifungals, azoles **(fluconazole, isavuconazole, posaconazole)** are predicted to increase the exposure to ribociclib. Moderate Study → Also see TABLE 9 p. 1336
- Antifungals, azoles **(itraconazole, ketoconazole, voriconazole)** are predicted to increase the exposure to ribociclib. Avoid or adjust **ribociclib** dose, p. 965. Moderate Study → Also see TABLE 9 p. 1336
- Antifungals, azoles **(itraconazole, posaconazole)** increase the concentration of rifabutin and rifabutin decreases the concentration of antifungals, azoles **(itraconazole, posaconazole)**. Avoid. Severe Study
- **Fluconazole** increases the risk of uveitis when given with rifabutin. Adjust dose. Severe Study
- Rifabutin is predicted to decrease the exposure to **isavuconazole**. Avoid. Severe Theoretical
- **Ketoconazole** is predicted to increase the concentration of rifabutin and rifabutin is predicted to decrease the concentration of **ketoconazole**. Avoid. Severe Theoretical
- **Miconazole** is predicted to increase the concentration of rifabutin. Use with caution and adjust dose. Moderate Theoretical
- Rifabutin decreases the concentration of **voriconazole** and **voriconazole** increases the concentration of rifabutin. Avoid or adjust **voriconazole** dose, p. 588. Severe Study
- Rifampicin slightly decreases the exposure to **fluconazole**. Adjust dose. Moderate Study
- Rifampicin is predicted to decrease the exposure to **isavuconazole**. Avoid. Severe Study
- Rifampicin markedly decreases the exposure to **itraconazole**. Avoid and for 14 days after stopping **rifampicin**. Moderate Study

- Rifampicin markedly decreases the exposure to **ketoconazole** and **ketoconazole** potentially decreases the exposure to rifampicin. Avoid. Moderate Study
- Rifampicin is predicted to decrease the exposure to **posaconazole**. Avoid. Moderate Anecdotal
- Rifampicin very markedly decreases the exposure to **voriconazole**. Avoid. Moderate Study
- **Itraconazole** is predicted to increase the exposure to riociguat. Avoid. Moderate Study
- **Ketoconazole** moderately increases the exposure to riociguat. Avoid. Moderate Study
- Antifungals, azoles **(itraconazole, ketoconazole, voriconazole)** are predicted to increase the exposure to risperidone. Adjust dose. Moderate Study → Also see TABLE 9 p. 1336
- Antifungals, azoles **(itraconazole, ketoconazole)** are predicted to moderately increase the exposure to rivaroxaban. Avoid. Severe Study
- Antifungals, azoles **(fluconazole, isavuconazole, posaconazole)** are predicted to increase the exposure to ruxolitinib. Moderate Theoretical
- Antifungals, azoles **(itraconazole, ketoconazole, voriconazole)** are predicted to increase the exposure to ruxolitinib. Adjust dose and monitor side effects. Moderate Study
- Antifungals, azoles **(fluconazole, isavuconazole, posaconazole)** are predicted to increase the exposure to saxagliptin. Mild Study
- Antifungals, azoles **(itraconazole, ketoconazole, voriconazole)** are predicted to increase the exposure to saxagliptin. Moderate Study
- **Fluconazole** is predicted to increase the exposure to selexipag. Unknown Theoretical
- Antifungals, azoles **(fluconazole, isavuconazole, itraconazole, ketoconazole, posaconazole, voriconazole)** are predicted to increase the exposure to simeprevir. Avoid. Severe Study
- Antifungals, azoles **(fluconazole, isavuconazole, posaconazole)** increase the concentration of sirolimus. Monitor and adjust dose. Moderate Study
- Antifungals, azoles **(itraconazole, ketoconazole, voriconazole)** are predicted to increase the concentration of sirolimus. Avoid. Severe Study
- **Miconazole** is predicted to increase the concentration of sirolimus. Monitor and adjust dose. Moderate Study
- Oral sodium bicarbonate decreases the absorption of **ketoconazole**. Moderate Study
- Antifungals, azoles **(itraconazole, ketoconazole, voriconazole)** are predicted to increase the exposure to solifenacin. Adjust **solifenacin**, p. 761 or **tamsulosin with solifenacin** p. 768 dose; avoid in hepatic and renal impairment. Severe Study
- **Voriconazole** is predicted to increase the exposure to SSRIs (citalopram). Severe Theoretical → Also see TABLE 9 p. 1336
- Antifungals, azoles **(fluconazole, isavuconazole, posaconazole)** are predicted to increase the exposure to SSRIs (dapoxetine). Adjust **dapoxetine** dose with moderate inhibitors of CYP3A4, p. 801. Moderate Theoretical
- Antifungals, azoles **(itraconazole, ketoconazole, voriconazole)** are predicted to moderately increase the exposure to SSRIs (dapoxetine). Avoid potent inhibitors of CYP3A4 or adjust **dapoxetine** dose, p. 801. Severe Study
- St John's Wort is predicted to decrease the exposure to **isavuconazole**. Avoid. Severe Theoretical
- St John's Wort moderately decreases the exposure to **voriconazole**. Avoid. Moderate Study
- **Miconazole** potentially increases the exposure to statins (atorvastatin). Severe Anecdotal
- Antifungals, azoles **(fluconazole, isavuconazole, posaconazole)** are predicted to increase the exposure to statins (atorvastatin). Monitor and adjust dose. Severe Study → Also see TABLE 1 p. 1334
- Antifungals, azoles **(itraconazole, ketoconazole, voriconazole)** are predicted to increase the exposure to statins (atorvastatin). Avoid or adjust dose and monitor rhabdomyolysis. Severe Study → Also see TABLE 1 p. 1334
- Antifungals, azoles **(fluconazole, miconazole)** are predicted to increase the exposure to statins (fluvastatin). Severe Theoretical → Also see TABLE 1 p. 1334

Antifungals, azoles (continued)

▶ **Miconazole** is predicted to increase the exposure to statins (simvastatin). Avoid. [Severe] Theoretical
▶ Antifungals, azoles **(fluconazole, isavuconazole, posaconazole)** are predicted to increase the exposure to statins (simvastatin). Use with caution and adjust **simvastatin** dose, p. 203. [Severe] Study → Also see TABLE 1 p. 1334
▶ Antifungals, azoles **(itraconazole, ketoconazole, voriconazole)** are predicted to increase the exposure to statins (simvastatin). Avoid. [Severe] Study → Also see TABLE 1 p. 1334
▶ Antifungals, azoles **(fluconazole, miconazole)** are predicted to increase the exposure to sulfonylureas. Use with caution and adjust dose. [Moderate] Study
▶ **Voriconazole** is predicted to increase the concentration of sulfonylureas. Use with caution and adjust dose. [Moderate] Study
▶ Antifungals, azoles **(fluconazole, isavuconazole, posaconazole)** are predicted to increase the exposure to sunitinib. [Moderate] Theoretical → Also see TABLE 9 p. 1336
▶ Antifungals, azoles **(itraconazole, ketoconazole, voriconazole)** are predicted to slightly increase the exposure to sunitinib. Avoid or adjust **sunitinib** dose, p. 967. [Moderate] Study → Also see TABLE 9 p. 1336
▶ Antifungals, azoles **(fluconazole, isavuconazole, posaconazole)** are predicted to increase the concentration of tacrolimus. [Severe] Study
▶ Antifungals, azoles **(itraconazole, ketoconazole, voriconazole)** are predicted to increase the concentration of tacrolimus. Monitor and adjust dose. [Severe] Study
▶ **Miconazole** is predicted to increase the concentration of tacrolimus. Monitor and adjust dose. [Severe] Theoretical
▶ Antifungals, azoles **(fluconazole, isavuconazole, posaconazole)** are predicted to increase the exposure to taxanes (cabazitaxel). [Moderate] Theoretical
▶ Antifungals, azoles **(itraconazole, ketoconazole, voriconazole)** are predicted to increase the exposure to taxanes (cabazitaxel). Avoid. [Severe] Study
▶ **Miconazole** is predicted to increase the concentration of taxanes (docetaxel). Use with caution and adjust dose. [Moderate] Theoretical
▶ Antifungals, azoles **(itraconazole, ketoconazole, voriconazole)** are predicted to moderately increase the exposure to taxanes (docetaxel). Avoid or adjust dose. [Severe] Study
▶ Antifungals, azoles **(itraconazole, ketoconazole, voriconazole)** are predicted to increase the exposure to taxanes (paclitaxel). [Severe] Theoretical
▶ Antifungals, azoles **(fluconazole, isavuconazole, posaconazole)** are predicted to increase the concentration of temsirolimus. [Moderate] Theoretical
▶ Antifungals, azoles **(itraconazole, ketoconazole, voriconazole)** are predicted to increase the concentration of temsirolimus. Avoid. [Severe] Theoretical
▶ Antifungals, azoles **(itraconazole, ketoconazole, voriconazole)** are predicted to markedly increase the exposure to ticagrelor. Avoid. [Severe] Study
▶ Antifungals, azoles **(fluconazole, itraconazole, ketoconazole, voriconazole)** are predicted to increase the exposure to tofacitinib. Adjust **tofacitinib** dose, p. 1072. [Moderate] Study
▶ **Isavuconazole** is predicted to increase the exposure to tofacitinib. [Moderate] Study
▶ **Posaconazole** is predicted to increase the exposure to tofacitinib. [Moderate] Theoretical
▶ Antifungals, azoles **(fluconazole, isavuconazole, posaconazole)** are predicted to increase the exposure to tolterodine. [Mild] Theoretical → Also see TABLE 9 p. 1336
▶ Antifungals, azoles **(itraconazole, ketoconazole, voriconazole)** are predicted to increase the exposure to tolterodine. Avoid. [Severe] Study → Also see TABLE 9 p. 1336
▶ Antifungals, azoles **(fluconazole, isavuconazole, posaconazole)** are predicted to increase the exposure to tolvaptan. Adjust dose. [Moderate] Study
▶ Antifungals, azoles **(itraconazole, ketoconazole, voriconazole)** are predicted to increase the exposure to tolvaptan. Adjust dose. [Severe] Study

▶ Antifungals, azoles **(itraconazole, ketoconazole)** are predicted to increase the exposure to topotecan. [Severe] Study
▶ Antifungals, azoles **(itraconazole, ketoconazole, posaconazole)** are predicted to increase the exposure to toremifene. [Moderate] Theoretical → Also see TABLE 9 p. 1336
▶ Antifungals, azoles **(itraconazole, ketoconazole, voriconazole)** are predicted to increase the exposure to trabectedin. Avoid or adjust dose. [Severe] Theoretical → Also see TABLE 1 p. 1334
▶ Antifungals, azoles **(itraconazole, ketoconazole)** are predicted to increase the concentration of trametinib. [Moderate] Theoretical
▶ Antifungals, azoles **(fluconazole, isavuconazole, posaconazole)** are predicted to increase the exposure to trazodone. [Moderate] Theoretical
▶ Antifungals, azoles **(itraconazole, ketoconazole, voriconazole)** are predicted to moderately increase the exposure to trazodone. Avoid or adjust dose. [Moderate] Study
▶ Antifungals, azoles **(fluconazole, isavuconazole, posaconazole)** are predicted to increase the exposure to ulipristal. Avoid if used for uterine fibroids. [Moderate] Study
▶ Antifungals, azoles **(itraconazole, ketoconazole, voriconazole)** are predicted to increase the exposure to ulipristal. Avoid if used for uterine fibroids. [Severe] Study
▶ Antifungals, azoles **(itraconazole, ketoconazole, voriconazole)** are predicted to increase the exposure to vemurafenib. [Severe] Theoretical → Also see TABLE 9 p. 1336
▶ Antifungals, azoles **(fluconazole, isavuconazole, posaconazole)** are predicted to increase the exposure to venetoclax. Avoid moderate inhibitors of CYP3A4 or adjust **venetoclax** dose, p. 974. [Severe] Study
▶ Antifungals, azoles **(itraconazole, ketoconazole, voriconazole)** are predicted to increase the exposure to venetoclax. Avoid potent inhibitors of CYP3A4 or adjust **venetoclax** dose, p. 974. [Severe] Study
▶ Antifungals, azoles **(itraconazole, ketoconazole, voriconazole)** are predicted to increase the exposure to venlafaxine. [Moderate] Study → Also see TABLE 9 p. 1336
▶ Antifungals, azoles **(fluconazole, isavuconazole, itraconazole, ketoconazole, posaconazole, voriconazole)** are predicted to increase the exposure to vinca alkaloids. [Severe] Theoretical → Also see TABLE 1 p. 1334 → Also see TABLE 9 p. 1336
▶ **Miconazole** is predicted to increase the concentration of vinca alkaloids. Use with caution and adjust dose. [Moderate] Theoretical
▶ Antifungals, azoles **(clotrimazole, ketoconazole)** are predicted to decrease the exposure to vitamin D substances (colecalciferol). [Moderate] Theoretical
▶ Antifungals, azoles **(itraconazole, ketoconazole, voriconazole)** are predicted to increase the exposure to vitamin D substances (paricalcitol). [Moderate] Study
▶ Antifungals, azoles **(fluconazole, isavuconazole, posaconazole)** are predicted to increase the exposure to zopiclone. Adjust dose. [Moderate] Study
▶ Antifungals, azoles **(itraconazole, ketoconazole, voriconazole)** are predicted to increase the exposure to zopiclone. Adjust dose. [Moderate] Theoretical

Antihistamines, non-sedating → see TABLE 9 p. 1336 (QT-interval prolongation)

acrivastine · azelastine · bilastine · cetirizine · desloratadine · fexofenadine · levocetirizine · loratadine · mizolastine · rupatadine

FOOD AND LIFESTYLE Apple juice and orange juice decrease the exposure to fexofenadine.

▶ Antacids decrease the absorption of **fexofenadine**. Separate administration by 2 hours. [Mild] Study
▶ Antiarrhythmics (dronedarone) are predicted to increase the exposure to **rupatadine**. Avoid. [Moderate] Study
▶ Antiarrhythmics (dronedarone) are predicted to increase the exposure to antihistamines, non-sedating **(fexofenadine, mizolastine)**. [Severe] Theoretical
▶ Antifungals, azoles (fluconazole, isavuconazole, itraconazole, ketoconazole, posaconazole, voriconazole) are predicted to increase the exposure to **rupatadine**. Avoid. [Moderate] Study
▶ Antifungals, azoles (fluconazole, isavuconazole, posaconazole) are predicted to increase the exposure to **mizolastine**. [Severe] Theoretical

▸ Antifungals, azoles (itraconazole, ketoconazole, voriconazole) are predicted to increase the exposure to **mizolastine**. Avoid. ⟨Severe⟩ Study

▸ Antifungals, azoles (miconazole) are predicted to increase the exposure to **mizolastine**. Avoid. ⟨Moderate⟩ Theoretical

▸ Aprepitant is predicted to increase the exposure to **mizolastine**. ⟨Severe⟩ Theoretical

▸ Aprepitant is predicted to increase the exposure to **rupatadine**. Avoid. ⟨Moderate⟩ Study

▸ **Antihistamines, non-sedating** are predicted to decrease the effects of betahistine. ⟨Moderate⟩ Theoretical

▸ Calcium channel blockers (diltiazem, verapamil) are predicted to increase the exposure to **mizolastine**. ⟨Severe⟩ Theoretical

▸ Calcium channel blockers (diltiazem, verapamil) are predicted to increase the exposure to **rupatadine**. Avoid. ⟨Moderate⟩ Study

▸ Ceritinib is predicted to increase the exposure to **fexofenadine**. ⟨Moderate⟩ Theoretical

▸ Cobicistat is predicted to increase the exposure to **mizolastine**. Avoid. ⟨Severe⟩ Study

▸ Cobicistat is predicted to increase the exposure to **rupatadine**. Avoid. ⟨Moderate⟩ Study

▸ Crizotinib is predicted to increase the exposure to **mizolastine**. Avoid. ⟨Severe⟩ Theoretical

▸ Crizotinib is predicted to increase the exposure to **rupatadine**. Avoid. ⟨Moderate⟩ Study

▸ **Mizolastine** is predicted to increase the risk of QT-prolongation when given with drugs that prolong the QT interval. Avoid. ⟨Severe⟩ Theoretical

▸ Eliglustat is predicted to increase the exposure to **fexofenadine**. Adjust dose. ⟨Moderate⟩ Study

▸ Grapefruit juice slightly decreases the exposure to **bilastine**. **Bilastine** should be taken 1 hour before or 2 hours after **grapefruit juice**. ⟨Moderate⟩ Study

▸ Grapefruit juice increases the exposure to **rupatadine**. Avoid. ⟨Moderate⟩ Study

▸ HIV-protease inhibitors are predicted to increase the exposure to **mizolastine**. Avoid. ⟨Severe⟩ Study

▸ HIV-protease inhibitors are predicted to increase the exposure to **rupatadine**. Avoid. ⟨Moderate⟩ Study

▸ Idelalisib is predicted to increase the exposure to **mizolastine**. Avoid. ⟨Severe⟩ Study

▸ Idelalisib is predicted to increase the exposure to **rupatadine**. Avoid. ⟨Moderate⟩ Study

▸ Imatinib is predicted to increase the exposure to **mizolastine**. Avoid. ⟨Severe⟩ Theoretical

▸ Imatinib is predicted to increase the exposure to **rupatadine**. Avoid. ⟨Moderate⟩ Study

▸ Lapatinib is predicted to increase the exposure to **fexofenadine**. ⟨Moderate⟩ Theoretical

▸ Macrolides (clarithromycin) are predicted to increase the exposure to **mizolastine**. Avoid. ⟨Severe⟩ Study

▸ Macrolides (clarithromycin, erythromycin) are predicted to increase the exposure to **rupatadine**. Avoid. ⟨Moderate⟩ Study

▸ Macrolides (erythromycin) are predicted to increase the exposure to **mizolastine**. ⟨Severe⟩ Theoretical

▸ Mirabegron is predicted to increase the exposure to **fexofenadine**. ⟨Mild⟩ Theoretical

▸ Monoamine-oxidase A and B inhibitors, irreversible are predicted to increase the risk of antimuscarinic side-effects when given with **antihistamines, non-sedating**. Avoid. ⟨Severe⟩ Theoretical

▸ Netupitant is predicted to increase the exposure to **mizolastine**. ⟨Severe⟩ Theoretical

▸ Netupitant is predicted to increase the exposure to **rupatadine**. Avoid. ⟨Moderate⟩ Study

▸ Nilotinib is predicted to increase the exposure to **mizolastine**. ⟨Severe⟩ Theoretical

▸ Nilotinib is predicted to increase the exposure to **rupatadine**. Avoid. ⟨Moderate⟩ Study

▸ Rifampicin is predicted to decrease the exposure to **bilastine**. ⟨Moderate⟩ Theoretical

▸ Rifampicin increases the clearance of **fexofenadine**. ⟨Moderate⟩ Study

▸ Velpatasvir is predicted to increase the exposure to **fexofenadine**. ⟨Severe⟩ Theoretical

Antihistamines, sedating → see TABLE 9 p. 1336 (QT-interval prolongation), TABLE 11 p. 1336 (CNS depressant effects), TABLE 10 p. 1336 (antimuscarinics)

alimemazine · antazoline · buclizine · chlorphenamine · cinnarizine · clemastine · cyclizine · cyproheptadine · hydroxyzine · ketotifen · pizotifen · promethazine

ROUTE-SPECIFIC INFORMATION Since systemic absorption can follow topical application of **ketotifen**, the possibility of interactions should be borne in mind.

▸ Hydroxyzine potentially increases the risk of overheating and dehydration when given with antiepileptics (zonisamide). Avoid in children. ⟨Severe⟩ Theoretical

▸ **Antihistamines, sedating** are predicted to decrease the effects of betahistine. ⟨Moderate⟩ Theoretical

▸ **Cyproheptadine** decreases the effects of metyrapone. Avoid. ⟨Moderate⟩ Study

▸ Monoamine-oxidase A and B inhibitors, irreversible are predicted to increase the risk of antimuscarinic side-effects when given with **antihistamines, sedating**. Avoid. ⟨Severe⟩ Theoretical

▸ **Antihistamines, sedating** are predicted to decrease the efficacy of pitolisant. ⟨Unknown⟩ Theoretical

▸ **Cyproheptadine** potentially decreases the effects of SSRIs. ⟨Moderate⟩ Anecdotal

Antimalarials → see TABLE 15 p. 1337 (myelosuppression), TABLE 9 p. 1336 (QT-interval prolongation)

artemether · artenimol · atovaquone · chloroquine · lumefantrine · mefloquine · piperaquine · primaquine · proguanil · pyrimethamine · quinine

PHARMACOLOGY Piperaquine has a long half-life; there is a potential for drug interactions to occur for up to 3 months after treatment has been stopped.

▸ **Chloroquine** is predicted to decrease the effects of agalsidase. Avoid. ⟨Moderate⟩ Theoretical

▸ Antimalarials (chloroquine, primaquine) are predicted to increase the risk of methaemoglobinaemia when given with topical anaesthetics, local (prilocaine). Use with caution or avoid. ⟨Severe⟩ Theoretical

▸ Antacids decrease the absorption of **chloroquine**. Separate administration by at least 4 hours. ⟨Moderate⟩ Study

▸ Antacids are predicted to decrease the absorption of **proguanil**. Separate administration by at least 2 hours. ⟨Moderate⟩ Study

▸ Antiarrhythmics (dronedarone) are predicted to increase the concentration of piperaquine. ⟨Severe⟩ Theoretical

▸ Antiepileptics (carbamazepine, fosphenytoin, phenobarbital, phenytoin, primidone) are predicted to decrease the exposure to **artemether** (with lumafantrine). Avoid. ⟨Severe⟩ Study

▸ Antiepileptics (carbamazepine, fosphenytoin, phenobarbital, phenytoin, primidone) are predicted to decrease the concentration of piperaquine. Avoid. ⟨Moderate⟩ Theoretical

▸ Antiepileptics (carbamazepine, phenobarbital, primidone) potentially increase the risk of toxicity when given with quinine. ⟨Unknown⟩ Study

▸ **Pyrimethamine** increases the risk of haematological toxicity when given with antiepileptics (fosphenytoin, phenytoin). ⟨Severe⟩ Study

▸ **Pyrimethamine** is predicted to increase the risk of haematological toxicity when given with antiepileptics (phenobarbital, primidone). ⟨Severe⟩ Study

▸ Antifungals, azoles (fluconazole, isavuconazole, itraconazole, ketoconazole, posaconazole, voriconazole) are predicted to increase the concentration of piperaquine. ⟨Severe⟩ Theoretical

▸ Antifungals, azoles (fluconazole, itraconazole, posaconazole, voriconazole) are predicted to increase the exposure to mefloquine. ⟨Moderate⟩ Study

▸ Antifungals, azoles (ketoconazole) increase the exposure to mefloquine. ⟨Moderate⟩ Study

▸ Antimalarials (proguanil) are predicted to increase the risk of side-effects when given with antimalarials (pyrimethamine). ⟨Severe⟩ Theoretical

▸ Aprepitant is predicted to increase the concentration of piperaquine. ⟨Severe⟩ Theoretical

Antimalarials (continued)

‣ **Mefloquine** is predicted to increase the risk of bradycardia when given with beta blockers, non-selective. Severe Theoretical

‣ **Mefloquine** is predicted to increase the risk of bradycardia when given with beta blockers, selective. Severe Theoretical

‣ **Mefloquine** is predicted to increase the risk of bradycardia when given with calcium channel blockers. Severe Theoretical

‣ Calcium channel blockers (diltiazem, verapamil) are predicted to increase the concentration of **piperaquine**. Severe Theoretical

‣ Calcium salts (calcium carbonate) decrease the absorption of **chloroquine**. Separate administration by at least 4 hours. Moderate Study

‣ Calcium salts (calcium carbonate) are predicted to decrease the absorption of **proguanil**. Separate administration by at least 2 hours. Moderate Study

‣ **Chloroquine** decreases the efficacy of oral cholera vaccine. Moderate Study

‣ Cobicistat is predicted to increase the concentration of **piperaquine**. Severe Theoretical

‣ Crizotinib is predicted to increase the concentration of **piperaquine**. Severe Theoretical

‣ Antimalarials (chloroquine, primaquine) are predicted to increase the risk of methaemoglobinaemia when given with dapsone. Severe Theoretical

‣ **Mefloquine** is predicted to increase the risk of bradycardia when given with digoxin. Severe Theoretical

‣ **Quinine** increases the concentration of digoxin. Monitor and adjust **digoxin** dose, p. 109. Severe Anecdotal

‣ **Mefloquine** is predicted to increase the risk of QT-prolongation when given with drugs that prolong the QT interval. Severe Theoretical

‣ Efavirenz decreases the concentration of **artemether**. Severe Study → Also see **TABLE 9** p. 1336

‣ Efavirenz moderately decreases the exposure to **atovaquone**. Avoid. Moderate Study

‣ Efavirenz affects the exposure to **proguanil**. Avoid. Moderate Study

‣ Enzalutamide is predicted to decrease the exposure to **artemether** (with lumefantrine). Avoid. Severe Study

‣ Enzalutamide is predicted to decrease the concentration of **piperaquine**. Avoid. Moderate Theoretical

‣ Etravirine decreases the exposure to **artemether**. Moderate Study

‣ Grapefruit juice increases the exposure to **artemether**. Unknown Study

‣ Grapefruit juice is predicted to increase the concentration of **piperaquine**. Severe Theoretical

‣ H_2 receptor antagonists (cimetidine) decrease the clearance of **chloroquine**. Moderate Study

‣ H_2 receptor antagonists (cimetidine) slightly increase the exposure to **quinine**. Moderate Study

‣ HIV-protease inhibitors decrease the exposure to **atovaquone**. Avoid if boosted with ritonavir. Moderate Study

‣ HIV-protease inhibitors are predicted to increase the concentration of **piperaquine**. Severe Theoretical

‣ HIV-protease inhibitors are predicted to decrease the exposure to **proguanil**. Avoid. Moderate Study

‣ HIV-protease inhibitors are predicted to affect the exposure to **quinine**. Severe Study → Also see **TABLE 9** p. 1336

‣ Idelalisib is predicted to increase the concentration of **piperaquine**. Severe Theoretical

‣ Imatinib is predicted to increase the concentration of **piperaquine**. Severe Theoretical

‣ Lanthanum is predicted to decrease the absorption of **chloroquine**. Separate administration by at least 2 hours. Moderate Theoretical

‣ **Chloroquine** is predicted to decrease the exposure to laronidase. Avoid simultaneous administration. Severe Theoretical

‣ Macrolides (clarithromycin, erythromycin) are predicted to increase the concentration of **piperaquine**. Severe Theoretical

‣ Mepacrine is predicted to increase the concentration of **primaquine**. Avoid. Moderate Theoretical

‣ Pyrimethamine is predicted to increase the risk of side-effects when given with methotrexate. Severe Theoretical → Also see **TABLE 15** p. 1337

‣ Metoclopramide decreases the concentration of **atovaquone**. Avoid. Moderate Study

‣ Mitotane is predicted to decrease the exposure to **artemether** (with lumefantrine). Avoid. Severe Study

‣ Mitotane is predicted to decrease the concentration of **piperaquine**. Avoid. Moderate Theoretical

‣ Netupitant is predicted to increase the concentration of **piperaquine**. Severe Theoretical

‣ Nilotinib is predicted to increase the concentration of **piperaquine**. Severe Theoretical

‣ Pyrimethamine is predicted to increase the risk of side-effects when given with pemetrexed. Severe Theoretical → Also see **TABLE 15** p. 1337

‣ **Chloroquine** is predicted to increase the risk of haematological toxicity when given with penicillamine. Avoid. Severe Theoretical

‣ **Chloroquine** moderately decreases the exposure to praziquantel. Use with caution and adjust dose. Moderate Study

‣ **Chloroquine** decreases the efficacy of rabies vaccine. Avoid. Moderate Study

‣ Rifabutin slightly decreases the exposure to **atovaquone**. Avoid. Moderate Study

‣ Rifampicin is predicted to decrease the exposure to **artemether** (with lumefantrine). Avoid. Severe Study

‣ Rifampicin moderately decreases the exposure to **atovaquone** and **atovaquone** slightly increases the exposure to rifampicin. Avoid. Moderate Study

‣ Rifampicin moderately decreases the exposure to **mefloquine**. Severe Study

‣ Rifampicin is predicted to decrease the concentration of **piperaquine**. Avoid. Moderate Theoretical

‣ Rifampicin decreases the exposure to **quinine**. Severe Study

‣ St John's Wort is predicted to decrease the concentration of **piperaquine**. Avoid. Moderate Theoretical

‣ Pyrimethamine increases the risk of side-effects when given with sulfonamides. Severe Study → Also see **TABLE 15** p. 1337

‣ Tetracyclines (tetracycline) decrease the concentration of **atovaquone**. Moderate Study

‣ Pyrimethamine increases the risk of side-effects when given with trimethoprim. Severe Study

‣ Pyrimethamine is predicted to increase the risk of side-effects when given with zidovudine. Severe Theoretical → Also see **TABLE 15** p. 1337

Apixaban → see **TABLE 3** p. 1334 (anticoagulant effects)

‣ Antiarrhythmics (dronedarone) are predicted to increase the exposure to **apixaban**. Moderate Theoretical

‣ Antiepileptics (carbamazepine, fosphenytoin, phenobarbital, phenytoin, primidone) are predicted to moderately decrease the exposure to **apixaban**. Use with caution or avoid. Severe Study

‣ Antifungals, azoles (itraconazole) are predicted to increase the exposure to **apixaban**. Avoid. Severe Theoretical

‣ Antifungals, azoles (ketoconazole) slightly to moderately increase the exposure to **apixaban**. Avoid. Severe Study

‣ Calcium channel blockers (verapamil) are predicted to increase the exposure to **apixaban**. Moderate Theoretical

‣ Enzalutamide is predicted to moderately decrease the exposure to **apixaban**. Use with caution or avoid. Severe Study

‣ HIV-protease inhibitors (ritonavir) are predicted to increase the exposure to **apixaban**. Avoid. Severe Theoretical

‣ Macrolides (clarithromycin) are predicted to increase the exposure to **apixaban**. Severe Theoretical

‣ Macrolides (erythromycin) are predicted to increase the exposure to **apixaban**. Moderate Theoretical

‣ Mitotane is predicted to moderately decrease the exposure to **apixaban**. Use with caution or avoid. Severe Study

‣ Rifampicin is predicted to moderately decrease the exposure to **apixaban**. Use with caution or avoid. Severe Study

‣ St John's Wort is predicted to decrease the exposure to **apixaban**. Use with caution or avoid. Moderate Theoretical

Apomorphine → see dopamine receptor agonists

Apraclonidine → see TABLE 6 p. 1335 (bradycardia), TABLE 8 p. 1335 (hypotension), TABLE 11 p. 1336 (CNS depressant effects)
▸ Amfetamines are predicted to decrease the effects of **apraclonidine**. Avoid. [Severe] Theoretical
▸ Methylphenidate is predicted to decrease the effects of **apraclonidine**. Avoid. [Severe] Theoretical
▸ Sympathomimetics, inotropic are predicted to decrease the effects of **apraclonidine**. Avoid. [Severe] Theoretical
▸ Sympathomimetics, vasoconstrictor are predicted to decrease the effects of **apraclonidine**. Avoid. [Severe] Theoretical

Apremilast
▸ Antiepileptics (carbamazepine, fosphenytoin, phenobarbital, phenytoin, primidone) moderately decrease the exposure to **apremilast**. Avoid. [Severe] Study
▸ Enzalutamide moderately decreases the exposure to **apremilast**. Avoid. [Severe] Study
▸ Mitotane moderately decreases the exposure to **apremilast**. Avoid. [Severe] Study
▸ Rifampicin moderately decreases the exposure to **apremilast**. Avoid. [Severe] Study
▸ St John's Wort is predicted to decrease the exposure to **apremilast**. Avoid. [Severe] Theoretical

Aprepitant
▸ **Aprepitant** is predicted to increase the exposure to aldosterone antagonists (eplerenone). Adjust **eplerenone** dose, p. 190. [Severe] Study
▸ **Aprepitant** is predicted to increase the exposure to alpha blockers (tamsulosin). [Moderate] Theoretical
▸ **Aprepitant** is predicted to increase the exposure to alprazolam. [Severe] Study
▸ **Aprepitant** increases the exposure to antiarrhythmics (dronedarone). [Severe] Theoretical
▸ **Aprepitant** is predicted to increase the exposure to antiarrhythmics (propafenone). Monitor and adjust dose. [Moderate] Study
▸ Antiepileptics (carbamazepine, fosphenytoin, phenobarbital, phenytoin, primidone) are predicted to markedly decrease the exposure to **aprepitant**. Avoid. [Moderate] Study
▸ Antifungals, azoles (itraconazole, ketoconazole, voriconazole) are predicted to markedly increase the exposure to **aprepitant**. [Moderate] Study
▸ **Aprepitant** is predicted to increase the exposure to antifungals, azoles (isavuconazole). [Moderate] Theoretical
▸ **Aprepitant** is predicted to increase the exposure to antihistamines, non-sedating (mizolastine). [Severe] Theoretical
▸ **Aprepitant** is predicted to increase the exposure to antihistamines, non-sedating (rupatadine). Avoid. [Moderate] Study
▸ **Aprepitant** is predicted to increase the concentration of antimalarials (piperaquine). [Severe] Theoretical
▸ **Aprepitant** is predicted to increase the exposure to axitinib. [Moderate] Theoretical
▸ **Aprepitant** is predicted to increase the exposure to bedaquiline. Avoid prolonged use. [Mild] Theoretical
▸ **Aprepitant** is predicted to increase the exposure to bosutinib. Avoid or adjust dose. [Severe] Theoretical
▸ **Aprepitant** is predicted to increase the exposure to buspirone. Use with caution and adjust dose. [Moderate] Study
▸ **Aprepitant** is predicted to increase the exposure to cabozantinib. [Moderate] Theoretical
▸ Calcium channel blockers (diltiazem, verapamil) are predicted to increase the exposure to **aprepitant** and **aprepitant** is predicted to increase the exposure to calcium channel blockers (diltiazem, verapamil). [Moderate] Study
▸ **Aprepitant** is predicted to increase the exposure to calcium channel blockers (amlodipine, felodipine, lacidipine, lercanidipine, nicardipine, nifedipine, nimodipine). Monitor and adjust dose. [Moderate] Study
▸ **Aprepitant** is predicted to increase the exposure to ceritinib. [Moderate] Theoretical
▸ **Aprepitant** increases the concentration of ciclosporin. [Severe] Study
▸ Cobicistat is predicted to markedly increase the exposure to **aprepitant**. [Moderate] Study
▸ **Aprepitant** is predicted to increase the exposure to cobimetinib. [Severe] Theoretical

▸ **Aprepitant** is predicted to increase the exposure to colchicine. Adjust **colchicine** dose with moderate inhibitors of CYP3A4, p. 1085. [Severe] Study
▸ **Aprepitant** is predicted to decrease the efficacy of combined hormonal contraceptives. For FSRH guidance, see Contraceptives, interactions p. 775. [Severe] Study
▸ **Aprepitant** moderately increases the exposure to corticosteroids (dexamethasone). Monitor and adjust dose. [Moderate] Study
▸ **Aprepitant** is predicted to increase the exposure to corticosteroids (methylprednisolone). Monitor and adjust dose. [Moderate] Study
▸ **Aprepitant** decreases the anticoagulant effect of coumarins. [Moderate] Study
▸ **Aprepitant** is predicted to slightly increase the exposure to darifenacin. [Moderate] Study
▸ **Aprepitant** is predicted to increase the exposure to dasatinib. [Severe] Study
▸ **Aprepitant** is predicted to decrease the efficacy of desogestrel. For FSRH guidance, see Contraceptives, interactions p. 775. [Severe] Theoretical
▸ **Aprepitant** increases the risk of QT-prolongation when given with domperidone. Avoid. [Severe] Study
▸ **Aprepitant** is predicted to increase the exposure to dopamine receptor agonists (bromocriptine). [Severe] Theoretical
▸ **Aprepitant** is predicted to increase the concentration of dopamine receptor agonists (cabergoline). [Moderate] Anecdotal
▸ **Aprepitant** is predicted to moderately increase the exposure to dutasteride. [Mild] Study
▸ **Aprepitant** is predicted to increase the exposure to eliglustat. Avoid or adjust dose—consult product literature. [Severe] Study
▸ Enzalutamide is predicted to markedly decrease the exposure to **aprepitant**. Avoid. [Moderate] Study
▸ **Aprepitant** is predicted to increase the risk of ergotism when given with ergometrine. [Severe] Theoretical
▸ **Aprepitant** is predicted to increase the risk of ergotism when given with ergotamine. [Severe] Theoretical
▸ **Aprepitant** is predicted to increase the exposure to erlotinib. [Moderate] Theoretical
▸ **Aprepitant** is predicted to decrease the efficacy of etonogestrel. For FSRH guidance, see Contraceptives, interactions p. 775. [Severe] Theoretical
▸ **Aprepitant** is predicted to increase the concentration of everolimus. Avoid or adjust dose. [Moderate] Study
▸ **Aprepitant** is predicted to increase the exposure to fesoterodine. Adjust **fesoterodine** dose with moderate inhibitors of CYP3A4 in hepatic and renal impairment, p. 759. [Mild] Study
▸ **Aprepitant** is predicted to increase the exposure to gefitinib. [Moderate] Theoretical
▸ **Aprepitant** is predicted to increase the concentration of guanfacine. Adjust **guanfacine** dose, p. 349. [Moderate] Theoretical
▸ HIV-protease inhibitors are predicted to markedly increase the exposure to **aprepitant**. [Moderate] Study
▸ **Aprepitant** is predicted to decrease the effects of hormone replacement therapy. [Moderate] Anecdotal
▸ **Aprepitant** is predicted to increase the exposure to ibrutinib. Adjust **ibrutinib** dose with moderate inhibitors of CYP3A4, p. 952. [Severe] Study
▸ Idelalisib is predicted to markedly increase the exposure to **aprepitant**. [Moderate] Study
▸ **Aprepitant** is predicted to increase the exposure to imatinib. [Moderate] Theoretical
▸ **Aprepitant** is predicted to increase the exposure to ivabradine. Adjust **ivabradine** dose, p. 210. [Severe] Theoretical
▸ **Aprepitant** is predicted to increase the exposure to ivacaftor. Adjust **ivacaftor** dose with moderate inhibitors of CYP3A4, p. 292. [Severe] Study
▸ **Aprepitant** is predicted to increase the exposure to lapatinib. [Moderate] Study
▸ **Aprepitant** is predicted to decrease the efficacy of levonorgestrel. For FSRH guidance, see Contraceptives, interactions p. 775. [Severe] Theoretical
▸ **Aprepitant** is predicted to increase the exposure to lomitapide. Avoid. [Moderate] Theoretical

Aprepitant (continued)
▸ **Aprepitant** is predicted to increase the exposure to lurasidone. Moderate Study
▸ **Macrolides** (clarithromycin) are predicted to markedly increase the exposure to **aprepitant**. Moderate Study
▸ **Aprepitant** is predicted to increase the exposure to midazolam. Monitor side effects and adjust dose. Severe Study
▸ **Aprepitant** is predicted to increase the exposure to midostaurin. Moderate Theoretical
▸ **Mitotane** is predicted to markedly decrease the exposure to **aprepitant**. Avoid. Moderate Study
▸ **Aprepitant** is predicted to increase the exposure to naloxegol. Adjust **naloxegol** dose and monitor side effects, p. 64. Moderate Study
▸ **Aprepitant** is predicted to increase the exposure to nilotinib. Moderate Theoretical
▸ **Aprepitant** is predicted to decrease the efficacy of norethisterone. For FSRH guidance, see Contraceptives, interactions p. 775. Severe Anecdotal
▸ **Aprepitant** is predicted to increase the exposure to olaparib. Avoid moderate inhibitors of CYP3A4 or adjust **olaparib** dose, p. 973. Moderate Theoretical
▸ **Aprepitant** is predicted to increase the exposure to opioids (alfentanil, buprenorphine, fentanyl, oxycodone). Monitor and adjust dose. Moderate Study
▸ **Aprepitant** is predicted to increase the exposure to opioids (methadone, sufentanil). Moderate Theoretical
▸ **Aprepitant** is predicted to increase the exposure to oxybutynin. Mild Theoretical
▸ **Aprepitant** is predicted to increase the exposure to pazopanib. Moderate Theoretical
▸ **Aprepitant** is predicted to increase the exposure to phosphodiesterase type-5 inhibitors (avanafil). Adjust **avanafil** dose, p. 794. Moderate Theoretical
▸ **Aprepitant** is predicted to increase the exposure to phosphodiesterase type-5 inhibitors (sildenafil). Monitor or adjust **sildenafil** dose with moderate inhibitors of CYP3A4, p. 794. Moderate Study
▸ **Aprepitant** is predicted to increase the exposure to phosphodiesterase type-5 inhibitors (tadalafil). Severe Theoretical
▸ **Aprepitant** is predicted to increase the exposure to phosphodiesterase type-5 inhibitors (vardenafil). Adjust dose. Severe Theoretical
▸ **Aprepitant** is predicted to increase the exposure to pimozide. Avoid. Severe Theoretical
▸ **Aprepitant** is predicted to increase the exposure to quetiapine. Avoid. Moderate Study
▸ **Aprepitant** is predicted to increase the exposure to ranolazine. Severe Study
▸ **Aprepitant** is predicted to increase the exposure to ribociclib. Moderate Study
▸ **Rifampicin** is predicted to markedly decrease the exposure to **aprepitant**. Avoid. Moderate Study
▸ **Aprepitant** is predicted to increase the exposure to ruxolitinib. Moderate Theoretical
▸ **Aprepitant** is predicted to increase the exposure to saxagliptin. Mild Study
▸ **Aprepitant** is predicted to increase the exposure to simeprevir. Avoid. Severe Study
▸ **Aprepitant** increases the concentration of sirolimus. Monitor and adjust dose. Moderate Study
▸ **Aprepitant** is predicted to increase the exposure to SSRIs (dapoxetine). Adjust **dapoxetine** dose with moderate inhibitors of CYP3A4, p. 801. Moderate Theoretical
▸ **St John's Wort** is predicted to decrease the exposure to **aprepitant**. Avoid. Moderate Theoretical
▸ **Aprepitant** is predicted to increase the exposure to statins (atorvastatin). Monitor and adjust dose. Severe Study
▸ **Aprepitant** is predicted to increase the exposure to statins (simvastatin). Use with caution and adjust **simvastatin** dose, p. 203. Severe Study
▸ **Aprepitant** is predicted to increase the exposure to sunitinib. Moderate Theoretical
▸ **Aprepitant** is predicted to increase the concentration of tacrolimus. Severe Study

▸ **Aprepitant** is predicted to increase the exposure to taxanes (cabazitaxel). Moderate Theoretical
▸ **Aprepitant** is predicted to increase the concentration of temsirolimus. Moderate Theoretical
▸ **Aprepitant** is predicted to increase the exposure to tofacitinib. Moderate Study
▸ **Aprepitant** is predicted to increase the exposure to tolterodine. Mild Theoretical
▸ **Aprepitant** is predicted to increase the exposure to tolvaptan. Adjust dose. Moderate Study
▸ **Aprepitant** is predicted to increase the exposure to trazodone. Moderate Theoretical
▸ **Aprepitant** decreases the efficacy of ulipristal. For FSRH guidance, see Contraceptives, interactions p. 775. Severe Anecdotal
▸ **Aprepitant** is predicted to increase the exposure to venetoclax. Avoid moderate inhibitors of CYP3A4 or adjust **venetoclax** dose, p. 974. Severe Study
▸ **Aprepitant** is predicted to increase the exposure to vinca alkaloids. Severe Theoretical
▸ **Aprepitant** is predicted to increase the exposure to zopiclone. Adjust dose. Moderate Study

Argatroban → see TABLE 3 p. 1334 (anticoagulant effects)
▸ **Ranibizumab** is predicted to increase the risk of bleeding events when given with **argatroban**. Severe Theoretical

Aripiprazole → see TABLE 8 p. 1335 (hypotension), TABLE 11 p. 1336 (CNS depressant effects)
▸ **Antiepileptics** (carbamazepine, fosphenytoin, phenobarbital, phenytoin, primidone) are predicted to moderately decrease the exposure to **aripiprazole**. Adjust **aripiprazole** dose, p. 391. Moderate Study → Also see TABLE 11 p. 1336
▸ **Antifungals, azoles** (itraconazole, ketoconazole, voriconazole) are predicted to slightly increase the exposure to **aripiprazole**. Adjust **aripiprazole** dose, p. 391. Moderate Study
▸ **Bupropion** is predicted to moderately increase the exposure to **aripiprazole**. Adjust **aripiprazole** dose, p. 391. Moderate Study
▸ **Cinacalcet** is predicted to moderately increase the exposure to **aripiprazole**. Adjust **aripiprazole** dose, p. 391. Moderate Study
▸ **Cobicistat** is predicted to slightly increase the exposure to **aripiprazole**. Adjust **aripiprazole** dose, p. 391. Moderate Study
▸ **Aripiprazole** is predicted to decrease the effects of dopamine receptor agonists. Moderate Theoretical → Also see TABLE 8 p. 1335
▸ **Enzalutamide** is predicted to moderately decrease the exposure to **aripiprazole**. Adjust **aripiprazole** dose, p. 391. Moderate Study
▸ **HIV-protease inhibitors** are predicted to slightly increase the exposure to **aripiprazole**. Adjust **aripiprazole** dose, p. 391. Moderate Study
▸ **Idelalisib** is predicted to slightly increase the exposure to **aripiprazole**. Adjust **aripiprazole** dose, p. 391. Moderate Study
▸ **Aripiprazole** is predicted to decrease the effects of levodopa. Severe Theoretical → Also see TABLE 8 p. 1335
▸ **Macrolides** (clarithromycin) are predicted to slightly increase the exposure to **aripiprazole**. Adjust **aripiprazole** dose, p. 391. Moderate Study
▸ **Mitotane** is predicted to moderately decrease the exposure to **aripiprazole**. Adjust **aripiprazole** dose, p. 391. Moderate Study
▸ **Rifampicin** is predicted to moderately decrease the exposure to **aripiprazole**. Adjust **aripiprazole** dose, p. 391. Moderate Study
▸ **SSRIs** (fluoxetine, paroxetine) are predicted to moderately increase the exposure to **aripiprazole**. Adjust **aripiprazole** dose, p. 391. Moderate Study
▸ **Terbinafine** is predicted to moderately increase the exposure to **aripiprazole**. Adjust **aripiprazole** dose, p. 391. Moderate Study

Arsenic trioxide → see TABLE 15 p. 1337 (myelosuppression), TABLE 9 p. 1336 (QT-interval prolongation)
Artemether → see antimalarials
Artenimol → see antimalarials
Articaine → see TABLE 11 p. 1336 (CNS depressant effects)
Ascorbic acid
▸ **Ascorbic acid** is predicted to increase the risk of cardiovascular side-effects when given with deferiprone. Severe Theoretical
▸ **Ascorbic acid** is predicted to increase the risk of cardiovascular side-effects when given with iron chelators (desferrioxamine). Severe Theoretical

Asenapine → see **TABLE 8** p. 1335 (hypotension), **TABLE 11** p. 1336 (CNS depressant effects)
- **Asenapine** is predicted to decrease the effects of dopamine receptor agonists. Adjust dose. Moderate Theoretical → Also see **TABLE 8** p. 1335
- **Asenapine** is predicted to decrease the effects of levodopa. Adjust dose. Severe Theoretical → Also see **TABLE 8** p. 1335
- SSRIs (fluvoxamine) increase the exposure to **asenapine**. Moderate Study
- SSRIs (paroxetine) moderately increase the exposure to **asenapine**. Moderate Study

Asparaginase → see **TABLE 1** p. 1334 (hepatotoxicity), **TABLE 15** p. 1337 (myelosuppression)
- **Asparaginase** is predicted to increase the risk of hepatotoxicity when given with imatinib. Severe Theoretical → Also see **TABLE 15** p. 1337
- **Asparaginase** affects the efficacy of methotrexate. Severe Anecdotal → Also see **TABLE 1** p. 1334 → Also see **TABLE 15** p. 1337
- **Asparaginase** potentially increases the risk of neurotoxicity when given with vinca alkaloids (vincristine). **Vincristine** should be taken 3 to 24 hours before **asparaginase**, p. 908. Severe Anecdotal → Also see **TABLE 1** p. 1334 → Also see **TABLE 15** p. 1337

Aspirin → see **TABLE 4** p. 1334 (antiplatelet effects)
- Acetazolamide increases the risk of severe toxic reaction when given with **aspirin** (high-dose). Severe Study
- Antacids decrease the absorption of **aspirin** (high-dose). Moderate Study
- **Aspirin** (high-dose) is predicted to increase the risk of gastrointestinal irritation when given with bisphosphonates (alendronic acid, ibandronic acid). Moderate Study
- **Aspirin** (high-dose) is predicted to increase the risk of renal impairment when given with bisphosphonates (sodium clodronate). Severe Theoretical
- Corticosteroids are predicted to decrease the concentration of **aspirin** (high-dose) and **aspirin** (high-dose) increases the risk of gastrointestinal bleeding when given with corticosteroids. Moderate Study
- **Aspirin** (high-dose) increases the risk of renal impairment when given with daptomycin. Moderate Theoretical
- Erlotinib is predicted to increase the risk of gastrointestinal perforation when given with **aspirin** (high-dose). Severe Theoretical
- **Aspirin** (high-dose) is predicted to increase the risk of gastrointestinal bleeds when given with iron chelators (deferasirox). Severe Theoretical
- **Aspirin** (high-dose) is predicted to increase the risk of toxicity when given with methotrexate. Severe Theoretical
- **Aspirin** is predicted to increase the risk of gastrointestinal perforation when given with nicorandil. Severe Theoretical
- **Aspirin** (high-dose) potentially increases the exposure to pemetrexed. Use with caution or avoid. Severe Theoretical
- **Aspirin** decreases the effects of sulfinpyrazone. Moderate Study → Also see **TABLE 4** p. 1334
- **Aspirin** (high-dose) increases the risk of acute renal failure when given with thiazide diuretics. Severe Theoretical
- Zidovudine increases the risk of haematological toxicity when given with **aspirin** (high-dose). Severe Study

Ataluren
- Ataluren increases the exposure to adefovir. Moderate Study
- Ataluren is predicted to increase the risk of nephrotoxicity when given with intravenous aminoglycosides. Avoid. Severe Study
- Rifampicin decreases the exposure to ataluren. Moderate Study

Atazanavir → see HIV-protease inhibitors

Atenolol → see beta blockers, selective

Atezolizumab → see monoclonal antibodies

Atomoxetine
- Amfetamines are predicted to increase the risk of side-effects when given with **atomoxetine**. Severe Theoretical
- **Atomoxetine** is predicted to increase the risk of cardiovascular side-effects when given with beta$_2$ agonists (high-dose). Moderate Study
- Bupropion is predicted to markedly increase the exposure to **atomoxetine**. Adjust dose. Severe Study

- Cinacalcet is predicted to markedly increase the exposure to **atomoxetine**. Adjust dose. Severe Study
- Eliglustat is predicted to increase the exposure to **atomoxetine**. Adjust dose. Moderate Theoretical
- Monoamine-oxidase A and B inhibitors, irreversible are predicted to increase the risk of side-effects when given with **atomoxetine**. Avoid and for 2 weeks after stopping the MAOI. Severe Theoretical
- Panobinostat is predicted to increase the exposure to **atomoxetine**. Monitor and adjust dose. Severe Theoretical
- SSRIs (fluoxetine, paroxetine) are predicted to markedly increase the exposure to **atomoxetine**. Adjust dose. Severe Study
- Terbinafine is predicted to markedly increase the exposure to **atomoxetine**. Adjust dose. Severe Study

Atorvastatin → see statins

Atovaquone → see antimalarials

Atracurium → see neuromuscular blocking drugs, non-depolarising

Atropine → see **TABLE 10** p. 1336 (antimuscarinics)
- **Atropine** increases the risk of severe hypertension when given with sympathomimetics, vasoconstrictor (phenylephrine). Severe Study

Avanafil → see phosphodiesterase type-5 inhibitors

Avelumab → see monoclonal antibodies

Axitinib → see **TABLE 15** p. 1337 (myelosuppression)
- Antiarrhythmics (dronedarone) are predicted to increase the exposure to **axitinib**. Moderate Theoretical
- Antiepileptics (carbamazepine, fosphenytoin, phenobarbital, phenytoin, primidone) are predicted to decrease the exposure to **axitinib**. Avoid or adjust dose. Moderate Study
- Antifungals, azoles (fluconazole, isavuconazole, posaconazole) are predicted to increase the exposure to **axitinib**. Moderate Theoretical
- Antifungals, azoles (itraconazole, ketoconazole, voriconazole) are predicted to increase the exposure to **axitinib**. Avoid or adjust dose. Moderate Study
- Aprepitant is predicted to increase the exposure to **axitinib**. Moderate Theoretical
- Bosentan is predicted to decrease the exposure to **axitinib**. Moderate Theoretical
- Calcium channel blockers (diltiazem, verapamil) are predicted to increase the exposure to **axitinib**. Moderate Theoretical
- Cobicistat is predicted to increase the exposure to **axitinib**. Avoid or adjust dose. Moderate Study
- **Axitinib** is predicted to increase the risk of bleeding events when given with coumarins. Severe Theoretical
- Crizotinib is predicted to increase the exposure to **axitinib**. Moderate Theoretical → Also see **TABLE 15** p. 1337
- Efavirenz is predicted to decrease the exposure to **axitinib**. Moderate Theoretical
- Enzalutamide is predicted to decrease the exposure to **axitinib**. Avoid or adjust dose. Moderate Study
- Grapefruit juice is predicted to increase the exposure to **axitinib**. Moderate Theoretical
- HIV-protease inhibitors are predicted to increase the exposure to **axitinib**. Avoid or adjust dose. Moderate Study
- Idelalisib is predicted to increase the exposure to **axitinib**. Avoid or adjust dose. Moderate Study → Also see **TABLE 15** p. 1337
- Imatinib is predicted to increase the exposure to **axitinib**. Moderate Theoretical → Also see **TABLE 15** p. 1337
- Macrolides (clarithromycin) are predicted to increase the exposure to **axitinib**. Avoid or adjust dose. Moderate Study
- Macrolides (erythromycin) are predicted to increase the exposure to **axitinib**. Moderate Theoretical
- Mitotane is predicted to decrease the exposure to **axitinib**. Avoid or adjust dose. Moderate Study → Also see **TABLE 15** p. 1337
- Netupitant is predicted to increase the exposure to **axitinib**. Moderate Theoretical
- Nevirapine is predicted to decrease the exposure to **axitinib**. Moderate Theoretical
- Nilotinib is predicted to increase the exposure to **axitinib**. Moderate Theoretical → Also see **TABLE 15** p. 1337
- **Axitinib** is predicted to increase the risk of bleeding events when given with phenindione. Severe Theoretical

Axitinib (continued)
- Rifampicin is predicted to decrease the exposure to **axitinib**. Avoid or adjust dose. Moderate Study
- St John's Wort is predicted to decrease the exposure to **axitinib**. Moderate Theoretical

Azacitidine → see TABLE 15 p. 1337 (myelosuppression)

Azathioprine → see TABLE 15 p. 1337 (myelosuppression)
- ACE inhibitors are predicted to increase the risk of anaemia and/or leucopenia when given with **azathioprine**. Severe Anecdotal
- Allopurinol potentially increases the risk of haematological toxicity when given with **azathioprine**. Adjust **azathioprine** dose, p. 816. Severe Study
- **Azathioprine** decreases the anticoagulant effect of coumarins. Moderate Study
- Febuxostat is predicted to increase the exposure to **azathioprine**. Avoid. Severe Theoretical
- Live vaccines are predicted to increase the risk of generalised infection (possibly life-threatening) when given with **azathioprine** (high-dose). Public Health England advises avoid (refer to Green Book). Severe Theoretical

Azelastine → see antihistamines, non-sedating

Azilsartan → see angiotensin-II receptor antagonists

Azithromycin → see macrolides

Bacillus Calmette-Guérin vaccine → see live vaccines

Bacitracin → see TABLE 2 p. 1334 (nephrotoxicity)

Baclofen → see TABLE 8 p. 1335 (hypotension), TABLE 11 p. 1336 (CNS depressant effects), TABLE 10 p. 1336 (antimuscarinics)
- **Baclofen** is predicted to increase the risk of side-effects when given with levodopa. Severe Anecdotal → Also see TABLE 8 p. 1335

Balsalazide → see TABLE 15 p. 1337 (myelosuppression)
- **Balsalazide** is predicted to decrease the concentration of digoxin. Moderate Theoretical

Bambuterol → see beta₂ agonists

Baricitinib
- Leflunomide potentially increases the exposure to **baricitinib**. Moderate Theoretical
- Live vaccines are predicted to increase the risk of generalised infection (possibly life-threatening) when given with **baricitinib**. Avoid. Severe Theoretical
- Teriflunomide potentially increases the exposure to **baricitinib**. Moderate Theoretical

Basiliximab → see monoclonal antibodies

Bazedoxifene
- Antiepileptics (carbamazepine, fosphenytoin, phenobarbital, phenytoin, primidone) are predicted to decrease the exposure to **bazedoxifene**. Moderate Theoretical
- Rifampicin is predicted to decrease the exposure to **bazedoxifene**. Moderate Theoretical

Beclometasone → see corticosteroids

Bedaquiline → see TABLE 9 p. 1336 (QT-interval prolongation)
- Antiarrhythmics (dronedarone) are predicted to increase the exposure to **bedaquiline**. Avoid prolonged use. Mild Theoretical → Also see TABLE 9 p. 1336
- Antiepileptics (carbamazepine, fosphenytoin, phenobarbital, phenytoin, primidone) decrease the exposure to **bedaquiline**. Avoid. Severe Study
- Antifungals, azoles (fluconazole, isavuconazole, posaconazole) are predicted to increase the exposure to **bedaquiline**. Avoid prolonged use. Mild Theoretical → Also see TABLE 9 p. 1336
- Antifungals, azoles (itraconazole, ketoconazole, voriconazole) are predicted to increase the exposure to **bedaquiline**. Avoid prolonged use. Mild Study → Also see TABLE 9 p. 1336
- Aprepitant is predicted to increase the exposure to **bedaquiline**. Avoid prolonged use. Mild Theoretical
- Bosentan is predicted to decrease the exposure to **bedaquiline**. Avoid. Severe Study
- Calcium channel blockers (diltiazem, verapamil) are predicted to increase the exposure to **bedaquiline**. Avoid prolonged use. Mild Theoretical
- Clofazimine potentially increases the risk of QT-prolongation when given with **bedaquiline**. Severe Study
- Cobicistat is predicted to increase the exposure to **bedaquiline**. Avoid prolonged use. Mild Study

- Crizotinib is predicted to increase the exposure to **bedaquiline**. Avoid prolonged use. Mild Theoretical → Also see TABLE 9 p. 1336
- Efavirenz is predicted to decrease the exposure to **bedaquiline**. Avoid. Severe Study → Also see TABLE 9 p. 1336
- Enzalutamide decreases the exposure to **bedaquiline**. Avoid. Severe Study
- Etravirine is predicted to increase the exposure to **bedaquiline**. Avoid. Severe Theoretical
- HIV-protease inhibitors are predicted to increase the exposure to **bedaquiline**. Avoid prolonged use. Mild Study → Also see TABLE 9 p. 1336
- Idelalisib is predicted to increase the exposure to **bedaquiline**. Avoid prolonged use. Mild Study
- Imatinib is predicted to increase the exposure to **bedaquiline**. Avoid prolonged use. Mild Theoretical
- Macrolides (clarithromycin) are predicted to increase the exposure to **bedaquiline**. Avoid prolonged use. Mild Study → Also see TABLE 9 p. 1336
- Macrolides (erythromycin) are predicted to increase the exposure to **bedaquiline**. Avoid prolonged use. Mild Theoretical → Also see TABLE 9 p. 1336
- Mitotane decreases the exposure to **bedaquiline**. Avoid. Severe Study
- Netupitant is predicted to increase the exposure to **bedaquiline**. Avoid prolonged use. Mild Theoretical
- Nevirapine is predicted to decrease the exposure to **bedaquiline**. Avoid. Severe Study
- Nilotinib is predicted to increase the exposure to **bedaquiline**. Avoid prolonged use. Mild Theoretical → Also see TABLE 9 p. 1336
- Rifampicin decreases the exposure to **bedaquiline**. Avoid. Severe Study
- St John's Wort is predicted to decrease the exposure to **bedaquiline**. Avoid. Severe Study

Bee venom extract

GENERAL INFORMATION Desensitising vaccines should be avoided in patients taking beta-blockers (adrenaline might be ineffective in case of a hypersensitivity reaction) or ACE inhibitors (risk of severe anaphylactoid reactions).

Belatacept
- Live vaccines are predicted to increase the risk of generalised infection (possibly life-threatening) when given with **belatacept**. Public Health England advises avoid (refer to Green Book). Severe Theoretical

Belimumab → see monoclonal antibodies

Bendamustine → see alkylating agents

Bendroflumethiazide → see thiazide diuretics

Benperidol → see TABLE 8 p. 1335 (hypotension), TABLE 11 p. 1336 (CNS depressant effects)
- **Benperidol** is predicted to decrease the effects of dopamine receptor agonists. Avoid. Moderate Theoretical → Also see TABLE 8 p. 1335
- **Benperidol** is predicted to decrease the effects of guanethidine. Moderate Theoretical → Also see TABLE 8 p. 1335
- **Benperidol** is predicted to decrease the effects of levodopa. Severe Study → Also see TABLE 8 p. 1335

Benralizumab → see monoclonal antibodies

Benzydamine → see NSAIDs

Benzylpenicillin → see penicillins

Beta blockers, non-selective → see TABLE 6 p. 1335 (bradycardia), TABLE 8 p. 1335 (hypotension), TABLE 9 p. 1336 (QT-interval prolongation)

carvedilol · labetalol · levobunolol · nadolol · oxprenolol · pindolol · propranolol · sotalol · timolol

ROUTE-SPECIFIC INFORMATION Since systemic absorption can follow topical application of **levobunolol**, and **timolol**, the possibility of interactions should be borne in mind.

- **Beta blockers, non-selective** are predicted to increase the risk of bronchospasm when given with aminophylline. Avoid. Severe Theoretical
- Antiarrhythmics (amiodarone, disopyramide, dronedarone, flecainide, lidocaine) are predicted to increase the risk of cardiovascular side-effects when given with **beta blockers, non-selective**. Use with caution or avoid. Severe Study → Also see TABLE 6 p. 1335 → Also see TABLE 9 p. 1336

▶ Antiarrhythmics (propafenone) increase the risk of cardiovascular side-effects when given with **propranolol**. Use with caution or avoid. [Severe] Study

▶ Antiarrhythmics (propafenone) are predicted to increase the exposure to **timolol** and **timolol** is predicted to increase the risk of cardiodepression when given with antiarrhythmics (propafenone). [Severe] Anecdotal

▶ Antiarrhythmics (propafenone) are predicted to increase the risk of cardiovascular side-effects when given with beta blockers, non-selective (**labetalol, levobunolol, nadolol, oxprenolol, pindolol, sotalol**). Use with caution or avoid. [Severe] Study

▶ Anticholinesterases, centrally acting are predicted to increase the risk of bradycardia when given with beta blockers, non-selective. [Moderate] Anecdotal → Also see TABLE 6 p. 1335

▶ Antiepileptics (phenobarbital, primidone) are predicted to decrease the exposure to **propranolol**. [Moderate] Study

▶ Antiepileptics (phenobarbital, primidone) are predicted to decrease the exposure to beta blockers, non-selective (**carvedilol, labetalol**). [Moderate] Theoretical

▶ Antifungals, azoles (itraconazole, ketoconazole) are predicted to increase the exposure to **nadolol**. [Moderate] Study

▶ Antimalarials (mefloquine) are predicted to increase the risk of bradycardia when given with beta blockers, non-selective. [Severe] Theoretical

▶ Calcium channel blockers (diltiazem) are predicted to increase the risk of cardiodepression when given with beta blockers, non-selective. [Severe] Study → Also see TABLE 6 p. 1335 → Also see TABLE 8 p. 1335

▶ Intravenous calcium channel blockers (verapamil) increase the risk of cardiovascular side-effects when given with beta blockers, non-selective. Avoid. [Severe] Study → Also see TABLE 6 p. 1335 → Also see TABLE 8 p. 1335

▶ Oral calcium channel blockers (verapamil) increase the risk of cardiovascular side-effects when given with beta blockers, non-selective. [Severe] Study → Also see TABLE 6 p. 1335 → Also see TABLE 8 p. 1335

▶ Ciclosporin is predicted to increase the exposure to **nadolol**. [Moderate] Study

▶ Eliglustat is predicted to increase the exposure to **propranolol**. Adjust dose. [Moderate] Study

▶ **Beta blockers, non-selective** are predicted to increase the risk of peripheral vasoconstriction when given with ergometrine. [Severe] Study

▶ **Beta blockers, non-selective** are predicted to increase the risk of peripheral vasoconstriction when given with ergotamine. [Severe] Study

▶ HIV-protease inhibitors (lopinavir, ritonavir, saquinavir) are predicted to increase the exposure to **nadolol**. [Moderate] Study

▶ **Beta blockers, non-selective** are predicted to increase the risk of bradycardia when given with lanreotide. [Moderate] Theoretical

▶ Lapatinib is predicted to increase the exposure to **nadolol**. [Moderate] Study

▶ Macrolides are predicted to increase the exposure to **nadolol**. [Moderate] Study

▶ Ranolazine is predicted to increase the exposure to **nadolol**. [Moderate] Study

▶ Rifampicin moderately decreases the exposure to **carvedilol**. [Moderate] Study

▶ Rifampicin decreases the exposure to **propranolol**. Monitor and adjust dose. [Moderate] Study

▶ **Propranolol** slightly to moderately increases the exposure to **rizatriptan**. Adjust rizatriptan dose and separate administration by at least 2 hours. [Moderate] Study

▶ SSRIs (fluvoxamine) moderately increase the concentration of **propranolol**. [Moderate] Study

▶ **Beta blockers, non-selective** increase the risk of hypertension and bradycardia when given with sympathomimetics, inotropic (dobutamine). [Severe] Theoretical

▶ **Beta blockers, non-selective** are predicted to increase the risk of hypertension and bradycardia when given with sympathomimetics, vasoconstrictor (adrenaline/epinephrine, noradrenaline/norepinephrine). [Severe] Study

▶ **Beta blockers, non-selective** are predicted to increase the risk of bronchospasm when given with theophylline. Avoid. [Severe] Theoretical

▶ Vemurafenib is predicted to increase the exposure to **nadolol**. [Moderate] Study

Beta blockers, selective → see TABLE 6 p. 1335 (bradycardia), TABLE 8 p. 1335 (hypotension)

acebutolol · atenolol · betaxolol · bisoprolol · celiprolol · esmolol · metoprolol · nebivolol

▶ Since systemic absorption can follow topical application of **betaxolol**, the possibility of interactions should be borne in mind.

▶ Orange juice greatly decreases the exposure to **celiprolol**.

▶ Abiraterone is predicted to increase the exposure to **metoprolol**. [Moderate] Study

▶ **Beta blockers, selective** are predicted to increase the risk of bronchospasm when given with aminophylline. Avoid. [Severe] Theoretical

▶ Antiarrhythmics (amiodarone, disopyramide, dronedarone, flecainide, lidocaine) are predicted to increase the risk of cardiovascular side-effects when given with beta blockers, selective. Use with caution or avoid. [Severe] Study → Also see TABLE 6 p. 1335

▶ Antiarrhythmics (propafenone) are predicted to increase the exposure to **metoprolol**. [Moderate] Study

▶ Antiarrhythmics (propafenone) are predicted to increase the exposure to **nebivolol** and **nebivolol** is predicted to increase the risk of cardiodepression when given with antiarrhythmics (propafenone). Avoid. [Severe] Theoretical

▶ Antiarrhythmics (propafenone) are predicted to increase the risk of cardiovascular side-effects when given with beta blockers, selective (**acebutolol, atenolol, betaxolol, bisoprolol, celiprolol, esmolol**). Use with caution or avoid. [Severe] Study

▶ Anticholinesterases, centrally acting are predicted to increase the risk of bradycardia when given with beta blockers, selective. [Moderate] Anecdotal → Also see TABLE 6 p. 1335

▶ Antiepileptics (phenobarbital, primidone) are predicted to decrease the exposure to beta blockers, selective (**acebutolol, bisoprolol, metoprolol, nebivolol**). [Moderate] Study

▶ Antimalarials (mefloquine) are predicted to increase the risk of bradycardia when given with **beta blockers, selective**. [Severe] Theoretical

▶ Bupropion is predicted to increase the exposure to beta blockers, selective (**metoprolol, nebivolol**). [Moderate] Study

▶ Calcium channel blockers (diltiazem) are predicted to increase the risk of cardiodepression when given with beta blockers, selective. [Severe] Study → Also see TABLE 6 p. 1335 → Also see TABLE 8 p. 1335

▶ Intravenous calcium channel blockers (verapamil) increase the risk of cardiovascular side-effects when given with beta blockers, selective. Avoid. [Severe] Study → Also see TABLE 6 p. 1335 → Also see TABLE 8 p. 1335

▶ Oral calcium channel blockers (verapamil) increase the risk of cardiovascular side-effects when given with beta blockers, selective. [Severe] Study → Also see TABLE 6 p. 1335 → Also see TABLE 8 p. 1335

▶ Cinacalcet is predicted to increase the exposure to beta blockers, selective (**metoprolol, nebivolol**). [Moderate] Study

▶ Duloxetine is predicted to increase the exposure to **metoprolol**. [Moderate] Study

▶ Eliglustat is predicted to increase the exposure to **metoprolol**. Adjust dose. [Moderate] Study

▶ **Beta blockers, selective** are predicted to increase the risk of peripheral vasoconstriction when given with ergometrine. [Severe] Study

▶ **Beta blockers, selective** are predicted to increase the risk of peripheral vasoconstriction when given with ergotamine. [Severe] Study

▶ Grapefruit juice greatly decreases the exposure to **celiprolol**. [Moderate] Study

▶ HIV-protease inhibitors (ritonavir) are predicted to increase the exposure to **metoprolol**. [Moderate] Study

▶ **Beta blockers, selective** are predicted to increase the risk of bradycardia when given with lanreotide. [Moderate] Theoretical

▶ Mirabegron is predicted to increase the exposure to **metoprolol**. [Moderate] Study

Beta blockers, selective (continued)

▸ Panobinostat is predicted to increase the exposure to **metoprolol**. Monitor and adjust dose. Moderate Theoretical
▸ Panobinostat is predicted to increase the exposure to **nebivolol**. Monitor and adjust dose. Mild Theoretical
▸ Rifampicin slightly decreases the exposure to beta blockers, selective **(bisoprolol, metoprolol)**. Mild Study
▸ Rifampicin moderately decreases the exposure to **celiprolol**. Moderate Study
▸ Rolapitant is predicted to moderately increase the exposure to **metoprolol**. Severe Study
▸ SSRIs (fluoxetine, paroxetine) are predicted to increase the exposure to beta blockers, selective **(metoprolol, nebivolol)**. Moderate Study
▸ **Beta blockers, selective** increase the risk of hypertension and bradycardia when given with sympathomimetics, inotropic (dobutamine). Moderate Theoretical
▸ **Beta blockers, selective** are predicted to increase the risk of hypertension and bradycardia when given with sympathomimetics, vasoconstrictor (adrenaline/epinephrine, noradrenaline/norepinephrine). Severe Study
▸ Terbinafine is predicted to increase the exposure to beta blockers, selective **(metoprolol, nebivolol)**. Moderate Study
▸ **Beta blockers, selective** are predicted to increase the risk of bronchospasm when given with theophylline. Avoid. Severe Theoretical

Beta₂ agonists → see TABLE 17 p. 1338 (reduced serum potassium)

bambuterol · formoterol · indacaterol · olodaterol · salbutamol · salmeterol · terbutaline · vilanterol

▸ Antifungals, azoles (itraconazole, ketoconazole, voriconazole) are predicted to increase the exposure to **salmeterol**. Avoid. Severe Study
▸ Atomoxetine is predicted to increase the risk of cardiovascular side-effects when given with **beta₂ agonists** (high-dose). Moderate Study
▸ Cobicistat is predicted to increase the exposure to **salmeterol**. Avoid. Severe Study
▸ HIV-protease inhibitors are predicted to increase the exposure to **salmeterol**. Avoid. Severe Study
▸ Idelalisib is predicted to increase the exposure to **salmeterol**. Avoid. Severe Study
▸ **Beta₂ agonists** are predicted to increase the risk of glaucoma when given with ipratropium. Moderate Anecdotal
▸ **Beta₂ agonists** are predicted to increase the risk of elevated blood pressure when given with linezolid. Avoid. Severe Theoretical
▸ Macrolides (clarithromycin) are predicted to increase the exposure to **salmeterol**. Severe Study
▸ Monoamine-oxidase A and B inhibitors, irreversible are predicted to increase the risk of cardiovascular side-effects when given with **beta₂ agonists**. Moderate Anecdotal
▸ Monoamine-oxidase B inhibitors (rasagiline, selegiline) are predicted to increase the risk of severe hypertension when given with **beta₂ agonists**. Avoid. Severe Theoretical
▸ Monoamine-oxidase B inhibitors (safinamide) are predicted to increase the risk of severe hypertension when given with **beta₂ agonists**. Severe Theoretical

Betahistine

▸ Antihistamines, non-sedating are predicted to decrease the effects of **betahistine**. Moderate Theoretical
▸ Antihistamines, sedating are predicted to decrease the effects of **betahistine**. Moderate Theoretical

Betamethasone → see corticosteroids
Betaxolol → see beta blockers, selective
Bevacizumab → see monoclonal antibodies
Bexarotene → see retinoids
Bezafibrate → see fibrates
Bicalutamide

▸ Bicalutamide is predicted to increase the exposure to lomitapide. Separate administration by 12 hours. Moderate Theoretical

Bilastine → see antihistamines, non-sedating
Bisoprolol → see beta blockers, selective
Bisphosphonates → see TABLE 2 p. 1334 (nephrotoxicity)

alendronic acid · ibandronic acid · pamidronate · risedronate · sodium clodronate · zoledronic acid

▸ Aminoglycosides increase the risk of hypocalcaemia when given with **bisphosphonates**. Moderate Anecdotal → Also see TABLE 2 p. 1334
▸ Antacids decrease the absorption of **alendronic acid**. Alendronic acid should be taken at least 30 minutes before **antacids**, p. 710. Moderate Study
▸ Antacids are predicted to decrease the absorption of **ibandronic acid**. Avoid **antacids** for at least 6 hours before or 1 hour after **ibandronic acid**. Moderate Theoretical
▸ Antacids decrease the absorption of **risedronate**. Separate administration by at least 2 hours. Moderate Study
▸ Antacids decrease the absorption of **sodium clodronate**. Avoid **antacids** for 2 hours before or 1 hour after **sodium clodronate**. Moderate Study
▸ Aspirin (high-dose) is predicted to increase the risk of gastrointestinal irritation when given with **bisphosphonates** **(alendronic acid, ibandronic acid)**. Moderate Study
▸ Aspirin (high-dose) is predicted to increase the risk of renal impairment when given with **sodium clodronate**. Severe Theoretical
▸ Oral calcium salts decrease the absorption of **alendronic acid**. Alendronic acid should be taken at least 30 minutes before **calcium salts**. Moderate Study
▸ Oral calcium salts are predicted to decrease the absorption of oral **ibandronic acid**. Avoid **calcium salts** for at least 6 hours before or 1 hour after **ibandronic acid**. Moderate Theoretical
▸ Oral calcium salts decrease the absorption of **risedronate**. Separate administration by at least 2 hours. Moderate Study
▸ Oral calcium salts are predicted to decrease the absorption of **sodium clodronate**. Avoid **calcium salts** for 2 hours before or 1 hour after **sodium clodronate**. Moderate Study
▸ Iron (oral) is predicted to decrease the absorption of oral **ibandronic acid**. Avoid **iron (oral)** for at least 6 hours before or 1 hour after **ibandronic acid**. Moderate Theoretical
▸ Iron (oral) decreases the absorption of **risedronate**. Separate administration by at least 2 hours. Moderate Study
▸ Iron (oral) decreases the absorption of **sodium clodronate**. Avoid **iron (oral)** for 2 hours before or 1 hour after **sodium clodronate**. Moderate Study
▸ **Bisphosphonates** are predicted to increase the risk of gastrointestinal bleeding when given with iron chelators (deferasirox). Severe Theoretical
▸ Oral magnesium decreases the absorption of **alendronic acid**. Alendronic acid should be taken at least 30 minutes before **magnesium**. Moderate Study
▸ Oral magnesium is predicted to decrease the absorption of oral **ibandronic acid**. Avoid **magnesium** for at least 6 hours before or 1 hour after **ibandronic acid**. Moderate Theoretical
▸ Oral magnesium decreases the absorption of **risedronate**. Separate administration by at least 2 hours. Moderate Study
▸ Oral magnesium decreases the absorption of **sodium clodronate**. Avoid **magnesium** for 2 hours before or 1 hour after **sodium clodronate**. Moderate Study
▸ NSAIDs are predicted to increase the risk of gastrointestinal irritation when given with bisphosphonates **(alendronic acid, ibandronic acid)**. Moderate Study
▸ NSAIDs are predicted to increase the risk of renal impairment when given with **sodium clodronate**. Severe Theoretical
▸ **Bisphosphonates** are predicted to decrease the effects of parathyroid hormone. Avoid. Moderate Study
▸ Oral zinc decreases the absorption of oral **alendronic acid**. Zinc should be taken at least 30 minutes before **alendronic acid**. Moderate Study
▸ Oral zinc is predicted to decrease the absorption of oral **ibandronic acid**. Avoid **zinc** for at least 6 hours before or 1 hour after **ibandronic acid**. Moderate Theoretical
▸ Oral zinc decreases the absorption of oral **risedronate**. Separate administration by at least 2 hours. Moderate Study
▸ Oral zinc decreases the absorption of oral **sodium clodronate**. Avoid **zinc** for 2 hours before or 1 hour after **sodium clodronate**. Moderate Study

Bivalirudin → see TABLE 3 p. 1334 (anticoagulant effects)

▸ Ranibizumab is predicted to increase the risk of bleeding events when given with **bivalirudin**. [Moderate] Theoretical

Bleomycin → see TABLE 15 p. 1337 (myelosuppression), TABLE 5 p. 1334 (thromboembolism)

▸ Live vaccines are predicted to increase the risk of generalised infection (possibly life-threatening) when given with **bleomycin**. Public Health England advises avoid (refer to Green Book). [Severe] Theoretical

▸ Monoclonal antibodies (brentuximab vedotin) increase the risk of pulmonary toxicity when given with **bleomycin**. Avoid. [Severe] Study → Also see TABLE 15 p. 1337

▸ Platinum compounds (cisplatin) increase the risk of pulmonary toxicity when given with **bleomycin**. [Severe] Study → Also see TABLE 15 p. 1337

Blinatumomab → see monoclonal antibodies

Bortezomib → see TABLE 8 p. 1335 (hypotension), TABLE 15 p. 1337 (myelosuppression), TABLE 12 p. 1337 (peripheral neuropathy)

▸ Antiepileptics (carbamazepine, fosphenytoin, phenobarbital, phenytoin, primidone) slightly decrease the exposure to **bortezomib**. Avoid. [Severe] Study → Also see TABLE 12 p. 1337

▸ Antifungals, azoles (itraconazole, ketoconazole, voriconazole) slightly increase the exposure to **bortezomib**. [Moderate] Study

▸ Cobicistat slightly increases the exposure to **bortezomib**. [Moderate] Study

▸ Enzalutamide slightly decreases the exposure to **bortezomib**. Avoid. [Severe] Study

▸ HIV-protease inhibitors slightly increase the exposure to **bortezomib**. [Moderate] Study

▸ Idelalisib slightly increases the exposure to **bortezomib**. [Moderate] Study → Also see TABLE 15 p. 1337

▸ Macrolides (clarithromycin) slightly increase the exposure to **bortezomib**. [Moderate] Study

▸ Mitotane slightly decreases the exposure to **bortezomib**. Avoid. [Severe] Study → Also see TABLE 15 p. 1337

▸ Rifampicin slightly decreases the exposure to **bortezomib**. Avoid. [Severe] Study

Bosentan

▸ **Bosentan** is predicted to decrease the exposure to antiarrhythmics (dronedarone). [Severe] Theoretical

▸ Antiepileptics (carbamazepine, fosphenytoin, phenobarbital, phenytoin, primidone) affect the exposure to **bosentan**. Avoid. [Severe] Study

▸ Antifungals, azoles (fluconazole) are predicted to increase the exposure to **bosentan**. Avoid. [Severe] Study

▸ Antifungals, azoles (itraconazole) are predicted to increase the exposure to **bosentan**. [Moderate] Theoretical

▸ Antifungals, azoles (ketoconazole) moderately increase the exposure to **bosentan**. [Moderate] Study

▸ Antifungals, azoles (voriconazole) are predicted to increase the exposure to **bosentan**. Avoid. [Severe] Theoretical

▸ **Bosentan** is predicted to decrease the exposure to antifungals, azoles (isavuconazole). Avoid. [Severe] Theoretical

▸ **Bosentan** is predicted to decrease the exposure to axitinib. [Moderate] Theoretical

▸ **Bosentan** is predicted to decrease the exposure to bedaquiline. Avoid. [Severe] Study

▸ **Bosentan** is predicted to decrease the exposure to bosutinib. Avoid. [Severe] Theoretical

▸ **Bosentan** is predicted to decrease the exposure to cabozantinib. [Moderate] Theoretical

▸ **Bosentan** is predicted to decrease the exposure to calcium channel blockers (amlodipine, felodipine, lacidipine, lercanidipine, nicardipine, nifedipine, nimodipine). Monitor and adjust dose. [Moderate] Theoretical

▸ **Bosentan** is predicted to decrease the exposure to calcium channel blockers (diltiazem, verapamil). [Moderate] Theoretical

▸ Cephalosporins (ceftobiprole) are predicted to increase the exposure to **bosentan**. [Moderate] Theoretical

▸ **Bosentan** moderately decreases the exposure to ciclosporin and ciclosporin moderately increases the exposure to **bosentan**. Avoid. [Severe] Study

▸ **Bosentan** is predicted to decrease the exposure to cobicistat. Avoid. [Severe] Theoretical

▸ **Bosentan** is predicted to decrease the exposure to cobimetinib. Avoid. [Severe] Theoretical

▸ **Bosentan** is predicted to decrease the efficacy of combined hormonal contraceptives. For FSRH guidance, see Contraceptives, interactions p. 775. [Severe] Study

▸ **Bosentan** decreases the anticoagulant effect of coumarins. [Moderate] Study

▸ **Bosentan** is predicted to decrease the exposure to crizotinib. Avoid. [Severe] Theoretical

▸ **Bosentan** is predicted to decrease the exposure to daclatasvir. Adjust **daclatasvir** dose, p. 614. [Moderate] Theoretical

▸ **Bosentan** is predicted to decrease the exposure to dasatinib. [Severe] Study

▸ **Bosentan** is predicted to decrease the efficacy of desogestrel. For FSRH guidance, see Contraceptives, interactions p. 775. [Severe] Theoretical

▸ **Bosentan** decreases the exposure to dolutegravir. Adjust dose. [Severe] Study

▸ **Bosentan** is predicted to moderately decrease the exposure to elbasvir. Avoid. [Severe] Study

▸ **Bosentan** is predicted to decrease the exposure to eliglustat. [Moderate] Theoretical

▸ **Bosentan** is predicted to decrease the concentration of elvitegravir. Avoid. [Severe] Theoretical

▸ Enzalutamide affects the exposure to **bosentan**. Avoid. [Severe] Study

▸ **Bosentan** is predicted to decrease the effects of ergotamine. [Moderate] Theoretical

▸ **Bosentan** is predicted to decrease the exposure to erlotinib. [Severe] Theoretical

▸ **Bosentan** is predicted to decrease the efficacy of etonogestrel. For FSRH guidance, see Contraceptives, interactions p. 775. [Severe] Theoretical

▸ **Bosentan** is predicted to decrease the exposure to etravirine. Avoid. [Severe] Study

▸ **Bosentan** is predicted to decrease the concentration of everolimus. Avoid or adjust dose. [Severe] Study

▸ **Bosentan** is predicted to decrease the exposure to gefitinib. Avoid. [Severe] Theoretical

▸ **Bosentan** is predicted to decrease the exposure to glecaprevir. Avoid. [Severe] Study

▸ **Bosentan** is predicted to markedly decrease the exposure to grazoprevir. Avoid. [Severe] Study

▸ **Bosentan** is predicted to decrease the concentration of guanfacine. Adjust dose. [Moderate] Theoretical

▸ HIV-protease inhibitors are predicted to increase the exposure to **bosentan**. [Severe] Study

▸ **Bosentan** is predicted to decrease the effects of hormone replacement therapy. [Moderate] Anecdotal

▸ **Bosentan** is predicted to decrease the exposure to idelalisib. Avoid. [Moderate] Theoretical

▸ **Bosentan** is predicted to decrease the exposure to imatinib. [Moderate] Study

▸ **Bosentan** is predicted to decrease the exposure to ivacaftor. [Severe] Theoretical

▸ **Bosentan** is predicted to decrease the exposure to lapatinib. Avoid. [Severe] Study

▸ **Bosentan** is predicted to decrease the efficacy of levonorgestrel. For FSRH guidance, see Contraceptives, interactions p. 775. [Severe] Theoretical

▸ **Bosentan** is predicted to decrease the exposure to lurasidone. Monitor and adjust dose. [Moderate] Theoretical

▸ Macrolides (clarithromycin) are predicted to increase the exposure to **bosentan**. [Moderate] Theoretical

▸ **Bosentan** is predicted to decrease the exposure to maraviroc. Avoid. [Moderate] Theoretical

▸ **Bosentan** is predicted to decrease the concentration of midazolam. Monitor and adjust dose. [Moderate] Theoretical

▸ Mitotane affects the exposure to **bosentan**. Avoid. [Severe] Study

▸ **Bosentan** is predicted to decrease the exposure to netupitant. [Moderate] Theoretical

▸ **Bosentan** is predicted to decrease the exposure to nilotinib. Avoid. [Severe] Theoretical

▸ **Bosentan** is predicted to decrease the efficacy of norethisterone. For FSRH guidance, see Contraceptives, interactions p. 775. [Severe] Anecdotal

Interactions | Appendix 1

A1

Bosentan (continued)

▶ **Bosentan** is predicted to decrease the exposure to olaparib. Avoid. Moderate Theoretical
▶ **Bosentan** decreases the exposure to opioids (methadone). Monitor and adjust dose. Severe Study
▶ **Bosentan** is predicted to decrease the exposure to osimertinib. Moderate Theoretical
▶ **Bosentan** is predicted to decrease the exposure to paritaprevir (with ritonavir and ombitasvir). Avoid. Severe Study
▶ **Bosentan** decreases the exposure to phosphodiesterase type-5 inhibitors. Moderate Study
▶ **Bosentan** is predicted to decrease the exposure to pibrentasvir. Avoid. Severe Study
▶ **Bosentan** is predicted to decrease the exposure to quetiapine. Moderate Study
▶ **Bosentan** is predicted to decrease the exposure to ribociclib. Moderate Study
▶ Rifampicin affects the exposure to **bosentan**. Avoid. Severe Study
▶ **Bosentan** is predicted to decrease the exposure to rilpivirine. Avoid. Severe Theoretical
▶ **Bosentan** is predicted to decrease the exposure to rolapitant. Avoid. Severe Study
▶ **Bosentan** is predicted to decrease the exposure to ruxolitinib. Monitor and adjust dose. Moderate Theoretical
▶ **Bosentan** is predicted to decrease the exposure to simeprevir. Avoid. Severe Study
▶ **Bosentan** is predicted to decrease the concentration of sirolimus and sirolimus potentially increases the concentration of **bosentan**. Avoid. Severe Theoretical
▶ St John's Wort is predicted to decrease the exposure to **bosentan**. Avoid. Moderate Theoretical
▶ **Bosentan** slightly decreases the exposure to statins (atorvastatin). Mild Study
▶ **Bosentan** moderately decreases the exposure to statins (simvastatin). Moderate Study
▶ **Bosentan** increases the risk of hepatotoxicity when given with sulfonylureas (glibenclamide). Avoid. Severe Study
▶ **Bosentan** is predicted to decrease the concentration of tacrolimus and tacrolimus potentially increases the concentration of **bosentan**. Avoid. Severe Theoretical
▶ **Bosentan** is predicted to decrease the exposure to taxanes (cabazitaxel). Avoid. Severe Study
▶ **Bosentan** is predicted to decrease the concentration of temsirolimus. Avoid. Severe Theoretical
▶ **Bosentan** is predicted to decrease the exposure to ticagrelor. Moderate Theoretical
▶ **Bosentan** is predicted to decrease the exposure to tofacitinib. Moderate Study
▶ **Bosentan** is predicted to decrease the exposure to tolvaptan. Moderate Theoretical
▶ **Bosentan** decreases the efficacy of ulipristal. For FSRH guidance, see Contraceptives, interactions p. 775. Severe Anecdotal
▶ **Bosentan** is predicted to decrease the exposure to velpatasvir. Avoid. Moderate Theoretical
▶ **Bosentan** is predicted to decrease the exposure to venetoclax. Avoid. Severe Study
▶ **Bosentan** is predicted to decrease the concentration of voxilaprevir. Avoid. Severe Study

Bosutinib → see TABLE 15 p. 1337 (myelosuppression), TABLE 9 p. 1336 (QT-interval prolongation)
▶ Antacids are predicted to decrease the absorption of **bosutinib**. **Bosutinib** should be taken at least 12 hours before **antacids**. Moderate Theoretical
▶ Antiarrhythmics (dronedarone) are predicted to increase the exposure to **bosutinib**. Avoid or adjust dose. Severe Theoretical → Also see TABLE 9 p. 1336
▶ Antiepileptics (carbamazepine, fosphenytoin, phenobarbital, phenytoin, primidone) are predicted to very markedly decrease the exposure to **bosutinib**. Avoid. Severe Study
▶ Antifungals, azoles (fluconazole, isavuconazole, posaconazole) are predicted to increase the exposure to **bosutinib**. Avoid or adjust dose. Severe Theoretical → Also see TABLE 9 p. 1336

▶ Antifungals, azoles (itraconazole, ketoconazole, voriconazole) are predicted to markedly increase the exposure to **bosutinib**. Avoid or adjust dose. Severe Study → Also see TABLE 9 p. 1336
▶ Aprepitant is predicted to increase the exposure to **bosutinib**. Avoid or adjust dose. Severe Theoretical
▶ Bosentan is predicted to decrease the exposure to **bosutinib**. Avoid. Severe Theoretical
▶ Calcium channel blockers (diltiazem, verapamil) are predicted to increase the exposure to **bosutinib**. Avoid or adjust dose. Severe Theoretical
▶ Cobicistat is predicted to markedly increase the exposure to **bosutinib**. Avoid or adjust dose. Severe Study
▶ **Bosutinib** is predicted to increase the risk of bleeding events when given with coumarins. Severe Theoretical
▶ Crizotinib is predicted to increase the exposure to **bosutinib**. Avoid or adjust dose. Severe Theoretical → Also see TABLE 15 p. 1337 → Also see TABLE 9 p. 1336
▶ Efavirenz is predicted to decrease the exposure to **bosutinib**. Avoid. Severe Theoretical → Also see TABLE 9 p. 1336
▶ Enzalutamide is predicted to very markedly decrease the exposure to **bosutinib**. Avoid. Severe Study
▶ Etravirine is predicted to decrease the exposure to **bosutinib**. Avoid. Severe Theoretical
▶ Fosaprepitant is predicted to increase the exposure to **bosutinib**. Severe Theoretical
▶ Grapefruit juice is predicted to increase the exposure to **bosutinib**. Avoid. Moderate Theoretical
▶ H_2 receptor antagonists are predicted to decrease the absorption of **bosutinib**. Moderate Theoretical
▶ HIV-protease inhibitors are predicted to markedly increase the exposure to **bosutinib**. Avoid or adjust dose. Severe Study → Also see TABLE 9 p. 1336
▶ Idelalisib is predicted to markedly increase the exposure to **bosutinib**. Avoid or adjust dose. Severe Study → Also see TABLE 15 p. 1337
▶ Imatinib is predicted to increase the exposure to **bosutinib**. Avoid or adjust dose. Severe Theoretical → Also see TABLE 15 p. 1337
▶ Macrolides (clarithromycin) are predicted to markedly increase the exposure to **bosutinib**. Avoid or adjust dose. Severe Study → Also see TABLE 9 p. 1336
▶ Macrolides (erythromycin) are predicted to increase the exposure to **bosutinib**. Avoid or adjust dose. Severe Theoretical → Also see TABLE 9 p. 1336
▶ Mitotane is predicted to very markedly decrease the exposure to **bosutinib**. Avoid. Severe Study → Also see TABLE 15 p. 1337
▶ Modafinil is predicted to decrease the exposure to **bosutinib**. Avoid. Severe Theoretical
▶ Netupitant is predicted to increase the exposure to **bosutinib**. Avoid or adjust dose. Severe Theoretical
▶ Nevirapine is predicted to decrease the exposure to **bosutinib**. Avoid. Severe Theoretical
▶ Nilotinib is predicted to increase the exposure to **bosutinib**. Avoid or adjust dose. Severe Theoretical → Also see TABLE 15 p. 1337 → Also see TABLE 9 p. 1336
▶ **Bosutinib** is predicted to increase the risk of bleeding events when given with phenindione. Severe Theoretical
▶ Pitolisant is predicted to decrease the exposure to **bosutinib**. Avoid. Severe Theoretical
▶ Proton pump inhibitors are predicted to decrease the absorption of **bosutinib**. Moderate Study
▶ Rifampicin is predicted to very markedly decrease the exposure to **bosutinib**. Avoid. Severe Study
▶ St John's Wort is predicted to decrease the exposure to **bosutinib**. Avoid. Severe Theoretical

Botulinum toxin type A → see TABLE 20 p. 1338 (neuromuscular blocking effects)

Botulinum toxin type B → see TABLE 20 p. 1338 (neuromuscular blocking effects)

Bowel cleansing preparations

> **SEPARATION OF ADMINISTRATION** Other oral drugs should not be taken 1 hour before, or after, administration of bowel cleansing preparations because absorption may be impaired. Consider withholding ACE inhibitors, angiotensin-II receptor antagonists, and NSAIDs on the day that bowel cleansing

preparations are given and for up to 72 hours after the procedure. Also consider withholding diuretics on the day that bowel cleansing preparations are given.

Brentuximab vedotin → see monoclonal antibodies

Brimonidine → see TABLE 6 p. 1335 (bradycardia), TABLE 8 p. 1335 (hypotension), TABLE 11 p. 1336 (CNS depressant effects)

Brinzolamide

ROUTE-SPECIFIC INFORMATION Since systemic absorption can follow topical application, the possibility of interactions should be borne in mind.

Brivaracetam → see antiepileptics

Brodalumab → see monoclonal antibodies

Bromfenac → see NSAIDs

Bromocriptine → see dopamine receptor agonists

Buclizine → see antihistamines, sedating

Budesonide → see corticosteroids

Bumetanide → see loop diuretics

Bupivacaine → see anaesthetics, local

Buprenorphine → see opioids

Bupropion → see TABLE 13 p. 1337 (serotonin syndrome)

▸ **Bupropion** is predicted to increase the exposure to anticholinesterases, centrally acting (galantamine). Monitor and adjust dose. Moderate Study

▸ Antiepileptics (carbamazepine, fosphenytoin, phenobarbital, phenytoin, primidone) are predicted to markedly decrease the exposure to **bupropion**. Severe Study

▸ Antiepileptics (valproate) increase the exposure to **bupropion**. Severe Study

▸ Antifungals, azoles (isavuconazole) slightly increase the exposure to **bupropion**. Adjust dose. Moderate Study

▸ **Bupropion** is predicted to moderately increase the exposure to aripiprazole. Adjust aripiprazole dose, p. 391. Moderate Study

▸ **Bupropion** is predicted to markedly increase the exposure to atomoxetine. Adjust dose. Severe Study

▸ **Bupropion** is predicted to increase the exposure to beta blockers, selective (metoprolol, nebivolol). Moderate Study

▸ **Bupropion** is predicted to slightly increase the exposure to darifenacin. Mild Study

▸ **Bupropion** increases the risk of side-effects when given with dopamine receptor agonists (amantadine). Moderate Study

▸ Efavirenz is predicted to decrease the exposure to **bupropion**. Moderate Study

▸ **Bupropion** is predicted to increase the exposure to eliglustat. Avoid or adjust dose—consult product literature. Severe Study

▸ HIV-protease inhibitors (ritonavir) are predicted to decrease the exposure to **bupropion**. Moderate Study

▸ **Bupropion** increases the risk of side-effects when given with levodopa. Moderate Study

▸ **Bupropion** is predicted to increase the risk of intraoperative hypertension when given with linezolid. Severe Anecdotal → Also see TABLE 13 p. 1337

▸ Methylthioninium chloride is predicted to increase the risk of severe hypertension when given with **bupropion**. Avoid. Severe Theoretical → Also see TABLE 13 p. 1337

▸ Moclobemide is predicted to increase the risk of severe hypertension when given with **bupropion**. Avoid. Severe Theoretical → Also see TABLE 13 p. 1337

▸ Monoamine-oxidase A and B inhibitors, irreversible are predicted to increase the risk of severe hypertension when given with **bupropion**. Avoid and for 14 days after stopping the MAOI. Severe Theoretical → Also see TABLE 13 p. 1337

▸ Monoamine-oxidase B inhibitors are predicted to increase the risk of severe hypertension when given with **bupropion**. Avoid. Moderate Theoretical → Also see TABLE 13 p. 1337

▸ **Bupropion** is predicted to decrease the efficacy of opioids (codeine). Moderate Theoretical

▸ **Bupropion** is predicted to decrease the efficacy of opioids (tramadol). Severe Study → Also see TABLE 13 p. 1337

▸ **Bupropion** is predicted to moderately increase the exposure to pitolisant. Use with caution and adjust dose. Moderate Study

▸ Rifampicin is predicted to decrease the exposure to **bupropion**. Moderate Study

▸ **Bupropion** is predicted to increase the exposure to risperidone. Adjust dose. Moderate Study

▸ **Bupropion** is predicted to increase the exposure to SSRIs (dapoxetine). Moderate Theoretical → Also see TABLE 13 p. 1337

▸ **Bupropion** is predicted to decrease the efficacy of tamoxifen. Avoid. Severe Study

▸ **Bupropion** is predicted to increase the exposure to tricyclic antidepressants. Monitor for toxicity and adjust dose. Severe Study → Also see TABLE 13 p. 1337

▸ **Bupropion** is predicted to increase the exposure to vortioxetine. Monitor and adjust dose. Moderate Study → Also see TABLE 13 p. 1337

Buspirone → see TABLE 13 p. 1337 (serotonin syndrome)

▸ Antiarrhythmics (dronedarone) are predicted to increase the exposure to **buspirone**. Use with caution and adjust dose. Moderate Study

▸ Antiepileptics (carbamazepine, fosphenytoin, phenobarbital, phenytoin, primidone) are predicted to decrease the exposure to **buspirone**. Use with caution and adjust dose. Severe Study

▸ Antifungals, azoles (fluconazole, isavuconazole, posaconazole) are predicted to increase the exposure to **buspirone**. Use with caution and adjust dose. Moderate Study

▸ Antifungals, azoles (itraconazole, ketoconazole, voriconazole) are predicted to increase the exposure to **buspirone**. Adjust **buspirone** dose, p. 338. Severe Study

▸ Antifungals, azoles (miconazole) are predicted to increase the concentration of **buspirone**. Use with caution and adjust dose. Moderate Theoretical

▸ Aprepitant is predicted to increase the exposure to **buspirone**. Use with caution and adjust dose. Moderate Study

▸ Calcium channel blockers (diltiazem, verapamil) are predicted to increase the exposure to **buspirone**. Use with caution and adjust dose. Moderate Study

▸ Cobicistat is predicted to increase the exposure to **buspirone**. Adjust **buspirone** dose, p. 338. Severe Study

▸ Crizotinib is predicted to increase the exposure to **buspirone**. Use with caution and adjust dose. Moderate Study

▸ Enzalutamide is predicted to decrease the exposure to **buspirone**. Use with caution and adjust dose. Severe Study

▸ Grapefruit juice increases the exposure to **buspirone**. Avoid. Mild Study

▸ HIV-protease inhibitors are predicted to increase the exposure to **buspirone**. Adjust **buspirone** dose, p. 338. Severe Study

▸ Idelalisib is predicted to increase the exposure to **buspirone**. Adjust **buspirone** dose, p. 338. Severe Study

▸ Imatinib is predicted to increase the exposure to **buspirone**. Use with caution and adjust dose. Moderate Study

▸ **Buspirone** is predicted to increase the risk of elevated blood pressure when given with linezolid. Avoid. Severe Theoretical → Also see TABLE 13 p. 1337

▸ Macrolides (clarithromycin) are predicted to increase the exposure to **buspirone**. Adjust **buspirone** dose, p. 338. Severe Study

▸ Macrolides (erythromycin) are predicted to increase the exposure to **buspirone**. Use with caution and adjust dose. Moderate Study

▸ Mitotane is predicted to decrease the exposure to **buspirone**. Use with caution and adjust dose. Severe Study

▸ **Buspirone** is predicted to increase the risk of elevated blood pressure when given with monoamine-oxidase A and B inhibitors, irreversible. Avoid. Severe Anecdotal → Also see TABLE 13 p. 1337

▸ Netupitant is predicted to increase the exposure to **buspirone**. Use with caution and adjust dose. Moderate Study

▸ Nilotinib is predicted to increase the exposure to **buspirone**. Use with caution and adjust dose. Moderate Study

▸ Rifampicin is predicted to decrease the exposure to **buspirone**. Use with caution and adjust dose. Severe Study

Busulfan → see alkylating agents

Cabazitaxel → see taxanes

Cabergoline → see dopamine receptor agonists

Cabozantinib → see TABLE 15 p. 1337 (myelosuppression), TABLE 9 p. 1336 (QT-interval prolongation)

▸ Antiarrhythmics (dronedarone) are predicted to increase the exposure to **cabozantinib**. Moderate Theoretical → Also see TABLE 9 p. 1336

Cabozantinib (continued)

▶ Antiepileptics (carbamazepine, fosphenytoin, phenobarbital, phenytoin, primidone) moderately decrease the exposure to **cabozantinib**. Avoid. Moderate Study

▶ Antifungals, azoles (fluconazole, isavuconazole, posaconazole) are predicted to increase the exposure to **cabozantinib**. Moderate Theoretical → Also see TABLE 9 p. 1336

▶ Antifungals, azoles (itraconazole, ketoconazole, voriconazole) slightly increase the exposure to **cabozantinib**. Moderate Study → Also see TABLE 9 p. 1336

▶ Aprepitant is predicted to increase the exposure to **cabozantinib**. Moderate Theoretical

▶ Bosentan is predicted to decrease the exposure to **cabozantinib**. Moderate Theoretical

▶ Calcium channel blockers (diltiazem, verapamil) are predicted to increase the exposure to **cabozantinib**. Moderate Theoretical

▶ Cobicistat slightly increases the exposure to **cabozantinib**. Moderate Study

▶ **Cabozantinib** is predicted to increase the risk of bleeding events when given with coumarins. Severe Theoretical

▶ Crizotinib is predicted to increase the exposure to **cabozantinib**. Moderate Theoretical → Also see TABLE 15 p. 1337 → Also see TABLE 9 p. 1336

▶ Efavirenz is predicted to decrease the exposure to **cabozantinib**. Moderate Theoretical → Also see TABLE 9 p. 1336

▶ Enzalutamide moderately decreases the exposure to **cabozantinib**. Avoid. Moderate Study

▶ Grapefruit juice is predicted to increase the exposure to **cabozantinib**. Moderate Theoretical

▶ HIV-protease inhibitors slightly increase the exposure to **cabozantinib**. Moderate Study → Also see TABLE 9 p. 1336

▶ Idelalisib slightly increases the exposure to **cabozantinib**. Moderate Study → Also see TABLE 15 p. 1337

▶ Imatinib is predicted to increase the exposure to **cabozantinib**. Moderate Theoretical → Also see TABLE 15 p. 1337

▶ Macrolides (clarithromycin) slightly increase the exposure to **cabozantinib**. Moderate Study → Also see TABLE 9 p. 1336

▶ Macrolides (erythromycin) are predicted to increase the exposure to **cabozantinib**. Moderate Theoretical → Also see TABLE 9 p. 1336

▶ Mitotane moderately decreases the exposure to **cabozantinib**. Avoid. Moderate Study → Also see TABLE 15 p. 1337

▶ Netupitant is predicted to increase the exposure to **cabozantinib**. Moderate Theoretical

▶ Nevirapine is predicted to decrease the exposure to **cabozantinib**. Moderate Theoretical

▶ Nilotinib is predicted to increase the exposure to **cabozantinib**. Moderate Theoretical → Also see TABLE 15 p. 1337 → Also see TABLE 9 p. 1336

▶ **Cabozantinib** is predicted to increase the risk of bleeding events when given with phenindione. Severe Theoretical

▶ Rifampicin moderately decreases the exposure to **cabozantinib**. Avoid. Moderate Study

▶ St John's Wort is predicted to decrease the exposure to **cabozantinib**. Moderate Theoretical

Caffeine citrate

▶ **Caffeine citrate** decreases the efficacy of antiarrhythmics (adenosine). Separate administration by 24 hours. Mild Study

▶ Antiepileptics (fosphenytoin, phenytoin) are predicted to moderately increase the clearance of **caffeine citrate**. Monitor and adjust dose. Moderate Study

▶ HIV-protease inhibitors (ritonavir) are predicted to moderately increase the clearance of **caffeine citrate**. Monitor and adjust dose. Moderate Study

▶ Leflunomide is predicted to moderately increase the clearance of **caffeine citrate**. Monitor and adjust dose. Moderate Study

▶ Rifampicin is predicted to moderately increase the clearance of **caffeine citrate**. Monitor and adjust dose. Moderate Study

▶ SSRIs (fluvoxamine) markedly decrease the clearance of **caffeine citrate**. Monitor and adjust dose. Severe Study

▶ Teriflunomide is predicted to moderately increase the clearance of **caffeine citrate**. Monitor and adjust dose. Moderate Study

▶ **Caffeine citrate** decreases the clearance of theophylline. Moderate Study

Calcipotriol → see vitamin D substances

Calcitonin (salmon)

▶ Calcitonin (salmon) decreases the concentration of lithium. Monitor concentration and adjust dose. Moderate Study

Calcitriol → see vitamin D substances

Calcium acetate → see calcium salts

Calcium carbonate → see calcium salts

Calcium channel blockers → see TABLE 6 p. 1335 (bradycardia), TABLE 8 p. 1335 (hypotension)

amlodipine · clevidipine · diltiazem · felodipine · lacidipine · lercanidipine · nicardipine · nifedipine · nimodipine · verapamil

▶ **Verapamil** is predicted to increase the exposure to afatinib. Separate administration by 12 hours. Moderate Study

▶ Calcium channel blockers (diltiazem, verapamil) are predicted to increase the exposure to aldosterone antagonists (eplerenone). Adjust eplerenone dose, p. 190. Severe Study → Also see TABLE 8 p. 1335

▶ **Verapamil** moderately increases the exposure to aliskiren. Moderate Study → Also see TABLE 8 p. 1335

▶ Calcium channel blockers (diltiazem, verapamil) are predicted to increase the exposure to alpha blockers (tamsulosin). Moderate Theoretical → Also see TABLE 8 p. 1335

▶ Calcium channel blockers (diltiazem, verapamil) are predicted to increase the exposure to alprazolam. Severe Study

▶ **Verapamil** moderately increases the exposure to anthracyclines (doxorubicin). Moderate Study

▶ Antiarrhythmics (disopyramide) are predicted to increase the risk of cardiodepression when given with **verapamil**. Severe Theoretical

▶ Antiarrhythmics (dronedarone) are predicted to increase the exposure to calcium channel blockers (amlodipine, felodipine, lacidipine, lercanidipine, nicardipine, nifedipine, nimodipine). Monitor and adjust dose. Moderate Study

▶ Antiarrhythmics (amiodarone) are predicted to increase the risk of cardiodepression when given with calcium channel blockers (diltiazem, verapamil). Avoid. Severe Theoretical → Also see TABLE 6 p. 1335

▶ Calcium channel blockers (diltiazem, verapamil) increase the exposure to antiarrhythmics (dronedarone) and antiarrhythmics (dronedarone) increase the exposure to calcium channel blockers (diltiazem, verapamil). Moderate Study

▶ **Verapamil** increases the risk of cardiodepression when given with antiarrhythmics (flecainide). Severe Anecdotal → Also see TABLE 6 p. 1335

▶ Calcium channel blockers (diltiazem, verapamil) are predicted to increase the exposure to antiarrhythmics (propafenone). Monitor and adjust dose. Moderate Study

▶ Calcium channel blockers (diltiazem, verapamil) increase the risk of bradycardia when given with anticholinesterases, centrally acting. Moderate Anecdotal → Also see TABLE 6 p. 1335

▶ Antiepileptics (carbamazepine, fosphenytoin, phenobarbital, phenytoin, primidone) are predicted to decrease the exposure to calcium channel blockers (amlodipine, felodipine, lacidipine, lercanidipine, nicardipine, nifedipine, nimodipine). Monitor and adjust dose. Moderate Study

▶ **Diltiazem** increases the concentration of antiepileptics (carbamazepine) and antiepileptics (carbamazepine) are predicted to decrease the exposure to **diltiazem**. Monitor concentration and adjust dose. Severe Anecdotal

▶ **Verapamil** increases the concentration of antiepileptics (carbamazepine) and antiepileptics (carbamazepine) are predicted to decrease the exposure to **verapamil**. Severe Anecdotal

▶ Antiepileptics (phenobarbital, primidone) are predicted to decrease the exposure to calcium channel blockers (diltiazem, verapamil). Severe Study

▶ Calcium channel blockers (diltiazem, verapamil) potentially increase the concentration of antiepileptics (fosphenytoin, phenytoin) and antiepileptics (fosphenytoin, phenytoin) are predicted to decrease the exposure to calcium channel blockers (diltiazem, verapamil). Severe Study

▶ Antifungals, azoles (itraconazole, ketoconazole, voriconazole) are predicted to markedly increase the exposure to lercanidipine. Avoid. Severe Study

- Antifungals, azoles (miconazole) are predicted to increase the exposure to calcium channel blockers (amlodipine, clevidipine, felodipine, lacidipine, lercanidipine, nicardipine, nifedipine, nimodipine, verapamil). Use with caution and adjust dose. Moderate Theoretical
- Antifungals, azoles (fluconazole, isavuconazole, posaconazole) are predicted to increase the exposure to calcium channel blockers (amlodipine, felodipine, lacidipine, lercanidipine, nicardipine, nifedipine, nimodipine). Monitor and adjust dose. Moderate Study
- Antifungals, azoles (itraconazole, ketoconazole, voriconazole) are predicted to increase the exposure to calcium channel blockers (amlodipine, felodipine, lacidipine, lercanidipine, nicardipine, nifedipine, nimodipine). Monitor and adjust dose. Moderate Study
- Antifungals, azoles (fluconazole) (high-dose) are predicted to increase the exposure to calcium channel blockers (diltiazem, verapamil). Moderate Theoretical
- Antifungals, azoles (itraconazole, ketoconazole, voriconazole) are predicted to increase the exposure to calcium channel blockers (diltiazem, verapamil). Severe Study
- Antifungals, azoles (posaconazole) are predicted to increase the exposure to calcium channel blockers (diltiazem, verapamil). Moderate Theoretical
- Calcium channel blockers (diltiazem, verapamil) are predicted to increase the exposure to antifungals, azoles (isavuconazole). Moderate Theoretical
- Calcium channel blockers (diltiazem, verapamil) are predicted to increase the exposure to antihistamines, non-sedating (mizolastine). Severe Theoretical
- Calcium channel blockers (diltiazem, verapamil) are predicted to increase the exposure to antihistamines, non-sedating (rupatadine). Avoid. Moderate Study
- Antimalarials (mefloquine) are predicted to increase the risk of bradycardia when given with calcium channel blockers. Severe Theoretical
- Calcium channel blockers (diltiazem, verapamil) are predicted to increase the concentration of antimalarials (piperaquine). Severe Theoretical
- Verapamil is predicted to increase the exposure to apixaban. Moderate Theoretical
- Calcium channel blockers (diltiazem, verapamil) are predicted to increase the exposure to aprepitant and aprepitant is predicted to increase the exposure to calcium channel blockers (diltiazem, verapamil). Moderate Study
- Aprepitant is predicted to increase the exposure to calcium channel blockers (amlodipine, felodipine, lacidipine, lercanidipine, nicardipine, nifedipine, nimodipine). Monitor and adjust dose. Moderate Study
- Calcium channel blockers (diltiazem, verapamil) are predicted to increase the exposure to axitinib. Moderate Theoretical
- Calcium channel blockers (diltiazem, verapamil) are predicted to increase the exposure to bedaquiline. Avoid prolonged use. Mild Theoretical
- Diltiazem is predicted to increase the risk of cardiodepression when given with beta blockers, non-selective. Severe Study → Also see TABLE 6 p. 1335 → Also see TABLE 8 p. 1335
- Intravenous verapamil increases the risk of cardiovascular side-effects when given with beta blockers, non-selective. Avoid. Severe Study → Also see TABLE 6 p. 1335 → Also see TABLE 8 p. 1335
- Oral verapamil increases the risk of cardiovascular side-effects when given with beta blockers, non-selective. Severe Study → Also see TABLE 6 p. 1335 → Also see TABLE 8 p. 1335
- Diltiazem is predicted to increase the risk of cardiodepression when given with beta blockers, selective. Severe Study → Also see TABLE 6 p. 1335 → Also see TABLE 8 p. 1335
- Intravenous verapamil increases the risk of cardiovascular side-effects when given with beta blockers, selective. Avoid. Severe Study → Also see TABLE 6 p. 1335 → Also see TABLE 8 p. 1335
- Oral verapamil increases the risk of cardiovascular side-effects when given with beta blockers, selective. Severe Study → Also see TABLE 6 p. 1335 → Also see TABLE 8 p. 1335
- Bosentan is predicted to decrease the exposure to calcium channel blockers (amlodipine, felodipine, lacidipine,

lercanidipine, nicardipine, nifedipine, nimodipine). Monitor and adjust dose. Moderate Theoretical
- Bosentan is predicted to decrease the exposure to calcium channel blockers (diltiazem, verapamil). Moderate Theoretical
- Calcium channel blockers (diltiazem, verapamil) are predicted to increase the exposure to bosutinib. Avoid or adjust dose. Severe Theoretical
- Calcium channel blockers (diltiazem, verapamil) are predicted to increase the exposure to buspirone. Use with caution and adjust dose. Moderate Study
- Calcium channel blockers (diltiazem, verapamil) are predicted to increase the exposure to cabozantinib. Moderate Theoretical
- Calcium channel blockers (diltiazem) are predicted to increase the exposure to calcium channel blockers (amlodipine, felodipine, lacidipine, lercanidipine, nicardipine, nifedipine, nimodipine). Monitor and adjust dose. Moderate Study → Also see TABLE 8 p. 1335
- Calcium channel blockers (verapamil) are predicted to increase the exposure to calcium channel blockers (amlodipine, felodipine, lacidipine, lercanidipine, nicardipine, nifedipine, nimodipine). Monitor and adjust dose. Moderate Study → Also see TABLE 8 p. 1335
- Calcium channel blockers (diltiazem) are predicted to increase the exposure to calcium channel blockers (felodipine, lacidipine, lercanidipine, nicardipine, nifedipine, nimodipine). Monitor and adjust dose. Moderate Study → Also see TABLE 8 p. 1335
- Calcium channel blockers (diltiazem, verapamil) are predicted to increase the exposure to ceritinib. Moderate Theoretical
- Calcium channel blockers (diltiazem, nicardipine, verapamil) increase the concentration of ciclosporin. Severe Study
- Ciclosporin moderately increases the exposure to lercanidipine. Use with caution or avoid. Severe Study
- Cobicistat is predicted to increase the exposure to calcium channel blockers (amlodipine, felodipine, lacidipine, nicardipine, nifedipine, nimodipine). Monitor and adjust dose. Moderate Study
- Cobicistat is predicted to increase the exposure to calcium channel blockers (diltiazem, verapamil). Severe Study
- Cobicistat is predicted to markedly increase the exposure to lercanidipine. Avoid. Severe Study
- Calcium channel blockers (diltiazem, verapamil) are predicted to increase the exposure to cobimetinib. Severe Theoretical
- Calcium channel blockers (diltiazem, verapamil) are predicted to increase the exposure to colchicine. Adjust colchicine dose with moderate inhibitors of CYP3A4, p. 1085. Severe Study
- Calcium channel blockers (diltiazem, verapamil) are predicted to increase the exposure to corticosteroids (methylprednisolone). Monitor and adjust dose. Moderate Study
- Crizotinib is predicted to increase the exposure to calcium channel blockers (amlodipine, felodipine, lacidipine, lercanidipine, nicardipine, nifedipine, nimodipine). Monitor and adjust dose. Moderate Study
- Verapamil increases the exposure to dabigatran. Adjust dabigatran dose, p. 135. Severe Study
- Intravenous dantrolene potentially increases the risk of acute hyperkalaemia and cardiovascular collapse when given with calcium channel blockers (diltiazem, verapamil). Avoid. Severe Anecdotal
- Calcium channel blockers (diltiazem, verapamil) are predicted to slightly increase the exposure to darifenacin. Moderate Study
- Calcium channel blockers (diltiazem, verapamil) are predicted to increase the exposure to dasatinib. Severe Study
- Calcium channel blockers (diltiazem, verapamil) increase the concentration of digoxin. Monitor and adjust dose. Severe Study → Also see TABLE 6 p. 1335
- Calcium channel blockers (diltiazem, verapamil) increase the risk of QT-prolongation when given with domperidone. Avoid. Severe Study
- Calcium channel blockers (diltiazem, verapamil) are predicted to increase the exposure to dopamine receptor agonists (bromocriptine). Severe Theoretical → Also see TABLE 8 p. 1335
- Calcium channel blockers (diltiazem, verapamil) are predicted to increase the concentration of dopamine receptor agonists (cabergoline). Moderate Anecdotal → Also see TABLE 8 p. 1335
- Calcium channel blockers (diltiazem, verapamil) are predicted to moderately increase the exposure to dutasteride. Mild Study

Calcium channel blockers (continued)

▶ **Verapamil** is predicted to slightly increase the exposure to edoxaban. Severe Theoretical

▶ **Efavirenz** is predicted to decrease the exposure to calcium channel blockers **(amlodipine, felodipine, lacidipine, lercanidipine, nicardipine, nifedipine, nimodipine)**. Monitor and adjust dose. Moderate Theoretical

▶ **Efavirenz** is predicted to decrease the exposure to calcium channel blockers **(diltiazem, verapamil)**. Moderate Theoretical

▶ Calcium channel blockers **(diltiazem, verapamil)** are predicted to increase the exposure to **eliglustat**. Avoid or adjust dose—consult product literature. Severe Study

▶ **Enzalutamide** is predicted to decrease the exposure to calcium channel blockers **(amlodipine, felodipine, lacidipine, lercanidipine, nicardipine, nifedipine, nimodipine)**. Monitor and adjust dose. Moderate Study

▶ **Enzalutamide** is predicted to decrease the exposure to calcium channel blockers **(diltiazem, verapamil)**. Severe Study

▶ Calcium channel blockers **(diltiazem, verapamil)** are predicted to increase the risk of ergotism when given with **ergometrine**. Severe Theoretical

▶ Calcium channel blockers **(diltiazem, verapamil)** are predicted to increase the risk of ergotism when given with **ergotamine**. Severe Theoretical

▶ Calcium channel blockers **(diltiazem, verapamil)** are predicted to increase the exposure to **erlotinib**. Moderate Theoretical

▶ Calcium channel blockers **(diltiazem, verapamil)** are predicted to increase the concentration of **everolimus**. Avoid or adjust dose. Moderate Study

▶ Calcium channel blockers **(diltiazem, verapamil)** are predicted to increase the exposure to **fesoterodine**. Adjust **fesoterodine** dose with moderate inhibitors of CYP3A4 in hepatic and renal impairment, p. 759. Mild Study

▶ **Verapamil** is predicted to increase the exposure to **fidaxomicin**. Avoid. Moderate Study

▶ Calcium channel blockers **(diltiazem, verapamil)** are predicted to increase the exposure to **fingolimod**. Avoid. Moderate Theoretical → Also see TABLE 6 p. 1335

▶ Calcium channel blockers **(diltiazem, verapamil)** are predicted to increase the exposure to **gefitinib**. Moderate Theoretical

▶ **Grapefruit juice** very slightly increases the exposure to **amlodipine**. Avoid. Mild Study

▶ **Grapefruit juice** increases the exposure to calcium channel blockers **(nifedipine, verapamil)**. Avoid. Mild Study

▶ **Grapefruit juice** increases the exposure to **felodipine**. Avoid. Moderate Study

▶ **Grapefruit juice** is predicted to increase the exposure to **lercanidipine**. Avoid. Moderate Theoretical

▶ **Grapefruit juice** increases the exposure to **nicardipine**. Mild Study

▶ Calcium channel blockers **(diltiazem, verapamil)** are predicted to increase the concentration of **guanfacine**. Adjust **guanfacine** dose, p. 349. Moderate Theoretical → Also see TABLE 8 p. 1335

▶ H_2 receptor antagonists **(cimetidine)** (high-dose) are predicted to increase the exposure to **lercanidipine**. Moderate Theoretical

▶ H_2 receptor antagonists **(cimetidine)** moderately increase the exposure to **nifedipine**. Monitor and adjust dose. Severe Study

▶ H_2 receptor antagonists **(cimetidine)** increase the exposure to **verapamil**. Moderate Study

▶ H_2 receptor antagonists **(cimetidine)** slightly increase the exposure to calcium channel blockers **(diltiazem, nimodipine)**. Monitor and adjust dose. Moderate Study

▶ **HIV-protease inhibitors** are predicted to increase the exposure to calcium channel blockers **(amlodipine, felodipine, lacidipine, nicardipine, nifedipine, nimodipine)**. Monitor and adjust dose. Moderate Study

▶ **HIV-protease inhibitors** are predicted to increase the exposure to calcium channel blockers **(diltiazem, verapamil)**. Severe Study

▶ **HIV-protease inhibitors** are predicted to markedly increase the exposure to **lercanidipine**. Avoid. Severe Study

▶ Calcium channel blockers **(diltiazem, verapamil)** are predicted to increase the exposure to **ibrutinib**. Adjust **ibrutinib** dose with moderate inhibitors of CYP3A4, p. 952. Severe Study

▶ **Idelalisib** is predicted to increase the exposure to calcium channel blockers **(amlodipine, felodipine, lacidipine, nicardipine,**

nifedipine, nimodipine)**. Monitor and adjust dose. Moderate Study

▶ **Idelalisib** is predicted to increase the exposure to calcium channel blockers **(diltiazem, verapamil)**. Severe Study

▶ **Idelalisib** is predicted to markedly increase the exposure to **lercanidipine**. Avoid. Severe Study

▶ Calcium channel blockers **(diltiazem, verapamil)** are predicted to increase the exposure to **imatinib**. Moderate Theoretical

▶ **Imatinib** is predicted to increase the exposure to calcium channel blockers **(amlodipine, felodipine, lacidipine, lercanidipine, nicardipine, nifedipine, nimodipine)**. Monitor and adjust dose. Moderate Study

▶ Calcium channel blockers **(diltiazem, verapamil)** are predicted to increase the exposure to **ivabradine**. Avoid. Moderate Study → Also see TABLE 6 p. 1335

▶ Calcium channel blockers **(diltiazem, verapamil)** are predicted to increase the exposure to **ivacaftor**. Adjust **ivacaftor** dose with moderate inhibitors of CYP3A4, p. 292. Severe Study

▶ Calcium channel blockers **(diltiazem, verapamil)** are predicted to increase the exposure to **lapatinib**. Moderate Study

▶ Calcium channel blockers **(diltiazem, verapamil)** are predicted to increase the risk of neurotoxicity when given with **lithium**. Severe Anecdotal

▶ Calcium channel blockers **(amlodipine, lacidipine)** are predicted to increase the exposure to **lomitapide**. Separate administration by 12 hours. Moderate Theoretical

▶ Calcium channel blockers **(diltiazem, verapamil)** are predicted to increase the exposure to **lomitapide**. Avoid. Moderate Theoretical

▶ Calcium channel blockers **(diltiazem, verapamil)** are predicted to increase the exposure to **lurasidone**. Moderate Study → Also see TABLE 8 p. 1335

▶ **Macrolides (clarithromycin)** are predicted to markedly increase the exposure to **lercanidipine**. Avoid. Severe Study

▶ **Macrolides (erythromycin)** are predicted to increase the exposure to **diltiazem**. Severe Theoretical

▶ **Macrolides (erythromycin)** are predicted to increase the exposure to **verapamil**. Severe Study

▶ **Macrolides (erythromycin)** are predicted to increase the exposure to calcium channel blockers **(amlodipine, felodipine, lacidipine, lercanidipine, nicardipine, nifedipine, nimodipine)**. Monitor and adjust dose. Moderate Study

▶ **Macrolides (clarithromycin)** are predicted to increase the exposure to calcium channel blockers **(amlodipine, felodipine, lacidipine, nicardipine, nifedipine, nimodipine)**. Monitor and adjust dose. Moderate Study

▶ **Macrolides (clarithromycin)** are predicted to increase the exposure to calcium channel blockers **(diltiazem, verapamil)**. Severe Study

▶ Intravenous **magnesium** potentially increases the risk of hypotension when given with calcium channel blockers **(amlodipine, clevidipine, felodipine, lacidipine, lercanidipine, nicardipine, nifedipine, nimodipine, verapamil)** (in pregnant women). Severe Anecdotal

▶ Calcium channel blockers **(diltiazem, verapamil)** are predicted to increase the exposure to **midazolam**. Monitor side effects and adjust dose. Severe Study

▶ Calcium channel blockers **(diltiazem, verapamil)** are predicted to increase the exposure to **midostaurin**. Moderate Theoretical

▶ **Mitotane** is predicted to decrease the exposure to calcium channel blockers **(amlodipine, felodipine, lacidipine, lercanidipine, nicardipine, nimodipine)**. Monitor and adjust dose. Moderate Study

▶ **Monoclonal antibodies (tocilizumab)** are predicted to decrease the exposure to **calcium channel blockers**. Monitor and adjust dose. Moderate Theoretical

▶ Calcium channel blockers **(diltiazem, verapamil)** are predicted to increase the exposure to **naloxegol**. Adjust **naloxegol** dose and monitor side effects, p. 64. Moderate Study

▶ **Netupitant** is predicted to increase the exposure to calcium channel blockers **(amlodipine, felodipine, lacidipine, lercanidipine, nicardipine, nifedipine, nimodipine)**. Monitor and adjust dose. Moderate Study

▶ **Nevirapine** is predicted to decrease the exposure to calcium channel blockers **(amlodipine, felodipine, lacidipine,**

lercanidipine, nicardipine, nifedipine, nimodipine). Monitor and adjust dose. Moderate Theoretical
▶ **Nevirapine** is predicted to decrease the exposure to calcium channel blockers (**diltiazem, verapamil**). Moderate Theoretical
▶ Calcium channel blockers (**diltiazem, verapamil**) are predicted to increase the exposure to nilotinib. Moderate Theoretical
▶ **Nilotinib** is predicted to increase the exposure to calcium channel blockers (**amlodipine, felodipine, lacidipine, lercanidipine, nicardipine, nifedipine, nimodipine**). Monitor and adjust dose. Moderate Study
▶ **Verapamil** is predicted to increase the exposure to nintedanib. Moderate Study
▶ Calcium channel blockers (**diltiazem, verapamil**) are predicted to increase the exposure to olaparib. Avoid moderate inhibitors of CYP3A4 or adjust **olaparib** dose, p. 973. Moderate Theoretical
▶ Calcium channel blockers (**diltiazem, verapamil**) are predicted to increase the exposure to opioids (alfentanil, buprenorphine, fentanyl, oxycodone). Monitor and adjust dose. Moderate Study → Also see TABLE 6 p. 1335
▶ Calcium channel blockers (**diltiazem, verapamil**) are predicted to increase the exposure to opioids (methadone, sufentanil). Moderate Theoretical → Also see TABLE 6 p. 1335
▶ Calcium channel blockers (**diltiazem, verapamil**) are predicted to increase the exposure to oxybutynin. Mild Theoretical
▶ **Verapamil** is predicted to increase the exposure to panobinostat. Adjust dose. Moderate Theoretical
▶ Calcium channel blockers (**diltiazem, verapamil**) are predicted to increase the exposure to pazopanib. Moderate Theoretical
▶ Calcium channel blockers (**diltiazem, verapamil**) are predicted to increase the exposure to phosphodiesterase type-5 inhibitors (avanafil). Adjust **avanafil** dose, p. 794. Moderate Theoretical → Also see TABLE 8 p. 1335
▶ Calcium channel blockers (**diltiazem, verapamil**) are predicted to increase the exposure to phosphodiesterase type-5 inhibitors (sildenafil). Monitor or adjust **sildenafil** dose with moderate inhibitors of CYP3A4, p. 794. Moderate Study → Also see TABLE 8 p. 1335
▶ Calcium channel blockers (**diltiazem, verapamil**) are predicted to increase the exposure to phosphodiesterase type-5 inhibitors (tadalafil). Severe Theoretical → Also see TABLE 8 p. 1335
▶ Calcium channel blockers (**diltiazem, verapamil**) are predicted to increase the exposure to phosphodiesterase type-5 inhibitors (vardenafil). Adjust dose. Severe Theoretical → Also see TABLE 8 p. 1335
▶ Calcium channel blockers (**diltiazem, verapamil**) are predicted to increase the exposure to pimozide. Avoid. Severe Theoretical → Also see TABLE 8 p. 1335
▶ Calcium channel blockers (**diltiazem, verapamil**) are predicted to increase the exposure to quetiapine. Avoid. Moderate Study → Also see TABLE 8 p. 1335
▶ Calcium channel blockers (**diltiazem, verapamil**) are predicted to increase the exposure to ranolazine. Severe Study
▶ Calcium channel blockers (**diltiazem, verapamil**) are predicted to increase the exposure to ribociclib. Moderate Study
▶ **Rifampicin** is predicted to decrease the exposure to calcium channel blockers (**amlodipine, felodipine, lacidipine, lercanidipine, nicardipine, nifedipine, nimodipine**). Monitor and adjust dose. Moderate Study
▶ **Rifampicin** greatly decreases the exposure to calcium channel blockers (**diltiazem, verapamil**). Severe Study
▶ **Rifampicin** moderately decreases the exposure to nifedipine. Avoid. Severe Study
▶ Calcium channel blockers (**diltiazem, verapamil**) are predicted to increase the exposure to ruxolitinib. Moderate Theoretical
▶ Calcium channel blockers (**diltiazem, verapamil**) are predicted to increase the exposure to saxagliptin. Mild Study
▶ Calcium channel blockers (**diltiazem, verapamil**) are predicted to increase the exposure to simeprevir. Avoid. Severe Study
▶ Calcium channel blockers (**diltiazem, verapamil**) increase the concentration of sirolimus. Monitor and adjust dose. Moderate Study
▶ Calcium channel blockers (**diltiazem, verapamil**) are predicted to increase the exposure to SSRIs (dapoxetine). Adjust **dapoxetine** dose with moderate inhibitors of CYP3A4, p. 801. Moderate Theoretical

▶ **St John's Wort** is predicted to decrease the exposure to calcium channel blockers (**amlodipine, felodipine, lacidipine, lercanidipine, nicardipine, nifedipine, nimodipine**). Monitor and adjust dose. Moderate Theoretical
▶ **St John's Wort** is predicted to decrease the exposure to calcium channel blockers (**diltiazem, verapamil**). Moderate Theoretical
▶ Calcium channel blockers (**diltiazem, verapamil**) are predicted to increase the exposure to statins (atorvastatin). Monitor and adjust dose. Severe Study
▶ **Amlodipine** slightly increases the exposure to statins (simvastatin). Adjust **simvastatin** dose, p. 203. Mild Study
▶ Calcium channel blockers (**diltiazem, verapamil**) are predicted to increase the exposure to statins (simvastatin). Use with caution and adjust **simvastatin** dose, p. 203. Severe Study
▶ **Sulfinpyrazone** decreases the exposure to **verapamil**. Moderate Study
▶ Calcium channel blockers (**diltiazem, verapamil**) are predicted to increase the exposure to sunitinib. Moderate Theoretical
▶ Calcium channel blockers (**diltiazem, verapamil**) are predicted to increase the concentration of tacrolimus. Severe Study
▶ **Nicardipine** potentially increases the concentration of tacrolimus. Monitor concentration and adjust dose. Severe Anecdotal
▶ Calcium channel blockers (**diltiazem, verapamil**) are predicted to increase the exposure to taxanes (cabazitaxel). Moderate Theoretical
▶ Calcium channel blockers (**diltiazem, verapamil**) are predicted to increase the concentration of temsirolimus. Moderate Theoretical
▶ Calcium channel blockers (**diltiazem, verapamil**) are predicted to increase the exposure to tofacitinib. Moderate Study
▶ Calcium channel blockers (**diltiazem, verapamil**) are predicted to increase the exposure to tolterodine. Mild Theoretical
▶ Calcium channel blockers (**diltiazem, verapamil**) are predicted to increase the exposure to tolvaptan. Adjust dose. Moderate Study
▶ **Verapamil** is predicted to increase the exposure to topotecan. Severe Study
▶ **Verapamil** is predicted to increase the concentration of trametinib. Moderate Theoretical
▶ Calcium channel blockers (**diltiazem, verapamil**) are predicted to increase the exposure to trazodone. Moderate Theoretical
▶ Calcium channel blockers (**diltiazem, verapamil**) are predicted to increase the exposure to ulipristal. Avoid if used for uterine fibroids. Moderate Study
▶ Calcium channel blockers (**diltiazem, verapamil**) are predicted to increase the exposure to venetoclax. Avoid moderate inhibitors of CYP3A4 or adjust **venetoclax** dose, p. 974. Severe Study
▶ Calcium channel blockers (**diltiazem, verapamil**) are predicted to increase the exposure to vinca alkaloids. Severe Theoretical
▶ Calcium channel blockers (**diltiazem, verapamil**) are predicted to increase the exposure to zopiclone. Adjust dose. Moderate Study

Calcium chloride → see calcium salts
Calcium gluconate → see calcium salts
Calcium lactate → see calcium salts
Calcium phosphate → see calcium salts
Calcium salts

calcium acetate · calcium carbonate · calcium chloride · calcium gluconate · calcium lactate · calcium phosphate

SEPARATION OF ADMINISTRATION Calcium carbonate-containing antacids should preferably not be taken at the same time as other drugs since they might impair absorption. Antacids might damage enteric coatings designed to prevent dissolution in the stomach.

▶ Oral **calcium salts** decrease the absorption of alkylating agents (estramustine). Severe Study
▶ **Calcium carbonate** decreases the absorption of antimalarials (chloroquine). Separate administration by at least 4 hours. Moderate Study
▶ **Calcium carbonate** is predicted to decrease the absorption of antimalarials (proguanil). Separate administration by at least 2 hours. Moderate Study

Calcium salts (continued)

▸ Oral **calcium salts** decrease the absorption of bisphosphonates (alendronic acid). **Alendronic acid** should be taken at least 30 minutes before **calcium salts**. Study

▸ Oral **calcium salts** are predicted to decrease the absorption of oral bisphosphonates (ibandronic acid). Avoid **calcium salts** for at least 6 hours before or 1 hour after **ibandronic acid**. Moderate Theoretical

▸ Oral **calcium salts** decrease the absorption of bisphosphonates (risedronate). Separate administration by at least 2 hours. Moderate Study

▸ Oral **calcium salts** decrease the absorption of bisphosphonates (sodium clodronate). Avoid **calcium salts** for 2 hours before or 1 hour after **sodium clodronate**. Moderate Study

▸ Cephalosporins (ceftriaxone) increase the risk of cardio-respiratory arrest when given with **calcium chloride**. Avoid. Severe Anecdotal

▸ Cephalosporins (ceftriaxone) increase the risk of cardio-respiratory arrest when given with intravenous **calcium gluconate**. Avoid. Severe Anecdotal

▸ Intravenous **calcium salts** increase the concentration of digoxin. Avoid. Moderate Anecdotal

▸ Oral **calcium salts** decrease the absorption of dolutegravir. **Dolutegravir** should be taken 2 hours before or 6 hours after **calcium salts**. Moderate Study

▸ Oral **calcium salts** decrease the absorption of eltrombopag. **Eltrombopag** should be taken 2 hours before or 4 hours after **calcium salts**. Severe Study

▸ **Calcium carbonate** decreases the absorption of hydroxychloroquine. Separate administration by at least 4 hours. Moderate Study

▸ **Calcium carbonate** decreases the absorption of iron (oral). **Calcium carbonate** should be taken 1 hour before or 2 hours after **iron (oral)**. Moderate Study

▸ **Calcium carbonate** is predicted to decrease the exposure to ledipasvir. Separate administration by 4 hours. Moderate Theoretical

▸ **Calcium carbonate** decreases the absorption of quinolones (ciprofloxacin). Separate administration by 2 hours. Moderate Study

▸ **Calcium carbonate** decreases the absorption of quinolones (norfloxacin). **Norfloxacin** should be taken 2 hours before or 4 hours after **calcium carbonate**. Moderate Study

▸ **Calcium carbonate** greatly decreases the exposure to raltegravir (high-dose). Avoid. Severe Study

▸ **Calcium carbonate** is predicted to slightly decrease the exposure to rilpivirine. **Calcium carbonate** should be taken 2 hours before or 4 hours after **rilpivirine**. Severe Theoretical

▸ **Calcium carbonate** is predicted to decrease the absorption of tetracyclines. Separate administration by 2 to 3 hours. Moderate Theoretical

▸ Thiazide diuretics increase the risk of hypercalcaemia when given with **calcium salts**. Severe Anecdotal

▸ Oral **calcium salts** are predicted to decrease the absorption of thyroid hormones (levothyroxine). Separate administration by at least 4 hours. Moderate Anecdotal

▸ **Calcium carbonate** is predicted to decrease the concentration of velpatasvir. Separate administration by 4 hours. Moderate Anecdotal

▸ Oral **calcium salts** decrease the absorption of zinc. Moderate Study

Canagliflozin → see TABLE 14 p. 1337 (antidiabetic drugs), TABLE 8 p. 1335 (hypotension)

▸ Rifampicin moderately decreases the exposure to **canagliflozin**. Adjust **canagliflozin** dose, p. 687. Moderate Study

Canakinumab → see monoclonal antibodies
Candesartan → see angiotensin-II receptor antagonists
Cangrelor → see TABLE 4 p. 1334 (antiplatelet effects)
Cannabis extract → see TABLE 11 p. 1336 (CNS depressant effects)

▸ Antiepileptics (carbamazepine, fosphenytoin, phenobarbital, phenytoin, primidone) are predicted to decrease the exposure to **cannabis extract**. Avoid. Severe Theoretical → Also see TABLE 11 p. 1336

▸ Antifungals, azoles (itraconazole, ketoconazole, voriconazole) are predicted to increase the exposure to **cannabis extract**. Use with caution and adjust dose. Moderate Theoretical

▸ Cobicistat is predicted to increase the exposure to **cannabis extract**. Use with caution and adjust dose. Moderate Theoretical

▸ Enzalutamide is predicted to decrease the exposure to **cannabis extract**. Avoid. Severe Theoretical

▸ HIV-protease inhibitors are predicted to increase the exposure to **cannabis extract**. Use with caution and adjust dose. Moderate Theoretical

▸ Idelalisib is predicted to increase the exposure to **cannabis extract**. Use with caution and adjust dose. Moderate Theoretical

▸ Macrolides (clarithromycin) are predicted to increase the exposure to **cannabis extract**. Use with caution and adjust dose. Moderate Theoretical

▸ Mitotane is predicted to decrease the exposure to **cannabis extract**. Avoid. Severe Theoretical

▸ Rifampicin is predicted to decrease the exposure to **cannabis extract**. Avoid. Severe Theoretical

Capecitabine → see TABLE 15 p. 1337 (myelosuppression)

▸ Allopurinol is predicted to decrease the effects of **capecitabine**. Avoid. Study

▸ **Capecitabine** increases the concentration of antiepileptics (fosphenytoin, phenytoin). Severe Anecdotal

▸ **Capecitabine** increases the effects of coumarins. Monitor INR and adjust dose. Moderate Anecdotal

▸ Folates are predicted to increase the risk of toxicity when given with **capecitabine**. Severe Anecdotal

▸ H_2 receptor antagonists (cimetidine) are predicted to slightly increase the exposure to **capecitabine**. Severe Theoretical

▸ Live vaccines are predicted to increase the risk of generalised infection (possibly life-threatening) when given with **capecitabine**. Public Health England advises avoid (refer to Green Book). Severe Theoretical

▸ Metronidazole is predicted to increase the risk of capecitabine toxicity when given with **capecitabine**. Severe Anecdotal

Capreomycin → see TABLE 2 p. 1334 (nephrotoxicity), TABLE 19 p. 1338 (ototoxicity)

Captopril → see ACE inhibitors
Carbamazepine → see antiepileptics
Carbapenems

ertapenem · imipenem · meropenem

▸ **Carbapenems** decrease the concentration of antiepileptics (valproate). Avoid. Severe Anecdotal

▸ Ganciclovir is predicted to increase the risk of seizures when given with **imipenem**. Avoid. Severe Anecdotal

▸ Valganciclovir is predicted to increase the risk of seizures when given with **imipenem**. Avoid. Severe Anecdotal

Carbidopa

▸ Iron (oral) is predicted to decrease the exposure to **carbidopa**. Moderate Theoretical

Carbimazole → see TABLE 15 p. 1337 (myelosuppression)

▸ **Carbimazole** affects the concentration of digoxin. Monitor and adjust dose. Moderate Theoretical

▸ **Carbimazole** decreases the effects of metyrapone. Avoid. Moderate Theoretical

Carboplatin → see platinum compounds
Carfilzomib → see TABLE 15 p. 1337 (myelosuppression)
Carmustine → see alkylating agents
Carvedilol → see beta blockers, non-selective
Caspofungin

▸ Antiepileptics (carbamazepine, fosphenytoin, phenytoin) are predicted to decrease the concentration of **caspofungin**. Adjust **caspofungin** dose, p. 582. Moderate Theoretical

▸ Ciclosporin slightly increases the exposure to **caspofungin**. Severe Study

▸ Corticosteroids (dexamethasone) are predicted to decrease the concentration of **caspofungin**. Adjust **caspofungin** dose, p. 582. Moderate Theoretical

▸ Efavirenz is predicted to decrease the concentration of **caspofungin**. Adjust dose. Moderate Study

▸ Nevirapine is predicted to decrease the concentration of **caspofungin**. Adjust dose. Moderate Theoretical

▸ Rifampicin decreases the concentration of **caspofungin**. Adjust **caspofungin** dose, p. 582. Moderate Study

Cefaclor → see cephalosporins
Cefadroxil → see cephalosporins
Cefalexin → see cephalosporins
Cefixime → see cephalosporins
Cefotaxime → see cephalosporins
Cefradine → see cephalosporins
Ceftaroline → see cephalosporins
Ceftazidime → see cephalosporins
Ceftobiprole → see cephalosporins
Ceftolozane → see cephalosporins
Ceftriaxone → see cephalosporins
Cefuroxime → see cephalosporins
Celecoxib → see NSAIDs
Celiprolol → see beta blockers, selective
Cephalosporins → see TABLE 2 p. 1334 (nephrotoxicity)

cefaclor · cefadroxil · cefalexin · cefixime · cefotaxime · cefradine · ceftaroline · ceftazidime · ceftobiprole · ceftolozane · ceftriaxone · cefuroxime

▸ **Ceftobiprole** is predicted to increase the exposure to bosentan. Moderate Theoretical
▸ **Ceftriaxone** increases the risk of cardio-respiratory arrest when given with calcium salts (calcium chloride). Avoid. Severe Anecdotal
▸ **Ceftriaxone** increases the risk of cardio-respiratory arrest when given with intravenous calcium salts (calcium gluconate). Avoid. Severe Anecdotal
▸ **Ceftriaxone** potentially increases the risk of bleeding events when given with coumarins. Severe Anecdotal
▸ **Ceftriaxone** potentially increases the risk of bleeding events when given with phenindione. Severe Anecdotal
▸ **Ceftobiprole** is predicted to increase the concentration of statins. Moderate Theoretical
▸ **Ceftobiprole** is predicted to increase the concentration of sulfonylureas (glibenclamide). Moderate Theoretical
Ceritinib → see TABLE 15 p. 1337 (myelosuppression), TABLE 9 p. 1336 (QT-interval prolongation)
▸ **Ceritinib** is predicted to increase the exposure to aliskiren. Moderate Theoretical
▸ Antacids are predicted to decrease the absorption of **ceritinib**. Separate administration by 2 hours. Moderate Theoretical
▸ Antiarrhythmics (amiodarone, dronedarone) are predicted to increase the exposure to **ceritinib**. Moderate Theoretical → Also see TABLE 9 p. 1336
▸ Antiepileptics (carbamazepine, fosphenytoin, phenobarbital, phenytoin, primidone) are predicted to decrease the exposure to **ceritinib**. Avoid. Severe Study
▸ Antifungals, azoles (fluconazole, isavuconazole, posaconazole) are predicted to increase the exposure to **ceritinib**. Moderate Theoretical → Also see TABLE 9 p. 1336
▸ Antifungals, azoles (itraconazole, ketoconazole, voriconazole) are predicted to increase the exposure to **ceritinib**. Avoid or adjust **ceritinib** dose, p. 945. Severe Study → Also see TABLE 9 p. 1336
▸ **Ceritinib** is predicted to increase the exposure to antihistamines, non-sedating (fexofenadine). Moderate Theoretical
▸ Aprepitant is predicted to increase the exposure to **ceritinib**. Moderate Theoretical
▸ Calcium channel blockers (diltiazem, verapamil) are predicted to increase the exposure to **ceritinib**. Moderate Theoretical
▸ **Ceritinib** is predicted to increase the exposure to ciclosporin. Avoid. Severe Theoretical
▸ Cobicistat is predicted to increase the exposure to **ceritinib**. Avoid or adjust **ceritinib** dose, p. 945. Severe Study
▸ **Ceritinib** is predicted to increase the exposure to colchicine. Moderate Theoretical
▸ **Ceritinib** is predicted to increase the exposure to coumarins (warfarin). Avoid. Severe Theoretical
▸ Crizotinib is predicted to increase the exposure to **ceritinib**. Moderate Theoretical → Also see TABLE 15 p. 1337 → Also see TABLE 9 p. 1336
▸ **Ceritinib** is predicted to increase the exposure to dabigatran. Moderate Theoretical
▸ **Ceritinib** is predicted to increase the risk of bradycardia when given with digoxin. Avoid. Severe Theoretical
▸ **Ceritinib** is predicted to increase the exposure to edoxaban. Moderate Theoretical

▸ Enzalutamide is predicted to decrease the exposure to **ceritinib**. Avoid. Severe Study
▸ **Ceritinib** is predicted to increase the exposure to ergotamine. Avoid. Severe Theoretical
▸ **Ceritinib** is predicted to increase the exposure to everolimus. Moderate Theoretical → Also see TABLE 15 p. 1337
▸ Grapefruit juice is predicted to increase the exposure to **ceritinib**. Avoid. Severe Theoretical
▸ H_2 receptor antagonists are predicted to decrease the absorption of **ceritinib**. Moderate Theoretical
▸ HIV-protease inhibitors are predicted to increase the exposure to **ceritinib**. Avoid or adjust **ceritinib** dose, p. 945. Severe Study → Also see TABLE 9 p. 1336
▸ Idelalisib is predicted to increase the exposure to **ceritinib**. Avoid or adjust **ceritinib** dose, p. 945. Severe Study → Also see TABLE 15 p. 1337
▸ Imatinib is predicted to increase the exposure to **ceritinib**. Moderate Theoretical → Also see TABLE 15 p. 1337
▸ Lapatinib is predicted to increase the exposure to **ceritinib**. Moderate Theoretical → Also see TABLE 9 p. 1336
▸ **Ceritinib** is predicted to increase the exposure to loperamide. Moderate Theoretical
▸ Macrolides (azithromycin, erythromycin) are predicted to increase the exposure to **ceritinib**. Moderate Theoretical → Also see TABLE 9 p. 1336
▸ Macrolides (clarithromycin) are predicted to increase the exposure to **ceritinib**. Avoid or adjust **ceritinib** dose, p. 945. Severe Study → Also see TABLE 9 p. 1336
▸ Mitotane is predicted to decrease the exposure to **ceritinib**. Avoid. Severe Study → Also see TABLE 15 p. 1337
▸ Netupitant is predicted to increase the exposure to **ceritinib**. Moderate Theoretical
▸ Nilotinib is predicted to increase the exposure to **ceritinib**. Moderate Theoretical → Also see TABLE 15 p. 1337 → Also see TABLE 9 p. 1336
▸ **Ceritinib** is predicted to increase the exposure to NSAIDs (celecoxib, diclofenac). Adjust dose. Moderate Theoretical
▸ **Ceritinib** is predicted to increase the exposure to opioids (alfentanil, fentanyl). Avoid. Severe Theoretical
▸ **Ceritinib** is predicted to increase the exposure to pimozide. Avoid. Severe Theoretical → Also see TABLE 9 p. 1336
▸ Proton pump inhibitors are predicted to decrease the absorption of **ceritinib**. Moderate Theoretical
▸ Ranolazine is predicted to increase the exposure to **ceritinib**. Moderate Theoretical → Also see TABLE 9 p. 1336
▸ Rifampicin is predicted to decrease the exposure to **ceritinib**. Avoid. Severe Study
▸ **Ceritinib** is predicted to increase the exposure to sirolimus. Avoid. Severe Theoretical
▸ St John's Wort is predicted to decrease the exposure to **ceritinib**. Avoid. Severe Theoretical
▸ **Ceritinib** is predicted to increase the exposure to sulfonylureas (glimepiride). Adjust dose. Moderate Theoretical
▸ **Ceritinib** is predicted to increase the exposure to tacrolimus. Avoid. Severe Theoretical
▸ **Ceritinib** is predicted to increase the exposure to taxanes (paclitaxel). Moderate Theoretical → Also see TABLE 15 p. 1337
▸ **Ceritinib** is predicted to increase the exposure to topotecan. Moderate Theoretical → Also see TABLE 15 p. 1337
Certolizumab pegol → see monoclonal antibodies
Cetirizine → see antihistamines, non-sedating
Cetuximab → see monoclonal antibodies
Chenodeoxycholic acid
▸ Oral antacids (aluminium hydroxide) decrease the absorption of **chenodeoxycholic acid**. Moderate Study
▸ Antiepileptics (phenobarbital, primidone) are predicted to affect the efficacy of **chenodeoxycholic acid**. Monitor and adjust dose. Moderate Theoretical
▸ Ciclosporin is predicted to affect the efficacy of **chenodeoxycholic acid**. Monitor and adjust dose. Moderate Theoretical
▸ Oral combined hormonal contraceptives potentially decrease the efficacy of **chenodeoxycholic acid**. Avoid. Moderate Theoretical

A1

Interactions | Appendix 1

Chenodeoxycholic acid (continued)

▶ Sirolimus is predicted to affect the efficacy of **chenodeoxycholic acid**. Monitor and adjust dose. [Moderate] Theoretical

Chloral hydrate → see TABLE 11 p. 1336 (CNS depressant effects)

▶ Intravenous loop diuretics (furosemide) potentially increase the risk of sweating, variable blood pressure, and tachycardia when given after **chloral hydrate**. [Moderate] Anecdotal

Chlorambucil → see alkylating agents

Chloramphenicol

ROUTE-SPECIFIC INFORMATION Since systemic absorption can follow topical application, the possibility of interactions should be borne in mind.

▶ Antiepileptics (phenobarbital, primidone) decrease the concentration of **chloramphenicol**. [Moderate] Study

▶ Intravenous **chloramphenicol** increases the concentration of antiepileptics (fosphenytoin, phenytoin) and antiepileptics (fosphenytoin, phenytoin) affect the concentration of intravenous **chloramphenicol**. Monitor concentration and adjust dose. [Severe] Study

▶ **Chloramphenicol** potentially increases the anticoagulant effect of coumarins. [Moderate] Anecdotal

▶ **Chloramphenicol** is predicted to increase the exposure to guanfacine. Adjust **guanfacine** dose, p. 349. [Moderate] Theoretical

▶ **Chloramphenicol** decreases the efficacy of intravenous iron (injectable). [Moderate] Anecdotal

▶ **Chloramphenicol** decreases the efficacy of oral iron (oral). [Moderate] Theoretical

▶ Rifampicin decreases the concentration of **chloramphenicol**. [Moderate] Study

▶ **Chloramphenicol** is predicted to increase the exposure to sulfonylureas. [Severe] Study

▶ **Chloramphenicol** increases the concentration of tacrolimus. [Severe] Study

Chlordiazepoxide → see TABLE 11 p. 1336 (CNS depressant effects)

▶ **Chlordiazepoxide** affects the concentration of antiepileptics (fosphenytoin, phenytoin). [Severe] Study

▶ Rifampicin is predicted to decrease the exposure to **chlordiazepoxide**. [Moderate] Theoretical

Chloroquine → see antimalarials

Chlorothiazide → see TABLE 18 p. 1338 (hyponatraemia), TABLE 8 p. 1335 (hypotension), TABLE 17 p. 1338 (reduced serum potassium)

Chlorphenamine → see antihistamines, sedating

Chlorpromazine → see phenothiazines

Chlortalidone → see thiazide diuretics

Cholera vaccine

▶ Antimalarials (chloroquine) decrease the efficacy of oral **cholera vaccine**. [Moderate] Study

▶ Hydroxychloroquine is predicted to decrease the efficacy of oral **cholera vaccine**. [Moderate] Theoretical

Cholic acid

▶ Antacids are predicted to decrease the absorption of **cholic acid**. Separate administration by 5 hours. [Mild] Theoretical

▶ Antiepileptics (phenobarbital) decrease the effects of **cholic acid**. Avoid. [Moderate] Study

▶ Ciclosporin affects the concentration of **cholic acid**. Avoid. [Moderate] Study

Choline salicylate

▶ Corticosteroids are predicted to decrease the concentration of **choline salicylate**. [Moderate] Study

Ciclesonide → see corticosteroids

Ciclosporin → see TABLE 2 p. 1334 (nephrotoxicity), TABLE 16 p. 1338 (increased serum potassium)

▶ Pomelo juice is predicted to increase ciclosporin exposure, and purple grape juice is predicted to decrease ciclosporin exposure.

▶ Since systemic absorption can follow topical application, the possibility of interactions should be borne in mind.

▶ **Ciclosporin** is predicted to increase the exposure to afatinib. Separate administration by 12 hours. [Moderate] Study

▶ **Ciclosporin** markedly increases the exposure to aliskiren. Avoid. [Severe] Study → Also see TABLE 16 p. 1338

▶ **Ciclosporin** moderately increases the exposure to ambrisentan. Adjust **ambrisentan** dose, p. 184. [Moderate] Study

▶ **Ciclosporin** increases the concentration of anthracyclines (daunorubicin, doxorubicin, epirubicin, idarubicin, mitoxantrone). [Severe] Study

▶ Antiarrhythmics (amiodarone) increase the concentration of **ciclosporin**. Monitor concentration and adjust dose. [Severe] Study

▶ Antiarrhythmics (dronedarone) increase the concentration of **ciclosporin**. [Severe] Study

▶ **Ciclosporin** increases the exposure to antiarrhythmics (dronedarone). Avoid. [Severe] Theoretical

▶ Antiepileptics (carbamazepine, fosphenytoin, phenobarbital, phenytoin, primidone) decrease the concentration of **ciclosporin**. [Severe] Study

▶ Antiepileptics (oxcarbazepine) decrease the concentration of **ciclosporin**. [Severe] Anecdotal

▶ Antifungals, azoles (fluconazole, isavuconazole, itraconazole, ketoconazole, posaconazole, voriconazole) increase the concentration of **ciclosporin**. [Severe] Study

▶ Antifungals, azoles (miconazole) increase the concentration of **ciclosporin**. Monitor and adjust dose. [Severe] Anecdotal

▶ Aprepitant increases the concentration of **ciclosporin**. [Severe] Study

▶ **Ciclosporin** is predicted to increase the exposure to beta blockers, non-selective (nadolol). [Moderate] Study

▶ Bosentan moderately decreases the exposure to **ciclosporin** and **ciclosporin** moderately increases the exposure to bosentan. Avoid. [Severe] Study

▶ Calcium channel blockers (diltiazem, nicardipine, verapamil) increase the concentration of **ciclosporin**. [Severe] Study

▶ **Ciclosporin** moderately increases the exposure to calcium channel blockers (lercanidipine). Use with caution or avoid. [Severe] Study

▶ **Ciclosporin** slightly increases the exposure to caspofungin. [Severe] Study

▶ Ceritinib is predicted to increase the exposure to **ciclosporin**. Avoid. [Severe] Theoretical

▶ **Ciclosporin** is predicted to affect the efficacy of chenodeoxycholic acid. Monitor and adjust dose. [Moderate] Theoretical

▶ **Ciclosporin** affects the concentration of cholic acid. Avoid. [Moderate] Study

▶ Cobicistat increases the concentration of **ciclosporin**. [Severe] Study

▶ **Ciclosporin** increases the exposure to colchicine. Avoid or adjust **colchicine** dose, p. 1085. [Severe] Study

▶ Crizotinib increases the concentration of **ciclosporin**. [Severe] Study

▶ **Ciclosporin** is predicted to increase the exposure to dabigatran. Avoid. [Severe] Theoretical

▶ Danazol increases the concentration of **ciclosporin**. [Severe] Study

▶ **Ciclosporin** is predicted to increase the risk of rhabdomyolysis when given with daptomycin. [Severe] Theoretical

▶ **Ciclosporin** is predicted to increase the exposure to darifenacin. Avoid. [Moderate] Theoretical

▶ **Ciclosporin** increases the concentration of digoxin. Monitor and adjust dose. [Severe] Theoretical

▶ **Ciclosporin** slightly increases the exposure to edoxaban. Adjust **edoxaban** dose, p. 125. [Severe] Study

▶ Efavirenz decreases the concentration of **ciclosporin**. Monitor concentration and adjust dose. [Moderate] Study

▶ **Ciclosporin** increases the exposure to eluxadoline. Avoid. [Moderate] Study

▶ Enzalutamide decreases the concentration of **ciclosporin**. [Severe] Study

▶ **Ciclosporin** is predicted to increase the exposure to erlotinib. [Moderate] Theoretical

▶ **Ciclosporin** increases the exposure to etoposide. Monitor and adjust dose. [Severe] Study

▶ **Ciclosporin** moderately increases the exposure to everolimus. Avoid or adjust dose. [Severe] Study

▶ **Ciclosporin** moderately increases the exposure to ezetimibe and ezetimibe slightly increases the exposure to **ciclosporin**. [Moderate] Study

► Fibrates (bezafibrate) are predicted to increase the risk of nephrotoxicity when given with **ciclosporin**. Severe Theoretical
► Fibrates (fenofibrate) increase the risk of nephrotoxicity when given with **ciclosporin**. Severe Study
► **Ciclosporin** is predicted to increase the exposure to fidaxomicin. Avoid. Moderate Study
► **Ciclosporin** increases the exposure to glecaprevir. Avoid or monitor. Severe Study
► Grapefruit juice increases the concentration of **ciclosporin**. Avoid. Severe Study
► **Ciclosporin** greatly increases the exposure to grazoprevir. Avoid. Severe Study
► H$_2$ receptor antagonists (cimetidine) increase the concentration of **ciclosporin**. Mild Study
► HIV-protease inhibitors increase the concentration of **ciclosporin**. Severe Study
► Idelalisib increases the concentration of **ciclosporin**. Severe Study
► Imatinib increases the concentration of **ciclosporin**. Severe Study
► Lanreotide is predicted to decrease the absorption of oral **ciclosporin**. Adjust dose. Severe Theoretical
► Live vaccines are predicted to increase the risk of generalised infection (possibly life-threatening) when given with **ciclosporin**. Public Health England advises avoid (refer to Green Book). Severe Theoretical
► **Ciclosporin** is predicted to increase the exposure to lomitapide. Separate administration by 12 hours. Moderate Theoretical
► Lumacaftor is predicted to decrease the exposure to **ciclosporin**. Avoid. Severe Theoretical
► Macrolides (clarithromycin, erythromycin) increase the concentration of **ciclosporin**. Severe Study
► **Ciclosporin** is predicted to decrease the efficacy of mifamurtide. Avoid. Severe Theoretical
► Mitotane decreases the concentration of **ciclosporin**. Severe Study
► Monoclonal antibodies (blinatumomab) are predicted to transiently increase the exposure to **ciclosporin**. Monitor and adjust dose. Moderate Theoretical
► Monoclonal antibodies (sarilumab) potentially affect the exposure to **ciclosporin**. Monitor and adjust dose. Moderate Theoretical
► Monoclonal antibodies (tocilizumab) are predicted to decrease the exposure to **ciclosporin**. Monitor and adjust dose. Moderate Theoretical
► Netupitant increases the concentration of **ciclosporin**. Severe Study
► Nevirapine is predicted to decrease the concentration of **ciclosporin**. Moderate Study
► Nilotinib increases the concentration of **ciclosporin**. Severe Study
► **Ciclosporin** is predicted to increase the exposure to nintedanib. Moderate Study
► **Ciclosporin** increases the concentration of NSAIDs (diclofenac). Severe Study → Also see TABLE 2 p. 1334 → Also see TABLE 16 p. 1338
► Octreotide decreases the absorption of oral **ciclosporin**. Adjust **ciclosporin** dose, p. 818. Severe Anecdotal
► Palbociclib is predicted to increase the exposure to **ciclosporin**. Adjust dose. Moderate Theoretical
► **Ciclosporin** is predicted to increase the exposure to panobinostat. Adjust dose. Moderate Theoretical
► Pasireotide is predicted to decrease the absorption of oral **ciclosporin**. Adjust dose. Severe Theoretical
► **Ciclosporin** increases the exposure to pibrentasvir. Avoid or monitor. Severe Study
► Pitolisant is predicted to decrease the exposure to **ciclosporin**. Avoid. Severe Theoretical
► **Ciclosporin** is predicted to increase the concentration of ranolazine and ranolazine is predicted to increase the concentration of **ciclosporin**. Moderate Theoretical
► **Ciclosporin** moderately increases the exposure to repaglinide. Moderate Study
► Ribociclib is predicted to increase the exposure to **ciclosporin**. Use with caution and adjust dose. Moderate Theoretical

► Rifampicin decreases the concentration of **ciclosporin**. Severe Study
► **Ciclosporin** very markedly increases the exposure to rifaximin. Severe Study
► **Ciclosporin** is predicted to increase the exposure to riociguat. Moderate Theoretical
► **Ciclosporin** moderately increases the exposure to sirolimus. Separate administration by 4 hours. Severe Study
► St John's Wort decreases the concentration of **ciclosporin**. Avoid. Moderate Study
► **Ciclosporin** very markedly increases the exposure to statins (atorvastatin). Avoid or adjust **atorvastatin** dose, p. 200. Severe Study
► **Ciclosporin** moderately increases the exposure to statins (fluvastatin). Severe Study
► **Ciclosporin** markedly to very markedly increases the exposure to statins (pravastatin). Adjust dose. Severe Study
► **Ciclosporin** markedly increases the exposure to statins (rosuvastatin, simvastatin). Avoid. Severe Study
► Sulfinpyrazone decreases the concentration of **ciclosporin**. Severe Study
► **Ciclosporin** increases the concentration of tacrolimus. Avoid. Severe Study → Also see TABLE 2 p. 1334 → Also see TABLE 16 p. 1338
► **Ciclosporin** is predicted to increase the exposure to ticagrelor. Use with caution or avoid. Severe Study
► **Ciclosporin** increases the exposure to tofacitinib. Avoid. Severe Study
► **Ciclosporin** is predicted to increase the exposure to topotecan. Severe Study
► **Ciclosporin** is predicted to increase the concentration of trametinib. Moderate Theoretical
► Ursodeoxycholic acid affects the concentration of **ciclosporin**. Use with caution and adjust dose. Severe Anecdotal
► **Ciclosporin** is predicted to increase the exposure to venetoclax. Avoid or monitor for toxicity. Severe Theoretical
► Vitamin E substances affect the exposure to **ciclosporin**. Moderate Study
► **Ciclosporin** increases the concentration of voxilaprevir. Avoid. Severe Study

Cilostazol → see TABLE 4 p. 1334 (antiplatelet effects)

GENERAL INFORMATION Concurrent use with 2 or more antiplatelets or anticoagulants is contra-indicated.

► Antiepileptics (carbamazepine, fosphenytoin, phenobarbital, phenytoin, primidone) are predicted to alter the effects of **cilostazol**. Moderate Theoretical
► Antifungals, azoles (fluconazole) are predicted to increase the exposure to **cilostazol**. Adjust **cilostazol** dose, p. 231. Moderate Theoretical
► Antifungals, azoles (itraconazole, ketoconazole, voriconazole) are predicted to moderately increase the exposure to **cilostazol**. Adjust **cilostazol** dose, p. 231. Moderate Study
► Antifungals, azoles (miconazole) are predicted to increase the exposure to **cilostazol**. Use with caution and adjust dose. Moderate Theoretical
► Cobicistat is predicted to moderately increase the exposure to **cilostazol**. Adjust **cilostazol** dose, p. 231. Moderate Study
► Enzalutamide is predicted to alter the effects of **cilostazol**. Moderate Theoretical
► HIV-protease inhibitors are predicted to moderately increase the exposure to **cilostazol**. Adjust **cilostazol** dose, p. 231. Moderate Study
► Idelalisib is predicted to moderately increase the exposure to **cilostazol**. Adjust **cilostazol** dose, p. 231. Moderate Study
► **Cilostazol** is predicted to increase the exposure to lomitapide. Separate administration by 12 hours. Moderate Theoretical
► Macrolides (clarithromycin) are predicted to moderately increase the exposure to **cilostazol**. Adjust **cilostazol** dose, p. 231. Moderate Study
► Macrolides (erythromycin) slightly increase the exposure to **cilostazol**. Adjust **cilostazol** dose, p. 231. Moderate Study
► Mitotane is predicted to alter the effects of **cilostazol**. Moderate Theoretical
► Moclobemide is predicted to increase the exposure to **cilostazol**. Moderate Theoretical

Cilostazol (continued)

▶ Proton pump inhibitors (esomeprazole) are predicted to increase the exposure to **cilostazol**. Moderate Theoretical
▶ Proton pump inhibitors (omeprazole) are predicted to increase the exposure to **cilostazol**. Adjust **cilostazol** dose, p. 231. Moderate Study
▶ Rifampicin is predicted to alter the effects of **cilostazol**. Moderate Theoretical
▶ SSRIs (fluoxetine, fluvoxamine) are predicted to increase the exposure to **cilostazol**. Adjust **cilostazol** dose, p. 231. Moderate Theoretical → Also see TABLE 4 p. 1334
▶ St John's Wort is predicted to alter the effects of **cilostazol**. Moderate Theoretical

Cimetidine → see H₂ receptor antagonists

Cinacalcet

FOOD AND LIFESTYLE Dose adjustment might be necessary if smoking started or stopped during treatment.

▶ Cinacalcet is predicted to increase the exposure to anticholinesterases, centrally acting (galantamine). Monitor and adjust dose. Moderate Study
▶ Antiepileptics (carbamazepine, fosphenytoin, phenobarbital, phenytoin, primidone) are predicted to decrease the exposure to **cinacalcet**. Monitor and adjust dose. Moderate Study
▶ Antifungals, azoles (itraconazole, ketoconazole, voriconazole) are predicted to moderately increase the exposure to **cinacalcet**. Adjust dose. Moderate Study
▶ **Cinacalcet** is predicted to moderately increase the exposure to aripiprazole. Adjust **aripiprazole** dose, p. 391. Moderate Study
▶ **Cinacalcet** is predicted to markedly increase the exposure to atomoxetine. Adjust dose. Severe Study
▶ **Cinacalcet** is predicted to increase the exposure to beta blockers, selective (metoprolol, nebivolol). Moderate Study
▶ Cobicistat is predicted to moderately increase the exposure to **cinacalcet**. Adjust dose. Moderate Study
▶ **Cinacalcet** is predicted to slightly increase the exposure to darifenacin. Mild Study
▶ **Cinacalcet** is predicted to increase the exposure to eliglustat. Avoid or adjust dose—consult product literature. Severe Study
▶ Enzalutamide is predicted to decrease the exposure to **cinacalcet**. Monitor and adjust dose. Moderate Study
▶ **Cinacalcet** increases the risk of hypocalcaemia when given with etelcalcetide. Avoid. Severe Theoretical
▶ HIV-protease inhibitors are predicted to moderately increase the exposure to **cinacalcet**. Adjust dose. Moderate Study
▶ Idelalisib is predicted to moderately increase the exposure to **cinacalcet**. Adjust dose. Moderate Study
▶ Macrolides (clarithromycin) are predicted to moderately increase the exposure to **cinacalcet**. Adjust dose. Moderate Study
▶ Mitotane is predicted to decrease the exposure to **cinacalcet**. Monitor and adjust dose. Moderate Study
▶ **Cinacalcet** is predicted to decrease the efficacy of opioids (codeine). Moderate Theoretical
▶ **Cinacalcet** is predicted to decrease the efficacy of opioids (tramadol). Severe Study
▶ **Cinacalcet** is predicted to moderately increase the exposure to pitolisant. Use with caution and adjust dose. Moderate Study
▶ Rifampicin is predicted to decrease the exposure to **cinacalcet**. Monitor and adjust dose. Moderate Study
▶ **Cinacalcet** is predicted to increase the exposure to risperidone. Adjust dose. Moderate Study
▶ SSRIs (fluvoxamine) are predicted to increase the exposure to **cinacalcet**. Adjust dose. Moderate Theoretical
▶ **Cinacalcet** is predicted to increase the exposure to SSRIs (dapoxetine). Moderate Theoretical
▶ **Cinacalcet** is predicted to decrease the efficacy of tamoxifen. Avoid. Severe Study
▶ **Cinacalcet** is predicted to increase the exposure to tricyclic antidepressants. Monitor for toxicity and adjust dose. Severe Study
▶ **Cinacalcet** is predicted to increase the exposure to vortioxetine. Monitor and adjust dose. Moderate Study

Cinnarizine → see antihistamines, sedating
Ciprofibrate → see fibrates
Ciprofloxacin → see quinolones

Cisatracurium → see neuromuscular blocking drugs, non-depolarising
Cisplatin → see platinum compounds
Citalopram → see SSRIs
Cladribine → see TABLE 15 p. 1337 (myelosuppression)

SEPARATION OF ADMINISTRATION Oral cladribine might affect the absorption of concurrently administered drugs—consider separating administration by at least 3 hours.

▶ Antiepileptics (carbamazepine) are predicted to increase the risk of haematological toxicity when given with oral **cladribine**. Moderate Theoretical
▶ Live vaccines are predicted to increase the risk of generalised infection (possibly life-threatening) when given with **cladribine**. Public Health England advises avoid (refer to Green Book). Severe Theoretical

Clarithromycin → see macrolides
Clavulanic acid → see TABLE 1 p. 1334 (hepatotoxicity)
Clemastine → see antihistamines, sedating
Clevidipine → see calcium channel blockers
Clindamycin

ROUTE-SPECIFIC INFORMATION Since systemic absorption can follow topical application, the possibility of interactions should be borne in mind.

▶ Clindamycin increases the effects of neuromuscular blocking drugs, non-depolarising. Severe Anecdotal
▶ Clindamycin increases the effects of suxamethonium. Severe Anecdotal

Clobazam → see TABLE 11 p. 1336 (CNS depressant effects)

▶ Antiepileptics (stiripentol) increase the concentration of **clobazam**. Severe Study
▶ **Clobazam** potentially affects the concentration of antiepileptics (fosphenytoin, phenytoin). Severe Anecdotal
▶ Antifungals, azoles (fluconazole, voriconazole) potentially increase the exposure to **clobazam**. Adjust dose. Moderate Theoretical
▶ Moclobemide potentially increases the exposure to **clobazam**. Adjust dose. Moderate Theoretical
▶ Proton pump inhibitors (esomeprazole, omeprazole) potentially increase the exposure to **clobazam**. Adjust dose. Moderate Theoretical
▶ SSRIs (fluoxetine, fluvoxamine) potentially increase the exposure to **clobazam**. Adjust dose. Moderate Theoretical

Clofarabine → see TABLE 15 p. 1337 (myelosuppression)

▶ Live vaccines are predicted to increase the risk of generalised infection (possibly life-threatening) when given with **clofarabine**. Public Health England advises avoid (refer to Green Book). Severe Theoretical

Clofazimine

▶ Clofazimine potentially increases the risk of QT-prolongation when given with bedaquiline. Severe Study

Clomethiazole → see TABLE 11 p. 1336 (CNS depressant effects)

▶ Alcohol (beverage) causes serious, potentially fatal, CNS depression when given with **clomethiazole**. Avoid. Severe Study → Also see TABLE 11 p. 1336
▶ Antiepileptics (carbamazepine, fosphenytoin, phenobarbital, phenytoin, primidone) decrease the exposure to **clomethiazole**. Monitor and adjust dose. Moderate Study → Also see TABLE 11 p. 1336
▶ Enzalutamide decreases the exposure to **clomethiazole**. Monitor and adjust dose. Moderate Study
▶ Mitotane decreases the exposure to **clomethiazole**. Monitor and adjust dose. Moderate Study
▶ Rifampicin decreases the exposure to **clomethiazole**. Monitor and adjust dose. Moderate Study

Clomipramine → see tricyclic antidepressants
Clonazepam → see TABLE 11 p. 1336 (CNS depressant effects)

▶ Clonazepam potentially affects the concentration of antiepileptics (fosphenytoin, phenytoin). Severe Anecdotal

Clonidine → see TABLE 6 p. 1335 (bradycardia), TABLE 8 p. 1335 (hypotension), TABLE 11 p. 1336 (CNS depressant effects)

▶ Tricyclic antidepressants decrease the antihypertensive effects of **clonidine**. Monitor and adjust dose. Moderate Anecdotal → Also see TABLE 8 p. 1335

Clopamide → see thiazide diuretics
Clopidogrel → see TABLE 4 p. 1334 (antiplatelet effects)

- Antifungals, azoles (fluconazole) are predicted to decrease the efficacy of **clopidogrel**. Avoid. Severe Theoretical
- Antifungals, azoles (voriconazole) are predicted to decrease the efficacy of **clopidogrel**. Avoid. Moderate Study
- **Clopidogrel** is predicted to increase the exposure to dabrafenib. Moderate Theoretical
- **Clopidogrel** moderately increases the exposure to enzalutamide. Avoid or adjust **enzalutamide** dose, p. 921. Severe Study
- Grapefruit juice markedly decreases the exposure to **clopidogrel**. Severe Study
- Moclobemide is predicted to decrease the efficacy of **clopidogrel**. Moderate Study
- **Clopidogrel** is predicted to moderately increase the exposure to montelukast. Moderate Study
- **Clopidogrel** increases the exposure to pioglitazone. Monitor blood glucose and adjust dose. Severe Study
- Proton pump inhibitors (esomeprazole, omeprazole) are predicted to decrease the efficacy of **clopidogrel**. Avoid. Moderate Study
- **Clopidogrel** increases the exposure to repaglinide. Avoid. Severe Study
- **Clopidogrel** is predicted to increase the exposure to retinoids (alitretinoin). Adjust **alitretinoin** dose, p. 1226. Moderate Theoretical
- **Clopidogrel** is predicted to increase the exposure to selexipag. Adjust dose. Moderate Study
- SSRIs (fluoxetine, fluvoxamine) are predicted to decrease the efficacy of **clopidogrel**. Avoid. Severe Theoretical → Also see **TABLE 4** p. 1334
- **Clopidogrel** increases the exposure to statins (rosuvastatin). Adjust **rosuvastatin** dose, p. 202. Moderate Study
- **Clopidogrel** is predicted to increase the concentration of taxanes (paclitaxel). Severe Anecdotal

Clotrimazole → see antifungals, azoles

Clozapine → see **TABLE 8** p. 1335 (hypotension), **TABLE 15** p. 1337 (myelosuppression), **TABLE 11** p. 1336 (CNS depressant effects), **TABLE 10** p. 1336 (antimuscarinics)

  ‣ Dose adjustment might be necessary if smoking started or stopped during treatment.
  ‣ Avoid concomitant use of clozapine with drugs that have a substantial potential for causing agranulocytosis.

- Antiepileptics (carbamazepine) are predicted to increase the risk of myelosuppression when given with **clozapine**. Avoid. Severe Anecdotal
- Antiepileptics (fosphenytoin, phenobarbital, phenytoin, primidone) are predicted to decrease the exposure to **clozapine**. Moderate Anecdotal → Also see **TABLE 11** p. 1336
- Combined hormonal contraceptives increase the concentration of **clozapine**. Monitor side effects and adjust dose. Severe Study
- **Clozapine** is predicted to decrease the effects of dopamine receptor agonists. Moderate Theoretical → Also see **TABLE 8** p. 1335 → Also see **TABLE 10** p. 1336
- Enzalutamide is predicted to decrease the exposure to **clozapine**. Moderate Theoretical
- HIV-protease inhibitors (ritonavir) are predicted to affect the exposure to **clozapine**. Avoid. Severe Theoretical
- Iron chelators (deferasirox) are predicted to increase the exposure to **clozapine**. Avoid. Moderate Theoretical
- Leflunomide is predicted to decrease the exposure to **clozapine**. Moderate Theoretical → Also see **TABLE 15** p. 1337
- **Clozapine** is predicted to decrease the effects of levodopa. Severe Theoretical → Also see **TABLE 8** p. 1335
- Macrolides (erythromycin) potentially increase the risk of toxicity when given with **clozapine**. Severe Anecdotal
- Quinolones (ciprofloxacin) increase the concentration of **clozapine**. Monitor side effects and adjust dose. Severe Study
- Rifampicin decreases the exposure to **clozapine**. Severe Anecdotal
- SSRIs (fluvoxamine) increase the concentration of **clozapine**. Monitor side effects and adjust dose. Severe Study
- Teriflunomide is predicted to decrease the concentration of **clozapine**. Moderate Theoretical

Co-trimoxazole → see sulfonamides

Cobicistat

- **Cobicistat** is predicted to increase the exposure to abiraterone. Severe Theoretical
- **Cobicistat** is predicted to markedly increase the exposure to aldosterone antagonists (eplerenone). Avoid. Severe Study
- **Cobicistat** increases the exposure to almotriptan. Mild Study
- **Cobicistat** is predicted to moderately increase the exposure to alpha blockers (alfuzosin, tamsulosin). Use with caution or avoid. Moderate Study
- **Cobicistat** is predicted to increase the exposure to alpha blockers (doxazosin). Moderate Study
- **Cobicistat** moderately increases the exposure to alprazolam. Avoid. Moderate Study
- **Cobicistat** very markedly increases the exposure to antiarrhythmics (dronedarone). Avoid. Severe Study
- **Cobicistat** is predicted to increase the exposure to antiarrhythmics (propafenone). Monitor and adjust dose. Severe Study
- **Cobicistat** is predicted to increase the exposure to anticholinesterases, centrally acting (galantamine). Monitor and adjust dose. Moderate Study
- Antiepileptics (carbamazepine, fosphenytoin, phenobarbital, phenytoin, primidone) are predicted to decrease the exposure to **cobicistat**. Avoid. Severe Theoretical
- Antiepileptics (oxcarbazepine) are predicted to decrease the concentration of **cobicistat**. Severe Theoretical
- **Cobicistat** is predicted to very slightly increase the exposure to antiepileptics (perampanel). Mild Study
- **Cobicistat** is predicted to increase the exposure to antifungals, azoles (fluconazole, posaconazole). Moderate Theoretical
- **Cobicistat** is predicted to increase the exposure to antifungals, azoles (isavuconazole). Avoid or monitor side effects. Severe Study
- **Cobicistat** is predicted to increase the exposure to antifungals, azoles (itraconazole, ketoconazole). Adjust dose. Moderate Theoretical
- **Cobicistat** is predicted to affect the exposure to antifungals, azoles (voriconazole). Avoid. Moderate Theoretical
- **Cobicistat** is predicted to increase the exposure to antihistamines, non-sedating (mizolastine). Avoid. Severe Study
- **Cobicistat** is predicted to increase the exposure to antihistamines, non-sedating (rupatadine). Avoid. Moderate Study
- **Cobicistat** is predicted to increase the concentration of antimalarials (piperaquine). Severe Theoretical
- **Cobicistat** is predicted to markedly increase the exposure to aprepitant. Moderate Study
- **Cobicistat** is predicted to slightly increase the exposure to aripiprazole. Adjust **aripiprazole** dose, p. 391. Moderate Study
- **Cobicistat** is predicted to increase the exposure to axitinib. Avoid or adjust dose. Moderate Study
- **Cobicistat** is predicted to increase the exposure to bedaquiline. Avoid prolonged use. Mild Study
- **Cobicistat** is predicted to increase the exposure to beta₂ agonists (salmeterol). Avoid. Severe Study
- **Cobicistat** slightly increases the exposure to bortezomib. Moderate Study
- Bosentan is predicted to decrease the exposure to **cobicistat**. Avoid. Severe Theoretical
- **Cobicistat** is predicted to markedly increase the exposure to bosutinib. Avoid or adjust dose. Severe Study
- **Cobicistat** is predicted to increase the exposure to buspirone. Adjust **buspirone** dose, p. 338. Severe Study
- **Cobicistat** slightly increases the exposure to cabozantinib. Moderate Study
- **Cobicistat** is predicted to increase the exposure to calcium channel blockers (amlodipine, felodipine, lacidipine, nicardipine, nifedipine, nimodipine). Monitor and adjust dose. Moderate Study
- **Cobicistat** is predicted to increase the exposure to calcium channel blockers (diltiazem, verapamil). Severe Study
- **Cobicistat** is predicted to markedly increase the exposure to calcium channel blockers (lercanidipine). Avoid. Severe Study
- **Cobicistat** is predicted to increase the exposure to cannabis extract. Use with caution and adjust dose. Moderate Theoretical

A1

Interactions | Appendix 1

Cobicistat (continued)

▸ **Cobicistat** is predicted to increase the exposure to ceritinib. Avoid or adjust **ceritinib** dose, p. 945. [Severe] Study
▸ **Cobicistat** increases the concentration of ciclosporin. [Severe] Study
▸ **Cobicistat** is predicted to moderately increase the exposure to cilostazol. Adjust **cilostazol** dose, p. 231. [Moderate] Study
▸ **Cobicistat** is predicted to moderately increase the exposure to cinacalcet. Adjust dose. [Moderate] Study
▸ **Cobicistat** is predicted to markedly increase the exposure to cobimetinib. Avoid or monitor for toxicity. [Severe] Study
▸ **Cobicistat** is predicted to increase the exposure to colchicine. Avoid potent inhibitors of CYP3A4 or adjust **colchicine** dose, p. 1085. [Severe] Study
▸ **Cobicistat** is predicted to decrease the efficacy of combined hormonal contraceptives. Avoid. [Severe] Study
▸ **Cobicistat** is predicted to increase the exposure to corticosteroids (beclometasone) (risk with beclometasone is likely to be lower than with other corticosteroids). [Moderate] Theoretical
▸ **Cobicistat** is predicted to increase the exposure to corticosteroids (betamethasone, budesonide, ciclesonide, deflazacort, dexamethasone, fludrocortisone, fluticasone, hydrocortisone, methylprednisolone, mometasone, prednisolone, prednisone, triamcinolone). Avoid or monitor side effects. [Severe] Study
▸ **Cobicistat** is predicted to moderately increase the exposure to crizotinib. Avoid. [Moderate] Study
▸ **Cobicistat** is predicted to increase the exposure to dabrafenib. Use with caution or avoid. [Moderate] Study
▸ **Cobicistat** is predicted to moderately increase the exposure to daclatasvir. Adjust **daclatasvir** dose, p. 614. [Moderate] Study
▸ **Cobicistat** is predicted to markedly to very markedly increase the exposure to darifenacin. Avoid. [Severe] Study
▸ **Cobicistat** is predicted to markedly increase the exposure to dasatinib. Avoid. [Severe] Study
▸ **Cobicistat** very slightly increases the exposure to delamanid. [Severe] Study
▸ **Cobicistat** increases the risk of QT-prolongation when given with domperidone. Avoid. [Severe] Study
▸ **Cobicistat** increases the exposure to dopamine receptor agonists (bromocriptine). [Severe] Study
▸ **Cobicistat** is predicted to increase the concentration of dopamine receptor agonists (cabergoline). [Moderate] Anecdotal
▸ **Cobicistat** is predicted to increase the exposure to dutasteride. Monitor side effects and adjust dose. [Moderate] Theoretical
▸ **Efavirenz** is predicted to decrease the exposure to cobicistat. Avoid. [Severe] Theoretical
▸ **Cobicistat** slightly to moderately increases the exposure to elbasvir. Avoid. [Moderate] Study
▸ **Cobicistat** is predicted to markedly increase the exposure to eletriptan. Avoid. [Severe] Study
▸ **Cobicistat** is predicted to increase the exposure to eliglustat. Avoid or adjust dose—consult product literature. [Severe] Study
▸ **Enzalutamide** is predicted to decrease the exposure to cobicistat. Avoid. [Severe] Theoretical
▸ **Cobicistat** is predicted to increase the risk of ergotism when given with ergometrine. Avoid. [Severe] Theoretical
▸ **Cobicistat** is predicted to increase the risk of ergotism when given with ergotamine. Avoid. [Severe] Theoretical
▸ **Cobicistat** is predicted to slightly increase the exposure to erlotinib. Use with caution and adjust dose. [Moderate] Study
▸ **Cobicistat** is predicted to increase the concentration of everolimus. Avoid. [Severe] Study
▸ **Cobicistat** is predicted to moderately increase the exposure to fesoterodine. Adjust **fesoterodine** dose with potent inhibitors of CYP3A4; avoid in hepatic and renal impairment, p. 759. [Severe] Study
▸ **Cobicistat** is predicted to increase the exposure to fosaprepitant. [Moderate] Theoretical
▸ **Cobicistat** is predicted to increase the exposure to gefitinib. [Moderate] Study
▸ **Cobicistat** potentially increases the exposure to glecaprevir. [Moderate] Theoretical

▸ **Cobicistat** is predicted to moderately to markedly increase the exposure to grazoprevir. Avoid. [Severe] Study
▸ **Cobicistat** is predicted to increase the exposure to guanfacine. Adjust **guanfacine** dose, p. 349. [Moderate] Study
▸ **Cobicistat** is predicted to very markedly increase the exposure to ibrutinib. Avoid potent inhibitors of CYP3A4 or adjust **ibrutinib** dose, p. 952. [Severe] Study
▸ **Cobicistat** is predicted to increase the exposure to imatinib. [Moderate] Study
▸ **Cobicistat** is predicted to increase the risk of toxicity when given with irinotecan. Avoid. [Moderate] Study
▸ **Cobicistat** is predicted to increase the exposure to ivabradine. Avoid. [Severe] Study
▸ **Cobicistat** is predicted to increase the exposure to ivacaftor. Adjust **ivacaftor** p. 292 or **lumacaftor with ivacaftor** p. 293 dose with potent inhibitors of CYP3A4. [Severe] Study
▸ **Cobicistat** is predicted to increase the exposure to lapatinib. Avoid. [Moderate] Study
▸ **Cobicistat** is predicted to markedly increase the exposure to lomitapide. Avoid. [Severe] Study
▸ **Cobicistat** is predicted to increase the exposure to lurasidone. Avoid. [Severe] Study
▸ **Cobicistat** is predicted to increase the exposure to macitentan. [Moderate] Study
▸ **Cobicistat** markedly increases the exposure to maraviroc. Refer to specialist literature. [Severe] Study
▸ **Cobicistat** is predicted to markedly to very markedly increase the exposure to midazolam. Avoid or adjust dose. [Severe] Study
▸ **Cobicistat** is predicted to very markedly increase the exposure to midostaurin. Avoid or monitor for toxicity. [Severe] Study
▸ **Cobicistat** is predicted to increase the exposure to mirabegron. Adjust **mirabegron** dose in hepatic and renal impairment, p. 763. [Moderate] Study
▸ **Cobicistat** is predicted to increase the exposure to mirtazapine. [Moderate] Study
▸ **Mitotane** is predicted to decrease the exposure to cobicistat. Avoid. [Severe] Theoretical
▸ **Cobicistat** is predicted to increase the exposure to modafinil. [Mild] Theoretical
▸ **Cobicistat** is predicted to increase the exposure to monoclonal antibodies (trastuzumab emtansine). Avoid. [Severe] Theoretical
▸ **Cobicistat** is predicted to markedly increase the exposure to naloxegol. Avoid. [Severe] Study
▸ **Cobicistat** is predicted to increase the exposure to netupitant. [Moderate] Study
▸ **Nevirapine** is predicted to decrease the exposure to cobicistat. Avoid. [Severe] Theoretical
▸ **Cobicistat** is predicted to moderately increase the exposure to nilotinib. Avoid. [Severe] Study
▸ **Cobicistat** is predicted to increase the exposure to nitisinone. Adjust dose. [Moderate] Theoretical
▸ **Cobicistat** is predicted to increase the exposure to olaparib. Avoid potent inhibitors of CYP3A4 or adjust **olaparib** dose, p. 973. [Moderate] Study
▸ **Cobicistat** is predicted to increase the exposure to opioids (alfentanil, buprenorphine, fentanyl, oxycodone, sufentanil). Monitor and adjust dose. [Severe] Study
▸ **Cobicistat** is predicted to increase the exposure to oxybutynin. [Mild] Study
▸ **Cobicistat** is predicted to increase the exposure to palbociclib. Avoid or adjust **palbociclib** dose, p. 961. [Severe] Study
▸ **Cobicistat** is predicted to increase the exposure to panobinostat. Adjust **panobinostat** dose; in hepatic impairment avoid, p. 911. [Moderate] Study
▸ **Cobicistat** is predicted to increase the exposure to paritaprevir (with ritonavir and ombitasvir). Avoid. [Severe] Theoretical
▸ **Cobicistat** is predicted to increase the exposure to pazopanib. Avoid or adjust **pazopanib** dose, p. 962. [Moderate] Study
▸ **Cobicistat** is predicted to increase the exposure to phosphodiesterase type-5 inhibitors (avanafil, vardenafil). Avoid. [Severe] Study
▸ **Cobicistat** is predicted to increase the exposure to phosphodiesterase type-5 inhibitors (sildenafil). Avoid potent inhibitors of CYP3A4 or adjust **sildenafil** dose, p. 794. [Severe] Study

▸ **Cobicistat** is predicted to increase the exposure to phosphodiesterase type-5 inhibitors (tadalafil). Use with caution or avoid. Severe Study

▸ **Cobicistat** is predicted to increase the exposure to pimozide. Avoid. Severe Study

▸ **Cobicistat** is predicted to slightly increase the exposure to ponatinib. Monitor and adjust **ponatinib** dose, p. 963. Moderate Study

▸ **Cobicistat** is predicted to moderately increase the exposure to praziquantel. Mild Study

▸ **Cobicistat** is predicted to increase the exposure to quetiapine. Avoid. Severe Study

▸ **Cobicistat** is predicted to increase the exposure to ranolazine. Avoid. Severe Study

▸ **Cobicistat** is predicted to increase the exposure to reboxetine. Avoid. Moderate Study

▸ **Cobicistat** is predicted to increase the exposure to regorafenib. Avoid. Moderate Study

▸ **Cobicistat** is predicted to increase the exposure to repaglinide. Moderate Study

▸ **Cobicistat** is predicted to increase the exposure to retinoids (alitretinoin). Adjust **alitretinoin** dose, p. 1226. Moderate Theoretical

▸ **Cobicistat** is predicted to increase the exposure to ribociclib. Avoid or adjust **ribociclib** dose, p. 965. Moderate Study

▸ Rifabutin decreases the concentration of **cobicistat** and **cobicistat** increases the exposure to rifabutin. Avoid or adjust dose. Severe Study

▸ Rifampicin is predicted to decrease the exposure to **cobicistat**. Avoid. Severe Theoretical

▸ **Cobicistat** is predicted to increase the exposure to risperidone. Adjust dose. Moderate Study

▸ **Cobicistat** is predicted to increase the exposure to ruxolitinib. Adjust dose and monitor side effects. Moderate Study

▸ **Cobicistat** is predicted to increase the exposure to saxagliptin. Moderate Study

▸ **Cobicistat** is predicted to increase the exposure to simeprevir. Avoid. Severe Study

▸ **Cobicistat** is predicted to increase the concentration of sirolimus. Avoid. Severe Study

▸ **Cobicistat** is predicted to increase the exposure to solifenacin. Adjust **solifenacin** p. 761 or **tamsulosin with solifenacin** p. 768 dose; avoid in hepatic and renal impairment. Severe Study

▸ **Cobicistat** is predicted to moderately increase the exposure to SSRIs (dapoxetine). Avoid potent inhibitors of CYP3A4 or adjust **dapoxetine** dose, p. 801. Severe Study

▸ St John's Wort is predicted to decrease the exposure to **cobicistat**. Avoid. Severe Theoretical

▸ **Cobicistat** is predicted to increase the exposure to statins (atorvastatin). Avoid or adjust dose and monitor rhabdomyolysis. Severe Study

▸ **Cobicistat** is predicted to increase the exposure to statins (simvastatin). Avoid. Severe Study

▸ **Cobicistat** is predicted to slightly increase the exposure to sunitinib. Avoid or adjust **sunitinib** dose, p. 967. Moderate Study

▸ **Cobicistat** is predicted to increase the concentration of tacrolimus. Monitor and adjust dose. Severe Study

▸ **Cobicistat** is predicted to increase the exposure to taxanes (cabazitaxel). Avoid. Severe Study

▸ **Cobicistat** is predicted to moderately increase the exposure to taxanes (docetaxel). Avoid or adjust dose. Severe Study

▸ **Cobicistat** is predicted to increase the exposure to taxanes (paclitaxel). Severe Theoretical

▸ **Cobicistat** is predicted to increase the concentration of temsirolimus. Avoid. Severe Theoretical

▸ **Cobicistat** is predicted to markedly increase the exposure to ticagrelor. Avoid. Severe Study

▸ **Cobicistat** is predicted to increase the exposure to tofacitinib. Adjust **tofacitinib** dose, p. 1072. Moderate Study

▸ **Cobicistat** is predicted to increase the exposure to tolterodine. Avoid. Severe Study

▸ **Cobicistat** is predicted to increase the exposure to tolvaptan. Adjust dose. Severe Study

▸ **Cobicistat** is predicted to increase the exposure to toremifene. Moderate Theoretical

▸ **Cobicistat** is predicted to increase the exposure to trabectedin. Avoid or adjust dose. Severe Theoretical

▸ **Cobicistat** is predicted to moderately increase the exposure to trazodone. Avoid or adjust dose. Moderate Study

▸ **Cobicistat** is predicted to slightly increase the exposure to tricyclic antidepressants. Mild Study

▸ **Cobicistat** is predicted to increase the exposure to ulipristal. Avoid if used for uterine fibroids. Severe Study

▸ **Cobicistat** is predicted to increase the exposure to vemurafenib. Severe Theoretical

▸ **Cobicistat** is predicted to increase the exposure to venetoclax. Avoid potent inhibitors of CYP3A4 or adjust **venetoclax** dose, p. 974. Severe Study

▸ **Cobicistat** is predicted to increase the exposure to venlafaxine. Moderate Study

▸ **Cobicistat** is predicted to increase the exposure to vinca alkaloids. Severe Theoretical

▸ **Cobicistat** is predicted to increase the exposure to vitamin D substances (paricalcitol). Moderate Study

▸ **Cobicistat** is predicted to increase the exposure to zopiclone. Adjust dose. Moderate Theoretical

Cobimetinib

▸ Antiarrhythmics (dronedarone) are predicted to increase the exposure to **cobimetinib**. Severe Theoretical

▸ Antiepileptics (carbamazepine, fosphenytoin, phenobarbital, phenytoin, primidone) are predicted to decrease the exposure to **cobimetinib**. Avoid. Severe Theoretical

▸ Antifungals, azoles (fluconazole, isavuconazole, miconazole, posaconazole) are predicted to increase the exposure to **cobimetinib**. Severe Theoretical

▸ Antifungals, azoles (itraconazole, ketoconazole, voriconazole) are predicted to markedly increase the exposure to **cobimetinib**. Avoid or monitor for toxicity. Severe Study

▸ Aprepitant is predicted to increase the exposure to **cobimetinib**. Severe Theoretical

▸ Bosentan is predicted to decrease the exposure to **cobimetinib**. Avoid. Severe Theoretical

▸ Calcium channel blockers (diltiazem, verapamil) are predicted to increase the exposure to **cobimetinib**. Severe Theoretical

▸ **Cobicistat** is predicted to markedly increase the exposure to **cobimetinib**. Avoid or monitor for toxicity. Severe Study

▸ Crizotinib is predicted to increase the exposure to **cobimetinib**. Severe Theoretical

▸ Efavirenz is predicted to decrease the exposure to **cobimetinib**. Avoid. Severe Theoretical

▸ Enzalutamide is predicted to decrease the exposure to **cobimetinib**. Avoid. Severe Theoretical

▸ Grapefruit juice is predicted to increase the exposure to **cobimetinib**. Avoid. Severe Theoretical

▸ HIV-protease inhibitors are predicted to markedly increase the exposure to **cobimetinib**. Avoid or monitor for toxicity. Severe Study

▸ Idelalisib is predicted to markedly increase the exposure to **cobimetinib**. Avoid or monitor for toxicity. Severe Study

▸ Imatinib is predicted to increase the exposure to **cobimetinib**. Severe Theoretical

▸ Macrolides (clarithromycin) are predicted to markedly increase the exposure to **cobimetinib**. Avoid or monitor for toxicity. Severe Study

▸ Macrolides (erythromycin) are predicted to increase the exposure to **cobimetinib**. Severe Theoretical

▸ Mitotane is predicted to decrease the exposure to **cobimetinib**. Avoid. Severe Theoretical

▸ Netupitant is predicted to increase the exposure to **cobimetinib**. Severe Theoretical

▸ Nevirapine is predicted to decrease the exposure to **cobimetinib**. Avoid. Severe Theoretical

▸ Nilotinib is predicted to increase the exposure to **cobimetinib**. Severe Theoretical

▸ Rifampicin is predicted to decrease the exposure to **cobimetinib**. Avoid. Severe Theoretical

▸ St John's Wort is predicted to decrease the exposure to **cobimetinib**. Avoid. Severe Theoretical

Codeine → see opioids

A1

Interactions | Appendix 1

Colchicine

▶ Antiarrhythmics (dronedarone) are predicted to increase the exposure to **colchicine**. Adjust **colchicine** dose with moderate inhibitors of CYP3A4, p. 1085. Severe Study

▶ Antifungals, azoles (fluconazole, isavuconazole, posaconazole) are predicted to increase the exposure to **colchicine**. Adjust **colchicine** dose with moderate inhibitors of CYP3A4, p. 1085. Severe Study

▶ Antifungals, azoles (itraconazole, ketoconazole, voriconazole) are predicted to increase the exposure to **colchicine**. Avoid potent inhibitors of CYP3A4 or adjust **colchicine** dose, p. 1085. Severe Study

▶ Aprepitant is predicted to increase the exposure to **colchicine**. Adjust **colchicine** dose with moderate inhibitors of CYP3A4, p. 1085. Severe Study

▶ Calcium channel blockers (diltiazem, verapamil) are predicted to increase the exposure to **colchicine**. Adjust **colchicine** dose with moderate inhibitors of CYP3A4, p. 1085. Severe Study

▶ Ceritinib is predicted to increase the exposure to **colchicine**. Moderate Theoretical

▶ Ciclosporin increases the exposure to **colchicine**. Avoid or adjust **colchicine** dose, p. 1085. Severe Study

▶ Cobicistat is predicted to increase the exposure to **colchicine**. Avoid potent inhibitors of CYP3A4 or adjust **colchicine** dose, p. 1085. Severe Study

▶ Crizotinib is predicted to increase the exposure to **colchicine**. Adjust **colchicine** dose with moderate inhibitors of CYP3A4, p. 1085. Severe Study

▶ Eliglustat is predicted to increase the exposure to **colchicine**. Avoid or adjust **colchicine** dose, p. 1085. Severe Theoretical

▶ Colchicine increases the risk of rhabdomyolysis when given with fibrates. Severe Anecdotal

▶ HIV-protease inhibitors are predicted to increase the exposure to **colchicine**. Avoid potent inhibitors of CYP3A4 or adjust **colchicine** dose, p. 1085. Severe Study

▶ Idelalisib is predicted to increase the exposure to **colchicine**. Avoid potent inhibitors of CYP3A4 or adjust **colchicine** dose, p. 1085. Severe Study

▶ Imatinib is predicted to increase the exposure to **colchicine**. Adjust **colchicine** dose with moderate inhibitors of CYP3A4, p. 1085. Severe Study

▶ Lapatinib is predicted to increase the exposure to **colchicine**. Avoid or adjust **colchicine** dose, p. 1085. Moderate Theoretical

▶ Macrolides (azithromycin) are predicted to increase the exposure to **colchicine**. Avoid or adjust **colchicine** dose, p. 1085. Severe Theoretical

▶ Macrolides (clarithromycin) are predicted to increase the exposure to **colchicine**. Avoid potent inhibitors of CYP3A4 or adjust **colchicine** dose, p. 1085. Severe Study

▶ Macrolides (erythromycin) are predicted to increase the exposure to **colchicine**. Adjust **colchicine** dose with moderate inhibitors of CYP3A4, p. 1085. Severe Study

▶ Mirabegron is predicted to increase the exposure to **colchicine**. Mild Theoretical

▶ Netupitant is predicted to increase the exposure to **colchicine**. Adjust **colchicine** dose with moderate inhibitors of CYP3A4, p. 1085. Severe Study

▶ Nilotinib is predicted to increase the exposure to **colchicine**. Adjust **colchicine** dose with moderate inhibitors of CYP3A4, p. 1085. Severe Study

▶ Ranolazine is predicted to increase the exposure to **colchicine**. Avoid or adjust **colchicine** dose, p. 1085. Severe Theoretical

▶ Rolapitant is predicted to increase the exposure to **colchicine**. Moderate Study

▶ Colchicine increases the risk of rhabdomyolysis when given with statins. Severe Anecdotal

▶ Velpatasvir is predicted to increase the exposure to **colchicine**. Severe Theoretical

▶ Vemurafenib is predicted to increase the exposure to **colchicine**. Avoid or adjust **colchicine** dose, p. 1085. Severe Theoretical

Colecalciferol → see vitamin D substances

Colesevelam

SEPARATION OF ADMINISTRATION Manufacturer advises take 4 hours before, or after, other drugs.

Colestipol

SEPARATION OF ADMINISTRATION Manufacturer advises take other drugs at least 1 hour before, or 4 hours after, colestipol.

Colestyramine

SEPARATION OF ADMINISTRATION Manufacturer advises take other drugs at least 1 hour before, or 4–6 hours after, colestyramine.

Colistimethate → see TABLE 2 p. 1334 (nephrotoxicity), TABLE 20 p. 1338 (neuromuscular blocking effects)

Combined hormonal contraceptives

▶ Combined hormonal contraceptives are predicted to increase the exposure to agomelatine. Moderate Study

▶ Combined hormonal contraceptives are predicted to increase the exposure to aminophylline. Adjust dose. Moderate Theoretical

▶ Combined hormonal contraceptives are predicted to increase the exposure to anagrelide. Moderate Theoretical

▶ Antiepileptics (carbamazepine, eslicarbazepine, fosphenytoin, oxcarbazepine, perampanel, phenobarbital, phenytoin, primidone, rufinamide, topiramate) are predicted to decrease the efficacy of **combined hormonal contraceptives**. For FSRH guidance, see Contraceptives, interactions p. 775. Severe Study

▶ Combined hormonal contraceptives alter the exposure to antiepileptics (lamotrigine). Adjust dose. Moderate Study

▶ Aprepitant is predicted to decrease the efficacy of **combined hormonal contraceptives**. For FSRH guidance, see Contraceptives, interactions p. 775. Severe Study

▶ Bosentan is predicted to decrease the efficacy of **combined hormonal contraceptives**. For FSRH guidance, see Contraceptives, interactions p. 775. Severe Study

▶ Oral **combined hormonal contraceptives** potentially decrease the efficacy of chenodeoxycholic acid. Avoid. Moderate Theoretical

▶ Combined hormonal contraceptives increase the concentration of clozapine. Monitor side effects and adjust dose. Severe Study

▶ Cobicistat is predicted to decrease the efficacy of **combined hormonal contraceptives**. Avoid. Severe Study

▶ Combined hormonal contraceptives increase the risk of raised liver function tests when given with dasabuvir. Avoid. Severe Study

▶ Combined hormonal contraceptives are predicted to increase the exposure to dopamine receptor agonists (ropinirole). Adjust dose. Moderate Study

▶ Efavirenz is predicted to decrease the efficacy of **combined hormonal contraceptives**. For FSRH guidance, see Contraceptives, interactions p. 775. Severe Study

▶ Combined hormonal contraceptives slightly increase the exposure to erlotinib. Monitor side effects and adjust dose. Moderate Study

▶ Fosaprepitant is predicted to decrease the efficacy of **combined hormonal contraceptives**. For FSRH guidance, see Contraceptives, interactions p. 775. Severe Study

▶ Griseofulvin potentially decreases the efficacy of **combined hormonal contraceptives**. For FSRH guidance, see Contraceptives, interactions p. 775. Severe Anecdotal

▶ HIV-protease inhibitors (atazanavir) (unboosted) increase the exposure to **combined hormonal contraceptives**. Adjust dose. Severe Study

▶ HIV-protease inhibitors (ritonavir) are predicted to decrease the efficacy of **combined hormonal contraceptives**. For FSRH guidance, see Contraceptives, interactions p. 775. Severe Study

▶ Combined hormonal contraceptives are predicted to increase the risk of venous thromboembolism when given with lenalidomide. Avoid. Severe Theoretical

▶ Oral **combined hormonal contraceptives** slightly increase the exposure to lomitapide. Separate administration by 12 hours. Moderate Theoretical

▶ Combined hormonal contraceptives are predicted to increase the exposure to loxapine. Avoid. Unknown Theoretical

▶ Lumacaftor is predicted to decrease the efficacy of **combined hormonal contraceptives**. Use additional contraceptive precautions. Severe Theoretical

▶ Combined hormonal contraceptives are predicted to increase the exposure to melatonin. Moderate Theoretical

- Combined hormonal contraceptives decrease the effects of metyrapone. Avoid. Moderate Theoretical
- Modafinil is predicted to decrease the efficacy of **combined hormonal contraceptives**. For FSRH guidance, see Contraceptives, interactions p. 775. Severe Study
- **Combined hormonal contraceptives** slightly increase the exposure to monoamine-oxidase B inhibitors (rasagiline). Moderate Study
- **Combined hormonal contraceptives** increase the exposure to monoamine-oxidase B inhibitors (selegiline). Avoid. Severe Study
- Monoclonal antibodies (sarilumab) potentially decrease the exposure to **combined hormonal contraceptives**. Severe Theoretical
- Nevirapine is predicted to decrease the efficacy of **combined hormonal contraceptives**. For FSRH guidance, see Contraceptives, interactions p. 775. Severe Study
- NSAIDs (etoricoxib) slightly increase the exposure to **combined hormonal contraceptives**. Moderate Study
- Paritaprevir (with ritonavir and ombitasvir) increases the risk of raised liver function tests when given with **combined hormonal contraceptives**. Avoid. Severe Study
- **Combined hormonal contraceptives** are predicted to increase the exposure to pirfenidone. Use with caution and adjust dose. Moderate Study
- Pitolisant is predicted to decrease the efficacy of **combined hormonal contraceptives**. Avoid. Severe Theoretical
- **Combined hormonal contraceptives** are predicted to increase the risk of venous thromboembolism when given with pomalidomide. Avoid. Severe Theoretical
- Rifabutin is predicted to decrease the efficacy of **combined hormonal contraceptives**. For FSRH guidance, see Contraceptives, interactions p. 775. Severe Study
- Rifampicin is predicted to decrease the efficacy of **combined hormonal contraceptives**. For FSRH guidance, see Contraceptives, interactions p. 775. Severe Study
- **Combined hormonal contraceptives** are predicted to increase the exposure to roflumilast. Moderate Theoretical
- St John's Wort decreases the efficacy of **combined hormonal contraceptives**. MHRA advises avoid. For FSRH guidance, see Contraceptives, interactions p. 775. Severe Anecdotal
- Sugammadex is predicted to decrease the exposure to oral **combined hormonal contraceptives**. Refer to patient information leaflet for missed pill advice. Severe Theoretical
- **Combined hormonal contraceptives** are predicted to increase the risk of venous thromboembolism when given with thalidomide. Avoid. Severe Study
- **Combined hormonal contraceptives** are predicted to increase the exposure to theophylline. Monitor and adjust dose. Moderate Theoretical
- **Combined hormonal contraceptives** increase the exposure to tizanidine. Avoid. Moderate Study
- Ulipristal is predicted to decrease the efficacy of **combined hormonal contraceptives**. Avoid. Severe Theoretical
- **Combined hormonal contraceptives** are predicted to increase the exposure to zolmitriptan. Adjust zolmitriptan dose, p. 475. Moderate Theoretical

Corticosteroids → see TABLE 17 p. 1338 (reduced serum potassium)

beclometasone · betamethasone · budesonide · ciclesonide · deflazacort · dexamethasone · fludrocortisone · fluticasone · hydrocortisone · methylprednisolone · mometasone · prednisolone · prednisone · triamcinolone

- Interactions do not generally apply to corticosteroids used for topical action (including inhalation) unless specified.
- With intravitreal use of **dexamethasone** in adults: caution with concurrent administration of anticoagulant or antiplatelet drugs—increased risk of haemorrhagic events.

- Antacids are predicted to decrease the absorption of **deflazacort**. Separate administration by 2 hours. Moderate Theoretical
- Antacids decrease the absorption of **dexamethasone**. Moderate Study
- Antiarrhythmics (dronedarone) are predicted to increase the exposure to **methylprednisolone**. Monitor and adjust dose. Moderate Study

- Antiepileptics (carbamazepine, fosphenytoin, phenobarbital, phenytoin, primidone) are predicted to decrease the exposure to fluticasone. Unknown Theoretical
- Antiepileptics (carbamazepine, fosphenytoin, phenobarbital, phenytoin, primidone) are predicted to decrease the exposure to corticosteroids (**budesonide, deflazacort, dexamethasone, fludrocortisone, hydrocortisone, methylprednisolone, prednisolone, prednisone, triamcinolone**). Monitor and adjust dose. Moderate Study
- Antifungals, azoles (fluconazole, isavuconazole, posaconazole) are predicted to increase the exposure to **methylprednisolone**. Monitor and adjust dose. Moderate Study
- Antifungals, azoles (itraconazole, ketoconazole, voriconazole) are predicted to increase the exposure to **beclometasone** (risk with beclometasone is likely to be lower than with other corticosteroids). Moderate Theoretical
- Antifungals, azoles (miconazole) are predicted to increase the concentration of **methylprednisolone**. Monitor and adjust dose. Moderate Theoretical
- Antifungals, azoles (itraconazole, ketoconazole, voriconazole) are predicted to increase the exposure to corticosteroids (**betamethasone, budesonide, ciclesonide, deflazacort, dexamethasone, fludrocortisone, fluticasone, hydrocortisone, methylprednisolone, mometasone, prednisolone, prednisone, triamcinolone**). Avoid or monitor side effects. Severe Study
- **Prednisone** potentially decreases the exposure to antifungals, azoles (isavuconazole). Use with caution or avoid. Moderate Theoretical
- Aprepitant moderately increases the exposure to **dexamethasone**. Monitor and adjust dose. Moderate Study
- Aprepitant is predicted to increase the exposure to **methylprednisolone**. Monitor and adjust dose. Moderate Study
- **Corticosteroids** are predicted to decrease the concentration of aspirin (high-dose) and aspirin (high-dose) increases the risk of gastrointestinal bleeding when given with **corticosteroids**. Moderate Study
- Calcium channel blockers (diltiazem, verapamil) are predicted to increase the exposure to **methylprednisolone**. Monitor and adjust dose. Moderate Study
- **Dexamethasone** is predicted to decrease the concentration of caspofungin. Adjust **caspofungin** dose, p. 582. Moderate Theoretical
- **Corticosteroids** are predicted to decrease the concentration of choline salicylate. Moderate Study
- Cobicistat is predicted to increase the exposure to **beclometasone** (risk with beclometasone is likely to be lower than with other corticosteroids). Moderate Theoretical
- Cobicistat is predicted to increase the exposure to corticosteroids (**betamethasone, budesonide, ciclesonide, deflazacort, dexamethasone, fludrocortisone, fluticasone, hydrocortisone, methylprednisolone, mometasone, prednisolone, prednisone, triamcinolone**). Avoid or monitor side effects. Severe Study
- **Corticosteroids** are predicted to increase the effects of coumarins. Moderate Study
- Crizotinib is predicted to increase the exposure to **methylprednisolone**. Monitor and adjust dose. Moderate Study
- Enzalutamide is predicted to decrease the exposure to corticosteroids (**budesonide, deflazacort, dexamethasone, fludrocortisone, hydrocortisone, methylprednisolone, prednisolone, prednisone, triamcinolone**). Monitor and adjust dose. Moderate Study
- Enzalutamide is predicted to decrease the exposure to fluticasone. Unknown Theoretical
- **Corticosteroids** increase the risk of gastrointestinal perforation when given with erlotinib. Severe Theoretical
- Fosaprepitant is predicted to increase the exposure to corticosteroids (**dexamethasone, methylprednisolone**). Monitor and adjust dose. Moderate Theoretical
- **Corticosteroids** potentially oppose the effects of glycerol phenylbutyrate. Moderate Theoretical
- Grapefruit juice moderately increases the exposure to oral **budesonide**. Avoid. Moderate Study

A1

Corticosteroids (continued)

▸ HIV-protease inhibitors are predicted to increase the exposure to **beclometasone** (risk with beclometasone is likely to be lower than with other corticosteroids). [Moderate] Theoretical

▸ HIV-protease inhibitors are predicted to increase the exposure to corticosteroids **(betamethasone, budesonide, ciclesonide, deflazacort, dexamethasone, fludrocortisone, fluticasone, hydrocortisone, methylprednisolone, mometasone, prednisolone, prednisone, triamcinolone)**. Avoid or monitor side effects. [Severe] Study

▸ Idelalisib is predicted to increase the exposure to **beclometasone** (risk with beclometasone is likely to be lower than with other corticosteroids). [Moderate] Theoretical

▸ Idelalisib is predicted to increase the exposure to corticosteroids **(betamethasone, budesonide, ciclesonide, deflazacort, dexamethasone, fludrocortisone, fluticasone, hydrocortisone, methylprednisolone, mometasone, prednisolone, prednisone, triamcinolone)**. Avoid or monitor side effects. [Severe] Study

▸ Imatinib is predicted to increase the exposure to **methylprednisolone**. Monitor and adjust dose. [Moderate] Study

▸ **Corticosteroids** are predicted to increase the risk of gastrointestinal bleeding when given with iron chelators (deferasirox). [Severe] Theoretical

▸ Live vaccines are predicted to increase the risk of generalised infection (possibly life-threatening) when given with **corticosteroids** (high-dose). Public Health England advises avoid (refer to Green Book). [Severe] Theoretical

▸ Lumacaftor is predicted to decrease the exposure to corticosteroids **(methylprednisolone, prednisone)**. Adjust dose. [Severe] Theoretical

▸ Macrolides (clarithromycin) are predicted to increase the exposure to **beclometasone** (risk with beclometasone is likely to be lower than with other corticosteroids). [Moderate] Theoretical

▸ Macrolides (clarithromycin) are predicted to increase the exposure to corticosteroids **(betamethasone, budesonide, ciclesonide, deflazacort, dexamethasone, fludrocortisone, fluticasone, hydrocortisone, methylprednisolone, mometasone, prednisolone, prednisone, triamcinolone)**. Avoid or monitor side effects. [Severe] Study

▸ Macrolides (erythromycin) are predicted to increase the exposure to **methylprednisolone**. Monitor and adjust dose. [Moderate] Study

▸ **Corticosteroids** are predicted to decrease the efficacy of mifamurtide. Avoid. [Severe] Theoretical

▸ Mifepristone is predicted to decrease the efficacy of **corticosteroids**. Use with caution and adjust dose. [Moderate] Theoretical

▸ Mitotane is predicted to decrease the exposure to corticosteroids **(budesonide, deflazacort, dexamethasone, fludrocortisone, hydrocortisone, methylprednisolone, prednisolone, prednisone, triamcinolone)**. Monitor and adjust dose. [Moderate] Study

▸ Mitotane is predicted to decrease the exposure to **fluticasone**. [Unknown] Theoretical

▸ Corticosteroids **(betamethasone, deflazacort, dexamethasone, hydrocortisone, methylprednisolone, prednisolone, prednisone)** are predicted to decrease the efficacy of monoclonal antibodies (atezolizumab, ipilimumab, nivolumab, pembrolizumab). Use with caution or avoid. [Severe] Theoretical

▸ Monoclonal antibodies (tocilizumab) are predicted to decrease the exposure to corticosteroids **(dexamethasone, methylprednisolone)**. Monitor and adjust dose. [Moderate] Theoretical

▸ Netupitant is predicted to increase the exposure to **dexamethasone**. Adjust dose. [Moderate] Study

▸ Netupitant is predicted to increase the exposure to **methylprednisolone**. Monitor and adjust dose. [Moderate] Study

▸ **Corticosteroids** are predicted to decrease the effects of neuromuscular blocking drugs, non-depolarising. [Severe] Anecdotal

▸ **Corticosteroids** increase the risk of gastrointestinal perforation when given with nicorandil. [Severe] Anecdotal

▸ Nilotinib is predicted to increase the exposure to **methylprednisolone**. Monitor and adjust dose. [Moderate] Study

▸ NSAIDs increase the risk of gastrointestinal bleeding when given with **corticosteroids**. [Severe] Study

▸ **Corticosteroids** are predicted to increase the effects of phenindione. [Moderate] Anecdotal

▸ **Dexamethasone** decreases the exposure to praziquantel. [Moderate] Study

▸ Rifampicin is predicted to decrease the exposure to corticosteroids **(budesonide, deflazacort, dexamethasone, fludrocortisone, hydrocortisone, methylprednisolone, prednisolone, prednisone, triamcinolone)**. Monitor and adjust dose. [Moderate] Study

▸ Rifampicin is predicted to decrease the exposure to **fluticasone**. [Unknown] Theoretical

▸ **Corticosteroids** potentially decrease the effects of sodium phenylbutyrate. [Moderate] Anecdotal

▸ **Corticosteroids** are predicted to decrease the effects of somatropin. [Moderate] Theoretical

▸ **Corticosteroids** are predicted to decrease the effects of suxamethonium. [Severe] Anecdotal

Coumarins → see TABLE 3 p. 1334 (anticoagulant effects)

acenocoumarol · warfarin

FOOD AND LIFESTYLE The effects of coumarins can be reduced or abolished by vitamin K, including that found in health foods, food supplements, enteral feeds, or large amounts of some green vegetables or green tea. Major changes in diet (especially involving salads and vegetables) and in alcohol consumption can affect anticoagulant control. Pomegranate increases the INR in response to **warfarin** and is predicted to increase the INR in response to **acenocoumarol**.

▸ Alcohol (beverage) (in those who drink heavily) potentially decreases the anticoagulant effect of **coumarins**. [Severe] Study

▸ Antiarrhythmics (amiodarone) increase the anticoagulant effect of **coumarins**. [Severe] Study

▸ Antiarrhythmics (propafenone) increase the anticoagulant effect of **coumarins**. Monitor INR and adjust dose. [Moderate] Study

▸ Antiepileptics (carbamazepine) decrease the effects of **coumarins**. Monitor and adjust dose. [Severe] Study

▸ Antiepileptics (fosphenytoin, phenytoin) are predicted to alter the anticoagulant effect of **coumarins**. [Moderate] Anecdotal

▸ Antiepileptics (phenobarbital, primidone) decrease the anticoagulant effect of **coumarins**. Monitor INR and adjust dose. [Moderate] Study

▸ Antifungals, azoles (fluconazole) increase the anticoagulant effect of **coumarins**. Monitor INR and adjust dose. [Severe] Study

▸ Antifungals, azoles (itraconazole) potentially increase the anticoagulant effect of **coumarins**. [Severe] Anecdotal

▸ Antifungals, azoles (ketoconazole) potentially increase the anticoagulant effect of **warfarin**. Monitor INR and adjust dose. [Severe] Anecdotal

▸ Antifungals, azoles (miconazole) greatly increase the anticoagulant effect of **coumarins**. MHRA advises avoid unless INR can be monitored closely; monitor for signs of bleeding. [Severe] Study

▸ Antifungals, azoles (voriconazole) increase the anticoagulant effect of **coumarins**. Monitor INR and adjust dose. [Moderate] Study

▸ Aprepitant decreases the anticoagulant effect of **coumarins**. [Moderate] Study

▸ Axitinib is predicted to increase the risk of bleeding events when given with **coumarins**. [Severe] Theoretical

▸ Azathioprine decreases the anticoagulant effect of **coumarins**. [Moderate] Study

▸ Bosentan decreases the anticoagulant effect of **coumarins**. [Moderate] Study

▸ Bosutinib is predicted to increase the risk of bleeding events when given with **coumarins**. [Severe] Theoretical

▸ Cabozantinib is predicted to increase the risk of bleeding events when given with **coumarins**. [Severe] Theoretical

▸ Capecitabine increases the effects of **coumarins**. Monitor INR and adjust dose. [Moderate] Anecdotal

▶ Cephalosporins (ceftriaxone) potentially increase the risk of bleeding events when given with **coumarins**. [Severe] Anecdotal

▶ Ceritinib is predicted to increase the exposure to **warfarin**. Avoid. [Severe] Theoretical

▶ Chloramphenicol potentially increases the anticoagulant effect of **coumarins**. [Moderate] Anecdotal

▶ Corticosteroids are predicted to increase the effects of **coumarins**. [Moderate] Study

▶ Cranberry juice potentially increases the anticoagulant effect of **warfarin**. Avoid. [Severe] Anecdotal

▶ Crizotinib is predicted to increase the risk of bleeding events when given with **coumarins**. [Severe] Theoretical

▶ Dabrafenib is predicted to decrease the anticoagulant effect of **coumarins**. [Severe] Theoretical

▶ Danazol potentially increases the anticoagulant effect of **coumarins**. [Severe] Anecdotal

▶ Dasatinib is predicted to increase the risk of bleeding events when given with **coumarins**. [Severe] Theoretical

▶ Disulfiram increases the anticoagulant effect of **coumarins**. Monitor and adjust dose. [Severe] Study

▶ Efavirenz is predicted to affect the concentration of **coumarins**. Adjust dose. [Moderate] Theoretical

▶ Elvitegravir is predicted to decrease the anticoagulant effect of **coumarins**. [Moderate] Theoretical

▶ Enteral feeds (vitamin-K containing) potentially decrease the anticoagulant effect of **coumarins**. [Severe] Anecdotal

▶ Enzalutamide potentially decreases the exposure to **coumarins**. Avoid or adjust dose and monitor INR. [Severe] Study

▶ Erlotinib increases the anticoagulant effect of **coumarins**. [Severe] Anecdotal

▶ Etravirine increases the anticoagulant effect of **coumarins**. [Moderate] Theoretical

▶ Fibrates are predicted to increase the anticoagulant effect of **coumarins**. Monitor INR and adjust dose. [Severe] Study

▶ Fluorouracil increases the anticoagulant effect of **coumarins**. [Severe] Anecdotal

▶ Fosaprepitant is predicted to decrease the anticoagulant effect of **coumarins**. [Moderate] Theoretical

▶ Gefitinib is predicted to increase the anticoagulant effect of **coumarins**. [Severe] Anecdotal

▶ Glucagon increases the anticoagulant effect of **warfarin**. [Severe] Study

▶ Glucosamine increases the anticoagulant effect of **warfarin**. Avoid. [Moderate] Anecdotal

▶ Griseofulvin potentially decreases the anticoagulant effect of **coumarins**. [Moderate] Anecdotal

▶ H₂ receptor antagonists (cimetidine) increase the anticoagulant effect of **coumarins**. [Severe] Study

▶ HIV-protease inhibitors are predicted to affect the anticoagulant effect of **coumarins**. [Moderate] Study

▶ Imatinib is predicted to increase the risk of bleeding events when given with **coumarins**. [Severe] Theoretical

▶ Ivacaftor is predicted to increase the anticoagulant effect of **warfarin**. [Severe] Theoretical

▶ Ivermectin potentially increases the anticoagulant effect of **coumarins**. [Severe] Anecdotal

▶ Lapatinib is predicted to increase the risk of bleeding events when given with **coumarins**. [Severe] Theoretical

▶ Leflunomide increases the anticoagulant effect of **coumarins**. [Severe] Anecdotal

▶ Lomitapide increases the exposure to **warfarin**. Monitor INR and adjust dose. [Severe] Study

▶ Macrolides (clarithromycin, erythromycin) increase the anticoagulant effect of **coumarins**. Monitor INR and adjust dose. [Severe] Anecdotal

▶ Mercaptopurine decreases the anticoagulant effect of **coumarins**. [Moderate] Anecdotal

▶ Metronidazole increases the anticoagulant effect of **coumarins**. Monitor INR and adjust dose. [Severe] Study

▶ Monoclonal antibodies (blinatumomab) are predicted to transiently increase the exposure to **warfarin**. Monitor and adjust dose. [Moderate] Theoretical

▶ Monoclonal antibodies (sarilumab) potentially affect the exposure to **warfarin**. Monitor and adjust dose. [Severe] Theoretical

▶ Monoclonal antibodies (tocilizumab) are predicted to decrease the exposure to **warfarin**. Monitor and adjust dose. [Moderate] Theoretical

▶ Nandrolone is predicted to increase the anticoagulant effect of **coumarins**. Monitor and adjust dose. [Severe] Theoretical

▶ Nevirapine potentially alters the anticoagulant effect of **coumarins**. [Severe] Anecdotal

▶ Nilotinib is predicted to increase the risk of bleeding events when given with **coumarins**. [Severe] Theoretical

▶ Obeticholic acid decreases the anticoagulant effect of **warfarin**. [Severe] Study

▶ Oxymetholone increases the anticoagulant effect of **coumarins**. [Severe] Anecdotal

▶ Paracetamol increases the anticoagulant effect of **coumarins**. [Moderate] Study

▶ Pazopanib is predicted to increase the risk of bleeding events when given with **coumarins**. [Severe] Theoretical

▶ Penicillins potentially alter the anticoagulant effect of **coumarins**. Monitor INR and adjust dose. [Severe] Anecdotal

▶ Pitolisant is predicted to decrease the exposure to **warfarin**. [Unknown] Theoretical

▶ Ponatinib is predicted to increase the risk of bleeding events when given with **coumarins**. [Severe] Theoretical

▶ Quinolones increase the anticoagulant effect of **coumarins**. [Severe] Anecdotal

▶ Ranibizumab increases the risk of bleeding events when given with **coumarins**. [Severe] Theoretical

▶ Regorafenib is predicted to increase the risk of bleeding events when given with **coumarins**. [Severe] Study

▶ Rifampicin decreases the anticoagulant effect of **coumarins**. [Severe] Study

▶ Ruxolitinib is predicted to increase the risk of bleeding events when given with **coumarins**. [Severe] Theoretical

▶ Sorafenib increases the anticoagulant effect of **coumarins**. [Severe] Anecdotal

▶ St John's Wort decreases the anticoagulant effect of **coumarins**. Avoid. [Severe] Anecdotal

▶ Statins (fluvastatin, rosuvastatin) increase the anticoagulant effect of **coumarins**. Monitor INR and adjust dose. [Severe] Study

▶ Sucralfate potentially decreases the effects of **warfarin**. Separate administration by 2 hours. [Moderate] Anecdotal

▶ Sulfinpyrazone increases the anticoagulant effect of **coumarins**. Avoid. [Severe] Study

▶ Sulfonamides (sulfadiazine) are predicted to increase the anticoagulant effect of **coumarins**. [Severe] Theoretical

▶ Sulfonamides (sulfamethoxazole) increase the anticoagulant effect of **coumarins**. [Severe] Study

▶ Sunitinib is predicted to increase the risk of bleeding events when given with **coumarins**. [Severe] Theoretical

▶ Tamoxifen increases the anticoagulant effect of **coumarins**. [Severe] Study

▶ Tegafur increases the anticoagulant effect of **coumarins**. [Moderate] Theoretical

▶ Teriflunomide affects the anticoagulant effect of **coumarins**. [Severe] Study

▶ Tetracyclines increase the risk of bleeding events when given with **coumarins**. [Moderate] Anecdotal

▶ Tinidazole is predicted to increase the anticoagulant effect of **coumarins**. Monitor INR and adjust dose. [Severe] Theoretical

▶ Toremifene is predicted to increase the anticoagulant effect of **coumarins**. [Severe] Theoretical

▶ Trimethoprim is predicted to increase the anticoagulant effect of **coumarins**. [Severe] Study

▶ Vandetanib is predicted to increase the risk of bleeding events when given with **coumarins**. [Severe] Theoretical

▶ Venetoclax slightly increases the exposure to **warfarin**. [Moderate] Study

Cranberry juice

▶ Cranberry juice potentially increases the anticoagulant effect of coumarins (warfarin). Avoid. [Severe] Anecdotal

Crisantaspase → see TABLE 1 p. 1334 (hepatotoxicity), **TABLE 15** p. 1337 (myelosuppression)

▶ **Crisantaspase** is predicted to increase the risk of hepatotoxicity when given with imatinib. [Severe] Theoretical → Also see **TABLE 15** p. 1337

A1

Interactions | Appendix 1

Crisantaspase (continued)

▸ **Crisantaspase** affects the efficacy of methotrexate. Severe
Anecdotal → Also see TABLE 1 p. 1334 → Also see TABLE 15 p. 1337

▸ **Crisantaspase** potentially increases the risk of neurotoxicity
when given with vinca alkaloids (vincristine). **Vincristine** should
be taken 3 to 24 hours before **crisantaspase**, p. 908. Severe
Anecdotal → Also see TABLE 1 p. 1334 → Also see TABLE 15 p. 1337

Crizotinib → see TABLE 6 p. 1335 (bradycardia), TABLE 15 p. 1337
(myelosuppression), TABLE 9 p. 1336 (QT-interval prolongation)

GENERAL INFORMATION Caution with concurrent use of drugs
that cause gastrointestinal perforation—discontinue
treatment if gastrointestinal perforation occurs.

▸ **Crizotinib** is predicted to increase the exposure to aldosterone
antagonists (eplerenone). Adjust **eplerenone** dose, p. 190. Severe
Study

▸ **Crizotinib** is predicted to increase the exposure to alpha
blockers (tamsulosin). Moderate Theoretical

▸ **Crizotinib** is predicted to increase the exposure to alprazolam.
Severe Study

▸ **Crizotinib** is predicted to increase the exposure to
antiarrhythmics (propafenone). Monitor and adjust dose.
Moderate Study

▸ Antiepileptics (carbamazepine, fosphenytoin, phenobarbital,
phenytoin, primidone) are predicted to markedly decrease the
exposure to **crizotinib**. Avoid. Severe Study

▸ Antifungals, azoles (itraconazole, ketoconazole, voriconazole) are
predicted to moderately increase the exposure to **crizotinib**.
Avoid. Moderate Study → Also see TABLE 9 p. 1336

▸ **Crizotinib** is predicted to increase the exposure to
antihistamines, non-sedating (mizolastine). Severe Theoretical

▸ **Crizotinib** is predicted to increase the exposure to
antihistamines, non-sedating (rupatadine). Avoid. Moderate Study

▸ **Crizotinib** is predicted to increase the concentration of
antimalarials (piperaquine). Severe Theoretical

▸ **Crizotinib** is predicted to increase the exposure to axitinib.
Moderate Theoretical → Also see TABLE 15 p. 1337

▸ **Crizotinib** is predicted to increase the exposure to bedaquiline.
Avoid prolonged use. Mild Theoretical → Also see TABLE 9 p. 1336

▸ Bosentan is predicted to decrease the exposure to **crizotinib**.
Avoid. Severe Theoretical

▸ **Crizotinib** is predicted to increase the exposure to bosutinib.
Avoid or adjust dose. Severe Theoretical → Also see TABLE 15
p. 1337 → Also see TABLE 9 p. 1336

▸ **Crizotinib** is predicted to increase the exposure to buspirone.
Use with caution and adjust dose. Moderate Study

▸ **Crizotinib** is predicted to increase the exposure to
cabozantinib. Moderate Theoretical → Also see TABLE 15 p. 1337 →
Also see TABLE 9 p. 1336

▸ **Crizotinib** is predicted to increase the exposure to calcium
channel blockers (amlodipine, felodipine, lacidipine,
lercanidipine, nicardipine, nifedipine, nimodipine). Monitor and
adjust dose. Moderate Study

▸ **Crizotinib** is predicted to increase the exposure to ceritinib.
Moderate Theoretical → Also see TABLE 15 p. 1337 → Also see TABLE 9
p. 1336

▸ **Crizotinib** increases the concentration of ciclosporin. Severe
Study

▸ Cobicistat is predicted to moderately increase the exposure to
crizotinib. Avoid. Moderate Study

▸ **Crizotinib** is predicted to increase the exposure to cobimetinib.
Severe Theoretical

▸ **Crizotinib** is predicted to increase the exposure to colchicine.
Adjust **colchicine** dose with moderate inhibitors of CYP3A4,
p. 1085. Severe Study

▸ **Crizotinib** is predicted to increase the exposure to
corticosteroids (methylprednisolone). Monitor and adjust dose.
Moderate Study

▸ **Crizotinib** is predicted to increase the risk of bleeding events
when given with coumarins. Severe Theoretical

▸ **Crizotinib** is predicted to slightly increase the exposure to
darifenacin. Moderate Study

▸ **Crizotinib** is predicted to increase the exposure to dasatinib.
Severe Study → Also see TABLE 15 p. 1337 → Also see TABLE 9 p. 1336

▸ **Crizotinib** increases the risk of QT-prolongation when given
with domperidone. Avoid. Severe Study

▸ **Crizotinib** is predicted to increase the exposure to dopamine
receptor agonists (bromocriptine). Severe Theoretical

▸ **Crizotinib** is predicted to increase the concentration of
dopamine receptor agonists (cabergoline). Moderate Anecdotal

▸ **Crizotinib** is predicted to moderately increase the exposure to
dutasteride. Mild Study

▸ Efavirenz is predicted to decrease the exposure to **crizotinib**.
Avoid. Severe Theoretical → Also see TABLE 15 p. 1336

▸ **Crizotinib** is predicted to increase the exposure to eliglustat.
Avoid or adjust dose—consult product literature. Severe Study

▸ Enzalutamide is predicted to markedly decrease the exposure
to **crizotinib**. Avoid. Severe Study

▸ **Crizotinib** is predicted to increase the risk of ergotism when
given with ergometrine. Severe Theoretical

▸ **Crizotinib** is predicted to increase the risk of ergotism when
given with ergotamine. Severe Theoretical

▸ **Crizotinib** is predicted to increase the exposure to erlotinib.
Moderate Theoretical

▸ **Crizotinib** is predicted to increase the concentration of
everolimus. Avoid or adjust dose. Moderate Study → Also see
TABLE 15 p. 1337

▸ **Crizotinib** is predicted to increase the exposure to
fesoterodine. Adjust **fesoterodine** dose with moderate
inhibitors of CYP3A4 in hepatic and renal impairment, p. 759.
Mild Study

▸ **Crizotinib** is predicted to increase the exposure to gefitinib.
Moderate Theoretical → Also see TABLE 15 p. 1337

▸ **Crizotinib** potentially decreases the exposure to glecaprevir.
Avoid. Severe Theoretical

▸ Grapefruit juice is predicted to increase the exposure to
crizotinib. Avoid. Moderate Theoretical

▸ **Crizotinib** is predicted to increase the concentration of
guanfacine. Adjust **guanfacine** dose, p. 349. Moderate Theoretical

▸ HIV-protease inhibitors are predicted to moderately increase
the exposure to **crizotinib**. Avoid. Moderate Study → Also see
TABLE 9 p. 1336

▸ **Crizotinib** is predicted to increase the exposure to ibrutinib.
Adjust **ibrutinib** dose with moderate inhibitors of CYP3A4,
p. 952. Severe Study → Also see TABLE 15 p. 1337

▸ Idelalisib is predicted to moderately increase the exposure to
crizotinib. Avoid. Moderate Study → Also see TABLE 15 p. 1337

▸ **Crizotinib** is predicted to increase the exposure to ivabradine.
Adjust **ivabradine** dose, p. 210. Severe Theoretical → Also see
TABLE 6 p. 1335

▸ **Crizotinib** is predicted to increase the exposure to ivacaftor.
Adjust **ivacaftor** dose with moderate inhibitors of CYP3A4,
p. 292. Severe Study

▸ **Crizotinib** is predicted to increase the exposure to lapatinib.
Moderate Study → Also see TABLE 9 p. 1336

▸ **Crizotinib** is predicted to increase the exposure to lomitapide.
Avoid. Moderate Theoretical

▸ **Crizotinib** is predicted to increase the exposure to lurasidone.
Moderate Study

▸ Macrolides (clarithromycin) are predicted to moderately
increase the exposure to **crizotinib**. Avoid. Moderate Study →
Also see TABLE 9 p. 1336

▸ **Crizotinib** is predicted to increase the exposure to midazolam.
Monitor side effects and adjust dose. Severe Study

▸ **Crizotinib** is predicted to increase the exposure to midostaurin.
Moderate Theoretical

▸ Mitotane is predicted to markedly decrease the exposure to
crizotinib. Avoid. Severe Study → Also see TABLE 15 p. 1337

▸ **Crizotinib** is predicted to increase the exposure to naloxegol.
Adjust **naloxegol** dose and monitor side effects, p. 64. Moderate
Study

▸ Nevirapine is predicted to decrease the exposure to **crizotinib**.
Avoid. Severe Theoretical

▸ **Crizotinib** is predicted to increase the exposure to olaparib.
Avoid moderate inhibitors of CYP3A4 or adjust **olaparib** dose,
p. 973. Moderate Theoretical → Also see TABLE 15 p. 1337

▸ **Crizotinib** is predicted to increase the exposure to opioids
(alfentanil, buprenorphine, fentanyl, oxycodone). Monitor and
adjust dose. Moderate Study → Also see TABLE 6 p. 1335

▸ **Crizotinib** is predicted to increase the exposure to opioids (methadone, sufentanil). Moderate Theoretical → Also see **TABLE 6** p. 1335 → Also see **TABLE 9** p. 1336

▸ **Crizotinib** is predicted to increase the exposure to oxybutynin. Mild Theoretical

▸ **Crizotinib** is predicted to increase the exposure to pazopanib. Moderate Theoretical → Also see **TABLE 15** p. 1337 → Also see **TABLE 9** p. 1336

▸ **Crizotinib** is predicted to increase the risk of bleeding events when given with phenindione. Severe Theoretical

▸ **Crizotinib** is predicted to increase the exposure to phosphodiesterase type-5 inhibitors (avanafil). Adjust **avanafil** dose, p. 794. Moderate Theoretical

▸ **Crizotinib** is predicted to increase the exposure to phosphodiesterase type-5 inhibitors (sildenafil). Monitor or adjust **sildenafil** dose with moderate inhibitors of CYP3A4, p. 794. Moderate Study → Also see **TABLE 9** p. 1336

▸ **Crizotinib** is predicted to increase the exposure to phosphodiesterase type-5 inhibitors (tadalafil). Severe Theoretical

▸ **Crizotinib** is predicted to increase the exposure to phosphodiesterase type-5 inhibitors (vardenafil). Adjust dose. Severe Theoretical → Also see **TABLE 9** p. 1336

▸ **Crizotinib** potentially decreases the exposure to pibrentasvir. Avoid. Severe Theoretical

▸ **Crizotinib** is predicted to increase the exposure to pimozide. Avoid. Severe Theoretical → Also see **TABLE 9** p. 1336

▸ Pitolisant is predicted to decrease the exposure to **crizotinib**. Avoid. Severe Theoretical

▸ **Crizotinib** is predicted to increase the exposure to quetiapine. Avoid. Moderate Study

▸ **Crizotinib** is predicted to increase the exposure to ranolazine. Severe Study → Also see **TABLE 9** p. 1336

▸ **Crizotinib** is predicted to increase the exposure to ribociclib. Moderate Study → Also see **TABLE 9** p. 1336

▸ Rifampicin is predicted to markedly decrease the exposure to **crizotinib**. Avoid. Severe Study

▸ **Crizotinib** is predicted to increase the exposure to ruxolitinib. Moderate Theoretical → Also see **TABLE 15** p. 1337

▸ **Crizotinib** is predicted to increase the exposure to saxagliptin. Mild Study

▸ **Crizotinib** is predicted to increase the exposure to simeprevir. Avoid. Severe Study

▸ **Crizotinib** increases the concentration of sirolimus. Monitor and adjust dose. Moderate Study

▸ **Crizotinib** is predicted to increase the exposure to SSRIs (dapoxetine). Adjust **dapoxetine** dose with moderate inhibitors of CYP3A4, p. 801. Moderate Theoretical

▸ St John's Wort is predicted to decrease the exposure to **crizotinib**. Avoid. Severe Theoretical

▸ **Crizotinib** is predicted to increase the exposure to statins (atorvastatin). Monitor and adjust dose. Severe Study

▸ **Crizotinib** is predicted to increase the exposure to statins (simvastatin). Use with caution and adjust **simvastatin** dose, p. 203. Severe Study

▸ **Crizotinib** is predicted to increase the exposure to sunitinib. Moderate Theoretical → Also see **TABLE 15** p. 1337 → Also see **TABLE 9** p. 1336

▸ **Crizotinib** is predicted to increase the concentration of tacrolimus. Severe Study

▸ **Crizotinib** is predicted to increase the exposure to taxanes (cabazitaxel). Moderate Theoretical → Also see **TABLE 15** p. 1337

▸ **Crizotinib** is predicted to increase the concentration of temsirolimus. Moderate Theoretical → Also see **TABLE 15** p. 1337

▸ **Crizotinib** is predicted to increase the exposure to tofacitinib. Moderate Study

▸ **Crizotinib** is predicted to increase the exposure to tolterodine. Mild Theoretical → Also see **TABLE 9** p. 1336

▸ **Crizotinib** is predicted to increase the exposure to tolvaptan. Adjust dose. Moderate Study

▸ **Crizotinib** is predicted to increase the exposure to trazodone. Moderate Theoretical

▸ **Crizotinib** is predicted to increase the exposure to ulipristal. Avoid if used for uterine fibroids. Moderate Study

▸ **Crizotinib** is predicted to increase the exposure to venetoclax. Avoid moderate inhibitors of CYP3A4 or adjust **venetoclax** dose, p. 974. Severe Study

▸ **Crizotinib** is predicted to increase the exposure to vinca alkaloids. Severe Theoretical → Also see **TABLE 15** p. 1337 → Also see **TABLE 9** p. 1336

▸ **Crizotinib** is predicted to increase the exposure to zopiclone. Adjust dose. Moderate Study

Cyclizine → see antihistamines, sedating

Cyclopenthiazide → see thiazide diuretics

Cyclopentolate → see **TABLE 10** p. 1336 (antimuscarinics)

Cyclophosphamide → see alkylating agents

Cycloserine

▸ **Cycloserine** increases the risk of CNS toxicity when given with isoniazid. Monitor and adjust dose. Moderate Study

Cyproheptadine → see antihistamines, sedating

Cytarabine → see **TABLE 15** p. 1337 (myelosuppression)

▸ **Cytarabine** decreases the concentration of flucytosine. Avoid. Severe Study

▸ Live vaccines are predicted to increase the risk of generalised infection (possibly life-threatening) when given with **cytarabine**. Public Health England advises avoid (refer to Green Book). Severe Theoretical

Dabigatran → see **TABLE 3** p. 1334 (anticoagulant effects)

▸ Antiarrhythmics (amiodarone) increase the exposure to **dabigatran**. Adjust **dabigatran** dose, p. 135. Moderate Study

▸ Antiarrhythmics (dronedarone) slightly increase the exposure to **dabigatran**. Avoid. Severe Study

▸ Antiepileptics (carbamazepine) are predicted to decrease the exposure to **dabigatran**. Avoid. Severe Study

▸ Antifungals, azoles (isavuconazole) are predicted to increase the exposure to **dabigatran**. Monitor and adjust dose. Moderate Study

▸ Antifungals, azoles (itraconazole, ketoconazole) are predicted to increase the exposure to **dabigatran**. Avoid. Severe Study

▸ Calcium channel blockers (verapamil) increase the exposure to **dabigatran**. Adjust **dabigatran** dose, p. 135. Severe Study

▸ Ceritinib is predicted to increase the exposure to **dabigatran**. Moderate Theoretical

▸ Ciclosporin is predicted to increase the exposure to **dabigatran**. Avoid. Severe Theoretical

▸ Elbasvir is predicted to increase the concentration of **dabigatran**. Moderate Theoretical

▸ Eliglustat is predicted to increase the exposure to **dabigatran**. Adjust dose. Moderate Study

▸ Glecaprevir (with pibrentasvir) increases the exposure to **dabigatran**. Avoid. Moderate Study

▸ HIV-protease inhibitors (lopinavir, ritonavir, saquinavir) are predicted to increase the exposure to **dabigatran**. Avoid. Severe Theoretical

▸ Lapatinib is predicted to increase the exposure to **dabigatran**. Severe Theoretical

▸ Macrolides are predicted to increase the exposure to **dabigatran**. Moderate Theoretical

▸ Mirabegron is predicted to increase the exposure to **dabigatran**. Severe Theoretical

▸ Pibrentasvir (with glecaprevir) increases the exposure to **dabigatran**. Avoid. Moderate Study

▸ Pitolisant is predicted to decrease the exposure to **dabigatran**. Unknown Theoretical

▸ Ranolazine is predicted to increase the exposure to **dabigatran**. Severe Theoretical

▸ Rifampicin is predicted to decrease the exposure to **dabigatran**. Avoid. Severe Study

▸ Rolapitant is predicted to increase the exposure to **dabigatran**. Moderate Study

▸ St John's Wort is predicted to decrease the exposure to **dabigatran**. Avoid. Severe Study

▸ Velpatasvir is predicted to increase the exposure to **dabigatran**. Severe Theoretical

▸ Vemurafenib increases the exposure to **dabigatran**. Use with caution and adjust dose. Severe Theoretical

▸ Voxilaprevir is predicted to increase the concentration of **dabigatran**. Avoid. Severe Study

Dabrafenib → see **TABLE 15** p. 1337 (myelosuppression)

Interactions | **Appendix 1**

Dabrafenib (continued)
▶ Antiepileptics **(carbamazepine, fosphenytoin, phenobarbital, phenytoin, primidone)** are predicted to decrease the exposure to **dabrafenib**. Avoid. [Moderate] Theoretical
▶ Antifungals, azoles **(itraconazole, ketoconazole, voriconazole)** are predicted to increase the exposure to **dabrafenib**. Use with caution or avoid. [Moderate] Study
▶ **Clopidogrel** is predicted to increase the exposure to **dabrafenib**. [Moderate] Theoretical
▶ **Cobicistat** is predicted to increase the exposure to **dabrafenib**. Use with caution or avoid. [Moderate] Study
▶ **Dabrafenib** is predicted to decrease the anticoagulant effect of coumarins. [Severe] Theoretical
▶ **Enzalutamide** is predicted to decrease the exposure to **dabrafenib**. Avoid. [Moderate] Theoretical
▶ **Fibrates (gemfibrozil)** are predicted to increase the exposure to **dabrafenib**. [Moderate] Theoretical
▶ **HIV-protease inhibitors** are predicted to increase the exposure to **dabrafenib**. Use with caution or avoid. [Moderate] Study
▶ **Idelalisib** is predicted to increase the exposure to **dabrafenib**. Use with caution or avoid. [Moderate] Study → Also see TABLE 15 p. 1337
▶ **Macrolides (clarithromycin)** are predicted to increase the exposure to **dabrafenib**. Use with caution or avoid. [Moderate] Study
▶ **Dabrafenib** decreases the exposure to midazolam. Monitor and adjust dose. [Moderate] Study
▶ **Mitotane** is predicted to decrease the exposure to **dabrafenib**. Avoid. [Moderate] Theoretical → Also see TABLE 15 p. 1337
▶ **Rifampicin** is predicted to decrease the exposure to **dabrafenib**. Avoid. [Moderate] Theoretical
Dacarbazine → see alkylating agents
Daclatasvir
▶ **Daclatasvir** is predicted to increase the risk of severe bradycardia or heart block when given with antiarrhythmics (amiodarone). Refer to specialist literature. [Severe] Anecdotal
▶ Antiepileptics **(carbamazepine, fosphenytoin, phenobarbital, phenytoin, primidone)** are predicted to moderately decrease the exposure to **daclatasvir**. Avoid. [Severe] Study
▶ Antiepileptics **(oxcarbazepine)** are predicted to decrease the exposure to **daclatasvir**. Avoid. [Severe] Theoretical
▶ Antifungals, azoles **(itraconazole, ketoconazole, voriconazole)** are predicted to moderately increase the exposure to **daclatasvir**. Adjust **daclatasvir** dose, p. 614. [Moderate] Study
▶ **Bosentan** is predicted to decrease the exposure to **daclatasvir**. Adjust **daclatasvir** dose, p. 614. [Moderate] Theoretical
▶ **Cobicistat** is predicted to moderately increase the exposure to **daclatasvir**. Adjust **daclatasvir** dose, p. 614. [Moderate] Study
▶ **Daclatasvir** slightly increases the concentration of digoxin. [Severe] Study
▶ **Efavirenz** is predicted to decrease the exposure to **daclatasvir**. Adjust dose. [Severe] Study
▶ **Enzalutamide** is predicted to moderately decrease the exposure to **daclatasvir**. Avoid. [Severe] Study
▶ **Etravirine** is predicted to decrease the exposure to **daclatasvir**. Avoid. [Moderate] Theoretical
▶ **HIV-protease inhibitors** are predicted to moderately increase the exposure to **daclatasvir**. Adjust **daclatasvir** dose, p. 614. [Moderate] Study
▶ **Idelalisib** is predicted to moderately increase the exposure to **daclatasvir**. Adjust **daclatasvir** dose, p. 614. [Moderate] Study
▶ **Macrolides (clarithromycin)** are predicted to moderately increase the exposure to **daclatasvir**. Adjust **daclatasvir** dose, p. 614. [Moderate] Study
▶ **Mitotane** is predicted to moderately decrease the exposure to **daclatasvir**. Avoid. [Severe] Study
▶ **Nevirapine** is predicted to decrease the exposure to **daclatasvir**. Avoid. [Severe] Theoretical
▶ **Rifampicin** is predicted to moderately decrease the exposure to **daclatasvir**. Avoid. [Severe] Study
▶ **St John's Wort** is predicted to decrease the exposure to **daclatasvir**. Avoid. [Severe] Theoretical
Dactinomycin → see TABLE 1 p. 1334 (hepatotoxicity), TABLE 15 p. 1337 (myelosuppression)

▶ **Live vaccines** are predicted to increase the risk of generalised infection (possibly life-threatening) when given with **dactinomycin**. Public Health England advises avoid (refer to Green Book). [Severe] Theoretical
Dairy products
▶ **Dairy products** are predicted to decrease the absorption of eltrombopag. Eltrombopag should be taken 2 hours before or 4 hours after **dairy products**. [Severe] Theoretical
▶ **Dairy products** decrease the exposure to tetracyclines (demeclocycline, oxytetracycline, tetracycline). Avoid. [Moderate] Study
Dalteparin → see low molecular-weight heparins
Danaparoid → see TABLE 3 p. 1334 (anticoagulant effects)
▶ **Ranibizumab** is predicted to increase the risk of bleeding events when given with **danaparoid**. [Severe] Theoretical
Danazol
▶ **Danazol** moderately increases the concentration of antiepileptics **(carbamazepine)**. Monitor and adjust dose. [Severe] Study
▶ **Danazol** increases the concentration of ciclosporin. [Severe] Study
▶ **Danazol** potentially increases the anticoagulant effect of coumarins. [Severe] Anecdotal
▶ **Danazol** is predicted to increase the risk of rhabdomyolysis when given with statins **(atorvastatin)**. [Severe] Theoretical
▶ **Danazol** increases the risk of rhabdomyolysis when given with statins **(simvastatin)**. Avoid. [Severe] Anecdotal
▶ **Danazol** potentially increases the concentration of tacrolimus. [Severe] Anecdotal
Dantrolene → see TABLE 1 p. 1334 (hepatotoxicity)
▶ Intravenous **dantrolene** potentially increases the risk of acute hyperkalaemia and cardiovascular collapse when given with calcium channel blockers **(diltiazem, verapamil)**. Avoid. [Severe] Anecdotal
Dapagliflozin → see TABLE 14 p. 1337 (antidiabetic drugs), TABLE 8 p. 1335 (hypotension)
Dapoxetine → see SSRIs
Dapsone
▶ **Aminosalicylic acid** is predicted to increase the risk of methaemoglobinaemia when given with **dapsone**. [Severe] Theoretical
▶ **Dapsone** is predicted to increase the risk of methaemoglobinaemia when given with topical anaesthetics, local **(prilocaine)**. Use with caution or avoid. [Severe] Theoretical
▶ Antiepileptics **(fosphenytoin, phenobarbital, phenytoin, primidone)** are predicted to increase the risk of methaemoglobinaemia when given with **dapsone**. [Severe] Theoretical
▶ Antimalarials **(chloroquine, primaquine)** are predicted to increase the risk of methaemoglobinaemia when given with **dapsone**. [Severe] Theoretical
▶ **Nitrates** are predicted to increase the risk of methaemoglobinaemia when given with **dapsone**. [Severe] Theoretical
▶ **Nitrofurantoin** is predicted to increase the risk of methaemoglobinaemia when given with **dapsone**. [Severe] Theoretical
▶ **Paracetamol** is predicted to increase the risk of methaemoglobinaemia when given with **dapsone**. [Severe] Theoretical
▶ **Rifabutin** decreases the exposure to **dapsone**. [Moderate] Study
▶ **Rifampicin** decreases the exposure to **dapsone**. [Moderate] Study
▶ **Sodium nitroprusside** is predicted to increase the risk of methaemoglobinaemia when given with **dapsone**. [Severe] Theoretical
▶ **Sulfonamides** are predicted to increase the risk of methaemoglobinaemia when given with **dapsone**. [Severe] Theoretical
▶ **Dapsone** increases the exposure to trimethoprim and trimethoprim increases the exposure to **dapsone**. [Severe] Study
Daptomycin
▶ **Aspirin** (high-dose) increases the risk of renal impairment when given with **daptomycin**. [Moderate] Theoretical
▶ **Ciclosporin** is predicted to increase the risk of rhabdomyolysis when given with **daptomycin**. [Severe] Theoretical

▸ Fibrates are predicted to increase the risk of rhabdomyolysis when given with **daptomycin**. [Severe] Theoretical

▸ NSAIDs increase the risk of renal impairment when given with **daptomycin**. [Moderate] Theoretical

▸ Statins are predicted to increase the risk of rhabdomyolysis when given with **daptomycin**. [Severe] Theoretical

Daratumumab → see monoclonal antibodies

Darbepoetin alfa → see TABLE 5 p. 1334 (thromboembolism), TABLE 16 p. 1338 (increased serum potassium)

Darifenacin → see TABLE 10 p. 1336 (antimuscarinics)

▸ Antiarrhythmics (dronedarone) are predicted to slightly increase the exposure to **darifenacin**. [Moderate] Study

▸ **Darifenacin** is predicted to increase the concentration of antiarrhythmics (flecainide). [Moderate] Theoretical

▸ Antiepileptics (carbamazepine, fosphenytoin, phenobarbital, phenytoin, primidone) are predicted to decrease the exposure to **darifenacin**. [Moderate] Theoretical

▸ Antifungals, azoles (fluconazole, isavuconazole, posaconazole) are predicted to slightly increase the exposure to **darifenacin**. [Moderate] Study

▸ Antifungals, azoles (itraconazole, ketoconazole, voriconazole) are predicted to markedly to very markedly increase the exposure to **darifenacin**. Avoid. [Severe] Study

▸ Aprepitant is predicted to slightly increase the exposure to **darifenacin**. [Moderate] Study

▸ Bupropion is predicted to slightly increase the exposure to **darifenacin**. [Mild] Study

▸ Calcium channel blockers (diltiazem, verapamil) are predicted to slightly increase the exposure to **darifenacin**. [Moderate] Study

▸ Ciclosporin is predicted to increase the exposure to **darifenacin**. Avoid. [Moderate] Theoretical

▸ Cinacalcet is predicted to slightly increase the exposure to **darifenacin**. [Mild] Study

▸ Cobicistat is predicted to markedly to very markedly increase the exposure to **darifenacin**. Avoid. [Severe] Study

▸ Crizotinib is predicted to slightly increase the exposure to **darifenacin**. [Moderate] Study

▸ Enzalutamide is predicted to decrease the exposure to **darifenacin**. [Moderate] Theoretical

▸ Grapefruit juice is predicted to increase the exposure to **darifenacin**. [Moderate] Study

▸ HIV-protease inhibitors are predicted to markedly to very markedly increase the exposure to **darifenacin**. Avoid. [Severe] Study

▸ Idelalisib is predicted to markedly to very markedly increase the exposure to **darifenacin**. Avoid. [Severe] Study

▸ Imatinib is predicted to slightly increase the exposure to **darifenacin**. [Moderate] Study

▸ Macrolides (clarithromycin) are predicted to markedly to very markedly increase the exposure to **darifenacin**. Avoid. [Severe] Study

▸ Macrolides (erythromycin) are predicted to slightly increase the exposure to **darifenacin**. [Moderate] Study

▸ Mitotane is predicted to decrease the exposure to **darifenacin**. [Moderate] Theoretical

▸ Netupitant is predicted to slightly increase the exposure to **darifenacin**. [Moderate] Study

▸ Nilotinib is predicted to slightly increase the exposure to **darifenacin**. [Moderate] Study

▸ Rifampicin is predicted to decrease the exposure to **darifenacin**. [Moderate] Theoretical

▸ SSRIs (fluoxetine, paroxetine) are predicted to slightly increase the exposure to **darifenacin**. [Mild] Study

▸ St John's Wort is predicted to decrease the exposure to **darifenacin**. [Moderate] Theoretical

▸ Terbinafine is predicted to slightly increase the exposure to **darifenacin**. [Mild] Study

▸ **Darifenacin** is predicted to increase the exposure to tricyclic antidepressants. [Moderate] Theoretical → Also see TABLE 10 p. 1336

Darunavir → see HIV-protease inhibitors

Dasabuvir

▸ Antiepileptics (carbamazepine, fosphenytoin, phenobarbital, phenytoin, primidone) are predicted to decrease the exposure to **dasabuvir**. Avoid. [Severe] Theoretical

▸ Combined hormonal contraceptives increase the risk of raised liver function tests when given with **dasabuvir**. Avoid. [Severe] Study

▸ Enzalutamide is predicted to decrease the exposure to **dasabuvir**. Avoid. [Severe] Theoretical

▸ Fibrates (gemfibrozil) very markedly increase the exposure to **dasabuvir**. Avoid. [Severe] Study

▸ **Dasabuvir** (with ombitasvir, paritaprevir and ritonavir) increases the concentration of loop diuretics (furosemide). Adjust dose. [Moderate] Study

▸ Rifampicin is predicted to decrease the exposure to **dasabuvir**. Avoid. [Severe] Study

▸ St John's Wort is predicted to decrease the exposure to **dasabuvir**. Avoid. [Severe] Theoretical

▸ **Dasabuvir** is predicted to increase the exposure to statins (rosuvastatin). Adjust rosuvastatin dose, p. 202. [Moderate] Study

Dasatinib → see TABLE 15 p. 1337 (myelosuppression), TABLE 9 p. 1336 (QT-interval prolongation), TABLE 4 p. 1334 (antiplatelet effects)

▸ Antacids decrease the absorption of **dasatinib**. Separate administration by at least 2 hours. [Moderate] Study

▸ Antiarrhythmics (dronedarone) are predicted to increase the exposure to **dasatinib**. [Severe] Study → Also see TABLE 9 p. 1336

▸ Antiepileptics (carbamazepine, fosphenytoin, phenobarbital, phenytoin, primidone) are predicted to markedly decrease the exposure to **dasatinib**. Avoid. [Severe] Study

▸ Antifungals, azoles (fluconazole, isavuconazole, posaconazole) are predicted to increase the exposure to **dasatinib**. [Severe] Study → Also see TABLE 9 p. 1336

▸ Antifungals, azoles (itraconazole, ketoconazole, voriconazole) are predicted to markedly increase the exposure to **dasatinib**. Avoid. [Severe] Study → Also see TABLE 9 p. 1336

▸ Aprepitant is predicted to increase the exposure to **dasatinib**. [Severe] Study

▸ Bosentan is predicted to decrease the exposure to **dasatinib**. [Severe] Study

▸ Calcium channel blockers (diltiazem, verapamil) are predicted to increase the exposure to **dasatinib**. [Severe] Study

▸ Cobicistat is predicted to markedly increase the exposure to **dasatinib**. Avoid. [Severe] Study

▸ **Dasatinib** is predicted to increase the risk of bleeding events when given with coumarins. [Severe] Theoretical

▸ Crizotinib is predicted to increase the exposure to **dasatinib**. [Severe] Study → Also see TABLE 15 p. 1337 → Also see TABLE 9 p. 1336

▸ Efavirenz is predicted to decrease the exposure to **dasatinib**. [Severe] Study → Also see TABLE 9 p. 1336

▸ Enzalutamide is predicted to markedly decrease the exposure to **dasatinib**. Avoid. [Severe] Study

▸ Grapefruit juice is predicted to increase the exposure to **dasatinib**. Avoid. [Moderate] Theoretical

▸ H₂ receptor antagonists are predicted to decrease the exposure to **dasatinib**. Avoid. [Moderate] Study

▸ HIV-protease inhibitors are predicted to markedly increase the exposure to **dasatinib**. Avoid. [Severe] Study → Also see TABLE 9 p. 1336

▸ Idelalisib is predicted to markedly increase the exposure to **dasatinib**. Avoid. [Severe] Study → Also see TABLE 15 p. 1337

▸ Imatinib is predicted to increase the exposure to **dasatinib**. [Severe] Study → Also see TABLE 15 p. 1337

▸ Macrolides (clarithromycin) are predicted to markedly increase the exposure to **dasatinib**. Avoid. [Severe] Study → Also see TABLE 9 p. 1336

▸ Macrolides (erythromycin) are predicted to increase the exposure to **dasatinib**. [Severe] Study → Also see TABLE 9 p. 1336

▸ Mitotane is predicted to markedly decrease the exposure to **dasatinib**. Avoid. [Severe] Study → Also see TABLE 15 p. 1337

▸ Netupitant is predicted to increase the exposure to **dasatinib**. [Severe] Study

▸ Nevirapine is predicted to decrease the exposure to **dasatinib**. [Severe] Study

▸ Nilotinib is predicted to increase the exposure to **dasatinib**. [Severe] Study → Also see TABLE 15 p. 1337 → Also see TABLE 9 p. 1336

▸ **Dasatinib** is predicted to increase the risk of bleeding events when given with phenindione. [Severe] Theoretical

▸ Pitolisant is predicted to decrease the exposure to **dasatinib**. Avoid. [Severe] Theoretical

A1

Interactions | Appendix 1

Dasatinib (continued)

▶ Proton pump inhibitors are predicted to slightly to moderately decrease the exposure to **dasatinib**. Avoid. Severe Study

▶ Rifampicin is predicted to markedly decrease the exposure to **dasatinib**. Avoid. Severe Study

▶ St John's Wort is predicted to decrease the exposure to **dasatinib**. Severe Study

▶ **Dasatinib** is predicted to increase the exposure to statins (simvastatin). Moderate Theoretical

Daunorubicin → see anthracyclines

Decitabine → see TABLE 15 p. 1337 (myelosuppression)

Deferasirox → see iron chelators

Deferiprone → see TABLE 15 p. 1337 (myelosuppression)

▶ Antacids (aluminium hydroxide) are predicted to decrease the absorption of **deferiprone**. Avoid. Moderate Theoretical

▶ Ascorbic acid is predicted to increase the risk of cardiovascular side-effects when given with **deferiprone**. Severe Theoretical

Deflazacort → see corticosteroids

Delamanid → see TABLE 9 p. 1336 (QT-interval prolongation)

▶ Antiepileptics (carbamazepine, fosphenytoin, phenobarbital, phenytoin, primidone) are predicted to slightly decrease the exposure to **delamanid**. Avoid. Moderate Study

▶ Antifungals, azoles (itraconazole, ketoconazole, voriconazole) very slightly increase the exposure to **delamanid**. Severe Study → Also see TABLE 9 p. 1336

▶ Cobicistat very slightly increases the exposure to **delamanid**. Severe Study

▶ Enzalutamide is predicted to slightly decrease the exposure to **delamanid**. Avoid. Moderate Study

▶ HIV-protease inhibitors very slightly increase the exposure to **delamanid**. Severe Study → Also see TABLE 9 p. 1336

▶ Idelalisib very slightly increases the exposure to **delamanid**. Severe Study

▶ Macrolides (clarithromycin) very slightly increase the exposure to **delamanid**. Severe Study → Also see TABLE 9 p. 1336

▶ Mitotane is predicted to slightly decrease the exposure to **delamanid**. Moderate Study

▶ Rifampicin is predicted to slightly decrease the exposure to **delamanid**. Avoid. Moderate Study

Demeclocycline → see tetracyclines

Desferrioxamine → see iron chelators

Desflurane → see volatile halogenated anaesthetics

Desloratadine → see antihistamines, non-sedating

Desmopressin → see TABLE 18 p. 1338 (hyponatraemia)

▶ Antiepileptics (lamotrigine) are predicted to increase the risk of hyponatraemia when given with **desmopressin**. Severe Theoretical

▶ Loperamide greatly increases the absorption of oral **desmopressin** (and possibly sublingual). Moderate Study

▶ Phenothiazines (chlorpromazine) are predicted to increase the risk of hyponatraemia when given with **desmopressin**. Severe Theoretical

Desogestrel

▶ Antiepileptics (carbamazepine, eslicarbazepine, fosphenytoin, oxcarbazepine, perampanel, phenobarbital, phenytoin, primidone, rufinamide, topiramate) are predicted to decrease the efficacy of **desogestrel**. For FSRH guidance, see Contraceptives, interactions p. 775. Severe Theoretical

▶ **Desogestrel** is predicted to increase the exposure to antiepileptics (lamotrigine). Moderate Study

▶ Aprepitant is predicted to decrease the efficacy of **desogestrel**. For FSRH guidance, see Contraceptives, interactions p. 775. Severe Theoretical

▶ Bosentan is predicted to decrease the efficacy of **desogestrel**. For FSRH guidance, see Contraceptives, interactions p. 775. Severe Theoretical

▶ Efavirenz is predicted to decrease the efficacy of **desogestrel**. For FSRH guidance, see Contraceptives, interactions p. 775. Severe Theoretical

▶ Fosaprepitant is predicted to decrease the efficacy of **desogestrel**. For FSRH guidance, see Contraceptives, interactions p. 775. Severe Theoretical

▶ Griseofulvin potentially decreases the efficacy of **desogestrel**. For FSRH guidance, see Contraceptives, interactions p. 775. Severe Anecdotal

▶ HIV-protease inhibitors (ritonavir) are predicted to decrease the efficacy of **desogestrel**. For FSRH guidance, see Contraceptives, interactions p. 775. Severe Theoretical

▶ Modafinil is predicted to decrease the efficacy of **desogestrel**. For FSRH guidance, see Contraceptives, interactions p. 775. Severe Theoretical

▶ Nevirapine is predicted to decrease the efficacy of **desogestrel**. For FSRH guidance, see Contraceptives, interactions p. 775. Severe Theoretical

▶ Rifabutin is predicted to decrease the efficacy of **desogestrel**. For FSRH guidance, see Contraceptives, interactions p. 775. Severe Theoretical

▶ Rifampicin is predicted to decrease the efficacy of **desogestrel**. For FSRH guidance, see Contraceptives, interactions p. 775. Severe Theoretical

▶ St John's Wort is predicted to decrease the efficacy of **desogestrel**. MHRA advises avoid. For FSRH guidance, see Contraceptives, interactions p. 775. Severe Theoretical

▶ Sugammadex is predicted to decrease the exposure to **desogestrel**. Refer to patient information leaflet for missed pill advice. Severe Theoretical

▶ Ulipristal is predicted to decrease the efficacy of **desogestrel**. Avoid. Severe Theoretical

Dexamethasone → see corticosteroids

Dexamfetamine → see amfetamines

Dexibuprofen → see NSAIDs

Dexketoprofen → see NSAIDs

Dexmedetomidine → see TABLE 11 p. 1336 (CNS depressant effects)

Dexrazoxane → see iron chelators

Diamorphine → see opioids

Diazepam → see TABLE 11 p. 1336 (CNS depressant effects)

▶ **Diazepam** potentially affects the concentration of antiepileptics (fosphenytoin, phenytoin). Monitor concentration and adjust dose. Severe Study

▶ Antifungals, azoles (fluconazole, voriconazole) moderately increase the exposure to **diazepam**. Monitor and adjust dose. Moderate Study

▶ HIV-protease inhibitors (ritonavir) are predicted to increase the exposure to **diazepam**. Avoid. Moderate Theoretical

▶ Monoclonal antibodies (tocilizumab) are predicted to decrease the exposure to **diazepam**. Monitor and adjust dose. Moderate Theoretical

▶ Rifampicin moderately decreases the exposure to **diazepam**. Avoid. Moderate Study

▶ SSRIs (fluvoxamine) moderately increase the exposure to **diazepam**. Moderate Study

Diazoxide → see TABLE 8 p. 1335 (hypotension)

▶ **Diazoxide** decreases the concentration of antiepileptics (fosphenytoin, phenytoin) and antiepileptics (fosphenytoin, phenytoin) are predicted to decrease the effects of **diazoxide**. Monitor concentration and adjust dose. Moderate Anecdotal

▶ **Diazoxide** increases the risk of severe hypotension when given with hydralazine. Severe Study → Also see TABLE 8 p. 1335

Diclofenac → see NSAIDs

Dicycloverine → see TABLE 10 p. 1336 (antimuscarinics)

Didanosine → see TABLE 1 p. 1334 (hepatotoxicity), TABLE 12 p. 1337 (peripheral neuropathy)

ROUTE-SPECIFIC INFORMATION Antacids in tablet formulation might affect absorption of other drugs—give at least 2 hours apart.

▶ Allopurinol moderately increases the exposure to **didanosine**. Avoid. Severe Study

▶ **Didanosine** (buffered) decreases the exposure to antifungals, azoles (itraconazole, ketoconazole). Separate administration by 2 hours. Severe Study → Also see TABLE 1 p. 1334

▶ Febuxostat is predicted to increase the exposure to **didanosine**. Severe Theoretical

▶ Ganciclovir is predicted to increase the exposure to **didanosine**. Moderate Study

▶ HIV-protease inhibitors (tipranavir) decrease the exposure to **didanosine**. Separate administration by 2 hours. Moderate Study

▶ **Didanosine** (buffered) decreases the exposure to HIV-protease inhibitors (atazanavir). **Didanosine** should be taken 2 hours after **atazanavir**. Severe Study

▶ **Didanosine** (buffered) is predicted to decrease the exposure to HIV-protease inhibitors (darunavir boosted with ritonavir). **Didanosine** should be taken 1 hour before or 2 hours after darunavir. Moderate Theoretical

▶ Hydroxycarbamide increases the risk of toxicity when given with **didanosine**. Avoid. Severe Study

▶ Isoniazid is predicted to increase the risk of peripheral neuropathy when given with **didanosine**. Theoretical → Also see TABLE 1 p. 1334 → Also see TABLE 12 p. 1337

▶ **Didanosine** is predicted to increase the risk of pancreatitis when given with pentamidine. Avoid. Severe Study

▶ **Didanosine** (buffered) is predicted to greatly decrease the exposure to oral quinolones. **Didanosine** should be taken 2 hours after quinolones. Moderate Study

▶ Ribavirin is predicted to increase the exposure to **didanosine**. Avoid. Severe Study

▶ **Didanosine** increases the risk of toxicity when given with stavudine. Avoid. Severe Study → Also see TABLE 12 p. 1337

▶ Tenofovir disoproxil increases the risk of toxicity when given with **didanosine**. Avoid. Severe Study

▶ Valganciclovir is predicted to increase the exposure to **didanosine**. Moderate Study

Digoxin → see TABLE 6 p. 1335 (bradycardia)

GENERAL INFORMATION Drugs that reduce serum potassium are predicted to increase the risk of digoxin toxicity, see TABLE 17 p. 1335.

▶ Acarbose decreases the concentration of **digoxin**. Moderate Study

▶ Aldosterone antagonists (eplerenone) very slightly increase the exposure to **digoxin**. Mild Study

▶ Aldosterone antagonists (spironolactone) increase the concentration of **digoxin**. Monitor and adjust dose. Moderate Study

▶ Aminoglycosides potentially increase the concentration of **digoxin**. Monitor and adjust dose. Mild Study

▶ Antacids decrease the absorption of **digoxin**. Separate administration by 2 hours. Mild Study

▶ Antiarrhythmics (amiodarone, dronedarone) are predicted to moderately increase the exposure to **digoxin**. Monitor and adjust **digoxin** dose, p. 109. Severe Study → Also see TABLE 6 p. 1335

▶ Antiarrhythmics (propafenone) increase the concentration of **digoxin**. Monitor and adjust dose. Severe Study

▶ Antiepileptics (fosphenytoin, phenytoin) are predicted to decrease the concentration of **digoxin**. Moderate Anecdotal

▶ Antifungals, azoles (isavuconazole) slightly increase the exposure to **digoxin**. Monitor and adjust dose. Moderate Study

▶ Antifungals, azoles (itraconazole) are predicted to markedly increase the concentration of **digoxin**. Monitor and adjust dose. Severe Study

▶ Antifungals, azoles (ketoconazole) are predicted to markedly increase the concentration of **digoxin**. Severe Study

▶ Antifungals, azoles (posaconazole) are predicted to increase the concentration of **digoxin**. Severe Study

▶ Antimalarials (mefloquine) are predicted to increase the risk of bradycardia when given with **digoxin**. Severe Theoretical

▶ Antimalarials (quinine) increase the concentration of **digoxin**. Monitor and adjust **digoxin** dose, p. 109. Severe Anecdotal

▶ Balsalazide is predicted to decrease the concentration of **digoxin**. Moderate Study

▶ Calcium channel blockers (diltiazem, verapamil) increase the concentration of **digoxin**. Monitor and adjust dose. Severe Study → Also see TABLE 6 p. 1335

▶ Intravenous calcium salts increase the concentration of **digoxin**. Avoid. Moderate Anecdotal

▶ Carbimazole affects the concentration of **digoxin**. Monitor and adjust dose. Moderate Theoretical

▶ Ceritinib is predicted to increase the risk of bradycardia when given with **digoxin**. Avoid. Severe Theoretical

▶ Ciclosporin increases the concentration of **digoxin**. Monitor and adjust dose. Severe Theoretical

▶ Daclatasvir slightly increases the concentration of **digoxin**. Severe Study

▶ Eliglustat increases the exposure to **digoxin**. Adjust dose. Moderate Study

▶ Glecaprevir (with pibrentasvir) increases the exposure to **digoxin**. Moderate Study

▶ HIV-protease inhibitors (ritonavir) increase the concentration of **digoxin**. Adjust dose and monitor concentration. Severe Study

▶ Ivacaftor slightly increases the exposure to **digoxin**. Moderate Study

▶ Lapatinib is predicted to increase the exposure to **digoxin**. Moderate Theoretical

▶ Macrolides increase the concentration of **digoxin**. Severe Anecdotal

▶ Mirabegron slightly increases the exposure to **digoxin**. Monitor concentration and adjust dose. Severe Study

▶ Neomycin decreases the absorption of **digoxin**. Moderate Study

▶ Neuromuscular blocking drugs, non-depolarising (pancuronium) are predicted to increase the risk of cardiovascular side-effects when given with **digoxin**. Severe Anecdotal

▶ NSAIDs (indometacin) increase the concentration of **digoxin**. Severe Study

▶ Penicillamine potentially decreases the concentration of **digoxin**. Separate administration by 2 hours. Severe Anecdotal

▶ Pibrentasvir (with glecaprevir) increases the exposure to **digoxin**. Moderate Study

▶ Pitolisant is predicted to decrease the exposure to **digoxin**. Unknown Theoretical

▶ Ranolazine increases the concentration of **digoxin**. Moderate Study

▶ Rifampicin decreases the concentration of **digoxin**. Moderate Study

▶ Rolapitant slightly increases the exposure to **digoxin**. Moderate Study

▶ St John's Wort decreases the concentration of **digoxin**. Avoid. Severe Anecdotal

▶ Sucralfate decreases the absorption of **digoxin**. Separate administration by 2 hours. Severe Anecdotal

▶ Sulfasalazine decreases the concentration of **digoxin**. Moderate Study

▶ Suxamethonium is predicted to increase the risk of cardiovascular side-effects when given with **digoxin**. Severe Anecdotal

▶ Thyroid hormones are predicted to affect the concentration of **digoxin**. Monitor and adjust dose. Moderate Theoretical

▶ Ticagrelor increases the concentration of **digoxin**. Moderate Study

▶ Tolvaptan increases the concentration of **digoxin**. Mild Study

▶ Trimethoprim increases the concentration of **digoxin**. Moderate Study

▶ Vandetanib slightly increases the exposure to **digoxin**. Monitor ECG and adjust dose. Moderate Study

▶ Velpatasvir is predicted to increase the exposure to **digoxin**. Severe Study

▶ Vitamin D substances are predicted to increase the risk of toxicity when given with **digoxin**. Severe Theoretical

Dihydrocodeine → see opioids

Dihydrotachysterol → see vitamin D substances

Diltiazem → see calcium channel blockers

Dimenhydrinate → see TABLE 10 p. 1336 (antimuscarinics)

Dimethyl fumarate

▶ Alcohol (beverage)(excessive consumption) potentially increases the risk of gastrointestinal side-effects when given with **dimethyl fumarate**. Avoid. Moderate Theoretical

▶ Live vaccines are predicted to increase the risk of generalised infection (possibly life-threatening) when given with **dimethyl fumarate**. Public Health England advises avoid (refer to Green Book). Severe Theoretical

Diphenoxylate → see opioids

Dipipanone → see opioids

Dipyridamole → see TABLE 8 p. 1335 (hypotension), TABLE 4 p. 1334 (antiplatelet effects)

▶ Antacids are predicted to decrease the absorption of **dipyridamole** (immediate release tablets). Moderate Theoretical

▶ **Dipyridamole** increases the exposure to antiarrhythmics (adenosine). Avoid or adjust dose. Severe Study

▶ H₂ receptor antagonists are predicted to decrease the absorption of **dipyridamole** (immediate release tablets). Moderate Theoretical

A1

Interactions | Appendix 1

Dipyridamole (continued)

▶ Proton pump inhibitors are predicted to decrease the absorption of **dipyridamole** (immediate release tablets). Moderate Theoretical

Disopyramide → see antiarrhythmics

Disulfiram → see TABLE 12 p. 1337 (peripheral neuropathy)

▶ Alcohol (beverage) causes an extremely unpleasant systemic reaction when given with **disulfiram**. Avoid for at least 24 hours before and up to 14 days after stopping treatment. Severe Study

▶ **Disulfiram** increases the concentration of antiepileptics (fosphenytoin, phenytoin). Monitor concentration and adjust dose. Severe Study → Also see TABLE 12 p. 1337

▶ **Disulfiram** increases the anticoagulant effect of coumarins. Monitor and adjust dose. Severe Study

▶ **Disulfiram** increases the risk of acute psychoses when given with metronidazole. Severe Study → Also see TABLE 12 p. 1337

▶ **Disulfiram** is predicted to increase the anticoagulant effect of phenindione. Severe Theoretical

Dobutamine → see sympathomimetics, inotropic

Docetaxel → see taxanes

Dolutegravir

▶ Antacids moderately decrease the exposure to **dolutegravir**. **Dolutegravir** should be taken 2 hours before or 6 hours after antacids. Moderate Study

▶ Antiepileptics (carbamazepine, fosphenytoin, phenobarbital, phenytoin, primidone) decrease the exposure to **dolutegravir**. Adjust dose. Severe Study

▶ Antiepileptics (oxcarbazepine) are predicted to decrease the exposure to **dolutegravir**. Adjust dose. Severe Theoretical

▶ Bosentan decreases the exposure to **dolutegravir**. Adjust dose. Severe Study

▶ Oral calcium salts decrease the absorption of **dolutegravir**. **Dolutegravir** should be taken 2 hours before or 6 hours after calcium salts. Moderate Study

▶ Efavirenz decreases the exposure to **dolutegravir**. Adjust dose. Severe Study

▶ Enzalutamide decreases the exposure to **dolutegravir**. Adjust dose. Severe Study

▶ Etravirine moderately decreases the exposure to **dolutegravir**. Avoid unless given with atazanavir, darunavir, or lopinavir (all boosted with ritonavir). Severe Study

▶ HIV-protease inhibitors (fosamprenavir boosted with ritonavir) slightly decrease the exposure to **dolutegravir**. Avoid if resistant to HIV-integrase inhibitors. Severe Study

▶ HIV-protease inhibitors (tipranavir) moderately decrease the exposure to **dolutegravir**. Refer to specialist literature. Severe Study

▶ Iron (oral) decreases the absorption of **dolutegravir**. **Dolutegravir** should be taken 2 hours before or 6 hours after iron (oral). Moderate Study

▶ **Dolutegravir** slightly to moderately increases the exposure to metformin. Use with caution and adjust dose. Severe Study

▶ Mitotane decreases the exposure to **dolutegravir**. Adjust dose. Severe Study

▶ Nevirapine decreases the exposure to **dolutegravir**. Adjust dose. Severe Study

▶ Rifampicin decreases the exposure to **dolutegravir**. Adjust dose. Severe Study

▶ St John's Wort decreases the exposure to **dolutegravir**. Adjust dose. Severe Study

▶ Sucralfate decreases the absorption of **dolutegravir**. Moderate Study

Domperidone → see TABLE 9 p. 1336 (QT-interval prolongation)

▶ Antiarrhythmics (dronedarone) increase the risk of QT-prolongation when given with **domperidone**. Avoid. Severe Study

▶ Antifungals, azoles (fluconazole, isavuconazole, itraconazole, ketoconazole, posaconazole, voriconazole) increase the risk of QT-prolongation when given with **domperidone**. Avoid. Severe Study

▶ Aprepitant increases the risk of QT-prolongation when given with **domperidone**. Avoid. Severe Study

▶ Calcium channel blockers (diltiazem, verapamil) increase the risk of QT-prolongation when given with **domperidone**. Avoid. Severe Study

▶ Cobicistat increases the risk of QT-prolongation when given with **domperidone**. Avoid. Severe Study

▶ Crizotinib increases the risk of QT-prolongation when given with **domperidone**. Avoid. Severe Study

▶ **Domperidone** is predicted to decrease the prolactin-lowering effect of dopamine receptor agonists (bromocriptine, cabergoline). Moderate Theoretical

▶ HIV-protease inhibitors increase the risk of QT-prolongation when given with **domperidone**. Avoid. Severe Study

▶ Idelalisib increases the risk of QT-prolongation when given with **domperidone**. Avoid. Severe Study

▶ Imatinib increases the risk of QT-prolongation when given with **domperidone**. Avoid. Severe Study

▶ Macrolides (clarithromycin, erythromycin) increase the risk of QT-prolongation when given with **domperidone**. Avoid. Severe Study

▶ Netupitant increases the risk of QT-prolongation when given with **domperidone**. Avoid. Severe Study

▶ Nilotinib increases the risk of QT-prolongation when given with **domperidone**. Avoid. Severe Study

Donepezil → see anticholinesterases, centrally acting

Dopamine → see sympathomimetics, inotropic

Dopamine receptor agonists → see TABLE 8 p. 1335 (hypotension), TABLE 9 p. 1336 (QT-interval prolongation), TABLE 10 p. 1336 (antimuscarinics)

amantadine · apomorphine · bromocriptine · cabergoline · pergolide · pramipexole · quinagolide · ropinirole · rotigotine

FOOD AND LIFESTYLE Dose adjustment might be necessary if smoking started or stopped during treatment with **ropinirole**.

▶ Amisulpride is predicted to decrease the effects of **dopamine receptor agonists**. Avoid. Moderate Theoretical → Also see TABLE 8 p. 1336

▶ Antiarrhythmics (dronedarone) are predicted to increase the exposure to **bromocriptine**. Severe Theoretical

▶ Antiarrhythmics (dronedarone) are predicted to increase the concentration of **cabergoline**. Severe Anecdotal

▶ Antifungals, azoles (fluconazole, isavuconazole, itraconazole, ketoconazole, posaconazole, voriconazole) are predicted to increase the concentration of **cabergoline**. Moderate Anecdotal

▶ Antifungals, azoles (fluconazole, isavuconazole, posaconazole) are predicted to increase the exposure to **bromocriptine**. Severe Theoretical

▶ Antifungals, azoles (itraconazole, ketoconazole, voriconazole) increase the exposure to **bromocriptine**. Severe Study

▶ Aprepitant is predicted to increase the exposure to **bromocriptine**. Severe Theoretical

▶ Aprepitant is predicted to increase the concentration of **cabergoline**. Moderate Anecdotal

▶ Aripiprazole is predicted to decrease the effects of **dopamine receptor agonists**. Moderate Theoretical → Also see TABLE 8 p. 1335

▶ Asenapine is predicted to decrease the effects of **dopamine receptor agonists**. Adjust dose. Moderate Theoretical → Also see TABLE 8 p. 1335

▶ Benperidol is predicted to decrease the effects of **dopamine receptor agonists**. Avoid. Moderate Theoretical → Also see TABLE 8 p. 1335

▶ Bupropion increases the risk of side-effects when given with amantadine. Moderate Study

▶ Calcium channel blockers (diltiazem, verapamil) are predicted to increase the exposure to **bromocriptine**. Severe Theoretical → Also see TABLE 8 p. 1335

▶ Calcium channel blockers (diltiazem, verapamil) are predicted to increase the concentration of **cabergoline**. Moderate Anecdotal → Also see TABLE 8 p. 1335

▶ Clozapine is predicted to decrease the effects of **dopamine receptor agonists**. Moderate Theoretical → Also see TABLE 8 p. 1335 → Also see TABLE 10 p. 1336

▶ Cobicistat increases the exposure to **bromocriptine**. Severe Study

▶ Cobicistat is predicted to increase the concentration of **cabergoline**. Moderate Anecdotal

- Combined hormonal contraceptives are predicted to increase the exposure to **ropinirole**. Adjust dose. Moderate Study
- Crizotinib is predicted to increase the exposure to **bromocriptine**. Severe Theoretical
- Crizotinib is predicted to increase the concentration of **cabergoline**. Moderate Anecdotal
- Domperidone is predicted to decrease the prolactin-lowering effect of dopamine receptor agonists **(bromocriptine, cabergoline)**. Moderate Theoretical
- Dopamine receptor agonists **(cabergoline)** are predicted to increase the risk of ergotism when given with dopamine receptor agonists **(bromocriptine)**. Avoid. Moderate Theoretical → Also see TABLE 8 p. 1335
- Dopamine receptor agonists **(bromocriptine, cabergoline)** are predicted to increase the risk of ergotism when given with dopamine receptor agonists **(pergolide)**. Avoid. Moderate Theoretical → Also see TABLE 8 p. 1335
- Dopamine receptor agonists **(amantadine)** are predicted to increase the exposure to dopamine receptor agonists **(pramipexole)**. Adjust dose. Moderate Theoretical → Also see TABLE 8 p. 1335
- Droperidol is predicted to decrease the effects of **dopamine receptor agonists**. Avoid. Moderate Theoretical → Also see TABLE 8 p. 1335 → Also see TABLE 9 p. 1336
- Ergometrine is predicted to increase the risk of ergotism when given with dopamine receptor agonists **(cabergoline, pergolide)**. Avoid. Moderate Theoretical
- Ergotamine is predicted to increase the risk of ergotism when given with dopamine receptor agonists **(bromocriptine, cabergoline)**. Avoid. Moderate Theoretical
- Ergotamine is predicted to increase the risk of ergotism when given with **pergolide**. Moderate Theoretical
- Flupentixol is predicted to decrease the effects of **dopamine receptor agonists**. Avoid. Moderate Theoretical → Also see TABLE 8 p. 1335
- Apomorphine is predicted to increase the risk of severe hypotension when given with granisetron. Severe Theoretical
- H₂ receptor antagonists **(cimetidine)** slightly increase the exposure to **pramipexole**. Adjust dose. Moderate Study
- Haloperidol is predicted to decrease the effects of **dopamine receptor agonists**. Avoid. Moderate Theoretical → Also see TABLE 8 p. 1335 → Also see TABLE 9 p. 1336 → Also see TABLE 10 p. 1336
- HIV-protease inhibitors increase the exposure to **bromocriptine**. Severe Study
- HIV-protease inhibitors are predicted to increase the concentration of **cabergoline**. Moderate Anecdotal
- Hormone replacement therapy decreases the clearance of **ropinirole**. Monitor and adjust dose. Moderate Study
- Idelalisib increases the exposure to **bromocriptine**. Severe Study
- Idelalisib is predicted to increase the concentration of **cabergoline**. Moderate Anecdotal
- Imatinib is predicted to increase the exposure to **bromocriptine**. Severe Theoretical
- Imatinib is predicted to increase the concentration of **cabergoline**. Moderate Anecdotal
- Loxapine is predicted to decrease the effects of **dopamine receptor agonists**. Moderate Theoretical → Also see TABLE 8 p. 1335 → Also see TABLE 10 p. 1336
- Macrolides **(clarithromycin)** increase the exposure to **bromocriptine**. Severe Study
- Macrolides **(clarithromycin, erythromycin)** are predicted to increase the concentration of **cabergoline**. Avoid. Severe Study
- Macrolides **(erythromycin)** are predicted to increase the exposure to **bromocriptine**. Severe Theoretical
- Amantadine increases the risk of CNS toxicity when given with memantine. Use with caution or avoid. Severe Theoretical
- Memantine is predicted to increase the effects of dopamine receptor agonists **(apomorphine, bromocriptine, cabergoline, pergolide, pramipexole, quinagolide, ropinirole, rotigotine)**. Moderate Theoretical
- Metoclopramide is predicted to decrease the effects of dopamine receptor agonists **(apomorphine, bromocriptine, cabergoline, pergolide, pramipexole, quinagolide, ropinirole, rotigotine)**. Avoid. Moderate Study

- Netupitant is predicted to increase the exposure to **bromocriptine**. Severe Theoretical
- Netupitant is predicted to increase the concentration of **cabergoline**. Moderate Anecdotal
- Nilotinib is predicted to increase the exposure to **bromocriptine**. Severe Theoretical
- Nilotinib is predicted to increase the concentration of **cabergoline**. Moderate Anecdotal
- Olanzapine is predicted to decrease the effects of **dopamine receptor agonists**. Avoid. Moderate Theoretical → Also see TABLE 8 p. 1335
- Apomorphine increases the risk of severe hypotension when given with ondansetron. Avoid. Severe Study → Also see TABLE 9 p. 1336
- Paliperidone is predicted to decrease the effects of **dopamine receptor agonists**. Avoid. Moderate Theoretical → Also see TABLE 8 p. 1335 → Also see TABLE 9 p. 1336
- Apomorphine is predicted to increase the risk of severe hypotension when given with palonosetron. Severe Theoretical
- Phenothiazines are predicted to decrease the effects of **dopamine receptor agonists**. Avoid. Moderate Theoretical → Also see TABLE 8 p. 1335 → Also see TABLE 9 p. 1336 → Also see TABLE 10 p. 1336
- Pimozide is predicted to decrease the effects of **dopamine receptor agonists**. Avoid. Moderate Theoretical → Also see TABLE 8 p. 1335 → Also see TABLE 9 p. 1336 → Also see TABLE 10 p. 1336
- Quetiapine is predicted to decrease the effects of **dopamine receptor agonists**. Avoid. Moderate Theoretical → Also see TABLE 8 p. 1335
- Quinolones **(ciprofloxacin)** are predicted to increase the exposure to **ropinirole**. Adjust dose. Moderate Study
- Risperidone is predicted to decrease the effects of **dopamine receptor agonists**. Avoid. Moderate Theoretical → Also see TABLE 8 p. 1335 → Also see TABLE 9 p. 1336
- SSRIs **(fluvoxamine)** are predicted to increase the exposure to **ropinirole**. Adjust dose. Moderate Study
- Sulpiride is predicted to decrease the effects of **dopamine receptor agonists**. Avoid. Moderate Theoretical → Also see TABLE 8 p. 1335 → Also see TABLE 9 p. 1336
- Sympathomimetics, vasoconstrictor **(isometheptene)** potentially increase the risk of side-effects when given with **bromocriptine**. Avoid. Severe Anecdotal
- Zuclopenthixol is predicted to decrease the effects of **dopamine receptor agonists**. Avoid. Moderate Theoretical → Also see TABLE 8 p. 1335 → Also see TABLE 9 p. 1336

Dorzolamide

ROUTE-SPECIFIC INFORMATION Since systemic absorption can follow topical application, the possibility of interactions should be borne in mind.

Dosulepin → see tricyclic antidepressants

Doxapram
- Aminophylline increases the risk of agitation when given with **doxapram**. Moderate Study
- Monoamine-oxidase A and B inhibitors, irreversible are predicted to increase the effects of **doxapram**. Moderate Theoretical
- Theophylline increases the risk of agitation when given with **doxapram**. Moderate Study

Doxazosin → see alpha blockers
Doxepin → see tricyclic antidepressants
Doxorubicin → see anthracyclines
Doxycycline → see tetracyclines
Dronedarone → see antiarrhythmics
Droperidol → see TABLE 8 p. 1335 (hypotension), TABLE 9 p. 1336 (QT-interval prolongation), TABLE 11 p. 1336 (CNS depressant effects)
- Droperidol is predicted to decrease the effects of **dopamine receptor agonists**. Avoid. Moderate Theoretical → Also see TABLE 8 p. 1335 → Also see TABLE 9 p. 1336
- Droperidol is predicted to decrease the effects of guanethidine. Monitor and adjust dose. Moderate Theoretical → Also see TABLE 8 p. 1335
- Droperidol decreases the effects of levodopa. Severe Study → Also see TABLE 8 p. 1335

Drospirenone → see TABLE 16 p. 1338 (increased serum potassium)

A1

Interactions | Appendix 1

Drospirenone (continued)

▸ Antifungals, azoles (ketoconazole) moderately increase the exposure to **drospirenone**. [Severe] Study

Dulaglutide → see TABLE 14 p. 1337 (antidiabetic drugs)

Duloxetine → see TABLE 18 p. 1338 (hyponatraemia), TABLE 13 p. 1337 (serotonin effects), TABLE 4 p. 1334 (antiplatelet effects)

▸ Antiepileptics (phenytoin) are predicted to decrease the exposure to **duloxetine**. [Moderate] Theoretical

▸ **Duloxetine** is predicted to increase the exposure to beta blockers, selective (metoprolol). [Moderate] Study

▸ **Duloxetine** is predicted to increase the exposure to eliglustat. Avoid or adjust dose—consult product literature. [Severe] Study

▸ HIV-protease inhibitors (ritonavir) are predicted to decrease the exposure to **duloxetine**. [Moderate] Theoretical

▸ Leflunomide is predicted to decrease the exposure to **duloxetine**. [Moderate] Theoretical

▸ **Duloxetine** is predicted to increase the exposure to pitolisant. Use with caution and adjust dose. [Moderate] Study

▸ Quinolones (ciprofloxacin) are predicted to increase the exposure to **duloxetine**. Avoid. [Moderate] Theoretical

▸ Rifampicin is predicted to increase the exposure to **duloxetine**. [Moderate] Theoretical

▸ SSRIs (fluvoxamine) markedly increase the exposure to **duloxetine**. Avoid. [Severe] Study → Also see TABLE 18 p. 1338 → Also see TABLE 13 p. 1337 → Also see TABLE 4 p. 1334

▸ Teriflunomide is predicted to decrease the exposure to **duloxetine**. [Moderate] Theoretical

Dupilumab → see monoclonal antibodies

Dutasteride

▸ Antiarrhythmics (dronedarone) are predicted to moderately increase the exposure to **dutasteride**. [Mild] Study

▸ Antifungals, azoles (fluconazole, isavuconazole, posaconazole) are predicted to moderately increase the exposure to **dutasteride**. [Mild] Study

▸ Antifungals, azoles (itraconazole, ketoconazole, voriconazole) are predicted to increase the exposure to **dutasteride**. Monitor side effects and adjust dose. [Moderate] Theoretical

▸ Aprepitant is predicted to moderately increase the exposure to **dutasteride**. [Mild] Study

▸ Calcium channel blockers (diltiazem, verapamil) are predicted to moderately increase the exposure to **dutasteride**. [Mild] Study

▸ Cobicistat is predicted to increase the exposure to **dutasteride**. Monitor side effects and adjust dose. [Moderate] Theoretical

▸ Crizotinib is predicted to moderately increase the exposure to **dutasteride**. [Mild] Study

▸ HIV-protease inhibitors are predicted to increase the exposure to **dutasteride**. Monitor side effects and adjust dose. [Moderate] Theoretical

▸ Idelalisib is predicted to increase the exposure to **dutasteride**. Monitor side effects and adjust dose. [Moderate] Theoretical

▸ Imatinib is predicted to moderately increase the exposure to **dutasteride**. [Mild] Study

▸ Macrolides (clarithromycin) are predicted to increase the exposure to **dutasteride**. Monitor side effects and adjust dose. [Moderate] Theoretical

▸ Macrolides (erythromycin) are predicted to moderately increase the exposure to **dutasteride**. [Mild] Study

▸ Netupitant is predicted to moderately increase the exposure to **dutasteride**. [Mild] Study

▸ Nilotinib is predicted to moderately increase the exposure to **dutasteride**. [Mild] Study

Eculizumab → see monoclonal antibodies

Edoxaban → see TABLE 3 p. 1334 (anticoagulant effects)

▸ Antiarrhythmics (amiodarone) slightly increase the exposure to **edoxaban**. [Severe] Study

▸ Antiarrhythmics (dronedarone) slightly increase the exposure to **edoxaban**. Adjust **edoxaban** dose, p. 125. [Severe] Study

▸ Antiepileptics (carbamazepine) are predicted to decrease the exposure to **edoxaban**. [Moderate] Study

▸ Antifungals, azoles (itraconazole) are predicted to slightly increase the exposure to **edoxaban**. [Severe] Theoretical

▸ Antifungals, azoles (ketoconazole) slightly increase the exposure to **edoxaban**. Adjust **edoxaban** dose, p. 125. [Severe] Study

▸ Calcium channel blockers (verapamil) are predicted to slightly increase the exposure to **edoxaban**. [Severe] Theoretical

▸ Ceritinib is predicted to increase the exposure to **edoxaban**. [Moderate] Theoretical

▸ Ciclosporin slightly increases the exposure to **edoxaban**. Adjust **edoxaban** dose, p. 125. [Severe] Study

▸ Eliglustat is predicted to increase the exposure to **edoxaban**. Adjust dose. [Moderate] Study

▸ HIV-protease inhibitors (lopinavir, ritonavir, saquinavir) are predicted to slightly increase the exposure to **edoxaban**. [Severe] Theoretical

▸ Lapatinib is predicted to slightly increase the exposure to **edoxaban**. [Severe] Theoretical

▸ Macrolides (azithromycin, clarithromycin) are predicted to slightly increase the exposure to **edoxaban**. [Severe] Theoretical

▸ Macrolides (erythromycin) slightly increase the exposure to **edoxaban**. Adjust **edoxaban** dose, p. 125. [Severe] Study

▸ Mirabegron is predicted to increase the exposure to **edoxaban**. [Mild] Theoretical

▸ Ranolazine is predicted to slightly increase the exposure to **edoxaban**. [Severe] Theoretical

▸ Rifampicin is predicted to decrease the exposure to **edoxaban**. [Moderate] Study

▸ St John's Wort is predicted to decrease the exposure to **edoxaban**. [Moderate] Study

▸ Velpatasvir is predicted to increase the exposure to **edoxaban**. [Severe] Theoretical

▸ Vemurafenib is predicted to slightly increase the exposure to **edoxaban**. [Severe] Theoretical

▸ Voxilaprevir is predicted to increase the concentration of **edoxaban**. Avoid. [Severe] Theoretical

Efavirenz → see TABLE 9 p. 1336 (QT-interval prolongation)

▸ **Efavirenz** is predicted to decrease the exposure to antiarrhythmics (dronedarone). [Severe] Theoretical → Also see TABLE 9 p. 1336

▸ Antiepileptics (carbamazepine) slightly decrease the exposure to **efavirenz** and **efavirenz** slightly decreases the exposure to antiepileptics (carbamazepine). [Severe] Study

▸ Antiepileptics (fosphenytoin, phenytoin) slightly decrease the exposure to **efavirenz** and **efavirenz** affects the concentration of antiepileptics (fosphenytoin, phenytoin). [Severe] Theoretical

▸ Antiepileptics (phenobarbital) are predicted to decrease the exposure to **efavirenz** and **efavirenz** affects the concentration of antiepileptics (phenobarbital). [Severe] Theoretical

▸ **Efavirenz** is predicted to affect the efficacy of antiepileptics (primidone) and antiepileptics (primidone) are predicted to slightly decrease the exposure to **efavirenz**. [Severe] Theoretical

▸ **Efavirenz** is predicted to decrease the exposure to antifungals, azoles (isavuconazole). Avoid. [Severe] Theoretical

▸ **Efavirenz** slightly decreases the exposure to antifungals, azoles (itraconazole). Avoid and for 14 days after stopping **efavirenz**. [Moderate] Study

▸ **Efavirenz** moderately decreases the exposure to antifungals, azoles (ketoconazole). [Severe] Study

▸ **Efavirenz** slightly decreases the exposure to antifungals, azoles (posaconazole). Avoid. [Moderate] Study

▸ **Efavirenz** moderately decreases the exposure to antifungals, azoles (voriconazole) and antifungals, azoles (voriconazole) slightly increase the exposure to **efavirenz**. Adjust dose. [Severe] Study → Also see TABLE 9 p. 1336

▸ **Efavirenz** decreases the concentration of antimalarials (artemether). [Severe] Study → Also see TABLE 9 p. 1336

▸ **Efavirenz** moderately decreases the exposure to antimalarials (atovaquone). Avoid. [Moderate] Study

▸ **Efavirenz** affects the exposure to antimalarials (proguanil). Avoid. [Moderate] Study

▸ **Efavirenz** is predicted to decrease the exposure to axitinib. [Moderate] Theoretical

▸ **Efavirenz** is predicted to decrease the exposure to bedaquiline. Avoid. [Severe] Study → Also see TABLE 9 p. 1336

▸ **Efavirenz** is predicted to decrease the exposure to bosutinib. Avoid. [Severe] Theoretical → Also see TABLE 9 p. 1336

▸ **Efavirenz** is predicted to decrease the exposure to bupropion. [Moderate] Study

▸ **Efavirenz** is predicted to decrease the exposure to cabozantinib. [Moderate] Theoretical → Also see TABLE 9 p. 1336

▸ **Efavirenz** is predicted to decrease the exposure to calcium channel blockers (amlodipine, felodipine, lacidipine, lercanidipine, nicardipine, nifedipine, nimodipine). Monitor and adjust dose. Moderate Theoretical

▸ **Efavirenz** is predicted to decrease the exposure to calcium channel blockers (diltiazem, verapamil). Moderate Theoretical

▸ **Efavirenz** is predicted to decrease the concentration of caspofungin. Adjust dose. Moderate Study

▸ **Efavirenz** decreases the concentration of ciclosporin. Monitor concentration and adjust dose. Moderate Study

▸ **Efavirenz** is predicted to decrease the exposure to cobicistat. Avoid. Severe Theoretical

▸ **Efavirenz** is predicted to decrease the exposure to cobimetinib. Avoid. Severe Theoretical

▸ **Efavirenz** is predicted to decrease the efficacy of combined hormonal contraceptives. For FSRH guidance, see Contraceptives, interactions p. 775. Severe Study

▸ **Efavirenz** is predicted to affect the concentration of coumarins. Adjust dose. Moderate Theoretical

▸ **Efavirenz** is predicted to decrease the exposure to crizotinib. Avoid. Severe Theoretical → Also see TABLE 9 p. 1336

▸ **Efavirenz** is predicted to decrease the exposure to daclatasvir. Adjust dose. Severe Study

▸ **Efavirenz** is predicted to decrease the exposure to dasatinib. Severe Study → Also see TABLE 9 p. 1336

▸ **Efavirenz** is predicted to decrease the efficacy of desogestrel. For FSRH guidance, see Contraceptives, interactions p. 775. Severe Theoretical

▸ **Efavirenz** decreases the exposure to dolutegravir. Adjust dose. Severe Study

▸ **Efavirenz** is predicted to moderately decrease the exposure to elbasvir. Avoid. Severe Study

▸ **Efavirenz** is predicted to decrease the exposure to eliglustat. Moderate Theoretical

▸ **Efavirenz** is predicted to decrease the concentration of elvitegravir. Avoid. Severe Theoretical

▸ **Efavirenz** is predicted to decrease the effects of ergotamine. Moderate Theoretical

▸ **Efavirenz** is predicted to decrease the exposure to erlotinib. Severe Theoretical

▸ **Efavirenz** is predicted to decrease the efficacy of etonogestrel. For FSRH guidance, see Contraceptives, interactions p. 775. Severe Theoretical

▸ **Efavirenz** is predicted to decrease the exposure to etravirine. Avoid. Severe Study

▸ **Efavirenz** is predicted to decrease the concentration of everolimus. Avoid or adjust dose. Severe Study

▸ **Efavirenz** is predicted to decrease the exposure to gefitinib. Avoid. Severe Theoretical

▸ **Efavirenz** is predicted to decrease the exposure to glecaprevir. Avoid. Severe Study

▸ **Efavirenz** is predicted to markedly decrease the exposure to grazoprevir. Avoid. Severe Study

▸ **Efavirenz** is predicted to decrease the concentration of guanfacine. Adjust dose. Moderate Theoretical

▸ **Efavirenz** decreases the exposure to HIV-protease inhibitors. Refer to specialist literature. Severe Study → Also see TABLE 9 p. 1336

▸ **Efavirenz** is predicted to decrease the effects of hormone replacement therapy. Moderate Anecdotal

▸ **Efavirenz** is predicted to decrease the exposure to idelalisib. Avoid. Moderate Theoretical

▸ **Efavirenz** is predicted to decrease the exposure to imatinib. Moderate Study

▸ **Efavirenz** is predicted to decrease the exposure to ivacaftor. Severe Theoretical

▸ **Efavirenz** is predicted to decrease the exposure to lapatinib. Avoid. Severe Study → Also see TABLE 9 p. 1336

▸ **Efavirenz** is predicted to decrease the efficacy of levonorgestrel. For FSRH guidance, see Contraceptives, interactions p. 775. Severe Theoretical

▸ **Efavirenz** is predicted to decrease the exposure to lurasidone. Monitor and adjust dose. Moderate Theoretical

▸ **Efavirenz** decreases the exposure to macrolides (clarithromycin). Moderate Study → Also see TABLE 9 p. 1336

▸ **Efavirenz** decreases the exposure to maraviroc. Refer to specialist literature. Severe Theoretical

▸ **Efavirenz** is predicted to alter the effects of midazolam. Avoid. Moderate Theoretical

▸ **Efavirenz** is predicted to decrease the exposure to netupitant. Moderate Theoretical

▸ Nevirapine decreases the concentration of **efavirenz**. Avoid. Severe Study

▸ **Efavirenz** is predicted to decrease the exposure to nilotinib. Avoid. Severe Theoretical → Also see TABLE 9 p. 1336

▸ **Efavirenz** is predicted to decrease the efficacy of norethisterone. For FSRH guidance, see Contraceptives, interactions p. 775. Severe Anecdotal

▸ **Efavirenz** is predicted to decrease the exposure to olaparib. Avoid. Moderate Theoretical

▸ **Efavirenz** decreases the exposure to opioids (methadone). Monitor and adjust dose. Severe Study → Also see TABLE 9 p. 1336

▸ **Efavirenz** is predicted to decrease the exposure to osimertinib. Moderate Theoretical → Also see TABLE 9 p. 1336

▸ **Efavirenz** is predicted to decrease the exposure to paritaprevir (with ritonavir and ombitasvir). Avoid. Severe Study

▸ **Efavirenz** is predicted to decrease the exposure to phosphodiesterase type-5 inhibitors. Moderate Theoretical → Also see TABLE 9 p. 1336

▸ **Efavirenz** is predicted to decrease the exposure to pibrentasvir. Avoid. Severe Study

▸ Pitolisant is predicted to decrease the exposure to **efavirenz**. Unknown Theoretical

▸ **Efavirenz** is predicted to decrease the exposure to quetiapine. Moderate Study

▸ **Efavirenz** is predicted to decrease the exposure to ribociclib. Moderate Study → Also see TABLE 9 p. 1336

▸ **Efavirenz** slightly decreases the exposure to rifabutin. Adjust dose. Severe Study

▸ Rifampicin slightly decreases the exposure to **efavirenz**. Adjust dose. Severe Study

▸ **Efavirenz** is predicted to decrease the exposure to rilpivirine. Avoid. Severe Theoretical

▸ **Efavirenz** is predicted to decrease the exposure to rolapitant. Avoid. Severe Study

▸ **Efavirenz** is predicted to decrease the exposure to ruxolitinib. Monitor and adjust dose. Moderate Theoretical

▸ **Efavirenz** is predicted to decrease the exposure to simeprevir. Avoid. Severe Study

▸ **Efavirenz** is predicted to decrease the concentration of sirolimus. Monitor and adjust dose. Moderate Theoretical

▸ St John's Wort is predicted to decrease the concentration of **efavirenz**. Avoid. Severe Theoretical

▸ **Efavirenz** slightly decreases the exposure to statins (atorvastatin). Mild Study

▸ **Efavirenz** moderately decreases the exposure to statins (simvastatin). Moderate Study

▸ **Efavirenz** is predicted to decrease the concentration of tacrolimus. Monitor and adjust dose. Moderate Theoretical

▸ **Efavirenz** is predicted to decrease the exposure to taxanes (cabazitaxel). Avoid. Severe Study

▸ **Efavirenz** is predicted to decrease the concentration of temsirolimus. Avoid. Severe Theoretical

▸ **Efavirenz** is predicted to decrease the exposure to ticagrelor. Moderate Theoretical

▸ **Efavirenz** is predicted to decrease the exposure to tofacitinib. Moderate Study

▸ **Efavirenz** is predicted to decrease the exposure to tolvaptan. Moderate Theoretical

▸ **Efavirenz** decreases the efficacy of ulipristal. For FSRH guidance, see Contraceptives, interactions p. 775. Severe Anecdotal

▸ **Efavirenz** is predicted to decrease the exposure to velpatasvir. Avoid. Moderate Theoretical

▸ **Efavirenz** is predicted to decrease the exposure to venetoclax. Avoid. Severe Study

▸ **Efavirenz** is predicted to decrease the concentration of voxilaprevir. Avoid. Severe Theoretical

A1

Elbasvir

▶ Antiepileptics (carbamazepine, fosphenytoin, phenobarbital, phenytoin, primidone) are predicted to decrease the exposure to elbasvir. Avoid. [Severe] Study
▶ Antifungals, azoles (itraconazole, ketoconazole, voriconazole) slightly to moderately increase the exposure to elbasvir. Avoid. [Moderate] Study
▶ Bosentan is predicted to moderately decrease the exposure to elbasvir. Avoid. [Severe] Study
▶ Cobicistat slightly to moderately increases the exposure to elbasvir. Avoid. [Moderate] Study
▶ Elbasvir is predicted to increase the concentration of dabigatran. Avoid. [Moderate] Theoretical
▶ Efavirenz is predicted to moderately decrease the exposure to elbasvir. Avoid. [Severe] Study
▶ Enzalutamide is predicted to decrease the exposure to elbasvir. Avoid. [Severe] Study
▶ Etravirine is predicted to decrease the exposure to elbasvir. Avoid. [Unknown] Theoretical
▶ HIV-protease inhibitors slightly to moderately increase the exposure to elbasvir. Avoid. [Moderate] Study
▶ Idelalisib slightly to moderately increases the exposure to elbasvir. Avoid. [Moderate] Study
▶ Macrolides (clarithromycin) slightly to moderately increase the exposure to elbasvir. Avoid. [Moderate] Study
▶ Mitotane is predicted to decrease the exposure to elbasvir. Avoid. [Severe] Study
▶ Modafinil is predicted to decrease the exposure to elbasvir. Avoid. [Unknown] Theoretical
▶ Nevirapine is predicted to moderately decrease the exposure to elbasvir. Avoid. [Severe] Study
▶ Rifampicin is predicted to decrease the exposure to elbasvir. Avoid. [Severe] Study
▶ St John's Wort is predicted to moderately decrease the exposure to elbasvir. Avoid. [Severe] Study
▶ Elbasvir potentially increases the exposure to statins (atorvastatin). Adjust atorvastatin dose, p. 200. [Moderate] Study
▶ Elbasvir is predicted to increase the exposure to statins (fluvastatin). Adjust fluvastatin dose, p. 201. [Unknown] Theoretical
▶ Elbasvir increases the exposure to statins (rosuvastatin). Adjust rosuvastatin dose, p. 202. [Moderate] Study
▶ Elbasvir is predicted to increase the exposure to statins (simvastatin). Adjust simvastatin dose, p. 203. [Unknown] Theoretical
▶ Elbasvir is predicted to increase the concentration of sunitinib. Use with caution and adjust dose. [Moderate] Theoretical

Eletriptan → see TABLE 13 p. 1337 (serotonin syndrome)

▶ Antifungals, azoles (itraconazole, ketoconazole, voriconazole) are predicted to markedly increase the exposure to eletriptan. Avoid. [Severe] Study
▶ Cobicistat is predicted to markedly increase the exposure to eletriptan. Avoid. [Severe] Study
▶ Eletriptan increases the risk of vasoconstriction when given with ergotamine. Separate administration by 24 hours. [Severe] Study
▶ HIV-protease inhibitors are predicted to markedly increase the exposure to eletriptan. Avoid. [Severe] Study
▶ Idelalisib is predicted to markedly increase the exposure to eletriptan. Avoid. [Severe] Study
▶ Macrolides (clarithromycin) are predicted to markedly increase the exposure to eletriptan. Avoid. [Severe] Study
▶ Macrolides (erythromycin) moderately increase the exposure to eletriptan. Avoid. [Moderate] Study

Eliglustat

▶ Abiraterone is predicted to increase the exposure to eliglustat. Avoid or adjust dose—consult product literature. [Severe] Study
▶ Eliglustat is predicted to increase the exposure to aliskiren. Adjust dose. [Moderate] Study
▶ Antiarrhythmics (dronedarone, propafenone) are predicted to increase the exposure to eliglustat. Avoid or adjust dose—consult product literature. [Severe] Study
▶ Antiepileptics (carbamazepine, fosphenytoin, phenobarbital, phenytoin, primidone) are predicted to decrease the exposure to eliglustat. Avoid. [Severe] Study

▶ Antifungals, azoles (fluconazole, isavuconazole, itraconazole, ketoconazole, posaconazole, voriconazole) are predicted to increase the exposure to eliglustat. Avoid or adjust dose—consult product literature. [Severe] Study
▶ Eliglustat is predicted to increase the exposure to antihistamines, non-sedating (fexofenadine). Adjust dose. [Moderate] Study
▶ Aprepitant is predicted to increase the exposure to eliglustat. Avoid or adjust dose—consult product literature. [Severe] Study
▶ Eliglustat is predicted to increase the exposure to atomoxetine. Adjust dose. [Moderate] Theoretical
▶ Eliglustat is predicted to increase the exposure to beta blockers, non-selective (propranolol). Adjust dose. [Moderate] Study
▶ Eliglustat is predicted to increase the exposure to beta blockers, selective (metoprolol). Adjust dose. [Moderate] Study
▶ Bosentan is predicted to decrease the exposure to eliglustat. [Moderate] Theoretical
▶ Bupropion is predicted to increase the exposure to eliglustat. Avoid or adjust dose—consult product literature. [Severe] Study
▶ Calcium channel blockers (diltiazem, verapamil) are predicted to increase the exposure to eliglustat. Avoid or adjust dose—consult product literature. [Severe] Study
▶ Cinacalcet is predicted to increase the exposure to eliglustat. Avoid or adjust dose—consult product literature. [Severe] Study
▶ Cobicistat is predicted to increase the exposure to eliglustat. Avoid or adjust dose—consult product literature. [Severe] Study
▶ Eliglustat is predicted to increase the exposure to colchicine. Avoid or adjust colchicine dose, p. 1085. [Severe] Theoretical
▶ Crizotinib is predicted to increase the exposure to eliglustat. Avoid or adjust dose—consult product literature. [Severe] Study
▶ Eliglustat is predicted to increase the exposure to dabigatran. Adjust dose. [Moderate] Study
▶ Eliglustat increases the exposure to digoxin. Adjust dose. [Moderate] Study
▶ Duloxetine is predicted to increase the exposure to eliglustat. Avoid or adjust dose—consult product literature. [Severe] Study
▶ Eliglustat is predicted to increase the exposure to edoxaban. Adjust dose. [Moderate] Study
▶ Efavirenz is predicted to decrease the exposure to eliglustat. [Moderate] Theoretical
▶ Enzalutamide is predicted to decrease the exposure to eliglustat. Avoid. [Severe] Study
▶ Eliglustat is predicted to increase the exposure to everolimus. Adjust dose. [Moderate] Study
▶ Grapefruit juice is predicted to increase the exposure to eliglustat. Avoid. [Severe] Theoretical
▶ HIV-protease inhibitors are predicted to increase the exposure to eliglustat. Avoid or adjust dose—consult product literature. [Severe] Study
▶ Idelalisib is predicted to increase the exposure to eliglustat. Avoid or adjust dose—consult product literature. [Severe] Study
▶ Imatinib is predicted to increase the exposure to eliglustat. Avoid or adjust dose—consult product literature. [Severe] Study
▶ Eliglustat is predicted to increase the exposure to loperamide. Adjust dose. [Moderate] Study
▶ Macrolides (clarithromycin, erythromycin) are predicted to increase the exposure to eliglustat. Avoid or adjust dose—consult product literature. [Severe] Study
▶ Mirabegron is predicted to increase the exposure to eliglustat. Avoid or adjust dose—consult product literature. [Severe] Study
▶ Mitotane is predicted to decrease the exposure to eliglustat. Avoid. [Severe] Study
▶ Moclobemide is predicted to increase the exposure to eliglustat. Avoid or adjust dose—consult product literature. [Severe] Theoretical
▶ Netupitant is predicted to increase the exposure to eliglustat. Avoid or adjust dose—consult product literature. [Severe] Study
▶ Nevirapine is predicted to decrease the exposure to eliglustat. [Moderate] Theoretical
▶ Nilotinib is predicted to increase the exposure to eliglustat. Avoid or adjust dose—consult product literature. [Severe] Study
▶ Eliglustat is predicted to increase the exposure to phenothiazines (perphenazine). Adjust dose. [Moderate] Theoretical

▶ Quinolones (**ciprofloxacin**) are predicted to increase the exposure to **eliglustat**. Avoid or adjust dose—consult product literature. Severe Theoretical

▶ **Rifampicin** is predicted to decrease the exposure to **eliglustat**. Avoid. Severe Study

▶ **Eliglustat** is predicted to increase the exposure to **sirolimus**. Adjust dose. Moderate Study

▶ **SSRIs** (**fluoxetine, paroxetine**) are predicted to increase the exposure to **eliglustat**. Avoid or adjust dose—consult product literature. Severe Study

▶ **St John's Wort** is predicted to increase the exposure to **eliglustat**. Avoid. Severe Study

▶ **Eliglustat** is predicted to increase the exposure to taxanes (**paclitaxel**). Adjust dose. Moderate Study

▶ **Terbinafine** is predicted to increase the exposure to **eliglustat**. Avoid or adjust dose—consult product literature. Severe Study

▶ **Eliglustat** is predicted to increase the exposure to **tolterodine**. Adjust dose. Moderate Theoretical

▶ **Eliglustat** is predicted to increase the exposure to **topotecan**. Adjust dose. Moderate Study

▶ **Eliglustat** is predicted to increase the exposure to tricyclic antidepressants (**nortriptyline**). Adjust dose. Moderate Theoretical

Elotuzumab → see monoclonal antibodies

Eltrombopag

▶ **Antacids** decrease the absorption of **eltrombopag**. **Eltrombopag** should be taken 2 hours before or 4 hours after **antacids**. Severe Study

▶ Oral **calcium salts** decrease the absorption of **eltrombopag**. **Eltrombopag** should be taken 2 hours before or 4 hours after **calcium salts**. Severe Study

▶ **Dairy products** are predicted to decrease the absorption of **eltrombopag**. **Eltrombopag** should be taken 2 hours before or 4 hours after **dairy products**. Severe Theoretical

▶ Iron (oral) is predicted to decrease the absorption of **eltrombopag**. **Eltrombopag** should be taken 2 hours before or 4 hours after **iron (oral)**. Severe Theoretical

▶ **Selenium** is predicted to decrease the absorption of **eltrombopag**. **Eltrombopag** should be taken 2 hours before or 4 hours after **selenium**. Severe Theoretical

▶ **Eltrombopag** is predicted to increase the exposure to **statins**. Monitor and adjust dose. Moderate Study

▶ **Zinc** is predicted to decrease the absorption of **eltrombopag**. **Eltrombopag** should be taken 2 hours before or 4 hours after **zinc**. Severe Theoretical

Eluxadoline

▶ **Ciclosporin** increases the exposure to **eluxadoline**. Avoid. Moderate Study

▶ Fibrates (**gemfibrozil**) are predicted to increase the exposure to **eluxadoline**. Avoid. Moderate Theoretical

▶ HIV-protease inhibitors (**atazanavir, lopinavir, ritonavir, saquinavir, tipranavir**) are predicted to increase the exposure to **eluxadoline**. Avoid. Moderate Theoretical

▶ **Rifampicin** is predicted to increase the exposure to **eluxadoline**. Avoid. Moderate Theoretical

▶ **Eluxadoline** is predicted to increase the exposure to **statins**. Moderate Study

Elvitegravir

▶ **Antacids** moderately decrease the exposure to **elvitegravir**. Separate administration by at least 4 hours. Moderate Study

▶ Antiepileptics (**carbamazepine, fosphenytoin, phenobarbital, phenytoin, primidone**) are predicted to decrease the concentration of **elvitegravir**. Avoid. Severe Theoretical

▶ **Bosentan** is predicted to decrease the concentration of **elvitegravir**. Avoid. Severe Theoretical

▶ **Elvitegravir** is predicted to decrease the anticoagulant effect of coumarins. Moderate Theoretical

▶ **Efavirenz** is predicted to decrease the concentration of **elvitegravir**. Avoid. Severe Theoretical

▶ **Enzalutamide** is predicted to decrease the concentration of **elvitegravir**. Avoid. Severe Theoretical

▶ HIV-protease inhibitors (**atazanavir, lopinavir**) (boosted with ritonavir) increase the concentration of **elvitegravir**. Refer to specialist literature. Moderate Study

▶ **Mitotane** is predicted to decrease the concentration of **elvitegravir**. Avoid. Severe Theoretical

▶ **Nevirapine** is predicted to decrease the concentration of **elvitegravir**. Avoid. Severe Theoretical

▶ **Rifampicin** is predicted to decrease the concentration of **elvitegravir**. Avoid. Severe Theoretical

▶ **St John's Wort** is predicted to decrease the concentration of **elvitegravir**. Avoid. Severe Theoretical

Empagliflozin → see TABLE 14 p. 1337 (antidiabetic drugs), TABLE 8 p. 1335 (hypotension)

Enalapril → see ACE inhibitors

Enoxaparin → see low molecular-weight heparins

Entacapone

▶ Iron (oral) is predicted to decrease the absorption of **entacapone**. Separate administration by at least 2 hours. Moderate Theoretical

▶ **Entacapone** increases the exposure to levodopa. Monitor side effects and adjust dose. Moderate Study

▶ **Entacapone** is predicted to increase the exposure to methyldopa. Moderate Theoretical

▶ **Entacapone** is predicted to increase the risk of elevated blood pressure when given with monoamine-oxidase A and B inhibitors, irreversible. Avoid. Severe Theoretical

▶ **Entacapone** is predicted to increase the risk of cardiovascular side-effects when given with sympathomimetics, inotropic. Moderate Theoretical

▶ **Entacapone** is predicted to increase the risk of cardiovascular side-effects when given with sympathomimetics, vasoconstrictor (**adrenaline/epinephrine, noradrenaline/norepinephrine**). Moderate Study

Enteral feeds

▶ Antacids (**aluminium hydroxide**) increase the risk of blocked enteral or nasogastric tubes when given with **enteral feeds**. Moderate Study

▶ **Enteral feeds** decrease the absorption of antiepileptics (**phenytoin**). Severe Study

▶ **Enteral feeds** (vitamin-K containing) potentially decrease the anticoagulant effect of coumarins. Severe Anecdotal

▶ **Enteral feeds** (vitamin-K containing) potentially decrease the effects of phenindione. Severe Theoretical

▶ **Enteral feeds** decrease the exposure to quinolones (**ciprofloxacin**). Moderate Study

▶ **Sucralfate** increases the risk of blocked enteral or nasogastric tubes when given with **enteral feeds**. Separate administration by 1 hour. Moderate Study

▶ **Enteral feeds** decrease the exposure to theophylline. Moderate Study

Enzalutamide

GENERAL INFORMATION Caution with concurrent chemotherapy—safety and efficacy not established.

▶ **Enzalutamide** is predicted to decrease the exposure to abiraterone. Avoid. Severe Theoretical

▶ **Enzalutamide** is predicted to decrease the exposure to aldosterone antagonists (**eplerenone**). Avoid. Moderate Theoretical

▶ **Enzalutamide** is predicted to decrease the exposure to alprazolam. Adjust dose. Moderate Theoretical

▶ **Enzalutamide** is predicted to decrease the exposure to antiarrhythmics (**disopyramide, dronedarone**). Avoid. Severe Study

▶ **Enzalutamide** is predicted to decrease the efficacy of antiarrhythmics (**propafenone**). Moderate Study

▶ **Enzalutamide** is predicted to decrease the exposure to anticholinesterases, centrally acting (**donepezil**). Mild Study

▶ **Enzalutamide** is predicted to slightly decrease the exposure to antiepileptics (**brivaracetam**). Moderate Theoretical

▶ **Enzalutamide** is predicted to decrease the exposure to antiepileptics (**perampanel**). Monitor and adjust dose. Moderate Study

▶ **Enzalutamide** is predicted to decrease the exposure to antifungals, azoles (**isavuconazole**). Avoid. Severe Study

▶ **Enzalutamide** is predicted to decrease the exposure to antimalarials (**artemether**) (with lumefantrine). Avoid. Severe Study

▶ **Enzalutamide** is predicted to decrease the concentration of antimalarials (**piperaquine**). Avoid. Moderate Theoretical

▶ **Enzalutamide** is predicted to moderately decrease the exposure to apixaban. Use with caution or avoid. Severe Study

Enzalutamide (continued)

▸ **Enzalutamide** moderately decreases the exposure to apremilast. Avoid. [Severe] Study

▸ **Enzalutamide** is predicted to markedly decrease the exposure to aprepitant. Avoid. [Moderate] Study

▸ **Enzalutamide** is predicted to moderately decrease the exposure to aripiprazole. Adjust **aripiprazole** dose, p. 391. [Moderate] Study

▸ **Enzalutamide** is predicted to decrease the exposure to axitinib. Avoid or adjust dose. [Moderate] Study

▸ **Enzalutamide** decreases the exposure to bedaquiline. Avoid. [Severe] Study

▸ **Enzalutamide** slightly decreases the exposure to bortezomib. Avoid. [Severe] Study

▸ **Enzalutamide** affects the exposure to bosentan. Avoid. [Severe] Study

▸ **Enzalutamide** is predicted to very markedly decrease the exposure to bosutinib. Avoid. [Severe] Study

▸ **Enzalutamide** is predicted to decrease the exposure to buspirone. Use with caution and adjust dose. [Severe] Study

▸ **Enzalutamide** moderately decreases the exposure to cabozantinib. Avoid. [Moderate] Study

▸ **Enzalutamide** is predicted to decrease the exposure to calcium channel blockers (amlodipine, felodipine, lacidipine, lercanidipine, nicardipine, nifedipine, nimodipine). Monitor and adjust dose. [Moderate] Study

▸ **Enzalutamide** is predicted to decrease the exposure to calcium channel blockers (diltiazem, verapamil). [Severe] Study

▸ **Enzalutamide** is predicted to decrease the exposure to cannabis extract. Avoid. [Severe] Theoretical

▸ **Enzalutamide** is predicted to decrease the exposure to ceritinib. Avoid. [Severe] Study

▸ **Enzalutamide** decreases the concentration of ciclosporin. [Severe] Study

▸ **Enzalutamide** is predicted to alter the effects of cilostazol. [Moderate] Theoretical

▸ **Enzalutamide** is predicted to decrease the exposure to cinacalcet. Monitor and adjust dose. [Moderate] Study

▸ **Enzalutamide** decreases the exposure to clomethiazole. Monitor and adjust dose. [Moderate] Study

▸ Clopidogrel moderately increases the exposure to **enzalutamide**. Avoid or adjust **enzalutamide** dose, p. 921. [Severe] Study

▸ **Enzalutamide** is predicted to decrease the exposure to clozapine. [Moderate] Theoretical

▸ **Enzalutamide** is predicted to decrease the exposure to cobicistat. Avoid. [Severe] Theoretical

▸ **Enzalutamide** is predicted to decrease the exposure to cobimetinib. Avoid. [Severe] Theoretical

▸ **Enzalutamide** is predicted to decrease the exposure to corticosteroids (budesonide, deflazacort, dexamethasone, fludrocortisone, hydrocortisone, methylprednisolone, prednisolone, prednisone, triamcinolone). Monitor and adjust dose. [Moderate] Study

▸ **Enzalutamide** is predicted to decrease the exposure to corticosteroids (fluticasone). [Unknown] Theoretical

▸ **Enzalutamide** potentially decreases the exposure to coumarins. Avoid or adjust dose and monitor INR. [Severe] Study

▸ **Enzalutamide** is predicted to markedly decrease the exposure to crizotinib. Avoid. [Severe] Study

▸ **Enzalutamide** is predicted to decrease the exposure to dabrafenib. Avoid. [Moderate] Theoretical

▸ **Enzalutamide** is predicted to moderately decrease the exposure to daclatasvir. Avoid. [Severe] Study

▸ **Enzalutamide** is predicted to decrease the exposure to darifenacin. [Moderate] Theoretical

▸ **Enzalutamide** is predicted to decrease the exposure to dasabuvir. Avoid. [Severe] Theoretical

▸ **Enzalutamide** is predicted to markedly decrease the exposure to dasatinib. Avoid. [Severe] Study

▸ **Enzalutamide** is predicted to slightly decrease the exposure to delamanid. Avoid. [Moderate] Study

▸ **Enzalutamide** decreases the exposure to dolutegravir. Adjust dose. [Severe] Study

▸ **Enzalutamide** is predicted to decrease the exposure to elbasvir. Avoid. [Severe] Study

▸ **Enzalutamide** is predicted to decrease the exposure to eliglustat. Avoid. [Severe] Study

▸ **Enzalutamide** is predicted to decrease the concentration of elvitegravir. Avoid. [Severe] Theoretical

▸ **Enzalutamide** is predicted to decrease the effects of ergotamine. [Moderate] Theoretical

▸ **Enzalutamide** is predicted to decrease the exposure to erlotinib. Avoid or adjust **erlotinib** dose, p. 949. [Severe] Study

▸ **Enzalutamide** is predicted to decrease the exposure to etravirine. Avoid. [Severe] Theoretical

▸ **Enzalutamide** is predicted to decrease the concentration of everolimus. Avoid or adjust dose. [Severe] Study

▸ **Enzalutamide** moderately decreases the exposure to exemestane. [Moderate] Study

▸ **Enzalutamide** is predicted to decrease the exposure to fesoterodine. Avoid. [Moderate] Study

▸ Fibrates (gemfibrozil) moderately increase the exposure to **enzalutamide**. Avoid or adjust **enzalutamide** dose, p. 921. [Severe] Study

▸ **Enzalutamide** is predicted to decrease the exposure to fingolimod. [Moderate] Study

▸ **Enzalutamide** is predicted to decrease the exposure to fosaprepitant. Avoid. [Moderate] Theoretical

▸ **Enzalutamide** is predicted to decrease the exposure to gefitinib. Avoid. [Severe] Study

▸ **Enzalutamide** is predicted to decrease the exposure to grazoprevir. Avoid. [Severe] Study

▸ **Enzalutamide** is predicted to decrease the concentration of guanfacine. Adjust **guanfacine** dose, p. 349. [Moderate] Study

▸ **Enzalutamide** decreases the concentration of haloperidol. Adjust dose. [Moderate] Study

▸ **Enzalutamide** is predicted to decrease the exposure to ibrutinib. Avoid or adjust **ibrutinib** dose, p. 952. [Severe] Study

▸ **Enzalutamide** is predicted to decrease the exposure to idelalisib. Avoid. [Severe] Study

▸ **Enzalutamide** is predicted to decrease the exposure to imatinib. Avoid. [Moderate] Study

▸ **Enzalutamide** is predicted to decrease the exposure to irinotecan. Avoid. [Severe] Study

▸ **Enzalutamide** is predicted to decrease the exposure to ivabradine. Adjust dose. [Moderate] Theoretical

▸ **Enzalutamide** is predicted to moderately to markedly decrease the exposure to ivacaftor. Avoid. [Severe] Study

▸ **Enzalutamide** is predicted to decrease the exposure to ixazomib. Avoid. [Severe] Study

▸ **Enzalutamide** is predicted to decrease the exposure to lapatinib. Avoid. [Severe] Study

▸ **Enzalutamide** is predicted to decrease the exposure to linagliptin. [Moderate] Study

▸ **Enzalutamide** is predicted to decrease the exposure to lomitapide. Monitor and adjust dose. [Moderate] Theoretical

▸ **Enzalutamide** is predicted to decrease the exposure to lurasidone. Avoid. [Moderate] Study

▸ **Enzalutamide** is predicted to decrease the exposure to macitentan. Avoid. [Severe] Study

▸ **Enzalutamide** is predicted to decrease the exposure to maraviroc. Adjust dose. [Severe] Study

▸ **Enzalutamide** is predicted to decrease the exposure to midazolam. Monitor and adjust dose. [Moderate] Study

▸ **Enzalutamide** is predicted to decrease the exposure to midostaurin. Avoid. [Severe] Study

▸ **Enzalutamide** is predicted to decrease the exposure to mirtazapine. Adjust dose. [Moderate] Study

▸ **Enzalutamide** is predicted to decrease the exposure to montelukast. [Mild] Study

▸ **Enzalutamide** is predicted to markedly decrease the exposure to naloxegol. Avoid. [Moderate] Study

▸ **Enzalutamide** is predicted to slightly decrease the exposure to nateglinide. [Mild] Study

▸ **Enzalutamide** is predicted to decrease the exposure to netupitant. Avoid. [Severe] Study

▸ **Enzalutamide** is predicted to moderately decrease the exposure to nilotinib. Avoid. [Severe] Study

- ► **Enzalutamide** is predicted to decrease the exposure to nitisinone. Adjust dose. Moderate Theoretical
- ► **Enzalutamide** is predicted to decrease the exposure to olaparib. Avoid. Moderate Theoretical
- ► **Enzalutamide** is predicted to decrease the exposure to ondansetron. Moderate Study
- ► **Enzalutamide** is predicted to decrease the exposure to opioids (alfentanil, fentanyl). Moderate Study
- ► **Enzalutamide** is predicted to decrease the exposure to opioids (buprenorphine). Monitor and adjust dose. Moderate Theoretical
- ► **Enzalutamide** decreases the exposure to opioids (methadone). Monitor and adjust dose. Severe Study
- ► **Enzalutamide** is predicted to decrease the exposure to opioids (oxycodone). Monitor and adjust dose. Moderate Study
- ► **Enzalutamide** is predicted to moderately decrease the exposure to osimertinib. Avoid. Moderate Study
- ► **Enzalutamide** is predicted to decrease the exposure to palbociclib. Avoid. Severe Study
- ► **Enzalutamide** is predicted to decrease the exposure to paliperidone. Monitor and adjust dose. Severe Study
- ► **Enzalutamide** is predicted to decrease the exposure to panobinostat. Avoid. Moderate Theoretical
- ► **Enzalutamide** is predicted to decrease the exposure to paritaprevir (with ritonavir and ombitasvir). Avoid. Severe Study
- ► **Enzalutamide** is predicted to decrease the exposure to pazopanib. Avoid. Severe Theoretical
- ► **Enzalutamide** is predicted to decrease the exposure to phosphodiesterase type-5 inhibitors (avanafil, tadalafil). Avoid. Severe Study
- ► **Enzalutamide** is predicted to decrease the exposure to phosphodiesterase type-5 inhibitors (sildenafil, vardenafil). Moderate Theoretical
- ► **Enzalutamide** is predicted to moderately to markedly decrease the exposure to pibrentasvir. Avoid. Severe Study
- ► **Enzalutamide** is predicted to moderately decrease the exposure to pitolisant. Moderate Study
- ► **Enzalutamide** is predicted to decrease the exposure to ponatinib. Avoid. Moderate Theoretical
- ► **Enzalutamide** is predicted to markedly decrease the exposure to praziquantel. Avoid. Moderate Study
- ► **Enzalutamide** is predicted to decrease the exposure to quetiapine. Moderate Study
- ► **Enzalutamide** is predicted to decrease the exposure to ranolazine. Avoid. Severe Study
- ► **Enzalutamide** is predicted to decrease the exposure to reboxetine. Moderate Anecdotal
- ► **Enzalutamide** is predicted to decrease the exposure to regorafenib. Avoid. Moderate Study
- ► **Enzalutamide** is predicted to decrease the exposure to repaglinide. Monitor blood glucose and adjust dose. Moderate Study
- ► **Enzalutamide** is predicted to markedly decrease the exposure to ribociclib. Avoid. Severe Study
- ► **Enzalutamide** markedly decreases the exposure to rilpivirine. Avoid. Severe Study
- ► **Enzalutamide** is predicted to decrease the exposure to risperidone. Adjust dose. Moderate Study
- ► **Enzalutamide** is predicted to moderately decrease the exposure to rivaroxaban. Avoid unless patient can be monitored for signs of thrombosis. Severe Study
- ► **Enzalutamide** is predicted to decrease the exposure to roflumilast. Avoid. Moderate Study
- ► **Enzalutamide** is predicted to markedly decrease the exposure to rolapitant. Avoid. Severe Study
- ► **Enzalutamide** is predicted to decrease the exposure to ruxolitinib. Monitor and adjust dose. Moderate Study
- ► **Enzalutamide** is predicted to moderately decrease the exposure to saxagliptin. Moderate Study
- ► **Enzalutamide** is predicted to decrease the exposure to simeprevir. Avoid. Severe Study
- ► **Enzalutamide** is predicted to decrease the concentration of sirolimus. Avoid. Severe Study
- ► **Enzalutamide** is predicted to decrease the exposure to solifenacin. Moderate Theoretical

- ► **Enzalutamide** is predicted to decrease the exposure to sorafenib. Moderate Theoretical
- ► **Enzalutamide** is predicted to decrease the exposure to statins (simvastatin). Severe Study
- ► **Enzalutamide** is predicted to decrease the exposure to sunitinib. Avoid or adjust **sunitinib** dose, p. 967. Moderate Study
- ► **Enzalutamide** decreases the concentration of tacrolimus. Monitor and adjust dose. Severe Study
- ► **Enzalutamide** is predicted to decrease the exposure to taxanes (cabazitaxel, paclitaxel). Avoid. Severe Study
- ► **Enzalutamide** is predicted to decrease the exposure to taxanes (docetaxel). Severe Theoretical
- ► **Enzalutamide** is predicted to decrease the concentration of temsirolimus. Avoid. Severe Study
- ► **Enzalutamide** decreases the exposure to tetracyclines (doxycycline). Monitor and adjust dose. Moderate Study
- ► **Enzalutamide** is predicted to markedly decrease the exposure to ticagrelor. Avoid. Severe Study
- ► **Enzalutamide** is predicted to decrease the exposure to tivozanib. Severe Study
- ► **Enzalutamide** is predicted to decrease the exposure to tofacitinib. Avoid. Severe Study
- ► **Enzalutamide** is predicted to decrease the exposure to tolvaptan. Avoid. Severe Study
- ► **Enzalutamide** is predicted to decrease the exposure to toremifene. Adjust dose. Moderate Study
- ► **Enzalutamide** is predicted to decrease the exposure to trabectedin. Avoid. Severe Theoretical
- ► **Enzalutamide** is predicted to markedly decrease the exposure to ulipristal. Avoid and for 4 weeks after stopping **ulipristal**. Severe Theoretical
- ► **Enzalutamide** is predicted to decrease the exposure to vandetanib. Avoid. Moderate Study
- ► **Enzalutamide** is predicted to moderately decrease the exposure to velpatasvir. Avoid. Severe Study
- ► **Enzalutamide** is predicted to decrease the exposure to vemurafenib. Avoid. Severe Theoretical
- ► **Enzalutamide** is predicted to decrease the exposure to venetoclax. Avoid. Severe Study
- ► **Enzalutamide** is predicted to decrease the exposure to vinca alkaloids (vinblastine, vincristine, vindesine). Severe Theoretical
- ► **Enzalutamide** is predicted to decrease the exposure to vinca alkaloids (vinflunine). Avoid. Severe Theoretical
- ► **Enzalutamide** is predicted to decrease the exposure to vinca alkaloids (vinorelbine). Use with caution or avoid. Severe Theoretical
- ► **Enzalutamide** is predicted to decrease the exposure to vismodegib. Avoid. Moderate Theoretical
- ► **Enzalutamide** is predicted to decrease the exposure to vortioxetine. Monitor and adjust dose. Moderate Study
- ► **Enzalutamide** is predicted to decrease the concentration of voxilaprevir. Avoid. Severe Study
- ► **Enzalutamide** is predicted to decrease the exposure to zopiclone. Adjust dose. Moderate Study

Ephedrine → see sympathomimetics, vasoconstrictor
Epirubicin → see anthracyclines
Eplerenone → see aldosterone antagonists
Epoetin alfa → see TABLE 5 p. 1334 (thromboembolism), TABLE 16 p. 1338 (increased serum potassium)
Epoetin beta → see TABLE 5 p. 1334 (thromboembolism), TABLE 16 p. 1338 (increased serum potassium)
Epoetin zeta → see TABLE 5 p. 1334 (thromboembolism), TABLE 16 p. 1338 (increased serum potassium)
Epoprostenol → see TABLE 4 p. 1334 (antiplatelet effects)
Eprosartan → see angiotensin-II receptor antagonists
Eptifibatide → see TABLE 4 p. 1334 (antiplatelet effects)
Ergocalciferol → see vitamin D substances
Ergometrine
- ► Antiarrhythmics (dronedarone) are predicted to increase the risk of ergotism when given with **ergometrine**. Severe Theoretical
- ► Antifungals, azoles (fluconazole, isavuconazole, posaconazole) are predicted to increase the risk of ergotism when given with **ergometrine**. Severe Theoretical

Ergometrine (continued)

► Antifungals, azoles (itraconazole, ketoconazole, voriconazole) are predicted to increase the risk of ergotism when given with **ergometrine**. Avoid. Severe Theoretical
► Antifungals, azoles (miconazole) are predicted to increase the exposure to **ergometrine**. Avoid. Moderate Theoretical
► Aprepitant is predicted to increase the risk of ergotism when given with **ergometrine**. Severe Theoretical
► Beta blockers, non-selective are predicted to increase the risk of peripheral vasoconstriction when given with **ergometrine**. Severe Study
► Beta blockers, selective are predicted to increase the risk of peripheral vasoconstriction when given with **ergometrine**. Severe Study
► Calcium channel blockers (diltiazem, verapamil) are predicted to increase the risk of ergotism when given with **ergometrine**. Severe Theoretical
► Cobicistat is predicted to increase the risk of ergotism when given with **ergometrine**. Avoid. Severe Theoretical
► Crizotinib is predicted to increase the risk of ergotism when given with **ergometrine**. Severe Theoretical
► **Ergometrine** is predicted to increase the risk of ergotism when given with dopamine receptor agonists (cabergoline, pergolide). Avoid. Moderate Theoretical
► Grapefruit juice is predicted to increase the exposure to **ergometrine**. Severe Theoretical
► HIV-protease inhibitors are predicted to increase the risk of ergotism when given with **ergometrine**. Avoid. Severe Theoretical
► Idelalisib is predicted to increase the risk of ergotism when given with **ergometrine**. Severe Theoretical
► Imatinib is predicted to increase the risk of ergotism when given with **ergometrine**. Severe Theoretical
► Macrolides (clarithromycin) are predicted to increase the risk of ergotism when given with **ergometrine**. Avoid. Severe Theoretical
► Macrolides (erythromycin) are predicted to increase the risk of ergotism when given with **ergometrine**. Severe Theoretical
► Netupitant is predicted to increase the risk of ergotism when given with **ergometrine**. Severe Theoretical
► Nilotinib is predicted to increase the risk of ergotism when given with **ergometrine**. Severe Theoretical
► **Ergometrine** potentially increases the risk of peripheral vasoconstriction when given with sympathomimetics, inotropic (dopamine). Avoid. Severe Anecdotal
► **Ergometrine** is predicted to increase the risk of peripheral vasoconstriction when given with sympathomimetics, vasoconstrictor (noradrenaline/norepinephrine). Severe Anecdotal

Ergotamine

► Almotriptan is predicted to increase the risk of vasoconstriction when given with **ergotamine**. **Ergotamine** should be taken at least 24 hours before or 6 hours after **almotriptan**. Severe Theoretical
► Antiarrhythmics (dronedarone) are predicted to increase the risk of ergotism when given with **ergotamine**. Severe Theoretical
► Antiepileptics (carbamazepine, fosphenytoin, phenobarbital, phenytoin, primidone) are predicted to decrease the effects of **ergotamine**. Moderate Theoretical
► Antifungals, azoles (fluconazole, isavuconazole, posaconazole) are predicted to increase the risk of ergotism when given with **ergotamine**. Severe Theoretical
► Antifungals, azoles (itraconazole, ketoconazole, voriconazole) are predicted to increase the risk of ergotism when given with **ergotamine**. Avoid. Severe Theoretical
► Antifungals, azoles (miconazole) are predicted to increase the exposure to **ergotamine**. Moderate Theoretical
► Aprepitant is predicted to increase the risk of ergotism when given with **ergotamine**. Severe Theoretical
► Beta blockers, non-selective are predicted to increase the risk of peripheral vasoconstriction when given with **ergotamine**. Severe Study
► Beta blockers, selective are predicted to increase the risk of peripheral vasoconstriction when given with **ergotamine**. Severe Study

► Bosentan is predicted to decrease the effects of **ergotamine**. Moderate Theoretical
► Calcium channel blockers (diltiazem, verapamil) are predicted to increase the risk of ergotism when given with **ergotamine**. Severe Theoretical
► Ceritinib is predicted to increase the exposure to **ergotamine**. Avoid. Moderate Theoretical
► Cobicistat is predicted to increase the risk of ergotism when given with **ergotamine**. Avoid. Severe Theoretical
► Crizotinib is predicted to increase the risk of ergotism when given with **ergotamine**. Severe Theoretical
► **Ergotamine** is predicted to increase the risk of ergotism when given with dopamine receptor agonists (bromocriptine, cabergoline). Avoid. Moderate Theoretical
► **Ergotamine** is predicted to increase the risk of ergotism when given with dopamine receptor agonists (pergolide). Moderate Theoretical
► Efavirenz is predicted to decrease the effects of **ergotamine**. Moderate Theoretical
► Eletriptan increases the risk of vasoconstriction when given with **ergotamine**. Separate administration by 24 hours. Severe Study
► Enzalutamide is predicted to decrease the effects of **ergotamine**. Moderate Theoretical
► Grapefruit juice is predicted to increase the exposure to **ergotamine**. Severe Theoretical
► HIV-protease inhibitors are predicted to increase the risk of ergotism when given with **ergotamine**. Avoid. Severe Theoretical
► Idelalisib is predicted to increase the risk of ergotism when given with **ergotamine**. Avoid. Severe Theoretical
► Imatinib is predicted to increase the risk of ergotism when given with **ergotamine**. Severe Theoretical
► Macrolides (clarithromycin) are predicted to increase the risk of ergotism when given with **ergotamine**. Avoid. Severe Theoretical
► Macrolides (erythromycin) are predicted to increase the risk of ergotism when given with **ergotamine**. Severe Theoretical
► Mitotane is predicted to decrease the effects of **ergotamine**. Moderate Theoretical
► Naratriptan is predicted to increase the risk of vasoconstriction when given with **ergotamine**. Separate administration by 24 hours. Severe Theoretical
► Netupitant is predicted to increase the risk of ergotism when given with **ergotamine**. Severe Theoretical
► Nevirapine is predicted to decrease the effects of **ergotamine**. Moderate Theoretical
► Nilotinib is predicted to increase the risk of ergotism when given with **ergotamine**. Severe Theoretical
► Palbociclib is predicted to increase the exposure to **ergotamine**. Adjust dose. Moderate Theoretical
► Ribociclib (high-dose) is predicted to increase the exposure to **ergotamine**. Avoid. Moderate Theoretical
► Rifampicin is predicted to decrease the effects of **ergotamine**. Moderate Theoretical
► Rizatriptan is predicted to increase the risk of vasoconstriction when given with **ergotamine**. **Ergotamine** should be taken at least 24 hours before or 6 hours after **rizatriptan**. Severe Theoretical
► St John's Wort is predicted to decrease the effects of **ergotamine**. Moderate Theoretical
► Sumatriptan increases the risk of vasoconstriction when given with **ergotamine**. **Ergotamine** should be taken at least 24 hours before or 6 hours after **sumatriptan**. Severe Study
► Ticagrelor is predicted to increase the exposure to **ergotamine**. Avoid. Severe Theoretical

Eribulin → see TABLE 15 p. 1337 (myelosuppression), TABLE 12 p. 1337 (peripheral neuropathy), TABLE 9 p. 1336 (QT-interval prolongation)

Erlotinib

FOOD AND LIFESTYLE Dose adjustment may be necessary if smoking started or stopped during treatment.

► Antacids are predicted to decrease the absorption of **erlotinib**. **Antacids** should be taken 4 hours before or 2 hours after **erlotinib**. Moderate Theoretical
► Antiarrhythmics (amiodarone, dronedarone) are predicted to increase the exposure to **erlotinib**. Moderate Theoretical

▸ Antiepileptics (carbamazepine, fosphenytoin, phenobarbital, phenytoin, primidone) are predicted to decrease the exposure to **erlotinib**. Avoid or adjust **erlotinib** dose, p. 949. Severe Study

▸ Antifungals, azoles (fluconazole, isavuconazole, posaconazole) are predicted to increase the exposure to **erlotinib**. Moderate Theoretical

▸ Antifungals, azoles (itraconazole, ketoconazole, voriconazole) are predicted to slightly increase the exposure to **erlotinib**. Use with caution and adjust dose. Moderate Study

▸ Aprepitant is predicted to increase the exposure to **erlotinib**. Moderate Theoretical

▸ **Erlotinib** is predicted to increase the risk of gastrointestinal perforation when given with aspirin (high-dose). Severe Theoretical

▸ Bosentan is predicted to decrease the exposure to **erlotinib**. Severe Theoretical

▸ Calcium channel blockers (diltiazem, verapamil) are predicted to increase the exposure to **erlotinib**. Moderate Theoretical

▸ Ciclosporin is predicted to increase the exposure to **erlotinib**. Moderate Theoretical

▸ Cobicistat is predicted to slightly increase the exposure to **erlotinib**. Use with caution and adjust dose. Moderate Study

▸ Combined hormonal contraceptives slightly increase the exposure to **erlotinib**. Monitor side effects and adjust dose. Moderate Study

▸ Corticosteroids increase the risk of gastrointestinal perforation when given with **erlotinib**. Severe Theoretical

▸ **Erlotinib** increases the anticoagulant effect of coumarins. Severe Anecdotal

▸ Crizotinib is predicted to increase the exposure to **erlotinib**. Moderate Theoretical

▸ Efavirenz is predicted to decrease the exposure to **erlotinib**. Severe Theoretical

▸ Enzalutamide is predicted to decrease the exposure to **erlotinib**. Avoid or adjust **erlotinib** dose, p. 949. Severe Study

▸ Grapefruit juice is predicted to increase the exposure to **erlotinib**. Moderate Theoretical

▸ H$_2$ receptor antagonists are predicted to decrease the exposure to **erlotinib**. **Erlotinib** should be taken 2 hours before or 10 hours after H$_2$ receptor antagonists. Moderate Study

▸ HIV-protease inhibitors are predicted to slightly increase the exposure to **erlotinib**. Use with caution and adjust dose. Moderate Study

▸ Idelalisib is predicted to slightly increase the exposure to **erlotinib**. Use with caution and adjust dose. Moderate Study

▸ Imatinib is predicted to increase the exposure to **erlotinib**. Moderate Theoretical

▸ Lapatinib is predicted to increase the exposure to **erlotinib**. Moderate Theoretical

▸ Macrolides (azithromycin, erythromycin) are predicted to increase the exposure to **erlotinib**. Moderate Theoretical

▸ Macrolides (clarithromycin) are predicted to slightly increase the exposure to **erlotinib**. Use with caution and adjust dose. Moderate Study

▸ Mitotane is predicted to decrease the exposure to **erlotinib**. Avoid or adjust **erlotinib** dose, p. 949. Severe Study

▸ Netupitant is predicted to increase the exposure to **erlotinib**. Moderate Theoretical

▸ Nevirapine is predicted to decrease the exposure to **erlotinib**. Severe Theoretical

▸ Nilotinib is predicted to increase the exposure to **erlotinib**. Moderate Theoretical

▸ **Erlotinib** is predicted to increase the risk of gastrointestinal perforation when given with NSAIDs. Severe Theoretical

▸ **Erlotinib** is predicted to increase the risk of bleeding events when given with phenindione. Severe Theoretical

▸ Proton pump inhibitors are predicted to slightly decrease the exposure to **erlotinib**. Avoid. Moderate Study

▸ Quinolones (ciprofloxacin) slightly increase the exposure to **erlotinib**. Monitor side effects and adjust dose. Moderate Study

▸ Ranolazine is predicted to increase the exposure to **erlotinib**. Moderate Theoretical

▸ Rifampicin is predicted to decrease the exposure to **erlotinib**. Avoid or adjust **erlotinib** dose, p. 949. Severe Study

▸ SSRIs (fluvoxamine) are predicted to increase the exposure to **erlotinib**. Monitor side effects and adjust dose. Moderate Theoretical

▸ St John's Wort is predicted to decrease the exposure to **erlotinib**. Severe Theoretical

▸ Vemurafenib is predicted to increase the exposure to **erlotinib**. Moderate Theoretical

Ertapenem → see carbapenems

Erythromycin → see macrolides

Escitalopram → see SSRIs

Eslicarbazepine → see antiepileptics

Esmolol → see beta blockers, selective

Esomeprazole → see proton pump inhibitors

Estramustine → see alkylating agents

Etanercept

▸ Live vaccines are predicted to increase the risk of generalised infection (possibly life-threatening) when given with etanercept. Public Health England advises avoid (refer to Green Book). Severe Theoretical

Etelcalcetide

▸ Cinacalcet increases the risk of hypocalcaemia when given with etelcalcetide. Avoid. Severe Theoretical

Ethambutol

▸ Isoniazid increases the risk of optic neuropathy when given with ethambutol. Severe Anecdotal

Ethosuximide → see antiepileptics

Etodolac → see NSAIDs

Etomidate → see TABLE 8 p. 1335 (hypotension), TABLE 11 p. 1336 (CNS depressant effects)

Etonogestrel

▸ Antiepileptics (carbamazepine, eslicarbazepine, fosphenytoin, oxcarbazepine, perampanel, phenobarbital, phenytoin, primidone, rufinamide, topiramate) are predicted to decrease the efficacy of **etonogestrel**. For FSRH guidance, see Contraceptives, interactions p. 775. Severe Theoretical

▸ Aprepitant is predicted to decrease the efficacy of **etonogestrel**. For FSRH guidance, see Contraceptives, interactions p. 775. Severe Theoretical

▸ Bosentan is predicted to decrease the efficacy of **etonogestrel**. For FSRH guidance, see Contraceptives, interactions p. 775. Severe Theoretical

▸ Efavirenz is predicted to decrease the efficacy of **etonogestrel**. For FSRH guidance, see Contraceptives, interactions p. 775. Severe Theoretical

▸ Fosaprepitant is predicted to decrease the efficacy of **etonogestrel**. For FSRH guidance, see Contraceptives, interactions p. 775. Severe Theoretical

▸ Griseofulvin decreases the efficacy of **etonogestrel**. For FSRH guidance, see Contraceptives, interactions p. 775. Severe Anecdotal

▸ HIV-protease inhibitors (ritonavir) are predicted to decrease the efficacy of **etonogestrel**. For FSRH guidance, see Contraceptives, interactions p. 775. Severe Theoretical

▸ Modafinil is predicted to decrease the efficacy of **etonogestrel**. For FSRH guidance, see Contraceptives, interactions p. 775. Severe Theoretical

▸ Nevirapine is predicted to decrease the efficacy of **etonogestrel**. For FSRH guidance, see Contraceptives, interactions p. 775. Severe Theoretical

▸ Rifabutin is predicted to decrease the efficacy of **etonogestrel**. For FSRH guidance, see Contraceptives, interactions p. 775. Severe Theoretical

▸ Rifampicin is predicted to decrease the efficacy of **etonogestrel**. For FSRH guidance, see Contraceptives, interactions p. 775. Severe Theoretical

▸ St John's Wort is predicted to decrease the efficacy of **etonogestrel**. MHRA advises avoid. For FSRH guidance, see Contraceptives, interactions p. 775. Severe Theoretical

▸ Sugammadex is predicted to decrease the efficacy of **etonogestrel**. Use additional contraceptive precautions. Severe Theoretical

▸ Ulipristal is predicted to decrease the efficacy of **etonogestrel**. Avoid. Severe Theoretical

Etoposide → see TABLE 15 p. 1337 (myelosuppression)

Etoposide (continued)

▸ Antiepileptics (carbamazepine, fosphenytoin, phenobarbital, phenytoin, primidone) are predicted to decrease the efficacy of etoposide. Moderate Study

▸ Ciclosporin increases the exposure to etoposide. Monitor and adjust dose. Severe Study

▸ Live vaccines are predicted to increase the risk of generalised infection (possibly life-threatening) when given with etoposide. Public Health England advises avoid (refer to Green Book). Severe Theoretical

Etoricoxib → see NSAIDs

Etravirine

▸ Antiepileptics (carbamazepine, fosphenytoin, phenobarbital, phenytoin, primidone) are predicted to decrease the exposure to etravirine. Avoid. Severe Theoretical

▸ Etravirine decreases the exposure to antimalarials (artemether). Moderate Study

▸ Etravirine is predicted to decrease the exposure to bedaquiline. Avoid. Severe Theoretical

▸ Bosentan is predicted to decrease the exposure to etravirine. Avoid. Severe Study

▸ Etravirine is predicted to decrease the exposure to bosutinib. Avoid. Severe Theoretical

▸ Etravirine increases the anticoagulant effect of coumarins. Moderate Theoretical

▸ Etravirine is predicted to decrease the exposure to daclatasvir. Avoid. Moderate Theoretical

▸ Etravirine moderately decreases the exposure to dolutegravir. Avoid unless given with atazanavir, darunavir, or lopinavir (all boosted with ritonavir). Severe Study

▸ Efavirenz is predicted to decrease the exposure to etravirine. Avoid. Severe Study

▸ Etravirine is predicted to decrease the exposure to elbasvir. Avoid. Unknown Theoretical

▸ Enzalutamide is predicted to decrease the exposure to etravirine. Avoid. Severe Theoretical

▸ Etravirine is predicted to decrease the exposure to grazoprevir. Avoid. Mild Theoretical

▸ HIV-protease inhibitors (tipranavir) decrease the exposure to etravirine. Severe Study

▸ Etravirine increases the exposure to HIV-protease inhibitors (fosamprenavir) (boosted with ritonavir). Refer to specialist literature. Moderate Study

▸ Etravirine decreases the exposure to macrolides (clarithromycin). Severe Study

▸ Etravirine (with a boosted protease inhibitor) increases the exposure to maraviroc. Avoid or adjust dose. Moderate Study

▸ Mitotane is predicted to decrease the exposure to etravirine. Avoid. Severe Theoretical

▸ Nevirapine is predicted to decrease the exposure to etravirine. Avoid. Severe Study

▸ Etravirine moderately decreases the exposure to phosphodiesterase type-5 inhibitors. Adjust dose. Moderate Study

▸ Rifabutin decreases the exposure to etravirine. Moderate Study

▸ Rifampicin is predicted to decrease the exposure to etravirine. Avoid. Severe Theoretical

▸ Etravirine is predicted to decrease the exposure to rilpivirine. Avoid. Severe Theoretical

▸ Etravirine is predicted to decrease the exposure to simeprevir. Avoid. Moderate Study

▸ St John's Wort is predicted to decrease the exposure to etravirine. Avoid. Severe Study

Everolimus → see TABLE 15 p. 1337 (myelosuppression)

▸ Antiarrhythmics (dronedarone) are predicted to increase the concentration of everolimus. Avoid or adjust dose. Moderate Study

▸ Antiepileptics (carbamazepine, fosphenytoin, phenobarbital, phenytoin, primidone) are predicted to decrease the concentration of everolimus. Avoid or adjust dose. Severe Study

▸ Antifungals, azoles (fluconazole, isavuconazole, posaconazole) are predicted to increase the concentration of everolimus. Avoid or adjust dose. Moderate Study

▸ Antifungals, azoles (itraconazole, ketoconazole, voriconazole) are predicted to increase the concentration of everolimus. Avoid. Severe Study

▸ Aprepitant is predicted to increase the concentration of everolimus. Avoid or adjust dose. Moderate Study

▸ Bosentan is predicted to decrease the concentration of everolimus. Avoid or adjust dose. Moderate Study

▸ Calcium channel blockers (diltiazem, verapamil) are predicted to increase the concentration of everolimus. Avoid or adjust dose. Moderate Study

▸ Ceritinib is predicted to increase the exposure to everolimus. Moderate Theoretical → Also see TABLE 15 p. 1337

▸ Ciclosporin moderately increases the exposure to everolimus. Avoid or adjust dose. Severe Study

▸ Cobicistat is predicted to increase the concentration of everolimus. Avoid. Severe Study

▸ Crizotinib is predicted to increase the concentration of everolimus. Avoid or adjust dose. Moderate Study → Also see TABLE 15 p. 1337

▸ Efavirenz is predicted to decrease the concentration of everolimus. Avoid or adjust dose. Severe Study

▸ Eliglustat is predicted to increase the exposure to everolimus. Adjust dose. Moderate Study

▸ Enzalutamide is predicted to decrease the concentration of everolimus. Avoid or adjust dose. Severe Study

▸ Grapefruit juice is predicted to increase the exposure to everolimus. Avoid. Severe Theoretical

▸ HIV-protease inhibitors are predicted to increase the concentration of everolimus. Avoid. Severe Study

▸ Idelalisib is predicted to increase the concentration of everolimus. Avoid. Severe Study → Also see TABLE 15 p. 1337

▸ Imatinib is predicted to increase the concentration of everolimus. Avoid or adjust dose. Moderate Study → Also see TABLE 15 p. 1337

▸ Lapatinib is predicted to increase the exposure to everolimus. Moderate Theoretical

▸ Live vaccines are predicted to increase the risk of generalised infection (possibly life-threatening) when given with everolimus. Public Health England advises avoid (refer to Green Book). Severe Theoretical

▸ Everolimus is predicted to increase the exposure to lomitapide. Separate administration by 12 hours. Moderate Theoretical

▸ Lumacaftor is predicted to decrease the exposure to everolimus. Avoid. Severe Theoretical

▸ Macrolides (clarithromycin) are predicted to increase the concentration of everolimus. Avoid. Severe Study

▸ Macrolides (erythromycin) are predicted to increase the concentration of everolimus. Avoid or adjust dose. Moderate Study

▸ Mirabegron is predicted to increase the exposure to everolimus. Mild Theoretical

▸ Mitotane is predicted to decrease the concentration of everolimus. Avoid or adjust dose. Severe Study → Also see TABLE 15 p. 1337

▸ Netupitant is predicted to increase the concentration of everolimus. Avoid or adjust dose. Moderate Study

▸ Nevirapine is predicted to decrease the concentration of everolimus. Avoid or adjust dose. Severe Study

▸ Nilotinib is predicted to increase the concentration of everolimus. Avoid or adjust dose. Moderate Study → Also see TABLE 15 p. 1337

▸ Palbociclib is predicted to increase the concentration of everolimus. Adjust dose. Moderate Theoretical

▸ Pitolisant is predicted to decrease the exposure to everolimus. Avoid. Severe Theoretical

▸ Ribociclib is predicted to increase the exposure to everolimus. Use with caution and adjust dose. Moderate Theoretical

▸ Rifampicin is predicted to decrease the concentration of everolimus. Avoid or adjust dose. Severe Study

▸ St John's Wort is predicted to decrease the concentration of everolimus. Avoid or adjust dose. Severe Study

▸ Velpatasvir is predicted to increase the exposure to everolimus. Severe Theoretical

Exemestane

▶ Antiepileptics (carbamazepine, fosphenytoin, phenobarbital, phenytoin, primidone) moderately decrease the exposure to **exemestane**. Moderate Study
▶ Enzalutamide moderately decreases the exposure to **exemestane**. Moderate Study
▶ Mitotane moderately decreases the exposure to **exemestane**. Moderate Study
▶ Rifampicin moderately decreases the exposure to **exemestane**. Moderate Study
▶ St John's Wort is predicted to decrease the exposure to **exemestane**. Moderate Theoretical

Exenatide → see TABLE 14 p. 1337 (antidiabetic drugs)

SEPARATION OF ADMINISTRATION With standard-release exenatide: some orally administered drugs should be taken at least 1 hour before, or 4 hours after, exenatide injection.

Ezetimibe

▶ Ciclosporin moderately increases the exposure to **ezetimibe** and **ezetimibe** slightly increases the exposure to ciclosporin. Moderate Study
▶ Fibrates are predicted to increase the risk of gallstones when given with **ezetimibe**. Severe Theoretical
▶ **Ezetimibe** potentially increases the risk of rhabdomyolysis when given with statins. Severe Anecdotal

Famotidine → see H₂ receptor antagonists

Fampridine

▶ H₂ receptor antagonists (cimetidine) increase the concentration of **fampridine**. Avoid. Severe Theoretical

Febuxostat

▶ **Febuxostat** is predicted to increase the exposure to azathioprine. Avoid. Severe Theoretical
▶ **Febuxostat** is predicted to increase the exposure to didanosine. Severe Theoretical
▶ **Febuxostat** is predicted to increase the exposure to mercaptopurine. Avoid. Severe Theoretical

Felbinac → see NSAIDs
Felodipine → see calcium channel blockers
Fenofibrate → see fibrates
Fenoprofen → see NSAIDs
Fentanyl → see opioids
Ferric carboxymaltose → see iron (injectable)
Ferric maltol → see iron (oral)
Ferrous fumarate → see iron (oral)
Ferrous gluconate → see iron (oral)
Ferrous sulfate → see iron (oral)
Fesoterodine → see TABLE 10 p. 1336 (antimuscarinics)

▶ Antiarrhythmics (dronedarone) are predicted to increase the exposure to **fesoterodine**. Adjust **fesoterodine** dose with moderate inhibitors of CYP3A4 in hepatic and renal impairment, p. 759. Mild Study
▶ Antiepileptics (carbamazepine, fosphenytoin, phenobarbital, phenytoin, primidone) are predicted to decrease the exposure to **fesoterodine**. Avoid. Moderate Study
▶ Antifungals, azoles (fluconazole, isavuconazole, posaconazole) are predicted to increase the exposure to **fesoterodine**. Adjust **fesoterodine** dose with moderate inhibitors of CYP3A4 in hepatic and renal impairment, p. 759. Mild Study
▶ Antifungals, azoles (itraconazole, ketoconazole, voriconazole) are predicted to moderately increase the exposure to **fesoterodine**. Adjust **fesoterodine** dose with potent inhibitors of CYP3A4; avoid in hepatic and renal impairment, p. 759. Severe Study
▶ Aprepitant is predicted to increase the exposure to **fesoterodine**. Adjust **fesoterodine** dose with moderate inhibitors of CYP3A4 in hepatic and renal impairment, p. 759. Mild Study
▶ Calcium channel blockers (diltiazem, verapamil) are predicted to increase the exposure to **fesoterodine**. Adjust **fesoterodine** dose with moderate inhibitors of CYP3A4 in hepatic and renal impairment, p. 759. Mild Study
▶ Cobicistat is predicted to moderately increase the exposure to **fesoterodine**. Adjust **fesoterodine** dose with potent inhibitors of CYP3A4; avoid in hepatic and renal impairment, p. 759. Severe Study
▶ Crizotinib is predicted to increase the exposure to **fesoterodine**. Adjust **fesoterodine** dose with moderate

inhibitors of CYP3A4 in hepatic and renal impairment, p. 759. Mild Study
▶ Enzalutamide is predicted to decrease the exposure to **fesoterodine**. Avoid. Moderate Study
▶ HIV-protease inhibitors are predicted to moderately increase the exposure to **fesoterodine**. Adjust **fesoterodine** dose with potent inhibitors of CYP3A4; avoid in hepatic and renal impairment, p. 759. Severe Study
▶ Idelalisib is predicted to moderately increase the exposure to **fesoterodine**. Adjust **fesoterodine** dose with potent inhibitors of CYP3A4; avoid in hepatic and renal impairment, p. 759. Severe Study
▶ Imatinib is predicted to increase the exposure to **fesoterodine**. Adjust **fesoterodine** dose with moderate inhibitors of CYP3A4 in hepatic and renal impairment, p. 759. Mild Study
▶ Macrolides (clarithromycin) are predicted to moderately increase the exposure to **fesoterodine**. Adjust **fesoterodine** dose with potent inhibitors of CYP3A4; avoid in hepatic and renal impairment, p. 759. Severe Study
▶ Macrolides (erythromycin) are predicted to increase the exposure to **fesoterodine**. Adjust **fesoterodine** dose with moderate inhibitors of CYP3A4 in hepatic and renal impairment, p. 759. Mild Study
▶ Mitotane is predicted to decrease the exposure to **fesoterodine**. Avoid. Moderate Study
▶ Netupitant is predicted to increase the exposure to **fesoterodine**. Adjust **fesoterodine** dose with moderate inhibitors of CYP3A4 in hepatic and renal impairment, p. 759. Mild Study
▶ Nilotinib is predicted to increase the exposure to **fesoterodine**. Adjust **fesoterodine** dose with moderate inhibitors of CYP3A4 in hepatic and renal impairment, p. 759. Mild Study
▶ Rifampicin is predicted to decrease the exposure to **fesoterodine**. Avoid. Moderate Study
▶ St John's Wort is predicted to decrease the exposure to **fesoterodine**. Avoid. Severe Theoretical

Fexofenadine → see antihistamines, non-sedating

Fibrates

bezafibrate · ciprofibrate · fenofibrate · gemfibrozil

▶ Antacids slightly to moderately decrease the exposure to gemfibrozil. Moderate Study
▶ **Bezafibrate** is predicted to increase the risk of nephrotoxicity when given with ciclosporin. Severe Theoretical
▶ **Fenofibrate** increases the risk of nephrotoxicity when given with ciclosporin. Severe Study
▶ Colchicine increases the risk of rhabdomyolysis when given with **fibrates**. Severe Anecdotal
▶ **Fibrates** are predicted to increase the anticoagulant effect of coumarins. Monitor INR and adjust dose. Severe Study
▶ **Gemfibrozil** is predicted to increase the exposure to dabrafenib. Moderate Theoretical
▶ **Fibrates** are predicted to increase the risk of rhabdomyolysis when given with daptomycin. Severe Theoretical
▶ **Gemfibrozil** very markedly increases the exposure to dasabuvir. Avoid. Severe Study
▶ **Gemfibrozil** is predicted to increase the exposure to eluxadoline. Avoid. Moderate Theoretical
▶ **Gemfibrozil** moderately increases the exposure to enzalutamide. Avoid or adjust enzalutamide dose, p. 921. Severe Study
▶ **Fibrates** are predicted to increase the risk of gallstones when given with ezetimibe. Severe Theoretical
▶ **Fibrates** are predicted to increase the risk of hypoglycaemia when given with insulins. Moderate Theoretical
▶ **Gemfibrozil** is predicted to moderately increase the exposure to montelukast. Moderate Study
▶ **Fibrates** are predicted to increase the anticoagulant effect of phenindione. Monitor INR and adjust dose. Severe Study
▶ **Gemfibrozil** increases the exposure to pioglitazone. Monitor blood glucose and adjust dose. Severe Study
▶ **Gemfibrozil** increases the exposure to repaglinide. Avoid. Severe Study
▶ **Gemfibrozil** is predicted to increase the exposure to retinoids (alitretinoin). Adjust alitretinoin dose, p. 1226. Moderate Theoretical

A1

Interactions | Appendix 1

Fibrates (continued)

▶ **Gemfibrozil** increases the concentration of retinoids (bexarotene). Avoid. Severe Study

▶ **Gemfibrozil** increases the exposure to selexipag. Avoid. Severe Study

▶ **Ciprofibrate** increases the risk of rhabdomyolysis when given with statins (atorvastatin). Avoid or adjust dose. Severe Study

▶ **Bezafibrate** increases the risk of rhabdomyolysis when given with statins (atorvastatin, fluvastatin). Severe Study

▶ **Fenofibrate** increases the risk of rhabdomyolysis when given with statins (atorvastatin, simvastatin). Adjust **fenofibrate** dose, p. 198. Severe Anecdotal

▶ **Ciprofibrate** increases the risk of rhabdomyolysis when given with statins (fluvastatin). Severe Study

▶ **Fenofibrate** is predicted to increase the risk of rhabdomyolysis when given with statins (fluvastatin). Adjust **fenofibrate** dose, p. 198. Severe Theoretical

▶ **Fenofibrate** is predicted to increase the risk of rhabdomyolysis when given with statins (pravastatin). Avoid. Severe Theoretical

▶ Fibrates (bezafibrate, ciprofibrate) increase the risk of rhabdomyolysis when given with statins (pravastatin). Avoid. Severe Study

▶ **Fenofibrate** increases the risk of rhabdomyolysis when given with statins (rosuvastatin). Adjust **fenofibrate** and **rosuvastatin** doses, p. 198, p. 202. Severe Anecdotal

▶ Fibrates (bezafibrate, ciprofibrate) increase the risk of rhabdomyolysis when given with statins (rosuvastatin). Adjust **rosuvastatin** dose, p. 202. Severe Study

▶ Fibrates (bezafibrate, ciprofibrate) increase the risk of rhabdomyolysis when given with statins (simvastatin). Adjust **simvastatin** dose, p. 203. Severe Study

▶ **Gemfibrozil** increases the risk of rhabdomyolysis when given with statins. Avoid. Severe Anecdotal

▶ Fibrates are predicted to increase the risk of hypoglycaemia when given with sulfonylureas. Moderate Theoretical

▶ **Gemfibrozil** is predicted to increase the concentration of taxanes (paclitaxel). Severe Anecdotal

▶ Fibrates are predicted to decrease the efficacy of ursodeoxycholic acid. Avoid. Severe Theoretical

Fidaxomicin

▶ Antiarrhythmics (amiodarone, dronedarone) are predicted to increase the exposure to **fidaxomicin**. Avoid. Moderate Study

▶ Antifungals, azoles (itraconazole, ketoconazole) are predicted to increase the exposure to **fidaxomicin**. Avoid. Moderate Study

▶ Calcium channel blockers (verapamil) are predicted to increase the exposure to **fidaxomicin**. Avoid. Moderate Study

▶ Ciclosporin is predicted to increase the exposure to **fidaxomicin**. Avoid. Moderate Study

▶ HIV-protease inhibitors (lopinavir, ritonavir, saquinavir) are predicted to increase the exposure to **fidaxomicin**. Avoid. Moderate Study

▶ Lapatinib is predicted to increase the exposure to **fidaxomicin**. Avoid. Moderate Study

▶ Macrolides are predicted to increase the exposure to **fidaxomicin**. Avoid. Moderate Study

▶ Ranolazine is predicted to increase the exposure to **fidaxomicin**. Avoid. Moderate Study

▶ Vemurafenib is predicted to increase the exposure to **fidaxomicin**. Avoid. Moderate Study

Fingolimod → see TABLE 6 p. 1335 (bradycardia), TABLE 9 p. 1336 (QT-interval prolongation)

▶ Antiepileptics (carbamazepine, fosphenytoin, phenobarbital, phenytoin, primidone) are predicted to decrease the exposure to **fingolimod**. Moderate Study

▶ Calcium channel blockers (diltiazem, verapamil) are predicted to increase the exposure to **fingolimod**. Moderate Theoretical → Also see TABLE 6 p. 1335

▶ Enzalutamide is predicted to decrease the exposure to **fingolimod**. Moderate Study

▶ Live vaccines are predicted to increase the risk of generalised infection (possibly life-threatening) when given with **fingolimod**. Public Health England advises avoid (refer to Green Book). Severe Theoretical

▶ Mitotane is predicted to decrease the exposure to **fingolimod**. Moderate Study

▶ Rifampicin is predicted to decrease the exposure to **fingolimod**. Moderate Study

▶ St John's Wort is predicted to decrease the exposure to **fingolimod**. Avoid. Moderate Theoretical

Flavoxate → see TABLE 10 p. 1336 (antimuscarinics)

Flecainide → see antiarrhythmics

Flucloxacillin → see penicillins

Fluconazole → see antifungals, azoles

Flucytosine

▶ Amphotericin increases the risk of toxicity when given with **flucytosine**. Severe Study

▶ Cytarabine decreases the concentration of **flucytosine**. Avoid. Severe Study

Fludarabine → see TABLE 15 p. 1337 (myelosuppression)

▶ Live vaccines are predicted to increase the risk of generalised infection (possibly life-threatening) when given with **fludarabine**. Public Health England advises avoid (refer to Green Book). Severe Theoretical

▶ **Fludarabine** increases the risk of pulmonary toxicity when given with pentostatin. Avoid. Severe Study → Also see TABLE 15 p. 1337

Fludrocortisone → see corticosteroids

Fluocinolone

ROUTE-SPECIFIC INFORMATION With intravitreal use in adults: caution with concurrent administration of anticoagulant or antiplatelet drugs (higher incidence of conjunctival haemorrhage).

Fluorouracil → see TABLE 15 p. 1337 (myelosuppression), TABLE 5 p. 1334 (thromboembolism)

ROUTE-SPECIFIC INFORMATION Since systemic absorption can follow topical application, the possibility of interactions should be borne in mind.

▶ **Fluorouracil** increases the concentration of antiepileptics (fosphenytoin, phenytoin). Monitor concentration and adjust dose. Severe Anecdotal

▶ **Fluorouracil** increases the anticoagulant effect of coumarins. Severe Anecdotal

▶ Folates (folic acid) are predicted to increase the risk of toxicity when given with **fluorouracil**. Avoid. Severe Theoretical

▶ Folates (folinic acid) are predicted to increase the risk of toxicity when given with **fluorouracil**. Monitor and adjust dose. Severe Theoretical

▶ H_2 receptor antagonists (cimetidine) slightly increase the exposure to **fluorouracil**. Severe Study

▶ Live vaccines are predicted to increase the risk of generalised infection (possibly life-threatening) when given with **fluorouracil**. Public Health England advises avoid (refer to Green Book). Severe Theoretical

▶ Metronidazole increases the risk of toxicity when given with **fluorouracil**. Severe Study

Fluoxetine → see SSRIs

Flupentixol → see TABLE 8 p. 1335 (hypotension), TABLE 11 p. 1336 (CNS depressant effects)

▶ **Flupentixol** is predicted to decrease the effects of dopamine receptor agonists. Avoid. Moderate Theoretical → Also see TABLE 8 p. 1335

▶ **Flupentixol** decreases the effects of levodopa. Avoid or monitor worsening parkinsonian symptoms. Severe Theoretical → Also see TABLE 8 p. 1335

Fluphenazine → see phenothiazines

Flurazepam → see TABLE 11 p. 1336 (CNS depressant effects)

▶ HIV-protease inhibitors (ritonavir) are predicted to increase the exposure to **flurazepam**. Avoid. Moderate Theoretical

Flurbiprofen → see NSAIDs

Fluticasone → see corticosteroids

Fluvastatin → see statins

Fluvoxamine → see SSRIs

Folates

folic acid · folinic acid · levofolinic acid

▶ **Folates** are predicted to decrease the concentration of antiepileptics (fosphenytoin, phenobarbital, phenytoin, primidone). Monitor concentration and adjust dose. Severe Study

- **Folates** are predicted to increase the risk of toxicity when given with capecitabine. Severe Anecdotal
- **Folic acid** is predicted to increase the risk of toxicity when given with fluorouracil. Avoid. Severe Theoretical
- **Folinic acid** is predicted to increase the risk of toxicity when given with fluorouracil. Monitor and adjust dose. Severe Theoretical
- **Folates** are predicted to alter the effects of raltitrexed. Avoid. Moderate Study
- Sulfasalazine is predicted to decrease the absorption of **folates**. Moderate Study
- **Folates** are predicted to increase the risk of toxicity when given with tegafur. Severe Theoretical

Folic acid → see folates
Folinic acid → see folates
Fondaparinux → see TABLE 3 p. 1334 (anticoagulant effects)
Formoterol → see beta₂ agonists
Fosamprenavir → see HIV-protease inhibitors
Fosaprepitant
- Antiepileptics (carbamazepine, fosphenytoin, phenobarbital, phenytoin, primidone) are predicted to decrease the exposure to **fosaprepitant**. Avoid. Moderate Theoretical
- Antifungals, azoles (itraconazole, ketoconazole, voriconazole) are predicted to increase the exposure to **fosaprepitant**. Moderate Theoretical
- **Fosaprepitant** is predicted to increase the exposure to bosutinib. Severe Theoretical
- Cobicistat is predicted to increase the exposure to **fosaprepitant**. Moderate Theoretical
- **Fosaprepitant** is predicted to decrease the efficacy of combined hormonal contraceptives. For FSRH guidance, see Contraceptives, interactions p. 775. Severe Study
- **Fosaprepitant** is predicted to increase the exposure to corticosteroids (dexamethasone, methylprednisolone). Monitor and adjust dose. Moderate Theoretical
- **Fosaprepitant** is predicted to decrease the anticoagulant effect of coumarins. Moderate Theoretical
- **Fosaprepitant** is predicted to decrease the efficacy of desogestrel. For FSRH guidance, see Contraceptives, interactions p. 775. Severe Theoretical
- Enzalutamide is predicted to decrease the exposure to **fosaprepitant**. Avoid. Moderate Theoretical
- **Fosaprepitant** is predicted to decrease the efficacy of etonogestrel. For FSRH guidance, see Contraceptives, interactions p. 775. Severe Theoretical
- **Fosaprepitant** is predicted to increase the concentration of guanfacine. Moderate Theoretical
- HIV-protease inhibitors are predicted to increase the exposure to **fosaprepitant**. Moderate Theoretical
- **Fosaprepitant** is predicted to decrease the effects of hormone replacement therapy. Moderate Anecdotal
- **Fosaprepitant** is predicted to slightly increase the exposure to ibrutinib. Moderate Theoretical
- Idelalisib is predicted to increase the exposure to **fosaprepitant**. Moderate Theoretical
- **Fosaprepitant** is predicted to decrease the efficacy of levonorgestrel. For FSRH guidance, see Contraceptives, interactions p. 775. Severe Theoretical
- **Fosaprepitant** is predicted to increase the exposure to lomitapide. Separate administration by 12 hours. Moderate Theoretical
- Macrolides (clarithromycin) are predicted to increase the exposure to **fosaprepitant**. Moderate Theoretical
- **Fosaprepitant** slightly increases the exposure to midazolam. Moderate Study
- Mitotane is predicted to decrease the exposure to **fosaprepitant**. Avoid. Moderate Theoretical
- **Fosaprepitant** is predicted to decrease the efficacy of norethisterone. For FSRH guidance, see Contraceptives, interactions p. 775. Severe Anecdotal
- **Fosaprepitant** is predicted to increase the exposure to pimozide. Avoid. Severe Theoretical
- Rifampicin is predicted to decrease the exposure to **fosaprepitant**. Moderate Theoretical

- St John's Wort is predicted to decrease the exposure to **fosaprepitant**. Avoid. Moderate Theoretical
- **Fosaprepitant** decreases the efficacy of ulipristal. For FSRH guidance, see Contraceptives, interactions p. 775. Severe Anecdotal

Foscarnet → see TABLE 2 p. 1334 (nephrotoxicity)
- **Foscarnet** increases the risk of hypocalcaemia when given with pentamidine. Severe Anecdotal → Also see TABLE 2 p. 1334
Fosinopril → see ACE inhibitors
Fosphenytoin → see antiepileptics
Frovatriptan → see TABLE 13 p. 1337 (serotonin syndrome)
- SSRIs (fluvoxamine) increase the concentration of **frovatriptan**. Severe Study → Also see TABLE 13 p. 1337
Fulvestrant → see TABLE 5 p. 1334 (thromboembolism)
Furosemide → see loop diuretics
Fusidic acid
- **Fusidic acid** increases the risk of rhabdomyolysis when given with statins. Avoid. Severe Anecdotal
Gabapentin → see antiepileptics
Galantamine → see anticholinesterases, centrally acting
Ganciclovir → see TABLE 15 p. 1337 (myelosuppression), TABLE 2 p. 1334 (nephrotoxicity)

ROUTE-SPECIFIC INFORMATION Since systemic absorption can follow topical application, the possibility of interactions should be borne in mind.

- **Ganciclovir** is predicted to increase the risk of seizures when given with carbapenems (imipenem). Avoid. Severe Anecdotal
- **Ganciclovir** is predicted to increase the exposure to didanosine. Moderate Study
- Mycophenolate is predicted to increase the risk of haematological toxicity when given with **ganciclovir**. Moderate Theoretical → Also see TABLE 15 p. 1337
Gefitinib → see TABLE 15 p. 1337 (myelosuppression)
- Antacids are predicted to slightly decrease the exposure to **gefitinib**. Moderate Theoretical
- Antiarrhythmics (dronedarone) are predicted to increase the exposure to **gefitinib**. Moderate Theoretical
- Antiepileptics (carbamazepine, fosphenytoin, phenobarbital, phenytoin, primidone) are predicted to decrease the exposure to **gefitinib**. Avoid. Severe Study
- Antifungals, azoles (fluconazole, isavuconazole, posaconazole) are predicted to increase the exposure to **gefitinib**. Moderate Theoretical
- Antifungals, azoles (itraconazole, ketoconazole, voriconazole) are predicted to increase the exposure to **gefitinib**. Moderate Study
- Aprepitant is predicted to increase the exposure to **gefitinib**. Moderate Theoretical
- Bosentan is predicted to decrease the exposure to **gefitinib**. Avoid. Severe Theoretical
- Calcium channel blockers (diltiazem, verapamil) are predicted to increase the exposure to **gefitinib**. Moderate Theoretical
- Cobicistat is predicted to increase the exposure to **gefitinib**. Moderate Study
- **Gefitinib** is predicted to increase the anticoagulant effect of coumarins. Severe Anecdotal
- Crizotinib is predicted to increase the exposure to **gefitinib**. Moderate Theoretical → Also see TABLE 15 p. 1337
- Efavirenz is predicted to decrease the exposure to **gefitinib**. Avoid. Severe Theoretical
- Enzalutamide is predicted to decrease the exposure to **gefitinib**. Avoid. Severe Study
- H₂ receptor antagonists are predicted to slightly to moderately decrease the exposure to **gefitinib**. Moderate Study
- HIV-protease inhibitors are predicted to increase the exposure to **gefitinib**. Moderate Study
- Idelalisib is predicted to increase the exposure to **gefitinib**. Moderate Study → Also see TABLE 15 p. 1337
- Imatinib is predicted to increase the exposure to **gefitinib**. Moderate Theoretical → Also see TABLE 15 p. 1337
- Macrolides (clarithromycin) are predicted to increase the exposure to **gefitinib**. Moderate Study
- Macrolides (erythromycin) are predicted to increase the exposure to **gefitinib**. Moderate Theoretical
- Mitotane is predicted to decrease the exposure to **gefitinib**. Avoid. Severe Study → Also see TABLE 15 p. 1337

A1

Interactions | Appendix 1

Gefitinib (continued)
▸ Netupitant is predicted to increase the exposure to **gefitinib**. Moderate Theoretical
▸ Nevirapine is predicted to decrease the exposure to **gefitinib**. Avoid. Severe Theoretical
▸ Nilotinib is predicted to increase the exposure to **gefitinib**. Moderate Theoretical → Also see **TABLE 15** p. 1337
▸ **Gefitinib** is predicted to increase the risk of bleeding events when given with phenindione. Severe Theoretical
▸ Proton pump inhibitors are predicted to decrease the exposure to **gefitinib**. Severe Theoretical
▸ Rifampicin is predicted to decrease the exposure to **gefitinib**. Avoid. Severe Study
▸ St John's Wort is predicted to decrease the exposure to **gefitinib**. Avoid. Severe Theoretical

Gemcitabine → see **TABLE 15** p. 1337 (myelosuppression)
▸ Live vaccines are predicted to increase the risk of generalised infection (possibly life-threatening) when given with **gemcitabine**. Public Health England advises avoid (refer to Green Book). Severe Theoretical

Gemfibrozil → see fibrates
Gentamicin → see aminoglycosides
Glecaprevir
▸ Antiarrhythmics (dronedarone) potentially increase the exposure to **glecaprevir**. Moderate Theoretical
▸ Antiepileptics (carbamazepine, fosphenytoin, phenobarbital, phenytoin, primidone) are predicted to moderately decrease the exposure to **glecaprevir**. Avoid. Severe Study
▸ Antiepileptics (eslicarbazepine, oxcarbazepine) potentially decrease the exposure to **glecaprevir**. Avoid. Severe Theoretical
▸ Antifungals, azoles (itraconazole, ketoconazole) potentially increase the exposure to **glecaprevir**. Moderate Theoretical
▸ Bosentan is predicted to decrease the exposure to **glecaprevir**. Avoid. Severe Study
▸ Ciclosporin increases the exposure to **glecaprevir**. Avoid or monitor. Severe Study
▸ Cobicistat potentially increases the exposure to **glecaprevir**. Moderate Theoretical
▸ Crizotinib potentially decreases the exposure to **glecaprevir**. Avoid. Severe Theoretical
▸ **Glecaprevir** (with pibrentasvir) increases the exposure to dabigatran. Avoid. Moderate Study
▸ **Glecaprevir** (with pibrentasvir) increases the exposure to digoxin. Moderate Study
▸ Efavirenz is predicted to decrease the exposure to **glecaprevir**. Avoid. Severe Study
▸ HIV-protease inhibitors (atazanavir, darunavir, lopinavir) (boosted with ritonavir) increase the exposure to **glecaprevir**. Avoid. Severe Study
▸ HIV-protease inhibitors (ritonavir) potentially increase the exposure to **glecaprevir**. Severe Theoretical
▸ Lumacaftor potentially decreases the exposure to **glecaprevir**. Avoid. Severe Theoretical
▸ Nevirapine is predicted to decrease the exposure to **glecaprevir**. Avoid. Severe Study
▸ Rifampicin markedly affects the exposure to **glecaprevir**. Avoid. Severe Study
▸ St John's Wort is predicted to decrease the exposure to **glecaprevir**. Avoid. Severe Study
▸ **Glecaprevir** (with pibrentasvir) increases the exposure to statins (atorvastatin, simvastatin). Avoid. Moderate Study
▸ **Glecaprevir** (with pibrentasvir) is predicted to increase the exposure to statins (fluvastatin). Moderate Theoretical
▸ **Glecaprevir** (with pibrentasvir) increases the exposure to statins (pravastatin). Use with caution and adjust **pravastatin** dose. Moderate Study
▸ **Glecaprevir** (with pibrentasvir) increases the exposure to statins (rosuvastatin). Use with caution and adjust **rosuvastatin** dose, p. 202. Moderate Study

Glibenclamide → see sulfonylureas
Gliclazide → see sulfonylureas
Glimepiride → see sulfonylureas
Glipizide → see sulfonylureas

Glucagon
▸ Glucagon increases the anticoagulant effect of coumarins (warfarin). Severe Study
Glucosamine
▸ Glucosamine increases the anticoagulant effect of coumarins (warfarin). Avoid. Moderate Anecdotal
Glucose → see **TABLE 3** p. 1334 (anticoagulant effects)
Glycerol phenylbutyrate
▸ Antiepileptics (valproate) potentially oppose the effects of **glycerol phenylbutyrate**. Moderate Theoretical
▸ Corticosteroids potentially oppose the effects of **glycerol phenylbutyrate**. Moderate Theoretical
▸ Haloperidol potentially opposes the effects of **glycerol phenylbutyrate**. Moderate Theoretical
Glyceryl trinitrate → see nitrates
Glycopyrronium → see **TABLE 10** p. 1336 (antimuscarinics)
Golimumab → see monoclonal antibodies
Granisetron → see **TABLE 13** p. 1337 (serotonin syndrome), **TABLE 9** p. 1336 (QT-interval prolongation)
▸ Dopamine receptor agonists (apomorphine) are predicted to increase the risk of severe hypotension when given with granisetron. Severe Theoretical

Grapefruit juice
▸ **Grapefruit juice** moderately decreases the exposure to aliskiren. Avoid. Severe Study
▸ **Grapefruit juice** increases the exposure to antiarrhythmics (amiodarone). Avoid. Moderate Study
▸ **Grapefruit juice** moderately increases the exposure to antiarrhythmics (dronedarone). Avoid. Severe Study
▸ **Grapefruit juice** increases the exposure to antiarrhythmics (propafenone). Monitor and adjust dose. Moderate Study
▸ **Grapefruit juice** slightly increases the exposure to antiepileptics (carbamazepine). Monitor and adjust dose. Moderate Study
▸ **Grapefruit juice** slightly decreases the exposure to antihistamines, non-sedating (bilastine). **Bilastine** should be taken 1 hour before or 2 hours after **grapefruit juice**. Moderate Study
▸ **Grapefruit juice** increases the exposure to antihistamines, non-sedating (rupatadine). Avoid. Moderate Study
▸ **Grapefruit juice** increases the exposure to antimalarials (artemether). Unknown Study
▸ **Grapefruit juice** is predicted to increase the concentration of antimalarials (piperaquine). Avoid. Severe Theoretical
▸ **Grapefruit juice** is predicted to increase the exposure to axitinib. Moderate Theoretical
▸ **Grapefruit juice** greatly decreases the exposure to beta blockers, selective (celiprolol). Moderate Study
▸ **Grapefruit juice** is predicted to increase the exposure to bosutinib. Avoid. Moderate Theoretical
▸ **Grapefruit juice** increases the exposure to buspirone. Avoid. Mild Study
▸ **Grapefruit juice** is predicted to increase the exposure to cabozantinib. Moderate Theoretical
▸ **Grapefruit juice** very slightly increases the exposure to calcium channel blockers (amlodipine). Avoid. Mild Study
▸ **Grapefruit juice** increases the exposure to calcium channel blockers (felodipine). Avoid. Moderate Study
▸ **Grapefruit juice** is predicted to increase the exposure to calcium channel blockers (lercanidipine). Avoid. Moderate Theoretical
▸ **Grapefruit juice** is predicted to increase the exposure to calcium channel blockers (nicardipine). Mild Study
▸ **Grapefruit juice** increases the exposure to calcium channel blockers (nifedipine, verapamil). Avoid. Mild Study
▸ **Grapefruit juice** is predicted to increase the exposure to ceritinib. Avoid. Severe Theoretical
▸ **Grapefruit juice** increases the concentration of ciclosporin. Avoid. Severe Study
▸ **Grapefruit juice** markedly decreases the exposure to clopidogrel. Severe Study
▸ **Grapefruit juice** is predicted to increase the exposure to cobimetinib. Avoid. Severe Theoretical
▸ **Grapefruit juice** moderately increases the exposure to oral corticosteroids (budesonide). Avoid. Moderate Study

▸ **Grapefruit juice** is predicted to increase the exposure to crizotinib. Avoid. [Moderate] Theoretical

▸ **Grapefruit juice** is predicted to increase the exposure to darifenacin. [Moderate] Study

▸ **Grapefruit juice** is predicted to increase the exposure to dasatinib. Avoid. [Moderate] Theoretical

▸ **Grapefruit juice** is predicted to increase the exposure to eliglustat. Avoid. [Severe] Theoretical

▸ **Grapefruit juice** is predicted to increase the exposure to ergometrine. [Severe] Theoretical

▸ **Grapefruit juice** is predicted to increase the exposure to ergotamine. [Severe] Theoretical

▸ **Grapefruit juice** is predicted to increase the exposure to erlotinib. [Moderate] Theoretical

▸ **Grapefruit juice** is predicted to increase the exposure to everolimus. Avoid. [Severe] Theoretical

▸ **Grapefruit juice** is predicted to increase the exposure to guanfacine. Avoid. [Moderate] Theoretical

▸ **Grapefruit juice** is predicted to increase the exposure to ibrutinib. Avoid. [Moderate] Theoretical

▸ **Grapefruit juice** is predicted to increase the exposure to imatinib. [Moderate] Theoretical

▸ **Grapefruit juice** is predicted to increase the exposure to ivabradine. [Moderate] Study

▸ **Grapefruit juice** is predicted to increase the exposure to ivacaftor. Avoid. [Moderate] Theoretical

▸ **Grapefruit juice** is predicted to increase the exposure to lapatinib. Avoid. [Moderate] Theoretical

▸ **Grapefruit juice** is predicted to increase the exposure to lomitapide. Separate administration by 12 hours. [Moderate] Theoretical

▸ **Grapefruit juice** is predicted to increase the exposure to lurasidone. Avoid. [Severe] Theoretical

▸ **Grapefruit juice** is predicted to increase the exposure to naloxegol. Avoid. [Moderate] Theoretical

▸ **Grapefruit juice** is predicted to increase the exposure to nilotinib. Avoid. [Moderate] Theoretical

▸ **Grapefruit juice** is predicted to increase the exposure to olaparib. Avoid. [Moderate] Theoretical

▸ **Grapefruit juice** is predicted to increase the exposure to palbociclib. Avoid. [Severe] Theoretical

▸ **Grapefruit juice** is predicted to increase the exposure to pazopanib. Avoid. [Severe] Theoretical

▸ **Grapefruit juice** is predicted to increase the exposure to phosphodiesterase type-5 inhibitors. Use with caution or avoid. [Moderate] Study

▸ **Grapefruit juice** increases the exposure to pimozide. Avoid. [Severe] Theoretical

▸ **Grapefruit juice** is predicted to increase the exposure to ponatinib. [Moderate] Theoretical

▸ **Grapefruit juice** is predicted to increase the exposure to praziquantel. [Moderate] Study

▸ **Grapefruit juice** is predicted to increase the exposure to quetiapine. Avoid. [Severe] Theoretical

▸ **Grapefruit juice** is predicted to increase the concentration of ranolazine. Avoid. [Severe] Theoretical

▸ **Grapefruit juice** is predicted to increase the exposure to regorafenib. Avoid. [Moderate] Theoretical

▸ **Grapefruit juice** is predicted to increase the exposure to ribociclib. Avoid. [Moderate] Theoretical

▸ **Grapefruit juice** is predicted to increase the exposure to ruxolitinib. [Severe] Theoretical

▸ **Grapefruit juice** is predicted to increase the exposure to saxagliptin. [Mild] Theoretical

▸ **Grapefruit juice** increases the concentration of sirolimus. Avoid. [Moderate] Study

▸ **Grapefruit juice** moderately increases the exposure to SSRIs (sertraline). Avoid. [Moderate] Study

▸ **Grapefruit juice** increases the exposure to statins (atorvastatin). [Mild] Study

▸ **Grapefruit juice** increases the exposure to statins (simvastatin). Avoid. [Severe] Study

▸ **Grapefruit juice** is predicted to increase the exposure to sunitinib. Avoid. [Moderate] Theoretical

▸ **Grapefruit juice** increases the concentration of tacrolimus. Avoid. [Severe] Study

▸ **Grapefruit juice** is predicted to increase the concentration of temsirolimus. Use with caution or avoid. [Moderate] Theoretical

▸ **Grapefruit juice** moderately increases the exposure to ticagrelor. [Moderate] Study

▸ **Grapefruit juice** increases the exposure to tolvaptan. Avoid. [Moderate] Study

▸ **Grapefruit juice** is predicted to increase the exposure to ulipristal. Avoid if used for uterine fibroids. [Moderate] Theoretical

▸ **Grapefruit juice** is predicted to increase the exposure to venetoclax. Avoid. [Severe] Theoretical

Grass pollen extract

GENERAL INFORMATION Desensitising vaccines should be avoided in patients taking beta-blockers (adrenaline might be ineffective in case of a hypersensitivity reaction) or ACE inhibitors (risk of severe anaphylactoid reactions).

Grazoprevir

▸ Antiepileptics (carbamazepine, fosphenytoin, phenobarbital, phenytoin, primidone) are predicted to decrease the exposure to **grazoprevir**. Avoid. [Severe] Study

▸ Antifungals, azoles (itraconazole, ketoconazole, voriconazole) are predicted to moderately to markedly increase the exposure to **grazoprevir**. Avoid. [Severe] Study

▸ Bosentan is predicted to markedly decrease the exposure to **grazoprevir**. Avoid. [Severe] Study

▸ Ciclosporin greatly increases the exposure to **grazoprevir**. Avoid. [Severe] Study

▸ Cobicistat is predicted to moderately to markedly increase the exposure to **grazoprevir**. Avoid. [Severe] Study

▸ Efavirenz is predicted to markedly decrease the exposure to **grazoprevir**. Avoid. [Severe] Study

▸ Enzalutamide is predicted to decrease the exposure to **grazoprevir**. Avoid. [Severe] Study

▸ Etravirine is predicted to decrease the exposure to **grazoprevir**. Avoid. [Mild] Theoretical

▸ HIV-protease inhibitors are predicted to moderately to markedly increase the exposure to **grazoprevir**. Avoid. [Severe] Study

▸ Idelalisib is predicted to moderately to markedly increase the exposure to **grazoprevir**. Avoid. [Severe] Study

▸ Macrolides (clarithromycin) are predicted to moderately to markedly increase the exposure to **grazoprevir**. Avoid. [Severe] Study

▸ Mitotane is predicted to decrease the exposure to **grazoprevir**. Avoid. [Severe] Study

▸ Modafinil is predicted to decrease the exposure to **grazoprevir**. Avoid. [Unknown] Study

▸ Nevirapine is predicted to markedly decrease the exposure to **grazoprevir**. Avoid. [Severe] Study

▸ Rifampicin is predicted to decrease the exposure to **grazoprevir**. Avoid. [Severe] Study

▸ St John's Wort is predicted to markedly decrease the exposure to **grazoprevir**. Avoid. [Severe] Study

▸ **Grazoprevir** increases the exposure to statins (atorvastatin). Adjust **atorvastatin** dose, p. 200. [Moderate] Study

▸ **Grazoprevir** is predicted to increase the exposure to statins (fluvastatin). Adjust **fluvastatin** dose, p. 201. [Unknown] Theoretical

▸ **Grazoprevir** increases the exposure to statins (rosuvastatin). Adjust **rosuvastatin** dose, p. 202. [Moderate] Study

▸ **Grazoprevir** is predicted to increase the exposure to statins (simvastatin). Adjust **simvastatin** dose, p. 203. [Unknown] Theoretical

▸ **Grazoprevir** is predicted to increase the concentration of sunitinib. Use with caution and adjust dose. [Moderate] Theoretical

▸ **Grazoprevir** increases the exposure to tacrolimus. [Moderate] Study

Griseofulvin

▸ Alcohol (beverage) potentially causes a disulfiram-like reaction when given with **griseofulvin**. [Moderate] Anecdotal

▸ Antiepileptics (phenobarbital, primidone) decrease the effects of **griseofulvin**. [Moderate] Study

A1

Interactions | Appendix 1

Griseofulvin (continued)
▸ **Griseofulvin** potentially decreases the efficacy of combined hormonal contraceptives. For FSRH guidance, see Contraceptives, interactions p. 775. [Severe] Anecdotal
▸ **Griseofulvin** potentially decreases the anticoagulant effect of coumarins. [Moderate] Anecdotal
▸ **Griseofulvin** potentially decreases the efficacy of desogestrel. For FSRH guidance, see Contraceptives, interactions p. 775. [Severe] Anecdotal
▸ **Griseofulvin** decreases the efficacy of etonogestrel. For FSRH guidance, see Contraceptives, interactions p. 775. [Severe] Anecdotal
▸ **Griseofulvin** potentially decreases the efficacy of oral levonorgestrel. For FSRH guidance, see Contraceptives, interactions p. 775. [Severe] Anecdotal
▸ **Griseofulvin** potentially decreases the efficacy of norethisterone. For FSRH guidance, see Contraceptives, interactions p. 775. [Severe] Anecdotal
▸ **Griseofulvin** potentially decreases the efficacy of ulipristal. For FSRH guidance, see Contraceptives, interactions p. 775. [Severe] Anecdotal

Guanethidine → see TABLE 8 p. 1335 (hypotension)
▸ Amfetamines (dexamfetamine) decrease the effects of **guanethidine**. [Severe] Study
▸ Benperidol is predicted to decrease the effects of **guanethidine**. [Moderate] Theoretical → Also see TABLE 8 p. 1335
▸ Droperidol is predicted to decrease the effects of **guanethidine**. Monitor and adjust dose. [Moderate] Theoretical → Also see TABLE 8 p. 1335
▸ Haloperidol is predicted to decrease the antihypertensive effects of **guanethidine**. Monitor and adjust dose. [Moderate] Theoretical → Also see TABLE 8 p. 1335
▸ Monoamine-oxidase A and B inhibitors, irreversible are predicted to decrease the antihypertensive effects of **guanethidine**. Avoid and for 14 days after stopping the MAOI. [Severe] Theoretical → Also see TABLE 8 p. 1335
▸ Phenothiazines are predicted to decrease the antihypertensive effects of **guanethidine**. [Moderate] Theoretical → Also see TABLE 8 p. 1335
▸ **Guanethidine** is predicted to increase the effects of sympathomimetics, inotropic (dopamine). [Severe] Theoretical
▸ **Guanethidine** is predicted to increase the effects of sympathomimetics, vasoconstrictor (adrenaline/epinephrine, noradrenaline/norepinephrine). [Moderate] Study
▸ **Guanethidine** increases the effects of sympathomimetics, vasoconstrictor (metaraminol). [Severe] Anecdotal
▸ **Guanethidine** increases the effects of sympathomimetics, vasoconstrictor (phenylephrine). [Severe] Study
▸ Tricyclic antidepressants are predicted to decrease the antihypertensive effects of **guanethidine**. [Moderate] Study → Also see TABLE 8 p. 1335

Guanfacine → see TABLE 8 p. 1335 (hypotension), TABLE 11 p. 1336 (CNS depressant effects)
▸ Antiarrhythmics (dronedarone) are predicted to increase the concentration of **guanfacine**. Adjust **guanfacine** dose, p. 349. [Moderate] Theoretical
▸ Antiepileptics (carbamazepine, fosphenytoin, phenobarbital, phenytoin, primidone) are predicted to decrease the concentration of **guanfacine**. Adjust **guanfacine** dose, p. 349. [Moderate] Study → Also see TABLE 11 p. 1336
▸ Antiepileptics (oxcarbazepine) are predicted to decrease the concentration of **guanfacine**. Monitor and adjust **guanfacine** dose, p. 349. [Moderate] Theoretical
▸ **Guanfacine** increases the concentration of antiepileptics (valproate). Monitor and adjust dose. [Moderate] Study
▸ Antifungals, azoles (fluconazole, isavuconazole, posaconazole) are predicted to increase the concentration of **guanfacine**. Adjust **guanfacine** dose, p. 349. [Moderate] Theoretical
▸ Antifungals, azoles (itraconazole, ketoconazole, voriconazole) are predicted to increase the exposure to **guanfacine**. Adjust **guanfacine** dose, p. 349. [Moderate] Study
▸ Aprepitant is predicted to increase the concentration of **guanfacine**. Adjust **guanfacine** dose, p. 349. [Moderate] Theoretical
▸ Bosentan is predicted to decrease the concentration of **guanfacine**. Adjust dose. [Moderate] Theoretical

▸ Calcium channel blockers (diltiazem, verapamil) are predicted to increase the concentration of **guanfacine**. Adjust **guanfacine** dose, p. 349. [Moderate] Theoretical → Also see TABLE 8 p. 1335
▸ Chloramphenicol is predicted to increase the exposure to **guanfacine**. Adjust **guanfacine** dose, p. 349. [Moderate] Theoretical
▸ Cobicistat is predicted to increase the exposure to **guanfacine**. Adjust **guanfacine** dose, p. 349. [Moderate] Study
▸ Crizotinib is predicted to increase the concentration of **guanfacine**. Adjust **guanfacine** dose, p. 349. [Moderate] Theoretical
▸ Efavirenz is predicted to decrease the concentration of **guanfacine**. Adjust dose. [Moderate] Theoretical
▸ Enzalutamide is predicted to decrease the concentration of **guanfacine**. Adjust **guanfacine** dose, p. 349. [Moderate] Study
▸ Fosaprepitant is predicted to increase the concentration of **guanfacine**. [Moderate] Theoretical
▸ Grapefruit juice is predicted to increase the exposure to **guanfacine**. Avoid. [Moderate] Theoretical
▸ HIV-protease inhibitors are predicted to increase the exposure to **guanfacine**. Adjust **guanfacine** dose, p. 349. [Moderate] Study
▸ Idelalisib is predicted to increase the exposure to **guanfacine**. Adjust **guanfacine** dose, p. 349. [Moderate] Study
▸ Imatinib is predicted to increase the concentration of **guanfacine**. Adjust **guanfacine** dose, p. 349. [Moderate] Theoretical
▸ Macrolides (clarithromycin) are predicted to increase the exposure to **guanfacine**. Adjust **guanfacine** dose, p. 349. [Moderate] Study
▸ Macrolides (erythromycin) are predicted to increase the concentration of **guanfacine**. Adjust **guanfacine** dose, p. 349. [Moderate] Theoretical
▸ Mitotane is predicted to decrease the concentration of **guanfacine**. Adjust **guanfacine** dose, p. 349. [Moderate] Study
▸ Netupitant is predicted to increase the concentration of **guanfacine**. Adjust **guanfacine** dose, p. 349. [Moderate] Theoretical
▸ Nevirapine is predicted to decrease the concentration of **guanfacine**. Adjust dose. [Moderate] Theoretical
▸ Nilotinib is predicted to increase the concentration of **guanfacine**. Adjust **guanfacine** dose, p. 349. [Moderate] Theoretical
▸ Rifampicin is predicted to decrease the concentration of **guanfacine**. Adjust **guanfacine** dose, p. 349. [Moderate] Study
▸ St John's Wort is predicted to decrease the concentration of **guanfacine**. Adjust dose. [Moderate] Theoretical

Guselkumab → see monoclonal antibodies

H₂ receptor antagonists

cimetidine · famotidine · nizatidine · ranitidine

▸ **Cimetidine** decreases the clearance of albendazole. [Moderate] Study
▸ **Cimetidine** increases the concentration of aminophylline. Adjust dose. [Severe] Study
▸ **Cimetidine** slightly increases the exposure to anthracyclines (epirubicin). Avoid. [Moderate] Study
▸ **Cimetidine** increases the exposure to antiarrhythmics (amiodarone). [Moderate] Study
▸ **Cimetidine** slightly increases the exposure to antiarrhythmics (flecainide). Monitor and adjust dose. [Mild] Study
▸ **Cimetidine** increases the exposure to antiarrhythmics (lidocaine). Monitor and adjust dose. [Moderate] Study
▸ **Cimetidine** is predicted to increase the exposure to antiarrhythmics (propafenone). Monitor and adjust dose. [Moderate] Theoretical
▸ **Cimetidine** transiently increases the concentration of antiepileptics (carbamazepine). Monitor concentration and adjust dose. [Moderate] Study
▸ **Cimetidine** increases the concentration of antiepileptics (fosphenytoin, phenytoin). Monitor concentration and adjust dose. [Severe] Study
▸ **H₂ receptor antagonists** are predicted to decrease the absorption of antifungals, azoles (itraconazole). Administer **itraconazole** capsules with an acidic beverage. [Moderate] Study
▸ **H₂ receptor antagonists** are predicted to decrease the absorption of antifungals, azoles (ketoconazole). Administer **ketoconazole** with an acidic beverage. [Moderate] Study
▸ **H₂ receptor antagonists** are predicted to decrease the exposure to antifungals, azoles (posaconazole). Avoid use of posaconazole oral suspension. [Moderate] Study

- **Cimetidine** decreases the clearance of antimalarials (chloroquine). Moderate Study
- **Cimetidine** slightly increases the exposure to antimalarials (quinine). Moderate Study
- **H₂ receptor antagonists** are predicted to decrease the absorption of bosutinib. Moderate Theoretical
- **Cimetidine** slightly increases the exposure to calcium channel blockers (diltiazem, nimodipine). Monitor and adjust dose. Moderate Study
- **Cimetidine** (high-dose) is predicted to increase the exposure to calcium channel blockers (lercanidipine). Moderate Theoretical
- **Cimetidine** moderately increases the exposure to calcium channel blockers (nifedipine). Monitor and adjust dose. Severe Study
- **Cimetidine** increases the exposure to calcium channel blockers (verapamil). Moderate Study
- **Cimetidine** is predicted to slightly increase the exposure to capecitabine. Severe Theoretical
- **H₂ receptor antagonists** are predicted to decrease the absorption of ceritinib. Moderate Theoretical
- **Cimetidine** increases the concentration of ciclosporin. Mild Study
- **Cimetidine** increases the anticoagulant effect of coumarins. Severe Study
- **H₂ receptor antagonists** are predicted to decrease the exposure to dasatinib. Avoid. Moderate Study
- **H₂ receptor antagonists** are predicted to decrease the absorption of dipyridamole (immediate release tablets). Moderate Theoretical
- **Cimetidine** slightly increases the exposure to dopamine receptor agonists (pramipexole). Adjust dose. Moderate Study
- **H₂ receptor antagonists** are predicted to decrease the exposure to erlotinib. **Erlotinib** should be taken 2 hours before or 10 hours after **H₂ receptor antagonists**. Moderate Study
- **Cimetidine** increases the concentration of fampridine. Avoid. Severe Theoretical
- **Cimetidine** slightly increases the exposure to fluorouracil. Severe Study
- **H₂ receptor antagonists** are predicted to slightly to moderately decrease the exposure to gefitinib. Moderate Study
- **H₂ receptor antagonists** decrease the exposure to HIV-protease inhibitors (atazanavir). Monitor and adjust dose. Moderate Study
- **Cimetidine** is predicted to decrease the clearance of hydroxychloroquine. Moderate Theoretical
- **H₂ receptor antagonists** are predicted to decrease the absorption of lapatinib. Avoid. Moderate Theoretical
- **H₂ receptor antagonists** are predicted to decrease the exposure to ledipasvir. Adjust dose, see ledipasvir with sofosbuvir p. 617. Moderate Study
- **H₂ receptor antagonists** (cimetidine, ranitidine) are predicted to increase the exposure to lomitapide. Separate administration by 12 hours. Moderate Theoretical
- **Cimetidine** slightly increases the exposure to macrolides (erythromycin). Moderate Study
- **Cimetidine** increases the concentration of mebendazole. Moderate Study
- **Cimetidine** slightly increases the exposure to metformin. Monitor and adjust dose. Moderate Study
- **Cimetidine** slightly increases the exposure to mirtazapine. Use with caution and adjust dose. Moderate Study
- **Cimetidine** increases the exposure to moclobemide. Adjust **moclobemide** dose, p. 359. Mild Study
- **H₂ receptor antagonists** are predicted to decrease the absorption of nilotinib. **H₂ receptor antagonists** should be taken 10 hours before or 2 hours after **nilotinib**. Mild Theoretical
- **Cimetidine** increases the concentration of opioids (alfentanil). Use with caution and adjust dose. Severe Study
- **Cimetidine** increases the exposure to opioids (fentanyl). Moderate Study
- **H₂ receptor antagonists** are predicted to decrease the exposure to pazopanib. **H₂ receptor antagonists** should be taken 10 hours before or 2 hours after **pazopanib**. Moderate Theoretical
- **Cimetidine** increases the exposure to phenindione. Severe Anecdotal

- **Cimetidine** moderately increases the exposure to praziquantel. Moderate Study
- **H₂ receptor antagonists** are predicted to decrease the exposure to rilpivirine. **H₂ receptor antagonists** should be taken 12 hours before or 4 hours after rilpivirine. Severe Study
- **Cimetidine** slightly increases the exposure to roflumilast. Moderate Study
- **H₂ receptor antagonists** potentially decrease the exposure to sofosbuvir. Adjust dose, see ledipasvir with sofosbuvir p. 617, sofosbuvir with velpatasvir p. 619, and sofosbuvir with velpatasvir and voxilaprevir p. 619. Moderate Study
- **Cimetidine** slightly increases the exposure to SSRIs (citalopram, escitalopram). Adjust dose. Moderate Study
- **Cimetidine** slightly increases the exposure to SSRIs (paroxetine, sertraline). Moderate Study
- **Cimetidine** is predicted to increase the risk of toxicity when given with tegafur. Severe Theoretical
- **Cimetidine** increases the concentration of theophylline. Adjust dose. Severe Study
- **Cimetidine** increases the exposure to tricyclic antidepressants. Moderate Study
- **H₂ receptor antagonists** are predicted to decrease the concentration of velpatasvir. Adjust dose, see sofosbuvir with velpatasvir p. 619. Moderate Study
- **Cimetidine** slightly increases the exposure to venlafaxine. Mild Study
- **Cimetidine** slightly increases the exposure to zolmitriptan. Adjust **zolmitriptan** dose, p. 475. Mild Study

Haloperidol → see TABLE 8 p. 1335 (hypotension), TABLE 9 p. 1336 (QT-interval prolongation), TABLE 11 p. 1336 (CNS depressant effects), TABLE 10 p. 1336 (antimuscarinics)

FOOD AND LIFESTYLE Dose adjustment might be necessary if smoking started or stopped during treatment.

- Antiepileptics (carbamazepine, fosphenytoin, phenobarbital, phenytoin, primidone) decrease the concentration of **haloperidol**. Adjust dose. Moderate Study → Also see TABLE 11 p. 1336
- **Haloperidol** potentially increases the risk of overheating and dehydration when given with antiepileptics (zonisamide). Avoid in children. Severe Theoretical
- Antifungals, azoles (itraconazole) increase the concentration of **haloperidol**. Moderate Study
- **Haloperidol** is predicted to decrease the effects of dopamine receptor agonists. Avoid. Moderate Theoretical → Also see TABLE 8 p. 1335 → Also see TABLE 9 p. 1336 → Also see TABLE 10 p. 1336
- Enzalutamide decreases the concentration of **haloperidol**. Adjust dose. Moderate Study
- **Haloperidol** potentially opposes the effects of glycerol phenylbutyrate. Moderate Theoretical
- **Haloperidol** is predicted to decrease the antihypertensive effects of guanethidine. Monitor and adjust dose. Moderate Theoretical → Also see TABLE 8 p. 1335
- HIV-protease inhibitors (ritonavir) are predicted to increase the exposure to **haloperidol**. Severe Theoretical
- **Haloperidol** decreases the effects of levodopa. Severe Study → Also see TABLE 8 p. 1335
- Mitotane decreases the concentration of **haloperidol**. Adjust dose. Moderate Study
- Rifampicin decreases the concentration of **haloperidol**. Adjust dose. Moderate Study
- **Haloperidol** potentially decreases the effects of sodium phenylbutyrate. Moderate Anecdotal
- SSRIs (fluoxetine) increase the concentration of **haloperidol**. Adjust dose. Moderate Anecdotal
- SSRIs (fluvoxamine) increase the concentration of **haloperidol**. Adjust dose. Moderate Study
- Venlafaxine slightly increases the exposure to **haloperidol**. Severe Study → Also see TABLE 9 p. 1336 → Also see TABLE 11 p. 1336

Heparin (unfractionated) → see TABLE 16 p. 1338 (increased serum potassium), TABLE 3 p. 1334 (anticoagulant effects)

- Ranibizumab increases the risk of bleeding events when given with heparin (unfractionated). Severe Theoretical

HIV-protease inhibitors → see TABLE 9 p. 1336 (QT-interval prolongation)

atazanavir · darunavir · fosamprenavir · lopinavir · ritonavir · saquinavir · tipranavir

- Caution on concurrent use of **atazanavir, lopinavir with ritonavir**, or **ritonavir** with drugs that prolong the PR interval.
- Concurrent use of **saquinavir** with drugs that prolong the PR interval is contra-indicated.
- Caution with concurrent use of **tipranavir** that increase risk of bleeding.

▸ **Tipranavir** slightly decreases the exposure to abacavir. Avoid. Severe Study
▸ **HIV-protease inhibitors** are predicted to increase the exposure to abiraterone. Severe Theoretical
▸ HIV-protease inhibitors **(lopinavir, ritonavir, saquinavir)** are predicted to increase the exposure to afatinib. Separate administration by 12 hours. Moderate Study
▸ **Ritonavir** is predicted to decrease the exposure to agomelatine. Moderate Theoretical
▸ **Ritonavir** decreases the exposure to albendazole. Moderate Study
▸ **HIV-protease inhibitors** are predicted to markedly increase the exposure to aldosterone antagonists **(eplerenone)**. Avoid. Severe Study
▸ HIV-protease inhibitors **(ritonavir, saquinavir)** are predicted to increase the exposure to aliskiren. Moderate Theoretical
▸ **HIV-protease inhibitors** increase the exposure to almotriptan. Mild Study
▸ **HIV-protease inhibitors** are predicted to moderately increase the exposure to alpha blockers **(alfuzosin, tamsulosin)**. Use with caution or avoid. Moderate Study
▸ **HIV-protease inhibitors** are predicted to increase the exposure to alpha blockers **(doxazosin)**. Moderate Study
▸ **HIV-protease inhibitors** moderately increase the exposure to alprazolam. Avoid. Moderate Study
▸ HIV-protease inhibitors **(ritonavir, tipranavir)** are predicted to increase the exposure to amfetamines. Severe Theoretical
▸ **Ritonavir** decreases the exposure to aminophylline. Adjust dose. Moderate Study
▸ **Ritonavir** is predicted to decrease the exposure to anaesthetics, local **(ropivacaine)**. Moderate Theoretical
▸ Antacids are predicted to decrease the absorption of atazanavir. **Atazanavir** should be taken 2 hours before or 1 hour after **antacids**. Severe Theoretical
▸ Antacids are predicted to decrease the absorption of tipranavir. Separate administration by 2 hours. Moderate Study
▸ **HIV-protease inhibitors** are predicted to increase the exposure to antiarrhythmics **(amiodarone)**. Avoid. Severe Theoretical → Also see TABLE 9 p. 1336
▸ **HIV-protease inhibitors** are predicted to increase the exposure to antiarrhythmics **(disopyramide)**. Severe Theoretical → Also see TABLE 9 p. 1336
▸ **HIV-protease inhibitors** very markedly increase the exposure to antiarrhythmics **(dronedarone)**. Avoid. Severe Study → Also see TABLE 9 p. 1336
▸ **HIV-protease inhibitors** are predicted to increase the exposure to antiarrhythmics **(lidocaine)**. Avoid. Severe Study
▸ **HIV-protease inhibitors** are predicted to increase the exposure to antiarrhythmics **(propafenone)**. Monitor and adjust dose. Severe Study
▸ **HIV-protease inhibitors** are predicted to increase the exposure to anticholinesterases, centrally acting **(galantamine)**. Monitor and adjust dose. Moderate Study
▸ **HIV-protease inhibitors** are predicted to increase the exposure to antiepileptics **(carbamazepine)** and antiepileptics **(carbamazepine)** are predicted to decrease the exposure to **HIV-protease inhibitors**. Monitor and adjust dose. Severe Theoretical
▸ **HIV-protease inhibitors** are predicted to affect the exposure to antiepileptics **(fosphenytoin, phenytoin)** and antiepileptics **(fosphenytoin, phenytoin)** decrease the concentration of **HIV-protease inhibitors**. Severe Theoretical

▸ **Ritonavir** slightly decreases the exposure to antiepileptics **(lamotrigine)**. Severe Study
▸ **HIV-protease inhibitors** are predicted to very slightly increase the exposure to antiepileptics **(perampanel)**. Mild Study
▸ **HIV-protease inhibitors** are predicted to affect the concentration of antiepileptics **(phenobarbital, primidone)** and antiepileptics **(phenobarbital, primidone)** are predicted to decrease the concentration of **HIV-protease inhibitors**. Severe Theoretical
▸ **Ritonavir** is predicted to decrease the concentration of antiepileptics **(valproate)**. Severe Anecdotal
▸ Antifungals, azoles **(fluconazole)** slightly increase the exposure to tipranavir. Avoid or adjust dose. Moderate Study
▸ Antifungals, azoles **(miconazole)** are predicted to increase the concentration of **HIV-protease inhibitors**. Use with caution and adjust dose. Moderate Theoretical
▸ Antifungals, azoles **(posaconazole)** are predicted to increase the exposure to **HIV-protease inhibitors**. Moderate Study
▸ **HIV-protease inhibitors** are predicted to increase the exposure to antifungals, azoles **(isavuconazole)**. Avoid or monitor side effects. Severe Study
▸ **HIV-protease inhibitors** are predicted to increase the exposure to antifungals, azoles **(itraconazole)**. Use with caution and adjust dose. Severe Study
▸ **HIV-protease inhibitors** are predicted to increase the exposure to antifungals, azoles **(ketoconazole)**. Use with caution and adjust dose. Moderate Study
▸ **HIV-protease inhibitors** are predicted to affect the exposure to antifungals, azoles **(voriconazole)** and antifungals, azoles **(voriconazole)** potentially affect the exposure to **HIV-protease inhibitors**. Severe Study → Also see TABLE 9 p. 1336
▸ **HIV-protease inhibitors** are predicted to increase the exposure to antihistamines, non-sedating **(mizolastine)**. Avoid. Severe Study
▸ **HIV-protease inhibitors** are predicted to increase the exposure to antihistamines, non-sedating **(rupatadine)**. Avoid. Moderate Study
▸ **HIV-protease inhibitors** decrease the exposure to antimalarials **(atovaquone)**. Avoid if boosted with ritonavir. Moderate Study
▸ **HIV-protease inhibitors** are predicted to increase the concentration of antimalarials **(piperaquine)**. Severe Theoretical
▸ **HIV-protease inhibitors** are predicted to decrease the exposure to antimalarials **(proguanil)**. Avoid. Moderate Study
▸ **HIV-protease inhibitors** are predicted to affect the exposure to antimalarials **(quinine)**. Severe Study → Also see TABLE 9 p. 1336
▸ **Ritonavir** is predicted to increase the exposure to apixaban. Avoid. Severe Theoretical
▸ **HIV-protease inhibitors** are predicted to markedly increase the exposure to aprepitant. Moderate Study
▸ **HIV-protease inhibitors** are predicted to slightly increase the exposure to aripiprazole. Adjust **aripiprazole** dose, p. 391. Moderate Study
▸ **HIV-protease inhibitors** are predicted to increase the exposure to axitinib. Avoid or adjust dose. Moderate Study
▸ **HIV-protease inhibitors** are predicted to increase the exposure to bedaquiline. Avoid prolonged use. Mild Study → Also see TABLE 9 p. 1336
▸ HIV-protease inhibitors **(lopinavir, ritonavir, saquinavir)** are predicted to increase the exposure to beta blockers, non-selective **(nadolol)**. Moderate Study
▸ **Ritonavir** is predicted to increase the exposure to beta blockers, selective **(metoprolol)**. Moderate Study
▸ **HIV-protease inhibitors** are predicted to increase the exposure to beta$_2$ agonists **(salmeterol)**. Avoid. Severe Study
▸ **HIV-protease inhibitors** slightly increase the exposure to bortezomib. Moderate Study
▸ **HIV-protease inhibitors** are predicted to increase the exposure to bosentan. Severe Study
▸ **HIV-protease inhibitors** are predicted to markedly increase the exposure to bosutinib. Avoid or adjust dose. Severe Study → Also see TABLE 9 p. 1336
▸ **Ritonavir** is predicted to decrease the exposure to bupropion. Moderate Study
▸ **HIV-protease inhibitors** are predicted to increase the exposure to buspirone. Adjust **buspirone** dose, p. 338. Severe Study

- HIV-protease inhibitors slightly increase the exposure to cabozantinib. [Moderate] Study → Also see TABLE 9 p. 1336
- Ritonavir is predicted to moderately increase the clearance of caffeine citrate. Monitor and adjust dose. [Moderate] Study
- HIV-protease inhibitors are predicted to increase the exposure to calcium channel blockers (amlodipine, felodipine, lacidipine, nicardipine, nifedipine, nimodipine). Monitor and adjust dose. [Moderate] Study
- HIV-protease inhibitors are predicted to increase the exposure to calcium channel blockers (diltiazem, verapamil). [Severe] Study
- HIV-protease inhibitors are predicted to markedly increase the exposure to calcium channel blockers (lercanidipine). Avoid. [Severe] Study
- HIV-protease inhibitors are predicted to increase the exposure to cannabis extract. Use with caution and adjust dose. [Moderate] Theoretical
- HIV-protease inhibitors are predicted to increase the exposure to ceritinib. Avoid or adjust **ceritinib** dose, p. 945. [Severe] Study → Also see TABLE 9 p. 1336
- HIV-protease inhibitors increase the concentration of ciclosporin. [Severe] Study
- HIV-protease inhibitors are predicted to moderately increase the exposure to cilostazol. Adjust **cilostazol** dose, p. 231. [Moderate] Study
- HIV-protease inhibitors are predicted to moderately increase the exposure to cinacalcet. Adjust dose. [Moderate] Study
- Ritonavir is predicted to affect the exposure to clozapine. Avoid. [Severe] Theoretical
- HIV-protease inhibitors are predicted to markedly increase the exposure to cobimetinib. Avoid or monitor for toxicity. [Severe] Study
- HIV-protease inhibitors are predicted to increase the exposure to colchicine. Avoid potent inhibitors of CYP3A4 or adjust **colchicine** dose, p. 1085. [Severe] Study
- Atazanavir (unboosted) increases the exposure to combined hormonal contraceptives. Adjust dose. [Severe] Study
- Ritonavir is predicted to decrease the efficacy of combined hormonal contraceptives. For FSRH guidance, see Contraceptives, interactions p. 775. [Severe] Study
- HIV-protease inhibitors are predicted to increase the exposure to corticosteroids (beclometasone) (risk with beclometasone is likely to be lower than with other corticosteroids). [Moderate] Theoretical
- HIV-protease inhibitors are predicted to increase the exposure to corticosteroids (betamethasone, budesonide, ciclesonide, deflazacort, dexamethasone, fludrocortisone, fluticasone, hydrocortisone, methylprednisolone, mometasone, prednisolone, prednisone, triamcinolone). Avoid or monitor side effects. [Severe] Study
- HIV-protease inhibitors are predicted to affect the anticoagulant effect of coumarins. [Moderate] Study
- HIV-protease inhibitors are predicted to moderately increase the exposure to crizotinib. Avoid. [Moderate] Study → Also see TABLE 9 p. 1336
- HIV-protease inhibitors (lopinavir, ritonavir, saquinavir) are predicted to increase the exposure to dabigatran. Avoid. [Severe] Theoretical
- HIV-protease inhibitors are predicted to increase the exposure to dabrafenib. Use with caution or avoid. [Moderate] Study
- HIV-protease inhibitors are predicted to moderately increase the exposure to daclatasvir. Adjust **daclatasvir** dose, p. 614. [Moderate] Study
- HIV-protease inhibitors are predicted to markedly to very markedly increase the exposure to darifenacin. Avoid. [Severe] Study
- HIV-protease inhibitors are predicted to markedly increase the exposure to dasatinib. Avoid. [Severe] Study → Also see TABLE 9 p. 1336
- HIV-protease inhibitors very slightly increase the exposure to delamanid. [Severe] Study → Also see TABLE 9 p. 1336
- Ritonavir is predicted to decrease the efficacy of desogestrel. For FSRH guidance, see Contraceptives, interactions p. 775. [Severe] Theoretical
- Ritonavir is predicted to increase the exposure to diazepam. Avoid. [Moderate] Theoretical

- Didanosine (buffered) decreases the exposure to atazanavir. Didanosine should be taken 2 hours after atazanavir. [Severe] Study
- Didanosine (buffered) is predicted to decrease the exposure to darunavir (boosted with ritonavir). Didanosine should be taken 1 hour before or 2 hours after darunavir. [Moderate] Theoretical
- Tipranavir decreases the exposure to didanosine. Separate administration by 2 hours. [Moderate] Study
- Ritonavir increases the concentration of digoxin. Adjust dose and monitor concentration. [Severe] Study
- Fosamprenavir (boosted with ritonavir) slightly decreases the exposure to dolutegravir. Avoid if resistant to HIV-integrase inhibitors. [Severe] Study
- Tipranavir moderately decreases the exposure to dolutegravir. Refer to specialist literature. [Severe] Study
- HIV-protease inhibitors increase the risk of QT-prolongation when given with domperidone. Avoid. [Severe] Study
- HIV-protease inhibitors increase the exposure to dopamine receptor agonists (bromocriptine). [Severe] Study
- HIV-protease inhibitors are predicted to increase the concentration of dopamine receptor agonists (cabergoline). [Moderate] Anecdotal
- Ritonavir is predicted to decrease the exposure to duloxetine. [Moderate] Theoretical
- HIV-protease inhibitors are predicted to increase the exposure to dutasteride. Monitor side effects and adjust dose. [Moderate] Theoretical
- HIV-protease inhibitors (lopinavir, ritonavir, saquinavir) are predicted to slightly increase the exposure to edoxaban. [Severe] Theoretical
- Efavirenz decreases the exposure to HIV-protease inhibitors. Refer to specialist literature. [Severe] Study → Also see TABLE 9 p. 1336
- HIV-protease inhibitors slightly to moderately increase the exposure to elbasvir. Avoid. [Moderate] Study
- HIV-protease inhibitors are predicted to markedly increase the exposure to eletriptan. Avoid. [Severe] Study
- HIV-protease inhibitors are predicted to increase the exposure to eliglustat. Avoid or adjust dose—consult product literature. [Severe] Study
- HIV-protease inhibitors (atazanavir, lopinavir, ritonavir, saquinavir, tipranavir) are predicted to increase the exposure to eluxadoline. Avoid. [Moderate] Theoretical
- HIV-protease inhibitors (atazanavir, lopinavir) (boosted with ritonavir) increase the concentration of elvitegravir. Refer to specialist literature. [Moderate] Study
- HIV-protease inhibitors are predicted to increase the risk of ergotism when given with ergometrine. Avoid. [Severe] Theoretical
- HIV-protease inhibitors are predicted to increase the risk of ergotism when given with ergotamine. Avoid. [Severe] Theoretical
- HIV-protease inhibitors are predicted to slightly increase the exposure to erlotinib. Use with caution and adjust dose. [Moderate] Study
- Ritonavir is predicted to decrease the efficacy of etonogestrel. For FSRH guidance, see Contraceptives, interactions p. 775. [Severe] Theoretical
- Etravirine increases the exposure to fosamprenavir (boosted with ritonavir). Refer to specialist literature. [Moderate] Study
- Tipranavir decreases the exposure to etravirine. Avoid. [Severe] Study
- HIV-protease inhibitors are predicted to increase the concentration of everolimus. Avoid. [Severe] Study
- HIV-protease inhibitors are predicted to moderately increase the exposure to fesoterodine. Adjust **fesoterodine** dose with potent inhibitors of CYP3A4; avoid in hepatic and renal impairment, p. 759. [Severe] Study
- HIV-protease inhibitors (lopinavir, ritonavir, saquinavir) are predicted to increase the exposure to fidaxomicin. Avoid. [Moderate] Study
- Ritonavir is predicted to increase the exposure to flurazepam. Avoid. [Moderate] Theoretical
- HIV-protease inhibitors are predicted to increase the exposure to fosaprepitant. [Moderate] Theoretical

HIV-protease inhibitors (continued)

▶ **HIV-protease inhibitors** are predicted to increase the exposure to gefitinib. Moderate Study

▶ HIV-protease inhibitors (**atazanavir, darunavir, lopinavir**) (boosted with ritonavir) increase the exposure to glecaprevir. Avoid. Severe Study

▶ **Ritonavir** potentially increases the exposure to glecaprevir. Severe Theoretical

▶ **HIV-protease inhibitors** are predicted to moderately to markedly increase the exposure to grazoprevir. Avoid. Severe Study

▶ **HIV-protease inhibitors** are predicted to increase the exposure to guanfacine. Adjust **guanfacine** dose, p. 349. Moderate Study

▶ H$_2$ receptor antagonists decrease the exposure to **atazanavir**. Monitor and adjust dose. Moderate Study

▶ **Ritonavir** is predicted to increase the exposure to haloperidol. Severe Theoretical

▶ **Ritonavir** is predicted to decrease the effects of hormone replacement therapy. Moderate Anecdotal

▶ **HIV-protease inhibitors** are predicted to very markedly increase the exposure to ibrutinib. Avoid potent inhibitors of CYP3A4 or adjust **ibrutinib** dose, p. 952. Severe Study

▶ **HIV-protease inhibitors** are predicted to increase the exposure to imatinib. Moderate Study

▶ **HIV-protease inhibitors** are predicted to increase the risk of toxicity when given with irinotecan. Avoid. Moderate Study

▶ **Ritonavir** is predicted to decrease the exposure to iron chelators (deferasirox). Monitor serum ferritin and adjust dose. Moderate Theoretical

▶ **HIV-protease inhibitors** are predicted to increase the exposure to ivabradine. Avoid. Severe Study

▶ **HIV-protease inhibitors** are predicted to increase the exposure to ivacaftor. Adjust **ivacaftor** p. 292 or **lumacaftor with ivacaftor** p. 293 dose with potent inhibitors of CYP3A4. Severe Study

▶ **HIV-protease inhibitors** are predicted to increase the exposure to lapatinib. Avoid. Moderate Study → Also see TABLE 9 p. 1336

▶ **Ritonavir** is predicted to decrease the efficacy of levonorgestrel. For FSRH guidance, see Contraceptives, interactions p. 775. Severe Theoretical

▶ **HIV-protease inhibitors** are predicted to markedly increase the exposure to lomitapide. Avoid. Severe Study

▶ **HIV-protease inhibitors** are predicted to increase the exposure to lurasidone. Avoid. Severe Study

▶ **HIV-protease inhibitors** are predicted to increase the exposure to macitentan. Moderate Study

▶ Macrolides (clarithromycin) increase the exposure to **saquinavir** and **saquinavir** increases the exposure to macrolides (clarithromycin). Avoid. Severe Study → Also see TABLE 9 p. 1336

▶ Macrolides (erythromycin) are predicted to increase the exposure to **saquinavir**. Avoid. Severe Theoretical → Also see TABLE 9 p. 1336

▶ **Atazanavir** is predicted to increase the exposure to macrolides (clarithromycin). Adjust dose in renal impairment. Severe Study

▶ **Ritonavir** increases the exposure to macrolides (clarithromycin). Adjust dose in renal impairment. Severe Study

▶ **Tipranavir** (boosted with ritonavir) increases the exposure to macrolides (clarithromycin) and macrolides (clarithromycin) increase the exposure to **tipranavir** (boosted with ritonavir). Monitor; adjust dose in renal impairment. Severe Study

▶ HIV-protease inhibitors (**darunavir, fosamprenavir, lopinavir**) (boosted with ritonavir) are predicted to increase the exposure to macrolides (clarithromycin). Adjust dose in renal impairment. Severe Study

▶ HIV-protease inhibitors (**atazanavir, darunavir, fosamprenavir, lopinavir, ritonavir, tipranavir**) are predicted to increase the exposure to macrolides (erythromycin). Severe Theoretical

▶ **Darunavir** (boosted with ritonavir) markedly increases the exposure to maraviroc. Refer to specialist literature. Severe Study

▶ Maraviroc potentially decreases the exposure to **fosamprenavir** and **fosamprenavir** potentially decreases the exposure to maraviroc. Avoid. Severe Study

▶ HIV-protease inhibitors (**atazanavir, saquinavir**) moderately to markedly increase the exposure to maraviroc. Refer to specialist literature. Severe Study

▶ **Lopinavir** (boosted with ritonavir) moderately increases the exposure to maraviroc. Refer to specialist literature. Severe Study

▶ **Ritonavir** markedly increases the exposure to maraviroc. Refer to specialist literature. Severe Study

▶ **Ritonavir** is predicted to decrease the exposure to melatonin. Moderate Theoretical

▶ **HIV-protease inhibitors** are predicted to markedly to very markedly increase the exposure to midazolam. Avoid or adjust dose. Severe Study

▶ **HIV-protease inhibitors** are predicted to very markedly increase the exposure to midostaurin. Avoid or monitor for toxicity. Severe Study

▶ **HIV-protease inhibitors** are predicted to increase the exposure to mirabegron. Adjust **mirabegron** dose in hepatic and renal impairment, p. 763. Moderate Study

▶ **HIV-protease inhibitors** are predicted to increase the exposure to mirtazapine. Moderate Study

▶ **HIV-protease inhibitors** are predicted to increase the exposure to modafinil. Mild Theoretical

▶ HIV-protease inhibitors (**lopinavir, ritonavir, saquinavir**) are predicted to increase the risk of neutropenia when given with monoclonal antibodies (brentuximab vedotin). Monitor and adjust dose. Severe Study

▶ **HIV-protease inhibitors** are predicted to increase the exposure to monoclonal antibodies (trastuzumab emtansine). Avoid. Severe Theoretical

▶ **HIV-protease inhibitors** are predicted to markedly increase the exposure to naloxegol. Avoid. Severe Study

▶ **HIV-protease inhibitors** are predicted to increase the exposure to netupitant. Moderate Study

▶ Nevirapine decreases the exposure to **HIV-protease inhibitors**. Refer to specialist literature. Moderate Study

▶ **HIV-protease inhibitors** are predicted to moderately increase the exposure to nilotinib. Avoid. Severe Study → Also see TABLE 9 p. 1336

▶ HIV-protease inhibitors (**lopinavir, ritonavir, saquinavir**) are predicted to increase the exposure to nintedanib. Moderate Study

▶ **HIV-protease inhibitors** are predicted to increase the exposure to nitisinone. Adjust dose. Moderate Theoretical

▶ **Ritonavir** is predicted to decrease the efficacy of norethisterone. For FSRH guidance, see Contraceptives, interactions p. 775. Severe Anecdotal

▶ **Ritonavir** is predicted to decrease the exposure to olanzapine. Monitor and adjust dose. Moderate Study

▶ **HIV-protease inhibitors** are predicted to increase the exposure to olaparib. Avoid potent inhibitors of CYP3A4 or adjust **olaparib** dose, p. 973. Moderate Study

▶ **HIV-protease inhibitors** are predicted to increase the exposure to opioids (alfentanil, buprenorphine, fentanyl, oxycodone, sufentanil). Monitor and adjust dose. Severe Study

▶ **HIV-protease inhibitors** (boosted with ritonavir) are predicted to decrease the exposure to opioids (methadone). Moderate Study → Also see TABLE 9 p. 1336

▶ **Ritonavir** is predicted to decrease the concentration of opioids (morphine). Moderate Theoretical

▶ **Ritonavir** increases the risk of CNS toxicity when given with opioids (pethidine). Avoid. Severe Study

▶ **HIV-protease inhibitors** are predicted to increase the exposure to oxybutynin. Mild Study

▶ **HIV-protease inhibitors** are predicted to increase the exposure to palbociclib. Avoid or adjust **palbociclib** dose, p. 961. Severe Study

▶ **HIV-protease inhibitors** are predicted to increase the exposure to panobinostat. Adjust **panobinostat** dose; in hepatic impairment avoid, p. 911. Moderate Study → Also see TABLE 9 p. 1336

▶ **HIV-protease inhibitors** are predicted to increase the exposure to paritaprevir (with ritonavir and ombitasvir). Avoid. Severe Theoretical

▶ **HIV-protease inhibitors** are predicted to increase the exposure to pazopanib. Avoid or adjust **pazopanib** dose, p. 962. Moderate Study → Also see TABLE 9 p. 1336

▸ **HIV-protease inhibitors** are predicted to increase the exposure to phosphodiesterase type-5 inhibitors (**avanafil, vardenafil**). Avoid. [Severe] Study →Also see TABLE 9 p. 1336

▸ **HIV-protease inhibitors** are predicted to increase the exposure to phosphodiesterase type-5 inhibitors (**sildenafil**). Avoid potent inhibitors of CYP3A4 or adjust **sildenafil** dose, p. 794. [Severe] Study →Also see TABLE 9 p. 1336

▸ **HIV-protease inhibitors** are predicted to increase the exposure to phosphodiesterase type-5 inhibitors (**tadalafil**). Use with caution or avoid. [Severe] Study

▸ HIV-protease inhibitors (**atazanavir, lopinavir**) (boosted with ritonavir) increase the exposure to pibrentasvir. Avoid. [Severe] Study

▸ **Ritonavir** potentially increases the exposure to pibrentasvir. [Severe] Theoretical

▸ **HIV-protease inhibitors** are predicted to increase the exposure to pimozide. Avoid. [Severe] Study →Also see TABLE 9 p. 1336

▸ **Ritonavir** is predicted to decrease the exposure to pirfenidone. [Moderate] Theoretical

▸ **Ritonavir** is predicted to increase the exposure to pitolisant. Use with caution and adjust dose. [Moderate] Study

▸ **HIV-protease inhibitors** are predicted to slightly increase the exposure to ponatinib. Monitor and adjust **ponatinib** dose, p. 963. [Moderate] Study

▸ **HIV-protease inhibitors** are predicted to moderately increase the exposure to praziquantel. [Mild] Study

▸ Proton pump inhibitors decrease the exposure to **atazanavir**. Avoid or adjust dose. [Severe] Study

▸ Proton pump inhibitors increase the exposure to **saquinavir**. Avoid. [Severe] Study

▸ **Tipranavir** decreases the exposure to proton pump inhibitors. Avoid. [Severe] Study

▸ **HIV-protease inhibitors** are predicted to increase the exposure to quetiapine. Avoid. [Severe] Study

▸ **Atazanavir** increases the exposure to raltegravir (high-dose). Avoid. [Moderate] Study

▸ **Darunavir** increases the risk of rash when given with raltegravir. [Moderate] Study

▸ **Fosamprenavir** (boosted with ritonavir) decreases the exposure to raltegravir and raltegravir decreases the exposure to **fosamprenavir** (boosted with ritonavir). Avoid. [Severe] Study

▸ **Tipranavir** (boosted with ritonavir) is predicted to decrease the exposure to raltegravir (high-dose). Avoid. [Moderate] Study

▸ **HIV-protease inhibitors** are predicted to increase the exposure to ranolazine. Avoid. [Severe] Study →Also see TABLE 9 p. 1336

▸ **HIV-protease inhibitors** are predicted to increase the exposure to reboxetine. Avoid. [Moderate] Study

▸ **HIV-protease inhibitors** are predicted to increase the exposure to regorafenib. Avoid. [Moderate] Study

▸ **HIV-protease inhibitors** are predicted to increase the exposure to repaglinide. [Moderate] Study

▸ **HIV-protease inhibitors** are predicted to increase the exposure to retinoids (**alitretinoin**). Adjust **alitretinoin** dose, p. 1226. [Moderate] Theoretical

▸ **HIV-protease inhibitors** are predicted to increase the exposure to ribociclib. Avoid or adjust **ribociclib** dose, p. 965. [Moderate] Study →Also see TABLE 9 p. 1336

▸ HIV-protease inhibitors (**atazanavir, darunavir, fosamprenavir, lopinavir, saquinavir, tipranavir**) (boosted with ritonavir) increase the exposure to rifabutin. Monitor and adjust dose. [Severe] Study →Also see TABLE 9 p. 1336

▸ **Ritonavir** markedly increases the exposure to rifabutin. Avoid or adjust dose. [Severe] Study

▸ Rifampicin is predicted to moderately to markedly decrease the exposure to HIV-protease inhibitors (**atazanavir, darunavir, fosamprenavir, lopinavir, saquinavir**). Avoid. [Severe] Study

▸ Rifampicin slightly decreases the exposure to **ritonavir**. [Severe] Study

▸ Rifampicin is predicted to decrease the exposure to **tipranavir**. Avoid. [Severe] Study

▸ **Ritonavir** is predicted to increase the exposure to riociguat. Avoid. [Moderate] Theoretical

▸ **HIV-protease inhibitors** are predicted to increase the exposure to risperidone. Adjust dose. [Moderate] Study →Also see TABLE 9 p. 1336

▸ Ritonavir moderately increases the exposure to rivaroxaban. Avoid. [Severe] Study

▸ **HIV-protease inhibitors** are predicted to increase the exposure to ruxolitinib. Adjust dose and monitor side effects. [Moderate] Study

▸ **HIV-protease inhibitors** are predicted to increase the exposure to saxagliptin. [Moderate] Study

▸ **HIV-protease inhibitors** are predicted to increase the exposure to simeprevir. Avoid. [Severe] Study

▸ **HIV-protease inhibitors** are predicted to increase the concentration of sirolimus. Avoid. [Severe] Study

▸ **Tipranavir** is predicted to decrease the exposure to sofosbuvir. Avoid. [Severe] Theoretical

▸ **HIV-protease inhibitors** are predicted to increase the exposure to solifenacin. Adjust **solifenacin** p. 761 or **tamsulosin with solifenacin** p. 768 dose; avoid in hepatic and renal impairment. [Severe] Study

▸ **HIV-protease inhibitors** are predicted to moderately increase the exposure to SSRIs (**dapoxetine**). Avoid potent inhibitors of CYP3A4 or adjust **dapoxetine** dose, p. 801. [Severe] Study

▸ St John's Wort is predicted to decrease the exposure to **HIV-protease inhibitors**. Avoid. [Severe] Study

▸ **HIV-protease inhibitors** are predicted to increase the exposure to statins (**atorvastatin**). Avoid or adjust dose and monitor rhabdomyolysis. [Severe] Study

▸ **HIV-protease inhibitors** slightly to moderately increase the exposure to statins (**rosuvastatin**). Avoid or adjust dose. [Severe] Study

▸ **HIV-protease inhibitors** are predicted to increase the exposure to statins (**simvastatin**). Avoid. [Severe] Study

▸ **HIV-protease inhibitors** are predicted to slightly increase the exposure to sunitinib. Avoid or adjust **sunitinib** dose, p. 967. [Moderate] Study →Also see TABLE 9 p. 1336

▸ **HIV-protease inhibitors** are predicted to increase the concentration of tacrolimus. Monitor and adjust dose. [Severe] Study

▸ **HIV-protease inhibitors** are predicted to increase the exposure to taxanes (**cabazitaxel**). Avoid. [Severe] Study

▸ **HIV-protease inhibitors** are predicted to moderately increase the exposure to taxanes (**docetaxel**). Avoid or adjust dose. [Severe] Study

▸ **HIV-protease inhibitors** are predicted to increase the exposure to taxanes (**paclitaxel**). [Severe] Theoretical

▸ **HIV-protease inhibitors** are predicted to increase the concentration of temsirolimus. Avoid. [Severe] Theoretical

▸ HIV-protease inhibitors (**atazanavir, darunavir**) increase the exposure to tenofovir alafenamide. Avoid. [Moderate] Study

▸ **Tipranavir** is predicted to affect the exposure to tenofovir alafenamide. Avoid. [Moderate] Theoretical

▸ **Ritonavir** is predicted to decrease the exposure to theophylline. Adjust dose. [Moderate] Study

▸ **HIV-protease inhibitors** are predicted to markedly increase the exposure to ticagrelor. Avoid. [Severe] Study

▸ **Ritonavir** moderately decreases the exposure to tizanidine. [Mild] Study

▸ **HIV-protease inhibitors** are predicted to increase the exposure to tofacitinib. Adjust **tofacitinib** dose, p. 1072. [Moderate] Study

▸ **HIV-protease inhibitors** are predicted to increase the exposure to tolterodine. Avoid. [Severe] Study →Also see TABLE 9 p. 1336

▸ **HIV-protease inhibitors** are predicted to increase the exposure to tolvaptan. Adjust dose. [Severe] Study

▸ HIV-protease inhibitors (**lopinavir, ritonavir, saquinavir**) are predicted to increase the exposure to topotecan. [Severe] Study

▸ **HIV-protease inhibitors** are predicted to increase the exposure to toremifene. [Moderate] Theoretical →Also see TABLE 9 p. 1336

▸ **HIV-protease inhibitors** are predicted to increase the exposure to trabectedin. Avoid or adjust dose. [Severe] Theoretical

▸ HIV-protease inhibitors (**lopinavir, ritonavir, saquinavir**) are predicted to increase the concentration of trametinib. [Moderate] Theoretical

▸ **HIV-protease inhibitors** are predicted to moderately increase the exposure to trazodone. Avoid or adjust dose. [Moderate] Study

Interactions | Appendix 1

HIV-protease inhibitors (continued)

▸ HIV-protease inhibitors **(ritonavir, tipranavir)** are predicted to increase the exposure to tricyclic antidepressants. Moderate Theoretical

▸ HIV-protease inhibitors **(atazanavir, darunavir, fosamprenavir, lopinavir, saquinavir, tipranavir)** are predicted to increase the exposure to ulipristal. Avoid if used for uterine fibroids. Severe Study

▸ **Ritonavir** decreases the efficacy of ulipristal. For FSRH guidance, see Contraceptives, interactions p. 775. Severe Anecdotal

▸ **HIV-protease inhibitors** are predicted to increase the exposure to vemurafenib. Severe Theoretical → Also see TABLE 9 p. 1336

▸ **HIV-protease inhibitors** are predicted to increase the exposure to venetoclax. Avoid potent inhibitors of CYP3A4 or adjust **venetoclax** dose, p. 974. Severe Study

▸ **HIV-protease inhibitors** are predicted to increase the exposure to venlafaxine. Moderate Study → Also see TABLE 9 p. 1336

▸ **HIV-protease inhibitors** are predicted to increase the exposure to vinca alkaloids. Severe Theoretical → Also see TABLE 9 p. 1336

▸ **HIV-protease inhibitors** are predicted to increase the exposure to vitamin D substances (paricalcitol). Moderate Study

▸ **Atazanavir** (boosted with ritonavir) increases the concentration of voxilaprevir. Avoid. Severe Study

▸ **Lopinavir** is predicted to increase the concentration of voxilaprevir. Avoid. Severe Theoretical

▸ **Tipranavir** slightly decreases the exposure to zidovudine. Avoid. Moderate Study

▸ **HIV-protease inhibitors** are predicted to increase the exposure to zopiclone. Adjust dose. Moderate Theoretical

Homatropine → see TABLE 10 p. 1336 (antimuscarinics)

Hormone replacement therapy

▸ Antiepileptics **(carbamazepine, eslicarbazepine, fosphenytoin, oxcarbazepine, perampanel, phenobarbital, phenytoin, primidone, rufinamide, topiramate)** are predicted to decrease the effects of **hormone replacement therapy**. Moderate Anecdotal

▸ **Hormone replacement therapy** is predicted to alter the exposure to antiepileptics **(lamotrigine)**. Moderate Theoretical

▸ **Aprepitant** is predicted to decrease the effects of **hormone replacement therapy**. Moderate Anecdotal

▸ **Bosentan** is predicted to decrease the effects of **hormone replacement therapy**. Moderate Anecdotal

▸ **Hormone replacement therapy** decreases the clearance of dopamine receptor agonists **(ropinirole)**. Monitor and adjust dose. Moderate Study

▸ **Efavirenz** is predicted to decrease the effects of **hormone replacement therapy**. Moderate Anecdotal

▸ **Fosaprepitant** is predicted to decrease the effects of **hormone replacement therapy**. Moderate Anecdotal

▸ HIV-protease inhibitors **(ritonavir)** are predicted to decrease the effects of **hormone replacement therapy**. Moderate Anecdotal

▸ **Hormone replacement therapy** is predicted to increase the risk of venous thromboembolism when given with lenalidomide. Severe Theoretical

▸ **Modafinil** is predicted to decrease the effects of **hormone replacement therapy**. Moderate Anecdotal

▸ **Hormone replacement therapy** is predicted to decrease the exposure to monoamine-oxidase B inhibitors **(selegiline)**. Avoid. Moderate Study

▸ **Nevirapine** is predicted to decrease the effects of **hormone replacement therapy**. Moderate Anecdotal

▸ NSAIDs **(etoricoxib)** slightly increase the exposure to **hormone replacement therapy**. Moderate Study

▸ **Hormone replacement therapy** is predicted to increase the risk of venous thromboembolism when given with pomalidomide. Severe Theoretical

▸ **Rifabutin** is predicted to decrease the effects of **hormone replacement therapy**. Moderate Anecdotal

▸ **Rifampicin** is predicted to decrease the effects of **hormone replacement therapy**. Moderate Anecdotal

▸ **St John's Wort** is predicted to decrease the efficacy of **hormone replacement therapy**. Moderate Theoretical

▸ **Hormone replacement therapy** is predicted to increase the risk of venous thromboembolism when given with thalidomide. Severe Theoretical

▸ Oral **hormone replacement therapy** is predicted to decrease the effects of thyroid hormones. Moderate Theoretical

Hydralazine → see TABLE 8 p. 1335 (hypotension)

▸ Diazoxide increases the risk of severe hypotension when given with hydralazine. Severe Study → Also see TABLE 8 p. 1335

Hydrochlorothiazide → see thiazide diuretics

Hydrocortisone → see corticosteroids

Hydroflumethiazide → see thiazide diuretics

Hydromorphone → see opioids

Hydroxycarbamide → see TABLE 15 p. 1337 (myelosuppression)

▸ **Hydroxycarbamide** increases the risk of toxicity when given with didanosine. Avoid. Severe Study

▸ Live vaccines are predicted to increase the risk of generalised infection (possibly life-threatening) when given with **hydroxycarbamide**. Public Health England advises avoid (refer to Green Book). Severe Theoretical

▸ **Hydroxycarbamide** increases the risk of toxicity when given with stavudine. Avoid. Severe Study

Hydroxychloroquine

▸ **Hydroxychloroquine** is predicted to decrease the effects of agalsidase. Moderate Theoretical

▸ Antacids decrease the absorption of **hydroxychloroquine**. Separate administration by at least 4 hours. Moderate Study

▸ Calcium salts **(calcium carbonate)** decrease the absorption of **hydroxychloroquine**. Separate administration by at least 4 hours. Moderate Study

▸ **Hydroxychloroquine** is predicted to decrease the efficacy of oral cholera vaccine. Moderate Theoretical

▸ H₂ receptor antagonists **(cimetidine)** are predicted to decrease the clearance of **hydroxychloroquine**. Moderate Theoretical

▸ Lanthanum is predicted to decrease the absorption of **hydroxychloroquine**. Separate administration by at least 2 hours. Moderate Theoretical

▸ **Hydroxychloroquine** is predicted to decrease the exposure to laronidase. Avoid simultaneous administration. Severe Theoretical

▸ **Hydroxychloroquine** is predicted to increase the risk of haematological toxicity when given with penicillamine. Avoid. Severe Theoretical

▸ **Hydroxychloroquine** is predicted to decrease efficacy rabies vaccine. Moderate Theoretical

Hydroxyzine → see antihistamines, sedating

Hyoscine → see TABLE 10 p. 1336 (antimuscarinics)

Ibandronic acid → see bisphosphonates

Ibrutinib → see TABLE 15 p. 1337 (myelosuppression), TABLE 4 p. 1334 (antiplatelet effects)

FOOD AND LIFESTYLE Avoid food or drink containing bitter (Seville) oranges as they are predicted to increase the exposure to ibrutinib.

▸ Antiarrhythmics **(amiodarone)** are predicted to increase the exposure to **ibrutinib**. Adjust **ibrutinib** dose, p. 952. Severe Theoretical

▸ Antiarrhythmics **(dronedarone)** are predicted to increase the exposure to **ibrutinib**. Adjust **ibrutinib** dose with moderate inhibitors of CYP3A4, p. 952. Severe Study

▸ Antiepileptics **(carbamazepine, fosphenytoin, phenobarbital, phenytoin, primidone)** are predicted to decrease the exposure to **ibrutinib**. Avoid or adjust **ibrutinib** dose, p. 952. Severe Study

▸ Antifungals, azoles **(fluconazole, isavuconazole, posaconazole)** are predicted to increase the exposure to **ibrutinib**. Adjust **ibrutinib** dose with moderate inhibitors of CYP3A4, p. 952. Severe Study

▸ Antifungals, azoles **(itraconazole, ketoconazole, voriconazole)** are predicted to very markedly increase the exposure to **ibrutinib**. Avoid potent inhibitors of CYP3A4 or adjust **ibrutinib** dose, p. 952. Severe Study

▸ Aprepitant is predicted to increase the exposure to **ibrutinib**. Adjust **ibrutinib** dose with moderate inhibitors of CYP3A4, p. 952. Severe Study

▸ Calcium channel blockers **(diltiazem, verapamil)** are predicted to increase the exposure to **ibrutinib**. Adjust **ibrutinib** dose with moderate inhibitors of CYP3A4, p. 952. Severe Study

▸ Cobicistat is predicted to very markedly increase the exposure to **ibrutinib**. Avoid potent inhibitors of CYP3A4 or adjust **ibrutinib** dose, p. 952. Severe Study

- ► Crizotinib is predicted to increase the exposure to **ibrutinib**. Adjust **ibrutinib** dose with moderate inhibitors of CYP3A4, p. 952. Severe Study → Also see TABLE 15 p. 1337
- ► Enzalutamide is predicted to decrease the exposure to **ibrutinib**. Avoid or adjust **ibrutinib** dose, p. 952. Severe Study
- ► Fosaprepitant is predicted to slightly increase the exposure to **ibrutinib**. Moderate Theoretical
- ► Grapefruit juice is predicted to increase the exposure to **ibrutinib**. Avoid. Moderate Theoretical
- ► HIV-protease inhibitors are predicted to very markedly increase the exposure to **ibrutinib**. Avoid potent inhibitors of CYP3A4 or adjust **ibrutinib** dose. Severe Study
- ► Idelalisib is predicted to very markedly increase the exposure to **ibrutinib**. Avoid potent inhibitors of CYP3A4 or adjust **ibrutinib** dose, p. 952. Severe Study → Also see TABLE 15 p. 1337
- ► Imatinib is predicted to increase the exposure to **ibrutinib**. Adjust **ibrutinib** dose with moderate inhibitors of CYP3A4, p. 952. Severe Study → Also see TABLE 15 p. 1337
- ► Macrolides (clarithromycin) are predicted to very markedly increase the exposure to **ibrutinib**. Avoid potent inhibitors of CYP3A4 or adjust **ibrutinib** dose, p. 952. Severe Study
- ► Macrolides (erythromycin) are predicted to increase the exposure to **ibrutinib**. Adjust **ibrutinib** dose with moderate inhibitors of CYP3A4, p. 952. Severe Study
- ► Mitotane is predicted to decrease the exposure to **ibrutinib**. Avoid or adjust **ibrutinib** dose, p. 952. Severe Study → Also see TABLE 15 p. 1337
- ► Netupitant is predicted to increase the exposure to **ibrutinib**. Adjust **ibrutinib** dose with moderate inhibitors of CYP3A4, p. 952. Severe Study
- ► Nilotinib is predicted to increase the exposure to **ibrutinib**. Adjust **ibrutinib** dose with moderate inhibitors of CYP3A4, p. 952. Severe Study → Also see TABLE 15 p. 1337
- ► Quinolones (ciprofloxacin) are predicted to increase the exposure to **ibrutinib**. Adjust **ibrutinib** dose, p. 952. Severe Theoretical
- ► Rifampicin is predicted to decrease the exposure to **ibrutinib**. Avoid or adjust **ibrutinib** dose, p. 952. Severe Study
- ► St John's Wort is predicted to decrease the exposure to **ibrutinib**. Avoid. Severe Theoretical

Ibuprofen → see NSAIDs

Icatibant
- ► ACE inhibitors are predicted to decrease the efficacy of **icatibant** and **icatibant** is predicted to decrease the efficacy of ACE inhibitors. Avoid. Moderate Theoretical

Idarubicin → see anthracyclines

Idelalisib → see TABLE 15 p. 1337 (myelosuppression)
- ► Idelalisib is predicted to increase the exposure to abiraterone. Severe Theoretical
- ► Idelalisib is predicted to markedly increase the exposure to aldosterone antagonists (eplerenone). Avoid. Severe Theoretical
- ► Idelalisib increases the exposure to almotriptan. Mild Study
- ► Idelalisib is predicted to moderately increase the exposure to alpha blockers (alfuzosin, tamsulosin). Use with caution or avoid. Moderate Study
- ► Idelalisib is predicted to increase the exposure to alpha blockers (doxazosin). Moderate Study
- ► Idelalisib moderately increases the exposure to alprazolam. Avoid. Moderate Study
- ► Idelalisib is predicted to increase the exposure to antiarrhythmics (amiodarone). Avoid. Moderate Theoretical
- ► Idelalisib very markedly increases the exposure to antiarrhythmics (dronedarone). Avoid. Severe Study
- ► Idelalisib is predicted to increase the exposure to antiarrhythmics (propafenone). Monitor and adjust dose. Severe Study
- ► Idelalisib is predicted to increase the exposure to anticholinesterases, centrally acting (galantamine). Monitor and adjust dose. Moderate Study
- ► Antiepileptics (carbamazepine, fosphenytoin, phenobarbital, phenytoin, primidone) are predicted to decrease the exposure to **idelalisib**. Avoid. Severe Study
- ► Idelalisib is predicted to very slightly increase the exposure to antiepileptics (perampanel). Mild Study

- ► Idelalisib is predicted to increase the exposure to antifungals, azoles (isavuconazole). Avoid or monitor side effects. Severe Study
- ► Idelalisib is predicted to increase the exposure to antihistamines, non-sedating (mizolastine). Avoid. Severe Study
- ► Idelalisib is predicted to increase the exposure to antihistamines, non-sedating (rupatadine). Avoid. Moderate Study
- ► Idelalisib is predicted to increase the concentration of antimalarials (piperaquine). Severe Theoretical
- ► Idelalisib is predicted to markedly increase the exposure to aprepitant. Moderate Study
- ► Idelalisib is predicted to slightly increase the exposure to aripiprazole. Adjust **aripiprazole** dose, p. 391. Moderate Study
- ► Idelalisib is predicted to increase the exposure to axitinib. Avoid or adjust dose. Moderate Study → Also see TABLE 15 p. 1337
- ► Idelalisib is predicted to increase the exposure to bedaquiline. Avoid prolonged use. Mild Study
- ► Idelalisib is predicted to increase the exposure to beta₂ agonists (salmeterol). Avoid. Severe Study
- ► Idelalisib slightly increases the exposure to bortezomib. Moderate Study → Also see TABLE 15 p. 1337
- ► Bosentan is predicted to decrease the exposure to **idelalisib**. Avoid. Moderate Theoretical
- ► Idelalisib is predicted to markedly increase the exposure to bosutinib. Avoid or adjust dose. Severe Study → Also see TABLE 15 p. 1337
- ► Idelalisib is predicted to increase the exposure to buspirone. Adjust **buspirone** dose, p. 338. Severe Study
- ► Idelalisib slightly increases the exposure to cabozantinib. Moderate Study → Also see TABLE 15 p. 1337
- ► Idelalisib is predicted to increase the exposure to calcium channel blockers (amlodipine, felodipine, lacidipine, nicardipine, nifedipine, nimodipine). Monitor and adjust dose. Moderate Study
- ► Idelalisib is predicted to increase the exposure to calcium channel blockers (diltiazem, verapamil). Severe Study
- ► Idelalisib is predicted to markedly increase the exposure to calcium channel blockers (lercanidipine). Avoid. Severe Study
- ► Idelalisib is predicted to increase the exposure to cannabis extract. Use with caution and adjust dose. Moderate Theoretical
- ► Idelalisib is predicted to increase the exposure to ceritinib. Avoid or adjust **ceritinib** dose, p. 945. Severe Study → Also see TABLE 15 p. 1337
- ► Idelalisib increases the concentration of ciclosporin. Severe Study
- ► Idelalisib is predicted to moderately increase the exposure to cilostazol. Adjust **cilostazol** dose, p. 231. Moderate Study
- ► Idelalisib is predicted to moderately increase the exposure to cinacalcet. Adjust dose. Moderate Study
- ► Idelalisib is predicted to markedly increase the exposure to cobimetinib. Avoid or monitor for toxicity. Severe Study
- ► Idelalisib is predicted to increase the exposure to colchicine. Avoid potent inhibitors of CYP3A4 or adjust **colchicine** dose, p. 1085. Severe Study
- ► Idelalisib is predicted to increase the exposure to corticosteroids (beclometasone) (risk with beclometasone is likely to be lower than with other corticosteroids). Moderate Theoretical
- ► Idelalisib is predicted to increase the exposure to corticosteroids (betamethasone, budesonide, ciclesonide, deflazacort, dexamethasone, fludrocortisone, fluticasone, hydrocortisone, methylprednisolone, mometasone, prednisolone, prednisone, triamcinolone). Avoid or monitor side effects. Severe Study
- ► Idelalisib is predicted to moderately increase the exposure to crizotinib. Avoid. Moderate Study → Also see TABLE 15 p. 1337
- ► Idelalisib is predicted to increase the exposure to dabrafenib. Use with caution or avoid. Moderate Study → Also see TABLE 15 p. 1337
- ► Idelalisib is predicted to moderately increase the exposure to daclatasvir. Adjust **daclatasvir** dose, p. 614. Moderate Study
- ► Idelalisib is predicted to markedly to very markedly increase the exposure to darifenacin. Avoid. Severe Study
- ► Idelalisib is predicted to markedly increase the exposure to dasatinib. Avoid. Severe Study → Also see TABLE 15 p. 1337

Idelalisib (continued)
- **Idelalisib** very slightly increases the exposure to delamanid. Severe Study
- **Idelalisib** increases the risk of QT-prolongation when given with domperidone. Avoid. Severe Study
- **Idelalisib** increases the exposure to dopamine receptor agonists (bromocriptine). Severe Study
- **Idelalisib** is predicted to increase the concentration of dopamine receptor agonists (cabergoline). Moderate Anecdotal
- **Idelalisib** is predicted to increase the exposure to dutasteride. Monitor side effects and adjust dose. Moderate Theoretical
- **Efavirenz** is predicted to decrease the exposure to idelalisib. Avoid. Moderate Theoretical
- **Idelalisib** slightly to moderately increases the exposure to elbasvir. Avoid. Moderate Study
- **Idelalisib** is predicted to markedly increase the exposure to eletriptan. Avoid. Severe Study
- **Idelalisib** is predicted to increase the exposure to eliglustat. Avoid or adjust dose—consult product literature. Severe Study
- **Enzalutamide** is predicted to decrease the exposure to idelalisib. Avoid. Severe Study
- **Idelalisib** is predicted to increase the risk of ergotism when given with ergometrine. Avoid. Severe Theoretical
- **Idelalisib** is predicted to increase the risk of ergotism when given with ergotamine. Avoid. Severe Theoretical
- **Idelalisib** is predicted to slightly increase the exposure to erlotinib. Use with caution and adjust dose. Moderate Study
- **Idelalisib** is predicted to increase the concentration of everolimus. Avoid. Severe Study → Also see TABLE 15 p. 1337
- **Idelalisib** is predicted to moderately increase the exposure to fesoterodine. Adjust **fesoterodine** dose with potent inhibitors of CYP3A4; avoid in hepatic and renal impairment, p. 759. Severe Study
- **Idelalisib** is predicted to increase the exposure to fosaprepitant. Moderate Theoretical
- **Idelalisib** is predicted to increase the exposure to gefitinib. Moderate Study → Also see TABLE 15 p. 1337
- **Idelalisib** is predicted to moderately to markedly increase the exposure to grazoprevir. Avoid. Severe Study
- **Idelalisib** is predicted to increase the exposure to guanfacine. Adjust **guanfacine** dose, p. 349. Moderate Study
- **Idelalisib** is predicted to very markedly increase the exposure to ibrutinib. Avoid potent inhibitors of CYP3A4 or adjust **ibrutinib** dose, p. 952. Severe Study → Also see TABLE 15 p. 1337
- **Idelalisib** is predicted to increase the exposure to imatinib. Moderate Study → Also see TABLE 15 p. 1337
- **Idelalisib** is predicted to increase the risk of toxicity when given with irinotecan. Avoid. Moderate Study → Also see TABLE 15 p. 1337
- **Idelalisib** is predicted to increase the exposure to ivabradine. Avoid. Severe Study
- **Idelalisib** is predicted to increase the exposure to ivacaftor. Adjust **ivacaftor** p. 292 or **lumacaftor with ivacaftor** p. 293 dose with potent inhibitors of CYP3A4. Severe Study
- **Idelalisib** is predicted to increase the exposure to lapatinib. Avoid. Moderate Study
- **Idelalisib** is predicted to markedly increase the exposure to lomitapide. Avoid. Severe Study
- **Idelalisib** is predicted to increase the exposure to lurasidone. Avoid. Severe Study
- **Idelalisib** is predicted to increase the exposure to macitentan. Moderate Study
- **Idelalisib** markedly increases the exposure to maraviroc. Adjust dose. Severe Theoretical
- **Idelalisib** is predicted to markedly to very markedly increase the exposure to midazolam. Avoid or adjust dose. Severe Study
- **Idelalisib** is predicted to very markedly increase the exposure to midostaurin. Avoid or monitor for toxicity. Severe Study
- **Idelalisib** is predicted to increase the exposure to mirabegron. Adjust **mirabegron** dose in hepatic and renal impairment, p. 763. Moderate Study
- **Idelalisib** is predicted to increase the exposure to mirtazapine. Moderate Study
- **Mitotane** is predicted to decrease the exposure to idelalisib. Avoid. Severe Study → Also see TABLE 15 p. 1337

- **Idelalisib** is predicted to increase the exposure to modafinil. Mild Theoretical
- **Idelalisib** is predicted to increase the exposure to monoclonal antibodies (trastuzumab emtansine). Avoid. Severe Theoretical → Also see TABLE 15 p. 1337
- **Idelalisib** is predicted to markedly increase the exposure to naloxegol. Avoid. Severe Study
- **Idelalisib** is predicted to increase the exposure to netupitant. Moderate Study
- **Nevirapine** is predicted to decrease the exposure to idelalisib. Avoid. Moderate Theoretical
- **Idelalisib** is predicted to moderately increase the exposure to nilotinib. Avoid. Severe Study → Also see TABLE 15 p. 1337
- **Idelalisib** is predicted to increase the exposure to nitisinone. Adjust dose. Moderate Theoretical
- **Idelalisib** is predicted to increase the exposure to olaparib. Avoid potent inhibitors of CYP3A4 or adjust **olaparib** dose, p. 973. Moderate Study → Also see TABLE 15 p. 1337
- **Idelalisib** is predicted to increase the exposure to opioids (alfentanil, buprenorphine, fentanyl, oxycodone, sufentanil). Monitor and adjust dose. Severe Study
- **Idelalisib** is predicted to increase the exposure to opioids (methadone). Severe Theoretical
- **Idelalisib** is predicted to increase the exposure to oxybutynin. Mild Study
- **Idelalisib** is predicted to increase the exposure to palbociclib. Avoid or adjust **palbociclib** dose, p. 961. Severe Study
- **Idelalisib** is predicted to increase the exposure to panobinostat. Adjust **panobinostat** dose; in hepatic impairment avoid, p. 911. Moderate Study → Also see TABLE 15 p. 1337
- **Idelalisib** is predicted to increase the exposure to paritaprevir (with ritonavir and ombitasvir). Avoid. Severe Theoretical
- **Idelalisib** is predicted to increase the exposure to pazopanib. Avoid or adjust **pazopanib** dose, p. 962. Moderate Study → Also see TABLE 15 p. 1337
- **Idelalisib** is predicted to increase the exposure to phosphodiesterase type-5 inhibitors (avanafil, vardenafil). Avoid. Severe Study
- **Idelalisib** is predicted to increase the exposure to phosphodiesterase type-5 inhibitors (sildenafil). Avoid potent inhibitors of CYP3A4 or adjust **sildenafil** dose, p. 794. Severe Study
- **Idelalisib** is predicted to increase the exposure to phosphodiesterase type-5 inhibitors (tadalafil). Use with caution or avoid. Severe Study
- **Idelalisib** is predicted to increase the exposure to pimozide. Avoid. Severe Study
- **Idelalisib** is predicted to slightly increase the exposure to ponatinib. Monitor and adjust **ponatinib** dose, p. 963. Moderate Study
- **Idelalisib** is predicted to moderately increase the exposure to praziquantel. Mild Study
- **Idelalisib** is predicted to increase the exposure to quetiapine. Avoid. Severe Study
- **Idelalisib** is predicted to increase the exposure to ranolazine. Avoid. Severe Study
- **Idelalisib** is predicted to increase the exposure to reboxetine. Avoid. Moderate Study
- **Idelalisib** is predicted to increase the exposure to regorafenib. Avoid. Moderate Study → Also see TABLE 15 p. 1337
- **Idelalisib** is predicted to increase the exposure to repaglinide. Moderate Study
- **Idelalisib** is predicted to increase the exposure to retinoids (alitretinoin). Adjust **alitretinoin** dose, p. 1226. Moderate Theoretical
- **Idelalisib** is predicted to increase the exposure to ribociclib. Avoid or adjust **ribociclib** dose, p. 965. Moderate Study
- **Rifampicin** is predicted to decrease the exposure to idelalisib. Avoid. Severe Study
- **Idelalisib** is predicted to increase the exposure to risperidone. Adjust dose. Moderate Study
- **Idelalisib** is predicted to increase the exposure to ruxolitinib. Adjust dose and monitor side effects. Moderate Study → Also see TABLE 15 p. 1337

▸ **Idelalisib** is predicted to increase the exposure to saxagliptin. Moderate Study
▸ **Idelalisib** is predicted to increase the exposure to simeprevir. Avoid. Severe Study
▸ **Idelalisib** is predicted to increase the concentration of sirolimus. Avoid. Severe Study
▸ **Idelalisib** is predicted to increase the exposure to solifenacin. Adjust **solifenacin** or tamsulosin with solifenacin p. 768 dose; avoid in hepatic and renal impairment, p. 761. Severe Study
▸ **Idelalisib** is predicted to moderately increase the exposure to SSRIs (dapoxetine). Avoid potent inhibitors of CYP3A4 or adjust **dapoxetine** dose, p. 801. Severe Study
▸ **St John's Wort** is predicted to decrease the exposure to **idelalisib**. Avoid. Moderate Theoretical
▸ **Idelalisib** is predicted to increase the exposure to statins (atorvastatin). Avoid or adjust dose and monitor rhabdomyolysis. Severe Study
▸ **Idelalisib** is predicted to increase the exposure to statins (simvastatin). Avoid. Severe Study
▸ **Idelalisib** is predicted to slightly increase the exposure to sunitinib. Avoid or adjust **sunitinib** dose, p. 967. Moderate Study → Also see TABLE 15 p. 1337
▸ **Idelalisib** is predicted to increase the concentration of tacrolimus. Monitor and adjust dose. Severe Study
▸ **Idelalisib** is predicted to increase the exposure to taxanes (cabazitaxel). Avoid. Severe Study → Also see TABLE 15 p. 1337
▸ **Idelalisib** is predicted to moderately increase the exposure to taxanes (docetaxel). Avoid or adjust dose. Severe Study → Also see TABLE 15 p. 1337
▸ **Idelalisib** is predicted to increase the exposure to taxanes (paclitaxel). Severe Theoretical → Also see TABLE 15 p. 1337
▸ **Idelalisib** is predicted to increase the concentration of temsirolimus. Avoid. Severe Theoretical → Also see TABLE 15 p. 1337
▸ **Idelalisib** is predicted to markedly increase the exposure to ticagrelor. Avoid. Severe Study
▸ **Idelalisib** is predicted to increase the exposure to tofacitinib. Adjust **tofacitinib** dose, p. 1072. Moderate Study
▸ **Idelalisib** is predicted to increase the exposure to tolterodine. Avoid. Severe Study
▸ **Idelalisib** is predicted to increase the exposure to tolvaptan. Adjust dose. Severe Study
▸ **Idelalisib** is predicted to increase the exposure to toremifene. Moderate Theoretical
▸ **Idelalisib** is predicted to increase the exposure to trabectedin. Avoid or adjust dose. Severe Theoretical → Also see TABLE 15 p. 1337
▸ **Idelalisib** is predicted to moderately increase the exposure to trazodone. Avoid or adjust dose. Moderate Study
▸ **Idelalisib** is predicted to increase the exposure to ulipristal. Avoid if used for uterine fibroids. Severe Study
▸ **Idelalisib** is predicted to increase the exposure to vemurafenib. Severe Theoretical
▸ **Idelalisib** is predicted to increase the exposure to venetoclax. Avoid potent inhibitors of CYP3A4 or adjust **venetoclax** dose, p. 974. Severe Study
▸ **Idelalisib** is predicted to increase the exposure to venlafaxine. Moderate Study
▸ **Idelalisib** is predicted to increase the exposure to vinca alkaloids. Severe Theoretical → Also see TABLE 15 p. 1337
▸ **Idelalisib** is predicted to increase the exposure to vitamin D substances (paricalcitol). Moderate Study
▸ **Idelalisib** is predicted to increase the exposure to zopiclone. Adjust dose. Moderate Theoretical

Ifosfamide → see alkylating agents
Iloprost → see TABLE 4 p. 1334 (antiplatelet effects)
Imatinib → see TABLE 15 p. 1337 (myelosuppression)
▸ **Imatinib** is predicted to increase the exposure to aldosterone antagonists (eplerenone). Adjust **eplerenone** dose, p. 190. Severe Study
▸ **Imatinib** is predicted to increase the exposure to alpha blockers (tamsulosin). Moderate Theoretical
▸ **Imatinib** is predicted to increase the exposure to alprazolam. Severe Study
▸ **Imatinib** is predicted to increase the exposure to antiarrhythmics (dronedarone). Severe Theoretical

▸ **Imatinib** is predicted to increase the exposure to antiarrhythmics (propafenone). Monitor and adjust dose. Moderate Study
▸ **Antiepileptics (carbamazepine, fosphenytoin, phenobarbital, phenytoin, primidone)** are predicted to decrease the exposure to imatinib. Avoid. Moderate Study
▸ **Antiepileptics (oxcarbazepine)** decrease the exposure to imatinib. Avoid. Moderate Study
▸ **Antifungals, azoles (fluconazole, posaconazole)** are predicted to increase the exposure to imatinib. Moderate Study
▸ **Antifungals, azoles (itraconazole, ketoconazole, voriconazole)** are predicted to increase the exposure to imatinib. Moderate Study
▸ **Imatinib** is predicted to decrease the exposure to antifungals, azoles (isavuconazole). Moderate Theoretical
▸ **Imatinib** is predicted to increase the exposure to antihistamines, non-sedating (mizolastine). Severe Theoretical
▸ **Imatinib** is predicted to increase the exposure to antihistamines, non-sedating (rupatadine). Avoid. Moderate Study
▸ **Imatinib** is predicted to increase the concentration of antimalarials (piperaquine). Severe Theoretical
▸ **Aprepitant** is predicted to increase the exposure to imatinib. Moderate Theoretical
▸ **Asparaginase** is predicted to increase the risk of hepatotoxicity when given with imatinib. Severe Theoretical → Also see TABLE 15 p. 1337
▸ **Imatinib** is predicted to increase the exposure to axitinib. Moderate Theoretical → Also see TABLE 15 p. 1337
▸ **Imatinib** is predicted to increase the exposure to bedaquiline. Avoid prolonged use. Mild Theoretical
▸ **Bosentan** is predicted to decrease the exposure to imatinib. Moderate Study
▸ **Imatinib** is predicted to increase the exposure to bosutinib. Avoid or adjust dose. Severe Theoretical → Also see TABLE 15 p. 1337
▸ **Imatinib** is predicted to increase the exposure to buspirone. Use with caution and adjust dose. Moderate Study
▸ **Imatinib** is predicted to increase the exposure to cabozantinib. Moderate Theoretical → Also see TABLE 15 p. 1337
▸ **Calcium channel blockers (diltiazem, verapamil)** are predicted to increase the exposure to imatinib. Moderate Theoretical
▸ **Imatinib** is predicted to increase the exposure to calcium channel blockers (amlodipine, felodipine, lacidipine, lercanidipine, nicardipine, nifedipine, nimodipine). Monitor and adjust dose. Moderate Study
▸ **Imatinib** is predicted to increase the exposure to ceritinib. Moderate Theoretical → Also see TABLE 15 p. 1337
▸ **Imatinib** increases the concentration of ciclosporin. Severe Study
▸ **Cobicistat** is predicted to increase the exposure to imatinib. Moderate Study
▸ **Imatinib** is predicted to increase the exposure to cobimetinib. Severe Theoretical
▸ **Imatinib** is predicted to increase the exposure to colchicine. Adjust **colchicine** dose with moderate inhibitors of CYP3A4, p. 1085. Severe Study
▸ **Imatinib** is predicted to increase the exposure to corticosteroids (methylprednisolone). Monitor and adjust dose. Moderate Study
▸ **Imatinib** is predicted to increase the risk of bleeding events when given with coumarins. Severe Theoretical
▸ **Crisantaspase** is predicted to increase the risk of hepatotoxicity when given with imatinib. Severe Theoretical → Also see TABLE 15 p. 1337
▸ **Imatinib** is predicted to slightly increase the exposure to darifenacin. Moderate Study
▸ **Imatinib** is predicted to increase the exposure to dasatinib. Severe Study → Also see TABLE 15 p. 1337
▸ **Imatinib** increases the risk of QT-prolongation when given with domperidone. Avoid. Severe Study
▸ **Imatinib** is predicted to increase the exposure to dopamine receptor agonists (bromocriptine). Severe Theoretical
▸ **Imatinib** is predicted to increase the concentration of dopamine receptor agonists (cabergoline). Moderate Anecdotal
▸ **Imatinib** is predicted to moderately increase the exposure to dutasteride. Mild Study

Imatinib (continued)

▸ Efavirenz is predicted to decrease the exposure to **imatinib**. Moderate Study

▸ **Imatinib** is predicted to increase the exposure to eliglustat. Avoid or adjust dose—consult product literature. Severe Study

▸ Enzalutamide is predicted to decrease the exposure to **imatinib**. Avoid. Moderate Study

▸ **Imatinib** is predicted to increase the risk of ergotism when given with ergometrine. Severe Theoretical

▸ **Imatinib** is predicted to increase the risk of ergotism when given with ergotamine. Severe Theoretical

▸ **Imatinib** is predicted to increase the exposure to erlotinib. Moderate Theoretical

▸ **Imatinib** is predicted to increase the concentration of everolimus. Avoid or adjust dose. Moderate Study → Also see TABLE 15 p. 1337

▸ **Imatinib** is predicted to increase the exposure to fesoterodine. Adjust **fesoterodine** dose with moderate inhibitors of CYP3A4 in hepatic and renal impairment, p. 759. Mild Study

▸ **Imatinib** is predicted to increase the exposure to gefitinib. Moderate Theoretical → Also see TABLE 15 p. 1337

▸ Grapefruit juice is predicted to increase the exposure to **imatinib**. Moderate Theoretical

▸ **Imatinib** is predicted to increase the concentration of guanfacine. Adjust **guanfacine** dose, p. 349. Moderate Theoretical

▸ HIV-protease inhibitors are predicted to increase the exposure to **imatinib**. Moderate Study

▸ **Imatinib** is predicted to increase the exposure to ibrutinib. Adjust **ibrutinib** dose with moderate inhibitors of CYP3A4, p. 952. Severe Study → Also see TABLE 15 p. 1337

▸ Idelalisib is predicted to increase the exposure to **imatinib**. Moderate Study → Also see TABLE 15 p. 1337

▸ **Imatinib** is predicted to increase the exposure to ivabradine. Adjust **ivabradine** dose, p. 210. Severe Theoretical

▸ **Imatinib** is predicted to increase the exposure to ivacaftor. Adjust **ivacaftor** dose with moderate inhibitors of CYP3A4, p. 292. Severe Study

▸ **Imatinib** is predicted to increase the exposure to lapatinib. Moderate Study

▸ **Imatinib** is predicted to increase the exposure to lomitapide. Avoid. Moderate Theoretical

▸ **Imatinib** is predicted to increase the exposure to lurasidone. Moderate Study

▸ Macrolides (clarithromycin) are predicted to increase the exposure to **imatinib**. Moderate Study

▸ Macrolides (erythromycin) are predicted to increase the exposure to **imatinib**. Moderate Theoretical

▸ **Imatinib** is predicted to increase the exposure to midazolam. Monitor side effects and adjust dose. Severe Study

▸ **Imatinib** is predicted to increase the exposure to midostaurin. Moderate Theoretical

▸ Mitotane is predicted to decrease the exposure to **imatinib**. Avoid. Moderate Study → Also see TABLE 15 p. 1337

▸ **Imatinib** is predicted to increase the exposure to naloxegol. Adjust **naloxegol** dose and monitor side effects, p. 64. Moderate Study

▸ Netupitant is predicted to increase the exposure to **imatinib**. Moderate Theoretical

▸ Nevirapine is predicted to decrease the exposure to **imatinib**. Moderate Study

▸ **Imatinib** is predicted to increase the exposure to olaparib. Avoid moderate inhibitors of CYP3A4 or adjust **olaparib** dose, p. 973. Moderate Theoretical → Also see TABLE 15 p. 1337

▸ **Imatinib** is predicted to increase the exposure to opioids (alfentanil, buprenorphine, fentanyl, oxycodone). Monitor and adjust dose. Moderate Study

▸ **Imatinib** is predicted to increase the exposure to opioids (methadone, sufentanil). Moderate Theoretical

▸ **Imatinib** is predicted to increase the exposure to oxybutynin. Mild Theoretical

▸ **Imatinib** increases the risk of hepatotoxicity when given with paracetamol. Severe Anecdotal

▸ **Imatinib** is predicted to increase the exposure to pazopanib. Moderate Theoretical → Also see TABLE 15 p. 1337

▸ Pegaspargase is predicted to increase the risk of hepatotoxicity when given with **imatinib**. Severe Theoretical → Also see TABLE 15 p. 1337

▸ **Imatinib** is predicted to increase the risk of bleeding events when given with phenindione. Severe Theoretical

▸ **Imatinib** is predicted to increase the exposure to phosphodiesterase type-5 inhibitors (avanafil). Adjust **avanafil** dose, p. 794. Moderate Theoretical

▸ **Imatinib** is predicted to increase the exposure to phosphodiesterase type-5 inhibitors (sildenafil). Monitor or adjust **sildenafil** dose with moderate inhibitors of CYP3A4, p. 794. Moderate Theoretical

▸ **Imatinib** is predicted to increase the exposure to phosphodiesterase type-5 inhibitors (tadalafil). Severe Theoretical

▸ **Imatinib** is predicted to increase the exposure to phosphodiesterase type-5 inhibitors (vardenafil). Adjust dose. Severe Theoretical

▸ **Imatinib** is predicted to increase the exposure to pimozide. Avoid. Severe Theoretical

▸ **Imatinib** is predicted to increase the exposure to quetiapine. Avoid. Moderate Study

▸ **Imatinib** is predicted to increase the exposure to ranolazine. Severe Study

▸ **Imatinib** is predicted to increase the exposure to ribociclib. Moderate Study

▸ Rifampicin is predicted to decrease the exposure to **imatinib**. Avoid. Moderate Study

▸ **Imatinib** is predicted to increase the exposure to ruxolitinib. Moderate Theoretical → Also see TABLE 15 p. 1337

▸ **Imatinib** is predicted to increase the exposure to saxagliptin. Mild Study

▸ **Imatinib** is predicted to increase the exposure to simeprevir. Avoid. Severe Study

▸ **Imatinib** increases the concentration of sirolimus. Monitor and adjust dose. Moderate Study

▸ **Imatinib** is predicted to increase the exposure to SSRIs (dapoxetine). Adjust **dapoxetine** dose with moderate inhibitors of CYP3A4, p. 801. Moderate Theoretical

▸ St John's Wort is predicted to decrease the exposure to **imatinib**. Moderate Study

▸ **Imatinib** is predicted to increase the exposure to statins (atorvastatin). Monitor and adjust dose. Severe Study

▸ **Imatinib** is predicted to increase the exposure to statins (simvastatin). Use with caution and adjust **simvastatin** dose, p. 203. Severe Study

▸ **Imatinib** is predicted to increase the exposure to sunitinib. Moderate Theoretical → Also see TABLE 15 p. 1337

▸ **Imatinib** is predicted to increase the concentration of tacrolimus. Severe Study

▸ **Imatinib** is predicted to increase the exposure to taxanes (cabazitaxel). Moderate Theoretical → Also see TABLE 15 p. 1337

▸ Tedizolid is predicted to increase the exposure to **imatinib**. Avoid. Moderate Theoretical

▸ **Imatinib** is predicted to increase the concentration of temsirolimus. Moderate Theoretical → Also see TABLE 15 p. 1337

▸ **Imatinib** is predicted to increase the exposure to tofacitinib. Moderate Study

▸ **Imatinib** is predicted to increase the exposure to tolterodine. Mild Theoretical

▸ **Imatinib** is predicted to increase the exposure to tolvaptan. Adjust dose. Moderate Study

▸ **Imatinib** is predicted to increase the exposure to trazodone. Moderate Theoretical

▸ **Imatinib** is predicted to increase the exposure to ulipristal. Avoid if used for uterine fibroids. Moderate Study

▸ **Imatinib** is predicted to increase the exposure to venetoclax. Avoid moderate inhibitors of CYP3A4 or adjust **venetoclax** dose, p. 974. Severe Study

▸ **Imatinib** is predicted to increase the exposure to vinca alkaloids. Severe Theoretical → Also see TABLE 15 p. 1337

▸ **Imatinib** is predicted to increase the exposure to zopiclone. Adjust dose. Moderate Study

Imidapril → see ACE inhibitors

Imipenem → see carbapenems

Imipramine → see tricyclic antidepressants

Indacaterol → see beta₂ agonists

Indacaterol → see beta$_2$ agonists
Indapamide → see thiazide diuretics
Indometacin → see NSAIDs
Indoramin → see alpha blockers
Infliximab → see monoclonal antibodies
Influenza vaccine (live) → see live vaccines
Inotuzumab ozogamicin → see monoclonal antibodies
Insulins → see TABLE 14 p. 1337 (antidiabetic drugs)
▸ Fibrates are predicted to increase the risk of hypoglycaemia when given with **insulins**. Moderate Theoretical
Interferon alfa → see interferons
Interferon beta → see interferons
Interferons → see TABLE 15 p. 1337 (myelosuppression)

interferon alfa · interferon beta · peginterferon alfa

▸ Interferons are predicted to slightly increase the exposure to aminophylline. Adjust dose. Moderate Theoretical
▸ Interferon alfa is predicted to increase the risk of peripheral neuropathy when given with telbivudine. Avoid. Severe Theoretical
▸ Peginterferon alfa increases the risk of peripheral neuropathy when given with telbivudine. Avoid. Severe Study
▸ Interferons slightly increase the exposure to theophylline. Adjust dose. Moderate Study

Ipilimumab → see monoclonal antibodies
Ipratropium → see TABLE 10 p. 1336 (antimuscarinics)
▸ Beta₂ agonists are predicted to increase the risk of glaucoma when given with **ipratropium**. Moderate Anecdotal
Irbesartan → see angiotensin-II receptor antagonists
Irinotecan → see TABLE 15 p. 1337 (myelosuppression)
▸ Antiepileptics (carbamazepine, fosphenytoin, phenobarbital, phenytoin, primidone) are predicted to decrease the exposure to **irinotecan**. Avoid. Severe Study
▸ Antifungals, azoles (itraconazole, ketoconazole, voriconazole) are predicted to increase the risk of toxicity when given with **irinotecan**. Avoid. Moderate Study
▸ Cobicistat is predicted to increase the risk of toxicity when given with **irinotecan**. Avoid. Moderate Study
▸ Enzalutamide is predicted to decrease the exposure to **irinotecan**. Avoid. Moderate Study
▸ HIV-protease inhibitors are predicted to increase the risk of toxicity when given with **irinotecan**. Avoid. Moderate Study
▸ Idelalisib is predicted to increase the risk of toxicity when given with **irinotecan**. Avoid. Moderate Study → Also see TABLE 15 p.1337
▸ Live vaccines are predicted to increase the risk of generalised infection (possibly life-threatening) when given with **irinotecan**. Public Health England advises avoid (refer to Green Book). Severe Theoretical
▸ Macrolides (clarithromycin) are predicted to increase the risk of toxicity when given with **irinotecan**. Avoid. Moderate Study
▸ Mitotane is predicted to decrease the exposure to **irinotecan**. Avoid. Severe Study → Also see TABLE 15 p. 1337
▸ Irinotecan is predicted to decrease the effects of neuromuscular blocking drugs, non-depolarising. Moderate Theoretical
▸ Pitolisant is predicted to decrease the exposure to **irinotecan**. Unknown Theoretical
▸ Rifampicin is predicted to decrease the exposure to **irinotecan**. Avoid. Severe Study
▸ Rolapitant is predicted to increase the exposure to **irinotecan**. Avoid or monitor. Moderate Study
▸ St John's Wort slightly decreases the exposure to **irinotecan**. Avoid. Severe Study
▸ Irinotecan is predicted to increase the risk of prolonged neuromuscular blockade when given with suxamethonium. Moderate Theoretical

Iron (injectable)

ferric carboxymaltose · iron dextran · iron isomaltoside 1000 · iron sucrose

▸ Chloramphenicol decreases the efficacy of intravenous **iron (injectable)**. Moderate Anecdotal

Iron (oral)

ferric maltol · ferrous fumarate · ferrous gluconate · ferrous sulfate · polysaccharide-iron complex · sodium feredetate

▸ Antacids decrease the absorption of **iron (oral)**. **Iron (oral)** should be taken 1 hour before or 2 hours after antacids. Moderate Study
▸ **Iron (oral)** is predicted to decrease the absorption of oral bisphosphonates (ibandronic acid). Avoid **iron (oral)** for at least 6 hours before or 1 hour after ibandronic acid. Moderate Theoretical
▸ **Iron (oral)** decreases the absorption of bisphosphonates (risedronate). Separate administration by at least 2 hours. Moderate Study
▸ **Iron (oral)** decreases the absorption of bisphosphonates (sodium clodronate). Avoid **iron (oral)** for 2 hours before or 1 hour after sodium clodronate. Moderate Study
▸ Calcium salts (calcium carbonate) decrease the absorption of **iron (oral)**. Calcium carbonate should be taken 1 hour before or 2 hours after **iron (oral)**. Moderate Study
▸ **Iron (oral)** is predicted to decrease the exposure to carbidopa. Moderate Theoretical
▸ Chloramphenicol decreases the efficacy of oral **iron (oral)**. Moderate Theoretical
▸ **Iron (oral)** decreases the absorption of dolutegravir. Dolutegravir should be taken 2 hours before or 6 hours after **iron (oral)**. Moderate Study
▸ **Iron (oral)** is predicted to decrease the absorption of eltrombopag. **Eltrombopag** should be taken 2 hours before or 4 hours after **iron (oral)**. Severe Theoretical
▸ **Iron (oral)** is predicted to decrease the absorption of entacapone. Separate administration by at least 2 hours. Moderate Theoretical
▸ **Iron (oral)** decreases the absorption of levodopa. Moderate Study
▸ **Iron (oral)** decreases the effects of methyldopa. Moderate Study
▸ **Iron (oral)** is predicted to decrease the absorption of penicillamine. Separate administration by at least 2 hours. Mild Study
▸ **Iron (oral)** decreases the exposure to quinolones. Separate administration by at least 2 hours. Moderate Study
▸ **Iron (oral)** decreases the absorption of tetracyclines. Tetracyclines should be taken 2 to 3 hours after **iron (oral)**. Moderate Study
▸ **Iron (oral)** decreases the absorption of thyroid hormones (levothyroxine). Separate administration by at least 4 hours. Moderate Study
▸ Trientine potentially decreases the absorption of **iron (oral)**. Moderate Theoretical
▸ Zinc is predicted to decrease the efficacy of **iron (oral)** and **iron (oral)** is predicted to decrease the efficacy of zinc. Moderate Study

Iron chelators

deferasirox · desferrioxamine · dexrazoxane

▸ **Deferasirox** is predicted to increase the exposure to aminophylline. Avoid. Moderate Theoretical
▸ Antacids (aluminium hydroxide) are predicted to decrease the exposure to **deferasirox**. Avoid. Moderate Theoretical
▸ Antiepileptics (carbamazepine, fosphenytoin, phenobarbital, phenytoin, primidone) are predicted to decrease the exposure to **deferasirox**. Monitor serum ferritin and adjust dose. Moderate Theoretical
▸ Ascorbic acid is predicted to increase the risk of cardiovascular side-effects when given with **desferrioxamine**. Severe Theoretical
▸ Aspirin (high-dose) is predicted to increase the risk of gastrointestinal bleeds when given with **deferasirox**. Severe Theoretical
▸ Bisphosphonates are predicted to increase the risk of gastrointestinal bleeding when given with **deferasirox**. Severe Theoretical
▸ **Deferasirox** is predicted to increase the exposure to clozapine. Avoid. Moderate Theoretical

Iron chelators (continued)

▸ Corticosteroids are predicted to increase the risk of gastrointestinal bleeding when given with **deferasirox**. Severe Theoretical

▸ HIV-protease inhibitors (ritonavir) are predicted to decrease the exposure to **deferasirox**. Monitor serum ferritin and adjust dose. Moderate Theoretical

▸ Live vaccines are predicted to increase the risk of generalised infection (possibly life-threatening) when given with **dexrazoxane**. Avoid. Severe Theoretical

▸ NSAIDs are predicted to increase the risk of gastrointestinal bleeding when given with **deferasirox**. Severe Theoretical

▸ **Deferasirox** moderately increases the exposure to repaglinide. Avoid. Study

▸ Rifampicin is predicted to decrease the exposure to **deferasirox**. Monitor serum ferritin and adjust dose. Moderate Study

▸ **Deferasirox** is predicted to increase the exposure to selexipag. Adjust dose. Moderate Study

▸ **Deferasirox** increases the exposure to theophylline. Avoid. Moderate Study

▸ **Deferasirox** is predicted to increase the exposure to tizanidine. Avoid. Moderate Theoretical

Iron dextran → see iron (injectable)
Iron isomaltoside 1000 → see iron (injectable)
Iron sucrose → see iron (injectable)
Isavuconazole → see antifungals, azoles
Isocarboxazid → see monoamine-oxidase A and B inhibitors, irreversible
Isoflurane → see volatile halogenated anaesthetics
Isometheptene → see sympathomimetics, vasoconstrictor
Isoniazid → see TABLE 1 p. 1334 (hepatotoxicity), TABLE 12 p. 1337 (peripheral neuropathy)

FOOD AND LIFESTYLE Avoid tyramine or histamine rich foods, as tachycardia, palpitation, hypotension, flushing, headache, dizziness, and sweating reported.

▸ **Isoniazid** is predicted to affect the clearance of aminophylline. Severe Theoretical

▸ **Isoniazid** markedly increases the concentration of antiepileptics (carbamazepine) and antiepileptics (carbamazepine) increase the risk of hepatotoxicity when given with **isoniazid**. Monitor concentration and adjust dose. Severe Study → Also see TABLE 1 p. 1334

▸ **Isoniazid** increases the concentration of antiepileptics (fosphenytoin, phenytoin). Moderate Study → Also see TABLE 12 p. 1337

▸ Cycloserine increases the risk of CNS toxicity when given with **isoniazid**. Monitor and adjust dose. Moderate Study

▸ **Isoniazid** is predicted to increase the risk of peripheral neuropathy when given with didanosine. Severe Theoretical → Also see TABLE 1 p. 1334 → Also see TABLE 12 p. 1337

▸ **Isoniazid** increases the risk of optic neuropathy when given with ethambutol. Severe Anecdotal

▸ **Isoniazid** decreases the effects of levodopa. Moderate Study

▸ **Isoniazid** is predicted to increase the exposure to lomitapide. Separate administration by 12 hours. Unknown Theoretical → Also see TABLE 1 p. 1334

▸ **Isoniazid** is predicted to increase the risk of peripheral neuropathy when given with stavudine. Severe Theoretical → Also see TABLE 12 p. 1337

▸ **Isoniazid** is predicted to affect the clearance of theophylline. Severe Anecdotal

▸ **Isoniazid** potentially increases the risk of nephrotoxicity when given with volatile halogenated anaesthetics (methoxyflurane). Avoid. Severe Theoretical

Isosorbide dinitrate → see nitrates
Isosorbide mononitrate → see nitrates
Isotretinoin → see retinoids
Itraconazole → see antifungals, azoles
Ivabradine → see TABLE 6 p. 1335 (bradycardia), TABLE 9 p. 1336 (QT-interval prolongation)

▸ Antiarrhythmics (dronedarone) are predicted to increase the exposure to **ivabradine**. Adjust **ivabradine** dose, p. 210. Severe Theoretical

▸ Antiepileptics (carbamazepine, fosphenytoin, phenobarbital, phenytoin, primidone) are predicted to decrease the exposure to **ivabradine**. Adjust dose. Moderate Theoretical

▸ Antifungals, azoles (fluconazole, isavuconazole, posaconazole) are predicted to increase the exposure to **ivabradine**. Adjust **ivabradine** dose, p. 210. Severe Theoretical

▸ Antifungals, azoles (itraconazole, ketoconazole, voriconazole) are predicted to increase the exposure to **ivabradine**. Avoid. Severe Study

▸ Aprepitant is predicted to increase the exposure to **ivabradine**. Adjust **ivabradine** dose, p. 210. Severe Theoretical

▸ Calcium channel blockers (diltiazem, verapamil) are predicted to increase the exposure to **ivabradine**. Avoid. Moderate Study → Also see TABLE 6 p. 1335

▸ Cobicistat is predicted to increase the exposure to **ivabradine**. Avoid. Severe Study

▸ Crizotinib is predicted to increase the exposure to **ivabradine**. Adjust **ivabradine** dose, p. 210. Severe Theoretical → Also see TABLE 6 p. 1335

▸ Enzalutamide is predicted to decrease the exposure to **ivabradine**. Adjust dose. Moderate Theoretical

▸ Grapefruit juice is predicted to increase the exposure to **ivabradine**. Avoid. Moderate Study

▸ HIV-protease inhibitors are predicted to increase the exposure to **ivabradine**. Avoid. Severe Study

▸ Idelalisib is predicted to increase the exposure to **ivabradine**. Avoid. Severe Study

▸ Imatinib is predicted to increase the exposure to **ivabradine**. Adjust **ivabradine** dose, p. 210. Severe Theoretical

▸ Macrolides (clarithromycin) are predicted to increase the exposure to **ivabradine**. Avoid. Severe Study

▸ Macrolides (erythromycin) are predicted to increase the exposure to **ivabradine**. Avoid. Severe Study

▸ Mitotane is predicted to decrease the exposure to **ivabradine**. Adjust dose. Moderate Theoretical

▸ Netupitant is predicted to increase the exposure to **ivabradine**. Adjust **ivabradine** dose, p. 210. Severe Theoretical

▸ Nilotinib is predicted to increase the exposure to **ivabradine**. Adjust **ivabradine** dose, p. 210. Severe Theoretical

▸ Rifampicin is predicted to decrease the exposure to **ivabradine**. Adjust dose. Moderate Study

▸ St John's Wort decreases the exposure to **ivabradine**. Avoid. Moderate Study

Ivacaftor

FOOD AND LIFESTYLE Avoid bitter (Seville) oranges as they are predicted to increase the exposure to ivacaftor.

▸ Antiarrhythmics (dronedarone) are predicted to increase the exposure to **ivacaftor**. Adjust **ivacaftor** dose with moderate inhibitors of CYP3A4, p. 292. Severe Study

▸ Antiepileptics (carbamazepine, fosphenytoin, phenobarbital, phenytoin, primidone) are predicted to moderately to markedly decrease the exposure to **ivacaftor**. Avoid. Severe Study

▸ Antifungals, azoles (fluconazole, isavuconazole, posaconazole) are predicted to increase the exposure to **ivacaftor**. Adjust **ivacaftor** dose with moderate inhibitors of CYP3A4, p. 292. Severe Study

▸ Antifungals, azoles (itraconazole, ketoconazole, voriconazole) are predicted to increase the exposure to **ivacaftor**. Adjust **ivacaftor** p. 292 or lumacaftor with ivacaftor p. 293 dose with potent inhibitors of CYP3A4. Severe Study

▸ Aprepitant is predicted to increase the exposure to **ivacaftor**. Adjust **ivacaftor** dose with moderate inhibitors of CYP3A4, p. 292. Severe Study

▸ Bosentan is predicted to decrease the exposure to **ivacaftor**. Severe Theoretical

▸ Calcium channel blockers (diltiazem, verapamil) are predicted to increase the exposure to **ivacaftor**. Adjust **ivacaftor** dose with moderate inhibitors of CYP3A4, p. 292. Severe Study

▸ Cobicistat is predicted to increase the exposure to **ivacaftor**. Adjust **ivacaftor** p. 292 or lumacaftor with ivacaftor p. 293 dose with potent inhibitors of CYP3A4. Severe Study

▸ **Ivacaftor** is predicted to increase the anticoagulant effect of coumarins (warfarin). Severe Theoretical

- ▸ Crizotinib is predicted to increase the exposure to **ivacaftor**. Adjust **ivacaftor** dose with moderate inhibitors of CYP3A4, p. 292. [Severe] Study
- ▸ **Ivacaftor** slightly increases the exposure to digoxin. [Moderate] Study
- ▸ Efavirenz is predicted to decrease the exposure to **ivacaftor**. [Severe] Theoretical
- ▸ Enzalutamide is predicted to moderately to markedly decrease the exposure to **ivacaftor**. Avoid. [Severe] Study
- ▸ Grapefruit juice is predicted to increase the exposure to **ivacaftor**. Avoid. [Moderate] Theoretical
- ▸ HIV-protease inhibitors are predicted to increase the exposure to **ivacaftor**. Adjust **ivacaftor** p. 292 or **lumacaftor with ivacaftor** p. 293 dose with potent inhibitors of CYP3A4,. [Severe] Study
- ▸ Idelalisib is predicted to increase the exposure to **ivacaftor**. Adjust **ivacaftor** p. 292 or **lumacaftor with ivacaftor** p. 293 dose with potent inhibitors of CYP3A4. [Severe] Study
- ▸ Imatinib is predicted to increase the exposure to **ivacaftor**. Adjust **ivacaftor** dose with moderate inhibitors of CYP3A4, p. 292. [Severe] Study
- ▸ **Ivacaftor** is predicted to increase the exposure to lomitapide. Separate administration by 12 hours. [Moderate] Theoretical
- ▸ Macrolides (clarithromycin) are predicted to increase the exposure to **ivacaftor**. Adjust **ivacaftor** p. 292 or **lumacaftor with ivacaftor** p. 293 dose with potent inhibitors of CYP3A4. [Severe] Study
- ▸ Macrolides (erythromycin) are predicted to increase the exposure to **ivacaftor**. Adjust **ivacaftor** dose with moderate inhibitors of CYP3A4, p. 292. [Severe] Study
- ▸ Mitotane is predicted to moderately to markedly decrease the exposure to **ivacaftor**. Avoid. [Severe] Study
- ▸ Netupitant is predicted to increase the exposure to **ivacaftor**. Adjust **ivacaftor** dose with moderate inhibitors of CYP3A4, p. 292. [Severe] Study
- ▸ Nevirapine is predicted to decrease the exposure to **ivacaftor**. [Severe] Theoretical
- ▸ Nilotinib is predicted to increase the exposure to **ivacaftor**. Adjust **ivacaftor** dose with moderate inhibitors of CYP3A4, p. 292. [Severe] Study
- ▸ Rifampicin is predicted to moderately to markedly decrease the exposure to **ivacaftor**. Avoid. [Severe] Study
- ▸ St John's Wort is predicted to decrease the exposure to **ivacaftor**. [Severe] Theoretical

Ivermectin
- ▸ **Ivermectin** potentially increases the anticoagulant effect of coumarins. [Severe] Anecdotal
- ▸ Levamisole increases the exposure to **ivermectin**. [Moderate] Study

Ixazomib
- ▸ Antiepileptics (carbamazepine, fosphenytoin, phenobarbital, phenytoin, primidone) are predicted to decrease the exposure to **ixazomib**. Avoid. [Severe] Study
- ▸ Enzalutamide is predicted to decrease the exposure to **ixazomib**. Avoid. [Severe] Study
- ▸ Mitotane is predicted to decrease the exposure to **ixazomib**. Avoid. [Severe] Study
- ▸ Rifampicin is predicted to decrease the exposure to **ixazomib**. Avoid. [Severe] Study
- ▸ St John's Wort is predicted to decrease the exposure to **ixazomib**. Avoid. [Severe] Study

Ixekizumab → see monoclonal antibodies

Kaolin
- ▸ **Kaolin** is predicted to decrease the absorption of tetracyclines. [Moderate] Theoretical

Ketamine → see TABLE 8 p. 1335 (hypotension), TABLE 11 p. 1336 (CNS depressant effects)
- ▸ Memantine is predicted to increase the risk of CNS side-effects when given with **ketamine**. Avoid. [Severe] Theoretical

Ketoconazole → see antifungals, azoles

Ketoprofen → see NSAIDs

Ketorolac → see NSAIDs

Ketotifen → see antihistamines, sedating

Labetalol → see beta blockers, non-selective

Lacidipine → see calcium channel blockers

Lacosamide → see antiepileptics

Lamivudine → see TABLE 12 p. 1337 (peripheral neuropathy)
- ▸ Trimethoprim slightly increases the exposure to **lamivudine**. [Moderate] Study

Lamotrigine → see antiepileptics

Lanreotide
- ▸ Beta blockers, non-selective are predicted to increase the risk of bradycardia when given with **lanreotide**. [Moderate] Theoretical
- ▸ Beta blockers, selective are predicted to increase the risk of bradycardia when given with **lanreotide**. [Moderate] Theoretical
- ▸ **Lanreotide** is predicted to decrease the absorption of oral ciclosporin. Adjust dose. [Severe] Theoretical

Lansoprazole → see proton pump inhibitors

Lanthanum
- ▸ **Lanthanum** is predicted to decrease the absorption of antifungals, azoles (ketoconazole). Separate administration by at least 2 hours. [Moderate] Theoretical
- ▸ **Lanthanum** is predicted to decrease the absorption of antimalarials (chloroquine). Separate administration by at least 2 hours. [Moderate] Theoretical
- ▸ **Lanthanum** is predicted to decrease the absorption of hydroxychloroquine. Separate administration by at least 2 hours. [Moderate] Theoretical
- ▸ **Lanthanum** moderately decreases the exposure to quinolones. Quinolones should be taken 2 hours before or 4 hours after **lanthanum**. [Moderate] Study
- ▸ **Lanthanum** is predicted to decrease the absorption of tetracyclines. Separate administration by 2 hours. [Moderate] Theoretical
- ▸ **Lanthanum** decreases the absorption of thyroid hormones. Separate administration by 2 hours. [Moderate] Study

Lapatinib → see TABLE 9 p. 1336 (QT-interval prolongation)
- ▸ **Lapatinib** is predicted to increase the exposure to afatinib. Separate administration by 12 hours. [Moderate] Study
- ▸ **Lapatinib** is predicted to increase the exposure to aliskiren. [Moderate] Theoretical
- ▸ Antacids are predicted to decrease the absorption of **lapatinib**. Avoid. [Moderate] Theoretical
- ▸ Antiarrhythmics (dronedarone) are predicted to increase the exposure to **lapatinib**. [Moderate] Study → Also see TABLE 9 p. 1336
- ▸ Antiepileptics (carbamazepine, fosphenytoin, phenobarbital, phenytoin, primidone) are predicted to decrease the exposure to **lapatinib**. Avoid. [Severe] Study
- ▸ Antifungals, azoles (fluconazole, isavuconazole, posaconazole) are predicted to increase the exposure to **lapatinib**. [Moderate] Study → Also see TABLE 9 p. 1336
- ▸ Antifungals, azoles (itraconazole, ketoconazole, voriconazole) are predicted to increase the exposure to **lapatinib**. Avoid. [Moderate] Study → Also see TABLE 9 p. 1336
- ▸ **Lapatinib** is predicted to increase the exposure to antihistamines, non-sedating (fexofenadine). [Moderate] Theoretical
- ▸ Aprepitant is predicted to increase the exposure to **lapatinib**. [Moderate] Study
- ▸ **Lapatinib** is predicted to increase the exposure to beta blockers, non-selective (nadolol). [Moderate] Study
- ▸ Bosentan is predicted to decrease the exposure to **lapatinib**. Avoid. [Severe] Study
- ▸ Calcium channel blockers (diltiazem, verapamil) are predicted to increase the exposure to **lapatinib**. [Moderate] Study
- ▸ **Lapatinib** is predicted to increase the exposure to ceritinib. [Moderate] Theoretical → Also see TABLE 9 p. 1336
- ▸ Cobicistat is predicted to increase the exposure to **lapatinib**. Avoid. [Moderate] Study
- ▸ **Lapatinib** is predicted to increase the exposure to colchicine. Avoid or adjust colchicine dose, p. 1085. [Moderate] Theoretical
- ▸ **Lapatinib** is predicted to increase the risk of bleeding events when given with coumarins. [Severe] Theoretical
- ▸ Crizotinib is predicted to increase the exposure to **lapatinib**. [Moderate] Study → Also see TABLE 9 p. 1336
- ▸ **Lapatinib** is predicted to increase the exposure to dabigatran. [Severe] Theoretical
- ▸ **Lapatinib** is predicted to increase the exposure to digoxin. [Moderate] Theoretical
- ▸ **Lapatinib** is predicted to slightly increase the exposure to edoxaban. [Severe] Theoretical

Lapatinib (continued)
▶ Efavirenz is predicted to decrease the exposure to **lapatinib**. Avoid. Severe Study → Also see TABLE 9 p. 1336
▶ Enzalutamide is predicted to decrease the exposure to **lapatinib**. Avoid. Severe Study
▶ **Lapatinib** is predicted to increase the exposure to erlotinib. Moderate Theoretical
▶ **Lapatinib** is predicted to increase the exposure to everolimus. Moderate Theoretical
▶ **Lapatinib** is predicted to increase the exposure to fidaxomicin. Avoid. Moderate Study
▶ Grapefruit juice is predicted to increase the exposure to **lapatinib**. Avoid. Moderate Study
▶ H_2 receptor antagonists are predicted to decrease the absorption of **lapatinib**. Avoid. Moderate Theoretical
▶ HIV-protease inhibitors are predicted to increase the exposure to **lapatinib**. Avoid. Moderate Study → Also see TABLE 9 p. 1336
▶ Idelalisib is predicted to increase the exposure to **lapatinib**. Avoid. Moderate Study
▶ Imatinib is predicted to increase the exposure to **lapatinib**. Moderate Study
▶ **Lapatinib** is predicted to increase the exposure to lomitapide. Separate administration by 12 hours. Moderate Theoretical
▶ **Lapatinib** is predicted to increase the exposure to loperamide. Moderate Theoretical
▶ Macrolides (clarithromycin) are predicted to increase the exposure to **lapatinib**. Avoid. Moderate Study → Also see TABLE 9 p. 1336
▶ Macrolides (erythromycin) are predicted to increase the exposure to **lapatinib**. Moderate Study → Also see TABLE 9 p. 1336
▶ Mitotane is predicted to decrease the exposure to **lapatinib**. Avoid. Severe Study
▶ Netupitant is predicted to increase the exposure to **lapatinib**. Moderate Study
▶ Nevirapine is predicted to decrease the exposure to **lapatinib**. Avoid. Severe Study
▶ Nilotinib is predicted to increase the exposure to **lapatinib**. Moderate Study → Also see TABLE 9 p. 1336
▶ **Lapatinib** is predicted to increase the exposure to nintedanib. Moderate Study
▶ **Lapatinib** is predicted to increase the exposure to panobinostat. Adjust dose. Moderate Theoretical → Also see TABLE 9 p. 1336
▶ **Lapatinib** is predicted to increase the risk of bleeding events when given with phenindione. Severe Theoretical
▶ Rifampicin is predicted to decrease the exposure to **lapatinib**. Avoid. Severe Study
▶ **Lapatinib** is predicted to increase the exposure to sirolimus. Moderate Theoretical
▶ St John's Wort is predicted to decrease the exposure to **lapatinib**. Avoid. Severe Study
▶ **Lapatinib** slightly increases the exposure to taxanes (paclitaxel). Severe Study
▶ Tedizolid is predicted to increase the exposure to **lapatinib**. Avoid. Moderate Theoretical
▶ **Lapatinib** is predicted to increase the exposure to topotecan. Severe Study
▶ **Lapatinib** is predicted to increase the concentration of trametinib. Moderate Theoretical
▶ **Lapatinib** is predicted to increase the exposure to venetoclax. Avoid or monitor for toxicity. Severe Theoretical

Laronidase
▶ Antimalarials (chloroquine) are predicted to decrease the exposure to **laronidase**. Avoid simultaneous administration. Severe Theoretical
▶ Hydroxychloroquine is predicted to decrease the exposure to **laronidase**. Avoid simultaneous administration. Severe Theoretical

Ledipasvir
▶ Antacids are predicted to decrease the exposure to **ledipasvir**. Separate administration by 4 hours. Moderate Theoretical
▶ **Ledipasvir** increases the risk of severe bradycardia or heart block when given with antiarrhythmics (amiodarone). Refer to specialist literature. Severe Anecdotal

▶ Antiepileptics (carbamazepine) are predicted to decrease the exposure to **ledipasvir**. Avoid. Severe Theoretical
▶ Calcium salts (calcium carbonate) are predicted to decrease the exposure to **ledipasvir**. Separate administration by 4 hours. Moderate Theoretical
▶ H_2 receptor antagonists are predicted to decrease the exposure to **ledipasvir**. Adjust dose, see ledipasvir with sofosbuvir p. 617. Moderate Study
▶ Proton pump inhibitors are predicted to decrease the exposure to **ledipasvir**. Adjust dose, see ledipasvir with sofosbuvir p. 617. Moderate Theoretical
▶ Rifampicin is predicted to decrease the exposure to **ledipasvir**. Avoid. Severe Theoretical
▶ **Ledipasvir** moderately increases the exposure to simeprevir and simeprevir slightly increases the exposure to **ledipasvir**. Avoid. Severe Study
▶ St John's Wort is predicted to decrease the exposure to **ledipasvir**. Avoid. Severe Theoretical
▶ **Ledipasvir** is predicted to increase the exposure to statins (atorvastatin, fluvastatin, pravastatin, simvastatin). Monitor and adjust dose. Moderate Theoretical
▶ **Ledipasvir** is predicted to increase the exposure to statins (rosuvastatin). Avoid. Severe Theoretical
▶ **Ledipasvir** (with sofosbuvir) slightly increases the exposure to tenofovir disoproxil. Moderate Study

Leflunomide → see TABLE 1 p. 1334 (hepatotoxicity), TABLE 15 p. 1337 (myelosuppression)

PHARMACOLOGY Leflunomide has a long half-life; washout procedure recommended before switching to other DMARDs (consult product literature).

▶ **Leflunomide** is predicted to decrease the exposure to agomelatine. Moderate Theoretical
▶ **Leflunomide** decreases the exposure to aminophylline. Adjust dose. Moderate Study
▶ **Leflunomide** is predicted to decrease the exposure to anaesthetics, local (ropivacaine). Moderate Theoretical
▶ **Leflunomide** potentially increases the exposure to baricitinib. Moderate Theoretical
▶ **Leflunomide** is predicted to moderately increase the clearance of caffeine citrate. Monitor and adjust dose. Moderate Study
▶ **Leflunomide** is predicted to decrease the exposure to clozapine. Moderate Theoretical → Also see TABLE 15 p. 1337
▶ **Leflunomide** increases the anticoagulant effect of coumarins. Severe Anecdotal
▶ **Leflunomide** is predicted to decrease the exposure to duloxetine. Moderate Theoretical
▶ Live vaccines are predicted to increase the risk of generalised infection (possibly life-threatening) when given with **leflunomide**. Public Health England advises avoid (refer to Green Book). Severe Theoretical
▶ **Leflunomide** is predicted to decrease the exposure to melatonin. Moderate Theoretical
▶ **Leflunomide** is predicted to increase the exposure to montelukast. Moderate Theoretical
▶ **Leflunomide** is predicted to decrease the exposure to olanzapine. Monitor and adjust dose. Moderate Study → Also see TABLE 15 p. 1337
▶ **Leflunomide** is predicted to increase the exposure to pioglitazone. Moderate Study
▶ **Leflunomide** is predicted to decrease the exposure to pirfenidone. Moderate Theoretical
▶ **Leflunomide** is predicted to increase the exposure to repaglinide. Moderate Study
▶ **Leflunomide** is predicted to increase the exposure to selexipag. Adjust dose. Moderate Theoretical
▶ **Leflunomide** is predicted to increase the exposure to statins (rosuvastatin). Adjust dose. Moderate Study → Also see TABLE 1 p. 1334
▶ **Leflunomide** is predicted to increase the concentration of taxanes (paclitaxel). Severe Anecdotal → Also see TABLE 15 p. 1337
▶ **Leflunomide** is predicted to decrease the exposure to theophylline. Adjust dose. Moderate Study
▶ **Leflunomide** moderately decreases the exposure to tizanidine. Mild Study

Lenalidomide → see TABLE 1 p. 1334 (hepatotoxicity), TABLE 15 p. 1337 (myelosuppression), TABLE 5 p. 1334 (thromboembolism)
► Combined hormonal contraceptives are predicted to increase the risk of venous thromboembolism when given with lenalidomide. Avoid. Severe Theoretical
► Hormone replacement therapy is predicted to increase the risk of venous thromboembolism when given with lenalidomide. Severe Theoretical

Lercanidipine → see calcium channel blockers

Levamisole
► Albendazole slightly decreases the exposure to levamisole and levamisole moderately decreases the exposure to albendazole. Moderate Study
► Alcohol (beverage) potentially causes a disulfiram-like reaction when given with levamisole. Moderate Study
► Levamisole increases the exposure to ivermectin. Moderate Study

Levetiracetam → see antiepileptics
Levobunolol → see beta blockers, non-selective
Levobupivacaine → see anaesthetics, local
Levocetirizine → see antihistamines, non-sedating
Levodopa → see TABLE 8 p. 1335 (hypotension)

GENERAL INFORMATION Drugs with antimuscarinic effects might reduce the absorption of levodopa, see TABLE 10 p. 1336

► Amisulpride is predicted to decrease the effects of levodopa. Avoid. Severe Theoretical
► Antiepileptics (fosphenytoin, phenytoin) decrease the effects of levodopa. Moderate Study
► Aripiprazole is predicted to decrease the effects of levodopa. Severe Theoretical → Also see TABLE 8 p. 1335
► Asenapine is predicted to decrease the effects of levodopa. Adjust dose. Severe Theoretical → Also see TABLE 8 p. 1335
► Baclofen is predicted to increase the risk of side-effects when given with levodopa. Severe Anecdotal → Also see TABLE 8 p. 1335
► Benperidol is predicted to decrease the effects of levodopa. Severe Study → Also see TABLE 8 p. 1335
► Bupropion increases the risk of side-effects when given with levodopa. Moderate Study
► Clozapine is predicted to decrease the effects of levodopa. Severe Theoretical → Also see TABLE 8 p. 1335
► Droperidol decreases the effects of levodopa. Severe Study → Also see TABLE 8 p. 1335
► Entacapone increases the exposure to levodopa. Monitor side effects and adjust dose. Moderate Study
► Flupentixol decreases the effects of levodopa. Avoid or monitor worsening parkinsonian symptoms. Severe Theoretical → Also see TABLE 8 p. 1335
► Haloperidol decreases the effects of levodopa. Severe Study → Also see TABLE 8 p. 1335
► Iron (oral) decreases the absorption of levodopa. Moderate Study
► Isoniazid decreases the effects of levodopa. Moderate Study
► Levodopa is predicted to increase the risk of elevated blood pressure when given with linezolid. Avoid. Severe Theoretical
► Loxapine is predicted to decrease the effects of levodopa. Severe Theoretical → Also see TABLE 8 p. 1335
► Lurasidone is predicted to decrease the effects of levodopa. Severe Theoretical → Also see TABLE 8 p. 1335
► Memantine is predicted to increase the effects of levodopa. Moderate Theoretical
► Metoclopramide decreases the effects of levodopa. Avoid. Moderate Study
► Levodopa increases the risk of side-effects when given with moclobemide. Moderate Study
► Levodopa increases the risk of a hypertensive crisis when given with monoamine-oxidase A and B inhibitors, irreversible. Avoid and for 14 days after stopping the MAOI. Severe Study → Also see TABLE 8 p. 1335
► Monoamine-oxidase B inhibitors are predicted to increase the effects of levodopa. Adjust dose. Mild Study → Also see TABLE 8 p. 1335
► Olanzapine decreases the effects of levodopa. Avoid or monitor worsening parkinsonian symptoms. Severe Anecdotal → Also see TABLE 8 p. 1335

► Opicapone increases the exposure to levodopa. Adjust dose. Moderate Study
► Paliperidone is predicted to decrease the effects of levodopa. Severe Theoretical → Also see TABLE 8 p. 1335
► Phenothiazines decrease the effects of levodopa. Avoid or monitor worsening parkinsonian symptoms. Severe Study → Also see TABLE 8 p. 1335
► Pimozide decreases the effects of levodopa. Severe Theoretical → Also see TABLE 8 p. 1335
► Quetiapine decreases the effects of levodopa. Severe Anecdotal → Also see TABLE 8 p. 1335
► Risperidone is predicted to decrease the effects of levodopa. Avoid or adjust dose. Severe Anecdotal → Also see TABLE 8 p. 1335
► Sulpiride is predicted to decrease the effects of levodopa. Avoid. Severe Theoretical → Also see TABLE 8 p. 1335
► Tetrabenazine is predicted to decrease the effects of levodopa. Use with caution or avoid. Moderate Theoretical
► Tolcapone increases the exposure to levodopa. Monitor and adjust dose. Moderate Study
► Tryptophan greatly decreases the concentration of levodopa. Moderate Study
► Zuclopenthixol is predicted to decrease the effects of levodopa. Avoid or monitor worsening parkinsonian symptoms. Severe Theoretical → Also see TABLE 8 p. 1335

Levofloxacin → see quinolones
Levofolinic acid → see folates
Levomepromazine → see phenothiazines
Levonorgestrel
► Antiepileptics (carbamazepine, eslicarbazepine, fosphenytoin, oxcarbazepine, perampanel, phenobarbital, phenytoin, primidone, rufinamide, topiramate) are predicted to decrease the efficacy of levonorgestrel. For FSRH guidance, see Contraceptives, interactions p. 775. Severe Theoretical
► Aprepitant is predicted to decrease the efficacy of levonorgestrel. For FSRH guidance, see Contraceptives, interactions p. 775. Severe Theoretical
► Bosentan is predicted to decrease the efficacy of levonorgestrel. For FSRH guidance, see Contraceptives, interactions p. 775. Severe Theoretical
► Efavirenz is predicted to decrease the efficacy of levonorgestrel. For FSRH guidance, see Contraceptives, interactions p. 775. Severe Theoretical
► Fosaprepitant is predicted to decrease the efficacy of levonorgestrel. For FSRH guidance, see Contraceptives, interactions p. 775. Severe Theoretical
► Griseofulvin potentially decreases the efficacy of oral levonorgestrel. For FSRH guidance, see Contraceptives, interactions p. 775. Severe Anecdotal
► HIV-protease inhibitors (ritonavir) are predicted to decrease the efficacy of levonorgestrel. For FSRH guidance, see Contraceptives, interactions p. 775. Severe Theoretical
► Lumacaftor is predicted to decrease the efficacy of levonorgestrel. Use additional contraceptive precautions. Severe Theoretical
► Modafinil is predicted to decrease the efficacy of levonorgestrel. For FSRH guidance, see Contraceptives, interactions p. 775. Severe Theoretical
► Nevirapine is predicted to decrease the efficacy of levonorgestrel. For FSRH guidance, see Contraceptives, interactions p. 775. Severe Theoretical
► Rifabutin is predicted to decrease the efficacy of levonorgestrel. For FSRH guidance, see Contraceptives, interactions p. 775. Severe Theoretical
► Rifampicin is predicted to decrease the efficacy of levonorgestrel. For FSRH guidance, see Contraceptives, interactions p. 775. Severe Theoretical
► St John's Wort is predicted to decrease the efficacy of levonorgestrel. MHRA advises avoid. For FSRH guidance, see Contraceptives, interactions p. 775. Severe Theoretical
► Sugammadex is predicted to decrease the exposure to levonorgestrel. Use additional contraceptive precautions. Severe Theoretical
► Ulipristal is predicted to decrease the efficacy of levonorgestrel. Avoid. Severe Theoretical

Levothyroxine → see thyroid hormones

A1

Interactions | Appendix 1

Lidocaine → see antiarrhythmics

Linagliptin → see TABLE 14 p. 1337 (antidiabetic drugs)

▶ Antiepileptics (carbamazepine, fosphenytoin, phenobarbital, phenytoin, primidone) are predicted to decrease the exposure to linagliptin. Moderate Study

▶ Enzalutamide is predicted to decrease the exposure to linagliptin. Moderate Study

▶ Linagliptin is predicted to increase the exposure to lomitapide. Separate administration by 12 hours. Moderate Theoretical

▶ Mitotane is predicted to decrease the exposure to linagliptin. Moderate Study

▶ Rifampicin is predicted to decrease the exposure to linagliptin. Moderate Study

Linezolid → see TABLE 15 p. 1337 (myelosuppression), TABLE 13 p. 1337 (serotonin syndrome)

FOOD AND LIFESTYLE Patients taking linezolid should avoid consuming large amounts of tyramine-rich foods (such as mature cheese, salami, pickled herring, *Bovril*®, *Oxo*®, *Marmite*® or any similar meat or yeast extract or fermented soya bean extract, and some beers, lagers or wines).

▶ Beta₂ agonists are predicted to increase the risk of elevated blood pressure when given with linezolid. Avoid. Severe Theoretical

▶ Bupropion is predicted to increase the risk of intraoperative hypertension when given with linezolid. Severe Anecdotal → Also see TABLE 13 p. 1337

▶ Buspirone is predicted to increase the risk of elevated blood pressure when given with linezolid. Avoid. Severe Theoretical → Also see TABLE 13 p. 1337

▶ Levodopa is predicted to increase the risk of elevated blood pressure when given with linezolid. Avoid. Severe Theoretical

▶ Macrolides (clarithromycin) increase the exposure to linezolid. Moderate Anecdotal

▶ Methylphenidate is predicted to increase the risk of elevated blood pressure when given with linezolid. Avoid. Severe Theoretical

▶ Moclobemide is predicted to increase the risk of side-effects when given with linezolid. Avoid and for 14 days after stopping moclobemide. Severe Theoretical → Also see TABLE 13 p. 1337

▶ Monoamine-oxidase A and B inhibitors, irreversible are predicted to increase the risk of side-effects when given with linezolid. Avoid and for 14 days after stopping the MAOI. Severe Theoretical → Also see TABLE 13 p. 1337

▶ Monoamine-oxidase B inhibitors (rasagiline, selegiline) are predicted to increase the risk of side-effects when given with linezolid. Avoid and for 14 days after stopping the MAOI. Severe Theoretical → Also see TABLE 13 p. 1337

▶ Monoamine-oxidase B inhibitors (safinamide) are predicted to increase the risk of side-effects when given with linezolid. Avoid and for 1 week after stopping safinamide. Severe Theoretical → Also see TABLE 13 p. 1337

▶ Reboxetine is predicted to increase the risk of a hypertensive crisis when given with linezolid. Avoid. Severe Theoretical

▶ Rifampicin slightly decreases the exposure to linezolid. Moderate Study

▶ Sympathomimetics, inotropic are predicted to increase the risk of elevated blood pressure when given with linezolid. Avoid. Severe Theoretical

▶ Sympathomimetics, vasoconstrictor (adrenaline/epinephrine, ephedrine, isometheptene, noradrenaline/norepinephrine, phenylephrine) are predicted to increase the risk of elevated blood pressure when given with linezolid. Avoid. Severe Theoretical

▶ Sympathomimetics, vasoconstrictor (pseudoephedrine) increase the risk of elevated blood pressure when given with linezolid. Avoid. Severe Study

Liothyronine → see thyroid hormones

Liraglutide → see TABLE 14 p. 1337 (antidiabetic drugs)

Lisdexamfetamine → see amfetamines

Lisinopril → see ACE inhibitors

Lithium → see TABLE 13 p. 1337 (serotonin syndrome), TABLE 9 p. 1336 (QT-interval prolongation)

▶ ACE inhibitors are predicted to increase the concentration of lithium. Monitor and adjust dose. Severe Anecdotal

▶ Acetazolamide alters the concentration of lithium. Anecdotal

▶ Aldosterone antagonists (eplerenone) potentially increase the concentration of lithium. Avoid. Moderate Theoretical

▶ Aldosterone antagonists (spironolactone) potentially increase the concentration of lithium. Moderate Study

▶ Aminophylline is predicted to decrease the concentration of lithium. Moderate Theoretical

▶ Angiotensin-II receptor antagonists potentially increase the concentration of lithium. Monitor concentration and adjust dose. Severe Anecdotal

▶ Antiepileptics (carbamazepine, oxcarbazepine) are predicted to increase the risk of neurotoxicity when given with lithium. Severe Anecdotal

▶ Calcitonin (salmon) decreases the concentration of lithium. Monitor concentration and adjust dose. Moderate Study

▶ Calcium channel blockers (diltiazem, verapamil) are predicted to increase the risk of neurotoxicity when given with lithium. Severe Anecdotal

▶ Loop diuretics increase the concentration of lithium. Monitor and adjust dose. Severe Study

▶ Methyldopa increases the risk of neurotoxicity when given with lithium. Severe Anecdotal

▶ NSAIDs increase the concentration of lithium. Monitor and adjust dose. Severe Study

▶ Phenothiazines potentially increase the risk of neurotoxicity when given with lithium. Severe Anecdotal → Also see TABLE 9 p. 1336

▶ Potassium-sparing diuretics (triamterene) potentially increase the clearance of lithium. Moderate Study

▶ Quetiapine potentially increases the risk of neurotoxicity when given with lithium. Severe Anecdotal

▶ Risperidone potentially increases the risk of neurotoxicity when given with lithium. Severe Anecdotal → Also see TABLE 9 p. 1336

▶ Sodium bicarbonate decreases the concentration of lithium. Severe Anecdotal

▶ Sulpiride potentially increases the risk of neurotoxicity when given with lithium. Severe Anecdotal → Also see TABLE 9 p. 1336

▶ Theophylline is predicted to decrease the concentration of lithium. Monitor concentration and adjust dose. Moderate Anecdotal

▶ Thiazide diuretics increase the concentration of lithium. Avoid or adjust dose and monitor concentration. Severe Study

▶ Tricyclic antidepressants potentially increase the risk of neurotoxicity when given with lithium. Severe Anecdotal → Also see TABLE 13 p. 1337 → Also see TABLE 9 p. 1336

▶ Zuclopenthixol potentially increases the risk of neurotoxicity when given with lithium. Severe Anecdotal → Also see TABLE 9 p. 1336

Live vaccines

Bacillus Calmette-Guérin vaccine · influenza vaccine (live) · measles, mumps and rubella vaccine, live · rotavirus vaccine · typhoid vaccine, oral · varicella-zoster vaccine · yellow fever vaccine, live

GENERAL INFORMATION Oral typhoid vaccine is inactivated by concurrent administration of antibacterials or antimalarials: antibacterials should be avoided for 3 days before and after oral typhoid vaccination; *mefloquine* should be avoided for at least 12 hours before or after oral typhoid vaccination; for other antimalarials oral typhoid vaccine vaccination should be completed at least 3 days before the first dose of the antimalarial (except proguanil hydrochloride with atovaquone, which can be given concurrently).

▶ Live vaccines are predicted to increase the risk of generalised infection (possibly life-threatening) when given with abatacept. Public Health England advises avoid (refer to Green Book). Severe Theoretical

▶ Live vaccines are predicted to increase the risk of generalised infection (possibly life-threatening) when given with alkylating agents. Public Health England advises avoid (refer to Green Book). Severe Theoretical

▶ Live vaccines are predicted to increase the risk of generalised infection (possibly life-threatening) when given with

A1

Interactions | Appendix 1

amsacrine. Public Health England advises avoid (refer to Green Book). [Severe] Theoretical
▸ **Live vaccines** are predicted to increase the risk of generalised infection (possibly life-threatening) when given with anakinra. Public Health England advises avoid (refer to Green Book). [Severe] Theoretical
▸ **Live vaccines** are predicted to increase the risk of generalised infection (possibly life-threatening) when given with anthracyclines. Public Health England advises avoid (refer to Green Book). [Severe] Theoretical
▸ **Live vaccines** are predicted to increase the risk of generalised infection (possibly life-threatening) when given with azathioprine (high-dose). Public Health England advises avoid (refer to Green Book). [Severe] Theoretical
▸ **Live vaccines** are predicted to increase the risk of generalised infection (possibly life-threatening) when given with baricitinib. Avoid. [Severe] Theoretical
▸ **Live vaccines** are predicted to increase the risk of generalised infection (possibly life-threatening) when given with belatacept. Public Health England advises avoid (refer to Green Book). [Severe] Theoretical
▸ **Live vaccines** are predicted to increase the risk of generalised infection (possibly life-threatening) when given with bleomycin. Public Health England advises avoid (refer to Green Book). [Severe] Theoretical
▸ **Live vaccines** are predicted to increase the risk of generalised infection (possibly life-threatening) when given with capecitabine. Public Health England advises avoid (refer to Green Book). [Severe] Theoretical
▸ **Live vaccines** are predicted to increase the risk of generalised infection (possibly life-threatening) when given with ciclosporin. Public Health England advises avoid (refer to Green Book). [Severe] Theoretical
▸ **Live vaccines** are predicted to increase the risk of generalised infection (possibly life-threatening) when given with cladribine. Public Health England advises avoid (refer to Green Book). [Severe] Theoretical
▸ **Live vaccines** are predicted to increase the risk of generalised infection (possibly life-threatening) when given with clofarabine. Public Health England advises avoid (refer to Green Book). [Severe] Theoretical
▸ **Live vaccines** are predicted to increase the risk of generalised infection (possibly life-threatening) when given with corticosteroids (high-dose). Public Health England advises avoid (refer to Green Book). [Severe] Theoretical
▸ **Live vaccines** are predicted to increase the risk of generalised infection (possibly life-threatening) when given with cytarabine. Public Health England advises avoid (refer to Green Book). [Severe] Theoretical
▸ **Live vaccines** are predicted to increase the risk of generalised infection (possibly life-threatening) when given with dactinomycin. Public Health England advises avoid (refer to Green Book). [Severe] Theoretical
▸ **Live vaccines** are predicted to increase the risk of generalised infection (possibly life-threatening) when given with dimethyl fumarate. Public Health England advises avoid (refer to Green Book). [Severe] Theoretical
▸ **Live vaccines** are predicted to increase the risk of generalised infection (possibly life-threatening) when given with etanercept. Public Health England advises avoid (refer to Green Book). [Severe] Theoretical
▸ **Live vaccines** are predicted to increase the risk of generalised infection (possibly life-threatening) when given with etoposide. Public Health England advises avoid (refer to Green Book). [Severe] Theoretical
▸ **Live vaccines** are predicted to increase the risk of generalised infection (possibly life-threatening) when given with everolimus. Public Health England advises avoid (refer to Green Book). [Severe] Theoretical
▸ **Live vaccines** are predicted to increase the risk of generalised infection (possibly life-threatening) when given with fingolimod. Public Health England advises avoid (refer to Green Book). [Severe] Theoretical
▸ **Live vaccines** are predicted to increase the risk of generalised infection (possibly life-threatening) when given with

fludarabine. Public Health England advises avoid (refer to Green Book). [Severe] Theoretical
▸ **Live vaccines** are predicted to increase the risk of generalised infection (possibly life-threatening) when given with fluorouracil. Public Health England advises avoid (refer to Green Book). [Severe] Theoretical
▸ **Live vaccines** are predicted to increase the risk of generalised infection (possibly life-threatening) when given with gemcitabine. Public Health England advises avoid (refer to Green Book). [Severe] Theoretical
▸ **Live vaccines** are predicted to increase the risk of generalised infection (possibly life-threatening) when given with hydroxycarbamide. Public Health England advises avoid (refer to Green Book). [Severe] Theoretical
▸ **Live vaccines** are predicted to increase the risk of generalised infection (possibly life-threatening) when given with irinotecan. Public Health England advises avoid (refer to Green Book). [Severe] Theoretical
▸ **Live vaccines** are predicted to increase the risk of generalised infection (possibly life-threatening) when given with iron chelators (dexrazoxane). Avoid. [Severe] Theoretical
▸ **Live vaccines** are predicted to increase the risk of generalised infection (possibly life-threatening) when given with leflunomide. Public Health England advises avoid (refer to Green Book). [Severe] Theoretical
▸ **Live vaccines** are predicted to increase the risk of generalised infection (possibly life-threatening) when given with mercaptopurine (high-dose). Public Health England advises avoid (refer to Green Book). [Severe] Theoretical
▸ **Live vaccines** are predicted to increase the risk of generalised infection (possibly life-threatening) when given with methotrexate (high-dose). Public Health England advises avoid (refer to Green Book). [Severe] Theoretical
▸ **Live vaccines** are predicted to increase the risk of generalised infection (possibly life-threatening) when given with mitomycin. Public Health England advises avoid (refer to Green Book). [Severe] Theoretical
▸ **Live vaccines** are predicted to increase the risk of generalised infection (possibly life-threatening) when given with monoclonal antibodies. Public Health England advises avoid (refer to Green Book). [Severe] Theoretical
▸ **Live vaccines** are predicted to increase the risk of generalised infection (possibly life-threatening) when given with mycophenolate. Public Health England advises avoid (refer to Green Book). [Severe] Theoretical
▸ **Live vaccines** are predicted to increase the risk of generalised infection (possibly life-threatening) when given with pemetrexed. Public Health England advises avoid (refer to Green Book). [Severe] Theoretical
▸ **Live vaccines** are predicted to increase the risk of generalised infection (possibly life-threatening) when given with platinum compounds. Public Health England advises avoid (refer to Green Book). [Severe] Theoretical
▸ **Live vaccines** are predicted to increase the risk of generalised infection (possibly life-threatening) when given with procarbazine. Public Health England advises avoid (refer to Green Book). [Severe] Theoretical
▸ **Live vaccines** are predicted to increase the risk of generalised infection (possibly life-threatening) when given with raltitrexed. Public Health England advises avoid (refer to Green Book). [Severe] Theoretical
▸ **Live vaccines** are predicted to increase the risk of generalised infection (possibly life-threatening) when given with sirolimus. Public Health England advises avoid (refer to Green Book). [Severe] Theoretical
▸ **Live vaccines** are predicted to increase the risk of generalised infection (possibly life-threatening) when given with tacrolimus. Public Health England advises avoid (refer to Green Book). [Severe] Theoretical
▸ **Live vaccines** are predicted to increase the risk of generalised infection (possibly life-threatening) when given with taxanes (docetaxel, paclitaxel). Public Health England advises avoid (refer to Green Book). [Severe] Theoretical

A1

Interactions | Appendix 1

Live vaccines (continued)

▶ **Live vaccines** are predicted to increase the risk of generalised infection (possibly life-threatening) when given with tegafur. Public Health England advises avoid (refer to Green Book). Severe Theoretical

▶ **Live vaccines** are predicted to increase the risk of generalised infection (possibly life-threatening) when given with temsirolimus. Public Health England advises avoid (refer to Green Book). Severe Theoretical

▶ **Live vaccines** are predicted to increase the risk of generalised infection (possibly life-threatening) when given with teriflunomide. Public Health England advises avoid (refer to Green Book). Severe Theoretical

▶ **Live vaccines** are predicted to increase the risk of generalised infection (possibly life-threatening) when given with tioguanine. Public Health England advises avoid (refer to Green Book). Severe Theoretical

▶ **Live vaccines** potentially increase the risk of generalised infection (possibly life-threatening) when given with tofacitinib. Avoid. Severe Theoretical

▶ **Live vaccines** are predicted to increase the risk of generalised infection (possibly life-threatening) when given with topotecan. Public Health England advises avoid (refer to Green Book). Severe Theoretical

▶ **Live vaccines** are predicted to increase the risk of generalised infection (possibly life-threatening) when given with trabectedin. Public Health England advises avoid (refer to Green Book). Severe Theoretical

▶ Venetoclax potentially decreases the efficacy of **live vaccines**. Avoid. Severe Theoretical

▶ **Live vaccines** are predicted to increase the risk of generalised infection (possibly life-threatening) when given with vinca alkaloids. Public Health England advises avoid (refer to Green Book). Severe Theoretical

Lixisenatide → see TABLE 14 p. 1337 (antidiabetic drugs)

SEPARATION OF ADMINISTRATION Some orally administered drugs should be taken at least 1 hour before, or 4 hours after, lixisenatide injection.

Lofepramine → see tricyclic antidepressants

Lofexidine → see TABLE 8 p. 1335 (hypotension), TABLE 9 p. 1336 (QT-interval prolongation), TABLE 11 p. 1336 (CNS depressant effects)

Lomitapide → see TABLE 1 p. 1334 (hepatotoxicity)

FOOD AND LIFESTYLE Bitter (Seville) orange is predicted to increase the exposure to lomitapide; separate administration by 12 hours.

▶ Alprazolam is predicted to increase the exposure to **lomitapide**. Separate administration by 12 hours. Moderate Theoretical

▶ Antiarrhythmics (amiodarone) are predicted to increase the exposure to **lomitapide**. Separate administration by 12 hours. Moderate Theoretical

▶ Antiarrhythmics (dronedarone) are predicted to increase the exposure to **lomitapide**. Avoid. Moderate Theoretical

▶ Antiepileptics (carbamazepine, fosphenytoin, phenobarbital, phenytoin, primidone) are predicted to decrease the exposure to **lomitapide**. Monitor and adjust dose. Moderate Theoretical → Also see TABLE 1 p. 1334

▶ Antifungals, azoles (clotrimazole) are predicted to increase the exposure to **lomitapide**. Separate administration by 12 hours. Moderate Theoretical

▶ Antifungals, azoles (fluconazole, isavuconazole, posaconazole) are predicted to increase the exposure to **lomitapide**. Avoid. Moderate Theoretical → Also see TABLE 1 p. 1334

▶ Antifungals, azoles (itraconazole, ketoconazole, voriconazole) are predicted to markedly increase the exposure to **lomitapide**. Avoid. Severe Study → Also see TABLE 1 p. 1334

▶ Aprepitant is predicted to increase the exposure to **lomitapide**. Avoid. Moderate Theoretical

▶ Bicalutamide is predicted to increase the exposure to **lomitapide**. Separate administration by 12 hours. Moderate Theoretical

▶ Calcium channel blockers (amlodipine, lacidipine) are predicted to increase the exposure to **lomitapide**. Separate administration by 12 hours. Moderate Theoretical

▶ Calcium channel blockers (diltiazem, verapamil) are predicted to increase the exposure to **lomitapide**. Avoid. Moderate Theoretical

▶ Ciclosporin is predicted to increase the exposure to **lomitapide**. Separate administration by 12 hours. Moderate Theoretical

▶ Cilostazol is predicted to increase the exposure to **lomitapide**. Separate administration by 12 hours. Moderate Theoretical

▶ Cobicistat is predicted to markedly increase the exposure to **lomitapide**. Avoid. Severe Study

▶ Oral combined hormonal contraceptives slightly increase the exposure to **lomitapide**. Separate administration by 12 hours. Moderate Theoretical

▶ **Lomitapide** increases the exposure to coumarins (warfarin). Monitor INR and adjust dose. Severe Study

▶ Crizotinib is predicted to increase the exposure to **lomitapide**. Avoid. Moderate Theoretical

▶ Enzalutamide is predicted to decrease the exposure to **lomitapide**. Monitor and adjust dose. Moderate Theoretical

▶ Everolimus is predicted to increase the exposure to **lomitapide**. Separate administration by 12 hours. Moderate Theoretical

▶ Fosaprepitant is predicted to increase the exposure to **lomitapide**. Separate administration by 12 hours. Moderate Theoretical

▶ Grapefruit juice is predicted to increase the exposure to **lomitapide**. Separate administration by 12 hours. Moderate Theoretical

▶ H₂ receptor antagonists (cimetidine, ranitidine) are predicted to increase the exposure to **lomitapide**. Separate administration by 12 hours. Moderate Theoretical

▶ HIV-protease inhibitors are predicted to markedly increase the exposure to **lomitapide**. Avoid. Severe Study

▶ Idelalisib is predicted to markedly increase the exposure to **lomitapide**. Avoid. Severe Study

▶ Imatinib is predicted to increase the exposure to **lomitapide**. Avoid. Moderate Theoretical

▶ Isoniazid is predicted to increase the exposure to **lomitapide**. Separate administration by 12 hours. Unknown Theoretical → Also see TABLE 1 p. 1334

▶ Ivacaftor is predicted to increase the exposure to **lomitapide**. Separate administration by 12 hours. Moderate Theoretical

▶ Lapatinib is predicted to increase the exposure to **lomitapide**. Separate administration by 12 hours. Moderate Theoretical

▶ Linagliptin is predicted to increase the exposure to **lomitapide**. Separate administration by 12 hours. Moderate Theoretical

▶ Macrolides (azithromycin) are predicted to increase the exposure to **lomitapide**. Separate administration by 12 hours. Moderate Theoretical

▶ Macrolides (clarithromycin) are predicted to markedly increase the exposure to **lomitapide**. Avoid. Severe Study

▶ Macrolides (erythromycin) are predicted to increase the exposure to **lomitapide**. Avoid. Moderate Theoretical

▶ Mitotane is predicted to decrease the exposure to **lomitapide**. Monitor and adjust dose. Moderate Theoretical

▶ Netupitant is predicted to increase the exposure to **lomitapide**. Avoid. Moderate Theoretical

▶ Nilotinib is predicted to increase the exposure to **lomitapide**. Avoid. Moderate Theoretical

▶ Pazopanib is predicted to increase the exposure to **lomitapide**. Separate administration by 12 hours. Moderate Theoretical

▶ Peppermint oil is predicted to increase the exposure to **lomitapide**. Separate administration by 12 hours. Moderate Theoretical

▶ Propiverine is predicted to increase the exposure to **lomitapide**. Separate administration by 12 hours. Moderate Theoretical

▶ Ranolazine is predicted to increase the exposure to **lomitapide**. Separate administration by 12 hours. Moderate Theoretical

▶ Rifampicin is predicted to decrease the exposure to **lomitapide**. Monitor and adjust dose. Moderate Theoretical

▶ SSRIs (fluoxetine) are predicted to increase the exposure to **lomitapide**. Separate administration by 12 hours. Unknown Theoretical

▶ SSRIs (fluvoxamine) are predicted to increase the exposure to **lomitapide**. Separate administration by 12 hours. Moderate Theoretical

‣ **Lomitapide** increases the exposure to statins (atorvastatin). Adjust **lomitapide** dose or separate administration by 12 hours. Mild Study → Also see **TABLE 1** p. 1334
‣ **Lomitapide** increases the exposure to statins (simvastatin). Monitor and adjust **simvastatin** dose, p. 203. Moderate Study → Also see **TABLE 1** p. 1334
‣ Tacrolimus is predicted to increase the exposure to **lomitapide**. Separate administration by 12 hours. Moderate Theoretical
‣ Ticagrelor is predicted to increase the exposure to **lomitapide**. Separate administration by 12 hours. Moderate Theoretical
‣ Tolvaptan is predicted to increase the exposure to **lomitapide**. Separate administration by 12 hours. Moderate Theoretical

Lomustine → see alkylating agents

Loop diuretics → see **TABLE 18** p. 1338 (hyponatraemia), **TABLE 8** p. 1335 (hypotension), **TABLE 19** p. 1338 (ototoxicity), **TABLE 17** p. 1338 (reduced serum potassium)

bumetanide · furosemide · torasemide

‣ Aliskiren slightly decreases the exposure to **furosemide**. Moderate Study → Also see **TABLE 8** p. 1335
‣ **Loop diuretics** increase the risk of nephrotoxicity when given with aminoglycosides. Avoid. Moderate Study → Also see **TABLE 19** p. 1338
‣ Antiepileptics (fosphenytoin, phenytoin) decrease the effects of **furosemide**. Moderate Study
‣ Intravenous **furosemide** potentially increases the risk of sweating, variable blood pressure, and tachycardia when given after chloral hydrate. Moderate Anecdotal
‣ Dasabuvir (with ombitasvir, paritaprevir and ritonavir) increases the concentration of **furosemide**. Adjust dose. Moderate Study
‣ **Loop diuretics** increase the concentration of lithium. Monitor and adjust dose. Severe Study
‣ Paritaprevir (with ritonavir and ombitasvir) is predicted to increase the exposure to **furosemide**. Adjust dose. Moderate Theoretical
‣ Reboxetine is predicted to increase the risk of hypokalaemia when given with **loop diuretics**. Moderate Theoretical

Loperamide

‣ Antiarrhythmics (dronedarone) are predicted to increase the exposure to **loperamide**. Severe Theoretical
‣ Ceritinib is predicted to increase the exposure to **loperamide**. Moderate Theoretical
‣ **Loperamide** greatly increases the absorption of oral desmopressin (and possibly sublingual). Moderate Study
‣ Eliglustat is predicted to increase the exposure to **loperamide**. Adjust dose. Moderate Study
‣ Lapatinib is predicted to increase the exposure to **loperamide**. Moderate Theoretical
‣ Mirabegron is predicted to increase the exposure to **loperamide**. Mild Theoretical
‣ Opicapone is predicted to increase the exposure to **loperamide**. Avoid. Moderate Study
‣ Velpatasvir is predicted to increase the exposure to **loperamide**. Severe Theoretical

Lopinavir → see HIV-protease inhibitors

Loprazolam → see **TABLE 11** p. 1336 (CNS depressant effects)

Loratadine → see antihistamines, non-sedating

Lorazepam → see **TABLE 11** p. 1336 (CNS depressant effects)

‣ Rifampicin increases the clearance of **lorazepam**. Moderate Study

Lormetazepam → see **TABLE 11** p. 1336 (CNS depressant effects)

Losartan → see angiotensin-II receptor antagonists

Low molecular-weight heparins → see **TABLE 16** p. 1338 (increased serum potassium), **TABLE 3** p. 1334 (anticoagulant effects)

dalteparin · enoxaparin · tinzaparin

‣ Ranibizumab increases the risk of bleeding events when given with **low molecular-weight heparins**. Severe Study

Loxapine → see **TABLE 8** p. 1335 (hypotension), **TABLE 11** p. 1336 (CNS depressant effects), **TABLE 10** p. 1336 (antimuscarinics)

‣ Combined hormonal contraceptives are predicted to increase the exposure to **loxapine**. Avoid. Unknown Theoretical
‣ **Loxapine** is predicted to decrease the effects of dopamine receptor agonists. Moderate Theoretical → Also see **TABLE 8** p. 1335 → Also see **TABLE 10** p. 1336

‣ **Loxapine** is predicted to decrease the effects of levodopa. Severe Theoretical → Also see **TABLE 8** p. 1335
‣ Quinolones (ciprofloxacin) are predicted to increase the exposure to **loxapine**. Avoid. Unknown Theoretical
‣ SSRIs (fluvoxamine) are predicted to increase the exposure to **loxapine**. Avoid. Unknown Theoretical

Lumacaftor

‣ **Lumacaftor** is predicted to decrease the exposure to antiepileptics (carbamazepine, fosphenytoin, phenobarbital, phenytoin, primidone). Avoid. Severe Theoretical
‣ **Lumacaftor** is predicted to decrease the exposure to antifungals, azoles (fluconazole). Adjust dose. Mild Theoretical
‣ **Lumacaftor** is predicted to decrease the exposure to antifungals, azoles (itraconazole, ketoconazole, posaconazole, voriconazole). Avoid or monitor efficacy. Moderate Theoretical
‣ **Lumacaftor** is predicted to decrease the exposure to ciclosporin. Avoid. Severe Theoretical
‣ **Lumacaftor** is predicted to decrease the efficacy of combined hormonal contraceptives. Use additional contraceptive precautions. Severe Theoretical
‣ **Lumacaftor** is predicted to decrease the exposure to corticosteroids (methylprednisolone, prednisone). Adjust dose. Severe Theoretical
‣ **Lumacaftor** is predicted to decrease the exposure to everolimus. Avoid. Severe Theoretical
‣ **Lumacaftor** potentially decreases the exposure to glecaprevir. Avoid. Severe Theoretical
‣ **Lumacaftor** is predicted to decrease the efficacy of levonorgestrel. Use additional contraceptive precautions. Severe Theoretical
‣ **Lumacaftor** is predicted to decrease the exposure to macrolides (clarithromycin, erythromycin). Moderate Theoretical
‣ **Lumacaftor** is predicted to decrease the exposure to midazolam. Severe Theoretical
‣ **Lumacaftor** potentially decreases the exposure to pibrentasvir. Avoid. Severe Theoretical
‣ **Lumacaftor** is predicted to decrease the exposure to rifabutin. Adjust dose. Moderate Theoretical
‣ **Lumacaftor** is predicted to decrease the exposure to sirolimus. Avoid. Severe Theoretical
‣ **Lumacaftor** is predicted to decrease the exposure to tacrolimus. Avoid. Severe Theoretical
‣ **Lumacaftor** is predicted to decrease the exposure to temsirolimus. Avoid. Severe Theoretical
‣ **Lumacaftor** is predicted to decrease the efficacy of ulipristal. Use additional contraceptive precautions. Severe Theoretical

Lumefantrine → see antimalarials

Lurasidone → see **TABLE 8** p. 1335 (hypotension), **TABLE 11** p. 1336 (CNS depressant effects)

‣ Antiarrhythmics (dronedarone) are predicted to increase the exposure to **lurasidone**. Moderate Study
‣ Antiepileptics (carbamazepine, fosphenytoin, phenobarbital, phenytoin, primidone) are predicted to decrease the exposure to **lurasidone**. Avoid. Moderate Study → Also see **TABLE 11** p. 1336
‣ Antifungals, azoles (fluconazole, isavuconazole, posaconazole) are predicted to increase the exposure to **lurasidone**. Moderate Study
‣ Antifungals, azoles (itraconazole, ketoconazole, voriconazole) are predicted to increase the exposure to **lurasidone**. Avoid. Severe Study
‣ Aprepitant is predicted to increase the exposure to **lurasidone**. Moderate Study
‣ Bosentan is predicted to decrease the exposure to **lurasidone**. Monitor and adjust dose. Moderate Theoretical
‣ Calcium channel blockers (diltiazem, verapamil) are predicted to increase the exposure to **lurasidone**. Moderate Study → Also see **TABLE 8** p. 1335
‣ Cobicistat is predicted to increase the exposure to **lurasidone**. Avoid. Severe Study
‣ Crizotinib is predicted to increase the exposure to **lurasidone**. Moderate Study
‣ Efavirenz is predicted to decrease the exposure to **lurasidone**. Monitor and adjust dose. Moderate Theoretical
‣ Enzalutamide is predicted to decrease the exposure to **lurasidone**. Avoid. Moderate Study

A1

Interactions | Appendix 1

Lurasidone (continued)
- Grapefruit juice is predicted to increase the exposure to **lurasidone**. Avoid. Severe Theoretical
- HIV-protease inhibitors are predicted to increase the exposure to **lurasidone**. Avoid. Severe Study
- Idelalisib is predicted to increase the exposure to **lurasidone**. Avoid. Severe Study
- Imatinib is predicted to increase the exposure to **lurasidone**. Moderate Study
- **Lurasidone** is predicted to decrease the effects of levodopa. Severe Theoretical → Also see TABLE 8 p. 1335
- Macrolides (clarithromycin) are predicted to increase the exposure to **lurasidone**. Avoid. Severe Study
- Macrolides (erythromycin) are predicted to increase the exposure to **lurasidone**. Moderate Study
- Mitotane is predicted to decrease the exposure to **lurasidone**. Avoid. Moderate Study
- Netupitant is predicted to increase the exposure to **lurasidone**. Moderate Study
- Nevirapine is predicted to decrease the exposure to **lurasidone**. Monitor and adjust dose. Moderate Theoretical
- Nilotinib is predicted to increase the exposure to **lurasidone**. Moderate Study
- Rifampicin is predicted to decrease the exposure to **lurasidone**. Avoid. Moderate Study
- St John's Wort is predicted to decrease the exposure to **lurasidone**. Monitor and adjust dose. Moderate Theoretical

Lymecycline → see tetracyclines

Macitentan
- Antiepileptics (carbamazepine, fosphenytoin, phenobarbital, phenytoin, primidone) are predicted to decrease the exposure to **macitentan**. Avoid. Severe Study
- Antifungals, azoles (itraconazole, ketoconazole, voriconazole) are predicted to increase the exposure to **macitentan**. Moderate Study
- Cobicistat is predicted to increase the exposure to **macitentan**. Moderate Study
- Enzalutamide is predicted to decrease the exposure to **macitentan**. Avoid. Severe Study
- HIV-protease inhibitors are predicted to increase the exposure to **macitentan**. Moderate Study
- Idelalisib is predicted to increase the exposure to **macitentan**. Moderate Study
- Macrolides (clarithromycin) are predicted to increase the exposure to **macitentan**. Moderate Study
- Mitotane is predicted to decrease the exposure to **macitentan**. Avoid. Severe Study
- Rifampicin is predicted to decrease the exposure to **macitentan**. Avoid. Severe Study
- St John's Wort is predicted to decrease the exposure to **macitentan**. Avoid. Severe Theoretical

Macrolides → see TABLE 9 p. 1336 (QT-interval prolongation)

azithromycin · clarithromycin · erythromycin

ROUTE-SPECIFIC INFORMATION Since systemic absorption can follow topical application, the possibility of interactions should be borne in mind.

- **Clarithromycin** is predicted to increase the exposure to abiraterone. Severe Theoretical
- **Macrolides** are predicted to increase the exposure to afatinib. Separate administration by 12 hours. Moderate Study
- **Clarithromycin** is predicted to markedly increase the exposure to aldosterone antagonists (eplerenone). Avoid. Severe Study
- **Erythromycin** is predicted to increase the exposure to aldosterone antagonists (eplerenone). Adjust eplerenone dose, p. 190. Severe Study
- **Azithromycin** is predicted to increase the exposure to aliskiren. Moderate Theoretical
- **Macrolides** (clarithromycin, erythromycin) are predicted to increase the exposure to aliskiren. Moderate Study
- **Clarithromycin** increases the exposure to almotriptan. Mild Study
- **Clarithromycin** is predicted to moderately increase the exposure to alpha blockers (alfuzosin, tamsulosin). Use with caution or avoid. Moderate Study

- **Clarithromycin** is predicted to increase the exposure to alpha blockers (doxazosin). Moderate Study
- **Erythromycin** is predicted to increase the exposure to alpha blockers (tamsulosin). Moderate Theoretical
- **Clarithromycin** moderately increases the exposure to alprazolam. Avoid. Moderate Study
- **Erythromycin** is predicted to increase the exposure to alprazolam. Severe Study
- **Azithromycin** is predicted to increase the exposure to aminophylline. Moderate Theoretical
- **Clarithromycin** is predicted to increase the exposure to aminophylline. Adjust dose. Moderate Theoretical
- **Aminophylline** is predicted to decrease the exposure to **erythromycin**. Adjust dose. Severe Study
- **Clarithromycin** very markedly increases the exposure to antiarrhythmics (dronedarone). Avoid. Severe Study → Also see TABLE 9 p. 1336
- **Erythromycin** is predicted to moderately increase the exposure to antiarrhythmics (dronedarone). Avoid. Severe Theoretical → Also see TABLE 9 p. 1336
- Macrolides (clarithromycin, erythromycin) are predicted to increase the exposure to antiarrhythmics (lidocaine). Moderate Theoretical
- **Clarithromycin** is predicted to increase the exposure to antiarrhythmics (propafenone). Monitor and adjust dose. Severe Study
- **Erythromycin** is predicted to increase the exposure to antiarrhythmics (propafenone). Monitor and adjust dose. Moderate Study
- **Clarithromycin** is predicted to increase the exposure to anticholinesterases, centrally acting (galantamine). Monitor and adjust dose. Moderate Study
- **Clarithromycin** slightly increases the concentration of antiepileptics (carbamazepine). Monitor concentration and adjust dose. Severe Study
- **Erythromycin** markedly increases the concentration of antiepileptics (carbamazepine). Monitor concentration and adjust dose. Severe Study
- **Clarithromycin** is predicted to very slightly increase the exposure to antiepileptics (perampanel). Mild Study
- **Clarithromycin** is predicted to increase the exposure to antifungals, azoles (isavuconazole). Avoid or monitor side effects. Severe Study
- **Erythromycin** is predicted to increase the exposure to antifungals, azoles (isavuconazole). Moderate Theoretical
- **Clarithromycin** is predicted to increase the exposure to antihistamines, non-sedating (mizolastine). Avoid. Severe Study
- **Erythromycin** is predicted to increase the exposure to antihistamines, non-sedating (mizolastine). Severe Theoretical
- Macrolides (clarithromycin, erythromycin) are predicted to increase the exposure to antihistamines, non-sedating (rupatadine). Avoid. Moderate Study
- Macrolides (clarithromycin, erythromycin) are predicted to increase the concentration of antimalarials (piperaquine). Severe Theoretical
- **Clarithromycin** is predicted to increase the exposure to apixaban. Severe Theoretical
- **Erythromycin** is predicted to increase the exposure to apixaban. Moderate Theoretical
- **Clarithromycin** is predicted to markedly increase the exposure to aprepitant. Moderate Study
- **Clarithromycin** is predicted to slightly increase the exposure to aripiprazole. Adjust aripiprazole dose, p. 391. Moderate Study
- **Clarithromycin** is predicted to increase the exposure to axitinib. Avoid or adjust dose. Moderate Study
- **Erythromycin** is predicted to increase the exposure to axitinib. Moderate Theoretical
- **Clarithromycin** is predicted to increase the exposure to bedaquiline. Avoid prolonged use. Mild Study → Also see TABLE 9 p. 1336
- **Erythromycin** is predicted to increase the exposure to bedaquiline. Avoid prolonged use. Mild Theoretical → Also see TABLE 9 p. 1336
- **Macrolides** are predicted to increase the exposure to beta blockers, non-selective (nadolol). Moderate Study

▶ **Clarithromycin** is predicted to increase the exposure to beta₂ agonists (salmeterol). Avoid. Severe Study

▶ **Clarithromycin** slightly increases the exposure to bortezomib. Moderate Study

▶ **Clarithromycin** is predicted to increase the exposure to bosentan. Moderate Theoretical

▶ **Clarithromycin** is predicted to markedly increase the exposure to bosutinib. Avoid or adjust dose. Severe Study → Also see **TABLE 9** p. 1336

▶ **Erythromycin** is predicted to increase the exposure to bosutinib. Avoid or adjust dose. Severe Theoretical → Also see **TABLE 9** p. 1336

▶ **Clarithromycin** is predicted to increase the exposure to buspirone. Adjust **buspirone** dose, p. 338. Severe Study

▶ **Erythromycin** is predicted to increase the exposure to buspirone. Use with caution and adjust dose. Moderate Study

▶ **Clarithromycin** slightly increases the exposure to cabozantinib. Moderate Study → Also see **TABLE 9** p. 1336

▶ **Erythromycin** is predicted to increase the exposure to cabozantinib. Moderate Theoretical → Also see **TABLE 9** p. 1336

▶ **Erythromycin** is predicted to increase the exposure to calcium channel blockers (amlodipine, felodipine, lacidipine, lercanidipine, nicardipine, nifedipine, nimodipine). Monitor and adjust dose. Moderate Study

▶ **Clarithromycin** is predicted to increase the exposure to calcium channel blockers (amlodipine, felodipine, lacidipine, nicardipine, nifedipine, nimodipine). Monitor and adjust dose. Moderate Study

▶ **Erythromycin** is predicted to increase the exposure to calcium channel blockers (diltiazem). Severe Theoretical

▶ **Clarithromycin** is predicted to increase the exposure to calcium channel blockers (diltiazem, verapamil). Severe Study

▶ **Clarithromycin** is predicted to markedly increase the exposure to calcium channel blockers (lercanidipine). Avoid. Severe Study

▶ **Erythromycin** is predicted to increase the exposure to calcium channel blockers (verapamil). Severe Study

▶ **Clarithromycin** is predicted to increase the exposure to cannabis extract. Use with caution and adjust dose. Moderate Theoretical

▶ **Clarithromycin** is predicted to increase the exposure to ceritinib. Avoid or adjust **ceritinib** dose, p. 945. Severe Study → Also see **TABLE 9** p. 1336

▶ Macrolides **(azithromycin, erythromycin)** are predicted to increase the exposure to ceritinib. Moderate Theoretical → Also see **TABLE 9** p. 1336

▶ Macrolides **(clarithromycin, erythromycin)** increase the concentration of ciclosporin. Severe Study

▶ **Clarithromycin** is predicted to moderately increase the exposure to cilostazol. Adjust **cilostazol** dose, p. 231. Moderate Study

▶ **Erythromycin** slightly increases the exposure to cilostazol. Adjust **cilostazol** dose, p. 231. Moderate Study

▶ **Clarithromycin** is predicted to moderately increase the exposure to cinacalcet. Adjust dose. Moderate Study

▶ **Erythromycin** potentially increases the risk of toxicity when given with clozapine. Severe Anecdotal

▶ **Clarithromycin** is predicted to markedly increase the exposure to cobimetinib. Avoid or monitor for toxicity. Severe Study

▶ **Erythromycin** is predicted to increase the exposure to cobimetinib. Severe Theoretical

▶ **Azithromycin** is predicted to increase the exposure to colchicine. Avoid or adjust **colchicine** dose, p. 1085. Severe Theoretical

▶ **Clarithromycin** is predicted to increase the exposure to colchicine. Avoid potent inhibitors of CYP3A4 or adjust **colchicine** dose, p. 1085. Severe Study

▶ **Erythromycin** is predicted to increase the exposure to colchicine. Adjust **colchicine** dose with moderate inhibitors of CYP3A4, p. 1085. Severe Study

▶ **Clarithromycin** is predicted to increase the exposure to corticosteroids (beclometasone) (risk with beclometasone is likely to be lower than with other corticosteroids). Moderate Theoretical

▶ **Clarithromycin** is predicted to increase the exposure to corticosteroids (betamethasone, budesonide, ciclesonide,

deflazacort, dexamethasone, fludrocortisone, fluticasone, hydrocortisone, methylprednisolone, mometasone, prednisolone, prednisone, triamcinolone). Avoid or monitor side effects. Severe Study

▶ **Erythromycin** is predicted to increase the exposure to corticosteroids (methylprednisolone). Monitor and adjust dose. Moderate Study

▶ Macrolides **(clarithromycin, erythromycin)** increase the anticoagulant effect of coumarins. Monitor INR and adjust dose. Severe Anecdotal

▶ **Clarithromycin** is predicted to moderately increase the exposure to crizotinib. Avoid. Moderate Study → Also see **TABLE 9** p. 1336

▶ Macrolides are predicted to increase the exposure to dabigatran. Moderate Theoretical

▶ **Clarithromycin** is predicted to increase the exposure to dabrafenib. Use with caution or avoid. Moderate Study

▶ **Clarithromycin** is predicted to moderately increase the exposure to daclatasvir. Adjust **daclatasvir** dose, p. 614. Moderate Study

▶ **Clarithromycin** is predicted to markedly to very markedly increase the exposure to darifenacin. Avoid. Severe Study

▶ **Erythromycin** is predicted to slightly increase the exposure to darifenacin. Moderate Study

▶ **Clarithromycin** is predicted to markedly increase the exposure to dasatinib. Avoid. Severe Study → Also see **TABLE 9** p. 1336

▶ **Erythromycin** is predicted to increase the exposure to dasatinib. Severe Study → Also see **TABLE 9** p. 1336

▶ **Clarithromycin** very slightly increases the exposure to delamanid. Severe Study → Also see **TABLE 9** p. 1336

▶ Macrolides increase the concentration of digoxin. Severe Anecdotal

▶ Macrolides **(clarithromycin, erythromycin)** increase the risk of QT-prolongation when given with domperidone. Avoid. Severe Study

▶ **Clarithromycin** increases the exposure to dopamine receptor agonists (bromocriptine). Severe Study

▶ **Erythromycin** is predicted to increase the exposure to dopamine receptor agonists (bromocriptine). Severe Theoretical

▶ Macrolides **(clarithromycin, erythromycin)** are predicted to increase the concentration of dopamine receptor agonists (cabergoline). Avoid. Severe Study

▶ **Clarithromycin** is predicted to increase the exposure to dutasteride. Monitor side effects and adjust dose. Moderate Theoretical

▶ **Erythromycin** is predicted to moderately increase the exposure to dutasteride. Mild Study

▶ **Erythromycin** slightly increases the exposure to edoxaban. Adjust **edoxaban** dose, p. 125. Severe Study

▶ Macrolides **(azithromycin, clarithromycin)** are predicted to slightly increase the exposure to edoxaban. Severe Theoretical

▶ **Efavirenz** decreases the exposure to **clarithromycin**. Moderate Study → Also see **TABLE 9** p. 1336

▶ **Clarithromycin** slightly to moderately increases the exposure to elbasvir. Avoid. Moderate Study

▶ **Clarithromycin** is predicted to markedly increase the exposure to eletriptan. Avoid. Severe Study

▶ **Erythromycin** moderately increases the exposure to eletriptan. Avoid. Moderate Study

▶ Macrolides **(clarithromycin, erythromycin)** are predicted to increase the exposure to eliglustat. Avoid or adjust dose—consult product literature. Severe Study

▶ **Clarithromycin** is predicted to increase the risk of ergotism when given with ergometrine. Avoid. Severe Theoretical

▶ **Erythromycin** is predicted to increase the risk of ergotism when given with ergometrine. Severe Theoretical

▶ **Clarithromycin** is predicted to increase the risk of ergotism when given with ergotamine. Avoid. Severe Theoretical

▶ **Erythromycin** is predicted to increase the risk of ergotism when given with ergotamine. Severe Theoretical

▶ **Clarithromycin** is predicted to slightly increase the exposure to erlotinib. Use with caution and adjust dose. Moderate Study

▶ Macrolides **(azithromycin, erythromycin)** are predicted to increase the exposure to erlotinib. Moderate Theoretical

Macrolides (continued)

▸ Etravirine decreases the exposure to **clarithromycin**. Severe Study

▸ **Clarithromycin** is predicted to increase the concentration of everolimus. Avoid. Severe Study

▸ **Erythromycin** is predicted to increase the concentration of everolimus. Avoid or adjust dose. Moderate Study

▸ **Clarithromycin** is predicted to moderately increase the exposure to fesoterodine. Adjust **fesoterodine** dose with potent inhibitors of CYP3A4; avoid in hepatic and renal impairment, p. 759. Severe Study

▸ **Erythromycin** is predicted to increase the exposure to fesoterodine. Adjust **fesoterodine** dose with moderate inhibitors of CYP3A4 in hepatic and renal impairment, p. 759. Mild Study

▸ **Macrolides** are predicted to increase the exposure to fidaxomicin. Avoid. Moderate Study

▸ **Clarithromycin** is predicted to increase the exposure to fosaprepitant. Moderate Theoretical

▸ **Clarithromycin** is predicted to increase the exposure to gefitinib. Moderate Study

▸ **Erythromycin** is predicted to increase the exposure to gefitinib. Moderate Theoretical

▸ **Clarithromycin** is predicted to moderately to markedly increase the exposure to grazoprevir. Avoid. Severe Study

▸ **Clarithromycin** is predicted to increase the exposure to guanfacine. Adjust **guanfacine** dose, p. 349. Moderate Study

▸ **Erythromycin** is predicted to increase the concentration of guanfacine. Adjust **guanfacine** dose, p. 349. Moderate Theoretical

▸ H₂ receptor antagonists (cimetidine) slightly increase the exposure to **erythromycin**. Moderate Study

▸ HIV-protease inhibitors (atazanavir) are predicted to increase the exposure to **clarithromycin**. Adjust dose in renal impairment. Severe Study

▸ HIV-protease inhibitors (atazanavir, darunavir, fosamprenavir, lopinavir, ritonavir, tipranavir) are predicted to increase the exposure to **erythromycin**. Severe Theoretical

▸ HIV-protease inhibitors (darunavir, fosamprenavir, lopinavir) (boosted with ritonavir) are predicted to increase the exposure to **clarithromycin**. Adjust dose in renal impairment. Severe Study

▸ HIV-protease inhibitors (ritonavir) increase the exposure to **clarithromycin**. Adjust dose in renal impairment. Severe Study

▸ HIV-protease inhibitors (tipranavir) (boosted with ritonavir) increase the exposure to **clarithromycin** and **clarithromycin** increases the exposure to HIV-protease inhibitors (tipranavir) (boosted with ritonavir). Monitor; adjust dose in renal impairment. Severe Study

▸ **Clarithromycin** increases the exposure to HIV-protease inhibitors (saquinavir) and HIV-protease inhibitors (saquinavir) increase the exposure to **clarithromycin**. Avoid. Study → Also see TABLE 9 p. 1336

▸ **Erythromycin** is predicted to increase the exposure to HIV-protease inhibitors (saquinavir). Avoid. Severe Theoretical → Also see TABLE 9 p. 1336

▸ **Clarithromycin** is predicted to very markedly increase the exposure to ibrutinib. Avoid potent inhibitors of CYP3A4 or adjust **ibrutinib** dose, p. 952. Severe Study

▸ **Erythromycin** is predicted to increase the exposure to ibrutinib. Adjust **ibrutinib** dose with moderate inhibitors of CYP3A4, p. 952. Severe Study

▸ **Clarithromycin** is predicted to increase the exposure to imatinib. Moderate Study

▸ **Erythromycin** is predicted to increase the exposure to imatinib. Moderate Theoretical

▸ **Clarithromycin** is predicted to increase the risk of toxicity when given with irinotecan. Avoid. Moderate Study

▸ **Clarithromycin** is predicted to increase the exposure to ivabradine. Avoid. Severe Study

▸ **Erythromycin** is predicted to increase the exposure to ivabradine. Avoid. Severe Theoretical

▸ **Clarithromycin** is predicted to increase the exposure to ivacaftor. Adjust **ivacaftor** p. 292 or **lumacaftor with ivacaftor** p. 293 dose with potent inhibitors of CYP3A4. Severe Study

▸ **Erythromycin** is predicted to increase the exposure to ivacaftor. Adjust **ivacaftor** dose with moderate inhibitors of CYP3A4, p. 292. Severe Study

▸ **Clarithromycin** is predicted to increase the exposure to lapatinib. Avoid. Moderate Study → Also see TABLE 9 p. 1336

▸ **Erythromycin** is predicted to increase the exposure to lapatinib. Moderate Study → Also see TABLE 9 p. 1336

▸ **Clarithromycin** increases the exposure to linezolid. Moderate Anecdotal

▸ **Azithromycin** is predicted to increase the exposure to lomitapide. Separate administration by 12 hours. Moderate Theoretical

▸ **Clarithromycin** is predicted to markedly increase the exposure to lomitapide. Avoid. Severe Study

▸ **Erythromycin** is predicted to increase the exposure to lomitapide. Avoid. Moderate Theoretical

▸ Lumacaftor is predicted to decrease the exposure to macrolides (**clarithromycin, erythromycin**). Moderate Theoretical

▸ **Clarithromycin** is predicted to increase the exposure to lurasidone. Avoid. Severe Study

▸ **Erythromycin** is predicted to increase the exposure to lurasidone. Moderate Study

▸ **Clarithromycin** is predicted to increase the exposure to macitentan. Moderate Study

▸ **Clarithromycin** is predicted to markedly increase the exposure to maraviroc. Adjust dose. Severe Study

▸ **Clarithromycin** is predicted to markedly to very markedly increase the exposure to midazolam. Avoid or adjust dose. Severe Study

▸ **Erythromycin** is predicted to increase the exposure to midazolam. Monitor side effects and adjust dose. Severe Study

▸ **Clarithromycin** is predicted to very markedly increase the exposure to midostaurin. Avoid or monitor for toxicity. Severe Study

▸ **Erythromycin** is predicted to increase the exposure to midostaurin. Moderate Theoretical

▸ **Clarithromycin** is predicted to increase the exposure to mirabegron. Adjust **mirabegron** dose in hepatic and renal impairment, p. 763. Moderate Study

▸ **Clarithromycin** is predicted to increase the exposure to mirtazapine. Moderate Study

▸ **Clarithromycin** is predicted to increase the exposure to modafinil. Mild Theoretical

▸ **Clarithromycin** increases the risk of neutropenia when given with monoclonal antibodies (brentuximab vedotin). Monitor and adjust dose. Severe Theoretical

▸ **Clarithromycin** is predicted to increase the exposure to monoclonal antibodies (trastuzumab emtansine). Avoid. Severe Theoretical

▸ **Clarithromycin** is predicted to markedly increase the exposure to naloxegol. Avoid. Severe Study

▸ **Erythromycin** is predicted to increase the exposure to naloxegol. Adjust **naloxegol** dose and monitor side effects, p. 64. Moderate Study

▸ **Clarithromycin** is predicted to increase the exposure to netupitant. Moderate Study

▸ Nevirapine decreases the exposure to **clarithromycin**. Moderate Study

▸ **Clarithromycin** is predicted to moderately increase the exposure to nilotinib. Avoid. Severe Study → Also see TABLE 9 p. 1336

▸ **Erythromycin** is predicted to increase the exposure to nilotinib. Moderate Theoretical → Also see TABLE 9 p. 1336

▸ **Macrolides** are predicted to increase the exposure to nintedanib. Moderate Study

▸ **Clarithromycin** is predicted to increase the exposure to nitisinone. Adjust dose. Moderate Theoretical

▸ **Clarithromycin** is predicted to increase the exposure to olaparib. Avoid potent inhibitors of CYP3A4 or adjust **olaparib** dose, p. 973. Moderate Study

▸ **Erythromycin** is predicted to increase the exposure to olaparib. Avoid moderate inhibitors of CYP3A4 or adjust **olaparib** dose, p. 973. Moderate Theoretical

▸ **Erythromycin** is predicted to increase the exposure to opioids (alfentanil, buprenorphine, fentanyl, oxycodone). Monitor and adjust dose. Moderate Study

▸ **Clarithromycin** is predicted to increase the exposure to opioids (alfentanil, buprenorphine, fentanyl, oxycodone, sufentanil). Monitor and adjust dose. Severe Study

▸ **Clarithromycin** is predicted to increase the concentration of opioids (methadone). Severe Theoretical → Also see **TABLE 9** p. 1336

▸ **Erythromycin** is predicted to increase the exposure to opioids (methadone, sufentanil). Moderate Theoretical → Also see **TABLE 9** p. 1336

▸ **Clarithromycin** is predicted to increase the exposure to oxybutynin. Mild Study

▸ **Erythromycin** is predicted to increase the exposure to oxybutynin. Mild Theoretical

▸ **Clarithromycin** is predicted to increase the exposure to palbociclib. Avoid or adjust **palbociclib** dose, p. 961. Severe Study

▸ **Clarithromycin** is predicted to increase the exposure to panobinostat. Adjust **panobinostat** dose; in hepatic impairment avoid, p. 911. Moderate Study → Also see **TABLE 9** p. 1336

▸ Macrolides **(azithromycin, erythromycin)** are predicted to increase the exposure to panobinostat. Adjust dose. Moderate Theoretical → Also see **TABLE 9** p. 1336

▸ **Clarithromycin** is predicted to increase the exposure to paritaprevir (with ritonavir and ombitasvir). Avoid. Severe Theoretical

▸ **Clarithromycin** is predicted to increase the exposure to pazopanib. Avoid or adjust **pazopanib** dose, p. 962. Moderate Study → Also see **TABLE 9** p. 1336

▸ **Erythromycin** is predicted to increase the exposure to pazopanib. Moderate Theoretical → Also see **TABLE 9** p. 1336

▸ **Erythromycin** is predicted to increase the exposure to phosphodiesterase type-5 inhibitors (avanafil). Adjust **avanafil** dose, p. 794. Moderate Theoretical

▸ **Clarithromycin** is predicted to increase the exposure to phosphodiesterase type-5 inhibitors (avanafil, vardenafil). Avoid. Severe Study → Also see **TABLE 9** p. 1336

▸ **Clarithromycin** is predicted to increase the exposure to phosphodiesterase type-5 inhibitors (sildenafil). Avoid potent inhibitors of CYP3A4 or adjust **sildenafil** dose, p. 794. Severe Study → Also see **TABLE 9** p. 1336

▸ **Erythromycin** is predicted to increase the exposure to phosphodiesterase type-5 inhibitors (sildenafil). Monitor or adjust **sildenafil** dose with moderate inhibitors of CYP3A4, p. 794. Moderate Study → Also see **TABLE 9** p. 1336

▸ **Clarithromycin** is predicted to increase the exposure to phosphodiesterase type-5 inhibitors (tadalafil). Use with caution or avoid. Severe Study

▸ **Erythromycin** is predicted to increase the exposure to phosphodiesterase type-5 inhibitors (tadalafil). Severe Theoretical

▸ **Erythromycin** is predicted to increase the exposure to phosphodiesterase type-5 inhibitors (vardenafil). Adjust dose. Severe Theoretical → Also see **TABLE 9** p. 1336

▸ **Clarithromycin** is predicted to increase the exposure to pimozide. Avoid. Severe Study → Also see **TABLE 9** p. 1336

▸ **Erythromycin** is predicted to increase the exposure to pimozide. Avoid. Severe Theoretical → Also see **TABLE 9** p. 1336

▸ **Clarithromycin** is predicted to slightly increase the exposure to ponatinib. Monitor and adjust **ponatinib** dose, p. 963. Moderate Study

▸ **Clarithromycin** is predicted to moderately increase the exposure to praziquantel. Mild Study

▸ **Clarithromycin** is predicted to increase the exposure to quetiapine. Avoid. Severe Study

▸ **Erythromycin** is predicted to increase the exposure to quetiapine. Avoid. Moderate Study

▸ **Clarithromycin** is predicted to increase the exposure to ranolazine. Avoid. Severe Study → Also see **TABLE 9** p. 1336

▸ **Erythromycin** is predicted to increase the exposure to ranolazine. Severe Study → Also see **TABLE 9** p. 1336

▸ **Clarithromycin** is predicted to increase the exposure to reboxetine. Avoid. Moderate Study

▸ **Clarithromycin** is predicted to increase the exposure to regorafenib. Avoid. Moderate Study

▸ **Clarithromycin** is predicted to increase the exposure to repaglinide. Moderate Study

▸ **Clarithromycin** is predicted to increase the exposure to retinoids (alitretinoin). Adjust **alitretinoin** dose, p. 1226. Moderate Theoretical

▸ **Clarithromycin** is predicted to increase the exposure to ribociclib. Avoid or adjust **ribociclib** dose, p. 965. Moderate Study → Also see **TABLE 9** p. 1336

▸ **Erythromycin** is predicted to increase the exposure to ribociclib. Moderate Study → Also see **TABLE 9** p. 1336

▸ **Azithromycin** increases the risk of neutropenia when given with rifabutin. Severe Study

▸ **Clarithromycin** increases the risk of uveitis when given with rifabutin. Adjust dose. Severe Study

▸ **Erythromycin** is predicted to increase the risk of uveitis when given with rifabutin. Adjust dose. Severe Study

▸ Rifampicin decreases the concentration of **clarithromycin**. Severe Study

▸ **Clarithromycin** is predicted to increase the exposure to risperidone. Adjust dose. Moderate Study → Also see **TABLE 9** p. 1336

▸ **Clarithromycin** is predicted to increase the exposure to ruxolitinib. Adjust dose and monitor side effects. Moderate Study

▸ **Erythromycin** is predicted to increase the exposure to ruxolitinib. Moderate Theoretical

▸ **Clarithromycin** is predicted to increase the exposure to saxagliptin. Moderate Study

▸ **Erythromycin** is predicted to increase the exposure to saxagliptin. Mild Study

▸ Macrolides **(clarithromycin, erythromycin)** are predicted to increase the exposure to simeprevir. Avoid. Severe Study

▸ **Clarithromycin** is predicted to increase the concentration of sirolimus. Avoid. Severe Study

▸ **Erythromycin** increases the concentration of sirolimus. Monitor and adjust dose. Moderate Study

▸ **Clarithromycin** is predicted to increase the exposure to solifenacin. Adjust **solifenacin** p. 761 or **tamsulosin with solifenacin** p. 768 dose; avoid in hepatic and renal impairment. Severe Study

▸ **Clarithromycin** is predicted to moderately increase the exposure to SSRIs (dapoxetine). Avoid potent inhibitors of CYP3A4 or adjust **dapoxetine** dose, p. 801. Severe Study

▸ **Erythromycin** is predicted to increase the exposure to SSRIs (dapoxetine). Adjust **dapoxetine** dose with moderate inhibitors of CYP3A4, p. 801. Moderate Theoretical

▸ **Clarithromycin** is predicted to increase the exposure to statins (atorvastatin). Avoid or adjust dose and monitor rhabdomyolysis. Severe Study

▸ **Erythromycin** is predicted to increase the exposure to statins (atorvastatin). Monitor and adjust dose. Severe Study

▸ **Clarithromycin** moderately increases the exposure to statins (pravastatin). Severe Study

▸ **Erythromycin** is predicted to increase the exposure to statins (pravastatin). Severe Study

▸ **Clarithromycin** is predicted to increase the exposure to statins (simvastatin). Avoid. Severe Study

▸ **Erythromycin** is predicted to increase the exposure to statins (simvastatin). Use with caution and adjust **simvastatin** dose, p. 203. Severe Study

▸ **Clarithromycin** is predicted to slightly increase the exposure to sulfonylureas. Moderate Theoretical

▸ **Clarithromycin** is predicted to slightly increase the exposure to sunitinib. Avoid or adjust **sunitinib** dose, p. 967. Moderate Study → Also see **TABLE 9** p. 1336

▸ **Erythromycin** is predicted to increase the exposure to sunitinib. Moderate Theoretical → Also see **TABLE 9** p. 1336

▸ **Clarithromycin** is predicted to increase the concentration of tacrolimus. Monitor and adjust dose. Severe Study

▸ **Erythromycin** is predicted to increase the concentration of tacrolimus. Severe Study

▸ **Clarithromycin** is predicted to increase the exposure to taxanes (cabazitaxel). Avoid. Severe Study

▸ **Erythromycin** is predicted to increase the exposure to taxanes (cabazitaxel). Moderate Theoretical

A1

Interactions | **Appendix 1**

Macrolides (continued)
▶ **Clarithromycin** is predicted to moderately increase the exposure to taxanes (docetaxel). Avoid or adjust dose. [Severe] Study
▶ **Clarithromycin** is predicted to increase the exposure to taxanes (paclitaxel). [Severe] Theoretical
▶ **Clarithromycin** is predicted to increase the concentration of temsirolimus. Avoid. [Severe] Theoretical
▶ **Erythromycin** is predicted to increase the concentration of temsirolimus. [Moderate] Theoretical
▶ **Erythromycin** decreases the clearance of theophylline and theophylline potentially decreases the clearance of **erythromycin**. Adjust dose. [Severe] Study
▶ Macrolides **(azithromycin, clarithromycin)** are predicted to increase the exposure to theophylline. Adjust dose. [Moderate] Anecdotal
▶ **Azithromycin** is predicted to increase the exposure to ticagrelor. Use with caution or avoid. [Severe] Study
▶ **Clarithromycin** is predicted to markedly increase the exposure to ticagrelor. Avoid. [Severe] Study
▶ **Clarithromycin** is predicted to increase the exposure to tofacitinib. Adjust **tofacitinib** dose, p. 1072. [Moderate] Study
▶ **Erythromycin** is predicted to increase the exposure to tofacitinib. [Moderate] Study
▶ **Clarithromycin** is predicted to increase the exposure to tolterodine. Avoid. [Severe] Study → Also see **TABLE 9** p. 1336
▶ **Erythromycin** is predicted to increase the exposure to tolterodine. [Mild] Theoretical → Also see **TABLE 9** p. 1336
▶ **Clarithromycin** is predicted to increase the exposure to tolvaptan. Adjust dose. [Severe] Study
▶ **Erythromycin** is predicted to increase the exposure to tolvaptan. Adjust dose. [Moderate] Study
▶ **Macrolides** are predicted to increase the exposure to topotecan. [Severe] Study
▶ **Clarithromycin** is predicted to increase the exposure to toremifene. [Moderate] Theoretical → Also see **TABLE 9** p. 1336
▶ **Clarithromycin** is predicted to increase the exposure to trabectedin. Avoid or adjust dose. [Severe] Theoretical
▶ **Macrolides** are predicted to increase the concentration of trametinib. [Moderate] Theoretical
▶ **Clarithromycin** is predicted to moderately increase the exposure to trazodone. Avoid or adjust dose. [Moderate] Study
▶ **Erythromycin** is predicted to increase the exposure to trazodone. [Moderate] Theoretical
▶ **Clarithromycin** is predicted to increase the exposure to ulipristal. Avoid if used for uterine fibroids. [Severe] Study
▶ **Erythromycin** is predicted to increase the exposure to ulipristal. Avoid if used for uterine fibroids. [Moderate] Study
▶ **Clarithromycin** is predicted to increase the exposure to vemurafenib. [Severe] Theoretical → Also see **TABLE 9** p. 1336
▶ **Azithromycin** decreases the exposure to venetoclax. [Mild] Study
▶ **Clarithromycin** is predicted to increase the exposure to venetoclax. Avoid potent inhibitors of CYP3A4 or adjust **venetoclax** dose, p. 974. [Severe] Study
▶ **Erythromycin** is predicted to increase the exposure to venetoclax. Avoid moderate inhibitors of CYP3A4 or adjust **venetoclax** dose, p. 974. [Severe] Study
▶ **Clarithromycin** is predicted to increase the exposure to venlafaxine. [Moderate] Study → Also see **TABLE 9** p. 1336
▶ Macrolides **(clarithromycin, erythromycin)** are predicted to increase the exposure to vinca alkaloids. [Severe] Theoretical → Also see **TABLE 9** p. 1336
▶ **Clarithromycin** is predicted to increase the exposure to vitamin D substances (paricalcitol). [Moderate] Study
▶ **Clarithromycin** decreases the absorption of zidovudine. Separate administration by at least 2 hours. [Moderate] Study
▶ **Clarithromycin** is predicted to increase the exposure to zopiclone. Adjust dose. [Moderate] Theoretical
▶ **Erythromycin** is predicted to increase the exposure to zopiclone. Adjust dose. [Moderate] Study

Magnesium
▶ Oral **magnesium** decreases the absorption of bisphosphonates (alendronic acid). **Alendronic acid** should be taken at least 30 minutes before **magnesium**. [Moderate] Study

▶ Oral **magnesium** is predicted to decrease the absorption of oral bisphosphonates (ibandronic acid). Avoid **magnesium** for at least 6 hours before or 1 hour after **ibandronic acid**. [Moderate] Theoretical
▶ Oral **magnesium** decreases the absorption of bisphosphonates (risedronate). Separate administration by at least 2 hours. [Moderate] Study
▶ Oral **magnesium** decreases the absorption of bisphosphonates (sodium clodronate). Avoid **magnesium** for 2 hours before or 1 hour after **sodium clodronate**. [Moderate] Study
▶ Intravenous **magnesium** potentially increases the risk of hypotension when given with calcium channel blockers (amlodipine, clevidipine, felodipine, lacidipine, lercanidipine, nicardipine, nifedipine, nimodipine, verapamil) (in pregnant women). [Severe] Anecdotal
▶ Intravenous **magnesium** increases the effects of neuromuscular blocking drugs, non-depolarising. [Moderate] Study
▶ Intravenous **magnesium** is predicted to increase the effects of suxamethonium. [Moderate] Study

Magnesium carbonate → see antacids
Magnesium trisilicate → see antacids
Maraviroc
▶ Antiepileptics **(carbamazepine, fosphenytoin, phenobarbital, phenytoin, primidone)** are predicted to decrease the exposure to maraviroc. Adjust dose. [Severe] Study
▶ Antifungals, azoles **(itraconazole, ketoconazole, voriconazole)** are predicted to markedly increase the exposure to maraviroc. Adjust dose. [Severe] Study
▶ Bosentan is predicted to decrease the exposure to maraviroc. Avoid. [Moderate] Theoretical
▶ Cobicistat markedly increases the exposure to maraviroc. Refer to specialist literature. [Severe] Study
▶ Efavirenz decreases the exposure to maraviroc. Refer to specialist literature. [Severe] Theoretical
▶ Enzalutamide is predicted to decrease the exposure to maraviroc. Adjust dose. [Severe] Study
▶ Etravirine (with a boosted protease inhibitor) increases the exposure to maraviroc. Avoid or adjust dose. [Moderate] Study
▶ HIV-protease inhibitors **(atazanavir, saquinavir)** moderately to markedly increase the exposure to maraviroc. Refer to specialist literature. [Severe] Study
▶ HIV-protease inhibitors **(darunavir)** (boosted with ritonavir) markedly increase the exposure to maraviroc. Refer to specialist literature. [Severe] Study
▶ HIV-protease inhibitors **(lopinavir)** (boosted with ritonavir) moderately increase the exposure to maraviroc. Refer to specialist literature. [Severe] Study
▶ HIV-protease inhibitors **(ritonavir)** markedly increase the exposure to maraviroc. Refer to specialist literature. [Severe] Study
▶ **Maraviroc** potentially decreases the exposure to HIV-protease inhibitors **(fosamprenavir)** and HIV-protease inhibitors (fosamprenavir) potentially decrease the exposure to maraviroc. Avoid. [Severe] Study
▶ Idelalisib markedly increases the exposure to maraviroc. Adjust dose. [Severe] Theoretical
▶ Macrolides **(clarithromycin)** are predicted to markedly increase the exposure to maraviroc. Adjust dose. [Severe] Study
▶ Mitotane is predicted to decrease the exposure to maraviroc. Adjust dose. [Severe] Study
▶ Rifampicin is predicted to decrease the exposure to maraviroc. Adjust dose. [Severe] Study
▶ St John's Wort is predicted to decrease the exposure to maraviroc. Avoid. [Severe] Theoretical

Measles, mumps and rubella vaccine, live → see live vaccines
Mebendazole
▶ H_2 receptor antagonists (cimetidine) increase the concentration of **mebendazole**. [Moderate] Study
Medroxyprogesterone
▶ Sugammadex is predicted to decrease the exposure to **medroxyprogesterone**. Use additional contraceptive precautions. [Severe] Theoretical
Mefenamic acid → see NSAIDs
Mefloquine → see antimalarials
Melatonin → see **TABLE 11** p. 1336 (CNS depressant effects)

▶ Antiepileptics (phenytoin) are predicted to decrease the exposure to **melatonin**. Moderate Theoretical
▶ Combined hormonal contraceptives are predicted to increase the exposure to **melatonin**. Moderate Theoretical
▶ HIV-protease inhibitors (ritonavir) are predicted to decrease the exposure to **melatonin**. Moderate Theoretical
▶ Leflunomide is predicted to decrease the exposure to **melatonin**. Moderate Theoretical
▶ Quinolones (ciprofloxacin) are predicted to increase the exposure to **melatonin**. Moderate Theoretical
▶ Rifampicin is predicted to decrease the exposure to **melatonin**. Moderate Theoretical
▶ SSRIs (fluvoxamine) very markedly increase the exposure to **melatonin**. Avoid. Severe Study
▶ Teriflunomide is predicted to decrease the exposure to **melatonin**. Moderate Theoretical

Meloxicam → see NSAIDs
Melphalan → see alkylating agents
Memantine
▶ Dopamine receptor agonists (amantadine) increase the risk of CNS toxicity when given with **memantine**. Use with caution or avoid. Severe Theoretical
▶ **Memantine** is predicted to increase the effects of dopamine receptor agonists (apomorphine, bromocriptine, cabergoline, pergolide, pramipexole, quinagolide, ropinirole, rotigotine). Moderate Theoretical
▶ **Memantine** is predicted to increase the risk of CNS side-effects when given with ketamine. Avoid. Severe Theoretical
▶ **Memantine** is predicted to increase the effects of levodopa. Moderate Theoretical
Mepacrine
▶ **Mepacrine** is predicted to increase the concentration of antimalarials (primaquine). Avoid. Moderate Theoretical
Mepivacaine → see anaesthetics, local
Meprobamate → see TABLE 11 p. 1336 (CNS depressant effects)
Meptazinol → see opioids
Mercaptopurine → see TABLE 1 p. 1334 (hepatotoxicity), TABLE 15 p. 1337 (myelosuppression)
▶ Allopurinol potentially increases the risk of haematological toxicity when given with **mercaptopurine**. Adjust mercaptopurine dose, p. 887. Severe Study
▶ **Mercaptopurine** decreases the anticoagulant effect of coumarins. Moderate Anecdotal
▶ Febuxostat is predicted to increase the exposure to mercaptopurine. Avoid. Severe Theoretical
▶ Live vaccines are predicted to increase the risk of generalised infection (possibly life-threatening) when given with mercaptopurine (high-dose). Public Health England advises avoid (refer to Green Book). Severe Theoretical
Meropenem → see carbapenems
Mesalazine

ROUTE-SPECIFIC INFORMATION The manufacturers of some mesalazine gastro-resistant and modified-release medicines (Asacol MR tablets, Ipocol, Salofalk granules) suggest that preparations that lower stool pH (e.g. lactulose) might prevent the release of mesalazine.

Metaraminol → see sympathomimetics, vasoconstrictor
Metformin → see TABLE 14 p. 1337 (antidiabetic drugs)
▶ Alcohol (beverage)(excessive consumption) potentially increases the risk of lactic acidosis when given with **metformin**. Avoid excessive alcohol consumption. Moderate Theoretical
▶ Dolutegravir slightly to moderately increases the exposure to **metformin**. Use with caution and adjust dose. Severe Study
▶ H₂ receptor antagonists (cimetidine) slightly increase the exposure to **metformin**. Monitor and adjust dose. Moderate Study
▶ Pitolisant is predicted to increase the exposure to **metformin**. Unknown Theoretical
▶ Vandetanib slightly increases the exposure to **metformin**. Monitor and adjust dose. Moderate Study
Methadone → see opioids
Methenamine
▶ Acetazolamide is predicted to decrease the efficacy of **methenamine**. Avoid. Moderate Theoretical

▶ Potassium citrate is predicted to decrease the efficacy of **methenamine**. Avoid. Moderate Theoretical
▶ Sodium bicarbonate is predicted to decrease the efficacy of **methenamine**. Avoid. Moderate Theoretical
▶ Sodium citrate is predicted to decrease the efficacy of **methenamine**. Avoid. Moderate Theoretical
Methocarbamol → see TABLE 11 p. 1336 (CNS depressant effects)
Methotrexate → see TABLE 1 p. 1334 (hepatotoxicity), TABLE 15 p. 1337 (myelosuppression), TABLE 2 p. 1334 (nephrotoxicity), TABLE 5 p. 1334 (thromboembolism)
▶ Acetazolamide increases the urinary excretion of **methotrexate**. Moderate Study
▶ **Methotrexate** is predicted to decrease the clearance of aminophylline. Moderate Theoretical
▶ Antiepileptics (levetiracetam) decrease the clearance of **methotrexate**. Severe Anecdotal
▶ Antimalarials (pyrimethamine) are predicted to increase the risk of side-effects when given with **methotrexate**. Severe Theoretical → Also see TABLE 15 p. 1337
▶ Asparaginase affects the efficacy of **methotrexate**. Severe Anecdotal → Also see TABLE 1 p. 1334 → Also see TABLE 15 p. 1337
▶ Aspirin (high-dose) is predicted to increase the risk of toxicity when given with **methotrexate**. Severe Theoretical
▶ Crisantaspase affects the efficacy of **methotrexate**. Severe Anecdotal → Also see TABLE 1 p. 1334 → Also see TABLE 15 p. 1337
▶ Live vaccines are predicted to increase the risk of generalised infection (possibly life-threatening) when given with **methotrexate** (high-dose). Public Health England advises avoid (refer to Green Book). Severe Theoretical
▶ NSAIDs are predicted to increase the risk of toxicity when given with **methotrexate**. Monitor and adjust dose. Severe Study → Also see TABLE 2 p. 1334
▶ Pegaspargase affects the efficacy of **methotrexate**. Severe Anecdotal → Also see TABLE 1 p. 1334 → Also see TABLE 15 p. 1337
▶ Penicillins are predicted to increase the risk of toxicity when given with **methotrexate**. Severe Theoretical → Also see TABLE 1 p. 1334
▶ Proton pump inhibitors decrease the clearance of **methotrexate** (high-dose). Use with caution or avoid. Severe Study
▶ Quinolones (ciprofloxacin) potentially increase the risk of toxicity when given with **methotrexate**. Avoid. Severe Anecdotal
▶ Regorafenib is predicted to increase the exposure to **methotrexate**. Severe Theoretical → Also see TABLE 15 p. 1337
▶ Retinoids (acitretin) are predicted to increase the concentration of **methotrexate**. Avoid. Moderate Anecdotal
▶ Rolapitant is predicted to increase the exposure to **methotrexate**. Avoid or monitor. Moderate Study
▶ **Methotrexate** is predicted to decrease the efficacy of sapropterin. Moderate Theoretical
▶ Sulfonamides are predicted to increase the exposure to **methotrexate**. Use with caution or avoid. Severe Theoretical → Also see TABLE 15 p. 1337
▶ Tedizolid is predicted to increase the exposure to **methotrexate**. Avoid. Moderate Theoretical
▶ **Methotrexate** is predicted to increase the risk of toxicity when given with tegafur. Severe Theoretical
▶ **Methotrexate** decreases the clearance of theophylline. Moderate Study
▶ Trimethoprim is predicted to increase the risk of side-effects when given with **methotrexate**. Avoid. Severe Theoretical → Also see TABLE 2 p. 1334
Methoxyflurane → see volatile halogenated anaesthetics
Methyldopa → see TABLE 8 p. 1335 (hypotension)
▶ Entacapone is predicted to increase the exposure to **methyldopa**. Moderate Theoretical
▶ Iron (oral) decreases the effects of **methyldopa**. Moderate Study
▶ **Methyldopa** increases the risk of neurotoxicity when given with lithium. Severe Anecdotal
▶ Monoamine-oxidase A and B inhibitors, irreversible are predicted to alter the antihypertensive effects of **methyldopa**. Avoid. Severe Theoretical → Also see TABLE 8 p. 1335
Methylphenidate
▶ **Methylphenidate** is predicted to decrease the effects of apraclonidine. Avoid. Severe Theoretical

A1

Interactions | Appendix 1

Methylphenidate (continued)
▸ **Methylphenidate** is predicted to increase the risk of elevated blood pressure when given with linezolid. Avoid. Severe Theoretical
▸ **Methylphenidate** is predicted to increase the risk of a hypertensive crisis when given with moclobemide. Severe Theoretical
▸ **Methylphenidate** is predicted to increase the risk of a hypertensive crisis when given with monoamine-oxidase A and B inhibitors, irreversible. Avoid and for 14 days after stopping the MAOI. Severe Theoretical
▸ Monoamine-oxidase B inhibitors (rasagiline, selegiline) are predicted to increase the risk of a hypertensive crisis when given with **methylphenidate**. Avoid. Severe Theoretical
▸ Risperidone increases the risk of dyskinesias when given with **methylphenidate**. Severe Anecdotal
Methylprednisolone → see corticosteroids
Methylthioninium chloride → see TABLE 13 p. 1337 (serotonin syndrome)
▸ **Methylthioninium chloride** is predicted to increase the risk of severe hypertension when given with bupropion. Avoid. Severe Theoretical → Also see TABLE 13 p. 1337
Metoclopramide
▸ **Metoclopramide** is predicted to increase the risk of methaemoglobinaemia when given with topical anaesthetics, local (prilocaine). Avoid. Severe Theoretical
▸ **Metoclopramide** potentially decreases the absorption of antifungals, azoles (posaconazole) (oral suspension). Moderate Study
▸ **Metoclopramide** decreases the concentration of antimalarials (atovaquone). Avoid. Moderate Study
▸ **Metoclopramide** is predicted to decrease the effects of dopamine receptor agonists (apomorphine, bromocriptine, cabergoline, pergolide, pramipexole, quinagolide, ropinirole, rotigotine). Avoid. Moderate Study
▸ **Metoclopramide** decreases the effects of levodopa. Avoid. Moderate Study
▸ **Metoclopramide** is predicted to increase the effects of neuromuscular blocking drugs, non-depolarising. Moderate Theoretical
▸ **Metoclopramide** increases the effects of suxamethonium. Moderate Study
Metolazone → see thiazide diuretics
Metoprolol → see beta blockers, selective
Metronidazole → see TABLE 12 p. 1337 (peripheral neuropathy)

ROUTE-SPECIFIC INFORMATION Since systemic absorption can follow topical application, the possibility of interactions should be borne in mind.

▸ Alcohol (beverage) potentially causes a disulfiram-like reaction when given with **metronidazole**. Avoid for at least 48 hours stopping treatment. Moderate Study
▸ **Metronidazole** increases the risk of toxicity when given with alkylating agents (busulfan). Severe Study
▸ Antiepileptics (phenobarbital, primidone) are predicted to decrease the exposure to **metronidazole**. Moderate Study
▸ **Metronidazole** is predicted to increase the risk of capecitabine toxicity when given with capecitabine. Severe Theoretical
▸ **Metronidazole** increases the anticoagulant effect of coumarins. Monitor INR and adjust dose. Severe Study
▸ Disulfiram increases the risk of acute psychoses when given with **metronidazole**. Severe Study → Also see TABLE 12 p. 1337
▸ **Metronidazole** increases the risk of toxicity when given with fluorouracil. Severe Study
Metyrapone
▸ Antiepileptics (fosphenytoin, phenobarbital, phenytoin, primidone) are predicted to decrease the effects of **metyrapone**. Avoid. Moderate Study
▸ Antihistamines, sedating (cyproheptadine) decrease the effects of **metyrapone**. Avoid. Moderate Study
▸ Carbimazole decreases the effects of **metyrapone**. Avoid. Moderate Theoretical
▸ Combined hormonal contraceptives decrease the effects of **metyrapone**. Avoid. Moderate Theoretical
▸ Phenothiazines (chlorpromazine) decrease the effects of **metyrapone**. Avoid. Moderate Theoretical

▸ Propylthiouracil is predicted to decrease the effects of **metyrapone**. Avoid. Moderate Theoretical
▸ Tricyclic antidepressants (amitriptyline) decrease the effects of **metyrapone**. Avoid. Moderate Theoretical
Mianserin → see TABLE 13 p. 1337 (serotonin syndrome), TABLE 11 p. 1336 (CNS depressant effects)
▸ Antiepileptics (carbamazepine) markedly decrease the exposure to **mianserin**. Adjust dose. Moderate Study
▸ Antiepileptics (phenobarbital, primidone) are predicted to decrease the exposure to **mianserin**. Moderate Study → Also see TABLE 11 p. 1336
▸ **Mianserin** is predicted to increase the risk of toxicity when given with moclobemide. Avoid and for 1 week after stopping mianserin. Severe Theoretical → Also see TABLE 13 p. 1337
▸ **Mianserin** is predicted to increase the risk of toxicity when given with monoamine-oxidase A and B inhibitors, irreversible. Avoid and for 14 days after stopping the MAOI. Severe Theoretical → Also see TABLE 13 p. 1337
▸ **Mianserin** is predicted to decrease the efficacy of pitolisant. Unknown Theoretical
▸ **Mianserin** decreases the effects of sympathomimetics, vasoconstrictor (ephedrine). Severe Anecdotal
Micafungin → see TABLE 1 p. 1334 (hepatotoxicity)
▸ **Micafungin** slightly increases the exposure to amphotericin. Avoid or monitor toxicity. Moderate Study
Miconazole → see antifungals, azoles
Midazolam → see TABLE 11 p. 1336 (CNS depressant effects)
▸ Antiarrhythmics (dronedarone) are predicted to increase the exposure to **midazolam**. Monitor side effects and adjust dose. Severe Study
▸ Antiepileptics (carbamazepine, fosphenytoin, phenobarbital, phenytoin, primidone) are predicted to decrease the exposure to **midazolam**. Monitor and adjust dose. Moderate Study → Also see TABLE 11 p. 1336
▸ Antifungals, azoles (fluconazole, isavuconazole, posaconazole) are predicted to increase the exposure to **midazolam**. Monitor side effects and adjust dose. Severe Study
▸ Antifungals, azoles (itraconazole, ketoconazole, voriconazole) are predicted to markedly to very markedly increase the exposure to **midazolam**. Avoid or adjust dose. Severe Study
▸ Antifungals, azoles (miconazole) are predicted to increase the exposure to intravenous **midazolam**. Use with caution and adjust dose. Moderate Theoretical
▸ Antifungals, azoles (miconazole) are predicted to increase the exposure to oral **midazolam**. Avoid. Moderate Theoretical
▸ Aprepitant is predicted to increase the exposure to **midazolam**. Monitor side effects and adjust dose. Severe Study
▸ Bosentan is predicted to decrease the concentration of **midazolam**. Monitor and adjust dose. Moderate Theoretical
▸ Calcium channel blockers (diltiazem, verapamil) are predicted to increase the exposure to **midazolam**. Monitor side effects and adjust dose. Severe Study
▸ Cobicistat is predicted to markedly to very markedly increase the exposure to **midazolam**. Avoid or adjust dose. Severe Study
▸ Crizotinib is predicted to increase the exposure to **midazolam**. Monitor side effects and adjust dose. Severe Study
▸ Dabrafenib decreases the exposure to **midazolam**. Monitor and adjust dose. Moderate Study
▸ Efavirenz is predicted to alter the effects of **midazolam**. Avoid. Moderate Study
▸ Enzalutamide is predicted to decrease the exposure to **midazolam**. Monitor and adjust dose. Moderate Study
▸ Fosaprepitant slightly increases the exposure to **midazolam**. Moderate Study
▸ HIV-protease inhibitors are predicted to markedly to very markedly increase the exposure to **midazolam**. Avoid or adjust dose. Severe Study
▸ Idelalisib is predicted to markedly to very markedly increase the exposure to **midazolam**. Avoid or adjust dose. Severe Study
▸ Imatinib is predicted to increase the exposure to **midazolam**. Monitor side effects and adjust dose. Severe Study
▸ Lumacaftor is predicted to decrease the exposure to **midazolam**. Avoid. Severe Theoretical

- Macrolides (clarithromycin) are predicted to markedly to very markedly increase the exposure to **midazolam**. Avoid or adjust dose. [Severe] Study
- Macrolides (erythromycin) are predicted to increase the exposure to **midazolam**. Monitor side effects and adjust dose. [Severe] Study
- Mitotane is predicted to decrease the exposure to **midazolam**. Monitor and adjust dose. [Moderate] Study
- Monoclonal antibodies (tocilizumab) are predicted to decrease the exposure to **midazolam**. Monitor and adjust dose. [Moderate] Theoretical
- Netupitant is predicted to increase the exposure to **midazolam**. Monitor side effects and adjust dose. [Severe] Study
- Nevirapine decreases the concentration of **midazolam**. Monitor and adjust dose. [Moderate] Study
- Nilotinib is predicted to increase the exposure to **midazolam**. Monitor side effects and adjust dose. [Severe] Study
- Palbociclib increases the exposure to **midazolam**. [Moderate] Study
- Ribociclib moderately increases the exposure to **midazolam**. Avoid. [Moderate] Study
- Rifampicin is predicted to decrease the exposure to **midazolam**. Monitor and adjust dose. [Moderate] Study
- St John's Wort moderately decreases the exposure to **midazolam**. Monitor and adjust dose. [Moderate] Study
- Telotristat ethyl decreases the exposure to **midazolam**. [Moderate] Study

Midodrine → see sympathomimetics, vasoconstrictor

Midostaurin
- Antiarrhythmics (dronedarone) are predicted to increase the exposure to **midostaurin**. [Moderate] Theoretical
- Antiepileptics (carbamazepine, fosphenytoin, phenobarbital, phenytoin, primidone) are predicted to decrease the exposure to **midostaurin**. Avoid. [Severe] Study
- Antifungals, azoles (fluconazole, isavuconazole, posaconazole) are predicted to increase the exposure to **midostaurin**. [Moderate] Theoretical
- Antifungals, azoles (itraconazole, ketoconazole, voriconazole) are predicted to very markedly increase the exposure to **midostaurin**. Avoid or monitor for toxicity. [Severe] Study
- Aprepitant is predicted to increase the exposure to **midostaurin**. [Moderate] Theoretical
- Calcium channel blockers (diltiazem, verapamil) are predicted to increase the exposure to **midostaurin**. [Moderate] Theoretical
- Cobicistat is predicted to very markedly increase the exposure to **midostaurin**. Avoid or monitor for toxicity. [Severe] Study
- Crizotinib is predicted to increase the exposure to **midostaurin**. [Moderate] Theoretical
- Enzalutamide is predicted to decrease the exposure to **midostaurin**. Avoid. [Severe] Study
- HIV-protease inhibitors are predicted to very markedly increase the exposure to **midostaurin**. Avoid or monitor for toxicity. [Severe] Study
- Idelalisib is predicted to very markedly increase the exposure to **midostaurin**. Avoid or monitor for toxicity. [Severe] Study
- Imatinib is predicted to increase the exposure to **midostaurin**. [Moderate] Theoretical
- Macrolides (clarithromycin) are predicted to very markedly increase the exposure to **midostaurin**. Avoid or monitor for toxicity. [Severe] Study
- Macrolides (erythromycin) are predicted to increase the exposure to **midostaurin**. [Moderate] Theoretical
- Mitotane is predicted to decrease the exposure to **midostaurin**. Avoid. [Severe] Study
- Netupitant is predicted to increase the exposure to **midostaurin**. [Moderate] Theoretical
- Nilotinib is predicted to increase the exposure to **midostaurin**. [Moderate] Theoretical
- Rifampicin is predicted to decrease the exposure to **midostaurin**. Avoid. [Severe] Study
- St John's Wort is predicted to decrease the exposure to **midostaurin**. Avoid. [Severe] Theoretical

Mifamurtide
- Ciclosporin is predicted to decrease the efficacy of **mifamurtide**. Avoid. [Severe] Theoretical

- Corticosteroids are predicted to decrease the efficacy of **mifamurtide**. Avoid. [Severe] Theoretical
- NSAIDs (high-dose) are predicted to decrease the efficacy of **mifamurtide**. Avoid. [Severe] Theoretical
- Pimecrolimus is predicted to decrease the efficacy of **mifamurtide**. Avoid. [Severe] Theoretical
- Sirolimus is predicted to decrease the efficacy of **mifamurtide**. Avoid. [Severe] Theoretical
- Tacrolimus is predicted to affect the efficacy of **mifamurtide**. Avoid. [Severe] Theoretical

Mifepristone
- Mifepristone is predicted to decrease the efficacy of corticosteroids. Use with caution and adjust dose. [Moderate] Theoretical

Minocycline → see tetracyclines
Minoxidil → see TABLE 8 p. 1335 (hypotension)
Mirabegron
- Mirabegron is predicted to increase the exposure to aliskiren. [Mild] Theoretical
- Antifungals, azoles (itraconazole, ketoconazole, voriconazole) are predicted to increase the exposure to **mirabegron**. Adjust mirabegron dose in hepatic and renal impairment, p. 763. [Moderate] Study
- Mirabegron is predicted to increase the exposure to antihistamines, non-sedating (fexofenadine). [Mild] Theoretical
- Mirabegron is predicted to increase the exposure to beta blockers, selective (metoprolol). [Moderate] Study
- Cobicistat is predicted to increase the exposure to **mirabegron**. Adjust mirabegron dose in hepatic and renal impairment, p. 763. [Moderate] Study
- Mirabegron is predicted to increase the exposure to colchicine. [Mild] Theoretical
- Mirabegron is predicted to increase the exposure to dabigatran. [Severe] Theoretical
- Mirabegron slightly increases the exposure to digoxin. Monitor concentration and adjust dose. [Severe] Study
- Mirabegron is predicted to increase the exposure to edoxaban. [Mild] Theoretical
- Mirabegron is predicted to increase the exposure to eliglustat. Avoid or adjust dose—consult product literature. [Severe] Study
- Mirabegron is predicted to increase the exposure to everolimus. [Mild] Theoretical
- HIV-protease inhibitors are predicted to increase the exposure to **mirabegron**. Adjust mirabegron dose in hepatic and renal impairment, p. 763. [Moderate] Study
- Idelalisib is predicted to increase the exposure to **mirabegron**. Adjust mirabegron dose in hepatic and renal impairment, p. 763. [Moderate] Study
- Mirabegron is predicted to increase the exposure to loperamide. [Mild] Theoretical
- Macrolides (clarithromycin) are predicted to increase the exposure to **mirabegron**. Adjust mirabegron dose in hepatic and renal impairment, p. 763. [Moderate] Study
- Mirabegron is predicted to increase the exposure to pitolisant. Use with caution and adjust dose. [Moderate] Study
- Mirabegron is predicted to increase the exposure to sirolimus. [Mild] Theoretical
- Mirabegron is predicted to increase the exposure to taxanes (paclitaxel). [Mild] Theoretical
- Mirabegron is predicted to increase the exposure to topotecan. [Mild] Theoretical

Mirtazapine → see TABLE 13 p. 1337 (serotonin syndrome), TABLE 11 p. 1336 (CNS depressant effects)
- Antiepileptics (carbamazepine, fosphenytoin, phenobarbital, phenytoin, primidone) are predicted to decrease the exposure to **mirtazapine**. Adjust dose. [Moderate] Study → Also see TABLE 11 p. 1336
- Antifungals, azoles (itraconazole, ketoconazole, voriconazole) are predicted to increase the exposure to **mirtazapine**. [Moderate] Study
- Cobicistat is predicted to increase the exposure to **mirtazapine**. [Moderate] Study
- Enzalutamide is predicted to decrease the exposure to **mirtazapine**. Adjust dose. [Moderate] Study

Mirtazapine (continued)

▸ H$_2$ receptor antagonists (cimetidine) slightly increase the exposure to **mirtazapine**. Use with caution and adjust dose. Moderate Theoretical

▸ HIV-protease inhibitors are predicted to increase the exposure to **mirtazapine**. Moderate Study

▸ Idelalisib is predicted to increase the exposure to **mirtazapine**. Moderate Study

▸ Macrolides (clarithromycin) are predicted to increase the exposure to **mirtazapine**. Moderate Study

▸ Mitotane is predicted to decrease the exposure to **mirtazapine**. Adjust dose. Moderate Study

▸ **Mirtazapine** is predicted to decrease the efficacy of pitolisant. Unknown Theoretical

▸ Rifampicin is predicted to decrease the exposure to **mirtazapine**. Adjust dose. Moderate Study

Mitomycin → see TABLE 15 p. 1337 (myelosuppression), TABLE 5 p. 1334 (thromboembolism)

▸ Live vaccines are predicted to increase the risk of generalised infection (possibly life-threatening) when given with **mitomycin**. Public Health England advises avoid (refer to Green Book). Severe Theoretical

Mitotane → see TABLE 15 p. 1337 (myelosuppression)

▸ **Mitotane** is predicted to decrease the exposure to abiraterone. Avoid. Severe Theoretical

▸ Aldosterone antagonists (spironolactone) are predicted to decrease the effects of **mitotane**. Avoid. Severe Anecdotal

▸ **Mitotane** is predicted to decrease the exposure to aldosterone antagonists (eplerenone). Avoid. Moderate Theoretical

▸ **Mitotane** is predicted to decrease the exposure to alprazolam. Adjust dose. Moderate Theoretical

▸ **Mitotane** is predicted to decrease the exposure to antiarrhythmics (disopyramide, dronedarone). Avoid. Severe Study

▸ **Mitotane** is predicted to decrease the efficacy of antiarrhythmics (propafenone). Moderate Study

▸ **Mitotane** is predicted to decrease the exposure to anticholinesterases, centrally acting (donepezil). Mild Study

▸ **Mitotane** is predicted to decrease the exposure to antiepileptics (perampanel). Monitor and adjust dose. Moderate Study

▸ **Mitotane** is predicted to decrease the exposure to antifungals, azoles (isavuconazole). Avoid. Severe Study

▸ **Mitotane** is predicted to decrease the exposure to antimalarials (artemether) (with lumefantrine). Avoid. Severe Study

▸ **Mitotane** is predicted to decrease the concentration of antimalarials (piperaquine). Avoid. Moderate Theoretical

▸ **Mitotane** is predicted to moderately decrease the exposure to apixaban. Use with caution or avoid. Severe Study

▸ **Mitotane** moderately decreases the exposure to apremilast. Avoid. Severe Study

▸ **Mitotane** is predicted to markedly decrease the exposure to aprepitant. Avoid. Moderate Study

▸ **Mitotane** is predicted to moderately decrease the exposure to aripiprazole. Adjust **aripiprazole** dose, p. 391. Moderate Study

▸ **Mitotane** is predicted to decrease the exposure to axitinib. Avoid or adjust dose. Moderate Study → Also see TABLE 15 p. 1337

▸ **Mitotane** decreases the exposure to bedaquiline. Avoid. Severe Study

▸ **Mitotane** slightly decreases the exposure to bortezomib. Avoid. Severe Study → Also see TABLE 15 p. 1337

▸ **Mitotane** affects the exposure to bosentan. Avoid. Severe Study

▸ **Mitotane** is predicted to very markedly decrease the exposure to bosutinib. Avoid. Severe Study → Also see TABLE 15 p. 1337

▸ **Mitotane** is predicted to decrease the exposure to buspirone. Use with caution and adjust dose. Severe Study

▸ **Mitotane** moderately decreases the exposure to cabozantinib. Avoid. Moderate Study → Also see TABLE 15 p. 1337

▸ **Mitotane** is predicted to decrease the exposure to calcium channel blockers (amlodipine, felodipine, lacidipine, lercanidipine, nicardipine, nimodipine). Monitor and adjust dose. Moderate Study

▸ **Mitotane** is predicted to decrease the exposure to cannabis extract. Avoid. Severe Theoretical

▸ **Mitotane** is predicted to decrease the exposure to ceritinib. Avoid. Severe Study → Also see TABLE 15 p. 1337

▸ **Mitotane** decreases the concentration of ciclosporin. Severe Study

▸ **Mitotane** is predicted to alter the effects of cilostazol. Moderate Theoretical

▸ **Mitotane** is predicted to decrease the exposure to cinacalcet. Monitor and adjust dose. Moderate Study

▸ **Mitotane** decreases the exposure to clomethiazole. Monitor and adjust dose. Moderate Study

▸ **Mitotane** is predicted to decrease the exposure to cobicistat. Avoid. Severe Theoretical

▸ **Mitotane** is predicted to decrease the exposure to cobimetinib. Avoid. Severe Theoretical

▸ **Mitotane** is predicted to decrease the exposure to corticosteroids (budesonide, deflazacort, dexamethasone, fludrocortisone, hydrocortisone, methylprednisolone, prednisolone, prednisone, triamcinolone). Monitor and adjust dose. Moderate Study

▸ **Mitotane** is predicted to decrease the exposure to corticosteroids (fluticasone). Unknown Theoretical

▸ **Mitotane** is predicted to markedly decrease the exposure to crizotinib. Avoid. Severe Study → Also see TABLE 15 p. 1337

▸ **Mitotane** is predicted to decrease the exposure to dabrafenib. Avoid. Moderate Theoretical → Also see TABLE 15 p. 1337

▸ **Mitotane** is predicted to moderately decrease the exposure to daclatasvir. Avoid. Severe Study

▸ **Mitotane** is predicted to decrease the exposure to darifenacin. Moderate Theoretical

▸ **Mitotane** is predicted to markedly decrease the exposure to dasatinib. Avoid. Severe Study → Also see TABLE 15 p. 1337

▸ **Mitotane** is predicted to slightly decrease the exposure to delamanid. Avoid. Moderate Study

▸ **Mitotane** decreases the exposure to dolutegravir. Adjust dose. Severe Study

▸ **Mitotane** is predicted to decrease the exposure to elbasvir. Avoid. Severe Study

▸ **Mitotane** is predicted to decrease the exposure to eliglustat. Avoid. Severe Study

▸ **Mitotane** is predicted to decrease the concentration of elvitegravir. Avoid. Severe Theoretical

▸ **Mitotane** is predicted to decrease the effects of ergotamine. Moderate Theoretical

▸ **Mitotane** is predicted to decrease the exposure to erlotinib. Avoid or adjust **erlotinib** dose, p. 949. Severe Study

▸ **Mitotane** is predicted to decrease the exposure to etravirine. Avoid. Severe Theoretical

▸ **Mitotane** is predicted to decrease the concentration of everolimus. Avoid or adjust dose. Severe Study → Also see TABLE 15 p. 1337

▸ **Mitotane** moderately decreases the exposure to exemestane. Moderate Study

▸ **Mitotane** is predicted to decrease the exposure to fesoterodine. Avoid. Moderate Study

▸ **Mitotane** is predicted to decrease the exposure to fingolimod. Moderate Study

▸ **Mitotane** is predicted to decrease the exposure to fosaprepitant. Avoid. Moderate Theoretical

▸ **Mitotane** is predicted to decrease the exposure to gefitinib. Avoid. Severe Study → Also see TABLE 15 p. 1337

▸ **Mitotane** is predicted to decrease the exposure to grazoprevir. Avoid. Severe Study

▸ **Mitotane** is predicted to decrease the concentration of guanfacine. Adjust **guanfacine** dose, p. 349. Moderate Study

▸ **Mitotane** decreases the concentration of haloperidol. Adjust dose. Moderate Study

▸ **Mitotane** is predicted to decrease the exposure to ibrutinib. Avoid or adjust **ibrutinib** dose, p. 952. Severe Study → Also see TABLE 15 p. 1337

▸ **Mitotane** is predicted to decrease the exposure to idelalisib. Avoid. Severe Study → Also see TABLE 15 p. 1337

▸ **Mitotane** is predicted to decrease the exposure to imatinib. Avoid. Moderate Study → Also see TABLE 15 p. 1337

▸ **Mitotane** is predicted to decrease the exposure to irinotecan. Avoid. Severe Study → Also see TABLE 15 p. 1337

▸ **Mitotane** is predicted to decrease the exposure to ivabradine. Adjust dose. Moderate Theoretical

▸ **Mitotane** is predicted to moderately to markedly decrease the exposure to ivacaftor. Avoid. [Severe] Study

▸ **Mitotane** is predicted to decrease the exposure to ixazomib. Avoid. [Severe] Study

▸ **Mitotane** is predicted to decrease the exposure to lapatinib. Avoid. [Severe] Study

▸ **Mitotane** is predicted to decrease the exposure to linagliptin. [Moderate] Study

▸ **Mitotane** is predicted to decrease the exposure to lomitapide. Monitor and adjust dose. [Moderate] Theoretical

▸ **Mitotane** is predicted to decrease the exposure to lurasidone. Avoid. [Moderate] Study

▸ **Mitotane** is predicted to decrease the exposure to macitentan. Avoid. [Severe] Study

▸ **Mitotane** is predicted to decrease the exposure to maraviroc. Adjust dose. [Severe] Study

▸ **Mitotane** is predicted to decrease the exposure to midazolam. Monitor and adjust dose. [Moderate] Study

▸ **Mitotane** is predicted to decrease the exposure to midostaurin. Avoid. [Severe] Study

▸ **Mitotane** is predicted to decrease the exposure to mirtazapine. Adjust dose. [Moderate] Study

▸ **Mitotane** is predicted to decrease the exposure to montelukast. [Mild] Study

▸ **Mitotane** is predicted to markedly decrease the exposure to naloxegol. Avoid. [Moderate] Study

▸ **Mitotane** is predicted to slightly decrease the exposure to nateglinide. [Mild] Study

▸ **Mitotane** is predicted to decrease the exposure to netupitant. Avoid. [Severe] Study

▸ **Mitotane** is predicted to moderately decrease the exposure to nilotinib. Avoid. [Severe] Study → Also see TABLE 15 p. 1337

▸ **Mitotane** is predicted to decrease the exposure to nitisinone. Adjust dose. [Moderate] Theoretical

▸ **Mitotane** is predicted to decrease the exposure to olaparib. Avoid. [Moderate] Theoretical → Also see TABLE 15 p. 1337

▸ **Mitotane** is predicted to decrease the exposure to ondansetron. [Moderate] Study

▸ **Mitotane** is predicted to decrease the exposure to opioids (alfentanil, fentanyl). [Moderate] Study

▸ **Mitotane** is predicted to decrease the exposure to opioids (buprenorphine). Monitor and adjust dose. [Moderate] Theoretical

▸ **Mitotane** decreases the exposure to opioids (methadone). Monitor and adjust dose. [Severe] Study

▸ **Mitotane** is predicted to decrease the exposure to opioids (oxycodone). Monitor and adjust dose. [Moderate] Study

▸ **Mitotane** is predicted to moderately decrease the exposure to osimertinib. Avoid. [Moderate] Study

▸ **Mitotane** is predicted to decrease the exposure to palbociclib. Avoid. [Severe] Study

▸ **Mitotane** is predicted to decrease the exposure to paliperidone. Monitor and adjust dose. [Severe] Study

▸ **Mitotane** is predicted to decrease the exposure to panobinostat. Avoid. [Moderate] Theoretical → Also see TABLE 15 p. 1337

▸ **Mitotane** is predicted to decrease the exposure to paritaprevir (with ritonavir and ombitasvir). Avoid. [Severe] Study

▸ **Mitotane** is predicted to decrease the exposure to pazopanib. Avoid. [Severe] Theoretical → Also see TABLE 15 p. 1337

▸ **Mitotane** is predicted to decrease the exposure to phosphodiesterase type-5 inhibitors (avanafil, tadalafil). Avoid. [Severe] Study

▸ **Mitotane** is predicted to decrease the exposure to phosphodiesterase type-5 inhibitors (sildenafil, vardenafil). [Moderate] Theoretical

▸ **Mitotane** is predicted to moderately to markedly decrease the exposure to pibrentasvir. Avoid. [Severe] Study

▸ **Mitotane** is predicted to moderately decrease the exposure to pitolisant. [Moderate] Study

▸ **Mitotane** is predicted to decrease the exposure to ponatinib. Avoid. [Moderate] Theoretical

▸ **Mitotane** is predicted to markedly decrease the exposure to praziquantel. Avoid. [Moderate] Study

▸ **Mitotane** is predicted to decrease the exposure to quetiapine. [Moderate] Study

▸ **Mitotane** is predicted to decrease the exposure to ranolazine. Avoid. [Severe] Study

▸ **Mitotane** is predicted to decrease the exposure to reboxetine. [Moderate] Anecdotal

▸ **Mitotane** is predicted to decrease the exposure to regorafenib. Avoid. [Moderate] Study → Also see TABLE 15 p. 1337

▸ **Mitotane** is predicted to decrease the exposure to repaglinide. Monitor blood glucose and adjust dose. [Moderate] Study

▸ **Mitotane** is predicted to markedly decrease the exposure to ribociclib. Avoid. [Severe] Study

▸ **Mitotane** markedly decreases the exposure to rilpivirine. Avoid. [Severe] Study

▸ **Mitotane** is predicted to decrease the exposure to risperidone. Adjust dose. [Moderate] Study

▸ **Mitotane** is predicted to moderately decrease the exposure to rivaroxaban. Avoid unless patient can be monitored for signs of thrombosis. [Severe] Study

▸ **Mitotane** is predicted to decrease the exposure to roflumilast. Avoid. [Moderate] Study

▸ **Mitotane** is predicted to markedly decrease the exposure to rolapitant. Avoid. [Severe] Study

▸ **Mitotane** is predicted to decrease the exposure to ruxolitinib. Monitor and adjust dose. [Moderate] Study → Also see TABLE 15 p. 1337

▸ **Mitotane** is predicted to moderately decrease the exposure to saxagliptin. [Moderate] Study

▸ **Mitotane** is predicted to decrease the exposure to simeprevir. Avoid. [Severe] Study

▸ **Mitotane** is predicted to decrease the concentration of sirolimus. Avoid. [Severe] Study

▸ **Mitotane** is predicted to decrease the exposure to solifenacin. [Moderate] Theoretical

▸ **Mitotane** is predicted to decrease the exposure to sorafenib. [Moderate] Theoretical → Also see TABLE 15 p. 1337

▸ **Mitotane** is predicted to decrease the exposure to statins (simvastatin). [Severe] Study

▸ **Mitotane** is predicted to decrease the exposure to sunitinib. Avoid or adjust **sunitinib** dose, p. 967. [Moderate] Study → Also see TABLE 15 p. 1337

▸ **Mitotane** decreases the concentration of tacrolimus. Monitor and adjust dose. [Severe] Study

▸ **Mitotane** is predicted to decrease the exposure to taxanes (cabazitaxel, paclitaxel). Avoid. [Severe] Study → Also see TABLE 15 p. 1337

▸ **Mitotane** is predicted to decrease the exposure to taxanes (docetaxel). [Severe] Theoretical → Also see TABLE 15 p. 1337

▸ **Mitotane** is predicted to decrease the concentration of temsirolimus. Avoid. [Severe] Study → Also see TABLE 15 p. 1337

▸ **Mitotane** decreases the exposure to tetracyclines (doxycycline). Monitor and adjust dose. [Moderate] Study

▸ **Mitotane** is predicted to markedly decrease the exposure to ticagrelor. Avoid. [Severe] Study

▸ **Mitotane** is predicted to decrease the exposure to tivozanib. [Severe] Study

▸ **Mitotane** is predicted to decrease the exposure to tofacitinib. Avoid. [Severe] Study

▸ **Mitotane** is predicted to decrease the exposure to tolvaptan. Avoid. [Severe] Study

▸ **Mitotane** is predicted to decrease the exposure to toremifene. Adjust dose. [Moderate] Study

▸ **Mitotane** is predicted to decrease the exposure to trabectedin. Avoid. [Severe] Theoretical → Also see TABLE 15 p. 1337

▸ **Mitotane** is predicted to decrease the exposure to vandetanib. Avoid. [Moderate] Study

▸ **Mitotane** is predicted to moderately decrease the exposure to velpatasvir. Avoid. [Severe] Study

▸ **Mitotane** is predicted to decrease the exposure to vemurafenib. Avoid. [Severe] Theoretical

▸ **Mitotane** is predicted to decrease the exposure to venetoclax. Avoid. [Severe] Study

▸ **Mitotane** is predicted to decrease the exposure to vinca alkaloids (vinblastine, vincristine, vindesine). [Severe] Theoretical → Also see TABLE 15 p. 1337

Mitotane (continued)

▶ **Mitotane** is predicted to decrease the exposure to vinca alkaloids (vinflunine). Avoid. Severe Theoretical → Also see TABLE 15 p. 1337
▶ **Mitotane** is predicted to decrease the exposure to vinca alkaloids (vinorelbine). Use with caution or avoid. Severe Theoretical → Also see TABLE 15 p. 1337
▶ **Mitotane** is predicted to decrease the exposure to vismodegib. Avoid. Moderate Theoretical → Also see TABLE 15 p. 1337
▶ **Mitotane** is predicted to decrease the exposure to vortioxetine. Monitor and adjust dose. Moderate Study
▶ **Mitotane** is predicted to decrease the concentration of voxilaprevir. Avoid. Severe Study
▶ **Mitotane** is predicted to decrease the exposure to zopiclone. Adjust dose. Moderate Study

Mitoxantrone → see anthracyclines
Mivacurium → see neuromuscular blocking drugs, non-depolarising
Mizolastine → see antihistamines, non-sedating
Moclobemide → see TABLE 13 p. 1337 (serotonin syndrome)

FOOD AND LIFESTYLE Moclobemide is claimed to cause less potentiation of the pressor effect of tyramine than the traditional (irreversible) MAOIs, but patients should avoid consuming large amounts of tyramine-rich foods (such as mature cheese, salami, pickled herring, *Bovril®*, *Oxo®*, *Marmite®* or any similar meat or yeast extract or fermented soya bean extract, and some beers, lagers or wines).

▶ **Moclobemide** is predicted to increase the risk of a hypertensive crisis when given with amfetamines. Avoid. Severe Theoretical → Also see TABLE 13 p. 1337
▶ **Moclobemide** is predicted to increase the risk of severe hypertension when given with bupropion. Avoid. Severe Theoretical → Also see TABLE 13 p. 1337
▶ **Moclobemide** is predicted to increase the exposure to cilostazol. Moderate Theoretical
▶ **Moclobemide** potentially increases the exposure to clobazam. Adjust dose. Moderate Theoretical
▶ **Moclobemide** is predicted to decrease the efficacy of clopidogrel. Avoid. Moderate Study
▶ **Moclobemide** is predicted to increase the exposure to eliglustat. Avoid or adjust dose—consult product literature. Severe Theoretical
▶ H₂ receptor antagonists (cimetidine) increase the exposure to moclobemide. Adjust **moclobemide** dose, p. 359. Mild Study
▶ Levodopa increases the risk of side-effects when given with **moclobemide**. Moderate Study
▶ **Moclobemide** is predicted to increase the risk of side-effects when given with linezolid. Avoid and for 14 days after stopping **moclobemide**. Severe Theoretical → Also see TABLE 13 p. 1337
▶ Methylphenidate is predicted to increase the risk of a hypertensive crisis when given with **moclobemide**. Severe Theoretical
▶ Mianserin is predicted to increase the risk of toxicity when given with **moclobemide**. Avoid and for 1 week after stopping **mianserin**. Severe Theoretical → Also see TABLE 13 p. 1337
▶ **Moclobemide** is predicted to increase the effects of monoamine-oxidase B inhibitors (rasagiline, selegiline). Avoid. Severe Theoretical → Also see TABLE 13 p. 1337
▶ **Moclobemide** is predicted to increase the risk of side-effects when given with monoamine-oxidase B inhibitors (safinamide). Avoid and for 1 week after stopping **safinamide**. Severe Theoretical → Also see TABLE 13 p. 1337
▶ Opicapone is predicted to increase the risk of elevated blood pressure when given with **moclobemide**. Avoid. Severe Theoretical
▶ **Moclobemide** increases the risk of side-effects when given with phenothiazines (levomepromazine). Moderate Study
▶ Reboxetine is predicted to increase the risk of a hypertensive crisis when given with **moclobemide**. Avoid. Severe Theoretical
▶ **Moclobemide** moderately increases the exposure to rizatriptan. Avoid. Moderate Study → Also see TABLE 13 p. 1337
▶ **Moclobemide** moderately increases the exposure to sumatriptan. Avoid. Moderate Study → Also see TABLE 13 p. 1337
▶ **Moclobemide** is predicted to increase the risk of a hypertensive crisis when given with sympathomimetics, vasoconstrictor

(ephedrine, isometheptene, phenylephrine, pseudoephedrine). Avoid. Severe Study
▶ Tricyclic antidepressants are predicted to increase the risk of severe toxic reaction when given with **moclobemide**. Avoid. Severe Theoretical → Also see TABLE 13 p. 1337
▶ **Moclobemide** slightly increases the exposure to zolmitriptan. Adjust zolmitriptan dose, p. 475. Moderate Study → Also see TABLE 13 p. 1337

Modafinil

▶ Antiepileptics (carbamazepine, phenobarbital, primidone) are predicted to decrease the exposure to **modafinil**. Mild Theoretical
▶ Antiepileptics (fosphenytoin, phenytoin) are predicted to decrease the exposure to **modafinil** and **modafinil** is predicted to increase the concentration of antiepileptics (fosphenytoin, phenytoin). Monitor concentration and adjust dose. Moderate Theoretical
▶ Antifungals, azoles (itraconazole, ketoconazole, voriconazole) are predicted to increase the exposure to **modafinil**. Mild Theoretical
▶ **Modafinil** is predicted to decrease the exposure to bosutinib. Avoid. Severe Theoretical
▶ Cobicistat is predicted to increase the exposure to **modafinil**. Mild Theoretical
▶ **Modafinil** is predicted to decrease the efficacy of combined hormonal contraceptives. For FSRH guidance, see Contraceptives, interactions p. 775. Severe Study
▶ **Modafinil** is predicted to decrease the efficacy of desogestrel. For FSRH guidance, see Contraceptives, interactions p. 775. Severe Theoretical
▶ **Modafinil** is predicted to decrease the exposure to elbasvir. Avoid. Unknown Theoretical
▶ **Modafinil** is predicted to decrease the efficacy of etonogestrel. For FSRH guidance, see Contraceptives, interactions p. 775. Severe Theoretical
▶ **Modafinil** is predicted to decrease the exposure to grazoprevir. Avoid. Unknown Theoretical
▶ HIV-protease inhibitors are predicted to increase the exposure to **modafinil**. Mild Theoretical
▶ **Modafinil** is predicted to decrease the effects of hormone replacement therapy. Moderate Anecdotal
▶ Idelalisib is predicted to increase the exposure to **modafinil**. Mild Theoretical
▶ **Modafinil** is predicted to decrease the efficacy of levonorgestrel. For FSRH guidance, see Contraceptives, interactions p. 775. Severe Theoretical
▶ Macrolides (clarithromycin) are predicted to increase the exposure to **modafinil**. Mild Theoretical
▶ **Modafinil** is predicted to decrease the efficacy of norethisterone. For FSRH guidance, see Contraceptives, interactions p. 775. Severe Anecdotal
▶ Rifampicin is predicted to decrease the exposure to **modafinil**. Moderate Theoretical
▶ **Modafinil** decreases the efficacy of ulipristal. For FSRH guidance, see Contraceptives, interactions p. 775. Severe Anecdotal
▶ **Modafinil** is predicted to decrease the concentration of voxilaprevir. Avoid. Severe Theoretical

Mometasone → see corticosteroids
Monoamine-oxidase A and B inhibitors, irreversible → see TABLE 8 p. 1335 (hypotension), TABLE 13 p. 1337 (serotonin syndrome)

isocarboxazid · phenelzine · tranylcypromine

FOOD AND LIFESTYLE Potentially life-threatening hypertensive crisis can develop in those taking MAOIs who eat tyramine-rich food (such as mature cheese, salami, pickled herring, *Bovril®*, *Oxo®*, *Marmite®* or any similar meat or yeast extract or fermented soya bean extract, and some beers, lagers or wines) or foods containing dopa (such as broad bean pods). Avoid tyramine-rich or dopa-rich food or drinks with, or for 2 to 3 weeks after stopping, the MAOI.

▶ **Monoamine-oxidase A and B inhibitors, irreversible** are predicted to increase the effects of alpha blockers (indoramin). Avoid. Severe Theoretical → Also see TABLE 8 p. 1335
▶ **Monoamine-oxidase A and B inhibitors, irreversible** are predicted to increase the risk of a hypertensive crisis when

given with amfetamines. Avoid and for 14 days after stopping the MAOI. Severe Anecdotal → Also see TABLE 13 p. 1337

▶ Antiepileptics (carbamazepine) are predicted to increase the risk of severe toxic reaction when given with **monoamine-oxidase A and B inhibitors, irreversible**. Avoid and for 14 days after stopping the MAOI. Severe Theoretical

▶ Antiepileptics (phenobarbital, primidone) are predicted to increase the effects of **monoamine-oxidase A and B inhibitors, irreversible**. Severe Theoretical

▶ **Monoamine-oxidase A and B inhibitors, irreversible** are predicted to increase the risk of antimuscarinic side-effects when given with antihistamines, non-sedating. Avoid. Severe Theoretical

▶ **Monoamine-oxidase A and B inhibitors, irreversible** are predicted to increase the risk of antimuscarinic side-effects when given with antihistamines, sedating. Avoid. Severe Theoretical

▶ **Monoamine-oxidase A and B inhibitors, irreversible** are predicted to increase the risk of side-effects when given with atomoxetine. Avoid and for 2 weeks after stopping the MAOI. Severe Theoretical

▶ **Monoamine-oxidase A and B inhibitors, irreversible** are predicted to increase the risk of cardiovascular side-effects when given with beta$_2$ agonists. Moderate Anecdotal

▶ **Monoamine-oxidase A and B inhibitors, irreversible** are predicted to increase the risk of severe hypertension when given with bupropion. Avoid and for 14 days after stopping the MAOI. Severe Theoretical → Also see TABLE 13 p. 1337

▶ Buspirone is predicted to increase the risk of elevated blood pressure when given with **monoamine-oxidase A and B inhibitors, irreversible**. Avoid. Severe Anecdotal → Also see TABLE 13 p. 1337

▶ **Monoamine-oxidase A and B inhibitors, irreversible** are predicted to increase the effects of doxapram. Moderate Theoretical

▶ Entacapone is predicted to increase the risk of elevated blood pressure when given with **monoamine-oxidase A and B inhibitors, irreversible**. Avoid. Severe Theoretical

▶ **Monoamine-oxidase A and B inhibitors, irreversible** are predicted to decrease the antihypertensive effects of guanethidine. Avoid and for 14 days after stopping the MAOI. Severe Theoretical → Also see TABLE 8 p. 1335

▶ Levodopa increases the risk of a hypertensive crisis when given with **monoamine-oxidase A and B inhibitors, irreversible**. Avoid and for 14 days after stopping the MAOI. Severe Study → Also see TABLE 8 p. 1335

▶ **Monoamine-oxidase A and B inhibitors, irreversible** are predicted to increase the risk of side-effects when given with linezolid. Avoid and for 14 days after stopping the MAOI. Severe Theoretical → Also see TABLE 13 p. 1337

▶ **Monoamine-oxidase A and B inhibitors, irreversible** are predicted to alter the antihypertensive effects of methyldopa. Avoid. Severe Theoretical → Also see TABLE 8 p. 1335

▶ Methylphenidate is predicted to increase the risk of a hypertensive crisis when given with **monoamine-oxidase A and B inhibitors, irreversible**. Avoid and for 14 days after stopping the MAOI. Severe Theoretical

▶ Mianserin is predicted to increase the risk of toxicity when given with **monoamine-oxidase A and B inhibitors, irreversible**. Avoid and for 14 days after stopping the MAOI. Severe Theoretical → Also see TABLE 13 p. 1337

▶ Monoamine-oxidase B inhibitors (rasagiline, selegiline) are predicted to increase the risk of side-effects when given with **monoamine-oxidase A and B inhibitors, irreversible**. Avoid and for 14 days after stopping the MAOI. Severe Theoretical → Also see TABLE 8 p. 1335 → Also see TABLE 13 p. 1337

▶ Monoamine-oxidase B inhibitors (safinamide) are predicted to increase the risk of side-effects when given with **monoamine-oxidase A and B inhibitors, irreversible**. Avoid and for 1 week after stopping safinamide. Severe Theoretical → Also see TABLE 13 p. 1337

▶ Nefopam is predicted to increase the risk of serious elevations in blood pressure when given with **monoamine-oxidase A and B inhibitors, irreversible**. Avoid. Severe Theoretical

▶ Opicapone is predicted to increase the risk of elevated blood pressure when given with **monoamine-oxidase A and B inhibitors, irreversible**. Avoid. Severe Theoretical

▶ Opioids are predicted to increase the risk of CNS excitation or depression when given with **monoamine-oxidase A and B inhibitors, irreversible**. Avoid. Severe Study → Also see TABLE 13 p. 1337

▶ **Monoamine-oxidase A and B inhibitors, irreversible** are predicted to increase the risk of neuroleptic malignant syndrome when given with phenothiazines. Severe Theoretical → Also see TABLE 8 p. 1335

▶ Pholcodine is predicted to increase the risk of CNS excitation or depression when given with **monoamine-oxidase A and B inhibitors, irreversible**. Avoid and for 14 days after stopping the MAOI. Severe Theoretical

▶ Reboxetine is predicted to increase the risk of a hypertensive crisis when given with **monoamine-oxidase A and B inhibitors, irreversible**. Avoid. Severe Theoretical

▶ **Monoamine-oxidase A and B inhibitors, irreversible** are predicted to increase the exposure to rizatriptan. Avoid and for 14 days after stopping the MAOI. Severe Theoretical → Also see TABLE 13 p. 1337

▶ **Monoamine-oxidase A and B inhibitors, irreversible** are predicted to increase the exposure to sumatriptan. Avoid and for 14 days after stopping the MAOI. Severe Theoretical → Also see TABLE 13 p. 1337

▶ **Monoamine-oxidase A and B inhibitors, irreversible** are predicted to increase the risk of a hypertensive crisis when given with sympathomimetics, inotropic. Avoid and for 14 days after stopping the MAOI. Severe Theoretical

▶ **Monoamine-oxidase A and B inhibitors, irreversible** are predicted to increase the risk of a hypertensive crisis when given with sympathomimetics, vasoconstrictor. Avoid and for 14 days after stopping the MAOI. Severe Study

▶ Tetrabenazine is predicted to increase the risk of CNS toxicity when given with **monoamine-oxidase A and B inhibitors, irreversible**. Avoid and for 14 days after stopping the MAOI. Severe Theoretical

▶ Tolcapone is predicted to increase the effects of **monoamine-oxidase A and B inhibitors, irreversible**. Avoid. Severe Theoretical

▶ Tricyclic antidepressants are predicted to increase the risk of severe toxic reaction when given with **monoamine-oxidase A and B inhibitors, irreversible**. Avoid and for 14 days after stopping the MAOI. Severe Theoretical → Also see TABLE 8 p. 1335 → Also see TABLE 13 p. 1337

▶ Tryptophan increases the risk of side-effects when given with **monoamine-oxidase A and B inhibitors, irreversible**. Anecdotal → Also see TABLE 13 p. 1337

▶ **Monoamine-oxidase A and B inhibitors, irreversible** are predicted to increase the exposure to zolmitriptan. Severe Theoretical → Also see TABLE 13 p. 1337

Monoamine-oxidase B inhibitors → see TABLE 6 p. 1335 (bradycardia), TABLE 8 p. 1335 (hypotension), TABLE 13 p. 1337 (serotonin syndrome)

rasagiline · safinamide · selegiline

FOOD AND LIFESTYLE Hypertension is predicted to occur when high-dose **selegiline** is taken with tyramine-rich foods (such as mature cheese, salami, pickled herring, *Bovril*®, *Oxo*®, *Marmite*® or any similar meat or yeast extract or fermented soya bean extract, and some beers, lagers or wines).

▶ Monoamine-oxidase B inhibitors (rasagiline, selegiline) are predicted to increase the risk of severe hypertension when given with amfetamines. Avoid. Severe Theoretical → Also see TABLE 13 p. 1337

▶ Safinamide is predicted to increase the risk of severe hypertension when given with amfetamines. Severe Theoretical → Also see TABLE 13 p. 1337

▶ Monoamine-oxidase B inhibitors (rasagiline, selegiline) are predicted to increase the risk of severe hypertension when given with beta$_2$ agonists. Avoid. Severe Theoretical

▶ Safinamide is predicted to increase the risk of severe hypertension when given with beta$_2$ agonists. Severe Theoretical

Monoamine-oxidase B inhibitors (continued)

▸ **Monoamine-oxidase B inhibitors** are predicted to increase the risk of severe hypertension when given with bupropion. Avoid. Moderate Theoretical → Also see TABLE 13 p. 1337

▸ Combined hormonal contraceptives slightly increase the exposure to **rasagiline**. Moderate Study

▸ Combined hormonal contraceptives increase the exposure to **selegiline**. Avoid. Severe Study

▸ Hormone replacement therapy is predicted to increase the exposure to **selegiline**. Avoid. Moderate Study

▸ **Monoamine-oxidase B inhibitors** are predicted to increase the effects of levodopa. Adjust dose. Mild Study → Also see TABLE 8 p. 1335

▸ Monoamine-oxidase B inhibitors (**rasagiline, selegiline**) are predicted to increase the risk of side-effects when given with linezolid. Avoid and for 14 days after stopping the MAOI. Severe Theoretical → Also see TABLE 13 p. 1337

▸ **Safinamide** is predicted to increase the risk of side-effects when given with linezolid. Avoid and for 1 week after stopping **safinamide**. Severe Theoretical → Also see TABLE 13 p. 1337

▸ Monoamine-oxidase B inhibitors (**rasagiline, selegiline**) are predicted to increase the risk of a hypertensive crisis when given with methylphenidate. Avoid. Severe Theoretical

▸ **Moclobemide** is predicted to increase the effects of monoamine-oxidase B inhibitors (**rasagiline, selegiline**). Avoid. Severe Theoretical → Also see TABLE 13 p. 1337

▸ **Moclobemide** is predicted to increase the risk of side-effects when given with **safinamide**. Avoid and for 1 week after stopping **safinamide**. Severe Theoretical → Also see TABLE 13 p. 1337

▸ Monoamine-oxidase B inhibitors (**rasagiline, selegiline**) are predicted to increase the risk of side-effects when given with monoamine-oxidase A and B inhibitors, irreversible. Avoid and for 14 days after stopping the MAOI. Severe Theoretical → Also see TABLE 8 p. 1335 → Also see TABLE 13 p. 1337

▸ **Safinamide** is predicted to increase the risk of side-effects when given with monoamine-oxidase A and B inhibitors, irreversible. Avoid and for 1 week after stopping **safinamide**. Severe Theoretical → Also see TABLE 13 p. 1337

▸ **Rasagiline** is predicted to increase the risk of side-effects when given with opioids (pethidine). Avoid and for 14 days after stopping **rasagiline**. Severe Theoretical → Also see TABLE 13 p. 1337

▸ **Safinamide** is predicted to increase the risk of side-effects when given with opioids (pethidine). Avoid and for 1 week after stopping **safinamide**. Severe Theoretical → Also see TABLE 13 p. 1337

▸ **Selegiline** increases the risk of side-effects when given with opioids (pethidine). Avoid. Severe Anecdotal → Also see TABLE 13 p. 1337

▸ Quinolones (ciprofloxacin) slightly increase the exposure to **rasagiline**. Moderate Study

▸ Reboxetine is predicted to increase the risk of a hypertensive crisis when given with monoamine-oxidase B inhibitors (**rasagiline, selegiline**). Avoid. Severe Theoretical

▸ **Monoamine-oxidase B inhibitors** are predicted to increase the risk of a hypertensive crisis when given with sympathomimetics, inotropic. Avoid. Severe Anecdotal

▸ **Monoamine-oxidase B inhibitors** are predicted to increase the risk of a hypertensive crisis when given with sympathomimetics, vasoconstrictor. Avoid. Severe Anecdotal

Monoclonal antibodies → see TABLE 15 p. 1337 (myelosuppression), TABLE 12 p. 1337 (peripheral neuropathy), TABLE 9 p. 1336 (QT-interval prolongation), TABLE 4 p. 1334 (antiplatelet effects)

adalimumab · alemtuzumab · atezolizumab · avelumab · basiliximab · belimumab · benralizumab · bevacizumab · blinatumomab · brentuximab vedotin · brodalumab · canakinumab · certolizumab pegol · cetuximab · daratumumab · dupilumab · eculizumab · elotuzumab · golimumab · guselkumab · infliximab · inotuzumab ozogamicin · ipilimumab · ixekizumab · natalizumab · necitumumab · nivolumab · obinutuzumab · ocrelizumab · ofatumumab · olaratumab · panitumumab · pembrolizumab · pertuzumab · ramucirumab · rituximab · sarilumab · secukinumab · siltuximab · tocilizumab · trastuzumab · trastuzumab emtansine · ustekinumab · vedolizumab

▸ **Tocilizumab** is predicted to decrease the exposure to alprazolam. Monitor and adjust dose. Moderate Theoretical

▸ **Blinatumomab** is predicted to transiently increase the exposure to aminophylline. Monitor and adjust dose. Moderate Theoretical

▸ **Sarilumab** potentially affects the exposure to aminophylline. Monitor and adjust dose. Moderate Theoretical

▸ **Tocilizumab** is predicted to decrease the exposure to aminophylline. Monitor and adjust dose. Moderate Theoretical

▸ Anthracyclines are predicted to increase the risk of cardiotoxicity when given with monoclonal antibodies (**trastuzumab, trastuzumab emtansine**). Avoid. Severe Theoretical → Also see TABLE 15 p. 1337

▸ Antiarrhythmics (dronedarone) increase the risk of neutropenia when given with **brentuximab vedotin**. Monitor and adjust dose. Severe Theoretical

▸ Antiepileptics (carbamazepine) are predicted to decrease the effects of **brentuximab vedotin**. Severe Theoretical

▸ **Tocilizumab** is predicted to decrease the exposure to antiepileptics (fosphenytoin, phenytoin). Monitor and adjust dose. Moderate Theoretical

▸ Antifungals, azoles (itraconazole, ketoconazole) increase the risk of neutropenia when given with **brentuximab vedotin**. Monitor and adjust dose. Severe Study

▸ Antifungals, azoles (itraconazole, ketoconazole, voriconazole) are predicted to increase the exposure to **trastuzumab emtansine**. Avoid. Severe Theoretical

▸ **Brentuximab vedotin** increases the risk of pulmonary toxicity when given with bleomycin. Avoid. Severe Study → Also see TABLE 15 p. 1337

▸ **Tocilizumab** is predicted to decrease the exposure to calcium channel blockers. Monitor and adjust dose. Moderate Theoretical

▸ **Blinatumomab** is predicted to transiently increase the exposure to ciclosporin. Monitor and adjust dose. Moderate Theoretical

▸ **Sarilumab** potentially affects the exposure to ciclosporin. Monitor and adjust dose. Moderate Theoretical

▸ **Tocilizumab** is predicted to decrease the exposure to ciclosporin. Monitor and adjust dose. Moderate Theoretical

▸ Cobicistat is predicted to increase the exposure to **trastuzumab emtansine**. Avoid. Severe Theoretical

▸ **Sarilumab** potentially decreases the exposure to combined hormonal contraceptives. Severe Theoretical

▸ Corticosteroids (betamethasone, deflazacort, dexamethasone, hydrocortisone, methylprednisolone, prednisolone, prednisone) are predicted to decrease the efficacy of monoclonal antibodies (**atezolizumab, ipilimumab, nivolumab, pembrolizumab**). Use with caution or avoid. Severe Theoretical

▸ **Tocilizumab** is predicted to decrease the exposure to corticosteroids (dexamethasone, methylprednisolone). Monitor and adjust dose. Moderate Theoretical

▸ **Blinatumomab** is predicted to transiently increase the exposure to coumarins (warfarin). Monitor and adjust dose. Moderate Theoretical

▸ **Sarilumab** potentially affects the exposure to coumarins (warfarin). Monitor and adjust dose. Severe Theoretical

▸ **Tocilizumab** is predicted to decrease the exposure to coumarins (warfarin). Monitor and adjust dose. Moderate Theoretical

▸ **Tocilizumab** is predicted to decrease the exposure to diazepam. Monitor and adjust dose. Moderate Theoretical

▸ HIV-protease inhibitors (lopinavir, ritonavir, saquinavir) are predicted to increase the risk of neutropenia when given with **brentuximab vedotin**. Monitor and adjust dose. Severe Study

▸ HIV-protease inhibitors are predicted to increase the exposure to **trastuzumab emtansine**. Avoid. Severe Theoretical

▸ Idelalisib is predicted to increase the exposure to **trastuzumab emtansine**. Avoid. Severe Theoretical → Also see TABLE 15 p. 1337

▸ Live vaccines are predicted to increase the risk of generalised infection (possibly life-threatening) when given with **monoclonal antibodies**. Public Health England advises avoid (refer to Green Book). Severe Theoretical

▸ Macrolides (clarithromycin) increase the risk of neutropenia when given with **brentuximab vedotin**. Monitor and adjust dose. Severe Theoretical

▸ Macrolides (clarithromycin) are predicted to increase the exposure to **trastuzumab emtansine**. Avoid. Severe Theoretical

- **Tocilizumab** is predicted to decrease the exposure to midazolam. Monitor and adjust dose. [Moderate] Theoretical
- Rifampicin decreases the effects of **brentuximab vedotin**. [Severe] Study
- **Sarilumab** potentially affects the exposure to sirolimus. Monitor and adjust dose. [Moderate] Theoretical
- **Sarilumab** is predicted to decrease the exposure to statins (atorvastatin, simvastatin). [Moderate] Study
- **Tocilizumab** is predicted to decrease the exposure to statins (atorvastatin, simvastatin). Monitor and adjust dose. [Moderate] Study
- **Sarilumab** potentially affects the exposure to tacrolimus. Monitor and adjust dose. [Moderate] Theoretical
- **Blinatumomab** is predicted to transiently increase the exposure to theophylline. Monitor and adjust dose. [Moderate] Theoretical
- **Sarilumab** potentially affects the exposure to theophylline. Monitor and adjust dose. [Moderate] Theoretical
- **Tocilizumab** is predicted to decrease the exposure to theophylline. Monitor and adjust dose. [Moderate] Theoretical

Montelukast

- Antiepileptics (carbamazepine, fosphenytoin, phenobarbital, phenytoin, primidone) are predicted to decrease the exposure to **montelukast**. [Mild] Study
- Clopidogrel is predicted to moderately increase the exposure to **montelukast**. [Moderate] Study
- Enzalutamide is predicted to decrease the exposure to **montelukast**. [Mild] Study
- Fibrates (gemfibrozil) are predicted to moderately increase the exposure to **montelukast**. [Moderate] Study
- Leflunomide is predicted to increase the exposure to **montelukast**. [Moderate] Theoretical
- Mitotane is predicted to decrease the exposure to **montelukast**. [Mild] Study
- Opicapone is predicted to increase the exposure to **montelukast**. Avoid. [Moderate] Study
- Rifampicin is predicted to decrease the exposure to **montelukast**. [Mild] Study
- Teriflunomide is predicted to increase the exposure to **montelukast**. [Moderate] Theoretical

Morphine → see opioids

Moxifloxacin → see quinolones

Moxisylyte → see TABLE 8 p. 1335 (hypotension)

Moxonidine → see TABLE 8 p. 1335 (hypotension), TABLE 11 p. 1336 (CNS depressant effects)

- Tricyclic antidepressants are predicted to decrease the effects of **moxonidine**. Avoid. [Moderate] Theoretical → Also see TABLE 8 p. 1335

Mycophenolate → see TABLE 15 p. 1337 (myelosuppression)

- **Mycophenolate** is predicted to increase the risk of haematological toxicity when given with aciclovir. [Moderate] Theoretical
- Antacids decrease the exposure to **mycophenolate**. [Moderate] Study
- Antifungals, azoles (isavuconazole) increase the exposure to **mycophenolate**. [Moderate] Study
- **Mycophenolate** is predicted to increase the risk of haematological toxicity when given with ganciclovir. [Moderate] Theoretical → Also see TABLE 15 p. 1337
- Live vaccines are predicted to increase the risk of generalised infection (possibly life-threatening) when given with **mycophenolate**. Public Health England advises avoid (refer to Green Book). [Severe] Theoretical
- Rifampicin decreases the concentration of **mycophenolate**. Monitor and adjust dose. [Severe] Study
- **Mycophenolate** is predicted to increase the risk of haematological toxicity when given with valaciclovir. [Moderate] Theoretical
- **Mycophenolate** is predicted to increase the risk of haematological toxicity when given with valganciclovir. [Moderate] Theoretical → Also see TABLE 15 p. 1337

Nabilone → see TABLE 11 p. 1336 (CNS depressant effects)

- **Nabilone** is predicted to increase the risk of cardiovascular side-effects when given with amfetamines. [Severe] Theoretical

Nabumetone → see NSAIDs

Nadolol → see beta blockers, non-selective

Nalmefene

GENERAL INFORMATION Discontinue treatment 1 week before anticipated use of opioids; if emergency analgesia is required during treatment, an increased dose of opioid analgesic might be necessary (monitor for opioid intoxication).

- **Nalmefene** is predicted to decrease the efficacy of opioids. Avoid. [Severe] Theoretical

Naloxegol

- Antiarrhythmics (dronedarone) are predicted to increase the exposure to **naloxegol**. Adjust **naloxegol** dose and monitor side effects, p. 64. [Moderate] Study
- Antiepileptics (carbamazepine, fosphenytoin, phenobarbital, phenytoin, primidone) are predicted to markedly decrease the exposure to **naloxegol**. Avoid. [Severe] Study
- Antifungals, azoles (fluconazole, isavuconazole, posaconazole) are predicted to increase the exposure to **naloxegol**. Adjust **naloxegol** dose and monitor side effects, p. 64. [Moderate] Study
- Antifungals, azoles (itraconazole, ketoconazole, voriconazole) are predicted to markedly increase the exposure to **naloxegol**. Avoid. [Severe] Study
- Aprepitant is predicted to increase the exposure to **naloxegol**. Adjust **naloxegol** dose and monitor side effects, p. 64. [Moderate] Study
- Calcium channel blockers (diltiazem, verapamil) are predicted to increase the exposure to **naloxegol**. Adjust **naloxegol** dose and monitor side effects, p. 64. [Moderate] Study
- Cobicistat is predicted to markedly increase the exposure to **naloxegol**. Avoid. [Severe] Study
- Crizotinib is predicted to increase the exposure to **naloxegol**. Adjust **naloxegol** dose and monitor side effects, p. 64. [Moderate] Study
- Enzalutamide is predicted to markedly decrease the exposure to **naloxegol**. Avoid. [Moderate] Study
- Grapefruit juice is predicted to increase the exposure to **naloxegol**. Avoid. [Moderate] Theoretical
- HIV-protease inhibitors are predicted to markedly increase the exposure to **naloxegol**. Avoid. [Severe] Study
- Idelalisib is predicted to markedly increase the exposure to **naloxegol**. Avoid. [Severe] Study
- Imatinib is predicted to increase the exposure to **naloxegol**. Adjust **naloxegol** dose and monitor side effects, p. 64. [Moderate] Study
- Macrolides (clarithromycin) are predicted to markedly increase the exposure to **naloxegol**. Avoid. [Severe] Study
- Macrolides (erythromycin) are predicted to increase the exposure to **naloxegol**. Adjust **naloxegol** dose and monitor side effects, p. 64. [Moderate] Study
- Mitotane is predicted to markedly decrease the exposure to **naloxegol**. Avoid. [Moderate] Study
- Netupitant is predicted to increase the exposure to **naloxegol**. Adjust **naloxegol** dose and monitor side effects, p. 64. [Moderate] Study
- Nilotinib is predicted to increase the exposure to **naloxegol**. Adjust **naloxegol** dose and monitor side effects, p. 64. [Moderate] Study
- Rifampicin is predicted to markedly decrease the exposure to **naloxegol**. Avoid. [Moderate] Study
- St John's Wort is predicted to decrease the exposure to **naloxegol**. [Moderate] Theoretical

Naltrexone

GENERAL INFORMATION Avoid concurrent use of opioids.

Nandrolone

- **Nandrolone** is predicted to increase the anticoagulant effect of coumarins. Monitor and adjust dose. [Severe] Theoretical
- **Nandrolone** is predicted to increase the anticoagulant effect of phenindione. Monitor and adjust dose. [Severe] Theoretical

Naproxen → see NSAIDs

Naratriptan → see TABLE 13 p. 1337 (serotonin syndrome)

- Naratriptan is predicted to increase the risk of vasoconstriction when given with ergotamine. Separate administration by 24 hours. [Severe] Theoretical

Natalizumab → see monoclonal antibodies

Nateglinide → see TABLE 14 p. 1337 (antidiabetic drugs)

Nateglinide (continued)
▶ Antiepileptics (carbamazepine, fosphenytoin, phenobarbital, phenytoin, primidone) are predicted to slightly decrease the exposure to **nateglinide**. Mild Study
▶ Enzalutamide is predicted to slightly decrease the exposure to **nateglinide**. Mild Study
▶ Mitotane is predicted to slightly decrease the exposure to **nateglinide**. Mild Study
▶ Rifampicin is predicted to slightly decrease the exposure to **nateglinide**. Mild Study
▶ Sulfinpyrazone slightly increases the exposure to **nateglinide**. Mild Study

Nebivolol → see beta blockers, selective
Necitumumab → see monoclonal antibodies
Nefopam → see TABLE 10 p. 1336 (antimuscarinics)
▶ Nefopam is predicted to increase the risk of serious elevations in blood pressure when given with monoamine-oxidase A and B inhibitors, irreversible. Avoid. Severe Theoretical

Nelarabine → see TABLE 15 p. 1337 (myelosuppression)
Neomycin → see TABLE 2 p. 1334 (nephrotoxicity), TABLE 19 p. 1338 (ototoxicity), TABLE 20 p. 1338 (neuromuscular blocking effects)
▶ Neomycin decreases the absorption of digoxin. Moderate Study
▶ Neomycin moderately decreases the exposure to sorafenib. Moderate Study

Neostigmine → see TABLE 6 p. 1335 (bradycardia), TABLE 20 p. 1338 (neuromuscular blocking effects)
▶ Aminoglycosides are predicted to decrease the effects of **neostigmine**. Moderate Theoretical → Also see TABLE 20 p. 1338

Nepafenac → see NSAIDs

Netupitant
▶ **Netupitant** is predicted to increase the exposure to aldosterone antagonists (eplerenone). Adjust **eplerenone** dose, p. 190. Severe Study
▶ **Netupitant** is predicted to increase the exposure to alpha blockers (tamsulosin). Moderate Theoretical
▶ **Netupitant** is predicted to increase the exposure to alprazolam. Severe Study
▶ **Netupitant** is predicted to increase the exposure to antiarrhythmics (propafenone). Monitor and adjust dose. Moderate Study
▶ Antiepileptics (carbamazepine, fosphenytoin, phenobarbital, phenytoin, primidone) are predicted to decrease the exposure to **netupitant**. Avoid. Severe Study
▶ Antifungals, azoles (itraconazole, ketoconazole, voriconazole) are predicted to increase the exposure to **netupitant**. Moderate Study
▶ **Netupitant** is predicted to decrease the exposure to antifungals, azoles (isavuconazole). Moderate Theoretical
▶ **Netupitant** is predicted to increase the exposure to antihistamines, non-sedating (mizolastine). Severe Theoretical
▶ **Netupitant** is predicted to increase the exposure to antihistamines, non-sedating (rupatadine). Avoid. Moderate Study
▶ **Netupitant** is predicted to increase the concentration of antimalarials (piperaquine). Severe Theoretical
▶ **Netupitant** is predicted to increase the exposure to axitinib. Moderate Theoretical
▶ **Netupitant** is predicted to increase the exposure to bedaquiline. Avoid prolonged use. Mild Theoretical
▶ Bosentan is predicted to decrease the exposure to **netupitant**. Moderate Theoretical
▶ **Netupitant** is predicted to increase the exposure to bosutinib. Avoid or adjust dose. Severe Theoretical
▶ **Netupitant** is predicted to increase the exposure to buspirone. Use with caution and adjust dose. Moderate Study
▶ **Netupitant** is predicted to increase the exposure to cabozantinib. Moderate Theoretical
▶ **Netupitant** is predicted to increase the exposure to calcium channel blockers (amlodipine, felodipine, lacidipine, lercanidipine, nicardipine, nifedipine, nimodipine). Monitor and adjust dose. Moderate Study
▶ **Netupitant** is predicted to increase the exposure to ceritinib. Moderate Theoretical
▶ **Netupitant** increases the concentration of ciclosporin. Severe Study

▶ Cobicistat is predicted to increase the exposure to **netupitant**. Moderate Study
▶ **Netupitant** is predicted to increase the exposure to cobimetinib. Severe Theoretical
▶ **Netupitant** is predicted to increase the exposure to colchicine. Adjust **colchicine** dose with moderate inhibitors of CYP3A4, p. 1085. Severe Study
▶ **Netupitant** is predicted to increase the exposure to corticosteroids (dexamethasone). Adjust dose. Moderate Study
▶ **Netupitant** is predicted to increase the exposure to corticosteroids (methylprednisolone). Monitor and adjust dose. Moderate Study
▶ **Netupitant** is predicted to slightly increase the exposure to darifenacin. Moderate Study
▶ **Netupitant** is predicted to increase the exposure to dasatinib. Severe Study
▶ **Netupitant** increases the risk of QT-prolongation when given with domperidone. Avoid. Severe Study
▶ **Netupitant** is predicted to increase the exposure to dopamine receptor agonists (bromocriptine). Severe Theoretical
▶ **Netupitant** is predicted to increase the concentration of dopamine receptor agonists (cabergoline). Moderate Anecdotal
▶ **Netupitant** is predicted to moderately increase the exposure to dutasteride. Mild Study
▶ Efavirenz is predicted to decrease the exposure to **netupitant**. Moderate Theoretical
▶ **Netupitant** is predicted to increase the exposure to eliglustat. Avoid or adjust dose—consult product literature. Severe Study
▶ Enzalutamide is predicted to decrease the exposure to **netupitant**. Avoid. Severe Study
▶ **Netupitant** is predicted to increase the risk of ergotism when given with ergometrine. Severe Theoretical
▶ **Netupitant** is predicted to increase the risk of ergotism when given with ergotamine. Severe Theoretical
▶ **Netupitant** is predicted to increase the exposure to erlotinib. Moderate Theoretical
▶ **Netupitant** is predicted to increase the concentration of everolimus. Avoid or adjust dose. Moderate Study
▶ **Netupitant** is predicted to increase the exposure to fesoterodine. Adjust **fesoterodine** dose with moderate inhibitors of CYP3A4 in hepatic and renal impairment, p. 759. Mild Study
▶ **Netupitant** is predicted to increase the exposure to gefitinib. Moderate Theoretical
▶ **Netupitant** is predicted to increase the concentration of guanfacine. Adjust **guanfacine** dose, p. 349. Moderate Theoretical
▶ HIV-protease inhibitors are predicted to increase the exposure to **netupitant**. Moderate Study
▶ **Netupitant** is predicted to increase the exposure to ibrutinib. Adjust **ibrutinib** dose with moderate inhibitors of CYP3A4, p. 952. Severe Study
▶ Idelalisib is predicted to increase the exposure to **netupitant**. Moderate Study
▶ **Netupitant** is predicted to increase the exposure to imatinib. Moderate Theoretical
▶ **Netupitant** is predicted to increase the exposure to ivabradine. Adjust **ivabradine** dose, p. 210. Severe Theoretical
▶ **Netupitant** is predicted to increase the exposure to ivacaftor. Adjust **ivacaftor** dose with moderate inhibitors of CYP3A4, p. 292. Severe Study
▶ **Netupitant** is predicted to increase the exposure to lapatinib. Moderate Study
▶ **Netupitant** is predicted to increase the exposure to lomitapide. Avoid. Moderate Theoretical
▶ **Netupitant** is predicted to increase the exposure to lurasidone. Moderate Study
▶ Macrolides (clarithromycin) are predicted to increase the exposure to **netupitant**. Moderate Study
▶ **Netupitant** is predicted to increase the exposure to midazolam. Monitor side effects and adjust dose. Severe Study
▶ **Netupitant** is predicted to increase the exposure to midostaurin. Moderate Theoretical
▶ Mitotane is predicted to decrease the exposure to **netupitant**. Avoid. Severe Study

▸ **Netupitant** is predicted to increase the exposure to naloxegol. Adjust **naloxegol** dose and monitor side effects, p. 64. Moderate Study

▸ **Nevirapine** is predicted to decrease the exposure to **netupitant**. Moderate Theoretical

▸ **Netupitant** is predicted to increase the exposure to nilotinib. Moderate Theoretical

▸ **Netupitant** is predicted to increase the exposure to olaparib. Avoid moderate inhibitors of CYP3A4 or adjust **olaparib** dose, p. 973. Moderate Theoretical

▸ **Netupitant** is predicted to increase the exposure to opioids (alfentanil, buprenorphine, fentanyl, oxycodone). Monitor and adjust dose. Moderate Study

▸ **Netupitant** is predicted to increase the exposure to opioids (methadone, sufentanil). Moderate Theoretical

▸ **Netupitant** is predicted to increase the exposure to oxybutynin. Mild Theoretical

▸ **Netupitant** is predicted to increase the exposure to pazopanib. Moderate Theoretical

▸ **Netupitant** is predicted to increase the exposure to phosphodiesterase type-5 inhibitors (avanafil). Adjust **avanafil** dose, p. 794. Moderate Theoretical

▸ **Netupitant** is predicted to increase the exposure to phosphodiesterase type-5 inhibitors (sildenafil). Monitor or adjust **sildenafil** dose with moderate inhibitors of CYP3A4, p. 794. Moderate Study

▸ **Netupitant** is predicted to increase the exposure to phosphodiesterase type-5 inhibitors (tadalafil). Severe Theoretical

▸ **Netupitant** is predicted to increase the exposure to phosphodiesterase type-5 inhibitors (vardenafil). Adjust dose. Severe Theoretical

▸ **Netupitant** is predicted to increase the exposure to pimozide. Avoid. Severe Theoretical

▸ **Netupitant** is predicted to increase the exposure to quetiapine. Avoid. Moderate Study

▸ **Netupitant** is predicted to increase the exposure to ranolazine. Severe Study

▸ **Netupitant** is predicted to increase the exposure to ribociclib. Moderate Study

▸ **Rifampicin** is predicted to decrease the exposure to **netupitant**. Avoid. Severe Study

▸ **Netupitant** is predicted to increase the exposure to ruxolitinib. Moderate Theoretical

▸ **Netupitant** is predicted to increase the exposure to saxagliptin. Mild Study

▸ **Netupitant** is predicted to increase the exposure to simeprevir. Avoid. Severe Study

▸ **Netupitant** increases the concentration of sirolimus. Monitor and adjust dose. Moderate Study

▸ **Netupitant** is predicted to increase the exposure to SSRIs (dapoxetine). Adjust **dapoxetine** dose with moderate inhibitors of CYP3A4, p. 801. Moderate Theoretical

▸ **St John's Wort** is predicted to decrease the exposure to **netupitant**. Moderate Theoretical

▸ **Netupitant** is predicted to increase the exposure to statins (atorvastatin). Monitor and adjust dose. Severe Study

▸ **Netupitant** is predicted to increase the exposure to statins (simvastatin). Use with caution and adjust **simvastatin** dose, p. 203. Severe Study

▸ **Netupitant** is predicted to increase the exposure to sunitinib. Moderate Theoretical

▸ **Netupitant** is predicted to increase the concentration of tacrolimus. Severe Study

▸ **Netupitant** is predicted to increase the exposure to taxanes (cabazitaxel). Moderate Theoretical

▸ **Netupitant** is predicted to increase the concentration of temsirolimus. Moderate Theoretical

▸ **Netupitant** is predicted to increase the exposure to tofacitinib. Moderate Study

▸ **Netupitant** is predicted to increase the exposure to tolterodine. Mild Theoretical

▸ **Netupitant** is predicted to increase the exposure to tolvaptan. Adjust dose. Moderate Study

▸ **Netupitant** is predicted to increase the exposure to trazodone. Moderate Theoretical

▸ **Netupitant** is predicted to increase the exposure to ulipristal. Avoid if used for uterine fibroids. Moderate Study

▸ **Netupitant** is predicted to increase the exposure to venetoclax. Avoid moderate inhibitors of CYP3A4 or adjust **venetoclax** dose, p. 974. Severe Study

▸ **Netupitant** is predicted to increase the exposure to vinca alkaloids. Severe Theoretical

▸ **Netupitant** is predicted to increase the exposure to zopiclone. Adjust dose. Moderate Study

Neuromuscular blocking drugs, non-depolarising → see TABLE 6 p. 1335 (bradycardia), TABLE 20 p. 1338 (neuromuscular effects)

atracurium · cisatracurium · mivacurium · pancuronium · rocuronium · vecuronium

▸ **Anticholinesterases, centrally acting** are predicted to decrease the effects of **neuromuscular blocking drugs, non-depolarising**. Moderate Theoretical → Also see TABLE 6 p. 1335

▸ **Antiepileptics (carbamazepine)** are predicted to decrease the effects of (but acute use increases the effects of) neuromuscular blocking drugs, non-depolarising (**atracurium, cisatracurium, pancuronium, rocuronium, vecuronium**). Monitor and adjust dose. Moderate Study

▸ **Antiepileptics (fosphenytoin, phenytoin)** decrease the effects of (but acute use increases the effects of) neuromuscular blocking drugs, non-depolarising (**atracurium, cisatracurium, pancuronium, rocuronium, vecuronium**). Moderate Study

▸ **Clindamycin** increases the effects of **neuromuscular blocking drugs, non-depolarising**. Severe Anecdotal

▸ **Corticosteroids** are predicted to decrease the effects of **neuromuscular blocking drugs, non-depolarising**. Severe Anecdotal

▸ **Pancuronium** is predicted to increase the risk of cardiovascular side-effects when given with digoxin. Severe Anecdotal

▸ **Irinotecan** is predicted to decrease the effects of **neuromuscular blocking drugs, non-depolarising**. Moderate Theoretical

▸ **Intravenous magnesium** increases the effects of **neuromuscular blocking drugs, non-depolarising**. Moderate Study

▸ **Metoclopramide** is predicted to increase the effects of **neuromuscular blocking drugs, non-depolarising**. Moderate Theoretical

▸ **Penicillins (piperacillin)** increase the effects of **neuromuscular blocking drugs, non-depolarising**. Moderate Study

▸ **SSRIs** potentially increase the risk of prolonged neuromuscular blockade when given with **mivacurium**. Unknown Theoretical

Nevirapine

▸ **Nevirapine** is predicted to decrease the exposure to antiarrhythmics (dronedarone). Severe Theoretical

▸ **Nevirapine** is predicted to decrease the concentration of antiepileptics (carbamazepine, fosphenytoin, phenobarbital, phenytoin, primidone) and antiepileptics (carbamazepine, fosphenytoin, phenobarbital, phenytoin, primidone) are predicted to decrease the concentration of **nevirapine**. Severe Study

▸ **Antifungals, azoles (fluconazole)** slightly to moderately increase the exposure to **nevirapine**. Moderate Study

▸ **Nevirapine** is predicted to decrease the exposure to antifungals, azoles (isavuconazole). Avoid. Severe Theoretical

▸ **Nevirapine** moderately decreases the exposure to antifungals, azoles (itraconazole). Avoid and for 14 days after stopping **nevirapine**. Moderate Study

▸ **Nevirapine** moderately decreases the exposure to antifungals, azoles (ketoconazole). Avoid. Severe Study

▸ **Nevirapine** is predicted to decrease the exposure to antifungals, azoles (voriconazole) and antifungals, azoles (voriconazole) increase the exposure to **nevirapine**. Monitor and adjust dose. Severe Theoretical

▸ **Nevirapine** is predicted to decrease the exposure to axitinib. Moderate Theoretical

▸ **Nevirapine** is predicted to decrease the exposure to bedaquiline. Avoid. Severe Study

▸ **Nevirapine** is predicted to decrease the exposure to bosutinib. Avoid. Severe Theoretical

▸ **Nevirapine** is predicted to decrease the exposure to cabozantinib. Moderate Theoretical

Nevirapine (continued)

▶ **Nevirapine** is predicted to decrease the exposure to calcium channel blockers (amlodipine, felodipine, lacidipine, lercanidipine, nicardipine, nifedipine, nimodipine). Monitor and adjust dose. Moderate Theoretical

▶ **Nevirapine** is predicted to decrease the exposure to calcium channel blockers (diltiazem, verapamil). Moderate Theoretical

▶ **Nevirapine** is predicted to decrease the concentration of caspofungin. Adjust dose. Moderate Theoretical

▶ **Nevirapine** is predicted to decrease the concentration of ciclosporin. Moderate Study

▶ **Nevirapine** is predicted to decrease the exposure to cobicistat. Avoid. Severe Theoretical

▶ **Nevirapine** is predicted to decrease the exposure to cobimetinib. Avoid. Severe Theoretical

▶ **Nevirapine** is predicted to decrease the efficacy of combined hormonal contraceptives. For FSRH guidance, see Contraceptives, interactions p. 775. Severe Study

▶ **Nevirapine** potentially alters the anticoagulant effect of coumarins. Severe Anecdotal

▶ **Nevirapine** is predicted to decrease the exposure to crizotinib. Avoid. Severe Theoretical

▶ **Nevirapine** is predicted to decrease the exposure to daclatasvir. Avoid. Severe Theoretical

▶ **Nevirapine** is predicted to decrease the exposure to dasatinib. Severe Study

▶ **Nevirapine** is predicted to decrease the efficacy of desogestrel. For FSRH guidance, see Contraceptives, interactions p. 775. Severe Theoretical

▶ **Nevirapine** decreases the exposure to dolutegravir. Adjust dose. Severe Study

▶ **Nevirapine** decreases the concentration of efavirenz. Avoid. Severe Study

▶ **Nevirapine** is predicted to moderately decrease the exposure to elbasvir. Avoid. Severe Study

▶ **Nevirapine** is predicted to decrease the exposure to eliglustat. Moderate Theoretical

▶ **Nevirapine** is predicted to decrease the concentration of elvitegravir. Avoid. Severe Theoretical

▶ **Nevirapine** is predicted to decrease the effects of ergotamine. Moderate Theoretical

▶ **Nevirapine** is predicted to decrease the exposure to erlotinib. Severe Theoretical

▶ **Nevirapine** is predicted to decrease the efficacy of etonogestrel. For FSRH guidance, see Contraceptives, interactions p. 775. Severe Theoretical

▶ **Nevirapine** is predicted to decrease the exposure to etravirine. Avoid. Severe Study

▶ **Nevirapine** is predicted to decrease the concentration of everolimus. Avoid or adjust dose. Severe Study

▶ **Nevirapine** is predicted to decrease the exposure to gefitinib. Avoid. Severe Theoretical

▶ **Nevirapine** is predicted to decrease the exposure to glecaprevir. Avoid. Severe Study

▶ **Nevirapine** is predicted to markedly decrease the exposure to grazoprevir. Avoid. Severe Study

▶ **Nevirapine** is predicted to decrease the concentration of guanfacine. Adjust dose. Moderate Theoretical

▶ **Nevirapine** decreases the exposure to HIV-protease inhibitors. Refer to specialist literature. Moderate Study

▶ **Nevirapine** is predicted to decrease the effects of hormone replacement therapy. Moderate Anecdotal

▶ **Nevirapine** is predicted to decrease the exposure to idelalisib. Avoid. Moderate Theoretical

▶ **Nevirapine** is predicted to decrease the exposure to imatinib. Moderate Study

▶ **Nevirapine** is predicted to decrease the exposure to ivacaftor. Severe Theoretical

▶ **Nevirapine** is predicted to decrease the exposure to lapatinib. Avoid. Severe Study

▶ **Nevirapine** is predicted to decrease the efficacy of levonorgestrel. For FSRH guidance, see Contraceptives, interactions p. 775. Severe Theoretical

▶ **Nevirapine** is predicted to decrease the exposure to lurasidone. Monitor and adjust dose. Moderate Theoretical

▶ **Nevirapine** decreases the exposure to macrolides (clarithromycin). Moderate Study

▶ **Nevirapine** decreases the concentration of midazolam. Monitor and adjust dose. Moderate Study

▶ **Nevirapine** is predicted to decrease the exposure to netupitant. Moderate Theoretical

▶ **Nevirapine** is predicted to decrease the exposure to nilotinib. Avoid. Severe Theoretical

▶ **Nevirapine** is predicted to decrease the efficacy of norethisterone. For FSRH guidance, see Contraceptives, interactions p. 775. Severe Anecdotal

▶ **Nevirapine** is predicted to decrease the exposure to olaparib. Avoid. Moderate Theoretical

▶ **Nevirapine** decreases the exposure to opioids (methadone). Monitor and adjust dose. Severe Study

▶ **Nevirapine** is predicted to decrease the exposure to osimertinib. Severe Theoretical

▶ **Nevirapine** is predicted to decrease the exposure to paritaprevir (with ritonavir and ombitasvir). Avoid. Severe Study

▶ **Nevirapine** is predicted to decrease the exposure to phosphodiesterase type-5 inhibitors. Moderate Theoretical

▶ **Nevirapine** is predicted to decrease the exposure to pibrentasvir. Avoid. Severe Study

▶ **Nevirapine** is predicted to decrease the exposure to quetiapine. Moderate Study

▶ **Nevirapine** is predicted to decrease the exposure to ribociclib. Moderate Study

▶ Rifampicin decreases the concentration of **nevirapine**. Avoid. Severe Study

▶ **Nevirapine** is predicted to decrease the exposure to rilpivirine. Avoid. Severe Theoretical

▶ **Nevirapine** is predicted to decrease the exposure to rolapitant. Avoid. Severe Study

▶ **Nevirapine** is predicted to decrease the exposure to ruxolitinib. Monitor and adjust dose. Moderate Theoretical

▶ **Nevirapine** is predicted to decrease the exposure to simeprevir. Avoid. Severe Study

▶ **Nevirapine** is predicted to decrease the concentration of sirolimus. Monitor and adjust dose. Moderate Theoretical

▶ St John's Wort is predicted to decrease the concentration of **nevirapine**. Avoid. Severe Theoretical

▶ **Nevirapine** slightly decreases the exposure to statins (atorvastatin). Mild Study

▶ **Nevirapine** moderately decreases the exposure to statins (simvastatin). Moderate Study

▶ **Nevirapine** is predicted to decrease the concentration of tacrolimus. Monitor and adjust dose. Moderate Theoretical

▶ **Nevirapine** is predicted to decrease the exposure to taxanes (cabazitaxel). Avoid. Severe Study

▶ **Nevirapine** is predicted to decrease the concentration of temsirolimus. Avoid. Severe Theoretical

▶ **Nevirapine** is predicted to decrease the exposure to ticagrelor. Moderate Theoretical

▶ **Nevirapine** is predicted to decrease the exposure to tofacitinib. Moderate Study

▶ **Nevirapine** is predicted to decrease the exposure to tolvaptan. Moderate Theoretical

▶ **Nevirapine** decreases the efficacy of ulipristal. For FSRH guidance, see Contraceptives, interactions p. 775. Severe Anecdotal

▶ **Nevirapine** is predicted to decrease the exposure to velpatasvir. Avoid. Moderate Theoretical

▶ **Nevirapine** is predicted to decrease the exposure to venetoclax. Avoid. Severe Study

▶ **Nevirapine** is predicted to decrease the concentration of voxilaprevir. Avoid. Severe Theoretical

▶ **Nevirapine** is predicted to decrease the concentration of zidovudine. Refer to specialist literature. Severe Theoretical

Nicardipine → see calcium channel blockers

Nicorandil → see TABLE 8 p. 1335 (hypotension)

▶ Aspirin is predicted to increase the risk of gastrointestinal perforation when given with **nicorandil**. Severe Theoretical

▶ Corticosteroids increase the risk of gastrointestinal perforation when given with **nicorandil**. Severe Anecdotal

► **Nicorandil** is predicted to increase the risk of gastrointestinal perforation when given with NSAIDs. Severe Theoretical
► **Nicorandil** is predicted to increase the risk of hypotension when given with phosphodiesterase type-5 inhibitors. Avoid. Severe Theoretical → Also see TABLE 8 p. 1335
Nicotinic acid → see TABLE 3 p. 1334 (anticoagulant effects)
► **Nicotinic acid** is predicted to increase the risk of rhabdomyolysis when given with statins. Severe Theoretical
Nifedipine → see calcium channel blockers
Nilotinib → see TABLE 15 p. 1337 (myelosuppression), TABLE 9 p. 1336 (QT-interval prolongation)
► **Nilotinib** is predicted to increase the exposure to aldosterone antagonists (eplerenone). Adjust **eplerenone** dose, p. 190. Severe Study
► **Nilotinib** is predicted to increase the exposure to alpha blockers (tamsulosin). Moderate Theoretical
► **Nilotinib** is predicted to increase the exposure to alprazolam. Severe Study
► Antacids are predicted to decrease the absorption of **nilotinib**. Separate administration by at least 2 hours. Moderate Theoretical
► **Nilotinib** is predicted to increase the exposure to antiarrhythmics (propafenone). Monitor and adjust dose. Moderate Study
► Antiepileptics (carbamazepine, fosphenytoin, phenobarbital, phenytoin, primidone) are predicted to moderately decrease the exposure to **nilotinib**. Avoid. Severe Study
► Antifungals, azoles (fluconazole, posaconazole) are predicted to increase the exposure to **nilotinib**. Moderate Theoretical → Also see TABLE 9 p. 1336
► Antifungals, azoles (itraconazole, ketoconazole, voriconazole) are predicted to moderately increase the exposure to **nilotinib**. Avoid. Severe Study → Also see TABLE 9 p. 1336
► **Nilotinib** is predicted to increase the exposure to antihistamines, non-sedating (mizolastine). Severe Theoretical
► **Nilotinib** is predicted to increase the exposure to antihistamines, non-sedating (rupatadine). Avoid. Moderate Study
► **Nilotinib** is predicted to increase the concentration of antimalarials (piperaquine). Severe Theoretical
► Aprepitant is predicted to increase the exposure to **nilotinib**. Moderate Theoretical
► **Nilotinib** is predicted to increase the exposure to axitinib. Moderate Theoretical → Also see TABLE 15 p. 1337
► **Nilotinib** is predicted to increase the exposure to bedaquiline. Avoid prolonged use. Mild Theoretical → Also see TABLE 9 p. 1336
► Bosentan is predicted to decrease the exposure to **nilotinib**. Avoid. Severe Theoretical
► **Nilotinib** is predicted to increase the exposure to bosutinib. Avoid or adjust dose. Severe Theoretical → Also see TABLE 15 p. 1337 → Also see TABLE 9 p. 1336
► **Nilotinib** is predicted to increase the exposure to buspirone. Use with caution and adjust dose. Moderate Study
► **Nilotinib** is predicted to increase the exposure to cabozantinib. Moderate Theoretical → Also see TABLE 15 p. 1337 → Also see TABLE 9 p. 1336
► Calcium channel blockers (diltiazem, verapamil) are predicted to increase the exposure to **nilotinib**. Moderate Theoretical
► **Nilotinib** is predicted to increase the exposure to calcium channel blockers (amlodipine, felodipine, lacidipine, lercanidipine, nicardipine, nifedipine, nimodipine). Monitor and adjust dose. Moderate Study
► **Nilotinib** is predicted to increase the exposure to ceritinib. Moderate Theoretical → Also see TABLE 15 p. 1337 → Also see TABLE 9 p. 1336
► **Nilotinib** increases the concentration of ciclosporin. Severe Study
► Cobicistat is predicted to moderately increase the exposure to **nilotinib**. Avoid. Severe Study
► **Nilotinib** is predicted to increase the exposure to cobimetinib. Severe Theoretical
► **Nilotinib** is predicted to increase the exposure to colchicine. Adjust **colchicine** dose with moderate inhibitors of CYP3A4, p. 1085. Severe Study
► **Nilotinib** is predicted to increase the exposure to corticosteroids (methylprednisolone). Monitor and adjust dose. Moderate Study

► **Nilotinib** is predicted to increase the risk of bleeding events when given with coumarins. Severe Theoretical
► **Nilotinib** is predicted to slightly increase the exposure to darifenacin. Moderate Study
► **Nilotinib** is predicted to increase the exposure to dasatinib. Severe Study → Also see TABLE 15 p. 1337 → Also see TABLE 9 p. 1336
► **Nilotinib** increases the risk of QT-prolongation when given with domperidone. Avoid. Severe Study
► **Nilotinib** is predicted to increase the exposure to dopamine receptor agonists (bromocriptine). Severe Theoretical
► **Nilotinib** is predicted to increase the concentration of dopamine receptor agonists (cabergoline). Moderate Anecdotal
► **Nilotinib** is predicted to moderately increase the exposure to dutasteride. Mild Study
► Efavirenz is predicted to decrease the exposure to **nilotinib**. Avoid. Severe Theoretical → Also see TABLE 9 p. 1336
► **Nilotinib** is predicted to increase the exposure to eliglustat. Avoid or adjust dose—consult product literature. Severe Study
► Enzalutamide is predicted to moderately decrease the exposure to **nilotinib**. Avoid. Severe Study
► **Nilotinib** is predicted to increase the risk of ergotism when given with ergometrine. Severe Theoretical
► **Nilotinib** is predicted to increase the risk of ergotism when given with ergotamine. Severe Theoretical
► **Nilotinib** is predicted to increase the exposure to erlotinib. Moderate Theoretical
► **Nilotinib** is predicted to increase the concentration of everolimus. Avoid or adjust dose. Moderate Study → Also see TABLE 15 p. 1337
► **Nilotinib** is predicted to increase the exposure to fesoterodine. Adjust **fesoterodine** dose with moderate inhibitors of CYP3A4 in hepatic and renal impairment, p. 759. Mild Study
► **Nilotinib** is predicted to increase the exposure to gefitinib. Moderate Theoretical → Also see TABLE 15 p. 1337
► Grapefruit juice is predicted to increase the exposure to **nilotinib**. Avoid. Severe Theoretical
► **Nilotinib** is predicted to increase the concentration of guanfacine. Adjust **guanfacine** dose, p. 349. Moderate Theoretical
► H_2 receptor antagonists are predicted to decrease the absorption of **nilotinib**. **H_2 receptor antagonists** should be taken 10 hours before or 2 hours after **nilotinib**. Mild Theoretical
► HIV-protease inhibitors are predicted to moderately increase the exposure to **nilotinib**. Avoid. Severe Study → Also see TABLE 9 p. 1336
► **Nilotinib** is predicted to increase the exposure to ibrutinib. Adjust **ibrutinib** dose with moderate inhibitors of CYP3A4, p. 952. Severe Study → Also see TABLE 15 p. 1337
► Idelalisib is predicted to moderately increase the exposure to **nilotinib**. Avoid. Severe Study → Also see TABLE 15 p. 1337
► **Nilotinib** is predicted to increase the exposure to ivabradine. Adjust **ivabradine** dose, p. 210. Severe Theoretical
► **Nilotinib** is predicted to increase the exposure to ivacaftor. Adjust **ivacaftor** dose with moderate inhibitors of CYP3A4, p. 292. Severe Study
► **Nilotinib** is predicted to increase the exposure to lapatinib. Moderate Study → Also see TABLE 9 p. 1336
► **Nilotinib** is predicted to increase the exposure to lomitapide. Avoid. Moderate Theoretical
► **Nilotinib** is predicted to increase the exposure to lurasidone. Moderate Theoretical
► Macrolides (clarithromycin) are predicted to moderately increase the exposure to **nilotinib**. Avoid. Severe Study → Also see TABLE 9 p. 1336
► Macrolides (erythromycin) are predicted to increase the exposure to **nilotinib**. Moderate Theoretical → Also see TABLE 9 p. 1336
► **Nilotinib** is predicted to increase the exposure to midazolam. Monitor side effects and adjust dose. Severe Study
► **Nilotinib** is predicted to increase the exposure to midostaurin. Moderate Theoretical
► Mitotane is predicted to moderately decrease the exposure to **nilotinib**. Avoid. Severe Study → Also see TABLE 15 p. 1337
► **Nilotinib** is predicted to increase the exposure to naloxegol. Adjust **naloxegol** dose and monitor side effects, p. 64. Moderate Study

A1

Interactions | Appendix 1

Nilotinib (continued)

► Netupitant is predicted to increase the exposure to **nilotinib**. Moderate Theoretical
► Nevirapine is predicted to decrease the exposure to **nilotinib**. Avoid. Severe Theoretical
► **Nilotinib** is predicted to increase the exposure to olaparib. Avoid moderate inhibitors of CYP3A4 or adjust olaparib dose, p. 973. Moderate Theoretical → Also see TABLE 15 p. 1337
► **Nilotinib** is predicted to increase the exposure to opioids (alfentanil, buprenorphine, fentanyl, oxycodone). Monitor and adjust dose. Moderate Study
► **Nilotinib** is predicted to increase the exposure to opioids (methadone, sufentanil). Moderate Theoretical → Also see TABLE 9 p. 1336
► **Nilotinib** is predicted to increase the exposure to oxybutynin. Mild Theoretical
► **Nilotinib** is predicted to increase the exposure to pazopanib. Moderate Theoretical → Also see TABLE 15 p. 1337 → Also see TABLE 9 p. 1336
► **Nilotinib** is predicted to increase the risk of bleeding events when given with phenindione. Severe Theoretical
► **Nilotinib** is predicted to increase the exposure to phosphodiesterase type-5 inhibitors (avanafil). Adjust avanafil dose, p. 794. Moderate Theoretical
► **Nilotinib** is predicted to increase the exposure to phosphodiesterase type-5 inhibitors (sildenafil). Monitor or adjust sildenafil dose with moderate inhibitors of CYP3A4, p. 794. Moderate Study → Also see TABLE 9 p. 1336
► **Nilotinib** is predicted to increase the exposure to phosphodiesterase type-5 inhibitors (tadalafil). Severe Theoretical
► **Nilotinib** is predicted to increase the exposure to phosphodiesterase type-5 inhibitors (vardenafil). Adjust dose. Severe Theoretical → Also see TABLE 9 p. 1336
► **Nilotinib** is predicted to increase the exposure to pimozide. Avoid. Severe Theoretical → Also see TABLE 9 p. 1336
► **Nilotinib** is predicted to increase the exposure to quetiapine. Avoid. Moderate Study
► **Nilotinib** is predicted to increase the exposure to ranolazine. Severe Study → Also see TABLE 9 p. 1336
► **Nilotinib** is predicted to increase the exposure to ribociclib. Moderate Study → Also see TABLE 9 p. 1336
► Rifampicin is predicted to moderately decrease the exposure to **nilotinib**. Avoid. Severe Study
► **Nilotinib** is predicted to increase the exposure to ruxolitinib. Moderate Theoretical → Also see TABLE 15 p. 1337
► **Nilotinib** is predicted to increase the exposure to saxagliptin. Mild Study
► **Nilotinib** is predicted to increase the exposure to simeprevir. Avoid. Severe Study
► **Nilotinib** increases the concentration of sirolimus. Monitor and adjust dose. Moderate Study
► **Nilotinib** is predicted to increase the exposure to SSRIs (dapoxetine). Adjust dapoxetine dose with moderate inhibitors of CYP3A4, p. 801. Moderate Theoretical
► St John's Wort is predicted to decrease the exposure to **nilotinib**. Avoid. Severe Theoretical
► **Nilotinib** is predicted to increase the exposure to statins (atorvastatin). Monitor and adjust dose. Severe Study
► **Nilotinib** is predicted to increase the exposure to statins (simvastatin). Use with caution and adjust simvastatin dose, p. 203. Severe Study
► **Nilotinib** is predicted to increase the exposure to sunitinib. Moderate Theoretical → Also see TABLE 15 p. 1337 → Also see TABLE 9 p. 1336
► **Nilotinib** is predicted to increase the concentration of tacrolimus. Severe Study
► **Nilotinib** is predicted to increase the exposure to taxanes (cabazitaxel). Moderate Theoretical → Also see TABLE 15 p. 1337
► **Nilotinib** is predicted to increase the concentration of temsirolimus. Moderate Theoretical → Also see TABLE 15 p. 1337
► **Nilotinib** is predicted to increase the exposure to tofacitinib. Moderate Study
► **Nilotinib** is predicted to increase the exposure to tolterodine. Mild Theoretical → Also see TABLE 9 p. 1336
► **Nilotinib** is predicted to increase the exposure to tolvaptan. Adjust dose. Moderate Study

► **Nilotinib** is predicted to increase the exposure to trazodone. Moderate Theoretical
► **Nilotinib** is predicted to increase the exposure to ulipristal. Avoid if used for uterine fibroids. Moderate Study
► **Nilotinib** is predicted to increase the exposure to venetoclax. Avoid moderate inhibitors of CYP3A4 or adjust venetoclax dose, p. 974. Severe Study
► **Nilotinib** is predicted to increase the exposure to vinca alkaloids. Severe Theoretical → Also see TABLE 15 p. 1337 → Also see TABLE 9 p. 1336
► **Nilotinib** is predicted to increase the exposure to zopiclone. Adjust dose. Moderate Study

Nimodipine → see calcium channel blockers

Nintedanib
► Antiarrhythmics (amiodarone, dronedarone) are predicted to increase the exposure to **nintedanib**. Moderate Study
► Antiepileptics (carbamazepine) are predicted to decrease the exposure to **nintedanib**. Moderate Study
► Antifungals, azoles (itraconazole, ketoconazole) are predicted to increase the exposure to **nintedanib**. Moderate Study
► Calcium channel blockers (verapamil) are predicted to increase the exposure to **nintedanib**. Moderate Study
► Ciclosporin is predicted to increase the exposure to **nintedanib**. Moderate Study
► HIV-protease inhibitors (lopinavir, ritonavir, saquinavir) are predicted to increase the exposure to **nintedanib**. Moderate Study
► Lapatinib is predicted to increase the exposure to **nintedanib**. Moderate Study
► Macrolides are predicted to increase the exposure to **nintedanib**. Moderate Study
► Ranolazine is predicted to increase the exposure to **nintedanib**. Moderate Study
► Rifampicin is predicted to decrease the exposure to **nintedanib**. Moderate Study
► St John's Wort is predicted to decrease the exposure to **nintedanib**. Moderate Study
► Vemurafenib is predicted to increase the exposure to **nintedanib**. Moderate Study

Nitisinone
► Antiepileptics (carbamazepine, fosphenytoin, phenobarbital, phenytoin, primidone) are predicted to decrease the exposure to **nitisinone**. Adjust dose. Moderate Theoretical
► Antifungals, azoles (itraconazole, ketoconazole, voriconazole) are predicted to increase the exposure to **nitisinone**. Adjust dose. Moderate Theoretical
► Cobicistat is predicted to increase the exposure to **nitisinone**. Adjust dose. Moderate Theoretical
► Enzalutamide is predicted to decrease the exposure to **nitisinone**. Adjust dose. Moderate Theoretical
► HIV-protease inhibitors are predicted to increase the exposure to **nitisinone**. Adjust dose. Moderate Theoretical
► Idelalisib is predicted to increase the exposure to **nitisinone**. Adjust dose. Moderate Theoretical
► Macrolides (clarithromycin) are predicted to increase the exposure to **nitisinone**. Adjust dose. Moderate Theoretical
► Mitotane is predicted to decrease the exposure to **nitisinone**. Adjust dose. Moderate Theoretical
► Rifampicin is predicted to decrease the exposure to **nitisinone**. Adjust dose. Moderate Theoretical

Nitrates → see TABLE 7 p. 1335 (first-dose hypotension), TABLE 8 p. 1335 (hypotension)

glyceryl trinitrate · isosorbide dinitrate · isosorbide mononitrate

PHARMACOLOGY Drugs with antimuscarinic effects can cause dry mouth, which can reduce the effectiveness of sublingual glyceryl trinitrate tablets.

► **Nitrates** are predicted to increase the risk of methaemoglobinaemia when given with topical anaesthetics, local (prilocaine). Avoid. Severe Theoretical
► **Nitrates** are predicted to increase the risk of methaemoglobinaemia when given with dapsone. Severe Theoretical

▶ **Nitrates** potentially increase the risk of hypotension when given with phosphodiesterase type-5 inhibitors. Avoid. Severe Study → Also see TABLE 8 p. 1335

Nitrazepam → see TABLE 11 p. 1336 (CNS depressant effects)

▶ Rifampicin increases the clearance of **nitrazepam**. Moderate Study

Nitrofurantoin → see TABLE 12 p. 1337 (peripheral neuropathy)

▶ **Nitrofurantoin** is predicted to increase the risk of methaemoglobinaemia when given with topical anaesthetics, local (prilocaine). Use with caution or avoid. Severe Theoretical

▶ Antacids (magnesium trisilicate) decrease the absorption of **nitrofurantoin**. Moderate Study

▶ **Nitrofurantoin** is predicted to increase the risk of methaemoglobinaemia when given with dapsone. Severe Theoretical

Nitrous oxide → see TABLE 8 p. 1335 (hypotension), TABLE 11 p. 1336 (CNS depressant effects)

Nivolumab → see monoclonal antibodies

Nizatidine → see H₂ receptor antagonists

Noradrenaline/norepinephrine → see sympathomimetics, vasoconstrictor

Norethisterone

▶ Antiepileptics (carbamazepine, eslicarbazepine, fosphenytoin, oxcarbazepine, perampanel, phenobarbital, phenytoin, primidone, rufinamide, topiramate) are predicted to decrease the efficacy of **norethisterone**. For FSRH guidance, see Contraceptives, interactions p. 775. Severe Anecdotal

▶ Aprepitant is predicted to decrease the efficacy of **norethisterone**. For FSRH guidance, see Contraceptives, interactions p. 775. Severe Anecdotal

▶ Bosentan is predicted to decrease the efficacy of **norethisterone**. For FSRH guidance, see Contraceptives, interactions p. 775. Severe Anecdotal

▶ Efavirenz is predicted to decrease the efficacy of **norethisterone**. For FSRH guidance, see Contraceptives, interactions p. 775. Severe Anecdotal

▶ Fosaprepitant is predicted to decrease the efficacy of **norethisterone**. For FSRH guidance, see Contraceptives, interactions p. 775. Severe Anecdotal

▶ Griseofulvin potentially decreases the efficacy of **norethisterone**. For FSRH guidance, see Contraceptives, interactions p. 775. Severe Anecdotal

▶ HIV-protease inhibitors (ritonavir) are predicted to decrease the efficacy of **norethisterone**. For FSRH guidance, see Contraceptives, interactions p. 775. Severe Anecdotal

▶ Modafinil is predicted to decrease the efficacy of **norethisterone**. For FSRH guidance, see Contraceptives, interactions p. 775. Severe Anecdotal

▶ Nevirapine is predicted to decrease the efficacy of **norethisterone**. For FSRH guidance, see Contraceptives, interactions p. 775. Severe Anecdotal

▶ Rifabutin is predicted to decrease the efficacy of **norethisterone**. For FSRH guidance, see Contraceptives, interactions p. 775. Severe Anecdotal

▶ Rifampicin is predicted to decrease the efficacy of **norethisterone**. For FSRH guidance, see Contraceptives, interactions p. 775. Severe Anecdotal

▶ St John's Wort is predicted to decrease the efficacy of **norethisterone**. MHRA advises avoid. For FSRH guidance, see Contraceptives, interactions p. 775. Severe Anecdotal

▶ Sugammadex is predicted to decrease the exposure to **norethisterone**. Use additional contraceptive precautions. Severe Theoretical

▶ Ulipristal is predicted to decrease the efficacy of **norethisterone**. Avoid. Severe Theoretical

Norfloxacin → see quinolones

Nortriptyline → see tricyclic antidepressants

NSAIDs → see TABLE 18 p. 1338 (hyponatraemia), TABLE 2 p. 1334 (nephrotoxicity), TABLE 16 p. 1338 (increased serum potassium), TABLE 4 p. 1334 (antiplatelet effects)

aceclofenac · acemetacin · benzydamine · bromfenac · celecoxib · dexibuprofen · dexketoprofen · diclofenac · etodolac · etoricoxib · felbinac · fenoprofen · flurbiprofen · ibuprofen · indometacin · ketoprofen · ketorolac · mefenamic acid · meloxicam · nabumetone · naproxen · nepafenac · parecoxib · piroxicam · sulindac · tenoxicam · tiaprofenic acid · tolfenamic acid ·

ROUTE-SPECIFIC INFORMATION Since systemic absorption can follow topical application, the possibility of interactions should be borne in mind.

▶ **Celecoxib** is predicted to increase the exposure to antiarrhythmics (flecainide, propafenone). Monitor and adjust dose. Moderate Theoretical

▶ Antifungals, azoles (fluconazole) moderately increase the exposure to **celecoxib**. Adjust **celecoxib** dose, p. 1097. Moderate Study

▶ Antifungals, azoles (fluconazole) increase the exposure to **parecoxib**. Monitor and adjust dose. Moderate Study

▶ Antifungals, azoles (voriconazole) slightly increase the exposure to **diclofenac**. Monitor and adjust dose. Moderate Study

▶ Antifungals, azoles (voriconazole) moderately increase the exposure to **ibuprofen**. Adjust dose. Moderate Study

▶ **NSAIDs** are predicted to increase the risk of gastrointestinal irritation when given with bisphosphonates (alendronic acid, ibandronic acid). Moderate Study

▶ **NSAIDs** are predicted to increase the risk of renal impairment when given with bisphosphonates (sodium clodronate). Severe Theoretical

▶ **Ceritinib** is predicted to increase the exposure to NSAIDs (celecoxib, diclofenac). Adjust dose. Moderate Theoretical

▶ **Ciclosporin** increases the concentration of **diclofenac**. Severe Study → Also see TABLE 2 p. 1334 → Also see TABLE 16 p. 1338

▶ **Etoricoxib** slightly increases the exposure to combined hormonal contraceptives. Moderate Study

▶ **NSAIDs** increase the risk of gastrointestinal bleeding when given with corticosteroids. Severe Study

▶ **NSAIDs** increase the risk of renal impairment when given with daptomycin. Moderate Theoretical

▶ **Indometacin** increases the concentration of digoxin. Severe Study

▶ **Erlotinib** is predicted to increase the risk of gastrointestinal perforation when given with **NSAIDs**. Severe Theoretical

▶ **Etoricoxib** slightly increases the exposure to hormone replacement therapy. Moderate Study

▶ **NSAIDs** are predicted to increase the risk of gastrointestinal bleeding when given with iron chelators (deferasirox). Severe Theoretical

▶ **NSAIDs** increase the concentration of lithium. Monitor and adjust dose. Severe Study

▶ **NSAIDs** are predicted to increase the risk of toxicity when given with methotrexate. Monitor and adjust dose. Severe Study → Also see TABLE 2 p. 1334

▶ **NSAIDs** (high-dose) are predicted to decrease the efficacy of mifamurtide. Avoid. Severe Theoretical

▶ **Nicorandil** is predicted to increase the risk of gastrointestinal perforation when given with **NSAIDs**. Severe Theoretical

▶ **NSAIDs** are predicted to increase the exposure to pemetrexed. Use with caution or avoid. Severe Theoretical → Also see TABLE 2 p. 1334

▶ **NSAIDs** potentially increase the risk of seizures when given with quinolones. Severe Theoretical

▶ **Regorafenib** is predicted to increase the exposure to **mefenamic acid**. Avoid. Moderate Theoretical → Also see TABLE 4 p. 1334

▶ **Rifampicin** moderately decreases the exposure to NSAIDs (celecoxib, diclofenac, etoricoxib). Moderate Study

▶ **NSAIDs** increase the risk of acute renal failure when given with thiazide diuretics. Severe Theoretical → Also see TABLE 18 p. 1338

▶ **Zidovudine** increases the risk of haematological toxicity when given with **NSAIDs**. Severe Study → Also see TABLE 2 p. 1334

Obeticholic acid

▶ **Obeticholic acid** decreases the anticoagulant effect of coumarins (warfarin). Severe Study

▶ **Obeticholic acid** is predicted to increase the exposure to theophylline. Severe Theoretical

▶ **Obeticholic acid** is predicted to increase the exposure to tizanidine. Severe Theoretical

Obinutuzumab → see monoclonal antibodies

Ocrelizumab → see monoclonal antibodies

Octreotide

▶ **Octreotide** decreases the absorption of oral ciclosporin. Adjust ciclosporin dose, p. 818. Severe Anecdotal

A1

Interactions | Appendix 1

Octreotide (continued)
▶ **Octreotide** (short-acting) decreases the exposure to telotristat ethyl. Telotristat ethyl should be taken at least 30 minutes before **octreotide**. Moderate Study
Ofatumumab → see monoclonal antibodies
Ofloxacin → see quinolones
Olanzapine → see TABLE 8 p. 1335 (hypotension), TABLE 15 p. 1337 (myelosuppression), TABLE 11 p. 1336 (CNS depressant effects)

FOOD AND LIFESTYLE Dose adjustment might be necessary if smoking started or stopped during treatment.

▶ Antiepileptics (carbamazepine) potentially decrease the exposure to **olanzapine**. Monitor and adjust dose. Moderate Study
▶ Antiepileptics (phenytoin) are predicted to decrease the exposure to **olanzapine**. Monitor and adjust dose. Moderate Study
▶ **Olanzapine** is predicted to decrease the effects of dopamine receptor agonists. Avoid. Moderate Theoretical → Also see TABLE 8 p. 1335
▶ HIV-protease inhibitors (ritonavir) are predicted to decrease the exposure to **olanzapine**. Monitor and adjust dose. Moderate Study
▶ Leflunomide is predicted to decrease the exposure to **olanzapine**. Monitor and adjust dose. Moderate Study → Also see TABLE 15 p. 1337
▶ **Olanzapine** decreases the effects of levodopa. Avoid or monitor worsening parkinsonian symptoms. Severe Anecdotal → Also see TABLE 8 p. 1335
▶ Rifampicin is predicted to decrease the exposure to **olanzapine**. Monitor and adjust dose. Moderate Study
▶ SSRIs (fluvoxamine) moderately increase the exposure to **olanzapine**. Adjust dose. Severe Anecdotal
▶ Teriflunomide is predicted to decrease the exposure to **olanzapine**. Monitor and adjust dose. Moderate Study
Olaparib → see TABLE 15 p. 1337 (myelosuppression)

FOOD AND LIFESTYLE Bitter (Seville) orange is predicted to increase the exposure to olaparib.

▶ Antiarrhythmics (dronedarone) are predicted to increase the exposure to **olaparib**. Avoid moderate inhibitors of CYP3A4 or adjust **olaparib** dose, p. 973. Moderate Theoretical
▶ Antiepileptics (carbamazepine, fosphenytoin, phenobarbital, phenytoin, primidone) are predicted to decrease the exposure to **olaparib**. Avoid. Moderate Theoretical
▶ Antifungals, azoles (fluconazole, isavuconazole, posaconazole) are predicted to increase the exposure to **olaparib**. Avoid moderate inhibitors of CYP3A4 or adjust **olaparib** dose, p. 973. Moderate Theoretical
▶ Antifungals, azoles (itraconazole, ketoconazole, voriconazole) are predicted to increase the exposure to **olaparib**. Avoid potent inhibitors of CYP3A4 or adjust **olaparib** dose, p. 973. Moderate Study
▶ Aprepitant is predicted to increase the exposure to **olaparib**. Avoid moderate inhibitors of CYP3A4 or adjust **olaparib** dose, p. 973. Moderate Theoretical
▶ Bosentan is predicted to decrease the exposure to **olaparib**. Avoid. Moderate Theoretical
▶ Calcium channel blockers (diltiazem, verapamil) are predicted to increase the exposure to **olaparib**. Avoid moderate inhibitors of CYP3A4 or adjust **olaparib** dose, p. 973. Moderate Theoretical
▶ Cobicistat is predicted to increase the exposure to **olaparib**. Avoid potent inhibitors of CYP3A4 or adjust **olaparib** dose, p. 973. Moderate Study
▶ Crizotinib is predicted to increase the exposure to **olaparib**. Avoid moderate inhibitors of CYP3A4 or adjust **olaparib** dose, p. 973. Moderate Theoretical → Also see TABLE 15 p. 1337
▶ Efavirenz is predicted to decrease the exposure to **olaparib**. Avoid. Moderate Theoretical
▶ Enzalutamide is predicted to decrease the exposure to **olaparib**. Avoid. Moderate Theoretical
▶ Grapefruit juice is predicted to increase the exposure to **olaparib**. Avoid. Moderate Theoretical
▶ HIV-protease inhibitors are predicted to increase the exposure to **olaparib**. Avoid potent inhibitors of CYP3A4 or adjust **olaparib** dose, p. 973. Moderate Study

▶ Idelalisib is predicted to increase the exposure to **olaparib**. Avoid potent inhibitors of CYP3A4 or adjust **olaparib** dose, p. 973. Moderate Study → Also see TABLE 15 p. 1337
▶ Imatinib is predicted to increase the exposure to **olaparib**. Avoid moderate inhibitors of CYP3A4 or adjust **olaparib** dose, p. 973. Moderate Theoretical → Also see TABLE 15 p. 1337
▶ Macrolides (clarithromycin) are predicted to increase the exposure to **olaparib**. Avoid potent inhibitors of CYP3A4 or adjust **olaparib** dose, p. 973. Moderate Study
▶ Macrolides (erythromycin) are predicted to increase the exposure to **olaparib**. Avoid moderate inhibitors of CYP3A4 or adjust **olaparib** dose, p. 973. Moderate Theoretical
▶ Mitotane is predicted to decrease the exposure to **olaparib**. Avoid. Moderate Theoretical → Also see TABLE 15 p. 1337
▶ Netupitant is predicted to increase the exposure to **olaparib**. Avoid moderate inhibitors of CYP3A4 or adjust **olaparib** dose, p. 973. Moderate Theoretical
▶ Nevirapine is predicted to decrease the exposure to **olaparib**. Avoid. Moderate Theoretical
▶ Nilotinib is predicted to increase the exposure to **olaparib**. Avoid moderate inhibitors of CYP3A4 or adjust **olaparib** dose, p. 973. Moderate Theoretical → Also see TABLE 15 p. 1337
▶ Rifampicin is predicted to decrease the exposure to **olaparib**. Avoid. Moderate Theoretical
▶ St John's Wort is predicted to decrease the exposure to **olaparib**. Avoid. Moderate Theoretical
Olaratumab → see monoclonal antibodies
Olmesartan → see angiotensin-II receptor antagonists
Olodaterol → see beta₂ agonists
Olsalazine → see TABLE 15 p. 1337 (myelosuppression)
Ombitasvir
▶ Antiepileptics (carbamazepine) are predicted to decrease the exposure to **ombitasvir**. Avoid. Severe Theoretical
▶ Rifampicin is predicted to decrease the exposure to **ombitasvir**. Avoid. Severe Theoretical
▶ St John's Wort is predicted to decrease the exposure to **ombitasvir**. Avoid. Severe Theoretical
Omega-3-acid ethyl esters → see TABLE 3 p. 1334 (anticoagulant effects)
Omeprazole → see proton pump inhibitors
Ondansetron → see TABLE 13 p. 1337 (serotonin syndrome), TABLE 9 p. 1336 (QT-interval prolongation)
▶ Antiepileptics (carbamazepine, fosphenytoin, phenobarbital, phenytoin, primidone) are predicted to decrease the exposure to **ondansetron**. Moderate Study
▶ Dopamine receptor agonists (apomorphine) increase the risk of severe hypotension when given with **ondansetron**. Avoid. Severe Study → Also see TABLE 9 p. 1336
▶ Enzalutamide is predicted to decrease the exposure to **ondansetron**. Moderate Study
▶ Mitotane is predicted to decrease the exposure to **ondansetron**. Moderate Study
▶ Rifampicin is predicted to decrease the exposure to **ondansetron**. Moderate Study
Opicapone
▶ **Opicapone** increases the exposure to levodopa. Adjust dose. Moderate Study
▶ **Opicapone** is predicted to increase the exposure to loperamide. Avoid. Moderate Study
▶ **Opicapone** is predicted to increase the risk of elevated blood pressure when given with moclobemide. Avoid. Severe Theoretical
▶ **Opicapone** is predicted to increase the risk of elevated blood pressure when given with monoamine-oxidase A and B inhibitors, irreversible. Avoid. Severe Theoretical
▶ **Opicapone** is predicted to increase the exposure to montelukast. Avoid. Moderate Study
▶ **Opicapone** is predicted to increase the exposure to pioglitazone. Avoid. Moderate Study
▶ **Opicapone** is predicted to increase the exposure to repaglinide. Avoid. Moderate Study
▶ **Opicapone** is predicted to increase the risk of cardiovascular side-effects when given with sympathomimetics, inotropic. Severe Theoretical

‣ **Opicapone** is predicted to increase the risk of cardiovascular side-effects when given with sympathomimetics, vasoconstrictor (adrenaline/epinephrine, noradrenaline/norepinephrine). [Severe] Theoretical

Opioids → see TABLE 6 p. 1335 (bradycardia), TABLE 13 p. 1337 (serotonin syndrome), TABLE 9 p. 1336 (QT-interval prolongation), TABLE 11 p. 1336 (CNS depressant effects)

alfentanil · buprenorphine · codeine · diamorphine · dihydrocodeine · diphenoxylate · dipipanone · fentanyl · hydromorphone · meptazinol · methadone · morphine · oxycodone · papaveretum · pentazocine · pethidine · remifentanil · sufentanil · tapentadol · tramadol

‣ **Alcohol** (beverage) causes rapid release of opioids **(hydromorphone, morphine)** (from extended-release preparations). Avoid. [Severe] Study → Also see TABLE 11 p. 1336

‣ **Antiarrhythmics** (amiodarone) are predicted to increase the concentration of **fentanyl**. [Moderate] Theoretical → Also see TABLE 6 p. 1335

‣ **Antiarrhythmics** (dronedarone) are predicted to increase the exposure to opioids **(alfentanil, buprenorphine, fentanyl, oxycodone)**. Monitor and adjust dose. [Moderate] Study

‣ **Antiarrhythmics** (dronedarone) are predicted to increase the exposure to opioids **(methadone, sufentanil)**. [Moderate] Theoretical → Also see TABLE 9 p. 1336

‣ **Antiepileptics** (carbamazepine) decrease the concentration of **tramadol**. Adjust dose. [Severe] Study

‣ **Antiepileptics** (carbamazepine, fosphenytoin, phenobarbital, phenytoin, primidone) are predicted to decrease the exposure to **buprenorphine**. Monitor and adjust dose. [Moderate] Theoretical → Also see TABLE 11 p. 1336

‣ **Antiepileptics** (carbamazepine, fosphenytoin, phenobarbital, phenytoin, primidone) decrease the exposure to **methadone**. Monitor and adjust dose. [Severe] Study → Also see TABLE 11 p. 1336

‣ **Antiepileptics** (carbamazepine, fosphenytoin, phenobarbital, phenytoin, primidone) are predicted to decrease the exposure to **oxycodone**. Monitor and adjust dose. [Moderate] Study → Also see TABLE 11 p. 1336

‣ **Antiepileptics** (carbamazepine, fosphenytoin, phenobarbital, phenytoin, primidone) are predicted to decrease the exposure to opioids **(alfentanil, fentanyl)**. [Moderate] Study → Also see TABLE 11 p. 1336

‣ **Antifungals**, azoles (itraconazole, ketoconazole, voriconazole) are predicted to increase the exposure to **methadone**. Adjust dose. [Severe] Theoretical → Also see TABLE 9 p. 1336

‣ **Antifungals**, azoles (miconazole) are predicted to increase the exposure to **alfentanil**. Use with caution and adjust dose. [Moderate] Theoretical

‣ **Antifungals**, azoles (fluconazole, isavuconazole, posaconazole) are predicted to increase the exposure to opioids **(alfentanil, buprenorphine, fentanyl, oxycodone)**. Monitor and adjust dose. [Moderate] Study

‣ **Antifungals**, azoles (itraconazole, ketoconazole, voriconazole) are predicted to increase the exposure to opioids **(alfentanil, buprenorphine, fentanyl, oxycodone, sufentanil)**. Monitor and adjust dose. [Severe] Study

‣ **Antifungals**, azoles (fluconazole, isavuconazole, posaconazole) are predicted to increase the exposure to opioids **(methadone, sufentanil)**. [Moderate] Theoretical → Also see TABLE 9 p. 1336

‣ **Aprepitant** is predicted to increase the exposure to opioids **(alfentanil, buprenorphine, fentanyl, oxycodone)**. Monitor and adjust dose. [Moderate] Study

‣ **Aprepitant** is predicted to increase the exposure to opioids **(methadone, sufentanil)**. [Moderate] Theoretical

‣ **Bosentan** decreases the exposure to **methadone**. Monitor and adjust dose. [Severe] Study

‣ **Bupropion** is predicted to decrease the efficacy of **codeine**. [Moderate] Theoretical

‣ **Bupropion** is predicted to decrease the efficacy of **tramadol**. [Severe] Study → Also see TABLE 13 p. 1337

‣ **Calcium channel blockers** (diltiazem, verapamil) are predicted to increase the exposure to opioids **(alfentanil, buprenorphine, fentanyl, oxycodone)**. Monitor and adjust dose. [Moderate] Study → Also see TABLE 6 p. 1335

‣ **Calcium channel blockers** (diltiazem, verapamil) are predicted to increase the exposure to opioids **(methadone, sufentanil)**. [Moderate] Theoretical → Also see TABLE 6 p. 1335

‣ **Ceritinib** is predicted to increase the exposure to opioids **(alfentanil, fentanyl)**. Avoid. [Severe] Theoretical

‣ **Cinacalcet** is predicted to decrease the efficacy of **codeine**. [Moderate] Theoretical

‣ **Cinacalcet** is predicted to decrease the efficacy of **tramadol**. [Severe] Study

‣ **Cobicistat** is predicted to increase the exposure to opioids **(alfentanil, buprenorphine, fentanyl, oxycodone, sufentanil)**. Monitor and adjust dose. [Severe] Study

‣ **Crizotinib** is predicted to increase the exposure to opioids **(alfentanil, buprenorphine, fentanyl, oxycodone)**. Monitor and adjust dose. [Moderate] Study → Also see TABLE 6 p. 1335

‣ **Crizotinib** is predicted to increase the exposure to opioids **(methadone, sufentanil)**. [Moderate] Theoretical → Also see TABLE 6 p. 1335 → Also see TABLE 9 p. 1336

‣ **Efavirenz** decreases the exposure to **methadone**. Monitor and adjust dose. [Severe] Study → Also see TABLE 9 p. 1336

‣ **Enzalutamide** is predicted to decrease the exposure to **buprenorphine**. Monitor and adjust dose. [Moderate] Theoretical

‣ **Enzalutamide** decreases the exposure to **methadone**. Monitor and adjust dose. [Severe] Study

‣ **Enzalutamide** is predicted to decrease the exposure to opioids **(alfentanil, fentanyl)**. [Moderate] Study

‣ **Enzalutamide** is predicted to decrease the exposure to **oxycodone**. Monitor and adjust dose. [Moderate] Study

‣ **H_2 receptor antagonists** (cimetidine) increase the concentration of **alfentanil**. Use with caution and adjust dose. [Severe] Study

‣ **H_2 receptor antagonists** (cimetidine) increase the exposure to **fentanyl**. [Moderate] Study

‣ **HIV-protease inhibitors** (boosted with ritonavir) are predicted to decrease the exposure to **methadone**. [Moderate] Study → Also see TABLE 9 p. 1336

‣ **HIV-protease inhibitors** (ritonavir) are predicted to decrease the concentration of **morphine**. [Moderate] Theoretical

‣ **HIV-protease inhibitors** (ritonavir) increase the risk of CNS toxicity when given with **pethidine**. Avoid. [Severe] Study

‣ **HIV-protease inhibitors** are predicted to increase the exposure to opioids **(alfentanil, buprenorphine, fentanyl, oxycodone, sufentanil)**. Monitor and adjust dose. [Severe] Study

‣ **Idelalisib** is predicted to increase the exposure to **methadone**. [Severe] Theoretical

‣ **Idelalisib** is predicted to increase the exposure to opioids **(alfentanil, buprenorphine, fentanyl, oxycodone, sufentanil)**. Monitor and adjust dose. [Severe] Study

‣ **Imatinib** is predicted to increase the exposure to opioids **(alfentanil, buprenorphine, fentanyl, oxycodone)**. Monitor and adjust dose. [Moderate] Study

‣ **Imatinib** is predicted to increase the exposure to opioids **(methadone, sufentanil)**. [Moderate] Theoretical

‣ **Macrolides** (clarithromycin) are predicted to increase the concentration of **methadone**. [Severe] Theoretical → Also see TABLE 9 p. 1336

‣ **Macrolides** (erythromycin) are predicted to increase the exposure to opioids **(alfentanil, buprenorphine, fentanyl, oxycodone)**. Monitor and adjust dose. [Moderate] Study

‣ **Macrolides** (clarithromycin) are predicted to increase the exposure to opioids **(alfentanil, buprenorphine, fentanyl, oxycodone, sufentanil)**. Monitor and adjust dose. [Severe] Study

‣ **Macrolides** (erythromycin) are predicted to increase the exposure to opioids **(methadone, sufentanil)**. [Moderate] Theoretical → Also see TABLE 9 p. 1336

‣ **Mitotane** is predicted to decrease the exposure to **buprenorphine**. Monitor and adjust dose. [Moderate] Theoretical

‣ **Mitotane** decreases the exposure to **methadone**. Monitor and adjust dose. [Severe] Study

‣ **Mitotane** is predicted to decrease the exposure to opioids **(alfentanil, fentanyl)**. [Moderate] Study

‣ **Mitotane** is predicted to decrease the exposure to **oxycodone**. Monitor and adjust dose. [Moderate] Study

‣ **Opioids** are predicted to increase the risk of CNS excitation or depression when given with monoamine-oxidase A and B inhibitors, irreversible. Avoid. [Severe] Study → Also see TABLE 13 p. 1337

Opioids (continued)
- Monoamine-oxidase B inhibitors (rasagiline) are predicted to increase the risk of side-effects when given with **pethidine**. Avoid and for 14 days after stopping **rasagiline**. Severe Theoretical → Also see TABLE 13 p. 1337
- Monoamine-oxidase B inhibitors (safinamide) are predicted to increase the risk of side-effects when given with **pethidine**. Avoid and for 1 week after stopping **safinamide**. Severe Theoretical → Also see TABLE 13 p. 1337
- Monoamine-oxidase B inhibitors (selegiline) increase the risk of side-effects when given with **pethidine**. Avoid. Severe Anecdotal → Also see TABLE 13 p. 1337
- **Nalmefene** is predicted to decrease the efficacy of **opioids**. Avoid. Severe Theoretical
- Netupitant is predicted to increase the exposure to opioids **(alfentanil, buprenorphine, fentanyl, oxycodone)**. Monitor and adjust dose. Moderate Study
- Netupitant is predicted to increase the exposure to opioids **(methadone, sufentanil)**. Moderate Theoretical
- Nevirapine decreases the exposure to **methadone**. Monitor and adjust dose. Severe Study
- Nilotinib is predicted to increase the exposure to opioids **(alfentanil, buprenorphine, fentanyl, oxycodone)**. Monitor and adjust dose. Moderate Study
- Nilotinib is predicted to increase the exposure to opioids **(methadone, sufentanil)**. Moderate Theoretical → Also see TABLE 9 p. 1336
- Opioids **(buprenorphine)** are predicted to increase the risk of opiate withdrawal when given with opioids **(alfentanil)**. Severe Theoretical → Also see TABLE 11 p. 1336
- Opioids **(pentazocine)** are predicted to increase the risk of opiate withdrawal when given with opioids **(alfentanil, codeine, diamorphine, dihydrocodeine, dipipanone, fentanyl, hydromorphone, meptazinol, methadone, morphine, oxycodone, papaveretum)**. Severe Theoretical → Also see TABLE 13 p. 1337 → Also see TABLE 11 p. 1336
- Opioids **(buprenorphine)** are predicted to increase the risk of opiate withdrawal when given with opioids **(codeine, diamorphine, dihydrocodeine, dipipanone, fentanyl, hydromorphone, meptazinol, methadone, morphine, oxycodone, papaveretum, pentazocine, pethidine, remifentanil, sufentanil, tapentadol, tramadol)**. Severe Theoretical → Also see TABLE 11 p. 1336 → Also see TABLE 13 p. 1337
- Opioids **(pentazocine)** are predicted to increase the risk of opiate withdrawal when given with opioids **(pethidine, remifentanil, tapentadol, tramadol)**. Severe Theoretical → Also see TABLE 11 p. 1336 → Also see TABLE 13 p. 1337
- Opioids **(pentazocine)** are predicted to increase the risk of opiate withdrawal when given with opioids **(sufentanil)**. Severe Anecdotal → Also see TABLE 11 p. 1336
- Palbociclib is predicted to increase the exposure to opioids **(alfentanil, fentanyl)**. Adjust dose. Moderate Theoretical
- Pitolisant is predicted to decrease the exposure to **morphine**. Unknown Theoretical
- Ribociclib is predicted to increase the exposure to opioids **(alfentanil, fentanyl)**. Use with caution and adjust dose. Moderate Theoretical
- Rifampicin is predicted to decrease the exposure to **buprenorphine**. Monitor and adjust dose. Moderate Theoretical
- Rifampicin decreases the exposure to **methadone**. Monitor and adjust dose. Severe Study
- Rifampicin is predicted to decrease the exposure to opioids **(alfentanil, fentanyl)**. Moderate Study
- Rifampicin decreases the exposure to opioids **(codeine, morphine)**. Moderate Study
- Rifampicin is predicted to decrease the exposure to **oxycodone**. Monitor and adjust dose. Moderate Study
- SSRIs (fluoxetine, paroxetine) are predicted to decrease the efficacy of **codeine**. Moderate Theoretical
- SSRIs (fluoxetine, paroxetine) are predicted to decrease the efficacy of **tramadol**. Severe Study → Also see TABLE 13 p. 1337
- St John's Wort decreases the exposure to **methadone**. Monitor and adjust dose. Severe Study → Also see TABLE 13 p. 1337
- St John's Wort moderately decreases the exposure to **oxycodone**. Adjust dose. Moderate Study

- Terbinafine is predicted to decrease the efficacy of **codeine**. Moderate Theoretical
- Terbinafine is predicted to decrease the efficacy of **tramadol**. Severe Study

Orlistat

SEPARATION OF ADMINISTRATION Orlistat might affect the absorption of concurrently administered drugs—consider separating administration. Particular care should be taken with antiepileptics, antiretrovirals, and drugs that have a narrow therapeutic index.

Orphenadrine → see TABLE 10 p. 1336 (antimuscarinics)
Osimertinib → see TABLE 9 p. 1336 (QT-interval prolongation)
- Antiepileptics (carbamazepine, fosphenytoin, phenobarbital, phenytoin, primidone) are predicted to moderately decrease the exposure to **osimertinib**. Avoid. Moderate Study
- Bosentan is predicted to decrease the exposure to **osimertinib**. Moderate Theoretical
- Efavirenz is predicted to decrease the exposure to **osimertinib**. Moderate Theoretical → Also see TABLE 9 p. 1336
- Enzalutamide is predicted to moderately decrease the exposure to **osimertinib**. Avoid. Moderate Study
- Mitotane is predicted to moderately decrease the exposure to **osimertinib**. Avoid. Moderate Study
- Nevirapine is predicted to decrease the exposure to **osimertinib**. Severe Theoretical
- Rifampicin is predicted to moderately decrease the exposure to **osimertinib**. Moderate Study
- St John's Wort is predicted to decrease the exposure to **osimertinib**. Avoid. Moderate Theoretical
- **Osimertinib** slightly increases the exposure to statins (rosuvastatin). Moderate Study

Oxaliplatin → see platinum compounds
Oxazepam → see TABLE 11 p. 1336 (CNS depressant effects)
Oxcarbazepine → see antiepileptics
Oxprenolol → see beta blockers, non-selective
Oxybuprocaine → see anaesthetics, local
Oxybutynin → see TABLE 10 p. 1336 (antimuscarinics)
- Antiarrhythmics (dronedarone) are predicted to increase the exposure to **oxybutynin**. Mild Theoretical
- **Oxybutynin** potentially increases the risk of overheating and dehydration when given with antiepileptics (zonisamide). Avoid in children. Severe Theoretical
- Antifungals, azoles (fluconazole, isavuconazole, posaconazole) are predicted to increase the exposure to **oxybutynin**. Mild Theoretical
- Antifungals, azoles (itraconazole, ketoconazole, voriconazole) are predicted to increase the exposure to **oxybutynin**. Mild Study
- Aprepitant is predicted to increase the exposure to **oxybutynin**. Mild Theoretical
- Calcium channel blockers (diltiazem, verapamil) are predicted to increase the exposure to **oxybutynin**. Mild Theoretical
- Cobicistat is predicted to increase the exposure to **oxybutynin**. Mild Theoretical
- Crizotinib is predicted to increase the exposure to **oxybutynin**. Mild Theoretical
- HIV-protease inhibitors are predicted to increase the exposure to **oxybutynin**. Mild Study
- Idelalisib is predicted to increase the exposure to **oxybutynin**. Mild Study
- Imatinib is predicted to increase the exposure to **oxybutynin**. Mild Theoretical
- Macrolides (clarithromycin) are predicted to increase the exposure to **oxybutynin**. Mild Study
- Macrolides (erythromycin) are predicted to increase the exposure to **oxybutynin**. Mild Theoretical
- Netupitant is predicted to increase the exposure to **oxybutynin**. Mild Theoretical
- Nilotinib is predicted to increase the exposure to **oxybutynin**. Mild Theoretical

Oxycodone → see opioids
Oxymetholone
- **Oxymetholone** increases the anticoagulant effect of coumarins. Severe Anecdotal
- **Oxymetholone** increases the anticoagulant effect of phenindione. Severe Anecdotal

Oxytetracycline → see tetracyclines
Paclitaxel → see taxanes
Palbociclib

▶ Antiepileptics (carbamazepine, fosphenytoin, phenobarbital, phenytoin, primidone) are predicted to decrease the exposure to palbociclib. Avoid. Severe Study
▶ Antifungals, azoles (itraconazole, ketoconazole, voriconazole) are predicted to increase the exposure to palbociclib. Avoid or adjust **palbociclib** dose, p. 961. Severe Study
▶ Palbociclib is predicted to increase the exposure to ciclosporin. Adjust dose. Moderate Theoretical
▶ Cobicistat is predicted to increase the exposure to palbociclib. Avoid or adjust **palbociclib** dose, p. 961. Severe Study
▶ Enzalutamide is predicted to decrease the exposure to palbociclib. Avoid. Severe Study
▶ Palbociclib is predicted to increase the exposure to ergotamine. Adjust dose. Moderate Theoretical
▶ Palbociclib is predicted to increase the exposure to everolimus. Adjust dose. Moderate Theoretical
▶ Grapefruit juice is predicted to increase the exposure to palbociclib. Avoid. Severe Theoretical
▶ HIV-protease inhibitors are predicted to increase the exposure to palbociclib. Avoid or adjust **palbociclib** dose, p. 961. Severe Study
▶ Idelalisib is predicted to increase the exposure to palbociclib. Avoid or adjust **palbociclib** dose, p. 961. Severe Study
▶ Macrolides (clarithromycin) are predicted to increase the exposure to palbociclib. Avoid or adjust **palbociclib** dose, p. 961. Severe Study
▶ Palbociclib increases the exposure to midazolam. Moderate Study
▶ Mitotane is predicted to decrease the exposure to palbociclib. Avoid. Severe Study
▶ Palbociclib is predicted to increase the exposure to opioids (alfentanil, fentanyl). Adjust dose. Moderate Theoretical
▶ Palbociclib is predicted to increase the exposure to pimozide. Adjust dose. Moderate Theoretical
▶ Rifampicin is predicted to decrease the exposure to palbociclib. Avoid. Severe Study
▶ Palbociclib is predicted to increase the exposure to sirolimus. Adjust dose. Moderate Theoretical
▶ St John's Wort is predicted to decrease the exposure to palbociclib. Avoid. Severe Theoretical
▶ Palbociclib is predicted to increase the exposure to tacrolimus. Adjust dose. Moderate Theoretical
Paliperidone → see TABLE 8 p. 1335 (hypotension), TABLE 9 p. 1336 (QT-interval prolongation), TABLE 11 p. 1336 (CNS depressant effects)

▶ Antiepileptics (carbamazepine, fosphenytoin, phenobarbital, phenytoin, primidone) are predicted to decrease the exposure to paliperidone. Monitor and adjust dose. Severe Study → Also see TABLE 11 p. 1336
▶ Antiepileptics (valproate) slightly increase the exposure to paliperidone. Adjust dose. Moderate Study
▶ Paliperidone is predicted to decrease the effects of dopamine receptor agonists. Avoid. Moderate Theoretical → Also see TABLE 8 p. 1335 → Also see TABLE 9 p. 1336
▶ Enzalutamide is predicted to decrease the exposure to paliperidone. Monitor and adjust dose. Severe Study
▶ Paliperidone is predicted to decrease the effects of levodopa. Severe Theoretical → Also see TABLE 8 p. 1335
▶ Mitotane is predicted to decrease the exposure to paliperidone. Monitor and adjust dose. Severe Study
▶ Rifampicin is predicted to decrease the exposure to paliperidone. Monitor and adjust dose. Severe Study
▶ St John's Wort is predicted to decrease the exposure to paliperidone. Severe Theoretical
Palonosetron → see TABLE 13 p. 1337 (serotonin syndrome), TABLE 9 p. 1336 (QT-interval prolongation)

▶ Dopamine receptor agonists (apomorphine) are predicted to increase the risk of severe hypotension when given with palonosetron. Severe Theoretical
Pamidronate → see bisphosphonates
Pancreatin

▶ Pancreatin is predicted to decrease the effects of acarbose. Avoid. Moderate Theoretical

Pancuronium → see neuromuscular blocking drugs, non-depolarising
Panitumumab → see monoclonal antibodies
Panobinostat → see TABLE 15 p. 1337 (myelosuppression), TABLE 9 p. 1336 (QT-interval prolongation)

FOOD AND LIFESTYLE Avoid pomegranate, pomegranate juice, and star fruit as they are predicted to increase panobinostat exposure.

▶ Antiarrhythmics (amiodarone, dronedarone) are predicted to increase the exposure to panobinostat. Adjust dose. Moderate Theoretical → Also see TABLE 9 p. 1336
▶ Antiepileptics (carbamazepine, fosphenytoin, phenobarbital, phenytoin, primidone) are predicted to decrease the exposure to panobinostat. Avoid. Moderate Theoretical
▶ Antifungals, azoles (itraconazole, ketoconazole, voriconazole) are predicted to increase the exposure to panobinostat. Adjust panobinostat dose; in hepatic impairment avoid, p. 911. Moderate Study → Also see TABLE 9 p. 1336
▶ Antifungals, azoles (posaconazole) are predicted to increase the exposure to panobinostat. Adjust dose. Moderate Theoretical
▶ Panobinostat is predicted to increase the exposure to atomoxetine. Monitor and adjust dose. Severe Theoretical
▶ Panobinostat is predicted to increase the exposure to beta blockers, selective (metoprolol). Monitor and adjust dose. Moderate Theoretical
▶ Panobinostat is predicted to increase the exposure to beta blockers, selective (nebivolol). Monitor and adjust dose. Mild Theoretical
▶ Calcium channel blockers (verapamil) are predicted to increase the exposure to panobinostat. Adjust dose. Moderate Theoretical
▶ Ciclosporin is predicted to increase the exposure to panobinostat. Adjust dose. Moderate Theoretical
▶ Cobicistat is predicted to increase the exposure to panobinostat. Adjust panobinostat dose; in hepatic impairment avoid, p. 911. Moderate Study
▶ Enzalutamide is predicted to decrease the exposure to panobinostat. Avoid. Moderate Theoretical
▶ HIV-protease inhibitors are predicted to increase the exposure to panobinostat. Adjust panobinostat dose; in hepatic impairment avoid, p. 911. Moderate Study → Also see TABLE 9 p. 1336
▶ Idelalisib is predicted to increase the exposure to panobinostat. Adjust panobinostat dose; in hepatic impairment avoid, p. 911. Moderate Study → Also see TABLE 15 p. 1337
▶ Lapatinib is predicted to increase the exposure to panobinostat. Adjust dose. Moderate Theoretical → Also see TABLE 9 p. 1336
▶ Macrolides (azithromycin, erythromycin) are predicted to increase the exposure to panobinostat. Moderate Theoretical → Also see TABLE 9 p. 1336
▶ Macrolides (clarithromycin) are predicted to increase the exposure to panobinostat. Adjust panobinostat dose; in hepatic impairment avoid, p. 911. Moderate Study → Also see TABLE 9 p. 1336
▶ Mitotane is predicted to decrease the exposure to panobinostat. Avoid. Moderate Theoretical → Also see TABLE 15 p. 1337
▶ Panobinostat is predicted to increase the exposure to phenothiazines (perphenazine). Monitor and adjust dose. Severe Theoretical
▶ Panobinostat is predicted to increase the exposure to pimozide. Avoid. Severe Theoretical → Also see TABLE 9 p. 1336
▶ Ranolazine is predicted to increase the exposure to panobinostat. Adjust dose. Moderate Theoretical → Also see TABLE 9 p. 1336
▶ Rifampicin is predicted to decrease the exposure to panobinostat. Avoid. Moderate Theoretical
▶ St John's Wort is predicted to decrease the exposure to panobinostat. Avoid. Moderate Theoretical
▶ Vemurafenib is predicted to increase the exposure to panobinostat. Adjust dose. Moderate Theoretical → Also see TABLE 9 p. 1336

Pantoprazole → see proton pump inhibitors
Papaveretum → see opioids
Paracetamol → see TABLE 1 p. 1334 (hepatotoxicity)

A1

Interactions | Appendix 1

Paracetamol (continued)

▸ Alcohol (beverage) (in those who drink heavily) causes severe liver damage when given with **paracetamol**. Severe Study → Also see TABLE 1 p. 1334

▸ **Paracetamol** is predicted to decrease the clearance of alkylating agents (busulfan). Moderate Theoretical

▸ **Paracetamol** is predicted to increase the risk of methaemoglobinaemia when given with topical anaesthetics, local (prilocaine). Use with caution or avoid. Severe Theoretical

▸ Antiepileptics (carbamazepine, fosphenytoin, phenobarbital, phenytoin, primidone) decrease the exposure to **paracetamol**. Moderate Study → Also see TABLE 1 p. 1334

▸ **Paracetamol** increases the anticoagulant effect of coumarins. Moderate Study

▸ **Paracetamol** is predicted to increase the risk of methaemoglobinaemia when given with dapsone. Severe Theoretical

▸ Imatinib increases the risk of hepatotoxicity when given with **paracetamol**. Severe Anecdotal

▸ **Paracetamol** is predicted to increase the anticoagulant effect of phenindione. Severe Theoretical

▸ Pitolisant is predicted to decrease the exposure to **paracetamol**. Unknown Theoretical

▸ Rifampicin decreases the exposure to **paracetamol**. Moderate Study

Paraldehyde → see antiepileptics

Parathyroid hormone

▸ Bisphosphonates are predicted to decrease the effects of parathyroid hormone. Avoid. Moderate Study

Parecoxib → see NSAIDs

Paricalcitol → see vitamin D substances

Paritaprevir

▸ Antiepileptics (carbamazepine, fosphenytoin, phenobarbital, phenytoin, primidone) are predicted to decrease the exposure to **paritaprevir** (with ritonavir and ombitasvir). Avoid. Severe Study

▸ Antifungals, azoles (itraconazole, ketoconazole, voriconazole) are predicted to increase the exposure to **paritaprevir** (with ritonavir and ombitasvir). Avoid. Severe Theoretical

▸ Antifungals, azoles (posaconazole) are predicted to increase the exposure to **paritaprevir** (with ritonavir and ombitasvir) and **paritaprevir** (with ritonavir and ombitasvir) is predicted to increase the exposure to antifungals, azoles (posaconazole). Avoid. Severe Theoretical

▸ Bosentan is predicted to decrease the exposure to **paritaprevir** (with ritonavir and ombitasvir). Avoid. Severe Study

▸ Cobicistat is predicted to increase the exposure to **paritaprevir** (with ritonavir and ombitasvir). Avoid. Severe Theoretical

▸ **Paritaprevir** (with ritonavir and ombitasvir) increases the risk of raised liver function tests when given with combined hormonal contraceptives. Avoid. Severe Study

▸ Efavirenz is predicted to decrease the exposure to **paritaprevir** (with ritonavir and ombitasvir). Avoid. Severe Study

▸ Enzalutamide is predicted to decrease the exposure to **paritaprevir** (with ritonavir and ombitasvir). Avoid. Severe Study

▸ HIV-protease inhibitors are predicted to increase the exposure to **paritaprevir** (with ritonavir and ombitasvir). Avoid. Severe Theoretical

▸ Idelalisib is predicted to increase the exposure to **paritaprevir** (with ritonavir and ombitasvir). Avoid. Severe Theoretical

▸ **Paritaprevir** (with ritonavir and ombitasvir) is predicted to increase the exposure to loop diuretics (furosemide). Adjust dose. Moderate Theoretical

▸ Macrolides (clarithromycin) are predicted to increase the exposure to **paritaprevir** (with ritonavir and ombitasvir). Avoid. Severe Theoretical

▸ Mitotane is predicted to decrease the exposure to **paritaprevir** (with ritonavir and ombitasvir). Avoid. Severe Study

▸ Nevirapine is predicted to decrease the exposure to **paritaprevir** (with ritonavir and ombitasvir). Avoid. Severe Study

▸ Rifampicin is predicted to decrease the exposure to **paritaprevir** (with ritonavir and ombitasvir). Avoid. Severe Study

▸ St John's Wort is predicted to decrease the exposure to **paritaprevir** (with ritonavir and ombitasvir). Avoid. Severe Study

▸ **Paritaprevir** (with ritonavir and ombitasvir) is predicted to increase the exposure to statins (fluvastatin). Avoid. Moderate Theoretical

▸ **Paritaprevir** (with ritonavir and ombitasvir) increases the exposure to statins (pravastatin). Adjust **pravastatin** dose. Moderate Study

▸ **Paritaprevir** (with ritonavir and ombitasvir) increases the exposure to statins (rosuvastatin). Adjust **rosuvastatin** dose, p. 202. Moderate Study

Paroxetine → see SSRIs

Pasireotide → see TABLE 6 p. 1335 (bradycardia), TABLE 9 p. 1336 (QT-interval prolongation)

▸ Pasireotide is predicted to decrease the absorption of oral ciclosporin. Adjust dose. Severe Theoretical

Patiromer

> SEPARATION OF ADMINISTRATION Manufacturer advises take 3 hours before, or after, other drugs.

Pazopanib → see TABLE 15 p. 1337 (myelosuppression), TABLE 9 p. 1336 (QT-interval prolongation)

▸ Antacids are predicted to decrease the absorption of **pazopanib**. **Pazopanib** should be taken 1 hour before or 2 hours after **antacids**. Moderate Theoretical

▸ Antiarrhythmics (dronedarone) are predicted to increase the exposure to **pazopanib**. Moderate Theoretical → Also see TABLE 9 p. 1336

▸ Antiepileptics (carbamazepine, fosphenytoin, phenobarbital, phenytoin, primidone) are predicted to decrease the exposure to **pazopanib**. Avoid. Severe Theoretical

▸ Antifungals, azoles (fluconazole, isavuconazole, posaconazole) are predicted to increase the exposure to **pazopanib**. Moderate Theoretical → Also see TABLE 9 p. 1336

▸ Antifungals, azoles (itraconazole, ketoconazole, voriconazole) are predicted to increase the exposure to **pazopanib**. Avoid or adjust **pazopanib** dose, p. 962. Moderate Study → Also see TABLE 9 p. 1336

▸ Aprepitant is predicted to increase the exposure to **pazopanib**. Moderate Theoretical

▸ Calcium channel blockers (diltiazem, verapamil) are predicted to increase the exposure to **pazopanib**. Moderate Theoretical

▸ Cobicistat is predicted to increase the exposure to **pazopanib**. Avoid or adjust **pazopanib** dose, p. 962. Moderate Study

▸ **Pazopanib** is predicted to increase the risk of bleeding events when given with coumarins. Severe Theoretical

▸ Crizotinib is predicted to increase the exposure to **pazopanib**. Moderate Theoretical → Also see TABLE 15 p. 1337 → Also see TABLE 9 p. 1336

▸ Enzalutamide is predicted to decrease the exposure to **pazopanib**. Avoid. Severe Theoretical

▸ Grapefruit juice is predicted to increase the exposure to **pazopanib**. Moderate Theoretical

▸ H_2 receptor antagonists are predicted to decrease the exposure to **pazopanib**. H_2 receptor antagonists should be taken 10 hours before or 2 hours after **pazopanib**. Moderate Theoretical

▸ HIV-protease inhibitors are predicted to increase the exposure to **pazopanib**. Avoid or adjust **pazopanib** dose, p. 962. Moderate Study → Also see TABLE 9 p. 1336

▸ Idelalisib is predicted to increase the exposure to **pazopanib**. Avoid or adjust **pazopanib** dose, p. 962. Moderate Study → Also see TABLE 15 p. 1337

▸ Imatinib is predicted to increase the exposure to **pazopanib**. Moderate Theoretical → Also see TABLE 15 p. 1337

▸ **Pazopanib** is predicted to increase the exposure to lomitapide. Separate administration by 12 hours. Moderate Theoretical

▸ Macrolides (clarithromycin) are predicted to increase the exposure to **pazopanib**. Avoid or adjust **pazopanib** dose, p. 962. Moderate Study → Also see TABLE 9 p. 1336

▸ Macrolides (erythromycin) are predicted to increase the exposure to **pazopanib**. Moderate Theoretical → Also see TABLE 9 p. 1336

▸ Mitotane is predicted to decrease the exposure to **pazopanib**. Avoid. Severe Theoretical → Also see TABLE 15 p. 1337

- Netupitant is predicted to increase the exposure to **pazopanib**. Moderate Theoretical
- Nilotinib is predicted to increase the exposure to **pazopanib**. Moderate Theoretical → Also see TABLE 15 p. 1337 → Also see TABLE 9 p. 1336
- **Pazopanib** is predicted to increase the risk of bleeding events when given with phenindione. Severe Theoretical
- Proton pump inhibitors are predicted to decrease the exposure to **pazopanib**. Avoid or administer concurrently without food. Moderate Study
- Rifampicin is predicted to decrease the exposure to **pazopanib**. Avoid. Severe Theoretical

Pegaspargase → see TABLE 1 p. 1334 (hepatotoxicity), TABLE 15 p. 1337 (myelosuppression)

- **Pegaspargase** is predicted to increase the risk of hepatotoxicity when given with imatinib. Severe Theoretical → Also see TABLE 15 p. 1337
- **Pegaspargase** affects the efficacy of methotrexate. Severe Anecdotal → Also see TABLE 1 p. 1334 → Also see TABLE 15 p. 1337
- **Pegaspargase** potentially increases the risk of neurotoxicity when given with vinca alkaloids (vincristine). Vincristine should be taken 3 to 24 hours before **pegaspargase**. Severe Anecdotal → Also see TABLE 1 p. 1334 → Also see TABLE 15 p. 1337

Peginterferon alfa → see interferons

Peginterferon beta-1a → see TABLE 15 p. 1337 (myelosuppression)

Pembrolizumab → see monoclonal antibodies

Pemetrexed → see TABLE 15 p. 1337 (myelosuppression), TABLE 2 p. 1334 (nephrotoxicity)

- Antimalarials (pyrimethamine) are predicted to increase the risk of side-effects when given with **pemetrexed**. Severe Theoretical → Also see TABLE 15 p. 1337
- Aspirin (high-dose) potentially increases the exposure to **pemetrexed**. Use with caution or avoid. Severe Theoretical
- Live vaccines are predicted to increase the risk of generalised infection (possibly life-threatening) when given with **pemetrexed**. Public Health England advises avoid (refer to Green Book). Severe Theoretical
- NSAIDs are predicted to increase the exposure to **pemetrexed**. Use with caution or avoid. Severe Theoretical → Also see TABLE 2 p. 1334

Penicillamine → see TABLE 2 p. 1334 (nephrotoxicity)

- Antacids decrease the absorption of **penicillamine**. Separate administration by 2 hours. Mild Study
- Antimalarials (chloroquine) are predicted to increase the risk of haematological toxicity when given with **penicillamine**. Avoid. Severe Theoretical
- **Penicillamine** potentially decreases the concentration of digoxin. Separate administration by 2 hours. Severe Anecdotal
- Hydroxychloroquine is predicted to increase the risk of haematological toxicity when given with **penicillamine**. Avoid. Severe Theoretical
- Iron (oral) is predicted to decrease the absorption of **penicillamine**. Separate administration by at least 2 hours. Mild Study
- Sodium aurothiomalate potentially increases the risk of side-effects when given with **penicillamine** (in those who have had previous adverse reactions to gold). Avoid. Severe Study
- Zinc is predicted to decrease the absorption of **penicillamine**. Mild Theoretical

Penicillins → see TABLE 1 p. 1334 (hepatotoxicity)

amoxicillin · ampicillin · benzylpenicillin · flucloxacillin · phenoxymethylpenicillin · piperacillin · pivmecillinam · temocillin · ticarcillin

- Allopurinol increases the risk of skin rash when given with penicillins **(amoxicillin, ampicillin)**. Moderate Study
- Antiepileptics (valproate) increase the risk of side-effects when given with **pivmecillinam**. Avoid. Severe Anecdotal
- **Penicillins** potentially alter the anticoagulant effect of coumarins. Monitor INR and adjust dose. Severe Anecdotal
- **Penicillins** are predicted to increase the risk of toxicity when given with methotrexate. Severe Theoretical → Also see TABLE 1 p. 1334
- **Piperacillin** increases the effects of neuromuscular blocking drugs, non-depolarising. Moderate Study

- **Penicillins** are predicted to increase the risk of bleeding events when given with phenindione. Severe Theoretical
- **Piperacillin** increases the effects of suxamethonium. Moderate Study

Pentamidine → see TABLE 15 p. 1337 (myelosuppression), TABLE 2 p. 1334 (nephrotoxicity), TABLE 9 p. 1336 (QT-interval prolongation)

- Didanosine is predicted to increase the risk of pancreatitis when given with **pentamidine**. Avoid. Severe Study
- Intravenous **pentamidine** potentially increases the risk of QT-prolongation when given with drugs that prolong the QT interval. Severe Anecdotal
- Foscarnet increases the risk of hypocalcaemia when given with **pentamidine**. Severe Anecdotal → Also see TABLE 2 p. 1334

Pentazocine → see opioids

Pentostatin → see TABLE 15 p. 1337 (myelosuppression), TABLE 5 p. 1334 (thromboembolism)

- Alkylating agents (cyclophosphamide) (high-dose) increase the risk of toxicity when given with **pentostatin**. Avoid. Severe Anecdotal → Also see TABLE 15 p. 1337 → Also see TABLE 5 p. 1334
- Fludarabine increases the risk of pulmonary toxicity when given with **pentostatin**. Avoid. Severe Study → Also see TABLE 15 p. 1337

Pentoxifylline

- **Pentoxifylline** is predicted to increase the concentration of aminophylline. Use with caution or avoid. Severe Theoretical
- Quinolones (ciprofloxacin) very slightly increase the exposure to **pentoxifylline**. Moderate Study
- SSRIs (fluvoxamine) are predicted to increase the exposure to **pentoxifylline**. Moderate Theoretical
- **Pentoxifylline** increases the concentration of theophylline. Monitor and adjust dose. Severe Study

Peppermint oil

- **Peppermint oil** is predicted to increase the exposure to lomitapide. Separate administration by 12 hours. Moderate Theoretical

Perampanel → see antiepileptics

Pergolide → see dopamine receptor agonists

Pericyazine → see phenothiazines

Perindopril → see ACE inhibitors

Perphenazine → see phenothiazines

Pertuzumab → see monoclonal antibodies

Pethidine → see opioids

Phenelzine → see monoamine-oxidase A and B inhibitors, irreversible

Phenindione → see TABLE 3 p. 1334 (anticoagulant effects)

FOOD AND LIFESTYLE　The effects of phenindione can be reduced or abolished by vitamin K, including that found in health foods, food supplements, enteral feeds, or large amounts of some green vegetables or green tea. Major changes in diet (especially involving salads and vegetables) and in alcohol consumption can affect anticoagulant control.

- Antiarrhythmics (propafenone) are predicted to increase the anticoagulant effect of **phenindione**. Monitor and adjust dose. Moderate Theoretical
- Antifungals, azoles (miconazole) greatly increase the anticoagulant effect of **phenindione**. Severe Theoretical
- Axitinib is predicted to increase the risk of bleeding events when given with **phenindione**. Severe Theoretical
- Bosutinib is predicted to increase the risk of bleeding events when given with **phenindione**. Severe Theoretical
- Cabozantinib is predicted to increase the risk of bleeding events when given with **phenindione**. Severe Theoretical
- Cephalosporins (ceftriaxone) potentially increase the risk of bleeding events when given with **phenindione**. Severe Anecdotal
- Corticosteroids are predicted to increase the effects of **phenindione**. Moderate Anecdotal
- Crizotinib is predicted to increase the risk of bleeding events when given with **phenindione**. Severe Theoretical
- Dasatinib is predicted to increase the risk of bleeding events when given with **phenindione**. Severe Theoretical
- Disulfiram is predicted to increase the anticoagulant effect of **phenindione**. Severe Theoretical
- Enteral feeds (vitamin-K containing) potentially decrease the effects of **phenindione**. Severe Theoretical
- Erlotinib is predicted to increase the risk of bleeding events when given with **phenindione**. Severe Theoretical

A1

Interactions | Appendix 1

Phenindione (continued)

▸ **Fibrates** are predicted to increase the anticoagulant effect of **phenindione**. Monitor INR and adjust dose. Severe Study

▸ **Gefitinib** is predicted to increase the risk of bleeding events when given with **phenindione**. Severe Theoretical

▸ H₂ receptor antagonists (cimetidine) increase the exposure to **phenindione**. Severe Anecdotal

▸ **Imatinib** is predicted to increase the risk of bleeding events when given with **phenindione**. Severe Theoretical

▸ **Lapatinib** is predicted to increase the risk of bleeding events when given with **phenindione**. Severe Theoretical

▸ **Nandrolone** is predicted to increase the anticoagulant effect of **phenindione**. Monitor and adjust dose. Severe Theoretical

▸ **Nilotinib** is predicted to increase the risk of bleeding events when given with **phenindione**. Severe Theoretical

▸ **Oxymetholone** increases the anticoagulant effect of **phenindione**. Severe Anecdotal

▸ **Paracetamol** is predicted to increase the anticoagulant effect of **phenindione**. Severe Theoretical

▸ **Pazopanib** is predicted to increase the risk of bleeding events when given with **phenindione**. Severe Theoretical

▸ **Penicillins** are predicted to increase the risk of bleeding events when given with **phenindione**. Severe Theoretical

▸ **Ponatinib** is predicted to increase the risk of bleeding events when given with **phenindione**. Severe Theoretical

▸ **Ranibizumab** is predicted to increase the risk of bleeding events when given with **phenindione**. Severe Theoretical

▸ **Regorafenib** is predicted to increase the risk of bleeding events when given with **phenindione**. Severe Theoretical

▸ **Ruxolitinib** is predicted to increase the risk of bleeding events when given with **phenindione**. Severe Theoretical

▸ **Sorafenib** is predicted to increase the risk of bleeding events when given with **phenindione**. Severe Theoretical

▸ **Statins** (rosuvastatin) are predicted to increase the anticoagulant effect of **phenindione**. Monitor INR and adjust dose. Severe Theoretical

▸ **Sunitinib** is predicted to increase the risk of bleeding events when given with **phenindione**. Severe Theoretical

▸ **Vandetanib** is predicted to increase the risk of bleeding events when given with **phenindione**. Severe Theoretical

Phenobarbital → see antiepileptics

Phenothiazines → see TABLE 8 p. 1335 (hypotension), TABLE 9 p. 1336 (QT-interval prolongation), TABLE 11 p. 1336 (CNS depressant effects), TABLE 10 p. 1336 (antimuscarinics)

chlorpromazine · fluphenazine · levomepromazine · pericyazine · perphenazine · prochlorperazine · promazine · trifluoperazine

▸ **Chlorpromazine** dose adjustment might be necessary if smoking started or stopped during treatment.

▸ **Fluphenazine** dose adjustment might be necessary if smoking started or stopped during treatment.

▸ **Amfetamines** are predicted to decrease the effects of **chlorpromazine**. Moderate Study

▸ **Phenothiazines** are predicted to decrease the effects of amfetamines. Moderate Study

▸ **Antacids** decrease the absorption of **phenothiazines**. Moderate Anecdotal

▸ **Chlorpromazine** decreases the concentration of antiepileptics (phenobarbital, primidone) and antiepileptics (phenobarbital, primidone) decrease the concentration of **chlorpromazine**. Moderate Study → Also see TABLE 11 p. 1336

▸ **Chlorpromazine** is predicted to increase the risk of hyponatraemia when given with desmopressin. Severe Theoretical

▸ **Phenothiazines** are predicted to decrease the effects of dopamine receptor agonists. Avoid. Moderate Theoretical → Also see TABLE 8 p. 1335 → Also see TABLE 9 p. 1336 → Also see TABLE 10 p. 1336

▸ **Eliglustat** is predicted to increase the exposure to perphenazine. Adjust dose. Moderate Theoretical

▸ **Phenothiazines** are predicted to decrease the antihypertensive effects of guanethidine. Moderate Theoretical → Also see TABLE 8 p. 1335

▸ **Phenothiazines** decrease the effects of levodopa. Avoid or monitor worsening parkinsonian symptoms. Severe Study → Also see TABLE 8 p. 1335

▸ **Phenothiazines** potentially increase the risk of neurotoxicity when given with lithium. Severe Anecdotal → Also see TABLE 9 p. 1336

▸ **Chlorpromazine** decreases the effects of metyrapone. Avoid. Moderate Theoretical

▸ **Moclobemide** increases the risk of side-effects when given with **levomepromazine**. Moderate Study

▸ **Monoamine-oxidase A and B inhibitors, irreversible** are predicted to increase the risk of neuroleptic malignant syndrome when given with **phenothiazines**. Severe Theoretical → Also see TABLE 8 p. 1335

▸ **Panobinostat** is predicted to increase the exposure to perphenazine. Monitor and adjust dose. Severe Theoretical

▸ SSRIs (paroxetine) markedly increase the exposure to perphenazine. Severe Study

Phenoxymethylpenicillin → see penicillins

Phenylephrine → see sympathomimetics, vasoconstrictor

Phenytoin → see antiepileptics

Pholcodine

▸ **Pholcodine** is predicted to increase the risk of CNS excitation or depression when given with monoamine-oxidase A and B inhibitors, irreversible. Avoid and for 14 days after stopping the MAOI. Severe Theoretical

Phosphodiesterase type-5 inhibitors → see TABLE 8 p. 1335 (hypotension), TABLE 9 p. 1336 (QT-interval prolongation)

avanafil · sildenafil · tadalafil · vardenafil

▸ **Alpha blockers** cause significant hypotensive effects when given with **phosphodiesterase type-5 inhibitors**. Patient should be stabilised on first drug then second drug should be added at the lowest recommended dose. Severe Study → Also see TABLE 8 p. 1335

▸ **Antiarrhythmics** (dronedarone) are predicted to increase the exposure to **avanafil**. Adjust **avanafil** dose, p. 794. Moderate Theoretical

▸ **Antiarrhythmics** (dronedarone) are predicted to increase the exposure to **sildenafil**. Monitor or adjust **sildenafil** dose with moderate inhibitors of CYP3A4, p. 794. Moderate Study → Also see TABLE 9 p. 1336

▸ **Antiarrhythmics** (dronedarone) are predicted to increase the exposure to **tadalafil**. Severe Theoretical

▸ **Antiarrhythmics** (dronedarone) are predicted to increase the exposure to **vardenafil**. Adjust dose. Severe Theoretical → Also see TABLE 9 p. 1336

▸ **Antiepileptics** (carbamazepine, fosphenytoin, phenobarbital, phenytoin, primidone) are predicted to decrease the exposure to phosphodiesterase type-5 inhibitors (**avanafil, tadalafil**). Avoid. Severe Study

▸ **Antiepileptics** (carbamazepine, fosphenytoin, phenobarbital, phenytoin, primidone) are predicted to decrease the exposure to phosphodiesterase type-5 inhibitors (**sildenafil, vardenafil**). Moderate Theoretical

▸ **Antifungals, azoles** (fluconazole, isavuconazole, posaconazole) are predicted to increase the exposure to **avanafil**. Adjust **avanafil** dose, p. 794. Moderate Theoretical

▸ **Antifungals, azoles** (fluconazole, isavuconazole, posaconazole) are predicted to increase the exposure to **sildenafil**. Monitor or adjust **sildenafil** dose with moderate inhibitors of CYP3A4, p. 794. Moderate Study → Also see TABLE 9 p. 1336

▸ **Antifungals, azoles** (fluconazole, isavuconazole, posaconazole) are predicted to increase the exposure to **tadalafil**. Severe Theoretical

▸ **Antifungals, azoles** (fluconazole, isavuconazole, posaconazole) are predicted to increase the exposure to **vardenafil**. Adjust dose. Severe Theoretical → Also see TABLE 9 p. 1336

▸ **Antifungals, azoles** (itraconazole, ketoconazole, voriconazole) are predicted to increase the exposure to **sildenafil**. Avoid potent inhibitors of CYP3A4 or adjust **sildenafil** dose, p. 794. Severe Study → Also see TABLE 9 p. 1336

▸ **Antifungals, azoles** (itraconazole, ketoconazole, voriconazole) are predicted to increase the exposure to **tadalafil**. Use with caution or avoid. Severe Study

▸ Antifungals, azoles (**miconazole**) are predicted to increase the exposure to **sildenafil**. Use with caution and adjust dose. Severe Theoretical

▸ Antifungals, azoles (**itraconazole, ketoconazole, voriconazole**) are predicted to increase the exposure to phosphodiesterase type-5 inhibitors (**avanafil, vardenafil**). Avoid. Severe Study → Also see **TABLE 9** p. 1336

▸ Aprepitant is predicted to increase the exposure to **avanafil**. Adjust **avanafil** dose, p. 794. Moderate Theoretical

▸ Aprepitant is predicted to increase the exposure to **sildenafil**. Monitor or adjust **sildenafil** dose with moderate inhibitors of CYP3A4, p. 794. Moderate Study

▸ Aprepitant is predicted to increase the exposure to **tadalafil**. Severe Theoretical

▸ Aprepitant is predicted to increase the exposure to **vardenafil**. Adjust dose. Severe Theoretical

▸ Bosentan decreases the exposure to **phosphodiesterase type-5 inhibitors**. Moderate Study

▸ Calcium channel blockers (**diltiazem, verapamil**) are predicted to increase the exposure to **avanafil**. Adjust **avanafil** dose, p. 794. Moderate Theoretical → Also see **TABLE 8** p. 1335

▸ Calcium channel blockers (**diltiazem, verapamil**) are predicted to increase the exposure to **sildenafil**. Monitor or adjust **sildenafil** dose with moderate inhibitors of CYP3A4, p. 794. Moderate Study → Also see **TABLE 8** p. 1335

▸ Calcium channel blockers (**diltiazem, verapamil**) are predicted to increase the exposure to **tadalafil**. Severe Theoretical → Also see **TABLE 8** p. 1335

▸ Calcium channel blockers (**diltiazem, verapamil**) are predicted to increase the exposure to **vardenafil**. Adjust dose. Severe Theoretical → Also see **TABLE 8** p. 1335

▸ Cobicistat is predicted to increase the exposure to phosphodiesterase type-5 inhibitors (**avanafil, vardenafil**). Avoid. Severe Study

▸ Cobicistat is predicted to increase the exposure to **sildenafil**. Avoid potent inhibitors of CYP3A4 or adjust **sildenafil** dose, p. 794. Severe Study

▸ Cobicistat is predicted to increase the exposure to **tadalafil**. Use with caution or avoid. Severe Study

▸ Crizotinib is predicted to increase the exposure to **avanafil**. Adjust **avanafil** dose, p. 794. Moderate Theoretical

▸ Crizotinib is predicted to increase the exposure to **sildenafil**. Monitor or adjust **sildenafil** dose with moderate inhibitors of CYP3A4, p. 794. Moderate Study → Also see **TABLE 9** p. 1336

▸ Crizotinib is predicted to increase the exposure to **tadalafil**. Severe Theoretical

▸ Crizotinib is predicted to increase the exposure to **vardenafil**. Adjust dose. Severe Theoretical → Also see **TABLE 9** p. 1336

▸ Efavirenz is predicted to increase the exposure to **phosphodiesterase type-5 inhibitors**. Moderate Theoretical → Also see **TABLE 9** p. 1336

▸ Enzalutamide is predicted to decrease the exposure to phosphodiesterase type-5 inhibitors (**avanafil, tadalafil**). Avoid. Severe Study

▸ Enzalutamide is predicted to decrease the exposure to phosphodiesterase type-5 inhibitors (**sildenafil, vardenafil**). Moderate Theoretical

▸ Etravirine moderately decreases the exposure to **phosphodiesterase type-5 inhibitors**. Adjust dose. Moderate Study

▸ Grapefruit juice is predicted to increase the exposure to **phosphodiesterase type-5 inhibitors**. Use with caution or avoid. Moderate Study

▸ HIV-protease inhibitors are predicted to increase the exposure to phosphodiesterase type-5 inhibitors (**avanafil, vardenafil**). Avoid. Severe Study → Also see **TABLE 9** p. 1336

▸ HIV-protease inhibitors are predicted to increase the exposure to **sildenafil**. Avoid potent inhibitors of CYP3A4 or adjust **sildenafil** dose, p. 794. Severe Study → Also see **TABLE 9** p. 1336

▸ HIV-protease inhibitors are predicted to increase the exposure to **tadalafil**. Use with caution or avoid. Severe Study

▸ Idelalisib is predicted to increase the exposure to phosphodiesterase type-5 inhibitors (**avanafil, vardenafil**). Avoid. Severe Study

▸ Idelalisib is predicted to increase the exposure to **sildenafil**. Avoid potent inhibitors of CYP3A4 or adjust **sildenafil** dose, p. 794. Severe Study

▸ Idelalisib is predicted to increase the exposure to **tadalafil**. Use with caution or avoid. Severe Study

▸ Imatinib is predicted to increase the exposure to **avanafil**. Adjust **avanafil** dose, p. 794. Moderate Theoretical

▸ Imatinib is predicted to increase the exposure to **sildenafil**. Monitor or adjust **sildenafil** dose with moderate inhibitors of CYP3A4, p. 794. Moderate Study

▸ Imatinib is predicted to increase the exposure to **tadalafil**. Severe Theoretical

▸ Imatinib is predicted to increase the exposure to **vardenafil**. Adjust dose. Severe Theoretical

▸ Macrolides (**clarithromycin**) are predicted to increase the exposure to **sildenafil**. Avoid potent inhibitors of CYP3A4 or adjust **sildenafil** dose, p. 794. Severe Study → Also see **TABLE 9** p. 1336

▸ Macrolides (**clarithromycin**) are predicted to increase the exposure to **tadalafil**. Use with caution or avoid. Severe Study

▸ Macrolides (**erythromycin**) are predicted to increase the exposure to **avanafil**. Adjust **avanafil** dose, p. 794. Moderate Theoretical

▸ Macrolides (**erythromycin**) are predicted to increase the exposure to **sildenafil**. Monitor or adjust **sildenafil** dose with moderate inhibitors of CYP3A4, p. 794. Moderate Study → Also see **TABLE 9** p. 1336

▸ Macrolides (**erythromycin**) are predicted to increase the exposure to **tadalafil**. Severe Theoretical

▸ Macrolides (**erythromycin**) are predicted to increase the exposure to **vardenafil**. Adjust dose. Severe Theoretical → Also see **TABLE 9** p. 1336

▸ Macrolides (**clarithromycin**) are predicted to increase the exposure to phosphodiesterase type-5 inhibitors (**avanafil, vardenafil**). Avoid. Severe Study → Also see **TABLE 9** p. 1336

▸ Mitotane is predicted to decrease the exposure to phosphodiesterase type-5 inhibitors (**avanafil, tadalafil**). Avoid. Severe Study

▸ Mitotane is predicted to decrease the exposure to phosphodiesterase type-5 inhibitors (**sildenafil, vardenafil**). Moderate Theoretical

▸ Netupitant is predicted to increase the exposure to **avanafil**. Adjust **avanafil** dose, p. 794. Moderate Theoretical

▸ Netupitant is predicted to increase the exposure to **sildenafil**. Monitor or adjust **sildenafil** dose with moderate inhibitors of CYP3A4, p. 794. Moderate Study

▸ Netupitant is predicted to increase the exposure to **tadalafil**. Severe Theoretical

▸ Netupitant is predicted to increase the exposure to **vardenafil**. Adjust dose. Severe Theoretical

▸ Nevirapine is predicted to decrease the exposure to **phosphodiesterase type-5 inhibitors**. Moderate Theoretical

▸ Nicorandil is predicted to increase the risk of hypotension when given with **phosphodiesterase type-5 inhibitors**. Avoid. Severe Theoretical → Also see **TABLE 8** p. 1335

▸ Nilotinib is predicted to increase the exposure to **avanafil**. Adjust **avanafil** dose, p. 794. Moderate Theoretical

▸ Nilotinib is predicted to increase the exposure to **sildenafil**. Monitor or adjust **sildenafil** dose with moderate inhibitors of CYP3A4, p. 794. Moderate Study → Also see **TABLE 9** p. 1336

▸ Nilotinib is predicted to increase the exposure to **tadalafil**. Severe Theoretical

▸ Nilotinib is predicted to increase the exposure to **vardenafil**. Adjust dose. Severe Theoretical → Also see **TABLE 9** p. 1336

▸ Nitrates potentially increase the risk of hypotension when given with **phosphodiesterase type-5 inhibitors**. Avoid. Severe Study → Also see **TABLE 8** p. 1335

▸ Ribociclib is predicted to increase the exposure to **sildenafil**. Avoid. Moderate Theoretical → Also see **TABLE 9** p. 1336

▸ Rifampicin is predicted to decrease the exposure to phosphodiesterase type-5 inhibitors (**avanafil, tadalafil**). Avoid. Severe Study

▸ Rifampicin is predicted to decrease the exposure to phosphodiesterase type-5 inhibitors (**sildenafil, vardenafil**). Moderate Theoretical

Phosphodiesterase type-5 inhibitors (continued)

▸ Riociguat is predicted to increase the risk of hypotension when given with **phosphodiesterase type-5 inhibitors**. Avoid. Severe Theoretical → Also see TABLE 8 p. 1335

▸ **Phosphodiesterase type-5 inhibitors** are predicted to increase the risk of hypotension when given with sapropterin. Moderate Theoretical → Also see TABLE 8 p. 1335

▸ St John's Wort is predicted to decrease the exposure to **phosphodiesterase type-5 inhibitors**. Moderate Theoretical

Pibrentasvir

▸ Antiarrhythmics (dronedarone) potentially increase the exposure to **pibrentasvir**. Moderate Theoretical

▸ Antiepileptics (carbamazepine, fosphenytoin, phenobarbital, phenytoin, primidone) are predicted to moderately to markedly decrease the exposure to **pibrentasvir**. Avoid. Severe Study

▸ Antiepileptics (eslicarbazepine, oxcarbazepine) potentially decrease the exposure to **pibrentasvir**. Avoid. Severe Theoretical

▸ Antifungals, azoles (itraconazole, ketoconazole) potentially increase the exposure to **pibrentasvir**. Moderate Theoretical

▸ Bosentan is predicted to decrease the exposure to **pibrentasvir**. Avoid. Severe Study

▸ Ciclosporin increases the exposure to **pibrentasvir**. Avoid or monitor. Severe Study

▸ Crizotinib potentially decreases the exposure to **pibrentasvir**. Avoid. Severe Theoretical

▸ **Pibrentasvir** (with glecaprevir) increases the exposure to dabigatran. Avoid. Moderate Study

▸ **Pibrentasvir** (with glecaprevir) increases the exposure to digoxin. Moderate Study

▸ Efavirenz is predicted to decrease the exposure to **pibrentasvir**. Avoid. Severe Study

▸ Enzalutamide is predicted to moderately to markedly decrease the exposure to **pibrentasvir**. Avoid. Severe Study

▸ HIV-protease inhibitors (atazanavir, lopinavir) (boosted with ritonavir) increase the exposure to **pibrentasvir**. Avoid. Severe Study

▸ HIV-protease inhibitors (ritonavir) potentially increase the exposure to **pibrentasvir**. Moderate Study

▸ Lumacaftor potentially decreases the exposure to **pibrentasvir**. Avoid. Severe Theoretical

▸ Mitotane is predicted to moderately to markedly decrease the exposure to **pibrentasvir**. Avoid. Severe Study

▸ Nevirapine is predicted to decrease the exposure to **pibrentasvir**. Avoid. Severe Study

▸ Rifampicin is predicted to moderately to markedly decrease the exposure to **pibrentasvir**. Avoid. Severe Study

▸ St John's Wort is predicted to decrease the exposure to **pibrentasvir**. Avoid. Severe Study

▸ **Pibrentasvir** (with glecaprevir) increases the exposure to statins (atorvastatin, simvastatin). Avoid. Moderate Study

▸ **Pibrentasvir** (with glecaprevir) is predicted to increase the exposure to statins (fluvastatin). Moderate Theoretical

▸ **Pibrentasvir** (with glecaprevir) increases the exposure to statins (pravastatin). Use with caution and adjust **pravastatin** dose. Moderate Study

▸ **Pibrentasvir** (with glecaprevir) increases the exposure to statins (rosuvastatin). Use with caution and adjust **rosuvastatin** dose, p. 202. Moderate Study

Pilocarpine

ROUTE-SPECIFIC INFORMATION Since systemic absorption can follow topical application, the possibility of interactions should be borne in mind.

Pimecrolimus

▸ Alcohol (beverage) increases the risk of facial flushing and skin irritation when given with topical **pimecrolimus**. Moderate Study

▸ **Pimecrolimus** is predicted to decrease the efficacy of mifamurtide. Avoid. Severe Theoretical

Pimozide → see TABLE 8 p. 1335 (hypotension), TABLE 9 p. 1336 (QT-interval prolongation), TABLE 11 p. 1336 (CNS depressant effects), TABLE 10 p. 1336 (antimuscarinics)

▸ Antiarrhythmics (dronedarone) are predicted to increase the exposure to **pimozide**. Avoid. Severe Theoretical → Also see TABLE 9 p. 1336

▸ Antifungals, azoles (fluconazole, isavuconazole, posaconazole) are predicted to increase the exposure to **pimozide**. Avoid. Severe Theoretical → Also see TABLE 9 p. 1336

▸ Antifungals, azoles (itraconazole, ketoconazole, voriconazole) are predicted to increase the exposure to **pimozide**. Avoid. Severe Study → Also see TABLE 9 p. 1336

▸ Antifungals, azoles (miconazole) are predicted to increase the exposure to **pimozide**. Moderate Theoretical

▸ Aprepitant is predicted to increase the exposure to **pimozide**. Avoid. Severe Theoretical

▸ Calcium channel blockers (diltiazem, verapamil) are predicted to increase the exposure to **pimozide**. Severe Theoretical → Also see TABLE 8 p. 1335

▸ Ceritinib is predicted to increase the exposure to **pimozide**. Avoid. Severe Theoretical → Also see TABLE 9 p. 1336

▸ Cobicistat is predicted to increase the exposure to **pimozide**. Avoid. Severe Study

▸ Crizotinib is predicted to increase the exposure to **pimozide**. Avoid. Severe Theoretical → Also see TABLE 9 p. 1336

▸ **Pimozide** is predicted to decrease the effects of dopamine receptor agonists. Avoid. Moderate Theoretical → Also see TABLE 8 p. 1335 → Also see TABLE 9 p. 1336 → Also see TABLE 10 p. 1336

▸ Fosaprepitant is predicted to increase the exposure to **pimozide**. Avoid. Severe Theoretical

▸ Grapefruit juice increases the exposure to **pimozide**. Avoid. Severe Theoretical

▸ HIV-protease inhibitors are predicted to increase the exposure to **pimozide**. Avoid. Severe Study → Also see TABLE 9 p. 1336

▸ Idelalisib is predicted to increase the exposure to **pimozide**. Avoid. Severe Study

▸ Imatinib is predicted to increase the exposure to **pimozide**. Avoid. Severe Theoretical

▸ **Pimozide** decreases the effects of levodopa. Severe Theoretical → Also see TABLE 8 p. 1335

▸ Macrolides (clarithromycin) are predicted to increase the exposure to **pimozide**. Avoid. Severe Study → Also see TABLE 9 p. 1336

▸ Macrolides (erythromycin) are predicted to increase the exposure to **pimozide**. Avoid. Severe Theoretical → Also see TABLE 9 p. 1336

▸ Netupitant is predicted to increase the exposure to **pimozide**. Avoid. Severe Theoretical

▸ Nilotinib is predicted to increase the exposure to **pimozide**. Avoid. Severe Theoretical → Also see TABLE 9 p. 1336

▸ Palbociclib is predicted to increase the exposure to **pimozide**. Adjust dose. Moderate Theoretical

▸ Panobinostat is predicted to increase the exposure to **pimozide**. Avoid. Severe Theoretical → Also see TABLE 9 p. 1336

▸ Pitolisant is predicted to decrease the effects of **pimozide**. Avoid. Severe Theoretical

▸ Ribociclib (high-dose) is predicted to increase the exposure to **pimozide**. Moderate Theoretical → Also see TABLE 9 p. 1336

▸ Rolapitant is predicted to increase the exposure to **pimozide**. Severe Study

Pindolol → see beta blockers, non-selective

Pioglitazone → see TABLE 14 p. 1337 (antidiabetic drugs)

▸ **Pioglitazone** potentially decreases the exposure to antifungals, azoles (isavuconazole). Use with caution or avoid. Moderate Theoretical

▸ Clopidogrel increases the exposure to **pioglitazone**. Monitor blood glucose and adjust dose. Severe Study

▸ Fibrates (gemfibrozil) increase the exposure to **pioglitazone**. Monitor blood glucose and adjust dose. Severe Study

▸ Leflunomide is predicted to increase the exposure to **pioglitazone**. Moderate Study

▸ Opicapone is predicted to increase the exposure to **pioglitazone**. Moderate Study

▸ Rifampicin moderately decreases the exposure to **pioglitazone**. Monitor and adjust dose. Moderate Study

▸ St John's Wort slightly decreases the exposure to **pioglitazone**. Mild Study

▸ Teriflunomide is predicted to increase the exposure to **pioglitazone**. Moderate Study

Piperacillin → see penicillins

Piperaquine → see antimalarials

Pirfenidone

FOOD AND LIFESTYLE Smoking increases pirfenidone clearance; patients should be encouraged to stop smoking before and during treatment with pirfenidone.

▸ Antiepileptics (fosphenytoin, phenytoin) are predicted to decrease the exposure to **pirfenidone**. Moderate Theoretical
▸ Combined hormonal contraceptives are predicted to increase the exposure to **pirfenidone**. Use with caution and adjust dose. Moderate Study
▸ HIV-protease inhibitors (ritonavir) are predicted to decrease the exposure to **pirfenidone**. Moderate Theoretical
▸ Leflunomide is predicted to decrease the exposure to **pirfenidone**. Moderate Theoretical
▸ Quinolones (ciprofloxacin) are predicted to increase the exposure to **pirfenidone**. Use with caution and adjust dose. Moderate Study
▸ Rifampicin is predicted to decrease the exposure to **pirfenidone**. Avoid. Moderate Theoretical
▸ SSRIs (fluvoxamine) are predicted to moderately increase the exposure to **pirfenidone**. Avoid. Moderate Study
▸ Teriflunomide is predicted to decrease the exposure to **pirfenidone**. Moderate Theoretical

Piroxicam → see NSAIDs

Pitolisant

▸ Abiraterone is predicted to increase the exposure to **pitolisant**. Use with caution and adjust dose. Moderate Study
▸ Antiarrhythmics (propafenone) are predicted to increase the exposure to **pitolisant**. Use with caution and adjust dose. Moderate Study
▸ Antiepileptics (carbamazepine, fosphenytoin, phenobarbital, phenytoin, primidone) are predicted to moderately decrease the exposure to **pitolisant**. Moderate Study
▸ Antihistamines, sedating are predicted to decrease the efficacy of **pitolisant**. Unknown Theoretical
▸ **Pitolisant** is predicted to decrease the exposure to bosutinib. Avoid. Severe Theoretical
▸ Bupropion is predicted to moderately increase the exposure to **pitolisant**. Use with caution and adjust dose. Moderate Study
▸ **Pitolisant** is predicted to decrease the exposure to ciclosporin. Avoid. Severe Theoretical
▸ Cinacalcet is predicted to increase the exposure to **pitolisant**. Use with caution and adjust dose. Moderate Study
▸ **Pitolisant** is predicted to decrease the efficacy of combined hormonal contraceptives. Avoid. Severe Theoretical
▸ **Pitolisant** is predicted to decrease the exposure to coumarins (warfarin). Unknown Theoretical
▸ **Pitolisant** is predicted to decrease the exposure to crizotinib. Avoid. Severe Theoretical
▸ **Pitolisant** is predicted to decrease the exposure to dabigatran. Unknown Theoretical
▸ **Pitolisant** is predicted to decrease the exposure to dasatinib. Avoid. Severe Theoretical
▸ **Pitolisant** is predicted to decrease the exposure to digoxin. Unknown Theoretical
▸ Duloxetine is predicted to increase the exposure to **pitolisant**. Use with caution and adjust dose. Moderate Study
▸ **Pitolisant** is predicted to decrease the exposure to efavirenz. Unknown Theoretical
▸ Enzalutamide is predicted to moderately decrease the exposure to **pitolisant**. Moderate Study
▸ **Pitolisant** is predicted to decrease the exposure to everolimus. Avoid. Severe Theoretical
▸ HIV-protease inhibitors (ritonavir) are predicted to increase the exposure to **pitolisant**. Use with caution and adjust dose. Moderate Study
▸ **Pitolisant** is predicted to decrease the exposure to irinotecan. Unknown Theoretical
▸ **Pitolisant** is predicted to increase the exposure to metformin. Unknown Theoretical
▸ Mianserin is predicted to decrease the efficacy of **pitolisant**. Unknown Theoretical
▸ Mirabegron is predicted to increase the exposure to **pitolisant**. Use with caution and adjust dose. Moderate Study
▸ Mirtazapine is predicted to decrease the efficacy of **pitolisant**. Unknown Theoretical

▸ Mitotane is predicted to moderately decrease the exposure to **pitolisant**. Moderate Study
▸ **Pitolisant** is predicted to decrease the exposure to opioids (morphine). Unknown Theoretical
▸ **Pitolisant** is predicted to decrease the exposure to paracetamol. Unknown Theoretical
▸ **Pitolisant** is predicted to decrease the exposure to pimozide. Avoid. Severe Theoretical
▸ **Pitolisant** is predicted to decrease the exposure to repaglinide. Unknown Theoretical
▸ Rifampicin is predicted to moderately decrease the exposure to **pitolisant**. Moderate Study
▸ **Pitolisant** is predicted to decrease the exposure to sirolimus. Avoid. Severe Theoretical
▸ SSRIs (fluoxetine, paroxetine) are predicted to moderately increase the exposure to **pitolisant**. Use with caution and adjust dose. Moderate Study
▸ St John's Wort is predicted to decrease the exposure to **pitolisant**. Monitor and adjust dose. Moderate Theoretical
▸ **Pitolisant** is predicted to decrease the exposure to tacrolimus. Avoid. Severe Theoretical
▸ **Pitolisant** is predicted to decrease the exposure to taxanes (docetaxel). Avoid. Severe Theoretical
▸ **Pitolisant** is predicted to decrease the exposure to temsirolimus. Avoid. Severe Theoretical
▸ Terbinafine is predicted to moderately increase the exposure to **pitolisant**. Use with caution and adjust dose. Moderate Study
▸ Tricyclic antidepressants are predicted to decrease the efficacy of **pitolisant**. Mild Theoretical

Pivmecillinam → see penicillins

Pixantrone → see anthracyclines

Pizotifen → see antihistamines, sedating

Platinum compounds → see TABLE 15 p. 1337 (myelosuppression), TABLE 2 p. 1334 (nephrotoxicity), TABLE 19 p. 1338 (ototoxicity), TABLE 12 p. 1337 (peripheral neuropathy)

carboplatin · cisplatin · oxaliplatin

▸ Cisplatin increases the risk of pulmonary toxicity when given with bleomycin. Severe Study → Also see TABLE 15 p. 1337
▸ Live vaccines are predicted to increase the risk of generalised infection (possibly life-threatening) when given with **platinum compounds**. Public Health England advises avoid (refer to Green Book). Severe Theoretical

Polymyxins → see TABLE 2 p. 1334 (nephrotoxicity), TABLE 20 p. 1338 (neuromuscular blocking effects)

Polysaccharide-iron complex → see iron (oral)

Polystyrene sulfonate

▸ Antacids increase the risk of metabolic alkalosis when given with **polystyrene sulfonate**. Severe Anecdotal
▸ Polystyrene sulfonate is predicted to decrease the absorption of thyroid hormones (levothyroxine). Separate administration by at least 4 hours. Moderate Theoretical

Pomalidomide → see TABLE 15 p. 1337 (myelosuppression), TABLE 5 p. 1334 (thromboembolism)

▸ Combined hormonal contraceptives are predicted to increase the risk of venous thromboembolism when given with **pomalidomide**. Avoid. Severe Theoretical
▸ Hormone replacement therapy is predicted to increase the risk of venous thromboembolism when given with **pomalidomide**. Severe Theoretical
▸ Quinolones (ciprofloxacin) are predicted to increase the exposure to **pomalidomide**. Adjust **pomalidomide** dose, p. 935. Moderate Theoretical
▸ SSRIs (fluvoxamine) moderately increase the exposure to **pomalidomide**. Adjust **pomalidomide** dose, p. 935. Moderate Study

Ponatinib

▸ Antiepileptics (carbamazepine, fosphenytoin, phenobarbital, phenytoin, primidone) are predicted to decrease the exposure to **ponatinib**. Avoid. Moderate Theoretical
▸ Antifungals, azoles (itraconazole, ketoconazole, voriconazole) are predicted to slightly increase the exposure to **ponatinib**. Monitor and adjust **ponatinib** dose, p. 963. Moderate Study
▸ Cobicistat is predicted to slightly increase the exposure to **ponatinib**. Monitor and adjust **ponatinib** dose, p. 963. Moderate Study

Ponatinib (continued)
- Ponatinib is predicted to increase the risk of bleeding events when given with coumarins. Severe Theoretical
- Enzalutamide is predicted to decrease the exposure to ponatinib. Avoid. Moderate Theoretical
- Grapefruit juice is predicted to increase the exposure to ponatinib. Moderate Theoretical
- HIV-protease inhibitors are predicted to slightly increase the exposure to ponatinib. Monitor and adjust ponatinib dose, p. 963. Moderate Study
- Idelalisib is predicted to slightly increase the exposure to ponatinib. Monitor and adjust ponatinib dose, p. 963. Moderate Study
- Macrolides (clarithromycin) are predicted to slightly increase the exposure to ponatinib. Monitor and adjust ponatinib dose, p. 963. Moderate Study
- Mitotane is predicted to decrease the exposure to ponatinib. Avoid. Moderate Theoretical
- Ponatinib is predicted to increase the risk of bleeding events when given with phenindione. Severe Theoretical
- Rifampicin is predicted to decrease the exposure to ponatinib. Avoid. Moderate Theoretical
- St John's Wort is predicted to decrease the exposure to ponatinib. Avoid. Severe Theoretical

Posaconazole → see antifungals, azoles
Potassium canrenoate → see TABLE 16 p. 1338 (increased serum potassium)
Potassium chloride → see TABLE 16 p. 1338 (increased serum potassium)
Potassium citrate
- Potassium citrate is predicted to decrease the efficacy of methenamine. Avoid. Moderate Theoretical
- Potassium citrate increases the risk of side-effects when given with sucralfate. Avoid. Moderate Theoretical
Potassium-sparing diuretics → see TABLE 18 p. 1338 (hyponatraemia), TABLE 16 p. 1338 (increased serum potassium)

amiloride · triamterene

- Triamterene potentially increases the clearance of lithium. Moderate Study

Pramipexole → see dopamine receptor agonists
Prasugrel → see TABLE 4 p. 1334 (antiplatelet effects)
Pravastatin → see statins
Praziquantel
- Antiepileptics (carbamazepine, fosphenytoin, phenobarbital, phenytoin, primidone) are predicted to markedly decrease the exposure to praziquantel. Avoid. Moderate Study
- Antifungals, azoles (itraconazole, ketoconazole, voriconazole) are predicted to moderately increase the exposure to praziquantel. Mild Study
- Antimalarials (chloroquine) moderately decrease the exposure to praziquantel. Use with caution and adjust dose. Moderate Study
- Cobicistat is predicted to moderately increase the exposure to praziquantel. Mild Study
- Corticosteroids (dexamethasone) decrease the exposure to praziquantel. Moderate Study
- Enzalutamide is predicted to markedly decrease the exposure to praziquantel. Avoid. Moderate Study
- Grapefruit juice is predicted to increase the exposure to praziquantel. Moderate Study
- H₂ receptor antagonists (cimetidine) moderately increase the exposure to praziquantel. Moderate Study
- HIV-protease inhibitors are predicted to moderately increase the exposure to praziquantel. Mild Study
- Idelalisib is predicted to moderately increase the exposure to praziquantel. Mild Study
- Macrolides (clarithromycin) are predicted to moderately increase the exposure to praziquantel. Mild Study
- Mitotane is predicted to markedly decrease the exposure to praziquantel. Avoid. Moderate Study
- Rifampicin is predicted to markedly decrease the exposure to praziquantel. Avoid. Moderate Study

Prazosin → see alpha blockers
Prednisolone → see corticosteroids
Prednisone → see corticosteroids

Pregabalin → see antiepileptics
Prilocaine → see anaesthetics, local
Primaquine → see antimalarials
Primidone → see antiepileptics
Procarbazine → see TABLE 15 p. 1337 (myelosuppression), TABLE 13 p. 1337 (serotonin syndrome)

> **FOOD AND LIFESTYLE** Procarbazine is a mild monoamine-oxidase inhibitor and might rarely interact with tyramine-rich foods (such as mature cheese, salami, pickled herring, *Bovril*®, *Oxo*®, *Marmite*® or any similar meat or yeast extract or fermented soya bean extract, and some beers, lagers or wines).

- Alcohol (beverage) potentially causes a disulfiram-like reaction when given with procarbazine. Moderate Anecdotal
- Antiepileptics (carbamazepine, phenobarbital, phenytoin, primidone) are predicted to increase the risk of hypersensitivity reactions when given with procarbazine. Severe Anecdotal
- Antiepileptics (fosphenytoin) are predicted to increase the risk of hypersensitivity when given with procarbazine. Severe Anecdotal
- Live vaccines are predicted to increase the risk of generalised infection (possibly life-threatening) when given with procarbazine. Public Health England advises avoid (refer to Green Book). Severe Theoretical

Prochlorperazine → see phenothiazines
Procyclidine → see TABLE 10 p. 1336 (antimuscarinics)
- SSRIs (paroxetine) slightly increase the exposure to procyclidine. Monitor and adjust dose. Moderate Study
Proguanil → see antimalarials
Promazine → see phenothiazines
Promethazine → see antihistamines, sedating
Propafenone → see antiarrhythmics
Propantheline → see TABLE 10 p. 1336 (antimuscarinics)
Propiverine → see TABLE 10 p. 1336 (antimuscarinics)
- Propiverine is predicted to increase the exposure to lomitapide. Separate administration by 12 hours. Moderate Theoretical
Propofol → see TABLE 8 p. 1335 (hypotension), TABLE 11 p. 1336 (CNS depressant effects)
- Antiepileptics (valproate) potentially increase the concentration of propofol. Adjust dose. Severe Theoretical
Propranolol → see beta blockers, non-selective
Propylthiouracil → see TABLE 15 p. 1337 (myelosuppression)
- Propylthiouracil is predicted to decrease the effects of metyrapone. Avoid. Moderate Theoretical
Proton pump inhibitors

esomeprazole · lansoprazole · omeprazole · pantoprazole · rabeprazole

- Antifungals, azoles (voriconazole) increase the exposure to proton pump inhibitors (esomeprazole, omeprazole). Adjust dose. Moderate Study
- Proton pump inhibitors decrease the absorption of antifungals, azoles (itraconazole). Administer **itraconazole** capsules with an acidic beverage. Moderate Study
- Proton pump inhibitors decrease the absorption of antifungals, azoles (ketoconazole). Administer **ketoconazole** with an acidic beverage. Moderate Study
- Proton pump inhibitors decrease the absorption of antifungals, azoles (posaconazole) (oral suspension). Avoid. Moderate Study
- Proton pump inhibitors are predicted to decrease the absorption of bosutinib. Moderate Study
- Proton pump inhibitors are predicted to decrease the absorption of ceritinib. Moderate Theoretical
- Esomeprazole is predicted to increase the exposure to cilostazol. Moderate Theoretical
- Omeprazole is predicted to increase the exposure to cilostazol. Adjust cilostazol dose, p. 231. Moderate Study
- Proton pump inhibitors (esomeprazole, omeprazole) potentially increase the exposure to clobazam. Adjust dose. Moderate Theoretical
- Proton pump inhibitors (esomeprazole, omeprazole) are predicted to decrease the efficacy of clopidogrel. Avoid. Moderate Study

▸ **Proton pump inhibitors** are predicted to slightly to moderately decrease the exposure to dasatinib. Avoid. Severe Study

▸ **Proton pump inhibitors** are predicted to decrease the absorption of dipyridamole (immediate release tablets). Moderate Theoretical

▸ **Proton pump inhibitors** are predicted to slightly decrease the exposure to erlotinib. Avoid. Moderate Study

▸ **Proton pump inhibitors** are predicted to decrease the exposure to gefitinib. Severe Theoretical

▸ HIV-protease inhibitors (tipranavir) decrease the exposure to **proton pump inhibitors**. Avoid. Severe Study

▸ **Proton pump inhibitors** decrease the exposure to HIV-protease inhibitors (atazanavir). Avoid or adjust dose. Severe Study

▸ **Proton pump inhibitors** increase the exposure to HIV-protease inhibitors (saquinavir). Avoid. Severe Study

▸ **Proton pump inhibitors** are predicted to decrease the exposure to ledipasvir. Adjust dose, see ledipasvir with sofosbuvir p. 617. Moderate Theoretical

▸ **Proton pump inhibitors** decrease the clearance of methotrexate (high-dose). Use with caution or avoid. Severe Study

▸ **Proton pump inhibitors** are predicted to decrease the exposure to pazopanib. Avoid or administer concurrently without food. Moderate Study

▸ **Proton pump inhibitors** are predicted to decrease the exposure to rilpivirine. Avoid. Severe Study

▸ **Proton pump inhibitors** potentially decrease the exposure to sofosbuvir. Adjust dose, see ledipasvir with sofosbuvir p. 617, sofosbuvir with velpatasvir p. 619, and sofosbuvir with velpatasvir and voxilaprevir p. 619. Moderate Study

▸ **Esomeprazole** is predicted to slightly to moderately increase the exposure to SSRIs (citalopram, escitalopram). Monitor and adjust dose. Severe Theoretical

▸ **Omeprazole** slightly to moderately increases the exposure to SSRIs (citalopram, escitalopram). Monitor and adjust dose. Severe Study

▸ **Proton pump inhibitors** are predicted to decrease the concentration of velpatasvir. Adjust dose, see sofosbuvir with velpatasvir p. 619. Moderate Study

▸ **Proton pump inhibitors** are predicted to decrease the exposure to voxilaprevir. Adjust dose, see sofosbuvir with velpatasvir and voxilaprevir p. 619. Moderate Study

Proxymetacaine → see anaesthetics, local
Pseudoephedrine → see sympathomimetics, vasoconstrictor
Pyrazinamide

▸ Allopurinol is predicted to increase the risk of hyperuricaemia when given with **pyrazinamide**. Moderate Theoretical

▸ **Pyrazinamide** is predicted to decrease the effects of sulfinpyrazone. Moderate Theoretical

Pyridostigmine → see TABLE 6 p. 1335 (bradycardia), TABLE 20 p. 1338 (neuromuscular blocking effects)

▸ Aminoglycosides are predicted to decrease the effects of **pyridostigmine**. Moderate Study → Also see TABLE 20 p. 1338

Pyrimethamine → see antimalarials
Quetiapine → see TABLE 8 p. 1335 (hypotension), TABLE 11 p. 1336 (CNS depressant effects)

▸ Antiarrhythmics (dronedarone) are predicted to increase the exposure to **quetiapine**. Avoid. Moderate Study

▸ Antiepileptics (carbamazepine, fosphenytoin, phenobarbital, phenytoin, primidone) are predicted to decrease the exposure to **quetiapine**. Moderate Study → Also see TABLE 11 p. 1336

▸ Antiepileptics (valproate) potentially increase the risk of neutropenia when given with **quetiapine**. Moderate Study

▸ Antifungals, azoles (fluconazole, isavuconazole, posaconazole) are predicted to increase the exposure to **quetiapine**. Avoid. Moderate Study

▸ Antifungals, azoles (itraconazole, ketoconazole, voriconazole) are predicted to increase the exposure to **quetiapine**. Avoid. Severe Study

▸ Aprepitant is predicted to increase the exposure to **quetiapine**. Avoid. Moderate Study

▸ Bosentan is predicted to decrease the exposure to **quetiapine**. Moderate Study

▸ Calcium channel blockers (diltiazem, verapamil) are predicted to increase the exposure to **quetiapine**. Avoid. Moderate Study → Also see TABLE 8 p. 1335

▸ Cobicistat is predicted to increase the exposure to **quetiapine**. Avoid. Moderate Study

▸ Crizotinib is predicted to increase the exposure to **quetiapine**. Avoid. Moderate Study

▸ **Quetiapine** is predicted to decrease the effects of dopamine receptor agonists. Avoid. Moderate Theoretical → Also see TABLE 8 p. 1335

▸ Efavirenz is predicted to decrease the exposure to **quetiapine**. Moderate Study

▸ Enzalutamide is predicted to decrease the exposure to **quetiapine**. Moderate Study

▸ Grapefruit juice is predicted to increase the exposure to **quetiapine**. Avoid. Severe Theoretical

▸ HIV-protease inhibitors are predicted to increase the exposure to **quetiapine**. Avoid. Severe Study

▸ Idelalisib is predicted to increase the exposure to **quetiapine**. Avoid. Severe Study

▸ Imatinib is predicted to increase the exposure to **quetiapine**. Avoid. Moderate Study

▸ **Quetiapine** decreases the effects of levodopa. Severe Anecdotal → Also see TABLE 8 p. 1335

▸ **Quetiapine** potentially increases the risk of neurotoxicity when given with lithium. Severe Anecdotal

▸ Macrolides (clarithromycin) are predicted to increase the exposure to **quetiapine**. Avoid. Severe Study

▸ Macrolides (erythromycin) are predicted to increase the exposure to **quetiapine**. Avoid. Moderate Study

▸ Mitotane is predicted to decrease the exposure to **quetiapine**. Moderate Study

▸ Netupitant is predicted to increase the exposure to **quetiapine**. Avoid. Moderate Study

▸ Nevirapine is predicted to decrease the exposure to **quetiapine**. Moderate Study

▸ Nilotinib is predicted to increase the exposure to **quetiapine**. Avoid. Moderate Study

▸ Ribociclib (high-dose) is predicted to increase the exposure to **quetiapine**. Avoid. Moderate Theoretical

▸ Rifampicin is predicted to decrease the exposure to **quetiapine**. Moderate Study

▸ St John's Wort is predicted to decrease the exposure to **quetiapine**. Moderate Study

Quinagolide → see dopamine receptor agonists
Quinapril → see ACE inhibitors
Quinine → see antimalarials
Quinolones → see TABLE 9 p. 1336 (QT-interval prolongation)

ciprofloxacin · levofloxacin · moxifloxacin · norfloxacin · ofloxacin

ROUTE-SPECIFIC INFORMATION Since systemic absorption can follow topical application, the possibility of interactions should be borne in mind.

▸ **Ciprofloxacin** is predicted to increase the exposure to agomelatine. Moderate Study

▸ Quinolones (ciprofloxacin, norfloxacin) are predicted to increase the exposure to aminophylline. Adjust dose. Moderate Theoretical

▸ **Ciprofloxacin** is predicted to increase the exposure to anagrelide. Moderate Theoretical

▸ Antacids decrease the absorption of **quinolones**. **Quinolones** should be taken 2 hours before or 4 hours after **antacids**. Moderate Study

▸ **Ciprofloxacin** slightly increases the exposure to antiarrhythmics (lidocaine). Mild Study

▸ **Ciprofloxacin** affects the concentration of antiepileptics (fosphenytoin, phenytoin). Monitor concentration and adjust dose. Severe Study

▸ Calcium salts (calcium carbonate) decrease the absorption of **ciprofloxacin**. Separate administration by 2 hours. Moderate Study

▸ Calcium salts (calcium carbonate) decrease the absorption of **norfloxacin**. Norfloxacin should be taken 2 hours before or 4 hours after **calcium carbonate**. Moderate Study

▸ **Ciprofloxacin** increases the concentration of clozapine. Monitor side effects and adjust dose. Severe Study

▸ **Quinolones** increase the anticoagulant effect of coumarins. Severe Anecdotal

A1

Interactions | Appendix 1

Quinolones (continued)

▸ Didanosine (buffered) is predicted to greatly decrease the exposure to oral **quinolones**. **Didanosine** should be taken 2 hours after quinolones. Moderate Study

▸ **Ciprofloxacin** is predicted to increase the exposure to dopamine receptor agonists (ropinirole). Adjust dose. Moderate Study

▸ **Ciprofloxacin** is predicted to increase the exposure to duloxetine. Avoid. Moderate Theoretical

▸ **Ciprofloxacin** is predicted to increase the exposure to eliglustat. Avoid or adjust dose—consult product literature. Severe Theoretical

▸ Enteral feeds decrease the exposure to **ciprofloxacin**. Moderate Study

▸ **Ciprofloxacin** slightly increases the exposure to erlotinib. Monitor side effects and adjust dose. Moderate Study

▸ **Ciprofloxacin** is predicted to increase the exposure to ibrutinib. Adjust **ibrutinib** dose, p. 952. Severe Theoretical

▸ Iron (oral) decreases the exposure to **quinolones**. Separate administration by at least 2 hours. Moderate Study

▸ Lanthanum moderately decreases the exposure to **quinolones**. **Quinolones** should be taken 2 hours before or 4 hours after lanthanum. Moderate Study

▸ **Ciprofloxacin** is predicted to increase the exposure to loxapine. Avoid. Unknown Theoretical

▸ **Ciprofloxacin** is predicted to increase the exposure to melatonin. Moderate Theoretical

▸ **Ciprofloxacin** potentially increases the risk of toxicity when given with methotrexate. Avoid. Severe Anecdotal

▸ **Ciprofloxacin** slightly increases the exposure to monoamine-oxidase B inhibitors (rasagiline). Moderate Study

▸ NSAIDs potentially increase the risk of seizures when given with **quinolones**. Severe Theoretical

▸ **Ciprofloxacin** very slightly increases the exposure to pentoxifylline. Moderate Study

▸ **Ciprofloxacin** is predicted to increase the exposure to pirfenidone. Use with caution and adjust dose. Moderate Study

▸ **Ciprofloxacin** is predicted to increase the exposure to pomalidomide. Adjust **pomalidomide** dose, p. 935. Moderate Theoretical

▸ **Ciprofloxacin** is predicted to increase the exposure to roflumilast. Moderate Theoretical

▸ Sucralfate decreases the exposure to **quinolones**. Separate administration by 2 hours. Moderate Study

▸ **Ciprofloxacin** is predicted to increase the exposure to theophylline. Monitor and adjust dose. Moderate Theoretical

▸ **Norfloxacin** is predicted to increase the exposure to theophylline. Adjust dose. Moderate Anecdotal

▸ **Ciprofloxacin** increases the exposure to tizanidine. Avoid. Moderate Study

▸ Zinc is predicted to decrease the exposure to **quinolones**. Separate administration by 2 hours. Moderate Study

▸ **Ciprofloxacin** is predicted to increase the exposure to zolmitriptan. Adjust **zolmitriptan** dose, p. 475. Moderate Theoretical

Rabeprazole → see proton pump inhibitors

Rabies vaccine

▸ Antimalarials (chloroquine) decrease the efficacy of **rabies vaccine**. Avoid. Moderate Study

▸ Hydroxychloroquine is predicted to decrease efficacy **rabies vaccine**. Moderate Theoretical

Raloxifene → see TABLE 5 p. 1334 (thromboembolism)

Raltegravir

▸ Antacids slightly decrease the exposure to **raltegravir**. Avoid. Moderate Study

▸ Antiepileptics (carbamazepine) are predicted to affect the exposure to **raltegravir**. Moderate Theoretical

▸ Antiepileptics (fosphenytoin, phenobarbital, phenytoin, primidone) are predicted to affect the exposure to **raltegravir**. Use with caution or avoid. Moderate Theoretical

▸ Calcium salts (calcium carbonate) greatly decrease the exposure to **raltegravir** (high-dose). Avoid. Severe Study

▸ HIV-protease inhibitors (atazanavir) increase the exposure to **raltegravir** (high-dose). Avoid. Moderate Study

▸ HIV-protease inhibitors (darunavir) increase the risk of rash when given with **raltegravir**. Moderate Study

▸ HIV-protease inhibitors (fosamprenavir) (boosted with ritonavir) decrease the exposure to **raltegravir** and **raltegravir** decreases the exposure to HIV-protease inhibitors (fosamprenavir) (boosted with ritonavir). Avoid. Severe Study

▸ HIV-protease inhibitors (tipranavir) (boosted with ritonavir) are predicted to decrease the exposure to **raltegravir** (high-dose). Avoid. Moderate Study

▸ Rifampicin slightly decreases the exposure to **raltegravir**. Avoid or adjust dose—consult product literature. Moderate Study

Raltitrexed → see TABLE 15 p. 1337 (myelosuppression)

▸ Folates are predicted to alter the effects of **raltitrexed**. Avoid. Moderate Study

▸ Live vaccines are predicted to increase the risk of generalised infection (possibly life-threatening) when given with **raltitrexed**. Public Health England advises avoid (refer to Green Book). Severe Theoretical

Ramipril → see ACE inhibitors

Ramucirumab → see monoclonal antibodies

Ranibizumab

▸ **Ranibizumab** is predicted to increase the risk of bleeding events when given with argatroban. Severe Theoretical

▸ **Ranibizumab** is predicted to increase the risk of bleeding events when given with bivalirudin. Moderate Theoretical

▸ **Ranibizumab** increases the risk of bleeding events when given with coumarins. Severe Theoretical

▸ **Ranibizumab** is predicted to increase the risk of bleeding events when given with danaparoid. Severe Theoretical

▸ **Ranibizumab** increases the risk of bleeding events when given with heparin (unfractionated). Severe Theoretical

▸ **Ranibizumab** is predicted to increase the risk of bleeding events when given with low molecular-weight heparins. Severe Theoretical

▸ **Ranibizumab** is predicted to increase the risk of bleeding events when given with phenindione. Severe Theoretical

Ranitidine → see H₂ receptor antagonists

Ranolazine → see TABLE 9 p. 1336 (QT-interval prolongation)

▸ **Ranolazine** is predicted to increase the exposure to afatinib. Separate administration by 12 hours. Moderate Study

▸ **Ranolazine** is predicted to increase the exposure to aliskiren. Moderate Theoretical

▸ Antiarrhythmics (dronedarone) are predicted to increase the exposure to **ranolazine**. Severe Study → Also see TABLE 9 p. 1336

▸ Antiepileptics (carbamazepine, fosphenytoin, phenobarbital, phenytoin, primidone) are predicted to decrease the exposure to **ranolazine**. Avoid. Severe Study

▸ Antifungals, azoles (fluconazole, isavuconazole, posaconazole) are predicted to increase the exposure to **ranolazine**. Severe Study → Also see TABLE 9 p. 1336

▸ Antifungals, azoles (itraconazole, ketoconazole, voriconazole) are predicted to increase the exposure to **ranolazine**. Avoid. Severe Study → Also see TABLE 9 p. 1336

▸ Aprepitant is predicted to increase the exposure to **ranolazine**. Severe Study

▸ **Ranolazine** is predicted to increase the exposure to beta blockers, non-selective (nadolol). Moderate Study

▸ Calcium channel blockers (diltiazem, verapamil) are predicted to increase the exposure to **ranolazine**. Severe Study

▸ **Ranolazine** is predicted to increase the exposure to ceritinib. Moderate Theoretical → Also see TABLE 9 p. 1336

▸ Ciclosporin is predicted to increase the concentration of **ranolazine** and **ranolazine** is predicted to increase the concentration of ciclosporin. Moderate Theoretical

▸ Cobicistat is predicted to increase the exposure to **ranolazine**. Avoid. Severe Study

▸ **Ranolazine** is predicted to increase the exposure to colchicine. Avoid or adjust **colchicine** dose, p. 1085. Severe Theoretical

▸ Crizotinib is predicted to increase the exposure to **ranolazine**. Severe Study → Also see TABLE 9 p. 1336

▸ **Ranolazine** is predicted to increase the exposure to dabigatran. Severe Theoretical

▸ **Ranolazine** increases the concentration of digoxin. Moderate Study

▸ **Ranolazine** is predicted to slightly increase the exposure to edoxaban. Severe Theoretical

- Enzalutamide is predicted to decrease the exposure to **ranolazine**. Avoid. [Severe] Study
- **Ranolazine** is predicted to increase the exposure to erlotinib. [Moderate] Theoretical
- **Ranolazine** is predicted to increase the exposure to fidaxomicin. Avoid. [Moderate] Study
- Grapefruit juice is predicted to increase the concentration of **ranolazine**. Avoid. [Severe] Theoretical
- HIV-protease inhibitors are predicted to increase the exposure to **ranolazine**. Avoid. [Severe] Study → Also see TABLE 9 p. 1336
- Idelalisib is predicted to increase the exposure to **ranolazine**. Avoid. [Severe] Study
- Imatinib is predicted to increase the exposure to **ranolazine**. [Severe] Study
- **Ranolazine** is predicted to increase the exposure to lomitapide. Separate administration by 12 hours. [Moderate] Theoretical
- Macrolides (clarithromycin) are predicted to increase the exposure to **ranolazine**. Avoid. [Severe] Study → Also see TABLE 9 p. 1336
- Macrolides (erythromycin) are predicted to increase the exposure to **ranolazine**. [Severe] Study → Also see TABLE 9 p. 1336
- Mitotane is predicted to decrease the exposure to **ranolazine**. Avoid. [Severe] Study
- Netupitant is predicted to increase the exposure to **ranolazine**. [Severe] Study
- Nilotinib is predicted to increase the exposure to **ranolazine**. [Severe] Study → Also see TABLE 9 p. 1336
- **Ranolazine** is predicted to increase the exposure to nintedanib. [Moderate] Study
- **Ranolazine** is predicted to increase the exposure to panobinostat. Adjust dose. [Moderate] Theoretical → Also see TABLE 9 p. 1336
- Rifampicin is predicted to decrease the exposure to **ranolazine**. Avoid. [Severe] Study
- St John's Wort is predicted to decrease the exposure to **ranolazine**. Avoid. [Severe] Study
- **Ranolazine** is predicted to increase the exposure to statins (atorvastatin). [Moderate] Theoretical
- **Ranolazine** slightly increases the exposure to statins (simvastatin). Adjust **simvastatin** dose, p. 203. [Moderate] Study
- **Ranolazine** increases the concentration of tacrolimus. Adjust dose. [Severe] Anecdotal
- **Ranolazine** is predicted to increase the exposure to ticagrelor. Use with caution or avoid. [Severe] Study
- **Ranolazine** is predicted to increase the exposure to topotecan. [Severe] Study
- **Ranolazine** is predicted to increase the concentration of trametinib. [Moderate] Theoretical
- **Ranolazine** is predicted to increase the exposure to venetoclax. Avoid or monitor for toxicity. [Severe] Theoretical

Rasagiline → see monoamine-oxidase B inhibitors

Reboxetine
- Antiepileptics (carbamazepine, fosphenytoin, phenobarbital, phenytoin, primidone) are predicted to decrease the exposure to **reboxetine**. [Moderate] Anecdotal
- Antifungals, azoles (itraconazole, ketoconazole, voriconazole) are predicted to increase the exposure to **reboxetine**. Avoid. [Moderate] Study
- Antifungals, azoles (miconazole) are predicted to increase the concentration of **reboxetine**. Use with caution and adjust dose. [Moderate] Theoretical
- Cobicistat is predicted to increase the exposure to **reboxetine**. Avoid. [Moderate] Study
- Enzalutamide is predicted to decrease the exposure to **reboxetine**. [Moderate] Anecdotal
- HIV-protease inhibitors are predicted to increase the exposure to **reboxetine**. Avoid. [Moderate] Study
- Idelalisib is predicted to increase the exposure to **reboxetine**. Avoid. [Moderate] Study
- **Reboxetine** is predicted to increase the risk of a hypertensive crisis when given with linezolid. Avoid. [Severe] Theoretical
- **Reboxetine** is predicted to increase the risk of hypokalaemia when given with loop diuretics. [Moderate] Theoretical
- Macrolides (clarithromycin) are predicted to increase the exposure to **reboxetine**. Avoid. [Moderate] Study

- Mitotane is predicted to decrease the exposure to **reboxetine**. [Moderate] Anecdotal
- **Reboxetine** is predicted to increase the risk of a hypertensive crisis when given with moclobemide. Avoid. [Severe] Theoretical
- **Reboxetine** is predicted to increase the risk of a hypertensive crisis when given with monoamine-oxidase A and B inhibitors, irreversible. Avoid. [Severe] Theoretical
- **Reboxetine** is predicted to increase the risk of a hypertensive crisis when given with monoamine-oxidase B inhibitors (rasagiline, selegiline). Avoid. [Severe] Theoretical
- Rifampicin is predicted to decrease the exposure to **reboxetine**. [Moderate] Anecdotal
- **Reboxetine** is predicted to increase the risk of hypokalaemia when given with thiazide diuretics. [Moderate] Anecdotal

Regorafenib → see TABLE 15 p. 1337 (myelosuppression), TABLE 4 p. 1334 (antiplatelet effects)
- Antiepileptics (carbamazepine, fosphenytoin, phenobarbital, phenytoin, primidone) are predicted to decrease the exposure to **regorafenib**. Avoid. [Moderate] Study
- Antifungals, azoles (itraconazole, ketoconazole, voriconazole) are predicted to increase the exposure to **regorafenib**. Avoid. [Moderate] Study
- Cobicistat is predicted to increase the exposure to **regorafenib**. Avoid. [Moderate] Study
- **Regorafenib** is predicted to increase the risk of bleeding events when given with coumarins. [Severe] Study
- Enzalutamide is predicted to decrease the exposure to **regorafenib**. Avoid. [Moderate] Study
- Grapefruit juice is predicted to increase the exposure to **regorafenib**. Avoid. [Moderate] Theoretical
- HIV-protease inhibitors are predicted to increase the exposure to **regorafenib**. Avoid. [Moderate] Study
- Idelalisib is predicted to increase the exposure to **regorafenib**. Avoid. [Moderate] Study → Also see TABLE 15 p. 1337
- Macrolides (clarithromycin) are predicted to increase the exposure to **regorafenib**. Avoid. [Moderate] Study
- **Regorafenib** is predicted to increase the exposure to methotrexate. [Severe] Theoretical → Also see TABLE 15 p. 1337
- Mitotane is predicted to decrease the exposure to **regorafenib**. Avoid. [Moderate] Study → Also see TABLE 15 p. 1337
- **Regorafenib** is predicted to increase the exposure to NSAIDs (mefenamic acid). Avoid. [Moderate] Theoretical → Also see TABLE 4 p. 1334
- **Regorafenib** is predicted to increase the risk of bleeding events when given with phenindione. [Severe] Theoretical
- Rifampicin is predicted to decrease the exposure to **regorafenib**. Avoid. [Moderate] Study
- **Regorafenib** is predicted to increase the exposure to statins (atorvastatin, fluvastatin, rosuvastatin). [Severe] Theoretical

Remifentanil → see opioids

Repaglinide → see TABLE 14 p. 1337 (antidiabetic drugs)
- Antiepileptics (carbamazepine, fosphenytoin, phenobarbital, phenytoin, primidone) are predicted to decrease the exposure to **repaglinide**. Monitor blood glucose and adjust dose. [Moderate] Study
- Antifungals, azoles (itraconazole, ketoconazole, voriconazole) are predicted to increase the exposure to **repaglinide**. [Moderate] Study
- Ciclosporin moderately increases the exposure to **repaglinide**. [Moderate] Study
- Clopidogrel increases the exposure to **repaglinide**. Avoid. [Severe] Study
- Cobicistat is predicted to increase the exposure to **repaglinide**. [Moderate] Study
- Enzalutamide is predicted to decrease the exposure to **repaglinide**. Monitor blood glucose and adjust dose. [Moderate] Study
- Fibrates (gemfibrozil) increase the exposure to **repaglinide**. Avoid. [Severe] Study
- HIV-protease inhibitors are predicted to increase the exposure to **repaglinide**. [Moderate] Study
- Idelalisib is predicted to increase the exposure to **repaglinide**. [Moderate] Study
- Iron chelators (deferasirox) moderately increase the exposure to **repaglinide**. Avoid. [Moderate] Study

Repaglinide (continued)

▶ Leflunomide is predicted to increase the exposure to **repaglinide**. Moderate Study
▶ Macrolides (clarithromycin) are predicted to increase the exposure to **repaglinide**. Moderate Study
▶ Mitotane is predicted to decrease the exposure to **repaglinide**. Monitor blood glucose and adjust dose. Moderate Study
▶ Opicapone is predicted to increase the exposure to **repaglinide**. Avoid. Moderate Study
▶ Pitolisant is predicted to decrease the exposure to **repaglinide**. Unknown Theoretical
▶ Rifampicin is predicted to decrease the exposure to **repaglinide**. Monitor blood glucose and adjust dose. Moderate Study
▶ Teriflunomide is predicted to increase the exposure to **repaglinide**. Moderate Study
▶ Trimethoprim slightly increases the exposure to **repaglinide**. Avoid or monitor blood glucose. Moderate Study

Retigabine → see antiepileptics
Retinoids → see TABLE 5 p. 1334 (thromboembolism)

acitretin · adapalene · alitretinoin · bexarotene · isotretinoin · tazarotene · tretinoin

▶ Avoid concomitant use of keratolytics in patients taking **acitretin** and **isotretinoin**.
▶ Since systemic absorption can follow topical application of **isotretinoin**, the possibility of interactions should be borne in mind.

▶ Alcohol (beverage) potentially increases the concentration of **acitretin**. Avoid and for 2 months after stopping **acitretin**, p. 1225. Moderate Study
▶ Antiarrhythmics (amiodarone) are predicted to increase the exposure to **alitretinoin**. Adjust **alitretinoin** dose, p. 1226. Moderate Theoretical
▶ Antifungals, azoles (fluconazole, itraconazole, ketoconazole, miconazole, voriconazole) are predicted to increase the exposure to **alitretinoin**. Adjust **alitretinoin** dose, p. 1226. Moderate Theoretical
▶ Antifungals, azoles (fluconazole, ketoconazole, voriconazole) are predicted to increase the risk of tretinoin toxicity when given with **tretinoin**. Moderate Study
▶ Clopidogrel is predicted to increase the exposure to **alitretinoin**. Adjust **alitretinoin** dose, p. 1226. Moderate Theoretical
▶ Cobicistat is predicted to increase the exposure to **alitretinoin**. Adjust **alitretinoin** dose, p. 1226. Moderate Theoretical
▶ Fibrates (gemfibrozil) are predicted to increase the exposure to **alitretinoin**. Adjust **alitretinoin** dose, p. 1226. Moderate Theoretical
▶ Fibrates (gemfibrozil) increase the concentration of **bexarotene**. Avoid. Severe Study
▶ HIV-protease inhibitors are predicted to increase the exposure to **alitretinoin**. Adjust **alitretinoin** dose, p. 1226. Moderate Theoretical
▶ Idelalisib is predicted to increase the exposure to **alitretinoin**. Adjust **alitretinoin** dose, p. 1226. Moderate Theoretical
▶ Macrolides (clarithromycin) are predicted to increase the exposure to **alitretinoin**. Adjust **alitretinoin** dose, p. 1226. Moderate Theoretical
▶ **Acitretin** is predicted to increase the concentration of methotrexate. Avoid. Moderate Anecdotal
▶ Sulfinpyrazone is predicted to increase the exposure to **alitretinoin**. Adjust **alitretinoin** dose, p. 1226. Moderate Theoretical
▶ Retinoids (acitretin, alitretinoin, isotretinoin, tretinoin) increase the risk of benign intracranial hypertension when given with tetracyclines. Avoid. Severe Anecdotal
▶ **Bexarotene** is predicted to increase the risk of toxicity when given with vitamin A. Adjust dose. Moderate Theoretical
▶ Retinoids (acitretin, alitretinoin, isotretinoin) are predicted to increase the risk of vitamin A toxicity when given with vitamin A. Avoid. Severe Theoretical
▶ **Tretinoin** is predicted to increase the risk of vitamin A toxicity when given with vitamin A. Avoid. Severe Study

Ribavirin

▶ **Ribavirin** is predicted to increase the exposure to didanosine. Avoid. Severe Study

▶ **Ribavirin** increases the risk of toxicity when given with stavudine. Avoid. Severe Study
▶ **Ribavirin** increases the risk of anaemia and/or leucopenia when given with zidovudine. Avoid. Severe Study

Ribociclib → see TABLE 9 p. 1336 (QT-interval prolongation)

FOOD AND LIFESTYLE Avoid concomitant use of pomegranate or pomegranate juice as it is predicted to increase ribociclib exposure.

▶ **Ribociclib** (high-dose) is predicted to increase the exposure to alpha blockers (alfuzosin). Avoid. Moderate Theoretical
▶ Antiarrhythmics (dronedarone) are predicted to increase the exposure to **ribociclib**. Moderate Study → Also see TABLE 9 p. 1336
▶ **Ribociclib** (high-dose) is predicted to increase the exposure to antiarrhythmics (amiodarone). Avoid. Moderate Theoretical → Also see TABLE 9 p. 1336
▶ Antiepileptics (carbamazepine, fosphenytoin, phenobarbital, phenytoin, primidone) are predicted to markedly decrease the exposure to **ribociclib**. Severe Study
▶ Antifungals, azoles (fluconazole, isavuconazole, posaconazole) are predicted to increase the exposure to **ribociclib**. Moderate Study → Also see TABLE 9 p. 1336
▶ Antifungals, azoles (itraconazole, ketoconazole, voriconazole) are predicted to increase the exposure to **ribociclib**. Avoid or adjust **ribociclib** dose, p. 965. Moderate Study → Also see TABLE 9 p. 1336
▶ Aprepitant is predicted to increase the exposure to **ribociclib**. Moderate Study
▶ Bosentan is predicted to decrease the exposure to **ribociclib**. Moderate Study
▶ Calcium channel blockers (diltiazem, verapamil) are predicted to increase the exposure to **ribociclib**. Moderate Study
▶ **Ribociclib** is predicted to increase the exposure to ciclosporin. Use with caution and adjust dose. Moderate Theoretical
▶ Cobicistat is predicted to increase the exposure to **ribociclib**. Avoid or adjust **ribociclib** dose, p. 965. Moderate Study
▶ Crizotinib is predicted to increase the exposure to **ribociclib**. Moderate Study → Also see TABLE 9 p. 1336
▶ Efavirenz is predicted to decrease the exposure to **ribociclib**. Moderate Study → Also see TABLE 9 p. 1336
▶ Enzalutamide is predicted to markedly decrease the exposure to **ribociclib**. Avoid. Severe Study
▶ **Ribociclib** (high-dose) is predicted to increase the exposure to ergotamine. Avoid. Moderate Theoretical
▶ **Ribociclib** is predicted to increase the exposure to everolimus. Use with caution and adjust dose. Moderate Theoretical
▶ Grapefruit juice is predicted to increase the exposure to **ribociclib**. Avoid. Moderate Theoretical
▶ HIV-protease inhibitors are predicted to increase the exposure to **ribociclib**. Avoid or adjust **ribociclib** dose, p. 965. Moderate Study → Also see TABLE 9 p. 1336
▶ Idelalisib is predicted to increase the exposure to **ribociclib**. Avoid or adjust **ribociclib** dose, p. 965. Moderate Study
▶ Imatinib is predicted to increase the exposure to **ribociclib**. Moderate Study
▶ Macrolides (clarithromycin) are predicted to increase the exposure to **ribociclib**. Avoid or adjust **ribociclib** dose, p. 965. Moderate Study → Also see TABLE 9 p. 1336
▶ Macrolides (erythromycin) are predicted to increase the exposure to **ribociclib**. Moderate Study → Also see TABLE 9 p. 1336
▶ **Ribociclib** moderately increases the exposure to midazolam. Avoid. Moderate Study
▶ Mitotane is predicted to markedly decrease the exposure to **ribociclib**. Avoid. Severe Study
▶ Netupitant is predicted to increase the exposure to **ribociclib**. Moderate Study
▶ Nevirapine is predicted to decrease the exposure to **ribociclib**. Moderate Study
▶ Nilotinib is predicted to increase the exposure to **ribociclib**. Moderate Study → Also see TABLE 9 p. 1336
▶ **Ribociclib** is predicted to increase the exposure to opioids (alfentanil, fentanyl). Use with caution and adjust dose. Moderate Theoretical
▶ **Ribociclib** is predicted to increase the exposure to phosphodiesterase type-5 inhibitors (sildenafil). Avoid. Moderate Theoretical → Also see TABLE 9 p. 1336

Interactions | Appendix 1

A1

- **Ribociclib** (high-dose) is predicted to increase the exposure to pimozide. Avoid. Moderate Theoretical → Also see TABLE 9 p. 1336
- **Ribociclib** (high-dose) is predicted to increase the exposure to quetiapine. Avoid. Moderate Theoretical
- **Rifampicin** is predicted to markedly decrease the exposure to **ribociclib**. Avoid. Severe Study
- **Ribociclib** is predicted to increase the exposure to sirolimus. Use with caution and adjust dose. Moderate Theoretical
- **St John's Wort** is predicted to decrease the exposure to **ribociclib**. Avoid. Severe Study
- **Ribociclib** (high-dose) is predicted to increase the exposure to statins (simvastatin). Avoid. Moderate Theoretical
- **Ribociclib** is predicted to increase the exposure to tacrolimus. Use with caution and adjust dose. Moderate Theoretical

Rifabutin

GENERAL INFORMATION Although some manufacturers class rifabutin as a potent inducer of CYP3A4, clinical data suggests it is potentially a weak inducer, and therefore the BNF does not extrapolate the interactions of potent CYP3A4 inducers to rifabutin. For those who wish to err on the side of caution, see the interactions of rifampicin but bear in mind other mechanisms might be involved.

- Antifungals, azoles (fluconazole) increase the risk of uveitis when given with **rifabutin**. Adjust dose. Severe Study
- Antifungals, azoles (itraconazole, posaconazole) increase the concentration of **rifabutin** and **rifabutin** decreases the concentration of antifungals, azoles (itraconazole, posaconazole). Avoid. Severe Study
- Antifungals, azoles (ketoconazole) are predicted to increase the concentration of **rifabutin** and **rifabutin** is predicted to decrease the concentration of antifungals, azoles (ketoconazole). Avoid. Severe Study
- Antifungals, azoles (miconazole) are predicted to increase the concentration of **rifabutin**. Use with caution and adjust dose. Moderate Theoretical
- **Rifabutin** is predicted to decrease the exposure to antifungals, azoles (isavuconazole). Avoid. Severe Theoretical
- **Rifabutin** decreases the concentration of antifungals, azoles (voriconazole) and antifungals, azoles (voriconazole) increase the concentration of **rifabutin**. Avoid or adjust **voriconazole** dose, p. 588. Severe Study
- **Rifabutin** slightly decreases the exposure to antimalarials (atovaquone). Avoid. Moderate Study
- **Rifabutin** is predicted to decrease the concentration of cobicistat and cobicistat increases the exposure to **rifabutin**. Avoid or adjust dose. Severe Study
- **Rifabutin** is predicted to decrease the efficacy of combined hormonal contraceptives. For FSRH guidance, see Contraceptives, interactions p. 775. Severe Study
- **Rifabutin** decreases the exposure to dapsone. Moderate Study
- **Rifabutin** is predicted to decrease the efficacy of desogestrel. For FSRH guidance, see Contraceptives, interactions p. 775. Severe Theoretical
- **Efavirenz** slightly decreases the exposure to **rifabutin**. Adjust dose. Severe Study
- **Rifabutin** is predicted to decrease the efficacy of etonogestrel. For FSRH guidance, see Contraceptives, interactions p. 775. Severe Theoretical
- **Rifabutin** decreases the exposure to etravirine. Moderate Study
- HIV-protease inhibitors (atazanavir, darunavir, fosamprenavir, lopinavir, saquinavir, tipranavir) (boosted with ritonavir) increase the exposure to **rifabutin**. Monitor and adjust dose. Severe Study
- HIV-protease inhibitors (ritonavir) markedly increase the exposure to **rifabutin**. Avoid or adjust dose. Severe Study
- **Rifabutin** is predicted to decrease the effects of hormone replacement therapy. Moderate Anecdotal
- **Rifabutin** is predicted to decrease the efficacy of levonorgestrel. For FSRH guidance, see Contraceptives, interactions p. 775. Severe Theoretical
- **Lumacaftor** is predicted to decrease the exposure to **rifabutin**. Adjust dose. Moderate Theoretical
- Macrolides (azithromycin) increase the risk of neutropenia when given with **rifabutin**. Severe Study
- Macrolides (clarithromycin) increase the risk of uveitis when given with **rifabutin**. Adjust dose. Severe Study
- Macrolides (erythromycin) are predicted to increase the risk of uveitis when given with **rifabutin**. Adjust dose. Severe Theoretical
- **Rifabutin** is predicted to decrease the efficacy of norethisterone. For FSRH guidance, see Contraceptives, interactions p. 775. Severe Anecdotal
- **Rifabutin** slightly decreases the exposure to rilpivirine. Adjust dose. Severe Study
- **Rifabutin** is predicted to decrease the exposure to rolapitant. Avoid. Moderate Theoretical
- **Rifabutin** is predicted to decrease the exposure to simeprevir. Avoid. Moderate Theoretical
- **Rifabutin** is predicted to decrease the exposure to tenofovir alafenamide. Avoid. Moderate Theoretical
- **Rifabutin** decreases the efficacy of ulipristal. For FSRH guidance, see Contraceptives, interactions p. 775. Severe Anecdotal
- **Rifabutin** is predicted to decrease the concentration of voxilaprevir. Avoid. Severe Theoretical

Rifampicin

- **Rifampicin** is predicted to decrease the exposure to abiraterone. Avoid. Severe Theoretical
- **Rifampicin** is predicted to decrease the exposure to afatinib. Moderate Study
- **Rifampicin** is predicted to decrease the exposure to agomelatine. Moderate Theoretical
- **Rifampicin** is predicted to decrease the exposure to aldosterone antagonists (eplerenone). Avoid. Moderate Theoretical
- **Rifampicin** decreases the exposure to aliskiren. Moderate Study
- **Rifampicin** is predicted to decrease the exposure to alprazolam. Adjust dose. Moderate Theoretical
- **Rifampicin** transiently increases the exposure to ambrisentan. Moderate Study
- **Rifampicin** decreases the exposure to aminophylline. Adjust dose. Moderate Study
- **Rifampicin** is predicted to decrease the exposure to anaesthetics, local (ropivacaine). Moderate Theoretical
- Antacids decrease the absorption of **rifampicin**. **Rifampicin** should be taken 1 hour before **antacids**. Moderate Study
- **Rifampicin** is predicted to decrease the exposure to antiarrhythmics (disopyramide, dronedarone). Avoid. Severe Study
- **Rifampicin** is predicted to decrease the efficacy of antiarrhythmics (propafenone). Moderate Study
- **Rifampicin** is predicted to decrease the exposure to anticholinesterases, centrally acting (donepezil). Mild Study
- Antiepileptics (phenobarbital, primidone) are predicted to decrease the exposure to **rifampicin** and **rifampicin** is predicted to decrease the exposure to antiepileptics (phenobarbital, primidone). Use with caution and adjust dose. Moderate Study
- **Rifampicin** slightly decreases the exposure to antiepileptics (brivaracetam). Adjust dose. Moderate Study
- **Rifampicin** decreases the concentration of antiepileptics (fosphenytoin, phenytoin). Use with caution and adjust dose. Moderate Study
- **Rifampicin** markedly increases the clearance of antiepileptics (lamotrigine). Adjust lamotrigine dose, p. 316. Moderate Study
- **Rifampicin** is predicted to decrease the exposure to antiepileptics (perampanel). Monitor and adjust dose. Moderate Study
- **Rifampicin** slightly decreases the exposure to antifungals, azoles (fluconazole). Adjust dose. Moderate Study
- **Rifampicin** is predicted to decrease the exposure to antifungals, azoles (isavuconazole). Avoid. Severe Study
- **Rifampicin** markedly decreases the exposure to antifungals, azoles (itraconazole). Avoid and for 14 days after stopping **rifampicin**. Moderate Study
- **Rifampicin** markedly decreases the exposure to antifungals, azoles (ketoconazole) and antifungals, azoles (ketoconazole) potentially decrease the exposure to **rifampicin**. Avoid. Moderate Study
- **Rifampicin** is predicted to decrease the exposure to antifungals, azoles (posaconazole). Avoid. Moderate Anecdotal

Rifampicin (continued)

▸ **Rifampicin** very markedly decreases the exposure to antifungals, azoles (**voriconazole**). Avoid. Moderate Study
▸ **Rifampicin** is predicted to decrease the exposure to antihistamines, non-sedating (**bilastine**). Moderate Theoretical
▸ **Rifampicin** increases the clearance of antihistamines, non-sedating (**fexofenadine**). Moderate Study
▸ **Rifampicin** is predicted to decrease the exposure to antimalarials (**artemether**) (with lumefantrine). Avoid. Severe Study
▸ **Rifampicin** moderately decreases the exposure to antimalarials (**atovaquone**) and antimalarials (**atovaquone**) slightly increase the exposure to **rifampicin**. Avoid. Moderate Study
▸ **Rifampicin** moderately decreases the exposure to antimalarials (**mefloquine**). Severe Study
▸ **Rifampicin** is predicted to decrease the concentration of antimalarials (**piperaquine**). Avoid. Moderate Theoretical
▸ **Rifampicin** decreases the exposure to antimalarials (**quinine**). Severe Study
▸ **Rifampicin** is predicted to moderately decrease the exposure to apixaban. Use with caution or avoid. Severe Study
▸ **Rifampicin** moderately decreases the exposure to apremilast. Avoid. Severe Study
▸ **Rifampicin** is predicted to markedly decrease the exposure to aprepitant. Avoid. Moderate Study
▸ **Rifampicin** is predicted to moderately decrease the exposure to aripiprazole. Adjust **aripiprazole** dose, p. 391. Moderate Study
▸ **Rifampicin** decreases the exposure to ataluren. Moderate Study
▸ **Rifampicin** is predicted to decrease the exposure to axitinib. Avoid or adjust dose. Moderate Study
▸ **Rifampicin** is predicted to decrease the exposure to bazedoxifene. Moderate Theoretical
▸ **Rifampicin** decreases the exposure to bedaquiline. Avoid. Severe Study
▸ **Rifampicin** moderately decreases the exposure to beta blockers, non-selective (**carvedilol**). Moderate Study
▸ **Rifampicin** decreases the exposure to beta blockers, non-selective (**propranolol**). Monitor and adjust dose. Moderate Study
▸ **Rifampicin** slightly decreases the exposure to beta blockers, selective (**bisoprolol, metoprolol**). Mild Study
▸ **Rifampicin** moderately decreases the exposure to beta blockers, selective (**celiprolol**). Moderate Study
▸ **Rifampicin** slightly decreases the exposure to bortezomib. Avoid. Severe Study
▸ **Rifampicin** affects the exposure to bosentan. Avoid. Severe Study
▸ **Rifampicin** is predicted to very markedly decrease the exposure to bosutinib. Avoid. Severe Study
▸ **Rifampicin** is predicted to decrease the exposure to bupropion. Moderate Study
▸ **Rifampicin** is predicted to decrease the exposure to buspirone. Use with caution and adjust dose. Severe Study
▸ **Rifampicin** moderately decreases the exposure to cabozantinib. Avoid. Moderate Study
▸ **Rifampicin** is predicted to moderately increase the clearance of caffeine citrate. Monitor and adjust dose. Moderate Study
▸ **Rifampicin** is predicted to decrease the exposure to calcium channel blockers (**amlodipine, felodipine, lacidipine, lercanidipine, nicardipine, nimodipine**). Monitor and adjust dose. Moderate Study
▸ **Rifampicin** greatly decreases the exposure to calcium channel blockers (**diltiazem, verapamil**). Severe Study
▸ **Rifampicin** moderately decreases the exposure to calcium channel blockers (**nifedipine**). Avoid. Severe Study
▸ **Rifampicin** moderately decreases the exposure to canagliflozin. Adjust **canagliflozin** dose, p. 687. Moderate Study
▸ **Rifampicin** is predicted to decrease the exposure to cannabis extract. Avoid. Severe Theoretical
▸ **Rifampicin** decreases the concentration of caspofungin. Adjust **caspofungin** dose, p. 582. Moderate Study
▸ **Rifampicin** is predicted to decrease the exposure to ceritinib. Avoid. Severe Study
▸ **Rifampicin** decreases the concentration of chloramphenicol. Moderate Study

▸ **Rifampicin** is predicted to decrease the exposure to chlordiazepoxide. Moderate Theoretical
▸ **Rifampicin** decreases the concentration of ciclosporin. Severe Study
▸ **Rifampicin** is predicted to alter the effects of cilostazol. Moderate Theoretical
▸ **Rifampicin** is predicted to decrease the exposure to cinacalcet. Monitor and adjust dose. Moderate Study
▸ **Rifampicin** decreases the exposure to clomethiazole. Monitor and adjust dose. Moderate Study
▸ **Rifampicin** decreases the exposure to clozapine. Severe Anecdotal
▸ **Rifampicin** is predicted to decrease the exposure to cobicistat. Avoid. Severe Theoretical
▸ **Rifampicin** is predicted to decrease the exposure to cobimetinib. Avoid. Severe Theoretical
▸ **Rifampicin** is predicted to decrease the efficacy of combined hormonal contraceptives. For FSRH guidance, see Contraceptives, interactions p. 775. Severe Study
▸ **Rifampicin** is predicted to decrease the exposure to corticosteroids (**budesonide, deflazacort, dexamethasone, fludrocortisone, hydrocortisone, methylprednisolone, prednisolone, prednisone, triamcinolone**). Monitor and adjust dose. Moderate Study
▸ **Rifampicin** is predicted to decrease the exposure to corticosteroids (**fluticasone**). Unknown Theoretical
▸ **Rifampicin** decreases the anticoagulant effect of coumarins. Severe Study
▸ **Rifampicin** is predicted to markedly decrease the exposure to crizotinib. Avoid. Severe Study
▸ **Rifampicin** is predicted to decrease the exposure to dabigatran. Avoid. Severe Study
▸ **Rifampicin** is predicted to decrease the exposure to dabrafenib. Avoid. Moderate Theoretical
▸ **Rifampicin** is predicted to moderately decrease the exposure to daclatasvir. Avoid. Severe Study
▸ **Rifampicin** decreases the exposure to dapsone. Moderate Study
▸ **Rifampicin** is predicted to decrease the exposure to darifenacin. Moderate Theoretical
▸ **Rifampicin** is predicted to decrease the exposure to dasabuvir. Avoid. Severe Theoretical
▸ **Rifampicin** is predicted to markedly decrease the exposure to dasatinib. Avoid. Severe Study
▸ **Rifampicin** is predicted to slightly decrease the exposure to delamanid. Avoid. Moderate Study
▸ **Rifampicin** is predicted to decrease the efficacy of desogestrel. For FSRH guidance, see Contraceptives, interactions p. 775. Severe Theoretical
▸ **Rifampicin** moderately decreases the exposure to diazepam. Avoid. Moderate Study
▸ **Rifampicin** decreases the concentration of digoxin. Moderate Study
▸ **Rifampicin** decreases the exposure to dolutegravir. Adjust dose. Severe Study
▸ **Rifampicin** is predicted to decrease the exposure to duloxetine. Moderate Theoretical
▸ **Rifampicin** is predicted to decrease the exposure to edoxaban. Moderate Study
▸ **Rifampicin** slightly decreases the exposure to efavirenz. Adjust dose. Severe Study
▸ **Rifampicin** is predicted to decrease the exposure to elbasvir. Avoid. Severe Study
▸ **Rifampicin** is predicted to decrease the exposure to eliglustat. Avoid. Severe Study
▸ **Rifampicin** is predicted to increase the exposure to eluxadoline. Avoid. Moderate Theoretical
▸ **Rifampicin** is predicted to decrease the concentration of elvitegravir. Avoid. Severe Theoretical
▸ **Rifampicin** is predicted to decrease the effects of ergotamine. Moderate Theoretical
▸ **Rifampicin** is predicted to decrease the exposure to erlotinib. Avoid or adjust **erlotinib** dose, p. 949. Severe Study
▸ **Rifampicin** is predicted to decrease the efficacy of etonogestrel. For FSRH guidance, see Contraceptives, interactions p. 775. Severe Theoretical

▶ **Rifampicin** is predicted to decrease the exposure to etravirine. Avoid. Severe Theoretical

▶ **Rifampicin** is predicted to decrease the concentration of everolimus. Avoid or adjust dose. Severe Study

▶ **Rifampicin** moderately decreases the exposure to exemestane. Moderate Study

▶ **Rifampicin** is predicted to decrease the exposure to fesoterodine. Avoid. Moderate Study

▶ **Rifampicin** is predicted to decrease the exposure to fingolimod. Moderate Study

▶ **Rifampicin** is predicted to decrease the exposure to fosaprepitant. Avoid. Moderate Theoretical

▶ **Rifampicin** is predicted to decrease the exposure to gefitinib. Avoid. Severe Study

▶ **Rifampicin** markedly affects the exposure to glecaprevir. Avoid. Severe Study

▶ **Rifampicin** is predicted to decrease the exposure to grazoprevir. Avoid. Severe Study

▶ **Rifampicin** is predicted to decrease the concentration of guanfacine. Adjust **guanfacine** dose, p. 349. Moderate Study

▶ **Rifampicin** decreases the concentration of haloperidol. Adjust dose. Moderate Study

▶ **Rifampicin** is predicted to moderately to markedly decrease the exposure to HIV-protease inhibitors (atazanavir, darunavir, fosamprenavir, lopinavir, saquinavir). Avoid. Severe Study

▶ **Rifampicin** slightly decreases the exposure to HIV-protease inhibitors (ritonavir). Severe Study

▶ **Rifampicin** is predicted to decrease the exposure to HIV-protease inhibitors (tipranavir). Avoid. Severe Study

▶ **Rifampicin** is predicted to decrease the effects of hormone replacement therapy. Moderate Anecdotal

▶ **Rifampicin** is predicted to decrease the exposure to ibrutinib. Avoid or adjust **ibrutinib** dose, p. 952. Severe Study

▶ **Rifampicin** is predicted to decrease the exposure to idelalisib. Avoid. Severe Study

▶ **Rifampicin** is predicted to decrease the exposure to imatinib. Avoid. Moderate Study

▶ **Rifampicin** is predicted to decrease the exposure to irinotecan. Avoid. Severe Study

▶ **Rifampicin** is predicted to decrease the exposure to iron chelators (deferasirox). Monitor serum ferritin and adjust dose. Moderate Study

▶ **Rifampicin** is predicted to decrease the exposure to ivabradine. Adjust dose. Moderate Theoretical

▶ **Rifampicin** is predicted to moderately to markedly decrease the exposure to ivacaftor. Avoid. Severe Study

▶ **Rifampicin** is predicted to decrease the exposure to ixazomib. Avoid. Severe Study

▶ **Rifampicin** is predicted to decrease the exposure to lapatinib. Avoid. Severe Study

▶ **Rifampicin** is predicted to decrease the exposure to ledipasvir. Avoid. Severe Theoretical

▶ **Rifampicin** is predicted to decrease the efficacy of levonorgestrel. For FSRH guidance, see Contraceptives, interactions p. 775. Severe Theoretical

▶ **Rifampicin** is predicted to decrease the exposure to linagliptin. Moderate Study

▶ **Rifampicin** slightly decreases the exposure to linezolid. Moderate Study

▶ **Rifampicin** is predicted to decrease the exposure to lomitapide. Monitor and adjust dose. Moderate Theoretical

▶ **Rifampicin** increases the clearance of lorazepam. Moderate Study

▶ **Rifampicin** is predicted to decrease the exposure to lurasidone. Avoid. Moderate Study

▶ **Rifampicin** is predicted to decrease the exposure to macitentan. Avoid. Severe Study

▶ **Rifampicin** decreases the concentration of macrolides (clarithromycin). Severe Study

▶ **Rifampicin** is predicted to decrease the exposure to maraviroc. Adjust dose. Severe Study

▶ **Rifampicin** is predicted to decrease the exposure to melatonin. Moderate Theoretical

▶ **Rifampicin** is predicted to decrease the exposure to midazolam. Monitor and adjust dose. Moderate Study

▶ **Rifampicin** is predicted to decrease the exposure to midostaurin. Avoid. Severe Study

▶ **Rifampicin** is predicted to decrease the exposure to mirtazapine. Adjust dose. Moderate Study

▶ **Rifampicin** is predicted to decrease the exposure to modafinil. Moderate Theoretical

▶ **Rifampicin** decreases the effects of monoclonal antibodies (brentuximab vedotin). Severe Study

▶ **Rifampicin** is predicted to decrease the exposure to montelukast. Mild Study

▶ **Rifampicin** decreases the concentration of mycophenolate. Monitor and adjust dose. Severe Study

▶ **Rifampicin** is predicted to markedly decrease the exposure to naloxegol. Avoid. Moderate Study

▶ **Rifampicin** is predicted to slightly decrease the exposure to nateglinide. Mild Study

▶ **Rifampicin** is predicted to decrease the exposure to netupitant. Avoid. Severe Study

▶ **Rifampicin** decreases the concentration of nevirapine. Avoid. Severe Study

▶ **Rifampicin** is predicted to moderately decrease the exposure to nilotinib. Avoid. Severe Study

▶ **Rifampicin** is predicted to decrease the exposure to nintedanib. Moderate Study

▶ **Rifampicin** is predicted to decrease the exposure to nitisinone. Adjust dose. Moderate Theoretical

▶ **Rifampicin** increases the clearance of nitrazepam. Moderate Study

▶ **Rifampicin** is predicted to decrease the efficacy of norethisterone. For FSRH guidance, see Contraceptives, interactions p. 775. Severe Anecdotal

▶ **Rifampicin** moderately decreases the exposure to NSAIDs (celecoxib, diclofenac, etoricoxib). Moderate Study

▶ **Rifampicin** is predicted to decrease the exposure to olanzapine. Monitor and adjust dose. Moderate Study

▶ **Rifampicin** is predicted to decrease the exposure to olaparib. Avoid. Moderate Theoretical

▶ **Rifampicin** is predicted to decrease the exposure to ombitasvir. Avoid. Severe Theoretical

▶ **Rifampicin** is predicted to decrease the exposure to ondansetron. Moderate Study

▶ **Rifampicin** is predicted to decrease the exposure to opioids (alfentanil, fentanyl). Moderate Study

▶ **Rifampicin** is predicted to decrease the exposure to opioids (buprenorphine). Monitor and adjust dose. Moderate Theoretical

▶ **Rifampicin** decreases the exposure to opioids (codeine, morphine). Moderate Study

▶ **Rifampicin** decreases the exposure to opioids (methadone). Monitor and adjust dose. Severe Study

▶ **Rifampicin** is predicted to decrease the exposure to opioids (oxycodone). Monitor and adjust dose. Moderate Study

▶ **Rifampicin** is predicted to moderately decrease the exposure to osimertinib. Avoid. Moderate Study

▶ **Rifampicin** is predicted to decrease the exposure to palbociclib. Avoid. Severe Study

▶ **Rifampicin** is predicted to decrease the exposure to paliperidone. Monitor and adjust dose. Severe Study

▶ **Rifampicin** is predicted to decrease the exposure to panobinostat. Avoid. Moderate Theoretical

▶ **Rifampicin** decreases the exposure to paracetamol. Moderate Study

▶ **Rifampicin** is predicted to decrease the exposure to paritaprevir (with ritonavir and ombitasvir). Avoid. Severe Study

▶ **Rifampicin** is predicted to decrease the exposure to pazopanib. Avoid. Severe Theoretical

▶ **Rifampicin** is predicted to decrease the exposure to phosphodiesterase type-5 inhibitors (avanafil, tadalafil). Avoid. Severe Study

▶ **Rifampicin** is predicted to decrease the exposure to phosphodiesterase type-5 inhibitors (sildenafil, vardenafil). Moderate Theoretical

▶ **Rifampicin** is predicted to moderately to markedly decrease the exposure to pibrentasvir. Avoid. Severe Study

Rifampicin (continued)
▶ **Rifampicin** moderately decreases the exposure to pioglitazone. Monitor and adjust dose. Moderate Study
▶ **Rifampicin** is predicted to decrease the exposure to pirfenidone. Avoid. Moderate Theoretical
▶ **Rifampicin** is predicted to moderately decrease the exposure to pitolisant. Moderate Study
▶ **Rifampicin** is predicted to decrease the exposure to ponatinib. Avoid. Moderate Theoretical
▶ **Rifampicin** is predicted to markedly decrease the exposure to praziquantel. Avoid. Moderate Study
▶ **Rifampicin** is predicted to decrease the exposure to quetiapine. Moderate Study
▶ **Rifampicin** slightly decreases the exposure to raltegravir. Avoid or adjust dose—consult product literature. Moderate Study
▶ **Rifampicin** is predicted to decrease the exposure to ranolazine. Avoid. Severe Study
▶ **Rifampicin** is predicted to decrease the exposure to reboxetine. Moderate Anecdotal
▶ **Rifampicin** is predicted to decrease the exposure to regorafenib. Avoid. Moderate Study
▶ **Rifampicin** is predicted to decrease the exposure to repaglinide. Monitor blood glucose and adjust dose. Moderate Study
▶ **Rifampicin** is predicted to markedly decrease the exposure to ribociclib. Avoid. Severe Study
▶ **Rifampicin** markedly decreases the exposure to rilpivirine. Avoid. Severe Study
▶ **Rifampicin** is predicted to decrease the exposure to risperidone. Adjust dose. Moderate Study
▶ **Rifampicin** is predicted to moderately decrease the exposure to rivaroxaban. Avoid unless patient can be monitored for signs of thrombosis. Severe Study
▶ **Rifampicin** is predicted to decrease the exposure to roflumilast. Avoid. Moderate Study
▶ **Rifampicin** is predicted to markedly decrease the exposure to rolapitant. Avoid. Severe Study
▶ **Rifampicin** is predicted to decrease the exposure to ruxolitinib. Monitor and adjust dose. Moderate Study
▶ **Rifampicin** is predicted to moderately decrease the exposure to saxagliptin. Moderate Study
▶ **Rifampicin** moderately decreases the exposure to the active metabolite of selexipag. Adjust dose. Moderate Study
▶ **Rifampicin** is predicted to decrease the exposure to simeprevir. Avoid. Severe Study
▶ **Rifampicin** is predicted to decrease the concentration of sirolimus. Avoid. Severe Study
▶ **Rifampicin** is predicted to decrease the exposure to sofosbuvir. Avoid. Severe Study
▶ **Rifampicin** is predicted to decrease the exposure to solifenacin. Moderate Theoretical
▶ **Rifampicin** is predicted to decrease the exposure to sorafenib. Moderate Theoretical
▶ **Rifampicin** markedly decreases the exposure to statins (atorvastatin). **Atorvastatin** should be taken at the same time as **rifampicin**, p. 200, p. 571. Moderate Study
▶ **Rifampicin** moderately decreases the exposure to statins (fluvastatin). Monitor and adjust dose. Moderate Study
▶ **Rifampicin** very markedly decreases the exposure to statins (simvastatin). Moderate Study
▶ **Rifampicin** is predicted to decrease the exposure to sulfonylureas. Moderate Study
▶ **Rifampicin** is predicted to decrease the exposure to sunitinib. Avoid or adjust **sunitinib** dose, p. 967. Moderate Study
▶ **Rifampicin** decreases the concentration of tacrolimus. Monitor and adjust dose. Severe Study
▶ **Rifampicin** markedly decreases the exposure to tamoxifen. Unknown Study
▶ **Rifampicin** is predicted to decrease the exposure to taxanes (cabazitaxel, paclitaxel). Avoid. Severe Study
▶ **Rifampicin** is predicted to decrease the exposure to taxanes (docetaxel). Severe Theoretical
▶ **Rifampicin** is predicted to decrease the concentration of temsirolimus. Avoid. Severe Study

▶ **Rifampicin** is predicted to decrease the exposure to tenofovir alafenamide. Avoid. Moderate Theoretical
▶ **Rifampicin** decreases the exposure to terbinafine. Adjust dose. Moderate Study
▶ **Rifampicin** decreases the exposure to tetracyclines (doxycycline). Monitor and adjust dose. Moderate Study
▶ **Rifampicin** is predicted to decrease the exposure to theophylline. Adjust dose. Moderate Study
▶ **Rifampicin** is predicted to markedly decrease the exposure to ticagrelor. Avoid. Severe Study
▶ **Rifampicin** is predicted to decrease the exposure to tivozanib. Severe Study
▶ **Rifampicin** moderately decreases the exposure to tizanidine. Mild Study
▶ **Rifampicin** is predicted to decrease the exposure to tofacitinib. Avoid. Severe Study
▶ **Rifampicin** is predicted to decrease the exposure to tolvaptan. Avoid. Severe Study
▶ **Rifampicin** is predicted to decrease the exposure to toremifene. Adjust dose. Moderate Study
▶ **Rifampicin** is predicted to decrease the exposure to trabectedin. Avoid. Severe Theoretical
▶ **Rifampicin** decreases the exposure to trimethoprim. Moderate Study
▶ **Rifampicin** decreases the efficacy of ulipristal. For FSRH guidance, see Contraceptives, interactions p. 775. Severe Anecdotal
▶ **Rifampicin** is predicted to decrease the exposure to vandetanib. Avoid. Moderate Study
▶ **Rifampicin** is predicted to moderately decrease the exposure to velpatasvir. Avoid. Severe Study
▶ **Rifampicin** is predicted to decrease the exposure to vemurafenib. Avoid. Severe Theoretical
▶ **Rifampicin** is predicted to decrease the exposure to venetoclax. Avoid. Severe Study
▶ **Rifampicin** is predicted to decrease the exposure to vinca alkaloids (vinblastine, vincristine, vindesine). Severe Theoretical
▶ **Rifampicin** is predicted to decrease the exposure to vinca alkaloids (vinflunine). Avoid. Severe Theoretical
▶ **Rifampicin** is predicted to decrease the exposure to vinca alkaloids (vinorelbine). Use with caution or avoid. Severe Theoretical
▶ **Rifampicin** is predicted to decrease the exposure to vismodegib. Avoid. Moderate Theoretical
▶ **Rifampicin** potentially increases the risk of nephrotoxicity when given with volatile halogenated anaesthetics (methoxyflurane). Avoid. Severe Theoretical
▶ **Rifampicin** is predicted to decrease the exposure to vortioxetine. Monitor and adjust dose. Moderate Study
▶ **Rifampicin** is predicted to decrease the concentration of voxilaprevir. Avoid. Severe Study
▶ **Rifampicin** markedly decreases the exposure to zaleplon. Moderate Study
▶ **Rifampicin** moderately decreases the exposure to zolpidem. Moderate Study
▶ **Rifampicin** is predicted to decrease the exposure to zopiclone. Adjust dose. Moderate Study

Rifaximin
▶ Ciclosporin very markedly increases the exposure to **rifaximin**. Severe Study

Rilpivirine
▶ Antacids are predicted to decrease the exposure to **rilpivirine**. **Antacids** should be taken 2 hours before or 4 hours after **rilpivirine**, p. 634. Severe Theoretical
▶ Antiepileptics (carbamazepine, fosphenytoin, phenobarbital, phenytoin, primidone) markedly decrease the exposure to **rilpivirine**. Avoid. Severe Study
▶ Antiepileptics (oxcarbazepine) are predicted to decrease the concentration of **rilpivirine**. Avoid. Severe Theoretical
▶ Bosentan is predicted to decrease the exposure to **rilpivirine**. Avoid. Severe Theoretical
▶ Calcium salts (calcium carbonate) are predicted to slightly decrease the exposure to **rilpivirine**. **Calcium carbonate** should be taken 2 hours before or 4 hours after **rilpivirine**. Severe Theoretical

- Efavirenz is predicted to decrease the exposure to **rilpivirine**. Avoid. Severe Theoretical
- Enzalutamide markedly decreases the exposure to **rilpivirine**. Avoid. Severe Study
- Etravirine is predicted to decrease the exposure to **rilpivirine**. Avoid. Severe Theoretical
- H₂ receptor antagonists are predicted to decrease the exposure to **rilpivirine**. H₂ **receptor antagonists** should be taken 12 hours before or 4 hours after **rilpivirine**. Severe Study
- Mitotane markedly decreases the exposure to **rilpivirine**. Avoid. Severe Study
- Nevirapine is predicted to decrease the exposure to **rilpivirine**. Avoid. Severe Theoretical
- Proton pump inhibitors are predicted to decrease the exposure to **rilpivirine**. Avoid. Severe Study
- Rifabutin slightly decreases the exposure to **rilpivirine**. Adjust dose. Severe Study
- Rifampicin markedly decreases the exposure to **rilpivirine**. Avoid. Severe Study
- St John's Wort is predicted to decrease the exposure to **rilpivirine**. Avoid. Severe Theoretical

Riluzole

> FOOD AND LIFESTYLE Charcoal-grilled foods are predicted to decrease the exposure to riluzole.

- SSRIs (fluvoxamine) are predicted to increase the exposure to **riluzole**. Moderate Theoretical

Riociguat → see TABLE 8 p. 1335 (hypotension)
- Antacids slightly decrease the exposure to **riociguat**. Antacids should be taken 2 hours before or 1 hour after **riociguat**. Mild Study
- Antifungals, azoles (itraconazole) are predicted to increase the exposure to **riociguat**. Avoid. Moderate Study
- Antifungals, azoles (ketoconazole) moderately increase the exposure to **riociguat**. Avoid. Moderate Study
- Ciclosporin is predicted to increase the exposure to **riociguat**. Moderate Theoretical
- HIV-protease inhibitors (ritonavir) are predicted to increase the exposure to **riociguat**. Avoid. Moderate Theoretical
- Riociguat is predicted to increase the risk of hypotension when given with phosphodiesterase type-5 inhibitors. Avoid. Severe Theoretical → Also see TABLE 8 p. 1335

Risedronate → see bisphosphonates
Risperidone → see TABLE 8 p. 1335 (hypotension), TABLE 9 p. 1336 (QT-interval prolongation), TABLE 11 p. 1336 (CNS depressant effects)
- Antiepileptics (carbamazepine, fosphenytoin, phenobarbital, phenytoin, primidone) are predicted to decrease the exposure to **risperidone**. Adjust dose. Moderate Study → Also see TABLE 11 p. 1336
- Antifungals, azoles (itraconazole, ketoconazole, voriconazole) are predicted to increase the exposure to **risperidone**. Adjust dose. Moderate Study → Also see TABLE 9 p. 1336
- Bupropion is predicted to increase the exposure to **risperidone**. Adjust dose. Moderate Study
- Cinacalcet is predicted to increase the exposure to **risperidone**. Adjust dose. Moderate Study
- Cobicistat is predicted to increase the exposure to **risperidone**. Adjust dose. Moderate Study
- Risperidone is predicted to decrease the effects of dopamine receptor agonists. Avoid. Moderate Theoretical → Also see TABLE 8 p. 1335 → Also see TABLE 9 p. 1336
- Enzalutamide is predicted to decrease the exposure to **risperidone**. Adjust dose. Moderate Study
- HIV-protease inhibitors are predicted to increase the exposure to **risperidone**. Adjust dose. Moderate Study → Also see TABLE 9 p. 1336
- Idelalisib is predicted to increase the exposure to **risperidone**. Adjust dose. Moderate Study
- Risperidone is predicted to decrease the effects of levodopa. Avoid or adjust dose. Severe Anecdotal → Also see TABLE 8 p. 1335
- Risperidone potentially increases the risk of neurotoxicity when given with lithium. Severe Anecdotal → Also see TABLE 9 p. 1336
- Macrolides (clarithromycin) are predicted to increase the exposure to **risperidone**. Adjust dose. Moderate Study → Also see TABLE 9 p. 1336

- Risperidone increases the risk of dyskinesias when given with methylphenidate. Severe Anecdotal
- Mitotane is predicted to decrease the exposure to **risperidone**. Adjust dose. Moderate Study
- Rifampicin is predicted to decrease the exposure to **risperidone**. Adjust dose. Moderate Study
- SSRIs (fluoxetine, paroxetine) are predicted to increase the exposure to **risperidone**. Adjust dose. Moderate Study
- Terbinafine is predicted to increase the exposure to **risperidone**. Adjust dose. Moderate Study

Ritonavir → see HIV-protease inhibitors
Rituximab → see monoclonal antibodies
Rivaroxaban → see TABLE 3 p. 1334 (anticoagulant effects)
- Antiarrhythmics (dronedarone) are predicted to increase the exposure to **rivaroxaban**. Avoid. Moderate Theoretical
- Antiepileptics (carbamazepine, fosphenytoin, phenobarbital, phenytoin, primidone) are predicted to moderately decrease the exposure to **rivaroxaban**. Avoid unless patient can be monitored for signs of thrombosis. Severe Study
- Antifungals, azoles (itraconazole, ketoconazole) are predicted to moderately increase the exposure to **rivaroxaban**. Avoid. Severe Study
- Enzalutamide is predicted to moderately decrease the exposure to **rivaroxaban**. Avoid unless patient can be monitored for signs of thrombosis. Severe Study
- HIV-protease inhibitors (ritonavir) moderately increase the exposure to **rivaroxaban**. Avoid. Severe Study
- Mitotane is predicted to moderately decrease the exposure to **rivaroxaban**. Avoid unless patient can be monitored for signs of thrombosis. Severe Study
- Rifampicin is predicted to moderately decrease the exposure to **rivaroxaban**. Avoid unless patient can be monitored for signs of thrombosis. Severe Study

Rivastigmine → see anticholinesterases, centrally acting
Rizatriptan → see TABLE 13 p. 1337 (serotonin syndrome)
- Beta blockers, non-selective (propranolol) slightly to moderately increase the exposure to **rizatriptan**. Adjust **rizatriptan** dose and separate administration by at least 2 hours. Moderate Study
- Rizatriptan is predicted to increase the risk of vasoconstriction when given with ergotamine. Ergotamine should be taken at least 24 hours before or 6 hours after **rizatriptan**. Severe Theoretical
- Moclobemide moderately increases the exposure to **rizatriptan**. Avoid. Moderate Study → Also see TABLE 13 p. 1337
- Monoamine-oxidase A and B inhibitors, irreversible are predicted to increase the exposure to **rizatriptan**. Avoid and for 14 days after stopping the MAOI. Severe Theoretical → Also see TABLE 13 p. 1337

Rocuronium → see neuromuscular blocking drugs, non-depolarising
Roflumilast
- Aminophylline is predicted to slightly increase the exposure to **roflumilast**. Avoid. Moderate Theoretical
- Antiepileptics (carbamazepine, fosphenytoin, phenobarbital, phenytoin, primidone) are predicted to decrease the exposure to **roflumilast**. Avoid. Moderate Study
- Combined hormonal contraceptives are predicted to increase the exposure to **roflumilast**. Moderate Theoretical
- Enzalutamide is predicted to decrease the exposure to **roflumilast**. Avoid. Moderate Study
- H₂ receptor antagonists (cimetidine) slightly increase the exposure to **roflumilast**. Moderate Study
- Mitotane is predicted to decrease the exposure to **roflumilast**. Avoid. Moderate Study
- Quinolones (ciprofloxacin) are predicted to increase the exposure to **roflumilast**. Moderate Theoretical
- Rifampicin is predicted to decrease the exposure to **roflumilast**. Avoid. Moderate Study
- SSRIs (fluvoxamine) are predicted to increase the exposure to **roflumilast**. Moderate Study
- Theophylline is predicted to slightly increase the exposure to **roflumilast**. Avoid. Moderate Theoretical

Rolapitant
- Rolapitant is predicted to increase the exposure to alkylating agents (bendamustine). Avoid or monitor. Moderate Study

Rolapitant (continued)

▶ **Rolapitant** is predicted to increase the exposure to anthracyclines (doxorubicin, mitoxantrone). Avoid or monitor. Moderate Study

▶ **Rolapitant** is predicted to increase the exposure to antiarrhythmics (propafenone). Severe Study

▶ Antiepileptics (carbamazepine, fosphenytoin, phenobarbital, phenytoin, primidone) are predicted to markedly decrease the exposure to **rolapitant**. Avoid. Severe Study

▶ **Rolapitant** is predicted to moderately increase the exposure to beta blockers, selective (metoprolol). Severe Study

▶ Bosentan is predicted to decrease the exposure to **rolapitant**. Avoid. Severe Study

▶ **Rolapitant** is predicted to increase the exposure to colchicine. Moderate Study

▶ **Rolapitant** is predicted to increase the exposure to dabigatran. Moderate Study

▶ **Rolapitant** slightly increases the exposure to digoxin. Moderate Study

▶ Efavirenz is predicted to decrease the exposure to **rolapitant**. Avoid. Severe Study

▶ Enzalutamide is predicted to markedly decrease the exposure to **rolapitant**. Avoid. Severe Study

▶ **Rolapitant** is predicted to increase the exposure to irinotecan. Avoid or monitor. Moderate Study

▶ **Rolapitant** is predicted to increase the exposure to methotrexate. Avoid or monitor. Moderate Study

▶ Mitotane is predicted to markedly decrease the exposure to **rolapitant**. Avoid. Severe Study

▶ Nevirapine is predicted to decrease the exposure to **rolapitant**. Avoid. Severe Study

▶ **Rolapitant** is predicted to increase the exposure to pimozide. Severe Study

▶ Rifabutin is predicted to decrease the exposure to **rolapitant**. Avoid. Moderate Theoretical

▶ Rifampicin is predicted to markedly decrease the exposure to **rolapitant**. Avoid. Severe Study

▶ St John's Wort is predicted to decrease the exposure to **rolapitant**. Avoid. Severe Study

▶ **Rolapitant** is predicted to increase the exposure to statins (rosuvastatin). Monitor and adjust dose. Severe Study

▶ **Rolapitant** increases the exposure to sulfasalazine. Severe Study

▶ **Rolapitant** is predicted to increase the exposure to tamoxifen. Severe Study

▶ **Rolapitant** is predicted to increase the exposure to topotecan. Avoid or monitor. Moderate Study

Ropinirole → see dopamine receptor agonists

Ropivacaine → see anaesthetics, local

Rosuvastatin → see statins

Rotavirus vaccine → see live vaccines

Rotigotine → see dopamine receptor agonists

Rufinamide → see antiepileptics

Rupatadine → see antihistamines, non-sedating

Ruxolitinib → see TABLE 15 p. 1337 (myelosuppression)

▶ Antiarrhythmics (dronedarone) are predicted to increase the exposure to **ruxolitinib**. Moderate Theoretical

▶ Antiepileptics (carbamazepine, fosphenytoin, phenobarbital, phenytoin, primidone) are predicted to decrease the exposure to **ruxolitinib**. Monitor and adjust dose. Moderate Study

▶ Antifungals, azoles (fluconazole, isavuconazole, posaconazole) are predicted to increase the exposure to **ruxolitinib**. Moderate Theoretical

▶ Antifungals, azoles (itraconazole, ketoconazole, voriconazole) are predicted to increase the exposure to **ruxolitinib**. Adjust dose and monitor side effects. Moderate Study

▶ Aprepitant is predicted to increase the exposure to **ruxolitinib**. Moderate Theoretical

▶ Bosentan is predicted to decrease the exposure to **ruxolitinib**. Monitor and adjust dose. Moderate Theoretical

▶ Calcium channel blockers (diltiazem, verapamil) are predicted to increase the exposure to **ruxolitinib**. Moderate Theoretical

▶ Cobicistat is predicted to increase the exposure to **ruxolitinib**. Adjust dose and monitor side effects. Moderate Study

▶ **Ruxolitinib** is predicted to increase the risk of bleeding events when given with coumarins. Severe Theoretical

▶ Crizotinib is predicted to increase the exposure to **ruxolitinib**. Moderate Theoretical → Also see TABLE 15 p. 1337

▶ Efavirenz is predicted to decrease the exposure to **ruxolitinib**. Monitor and adjust dose. Moderate Theoretical

▶ Enzalutamide is predicted to decrease the exposure to **ruxolitinib**. Monitor and adjust dose. Moderate Study

▶ Grapefruit juice is predicted to increase the exposure to **ruxolitinib**. Severe Theoretical

▶ HIV-protease inhibitors are predicted to increase the exposure to **ruxolitinib**. Adjust dose and monitor side effects. Moderate Study

▶ Idelalisib is predicted to increase the exposure to **ruxolitinib**. Adjust dose and monitor side effects. Moderate Study → Also see TABLE 15 p. 1337

▶ Imatinib is predicted to increase the exposure to **ruxolitinib**. Moderate Theoretical → Also see TABLE 15 p. 1337

▶ Macrolides (clarithromycin) are predicted to increase the exposure to **ruxolitinib**. Adjust dose and monitor side effects. Moderate Study

▶ Macrolides (erythromycin) are predicted to increase the exposure to **ruxolitinib**. Moderate Theoretical

▶ Mitotane is predicted to decrease the exposure to **ruxolitinib**. Monitor and adjust dose. Moderate Study → Also see TABLE 15 p. 1337

▶ Netupitant is predicted to increase the exposure to **ruxolitinib**. Moderate Theoretical

▶ Nevirapine is predicted to decrease the exposure to **ruxolitinib**. Monitor and adjust dose. Moderate Theoretical

▶ Nilotinib is predicted to increase the exposure to **ruxolitinib**. Moderate Theoretical → Also see TABLE 15 p. 1337

▶ **Ruxolitinib** is predicted to increase the risk of bleeding events when given with phenindione. Severe Theoretical

▶ Rifampicin is predicted to decrease the exposure to **ruxolitinib**. Monitor and adjust dose. Moderate Study

▶ St John's Wort is predicted to decrease the exposure to **ruxolitinib**. Monitor and adjust dose. Moderate Theoretical

Sacubitril → see TABLE 8 p. 1335 (hypotension)

▶ Sacubitril is predicted to increase the exposure to statins. Severe Study

Safinamide → see monoamine-oxidase B inhibitors

Salbutamol → see beta$_2$ agonists

Salmeterol → see beta$_2$ agonists

Sapropterin → see TABLE 8 p. 1335 (hypotension)

▶ Methotrexate is predicted to decrease the efficacy of **sapropterin**. Moderate Theoretical

▶ Phosphodiesterase type-5 inhibitors are predicted to increase the risk of hypotension when given with **sapropterin**. Moderate Theoretical → Also see TABLE 8 p. 1335

▶ Trimethoprim is predicted to decrease the efficacy of **sapropterin**. Moderate Theoretical

Saquinavir → see HIV-protease inhibitors

Sarilumab → see monoclonal antibodies

Saxagliptin → see TABLE 14 p. 1337 (antidiabetic drugs)

▶ Antiarrhythmics (dronedarone) are predicted to increase the exposure to **saxagliptin**. Mild Study

▶ Antiepileptics (carbamazepine, fosphenytoin, phenobarbital, phenytoin, primidone) are predicted to moderately decrease the exposure to **saxagliptin**. Moderate Study

▶ Antifungals, azoles (fluconazole, isavuconazole, posaconazole) are predicted to increase the exposure to **saxagliptin**. Mild Study

▶ Antifungals, azoles (itraconazole, ketoconazole, voriconazole) are predicted to increase the exposure to **saxagliptin**. Moderate Study

▶ Aprepitant is predicted to increase the exposure to **saxagliptin**. Mild Study

▶ Calcium channel blockers (diltiazem, verapamil) are predicted to increase the exposure to **saxagliptin**. Mild Study

▶ Cobicistat is predicted to increase the exposure to **saxagliptin**. Moderate Study

▶ Crizotinib is predicted to increase the exposure to **saxagliptin**. Mild Study

▶ Enzalutamide is predicted to moderately decrease the exposure to **saxagliptin**. Moderate Study

▸ Grapefruit juice is predicted to increase the exposure to **saxagliptin**. [Mild] Theoretical

▸ HIV-protease inhibitors are predicted to increase the exposure to **saxagliptin**. [Moderate] Study

▸ Idelalisib is predicted to increase the exposure to **saxagliptin**. [Moderate] Study

▸ Imatinib is predicted to increase the exposure to **saxagliptin**. [Mild] Study

▸ Macrolides (clarithromycin) are predicted to increase the exposure to **saxagliptin**. [Moderate] Study

▸ Macrolides (erythromycin) are predicted to increase the exposure to **saxagliptin**. [Mild] Study

▸ Mitotane is predicted to moderately decrease the exposure to **saxagliptin**. [Moderate] Study

▸ Netupitant is predicted to increase the exposure to **saxagliptin**. [Mild] Study

▸ Nilotinib is predicted to increase the exposure to **saxagliptin**. [Mild] Study

▸ Rifampicin is predicted to moderately decrease the exposure to **saxagliptin**. [Moderate] Study

Secukinumab → see monoclonal antibodies

Selegiline → see monoamine-oxidase B inhibitors

Selenium

▸ **Selenium** is predicted to decrease the absorption of eltrombopag. **Eltrombopag** should be taken 2 hours before or 4 hours after **selenium**, p. 1001, p. 1037. [Severe] Theoretical

Selexipag

▸ Antiepileptics (carbamazepine, fosphenytoin, phenytoin) are predicted to decrease the exposure to the active metabolite of **selexipag**. Adjust dose. [Moderate] Study

▸ Antiepileptics (valproate) are predicted to increase the exposure to **selexipag**. [Unknown] Theoretical

▸ Antifungals, azoles (fluconazole) are predicted to increase the exposure to **selexipag**. [Unknown] Theoretical

▸ Clopidogrel is predicted to increase the exposure to **selexipag**. Adjust dose. [Moderate] Study

▸ Fibrates (gemfibrozil) increase the exposure to **selexipag**. Avoid. [Severe] Study

▸ Iron chelators (deferasirox) are predicted to increase the exposure to **selexipag**. Adjust dose. [Moderate] Study

▸ Leflunomide is predicted to increase the exposure to **selexipag**. Adjust dose. [Moderate] Theoretical

▸ Rifampicin moderately decreases the exposure to the active metabolite of **selexipag**. Adjust dose. [Moderate] Study

▸ Teriflunomide is predicted to increase the exposure to **selexipag**. Adjust dose. [Moderate] Theoretical

Sertraline → see SSRIs

Sevoflurane → see volatile halogenated anaesthetics

Sildenafil → see phosphodiesterase type-5 inhibitors

Siltuximab → see monoclonal antibodies

Silver sulfadiazine

PHARMACOLOGY Silver might inactivate enzymatic debriding agents—concurrent use might not be appropriate.

Simeprevir

▸ Antiarrhythmics (dronedarone) are predicted to increase the exposure to **simeprevir**. Avoid. [Severe] Study

▸ Simeprevir is predicted to increase the concentration of antiarrhythmics (amiodarone). Refer to specialist literature. [Severe] Anecdotal

▸ Antiepileptics (carbamazepine, fosphenytoin, phenobarbital, phenytoin, primidone) are predicted to decrease the exposure to **simeprevir**. Avoid. [Severe] Study

▸ Antiepileptics (oxcarbazepine) are predicted to decrease the exposure to **simeprevir**. Avoid. [Severe] Theoretical

▸ Antifungals, azoles (fluconazole, isavuconazole, itraconazole, ketoconazole, posaconazole, voriconazole) are predicted to increase the exposure to **simeprevir**. Avoid. [Severe] Study

▸ Aprepitant is predicted to increase the exposure to **simeprevir**. Avoid. [Severe] Study

▸ Bosentan is predicted to decrease the exposure to **simeprevir**. Avoid. [Severe] Study

▸ Calcium channel blockers (diltiazem, verapamil) are predicted to increase the exposure to **simeprevir**. Avoid. [Severe] Study

▸ Cobicistat is predicted to increase the exposure to **simeprevir**. Avoid. [Severe] Study

▸ Crizotinib is predicted to increase the exposure to **simeprevir**. Avoid. [Severe] Study

▸ Efavirenz is predicted to decrease the exposure to **simeprevir**. Avoid. [Severe] Study

▸ Enzalutamide is predicted to decrease the exposure to **simeprevir**. Avoid. [Severe] Study

▸ Etravirine is predicted to decrease the exposure to **simeprevir**. Avoid. [Moderate] Study

▸ HIV-protease inhibitors are predicted to increase the exposure to **simeprevir**. Avoid. [Severe] Study

▸ Idelalisib is predicted to increase the exposure to **simeprevir**. Avoid. [Severe] Study

▸ Imatinib is predicted to increase the exposure to **simeprevir**. Avoid. [Severe] Study

▸ Ledipasvir moderately increases the exposure to **simeprevir** and **simeprevir** slightly increases the exposure to ledipasvir. Avoid. [Severe] Study

▸ Macrolides (clarithromycin, erythromycin) are predicted to increase the exposure to **simeprevir**. Avoid. [Severe] Study

▸ Mitotane is predicted to decrease the exposure to **simeprevir**. Avoid. [Severe] Study

▸ Netupitant is predicted to increase the exposure to **simeprevir**. Avoid. [Severe] Study

▸ Nevirapine is predicted to decrease the exposure to **simeprevir**. Avoid. [Severe] Study

▸ Nilotinib is predicted to increase the exposure to **simeprevir**. Avoid. [Severe] Study

▸ Rifabutin is predicted to decrease the exposure to **simeprevir**. Avoid. [Moderate] Theoretical

▸ Rifampicin is predicted to decrease the exposure to **simeprevir**. Avoid. [Severe] Study

▸ St John's Wort is predicted to decrease the exposure to **simeprevir**. Avoid. [Severe] Study

▸ Simeprevir moderately increases the exposure to statins (atorvastatin). Monitor and adjust dose. [Moderate] Study

▸ Simeprevir is predicted to increase the exposure to statins (pravastatin). Monitor and adjust dose. [Severe] Theoretical

▸ Simeprevir moderately increases the exposure to statins (rosuvastatin). Adjust **rosuvastatin** dose, p. 202. [Moderate] Study

▸ Simeprevir slightly increases the exposure to statins (simvastatin). Monitor and adjust dose. [Moderate] Study

Simvastatin → see statins

Sirolimus

▸ Antiarrhythmics (amiodarone) are predicted to increase the concentration of **sirolimus**. [Severe] Anecdotal

▸ Antiarrhythmics (dronedarone) increase the concentration of **sirolimus**. Monitor and adjust dose. [Moderate] Study

▸ Antiepileptics (carbamazepine, fosphenytoin, phenobarbital, phenytoin, primidone) are predicted to decrease the concentration of **sirolimus**. Avoid. [Severe] Study

▸ Antifungals, azoles (fluconazole, isavuconazole, posaconazole) increase the concentration of **sirolimus**. Monitor and adjust dose. [Moderate] Study

▸ Antifungals, azoles (itraconazole, ketoconazole, voriconazole) are predicted to increase the concentration of **sirolimus**. Avoid. [Severe] Study

▸ Antifungals, azoles (miconazole) are predicted to increase the concentration of **sirolimus**. Monitor and adjust dose. [Moderate] Study

▸ Aprepitant increases the concentration of **sirolimus**. Monitor and adjust dose. [Moderate] Study

▸ Bosentan is predicted to decrease the concentration of **sirolimus** and **sirolimus** potentially increases the concentration of bosentan. Avoid. [Severe] Theoretical

▸ Calcium channel blockers (diltiazem, verapamil) increase the concentration of **sirolimus**. Monitor and adjust dose. [Moderate] Study

▸ Ceritinib is predicted to increase the exposure to **sirolimus**. Avoid. [Severe] Theoretical

▸ Sirolimus is predicted to affect the efficacy of chenodeoxycholic acid. Monitor and adjust dose. [Moderate] Theoretical

▸ Ciclosporin moderately increases the exposure to **sirolimus**. Separate administration by 4 hours. [Severe] Study

▸ Cobicistat is predicted to increase the concentration of **sirolimus**. Avoid. [Severe] Study

Sirolimus (continued)
▸ Crizotinib increases the concentration of **sirolimus**. Monitor and adjust dose. Moderate Study
▸ Efavirenz is predicted to decrease the concentration of **sirolimus**. Monitor and adjust dose. Moderate Theoretical
▸ Eliglustat is predicted to increase the exposure to **sirolimus**. Adjust dose. Moderate Study
▸ Enzalutamide is predicted to decrease the concentration of **sirolimus**. Avoid. Severe Study
▸ Grapefruit juice increases the concentration of **sirolimus**. Avoid. Moderate Study
▸ HIV-protease inhibitors are predicted to increase the concentration of **sirolimus**. Avoid. Severe Study
▸ Idelalisib is predicted to increase the concentration of **sirolimus**. Avoid. Severe Study
▸ Imatinib increases the concentration of **sirolimus**. Monitor and adjust dose. Moderate Study
▸ Lapatinib is predicted to increase the exposure to **sirolimus**. Moderate Theoretical
▸ Live vaccines are predicted to increase the risk of generalised infection (possibly life-threatening) when given with **sirolimus**. Public Health England advises avoid (refer to Green Book). Severe Theoretical
▸ Lumacaftor is predicted to decrease the exposure to **sirolimus**. Avoid. Severe Theoretical
▸ Macrolides (clarithromycin) are predicted to increase the concentration of **sirolimus**. Avoid. Severe Study
▸ Macrolides (erythromycin) increase the concentration of **sirolimus**. Monitor and adjust dose. Moderate Study
▸ **Sirolimus** is predicted to decrease the efficacy of mifamurtide. Avoid. Severe Theoretical
▸ Mirabegron is predicted to increase the exposure to **sirolimus**. Mild Theoretical
▸ Mitotane is predicted to decrease the concentration of **sirolimus**. Avoid. Severe Study
▸ Monoclonal antibodies (sarilumab) potentially affect the exposure to **sirolimus**. Monitor and adjust dose. Moderate Theoretical
▸ Netupitant increases the concentration of **sirolimus**. Monitor and adjust dose. Moderate Study
▸ Nevirapine is predicted to decrease the concentration of **sirolimus**. Monitor and adjust dose. Moderate Theoretical
▸ Nilotinib increases the concentration of **sirolimus**. Monitor and adjust dose. Moderate Study
▸ Palbociclib is predicted to increase the exposure to **sirolimus**. Adjust dose. Moderate Theoretical
▸ Pitolisant is predicted to decrease the exposure to **sirolimus**. Avoid. Moderate Theoretical
▸ Ribociclib is predicted to increase the exposure to **sirolimus**. Use with caution and adjust dose. Moderate Theoretical
▸ Rifampicin is predicted to decrease the concentration of **sirolimus**. Avoid. Severe Study
▸ St John's Wort is predicted to decrease the concentration of **sirolimus**. Monitor and adjust dose. Severe Theoretical
▸ **Sirolimus** is predicted to decrease the concentration of tacrolimus and tacrolimus increases the exposure to **sirolimus**. Severe Study
▸ Velpatasvir is predicted to increase the exposure to **sirolimus**. Severe Theoretical

Sitagliptin → see TABLE 14 p. 1337 (antidiabetic drugs)

Sodium aurothiomalate
▸ ACE inhibitors are predicted to increase the risk of hypersensitivity when given with **sodium aurothiomalate**. Severe Anecdotal
▸ **Sodium aurothiomalate** potentially increases the risk of side-effects when given with penicillamine (in those who have had previous adverse reactions to gold). Avoid. Severe Study

Sodium bicarbonate
▸ Oral **sodium bicarbonate** decreases the absorption of antifungals, azoles (ketoconazole). Moderate Study
▸ **Sodium bicarbonate** decreases the concentration of lithium. Severe Anecdotal
▸ **Sodium bicarbonate** is predicted to decrease the efficacy of methenamine. Avoid. Moderate Theoretical

Sodium citrate
▸ **Sodium citrate** is predicted to decrease the efficacy of methenamine. Avoid. Moderate Theoretical
▸ **Sodium citrate** is predicted to increase the risk of side-effects when given with sucralfate. Avoid. Moderate Theoretical

Sodium clodronate → see bisphosphonates

Sodium feredetate → see iron (oral)

Sodium nitroprusside → see TABLE 8 p. 1335 (hypotension)
▸ **Sodium nitroprusside** is predicted to increase the risk of methaemoglobinaemia when given with topical anaesthetics, local (prilocaine). Use with caution or avoid. Severe Theoretical
▸ **Sodium nitroprusside** is predicted to increase the risk of methaemoglobinaemia when given with dapsone. Severe Theoretical

Sodium oxybate → see TABLE 8 p. 1335 (hypotension), TABLE 11 p. 1336 (CNS depressant effects)
▸ Antiepileptics (valproate) increase the exposure to **sodium oxybate**. Adjust **sodium oxybate** dose, p. 484. Moderate Study

Sodium phenylbutyrate
▸ Antiepileptics (valproate) potentially decrease the effects of **sodium phenylbutyrate**. Moderate Anecdotal
▸ Corticosteroids potentially decrease the effects of **sodium phenylbutyrate**. Moderate Anecdotal
▸ Haloperidol potentially decreases the effects of **sodium phenylbutyrate**. Moderate Anecdotal

Sodium picosulfate → see TABLE 18 p. 1338 (hyponatraemia)

Sodium stibogluconate
▸ **Sodium stibogluconate** increases the risk of cardiovascular side-effects when given with amphotericin. Separate administration by 14 days. Severe Study

Sofosbuvir
▸ **Sofosbuvir** is predicted to increase the risk of severe bradycardia or heart block when given with antiarrhythmics (amiodarone). Refer to specialist literature. Severe Anecdotal
▸ Antiepileptics (carbamazepine) are predicted to decrease the exposure to **sofosbuvir**. Avoid. Severe Study
▸ Antiepileptics (fosphenytoin, oxcarbazepine, phenobarbital, phenytoin, primidone) are predicted to decrease the exposure to **sofosbuvir**. Avoid. Severe Theoretical
▸ H₂ receptor antagonists potentially decrease the exposure to **sofosbuvir**. Adjust dose, see ledipasvir with sofosbuvir p. 617, sofosbuvir with velpatasvir p. 619, and sofosbuvir with velpatasvir and voxilaprevir p. 619. Moderate Study
▸ HIV-protease inhibitors (tipranavir) are predicted to decrease the exposure to **sofosbuvir**. Avoid. Severe Theoretical
▸ Proton pump inhibitors potentially decrease the exposure to **sofosbuvir**. Adjust dose, see ledipasvir with sofosbuvir p. 617, sofosbuvir with velpatasvir p. 619, and sofosbuvir with velpatasvir and voxilaprevir p. 619. Moderate Study
▸ Rifampicin is predicted to decrease the exposure to **sofosbuvir**. Avoid. Severe Study
▸ St John's Wort is predicted to decrease the exposure to **sofosbuvir**. Avoid. Severe Study

Solifenacin → see TABLE 10 p. 1336 (antimuscarinics)
▸ Antiepileptics (carbamazepine, fosphenytoin, phenobarbital, phenytoin, primidone) are predicted to decrease the exposure to **solifenacin**. Moderate Theoretical
▸ Antifungals, azoles (itraconazole, ketoconazole, voriconazole) are predicted to increase the exposure to **solifenacin**. Adjust **solifenacin** p. 761 or **tamsulosin with solifenacin** p. 768 dose; avoid in hepatic and renal impairment. Severe Study
▸ Cobicistat is predicted to increase the exposure to **solifenacin**. Adjust **solifenacin** p. 761 or **tamsulosin with solifenacin** p. 768 dose; avoid in hepatic and renal impairment. Severe Study
▸ Enzalutamide is predicted to decrease the exposure to **solifenacin**. Moderate Theoretical
▸ HIV-protease inhibitors are predicted to increase the exposure to **solifenacin**. Adjust **solifenacin** p. 761 or **tamsulosin with solifenacin** p. 768 dose; avoid in hepatic and renal impairment. Severe Study
▸ Idelalisib is predicted to increase the exposure to **solifenacin**. Adjust **solifenacin** p. 761 or **tamsulosin with solifenacin** p. 768 dose; avoid in hepatic and renal impairment. Severe Study
▸ Macrolides (clarithromycin) are predicted to increase the exposure to **solifenacin**. Adjust **solifenacin** p. 761 or **tamsulosin**

with solifenacin p. 768 dose; avoid in hepatic and renal impairment. Severe Study
▸ Mitotane is predicted to decrease the exposure to **solifenacin**. Moderate Theoretical
▸ Rifampicin is predicted to decrease the exposure to **solifenacin**. Moderate Theoretical

Somatropin
▸ Corticosteroids are predicted to decrease the effects of **somatropin**. Moderate Theoretical

Sorafenib → see TABLE 15 p. 1337 (myelosuppression), TABLE 9 p. 1336 (QT-interval prolongation)
▸ Antiepileptics (carbamazepine, fosphenytoin, phenobarbital, phenytoin, primidone) are predicted to decrease the exposure to **sorafenib**. Moderate Theoretical
▸ Sorafenib increases the anticoagulant effect of coumarins. Severe Anecdotal
▸ Enzalutamide is predicted to decrease the exposure to **sorafenib**. Moderate Theoretical
▸ Mitotane is predicted to decrease the exposure to **sorafenib**. Moderate Theoretical → Also see TABLE 15 p. 1337
▸ Neomycin moderately decreases the exposure to **sorafenib**. Moderate Study
▸ **Sorafenib** is predicted to increase the risk of bleeding events when given with phenindione. Severe Theoretical
▸ Rifampicin is predicted to decrease the exposure to **sorafenib**. Moderate Theoretical

Sotalol → see beta blockers, non-selective
Spironolactone → see aldosterone antagonists
SSRIs → see TABLE 18 p. 1338 (hyponatraemia), TABLE 13 p. 1337 (serotonin syndrome), TABLE 9 p. 1336 (QT-interval prolongation), TABLE 4 p. 1334 (antiplatelet effects)

citalopram · dapoxetine · escitalopram · fluoxetine · fluvoxamine · paroxetine · sertraline

▸ **Fluvoxamine** very markedly increases the exposure to agomelatine. Avoid. Severe Study
▸ **Fluvoxamine** moderately increases the exposure to alprazolam. Adjust dose. Moderate Study
▸ SSRIs **(fluoxetine, paroxetine)** are predicted to increase the exposure to amfetamines. Severe Theoretical → Also see TABLE 13 p. 1337
▸ **Fluvoxamine** moderately to markedly increases the exposure to aminophylline. Avoid. Severe Study
▸ **Fluvoxamine** decreases the clearance of anaesthetics, local (ropivacaine). Avoid prolonged use. Moderate Study
▸ **Fluvoxamine** is predicted to increase the exposure to anagrelide. Moderate Theoretical → Also see TABLE 4 p. 1334
▸ Antiarrhythmics (dronedarone) are predicted to increase the exposure to **dapoxetine**. Adjust **dapoxetine** dose with moderate inhibitors of CYP3A4, p. 801. Moderate Theoretical
▸ Antiarrhythmics (dronedarone) are predicted to increase the exposure to SSRIs **(citalopram, escitalopram, fluoxetine, fluvoxamine, paroxetine, sertraline)**. Severe Theoretical → Also see TABLE 9 p. 1336
▸ **Fluvoxamine** is predicted to increase the exposure to antiarrhythmics (propafenone). Monitor and adjust dose. Moderate Study
▸ SSRIs **(fluoxetine, paroxetine)** are predicted to increase the exposure to anticholinesterases, centrally acting (galantamine). Monitor and adjust dose. Moderate Study
▸ Antiepileptics (fosphenytoin, phenytoin) decrease the concentration of **paroxetine**. Moderate Study
▸ **Sertraline** potentially increases the risk of toxicity when given with antiepileptics (fosphenytoin, phenytoin). Monitor concentration and adjust dose. Severe Anecdotal
▸ SSRIs **(fluoxetine, fluvoxamine)** are predicted to increase the concentration of antiepileptics (fosphenytoin, phenytoin). Monitor and adjust dose. Severe Anecdotal
▸ Antifungals, azoles (fluconazole, isavuconazole, posaconazole) are predicted to increase the exposure to **dapoxetine**. Adjust **dapoxetine** dose with moderate inhibitors of CYP3A4, p. 801. Moderate Theoretical
▸ Antifungals, azoles (itraconazole, ketoconazole, voriconazole) are predicted to moderately increase the exposure to **dapoxetine**. Avoid potent inhibitors of CYP3A4 or adjust **dapoxetine** dose, Severe Study

▸ Antifungals, azoles (voriconazole) are predicted to increase the exposure to **citalopram**. Severe Theoretical → Also see TABLE 9 p. 1336
▸ Antihistamines, sedating (cyproheptadine) potentially decrease the effects of **SSRIs**. Moderate Anecdotal
▸ Aprepitant is predicted to increase the exposure to **dapoxetine**. Adjust **dapoxetine** dose with moderate inhibitors of CYP3A4, p. 801. Moderate Theoretical
▸ SSRIs **(fluoxetine, paroxetine)** are predicted to moderately increase the exposure to aripiprazole. Adjust **aripiprazole** dose, p. 391. Moderate Study
▸ **Fluvoxamine** increases the exposure to asenapine. Moderate Study
▸ **Paroxetine** moderately increases the exposure to asenapine. Moderate Study
▸ SSRIs **(fluoxetine, paroxetine)** are predicted to markedly increase the exposure to atomoxetine. Adjust dose. Severe Study
▸ **Fluvoxamine** moderately increases the concentration of beta blockers, non-selective (propranolol). Moderate Study
▸ SSRIs **(fluoxetine, paroxetine)** are predicted to increase the exposure to beta blockers, selective (metoprolol, nebivolol). Moderate Study
▸ Bupropion is predicted to increase the exposure to **dapoxetine**. Moderate Theoretical → Also see TABLE 13 p. 1337
▸ **Fluvoxamine** markedly decreases the clearance of caffeine citrate. Monitor and adjust dose. Severe Study
▸ Calcium channel blockers (diltiazem, verapamil) are predicted to increase the exposure to **dapoxetine**. Adjust **dapoxetine** dose with moderate inhibitors of CYP3A4, p. 801. Moderate Theoretical
▸ SSRIs **(fluoxetine, fluvoxamine)** are predicted to increase the exposure to cilostazol. Adjust **cilostazol** dose, p. 231. Moderate Theoretical → Also see TABLE 4 p. 1334
▸ Cinacalcet is predicted to increase the exposure to **dapoxetine**. Moderate Theoretical
▸ **Fluvoxamine** is predicted to increase the exposure to cinacalcet. Adjust dose. Moderate Theoretical
▸ SSRIs **(fluoxetine, fluvoxamine)** potentially increase the exposure to clobazam. Adjust dose. Moderate Theoretical
▸ SSRIs **(fluoxetine, fluvoxamine)** are predicted to decrease the efficacy of clopidogrel. Avoid. Severe Theoretical → Also see TABLE 4 p. 1334
▸ **Fluvoxamine** increases the concentration of clozapine. Monitor side effects and adjust dose. Severe Study
▸ Cobicistat is predicted to moderately increase the exposure to **dapoxetine**. Avoid potent inhibitors of CYP3A4 or adjust **dapoxetine** dose, p. 801. Severe Study
▸ Crizotinib is predicted to increase the exposure to **dapoxetine**. Adjust **dapoxetine** dose with moderate inhibitors of CYP3A4, p. 801. Moderate Theoretical
▸ SSRIs **(fluoxetine, paroxetine)** are predicted to slightly increase the exposure to darifenacin. Mild Study
▸ **Fluvoxamine** moderately increases the exposure to diazepam. Moderate Study
▸ **Fluvoxamine** is predicted to increase the exposure to dopamine receptor agonists (ropinirole). Adjust dose. Moderate Study
▸ **Fluvoxamine** markedly increases the exposure to duloxetine. Avoid. Severe Study → Also see TABLE 18 p. 1338 → Also see TABLE 13 p. 1337 → Also see TABLE 4 p. 1334
▸ SSRIs **(fluoxetine, paroxetine)** are predicted to increase the exposure to eliglustat. Avoid or adjust dose—consult product literature. Severe Study
▸ **Fluvoxamine** is predicted to increase the exposure to erlotinib. Monitor side effects and adjust dose. Moderate Theoretical
▸ **Fluvoxamine** increases the concentration of frovatriptan. Severe Study → Also see TABLE 13 p. 1337
▸ Grapefruit juice moderately increases the exposure to **sertraline**. Avoid. Moderate Study
▸ H_2 receptor antagonists (cimetidine) slightly increase the exposure to SSRIs **(citalopram, escitalopram)**. Adjust dose. Moderate Study
▸ H_2 receptor antagonists (cimetidine) slightly increase the exposure to SSRIs **(paroxetine, sertraline)**. Moderate Study
▸ **Fluoxetine** increases the concentration of haloperidol. Adjust dose. Moderate Anecdotal

SSRIs (continued)

▸ **Fluvoxamine** increases the concentration of haloperidol. Adjust dose. Moderate Study

▸ HIV-protease inhibitors are predicted to moderately increase the exposure to **dapoxetine**. Avoid potent inhibitors of CYP3A4 or adjust **dapoxetine** dose, p. 801. Severe Study

▸ Idelalisib is predicted to moderately increase the exposure to **dapoxetine**. Avoid potent inhibitors of CYP3A4 or adjust **dapoxetine** dose, p. 801. Severe Study

▸ Imatinib is predicted to increase the exposure to **dapoxetine**. Adjust **dapoxetine** dose with moderate inhibitors of CYP3A4, p. 801. Moderate Theoretical

▸ **Fluoxetine** is predicted to increase the exposure to lomitapide. Separate administration by 12 hours. Unknown Theoretical

▸ **Fluvoxamine** is predicted to increase the exposure to lomitapide. Separate administration by 12 hours. Moderate Theoretical

▸ **Fluvoxamine** is predicted to increase the exposure to loxapine. Avoid. Unknown Theoretical

▸ Macrolides (clarithromycin) are predicted to moderately increase the exposure to **dapoxetine**. Avoid potent inhibitors of CYP3A4 or adjust **dapoxetine** dose, p. 801. Severe Study

▸ Macrolides (erythromycin) are predicted to increase the exposure to **dapoxetine**. Adjust **dapoxetine** dose with moderate inhibitors of CYP3A4, p. 801. Moderate Theoretical

▸ **Fluvoxamine** very markedly increases the exposure to melatonin. Avoid. Severe Study

▸ Netupitant is predicted to increase the exposure to **dapoxetine**. Adjust **dapoxetine** dose with moderate inhibitors of CYP3A4, p. 801. Moderate Theoretical

▸ **SSRIs** potentially increase the risk of prolonged neuromuscular blockade when given with neuromuscular blocking drugs, non-depolarising (mivacurium). Unknown Theoretical

▸ Nilotinib is predicted to increase the exposure to **dapoxetine**. Adjust **dapoxetine** dose with moderate inhibitors of CYP3A4, p. 801. Moderate Theoretical

▸ **Fluvoxamine** moderately increases the exposure to olanzapine. Adjust dose. Severe Anecdotal

▸ **SSRIs (fluoxetine, paroxetine)** are predicted to decrease the efficacy of opioids (codeine). Moderate Theoretical

▸ **SSRIs (fluoxetine, paroxetine)** are predicted to decrease the efficacy of opioids (tramadol). Severe Study → Also see TABLE 13 p. 1337

▸ **Fluvoxamine** is predicted to increase the exposure to pentoxifylline. Moderate Theoretical

▸ **Paroxetine** markedly increases the exposure to phenothiazines (perphenazine). Severe Study

▸ **Fluvoxamine** is predicted to moderately increase the exposure to pirfenidone. Avoid. Moderate Study

▸ **SSRIs (fluoxetine, paroxetine)** are predicted to moderately increase the exposure to pitolisant. Use with caution and adjust dose. Moderate Study

▸ **Fluvoxamine** moderately increases the exposure to pomalidomide. Adjust **pomalidomide** dose, p. 935. Moderate Study

▸ **Paroxetine** slightly increases the exposure to procyclidine. Monitor and adjust dose. Moderate Study

▸ Proton pump inhibitors (esomeprazole) are predicted to slightly to moderately increase the exposure to SSRIs (**citalopram, escitalopram**). Monitor and adjust dose. Severe Theoretical

▸ Proton pump inhibitors (omeprazole) slightly to moderately increase the exposure to SSRIs (**citalopram, escitalopram**). Monitor and adjust dose. Severe Study

▸ **Fluvoxamine** is predicted to increase the exposure to riluzole. Moderate Theoretical

▸ **SSRIs (fluoxetine, paroxetine)** are predicted to increase the exposure to risperidone. Adjust dose. Moderate Study

▸ **Fluvoxamine** is predicted to increase the exposure to roflumilast. Moderate Study

▸ **SSRIs (fluoxetine, paroxetine)** are predicted to increase the exposure to SSRIs (**dapoxetine**). Moderate Theoretical → Also see TABLE 18 p. 1338 → Also see TABLE 13 p. 1337 → Also see TABLE 4 p. 1334

▸ **SSRIs** potentially increase the risk of prolonged neuromuscular blockade when given with suxamethonium. Unknown Theoretical

▸ **SSRIs (fluoxetine, paroxetine)** are predicted to decrease the efficacy of tamoxifen. Avoid. Severe Study

▸ Terbinafine is predicted to increase the exposure to **fluoxetine**. Adjust dose. Moderate Theoretical

▸ Terbinafine moderately increases the exposure to **paroxetine**. Moderate Study

▸ Terbinafine is predicted to increase the exposure to SSRIs (**citalopram, dapoxetine, escitalopram, fluvoxamine, sertraline**). Moderate Theoretical

▸ **Fluvoxamine** moderately to markedly increases the exposure to theophylline. Avoid. Severe Study

▸ **Fluvoxamine** very markedly increases the exposure to tizanidine. Avoid. Severe Study

▸ **SSRIs (fluoxetine, paroxetine)** are predicted to increase the exposure to tricyclic antidepressants. Monitor for toxicity and adjust dose. Severe Study → Also see TABLE 18 p. 1338 → Also see TABLE 13 p. 1337

▸ **Fluvoxamine** increases the exposure to tricyclic antidepressants (amitriptyline, imipramine). Adjust dose. Severe Study → Also see TABLE 18 p. 1338 → Also see TABLE 13 p. 1337

▸ **Fluvoxamine** markedly increases the exposure to tricyclic antidepressants (clomipramine). Adjust dose. Severe Study → Also see TABLE 18 p. 1338 → Also see TABLE 13 p. 1337

▸ **SSRIs (fluoxetine, paroxetine)** are predicted to increase the exposure to vortioxetine. Monitor and adjust dose. Moderate Study → Also see TABLE 13 p. 1337 → Also see TABLE 4 p. 1334

▸ **Fluvoxamine** is predicted to increase the exposure to zolmitriptan. Adjust **zolmitriptan** dose, p. 475. Severe Theoretical → Also see TABLE 13 p. 1337

St John's Wort → see TABLE 13 p. 1337 (serotonin syndrome)

▸ **St John's Wort** is predicted to decrease the exposure to afatinib. Moderate Study

▸ **St John's Wort** is predicted to slightly decrease the exposure to aldosterone antagonists (**eplerenone**). Avoid. Moderate Study

▸ **St John's Wort** decreases the exposure to aliskiren. Moderate Study

▸ **St John's Wort** moderately decreases the exposure to alprazolam. Moderate Study

▸ **St John's Wort** is predicted to decrease the concentration of aminophylline. Severe Theoretical

▸ **St John's Wort** is predicted to decrease the exposure to antiarrhythmics (**dronedarone**). Avoid. Severe Theoretical

▸ **St John's Wort** is predicted to decrease the exposure to antiepileptics (**brivaracetam**). Moderate Theoretical

▸ **St John's Wort** is predicted to decrease the exposure to antiepileptics (**carbamazepine**). Monitor and adjust dose. Moderate Theoretical

▸ **St John's Wort** is predicted to decrease the concentration of antiepileptics (**fosphenytoin, phenobarbital, phenytoin, primidone**). Avoid. Severe Theoretical

▸ **St John's Wort** is predicted to decrease the exposure to antiepileptics (**perampanel**). Monitor and adjust dose. Moderate Theoretical

▸ **St John's Wort** is predicted to decrease the exposure to antiepileptics (**tiagabine**). Avoid. Mild Theoretical

▸ **St John's Wort** is predicted to decrease the exposure to antifungals, azoles (**isavuconazole**). Avoid. Severe Theoretical

▸ **St John's Wort** moderately decreases the exposure to antifungals, azoles (**voriconazole**). Avoid. Moderate Study

▸ **St John's Wort** is predicted to decrease the concentration of antimalarials (**piperaquine**). Avoid. Moderate Theoretical

▸ **St John's Wort** is predicted to decrease the exposure to apixaban. Use with caution or avoid. Moderate Theoretical

▸ **St John's Wort** is predicted to decrease the exposure to apremilast. Avoid. Severe Theoretical

▸ **St John's Wort** is predicted to decrease the exposure to aprepitant. Avoid. Moderate Theoretical

▸ **St John's Wort** is predicted to decrease the exposure to axitinib. Moderate Theoretical

▸ **St John's Wort** is predicted to decrease the exposure to bedaquiline. Avoid. Severe Study

- **St John's Wort** is predicted to decrease the exposure to bosentan. Avoid. Moderate Theoretical
- **St John's Wort** is predicted to decrease the exposure to bosutinib. Avoid. Severe Theoretical
- **St John's Wort** is predicted to decrease the exposure to cabozantinib. Moderate Theoretical
- **St John's Wort** is predicted to decrease the exposure to calcium channel blockers (amlodipine, felodipine, lacidipine, lercanidipine, nicardipine, nifedipine, nimodipine). Monitor and adjust dose. Moderate Theoretical
- **St John's Wort** is predicted to decrease the exposure to calcium channel blockers (diltiazem, verapamil). Moderate Theoretical
- **St John's Wort** is predicted to decrease the exposure to ceritinib. Avoid. Severe Theoretical
- **St John's Wort** decreases the concentration of ciclosporin. Avoid. Moderate Study
- **St John's Wort** is predicted to alter the effects of cilostazol. Moderate Theoretical
- **St John's Wort** is predicted to decrease the exposure to cobicistat. Avoid. Severe Theoretical
- **St John's Wort** is predicted to decrease the exposure to cobimetinib. Avoid. Severe Theoretical
- **St John's Wort** decreases the efficacy of combined hormonal contraceptives. MHRA advises avoid. For FSRH guidance, see Contraceptives, interactions p. 775. Severe Anecdotal
- **St John's Wort** decreases the anticoagulant effect of coumarins. Avoid. Severe Anecdotal
- **St John's Wort** is predicted to decrease the exposure to crizotinib. Avoid. Severe Theoretical
- **St John's Wort** is predicted to decrease the exposure to dabigatran. Avoid. Severe Study
- **St John's Wort** is predicted to decrease the exposure to daclatasvir. Avoid. Severe Theoretical
- **St John's Wort** is predicted to decrease the exposure to darifenacin. Moderate Theoretical
- **St John's Wort** is predicted to decrease the exposure to dasabuvir. Avoid. Severe Theoretical
- **St John's Wort** is predicted to decrease the exposure to dasatinib. Severe Study
- **St John's Wort** is predicted to decrease the efficacy of desogestrel. MHRA advises avoid. For FSRH guidance, see Contraceptives, interactions p. 775. Severe Theoretical
- **St John's Wort** decreases the concentration of digoxin. Avoid. Severe Anecdotal
- **St John's Wort** decreases the exposure to dolutegravir. Adjust dose. Severe Study
- **St John's Wort** is predicted to decrease the exposure to edoxaban. Moderate Study
- **St John's Wort** is predicted to decrease the concentration of efavirenz. Avoid. Severe Theoretical
- **St John's Wort** is predicted to moderately decrease the exposure to elbasvir. Avoid. Severe Study
- **St John's Wort** is predicted to increase the exposure to eliglustat. Avoid. Severe Study
- **St John's Wort** is predicted to decrease the concentration of elvitegravir. Avoid. Severe Theoretical
- **St John's Wort** is predicted to decrease the effects of ergotamine. Moderate Theoretical
- **St John's Wort** is predicted to decrease the exposure to erlotinib. Severe Theoretical
- **St John's Wort** is predicted to decrease the efficacy of etonogestrel. MHRA advises avoid. For FSRH guidance, see Contraceptives, interactions p. 775. Severe Theoretical
- **St John's Wort** is predicted to decrease the exposure to etravirine. Avoid. Severe Study
- **St John's Wort** is predicted to decrease the concentration of everolimus. Avoid or adjust dose. Severe Study
- **St John's Wort** is predicted to decrease the exposure to exemestane. Moderate Theoretical
- **St John's Wort** is predicted to decrease the exposure to fesoterodine. Avoid. Severe Theoretical
- **St John's Wort** is predicted to decrease the exposure to fingolimod. Avoid. Moderate Theoretical
- **St John's Wort** is predicted to decrease the exposure to fosaprepitant. Avoid. Moderate Theoretical

- **St John's Wort** is predicted to decrease the exposure to gefitinib. Avoid. Severe Theoretical
- **St John's Wort** is predicted to decrease the exposure to glecaprevir. Avoid. Severe Study
- **St John's Wort** is predicted to markedly decrease the exposure to grazoprevir. Avoid. Severe Study
- **St John's Wort** is predicted to decrease the concentration of guanfacine. Adjust dose. Moderate Theoretical
- **St John's Wort** is predicted to decrease the exposure to HIV-protease inhibitors. Avoid. Severe Study
- **St John's Wort** is predicted to decrease the efficacy of hormone replacement therapy. Moderate Theoretical
- **St John's Wort** is predicted to decrease the exposure to ibrutinib. Avoid. Severe Theoretical
- **St John's Wort** is predicted to decrease the exposure to idelalisib. Avoid. Moderate Theoretical
- **St John's Wort** is predicted to decrease the exposure to imatinib. Moderate Study
- **St John's Wort** slightly decreases the exposure to irinotecan. Avoid. Severe Study
- **St John's Wort** decreases the exposure to ivabradine. Avoid. Moderate Study
- **St John's Wort** is predicted to decrease the exposure to ivacaftor. Moderate Theoretical
- **St John's Wort** is predicted to decrease the exposure to ixazomib. Avoid. Severe Theoretical
- **St John's Wort** is predicted to decrease the exposure to lapatinib. Avoid. Severe Study
- **St John's Wort** is predicted to decrease the exposure to ledipasvir. Avoid. Severe Theoretical
- **St John's Wort** is predicted to decrease the efficacy of levonorgestrel. MHRA advises avoid. For FSRH guidance, see Contraceptives, interactions p. 775. Severe Theoretical
- **St John's Wort** is predicted to decrease the exposure to lurasidone. Monitor and adjust dose. Moderate Theoretical
- **St John's Wort** is predicted to decrease the exposure to macitentan. Avoid. Severe Theoretical
- **St John's Wort** is predicted to decrease the exposure to maraviroc. Avoid. Severe Theoretical
- **St John's Wort** moderately decreases the exposure to midazolam. Monitor and adjust dose. Moderate Study
- **St John's Wort** is predicted to decrease the exposure to midostaurin. Avoid. Severe Theoretical
- **St John's Wort** is predicted to decrease the exposure to naloxegol. Avoid. Moderate Theoretical
- **St John's Wort** is predicted to decrease the exposure to netupitant. Moderate Theoretical
- **St John's Wort** is predicted to decrease the concentration of nevirapine. Avoid. Severe Theoretical
- **St John's Wort** is predicted to decrease the exposure to nilotinib. Avoid. Severe Theoretical
- **St John's Wort** is predicted to decrease the exposure to nintedanib. Moderate Study
- **St John's Wort** is predicted to decrease the efficacy of norethisterone. MHRA advises avoid. For FSRH guidance, see Contraceptives, interactions p. 775. Severe Anecdotal
- **St John's Wort** is predicted to decrease the exposure to olaparib. Avoid. Moderate Theoretical
- **St John's Wort** is predicted to decrease the exposure to ombitasvir. Avoid. Severe Theoretical
- **St John's Wort** decreases the exposure to opioids (methadone). Monitor and adjust dose. Severe Study → Also see TABLE 13 p. 1337
- **St John's Wort** moderately decreases the exposure to opioids (oxycodone). Adjust dose. Moderate Study
- **St John's Wort** is predicted to decrease the exposure to osimertinib. Avoid. Moderate Theoretical
- **St John's Wort** is predicted to decrease the exposure to palbociclib. Avoid. Severe Theoretical
- **St John's Wort** is predicted to decrease the exposure to paliperidone. Severe Theoretical
- **St John's Wort** is predicted to decrease the exposure to panobinostat. Avoid. Moderate Theoretical
- **St John's Wort** is predicted to decrease the exposure to paritaprevir (with ritonavir and ombitasvir). Avoid. Severe Study

St John's Wort (continued)

▸ **St John's Wort** is predicted to decrease the exposure to phosphodiesterase type-5 inhibitors. Moderate Theoretical
▸ **St John's Wort** is predicted to decrease the exposure to pibrentasvir. Avoid. Severe Study
▸ **St John's Wort** slightly decreases the exposure to pioglitazone. Mild Study
▸ **St John's Wort** is predicted to decrease the exposure to pitolisant. Monitor and adjust dose. Moderate Theoretical
▸ **St John's Wort** is predicted to decrease the exposure to ponatinib. Avoid. Severe Theoretical
▸ **St John's Wort** is predicted to decrease the exposure to quetiapine. Moderate Study
▸ **St John's Wort** is predicted to decrease the exposure to ranolazine. Avoid. Severe Study
▸ **St John's Wort** is predicted to decrease the exposure to ribociclib. Avoid. Severe Study
▸ **St John's Wort** is predicted to decrease the exposure to rilpivirine. Avoid. Severe Theoretical
▸ **St John's Wort** is predicted to decrease the exposure to rolapitant. Avoid. Severe Study
▸ **St John's Wort** is predicted to decrease the exposure to ruxolitinib. Monitor and adjust dose. Moderate Theoretical
▸ **St John's Wort** is predicted to decrease the exposure to simeprevir. Avoid. Severe Study
▸ **St John's Wort** is predicted to decrease the concentration of sirolimus. Monitor and adjust dose. Severe Theoretical
▸ **St John's Wort** is predicted to decrease the exposure to sofosbuvir. Avoid. Severe Study
▸ **St John's Wort** slightly decreases the exposure to statins (atorvastatin). Mild Study
▸ **St John's Wort** moderately decreases the exposure to statins (simvastatin). Moderate Study
▸ **St John's Wort** decreases the concentration of tacrolimus. Avoid. Severe Study
▸ **St John's Wort** is predicted to decrease the exposure to taxanes (cabazitaxel). Avoid. Severe Study
▸ **St John's Wort** is predicted to decrease the concentration of temsirolimus. Avoid. Severe Theoretical
▸ **St John's Wort** is predicted to decrease the exposure to tenofovir alafenamide. Avoid. Moderate Theoretical
▸ **St John's Wort** potentially decreases the exposure to theophylline. Severe Anecdotal
▸ **St John's Wort** is predicted to decrease the exposure to ticagrelor. Moderate Theoretical
▸ **St John's Wort** is predicted to decrease the exposure to tivozanib. Avoid. Severe Study
▸ **St John's Wort** is predicted to decrease the exposure to tofacitinib. Moderate Study
▸ **St John's Wort** is predicted to decrease the exposure to tolvaptan. Moderate Theoretical
▸ **St John's Wort** is predicted to decrease the exposure to topotecan. Severe Theoretical
▸ **St John's Wort** is predicted to decrease the exposure to velpatasvir. Avoid. Moderate Theoretical
▸ **St John's Wort** is predicted to decrease the exposure to venetoclax. Avoid. Severe Study
▸ **St John's Wort** is predicted to decrease the exposure to vismodegib. Avoid. Moderate Theoretical
▸ **St John's Wort** is predicted to decrease the concentration of voxilaprevir. Avoid. Severe Theoretical

Statins → see TABLE 1 p. 1334 (hepatotoxicity)

atorvastatin · fluvastatin · pravastatin · rosuvastatin · simvastatin

▸ **Atorvastatin** slightly to moderately increases the exposure to aliskiren. Moderate Study
▸ Antacids moderately decrease the absorption of **rosuvastatin**. Separate administration by 2 hours. Moderate Study
▸ Antiarrhythmics (amiodarone) are predicted to increase the risk of rhabdomyolysis when given with **atorvastatin**. Monitor and adjust dose. Moderate Theoretical
▸ Antiarrhythmics (amiodarone) are predicted to increase the exposure to **fluvastatin**. Severe Theoretical
▸ Antiarrhythmics (amiodarone) increase the risk of rhabdomyolysis when given with **simvastatin**. Adjust **simvastatin** dose, p. 203. Severe Study

▸ Antiarrhythmics (dronedarone) are predicted to increase the exposure to **atorvastatin**. Monitor and adjust dose. Severe Study
▸ Antiarrhythmics (dronedarone) slightly increase the exposure to **rosuvastatin**. Adjust dose. Severe Study
▸ Antiarrhythmics (dronedarone) are predicted to increase the exposure to **simvastatin**. Use with caution and adjust **simvastatin** dose, p. 203. Severe Study
▸ Antiepileptics (carbamazepine) moderately decrease the exposure to **simvastatin**. Monitor and adjust dose. Severe Study → Also see TABLE 1 p. 1334
▸ Antiepileptics (carbamazepine, eslicarbazepine) are predicted to decrease the exposure to **atorvastatin**. Monitor and adjust dose. Moderate Theoretical → Also see TABLE 1 p. 1334
▸ Antiepileptics (eslicarbazepine) moderately decrease the exposure to **simvastatin**. Monitor and adjust dose. Moderate Study
▸ Antiepileptics (fosphenytoin, phenytoin) potentially decrease the exposure to statins (**atorvastatin, simvastatin**). Moderate Anecdotal
▸ Antifungals, azoles (fluconazole, isavuconazole, posaconazole) are predicted to increase the exposure to **atorvastatin**. Monitor and adjust dose. Severe Study → Also see TABLE 1 p. 1334
▸ Antifungals, azoles (fluconazole, isavuconazole, posaconazole) are predicted to increase the exposure to **simvastatin**. Use with caution and adjust **simvastatin** dose, p. 203. Severe Study → Also see TABLE 1 p. 1334
▸ Antifungals, azoles (fluconazole, miconazole) are predicted to increase the exposure to **fluvastatin**. Severe Theoretical → Also see TABLE 1 p. 1334
▸ Antifungals, azoles (itraconazole, ketoconazole, voriconazole) are predicted to increase the exposure to **atorvastatin**. Avoid or adjust dose and monitor rhabdomyolysis. Severe Study → Also see TABLE 1 p. 1334
▸ Antifungals, azoles (itraconazole, ketoconazole, voriconazole) are predicted to increase the exposure to **simvastatin**. Avoid. Severe Study → Also see TABLE 1 p. 1334
▸ Antifungals, azoles (miconazole) potentially increase the exposure to **atorvastatin**. Severe Anecdotal
▸ Antifungals, azoles (miconazole) are predicted to increase the exposure to **simvastatin**. Avoid. Severe Theoretical
▸ Aprepitant is predicted to increase the exposure to **atorvastatin**. Monitor and adjust dose. Severe Study
▸ Aprepitant is predicted to increase the exposure to **simvastatin**. Use with caution and adjust **simvastatin** dose, p. 203. Severe Study
▸ Bosentan slightly decreases the exposure to **atorvastatin**. Mild Study
▸ Bosentan moderately decreases the exposure to **simvastatin**. Moderate Study
▸ Calcium channel blockers (amlodipine) slightly increase the exposure to **simvastatin**. Adjust **simvastatin** dose, p. 203. Mild Study
▸ Calcium channel blockers (diltiazem, verapamil) are predicted to increase the exposure to **atorvastatin**. Monitor and adjust dose. Severe Study
▸ Calcium channel blockers (diltiazem, verapamil) are predicted to increase the exposure to **simvastatin**. Use with caution and adjust **simvastatin** dose, p. 203. Severe Study
▸ Cephalosporins (ceftobiprole) are predicted to increase the concentration of statins. Moderate Theoretical
▸ Ciclosporin very markedly increases the exposure to **atorvastatin**. Avoid or adjust **atorvastatin** dose, p. 200. Severe Study
▸ Ciclosporin moderately increases the exposure to **fluvastatin**. Severe Study
▸ Ciclosporin markedly to very markedly increases the exposure to **pravastatin**. Adjust dose. Severe Study
▸ Ciclosporin markedly increases the exposure to statins (**rosuvastatin, simvastatin**). Avoid. Severe Study
▸ Clopidogrel increases the exposure to **rosuvastatin**. Adjust **rosuvastatin** dose, p. 202. Moderate Study
▸ Cobicistat is predicted to increase the exposure to **atorvastatin**. Avoid or adjust dose and monitor rhabdomyolysis. Severe Study

▸ Cobicistat is predicted to increase the exposure to **simvastatin**. Avoid. [Severe] Study

▸ Colchicine increases the risk of rhabdomyolysis when given with **statins**. [Severe] Anecdotal

▸ Statins **(fluvastatin, rosuvastatin)** increase the anticoagulant effect of coumarins. Monitor INR and adjust dose. [Severe] Study

▸ Crizotinib is predicted to increase the exposure to **atorvastatin**. Monitor and adjust dose. [Severe] Study

▸ Crizotinib is predicted to increase the exposure to **simvastatin**. Use with caution and adjust **simvastatin** dose, p. 203. [Severe] Study

▸ Danazol is predicted to increase the risk of rhabdomyolysis when given with **atorvastatin**. [Severe] Theoretical

▸ Danazol increases the risk of rhabdomyolysis when given with **simvastatin**. Avoid. [Severe] Anecdotal

▸ Statins are predicted to increase the risk of rhabdomyolysis when given with **daptomycin**. [Severe] Theoretical

▸ Dasabuvir increases the exposure to **rosuvastatin**. Adjust **rosuvastatin** dose, p. 202. [Moderate] Study

▸ Dasatinib is predicted to increase the exposure to **simvastatin**. [Moderate] Theoretical

▸ Efavirenz slightly decreases the exposure to **atorvastatin**. [Mild] Study

▸ Efavirenz moderately decreases the exposure to **simvastatin**. [Moderate] Study

▸ Elbasvir potentially increases the exposure to **atorvastatin**. Adjust **atorvastatin** dose, p. 200. [Moderate] Study

▸ Elbasvir is predicted to increase the exposure to **fluvastatin**. Adjust **fluvastatin** dose, p. 201. [Unknown] Theoretical

▸ Elbasvir increases the exposure to **rosuvastatin**. Adjust **rosuvastatin** dose, p. 202. [Moderate] Study

▸ Elbasvir is predicted to increase the exposure to **simvastatin**. Adjust **simvastatin** dose, p. 203. [Unknown] Theoretical

▸ Eltrombopag is predicted to increase the exposure to **statins**. Monitor and adjust dose. [Moderate] Study

▸ Eluxadoline is predicted to increase the exposure to **statins**. [Moderate] Study

▸ Enzalutamide is predicted to decrease the exposure to **simvastatin**. [Severe] Study

▸ Ezetimibe potentially increases the risk of rhabdomyolysis when given with **statins**. [Severe] Anecdotal

▸ Fibrates (bezafibrate, ciprofibrate) increase the risk of rhabdomyolysis when given with **pravastatin**. Avoid. [Severe] Study

▸ Fibrates (bezafibrate, ciprofibrate) increase the risk of rhabdomyolysis when given with **rosuvastatin**. Adjust **rosuvastatin** dose, p. 202. [Severe] Study

▸ Fibrates (bezafibrate, ciprofibrate) increase the risk of rhabdomyolysis when given with **simvastatin**. Adjust **simvastatin** dose, p. 203. [Severe] Study

▸ Fibrates (ciprofibrate) increase the risk of rhabdomyolysis when given with **atorvastatin**. Avoid or adjust dose. [Severe] Study

▸ Fibrates (ciprofibrate) increase the risk of rhabdomyolysis when given with **fluvastatin**. [Severe] Study

▸ Fibrates (fenofibrate) are predicted to increase the risk of rhabdomyolysis when given with **fluvastatin**. Adjust **fenofibrate** dose, p. 198. [Severe] Theoretical

▸ Fibrates (fenofibrate) are predicted to increase the risk of rhabdomyolysis when given with **pravastatin**. Avoid. [Severe] Theoretical

▸ Fibrates (fenofibrate) increase the risk of rhabdomyolysis when given with **rosuvastatin**. Adjust **fenofibrate** and **rosuvastatin** doses, p. 198, p. 202. [Severe] Anecdotal

▸ Fibrates (gemfibrozil) increase the risk of rhabdomyolysis when given with **statins**. Avoid. [Severe] Anecdotal

▸ Fibrates (bezafibrate) increase the risk of rhabdomyolysis when given with statins **(atorvastatin, fluvastatin)**. [Severe] Study

▸ Fibrates (fenofibrate) increase the risk of rhabdomyolysis when given with statins **(atorvastatin, simvastatin)**. Adjust **fenofibrate** dose, p. 198. [Severe] Anecdotal

▸ Fusidic acid increases the risk of rhabdomyolysis when given with **statins**. Avoid. [Severe] Anecdotal

▸ Glecaprevir (with pibrentasvir) is predicted to increase the exposure to **fluvastatin**. [Moderate] Theoretical

▸ Glecaprevir (with pibrentasvir) increases the exposure to **pravastatin**. Use with caution and adjust **pravastatin** dose, p. 202. [Moderate] Study

▸ Glecaprevir (with pibrentasvir) increases the exposure to **rosuvastatin**. Use with caution and adjust **rosuvastatin** dose, p. 202. [Moderate] Study

▸ Glecaprevir (with pibrentasvir) increases the exposure to statins **(atorvastatin, simvastatin)**. Avoid. [Moderate] Study

▸ Grapefruit juice increases the exposure to **atorvastatin**. [Mild] Study

▸ Grapefruit juice increases the exposure to **simvastatin**. Avoid. [Severe] Study

▸ Grazoprevir increases the exposure to **atorvastatin**. Adjust **atorvastatin** dose, p. 200. [Moderate] Study

▸ Grazoprevir is predicted to increase the exposure to **fluvastatin**. Adjust **fluvastatin** dose, p. 201. [Unknown] Theoretical

▸ Grazoprevir increases the exposure to **rosuvastatin**. Adjust **rosuvastatin** dose, p. 202. [Moderate] Study

▸ Grazoprevir is predicted to increase the exposure to **simvastatin**. Adjust **simvastatin** dose, p. 203. [Unknown] Theoretical

▸ HIV-protease inhibitors are predicted to increase the exposure to **atorvastatin**. Avoid or adjust dose and monitor rhabdomyolysis. [Severe] Study

▸ HIV-protease inhibitors slightly to moderately increase the exposure to **rosuvastatin**. Avoid or adjust dose. [Severe] Study

▸ HIV-protease inhibitors are predicted to increase the exposure to **simvastatin**. Avoid. [Severe] Study

▸ Idelalisib is predicted to increase the exposure to **atorvastatin**. Avoid or adjust dose and monitor rhabdomyolysis. [Severe] Study

▸ Idelalisib is predicted to increase the exposure to **simvastatin**. Avoid. [Severe] Study

▸ Imatinib is predicted to increase the exposure to **atorvastatin**. Monitor and adjust dose. [Severe] Study

▸ Imatinib is predicted to increase the exposure to **simvastatin**. Use with caution and adjust **simvastatin** dose, p. 203. [Severe] Study

▸ Ledipasvir is predicted to increase the exposure to **rosuvastatin**. Avoid. [Severe] Theoretical

▸ Ledipasvir is predicted to increase the exposure to statins **(atorvastatin, fluvastatin, pravastatin, simvastatin)**. Monitor and adjust dose. [Moderate] Theoretical

▸ Leflunomide is predicted to increase the exposure to **rosuvastatin**. Adjust dose. [Moderate] Study → Also see TABLE 1 p. 1334

▸ Lomitapide increases the exposure to **atorvastatin**. Adjust **lomitapide** dose or separate administration by 12 hours, p. 206. [Mild] Study → Also see TABLE 1 p. 1334

▸ Lomitapide increases the exposure to **simvastatin**. Monitor and adjust **simvastatin** dose, p. 203. [Moderate] Study → Also see TABLE 1 p. 1334

▸ Macrolides **(clarithromycin)** are predicted to increase the exposure to **atorvastatin**. Avoid or adjust dose and monitor rhabdomyolysis. [Severe] Study

▸ Macrolides **(clarithromycin)** moderately increase the exposure to **pravastatin**. [Severe] Study

▸ Macrolides **(clarithromycin)** are predicted to increase the exposure to **simvastatin**. Avoid. [Severe] Study

▸ Macrolides **(erythromycin)** are predicted to increase the exposure to **atorvastatin**. Monitor and adjust dose. [Severe] Study

▸ Macrolides **(erythromycin)** are predicted to increase the exposure to **pravastatin**. [Severe] Study

▸ Macrolides **(erythromycin)** are predicted to increase the exposure to **simvastatin**. Use with caution and adjust **simvastatin** dose, p. 203. [Severe] Study

▸ Mitotane is predicted to decrease the exposure to **simvastatin**. [Severe] Study

▸ Monoclonal antibodies **(sarilumab)** are predicted to decrease the exposure to statins **(atorvastatin, simvastatin)**. [Moderate] Study

▸ Monoclonal antibodies **(tocilizumab)** are predicted to decrease the exposure to statins **(atorvastatin, simvastatin)**. Monitor and adjust dose. [Moderate] Study

▸ Netupitant is predicted to increase the exposure to **atorvastatin**. Monitor and adjust dose. [Severe] Study

Statins (continued)

▶ Netupitant is predicted to increase the exposure to **simvastatin**. Use with caution and adjust **simvastatin** dose, p. 203. Severe Study

▶ Nevirapine slightly decreases the exposure to **atorvastatin**. Mild Study

▶ Nevirapine moderately decreases the exposure to **simvastatin**. Moderate Study

▶ Nicotinic acid is predicted to increase the risk of rhabdomyolysis when given with **statins**. Severe Theoretical

▶ Nilotinib is predicted to increase the exposure to **atorvastatin**. Monitor and adjust dose. Severe Study

▶ Nilotinib is predicted to increase the exposure to **simvastatin**. Use with caution and adjust **simvastatin** dose, p. 203. Severe Study

▶ Osimertinib slightly increases the exposure to **rosuvastatin**. Moderate Study

▶ Paritaprevir (with ritonavir and ombitasvir) is predicted to increase the exposure to **fluvastatin**. Avoid. Moderate Theoretical

▶ Paritaprevir (with ritonavir and ombitasvir) increases the exposure to **pravastatin**. Adjust **pravastatin** dose, p. 202. Moderate Study

▶ Paritaprevir (with ritonavir and ombitasvir) increases the exposure to **rosuvastatin**. Adjust **rosuvastatin** dose, p. 202. Moderate Study

▶ **Rosuvastatin** is predicted to increase the anticoagulant effect of phenindione. Monitor INR and adjust dose. Severe Theoretical

▶ Pibrentasvir (with glecaprevir) is predicted to increase the exposure to **fluvastatin**. Moderate Theoretical

▶ Pibrentasvir (with glecaprevir) increases the exposure to **pravastatin**. Use with caution and adjust **pravastatin** dose, p. 202. Moderate Study

▶ Pibrentasvir (with glecaprevir) increases the exposure to **rosuvastatin**. Use with caution and adjust **rosuvastatin** dose, p. 202. Moderate Study

▶ Pibrentasvir (with glecaprevir) increases the exposure to **statins (atorvastatin, simvastatin)**. Avoid. Moderate Study

▶ Ranolazine is predicted to increase the exposure to **atorvastatin**. Moderate Theoretical

▶ Ranolazine slightly increases the exposure to **simvastatin**. Adjust **simvastatin** dose, p. 203. Moderate Study

▶ Regorafenib is predicted to increase the exposure to **statins (atorvastatin, fluvastatin, rosuvastatin)**. Severe Theoretical

▶ Ribociclib (high-dose) is predicted to increase the exposure to **simvastatin**. Avoid. Moderate Theoretical

▶ Rifampicin markedly decreases the exposure to **atorvastatin**. **Atorvastatin** should be taken at the same time as rifampicin, p. 200, p. 571. Moderate Study

▶ Rifampicin moderately decreases the exposure to **fluvastatin**. Monitor and adjust dose. Moderate Study

▶ Rifampicin very markedly decreases the exposure to **simvastatin**. Moderate Study

▶ Rolapitant is predicted to increase the exposure to **rosuvastatin**. Monitor and adjust dose. Severe Study

▶ Sacubitril is predicted to increase the exposure to **statins**. Severe Study

▶ Simeprevir moderately increases the exposure to **atorvastatin**. Monitor and adjust dose. Moderate Study

▶ Simeprevir is predicted to increase the exposure to **pravastatin**. Monitor and adjust dose. Severe Theoretical

▶ Simeprevir moderately increases the exposure to **rosuvastatin**. Adjust **rosuvastatin** dose, p. 202. Moderate Study

▶ Simeprevir slightly increases the exposure to **simvastatin**. Monitor and adjust dose. Moderate Study

▶ St John's Wort slightly decreases the exposure to **atorvastatin**. Mild Study

▶ St John's Wort moderately decreases the exposure to **simvastatin**. Moderate Study

▶ Sulfinpyrazone is predicted to increase the exposure to **fluvastatin**. Severe Theoretical

▶ **Fluvastatin** slightly increases the exposure to sulfonylureas (glibenclamide). Mild Study

▶ Tedizolid increases the exposure to **rosuvastatin**. Avoid. Moderate Study

▶ Teriflunomide moderately increases the exposure to **rosuvastatin**. Adjust **rosuvastatin** dose, p. 202. Moderate Study

▶ Ticagrelor slightly increases the exposure to **simvastatin**. Adjust **simvastatin** dose, p. 203. Moderate Study

▶ Tivozanib is predicted to decrease the exposure to **rosuvastatin**. Moderate Theoretical

▶ Velpatasvir increases the exposure to **rosuvastatin**. Adjust **rosuvastatin** dose and monitor side effects, p. 202. Severe Study

▶ Velpatasvir is predicted to increase the exposure to statins **(atorvastatin, simvastatin)**. Monitor side effects and adjust dose. Severe Theoretical

▶ Voxilaprevir is predicted to increase the exposure to **pravastatin**. Monitor and adjust **pravastatin** dose, p. 202. Severe Study

▶ Voxilaprevir is predicted to increase the exposure to **rosuvastatin**. Avoid. Severe Study

▶ Voxilaprevir is predicted to increase the exposure to statins **(atorvastatin, fluvastatin, simvastatin)**. Avoid. Severe Theoretical

Stavudine → see TABLE 12 p. 1337 (peripheral neuropathy)

▶ Didanosine increases the risk of toxicity when given with **stavudine**. Avoid. Severe Study → Also see TABLE 12 p. 1337

▶ Hydroxycarbamide increases the risk of toxicity when given with **stavudine**. Avoid. Severe Study

▶ Isoniazid is predicted to increase the exposure to peripheral neuropathy when given with **stavudine**. Severe Theoretical → Also see TABLE 12 p. 1337

▶ Ribavirin increases the risk of toxicity when given with **stavudine**. Avoid. Severe Study

▶ Zidovudine is predicted to decrease the efficacy of **stavudine**. Avoid. Severe Theoretical

Stiripentol → see antiepileptics

Streptokinase → see TABLE 3 p. 1334 (anticoagulant effects)

Streptomycin → see aminoglycosides

Sucralfate

▶ **Sucralfate** potentially decreases the effects of coumarins (warfarin). Separate administration by 2 hours. Moderate Anecdotal

▶ **Sucralfate** decreases the absorption of digoxin. Separate administration by 2 hours. Severe Anecdotal

▶ **Sucralfate** decreases the absorption of dolutegravir. Moderate Study

▶ **Sucralfate** increases the risk of blocked enteral or nasogastric tubes when given with enteral feeds. Separate administration by 1 hour. Moderate Study

▶ Potassium citrate increases the risk of side-effects when given with **sucralfate**. Avoid. Moderate Theoretical

▶ **Sucralfate** decreases the exposure to quinolones. Separate administration by 2 hours. Moderate Study

▶ Sodium citrate is predicted to increase the risk of side-effects when given with **sucralfate**. Avoid. Moderate Theoretical

▶ **Sucralfate** decreases the absorption of sulpiride. Separate administration by 2 hours. Moderate Study

▶ **Sucralfate** potentially decreases the absorption of theophylline. Separate administration by at least 2 hours. Moderate Study

▶ **Sucralfate** decreases the absorption of thyroid hormones (levothyroxine). Separate administration by at least 4 hours. Moderate Study

▶ **Sucralfate** is predicted to decrease the absorption of tricyclic antidepressants. Moderate Study

Sufentanil → see opioids

Sugammadex

▶ **Sugammadex** is predicted to decrease the exposure to oral combined hormonal contraceptives. Refer to patient information leaflet for missed pill advice. Severe Theoretical

▶ **Sugammadex** is predicted to decrease the exposure to desogestrel. Refer to patient information leaflet for missed pill advice. Severe Theoretical

▶ **Sugammadex** is predicted to decrease the efficacy of etonogestrel. Use additional contraceptive precautions. Severe Theoretical

▶ **Sugammadex** is predicted to decrease the exposure to levonorgestrel. Use additional contraceptive precautions. Severe Theoretical

- **Sugammadex** is predicted to decrease the exposure to medroxyprogesterone. Use additional contraceptive precautions. [Severe] Theoretical
- **Sugammadex** is predicted to decrease the exposure to norethisterone. Use additional contraceptive precautions. [Severe] Theoretical

Sulfadiazine → see sulfonamides

Sulfadoxine → see sulfonamides

Sulfamethoxazole → see sulfonamides

Sulfasalazine → see TABLE 1 p. 1334 (hepatotoxicity), TABLE 15 p. 1337 (myelosuppression)
- **Sulfasalazine** decreases the concentration of digoxin. [Moderate] Study
- **Sulfasalazine** is predicted to decrease the absorption of folates. [Moderate] Study
- Rolapitant increases the exposure to **sulfasalazine**. [Severe] Study
- Tedizolid is predicted to increase the exposure to **sulfasalazine**. Avoid. [Moderate] Theoretical

Sulfinpyrazone → see TABLE 4 p. 1334 (antiplatelet effects)
- **Sulfinpyrazone** increases the concentration of antiepileptics (fosphenytoin, phenytoin). [Moderate] Study
- Aspirin decreases the effects of **sulfinpyrazone**. [Moderate] Study → Also see TABLE 4 p. 1334
- **Sulfinpyrazone** decreases the exposure to calcium channel blockers (verapamil). [Moderate] Study
- **Sulfinpyrazone** decreases the concentration of ciclosporin. [Severe] Study
- **Sulfinpyrazone** increases the anticoagulant effect of coumarins. Avoid. [Severe] Study
- **Sulfinpyrazone** slightly increases the exposure to nateglinide. [Mild] Study
- Pyrazinamide is predicted to decrease the effects of **sulfinpyrazone**. [Moderate] Theoretical
- **Sulfinpyrazone** is predicted to increase the exposure to retinoids (alitretinoin). Adjust **alitretinoin** dose, p. 1226. [Moderate] Theoretical
- **Sulfinpyrazone** is predicted to increase the exposure to statins (fluvastatin). [Severe] Theoretical
- **Sulfinpyrazone** is predicted to increase the exposure to sulfonylureas. Use with caution and adjust dose. [Moderate] Study

Sulfonamides → see TABLE 15 p. 1337 (myelosuppression)

co-trimoxazole · sulfadiazine · sulfadoxine · sulfamethoxazole

- **Sulfonamides** potentially increase the risk of methaemoglobinaemia when given with topical anaesthetics, local (prilocaine). Use with caution or avoid. [Severe] Anecdotal
- **Sulfadiazine** is predicted to increase the concentration of antiepileptics (fosphenytoin). Monitor and adjust dose. [Moderate] Study
- **Sulfadiazine** increases the concentration of antiepileptics (phenytoin). Monitor and adjust dose. [Moderate] Study
- Antimalarials (pyrimethamine) increase the risk of side-effects when given with **sulfonamides**. [Severe] Study → Also see TABLE 15 p. 1337
- **Sulfadiazine** is predicted to increase the anticoagulant effect of coumarins. [Severe] Theoretical
- **Sulfamethoxazole** increases the anticoagulant effect of coumarins. [Severe] Study
- **Sulfonamides** are predicted to increase the risk of methaemoglobinaemia when given with dapsone. [Severe] Theoretical
- **Sulfonamides** are predicted to increase the exposure to methotrexate. Use with caution or avoid. [Severe] Theoretical → Also see TABLE 15 p. 1337
- **Sulfonamides** are predicted to increase the exposure to sulfonylureas. [Moderate] Study
- **Sulfonamides** are predicted to increase the effects of thiopental. [Moderate] Study

Sulfonylureas → see TABLE 14 p. 1337 (antidiabetic drugs)

glibenclamide · gliclazide · glimepiride · glipizide · tolbutamide

- Antiarrhythmics (amiodarone) are predicted to increase the exposure to **sulfonylureas**. Use with caution and adjust dose. [Moderate] Study

- Antifungals, azoles (fluconazole, miconazole) are predicted to increase the exposure to **sulfonylureas**. Use with caution and adjust dose. [Moderate] Study
- Antifungals, azoles (voriconazole) are predicted to increase the concentration of **sulfonylureas**. Use with caution and adjust dose. [Moderate] Study
- Bosentan increases the risk of hepatotoxicity when given with **glibenclamide**. Avoid. [Severe] Study
- Cephalosporins (ceftobiprole) are predicted to increase the concentration of **glibenclamide**. [Moderate] Theoretical
- Ceritinib is predicted to increase the exposure to **glimepiride**. Adjust dose. [Moderate] Theoretical
- Chloramphenicol is predicted to increase the exposure to **sulfonylureas**. [Severe] Study
- Fibrates are predicted to increase the risk of hypoglycaemia when given with **sulfonylureas**. [Moderate] Theoretical
- Macrolides (clarithromycin) are predicted to slightly increase the exposure to **sulfonylureas**. [Moderate] Theoretical
- Rifampicin is predicted to decrease the exposure to **sulfonylureas**. [Moderate] Study
- Statins (fluvastatin) slightly increase the exposure to **glibenclamide**. [Mild] Study
- Sulfinpyrazone is predicted to increase the exposure to **sulfonylureas**. Use with caution and adjust dose. [Moderate] Study
- Sulfonamides are predicted to increase the exposure to **sulfonylureas**. [Moderate] Study

Sulindac → see NSAIDs

Sulpiride → see TABLE 8 p. 1335 (hypotension), TABLE 9 p. 1336 (QT-interval prolongation), TABLE 11 p. 1336 (CNS depressant effects)
- Antacids decrease the absorption of **sulpiride**. Separate administration by 2 hours. [Moderate] Study
- **Sulpiride** is predicted to decrease the effects of dopamine receptor agonists. Avoid. [Moderate] Theoretical → Also see TABLE 8 p. 1335 → Also see TABLE 9 p. 1336
- **Sulpiride** is predicted to decrease the effects of levodopa. Avoid. [Severe] Theoretical → Also see TABLE 8 p. 1335
- **Sulpiride** potentially increases the risk of neurotoxicity when given with lithium. [Severe] Anecdotal → Also see TABLE 9 p. 1336
- Sucralfate decreases the absorption of **sulpiride**. Separate administration by 2 hours. [Moderate] Study

Sumatriptan → see TABLE 13 p. 1337 (serotonin syndrome)
- **Sumatriptan** increases the risk of vasoconstriction when given with ergotamine. **Ergotamine** should be taken at least 24 hours before or 6 hours after **sumatriptan**. [Severe] Study
- Moclobemide moderately increases the exposure to **sumatriptan**. Avoid. [Moderate] Study → Also see TABLE 13 p. 1337
- Monoamine-oxidase A and B inhibitors, irreversible are predicted to increase the exposure to **sumatriptan**. Avoid and for 14 days after stopping the MAOI. [Severe] Theoretical → Also see TABLE 13 p. 1337

Sunitinib → see TABLE 15 p. 1337 (myelosuppression), TABLE 9 p. 1336 (QT-interval prolongation)
- Antiarrhythmics (dronedarone) are predicted to increase the exposure to **sunitinib**. [Moderate] Theoretical → Also see TABLE 9 p. 1336
- Antiepileptics (carbamazepine, fosphenytoin, phenobarbital, phenytoin, primidone) are predicted to decrease the exposure to **sunitinib**. Avoid or adjust **sunitinib** dose, p. 967. [Moderate] Study
- Antifungals, azoles (fluconazole, isavuconazole, posaconazole) are predicted to increase the exposure to **sunitinib**. [Moderate] Theoretical → Also see TABLE 9 p. 1336
- Antifungals, azoles (itraconazole, ketoconazole, voriconazole) are predicted to slightly increase the exposure to **sunitinib**. Avoid or adjust **sunitinib** dose, p. 967. [Moderate] Study → Also see TABLE 9 p. 1336
- Aprepitant is predicted to increase the exposure to **sunitinib**. [Moderate] Theoretical
- Calcium channel blockers (diltiazem, verapamil) are predicted to increase the exposure to **sunitinib**. [Moderate] Theoretical
- Cobicistat is predicted to slightly increase the exposure to **sunitinib**. Avoid or adjust **sunitinib** dose, p. 967. [Moderate] Study
- **Sunitinib** is predicted to increase the risk of bleeding events when given with coumarins. [Severe] Theoretical

Sunitinib (continued)
▶ Crizotinib is predicted to increase the exposure to **sunitinib**. Moderate Theoretical → Also see TABLE 15 p. 1337 → Also see TABLE 9 p. 1336
▶ Elbasvir is predicted to increase the concentration of **sunitinib**. Use with caution and adjust dose. Moderate Theoretical
▶ Enzalutamide is predicted to decrease the exposure to **sunitinib**. Avoid or adjust **sunitinib** dose, p. 967. Moderate Study
▶ Grapefruit juice is predicted to increase the exposure to **sunitinib**. Avoid. Moderate Theoretical
▶ Grazoprevir is predicted to increase the concentration of **sunitinib**. Use with caution and adjust dose. Moderate Theoretical
▶ HIV-protease inhibitors are predicted to slightly increase the exposure to **sunitinib**. Avoid or adjust **sunitinib** dose, p. 967. Moderate Study → Also see TABLE 9 p. 1336
▶ Idelalisib is predicted to slightly increase the exposure to **sunitinib**. Avoid or adjust **sunitinib** dose, p. 967. Moderate Study → Also see TABLE 15 p. 1337
▶ Imatinib is predicted to increase the exposure to **sunitinib**. Moderate Theoretical → Also see TABLE 15 p. 1337
▶ Macrolides (clarithromycin) are predicted to slightly increase the exposure to **sunitinib**. Avoid or adjust **sunitinib** dose, p. 967. Moderate Study → Also see TABLE 9 p. 1336
▶ Macrolides (erythromycin) are predicted to increase the exposure to **sunitinib**. Moderate Theoretical → Also see TABLE 9 p. 1336
▶ Mitotane is predicted to decrease the exposure to **sunitinib**. Avoid or adjust **sunitinib** dose, p. 967. Moderate Study → Also see TABLE 15 p. 1337
▶ Netupitant is predicted to increase the exposure to **sunitinib**. Moderate Theoretical
▶ Nilotinib is predicted to increase the exposure to **sunitinib**. Moderate Theoretical → Also see TABLE 15 p. 1337 → Also see TABLE 9 p. 1336
▶ **Sunitinib** is predicted to increase the risk of bleeding events when given with phenindione. Severe Theoretical
▶ Rifampicin is predicted to decrease the exposure to **sunitinib**. Avoid or adjust **sunitinib** dose, p. 967. Moderate Study

Suxamethonium → see TABLE 20 p. 1338 (neuromuscular blocking effects)
▶ Alkylating agents (cyclophosphamide) increase the risk of prolonged neuromuscular blockade when given with **suxamethonium**. Moderate Study
▶ Antiarrhythmics (lidocaine) are predicted to increase the effects of **suxamethonium**. Moderate Study
▶ Anticholinesterases, centrally acting increase the effects of **suxamethonium**. Moderate Theoretical
▶ Antiepileptics (carbamazepine) increase the risk of prolonged neuromuscular blockade when given with **suxamethonium**. Moderate Study
▶ Antiepileptics (fosphenytoin, phenytoin) increase the effects of **suxamethonium**. Moderate Study
▶ Clindamycin increases the effects of **suxamethonium**. Severe Anecdotal
▶ Corticosteroids are predicted to decrease the effects of **suxamethonium**. Severe Anecdotal
▶ **Suxamethonium** is predicted to increase the risk of cardiovascular side-effects when given with digoxin. Severe Anecdotal
▶ Irinotecan is predicted to increase the risk of prolonged neuromuscular blockade when given with **suxamethonium**. Moderate Theoretical
▶ Intravenous magnesium is predicted to increase the effects of **suxamethonium**. Moderate Study
▶ Metoclopramide increases the effects of **suxamethonium**. Moderate Study
▶ Penicillins (piperacillin) increase the effects of **suxamethonium**. Moderate Study
▶ SSRIs potentially increase the risk of prolonged neuromuscular blockade when given with **suxamethonium**. Unknown Theoretical

Sympathomimetics, inotropic

dobutamine · dopamine

▶ **Sympathomimetics, inotropic** are predicted to decrease the effects of apraclonidine. Avoid. Severe Theoretical
▶ Beta blockers, non-selective increase the risk of hypertension and bradycardia when given with dobutamine. Severe Theoretical
▶ Beta blockers, selective increase the risk of hypertension and bradycardia when given with dobutamine. Moderate Theoretical
▶ Entacapone is predicted to increase the risk of cardiovascular side-effects when given with **sympathomimetics, inotropic**. Moderate Theoretical
▶ Ergometrine potentially increases the risk of peripheral vasoconstriction when given with dopamine. Avoid. Severe Anecdotal
▶ Guanethidine is predicted to increase the effects of dopamine. Severe Theoretical
▶ **Sympathomimetics, inotropic** are predicted to increase the risk of elevated blood pressure when given with linezolid. Avoid. Severe Theoretical
▶ Monoamine-oxidase A and B inhibitors, irreversible are predicted to increase the risk of a hypertensive crisis when given with **sympathomimetics, inotropic**. Avoid and for 14 days after stopping the MAOI. Severe Theoretical
▶ Monoamine-oxidase B inhibitors are predicted to increase the risk of a hypertensive crisis when given with **sympathomimetics, inotropic**. Avoid. Severe Anecdotal
▶ Opicapone is predicted to increase the risk of cardiovascular side-effects when given with **sympathomimetics, inotropic**. Severe Theoretical
▶ Tolcapone is predicted to increase the risk of cardiovascular side-effects when given with **sympathomimetics, inotropic**. Moderate Theoretical

Sympathomimetics, vasoconstrictor

adrenaline/epinephrine · ephedrine · isometheptene · metaraminol · midodrine · noradrenaline/norepinephrine · phenylephrine · pseudoephedrine · xylometazoline

ROUTE-SPECIFIC INFORMATION Since systemic absorption can follow topical application, the possibility of interactions should be borne in mind.

▶ Ephedrine increases the risk of side-effects when given with aminophylline. Avoid in children. Moderate Study
▶ **Sympathomimetics, vasoconstrictor** are predicted to decrease the effects of apraclonidine. Avoid. Severe Theoretical
▶ Atropine increases the risk of severe hypertension when given with phenylephrine. Severe Study
▶ Beta blockers, non-selective are predicted to increase the risk of hypertension and bradycardia when given with sympathomimetics, vasoconstrictor (**adrenaline/epinephrine, noradrenaline/norepinephrine**). Severe Study
▶ Beta blockers, selective are predicted to increase the risk of hypertension and bradycardia when given with sympathomimetics, vasoconstrictor (**adrenaline/epinephrine, noradrenaline/norepinephrine**). Severe Study
▶ Isometheptene potentially increases the risk of side-effects when given with dopamine receptor agonists (bromocriptine). Avoid. Severe Anecdotal
▶ Entacapone is predicted to increase the risk of cardiovascular side-effects when given with sympathomimetics, vasoconstrictor (**adrenaline/epinephrine, noradrenaline/norepinephrine**). Moderate Study
▶ Ergometrine is predicted to increase the risk of peripheral vasoconstriction when given with noradrenaline/norepinephrine. Severe Anecdotal
▶ Guanethidine increases the effects of metaraminol. Severe Anecdotal
▶ Guanethidine increases the effects of phenylephrine. Severe Study
▶ Guanethidine is predicted to increase the effects of sympathomimetics, vasoconstrictor (**adrenaline/epinephrine, noradrenaline/norepinephrine**). Moderate Study
▶ Pseudoephedrine increases the risk of elevated blood pressure when given with linezolid. Avoid. Severe Study
▶ Sympathomimetics, vasoconstrictor (**adrenaline/epinephrine, ephedrine, isometheptene, noradrenaline/norepinephrine, phenylephrine**) are predicted to increase the risk of elevated

blood pressure when given with linezolid. Avoid. [Severe] Theoretical

▸ Mianserin decreases the effects of **ephedrine**. [Severe] Anecdotal

▸ Moclobemide is predicted to increase the risk of a hypertensive crisis when given with sympathomimetics, vasoconstrictor (**ephedrine, isometheptene, phenylephrine, pseudoephedrine**). Avoid. [Severe] Study

▸ Monoamine-oxidase A and B inhibitors, irreversible are predicted to increase the risk of a hypertensive crisis when given with **sympathomimetics, vasoconstrictor**. Avoid and for 14 days after stopping the MAOI. [Severe] Study

▸ Monoamine-oxidase B inhibitors are predicted to increase the risk of a hypertensive crisis when given with **sympathomimetics, vasoconstrictor**. Avoid. [Severe] Anecdotal

▸ Opicapone is predicted to increase the risk of cardiovascular side-effects when given with sympathomimetics, vasoconstrictor (**adrenaline/epinephrine, noradrenaline/norepinephrine**). [Severe] Theoretical

▸ **Ephedrine** increases the risk of side-effects when given with theophylline. Avoid in children. [Moderate] Study

▸ Tolcapone is predicted to increase the effects of sympathomimetics, vasoconstrictor (**adrenaline/epinephrine, noradrenaline/norepinephrine**). [Moderate] Theoretical

▸ Tricyclic antidepressants are predicted to decrease the effects of **ephedrine**. Avoid. [Severe] Study

▸ Tricyclic antidepressants increase the effects of sympathomimetics, vasoconstrictor (**adrenaline/epinephrine, noradrenaline/norepinephrine, phenylephrine**). Avoid. [Severe] Study

Tacalcitol → see vitamin D substances

Tacrolimus → see TABLE 2 p. 1334 (nephrotoxicity), TABLE 16 p. 1338 (increased serum potassium)

▸ Pomelo might greatly increase the concentration of tacrolimus.

▸ Since systemic absorption can follow topical application, the possibility of interactions should be borne in mind.

▸ Alcohol (beverage) increases the risk of facial flushing and skin irritation when given with topical **tacrolimus**. [Moderate] Study

▸ Antiarrhythmics (amiodarone) are predicted to increase the concentration of **tacrolimus**. [Severe] Anecdotal

▸ Antiarrhythmics (dronedarone) are predicted to increase the concentration of **tacrolimus**. [Severe] Study

▸ Antiepileptics (carbamazepine, fosphenytoin, phenobarbital, phenytoin, primidone) decrease the concentration of **tacrolimus**. Monitor and adjust dose. [Severe] Study

▸ Antifungals, azoles (fluconazole, isavuconazole, posaconazole) are predicted to increase the concentration of **tacrolimus**. [Severe] Study

▸ Antifungals, azoles (itraconazole, ketoconazole, voriconazole) are predicted to increase the concentration of **tacrolimus**. Monitor and adjust dose. [Severe] Study

▸ Antifungals, azoles (miconazole) are predicted to increase the concentration of **tacrolimus**. Monitor and adjust dose. [Severe] Theoretical

▸ Aprepitant is predicted to increase the concentration of **tacrolimus**. [Severe] Study

▸ Bosentan is predicted to decrease the concentration of **tacrolimus** and **tacrolimus** potentially increases the concentration of bosentan. Avoid. [Severe] Theoretical

▸ Calcium channel blockers (diltiazem, verapamil) are predicted to increase the concentration of **tacrolimus**. [Severe] Study

▸ Calcium channel blockers (nicardipine) potentially increase the concentration of **tacrolimus**. Monitor concentration and adjust dose. [Severe] Anecdotal

▸ Ceritinib is predicted to increase the exposure to **tacrolimus**. Avoid. [Severe] Theoretical

▸ Chloramphenicol increases the concentration of **tacrolimus**. [Severe] Study

▸ Ciclosporin increases the concentration of **tacrolimus**. Avoid. [Severe] Study → Also see TABLE 2 p. 1334 → Also see TABLE 16 p. 1338

▸ Cobicistat is predicted to increase the concentration of **tacrolimus**. Monitor and adjust dose. [Severe] Study

▸ Crizotinib is predicted to increase the concentration of **tacrolimus**. [Severe] Study

▸ Danazol potentially increases the concentration of **tacrolimus**. [Severe] Anecdotal

▸ Efavirenz is predicted to decrease the concentration of **tacrolimus**. Monitor and adjust dose. [Moderate] Theoretical

▸ Enzalutamide decreases the concentration of **tacrolimus**. Monitor and adjust dose. [Severe] Study

▸ Grapefruit juice increases the concentration of **tacrolimus**. Avoid. [Moderate] Study

▸ Grazoprevir increases the exposure to **tacrolimus**. [Moderate] Study

▸ HIV-protease inhibitors are predicted to increase the concentration of **tacrolimus**. Monitor and adjust dose. [Severe] Study

▸ Idelalisib is predicted to increase the concentration of **tacrolimus**. Monitor and adjust dose. [Severe] Study

▸ Imatinib is predicted to increase the concentration of **tacrolimus**. [Severe] Study

▸ Live vaccines are predicted to increase the risk of generalised infection (possibly life-threatening) when given with **tacrolimus**. Public Health England advises avoid (refer to Green Book). [Severe] Theoretical

▸ **Tacrolimus** is predicted to increase the exposure to lomitapide. Separate administration by 12 hours. [Moderate] Theoretical

▸ Lumacaftor is predicted to decrease the exposure to **tacrolimus**. Avoid. [Severe] Theoretical

▸ Macrolides (clarithromycin) are predicted to increase the concentration of **tacrolimus**. Monitor and adjust dose. [Severe] Study

▸ Macrolides (erythromycin) are predicted to increase the concentration of **tacrolimus**. [Severe] Study

▸ **Tacrolimus** is predicted to affect the efficacy of mifamurtide. Avoid. [Severe] Theoretical

▸ Mitotane decreases the concentration of **tacrolimus**. Monitor and adjust dose. [Severe] Study

▸ Monoclonal antibodies (sarilumab) potentially affect the exposure to **tacrolimus**. Monitor and adjust dose. [Moderate] Theoretical

▸ Netupitant is predicted to increase the concentration of **tacrolimus**. [Severe] Study

▸ Nevirapine is predicted to decrease the concentration of **tacrolimus**. Monitor and adjust dose. [Moderate] Theoretical

▸ Nilotinib is predicted to increase the concentration of **tacrolimus**. [Severe] Study

▸ Palbociclib is predicted to increase the exposure to **tacrolimus**. Adjust dose. [Moderate] Theoretical

▸ Pitolisant is predicted to decrease the exposure to **tacrolimus**. Avoid. [Severe] Theoretical

▸ Ranolazine increases the concentration of **tacrolimus**. Adjust dose. [Severe] Anecdotal

▸ Ribociclib is predicted to increase the exposure to **tacrolimus**. Use with caution and adjust dose. [Moderate] Theoretical

▸ Rifampicin decreases the concentration of **tacrolimus**. Monitor and adjust dose. [Severe] Study

▸ Sirolimus is predicted to decrease the concentration of **tacrolimus** and **tacrolimus** increases the exposure to sirolimus. [Severe] Study

▸ St John's Wort decreases the concentration of **tacrolimus**. Avoid. [Severe] Study

▸ **Tacrolimus** increases the exposure to tofacitinib. Avoid. [Severe] Study

▸ **Tacrolimus** potentially increases the risk of serotonin syndrome when given with venlafaxine. [Severe] Anecdotal

Tadalafil → see phosphodiesterase type-5 inhibitors

Tamoxifen → see TABLE 5 p. 1334 (thromboembolism)

▸ Bupropion is predicted to decrease the efficacy of **tamoxifen**. Avoid. [Severe] Study

▸ Cinacalcet is predicted to decrease the efficacy of **tamoxifen**. Avoid. [Severe] Study

▸ **Tamoxifen** increases the anticoagulant effect of coumarins. [Severe] Study

▸ Rifampicin markedly decreases the exposure to **tamoxifen**. [Unknown] Study

▸ Rolapitant is predicted to increase the exposure to **tamoxifen**. [Severe] Study

Tamoxifen (continued)
▸ SSRIs (fluoxetine, paroxetine) are predicted to decrease the efficacy of **tamoxifen**. Avoid. Severe Study
▸ Terbinafine is predicted to decrease the efficacy of **tamoxifen**. Avoid. Severe Study

Tamsulosin → see alpha blockers

Tapentadol → see opioids

Taxanes → see TABLE 15 p. 1337 (myelosuppression), TABLE 12 p. 1337 (peripheral neuropathy)

cabazitaxel · docetaxel · paclitaxel

▸ Antiarrhythmics (dronedarone) are predicted to increase the exposure to **cabazitaxel**. Moderate Theoretical
▸ Antiarrhythmics (dronedarone) are predicted to increase the exposure to **paclitaxel**. Severe Theoretical
▸ Antiepileptics (carbamazepine, fosphenytoin, phenobarbital, phenytoin, primidone) are predicted to decrease the exposure to **docetaxel**. Severe Theoretical → Also see TABLE 12 p. 1337
▸ Antiepileptics (carbamazepine, fosphenytoin, phenobarbital, phenytoin, primidone) are predicted to decrease the exposure to taxanes (**cabazitaxel, paclitaxel**). Avoid. Severe Study → Also see TABLE 12 p. 1337
▸ Antifungals, azoles (fluconazole, isavuconazole, posaconazole) are predicted to increase the exposure to **cabazitaxel**. Moderate Theoretical
▸ Antifungals, azoles (itraconazole, ketoconazole, voriconazole) are predicted to increase the exposure to **cabazitaxel**. Avoid. Severe Study
▸ Antifungals, azoles (itraconazole, ketoconazole, voriconazole) are predicted to moderately increase the exposure to **docetaxel**. Avoid or adjust dose. Severe Study
▸ Antifungals, azoles (itraconazole, ketoconazole, voriconazole) are predicted to increase the exposure to **paclitaxel**. Severe Theoretical
▸ Antifungals, azoles (miconazole) are predicted to increase the concentration of **docetaxel**. Use with caution and adjust dose. Moderate Theoretical
▸ Aprepitant is predicted to increase the exposure to **cabazitaxel**. Moderate Theoretical
▸ Bosentan is predicted to decrease the exposure to **cabazitaxel**. Avoid. Severe Study
▸ Calcium channel blockers (diltiazem, verapamil) are predicted to increase the exposure to **cabazitaxel**. Moderate Theoretical
▸ Ceritinib is predicted to increase the exposure to **paclitaxel**. Moderate Theoretical → Also see TABLE 15 p. 1337
▸ Clopidogrel is predicted to increase the concentration of **paclitaxel**. Severe Anecdotal
▸ Cobicistat is predicted to increase the exposure to **cabazitaxel**. Avoid. Severe Study
▸ Cobicistat is predicted to moderately increase the exposure to **docetaxel**. Avoid or adjust dose. Severe Study
▸ Cobicistat is predicted to increase the exposure to **paclitaxel**. Severe Theoretical
▸ Crizotinib is predicted to increase the exposure to **cabazitaxel**. Moderate Theoretical → Also see TABLE 15 p. 1337
▸ Efavirenz is predicted to decrease the exposure to **cabazitaxel**. Avoid. Severe Study
▸ Eliglustat is predicted to increase the exposure to **paclitaxel**. Adjust dose. Moderate Study
▸ Enzalutamide is predicted to decrease the exposure to **docetaxel**. Severe Theoretical
▸ Enzalutamide is predicted to decrease the exposure to taxanes (**cabazitaxel, paclitaxel**). Avoid. Severe Study
▸ Fibrates (gemfibrozil) are predicted to increase the concentration of **paclitaxel**. Severe Anecdotal
▸ HIV-protease inhibitors are predicted to increase the exposure to **cabazitaxel**. Avoid. Severe Study
▸ HIV-protease inhibitors are predicted to moderately increase the exposure to **docetaxel**. Avoid or adjust dose. Severe Study
▸ HIV-protease inhibitors are predicted to increase the exposure to **paclitaxel**. Severe Theoretical
▸ Idelalisib is predicted to increase the exposure to **cabazitaxel**. Avoid. Severe Study → Also see TABLE 15 p. 1337
▸ Idelalisib is predicted to moderately increase the exposure to **docetaxel**. Avoid or adjust dose. Severe Study → Also see TABLE 15 p. 1337

▸ Idelalisib is predicted to increase the exposure to **paclitaxel**. Severe Theoretical → Also see TABLE 15 p. 1337
▸ Imatinib is predicted to increase the exposure to **cabazitaxel**. Moderate Theoretical → Also see TABLE 15 p. 1337
▸ Lapatinib slightly increases the exposure to **paclitaxel**. Severe Study
▸ Leflunomide is predicted to increase the concentration of **paclitaxel**. Severe Anecdotal → Also see TABLE 15 p. 1337
▸ Live vaccines are predicted to increase the risk of generalised infection (possibly life-threatening) when given with taxanes (**docetaxel, paclitaxel**). Public Health England advises avoid (refer to Green Book). Severe Theoretical
▸ Macrolides (clarithromycin) are predicted to increase the exposure to **cabazitaxel**. Avoid. Severe Study
▸ Macrolides (clarithromycin) are predicted to moderately increase the exposure to **docetaxel**. Avoid or adjust dose. Severe Study
▸ Macrolides (clarithromycin) are predicted to increase the exposure to **paclitaxel**. Severe Theoretical
▸ Macrolides (erythromycin) are predicted to increase the exposure to **cabazitaxel**. Moderate Theoretical
▸ Mirabegron is predicted to increase the exposure to **paclitaxel**. Mild Theoretical
▸ Mitotane is predicted to decrease the exposure to **docetaxel**. Severe Theoretical → Also see TABLE 15 p. 1337
▸ Mitotane is predicted to decrease the exposure to taxanes (**cabazitaxel, paclitaxel**). Avoid. Severe Study → Also see TABLE 15 p. 1337
▸ Netupitant is predicted to increase the exposure to **cabazitaxel**. Moderate Theoretical
▸ Nevirapine is predicted to decrease the exposure to **cabazitaxel**. Avoid. Severe Study
▸ Nilotinib is predicted to increase the exposure to **cabazitaxel**. Moderate Theoretical → Also see TABLE 15 p. 1337
▸ Pitolisant is predicted to decrease the exposure to **docetaxel**. Avoid. Severe Theoretical
▸ Rifampicin is predicted to decrease the exposure to **docetaxel**. Severe Theoretical
▸ Rifampicin is predicted to decrease the exposure to taxanes (**cabazitaxel, paclitaxel**). Avoid. Severe Study
▸ St John's Wort is predicted to decrease the exposure to **cabazitaxel**. Avoid. Severe Study
▸ Teriflunomide is predicted to increase the concentration of **paclitaxel**. Severe Anecdotal
▸ Velpatasvir is predicted to increase the exposure to **paclitaxel**. Severe Theoretical

Tazarotene → see retinoids

Tedizolid
▸ Tedizolid is predicted to increase the exposure to imatinib. Avoid. Moderate Theoretical
▸ Tedizolid is predicted to increase the exposure to lapatinib. Avoid. Moderate Theoretical
▸ Tedizolid is predicted to increase the exposure to methotrexate. Avoid. Moderate Theoretical
▸ Tedizolid increases the exposure to statins (rosuvastatin). Avoid. Moderate Study
▸ Tedizolid is predicted to increase the exposure to sulfasalazine. Avoid. Moderate Theoretical
▸ Tedizolid is predicted to increase the exposure to topotecan. Avoid. Moderate Theoretical

Tegafur
▸ **Tegafur** potentially increases the concentration of antiepileptics (fosphenytoin, phenytoin). Monitor concentration and adjust dose. Severe Anecdotal
▸ **Tegafur** increases the anticoagulant effect of coumarins. Moderate Theoretical
▸ Folates are predicted to increase the risk of toxicity when given with **tegafur**. Severe Theoretical
▸ H₂ receptor antagonists (cimetidine) are predicted to increase the risk of toxicity when given with **tegafur**. Severe Theoretical
▸ Live vaccines are predicted to increase the risk of generalised infection (possibly life-threatening) when given with **tegafur**. Public Health England advises avoid (refer to Green Book). Severe Theoretical

▸ Methotrexate is predicted to increase the risk of toxicity when given with **tegafur**. [Severe] Theoretical

Teicoplanin

GENERAL INFORMATION If other nephrotoxic or neurotoxic drugs are given, monitor renal and auditory function on prolonged administration.

Telavancin → see TABLE 2 p. 1334 (nephrotoxicity), **TABLE 19** p. 1338 (ototoxicity), **TABLE 9** p. 1336 (QT-interval prolongation)

Telbivudine

▸ Interferons (interferon alfa) are predicted to increase the risk of peripheral neuropathy when given with **telbivudine**. Avoid. [Severe] Theoretical

▸ Interferons (peginterferon alfa) increase the risk of peripheral neuropathy when given with **telbivudine**. Avoid. [Severe] Study

Telmisartan → see angiotensin-II receptor antagonists

Telotristat ethyl

▸ **Telotristat ethyl** decreases the exposure to midazolam. [Moderate] Study

▸ Octreotide (short-acting) decreases the exposure to **telotristat ethyl**. **Telotristat ethyl** should be taken at least 30 minutes before octreotide, p. 864, p. 924. [Moderate] Study

Temazepam → see TABLE 11 p. 1336 (CNS depressant effects)

Temocillin → see penicillins

Temozolomide → see alkylating agents

Temsirolimus → see TABLE 15 p. 1337 (myelosuppression)

▸ Antiarrhythmics (dronedarone) are predicted to increase the concentration of **temsirolimus**. [Moderate] Theoretical

▸ Antiepileptics (carbamazepine, fosphenytoin, phenobarbital, phenytoin, primidone) are predicted to decrease the concentration of **temsirolimus**. Avoid. [Severe] Study

▸ Antifungals, azoles (fluconazole, isavuconazole, posaconazole) are predicted to increase the concentration of **temsirolimus**. [Moderate] Theoretical

▸ Antifungals, azoles (itraconazole, ketoconazole, voriconazole) are predicted to increase the concentration of **temsirolimus**. Avoid. [Severe] Theoretical

▸ Aprepitant is predicted to increase the concentration of **temsirolimus**. [Moderate] Theoretical

▸ Bosentan is predicted to decrease the concentration of **temsirolimus**. Avoid. [Severe] Theoretical

▸ Calcium channel blockers (diltiazem, verapamil) are predicted to increase the concentration of **temsirolimus**. [Moderate] Theoretical

▸ Cobicistat is predicted to increase the concentration of **temsirolimus**. Avoid. [Severe] Theoretical

▸ Crizotinib is predicted to increase the concentration of **temsirolimus**. [Moderate] Theoretical → Also see TABLE 15 p. 1337

▸ Efavirenz is predicted to decrease the concentration of **temsirolimus**. Avoid. [Severe] Theoretical

▸ Enzalutamide is predicted to decrease the concentration of **temsirolimus**. Avoid. [Severe] Study

▸ Grapefruit juice is predicted to increase the concentration of **temsirolimus**. Use with caution or avoid. [Moderate] Theoretical

▸ HIV-protease inhibitors are predicted to increase the concentration of **temsirolimus**. Avoid. [Severe] Theoretical

▸ Idelalisib is predicted to increase the concentration of **temsirolimus**. Avoid. [Severe] Theoretical → Also see TABLE 15 p. 1337

▸ Imatinib is predicted to increase the concentration of **temsirolimus**. [Moderate] Theoretical → Also see TABLE 15 p. 1337

▸ Live vaccines are predicted to increase the risk of generalised infection (possibly life-threatening) when given with **temsirolimus**. Public Health England advises avoid (refer to Green Book). [Severe] Theoretical

▸ Lumacaftor is predicted to decrease the exposure to **temsirolimus**. Avoid. [Severe] Theoretical

▸ Macrolides (clarithromycin) are predicted to increase the concentration of **temsirolimus**. Avoid. [Severe] Theoretical

▸ Macrolides (erythromycin) are predicted to increase the concentration of **temsirolimus**. [Moderate] Theoretical

▸ Mitotane is predicted to decrease the concentration of **temsirolimus**. Avoid. [Severe] Study → Also see TABLE 15 p. 1337

▸ Netupitant is predicted to increase the concentration of **temsirolimus**. [Moderate] Theoretical

▸ Nevirapine is predicted to decrease the concentration of **temsirolimus**. Avoid. [Severe] Theoretical

▸ Nilotinib is predicted to increase the concentration of **temsirolimus**. [Moderate] Theoretical → Also see TABLE 15 p. 1337

▸ Pitolisant is predicted to decrease the exposure to **temsirolimus**. Avoid. [Severe] Theoretical

▸ Rifampicin is predicted to decrease the concentration of **temsirolimus**. Avoid. [Severe] Study

▸ St John's Wort is predicted to decrease the concentration of **temsirolimus**. Avoid. [Severe] Theoretical

Tenecteplase → see TABLE 3 p. 1334 (anticoagulant effects)

Tenofovir alafenamide

▸ Antiepileptics (carbamazepine, fosphenytoin, oxcarbazepine, phenobarbital, phenytoin, primidone) are predicted to decrease the exposure to **tenofovir alafenamide**. Avoid. [Moderate] Theoretical

▸ HIV-protease inhibitors (atazanavir, darunavir) increase the exposure to **tenofovir alafenamide**. Avoid. [Moderate] Study

▸ HIV-protease inhibitors (tipranavir) are predicted to affect the exposure to **tenofovir alafenamide**. Avoid. [Moderate] Theoretical

▸ Rifabutin is predicted to decrease the exposure to **tenofovir alafenamide**. Avoid. [Moderate] Theoretical

▸ Rifampicin is predicted to decrease the exposure to **tenofovir alafenamide**. Avoid. [Moderate] Theoretical

▸ St John's Wort is predicted to decrease the exposure to **tenofovir alafenamide**. Avoid. [Moderate] Theoretical

Tenofovir disoproxil → see TABLE 2 p. 1334 (nephrotoxicity)

▸ **Tenofovir disoproxil** increases the risk of toxicity when given with didanosine. Avoid. [Severe] Study

▸ Ledipasvir (with sofosbuvir) slightly increases the exposure to **tenofovir disoproxil**. [Moderate] Study

▸ Velpatasvir is predicted to increase the exposure to **tenofovir disoproxil**. [Severe] Study

▸ Voxilaprevir is predicted to increase the exposure to **tenofovir disoproxil**. [Severe] Study

Tenoxicam → see NSAIDs

Terazosin → see alpha blockers

Terbinafine

ROUTE-SPECIFIC INFORMATION Since systemic absorption can follow topical application, the possibility of interactions should be borne in mind.

▸ **Terbinafine** is predicted to increase the exposure to anticholinesterases, centrally acting (galantamine). Monitor and adjust dose. [Moderate] Study

▸ **Terbinafine** is predicted to moderately increase the exposure to aripiprazole. Adjust **aripiprazole** dose, p. 391. [Moderate] Study

▸ **Terbinafine** is predicted to markedly increase the exposure to atomoxetine. Adjust dose. [Severe] Study

▸ **Terbinafine** is predicted to increase the exposure to beta blockers, selective (metoprolol, nebivolol). [Moderate] Study

▸ **Terbinafine** is predicted to slightly increase the exposure to darifenacin. [Mild] Study

▸ **Terbinafine** is predicted to increase the exposure to eliglustat. Avoid or adjust dose—consult product literature. [Severe] Study

▸ **Terbinafine** is predicted to decrease the efficacy of opioids (codeine). [Moderate] Theoretical

▸ **Terbinafine** is predicted to decrease the efficacy of opioids (tramadol). [Severe] Study

▸ **Terbinafine** is predicted to moderately increase the exposure to pitolisant. Use with caution and adjust dose. [Moderate] Study

▸ Rifampicin decreases the exposure to **terbinafine**. Adjust dose. [Moderate] Study

▸ **Terbinafine** is predicted to increase the exposure to risperidone. Adjust dose. [Moderate] Study

▸ **Terbinafine** is predicted to increase the exposure to SSRIs (citalopram, dapoxetine, escitalopram, fluvoxamine, sertraline). [Moderate] Theoretical

▸ **Terbinafine** is predicted to increase the exposure to SSRIs (fluoxetine). Adjust dose. [Moderate] Theoretical

▸ **Terbinafine** moderately increases the exposure to SSRIs (paroxetine). [Moderate] Study

▸ **Terbinafine** is predicted to decrease the efficacy of tamoxifen. Avoid. [Severe] Study

▸ **Terbinafine** is predicted to increase the exposure to tricyclic antidepressants. Monitor for toxicity and adjust dose. [Severe] Study

A1

Interactions | Appendix 1

Terbinafine (continued)
▶ Terbinafine is predicted to increase the exposure to vortioxetine. Monitor and adjust dose. Moderate Study
Terbutaline → see beta₂ agonists
Teriflunomide
▶ Teriflunomide is predicted to decrease the exposure to agomelatine. Moderate Theoretical
▶ Teriflunomide decreases the exposure to aminophylline. Adjust dose. Moderate Study
▶ Teriflunomide is predicted to decrease the exposure to anaesthetics, local (ropivacaine). Moderate Theoretical
▶ Teriflunomide potentially increases the exposure to baricitinib. Moderate Theoretical
▶ Teriflunomide is predicted to moderately increase the clearance of caffeine citrate. Monitor and adjust dose. Moderate Study
▶ Teriflunomide is predicted to decrease the exposure to clozapine. Moderate Theoretical
▶ Teriflunomide affects the anticoagulant effect of coumarins. Severe Study
▶ Teriflunomide is predicted to decrease the exposure to duloxetine. Moderate Theoretical
▶ Live vaccines are predicted to increase the risk of generalised infection (possibly life-threatening) when given with teriflunomide. Public Health England advises avoid (refer to Green Book). Severe Theoretical
▶ Teriflunomide is predicted to decrease the exposure to melatonin. Moderate Theoretical
▶ Teriflunomide is predicted to increase the exposure to montelukast. Moderate Theoretical
▶ Teriflunomide is predicted to decrease the exposure to olanzapine. Monitor and adjust dose. Moderate Study
▶ Teriflunomide is predicted to increase the exposure to pioglitazone. Moderate Study
▶ Teriflunomide is predicted to decrease the exposure to pirfenidone. Moderate Theoretical
▶ Teriflunomide is predicted to increase the exposure to repaglinide. Moderate Study
▶ Teriflunomide is predicted to increase the exposure to selexipag. Adjust dose. Moderate Theoretical
▶ Teriflunomide moderately increases the exposure to statins (rosuvastatin). Adjust rosuvastatin dose, p. 202. Moderate Study
▶ Teriflunomide is predicted to increase the concentration of taxanes (paclitaxel). Severe Anecdotal
▶ Teriflunomide is predicted to decrease the exposure to theophylline. Adjust dose. Moderate Study
▶ Teriflunomide moderately decreases the exposure to tizanidine. Mild Study
Tetrabenazine → see TABLE 9 p. 1336 (QT-interval prolongation)
▶ Tetrabenazine is predicted to decrease the effects of levodopa. Use with caution or avoid. Moderate Theoretical
▶ Tetrabenazine is predicted to increase the risk of CNS toxicity when given with monoamine-oxidase A and B inhibitors, irreversible. Avoid and for 14 days after stopping the MAOI. Severe Theoretical
Tetracaine → see anaesthetics, local
Tetracycline → see tetracyclines
Tetracyclines → see TABLE 1 p. 1334 (hepatotoxicity)

demeclocycline · doxycycline · lymecycline · minocycline · oxytetracycline · tetracycline · tigecycline

▶ ACE inhibitors (quinapril) (tablet) decrease the absorption of oral tetracycline. Avoid. Moderate Study
▶ Antacids decrease the absorption of tetracyclines. Separate administration by 2 to 3 hours. Moderate Study
▶ Antiepileptics (carbamazepine, fosphenytoin, phenobarbital, phenytoin, primidone) decrease the exposure to doxycycline. Monitor and adjust dose. Moderate Study → Also see TABLE 1 p. 1334
▶ Tetracycline decreases the concentration of antimalarials (atovaquone). Moderate Study
▶ Calcium salts (calcium carbonate) are predicted to decrease the absorption of tetracyclines. Separate administration by 2 to 3 hours. Moderate Theoretical
▶ Tetracyclines increase the risk of bleeding events when given with coumarins. Moderate Anecdotal

▶ Dairy products decrease the exposure to tetracyclines (demeclocycline, oxytetracycline, tetracycline). Avoid. Moderate Study
▶ Enzalutamide decreases the exposure to doxycycline. Monitor and adjust dose. Moderate Study
▶ Iron (oral) decreases the absorption of tetracyclines. Tetracyclines should be taken 2 to 3 hours after iron (oral). Moderate Study
▶ Kaolin is predicted to decrease the absorption of tetracyclines. Moderate Theoretical
▶ Lanthanum is predicted to decrease the absorption of tetracyclines. Separate administration by 2 hours. Moderate Theoretical
▶ Mitotane decreases the exposure to doxycycline. Monitor and adjust dose. Moderate Study
▶ Retinoids (acitretin, alitretinoin, isotretinoin, tretinoin) increase the risk of benign intracranial hypertension when given with tetracyclines. Avoid. Severe Anecdotal
▶ Rifampicin decreases the exposure to doxycycline. Monitor and adjust dose. Moderate Study
▶ Oral zinc is predicted to decrease the absorption of tetracyclines. Separate administration by 2 to 3 hours. Moderate Theoretical
Thalidomide → see TABLE 6 p. 1335 (bradycardia), TABLE 15 p. 1337 (myelosuppression), TABLE 12 p. 1337 (peripheral neuropathy), TABLE 5 p. 1334 (thromboembolism), TABLE 11 p. 1336 (CNS depressant effects)
▶ Combined hormonal contraceptives are predicted to increase the risk of venous thromboembolism when given with thalidomide. Avoid. Severe Study
▶ Hormone replacement therapy is predicted to increase the risk of venous thromboembolism when given with thalidomide. Severe Theoretical
Theophylline → see TABLE 17 p. 1338 (reduced serum potassium)

FOOD AND LIFESTYLE Smoking can increase theophylline clearance and increased doses of theophylline are therefore required; dose adjustments are likely to be necessary if smoking started or stopped during treatment.

▶ Aciclovir is predicted to increase the exposure to theophylline. Monitor and adjust dose. Severe Theoretical
▶ Theophylline decreases the efficacy of antiarrhythmics (adenosine). Separate administration by 24 hours. Mild Study
▶ Antiepileptics (carbamazepine) potentially increase the clearance of theophylline and theophylline decreases the exposure to antiepileptics (carbamazepine). Adjust dose. Moderate Anecdotal
▶ Antiepileptics (fosphenytoin, phenytoin) are predicted to decrease the exposure to theophylline. Adjust dose. Moderate Study
▶ Antiepileptics (phenobarbital, primidone) are predicted to increase the clearance of theophylline. Adjust dose. Moderate Theoretical
▶ Antiepileptics (stiripentol) are predicted to increase the exposure to theophylline. Avoid. Moderate Theoretical
▶ Beta blockers, non-selective are predicted to increase the risk of bronchospasm when given with theophylline. Avoid. Severe Theoretical
▶ Beta blockers, selective are predicted to increase the risk of bronchospasm when given with theophylline. Avoid. Severe Theoretical
▶ Caffeine citrate decreases the clearance of theophylline. Moderate Study
▶ Combined hormonal contraceptives are predicted to increase the exposure to theophylline. Monitor and adjust dose. Moderate Theoretical
▶ Theophylline increases the risk of agitation when given with doxapram. Moderate Study
▶ Enteral feeds decrease the exposure to theophylline. Moderate Study
▶ H₂ receptor antagonists (cimetidine) increase the concentration of theophylline. Adjust dose. Severe Study
▶ HIV-protease inhibitors (ritonavir) are predicted to decrease the exposure to theophylline. Adjust dose. Moderate Study
▶ Interferons slightly increase the exposure to theophylline. Adjust dose. Moderate Study

▸ Iron chelators (deferasirox) increase the exposure to **theophylline**. Avoid. Moderate Study

▸ Isoniazid is predicted to affect the clearance of **theophylline**. Severe Anecdotal

▸ Leflunomide is predicted to decrease the exposure to **theophylline**. Adjust dose. Moderate Study

▸ **Theophylline** is predicted to decrease the concentration of lithium. Monitor concentration and adjust dose. Moderate Anecdotal

▸ Macrolides (azithromycin, clarithromycin) are predicted to increase the exposure to **theophylline**. Adjust dose. Moderate Anecdotal

▸ Macrolides (erythromycin) decrease the clearance of **theophylline** and **theophylline** potentially decreases the clearance of macrolides (erythromycin). Adjust dose. Severe Study

▸ Methotrexate decreases the clearance of **theophylline**. Moderate Study

▸ Monoclonal antibodies (blinatumomab) are predicted to transiently increase the exposure to **theophylline**. Monitor and adjust dose. Moderate Theoretical

▸ Monoclonal antibodies (sarilumab) potentially affect the exposure to **theophylline**. Monitor and adjust dose. Moderate Theoretical

▸ Monoclonal antibodies (tocilizumab) are predicted to decrease the exposure to **theophylline**. Monitor and adjust dose. Moderate Theoretical

▸ Obeticholic acid is predicted to increase the exposure to **theophylline**. Severe Theoretical

▸ Pentoxifylline increases the concentration of **theophylline**. Monitor and adjust dose. Severe Study

▸ Quinolones (ciprofloxacin) are predicted to increase the exposure to **theophylline**. Monitor and adjust dose. Moderate Theoretical

▸ Quinolones (norfloxacin) are predicted to increase the exposure to **theophylline**. Adjust dose. Moderate Anecdotal

▸ Rifampicin is predicted to decrease the exposure to **theophylline**. Adjust dose. Moderate Study

▸ **Theophylline** is predicted to slightly increase the exposure to roflumilast. Moderate Theoretical

▸ SSRIs (fluvoxamine) moderately to markedly increase the exposure to **theophylline**. Avoid. Severe Study

▸ St John's Wort potentially decreases the exposure to **theophylline**. Severe Anecdotal

▸ Sucralfate potentially decreases the absorption of **theophylline**. Separate administration by at least 2 hours. Moderate Study

▸ Sympathomimetics, vasoconstrictor (ephedrine) increase the risk of side-effects when given with **theophylline**. Avoid in children. Moderate Study

▸ Teriflunomide is predicted to decrease the exposure to **theophylline**. Adjust dose. Moderate Study

▸ Valaciclovir is predicted to increase the exposure to **theophylline**. Severe Theoretical

Thiazide diuretics → see TABLE 18 p. 1338 (hyponatraemia), TABLE 8 p. 1335 (hypotension), TABLE 17 p. 1338 (reduced serum potassium)

bendroflumethiazide · chlortalidone · clopamide · cyclopenthiazide · hydrochlorothiazide · hydroflumethiazide · indapamide · metolazone · xipamide

▸ **Thiazide diuretics** are predicted to increase the risk of hypersensitivity reactions when given with allopurinol. Severe Theoretical

▸ Aspirin (high-dose) increases the risk of acute renal failure when given with **thiazide diuretics**. Severe Theoretical

▸ **Thiazide diuretics** increase the risk of hypercalcaemia when given with calcium salts. Severe Anecdotal

▸ **Thiazide diuretics** increase the concentration of lithium. Avoid or adjust dose and monitor concentration. Severe Study

▸ NSAIDs increase the risk of acute renal failure when given with **thiazide diuretics**. Severe Theoretical → Also see TABLE 18 p. 1338

▸ Reboxetine is predicted to increase the risk of hypokalaemia when given with **thiazide diuretics**. Moderate Anecdotal

▸ **Thiazide diuretics** are predicted to increase the risk of hypercalcaemia when given with toremifene. Severe Theoretical

▸ **Thiazide diuretics** increase the risk of hypercalcaemia when given with vitamin D substances. Moderate Theoretical

Thiopental → see TABLE 8 p. 1335 (hypotension), TABLE 11 p. 1336 (CNS depressant effects)

▸ Sulfonamides are predicted to increase the effects of **thiopental**. Moderate Theoretical

▸ Tricyclic antidepressants increase the risk of cardiac arrhythmias and hypotension when given with **thiopental**. Moderate Study → Also see TABLE 8 p. 1335

Thiotepa → see alkylating agents

Thyroid hormones

levothyroxine · liothyronine

▸ Antacids are predicted to decrease the absorption of **levothyroxine**. Separate administration by at least 4 hours. Moderate Anecdotal

▸ Antiarrhythmics (amiodarone) are predicted to increase the risk of thyroid dysfunction when given with **thyroid hormones**. Avoid. Moderate Study

▸ Antiepileptics (carbamazepine, fosphenytoin, phenytoin) are predicted to increase the risk of hypothyroidism when given with **thyroid hormones**. Moderate Study

▸ Antiepileptics (phenobarbital, primidone) are predicted to decrease the effects of **thyroid hormones**. Moderate Theoretical

▸ Oral calcium salts are predicted to decrease the absorption of **levothyroxine**. Separate administration by at least 4 hours. Moderate Anecdotal

▸ **Thyroid hormones** are predicted to affect the concentration of digoxin. Monitor and adjust dose. Moderate Theoretical

▸ Oral hormone replacement therapy is predicted to decrease the effects of **thyroid hormones**. Moderate Theoretical

▸ Iron (oral) decreases the absorption of **levothyroxine**. Separate administration by at least 4 hours. Moderate Study

▸ Lanthanum decreases the absorption of **thyroid hormones**. Separate administration by 2 hours. Moderate Study

▸ Polystyrene sulfonate is predicted to decrease the absorption of **levothyroxine**. Separate administration by at least 4 hours. Moderate Theoretical

▸ Sucralfate decreases the absorption of **levothyroxine**. Separate administration by at least 4 hours. Moderate Study

Tiagabine → see antiepileptics

Tiaprofenic acid → see NSAIDs

Tibolone → see TABLE 5 p. 1334 (thromboembolism)

Ticagrelor → see TABLE 4 p. 1334 (antiplatelet effects)

▸ Antiarrhythmics (amiodarone) are predicted to increase the exposure to **ticagrelor**. Use with caution or avoid. Severe Study

▸ Antiepileptics (carbamazepine, fosphenytoin, phenobarbital, phenytoin, primidone) are predicted to markedly decrease the exposure to **ticagrelor**. Avoid. Severe Study

▸ Antifungals, azoles (itraconazole, ketoconazole, voriconazole) are predicted to markedly increase the exposure to **ticagrelor**. Avoid. Severe Study

▸ Bosentan is predicted to decrease the exposure to **ticagrelor**. Moderate Theoretical

▸ Ciclosporin is predicted to increase the exposure to **ticagrelor**. Use with caution or avoid. Severe Study

▸ Cobicistat is predicted to markedly increase the exposure to **ticagrelor**. Avoid. Severe Study

▸ **Ticagrelor** increases the concentration of digoxin. Moderate Study

▸ Efavirenz is predicted to decrease the exposure to **ticagrelor**. Moderate Theoretical

▸ Enzalutamide is predicted to markedly decrease the exposure to **ticagrelor**. Avoid. Severe Study

▸ **Ticagrelor** is predicted to increase the exposure to ergotamine. Avoid. Severe Theoretical

▸ Grapefruit juice moderately increases the exposure to **ticagrelor**. Moderate Study

▸ HIV-protease inhibitors are predicted to markedly increase the exposure to **ticagrelor**. Avoid. Severe Study

▸ Idelalisib is predicted to markedly increase the exposure to **ticagrelor**. Avoid. Severe Study

▸ **Ticagrelor** is predicted to increase the exposure to lomitapide. Separate administration by 12 hours. Moderate Theoretical

▸ Macrolides (azithromycin) are predicted to increase the exposure to **ticagrelor**. Use with caution or avoid. Severe Study

Ticagrelor (continued)

▶ Macrolides (clarithromycin) are predicted to markedly increase the exposure to **ticagrelor**. Avoid. Severe Study

▶ Mitotane is predicted to markedly decrease the exposure to **ticagrelor**. Avoid. Severe Study

▶ Nevirapine is predicted to decrease the exposure to **ticagrelor**. Moderate Theoretical

▶ Ranolazine is predicted to increase the exposure to **ticagrelor**. Use with caution or avoid. Severe Study

▶ Rifampicin is predicted to markedly decrease the exposure to **ticagrelor**. Avoid. Severe Study

▶ St John's Wort is predicted to decrease the exposure to **ticagrelor**. Moderate Theoretical

▶ **Ticagrelor** slightly increases the exposure to statins (simvastatin). Adjust **simvastatin** dose, p. 203. Moderate Study

▶ Vemurafenib is predicted to increase the exposure to **ticagrelor**. Use with caution or avoid. Severe Study

Ticarcillin → see penicillins

Tigecycline → see tetracyclines

Timolol → see beta blockers, non-selective

Tinidazole

▶ Alcohol (beverage) potentially causes a disulfiram-like reaction when given with **tinidazole**. Avoid for 72 hours stopping treatment. Moderate Theoretical

▶ **Tinidazole** is predicted to increase the anticoagulant effect of coumarins. Monitor INR and adjust dose. Severe Theoretical

Tinzaparin → see low molecular-weight heparins

Tioguanine → see TABLE 15 p. 1337 (myelosuppression)

▶ Live vaccines are predicted to increase the risk of generalised infection (possibly life-threatening) when given with **tioguanine**. Public Health England advises avoid (refer to Green Book). Severe Theoretical

Tiotropium → see TABLE 10 p. 1336 (antimuscarinics)

Tipranavir → see HIV-protease inhibitors

Tirofiban → see TABLE 4 p. 1334 (antiplatelet effects)

Tivozanib

▶ Antiepileptics (carbamazepine, fosphenytoin, phenobarbital, phenytoin, primidone) are predicted to decrease the exposure to **tivozanib**. Severe Study

▶ Enzalutamide is predicted to decrease the exposure to **tivozanib**. Severe Study

▶ Mitotane is predicted to decrease the exposure to **tivozanib**. Severe Study

▶ Rifampicin is predicted to decrease the exposure to **tivozanib**. Severe Study

▶ St John's Wort is predicted to decrease the exposure to **tivozanib**. Avoid. Severe Study

▶ **Tivozanib** is predicted to decrease the exposure to statins (rosuvastatin). Moderate Theoretical

Tizanidine → see TABLE 6 p. 1335 (bradycardia), TABLE 8 p. 1335 (hypotension), TABLE 9 p. 1336 (QT-interval prolongation), TABLE 11 p. 1336 (CNS depressant effects)

▶ Antiepileptics (fosphenytoin, phenytoin) moderately decrease the exposure to **tizanidine**. Mild Study

▶ Combined hormonal contraceptives increase the exposure to **tizanidine**. Avoid. Moderate Study

▶ HIV-protease inhibitors (ritonavir) moderately decrease the exposure to **tizanidine**. Mild Study

▶ Iron chelators (deferasirox) are predicted to increase the exposure to **tizanidine**. Avoid. Moderate Theoretical

▶ Leflunomide moderately decreases the exposure to **tizanidine**. Mild Study

▶ Obeticholic acid is predicted to increase the exposure to **tizanidine**. Severe Theoretical

▶ Quinolones (ciprofloxacin) increase the exposure to **tizanidine**. Avoid. Moderate Study

▶ Rifampicin moderately decreases the exposure to **tizanidine**. Mild Study

▶ SSRIs (fluvoxamine) very markedly increase the exposure to **tizanidine**. Avoid. Severe Study

▶ Teriflunomide moderately decreases the exposure to **tizanidine**. Mild Study

Tobramycin → see aminoglycosides

Tocilizumab → see monoclonal antibodies

Tofacitinib

▶ Antiarrhythmics (dronedarone) are predicted to increase the exposure to **tofacitinib**. Moderate Study

▶ Antiepileptics (carbamazepine, fosphenytoin, phenobarbital, phenytoin, primidone) are predicted to decrease the exposure to **tofacitinib**. Avoid. Severe Study

▶ Antifungals, azoles (fluconazole, itraconazole, ketoconazole, voriconazole) are predicted to increase the exposure to **tofacitinib**. Adjust **tofacitinib** dose, p. 1072. Moderate Study

▶ Antifungals, azoles (isavuconazole) are predicted to increase the exposure to **tofacitinib**. Moderate Study

▶ Antifungals, azoles (posaconazole) are predicted to increase the exposure to **tofacitinib**. Moderate Theoretical

▶ Aprepitant is predicted to increase the exposure to **tofacitinib**. Moderate Study

▶ Bosentan is predicted to decrease the exposure to **tofacitinib**. Moderate Study

▶ Calcium channel blockers (diltiazem, verapamil) are predicted to increase the exposure to **tofacitinib**. Moderate Study

▶ Ciclosporin increases the exposure to **tofacitinib**. Avoid. Severe Study

▶ Cobicistat is predicted to increase the exposure to **tofacitinib**. Adjust **tofacitinib** dose, p. 1072. Moderate Study

▶ Crizotinib is predicted to increase the exposure to **tofacitinib**. Moderate Study

▶ Efavirenz is predicted to decrease the exposure to **tofacitinib**. Moderate Study

▶ Enzalutamide is predicted to decrease the exposure to **tofacitinib**. Avoid. Severe Study

▶ HIV-protease inhibitors are predicted to increase the exposure to **tofacitinib**. Adjust **tofacitinib** dose, p. 1072. Moderate Study

▶ Idelalisib is predicted to increase the exposure to **tofacitinib**. Adjust **tofacitinib** dose, p. 1072. Moderate Study

▶ Imatinib is predicted to increase the exposure to **tofacitinib**. Moderate Study

▶ Live vaccines potentially increase the risk of generalised infection (possibly life-threatening) when given with **tofacitinib**. Avoid. Severe Theoretical

▶ Macrolides (clarithromycin) are predicted to increase the exposure to **tofacitinib**. Adjust **tofacitinib** dose, p. 1072. Moderate Study

▶ Macrolides (erythromycin) are predicted to increase the exposure to **tofacitinib**. Moderate Study

▶ Mitotane is predicted to decrease the exposure to **tofacitinib**. Avoid. Severe Study

▶ Netupitant is predicted to increase the exposure to **tofacitinib**. Moderate Study

▶ Nevirapine is predicted to decrease the exposure to **tofacitinib**. Moderate Study

▶ Nilotinib is predicted to increase the exposure to **tofacitinib**. Moderate Study

▶ Rifampicin is predicted to decrease the exposure to **tofacitinib**. Avoid. Severe Study

▶ St John's Wort is predicted to decrease the exposure to **tofacitinib**. Moderate Study

▶ Tacrolimus increases the exposure to **tofacitinib**. Avoid. Severe Study

Tolbutamide → see sulfonylureas

Tolcapone

▶ Tolcapone increases the exposure to levodopa. Monitor and adjust dose. Moderate Study

▶ **Tolcapone** is predicted to increase the effects of monoamine-oxidase A and B inhibitors, irreversible. Avoid. Severe Theoretical

▶ **Tolcapone** is predicted to increase the risk of cardiovascular side-effects when given with sympathomimetics, inotropic. Moderate Theoretical

▶ **Tolcapone** is predicted to increase the effects of sympathomimetics, vasoconstrictor (adrenaline/epinephrine, noradrenaline/norepinephrine). Moderate Theoretical

Tolfenamic acid → see NSAIDs

Tolterodine → see TABLE 9 p. 1336 (QT-interval prolongation), TABLE 10 p. 1336 (antimuscarinics)

▶ Antiarrhythmics (dronedarone) are predicted to increase the exposure to **tolterodine**. Mild Theoretical → Also see TABLE 9 p. 1336

- Antifungals, azoles (fluconazole, isavuconazole, posaconazole) are predicted to increase the exposure to **tolterodine**. Mild Theoretical → Also see TABLE 9 p. 1336
- Antifungals, azoles (itraconazole, ketoconazole, voriconazole) are predicted to increase the exposure to **tolterodine**. Avoid. Severe Study → Also see TABLE 9 p. 1336
- Aprepitant is predicted to increase the exposure to **tolterodine**. Mild Theoretical
- Calcium channel blockers (diltiazem, verapamil) are predicted to increase the exposure to **tolterodine**. Mild Theoretical
- Cobicistat is predicted to increase the exposure to **tolterodine**. Avoid. Severe Study
- Crizotinib is predicted to increase the exposure to **tolterodine**. Mild Theoretical → Also see TABLE 9 p. 1336
- Eliglustat is predicted to increase the exposure to **tolterodine**. Adjust dose. Moderate Theoretical
- HIV-protease inhibitors are predicted to increase the exposure to **tolterodine**. Avoid. Severe Study → Also see TABLE 9 p. 1336
- Idelalisib is predicted to increase the exposure to **tolterodine**. Avoid. Severe Study
- Imatinib is predicted to increase the exposure to **tolterodine**. Mild Theoretical
- Macrolides (clarithromycin) are predicted to increase the exposure to **tolterodine**. Avoid. Severe Study → Also see TABLE 9 p. 1336
- Macrolides (erythromycin) are predicted to increase the exposure to **tolterodine**. Mild Theoretical → Also see TABLE 9 p. 1336
- Netupitant is predicted to increase the exposure to **tolterodine**. Mild Theoretical
- Nilotinib is predicted to increase the exposure to **tolterodine**. Mild Theoretical → Also see TABLE 9 p. 1336

Tolvaptan → see TABLE 16 p. 1338 (increased serum potassium)

GENERAL INFORMATION Avoid concurrent use of drugs that increase serum-sodium concentrations.

- Antiarrhythmics (dronedarone) are predicted to increase the exposure to **tolvaptan**. Adjust dose. Moderate Study
- Antiepileptics (carbamazepine, fosphenytoin, phenobarbital, phenytoin, primidone) are predicted to decrease the exposure to **tolvaptan**. Avoid. Severe Study
- Antifungals, azoles (fluconazole, isavuconazole, posaconazole) are predicted to increase the exposure to **tolvaptan**. Adjust dose. Moderate Study
- Antifungals, azoles (itraconazole, ketoconazole, voriconazole) are predicted to increase the exposure to **tolvaptan**. Adjust dose. Severe Study
- Aprepitant is predicted to increase the exposure to **tolvaptan**. Adjust dose. Moderate Study
- Bosentan is predicted to decrease the exposure to **tolvaptan**. Moderate Theoretical
- Calcium channel blockers (diltiazem, verapamil) are predicted to increase the exposure to **tolvaptan**. Adjust dose. Moderate Study
- Cobicistat is predicted to increase the exposure to **tolvaptan**. Adjust dose. Severe Study
- Crizotinib is predicted to increase the exposure to **tolvaptan**. Adjust dose. Moderate Study
- **Tolvaptan** increases the concentration of digoxin. Mild Study
- Efavirenz is predicted to decrease the exposure to **tolvaptan**. Moderate Theoretical
- Enzalutamide is predicted to decrease the exposure to **tolvaptan**. Avoid. Severe Study
- Grapefruit juice increases the exposure to **tolvaptan**. Avoid. Moderate Study
- HIV-protease inhibitors are predicted to increase the exposure to **tolvaptan**. Adjust dose. Severe Study
- Idelalisib is predicted to increase the exposure to **tolvaptan**. Adjust dose. Severe Study
- Imatinib is predicted to increase the exposure to **tolvaptan**. Adjust dose. Moderate Study
- **Tolvaptan** is predicted to increase the exposure to lomitapide. Separate administration by 12 hours. Moderate Theoretical
- Macrolides (clarithromycin) are predicted to increase the exposure to **tolvaptan**. Adjust dose. Severe Study

- Macrolides (erythromycin) are predicted to increase the exposure to **tolvaptan**. Adjust dose. Moderate Study
- Mitotane is predicted to decrease the exposure to **tolvaptan**. Avoid. Severe Study
- Netupitant is predicted to increase the exposure to **tolvaptan**. Adjust dose. Moderate Study
- Nevirapine is predicted to decrease the exposure to **tolvaptan**. Moderate Theoretical
- Nilotinib is predicted to increase the exposure to **tolvaptan**. Adjust dose. Moderate Study
- Rifampicin is predicted to decrease the exposure to **tolvaptan**. Avoid. Severe Study
- St John's Wort is predicted to decrease the exposure to **tolvaptan**. Moderate Theoretical

Topiramate → see antiepileptics

Topotecan → see TABLE 15 p. 1337 (myelosuppression)

- Antiarrhythmics (amiodarone, dronedarone) are predicted to increase the exposure to **topotecan**. Severe Study
- Antiepileptics (fosphenytoin, phenytoin) increase the clearance of **topotecan**. Moderate Study
- Antifungals, azoles (itraconazole, ketoconazole) are predicted to increase the exposure to **topotecan**. Severe Study
- Calcium channel blockers (verapamil) are predicted to increase the exposure to **topotecan**. Severe Study
- Ceritinib is predicted to increase the exposure to **topotecan**. Moderate Theoretical → Also see TABLE 15 p. 1337
- Ciclosporin is predicted to increase the exposure to **topotecan**. Severe Study
- Eliglustat is predicted to increase the exposure to **topotecan**. Adjust dose. Moderate Study
- HIV-protease inhibitors (lopinavir, ritonavir, saquinavir) are predicted to increase the exposure to **topotecan**. Severe Study
- Lapatinib is predicted to increase the exposure to **topotecan**. Severe Study
- Live vaccines are predicted to increase the risk of generalised infection (possibly life-threatening) when given with **topotecan**. Public Health England advises avoid (refer to Green Book). Severe Theoretical
- Macrolides are predicted to increase the exposure to **topotecan**. Severe Study
- Mirabegron is predicted to increase the exposure to **topotecan**. Mild Theoretical
- Ranolazine is predicted to increase the exposure to **topotecan**. Severe Study
- Rolapitant is predicted to increase the exposure to **topotecan**. Avoid or monitor. Moderate Study
- St John's Wort is predicted to decrease the exposure to **topotecan**. Severe Theoretical
- Tedizolid is predicted to increase the exposure to **topotecan**. Avoid. Moderate Theoretical
- Velpatasvir is predicted to increase the exposure to **topotecan**. Severe Theoretical
- Vemurafenib is predicted to increase the exposure to **topotecan**. Severe Study

Torasemide → see loop diuretics

Toremifene → see TABLE 5 p. 1334 (thromboembolism), TABLE 9 p. 1336 (QT-interval prolongation)

- Antiepileptics (carbamazepine, fosphenytoin, phenobarbital, phenytoin, primidone) are predicted to decrease the exposure to **toremifene**. Adjust dose. Moderate Study
- Antifungals, azoles (itraconazole, ketoconazole, voriconazole) are predicted to increase the exposure to **toremifene**. Moderate Theoretical → Also see TABLE 9 p. 1336
- Cobicistat is predicted to increase the exposure to **toremifene**. Moderate Theoretical
- **Toremifene** is predicted to increase the anticoagulant effect of coumarins. Severe Theoretical
- Enzalutamide is predicted to decrease the exposure to **toremifene**. Adjust dose. Moderate Study
- HIV-protease inhibitors are predicted to increase the exposure to **toremifene**. Moderate Theoretical → Also see TABLE 9 p. 1336
- Idelalisib is predicted to increase the exposure to **toremifene**. Moderate Theoretical

Toremifene (continued)

▶ Macrolides (clarithromycin) are predicted to increase the exposure to **toremifene**. Moderate Theoretical → Also see TABLE 9 p. 1336

▶ Mitotane is predicted to decrease the exposure to **toremifene**. Adjust dose. Moderate Study

▶ Rifampicin is predicted to decrease the exposure to **toremifene**. Adjust dose. Moderate Study

▶ Thiazide diuretics are predicted to increase the risk of hypercalcaemia when given with **toremifene**. Severe Theoretical

Trabectedin → see TABLE 1 p. 1334 (hepatotoxicity), TABLE 15 p. 1337 (myelosuppression)

▶ Antiepileptics (carbamazepine, fosphenytoin, phenobarbital, phenytoin, primidone) are predicted to decrease the exposure to **trabectedin**. Avoid. Severe Theoretical → Also see TABLE 1 p. 1334

▶ Antifungals, azoles (itraconazole, ketoconazole, voriconazole) are predicted to increase the exposure to **trabectedin**. Avoid or adjust dose. Severe Theoretical → Also see TABLE 1 p. 1334

▶ Cobicistat is predicted to increase the exposure to **trabectedin**. Avoid or adjust dose. Severe Theoretical

▶ Enzalutamide is predicted to decrease the exposure to **trabectedin**. Avoid. Severe Theoretical

▶ HIV-protease inhibitors are predicted to increase the exposure to **trabectedin**. Avoid or adjust dose. Severe Theoretical

▶ Idelalisib is predicted to increase the exposure to **trabectedin**. Avoid or adjust dose. Severe Theoretical → Also see TABLE 15 p. 1337

▶ Live vaccines are predicted to increase the risk of generalised infection (possibly life-threatening) when given with **trabectedin**. Public Health England advises avoid (refer to Green Book). Severe Theoretical

▶ Macrolides (clarithromycin) are predicted to increase the exposure to **trabectedin**. Avoid or adjust dose. Severe Theoretical

▶ Mitotane is predicted to decrease the exposure to **trabectedin**. Avoid. Severe Theoretical → Also see TABLE 15 p. 1337

▶ Rifampicin is predicted to decrease the exposure to **trabectedin**. Avoid. Severe Theoretical

Tramadol → see opioids

Trametinib

▶ Antiarrhythmics (amiodarone, dronedarone) are predicted to increase the concentration of **trametinib**. Moderate Theoretical

▶ Antifungals, azoles (itraconazole, ketoconazole) are predicted to increase the concentration of **trametinib**. Moderate Theoretical

▶ Calcium channel blockers (verapamil) are predicted to increase the concentration of **trametinib**. Moderate Theoretical

▶ Ciclosporin is predicted to increase the concentration of **trametinib**. Moderate Theoretical

▶ HIV-protease inhibitors (lopinavir, ritonavir, saquinavir) are predicted to increase the concentration of **trametinib**. Moderate Theoretical

▶ Lapatinib is predicted to increase the concentration of **trametinib**. Moderate Theoretical

▶ Macrolides are predicted to increase the concentration of **trametinib**. Moderate Theoretical

▶ Ranolazine is predicted to increase the concentration of **trametinib**. Moderate Theoretical

▶ Vemurafenib is predicted to increase the concentration of **trametinib**. Moderate Theoretical

Trandolapril → see ACE inhibitors

Tranexamic acid → see TABLE 5 p. 1334 (thromboembolism)

Tranylcypromine → see monoamine-oxidase A and B inhibitors, irreversible

Trastuzumab → see monoclonal antibodies

Trastuzumab emtansine → see monoclonal antibodies

Trazodone → see TABLE 13 p. 1337 (serotonin syndrome), TABLE 11 p. 1336 (CNS depressant effects)

▶ Antiarrhythmics (dronedarone) are predicted to increase the exposure to **trazodone**. Moderate Theoretical

▶ Antiepileptics (carbamazepine) decrease the concentration of **trazodone**. Adjust dose. Moderate Anecdotal

▶ Antifungals, azoles (fluconazole, isavuconazole, posaconazole) are predicted to increase the exposure to **trazodone**. Moderate Theoretical

▶ Antifungals, azoles (itraconazole, ketoconazole, voriconazole) are predicted to moderately increase the exposure to **trazodone**. Avoid or adjust dose. Moderate Study

▶ Aprepitant is predicted to increase the exposure to **trazodone**. Moderate Theoretical

▶ Calcium channel blockers (diltiazem, verapamil) are predicted to increase the exposure to **trazodone**. Moderate Theoretical

▶ Cobicistat is predicted to moderately increase the exposure to **trazodone**. Avoid or adjust dose. Moderate Study

▶ Crizotinib is predicted to increase the exposure to **trazodone**. Moderate Theoretical

▶ HIV-protease inhibitors are predicted to moderately increase the exposure to **trazodone**. Avoid or adjust dose. Moderate Study

▶ Idelalisib is predicted to moderately increase the exposure to **trazodone**. Avoid or adjust dose. Moderate Study

▶ Imatinib is predicted to increase the exposure to **trazodone**. Moderate Theoretical

▶ Macrolides (clarithromycin) are predicted to moderately increase the exposure to **trazodone**. Avoid or adjust dose. Moderate Study

▶ Macrolides (erythromycin) are predicted to increase the exposure to **trazodone**. Moderate Theoretical

▶ Netupitant is predicted to increase the exposure to **trazodone**. Moderate Theoretical

▶ Nilotinib is predicted to increase the exposure to **trazodone**. Moderate Theoretical

Tree pollen extract

> **GENERAL INFORMATION** Desensitising vaccines should be avoided in patients taking beta-blockers (adrenaline might be ineffective in case of a hypersensitivity reaction) or ACE inhibitors (risk of severe anaphylactoid reactions).

Treosulfan → see alkylating agents

Tretinoin → see retinoids

Triamcinolone → see corticosteroids

Triamterene → see potassium-sparing diuretics

Tricyclic antidepressants → see TABLE 18 p. 1338 (hyponatraemia), TABLE 8 p. 1335 (hypotension), TABLE 13 p. 1337 (serotonin syndrome), TABLE 9 p. 1336 (QT-interval prolongation), TABLE 10 p. 1336 (antimuscarinics)

> amitriptyline · clomipramine · dosulepin · doxepin · imipramine · lofepramine · nortriptyline · trimipramine

▶ Antiarrhythmics (dronedarone) are predicted to increase the exposure to **tricyclic antidepressants**. Avoid. Severe Theoretical → Also see TABLE 9 p. 1336

▶ Antiarrhythmics (propafenone) are predicted to increase the concentration of **tricyclic antidepressants**. Moderate Theoretical → Also see TABLE 10 p. 1336

▶ Antiepileptics (carbamazepine) decrease the exposure to **tricyclic antidepressants**. Adjust dose. Moderate Study → Also see TABLE 18 p. 1338

▶ Antiepileptics (phenobarbital, primidone) are predicted to decrease the exposure to **tricyclic antidepressants**. Moderate Study

▶ Tricyclic antidepressants (clomipramine, imipramine) potentially increase the risk of overheating and dehydration when given with antiepileptics (zonisamide). Avoid in children. Severe Theoretical

▶ Bupropion is predicted to increase the exposure to **tricyclic antidepressants**. Monitor for toxicity and adjust dose. Severe Study → Also see TABLE 13 p. 1337

▶ Cinacalcet is predicted to increase the exposure to **tricyclic antidepressants**. Monitor for toxicity and adjust dose. Severe Study

▶ Tricyclic antidepressants decrease the antihypertensive effects of clonidine. Monitor and adjust dose. Moderate Anecdotal → Also see TABLE 8 p. 1335

▶ Cobicistat is predicted to slightly increase the exposure to **tricyclic antidepressants**. Mild Study

▶ Darifenacin is predicted to increase the exposure to **tricyclic antidepressants**. Moderate Theoretical → Also see TABLE 10 p. 1336

▶ Eliglustat is predicted to increase the exposure to **nortriptyline**. Adjust dose. Moderate Theoretical

- **Tricyclic antidepressants** are predicted to decrease the antihypertensive effects of guanethidine. Moderate Study → Also see TABLE 8 p. 1335
- ▸ H₂ receptor antagonists (cimetidine) increase the exposure to **tricyclic antidepressants**. Moderate Study
- ▸ HIV-protease inhibitors (ritonavir, tipranavir) are predicted to increase the exposure to **tricyclic antidepressants**. Moderate Theoretical
- **Tricyclic antidepressants** potentially increase the risk of neurotoxicity when given with lithium. Severe Anecdotal → Also see TABLE 8 p. 1337 → Also see TABLE 9 p. 1336
- **Amitriptyline** decreases the effects of metyrapone. Avoid. Moderate Theoretical
- **Tricyclic antidepressants** are predicted to increase the risk of severe toxic reaction when given with moclobemide. Avoid. Severe Theoretical → Also see TABLE 13 p. 1337
- **Tricyclic antidepressants** are predicted to increase the risk of severe toxic reaction when given with monoamine-oxidase A and B inhibitors, irreversible. Avoid and for 14 days after stopping the MAOI. Severe Theoretical → Also see TABLE 8 p. 1335 → Also see TABLE 13 p. 1337
- **Tricyclic antidepressants** are predicted to decrease the effects of moxonidine. Avoid. Moderate Theoretical → Also see TABLE 8 p. 1335
- **Tricyclic antidepressants** are predicted to decrease the efficacy of pitolisant. Mild Theoretical
- ▸ SSRIs (fluoxetine, paroxetine) are predicted to increase the exposure to **tricyclic antidepressants**. Monitor for toxicity and adjust dose. Severe Study → Also see TABLE 18 p. 1338 → Also see TABLE 13 p. 1337
- ▸ SSRIs (fluvoxamine) markedly increase the exposure to **clomipramine**. Adjust dose. Severe Study → Also see TABLE 18 p. 1338 → Also see TABLE 13 p. 1337
- ▸ SSRIs (fluvoxamine) increase the exposure to tricyclic antidepressants (amitriptyline, imipramine). Adjust dose. Severe Study → Also see TABLE 18 p. 1338 → Also see TABLE 13 p. 1337
- **Sucralfate** is predicted to decrease the absorption of **tricyclic antidepressants**. Moderate Study
- **Tricyclic antidepressants** increase the effects of sympathomimetics, vasoconstrictor (adrenaline/epinephrine, noradrenaline/norepinephrine, phenylephrine). Avoid. Severe Study
- **Tricyclic antidepressants** are predicted to decrease the effects of sympathomimetics, vasoconstrictor (ephedrine). Avoid. Severe Study
- **Terbinafine** is predicted to increase the exposure to **tricyclic antidepressants**. Monitor for toxicity and adjust dose. Severe Study
- **Tricyclic antidepressants** increase the risk of cardiac arrhythmias and hypotension when given with thiopental. Moderate Study → Also see TABLE 8 p. 1335

Trientine
- **Trientine** potentially decreases the absorption of iron (oral). Moderate Theoretical
- **Trientine** potentially decreases the absorption of zinc. Moderate Theoretical

Trifluoperazine → see phenothiazines
Trihexyphenidyl → see TABLE 10 p. 1336 (antimuscarinics)
Trimethoprim → see TABLE 18 p. 1338 (hyponatraemia), TABLE 2 p. 1334 (nephrotoxicity), TABLE 16 p. 1338 (increased serum potassium)
- **Trimethoprim** increases the concentration of antiepileptics (fosphenytoin, phenytoin). Moderate Study
- ▸ Antimalarials (pyrimethamine) increase the risk of side-effects when given with **trimethoprim**. Severe Study
- **Trimethoprim** is predicted to increase the anticoagulant effect of coumarins. Severe Study
- **Dapsone** increases the exposure to **trimethoprim** and **trimethoprim** increases the exposure to dapsone. Severe Study
- **Trimethoprim** increases the concentration of digoxin. Moderate Study
- **Trimethoprim** slightly increases the exposure to lamivudine. Moderate Study
- **Trimethoprim** is predicted to increase the risk of side-effects when given with methotrexate. Avoid. Severe Theoretical → Also see TABLE 2 p. 1334

- **Trimethoprim** slightly increases the exposure to repaglinide. Avoid or monitor blood glucose. Moderate Study
- **Rifampicin** decreases the exposure to **trimethoprim**. Moderate Study
- **Trimethoprim** is predicted to decrease the efficacy of sapropterin. Moderate Theoretical
Trimipramine → see tricyclic antidepressants
Tropicamide → see TABLE 10 p. 1336 (antimuscarinics)
Trospium → see TABLE 10 p. 1336 (antimuscarinics)
Tryptophan → see TABLE 13 p. 1337 (serotonin syndrome)
- **Tryptophan** greatly decreases the concentration of levodopa. Moderate Study
- **Tryptophan** increases the risk of side-effects when given with monoamine-oxidase A and B inhibitors, irreversible. Severe Anecdotal → Also see TABLE 13 p. 1337
Typhoid vaccine, oral → see live vaccines
Ulipristal
- ▸ Antiarrhythmics (dronedarone) are predicted to increase the exposure to **ulipristal**. Avoid if used for uterine fibroids. Moderate Study
- ▸ Antiepileptics (carbamazepine, eslicarbazepine, fosphenytoin, oxcarbazepine, perampanel, phenobarbital, phenytoin, primidone, rufinamide, topiramate) decrease the efficacy of **ulipristal**. For FSRH guidance, see Contraceptives, interactions p. 775. Severe Anecdotal
- ▸ Antifungals, azoles (fluconazole, isavuconazole, posaconazole) are predicted to increase the exposure to **ulipristal**. Avoid if used for uterine fibroids. Moderate Study
- ▸ Antifungals, azoles (itraconazole, ketoconazole, voriconazole) are predicted to increase the exposure to **ulipristal**. Avoid if used for uterine fibroids. Severe Study
- **Aprepitant** decreases the efficacy of **ulipristal**. For FSRH guidance, see Contraceptives, interactions p. 775. Severe Anecdotal
- **Bosentan** decreases the efficacy of **ulipristal**. For FSRH guidance, see Contraceptives, interactions p. 775. Severe Anecdotal
- ▸ Calcium channel blockers (diltiazem, verapamil) are predicted to increase the exposure to **ulipristal**. Avoid if used for uterine fibroids. Moderate Study
- **Cobicistat** is predicted to increase the exposure to **ulipristal**. Avoid if used for uterine fibroids. Severe Study
- **Ulipristal** is predicted to decrease the efficacy of combined hormonal contraceptives. Avoid. Severe Theoretical
- **Crizotinib** is predicted to increase the exposure to **ulipristal**. Avoid if used for uterine fibroids. Moderate Study
- **Ulipristal** is predicted to decrease the efficacy of desogestrel. Avoid. Severe Theoretical
- **Efavirenz** decreases the efficacy of **ulipristal**. For FSRH guidance, see Contraceptives, interactions p. 775. Severe Anecdotal
- **Enzalutamide** is predicted to markedly decrease the exposure to **ulipristal**. Avoid and for 4 weeks after stopping **ulipristal**, p. 785. Severe Theoretical
- **Ulipristal** is predicted to decrease the efficacy of etonogestrel. Avoid. Severe Theoretical
- **Fosaprepitant** decreases the efficacy of **ulipristal**. For FSRH guidance, see Contraceptives, interactions p. 775. Severe Anecdotal
- ▸ Grapefruit juice is predicted to increase the exposure to **ulipristal**. Avoid if used for uterine fibroids. Moderate Theoretical
- **Griseofulvin** potentially decreases the efficacy of **ulipristal**. For FSRH guidance, see Contraceptives, interactions p. 775. Severe Anecdotal
- ▸ HIV-protease inhibitors (atazanavir, darunavir, fosamprenavir, lopinavir, saquinavir, tipranavir) are predicted to increase the exposure to **ulipristal**. Avoid if used for uterine fibroids. Severe Study
- ▸ HIV-protease inhibitors (ritonavir) decrease the efficacy of **ulipristal**. For FSRH guidance, see Contraceptives, interactions p. 775. Severe Anecdotal
- **Idelalisib** is predicted to increase the exposure to **ulipristal**. Avoid if used for uterine fibroids. Severe Study
- **Imatinib** is predicted to increase the exposure to **ulipristal**. Avoid if used for uterine fibroids. Moderate Study

Ulipristal (continued)
▶ **Ulipristal** is predicted to decrease the efficacy of levonorgestrel. Avoid. [Severe] Theoretical
▶ **Lumacaftor** is predicted to decrease the efficacy of **ulipristal**. Use additional contraceptive precautions. [Severe] Theoretical
▶ Macrolides (**clarithromycin**) are predicted to increase the exposure to **ulipristal**. Avoid if used for uterine fibroids. [Severe] Study
▶ Macrolides (**erythromycin**) are predicted to increase the exposure to **ulipristal**. Avoid if used for uterine fibroids. [Moderate] Study
▶ **Modafinil** decreases the efficacy of **ulipristal**. For FSRH guidance, see Contraceptives, interactions p. 775. [Severe] Anecdotal
▶ **Netupitant** is predicted to increase the exposure to **ulipristal**. Avoid if used for uterine fibroids. [Moderate] Study
▶ **Nevirapine** decreases the efficacy of **ulipristal**. For FSRH guidance, see Contraceptives, interactions p. 775. [Severe] Anecdotal
▶ **Nilotinib** is predicted to increase the exposure to **ulipristal**. Avoid if used for uterine fibroids. [Moderate] Study
▶ **Ulipristal** is predicted to decrease the efficacy of norethisterone. Avoid. [Severe] Theoretical
▶ **Rifabutin** decreases the efficacy of **ulipristal**. For FSRH guidance, see Contraceptives, interactions p. 775. [Severe] Anecdotal
▶ **Rifampicin** decreases the efficacy of **ulipristal**. For FSRH guidance, see Contraceptives, interactions p. 775. [Severe] Anecdotal

Umeclidinium → see TABLE 10 p. 1336 (antimuscarinics)
Urokinase → see TABLE 3 p. 1334 (anticoagulant effects)
Ursodeoxycholic acid
▶ **Antacids** are predicted to decrease the absorption of **ursodeoxycholic acid**. Separate administration by 2 hours. [Moderate] Theoretical
▶ **Ursodeoxycholic acid** affects the concentration of ciclosporin. Use with caution and adjust dose. [Severe] Anecdotal
▶ **Fibrates** are predicted to decrease the efficacy of **ursodeoxycholic acid**. Avoid. [Severe] Theoretical

Ustekinumab → see monoclonal antibodies
Valaciclovir → see TABLE 2 p. 1334 (nephrotoxicity)
▶ **Valaciclovir** is predicted to increase the exposure to aminophylline. [Severe] Anecdotal
▶ **Mycophenolate** is predicted to increase the risk of haematological toxicity when given with **valaciclovir**. [Moderate] Theoretical
▶ **Valaciclovir** is predicted to increase the exposure to theophylline. [Severe] Theoretical

Valganciclovir → see TABLE 15 p. 1337 (myelosuppression), TABLE 2 p. 1334 (nephrotoxicity)
▶ **Valganciclovir** is predicted to increase the risk of seizures when given with carbapenems (**imipenem**). Avoid. [Severe] Anecdotal
▶ **Valganciclovir** is predicted to increase the exposure to didanosine. [Moderate] Study
▶ **Mycophenolate** is predicted to increase the risk of haematological toxicity when given with **valganciclovir**. [Moderate] Theoretical → Also see TABLE 15 p. 1337

Valproate → see antiepileptics
Valsartan → see angiotensin-II receptor antagonists
Vancomycin → see TABLE 2 p. 1334 (nephrotoxicity), TABLE 19 p. 1338 (ototoxicity)
Vandetanib → see TABLE 9 p. 1336 (QT-interval prolongation)
▶ Antiepileptics (**carbamazepine, fosphenytoin, phenobarbital, phenytoin, primidone**) are predicted to decrease the exposure to **vandetanib**. Avoid. [Moderate] Study
▶ **Vandetanib** is predicted to increase the risk of bleeding events when given with coumarins. [Severe] Theoretical
▶ **Vandetanib** slightly increases the exposure to digoxin. Monitor ECG and adjust dose. [Moderate] Study
▶ **Enzalutamide** is predicted to decrease the exposure to **vandetanib**. Avoid. [Moderate] Study
▶ **Vandetanib** slightly increases the exposure to metformin. Monitor and adjust dose. [Moderate] Study
▶ **Mitotane** is predicted to decrease the exposure to **vandetanib**. Avoid. [Moderate] Study

▶ **Vandetanib** is predicted to increase the risk of bleeding events when given with phenindione. [Severe] Theoretical
▶ **Rifampicin** is predicted to decrease the exposure to **vandetanib**. Avoid. [Moderate] Study

Vardenafil → see phosphodiesterase type-5 inhibitors
Varicella-zoster vaccine → see live vaccines
Vecuronium → see neuromuscular blocking drugs, non-depolarising
Vedolizumab → see monoclonal antibodies
Velpatasvir
▶ **Velpatasvir** is predicted to increase the exposure to aliskiren. [Severe] Theoretical
▶ **Antacids** are predicted to decrease the concentration of **velpatasvir**. Separate administration by 4 hours. [Moderate] Theoretical
▶ Antiarrhythmics (**amiodarone**) are predicted to increase the concentration of **velpatasvir**. Avoid or monitor. [Moderate] Theoretical
▶ Antiepileptics (**carbamazepine, fosphenytoin, phenobarbital, phenytoin, primidone**) are predicted to moderately decrease the exposure to **velpatasvir**. Avoid. [Severe] Study
▶ Antiepileptics (**oxcarbazepine**) are predicted to decrease the exposure to **velpatasvir**. Avoid. [Severe] Theoretical
▶ **Velpatasvir** is predicted to increase the exposure to antihistamines, non-sedating (**fexofenadine**). [Severe] Theoretical
▶ **Bosentan** is predicted to decrease the exposure to **velpatasvir**. Avoid. [Moderate] Theoretical
▶ Calcium salts (**calcium carbonate**) are predicted to decrease the concentration of **velpatasvir**. Separate administration by 4 hours. [Moderate] Anecdotal
▶ **Velpatasvir** is predicted to increase the exposure to colchicine. [Severe] Theoretical
▶ **Velpatasvir** is predicted to increase the exposure to dabigatran. [Severe] Theoretical
▶ **Velpatasvir** is predicted to increase the exposure to digoxin. [Severe] Study
▶ **Velpatasvir** is predicted to increase the exposure to edoxaban. [Severe] Theoretical
▶ **Efavirenz** is predicted to decrease the exposure to **velpatasvir**. Avoid. [Moderate] Theoretical
▶ **Enzalutamide** is predicted to moderately decrease the exposure to **velpatasvir**. Avoid. [Severe] Study
▶ **Velpatasvir** is predicted to increase the exposure to everolimus. [Severe] Theoretical
▶ H₂ receptor antagonists are predicted to decrease the concentration of **velpatasvir**. Adjust dose, see sofosbuvir with velpatasvir p. 619. [Moderate] Study
▶ **Velpatasvir** is predicted to increase the exposure to loperamide. [Severe] Theoretical
▶ **Mitotane** is predicted to moderately decrease the exposure to **velpatasvir**. Avoid. [Severe] Study
▶ **Nevirapine** is predicted to decrease the exposure to **velpatasvir**. Avoid. [Moderate] Theoretical
▶ Proton pump inhibitors are predicted to decrease the concentration of **velpatasvir**. Adjust dose, see sofosbuvir with velpatasvir p. 619. [Moderate] Study
▶ **Rifampicin** is predicted to moderately decrease the exposure to **velpatasvir**. Avoid. [Severe] Study
▶ **Velpatasvir** is predicted to increase the exposure to sirolimus. [Severe] Theoretical
▶ **St John's Wort** is predicted to decrease the exposure to **velpatasvir**. Avoid. [Moderate] Theoretical
▶ **Velpatasvir** is predicted to increase the exposure to statins (atorvastatin, simvastatin). Monitor side effects and adjust dose. [Severe] Theoretical
▶ **Velpatasvir** increases the exposure to statins (rosuvastatin). Adjust rosuvastatin dose and monitor side effects, p. 202. [Severe] Study
▶ **Velpatasvir** is predicted to increase the exposure to taxanes (paclitaxel). [Severe] Theoretical
▶ **Velpatasvir** is predicted to increase the exposure to tenofovir disoproxil. [Severe] Study
▶ **Velpatasvir** is predicted to increase the exposure to topotecan. [Severe] Theoretical

Vemurafenib → see TABLE 9 p. 1336 (QT-interval prolongation)

- **Vemurafenib** is predicted to increase the exposure to afatinib. Separate administration by 12 hours. [Moderate] Study
- **Vemurafenib** is predicted to increase the exposure to aliskiren. Use with caution and adjust dose. [Moderate] Theoretical
- Antiepileptics (carbamazepine, fosphenytoin, phenobarbital, phenytoin, primidone) are predicted to decrease the exposure to **vemurafenib**. Avoid. [Severe] Theoretical
- Antifungals, azoles (itraconazole, ketoconazole, voriconazole) are predicted to increase the exposure to **vemurafenib**. [Severe] Theoretical → Also see TABLE 9 p. 1336
- **Vemurafenib** is predicted to increase the exposure to beta blockers, non-selective (nadolol). [Moderate] Study
- Cobicistat is predicted to increase the exposure to **vemurafenib**. [Severe] Theoretical
- **Vemurafenib** is predicted to increase the exposure to colchicine. Avoid or adjust **colchicine** dose, p. 1085. [Severe] Theoretical
- **Vemurafenib** increases the exposure to dabigatran. Use with caution and adjust dose. [Severe] Theoretical
- **Vemurafenib** is predicted to slightly increase the exposure to edoxaban. [Severe] Theoretical
- Enzalutamide is predicted to decrease the exposure to **vemurafenib**. Avoid. [Severe] Theoretical
- **Vemurafenib** is predicted to increase the exposure to erlotinib. [Moderate] Theoretical
- **Vemurafenib** is predicted to increase the exposure to fidaxomicin. Avoid. [Moderate] Study
- HIV-protease inhibitors are predicted to increase the exposure to **vemurafenib**. [Severe] Theoretical → Also see TABLE 9 p. 1336
- Idelalisib is predicted to increase the exposure to **vemurafenib**. [Severe] Theoretical
- Macrolides (clarithromycin) are predicted to increase the exposure to **vemurafenib**. [Severe] Theoretical → Also see TABLE 9 p. 1336
- Mitotane is predicted to decrease the exposure to **vemurafenib**. Avoid. [Severe] Theoretical
- **Vemurafenib** is predicted to increase the exposure to nintedanib. [Moderate] Study
- **Vemurafenib** is predicted to increase the exposure to panobinostat. Adjust dose. [Moderate] Theoretical → Also see TABLE 9 p. 1336
- Rifampicin is predicted to decrease the exposure to **vemurafenib**. Avoid. [Severe] Theoretical
- **Vemurafenib** is predicted to increase the exposure to ticagrelor. Use with caution or avoid. [Severe] Study
- **Vemurafenib** is predicted to increase the exposure to topotecan. [Severe] Study
- **Vemurafenib** is predicted to increase the concentration of trametinib. [Moderate] Theoretical
- **Vemurafenib** is predicted to increase the exposure to venetoclax. Avoid or monitor for toxicity. [Severe] Theoretical

Venetoclax

FOOD AND LIFESTYLE Avoid Seville (bitter orange) and star fruit as they might increase the exposure to venetoclax.

- Antiarrhythmics (amiodarone) are predicted to increase the exposure to **venetoclax**. Avoid or monitor for toxicity. [Severe] Theoretical
- Antiarrhythmics (dronedarone) are predicted to increase the exposure to **venetoclax**. Avoid moderate inhibitors of CYP3A4 or adjust **venetoclax** dose, p. 974. [Severe] Study
- Antiepileptics (carbamazepine, fosphenytoin, phenobarbital, phenytoin, primidone) are predicted to decrease the exposure to **venetoclax**. Avoid. [Severe] Study
- Antifungals, azoles (fluconazole, isavuconazole, posaconazole) are predicted to increase the exposure to **venetoclax**. Avoid moderate inhibitors of CYP3A4 or adjust **venetoclax** dose, p. 974. [Severe] Study
- Antifungals, azoles (itraconazole, ketoconazole, voriconazole) are predicted to increase the exposure to **venetoclax**. Avoid potent inhibitors of CYP3A4 or adjust **venetoclax** dose, p. 974. [Severe] Study
- Aprepitant is predicted to increase the exposure to **venetoclax**. Avoid moderate inhibitors of CYP3A4 or adjust **venetoclax** dose, p. 974. [Severe] Study
- Bosentan is predicted to decrease the exposure to **venetoclax**. Avoid. [Severe] Study
- Calcium channel blockers (diltiazem, verapamil) are predicted to increase the exposure to **venetoclax**. Avoid moderate inhibitors of CYP3A4 or adjust **venetoclax** dose, p. 974. [Severe] Study
- Ciclosporin is predicted to increase the exposure to **venetoclax**. Avoid or monitor for toxicity. [Severe] Theoretical
- Cobicistat is predicted to increase the exposure to **venetoclax**. Avoid potent inhibitors of CYP3A4 or adjust **venetoclax** dose, p. 974. [Severe] Study
- **Venetoclax** slightly increases the exposure to coumarins (warfarin). [Moderate] Study
- Crizotinib is predicted to increase the exposure to **venetoclax**. Avoid moderate inhibitors of CYP3A4 or adjust **venetoclax** dose, p. 974. [Severe] Study
- Efavirenz is predicted to decrease the exposure to **venetoclax**. Avoid. [Severe] Study
- Enzalutamide is predicted to decrease the exposure to **venetoclax**. Avoid. [Severe] Study
- Grapefruit juice is predicted to increase the exposure to **venetoclax**. Avoid. [Severe] Theoretical
- HIV-protease inhibitors are predicted to increase the exposure to **venetoclax**. Avoid potent inhibitors of CYP3A4 or adjust **venetoclax** dose, p. 974. [Severe] Study
- Idelalisib is predicted to increase the exposure to **venetoclax**. Avoid potent inhibitors of CYP3A4 or adjust **venetoclax** dose, p. 974. [Severe] Study
- Imatinib is predicted to increase the exposure to **venetoclax**. Avoid moderate inhibitors of CYP3A4 or adjust **venetoclax** dose, p. 974. [Severe] Study
- Lapatinib is predicted to increase the exposure to **venetoclax**. Avoid or monitor for toxicity. [Severe] Theoretical
- **Venetoclax** potentially decreases the efficacy of live vaccines. Avoid. [Severe] Theoretical
- Macrolides (azithromycin) decrease the exposure to **venetoclax**. [Mild] Study
- Macrolides (clarithromycin) are predicted to increase the exposure to **venetoclax**. Avoid potent inhibitors of CYP3A4 or adjust **venetoclax** dose, p. 974. [Severe] Study
- Macrolides (erythromycin) are predicted to increase the exposure to **venetoclax**. Avoid moderate inhibitors of CYP3A4 or adjust **venetoclax** dose, p. 974. [Severe] Study
- Mitotane is predicted to decrease the exposure to **venetoclax**. Avoid. [Severe] Study
- Netupitant is predicted to increase the exposure to **venetoclax**. Avoid moderate inhibitors of CYP3A4 or adjust **venetoclax** dose, p. 974. [Severe] Study
- Nevirapine is predicted to decrease the exposure to **venetoclax**. Avoid. [Severe] Study
- Nilotinib is predicted to increase the exposure to **venetoclax**. Avoid moderate inhibitors of CYP3A4 or adjust **venetoclax** dose, p. 974. [Severe] Study
- Ranolazine is predicted to increase the exposure to **venetoclax**. Avoid or monitor for toxicity. [Severe] Theoretical
- Rifampicin is predicted to decrease the exposure to **venetoclax**. Avoid. [Severe] Study
- St John's Wort is predicted to decrease the exposure to **venetoclax**. Avoid. [Severe] Study
- Vemurafenib is predicted to increase the exposure to **venetoclax**. Avoid or monitor for toxicity. [Severe] Theoretical

Venlafaxine → see TABLE 13 p. 1337 (serotonin syndrome), TABLE 9 p. 1336 (QT-interval prolongation), TABLE 11 p. 1336 (CNS depressant effects), TABLE 4 p. 1334 (antiplatelet effects)

- Abiraterone potentially increases the exposure to **venlafaxine**. [Severe] Theoretical
- Antifungals, azoles (itraconazole, ketoconazole, voriconazole) are predicted to increase the exposure to **venlafaxine**. [Moderate] Study → Also see TABLE 9 p. 1336
- Cobicistat is predicted to increase the exposure to **venlafaxine**. [Moderate] Study
- H₂ receptor antagonists (cimetidine) slightly increase the exposure to **venlafaxine**. [Mild] Study
- **Venlafaxine** slightly increases the exposure to haloperidol. [Severe] Study → Also see TABLE 9 p. 1336 → Also see TABLE 11 p. 1336

Venlafaxine (continued)
▸ HIV-protease inhibitors are predicted to increase the exposure to **venlafaxine**. [Moderate] Study → Also see TABLE 9 p. 1336
▸ Idelalisib is predicted to increase the exposure to **venlafaxine**. [Moderate] Study
▸ Macrolides (clarithromycin) are predicted to increase the exposure to **venlafaxine**. [Moderate] Study → Also see TABLE 9 p. 1336
▸ Tacrolimus potentially increases the risk of serotonin syndrome when given with **venlafaxine**. [Severe] Anecdotal

Verapamil → see calcium channel blockers

Verteporfin

GENERAL INFORMATION Caution on concurrent use with other photosensitising drugs.

Vigabatrin → see antiepileptics
Vilanterol → see beta₂ agonists
Vildagliptin → see TABLE 14 p. 1337 (antidiabetic drugs)
Vinblastine → see vinca alkaloids
Vinca alkaloids → see TABLE 1 p. 1334 (hepatotoxicity), TABLE 15 p. 1337 (myelosuppression), TABLE 19 p. 1338 (ototoxicity), TABLE 12 p. 1337 (peripheral neuropathy), TABLE 5 p. 1334 (thromboembolism), TABLE 9 p. 1336 (QT-interval prolongation)

vinblastine · vincristine · vindesine · vinflunine · vinorelbine

▸ Antiarrhythmics (dronedarone) are predicted to increase the exposure to **vinca alkaloids**. [Severe] Theoretical → Also see TABLE 9 p. 1336
▸ Antiepileptics (carbamazepine, fosphenytoin, phenobarbital, phenytoin, primidone) are predicted to decrease the exposure to **vinflunine**. Avoid. [Severe] Theoretical → Also see TABLE 12 p. 1337
▸ Antiepileptics (carbamazepine, fosphenytoin, phenobarbital, phenytoin, primidone) are predicted to decrease the exposure to **vinorelbine**. Use with caution or avoid. [Severe] Theoretical → Also see TABLE 12 p. 1337
▸ Antiepileptics (carbamazepine, fosphenytoin, phenobarbital, phenytoin, primidone) are predicted to decrease the exposure to **vinca alkaloids** (vinblastine, vincristine, vindesine). [Severe] Theoretical → Also see TABLE 1 p. 1334 → Also see TABLE 12 p. 1337
▸ Antifungals, azoles (fluconazole, isavuconazole, itraconazole, ketoconazole, posaconazole, voriconazole) are predicted to increase the exposure to **vinca alkaloids**. [Severe] Theoretical → Also see TABLE 1 p. 1334 → Also see TABLE 9 p. 1336
▸ Antifungals, azoles (miconazole) are predicted to increase the concentration of **vinca alkaloids**. Use with caution and adjust dose. [Moderate] Theoretical
▸ Aprepitant is predicted to increase the exposure to **vinca alkaloids**. [Severe] Theoretical
▸ Asparaginase potentially increases the risk of neurotoxicity when given with **vincristine**. Vincristine should be taken 3 to 24 hours before asparaginase. [Severe] Anecdotal → Also see TABLE 1 p. 1334 → Also see TABLE 15 p. 1337
▸ Calcium channel blockers (diltiazem, verapamil) are predicted to increase the exposure to **vinca alkaloids**. [Severe] Theoretical
▸ Cobicistat is predicted to increase the exposure to **vinca alkaloids**. [Severe] Theoretical
▸ Crisantaspase potentially increases the risk of neurotoxicity when given with **vincristine**. Vincristine should be taken 3 to 24 hours before crisantaspase. [Severe] Anecdotal → Also see TABLE 1 p. 1334 → Also see TABLE 15 p. 1337
▸ Crizotinib is predicted to increase the exposure to **vinca alkaloids**. [Severe] Theoretical → Also see TABLE 15 p. 1337 → Also see TABLE 9 p. 1336
▸ Enzalutamide is predicted to decrease the exposure to **vinca alkaloids** (vinblastine, vincristine, vindesine). [Severe] Theoretical
▸ Enzalutamide is predicted to decrease the exposure to **vinflunine**. Avoid. [Severe] Theoretical
▸ Enzalutamide is predicted to decrease the exposure to **vinorelbine**. Use with caution or avoid. [Severe] Theoretical
▸ HIV-protease inhibitors are predicted to increase the exposure to **vinca alkaloids**. [Severe] Theoretical → Also see TABLE 9 p. 1336
▸ Idelalisib is predicted to increase the exposure to **vinca alkaloids**. [Severe] Theoretical → Also see TABLE 15 p. 1337
▸ Imatinib is predicted to increase the exposure to **vinca alkaloids**. [Severe] Theoretical → Also see TABLE 15 p. 1337

▸ Live vaccines are predicted to increase the risk of generalised infection (possibly life-threatening) when given with **vinca alkaloids**. Public Health England advises avoid (refer to Green Book). [Severe] Theoretical
▸ Macrolides (clarithromycin, erythromycin) are predicted to increase the exposure to **vinca alkaloids**. [Severe] Theoretical → Also see TABLE 9 p. 1336
▸ Mitotane is predicted to decrease the exposure to **vinca alkaloids** (vinblastine, vincristine, vindesine). [Severe] Theoretical → Also see TABLE 15 p. 1337
▸ Mitotane is predicted to decrease the exposure to **vinflunine**. Avoid. [Severe] Theoretical → Also see TABLE 15 p. 1337
▸ Mitotane is predicted to decrease the exposure to **vinorelbine**. Use with caution or avoid. [Severe] Theoretical → Also see TABLE 15 p. 1337
▸ Netupitant is predicted to increase the exposure to **vinca alkaloids**. [Severe] Theoretical
▸ Nilotinib is predicted to increase the exposure to **vinca alkaloids**. [Severe] Theoretical → Also see TABLE 15 p. 1337 → Also see TABLE 9 p. 1336
▸ Pegaspargase potentially increases the risk of neurotoxicity when given with **vincristine**. Vincristine should be taken 3 to 24 hours before pegaspargase. [Severe] Anecdotal → Also see TABLE 1 p. 1334 → Also see TABLE 15 p. 1337
▸ Rifampicin is predicted to decrease the exposure to **vinca alkaloids** (vinblastine, vincristine, vindesine). [Severe] Theoretical
▸ Rifampicin is predicted to decrease the exposure to **vinflunine**. Avoid. [Severe] Theoretical
▸ Rifampicin is predicted to decrease the exposure to **vinorelbine**. Use with caution or avoid. [Severe] Theoretical

Vincristine → see vinca alkaloids
Vindesine → see vinca alkaloids
Vinflunine → see vinca alkaloids
Vinorelbine → see vinca alkaloids
Vismodegib → see TABLE 15 p. 1337 (myelosuppression)
▸ Antiepileptics (carbamazepine, fosphenytoin, phenobarbital, phenytoin, primidone) are predicted to decrease the exposure to **vismodegib**. Avoid. [Moderate] Theoretical
▸ Enzalutamide is predicted to decrease the exposure to **vismodegib**. Avoid. [Moderate] Theoretical
▸ Mitotane is predicted to decrease the exposure to **vismodegib**. Avoid. [Moderate] Theoretical → Also see TABLE 15 p. 1337
▸ Rifampicin is predicted to decrease the exposure to **vismodegib**. Avoid. [Moderate] Theoretical
▸ St John's Wort is predicted to decrease the exposure to **vismodegib**. Avoid. [Moderate] Theoretical

Vitamin A
▸ Retinoids (acitretin, alitretinoin, isotretinoin) are predicted to increase the risk of vitamin A toxicity when given with **vitamin A**. Avoid. [Severe] Theoretical
▸ Retinoids (bexarotene) are predicted to increase the risk of toxicity when given with **vitamin A**. Adjust dose. [Moderate] Theoretical
▸ Retinoids (tretinoin) are predicted to increase the risk of vitamin A toxicity when given with **vitamin A**. Avoid. [Severe] Study

Vitamin D substances

alfacalcidol · calcipotriol · calcitriol · colecalciferol · dihydrotachysterol · ergocalciferol · paricalcitol · tacalcitol

▸ Antiepileptics (carbamazepine) are predicted to decrease the effects of **vitamin D substances**. [Moderate] Study
▸ Antiepileptics (fosphenytoin, phenytoin) decrease the effects of **vitamin D substances**. [Moderate] Study
▸ Antiepileptics (phenobarbital, primidone) are predicted to decrease the effects of **vitamin D substances**. [Moderate] Theoretical
▸ Antifungals, azoles (clotrimazole, ketoconazole) are predicted to decrease the exposure to **colecalciferol**. [Moderate] Theoretical
▸ Antifungals, azoles (itraconazole, ketoconazole, voriconazole) are predicted to increase the exposure to **paricalcitol**. [Moderate] Study
▸ Cobicistat is predicted to increase the exposure to **paricalcitol**. [Moderate] Study
▸ **Vitamin D substances** are predicted to increase the risk of toxicity when given with digoxin. [Severe] Theoretical

- HIV-protease inhibitors are predicted to increase the exposure to **paricalcitol**. Moderate Study
- **Idelalisib** is predicted to increase the exposure to **paricalcitol**. Moderate Study
- Macrolides (clarithromycin) are predicted to increase the exposure to **paricalcitol**. Moderate Study
- Thiazide diuretics increase the risk of hypercalcaemia when given with **vitamin D substances**. Moderate Theoretical

Vitamin E substances

alpha tocopherol · alpha tocopheryl acetate

- **Vitamin E substances** affect the exposure to ciclosporin. Moderate Study

Volatile halogenated anaesthetics → see TABLE 8 p. 1335
(hypotension), **TABLE 11** p. 1336 (CNS depressant effects)

desflurane · isoflurane · methoxyflurane · sevoflurane

- Antiepileptics (phenobarbital, primidone) potentially increase the risk of nephrotoxicity when given with **methoxyflurane**. Avoid. Severe Theoretical → Also see **TABLE 11** p. 1336
- Isoniazid potentially increases the risk of nephrotoxicity when given with **methoxyflurane**. Avoid. Severe Theoretical
- Rifampicin potentially increases the risk of nephrotoxicity when given with **methoxyflurane**. Avoid. Severe Theoretical

Voriconazole → see antifungals, azoles

Vortioxetine → see TABLE 13 p. 1337 (serotonin syndrome), **TABLE 4** p. 1334 (antiplatelet effects)

- Antiepileptics (carbamazepine, fosphenytoin, phenobarbital, phenytoin, primidone) are predicted to decrease the exposure to **vortioxetine**. Monitor and adjust dose. Moderate Study
- Bupropion is predicted to increase the exposure to **vortioxetine**. Monitor and adjust dose. Moderate Study → Also see **TABLE 13** p. 1337
- Cinacalcet is predicted to increase the exposure to **vortioxetine**. Monitor and adjust dose. Moderate Study
- Enzalutamide is predicted to decrease the exposure to **vortioxetine**. Monitor and adjust dose. Moderate Study
- Mitotane is predicted to decrease the exposure to **vortioxetine**. Monitor and adjust dose. Moderate Study
- Rifampicin is predicted to decrease the exposure to **vortioxetine**. Monitor and adjust dose. Moderate Study
- SSRIs (fluoxetine, paroxetine) are predicted to increase the exposure to **vortioxetine**. Monitor and adjust dose. Moderate Study → Also see **TABLE 13** p. 1337 → Also see **TABLE 4** p. 1334
- Terbinafine is predicted to increase the exposure to **vortioxetine**. Monitor and adjust dose. Moderate Study

Voxilaprevir

- Antiepileptics (carbamazepine, fosphenytoin, phenobarbital, phenytoin, primidone) are predicted to decrease the concentration of **voxilaprevir**. Avoid. Severe Study
- Antiepileptics (oxcarbazepine) are predicted to decrease the concentration of **voxilaprevir**. Avoid. Severe Theoretical
- Bosentan is predicted to decrease the concentration of **voxilaprevir**. Severe Theoretical
- Ciclosporin increases the concentration of **voxilaprevir**. Avoid. Severe Study
- **Voxilaprevir** is predicted to increase the concentration of dabigatran. Avoid. Severe Study
- **Voxilaprevir** is predicted to increase the concentration of edoxaban. Avoid. Severe Theoretical
- Efavirenz is predicted to decrease the concentration of **voxilaprevir**. Avoid. Severe Theoretical
- Enzalutamide is predicted to decrease the concentration of **voxilaprevir**. Avoid. Severe Study
- HIV-protease inhibitors (atazanavir) (boosted with ritonavir) increase the concentration of **voxilaprevir**. Avoid. Severe Study
- HIV-protease inhibitors (lopinavir) are predicted to increase the concentration of **voxilaprevir**. Avoid. Severe Theoretical
- Mitotane is predicted to decrease the concentration of **voxilaprevir**. Avoid. Severe Study
- Modafinil is predicted to decrease the concentration of **voxilaprevir**. Avoid. Severe Study
- Nevirapine is predicted to decrease the concentration of **voxilaprevir**. Avoid. Severe Theoretical

- Proton pump inhibitors are predicted to decrease the exposure to **voxilaprevir**. Adjust dose, see sofosbuvir with velpatasvir and voxilaprevir p. 619. Moderate Study
- Rifabutin is predicted to decrease the concentration of **voxilaprevir**. Avoid. Severe Theoretical
- Rifampicin is predicted to decrease the concentration of **voxilaprevir**. Avoid. Severe Study
- St John's Wort is predicted to decrease the concentration of **voxilaprevir**. Avoid. Severe Theoretical
- **Voxilaprevir** is predicted to increase the exposure to statins (atorvastatin, fluvastatin, simvastatin). Avoid. Severe Theoretical
- **Voxilaprevir** is predicted to increase the exposure to statins (pravastatin). Monitor and adjust **pravastatin** dose. Severe Study
- **Voxilaprevir** is predicted to increase the exposure to statins (rosuvastatin). Avoid. Severe Study
- **Voxilaprevir** is predicted to increase the exposure to tenofovir disoproxil. Severe Study

Warfarin → see coumarins

Wasp venom extract

GENERAL INFORMATION Desensitising vaccines should be avoided in patients taking beta-blockers (adrenaline might be ineffective in case of a hypersensitivity reaction) or ACE inhibitors (risk of severe anaphylactoid reactions).

Xipamide → see thiazide diuretics
Xylometazoline → see sympathomimetics, vasoconstrictor
Yellow fever vaccine, live → see vaccines
Zaleplon → see TABLE 11 p. 1336 (CNS depressant effects)
- Rifampicin markedly decreases the exposure to **zaleplon**. Moderate Study

Zidovudine → see TABLE 15 p. 1337 (myelosuppression), **TABLE 2** p. 1334 (nephrotoxicity)
- Antiepileptics (valproate) slightly increase the exposure to **zidovudine**. Moderate Study
- Antimalarials (pyrimethamine) are predicted to increase the risk of side-effects when given with **zidovudine**. Severe Theoretical → Also see **TABLE 15** p. 1337
- **Zidovudine** increases the risk of haematological toxicity when given with aspirin (high-dose). Severe Study
- HIV-protease inhibitors (tipranavir) slightly decrease the exposure to **zidovudine**. Avoid. Moderate Study
- Macrolides (clarithromycin) decrease the absorption of **zidovudine**. Separate administration by at least 2 hours. Moderate Study
- Nevirapine is predicted to decrease the concentration of **zidovudine**. Refer to specialist literature. Severe Theoretical
- **Zidovudine** increases the risk of haematological toxicity when given with NSAIDs. Severe Study → Also see **TABLE 2** p. 1334
- Ribavirin increases the risk of anaemia and/or leucopenia when given with **zidovudine**. Avoid. Severe Study
- **Zidovudine** is predicted to decrease the efficacy of stavudine. Avoid. Severe Theoretical

Zinc

- Oral **zinc** decreases the absorption of oral bisphosphonates (alendronic acid). **Zinc** should be taken at least 30 minutes before **alendronic acid**. Moderate Study
- Oral **zinc** is predicted to decrease the absorption of oral bisphosphonates (ibandronic acid). Avoid **zinc** for at least 6 hours before or 1 hour after **ibandronic acid**. Moderate Theoretical
- Oral **zinc** decreases the absorption of oral bisphosphonates (risedronate). Separate administration by at least 2 hours. Moderate Study
- Oral **zinc** decreases the absorption of oral bisphosphonates (sodium clodronate). Avoid **zinc** for 2 hours before or 1 hour after **sodium clodronate**. Moderate Study
- Oral calcium salts decrease the absorption of **zinc**. Moderate Study
- **Zinc** is predicted to decrease the absorption of eltrombopag. **Eltrombopag** should be taken 2 hours before or 4 hours after **zinc**. Severe Theoretical
- **Zinc** is predicted to decrease the efficacy of iron (oral) and iron (oral) is predicted to decrease the efficacy of **zinc**. Moderate Study

A1

Interactions | Appendix 1

Zinc (continued)

▸ **Zinc** is predicted to decrease the absorption of penicillamine. Mild Theoretical

▸ **Zinc** is predicted to decrease the exposure to quinolones. Separate administration by 2 hours. Moderate Study

▸ Oral **zinc** is predicted to decrease the absorption of tetracyclines. Separate administration by 2 to 3 hours. Moderate Theoretical

▸ Trientine potentially decreases the absorption of **zinc**. Moderate Theoretical

Zoledronic acid → see bisphosphonates

Zolmitriptan → see TABLE 13 p. 1337 (serotonin syndrome)

▸ Combined hormonal contraceptives are predicted to increase the exposure to **zolmitriptan**. Adjust **zolmitriptan** dose, p. 475. Moderate Theoretical

▸ H₂ receptor antagonists (cimetidine) slightly increase the exposure to **zolmitriptan**. Adjust **zolmitriptan** dose, p. 475. Mild Study

▸ Moclobemide slightly increases the exposure to **zolmitriptan**. Adjust **zolmitriptan** dose, p. 475. Moderate Study → Also see TABLE 13 p. 1337

▸ Monoamine-oxidase A and B inhibitors, irreversible are predicted to increase the exposure to **zolmitriptan**. Severe Theoretical → Also see TABLE 13 p. 1337

▸ Quinolones (ciprofloxacin) are predicted to increase the exposure to **zolmitriptan**. Adjust **zolmitriptan** dose, p. 475. Moderate Theoretical

▸ SSRIs (fluvoxamine) are predicted to increase the exposure to **zolmitriptan**. Adjust **zolmitriptan** dose, p. 475. Severe Theoretical → Also see TABLE 13 p. 1337

Zolpidem → see TABLE 11 p. 1336 (CNS depressant effects)

▸ Antiepileptics (carbamazepine) moderately decrease the exposure to **zolpidem**. Moderate Study

▸ Rifampicin moderately decreases the exposure to **zolpidem**. Moderate Study

Zonisamide → see antiepileptics

Zopiclone → see TABLE 11 p. 1336 (CNS depressant effects)

▸ Antiarrhythmics (dronedarone) are predicted to increase the exposure to **zopiclone**. Adjust dose. Moderate Study

▸ Antiepileptics (carbamazepine, fosphenytoin, phenobarbital, phenytoin, primidone) are predicted to decrease the exposure to **zopiclone**. Adjust dose. Moderate Study → Also see TABLE 11 p. 1336

▸ Antifungals, azoles (fluconazole, isavuconazole, posaconazole) are predicted to increase the exposure to **zopiclone**. Adjust dose. Moderate Study

▸ Antifungals, azoles (itraconazole, ketoconazole, voriconazole) are predicted to increase the exposure to **zopiclone**. Adjust dose. Moderate Theoretical

▸ Aprepitant is predicted to increase the exposure to **zopiclone**. Adjust dose. Moderate Study

▸ Calcium channel blockers (diltiazem, verapamil) are predicted to increase the exposure to **zopiclone**. Adjust dose. Moderate Study

▸ Cobicistat is predicted to increase the exposure to **zopiclone**. Adjust dose. Moderate Theoretical

▸ Crizotinib is predicted to increase the exposure to **zopiclone**. Adjust dose. Moderate Study

▸ Enzalutamide is predicted to decrease the exposure to **zopiclone**. Adjust dose. Moderate Study

▸ HIV-protease inhibitors are predicted to increase the exposure to **zopiclone**. Adjust dose. Moderate Theoretical

▸ Idelalisib is predicted to increase the exposure to **zopiclone**. Adjust dose. Moderate Theoretical

▸ Imatinib is predicted to increase the exposure to **zopiclone**. Adjust dose. Moderate Study

▸ Macrolides (clarithromycin) are predicted to increase the exposure to **zopiclone**. Adjust dose. Moderate Theoretical

▸ Macrolides (erythromycin) are predicted to increase the exposure to **zopiclone**. Adjust dose. Moderate Study

▸ Mitotane is predicted to decrease the exposure to **zopiclone**. Adjust dose. Moderate Study

▸ Netupitant is predicted to increase the exposure to **zopiclone**. Adjust dose. Moderate Study

▸ Nilotinib is predicted to increase the exposure to **zopiclone**. Adjust dose. Moderate Study

▸ Rifampicin is predicted to decrease the exposure to **zopiclone**. Adjust dose. Moderate Study

Zuclopenthixol → see TABLE 8 p. 1335 (hypotension), TABLE 9 p. 1336 (QT-interval prolongation), TABLE 11 p. 1336 (CNS depressant effects)

▸ **Zuclopenthixol** is predicted to decrease the effects of dopamine receptor agonists. Avoid. Moderate Theoretical → Also see TABLE 8 p. 1335 → Also see TABLE 9 p. 1336

▸ **Zuclopenthixol** is predicted to decrease the effects of levodopa. Avoid or monitor worsening parkinsonian symptoms. Severe Theoretical → Also see TABLE 8 p. 1335

▸ **Zuclopenthixol** potentially increases the risk of neurotoxicity when given with lithium. Severe Anecdotal → Also see TABLE 9 p. 1336

Appendix 2
Borderline substances

CONTENTS

In certain conditions some foods (and toilet preparations) have characteristics of drugs and the Advisory Committee on Borderline Substances (ACBS) advises as to the circumstances in which such substances may be regarded as drugs. Prescriptions issued in accordance with the Committee's advice and endorsed 'ACBS' will normally not be investigated.

Information

General Practitioners are reminded that the ACBS recommends products on the basis that they may be regarded as drugs for the management of specified conditions. Doctors should satisfy themselves that the products can safely be prescribed, that patients are adequately monitored and that, where necessary, expert hospital supervision is available.

Foods which may be prescribed on FP10, GP10 (Scotland), or WP10 (Wales)

All the food products listed in this appendix have ACBS approval. The clinical condition for which the product has been approved is included with each entry.
Note Foods included in this appendix may contain cariogenic sugars and patients should be advised to take appropriate oral hygiene measures.

Enteral feeds and supplements

For most enteral feeds and nutritional supplements, the main source of **carbohydrate** is either maltodextrin or glucose syrup; other carbohydrate sources are listed in the relevant table, below. Feeds containing residual lactose (less than 1 g lactose/100 mL formula) are described as 'clinically lactose-free' or 'lactose-free' by some manufacturers. The presence of lactose (including residual lactose) in feeds is indicated in the relevant table, below. The primary sources of **protein** or **amino acids** are included with each product entry. The **fat** or **oil** content is derived from a variety of sources such as vegetables, soya bean, corn, palm nuts, and seeds; where the fat content is derived from animal or fish sources, this information is included in the relevant table,

below. The presence of medium chain triglycerides (MCT) is also noted where the quantity exceeds 30% of the fat content.
Enteral feeds and nutritional supplements can contain varying amounts of **vitamins**, **minerals**, and **trace elements**—the manufacturer's product literature should be consulted for more detailed information. Feeds containing vitamin K may affect the INR in patients receiving warfarin. The suitability of food products for patients requiring a vegan, kosher, halal, or other compliant diet should be confirmed with individual manufacturers.
Note Feeds containing more than 6 g/100 mL protein or 2 g/100 mL fibre should be avoided in children unless recommended by an appropriate specialist or dietician.

Nutritional values

Nutritional values of products vary with flavour and pack size—consult product literature.

Other conditions for which ACBS products can be prescribed

This is a list of clinical conditions for which the ACBS has approved toilet preparations.
Birthmarks
Dermatitis
Excema and Pruritus
Aveeno® Bath Oil; *Aveeno*® Cream; *Aveeno*® Lotion; *E45*® Emollient Bath Oil; *E45*® Emollient Wash Cream; *E45*® Lotion
Disfiguring skin lesions (birthmarks, mutilating lesions, scars, vitiligo)
Covermark® classic foundation and finishing powder; *Dermablend*® *Ultra* corrective foundation; *Dermacolor*® Camouflage cream and fixing powder; *Keromask*® masking cream and finishing powder; *Veil*® Cover cream and Finishing Powder. (Cleansing Creams, Cleansing Milks, and Cleansing Lotions are excluded).
Disinfectants (antiseptics)
May be prescribed on an FP10 only when ordered in such quantities and with such directions as are appropriate for

the treatment of patients, but not for general hygenic purposes.

Dry mouth (xerostomia)

For patients suffering from dry mouth as a result of having (or having undergone) radiotherapy, or sicca syndrome.

AS Saliva Orthana®; *Biotène Oralbalance*®; *Glandosane*®; *Saliveze*®

Photodermatoses (skin protection in)

Anthelios® XL SPF 50+ Melt-in cream; *Sunsense*® Ultra; *Uvistat*® Lipscreen SPF 50, *Uvistat*® Suncream SPF 30 and 50

Standard ACBS indications: Disease-related malnutrition, intractable malabsorption, pre-operative preparation of malnourished patients, dysphagia, proven inflammatory bowel disease, following total gastrectomy, short-bowel syndrome, bowel fistula

Table 1 Enteral feeds (non-disease specific)

Less than 5 g protein/100 mL

Enteral feeds: 1 kcal/mL and less than 5 g protein/100 mL

Not suitable for use in child under 1 year unless otherwise stated; not recommended for child 1-6 years

Product	Formulation	Energy	Protein	Carbohydrate	Fat	Fibre	Special Characteristics	ACBS Indications	Presentation & Flavour
Fresubin® 1500 Complete (Fresenius Kabi Ltd)	Liquid (tube feed) per 100 mL	420 kJ (100 kcal)	3.8 g cows' milk soya	13 g (sugars 0.9 g)	3.4 g	1.5 g	Gluten-free Residual lactose Contains fish oil	Borderline substances standard ACBS indications p. 1500 except bowel fistula and pre-operative preparation of malnourished patients. Not suitable for child under 2 years	Fresubin 1500 Complete liquid: 1.5 litre = £14.05
Fresubin® Original (Fresenius Kabi Ltd)	Liquid (sip or tube feed) per 100 mL	420 kJ (100 kcal)	3.8 g cows' milk soya	13.8 g (sugars 3.5 g)	3.4 g	Nil	Gluten-free Residual lactose Contains fish gelatin Feed in flexible pack contains fish oil and fish gelatin	Borderline substances standard ACBS indications p. 1500	Fresubin Original drink: blackcurrant, chocolate, nut, peach, vanilla 200 ml = £2.28; Fresubin Original tube feed liquid: 1000 ml = £8.74; 1500 ml = £13.10; 500 ml = £4.41
Fresubin® Original Fibre (Fresenius Kabi Ltd)	Liquid (tube feed) per 100 mL	420 kJ (100 kcal)	3.8 g cows' milk soya	13 g (sugars 0.9 g)	3.4 g	1.5 g	Gluten-free Residual lactose Contains fish oil	Borderline substances standard ACBS indications p. 1500 except bowel fistula and pre-operative preparation of malnourished patients. Not suitable for child under 2 years	Fresubin Original Fibre liquid: 500 ml = £4.99; 1000 ml = £9.96
Jevity® (Abbott Laboratories Ltd)	Liquid (tube feed) per 100 mL	449 kJ (107 kcal)	4 g caseinates	14.1 g (sugars 470 mg)	3.47 g	1.76 g	Gluten-free Residual lactose	Borderline substances standard ACBS indications p. 1500 except bowel fistula. Not suitable for child under 2 years	Jevity liquid: 1000 ml = £10.59; 1500 ml = £15.85; 500 ml = £5.62
Nutrison® (Nutricia Ltd)	Liquid (tube feed) per 100 mL	420 kJ (100 kcal)	4 g cows' milk	12.3 g (sugars 1 g)	3.9 g	Nil	Gluten-free Residual lactose	Borderline substances standard ACBS indications p. 1500	Nutrison liquid: 500 ml = £5.20; 500 ml = £4.68; 1000 ml = £9.12; 1500 ml = £13.68
Nutrison® Multi Fibre (Nutricia Ltd)	Liquid (tube feed) per 100 mL	420 kJ (100 kcal)	4 g cows' milk	12.3 g (sugars 1 g)	3.9 g	1.5 g	Gluten-free Residual lactose	Borderline substances standard ACBS indications p. 1500 except bowel fistula	Nutrison Multi Fibre liquid: 1500 ml = £15.83; 500 ml = £5.62; 500 ml = £5.27; 1000 ml = £10.57
Osmolite® (Abbott Laboratories Ltd)	Liquid (tube feed) per 100 mL	424 kJ (100 kcal)	4 g caseinates soy isolate	13.6 g (sugars 630 mg)	3.4 g	Nil	Gluten-free Residual lactose	Borderline substances standard ACBS indications p. 1500	Osmolite liquid: 500 ml = £5.21; 1000 ml = £9.14; 1500 ml = £13.71

SOYA PROTEIN FORMULA

Product	Formulation	Energy	Protein	Carbohydrate	Fat	Fibre	Special Characteristics	ACBS Indications	Presentation & Flavour
Fresubin® Soya Fibre (Fresenius Kabi Ltd)	Liquid (tube feed) per 100 mL	420 kJ (100 kcal)	3.8 g soya protein	13.3 g (sugars 4.1 g)	3.6 g	2 g	Gluten-free Lactose-free Contains fish oil	Borderline substances standard ACBS indications p. 1500; also cows' milk protein intolerance, lactose intolerance	Fresubin Soya Fibre liquid: 500 ml = £5.16
Nutrison® Soya (Nutricia Ltd)	Liquid (tube feed) per 100 mL	420 kJ (100 kcal)	4 g soy isolate	12.3 g (sugars 1 g)	3.9 g	Nil	Gluten-free Residual lactose Milk protein-free	Borderline substances standard ACBS indications p. 1500; also cows' milk protein and lactose intolerance	Nutrison Soya liquid: 500 ml = £5.61; 1000 ml = £11.23
Nutrison® Soya Multi Fibre (Nutricia Ltd)	Liquid (tube feed) per 100 mL	420 kJ (100 kcal)	4 g soy isolate	12.3 g (sugars 700 mg)	3.9 g	1.5 g	Gluten-free Residual lactose Milk protein-free	Borderline substances standard ACBS indications p. 1500 except bowel fistula; also cows' milk protein and lactose intolerance	Nutrison Soya Multi Fibre liquid: 1.5 litre = £18.68

PEPTIDE-BASED FORMULA

Product	Formulation	Energy	Protein	Carbohydrate	Fat	Fibre	Special Characteristics	ACBS Indications	Presentation & Flavour
Nutrison® Peptisorb (Nutricia Ltd)	Liquid (tube feed) per 100 mL	425 kJ (100 kcal)	4 g whey protein hydrolysate	17.6 g (sugars 1.7 g)	1.7 g (MCT 47 %)	Nil	Gluten-free Residual lactose	Short bowel syndrome, intractable malabsorption, proven inflammatory bowel disease, bowel fistula	Nutrison Peptisorb liquid: 500 ml = £7.44; 1000 ml = £14.74; 500 ml = £8.18
Peptamen® (Nestle Health Science)	Liquid (sip or tube feed) per 100 mL	420 kJ (100 kcal)	4 g whey peptides	12.7 g (sugars 480 mg)	3.7 g (MCT 70 %)	Nil	Gluten-free Residual lactose	Short bowel syndrome, intractable malabsorption, proven inflammatory bowel disease, bowel fistula	Peptamen liquid: vanilla 800 ml = £12.56; unflavoured 500 ml = £7.06; 1000 ml = £13.25
Survimed® OPD (Fresenius Kabi Ltd)	Liquid (tube feed) per 100 mL	420 kJ (100 kcal)	4.5 g whey protein hydrolysate	14.3 g (sugars 1.1 g)	2.8 g (MCT 51 %)	0.1 g	Gluten-free Residual lactose Contains fish oil	Borderline substances standard ACBS indications p. 1500; also growth failure	Survimed OPD: liquid 500 ml = £7.36; 800 ml = £13.60; 1000 ml = £7.09; HN liquid 500 ml = £14.72

Enteral feeds: Less than 1 kcal/mL and less than 5 g protein/100 mL

AMINO ACID FORMULA (ESSENTIAL AND NON-ESSENTIAL AMINO ACIDS)

Not suitable for use in child under 1 year unless otherwise stated; not recommended for child 1-6 years

Product	Formulation	Energy	Protein	Carbohydrate	Fat	Fibre	Special Characteristics	ACBS Indications	Presentation & Flavour
Elemental 028® Extra (Nutricia Ltd)	Liquid (sip feed) per 100 mL	360 kJ (86 kcal)	2.5 g (protein equivalent)	11 g (sugars 4.7 g)	3.5 g (MCT 35 %)	Nil		Short bowel syndrome, intractable malabsorption, proven inflammatory bowel disease, bowel fistula	Elemental 028 Extra liquid: orange & pineapple, grapefruit, summer fruits 250 ml = £3.86
	Standard dilution (20 %) of powder (sip or tube feed) per 100 mL	374 kJ (89 kcal)	2.5 g (protein equivalent)	11.8 g (sugars 1.8 g)	3.5 g (MCT 35 %)	Nil		Short bowel syndrome, intractable malabsorption, proven inflammatory bowel disease, bowel fistula.	Elemental 028 Extra powder: plain, orange, banana 100 gram = £7.49

Powder provides protein equivalent 12.5 g, carbohydrate 59 g, fat 17.45 g, energy 1871 kJ (443 kcal)/100 g.

A2

Borderline substances | **Appendix 2**

A2

Enteral feeds (non-disease specific): 5 g (or more) protein/100 mL

Enteral feeds: 1.5 kcal/mL and 5 g (or more) protein/100 mL

Not suitable for use in child under 1 year unless otherwise stated; not recommended for child 1–6 years

Product	Formulation	Energy	Protein	Carbohydrate	Fat	Fibre	Special Characteristics	ACBS Indications	Presentation & Flavour
Fresubin® 2250 Complete (Fresenius Kabi Ltd)	Liquid (tube feed) per 100 mL	630 kJ (150 kcal)	5.6 g cows' milk	18.8 g (sugars 1.5 g)	5.8 g	2 g	Gluten-free; Residual lactose; Contains fish oil and fish gelatin	Borderline substances standard ACBS indications p. 1500	Fresubin 2250 Complete liquid: 1.5 litre = £15.68
Fresubin® Energy (Fresenius Kabi Ltd)	Liquid (sip feed) per 100 mL	630 kJ (150 kcal)	5.6 g cows' milk	18.8 g (sugars content varies with flavour)	5.8 g	Nil	Gluten-free; Residual lactose; Contains fish gelatin; Strawberry flavour may contain traces of wheat starch and egg.	Borderline substances standard ACBS indications p. 1500	Fresubin Energy liquid: banana, blackcurrant, cappuccino, chocolate, lemon, strawberry, tropical fruits, vanilla 200 ml = £1.40, unflavoured 200 ml = £1.40; 500 ml = £5.40
	Liquid (tube feed) per 100 mL	630 kJ (150 kcal)	5.6 g cows' milk	18.8 g (sugars 1.4 g)	5.8 g	Nil	Gluten-free; Residual lactose; Contains fish oil and fish gelatin	Borderline substances standard ACBS indications p. 1500	Fresubin Energy liquid: 1000 ml = £10.61; 1500 ml = £14.23
Fresubin® Energy Fibre (Fresenius Kabi Ltd)	Liquid (sip feed) per 100 mL	630 kJ (150 kcal)	5.6 g cows' milk	18.8 g (sugars content varies with flavour)	5.8 g	2 g	Gluten-free; Residual lactose; Contains fish gelatin	Borderline substances standard ACBS indications p. 1500	Fresubin Energy Fibre liquid: unflavoured 500 ml = £5.92; 1000 ml = £11.30; banana, caramel, cherry, chocolate, strawberry 200 ml = £2.17
	Liquid (tube feed) per 100 mL	630 kJ (150 kcal)	5.6 g cows' milk	18.8 g (sugars 1.5 g)	5.8 g	2 g	Gluten-free; Residual lactose; Contains fish oil and fish gelatin	Borderline substances standard ACBS indications p. 1500	Fresubin Energy Fibre liquid unflavoured: 500 ml = £5.92; 1000 ml = £11.30
Fresubin® HP Energy (Fresenius Kabi Ltd)	Liquid (tube feed) per 100 mL	630 kJ (150 kcal)	7.5 g cows' milk	17 g (sugars 1 g)	5.8 g (MCT 57%)	Nil	Gluten-free; Residual lactose; Contains fish oil and fish gelatin	Borderline substances standard ACBS indications p. 1500; also CAPD and haemodialysis	Fresubin HP Energy liquid: 500 ml = £5.50; 1000 ml = £11.00
Jevity® 1.5kcal (Abbott Laboratories Ltd)	Liquid (tube feed) per 100 mL	649 kJ (154 kcal)	6.38 g caseinates and soy isolate	20.1 g (sugars 1.47 g)	4.9 g	2.2 g	Gluten-free; Residual lactose	Borderline substances standard ACBS indications p. 1500. Not suitable for child under 2 years; not recommended for child 2–10 years	Jevity 1.5kcal liquid: 1500 ml = £19.55; 500 ml = £6.73; 1000 ml = £12.67
Nutrison® Energy (Nutricia Ltd)	Liquid (tube feed) per 100 mL	630 kJ (150 kcal)	6 g cows' milk	18.5 g (sugars 1.5 g)	5.8 g	Nil	Gluten-free; Residual lactose	Borderline substances standard ACBS indications p. 1500	Nutrison Energy liquid: 1000 ml = £11.39; 500 ml = £6.05; 1500 ml = £17.03; 500 ml = £5.66
Nutrison® Energy Multi Fibre (Nutricia Ltd)	Liquid (tube feed) per 100 mL	630 kJ (150 kcal)	6 g cows' milk	18.5 g (sugars 1.5 g)	5.8 g	1.5 g	Gluten-free; Residual lactose	Borderline substances standard ACBS indications p. 1500	Nutrison Energy Multi Fibre liquid: 500 ml = £6.33; 1000 ml = £12.64; 500 ml = £6.72; 1500 ml = £19.51
Osmolite® 1.5kcal (Abbott Laboratories Ltd)	Liquid (tube feed) per 100 mL	632 kJ (150 kcal)	6.25 g cows' milk soya protein isolate	20 g (sugars 4.9 g)	5 g	Nil	Gluten-free; Residual lactose	Borderline substances standard ACBS indications p. 1500	Osmolite 1.5kcal tube feed liquid: 1000 ml = £11.41; 500 ml = £6.06; 1500 ml = £17.07

Product	Formulation	Energy	Protein	Carbohydrate	Fat	Fibre	Special Characteristics	ACBS Indications	Presentation & Flavour
Resource® Energy (Nestle Health Science)	Liquid (sip feed) per 100 mL	630 kJ (150 kcal)	5.6 g cows' milk	21 g (sugars 5.2 g)	5 g	less than 0.5 g	Gluten-free Residual lactose	Borderline substances standard ACBS Indications p. 1500 Not suitable for use in child under 3 years	Resource Energy liquid: apricot, banana, chocolate, coffee, strawberry & raspberry, vanilla 800 ml = £7.93
Vital 1.5 kcal (Abbott Laboratories Ltd)	Liquid (sip or tube feed) per 100 mL	631 kJ (150 kcal)	6.75 g caseinate whey protein hydrolysate	18.4 g (sugars 3.6 g)	5.5 g (MCT 64%)	Nil	Gluten-free Residual lactose	Borderline substances standard ACBS Indications p. 1500; except proven inflammatory bowel disease and following total gastrectomy; not recommended for use in children	Vital 1.5kcal liquid vanilla: 1000 ml = £16.20; 200 ml = £3.17

Enteral feeds: Less than 1.5 kcal/mL and 5 g (or more) protein/100 mL

Not suitable for use in child under 1 year unless otherwise stated; not recommended for child 1-6 years

Product	Formulation	Energy	Protein	Carbohydrate	Fat	Fibre	Special Characteristics	ACBS Indications	Presentation & Flavour
Fresubin® 1000 Complete (Fresenius Kabi Ltd)	Liquid (tube feed) per 100 mL	420 kJ (100 kcal)	5.5 g cows' milk	12.5 g (sugars 1.1 g)	3.1 g	2 g	Gluten-free Residual lactose Contains fish oil	Borderline substances standard ACBS Indications p. 1500	Fresubin 1000 Complete liquid: 1 litre = £11.30
Fresubin® 1200 Complete (Fresenius Kabi Ltd)	Liquid (tube feed) per 100 mL	500 kJ (120 kcal)	6 g cows' milk	15 g (sugars 1.22 g)	4.1 g	2 g	Gluten-free Residual lactose Contains fish oil	Borderline substances standard ACBS Indications p. 1500	Fresubin 1200 Complete liquid: 1 litre = £14.38
Fresubin® 1800 Complete (Fresenius Kabi Ltd)	Liquid (tube feed) per 100 mL	500 kJ (120 kcal)	6 g cows' milk	15 g (sugars 1.22 g)	4.1 g	2 g	Gluten-free Residual lactose Contains fish oil	Borderline substances standard ACBS Indications p. 1500	Fresubin 1800 Complete liquid: 1.5 litre = £14.38
Jevity® Plus (Abbott Laboratories Ltd)	Liquid (tube feed) per 100 mL	514 kJ (122 kcal)	5.5 g caseinates soy isolates	15.1 g (sugars 890 mg)	3.93 g	2.2 g	Gluten-free Residual lactose	Borderline substances standard ACBS Indications p. 1500 Not suitable for child under 2 years; not recommended for child 2-10 years	Jevity Plus liquid: 1500 ml = £18.34; 1000 ml = £12.27; 500 ml = £6.74
Jevity® Plus HP (Abbott Laboratories Ltd)	Liquid (tube feed) per 100 mL	551 kJ (131 kcal)	8.13 g cows' milk soy isolates	14.2 g (sugars 950 mg)	4.33 g	1.5 g	Gluten-free Residual lactose	Borderline substances standard ACBS Indications p. 1500; also CAPD, haemodialysis Not suitable for child under 2 years; not recommended for child 2-10 years	Jevity Plus HP gluten free liquid: 500 ml = £6.60
Jevity® Promote (Abbott Laboratories Ltd)	Liquid (tube feed) per 100 mL	434 kJ (103 kcal)	5.55 g caseinates soy isolates	12 g (sugars 670 mg)	3.32 g	1.7 g	Gluten-free Residual lactose	Borderline substances standard ACBS Indications p. 1500 Not suitable for child under 2 years; not recommended for child 2-10 years	Jevity Promote liquid: 1 litre = £11.74
Nutrison® 800 Complete Multi Fibre (Nutricia Ltd)	Liquid (tube feed) per 100 mL	345 kJ (83 kcal)	5.5 g cows' milk pea protein soya protein	8.8 g (sugars 600 mg)	2.5 g	1.5 g	Gluten-free Residual lactose Contains fish oil	Borderline substances standard ACBS Indications p. 1500 except bowel fistula Not suitable for child under 6 years; not recommended for child 6-12 years	Nutrison 800 Complete Multi Fibre liquid: 1 litre = £11.05
Nutrison® 1000 Complete Multi Fibre (Nutricia Ltd)	Liquid (tube feed) per 100 mL	420 kJ (100 kcal)	5.5 g cows' milk	11.3 g (sugars 700 mg)	3.7 g	2 g	Gluten-free Residual lactose	Disease related malnutrition in patients with low energy and/or low fluid requirements	Nutrison 1000 Complete Multi Fibre liquid: 1 litre = £11.72

Borderline substances | **Appendix 2**

A2

Enteral feeds: Less than 1.5 kcal/mL and 5 g (or more) protein/100 mL (product list continued)

Not suitable for use in child under 1 year unless otherwise stated; not recommended for child 1-6 years

Product	Formulation	Energy	Protein	Carbohydrate	Fat	Fibre	Special Characteristics	ACBS Indications	Presentation & Flavour
Nutrison® 1200 Complete Multi Fibre (Nutricia Ltd)	Liquid (tube feed) per 100 mL	505 kJ (120 kcal)	5.5 g cows' milk	15 g (sugars 1.2 g)	4.3 g	2 g	Gluten-free Residual lactose	Borderline substances standard ACBS indications p. 1500 except bowel fistula	Nutrison 1200 Complete Multi Fibre liquid: 1500 ml = £18.62; 1000 ml = £12.40
Nutrison® MCT (Nutricia Ltd)	Liquid (tube feed) per 100 mL	420 kJ (100 kcal)	5 g cows' milk	12.6 g (sugars 1 g)	3.3 g (MCT 61%)	Nil	Gluten-free Residual lactose	Borderline substances standard ACBS indications p. 1500	Nutrison MCT liquid: 1000 ml = £10.56
Nutrison® Protein Plus (Nutricia Ltd)	Liquid (tube feed) per 100 mL	525 kJ (125 kcal)	6.3 g cows' milk	14.2 g (sugars 1.1 g)	4.9 g	Nil	Gluten-free Residual lactose	Borderline substances standard ACBS indications p. 1500	Nutrison Protein Plus liquid: 1 litre = £10.84
Nutrison® Protein Plus Multi Fibre (Nutricia Ltd)	Liquid (tube feed) per 100 mL	535 kJ (128 kcal)	6.3 g cow's milk	14.1 g (sugars 1.0 g)	4.9 g	1.5 g	Gluten-free Residual lactose	Disease related malnutrition	Nutrison Protein Plus Multifibre liquid: 1 litre = £12.08
Osmolite® Plus (Abbott Laboratories Ltd)	Liquid (tube feed) per 100 mL	508 kJ (121 kcal)	5.55 g caseinates	15.8 g (sugars 730 mg)	3.93 g	Nil	Gluten-free Residual lactose	Borderline substances standard ACBS indications p. 1500 Not suitable for child under 10 years	Osmolite Plus liquid: 1000 ml = £10.29; 500 ml = £5.66; 1500 ml = £15.39
Peptamen® HN (Nestle Health Science)	Liquid (tube feed) per 100 mL	556 kJ (133 kcal)	6.6 g whey protein hydrolysates	15.6 g (sugars 1.4 g)	4.9 g (MCT 70%)	Nil	Gluten-free Residual lactose Hydrolysed with pork trypsin	Short bowel syndrome, intractable malabsorption, proven inflammatory bowel disease, bowel fistula Not suitable for child under 3 years	Peptamen HN liquid: 500 ml = £7.60
Perative® (Abbott Laboratories Ltd)	Liquid (sip or tube feed) per 100 mL	552 kJ (131 kcal)	6.7 g caseinate whey protein hydrolysates	17.7 g (sugars 660 mg)	3.7 g (MCT 42%)	Nil	Gluten-free Residual lactose	Borderline substances standard ACBS indications p. 1500 Not suitable for child under 5 years	Perative liquid: 1000 ml = £14.77; 500 ml = £8.00

Enteral feeds: More than 1.5 kcal/mL and 5 g (or more) protein/100 mL

Not suitable for use in child under 1 year unless otherwise stated; not recommended for child 1-6 years

Product	Formulation	Energy	Protein	Carbohydrate	Fat	Fibre	Special Characteristics	ACBS Indications	Presentation & Flavour
Ensure® TwoCal (Abbott Laboratories Ltd)	Liquid (sip or tube feed) per 100 mL	838 kJ (200 kcal)	8.4 g cows' milk	21 g (sugars 4.5 g)	8.9 g	1 g	Gluten-free Residual lactose	Borderline substances standard ACBS indications p. 1500; also haemodialysis and CAPD	Ensure TwoCal liquid: banana, neutral, strawberry, vanilla 200 ml = £2.22
TwoCal® (Abbott Laboratories Ltd)	Liquid (tube feed) per 100 mL	837 kJ (200 kcal)	8.4 g cows' milk caseinates	21 g (sugars 4.5 g)	8.9 g	1 g	Gluten-free Residual lactose	Adults with or at risk of disease-related malnutrition, catabolic or fluid-restricted patients, and other patients requiring a 2 kcal/mL feed	TwoCal liquid: 1 litre = £16.58; 200 ml = £3.19

Enteral feeds (non-disease specific): Child under 12 years see *BNF for Children*

Table 2 Nutritional supplements (non-disease specific)

Nutritional supplements: less than 5 g protein/100 mL

Nutritional supplements: 1 kcal/mL and less than 5 g protein/100 mL
Not suitable for use in child under 1 year; use with caution in child 1-5 years unless stated otherwise

Product	Formulation	Energy	Protein	Carbohydrate	Fat	Fibre	Special Characteristics	ACBS Indications	Presentation & Flavour
Ensure® (Abbott Laboratories Ltd)	Liquid (sip or tube feed) per 100 mL	423 kJ (100 kcal)	4 g caseinates soy isolate	13.6 g (sugars 3.93 g)	3.36 g	Nil	Gluten-free Residual lactose	Borderline substances standard ACBS indications p. 1500	Ensure liquid: vanilla, chocolate, coffee 250 ml = £2.31

Nutritional supplements: More than 1 kcal/mL and less than 5 g protein/100 mL
Not suitable for use in child under 1 year unless stated otherwise; use with caution in child 1-5 years

Product	Formulation	Energy	Protein	Carbohydrate	Fat	Fibre	Special Characteristics	ACBS Indications	Presentation & Flavour
AYMES® Shake (Aymes International Ltd)	Standard dilution of powder (57 g in 200 mL water) (sip feed) per 100 mL	530.5 kJ (126 kcal)	4.5 g cows' milk	17.5 g (sugars 8.4 g)	4.2 g	Nil	Gluten-free Contains lactose	Borderline substances standard ACBS indications p. 1500. Use with caution in child 1-6 years.	Aymes Shake Sample Pack powder: 285 gram = £4.78; Aymes Shake powder: chocolate, vanilla 399 gram = £4.20; banana, neutral, strawberry 399 gram = £4.20

Powder 57 g reconstituted with 200 mL whole milk provides: protein 15.8 g, carbohydrate 44.1 g, fat 16.4 g, energy 1625 kJ (388 kcal).

Product	Formulation	Energy	Protein	Carbohydrate	Fat	Fibre	Special Characteristics	ACBS Indications	Presentation & Flavour
Ensure® Plus Juce (Abbott Laboratories Ltd)	Liquid (sip feed) per 100 mL	638 kJ (150 kcal)	4.8 g whey protein isolate	32.7 g (sugars 9.4 g)	Nil	Nil	Gluten-free Residual lactose Non-milk taste	Borderline substances standard ACBS indications p. 1500	Ensure Plus Juce liquid: assorted 880 ml = no price available; apple, fruit punch, lemon & lime, orange, peach, strawberry 220 ml = £1.97
Fortijuce® (Nutricia Ltd)	Liquid (sip feed) per 100 mL	640 kJ (150 kcal)	4.0 g cows' milk	33.5 g (sugars 13.1 g)	Nil	Nil	Gluten-free Residual lactose Non-milk taste	Borderline substances standard ACBS indications p. 1500 Not suitable for child under 3 years	Fortijuce Starter Pack liquid: 800 ml = £8.08; Fortijuce liquid: apple, blackcurrant, lemon, orange, strawberry, tropical 200 ml = £2.02; forest fruits 200 ml = £2.02
Fresubin® Jucy Drink (Fresenius Kabi Ltd)	Liquid (sip feed) per 100 mL	630 kJ (150 kcal)	4 g whey protein	33.5 g (sugars 8 g)	Nil	Nil	Gluten-free Residual lactose	Borderline substances standard ACBS indications p. 1500; also CAPD, haemodialysis	Fresubin Jucy drink: blackcurrant, cherry, pineapple 800 ml = £8.04; orange 800 ml = £8.04; apple 800 ml = £8.04

Nutritional supplements: 1.5 kcal/mL and 5 g (or more) protein/100 mL

Nutritional supplements: 1.5 kcal/mL and 5 g (or more) protein/100 mL
Not suitable for use in child under 1 year; use with caution in child 1-5 years unless otherwise stated.

Product	Formulation	Energy	Protein	Carbohydrate	Fat	Fibre	Special Characteristics	ACBS Indications	Presentation & Flavour
Altraplen® Protein (Nualtra Ltd)	Liquid (sip feed) per 100 mL	632 kJ (150 kcal)	10 g cows' milk soya protein	15 g (sugars 4.6 g)	5.6 g	Nil	Gluten-free Residual lactose	Borderline substances standard ACBS indications p. 1500 Not suitable for child under 3 years; use with caution in child 3-6 years	Altraplen Protein liquid: strawberry 800 ml = £6.36; vanilla 800 ml = £6.36

A2

Borderline substances | **Appendix 2**

Borderline substances | **Appendix 2**

Nutritional supplements: 1.5 kcal/mL and 5 g (or more) protein/100 mL (product list continued)

Not suitable for use in child under 1 year; use with caution in child 1-5 years unless stated otherwise.

Product	Formulation	Energy	Protein	Carbohydrate	Fat	Fibre	Special Characteristics	ACBS Indications	Presentation & Flavour
Ensure® Plus Advance (Abbott Laboratories Ltd)	Liquid (sip or tube feed) per 100 mL	631 kJ (150 kcal)	9.1 g cows' milk soya protein isolate whey protein concentrate	16.8 g (sugars 6.8 g)	4.8 g	0.75 g	Gluten-free Residual lactose	Frail elderly people (this is defined as older than 65 years with BMI less than or equal to 23 kg/m² where clinical assessment and nutritional screening show the individual to be at risk of undernutrition). Not suitable as the sole source of nutrition.	Ensure Plus Advance liquid: banana, chocolate, coffee, strawberry, vanilla 200 ml = £2.08
Ensure® Plus Commence (Abbott Laboratories Ltd)	Starter pack (5-10 day's supply), contains *Ensure® Plus Commence* (various flavours), 1 pack (10 × 200ml) = £11.10								
Ensure® Plus Fibre (Abbott Laboratories Ltd)	Liquid (sip or tube feed) per 100 mL	652 kJ (155 kcal)	6.25 g cows' milk soya protein isolate	20.2 g (sugars 5.5 g)	4.92 g	2.5 g	Gluten-free Residual lactose	Borderline substances standard ACBS indications p. 1500; also CAPD, haemodialysis.	Ensure Plus Fibre liquid: banana, chocolate, raspberry, strawberry, vanilla 200 ml = £2.07
Ensure® Plus Milkshake style (Abbott Laboratories Ltd)	Liquid (sip or tube feed) per 100 mL	632 kJ (150 kcal)	6.25 g cows' milk soya protein isolate	20.2 g (sugars 6.89 g)	4.92 g	Nil	Gluten-free Residual lactose	Borderline substances standard ACBS indications p. 1500; also CAPD, haemodialysis	Ensure Plus milkshake style liquid: banana, chocolate, coffee, fruits of the forest, neutral, peach, raspberry, strawberry, vanilla 200 ml = £1.11
Ensure® Plus Savoury (Abbott Laboratories Ltd)	Liquid (sip or tube feed) per 100 mL	632 kJ (150 kcal)	6.25 g cows' milk soy protein isolate	20.2 g (sugars 1.13 g)	4.92 g	Nil	Gluten-free Residual lactose	Borderline substances standard ACBS indications p. 1500; also CAPD, haemodialysis.	Ensure Plus savoury liquid: chicken, 200 ml = £1.11
Ensure® Plus Yoghurt style (Abbott Laboratories Ltd)	Liquid (sip feed) per 100 mL	632 kJ (150 kcal)	6.25 g cows' milk	20.2 g (sugars 11.7 g)	4.92 g	Nil	Gluten-free Residual lactose	Borderline substances standard ACBS indications p. 1500; also CAPD, haemodialysis.	Ensure Plus yoghurt style liquid: orchard peach, strawberry swirl 200 ml = £1.11
Fortisip® Bottle (Nutricia Ltd)	Liquid (sip feed) per 100 mL	630 kJ (150 kcal)	6 g cows' milk	18.4 g	5.8 g	Nil	Gluten-free Residual lactose	Borderline substances standard ACBS indications p. 1500 Not suitable for child under 3 years; use with caution in child 3-5 years.	Fortisip Bottle: banana, caramel, chocolate, neutral, orange, strawberry, tropical fruit, vanilla 200 ml = £1.12
Fortisip® Range (Nutricia Ltd)	Starter pack contains 4 × Fortisip® Bottle, 4 × Fortijuice® 2, 2 × Fortisip® Yoghurt Style, 1 pack (10 × 200ml) = £20.20								
Fortisip® Yoghurt Style (Nutricia Ltd)	Liquid (sip feed) per 100 mL	630 kJ (150 kcal)	6 g cows' milk	18.7 g (sugars 10.8 g)	5.8 g	0.2 g	Gluten-free Contains lactose	Borderline substances standard ACBS indications p. 1500 Not suitable for child under 3 years	Fortisip Yogurt Style liquid: vanilla & lemon, raspberry 200 ml = £2.14
Fresubin® Protein Energy Drink (Fresenius Kabi Ltd)	Liquid (sip feed) per 100 mL	630 kJ (150 kcal)	10 g cows' milk	12.4 g (sugars 6.4 g)	6.7 g	Nil	Gluten-free Residual lactose Contains fish gelatin	Borderline substances standard ACBS indications p. 1500; also CAPD, haemodialysis.	Fresubin Protein Energy drink: cappuccino, chocolate, tropical fruits, vanilla, wild strawberry 200 ml = £2.10

A2

Product	Formulation	Energy	Protein	Carbohydrate	Fat	Fibre	Special Characteristics	ACBS Indications	Presentation & Flavour
Fresubin® Thickened (Fresenius Kabi Ltd)	Liquid (sip feed) per 100 mL	630 kJ (150 kcal)	10 g cows' milk	12.2 g (sugars 7.1 g)	6.7 g	0.48 g	Gluten-free Residual lactose	Dysphagia or disease-related malnutrition. Not suitable for child under 3 years; use with caution in child 3-4 years.	Fresubin Thickened Stage 1 syrup: vanilla, wild strawberry 800 ml = £9.40; Fresubin Thickened Stage 2 custard: vanilla, wild strawberry 800 ml = £9.40
Fresubin® YOcrème (Fresenius Kabi Ltd)	Semi-solid per 100 g	630 kJ (150 kcal)	7.5 g whey protein	19.5 g (sugars 16.8 g)	4.7 g	Nil	Gluten-free Contains lactose	Dysphagia, or presence or risk of malnutrition Not suitable for child under 3 years	Fresubin YOcreme dessert: apricot-peach, biscuit, lemon, raspberry 500 gram = £8.16

Nutritional supplements: Less than 1.5 kcal/mL and 5 g (or more) protein/100 mL

Not suitable for use in child under 1 year; use with caution in child 1-5 years unless otherwise stated.

Product	Formulation	Energy	Protein	Carbohydrate	Fat	Fibre	Special Characteristics	ACBS Indications	Presentation & Flavour
Ensure® Plus Crème (Abbott Laboratories Ltd)	Semi-solid per 100 g	574 kJ (137 kcal)	5.68 g cow's milk soy protein isolates	18.4 g (sugars 12.4 g)	4.47 g	Nil	Gluten-free Residual lactose Contains soya	Borderline substances standard ACBS Indications p. 1500; also CAPD, haemodialysis. Not suitable for child under 3 years; use with caution in child 3-5 years.	Ensure Plus Creme: banana, chocolate, neutral, vanilla 500 gram = £7.72
Nutilis® Fruit Stage 3 (Nutricia Ltd)	Semi-Solid per 100 g	560 kJ (133 kcal)	7 g whey isolate	16.7 g (sugars 11.3 g)	4 g	2.6 g	Gluten-free Residual lactose	Borderline substances standard ACBS Indications p. 1500 except bowel fistula; also CAPD, haemodialysis. Not suitable for child under 3 years; use with caution in child 3-5 years.	Nutilis Fruit Stage 3: apple, strawberry 450 gram = £7.35
Oral Impact® (Nestle Health Science)	Standard dilution of powder (74 g in 250 mL water) (sip feed) per 100 mL	425 kJ (101 kcal)	5.6 g cows' milk	13.4 g (sugars 7.4 g)	2.8 g	1 g	Residual lactose Contains fish oil	Pre-operative nutritional supplement for malnourished patients or patients at risk of malnourishment Not suitable for child under 3 years; use with caution in child 3-5 years.	Oral Impact oral powder 74g sachets: citrus, tropical 5 sachet = £17.62

Powder provides: protein 16.8 g, carbohydrate 40.2 g, fat 8.3 g, fibre 3 g, energy 1276 kJ (303 kcal)/74 g.

Nutritional supplements: More than 1.5 kcal/mL and 5 g (or more) protein/100 mL

Not suitable for use in child under 1 year; use with caution in child 1-5 years unless otherwise stated.

Product	Formulation	Energy	Protein	Carbohydrate	Fat	Fibre	Special Characteristics	ACBS Indications	Presentation & Flavour
Altraplen® Compact (Nualtra Ltd)	Liquid (sip feed) per 100 mL	1008 kJ (240 kcal)	9.6 g cows' milk soya protein	28.8 g (sugars 11.6 g)	9.6 g	Nil	Gluten-free Residual lactose	Borderline substances standard ACBS Indications p. 1500 Not suitable for child under 3 years; use with caution in child 3-6 years.	Altraplen Compact liquid: vanilla 500 ml = £5.32; strawberry 500 ml = £5.32
Complan® Shake (Nutricia Ltd)	Powder per 57 g	1057 kJ (251 kcal)	8.8 g cows' milk	35.2 g (sugars 22.7 g)	8.4 g	Trace	Gluten-free Contains lactose	Borderline substances standard ACBS Indications p. 1500	Complan Shake Starter Pack sachets: 5 sachet = £4.39; Complan Shake oral powder 57 g sachets: strawberry, vanilla 4 sachet = £2.80; banana, chocolate, milk 4 sachet = £2.80

Powder 57 g reconstituted with 200 mL whole milk provides: protein 15.6 g, carbohydrate 44.5 g, fat 16.4 g, energy 1621 kJ (387 kcal).

A2

Borderline substances | **Appendix 2**

A2

Nutritional supplements: More than 1.5 kcal/mL and 5 g (or more) protein/100 mL (product list continued)

Not suitable for use in child under 1 year; use with caution in child 1–5 years unless otherwise stated.

Product	Formulation	Energy	Protein	Carbohydrate	Fat	Fibre	Special Characteristics	ACBS Indications	Presentation & Flavour
Ensure® Compact (Abbott Laboratories Ltd)	Liquid (sip or tube feed) per 100 mL	1008 kJ (240 kcal)	10.2 g cows' milk	28.8 g (sugars 6.2 g)	9.35 g	Nil	Gluten-free Residual lactose	As a sole source of nutrition or as a nutritional supplement for the dietary management of patient with, or at risk of developing disease-related malnutrition.	Ensure Compact liquid: banana, strawberry, vanilla 4 × 125 ml = £5.40
Ensure® Shake (Abbott Laboratories Ltd)	Powder per 100 g	1852 kJ (443 kcal)	17.8 g cows' milk whey protein concentrate	59 g (sugars 33.7 g)	15.1 g	Nil	Gluten-free Residual lactose	Borderline substances standard ACBS indications p. 1500	Ensure Shake oral powder 57 g sachets: banana, chocolate, strawberry, vanilla 7 sachet = £4.20
Powder 57 g reconstituted with 200 mL whole milk provides: protein 17 g, carbohydrate 43.2 g, fat 16.6 g, energy 1626 kJ (389 kcal)									
Foodlink® Complete (Nualtra Ltd)	Powder per 100 g	1842 kJ (437 kcal)	20.3 g cows' milk soya protein	58.7 g (sugars 42.7 g)	13.5 g	Nil	Contains lactose Gluten-free	Borderline substances standard ACBS indications p. 1500	Foodlink Complete powder: banana, chocolate, natural, strawberry, vanilla 399 gram = £4.20
Recommended serving = the contents of a 57-g sachet in 200 mL full cream milk provides: protein 18.4 g, carbohydrate 43 g, fat 15.7 g, energy 1614 kJ (385kcal).									
Foodlink® Complete with Fibre (Nualtra Ltd)	Powder per 100 g	1899 kJ (452 kcal)	20.3 g cows' milk soya protein	58.6 g (sugars 42.6 g)	13.5 g	7.2 g	Contains lactose Gluten-free	Borderline substances standard ACBS indications p. 1500	Foodlink Complete powder with fibre: vanilla 441 gram = £4.97
Recommended serving = the contents of a 63-g sachet in 200 mL full cream milk provides: protein 19.6 g, carbohydrate 46.4 g, fat 16.5 g, fibre 4.5 g, energy 1760 kJ (421 kcal).									
Forticreme® Complete (Nutricia Ltd)	Semi-solid per 100 g	675 kJ (160 kcal)	9.5 g cows' milk	19.2 g (sugars 10.6 g)	5 g	0.1 g	Gluten-free Residual lactose	Borderline substances p. 1500; also CAPD, haemodialysis. Not suitable for child under 3 years; use with caution in child 3–5 years.	Forticreme Complete dessert: banana, chocolate, forest fruits, vanilla 500 gram = £7.84
Fortisip® Compact (Nutricia Ltd)	Liquid (sip feed) per 100 mL	1010 kJ (240 kcal)	9.6 g cows' milk	29.7 g (sugars 15 g)	9.3 g	Nil	Residual lactose	Borderline substances standard ACBS indications p. 1500 Not suitable for child under 3 years; use with caution in child 3–5 years.	Fortisip Compact liquid: apricot, mocha 500 ml = £5.80; chocolate 500 ml = £5.80; banana, forest fruit, strawberry, vanilla 500 ml = £5.80
Fortisip® Compact Fibre (Nutricia Ltd)	Liquid (sip feed) per 100 mL	1000 kJ (240 kcal)	9.4 g cows' milk	25.2 g (sugars 13.9 g)	10.4 g	3.6 g	Gluten-free Residual lactose	Borderline substances standard ACBS indications p. 1500 Not suitable for child under 3 years; use with caution in child 3–5 years.	Fortisip Compact Fibre Starter Pack liquid: 500 ml = £8.36; Fortisip Compact Fibre liquid: mocha, strawberry, vanilla 500 ml = £8.36
Fortisip® Compact Protein (Nutricia Ltd)	Liquid (sip feed) per 100 mL	1010 kJ (240 kcal)	14.4 g cows' milk	24.4 g (sugars 13.3 g)	9.4 g	Nil	Gluten-free Residual lactose	Borderline substances standard ACBS indications p. 1500 Not suitable for child under 3 years; use with caution in child 3–5 years.	Fortisip Compact Protein Starter Pack liquid: 750 ml = £12.00; Fortisip Compact Protein liquid: banana, mocha, strawberry, vanilla 500 ml = £8.00
Fortisip® Extra (Nutricia Ltd)	Liquid (sip feed) per 100 mL	675 kJ (160 kcal)	10 g cows' milk	18.1 g (sugars 9 g)	5.3 g	Nil	Gluten-free Contains lactose	Borderline substances standard ACBS indications p. 1500 Not suitable for child under 3 years; use with caution in child 3–5 years.	Fortisip Extra liquid: strawberry, vanilla 200 ml = £2.30

Product	Formulation	Energy	Protein	Carbohydrate	Fat	Fibre		Notes	Flavours/price
Fresubin® 2 kcal Drink (Fresenius Kabi Ltd)	Liquid (sip feed) per 100 mL	840 kJ (200 kcal)	10 g cows' milk	22.5 g (sugars 5.8 g)	7.8 g	Nil	Gluten-free Residual lactose	Borderline substances standard ACBS indications p. 1500; also CAPD, haemodialysis. Not suitable for use in child under 1 year; use with caution in child 1–5 years.	Fresubin 2kcal drink: apricot-peach, cappuccino, fruits of the forest, neutral, toffee, vanilla 200 ml = £2.10
Fresubin® 2 kcal Fibre Drink (Fresenius Kabi Ltd)	Liquid (sip feed) per 100 mL	840 kJ (200 kcal)	10 g cows' milk	22.5 g (sugars 5.8 g)	7.8 g	1.6 g	Gluten-free Residual lactose	Borderline substances standard ACBS indications p. 1500; also CAPD, haemodialysis. Not suitable for use in child under 1 year; use with caution in child 1–5 years.	Fresubin 2kcal Fibre drink: apricot-peach, cappuccino, chocolate, lemon, neutral 200 ml = £2.10
Fresubin® Powder Extra (Fresenius Kabi Ltd)	Powder per 100 g	1764 kJ (420 kcal)	17.5 g cows' milk whey protein	63 g (sugars 24.7 g)	10.9 g	Nil	Gluten-free Contains lactose	Borderline substances standard ACBS indications p. 1500 Not suitable for child under 1 year; use with caution in child 1–5 years.	Fresubin Powder Extra oral powder 62g sachets: neutral, strawberry 7 sachet = £4.90; chocolate, vanilla 7 sachet = £4.90

Powder 62 g reconstituted with 200 ml whole milk provides: protein 17.7 g, carbohydrate 48.5 g, fat 14.8 g, energy 1658 kJ (397 kcal).

Product	Formulation	Energy	Protein	Carbohydrate	Fat	Fibre		Notes	Flavours/price
Nutilis® Complete Stage 1 (Nutricia Ltd)	Liquid (pre-thickened) per 100 mL	1010 kJ (240 kcal)	9.6 g cows' milk	29.1 g (sugars 5.4 g)	9.3 g	3.2 g	Residual lactose	Borderline substances standard ACBS indications p. 1500 Not suitable for child under 3 years; use with caution in child 3–5 years.	Nutilis Complete Stage 1 liquid: strawberry, vanilla 500 ml = £8.84
Nutilis® Complete Stage 2 (Nutricia Ltd)	Semi-solid per 100 g	1030 kJ (245 kcal)	9.6 g cows' milk	29.1 g (sugars 11.8 g)	9.4 g	3.2 g	Gluten-free Residual lactose	Borderline substances standard ACBS indications p. 1500 Not suitable for child under 3 years; use with caution in child 3–6 years.	Nutilis Complete Stage 2 custard: chocolate, strawberry, vanilla 500 gram = £8.84
Nutricrem® (Nualtra Ltd)	Semi-solid per 100 g	756 kJ (180 kcal)	10 g cows' milk soya protein	18.8 g (sugars 9.7 g)	7.2 g	Nil	Gluten-free Residual lactose	Borderline substances standard ACBS indications p. 1500 Not suitable for child under 3 years; use with caution in child 3–6 years.	Nutricrem dessert: strawberry, vanilla 500 gram = £6.36
Renilon® 7.5 (Nutricia Ltd)	Liquid (sip feed) per 100 mL	840 kJ (200 kcal)	7.5 g cows' milk	20 g (sugars 4.8 g)	10 g	Nil	Gluten-free Residual lactose	Borderline substances standard ACBS indications p. 1500 Not suitable for child under 3 years; use with caution in child 3–5 years.	Renilon 7.5 liquid: apricot, caramel 500 ml = £9.12
Resource® 2.0 Fibre (Nestlé Health Science)	Liquid (sip feed) per 100 mL	836 kJ (200 kcal)	9 g cows' milk	21.4 g (sugars 5.5 g)	8.7 g	2.5 g	Gluten-free Residual lactose	Borderline substances standard ACBS indications p. 1500 Not suitable for child under 6 years; use with caution in child 6–10 years.	Resource Fibre 2.0 liquid: apricot, coffee, neutral, strawberry, summer fruit, vanilla 200 ml = £1.95

Borderline substances | **Appendix 2**

A2

Table 3 Specialised formulas

Specialised formulas: Infant and child see *BNF for Children*

Specialised formulas for specific clinical conditions

Product	Formulation	Energy	Protein	Carbohydrate	Fat	Fibre	Special Characteristics	ACBS Indications	Presentation & Flavour
Alicalm® (Nutricia Ltd)	Standard dilution (30%) of powder per 100 mL	567 kJ (135 kcal)	4.5 g caseinate whey	17.4 g (sugars 3.2 g)	5.3 g	Nil	Residual lactose	Crohn's disease Not suitable for child under 1 year; use as nutritional supplement only in children 1–6 years.	Alicalm oral powder: 400 gram = £22.53

Powder provides: protein 15 g, carbohydrate 58 g, fat 17.5 g, energy 1889 kJ (450 kcal)/100 g.

Product	Formulation	Energy	Protein	Carbohydrate	Fat	Fibre	Special Characteristics	ACBS Indications	Presentation & Flavour
Forticare® (Nutricia Ltd)	Liquid (sip feed) per 100 mL.	675 kJ (160 kcal)	9 g cows' milk	19.1 g (sugars 13.6 g)	5.3 g	2.1 g	Gluten-free Residual lactose Contains fish oil	Nutritional supplement in patients with lung cancer undergoing chemotherapy, or with pancreatic cancer Not suitable in child under 3 years	Forticare liquid: cappuccino, orange & lemon, peach & ginger 500 ml = £9.40
Heparon® Junior (Nutricia Ltd)	Standard dilution (18%) of powder per 100 mL	363 kJ (86 kcal)	2 g cows' milk	11.6 g (sugars 2.9 g)	3.6 g	Nil	Contains lactose Electrolytes/100 mL: Na⁺ 0.56 mmol K⁺ 1.9 mmol Ca²⁺ 2.3 mmol P⁺ 1.6 mmol	Enteral feed or nutritional supplement for children with acute or chronic liver failure	Heparon Junior powder: 400 gram = £22.70

Powder provides: protein 11.1 g, carbohydrate 64.2 g, fat 19.9 g, energy 2016 kJ (480 kcal)/100 g.

Product	Formulation	Energy	Protein	Carbohydrate	Fat	Fibre	Special Characteristics	ACBS Indications	Presentation & Flavour
KetoCal® (Nutricia Ltd)	Standard dilution (20 %) of powder per 100 mL	602 kJ (146 kcal)	3.1 g cows' milk with additional amino acids	600 mg (sugars 120 mg)	14.6 g (LCT 100 %)	Nil	Electrolytes/100 mL: Na⁺ 4.3 mmol K⁺ 4.1 mmol Ca²⁺ 2.15 mmol P⁺ 2.77 mmol	Enteral feed or nutritional supplement as part of ketogenic diet in management of epilepsy resistant to drug therapy, in children over 1 year, only on the advice of secondary care physician with experience of ketogenic diet.	KetoCal 4:1 powder: unflavoured, vanilla 300 gram = £31.96

Powder provides: protein 15.25 g, carbohydrate 3 g, fat 73 g, energy 3011 kJ (730 kcal)/100 g.

Product	Formulation	Energy	Protein	Carbohydrate	Fat	Fibre	Special Characteristics	ACBS Indications	Presentation & Flavour
KetoCal® 3:1 (Nutricia Ltd)	Standard dilution (9.5%) of powder per 100 mL	276 kJ (66 kcal)	1.5 g	680 mg (sugars 570 mg)	6.4 g	Nil	Electrolytes/100 mL: Na⁺ 1.3 mmol K⁺ 2.4 mmol Ca²⁺ 2 mmol P⁺ 1.7 mmol	Enteral feed or nutritional supplement as part of ketogenic diet in management of drug resistant epilepsy or other conditions for which a ketogenic diet is indicated in children from birth to 6 years; as a nutritional supplement in children over 6 years.	KetoCal 3:1 powder: 300 gram = £30.93

Powder provides: protein 15.3 g, carbohydrate 7.2 g, fat 67.7 g, energy 2927 kJ (699 kcal)/100 g.

Product	Formulation	Energy	Protein	Carbohydrate	Fat	Fibre	Special Characteristics	ACBS Indications	Presentation & Flavour
KetoCal® 4:1 LQ (Nutricia Ltd)	Liquid (sip or tube feed) per 100 mL	620 kJ (150 kcal)	3.09 g casein and whey with additional amino acids	610 mg (sugars 230 mg)	14.8 g (LCT 100 %)	1.12 g	Residual lactose Electrolytes/100 mL: Na⁺ 4.9 mmol K⁺ 4.7 mmol Ca²⁺ 2.4 mmol P⁺ 3.1 mmol	Enteral feed or nutritional supplement as part of ketogenic diet in management of drug resistant epilepsy or other conditions for which a ketogenic diet is indicated in children 1–10 years; as a nutritional supplement in children over 10 years.	KetoCal 4:1 LQ liquid: unflavoured, vanilla 200 ml = £4.56

Product	Form/dilution	Energy	Protein	Carbohydrate	Fat		Characteristics / Electrolytes	Indication	Price
Kindergen® (Nutricia Ltd)	Standard dilution (20 %) of powder per 100 mL	421 kJ (101 kcal)	1.5 g whey protein	11.8 g (sugars 1.2 g)	5.3 g (LCT 93%)	Nil	Electrolytes/100 mL: Na⁺ 2 mmol, K⁺ 0.6 mmol, Ca²⁺ 2.8 mmol, P 3 mmol, Low Vitamin A	Enteral feed or nutritional supplement for children with chronic renal failure receiving peritoneal rapid overnight dialysis.	Kindergen powder: 400 gram = £30.47

Powder provides: protein 7.5 g, carbohydrate 59 g, fat 26.3 g, energy 2104 kJ (504 kcal)/100 g.

| Modulen IBD® (Nestle Health Science) | Standard dilution (20%) of powder (sip or tube feed) per 100 mL | 420 kJ (100 kcal) | 3.6 g casein | 11 g (sugars 3.98 g) | 4.7 g | Nil | Gluten-free, Residual lactose | Crohn's disease active phase, and in remission if malnourished | Modulen IBD powder: 400 gram = £15.59 |

Powder provides: protein 18 g, carbohydrate 54 g, fat 23 g, energy 2070 kJ (500 kcal)/100 g.

| ProSure® (Abbott Laboratories Ltd) | Liquid (sip or tube feed) per 100 mL | 536 kJ (127 kcal) | 6.65 g cows' milk | 18.3 g (sugars 2.95 g) | 2.56 g | 2.07 g | Gluten-free, Residual lactose, Contains fish oil | Nutritional supplement for patients with pancreatic cancer. Not suitable for child under 1 year; use with caution in child 1-4 years. | ProSure liquid: 220 ml = £3.47 |

| Renamil® (Stanningley Pharma Ltd) | Powder (sip or tube feed when reconstituted) per 100 g | 2003 kJ (477 kcal) | 4.6 g cows' milk | 70.8 g | 19.3 g | Nil | Contains lactose, Gluten-free, Electrolytes/100 g: Na⁺ 1.04 mmol, K⁺ 0.13 mmol, Ca²⁺ 10.22 mmol, P 1.06 mmol, Contains no vitamin A or vitamin D | Enteral feed or nutritional supplement for adults and children over 1 year with chronic renal failure. | Renamil powder: 1000 gram = £25.40 |

| Renapro® (Stanningley Pharma Ltd) | Powder per 100 g | 1580 kJ (372 kcal) | 90 g whey protein | 800 mg | 1 g | Nil | Gluten-free, Residual lactose, Electrolytes/100 g: Na⁺ 23 mmol, K⁺ 2 mmol, P 4.84 mmol | Nutritional supplement for biochemically proven hypoproteinaemia and patients undergoing dialysis. Not suitable for child under 1 year. | Renapro powder: 600 gram = £69.60 |

Powder provides: protein 18 g, energy 316 kJ (74 kcal)/20-g sachet.

| Renastart® (Vitaflo International Ltd) | Standard dilution (20%) of powder per 100 mL | 414 kJ (99 kcal) | 1.5 g cows' milk soya | 12.5 g (sugars 1.3 g) | 4.8 g | Nil | Contains lactose, Electrolytes/100 mL: Na⁺ 2.1 mmol, K⁺ 0.6 mmol, Ca²⁺ 0.6 mmol, P 0.6 mmol | Dietary management of renal failure in child from birth to 10 years. | Renastart powder: 400 gram = £27.92 |

Powder provides: protein 7.5 g, carbohydrate 62.5 g, fat 23.8 g, energy 2071 kJ (494 kcal)/100 g.

Borderline substances | **Appendix 2**

A2

Specialised formulas for specific clinical conditions (product list continued)

Product	Formulation	Energy	Protein	Carbohydrate	Fat	Fibre	Special Characteristics	ACBS Indications	Presentation & Flavour
Respifor® (Nutricia Ltd)	Liquid (sip feed) per 100 mL	633 kJ (150 kcal)	7.5 g cows' milk	22.5 g (sugars 6.4 g)	3.3 g	Nil	Contains lactose	Nutritional supplement for dietary management of disease-related malnutrition in patients with chronic obstructive pulmonary disease and body-mass index less than 20.	Respifor milkshake style liquid: chocolate, strawberry, vanilla 500 ml = £8.96
Supportan® (Fresenius Kabi Ltd)	Liquid (sip feed) per 100 mL	630 kJ (150 kcal)	10 g cows' milk	12.4 g (sugars 7.5 g)	6.7 g	1.5 g	Gluten-free Residual lactose Contains fish oil	Nutritional supplement in patients with pancreatic cancer or with lung cancer undergoing chemotherapy Not suitable for child under 1 year; use with caution in child 1–4 years	Supportan drink: cappuccino, tropical fruits 800 ml = £11.28

Table 4 Feed supplements

High-energy supplements

High-energy supplements: carbohydrate

Flavoured carbohydrate supplements are not suitable for child under 1 year; liquid supplements should be diluted before use in child under 5 years.

Product	Formulation	Energy	Protein	Carbohydrate	Fat	Fibre	Special Characteristics	ACBS Indications	Presentation & Flavour
Maxijul® Super Soluble (Nutricia Ltd)	Powder per 100 g	1615 kJ (380 kcal)	Nil	95 g Glucose polymer (sugars 8.6 g)	Nil	Nil	Gluten-free Lactose-free	Disease-related malnutrition, malabsorption states, or other conditions requiring fortification with a high or readily available carbohydrate supplement.	Maxijul Super Soluble powder: 200 gram = £2.73; 528 gram = £6.80; 25000 gram = £163.10
Polycal® (Nutricia Ltd)	Liquid per 100 mL	1050 kJ (247 kcal)	Nil	61.9 g Maltodextrin (sugars 12.2 g)	Nil	Nil	Gluten-free Lactose-free	Disease-related malnutrition, malabsorption states, or other conditions requiring fortification with a high or readily available carbohydrate supplement. Liquid not suitable for child under 3 years.	Polycal liquid: neutral, orange 200 ml = £1.81
	Powder per 100 g	1630 kJ (384 kcal)	Nil	96 g Maltodextrin (sugars 6 g)	Nil	Nil	Gluten-free Lactose-free	Disease-related malnutrition, malabsorption states, or other conditions requiring fortification with a high or readily available carbohydrate supplement.	Polycal powder: 400 gram = £4.53
S.O.S.® (Vitaflo International Ltd)	Powder per 100 g	1590 kJ (380 kcal)	Nil	95 g (sugars 9 g)	Nil	Nil	S.O.S. products are age-range specific—consult product literature	For use as an emergency regimen in the dietary management of inborn errors of metabolism in adults and children from birth.	S.O.S.: 10 oral powder 21g sachets 30 sachet = £7.74; 15 oral powder 31g sachets 30 sachet = £11.43; 20 oral powder 42g sachets 30 sachet = £15.48; 25 oral powder 52g sachets 30 sachet = £19.15

Contents of each sachet should be reconstituted with water to a total volume of 200ml

Product	Formulation	Energy	Protein	Carbohydrate	Fat	Fibre	Special Characteristics	ACBS Indications	Presentation & Flavour
Vitajoule® (Vitaflo International Ltd)	Powder per 100 g	1590 kJ (380 kcal)	Nil	95 g Dried glucose syrup (sugars 9 g)	Nil	Nil	Gluten-free Lactose-free	Disease-related malnutrition, malabsorption states, or other conditions requiring fortification with a high or readily available carbohydrate supplement.	Vitajoule powder: 500 gram = £4.63

High-energy supplements: fat

Liquid supplements should be diluted before use in child under 5 years

Product	Formulation	Energy	Protein	Carbohydrate	Fat	Fibre	Special Characteristics	ACBS Indications	Presentation & Flavour
Calogen® (Nutricia Ltd)	Liquid (emulsion) per 100 mL	1850 kJ (450 kcal)	Nil	100 mg	50 g (LCT 100 %)	Nil	Gluten-free Lactose-free	Disease-related malnutrition, malabsorption states, or other conditions requiring fortification with a high fat (or fat and carbohydrate) supplement.	Calogen emulsion: banana 500 ml = £11.33; neutral 200 ml = £4.61; 500 ml = £11.33; strawberry 200 ml = £4.61; 500 ml = £11.33
Fresubin® 5 kcal Shot (Fresenius Kabi Ltd)	Liquid (emulsion) per 100 mL	2100 kJ (500 kcal)	Nil	4.0 g (sucrose)	53.8 g	400 mg	Gluten-free Lactose-free	Disease-related malnutrition, malabsorption states, or other conditions requiring fortification with a high fat (or fat and carbohydrate) supplement. Not suitable for child under 3 years.	Fresubin 5kcal shot drink: lemon, neutral 480 ml = £11.84
Liquigen® (Nutricia Ltd)	Liquid (emulsion) per 100 mL	1850 kJ (450 kcal)	Nil	Nil	50 g (MCT 97%) Fractionated coconut oil	Nil	Gluten-free Lactose-free	Steatorrhoea associated with cystic fibrosis of the pancreas, intestinal lymphangiectasia, intestinal surgery, chronic liver disease, liver cirrhosis, other proven malabsorption syndromes, ketogenic diet in epilepsy, and in type 1 lipoproteinaemia Not suitable for child under 1 year	Liquigen emulsion: 250 ml = £9.71
Medium-chain Triglyceride (MCT) Oil (Nutricia Ltd)	Liquid per 100 mL	3515 kJ (855 kcal)	Nil	Nil	MCT 100 %	Nil		Nutritional supplement for steatorrhoea associated with cystic fibrosis of the pancreas, intestinal lymphangiectasia, intestinal surgery, chronic liver disease and liver cirrhosis, other proven malabsorption syndromes, ketogenic diet in management of epilepsy, type 1 hyperlipoproteinaemia	MCT oil: 500 ml = £15.40

A2

Borderline substances | **Appendix 2**

A2

FAT AND CARBOHYDRATE

Product	Formulation	Energy	Protein	Carbohydrate	Fat	Fibre	Special Characteristics	ACBS Indications	Presentation & Flavour
Duocal® Super Soluble (Nutricia Ltd)	Powder **per 100 g**	2061 kJ (492 kcal)	Nil	72.7 g (sugars 6.5 g)	22.3 g (MCT 35%)	Nil	Gluten-free Lactose-free	Disease-related malnutrition, malabsorption states, or other conditions requiring fortification with a high fat (or fat and carbohydrate) supplement.	Duocal Super Soluble powder: 400 gram = £18.96
Energivit® (Nutricia Ltd)	Standard dilution (15%) of powder per 100 mL	309 kJ (74 kcal)	Nil	10 g (sugars 900 mg)	3.75 g	Nil	Lactose-free With vitamins, minerals, and trace elements	For children requiring additional energy, vitamins, minerals, and trace elements following a protein-restricted diet	Energivit powder: 400 gram = £23.06

Powder provides: carbohydrate 66.7 g, fat 25 g, energy 2059 kJ (492 kcal)/100 g.

High-energy supplements: protein

Product	Formulation	Energy	Protein	Carbohydrate	Fat	Fibre	Special Characteristics	ACBS Indications	Presentation & Flavour
ProSource® Jelly (Nutrinovo Ltd)	Semi-solid **per 100 mL**	315 kJ (75 kcal)	16.9 g collagen protein hydrolysate whey protein isolate	Less than 1 g	Nil	Less than 1 g	Gluten-free Lactose-free Contains porcine derivatives	Hypoproteinaemia Not recommended for child under 3 years	ProSource jelly: fruit punch, orange 118 ml = £1.87
Protifar® (Nutricia Ltd)	Powder **per 100 g**	1580 kJ (373 kcal)	88.5 g cows' milk	less than 1.5 g	1.6 g	Nil	Gluten-free Residual lactose Electrolytes/100 mL: Na⁺ 1.3 mmol K⁺ 1.28 mmol Ca²⁺ 33.75 mmol P⁻ 22.58 mmol	Nutritional supplement for use in biochemically proven hypoproteinaemia.	Protifar powder: 225 gram = £9.20

Powder provides: protein 2.2 g per 2.5 g scoopful.

PROTEIN AND CARBOHYDRATE

Product	Formulation	Energy	Protein	Carbohydrate	Fat	Fibre	Special Characteristics	ACBS Indications	Presentation & Flavour
Dialamine® (Nutricia Ltd)	Standard dilution (20%) of powder per 100 mL	264 kJ (62 kcal)	4.3 g protein equivalent (essential and non-essential amino acids)	11.2 g (sugars 10.2 g)	Nil	Nil	Contains vitamin C	Hypoproteinaemia, chronic renal failure, wound fistula leakage with excessive protein loss, conditions requiring a controlled nitrogen intake, and haemodialysis. Not suitable for child under 6 months.	Dialamine powder: 400 gram = £77.02
ProSource® Liquid (Nutrinovo Ltd)	Liquid **per 30 mL**	420 kJ (100 kcal)	10 g collagen protein whey protein isolate	15 g (sugars 8 g)	Nil	Nil	Gluten-free Lactose-free May contain porcine derivatives	Biochemically proven hypoproteinaemia Not recommended for child under 3 years.	ProSource liquid 30ml sachets: citrus berry, lemon, orange creme, neutral 100 sachet = £101.16

Powder provides: protein equivalent 25 g, carbohydrate 65 g, vitamin C 125 mg, energy 1530 kJ (360 kcal)/100 g.

Product	Formulation	Energy	Protein	Carbohydrate	Fat	Fibre	Special Characteristics	ACBS Indications	Presentation & Flavour
ProSource® Plus (Nutrinovo Ltd)	Liquid per 30 mL	420 kJ (100 kcal)	15 g collagen whey protein isolate	11 g (sugars 10 g)	Nil	Nil	Gluten-free Lactose-free May contain porcine derivatives	Hypoproteinaemia Not recommended for child under 3 years	ProSource Plus liquid 30ml sachets neutral: 100 sachet = £143.90

PROTEIN, FAT, AND CARBOHYDRATE

Product	Formulation	Energy	Protein	Carbohydrate	Fat	Fibre	Special Characteristics	ACBS Indications	Presentation & Flavour
Calogen® Extra (Nutricia Ltd)	Liquid per 100 mL	1650 kJ (400 kcal)	5 g cows' milk	4.5 g (sugars 3.5 g)	40.3 g	Nil	Gluten-free Residual lactose Contains vitamins and minerals	Disease-related malnutrition, malabsorption states, or other conditions requiring fortification with a high fat or carbohydrate (with protein) supplement. Not suitable for child under 3 years; use with caution in child 3–6 years. May require dilution for child 3–5 years.	Calogen Extra emulsion: neutral, strawberry 200 ml = £4.98
Calogen® Extra Shots (Nutricia Ltd)	Liquid per 100 mL	1650 kJ (400 kcal)	5 g cows' milk	4.5 g (sugars 3.5 g)	40.3 g	Nil	Gluten-free Residual lactose With vitamins and minerals	Disease-related malnutrition, malabsorption states, or other conditions requiring fortification with a high fat or carbohydrate (with protein) supplement. Not suitable for child under 3 years; use with caution in child 3–6 years. May require dilution for child 3–5 years.	Calogen Extra Shots emulsion: neutral, strawberry 240 ml = £5.75
Calshake® (Fresenius Kabi Ltd)	Powder per 87 g	1841 kJ (439 kcal)	4.1 g cows' milk	56.4 g (sugars 20 g)	22 g	Nil	Contains lactose Gluten-free	Disease-related malnutrition, malabsorption states, or other conditions requiring fortification with a high fat or carbohydrate (with protein) supplement. Not suitable for child under 1 year.	Calshake powder: banana, neutral, strawberry, vanilla 609 gram = £17.71; chocolate 630 gram = £17.71

Powder: one sachet reconstituted with 240 mL whole milk provides approx. 2 kcal/mL and protein 12 g.

Product	Formulation	Energy	Protein	Carbohydrate	Fat	Fibre	Special Characteristics	ACBS Indications	Presentation & Flavour
Enshake® (Abbott Laboratories Ltd)	Powder per 100 g	1893 kJ (450 kcal)	8.4 g cows' milk, soy protein isolate	69 g (sugars 14.5 g)	15.6 g	Nil	Residual lactose Contains vitamins and minerals	Disease-related malnutrition, malabsorption states, or other conditions requiring fortification with a high fat or carbohydrate (with protein) supplement. Not suitable for child under 1 year; use with caution in child 1–6 years.	Enshake oral powder 96.5g sachets: banana, chocolate, strawberry, vanilla 6 sachet = £14.68

Powder: 96.5 g reconstituted with 240 mL whole milk provides approx. 2 kcal/mL and protein 16 g.

Product	Formulation	Energy	Protein	Carbohydrate	Fat	Fibre	Special Characteristics	ACBS Indications	Presentation & Flavour
MCT Procal® (Vitaflo International Ltd)	Powder per 100 g	2742 kJ (657 kcal)	12.5 g cows' milk	20.6 g (sugars 3.1 g)	63.1 g (MCT 99%)	Nil	Contains lactose	Dietary management of disorders of long-chain fatty acid oxidation, fat malabsorption, and other disorders requiring a low LCT, high MCT supplement. Not suitable for child under 1 year.	MCT procal oral powder 16g sachets: 30 sachet = £25.15

Powder 16 g provides: protein 2 g, carbohydrate 3.3 g, fat 10.1 g, energy 439 kJ (105 kcal).

A2

Borderline substances | **Appendix 2**

High-energy supplements: protein

Product	Formulation	Energy	Protein	Carbohydrate	Fat	Fibre	Special Characteristics	ACBS Indications	Presentation & Flavour
Pro-Cal® (Vitaflo International Ltd)	Powder per 100 g	2787 kJ (667 kcal)	13.6 g cows' milk	28.2 g (sugars 16 g)	55.5 g	Nil	Contains lactose Gluten-free	Disease-related malnutrition, malabsorption states, or other conditions requiring fortification with a high fat or carbohydrate (with protein) supplement. Not suitable for child under 1 year; use with caution in child 1-5 years.	Pro-Cal powder: 12500 gram = £224.84; 375 gram = £16.76; 510 gram = £15.53; 1500 gram = £31.64; 3000 gram = £74.68

Powder 15 g provides: protein 2 g, carbohydrate 4.2 g, fat 8.3 g, energy 418 kJ (100 kcal).

Product	Formulation	Energy	Protein	Carbohydrate	Fat	Fibre	Special Characteristics	ACBS Indications	Presentation & Flavour
Pro-Cal® Shot (Vitaflo International Ltd)	Liquid per 100 mL	1385 kJ (334 kcal)	6.7 g cows' milk	13.4 g (sugars 13.3 g)	28.2 g	Nil	Contains lactose Gluten-free Contains soya	Disease-related malnutrition, malabsorption states, or other conditions requiring fortification with a high fat or carbohydrate (with protein) supplement. Not suitable for child under 3 years.	Pro-Cal: shot starter pack 360 ml = £7.37; shot strawberry 720 ml = £14.71; shot banana, shot neutral 720 ml = £14.71
Scandishake® Mix (Nutricia Ltd)	Powder per 100 g	2099 kJ (500 kcal)	4.7 g cows' milk	65 g (sugars 14.3 g)	24.7 g	Nil	Gluten-free Contains lactose	Disease-related malnutrition, malabsorption states, or other conditions requiring fortification with a high fat or carbohydrate (with protein) supplement. Not suitable for child under 3 years.	Scandishake Mix oral powder 85g sachets: banana, caramel, chocolate, strawberry, unflavoured, vanilla 6 sachet = £15.54

Powder: 85 g reconstituted with 240 mL whole milk provides: protein 11.7 g, carbohydrate 66.8 g, fat 30.4 g, energy 2457 kJ (588 kcal).

Product	Formulation	Energy	Protein	Carbohydrate	Fat	Fibre	Special Characteristics	ACBS Indications	Presentation & Flavour
Vitasavoury® (Vitaflo International Ltd)	Powder per 100 g	2562 kJ (619 kcal)	12 g cows' milk	22.5 g (sugars 1.4 g)	52 g	6.4 g	Contains lactose Contains soya (chicken flavour)	Disease-related malnutrition, malabsorption states, or other conditions requiring fortification with a high fat or carbohydrate (with protein) supplement. Not suitable for child under 3 years.	Vitasavoury powder: chicken, golden vegetable, leek & potato, mushroom 500 g = £20.08

Fibre, vitamin, and mineral supplements

High-fibre supplements

Product	Formulation	Energy	Protein	Carbohydrate	Fat	Fibre	Special Characteristics	ACBS Indications	Presentation & Flavour
Resource® Optifibre® (Nestle Health Science)	Powder per 100 g	323 kJ (76 kcal)	Nil	19 g guar gum, partially hydrolysed	Nil	78 g	Gluten-free Lactose-free	Borderline substances standard ACBS indications p. 1500 except dysphagia Not suitable for child under 5 years	Resource Optifibre powder: 80 gram = £4.33; 250 gram = £10.64

Vitamin and Mineral supplements

Product	Formulation	Energy	Protein	Carbohydrate	Fat	Fibre	Special Characteristics	ACBS Indications	Presentation & Flavour
FruitiVits® (Vitaflo International Ltd)	Powder per 100 g	133 kJ (33 kcal)	Nil	8.3 g (sugars 400 mg)	less than 100 mg	3.3 g		Vitamin, mineral, and trace element supplement in children 3–10 years with restrictive therapeutic diets	FruitiVits oral powder 6g sachets: 30 sachet = £68.00
Paediatric Seravit® (Nutricia Ltd)	Powder per 100 g	1275 kJ (300 kcal)	Nil	75 g (sugars 6.75 g)	Nil	Nil	Pineapple flavour not suitable for child under 6 months	Vitamin, mineral, and trace element supplement in infants and children with restrictive therapeutic diets.	Seravit Paediatric powder: unflavoured 200 gram = £18.78; pineapple 200 gram = £20.01
Renavit® (Stanningley Pharma Ltd)	Tablet per 450 mg	3.15 kJ (0.75 kcal)	Nil	170 mg	Nil	Nil		Dietary management of water-soluble vitamin deficiency in adults with renal failure on dialysis	Renavit tablets: 100 tablet = £12.50

A2

Borderline substances | **Appendix 2**

Feed additives

Special additives for conditions of intolerance

Colief ®
▸ For the relief of symptoms associated with lactose intolerance in infants, provided that lactose intolerance is confirmed by the presence of reducing substances and/or excessive acid in stools, a low concentration of the corresponding disaccharide enzyme on intestinal biopsy or by breath hydrogen test or lactose intolerance test. For dosage and administration details, consult product literature.
LIQUID, lactase 50 000 units/g

Colief 50,000units/g infant drops (Forum Health Products Ltd)
7 ml (ACBS) · NHS indicative price = £8.40

Fructose
▸ (Laevulose) For proven glucose/galactose intolerance

Glucose
▸ (Dextrose monohydrate) For use as an energy supplement in sucrose-isomaltase deficiency

VSL#3 ®
▸ Nutritional supplement for use under the supervision of a physician, for the maintenance of remission of ileoanal pouchitis induced by antibacterials in adults. For dosage and administration details, consult product literature.
POWDER, containing 8 strains of live, freeze-dried, lactic acid bacteria. Contains traces of soya, gluten, and lactose.

VSL#3 Probiotic Food Supplement oral powder 4.4g sachets (Ferring Pharmaceuticals Ltd)
30 sachet (ACBS) · NHS indicative price = £34.36

Feed thickeners and pre-thickened drinks

Carobel, Instant ®
▸ For thickening feeds in the treatment of vomiting.
POWDER, carob seed flour.

Instant Carobel powder (Cow & Gate Ltd)
135 gram (ACBS) · NHS indicative price = £2.91

Multi-thick ®
▸ For thickening of liquids and foods in dysphagia. Not suitable for children under 1 year except in cases of failure to thrive.
POWDER, modified maize starch, gluten- and lactose-free.

Multi-thick powder (Abbott Laboratories Ltd)
250 gram (ACBS) · NHS indicative price = £4.83

Nutilis ® Clear
▸ For thickening of liquids or foods in dysphagia. Not suitable for children under 3 years.
POWDER, maltodextrin, xanthan gum, guar gum, gluten- and lactose-free.

Nutilis Clear powder (Nutricia Ltd)
72 gram (ACBS) · NHS indicative price = £11.04 | 175 gram (ACBS) · NHS indicative price = £8.46

Nutilis ® Powder
▸ For thickening of foods in dysphagia. Not suitable for child under 3 years.
POWDER, carbohydrate 86 g, energy 1520 kJ (358 kcal)/100 g, modified maize starch, gluten- and lactose-free.

Nutilis powder (Nutricia Ltd)
240 gram (ACBS) · NHS indicative price = £7.00 | 300 gram (ACBS) · NHS indicative price = £5.30

Resource ® Thickened Drink
▸ For dysphagia. Not suitable for children under 1 year.
LIQUID, carbohydrate 22 g, energy: orange 382 kJ (90 kcal); apple 376 kJ (89 kcal)/100 mL. Gluten- and lactose-free.

Resource Thickened Drink custard apple (Nestle Health Science)
114 ml (ACBS) · NHS indicative price = £0.75

Resource Thickened Drink custard orange (Nestle Health Science)
114 ml (ACBS) · NHS indicative price = £0.75

Resource Thickened Drink syrup apple (Nestle Health Science)
114 ml (ACBS) · NHS indicative price = £0.75

Resource Thickened Drink syrup orange (Nestle Health Science)
114 ml (ACBS) · NHS indicative price = £0.75

Resource ® ThickenUp Clear
▸ For thickening of liquids or foods in dysphagia. Not suitable for children under 3 years.
POWDER, maltodextrin, xanthum gum, gluten- and lactose-free.

Resource ThickenUp Clear powder (Nestle Health Science)
28.8 gram (ACBS) · NHS indicative price = £5.28 | 127 gram (ACBS) · NHS indicative price = £8.46

Resource ® ThickenUp ®
▸ For thickening of foods in dysphagia. Not suitable for children under 1 year.
POWDER, modified maize starch. Gluten- and lactose-free.

Resource ThickenUp powder (Nestle Health Science)
227 gram (ACBS) · NHS indicative price = £4.66 | 337.5 gram (ACBS) · NHS indicative price = £18.49

SLO Drinks ®
▸ Nutritional supplement for patient hydration in the dietary management of dysphagia. Not suitable for children under 3 years.
POWDER, carbohydrate content varies with flavour and chosen consistency (3 consistencies available), see product literature.

SLO Drink 1 oral powder blackcurrant (SLO Drinks Ltd)
25 cup (ACBS) · NHS indicative price = £7.50

SLO Drink 1 oral powder orange (SLO Drinks Ltd)
25 cup (ACBS) · NHS indicative price = £7.50

SLO Drink 2 oral powder blackcurrant (SLO Drinks Ltd)
25 cup (ACBS) · NHS indicative price = £7.50

SLO Drink 2 oral powder orange (SLO Drinks Ltd)
25 cup (ACBS) · NHS indicative price = £7.50

SLO Milkshakes+ ®
▸ Nutritional supplement in the dietary management of dysphagia. Not suitable for children under 3 years.
POWDER, carbohydrate content varies with flavour and chosen consistency (2 consistencies available), see product literature.

SLO Milkshake+ 1 oral powder chocolate (SLO Drinks Ltd)
7 × 50 gram (ACBS) · NHS indicative price = £5.88

SLO Milkshake+ 1 oral powder strawberry (SLO Drinks Ltd)
7 × 50 gram (ACBS) · NHS indicative price = £5.88

SLO Milkshake+ 2 oral powder chocolate (SLO Drinks Ltd)
7 × 50 gram (ACBS) · NHS indicative price = £5.88

SLO Milkshake+ 2 oral powder strawberry (SLO Drinks Ltd)
7 × 50 gram (ACBS) · NHS indicative price = £5.88

Thick and Easy ®
▸ For thickening of foods in dysphagia. Not suitable for children under 1 year except in cases of failure to thrive.
POWDER, modified maize starch

Thick & Easy powder (Fresenius Kabi Ltd)
225 gram (ACBS) · NHS indicative price = £5.21 | 900 gram (ACBS) · NHS indicative price = £33.00 | 4540 gram (ACBS) · NHS indicative price = £90.58

Thicken Aid ®
▸ For thickening of foods in dysphagia. Not suitable for children under 1 year.
POWDER, modified maize starch, maltodextrin, gluten- and lactose-free.

Thicken Aid powder (M & A Pharmachem Ltd)
225 gram (ACBS) · NHS indicative price = £3.71 | 900 gram (ACBS) · NHS indicative price = £22.40

Thixo-D ®
▸ For thickening of foods in dysphagia. Not suitable for children under 1 year except in cases of failure to thrive.
POWDER, modified maize starch, gluten-free.

Thixo-D powder (Sutherland Health Ltd)
375 gram (ACBS) · NHS indicative price = £8.10

Thixo-D Cal-Free powder (Sutherland Health Ltd)
30 gram · NHS indicative price = £3.00

Vitaquick ®
▸ For thickening of foods in dysphagia. Not suitable for children under 1 year except in cases of failure to thrive.
POWDER. Modified maize starch.

Vitaquick powder (Vitaflo International Ltd)
300 gram (ACBS) · NHS indicative price = £7.55

Flavouring preparations

FlavourPac ®
▸ For use with Vitaflo's range of unflavoured protein substitutes for metabolic diseases; not suitable for child under 3 years.
POWDER

FlavourPac oral powder 4g sachets blackcurrant (Vitaflo International Ltd)
30 sachet (ACBS) · NHS indicative price = £14.60

FlavourPac oral powder 4g sachets lemon (Vitaflo International Ltd)
30 sachet (ACBS) · NHS indicative price = £14.60

FlavourPac oral powder 4g sachets orange (Vitaflo International Ltd)
30 sachet (ACBS) · NHS indicative price = £14.60

FlavourPac oral powder 4g sachets raspberry (Vitaflo International Ltd)
30 sachet (ACBS) · NHS indicative price = £14.60

FlavourPac oral powder 4g sachets tropical (Vitaflo International Ltd)
30 sachet (ACBS) · NHS indicative price = £14.60

Foods for special diets

Gluten-free foods

ACBS indications: established gluten-sensitive enteropathies including steatorrhoea due to gluten sensitivity, coeliac disease, and dermatitis herpetiformis.

Bread
LOAVES

Barkat ® **Loaf**
GLUTEN-FREE

Barkat gluten free brown rice bread (Gluten Free Foods Ltd)
500 gram (ACBS) · NHS indicative price = £5.84

Barkat gluten free par baked white bread sliced (Gluten Free Foods Ltd)
300 gram (ACBS) · NHS indicative price = £4.21

Barkat gluten free home fresh country loaf (Gluten Free Foods Ltd)
250 gram (ACBS) · NHS indicative price = £4.43

Barkat gluten free wheat free multigrain bread (Gluten Free Foods Ltd)
500 gram (ACBS) · NHS indicative price = £5.84

Barkat gluten free wholemeal bread sliced (Gluten Free Foods Ltd)
500 gram (ACBS) · NHS indicative price = £4.05

Barkat gluten free white rice bread (Gluten Free Foods Ltd)
500 gram (ACBS) · NHS indicative price = £5.84

Ener-G ® **Loaves**
GLUTEN-FREE

Ener-G gluten free brown rice bread (General Dietary Ltd)
474 gram (ACBS) · NHS indicative price = £5.47

Ener-G gluten free tapioca bread (General Dietary Ltd)
480 gram (ACBS) · NHS indicative price = £5.47

Ener-G gluten free rice loaf (General Dietary Ltd)
612 gram (ACBS) · NHS indicative price = £5.47

Ener-G gluten free Seattle brown loaf (General Dietary Ltd)
454 gram (ACBS) · NHS indicative price = £6.22

Ener-G gluten free white rice bread (General Dietary Ltd)
456 gram (ACBS) · NHS indicative price = £5.47

Genius Gluten Free ® **Loaf**
GLUTEN-FREE

Genius gluten free brown sandwich bread sliced (Genius Foods Ltd)
535 gram (ACBS) · NHS indicative price = £3.80

Genius gluten free white sandwich bread sliced (Genius Foods Ltd)
535 gram (ACBS) · NHS indicative price = £3.80

Glutafin ® **Loaves**
GLUTEN-FREE

Glutafin gluten free fibre loaf sliced (Dr Schar UK Ltd)
300 gram (ACBS) · NHS indicative price = £2.89

Glutafin gluten free white loaf sliced (Dr Schar UK Ltd)
300 gram (ACBS) · NHS indicative price = £2.89

Glutafin ® **Select Loaves**
GLUTEN-FREE

Glutafin gluten free Select fibre loaf sliced (Dr Schar UK Ltd)
400 gram (ACBS) · NHS indicative price = £3.43

Glutafin gluten free Select fresh brown loaf sliced (Dr Schar UK Ltd)
400 gram (ACBS) · NHS indicative price = £3.43

Glutafin gluten free Select fresh white loaf sliced (Dr Schar UK Ltd)
400 gram (ACBS) · NHS indicative price = £3.43

Glutafin gluten free Select seeded loaf sliced (Dr Schar UK Ltd)
400 gram (ACBS) · NHS indicative price = £3.72

Glutafin gluten free Select white loaf sliced (Dr Schar UK Ltd)
400 gram (ACBS) · NHS indicative price = £3.43

Juvela ® **Loaf**
GLUTEN-FREE

Juvela gluten free fresh fibre loaf sliced (Hero UK Ltd)
400 gram (ACBS) · NHS indicative price = £3.39

Juvela gluten free fresh white loaf sliced (Hero UK Ltd)
400 gram (ACBS) · NHS indicative price = £3.69

Juvela gluten free fibre loaf sliced (Hero UK Ltd)
400 gram (ACBS) · NHS indicative price = £3.54

Juvela gluten free part baked loaf (Hero UK Ltd)
400 gram (ACBS) · NHS indicative price = £3.95

Juvela gluten free part baked fibre loaf (Hero UK Ltd)
400 gram (ACBS) · NHS indicative price = £3.80

Juvela gluten free loaf unsliced (Hero UK Ltd)
400 gram (ACBS) · NHS indicative price = £3.54

Juvela gluten free fibre loaf unsliced (Hero UK Ltd)
400 gram (ACBS) · NHS indicative price = £3.54

Lifestyle ® **Loaf**
GLUTEN-FREE

Lifestyle gluten free brown bread sliced (Ultrapharm Ltd)
400 gram (ACBS) · NHS indicative price = £2.82

Lifestyle gluten free high fibre bread sliced (Ultrapharm Ltd)
400 gram · NHS indicative price = £2.82

Lifestyle gluten free white bread sliced (Ultrapharm Ltd)
400 gram (ACBS) · NHS indicative price = £2.82

Warburtons ® **Loaf**
GLUTEN-FREE

Warburtons gluten free brown bread sliced (Warburtons Ltd)
400 gram (ACBS) · NHS indicative price = £3.06

Warburtons gluten free white bread sliced (Warburtons Ltd)
400 gram (ACBS) · NHS indicative price = £3.06

Wellfoods ® **Loaf**
GLUTEN-FREE

Wellfoods gluten free loaf sliced (Wellfoods Ltd)
600 gram (ACBS) · NHS indicative price = £5.05

Wellfoods gluten free loaf unsliced (Wellfoods Ltd)
600 gram (ACBS) · NHS indicative price = £4.95

BAGUETTES, BUNS AND ROLLS

Barkat ® **Baguettes and rolls**
GLUTEN-FREE

Barkat gluten free par baked rolls (Gluten Free Foods Ltd)
200 gram (ACBS) · NHS indicative price = £4.05

Barkat gluten free par baked baguettes (Gluten Free Foods Ltd)
200 gram (ACBS) · NHS indicative price = £4.05

Ener-G ® **Rolls**
GLUTEN-FREE

Ener-G gluten free dinner rolls (General Dietary Ltd)
280 gram (ACBS) · NHS indicative price = £3.71

Ener-G gluten free white round rolls (General Dietary Ltd)
220 gram (ACBS) · NHS indicative price = £2.98

Ener-G gluten free white long rolls (General Dietary Ltd)
220 gram (ACBS) · NHS indicative price = £2.98

Glutafin ® Baguettes and rolls
GLUTEN-FREE

Glutafin gluten free baguettes (Dr Schar UK Ltd)
350 gram (ACBS) · NHS indicative price = £3.51

Glutafin gluten free 4 white rolls (Dr Schar UK Ltd)
200 gram (ACBS) · NHS indicative price = £3.68

Glutafin gluten free part baked 4 fibre rolls (Dr Schar UK Ltd)
200 gram (ACBS) · NHS indicative price = £3.68

Glutafin ® Select Rolls
GLUTEN-FREE

Glutafin gluten free part baked 4 white rolls (Dr Schar UK Ltd)
200 gram (ACBS) · NHS indicative price = £3.68

Glutafin gluten free part baked 2 long white rolls (Dr Schar UK Ltd)
150 gram (ACBS) · NHS indicative price = £2.81

Juvela ® Rolls
GLUTEN-FREE

Juvela gluten free fresh fibre rolls (Hero UK Ltd)
425 gram (ACBS) · NHS indicative price = £4.42

Juvela gluten free fresh white rolls (Hero UK Ltd)
425 gram (ACBS) · NHS indicative price = £4.42

Juvela gluten free fibre bread rolls (Hero UK Ltd)
425 gram (ACBS) · NHS indicative price = £4.77

Juvela gluten free bread rolls (Hero UK Ltd)
425 gram (ACBS) · NHS indicative price = £4.77

Juvela gluten free part baked fibre bread rolls (Hero UK Ltd)
375 gram (ACBS) · NHS indicative price = £4.94

Juvela gluten free part baked white bread rolls (Hero UK Ltd)
375 gram (ACBS) · NHS indicative price = £4.94

Lifestyle ® Rolls
GLUTEN-FREE

Lifestyle gluten free brown bread rolls (Ultrapharm Ltd)
400 gram (ACBS) · NHS indicative price = £2.82

Lifestyle gluten free high fibre bread rolls (Ultrapharm Ltd)
400 gram (ACBS) · NHS indicative price = £2.82

Lifestyle gluten free white bread rolls (Ultrapharm Ltd)
400 gram (ACBS) · NHS indicative price = £2.82

Proceli ® Baguettes, buns and rolls
GLUTEN-FREE

Proceli gluten free part baked baguettes (Ambe Ltd)
250 gram (ACBS) · NHS indicative price = £3.24

Warburtons ® Baguettes and rolls
GLUTEN-FREE

Warburtons gluten free brown rolls (Warburtons Ltd)
220 gram (ACBS) · NHS indicative price = £2.55

Warburtons gluten free white rolls (Warburtons Ltd)
220 gram (ACBS) · NHS indicative price = £2.55

Wellfoods ® Buns and rolls
GLUTEN-FREE

Wellfoods gluten free burger buns (Wellfoods Ltd)
380 gram (ACBS) · NHS indicative price = £4.03

Wellfoods gluten free rolls (Wellfoods Ltd)
360 gram (ACBS) · NHS indicative price = £3.73

Cereals

Juvela ® Fibre flakes and oats
GLUTEN-FREE

Juvela gluten free fibre flakes (Hero UK Ltd)
300 gram (ACBS) · NHS indicative price = £2.78

Juvela gluten free flakes (Hero UK Ltd)
300 gram (ACBS) · NHS indicative price = £2.78

Juvela gluten free pure oats (Hero UK Ltd)
500 gram (ACBS) · NHS indicative price = £2.78

Nairns ® Porridge
GLUTEN-FREE

Nairn's gluten free oat porridge (Nairn's Oatcakes Ltd)
500 gram (ACBS) · NHS indicative price = £3.05

Cookies and biscuits

Barkat ® Biscuits
GLUTEN-FREE

Barkat gluten free digestive biscuits (Gluten Free Foods Ltd)
175 gram (ACBS) · NHS indicative price = £2.66

Barkat gluten free coffee biscuits (Gluten Free Foods Ltd)
200 gram (ACBS) · NHS indicative price = £3.44

Ener-G ® Cookies
GLUTEN-FREE

Ener-G gluten free vanilla cookies (General Dietary Ltd)
435 gram (ACBS) · NHS indicative price = £6.23

Glutafin ® Cookies and biscuits
GLUTEN-FREE

Glutafin gluten free tea biscuits (Dr Schar UK Ltd)
150 gram (ACBS) · NHS indicative price = £2.09

Glutafin gluten free digestive biscuits (Dr Schar UK Ltd)
150 gram (ACBS) · NHS indicative price = £2.13

Glutafin gluten free shortbread biscuits (Dr Schar UK Ltd)
100 gram (ACBS) · NHS indicative price = £1.73

Juvela ® Biscuits
GLUTEN-FREE

Juvela gluten free digestive biscuits (Hero UK Ltd)
150 gram (ACBS) · NHS indicative price = £3.05

Juvela gluten free savoury biscuits (Hero UK Ltd)
150 gram (ACBS) · NHS indicative price = £3.82

Juvela gluten free sweet biscuits (Hero UK Ltd)
150 gram (ACBS) · NHS indicative price = £2.88

Juvela gluten free tea biscuits (Hero UK Ltd)
150 gram (ACBS) · NHS indicative price = £3.05

Crackers, crispbreads, and breadsticks

Barkat ® Crackers
GLUTEN-FREE

Barkat gluten free matzo crackers (Gluten Free Foods Ltd)
200 gram (ACBS) · NHS indicative price = £3.59

Glutafin ® Crackers
GLUTEN-FREE

Glutafin gluten free crackers (Dr Schar UK Ltd)
200 gram (ACBS) · NHS indicative price = £3.46

Glutafin gluten free mini crackers (Dr Schar UK Ltd)
175 gram (ACBS) · NHS indicative price = £2.96

Juvela ® Crispbread
GLUTEN-FREE

Juvela gluten free crispbread (Hero UK Ltd)
200 gram (ACBS) · NHS indicative price = £4.64

Warburtons ® Crackers
GLUTEN-FREE

Warburtons gluten free bran crackers (Warburtons Ltd)
150 gram (ACBS) · NHS indicative price = £2.34

Flour mixes and xanthan gum
FLOUR MIXES

Barkat ® Flour mix
GLUTEN-FREE

Barkat gluten free bread mix (Gluten Free Foods Ltd)
500 gram (ACBS) · NHS indicative price = £6.94

Barkat gluten free high fibre bread mix (Gluten Free Foods Ltd)
500 gram (ACBS) · NHS indicative price = £9.13

Barkat gluten free all purpose flour mix (Gluten Free Foods Ltd)
500 gram (ACBS) · NHS indicative price = £4.74

Finax ® Flour mix
GLUTEN-FREE

Finax gluten free coarse flour mix (Drossa Ltd)
900 gram (ACBS) · NHS indicative price = £8.85

Finax gluten free fibre bread mix (Drossa Ltd)
1000 gram (ACBS) · NHS indicative price = £10.14

Finax gluten free flour mix (Drossa Ltd)
900 gram (ACBS) · NHS indicative price = £8.85

Glutafin Select ® Flour mix
GLUTEN-FREE

Glutafin gluten free Select bread mix (Dr Schar UK Ltd)
500 gram (ACBS) · NHS indicative price = £6.66

Glutafin gluten free Select fibre bread mix (Dr Schar UK Ltd)
500 gram (ACBS) · NHS indicative price = £6.66

Glutafin gluten free Select multipurpose fibre mix (Dr Schar UK Ltd)
500 gram (ACBS) · NHS indicative price = £6.66

Glutafin gluten free Select multipurpose white mix (Dr Schar UK Ltd)
500 gram (ACBS) · NHS indicative price = £6.66

Glutafin ® Flour mix
GLUTEN-FREE

Glutafin gluten free multipurpose white mix (Dr Schar UK Ltd)
500 gram (ACBS) · NHS indicative price = £6.66

Heron Foods ® Flour mix
GLUTEN-FREE

Heron Hi-Fibre gluten free organic bread mix (Gluten Free Foods Ltd)
500 gram (ACBS) · NHS indicative price = £9.13

Juvela ® Flour mix
GLUTEN-FREE

Juvela gluten free fibre mix (Hero UK Ltd)
500 gram (ACBS) · NHS indicative price = £7.35

Juvela gluten free harvest mix (Hero UK Ltd)
500 gram (ACBS) · NHS indicative price = £7.35

Juvela gluten free mix (Hero UK Ltd)
500 gram (ACBS) · NHS indicative price = £7.35

Mrs Crimbles ® Flour mixes
GLUTEN-FREE

Mrs Crimble's gluten free bread mix (Stiletto Foods (UK) Ltd)
275 gram (ACBS) · NHS indicative price = £1.09

Mrs Crimble's gluten free pastry mix (Stiletto Foods (UK) Ltd)
200 gram (ACBS) · NHS indicative price = £1.09

Orgran ® Flour mix
GLUTEN-FREE

Orgran gluten free pizza & pastry mix (Naturally Good Food Ltd)
375 gram (ACBS) · NHS indicative price = £3.80

Orgran gluten free self-raising flour (Naturally Good Food Ltd)
500 gram (ACBS) · NHS indicative price = £3.10

Orgran gluten free all purpose plain flour (Naturally Good Food Ltd)
500 gram · NHS indicative price = £3.10

Proceli ® Flour mix
GLUTEN-FREE

Proceli gluten free white plain flour (Ambe Ltd)
1000 gram (ACBS) · NHS indicative price = £9.95

Pure ® Flour mix
GLUTEN-FREE

Innovative Solutions Pure gluten free blended flour (Innovative Solutions (UK) Ltd)
1000 gram (ACBS) · NHS indicative price = £4.52

Innovative Solutions Pure gluten free brown rice flour (Innovative Solutions (UK) Ltd)
500 gram (ACBS) · NHS indicative price = £1.69

Innovative Solutions Pure gluten free white rice flour (Innovative Solutions (UK) Ltd)
500 gram (ACBS) · NHS indicative price = £1.73

Innovative Solutions Pure gluten free potato flour (Innovative Solutions (UK) Ltd)
500 gram (ACBS) · NHS indicative price = £1.73

Innovative Solutions Pure gluten free tapioca flour (Innovative Solutions (UK) Ltd)
500 gram (ACBS) · NHS indicative price = £2.42

Innovative Solutions Pure gluten free brown teff flour (Innovative Solutions (UK) Ltd)
1000 gram (ACBS) · NHS indicative price = £5.10

Innovative Solutions Pure gluten free white teff flour (Innovative Solutions (UK) Ltd)
1000 gram (ACBS) · NHS indicative price = £5.10

Tobia ® Flour mix
GLUTEN-FREE

Tobia Teff gluten free brown teff flour (Tobia Teff UK Ltd)
1000 gram (ACBS) · NHS indicative price = £3.60

Tobia Teff gluten free white teff flour (Tobia Teff UK Ltd)
1000 gram (ACBS) · NHS indicative price = £3.60

Tritamyl ® Flour mix
GLUTEN-FREE

Tritamyl gluten free brown bread mix (Gluten Free Foods Ltd)
1000 gram (ACBS) · NHS indicative price = £7.24

Tritamyl gluten free flour mix (Gluten Free Foods Ltd)
2000 gram (ACBS) · NHS indicative price = £14.54

Tritamyl gluten free white bread mix (Gluten Free Foods Ltd)
2000 gram (ACBS) · NHS indicative price = £14.54

Wellfoods ® Flour mix
GLUTEN-FREE

Wellfoods gluten free flour alternative (Wellfoods Ltd)
1000 gram (ACBS) · NHS indicative price = £7.80

XANTHAN GUM

Ener-G ® Xanthan gum
GLUTEN-FREE

Ener-G xanthan gum (General Dietary Ltd)
170 gram (ACBS) · NHS indicative price = £8.63

Pure ® Xanthan gum
GLUTEN-FREE

Innovative Solutions Pure xanthan gum (Innovative Solutions (UK) Ltd)
100 gram (ACBS) · NHS indicative price = £6.85

Pasta

Barkat ® Pasta
GLUTEN-FREE

Barkat gluten free pasta animal shapes (Gluten Free Foods Ltd)
500 gram (ACBS) · NHS indicative price = £5.99

Barkat gluten free pasta macaroni (Gluten Free Foods Ltd)
500 gram (ACBS) · NHS indicative price = £5.99

Barkat gluten free pasta spaghetti (Gluten Free Foods Ltd)
500 gram (ACBS) · NHS indicative price = £5.99

Barkat gluten free pasta spirals (Gluten Free Foods Ltd)
500 gram (ACBS) · NHS indicative price = £5.99

Barkat gluten free pasta tagliatelle (Gluten Free Foods Ltd)
500 gram (ACBS) · NHS indicative price = £5.99

Barkat gluten free pasta buckwheat penne (Gluten Free Foods Ltd)
250 gram (ACBS) · NHS indicative price = £2.98

Barkat gluten free pasta buckwheat spirals (Gluten Free Foods Ltd)
250 gram (ACBS) · NHS indicative price = £2.98

BiAlimenta ® Pasta
GLUTEN-FREE

BiAlimenta gluten free pasta formati misti (Drossa Ltd)
3000 gram (ACBS) · NHS indicative price = £36.63

BiAlimenta gluten free pasta sagnette (Drossa Ltd)
500 gram (ACBS) · NHS indicative price = £6.11

BiAlimenta gluten free pasta spirali (Drossa Ltd)
500 gram (ACBS) · NHS indicative price = £6.11

Ener-G ® Pasta
GLUTEN-FREE

General Dietary gluten free macaroni (General Dietary Ltd)
454 gram (ACBS) · NHS indicative price = £5.03

General Dietary gluten free spaghetti (General Dietary Ltd)
454 gram (ACBS) · NHS indicative price = £5.03

General Dietary gluten free vermicelli (General Dietary Ltd)
300 gram (ACBS) · NHS indicative price = £5.03

Glutafin ® Pasta
GLUTEN-FREE

Glutafin gluten free pasta macaroni penne (Dr Schar UK Ltd)
500 gram (ACBS) · NHS indicative price = £6.73

Glutafin gluten free pasta shells (Dr Schar UK Ltd)
500 gram (ACBS) · NHS indicative price = £6.73

Glutafin gluten free pasta spirals (Dr Schar UK Ltd)
500 gram (ACBS) · NHS indicative price = £6.73

Glutafin gluten free pasta long-cut spaghetti (Dr Schar UK Ltd)
500 gram (ACBS) · NHS indicative price = £6.73

Juvela ® Pasta
GLUTEN-FREE

Juvela gluten free fibre penne (Hero UK Ltd)
500 gram (ACBS) · NHS indicative price = £6.61

Juvela gluten free pasta fusilli (Hero UK Ltd)
500 gram (ACBS) · NHS indicative price = £7.21

Juvela gluten free pasta lasagne (Hero UK Ltd)
250 gram (ACBS) · NHS indicative price = £3.68

Juvela gluten free pasta macaroni (Hero UK Ltd)
500 gram (ACBS) · NHS indicative price = £7.21

Juvela gluten free pasta spaghetti (Hero UK Ltd)
500 gram (ACBS) · NHS indicative price = £7.21

Juvela gluten free pasta tagliatelle (Hero UK Ltd)
250 gram (ACBS) · NHS indicative price = £3.47

Orgran ® Pasta
GLUTEN-FREE

Orgran gluten free pasta rice & corn lasagne (Naturally Good Food Ltd)
200 gram (ACBS) · NHS indicative price = £3.13

Orgran gluten free pasta rice & corn macaroni (Naturally Good Food Ltd)
250 gram (ACBS) · NHS indicative price = £2.42

Orgran gluten free pasta buckwheat spirals (Naturally Good Food Ltd)
250 gram (ACBS) · NHS indicative price = £2.42

Orgran gluten free pasta corn spirals (Naturally Good Food Ltd)
250 gram (ACBS) · NHS indicative price = £2.42

Orgran gluten free pasta brown rice spirals (Naturally Good Food Ltd)
250 gram (ACBS) · NHS indicative price = £2.42

Orgran gluten free pasta rice & corn spirals (Naturally Good Food Ltd)
250 gram (ACBS) · NHS indicative price = £2.42

Orgran gluten free pasta rice & millet spirals (Naturally Good Food Ltd)
250 gram (ACBS) · NHS indicative price = £2.42

Rizopia ® Pasta
GLUTEN-FREE

Rizopia gluten free organic brown rice pasta fusilli (PGR Health Foods Ltd)
500 gram (ACBS) · NHS indicative price = £2.72

Rizopia gluten free organic brown rice pasta lasagne (PGR Health Foods Ltd)
375 gram (ACBS) · NHS indicative price = £2.72

Rizopia gluten free organic brown rice pasta penne (PGR Health Foods Ltd)
500 gram (ACBS) · NHS indicative price = £2.72

Rizopia gluten free organic brown rice pasta spaghetti (PGR Health Foods Ltd)
500 gram (ACBS) · NHS indicative price = £2.72

Pizza bases

Barkat ®, Pizza crust
GLUTEN-FREE

Barkat gluten free brown rice pizza crust (Gluten Free Foods Ltd)
150 gram (ACBS) · NHS indicative price = £5.10

Barkat gluten free white rice pizza crust (Gluten Free Foods Ltd)
150 gram (ACBS) · NHS indicative price = £5.10

Glutafin ® Pizza base
GLUTEN-FREE

Glutafin gluten free pizza base (Dr Schar UK Ltd)
300 gram (ACBS) · NHS indicative price = £6.56

Juvela ® Pizza base
GLUTEN-FREE

Juvela gluten free pizza base (Hero UK Ltd)
360 gram (ACBS) · NHS indicative price = £8.78

Proceli ® Pizza base
GLUTEN-FREE

Proceli gluten free pizza base (Ambe Ltd)
250 gram (ACBS) · NHS indicative price = £3.90

Wellfoods ® Pizza base
GLUTEN-FREE

Wellfoods gluten free pizza base (Wellfoods Ltd)
600 gram (ACBS) · NHS indicative price = £9.13

Gluten- and wheat-free foods

ACBS indications: established gluten-sensitive enteropathies with coexisting established wheat sensitivity only.

Ener-G ® Bread loaves, rolls and pizza bases
GLUTEN-FREE, WHEAT-FREE

Ener-G gluten free Seattle brown hamburger rolls (General Dietary Ltd)
320 gram (ACBS) · NHS indicative price = £4.08

Ener-G gluten free Seattle brown hot dog rolls (General Dietary Ltd)
320 gram (ACBS) · NHS indicative price = £4.08

Glutafin ® Flour mix, fibre and crispbread
GLUTEN-FREE, WHEAT-FREE

Glutafin gluten free crispbread (Dr Schar UK Ltd)
150 gram (ACBS) · NHS indicative price = £3.25

Glutafin gluten free bread mix (Dr Schar UK Ltd)
500 gram (ACBS) · NHS indicative price = £6.66

Glutafin gluten free fibre bread mix (Dr Schar UK Ltd)
500 gram (ACBS) · NHS indicative price = £6.66

Glutafin gluten free wheat free fibre mix (Dr Schar UK Ltd)
500 gram (ACBS) · NHS indicative price = £6.66

Heron Foods ® Flour mixes
GLUTEN-FREE, WHEAT-FREE

Barkat gluten free bread and cake mix (Gluten Free Foods Ltd)
500 gram (ACBS) · NHS indicative price = £9.13

Heron gluten free organic bread mix (Gluten Free Foods Ltd)
500 gram (ACBS) · NHS indicative price = £9.13

Low-protein foods

ACBS indications: inherited metabolic disorders, renal or liver failure, requiring a low-protein diet.

Bread

Ener-G ® Rice bread
LOW PROTEIN

Ener-G low protein rice bread (General Dietary Ltd)
600 gram (ACBS) · NHS indicative price = £5.60

Juvela ® Loaf and rolls
LOW PROTEIN

Juvela gluten free loaf sliced (Hero UK Ltd)
400 gram (ACBS) · NHS indicative price = £3.54

Juvela low protein bread rolls (Hero UK Ltd)
350 gram (ACBS) · NHS indicative price = £4.52

Juvela low protein loaf sliced (Hero UK Ltd)
400 gram (ACBS) · NHS indicative price = £3.64

Loprofin ® Bread
LOW-PROTEIN

Loprofin low protein part baked bread rolls (Nutricia Ltd)
260 gram (ACBS) · NHS indicative price = £4.34
Loprofin low protein part baked loaf sliced (Nutricia Ltd)
400 gram (ACBS) · NHS indicative price = £4.12
PK Foods ® Loaf
LOW PROTEIN
PK Foods low protein white bread sliced (Gluten Free Foods Ltd)
300 gram · NHS indicative price = £4.84

Cake, biscuits, and snacks

Juvela ® Cookies
LOW-PROTEIN
Juvela low protein cinnamon cookies (Hero UK Ltd)
125 gram (ACBS) · NHS indicative price = £7.62
Juvela low protein chocolate chip cookies (Hero UK Ltd)
110 gram (ACBS) · NHS indicative price = £7.62
Juvela low protein orange cookies (Hero UK Ltd)
125 gram (ACBS) · NHS indicative price = £7.62
Loprofin ® Wafers
LOW-PROTEIN
Loprofin low protein crackers (Nutricia Ltd)
150 gram (ACBS) · NHS indicative price = £3.79
Loprofin low protein herb crackers (Nutricia Ltd)
150 gram (ACBS) · NHS indicative price = £3.79
PK Foods ® Biscuits
LOW-PROTEIN
PK Foods Aminex low protein biscuits (Gluten Free Foods Ltd)
200 gram (ACBS) · NHS indicative price = £5.14
PK Foods Aminex low protein cookies (Gluten Free Foods Ltd)
150 gram (ACBS) · NHS indicative price = £5.14
PK Foods Aminex low protein rusks (Gluten Free Foods Ltd)
200 gram (ACBS) · NHS indicative price = £5.14
PK Foods low protein chocolate chip cookies (Gluten Free Foods Ltd)
150 gram (ACBS) · NHS indicative price = £5.14
PK Foods low protein cinnamon cookies (Gluten Free Foods Ltd)
150 gram (ACBS) · NHS indicative price = £5.14
PK Foods low protein crispbread (Gluten Free Foods Ltd)
75 gram (ACBS) · NHS indicative price = £2.46
PK Foods low protein orange cookies (Gluten Free Foods Ltd)
150 gram (ACBS) · NHS indicative price = £5.14
Promin ® Cooked and flavoured pasta snax
LOW-PROTEIN
Promin low protein Snax salt & vinegar 25g sachets (Firstplay Dietary Foods Ltd)
3 sachet · No NHS indicative price available | 12 sachet (ACBS)
· NHS indicative price = £10.58
Promin low protein Snax ready salted 25g sachets (Firstplay Dietary Foods Ltd)
3 sachet · No NHS indicative price available | 12 sachet (ACBS)
· NHS indicative price = £10.58
Promin low protein Snax jalapeno 25g sachets (Firstplay Dietary Foods Ltd)
3 sachet · No NHS indicative price available | 12 sachet (ACBS)
· NHS indicative price = £10.58
Promin low protein Snax cheese & onion 25g sachets (Firstplay Dietary Foods Ltd)
3 sachet · No NHS indicative price available | 12 sachet (ACBS)
· NHS indicative price = £10.58
Taranis ® Cake bars
LOW-PROTEIN
Taranis low protein apricot cake (Lactalis Nutrition Sante)
240 gram (ACBS) · NHS indicative price = £6.08
Taranis low protein lemon cake (Lactalis Nutrition Sante)
240 gram (ACBS) · NHS indicative price = £6.08
Taranis low protein pear cake (Lactalis Nutrition Sante)
240 gram (ACBS) · NHS indicative price = £6.08
Vita Bite ®
▸ Not recommended for any child under 1 year.
LOW PROTEIN.

Bar, protein 30 mg (less than 2.5 mg phenylalanine),
carbohydrate 15.35 g, fat 8.4 g, energy 572 kJ (137 kcal)/25 g.
VitaBite bar (Vitaflo International Ltd)
175 gram (ACBS) · NHS indicative price = £9.11
Vitaflo Choices ® Mini crackers
LOW-PROTEIN
Vitaflo Choices mini crackers (Vitaflo International Ltd)
40 gram (ACBS) · NHS indicative price = £0.90

Cereals

Loprofin ® Breakfast cereal
LOW-PROTEIN
Loprofin low protein breakfast cereal flakes apple (Nutricia Ltd)
375 gram (ACBS) · NHS indicative price = £8.37
Loprofin low protein breakfast cereal flakes chocolate (Nutricia Ltd)
375 gram (ACBS) · NHS indicative price = £8.37
Loprofin low protein breakfast cereal flakes strawberry (Nutricia Ltd)
375 gram (ACBS) · NHS indicative price = £8.37
Loprofin low protein breakfast cereal loops (Nutricia Ltd)
375 gram (ACBS) · NHS indicative price = £8.68
Promin ® Hot breakfast
LOW-PROTEIN
Promin low protein hot breakfast powder sachets apple & cinnamon (Firstplay Dietary Foods Ltd)
342 gram (ACBS) · NHS indicative price = £8.09
Promin low protein hot breakfast powder sachets banana (Firstplay Dietary Foods Ltd)
342 gram (ACBS) · NHS indicative price = £8.09
Promin low protein hot breakfast powder sachets chocolate (Firstplay Dietary Foods Ltd)
342 gram (ACBS) · NHS indicative price = £8.09
Promin low protein hot breakfast powder sachets original (Firstplay Dietary Foods Ltd)
336 gram (ACBS) · NHS indicative price = £8.09

Desserts

PK Foods ® Jelly
LOW-PROTEIN
PK Foods low protein jelly mix dessert cherry (Gluten Free Foods Ltd)
320 gram (ACBS) · NHS indicative price = £8.19
PK Foods low protein jelly mix dessert orange (Gluten Free Foods Ltd)
320 gram (ACBS) · NHS indicative price = £8.19
Promin ® Desserts
LOW-PROTEIN
Promin low protein imitation rice pudding apple (Firstplay Dietary Foods Ltd)
276 gram (ACBS) · NHS indicative price = £6.33
Promin low protein imitation rice pudding banana (Firstplay Dietary Foods Ltd)
276 gram (ACBS) · NHS indicative price = £6.33
Promin low protein imitation rice pudding original (Firstplay Dietary Foods Ltd)
276 gram (ACBS) · NHS indicative price = £6.33
Promin low protein imitation rice pudding strawberry (Firstplay Dietary Foods Ltd)
276 gram (ACBS) · NHS indicative price = £6.33

Flour mixes and egg substitutes

Ener-G ® Egg replacer
LOW-PROTEIN
Ener-G low protein egg replacer (General Dietary Ltd)
454 gram (ACBS) · NHS indicative price = £5.17
Fate ® Flour mix
LOW PROTEIN
Fate low protein all purpose mix (Fate Special Foods)
500 gram (ACBS) · NHS indicative price = £6.97

Fate low protein chocolate cake mix (Fate Special Foods)
500 gram (ACBS) · NHS indicative price = £6.97

Fate low protein plain cake mix (Fate Special Foods)
500 gram (ACBS) · NHS indicative price = £6.97

Juvela ® Mix
LOW-PROTEIN

Juvela low protein mix (Hero UK Ltd)
500 gram (ACBS) · NHS indicative price = £7.79

Loprofin ® Flour mixes and egg substitutes
LOW-PROTEIN

Loprofin low protein egg replacer (Nutricia Ltd)
500 gram (ACBS) · NHS indicative price = £16.26

Loprofin low protein egg white replacer (Nutricia Ltd)
100 gram (ACBS) · NHS indicative price = £10.46

Loprofin low protein cake mix chocolate (Nutricia Ltd)
500 gram (ACBS) · NHS indicative price = £9.37

Loprofin low protein mix (Nutricia Ltd)
500 gram (ACBS) · NHS indicative price = £8.72

PK Foods ® Flour mix and egg substitute
LOW-PROTEIN

PK Foods low protein egg replacer (Gluten Free Foods Ltd)
200 gram (ACBS) · NHS indicative price = £4.16

PK Foods low protein flour mix (Gluten Free Foods Ltd)
750 gram (ACBS) · NHS indicative price = £10.92

Pasta

Loprofin ® Pasta
LOW-PROTEIN

Loprofin low protein pasta animal shapes (Nutricia Ltd)
500 gram (ACBS) · NHS indicative price = £8.90

Loprofin low protein pasta lasagne (Nutricia Ltd)
250 gram (ACBS) · NHS indicative price = £4.50

Loprofin low protein pasta penne (Nutricia Ltd)
500 gram (ACBS) · NHS indicative price = £9.24

Loprofin low protein pasta tagliatelle (Nutricia Ltd)
250 gram (ACBS) · NHS indicative price = £4.45

Loprofin low protein pasta macaroni elbows (Nutricia Ltd)
250 gram (ACBS) · NHS indicative price = £4.45

Loprofin low protein rice (Nutricia Ltd)
500 gram (ACBS) · NHS indicative price = £8.98

Loprofin low protein pasta long cut spaghetti (Nutricia Ltd)
500 gram (ACBS) · NHS indicative price = £9.24

Promin ® Pasta
LOW-PROTEIN

Promin low protein pasta alphabets (Firstplay Dietary Foods Ltd)
500 gram (ACBS) · NHS indicative price = £6.99

Promin Plus low protein pasta macaroni (Firstplay Dietary Foods Ltd)
500 gram (ACBS) · NHS indicative price = £6.99

Promin Plus low protein pasta flat noodles (Firstplay Dietary Foods Ltd)
500 gram (ACBS) · NHS indicative price = £6.99

Promin low protein pasta shells (Firstplay Dietary Foods Ltd)
500 gram (ACBS) · NHS indicative price = £6.99

Promin low protein pasta short cut spaghetti (Firstplay Dietary Foods Ltd)
500 gram (ACBS) · NHS indicative price = £6.99

Promin low protein tricolour pasta spirals (Firstplay Dietary Foods Ltd)
500 gram (ACBS) · NHS indicative price = £6.99

Promin low protein pasta spirals (Firstplay Dietary Foods Ltd)
500 gram (ACBS) · NHS indicative price = £6.99

Promin low protein imitation rice (Firstplay Dietary Foods Ltd)
500 gram (ACBS) · NHS indicative price = £6.99

Promin low protein tricolour pasta alphabets (Firstplay Dietary Foods Ltd)
500 gram (ACBS) · NHS indicative price = £6.99

Promin low protein tricolour pasta shells (Firstplay Dietary Foods Ltd)
500 gram (ACBS) · NHS indicative price = £6.99

Promin low protein lasagne sheets (Firstplay Dietary Foods Ltd)
200 gram (ACBS) · NHS indicative price = £3.03

Pizza bases

Juvela ® Pizza base
LOW-PROTEIN

Juvela low protein pizza base (Hero UK Ltd)
360 gram (ACBS) · NHS indicative price = £8.61

Savoury meals and mixes

Promin ® Savoury meals and mixes
LOW-PROTEIN

Promin low protein burger mix (Firstplay Dietary Foods Ltd)
248 gram (ACBS) · NHS indicative price = £12.72

Promin low protein cous cous (Firstplay Dietary Foods Ltd)
500 gram (ACBS) · NHS indicative price = £6.99

Promin low protein pasta elbows (Firstplay Dietary Foods Ltd)
500 gram · NHS indicative price = £6.99

Promin low protein pastameal (Firstplay Dietary Foods Ltd)
500 gram (ACBS) · NHS indicative price = £6.99

Promin low protein pasta macaroni (Firstplay Dietary Foods Ltd)
500 gram (ACBS) · NHS indicative price = £6.99

Promin Plus low protein pasta spirals (Firstplay Dietary Foods Ltd)
500 gram (ACBS) · NHS indicative price = £6.99

Promin low protein lamb and mint burger mix (Firstplay Dietary Foods Ltd)
248 gram (ACBS) · NHS indicative price = £12.72

Promin low protein sausage mix apple and sage (Firstplay Dietary Foods Ltd)
120 gram (ACBS) · NHS indicative price = £7.15

Promin low protein sausage mix original (Firstplay Dietary Foods Ltd)
120 gram (ACBS) · NHS indicative price = £7.15

Promin low protein sausage mix tomato and basil (Firstplay Dietary Foods Ltd)
120 gram (ACBS) · NHS indicative price = £7.15

Promin low protein pasta in cheese and broccoli sauce (Firstplay Dietary Foods Ltd)
264 gram (ACBS) · NHS indicative price = £8.31

Promin low protein pasta spirals in Moroccan sauce (Firstplay Dietary Foods Ltd)
288 gram (ACBS) · NHS indicative price = £8.31

Promin low protein pasta in tomato, pepper and herb sauce (Firstplay Dietary Foods Ltd)
288 gram (ACBS) · NHS indicative price = £8.31

Promin low protein potato pot with croutons onion (Firstplay Dietary Foods Ltd)
200 gram (ACBS) · NHS indicative price = £16.40

Promin low protein potato pot with croutons cabbage & bacon (Firstplay Dietary Foods Ltd)
200 gram (ACBS) · NHS indicative price = £16.40

Promin low protein potato pot with croutons sausage (Firstplay Dietary Foods Ltd)
200 gram (ACBS) · NHS indicative price = £16.40

Promin low protein X-Pot all day scramble (Firstplay Dietary Foods Ltd)
240 gram (ACBS) · NHS indicative price = £20.94

Promin low protein X-Pot beef & tomato (Firstplay Dietary Foods Ltd)
240 gram (ACBS) · NHS indicative price = £20.94

Promin low protein X-Pot chip shop curry (Firstplay Dietary Foods Ltd)
240 gram (ACBS) · NHS indicative price = £20.94

Promin low protein X-Pot rogan style curry (Firstplay Dietary Foods Ltd)
240 gram (ACBS) · NHS indicative price = £20.94

Spreads

Taranis ® Spread
LOW-PROTEIN

Taranis low protein hazelnut spread (Lactalis Nutrition Sante)
230 gram (ACBS) · NHS indicative price = £7.87

Nutritional supplements for metabolic diseases

Glutaric aciduria (type 1)

GA Gel ®
▸ Nutritional supplement for dietary management of type 1
glutaric aciduria in children 6 months–10 years.
GEL, protein equivalent (essential and non-essential amino
acids except lysine, and low tryptophan) 10 g, carbohydrate
10.3 g, fat trace, energy 339 kJ (81 kcal)/24 g, with vitamins,
minerals, and trace elements. To flavour unflavoured products,
see FlavourPac p. 1521.

GA gel oral powder 24g sachets (Vitaflo International Ltd)
30 sachet (ACBS) · NHS indicative price = £224.92

GA1 Anamix ® Infant
▸ Nutritional supplement for the dietary management of proven
glutaric aciduria (type 1) in children from birth to 3 years.
POWDER, protein equivalent (essential and non-essential amino
acids except lysine, and low tryptophan) 13.1 g, carbohydrate
49.5 g, fat 23 g, fibre 5.3 g, energy 1915 kJ (457 kcal)/100 g, with
vitamins, minerals, and trace elements; standard dilution (15%)
provides protein equivalent 2 g, carbohydrate 7.4 g, fat 3.5 g,
fibre 800 mg, energy 287 kJ (69 kcal)/100 mL.

GA1 Anamix Infant powder (Nutricia Ltd)
400 gram (ACBS) · NHS indicative price = £40.79

GA1 Maxamaid ®
▸ Nutritional supplement for the dietary management of type 1
glutaric aciduria.
POWDER, protein equivalent (essential and non-essential amino
acids except lysine, and low tryptophan) 25 g, carbohydrate
51 g, fat less than 500 mg, energy 1311 kJ (309 kcal)/100 g, with
vitamins, minerals, and trace elements. Maxamaid products are
generally intended for use in children 1–8 years.

GA1 Maxamaid powder (Nutricia Ltd)
500 gram (ACBS) · NHS indicative price = £103.00

XLYS, TRY Glutaridon ®
▸ Nutritional supplement for the dietary management of type 1
glutaric aciduria in children and adults; requires additional
source of vitamins, minerals, and trace elements.
POWDER, protein equivalent (essential and non-essential amino
acids except lysine and tryptophan) 79 g, carbohydrate 4 g,
energy 1411 kJ (332 kcal)/100 g.

XLYS TRY Glutaridon powder (Nutricia Ltd)
500 gram (ACBS) · NHS indicative price = £195.11

Glycogen storage disease

Corn flour and corn starch
▸ For glycogen storage disease

Glycosade ®
▸ A nutritional supplement for use in the dietary management of
glycogen storage disease and other metabolic conditions where
a constant supply of glucose is essential. Not suitable for use in
children under 2 years.
POWDER, protein 200 mg, carbohydrate (maize starch) 47.6 g,
fat 100 mg, fibre less than 600 mg, energy 803 kJ (192 kcal)/60 g.

Glycosade oral powder 60g sachets (Vitaflo International Ltd)
30 sachet (ACBS) · NHS indicative price = £118.21

Homocystinuria or hypermethioninaemia

HCU Anamix ® Infant
▸ Nutritional supplement for the dietary management of proven
vitamin B6 non-responsive homocystinuria or
hypermethioninaemia in children from birth to 3 years.
POWDER, protein equivalent (essential and non-essential amino
acids except methionine) 13.1 g, carbohydrate 49.5 g, fat 23 g,
fibre 5.3 g, energy 1915 kJ (457 k...
minerals, and trace elements; sta...
protein equivalent 2 g, carbohydr...
800 mg, energy 287 kJ (69 kcal)/10...

HCU Anamix Infant powder (Nutricia...
400 gram (ACBS) · NHS indicative p...

HCU cooler ® 15
▸ A methionine-free protein substitut...
supplement in children over 3 years ...
LIQUID, protein (essential and non-e...
methionine) 15 g, carbohydrate 7 g, fa...
(92 kcal)/130 mL, with vitamins, miner...

HCU orange cooler 15 liquid (Vitaflo Intern...
130 ml (ACBS) · NHS indicative price = ...

HCU Express ® 15
▸ A methionine-free protein substitute for...
supplement in children over 8 years with...
POWDER, protein (essential and non-esser...
except methionine) 15 g, carbohydrate 3.8...
315 kJ (75.3 kcal)/25 g with vitamins, miner...
elements. To flavour unflavoured products, ...
p. 1521.

HCU express 15 oral powder 25g sachets (Vitafl...
30 sachet (ACBS) · NHS indicative price = £3...

HCU Express ® 20
▸ A methionine-free protein substitute for use as a ...
supplement in children over 8 years with homocysti...
POWDER, protein (essential and non-essential amino a...
except methionine) 20 g, carbohydrate 4.7 g, fat 70 mg, ene...
416 kJ (99 kcal)/34 g with vitamins, minerals, and trace
elements. To flavour unflavoured products, see FlavourPac
p. 1521

HCU express 20 oral powder 34g sachets (Vitaflo International Ltd)
30 sachet (ACBS) · NHS indicative price = £451.25

HCU gel ®
▸ A methionine-free protein substitute for use as a nutritional
supplement for the dietary management of children 1–10 years
with homocystinuria.
POWDER, protein (essential and non-essential amino acids
except methionine) 10 g, carbohydrate 10.3 g, fat 20 mg, energy
339 kJ (81 kcal)/24 g with vitamins, minerals, and trace
elements. To flavour unflavoured products, see FlavourPac
p. 1521.

HCU gel oral powder 24g sachets (Vitaflo International Ltd)
30 sachet (ACBS) · NHS indicative price = £224.86

HCU Lophlex ® LQ 20
▸ Nutritional supplement for the dietary management of
homocystinuria in children over 3 years.
LIQUID, protein equivalent (essential and non-essential amino
acids except methionine) 20 g, carbohydrate 8.8 g, fat 440 mg,
energy 509 kJ (120 kcal)/125 mL, with vitamins, minerals, and
trace elements.

HCU Lophlex LQ 20 liquid (Nutricia Ltd)
125 ml (ACBS) · NHS indicative price = £16.82

HCU LV ®
▸ Nutritional supplement for the dietary management of
hypermethioninaemia or vitamin B6 non-responsive
homocystinuria in children over 8 years.
POWDER, protein (essential and non-essential amino acids
except methionine) 20 g, carbohydrate 2.5 g, fat 190 mg, energy
390 kJ (92 kcal)/27.8-g sachet, with vitamins, minerals, and
trace elements.

HCU-LV oral powder 27.8g sachets tropical (Nutricia Ltd)
30 sachet (ACBS) · NHS indicative price = £517.20

HCU-LV oral powder 27.8g sachets unflavoured (Nutricia Ltd)
30 sachet (ACBS) · NHS indicative price = £517.20

XMET Homidon ®
▸ Nutritional supplement for the dietary management of
hypermethioninaemia or homocystinuria in children and
adults.

Borderline subst?

A2 Appendix 2

(essential and non-essential amino ... g, carbohydrate 4.5 g, fat nil, ...0 g.

POWDER, protein equiv... acids, except methi... (Nutricia Ltd)
energy 1386 kJ) indicative price = £195.11

XMET Homi... ...nt for the dietary management of
500 gram ...a or homocystinuria.

HCU ...onine) 39 g, carbohydrate 34 g, fat less than
Nu...60 kJ (297 kcal)/100 g, with vitamins,
...ace elements. Maxamum products are generally
...e in children over 8 years.

...m powder (Nutricia Ltd)
CBS) · NHS indicative price = £165.09

...sinaemia

...LYS Anamix ® Infant
...onal supplement for the dietary management of proven
...lysinaemia in children from birth to 3 years.
...DER, protein equivalent (essential and non-essential amino
...ds except lysine) 13.1 g, carbohydrate 49.5 g, fat 23 g, fibre
...3 g, energy 1915 kJ (457 kcal)/100 g, with vitamins, minerals,
...and trace elements; standard dilution (15%) provides protein
equivalent 2 g, carbohydrate 7.4 g, fat 3.5 g, fibre 800 mg, energy
287 kJ (69 kcal)/100 mL.

HYPER LYS Anamix Infant powder (Nutricia Ltd)
400 gram (ACBS) · NHS indicative price = £40.79

HYPER LYS Maxamaid ®
▶ Nutritional supplement for the dietary management of
hyperlysinaemia.
POWDER, protein equivalent (essential and non-essential amino
acids except lysine) 25 g, carbohydrate 51 g, fat less than
500 mg, energy 1311 kJ (309 kcal)/100 g with vitamins, minerals,
and trace elements. Maxamaid products are generally intended
for use in children 1-8 years.

HYPER LYS Maxamaid powder (Nutricia Ltd)
500 gram (ACBS) · NHS indicative price = £103.00

Isovaleric acidaemia

IVA Anamix ® Infant
▶ Nutritional supplement for the dietary management of proven
isovaleric acidaemia or other proven disorders of leucine
metabolism in children from birth to 3 years.
POWDER, protein equivalent (essential and non-essential amino
acids except leucine) 13.1 g, carbohydrate 49.5 g, fat 23 g, fibre
5.3 g, energy 1915 kJ (457 kcal)/100 g, with vitamins, minerals,
and trace elements; standard dilution (15%) provides protein
equivalent 2 g, carbohydrate 7.4 g, fat 3.5 g, fibre 800 mg, energy
287 kJ (69 kcal)/100 mL.

IVA Anamix Infant powder (Nutricia Ltd)
400 gram (ACBS) · NHS indicative price = £40.79

Maple syrup urine disease

MSUD Aid III ®
▶ Nutritional supplement for the dietary management of maple
syrup urine disease and related conditions in children and
adults where it is necessary to limit the intake of branched
chain amino acids.
POWDER, protein equivalent (essential and non-essential amino
acids except isoleucine, leucine, and valine) 77 g, carbohydrate
4.5 g, fat nil, energy 1386 kJ (326 kcal)/100 g.

MSUD Aid 111 powder (Nutricia Ltd)
500 gram (ACBS) · NHS indicative price = £195.11

MSUD Anamix ® Infant
▶ Nutritional supplement for the dietary management of proven
maple syrup urine disease in children from birth to 3 years.
POWDER, protein equivalent (essential and non-essential amino
acids except isoleucine, leucine, and valine) 13.1 g,

carbohydrate 49.5 g, fat 23 g, fibre 5.3 g, energy 1915 kJ
(457 kcal)/100 g, with vitamins, minerals, and trace elements;
standard dilution (15%) provides protein equivalent 2 g,
carbohydrate 7.4 g, fat 3.5 g, fibre 800 mg, energy 287 kJ
(69 kcal)/100 mL.

MSUD Anamix Infant powder (Nutricia Ltd)
400 gram (ACBS) · NHS indicative price = £40.79

MSUD Anamix ® Junior
▶ Nutritional supplement for the dietary management of maple
syrup urine disease in children 1–10 years.
POWDER, protein equivalent (essential and non-essential amino
acids except isoleucine, leucine, and valine) 8.4 g, carbohydrate
11 g, fat 3.9 g, energy 474 kJ (113 kcal)/29-g sachet, with
vitamins, minerals, and trace elements.

MSUD Anamix Junior oral powder 36 g sachets (Nutricia Ltd)
30 sachet (ACBS) · NHS indicative price = £218.10

MSUD Anamix ® Junior LQ
▶ Nutritional supplement for the dietary management of maple
syrup urine disease in children 1–10 years.
LIQUID, protein equivalent (essential and non-essential amino
acids except isoleucine, leucine, and valine) 10 g, carbohydrate
8.8 g, fat 4.8 g, fibre 310 mg, energy 497 kJ (118 kcal)/125 mL,
with vitamins, minerals, and trace elements. Lactose-free.

MSUD Anamix Junior LQ liquid (Nutricia Ltd)
125 ml (ACBS) · NHS indicative price = £9.46

MSUD cooler ® 15
▶ Nutritional supplement for the dietary management of maple
syrup urine disease in children over 3 years and adults.
LIQUID, protein equivalent (essential and non-essential amino
acids except leucine, isoleucine, and valine) 15 g, carbohydrate
7 g, fat 500 mg, energy 393 kJ (92 kcal)/130-mL pouch, with
vitamins, minerals, and trace elements.

MSUD orange cooler 15 liquid (Vitaflo International Ltd)
130 ml (ACBS) · NHS indicative price = £11.87

MSUD red cooler 15 liquid (Vitaflo International Ltd)
130 ml (ACBS) · NHS indicative price = £11.87

MSUD express ® 15
▶ Nutritional supplement for the dietary management of maple
syrup urine disease in children over 8 years and adults.
POWDER, protein equivalent (essential and non-essential amino
acids except leucine, isoleucine, and valine) 15 g, carbohydrate
3.8 g, fat less than 100 mg, energy 315 kJ (75 kcal)/25 g, with
vitamins, minerals, and trace elements. To flavour unflavoured
products, see FlavourPac p. 1521.

MSUD express 15 oral powder 25g sachets (Vitaflo International Ltd)
30 sachet (ACBS) · NHS indicative price = £349.27

MSUD express ® 20
▶ Nutritional supplement for the dietary management of maple
syrup urine disease in children over 8 years and adults.
POWDER, protein equivalent (essential and non-essential amino
acids except leucine, isoleucine, and valine) 20 g, carbohydrate
4.7 g, fat less than 100 mg, energy 416 kJ (99 kcal)/34 g, with
vitamins, minerals, and trace elements. To flavour unflavoured
products, see FlavourPac p. 1521.

MSUD express 20 oral powder 34g sachets (Vitaflo International Ltd)
30 sachet (ACBS) · NHS indicative price = £451.25

MSUD Gel ®
▶ Nutritional supplement for the dietary management of maple
syrup urine disease in children 1–10 years.
POWDER, protein equivalent (essential and non-essential amino
acids except leucine, isoleucine, and valine) 10 g, carbohydrate
10.3 g, fat less than 100 mg, energy 339 kJ (81 kcal)/24 g, with
vitamins, minerals, and trace elements. To flavour unflavoured
products, see FlavourPac p. 1521.

MSUD gel 24g sachets (Vitaflo International Ltd)
30 sachet (ACBS) · NHS indicative price = £227.50

MSUD Lophlex ® LQ 20
▶ Nutritional supplement for the dietary management of maple
syrup urine disease in children over 3 years.

LIQUID, protein equivalent (essential and non-essential amino acids except isoleucine, leucine, and valine) 20 g, carbohydrate 8.8 g, fat less than 500 mg, energy 509 kJ (120 kcal)/125 mL, with vitamins, minerals, and trace elements.

MSUD Lophlex LQ 20 liquid (Nutricia Ltd)
125 ml (ACBS) · NHS indicative price = £16.82

MSUD Maxamum ®
▸ Nutritional supplement for the dietary management of maple syrup urine disease.
POWDER, protein equivalent (essential and non-essential amino acids except isoleucine, leucine, and valine) 39 g, carbohydrate 34 g, fat less than 500 mg, energy 1260 kJ (297 kcal)/100 g, with vitamins, minerals, and trace elements. Maxamum products are generally intended for use in children over 8 years.

MSUD Maxamum powder orange (Nutricia Ltd)
500 gram (ACBS) · NHS indicative price = £165.09

MSUD Maxamum powder unflavoured (Nutricia Ltd)
500 gram (ACBS) · NHS indicative price = £165.09

Methylmalonic or propionic acidaemia

MMA/PA Anamix ® **Infant**
▸ Nutritional supplement for the dietary management of proven methylmalonic acidaemia or propionic acidaemia in children from birth to 3 years.
POWDER, protein equivalent (essential and non-essential amino acids except methionine, threonine, and valine, and low isoleucine) 13.1 g, carbohydrate 49.5 g, fat 23 g, fibre 5.3 g, energy 1915 kJ (457 kcal)/100 g, with vitamins, minerals, and trace elements; standard dilution (15%) provides protein equivalent 2 g, carbohydrate 7.4 g, fat 3.5 g, fibre 800 mg, energy 287 kJ (69 kcal)/100 mL.

MMA / PA Anamix Infant powder (Nutricia Ltd)
400 gram (ACBS) · NHS indicative price = £40.79

XMTVI Asadon ®
▸ Nutritional supplement for the dietary management of methylmalonic acidaemia or propionic acidaemia in children and adults.
POWDER, protein equivalent (essential and non-essential amino acids except methionine, threonine, and valine, and low isoleucine) 77 g, carbohydrate 4.5 g, fat nil, energy 1386 kJ (326 kcal)/100 g.

XMTVI Asadon powder (Nutricia Ltd)
200 gram (ACBS) · NHS indicative price = £78.04

MMA/PA Maxamum ®
▸ Nutritional supplement for the dietary management of methylmalonic acidaemia or propionic acidaemia.
POWDER, protein equivalent (essential and non-essential amino acids except methionine, threonine, and valine, and low isoleucine) 39 g, carbohydrate 34 g, fat less than 500 mg, energy 1260 kJ (297 kcal)/100 g, with vitamins, minerals, and trace elements. Maxamum products are generally intended for use in children over 8 years.

MMA/PA Maxamum powder (Nutricia Ltd)
500 gram (ACBS) · NHS indicative price = £165.09

Other inborn errors of metabolism

Cystine500 ®
▸ Nutritional supplement for the dietary management of inborn errors of amino acid metabolism in adults and children from birth.
POWDER, cystine 500 mg, carbohydrate 3.3 g, fat nil, energy 63 kJ (15 kcal)/4 g

Cystine500 oral powder sachets (Vitaflo International Ltd)
30 sachet (ACBS) · NHS indicative price = £57.14

DocOmega ®
▸ Nutritional supplement for the dietary management of inborn errors of metabolism for adults and children from birth.

POWDER, protein (cows' milk, soya) 100 mg, carbohydrate 3.2 g, fat 500 mg (of which docosahexaenoic acid 200 mg), fibre nil, energy 74 kJ (18 kcal)/4 g, with minerals

DocOmega oral powder 4g sachets (Vitaflo International Ltd)
30 sachet (ACBS) · NHS indicative price = £41.35

EAA ® **Supplement**
▸ Nutritional supplement for the dietary management of disorders of protein metabolism including urea cycle disorders in children over 3 years.
POWDER, protein equivalent (essential amino acids) 5 g, carbohydrate 4 g, fat nil, energy 151 kJ (36 kcal)/12.5 g, with vitamins, minerals, and trace elements.

EAA Supplement oral powder 12.5g sachets (Vitaflo International Ltd)
50 sachet (ACBS) · NHS indicative price = £215.60

Isoleucine50 ®
▸ Nutritional supplement for use in the dietary management of inborn errors of amino acid metabolism in adults and children from birth.
POWDER, isoleucine 50 mg, carbohydrate 3.8 g, fat nil, energy 63 kJ (15 kcal)/4 g

Isoleucine50 oral powder 4g sachets (Vitaflo International Ltd)
30 sachet (ACBS) · NHS indicative price = £57.14

KeyOmega ®
▸ Nutritional supplement for the dietary management of inborn errors of metabolism.
POWDER, protein (cows' milk, soya) 170 mg, carbohydrate 2.8 g, fat 800 mg (of which arachidonic acid 200 mg, docosahexaenoic acid 100 mg), energy 80 kJ (19 kcal)/4 g.

KeyOmega oral powder 4g sachets (Vitaflo International Ltd)
30 sachet (ACBS) · NHS indicative price = £42.29

Leucine100 ®
▸ Nutritional supplement for the dietary management of inborn errors of amino acid metabolism in adults and children from birth.
POWDER, leucine 100 mg, carbohydrate 3.7 g, fat nil, energy 63 kJ (15 kcal)/4 g

Leucine100 oral powder sachets (Vitaflo International Ltd)
30 sachet (ACBS) · NHS indicative price = £57.14

Low protein drink
▸ Nutritional supplement for the dietary management of inborn errors of amino acid metabolism in adults and children over 1 year.
POWDER, protein (cows' milk) 4.5 g (phenylalanine 100 mg), carbohydrate 59.5 g, fat 29.9 g, fibre nil, energy 2194 kJ (528 kcal)/100 g, with vitamins, minerals, and trace elements. Contains lactose.
Termed *Milupa® lp-drink* by manufacturer.

Milupa LP drink (Nutricia Ltd)
400 gram (ACBS) · NHS indicative price = £9.68

Phenylalanine50 ®
▸ Nutritional supplement for use in the dietary management of inborn errors of metabolism in adults and children from birth.
POWDER, phenylalanine 50 mg, carbohydrate 3.8 g, fat nil, energy 63 kJ (15 kcal)/4 g

Phenylalanine50 oral powder sachets (Vitaflo International Ltd)
30 sachet (ACBS) · NHS indicative price = £55.48

ProZero ®
▸ A protein-free nutritional supplement for the dietary management of inborn errors of metabolism in children over 6 months and adults.
LIQUID, carbohydrate 8.1 g (of which sugars 3.5 g), fat 3.8 g, energy 278 kJ (66 kcal)/100 mL. Contains lactose.

ProZero liquid (Vitaflo International Ltd)
250 ml (ACBS) · NHS indicative price = £1.52 | 1000 ml (ACBS) · NHS indicative price = £6.09

Tyrosine1000 ®
▸ Nutritional supplement for the dietary management of inborn errors of amino acid metabolism in adults and children from birth.

POWDER, tyrosine 1 g, carbohydrate 2.9 g, fat nil, energy 63 kJ (15 kcal)/4-g sachet.

Tyrosine1000 oral powder 4g sachets (Vitaflo International Ltd)
30 sachet (ACBS) · NHS indicative price = £5.23

Valine50 ®
▸ Nutritional supplement for the dietary management of inborn errors of amino acid metabolism in adults and children from birth.
POWDER, valine 50 mg, carbohydrate 3.8 g, fat nil, energy 63 kJ (15 kcal)/4 g

Valine50 oral powder 4g sachets (Vitaflo International Ltd)
30 sachet (ACBS) · NHS indicative price = £57.14

Phenylketonuria

Add-Ins ®
▸ Nutritional supplement for the dietary management of proven phenylketonuria in children over 4 years.
POWDER, protein equivalent (containing essential and non-essential amino acids except phenylalanine) 10 g, carbohydrate nil, fat 5.1 g, energy 359 kJ (86 kcal)/18.2-g sachet, with vitamins, minerals, and trace elements.

Add Ins oral powder 18.2g sachets (Nutricia Ltd)
60 sachet (ACBS) · NHS indicative price = £394.20

Easiphen ®
▸ Nutritional supplement for the dietary management of proven phenylketonuria in children over 8 years.
LIQUID, protein equivalent (containing essential and non-essential amino acids except phenylalanine) 6.7 g, carbohydrate 5.1 g, fat 2 g, energy 275 kJ (65 kcal)/100 mL with vitamins, minerals, and trace elements.

Easiphen liquid (Nutricia Ltd)
250 ml (ACBS) · NHS indicative price = £10.12

L-Tyrosine
▸ Nutritional supplement for the dietary management of phenylketonuria in pregnant women with low plasma tyrosine concentrations.
POWDER, L-tyrosine 20 g, carbohydrate 76.8 g, fat nil, energy 1612 kJ (379 kcal)/100 g.

L-Tyrosine powder (Nutricia Ltd)
100 gram (ACBS) · NHS indicative price = £22.98

Lophlex ®
▸ Nutritional supplement for the dietary management of proven phenylketonuria in children over 8 years and adults including pregnant women.
POWDER, protein equivalent (essential and non-essential amino acids except phenylalanine) 20 g, carbohydrate 2.5 g, fat 60 mg, fibre 220 mg, energy 385 kJ (91 kcal)/27.8-g sachet, with vitamins, minerals, and trace elements.

Lophlex powder 27.8g sachets berry (Nutricia Ltd)
30 sachet (ACBS) · NHS indicative price = £303.90

Lophlex powder 27.8g sachets orange (Nutricia Ltd)
30 sachet (ACBS) · NHS indicative price = £303.90

Lophlex powder 27.8g sachets unflavoured (Nutricia Ltd)
30 sachet (ACBS) · NHS indicative price = £303.90

Loprofin ® **PKU Drink**
▸ Nutritional supplement for the dietary management of phenylketonuria in children over 1 year and adults.
LIQUID, protein (cows' milk) 400 mg (phenylalanine 10 mg), lactose 9.4 g, fat 2 g, energy 165 kJ (40 kcal)/100 mL.

Loprofin PKU drink (Nutricia Ltd)
200 ml (ACBS) · NHS indicative price = £0.79

Loprofin ® **Sno-Pro**
▸ Nutritional supplement for the dietary management of phenylketonuria, chronic renal failure and other inborn errors of amino acid metabolism.
LIQUID, protein (cows' milk) 220 mg (phenylalanine 12.5 mg), carbohydrate 8 g, fat 3.8 g, energy 273 kJ (65 kcal)/100 mL. Contains lactose.

Loprofin SNO-PRO drink (Nutricia Ltd)
200 ml (ACBS) · NHS indicative price = £1.31

Phlexy-10 ® **Exchange System**
▸ Nutritional supplement for the dietary management of phenylketonuria.
CAPSULES, protein equivalent (essential and non-essential amino acids except phenylalanine) 416.5 mg/capsule.

Phlexy-10 500mg capsules (Nutricia Ltd)
200 capsule (ACBS) · NHS indicative price = £45.49
TABLETS, protein equivalent (essential and non-essential amino acids except phenylalanine) 833 mg tablet.

Phlexy-10 tablets (Nutricia Ltd)
75 tablet (ACBS) · NHS indicative price = £29.25
DRINK MIX, powder, protein equivalent (essential and non-essential amino acids except phenylalanine) 8.33 g, carbohydrate 8.8 g/20-g sachet.

Phlexy-10 drink mix apple & blackcurrant (Nutricia Ltd)
600 gram (ACBS) · NHS indicative price = £134.70

Phlexy-10 drink mix citrus burst (Nutricia Ltd)
600 gram (ACBS) · NHS indicative price = £134.70

Phlexy-10 drink mix tropical surprise (Nutricia Ltd)
600 gram (ACBS) · NHS indicative price = £134.70

Phlexy-Vits ®
▸ For use as a vitamin and mineral component of restricted therapeutic diets in children over 11 years and adults with phenylketonuria and similar amino acid abnormalities.
POWDER, vitamins, minerals, and trace elements

Phlexy-Vits powder (Nutricia Ltd)
210 gram (ACBS) · NHS indicative price = £74.70
TABLETS, vitamins, minerals, and trace elements

Phlexy-Vits tablets (Nutricia Ltd)
180 tablet (ACBS) · NHS indicative price = £85.60

PK Aid 4 ®
▸ Nutritional supplement for the dietary management of phenylketonuria in children and adults.
POWDER, protein equivalent (essential and non-essential amino acids except phenylalanine) 79 g, carbohydrate 4.5 g, fat nil, energy 1420 kJ (334 kcal)/100 g.

PK Aid 4 powder (Nutricia Ltd)
500 gram (ACBS) · NHS indicative price = £149.97

PKU Anamix Junior LQ ®
LIQUID, protein equivalent (essential and non-essential amino acids except phenylalanine) 10 g, carbohydrate 8.8 g, fat 4.8 g, fibre 310 mg, energy 497 kJ (118 kcal)/125 mL, with vitamins, minerals, and trace elements. Lactose-free.

PKU Anamix Junior LQ liquid berry (Nutricia Ltd)
125 ml (ACBS) · NHS indicative price = £5.88

PKU Anamix ® **Infant**
▸ Nutritional supplement for the dietary management of proven phenylketonuria in children from birth to 3 years.
POWDER, protein equivalent (essential and non-essential amino acids except phenylalanine) 13.1 g, carbohydrate 49.5 g, fat 23 g, fibre 5.3 g, energy 1915 kJ (457 kcal)/100 g, with vitamins, minerals, and trace elements; standard dilution (15%) provides protein equivalent 2 g, carbohydrate 7.4 g, fat 3.5 g, fibre 800 mg, energy 287 kJ (69 kcal)/100 mL

PKU Anamix Infant powder (Nutricia Ltd)
400 gram (ACBS) · NHS indicative price = £37.08

PKU Anamix ® **Junior**
▸ Nutritional supplement for the dietary management of phenylketonuria in children 1–10 years.
POWDER, protein equivalent (essential and non-essential amino acids except phenylalanine) 8.4 g, carbohydrate 9.9 g, fat 3.9 g, energy 455 kJ (108 kcal)/29-g sachet, with vitamins, minerals, and trace elements

PKU Anamix Junior powder chocolate (Nutricia Ltd)
1080 gram (ACBS) · NHS indicative price = £132.60

PKU Anamix Junior powder neutral (Nutricia Ltd)
1080 gram (ACBS) · NHS indicative price = £132.60

PKU Anamix ® Junior LQ
▸ Nutritional supplement for the dietary supplement of phenyketonuria in children 1–10 years.
LIQUID, protein equivalent (essential and non-essential amino acids except phenylalanine) 10 g, carbohydrate 8.8 g, fat 4.8 g, fibre 310 mg, energy 497 kJ (118 kcal)/125 mL, with vitamins, minerals, and trace elements. Lactose-free.
PKU Anamix Junior LQ liquid berry (Nutricia Ltd)
125 ml (ACBS) · NHS indicative price = £5.88
PKU Anamix Junior LQ liquid orange (Nutricia Ltd)
125 ml (ACBS) · NHS indicative price = £5.88

PKU cooler10 ®
▸ Nutritional supplement for the dietary management of phenylketonuria in children over 3 years.
LIQUID, protein equivalent (essential and non-essential amino acids except phenylalanine) 10 g, carbohydrate 5.1 g, energy 258 kJ (62 kcal)/87-mL pouch, with vitamins, minerals, and trace elements.
PKU orange cooler 10 liquid (Vitaflo International Ltd)
87 ml (ACBS) · NHS indicative price = £4.83
PKU purple cooler 10 liquid (Vitaflo International Ltd)
87 ml (ACBS) · NHS indicative price = £4.83
PKU red cooler 10 liquid (Vitaflo International Ltd)
87 ml (ACBS) · NHS indicative price = £4.83
PKU white cooler 10 liquid (Vitaflo International Ltd)
87 ml (ACBS) · NHS indicative price = £4.83

PKU cooler15 ®
▸ Nutritional supplement for the dietary management of phenylketonuria in children over 3 years.
LIQUID, protein equivalent (essential and non-essential amino acids except phenylalanine) 15 g, carbohydrate 7.8 g, energy 386 kJ (92 kcal)/130-mL pouch, with vitamins, minerals, and trace elements.
PKU orange cooler 15 liquid (Vitaflo International Ltd)
130 ml (ACBS) · NHS indicative price = £7.19
PKU purple cooler 15 liquid (Vitaflo International Ltd)
130 ml (ACBS) · NHS indicative price = £7.19
PKU red cooler 15 liquid (Vitaflo International Ltd)
130 ml (ACBS) · NHS indicative price = £7.19
PKU white cooler 15 liquid (Vitaflo International Ltd)
130 ml (ACBS) · NHS indicative price = £7.19

PKU cooler20 ®
▸ Nutritional supplement for the dietary management of phenylketonuria in children over 3 years.
LIQUID, protein equivalent (essential and non-essential amino acids except phenylalanine) 20 g, carbohydrate 10.2 g, energy 517 kJ (124 kcal)/174-mL pouch, with vitamins, minerals, and trace elements.
PKU orange cooler 20 liquid (Vitaflo International Ltd)
174 ml (ACBS) · NHS indicative price = £9.66
PKU purple cooler 20 liquid (Vitaflo International Ltd)
174 ml (ACBS) · NHS indicative price = £9.66
PKU red cooler 20 liquid (Vitaflo International Ltd)
174 ml (ACBS) · NHS indicative price = £9.66
PKU white cooler 20 liquid (Vitaflo International Ltd)
174 ml (ACBS) · NHS indicative price = £9.66

PKU express15 ®
▸ Nutritional supplement for the dietary management of phenylketonuria. Not recommended for children under 3 years.
POWDER, protein equivalent (essential and non-essential amino acids except phenylalanine) 15 g, carbohydrate 2.4 g, energy 293 kJ (70 kcal)/25 g, with vitamins, minerals, and trace elements. To flavour unflavoured products, see FlavourPac p. 1521.
PKU express 15 powder lemon (Vitaflo International Ltd)
750 gram (ACBS) · NHS indicative price = £211.75
PKU express 15 powder orange (Vitaflo International Ltd)
750 gram (ACBS) · NHS indicative price = £211.75

PKU express 15 powder tropical (Vitaflo International Ltd)
750 gram (ACBS) · NHS indicative price = £211.75
PKU express 15 powder unflavoured (Vitaflo International Ltd)
750 gram (ACBS) · NHS indicative price = £211.75

PKU express20 ®
▸ Nutritional supplement for the dietary management of phenylketonuria. Not recommended for children under 3 years.
POWDER, protein equivalent (essential and non-essential amino acids except phenylalanine) 20 g, carbohydrate 3.3 g, energy 389 kJ (93 kcal)/34 g, with vitamins, minerals, and trace elements. To flavour unflavoured products, see FlavourPac p. 1521.
PKU express 20 powder lemon (Vitaflo International Ltd)
1020 gram (ACBS) · NHS indicative price = £273.57
PKU express 20 powder orange (Vitaflo International Ltd)
1020 gram (ACBS) · NHS indicative price = £273.57
PKU express 20 powder tropical (Vitaflo International Ltd)
1020 gram (ACBS) · NHS indicative price = £273.57
PKU express 20 powder unflavoured (Vitaflo International Ltd)
1020 gram (ACBS) · NHS indicative price = £273.57

PKU gel ®
▸ For use as part of the low-protein dietary management of phenylketonuria in children 1–10 years
POWDER, protein equivalent (essential and non-essential amino acids except phenylalanine) 10 g, carbohydrate 8.9 g, fat less than 100 mg, energy 318 kJ (76 kcal)/24 g, with vitamins, minerals, and trace elements. To flavour unflavoured products, see FlavourPac p. 1521.
PKU gel powder orange (Vitaflo International Ltd)
720 gram (ACBS) · NHS indicative price = £146.49
PKU gel powder raspberry (Vitaflo International Ltd)
720 gram (ACBS) · NHS indicative price = £146.49
PKU gel powder unflavoured (Vitaflo International Ltd)
720 gram (ACBS) · NHS indicative price = £146.49

PKU Lophlex ® LQ 10
▸ Nutritional supplement for the dietary management of phenylketonuria in children over 4 years and adults including pregnant women.
LIQUID, protein equivalent (essential and non-essential amino acids except phenylalanine) 10 g, carbohydrate 4.4 g, fibre 250 mg, energy 245 kJ (58 kcal)/62.5 mL, with vitamins, minerals, and trace elements.
PKU Lophlex LQ 10 liquid berry (Nutricia Ltd)
62.5 ml (ACBS) · NHS indicative price = £5.43
PKU Lophlex LQ 10 liquid juicy berries (Nutricia Ltd)
62.5 ml (ACBS) · NHS indicative price = £5.43
PKU Lophlex LQ 10 liquid juicy orange (Nutricia Ltd)
62.5 ml (ACBS) · NHS indicative price = £5.43

PKU Lophlex ® LQ 20
▸ Nutritional supplement for the dietary management of phenylketonuria in children over 4 years and adults including pregnant women.
LIQUID, protein equivalent (essential and non-essential amino acids except phenylalanine) 20 g, carbohydrate 8.8 g, fibre 340 mg, energy 490 kJ (115 kcal)/125 mL, with vitamins, minerals, and trace elements.
PKU Lophlex LQ 20 liquid berry (Nutricia Ltd)
125 ml (ACBS) · NHS indicative price = £10.83
PKU Lophlex LQ 20 liquid juicy berries (Nutricia Ltd)
125 ml (ACBS) · NHS indicative price = £10.83
PKU Lophlex LQ 20 liquid juicy orange (Nutricia Ltd)
125 ml (ACBS) · NHS indicative price = £10.83
PKU Lophlex LQ 20 liquid orange (Nutricia Ltd)
125 ml (ACBS) · NHS indicative price = £10.83

PKU Lophlex ® Sensation 20
▸ Nutritional supplement for the dietary management of phenylketonuria in children over 4 years and adults including pregnant women.
SEMI-SOLID, protein equivalent (containing essential and non-essential amino acids except phenylalanine) 20 g, carbohydrate

A2

Borderline substances | Appendix 2

20.2 g, fibre 1 g, energy 706 kJ (166 kcal)/109 g, with vitamins, minerals, and trace elements.

PKU Lophlex Sensation 20 berries (Nutricia Ltd)
327 gram (ACBS) · NHS indicative price = £34.59

PKU squeezie ®
▸ Nutritional supplement for the dietary management of phenylketonuria in children from 6 months to 10 years.
LIQUID, protein equivalent (essential and non-essential amino acids except phenylalanine) 10 g, carbohydrate 22.5 g, fat 500 mg, energy 565 kJ (135 kcal)/85 g, with vitamins, minerals, and trace elements.

PKU squeezie liquid (Vitaflo International Ltd)
2550 gram (ACBS) · NHS indicative price = £140.04

PKU Maxamum ®
▸ Nutritional supplement for the dietary management of phenylketonuria in children over 8 years and adults.
POWDER, protein equivalent (essential and non-essential amino acids except phenylalanine) 39 g, carbohydrate 34 g, fat less than 500 mg, energy 1260 kJ (297 kcal)/100 g, with vitamins, minerals, and trace elements.

PKU Maxamum oral powder 50g sachets orange (Nutricia Ltd)
30 sachet (ACBS) · NHS indicative price = £282.60

PKU Maxamum oral powder 50g sachets unflavoured (Nutricia Ltd)
30 sachet (ACBS) · NHS indicative price = £282.60

PKU Maxamum powder orange (Nutricia Ltd)
500 gram (ACBS) · NHS indicative price = £94.24

PKU Maxamum powder unflavoured (Nutricia Ltd)
500 gram (ACBS) · NHS indicative price = £94.24

Tyrosinaemia

Methionine-free TYR Anamix ® Infant
▸ Nutritional supplement for the dietary management of proven tyrosinaemia type 1 in children from birth to 3 years.
POWDER, protein equivalent (essential and non-essential amino acids except methionine, phenylalanine, and tyrosine) 13.1 g, carbohydrate 49.5 g, fat 23 g, fibre 5.3 g, energy 1915 kJ (457 kcal)/100 g, with vitamins, minerals, and trace elements; standard dilution (15%) provides protein equivalent 2 g, carbohydrate 7.4 g, fat 3.5 g, fibre 800 mg, energy 287 kJ (69 kcal)/100 mL.

TYR Anamix Infant methionine free powder (Nutricia Ltd)
400 gram (ACBS) · NHS indicative price = £40.79

TYR Anamix ® Infant
▸ Nutritional supplement for the dietary management of proven tyrosinaemia where plasma-methionine concentrations are normal in children from birth to 3 years.
POWDER, protein equivalent (essential and non-essential amino acids except phenylalanine and tyrosine) 13.1 g, carbohydrate 49.5 g, fat 23 g, fibre 5.3 g, energy 1915 kJ (457 kcal)/100 g, with vitamins, minerals, and trace elements; standard dilution (15%) provides protein equivalent 2 g, carbohydrate 7.4 g, fat 3.5 g, fibre 800 mg, energy 287 kJ (69 kcal)/100 mL.

TYR Anamix Infant methionine free powder (Nutricia Ltd)
400 gram (ACBS) · NHS indicative price = £40.79

TYR Anamix Infant powder (Nutricia Ltd)
400 gram (ACBS) · NHS indicative price = £40.79

TYR Anamix ® Junior
▸ Nutritional supplement for the dietary management of proven tyrosinaemia in children 1–10 years.
POWDER, protein equivalent (essential and non-essential amino acids except phenylalanine and tyrosine) 8.4 g, carbohydrate 11 g, fat 3.9 g, energy 475 kJ (113 kcal)/29-g sachet, with vitamins, minerals, and trace elements.

TYR Anamix Junior oral powder 29g sachets (Nutricia Ltd)
30 sachet (ACBS) · NHS indicative price = £206.40

TYR Anamix ® Junior LQ
▸ Nutritional supplement for the dietary management of tyrosinaemia type 1 (when nitisinone (NTBC) is used, see nitisinone p. 1035), type II, and type III, in children over 1 year.

LIQUID, protein equivalent (essential and non-essential amino acids except phenylalanine and tyrosine) 10 g, carbohydrate 8.8 g, fat 4.8 g, fibre 310 mg, energy 500 kJ (119 kcal)/125 mL, with vitamins, minerals and trace elements.

TYR Anamix Junior LQ liquid (Nutricia Ltd)
125 ml (ACBS) · NHS indicative price = £9.46

TYR cooler ® 15
▸ Nutritional supplement for the dietary management of tyrosinaemia in children over 3 years and adults.
LIQUID, protein equivalent (essential and non-essential amino acids except tyrosine and phenylalanine) 15 g, carbohydrate 7 g, fat 500 mg, energy 393 kJ (92 kcal)/130 mL, with vitamins, minerals, and trace elements.

TYR orange cooler 15 liquid (Vitaflo International Ltd)
130 ml (ACBS) · NHS indicative price = £11.87

TYR red cooler 10 liquid (Vitaflo International Ltd)
87 ml (ACBS) · NHS indicative price = £7.60

TYR red cooler 15 liquid (Vitaflo International Ltd)
130 ml (ACBS) · NHS indicative price = £11.87

TYR red cooler 20 liquid (Vitaflo International Ltd)
174 ml (ACBS) · NHS indicative price = £15.89

TYR express15 ®
▸ Nutritional supplement for the dietary management of tyrosinaemia in children over 8 years and adults.
POWDER, protein equivalent (essential and non-essential amino acids except tyrosine and phenylalanine) 15 g, carbohydrate 3.4 g, fat less than 100 mg, energy 310 kJ (74 kcal)/25 g, with vitamins, minerals, and trace elements. To flavour unflavoured products, see FlavourPac p. 1521.

TYR express 15 oral powder 25g sachets (Vitaflo International Ltd)
30 sachet (ACBS) · NHS indicative price = £349.27

TYR express20 ®
▸ Nutritional supplement for the dietary management of tyrosinaemia in children over 8 years.
POWDER, protein equivalent (essential and non-essential amino acids except tyrosine and phenylalanine) 20 g, carbohydrate 4.7 g, fat less than 100 mg, energy 416 kJ (99 kcal)/34 g, with vitamins, minerals, and trace elements. To flavour unflavoured products, see FlavourPac p. 1521.

TYR express 20 oral powder 34g sachets (Vitaflo International Ltd)
30 sachet (ACBS) · NHS indicative price = £451.25

TYR Gel ®
▸ Nutritional supplement for the dietary management of tyrosinaemia in children 1–10 years.
GEL, protein equivalent (essential and non-essential amino acids except tyrosine and phenylalanine) 10 g, carbohydrate 10.3 g, fat less than 100 mg, energy 339 kJ (81 kcal)/24 g, with vitamins, minerals and trace elements. To flavour unflavoured products, see FlavourPac p. 1521.

TYR gel oral powder 24g sachets (Vitaflo International Ltd)
30 sachet (ACBS) · NHS indicative price = £224.86

TYR Lophlex ® LQ 20
▸ Nutritional supplement for the dietary management of tyrosinaemia in children over 3 years and adults.
LIQUID, protein equivalent (essential and non-essential amino acids except tyrosine and phenylalanine) 20 g, carbohydrate 8.8 g, fat less than 500 mg, fibre 500 mg, energy 509 kJ (120 kcal)/125 mL, with vitamins, minerals, and trace elements.

TYR Lophlex LQ 20 liquid (Nutricia Ltd)
125 ml (ACBS) · NHS indicative price = £16.82

XPHEN TYR Tyrosidon ®
▸ Nutritional supplement for the management of tyrosinaemia in children and adults where plasma-methionine concentrations are normal.
POWDER, protein equivalent (essential and non-essential amino acids except phenylalanine and tyrosine) 77 g, carbohydrate 4.5 g, fat nil, energy 1386 kJ (326 kcal)/100 g.

XPHEN TYR Tyrosidon Free AA Mix powder (Nutricia Ltd)
500 gram (ACBS) · NHS indicative price = £195.11

XPTM Tyrosidon ®

▸ Nutritional supplement for the dietary management of tyrosinaemia type I in children and adults where plasma-methionine concentrations are above normal.

POWDER, protein equivalent (essential and non-essential amino acids except methionine, phenylalanine, and tyrosine) 77 g, carbohydrate 4.5 g, fat nil, energy 1386 kJ (326 kcal)/100 g.

XPTM Tyrosidon powder (Nutricia Ltd)
500 gram · NHS indicative price = £91.31

Appendix 3
Cautionary and advisory labels for dispensed medicines

Guidance for cautionary and advisory labels

Medicinal forms within BNF publications include code numbers of the cautionary labels that pharmacists are recommended to add when dispensing. It is also expected that pharmacists will counsel patients and carers when necessary.

Counselling needs to be related to the age, experience, background, and understanding of the individual patient or carer. The pharmacist should ensure understanding of how to take or use the medicine and how to follow the correct dosage schedule. Any effects of the medicine on co-ordination, performance of skilled tasks (e.g. driving or work), any foods or medicines to be avoided, and what to do if a dose is missed should also be explained. Other matters, such as the possibility of staining of the clothes or skin, or discolouration of urine or stools by a medicine should also be mentioned.

For some medicines there is a special need for counselling, such as an unusual method or time of administration or a potential interaction with a common food or domestic remedy, and this should be mentioned where necessary.

Original packs

Most preparations are dispensed in unbroken original packs that include further advice for the patient in the form of patient information leaflets. Label 10 may be of value where appropriate. More general leaflets advising on the administration of preparations such as eye drops, eye ointments, inhalers, and suppositories are also available.

Scope of labels

In general no label recommendations have been made for injections on the assumption that they will be administered by a healthcare professional or a well-instructed patient. The labelling is not exhaustive and pharmacists are recommended to use their professional discretion in labelling new preparations and those for which no labels are shown.

Individual labelling advice is not given on the administration of the large variety of antacids. In the absence of instructions from the prescriber, and if on enquiry the patient has had no verbal instructions, the directions given under 'Dose' should be used on the label.

It is recognised that there may be occasions when pharmacists will use their knowledge and professional discretion and decide to omit one or more of the recommended labels for a particular patient. In this case counselling is of the utmost importance. There may also be an occasion when a prescriber does not wish additional cautionary labels to be used, in which case the prescription should be endorsed 'NCL' (no cautionary labels). The exact wording that is required instead should then be specified on the prescription.

Pharmacists label medicines with various wordings in addition to those directions specified on the prescription. Such labels include 'Shake the bottle', 'For external use only', and 'Store in a cool place', as well as 'Discard.... days after opening' and 'Do not use after....', which apply particularly to antibiotic mixtures, diluted liquid and topical preparations, and to eye-drops. Although not listed in the BNF these labels should continue to be used when appropriate; indeed, 'For external use only' is a legal requirement on external liquid preparations, while 'Keep out of the reach of children' is a legal requirement on all dispensed medicines. Care should be taken not to obscure other relevant information with adhesive labelling.

It is the usual practice for patients to take standard tablets with water or other liquid and for this reason no separate label has been recommended.

The label wordings recommended by the BNF apply to medicines dispensed against a prescription. Patients should be aware that a dispensed medicine should never be taken by, or shared with, anyone other than for whom the prescriber intended it. Therefore, the BNF does not include warnings against the use of a dispensed medicine by persons other than for whom it was specifically prescribed.

The label or labels for each preparation are recommended after careful consideration of the information available. However, it is recognised that in some cases this information may be either incomplete or open to a different interpretation. The BNF will therefore be grateful to receive any constructive comments on the labelling suggested for any preparation.

Recommended label wordings

For BNF 61 (March 2011), a revised set of cautionary and advisory labels were introduced. All of the existing labels were user-tested, and the revised wording selected reflects terminology that is better understood by patients.

Wordings which can be given as separate warnings are labels 1–19, 29–30, and 32. Wordings which can be incorporated in an appropriate position in the directions for dosage or administration are labels 21–28. A label has been omitted for number 20; labels 31 and 33 no longer apply to any medicines in the BNF and have therefore been deleted.

If separate labels are used it is recommended that the wordings be used without modification. If changes are made to suit computer requirements, care should be taken to retain the sense of the original.

Welsh labels

Comprehensive Welsh translations are available for each cautionary and advisory label.

Labels

1   **Warning: This medicine may make you sleepy**

   Rhybudd: Gall y feddyginiaeth hon eich gwneud yn gysglyd
   To be used on *preparations for children* containing antihistamines, or other preparations given to children where the warnings of label 2 on driving or alcohol would not be appropriate.

2   **Warning: This medicine may make you sleepy. If this happens, do not drive or use tools or machines. Do not drink alcohol**

   Rhybudd: Gall y feddyginiaeth hon eich gwneud yn gysglyd. Peidiwch â gyrru, defnyddio offer llaw neu beiriannau os yw hyn yn digwydd. Peidiwch ag yfed alcohol
   To be used on *preparations for adults that can cause drowsiness*, thereby affecting coordination and the ability to drive and operate hazardous machinery; label 1 is more appropriate for children. *It is an offence to drive while under the influence of drink or drugs.*

   Some of these preparations only cause drowsiness in the first few days of treatment and some only cause drowsiness in higher doses.

   In such cases the patient should be told that the advice applies until the effects have worn off. However many of these preparations can produce a slowing of reaction time and a loss of mental concentration that can have the same effects as drowsiness.

   Avoidance of alcoholic drink is recommended because the effects of CNS depressants are enhanced by alcohol. Strict prohibition however could lead to some patients not taking the medicine. Pharmacists should therefore explain the risk and encourage compliance, particularly in patients who may think they already tolerate the effects of alcohol (see also label 3). Queries from patients with epilepsy regarding fitness to drive should be referred back to the patient's doctor.

Side-effects unrelated to drowsiness that may affect a patient's ability to drive or operate machinery safely include *blurred vision, dizziness, or nausea*. In general, no label has been recommended to cover these cases, but the patient should be suitably counselled.

3 **Warning: This medicine may make you sleepy. If this happens, do not drive or use tools or machines**

Rhybudd: Gall y feddyginiaeth hon eich gwneud yn gysglyd. Peidiwch â gyrru, defnyddio offer llaw neu beiriannau os yw hyn yn digwydd
To be used on *preparations containing monoamine-oxidase inhibitors*; the warning to avoid alcohol and dealcoholised (low alcohol) drink is covered by the patient information leaflet.

Also to be used as for label 2 but where alcohol is not an issue.

4 **Warning: Do not drink alcohol**

Rhybudd: Peidiwch ag yfed alcohol
To be used on *preparations where a reaction such as flushing may occur if alcohol is taken* (e.g. metronidazole). Alcohol may also enhance the hypoglycaemia produced by some oral antidiabetic drugs but routine application of a warning label is not considered necessary.

Patients should be advised not to drink alcohol for as long as they are receiving/using a course of medication, and in some cases for a period of time after the course is finished.

5 **Do not take indigestion remedies 2 hours before or after you take this medicine**

Peidiwch â chymryd meddyginiaethau camdreuliad 2 awr cyn neu ar ôl y feddyginiaeth hon
To be used with label 25 on *preparations coated to resist gastric acid* (e.g. enteric-coated tablets). This is to avoid the possibility of premature dissolution of the coating in the presence of an alkaline pH.

Label 5 also applies to drugs such as gabapentin *where the absorption is significantly affected by antacids*. Pharmacists will be aware (from a knowledge of physiology) that the usual time during which indigestion remedies should be avoided is at least 2 hours before and after the majority of medicines have been taken; when a manufacturer advises a different time period, this can be followed, and should be explained to the patient.

6 **Do not take indigestion remedies, or medicines containing iron or zinc, 2 hours before or after you take this medicine**

Peidiwch â chymryd meddyginiaethau camdreuliad neu feddyginiaethau sy'n cynnwys haearn neu sinc, 2 awr cyn neu ar ôl y feddyginiaeth hon
To be used on *preparations containing ofloxacin and some other quinolones, doxycycline, lymecycline, minocycline, and penicillamine* . These drugs chelate calcium, iron, and zinc and are less well absorbed when taken with calcium-containing antacids or preparations containing iron or zinc. Pharmacists will be aware (from a knowledge of physiology) that these incompatible preparations should be taken at least 2 hours apart for the majority of medicines; when a manufacturer advises a different time period, this can be followed, and should be explained to the patient.

7 **Do not take milk, indigestion remedies, or medicines containing iron or zinc, 2 hours before or after you take this medicine**

Peidiwch â chymryd llaeth, meddyginiaethau camdreuliad, neu feddyginiaeth sy'n cynnwys haearn neu sinc, 2 awr cyn neu ar ôl cymryd y feddyginiaeth hon
To be used on *preparations containing ciprofloxacin, norfloxacin, or tetracyclines that chelate calcium, iron, magnesium, and zinc,* and are thus less available for absorption. Pharmacists will be aware (from a knowledge of

physiology) that these incompatible preparations should be taken at least 2 hours apart for the majority of medicines; when a manufacturer advises a different time period, this can be followed, and should be explained to the patient. Doxycycline, lymecycline, and minocycline are less liable to form chelates and therefore only require label 6 (see above).

8 **Warning: Do not stop taking this medicine unless your doctor tells you to stop**

Rhybudd: Peidiwch â stopio cymryd y feddyginiaeth hon, oni bai fod eich meddyg yn dweud wrthych am stopio
To be used on *preparations that contain a drug which is required to be taken over long periods without the patient necessarily perceiving any benefit* (e.g. antituberculous drugs).

Also to be used on *preparations that contain a drug whose withdrawal is likely to be a particular hazard* (e.g. clonidine for hypertension). Label 10 (see below) is more appropriate for corticosteroids.

9 **Space the doses evenly throughout the day. Keep taking this medicine until the course is finished, unless you are told to stop**

Gadewch yr un faint o amser rhwng pob dôs yn ystod y dydd. Parhewch i gymryd y feddyginiaeth nes bod y cyfan wedi'i orffen, oni bai eich bod yn cael cyngor i stopio
To be used on *preparations where a course of treatment should be completed* to reduce the incidence of relapse or failure of treatment.

The preparations are antimicrobial drugs given by mouth. Very occasionally, some may have severe side-effects (e.g. diarrhoea in patients receiving clindamycin) and in such cases the patient may need to be advised of reasons for stopping treatment quickly and returning to the doctor.

10 **Warning: Read the additional information given with this medicine**

Rhybudd: Darllenwch y wybodaeth ychwanegol gyda'r feddyginiaeth hon
To be used particularly on *preparations containing anticoagulants, lithium, and oral corticosteroids* . The appropriate treatment card should be given to the patient and any necessary explanations given.

This label may also be used on other preparations to remind the patient of the instructions that have been given.

11 **Protect your skin from sunlight—even on a bright but cloudy day. Do not use sunbeds**

Diogelwch eich croen rhag golau'r haul, hyd yn oed ar ddiwrnod braf ond cymylog. Peidiwch â defnyddio gwely haul
To be used on *preparations that may cause phototoxic or photoallergic reactions* if the patient is exposed to ultraviolet radiation. Exposure to high intensity ultraviolet radiation from sunray lamps and sunbeds is particularly likely to cause reactions.

12 **Do not take anything containing aspirin while taking this medicine**

Peidiwch â chymryd unrhyw beth sy'n cynnwys aspirin gyda'r feddyginiaeth hon
To be used on *preparations containing sulfinpyrazone* whose activity is reduced by aspirin.

Label 12 should not be used for anticoagulants since label 10 is more appropriate.

13 **Dissolve or mix with water before taking**

Gadewch i ddoddi mewn dŵr cyn ei gymryd
To be used on *preparations that are intended to be dissolved in water* (e.g. soluble tablets) or *mixed with water* (e.g. powders, granules) before use. In a few cases other liquids such as fruit juice or milk may be used.

14 **This medicine may colour your urine. This is harmless**

Gall y feddyginiaeth hon liwio eich dŵr. Nid yw hyn yn arwydd o ddrwg
To be used on *preparations that may cause the patient's urine to turn an unusual colour* . These include triamterene (blue under some lights), levodopa (dark reddish), and rifampicin (red).

15 Caution: flammable. Keep your body away from fire or flames after you have put on the medicine

Rhybudd: Fflamadwy. Ar ôl rhoi'r feddyginiaeth ymlaen, cadwch yn glir o dân neu fflamau

To be used on *preparations containing sufficient flammable solvent to render them flammable if exposed to a naked flame* .

16 Dissolve the tablet under your tongue—do not swallow. Store the tablets in this bottle with the cap tightly closed. Get a new supply 8 weeks after opening

Rhowch y dabled i doddi dan eich tafod - peidiwch â'i lyncu. Cadwch y tabledi yn y botel yma gyda'r caead wedi'i gau yn dynn. Gofynnwch am dabledi newydd 8 wythnos ar ôl ei hagor

To be used on *glyceryl trinitrate tablets* to remind the patient not to transfer the tablets to plastic or less suitable containers.

17 Do not take more than... in 24 hours

Peidiwch â chymryd mwy na... mewn 24 awr

To be used on *preparations for the treatment of acute migraine* except those containing ergotamine, for which label 18 is used. The dose form should be specified, e.g. tablets or capsules.

It may also be used on preparations for which no dose has been specified by the prescriber.

18 Do not take more than... in 24 hours. Also, do not take more than... in any one week

Peidiwch â chymryd mwy na... mewn 24 awr. Hefyd, peidiwch â chymryd mwy na... mewn wythnos

To be used on preparations containing ergotamine. The dose form should be specified, e.g. tablets or suppositories.

19 Warning: This medicine makes you sleepy. If you still feel sleepy the next day, do not drive or use tools or machines. Do not drink alcohol

Rhybudd: Bydd y feddyginiaeth hon yn eich gwneud yn gysglyd. Os ydych yn dal i deimlo'n gysglyd drannoeth, peidiwch â gyrru, defnyddio offer llaw neu beiriannau. Peidiwch ag yfed alcohol

To be used on *preparations containing hypnotics (or some other drugs with sedative effects) prescribed to be taken at night* . On the rare occasions when hypnotics are prescribed for daytime administration (e.g. nitrazepam in epilepsy), this label would clearly not be appropriate. Also to be used as an *alternative* to the label 2 wording (the choice being at the discretion of the pharmacist) *for anxiolytics prescribed to be taken at night*.

It is hoped that this wording will convey adequately the problem of residual morning sedation after taking 'sleeping tablets'.

21 Take with or just after food, or a meal

Cymerwch gyda neu ar ôl bwyd

To be used on *preparations that are liable to cause gastric irritation, or those that are better absorbed with food* .

Patients should be advised that a *small amount of food is sufficient*.

22 Take 30 to 60 minutes before food

Cymerwch 30 i 60 munud cyn bwyd

To be used on some preparations *whose absorption is thereby improved*.

Most oral antibacterials require label 23 instead (see below).

23 Take this medicine when your stomach is empty. This means an hour before food or 2 hours after food

Cymerwch y feddyginiaeth hon ar stumog wag. Mae hyn yn golygu awr cyn, neu 2 awr ar ôl bwyd

To be used on *oral antibacterials whose absorption may be reduced by the presence of food and acid in the stomach* .

24 Suck or chew this medicine

Bydd angen cnoi neu sugno'r feddyginiaeth hon

To be used on *preparations that should be sucked or chewed*.

The pharmacist should use discretion as to which of these words is appropriate.

25 Swallow this medicine whole. Do not chew or crush

Llyncwch yn gyfan. Peidiwch â chnoi neu falu'n fân

To be used on *preparations that are enteric-coated or designed for modified-release*.

Also to be used on *preparations that taste very unpleasant or may damage the mouth* if not swallowed whole.

Patients should be advised (where relevant) that some modified-release preparations can be broken in half, but that the halved tablet should still be swallowed whole, and not chewed or crushed.

26 Dissolve this medicine under your tongue

Gadewch i'r feddyginiaeth hon doddi o dan y tafod

To be used on *preparations designed for sublingual use*. Patients should be advised to hold under the tongue and avoid swallowing until dissolved. The buccal mucosa between the gum and cheek is occasionally specified by the prescriber.

27 Take with a full glass of water

Cymerwch gyda llond gwydr o ddŵr

To be used on *preparations that should be well diluted* (e.g. chloral hydrate), *where a high fluid intake is required* (e.g. sulfonamides), or *where water is required to aid the action* (e.g. methylcellulose). The patient should be advised that 'a full glass' means at least 150 mL. In most cases fruit juice, tea, or coffee may be used.

28 Spread thinly on the affected skin only

Taenwch yn denau ar y croen sydd wedi'i effeithio yn unig

To be used on *external preparations* that should be applied sparingly (e.g. corticosteroids, dithranol).

29 Do not take more than 2 at any one time. Do not take more than 8 in 24 hours

Peidiwch â chymryd mwy na 2 ar unrhyw un adeg. Peidiwch â chymryd mwy nag 8 mewn 24 awr

To be used on containers of dispensed *solid dose preparations containing paracetamol for adults when the instruction on the label indicates that the dose can be taken on an 'as required' basis* . The dose form should be specified, e.g. tablets or capsules.

This label has been introduced because of the serious consequences of overdosage with paracetamol.

30 Contains paracetamol. Do not take anything else containing paracetamol while taking this medicine. Talk to a doctor at once if you take too much of this medicine, even if you feel well

Yn cynnwys paracetamol. Peidiwch â chymryd unrhyw beth arall sy'n cynnwys paracetamol tra'n cymryd y feddyginiaeth hon. Siaradwch gyda'ch meddyg ar unwaith os ydych yn cymryd gormod, hyd yn oed os ydych yn teimlo'n iawn

To be used on all containers of dispensed *preparations containing paracetamol*.

32 Contains aspirin. Do not take anything else containing aspirin while taking this medicine

Yn cynnwys aspirin. Peidiwch â chymryd unrhyw beth arall sy'n cynnwys aspirin tra'n cymryd y feddyginiaeth hon

To be used on containers of dispensed *preparations containing aspirin when the name on the label does not include the word 'aspirin'* .

Appendix 4
Wound management products and elasticated garments

CONTENTS

A4

Wound management | **Appendix 4**

The correct dressing for wound management depends not only on the type of wound but also on the stage of the healing process. The principal stages of healing are: cleansing, removal of debris; granulation, vascularisation; epithelialisation. The ideal dressing for moist wound healing needs to ensure that the wound remains: moist with exudate, but not macerated; free of clinical infection and excessive slough; free of toxic chemicals, particles or fibres; at the optimum temperature for healing; undisturbed by the need for frequent changes; at the optimum pH value. As wound healing passes through its different stages, different types of dressings may be required to satisfy better one or other of these requirements. Under normal circumstances, a moist environment is a necessary part of the wound healing process; exudate provides a moist environment and promotes healing, but excessive exudate can cause maceration of the wound and surrounding healthy tissue. The volume and viscosity of exudate changes as the wound heals. There are certain circumstances where moist wound healing is not appropriate (e.g. gangrenous toes associated with vascular disease).

Advanced wound dressings are designed to control the environment for wound healing, for example to donate fluid (hydrogels), maintain hydration (hydrocolloids), or to absorb wound exudate (alginates, foams).

Practices such as the use of irritant cleansers and desloughing agents may be harmful and are largely obsolete; removal of debris and dressing remnants should need minimal irrigation with lukewarm sterile sodium chloride 0.9% solution or water.

Hydrogel, hydrocolloid, and medical grade honey dressings can be used to deslough wounds by promoting autolytic debridement; there is insufficient evidence to support any particular method of debridement for difficult-to-heal surgical wounds. Sterile larvae (maggots) are also available for biosurgical removal of wound debris.

There have been few clinical trials able to establish a clear advantage for any particular product. The choice between different dressings depends not only on the type and stage of the wound, but also on patient preference or tolerance, site of the wound, and cost. For further information, see Buyers' Guide: Advanced wound dressings (October 2008); NHS Purchasing and Supply Agency, Centre for Evidence-based Purchasing.

Prices quoted in Appendix 4 are basic NHS net prices; for further information see *Prices in the BNF* under How to use the BNF.

The table below gives suggestions for choices of primary dressing depending on the type of wound (a secondary dressing may be needed in some cases).

Basic wound contact dressings

Low adherence dressing

Low adherence dressings are used as interface layers under secondary absorbent dressings. Placed directly on the wound bed, non-absorbent, low adherence dressings are suitable for clean, granulating, lightly exuding wounds without necrosis, and protect the wound bed from direct contact with secondary dressings. Care must be taken to avoid granulation tissue growing into the weave of these dressings.

Wound contact material for different types of wounds

Wound PINK (epithelialising)

Low Exudate	Moderate Exudate
Low adherence p. 1537	Soft ploymer p. 1542
Vapour-permeable film p. 1541	Foam, low absorbent p. 1545
Soft polymer p. 1542	Alginate p. 1547
Hydrocolloid p. 1544	

Wound RED (granulating)
Symptoms or signs of infection, see Wounds with signs of infection

Low Exudate	Moderate Exudate	Heavy Exudate
Low adherence p. 1537	Hydrocolloid-fibrous p. 1544	Foam with extra absorbency p. 1545
Soft polymer p. 1542	Foam p. 1545	Hydrocolloid-fibrous p. 1544
Hydrocolloid p. 1544	Alginate p. 1547	Alginate p. 1547
Foam, low absorbent p. 1545		

Wound YELLOW (Sloughy) (granulating)
Symptoms or signs of infection, see Wounds with signs of infection

Low Exudate	Moderate Exudate	Heavy Exudate
Hydrogel p. 1540	Hydrocolloid-fibrous p. 1544	Hydrocolloid-fibrous p. 1544
Hydrocolloid p. 1544	Alginate p. 1547	Alginate p. 1547
		Capillary-action p. 1547

Wound BLACK (Necrotic/ Eschar)
Consider mechanical debridement alongside autolytic debridement

Low Exudate	Moderate Exudate	Heavy Exudate
Hydrogel p. 1540	Hydrocolloid p. 1544	Seek advice from wound care specialist
Hydrocolloid p. 1544	Hydrocolloid-fibrous p. 1544	
	Foam p. 1545	

Wounds with signs of infection
Consider systemic antibacterials if appropriate; also consider odour-absorbent dressings. For malodourous wounds with slough or necrotic tissue, consider mechanical or autolytic debridement

Low Exudate	Moderate Exudate	Heavy Exudate
Low adherence with honey p. 1548	Hydrocolloid-fibrous with silver p. 1550	Hydrocolloid-fibrous with silver p. 1550
Low adherence with iodine p. 1548	Foam with silver p. 1550	Foam extra absorbent, with silver p. 1550
Low adherence with silver p. 1550	Alginate with silver p. 1549	Alginate with honey p. 1548
Hydrocolloid with silver p. 1550	Honey-topical p. 1548	Alginate with silver p. 1549
	Cadexomer-iodine p. 1548	

Note In each section of this table the dressings are listed in order of increasing absorbency.
Some wound contact (primary) dressings require a secondary dressing

Tulle dressings are manufactured from cotton or viscose fibres which are impregnated with white or yellow soft paraffin to prevent the fibres from sticking, but this is only partly successful and it may be necessary to change the dressings frequently. The paraffin reduces absorbency of the dressing. Dressings with a reduced content (light loading) of soft paraffin are less liable to interfere with absorption; dressings with 'normal loading' (such as Jelonet ®) have been used for skin graft transfer. Knitted viscose primary dressing is an alternative to tulle dressings for exuding wounds; it can be used as the initial layer of multi-layer compression bandaging in the treatment of venous leg ulcers.

Knitted polyester primary dressing
Atrauman
Non-adherent knitted polyester primary dressing impregnated with neutral triglycerides
Atrauman dressing (Paul Hartmann Ltd) 10cm × 20cm= £0.80, 20cm × 30cm= £2.20, 5cm × 5cm £0.34, 7.5cm × 10cm= £0.35

Knitted viscose primary dressing
N-A Dressing
Warp knitted fabric manufactured from a bright viscose monofilament.
N-A dressing (Systagenix Wound Management Ltd) 19cm × 9.5cm= £0.67, 9.5cm × 9.5cm= £0.35

N-A Ultra
Warp knitted fabric manufactured from a bright viscose monofilament.

N-A Ultra dressing (Systagenix Wound Management Ltd) 19cm × 9.5cm= £0.63, 9.5cm × 9.5cm= £0.33

Profore
Warp knitted fabric manufactured from a bright viscose monofilament.
Profore (Smith & Nephew Healthcare Ltd) wound contact layer 14cm × 20cm= £0.32

Tricotex
Warp knitted fabric manufactured from a bright viscose monofilament.
Tricotex dressing (Smith & Nephew Healthcare Ltd) 9.5cm × 9.5cm= £0.35

Paraffin Gauze Dressing
Cuticell
(Tulle Gras). Fabric of leno weave, weft and warp threads of cotton and/or viscose yarn, impregnated with white or yellow soft paraffin; for light or normal loading
Cuticell (BSN medical Ltd) Classic dressing 10cm × 10cm= £0.29

Jelonet
(Tulle Gras). Fabric of leno weave, weft and warp threads of cotton and/or viscose yarn, impregnated with white or yellow soft paraffin; for light or normal loading
Jelonet dressing (Smith & Nephew Healthcare Ltd) 10cm × 10cm= £0.42

Neotulle

(Tulle Gras). Fabric of leno weave, weft and warp threads of cotton and/or viscose yarn, impregnated with white or yellow soft paraffin; for light or normal loading

Neotulle (Neomedic Ltd) dressing 10cm × 10cm= £0.29

Absorbent dressings

Perforated film absorbent dressings are suitable only for wounds with mild to moderate amounts of exudate; they are not appropriate for leg ulcers or for other lesions that produce large quantities of viscous exudate. Dressings with an absorbent cellulose or polymer wadding layer are suitable for use on moderately to heavily exuding wounds.

Absorbent cellulose dressing

CelluDress

Absorbent Cellulose Dressing with Fluid Repellent Backing

CelluDress dressing (Medicareplus International Ltd) 10cm × 10cm= £0.19, 10cm × 15cm= £0.20, 10cm × 20cm= £0.22, 15cm × 20cm= £0.30, 20cm × 25cm= £0.40, 20cm × 30cm= £0.85

Eclypse

Absorbent Cellulose Dressing with Fluid Repellent Backing

Eclypse (Advancis Medical) Boot dressing 60cm × 70cm= £13.88, dressing 15cm × 15cm= £0.98, 20cm × 30cm= £2.16, 60cm × 40cm= £8.21

Exu-Dry

Absorbent Cellulose Dressing with Fluid Repellent Backing

Exu-Dry dressing (Smith & Nephew Healthcare Ltd) 10cm × 15cm= £1.15, 15cm × 23cm= £2.34, 23cm × 38cm= £5.44

Mesorb

Cellulose wadding pad with gauze wound contact layer and non-woven repellent backing

Mesorb dressing (Molnlycke Health Care Ltd) 10cm × 10cm= £0.63, 10cm × 15cm= £0.82, 10cm × 20cm= £1.01, 15cm × 20cm= £1.44, 20cm × 20cm= £2.27, 20cm × 30cm= £2.57

Zetuvit E

Absorbent Cellulose Dressing with Fluid Repellent Backing; sterile or non-sterile

Zetuvit (Paul Hartmann Ltd) E non-sterile dressing 10cm × 10cm= £0.07, 10cm × 20cm= £0.09, 20cm × 20cm= £0.15, 20cm × 40cm= £0.28, sterile dressing 10cm × 10cm= £0.22, 10cm × 20cm= £0.25, 20cm × 20cm= £0.40, 20cm × 40cm= £1.12

Absorbent perforated dressing

Adpore

Low-adherence primary dressing consisting of viscose and rayon absorbent pad with adhesive border.

Adpore dressing (Medicareplus International Ltd) 10cm × 10cm= £0.10, 10cm × 15cm= £0.16, 10cm × 20cm= £0.30, 10cm × 25cm= £0.34, 10cm × 30cm= £0.42, 10cm × 35cm= £0.50, 7cm × 8cm= £0.08

Cosmopore E

Low-adherence primary dressing consisting of viscose and rayon absorbent pad with adhesive border.

Cosmopor E dressing (Paul Hartmann Ltd) 10cm × 20cm= £0.46, 10cm × 25cm= £0.57, 10cm × 35cm= £0.79, 5cm × 7.2cm= £0.08, 8cm × 10cm= £0.18, 8cm × 15cm= £0.28

Cutiplast Steril

Low-adherence primary dressing consisting of viscose and rayon absorbent pad with adhesive border.

Cutiplast Steril dressing (Smith & Nephew Healthcare Ltd) 10cm × 20cm= £0.31, 10cm × 25cm= £0.32, 10cm × 30cm= £0.43, 8cm × 10cm= £0.11, 8cm × 15cm= £0.25

Leukomed

Low-adherence primary dressing consisting of viscose and rayon absorbent pad with adhesive border.

Leukomed dressing (BSN medical Ltd) 10cm × 20cm= £0.44, 10cm × 25cm= £0.49, 10cm × 30cm= £0.64, 10cm × 35cm= £0.74, 5cm × 7.2cm= £0.09, 8cm × 10cm= £0.19, 8cm × 15cm= £0.33

Medipore + Pad

Low-adherence primary dressing consisting of viscose and rayon absorbent pad with adhesive border.

Medipore + Pads dressing (3M Health Care Ltd) 10cm × 10cm= £0.15, 10cm × 15cm= £0.25, 10cm × 20cm= £0.37, 10cm × 25cm= £0.46, 10cm × 35cm= £0.64, 5cm × 7.2cm= £0.07

Medisafe

Low-adherence primary dressing consisting of viscose and rayon absorbent pad with adhesive border.

Medisafe dressing (Neomedic Ltd) 6cm × 8cm= £0.08, 8cm × 10cm= £0.13, 8cm × 12cm= £0.23, 9cm × 15cm= £0.29, 9cm × 20cm= £0.34, 9cm × 25cm= £0.36

Mepore

Low-adherence primary dressing consisting of viscose and rayon absorbent pad with adhesive border.

Mepore dressing (Molnlycke Health Care Ltd) 10cm × 11cm= £0.22, 11cm × 15cm= £0.36, 7cm × 8cm= £0.11, 9cm × 20cm= £0.44, 9cm × 25cm= £0.61, 9cm × 30cm= £0.70, 9cm × 35cm= £0.76

PremierPore

Low-adherence primary dressing consisting of viscose and rayon absorbent pad with adhesive border.

PremierPore dressing (Shermond) 10cm × 10cm= £0.12, 10cm × 15cm= £0.18, 10cm × 20cm= £0.32, 10cm × 25cm= £0.36, 10cm × 30cm= £0.45, 10cm × 35cm= £0.52, 5cm × 7cm= £0.05

Primapore

Low-adherence primary dressing consisting of viscose and rayon absorbent pad with adhesive border.

Primapore dressing (Smith & Nephew Healthcare Ltd) 10cm × 20cm= £0.44, 10cm × 25cm= £0.51, 10cm × 30cm= £0.64, 10cm × 35cm= £0.98, 6cm × 8.3cm= £0.18, 8cm × 10cm= £0.20, 8cm × 15cm= £0.34

Softpore

Low-adherence primary dressing consisting of viscose and rayon absorbent pad with adhesive border.

Softpore dressing (Richardson Healthcare Ltd) 10cm × 10cm= £0.13, 10cm × 15cm= £0.20, 10cm × 20cm= £0.35, 10cm × 25cm= £0.40, 10cm × 30cm= £0.49, 10cm × 35cm= £0.58, 6cm × 7cm= £0.06

Telfa Island

Low-adherence primary dressing consisting of viscose and rayon absorbent pad with adhesive border.

Telfa Island dressing (H & R Healthcare Ltd) 10cm × 12.5cm= £0.27, 10cm × 20cm= £0.35, 10cm × 25.5cm= £0.45, 10cm × 35cm= £0.62, 5cm × 10cm= £0.08

Absorbent perforated plastic film faced dressing

Absopad

Low-adherence primary dressing consisting of 3 layers—perforated polyester film wound contact layer, absorbent cotton pad, and hydrophobic backing.

Absopad dressing (Medicareplus International Ltd) 10cm × 10cm= £0.13, 20cm × 10cm= £0.28

Askina Pad

Low-adherence primary dressing consisting of 3 layers—perforated polyester film wound contact layer, absorbent cotton pad, and hydrophobic backing.

Askina (B.Braun Medical Ltd) Pad dressing 10cm × 10cm= £0.21

Melolin

Low-adherence primary dressing consisting of 3 layers—perforated polyester film wound contact layer, absorbent cotton pad, and hydrophobic backing.

Melolin dressing (Smith & Nephew Healthcare Ltd) 10cm × 10cm= £0.28, 20cm × 10cm= £0.55, 5cm × 5cm= £0.17

Skintact

Low-adherence primary dressing consisting of 3 layers—perforated polyester film wound contact layer, absorbent cotton pad, and hydrophobic backing.

Skintact dressing (Robinson Healthcare) 10cm × 10cm= £0.17, 20cm × 10cm= £0.34, 5cm × 5cm= £0.10

Solvaline N

Low-adherence primary dressing consisting of 3 layers—perforated polyester film wound contact layer, absorbent cotton pad, and hydrophobic backing.

Solvaline N dressing (Lohmann & Rauscher) 10cm × 10cm= £0.18, 20cm × 10cm= £0.36, 5cm × 5cm= £0.10

Telfa
Low-adherence primary dressing consisting of 3 layers—
perforated polyester film wound contact layer, absorbent
cotton pad, and hydrophobic backing.
Telfa dressing (H & R Healthcare Ltd) 10cm × 7.5cm= £0.16, 15cm ×
7.5cm= £0.18, 20cm × 7.5cm= £0.29, 7.5cm × 5cm= £0.12

Super absorbent cellulose and polymer primary dressing
Curea P1
Super absorbent cellulose and polymer primary dressing.
Curea P1 dressing (Charles S. Bullen Stomacare Ltd) 10cm × 10cm
square= £2.15, 10cm × 20cm rectangular= £3.64, 10cm × 30cm
rectangular= £5.20, 12cm × 12cm square= £2.65, 20cm × 20cm
square= £6.89, 20cm × 30cm rectangular= £10.03, 7.5cm ×
7.5cm square= £1.72

Curea P2
Super absorbent cellulose and polymer primary dressing
(non-adherent)
Curea P2 dressing (Charles S. Bullen Stomacare Ltd) 10cm × 20cm
rectangular= £4.49, 11cm × 11cm square= £2.47, 20cm × 20cm
square= £7.82, 20cm × 30cm rectangular= £10.60

Cutisorb Ultra
Super absorbent cellulose and polymer primary dressing
Cutisorb Ultra dressing (BSN medical Ltd) 10cm × 10cm square=
£2.13, 10cm × 20cm rectangular= £3.56, 20cm × 20cm square=
£6.68, 20cm × 30cm rectangular= £10.06

DryMax Extra
Super absorbent cellulose and polymer primary dressing
DryMax Extra Soft dressing (Espere Healthcare Ltd) 10cm × 10cm
square= £0.87, 10cm × 20cm rectangular= £1.04, 20cm × 20cm
square= £1.84, 20cm × 30cm rectangular= £2.33

Zetuvit Plus
Super absorbent cellulose primary dressing
Zetuvit Plus dressing (Paul Hartmann Ltd) 10cm × 10cm= £0.83,
10cm × 20cm= £1.15, 15cm × 20cm= £1.32, 20cm × 25cm=
£1.80, 20cm × 40cm= £2.79

Super absorbent hydroconductive dressing
Drawtex
Super absorbent hydroconductive dressing with absorbent,
cross-action structures of viscose, polyester and cotton
Drawtex dressing (Martindale Pharmaceuticals Ltd) 10cm × 1.3m=
£16.00, 10cm × 10cm= £2.24, 10cm × 1m= £16.00, 15cm ×
20cm= £6.00, 20cm × 1m= £25.00, 20cm × 20cm= £6.98, 5cm ×
5cm= £0.95, 7.5cm × 1m= £15.50, 7.5cm × 7.5cm= £1.77

Advanced wound dressings

Advanced wound dressings can be used for both acute and
chronic wounds. Categories for dressings in this section start
with the least absorptive, moisture-donating hydrogel
dressings, followed by increasingly more absorptive
dressings. These dressings are classified according to their
primary component; some dressings are comprised of several
components.

Hydrogel dressings
Hydrogel dressings are most commonly supplied as an
amorphous, cohesive topical application that can take up the
shape of a wound. A secondary, non-absorbent dressing is
needed. These dressings are generally used to donate liquid
to dry sloughy wounds and facilitate autolytic debridement
of necrotic tissue; some also have the ability to absorb very
small amounts of exudate. Hydrogel products that do not
contain propylene glycol should be used if the wound is to be
treated with larval therapy. Hydrogel sheets have a fixed
structure and limited fluid-handling capacity; hydrogel sheet
dressings are best avoided in the presence of infection, and
are unsuitable for heavily exuding wounds.

Hydrogel application (amorphous)
ActivHeal Hydrogel
Hydrogel containing guar gum and propylene glycol
ActivHeal (Advanced Medical Solutions Ltd) Hydrogel dressing= £1.41

Aquaform
Hydrogel containing modified starch copolymer
AquaForm (Aspen Medical Europe Ltd) Hydrogel dressing= £2.04

Askina Gel
Hydrogel containing modified starch and glycerol
Askina (B.Braun Medical Ltd) Gel dressing= £2.05

Cutimed
Hydrogel
Cutimed (BSN medical Ltd) Gel dressing= £3.08

Flexigran
Hydrogel containing modified starch and glycerol
Flexigran (A1 Pharmaceuticals) Gel dressing= £1.90

GranuGel
Hydrogel containing carboxymethylcellulose, pectin and
propylene glycol
GranuGEL (ConvaTec Ltd) Hydrocolloid Gel dressing= £2.37

Intrasite Gel
Hydrogel containing modified carmellose polymer and
propylene glycol
IntraSite (Smith & Nephew Healthcare Ltd) Gel dressing= £3.65

Nu-Gel
Hydrogel containing alginate and propylene glycol
Nu-Gel (Systagenix Wound Management Ltd) dressing= £2.09

Purilon Gel
Hydrogel containing carboxymethylcellulose and calcium
alginate
Purilon (Coloplast Ltd) Gel dressing= £2.31

Hydrogel sheet dressings
ActiFormCool
Hydrogel dressing
ActiFormCool sheet (L&R Medical UK Ltd) 10cm × 10cm square=
£2.68, 10cm × 15cm rectangular= £3.86, 20cm × 20cm square=
£8.08, 5cm × 6.5cm rectangular= £1.83

Aquaflo
Hydrogel dressing
Aquaflo (Covidien (UK) Commercial Ltd) sheet 7.5cm discs= £2.60

Coolie
Hydrogel dressing (without adhesive border)
Coolie (Zeroderma Ltd) sheet 7cm discs= £1.96

Gel FX
Hydrogel dressing (without adhesive border)
Gel FX sheet (Synergy Health (UK) Ltd) 10cm × 10cm square= £1.60,
15cm × 15cm square= £3.20

Geliperm
Hydrogel sheets
Geliperm (Geistlich Sons Ltd) sheet 10cm × 10cm square= £2.53

Hydrosorb
Absorbent, transparent, hydrogel sheets containing
polyurethane polymers covered with a semi-permeable film
Hydrosorb sheet (Paul Hartmann Ltd) 10cm × 10cm square= £2.29,
20cm × 20cm square= £6.87, 5cm × 7.5cm rectangular= £1.60

Hydrosorb Comfort
Absorbent, transparent, hydrogel sheets containing
polyurethane polymers covered with a semi-permeable film
(with adhesive border, waterproof)
Hydrosorb Comfort sheet (Paul Hartmann Ltd) 12.5cm × 12.5cm
square= £3.66, 4.5cm × 6.5cm rectangular= £1.90, 7.5cm ×
10cm rectangular= £2.52

Intrasite Conformable
Soft non-woven dressing impregnated with Intrasite ® gel
IntraSite Conformable dressing (Smith & Nephew Healthcare Ltd) 10cm
× 10cm square= £1.84, 10cm × 20cm rectangular= £2.48, 10cm
× 40cm rectangular= £4.43

Novogel
Glycerol-based hydrogel sheets (standard or thin)
Novogel sheet (Ford Medical Associates Ltd) 10cm × 10cm square=
£3.18, 15cm × 20cm rectangular= £6.07, 20cm × 40cm
rectangular= £11.56, 30cm × 30cm (0.15cm thickness) square=
£12.71, (0.30cm thickness) square= £13.47, 5cm × 7.5cm
rectangular= £1.99, 7.5cm diameter circular= £2.89

SanoSkin NET
Hydrogel sheet (without adhesive border)
SanoSkin (Ideal Medical Solutions Ltd) NET sheet 8.5cm × 12cm rectangular= £2.28

Vacunet
Non-adherent, hydrogel coated polyester net dressing
Vacunet dressing (Protex Healthcare Ltd) 10cm × 10cm square= £1.93, 10cm × 15cm rectangular= £2.86

Sodium hyaluronate dressings
The hydrating properties of sodium hyaluronate promote wound healing, and dressings can be applied directly to the wound, or to a primary dressing (a secondary dressing should also be applied). The iodine and potassium iodide in these dressings prevent the bacterial decay of sodium hyaluronate in the wound.
Hyiodine® should be used with caution in thyroid disorders.

Hyiodine
Sodium hyaluronate 1.5%, potassium iodide 0.15%, iodine 0.1%, in a viscous solution

Vapour-permeable films and membranes
Vapour-permeable films and membranes allow the passage of water vapour and oxygen but are impermeable to water and micro-organisms, and are suitable for lightly exuding wounds. They are highly conformable, provide protection, and a moist healing environment; transparent film dressings permit constant observation of the wound. Water vapour loss can occur at a slower rate than exudate is generated, so that fluid accumulates under the dressing, which can lead to tissue maceration and to wrinkling at the adhesive contact site (with risk of bacterial entry). Newer versions of these dressings have increased moisture vapour permeability. Despite these advances, vapour-permeable films and membranes are unsuitable for infected, large heavily exuding wounds, and chronic leg ulcers. Vapour-permeable films and membranes are suitable for partial-thickness wounds with minimal exudate, or wounds with eschar. Most commonly, they are used as a secondary dressing over alginates or hydrogels; film dressings can also be used to protect the fragile skin of patients at risk of developing minor skin damage caused by friction or pressure.

Non-woven fabric dressing with viscose-rayon pad.
Niko Fix
For intravenous and subcutaneous catheter sites
Niko (Unomedical Ltd) Fix dressing 7cm × 8.5cm= £0.20

Vapour-permeable Adhesive Film Dressing (Semi-permeable Adhesive Dressing)
Extensible, waterproof, water vapour-permeable polyurethane film coated with synthetic adhesive mass; transparent. Supplied in single-use pieces.

Askina Derm
Extensible, waterproof, water vapour-permeable polyurethane film coated with synthetic adhesive mass; transparent. Supplied in single-use pieces
Askina Derm dressing (B.Braun Medical Ltd) 10cm × 12cm= £1.10, 10cm × 20cm= £2.10, 15cm × 20cm= £2.54, 20cm × 30cm= £4.55, 6cm × 7cm= £0.38

C-View
Extensible, waterproof, water vapour-permeable polyurethane film coated with synthetic adhesive mass; transparent. Supplied in single-use pieces
C-View dressing (Aspen Medical Europe Ltd) 10cm × 12cm= £1.03, 12cm × 12cm= £1.10, 15cm × 20cm= £2.38, 6cm × 7cm= £0.38

Dressfilm
Extensible, waterproof, water vapour-permeable polyurethane film coated with synthetic adhesive mass; transparent. Supplied in single-use pieces
Dressfilm (St Georges Medical Ltd) dressing 15cm × 20cm= £1.90

Hydrofilm
Extensible, waterproof, water vapour-permeable polyurethane film coated with synthetic adhesive mass; transparent. Supplied in single-use pieces
Hydrofilm dressing (Paul Hartmann Ltd) 10cm × 12.5cm= £0.43, 10cm × 15cm= £0.54, 10cm × 25cm= £0.83, 12cm × 25cm= £0.88, 15cm × 20cm= £0.99, 20cm × 30cm= £1.63, 6cm × 7cm= £0.23

Hypafix Transparent
Extensible, waterproof, water vapour-permeable polyurethane film coated with synthetic adhesive mass; transparent. Supplied in single-use pieces
Hypafix Transparent (BSN medical Ltd) dressing 10cm × 2m= £8.95

Leukomed T
Extensible, waterproof, water vapour-permeable polyurethane film coated with synthetic adhesive mass; transparent. Supplied in single-use pieces
Leukomed T dressing (BSN medical Ltd) 10cm × 12.5cm= £1.04, 11cm × 14cm= £1.26, 15cm × 20cm= £2.42, 15cm × 25cm= £2.58, 7.2cm × 5cm= £0.38, 8cm × 10cm= £0.71

Mepitel Film
Extensible, waterproof, water vapour-permeable polyurethane film coated with synthetic adhesive mass; transparent. Supplied in single-use pieces
Mepitel Film dressing (Molnlycke Health Care Ltd) 10.5cm × 12cm= £1.32, 10.5cm × 25cm= £2.57, 15.5cm × 20cm= £3.26, 6.5cm × 7cm= £0.49

Mepore Film
Extensible, waterproof, water vapour-permeable polyurethane film coated with synthetic adhesive mass; transparent. Supplied in single-use pieces
Mepore Film dressing (Molnlycke Health Care Ltd) 10cm × 12cm= £1.24, 10cm × 25cm= £2.41, 15cm × 20cm= £3.06, 6cm × 7cm= £0.46

OpSite Flexifix
Extensible, waterproof, water vapour-permeable polyurethane film coated with synthetic adhesive mass; transparent. Supplied in single-use pieces
OpSite Flexifix dressing (Smith & Nephew Healthcare Ltd) 10cm × 1m= £6.72, 5cm × 1m= £3.98

OpSite Flexigrid
Extensible, waterproof, water vapour-permeable polyurethane film coated with synthetic adhesive mass; transparent. Supplied in single-use pieces
OpSite Flexigrid dressing (Smith & Nephew Healthcare Ltd) 12cm × 12cm= £1.15, 15cm × 20cm= £2.91, 6cm × 7cm= £0.40

Polyskin II
Extensible, waterproof, water vapour-permeable polyurethane film coated with synthetic adhesive mass; transparent. Supplied in single-use pieces
Kendall Film dressing (H & R Healthcare Ltd) 10cm × 12cm= £1.03, 10cm × 20cm= £2.04, 15cm × 20cm= £2.35, 20cm × 25cm= £4.11, 4cm × 4cm= £0.36, 5cm × 7cm= £0.40

ProtectFilm
Extensible, waterproof, water vapour-permeable polyurethane film coated with synthetic adhesive mass; transparent. Supplied in single-use pieces
ProtectFilm dressing (Wallace, Cameron & Company Ltd) 10cm × 12cm= £0.20, 15cm × 20cm= £0.40, 6cm × 7cm= £0.11

Suprasorb F
Extensible, waterproof, water vapour-permeable polyurethane film coated with synthetic adhesive mass; transparent. Supplied in single-use pieces
Suprasorb F dressing (Lohmann & Rauscher) 10cm × 12cm= £0.82, 15cm × 20cm= £2.56, 5cm × 7cm= £0.34

Tegaderm
Extensible, waterproof, water vapour-permeable polyurethane film coated with synthetic adhesive mass; transparent. Supplied in single-use pieces
Tegaderm Film dressing (3M Health Care Ltd) 12cm × 12cm= £1.11, 15cm × 20cm= £2.41, 6cm × 7cm= £0.39

A4

Wound management | Appendix 4

Tegaderm diamond

Extensible, waterproof, water vapour-permeable polyurethane film coated with synthetic adhesive mass; transparent. Supplied in single-use pieces

Tegaderm Diamond dressing (3M Health Care Ltd) 10cm × 12cm= £1.21, 6cm × 7cm= £0.45

Vellafilm

Extensible, waterproof, water vapour-permeable polyurethane film coated with synthetic adhesive mass; transparent. Supplied in single-use pieces

Vellafilm dressing (Advancis Medical) 12cm × 12cm= £1.11, 12cm × 35cm= £2.77, 15cm × 20cm= £2.12

Vapour-permeable Adhesive Film Dressing with absorbent pad
Adpore Ultra

Film dressing with adsorbent pad

Adpore Ultra dressing (Medicareplus International Ltd) 10cm × 10cm= £0.14, 10cm × 15cm= £0.22, 10cm × 20cm= £0.33, 10cm × 25cm= £0.35, 10cm × 30cm= £0.52, 7cm × 8cm= £0.12

Vapour-permeable Adhesive Film Dressing with absorbent pad
Alldress

Film dressing with adsorbent pad

Alldress dressing (Molnlycke Health Care Ltd) 10cm × 10cm= £0.97, 15cm × 15cm= £2.11, 15cm × 20cm= £2.61

C-View Post-Op

Film dressing with adsorbent pad

C-View Post-Op dressing (Aspen Medical Europe Ltd) 10cm × 12cm= £1.11, 10cm × 25cm= £1.61, 10cm × 35cm= £2.62, 6cm × 7cm= £0.40

Clearpore

Film dressing with adsorbent pad

Clearpore dressing (Richardson Healthcare Ltd) 10cm × 10cm= £0.20, 10cm × 15cm= £0.24, 10cm × 20cm= £0.36, 10cm × 25cm= £0.40, 10cm × 30cm= £0.65, 6cm × 10cm= £0.15, 6cm × 7cm= £0.12

Hydrofilm Plus

Film dressing with adsorbent pad

Hydrofilm Plus dressing (Paul Hartmann Ltd) 10cm × 20cm= £0.46, 10cm × 25cm= £0.61, 10cm × 30cm= £0.69, 7.2cm × 5cm= £0.18, 9cm × 10cm= £0.27, 9cm × 15cm= £0.30

Leukomed T Plus

Film dressing with adsorbent pad

Leukomed T plus dressing (BSN medical Ltd) 10cm × 20cm= £1.37, 10cm × 25cm= £1.54, 10cm × 30cm= £2.58, 10cm × 35cm= £3.13, 7.2cm × 5cm= £0.27, 8cm × 10cm= £0.55, 8cm × 15cm= £0.82

Mepore Film & Pad

Film dressing with adsorbent pad

Mepore Film & Pad dressing (Molnlycke Health Care Ltd) 4cm × 5cm= £0.24, 5cm × 7cm= £0.25, 9cm × 10cm= £0.63, 9cm × 15cm= £0.92, 9cm × 20cm= £1.37, 9cm × 25cm= £1.51, 9cm × 30cm= £2.03, 9cm × 35cm= £2.52

Mepore Ultra

Film dressing with adsorbent pad

Mepore Ultra dressing (Molnlycke Health Care Ltd) 10cm × 11cm= £0.81, 11cm × 15cm= £1.19, 7cm × 8cm= £0.41, 9cm × 20cm= £1.52, 9cm × 30cm= £1.68, 9cm × 30cm= £2.77

OpSite Plus

Film dressing with adsorbent pad

OpSite Plus dressing (Smith & Nephew Healthcare Ltd) 10cm × 12cm= £1.22, 10cm × 20cm= £2.06, 10cm × 35cm= £3.41, 6.5cm × 5cm= £0.33, 8.5cm × 9.5cm= £0.90

OpSite Post-op

Film dressing with adsorbent pad

OpSite Post-Op dressing (Smith & Nephew Healthcare Ltd) 10cm × 12cm= £1.20, 10cm × 20cm= £2.01, 10cm × 25cm= £2.54, 10cm × 30cm= £3.01, 10cm × 35cm= £3.34, 8.5cm × 15.5cm= £1.22, 8.5cm × 9.5cm= £0.88

Pharmapore-PU

Film dressing with adsorbent pad

Pharmapore-PU dressing (Wallace, Cameron & Company Ltd) 10cm × 25cm= £0.38, 10cm × 30cm= £0.58, 8.5cm × 15.5cm= £0.20

PremierPore VP

Film dressing with adsorbent pad

PremierPore VP dressing (Shermond) 10cm × 10cm= £0.16, 10cm × 15cm= £0.24, 10cm × 20cm= £0.36, 10cm × 25cm= £0.38, 10cm × 30cm= £0.57, 10cm × 35cm= £0.70, 5cm × 7cm= £0.13

Tegaderm

Film dressing with adsorbent pad

Tegaderm + Pad dressing (3M Health Care Ltd) 5cm × 7cm= £0.26, 9cm × 10cm= £0.65, 9cm × 15cm= £0.95, 9cm × 20cm= £1.40, 9cm × 25cm= £1.57, 9cm × 35cm= £2.60

Tegaderm Absorbent Clear

Film dressing with clear acrylic polymer oval-shaped pad or rectangular-shaped pad

Tegaderm Absorbent Clear Acrylic dressing (3M Health Care Ltd) 11.1cm × 12.7cm oval= £4.11, 14.2cm × 15.8cm oval= £5.78, 14.9cm × 15.2cm rectangular= £8.66, 16.8cm × 19cm sacral= £10.37, 20cm × 20.3cm rectangular= £13.91, 7.6cm × 9.5cm oval= £3.17

Vapour-permeable transparent film dressing with adhesive foam border.
Central Gard

For intravenous and subcutaneous catheter sites

Central Gard dressing (Unomedical Ltd) 16cm × 7cm= £0.97, 16cm × 8.8cm= £1.06

EasI-V

For intravenous and subcutaneous catheter sites

EasI-V (ConvaTec Ltd) dressing 7cm × 7.5cm= £0.38

Vapour-permeable transparent, adhesive film dressing.
Hydrofilm I.V. Control

For intravenous and subcutaneous catheter sites

Hydrofilm (Paul Hartmann Ltd) I.V. Control dressing 7cm × 9cm= £0.31

Vapour-permeable, transparent, adhesive film dressing.
IV3000

For intravenous and subcutaneous catheter sites

IV3000 dressing (Smith & Nephew Healthcare Ltd) 10cm × 12cm= £1.42, 5cm × 6cm= £0.43, 6cm × 7cm= £0.57, 7cm × 9cm= £0.74, 9cm × 12cm= £1.48

Mepore IV

For intravenous and subcutaneous catheter sites

Mepore IV dressing (Molnlycke Health Care Ltd) 10cm × 11cm= £1.08, 5cm × 5.5cm= £0.31, 8cm × 9cm= £0.40

Pharmapore-PU IV

For intravenous and subcutaneous catheter sites

Pharmapore-PU-I.V dressing (Wallace, Cameron & Company Ltd) 6cm × 7cm= £0.08, 7cm × 8.5cm= £0.07, 7cm × 10cm= £0.17

Tegaderm IV

For intravenous and subcutaneous catheter sites

Tegaderm IV dressing with securing tapes (3M Health Care Ltd) 10cm × 15.5cm= £1.67, 7cm × 8.5cm= £0.59

Soft polymer dressings

Dressings with soft polymer, often a soft silicone polymer, in a non-adherent or gently adherent layer are suitable for use on lightly to moderately exuding wounds. For moderately to heavily exuding wounds, an absorbent secondary dressing can be added, or a soft polymer dressing with an absorbent pad can be used. Wound contact dressings coated with soft silicone have gentle adhesive properties and can be used on fragile skin areas or where it is beneficial to reduce the frequency of primary dressing changes. Soft polymer dressings should not be used on heavily bleeding wounds; blood clots can cause the dressing to adhere to the wound surface. For silicone keloid dressings see under Specialised dressings.

Cellulose dressings
Sorbion Sachet Border

Absorbent polymers in cellulose matrix, hypoallergenic polypropylene envelope, with adhesive border

Cutimed Sorbion Sachet Border dressing (BSN medical Ltd) 10cm × 10cm square= £3.01, 15cm × 15cm square= £4.57, 25cm × 15cm rectangular= £7.12

Sorbion Sachet EXTRA

Absorbent polymers in cellulose matrix, hypoallergenic polypropylene envelope

Cutimed Sorbion Sachet Extra dressing (BSN medical Ltd) 10cm × 10cm= £2.29, 20cm × 10cm= £3.80, 20cm × 20cm= £7.14, 30cm × 20cm= £10.18, 5cm × 5cm= £1.48, 7.5cm × 7.5cm= £1.81

Sorbion Sachet Multi Star

Absorbent polymers in cellulose matrix, hypoallergenic polypropylene envelope

Cutimed Sorbion Sachet Multi Star dressing (BSN medical Ltd) 14cm × 14cm= £4.98, 8cm × 8cm= £3.05

Sorbion Sachet S Drainage

Absorbent polymers in cellulose matrix, hypoallergenic polypropylene envelope ('v' shaped dressing)

Cutimed (BSN medical Ltd) Sorbion Sachet S drainage dressing 10cm × 10cm= £2.69

Suprasorb X

Biosynthetic cellulose fibre dressing

Suprasorb X dressing (Lohmann & Rauscher) 14cm × 20cm rectangular= £8.59, 2cm × 21cm rope= £6.67, 5cm × 5cm square= £2.08, 9cm × 9cm square= £4.33

With absorbent pad

Advazorb Border

Soft silicone wound contact dressing with polyurethane foam film backing and adhesive border

Advazorb Border dressing (Advancis Medical) 10cm × 10cm= £2.12, 10cm × 20cm= £2.92, 10cm × 30cm= £4.28, 12.5cm × 12.5cm= £2.60, 15cm × 15cm= £3.17, 20cm × 20cm= £5.50, 7.5cm × 7.5cm= £1.20

Advazorb Border Lite

Soft silicone wound contact dressing with polyurethane foam film backing and adhesive border

Advazorb Border Lite dressing (Advancis Medical) 10cm × 10cm= £1.90, 10cm × 20cm= £2.63, 10cm × 30cm= £3.86, 12.5cm × 12.5cm= £2.34, 15cm × 15cm= £2.86, 20cm × 20cm= £4.95, 7.5cm × 7.5cm= £1.08

Advazorb Silfix

Soft silicone wound contact dressing with polyurethane foam film backing

Advazorb Silfix dressing (Advancis Medical) 10cm × 10cm= £1.86, 10cm × 20cm= £3.20, 12.5cm × 12.5cm= £2.61, 15cm × 15cm= £3.38, 20cm × 20cm= £5.02, 7.5cm × 7.5cm= £1.00

Advazorb Silfix Lite

Soft silicone wound contact dressing with polyurethane foam film backing

Advazorb Silfix Lite dressing (Advancis Medical) 10cm × 10cm= £1.68, 10cm × 20cm= £2.88, 12.5cm × 12.5cm= £2.35, 15cm × 15cm= £3.04, 20cm × 20cm= £4.51, 7.5cm × 7.5cm= £0.90

Allevyn Gentle

Soft gel wound contact dressing, with polyurethane foam film backing

Allevyn Gentle dressing (Smith & Nephew Healthcare Ltd) 10cm × 10cm= £2.55, 10cm × 20cm= £4.10, 15cm × 15cm= £4.28, 20cm × 20cm= £6.84, 5cm × 5cm= £1.29

Allevyn Gentle Border

Silicone gel wound contact dressing, with polyurethane foam film backing

Allevyn Gentle Border (Smith & Nephew Healthcare Ltd) Heel dressing 23cm × 23.2cm= £9.82, dressing 10cm × 10cm= £2.23, 12.5cm × 12.5cm= £2.73, 17.5cm × 17.5cm= £5.38, 7.5cm × 7.5cm= £1.52

Allevyn Gentle Border Lite

Silicone gel wound contact dressing, with polyurethane foam film backing

Allevyn Gentle Border Lite dressing (Smith & Nephew Healthcare Ltd) 10cm × 10cm= £2.20, 15cm × 15cm= £3.88, 5.5cm × 12cm= £1.88, 5cm × 5cm= £0.91, 8cm × 15cm= £3.49

Allevyn Life

Soft silicone wound contact dressing, with central mesh screen, polyurethane foam film backing and adhesive border

Allevyn Life dressing (Smith & Nephew Healthcare Ltd) 10.3cm × 10.3cm= £1.72, 12.9cm × 12.9cm= £2.53, 15.4cm × 15.4cm= £3.09, 21cm × 21cm= £6.09

Cutimed Siltec

Soft silicone wound contact dressing, with polyurethane foam film backing

Cutimed Siltec (BSN medical Ltd) Sacrum dressing 17.5cm × 17.5cm= £4.54, 23cm × 23cm= £6.20, dressing 10cm × 10cm= £2.26, 10cm × 20cm= £3.73, 15cm × 15cm= £4.22, 20cm × 20cm= £6.40, 5cm × 6cm= £1.21

Cutimed Siltec B

Soft silicone wound contact dressing, with polyurethane foam film backing, with adhesive border, for lightly to moderately exuding wounds

Cutimed Siltec B dressing (BSN medical Ltd) 12.5cm × 12.5cm= £2.30, 15cm × 15cm= £3.06, 17.5cm × 17.5cm= £4.95, 22.5cm × 22.5cm= £6.04, 7.5cm × 7.5cm= £1.35

Cutimed Siltec L

Soft silicone wound contact dressing, with polyurethane foam film backing, for lightly to moderately exuding wounds

Cutimed Siltec L dressing (BSN medical Ltd) 10cm × 10cm= £1.57, 15cm × 15cm= £3.45, 5cm × 6cm= £1.07

Eclypse Adherent

Soft silicone wound contact layer with absorbent pad and film backing

Eclypse Adherent dressing (Advancis Medical) 10cm × 10cm= £3.01, 10cm × 20cm= £3.78, 15cm × 15cm= £5.03, 20cm × 30cm= £10.06, 17cm × 19cm sacral= £3.79, 22cm × 23cm sacral= £6.28

Flivasorb

Absorbent polymer dressing with non-adherent wound contact layer

Flivasorb dressing (Lohmann & Rauscher) 10cm × 10cm square= £0.89, 10cm × 20cm rectangular= £1.06, 20cm × 20cm square= £1.88, 20cm × 30cm rectangular= £2.37

Flivasorb Adhesive

Absorbent polymer dressing with non-adherent wound contact layer and adhesive border

Flivasorb Adhesive dressing (Lohmann & Rauscher) 12cm × 12cm square= £3.39, 15cm × 15cm square= £4.65

Mepilex

Absorbent soft silicone dressing with polyurethane foam film backing

Mepilex (Molnlycke Health Care Ltd) Heel dressing 13cm × 20cm= £5.45, 15cm × 22cm= £6.31, XT dressing 10cm × 11cm= £2.68, 11cm × 20cm= £4.43, 15cm × 16cm= £4.86, 20cm × 21cm= £7.34, dressing 5cm × 5cm= £1.22

Mepilex Border

Absorbent soft silicone dressing with polyurethane foam film backing and adhesive border

Mepilex Border (Molnlycke Health Care Ltd) Heel dressing 18.5cm × 24cm= £6.63, Sacrum dressing 18cm × 18cm= £4.85, 23cm × 23cm= £7.91, dressing 10cm × 12.5cm= £2.72, 10cm × 20cm= £3.72, 10cm × 30cm= £5.58, 15cm × 17.5cm= £4.18, 17cm × 20cm= £6.07

Mepilex Border Lite

Thin absorbent soft silicone dressing with polyurethane foam film backing and adhesive border

Mepilex Border Lite dressing (Molnlycke Health Care Ltd) 15cm × 15cm= £3.94, 4cm × 5cm= £0.92, 5cm × 12.5cm= £2.01, 7.5cm × 7.5cm= £1.35

Mepilex Lite

Thin absorbent soft silicone dressing with polyurethane foam film backing

Mepilex Lite dressing (Molnlycke Health Care Ltd) 10cm × 10cm= £2.17, 15cm × 15cm= £4.22, 20cm × 50cm= £26.66, 6cm × 8.5cm= £1.82

Mepilex Transfer

Soft silicone exudate transfer dressing

Mepilex Transfer dressing (Molnlycke Health Care Ltd) 10cm × 12cm= £3.54, 15cm × 20cm= £10.72, 20cm × 50cm= £27.39, 7.5cm × 8.5cm= £2.25

A4

Wound management | Appendix 4

Sorbion Sana

Non-adherent polyethylene wound contact dressing with absorbent core

Cutimed Sorbion Sana Gentle dressing (BSN medical Ltd) 12cm × 12cm= £2.54, 12cm × 22cm= £4.57, 22cm × 22cm= £8.14, 8.5cm × 8.5cm= £2.03

Urgotul Duo

Non-adherent soft polymer wound contact dressing with absorbent pad

UrgotulDuo dressing (Urgo Ltd) 10cm × 12cm= £3.90, 15cm × 20cm= £9.06, 5cm × 10cm= £2.52

Without absorbent pad

Adaptic Touch

Non-adherent soft silicone wound contact dressing

Adaptic Touch dressing (Systagenix Wound Management Ltd) 12.7cm × 15cm= £4.65, 20cm × 32cm= £12.50, 5cm × 7.6cm= £1.13, 7.6cm × 11cm= £2.25

Askina SilNet

Soft silicone-coated wound contact dressing

Askina SilNet dressing (B.Braun Medical Ltd) 10cm × 18cm= £5.08, 20cm × 30cm= £12.42, 5cm × 7.5cm= £1.15, 7.5cm × 10cm= £2.33

Mepitel

Soft silicone, semi-transparent wound contact dressing

Mepitel dressing (Molnlycke Health Care Ltd) 12cm × 15cm= £5.60, 5cm × 7cm= £1.40, 8cm × 10cm= £2.80

Mepitel One

Soft silicone, thin, transparent wound contact dressing

Mepitel One dressing (Molnlycke Health Care Ltd) 13cm × 15cm= £4.98, 24cm × 27.5cm= £14.25, 6cm × 7cm= £1.22, 9cm × 10cm= £2.41

Physiotulle

Non-adherent soft polymer wound contact dressing

Physiotulle dressing (Coloplast Ltd) 10cm × 10cm= £2.30, 15cm × 20cm= £7.02

Silflex

Soft silicone-coated polyester wound contact dressing

Silflex dressing (Advancis Medical) 12cm × 15cm= £4.61, 20cm × 30cm= £11.88, 35cm × 60cm= £39.83, 5cm × 7cm= £1.12, 8cm × 10cm= £2.29

Silon-TSR

Soft silicone polymer wound contact dressing

Silon-TSR dressing (Bio Med Sciences) 13cm × 13cm= £3.52, 13cm × 25cm= £5.47, 28cm × 30cm= £7.37

Sobion Contact

Non-adherent soft polymer wound contact dressing

Cutimed Sorbion Contact dressing (BSN medical Ltd) 10cm × 10cm= £2.03, 10cm × 20cm= £4.06, 20cm × 20cm= £7.12, 20cm × 30cm= £10.18, 7.5cm × 7.5cm= £1.52

Tegaderm Contact

Non-adherent soft polymer wound contact dressing

Tegaderm Contact dressing (3M Health Care Ltd) 20cm × 25cm= £10.86, 7.5cm × 10cm= £2.27

Urgotul

Non-adherent soft polymer wound contact dressing

Urgotul dressing (Urgo Ltd) 10cm × 10cm= £3.13, 10cm × 40cm= £10.53, 15cm × 15cm= £6.66, 15cm × 20cm= £8.86, 20cm × 30cm= £14.25, 5cm × 5cm= £1.57

Hydrocolloid dressings

Hydrocolloid dressings are usually presented as a hydrocolloid layer on a vapour-permeable film or foam pad. Semi-permeable to water vapour and oxygen, these dressings form a gel in the presence of exudate to facilitate rehydration in lightly to moderately exuding wounds and promote autolytic debridement of dry, sloughy, or necrotic wounds; they are also suitable for promoting granulation. Hydrocolloid-fibrous dressings made from modified carmellose fibres resemble alginate dressings; hydrocolloid-fibrous dressings are more absorptive and suitable for moderately to heavily exuding wounds.

Hydrocolloid-fibrous dressings

Aquacel

Soft non-woven pad containing hydrocolloid-fibres

Aquacel (ConvaTec Ltd) Ribbon dressing 1cm × 45cm= £1.88, 2cm × 45cm= £2.50, dressing 10cm × 10cm square= £2.47, 15cm × 15cm square= £4.64, 4cm × 10cm rectangular= £1.33, 4cm × 20cm rectangular= £1.95, 4cm × 30cm rectangular= £2.94, 5cm × 5cm square= £1.04

Aquacel Foam

Soft non-woven pad containing hydrocolloid-fibres with foam layer; with or without adhesive border

Aquacel Foam dressing (adhesive) (ConvaTec Ltd) 10cm × 10cm= £2.18, 12.5cm × 12.5cm= £2.70, 17.5cm × 17.5cm= £5.40, 19.8cm × 14cm heel= £5.53, 20cm × 16.9cm sacral= £4.96, 21cm × 21cm= £7.91, 25cm × 30cm= £10.24, 8cm × 8cm= £1.42, (non-adhesive) 10cm × 10cm= £2.58, 15cm × 15cm= £4.33, 15cm × 20cm= £5.92, 20cm × 20cm= £7.07

UrgoClean Pad

Pad, hydrocolloid fibres coated with soft-adherent lipo-colloidal wound contact layer

UrgoClean Pad dressing (Urgo Ltd) 10cm × 10cm square= £2.16, 20cm × 15cm rectangular= £4.06, 6cm × 6cm square= £0.97

UrgoClean Rope

Rope, non-woven rope containing hydrocolloid fibres

UrgoClean rope dressing (Urgo Ltd) 2.5cm × 40cm= £2.43, 5cm × 40cm= £3.21

Polyurethane matrix dressing

Cutinova Hydro

Polyurethane matrix with absorbent particles and waterproof polyurethane film

Cutinova Hydro dressing (Smith & Nephew Healthcare Ltd) 10cm × 10cm square= £2.59, 15cm × 20cm rectangular= £5.48, 5cm × 6cm rectangular= £1.29

With adhesive border

Biatain Super

Semi-permeable hydrocolloid dressing; without adhesive border

Biatain Super dressing (adhesive) (Coloplast Ltd) 10cm × 10cm square= £2.21, 12.5cm × 12.5cm square= £3.66, 12cm × 20cm rectangular= £3.67, 15cm × 15cm square= £4.41, 20cm × 20cm square= £6.87

Granuflex Bordered

Hydrocolloid wound contact layer bonded to plastic foam layer, with outer semi-permeable polyurethane film

Granuflex Bordered dressing (ConvaTec Ltd) 10cm × 10cm square= £3.39, 10cm × 13cm triangular= £4.01, 15cm × 15cm square= £6.48, 15cm × 18cm triangular= £6.24, 6cm × 6cm square= £1.79

Hydrocoll Border

Hydrocolloid dressing with adhesive border and absorbent wound contact pad

Hydrocoll Border (bevelled edge) dressing (Paul Hartmann Ltd) 10cm × 10cm square= £2.46, 12cm × 18cm sacral= £3.69, 15cm × 15cm square= £4.63, 5cm × 5cm square= £1.03, 7.5cm × 7.5cm square= £1.69, 8cm × 12cm concave= £2.17

Tegaderm Hydrocolloid

Hydrocolloid dressing with adhesive border; normal or thin

Tegaderm Hydrocolloid (3M Health Care Ltd) Thin dressing 10cm × 12cm oval= £1.55, 13cm × 15cm oval= £2.89, dressing 10cm × 12cm oval= £2.33, 13cm × 15cm oval= £4.34, 17.1cm × 16.1cm sacral= £4.85

Ultec Pro

Semi-permeable hydrocolloid dressing with adhesive border

Ultec Pro dressing (adhesive) (Covidien (UK) Commercial Ltd) 15cm × 18cm sacral= £3.30, 19.5cm × 23cm sacral= £4.98, 21cm × 21cm square= £4.67

Without adhesive border

ActiVHeal Hydrocolloid

Semi-permeable polyurethane film backing, hydrocolloid wound contact layer, with or without polyurethane foam later

ActivHeal Hydrocolloid (Advanced Medical Solutions Ltd) dressing
10cm × 10cm square= £1.58, 15cm × 15cm square= £3.43, 15cm
× 18cm sacral= £3.98, 5cm × 7.5cm rectangular= £0.78, foam
backed dressing 10cm × 10cm square= £1.55, 15cm × 15cm
square= £2.91, 15cm × 18cm sacral= £3.36, 5cm × 7.5cm
rectangular= £0.97

Askina Biofilm Transparent
Semi-permeable, polyurethane film dressing with
hydrocolloid adhesive
Askina Biofilm Transparent dressing (B.Braun Medical Ltd) 10cm ×
10cm square= £1.09, 20cm × 20cm square= £3.22

Biatain Super
Semi-permeable, hydrocolloid film dressing without
adhesive border
Biatain Super dressing (non-adhesive) (Coloplast Ltd) 10cm × 10cm
square= £2.21, 12.5cm × 12.5cm square= £3.66, 12cm × 20cm
rectangular= £3.67, 15cm × 15cm square= £4.41, 20cm × 20cm
square= £6.87

Comfeel Plus Contour
Hydrocolloid dressings containing carmellose sodium and
calcium alginate
Comfeel Plus Contour dressing (Coloplast Ltd) 6cm × 8cm= £2.24,
9cm × 11cm= £3.89

Comfeel Plus Pressure Relieving
Hydrocolloid dressings containing carmellose sodium and
calcium alginate
Comfeel Plus Pressure Relief dressing (Coloplast Ltd) 10cm diameter
circular= £4.69, 15cm diameter circular= £7.06, 7cm diameter
circular= £3.50

Comfeel Plus Transparent
Hydrocolloid dressings containing carmellose sodium and
calcium alginate
Comfeel Plus Transparent dressing (Coloplast Ltd) 10cm × 10cm
square= £1.29, 15cm × 15cm square= £3.37, 15cm × 20cm
rectangular= £3.42, 20cm × 20cm square= £3.44, 5cm × 15cm
rectangular= £1.60, 5cm × 25cm rectangular= £2.61, 5cm ×
7cm rectangular= £0.68, 9cm × 14cm rectangular= £2.46, 9cm
× 25cm rectangular= £3.49

Comfeel Plus Ulcer
Hydrocolloid dressings containing carmellose sodium and
calcium alginate
Comfeel Plus dressing (Coloplast Ltd) 10cm × 10cm square= £2.48,
20cm × 20cm square= £7.64, 4cm × 6cm rectangular= £0.97

DuoDERM Extra Thin
Semi-permeable hydrocolloid dressing
DuoDERM Extra Thin dressing (ConvaTec Ltd) 10cm × 10cm square=
£1.34, 15cm × 15cm square= £2.90, 5cm × 10cm rectangular=
£0.78, 7.5cm × 7.5cm square= £0.81, 9cm × 15cm rectangular=
£1.80, 9cm × 25cm rectangular= £2.87, 9cm × 35cm
rectangular= £4.02

DuoDERM Signal
Semi-permeable hydrocolloid dressing with 'Time to change'
indicator
DuoDERM Signal dressing (ConvaTec Ltd) 10cm × 10cm square=
£2.16, 11cm × 19cm oval= £3.31, 14cm × 14cm square= £3.78,
18.5cm × 19.5cm heel= £5.29, 20cm × 20cm square= £7.52,
22.5cm × 20cm sacral= £6.18

Flexigran
Semi-permeable hydrocolloid dressing without adhesive
border; normal or thin
Flexigran (A1 Pharmaceuticals) Thin dressing 10cm × 10cm
square= £1.08, dressing 10cm × 10cm square= £2.19

Granuflex
Hydrocolloid wound contact layer bonded to plastic foam
layer, with outer semi-permeable polyurethane film
Granuflex (modified) dressing (ConvaTec Ltd) 10cm × 10cm square=
£2.85, 15cm × 15cm square= £5.40, 15cm × 20cm rectangular=
£5.86, 20cm × 20cm square= £8.13

Hydrocoll Basic
Hydrocolloid dressing with absorbent wound contact pad
Hydrocoll (Paul Hartmann Ltd) Basic dressing 10cm × 10cm square=
£2.50

Hydrocoll Thin Film
Thin hydrocolloid dressing with absorbent wound contact
pad
Hydrocoll Thin Film dressing (Paul Hartmann Ltd) 10cm × 10cm
square= £1.18, 15cm × 15cm square= £2.65, 7.5cm × 7.5cm
square= £0.71

Nu-Derm
Semi-permeable hydrocolloid dressing (normal and thin)
Nu-Derm dressing (Systagenix Wound Management Ltd) 10cm × 10cm
square= £1.56, 15cm × 15cm square= £3.18, 15cm × 18cm
sacral= £4.45, 20cm × 20cm square= £6.36, 5cm × 5cm square=
£0.85, 8cm × 12cm heel/elbow= £3.18, thin 10cm × 10cm
square= £1.06

Tegaderm Hydrocolloid
Hydrocolloid dressing without adhesive border; normal and
thin
Tegaderm Hydrocolloid (3M Health Care Ltd) Thin dressing 10cm ×
10cm square= £1.55, dressing 10cm × 10cm square= £2.37

Ultec Pro
Semi-permeable hydrocolloid dressing; without adhesive
border
Ultec Pro dressing (Covidien (UK) Commercial Ltd) 10cm × 10cm
square= £2.28, 15cm × 15cm square= £4.44, 20cm × 20cm
square= £6.69

Foam dressings
Dressings containing hydrophilic polyurethane foam
(adhesive or non-adhesive), with or without plastic film-
backing, are suitable for all types of exuding wounds, but not
for dry wounds; some foam dressings have a moisture-
sensitive film backing with variable permeability dependant
on the level of exudate Foam dressings vary in their ability to
absorb exudate; some are suitable only for lightly to
moderately exuding wounds, others have greater fluid-
handing capacity and are suitable for heavily exuding
wounds. Saturated foam dressings can cause maceration of
healthy skin if left in contact with the wound. Foam
dressings can be used in combination with other primary
wound contact dressings. If used under compression
bandaging or compression garments, the fluid-handling
capacity of the foam dressing may be reduced. Foam
dressings can also be used to provide a protective cushion for
fragile skin. A foam dressing containing ibuprofen is
available and may be useful for treating painful exuding
wounds.

Cavi-Care
Soft, conforming cavity wound dressing prepared by mixing
thoroughly for 15 seconds immediately before use and
allowing to expand its volume within the cavity

Polyurethane Foam Dressing
Cutimed Cavity
Cutimed Cavity dressing (BSN medical Ltd) 10cm × 10cm= £3.17,
15cm × 15cm= £4.77, 5cm × 6cm= £1.91

Kendall
Kendall Foam dressing (H & R Healthcare Ltd) 10cm × 10cm square=
£1.06, 10cm × 20cm rectangular= £2.05, 12.5cm × 12.5cm
square= £1.80, 15cm × 15cm square= £2.60, 20cm × 20cm
square= £3.01, 5cm × 5cm square= £0.71, 7.5cm × 7.5cm
square= £1.21, 8.5cm × 7.5cm rectangular (fenestrated)= £0.91

Polyurethane Foam Film Dressing with Adhesive Border
ActivHeal Foam Adhesive
ActivHeal Foam Adhesive dressing (Advanced Medical Solutions Ltd)
10cm × 10cm square= £1.63, 12.5cm × 12.5cm square= £1.68,
15cm × 15cm square= £2.15, 20cm × 20cm square= £4.50, 7.5cm
× 7.5cm square= £1.18

A4

Wound management | Appendix 4

Allevyn Adhesive
Allevyn Adhesive dressing (Smith & Nephew Healthcare Ltd) 10cm ×
10cm square= £2.22, 12.5cm × 12.5cm square= £2.72, 12.5cm ×
22.5cm rectangular= £4.23, 17.5cm × 17.5cm square= £5.37,
17cm × 17cm anatomically shaped sacral= £4.04, 22.5cm ×
22.5cm square= £7.82, 22cm × 22cm anatomically shaped
sacral= £5.81, 7.5cm × 7.5cm square= £1.52

Biatain Adhesive
Biatain Adhesive dressing (Coloplast Ltd) 10cm × 10cm square=
£1.79, 12.5cm × 12.5cm square= £2.60, 17cm diameter contour=
£5.05, 18cm × 18cm square= £5.25, 18cm × 28cm rectangular=
£7.78, 19cm × 20cm heel= £5.25, 23cm × 23cm sacral= £4.49

Biatain Silicone
Biatain Silicone dressing (Coloplast Ltd) 7.5cm × 7.5cm= £1.48,
10cm × 10cm= £2.18, 12.5cm × 12.5cm= £2.67, 15cm × 15cm=
£3.96, 17.5cm × 17.5cm= £5.26

Kendall Island
Kendall Foam Island dressing (H & R Healthcare Ltd) 10cm × 10cm
square= £1.54, 15cm × 15cm square= £2.90, 20cm × 20cm
square= £5.46

PermaFoam
PermaFoam dressing (adhesive) (Paul Hartmann Ltd) 16.5cm × 18cm
concave= £4.12, 18cm × 18cm sacral= £3.39, 22cm × 22cm
sacral= £3.89

PermaFoam Comfort
PermaFoam Comfort dressing (Paul Hartmann Ltd) 10cm × 20cm
rectangular= £3.43, 11cm × 11cm square= £2.17, 15cm × 15cm
square= £3.55, 20cm × 20cm square= £5.15, 8cm × 8cm square=
£1.14

PolyMem
PolyMem dressing (Aspen Medical Europe Ltd) 5cm × 5cm square=
£0.52, 16.5cm × 20.9cm oval= £6.79, 18.4cm × 20cm sacral=
£4.56, 5cm × 7.6cm oval= £1.16, 8.8cm × 12.7cm oval= £2.06

Tegaderm Foam Adhesive
Tegaderm Foam dressing (adhesive) (3M Health Care Ltd) 10cm ×
11cm oval= £2.39, 13.9cm × 13.9cm circular (heel)= £4.22,
14.3cm × 14.3cm square= £3.54, 14.3cm × 15.6cm oval= £4.24,
19cm × 22.2cm oval= £6.96, 6.9cm × 6.9cm soft cloth border=
£1.71, 6.9cm × 7.6cm oval= £1.46

Tielle
Tielle (Systagenix Wound Management Ltd) Lite dressing 11cm ×
11cm square= £2.28, dressing 15cm × 15cm square= £3.89, 15cm
× 20cm rectangular= £4.87, 18cm × 18cm square= £4.95, 7cm
× 9cm rectangular= £1.28

Tielle Lite
Tielle Lite dressing (Systagenix Wound Management Ltd) 11cm × 11cm
square= £2.28, 7cm × 9cm rectangular= £1.21, 8cm × 15cm
rectangular= £2.81, 8cm × 20cm rectangular= £2.97

Tielle Plus
Tielle Plus dressing (Systagenix Wound Management Ltd) 11cm × 11cm
square= £2.63, 15cm × 15cm sacrum= £3.13, square= £4.30,
15cm × 20cm rectangular= £5.39, 20cm × 26.5cm heel= £4.45

Polyurethane Foam Film Dressing without Adhesive Border
ActivHeal Foam Non-Adhesive
ActivHeal Non-Adhesive Foam polyurethane dressing (Advanced
Medical Solutions Ltd) 10cm × 10cm square= £1.13, 10cm × 20cm
rectangular= £2.34, 20cm × 20cm square= £3.92, 5cm × 5cm
square= £0.75

Advazorb
Advazorb (Advancis Medical) Heel dressing 17cm × 21cm= £4.78,
dressing 10cm × 10cm square= £1.09, 10cm × 20cm
rectangular= £3.37, 12.5cm × 12.5cm square= £1.60, 15cm ×
15cm square= £2.12, 20cm × 20cm square= £3.78, 5cm × 5cm
square= £0.65, 7.5cm × 7.5cm square= £0.79

Advazorb Lite
Advazorb Lite dressing (Advancis Medical) 10cm × 10cm square=
£0.98, 10cm × 20cm rectangular= £3.04, 12.5cm × 12.5cm
square= £1.44, 15cm × 15cm square= £1.90, 20cm × 20cm
square= £3.40, 7.5cm × 7.5cm square= £0.71

Allevyn Non-Adhesive
Allevyn dressing (non-adhesive) (Smith & Nephew Healthcare Ltd)
10.5cm × 13.5cm heel (cup shaped)= £5.20, 10cm × 10cm
square= £2.54, 10cm × 20cm rectangular= £4.08, 20cm × 20cm
square= £6.82, 5cm × 5cm square= £1.28

Askina Foam
Askina (B.Braun Medical Ltd) Foam Cavity dressing 2.4cm × 40cm=
£2.49, Foam dressing 10cm × 10cm square= £2.23, 10cm ×
20cm rectangular= £3.52, 20cm × 20cm square= £5.88, Heel
dressing 12cm × 20cm= £4.76

Biatain -Ibu Non-Adhesive
Biatain-Ibu Non-Adhesive dressing (Coloplast Ltd) 10cm × 12cm
rectangular= £3.37, 10cm × 22.5cm rectangular= £5.30, 15cm ×
15cm square= £5.30, 20cm × 20cm square= £9.02, 5cm × 7cm
rectangular= £1.75

Biatain-Ibu Soft-Hold
Biatain-Ibu Soft-Hold dressing (Coloplast Ltd) 10cm × 12cm
rectangular= £3.37, 10cm × 22.5cm rectangular= £5.30, 15cm ×
15cm square= £5.30

Biatain Non-Adhesive
Biatain Non-Adhesive dressing (Coloplast Ltd) 10cm × 10cm
square= £2.42, 10cm × 20cm rectangular= £4.00, 15cm × 15cm
square= £4.46, 20cm × 20cm square= £6.62, 5cm × 7cm
rectangular= £1.33

Biatain Soft-Hold
Biatain Soft-Hold dressing (Coloplast Ltd) 10cm × 10cm square=
£2.63, 10cm × 20cm rectangular= £4.00, 15cm × 15cm square=
£4.37, 5cm × 7cm rectangular= £1.33

Kendall Plus
Kendall Foam Plus dressing (H & R Healthcare Ltd) 10cm × 10cm
square= £1.47, 10cm × 20cm rectangular= £2.69, 15cm × 15cm
square= £3.38, 20cm × 20cm square= £4.04, 5cm × 5cm square=
£0.82, 7.5cm × 7.5cm square= £1.42, 8.5cm × 7.5cm rectangular
(fenestrated)= £1.24

Kerraheel
Kerraheel (Crawford Healthcare Ltd) dressing 12cm × 20cm heel=
£4.72

Lyofoam Max
Lyofoam Max dressing (Molnlycke Health Care Ltd) 10cm × 10cm
square= £1.15, 10cm × 20cm rectangular= £2.03, 15cm × 15cm
square= £2.16, 15cm × 20cm rectangular= £2.73, 20cm × 20cm
square= £4.01, 7.5cm × 8.5cm rectangular= £1.10

PermaFoam
PermaFoam (Paul Hartmann Ltd) Cavity dressing 10cm × 10cm=
£2.06, dressing (non-adhesive) 10cm × 10cm square= £2.17,
10cm × 20cm rectangular= £3.72, 15cm × 15cm square= £4.12,
20cm × 20cm square= £6.29, 6cm diameter circular= £1.12, 8cm
× 8cm square (fenestrated)= £1.28

PolyMem
PolyMem dressing (Aspen Medical Europe Ltd) 7cm × 7cm tube=
£1.73, 9cm × 9cm tube= £2.19, finger/toe size 1= £2.52, 2=
£2.52, 3= £2.52

PolyMem
PolyMem dressing (non-adhesive) (Aspen Medical Europe Ltd) 10cm ×
10cm square= £2.49, 10cm × 61cm rectangular= £13.20, 13cm ×
13cm square= £4.15, 17cm × 19cm rectangular= £6.13, 20cm ×
60cm rectangular= £31.13, 8cm × 8cm square= £1.60

PolyMem Max
PolyMem Max dressing (Aspen Medical Europe Ltd) 11cm × 11cm
square= £2.99, 20cm × 20cm square= £11.77

PolyMem WIC
PolyMem (Aspen Medical Europe Ltd) WIC dressing 8cm × 8cm=
£3.72

Tegaderm Foam
Tegaderm Foam dressing (3M Health Care Ltd) 10cm × 10cm
square= £2.19, 10cm × 20cm rectangular= £3.71, 10cm × 60cm
rectangular= £12.54, 20cm × 20cm square= £5.92, 8.8cm ×
8.8cm square (fenestrated)= £2.23

Transorbent

Transorbent dressing (adhesive) (B.Braun Medical Ltd) 10cm × 10cm square= £2.00, 15cm × 15cm square= £3.68, 20cm × 20cm square= £5.87, 5cm × 7cm rectangular= £1.06

UrgoCell TLC

UrgoTul Absorb dressing (Urgo Ltd) 10cm × 10cm= £2.38, 15cm × 20cm= £4.20, 6cm × 6cm= £1.21, 12cm × 19cm heel= £4.80

Alginate dressings

Non-woven or fibrous, non-occlusive, alginate dressings, made from calcium alginate, or calcium sodium alginate, derived from brown seaweed, form a soft gel in contact with wound exudate. Alginate dressings are highly absorbent and suitable for use on exuding wounds, and for the promotion of autolytic debridement of debris in very moist wounds. Alginate dressings also act as a haemostatic, but caution is needed because blood clots can cause the dressing to adhere to the wound surface. Alginate dressings should not be used if bleeding is heavy and extreme caution is needed if used for tumours with friable tissue. Alginate sheets are suitable for use as a wound contact dressing for moderately to heavily exuding wounds and can be layered into deep wounds; alginate rope can be used in sinus and cavity wounds to improve absorption of exudate and prevent maceration. If the dressing does not have an adhesive border or integral adhesive plastic film backing, a secondary dressing will be required.

ActivHeal Alginate

Calcium sodium alginate dressing

ActivHeal Alginate dressing (Advanced Medical Solutions Ltd) 10cm × 10cm= £1.15, 10cm × 20cm= £2.83, 5cm × 5cm= £0.59

ActivHeal Aquafiber

Non-woven, calcium sodium alginate dressing

ActivHeal Aquafiber (Advanced Medical Solutions Ltd) Rope dressing 2cm × 42cm= £1.81, dressing 10cm × 10cm= £1.80, 15cm × 15cm= £3.40, 5cm × 5cm= £0.76

Algisite M

Calcium alginate fibre, non-woven dressing

Algisite M (Smith & Nephew Healthcare Ltd) Rope dressing 2cm × 30cm= £3.53, dressing 10cm × 10cm= £1.95, 15cm × 20cm= £5.23, 5cm × 5cm= £0.94

Algosteril

Calcium alginate dressing

Algosteril (Smith & Nephew Healthcare Ltd) Rope dressing 2g= £3.86, dressing 10cm × 10cm= £2.14, 10cm × 20cm= £3.61, 5cm × 5cm= £0.93

Biatain Alginate

Alginate and carboxymethylcellulose dressing, highly absorbent, gelling dressing

Biatain Alginate dressing (Coloplast Ltd) 10cm × 10cm= £2.35, 15cm × 15cm= £4.46, 44cm= £2.77, 5cm × 5cm= £0.99

Cutimed Alginate

Calcium sodium alginate dressing

Cutimed Alginate dressing (BSN medical Ltd) 10cm × 10cm= £1.59, 10cm × 20cm= £3.00, 5cm × 5cm= £0.76

Kaltostat

Calcium alginate fibre, non-woven

Kaltostat dressing (ConvaTec Ltd) 10cm × 20cm= £4.15, 15cm × 25cm= £7.14, 2g= £3.89, 5cm × 5cm= £0.97, 7.5cm × 12cm= £2.12

Kendall

Calcium alginate dressing

Kendall Calcium Alginate (H & R Healthcare Ltd) Rope dressing 30cm= £2.89, 61cm= £5.07, 91cm= £5.46, dressing 10cm × 10cm= £1.52, 10cm × 14cm= £2.45, 10cm × 20cm= £2.98, 15cm × 25cm= £5.25, 30cm × 61cm= £27.56, 5cm × 5cm= £0.72

Kendall Plus

Calcium alginate dressing

Kendall (H & R Healthcare Ltd) Foam Plus dressing 10cm × 10cm square= £1.47

Melgisorb

Calcium sodium alginate fibre, highly absorbent, gelling dressing, non-woven

Melgisorb (Molnlycke Health Care Ltd) Cavity dressing 2.2cm × 32cm= £3.55, dressing 10cm × 10cm= £1.88, 10cm × 20cm= £3.52, 5cm × 5cm= £0.90

Sorbalgon

Calcium alginate dressing

Sorbalgon (Paul Hartmann Ltd) T dressing 2g= £3.56, dressing 10cm × 10cm= £1.74, 5cm × 5cm= £0.83

Sorbsan Flat

Calcium alginate fibre, highly absorbent, flat non-woven pads

Sorbsan Flat dressing (Aspen Medical Europe Ltd) 10cm × 10cm= £1.72, 10cm × 20cm= £3.22, 5cm × 5cm= £0.82

Sorbsan Plus

Alginate dressing bonded to a secondary absorbent viscose pad

Sorbsan Plus dressing (Aspen Medical Europe Ltd) 10cm × 15cm= £3.12, 10cm × 20cm= £3.98, 15cm × 20cm= £5.53, 7.5cm × 10cm= £1.77

Sorbsan Ribbon

Alginate dressing bonded to a secondary absorbent viscose pad

Sorbsan (Aspen Medical Europe Ltd) Ribbon dressing 40cm= £2.06

Sorbsan Surgical Packing

Alginate dressing bonded to a secondary absorbent viscose pad

Sorbsan (Aspen Medical Europe Ltd) Packing dressing 2g= £3.50

Suprasorb A

Calcium alginate dressing

Suprasorb A (Lohmann & Rauscher) alginate dressing 10cm × 10cm= £1.25, 5cm × 5cm= £0.64, cavity dressing 2g= £2.32

Tegaderm Alginate

Calcium alginate dressing

Tegaderm Alginate dressing (3M Health Care Ltd) 10cm × 10cm= £1.72, 2cm × 30.4cm= £2.87, 5cm × 5cm= £0.81

Urgosorb

Alginate and carboxymethylcellulose dressing without adhesive border

Urgosorb (Urgo Ltd) Pad dressing 10cm × 10cm= £2.15, 10cm × 20cm= £3.94, 5cm × 5cm= £0.90, Rope dressing 30cm= £2.81

Capillary-acting dressings

Vacutex

Low-adherent dressing consisting of two external polyester wound contact layers with central wicking polyester/cotton mix absorbent layer

Vacutex dressing (Haddenham Healthcare Ltd) 10cm × 10cm= £1.69, 10cm × 15cm= £2.27, 10cm × 20cm= £2.72, 5cm × 5cm= £0.95

Odour absorbent dressings

Dressings containing activated charcoal are used to absorb odour from wounds. The underlying cause of wound odour should be identified. Wound odour is most effectively reduced by debridement of slough, reduction in bacterial levels, and frequent dressing changes. Fungating wounds and chronic infected wounds produce high volumes of exudate which can reduce the effectiveness of odour absorbent dressings. Many odour absorbent dressings are intended for use in combination with other dressings; odour absorbent dressings with a suitable wound contact layer can be used as a primary dressing.

Askina Carbosorb

Activated charcoal and non-woven viscose rayon dressing

Askina Carbosorb dressing (B.Braun Medical Ltd) 10cm × 10cm= £2.95, 10cm × 20cm= £5.68

CarboFLEX

Dressing in 5 layers: wound-facing absorbent layer containing alginate and hydrocolloid; water-resistant second layer; third layer containing activated charcoal; non-woven absorbent fourth layer; water-resistant backing layer

CarboFlex dressing (ConvaTec Ltd) 10cm × 10cm= £3.27, 15cm × 20cm= £7.44, 8cm × 15cm oval= £3.92

A4

Wound management | Appendix 4

Carbopad VC
Activated charcoal non-absorbent dressing
Carbopad VC dressing (Synergy Health (UK) Ltd) 10cm × 10cm=
£1.62, 10cm × 20cm= £2.19

CliniSorb Odour Control Dressings
Activated charcoal cloth enclosed in viscose rayon with outer
polyamide coating
CliniSorb dressing (CliniMed Ltd) 10cm × 10cm= £1.92, 10cm ×
20cm= £2.56, 15cm × 25cm= £4.12

Antimicrobial dressings

Spreading infection at the wound site requires treatment
with systemic antibacterials. For local wound infection, a
topical antimicrobial dressing can be used to reduce the level
of bacteria at the wound surface but will not eliminate a
spreading infection. Some dressings are designed to release
the antimicrobial into the wound, others act upon the
bacteria after absorption from the wound. The amount of
exudate present and the level of infection should be taken
into account when selecting an antimicrobial dressing.
Medical grade honey has antimicrobial and anti-
inflammatory properties. Dressings impregnated with iodine
can be used to treat clinically infected wounds. Dressings
containing silver should be used only when clinical signs or
symptoms of infection are present. Dressings containing
other antimicrobials such as polihexanide
(polyhexamethylene biguanide) or dialkylcarbamoyl chloride
are available for use on infected wounds. Although
hypersensitivity is unlikely with chlorhexidine impregnated
tulle dressing, the antibacterial efficacy of these dressings
has not been established.

Honey
Medical grade honey has antimicrobial and anti-
inflammatory properties and can be used for acute or chronic
wounds. Medical grade honey has osmotic properties,
producing an environment that promotes autolytic
debridement; it can help control wound malodour. Honey
dressings should not be used on patients with extreme
sensitivity to honey, bee stings or bee products. Patients
with diabetes should be monitored for changes in blood-
glucose concentrations during treatment with topical honey
or honey-impregnated dressings.
For *Activon Tulle* ®, where no size is stated by the prescriber
the 5 cm size is to be supplied.
Medihoney ® *Antimicrobial Wound Gel* is not recommended for
use in deep wounds or body cavities where removal of waxes
may be difficult.

Honey-based topical application
Activon Honey
Medical grade manuka honey
Activon Medical Grade Manuka Honey dressing (Advancis Medical)
25 gram= £2.77

L-Mesitran SOFT ointment dressing
Honey (medical grade) 40%
L-Mesitran (Aspen Medical Europe Ltd) SOFT ointment dressing=
£3.62

MANUKApli Honey
Medical grade manuka honey
MANUKApli (Manuka Medical Ltd) dressing= £5.90

Medihoney Antibacterial Medical Honey
Medical grade, Leptospermum sp.
Medihoney (Derma Sciences Europe, Ltd) Antibacterial Medical
Honey dressing= £9.97

Medihoney Antibacterial Wound Gel
Medical grade, Leptospermum sp. 80% in natural waxes and
oils
Medihoney (Derma Sciences Europe, Ltd) Antibacterial Wound Gel
dressing= £4.05

Sheet dressing
Actilite
Knitted viscose impregnated with medical grade manuka
honey and manuka oil
Actilite gauze dressing (Advancis Medical) 10cm × 10cm= £1.23,
10cm × 20cm= £2.38, 5cm × 5cm= £0.71

Activon Tulle
Knitted viscose impregnated with medical grade manuka
honey
Activon Tulle gauze dressing (Advancis Medical) 10cm × 10cm=
£3.71, 5cm × 5cm= £2.25

Algivon
Absorbent, non-adherent calcium alginate dressing
impregnated with medical grade manuka honey
Algivon dressing (Advancis Medical) 10cm × 10cm= £4.25, 5cm ×
5cm= £2.48

Algivon Plus
Reinforced calcium alginate dressing impregnated with
medical grade manuka honey
Algivon Plus (Advancis Medical) Ribbon dressing 2.5cm × 20cm=
£4.20, dressing 10cm × 10cm=£4.20, 5cm × 5cm= £2.45

L-Mesitran Border
Hydrogel, semi-permeable dressing impregnated with
medical grade honey, with adhesive border
L-Mesitran (Aspen Medical Europe Ltd) Border sheet 10cm × 10cm
square= £2.76

L-Mesitran Hydro
Hydrogel, semi-permeable dressing impregnated with
medical grade honey, without adhesive border
L-Mesitran Hydro sheet (Aspen Medical Europe Ltd) 10cm × 10cm
square= £2.65, 15cm × 20cm rectangular= £5.48

L-Mesitran Net
Hydrogel, non-adherent wound contact layer, without
adhesive border
L-Mesitran (Aspen Medical Europe Ltd) Net sheet 10cm × 10cm
square= £2.55

Medihoney Antibacterial Honey Apinate
Non-adherent calcium alginate dressing, impregnated with
medical grade honey
Medihoney Antibacterial Honey Apinate (Derma Sciences Europe, Ltd)
dressing 10cm × 10cm square= £3.42, 5cm × 5cm square=
£2.01, rope dressing 1.9cm × 30cm= £4.23

Medihoney Antibacterial Honey Tulle
Woven fabric impregnated with medical grade manuka
honey
Medihoney (Derma Sciences Europe, Ltd) Tulle dressing 10cm x10cm=
£3.00

Medihoney Gel sheet
Sodium alginate dressing impregnated with medical grade
honey
Medihoney Gel Sheet dressing (Derma Sciences Europe, Ltd) 10cm ×
10cm= £4.23, 5cm × 5cm= £1.76

MelMax
Acetate wound contact layer impregnated with buckwheat
honey 75% in ointment basis
MelMax dressing (DoubleWing Medical) 5cm × 6cm rectangular=
£1.68, 8cm × 10cm rectangular= £2.00, 8cm × 20cm
rectangular= £3.75

Melladerm Plus Tulle
Knitted viscose impregnated with medical grade honey
(Bulgarian, mountain flower) 45% in a basis containing
polyethylene glycol
Melladerm (SanoMed Manufacturing BV) Plus Tulle dressing 10cm ×
10cm= £2.10

Iodine
Cadexomer–iodine, like povidone–iodine, releases free
iodine when exposed to wound exudate. The free iodine acts
as an antiseptic on the wound surface, the cadexomer
absorbs wound exudate and encourages de-sloughing. Two-
component hydrogel dressings containing glucose oxidase
and iodide ions generate a low level of free iodine in the

presence of moisture and oxygen. Povidone–iodine fabric dressing is a knitted viscose dressing with povidone–iodine incorporated in a hydrophilic polyethylene glycol basis; this facilitates diffusion of the iodine into the wound and permits removal of the dressing by irrigation. The iodine has a wide spectrum of antimicrobial activity but it is rapidly deactivated by wound exudate. Systemic absorption of iodine may occur, particularly from large wounds or with prolonged use.

Iodoflex ® and *Iodosorb* ® are used for the treatment of chronic exuding wounds; max. single application 50 g, max. weekly application 150 g; max. duration up to 3 months in any single course of treatment. They are contra-indicated in patients receiving lithium, in thyroid disorders, in pregnancy and breast feeding, and in children; they should be used with caution in patients with severe renal impairment or history of thyroid disorder.

Iodozyme ® is an antimicrobial dressing used for lightly to moderately exuding wounds. It is contra-indicated in thyroid disorders and in patients receiving lithium; it should be used with caution in children and in women who are pregnant or breast-feeding.

Oxyzyme ® is used for non-infected, dry to moderately exuding wounds. It is contra-indicated in thyroid disorders and in patients receiving lithium; it should be used with caution in children and in women who are pregnant or breast-feeding.

Povidone-iodine Fabric Dressing is used as a wound contact layer for abrasions and superficial burns. It is contra-indicated in patients with severe renal impairment and in women who are pregnant or breast-feeding; it should be used with caution in patients with thyroid disease and in children under 6 months.

Iodoflex Paste

Iodine 0.9% as cadexomer–iodine in a paste basis with gauze backing

Iodoflex paste dressing (Smith & Nephew Healthcare Ltd) 5 gram= £4.19, 10 gram= £8.37, 17 gram= £13.25

Iodosorb Ointment

Iodine 0.9% as cadexomer–iodine in an ointment basis

Iodosorb (Smith & Nephew Healthcare Ltd) ointment dressing= £9.25

Iodosorb Powder

Iodine 0.9% as cadexomer–iodine microbeads, 3-g sachet

Iodosorb (Smith & Nephew Healthcare Ltd) powder dressing sachets= £1.98

Povidone-iodine fabric dressing

Inadine

(Drug Tariff specification 43). Knitted viscose primary dressing impregnated with povidone–iodine ointment 10%

Inadine dressing (Systagenix Wound Management Ltd) 5cm × 5cm= £0.33, 9.5cm × 9.5cm= £0.49

Silver

Antimicrobial dressings containing silver should be used only when infection is suspected as a result of clinical signs or symptoms (see also notes above). Silver ions exert an antimicrobial effect in the presence of wound exudate; the volume of wound exudate as well as the presence of infection should be considered when selecting a silver-containing dressing. Silver-impregnated dressings should not be used routinely for the management of uncomplicated ulcers. It is recommended that these dressings should not be used on acute wounds as there is some evidence to suggest they delay wound healing. Dressings impregnated with silver sulfadiazine have broad antimicrobial activity; if silver sulfadiazine is applied to large areas, or used for prolonged periods, there is a risk of blood disorders and skin discoloration. The use of silver sulfadiazine-impregnated dressings is contra-indicated in neonates, in pregnancy, and in patients with significant renal or hepatic impairment, sensitivity to sulfonamides, or G6PD deficiency. Large amounts of silver sulfadiazine applied topically may interact with other drugs—see Appendix 1 (sulfonamides).

Alginate dressings

Algisite Ag

Calcium alginate dressing, with silver

Algisite Ag dressing (Smith & Nephew Healthcare Ltd) 10cm × 10cm= £4.23, 10cm × 20cm= £7.79, 2g= £5.85, 5cm × 5cm= £1.69

Askina Calgitrol Ag

Calcium alginate and silver alginate dressing with polyurethane foam backing

Askina Calgitrol Ag dressing (B.Braun Medical Ltd) 10cm × 10cm square= £3.26, 15cm × 15cm square= £6.32, 20cm × 20cm square= £14.74

Askina Calgitrol Thin

Calcium alginate and silver alginate matrix, for use with absorptive secondary dressings

Askina Calgitrol Thin dressing (B.Braun Medical Ltd) 10cm × 10cm square= £4.16, 15cm × 15cm square= £9.33, 20cm × 20cm square= £16.48, 5cm × 5cm square= £2.00

Melgisorb Ag

Alginate and carboxymethylcellulose dressing, with ionic silver

Melgisorb Ag (Molnlycke Health Care Ltd) Cavity dressing 3cm × 44cm= £4.57, dressing 10cm × 10cm= £3.67, 15cm × 15cm= £7.76, 5cm × 5cm= £1.83

Silvercel

Alginate and carboxymethylcellulose dressing impregnated with silver

Silvercel dressing (Systagenix Wound Management Ltd) 10cm × 20cm rectangular= £7.68, 11cm × 11cm square= £4.14, 2.5cm × 30.5cm rectangular= £4.45, 5cm × 5cm square= £1.68

Silvercel Non-adherent

Alginate and carboxymethylcellulose dressing with film wound contact layer, impregnated with silver

Silvercel Non-Adherent (Systagenix Wound Management Ltd) cavity dressing 2.5cm × 30.5cm= £3.94, dressing 10cm × 20cm rectangular= £7.25, 11cm × 11cm square= £3.89, 5cm × 5cm square= £1.62

Sorbsan Silver Flat

Calcium alginate fibre, highly absorbent, flat non-woven pads, with silver

Sorbsan Silver Flat dressing (Aspen Medical Europe Ltd) 10cm × 10cm= £4.00, 10cm × 20cm= £7.31, 5cm × 5cm= £1.58

Sorbsan Silver Plus

Calcium alginate dressing with absorbent backing, with silver

Sorbsan Silver Plus dressing (Aspen Medical Europe Ltd) 10cm × 15cm= £5.60, 10cm × 20cm= £6.82, 15cm × 20cm= £9.15, 7.5cm × 10cm= £3.37

Sorbsan Silver Ribbon

With silver

Sorbsan (Aspen Medical Europe Ltd) Silver Ribbon dressing 1g= £4.18

Sorbsan Silver Surgical Packing

With silver

Sorbsan (Aspen Medical Europe Ltd) Silver Packing dressing 2g= £5.80

Suprasorb A + Ag

Calcium alginate dressing, with silver

Suprasorb A + Ag (Lohmann & Rauscher) dressing 10cm × 10cm= £4.17, 10cm × 20cm= £7.70, 5cm × 5cm= £1.66, rope dressing 2g= £6.17

Tegaderm Alginate Ag

Calcium alginate and carboxymethylcellulose dressing, with silver

Tegaderm Alginate Ag dressing (3M Health Care Ltd) 10cm × 10cm= £3.24, 3cm × 30cm= £3.70, 5cm × 5cm= £1.39

Urgosorb Silver

Alginate and carboxymethylcellulose dressing, impregnated with silver

Urgosorb Silver (Urgo Ltd) Rope dressing 2.5cm × 30cm= £3.74, dressing 10cm × 10cm= £3.71, 10cm × 20cm= £7.00, 5cm × 5cm= £1.56

Foam dressings

Acticoat Moisture Control

Three layer polyurethane dressing consisting of a silver coated layer, a foam layer, and a waterproof layer

Acticoat Moisture Control dressing (Smith & Nephew Healthcare Ltd) 10cm × 10cm square= £17.09, 10cm × 20cm rectangular= £33.31, 5cm × 5cm square= £7.31

Allevyn Ag

Silver sulfadiazine impregnated polyurethane foam film dressing with or without adhesive border

Allevyn Ag (Smith & Nephew Healthcare Ltd) (Adhesive dressing) 10cm × 10cm square= £5.60, 12.5cm × 12.5cm square= £7.36, 17.5cm × 17.5cm square= £14.16, 17cm × 17cm sacral= £11.05, 22cm × 22cm sacral= £14.81, 7.5cm × 7.5cm square= £3.56, Heel Non-Adhesive dressing 10.5cm × 13.5cm= £10.96, (Non-Adhesive dressing) 10cm × 10cm square= £6.25, 15cm × 15cm square= £11.85, 20cm × 20cm square= £17.36, 5cm × 5cm square= £3.32

Biatain Ag

Silver impregnated polyurethane foam film dressing, with or without adhesive border

Biatain Ag (Coloplast Ltd) cavity dressing 5cm × 8cm= £4.10, dressing 10cm × 10cm square= £8.23, 10cm × 20cm rectangular= £15.12, 12.5cm × 12.5cm square= £9.41, 15cm × 15cm square= £16.51, 18cm × 18cm square= £18.88, 19cm × 20cm heel= £18.62, 20cm × 20cm square= £23.29, 23cm × 23cm sacral= £19.79, 5cm × 7cm rectangular= £3.38

PolyMem Silver

Silver impregnated polyurethane foam film dressing, with or without adhesive border

PolyMem Silver (Aspen Medical Europe Ltd) WIC dressing 8cm × 8cm= £7.10, dressing 10.8cm × 10.8cm square= £8.93, 12.7cm × 8.8cm oval= £5.64, 17cm × 19cm rectangular= £17.89, 5cm × 7.6cm oval= £2.29

UrgoCell Silver

Non-adherent, polyurethane foam film dressing with silver in wound contact layer

UrgoCell Silver dressing (Urgo Ltd) 10cm × 10cm= £6.00, 15cm × 20cm= £10.99, 6cm × 6cm= £4.36

Hydrocolloid dressings

Aquacel Ag

Soft non-woven pad containing hydrocolloid fibres, (silver impregnated),

Aquacel Ag (ConvaTec Ltd) Ribbon dressing 1cm × 45cm= £3.14, 2cm × 45cm= £4.80, dressing 10cm × 10cm square= £4.77, 15cm × 15cm square= £8.99, 20cm × 30cm rectangular= £22.30, 4cm × 10cm rectangular= £2.91, 4cm × 20cm rectangular= £3.79, 4cm × 30cm rectangular= £5.67

Physiotulle Ag

Non-adherent polyester fabric with hydrocolloid and silver sulfadiazine

Physiotulle (Coloplast Ltd) dressing 10cm × 10cm= £2.30

Low adherence dressing

Acticoat

Three-layer antimicrobial barrier dressing consisting of a polyester core between low adherent silver-coated high density polyethylene mesh (for 3-day wear)

Acticoat dressing (Smith & Nephew Healthcare Ltd) 10cm × 10cm square= £8.72, 10cm × 20cm rectangular= £13.64, 20cm × 40cm rectangular= £46.66, 5cm × 5cm square= £3.57

Acticoat 7

Five-layer antimicrobial barrier dressing consisting of a polyester core between low adherent silver-coated high density polyethylene mesh (for 7-day wear)

Acticoat 7 dressing (Smith & Nephew Healthcare Ltd) 10cm × 12.5cm rectangular= £18.49, 15cm × 15cm square= £33.24, 5cm × 5cm square= £6.21

Acticoat Flex 3

Conformable antimicrobial barrier dressing consisting of a polyester core between low adherent silver-coated high density polyethylene mesh (for 3-day wear)

Acticoat Flex 3 dressing (Smith & Nephew Healthcare Ltd) 10cm × 10cm square= £8.80, 10cm × 20cm rectangular= £13.75, 20cm × 40cm rectangular= £47.07, 5cm × 5cm square= £3.60

Acticoat Flex 7

Conformable antimicrobial barrier dressing consisting of a polyester core between low adherent silver-coated high density polyethylene mesh (for 7-day wear)

Acticoat Flex 7 dressing (Smith & Nephew Healthcare Ltd) 10cm × 12.5cm rectangular= £18.65, 15cm × 15cm square= £33.54, 5cm × 5cm square= £6.26

Atrauman Ag

Non-adherent polyamide fabric impregnated with silver and neutral triglycerides

Atrauman Ag dressing (Paul Hartmann Ltd) 10cm × 10cm= £1.28, 10cm × 20cm= £2.51, 5cm × 5cm= £0.53

Soft polymer dressings

Allevyn Ag Gentle

Soft polymer wound contact dressing, with silver sulfadiazine impregnated polyurethane foam layer, with or without adhesive border

Allevyn Ag Gentle (Smith & Nephew Healthcare Ltd) Border dressing 10cm × 10cm= £6.48, 12.5cm × 12.5cm= £8.33, 17.5cm × 17.5cm= £15.87, 7.5cm × 7.5cm= £4.31, dressing 10cm × 10cm= £6.29, 10cm × 20cm= £10.40, 15cm × 15cm= £11.70, 20cm × 20cm= £17.33, 5cm × 5cm= £3.38

Mepilex Ag

Soft silicone wound contact dressing with polyurethane foam film backing, with silver, with or without adhesive border

Mepilex (Molnlycke Health Care Ltd) Ag dressing 10cm × 10cm= £6.17, 10cm × 20cm= £10.17, 15cm × 15cm= £11.44, 20cm × 20cm= £16.96, 20cm × 50cm= £63.64, Border Ag dressing 10cm × 12.5cm= £6.21, 10cm × 20cm= £9.03, 10cm × 30cm= £13.55, 15cm × 17.5cm= £11.39, 17cm × 20cm= £14.76, 7cm × 7.5cm= £3.43, Border Sacrum Ag dressing 18cm × 18cm= £11.91, 20cm × 20cm= £14.48, 23cm × 23cm= £19.02, Heel Ag dressing 13cm × 20cm= £12.87, 15cm × 22cm= £14.42

Urgotul Silver

Non-adherent soft polymer wound contact dressing, with silver

Urgotul Silver dressing (Urgo Ltd) 10cm × 12cm= £3.61, 15cm × 20cm= £9.83

With charcoal

Actisorb Silver 220

Knitted fabric of activated charcoal, with one-way stretch, with silver residues, within spun-bonded nylon sleeve

Actisorb Silver 220 dressing (Systagenix Wound Management Ltd) 10.5cm × 10.5cm= £2.58, 10.5cm × 19cm= £4.70, 6.5cm × 9.5cm= £1.64

Other antimicrobials

Cutimed Siltec Sorbact

Polyurethane foam dressing with acetate fabric coated with dialkylcarbamoyl chloride, with adhesive border

Cutimed Siltec Sorbact dressing (BSN medical Ltd) 12.5cm × 12.5cm= £6.56, 15cm × 15cm= £8.13, 17.5cm × 17.5cm= £11.38, 22.5cm × 22.5cm= £17.31, 7.5cm × 7.5cm= £2.56, 17.5cm × 17.5cm sacral= £8.22, 23cm × 23cm sacral= £12.36

Cutimed Sorbact

Low adherence acetate tissue impregnated with dialkylcarbamoyl chloride; dressing pad, swabs, round swabs or ribbon gauze, cotton

Cutimed Sorbact (BSN medical Ltd) Ribbon dressing 2cm × 50cm= £4.11, 5cm × 200cm= £8.10, Round swab 3cm= £3.36, dressing pad 10cm × 10cm= £5.60, 10cm × 20cm= £8.74, 7cm × 9cm= £3.58, swab 4cm × 6cm= £1.68, 7cm × 9cm= £2.80

Cutimed Sorbact Gel
Hydrogel dressing impregnated with dialkylcarbamoyl chloride
Cutimed Sorbact Gel dressing (BSN medical Ltd) 7.5cm × 15cm rectangular= £4.56, 7.5cm × 7.5cm square= £2.70

Cutimed Sorbact Hydroactive
Non-adhesive gel dressing with hydropolymer matrix and acetate fabric coated with dialkylcarbamoyl chloride
Cutimed Sorbact Hydroactive dressing (BSN medical Ltd) 14cm × 14cm= £5.47, 14cm × 24cm= £8.76, 19cm × 19cm= £10.29, 24cm × 24cm= £15.60, 7cm × 8.5cm= £3.75

Cutimed Sorbact Hydroactive B
Gel dressing with hydropolymer matrix and acetate fabric coated with dialkylcarbamoyl chloride, with adhesive border
Cutimed Sorbact Hydroactive B dressing (BSN medical Ltd) 10cm × 10cm= £7.22, 10cm × 20cm= £11.56, 15cm × 15cm= £13.58, 5cm × 6.5cm= £4.05

Flaminal Forte gel
Alginate with glucose oxidase and lactoperoxidase, for moderately to heavily exuding wounds
Flaminal Forte gel dressing (Flen Health UK Ltd) 15g= £7.79, 50g= £25.78

Flaminal Hydro gel
Alginate with glucose oxidase and lactoperoxidase, for lightly to moderately exuding wounds
Flaminal Hydro gel dressing (Flen Health UK Ltd) 15g= £7.79, 50g= £25.78

Kendall AMD
Foam dressing with polihexanide, without adhesive border
Kendall AMD Antimicrobial foam dressing (H & R Healthcare Ltd) 10cm × 10cm square= £4.71, 10cm × 20cm rectangular= £8.92, 15cm × 15cm square= £8.92, 20cm × 20cm square= £13.07, 5cm × 5cm square= £2.50, 8.8cm × 7.5cm rectangular (fenestrated)= £4.23

Kendall AMD Plus
Foam dressing with polihexanide, without adhesive border
Kendall AMD Antimicrobial Plus foam dressing (H & R Healthcare Ltd) 10cm × 10cm square= £4.94, 8.8cm × 7.5cm rectangular (fenestrated)= £4.43

Octenilin Wound gel
Wound gel, hydroxyethylcellulose and propylene glycol, with octenidine hydrochloride
Octenilin Wound Gel dressing (Schulke & Mayr Ltd) 20ml= £4.78

Prontosan Wound Gel
Hydrogel containing betaine surfactant and polihexanide
Prontosan Wound Gel dressing (B.Braun Medical Ltd) 30ml= £6.50

Suprasorb X + PHMB
Biosynthetic cellulose fibre dressing with polihexanide
Suprasorb X + PHMB dressing (Lohmann & Rauscher) 14cm × 20cm rectangular= £11.80, 2cm × 21cm rope= £7.35, 5cm × 5cm square= £2.61, 9cm × 9cm square= £5.19

Telfa AMD
Low adherence absorbent perforated plastic film faced dressing with polihexanide
Telfa AMD dressing (H & R Healthcare Ltd) 10cm × 7.5cm= £0.18, 20cm × 7.5cm= £0.28

Telfa AMD Island
Low adherence dressing with adhesive border and absorbent pad, with polihexanide
Telfa AMD Island dressing (H & R Healthcare Ltd) 10cm × 12.5cm= £0.59, 10cm × 20cm= £0.86, 10cm × 25.5cm= £0.98, 10cm × 35cm= £1.22

Chlorhexidine gauze dressing
Bactigras
Fabric of leno weave, weft and warp threads of cotton and/or viscose yarn, impregnated with ointment containing chlorhexidine acetate
Bactigras gauze dressing (Smith & Nephew Healthcare Ltd) 10cm × 10cm= no price available, 5cm × 5cm= no price available

Irrigation fluids
Octenilin Wound irrigation solution
Aqueous solution containing glycerol, ethylhexylglycerin and octenidine hydrochloride
Octenilin irrigation solution (Schulke & Mayr Ltd) 350mL bottles= £4.60

Prontosan Wound Irrigation Solution
Aqueous solution containing betaine surfactant and polihexanide
Prontosan irrigation solution (B.Braun Medical Ltd) 350ml bottles= £4.86, 40ml unit dose= £14.45

Specialised dressings

Protease-modulating matrix dressings
Cadesorb Ointment
Cadesorb (Smith & Nephew Healthcare Ltd) ointment= £9.40

Catrix
Catrix dressing (Cranage Healthcare Ltd) sachets= £3.80

Promogran
Collagen and oxidised regenerated cellulose matrix, applied directly to wound and covered with suitable dressing
Promogran dressing (Systagenix Wound Management Ltd) 123 square cm= £15.62, 28 square cm= £5.19

Promogran Prisma Matrix
Collagen, silver and oxidised regenerated cellulose matrix, applied directly to wound and covered with suitable dressing
Promogran Prisma dressing (Systagenix Wound Management Ltd) 123 square cm= £17.98, 28 square cm= £6.31

UrgoStart
Soft adherent polymer matrix containing nano-oligosaccharide factor (NOSF), with polyurethane foam film backing
UrgoStart dressing (Urgo Ltd) 10cm × 10cm= £6.21, 15cm × 20cm= £11.17, 6cm × 6cm= £4.49, 12cm × 19cm heel= £8.56

UrgoStart Contact
Non-adherent soft polymer wound contact dressing containing nano-oligosaccharide factor (NOSF)
UrgoStart (Urgo Ltd) Contact dressing 5cm × 7cm= £3.03

Silicone keloid dressings
Silicone gel and gel sheets are used to reduce or prevent hypertrophic and keloid scarring. They should not be used on open wounds. Application times should be increased gradually. Silicone sheets can be washed and reused.

Silicone gel
Bapscarcare
Silicone gel
Bapscarcare (Espere Healthcare Ltd) gel= £17.12

Ciltech
Silicone gel
Ciltech (Su-Med International (UK) Ltd) gel= £50.00

Dermatix
Silicone gel
Dermatix gel (Meda Pharmaceuticals Ltd) = £60.53

Kelo-cote UV
Silicone gel with SPF 30 UV protection
Kelo-cote (Alliance Pharmaceuticals Ltd) UV gel= £17.88

Kelo-cote gel
Silicone gel
Kelo-cote (Alliance Pharmaceuticals Ltd) gel= £51.00

Kelo-cote spray
Silicone spray
Kelo-cote (Alliance Pharmaceuticals Ltd) spray= £51.00

NewGel+E
Silicone gel with vitamin E
NewGel+E (Advantech Surgical Ltd) gel= £17.70

ScarSil
Silicone gel
ScarSil (Jobskin Ltd) gel= £15.19

A4

Wound management | Appendix 4

Silgel STC-SE
Silicone gel
Silgel (Nagor Ltd) STC-SE gel= £19.00

Silicone sheets
Advasil Conform
Self-adhesive silicone gel sheet with polyurethane film
backing
Advasil Conform sheet (Advancis Medical) 10cm × 10cm square=
£5.24, 15cm × 10cm rectangular= £9.24

Bapscarcare T
Self-adhesive silicone gel sheet
Bapscarcare T sheet (Espere Healthcare Ltd) 10cm × 15cm
rectangular= £9.07, 5cm × 30cm rectangular= £9.07, 5cm ×
7cm rectangular= £3.17

Cica-Care
Soft, self-adhesive, semi-occlusive silicone gel sheet with
backing
Cica-Care sheet (Smith & Nephew Healthcare Ltd) 15cm × 12cm
rectangular= £29.06, 6cm × 12cm rectangular= £14.91

Ciltech
Silicone gel sheet
Ciltech sheet (Su-Med International (UK) Ltd) 10cm × 10cm square=
£7.50, 10cm × 20cm rectangular= £12.50, 15cm × 15cm square=
£14.00

Dermatix
Self-adhesive silicone gel sheet (clear- or fabric-backed)
Dermatix (Meda Pharmaceuticals Ltd) Clear sheet 13cm × 13cm
square= £15.79, 13cm × 25cm rectangular= £28.53, 20cm ×
30cm rectangular= £51.97, 4cm × 13cm rectangular= £6.88,
Fabric sheet 13cm × 13cm square= £15.79, 13cm × 25cm
rectangular= £28.53, 20cm × 30cm rectangular= £51.97, 4cm ×
13cm rectangular= £6.88

Mepiform
Self-adhesive silicone gel sheet with polyurethane film
backing
Mepiform sheet (Molnlycke Health Care Ltd) 4cm × 31cm
rectangular= £11.10, 5cm × 7cm rectangular= £3.51, 9cm ×
18cm rectangular= £13.75

Scar FX
Self-adhesive, transparent, silicone gel sheet
Scar Fx sheet (Jobskin Ltd) 10cm × 20cm rectangular= £16.00,
22.5cm × 14.5cm shaped= £12.00, 25.5cm × 30.5cm
rectangular= £60.00, 3.75cm × 22.5cm rectangular= £12.00,
7.5cm diameter shaped= £8.50

Silgel
Silicone gel sheet
Silgel sheet (Nagor Ltd) 10cm × 10cm square= £13.50, 10cm ×
30cm rectangular= £31.50, 10cm × 5cm rectangular= £7.50,
15cm × 10cm rectangular= £19.50, 20cm × 20cm square=
£40.00, 25cm × 15cm shaped= £21.12, 30cm × 5cm rectangular=
£19.50, 40cm × 40cm square= £144.00, 46cm × 8.5cm shaped=
£39.46, 5.5cm diameter shaped= £4.00

Adjunct dressings and appliances

Surgical absorbents
Surgical absorbents applied directly to the wound have many
disadvantages—dehydration of and adherence to the wound,
shedding of fibres, and the leakage of exudate ('strike
through') with an associated risk of infection. Gauze and
cotton absorbent dressings can be used as secondary layers
in the management of heavily exuding wounds (but see also
Capillary-action dressings). Absorbent cotton gauze fabric
can be used for swabbing and cleaning skin. Ribbon gauze
can be used post-operatively to pack wound cavities, but
adherence to the wound bed will cause bleeding and tissue
damage on removal of the dressing—an advanced wound
dressing (e.g. hydrocolloid-fibrous, foam, or alginate)
layered into the cavity is often more suitable.

Cotton
Absorbent Cotton, BP
Carded cotton fibres of not less than 10 mm average staple
length, available in rolls and balls
Absorbent (Robert Bailey & Son Plc) cotton BP 1988

Absorbent Cotton, Hospital Quality
As for absorbent cotton but lower quality materials, shorter
staple length etc.
Absorbent (Robert Bailey & Son Plc) cotton hospital quality

Gauze and cotton tissue
Gamgee Tissue (blue)
Consists of absorbent cotton enclosed in absorbent cotton
gauze type 12 or absorbent cotton and viscose gauze type 2
Gamgee (Robinson Healthcare) tissue blue label

Gamgee Tissue (pink)
Consists of absorbent cotton enclosed in absorbent cotton
gauze type 12 or absorbent cotton and viscose gauze type 2
Gamgee (Robinson Healthcare) tissue pink label DT

Gauze and tissue
Absorbent Cotton Gauze, BP 1988
Cotton fabric of plain weave, in rolls and as swabs (see
below), usually Type 13 light, sterile
Absorbent (Robert Bailey & Son Plc) cotton BP 1988
Alvita (Alliance Healthcare (Distribution) Ltd) absorbent cotton BP
1988
Clini (CliniSupplies Ltd) absorbent cotton BP 1988
Vernaid (Synergy Health (UK) Ltd) absorbent cotton BP 1988

Absorbent Cotton and Viscose Ribbon Gauze, BP 1988
Woven fabric in ribbon form with fast selvedge edges, warp
threads of cotton, weft threads of viscose or combined
cotton and viscose yarn, sterile
Vernaid Fast Edge ribbon gauze sterile (Synergy Health (UK) Ltd)
1.25cm, 2.5cm

Lint
Absorbent Lint, BPC
Cotton cloth of plain weave with nap raised on one side from
warp yarns
Absorbent (Robinson Healthcare) lint
Alvita (Alliance Healthcare (Distribution) Ltd) absorbent lint BPC
Clini (CliniSupplies Ltd) absorbent lint BPC

Pads
Drisorb
Absorbent Dressing Pads, Sterile
Drisorb (Synergy Health (UK) Ltd) dressing pad 10cm × 20cm= £0.17

PremierPad
Absorbent Dressing Pads, Sterile
PremierPad dressing pad (Shermond) 10cm × 20cm= £0.18, 20cm
× 20cm= £0.25

XuPad
Absorbent Dressing Pads, Sterile
Xupad dressing pad (Richardson Healthcare Ltd) 10cm × 20cm=
£0.17, 20cm × 20cm= £0.28, 20cm × 40cm= £0.40

Wound drainage pouches
Wound drainage pouches can be used in the management of
wounds and fistulas with significant levels of exudate.

Biotrol Draina S
Wound drainage pouch
Biotrol Draina S wound drainage bag (B.Braun Medical Ltd) large
(Transparent)= £97.23, medium (Transparent)= £79.06, mini
(Transparent)= £79.30

Biotrol Draina S Vision
Wound drainage pouch
Draina S Vision (B.Braun Medical Ltd) 100 wound drainage bag=
£126.25, 50 wound drainage bag= £103.00, 75 wound drainage
bag= £108.81

Eakin Access window
For use with Eakin ® pouches
Eakin (Pelican Healthcare Ltd) access window large= £38.45

Eakin Wound pouch, bung closure

Wound pouch, bung closure

Eakin wound drainage bag with bung closure (Pelican Healthcare Ltd) large= £104.36, medium= £76.90, small= £54.93, and access window for horizontal wounds, extra large= £104.36, for horizontal wounds, extra large= £93.38, for vertical incision wounds, extra large= £93.38, wounds, extra large= £93.38

Eakin Wound pouch, fold and tuck closure

Wound pouch, fold and tuck closure

Eakin wound drainage bag with fold and tuck closure (Pelican Healthcare Ltd) large= £93.38, medium= £71.41, small= £49.44, extra large= £82.39

Option Wound Manager

Wound drainage bag

Option wound manager bag (Oakmed Ltd) large= £161.34, medium= £135.36, small= £132.42, square= £141.25, extra small= £119.06

Option Wound Manager with access port

Wound drainage bag, with access port

Option wound manager bag with access port (Oakmed Ltd) large= £172.46, medium= £141.25, small= £138.31, square= £147.13, extra small= £130.18

Option Wound Manager, cut to fit

Wound drainage bag, cut to fit

Option wound manager bag (Oakmed Ltd) large= £84.82, medium= £80.98, small= £73.10

Welland Fistula bag

Wound drainage bag, cut-to-fit

Welland (Welland Medical Ltd) Fistula wound drainage bag= £83.60

Physical debridement pads

DebriSoft ® is a pad that is used for the debridement of superficial wounds containing loose slough and debris, and for the removal of hyperkeratosis from the skin. DebriSoft ® must be fully moistened with a wound cleansing solution before use and is not appropriate for use as a wound dressing.

DebriSoft Pad

Polyester fibres with bound edges and knitted outer surface coated with polyacrylate

DebriSoft (Lohmann & Rauscher) pad 10cm × 10cm= £6.55

Complex adjunct therapies

Topical negative pressure therapy

Accessories

Renasys

Soft port and connector

Renasys (Smith & Nephew Healthcare Ltd) Soft Port= £11.38, connector for use with soft port= £3.31

V.A.C.

Drape, gel for canister, Sensa T.R.A.C. Pad

SensaT.R.A.C. (KCI Medical Ltd) pad= £10.95

T.R.A.C. (KCI Medical Ltd) connector= £3.13

V.A.C. (KCI Medical Ltd) drape= £9.39, gel strips= £3.76

Venturi

Gel patches, adhesive, and connector

Venturi (Talley Group Ltd) adhesive gel patch= £15.00, connector= £15.00

WoundASSIST gel strip

WoundASSIST (Huntleigh Healthcare Ltd) TNP gel strip= £3.37

Vacuum assisted closure products

Exsu-Fast kit 1

Dressing Kit

Exsu-Fast (Synergy Health (UK) Ltd) dressing kit 1= £28.04

Exsu-Fast kit 2

Dressing Kit

Exsu-Fast (Synergy Health (UK) Ltd) dressing kit 2= £35.83

Exsu-Fast kit 3

Dressing Kit

Exsu-Fast (Synergy Health (UK) Ltd) dressing kit 3= £35.83

Exsu-Fast kit 4

Dressing Kit

Exsu-Fast (Synergy Health (UK) Ltd) dressing kit 4= £28.04

V.A.C GranuFoam

Polyurethane foam dressing (with adhesive drapes and pad connector); with or without silver

V.A.C. GranuFoam (KCI Medical Ltd) Bridge dressing kit= £32.04, Silver with SensaT.R.A.C dressing kit medium= £38.04, small= £32.79, dressing kit large= £31.70, medium= £27.32, small= £22.95

V.A.C Simplace

Spiral-cut polyurethane foam dressings, vapour-permeable adhesive film dressings (with adhesive drapes and pad connector)

V.A.C. Simplace EX dressing kit (KCI Medical Ltd) medium= £30.58, small= £26.60

V.A.C WhiteFoam

Polyvinyl alcohol foam dressing or dressing kit

V.A.C. WhiteFoam dressing (KCI Medical Ltd) large= £17.04, small= £10.64, kit large= £33.54, small= £25.91

Venturi

Wound sealing kit, flat drain; with or without channel drain

Venturi wound sealing kit with (Talley Group Ltd) channel drain= £15.00, flat drain, large= £17.50, standard= £15.00

WoundASSIST

Wound pack and channel drain

WoundASSIST TNP dressing pack (Huntleigh Healthcare Ltd) medium/large= £23.85, small/medium= £20.81, channel drain medium/large= £23.85, small/medium= £20.81, extra large= £34.05

Wound drainage collection devices

ActiV.A.C.

Canister with gel

ActiV.A.C (KCI Medical Ltd) canister with gel= £28.42

S-Canister

Canister kit

S-Canister (Smith & Nephew Healthcare Ltd) kit= £19.00

V.A.C Freedom

Canister with gel

V.A.C.(KCI Medical Ltd) Freedom Canister with gel= £28.85

Venturi

Canister kit with solidifier

Venturi (Talley Group Ltd) Compact canister kit= £12.50, canister kit= £12.50

WoundASSIST wound pack

Canister

WoundASSIST (Huntleigh Healthcare Ltd) TNP canister= £20.30

Wound care accessories

Dressing packs

The role of dressing packs is very limited. They are used to provide a clean or sterile working surface; some packs shown below include cotton wool balls, which are not recommended for use on wounds.

Multiple Pack Dressing No. 1

Contains absorbent cotton, absorbent cotton gauze type 13 light (sterile), open-wove bandages (banded)

Vernaid (Synergy Health (UK) Ltd) multiple pack dressing

Non-drug tariff specification sterile dressing packs

Dressit

Vitrex gloves, large apron, disposable bag, paper towel, softswabs, absorbent pad, sterile field

Dressit sterile dressing pack (Richardson Healthcare Ltd) with medium/large gloves= £0.60, small/medium gloves= £0.60

Nurse It

Contains latex-free, powder-free nitrile gloves, sterile laminated paper sheet, large apron, non-woven swabs, paper towel, disposable bag, compartmented tray, disposable forceps, paper measuring tape

Nurse It sterile dressing pack (Medicareplus International Ltd) with medium/large gloves= £0.55, small/medium gloves= £0.55

A4

Wound management | **Appendix 4**

Polyfield Nitrile Patient Pack

Contains powder-free nitrile gloves, laminate sheet, non-woven swabs, towel, polythene disposable bag, apron
Polyfield Nitrile Patient Pack (Shermond) with large gloves= £0.52, medium gloves= £0.52, small gloves= £0.52

Sterile Dressing Pack with Non-Woven Pads
Vernaid

(Drug Tariff specification 35). Contains non-woven fabric covered dressing pad, non-woven fabric swabs, absorbent cotton wool balls, absorbent paper towel, water repellent inner wrapper
Vernaid (Synergy Health (UK) Ltd) sterile dressing pack with non-woven pads

Sterile dressing packs
Vernaid

(Drug Tariff specification 10). Contains gauze and cotton tissue pad, gauze swabs, absorbent cotton wool balls, absorbent paper towel, water repellent inner wrapper
Vernaid (Synergy Health (UK) Ltd) sterile dressing pack

Woven and fabric swabs
Gauze Swab, PB 1988

Consists of absorbent cotton gauze type 13 light or absorbent cotton and viscose gauze type 1 folded into squares or rectangles of 8-ply with no cut edges exposed, sterile or non-sterile
Alvita gauze swab 8ply (Alliance Healthcare (Distribution) Ltd) non-sterile 10cm × 10cm, sterile 7.5cm × 7.5cm
CS (CliniSupplies Ltd) gauze swab 8ply non-sterile 10cm × 10cm
Clini gauze swab 8ply (CliniSupplies Ltd) non-sterile 10cm × 10cm, sterile 7.5cm × 7.5cm
Gauze (Robert Bailey & Son Plc) swab 8ply non-sterile 10cm × 10cm
MeCoBo gauze swab 8ply (MeCoBo Ltd) non-sterile 10cm × 10cm, sterile 7.5cm × 7.5cm
Propax gauze (BSN medical Ltd) swab 8ply sterile 7.5cm × 7.5cm
Sovereign (Waymade Healthcare Plc) gauze swab 8ply sterile 7.5cm × 7.5cm
Steraid (Robert Bailey & Son Plc) gauze swab 8ply sterile 7.5cm × 7.5cm
Vernaid gauze swab 8ply (Synergy Health (UK) Ltd) non-sterile 10cm × 10cm, sterile 7.5cm × 7.5cm

Non-woven Fabric Swab

(Drug Tariff specification 28). Consists of non-woven fabric folded 4-ply; alternative to gauze swabs, type 13 light, sterile or non-sterile
CS (CliniSupplies Ltd) non-woven fabric swab 4ply non-sterile 10cm × 10cm
Clini non-woven fabric swab 4ply (CliniSupplies Ltd) non-sterile 10cm × 10cm, sterile 7.5cm × 7.5cm
CliniMed (CliniMed Ltd) non-woven fabric swab 4ply non-sterile 10cm × 10cm
MeCoBo (MeCoBo Ltd) non-woven fabric swab 4ply non-sterile 10cm × 10cm
Multisorb (BSN medical Ltd) non-woven fabric swab 4ply sterile 7.5cm × 7.5cm
Sofsorb non-woven fabric swab 4ply (Synergy Health (UK) Ltd) non-sterile 10cm × 10cm, sterile 7.5cm × 7.5cm
Softswab non-woven fabric swab 4ply (Richardson Healthcare Ltd) non-sterile 10cm × 10cm, sterile 7.5cm × 7.5cm
Topper 8 non-woven fabric swab 4ply (Systagenix Wound Management Ltd) non-sterile 10cm × 10cm, sterile 7.5cm × 7.5cm

Filmated non-woven Fabric Swab
Regal

(Drug Tariff specification 29). Film of viscose fibres enclosed within non-woven viscose fabric folded 8-ply, non-sterile
Regal (Systagenix Wound Management Ltd) filmated swab 8ply 10cm × 10cm

Surgical adhesive tapes

Adhesive tapes are useful for retaining dressings on joints or awkward body parts. These tapes, particularly those containing rubber, can cause irritant and allergic reactions in susceptible patients; synthetic adhesives have been developed to overcome this problem, but they, too, may sometimes be associated with reactions. Synthetic adhesive, or silicon adhesive, tapes can be used for patients with skin reactions to plasters and strapping containing rubber, or undergoing prolonged treatment.

Adhesive tapes that are occlusive may cause skin maceration. Care is needed not to apply these tapes under tension, to avoid creating a tourniquet effect. If applied over joints they need to be orientated so that the area of maximum extensibility of the fabric is in the direction of movement of the limb.

Occlusive adhesive tapes
Blenderm

(Impermeable Plastic Adhesive Tape, BP 1988). Extensible water-impermeable plastic film spread with a polymericadhesive mass
Blenderm tape (3M Health Care Ltd) 2.5cm= £1.77, 5cm= £3.37

Sleek

(Impermeable Plastic Adhesive Tape, BP 1988). Extensible water-impermeable plastic film spread with an adhesive mass
Leukoplast Sleek tape (BSN medical Ltd) 2.5cm, 5cm, 7.5cm

Permeable adhesive tapes
3m Kind Removal Silicone Tape

Soft silicone, water-resistant, knitted fabric, polyurethane film adhesive tape
3M Micropore Silicone tape (3M Health Care Ltd) 2.5cm= £3.58, 5cm= £6.48

Chemifix

(Permeable, Apertured Non-Woven Synthetic Adhesive Tape, BP 1988). Non-woven fabric with a polyacrylate adhesive
Chemifix tape (Medicareplus International Ltd) 10cm= £2.10, 2.5cm= £0.90, 5cm= £1.40

Chemipore

(Permeable Non-Woven Synthetic Adhesive Tape, BP 1988). Backing of paper-based or non-woven textile material spread with a polymeric adhesive mass
Chemipore tape (Medicareplus International Ltd) 1.25cm= £0.27, 2.5cm= £0.70, 5cm= £0.95

Clinipore

(Permeable Non-Woven Synthetic Adhesive Tape, BP 1988). Backing of paper-based or non-woven textile material spread with a polymeric adhesive mass
Clinipore tape (CliniSupplies Ltd) 1.25cm= £0.35, 2.5cm= £0.74, 5cm= £1.00

Elastoplast

(Elastic Adhesive Tape, BP 1988). Woven fabric, elastic in warp (crepe-twisted cotton threads), weft of cotton and/or viscose threads, spread with adhesive mass containing zinc oxide
Tensoplast (BSN medical Ltd) elastic adhesive tape 2.5cm

Hypafix

(Permeable, Apertured Non-Woven Synthetic Adhesive Tape, BP 1988). Non-woven fabric with a polyacrylate adhesive
Hypafix tape (BSN medical Ltd) 10cm= £4.76, 15cm= £7.05, 2.5cm= £1.72, 20cm= £9.35, 30cm= £13.52, 5cm= £2.73

Insil

Soft silicone, water-resistant, knitted fabric, polyurethane film adhesive tape
Insil tape (Insight Medical Products Ltd) 2cm= £5.77, 4cm= £5.77

Leukofix

(Permeable Non-Woven Synthetic Adhesive Tape, BP 1988). Backing of paper-based or non-woven textile material spread with a polymeric adhesive mass
Leukofix tape (BSN medical Ltd) 1.25cm= £0.56, 2.5cm= £0.91, 5cm= £1.60

Leukopor
(Permeable Non-Woven Synthetic Adhesive Tape, BP 1988). Backing of paper-based or non-woven textile material spread with a polymeric adhesive mass
Leukopor tape (BSN medical Ltd) 1.25cm= £0.50, 2.5cm= £0.78, 5cm= £1.38

Mediplast
(Permeable Non-Woven Synthetic Adhesive Tape, BP 1988). Backing of paper-based or non-woven textile material spread with a polymeric adhesive mass
Mediplast tape (Neomedic Ltd) 1.25cm= £0.30, 2.5cm= £0.50

Mediplast
Fabric, plain weave, warp and weft of cotton and /or viscose, spread with an adhesive containing zinc oxide
Mediplast Zinc Oxide plaster (Neomedic Ltd) 1.25cm= £0.82, 2.5cm= £1.19, 5cm= £1.99, 7.5cm= £2.99

Mefix
(Permeable, Apertured Non-Woven Synthetic Adhesive Tape, BP 1988). Non-woven fabric with a polyacrylate adhesive
Mefix tape (Molnlycke Health Care Ltd) 10cm= £2.92, 15cm= £3.98, 2.5cm= £1.03, 20cm= £5.10, 30cm= £7.32, 5cm= £1.83

Mepitac
Soft silicone, water-resistant, knitted fabric, polyurethane film adhesive tape
Mepitac tape (Molnlycke Health Care Ltd) 2cm= £7.01, 4cm= £7.01

Micropore
(Permeable Non-Woven Synthetic Adhesive Tape, BP 1988). Backing of paper-based or non-woven textile material spread with a polymeric adhesive mass
Micropore tape (3M Health Care Ltd) 1.25cm= £0.62, 2.5cm= £0.92, 5cm= £1.62

Omnifix
(Permeable, Apertured Non-Woven Synthetic Adhesive Tape, BP 1988). Non-woven fabric with a polyacrylate adhesive
Omnifix tape (Paul Hartmann Ltd) 10cm= £4.14, 15cm= £6.11, 5cm= £2.46

OpSite Flexifix Gentle
Soft silicone, water-resistant, knitted fabric, polyurethane film adhesive tape
OpSite Flexifix Gentle tape (Smith & Nephew Healthcare Ltd) 2.5cm= £10.49, 5cm= £19.67

Primafix
(Permeable, Apertured Non-Woven Synthetic Adhesive Tape, BP 1988). Non-woven fabric with a polyacrylate adhesive
Primafix tape (Smith & Nephew Healthcare Ltd) 10cm= £2.38, 15cm= £3.51, 20cm= £4.32, 5cm= £1.62

Scanpor
(Permeable Non-Woven Synthetic Adhesive Tape, BP 1988). Backing of paper-based or non-woven textile material spread with a polymeric adhesive mass
Scanpor tape (Bio-Diagnostics Ltd) 1.25cm= £0.55, 2.5cm= £0.92, 5cm= £1.75, 7.5cm= £2.56

Siltape
Soft silicone, water-resistant, knitted fabric, polyurethane film adhesive tape
Siltape (Advancis Medical) 2cm= £5.64, 4cm= £5.64

Strappal
Fabric, plain weave, warp and weft of cotton and /or viscose, spread with an adhesive containing zinc oxide
Strappal adhesive tape (BSN medical Ltd) 2.5cm= £1.41, 5cm= £2.39, 7.5cm= £3.59

Transpore
(Permeable Non-Woven Synthetic Adhesive Tape, BP 1988). Backing of paper-based or non-woven textile material spread with a polymeric adhesive mass
Transpore tape (3M Health Care Ltd) 2.5cm= £0.84, 5cm= £1.48

Zinc Oxide Adhesive Tape, BP 1988
Fabric, plain weave, warp and weft of cotton and /or viscose, spread with an adhesive containing zinc oxide
Fast Aid zinc oxide adhesive tape (Robinson Healthcare) 1.25cm, 2.5cm, 5cm, 7.5cm

Skin closure dressings
Skin closure strips are used as an alternative to sutures for minor cuts and lacerations. Skin tissue adhesive can be used for closure of minor skin wounds and for additional suture support.

Skin closure strips, sterile
Leukostrip
Drug Tariff specifies that these are specifically for personal administration by the prescriber
Leukostrip (Smith & Nephew Healthcare Ltd) skin closure strips 6.4mm × 76mm= £6.43

Omnistrip
Drug Tariff specifies that these are specifically for personal administration by the prescriber
Omnistrip (Paul Hartmann Ltd) skin closure strips sterile 6mm × 76mm= £24.68

Steri-strip
Drug Tariff specifies that these are specifically for personal administration by the prescriber
Steri-strip (3M Health Care Ltd) skin closure strips 6mm × 75mm= £8.77

Bandages

Non-extensible bandages
Skin closure strips are used as an alternative to sutures for minor cuts and lacerations. Skin tissue adhesive can be used for closure of minor skin wounds and for additional suture support.

Open-wove Bandage, Type 1 BP 1988
Cotton cloth, plain weave, warp of cotton, weft of cotton, viscose, or combination, one continuous length
Clini open wove bandage Type 1 BP 1988 (CliniSupplies Ltd) 10cm × 5m, 2.5cm × 5m, 5cm × 5m, 7.5cm × 5m
Vernaid white open wove bandage (Synergy Health (UK) Ltd) 10cm × 5m, 2.5cm × 5m, 5cm × 5m, 7.5cm × 5m
White open wove bandage (Robert Bailey & Son Plc) 10cm × 5m, 2.5cm × 5m, 5cm × 5m, 7.5cm × 5m

Triangular Calico Bandage, BP 1980
Unbleached calico right-angled triangle
Clini (CliniSupplies Ltd) triangular calico bandage BP 1980 90cm × 127cm
Triangular (BSN medical Ltd) calico bandage 90cm × 127cm

Light-weight conforming bandages
Lightweight conforming bandages are used for dressing retention, with the aim of keeping the dressing close to the wound without inhibiting movement or restricting blood flow. The elasticity of conforming-stretch bandages (also termed contour bandages) is greater than that of cotton conforming bandages.

Acti-Wrap
Fabric, plain weave, warp of polyamide filament, weft of cotton or viscose, fast edges, one continuous length, 4 m stretched (all)
Acti-Wrap (cohesive/latex free) bandage (L&R Medical UK Ltd) 10cm × 4m= £0.82, 6cm × 4m= £0.47, 8cm × 4m= £0.69

Cotton Conforming Bandage, BP 1988
Cotton fabric, plain weave, treated to impart some elasticity to warp and weft
Easifix Crinx bandage (BSN medical Ltd) 10cm × 3.5m= £1.05, 15cm × 3.5m= £1.43, 5cm × 3.5m= £0.69, 7.5cm × 3.5m= £0.85

Easifix
Fabric, plain weave, warp of polyamide filament, weft of cotton or viscose, fast edges, one continuous length, 4 m stretched (all)
Easifix bandage (BSN medical Ltd) 10cm × 4m= £0.52, 15cm × 4m= £0.88, 5cm × 4m= £0.36, 7.5cm × 4m= £0.43

Easifix K

Fabric, knitted warp of polyamide filament, weft of cotton or viscose, fast edges, one continuous length. 4 m stretched

Easifix K bandage (BSN medical Ltd) 10cm × 4m= £0.19, 15cm × 4m= £0.33, 2.5cm × 4m= £0.10, 5cm × 4m= £0.11, 7.5cm × 4m= £0.16

Hospiform

Fabric, plain weave, warp of polyamide, weft of viscose

Hospiform bandage (Paul Hartmann Ltd) 10cm × 4m= £0.19, 12cm × 4m= £0.24, 6cm × 4m= £0.14, 8cm × 4m= £0.17

K-Band

Fabric, knitted warp of polyamide filament, weft of cotton or viscose, fast edges, one continuous length. 4 m stretched

K-Band bandage (Urgo Ltd) 10cm × 4m= £0.29, 15cm × 4m= £0.50, 5cm × 4m= £0.21, 7cm × 4m= £0.26

Knit Fix

Fabric, knitted warp of polyamide filament, weft of cotton or viscose, fast edges, one continuous length. 4 m stretched

Knit Fix bandage (Robert Bailey & Son Plc) 10cm × 4m= £0.17, 15cm × 4m= £0.33, 5cm × 4m= £0.12, 7cm × 4m= £0.17

Knit-Band

Fabric, knitted warp of polyamide filament, weft of cotton or viscose, fast edges, one continuous length. 4 m stretched

Knit-Band bandage (CliniSupplies Ltd) 10cm × 4m= £0.17, 15cm × 4m= £0.31, 5cm × 4m= £0.10, 7cm × 4m= £0.15

Kontour

Fabric, plain weave, warp of polyamide filament, weft of cotton or viscose, fast edges, one continuous length, 4 m stretched (all)

Kontour bandage (Easigrip Ltd) 10cm × 4m= £0.40, 15cm × 4m= £0.66, 5cm × 4m= £0.28, 7.5cm × 4m= £0.35

Mollelast

Fabric, plain weave, warp of polyamide filament, weft of cotton or viscose, fast edges, one continuous length, 4 m stretched (all)

Mollelast (Lohmann & Rauscher) bandage 4cm × 4m= £0.31

Peha-haft

Polyamide and Cellulose Contour Bandage, cohesive, latex-free

Peha-haft bandage (Paul Hartmann Ltd) 10cm × 4m= £0.78, 12cm × 4m= £0.92, 2.5cm × 4m= £0.75, 4cm × 4m= £0.48, 6cm × 4m= £0.57, 8cm × 4m= £0.68

PremierBand

Polyamide and Cellulose Contour Bandage

PremierBand bandage (Shermond) 10cm × 4m= £0.17, 15cm × 4m= £0.25, 5cm × 4m= £0.12, 7.5cm × 4m= £0.14

Slinky

Fabric, plain weave, warp of polyamide filament, weft of cotton or viscose, fast edges, one continuous length, 4 m stretched (all)

Slinky bandage (Molnlycke Health Care Ltd) 10cm × 4m= £0.72, 15cm × 4m= £1.05, 7.5cm × 4m= £0.60

Stayform

Fabric, plain weave, warp of polyamide filament, weft of cotton or viscose, fast edges, one continuous length, 4 m stretched (all)

Stayform bandage (Robinson Healthcare) 10cm × 4m= £0.40, 15cm × 4m= £0.68, 5cm × 4m= £0.29, 7.5cm × 4m= £0.36

Tubular bandages and garments

Tubular bandages are available in different forms, according to the function required of them. Some are used under orthopaedic casts and some are suitable for protecting areas to which creams or ointments (other than those containing potent corticosteroids) have been applied. The conformability of the elasticated versions makes them particularly suitable for retaining dressings on difficult parts of the body or for soft tissue injury, but their use as the only means of applying pressure to an oedematous limb or to a varicose ulcer is not appropriate, since the pressure they exert is inadequate. Compression hosiery reduces the recurrence of venous leg ulcers and should be considered for use after wound healing. Silk clothing is available as an alternative to elasticated viscose stockinette garments, for use in the management of severe eczema and allergic skin conditions.

Elasticated Surgical Tubular Stockinette, Foam padded is used for relief of pressure and elimination of friction in relevant area; porosity of foam lining allows normal water loss from skin surface.

For *Elasticated Tubular Bandage, BP* 1993, where no size stated by the prescriber, the 50 cm length should be supplied and width endorsed.

Non-elasticated Cotton Stockinette, Bleached, BP 1988 1m lengths is used as basis (with wadding) for Plaster of Paris bandages etc.; 6 m length, compression bandage.

For *Non-elasticated Ribbed Cotton and Viscose Surgical Tubular Stockinette, BP* 1988, the Drug Tariff specifies various combinations of sizes to provide sufficient material for part or full body coverage. It is used as protective dressings with tar-based and other steroid ointments.

Elasticated

Acti-Fast

(Drug Tariff specification 46). Lightweight plain-knitted elasticated tubular bandage

Acti-Fast 2-way stretch stockinette (L&R Medical UK Ltd) 10.75cm= £6.04, 17.5cm= £1.83, 20cm= £3.20, 3.5cm= £0.56, 5cm= £0.58, 7.5cm= £0.77

Clinifast

(Drug Tariff specification 46). Lightweight plain-knitted elasticated tubular bandage; various colours and sizes

CliniFast stockinette (CliniSupplies Ltd) 10.75cm= £6.04, 17.5cm= £1.83, 3.5cm= £0.56, 5cm= £0.58, 7.5cm= £0.77, clava 5-14 years= £6.75, 6 months-5 years= £5.85, cycle shorts large adult= £16.37, medium adult= £14.35, small adult= £12.59, gloves large adult= £5.03, child/small adult= £5.03, gloves medium adult= £5.03, child= £5.03, gloves small child= £5.03, leggings 11-14 years= £11.88, leggings 2-5 (Blue, Pink, White) years= £9.57, years= £9.50, leggings 5-8 (Blue, Pink, White) years= £10.77, years= £10.69, leggings 8-11 years= £11.88, mittens 2-8 years= £2.97, 8-14 years= £2.97, up to 24 months= £2.97, socks 8-14 years= £2.99, up to 8 years= £2.97, tights 6-24 (Blue, Pink, White) months= £7.18, months= £7.13, vest long sleeve 11-14 years= £11.88, vest long sleeve 2-5 (Blue, Pink, White) years= £9.57, years= £9.50, vest long sleeve 5-8 (Blue, Pink, White) years= £10.77, years= £10.69, vest long sleeve 6-24 (Blue, Pink, White) months= £7.13, months= £7.18, vest long sleeve 8-11 years= £11.88, vest short sleeve large adult= £16.37, medium adult= £14.35, small adult= £12.59

Comfifast

(Drug Tariff specification 46). Lightweight plain-knitted elasticated tubular bandage; various colours and sizes

Comfifast stockinette (Synergy Health (UK) Ltd) 10.75cm= £6.04, 17.5cm= £1.83, 3.5cm= £0.56, 5cm= £0.58, 7.5cm= £0.77

Comfifast Easywrap

(Drug Tariff specification 46). Lightweight plain-knitted elasticated tubular bandage; various colours and sizes

Comfifast Easywrap stockinette (Synergy Health (UK) Ltd) clava 5-14 years= £6.75, 6 months-5 years= £5.85, leggings 11-14 years= £11.88, 2-5 years= £9.50, 5-8 years= £10.69, 8-11 years= £11.88, mittens 2-8 years= £2.97, 8-14 years= £2.97, up to 24 months= £2.97, socks 8-14 years= £2.97, up to 8 years= £2.97, tights 6-24 months= £7.13, vest long sleeve 11-14 years= £11.88, 2-5 years= £9.50, 5-8 years= £10.69, 6-24 months= £7.13, 8-11years= £11.88

Comfifast Multistretch

(Drug Tariff specification 46). Lightweight plain-knitted elasticated tubular bandage; various colours and sizes

Comfifast MultiStretch 2-way stretch stockinette (Synergy Health (UK) Ltd) 10.75cm= £6.45, 17.5cm= £2.49, 3.5cm= £0.61, 5cm= £0.63, 7.5cm= £0.83

Coverflex

(Drug Tariff specification 46). Lightweight plain-knitted elasticated tubular bandage; various colours and sizes
Coverflex stockinette (Paul Hartmann Ltd) 10.75cm= £9.65, 17.5cm= £2.54, 3.5cm= £0.83, 5cm= £0.87, 7.5cm= £5.72

Easifast

(Drug Tariff specification 46). Lightweight plain-knitted elasticated tubular bandage; various colours and sizes
Easifast stockinette (Easigrip Ltd) 10.75cm= £7.23, 17.5cm= £1.91, 3.5cm= £0.65, 5cm= £0.69, 7.5cm= £0.94

Elasticated Surgical Tubular Stockinette, Foam padded or Tupipad

(Drug Tariff specification 25). Fabric as for Elasticated Tubular Bandage with polyurethane foam lining.

Elasticated Tubular Bandage, BP 1993

(Drug Tariff specification 25). Fabric as for Elasticated Tubular Bandage with polyurethane foam lining; lenghts 50 cm and 1 m
CLINIgrip bandage (CliniSupplies Ltd) 10cm size F= £0.74, 12cm size G= £0.77, 6.25cm size B= £0.61, 6.75cm size C= £0.65, 7.5cm size D= £0.66, 8.75cm size E= £0.74
Comfigrip bandage (Synergy Health (UK) Ltd) 10cm size F= £0.74, 12cm size G= £0.77, 6.25cm size B= £0.61, 6.75cm size C= £0.65, 7.5cm size D= £0.66, 8.75cm size E= £0.74
Eesiban ESTS bandage (E Sallis Ltd) 10cm size F= £1.80, 12cm size G= £2.09, 6.25cm size B= £0.87, 6.75cm size C= £0.95, 7.5cm size D= £0.95, 8.75cm size E= £1.80
Tubigrip bandage (Molnlycke Health Care Ltd) 10cm size F= £2.05, 12cm size G= £2.37, 6.25cm size B= £0.99, 6.75cm size C= £1.89, 7.5cm size D= £1.89, 8.75cm size E= £2.05
easiGRIP bandage (Easigrip Ltd) 10cm size F= £0.75, 12cm size G= £0.78, 6.25cm size B= £0.62, 6.75cm size C= £0.66, 7.5cm size D= £0.68, 8.75cm size E= £0.75

Skinnies

(Drug Tariff specification 46). Lightweight plain-knitted elasticated tubular bandage; various colours and sizes
Skinnies Viscose stockinette (Dermacea Ltd) body suit (Blue, Ecru, Pink) 3-6 months= £16.18, 6-12 months= £18.21, premature= £16.18, up to 3 months= £16.18, clava (Blue, Ecru, Pink) 5-14 years= £7.73, 6 months-5 years= £6.74, gloves large (Beige, Blue, Ecru, Grey, Pink) adult= £5.34, child= £5.34, gloves medium (Beige, Blue, Ecru, Grey, Pink) adult= £5.34, child= £5.34, gloves small (Blue, Ecru, Grey, Pink) adult= £5.29, child= £5.29, knee socks extra (Black, Natural, White) large adult 11+= £13.94, knee socks large (Black, Natural, White) adult 8-11= £13.94, child 2-4= £13.94, knee socks medium (Black, Natural, White) adult 6-8= £13.94, child 1-2= £13.94, knee socks small (Black, Natural, White) adult 4-6= £13.94, child 0-1= £13.94, leggings (Beige, Blue, Ecru, Grey, Pink) 11-14 years= £17.20, 2-5 years= £13.74, 5-8 years= £15.52, 6-24 months= £10.48, 8-11 years= £17.20, large adult= £25.13, medium adult= £23.20, small adult= £21.27, mittens (Blue, Ecru, Pink) 2-8 years= £3.87, 8-14 years= £3.87, up to 24 months= £3.87, socks (Blue, Ecru, Pink) 6 months-8 years= £4.27, 8-14 years= £4.27, vest long sleeve (Beige, Blue, Ecru, Grey, Pink) 11-14 years= £17.20, 2-5 years= £13.74, 5-8 years= £15.52, 6-24 months= £10.48, 8-11 years= £17.20, large adult= £25.13, medium adult= £23.20, small adult= £21.27, vest short sleeve (White) 11-14 years= £17.09, 2-5 years= £13.63, 5-8 years= £15.36, 6-24 months= £10.38, 8-11 years= £17.09, large adult= £25.03, medium adult= £23.10, small adult= £21.16, vest sleeveless (White) 11-14 years= £17.09, 2-5 years= £13.63, 5-8 years= £15.42, 6-24 months= £10.38, 8-11 years= £17.09, large adult= £25.03, medium adult= £23.10, small adult= £21.16

Tubifast 2-way stretch

(Drug Tariff specification 46). Lightweight plain-knitted elasticated tubular bandage; various colours and sizes
Tubifast 2-way stretch stockinette (Molnlycke Health Care Ltd) 10.75cm= £5.74, 20cm= £3.20, 3.5cm= £0.61, 5cm= £0.63, 7.5cm= £0.77, gloves extra small child= £5.73, medium/large adult= £5.73, small child= £5.73, small/medium adult, medium/large child= £5.73, leggings 2-5 years= £15.25, 5-8 years= £17.16, 8-11 years= £19.06, socks (one size)= £4.83, tights 6-24 months=

£11.44, vest long sleeve 11-14 years= £19.06, 2-5 years= £15.25, 5-8 years= £17.16, 6-24 months= £11.44, 8-11 years= £19.06

Non-elasticated
Cotton Stockinette, Bleached, BP 1988
Knitted fabric, cotton yarn, tubular length, 1m
Cotton stockinette bleached heavyweight (E Sallis Ltd) 10cm, 2.5cm, 5cm, 7.5cm

Silk Clothing
DermaSilk
Knitted silk fabric, hypoallergenic, sericin-free
DermaSilk (Espere Healthcare Ltd) medium/large= £42.37, medium-large= £31.53, body suit 0-3 months= £38.81, 12-18 months= £41.12, 18-24 months= £42.16, 24-36 months= £42.24, 3-6 months= £38.90, 6-9 months= £40.01, 9-12 months= £41.04, boxer shorts male adult extra large/XX large= £42.37, small/small= £42.37, briefs female adult extra large-XX large= £31.53, small-small= £31.53, facial mask adult= £21.29, child= £16.69, infant= £16.69, teen= £21.29, gloves extra large adult= £21.05, gloves large adult= £21.09, gloves medium adult= £21.09, child= £15.02, gloves small adult= £21.09, child= £15.02, leggings 0-3 months= £27.71, leggings 12-18 months= £29.99, leggings 18-24 months= £31.05, leggings 3-4 years= £32.22, leggings 3-6 months= £27.77, leggings 6-9 months= £28.88, leggings 9-12 months= £29.93, leggings adult female XX large= £79.71, extra large= £79.71, large= £79.71, medium= £79.71, small= £79.71, leggings adult male XX large= £79.71, extra large= £79.71, large= £79.71, medium= £79.71, small= £79.71, pyjamas 10-12 years= £83.41, 3-4 years= £72.28, 5-6 years= £76.74, 7-8 years= £80.07, roll neck shirt 10-12 years= £55.40, 3-4 years= £47.93, 5-6 years= £51.13, 7-8 years= £53.26, round neck shirt adult female XX large= £78.78, extra large= £78.78, large= £78.78, medium= £78.78, small= £78.78, round neck shirt adult male XX large= £78.78, extra large= £78.78, large= £78.78, medium= £78.78, small= £78.78, tubular sleeves= £34.27, sleeves= £27.77, undersocks adult 11-13= £18.75, 5 1/2 - 6 1/2= £18.75, 7 - 8 1/2= £18.75, 9 - 10 1/2= £18.75, undersocks child 2-5= £18.75, 3-8= £18.75, 9-1= £18.75, unisex roll neck shirt adult XX large= £78.78, extra large= £78.78, large= £78.78, medium= £78.78, small= £78.78

DreamSkin
Knitted silk fabric, hypoallergenic, sericin-free, with methyacrylate copolymer and zinc-chelate antibacterial
DreamSkin (DreamSkin Health Ltd) baby leggings with foldaway feet 0-3 months= £25.66, 12-18 months= £28.59, 18-24 months= £29.13, 3-4 years= £30.72, 3-6 months= £26.17, 6-9 months= £27.53, 9-12 months= £28.06, body suit 0-3 months= £36.15, 12-18 months= £39.20, 18-24 months= £39.74, 3-4 years= £41.33, 3-6 months= £36.66, 6-9 months= £38.14, 9-12 months= £38.70, boxer shorts 11-12 years= £21.79, boxer shorts 3-4 years= £21.79, boxer shorts 5-6 years= £21.79, boxer shorts 7-8 years= £21.79, boxer shorts 9-10 years= £21.79, boxer shorts male adult XX large= £34.27, extra large= £34.27, large= £34.27, medium= £34.27, small= £34.27, briefs 11-12 years= £21.79, briefs 3-4 years= £21.79, briefs 5-6 years= £21.79, briefs 7-8 years= £21.79, briefs 9-10 years= £21.79, briefs female adult XX large= £32.19, extra large= £32.19, large= £32.19, medium= £32.19, small= £32.19, eye mask= £10.35, footless leggings 11-12 years= £33.80, footless leggings 3-4 years= £30.72, footless leggings 5-6 years= £32.24, footless leggings 7-8 years= £32.76, footless leggings 9-10 years= £33.28, footless leggings adult female XX large= £77.74, extra large= £77.74, large= £77.74, medium= £77.74, small= £77.74, footless leggings adult male XX large= £77.74, extra large= £77.74, large= £77.74, medium= £77.74, small= £77.74, gloves extra large adult= £20.41, gloves large adult= £20.41, gloves medium adult= £20.41, child= £14.54, gloves small adult= £20.41, child= £14.54, head mask= £15.91, infant= £15.91, teenager= £20.76, heel-less undersocks= £24.05, liner socks adult female 4 - 5 1/2= £18.29, 6 - 8 1/2= £18.29, liner socks adult male 6 - 8 1/2= £18.29, 9 - 11= £18.29, liner socks child 12 1/2 - 3 1/2= £18.29, 3 - 5 1/2= £18.29, 4 - 5 1/2= £18.29, 6 - 8 1/2= £18.29, 9 - 12= £18.29, polo neck shirt 11-12 years= £54.03, polo neck shirt 3-4 years= £46.75, polo neck shirt 5-6 years= £49.87, polo neck shirt 7-8 years= £51.95, polo neck shirt 9-10 years= £52.99, polo neck shirt adult female XX large= £76.84,

extra large= £76.84, large= £76.84, medium= £76.84, small= £76.84, polo neck shirt adult male XX large= £76.84, extra large= £76.84, large= £76.84, medium= £76.84, small= £76.84, pyjamas 11-12 years= £79.52, 3-4 years= £68.91, 5-6 years= £73.16, 7-8 years= £76.34, 9-10 years= £77.96, round neck shirt 3-4 years= £46.76, round neck shirt 5-6 years= £48.84, round neck shirt 7-8 years= £50.92, round neck shirt 9-10 years= £51.96, round neck shirt adult female XX large= £76.84, extra large= £76.84, large= £76.84, medium= £76.84, small= £76.84, round neck shirt adult male XX large= £76.84, extra large= £76.84, large= £76.84, medium= £76.84, small= £76.84, tubular sleeves= £33.42, sleeves= £26.87

Support bandages

Light support bandages, which include the various forms of crepe bandage, are used in the prevention of oedema; they are also used to provide support for mild sprains and joints but their effectiveness has not been proven for this purpose. Since they have limited extensibility, they are able to provide light support without exerting undue pressure. For a warning against injudicious compression see Compression bandages.

CliniLite
Knitted fabric, viscose and elastomer yarn. Type 2 (light support bandage)
CliniLite bandage (CliniSupplies Ltd) 10cm × 4.5m= £0.81, 15cm × 4.5m= £1.17, 5cm × 4.5m= £0.44, 7.5cm × 4.5m= £0.61

CliniPlus
Knitted fabric, viscose and elastomer yarn. Type 2 (light support bandage)
CliniPlus (CliniSupplies Ltd) bandage 10cm × 8.7m= £1.81

Cotton Crepe Bandage
Light support bandage, 4.5 m stretched (all)
Hospicrepe 239 bandage (Paul Hartmann Ltd) 10cm × 4.5m= £0.81, 15cm × 4.5m= £1.18, 5cm × 4.5m= £0.44, 7.5cm × 4.5m= £0.63

Cotton Crepe Bandage, BP 1988
Fabric, plain weave, warp of crepe-twisted cotton threads, weft of cotton and/or viscose threads; stretch bandage. 4.5 m stretched (both)
Elastocrepe bandage (BSN medical Ltd) 10cm × 4.5m, 7.5cm × 4.5m
Flexocrepe bandage (Robinson Healthcare) 10cm × 4.5m, 7.5cm × 4.5m
Sterocrepe bandage (Steroplast Healthcare Ltd) 10cm × 4.5m, 7.5cm × 4.5m

Cotton Suspensory Bandage
(Drug Tariff). Type 1: cotton net bag with draw tapes and webbing waistband; small, medium, and large (all)

Crepe Bandage, BP 1988
Fabric, plain weave, warp of wool threads and crepe-twisted cotton threads, weft of cotton threads; stretch bandage; 4.5 m stretched
Alvita crepe bandage (Alliance Healthcare (Distribution) Ltd) 10cm × 4.5m, 15cm × 4.5m, 5cm × 4.5m, 7.5cm × 4.5m
Clinicrepe bandage (CliniSupplies Ltd) 10cm × 4.5m, 15cm × 4.5m, 5cm × 4.5m, 7.5cm × 4.5m
Crepe bandage (Robert Bailey & Son Plc) 10cm × 4.5m, 15cm × 4.5m, 5cm × 4.5m, 7.5cm × 4.5m
Propax crepe bandage (BSN medical Ltd) 10cm × 4.5m, 15cm × 4.5m, 5cm × 4.5m, 7.5cm × 4.5m
Vernaid crepe bandage (Synergy Health (UK) Ltd) 10cm × 4.5m, 15cm × 4.5m, 5cm × 4.5m, 7.5cm × 4.5m

Elset
Knitted fabric, viscose and elastomer yarn. Type 2 (light support bandage)
Elset (Molnlycke Health Care Ltd) S bandage 15cm × 12m=£5.64, bandage 10cm × 6m=£2.63, 10cm × 8m=£3.37, 15cm × 6m= £2.82

Hospicrepe 233
Fabric, plain weave, warp of crepe-twisted cotton threads, weft of cotton threads; stretch bandage, lighter than cotton crepe, 4.5 m stretched (all)
Hospicrepe 233 bandage (Paul Hartmann Ltd) 10cm × 4.5m= £0.96, 15cm × 4.5m= £1.36, 5cm × 4.5m= £0.52, 7.5cm × 4.5m= £0.72

Hospilite
Fabric, cotton, polyamide, and elastane; light support bandage (Type 2), 4.5 m stretched (all)
Hospilite bandage (Paul Hartmann Ltd) 10cm × 4.5m= £0.63, 15cm × 4.5m= £0.92, 5cm × 4.5m= £0.37, 7.5cm × 4.5m= £0.52

K-Lite
Knitted fabric, viscose and elastomer yarn. Type 2 (light support bandage)
K-Lite (Urgo Ltd) Long bandage 10cm × 5.25m=£1.16, bandage 10cm × 4.5m=£1.02, 15cm × 4.5m=£1.47, 5cm × 4.5m=£0.56, 7cm × 4.5m=£0.78

K-Plus
Knitted fabric, viscose and elastomer yarn. Type 2 (light support bandage)
K-Plus (Urgo Ltd) Long bandage 10cm × 10.25m= £2.67, bandage 10cm × 8.7m= £2.31

Knit-Firm
Knitted fabric, viscose and elastomer yarn. Type 2 (light support bandage)
Knit-Firm bandage (Millpledge Healthcare) 10cm × 4.5m= £0.66, 15cm × 4.5m= £0.96, 5cm × 4.5m= £0.36, 7cm × 4.5m= £0.51

L3
Knitted fabric, viscose and elastomer yarn. Type 2 (light support bandage)
L3 (Smith & Nephew Healthcare Ltd) bandage 10cm × 8.6m= £2.24

Neosport
Fabric, cotton, polyamide, and elastane; light support bandage (Type 2), 4.5 m stretched (all)
Neosport bandage (Neomedic Ltd) 10cm × 4.5m= £0.91, 15cm × 4.5m= £1.12, 5cm × 4.5m= £0.54, 7.5cm × 4.5m= £0.73

PremierBand
Fabric, plain weave, warp of crepe-twisted cotton threads, weft of cotton threads; stretch bandage, lighter than cotton crepe, 4.5 m stretched (all)
PremierBand bandage (Shermond) 10cm × 4.5m= £0.79, 15cm × 4.5m= £1.18, 5cm × 4.5m= £0.45, 7.5cm × 4.5m= £0.63

Profore #2
Fabric, cotton, polyamide, and elastane; light support bandage (Type 2), 4.5 m stretched (all)
Profore #2 (Smith & Nephew Healthcare Ltd) bandage 10cm × 4.5m= £1.37, latex free bandage 10cm × 4.5m= £1.46

Profore #3
Knitted fabric, viscose and elastomer yarn. Type 2 (light support bandage)
Profore #3 (Smith & Nephew Healthcare Ltd) bandage 10cm × 8.7m= £4.00, latex free bandage 10cm × 8.7m= £4.34

Setocrepe
Fabric, cotton, polyamide, and elastane; light support bandage (Type 2), 4.5 m stretched (all)
Setocrepe (Molnlycke Health Care Ltd) bandage 10cm × 4.5m= £1.21

Soffcrepe
Fabric, cotton, polyamide, and elastane; light support bandage (Type 2), 4.5 m stretched (all)
Soffcrepe bandage (BSN medical Ltd) 10cm × 4.5m= £1.26, 15cm × 4.5m= £1.84, 5cm × 4.5m= £0.71, 7.5cm × 4.5m= £1.00

Adhesive bandages

Elastic adhesive bandages are used to provide compression in the treatment of varicose veins and for the support of injured joints; they should no longer be used for the support of fractured ribs and clavicles. They have also been used with zinc paste bandage in the treatment of venous ulcers, but they can cause skin reactions in susceptible patients and may not produce sufficient pressures for healing (significantly lower than those provided by other compression bandages).

Elastic Adhesive Bandage, BP 1993
Woven fabric, elastic in warp (crepe-twisted cotton threads), weft of cotton and/or viscose threads spread with adhesive mass containing zinc oxide. 4.5 m stretched

Tensoplast bandage (BSN medical Ltd) 10cm × 4.5m, 5cm × 4.5m, 7.5cm × 4.5m

Cohesive bandages

Cohesive bandages adhere to themselves, but not to the skin, and are useful for providing support for sports use where ordinary stretch bandages might become displaced and adhesive bandages are inappropriate. Care is needed in their application, however, since the loss of ability for movement between turns of the bandage to equalise local areas of high tension carries the potential for creating a tourniquet effect. Cohesive bandages can be used to support sprained joints and as an outer layer for multi-layer compression bandaging; they should not be used if arterial disease is suspected.

Cohesive extensible bandages
Coban
Bandage
Coban (3M Health Care Ltd) self-adherent bandage 10cm × 6m= £2.93

K Press
Bandage
K Press bandage (Urgo Ltd) 10cm × 6.5m= £2.96, 10cm × 7.5m= £3.45, 12cm × 7.5m= £4.34, 8cm × 7.5cm= £3.25

Profore #4
Bandage
Profore #4 (Smith & Nephew Healthcare Ltd) bandage 10cm × 2.5m= £3.30, latex free bandage 10cm × 2.5m= £3.59

Ultra Fast
Bandage
Ultra (Robinson Healthcare) Fast cohesive bandage 10cm × 6.3m= £2.59

Compression bandages

High compression products are used to provide the high compression needed for the management of gross varices, post-thrombotic venous insufficiency, venous leg ulcers, and gross oedema in average-sized limbs. Their use calls for an expert knowledge of the elastic properties of the products and experience in the technique of providing careful graduated compression. Incorrect application can lead to uneven and inadequate pressures or to hazardous levels of pressure. In particular, injudicious use of compression in limbs with arterial disease has been reported to cause severe skin and tissue necrosis (in some instances calling for amputation). Doppler testing is required before treatment with compression. Oral pentoxifylline p. 233 can be used as adjunct therapy if a chronic venous leg ulcer does not respond to compression bandaging [unlicensed indication].

High compression bandages
High Compression Bandage
Cotton, viscose, nylon, and Lycra® extensible bandage, 3 m (unstretched)
K-ThreeC (Urgo Ltd) bandage 10cm × 3m= £2.87
SurePress (ConvaTec Ltd) bandage 10cm × 3m= £3.68

PEC High Compression Bandages
Polyamide, elastane, and cotton compression (high) extensible bandage, 3.5 m unstretched
Setopress (Molnlycke Health Care Ltd) bandage 10cm × 3.5m= £3.58

VEC High Compression Bandages
Viscose, elastane, and cotton compression (high) extensible bandage, 3 m unstretched (both)
Tensopress bandage (BSN medical Ltd) 10cm × 3m= £3.51, 7.5cm × 3m= £2.73

Short stretch compression bandages
Actico
Bandage
Actico bandage (L&R Medical UK Ltd) 10cm × 6m= £3.41, 12cm × 6m= £4.34, 4cm × 6m= £2.44, 6cm × 6m= £2.85, 8cm × 6m= £3.28

Comprilan
Bandage
Comprilan bandage (BSN medical Ltd) 10cm × 5m= £3.44, 12cm × 5m= £4.19, 6cm × 5m= £2.72, 8cm × 5m= £3.20

Rosidal K
Bandage
Rosidal K bandage (Lohmann & Rauscher) 10cm × 10m= £6.11, 10cm × 5m= £3.51, 12cm × 5m= £4.26, 6cm × 5m= £2.69, 8cm × 5m= £3.21

Sub-compression wadding bandage
Cellona Undercast Padding
Padding
Cellona Undercast padding bandage (Lohmann & Rauscher) 10cm × 2.75m= £0.48, 15cm × 2.75m= £0.61, 5cm × 2.75m= £0.32, 7.5cm × 2.75m= £0.39

Flexi-Ban
Padding
Flexi-Ban (L&R Medical UK Ltd) bandage 10cm × 3.5m= £0.51

K Tech Reduced
Padding
K Tech Reduced bandage 10cm x (Urgo Ltd) 6m= £4.79, 7.3m= £5.23

K-Soft
Padding
K-Soft (Urgo Ltd) Long bandage 10cm × 4.5m= £0.58, bandage 10cm × 3.5m= £0.46

K-Tech (K Tech in DMD)
Padding
K Tech (Urgo Ltd) Reduced bandage 10cm × 7.3m= £5.23, bandage 10cm × 5m= £3.99, 10cm × 6m= £4.79, 12cm × 6m= £6.04, 12cm × 7.3m= £6.60, 8cm × 6m= £4.52, 8cm × 7.3m= £4.93

Ortho-Band Plus
Padding
Ortho-Band (Millpledge Healthcare) Plus bandage 10cm × 3.5m= £0.37

Profore #1
Padding
Profore #1 (Smith & Nephew Healthcare Ltd) bandage 10cm × 3.5m= £0.72, latex free bandage 10cm × 3.5m= £0.77

Softexe
Padding
Softexe (Molnlycke Health Care Ltd) bandage 10cm × 3.5m= £0.62

SurePres
Padding
SurePress (ConvaTec Ltd) bandage 10cm × 3m= £3.68

Ultra Soft
Padding
Ultra (Robinson Healthcare) Soft wadding bandage 10cm × 3.5m= £0.39

Velband
Padding
Velband (BSN medical Ltd) absorbent padding bandage 10cm × 4.5m= £0.74

Multi-layer compression bandaging

Multi-layer compression bandaging systems are an alternative to High Compression Bandages for the treatment of venous leg ulcers. Compression is achieved by the combined effects of two or three extensible bandages applied over a layer of orthopaedic wadding and a wound contact dressing.

Four layer systems
K-Four
Padding

K-Four
Multi-layer compression bandaging kit, four layer system
K-Four (Urgo Ltd) Reduced Compression multi-layer compression bandage kit 18cm+ ankle circumference = £4.55, multi-layer compression bandage kit 18cm-25cm ankle circumference= £6.96, 25cm-30cm ankle circumference= £6.96, greater than 30cm ankle circumference= £9.58, less than 18cm ankle circumference= £7.27

Profore
Wound contact layer

Profore
Multi-layer compression bandaging kit, four layer system
Profore (Smith & Nephew Healthcare Ltd) Lite latex free multi-layer
compression bandage kit= £6.05, multi-layer compression
bandage kit= £5.57, latex free multi-layer compression bandage
kit 18cm-25cm ankle circumference = £10.30, multi-layer
compression bandage kit 18cm-25cm ankle circumference=
£9.64, 25cm-30cm ankle circumference= £8.00, above 30cm
ankle circumference= £11.99, up to 18cm ankle circumference=
£10.35

Ultra Four
Wound contact layer

Ultra Four
Multi-layer compression bandaging kit, four layer system
Ultra Four (Robinson Healthcare) Reduced Compression multi-
layer compression bandage kit= £4.14, multi-layer compression
bandage kit 18cm-25cm ankle circumference= £5.67, up to 18cm
ankle circumference= £6.41

Two layer systems
Coban 2
Multi-layer compression bandaging kit, two layer system
(latex-free, foam bandage and cohesive compression
bandage)
Coban 2 (3M Health Care Ltd) Lite multi-layer compression bandage
kit= £8.24, multi-layer compression bandage kit= £8.24

K Two
Multi-layer compression bandaging kit, two layer system
UrgoKTwo (Urgo Ltd) Reduced latex free multi-layer compression
bandage kit (10cm) 18cm-25cm ankle circumference= £8.75,
25cm-32cm ankle circumference= £9.56, Reduced multi-layer
compression bandage kit 18cm-25cm ankle circumference=
£8.24, 25cm-32cm ankle circumference= £9.01, latex free multi-
layer compression bandage kit (10cm) 18cm-25cm ankle
circumference= £8.75, 25cm-32cm ankle circumference= £9.56,
multi-layer compression bandage kit (10cm) 18cm-25cm ankle
circumference= £8.24, 25cm-32cm ankle circumference= £9.00,
multi-layer compression bandage kit (12cm) 18cm-25cm ankle
circumference= £10.39, 25cm-32cm ankle circumference=
£11.35, multi-layer compression bandage kit (8cm) 18cm-25cm
ankle circumference= £7.77, 25cm-32cm ankle circumference=
£8.45, multi-layer compression bandage kit size 0 short 18cm-
25cm ankle circumference= £6.95, with UrgoStart multi-layer
compression bandage kit 18cm-25cm ankle circumference=
£10.27, 25cm-32cm ankle circumference= £10.95

Medicated bandages
Zinc Paste Bandage has been used with compression
bandaging for the treatment of venous leg ulcers. However,
paste bandages are associated with hypersensitivity
reactions and should be used with caution. Zinc paste
bandages are also used with coal tar or ichthammol in
chronic lichenified skin conditions such as chronic eczema
(ichthammol often being preferred since its action is
considered to be milder). They are also used with calamine in
milder eczematous skin conditions.
Zipzoc® can be used under appropriate compression
bandages or hosiery in chronic venous insufficiency.

Zinc Paste Bandage, BP 1993
Cotton fabric, plain weave, impregnated with suitable paste
containing zinc oxide; requires additional bandaging
Excipients: may include cetostearyl alcohol,
hydroxybenzoates
Viscopaste (Evolan Pharma AB) PB7 bandage 7.5cm × 6m= £3.72

Zinc Paste and Ichthammol Bandage, BP 1993
Cotton fabric, plain weave, impregnated with suitable paste
containing zinc oxide and ichthammol; requires additional
bandaging
Excipients: may include cetostearyl alcohol
Ichthopaste (Evolan Pharma AB) bandage 7.5cm × 6m= £3.75

Medicated stocking
Zipzoc
Sterile rayon stocking impregnated with ointment
containing zinc oxide 20%
Zipzoc (Evolan Pharma AB) stockings= £34.70

Compression hosiery and garments

Compression (elastic) hosiery is used to treat conditions
associated with chronic venous insufficiency, to prevent
recurrence of thrombosis, or to reduce the risk of further
venous ulceration after treatment with compression
bandaging. Doppler testing to confirm arterial sufficiency is
required before recommending the use of compression
hosiery.
Before elastic hosiery can be dispensed, the quantity (single
or pair), article (including accessories), and compression
class must be specified by the prescriber. There are different
compression values for graduated compression hosiery and
lymphoedema garments (see table below). All dispensed
elastic hosiery articles must state on the packaging that they
conform with Drug Tariff technical specification No. 40, for
further details see Drug Tariff.
Graduated Compression hosiery, Class 1 Light Support is used
for superficial or early varices, varicosis during pregnancy.
Graduated Compression hosiery, Class 2 Medium Support is
used for varices of medium severity, ulcer treatment and
prophylaxis, mild oedema, varicosis during pregnancy.
Graduated Compression hosiery, Class 3 Strong Support is used
for gross varices, post thrombotic venous insufficiency, gross
oedema, ulcer treatment and prophylaxis.
**Compression values for hosiery and lymphoedema
garments** *Class* 1: Compression hosiery (British standard)
14–17 mmHg, lymphoedema garments (European
classification) 18–21 mmHg; *Class* 2 Compression hosiery
(British standard) 18–24 mmHg, lymphoedema garments
(European classification) 23–32 mmHg; *Class* 3 Compression
hosiery (British standard) 25–35 mmHg, lymphoedema
garments (European classification) 34–46 mmHg; *Class* 4
Compression hosiery (British standard)—not available,
lymphoedema garments (European classification) 49–70
mmHg; *Class 4 super* Compression hosiery (British
standard)—not available, lymphoedema garments (European
classification) 60–90 mmHg.

Graduated compression hosiery
Class 1 Light Support
Hosiery, compression at ankle 14–17 mmHg, thigh length or
below knee with knitted in heel

Class 2 Light Support
Hosiery, compression at ankle 14–17 mmHg, thigh length or
below knee with knitted in heel

Accessories
Suspender
Suspender, for thigh stockings

Anklets
Class 2 Medium Support
Anklets, compression 18–24 mmHg, circular knit (standard
and made-to-measure)

Class 3 Strong Support
Anklets, compression 18–24 mmHg, circular knit (standard
and made-to-measure)

Knee caps
Class 2 Medium Support
Kneecaps, compression 18–24 mmHg, circular knit (standard
and made-to-measure)

Class 3 Strong Support
Kneecaps, compression 18–24 mmHg, circular knit (standard
and made-to-measure)

Lymphoedema garments
Lymphoedema compression garments are used to maintain
limb shape and prevent additional fluid retention. Either

flat-bed or circular knitting methods are used in the manufacture of elasticated compression garments. Seamless, circular-knitted garments (in standard sizes) can be used to prevent swelling if the lymphoedema is well controlled and if the limb is in good shape and without skin folds. Flat-knitted garments (usually made-to-measure) with a seam, provide greater rigidity and stiffness to maintain reduction of lymphoedema following treatment with compression bandages. A standard range of light, medium, or high compression garments are available, as well as low compression (12–16 mmHg) armsleeves, made-to-measure garments up to compression 90 mmHg, and accessories—see Drug Tariff for details. Note: There are different compression values for lymphoedema garments and graduated compression hosiery, see Compression hosiery and garments p. 1560.

A4

Dental Practitioners' Formulary

List of Dental Preparations

The following list has been approved by the appropriate Secretaries of State, and the preparations therein may be prescribed by dental practitioners on form FP10D (GP14 in Scotland, WP10D in Wales).

Licensed **sugar-free** versions, where available, are preferred. Licensed **alcohol-free** mouthwashes, where available, are preferred.

Aciclovir Cream, BP
Aciclovir Oral Suspension, BP, 200 mg/5 mL
Aciclovir Tablets, BP, 200 mg
Aciclovir Tablets, BP, 800 mg
Amoxicillin Capsules, BP
Amoxicillin Oral Powder, DPF
Amoxicillin Oral Suspension, BP
Artificial Saliva Gel, DPF
Artificial Saliva Oral Spray, DPF
Artificial Saliva Pastilles, DPF
Artificial Saliva Protective Spray, DPF
Artificial Saliva Substitutes as listed below (to be prescribed only for indications approved by ACBS (patients suffering from dry mouth as a result of having or, having undergone, radiotherapy or sicca syndrome):
  BioXtra ® Gel Mouthspray
  BioXtra ® Moisturising Gel
  Glandosane ®
  Saliveze ®
Artificial Saliva Substitute Spray, DPF
Aspirin Tablets, Dispersible, BP
Azithromycin Capsules, 250 mg, DPF
Azithromycin Oral Suspension, 200 mg/5 mL, DPF
Azithromycin Tablets, 250 mg, DPF
Azithromycin Tablets, 500 mg, DPF
Beclometasone Pressurised Inhalation, BP, 50 micrograms/metered inhalation, CFC-free, as:
  Clenil Modulite ®
Benzydamine Mouthwash, BP 0.15%
Benzydamine Oromucosal Spray, BP 0.15%
Betamethasone Soluble Tablets, 500 micrograms, DPF
Carbamazepine Tablets, BP
Cefalexin Capsules, BP
Cefalexin Oral Suspension, BP
Cefalexin Tablets, BP
Cefradine Capsules, BP
Cetirizine Oral Solution, BP, 5 mg/5 mL
Cetirizine Tablets, BP, 10 mg
Chlorhexidine Gluconate Gel, BP
Chlorhexidine Mouthwash, BP
Chlorhexidine Oral Spray, DPF
Chlorphenamine Oral Solution, BP
Chlorphenamine Tablets, BP
Choline Salicylate Dental Gel, BP
Clarithromycin Oral Suspension, 125 mg/5 mL, DPF
Clarithromycin Oral Suspension, 250 mg/5 mL, DPF
Clarithromycin Tablets, BP
Clindamycin Capsules, BP
Co-amoxiclav Tablets, BP, 250/125 (amoxicillin 250 mg as trihydrate, clavulanic acid 125 mg as potassium salt)
Co-amoxiclav Oral Suspension, BP, 125/31 (amoxicillin 125 mg as trihydrate, clavulanic acid 31.25 mg as potassium salt)/5 mL
Co-amoxiclav Oral Suspension, BP, 250/62 (amoxicillin 250 mg as trihydrate, clavulanic acid 62.5 mg as potassium salt)/5 mL
Diazepam Oral Solution, BP, 2 mg/5 mL
Diazepam Tablets, BP

Diclofenac Sodium Tablets, Gastro-resistant, BP
Dihydrocodeine Tablets, BP, 30 mg
Doxycycline Tablets, Dispersible, BP
Doxycycline Capsules, BP, 100 mg
Doxycycline Tablets, 20 mg, DPF
Ephedrine Nasal Drops, BP
Erythromycin Ethyl Succinate Oral Suspension, BP
Erythromycin Ethyl Succinate Tablets, BP
Erythromycin Stearate Tablets, BP
Erythromycin Tablets, Gastro-resistant, BP
Fluconazole Capsules, 50 mg, DPF
Fluconazole Oral Suspension, 50 mg/5 mL, DPF
Hydrocortisone Cream, BP, 1%
Hydrocortisone Oromucosal Tablets, BP
Hydrogen Peroxide Mouthwash, BP, 6%
Ibuprofen Oral Suspension, BP, sugar-free
Ibuprofen Tablets, BP
Lansoprazole Capsules, Gastro-resistant, BP
Lidocaine Ointment, BP, 5%
Lidocaine Spray 10%, DPF
Loratadine Syrup, 5 mg/5 mL, DPF
Loratadine Tablets, BP, 10 mg
Menthol and Eucalyptus Inhalation, BP 1980
Metronidazole Oral Suspension, BP
Metronidazole Tablets, BP
Miconazole Cream, BP
Miconazole Oromucosal Gel, BP
Miconazole and Hydrocortisone Cream, BP
Miconazole and Hydrocortisone Ointment, BP
Nystatin Oral Suspension, BP
Omeprazole Capsules, Gastro-resistant, BP
Oxytetracycline Tablets, BP
Paracetamol Oral Suspension, BP
Paracetamol Tablets, BP
Paracetamol Tablets, Soluble, BP
Phenoxymethylpenicillin Oral Solution, BP
Phenoxymethylpenicillin Tablets, BP
Promethazine Hydrochloride Tablets, BP
Promethazine Oral Solution, BP
Saliva Stimulating Tablets, DPF
Sodium Chloride Mouthwash, Compound, BP
Sodium Fluoride Mouthwash, BP
Sodium Fluoride Oral Drops, BP
Sodium Fluoride Tablets, BP
Sodium Fluoride Toothpaste 0.619%, DPF
Sodium Fluoride Toothpaste 1.1%, DPF
Sodium Fusidate Ointment, BP
Temazepam Oral Solution, BP
Temazepam Tablets, BP
Tetracycline Tablets, BP

Preparations in this list which are not included in the BP or BPC are described under Details of DPF preparations. For details of preparations that can be prescribed, see individual entries under the relevant drug monographs throughout the BNF publications.

Details of DPF preparations

Preparations on the List of Dental Preparations which are specified as DPF are described as follows in the DPF. Although brand names have sometimes been included for identification purposes preparations on the list should be prescribed by non-proprietary name.

Amoxicillin Oral Powder

amoxicillin (as trihydrate) 3 g sachet

Artificial Saliva Gel
(proprietary product: *Biotene Oralbalance*), lactoperoxidase, lactoferrin, lysozyme, glucose oxidase, xylitol in a gel basis

Artificial Saliva Oral Spray
(proprietary product: *Xerotin*) consists of water, sorbitol, carmellose (carboxymethylcellulose), potassium chloride, sodium chloride, potassium phosphate, magnesium chloride, calcium chloride and other ingredients, pH neutral

Artificial Saliva Pastilles
(proprietary product: *Salivix*), consists of acacia, malic acid, and other ingredients

Artificial Saliva Protective Spray
(proprietary product: *Aquoral*) consists of oxidised glycerol triesters, silicon dioxide, flavouring agents, aspartame

Artificial Saliva Substitute Spray
(proprietary product: *AS Saliva Orthana Spray*) consists of mucin, methylparaben, benzalkonium chloride, EDTA, xylitol, peppermint oil, spearmint oil, mineral salts

Azithromycin Capsules
azithromycin 250 mg

Azithromycin Oral Suspension 200 mg/5 mL
azithromycin 200 mg/5 mL when reconstituted with water

Azithromycin Tablets
azithromycin 250 mg and 500 mg

Betamethasone Soluble Tablets 500 micrograms
betamethasone (as sodium phosphate) 500 micrograms

Chlorhexidine Oral Spray
(proprietary product: *Corsodyl Oral Spray*), chlorhexidine gluconate 0.2%

Clarithromycin Oral Suspension 125 mg/5 mL
clarithromycin 125 mg/5 mL when reconstituted with water

Clarithromycin Oral Suspension 250 mg/5 mL
clarithromycin 250 mg/5 mL when reconstituted with water

Doxycycline Tablets 20 mg
(proprietary product: *Periostat*), doxycycline (as hyclate) 20 mg

Fluconazole Capsules 50 mg
fluconazole 50 mg

Fluconazole Oral Suspension 50 mg/5 mL
(proprietary product: *Diflucan*), fluconazole 50 mg/5 mL when reconstituted with water

Lidocaine Spray 10%
(proprietary product: *Xylocaine Spray*), lidocaine 10% supplying 10 mg lidocaine/spray

Loratadine Syrup 5 mg/5 mL
loratadine 5 mg/5 mL

Saliva Stimulating Tablets
(proprietary product: *SST*), citric acid, malic acid and other ingredients in a sorbitol base

Sodium Fluoride Toothpaste 0.619%
(proprietary product: *Duraphat '2800 ppm' Toothpaste*), sodium fluoride 0.619%

Sodium Fluoride Toothpaste 1.1%
(proprietary product: *Duraphat '5000 ppm' Toothpaste*), sodium fluoride 1.1%

Nurse Prescribers' Formulary

Nurse Prescribers' Formulary for Community Practitioners

List of preparations approved by the Secretary of State which may be prescribed on form FP10P (form HS21(N) in Northern Ireland, form GP10(N) in Scotland, forms WP10CN and WP10PN in Wales) by Nurses for National Health Service patients.

Community practitioners who have completed the necessary training may only prescribe items appearing in the nurse prescribers' list set out below. Community Practitioner Nurse Prescribers are recommended to prescribe generically, except where this would not be clinically appropriate or where there is no approved generic name.

Medicinal Preparations

Preparations on this list which are not included in the BP or BPC are described under Details of NPF preparations.

Almond Oil Ear Drops, BP
Arachis Oil Enema, NPF
Aspirin Tablets, Dispersible, 300 mg, BP (max. 96 tablets; max. pack size 32 tablets)
Bisacodyl Suppositories, BP (includes 5-mg and 10-mg strengths)
Bisacodyl Tablets, BP
Catheter Maintenance Solution, Sodium Chloride, NPF
Catheter Maintenance Solution, 'Solution G', NPF
Catheter Maintenance Solution, 'Solution R', NPF
Chlorhexidine Gluconate Alcoholic Solutions containing at least 0.05%
Chlorhexidine Gluconate Aqueous Solutions containing at least 0.05%
Choline Salicylate Dental Gel, BP
Clotrimazole Cream 1%, BP
Co-danthramer Capsules, NPF
Co-danthramer Capsules, Strong, NPF
Co-danthramer Oral Suspension, NPF
Co-danthramer Oral Suspension, Strong, NPF
Co-danthrusate Capsules, NPF
Co-danthrusate Oral Suspension, NPF
Crotamiton Cream, BP
Crotamiton Lotion, BP
Dimeticone barrier creams containing at least 10%
Dimeticone Lotion, NPF
Docusate Capsules, BP
Docusate Enema, NPF
Docusate Oral Solution, BP
Docusate Oral Solution, Paediatric, BP
Econazole Cream 1%, BP
Emollients as listed below:
　Aquadrate ® 10% w/w Cream
　Arachis Oil, BP
　Balneum ® Plus Cream
　Cetraben ® Emollient Cream
　Dermamist ®
　Diprobase ® Cream
　Diprobase ® Ointment
　Doublebase ®
　Doublebase ® Dayleve Gel
　E45 ® Cream
　E45 ® Itch Relief Cream
　Emulsifying Ointment, BP
　Eucerin ® Intensive 10% w/w Urea Treatment Cream
　Eucerin ® Intensive 10% w/w Urea Treatment Lotion
　Hydromol ® Cream

　Hydromol ® Intensive
　Hydrous Ointment, BP
　Lipobase ®
　Liquid and White Soft Paraffin Ointment, NPF
　Neutrogena ® Norwegian Formula Dermatological Cream
　Nutraplus ® Cream
　Oilatum ® Cream
　Oilatum ® Junior Cream
　Paraffin, White Soft, BP
　Paraffin, Yellow Soft, BP
　Ultrabase ®
　Unguentum M ®
Emollient Bath and Shower Preparations as listed below:
　Aqueous Cream, BP
　Balneum ® (except pack sizes that are not to be prescribed under the NHS (see Part XVIIIA of the Drug Tariff, Part XI of the Northern Ireland Drug Tariff))
　Balneum Plus ® Bath Oil (except pack sizes that are not to be prescribed under the NHS (see Part XVIIIA of the Drug Tariff, Part XI of the Northern Ireland Drug Tariff))
　Cetraben ® Emollient Bath Additive
　Dermalo ® Bath Emollient
　Doublebase ® Emollient Bath Additive
　Doublebase ® Emollient Shower Gel
　Doublebase ® Emollient Wash Gel
　Hydromol ® Bath and Shower Emollient
　Oilatum ® Emollient
　Oilatum ® Gel
　Oilatum ® Junior Bath Additive
　Zerolatum ® Emollient Medicinal Bath Oil
Folic Acid Tablets 400 micrograms, BP
Glycerol Suppositories, BP
Ibuprofen Oral Suspension, BP (except for indications and doses that are prescription-only)
Ibuprofen Tablets, BP (except for indications and doses that are prescription-only)
Ispaghula Husk Granules, BP
Ispaghula Husk Granules, Effervescent, BP
Ispaghula Husk Oral Powder, BP
Lactulose Solution, BP
Lidocaine Ointment, BP
Lidocaine and Chlorhexidine Gel, BP
Macrogol Oral Liquid, Compound, NPF
Macrogol Oral Powder, Compound, NPF
Macrogol Oral Powder, Compound, Half-strength, NPF
Magnesium Hydroxide Mixture, BP
Magnesium Sulfate Paste, BP
Malathion aqueous lotions containing at least 0.5%
Mebendazole Oral Suspension, NPF
Mebendazole Tablets, NPF
Methylcellulose Tablets, BP
Miconazole Cream 2%, BP
Miconazole Oromucosal Gel, BP
Mouthwash Solution-tablets, NPF
Nicotine Inhalation Cartridge for Oromucosal Use, NPF
Nicotine Lozenge, NPF
Nicotine Medicated Chewing Gum, NPF
Nicotine Nasal Spray, NPF
Nicotine Oral Spray, NPF
Nicotine Sublingual Tablets, NPF
Nicotine Transdermal Patches, NPF
Nystatin Oral Suspension, BP
Olive Oil Ear Drops, BP
Paracetamol Oral Suspension, BP (includes 120 mg/5 mL and 250 mg/5 mL strengths—both of which are available as sugar-free formulations)

Paracetamol Tablets, BP (max. 96 tablets; max. pack size 32 tablets)
Paracetamol Tablets, Soluble, BP (includes 120-mg and 500-mg tablets; max. 96 tablets; max. pack size 32 tablets)
Permethrin Cream, NPF
Phosphates Enema, BP
Povidone–Iodine Solution, BP
Senna Oral Solution, NPF
Senna Tablets, BP
Senna and Ispaghula Granules, NPF
Sodium Chloride Solution, Sterile, BP
Sodium Citrate Compound Enema, NPF
Sodium Picosulfate Capsules, NPF
Sodium Picosulfate Elixir, NPF
Spermicidal contraceptives as listed below:
  Gygel ® Contraceptive Jelly
Sterculia Granules, NPF
Sterculia and Frangula Granules, NPF
Titanium Ointment, BP
Water for Injections, BP
Zinc and Castor Oil Ointment, BP
Zinc Oxide and Dimeticone Spray, NPF
Zinc Oxide Impregnated Medicated Bandage, NPF
Zinc Oxide Impregnated Medicated Stocking, NPF
Zinc Paste Bandage, BP 1993
Zinc Paste and Ichthammol Bandage, BP 1993

Appliances and Reagents (including Wound Management Products)

Community Practitioner Nurse Prescribers in England, Wales and Northern Ireland can prescribe any appliance or reagent in the relevant Drug Tariff. In the Scottish Drug Tariff, Appliances and Reagents which may **not** be prescribed by Nurses are annotated **Nx**.

Appliances (including Contraceptive Devices) as listed in Part IXA of the Drug Tariff (Part III of the Northern Ireland Drug Tariff, Part 3 (Appliances) and Part 2 (Dressings) of the Scottish Drug Tariff). (Where it is not appropriate for nurse prescribers in family planning clinics to prescribe contraceptive devices using form FP10(P) (forms WP10CN and WP10PN in Wales), they may prescribe using the same system as doctors in the clinic.)

Incontinence Appliances as listed in Part IXB of the Drug Tariff (Part III of the Northern Ireland Drug Tariff, Part 5 of the Scottish Drug Tariff).

Stoma Appliances and Associated Products as listed in Part IXC of the Drug Tariff (Part III of the Northern Ireland Drug Tariff, Part 6 of the Scottish Drug Tariff).

Chemical Reagents as listed in Part IXR of the Drug Tariff (Part II of the Northern Ireland Drug Tariff, Part 9 of the Scottish Drug Tariff).

The Drug Tariffs can be accessed online at:
National Health Service Drug Tariff for England and Wales: www.ppa.org.uk/ppa/edt_intro.htm
Health and Personal Social Services for Northern Ireland Drug Tariff: www.hscbusiness.hscni.net/services/2034.htm
Scottish Drug Tariff: www.isdscotland.org/Health-topics/Prescribing-and-Medicines/Scottish-Drug-Tariff/

Details of NPF preparations

Preparations on the Nurse Prescribers' Formulary which are not included in the BP or BPC are described as follows in the Nurse Prescribers' Formulary. Although brand names have sometimes been included for identification purposes, it is recommended that non-proprietary names should be used for prescribing medicinal preparations in the NPF except where a non-proprietary name is not available.

Arachis Oil Enema
arachis oil 100%
Catheter Maintenance Solution, Sodium Chloride
(proprietary products: *OptiFlo S; Uro-Tainer Sodium Chloride; Uriflex-S*), sodium chloride 0.9%
Catheter Maintenance Solution, 'Solution G'
(proprietary products: *OptiFlo G; Uro-Tainer Suby G; Uriflex G*), citric acid 3.23%, magnesium oxide 0.38%, sodium bicarbonate 0.7%, disodium edetate 0.01%
Catheter Maintenance Solution, 'Solution R'
(proprietary product: *OptiFlo R; Uro-Tainer Solution R; Uriflex R*), citric acid 6%, gluconolactone 0.6%, magnesium carbonate 2.8%, disodium edetate 0.01%
Chlorhexidine gluconate alcoholic solutions
(proprietary products: *ChloraPrep; Hydrex Solution; Hydrex spray*), chlorhexidine gluconate in alcoholic solution
Chlorhexidine gluconate aqueous solutions
(proprietary product: *Unisept*), chlorhexidine gluconate in aqueous solution
Co-danthramer Capsules PoM
co-danthramer 25/200 (dantron 25 mg, poloxamer '188' 200 mg)
Co-danthramer Capsules, Strong PoM
co-danthramer 37.5/500 (dantron 37.5 mg, poloxamer '188' 500 mg)
Co-danthramer Oral Suspension PoM
(proprietary product: *Codalax*), co-danthramer 25/200 in 5 mL (dantron 25 mg, poloxamer '188' 200 mg/5 mL)
Co-danthramer Oral Suspension, Strong PoM
(proprietary product: *Codalax Forte*), co-danthramer 75/1000 in 5 mL (dantron 75 mg, poloxamer '188' 1 g/5 mL)
Co-danthrusate Oral Suspension PoM
(proprietary product: *Normax*), co-danthrusate 50/60 (dantron 50 mg, docusate sodium 60 mg/5 mL)
Dimeticone barrier creams
(proprietary products *Conotrane Cream*, dimeticone '350' 22%; *Siopel Barrier Cream*, dimeticone '1000' 10%), dimeticone 10–22%
Dimeticone Lotion
(proprietary product: *Hedrin*), dimeticone 4%
Docusate Enema
(proprietary product: *Norgalax Micro-enema*), docusate sodium 120 mg in 10 g
Liquid and White Soft Paraffin Ointment
liquid paraffin 50%, white soft paraffin 50%
Macrogol Oral Liquid, Compound
(proprietary product: *Movicol Liquid*), macrogol '3350' (polyethylene glycol '3350') 13.125 g, sodium bicarbonate 178.5 mg, sodium chloride 350.7 mg, potassium chloride 46.6 mg/25 mL
Macrogol Oral Powder, Compound
(proprietary products: *Laxido Orange, Molaxole, Movicol*), macrogol '3350' (polyethylene glycol '3350') 13.125 g, sodium bicarbonate 178.5 mg, sodium chloride 350.7 mg, potassium chloride 46.6 mg/sachet; (amount of potassium chloride varies according to flavour of *Movicol* as follows: plain-flavour (sugar-free) = 50.2 mg/sachet; lime and lemon flavour = 46.6 mg/sachet; chocolate flavour = 31.7 mg/sachet. 1 sachet when reconstituted with 125 mL water provides K^+ 5.4 mmol/litre)
Macrogol Oral Powder, Compound, Half-strength
(proprietary product: *Movicol-Half*), macrogol '3350' (polyethylene glycol '3350') 6.563 g, sodium bicarbonate 89.3 mg, sodium chloride 175.4 mg, potassium chloride 23.3 mg/sachet
Malathion aqueous lotions
(proprietary products: *Derbac-M Liquid*), malathion 0.5% in an aqueous basis
Mebendazole Oral Suspension PoM
(proprietary product: *Vermox*), mebendazole 100 mg/5 mL

Mebendazole Tablets PoM
(proprietary products: *Ovex, Vermox*), mebendazole 100 mg
(can be supplied for oral use in the treatment of enterobiasis
in adults and children over 2 years provided its container or
package is labelled to show a max. single dose of 100 mg and
it is supplied in a container or package containing not more
than 800 mg)

Mouthwash Solution-tablets
consist of tablets which may contain antimicrobial,
colouring and flavouring agents in a suitable soluble
effervescent basis to make a mouthwash

Nicotine Inhalation Cartridge for Oromucosal Use
(proprietary products: *NicAssist Inhalator, Nicorette
Inhalator*), nicotine 15 mg (for use with inhalation
mouthpiece; to be prescribed as either a starter pack
(6 cartridges with inhalator device and holder) or refill pack
(42 cartridges with inhalator device)

Nicotine Lozenge
nicotine (as bitartrate) 1 mg or 2 mg (proprietary product:
Nicorette Mint Lozenge, Nicotinell Mint Lozenge), or nicotine
(as resinate) 1.5 mg, 2 mg, or 4 mg (proprietary product:
NiQuitin Lozenges, NiQuitin Minis, NiQuitin Pre-quit)

Nicotine Medicated Chewing Gum
(proprietary products: *NicAssist Gum, Nicorette Gum,
Nicotinell Gum, NiQuitin Gum*), nicotine 2 mg or 4 mg

Nicotine Nasal Spray
(proprietary product: *NicAssist Nasal Spray, Nicorette Nasal
Spray*), nicotine 500 micrograms/metered spray

Nicotine Oral Spray
(proprietary product: *Nicorette Quickmist*), nicotine
1 mg/metered spray

Nicotine Sublingual Tablets
(proprietary product: *NicAssist Microtab, Nicorette Microtab*),
nicotine (as a cyclodextrin complex) 2 mg (to be prescribed
as either a starter pack (2 × 15-tablet discs with dispenser)
or refill pack (7 × 15-tablet discs))

Nicotine Transdermal Patches
releasing in each 16 hours, nicotine approx. 5 mg, 10 mg, or
15 mg (proprietary products: *Boots NicAssist Patch, Nicorette
Patch*), or releasing in each 16 hours approx. 10 mg, 15 mg, or
25 mg (proprietary products: *NicAssist Translucent Patch,
Nicorette Invisi Patch*), or releasing in each 24 hours nicotine
approx. 7 mg, 14 mg, or 21 mg (proprietary products:
Nicopatch, Nicotinell TTS, NiQuitin, NiQuitin Clear)
(prescriber should specify the brand to be dispensed)

Permethrin Cream
(proprietary product: *Lyclear Dermal Cream*), permethrin 5%

Senna Oral Solution
(proprietary product: *Senokot Syrup*), sennosides 7.5 mg/5 mL

Senna and Ispaghula Granules
(proprietary product: *Manevac Granules*), senna fruit 12.4%,
ispaghula 54.2%

Sodium Citrate Compound Enema
(proprietary products: *Micolette Micro-enema; Micralax
Micro-enema; Relaxit Micro-enema*),sodium citrate 450 mg
with glycerol, sorbitol and an anionic surfactant

Sodium Picosulfate Capsules
(proprietary products: *Dulcolax Perles*), sodium picosulfate
2.5 mg

Sodium Picosulfate Elixir
(proprietary product: *Dulcolax Liquid*), sodium picosulfate
5 mg/5 mL

Sterculia Granules
(proprietary product: *Normacol Granules*), sterculia 62%

Sterculia and Frangula Granules
(proprietary product: *Normacol Plus Granules*), sterculia 62%,
frangula (standardised) 8%

Zinc Oxide and Dimeticone Spray
(proprietary product: *Sprilon*), dimeticone 1.04%, zinc oxide
12.5% in a pressurised aerosol unit

Zinc Oxide Impregnated Medicated Bandage
(proprietary product: *Steripaste*), sterile cotton bandage
impregnated with paste containing zinc oxide 15%

Zinc Oxide Impregnated Medicated Stocking
(proprietary product: *Zipzoc*), sterile rayon stocking
impregnated with ointment containing zinc oxide 20%

Non-medical prescribing

Overview

A range of non-medical healthcare professionals can prescribe medicines for patients as either Independent or Supplementary Prescribers.

Independent prescribers are practitioners responsible and accountable for the assessment of patients with previously undiagnosed or diagnosed conditions and for decisions about the clinical management required, including prescribing. They are recommended to prescribe generically, except where this would not be clinically appropriate or where there is no approved non-proprietary name.

Supplementary prescribing is a partnership between an independent prescriber (a doctor or a dentist) and a supplementary prescriber to implement an agreed Clinical Management Plan for an individual patient with that patient's agreement.

Independent and Supplementary Prescribers are identified by an annotation next to their name in the relevant professional register.

Information and guidance on non-medical prescribing is available on the Department of Health website at www.dh. gov.uk/health/2012/04/prescribing-change.

For information on the mixing of medicines by Independent and Supplementary Prescribers, see *Mixing of medicines prior to administration in clinical practice: medical and non-medical prescribing*, National Prescribing Centre, May 2010 (available at www.gov.uk/government/uploads/ system/uploads/attachment_data/file/213885/dh_116360.pdf).

For information on the supply and administration of medicines to groups of patients using Patient Group Directions see Guidance on prescribing p. 1.

In order to protect patient safety, the initial prescribing and supply of medicines prescribed should normally remain separate functions performed by separate healthcare professionals.

Nurses

Nurse Independent Prescribers (formerly known as Extended Formulary Nurse Prescribers) are able to prescribe any medicine for any medical condition. Unlicensed medicines are excluded from the Nurse Prescribing Formulary in Scotland.

Nurse Independent Prescribers are able to prescribe, administer, and give directions for the administration of Schedule 2, 3, 4, and 5 Controlled Drugs. This extends to diamorphine hydrochloride p. 449, dipipanone, or cocaine for treating organic disease or injury, but not for treating addiction.

Nurse Independent Prescribers must work within their own level of professional competence and expertise.

The Nurse Prescribers' Formulary p. 1564 for Community Practitioners provides information on prescribing.

Pharmacists

Pharmacist Independent Prescribers can prescribe any medicine for any medical condition. This includes unlicensed medicines, subject to accepted clinical good practice.

They are also able to prescribe, administer, and give directions for the administration of Schedule 2, 3, 4, and 5 Controlled Drugs. This extends to diamorphine hydrochloride p. 449, dipipanone, or cocaine for treating organic disease or injury, but not for treating addiction.

Pharmacist Independent Prescribers must work within their own level of professional competence and expertise.

Physiotherapists

Physiotherapist Independent Prescribers can prescribe any medicine for any medical condition. This includes "off-label" medicines subject to accepted clinical good practice. They are also allowed to prescribe the following Controlled Drugs: oral or injectable morphine p. 456, transdermal fentanyl p. 451 and oral diazepam p. 340, dihydrocodeine tartrate p. 450, lorazepam p. 335, oxycodone hydrochloride p. 459 or temazepam p. 481.

Physiotherapist Independent Prescribers must work within their own level of professional competence and expertise.

Therapeutic radiographers

Therapeutic Radiographer Independent Prescribers can prescribe any medicine for any medical condition. This includes "off-label" medicines subject to accepted clinical good practice. Therapeutic Radiographer Independent Prescribers must work within their own level of professional competence and expertise.

Optometrists

Optometrist Independent Prescribers can prescribe any licensed medicine for ocular conditions affecting the eye and the tissues surrounding the eye, except Controlled Drugs or medicines for parenteral administration. Optometrist Independent Prescribers must work within their own level of professional competence and expertise.

Podiatrists

Podiatrist Independent Prescribers can prescribe any medicine for any medical condition. This includes "off-label" medicines subject to accepted clinical good practice. They are also allowed to prescribe the following Controlled Drugs for oral administration: diazepam p. 340, dihydrocodeine tartrate p. 450, lorazepam p. 335 and temazepam p. 481.

Podiatrist Independent Prescribers must work within their own level of professional competence and expertise.

Further Information

For further details about the different types of prescribers, see *Medicines, Ethics and Practice*, London, Pharmaceutical Press (always consult latest edition).

Index of proprietary manufacturers

The following is an alphabetical list of manufacturers and other companies referenced in the BNF, with their medicines information or general contact details. For information on 'special-order' manufacturers and specialist importing companies see 'Special-order manufacturers'.

3M Health Care Ltd, Tel: (01509) 611 611

A1 Pharmaceuticals Plc, Tel: (01708) 528 900, sales@a1plc.co.uk

Abbot Medical Optics, Tel: 0800 376 7950

Abbott, Tel: (01628) 773 355

Abbott Healthcare Products Ltd, Tel: (01628) 773 355, medinfo.shl@abbott.com

AbbVie Ltd, Tel: (01628) 561 090, ukmedinfo@abbvie.com

Abraxis BioScience Ltd, Tel: (020) 7081 0850, abraxismedical@idispharma.com

Acorus Therapeutics Ltd, Tel: (01244) 625 152

Actavis UK Ltd, a subsidary of Accord Healthcare Ltd, Tel: (01271) 385 257, medinfo@accord-healthcare.com

Actelion Pharmaceuticals UK Ltd, Tel: (020) 8987 3333, medinfo_uk@actelion.com

Activa Healthcare, Tel: 0845 060 6707, advice@activahealthcare.co.uk

Adienne Pharma and Biotech, Tel: 0039 (0) 335 873 8731

ADI Medical UK, Tel: (01628) 485159, info@adimedical.co.uk

Advanced Medical Solutions Group Plc, Tel: (01606) 863 500

Advancis Medical Ltd, Tel: (01623) 751 500, info@advancis.co.uk

Advantech Surgical Ltd, Tel: 0845 130 5866, customerservice@newgel.co.uk

Aegerion Pharmaceuticals Ltd, Tel: 00800 2343 7466, medinfo.emea@aegerion.com

AgaMatrix Europe Ltd, Tel: (01235) 838 639, info@wavesense.co.uk

Agepha GmbH, Tel: (020) 3239 6241, uk@agepha.com

Aguettant Ltd, Tel: (01275) 463 691, info@aguettant.co.uk

Air Products plc, Tel: 0800 373 580

Alan Pharmaceuticals, Tel: (020) 7284 2887, info@alanpharmaceuticals.com

Alcon Laboratories (UK) Ltd, Tel: 0345 266 9363, gbmedicaldepartment@alcon.com

Alexion Pharma UK Ltd, Tel: (01932) 359 220, alexion.uk@alxn.com

Alimera Sciences Limited, Tel: 0800 019 1253, medicalinformation@alimerasciences.com

Alissa Healthcare, Tel: (01489) 80 759, enquiries@alissahealthcare.com

ALK-Abelló (UK) Ltd, Tel: (0118) 903 7940, info@uk.alk-abello.com

Alkopharma Sarl, Tel: (0041) 277 206 969, regulatory@alkopharma.com

Allen & Hanburys Ltd, Tel: 0800 221 441, customercontactuk@gsk.com

Allergan Ltd, Tel: (01628) 494 026

Allergy Therapeutics Ltd, Tel: (01903) 844 702

Alliance Pharmaceuticals Ltd, Tel: (01249) 466 966, info@alliancepharma.co.uk

Almirall Ltd, Tel: 0800 008 7399, medinfouk@almirall.com

Altacor Ltd, Tel: (01223) 421 411, info@altacor-pharma.com

Amdipharm Mercury Company Ltd, Tel: 08700 70 30 33, medicalinformation@amcolimited.com

Amgen Ltd, Tel: (01223) 420 305, gbinfoline@amgen.com

Amred Healthcare Ltd, Tel: (0330) 333 0079, info@amredhealthcare.com

Amryt Pharma, Tel: 00800 234 37466, medinfo@amrytpharma.com

Apollo Medical Technologies Ltd, Tel: (01636) 831 201, supercheck2@btinternet.com

Archimed, Tel: 0800 756 9951, enquiries@archimed.co.uk

Archimedes Pharma UK Ltd, Tel: (0118) 931 5094, medicalinformationuk@archimedespharma.com

Arctic Medical Ltd, Tel: (01303) 277 751, sales@arcticmedical.co.uk

Ardana Bioscience Ltd, Tel: (0131) 226 8550

ARIAD Pharma UK Ltd, Tel: 0800 0002 7423, eumedinfo@ariad.com

Ark Therapeutics Group Plc, Tel: (020) 7388 7722, info@arktherapeutics.com

Aspen, Tel: 0800 008 7392, aspenmedinfo@professionalinformation.co.uk

Aspen Medical Europe Ltd, Tel: (01527) 587 728, customers@aspenmedicaleurope.com

AS Pharma Ltd, Tel: 0870 066 4117, info@aspharma.co.uk

Aspire Pharma Ltd, Tel: (01730) 231 148, info@aspirepharma.co.uk

Astellas Pharma Ltd, Tel: (020) 3379 8000, medinfo.gb@astellas.com

AstraZeneca UK Ltd, Tel: 0800 783 0033, medical.informationuk@astrazeneca.com

Auden Mckenzie (Pharma Division) Ltd, Tel: (01895) 627 420

Auxilium, Tel: 0845 017 2315, auxilium@pilglobal.com

Axcan Pharma SA, Tel: (0033) 130 461 900

AYMES International Ltd, Tel: 0845 6805 496, info@aymes.com

Ayrton Saunders Ltd, Tel: (0151) 709 2074, info@ayrtons.com

BAP Medical UK Ltd, Tel: 0844 879 7689

Bard Ltd, Tel: (01293) 527 888

Basilea Pharmaceuticals Ltd, Tel: (01483) 790 023, ukmedinfo@basilea.com

Bausch & Lomb UK Ltd, Tel: (01748) 828 864, medicalinformationuk@bausch.com

Baxalta UK Limited, Tel: (01635) 798 777, medinfo.emea@baxalta.com

Baxter Healthcare Ltd, Tel: (01635) 206 345, surecall@baxter.com

Bayer, Tel: (01635) 563 000, medical.information@bayer.co.uk

Bayer Consumer Care, Tel: (01635) 563 000, medical.information@bayer.co.uk

Bayer Diabetes Care, Tel: (01635) 563 000, medical.information@bayer.co.uk

Bayer Diagnostics, Tel: (01635) 563 000, medical.information@bayer.co.uk

BBI Healthcare, Tel: (01792) 229 333, info@bbihealthcare.com

B. Braun Medical Ltd, Tel: (0114) 225 9000, info.bbmuk@bbraun.com

Beacon Pharmaceuticals Ltd, Tel: (01892) 600 930, info@beaconpharma.co.uk

Beiersdorf UK Ltd, Tel: (0121) 329 8800

Besins Healthcare (UK) Ltd, Tel: (01748) 828 789, information@besins-healthcare.com

BGP Products Ltd, Tel: (01707) 853 000, medinfo.shl@mylan.com

BHR Pharmaceuticals Ltd, Tel: (024) 7637 7210, info@bhr.co.uk

Bial Pharma UK Ltd, Tel: 01753 916 010, medinfo.uk@bial.com

Biogen Idec Ltd, Tel: 0800 008 7401

Biolitec Pharma Ltd, Tel: (00353) 1463 7415

BioMarin Europe Ltd, Tel: (020) 7420 0800, biomarin-europe@bmrn.com

BioMonde, Tel: 0845 230 1810, info@biomonde.com

Bio Products Laboratory Ltd, Tel: (020) 8957 2255, medinfo@bpl.co.uk

Biotest (UK) Ltd, Tel: (0121) 733 3393, medicinesinformation@biotestuk.com

Blackwell Supplies Ltd, Tel: (01634) 877 620

BOC Medical, Tel: 0800 111 333

Boehringer Ingelheim Ltd, Tel: (01344) 424 600, medinfo@bra.boehringer-ingelheim.com

The Boots Company PLC, Tel: (0115) 959 5165

BPC 100 Ltd, Tel: 01942 852085

Brancaster Pharma Ltd, Tel: (01737) 243 407, enquiries@brancasterpharma.com

Bray Healthcare, Tel: (01367) 240 736, info@bray-healthcare.com

Bristol Laboratories Ltd, Tel: (0) 1442 200 922, info@bristol-labs.co.uk

Bristol-Myers Squibb Pharmaceuticals Ltd, Tel: (01895) 523 000, medical.information@bms.com

Britannia Pharmaceuticals, Tel: 0870 851 0207, enquiries@medinformation.co.uk

BSN Medical Ltd, Tel: 0845 122 3600

BTG International Ltd, Tel: (0207) 575 0000, medical.services@btgplc.com

Bullen Healthcare, Tel: 0800 269 327

Cambridge Healthcare Supplies Ltd, Tel: (01953) 607 856, customerservices@cambridge-healthcare.co.uk

Cambridge Medical Aesthetics Ltd, Tel: (01733) 396171, info@cambridgemedicalaesthetics.com

Cambridge Sensors Ltd, Tel: (01480) 482 920, sales-orders@cs-limited.co.uk

CareFusion UK 244 Ltd, Tel: 0800 043 7546, enquiries@chloraprep.co.uk

Casen-Fleet, Tel: (0034) 913 518 800

C D Medical Ltd, Tel: (01942) 816 184

Celgene Ltd, Tel: 0844 801 0045, medinfo.uk.ire@celgene.com

Chanelle Medical UK Ltd, Tel: (01233) 822 297

Chattem UK Ltd, Tel: (01256) 844 144

Chefaro UK Ltd, Tel: (01748) 828 860, info@omegapharma.co.uk

Chemidex Pharma Ltd, Tel: (01784) 477 167, info@chemidex.co.uk

Chiesi Ltd, Tel: (0161) 488 5555, medinfo.uk@chiesi.com

Chugai Pharma UK Ltd, Tel: (020) 8987 5680

Clement Clarke International Ltd, Tel: (01279) 414 969, resp@clement-clarke.com

Clinigen Group Plc, Tel: (01748) 828 375, clinigeneu@professionalinformation.co.uk

CliniMed Ltd, Tel: (01628) 535 250

Clinisupplies Ltd, Tel: (020) 8863 4168, info@clinisupplies.co.uk

Colgate-Palmolive Ltd, Tel: (01483) 302 222

Coloplast Ltd, Tel: (01733) 392 000

Community Foods Ltd, Tel: (020) 8450 9411, email@communityfoods.co.uk

Complan Foods Ltd, Tel: (020) 7395 7565

Consilient Health UK Ltd, Tel: (020) 8956 2310, drugsafety@consilienthealth.com

ConvaTec Ltd, Tel: 01244 584 300

Co-Pharma Ltd, Tel: 0870 851 0207

Correvio GmbH, Tel: (020) 3002 8114, info@correvio.com

Covidien UK Commercial Ltd, Tel: (01329) 224 226

Cow & Gate, Tel: 0845 762 3624

Cranage Healthcare Ltd, Tel: (01477) 549 392, db@cranagehealth.com

Crawford Healthcare Ltd, Tel: (01565) 654 920

Crescent Pharma, Tel: (01256) 772 730, info@crescentpharma.com

Crucell (UK) Ltd, Tel: 0844 800 3907, info@crucell.co.uk

CSL Behring UK Ltd, Tel: (01444) 447 400, medinfo@cslbehring.com

CTI Life Sciences Ltd, Tel: (01628) 643 974

Laboratoires CTRS, ctrsgb@pi-arm.co.uk

Daiichi Sankyo UK Ltd, Tel: (01753) 482 771, medinfo@daiichi-sankyo.co.uk

Danetre Health Products Ltd, Tel: (01327) 310 909, enquiries@danetrehealthproducts.com

DDD Ltd, Tel: (01923) 229 251

Dee Pharmaceuticals Ltd, Tel: (01978) 661993, enquiries@deepharmaceuticalsltd.co.uk

Dental Health Products Ltd, Tel: (01622) 749 222

Dentsply Ltd, Tel: (01932) 837 279

Dermal Laboratories Ltd, Tel: (01462) 458 866

Dermato Logical Ltd, Tel: (0208) 449 2931, enquiries@aqua-max.co.uk

Dermatonics Ltd, Tel: (01480) 462 910, sales@dermatonics.co.uk

Derma Sciences Europe Ltd, Tel: (01628) 625 916, cs@dermasciences.com

Derma UK Ltd, Tel: (01462) 733 500, info@dermauk.co.uk

Desitin Pharma Ltd, Tel: (01908) 488 817, medinfo@desitin.co.uk

DeVilbiss Healthcare UK Ltd, Tel: (01384) 446 688

Dexcel-Pharma Ltd, Tel: (01327) 312 266, office@dexcelpharma.co.uk

DHP Healthcare Ltd, Tel: (01622) 749 222, sales@dhphealthcare.co.uk

DiME, Tel: (01483) 715 008, info@dime-med.com

Dreamskin Health Ltd, Tel: (01707) 228 688

Dr Falk Pharma UK Ltd, Tel: (01628) 536 600

Drossa Ltd, Tel: (020) 3393 0859, info@drossa.co.uk

Durbin plc, Tel: (020) 8869 6500, info@durbin.co.uk

T G Eakin, Tel: (028) 9187 1000, mail@eakin.co.uk

Easigrip Ltd, Tel: (01926) 497 108, enquiry@easigrip.co.uk

Ecolab UK, Tel: (0113) 232 0066, info.healthcare@ecolab.co.uk

Egis Pharmaceuticals UK Ltd, Tel: (020) 7266 2669, enquiries@medimpexuk.com

Eisai Ltd, Tel: (020) 8600 1400, eumedinfo@eisai.net

Eli Lilly & Co Ltd, Tel: (01256) 315 000, ukmedinfo@lilly.com

Encysive (UK) Ltd, Tel: (01895) 876 168

Entra Health Systems, Tel: (0113) 815 5108

Espere Healthcare Ltd, Tel: (01462) 346 100, info@esperehealth.co.uk

Essential Pharmaceuticals Ltd, Tel: (01784) 477 167, info@essentialpharmaceuticals.com

Ethicon Ltd, Tel: (01506) 594 500

Eumedica S.A., Tel: (020) 8444 3377, enquiries@eumedica.com

Eurocept, Tel: +31 (0) 35 528 83 77, info@eurocept.nl

European Pharma Group, Tel: 0031 (0) 20 316 0140, info@insujet.com

EUSA Pharma (Europe) Ltd, Tel: (01438) 740 720, medinfo-uk@eusapharma.com

Pierre Fabre Ltd, Tel: (01962) 874 435, medicalinformation@pierre-fabre.co.uk

Fannin (UK) Ltd, Tel: (0) 1233 506 574, medical@athlone-laboratories.com

Fate Special Foods, Tel: (01215) 224 433

Fenton Pharmaceuticals Ltd, Tel: (020) 7224 1388, mail@fent-pharm.co.uk

Ferndale Pharmaceuticals Ltd, Tel: (01937) 541 122, info@ferndalepharma.co.uk

Ferring Pharmaceuticals (UK), Tel: 0844 931 0050, medical@ferring.com

Finox Biotech AG, Tel: 00 800 3466 9246, finoxEY@piglobal.com

Firstplay Dietary Foods Ltd, Tel: (0161) 474 7576

Flynn Pharma Ltd, Tel: (01438) 727 822, medinfo@flynnpharma.com

Focus Pharmaceuticals Ltd, Tel: (01283) 495 280, medinfo@focuspharma.co.uk

Foodlink (UK) Ltd, Tel: (01752) 344 544, info@foodlinkltd.co.uk

Ford Medical Associates Ltd, Tel: (01233) 633 224, enquiries@fordmedical.co.uk

Forest Laboratories UK Ltd, Tel: (01322) 421 800, medinfo@forest-labs.co.uk

Forum Health Products Ltd, Tel: (01737) 857 700, enquiries@forumgroup.co.uk

C. H. Fox Ltd, Tel: (020) 7240 3111

Fresenius Biotech GmbH, Tel: 0049 (0) 893 065 9311, med.info@fresenius-biotech.com

Fresenius Kabi Ltd, Tel: (01928) 533 533, med.info-uk@fresenius-kabi.com

Fresenius Medical Care UK Ltd, Tel: (01623) 445 171, medinfo-uk@fmc-ag.com

Frontier Multigate, Tel: (01495) 233 050, multigate@frontier-group.co.uk

Fyne Dynamics Ltd, Tel: (01279) 423 423, info@fyne-dynamics.com

Galderma (UK) Ltd, Tel: (01923) 208 950, medinfo.uk@galderma.com

Galen Ltd, Tel: (028) 3833 4974, customer.services@galen.co.uk

Gedeon Richter UK Ltd, Tel: (020) 7604 8806, drugsafety.uk@gedeonrichter.eu

GE Healthcare, Tel: (01494) 544 000

Geistlich Pharma, Tel: (01244) 347 534

General Dietary Ltd, Tel: (0203) 044 2933, info@generaldietary.com

Genius Foods Ltd, Tel: 0845 874 4000, info@geniusglutenfree.com

Laboratoires Genopharm, Tel: (0808) 234 2664, info@genopharm.eu

Genus Pharmaceuticals, Tel: (01635) 568 400, info@genuspharma.com

Genzyme Therapeutics, Tel: (01865) 405 200, ukmedinfo@genzyme.com

GF Foods Ltd, Tel: (01757) 289 207, admin@gffdirect.co.uk

Gilead Sciences Ltd, Tel: 0800 011 3700, ukmedinfo@gilead.com

GlaxoSmithKline, Tel: 0800 221 441, customercontactuk@gsk.com

GlaxoSmithKline Consumer Healthcare, Tel: 0800 783 8881, customer.relations@gsk.com

Glenwood GmbH, Tel: (0049) 815 199 8790, info@glenwood.de

GlucoRx Ltd, Tel: (01483) 755 133, info@glucorx.co.uk

Gluten Free Foods Ltd, Tel: (020) 8953 4444, info@glutenfree-foods.co.uk

Grifols UK Ltd, Tel: (01223) 395 700, medinfo.uk@grifols.com

Grünenthal Ltd, Tel: 0870 351 8960, medicalinformationuk@grunenthal.com

H&R Healthcare Ltd, Tel: (01482) 631 606, info@hrhealthcare.co.uk

Hameln Pharmaceuticals Ltd, Tel: (01452) 621 661, drugsafety@hameln.co.uk

Paul Hartmann Ltd, Tel: (01706) 363 200, info@uk.hartmann.info

Henleys Medical Supplies Ltd, Tel: (01707) 333 164

Hennig Arzneimittel GmbH & Co., Tel: 0844 504 0866

HFA Healthcare Ltd, Tel: 0844 335 8270

HK Pharma Ltd, Tel: 0845 519 1609

Hollister Ltd, Tel: (0118) 989 5000

Horizon Pharma, medicalinformation@horizonpharma.com

Hospira UK Ltd, Tel: 0800 088 5133, hospirami@pi-arm.co.uk

HRA Pharma UK & Ireland Ltd, Tel: 0800 917 9548, med.info.uk@hra-pharma.com

Huntleigh Healthcare Ltd, Tel: (01582) 413 104

Huxley Europe Ltd, Tel: (0161) 773 0485

Idis Ltd, Tel: (01932) 824 000, mi@idispharma.com

iMed Systems Ltd, Tel: (0203) 397 8020, emerade@imed-systems.com

INCA-Pharm UK, Tel: (01748) 828 812, info@inca-pharm.com

Infai UK Ltd, Tel: (01904) 435 228, info@infai.co.uk

Injex UK Ltd, Tel: 0845 126 8900, enquiries@injexuk.com

Innovative Solutions UK Ltd, Tel: (01706) 746 713, enquiries@innovative-solutions.org.uk

Insight Medical Products Ltd, Tel: (01666) 500 055, info@insightmedical.ne

InterMune, Tel: (03308) 080 960, med-info@intermune.co.uk

Internis Pharmaceuticals Ltd, Tel: 0870 851 0207, enquiries@medinformation.co.uk

Intrapharm Laboratories Ltd, Tel: (01628) 771 800, sales@intrapharmlabs.com

Ipsen Ltd, Tel: (01753) 627 777, medical.information.uk@ipsen.com

Iroko Cardio GmbH, Tel: (020) 3002 8114, info@irokocardio.com

Janssen-Cilag Ltd, Tel: 0800 731 8450, medinfo@its.jnj.com

Jobskin Ltd, Tel: (0115) 973 4300, dw@jobskin.co.uk

Johnson & Johnson Ltd, Tel: (01628) 822 222, medinfo@congb.jnj.com

Juvela (Hero UK) Ltd, Tel: (0151) 432 5300, info@juvela.co.uk

KCI Medical Ltd, Tel: (01865) 840 600

Kestrel Ophthalmics Ltd, Tel: (01202) 658 444, info@kestrelophthalmics.co.uk

King Pharmaceuticals Ltd, Tel: (01438) 356 924

K/L Pharmaceuticals Ltd, Tel: (01294) 215 951

KoRa Healthcare Ltd, Tel: 0845 303 8631, info@kora.ie

Kyowa Kirin Ltd, Tel: (01896) 664 000, medinfo@kyowakirin.com

Labopharm Europe Ltd, Tel: 0800 028 0037, medinfo@paladin-labs.com

LaCorium Health (UK) Ltd, Tel: 0800 158 8233, ukinfo@flexitol.com

Lantor UK Ltd, Tel: (01204) 855 000, help@lantor.co.uk

LEO Laboratories Ltd, Tel: (01844) 347 333, medical-info.uk@leo-pharma.com

LifeScan, Tel: 0800 001 210

Lincoln Medical Ltd, Tel: (01722) 742 900, info@lincolnmedical.co.uk

Linderma Ltd, Tel: (01942) 816 184, linderma@virgin.ne

Lipomed GmbH, Tel: (0041) 6170 20200, save@lipomed.com

Livwell Ltd, Tel: 0845 120 0038, info@livwell.eu

LogixX Pharma Solutions Ltd, Tel: (01189) 011 747, medinfo@logixxpharma.com

L'Oréal Active Cosmetics UK, Tel: 0800 055 6822

Lornamead UK Ltd, Tel: (01276) 674000, lornamead@dhl.com

LPC Pharmaceuticals Ltd, Tel: (01582) 560 393, info@lpcpharma.com

Lucane Pharma, Tel: 0033 (0) 153 868 750, info@lucanepharma.com

Lundbeck Ltd, Tel: (01908) 649 966, ukmedicalinformation@lundbeck.com

M & A Pharmachem Ltd, Tel: (01942) 816 184

Manuka Medical Ltd, Tel: (01623) 600 669

Manx Healthcare, Tel: (01926) 482 511, info@manxhealthcare.com

Marlborough Pharmaceuticals, Tel: (01279) 406 759, info@marlborough-pharma.co.uk

Martindale Pharma, Tel: (01277) 266 600, medinfo@martindalepharma.co.uk

MASTA, Tel: (0113) 238 7500, medical@masta.org

McNeil Products Ltd, Tel: (01628) 822 222

Medical Diagnostics Europe Ltd, Tel: 0845 370 8077, info@mdediagnostic.co.uk

Mead Johnson Nutrition, Tel: (01895) 230 575

Meadow Laboratories Ltd, Tel: (020) 8597 1203

Meda Pharmaceuticals Ltd, Tel: (01748) 828 810, meda@professionalinformation.co.uk

Medac (UK), Tel: (01786) 458 086, info@medac-uk.co.uk

Medical Developments UK Ltd, Tel: 0870 850 1234, enquiries@ashfieldin2focus.com

Medicare Plus International Ltd, Tel: (020) 8810 8811, info@medicare-plus.com

The Medicines Company, Tel: 00800 8436 3326, medical.information@themedco.com

Medicom Healthcare Ltd, Tel: (01489) 574 119, info@medicomhealthcare.com

Medihoney (Europe) Ltd, Tel: 0800 071 3912

Medisana, Tel: +49 (0) 2131/36 68 0

Medlock Medical Ltd, Tel: (0161) 621 2100

MedLogic Global Ltd, Tel: (01752) 209 955, enquiries@mlgl.co.uk

A. Menarini Farmaceutica Internazionale SRL, Tel: (01628) 856 400, menarini@medinformation.co.uk

A. Menarini Diagnostics, Tel: (0118) 944 4100

Merck Serono Ltd, Tel: (020) 8818 7200, medinfo.uk@merckserono.net

Merus Labs, Tel: 00352 (0) 2637 5878, qchs.mi@quintiles.com

Merz Pharma UK Ltd, Tel: (020) 8236 0000, info@merzpharma.co.uk

Micro Medical Ltd, Tel: (01634) 893 500

Milupa Aptamil, Tel: 0845 762 3676, careline@aptamil4hcps.co.uk

Mitsubishi Pharma, Tel: (0207) 382 9000, medinfo@mitsubishi-pharma.eu

Mölnlycke Health Care Ltd, Tel: (0161) 777 2628, info.uk@molnlycke.net

Moorfields Pharmaceuticals, Tel: (020) 7684 9090

Morningside Healthcare Ltd, Tel: (0116) 204 5950

Movianto UK, Tel: (01234) 248 500, movianto.uk@movianto.com

Mylan, Tel: (01707) 853 000, info@mylan.co.uk

Nagor Ltd, Tel: (01624) 625 556, enquiries@nagor.com

Nairn's Oatcakes Ltd, Tel: (0131) 620 7000

Napp Pharmaceuticals Ltd, Tel: (01223) 424 444

Neoceuticals Ltd, Tel: (01748) 828 865

Neolab Ltd, Tel: (01256) 704 110, info@neolab.co.uk

Neomedic Ltd, Tel: (01923) 836 379, marketing@neomedic.co.uk

Neon Diagnostics Ltd, Tel: (01376) 500 720

Nestlé Nutrition, Tel: 00800 6887 4846, nestlehealthcarenutrition@uk.nestle.com

Newport Pharmaceuticals, Tel: (00353) 1890 3011

Nicox Pharma, Tel: (01483) 549 211, ukmedicalinformation@nicox.com

Nipro Diagnostics (UK) Ltd, Tel: 0800 08 588 08, info@homediagnostics-uk.com

Nordic Pharma UK Ltd, Tel: (0118) 929 8233, info@nordicpharma.co.uk

Norgine Pharmaceuticals Ltd, Tel: (01895) 826 600, medinfo@norgine.com

Northern Ireland Blood Transfusion Service, Tel: (028) 9032 1414, inet@nibts.hscni.net

Nova Laboratories Ltd, Tel: 08707 120 655, xaluprine@aptivsolutions.com

Novartis Consumer Health, Tel: (01276) 687 202, medicalaffairs.uk@novartis.com

Novartis Pharmaceuticals UK Ltd, Tel: (01276) 692 255, medinfo.uk@novartis.com

Novartis Vaccines Ltd, Tel: 0845 745 1500, service.uk@novartis.com

Novo Nordisk Ltd, Tel: (01293) 613 555

nSPIRE Health Ltd, Tel: (01992) 526 300, info@nspirehealth.com

Nualtra Ltd, Tel: 0808 101 0926, support@nualtra.co.uk

Nutricia, Tel: (01225) 751 098, resourcecentre@nutricia.com

Nutrinovo Ltd, Tel: (01304) 829 068, info@nutrinovo.com

Nutrition Point Ltd, Tel: (07041) 544 044, info@nutritionpoint.co.uk

Nycomed UK Ltd, Tel: (01628) 646 4397, medinfo@nycomed.com

OakMed Ltd, Tel: 0800 592 786, orders@oakmed.co.uk

Octapharma Ltd, Tel: (0161) 837 3770, octapharma@octapharma.co.uk

Omega Pharma, Tel: (01748) 828 860, omega@professionalinformation.co.uk

Omron Healthcare (UK) Ltd, Tel: 0870 750 2771, info.omronhealthcare.uk@eu.omron.com

Organon, Tel: (01992) 467 272, medicalinformationuk@merck.com

Orion Pharma (UK) Ltd, Tel: (01635) 520 300, medicalinformation@orionpharma.com

Orphan Europe (UK) Ltd, Tel: (01491) 414 333, infouk@orphan-europe.com

Otsuka Novel Products GmbH, Tel: (0049) 892 0602 0500, medical@otsuka-onpg.com

Otsuka Pharmaceuticals (UK) Ltd, Tel: (020) 3747 5300, ukmedinfo@otsuka.co.uk

Ovation Healthcare International Ltd, Tel: (00353) 1613 9707

Owen Mumford Ltd, Tel: (01993) 812 021, customerservices@owenmumford.co.uk

Oxbridge Pharma Ltd, Tel: (020) 8335 4110, enquiries@oxbridgepharma.com

Oxford Nutrition Ltd, Tel: (01626) 832 067, info@nutrinox.com

PARI Medical Ltd, Tel: (01932) 341 122, infouk@pari.de

Parkside Healthcare, Tel: (0161) 795 2792

PaxVax, Tel: 0800 088 5449, medicalinformation@paxvax.com

Peckforton Pharmaceuticals Ltd, Tel: (01270) 582 255, info@peckforton.com

Penn Pharmaceuticals Services Ltd, Tel: (01495) 711 222, penn@pennpharm.co.uk

Pfizer Ltd, Tel: (01304) 616 161, eumedinfo@pfizer.com

PGR Health Foods Ltd, Tel: (01992) 581 715, info@pgrhealthfoods.co.uk

Pharmacia, Tel: (01304) 616 161, eumedinfo@pfizer.com

Pharmacosmos UK Ltd, Tel: (01844) 269 007, info@vitalineuk.co.uk

Pharma Mar, Tel: (01932) 824 000, mi@idispharma.com

Pharma Nord (UK) Ltd, Tel: (01670) 519 989, uksales@pharmanord.co.uk

Pharmasure Ltd, Tel: (01923) 233 466, info@pharmasure.co.uk

Pharmaxis Pharmaceuticals Ltd, Tel: (01628) 902 053, med.info@pharmaxis.com.au

PharSafer Associates Ltd, Tel: 01483 212151, medinfoenquiries@pharsafer.com

Phoenix Labs, Tel: (00353) 1468 8917, medicalinformation@phoenixlabs.ie

Pinewood Healthcare, Tel: (00353) 523 6253, info@pinewood.ie

Pinnacle Biologics Inc., Tel: 1-866-248-2039, pinnaclemedinfo@optum.com

Potters Herbal Medicines, Tel: (01942) 219 960

Proceli, Tel: (01226) 713 044, admin@proceli.co.uk

Procter & Gamble (Health and Beauty Care) Ltd, Tel: (0191) 297 5000

Profile Pharma Ltd, Tel: 0800 0288 942, info.profilepharma@zambongroup.com

Protex Healthcare (UK) Ltd, Tel: 0870 011 4112, orders@protexhealthcare.co.uk

PTC Therapeutics Ltd, Tel: (0)1483 246 865, medinfo@ptcbio.com

Qdem, Tel: (01223) 426 929, medicalinformationukqdem@qdem.co.uk

Ranbaxy UK Ltd, Tel: (020) 8280 1986, medinfoeurope@ranbaxy.com

Ransom Consumer Healthcare, Tel: (01462) 437 615, info@williamransom.com

Ratiopharm UK Ltd, Tel: (023) 9231 3592, info@ratiopharm.co.uk

Reckitt Benckiser Healthcare, Tel: (01482) 326 151, info.miu@reckittbenckiser.com

Recordati Pharmaceuticals Ltd, Tel: (01491) 576 336, medinfo@recordati.co.uk

ReSource Medical UK Ltd, Tel: (01484) 531 489, info@resource-medical.co.uk

Philips Respironics (UK) Ltd, Tel: 0800 130 0840, rukmarketing@respironics.com

RF Medical Supplies Ltd, Tel: (0151) 493 1473, enquiries@rfmedicalsupplies.co.uk

Richardson Healthcare Ltd, Tel: 0800 170 1126, info@richardsonhealthcare.com

Riemser Arzneimittel AG, Tel: (0049) 383 517 6679, info@riemser.de

RIS Products Ltd, Tel: (01438) 840 135

Robinson Healthcare Ltd, Tel: (01909) 735 064, enquiry@robinsonhealthcare.com

Roche Diagnostics Ltd, Tel: (01444) 256 000

Roche Products Ltd, Tel: 0800 328 1629, medinfo.uk@roche.com

Rosemont Pharmaceuticals Ltd, Tel: 0800 919 312, rosemont.infodesk@perrigouk.com

Rowa Pharmaceuticals Ltd, Tel: (00353) 275 0077, rowa@rowa-pharma.ie

RPH Pharmaceuticals Ltd, Tel: (01483) 212 151, medinfoenquiries@pharsafer.com

Sallis Healthcare Ltd, Tel: (0115) 978 7841

Sandoz Ltd, Tel: (01276) 698 020, sandoz@professionalinformation.co.uk

Sanochemia Diagnostics UK Ltd, Tel: (0117) 906 3562

Sanofi-Aventis Ltd, Tel: 0845 372 7101, uk-medicalinformation@sanofi-aventis.com

Sanofi Pasteur MSD Ltd, Tel: (01628) 785 291

SanoMed Manufacturing bv, Tel: +32 503 93627, info@sanomed.nl

Santen UK Limited, Tel: (0345) 075 4863, medinfo@santen.co.uk

Santhera (UK) Ltd, Tel: (0)203 434 5740, santhera@pi-arm.co.uk

Schering-Plough, Tel: (01992) 467 272, medicalinformationuk@merck.com

Schuco International Ltd, Tel: (020) 8368 1642, sales@schuco.co.uk

Schülke UK, Tel: (0114) 254 3500, mail.uk@schuelke.com

Scope Ophthamics Ltd, Tel: (01293) 897 209, info@scopeophthalmics.com

Scottish National Blood Transfusion Service, Tel: (0131) 536 5700, contact.pfc@snbts.csa.scot.nhs.uk

SD Biosensor, Inc., Tel: 0082 31 300 0475, sales@sdbiosensor.com

SD Healthcare, Tel: (0161) 776 7626, sales@sdhealthcare.com

Seahorse Laboratories Ltd, Tel: (020) 8257 8412, info@seahorse-labs.com

Septodont Ltd, Tel: (01622) 695 520

Servier Laboratories Ltd, Tel: (01753) 666 409, medical.information-uk@servier.com

Seven Seas Ltd, Tel: (01482) 375 234

Shermond, Tel: 0870 242 7701, sales@shermond.com

Shield TX, Tel: (01915) 118500, medinfo@shieldtx.com

Shire Pharmaceuticals Ltd, Tel: 0800 055 6614, medinfouk@shire.com

Shire Human Genetic Therapies, Tel: (01256) 894 000, hgtmedcomm@shire.com

SHS International Ltd, Tel: (0151) 228 8161

Siemens Healthcare Diagnostics Ltd, Tel: 0845 600 1966, dx-diag_sales-uk.med@siemens.com

Sigma-Tau Pharma Ltd (UK), Tel: 0800 043 1268, medical.information@sigma-tau.co.uk

SilDerm Ltd, Tel: (01260) 271 666

Sinclair IS Pharma, Tel: (01244) 625 152, enquiries@ispharma.plc.uk

The Skin Camouflage Company Ltd, Tel: (01507) 343 091, smjcovermark@aol.com

Skinnies UK, Tel: (01562) 546 123, info@skinniesuk.com

SLO Drinks Ltd, Tel: 0345 222 205, info@slodrinks.com

SMA Nutrition, Tel: (01628) 604 377, eumedinfo@pfizer.com

Smith & Nephew Healthcare Ltd, Tel: (01482) 222 200, advice@smith-nephew.com

Sound Opinion, Tel: 0870 192 3283, enquiries@medinformation.co.uk

Speciality European Pharma Ltd, Tel: (020) 7421 7400, info@spepharma.com

SpePharm UK Ltd, Tel: 0844 800 7579, medinfo.uk@spepharm.com

Spirit Healthcare Ltd, Tel: 0800 881 5423, cs@spirit-healthcare.co.uk

Squibb Pharmaceuticals Ltd, Tel: (01895) 523 000, medical.information@bms.com

SSL International plc, Tel: 0870 122 2690

Stanningley Pharma Ltd, Tel: (01159) 124 253, medinfo@stanningleypharma.co.uk

STD Pharmaceutical Products Ltd, Tel: (01432) 373 555, enquiries@stdpharm.co.uk

Steraid (Gainsborough) Ltd, Tel: (01427) 677 559

St George's Medical, Tel: (020) 7582 1015

Stiefel (a GSK company), Tel: 0800 221 441

Stiletto Foods UK Ltd, Tel: 0845 130 0869

Stragen UK Ltd, Tel: 0870 351 8744, info@stragenuk.com

Sucampo Pharma, Tel: 0800 756 3416, infoeu@sucampo.com

Su-Med International UK Ltd, Tel: (01457) 890 980, sales@sumed.co.uk

Sunovion Pharmaceuticals Europe Ltd, Tel: (020) 7821 2840, medinfo@sunovion.eu

Sutherland Health Ltd, Tel: (01635) 874 488

Swedish Orphan Biovitrum Ltd, Tel: (01638) 722 380, medical.info@sobi.com

Synergy Healthcare (UK) Ltd, Tel: (0161) 624 5641, healthcaresolutions@synergyhealthplc.com

Syner-Med (Pharmaceutical Products) Ltd, Tel: 0845 634 2100, mail@syner-med.com

Systagenix Wound Management, Tel: (01293) 842 000

Takeda UK Ltd, Tel: (01628) 537 900, medinfo@takeda.co.uk

Talley Group Ltd, Tel: (01794) 503 500

Taro Pharmaceuticals (UK) Ltd, Tel: 0870 736 9544, customerservice@taropharma.co.uk

Teofarma S.r.l., servizioclienti@teofarma.it

TEVA UK Ltd, Tel: 0870 502 0304, (020) 7540 7117, medinfo@tevauk.com

Thea Pharmaceuticals, Tel: 0870 192 3283, thea-pharma@medinformation.co.uk

Therabel Pharma UK Ltd, Tel: 0800 066 5446, info@therabel.co.uk

Thomas Blake Cosmetic Creams Ltd, Tel: (01207) 272 311, sales@veilcover.com

Thornton & Ross Ltd, Tel: (01484) 842 217

Tillomed Laboratories Ltd, Tel: (01480) 402 400, info@tillomed.co.uk

Tillotts Pharma UK Ltd, Tel: 01522 813 500, ukmedinfo@tillotts.com

TMC Pharma Services Ltd, Tel: (01252) 842 255, info@tmcpharma.com

Tobia Teff UK Ltd, Tel: (020) 7328 2045, info@tobiateff.co.uk

Torbet Laboratories Ltd, Tel: (01953) 607 856, customerservices@cambridge-healthcare.co.uk

Transdermal Ltd, Tel: (020) 8654 2251, info@transdermal.co.uk

TRB Chemedica (UK) Ltd, Tel: 0845 330 7556

Typharm Ltd, Tel: (01603) 722 480, customerservices@typharm.com

UCB Pharma Ltd, Tel: (01753) 534 655, medicalinformationuk@ucb.com

Ultrapharm Ltd, Tel: (01491) 578 016

Univar Ltd, Tel: (01908) 362 200, trientine@univareurope.com

Unomedical Ltd, Tel: (01527) 587 700

Urgo Ltd, Tel: (01509) 502 051, woundcare@uk.urgo.com

The Urology Company Ltd, Tel: (020) 3077 5411, info@theurologyco.com

Vegenat, Tel: 0870 803 2484

Vertex Pharmaceuticals (UK) Ltd, Tel: 0800 028 2616, eumedicalinfo@vrtx.com

Vifor Pharma UK Ltd, Tel: (01276) 853 633, medicalinfo_uk@viforpharma.com

ViiV Healthcare UK Ltd, Tel: 0800221441, customercontactuk@gsk.com

Viridian Pharma Ltd, Tel: (01633) 400 335, info@viridianpharma.co.uk

ViroPharma Ltd, Tel: (020) 7572 1222

Vitaflo International Ltd, Tel: (0151) 709 9020, vitaflo@vitaflo.co.uk

Vitalograph Ltd, Tel: (01280) 827 110, sales@vitalograph.co.uk

Wallace Cameron Ltd, Tel: (01698) 354 600, sales@wallacecameron.com

Wallace Manufacturing Chemists Ltd, Tel: (01235) 538 700, info@alinter.co.uk

Warburtons, Tel: (01204) 513 004

Warner Chilcott UK Ltd, Tel: (01932) 824 700

Wellfoods Ltd, Tel: (01226) 381 712, wellfoods@wellfoods.co.uk

Welsh Blood Service, Tel: (01443) 622 000, donor.care@wales.nhs.uk

Williams Medical Supplies Ltd, Tel: (01685) 844 739

Wockhardt UK Ltd, Tel: (01978) 661 261

Wyeth Pharmaceuticals, Tel: (01628) 604 377, eumedinfo@pfizer.com

Wynlit Laboratories, Tel: (07903) 370 130

Wyvern Medical Ltd, Tel: (01531) 631 105

Zentiva, Tel: (01483) 554 101, gb-zentivamedicalinformation@sanofi.com

Zeroderma Ltd, Tel: (01858) 525 643

Special-order manufacturers

Unlicensed medicines are available from 'special-order' manufacturers and specialist-importing companies; the MHRA maintains a register of these companies at tinyurl.com/cdslke.

Licensed **hospital manufacturing units** also manufacture 'special-order' products as unlicensed medicines, the principal NHS units are listed below. A database (*Pro-File*; www.pro-file.nhs.uk) provides information on medicines manufactured in the NHS; access is restricted to NHS pharmacy staff.

The Association of Pharmaceutical Specials Manufacturers may also be able to provide further information about commercial companies (www.apsm-uk. com).

The MHRA recommends that an unlicensed medicine should only be used when a patient has special requirements that cannot be met by use of a licensed medicine.

As well as being available direct from the hospital manufacturer(s) concerned, many NHS-manufactured Specials may be bought from the Oxford Pharmacy Store, owned and operated by Oxford Health NHS Foundation Trust.

England

London

Barts and the London NHS Trust
Mr J. A. Rickard, Head of Barts Health Pharmaceuticals
Barts Health NHS Trust
The Royal London Hospital
Pathology and Pharmacy Building
80 Newark St
Whitechapel
London
E1 2ES
(020) 3246 0394 (order/enquiry)
barts.pharmaceuticals@bartshealth.nhs.uk

Guy's and St. Thomas' NHS Foundation Trust
Mr P. Forsey, Associate Chief Pharmacist
Guy's and St. Thomas' NHS Foundation Trust
Guy's Hospital
Pharmacy Department
Great Maze Pond
London
SE1 9RT
(020) 7188 4992 (order)
(020) 7188 5003 (enquiry)
Fax: (020) 7188 5013
paul.forsey@gstt.nhs.uk

Moorfields Pharmaceuticals
Mr. T. Record, Technical Director
Moorfields Pharmaceuticals
25 Provost St
London
N1 7NH
(020) 7684 9090 (order/enquiry)
Fax: (020) 7502 2332

London North West Healthcare NHS Trust
Mr K. Wong,
London North West Healthcare NHS Trust
Northwick Park Hospital
Watford Rd
Harrow
Middlesex
HA1 3UJ
(020) 8869 2295 (order)
(020) 8869 2204/2223 (enquiry)
kwong@nhs.net

Royal Free Hampstead NHS Trust
Ms C. Trehane, Production Manager
Royal Free Hampstead NHS Trust
Pond St
London
NW3 2QG
(020) 7830 2424 (order)
(020) 7830 2282 (enquiry)
Fax: (020) 7794 1875
christine.trehane@nhs.net

St George's Healthcare NHS Trust
Mr V. Kumar, Assistant Chief Pharmacist
St George's Hospital
Technical Services
Blackshaw Rd
Tooting
London
SW17 0QT
(020) 8725 1770/1768
Fax: (020) 8725 3947
vinodh.kumar@stgeorges.nhs.uk

University College Hospital NHS Foundation Trust
Mr T. Murphy, Production Manager
University College Hospital
235 Euston Rd
London
NW1 2BU
(020) 7380 9723 (order)
(020) 7380 9472 (enquiry)
Fax: (020) 7380 9726
tony.murphy@uclh.nhs.uk

Midlands and Eastern

Barking, Havering and Redbridge University Trust
Mr N. Fisher, Senior Principal Pharmacist
Queen's Hospital
Pharmacy Department
Romford
Essex
RM7 0AG
(01708) 435 463 (order)
(01708) 435 042 (enquiry)
neil.fisher@bhrhospitals.nhs.uk

Burton Hospitals NHS Foundation Trust
Mr D. Raynor, Head of Pharmacy Manufacturing Unit
Queens Hospital
Burton Hospitals NHS Foundation Trust
Pharmacy Manufacturing Unit
Belvedere Rd
Burton-on-Trent
DE13 0RB
(01283) 511 511 ext: 5275 (order/enquiry)
Fax: (01283) 593 036
david.raynor@burtonft.nhs.uk

Colchester Hospital University NHS Foundation Trust
Mr S. Pullen, Pharmacy Production Manager
Colchester General Hospital
Main Pharmacy
Turner Rd
Colchester
Essex
CO4 5JL
(01206) 742 007 (order)
(01206) 744 208 (enquiry)
Fax: (01206) 841 249
pharmacy.stores@colchesterhospital.nhs.uk (order)
psu.enquiries@colchesterhospital.nhs.uk (enquiry)

Ipswich Hospital NHS Trust
Dr J. Harwood, Production Manager
Ipswich Hospital NHS Trust
Pharmacy Manufacturing Unit
Heath Rd
Ipswich,
IP4 5PD
(01473) 703 440 (order)
(01473) 703 603 (enquiry)
Fax: (01473) 703 609
john.harwood@ipswichhospital.nhs.uk

Nottingham University Hospitals NHS Trust
Mr J. Graham, Senior Pharmacist, Production
Nottingham University Hospitals NHS Trust
Pharmacy Production Units
Queens Medical Centre Campus
Nottingham
NG7 2UH
(0115) 924 9924 ext: 66521 (enquiry/order)
Fax: (0115) 970 9780
jeff.graham@nuh.nhs.uk

University Hospital of North Staffordshire NHS Trust
Ms K. Ferguson, Chief Technician
University Hospital of North Staffordshire NHS Trust
Pharmacy Technical Services
City General Site
Stoke-on-Trent
ST4 6QG
(01782) 674 568 (order)
(01782) 674 568 (enquiry)
Fax: (01782) 674 575
caroline.ferguson@uhns.nhs.uk

North East

The Newcastle upon Tyne Hospitals NHS Foundation Trust
Mr Y. Hunter-Blair, Production Manager
Royal Victoria Infirmary
Newcastle Specials
Pharmacy Production Unit
Queen Victoria Rd
Newcastle-upon-Tyne
NE1 4LP
(0191) 282 0395 (order)
(0191) 282 0389 (enquiry)
Fax: (0191) 282 0469
yan.hunter-blair@nuth.nhs.uk

North West

Preston Pharmaceuticals

Ms A. Bolch, Deputy Chief Pharmacist (PMU)
Preston Pharmaceuticals
Royal Preston Hospital
Fulwood
Preston
PR2 9HT
(01772) 523 617 (order)
(01772) 522 593 (enquiry)
Fax: (01772) 523 645
angela.bolch@lthtr.nhs.uk

Stockport Pharmaceuticals

Mr A. Singleton, Head of Production
Stepping Hill Hospital
Stockport NHS Foundation Trust
Stockport Pharmaceuticals
Stockport
SK2 7JE
(0161) 419 5666 (order)
(0161) 419 5657 (enquiry)
Fax: (0161) 419 5426
andrew.singleton@stockport.nhs.uk

South

Portsmouth Hospitals NHS Trust

Mr R. Lucas, Product Development Manager
Portsmouth Hospitals NHS Trust
Pharmacy Manufacturing Unit
Unit D2, Railway Triangle Industrial Estate
Walton Road
Farlington
Portsmouth
PO6 1TF
(02392) 389 078 (order)
(02392) 316 312 (enquiry)
Fax: (02392) 316 316
robert.lucas@porthosp.nhs.uk

South East

East Sussex Healthcare NHS Trust

Mr P. Keen, Business Manager
Eastbourne District General Hospital
East Sussex Hospitals NHS Trust
Eastbourne Pharmaceuticals
Kings Drive
Eastbourne
BN21 2UD
(01323) 414 906 (order)
(01323) 417 400 ext: 3076 (enquiry)
Fax: (01323) 414 931
paul.keen@esht.nhs.uk

South West

Torbay Pharmaceuticals

Ms J. Bamby, Pharmacy Manufacturing Services Manager
South Devon Healthcare NHS Foundation Trust
Torbay Pharmaceuticals
Kemmings Close, Long Rd
Paignton
TQ4 7TW
(01803) 664 707
Fax: (01803) 664 354
jane.bamby@nhs.net

Yorkshire

Calderdale and Huddersfield NHS Foundation Trust

Dr B. Grewal, Managing Director
Calderdale and Huddersfield NHS Foundation Trust
Huddersfield Pharmacy Specials
Gate 2 - Acre Mills, School St West
Huddersfield
HD3 3ET
(01484) 355 388 (order/enquiry)
info.hps@cht.nhs.uk

Northern Ireland

Victoria Pharmaceuticals

Mr S. Cameron, Production Manager - Pharmacy
Victoria Pharmaceuticals
Royal Hospitals
Plenum Building
Grosvenor Road
Belfast
BT12 6BA
(028) 9063 0070 (order/enquiry)
Fax: (028) 9063 5282 (order/enquiry)
samuel.cameron@belfasttrust.hscni.net

Scotland

NHS Greater Glasgow and Clyde

Ms K. Pollock, Acting Production Manager
Pharmacy Production Unit
University Place
Glasgow
G12 8TA
(0141) 451 5820 (order)
(0141) 451 5822 (enquiry)
Fax: (0141) 334 9137
pharmacyproductionunit@ggc.scot.nhs.uk

Tayside Pharmaceuticals

Mr S. Bath, Production Manager
Ninewells Hospital
Tayside Pharmaceuticals
Dundee
DD1 9SY
(01382) 632 052 (order)
(01382) 632 273 (enquiry)
Fax: (01382) 632 060
sbath@nhs.net

Wales

Cardiff and Vale University Health Board

Mr P. Spark, Principal Pharmacist (Production)
Cardiff and Vale University Health Board
20 Fieldway
Cardiff
CF14 4HY
(029) 2074 8120
Fax: (029) 2074 8130
paul.spark@wales.nhs.uk

Index

In Confidence

YellowCard
COMMISSION ON HUMAN MEDICINES (CHM)

MHRA
Regulating Medicines and Medical Devices

It's easy to report online at:
www.mhra.gov.uk/yellowcard

REPORT OF SUSPECTED ADVERSE DRUG REACTIONS

If you suspect an adverse reaction may be related to one or more drugs/vaccines/complementary remedies, please complete this Yellow Card. See 'Adverse reactions to drugs' section in BNF or **www.mhra.gov.uk/yellowcard** for guidance. Do not be put off reporting because some details are not known.

PATIENT DETAILS

Patient Initials: _____   Sex: M / F   Is the patient pregnant? Y / N   Ethnicity: _____

Age (at time of reaction): _____   Weight (kg): _____   Identification number (e.g. Practice or Hospital Ref): _____

SUSPECTED DRUG(S)/VACCINE(S)

Drug/Vaccine (Brand if known)	Batch	Route	Dosage	Date started	Date stopped	Prescribed for

SUSPECTED REACTION(S)

Please describe the reaction(s) and any treatment given. (Please attach additional pages if necessary):

Outcome

☐ Recovered
☐ Recovering
☐ Continuing
☐ Other

Date reaction(s) started: _____   Date reaction(s) stopped: _____

Do you consider the reactions to be serious?   Yes / No

If yes, please indicate why the reaction is considered to be serious (please tick all that apply):

☐ Patient died due to reaction
☐ Life threatening
☐ Congenital abnormality

☐ Involved or prolonged inpatient hospitalisation
☐ Involved persistent or significant disability or incapacity
☐ Medically significant; please give details: _____

If the reactions were not serious according to the categories above, how bad was the suspected reaction?

☐ Mild   ☐ Unpleasant, but did not affect everyday activities   ☐ Bad enough to affect everyday activities

It's easy to report online: www.mhra.gov.uk/yellowcard

OTHER DRUG(S) (including self-medication and complementary remedies)

Did the patient take any other medicines/vaccines/complementary remedies in the last 3 months prior to the reaction? Yes / No

If yes, please give the following information if known:

Drug/Vaccine (Brand if known)	Batch	Route	Dosage	Date started	Date stopped	Prescribed for

Additional relevant information e.g. medical history, test results, known allergies, rechallenge (if performed). For reactions relating to use of a medicine during pregnancy please state all other drugs taken during pregnancy, the last menstrual period, information on previous pregnancies, ultrasound scans, any delivery complications, birth defects or developmental concerns.

Please list any medicines obtained from the internet:

REPORTER DETAILS
Name and Professional Address:

Postcode: _____ Tel No:_____
Email:
Speciality:
Signature: _____ Date:_____

CLINICIAN (if not the reporter)
Name and Professional Address:

Postcode: _____ Tel No:_____
Email:
Speciality:
Date:

Information on adverse drug reactions received by the MHRA can be downloaded at **www.mhra.gov.uk/daps**
Stay up-to-date on the latest advice for the safe use of medicines with our monthly bulletin *Drug Safety Update* at: **www.mhra.gov.uk/drugsafetyupdate**

Please attach additional pages if necessary. Send to: FREEPOST YELLOW CARD (no other address details required)

In Confidence

BNF

YellowCard

COMMISSION ON HUMAN MEDICINES (CHM)

It's easy to report online at:
www.mhra.gov.uk/yellowcard

 MHRA
Regulating Medicines and Medical Devices

REPORT OF SUSPECTED ADVERSE DRUG REACTIONS

If you suspect an adverse reaction may be related to one or more drugs/vaccines/complementary remedies, please complete this Yellow Card. See 'Adverse reactions to drugs' section in BNF or **www.mhra.gov.uk/yellowcard** for guidance. Do not be put off reporting because some details are not known.

PATIENT DETAILS
Patient Initials: _____ Sex: M / F   Is the patient pregnant? Y / N   Ethnicity: _____

Age (at time of reaction): _____ Weight (kg): _____ Identification number (e.g. Practice or Hospital Ref): _____

SUSPECTED DRUG(S)/VACCINE(S)

Drug/Vaccine (Brand if known)	Batch	Route	Dosage	Date started	Date stopped	Prescribed for

SUSPECTED REACTION(S) Please describe the reaction(s) and any treatment given. (Please attach additional pages if necessary):

Outcome

- Recovered ☐
- Recovering ☐
- Continuing ☐
- Other ☐

Date reaction(s) started: _____   Date reaction(s) stopped: _____

Do you consider the reactions to be serious?   Yes / No

If yes, please indicate why the reaction is considered to be serious (please tick all that apply):

- ☐ Patient died due to reaction
- ☐ Life threatening
- ☐ Congenital abnormality
- ☐ Involved or prolonged inpatient hospitalisation
- ☐ Involved persistent or significant disability or incapacity
- ☐ Medically significant; please give details: _____

If the reactions were not serious according to the categories above, how bad was the suspected reaction?

☐ Mild   ☐ Unpleasant, but did not affect everyday activities   ☐ Bad enough to affect everyday activities

It's easy to report online: www.mhra.gov.uk/yellowcard

OTHER DRUG(S) (including self-medication and complementary remedies)

Did the patient take any other medicines/vaccines/complementary remedies in the last 3 months prior to the reaction? Yes / No

If yes, please give the following information if known:

Drug/Vaccine (Brand if known)	Batch	Route	Dosage	Date started	Date stopped	Prescribed for

Additional relevant information e.g. medical history, test results, known allergies, rechallenge (if performed). For reactions relating to use of a medicine during pregnancy please state all other drugs taken during pregnancy, the last menstrual period, information on previous pregnancies, ultrasound scans, any delivery complications, birth defects or developmental concerns.

Please list any medicines obtained from the internet:

REPORTER DETAILS

Name and Professional Address:

Postcode: _____ Tel No:_____

Email:

Speciality:

Signature: _____ Date:

CLINICIAN (if not the reporter)

Name and Professional Address:

Postcode:_____ Tel No:_____

Email:

Speciality:

Date:

Information on adverse drug reactions received by the MHRA can be downloaded at **www.mhra.gov.uk/daps**

Stay up-to-date on the latest advice for the safe use of medicines with our monthly bulletin *Drug Safety Update* at: **www.mhra.gov.uk/drugsafetyupdate**

Please attach additional pages if necessary. Send to: FREEPOST YELLOW CARD (no other address details required)

Adult Advanced Life Support Algorithm

 Resuscitation Council (UK) **Adult Advanced Life Support**

Unresponsive and not breathing normally

→ Call resuscitation team

CPR 30:2
Attach defibrillator/monitor
Minimise interruptions

↓

Assess rhythm

Shockable (VF/Pulseless VT)

Return of spontaneous circulation

Non-shockable (PEA/Asystole)

---

1 Shock
Minimise interruptions

Immediate post cardiac arrest treatment
- Use ABCDE approach
- Aim for SpO$_2$ of 94-98%
- Aim for normal PaCO$_2$
- 12-lead ECG
- Treat precipitating cause
- Targeted temperature management

Immediately resume **CPR for 2 min**
Minimise interruptions

Immediately resume **CPR for 2 min**
Minimise interruptions

During CPR
- Ensure high quality chest compressions
- Minimise interruptions to compressions
- Give oxygen
- Use waveform capnography
- Continuous compressions when advanced airway in place
- Vascular access (intravenous or intraosseous)
- Give adrenaline every 3-5 min
- Give amiodarone after 3 shocks

Treat Reversible Causes
- Hypoxia
- Hypovolaemia
- Hypo-/hyperkalaemia/metabolic
- Hypothermia

- Thrombosis - coronary or pulmonary
- Tension pneumothorax
- Tamponade – cardiac
- Toxins

Consider
- Ultrasound imaging
- Mechanical chest compressions to facilitate transfer/treatment
- Coronary angiography and percutaneous coronary intervention
- Extracorporeal CPR

Medical emergencies in the community

Overview
Drug treatment outlined below is intended for use by appropriately qualified healthcare professionals. Only drugs that are used for immediate relief are shown; advice on supporting care is not given. Where the patient's condition requires investigation and further treatment, the patient should be transferred to hospital promptly.

Acute coronary syndromes

▶ **ANGINA: UNSTABLE**
Aspirin dispersible tablets p. 121 (75 mg, 300 mg)
BY MOUTH (DISPERSED IN WATER OR CHEWED)
  ▶ Adult: 300 mg

▶ PLUS

▶ EITHER **Glyceryl trinitrate aerosol spray p. 217**
(400 micrograms/metered dose)
SUBLINGUALLY
  ▶ Adult: 1–2 sprays, repeated as required

▶ OR **Glyceryl trinitrate tablets** (300 micrograms, 500 micrograms, 600 micrograms)
SUBLINGUALLY
  ▶ Adult: 0.3–1 mg, repeated as required

▶ **MYOCARDIAL INFARCTION: NON-ST-SEGMENT ELEVATION**
Treat as for Angina: unstable

▶ **MYOCARDIAL INFARCTION: ST-SEGMENT ELEVATION**
Aspirin dispersible tablets (75 mg, 300 mg)
BY MOUTH (DISPERSED IN WATER OR CHEWED)
  ▶ Adult: 300 mg

Glyceryl trinitrate aerosol spray (400 micrograms/metered dose)
SUBLINGUALLY
  ▶ Adult: 1–2 sprays, repeated as required

▶ OR **Glyceryl trinitrate tablets** (300 micrograms, 500 micrograms, 600 micrograms)
SUBLINGUALLY
  ▶ Adult: 0.3–1 mg, repeated as required

Metoclopramide hydrochloride injection p. 426 (5 mg/mL)
BY INTRAVENOUS INJECTION
  ▶ Adult 18-19 years (body-weight up to 60 kg): 5 mg
  ▶ Adult 18-19 years (body-weight 60 kg and over): 10 mg
  ▶ Adult over 19 years: 10 mg

Diamorphine hydrochloride injection p. 449 (5 mg powder for reconstitution)
BY SLOW INTRAVENOUS INJECTION (1-2 MG/MINUTE)
  ▶ Adult: 5 mg followed by a further 2.5–5 mg if necessary
  ▶ Elderly or frail patients: reduce dose by half

▶ OR **Morphine sulfate injection p. 456** (10 mg/mL)
BY SLOW INTRAVENOUS INJECTION (1-2 MG/MINUTE)
  ▶ Adult: 5–10 mg followed by a further 5–10 mg if necessary
  ▶ Elderly or frail patients: reduce dose by half
Oxygen, if appropriate

Airways disease, obstructive

▶ **ASTHMA: ACUTE**
Regard each emergency consultation as being for **severe acute asthma** until shown otherwise; failure to respond adequately **at any time** requires immediate transfer to hospital

▶ EITHER **Salbutamol aerosol inhaler p. 252**
(100 micrograms/metered inhalation)
BY AEROSOL INHALATION VIA LARGE-VOLUME SPACER
(AND A CLOSE-FITTING FACE MASK IF CHILD UNDER 3 YEARS)
  ▶ Adult and child: 2–10 puffs each inhaled separately, repeated every 10–20 minutes or as necessary

▶ OR **Salbutamol nebuliser solution** (1 mg/mL, 2 mg/mL)
BY INHALATION OF NEBULISED SOLUTION (VIA OXYGEN-DRIVEN NEBULISER IF AVAILABLE)
  ▶ Child 4 years and below: 2.5 mg every 20–30 minutes or as necessary
  ▶ Child 5-11 years: 2.5–5 mg every 20–30 minutes or as necessary
  ▶ Child 12-17 years: 5 mg every 20–30 minutes or as necessary
  ▶ Adult: 5 mg every 20–30 minutes or as necessary

▶ OR **Terbutaline sulfate nebuliser solution p. 254** (2.5 mg/mL)
BY INHALATION OF NEBULISED SOLUTION (VIA OXYGEN-DRIVEN NEBULISER IF AVAILABLE)
  ▶ Child 4 years and below: 5 mg every 20–30 minutes or as necessary
  ▶ Child 5-11 years: 5–10 mg every 20–30 minutes or as necessary
  ▶ Child 12-17 years: 10 mg every 20–30 minutes or as necessary
  ▶ Adult: 10 mg every 20–30 minutes or as necessary

▶ PLUS **(in all cases)**

▶ EITHER **Prednisolone tablets p. 664 (or prednisolone soluble tablets)** (5 mg)
BY MOUTH
  ▶ Child 11 years and below: 1–2 mg/kg (max. 40 mg) once daily for up to 3 days or longer if necessary; if child has been taking an oral corticosteroid for more than a few days, give prednisolone 2 mg/kg (max. 60 mg) once daily
  ▶ Child 12-17 years: 40–50 mg once daily for at least 5 days
  ▶ Adult: 40–50 mg once daily for at least 5 days

▶ OR **Hydrocortisone p. 662 (preferably as sodium succinate)**
BY INTRAVENOUS INJECTION
  ▶ Child 17 years and below: 4 mg/kg (max. 100 mg) every 6 hours until conversion to oral prednisolone is possible; alternative dose if weight unavailable:
  ▶ Child 1 year and below: 25 mg
  ▶ Child 2-4 years: 50 mg
  ▶ Child 5-17 years: 100 mg
  ▶ Adult: 100 mg every 6 hours until conversion to oral prednisolone is possible

High-flow **oxygen** should be given if available (via face mask in children)

Monitor response 15 to 30 minutes after nebulisation; if any signs of acute asthma persist, arrange hospital admission. While awaiting ambulance, repeat **nebulised beta₂ agonist** (as above) and give with

Ipratropium bromide nebuliser solution p. 246
(250 micrograms/mL)
BY INHALATION OF NEBULISED SOLUTION (VIA OXYGEN-DRIVEN
NEBULISER IF AVAILABLE)
▸ Child 11 years and below: 250 micrograms, repeated every
20–30 minutes for the first 2 hours, then every
4–6 hours as necessary
▸ Child 12-17 years: 500 micrograms every 4–6 hours as
necessary
▸ Adult: 500 micrograms every 4–6 hours as necessary

▸ **CROUP**
Dexamethasone oral solution p. 660 (2 mg/5 mL)
BY MOUTH
▸ Child 1 month-2 years: 150 micrograms/kg as a single dose

Anaphylaxis

▸ **ANAPHYLAXIS**
Adrenaline/epinephrine injection p. 221 (1 mg/mL (1 in 1000))
BY INTRAMUSCULAR INJECTION
▸ Child 5 years and below: 150 micrograms (0.15 mL),
repeated every 5 minutes if necessary
▸ Child 6-11 years: 300 micrograms (0.3 mL), repeated every
5 minutes if necessary
▸ Child 12-17 years: 500 micrograms (0.5 mL), repeated
every 5 minutes if necessary; 300 micrograms (0.3 mL)
should be given if child is small or prepubertal
▸ Adult: 500 micrograms (0.5 mL), repeated every
5 minutes if necessary

High-flow **oxygen** and **intravenous fluids** should be given
as soon as available.

Chlorphenamine maleate injection p. 283
BY INTRAMUSCULAR OR INTRAVENOUS INJECTION
May help counter histamine-mediated vasodilation and
bronchoconstriction.

Hydrocortisone(preferably as sodium succinate)
BY INTRAVENOUS INJECTION
Has delayed action but should be given to severely affected
patients to prevent further deterioration.

Bacterial infection

▸ **MENINGOCOCCAL DISEASE**
Benzylpenicillin sodium injection p. 537 (600 mg, 1.2 g)
BY INTRAVENOUS INJECTION (OR BY INTRAMUSCULAR INJECTION IF
VENOUS ACCESS NOT AVAILABLE)
▸ Neonate: 300 mg
▸ Child 1 month-11 months: 300 mg
▸ Child 1-9 years: 600 mg
▸ Child 10-17 years: 1.2 g
▸ Adult: 1.2 g
NOTE A single dose should be given before urgent transfer to
hospital, so long as this does not delay the transfer.

▸ OR **if history of allergy to penicillin**
Cefotaxime injection p. 519 (1 g)
BY INTRAVENOUS INJECTION (OR BY INTRAMUSCULAR INJECTION IF
VENOUS ACCESS NOT AVAILABLE)
▸ Neonate: 50 mg/kg
▸ Child 1 month-11 years: 50 mg/kg (max. 1 g)
▸ Child 12-17 years: 1 g
▸ Adult: 1 g
NOTE A single dose can be given before urgent transfer to
hospital, so long as this does not delay the transfer.

▸ OR **if history of immediate hypersensitivity reaction
(including anaphylaxis, angioedema, urticaria, or rash
immediately after administration) to penicillin or to
cephalosporins**
Chloramphenicol injection p. 558 (1 g)
BY INTRAVENOUS INJECTION
▸ Child: 12.5–25 mg/kg
▸ Adult: 12.5–25 mg/kg
NOTE A single dose can be given before urgent transfer to
hospital, so long as this does not delay the transfer.
See also Central nervous system infections, antibacterial
therapy p. 504.

Hypoglycaemia

▸ **DIABETIC HYPOGLYCAEMIA**
Glucose or sucrose
BY MOUTH
▸ Adult and child over 2 years: approx. 10–20 g
(110–220 mL *Lucozade® Energy Original* or 100–200 mL
Coca-Cola®—both non-diet versions *or*
2–4 teaspoonfuls of sugar *or* 3–6 sugar lumps)
repeated after 10–15 minutes if necessary

▸ OR **if hypoglycaemia unresponsive *or* if oral route
cannot be used**
Glucagon injection p. 707 (1 mg/mL)
BY SUBCUTANEOUS OR INTRAMUSCULAR INJECTION
▸ Child body-weight up to 25 kg: 500 micrograms (0.5 mL)
▸ Child body-weight 25 kg and over: 1 mg (1 mL)
▸ Adult: 1 mg (1 mL)

▸ OR **if hypoglycaemia prolonged *or* unresponsive to glucagon
after 10 minutes**
Glucose intravenous infusion p. 1009 (10%)
BY INTRAVENOUS INJECTION INTO LARGE VEIN
▸ Child: 5 mL/kg (glucose 500 mg/kg)

Glucose intravenous infusion (20%)
BY INTRAVENOUS INJECTION INTO LARGE VEIN
▸ Adult: 50 mL

Seizures

▸ **CONVULSIVE (INCLUDING FEBRILE) SEIZURES LASTING
LONGER THAN 5 MINUTES**
▸ EITHER **Diazepam rectal solution p. 340** (2 mg/mL, 4 mg/mL)
BY RECTUM
▸ Neonate: 1.25–2.5 mg, repeated once after
10–15 minutes if necessary
▸ Child 1 month-1 year: 5 mg, repeated once after
10–15 minutes if necessary
▸ Child 2-11 years: 5–10 mg, repeated once after
10–15 minutes if necessary
▸ Child 12-17 years: 10–20 mg, repeated once after
10–15 minutes if necessary
▸ Adult: 10–20 mg, repeated once after 10–15 minutes if
necessary
▸ Elderly: 10 mg, repeated once after 10–15 minutes if
necessary

▸ OR **Midazolam oromucosal solution p. 336**
BY BUCCAL ADMINISTRATION, REPEATED ONCE AFTER 10 MINUTES IF
NECESSARY
▸ Neonate: 300 micrograms/kg [unlicensed]
▸ Child 1-2 months: 300 micrograms/kg (max. 2.5 mg)
[unlicensed]
▸ Child 3 months-11 months: 2.5 mg
▸ Child 1-4 years: 5 mg
▸ Child 5-9 years: 7.5 mg
▸ Child 10-17 years: 10 mg
▸ Adult: 10 mg [unlicensed]

Approximate Conversions and Units

Conversion of pounds to kilograms

lb	kg
1	0.45
2	0.91
3	1.36
4	1.81
5	2.27
6	2.72
7	3.18
8	3.63
9	4.08
10	4.54
11	4.99
12	5.44
13	5.90
14	6.35

Conversion of stones to kilograms

stones	kg
1	6.35
2	12.70
3	19.05
4	25.40
5	31.75
6	38.10
7	44.45
8	50.80
9	57.15
10	63.50
11	69.85
12	76.20
13	82.55
14	88.90
15	95.25

Conversion from millilitres to fluid ounces

mL	fl oz
50	1.8
100	3.5
150	5.3
200	7.0
500	17.6
1000	35.2

Length

1 metre (m) = 1000 millimetres (mm)
1 centimetre (cm) = 10 mm
1 inch (in) = 25.4 mm
1 foot (ft) = 12 inches
12 inches = 304.8 mm

Mass

1 kilogram (kg) = 1000 grams (g)
1 gram (g) = 1000 milligrams (mg)
1 milligram (mg) = 1000 micrograms
1 microgram = 1000 nanograms
1 nanogram = 1000 picograms

Volume

1 litre = 1000 millilitres (mL)
1 millilitre (1 mL) = 1000 microlitres
1 pint ≈ 568 mL

Other units

1 kilocalorie (kcal) = 4186.8 joules (J)
1000 kilocalories (kcal) = 4.1868 megajoules (MJ)
1 megajoule (MJ) = 238.8 kilocalories (kcal)
1 millimetre of mercury (mmHg) = 133.3 pascals (Pa)
1 kilopascal (kPa) = 7.5 mmHg (pressure)

Plasma-drug concentrations

Plasma-drug concentrations in BNF publications are expressed in mass units per litre (e.g. mg/litre). The approximate equivalent in terms of amount of substance units (e.g. micromol/litre) is given in brackets.

Prescribing for children: weight, height, and gender

The table below shows the **mean values** for weight, height, and gender by age; these values have been derived from the UK-WHO growth charts 2009 and UK1990 standard centile charts, by extrapolating the 50th centile, and may be used to calculate doses in the absence of measurements. However, an individual's weight and height might vary considerably from the values in the table and it is important to ensure that the value chosen is appropriate. In most cases the actual measurement should be obtained as soon as possible and the dose re-calculated.

Age	Weight (kg)	Height (cm)
Full-term neonate	3.5	51
1 month	4.3	55
2 months	5.4	58
3 months	6.1	61
4 months	6.7	63
6 months	7.6	67
1 year	9	75
3 years	14	96
5 years	18	109
7 years	23	122
10 years	32	138
12 years	39	149
14 year old boy	49	163
14 year old girl	50	159
Adult male	68	176
Adult female	58	164

Recommended wording of cautionary and advisory labels

For details including Welsh Language translation see p. 1534

1   Warning: This medicine may make you sleepy

2   Warning: This medicine may make you sleepy. If this happens, do not drive or use tools or machines. Do not drink alcohol

3   Warning: This medicine may make you sleepy. If this happens, do not drive or use tools or machines

4   Warning: Do not drink alcohol

5   Do not take indigestion remedies 2 hours before or after you take this medicine

6   Do not take indigestion remedies, or medicines containing iron or zinc, 2 hours before or after you take this medicine

7   Do not take milk, indigestion remedies, or medicines containing iron or zinc, 2 hours before or after you take this medicine

8   Warning: Do not stop taking this medicine unless your doctor tells you to stop

9   Space the doses evenly throughout the day. Keep taking this medicine until the course is finished, unless you are told to stop

10 Warning: Read the additional information given with this medicine

11 Protect your skin from sunlight—even on a bright but cloudy day. Do not use sunbeds

12 Do not take anything containing aspirin while taking this medicine

13 Dissolve or mix with water before taking

14 This medicine may colour your urine. This is harmless

15 Caution: flammable. Keep your body away from fire or flames after you have put on the medicine

16 Dissolve the tablet under your tongue—do not swallow. Store the tablets in this bottle with the cap tightly closed. Get a new supply 8 weeks after opening

17 Do not take more than... in 24 hours

18 Do not take more than... in 24 hours. Also, do not take more than... in any one week

19 Warning: This medicine makes you sleepy. If you still feel sleepy the next day, do not drive or use tools or machines. Do not drink alcohol

21 Take with or just after food, or a meal

22 Take 30 to 60 minutes before food

23 Take this medicine when your stomach is empty. This means an hour before food or 2 hours after food

24 Suck or chew this medicine

25 Swallow this medicine whole. Do not chew or crush

26 Dissolve this medicine under your tongue

27 Take with a full glass of water

28 Spread thinly on the affected skin only

29 Do not take more than 2 at any one time. Do not take more than 8 in 24 hours

30 Contains paracetamol. Do not take anything else containing paracetamol while taking this medicine. Talk to a doctor at once if you take too much of this medicine, even if you feel well

32 Contains aspirin. Do not take anything else containing aspirin while taking this medicine